Laboratory	Conventional Units	Conversion Factor	SI Units
CD8 lymphocyte count	18–39% of total lymphocytes		
Cerebrospinal fluid (CSF)			
Pressure	75–175 mm H_2O		
Glucose	40–70 mg/dL	0.0555	2.2–3.9 mmol/L
Protein	15–45 mg/dL	0.01	0.15–0.45 g/L
WBC	Less than 10/mm³		
Ceruloplasmin	18–45 mg/dL	10	180–450 mg/L
		0.063	1.1–2.8 μmol/L
Chloride	97–110 mEq/L	1	97–110 mmol/L
Cholesterol			
Desirable	Less than 200 mg/dL	0.0259	Less than 5.18 mmol/L
Borderline high	200–239 mg/dL	0.0259	5.18–6.19 mmol/L
High	Greater than or equal to 240 mg/dL	0.0259	Greater than or equal to 6.2 mmol/L
Chorionic gonadotropin (β-hCG)	Less than 5 milliunits/mL	1	Less than 5 units/L
Clozapine	Minimum trough 300–350 ng/mL or mcg/L	3.06	918–1071 nmol/L
CO_2 content	22–30 mEq/L	1	22–30 mmol/L
Complement component 3 (C3)	70–160 mg/dL	0.01	0.7–1.6 g/L
Complement component 4 (C4)	20–40 mg/dL	0.01	0.2–0.4 g/L
Copper	70–150 mcg/dL	0.157	11–24 μmol/L
Cortisol (fasting, morning)	5–25 mcg/dL	27.6	138–690 nmol/L
Cortisol (free, urinary)	10–100 mcg/day	2.76	28–276 nmol/day
Creatine kinase			
Male	30–200 IU/L	0.01667	0.50–3.33 μkat/L
Female	20–170 IU/L	0.01667	0.33–2.83 μkat/L
MB fraction	0–7 IU/L	0.01667	0.0–0.12 μkat/L
Creatinine clearance (CrCl) (urine)	85–135 mL/minute/1.73 m²	0.00963	0.82–1.3 mL/s/m²
Creatinine			
Male 4–20 years	0.2–1.0 mg/dL	88.4	18–88 μmol/L
Female 4–20 years	0.2–1.0 mg/dL	88.4	18–88 μmol/L
Male (adults)	0.7–1.3 mg/dL	88.4	62–115 μmol/L
Female (adults)	0.6–1.1 mg/dL	88.4	53–97 μmol/L
Cyclosporine			
Renal transplant	100–300 ng/mL or mcg/L	0.832	83–250 nmol/L
Cardiac, liver, or pancreatic transplant	200–350 ng/mL or mcg/L	0.832	166–291 nmol/L
Hematopoietic stem cell transplant	150–450 ng/mL or mcg/L		
Cryptococcal antigen	Negative		
D-dimers	Less than 250 ng/mL	1	Less than 250 mcg/L
Desipramine	75–300 ng/mL or mcg/L	3.75	281–1125 mmol/L
Dexamethasone suppression test (DST) (overnight)	8:00 am cortisol less than 5 mcg/dL	0.0276	Less than 0.14 μmol/L
DHEAS			
Male	170–670 mcg/dL	0.0271	4.6–18.2 μmol/L
Female			
Premenopausal	50–540 mcg/dL	0.0271	1.4–14.7 μmol/L
Postmenopausal	30–260 mcg/dL	0.0271	0.8–7.1 μmol/L
Digoxin, therapeutic	0.5–1.0 ng/mL or mcg/L	1.28	0.6–1.3 nmol/L
Erythrocyte count (blood) See under Red blood cell count			
Erythrocyte sedimentation rate (ESR)			
Westergren			
Male	0–20 mm/hour		
Female	0–30 mm/hour		
Wintrobe			
Male	0–9 mm/hour		
Female	0–15 mm/hour		
Erythropoietin	2–25 mIU/mL	1	2–25 IU/L
Estradiol			
Male	10–36 pg/mL	3.67	37–132 pmol/L
Female	34–170 pg/mL	3.67	125–624 pmol/L
Ethanol, legal intoxication	Greater than or equal to 50–100 mg/dL	0.217	10.9–21.7 mmol/L
	Greater than or equal to 0.05–0.1%	217	
Ethosuccimide, therapeutic	40–100 mg/L or mcg/mL	7.08	283–708 μmol/L
Factor VIII or factor IX			
Severe hemophilia	Less than 1 IU/dL	0.01	Less than 0.01 units/mL
Moderate hemophilia	1–5 IU/dL	0.01	0.01–0.05 units/mL
Mild hemophilia	Greater than 5 IU/dL	0.01	Greater than 0.05 units/mL
Usual adult levels	60–140 IU/dL	0.01	0.60–1.40 units/mL
Ferritin			
Male	20–250 ng/mL	1	20–250 mcg/L
Female	10–150 ng/mL	1	10–150 mcg/L
Fibrin degradation products (FDP)	2–10 mg/L		
Fibrinogen	200–400 mg/dL	0.01	2.0–4.0 g/L
Folate (plasma)	3.1–12.4 ng/mL	2.266	7.0–28.1 nmol/L
Folic acid (RBC)	125–600 ng/mL	2.266	283–1360 nmol/L
Follicle-stimulating hormone (FSH)			
Male	1–7 mIU/mL	1	1–7 IU/L
Female			
Follicular phase	1–9 mIU/mL	1	1–9 IU/L
Midcycle	6–26 mIU/mL	1	6–26 IU/L
Luteal phase	1–9 mIU/mL	1	1–9 IU/L
Postmenopausal	30–118 mIU/mL	1	30–118 IU/L
Free thyroxine index (FT_4I)	6.5–12.5		
Gamma glutamyl transferase (GGT)	0–30 IU/L	0.01667	0–0.5 μkat/L
Gastrin (fasting)	0–130 pg/mL	1	0–130 ng/L
Gentamicin, therapeutic	4–10 mg/L peak	2.09	8.4–21 μmol/L peak
	Less than or equal to 2 mg/L trough		Less than or equal to 4.2 μmol/L trough
Globulin	2.3–3.5 g/dL	10	23–35 g/L
Glucose (fasting, plasma)	65–109 mg/dL	0.0555	3.6–6.00 mmol/L
Glucose, two hour postprandial blood (PPBG)	Less than 140 mg/dL	0.0555	Less than 7.8 mmol/L
Granulocyte count	$1.8–6.6 \times 10^3/\mu L$	10^6	$1.8–6.6 \times 10^9/L$
Growth hormone (fasting)			
Male	Less than 5 ng/mL	1	Less than 5 mcg/L
Female	Less than 10 ng/mL	1	Less than 10 mcg/L

(continued on back inside cover)

9TH EDITION

PHARMACOTHERAPY

A PATHOPHYSIOLOGIC APPROACH

Notice

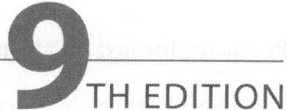

PHARMACOTHERAPY

A PATHOPHYSIOLOGIC APPROACH

Joseph T. DiPiro, PharmD, FCCP
Executive Dean and Professor, South Carolina College of Pharmacy, University of South Carolina and Medical University of South Carolina, Charleston and Columbia, South Carolina

Robert L. Talbert, PharmD, FCCP, BCPS, FAHA
Professor, Pharmacotherapy Division, College of Pharmacy, University of Texas at Austin, Professor, Department of Medicine, School of Medicine, University of Texas Health Science Center at San Antonio, San Antonio, Texas

Gary C. Yee, PharmD, FCCP, BCOP
Professor and Associate Dean, Department of Pharmacy Practice, College of Pharmacy, University of Nebraska Medical Center, Omaha, Nebraska

Gary R. Matzke, PharmD, FCP, FCCP, FASN, FNAP
Professor and Director, Pharmacy Practice Transformation Initiatives and Founding Director, ACCP/ASHP/VCU Congressional Health Care Policy Fellow Program, Department of Pharmacotherapy and Outcome Sciences, School of Pharmacy, Virginia Commonwealth University, Richmond, Virginia

Barbara G. Wells, PharmD, FCCP, FASHP
Dean Emeritus and Professor Emeritus, Department of Pharmacy Practice, University of Mississippi, School of Pharmacy, Oxford, Mississippi

L. Michael Posey, BSPharm, MA
Associate Vice President, Periodicals Department, American Pharmacists Association, Washington, District of Columbia

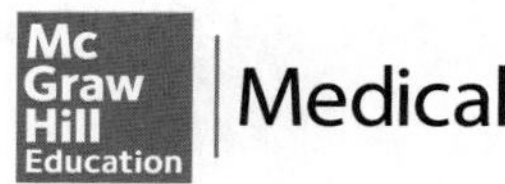

New York Chicago San Francisco Athens Lisbon Madrid
Mexico City Milan New Delhi Singapore Sydney Toronto

Pharmacotherapy: A Pathophysiologic Approach, Ninth Edition

1 2 3 4 5 6 7 8 9 0 DOW/DOW 18 17 16 15 14

ISBN 978-0-07-180053-2
MHID 0-07-180053-0

This book was set in Times LT Std Roman by Thomson Digital.
The editors were Michael Weitz and Brian Kearns.
The production supervisor was Catherine H. Saggese.
Project management was provided by Saloni Narang, Thomson Digital.
The interior designer was Elise Lansdon.
The cover designer was Thomas De Pierro.
Cover image credit: © Dennis Kunkel Microscopy, Inc./Visuals Unlimited/Corbis.
Caption: White Blood Cell Attacking E. coli.
RR Donnelley was printer and binder.

This book is printed on acid-free paper.

Library of Congress Cataloging-in-Publication Data

Pharmacotherapy (New York)
Pharmacotherapy : a pathophysiologic approach / [edited] by Joseph T. DiPiro, Robert L. Talbert, Gary C. Yee, Gary R. Matzke, Barbara G. Wells, L. Michael Posey.—9/E.
p. ; cm.
ISBN 978-0-07-180053-2 (hbk. : alk. paper)—ISBN 0-07-180053-0 (hbk. : alk. paper)
I. DiPiro, Joseph T., editor of compilation. II. Talbert, Robert L., editor of compilation. III. Yee, Gary C., editor of compilation. IV. Matzke, Gary R., editor of compilation. V. Wells, Barbara G., editor of compilation. VI. Posey, L. Michael, editor of compilation. VII. Title.
[DNLM: 1. Drug Therapy. WB 330]
RM263
615.5'8—dc23

2013038907

Dedication

To our patients, who have challenged and inspired us and given meaning to all our endeavors.

To practitioners who continue to improve patient health outcomes and thereby serve as role models for their colleagues and students while clinging tenaciously to the highest standards of practice.

To our mentors, whose vision provided educational and training programs that encouraged our professional growth and challenged us to be innovators in our patient care, research, and education.

To our faculty colleagues for their efforts and support for our mission to provide a comprehensive and challenging educational foundation for the pharmacists of the future.

And finally to our families for the time that they have sacrificed so that this ninth edition would become a reality.

No other text helps you achieve optimal patient outcomes through evidence-based medication therapy like DiPiro's

Pharmacotherapy: A Pathophysiologic Approach, Ninth Edition

KEY FEATURES

- Goes beyond drug indications and doses to include drug selection, administration, and monitoring
- Enriched by more than 300 expert contributors
- Revised and updated to reflect the latest evidence-based information and recommendations
- Includes valuable learning aids such Key Concepts at the beginning of each chapter, Clinical Presentation tables that summarize disease signs and symptoms, and Clinical Controversies boxes that examine the complicated issues faced by students and clinicians in providing drug therapy

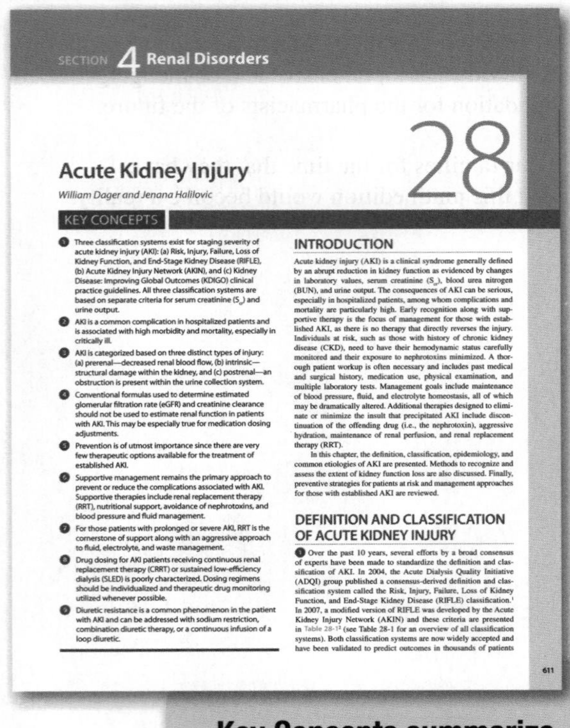

SECTION 4 Renal Disorders

28

Acute Kidney Injury

William Dager and Jenana Halilovic

KEY CONCEPTS

1. Three classification systems exist for staging severity of acute kidney injury (AKI): (a) Risk, Injury, Failure, Loss of Kidney Function, and End-Stage Kidney Disease (RIFLE), (b) Acute Kidney Injury Network (AKIN), and (c) Kidney Disease: Improving Global Outcomes (KDIGO) clinical practice guidelines. All three classification systems are based on separate criteria for serum creatinine (S_{cr}) and urine output.
2. AKI is a common complication in hospitalized patients and is associated with high morbidity and mortality, especially in critically ill.
3. AKI is categorized based on three distinct types of injury: (a) prerenal—decreased renal blood flow, (b) intrinsic—structural damage within the kidney, and (c) postrenal—an obstruction is present within the urine collection system.
4. Conventional formulas used to determine estimated glomerular filtration rate (eGFR) and creatinine clearance should not be used to estimate renal function in patients with AKI. This may be especially true for medication dosing adjustments.
5. Prevention is of utmost importance since there are very few therapeutic options available for the treatment of established AKI.
6. Supportive management remains the primary approach to prevent or reduce the complications associated with AKI. Supportive therapies include renal replacement therapy (RRT), nutritional support, avoidance of nephrotoxins, and blood pressure and fluid management.
7. For those patients with prolonged or severe AKI, RRT is the cornerstone of support along with an aggressive approach to fluid, electrolyte, and waste management.
8. Drug dosing for AKI patients receiving continuous renal replacement therapy (CRRT) or sustained low-efficiency dialysis (SLED) is poorly characterized. Dosing regimens should be individualized and therapeutic drug monitoring utilized whenever possible.
9. Diuretic resistance is a common phenomenon in the patient with AKI and can be addressed with sodium restriction, combination diuretic therapy, or a continuous infusion of a loop diuretic.

INTRODUCTION

Acute kidney injury (AKI) is a clinical syndrome generally defined by an abrupt reduction in kidney function as evidenced by changes in laboratory values, serum creatinine (S_{cr}), blood urea nitrogen (BUN), and urine output. The consequences of AKI can be serious, especially in hospitalized patients, among whom complications and mortality are particularly high. Early recognition along with supportive therapy is the focus of management for those with established AKI, as there is no therapy that directly reverses the injury. Individuals at risk, such as those with history of chronic kidney disease (CKD), need to have their hemodynamic status carefully monitored and their exposure to nephrotoxins minimized. A thorough patient workup is often necessary and includes past medical and surgical history, medication use, physical examination, and multiple laboratory tests. Management goals include maintenance of blood pressure, fluid, and electrolyte homeostasis, all of which may be dramatically altered. Additional therapies designed to eliminate or minimize the insult that precipitated AKI include discontinuation of the offending drug (i.e., the nephrotoxin), aggressive hydration, maintenance of renal perfusion, and renal replacement therapy (RRT).

In this chapter, the definition, classification, epidemiology, and common etiologies of AKI are presented. Methods to recognize and assess the extent of kidney function loss are also discussed. Finally, preventive strategies for patients at risk and management approaches for those with established AKI are reviewed.

DEFINITION AND CLASSIFICATION OF ACUTE KIDNEY INJURY

1 Over the past 10 years, several efforts by a broad consensus of experts have been made to standardize the definition and classification of AKI. In 2004, the Acute Dialysis Quality Initiative (ADQI) group published a consensus-derived definition and classification system called the Risk, Injury, Failure, Loss of Kidney Function, and End-Stage Kidney Disease (RIFLE) classification.[1] In 2007, a modified version of RIFLE was developed by the Acute Kidney Injury Network (AKIN) and these criteria are presented in Table 28-1[2] (see Table 28-1 for an overview of all classification systems). Both classification systems are now widely accepted and have been validated to predict outcomes in thousands of patients

611

Key Concepts summarize must-know information in each chapter

NEW TO THIS EDITION

- A section on personalized pharmacotherapy appears in most sections
- All diagnostic flow diagrams, treatment algorithms, dosing guideline recommendations, and monitoring approaches have been updated in full color to clearly distinguish treatment pathways
- New drug monitoring tables have been added
- Most of the disease-oriented chapters have incorporated evidence-based treatment guidelines when available, include ratings of the level of evidence to support the key therapeutic approaches
- Twenty-four online-only chapters are available at www.pharmacotherapyonline.com

Valuable tables encapsulate important information

TABLE 75-4 Topical Drugs Used in the Treatment of Open-Angle Glaucoma

Drug	Pharmacologic Properties	Common Brand Names	Dose Form	Strength (%)	Usual Dose[a]	Mechanism of Action
β-Adrenergic Blocking Agents						
Betaxolol	Relative β_1-selective	Generic	Solution	0.5	One drop twice a day	All reduce aqueous production of ciliary body
		Betoptic-S	Suspension	0.25	One drop twice a day	
Carteolol	Nonselective, intrinsic sympathomimetic activity	Generic	Solution	1	One drop twice a day	
Levobunolol	Nonselective	Betagan	Solution	0.25, 0.5	One drop twice a day	
Metipranolol	Nonselective	OptiPranolol	Solution	0.3	One drop twice a day	
Timolol	Nonselective	Timoptic, Betimol, Istalol	Solution	0.25, 0.5	One drop every day—one to two times a day	
		Timoptic-XE	Gelling solution	0.25, 0.5	One drop every day[a]	
Nonspecific Adrenergic Agonists						
Dipivefrin	Epinephrine prodrug	Propine	Solution	0.1	One drop twice a day	Increased aqueous humor outflow
α_2-Adrenergic Agonists						
Apraclonidine	Specific α_2-agonists	Iopidine	Solution	0.5, 1	One drop two to three times a day	Both reduce aqueous humor production; brimonidine known to also increase uveoscleral outflow; only brimonidine has primary indication
Brimonidine		Alphagan P	Solution	0.15, 0.1	One drop two to three times a day	
Cholinergic Agonists Direct Acting						
Carbachol	Irreversible	Carboptic, Isopto Carbachol	Solution	1.5, 3	One drop two to three times a day	All increase aqueous humor outflow through trabecular meshwork
Pilocarpine	Irreversible	Isopto Carpine, Pilocar	Solution	0.25, 0.5, 1, 2, 4, 6, 8, 10	One drop two to three times a day	
					One drop four times a day	
		Pilopine HS	Gel	4	Every 24 hours at bedtime	
Cholinesterase Inhibitors						
Echothiophate		Phospholine Iodide	Solution	0.125	Once or twice a day	
Carbonic Anhydrase Inhibitors						
Topical						
Brinzolamide	Carbonic anhydrase type II inhibition	Azopt	Suspension	1	Two to three times a day	All reduce aqueous humor production of ciliary body
Dorzolamide		Trusopt Generic	Solution	2	Two to three times a day	
Systemic						
Acetazolamide		Generic	Tablet	125 mg, 250 mg	125–250 mg two to four times a day	
		Injection	500 mg/vial	250–500 mg		
		Diamox Sequels	Capsule	500 mg	500 mg twice a day	
Methazolamide		Generic	Tablet	25 mg, 50 mg	25–50 mg two to three times a day	
Prostaglandin Analogs						
Latanoprost	Prostanoid agonist	Xalatan	Solution	0.005	One drop every night	Increases aqueous uveoscleral outflow and to a lesser extent trabecular outflow
Bimatoprost	Prostamide agonist	Lumigan	Solution	0.01, 0.03	One drop every night	
Travoprost	Prostanoid agonist	Travatan Z	Solution	0.004	One drop every night	
Tafluprost	Prostanoid agonist	Zioptan	Preservative free solution	0.0015%	One drop every night	
Combinations						
Timolol–dorzolamide		Cosopt Generic	Solution	Timolol 0.5% dorzolamide 2%	One drop twice daily	
Timolol–brimonidine		Combigan	Solution	Timolol 0.5% brimonide 0.2%	One drop twice daily	
Brinzolamide–brimonidine		Simrinza		Brinzolamide 1% brimonidine 0.2%	One drop three times daily	

[a]Use of nasolacrimal occlusion will increase the number of patients successfully treated with longer dosage intervals.

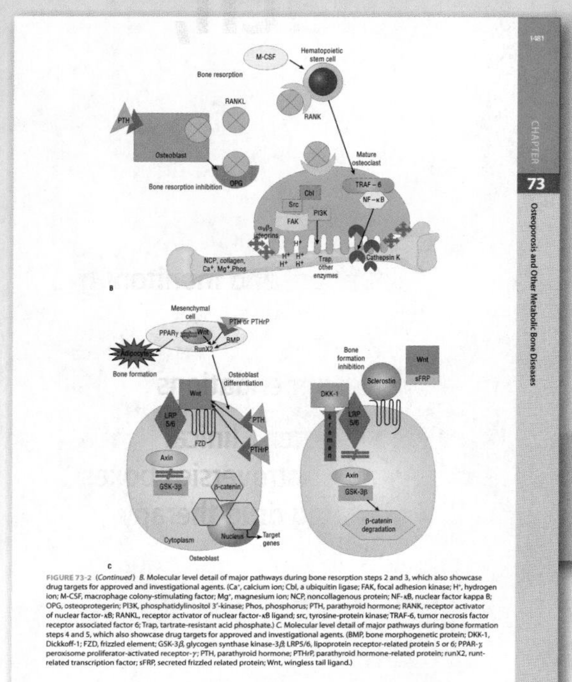

FIGURE 73-2 (*Continued*) *B.* Molecular level detail of major pathways during bone resorption steps 2 and 3, which also showcase drug targets for approved and investigational agents. (Ca^+, calcium ion; Cbl, a ubiquitin ligase; FAK, focal adhesion kinase; H^+, hydrogen ion; M-CSF, macrophage colony-stimulating factor; Mg^+, magnesium ion; NCP, noncollagenous protein; NF-κB, nuclear factor kappa B; OPG, osteoprotegerin; PI3K, phosphatidylinositol 3′-kinase; Phos, phosphorus; PTH, parathyroid hormone; RANK, receptor activator of nuclear factor-κB; RANKL, receptor activator of nuclear factor-κB ligand; src, tyrosine-protein kinase; TRAF-6, tumor necrosis factor receptor associated factor 6; Trap, tartrate-resistant acid phosphate.) *C.* Molecular level detail of major pathways during bone formation steps 4 and 5, which also showcase drug targets for approved and investigational agents. (BMP, bone morphogenetic protein; DKK-1, Dickkoff-1; FZD, frizzled element; GSK-3*β*, glycogen synthase kinase-3*β*; LRP5/6, lipoprotein receptor-related protein 5 or 6; PPAR-*γ*, peroxisome proliferator-activated receptor-*γ*; PTH, parathyroid hormone; PTHrP, parathyroid hormone-related protein; runX2, runt-related transcription factor; sFRP, secreted frizzled related protein; Wnt, wingless tail ligand.)

Full-color illustrations enhance and clarify the text

Clinical Presentation tables summarize disease signs and symptoms

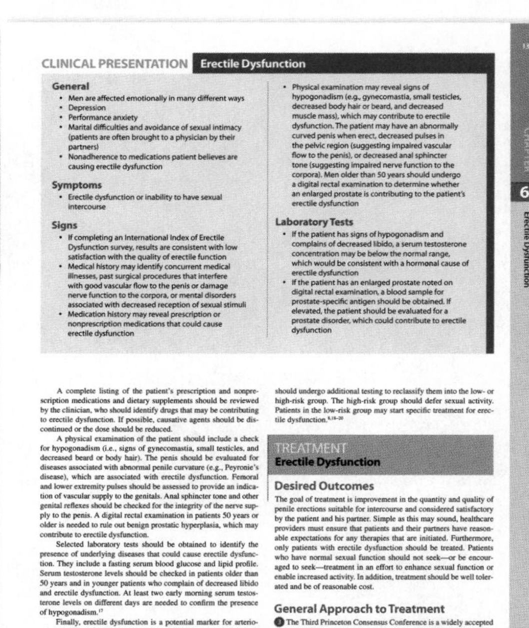

CLINICAL PRESENTATION **Erectile Dysfunction**

General

- Men are affected emotionally in many different ways
- Depression
- Performance anxiety
- Marital difficulties and avoidance of sexual intimacy (patients are often brought to a physician by their partners)
- Nonadherence to medications patient believes are causing erectile dysfunction

Symptoms

- Erectile dysfunction or inability to have sexual intercourse

Signs

- If completing an International Index of Erectile Dysfunction survey, results are consistent with low satisfaction with the quality of erectile function
- Medical history may identify concurrent medical illnesses, past surgical procedures that interfere with good vascular flow to the penis or damage nerve function to the corpora, or mental disorders associated with decreased reception of sexual stimuli
- Medication history may reveal prescription or nonprescription medications that could cause erectile dysfunction
- Physical examination may reveal signs of hypogonadism (e.g., gynecomastia, small testicles, decreased body hair or beard, and decreased muscle mass), which may contribute to erectile dysfunction. The patient may have an abnormally curved penis when erect, decreased pulses in the pelvic region (suggesting impaired vascular flow to the penis), or decreased anal sphincter tone (suggesting impaired nerve function to the corpora). Men older than 50 years should undergo a digital rectal examination to determine whether an enlarged prostate is contributing to the patient's erectile dysfunction

Laboratory Tests

- If the patient has signs of hypogonadism and complains of decreased libido, a serum testosterone concentration may be below the normal range, which would be consistent with a hormonal cause of erectile dysfunction
- If the patient has an enlarged prostate noted on digital rectal examination, a blood sample for prostate-specific antigen should be obtained. If elevated, the patient should be evaluated for a prostate disorder, which could contribute to erectile dysfunction

A complete listing of the patient's prescription and nonprescription medications and dietary supplements should be reviewed by the clinician, who should identify drugs that may be contributing to erectile dysfunction. If possible, causative agents should be discontinued or the dose should be reduced.

A physical examination of the patient should include a check for hypogonadism (i.e., signs of gynecomastia, small testicles, and decreased beard or body hair). The penis should be evaluated for diseases associated with abnormal penile curvature (e.g., Peyronie's disease), which are associated with erectile dysfunction. Femoral and lower extremity pulses should be assessed to provide an indication of vascular supply to the genitals. Anal sphincter tone and other genital reflexes should be checked for the integrity of the nerve supply to the penis. A digital rectal examination in patients 50 years or older is needed to rule out benign prostatic hyperplasia, which may contribute to erectile dysfunction.

Selected laboratory tests should be obtained to identify the presence of underlying diseases that could cause erectile dysfunction. They include a fasting serum blood glucose and lipid profile. Serum testosterone levels should be checked in patients older than 50 years and in younger patients who complain of decreased libido and erectile dysfunction. At least two early morning serum testosterone levels on different days are needed to confirm the presence of hypogonadism.[17]

Finally, erectile dysfunction is a potential marker for arteriosclerosis. Therefore, older patients and those at intermediate and high risk for cardiovascular disease should undergo a cardiovascular risk assessment before starting on drug treatment for erectile dysfunction. By doing so, patients will be categorized into low-, intermediate-, or high-risk groups for cardiovascular morbidity related to sexual intercourse. Patients in the intermediate-risk group should undergo additional testing to reclassify them into the low- or high-risk group. The high-risk group should defer sexual activity. Patients in the low-risk group may start specific treatment for erectile dysfunction.[8,18–20]

TREATMENT
Erectile Dysfunction

Desired Outcomes

The goal of treatment is improvement in the quantity and quality of penile erections suitable for intercourse and considered satisfactory by the patient and his partner. Simple as this may sound, healthcare providers must ensure that patients and their partners have reasonable expectations for any therapies that are initiated. Furthermore, only patients with erectile dysfunction should be treated. Patients who have normal sexual function should not seek—or be encouraged to seek—treatment in an effort to enhance sexual function or enable increased activity. In addition, treatment should be well tolerated and be of reasonable cost.

General Approach to Treatment

3 The Third Princeton Consensus Conference is a widely accepted multidisciplinary approach to managing erectile dysfunction that maps out a stepwise treatment plan.[20–22] The first step in clinical management of erectile dysfunction is to identify and, if possible, reverse underlying causes. Risk factors for erectile dysfunction, including hypertension, coronary artery disease, dyslipidemia, diabetes mellitus, smoking, or chronic ethanol abuse, should be

- *Pharmacotherapy Casebook* provides the case studies students need to learn how to identify and resolve the drug therapy problems most likely encountered in real-world practice. This new edition is packed with patient cases and makes the ideal study companion to the 9th edition of DiPiro's *Pharmacotherapy: A Pathophysiologic Approach*.
- Online Learning Center is designed to benefit the student and faculty. Both learning objectives and self-assessment questions for each chapter are available online at www.accesspharmacy.com

Contents

e|CHAPTERS **To access the eChapters please go to www.mhpharmacotherapy.com**

McGraw-Hill reserves the right to change the manner of distribution of these chapters to the customer.

SECTION 4 Renal Disorders 611

Section Editor: *Gary R. Matzke*

SECTION 5 Neurologic Disorders 817

Section Editor: *Barbara G. Wells*

SECTION 6 Psychiatric Disorders 959

Section Editor: *Barbara G. Wells*

SECTION 7 Endocrinologic Disorders 1143

Section Editor: *Robert L. Talbert*

SECTION 8 Gynecologic and Obstetric Disorders 1253

Section Editor: *Barbara G. Wells*

SECTION 9 Urologic Disorders 1337

Section Editor: *L. Michael Posey*

SECTION 10 Immunologic Disorders 1397

Section Editors: *Gary R. Matzke and Gary C. Yee*

SECTION 11 Rheumatologic Disorders 1437

Section Editor: *L. Michael Posey*

SECTION 12 Ophthalmic and Otolaryngological Disorders 1525

Section Editor: *L. Michael Posey*

SECTION 13 Dermatologic Disorders 1555

Section Editor: *L. Michael Posey*

SECTION 14 Hematologic Disorders 1605

Section Editor: *Gary C. Yee*

SECTION 15 Infectious Diseases 1661

Section Editor: *Joseph T. DiPiro*

CONTENTS

Contributors

Val R. Adams, PharmD, FCCP, BCOP
Associate Professor
Department of Pharmacy Practice and Science
College of Pharmacy
University of Kentucky
Lexington, Kentucky
Chapter 106

Jeffrey R. Aeschlimann, PharmD
Associate Professor
Department of Pharmacy Practice
School of Pharmacy
University of Connecticut
Storrs, Connecticut
eChapter 25

Ahmed Alhusban, PharmD, PhD
Assistant Professor
Department of Clinical Pharmacy
Jordan University of Science and Technology
Irbid, Jordan
eChapter 19

Rondall E. Allen, PharmD
Clinical Associate Professor
Associate Dean for Student Affairs
Division of Clinical and Administrative Sciences
Xavier University of Louisiana College of Pharmacy
New Orleans, Louisiana
eChapter 17

Carlos A. Alvarez, PharmD, MSc, MSCS, BCPS
Assistant Professor
Department of Pharmacy Practice
Texas Tech University Health Sciences Center
Dallas, Texas
Chapter 57

JV Anandan, PharmD
Adjunct Associate Professor
Eugene Applebaum College of Pharmacy
Wayne State University, Detroit
Pharmacy Specialist
Center for Drug Use Analysis and Information
Henry Ford Hospital
Department of Pharmacy Services
Detroit, Michigan
Chapter 93

Peter L. Anderson, PharmD
Associate Professor
Department of Pharmaceutical Sciences
Skaggs School of Pharmacy and Pharmaceutical Sciences
University of Colorado Anschutz Medical Campus
Aurora, Colorado
Chapter 103

Tami R. Argo, PharmD, MS
Clinical Pharmacy Specialist-Psychiatry
Department of Pharmacy
Iowa City Veterans Affairs Health Care System
Iowa City, Iowa
Chapter 50

Edward P. Armstrong, PharmD
Professor
Department of Pharmacy Practice and Science
College of Pharmacy
University of Arizona
Tucson, Arizona
Chapter 96

Susanne M. Arnold, MD
Professor
Department of Internal Medicine
Division of Medical Oncology
Markey Cancer Center
University of Kentucky
Lexington, Kentucky
Chapter 106

Jill Astolfi, PharmD
Philadelphia, Pennsylvania
eChapter 9

Rebecca L. Attridge, PharmD, MSc, BCPS
Assistant Professor
Department of Pharmacy Practice
University Incarnate Word Feik School of Pharmacy
Adjunct Assistant Professor
The University of Texas Health Science Center at San Antonio
Division of Pulmonary Diseases and Critical Care Medicine
San Antonio, Texas
Chapter 17

Jacquelyn L. Bainbridge, PharmD, FCCP
Professor
Department of Clinical Pharmacy and Neurology
University of Colorado
Anschutz Medical Campus
Skaggs School of Pharmacy and Pharmaceutical Sciences
Aurora, Colorado
Chapter 39

Jeffrey F. Barletta, PharmD, FCCM
Associate Professor and Vice Chair
Department of Pharmacy Practice
Midwestern University
College of Pharmacy
Glendale, Arizona
Chapter 2

Chad M. Barnett, PharmD, BCOP
Clinical Pharmacy Specialist-Breast Oncology
Division of Pharmacy
Clinical Pharmacy Services
University of Texas MD Anderson Cancer Center
Houston, Texas
Chapter 105

Larry A. Bauer, PharmD, FCP, FCCP
Professor
Department of Pharmacy
School of Pharmacy
Adjunct Professor
Department of Laboratory Medicine
School of Medicine
University of Washington
Seattle, Washington
eChapter 5

Jerry L. Bauman, PharmD, FCCP, FACC
Dean
College of Pharmacy, University of Illinois at Chicago
Professor
Departments of Pharmacy Practice and Medicine, Section of Cardiology
Colleges of Pharmacy and Medicine, University of Illinois at Chicago
Chicago, Illinois
Chapter 8

Terry J. Baumann, PharmD, BCPS
Clinical Manager, Pain Practitioner
Department of Pharmacy
Munson Medical Center
Traverse City, Michigan
Chapter 44

Oralia V. Bazaldua, PharmD, FCCP, BCPS
Associate Professor
Department of Family and Community Medicine
The University of Texas Health Science Center at San Antonio
San Antonio, Texas
eChapter 1

Martha G. Blackford, PharmD
Clinical Pharmacologist & Toxicologist
Clinical Pharmacology and Toxicology
Department of Pediatrics
Akron Children's Hospital
Akron, Ohio
Chapter 85

Scott Bolesta, PharmD, BCPS
Associate Professor
Department of Pharmacy Practice
Wilkes University
Wilkes-Bare, Pennsylvania
Clinical Pharmacist
Regional Hospital of Scranton
Scranton, Pennsylvania
Chapter 25

Jill S. Borchert, PharmD, BCPS, FCCP
Professor and Vice Chair
Department of Pharmacy Practice
Midwestern University Chicago College of Pharmacy
Downers Grove, Illinois
Chapter 73

Bradley A. Boucher, PharmD, FCCP, FCCM
Professor of Clinical Pharmacy and Associate Professor of Neurosurgery
Department of Clinical Pharmacy
University of Tennessee Health Science Center
Memphis, Tennessee
Chapter 42

Sharya V. Bourdet, PharmD, BCPS
Critical Care Pharmacist/Clinical Inpatient Program Manager
Pharmacy Service
Veterans Affairs Medical Center
Health Sciences Clinical Associate Professor
Department of Clinical Pharmacy
School of Pharmacy, University of California
San Francisco, California
Chapter 16

Nancy C. Brahm, PharmD, MS, BCPP, CGP
Clinical Professor
The University of Oklahoma, College of Pharmacy
Tulsa, Oklahoma
Chapter 56

Donald F. Brophy, PharmD, MSc, FCCP, FASN, BCPS
McFarlane Professor and Chairman
Department of Pharmacotherapy and Outcomes Sciences
Virginia Commonwealth University School of Pharmacy
Richmond, Virginia
Chapter 36

Jason E. Brouillard, PharmD, MBA
Clinical Pharmacy Advisor
TheraDoc
Hospira, Inc.
Spokane, Washington
eChapter 11

Thomas E. R. Brown, PharmD
Associate Professor
Leslie Dan Faculty of Pharmacy
University of Toronto and Women's College Hospital
Toronto, Ontario, Canada
Chapter 98

Peter F. Buckley, MD
Dean
Medical College of Georgia
Georgia Regents University
Augusta, Georgia
Chapter 50

David S. Burgess, PharmD, FCCP
Professor and Chair
Department of Pharmacy Practice and Science
College of Pharmacy, University of Kentucky
Lexington, Kentucky
Chapter 83

Lucinda M. Buys, PharmD, BCPS
Associate Professor
Department of Pharmacy Practice and Science
University of Iowa
College of Pharmacy and The Siouxland Medical Education Foundation
Sioux City, Iowa
Chapter 71

Karim Anton Calis, PharmD, MPH, FASHP, FCCP
Clinical Investigator
Office of the Clinical Director
Eunice Kennedy Shriver National Institute of Child Health and Human Development
National Institutes of Health
Bethesda, Maryland
Clinical Professor
Department of Pharmacy Practice and Science
School of Pharmacy, University of Maryland
Baltimore, Maryland
Clinical Professor
Department of Pharmacotherapy and Outcomes Science
School of Pharmacy
Virginia Commonwealth University
Richmond, Virginia
Chapters 60, 65, and 121

Peggy L. Carver, PharmD, FCCP
Associate Professor of Pharmacy
Clinical Pharmacist, Infectious Diseases
Department of Clinical, Social, and Administrative Sciences
University of Michigan College of Pharmacy and University of Michigan Health System
Ann Arbor, Michigan
Chapter 99

Larisa H. Cavallari, PharmD
Associate Professor
Department of Pharmacy Practice
University of Illinois at Chicago
Chicago, Illinois
eChapter 6
Chapter 4

Jose E. Cavazos, MD, PhD
Professor
Departments of Neurology, Pharmacology and Physiology
Assistant Dean for MD/PhD Program
The University of Texas Health Science Center at San Antonio
San Antonio, Texas
Chapter 40

Alexandre Chan, PharmD, MPH, BCPS, BCOP
Associate Professor
Department of Pharmacy
Faculty of Science
National University of Singapore
Associate Consultant Clinical Pharmacist
Department of Pharmacy
National Cancer Centre Singapore
Singapore, Singapore
Chapter 109

C. Y. Jennifer Chan, PharmD
Clinical Assistant Professor of Pharmacy
Pharmacotherapy Education and Research Center
University of Texas at Austin College of Pharmacy
Adjunct Associate Professor of Pediatrics
Department of Pediatrics
University of Texas Health Science Center
San Antonio, Texas
Chapter 82

Jack J. Chen, PharmD, BCPS
Associate Professor
Department of Neurology
Movement Disorders Clinic
Schools of Medicine and Pharmacy
Loma Linda University
Loma Linda, California
Chapter 43

Judy T. Chen, PharmD, BCPS
Clinical Associate Professor
Department of Pharmacy Practice
Purdue University College of Pharmacy
Clinical Pharmacy Specialist
The Jane Pauley Community Health Center, Inc.
Indianapolis, Indiana
Chapter 121

Katherine Hammond Chessman, BSPharm, PharmD
Professor
Clinical Pharmacy and Outcomes Sciences
South Carolina College of Pharmacy, MUSC Campus
Clinical Pharmacy Specialist, Pediatrics/Pediatric Surgery
Department of Pharmacy Services
The Children's Hospital of South Carolina
Charleston, South Carolina
Chapters 34, 118, and 120

Elaine Chiquette
San Antonio, Texas
eChapter 4

Mariann D. Churchwell, PharmD, BCPS
Associate Professor
University of Toledo College of Pharmacy
Toledo, Ohio
Chapter 30

Peter A. Chyka, PharmD, FAACT, DPNAP, DABAT
Professor and Executive Associate Dean
Department of Clinical Pharmacy
University of Tennessee Health Science Center
College of Pharmacy
Knoxville, Tennessee
eChapter 10

Elizabeth C. Clark, MD, MPH
Assistant Professor
Family Medicine and Community Health
Rutgers University, Robert Wood Johnson Medical School
New Brunswick, New Jersey
Chapter 74

Nathan P. Clark, PharmD, BCPS
Clinical Pharmacy Supervisor
Clinical Pharmacy
Anticoagulation and Anemia Service
Kaiser Permanente
Aurora, Colorado
Chapter 9

Kristen Cook, PharmD, BCPS
Assistant Professor
Department of Pharmacy Practice
College of Pharmacy
University of Nebraska Medical Center
Omaha, Nebraska
Chapter 80

John R. Corboy, MD
Professor
Department of Neurology
University of Colorado School of Medicine
Co-Director
Rocky Mountain MS Center
University of Colorado
Anschutz Medical Campus
Aurora, Colorado
Chapter 39

Lisa T. Costanigro, PharmD, BCPS
Staff Pharmacist
Poudre Valley Health System
Fort Collins, Colorado
eChapter 11

Elizabeth A. Coyle, PharmD, FCCM, BCPS
Assistant Dean of Assessment
Clinical Professor
University of Houston
College of Pharmacy
Houston, Texas
Chapter 94

Catherine M. Crill, PharmD, BCPS, BCNSP, FCCP
Associate Professor
Departments of Clinical Pharmacy and Pediatrics
The University of Tennessee Health Science Center
Memphis, Tennessee
Chapter 119

M. Lynn Crismon, PharmD
Dean
James T. Doluisio Regents Chair and Behrens Centennial Professor
College of Pharmacy
The University of Texas at Austin
Austin, Texas
Chapter 50

Michael A. Crouch, PharmD, FASHP, BCPS
Executive Associate Dean and Professor
Department of Pharmacy Practice
Gatton College of Pharmacy
East Tennessee State University
Johnson City, Tennessee
Chapter 89

William Dager, PharmD, BCPS (AQ Cardiology)
Pharmacist Specialist
UC Davis Medical Center
Clinical Professor of Pharmacy
UC San Francisco School of Pharmacy
Clinical Professor of Medicine
UC Davis School of Medicine
Clinical Professor of Pharmacy
Touro School of Pharmacy
Sacramento, California
Chapter 28

Devra K. Dang, PharmD, BCPS, CDE
Associate Clinical Professor
University of Connecticut
School of Pharmacy
Storrs, Connecticut
Chapter 65

Joseph F. Dasta, MSc, FCCM, FCCP
Adjunct Professor
The University of Texas
Professor Emeritus
The Ohio State University
Austin, Texas
Chapter 13

Dewayne A. Davidson, PharmD
Assistant Professor
Department of Family and Community Medicine
The University of Texas Health Science Center at San Antonio
San Antonio, Texas
eChapter 1

Lisa E. Davis, BS, PharmD
Professor of Clinical Pharmacy
Philadelphia College of Pharmacy
University of the Sciences in Philadelphia
Philadelphia, Pennsylvania
Chapter 107

Brian S. Decker, MD, PharmD, MS
Assistant Professor of Clinical Medicine
Department of Medicine, Division of Nephrology
Indiana University School of Medicine
Indianapolis, Indiana
Chapter 30

Timothy Dellenbaugh, MD
Associate Professor
Department of Psychiatry
University of Missouri-Kansas City
Center for Behavioral Medicine
Kansas City, Missouri
eChapter 20

Paulina Deming, PharmD
Associate Professor
Department of Pharmacy Practice
College of Pharmacy
University of New Mexico Health Sciences Center
Albuquerque, New Mexico
Chapter 26

Simon de Denus, B.Pharm, MSc, PhD
Research Pharmacist
Montreal Heart Institute
Associate Professor
Faculty of Pharmacy Université de Montréal
Université de Montréal Beaulieu-Saucier Chair in Pharmacogenomics
Montreal, Quebec
Chapter 7

John W. Devlin, PharmD, FCCP, FCCM
Associate Professor
Department of Pharmacy Practice
Bouve College of Health Professions
Northeastern University
Boston, Massachusetts
Chapter 37

Eric Dietrich, PharmD
Post Doctoral Fellow
Family Medicine College of Pharmacy and Medicine
University of Florida
Gainesville, Florida
Chapter 59

Cecily V. DiPiro, PharmD
Consultant Pharmacist
Mount Pleasant, South Carolina
Chapter 22

Joseph T. DiPiro, PharmD, FCCP
Executive Dean and Professor
South Carolina College of Pharmacy
University of South Carolina and Medical University of South Carolina
Charleston and Columbia, South Carolina
Chapter 92

Paul L. Doering, MS
Distinguished Service Professor of Pharmacy Practice Emeritus
Department of Pharmacotherapy and Translational Research
College of Pharmacy
University of Florida
Gainesville, Florida
Chapters 48 and 49

Julie A. Dopheide, PharmD, BCPP
Associate Professor of Clinical Pharmacy, Psychiatry and the Behavioral Sciences
University of Southern California School of Pharmacy and Keck School of Medicine
Los Angeles, California
Chapter 46

John M. Dopp, PharmD
Associate Professor
School of Pharmacy
University of Wisconsin
Madison, Wisconsin
Chapter 55

Thomas C. Dowling, PharmD, PhD, FCP
Associate Professor and Vice Chair
Department of Pharmacy Practice and Science
University of Maryland School of Pharmacy
Baltimore, Maryland
eChapter 18

Shannon J. Drayton, PharmD, BCPP
Associate Professor
Clinical Pharmacy and Outcomes Sciences
South Carolina College of Pharmacy
Medical University of South Carolina
Charleston, South Carolina
Chapter 52

Linda D. Dresser, PharmD, FCSHP
Assistant Professor
Leslie Dan Faculty of Pharmacy
University of Toronto
University Health Network, Toronto
Ontario, Canada
Chapter 98

Deepak P. Edward, MD
Jonas S Friedenwald Professor of Ophthalmology and Pathology
Department of Ophthalmology
Wilmer Eye Institute
Johns Hopkins University
Baltimore, Maryland
Chapter 75

Mary Elizabeth Elliott, PharmD, PhD
Associate Professor
Pharmacy Practice Division
School of Pharmacy
University of Wisconsin
Madison, Wisconsin
Chapter 71

Ramy H. Elshaboury, PharmD
Pharmacy Resident in Infectious Diseases
Department of Pharmacy
Abbott Northwestern Hospital, Part of Allina Health
Minneapolis, Minnesota
Chapter 84

Michael E. Ernst, PharmD
Professor (Clinical)
Department of Pharmacy Practice and Science
College of Pharmacy and Department of Family Medicine
Carver College of Medicine
The University of Iowa
Iowa City, Iowa
Chapter 74

Brian L. Erstad, PharmD, FCCM, FCCP, FASHP
Professor
Department of Pharmacy Practice and Science
University of Arizona College of Pharmacy
Tucson, Arizona
Chapter 14

Francisco J. Esteva, MD, PhD
Director
Breast Medical Oncology Program
Division of Hematology-Oncology
Department of Medicine
Associate Director of Clinical Investigation
New York University Cancer Institute
New York University Langone Medical Center
New York, New York
Chapter 105

Patricia H. Fabel, PharmD
Clinical Assistant Professor
Clinical Pharmacy and Outcomes Sciences
South Carolina College of Pharmacy, University of South Carolina Campus
Columbia, South Carolina
Chapter 23

Susan C. Fagan, PharmD, BCPS, FCCP
Jowdy Professor, Assistant Dean
Department of Clinical and Administrative Pharmacy
University of Georgia College of Pharmacy
Augusta, Georgia
eChapter 19
Chapter 10

Christopher A. Fausel, PharmD, MHA, BCOP
Clinical Manager, Oncology Pharmacy
Department of Pharmacy
Indiana University Simon Cancer Center
Indianapolis, Indiana
Chapter 112

Richard G. Fiscella, PharmD, MPH
Clinical Professor Emeritus
Department of Pharmacy Practice
University of Illinois at Chicago
Chicago, Illinois
Chapter 75

Douglas N. Fish, PharmD
Professor and Chair
Department of Clinical Pharmacy
Skaggs School of Pharmacy and Pharmaceutical Sciences
University of Colorado Anschutz Medical Campus
Clinical Specialist in Infectious Diseases/Critical Care
University of Colorado Hospital
Aurora, Colorado
Chapters 88 and 100

Courtney V. Fletcher, PharmD
Dean and Professor
Departments of Pharmacy Practice and Medicine
College of Pharmacy
University of Nebraska Medical Center
Omaha, Nebraska
Chapter 103

Michelle A. Fravel, PharmD
Assistant Professor (Clinical)
Department of Pharmacy Practice and Science and Department of Pharmaceutical Care
University of Iowa College of Pharmacy and University of Iowa Hospitals and Clinics
Iowa City, Iowa
Chapter 74

Bradi Frei, PharmD, MS, BCPS, BCOP
Associate Professor
Department of Pharmacy Practice
Feik School of Pharmacy
University of the Incarnate Word
San Antonio, Texas
Chapter 86

Christopher Frei, PharmD, MS, BCPS
Associate Professor
Division of Pharmacotherapy
College of Pharmacy
The University of Texas at Austin
Austin, Texas
Chapter 86

Melissa Frei-Jones, MD, MSCI
Assistant Professor
Department of Pediatrics
Division of Hematology/Oncology
School of Medicine
University of Texas Health Science Center
San Antonio, Texas
Chapter 82

Mark L. Glover, PharmD
Medical Writer
Global Medical Writing
PPD
Wilmington, North Carolina
Chapter 85

Shelly L. Gray, PharmD, MS
Professor and Vice Chair for Curriculum and Instruction
Department of Pharmacy
Director
Geriatric Pharmacy Program and Plein Certificate
School of Pharmacy
University of Washington
Seattle, Washington
eChapter 8

Alan E. Gross, PharmD, BCPS
Clinical Assistant Professor
Department of Pharmacy Practice
College of Pharmacy
University of Nebraska Medical Center
Adjunct Assistant Professor
Department of Medicine
College of Medicine
Section of Infectious Diseases
University of Nebraska Medical Center
Omaha, Nebraska
Chapter 92

Wayne P. Gulliver, MD, FRCPC
Professor of Dermatology and Medicine
Memorial University of Newfoundland
St. John's Newfoundland and Labrador
Canada
Chapter 78

John G. Gums, PharmD, FCCP
Professor of Pharmacy and Translational Research
Department of Family Medicine
College of Pharmacy and Medicine
University of Florida
Gainesville, Florida
Chapter 59

Emily R. Hajjar, PharmD, BCPS, BCAP, CGP
Associate Professor
Department of Pharmacy Practice
Jefferson School of Pharmacy
Thomas Jefferson University
Philadelphia, Pennsylvania
eChapter 8

Jenana Halilovic, PharmD, BCPS, AAHIVP
Assistant Professor
Department of Pharmacy Practice
Thomas J Long School of Pharmacy and Health Sciences
Stockton, California
Chapter 28

Philip D. Hall, PharmD, FCCP, BCPS, BCOP
Campus Dean and Professor
South Carolina College of Pharmacy
Medical University of South Carolina
Charleston, South Carolina
eChapter 21

Joseph T. Hanlon, PharmD, MS
Professor
Department of Medicine, Pharmacy and Therapeutics, and Epidemiology
University of Pittsburgh
Pittsburgh, Pennsylvania
eChapter 8

Michelle Harkins, MD
Associate Professor of Medicine
Department of Internal Medicine
University of New Mexico Health Sciences Center
Albuquerque, New Mexico
eChapter 15

Mary S. Hayney, PharmD, MPH, FCCP, BCPS
Professor of Pharmacy
University of Wisconsin School of Pharmacy
Madison, Wisconsin
Chapter 102

Brian A. Hemstreet, PharmD, FCCP, BCPS
Associate Professor
Department of Clinical Pharmacy
University of Colorado Skaggs School of Pharmacy and Pharmaceutical Sciences
Aurora, Colorado
Chapter 21

Elizabeth D. Hermsen, PharmD, MBA, BCPS-ID
Clinical Scientific Director
Cubist Pharmaceuticals, Inc.
Lexington, Massachusetts
Adjunct Associate Professor
Department of Pharmacy Practice
College of Pharmacy, University of Nebraska Medical Center
Omaha, Nebraska
Chapters 84 and 87

Chris M. Herndon, PharmD, BCPS, CPE
Associate Professor
Department of Pharmacy Practice
Southern Illinois University Edwardsville
Edwardsville, Illinois
Chapter 44

Lauren R. Hersh, MD
Instructor
Department of Family and Community Medicine
Thomas Jefferson University
Philadelphia, Pennsylvania
eChapter 8

David C. Hess, MD
Professor and Chairman
Department of Neurology
Medical College of Georgia
Augusta, Georgia
Chapter 10

Angela Massey Hill, PharmD, BCPP, CPH
Professor and Chair
Department of Pharmacotherapeutics
University of South Florida College of Pharmacy
Tampa, Florida
Chapter 38

L. David Hillis, MD
Professor and Chair
Department of Medicine
University of Texas Health Science Center
San Antonio, Texas
eChapter 13
Chapter 1

Barbara J. Hoeben, PharmD, MSPharm, BCPS
Pharmacy Flight Commander
Davis-Monthan Air Force Base
Tucson, Arizona
Chapter 12

Jessica S. Holt, PharmD, BCPS (AQ-ID)
Infectious Diseases Pharmacy Coordinator
Department of Pharmacy
Abbott Northwestern Hospital, Part of Allina Health
Minneapolis, Minnesota
Chapter 84

Joanna Q. Hudson, PharmD, BCPS, FASN, FCCP
Associate Professor
Departments of Clinical Pharmacy and Medicine (Nephrology)
The University of Tennessee Health Science Center
Memphis, Tennessee
Chapter 29

Grant F. Hutchins, MD
Assistant Professor, Internal Medicine
Division of Gastroenterology-Hepatology
University of Nebraska Medical Center
Omaha, Nebraska
eChapter 16

Robert J. Ignoffo, PharmD, FASHP, FCSHP
Professor of Pharmacy
Touro University California
Clinical Professor Emeritus
University of California
San Francisco, California
Chapter 22

Arthur A. Islas, MD, MPH
Associate Professor and Director of Sports Medicine
Department of Family and Community Medicine
Paul L. Foster School of Medicine
Texas Tech University Health Sciences Center-El Paso
El Paso, Texas
eChapter 2

Heather J. Johnson, PharmD, BCPS
Assistant Professor
Department of Pharmacy and Therapeutics
University of Pittsburgh School of Pharmacy
Pittsburgh, Pennsylvania
Chapter 70

Shawn E. Johnson, PharmD, MPH
Clinical Generalist Pharmacist
Department of Pharmacy
The Ohio State University Wexner Medical Center
Columbus, Ohio
eChapter 3

Jacqueline Jonklaas, MD, PhD
Associate Professor
Division of Endocrinology
Department of Medicine
Georgetown University
Washington, District of Columbia
Chapter 58

Joseph K. Jordan, PharmD
Associate Professor
Drug Information Specialist
Department of Pharmacy Practice
Butler University College of Pharmacy and Health Sciences
Indiana University Health
Indianapolis, Indiana
Chapter 60

Rose Jung, PharmD, MPH, BCPS
Clinical Associate Professor
Department of Pharmacy Practice
College of Pharmacy and Pharmaceutical Sciences
University of Toledo
Toledo, Ohio
Chapter 91

Thomas N. Kakuda, PharmD
Scientific Director
Department of Clinical Pharmacology
Janssen Research & Development, LLC
Titusville, New Jersey
Chapter 103

Sophia N. Kalantaridou, MD, PhD
Professor of Obstetrics and Gynecology
Department of Obstetrics and Gynecology
University of Ioannina Medical School
Ioannina, Greece
Chapter 65

Judith C. Kando, PharmD, BCPP
Senior Ana Medical Specialist
Sunovion Pharmaceuticals Inc.
Marlborough, Massachusetts
Chapter 51

S. Lena Kang-Birken, PharmD, FCCP
Associate Professor
Department of Pharmacy Practice
School of Pharmacy and Health Sciences
University of the Pacific
Stockton, California
Chapter 97

Salmaan Kanji, PharmD, BSc, Pharm, ACPR
Clinical Pharmacy Specialist
The Ottawa Hospital
Associate Scientist
Ottawa Hospital Research Institute
Adjunct Professor of Pharmacy
University of Montreal
Assistant Professor of Medicine
University of Ottawa
Pharmacy, Clinical Epidemiology
Ottawa, Ontario, Canada
Chapter 101

H. William Kelly, PharmD
Professor Emeritus Pediatrics
Department of Pediatrics
University of New Mexico Health Sciences Center
Albuquerque, New Mexico
Chapter 15

Patrick J. Kiel, PharmD, BCPS, BCOP
Clinical Pharmacy Specialist, Hematology/Stem Cell Transplant
Department of Pharmacy
Indiana University Simon Cancer Center
Indianapolis, Indiana
Chapter 112

William R. Kirchain, PharmD, CDE
Wilbur and Mildred Robichaux Endowed Professorship
Division of Clinical and Administrative Sciences
Xavier University of Louisiana
College of Pharmacy
New Orleans, Louisiana
eChapter 17

Cynthia K. Kirkwood, PharmD, BCPP
Professor
Vice Chair for Education
Department of Pharmacotherapy and Outcomes Science
School of Pharmacy
Virginia Commonwealth University
Richmond, Virginia
Chapters 53 and 54

Jacqueline Klootwyk, PharmD, BCPS
Assistant Professor of Pharmacy Practice
Jefferson School of Pharmacy
Thomas Jefferson University
Philadelphia, Pennsylvania
Chapter 63

Leroy C. Knodel, PharmD
Associate Professor
Department of Surgery
The University of Texas Health Science Center
San Antonio, Texas
Clinical Professor
College of Pharmacy
The University of Texas at Austin
Austin, Texas
Chapter 95

Jill M. Kolesar, PharmD, BCPS, FCCP
Professor
School of Pharmacy
University of Wisconsin
Madison, Wisconsin
Chapter 108

Sunil Kripalani, MD, MSc
Associate Professor
Section of Hospital Medicine
Division of General Internal Medicine and Public Health
Department of Medicine
Vanderbilt University
Nashville, Tennessee
eChapter 1

Vanessa J. Kumpf, PharmD, BCNSP
Clinical Specialist, Nutrition Support
Center for Human Nutrition
Vanderbilt Medical Center
Nashville, Tennessee
Chapters 118 and 120

Po Gin Kwa, MD, FRCPC
Clinical Assistant, Professor of Pediatrics
Faculty of Medicine
Memorial University of Newfoundland and Pediatrician
Eastern Health
St. John's, Newfoundland, Canada
Chapter 79

Sum Lam, PharmD, CGP, BCPS, FASCP
Associate Clinical Professor
Department of Clinical Pharmacy Practice
St. John's University
Queens, New York
Chapter 68

Y. W. Francis Lam, PharmD, FCCP
Professor of Pharmacology and Medicine
Department of Pharmacology
The University of Texas Health Science Center at San Antonio
San Antonio, Texas
Clinical Associate Professor of Pharmacy
University of Texas at Austin
Austin, Texas
eChapter 6

Richard A. Lange, MD, MBA
Professor and Executive Vice Chairman
Department of Medicine
The University of Texas Health Science Center
San Antonio, Texas
eChapter 13
Chapter 1

Kerry L. LaPlante, PharmD, BS
Associate Professor of Pharmacy
Department of Pharmacy Practice
University of Rhode Island College of Pharmacy
Infectious Diseases Pharmacotherapy Specialist
Pharmacy Services
Providence Veterans Affairs Medical Center
Adjunct Associate Professor of Medicine
Division of Infectious Diseases
Warren Alpert School of Medicine
Brown University
Kingston, Rhode Island
eChapter 25

Alan H. Lau, PharmD, FCCP
Professor
Department of Pharmacy Practice
Director, International Clinical Pharmacy Education
University of Illinois at Chicago, College of Pharmacy
Chicago, Illinois
Chapter 32

Michael Lauzardo, MD, MSc
Chief
Division of Infectious Diseases and Global Medicine
Director
Southeastern National Tuberculosis Center
College of Medicine
University of Florida
Gainesville, Florida
Chapter 90

David T.S. Law, BSc, MD, PhD, CCFP
Assistant Professor
Department of Family and Community Medicine
Faculty of Medicine
University of Toronto
Staff, Department of Family Practice
The Scarborough Hospital and Rouge Valley Health System
Scarborough, Ontario, Canada
eChapter 23

Rebecca M. Law, PharmD
School of Pharmacy and Discipline of Family Medicine
Faculty of Medicine
Memorial University of Newfoundland
St. John's Newfoundland, Canada
eChapter 23
Chapters 78 and 79

Grace C. Lee, PharmD, BCPS
Clinical Instructor
Division of Pharmacotherapy
College of Pharmacy
University of Texas at Austin
Austin, Texas
Chapter 83

Mary Lee, PharmD, BCPS, FCCP
Professor of Pharmacy Practice
Chicago College of Pharmacy
Midwestern University
Downers Grove, Illinois
Chapters 66 and 67

Timothy S. Lesar, PharmD
Director of Clinical Pharmacy Services
Patient Care Services Director
Department of Pharmacy
Albany Medical Center
Albany, New York
Chapter 75

Deborah J. Levine, MD, FCCP
Associate Professor of Medicine
Division of Pulmonary and Critical Care
University of Texas
San Antonio, Texas
Chapter 17

Stephanie M. Levine, MD
Professor of Medicine
Division of Pulmonary Diseases and Critical Care Medicine
The University of Texas Health Science Center
San Antonio, Texas
eChapter 14

Robin Moorman Li, PharmD, BCACP
Assistant Director
Jacksonville Campus
Clinical Assistant Professor
Department of Pharmacotherapy and Translational Research
University of Florida, College of Pharmacy
Gainesville, Florida
Chapters 48 and 49

Susanne Liewer, PharmD, BCOP
Clinical Pharmacy Coordinator, Stem Cell Transplant
Department of Pharmaceutical and Nutrition Care
The Nebraska Medical Center
Clinical Assistant Professor
Department of Pharmacy Practice
College of Pharmacy
University of Nebraska Medical Center
Omaha, Nebraska
Chapter 117

Bryan L. Love, PharmD
Associate Professor
Department of Clinical Pharmacy and Outcomes Science
South Carolina College of Pharmacy
Clinical Pharmacy Specialist
Departments of Pharmacy and Gastroenterology/Hepatology
William Jennings Bryan Dorn Veterans Affairs Medical Center
Columbia, South Carolina
Chapter 20

Amanda M. Loya, PharmD
Clinical Associate Professor
University of Texas at El Paso
UT Austin Cooperative Pharmacy Program
University of Texas at El Paso College of Health Sciences
University of Texas at Austin College of Pharmacy
Adjunct Clinical Assistant Professor
Department of Family and Community Medicine
Texas Tech University Health Sciences Center—El Paso
El Paso, Texas
eChapter 2

William L. Lyons, MD
Associate Professor
Section of Geriatrics
Department of Internal Medicine
University of Nebraska Medical Center
Omaha, Nebraska
Chapter 80

Robert MacLaren, BBSc, PharmD, MPH, FCCM, FCCP
Professor
Department of Clinical Pharmacy
Skaggs School of Pharmacy and Pharmaceutical Sciences
University of Colorado Denver
Aurora, Colorado
Chapter 13

Eric J. MacLaughlin, PharmD, FASHP, FCCP, BCPS
Professor and Interim Chair
Department of Pharmacy Practice
Professor
Departments of Family Medicine and Internal Medicine
Texas Tech University Health Sciences Center School of Pharmacy
Amarillo, Texas
Chapter 3

Robert L. Maher Jr, PharmD, CGP
Assistant Professor of Pharmacy Practice
Clinical, Social, and Administrative Sciences Division
Duquesne University Mylan School of Pharmacy
Pittsburgh, Pennsylvania
eChapter 8

Robert A. Mangione, EdD, RPh
Provost and Professor of Pharmacy
Office of the Provost
St. John's University
Queens, New York
Chapter 27

Steven Martin, PharmD
Professor and Chairman
Department of Pharmacy Practice
College of Pharmacy and Pharmaceutical Sciences
The University of Toledo
Toledo, Ohio
Chapter 91

Todd W. Mattox, PharmD, BCNSP
Critical Care
Nutrition Support Pharmacy Specialist
Department of Pharmacy
Moffitt Cancer Center
Tampa, Florida
Chapter 119

Gary R. Matzke, PharmD, FCP, FCCP, FASN, FNAP
Professor and Director
Pharmacy Practice Transformation Initiatives
and Founding Director
ACCP/ASHP/VCU Congressional Health Care Policy
Fellow Program
Department of Pharmacotherapy and Outcome Sciences
School of Pharmacy, Virginia Commonwealth University
Richmond, Virginia
Chapters 33, 34, and 37

Dianne B. May, PharmD, BCPS
Clinical Associate Professor
Department of Clinical and Administrative Pharmacy
Division of Experience Programs
College of Pharmacy
University of Georgia
Augusta, Georgia
Chapter 19

J. Russell May, PharmD
Clinical Professor
Department of Clinical and Administrative Pharmacy
University of Georgia College of Pharmacy
Augusta, Georgia
Chapter 76

Kristen B. McCullough, PharmD, BCPS, BCOP
Clinical Pharmacist
Department of Pharmacy Services
Mayo Clinic
Rochester, Minnesota
Chapter 114

Timothy R. McGuire, PharmD, FCCP, BCOP
Associate Professor
Department of Pharmacy Practice
College of Pharmacy
University of Nebraska Medical Center
Omaha, Nebraska
Chapter 113

Jerry R. McKee, PharmD, MS, BCPP
Regional Dean
Associate Professor of Pharmacy
Wingate University Hendersonville Campus
Hendersonville, North Carolina
Chapter 56

Patrick J. Medina, PharmD, BCOP
Associate Professor
The University of Oklahoma
College of Pharmacy
Oklahoma City, Oklahoma
Chapters 104 and 107

Sarah T. Melton, PharmD, BCPP, BCACP, CGP, FASCP
Associate Professor of Pharmacy Practice
Department of Pharmacy Practice
Gatton College of Pharmacy at East Tennessee State University
Johnson City, Tennessee
Chapters 53 and 54

Julianna A. Merten, PharmD, BCPS, BCOP
Clinical Pharmacy Specialist
Department of Pharmacy Services
Mayo Clinic
Rochester, Minnesota
Chapter 114

Laura Boehnke Michaud, PharmD, BCOP, FASHP
Manager, Clinical Pharmacy Services
Division of Pharmacy
Clinical Pharmacy Services
The University of Texas M. D. Anderson Cancer Center
Houston, Texas
Chapter 105

Deborah S. Minor, PharmD
Executive Vice Chair and Professor
Department of Medicine, School of Medicine
Associate Professor, School of Pharmacy
University of Mississippi Medical Center
Jackson, Mississippi
Chapter 45

Augusto Miravalle, MD
Assistant Professor
Department of Neurology
University of Colorado School of Medicine
Associate Director
Neurology Residency Program
University of Colorado
Anschutz Medical Campus
Aurora, Colorado
Chapter 39

Isaac F. Mitropoulos, BS, PharmD
Senior Medical Education and Research Liaison
Department of Medical Affairs
Optimer Pharmaceuticals, Inc.
Chapel Hill, North Carolina
Chapter 84

Rima A. Mohammad, PharmD, BCPS
Assistant Professor
Department of Pharmacy and Therapeutics
School of Pharmacy
University of Pittsburgh
Pittsburgh, Pennsylvania
Chapter 33

Patricia A. Montgomery, PharmD
Adjunct Professor
Thomas J. Long School of Pharmacy and Health Sciences
University of the Pacific
Sacramento, California
Chapter 25

Rebecca Moote, PharmD, MSc, BCPS
Assistant Professor
Department of Pharmacy Practice
Regis University School of Pharmacy
Denver, Colorado
Chapter 17

Scott W. Mueller, PharmD
Assistant Professor
Department of Clinical Pharmacy
Skaggs School of Pharmacy and Pharmaceutical Sciences
University of Colorado Anschutz Medical Campus
Clinical Specialist in Critical Care
University of Colorado Hospital
Aurora, Colorado
Chapter 100

Milap C. Nahata, PharmD, MS, FCCP
Professor of Pharmacy
Pediatrics and Internal Medicine
Division Chair
Pharmacy Practice and Administration College of Pharmacy
Ohio State University
Associate Director of Pharmacy
The Ohio State University Medical Center
Columbus, Ohio
eChapter 7

Rocsanna Namdar, PharmD, BCPS
Assistant Professor
Department of Clinical Pharmacy
University of Colorado
Skaggs School of Pharmacy and Pharmaceutical Sciences
Aurora, Colorado
Chapter 90

Jean M. Nappi, BS, PharmD, FCCP, BCPS
Professor
Department of Clinical Pharmacy and Outcome Sciences
South Carolina College of Pharmacy—MUSC Campus
Professor
Department of Medicine
Medical University of South Carolina
Charleston, South Carolina
Chapter 4

Leigh Anne Nelson, PharmD, BCPP
Associate Professor
Division of Pharmacy Practice and Administration
School of Pharmacy
University of Missouri-Kansas City
Kansas City, Missouri
eChapter 20

Fenwick T. Nichols III, MD
Professor of Neurology
Medical College of Georgia
Augusta, Georgia
eChapter 19

Jessica C. Njoku, PharmD, BCPS
Infectious Diseases and Antimicrobial Stewardship Coordinator
Department of Pharmacy
Baylor University Medical Center
Dallas, Texas
Chapter 87

Thomas D. Nolin, PharmD, PhD, FCCP, FCP, FASN
Assistant Professor
Department of Pharmacy and Therapeutics
Center for Clinical Pharmaceutical Sciences
Department of Medicine, Renal-Electrolyte Division
University of Pittsburgh Schools of Pharmacy and Medicine
Pittsburgh, Pennsylvania
Chapter 31

LeAnn B. Norris, PharmD, BCPS, BCOP
Assistant Professor
Clinical Pharmacy and Outcomes Sciences
South Carolina College of Pharmacy
Columbia, South Carolina
Chapter 108

Barbara M. O'Brien, MD
Assistant Professor
Division of MFM
Director
Perinatal Genetics
Co-Director Prenatal Diagnosis Center
Associate Director
Core Clerkship in Obstetrics and Gynecology
Providence, Rhode Island
Chapter 61

Cindy L. O'Bryant, PharmD, BCOP
Associate Professor
Department of Clinical Pharmacy
Skaggs School of Pharmacy and Pharmaceutical Sciences
Clinical Specialist in Oncology
University of Colorado Cancer Center
Aurora, Colorado
Chapter 116

Mary Beth O'Connell, PharmD, BCPS, FASHP, FCCP
Associate Professor
Department of Pharmacy Practice
Eugene Applebaum College of Pharmacy and Health Sciences
Wayne State University
Detroit, Michigan
Chapter 73

Brian L. Odle, PharmD
Assistant Professor
Department of Pharmacy Practice
Gatton College of Pharmacy
East Tennessee State University
Johnson City, Tennessee
Chapter 89

Keith M. Olsen, PharmD, FCCP, FCCM
Professor and Chair
Department of Pharmacy Practice
College of Pharmacy
University of Nebraska Medical Center
Omaha, Nebraska
eChapter 16
Chapter 92

Amy Barton Pai, PharmD, BCPS, FASN, FCCP
Associate Professor
Department of Pharmacy Practice
Albany College of Pharmacy and Health Sciences
Albany, New York
Chapter 35

Robert B. Parker, PharmD, FCCP
Professor
Department of Clinical Pharmacy
University of Tennessee College of Pharmacy
Memphis, Tennessee
Chapter 4

Priti N. Patel, PharmD, BCPS
Associate Clinical Professor
College of Pharmacy and Health Sciences
St. John's University
Queens, New York
Chapter 27

Mrinal M. Patnaik, MBBS, MD
Assistant Professor of Oncology and Internal Medicine
Division of Hematology
Department of Internal Medicine
Mayo Clinic
Rochester, Minnesota
Chaper 114

Christine M. Pelic, MD
Assistant Professor
Department of Psychiatry
Medical University of South Carolina
Charleston, South Carolina
Chapter 52

Charles A. Peloquin, PharmD
Professor
College of Pharmacy and Emerging Pathogens Institute
University of Florida
Gainesville, Florida
Chapter 90

Susan L. Pendland, MS, PharmD
Adjunct Associate Professor of Pharmacy Practice
University of Illinois at Chicago
Chicago, Illinois
Clinical Staff Pharmacist, St. Joseph Berea Hospital
Berea, Kentucky
Chapter 88

Janelle Perkins, PharmD, BCOP
Associate Professor
Departments of Pharmacotherapeutics, Clinical Research and Oncologic Sciences
Colleges of Pharmacy and Medicine
University of South Florida
Tampa, Florida
Chapter 117

Emily P. Peron, PharmD, MS, BCPS, FASCP
Assistant Professor
Geriatric Pharmacotherapy Program
Department of Pharmacotherapy and Outcomes Science
Virginia Commonwealth University
School of Pharmacy
Richmond, Virginia
Chapter 38

Jay I. Peters, MD
Professor and Chief
Division of Pulmonary Critical Care
University of Texas Health Science Center
San Antonio, Texas
eChapter 14

Stephanie J. Phelps, PharmD, BSPharm
Professor
Clinical Pharmacy and Pediatrics
College of Pharmacy and Pediatrics
The University of Tennessee Health Science Center
Memphis, Tennessee
Chapter 41

Bradley G. Phillips, PharmD, BCPS, FCCP
Milliken-Reeve Professor and Head
Department of Clinical and Administrative Pharmacy
University of Georgia College of Pharmacy
Athens, Georgia
Chapter 55

Nicole Weimert Pilch, PharmD, MSCR, BCPS
Clinical Specialist
Solid Organ Transplantation
Clinical Assistant Professor
Department of Pharmacy and Clinical Sciences
South Carolina College of Pharmacy
MUSC Campus
Medical University of South Carolina
Department of Pharmacy Services
Charleston, South Carolina
eChapter 21

Kathleen J. Pincus, PharmD, BCPS
Assistant Professor
Department of Pharmacy Practice and Sciences
University of Maryland
School of Pharmacy
Baltimore, Maryland
Chapter 64

Stephen R. Pliszka, MD
Professor and Chief
Division of Child and Adolescent Psychiatry
Department of Psychiatry
The University of Texas Health Science Center at San Antonio
San Antonio, Texas
Chapter 46

Betsy Bickert Poon, PharmD
Assistant Director of Pharmacy
Pediatric Hematology/Oncology/Stem Cell Transplant Specialist
Walt Disney Pavilion at Florida Hospital for Children
Orlando, Florida
Chapters 81 and 111

L. Michael Posey, BSPharm, MA
Associate Vice President
Periodicals Department
American Pharmacists Association
Washington, District of Columbia
eChapter 4

Jamie C. Poust, PharmD, BCOP
Oncology Pharmacy Specialist
Department of Pharmacy
University of Colorado Hospital
Anschutz Inpatient Pavilion
Aurora, Colorado
Chapter 116

Randall A. Prince, PharmD, PhD
Professor
University of Houston College of Pharmacy
Houston, Texas
Chapter 94

Jane Pruemer, PharmD, BCOP
Professor of Clinical Pharmacy Practice
Department of Pharmacy Practice and Administrative Sciences
James L. Winkle College of Pharmacy
University of Cincinnati
Cincinnati, Ohio
Chapter 81

Kelly R. Ragucci, PharmD, FCCP, BCPS, CDE
Professor and Chair
Clinical Pharmacy and Outcomes Sciences
South Carolina College of Pharmacy
Medical University of South Carolina Campus
Charleston, South Carolina
Chapter 62

Hengameh H. Raissy, PharmD
Research Associate Professor of Pediatrics
Pulmonary Division
School of Medicine
University of New Mexico
Albuquerque, New Mexico
eChapter 15

Kamakshi V. Rao, PharmD, BCOP, CPP, FASHP
Clinical Pharmacist Practitioner
Oncology/Bone Marrow Transplant
University of North Carolina Hospitals and Clinics
Clinical Assistant Professor
Division of Practice Advancement and Clinical Education
University of North Carolina Eshelman School of Pharmacy
Chapel Hill, North Carolina
eChapter 24

Satish SC Rao, MD, PhD, FRCP
Professor of Medicine
Chief, Section of Gastroenterology/Hepatology
Director
Digestive Health Center
Department of Medicine
Georgia Regents University
Medical College of Georgia
Augusta, Georgia
Chapter 19

Brent N. Reed, PharmD, BCPS
Assistant Professor
Department of Pharmacy Practice and Science
University of Maryland School of Pharmacy
Clinical Pharmacy Specialist
Department of Pharmacy
University of Maryland Medical Center
Baltimore, Maryland
Chapter 5

Michael D. Reed, PharmD
Director
Department of Clinical Pharmacology and Toxicology
The Rebecca D. Considine Research Institute
Akron Children's Hospital
Akron, Ohio
Chapter 85

Thomas Repas, DO, FACP, FACOI, FNLA, FACE, CDE
Clinical Assistant Professor
Department of Internal Medicine
Sanford School of Medicine
University of South Dakota
Sioux Falls, South Dakota
Chapter 57

Beth H. Resman-Targoff, PharmD, FCCP
Clinical Professor
Department of Pharmacy
Clinical and Administrative Sciences
University of Oklahoma College of Pharmacy
Oklahoma City, Oklahoma
Chapter 69

José O. Rivera, PharmD
Director and Clinical Professor
University of Texas at El Paso
UT Austin Cooperative Pharmacy Program
University of Texas at El Paso College of Health Sciences
University of Texas at Austin College of Pharmacy
Assistant Dean and Clinical Professor
El Paso, Texas
eChapter 2

Jo E. Rodgers, PharmD, FCCP, BCPS
Clinical Associate Professor
Division of Pharmacotherapy and Experimental Therapeutics
UNC Eshelman School of Pharmacy
Chapel Hill, North Carolina
Chapter 5

Susan J. Rogers, PharmD, BCPS
Assistant Clinical Professor at Austin
Clinical Pharmacy Specialist Neurology
South Texas Healthcare System
Audie L. Murphy Memorial Veterans Hospital
San Antonio, Texas
Chapter 40

John C. Rotschafer, PharmD, FCCP
Professor
Experimental and Clinical Pharmacology
University of Minnesota
College of Pharmacy
Minneapolis, Minnesota
Chapter 84

Eric S. Rovner, MD
Professor of Urology
Department of Urology
Medical University of South Carolina
Charleston, South Carolina
Chapter 68

Valerie L. Ruehter, PharmD, BCPP
Clinical Assistant Professor
Director of Experiential Learning
University of Missouri-Kansas City School of Pharmacy
Kansas City, Missouri
Chapter 47

Michael J. Rybak, PharmD, MPH
Professor of Pharmacy and Medicine
Director
Anti Infective Research Laboratory
Department of Pharmacy Practice
Eugene Applebaum College of Pharmacy
Wayne State University
Detroit, Michigan
eChapter 25

Cynthia A. Sanoski, PharmD, BCPS, FCCP
Chair
Department of Pharmacy Practice
Jefferson School of Pharmacy
Thomas Jefferson University
Philadelphia, Pennsylvania
Chapter 8

Joseph J. Saseen, PharmD, FASHP, FCCP, BCPS
Professor and Vice Chair
Department of Clinical Pharmacy
Professor
Department of Family Medicine
University of Colorado Anschutz Medical Campus
Skaggs School of Pharmacy and Pharmaceutical Sciences
Aurora, Colorado
Chapter 3

Mark E. Schneiderhan, PharmD, BCPP
Associate Professor
Department of Pharmacy Practice and Pharmaceutical Sciences
Department of Psychiatry
University of Minnesota, College of Pharmacy
Duluth/Human Development Center
Duluth, Minnesota
eChapter 20

Kristine S. Schonder, PharmD
Assistant Professor
Department of Pharmacy and Therapeutics
University of Pittsburgh School of Pharmacy
Pittsburgh, Pennsylvania
Chapter 70

Arthur A. Schuna, MS, BCACP
Clinical Coordinator
Department of Pharmacy Service
William S. Middleton VA Hospital
Clinical Professor
Department of Pharmacy Practice
University of Wisconsin School of Pharmacy
Madison, Wisconsin
Chapter 72

Richard B. Schwartz, MD
Professor and Chair
Department of Emergency Medicine
Medical College of Georgia
Augusta, Georgia
eChapter 12

Julie M. Sease, PharmD, BCPS, BCACP
Associate Professor
Department of Pharmacy Practice
Presbyterian College School of Pharmacy
Clinton, South Carolina
Chapter 24

Amy Hatfield Seung, PharmD, BCOP
Oncology Pharmacy Clinical Specialist
PGY2 Oncology Residency Director
Department of Pharmacy
Sidney Kimmel Comprehensive Cancer Center
Johns Hopkins Hospital
Baltimore, Maryland
Chapter 111

Kayce M. Shealy, PharmD
Assistant Professor
Department of Pharmacy Practice
Presbyterian College School of Pharmacy
Clinton, South Carolina
Chapter 23

Amy Heck Sheehan, PharmD
Associate Professor
Department of Pharmacy Practice
Purdue University College of Pharmacy
Drug Information Specialist
Indiana University Health System
Indianapolis, Indiana
Chapters 60 and 121

Ziad Shehab, MD
Professor
Departments of Pediatrics and Pathology
University of Arizona College of Medicine
Tucson, Arizona
Chapter 96

Greene Shepherd, PharmD
Clinical Professor
Department of Practice Advancement and Clinical Education
UNC Eshelman School of Pharmacy
Asheville, North Carolina
eChapter 12

Stacy S. Shord, PharmD, BCOP, FCCP
Reviewer
Office of Clinical Pharmacology
Office of Translational Science
Center for Drug Evaluation and Research
U.S. Food and Drug Administration
Silver Spring, Maryland
Chapter 104

Sarah P. Shrader, PharmD, BCPS, CDE
Clinical Associate Professor
Department of Pharmacy Practice
University of Kansas
School of Pharmacy
Lawrence, Kansas
Chapter 62

Jeri J. Sias, PharmD, MPH
Clinical Associate Professor
University of Texas at El Paso
UT Austin Cooperative Pharmacy Program
University of Texas at El Paso College of Health Sciences
University of Texas at Austin College of Pharmacy
Adjunct Clinical Assistant Professor
Department of Family and Community Medicine
Texas Tech University Health Sciences Center—El Paso
El Paso, Texas
eChapter 2

Debra Sibbald, BScPhm, RPh, ACPR, MA, PhD
Senior Lecturer
Division of Pharmacy Practice
Leslie Dan Faculty of Pharmacy
University of Toronto
Director
Department of Assessment Services
Centre for the Evaluation of Health Professionals Educated Abroad
Toronto, Ontario
Chapter 77

Ashley E. Simmons, PharmD
Post-Doctoral Fellow
Division of Pharmacotherapy and Experimental Therapeutics
University of North Carolina Eshelman School of Pharmacy
University of North Carolina
Chapel Hill, North Carolina
Chapter 115

Tamara D. Simpson, MD
Associate Professor of Medicine
Division of Pulmonary and Critical Care
University of Texas Health Science Center at San Antonio
San Antonio, Texas
eChapter 14

Patricia W. Slattum, PharmD, PhD
Director, Geriatric Pharmacotherapy Program
Department of Pharmacotherapy and Outcomes Science
Virginia Commonwealth University, School of Pharmacy
Richmond, Virginia
eChapter 8
Chapter 38

Judith A. Smith, PharmD, BCOP, CPHQ, FCCP, FISOPP
Associate Professor and Director, Pharmacology Research
Department of Gynecologic Oncology and Reproductive Medicine
Division of Surgery
Program Director, Oncology Translational Research Fellowship
Division of Pharmacy
University of Texas M.D. Anderson Cancer Center
Houston, Texas
Chapter 110

Philip H. Smith, MD
Assistant Professor
Department of Allergy and Immunology
Medical College of Georgia School of Medicine
Augusta, Georgia
Chapter 76

Steven M. Smith, PharmD, MPH
Assistant Professor
Department of Clinical Pharmacy
Skaggs School of Pharmacy and Pharmaceutical Sciences
University of Colorado
Aurora, Colorado
Chapter 59

Christine A. Sorkness, PharmD
Professor of Pharmacy and Medicine
Department of Pharmacy Practice
University of Wisconsin School of Pharmacy
Madison, Wisconsin
Chapter 15

Kevin M. Sowinski, PharmD, FCCP
Professor and Associate Head for Faculty Affairs
Department of Pharmacy Practice
School of Pharmacy and Pharmaceutical Sciences
Purdue University, West Lafayette and Indianapolis, Indiana
Adjunct Professor
Department of Medicine
School of Medicine
Indiana University
Indianapolis, Indiana
Chapter 30

Sarah A. Spinler, PharmD, FCCP, FAHA, BCPS
Professor of Clinical Pharmacy
Philadelphia College of Pharmacy
University of the Sciences in Philadelphia
Philadelphia, Pennsylvania
Chapter 7

Catherine I. Starner, PharmD, BCPS
Senior Health Outcomes Researcher
Medication Therapy Management
Prime Therapeutics, LLC
Adjunct Assistant Professor
Experimental and Clinical Pharmacology
College of Pharmacy
University of Minnesota
Minneapolis, Minnesota
eChapter 8

Douglas W. Stewart, DO, MPH
Associate Professor
Department of Pediatrics
School of Community Medicine
The University of Oklahoma
Tulsa, Oklahoma
Chapter 56

Steven C. Stoner, PharmD, BCPP
Clinical Professor and Chair
UMKC School of Pharmacy
Division of Pharmacy Practice and Administration
Kansas City, Missouri
Chapter 47

Jennifer M. Strickland, PharmD, BCPS
Director of Clinical Strategy
Millennium Laboratories
Assistant Clinical Professor
University of Florida
College of Pharmacy
Lakeland, Florida
Chapter 44

Deborah A. Sturpe, PharmD, BCPS, MA
Associate Professor
Department of Pharmacy Practice and Science
University of Maryland School of Pharmacy
Baltimore, Maryland
Chapter 64

Weijing Sun, MD, FACP
Professor
Department of Medicine
School of Medicine
University of Pittsburgh Cancer Institute
Pittsburgh, Pennsylvania
Chapter 107

David M. Swope, MD
Associate Professor
Department of Neurology
School of Medicine
Loma Linda University
Loma Linda, California
Chapter 43

Lynne M. Sylvia, PharmD
Senior Clinical Pharmacy Specialist—Cardiology
Department of Pharmacy
Tufts Medical Center
Clinical Professor
Northeastern University
School of Pharmacy
Boston, Massachusetts
eChapter 22

Carol Taketomo, PharmD
Director of Pharmacy and Clinical Nutrition
Children's Hospital of Los Angeles
Adjunct Assistant Professor of Pharmacy Practice
University of Southern California
School of Pharmacy
Los Angeles, California
eChapter 7

Robert L. Talbert, PharmD, FCCP, BCPS, FAHA
Professor
Pharmacotherapy Division
College of Pharmacy
University of Texas at Austin
Professor
Department of Medicine
School of Medicine
University of Texas Health Science Center at San Antonio
San Antonio, Texas
Chapters 6, 11, 12, and 58

Colleen M. Terriff, PharmD, BCPS (AQ-ID), AAHIVP, MPH International Medicine
Clinical Associate Professor
Department of Pharmacotherapy
Washington State University, College of Pharmacy
Deaconess Hospital
Spokane, Washington
eChapter 11

Christian J. Teter, PharmD, BCPP
Assistant Professor, Psychopharmacology
College of Pharmacy
University of New England
Portland, Maine
Chapter 51

Matthew N. Thoma, MD
Assistant Professor of Clinical Medicine
Department of Internal Medicine
University of South Carolina School of Medicine
Staff Gastroenterologist
Department of Gastroenterology/Hepatology
WJB Dorn VA Medical Center
Columbia, South Carolina
Chapter 20

Curtis L. Triplitt, PharmD, CDE
Clinical Assistant Professor
Department of Medicine
Division of Diabetes
University of Texas Health Science Center at San Antonio
Texas Diabetes Institute
University Health System
San Antonio, Texas
Chapter 57

Elena M. Umland, BS, PharmD
Associate Dean for Academic Affairs
Professor of Pharmacy Practice
Jefferson School of Pharmacy
Thomas Jefferson University
Philadelphia, Pennsylvania
Chapter 63

Yolanda Y. Vera, PharmD
Pediatric Patient Care Pharmacist
Department of Pharmacy
McLane Children's Hospital
Temple, Texas
Chapter 18

Angie Veverka, PharmD, BCPS
PGY1 Pharmacy Residency Director, Clinical Specialist, Internal Medicine
Department of Pharmacy
Carolinas Medical Center
Charlotte, North Carolina
Chapter 89

Kimberly Wahl, PharmD
Ambulatory Care Clinical Pharmacist
Department of Pharmacy
Ralph H. Johnson VA Medical Center, Myrtle Beach CBOC
Myrtle Beach, South Carolina
Chapter 72

Christine M. Walko, PharmD, BCOP
Assistant Professor
Division of Pharmacotherapy and Experimental Therapeutics
Institute of Pharmacogenomics and Individualized Therapy
University of North Carolina Eshelman School of Pharmacy
Lineberger Comprehensive Cancer Center
University of North Carolina
Chapel Hill, North Carolina
Chapter 115

Kristina E. Ward, BS, PharmD, BCPS
Clinical Associate Professor of Pharmacy Practice
Director, Drug Information Services
Department of Pharmacy Practice
University of Rhode Island
College of Pharmacy
Kingston, Rhode Island
Chapter 61

Lori D. Wazny, PharmD
Clinical Pharmacist
Manitoba Renal Program
Winnipeg, Manitoba, Canada
Chapter 29

Robert J. Weber, PharmD, MS
Senior Director, Pharmaceutical Services
Department of Pharmacy
The Ohio State University Wexner Medical Center
Columbus, Ohio
eChapter 3

Barbara G. Wells, PharmD, FCCP, FASHP
Dean Emeritus and Professor Emeritus
Department of Pharmacy Practice
University of Mississippi, School of Pharmacy
Oxford, Mississippi
Chapters 51 and 54

James W. Wheless, MD
Professor and Chief of Pediatric Neurology
LeBonheur Chair in Pediatric Neurology
University of Tennessee Health Science Center
Director
LeBonheur Comprehensive Epilepsy Program and Neuroscience Institute
LeBonheur Children's Hospital
Memphis, Tennessee
Chapter 41

Casey B. Williams, PharmD, BCOP
Director of Clinical Research
Sanford Research/University of South Dakota
Assistant Clinical Professor
Department of Internal Medicine
University of South Dakota Sanford School of Medicine
Adjunct Assistant Clinical Professor
Department of Pharmacy Practice
University of Kansas School of Pharmacy
Sioux Falls, South Dakota
Chapter 113

Dennis M. Williams, PharmD, BCPS, AE-C
Associate Professor and Vice Chair
Division of Pharmacotherapy and Experimental Therapeutics
University of North Carolina Eshelman School of Pharmacy
Chapel Hill, North Carolina
Chapter 16

Jeffrey L. Wilt, MD, FACP, FCCP
Director
Department of Medical Critical Care Services
Borgess Medical Center
Department of Pulmonary Curriculum
Western Michigan University School of Medicine
Kalamazoo, Michigan
Chapter 2

Char Witmer, MD, MSCE
Assistant Professor
Department of Pediatrics
The Children's Hospital of Philadelphia
Philadelphia, Pennsylvania
Chapter 81

Daniel M. Witt, PharmD, FCCP, BCPS
Senior Director Clinical Pharmacy Research and Applied Pharmacogenomics
Kaiser Permanente Colorado
Department of Pharmacy
Clinical Associate Professor
University of Colorado
Skaggs School of Pharmacy and Pharmaceutical Sciences
Aurora, Colorado
Chapter 9

Marion R. Wofford, MD, MPH
Professor
Department of Medicine
University of Mississippi Medical Center
Jackson, Mississippi
Chapter 45

Judith K. Wolf, MD
Adjunct Professor of Gynecologic Oncology
Division Chief of Surgery
Banner MD Anderson Cancer Center
Clinical Professor
University of Texas MD Anderson Cancer Center
Gilbert, Arizona
Chapter 110

G. Christopher Wood, PharmD, FCCP, FCCM, BCPS
Associate Professor of Clinical Pharmacy
Department of Clinical Pharmacy
University of Tennessee Health Science Center
Memphis, Tennessee
Chapter 42

Chanin C. Wright, PharmD
Assistant Professor
Department of Pediatrics
Texas A&M College of Pharmacy
McLane Children's Hospital and Clinics Scott & White
Temple, Texas
Chapter 18

Jean Wyman, MN, PhD
Professor
Cora Meidl Siehl Chair in Nursing Research
Adult and Gerontological Health Cooperative
School of Nursing
University of Minnesota
Minneapolis, Minnesota
Chapter 68

Jack A. Yanovski, MD, PhD
Chief, Section on Growth and Obesity
Program in Developmental Endocrinology and Genetics
Eunice Kennedy Shriver National Institute of Child Health and Human Development
National Institutes of Health
Bethesda, Maryland
Chapters 60 and 121

Gary C. Yee, PharmD, FCCP, BCOP
Professor and Associate Dean
Department of Pharmacy Practice
College of Pharmacy
University of Nebraska Medical Center
Omaha, Nebraska
Chapter 109

Foreword

This edition of *Pharmacotherapy: A Pathophysiologic Approach* comes at a time of unprecedented change in health care. While some would argue that the health care system has been slow to change, the environment of today is rapidly evolving. This requires that health care professionals, including pharmacists, are not only responsive and adaptive to change, but able to identify innovative strategies and new approaches to delivering care that contribute meaningfully to the transformation that is needed.

There are significant deficiencies in the way health care is delivered, including poor coordination, variation in quality, and an inability to integrate team-based approaches, all of which impact the quality of care provided to individuals and contribute to rising health care costs. This is especially true in caring for individuals and populations living with chronic disease, which is the leading cost driver in the U.S. health care system. This edition of *Pharmacotherapy: A Pathophysiologic Approach* will prepare future practitioners with the foundational knowledge critical in the management of these diseases.

Medications remain the most common and powerful of all health care interventions, yet are associated with serious harm. In 2011, more than 4 billion prescriptions were written annually in the U.S with prescription spending reaching nearly $320 billion. The adverse consequences of medication use are a major contributor to poor quality care and cost the health care industry billions of dollars each year. In 2007, hospital-based adverse drug events were estimated to be nearly 450,000 per year, with higher numbers in long-term care facilities (800,000), and the outpatient setting (550,000). While this imposes serious impact on the health of patients and the health care system as a whole, most troubling is that medication-related harm occurs at every step in the medication use process—manufacturing, purchasing, prescribing, dispensing, administering, and monitoring—and is largely preventable. It is not surprising that in a 2007 Institute of Medicine report, the appropriate use and management of drug therapy was acknowledged as a critical issue that must be addressed to improve national health care. This is important for the profession of pharmacy as we strive to position ourselves to contribute meaningfully to the delivery of high-quality patient care and play an integral role in transforming our health care system.

Patient-centered medical homes (PCMHs) and accountable care organizations (ACOs) are among the most promising approaches to delivering higher-quality, cost-effective care and present unique opportunities for improving drug therapy outcomes. Central to the PCMH is the patient having a personal physician and collaborative team to provide continuous and coordinated primary care that takes a whole person orientation. ACOs are healthcare organizations centered around the provision of coordinated care and characterized by a payment model that seeks to tie reimbursements to quality metrics and reductions in the total cost of care for a population of patients. PCMHs will require pharmacists to serve as integral members of the collaborative team, responsible for ensuring the safe, effective, and affordable use of medications. Likewise, the ACO model strives to improve quality and reduce total cost of care within health care organizations. Innovative and targeted strategies to improve drug therapy outcomes will be critical in any effort to improve total quality of care. Further, the ACO model provides a unique opportunity for pharmacy to demonstrate the true value-added proposition of pharmacists in health care, thereby informing payment reform and sustainability of clinical pharmacy services.

Numerous opportunities to transform health care delivery exist today; however, to ensure continued improvement of health and health care will require that health professions education be reengineered to better prepare students to meet the future needs of society. Education must be restructured to reduce the almost exclusive focus on the acquisition of knowledge and to place greater emphasis on the skills and behaviors that will be essential for students to survive in a rapidly changing health care environment. In pharmacy education, students must have an in-depth understanding of the foundations of pharmacy, the pharmaceutical sciences, and pharmacotherapy, but they must also be given ample opportunity to think critically, solve complex problems, communicate clearly, and work with others. Students must spend more time in real-world patient care settings and be immersed in complex systems of care, interacting with others to achieve shared goals and functioning in and leading teams toward improvement and change. In Flexner's 1910 report on medical education, he noted that just as scientists must inquire, analyze, identify solutions, and continually refine their approach toward discovery, so, too, must practitioners if they are to advance the practice of medicine and health care. To cultivate these "habits of mind," students must learn how to approach and solve complex problems through engagement in inquiry, discovery, and innovation rather than relying on memorization of facts. As schools of pharmacy move forward with new and innovative curricular designs as outlined in the 2011–2012 Argus Commission Report, authoritative textbooks like *Pharmacotherapy: A Pathophysiologic Approach* will become an important and integral part of student foundational learning.

Building a solid foundation and expertise that is deeply rooted in the pharmaceutical sciences and pharmacotherapy is critical to ensuring that pharmacists are well positioned to improve drug therapy outcomes. It is this unique expertise that differentiates us, as pharmacists, from any other profession. This edition of *Pharmacotherapy: A Pathophysiologic Approach* will equip pharmacy students and practitioners with the knowledge and perspective to be the health care professional most skilled in the provision of drug therapy management. As students and practitioners we must not lose sight of the opportunity we have to influence and shape health care delivery both now and in the future. Just as we take measureable steps to optimize and personalize one's drug therapy, so, too, must each of us take measureable steps toward transforming our health care system. These are unprecedented times of change and opportunity for the profession of pharmacy to shape the future of health care and improve drug therapy outcomes for patients and society.

Robert A. Blouin, PharmD
Professor and Dean
UNC Eshelman School of Pharmacy
University of North Carolina at Chapel Hill
Chapel Hill, North Carolina

Mary Roth McClurg, PharmD, MHS
Associate Professor
Executive Director, The Academy
UNC Eshelman School of Pharmacy
University of North Carolina at Chapel Hill
Chapel Hill, North Carolina

Foreword to the First Edition

Evidence of the maturity of a profession is not unlike that characterizing the maturity of an individual; a child's utterances and behavior typically reveal an unrealized potential for attainment, eventually, of those attributes characteristic of an appropriately confident, independently competent, socially responsible, sensitive, and productive member of society.

Within a period of perhaps 15 or 20 years, we have witnessed a profound maturation within the profession of pharmacy. The utterances of the profession, as projected in its literature, have evolved from mostly self-centered and self-serving issues of trade protection to a composite of expressed professional interests that prominently include responsible explorations of scientific/technological questions and ethical issues that promote the best interests of the clientele served by the profession. With the publication of *Pharmacotherapy: A Pathophysiologic Approach,* pharmacy's utterances bespeak a matured practitioner who is able to call upon unique knowledge and skills so as to function as an appropriately confident, independently competent pharmacotherapeutics expert.

In 1987, the Board of Pharmaceutical Specialties (BPS), in denying the petition filed by the American College of Clinical Pharmacy (ACCP) to recognize "clinical pharmacy" as a specialty, conceded nonetheless that the petitioning party had documented in its petition a specialist who does in fact exist within the practice of pharmacy and whose expertise clearly can be extricated from the performance characteristics of those in general practice. A refiled petition from ACCP requests recognition of "pharmacotherapy" as a Specialty Area of Pharmacy Practice. While the BPS had issued no decision when this book went to press, it is difficult to comprehend the basis for a rejection of the second petition.

Within this book one will find the scientific foundation for the essential knowledge required of one who may aspire to specialty practice as a pharmacotherapist. As is the case with any such publication, its usefulness to the practitioner or the future practitioner is limited to providing such a foundation. To be socially and professionally responsible in practice, the pharmacotherapist's foundation must be continually supplemented and complemented by the flow of information appearing in the primary literature. Of course this is not unique to the general or specialty practice of pharmacy; it is essential to the fulfillment of obligations to clients in any occupation operating under the code of professional ethics.

Because of the growing complexity of pharmacotherapeutic agents, their dosing regimens, and techniques for delivery, pharmacy is obligated to produce, recognize, and remunerate specialty practitioners who can fulfill the profession's responsibilities to society for service expertise where the competence required in a particular case exceeds that of the general practitioner. It simply is a component of our covenant with society and is as important as any other facet of that relationship existing between a profession and those it serves.

The recognition by BPS of pharmacotherapy as an area of specialty practice in pharmacy will serve as an important statement by the profession that we have matured sufficiently to be competent and willing to take unprecedented responsibilities in the collaborative, pharmacotherapeutic management of patient-specific problems. It commits pharmacy to an intention that will not be uniformly or rapidly accepted within the established health care community. Nonetheless, this formal action places us on the road to an avowed goal, and acceptance will be gained as the pharmacotherapists proliferate and establish their importance in the provision of optimal, cost-effective drug therapy.

Suspecting that other professions in other times must have faced similar quests for recognition of their unique knowledge and skills I once searched the literature for an example that might parallel pharmacy's modern-day aspirations. Writing in the *Philadelphia Medical Journal,* May 27, 1899, D. H. Galloway, MD, reflected on the need for specialty training and practice in a field of medicine lacking such expertise at that time. In an article entitled "The Anesthetizer as a Speciality," Galloway commented:

> The anesthetizer will have to make his own place in medicine: the profession will not make a place for him, and not until he has demonstrated the value of his services will it concede him the position which the importance of his duties entitles him to occupy. He will be obliged to define his own rights, duties and privileges, and he must not expect that his own estimate of the importance of his position will be conceded without opposition. There are many surgeons who are unwilling to share either the credit or the emoluments of their work with anyone, and their opposition will be overcome only when they are shown that the importance of their work will not be lessened, but enhanced, by the increased safety and dispatch with which operations may be done. . . .

It has been my experience that, given the opportunity for one-on-one, collaborative practice with physicians and other health professionals, pharmacy practitioners who have been educated and trained to perform at the level of pharmacotherapeutics specialists almost invariably have convinced the former that "the importance of their work will not be lessened, but enhanced, by the increased safety and dispatch with which" individualized problems of drug therapy could be managed in collaboration with clinical pharmacy practitioners.

It is fortuitous—the coinciding of the release of *Pharmacotherapy: A Pathophysiologic Approach* with ACCP's petitioning of BPS for recognition of the pharmacotherapy specialist. The utterances of a maturing profession as revealed in the contents of this book, and the intraprofessional recognition and acceptance of a higher level of responsibility in the safe, effective, and economical use of drugs and drug products, bode well for the future of the profession and for the improvement of patient care with drugs.

Charles A. Walton, PhD
San Antonio, Texas

Preface

With each edition of *Pharmacotherapy: A Pathophysiologic Approach* the pace of change in health care seems to accelerate, and this continues to be true for the 9th edition. At this time, pharmacists across the United States are actively contributing their expertise as integrated and virtual members of the new health care delivery models that are being implemented as part of the Affordable Care Act through accountable care organizations and patient-centered medical homes. These emerging care models have improved outcomes for Medicare and Medicaid beneficiaries and now are poised to affect the care of most individuals. Pharmacists throughout the world are recognizing their potential to improve access to affordable high-quality care in their country. As expectations and opportunities for pharmacists expand, the need for state-of-the-art, patient-centered education and training becomes more acute. The Editors and authors of PAPA continue to strive to make this text relevant to patient-focused pharmacists and other health care providers in this dynamic era.

The 9th edition of *Pharmacotherapy: A Pathophysiologic Approach* is the product of the editorial team's reflection on what are the core pathophysiological and therapeutic elements that students and young practioners need. As a result, we have streamlined the offerings in this edition and placed a portion of the foundational chapters on the web to make them accessible to a broader audience. Most importantly, each chapter of the book has been revised and updated to reflect the latest in evidence-based information and recommendations. We trust that you will find that this edition balances the need for accurate, thorough, and unbiased information about the treatment of diseases by presenting concise illustrative analyses of the multiplicity of therapeutic options.

With each edition, the editors recommit to our founding precepts:

- Advance the quality of patient care through evidence-based medication therapy management based on sound pharmacotherapeutic principles.
- Enhance the health of our communities by incorporating contemporary health promotion and disease-prevention strategies in our practice environments.
- Motivate young practitioners to enhance the breadth, depth, and quality of care they provide to their patients.
- Challenge established pharmacists and other primary-care providers to learn new concepts and refine their understanding of the pathophysiologic tenets that undergird the development of individualized therapeutic regimens.
- Present the pharmacy and health care communities with innovative patient assessment, triage, and pharmacotherapy management skills.

The ninth edition builds on and expands the foundation of previous editions. Most of the disease-oriented chapters have incorporated updated evidence-based treatment guidelines that include, when available, ratings of the level of evidence to support the key therapeutic approaches. Also, in this edition new features have been added:

- Most chapters have a section on personalized pharmacotherapy.
- The diagnostic flow diagrams, treatment algorithms, dosing guideline recommendations, and monitoring approaches that were present in the last edition have been revised with color codes to clearly distinguish treatment pathways.
- The Drug Dosing tables have been reformatted for clarity and consistency.
- New Drug Monitoring tables have been added.

The text's digital home, Access Pharmacy (www.accesspharmacy.com), has become the primary access point for many in the United States and around the world. Users of Access Pharmacy will find many features to enhance their learning and information retrieval. Thoughtful and provocative updates to PAPA chapters are added as new information mandates to keep our readers relevant in these times of rapid advancements. Also, the site has many new features such as education guides, Goodman & Gilman's animations, virtual cases, and many other textbooks. As in previous editions, the text coordinates well with *Pharmacotherapy: A Patient-focused Approach*, which includes in-depth patient cases with questions and answers.

Twenty-four chapters of this edition are being published online and are available to all users in the Online Learning Center at www.pharmacotherapyonline.com The chapters chosen for online publication include seven, which describe and critique the available means to assess major organ system function, and five, which characterize the adverse effects of drugs on organ systems. They join the 12 foundational chapters, which provide overviews of pharmacy skills in medication safety, pharmacokinetics, and pharmacogenetics, and patient-centered considerations such as health literacy, cultural competency, pediatrics, and geriatrics; finally, there are three chapters that address public health, clinical toxicology, and emergency preparedness. The Online Learning Center continues to provide unique features designed to benefit students, practitioners, and faculty around the world. The site includes learning objectives and self-assessment questions for each chapter. In closing, we acknowledge the many hours that *Pharmacotherapy's* more than 300 authors contributed to this labor of love. Without their devotion to the cause of improved pharmacotherapy and dedication in maintaining the accuracy, clarity, and relevance of their chapters, this text would unquestionably not be possible. In addition, we thank Michael Weitz, Brian Kearns, and James Shanahan and their colleagues at McGraw-Hill for their consistent support of the *Pharmacotherapy* family of resources, insights into trends in publishing and higher education, and the critical attention to detail so necessary in pharmacotherapy.

The Editors
March 2014

1

Cardiovascular Testing

Richard A. Lange and L. David Hillis

KEY CONCEPTS

1. A careful history and physical examination are extremely important in diagnosing cardiovascular disease; they should be performed before any testing.
2. Elevated jugular venous pressure is an important sign of heart failure and may be used to assess its severity and the response to therapy.
3. Heart sounds and heart murmurs are important in identifying heart valve abnormalities and other structural cardiac defects.
4. Electrocardiography is useful for determining rhythm disturbances (tachyarrhythmias or bradyarrhythmias).
5. Exercise stress testing provides important information concerning the presence and severity of coronary artery disease; changes in heart rate, blood pressure, and the electrocardiogram are used to assess the response to exercise.
6. Echocardiography is used to assess valve structure and function as well as ventricular wall motion; transesophageal echocardiography is more sensitive than transthoracic echocardiography for detecting thrombus and vegetations.
7. Radionuclides, such as technetium-99m and thallium-201, are used to assess wall motion and myocardial viability in patients with coronary artery disease and heart failure.
8. When patients cannot exercise, pharmacologic stress testing is used to assess the likelihood of coronary artery disease.
9. Cardiac catheterization and angiography are used to assess coronary anatomy and ventricular performance.

INTRODUCTION

In the United States, cardiovascular disease (CVD) afflicts an estimated 83 million people (i.e., approximately one in three adults) and accounts for 33% of all deaths. One of every six hospital stays results from CVD. In 2008, the estimated direct and indirect cost of CVD—which includes hypertension, coronary heart disease, heart failure, and stroke—was $297.7 billion.[1]

Atherosclerosis, the cause of most CVD events, is typically present for decades before symptoms appear. With a thorough history, comprehensive physical examination, and appropriate testing, the individual with subclinical CVD usually can be identified, and the subject with symptomatic CVD can be assessed for the risk of an adverse event and can be managed appropriately.

THE HISTORY

The elements of a comprehensive history include the chief complaint, current symptoms, past medical history, family history, social history, and review of systems.

The chief complaint is a brief statement describing the reason the patient is seeking medical attention. The patient is asked to describe his or her current symptoms, including their duration, quality, frequency, severity, progression, precipitating and relieving factors, associated symptoms, and impact on daily activities.

The past medical history may reveal previous cardiovascular problems, conditions that predispose the patient to develop CVD (i.e., hypertension, hyperlipidemia, or diabetes mellitus) (Table 1-1), or comorbid conditions that influence the identification or management of CVD. The patient should be asked about social habits that affect the cardiovascular system, including diet, amount of regular physical activity, tobacco use, alcohol intake, and illicit drug use. At present, family history of early onset CVD is the best available screening tool to identify patients with a genetic predisposition for CVD.

Cardiovascular History

1 Chest pain is a frequent symptom and may occur as a result of myocardial ischemia (angina pectoris) or infarction or a variety of noncardiac conditions, such as esophageal, pulmonary, or musculoskeletal disorders. The quality of chest pain, its location and duration, and the factors that provoke or relieve it are important in ascertaining its etiology.

Typically, patients with angina describe a sensation of heaviness or pressure in the retrosternal area that may radiate to the jaw, left shoulder, back, or left arm. It is precipitated by exertion, emotional stress, eating, smoking a cigarette, or exposure to cold, and it is usually relieved within minutes with rest or a sublingual nitroglycerin, although the latter also is effective in relieving chest pain due to esophageal spasm. Angina that is increasing in severity, longer in duration, or occurring at rest is called unstable angina; it should prompt the patient to seek medical attention expeditiously.

TABLE 1-1 Risk Factors for Cardiovascular Disease

Nonmodifiable
Advancing age
Male
Family history of early onset CVD
Postmenopausal status
Modifiable
Hypertension
Diabetes mellitus
Dyslipidemia
Cigarette smoking
Obesity
Physical inactivity
Excessive alcohol
Stress
Chronic inflammation (i.e., gingivitis, arthritis, elevated C-reactive protein, etc.)
Illicit drug use (e.g., cocaine or methamphetamine)

The patient with congestive heart failure and pulmonary vascular congestion may complain of shortness of breath (dyspnea) with exertion or even at rest, orthopnea, paroxysmal nocturnal dyspnea, and nocturia. The patient with congestive heart failure and peripheral venous congestion may report abdominal swelling (from hepatic congestion or ascites), nausea, vomiting, lower extremity edema, fatigue, and dyspnea.

The New York Heart Association (NYHA) grading system is used to indicate whether a patient has angina or symptoms of congestive heart failure with vigorous (class I), moderate (class II), mild (class III), or minimal/no (class IV) exertion.

PHYSICAL EXAMINATION

The patient with suspected heart disease should undergo a comprehensive physical examination, with particular attention to the cardiovascular system. This should include an assessment of the jugular venous pulse (JVP), carotid and peripheral arterial pulses, examination of the heart and lungs (i.e., palpation, percussion, and auscultation), and inspection of the abdomen and extremities.

Jugular Venous Pressure

2 The JVP is an indirect assessment of right atrial pressure. With the patient lying supine at 30° and his/her head rotated slightly to the left, the height of the fluid wave in the right internal jugular vein is determined relative to the sternal angle. The normal JVP is 1 to 2 cm above the sternal angle. The JVP typically is elevated in the patient with heart failure. The extent of elevation can be used to assess the severity of peripheral venous congestion, and its diminution can be used to assess the response to therapy.

Arterial Pulses

The carotid arterial pulse is examined for its intensity and, concurrently with the apical impulse, for concordance within the cardiac cycle. Diminished carotid arterial pulsations may be the result of a reduced stroke volume, atherosclerotic narrowing of the carotid artery, or obstruction to left ventricular outflow due to aortic valve stenosis or hypertrophic obstructive cardiomyopathy. Conversely, very forceful, hyperdynamic, "bounding" carotid arterial pulsations may be palpated in the patient with an increased stroke volume and suggest the presence of chronic aortic valve regurgitation or a high cardiac output due, for example, to hyperthyroidism, an arteriovenous shunt, or marked anemia.

The pulses in the arms and legs also are examined. Diminished peripheral pulses suggest the presence of a reduced stroke volume or atherosclerotic peripheral arterial disease (PAD). Concomitant pallor, skin atrophy, hair loss, or ulcerations are consistent with PAD, which often coexists with coronary artery disease (CAD). To quantify the severity of PAD, systolic arterial pressure is measured in all four extremities. Normally, the systolic arterial pressure in the feet should be similar or even slightly higher than the pressure in the arms. Thus, the ratio of the systolic arterial pressures in the foot and arm (the so-called ankle-brachial index [ABI]) is normally greater than 1. An ABI less than 0.9 suggests PAD.[2]

Chest

In the patient with chest pain, a thorough lung examination should be performed to exclude a pulmonary cause. The anterior chest wall is palpated to assess for the presence of tenderness in the sternal area, which may indicate that the patient has costochondritis. Percussion of the posterior chest is done to determine if a pleural effusion is present. Auscultation of the anterior and posterior lung fields is performed to assess for the presence of findings suggestive of pneumonia, airway obstruction, pneumothorax, pleural effusion, or pulmonary edema.

Heart Sounds

3 The typical "lub-dub" sound of the normal heart consists of the first heart sound (S_1), which precedes ventricular contraction and is due to closure of the mitral and tricuspid valves, and the second heart sound (S_2), which follows ventricular contraction and is due to closure of the aortic and pulmonic valves. Other heart sounds, which are normally not present (i.e., a third heart sound [S_3], fourth heart sound [S_4], or murmur), may indicate the presence of underlying heart disease (Fig. 1-1).

The S_3, a so-called ventricular gallop, is a low-pitched sound usually heard at the cardiac apex in early diastole (i.e., immediately after S_2). It is caused by the vibrations that occur when blood rapidly rushes from the atrium into a volume-loaded ventricle. Thus, it is usually associated with decompensated congestive heart failure or intravascular volume overload. A so-called "physiologic" S_3 is heard commonly in healthy children (who often have an increased cardiac output) and may persist into young adulthood.

The S_4 is a dull, low-pitched sound that is caused by the vibrations that occur when atrial contraction forces blood into a stiff, noncompliant ventricle. It is audible at the cardiac apex just before ventricular contraction (i.e., just before S_1); it is not present in the subject with a normal heart. An S_4 may be present in the patient with aortic stenosis, systemic arterial hypertension, hypertrophic cardiomyopathy, or CAD.

Murmurs are auditory vibrations resulting from turbulent blood flow within the heart chambers or across the valves. They are classified by their timing and duration within the cardiac cycle (systolic, diastolic, or continuous), location on the chest wall, intensity (grade 1 to 6, from softest to loudest), pitch (high or low frequency), and radiation (Fig. 1-2 and Table 1-2). Some murmurs are said to be "innocent" or "physiologic" and result from rapid, turbulent blood flow in the absence of cardiac disease. Fever, anxiety, anemia, hyperthyroidism, and pregnancy increase the intensity of a physiologic murmur.

Systolic murmurs occur during ventricular contraction. They begin with or after S_1 and end at or before S_2, depending on the origin of the murmur. They are classified based on time of onset and termination within systole: midsystolic or holosystolic (pansystolic). Examples of midsystolic murmurs include pulmonic stenosis, aortic stenosis, and hypertrophic obstructive cardiomyopathy.

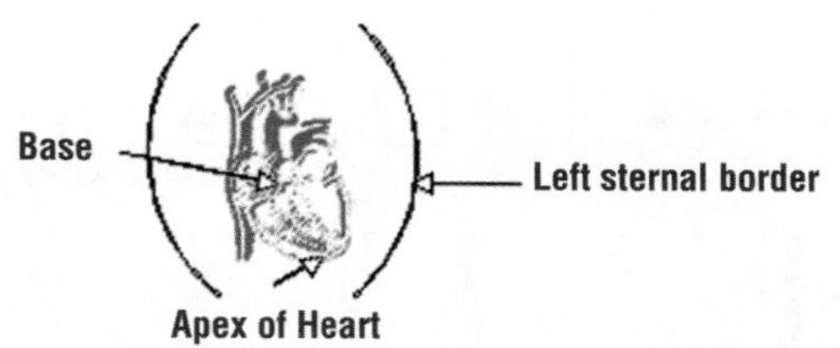

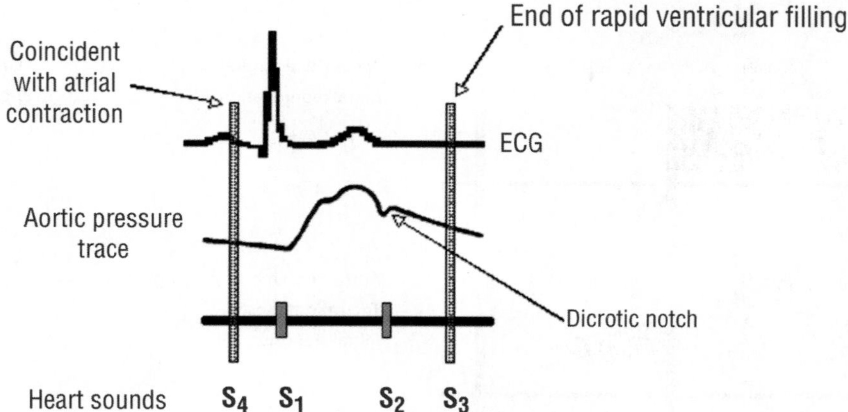

FIGURE 1-1 Correlation of the electrocardiogram (ECG) with an aortic pressure tracing and heart sounds. Normal heart sounds are S_1 (mitral and tricuspid valve closure) and S_2 (aortic and pulmonic valve closure). The S_3 and S_4 "gallops" are usually abnormal. The S_3 occurs in early diastole as blood rapidly rushes into a volume-loaded ventricle (e.g., with decompensated congestive heart failure). The S_4 occurs in late diastole and is caused by atrial contraction into a stiff, noncompliant ventricle (e.g., hypertrophy due to hypertension).

Holosystolic murmurs occur when blood flows from a chamber of higher pressure to one of lower pressure throughout systole, such as occurs with mitral or tricuspid valve regurgitation or a ventricular septal defect.

Diastolic murmurs occur during ventricular filling. They begin with or after S_2, depending on the origin of the murmur. Aortic or pulmonic valve regurgitation causes a high-pitched diastolic murmur that begins with S_2, whereas stenosis of the mitral or tricuspid valves causes a low-pitched, "rumbling" diastolic murmur.

Continuous murmurs begin in systole and continue without interruption into all or part of diastole. Such murmurs are mainly a result of aortopulmonary connections (e.g., patent ductus arteriosus) or arteriovenous connections (e.g., arteriovenous fistula, coronary artery fistula, or arteriovenous malformation).

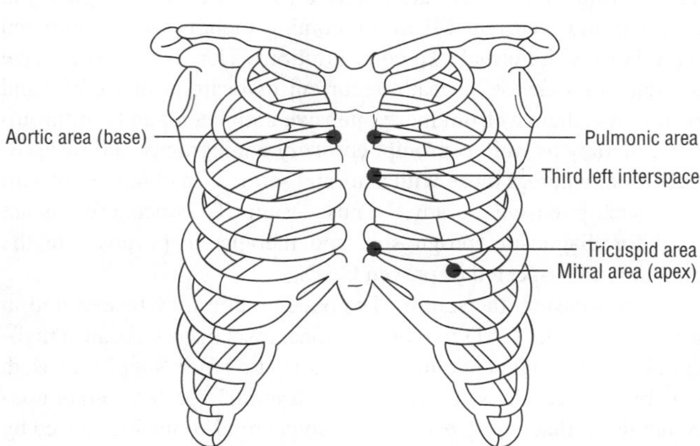

FIGURE 1-2 Schematic illustrations of topographic areas on the precordium for cardiac auscultation. Auscultatory areas do not correspond to anatomic locations of the valves but to the sites at which particular valvular sounds are heard best. *(Redrawn from Kinney MR, Packa DR, eds. Andreoli's Comprehensive Cardiac Care, 8th ed. St. Louis, MO: Mosby, 1996, with permission.)*

When a murmur is heard, the cardiac abnormality underlying it usually can be confirmed and assessed with echocardiography or other imaging modalities, such as cardiac angiography or magnetic resonance imaging (MRI) (see below).

PRACTICE GUIDELINES FOR DIAGNOSTIC AND PROGNOSTIC TESTING IN CARDIOVASCULAR DISEASE TESTING

The American Heart Association (AHA) and American College of Cardiology (ACC) Task Force on Practice Guidelines provide the indications and utility of various diagnostic cardiac tests (Fig. 1-3). Class I indications have unequivocal evidence or agreement that the specific procedure is useful and effective. Class II indications are those for which a divergence of opinion concerning the usefulness of the test is present: class IIa indications are those for which evidence or opinion in favor of the test exists, whereas class IIb indications are those for which less evidence favoring the test is present. Class III indications are those for which evidence or agreement exists that a diagnostic test is not useful.

For a specific clinical scenario, the guidelines also indicate the level of evidence for the recommendation. Level A evidence is said to be present if the recommendation is based on the results of multiple randomized clinical trials. Level B evidence is said to exist if only a single randomized trial or multiple nonrandomized trials exist. Level C evidence is said to be present if the recommendation is made solely on expert opinion.

TABLE 1-2 Characteristic Murmurs

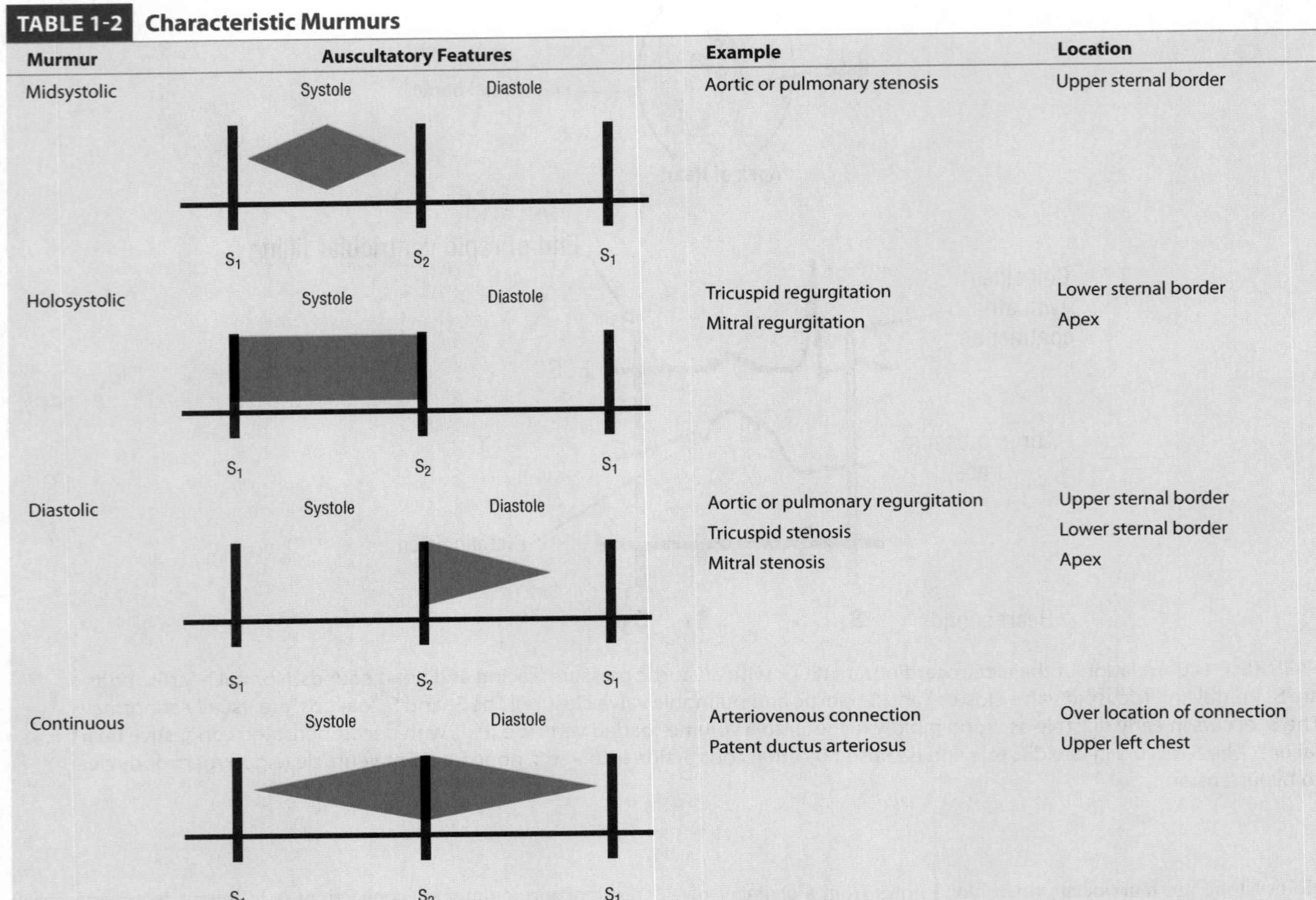

Murmur	Auscultatory Features	Example	Location
Midsystolic	Systole, Diastole; S_1 S_2 S_1	Aortic or pulmonary stenosis	Upper sternal border
Holosystolic	Systole, Diastole; S_1 S_2 S_1	Tricuspid regurgitation Mitral regurgitation	Lower sternal border Apex
Diastolic	Systole, Diastole; S_1 S_2 S_1	Aortic or pulmonary regurgitation Tricuspid stenosis Mitral stenosis	Upper sternal border Lower sternal border Apex
Continuous	Systole, Diastole; S_1 S_2 S_1	Arteriovenous connection Patent ductus arteriosus	Over location of connection Upper left chest

TESTING MODALITIES

Biomarkers

Blood tests are available for several substances that suggest the presence of myonecrosis (i.e., recent death of myocardial cells), inflammation, or hemodynamic stress (Fig. 1-4).[3–5]

Markers of Myonecrosis

When myocardial infarction (myonecrosis) occurs, proteins from the recently necrotic myocytes are released into the peripheral blood, where they can be detected using specific biochemical assays. These biomarkers of myonecrosis (a) aid in the diagnosis (or exclusion) of myocardial infarction as the cause of chest pain; (b) facilitate triage and risk stratification of patients with chest discomfort; and (c) identify patients who are appropriate candidates for specific therapeutic strategies or interventions. Cardiac troponin (cTn) is the preferred biomarker for the diagnosis of myonecrosis.[5] Other available biomarkers of necrosis include creatine kinase-MB (CK-MB) and myoglobin.

Troponin (Tn) I and T are contractile proteins found only in cardiac myocytes. In the patient with myocardial infarction, cTn is detectable in the blood 2 to 4 hours after the onset of symptoms and remains detectable for 5 to 10 days (Fig. 1-5). cTn is the preferred marker for evaluating the patient suspected of having a myocardial infarction, since it is the most sensitive and tissue-specific biomarker available. In the patient with ischemic chest pain and electrocardiographic (e.g., ST segment) abnormalities, the presence of an elevated serum cTn concentration establishes the diagnosis of myocardial infarction, and the absence of such an elevation excludes it. The use of high-sensitive cTn assays improves the early diagnosis of patients with suspected myocardial infarction, particularly the early exclusion of it.[6]

In the patient with an acute coronary syndrome, detection and quantitation of cTn in the blood provide prognostic information and guide management. Acute coronary syndrome patients with an elevated serum cTn concentration have a roughly fourfold higher risk of death and recurrent MI in the coming months when compared with those with normal cTn concentrations. They benefit (i.e., have a reduced incidence of death, recurrent myocardial infarction, and recurrent ischemia) from more intensive antiplatelet and antithrombotic therapy as well as prompt coronary angiography and revascularization, whereas those with a normal serum cTn obtain no benefit from such intensive therapy.[7,8] Thus, serum cTn concentrations are used for diagnostic, prognostic, and therapeutic purposes in the patient with suspected or proven CAD.

On occasion, the serum cTn concentration may be elevated in a patient without CAD in whom myonecrosis occurs because myocardial oxygen demands markedly exceed oxygen supply (caused, e.g., by tachycardia or severe systemic arterial hypertension) or nonischemic cardiac injury occurs (i.e., myocardial contusion caused by blunt trauma to the chest) (Table 1-3). In the patient with an elevated serum cTn concentration, the clinician must decide if the observed abnormal serum cTn concentration is the result of CAD or another condition.

When serum cTn measurements are not available, the best alternative is the MB isoenzyme of creatine kinase (CK-MB), which is a cytosolic carrier protein for high-energy phosphates that is released

Size of treatment effect

Estimate of certainty (precision) of treatment effect	Class I	Class IIa	Class IIb	Class III
	Benefit >>> Risk Procedure/Treatment SHOULD be performed/ administered	Benefit >>> Risk Additional studies with focused objectives needed **IT IS REASONABLE to perform procedure/ administer treatment**	Benefit ≥ Risk Additional studies with broad objectives needed; Additional registry data would be helpful **IT IS NOT UNREASONABLE to perform procedure/ administer treatment**	Risk ≥ Benefit No additional studies needed **Procedure/Treatment should NOT be performed/ administered SINCE IT IS NOT HELPFUL AND MAY BE HARMFUL**
Level A Multiple (3–5) population risk strata evaluated General consistency of direction and magnitude of effect	• Recommendation that procedure or treatment is useful/effective • Sufficient evidence from multiple randomized trials or meta analyses	• Recommendation in favor of treatment or procedure being useful/effective • Some conflicting evidence from multiple randomized trials or meta analyses	• Recommendation's usefulness/efficacy less well established • Greater conflicting evidence from multiple randomized trials or meta analyses	• Recommendation that procedure or treatment not useful/effective and may be harmful • Sufficient evidence from multiple randomized trials or meta analyses
Level B Limited (2–3) population risk strata evaluated	• Recommendation that procedure or treatment is useful/effective • Limited evidence from single randomized trial or non randomized studies	• Recommendation in favor of treatment or procedure being useful/effective • Some conflicting evidence from single randomized trial or non randomized studies	• Recommendation's usefulness/efficacy less well established • Greater conflicting evidence from single randomized trial or non randomized studies	• Recommendation that procedure or treatment not useful/effective and may be harmful • Limited evidence from single randomized trial or non randomized studies
Level C Very limited (1–2) population risk strata evaluated	• Recommendation that procedure or treatment is useful/effective • Only expert opinion, case studies, or standard-of-care	• Recommendation in favor of treatment or procedure being useful/effective • Only diverging expert opinion, case studies, or standard-of-care	• Recommendation's usefulness/efficacy less well established • Only diverging expert opinion, case studies, or standard-of-care	• Recommendation that procedure or treatment not useful/effective and may be harmful • Only expert opinion, case studies, or standard-of-care

FIGURE 1-3 Classification of recommendations and level of evidence.

into the blood when myonecrosis occurs. Although it was initially thought to be cardiac specific, CK-MB is now known to be present in small amounts in skeletal muscle; as a result, it may be detectable in the blood of patients with massive muscle injury, as occurs with rhabdomyolysis or myositis.

In the patient with a myocardial infarction, CK-MB can be detected in the blood 2 to 4 hours after symptom onset; its serum concentration peaks within 24 hours, and it remains detectable in the blood for 48 to 72 hours. To document the characteristic rise and fall of CK-MB concentrations, blood samples should be obtained every 4 to 8 hours. Although CK-MB is not as sensitive or cardiac-specific a biomarker as cTn, its blood concentration declines more rapidly than cTn, which makes it the preferred biomarker for evaluating suspected recurrent infarction in the patient who experiences recurrent chest pain within several days of myocardial infarction. With recurrent infarction, the typical rise and fall of the serum CK-MB concentration is interrupted by a second elevation. Conversely, serum cTn concentrations decline slowly following myocardial infarction; hence, they are not as sensitive as CK-MB for diagnosing recurrent infarction.

The serum myoglobin concentration is elevated in the patient with myonecrosis, but it has a low specificity for myocardial infarction because of its high concentration in skeletal muscle. Because of its small molecular size and consequent rapid release (within 1 hour) following the onset of myonecrosis, it is utilized as a very early marker of myocardial infarction. When it is combined with a more

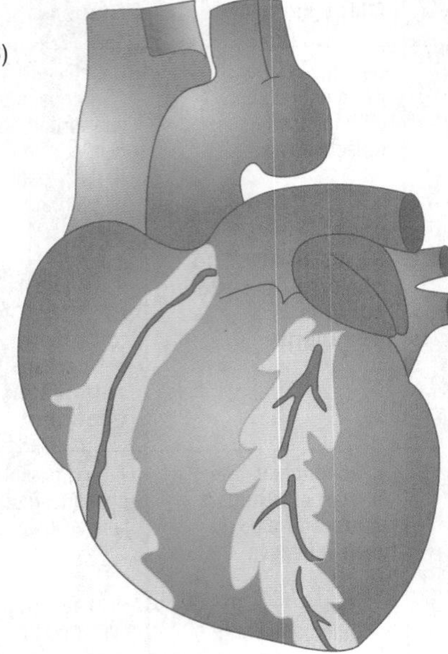

FIGURE 1-4 Cardiac biomarkers classified according to the different pathologic processes they indicate.

specific marker of myonecrosis, such as cTn or CK-MB, myoglobin is useful for the early exclusion of myocardial infarction.

Markers of Inflammation

Inflammatory processes participate in the development of atherosclerosis and contribute to the destabilization of atherosclerotic plaques, which may ultimately lead to an acute coronary syndrome. Several mediators of the inflammatory response, including acute-phase proteins, cytokines, and cellular adhesion molecules, have been evaluated as potential indicators of underlying atherosclerosis and as predictors of acute cardiovascular events.

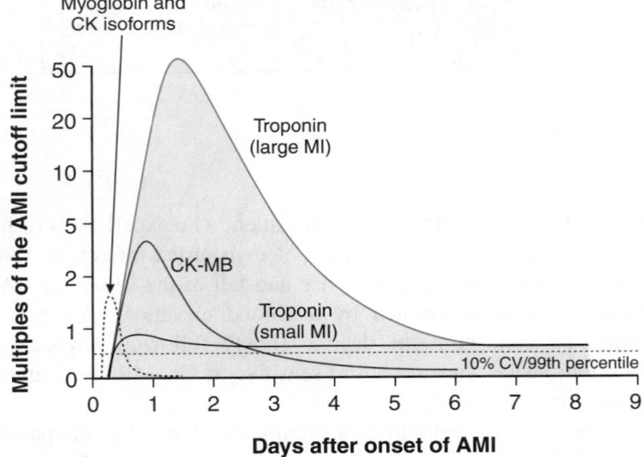

FIGURE 1-5 Time course of the appearance of various markers in the blood after acute myocardial infarction. *(Reprinted from Jaffe AS, Babuin L, Apple FS. Biomarkers in acute cardiac disease—The present and the future. J Am Coll Cardiol 2006;48:4. Copyright © 2006, with permission from Elsevier.)*

C-reactive protein (CRP) is an acute-phase reactant protein produced by the liver.[9] Although a receptor for CRP is present on endothelial cells, controversy exists regarding whether CRP is simply a marker for systemic inflammation or participates actively in atheroma formation.[10,11] In the absence of acute illness or myocardial infarction, serum concentrations of CRP are relatively stable, although they are influenced by gender and ethnicity.

Epidemiologic studies have shown that the relative risk of future vascular events increases as the serum high-sensitive CRP (hs-CRP) concentration increases.[9] Values greater than 3 mg/L are associated with an increased risk for developing CVD; conversely, values less than 1 mg/L are associated with a low risk. Those between 1 and 3 mg/L are considered to be at intermediate risk. To measure serum CRP concentrations accurately, a hs-CRP assay is required. In an individual with an elevated serum hs-CRP concentration, the measurement should be repeated several weeks later to exclude the possibility that an acute illness was responsible for the elevation.

TABLE 1-3 Conditions Associated with an Increased Serum Troponin Concentration

Myocardial infarction	Pulmonary embolism
Acute coronary syndrome	Strenuous exercise
Coronary intervention	Chemotherapy
Pericarditis	Severe asthma
Congestive heart failure	Respiratory distress
Cardiac defibrillation	Infiltrative disorders
Cardiac ablation	Acute limb ischemia
Cardiac contusion	Inflammatory disease
Tachycardia	Influenza
Aortic dissection	Hemodialysis
Stroke	Sepsis
Renal failure	Shock
Hypertension or hypotension	Rhabdomyolysis

Measurements should not be taken when subjects are acutely ill (e.g., with any acute febrile illness) or have a known autoimmune or rheumatologic disorder. Serum CRP concentrations above 10 mg/L are likely caused by an acute or chronic systemic illness.

Although the relative risk of future vascular events increases as the serum concentration of hs-CRP increases, controversy continues as to whether hs-CRP concentrations provide sufficient incremental information above traditional risk factors to warrant routine testing in subjects without known CVD in an attempt to prevent an adverse event (so-called primary prevention).[9,12,13] Recent guidelines have suggested that CRP is useful in patients who are considered (on the basis of traditional risk factors) to be at intermediate risk for CAD in an attempt to guide the intensity with which their risk factors are modified.[9,12] Only limited data have suggested that interventions that lower CRP concentrations (i.e., aspirin and statins) are beneficial.[14–16]

Clinical **Controversy...**

Assessing an individual's risk for CVD is important in guiding treatment. Many risk factors for CVD have been identified (i.e., hypertension, hyperlipidemia, diabetes mellitus, cigarette smoking, and family history of CVD). Whether hs-CRP concentrations provide sufficient incremental information above traditional risk factors to warrant routine testing in subjects without known CVD in an attempt to prevent an adverse event (so-called primary prevention) is unknown.

Multiple studies[17,18] of patients with acute coronary syndromes have demonstrated the capacity of hs-CRP concentrations—measured at the time of hospitalization or hospital discharge—to help to predict cardiovascular outcomes during the hospitalization or during long-term followup. This prognostic information appears to be independent of and complementary to data obtained from the history and electrocardiogram (ECG). hs-CRP concentrations may be useful for monitoring the response to statin therapy, in that those with low hs-CRP concentrations after statin therapy have better clinical outcomes than those in whom these concentrations are high.[14,16] Based on these data, the measurement of serum hs-CRP concentrations in patients with acute coronary syndromes is recommended as reasonable (class IIa) for risk stratification when additional prognostic information is desired.[5] In contrast, its routine use is not recommended in the absence of compelling data identifying its role in guiding specific therapy.

Other novel markers of inflammation and/or plaque stabilization that have been shown to provide prognostic information in patients with an acute coronary syndrome are myeloperoxidase, CD40 ligand, P-selectin, pregnancy-associated plasma protein A, interleukin 6, matrix metalloproteinase-9, soluble intercellular adhesion molecule 1, and fibrinogen.[3,5,19]

Markers of Hemodynamic Stress

B-type natriuretic peptide (BNP) and its precursor, N-terminal probrain natriuretic protein (NT-proBNP), are released from ventricular myocytes in response to increases in wall stress. As a result, their serum concentrations typically are increased in patients with congestive heart failure. They may also be elevated in patients with an acute coronary syndrome as a result of left ventricular systolic dysfunction, impairment of ventricular relaxation, and myocardial stunning.[5,20]

Since serum BNP and NT-proBNP concentrations manifest substantial biologic variability, their serum concentrations in an individual subject must increase or decrease at least twofold to provide assurance that a "real" change has occurred. In addition, when considering the normal range for an individual, one must be aware that considerable variation in serum concentrations exists according to age, gender, weight, and renal function. Women and older patients have a higher normal range, whereas obese patients have lower values than the nonobese. Patients with renal failure often have substantially higher values.

Elevated BNP and NT-proBNP concentrations support a suspected diagnosis of heart failure or lead to a suspicion of heart failure when a diagnosis is unclear. Conversely, a normal value (BNP less than 100 pg/mL [100 ng/L; 28.9 pmol/L] or NT-proBNP less than 300 pg/mL [300 ng/L; 35.4 pmol/L]) in an untreated patient strongly suggests that heart failure is not present.[20,21] In a study of 1,568 patients seeking medical attention after the abrupt onset of dyspnea, plasma BNP was significantly higher in those with clinically diagnosed heart failure than in those without (mean value, 675 pg/mL [675 ng/L; 195.1 pmol/L] compared with 110 pg/mL [110 ng/L; 31.8 pmol/L], respectively); those with known heart failure but with a noncardiac cause of dyspnea had intermediate values (mean, 346 pg/mL [346 ng/L; 100 pmol/L]).[22]

Plasma BNP concentrations provide prognostic information in patients with acute decompensated heart failure: in-hospital mortality is threefold higher in those in the highest BNP quartile when compared with the lowest quartile.[23] Similarly, in patients with compensated CHF, plasma BNP concentrations provide valuable prognostic information, in that each 100 pg/mL (100 ng/L; 28.9 pmol/L) increase in plasma BNP in these subjects is associated with a 35% increase in the relative risk of death.[24] Although the measurement of BNP can be used for prognostic purposes in patients with CHF, its role in assessing treatment efficacy and modifying drug therapy is not clearly established.

Elevated plasma concentrations of BNP and NT-proBNP have been observed in subjects with heart failure with depressed left ventricular systolic function, heart failure with preserved left ventricular systolic function, elevated left ventricular filling pressures, left ventricular hypertrophy, atrial fibrillation, and myocardial ischemia. They may be elevated in certain noncardiac conditions, including pulmonary embolism, chronic obstructive pulmonary disease, hypoxemia, sepsis, cirrhosis, and renal failure. As a result, values of BNP or NT-proBNP should not be used in isolation either to confirm or to refute a diagnosis of heart failure.

Elevated serum concentrations of BNP and NT-proBNP may be detected in patients with an acute coronary syndrome. Data from more than 30 studies have indicated that BNP and NT-proBNP are among the most robust predictors of death and heart failure in patients hospitalized with an acute coronary syndrome.[5,25–27] Nonetheless, data regarding the potential for these substances to guide specific therapeutic decisions, such as whether to perform coronary angiography and revascularization, have been mixed. At present, therefore, the use of BNP and NT-proBNP in patients with an acute coronary syndrome is limited to risk stratification, for which they can be used to help in the assessment of prognosis.

Chest Radiography

The chest x-ray provides supplemental information to the physical examination. Although it does not provide detailed information about internal cardiac structures, it can provide information about the position and size of the heart and its chambers as well as adjacent structures. The standard chest x-rays for evaluation of the lungs and heart are standing posteroanterior and lateral views taken with maximal inspiration; portable chest x-rays usually are less helpful. When possible, previous x-rays should be obtained for comparison.

The posteroanterior chest x-ray outlines the superior vena cava, right atrium, aortic knob, main pulmonary artery, left atrial appendage (especially if enlarged), and left ventricle. The lateral chest x-ray allows one to assess the right ventricle, inferior vena cava, and left ventricle. These structures are visualized as shadows of differing density rather than as discrete entities.

Cardiac enlargement is determined by the cardiothoracic ratio (CTR), which is the maximal transverse diameter of the heart divided by the maximal transverse diameter of the thorax on the posteroanterior view. The CTR normally is less than or equal to 0.45, but it may be higher (i.e., less than or equal to 0.55) in subjects with a large stroke volume (e.g., highly conditioned athletes). Certain cardiac conditions, such as heart failure and hypertension, may cause cardiac enlargement, with a resultant high CTR. Individual chamber enlargement can be seen on the chest x-ray. Left atrial enlargement is suspected if the left bronchus is elevated or the atrial appendage is enlarged. Left ventricular enlargement is the most common feature identified on chest x-ray and is seen as a lateral and downward displacement of the cardiac apex. Right ventricular enlargement is best seen on the lateral film, on which the heart appears to occupy the retrosternal space. A large pericardial effusion may appear as a large heart on a chest x-ray, but, in contrast to heart failure, pulmonary vascular congestion is not present (see below).

The pulmonary vessels are examined for size and filling. With diminished pulmonary blood flow, as would be present in the patient with tetralogy of Fallot or pulmonic valvular stenosis, the peripheral pulmonary vessels are small in caliber and underfilled. Increased pulmonary blood flow, as occurs with a high cardiac output or left-to-right intracardiac shunting, may lead to enlargement and tortuosity of the central and peripheral pulmonary vessels. Pulmonary arterial hypertension (increased pulmonary resistance) is identified by enlargement of the central pulmonary arteries and diminished peripheral perfusion. Elevated pulmonary venous pressure—usually the result of an elevated left atrial pressure—is characterized by dilation of vessels in the upper lung zones (e.g., cephalization of flow), owing to recruitment of upper lung vessels when blood is diverted from the constricted vessels in the lower lung zones.

Congestive heart failure causes Kerley B lines (edema of interlobular septae), which appear as thin, horizontal reticular lines in the costophrenic angles. As pulmonary venous pressure increases, alveolar edema becomes evident, and pleural effusions may appear as blunting of the costophrenic angles.

Electrocardiography

❹ The ECG is a graphic recording of the electrical potentials generated by the heart. The signals are detected by using electrodes attached to the extremities and chest wall (Figs. 1-6 and 1-7), which are then amplified and recorded (Fig. 1-8). The ECG leads display the instantaneous differences in potential between electrodes. As electrical activity approaches the positive electrode of the lead, it registers a positive (upright) deflection on the ECG, whereas electrical activity in the opposite direction of the positive electrode of the lead registers a negative (downward) deflection.

The ECG can be used to detect arrhythmias, conduction disturbances, myocardial ischemia or infarction, metabolic disturbances that may result in lethal arrhythmias (e.g., hyperkalemia), and increased susceptibility to sudden cardiac death (e.g., prolonged QT interval). It is simple to perform, noninvasive, and inexpensive.

Depolarization of the heart initiates cardiac contraction. The electrical current that depolarizes the heart originates in special cardiac pacemaker cells located in the sinoatrial (SA) node, or sinus node, which is located in the upper right atrium near the insertion of the superior vena cava (Fig. 1-9). The depolarization wave is transmitted through the atria, which initiates atrial contraction. Subsequently, the impulse is transmitted through specialized conduction tissues in (a) the atrioventricular (AV) node, which is located in the inferior right atrium near the tricuspid valve; (b) the bundle of His, which is located in the interventricular septum; and (c) the right and left

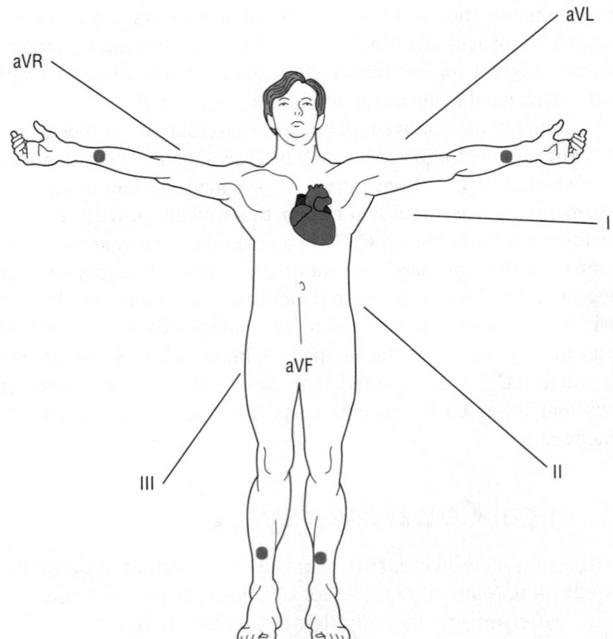

FIGURE 1-6 With electrodes (depicted as dots) attached to each arm and leg, electrical activity on the torso (i.e., frontal plane) is recorded from six different directions. These are known as the limb leads: leads I, II, III, aVF, aVL, and aVR. *(Source: Longo DL, Fauci AS, Kasper DL, Hauser SL, Jameson JL, Loscalzo J. Harrison's Principles of Internal Medicine, 18th ed. Figure 245-2, www.accessmedicine.com . Copyright © The McGraw-Hill Companies, Inc. All rights reserved.)*

bundles, which rapidly conduct the electrical impulse to the right and left ventricular myocardium via (d) the Purkinje fibers. The depolarization wave front then spreads through the ventricular muscle, from endocardium to epicardium, triggering ventricular contraction.

The ECG waveforms (Fig. 1-10), which are recorded during electrical depolarization of the heart, are labeled alphabetically and are read from left to right, beginning with the P wave, which represents depolarization of the atria. The normal duration of the P wave is up to 0.12 second. The *PR segment*, created by passage of the impulse through the AV node and the bundle of His and its branches, has a duration of 0.12 to 0.20 second. The *QRS complex* represents electrical depolarization of the ventricles. Initially, a negative deflection (the Q wave) appears, followed by a positive deflection, the R wave, and finally a negative deflection, the S wave. The normal duration of the QRS complex is less than 0.12 second. Since the left ventricle is much thicker than the right ventricle, most of the electrical wave front is directed toward the former. Accordingly, the precordial leads positioned over the left ventricle (leads V_5 and V_6) demonstrate a positive (upright) QRS complex, whereas those positioned over the right ventricle (V_1 and V_2) record a negative (downward) QRS complex.

Following the QRS complex is a plateau phase called the *ST segment*, which extends from the end of the QRS complex (called the *J point*) to the beginning of the T wave. When ischemia occurs, one may observe depression of the ST segment (Fig. 1-11A). When infarction from total obstruction of a coronary artery occurs, ST segment elevation may be observed (Fig. 1-11B). Repolarization of the ventricle leads to the T wave. The T wave usually goes in the same direction as the QRS complex.

The *QT interval*—measured from the beginning of the QRS complex to the end of the T wave—includes the time required for ventricular depolarization and repolarization, and it varies inversely with heart rate. A rate-related ("corrected") QT interval (QTc) can be calculated as $QT\sqrt{R-R}$ interval; it should be less than 0.44 second.

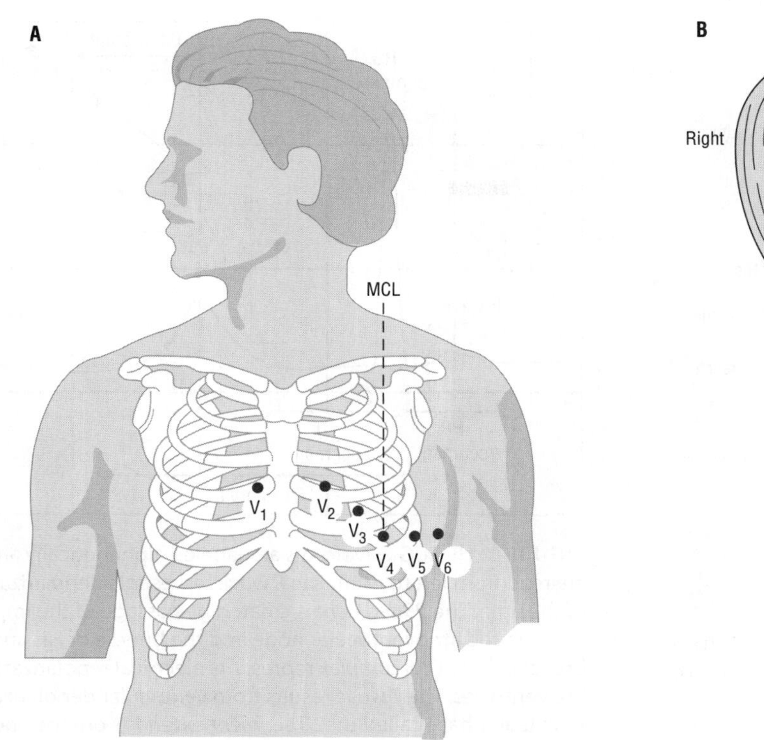

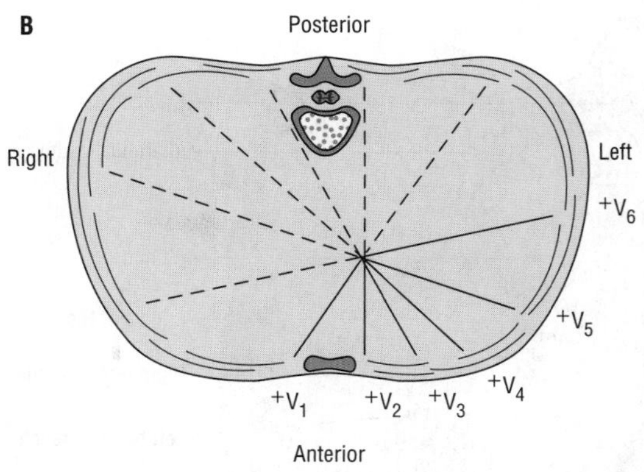

FIGURE 1-7 *A.* Electrode positions of the precordial leads. (MCL, midclavicular line; V_1, fourth intercostal space at the right sternal border; V_2, fourth intercostal space at the left sternal border; V_3, halfway between V_2 and V_4; V_4, fifth intercostal space at the midclavicular line; V_5, anterior axillary line directly lateral to V_4; V_6, anterior axillary space directly lateral to V_5.) *B.* The precordial reference figure. Leads V_1 and V_2 are called right-sided precordial leads; leads V_3 and V_4, midprecordial leads; and leads V_5 and V_6, left-sided precordial leads. *(Redrawn from Kinney MR, Packa DR, eds. Andreoli's Comprehensive Cardiac Care, 8th ed. St. Louis, MO: Mosby, 1996, with permission.)*

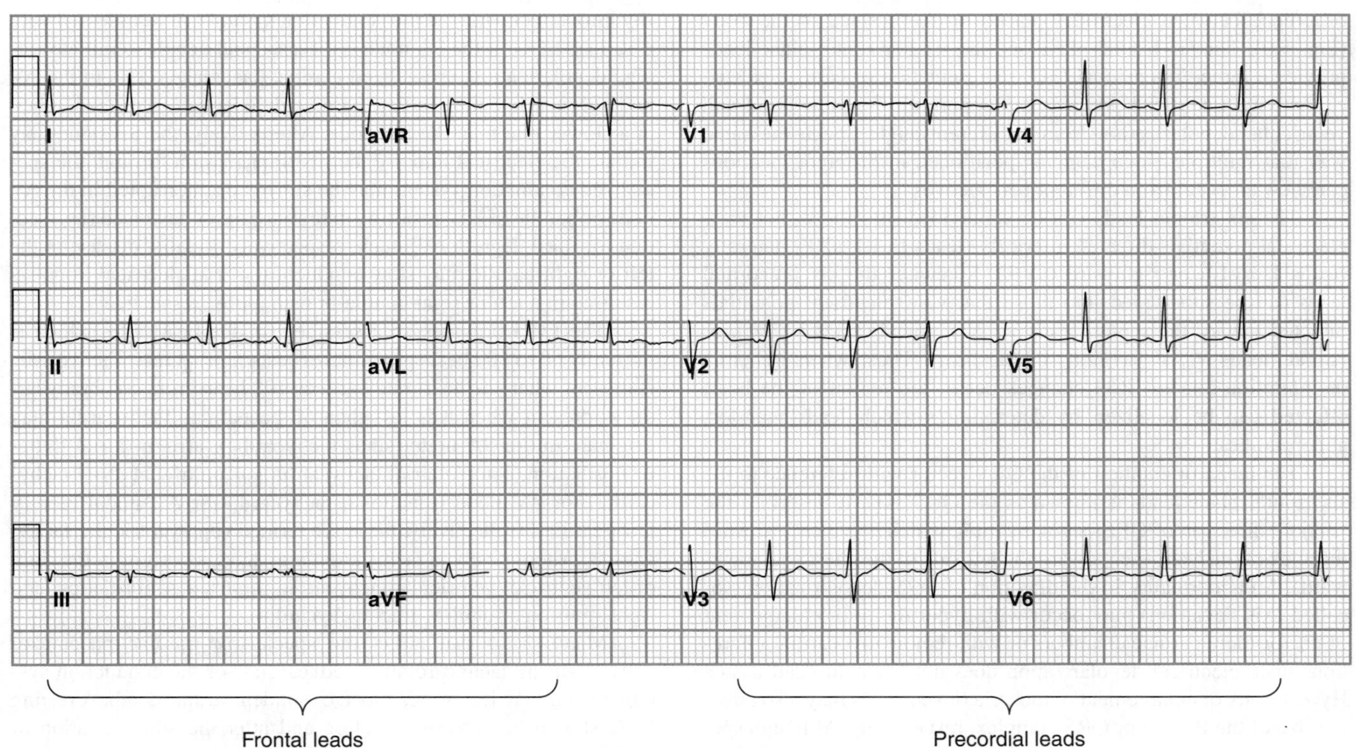

FIGURE 1-8 Standard 12-lead electrocardiogram, with six frontal and six precordial leads.

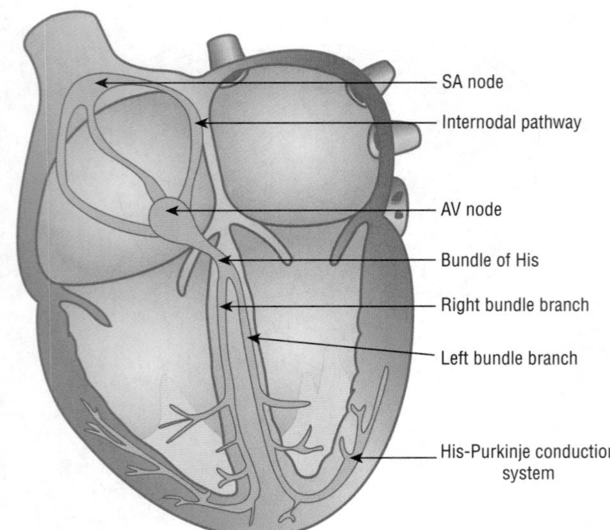

FIGURE 1-9 Schematic representation of the cardiac conduction system. (AV, atrioventricular; SA, sinoatrial.)

(From Vijayaraman P, Ellenbogen KA. Bradyarrhythmias and pacemakers. In: Fuster V, O'Rourke RA, Walsh RA, Poole-Wilson P, eds. Hurst's the Heart, 12th ed. New York: McGraw-Hill, 2004:1021.)

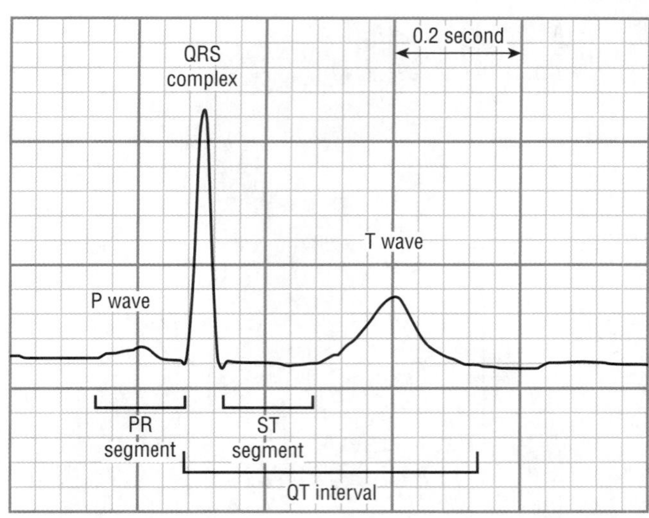

FIGURE 1-10 ECG waveforms are labeled alphabetically and are read from left to right. The *P wave* represents depolarization of the atria. The *PR segment* is created by passage of the impulse through the atrioventricular node and the bundle of His and its branches. The *QRS complex* represents electrical repolarization of the ventricles. The *T wave* results from ventricular depolarization. A plateau phase called the *ST segment* extends from the end of the QRS complex to the beginning of the T wave. The ST segment elevates with transmural (full thickness) ischemia and depresses with ischemia. The *QT interval*—measured from the beginning of the QRS complex to the end of the T wave—includes the time required for ventricular depolarization and repolarization.

A prolonged QTc interval is caused by abnormalities in depolarization or repolarization that are associated with sudden cardiac death. QTc prolongation may be due to genetic defects in action potential ion channels (e.g., congenital long QT syndrome), drugs (Table 1-4), or electrolyte disturbances (i.e., hypokalemia, hypocalcemia, hypomagnesemia). Regardless of the cause, QT prolongation increases susceptibility to a potentially lethal arrhythmia, torsades de pointes (a type of ventricular tachycardia).

The 12 conventional ECG leads record the electrical potential difference between electrodes placed on the surface of the body (Fig. 1-9). The six frontal plane and the six horizontal plane leads provide a three-dimensional (3D) representation of cardiac electrical activity. Each lead provides the opportunity to view atrial and ventricular depolarization from a different angle, much the same way that multiple video cameras positioned in different locations can view an event from different perspectives.

The six frontal leads can be subdivided into those that view electrical potentials directed inferiorly (leads II, III, aVF), laterally (leads I, aVL), or rightward (aVR). Likewise, the six precordial leads can be subdivided into those that view electrical potentials directed toward the septal (leads V_1, V_2), apical (leads V_3, V_4), or lateral (leads V_5, V_6) regions of the heart. Thus, when ischemia or infarction-related ECG changes occur, the region of the heart affected can be localized by determining which leads manifest abnormalities.

The mean orientation of the QRS vector with reference to the six frontal plane leads is known as the QRS axis. It describes the "major" direction of QRS depolarization, which is typically toward the apex of the heart (i.e., toward the left side of the chest and downward). An abnormality in the direction of QRS depolarization (so-called axis deviation) may occur with hypertrophy or enlargement of one or more cardiac chambers or with remote myocardial infarction, since electrical depolarization does not occur in dead tissue. Hypertrophy or enlargement of the atria or ventricles may also affect the size of the P wave or QRS complex, respectively. Although specific ECG criteria have been developed for diagnosing hypertrophy, the ECG is neither sensitive nor specific for establishing the presence of atrial dilation or ventricular hypertrophy. Other noninvasive modalities (i.e., echocardiography or MRI) are superior to the ECG for evaluating these conditions.

The origin of the electrical impulses (the so-called cardiac rhythm) and integrity of the conduction system can be assessed with a 12-lead ECG. If the SA node is diseased and unable to initiate cardiac depolarization, specialized cardiac pacemaker cells in the AV node or ventricle may initiate cardiac depolarization instead, albeit at a slower rate than the SA node. Alternatively, the SA node may initiate the electrical impulse, but its transmission through the specialized conduction system may be slowed or interrupted in the AV node or bundle of His, resulting in first-degree or advanced (i.e., second- or third-degree) AV block, respectively. Finally, disease in the left or right bundle may slow conduction of the electrical impulse, resulting in a left or right bundle-branch block, respectively.

The ECG provides an assessment of the heart rate, which is normally 60 to 100 beats per minute (beats/min) at rest. Tachycardia is present when the heart rate exceeds 100 beats/min, and bradycardia is present when it is less than 60 beats/min. Tachycardia may originate in the SA node (sinus tachycardia), atrium (atrial flutter or fibrillation, ectopic atrial tachycardia, or multifocal atrial tachycardia), or AV node (junctional tachycardia or AV nodal reentry tachycardia). Collectively, these are termed supraventricular tachycardias. Alternatively, a tachycardia may have its origin in the right or left ventricle (ventricular tachycardia, ventricular fibrillation, and right ventricular outflow tract tachycardia).

Many drugs can affect the specialized cardiac pacemaker cells—causing tachycardia or bradycardia—or the conduction system, which may lead to AV block or sudden cardiac death. A resting ECG should be performed before and after the administration of such drugs, with examination of the rhythm, heart rate, and various intervals (i.e., PR, QRS, and QT) to determine if substantial changes have occurred.

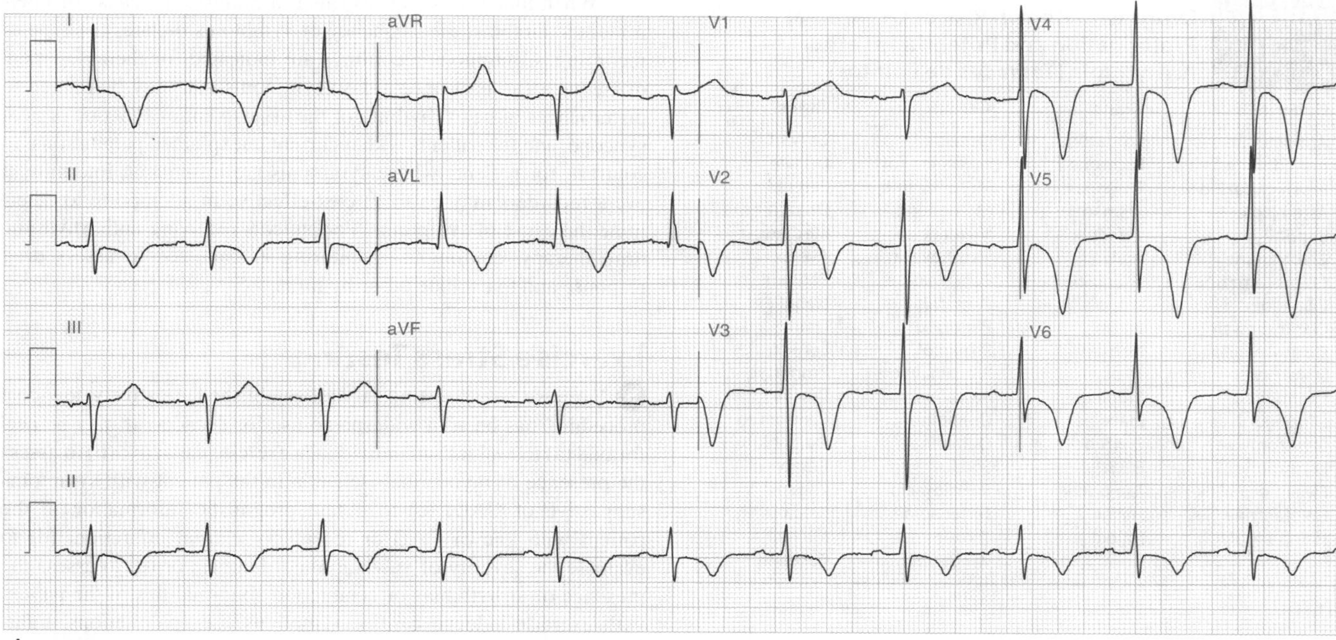

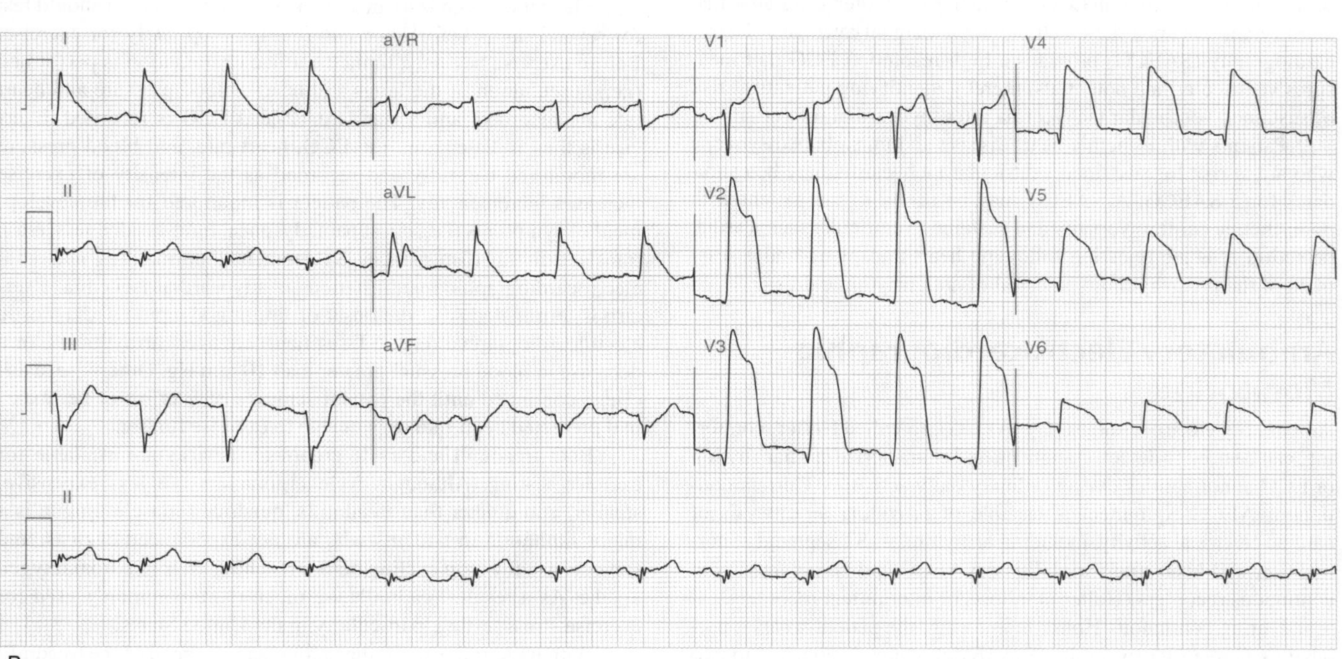

FIGURE 1-11 *A.* Anterior wall ischemia with deep T-wave inversions and ST segment depressions in leads I, aVL, and V_3 to V_6. *(Source: Longo DL, Fauci AS, Kasper DL, Hauser SL, Jameson JL, Loscalzo J. Harrison's Principles of internal Medicine, 18th ed. Figure e28-1, www.accessmedicine.com. Copyright © The McGraw-Hill Companies, Inc. All rights reserved.)* *B.* Extensive anterior MI with marked ST elevations in leads I, aVL, V_1 to V_6, and small pathologic Q waves in V_3 to V_6. Marked reciprocal ST segment depressions in leads III and aVF. *(Source: Longo DL, Fauci AS, Kasper DL, Hauser SL, Jameson JL, Loscalzo J. Harrison's Principles of Internal Medicine, 18th ed. Figure e28-5, www.accessmedicine.com. Copyright © The McGraw-Hill Companies, Inc. All rights reserved.)*

In the patient with chest pain, the resting ECG is examined for ST segment abnormalities that may indicate myocardial ischemia or infarction (i.e., ST segment depression or elevation). In addition, the resting ECG may indicate if the patient has had a remote myocardial infarction.

The ECG is used often in conjunction with other diagnostic tests to provide additional data, monitor the patient, or determine if symptoms correlate with what is observed on the ECG. For example, the patient suspected of having CAD may undergo stress testing with ECG monitoring to assess the presence of provocable ischemia.

Signal-Averaged ECG

Survivors of myocardial infarction may be at risk for life-threatening arrhythmias. In these individuals, myocardial scar tissue creates zones of slow conduction that appear as low-amplitude, high-frequency signals that are continuous with the QRS complex. These small electrical currents (so-called late potentials) are not detectable

TABLE 1-4 Drugs with Known Risk of QT Interval Prolongation and Potentially Lethal Arrhythmia (Torsades de Pointes)

Generic	Brand	Generic	Brand
Amiodarone	Cordarone	Ibutilide	Corvert
Amiodarone	Pacerone	Levomethadyl	Orlaam
Arsenic trioxide	Trisenox	Mesoridazine	Serentil
Astemizole	Hismanal	Methadone	Dolophine
Bepridil	Vascor	Methadone	Methadose
Chloroquine	Aralen	Moxifloxacin	Avelox
Chlorpromazine	Thorazine	Pentamidine	Pentam
Cisapride	Propulsid	Pentamidine	NebuPent
Clarithromycin	Biaxin	Pimozide	Orap
Disopyramide	Norpace	Probucol	Lorelco
Dofetilide	Tikosyn	Procainamide	Pronestyl
Domperidone	Motilium	Procainamide	Procan
Droperidol	Inapsine	Quinidine	Cardioquin
Erythromycin	Erythrocin	Quinidine	Quinaglute
Erythromycin	E.E.S.	Sotalol	Betapace
Flecanide	Tambocor	Sparfloxacin	Zagam
Halofantrine	Halfan	Terfenadine	Seldane
Haloperidol	Haldol	Thioridazine	Mellaril
		Vandetanib	Caprelsa

on a routine, traditional ECG. By using computer programs that amplify and enhance the electrical signal, signal-averaged electrocardiography (SAECG) provides a high-resolution ECG that measures ventricular late potentials, thereby identifying patients at risk of sustained ventricular tachycardia after myocardial infarction.[28]

Patients with ischemic heart disease and unexplained syncope who are at risk for sustained ventricular tachycardia may be candidates for a SAECG. A SAECG may be useful in the patient with nonischemic cardiomyopathy and sustained ventricular tachycardia, detection of acute rejection following heart transplant, and assessment of the proarrhythmic potential of antiarrhythmic drugs.

Ambulatory Electrocardiographic Monitoring

Ambulatory electrocardiography (AECG), so-called Holter monitoring, can be used to detect, document, and characterize cardiac rhythm or ECG abnormalities during ordinary daily activities. Current continuous AECG equipment is capable of providing an analysis of cardiac electrical activity, including arrhythmias, ST segment abnormalities, and heart rate variability. An AECG can be obtained with continuous recorders (Holter monitors) or intermittent recorders.

During continuous Holter monitoring, the patient wears a portable ECG recorder (weighing 8 to 16 oz), which is attached to two to four leads placed on the chest wall. During monitoring, the patient maintains a diary, in which he/she records the occurrence, duration, and severity of symptoms (e.g., light-headedness, chest pain, palpitations, etc.). The device is typically worn for 24 to 48 hours, after which the continuous ECG recording is scanned by computer to detect arrhythmias or ST segment abnormalities to determine if they are responsible for the patient's symptoms.

Intermittent recorders (also known as event monitors or loop recorders) are worn for longer periods of time (weeks to months). Although they continuously monitor the ECG, only brief (minutes) segments of it are recorded when the patient activates the device (i.e., when symptoms occur) or a preprogrammed abnormal ECG event occurs. Some intermittent event recorders incorporate a memory loop that permits capture of a rhythm recording during fleeting symptoms, tachycardia onset, and, in some cases, syncope that occurs infrequently. When the patient activates a looping monitor, it records several minutes of the preceding rhythm as well as the subsequent rhythm.

When monitoring is performed to evaluate the cause of intermittent symptoms, the frequency of symptoms dictates the type of recording. Continuous recordings are indicated for the assessment of frequent (at least once a day) symptoms that may be related to disturbances of heart rhythm, for the assessment of syncope or near syncope, and for patients with recurrent unexplained palpitations. In contrast, for patients whose symptoms are infrequent, intermittent event recorders may be more cost-effective in attempting to determine the cause of symptoms. For patients receiving antiarrhythmic drug therapy, continuous monitoring is indicated to assess drug response and to exclude proarrhythmia.

Exercise Stress Testing

5 Exercise stress testing, a well-established, relatively low-cost procedure, has been in widespread use for decades. It may be performed (a) to evaluate an individual's exercise capacity; (b) to assess the presence of myocardial ischemia in the patient with symptoms suggestive of CAD; (c) to obtain prognostic information in the patient with known CAD or recent myocardial infarction; (d) to evaluate the severity of valvular abnormalities; or (e) to assess the presence of arrhythmias or conduction abnormalities in the patient with exercise-induced cardiac symptoms (i.e., palpitations, light-headedness, or syncope).

The patient who is to undergo an exercise stress test should fast for several hours beforehand and dress appropriately for exercise. Before exercise begins, a limited cardiac examination is performed (i.e., auscultation of the lungs and heart), blood pressure and heart rate are recorded, and a standard 12-lead ECG is recorded. Exercise is then initiated, and the ECG, heart rate, and blood pressure are monitored carefully and recorded as the intensity of exercise increases incrementally. The patient is monitored for the development of symptoms (i.e., chest pain, dyspnea, light-headedness, etc.), transient rhythm disturbances, ST segment abnormalities, and other electrocardiographic manifestations of myocardial ischemia. Exercise is terminated with the onset of limiting symptoms, diagnostic electrocardiographic (e.g., ST segment) changes, arrhythmias, or a decrease in blood pressure greater than 10 mm Hg. Otherwise, exercise is continued until the patient achieves 85% of his or her maximal predicted heart rate or is unable to exercise further.

Both treadmill and cycle ergometer devices are available for exercise testing. Although cycle ergometers are less expensive, smaller, and quieter than treadmills, quadricep muscle fatigue is a major limitation in patients who are not experienced cyclists, and subjects usually stop cycling before reaching their maximal oxygen uptake. As a result, treadmills are much more commonly used for exercise stress testing, particularly in the United States.

With treadmill testing, the incline and/or speed of the treadmill is increased incrementally every 2 to 3 minutes. Several treadmill exercise protocols have been developed to accommodate the variations in fitness, age, and mobility of individuals. Accordingly, if the exercise capacity is reported in minutes, the details of the protocol should be specified. Alternatively, the translation of exercise duration or workload into metabolic equivalents (METs) (oxygen uptake expressed in multiples of basal oxygen uptake, 3.5 mL O_2/kg/min) has the advantage of providing a common measure of performance regardless of the type of exercise test or protocol used. Most domestic chores and activities require less than 5 METs, whereas participation in strenuous sports, such as swimming, singles tennis, football, basketball, or skiing, requires greater than 10 METs.

Interpretation of the results of exercise testing should include exercise capacity as well as the clinical, hemodynamic, and electrocardiographic responses. The occurrence of chest pain consistent with angina is important, particularly if it results in termination of the test. Abnormalities in exercise capacity, the response of systolic blood pressure to exercise, and the response of heart rate to

TABLE 1-5 Meta-Analyses of Exercise Testing

Grouping	Number of Studies	Total Number of Patients	Sens (%)	Spec (%)	Predictive Accuracy (%)
Meta-analysis of standard exercise test	147	24,047	68	77	73
Meta-analysis without MI	58	11,691	67	72	69
Meta-analysis without workup bias	3	>1,000	50	90	69
Meta-analysis with ST depression	22	9,153	69	70	69
Meta-analysis without ST depression	3	840	67	84	75
Meta-analysis with digoxin	15	6,338	68	74	71
Meta-analysis without digoxin	9	3,548	72	69	70
Meta-analysis with LVH	15	8,016	68	69	68
Meta-analysis without LVH	10	1,977	72	77	74

Sens, sensitivity; Spec, specificity; MI, myocardial infarction; LVH, left ventricular hypertrophy.

From Gibbons RJ, Balady GJ, Bricker JT, et al. ACC/AHA 2002 Guideline Update for Exercise Testing: A Report of the American College of Cardiology/American Heart Association Task Force on Practice Guidelines (Committee on Exercise Testing). 2002. American College of Cardiology Website, www.acc.org/clinical/guidelines/exercise/dirIndex.htm.

exercise and recovery may provide valuable information. The most important electrocardiographic findings are ST segment depression and elevation. A positive exercise test is said to have occurred if the ECG shows at least 1 mm of horizontal or downsloping ST segment depression or elevation for at least 60 to 80 milliseconds after the end of the QRS complex.

ST segment changes suggestive of myocardial ischemia that occur at a low level of exercise (less than 6 minutes of exercise or less than 5 METs) are associated with more severe CAD and a worse prognosis than those that occur at a higher workload. An estimate of myocardial oxygen demands can be obtained by calculating the so-called "rate–pressure product" (double product) (i.e., heart rate × systolic arterial pressure).

Most treadmill exercise testing is performed in adults with symptoms of known or suspected ischemic heart disease. In patients for whom the diagnosis of CAD is certain, stress testing is often used for risk stratification or prognostic assessment to determine the need for possible coronary angiography or revascularization. Patients who are candidates for exercise testing may (a) have stable chest pain; (b) be stabilized with medical therapy following an episode of unstable chest pain; or (c) be post–myocardial infarction or post-revascularization.

The ability of the exercise stress test to identify (or to exclude) individuals with CAD is influenced by (a) their exercise capacity (i.e., can the individual perform maximal or nearly maximal exercise?); (b) the presence of baseline electrocardiographic abnormalities (i.e., bundle-branch block or ST segment depression); (c) medications that affect the ECG or the hemodynamic response to exercise (i.e., digoxin and β-adrenergic blocking agents, respectively); and (d) concomitant cardiac conditions that are associated with electrocardiographic abnormalities (i.e., left ventricular hypertrophy, paced rhythm, preexcitation) (Table 1-5). Thus, patients who are unable to exercise or who have baseline ECG abnormalities require imaging (i.e., radionuclide or echocardiographic) stress testing to detect (or to exclude) CAD, since routine stress testing is unreliable in these individuals.

The ability of the exercise stress test to identify the presence of CAD is influenced by the pretest probability of CAD in the population tested. For example, exercise-induced ST segment depression in a 60-year-old man with typical anginal chest pain and multiple risk factors for atherosclerosis (i.e., a high pretest probability) is considered a "true positive" stress test, whereas the presence of same findings in a 30-year-old woman with chest pain believed to be atypical for angina (i.e., a low pretest probability) is most likely to be a "false-positive" test. The relatively poor accuracy of the exercise ECG for diagnosing CAD in asymptomatic subjects has led to the recommendation that exercise testing not be used as a screening tool,[29] since false-positive tests are common among asymptomatic adults, especially women, and may lead to unnecessary testing and treatment. Controversy exists as to whether exercise testing should be performed in asymptomatic individuals at increased risk of CAD (i.e., diabetics).

Clinical **Controversy. . .**

The relatively poor accuracy of the exercise ECG for diagnosing CAD in asymptomatic subjects has led to the recommendation that exercise testing not be used as a screening tool, since false-positive tests are common among asymptomatic adults, particularly women, and may lead subsequently to unnecessary testing and treatment. However, controversy exists as to whether exercise testing should be routinely performed in asymptomatic individuals at increased risk of CVD (i.e., diabetics) to identify "silent" (asymptomatic) myocardial ischemia.

The ACC and AHA have jointly developed guidelines describing the indications for exercise stress testing.[29,30]

Exercise stress testing is relatively safe, with an estimated risk of myocardial infarction or death of 1 per 2,500 tests. It should be supervised by a physician or a properly trained health professional working directly under the supervision of a physician, who should be in the immediate vicinity and available for emergencies. Exercise stress testing is contraindicated in subjects who are unable to exercise or who should not exercise because of physiologic or psychological limitations (Table 1-6). Although unstable angina is usually a contraindication to exercise stress testing, it can be performed safely once the patient has responded appropriately to intensive medical therapy. Exercise testing is contraindicated in patients with untreated life-threatening arrhythmias or congestive heart failure. Patients with comorbid diseases, such as chronic obstructive pulmonary disease or peripheral vascular disease, may be limited in their exercise capacity. For patients with disabilities or other medical conditions that limit their exercise capacity, pharmacologic stress testing (with dipyridamole, adenosine, regadenoson, or dobutamine) is an alternative (see Pharmacologic Stress Testing below).

Drug therapy is not routinely altered before exercise stress testing, since few data suggest that doing so improves its diagnostic accuracy. Although patients receiving a β-adrenergic or calcium channel blocker may have a blunted increase in heart rate and blood pressure with exercise, exercise stress testing in such patients nonetheless provides information regarding exercise capacity and ischemic ECG alterations. Nitrates do not directly alter exercise

TABLE 1-6 Contraindications to Exercise Testing

Absolute
Acute myocardial infarction (within 2 days)
High-risk unstable angina
Uncontrolled cardiac arrhythmias causing symptoms or hemodynamic compromise
Symptomatic severe aortic stenosis
Uncontrolled symptomatic heart failure
Acute pulmonary embolus or pulmonary infarction
Acute myocarditis or pericarditis
Acute aortic dissection
Relative
Left main coronary stenosis
Moderate stenotic valvular heart disease
Electrolyte abnormalities
Severe arterial hypertension
Tachyarrhythmias or bradyarrhythmias
Hypertrophic cardiomyopathy and other forms of outflow tract obstruction
Mental or physical impairment leading to inability to exercise adequately
High-degree atrioventricular block

Adapted from AHA/ACC guidelines.

capacity, but they may increase the patient's exercise capacity by preventing or relieving exercise-induced angina. Digoxin produces an abnormal ST segment response to exercise in 25% to 40% of healthy subjects. Because of its long half-life, digoxin should be discontinued for 2 weeks before exercise stress testing to avoid such drug-induced ST segment changes.[30]

Echocardiography

6 Using echocardiography, one can evaluate cardiac function and structure with images produced by ultrasound. High-frequency sound waves transmitted from a handheld transducer "bounce" off tissue and are reflected back to the transducer, where the waves are collected and used to construct a real-time image of the heart.

With the exception of the ECG, echocardiography is the most frequently performed cardiovascular test. It is noninvasive, relatively inexpensive, safe, devoid of ionizing radiation, and portable, so that it can be done at the patient's bedside, in the operating room, or in a physician's office. Serial echocardiograms can be performed, especially following a cardiac procedure or a change in clinical condition, as well as to follow the progression of the underlying cardiac disease over time. Echocardiography is the procedure of choice for the diagnosis and evaluation of many cardiac conditions, including valvular abnormalities, intracardiac thrombi, pericardial effusions, and congenital abnormalities. It often is used to assess chamber sizes, function, and wall thickness. In the patient suspected of having CAD, echocardiography can be performed before, during, and immediately after exercise or pharmacologic stress (e.g., dobutamine) to evaluate the presence of ischemia-induced ventricular wall motion abnormalities.

Two approaches to echocardiography are used in clinical practice. Transthoracic echocardiography (TTE) is performed with the transducer positioned on the anterior chest wall, whereas transesophageal echocardiography (TEE) is performed with the transducer positioned in the esophagus. Following transducer placement, several modes of operation are possible: M-mode (motion), two-dimensional (2D), 3D, and Doppler imaging.

With M-mode echocardiography, a transducer placed at a site on the anterior chest (usually along the sternal border) records the images of cardiac structures in one plane, producing a static picture of a small region of the heart, a so-called "ice pick view" (Fig. 1-12). Results depend on the exact placement of the transducer with respect to the underlying structures. Conventional M-mode echocardiography provides visualization of the right ventricle, left ventricle, and posterior left ventricular wall and pericardium. If the transducer is swept in an arc from the apex to the base of the heart, virtually the whole heart can be visualized, including the valves and left atrium.

2D echocardiography employs multiple windows of the heart, and each view provides a wedge-shaped image (Figs. 1-13 and 1-14). These views are processed to produce a motion picture of the beating heart. When compared with M-mode echocardiography, 2D echocardiography provides increased accuracy in calculating ventricular volumes, wall thickness, and the severity of valvular stenoses.

3D echocardiography, which uses an ultrasound probe with an array of transducers and an appropriate processing system, enables

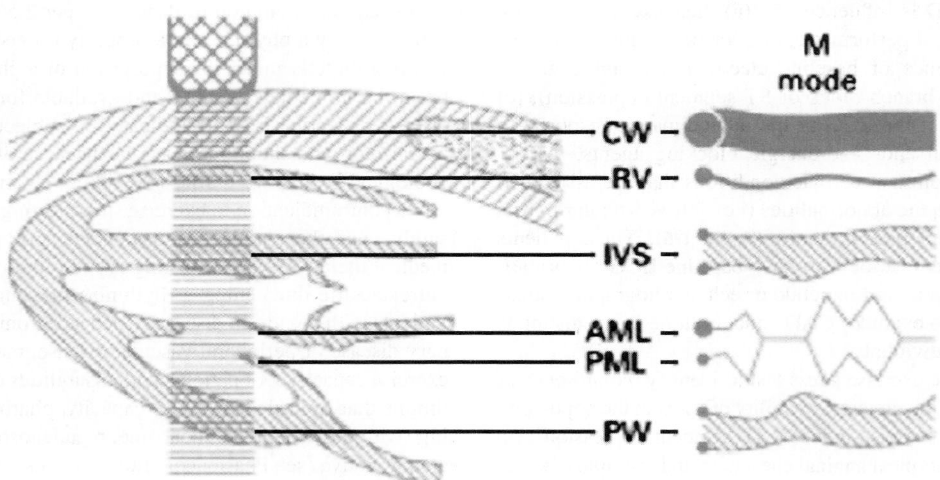

FIGURE 1-12 M-mode echocardiogram. The transducer emits an ultrasound beam, which reflects at each anatomic interface. The reflected wave fronts are detected by the probe, which records the images of cardiac structures in one plane, producing a static picture of a small region of the heart, a so-called "ice pick view." (AML, anterior mitral leaflet; CW, chest wall; IVS, interventricular septum; PML, posterior mitral leaflet; PW, posterior wall; RV, right ventricle.) *(Modified from Hagan AD, DeMaria AN. Clinical Applications of Two-Dimensional Echocardiography and Cardiac Doppler. Boston, MA: Little, Brown, 1989, with permission. From Fuster V, O'Rourke RA, Walsh RA, Poole-Wilson P, eds. Hurst's the Heart, 12th ed., http://www.accessmedicine.com. Copyright © The McGraw-Hill Companies, Inc. All rights reserved.)*

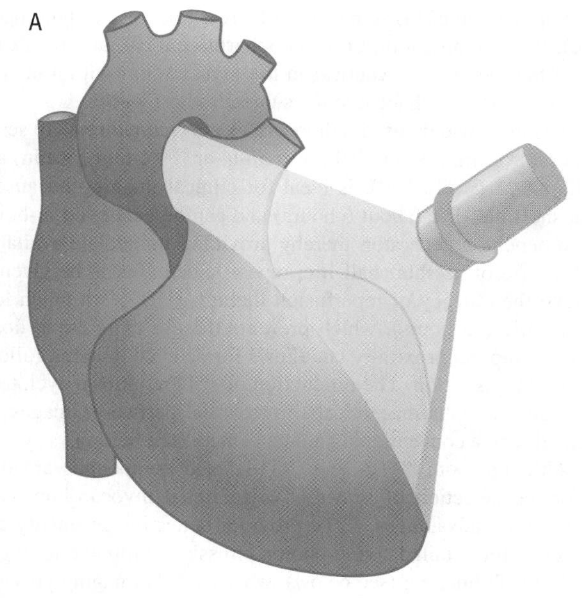

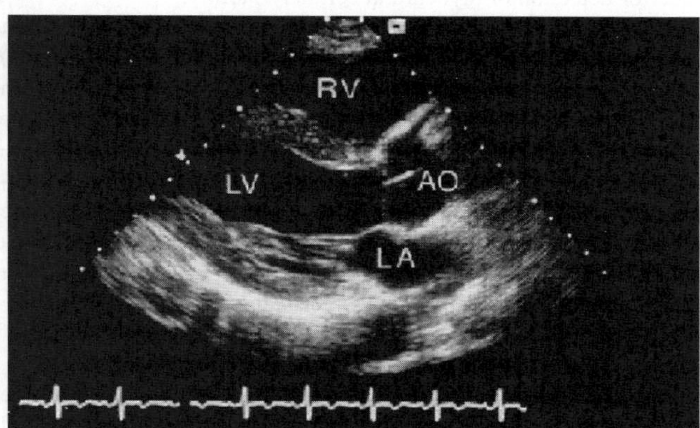

FIGURE 1-13 2D transthoracic echocardiography. *A.* Orientation of the sector beam and transducer position for the parasternal long-axis view of the left ventricle. *B.* 2D image of the heart, parasternal long-axis view. (Ao, aorta; LA, left atrium; LV, left ventricle; RV, right ventricle.) *(From DeMaria AN, Daniel G, Blanchard DG. Echocardiography. In: Fuster V, O'Rourke RA, Walsh RA, Poole-Wilson P, eds. Hurst's the Heart, 12th ed. New York: McGraw-Hill, 2004:369.)*

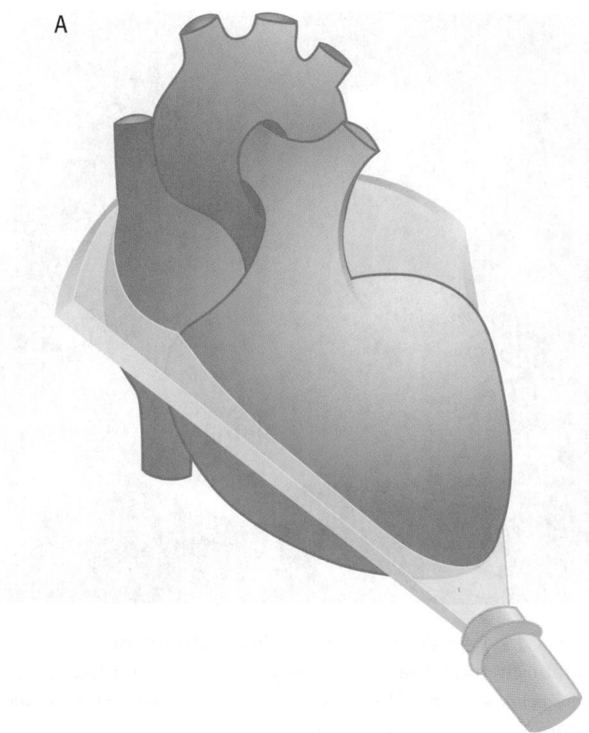

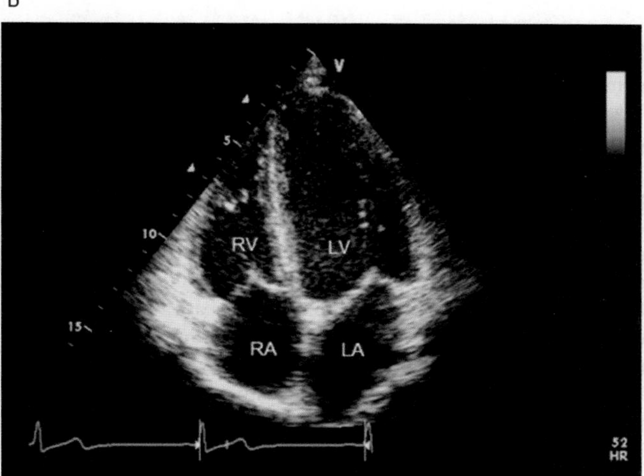

FIGURE 1-14 2D transthoracic echocardiography. *A.* Orientation of the sector beam and transducer position for the apical four-chamber plane. *B.* 2D image of the apical four-chamber plane. (LA, left atrium; LV, left ventricle; RA, right atrium; RV, right ventricle.) *(From DeMaria AN, Daniel G, Blanchard DG. Echocardiography. In: Fuster V, O'Rourke RA, Walsh RA, Poole-Wilson P, eds. Hurst's the Heart, 12th ed. New York: McGraw-Hill, 2004:372.)*

a detailed assessment of cardiac anatomy and pathology, particularly valvular abnormalities as well as ventricular size and function (Fig. 1-15). The ability to "slice" the heart in an infinite number of planes in an anatomically appropriate manner and to reconstruct 3D images of anatomic structures makes this technique very powerful in understanding congenital cardiac conditions.[31]

Doppler echocardiography is used to detect the velocity and direction of blood flow by measuring the change in frequency produced when ultrasound waves are reflected from red blood cells. Color enhancement allows blood flow direction and velocity to be visualized, with different colors used for antegrade and retrograde flow. Blood flow moving toward the transducer is displayed in red, and flow moving away from the transducer is displayed in blue; increasing velocity is depicted in brighter shades of each color. Thus, with Doppler echocardiography, information regarding the presence, direction, velocity, and turbulence of blood flow can be acquired. Cardiac hemodynamic variables (e.g., intracardiac pressures) and the presence and severity of valvular disease can be assessed noninvasively with Doppler echocardiography.

When TTE is performed, the transducer is placed on the anterior chest wall, and imaging is performed in three orthogonal planes: long axis (from aortic root to apex), short axis (perpendicular to the long axis), and four-chamber (visualizing both ventricles and atria through the mitral and tricuspid valves) (Figs. 1-13 and 1-14). Sound energy is poorly transmitted through air and bone, and the ability to record adequate images is dependent on a thoracic window that gives the ultrasound beam adequate access to cardiac structures. Accordingly, in approximately 15% of subjects, suboptimal TTE images are obtained, particularly those with large lung volumes (i.e., chronic lung disease or those being ventilated mechanically) or marked obesity. In addition, TTE may not provide adequate or

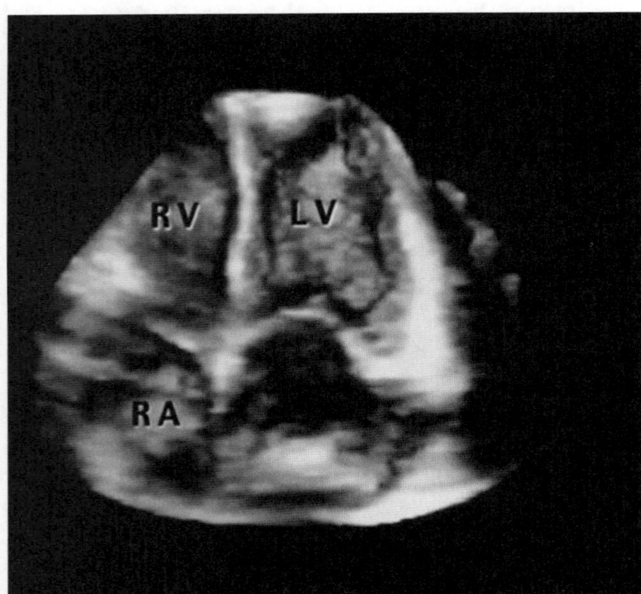

FIGURE 1-15 Real-time 3D echocardiography image, apical four-chamber plane. *(From DeMaria AN, Daniel G, Blanchard DG. Echocardiography. In: Fuster V, O'Rourke RA, Walsh RA, Poole-Wilson P, eds. Hurst's the Heart, 12th ed. New York: McGraw-Hill, 2004:374.)*

complete images of the posterior cardiac structures (i.e., left atrium, left atrial appendage, mitral valve, interatrial septum, descending aorta, etc.) that are located far away from the transducer.

With TEE, a flexible transducer is advanced into the esophagus and rests just behind the heart, adjacent to the left atrium and descending aorta. When compared with TTE, TEE provides clearer and more detailed images of the mitral valve, left atrium, left atrial appendage, pulmonary veins, and descending thoracic aorta. Because of the transducer's proximity to the heart, TEE allows one to delineate small cardiac structures (i.e., vegetations and thrombi less than 3 mm in diameter) that may not be seen with TTE. As a result, TEE often is used to assess the presence of (a) mitral valve vegetations, (b) endocarditis complications (e.g., myocardial abscess), (c) left atrial appendage thrombus in the patient with a stroke or under consideration for an elective cardioversion, and (d) aortic dissection.[32–38] In addition, the transducer can be advanced into the fundus of the stomach to obtain images of the ventricles. TEE is widely utilized intraoperatively to assess the success of mitral valve repair or replacement and to delineate cardiac anatomy in subjects with congenital heart disease at the time of surgical repair.

Although TEE is a low-risk invasive procedure, complications, such as tearing or perforation of the esophagus, esophageal burns, transient ventricular tachycardia, minor throat irritation, and transient vocal cord paralysis, occur rarely. TEE-related complications in ambulatory, nonoperative settings range from 0.2% to 0.5%, and mortality is less than 0.01%.[39] TEE is contraindicated in patients with esophageal abnormalities, in whom passage of the transducer may be difficult or hazardous (e.g., esophageal strictures, tear, tumor, or varices).

The ACC/AHA Task Force has published guidelines for application of echocardiography and stress echocardiography.[35,40,41]

Nuclear Cardiology

7 Myocardial perfusion imaging, the most commonly performed nuclear cardiology procedure, is used to assess the presence, location, and severity of ischemic or infarcted myocardium. It consists of a combination of (a) some form of stress (exercise or pharmacologic), (b) administration of a radiopharmaceutical, and (c) detection of the radiopharmaceutical in the myocardium with a nuclear camera positioned adjacent to the subject's chest wall.

The most widely used radionuclides are technetium (Tc) sestamibi or tetrofosmin-99m (^{99m}Tc-sestamibi or ^{99m}Tc-tetrofosmin) and thallium-201 (^{201}Tl). ^{99m}Tc is ideal for clinical imaging because it has a short half-life (about 6 hours) and can be generated in-house with a benchtop generator, thereby providing immediate availability. Because of its short half-life, repeat injections can be given to evaluate the efficacy of reperfusion therapy. ^{201}Tl has a much longer half-life (73 hours), which prevents the use of multiple doses in close temporal proximity but allows for delayed imaging following its administration. The production of ^{201}Tl requires a cyclotron. With both radiopharmaceuticals, myocardial perfusion images are obtained with a conventional gamma camera (see below).

Although both ^{99m}Tc- and ^{201}Tl-labeled compounds are useful for the detection of ischemic or infarcted myocardium, each offers certain advantages. ^{99m}Tc provides better image quality and is superior for detailed single-photon emission computed tomography (SPECT) imaging (see below), whereas ^{201}Tl imaging provides superior detection of myocardial cellular viability.

With ^{201}Tl imaging, the radioisotope is injected IV as the patient is completing exercise or pharmacologic stress. Since thallium (Tl) is a potassium analogue, it enters normal myocytes that have an active sodium–potassium ATPase pump (i.e., viable myocytes). The intracellular concentration of Tl depends on the perfusion of the tissue and its viability. In the normal heart, homogeneous distribution of Tl occurs in myocardial tissue. Conversely, regions that are scarred due to previous infarction or have stress-induced ischemia do not accumulate as much Tl as normal muscle; as a result, these areas appear as "cold" spots on the perfusion scan.

When evaluating for myocardial ischemia, an initial set of images is obtained immediately after stress and ^{201}Tl injection, and the images are examined for regions of decreased radioisotope uptake. Delayed images are obtained 3 to 4 hours later, since ^{201}Tl accumulation does not remain fixed in myocytes. Continuous redistribution of the isotope occurs across the cell membrane, with (a) differential washout rates between hypoperfused but viable myocardium and normal zones and (b) wash in to previously hypoperfused zones. Thus, when additional images are obtained after 3 to 4 hours of redistribution, viable myocytes have similar concentrations of ^{201}Tl. Consequently, any uptake abnormalities that were caused by myocardial ischemia will have resolved (i.e., "filled in") on the delayed scan and are termed "reversible" defects, whereas those representing scarred or infarcted myocardium will persist as cold spots.

Myocardial segments that demonstrate persistent ^{201}Tl hypoperfusion with stress and redistribution imaging may represent so-called "hibernating myocardium." This markedly hypoperfused myocardium is chronically ischemic and noncontractile but metabolically active; as a result, it has the potential to regain function if perfusion is restored. Hibernating myocardium can often be differentiated from irreversibly scarred myocardium by injecting additional ^{201}Tl to enhance uptake by viable myocytes, and then repeating the images 24 hours later.[42,43]

^{99m}Tc-sestamibi—also known as methoxy-isobutyl isonitrile (Tc-MIBI)—is the most widely used ^{99m}Tc-labeled compound. Similar to Tl, its uptake in the myocardium is proportional to blood flow, but its mechanism of myocyte uptake is different, in that it occurs passively, driven by the negative membrane potential. Once intracellular, it accumulates in the mitochondria, where it remains, not redistributing with the passage of time. Therefore, the myocardial distribution of sestamibi reflects perfusion at the moment of its injection. Performing a ^{99m}Tc-sestamibi procedure provides more flexibility than a ^{201}Tl procedure, in that images can be obtained for up to 4 to 6 hours after radioisotope injection and acquired again as

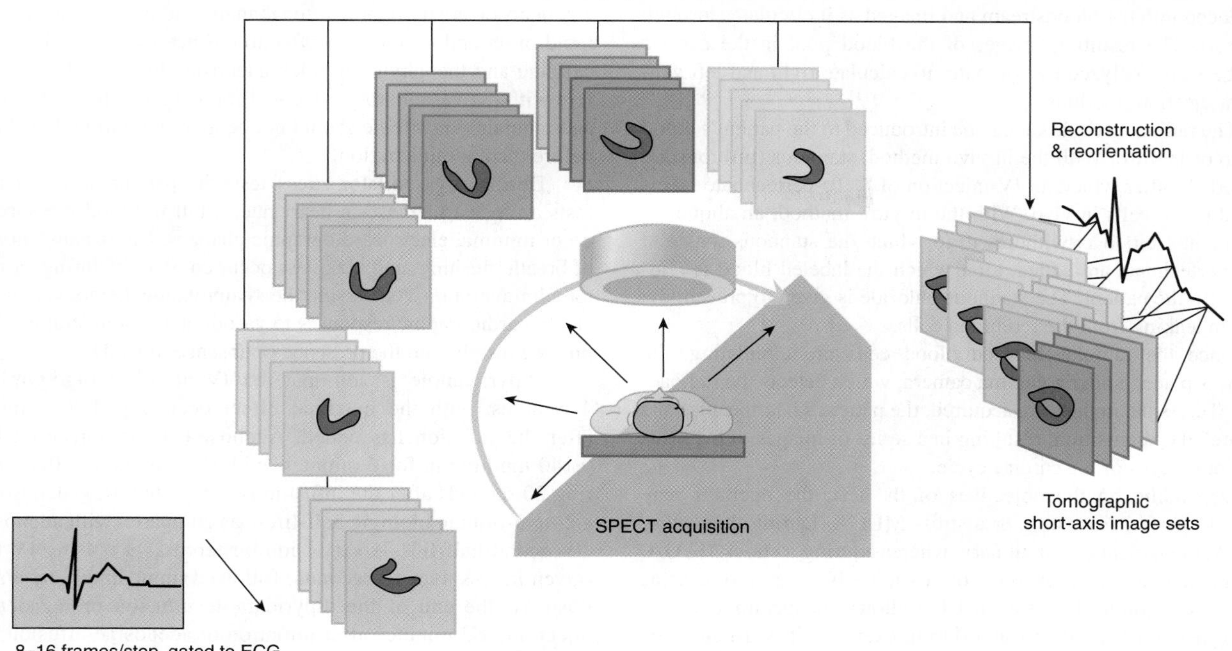

FIGURE 1-16 Schematic representation of ECG-gated SPECT imaging and acquisition. *(From Berman DS, Hachamovitch R, Shaw LJ, et al. Nuclear cardiology. In: Fuster V, O'Rourke RA, Walsh RA, Poole-Wilson P, eds. Hurst's the Heart, 12th ed. New York: McGraw-Hill, 2004:545.)*

necessary. A ^{99m}Tc-sestamibi study is usually performed as a 1-day protocol, with which an initial injection with a small tracer dose and imaging are performed at rest, after which (a few hours later) the patient undergoes a stress test, and repeat imaging is performed after injection of a larger tracer dose.

Myocardial perfusion imaging can be performed with either planar or SPECT approaches. The planar technique consists of three 2D image acquisitions, usually for 10 to 15 minutes each. With SPECT, the camera detectors rotate around the patient in a circular or elliptical fashion, collecting a series of planar projection images at regular angular intervals (Fig. 1-16). The 3D distribution of radioactivity in the myocardium is then "reconstructed" by computer from the 2D projections. Gated SPECT is a further refinement of the process, whereby the projection images are acquired in specific phases of the cardiac cycle based on ECG triggering (so-called "gating"). With gated SPECT, myocardial perfusion and function can be evaluated.

Although stress perfusion imaging with ^{99m}Tc- or ^{201}Tl-labeled compounds offers greater sensitivity and specificity than standard exercise electrocardiography for the detection of ischemia (Fig. 1-17),[43] they are considerably more expensive and expose the patient to ionizing radiation. As a result, they should be used judiciously. Stress perfusion scans are particularly useful in patients with an underlying ECG abnormality that precludes its accurate interpretation during conventional exercise stress testing, such as patients with a bundle-branch block, previous myocardial infarction, baseline ST segment abnormalities, or taking medications that affect the ST segments (e.g., digoxin).[44] When compared with standard exercise testing, nuclear perfusion imaging also provides more accurate anatomic localization of ischemia and quantitation of the extent of ischemia.[45]

Technetium Scanning

Tc scanning is used for the evaluation of cardiac function, myocardial perfusion, and the presence of infarcted myocardium.[43,46]

Radionuclide ventriculography—so-called multigated acquisition (MUGA) scanning—is a noninvasive method for determining right and left ventricular systolic function, detecting intracardiac shunting, estimating ventricular volumes, and assessing regional wall motion. For the most part, it has been replaced by other noninvasive techniques (i.e., echocardiography and MRI) that provide similar information without ionizing radiation. Nonetheless, it may be performed in the subject in whom suitable echocardiographic images cannot be obtained or who is unable to undergo an MRI study.

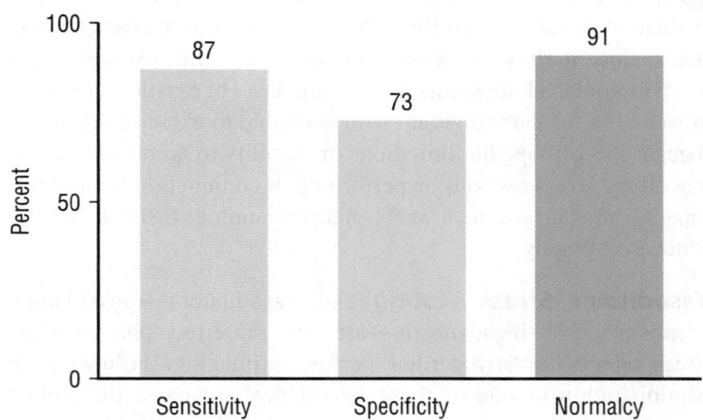

FIGURE 1-17 Detection of CAD by exercise SPECT: pooled analysis of 33 studies (≥50% stenoses). Sensitivity, specificity, and normalcy rates from a pooled analysis of 33 studies in the literature using exercise single-photon emission computed tomography (SPECT) myocardial perfusion imaging for detection of coronary artery disease (CAD). Note that the normalcy rate, which is derived from the percentage of patients with normal scans who have less than 5% pretest likelihood of CAD, is shown. This normalcy rate of 91% is significantly higher than specificity.[43]

During radionuclide ventriculography, ^{99m}Tc-pertechnate is introduced into the bloodstream and imaged as it circulates through the heart. The resulting images of the blood pool in the cardiac chambers are analyzed by computer to calculate right and left ventricular ejection fractions.

The radioactive marker can be introduced to the patient's blood in vivo or in vitro. With the in vivo method, stannous (tin) ions are injected IV, after which an IV injection of ^{99m}Tc-pertechnate labels the red blood cells in vivo. With the in vitro method, an aliquot of the patient's blood is withdrawn, to which the stannous ions and ^{99m}Tc-pertechnate are added, after which the labeled blood is reinfused into the patient. The stannous chloride is given to prevent the Tc from leaking from the red blood cells.

Once the radiolabeled red blood cells are circulating, the patient is placed under a gamma camera, which detects the radioactive ^{99m}Tc. As the images are acquired, the patient's heartbeat is used to "gate" the acquisition, resulting in a series of images of the heart at various stages of the cardiac cycle.

Depending on the objectives of the test, the operator may decide to perform a resting or a stress MUGA. During the resting MUGA, the patient lies stationary, whereas during a stress MUGA, the patient is asked to exercise on a supine bicycle ergometer as images are acquired. The stress MUGA allows the operator to assess cardiac performance at rest and during exercise. It is usually performed to assess the presence of suspected CAD.

Infarct-avid radionuclides, such as technetium pyrophosphate (^{99m}Tc-PYP), are used to assess the presence and extent of infarcted myocardium. Since ^{99m}Tc-PYP binds to calcium that is deposited in the infarcted area, it is known as *hot-spot scanning*. Hot spots appear where necrotic myocardial tissue is present, which may occur with recent myocardial infarction, myocarditis, myocardial abscesses, and myocardial trauma. Additionally, ^{99m}Tc-PYP uptake has been observed on occasion in patients with unstable angina, severe diabetes mellitus, and cardiac amyloidosis.

Uptake of ^{99m}Tc-PYP by necrotic myocardium is first detectable about 12 hours after the onset of myocardial infarction, with a peak intensity of ^{99m}Tc-PYP at 48 hours. Washout occurs over 5 to 7 days, so ^{99m}Tc-PYP is a useful late marker of infarction, especially in the patient suspected of having a painless (e.g., "silent") infarction.

Pharmacologic Stress Testing

8 In the patient undergoing myocardial perfusion imaging for the evaluation of CAD, exercise stress is preferred over pharmacologic stress, since it allows an assessment of the patient's exercise capacity, symptoms, ST segment changes, and level of exertion that results in ischemia. In the individual who is unable to exercise adequately (because of orthopedic limitations or inability to ambulate), a pharmacologic stress test can be performed in conjunction with various imaging modalities, such as Tl planar scanning, SPECT, MRI, or echocardiography.[43–45]

Vasodilator Stress Testing The vasodilators—dipyridamole, adenosine, and regadenoson—are the preferred pharmacologic stress agents for myocardial perfusion imaging. Following the administration of one of these, blood flow increases threefold to fivefold in undiseased coronary arteries and minimally, or not at all, in arteries with flow-limiting stenoses. Since radioisotope uptake by the myocardium is directly related to coronary arterial blood flow, the region of myocardium perfused by an artery with a flow-limiting stenosis appears as a "cold spot" on the nuclear perfusion scan following vasodilator administration.

Adenosine and regadenoson dilate coronary arteries by binding to specific adenosine receptors on smooth muscle cells in the coronary arterial media. Dipyridamole causes coronary vasodilation by blocking the cellular uptake of adenosine, thereby increasing the extracellular adenosine concentration. Currently, adenosine and regadenoson are used more often than dipyridamole because of their rapid onset and termination of action. Since methylxanthines (i.e., caffeine and theophylline) block adenosine binding and can interfere with the vasodilatory effects of these agents, foods and beverages containing caffeine should not be ingested during the 24 hours before their administration.

During a vasodilator stress test, the patient normally manifests a modest increase in heart rate, a fall in blood pressure, and no or minimal electrocardiographic changes. Chest pain, shortness of breath, flushing, and dizziness occur commonly during vasodilator administration. As a result, the symptomatic, hemodynamic, and electrocardiographic responses to vasodilator administration do not provide insight into the presence or absence of CAD.

Dipyridamole is administered IV at 0.142 mg/kg/min for 4 minutes, with the maximal effect occurring 3 to 4 minutes after the infusion has ended. Adenosine is administered IV at 0.140 mg/kg/min for 6 minutes, with the maximum effect occurring 30 seconds after the infusion is completed. Regadenoson has a 2- to 3-minute biologic half-life—as compared with adenosine's 30-second half-life—so it is administered as a 0.4 mg IV bolus (given in less than 10 seconds) followed immediately by a saline flush. At the end of the dipyridamole infusion or regadenoson injection or 3 minutes after initiation of adenosine infusion, Tl is administered, after which nuclear imaging follows immediately and can be repeated 24 hours later to distinguish scarred from hibernating myocardium.

Since these agents may induce severe bronchospasm in subjects with a history of asthma, they should not be administered to such individuals. With adenosine and regadenoson, advanced AV block may occur. Fortunately, severe side effects are rare, occurring in only 1 in 10,000 patients receiving these agents, and they usually are reversed with IV aminophylline, 75 to 125 mg.

In the patient referred for stress testing to assess the presence of CAD, pharmacologic stress is indicated for those unable or with a contraindication to exercise. This includes patients with (a) a chronic debilitating illness, such as pulmonary, liver, or kidney disease; (b) older age and decreased functional capacity; (c) limited exercise capacity due to injury, arthritis, orthopedic problems, neurologic disorders, myopathic diseases, or peripheral vascular disease; (d) an acute coronary syndrome; (e) postoperative state; and (f) β-blocker or other negative chronotropic agents that interfere with the subject's ability to achieve an adequate increase in heart rate in response to exercise.

Pharmacologic stress testing has a similar sensitivity and specificity to exercise stress testing (Fig. 1-18). In an analysis of 17 studies of almost 2,000 patients, pharmacologic stress testing had a sensitivity of 89% and a specificity of 75% for detecting ischemic heart disease.[43] As with routine stress testing, the sensitivity and specificity are affected by the prevalence and pretest likelihood of CAD in the population being studied.

Dobutamine Stress Testing The patient who is not a candidate for vasodilator stress testing (because of a history of bronchospasm, advanced AV block, or recent caffeine ingestion) or does not desire infusion of a radiopharmaceutical may undergo a dobutamine stress test with echocardiographic imaging. Dobutamine, a synthetic catecholamine, is an inotropic agent that increases heart rate and myocardial contractility, thereby increasing myocardial oxygen demands. In regions of the heart where myocardial oxygen supply is insufficient to meet the increased demands (because of a flow-limiting stenosis in the coronary artery supplying that region), ischemia develops and causes regional abnormalities in contraction that may be observed with echocardiography.

When used for stress testing, dobutamine is infused at 5 mcg/kg/min for 3 minutes, followed by infusions of 10, 20, 30,

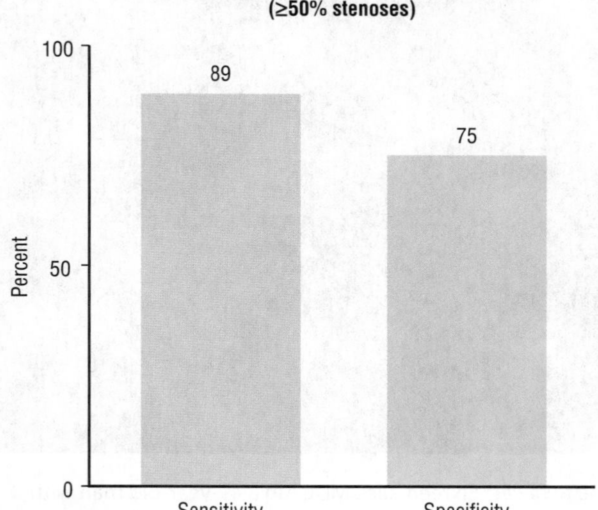

FIGURE 1-18 Detection of CAD by vasodilator SPECT (stenoses of 50% or greater). Sensitivity and specificity for detection of coronary artery disease (CAD) by vasodilator stress. The definition of a significant lesion was 50% or greater stenosis by coronary angiography. These data represent a pooled analysis from the literature.[43] (SPECT, single-photon emission computed tomography.)

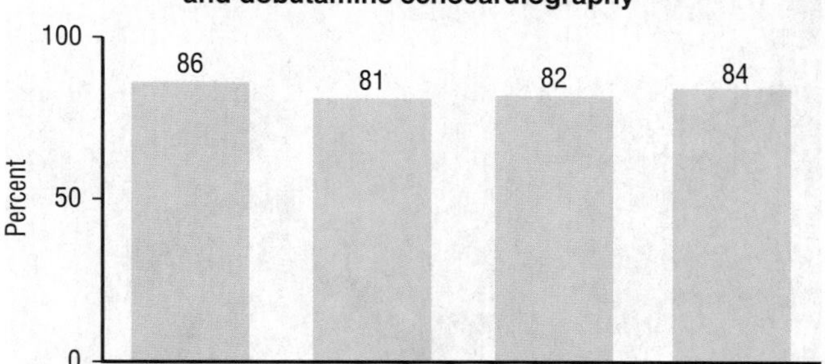

FIGURE 1-19 Sensitivity and specificity for exercise and dobutamine echocardiography. Note a slightly higher sensitivity for exercise echo compared with dobutamine echo.[47]

and 40 mcg/kg/min each at 3 minutes until a target heart rate is achieved. To achieve a further increase in myocardial oxygen demands, atropine (0.5 to 1 mg) may be injected to augment the dobutamine-induced increase in heart rate, and handgrip exercise may be performed concomitantly to achieve an increase in blood pressure. The ECG and blood pressure are monitored throughout the test, and echocardiographic images are obtained during the last minute of each dobutamine dose infusion and during recovery. For the patient with suboptimal echocardiographic images, dobutamine stress testing may be combined with radionuclide perfusion imaging, in which case Tl is injected 2 to 3 minutes before completion of the dobutamine infusion.

Since β-blocker and calcium channel blocker therapy may interfere with the heart rate response to dobutamine, it is recommended that they be discontinued before the test. Dobutamine stress testing is relatively well tolerated, with ventricular irritability occurring rarely (0.05%). The dobutamine infusion is discontinued with the appearance of severe chest pain, extensive new wall motion abnormalities, ST segment changes suggestive of severe ischemia, tachyarrhythmias, or a symptomatic fall in systemic arterial pressure. β-Blockers can be used to reverse most adverse effects if they persist. Dobutamine stress testing is contraindicated in patients with aortic stenosis, uncontrolled hypertension, and severe ventricular arrhythmias.

A review of 37 studies of 3,280 patients reported that dobutamine stress testing had a sensitivity of 82% and a specificity of 84% for detecting CAD (Fig. 1-19). The sensitivity was highest in subjects with three-vessel CAD (92%).[47]

Computed Tomography

Computed tomographic (CT) scanning is becoming increasingly popular as a primary screening procedure in the evaluation of individuals with suspected or known CVD, since it provides similar information as other diagnostic modalities, such as echocardiography and catheterization, yet it is less invasive than the latter.[48–50] In recent years, technologic advances have enhanced CT's definition and spatial resolution of cardiac structures, such as coronary arteries, valves, pericardium, and cardiac masses. In addition, CT provides an accurate measurement of chamber volumes and sizes as well as wall thickness.

CT scanners produce images by rotating an x-ray beam around a circular gantry (e.g., opening), through which the patient advances on a moving couch. Two types of CT scanners are used for cardiac imaging: electron beam computed tomography (EBCT) and mechanical CT.[50] With EBCT, the electron x-ray tube remains stationary, and the electron beam is swept electronically around the patient. With mechanical or conventional CT, the x-ray tube itself rotates around the patient, and the use of multirow detector system rays (i.e., multislice CT) allows acquisition of up to 320 simultaneous images, each 0.5 mm in thickness. With either type of CT, the image acquisition is gated to the ECG to minimize radiation exposure, and cardiac images are obtained at end inspiration (i.e., during a breath hold) to minimize artifact caused by cardiac motion.

Since EBCT has no moving parts, it requires a shorter image acquisition time and exposes the patient to less radiation when compared with conventional CT (less than 1 rad [10 mGy] vs. 15 rad [150 mGy], respectively). With EBCT, image resolution is sufficient to assess global and regional ventricular function and coronary anatomy, but it is insufficient to provide an accurate assessment of the presence and severity of CAD. However, it can reliably detect the presence and extent of coronary arterial calcification, which is expressed as a coronary artery calcium (CAC) score in Agatston units (Fig. 1-20). Although the presence of coronary arterial calcification correlates with the total atherosclerotic plaque burden in epicardial coronary arteries, it does not predict the presence or location of flow-limiting (greater than 50% luminal diameter narrowing) coronary arterial stenoses, nor does the lack of coronary arterial calcium exclude the presence of atherosclerotic plaque.[48–50]

The distribution of calcification scores in populations of individuals without known heart disease has been studied extensively. These studies have shown that the amount of coronary arterial calcification increases with age, and men typically develop calcification 10 to 15 years earlier than women.[50] Coronary arterial calcification is detectable in the majority of asymptomatic men over 55 years of age and women over 65 years of age. The person who undergoes coronary calcium screening with EBCT receives a score in Agatston units as well as a calcium score percentile, with which his/her score is compared with a population of subjects of similar age and gender.

Unlike EBCT, multislice CT has sufficient resolution to visualize the coronary arteries (Fig. 1-21). To accomplish this, radiographic

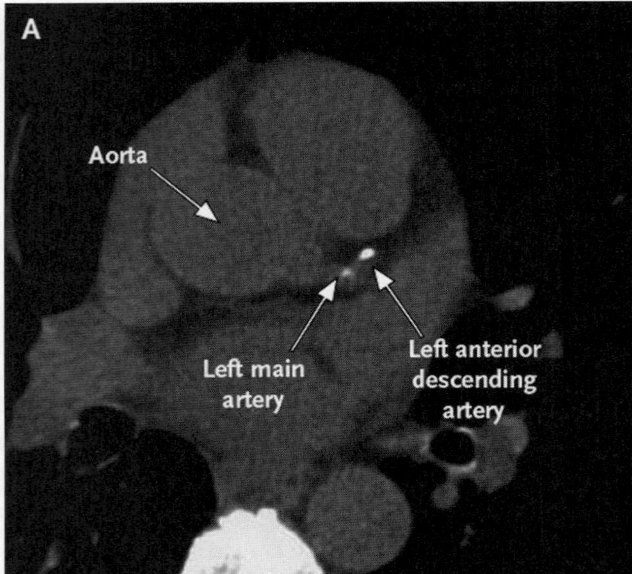

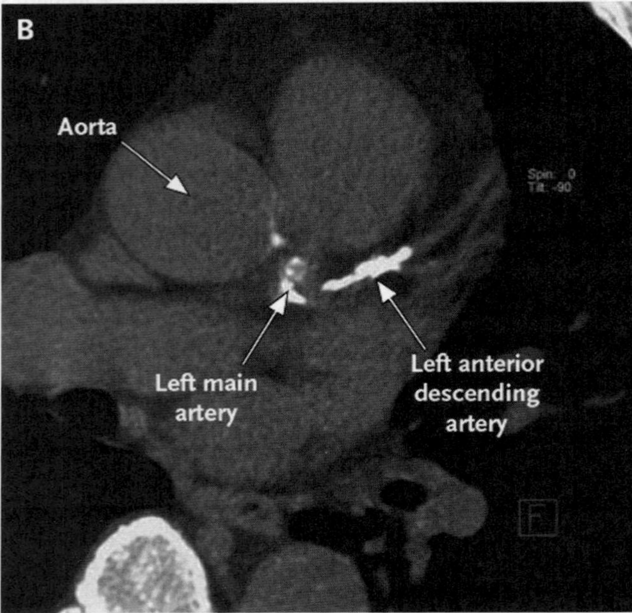

FIGURE 1-20 CT scans of the left coronary artery in two asymptomatic men. Two asymptomatic men, 51 and 81 years of age, underwent coronary artery calcium (CAC) imaging with multidetector CT. There is calcification of the left main and proximal left anterior descending coronary arteries in both the younger patient (*A*) and the older patient (*B*). The CAC score for the younger man, although relatively low at 80, places him in the 85th percentile for severity of CAC for men in his age group. The older man's CAC score is higher, at 1,054, but the severity of his CAC relative to that for men in his age group is lower—in the 70th percentile. *(From Bonow RO. Should coronary calcium screening be used in cardiovascular prevention strategies? N Engl J Med 2009;361:990–997. Copyright © 2009 Massachusetts Medical Society. All rights reserved.)*

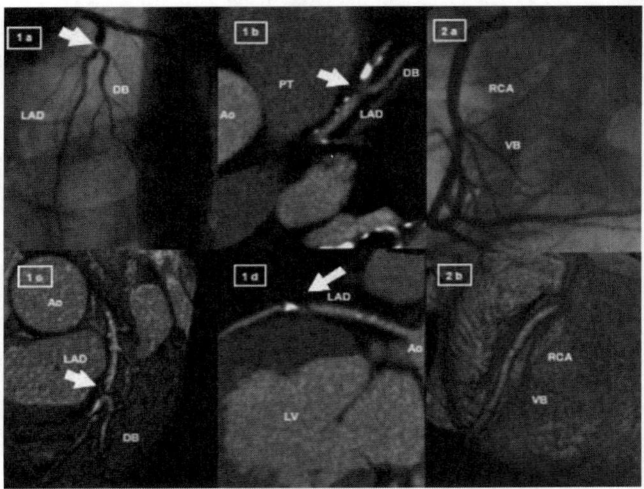

FIGURE 1-21 Sixteen-slice MDCT in a 49-year-old man with chest pain. (*1a*) Coronary angiography showing a severe stenosis in the left anterior descending (LAD) artery. (*1b*) MDCT axial slice visualizing high-grade stenosis (arrow) and calcification. (*1c*) MDCT three-dimensional volume-rendering technique showing the LAD stenosis. (*1d*) MDCT curved multiplanar reconstruction of the LAD. (*2a*) Coronary angiography of the right coronary artery (RCA), which is normal. (*2b*) MDCT volume-rendering technique of RCA. (Ao, aorta; DB, diagonal branch; LV, left ventricle; MDCT, multidetector computed tomography; PT, pulmonary trunk; VB, ventricular branch.) *(Reproduced with permission from Berman DS, Hachamovitch R, Shaw LJ, et al. Roles of nuclear cardiology, cardiac computed tomography, and cardiac magnetic resonance: Assessment of patients with suspected coronary artery disease. J Nucl Med 2006;47:74–82.)*

contrast material is administered IV, and a β-blocker is given to slow the heart rate to less than 70 beats/min in order to minimize motion artifact. Compared with conventional coronary angiography, cardiac CT has a sensitivity of 85%, a specificity of 90%, a positive predictive value of 91%, and a negative predictive value of 83% for detecting or excluding a coronary arterial stenosis of 50% or more luminal diameter narrowing.[51] It has limited diagnostic utility in patients with extensive coronary arterial calcification or a rapid heart rate, due to artifacts caused by high-density calcified coronary arterial stenoses or cardiac motion, respectively. Vessels with a luminal diameter less than 1.5 mm cannot be assessed reliably with cardiac CT, since the resolution is insufficient. Recent advances in cardiac CT technology have enabled the assessment of the physiologic significance of coronary arterial stenoses using myocardial CT perfusion imaging.[52]

Independent of its use in assessing coronary arteries, cardiac CT often is used in the subject with suspected aortic dissection, in whom its accuracy in detecting dissection is greater than 90%. In the patient with possible constrictive pericarditis, the pericardium can be evaluated for thickening and calcification. In the patient with a possible cardiac mass, CT scanning allows one to assess the size and location of the mass, and tissue density differentiation may aid in its characterization. Cardiac CT can be used to calculate left ventricular volumes, ejection fraction, and mass, and these measurements obtained with CT scanning are superior in accuracy and reproducibility to those obtained with echocardiography or angiography. CT scans allow visualization of congenital heart defects. Although MRI may provide similar information without exposing the patient to ionizing radiation, many patients have contraindications to MRI (i.e., those with an implanted metallic device). In such patients, cardiac CT is an alternative method for visualizing cardiac anatomy.

Positron Emission Tomography

Positron emission tomography (PET) is a relatively new modality for diagnostic imaging in patients with suspected or known CVD. Among imaging techniques, it is unique in its ability (a) to provide

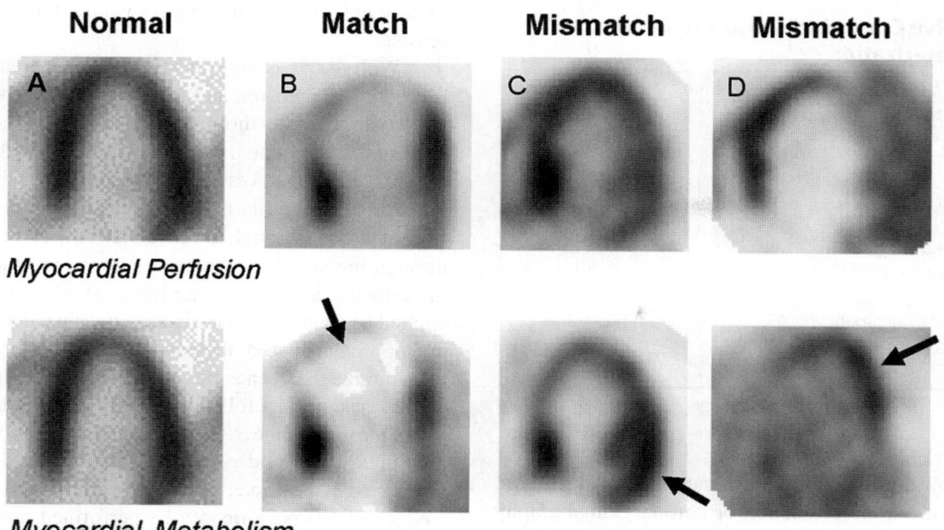

FIGURE 1-22 Patterns of myocardial perfusion (*upper panel*) and metabolism (with ^{18}F-FDG; *lower panel*). *A.* Normal myocardial perfusion and metabolism. *B.* Severely reduced myocardial perfusion in the anterior wall associated with a concordant reduction in ^{18}F-FDG uptake (arrow), corresponding to a match. *C.* Mildly reduced perfusion in the lateral and posterior lateral wall associated with a segmental increase in glucose metabolism (mismatch). *D.* Severely reduced myocardial perfusion in the lateral wall with a segmental increase in ^{18}F-FDG uptake (arrow), reflecting a perfusion metabolism mismatch. *(From Schelbert HR. Positron emission tomography for the noninvasive study and quantitation of myocardial blood flow and metabolism in cardiovascular disease. In: Fuster V, O'Rourke RA, Walsh RA, Poole-Wilson P, eds. Hurst's the Heart, 12th ed. New York: McGraw-Hill, 2004:675.)*

quantitative imaging with high temporal resolution; (b) to image a large number of physiologically active radiotracers; and (c) to apply tracer kinetic principles so that in vivo imaging can be performed. With PET, myocardial metabolic activity, perfusion, and viability can be assessed.[42,43] Using appropriate positron-emitting biologically active tracers, PET can measure regional myocardial uptake of exogenous glucose and fatty acids, quantitate free fatty acid metabolism, ascertain myocardial energy substrates, and evaluate myocardial chemoreceptor sites.

In the fasting state (i.e., low serum glucose and insulin concentrations), fatty acids are the preferred energy source of the myocardium. Following the ingestion of carbohydrate, serum glucose and insulin concentrations increase, and glucose becomes the preferred myocardial fuel. Glucose also is the major myocardial fuel during ischemia, since ischemia impairs mitochondrial fatty acid oxidation. Using positron-emitting isotopes, such as oxygen-15 (^{15}O-oxygen), carbon-11 (^{11}C-palmitate or ^{11}C acetate), and fluoride-18 (^{18}F-fluorodeoxyglucose), myocardial oxygen consumption and substrate utilization can be measured, from which ischemic and nonischemic regions of the heart can be identified.[42] PET usually is used in conjunction with pharmacologic stress testing to provoke ischemia, with images obtained before and after stress.

Tracers such as rubidium-82 (^{82}Rb) and nitrogen-13 (^{13}N) are retained in the myocardium in proportion to blood flow. PET imaging with these agents allows one to measure myocardial blood flow at rest and during pharmacologically induced hyperemia. Thus, PET can be used to assess the physiologic significance of coronary arterial stenoses, which is useful when attempting to determine if a luminal diameter narrowing of intermediate severity (50% to 70%) is causing ischemia.

In the patient with noncontractile myocardium, PET is considered to be the "gold standard" technique for distinguishing infarcted myocardium from chronically ischemic, metabolically active myocardium that has the potential to regain function if perfusion is restored (so-called "hibernating myocardium").[42] Myocardial infarction and ischemia can be distinguished by analysis of PET images of the glucose analogue ^{8}F-fluorodeoxyglucose (FDG), which is injected after glucose administration, and the perfusion tracer ^{13}N-ammonia. Regions that show a concordant reduction in myocardial blood flow and FDG uptake ("flow–metabolism match") are considered to be irreversibly injured, whereas regions in which FDG uptake is relatively preserved or increased despite a perfusion defect ("flow–metabolism mismatch") are considered to be ischemic (Fig. 1-22). This approach more accurately predicts recovery of regional function after revascularization than does SPECT imaging. The magnitude of improvement in heart failure symptoms after revascularization in patients with left ventricular dysfunction correlates with the preoperative extent of FDG "mismatch."[53]

The main strengths of PET compared with SPECT are its superior spatial resolution and ability to assess myocardial viability accurately.[42,43] The limited availability of PET scanners and the need for a cyclotron on site are its main limitations.

Cardiac Catheterization and Angiography

9 Cardiac catheterization plays a pivotal role in the evaluation of patients with suspected or known cardiac disease; in addition, it has become an important therapeutic alternative to cardiac surgery in many patients who require nonmedical therapy.

Indications

Diagnostic cardiac catheterization is appropriate under several conditions. First, it is often performed to confirm or to exclude the presence of a cardiac condition that is suspected from the patient's history, physical examination, or noninvasive evaluation. In such a circumstance, it allows an assessment of the presence and severity of cardiac disease. For example, in a subject with progressive angina pectoris or a positive exercise stress test, coronary angiography allows the physician to visualize the coronary arteries sufficiently to assess the presence and extent of CAD. Second, catheterization is often helpful in the patient with a confusing or difficult clinical

TABLE 1-7 Relative Contraindications to Cardiac Catheterization

Decompensated heart failure (e.g., pulmonary edema)
Uncontrolled ventricular irritability
Uncontrolled systemic arterial hypertension
Acute or severe renal insufficiency
Difficulty with vascular access
Electrolyte imbalance (i.e., hypokalemia or hyperkalemia)
Digitalis intoxication
Active infection or febrile illness
Uncorrected bleeding diathesis
Severe anemia
Active bleeding from internal organ
Severe allergy to radiographic contrast material
Mental incompetence

presentation in whom the noninvasive evaluation is inconclusive. For instance, a hemodynamic evaluation or coronary angiography may be useful in the patient with unexplained dyspnea. Third, data obtained at catheterization may provide prognostic information that is helpful in guiding therapy. Such is the case, for example, in the patient with cardiomyopathy, in whom the hemodynamic data obtained at catheterization are used to guide medical therapy and to assess the need for and timing of cardiac transplantation.

Contraindications

The only absolute contraindication to catheterization is the refusal of a mentally competent subject to provide informed consent. Relative contraindications (Table 1-7) mostly involve conditions in which the risks of the procedure are increased or the information obtained from it is potentially unreliable. In these circumstances, the benefits of having the data that are obtained at catheterization must be weighed against the procedure's increased risks. Catheterization usually is not performed in the patient who refuses therapy for the condition for which diagnostic catheterization is recommended.

Complications

Because catheterization is an invasive procedure, its performance is associated with major and minor risks. The incidence of a major complication (death, myocardial infarction, or cerebrovascular accident) during or within 24 hours of diagnostic catheterization is 0.2% to 0.3%. Deaths, which occur in 0.1% to 0.2% of patients, may be caused by perforation of the heart or great vessels, cardiac arrhythmias, acute myocardial infarction (AMI), or anaphylaxis to radiographic contrast material.

Numerous minor complications may cause morbidity but exert no effect on mortality. Local vascular complications occur in 0.5% to 1.5% of patients. The injection of radiographic contrast material occasionally is associated with allergic reactions of varying severity, and a rare individual has anaphylaxis. Of patients with a known allergy to contrast material, only about 15% have an adverse reaction with its repeat administration, and most of these reactions are minor (e.g., urticaria, nausea, vomiting). In most patients with a previous allergic reaction to radiographic contrast material, angiography can be performed safely, but premedication with glucocorticosteroids and antihistamines and the use of a different contrast material usually are recommended. Use of excessive quantities of radiographic contrast material may result in renal insufficiency, particularly in patients with preexisting renal dysfunction and diabetes mellitus.

Techniques

Cardiac catheterization is generally performed with the patient in the fasting state and mildly sedated. Anticoagulants are discontinued before the procedure (warfarin for several days, heparin for 4 to 6 hours). Cardiac catheterization requires vascular access, which is usually obtained percutaneously via the femoral, brachial, or radial vessels.

With the *percutaneous approach*, the area overlying the vessel is aseptically prepared and locally anesthetized. The vessel is punctured with a needle, through which a flexible metal wire is advanced into the vessel's lumen, over which a sheath with a sideport extension is advanced into the vessel. The sideport extension allows continuous monitoring of arterial pressure (through an arterial sheath) or infusion of fluids (through a venous sheath) as catheters are advanced through the sheath to the heart. When the procedure is completed, the catheters and sheaths are removed, after which local pressure is applied or a closure device is used to achieve hemostasis. If the femoral approach is used, the patient remains at bedrest for 2 to 8 hours to minimize the chance of hemorrhage. With the radial and brachial approaches, bedrest following sheath removal is not necessary.

During routine right heart catheterization, measurements of pressures and blood oxygen saturations in the vena cavae, right atrium, right ventricle, pulmonary artery, and pulmonary capillary wedge (PCW) position can be performed, and cardiac output can be quantified (Table 1-8 lists normal values). The measurement of right-sided pressures helps the physician to evaluate the severity of tricuspid or pulmonic stenosis, to assess the presence and severity of pulmonary hypertension, and to calculate pulmonary vascular resistance. In the absence of pulmonary vein stenosis (a rare condition), the PCW pressure accurately reflects the left atrial pressure. Occasionally angiography is performed to define right-sided anatomic abnormalities or to evaluate the severity of right-sided valvular regurgitation.

With left heart catheterization, mitral and aortic valvular function, left ventricular pressures and function, systemic vascular resistance, and coronary arterial anatomy can be assessed. To perform

TABLE 1-8 Normal Hemodynamic Values

Measurement	Value
Flows	
Cardiac index (L/min/m²)	2.6–4.2
Stroke volume index (mL/m²)	35–55
Pressures (mm Hg)	
Aorta/systemic artery	
Peak systolic/end-diastolic	100–140/60–90
Mean	70–105
Left ventricle	
Peak systolic/end-diastolic	100–140/3–12
Left atrium (PCW)	
Mean	1–10
a wave	3–15
v wave	3–15
Pulmonary artery	
Peak systolic/end-diastolic	16–30/4–12
Mean	10–16
Right ventricle	
Peak systolic/end-diastolic	16–30/0–8
Right atrium	
Mean	0–8
a wave	2–10
v wave	2–10
Resistances	
Systemic vascular resistance	
Wood units	10–20
dyne/s/cm⁵	770–1,500
Pulmonary vascular resistance	
Wood units	0.25–1.5
dyne/s/cm⁵	20–120
Oxygen consumption (mL/min/m²)	110–150
AV O_2 difference (mL/dL)	3–4.5

AV, arteriovenous; PCW, pulmonary capillary wedge.

angiography or to measure the pressure in the left ventricle, a catheter is usually advanced retrograde across the aortic valve.

Hemodynamic Measurements

Cardiac Output The blood flow measurement most often performed during catheterization is the quantitation of cardiac output. This variable allows an assessment of overall cardiovascular function, vascular resistances, valve orifice areas, and valvular regurgitation. In the catheterization laboratory, the three common methods of measuring cardiac output are the Fick principle, the indicator dilution technique, and angiography.

Fick Principle The Fick principle is based on the fact that when a substance is consumed by an organ, its concentration is the product of blood flow to the organ and the substance's arteriovenous difference across the organ. Using the lungs as the organ of interest and oxygen as the substance, one can calculate pulmonary blood flow (e.g., cardiac output) using the following formula:

$$\text{Cardiac output (L/min)} = \frac{\text{oxygen consumption (mL/min)}}{\text{arteriovenous oxygen difference (mL/L)}}$$

Oxygen consumption is measured by analyzing the patient's exhaled air, and the arteriovenous oxygen difference is calculated by measuring the oxygen content in a blood sample procured from the aorta and the pulmonary artery.

Dilution Method With indicator dilution, a known amount of indicator is injected as a bolus into the circulation and allowed to mix completely in the blood, after which its concentration is measured. A time–concentration curve is generated, and a minicomputer calculates the cardiac output from the area of the inscribed curve. The most widely used indicator for the measurement of cardiac output is cold solution. A balloon-tipped, flow-directed, polyvinyl chloride catheter (a so-called "Swan-Ganz catheter") with a thermistor at its tip and an opening 25 to 30 cm proximal to the tip is inserted into a vein and advanced to the pulmonary artery, so that the proximal opening is located in the vena cavae or right atrium and the thermistor is in the pulmonary artery. A known amount of cold fluid is injected through the proximal port; it mixes completely in the right ventricle and causes a change in blood temperature, which is detected by the thermistor. The thermodilution method is relatively inexpensive and easy to perform, and does not require arterial sampling or blood withdrawal.

Angiographic Method From the left ventriculogram, the volume of blood ejected with each heartbeat (stroke volume) can be determined. It is then multiplied by the heart rate, yielding the angiographic cardiac output. The measurement of cardiac output by the angiographic method is potentially erroneous in patients with extensive segmental wall motion abnormalities or misshapen ventricles, in whom the determination of stroke volume may be inaccurate.

Pressures One of the most important functions of cardiac catheterization is to measure intracardiac pressures. Once a catheter is positioned in a cardiac chamber, it is connected through fluid-filled, stiff, plastic tubing to a pressure transducer, which transforms the pressure signal into an electrical signal that is recorded. During catheterization, pressures are usually measured directly from each of the cardiac chambers: right atrium, right ventricle, pulmonary artery, ascending aorta, and left ventricle. Because the left atrial pressure is transmitted to the pulmonary capillaries, it can be recorded "indirectly" as the pulmonary capillary "wedge" pressure. In addition to measuring pressures from each cardiac chamber, pressures from certain chambers are examined simultaneously to identify or to exclude a gradient between them indicative of valvular stenosis.

Resistances The resistance of a vascular bed is calculated by dividing the pressure gradient across the bed by the blood flow through it. Thus:

$$\begin{array}{c}\text{Systemic} \\ \text{vascular resistance}\end{array} = \frac{\begin{array}{c}\text{mean systemic arterial pressure} \\ -\text{ mean right atrial pressure}\end{array}}{\text{sytemic blood flow}}$$

and

$$\begin{array}{c}\text{Pulmonary} \\ \text{vascular resistance}\end{array} = \frac{\begin{array}{c}\text{mean pulmonary arterial pressure} \\ -\text{ mean left atrial pressure}\end{array}}{\text{pulmonary blood flow}}$$

Because a properly obtained PCW pressure is similar to left atrial pressure, it can be substituted for it in the above equation. These formulae express resistances in arbitrary resistance units. Most often, these values are multiplied by 80 to express them in metric units of dyne/s/cm^5. Normal values are displayed in Table 1-8.

An elevated systemic vascular resistance is often present in the patient with systemic arterial hypertension. It may also be observed in patients with a reduced forward cardiac output and compensatory arteriolar vasoconstriction (often seen in patients with heart failure). Conversely, systemic vascular resistance may be reduced in patients with arteriolar vasodilation (due, e.g., to sepsis) or those with an increased cardiac output (due, e.g., to an arteriovenous fistula, severe anemia, fever, or thyrotoxicosis). An elevated pulmonary vascular resistance often is observed in patients with primary lung disease, pulmonary vascular disease, and a greatly elevated pulmonary venous pressure resulting from left-sided myocardial or valvular dysfunction.

Angiography

During angiography, radiographic contrast material is injected into the cardiovascular structure of interest, and the images are digitally recorded and stored on a computer-accessible medium (i.e., CD-ROM, DVD, external memory drives, etc.). The resultant angiogram permits the study of cardiac structures in real time, in slow motion, or by single frame.

Left Ventriculography

With angiography of the left ventricle, global and segmental left ventricular function, left ventricular volumes and ejection fraction, and the presence and severity of mitral regurgitation can be assessed. A segment of the left ventricular wall with reduced systolic motion is said to be hypokinetic, a segment that does not move is akinetic, and a segment that moves paradoxically during systole is dyskinetic.

Coronary Angiography

Selective coronary angiography is usually performed to determine the presence and severity of fixed, atherosclerotic CAD and to guide subsequent percutaneous (e.g., angioplasty with or without stent placement) or surgical (e.g., bypass grafting) therapy. Under fluoroscopic guidance, the ostia of the native right and left coronary arteries or bypass grafts are engaged selectively with a catheter, and radiographic contrast material is injected manually during digital image recording. Because atherosclerotic coronary arterial stenoses are often eccentric and the coronary vessels often overlap one another, images are obtained in multiple obliquities, thereby ensuring a complete angiographic assessment of each arterial segment.

Coronary angiography provides radiographic images of the coronary lumina but does not visualize the actual arterial walls. A stenosis is present when a discrete reduction in luminal diameter is noted, and its severity is assessed by comparing it with presumably normal adjacent segments of the same artery. Thus, if atherosclerosis is diffuse and involves the entire artery, angiography may lead to an underestimation of the severity of disease.

Aortography

Aortography is accomplished with the rapid injection of radiographic contrast material into the aorta. With proximal aortography, the severity of aortic valve regurgitation, the location of saphenous vein bypass grafts, and the anatomy of the proximal aorta and its branches can be assessed. Distal aortography usually is performed to assess the presence of vascular abnormalities, such as aneurysm, dissection, intraluminal thrombus, or branch vessel stenosis.

Valvular Stenosis or Regurgitation

In patients with valvular stenosis, the effective valve orifice area can be calculated with data obtained during catheterization using principles of standard fluid dynamics. The pressures on either side of a stenotic valve are recorded simultaneously, and the flow across it is measured, after which the valve area is calculated.

The presence and severity of valvular regurgitation may be evaluated qualitatively by observing the amount of radiographic contrast material that regurgitates in a retrograde direction across the valve. The magnitude of regurgitation is estimated as trivial (1+), mild (2+), moderate (3+), or severe (4+).

Endomyocardial Biopsy

Through a long sheath positioned across the tricuspid valve, a bioptome can be advanced to obtain small pieces (1 to 2 mm in diameter) of myocardial tissue from the right ventricular side of the interventricular septum. Endomyocardial biopsy is used most often to detect transplant rejection and to monitor immunosuppressive therapy in survivors of cardiac transplantation. Less commonly, it is undertaken in the patient with suspected infiltrative cardiomyopathy or active inflammation of the heart (e.g., myocarditis). In experienced hands, complications are uncommon: cardiac perforation occurs in only 0.3% to 0.5%, and the procedure-related mortality is only 0.05%.

Fractional Flow Reserve

Although coronary angiography can identify the presence of a coronary arterial stenosis, it does not provide information regarding its functional significance (i.e., whether it potentially may cause myocardial ischemia). The measurement of fractional flow reserve (FFR) is performed to assess the physiologic significance of a stenosis.[54] With this technique, the intraluminal pressure is measured proximal and distal to the stenosis during maximal blood flow (i.e., hyperemia). FFR is defined as the mean pressure distal to the stenosis relative to the pressure proximal to the stenosis. For example, an FFR of 0.50 means that a 50% drop in pressure across the stenosis was noted.

During coronary angiography, a catheter is inserted into the ostia of the coronary artery, through which a wire with a small sensor transducer positioned at its tip is advanced past the stenosis. The mean pressure distal to the stenosis is compared with the mean pressure proximal to it (measured through the catheter) both at rest and after hyperemia (which is induced by injecting a vasodilator, such as adenosine or papaverine). FFR is calculated as the ratio of mean arterial pressure distal to the stenosis and mean aortic pressure under conditions of maximal myocardial hyperemia (Fig. 1-23). An FFR of

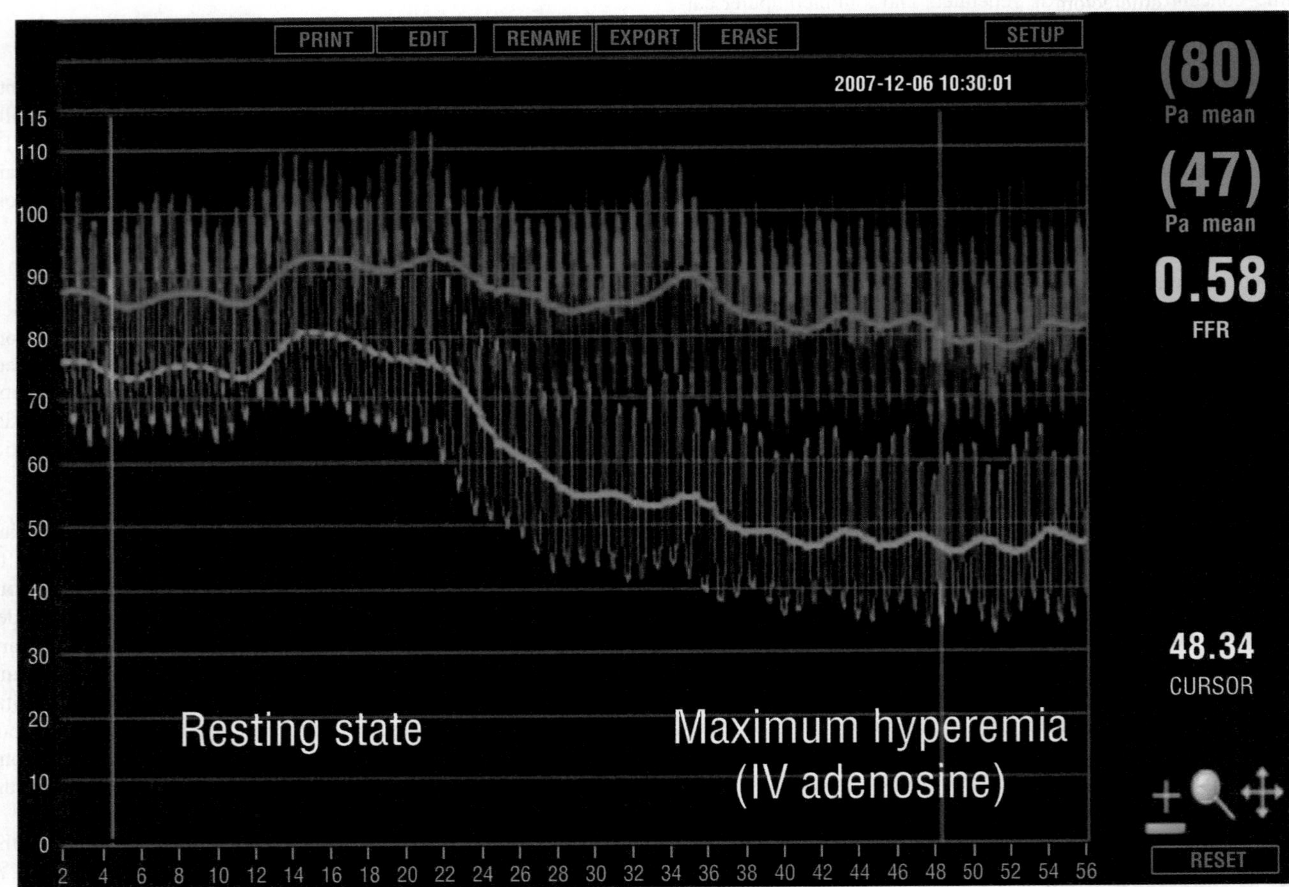

FIGURE 1-23 Simultaneous phasic and mean aortic pressure (Pa, shown in red) and distal coronary arterial pressure (Pd, shown in green) recordings at rest and during maximal hyperemia induced by an IV infusion of adenosine. Fractional flow reserve (FFR) is calculated as the ratio of mean Pd and Pa during maximal hyperemia, which in this case is 47/80 or 0.58. *(Reproduced with permission from Pijls NHJ, Sels JE. Functional measurement of coronary stenosis. J Am Coll Cardiol 2012;59:1045–1057.)*

1 is normal. An FFR below 0.75 to 0.80 is associated with myocardial ischemia. At this time, it is uncertain if coronary revascularization should be recommended or performed based on an abnormal FFR alone (in the absence of symptoms or other well-established indications).

Clinical **Controversy. . .**

In the patient with minimal or no symptoms, it is unknown if the presence of myocardial ischemia is an indication for coronary revascularization.

Intravascular Ultrasound

Intravascular ultrasound (IVUS) employs a small catheter-mounted ultrasound transducer to provide detailed images of the coronary arterial wall and lumen. In contrast to coronary angiography, which does not visualize the actual arterial wall, IVUS provides quantitative information from within the vessel regarding vessel diameter, circumference, luminal diameter, plaque volume, and percent narrowing. Qualitative information regarding the amount of plaque stenosis, plaque composition (e.g., calcific, fibrous, or fatty plaque), and the presence of plaque versus thrombus, thrombus versus tumor, and aneurysm and hematoma can be provided by IVUS. IVUS is used as a therapeutic adjunct to percutaneous coronary intervention (PCI), atherectomy, stent or graft placement, and fibrinolysis, although its routine use with these modalities may not be justified. These combination procedures may be monitored in real time as the procedure (e.g., atherectomy) is being performed. In recent studies, IVUS has been helpful in the evaluation of the progression or regression of atherosclerosis. Current trials are testing medications for atherosclerosis regression and changes in plaque morphology.

Intravascular optical coherence tomography provides high-resolution, cross-sectional images of tissue with an axial resolution of 10 μm and a lateral resolution of 20 μm. Optical coherence tomographic images of human coronary atherosclerotic plaques are much more structurally detailed than those obtained with IVUS. Clinically, the detection of thin fibrous caps (vulnerable atheromas) (less than 65 μm) is below the resolution of the current 40-MHz IVUS (100 to 200 μm). A summary of testing modalities used in cardiovascular medicine is provided in Appendices 1-1 and 1-2.

ABBREVIATIONS

ABI	ankle-brachial index
ACC	American College of Cardiology
AECG	ambulatory electrocardiography
AHA	American Heart Association
AMI	acute myocardial infarction
AV	atrioventricular
beats/min	beats per minute
BNP	B-type natriuretic protein
CAC	coronary artery calcium
CAD	coronary artery disease
CK-MB	creatine kinase-MB
CRP	C-reactive protein
CT	computed tomography
cTn	cardiac troponin
CTR	cardiothoracic ratio
CVD	cardiovascular disease
2D	two-dimensional
3D	three-dimensional
EBCT	electron beam computed tomography
ECG	electrocardiogram
FDG	fluorodeoxyglucose
FFR	fractional flow reserve
hs-CRP	high-sensitivity C-reactive protein
IVUS	intravascular ultrasound
JVP	jugular venous pressure
MET	metabolic equivalent
MRI	magnetic resonance imaging
MUGA	multigated acquisition
NT-proBNP	N-terminal pro-brain-type natriuretic protein
NYHA	New York Heart Association
PAD	peripheral arterial disease
PCI	percutaneous coronary intervention
PCW	pulmonary capillary wedge
PET	positron emission tomography
QTc	rate-related ("corrected") QT interval
S_1	first heart sound
S_2	second heart sound
S_3	third heart sound
S_4	fourth heart sound
SA	sinoatrial
SAECG	signal-averaged electrocardiography
SPECT	single-photon emission computed tomography
Tc	technetium
Tc-MIBI	methoxy-isobutyl isonitrile
Tc-PYP	technetium pyrophosphate
Tl	thallium
Tn	troponin
TEE	transesophageal echocardiography
TTE	transthoracic echocardiography

REFERENCES

1. Roger VL, Go AS, Lloyd Jones DM, et al. Heart disease and stroke statistics—2012 update. Circulation 2012;125: e2–e220.
2. Grenon SM, Gagnon J, Hsian Y. Ankle-brachial index for assessment of peripheral arterial disease. N Engl J Med 2009;361:e40.
3. Tang WHW, Francis GS, Morrow DA, et al. National Academy of Clinical Biochemistry laboratory medicine practice guidelines: Clinical utilization of cardiac biomarker testing in heart failure. Circulation 2007;116:e99–e109.
4. van Kimmeade RRJ, Januzzi JL. Emerging biomarkers in heart failure. Clin Chem 2012;58:127–138.
5. Morrow DA, Cannon CP, Jesse RL, et al. National Academy of Clinical Biochemistry laboratory medicine practice guidelines: Clinical characteristics and utilization of biochemical markers in acute coronary syndromes. Circulation 2007;115:e356–e375.
6. Twerenbold R Jaffe A, Reichlin T, et al. High-sensitive troponin T measurements: What do we gain and what are the challenges? Eur Heart J 2012;33:579–586.
7. Jneid H, Anderson JL, Wright RS, et al. 2012 ACCF/AHA focused update of the guideline for the management of patients with unstable angina/non–ST-elevation myocardial infarction (updating the 2007 guideline and replacing the 2011 focused update): A report of the American College of Cardiology Foundation/American Heart Association Task Force on Practice Guidelines. Circulation 2012;126: 875–910.
8. Hillis LD, Lange RA. Optimal management of acute coronary syndromes. N Engl J Med 2009;360:2237–2240.
9. Musunuru K, Kral BG, Blumenthal RS, et al. The use of high-sensitivity assays for C-reactive protein in clinical practice. Nat Clin Pract Cardiovasc Med 2008;5:621–635.

10. Schunkert H, Samani NJ. Elevated C-reactive protein in atherosclerosis—Chicken or egg? N Engl J Med 2008;359:1953–1955.
11. Zacho J, Tybjaerg-Hansen A, Jensen JS, Grande P, Sillesen H, Nordestgaard BG. Genetically elevated C-reactive protein and ischemic vascular disease. N Engl J Med 2008;359:1897–1908.
12. Greenland P, Alpert JS, Beller GA, et al. 2010 ACCF/AHA guideline for assessment of cardiovascular risk in asymptomatic adults: A report of the American College of Cardiology Foundation/American Heart Association Task Force on Practice Guidelines. J Am Coll Cardiol 2010;56:e50–e103.
13. Helfand M, Buckley DI, Freeman M, et al. Emerging risk factors for coronary heart disease: A summary of systematic reviews conducted for the U.S. Preventive Services Task Force. Ann Intern Med 2009;151:496–507.
14. Ridker PM, Danielson E, Fonseca FA, et al. Rosuvastatin to prevent vascular events in men and women with elevated C-reactive protein. N Engl J Med 2008;359:2195–2207.
15. Prasad K. C-reactive protein (CRP)-lowering agents. Cardiovasc Drug Rev 2006;24:33–50.
16. Ridker PM, MacFadyen J, Libby P, Glynn RJ. Relation of baseline high-sensitivity C-reactive protein level to cardiovascular outcomes with rosuvastatin in the Justification for Use of statins in Prevention: An Intervention Trial Evaluating Rosuvastatin (JUPITER). Am J Cardiol 2010;106:204–209.
17. He LP, Tang XY, Ling WH, et al. Early C-reactive protein in the prediction of long-term outcomes after acute coronary syndromes: A meta-analysis of longitudinal studies. Heart 2010;96:339–346.
18. Caixeta A, Stone GW, Mehran R, et al. Predictive value of C-reactive protein on 30-day and 1-year mortality in acute coronary syndromes: An analysis from the ACUITY trial. J Thromb Thrombolysis 2011;31:154–164.
19. Hochholzer W, Morrow DA, Giugliano RP. Novel biomarkers in cardiovascular disease: Update 2010. Am Heart J 2010;160:583–594.
20. Maisel AS, Daniels LB. Breathing not properly 10 years later: What we have learned and what we still need to learn. J Am Coll Cardiol 2012;60:277–282.
21. Maisel A, Mueller C, Adams K Jr, et al. State of the art: Using natriuretic peptide levels in clinical practice. Eur J Heart Fail 2008;10:824–839.
22. Maisel AS, Krishnaswamy P, Nowak RM, et al. Rapid measurement of B-type natriuretic peptide in the emergency diagnosis of heart failure. N Engl J Med 2002;347:161–167.
23. Fonarow GC, Peacock WF, Phillips CO, Givertz MM, Lopatin M. Admission B-type natriuretic peptide levels and in-hospital mortality in acute decompensated heart failure. J Am Coll Cardiol 2007;49:1943–1950.
24. Felker GM, Petersen JW, Mark DB. Natriuretic peptides in the diagnosis and management of heart failure. CMAJ 2006;175:611–617.
25. McCullough PA, Peacock WF, O'Neil B, et al. An evidence-based algorithm for the use of B-type natriuretic testing in acute coronary syndromes. Rev Cardiovasc Med 2010;11:S51–S65.
26. James SK, Lindback J, Tilly J, et al. Troponin-T and N-terminal pro-B-type natriuretic peptide predict mortality benefit from coronary revascularization in acute coronary syndromes: A GUSTO-IV substudy. J Am Coll Cardiol 2006;48:1146–1154.
27. Morrow DA, de Lemos JA, Sabatine MS, et al. Evaluation of B-type natriuretic peptide for risk assessment in unstable angina/non-ST-elevation myocardial infarction: B-type natriuretic peptide and prognosis in TACTICS-TIMI 18. J Am Coll Cardiol 2003;41:1264–1272.
28. Goldberger JJ, Cain ME, Hohnloser SH, et al. American Heart Association/American College of Cardiology Foundation/Heart Rhythm Society scientific statement on noninvasive risk stratification techniques for identifying patients at risk for sudden cardiac death: A scientific statement from the American Heart Association Council on Clinical Cardiology Committee on Electrocardiography and Arrhythmias and Council on Epidemiology and Prevention. Circulation 2008;118:1497–1518.
29. Lauer M, Froelicher ES, Williams M, Kligfield P. Exercise testing in asymptomatic adults: A statement for professionals from the American Heart Association Council on Clinical Cardiology, Subcommittee on Exercise, Cardiac Rehabilitation, and Prevention. Circulation 2005;112:771–776.
30. Gibbons RJ, Balady GJ, Bricker JT, et al. ACC/AHA 2002 guideline update for exercise testing: Summary article: A report of the American College of Cardiology/American Heart Association Task Force on Practice Guidelines (Committee to Update the 1997 Exercise Testing Guidelines). Circulation 2002;106:1883–1892.
31. Marwick TH. The future of echocardiography. Eur J Echocardiogr 2009;10:594–601.
32. Ayres NA, Miller-Hance W, Fyfe DA, et al. Indications and guidelines for performance of transesophageal echocardiography in the patient with pediatric acquired or congenital heart disease: Report from the Task Force of the Pediatric Council of the American Society of Echocardiography. J Am Soc Echocardiogr 2005;18:91–98.
33. Baddour LM, Wilson WR, Bayer AS, et al. Infective endocarditis: Diagnosis, antimicrobial therapy, and management of complications: A statement for healthcare professionals from the Committee on Rheumatic Fever, Endocarditis, and Kawasaki Disease, Council on Cardiovascular Disease in the Young, and the Councils on Clinical Cardiology, Stroke, and Cardiovascular Surgery and Anesthesia, American Heart Association: Endorsed by the Infectious Diseases Society of America. Circulation 2005;111:e394–e434.
34. Baumgartner H, Hung J, Bermejo J, et al. Echocardiographic assessment of valve stenosis: EAE/ASE recommendations for clinical practice. J Am Soc Echocardiogr 2009;22:1–23 [quiz 101–102].
35. Douglas PS, Khandheria B, Stainback RF, et al. ACCF/ASE/ACEP/ASNC/SCAI/SCCT/SCMR 2007 appropriateness criteria for transthoracic and transesophageal echocardiography: A report of the American College of Cardiology Foundation Quality Strategic Directions Committee Appropriateness Criteria Working Group, American Society of Echocardiography, American College of Emergency Physicians, American Society of Nuclear Cardiology, Society for Cardiovascular Angiography and Interventions, Society of Cardiovascular Computed Tomography, and the Society for Cardiovascular Magnetic Resonance endorsed by the American College of Chest Physicians and the Society of Critical Care Medicine. J Am Coll Cardiol 2007;50:187–204.
36. Singer DE, Albers GW, Dalen JE, et al. Antithrombotic therapy in atrial fibrillation: American College of Chest Physicians evidence-based clinical practice guidelines (8th edition). Chest 2008;133:546S–592S.
37. Vahanian A, Baumgartner H, Bax J, et al. Guidelines on the management of valvular heart disease: The Task Force on

the Management of Valvular Heart Disease of the European Society of Cardiology. Eur Heart J 2007;28:230–268.
38. Warnes CA, Williams RG, Bashore TM, et al. ACC/AHA 2008 guidelines for the management of adults with congenital heart disease: A report of the American College of Cardiology/American Heart Association Task Force on Practice Guidelines (Writing Committee to Develop Guidelines on the Management of Adults with Congenital Heart Disease). Circulation 2008;118:e714–e833.
39. Hilberath JN, Oakes DA, Shernan SK. Safety of transesophageal echocardiography. J Am Soc Echocardiogr 2010;23:1115–1127.
40. Douglas PS, Khandheria B, Stainback RF, et al. ACCF/ASE/ACEP/AHA/ASNC/SCAI/SCCT/SCMR 2008 appropriateness criteria for stress echocardiography: A report of the American College of Cardiology Foundation Appropriateness Criteria Task Force, American Society of Echocardiography, American College of Emergency Physicians, American Heart Association, American Society of Nuclear Cardiology, Society for Cardiovascular Angiography and Interventions, Society of Cardiovascular Computed Tomography, and Society for Cardiovascular Magnetic Resonance: Endorsed by the Heart Rhythm Society and the Society of Critical Care Medicine. Circulation 2008;117:1478–1497.
41. Douglas PS, Garcia MJ, Haines DE, et al. ACCF/ASE/AHA/ASNC/HFSA/HRS/SCAI/SCCM/SCCT/SCMR 2011 appropriate use criteria for echocardiography. A report of the American College of Cardiology Foundation Appropriate Use Criteria Task Force, American Society of Echocardiography, American Heart Association, American Society of Nuclear Cardiology, Heart Failure Society of America, Heart Rhythm Society, Society for Cardiovascular Angiography and Interventions, Society of Critical Care Medicine, Society of Cardiovascular Computed Tomography, Society for Cardiovascular Magnetic Resonance American College of Chest Physicians. J Am Soc Echocardiogr 2011;24:229–267.
42. Camici PG, Prasad SK, Rimoldi OE. Stunning, hibernation, and assessment of myocardial viability. Circulation 2008;117:103–114.
43. Klocke FJ, Baird MG, Lorell BH, et al. ACC/AHA/ASNC guidelines for the clinical use of cardiac radionuclide imaging—Executive summary: A report of the American College of Cardiology/American Heart Association Task Force on Practice Guidelines (ACC/AHA/ASNC Committee to Revise the 1995 Guidelines for the Clinical Use of Cardiac Radionuclide Imaging). Circulation 2003;108:1404–1418.
44. Hendel RC, Berman DS, Di Carli MF, et al. ACCF/ASNC/ACR/AHA/ASE/SCCT/SCMR/SNM 2009 appropriate use criteria for cardiac radionuclide imaging: A report of the American College of Cardiology Foundation Appropriate Use Criteria Task Force, the American Society of Nuclear Cardiology, the American College of Radiology, the American Heart Association, the American Society of Echocardiography, the Society of Cardiovascular Computed Tomography, the Society for Cardiovascular Magnetic Resonance, and the Society of Nuclear Medicine. Endorsed by the American College of Emergency Physicians. J Am Coll Cardiol 2009;53:2201–2229.
45. de Jong MC, Genders TS, van Geuns RJ, et al. Diagnostic performance of stress myocardial perfusion imaging for coronary artery disease: A systematic review and meta-analysis. Eur Radiol 2012;9:1881.
46. Somsen GA, Verberne HJ, Burri H, Ratib O, Righetti A. Ventricular mechanical dyssynchrony and resynchronization therapy in heart failure: A new indication for Fourier analysis of gated blood-pool radionuclide ventriculography. Nucl Med Commun 2006;27:105–112.
47. Cheitlin MD, Armstrong WF, Aurigemma GP, et al. ACC/AHA/ASE 2003 guideline update for the clinical application of echocardiography: Summary article: A report of the American College of Cardiology/American Heart Association Task Force on Practice Guidelines (ACC/AHA/ASE Committee to Update the 1997 Guidelines for the Clinical Application of Echocardiography). Circulation 2003;108:1146–1162.
48. Berman DS, Hachamovitch R, Shaw LJ, et al. Roles of nuclear cardiology, cardiac computed tomography, and cardiac magnetic resonance: Assessment of patients with suspected coronary artery disease. J Nucl Med 2006;47:74–82.
49. Bluemke DA, Achenbach S, Budoff M, et al. Noninvasive coronary artery imaging: Magnetic resonance angiography and multidetector computed tomography angiography: A scientific statement from the American Heart Association Committee on Cardiovascular Imaging and Intervention of the Council on Cardiovascular Radiology and Intervention, and the Councils on Clinical Cardiology and Cardiovascular Disease in the Young. Circulation 2008;118:586–606.
50. Budoff MJ, Achenbach S, Fayad Z, et al. Task Force 12: Training in advanced cardiovascular imaging (computed tomography): Endorsed by the American Society of Nuclear Cardiology, Society for Cardiovascular Angiography and Interventions, Society of Atherosclerosis Imaging and Prevention, and Society of Cardiovascular Computed Tomography. J Am Coll Cardiol 2006;47:915–920.
51. Miller JM, Rochitte CE, Dewey M, et al. Diagnostic performance of coronary angiography by 64-row CT. N Engl J Med 2008;359:2324–2336.
52. George RT, Arbab-Zadeh A, Miller JM, et al. Computed tomography myocardial perfusion imaging with 320-row detector computed tomography accurately detects myocardial ischemia in patients with obstructive coronary artery disease. Circ Cardiovasc Imaging 2012;5:333–340.
53. Slart RH, Bax JJ, van Veldhuisen DJ, et al. Prediction of functional recovery after revascularization in patients with coronary artery disease and left ventricular dysfunction by gated FDG-PET. J Nucl Cardiol 2006;13:210–219.
54. Pijls NHJ, Sels JE. Functional measurement of coronary stenosis. J Am Coll Cardiol 2012;59:1045–1057.

Appendix 1-1

Types of Tests Used to Evaluate the Cardiovascular System

	Cardiac Function[a]			
	Myocardial Perfusion	**Pump**	**Electrical Rhythm**	**Anatomy**
Types of tests	Stress tests Nuclear imaging Angiography Echocardiography Fractional flow reserve	Angiography MUGA Echocardiography	ECG Electrophysiologic studies Holter monitoring	Echocardiography Angiography Intravascular ultrasound
Parameters evaluated	Coronary anatomy and blood flow Myocardial perfusion	Cardiac output Ejection fraction Valvular function Shunts	Rhythm Rate Conduction pathways	Chamber size Wall motion Valve function Valve structure Pericardium Coronary anatomy

ECG, electrocardiogram; MUGA, multigated acquisition.

[a]Not all tests for any one cardiac function are used to evaluate all parameters listed.

Appendix 1-2

Types of Tests for Various Cardiac Diseases or Features

Feature/Disorder	CXR	Echo	Angiography	Nuclear Scan	CT	MRI	ET	ECG	PET
Ischemic	–	+++	++++	+++	++/++	++	++	++	+++
Valvular	+	++++	+++	+	+++	+++	++	+	+
Congenital	++	++++	+++	+	+++	++++	+	+	+
Anatomy	+	+++	++	+	+++	++++	–	+	+
Cardiomyopathy	+	++++	+++	++	+++	+++	–	–	++
Pericardial	+	++++	++	–	++++	++++	–	±	–
Endocarditis	–	++++[a]	+	–	++	+++	–	±	–
Masses	–	++++	+	–	+++	++++	–	–	+
Metabolism	–	–	–	+	–	–	–	–	++++
Graft patency	–	±	+++	++	+++	++	++	+	+++
CA anatomy	–	–	++++	++	+++	++	++	+	+
Ventricular function	–	++++	+++	++	+++	++++	+	–	++

CA, coronary artery; CT, computed tomography; CXR, chest radiograph; ECG, electrocardiogram; echo, echocardiography; ET, exercise testing; PET, positron emission tomography.

[a]Transesophageal echocardiography is superior to transthoracic echocardiography.

2

Cardiac Arrest

Jeffrey F. Barletta and Jeffrey L. Wilt

KEY CONCEPTS

1. High-quality cardiopulmonary resuscitation (CPR) with minimal interruptions in chest compressions should be emphasized in all patients following cardiac arrest.
2. The AHA algorithm for basic life support following cardiac arrest now emphasizes circulation, airway, and breathing forming the pneumonic "CAB" versus the historic pneumonic "ABC."
3. The purpose of using vasopressor therapy following cardiac arrest is to augment low coronary and cerebral perfusion pressures encountered during CPR.
4. Despite several theoretical advantages with vasopressin, clinical trials have not consistently demonstrated superior results over that achieved with epinephrine.
5. Amiodarone remains the preferred antiarrhythmic during cardiac arrest with lidocaine considered as an alternative.
6. Successful treatment of both pulseless electrical activity (PEA) and asystole depends almost entirely on diagnosis of the underlying cause.
7. Intraosseous administration is the preferred alternative route for administration if IV access cannot be achieved.

CARDIAC ARREST

Cardiac arrest is defined as the cessation of cardiac mechanical activity as confirmed by the absence of signs of circulation (e.g., a detectable pulse, unresponsiveness, and apnea).[1] While there is wide variation in the reported incidence of cardiac arrest, it is estimated that there are 350,000 people in North America each year who suffer a cardiac arrest and receive attempted resuscitation.[2] Approximately half of those are in an outpatient setting. Unfortunately, survival rates have not significantly improved over 30 years, ranging between 6.7% and 8.4%, despite enormous efforts in research and development.[3] Survival following in-hospital cardiac arrest is somewhat higher (approximately 18%), with higher rates being observed in victims with a shockable first documented rhythm.[4]

EPIDEMIOLOGY

In adult patients, cardiac arrest usually results from the development of an arrhythmia.[5] Historically, ventricular fibrillation (VF) and pulseless ventricular tachycardia (PVT) have been the most common initial rhythm accounting for 40% to 60% of out-of-hospital arrests, but their incidence now is estimated to be only about 25%.[2,6] In fact, one study of out-of-hospital arrests reported VF/PVT as the first recorded rhythm in only 13% of patients.[7] The reason for this change has not been firmly established. Possible explanations include the influence of noncardiac causes of arrest that typically present with apnea leading to bradycardia and then pulseless electrical activity (PEA) or asystole. A second explanation is the increasing role of implantable pacemakers and defibrillators.[8] Finally, it has been suggested that β-blockers and ACE inhibitors may shorten the duration of VF and the expanded use of these drug classes for ischemic heart disease and heart failure may account for the increased occurrence of non-VF/PVT rhythms.[6] Nonetheless, this declining incidence is particularly concerning as survival rates are substantially higher with shockable rhythms such as VF and PVT compared with those with nonshockable rhythms such as PEA and asystole. Survival rates with VF/PVT are roughly 15% to 23% versus 0% to 5% with asystole.[3]

A similar finding has been observed with in-hospital cardiac arrest. One study of 411 U.S. hospitals including approximately 52,000 adult patients revealed the incidence of VF and PVT to be 7.3% and 16.8%, respectively.[4] In this trial, survival rates were 37% for both VF and PVT compared with 12% (PEA) and 11% (asystole). Patients with VF/PVT were more likely to have myocardial infarction (MI) as the immediate factor prearrest, while acute respiratory failure and hypotension were the immediate factors more commonly found in patients with PEA/asystole.

In pediatric patients, cardiac arrest typically results from respiratory failure and asphyxiation. As such, the initial rhythm most often encountered in out-of-hospital arrest is PEA or asystole.[9] This could explain the dismal survival rates with out-of-hospital, pediatric cardiac arrest (approximately 6%), with the lowest being observed in infants compared with children and adolescents (4%, 10%, and 13%, respectively).[10] Survival following in-hospital cardiac arrest appears higher with an overall rate of 27%. In fact, children are more likely to survive in-hospital arrest versus adults and infants have a higher survival rate than children.[10]

ETIOLOGY

The most common clinical finding in adult patients who suffer cardiac arrest is coronary artery disease accounting for roughly 80% of sudden cardiac deaths.[5] Approximately 10% to 15% of sudden cardiac deaths occur in patients with cardiomyopathies (e.g., hypertrophic cardiomyopathy, dilated cardiomyopathy), and the remaining 5% to 10% are composed of either structurally abnormal congenital cardiac conditions or patients with structurally normal but electrically abnormal heart. Unfortunately, in many patients (approximately two thirds), cardiac arrest is the first clinical sign of coronary artery disease with no preceding signs or symptoms.[11]

In pediatric patients, cardiac arrest is often the terminal event of respiratory failure or progressive shock.[12] Out-of-hospital arrests frequently are associated with trauma, sudden infant death syndrome, drowning, poisoning, choking, severe asthma, and pneumonia. In-hospital arrests, on the other hand, are associated with sepsis, respiratory failure, drug toxicity, metabolic disorders, and arrhythmias.

PATHOPHYSIOLOGY OF CARDIAC ARREST

There are two distinctly different pathophysiologic conditions associated with cardiac arrest. The first is primary cardiac arrest whereby arterial blood is typically fully oxygenated at the time of arrest. The second is cardiac arrest secondary to respiratory failure in which lack of ventilation leads to severe hypoxemia, hypotension, and secondary cardiac arrest. It is important to understand specific condition at hand as different treatment approaches are likely necessary.[13]

CLINICAL PRESENTATION

Cardiac arrest is characterized by the cessation of cardiac mechanical activity; therefore, signs and symptoms are consistent with those encountered when there is no circulation. In the setting of cardiac causes of arrest, anxiety, crushing chest pain, nausea, vomiting, and diaphoresis can precede the event. Following an arrest, individuals are unresponsive, apneic, and hypotensive and do not have a detectable pulse. Extremities are cold and clammy and cyanosis is common.

TREATMENT

Cardiopulmonary resuscitation (CPR) is an attempt to restore spontaneous circulation by performing chest compressions (to restore threshold blood flows, particularly to the heart and brain) with or without ventilations. There are two proposed theories describing the mechanism of blood flow during CPR.[14] The original theory is known as the cardiac pump theory and is based on the active compression of the heart between the sternum and vertebrae thereby creating forward flow. Echocardiography, however, has revealed that left ventricular size does not always change with compressions and the mitral valve may, in fact, be open.[14] The second theory is the thoracic pump theory. This theory is based on intrathoracic pressure alterations induced by chest compressions and the differential compressibility of the arteries and veins. In this model, the heart merely acts as a passive conduit for flow. It is likely that both models contribute to the mechanism of blood flow with CPR.

High-quality CPR continues to be emphasized in the latest guidelines published by the American Heart Association (AHA). Clinicians must focus on proper technique, including adequate rate and depth of compressions, allowance of chest recoil after each compression, avoiding excessive ventilation, and minimizing interruptions.[2] One study, in patients suffering out-of-hospital VF, reported an increased chance of survival as chest compression fraction increased (e.g., the proportion of resuscitation time without spontaneous circulation where chest compressions were administered).[15] Unfortunately, the provision of high-quality CPR is frequently suboptimal particularly when rescuers become fatigued.[10,16] There are several devices available that provide prompts and/or feedback in "real time"; however, data illustrating improvement in survival are lacking.[16] Additionally, mechanical devices designed to improve hemodynamics have been studied but inconsistent results limit their applicability in routine practice.[17]

Desired Outcome

The global goals of resuscitation are to preserve life, restore health, relieve suffering, limit disability, and respect the individual's decisions, rights, and privacy.[18] This can be accomplished via CPR by the return of spontaneous circulation (ROSC) with effective perfusion and ventilation as quickly as possible to minimize hypoxic damage to vital organs. Survival to hospital discharge with good neurologic function should be considered the primary treatment outcome sought by clinicians. Survival to hospital discharge in a vegetative or comatose state cannot be classified as a success and can impose a tremendous economic burden on the healthcare system. Additionally, most patients would choose not to continue living in a massively disabled state.[19]

The presence of a healthcare advanced directive allows patients to communicate their wishes and preferences regarding medical care and may lead to a "do not attempt resuscitation (DNAR)" order. As many cardiac arrests occur following terminal illnesses and end-of-life care, "allow natural death (AND)" has become a preferred term to replace DNAR.[18] These orders should explicitly state the resuscitation interventions that are to be performed and have clearly been communicated by the patient, his or her family, or a surrogate decision maker.

General Approach to Treatment

Cardiopulmonary Resuscitation

Resuscitation techniques have been studied for many years. The first landmark article was published in 1960 and described the outcome of 20 patients who were given closed chest compressions at a rate of 60/min.[20] Artificial ventilation was used to augment the compressions, and three patients were given defibrillation for VF. In this landmark article, all 20 patients had ROSC, and 14 lived for an extended period of time, with reported good neurologic status. Initial descriptions after this started to integrate the approach to cardiac arrest, including three phases.[21]

In 1966, the AHA first published guidelines for the treatment of cardiac arrest.[22] Since then, national conferences and organized committees have played a major role in encouraging widespread competency in CPR technique. There have been tremendous revisions of the guidelines over the years, and this is true of the most recent guidelines, published in 2010.[2] These guidelines continue to emphasize the "chain of survival" to highlight the treatment approach and illustrate the importance of a timely response. The updated guidelines list five links in the chain of survival:

1. Immediate recognition of cardiac arrest and activation of emergency medical services (EMS)
2. Early CPR with an emphasis on chest compressions
3. Rapid defibrillation
4. Effective advanced life support
5. Integrated postcardiac arrest care

While all five links of the chain of survival are important, the most crucial would seem to be the first three, particularly early CPR with good chest compressions.[2] When used together, survival rates can approach 50% following witnessed out-of-hospital VF arrest.[23] CPR provides critical blood flow to the heart and brain, prolongs the time VF is present (prior to the deterioration to asystole), and increases the likelihood that a shock will terminate VF resulting in a rhythm compatible with life.[2] For every minute that elapsed from collapse to successful defibrillation during witnessed VF arrests, survival rates decrease by 7% to 10% if no CPR is provided.[24] If immediate CPR is added, the decrease in survival is more gradual (down to 3% to 4% per minute postcollapse).[25] In effect, CPR can increase the likelihood of survival threefold from arrest to survival. Basic CPR alone, however, is not likely to terminate VF and lead to ROSC. Thus, the 2010 AHA guidelines emphasize the integration of early CPR and defibrillation, especially mentioning the use of automatic external defibrillators.[25]

1 As in the 2005 AHA guidelines for CPR and emergency cardiovascular care (ECC), the AHA continues to emphasize the provision of high-quality CPR with minimal interruptions in chest compressions. In addition, algorithms seem to be more simplified, and there is emphasis on the use of end-tidal carbon dioxide ($ETCO_2$) to guide resuscitation.[26] Furthermore, there is growing importance of postarrest care, reflecting that optimization of many organ systems may help improve outcomes.[27] The use of drug therapy and airway adjuncts, on the other hand, have continued to devolve to a minimal role as survival to hospital discharge does not appear to be impacted.

Basic Life Support The 2010 AHA guidelines represent a paradigm shift in the provision of basic life support (BLS). Historically, BLS and advanced cardiac life support (ACLS) providers have been taught the pneumonic "ABC," representing, respectively, airway, breathing, and circulation for the CPR sequence. 2 The 2010 guidelines have changed this to "CAB," or circulation, airway, and breathing.[28]

When first encountering a victim of cardiac arrest, the initial action is to determine responsiveness of the patient. If there is no response, the rescuer should immediately activate the emergency medical response team, and obtain (or call for) an automated external defibrillator (AED) (if one is available) and then immediately start CPR with chest compressions. A true cardiac arrest victim will be unresponsive, and agonal respirations can be confused with normal breathing. Thus, the "look, listen, and feel" for respirations that has been a standard protocol for initial assessment is no longer recommended.[2] Similarly, pulse recognition is often inaccurate, and it is now recommended that lay rescuers not check for a pulse. Healthcare providers should assess for a pulse but take no more than 10 seconds to do so. If one is not detected within this short time frame, then chest compressions should be initiated immediately.[28,29]

The prompt provision of chest compressions is thus of paramount importance, and rescuers should attempt them regardless of rescuer experience or skill level. The teaching of BLS now focuses on delivering high-quality CPR with a rate of at least 100/min, adequate depth (at least 2 in [5 cm] in an adult), allowing full chest recoil, minimizing interruptions in compressions, and avoiding excessive ventilation.

While it is true that opening the airway has the potential to improve oxygenation and allow for better attempts at ventilation, this can be very challenging, especially if the rescuer is alone and is a novice. Thus, the simplified adult BLS algorithm calls for the initiation of CPR, with rhythm check every 2 minutes, shocking if indicated, with continued repetition.

Once chest compressions have been started, it is then appropriate for a trained rescuer to attempt to deliver rescue breaths, either by mouth-to-mouth or preferentially by bag-mask ventilation. The current guidelines recommend delivering a breath over 1 second, using enough volume to elicit a visible chest rise, and using a compression-to-ventilation ratio of 30:2 for one rescuer.[28]

The 2010 AHA guidelines for CPR and ECC continue to stress that there should be minimal interruptions in chest compressions. If there is no AED available, then cycles of compressions/breaths should continue, with pulse checks every 2 minutes until help arrives or the patient regains spontaneous circulation. If there is an AED available, then the rhythm should be checked to determine if defibrillation is advised. If so, then one shock should be delivered with the immediate resumption of chest compressions (and rescue breaths, if being provided). After 2 minutes (five cycles of 30:2 compression-to-ventilation), the rhythm should be reevaluated to determine the need for defibrillation. This algorithm should be repeated until help arrives, or the rhythm is no longer "shockable." If the rhythm is not shockable, then chest compressions and rescue breath cycles should be continued until help arrives, or the victim recovers spontaneous circulation (Fig. 2-1).

Despite widespread dissemination of cardiac arrest guidelines and the ongoing education even of healthcare providers, there is ample evidence that chest compression quality remains poor in general. Furthermore, it has been reported that only 20% to 30% of adults with out-of-hospital cardiac arrest receive bystander CPR.[28] This has led to further educational interventions in an attempt to increase quality of CPR, and EMS dispatchers will often attempt to give instructions over the phone when EMS is activated.

There is now a push for hands-only CPR for lay persons, given data that show similar survival compared with the addition of rescue breaths. There has been reluctance on many bystanders to consider mouth-to-mouth, although one data set cites panic as a reason not to pursue bystander CPR rather than actual reluctance.[30]

Advanced Cardiac Life Support Once ACLS providers arrive, then further definitive therapy is given. An advanced airway (endotracheal tube, laryngeal mask airway, or even bag-valve mask) can be utilized to provide ventilation. When this occurs, the rescuers no longer need to provide the cycles of 30:2 compression-to-ventilation. Instead, continuous chest compressions are recommended without pauses for ventilations, and the rescuer providing the ventilations needs to deliver a breath once every 6 to 8 seconds.

Monitoring during CPR has also evolved over time. Animal and human studies have shown that monitoring of $ETCO_2$, coronary perfusion pressure (CPP), and central venous oxygen saturation ($ScvO_2$) can provide valuable information as to the success of resuscitation.[26] Surprisingly, no study has ever shown the validity of checking a pulse during ongoing CPR. $ETCO_2$ is the concentration of carbon dioxide in exhaled air at the end of expiration. During cardiac arrest, the level of $ETCO_2$ decreases because there is no flow through the pulmonary circulation. Thus, a persistently low $ETCO_2$ (i.e., <10 mm Hg [<1.3 kPa]) during CPR in intubated patients suggests that ROSC is unlikely.[26] In fact, the return of $ETCO_2$ abruptly to a normal level is likely to correlate with ROSC. In patients without ROSC and persistently decreased $ETCO_2$, it is advised to evaluate the effectiveness of CPR, since good chest compressions can increase $ETCO_2$ somewhat. The latest guidelines convincingly recommend $ETCO_2$ monitoring during CPR if at all possible.[26]

CPP and $ScvO_2$ require more invasive monitoring and will not be covered.

If the cardiac rhythm is not deemed to be shockable, then it is likely to be either asystole or PEA (Fig. 2-2). For PEA, the rescuer must consider reversible causes. If the person is in VF or PVT, then one shock should be delivered (appropriate to the available electrical device), with the immediate resumption of chest compressions (utilizing 30 compressions to 2 breaths for 5 cycles, or 2 minutes of continuous compressions with assisted ventilations) prior to rechecking the rhythm or pulse. If there is still a shockable rhythm, then one shock should be delivered, and at this time pharmacologic intervention can be considered. After the first unsuccessful shock, vasopressors are the initially recommended pharmacologic intervention (before or after the second shock), and after the second unsuccessful shock, antiarrhythmics can be considered (before or after the third shock). Chest compressions for 2 minutes (five cycles of chest compressions-to-breaths) should be performed in between attempts at defibrillation. This algorithm will repeat until a pulse

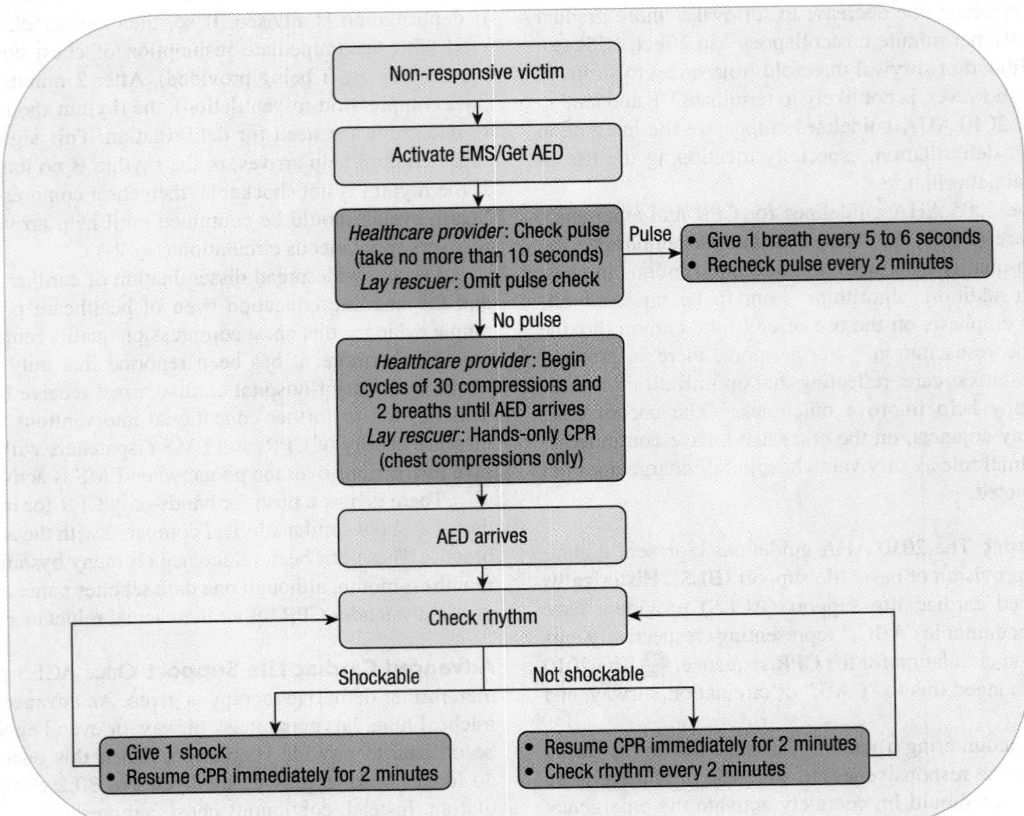

FIGURE 2-1 Treatment algorithm for adult cardiac arrest: basic life support (BLS).

is obtained with effective circulation, the rhythm changes, or the patient expires. For completeness, please refer to the guidelines published by the AHA.[26]

Cardiocerebral Resuscitation

It was interesting that after the previous AHA publication of guidelines in 2005, there was very quick questioning of appropriateness. Authors at the time seemed to favor a concept known as cardiocerebral resuscitation (CCR).[13] This "clarion call for change" was made in light of the suboptimal outcomes observed with the ECC guidelines as well as several limitations with the guideline process.[31] CCR has been embraced by the new 2010 AHA guidelines, and consists of three major components: (a) continuous chest compressions for bystander resuscitation, (b) simplified BLS and ACLS algorithm for providers, and (c) aggressive postresuscitation care including therapeutic hypothermia and early catheterization/intervention.

CCR initially advocated continuous chest compressions without mouth-to-mouth ventilations for witnessed cardiac arrests, and has led to updated guidelines as listed above. Chest compressions deliver a small but critical amount of oxygen to the brain and myocardium. Cerebral and CPPs, however, build up slowly once chest compressions are begun. These perfusion pressures are lost if chest compressions are stopped to deliver mouth-to-mouth ventilation. In fact, in earlier studies, approximately 16 seconds were required to deliver two breaths as recommended by earlier ECC guidelines.[32] The loss of perfusion during this time period has been shown to be extremely detrimental as ROSC is closely related to perfusion pressures generated during chest compressions.[33]

The second component of CCR is a new simplified algorithm. This protocol is based on the three-phase time-sensitive model of cardiac arrest.[34] The first phase is the electrical phase (0 to 5 minutes), where prompt defibrillation is the most important intervention. The second phase is the hemodynamic phase (5 to 15 minutes), where adequate coronary and cerebral perfusion pressures, before and after defibrillation, are crucial. In fact, defibrillation prior to CPR in this phase commonly leads to asystole or PEA. This is likely due to the presence of global tissue ischemia and the need for blood flow (via chest compressions) to "flush out" deleterious metabolic factors that have accumulated during ischemia. The third phase is the metabolic phase (beyond 15 minutes) in which survival is very low and hypothermia may be the most beneficial approach.

The third component of CCR is aggressive postresuscitation care. This consists of the use of hypothermia for all comatose patients and emergent cardiac catheterization and percutaneous coronary intervention (PCI) for patients with myocardial ischemia as a potential cause of their arrest. Since its conception in 2003, clinical studies evaluating CCR have demonstrated an improvement in survival of 250% to 300% compared with conventional CPR.[13]

Articles are starting to appear showing that this approach is most favorable. In one study, those who received CCR had better outcomes across age groups. For those who suffered VF arrest and were under 40 years of age, the survival increased from 3.7% (standard advanced life support) to 19% (CCR patients) (odds ratio [OR] 5.94; 95% confidence interval [CI] 1.82 to 19.26).[35]

Ventricular Fibrillation/Pulseless Ventricular Tachycardia

Nonpharmacologic Therapy

Electrical defibrillation is the only effective method of restoring a perfusing cardiac rhythm in either VF or PVT; therefore, it is a crucial link in the "chain of survival," especially for a witnessed arrest.[25] The probability of successful defibrillation is directly related to the time interval between the onset of VF and the delivery of the first

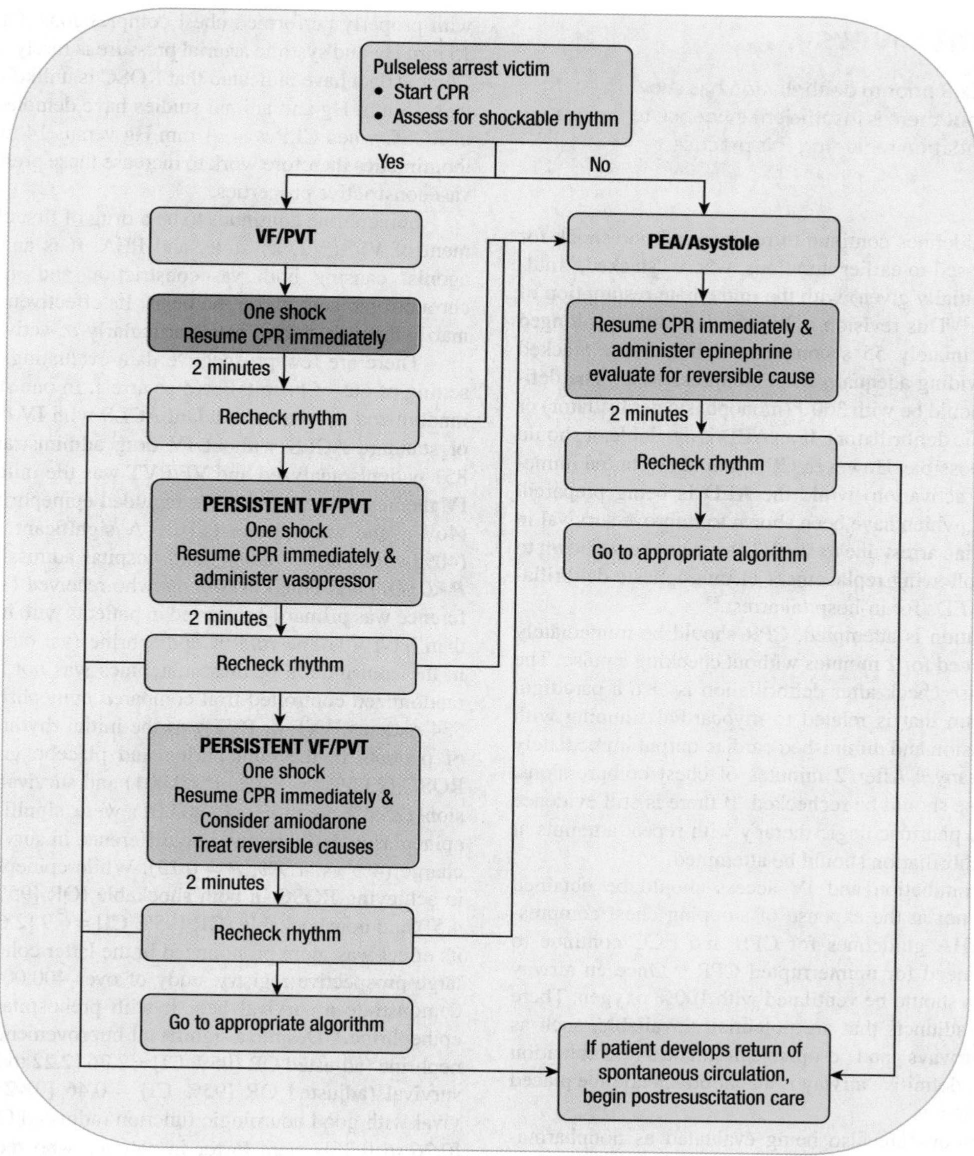

FIGURE 2-2 Treatment algorithm for adult cardiac arrest: advanced cardiac life support (ACLS).

shock.[25] In one study, a 23% relative improvement in survival was observed with each 1 minute reduction in the time to defibrillation (OR 0.77 [95% CI 0.73 to 0.81]).[36] If fact, survival decreases an estimated 7% to 10% for each minute after arrest to defibrillation if no CPR is given.[24] When bystander CPR is delivered, this decrease in survival is cut almost in half.[25]

Although early defibrillation is crucial for survival following cardiac arrest, several studies have suggested that CPR prior to defibrillation (consistent with the CCR model) may lead to more successful outcomes. This was reviewed extensively in the 2010 guidelines. For in-hospital cardiac arrest, if an AED is available, CPR should begin while the AED is being placed. With out-of-hospital cardiac arrest, there is growing evidence that CPR before defibrillation is, for the most part, beneficial. In studies where EMS arrivals were delayed more than 4 to 5 minutes, CPR before defibrillation increased ROSC, survival to discharge, and 1-year survival.[25,37,38] In one trial, the provision of roughly 90 seconds of CPR prior to defibrillation was associated with an increased rate of hospital survival (compared with a historical control group) when response intervals were 4 minutes or longer (27% vs. 17%; $P = 0.01$).[37] A second trial reported higher survival rates in patients with response intervals greater than 5 minutes when 3 minutes of CPR was administered prior to defibrillation (22% vs. 4%; $P = 0.006$).[38] In a study where each defibrillation, including the first, was preceded by 200 uninterrupted chest compressions, an increase in total survival (57% [19/33] vs. 20% [18/92], $P = 0.001$) and neurologically normal survival (48% [16/33] vs. 15% [14/92], $P = 0.001$) was reported compared with standard CPR practices.[39] Finally, one study noted an improvement in hospital survival (from 22% to 44%, $P = 0.0024$) in patients with witnessed VF using a modified resuscitation protocol that included 200 preshock chest compressions.[40] In lieu of these results, the AHA guidelines continue to offer that EMS personnel may give 2 minutes of chest compressions prior to attempting defibrillation. Recommendations are similar for victims in the metabolic phase; recognizing the likelihood of achieving ROSC, however, is drastically lower.

However, as in any topic in medicine, there are data sets that can contradict standard acceptance. Koike et al. in 2011 described no better outcome with CPR before attempted defibrillation in either 1-month survival or neurologically favorable 1-month outcome.[41] Thus, this is an issue of ongoing debate and study.

Clinical **Controversy...**

The provision of CPR prior to defibrillation has shown benefit in some studies, but there is insufficient evidence to make a strong recommendation regarding this practice.

The current guidelines continue to recommend one shock for VF or PVT (as opposed to earlier iterations, where "stacked," multiple shocks were initially given) with the immediate resumption of chest compressions.[25] This revision is largely due to the prolonged time noted (approximately 55 seconds) to deliver three stacked shocks without providing adequate chest compressions.[42] The defibrillation attempt should be with 360 J (monophasic defibrillator) or 150 to 200 J (biphasic defibrillator). If an AED is available, it should be used as soon as possible. However, CPR should be started immediately (after EMS activation) while the AED is being prepared. Interestingly, AEDs, which have been shown to improve survival in out-of-hospital cardiac arrest due to VF/VT, have not been shown to improve outcome following replacement of monophasic defibrillators with biphasic AEDs for in-hospital arrest.[43]

After defibrillation is attempted, CPR should be immediately restarted and continued for 2 minutes without checking a pulse. The omission of the pulse check after defibrillation is also a paradigm shift in the algorithm that is related to myocardial stunning with resultant poor perfusion and diminished cardiac output immediately after electrical therapy.[25] After 2 minutes of chest compressions, the rhythm and pulse should be rechecked. If there is still evidence of VF or PVT, then pharmacologic therapy with repeat attempts at single-discharge defibrillation should be attempted.

Endotracheal intubation and IV access should be obtained when feasible, but not at the expense of stopping chest compressions. The 2010 AHA guidelines for CPR and ECC continue to strongly stress the need for uninterrupted CPR.[28] Once an airway is achieved, patients should be ventilated with 100% oxygen. There are several airway adjuncts that are potentially available, such as laryngeal mask airways and esophageal–tracheal combination tubes. However, the definitive airway is an endotracheal tube placed with direct laryngoscopy.

Other interventions are also being evaluated as nonpharmacologic therapy. In a porcine model of VF arrest, a percutaneously placed left ventricular assist device (LVAD) was shown to sustain vital organ perfusion.[44] As well, the performance of angiography and PCI during suspected MI has been studied both in animals and anecdotally in humans refractory to traditional ACLS protocol without ROSC. A review of this topic suggests that this intervention is feasible and that further investigation is warranted.[45] Extracorporeal membrane oxygenation (ECMO) has also been evaluated and has been shown to improve outcomes in some series, but the logistics of widespread implementation is daunting.[46] While there are no conclusive human data regarding these issues, they do raise interesting concepts to deliberate and to research.

Pharmacologic Therapy

Sympathomimetics Sympathomimetics continue to be the first pharmacologic agents administered in the setting of cardiac arrest despite limited evidence demonstrating their ability to increase neurologically intact survival to hospital discharge. Nevertheless, sympathomimetics have been associated with an increased rate of ROSC and play a major role in the pharmacotherapy of cardiac arrest.

3 The primary goal of sympathomimetic therapy is to augment low coronary and cerebral perfusion pressures encountered during CPR. Chest compressions (via CPR) can provide some degree of blood flow to the heart and the brain but it is only about 25% of that encountered under basal conditions.[47] In fact, even with properly performed chest compressions, CPPs are only 10 to 15 mm Hg and systolic arterial pressure is rarely above 80 mm Hg.[48] Clinical data have indicated that ROSC is unlikely when CPP is less than 15 mm Hg and animal studies have demonstrated higher rates of ROSC when CPP was 31 mm Hg versus 14 mm Hg.[49,50] Sympathomimetics therefore work to increase these pressures through their vasoconstrictive properties.

Epinephrine continues to be a drug of first choice for the treatment of VF, PVT, asystole, and PEA. It is an α- and β-receptor agonist causing both vasoconstriction and increased inotropic/chronotropic activity on the heart. Its effectiveness however is primarily through its α effects, particularly α_2-activity.[51]

There are few prospective data evaluating epinephrine in the setting of out-of-hospital cardiac arrest. In one study, patients were randomized to receive standard ACLS with IV drug administration or standard ACLS without IV drug administration.[52] There were 851 patients analyzed and VF/PVT was the initial rhythm in 34%. IV medications administered included epinephrine (79%), atropine (46%), and amiodarone (17%). A significant increase in ROSC (40% vs. 25%, P <0.001) and hospital admission (43% vs. 29%, P <0.001) was noted in patients who received IV therapy. This difference was primarily observed in patients with initial rhythms other than VF/PVT. The role of epinephrine (vs. other IV medications) in the contribution of these outcomes was not assessed. A second randomized controlled trial compared epinephrine with placebo in 534 patients.[53] VF or PVT was the initial rhythm in 44% and 48% of patients in the epinephrine and placebo groups, respectively. ROSC (23.5% vs. 8.4%, P <0.001) and survival to hospital admission (25.4% vs. 13%, P <0.001) were significantly higher with epinephrine, but there was no difference in survival to hospital discharge (4% vs. 1.9%, P = 0.15). While epinephrine was effective in achieving ROSC in both shockable (OR [95% CI] = 2.5 [1.2 to 4.5]) and nonshockable (OR [95% CI] = 6.9 [2.6 to 18.4]) rhythms, its effect was more pronounced in the latter cohort. In contrast, one large prospective registry study of over 400,000 patients failed to demonstrate a survival benefit with prehospital administration of epinephrine.[54] Despite a significant improvement in ROSC with epinephrine (adjusted OR [95% CI] = 2.36 [2.22 to 2.5]), both 1-month survival (adjusted OR [95% CI] = 0.46 [0.42 to 0.51]) and survival with good neurologic function (adjusted OR [95% CI] = 0.31 [0.26 to 0.36]) were lower in patients who received epinephrine. These findings were confirmed through various sensitivity analyses accounting for in-hospital epinephrine use and CPR duration. Given the disparate results with epinephrine in clinical trials, it can be considered both a cure and a curse in cardiac arrest. One potential approach, which will require validation through clinical trials, is to administer epinephrine only in settings where aortic diastolic pressure is low (i.e., less than 30 to 40 mm Hg) recognizing that a vasoconstrictive agent will provide minimal benefit (and possible harm) when perfusion pressures are adequate.[55]

Clinical **Controversy...**

Given the disparate results with epinephrine in clinical trials, it can be considered both a cure and a curse in cardiac arrest.

One possible explanation for the negative effects of epinephrine is related to its mechanism of action. Epinephrine causes α-mediated vasoconstriction that increases coronary perfusion but can decrease perfusion to other vital organs. In fact, animal research has linked epinephrine to a decrease in cerebral microvascular blood flow and increase in brain tissue ischemia during and after CPR.[56] Epinephrine also stimulates β-receptors that can increase myocardial oxygen demand, impair lactate clearance, and advance the severity of postresuscitation myocardial dysfunction.[57] This has led some investigators to evaluate simultaneous adrenergic antagonist administration in conjunction with epinephrine therapy (thereby isolating the α_2 effects) using an animal model.[58] This approach has not been extensively studied in humans.

Several studies have compared epinephrine with other adrenergic agonists such as pure α_1-agonists (phenylephrine and methoxamine) and agents with more potent α-activity (norepinephrine).[59] When compared with pure α_1-agonists, no advantage in long-term survival could be reported. One potential reason could be the potent α_2 effects with epinephrine and the fact that these receptors lie extrajunctionally in the intima of the blood vessels making them more accessible to circulating catecholamines.[60] Furthermore, during ischemia, the number of postsynaptic α_1-receptors decreases, which suggests a greater role for α_2-agonists during CPR.[61] Epinephrine has also been compared with norepinephrine, a potent α-agonist (both α_1 and α_2) with some β_1 effects. In the only large-scale randomized, double-blind, prospective trial in out-of-hospital cardiac arrest, there were no significant differences in ROSC, hospital admission, or discharge.[62] A second, smaller study demonstrated higher resuscitation rates with norepinephrine compared with those with epinephrine (64% vs. 32%) but no significant difference in hospital discharge.[63] Since the use of epinephrine has been established for many decades in evidence-based guidelines, strong outcome-related data (e.g., survival to hospital discharge) would be required for an alternative to replace it. Consequently, epinephrine remains the first-line sympathomimetic for CPR.

The recommended dose for epinephrine is 1 mg administered by IV or intraosseous (IO) injection every 3 to 5 minutes[26] (Table 2-1). Higher doses may be administered to treat specific disorders such as β-blocker or calcium channel blocker overdose. Additionally, higher doses can be considered if indicated through arterial diastolic pressure (or CPP) monitoring. The recommended dose for epinephrine was derived from animal studies (0.1 mg/kg in a 10-kg dog) and equates to approximately 0.015 mg/kg for a 70-kg human.[64] Both animal and human studies have demonstrated a positive dose–response relationship with epinephrine suggesting that higher doses might be necessary to improve hemodynamics and achieve successful resuscitation.[59] These results, however, have not been replicated in human studies. In fact, some studies have reported increased morbidity with high epinephrine doses, indicative of catecholamine toxicity, including decreased cardiac indices, left ventricular dysfunction, and decreased oxygen consumption and delivery. This discrepancy between animal and human studies could be related to most victims of cardiac arrest having coronary artery disease, which is not encountered in an animal model. Additionally, atherosclerotic plaques (in humans) can aggravate the balance between myocardial oxygen supply and demand and the interval from arrest to treatment is longer in human studies than that encountered in an animal model.

Vasopressin Vasopressin, also known as antidiuretic hormone, is a potent, nonadrenergic vasoconstrictor that increases blood pressure and systemic vascular resistance. Although it acts on various receptors throughout the body, its vasoconstrictive properties are due primarily to its effects on the V_1 receptor. Measurement of vasopressin levels in patients undergoing CPR has shown a high correlation between the levels of endogenous vasopressin released and the potential for ROSC.[65] In fact, in one study, plasma vasopressin concentrations were approximately three times as high in survivors compared with those in nonsurvivors, suggesting that vasopressin is released as an adjunct vasopressor to epinephrine in life-threatening events such as cardiac arrest.[66]

Vasopressin may have several advantages over epinephrine. First, the metabolic acidosis that frequently accompanies cardiac arrest can blunt the vasoconstrictive effect of adrenergic agents

TABLE 2-1 Evidence-Based Recommendations

Recommendations	Recommendation Grades[a]
Immediate Bystander CPR	
High-quality CPR should be performed with minimal interruption in chest compressions and defibrillation as soon as it can be accomplished	Class I
Epinephrine	
One milligram IV/IO should be administered every 3–5 minutes in patients with cardiac arrest	Class IIb, LOE A
Vasopressin	
Forty units IV/IO may replace either the first or second dose of epinephrine in patients with cardiac arrest	Class IIb, LOE A
Amiodarone	
Three hundred milligrams IV/IO can be followed by 150 mg IV/IO in patients with VF/PVT unresponsive to CPR, shock, and a vasopressor	Class IIb, LOE B
Lidocaine	
Lidocaine can be considered in patients with VF/PVT as alternative if amiodarone is not available. The initial dose is 1–1.5 mg/kg IV. Additional doses of 0.5–0.75 mg/kg can be administered at 5- to 10-minute intervals to a maximum dose of 3 mg/kg if VF/PVT persists	Class IIb, LOE B
Magnesium	
Magnesium is recommended for VF/PVT that is caused by torsade de pointes. One to 2 g diluted in 10 mL D_5W should be administered IV/IO push over 15 minutes	Class IIb, LOE C
Routine administration of magnesium sulfate in cardiac arrest is not recommended	Class III, LOE A
Fibrinolysis	
Fibrinolytic therapy should not be used routinely in cardiac arrest	Class III, LOE B
When pulmonary embolism is presumed or known to be the cause, empirical fibrinolytic therapy can be considered	Class IIa, LOE B
Hypothermia	
Comatose adult patients with ROSC after out-of-hospital VF cardiac arrest should be cooled to 32–34°C (89.6–93.2°F) for 12–24 hours	Class I, LOE B
Induced hypothermia can be considered for comatose adult patients with ROSC after in-hospital cardiac arrest of any initial rhythm or after out-of-hospital cardiac arrest with an initial rhythm of PEA or asystole	Class IIb, LOE B

CPR, cardiopulmonary resuscitation; IO, intraosseous; VF, ventricular fibrillation; PVT, pulseless ventricular tachycardia; PEA, pulseless electrical activity; D_5W, dextrose 5% in water; LOE, Level of Evidence.

[a]Key for evidence-based classifications:

Class of recommendations:
Class I: High-level prospective studies support the action or therapy, and the benefit substantially outweighs the potential for harm. The treatment should be administered.
Class IIa: The weight of evidence supports the action or therapy, and the therapy is considered acceptable and useful. It is reasonable to administer the treatment.
Class IIb: The evidence documented only short-term benefits, or weakly positive or mixed results. Class IIb recommendations are identified by terms such as "may be useful" or "can be considered."
Class III: The risk outweighs the benefit for a particular treatment. The treatment should not be administered and may be harmful.

Levels of Evidence (LOE):
Level A: Data derived from multiple randomized clinical trials or meta analyses
Level B: Data derived from a single randomized trial or nonrandomized studies
Level C: Only consensus opinion of experts, case studies, or standard of care

TABLE 2-2 Prospective Randomized Controlled Trials with Vasopressin in Cardiac Arrest

					Initial Resuscitation		Hospital Discharge	
Author	**Setting**	**Initial Rhythm**	**Intervention**	***N***	**Vasopressin**	**Epinephrine**	**Vasopressin**	**Epinephrine**
Lindner et al.[67]	OOH	VF: 100%	Vasopressin 40 units versus epinephrine 1 mg for initial drug treatment	40	16/20 (80%)	11/20 (55%)	8/20 (40%)	3/20 (15%)
Stiell et al.[68]	IH	VF/PVT: 21% PEA: 48% Asystole: 31%	Vasopressin 40 units versus epinephrine 1 mg for initial drug treatment	200	62/104 (60%)	57/96 (59%)	12/104 (12%)	13/96 (14%)
Wenzel et al.[69]	OOH	VF/PVT: 40% PEA: 16% Asystole: 45%	Vasopressin 40 units versus epinephrine 1 mg for two doses as initial drug treatment	1,186	145/589 (25%)	167/597 (28%)	57/578 (10%)	58/588 (10%)
Callaway et al.[70]	OOH	VF: 15% PEA: 22% Asystole: 50%	Vasopressin 40 units or placebo as soon as possible after the first dose of epinephrine 1 mg	325	52/167 (31%)	48/158 (30%)	NR	NR
Gueugniaud et al.[71]	OOH	VF: 9% PEA: 8% Asystole: 83%	Epinephrine 1 mg followed by vasopressin 40 units (<10 seconds apart) versus epinephrine alone for two doses	2,894	413/1,442 (29%)	428/1,452 (30%)	24/1,439 (1.7%)	33/1,448 (2.3%)
Mentzelopoulos et al.[72]	IH	VF/PVT: 14% PEA: 25% Asystole: 61%	Vasopressin 20 units + epinephrine 1 mg + methylprednisolone 40 mg (vasopressin + epinephrine were repeated during each of four subsequent CPR cycles vs. epinephrine 1 mg) versus epinephrine 1 mg	100	39/48 (81%)[a]	27/52 (52%)	9/48 (19%)[a]	2/52 (4%)
Mukoyama et al.[73]	OOH	VF: 24% Asystole/PEA: 76%	Vasopressin 40 units versus epinephrine 1 mg for a maximum of four doses	336	51/178 (29%)	42/158 (27%)	10/178 (5.6%)	6/158 (3.8%)
Ong et al.[74]	OOH	VF/PVT: 8% PEA: 20% Asystole: 72%	Vasopressin 40 units versus epinephrine 1 mg	727	119/374 (32%)	106/353 (30%)	11/374 (2.9%)	8/353 (2.3%)

OOH, out-of-hospital; IH, in-hospital; VF, ventricular fibrillation; PVT, pulseless ventricular tachycardia; PEA, pulseless electrical activity; NR, not reported.

[a]$P < 0.05$.

such as epinephrine. This effect does not occur with vasopressin. Second, the stimulation of β-receptors caused by epinephrine can increase myocardial oxygen demand and complicate the postresuscitative phase of CPR. Because vasopressin does not act on β-receptors, this effect does not occur with its use. Vasopressin also may have a beneficial effect on renal blood flow by stimulating V_2 receptors in the kidney, causing vasodilation and increased water reabsorption. With regard to splanchnic blood flow, however, vasopressin has a detrimental effect when compared with epinephrine.[65]

Despite these theoretical advantages with vasopressin, clinical trials have not consistently demonstrated superior results over that achieved with epinephrine (Table 2-2). In one large trial of out-of-hospital arrest, no significant differences were noted in ROSC, hospital admission rate, or discharge rate.[69] Although when patients were stratified according to their initial rhythm, patients with asystole had a significantly higher rate of hospital admission (29% vs. 20%; $P = 0.02$) and discharge (4.7% vs. 1.5%; $P = 0.04$) with vasopressin compared with that with epinephrine. In addition, a subgroup analysis of 732 patients who required additional epinephrine therapy despite the two doses of study drug revealed significant benefits in ROSC (37% vs. 26%; $P = 0.002$), hospital admission rate (26% vs. 16%; $P = 0.002$), and discharge rate (6.2% vs. 1.7%; $P = 0.002$) with vasopressin. There was a trend, however, toward a poorer neurologic state or coma among the patients who survived to discharge and received vasopressin.

The favorable results observed in the subgroup analysis led to a prospective study evaluating the combination of vasopressin and epinephrine versus epinephrine alone.[71] In this study, patients were randomized to receive either 1 mg of epinephrine followed by 40 units of vasopressin (in less than 10 seconds) or 1 mg of epinephrine plus saline placebo. Unfortunately, there were no significant differences between the combination therapy group and epinephrine-only group in any of the outcome measures studied (ROSC, survival to hospital admission, survival to hospital discharge, 1-year survival, and good neurologic recovery at discharge). In contrast, a post hoc subgroup analysis revealed a lower rate of survival (0% vs. 5.8%, $P = 0.02$) with combination therapy when the initial rhythm was PEA.

One study evaluated a multidrug regimen that also included corticosteroids for patients with in-hospital cardiac arrest.[72] In this study, patients were randomized to receive either epinephrine alone or 20 units of vasopressin plus 1 mg of epinephrine and 40 mg of methylprednisolone (followed by hydrocortisone in the postresuscitative phase). Vasopressin 20 units plus epinephrine 1 mg was repeated during each of four subsequent CPR cycles. This study marks the first to include corticosteroids as part of drug therapy during CPR. The rationale is based on the hemodynamic effects of steroids alone with their potential to impact the intensity of the postresuscitation systemic inflammatory response and organ dysfunction. Significant benefits were observed in ROSC (81% vs. 52%, $P = 0.003$) and survival to hospital discharge (19% vs. 4%, $P = 0.02$) with combination therapy including corticosteroids. Future studies are required to determine the role of vasopressin and corticosteroids for cardiac arrest.

In lieu of the conflicting results across numerous randomized controlled trials, a meta analysis was performed to further define the role of vasopressin.[75] Six studies were chosen for analysis (4, out-of-hospital arrest; 2, in-hospital arrest) including 4,745 patients. No significant improvements were noted with vasopressin therapy in ROSC (OR [95% CI] = 1.25 [0.9 to 1.74]), long-term survival (OR [95% CI] = 1.13 [0.71 to 1.78]), or favorable neurologic outcome (OR [95% CI] = 0.87 [0.49 to 1.52]). When patients were stratified based on the presence of VF/PVT as their initial rhythm, the incidence of ROSC (OR [95% CI] = 1.18 [0.82 to 1.69]) and long-term survival (OR [95% CI] = 0.95 [0.66 to 1.37]) were similar with vasopressin. Interestingly, in patients with asystole, vasopressin was associated with superior long-term survival rates relative to control (OR [95% CI] = 1.8 [1.04 to 3.12]).

❹ In summary, vasopressin appears to offer no benefit over epinephrine when used as an alternative to or when coadministered with epinephrine. Future prospective trials are needed to validate the role of vasopressin in certain subpopulations (e.g., asystole) or when combined with corticosteroids. The current recommendations for vasopressin are that one dose (40 units) administered IV/IO may replace either the first or second dose of epinephrine in the treatment of cardiac arrest.

Clinical **Controversy. . .**

Vasopressin could have some potential benefit in patients with initial rhythms that are nonshockable.

Antiarrhythmics The purpose of antiarrhythmic drug therapy following unsuccessful defibrillation and vasopressor administration is to prevent the development or recurrence of VF and PVT by raising the fibrillation threshold. Clinical evidence demonstrating improved survival to hospital discharge however is lacking.[76]

❺ Amiodarone is the recommended antiarrhythmic in patients with VF or PVT, unresponsive to CPR, defibrillation, and vasopressor therapy. Amiodarone is classified as a Class III antiarrhythmic but possesses electrophysiologic characteristics of all four Vaughan Williams classifications. A large, randomized, double-blind trial in patients with out-of-hospital cardiac arrest secondary to VF or PVT (referred to as the ARREST trial) randomized individuals to receive either amiodarone 300 mg or placebo.[77] Recipients of amiodarone were more likely to be resuscitated and survive to hospital admission (44% vs. 34%, $P = 0.03$), but there was no difference in survival to hospital discharge (13.4% vs. 13.2%, P = NS). This was the first trial to demonstrate the benefit of an antiarrhythmic agent over placebo in patients with out-of-hospital cardiac arrest.

A subsequent trial (known as the ALIVE trial) compared amiodarone 5 mg/kg with lidocaine 1.5 mg/kg in patients with out-of-hospital cardiac arrest due to VF.[78] In this trial, amiodarone was associated with a relative improvement of 90% in survival to hospital admission compared with lidocaine (22.8% vs. 12%; OR 2.17 [95% CI 1.21 to 3.83]; $P = 0.009$). Similar to the ARREST trial, there was no difference in survival to hospital discharge (amiodarone, 5% vs. lidocaine, 3%; $P = 0.34$).

Amiodarone and lidocaine have also been compared in patients following in-hospital cardiac arrest. In a multicentered, retrospective review, 194 patients with VF or PVT who received amiodarone ($n = 74$), lidocaine ($n = 79$), or both ($n = 41$) were evaluated.[79] The rate of survival at 24 hours was 55%, 63%, and 50% for patients receiving amiodarone, lidocaine, or both, respectively ($P = 0.39$). There was no difference in survival to hospital discharge (amiodarone, 39%; lidocaine, 45%; both, 42%; $P = 0.72$). After adjusting for multiple covariates, Cox's regression analysis revealed higher survival to 24 hours (HR [95% CI] = 3.15 [1.68 to 5.92], $P < 0.001$) and hospital discharge (HR [95% CI] = 3.25 [1.22 to 8.65], $P = 0.02$) in those patients who received lidocaine compared with that in those patients who received amiodarone. The mean initial dose of amiodarone, though, was 190 mg, and only 25% of patients received the recommended dose of 300 mg. Additionally, the time to first dose of antiarrhythmic was significantly longer in the amiodarone group than in the lidocaine group (14 minutes vs. 6 minutes, $P < 0.001$).

Adverse effects of amiodarone encountered in cardiac arrest include hypotension and bradycardia.[26] The effects however are largely due to the IV vehicle, polysorbate 80, and benzyl alcohol. A formulation of amiodarone exists that does not contain these solvents and adverse hemodynamic effects appear to be minimized. Nevertheless, administration of a vasoconstrictor prior to amiodarone can potentially prevent hypotension.

Lidocaine is currently recommended as an alternative to amiodarone, if amiodarone is not available. Minimal evidence exists supporting lidocaine use for VF/PVT. In the only published case–control trial where patients were classified according to whether they received lidocaine, no significant difference was noted in ROSC, admission to the hospital, or survival to hospital discharge between groups.[80] Similarly, a prospective study comparing the effectiveness of lidocaine with that of standard-dose epinephrine showed not only a lack of benefit with lidocaine but also a higher tendency to promote asystole.[81] In contrast, a retrospective analysis in patients with VF indicated that lidocaine was associated with a higher rate of ROSC and hospitalization ($P < 0.01$) but not an increase in the hospital discharge rate.[82]

Magnesium Severe hypomagnesemia has been associated with VF/PVT, but routine administration of magnesium during a cardiac arrest has not demonstrated any benefit in clinical outcome. Two observation trials, though, have noted an improvement in ROSC in patients with arrests associated with torsade de pointes.[26] Therefore, magnesium administration should only be administered to those patients.

Thrombolytics Since most cardiac arrests are related to either MI or pulmonary embolism (PE), several investigators have evaluated the role of thrombolytics during CPR. Earlier smaller studies have demonstrated some benefit with their use, but in the two largest randomized controlled trials, no difference was noted.[26] In the first, 233 patients with PEA were randomized to receive either tissue plasminogen activator (tPA) or placebo.[83] The proportion of patients with ROSC was 21.4% and 23.3% for tPA- and placebo-treated patients, respectively. There was no significant difference in hemorrhage rates. The second study randomized patients with out-of-hospital cardiac arrest to receive either tenecteplase or placebo.[84] After a blinded review by the data and safety monitoring board, criteria for futility were met and enrollment was terminated. A total of 1,050 patients were analyzed, and both ROSC (tenecteplase, 55% vs. placebo, 55%; $P = 0.96$) and survival to hospital discharge (tenecteplase, 15.1% vs. placebo, 17.5%, $P = 0.33$) were similar between groups. Furthermore, the incidence of intracranial hemorrhage was significantly greater with tenecteplase versus placebo (2.7% vs. 0.4%, $P = 0.006$). Potential reasons for failure in this study include the omission of antiplatelet and antithrombin medication administration during CPR and decreased delivery of the thrombolytic to the coronary arteries (where the clots exist) due to impaired flow and perfusion. Given these results, fibrinolytic therapy should not be used routinely in cardiac arrest but when PE is presumed (or known) to be the cause, their use can be considered.

Pulseless Electrical Activity and Asystole

Nonpharmacologic Therapy

PEA is defined as the absence of a detectable pulse and the presence of some type of electrical activity other than VF or PVT. Several studies have documented that patients with PEA actually have mechanical cardiac contractions, but they are too weak to produce a palpable pulse or blood pressure. Although PEA is still classified as a "rhythm of survival," the success rate of treatment is much lower than the rates seen with VF/PVT.[85] PEA is often caused by treatable conditions, and the resuscitation team needs to identify and correct these conditions emergently if the resuscitation is to be successful (Table 2-3). Asystole is defined as the presence of a flat line on the ECG monitor and often represents confirmation of death rather than a rhythm to be treated. Therefore, withdrawal of efforts must be strongly considered if there is not a rapid ROSC.[26] 6 Like PEA, successful treatment of asystole depends almost entirely on diagnosis of the underlying cause.

The algorithm for treatment of PEA is the same as that for the treatment of asystole. Both conditions require CPR, airway control, and IV access. Asystole should be reconfirmed by checking a second lead on the cardiac monitor. Defibrillation should be avoided in patients with asystole because the parasympathetic discharge that occurs with defibrillation may reduce the chance of ROSC and worsen the chance of survival. The emphasis in resuscitation is good-quality CPR without interruption, and to try to identify a correctable cause. If available, transcutaneous pacing can be attempted.

Much like VF/PVT, there is an interest in hypothermia in these postarrest patients. Metabolic parameters (e.g., lactate and O_2 extraction) have been shown to be improved when postarrest comatose adults survived their arrest and were treated with hypothermia. Further studies are warranted in this area.[86]

Pharmacologic Therapy

The primary pharmacologic agents used in the treatment of asystole or PEA are epinephrine and vasopressin. While there are no studies evaluating these therapies solely in patients with asystole or PEA, these rhythms represent a majority of patients included in clinical trials. For example, in the largest observational trial evaluating the role of epinephrine, 93% had either PEA or systole as the first documented rhythm.[54] Epinephrine was associated with a significant improvement in ROSC, but 1-month survival and survival with good neurologic function were lower with epinephrine. In contrast, in a subgroup analysis of a randomized controlled trial comparing epinephrine with placebo, higher rates of ROSC and survival to hospital admission were observed with epinephrine in patients with nonshockable rhythms.[53]

Inconsistent results have also been reported with vasopressin. In a post hoc subgroup analysis of patients with out-of-hospital arrest and asystole as the first identified rhythm, survival to hospital admission (29% vs. 20%, $P = 0.02$) and discharge (4.7% vs. 1.5%, $P = 0.04$) were significantly higher with vasopressin compared with those with epinephrine.[69] There was, however, a nonstatistically significant increase in coma/vegetative state with vasopressin (40% vs. 0%, $P = 0.14$). Similar findings were cited in a meta analysis of randomized controlled trials comparing vasopressin with control.[75] Patients with asystole who had study drug administered within 20 minutes had higher rates of ROSC (OR [95% CI] = 1.7 [1.17 to 2.47]) and long-term survival (OR [95% CI] = 2.84 [1.19 to 6.79]). These results were largely influenced by the aforementioned trial

TABLE 2-3 Underlying Causes of Pulseless Electrical Activity and Asystole

Condition	Clues	Treatment
Hypovolemia	History, flat neck veins	IV fluids
Hypoxia	Cyanosis, blood gases, airway problems	Ventilation, oxygen
Hydrogen ion (acidosis)	History of bicarbonate-responsive preexisting acidosis	Sodium bicarbonate, hyperventilation
Hyperkalemia (hypokalemia)	History of renal failure, diabetes, recent dialysis, dialysis fistulas, medications	Calcium chloride, insulin, glucose, sodium bicarbonate, sodium polystyrene sulfonate, dialysis
Hypothermia	History of exposure to cold, central body temperature	Rewarming, oxygen, IV fluids
Hypoglycemia	History of diabetes	Glucose infusion
Toxin (drug overdose)	Bradycardia, history of ingestion, empty bottles at the scene, pupils, neurologic exam	Drug screens, intubation, lavage, activated charcoal
Tamponade (cardiac)	History (trauma, renal failure, thoracic malignancy), no pulse with CPR, vein distention, impending tamponade–tachycardia, hypotension, low pulse pressure changing to sudden bradycardia as terminal event	Pericardiocentesis
Tension pneumothorax	History (asthma, ventilator, chronic obstructive pulmonary disease, trauma), no pulse with CPR, neck vein distention, tracheal deviation	Needle decompression
Thrombosis, coronary	History, ECG, enzymes	PCI, thrombolytics, oxygen, nitroglycerin, heparin, aspirin, morphine
Thrombosis, pulmonary	History, no pulse with CPR, distended neck veins	Pulmonary arteriogram, surgical embolectomy, thrombolytics
Trauma	History, examination	Volume infusion, intracranial pressure monitoring, bleeding control, surgical intervention

Data from reference 26.

that accounted for a majority of the weight in those statistics. In contrast to these findings, one randomized controlled trial that evaluated combination therapy with vasopressin and epinephrine did not report an advantage with vasopressin in patients with asystole.[71] In fact, a post hoc subgroup analysis of patients with PEA as the initial rhythm revealed a lower rate of survival (0% vs. 5.8%, $P = 0.02$) with combination therapy compared with that with epinephrine alone.

One agent that is no longer recommended in the setting of PEA or asystole is atropine.[26] Atropine is an antimuscarinic agent that blocks the depressant effect of acetylcholine on both heart rate and atrioventricular nodal conduction, thus decreasing parasympathetic tone. During asystole, parasympathetic tone may increase because of the vagal stimulation that occurs secondary to intubation, the effects of hypoxia and acidosis, or alterations in the balance of parasympathetic and sympathetic control.[87] Nevertheless, there are no prospective controlled trials showing benefit from atropine for the treatment of asystole or PEA and conflicting evidence exists across retrospective and observational reports. Therefore, atropine should not be routinely administered in this setting.

Acid/Base Management

Acidosis seen during cardiac arrest is the result of decreased blood flow (leading to anaerobic metabolism) or inadequate ventilation. Chest compressions generate only approximately 20% to 30% of normal cardiac output, leading to inadequate organ perfusion, tissue hypoxia, and metabolic acidosis. In addition, the lack of ventilation causes retention of carbon dioxide, leading to respiratory acidosis. This combined acidosis produces not only reduced myocardial contractility and negative inotropic effect but also the appearance of arrhythmias because of a lower fibrillation threshold. In early cardiac arrest, adequate alveolar ventilation has been considered the mainstay of control to limit the accumulation of carbon dioxide and control the acid–base imbalance.[26] With the evolution to CCR, however, there are experts arguing against ventilation because of the negative effects it can have on the effectiveness of CPR. This has led to evidence showing no negative effects if compression-only CPR is used for out-of-hospital cardiac arrest (exceptions being pediatric arrest, drowning, trauma, airway obstruction, noncardiac etiology, or due to acute respiratory disease).[88] With arrests of long duration, buffer therapy is often considered; however, few data support its use during cardiac arrest.

Although sodium bicarbonate was once given routinely to reduce the detrimental effects associated with acidosis (e.g., reduced myocardial contractility), enhance the effect of epinephrine, and improve the rate of defibrillation, there are few clinical data supporting its use.[89] In fact, sodium bicarbonate may have some detrimental effects.[89,90] The effect of sodium bicarbonate can be described by the following reaction:

$$[HCO_3^-] + [H^+] \leftrightarrow [H_2O] + [CO_2]$$

When sodium bicarbonate is added to an acidic environment, this reaction will shift to the right, thereby increasing tissue and venous hypercarbia. The carbon dioxide generated by this reaction will diffuse into the cell and decrease intracellular pH. The accumulation of intracellular carbon dioxide, specifically within the myocardium, is inversely correlated with CPP produced by CPR. Intracellular acidosis also will decrease myocardial contractility, further complicating the low-flow state associated with CPR.[89] Furthermore, treatment with sodium bicarbonate often overcorrects extracellular pH because sodium bicarbonate has a greater effect when the pH is closer to normal.[90] The induced alkalosis causes an increase in the affinity of oxygen to hemoglobin ("left shift"), thus interfering with oxygen release into the tissues. More recently, the early administration of bicarbonate (1 mEq/kg) had no effect on survival in prehospital cardiac arrest. There was a slight trend toward improvement in prolonged arrest (>15 minutes) with a twofold improvement in survival (32.8% vs. 15.4%).[91]

Sodium bicarbonate can be used in special circumstances (i.e., underlying metabolic acidosis, hyperkalemia, salicylate overdose, or tricyclic antidepressant overdose); however, the dosage should be guided by laboratory analysis if possible. Tromethamine (THAM) is an alternative buffering agent that acts as a proton acceptor, but there is a dearth of clinical experience with this agent in cardiac arrest and outcome studies are not currently available.[26]

Postresuscitative Care

Following the ROSC from a cardiac arrest, a complex phase of resuscitation begins that has been termed postcardiac arrest syndrome.[92] There are four main components of postcardiac arrest syndrome highlighting succinct pathophysiologic processes and potential areas for treatment and include postcardiac arrest brain injury, myocardial dysfunction, systemic ischemia/reperfusion response, and persistent precipitating pathology. In general, many of the concepts within these four components surround the principles of basic ICU care (e.g., early hemodynamic optimization, circulatory support, sedation, etc.). Postarrest care has the significant potential to reduce early mortality from altered hemodynamics and later morbidity and mortality from multiple organ dysfunction and CNS injury.[27,92,93]

After ROSC, it is imperative to ensure adequate airway and oxygenation. Securing the airway to prevent inadvertent loss is an important step. If there is any question of cervical spine injury, the patient should have a cervical collar placed, with subsequent appropriate evaluation. The head of the bed should be raised to 30° (if this can be tolerated hemodynamically) to reduce the risk for aspiration, ventilator-associated pneumonia, and cerebral edema. Usually 100% oxygen is used during the initial resuscitation effort. If ROSC is obtained and the patient is placed on a mechanical ventilator, the healthcare team should titrate the oxygen fraction down as tolerated to avoid oxygen toxicity. Overventilation is common in the postresuscitation time frame; the advent of widespread $ETCO_2$ usage can avoid this pitfall (i.e., targeting an $ETCO_2$ of 40 to 45 mm Hg [5.3 to 6.0 kPa]).

Because the most common cause of cardiac arrest is ischemia, a rapid search for electrocardiographic changes consistent with acute MI should be undertaken as soon as possible in the postarrest time frame.[94] If there is an acute MI present, urgent revascularization should be enacted immediately.

Many patients do not regain consciousness immediately after a cardiac arrest. It is recommended that they be transferred to a facility with a comprehensive care plan for advanced cardiac care, advanced neurologic monitoring, and postarrest therapeutic hypothermia.[27]

Restoration of blood flow following cardiac arrest can lead to several chemical cascades and destructive enzymatic reactions that can result in cerebral injury. These reactions include free radical production, excitatory amino acid release, and calcium shifts, which ultimately lead to mitochondrial damage and apoptosis (programmed cell death).[95] Hypothermia can protect from cerebral injury by suppressing these chemical reactions, thereby reducing the production of free radicals. Various animal models have demonstrated improved functional recovery and reduced cerebral deficits with the induction of mild therapeutic hypothermia.[96] Recent data have attempted to refine this concept and even expand upon the organ systems protected. In a pig model of VF treated after 10 minutes, rapid head cooling led to more beneficial effects than surface cooling in terms of postresuscitation myocardial dysfunction.[97] In addition, a similar pig model of cardiac arrest showed that delayed surface cooling led to less favorable survival and neurologic outcome than early head cooling.[98]

Interestingly, hypothermia as a therapeutic endeavor in humans has been described since antiquity. It is reported that Hippocrates advocated for bleeding patients to be packed in snow and ice. Later, a chief battlefield surgeon for Napoleon Bonaparte noticed that survival rates were lower in wounded soldiers who were rewarmed versus survival rates in those who were left in the cold.[99,100] These early human observations, as well as current animal model investigations, have been parlayed into the clinical bedside in human trials, and literature continues to accumulate.

Early human success with hypothermia was described in two pivotal trials.[101,102] The first trial was conducted in nine centers in five European countries.[101] In this study, patients who had been resuscitated after cardiac arrest due to VF but remained comatose were assigned randomly to undergo therapeutic hypothermia, targeting a temperature of 32°C to 34°C (89.6°F to 93.2°F), for 24 hours. The primary end point was neurologic outcome within 6 months of cardiac arrest. Secondary end points were mortality (within 6 months) and complication rate within 7 days. A favorable neurologic outcome was achieved in 55% of patients in the hypothermia group as opposed to 39% in the normothermia group ($P = 0.009$). Additionally, mortality rates were improved significantly in the hypothermia group (41% vs. 55%; $P = 0.02$). Based on this difference, seven patients would need to be treated with hypothermia to prevent one death. The rate of complications (e.g., bleeding, pneumonia, sepsis, and renal failure) did not differ between the two groups (73% for the hypothermia group and 70% for the normothermia group; $P = 0.70$).

The second trial was conducted in four hospitals in Melbourne, Australia.[102] Entry criteria were similar to the previous trial, but the target temperature for hypothermia was 33°C (91.4°F), which was maintained for 12 hours. The primary outcome measure was survival to hospital discharge with good neurologic function. Forty-nine percent of patients in the hypothermia group had good neurologic function on discharge (to either home or a rehabilitation facility) compared with 26% of patients in the normothermia group ($P = 0.046$). Mortality rates were similar between the two groups (51% for the hypothermia group and 68% for the normothermia group; $P = 0.145$). Hypothermia was associated with a lower cardiac index, higher systemic vascular resistance, and hyperglycemia. It is important to note that only 8% of patients with cardiac arrest were selected for therapeutic hypothermia in these two studies.

Since that time, further data have continued to accumulate, including studies in arrests caused by rhythms other than VF. In one study, therapeutic hypothermia (combined with PCI, tight glycemic control, and seizure control) doubled the 1-year survival rate (reportedly with good brain function) from 26% to 56%.[103] The implementation of therapeutic hypothermia in clinical practice (i.e., outside of the context of a clinical trial) has also been evaluated. A review of this topic showed that there is a significant variation in reported protocols, but that survival and neurologic outcomes benefit from postarrest hypothermia and "are robust when compared over a wide range of studies of actual implementation" (OR [95% CI] = 2.5 [1.8 to 3.3]).[104] Nevertheless, there remains significant debate about hypothermia including when to consider limitation of care given a predicted poor outcome.[105] Initially hypothermia was described with only VF without sustained circulatory shock. As part of the "cardiocerebral" concept described above, investigations have expanded to non-VF arrests since similar benefit is being found.[27,106] In addition, there are case series of using therapeutic hypothermia in combination with emergent percutaneous coronary angioplasty.[27,107]

Methods of inducing hypothermia also continue to be in evaluation. There is debate over how quickly to achieve a therapeutic temperature, and in at least one animal model, a novel immersion device showed an average time to reach target temperature of only 9 minutes.[108] As well, simple maneuvers, such as iced saline infusion, can be used even in the prehospital setting with subsequent cooling by other means.[27,109] There were editorials clamoring for ongoing studies regarding methodologies and outcomes.[110,111] However, there is no consensus on the optimal method to induce hypothermia. Main methods currently in use include cold water immersion, endovascular cooling catheters, and surface cooling devices.[27]

In light of these accumulating data, unconscious adult patients with spontaneous circulation after out-of-hospital cardiac arrest should be cooled to 32°C to 34°C (89.6°F to 93.2°F) for 12 to 24 hours.[27,112] This is particularly true of VF arrest (Class I recommendation; Level of Evidence B).[27] There is less robust evidence for other arrests, but per the guidelines, hypothermia should be considered for comatose adult patients with ROSC after in-hospital cardiac arrest with any rhythm, and/or out-of-hospital cardiac arrest with an initial rhythm of PEA (Class IIb recommendation; Level of Evidence B).[27] However, given clinical experience that has been gained, most intensive care practitioners will use therapeutic hypothermia in the postarrest time frame regardless of the rhythm.

Hypothermia must be used with caution, however, as there are several complications that can develop. Coagulopathy, dysrhythmias, hyperglycemia, increased incidence of pneumonia, as well as sepsis have been described.[27,102,113] In addition, hypothermia can have profound effects on drug distribution and elimination.[114] Although the duration of hypothermia is typically short, careful monitoring during this time period is necessary, particularly with vasoactive agents. Further research is required in this area.

Special Populations

Asthma

Asthma is a very common disorder, and despite modern therapies, there are still in excess of 2 million emergency room visits yearly.[115] Despite improvements in mechanical ventilation strategies, there are still 5,000 to 6,000 asthma-related deaths annually in the United States.[115] True cardiac arrest in asthma is infrequent, as the primary pathophysiology is respiratory compromise and the inability to ventilate.[116] Asthma exacerbations are a combination of bronchoconstriction, airway inflammation, and mucous plugging. This leads to severe air trapping, hyperinflation, and hemodynamic compromise. While wheezing is common in an asthma exacerbation, it does not correlate with the degree of airway obstruction. In contrast, as the airflow decreases with worsening disease, wheezing can disappear. In addition, several other disease states cause wheezing, including pulmonary edema, pneumonia, anaphylaxis, foreign bodies, and tumors.[115]

Patients with life-threatening asthma need to be treated aggressively with bronchodilators and corticosteroids. Adjunctive therapies include anticholinergics, magnesium sulfate, ketamine, helium/oxygen mixtures, or even inhaled anesthetics.[117–121] Noninvasive ventilation can be attempted if the patient is deteriorating and still awake for short-term support, and may prevent the need for mechanical ventilation.[122] The decision to intubate an asthmatic is a clinical judgment; the clinician needs to remain keenly aware that the endotracheal tube will not solve the airway problem, and that ongoing aggressive asthma management needs to continue after intubation. Mechanical ventilation in the asthmatic can be very difficult, and the intubation and positive pressure can trigger further bronchoconstriction or hemodynamic compromise.

The provision of BLS in asthma is unchanged. Similarly, standard ACLS measures should be followed.[115] However, since the effect of auto-positive end-expiratory pressure (PEEP), known as breath stacking, in an asthmatic with cardiac arrest is likely to be severe, a strategy of low respiratory rate and volume ventilation may be appropriate.[115] Similarly, for cardiac arrest in asthma, especially when ventilation is difficult, tension pneumothorax should be strongly considered (Class I recommendation; Level of Evidence C).[115]

Anaphylaxis

Anaphylaxis is a severe allergic reaction involving most organs, and can lead to airway obstruction and cardiovascular collapse.[115] It still accounts for between 500 and 1,000 deaths annually in the United States.[123] The initial signs can be nonspecific, but with a severe reaction a "sense of impending doom" is common.[115] Rhinitis often leads to laryngeal edema with stridor in the upper airway, and bronchoconstriction often mimics an acute asthma attack as described above.

Cardiovascular collapse is common in severe reactions due to vasodilation and increased capillary permeability. This can rapidly lead to myocardial hypoperfusion and ischemia and to full cardiac arrest. There are no randomized trials of algorithms for arrest due to anaphylaxis.[115] Because of this lack of evidence, standard BLS and advanced life support should be provided.

Early advanced airway management is recommended due to the potential for rapid edema development. Epinephrine has been the mainstay of treatment for years, and continues to be listed first in the latest guidelines.[115] The recommended dose is 0.2 to 0.5 mg and should be administered via intramuscular injection to all patients with signs of systemic allergic reaction (Class I recommendation; Level of Evidence C).[115] This can be repeated every 5 to 15 minutes in the absence of clinical improvement. Vasopressin has been used successfully in patients who did not respond to standard therapy.[124] Fluid resuscitation is usually required for restoration of circulation and has been evaluated in one study where hypotension did not respond immediately to vasoactive drugs.[125] There are no prospective trials evaluating other agents in anaphylactic shock or arrest. Antihistamines, inhaled β-agonists, and IV corticosteroids have been used successfully in anaphylaxis and may be considered in cardiac arrest due to anaphylaxis.[115]

Pregnancy

Pregnancy is a unique situation in that survival of both the fetus and the mother depends on CPR. Despite the fact that pregnant patients are younger than the traditional cardiac arrest patient, the incidence of cardiac arrest in pregnancy seems to be on the rise, from 1 in 30,000 to 1 in 20,000.[115] In addition, the mortality rate of cardiac arrest with pregnancy seems to be higher, with one series reporting a survival rate of just 6.9%.[115,126]

The best hope for survival of the fetus is maternal survival. Because of the gravid uterus, resuscitation needs to be modified. Since the vena cava and aorta can be obstructed by a uterus of approximately 20 weeks gestation or later, it is appropriate to position the patient approximately 15° to 30° back from the left lateral decubitus position, or to pull the uterus to the side.[127] The optimal angle has been cited to be 27°, and has led to the development of the "Cardiff resuscitation wedge," which has been specifically designed for performing CPR on pregnant patients.[128] However, there are studies that suggest that manual left uterine displacement (with the patient supine) is as good as or better than lateral positioning.[129] Thus, the current guidelines suggest that manual left uterine displacement in the supine position be attempted to optimize CPR quality, and if this is unsuccessful, transitioning to a left lateral tilt position be attempted.[115]

Airway control is important in the pregnant patient. The airway may be smaller because of the hormonal changes and edema that accompany pregnancy.[128] Similarly, because of increased intraabdominal pressure exerted by the uterus, as well as hormonal changes that change the resting state of the gastroesophageal sphincter, clinicians need to be acutely aware of the increased risk of aspiration. Because of this, cricoid pressure needs to be maintained continuously during airway manipulation. The rescuer may need to give smaller tidal volumes than normal because of the diaphragm elevation that accompanies the later stages of pregnancy. Because of the increased ventilatory needs in pregnancy as well as the anatomic changes, some authors have suggested that it is important to perform early intubation during cardiac arrest in pregnancy and cite this rapid intubation as a difference from nonpregnant patients.[128] Similarly, circulatory support also has to be adjusted. In particular, chest compressions need to be administered slightly above the center of the sternum to adjust for the anatomic changes of the pregnant uterus.[115]

In an arrest situation during pregnancy the ACLS provider needs to follow the standard guidelines, including the same use of defibrillation and medications. While it is true that vasoactive agents, such as epinephrine, can diminish uterine blood flow, safer alternatives do not exist.[115] Available literature, though scant, suggests that the energy requirements for defibrillation do not change in pregnancy.[130]

While etiologies of arrest in pregnancy are often the same as in the nonpregnant patient, there are several unique situations that need to be considered in the differential diagnosis of a pregnancy arrest. These include excess magnesium sulfate administration (i.e., iatrogenic from treating eclampsia) in which case the therapeutic administration of calcium gluconate can be lifesaving; amniotic embolism, which is associated with complete cardiovascular collapse during labor and delivery (cardiopulmonary bypass has been reportedly successful in salvaging this condition); preeclampsia/eclampsia developing after the 20th week of gestation producing hypertension and multiple organ dysfunction; as well as vascular events including acute coronary syndromes and acute PE.[128,131,132]

It is paramount to remember that unless circulation is restored to the mother, both the mother and the fetus will succumb, especially if standard therapy is not used correctly and promptly. Because of this, the resuscitation leader should consider the need for emergent hysterotomy (i.e., Cesarean delivery) and delivery as soon as the arrest happens or if there is not immediate response after lateral uterine displacement and CPR. The best survival reported for infants >24 weeks gestation happens when delivery occurs no more than 5 minutes after the arrest of the mother.[115]

Hypothermia

Unintentional hypothermia (as opposed to the therapeutic hypothermia used postarrest, described above) is defined by a body temperature <30°C (86°F), and is associated with marked derangements in body function. Because it can depress virtually every body system, including pulse and respiration, the patient may appear to be dead on the initial evaluation. Hypothermia may lead to benefit on brain recovery after cardiac arrest (discussed earlier); thus, aggressive intervention is clearly indicated when there is a hypothermic arrest victim.

If the patient still has a perfusing rhythm, therapy is mainly based on rewarming techniques. For mild hypothermia (i.e., >34°C [>93.2°F]), passive rewarming is recommended. For moderate hypothermia (i.e., 30°C to 34°C [86°F to 93.2°F]), active external rewarming is recommended, and for severe hypothermia (i.e., <30°C [<86°F]), active internal rewarming is recommended. These patients need to be manipulated very gently as VF is sometimes precipitated by movement.[133]

If the patient is in cardiac arrest, then the standard BLS algorithm should be followed. However, there are some modifications that the rescuer needs to consider. The rescuer should evaluate for pulse for a longer time frame, since the heart rate may be slow or very difficult to palpate. If there is no pulse, then chest compressions and rescue breaths should ensue. If the patient is in VF or PVT, then electrical therapy should be given in a standard manner. However, the hypothermic heart may be less responsive to medications or defibrillation, and thus there have been worries about the optimal temperature at which to start defibrillation attempts.[115] There are no published consensus guidelines regarding this, but animal data support medications during CPR in cardiac arrest associated with hypothermia.[134] Immediately after defibrillation, CPR should resume as in the standard manner. During CPR, continued attempts at rewarming are of paramount importance. Included in this concept is preventing further heat loss (i.e., removal of wet clothing, protection from the environment, etc.). Patients often require significant volume challenges during the rewarming process. The use of steroids, antibiotics, and barbiturates has been proposed, but none of these agents have ever been shown to increase survival rates.[115]

It is debatable when to stop resuscitative efforts in the hypothermic patient. Many authors have proposed that a patient should not be pronounced dead until the core temperature has been restored to near normal.[115] Once the patient is in the hospital, it is still the judgment of the treating physician when efforts should be terminated.

Trauma

Cardiac resuscitation of the trauma arrest patient is basically performed with the same guidelines as with any other arrest. There are some specific etiologies to rapidly consider, however, since the survival of an out-of-hospital cardiac arrest due to trauma is rare.[115] The rescuer needs to consider airway obstruction, pneumothorax, tracheobronchial injury, cardiac or large arterial injury, cardiac tamponade, severe head injury with secondary cardiac collapse, and other injuries specific to the particular trauma.[115] The best survival seems to be in young patients with treatable penetrating injuries.

Trauma patients often suffer head or cervical injuries; thus, cervical spine precautions should be used in these patients. A jaw thrust maneuver is the preferred way to open the airway, with in-line stabilization during attempts at advanced airway placement.[115] The rescuer must be vigilant for the development of tension pneumothorax during ventilation. Inadequate ventilation of one side is usually due to tube malposition, tension pneumothorax, or hemothorax. These conditions are usually treated by medical personnel at the hospital after transport.

Chest compressions should be performed in a standard manner. Any visible hemorrhage should be controlled with direct pressure. Fluid resuscitation is done with a goal of adequate blood pressure and organ perfusion. The specific details of fluid resuscitation are highly controversial, however, and the optimal volume infusion for trauma resuscitation is a subject of ongoing debate.

Open thoracotomy for trauma-induced arrest has been performed in many instances. For penetrating chest trauma patients who arrest immediately before arrival or in the emergency department, open thoracotomy can allow relief of tamponade, control of major vessel hemorrhage, or direct repair of cardiac insult.[115] Furthermore, some have suggested that a physician-led, out-of-hospital thoracotomy for penetrating trauma may have a higher chance of survival.[135] In the case of blunt trauma, however, open thoracotomy has not been shown to definitively improve outcome.

A unique phenomenon of cardiac arrest (usually VF) caused by a blow to the anterior chest or sternum during the repolarization part of the cardiac cycle is called "commotio cordis."[136] These events are commonly seen in young athletes, and can be caused by a myriad of mechanisms, from falling directly on the sternum to the strike of a baseball or hockey puck. Prompt recognition is of paramount importance, as rapid defibrillation is often lifesaving. Provision of BLS, the use of an automatic external defibrillator, and standard ACLS are appropriate for this type of arrest.

For definitive postarrest care, trauma patients should be rapidly transferred to a facility with expertise in the provision of trauma care, and practitioners should consult guidelines for terminating efforts of cardiac arrest published by the National Association of EMS Physicians and the American College of Surgeons Committee on Trauma.[115,137]

Drowning

Drowning is a process resulting in primary respiratory impairment from immersion in a liquid. It is a common, preventable cause of morbidity and mortality. The most important inciting event is the hypoxia induced by submersion. Thus, early care of the drowning patient includes immediate rescue breathing, even before he or she is removed from the water. Prompt initiation of this therapy increases chance of survival.[138] Once the victim is removed from the water, immediate chest compressions should be started if he or she is pulseless. Drowning victims can present with any of the pulseless rhythms; standard guidelines need to be followed for therapy of these rhythms.

Electrocution/Lightning

There are many etiologies of electrical shock injuries, from lightning strike (mortality estimated to be 30%, with 70% of survivors sustaining significant morbidity) to high-tension current, to household current.[115] The severity of injury depends on the site, type of current, duration of contact, pathway, and the magnitude of delivered electricity.

Cardiac arrest is common in electrical injury due to current passing through the heart during the "vulnerable period" of the cardiac cycle. In large-current events, such as lightning strike, the heart undergoes massive depolarization simultaneously.[139] Sometimes the intrinsic pacemaker can restore an organized cardiac electrical cycle, but because of injury to other muscles, specifically the thoracic musculature, the patient cannot retain or sustain viable circulation due to the lack of ventilation and oxygenation.[140]

When approaching a victim of electrocution, the rescuer must first be certain of his or her own safety. Thereafter, standard BLS, prompt CPR, and ACLS when available are indicated. Electric shock is often associated with multiple trauma, including spinal injury, multiple injuries to the skeletal muscles, as well as fractures. These factors need to be evaluated by the resuscitation team.

Airway control may be difficult due to the edema that often accompanies such injuries; thus, an advanced airway early in the treatment process is recommended.[115] With soft-tissue swelling, there is often a need for aggressive fluid resuscitation in these patients. The underlying tissue, or visceral organ damage, is often worse than the external appearance. It is usually recommended that these patients be transferred to centers with expertise in dealing with these types of injuries.

Drug Administration

The routes of administration that are available for drug delivery during CPR include IV (both central and peripheral access), IO, and endotracheal. The chosen route represents a compromise between the availability of access and their apparent efficacy in introducing the drug into the central circulation. When selecting a route for drug administration, it is of utmost importance to minimize any interruptions in chest compressions during CPR.

Central venous access will result in a faster and higher peak drug concentration than peripheral access, but central line access is not needed in most resuscitation attempts. If a central line is already present, however, it should be the access site of choice. An appropriately trained provider may consider placing a central line if one is not present, but CPR should not be interrupted. Central lines located above the diaphragm are preferable to those located below the diaphragm because of poor blood flow during CPR.[141] If IV access (either central or peripheral) has not been established, a large peripheral venous catheter should be inserted. It has been suggested that only one attempt at peripheral IV insertion be allowed.[142] If this is not successful, an IO device should be inserted. Peripheral drug administration yields a peak concentration in the major systemic arteries in roughly 1.5 to 3 minutes, but circulation time can be shortened by up to 40% if the drug is followed by a 20-mL fluid bolus with elevation of the extremity.[141]

7 IO administration is the preferred alternative route for administration if IV access cannot be achieved.[26] Several studies have documented the effectiveness and safety of this administration route in both adults and children.[143] Pharmacokinetic data have demonstrated similar areas under the curve and times to peak concentration for sternal IO and central IV administration.[144] There appears to be variability, though, based on the anatomic site for insertion as IO administration via the tibia delivered only 65% of the dose compared with that via the sternum. Potential anatomic sites for insertion for an IO needle are the distal tibia, the proximal tibia, the distal femur, the sternum, and the humerus.[143,144] There are several IO access devices that are commercially available allowing for rapid insertion and are easy to use. In fact, clinical trials have documented success rates of approximately 80% with placement times of roughly 1 to 2 minutes.[143] The high success rates for achieving vascular access (on first attempt) allow for more rapid drug administration (vs. IV therapy) and could offset the pharmacokinetic differences observed with this approach. Future pharmacokinetic studies are needed to identify the most optimal anatomic site for IO placement and if current dosing recommendations are appropriate.

In the event that neither IV nor IO access can be established, a few drugs can be administered through an endotracheal tube. These drugs are atropine, lidocaine, epinephrine, naloxone, and vasopressin.[26] There are no data with amiodarone. Medications administered through the endotracheal route, however, will have both a lower and a delayed peak concentration than when they are administered by the IV or IO routes. In fact, animal studies have suggested that the lower epinephrine concentrations achieved with endotracheal administration may lead to vasodilation through β-receptor activity. Clinical trials in humans have also failed to demonstrate any benefit with using the endotracheal route.[145,146] In one clinical trial, a lower rate of ROSC (15% vs. 27%, $P \leq 0.01$), hospital admission (9% vs. 20%, $P \leq 0.02$), and hospital discharge (0% vs. 5%, $P \leq 0.02$) was observed with endotracheal drug administration compared with that with IV.[146] If the endotracheal route is to be used, the recommended medication dose is 2 to 2.5 times larger than the IV/IO dose. Providers should dilute the medication in 5 to 10 mL of either sterile water or normal saline, but better drug absorption may be achieved with sterile water.[26]

Personalized Pharmacotherapy

Several investigators have evaluated factors associated with good neurologic outcome following a cardiac arrest in an attempt to better predict prognosis, optimize resources, and decrease the percentage of patients who are left neurologically devastated. Many factors have been identified that are related to survival to hospital discharge. These include age, the occurrence of a witnessed arrest, rapid implementation of bystander CPR, presence of VF/PVT as the initial rhythm, early defibrillation therapy, achievement of ROSC in the field, and time to ROSC.[3,147–149] In fact, one group developed a statistical prediction model whereby the probability for a good neurologic outcome was = $\exp(B)/1 + \exp(B)$, where $B = -0.02$ (age in years) − 0.109 (time to ROSC in minutes) + 0.677 (ROSC prior to hospital arrival; 1 if yes, 0 if no) + 2.442 in patients with VF.[147] For patients with PEA/asystole, $B = -0.037$ (age in years) − 0.076 (time to ROSC in minutes) + 1.735 (ROSC prior to hospital arrival; 1 if yes, 0 if no) + 1.462 (conversion to VF; 1 if yes, 0 if no) + 1.101. Areas under the receiver-operating characteristic curve were 0.867 for VF and 0.873 for PEA/asystole, indicating a high predictive ability.

Other studies have evaluated prognostic indicators to identify scenarios whereby little or no chance of survival may be evident and prehospital termination of resuscitation would be appropriate.[150–152] From these data, two rules have been developed. The first rule, referred to as the BLS rule, has three criteria: (a) the event was not witnessed by EMS personnel, (b) no AED was used or manual shock applied, and (c) ROSC was not achieved in the out-of-hospital setting. The second rule, referred to as the advanced life support rule, consists of the BLS criteria plus (a) the arrest was not witnessed by a bystander and (b) no bystander CPR was administered. In one validation study of 5,505 patients, these rules accurately identified patients who were unlikely to benefit from rapid transport to a hospital with a positive predictive value of 0.998 (BLS rule) and 1 (ALS rule) when all criteria were met, respectively.[153]

Most patients who achieve ROSC and hospital admission ultimately do not survive to discharge; therefore, factors encountered in the ICU setting have tremendous impact on the clinical outcome obtained. In fact, postcardiac arrest care has now been added as the fifth link in the "chain of survival."[27] In one study, the significance of hypotension following ROSC was evaluated.[154] Overall, the incidence of post-ROSC hypotension was 47% with higher mortality (65% vs. 37%, $P < 0.001$) and a decline in functional status (49% vs. 38%, $P < 0.001$) being noted among survivors. On multivariate analysis and adjustment for confounding variables, post-ROSC hypotension had an OR (95% CI) for mortality of 2.69 (2.45 to 2.96, $P < 0.001$). This represents an important area for bedside evaluation and potential target for therapy in the postresuscitation phase of cardiac arrest.

Prediction models have also been investigated for in-hospital cardiac arrest. One large analysis used data from more than 42,000 patients admitted over a 10-year period to develop a score card with 11 variables that were identified in a multivariate analysis[155] (Table 2-4). This model was highly successful in predicting survival with favorable neurologic outcome ranging from 70% in the top decile to 2.8% in the bottom decile. While this scoring system was not designed to identify scenarios where resuscitation may be futile, it can provide useful prognostic information for the medical team, patients, and families.

EVALUATION OF THERAPEUTIC OUTCOMES

To measure the success of resuscitation outcomes, therapeutic outcome monitoring should occur both during the resuscitation attempt and in the postresuscitation phase. The optimal outcome following CPR is an awake, responsive, spontaneously breathing patient. Patients must remain neurologically intact with minimal morbidity following the resuscitation if it is to be truly classified as a success.

Unfortunately, there are no reliable surrogate markers that can be used at the bedside to gauge the efficacy of CPR and a positive outcome. Nonetheless, heart rate, cardiac rhythm, and blood pressure should be assessed and documented throughout the resuscitation attempt and subsequent to each intervention. Determination of the presence or absence of a pulse is paramount to deciding which interventions may be appropriate. However, clinicians must be cautious to not exceed 10 seconds when checking for a pulse. Palpating a pulse to determine the efficacy of blood flow during CPR has not been shown to be useful.

CPP (= aortic diastolic pressure − right atrial diastolic pressure) and $ScvO_2$ correlate with cardiac output and myocardial blood flow and can provide information on the patient's response to therapy. Moreover, thresholds have been identified that are associated with poor achievement of ROSC (<15 mm Hg for CPP, <30% [0.30] for $ScvO_2$).[26] Because CPPs are not routinely available during CPR, arterial diastolic pressure can be used as a reasonable surrogate. Arterial diastolic pressure values less than 20 mm Hg are generally considered suboptimal.[26] $ETCO_2$ monitoring is another useful method to assess cardiac output during CPR and has been

TABLE 2-4 Cardiac Arrest Survival Postresuscitation In-Hospital (CASPRI) Score Card

Predictor	Points
Age group (years)	
<50	0
50–59	0
60–69	1
70–79	2
≥80	4
Initial arrest rhythm	
VF/PVT time to defibrillation (minutes)	
≤2	0
3	0
4–5	2
>5	3
PEA	6
Asystole	7
Prearrest CPC score	
1	0
2	2
3	9
≥4	9
Hospital location	
Telemetry unit	0
Intensive care unit	1
Nonmonitored unit	3
Duration of resuscitation (minutes)	
<2	0
2–4	0
5–9	3
10–14	5
15–19	6
20–24	6
25–29	6
≥30	8
Mechanical ventilation	3
Renal insufficiency	2
Hepatic insufficiency	4
Sepsis	3
Malignant disease	4
Hypotension	3

Interpretation

Score	Survival (%)
0–4	83
5–9	67
10–14	42
15–19	23
20–24	12
25–29	5.2
30–34	2.1
35–39	0
≥40	0

VF, ventricular fibrillation; PVT, pulseless ventricular tachycardia; CPC, cerebral performance category.

Data from reference 155.

associated with ROSC. The main determinant for carbon dioxide excretion is the rate of delivery from the peripheral sites (where it is produced) to the lungs. Increasing cardiac output (through effective CPR) will yield higher $ETCO_2$ levels as delivery of carbon dioxide to the lungs increases. Persistently low $ETCO_2$ values (<10 mm Hg [<1.3 kPa]) during CPR in intubated patients suggest ROSC is unlikely.[26]

ABBREVIATIONS

ACLS	advanced cardiac life support
AED	automated external defibrillator
AHA	American Heart Association
AND	allow natural death
BLS	basic life support
CCR	cardiocerebral resuscitation
CI	confidence interval
CPP	coronary perfusion pressure
CPR	cardiopulmonary resuscitation
DNAR	do not attempt resuscitation
ECC	emergency cardiovascular care
ECMO	extracorporeal membrane oxygenation
EMS	emergency medical services
$ETCO_2$	end-tidal carbon dioxide
IO	intraosseous
LVAD	left ventricular assist device
MI	myocardial infarction
OR	odds ratio
PCI	percutaneous coronary intervention
PE	pulmonary embolism
PEEP	positive end-expiratory pressure
PEA	pulseless electrical activity
PVT	pulseless ventricular tachycardia
ROSC	return of spontaneous circulation
$ScvO_2$	central venous oxygen saturation
THAM	tromethamine
tPA	tissue plasminogen activator
VF	ventricular fibrillation

REFERENCES

1. Sandroni C, Nolan J, Cavallaro F, Antonelli M. In-hospital cardiac arrest: Incidence, prognosis and possible measures to improve survival. Intensive Care Med 2007;33:237–245.
2. Travers AH, Rea TD, Bobrow BJ, et al. Part 4: CPR overview: 2010 American Heart Association guidelines for cardiopulmonary resuscitation and emergency cardiovascular care. Circulation 2010;122:S676–S684.
3. Sasson C, Rogers MA, Dahl J, Kellermann AL. Predictors of survival from out-of-hospital cardiac arrest: A systematic review and meta-analysis. Circ Cardiovasc Qual Outcomes 2010;3:63–81.
4. Meaney PA, Nadkarni VM, Kern KB, Indik JH, Halperin HR, Berg RA. Rhythms and outcomes of adult in-hospital cardiac arrest. Crit Care Med 2010;38:101–108.
5. Chugh SS, Reinier K, Teodorescu C, et al. Epidemiology of sudden cardiac death: Clinical and research implications. Prog Cardiovasc Dis 2008;51:213–228.
6. Weil MH, Tang W. Rhythms and outcomes of cardiac arrest. Crit Care Med 2010;38:310.
7. Nichol G, Thomas E, Callaway CW, et al. Regional variation in out-of-hospital cardiac arrest incidence and outcome. JAMA 2008;300:1423–1431.
8. Weil MH, Fries M. In-hospital cardiac arrest. Crit Care Med 2005;33:2825–2830.
9. Atkins DL, Everson-Stewart S, Sears GK, et al. Epidemiology and outcomes from out-of-hospital cardiac arrest in children: The Resuscitation Outcomes Consortium Epistry-Cardiac Arrest. Circulation 2009;119:1484–1491.
10. Berg MD, Schexnayder SM, Chameides L, et al. Part 13: Pediatric basic life support: 2010 American Heart Association guidelines for cardiopulmonary resuscitation and emergency cardiovascular care. Circulation 2010;122:S862–S875.

11. Myerburg RJ, Castellanos A. Emerging paradigms of the epidemiology and demographics of sudden cardiac arrest. Heart Rhythm 2006;3:235–239.
12. Kleinman ME, Chameides L, Schexnayder SM, et al. Part 14: Pediatric advanced life support: 2010 American Heart Association guidelines for cardiopulmonary resuscitation and emergency cardiovascular care. Circulation 2010;122:S876–S908.
13. Ewy GA, Kern KB. Recent advances in cardiopulmonary resuscitation: Cardiocerebral resuscitation. J Am Coll Cardiol 2009;53:149–157.
14. Cooper JA, Cooper JD, Cooper JM. Cardiopulmonary resuscitation: History, current practice, and future direction. Circulation 2006;114:2839–2849.
15. Christenson J, Andrusiek D, Everson-Stewart S, et al. Chest compression fraction determines survival in patients with out-of-hospital ventricular fibrillation. Circulation 2009;120:1241–1247.
16. Soar J, Edelson DP, Perkins GD. Delivering high-quality cardiopulmonary resuscitation in-hospital. Curr Opin Crit Care 2011;17:225–230.
17. Cave DM, Gazmuri RJ, Otto CW, et al. Part 7: CPR techniques and devices: 2010 American Heart Association guidelines for cardiopulmonary resuscitation and emergency cardiovascular care. Circulation 2010;122:S720–S728.
18. Morrison LJ, Kierzek G, Diekema DS, et al. Part 3: Ethics: 2010 American Heart Association guidelines for cardiopulmonary resuscitation and emergency cardiovascular care. Circulation 2010;122:S665–S675.
19. Young GB. Clinical practice. Neurologic prognosis after cardiac arrest. N Engl J Med 2009;361:605–611.
20. Kouwenhoven WB, Jude JR, Knickerbocker GG. Closed-chest cardiac massage. JAMA 1960;173:1064–1067.
21. Safar P. Community-wide cardiopulmonary resuscitation. J Iowa Med Soc 1964;54:629–635.
22. Cardiopulmonary resuscitation. JAMA 1966;198:372–379.
23. Rea TD, Helbock M, Perry S, et al. Increasing use of cardiopulmonary resuscitation during out-of-hospital ventricular fibrillation arrest: Survival implications of guideline changes. Circulation 2006;114:2760–2765.
24. Larsen MP, Eisenberg MS, Cummins RO, Hallstrom AP. Predicting survival from out-of-hospital cardiac arrest: A graphic model. Ann Emerg Med 1993;22:1652–1658.
25. Link MS, Atkins DL, Passman RS, et al. Part 6: Electrical therapies: Automated external defibrillators, defibrillation, cardioversion, and pacing: 2010 American Heart Association guidelines for cardiopulmonary resuscitation and emergency cardiovascular care. Circulation 2010;122:S706–S719.
26. Neumar RW, Otto CW, Link MS, et al. Part 8: Adult advanced cardiovascular life support: 2010 American Heart Association guidelines for cardiopulmonary resuscitation and emergency cardiovascular care. Circulation 2010;122:S729–S767.
27. Peberdy MA, Callaway CW, Neumar RW, et al. Part 9: Post-cardiac arrest care: 2010 American Heart Association guidelines for cardiopulmonary resuscitation and emergency cardiovascular care. Circulation 2010;122:S768–S786.
28. Berg RA, Hemphill R, Abella BS, et al. Part 5: Adult basic life support: 2010 American Heart Association guidelines for cardiopulmonary resuscitation and emergency cardiovascular care. Circulation 2010;122:S685–S705.
29. Eberle B, Dick WF, Schneider T, Wisser G, Doetsch S, Tzanova I. Checking the carotid pulse check: Diagnostic accuracy of first responders in patients with and without a pulse. Resuscitation 1996;33:107–116.
30. Swor R, Khan I, Domeier R, Honeycutt L, Chu K, Compton S. CPR training and CPR performance: Do CPR-trained bystanders perform CPR? Acad Emerg Med 2006;13:596–601.
31. Ewy GA. A clarion call for change. Curr Opin Crit Care 2009;15:181–184.
32. Assar D, Chamberlain D, Colquhoun M, et al. Randomised controlled trials of staged teaching for basic life support. 1. Skill acquisition at bronze stage. Resuscitation 2000;45:7–15.
33. Ewy GA. Cardiocerebral resuscitation: The new cardiopulmonary resuscitation. Circulation 2005;111: 2134–2142.
34. Weisfeldt ML, Becker LB. Resuscitation after cardiac arrest: A 3-phase time-sensitive model. JAMA 2002;288:3035–3038.
35. Mosier J, Itty A, Sanders A, et al. Cardiocerebral resuscitation is associated with improved survival and neurologic outcome from out-of-hospital cardiac arrest in elders. Acad Emerg Med 2010;17:269–275.
36. De Maio VJ, Stiell IG, Wells GA, Spaite DW. Optimal defibrillation response intervals for maximum out-of-hospital cardiac arrest survival rates. Ann Emerg Med 2003;42:242–250.
37. Cobb LA, Fahrenbruch CE, Walsh TR, et al. Influence of cardiopulmonary resuscitation prior to defibrillation in patients with out-of-hospital ventricular fibrillation. JAMA 1999;281:1182–1188.
38. Wik L, Hansen TB, Fylling F, et al. Delaying defibrillation to give basic cardiopulmonary resuscitation to patients with out-of-hospital ventricular fibrillation: A randomized trial. JAMA 2003;289:1389–1395.
39. Kellum MJ, Kennedy KW, Ewy GA. Cardiocerebral resuscitation improves survival of patients with out-of-hospital cardiac arrest. Am J Med 2006;119:335–340.
40. Garza AG, Gratton MC, Salomone JA, Lindholm D, McElroy J, Archer R. Improved patient survival using a modified resuscitation protocol for out-of-hospital cardiac arrest. Circulation 2009;119:2597–2605.
41. Koike S, Tanabe S, Ogawa T, et al. Immediate defibrillation or defibrillation after cardiopulmonary resuscitation. Prehosp Emerg Care 2011;15:393–400.
42. Valenzuela TD, Roe DJ, Nichol G, Clark LL, Spaite DW, Hardman RG. Outcomes of rapid defibrillation by security officers after cardiac arrest in casinos. N Engl J Med 2000;343:1206–1209.
43. Forcina MS, Farhat AY, O'Neil WW, Haines DE. Cardiac arrest survival after implementation of automated external defibrillator technology in the in-hospital setting. Crit Care Med 2009;37:1229–1236.
44. Tuseth V, Salem M, Pettersen R, et al. Percutaneous left ventricular assist in ischemic cardiac arrest. Crit Care Med 2009;37:1365–1372.
45. Sunde K. Experimental and clinical use of ongoing mechanical cardiopulmonary resuscitation during angiography and percutaneous coronary intervention. Crit Care Med 2008;36:S405–S408.
46. Varon J, Acosta P. Extracorporeal membrane oxygenation in cardiopulmonary resuscitation: Are we there yet? Crit Care Med 2008;36:2685–2686.
47. Chamberlain D, Frenneaux M, Fletcher D. The primacy of basics in advanced life support. Curr Opin Crit Care 2009;15:198–202.
48. Robinson LA, Brown CG, Jenkins J, et al. The effect of norepinephrine versus epinephrine on myocardial hemodynamics during CPR. Ann Emerg Med 1989; 18:336–340.

49. Paradis NA, Martin GB, Rivers EP, et al. Coronary perfusion pressure and the return of spontaneous circulation in human cardiopulmonary resuscitation. JAMA 1990;263:1106–1113.
50. Reynolds JC, Salcido DD, Menegazzi JJ. Conceptual models of coronary perfusion pressure and their relationship to defibrillation success in a porcine model of prolonged out-of-hospital cardiac arrest. Resuscitation 2012;83:900–906.
51. Attaran RR, Ewy GA. Epinephrine in resuscitation: Curse or cure? Future Cardiol 2010;6:473–482.
52. Olasveengen TM, Sunde K, Brunborg C, Thowsen J, Steen PA, Wik L. Intravenous drug administration during out-of-hospital cardiac arrest: A randomized trial. JAMA 2009;302:2222–2229.
53. Jacobs IG, Finn JC, Jelinek GA, Oxer HF, Thompson PL. Effect of adrenaline on survival in out-of-hospital cardiac arrest: A randomised double-blind placebo-controlled trial. Resuscitation 2011;82:1138–1143.
54. Hagihara A, Hasegawa M, Abe T, Nagata T, Wakata Y, Miyazaki S. Prehospital epinephrine use and survival among patients with out-of-hospital cardiac arrest. JAMA 2012;307:1161–1168.
55. Sutton RM, Berg RA, Helfaer MA. Epinephrine for resuscitation from cardiac arrest: A double-edged sword? Crit Care Med 2009;37:1518–1520.
56. Ristagno G, Tang W, Huang L, et al. Epinephrine reduces cerebral perfusion during cardiopulmonary resuscitation. Crit Care Med 2009;37:1408–1415.
57. Rivers EP, Wortsman J, Rady MY, Blake HC, McGeorge FT, Buderer NM. The effect of the total cumulative epinephrine dose administered during human CPR on hemodynamic, oxygen transport, and utilization variables in the postresuscitation period. Chest 1994;106:1499–1507.
58. Huang L, Sun S, Fang X, Tang W, Weil MH. Simultaneous blockade of alpha1- and beta-actions of epinephrine during cardiopulmonary resuscitation. Crit Care Med 2006;34:S483–S485.
59. Larabee TM, Liu KY, Campbell JA, Little CM. Vasopressors in cardiac arrest: A systematic review. Resuscitation 2012;83:932–939.
60. Ornato JP. Use of adrenergic agonists during CPR in adults. Ann Emerg Med 1993;22:411–416.
61. Brown C, Wiklund L, Bar-Joseph G, et al. Future directions for resuscitation research. IV. Innovative advanced life support pharmacology. Resuscitation 1996;33:163–177.
62. Callaham M, Madsen CD, Barton CW, Saunders CE, Pointer J. A randomized clinical trial of high-dose epinephrine and norepinephrine vs standard-dose epinephrine in prehospital cardiac arrest. JAMA 1992;268:2667–2672.
63. Lindner KH, Ahnefeld FW, Grunert A. Epinephrine versus norepinephrine in prehospital ventricular fibrillation. Am J Cardiol 1991;67:427–428.
64. Redding JS, Pearson JW. Evaluation of drugs for cardiac resuscitation. Anesthesiology 1963;24:203–207.
65. Wenzel V, Raab H, Dunser MW. Role of arginine vasopressin in the setting of cardiopulmonary resuscitation. Best Pract Res Clin Anaesthesiol 2008;22:287–297.
66. Lindner KH, Haak T, Keller A, Bothner U, Lurie KG. Release of endogenous vasopressors during and after cardiopulmonary resuscitation. Heart 1996;75: 145–150.
67. Lindner KH, Dirks B, Strohmenger HU, Prengel AW, Lindner IM, Lurie KG. Randomised comparison of epinephrine and vasopressin in patients with out-of-hospital ventricular fibrillation. Lancet 1997;349:535–537.
68. Stiell IG, Hebert PC, Wells GA, et al. Vasopressin versus epinephrine for inhospital cardiac arrest: A randomised controlled trial. Lancet 2001;358:105–109.
69. Wenzel V, Krismer AC, Arntz HR, Sitter H, Stadlbauer KH, Lindner KH. A comparison of vasopressin and epinephrine for out-of-hospital cardiopulmonary resuscitation. N Engl J Med 2004;350:105–113.
70. Callaway CW, Hostler D, Doshi AA, et al. Usefulness of vasopressin administered with epinephrine during out-of-hospital cardiac arrest. Am J Cardiol 2006;98:1316–1321.
71. Gueugniaud PY, David JS, Chanzy E, et al. Vasopressin and epinephrine vs. epinephrine alone in cardiopulmonary resuscitation. N Engl J Med 2008;359:21–30.
72. Mentzelopoulos SD, Zakynthinos SG, Tzoufi M, et al. Vasopressin, epinephrine, and corticosteroids for in-hospital cardiac arrest. Arch Intern Med 2009;169:15–24.
73. Mukoyama T, Kinoshita K, Nagao K, Tanjoh K. Reduced effectiveness of vasopressin in repeated doses for patients undergoing prolonged cardiopulmonary resuscitation. Resuscitation 2009;80:755–761.
74. Ong ME, Tiah L, Leong BS, et al. A randomised, double-blind, multi-centre trial comparing vasopressin and adrenaline in patients with cardiac arrest presenting to or in the emergency department. Resuscitation 2012;83:953–960 [Epub ahead of print].
75. Mentzelopoulos SD, Zakynthinos SG, Siempos I, Malachias S, Ulmer H, Wenzel V. Vasopressin for cardiac arrest: Meta-analysis of randomized controlled trials. Resuscitation 2012;83:32–39.
76. Ong ME, Pellis T, Link MS. The use of antiarrhythmic drugs for adult cardiac arrest: A systematic review. Resuscitation 2011;82:665–670.
77. Kudenchuk PJ, Cobb LA, Copass MK, et al. Amiodarone for resuscitation after out-of-hospital cardiac arrest due to ventricular fibrillation. N Engl J Med 1999;341:871–878.
78. Dorian P, Cass D, Schwartz B, Cooper R, Gelaznikas R, Barr A. Amiodarone as compared with lidocaine for shock-resistant ventricular fibrillation. N Engl J Med 2002;346:884–890.
79. Rea RS, Kane-Gill SL, Rudis MI, et al. Comparing intravenous amiodarone or lidocaine, or both, outcomes for inpatients with pulseless ventricular arrhythmias. Crit Care Med 2006;34:1617–1623.
80. Harrison EE. Lidocaine in prehospital countershock refractory ventricular fibrillation. Ann Emerg Med 1981;10:420–423.
81. Weaver WD, Fahrenbruch CE, Johnson DD, Hallstrom AP, Cobb LA, Copass MK. Effect of epinephrine and lidocaine therapy on outcome after cardiac arrest due to ventricular fibrillation. Circulation 1990;82:2027–2034.
82. Herlitz J, Ekstrom L, Wennerblom B, et al. Lidocaine in out-of-hospital ventricular fibrillation. Does it improve survival? Resuscitation 1997;33:199–205.
83. Abu-Laban RB, Christenson JM, Innes GD, et al. Tissue plasminogen activator in cardiac arrest with pulseless electrical activity. N Engl J Med 2002;346:1522–1528.
84. Bottiger BW, Arntz HR, Chamberlain DA, et al. Thrombolysis during resuscitation for out-of-hospital cardiac arrest. N Engl J Med 2008;359:2651–2662.
85. Nadkarni VM, Larkin GL, Peberdy MA, et al. First documented rhythm and clinical outcome from in-hospital cardiac arrest among children and adults. JAMA 2006;295:50–57.
86. Hachimi-Idrissi S, Corne L, Ebinger G, Michotte Y, Huyghens L. Mild hypothermia induced by a helmet device: A clinical feasibility study. Resuscitation 2001;51:275–281.

87. Gonzalez ER. Pharmacologic controversies in CPR. Ann Emerg Med 1993;22:317–323.
88. Bohm K, Rosenqvist M, Herlitz J, Hollenberg J, Svensson L. Survival is similar after standard treatment and chest compression only in out-of-hospital bystander cardiopulmonary resuscitation. Circulation 2007;116: 2908–2912.
89. Levy MM. An evidence-based evaluation of the use of sodium bicarbonate during cardiopulmonary resuscitation. Crit Care Clin 1998;14:457–483.
90. Bjerneroth G. Tribonat—A comprehensive summary of its properties. Crit Care Med 1999;27:1009–1013.
91. Vukmir RB, Katz L, Sodium Bicarbonate Study Group. Sodium bicarbonate improves outcome in prolonged prehospital cardiac arrest. Am J Emerg Med 2006;24: 156–161.
92. Neumar RW, Nolan JP, Adrie C, et al. Post-cardiac arrest syndrome: Epidemiology, pathophysiology, treatment, and prognostication. A consensus statement from the International Liaison Committee on Resuscitation (American Heart Association, Australian and New Zealand Council on Resuscitation, European Resuscitation Council, Heart and Stroke Foundation of Canada, InterAmerican Heart Foundation, Resuscitation Council of Asia, and the Resuscitation Council of Southern Africa); the American Heart Association Emergency Cardiovascular Care Committee; the Council on Cardiovascular Surgery and Anesthesia; the Council on Cardiopulmonary, Perioperative, and Critical Care; the Council on Clinical Cardiology; and the Stroke Council. Circulation 2008;118:2452–2483.
93. Safar P. Resuscitation from clinical death: Pathophysiologic limits and therapeutic potentials. Crit Care Med 1988;16:923–941.
94. Anyfantakis ZA, Baron G, Aubry P, et al. Acute coronary angiographic findings in survivors of out-of-hospital cardiac arrest. Am Heart J 2009;157:312–318.
95. Nolan JP, Morley PT, Vanden Hoek TL, et al. Therapeutic hypothermia after cardiac arrest: An advisory statement by the advanced life support task force of the International Liaison Committee on Resuscitation. Circulation 2003;108:118–121.
96. Safar P, Xiao F, Radovsky A, et al. Improved cerebral resuscitation from cardiac arrest in dogs with mild hypothermia plus blood flow promotion. Stroke 1996;27:105–113.
97. Tsai M, Barbut D, Wang H, et al. Intra-arrest rapid head cooling improves postresuscitation myocardial function in comparison with delayed postresuscitation surface cooling. Crit Care Med 2008;36:S434–S439.
98. Guan J, Barbut D, Wang H, et al. A comparison between head cooling begun during cardiopulmonary resuscitation and surface cooling after resuscitation in a pig model of cardiac arrest. Crit Care Med 2008;36:S428–S433.
99. Dine CJ, Abella BS. Therapeutic hypothermia for neuroprotection. Emerg Med Clin North Am 2009;27: 137–149.
100. O'Sullivan ST, O'Shaughnessy M, O'Connor TP. Baron Larrey and cold injury during the campaigns of Napoleon. Ann Plast Surg 1995;34:446–449.
101. Hypothermia After Cardiac Arrest Study Group. Mild therapeutic hypothermia to improve the neurologic outcome after cardiac arrest. N Engl J Med 2002;346:549–556.
102. Bernard SA, Gray TW, Buist MD, et al. Treatment of comatose survivors of out-of-hospital cardiac arrest with induced hypothermia. N Engl J Med 2002;346:557–563.
103. Sunde K, Pytte M, Jacobsen D, et al. Implementation of a standardised treatment protocol for post resuscitation care after out-of-hospital cardiac arrest. Resuscitation 2007;73:29–39.
104. Sagalyn E, Band RA, Gaieski DF, Abella BS. Therapeutic hypothermia after cardiac arrest in clinical practice: Review and compilation of recent experiences. Crit Care Med 2009;37:S223–S226.
105. Sunde K, Steen PA. Studies in hypothermia-treated cardiac arrest patients are needed to establish the accuracy of proposed outcome predictors. Crit Care Med 2009;37: 2485–2486.
106. Oddo M, Ribordy V, Feihl F, et al. Early predictors of outcome in comatose survivors of ventricular fibrillation and non-ventricular fibrillation cardiac arrest treated with hypothermia: A prospective study. Crit Care Med 2008;36:2296–2301.
107. Hovdenes J, Laake JH, Aaberge L, Haugaa H, Bugge JF. Therapeutic hypothermia after out-of-hospital cardiac arrest: Experiences with patients treated with percutaneous coronary intervention and cardiogenic shock. Acta Anaesthesiol Scand 2007;51:137–142.
108. Janata A, Weihs W, Bayegan K, et al. Therapeutic hypothermia with a novel surface cooling device improves neurologic outcome after prolonged cardiac arrest in swine. Crit Care Med 2008;36:895–902.
109. Kim F, Olsufka M, Carlbom D, et al. Pilot study of rapid infusion of 2 L of 4 degrees C normal saline for induction of mild hypothermia in hospitalized, comatose survivors of out-of-hospital cardiac arrest. Circulation 2005;112:715–719.
110. Drabek T, Kochanek PM. In quest of the optimal cooling device: Isn't faster "too fast"? Crit Care Med 2008;36: 1018–1020.
111. Levine RL. Cardiocerebral resuscitation: Few answers, more questions. Crit Care Med 2009;37:747–748.
112. Gaieski DF, Abella BS, Goyal M. CPR and postarrest care: Overview, documentation, and databases. Chest 2012;141: 1082–1089.
113. Bunch TJ, White RD, Gersh BJ, et al. Long-term outcomes of out-of-hospital cardiac arrest after successful early defibrillation. N Engl J Med 2003;348:2626–2633.
114. Arpino PA, Greer DM. Practical pharmacologic aspects of therapeutic hypothermia after cardiac arrest. Pharmacotherapy 2008;28:102–111.
115. Vanden Hoek TL, Morrison LJ, Shuster M, et al. Part 12: Cardiac arrest in special situations: 2010 American Heart Association guidelines for cardiopulmonary resuscitation and emergency cardiovascular care. Circulation 2010;122: S829–S861.
116. McFadden ER Jr, Warren EL. Observations on asthma mortality. Ann Intern Med 1997;127:142–147.
117. Hess DR, Acosta FL, Ritz RH, Kacmarek RM, Camargo CA Jr. The effect of heliox on nebulizer function using a beta-agonist bronchodilator. Chest 1999;115:184–189.
118. Petrillo TM, Fortenberry JD, Linzer JF, Simon HK. Emergency department use of ketamine in pediatric status asthmaticus. J Asthma 2001;38:657–664.
119. Rodrigo GJ, Castro-Rodriguez JA. Anticholinergics in the treatment of children and adults with acute asthma: A systematic review with meta-analysis. Thorax 2005;60: 740–746.
120. Schultz TE. Sevoflurane administration in status asthmaticus: A case report. AANA J 2005;73:35–36.
121. Silverman RA, Osborn H, Runge J, et al. IV magnesium sulfate in the treatment of acute severe asthma: A multicenter randomized controlled trial. Chest 2002;122:489–497.

122. Soroksky A, Stav D, Shpirer I. A pilot prospective, randomized, placebo-controlled trial of bilevel positive airway pressure in acute asthmatic attack. Chest 2003;123:1018–1025.
123. Neugut AI, Ghatak AT, Miller RL. Anaphylaxis in the United States: An investigation into its epidemiology. Arch Intern Med 2001;161:15–21.
124. Schummer C, Wirsing M, Schummer W. The pivotal role of vasopressin in refractory anaphylactic shock. Anesth Analg 2008;107:620–624.
125. Brown SG, Blackman KE, Stenlake V, Heddle RJ. Insect sting anaphylaxis; prospective evaluation of treatment with intravenous adrenaline and volume resuscitation. Emerg Med J 2004;21:149–154.
126. Dijkman A, Huisman CM, Smit M, et al. Cardiac arrest in pregnancy: Increasing use of perimortem caesarean section due to emergency skills training? BJOG 2010;117:282–287.
127. Goodwin AP, Pearce AJ. The human wedge. A manoeuvre to relieve aortocaval compression during resuscitation in late pregnancy. Anaesthesia 1992;47:433–434.
128. Atta E, Gardner M. Cardiopulmonary resuscitation in pregnancy. Obstet Gynecol Clin North Am 2007;34:585–597.
129. Kundra P, Khanna S, Habeebullah S, Ravishankar M. Manual displacement of the uterus during Caesarean section. Anaesthesia 2007;62:460–465.
130. Nanson J, Elcock D, Williams M, Deakin CD. Do physiological changes in pregnancy change defibrillation energy requirements? Br J Anaesth 2001;87:237–239.
131. Munro PT. Management of eclampsia in the accident and emergency department. J Accid Emerg Med 2000;17:7–11.
132. Stanten RD, Iverson LI, Daugharty TM, Lovett SM, Terry C, Blumenstock E. Amniotic fluid embolism causing catastrophic pulmonary vasoconstriction: Diagnosis by transesophageal echocardiogram and treatment by cardiopulmonary bypass. Obstet Gynecol 2003;102:496–498.
133. Hanania NA, Zimmerman JL. Accidental hypothermia. Crit Care Clin 1999;15:235–249.
134. Wira CR, Becker JU, Martin G, Donnino MW. Anti-arrhythmic and vasopressor medications for the treatment of ventricular fibrillation in severe hypothermia: A systematic review of the literature. Resuscitation 2008;78:21–29.
135. Lockey D, Crewdson K, Davies G. Traumatic cardiac arrest: Who are the survivors? Ann Emerg Med 2006;48: 240–244.
136. Link MS, Maron BJ, Wang PJ, VanderBrink BA, Zhu W, Estes NA 3rd. Upper and lower limits of vulnerability to sudden arrhythmic death with chest-wall impact (commotio cordis). J Am Coll Cardiol 2003;41:99–104.
137. Hopson LR, Hirsh E, Delgado J, et al. Guidelines for withholding or termination of resuscitation in prehospital traumatic cardiopulmonary arrest. J Am Coll Surg 2003;196:475–481.
138. Kyriacou DN, Arcinue EL, Peek C, Kraus JF. Effect of immediate resuscitation on children with submersion injury. Pediatrics 1994;94:137–142.
139. Browne BJ, Gaasch WR. Electrical injuries and lightning. Emerg Med Clin North Am 1992;10:211–229.
140. Milzman DP, Moskowitz L, Hardel M. Lightning strikes at a mass gathering. South Med J 1999;92:708–710.
141. Vincent R. Drugs in modern resuscitation. Br J Anaesth 1997;79:188–197.
142. Kellum MJ. Improving performance of emergency medical services personnel during resuscitation of cardiac arrest patients: The McMAID approach. Curr Opin Crit Care 2009;15:216–220.
143. Weiser G, Hoffmann Y, Galbraith R, Shavit I. Current advances in intraosseous infusion—A systematic review. Resuscitation 2012;83:20–26.
144. Hoskins SL, do Nascimento P Jr, Lima RM, Espana-Tenorio JM, Kramer GC. Pharmacokinetics of intraosseous and central venous drug delivery during cardiopulmonary resuscitation. Resuscitation 2012;83:107–112.
145. Niemann JT, Stratton SJ. Endotracheal versus intravenous epinephrine and atropine in out-of-hospital "primary" and postcountershock asystole. Crit Care Med 2000;28: 1815–1819.
146. Niemann JT, Stratton SJ, Cruz B, Lewis RJ. Endotracheal drug administration during out-of-hospital resuscitation: Where are the survivors? Resuscitation 2002;53:153–157.
147. Hayakawa K, Tasaki O, Hamasaki T, et al. Prognostic indicators and outcome prediction model for patients with return of spontaneous circulation from cardiopulmonary arrest: The Utstein Osaka Project. Resuscitation 2011;82:874–880.
148. Herlitz J, Engdahl J, Svensson L, Angquist KA, Young M, Holmberg S. Factors associated with an increased chance of survival among patients suffering from an out-of-hospital cardiac arrest in a national perspective in Sweden. Am Heart J 2005;149:61–66.
149. Stiell IG, Wells GA, Field B, et al. Advanced cardiac life support in out-of-hospital cardiac arrest. N Engl J Med 2004;351:647–656.
150. Morrison LJ, Verbeek PR, Vermeulen MJ, et al. Derivation and evaluation of a termination of resuscitation clinical prediction rule for advanced life support providers. Resuscitation 2007;74:266–275.
151. Morrison LJ, Visentin LM, Kiss A, et al. Validation of a rule for termination of resuscitation in out-of-hospital cardiac arrest. N Engl J Med 2006;355:478–487.
152. Verbeek PR, Vermeulen MJ, Ali FH, Messenger DW, Summers J, Morrison LJ. Derivation of a termination-of-resuscitation guideline for emergency medical technicians using automated external defibrillators. Acad Emerg Med 2002;9:671–678.
153. Sasson C, Hegg AJ, Macy M, et al. Prehospital termination of resuscitation in cases of refractory out-of-hospital cardiac arrest. JAMA 2008;300:1432–1438.
154. Trzeciak S, Jones AE, Kilgannon JH, et al. Significance of arterial hypotension after resuscitation from cardiac arrest. Crit Care Med 2009;37:2895–2903 [quiz 904].
155. Chan PS, Spertus JA, Krumholz HM, et al. A validated prediction tool for initial survivors of in-hospital cardiac arrest. Arch Intern Med 2012;172:947–953.

3

Hypertension

Joseph J. Saseen and Eric J. MacLaughlin

KEY CONCEPTS

1. The risk of cardiovascular (CV) morbidity and mortality is directly correlated with blood pressure (BP).
2. Evidence from clinical trials have shown that antihypertensive drug therapy substantially reduces the risks of CV events and death in patients with high BP.
3. Essential hypertension is usually an asymptomatic disease. A diagnosis cannot be made based on one elevated BP measurement. An elevated value from the average of two or more measurements, present during two or more clinical encounters, is needed to diagnose hypertension.
4. The overall goal of treating hypertension is to reduce hypertension-associated morbidity and mortality from CV events. These are considered hypertension-associated complications. The selection of specific drug therapy should be based on evidence that demonstrates CV risk reduction.
5. A goal BP of <140/90 mm Hg is appropriate for general prevention of CV events and CV risk reduction in most patients. For some patients (e.g., diabetes and/or significant chronic kidney disease) lower goal BP values may be appropriate on a patient-specific basis.
6. Magnitude of BP elevation should be used to guide determination of the number of agents to start when implementing drug therapy. Most patients with stage 1 hypertension should be started on one drug, with the option of starting two for some patients. However, most patients presenting with stage 2 hypertension should be started on two drugs.
7. Lifestyle modifications should be prescribed in all patients, especially those with prehypertension and hypertension. However, they should never be used as a replacement for antihypertensive drug therapy for patients with hypertension, especially in those with additional CV risk factors.
8. Angiotensin-converting enzyme (ACE) inhibitors, angiotensin II receptor blockers (ARBs), calcium channel blockers (CCBs), and thiazide diuretics are all first-line agents for most patients with hypertension for general prevention of CV events and CV risk reduction. These first-line options are for patients with hypertension who do not have any compelling indications for a specific antihypertensive drug class.
9. For general prevention of CV events and CV risk reduction in most patients with hypertension, β-blockers do not reduce CV events to the extent that has been proven with thiazide-type diuretics, ACE inhibitors, ARBs, CCBs, or thiazide diuretics.
10. Compelling indications are comorbid conditions where specific antihypertensive drug classes have been shown in clinical trials to provide unique long-term benefits (reducing the risk of CV events).
11. Patients with diabetes are at high risk for CV events. All patients with diabetes and hypertension should ideally be managed with either an ACE inhibitor or an ARB. These are typically in combination with one or more other antihypertensive agents because multiple agents frequently are needed to control BP.
12. Older patients are often at risk for orthostatic hypotension when antihypertensive drug therapy is started. Although overall antihypertensive drug therapy should be the same as in younger patients, low initial doses should be used and dosage titrations should be gradual to minimize risk of orthostatic hypotension.
13. Alternative antihypertensive agents have not been proven to reduce the risk of CV events to the same extent compared with first-line antihypertensive agents. They should be used primarily in combination with first-line agents to provide additional BP lowering.
14. Initial therapy with the combination of two antihypertensive agents should be used in most patients presenting with stage 2 hypertension. This is also an option for patients presenting with stage 1 hypertension. Most patients require combination therapy to achieve goal BP.
15. Patients have resistant hypertension when they fail to attain goal BP values while adherent to a regimen that includes at least three agents at maximum dose, one of which includes a diuretic, or when four or more agents are needed to treat hypertension.
16. Hypertensive urgency is ideally managed by adjusting maintenance therapy, adding a new antihypertensive, and/or increasing the dose of a present medication. This provides a gradual reduction in BP, which is a safer treatment approach than rapid reductions in BP.

Hypertension is a common disease that is simply defined as persistently elevated arterial blood pressure (BP). Although elevated BP was perceived to be "essential" for adequate perfusion of vital organs during the early and middle 1900s, it is now identified as one of the most significant risk factors for cardiovascular (CV) disease. Increasing awareness and diagnosis of hypertension, and improving control of BP with appropriate treatment are considered critical public health initiatives to reduce CV morbidity and mortality.

The Seventh Report of the Joint National Committee on Prevention, Detection, Evaluation, and Treatment of High Blood Pressure (JNC7) is the most prominent evidence-based clinical guideline in the United States for the management of hypertension.[1] The Eighth Report of the Joint National Committee was under development for several years. In 2013, the sponsoring organization

(National Heart Lung and Blood Institute [NHLBI]) decided that the work of the JNC8 groups will be published as evidentiary reviews, not a guideline. However, the NHLBI will subsequently collaborate with another organization to prepare and issue an updated hypertension clinical practice guideline sometime after 2013. Once available, this will likely be viewed as the preeminent hypertension clinical guideline in the United States. The 2007 American Heart Association (AHA) Scientific Statement on the treatment of hypertension provides additional insight regarding pharmacotherapy for hypertension.[2] This chapter reviews relevant components of both these consensus documents and additional evidence from clinical trials, with a focus on the pharmacotherapy of hypertension.

The National Health and Nutrition Examination Survey and the National Center for Health Statistics regularly assess hypertension in the United States.[3] Data from 2007 to 2010 indicate that 77.9 million Americans aged 20 years and above have hypertension. Predictions indicate that by 2030 the prevalence of hypertension will increase by 7.2%. Approximately half of all patients with hypertension are at their goal BP value. While this control rate is substantially higher than in the past, there remain many opportunities for clinicians to improve the care of patients with hypertension.

EPIDEMIOLOGY

Approximately 1 in 3 adult Americans (77.9 million people) have elevated BP, defined as ≥140/90 mm Hg.[3] The overall incidence is similar between men and women, but varies depending on age. The percentage of men with high BP is higher than that of women before the age of 55 and is similar to that of women between the ages 55 and 64. However, after the age of 64, a much higher percentage of women have high BP than men.[3] Prevalence rates are highest in non-Hispanic blacks (47% in women, 43% in men), followed by non-Hispanic whites (31% in women, 33% in men), and Mexican Americans (29% in women, 30% in men).[3] With regard to BP control, 54.9% of non-Hispanic whites have controlled hypertension in contrast to 47.6% of non-Hispanic blacks and 39.3% in Mexican Americans.[3]

BP values increase with age, and hypertension (persistently elevated BP values) is very common in the elderly. The lifetime risk of developing hypertension among those 55 years of age and older who are normotensive is 90%.[1] Most patients have prehypertension before they are diagnosed with hypertension, with most diagnoses occurring between the third and fifth decades of life.

TABLE 3-1 Secondary Causes of Hypertension

Disease	Drugs and Other Products Associated with Hypertension[a]
Chronic kidney disease Cushing's syndrome Coarctation of the aorta Obstructive sleep apnea Parathyroid disease Pheochromocytoma Primary aldosteronism Renovascular disease Thyroid disease	**Prescription drugs** • Amphetamines (amphetamine, dexmethylphenidate, dextroamphetamine, lisdexamfetamine, methylphenidate, phendimetrazine, phentermine) and anorexiants (sibutramine) • Antivascular endothelin growth factor agents (bevacizumab, sorafenib, sunitinib) • Corticosteroids (cortisone, dexamethasone, fludrocortisone, hydrocortisone, methylprednisolone, prednisolone, prednisone, triamcinolone • Calcineurin inhibitors (cyclosporine, tacrolimus) • Decongestants (pseudoephedrine, phenylephrine) • Ergot alkaloids (ergonovine, methysergide) • Erythropoiesis-stimulating agents (erythropoietin, darbepoetin) • Estrogen-containing oral contraceptives • Nonsteroidal antiinflammatory drugs—cyclooxygenase-2 selective (celecoxib) and nonselective (aspirin, choline magnesium trisalicylate, diclofenac, diflunisal, etodolac, fenoprofen, flurbiprofen, ibuprofen, indomethacin, ketoprofen, ketorolac, meclofenamate, mefenamic acid, meloxicam, nabumetone, naproxen, naproxen sodium, oxaprozin, piroxicam, salsalate, sulindac, tolmetin) • Others: desvenlafaxine, venlafaxine, bupropion Situations: β-blocker or centrally acting α-agonists (when abruptly discontinued); β-blocker without α-blocker first when treating pheochromocytoma; use of a monoamine oxidase inhibitor (isocarboxazid, phenelzine, tranylcypromine) with tyramine-containing foods or certain drugs **Street drugs and other products** Cocaine and cocaine withdrawal Ephedra alkaloids (e.g., Ma huang), "herbal ecstasy," other analogues Nicotine and withdrawal, anabolic steroids, narcotic withdrawal, ergot-containing herbal products, St. John's wort **Food substances** Sodium Ethanol Licorice

[a]Agents of most clinical importance.

ETIOLOGY

In most patients, hypertension results from unknown pathophysiologic etiology (*essential* or *primary hypertension*). This form of hypertension cannot be cured, but it can be controlled. A small percentage of patients have a specific cause of their hypertension (*secondary hypertension*). There are many potential secondary causes that either are concurrent medical conditions or are endogenously induced. If the cause can be identified, hypertension in these patients can be mitigated or potentially be cured.

Essential Hypertension

Over 90% of individuals with high BP have essential hypertension.[1] Numerous mechanisms have been identified that may contribute to the pathogenesis of this form of hypertension, so identifying the exact underlying abnormality is not possible. Genetic factors may play an important role in the development of essential hypertension. There are monogenic and polygenic forms of BP dysregulation that may be responsible for essential hypertension.[4] Many of these genetic traits feature genes that affect sodium balance, but genetic mutations altering urinary kallikrein excretion, nitric oxide release, and excretion of aldosterone, other adrenal steroids, and angiotensinogen are also documented.[4] In the future, genetic testing for these traits could lead to alternative approaches to preventing or treating hypertension; however, this is not currently recommended.

Secondary Hypertension

Fewer than 10% of patients have secondary hypertension where either a comorbid disease or a drug (or other product) is responsible for elevating BP (see Table 3-1).[1,5] In most of these cases, renal dysfunction resulting from severe chronic kidney disease (CKD) or renovascular disease is the most common secondary cause. Certain drugs (or other products), either directly or indirectly, can cause hypertension or exacerbate hypertension by increasing BP. The most common agents are listed in Table 3-1. When a secondary cause is identified, removing the offending agent (when feasible) or treating/correcting the underlying comorbid condition should be the first step in management.

PATHOPHYSIOLOGY

Multiple factors that control BP are potential contributing components in the development of essential hypertension.[4,6] These include malfunctions in either humoral (i.e., the renin–angiotensin–aldosterone system [RAAS]) or vasodepressor mechanisms, abnormal neuronal mechanisms, defects in peripheral autoregulation, and disturbances in sodium, calcium, and natriuretic hormone. Many of these factors are cumulatively affected by the multifaceted RAAS, which ultimately regulates arterial BP. It is probable that no one factor is solely responsible for essential hypertension.

Arterial BP

Arterial BP is the pressure in the arterial wall measured in millimeters of mercury (mm Hg). The two typical arterial BP values are *systolic BP* (SBP) and *diastolic BP* (DBP). SBP represents the peak value, which is achieved during cardiac contraction. DBP is achieved after contraction when the cardiac chambers are filling, and represents the nadir value. The difference between SBP and DBP is called the pulse pressure and is a measure of arterial wall tension. Mean arterial pressure (MAP) is the average pressure throughout the cardiac cycle of contraction. It is sometimes used clinically to represent overall arterial BP, especially in hypertensive emergency. During a cardiac cycle, two thirds of the time is spent in diastole and one third in systole. Therefore, the MAP is calculated by using the following equation:

$$\text{MAP} = \left(\text{SBP} \times \frac{1}{3}\right) + \left(\text{DBP} \times \frac{2}{3}\right)$$

Arterial BP is hemodynamically generated by the interplay between blood flow and the resistance to blood flow. It is mathematically defined as the product of cardiac output (CO) and total peripheral resistance (TPR) according to the following equation:

$$\text{BP} = \text{CO} \times \text{TPR}$$

CO is the major determinant of SBP, whereas TPR largely determines DBP. In turn, CO is a function of stroke volume, heart rate, and venous capacitance. Table 3-2 lists physiologic causes of increased CO and TPR and correlates them to potential mechanisms of pathogenesis.

TABLE 3-2 Potential Mechanisms of Pathogenesis

Blood pressure (BP) is the mathematical product of cardiac output and peripheral resistance. Elevated BP can result from increased cardiac output and/or increased total peripheral resistance.

Increased cardiac output	Increased cardiac preload: • Increased fluid volume from excess sodium intake or renal sodium retention (from reduced number of nephrons or decreased glomerular filtration) Venous constriction: • Excess stimulation of the renin–angiotensin–aldosterone system (RAAS) • Sympathetic nervous system overactivity
Increased peripheral resistance	Functional vascular constriction: • Excess stimulation of the RAAS • Sympathetic nervous system overactivity • Genetic alterations of cell membranes • Endothelial-derived factors Structural vascular hypertrophy: • Excess stimulation of the RAAS • Sympathetic nervous system overactivity • Genetic alterations of cell membranes • Endothelial-derived factors • Hyperinsulinemia resulting from the metabolic syndrome

TABLE 3-3 Classification of Blood Pressure in Adults (Age ≥18 Years)[a]

Classification	Systolic Blood Pressure (mm Hg)		Diastolic Blood Pressure (mm Hg)
Normal	<120	and	<80
Prehypertension[b]	120–139	or	80–89
Stage 1 hypertension	140–159	or	90–99
Stage 2 hypertension	≥160	or	≥100

[a]Classification determined based on the average of two or more properly measured seated BP values from two or more clinical encounters. If systolic and diastolic BP values yield different classifications, the highest category is used for the purpose of determining a classification.
[b]For certain patients, BP values within the prehypertension range are considered above goal (see Box 3-2).

Under normal physiologic conditions, arterial BP fluctuates throughout the day following a circadian rhythm. BP decreases to its lowest daily values during sleep followed by a sharp rise starting a few hours prior to awakening with the highest values occurring midmorning. BP is also increased acutely during physical activity or emotional stress.

Classification

The classification of BP in adults (age 18 years and older) is based on the average of two or more properly measured BP values from two or more clinical encounters (Table 3-3).[1] It includes four categories: normal, prehypertension, stage 1 hypertension, and stage 2 hypertension. Prehypertension is not considered a disease category but identifies patients whose BP is likely to increase into the classification of hypertension in the future.

Hypertensive crises are clinical situations where BP values are very elevated, typically >180/120 mm Hg.[6] They are categorized as either *hypertensive emergency* or *hypertensive urgency*. Hypertensive emergencies are extreme elevations in BP that are accompanied by acute or progressing target-organ damage. Hypertensive urgencies are high elevations in BP without acute or progressing target-organ injury.

Cardiovascular Risk and Blood Pressure

1 Epidemiologic data demonstrate a strong correlation between BP and CV morbidity and mortality.[7] Risk of stroke, myocardial infarction (MI), angina, heart failure, kidney failure, or early death from a CV cause is directly correlated with BP. Starting at a BP of 115/75 mm Hg, risk of CV disease doubles with every 20/10 mm Hg increase.[1] Even patients with prehypertension have an increased risk of CV disease.

2 Treating patients with hypertension with antihypertensive drug therapy provides significant clinical benefits. Evidence from large-scale placebo-controlled clinical trials have shown that the increased risks of CV events and death associated with elevated BP are reduced substantially by antihypertensive therapy.[8–11] This is discussed in Treatment section of this chapter.

SBP is a stronger predictor of CV disease than DBP in adults aged 50 years and older; it is the most important clinical BP parameter for most patients.[1] Patients are considered to have *isolated systolic hypertension* when their SBP values are elevated (i.e., ≥140 mm Hg) and DBP values are not (i.e., <90 mm Hg, but commonly <80 mm Hg). Isolated systolic hypertension is believed to result from pathophysiologic changes in the arterial vasculature consistent with aging. These changes decrease the compliance of the arterial wall and portend an increased risk of CV morbidity and mortality. The elevated pulse pressure (SBP minus DBP) is believed to reflect extent of atherosclerotic disease in the elderly and is a measure of increased arterial stiffness. Higher pulse pressure values seen in those with isolated systolic hypertension are directly correlated with risk of CV mortality.

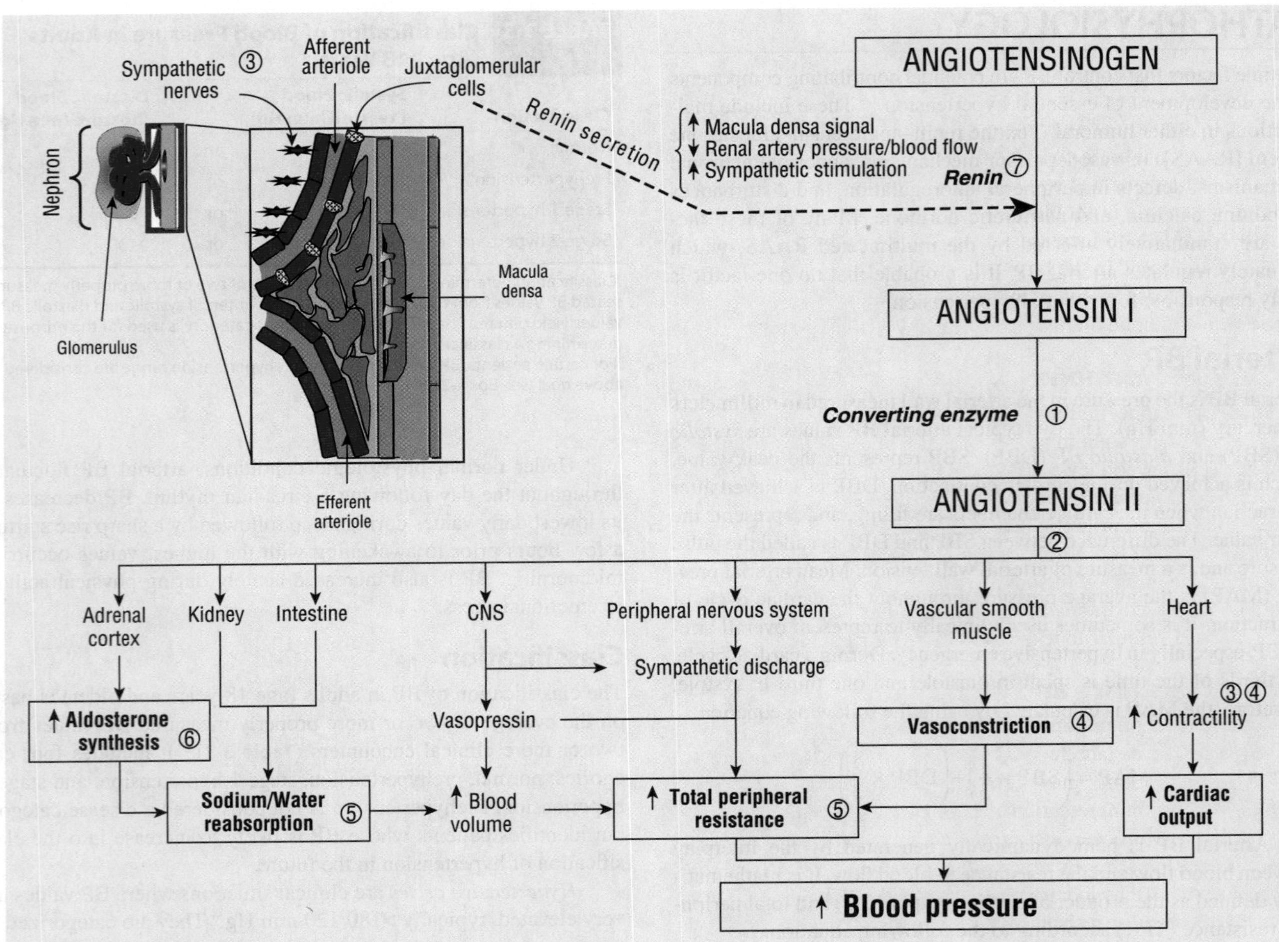

FIGURE 3-1 Diagram representing the renin–angiotensin–aldosterone system. The interrelationship between the kidney, angiotensin II, and regulation of blood pressure is depicted. Renin secretion from the juxtaglomerular cells in the afferent arterioles is regulated by three major factors to trigger conversion of angiotensinogen to angiotensin 1. The primary sites of action for major antihypertensive agents are included: ① ACE inhibitors; ② angiotensin II receptor blockers; ③ β-blockers; ④ calcium channel blockers; ⑤ diuretics; ⑥ aldosterone antagonists; ⑦ direct renin inhibitor.

Humoral Mechanisms

Several humoral abnormalities involving the RAAS, natriuretic hormone, and hyperinsulinemia may be involved in the development of essential hypertension.

The Renin–Angiotensin–Aldosterone System

The RAAS is a complex endogenous system involved with most regulatory components of arterial BP. Activation and regulation is primarily governed by the kidney (see Fig. 3-1). The RAAS regulates sodium, potassium, and blood volume. Therefore, this system significantly influences vascular tone and sympathetic nervous system activity, and is the most influential contributor to the homeostatic regulation of BP.

Renin is an enzyme that is stored in the juxtaglomerular cells, which are located in the afferent arterioles of the kidney. The release of renin is modulated by several factors: intrarenal factors (e.g., renal perfusion pressure, catecholamines, angiotensin II) and extrarenal factors (e.g., sodium, chloride, and potassium).

Juxtaglomerular cells function as a baroreceptor-sensing device. Decreased renal artery pressure and kidney blood flow is sensed by these cells and stimulates secretion of renin. The juxtaglomerular apparatus also includes a group of specialized distal tubule cells referred to collectively as the *macula densa*. A decrease in sodium and chloride delivered to the distal tubule stimulates renin release. Catecholamines increase renin release probably by directly stimulating sympathetic nerves on the afferent arterioles that in turn activate the juxtaglomerular cells.

Renin catalyzes the conversion of angiotensinogen to angiotensin I in the blood. Angiotensin I is then converted to angiotensin II by angiotensin-converting enzyme (ACE). After binding to specific receptors (classified as either angiotensin II type 1 [AT_1] or angiotensin II type 2 [AT_2] subtypes), angiotensin II exerts biologic effects in several tissues. The AT_1 receptor is located in brain, kidney, myocardium, peripheral vasculature, and the adrenal glands. These receptors mediate most responses that are critical to CV and kidney function. The AT_2 receptor is located in adrenal medullary tissue, uterus, and brain. Stimulation of the AT_2 receptor does not influence BP regulation.

Circulating angiotensin II can elevate BP through pressor and volume effects. Pressor effects include direct vasoconstriction, stimulation of catecholamine release from the adrenal medulla, and centrally mediated increases in sympathetic nervous system activity. Angiotensin II also stimulates aldosterone synthesis from the adrenal cortex. This leads to sodium and water reabsorption that increases plasma volume, TPR, and ultimately BP. Aldosterone also has a deleterious role in the pathophysiology of other CV diseases (e.g., heart failure, MI, kidney disease) by promoting tissue remodeling leading to myocardial fibrosis and vascular dysfunction. Clearly, any disturbance in the body that leads to activation of the RAAS could explain chronic hypertension.

The heart and brain contain a local RAAS. In the heart, angiotensin II is also generated by angiotensin I convertase (human chymase). This enzyme is not blocked by ACE inhibition. Activation of the myocardial RAAS increases cardiac contractility and stimulates cardiac hypertrophy. In the brain, angiotensin II modulates the production and release of hypothalamic and pituitary hormones, and enhances sympathetic outflow from the medulla oblongata.

Natriuretic Hormone

Natriuretic hormone inhibits sodium and potassium-ATPase and thus interferes with sodium transport across cell membranes. Inherited defects in the kidney's ability to eliminate sodium can cause increased blood volume. A compensatory increase in the concentration of circulating natriuretic hormone theoretically could increase urinary excretion of sodium and water. However, this hormone might block the active transport of sodium out of arteriolar smooth muscle cells. The increased intracellular sodium concentration ultimately would increase vascular tone and BP.

Insulin Resistance and Hyperinsulinemia

The combination of multiple CV and metabolic abnormalities is referred to as the metabolic syndrome.[12] Hypothetically, increased insulin concentrations may lead to hypertension because of increased renal sodium retention and enhanced sympathetic nervous system activity. Moreover, insulin has growth hormone–like actions that can induce hypertrophy of vascular smooth muscle cells. Insulin also may elevate BP by increasing intracellular calcium, which leads to increased vascular resistance. The exact mechanism by which insulin resistance and hyperinsulinemia occur in hypertension is unknown. However, this association is strong because many of the criteria used to define this population (i.e., elevated BP, abdominal obesity, high triglycerides, low high-density lipoprotein cholesterol, and elevated fasting glucose) are often present in patients with hypertension.[12]

Neuronal Regulation

Central and autonomic nervous systems are intricately involved in the regulation of arterial BP. Many receptors that either enhance or inhibit norepinephrine release are located on the presynaptic surface of sympathetic terminals. The α and β presynaptic receptors play a role in negative and positive feedback to the norepinephrine-containing vesicles. Stimulation of presynaptic α-receptors (α_2) exerts a negative inhibition on norepinephrine release. Stimulation of presynaptic β-receptors facilitates norepinephrine release.

Sympathetic neuronal fibers located on the surface of effector cells innervate the α- and β-receptors. Stimulation of postsynaptic α-receptors (α_1) on arterioles and venules results in vasoconstriction. There are two types of postsynaptic β-receptors, β_1 and β_2. Both are present in all tissues innervated by the sympathetic nervous system. However, in some tissues β_1-receptors predominate (e.g., heart), and in other tissues β_2-receptors predominate (e.g., bronchioles). Stimulation of β_1-receptors in the heart results in an increase in heart rate (chronotropy) and force of contraction (ionotropy), whereas stimulation of β_2-receptors in the arterioles and venules causes vasodilation.

The baroreceptor reflex system is the major negative feedback mechanism that controls sympathetic activity. Baroreceptors are nerve endings lying in the walls of large arteries, especially in the carotid arteries and aortic arch. Changes in arterial BP rapidly activate baroreceptors that then transmit impulses to the brain stem through the ninth cranial nerve and vagus nerve. In this reflex system, a decrease in arterial BP stimulates baroreceptors, causing reflex vasoconstriction and increased heart rate and force of cardiac contraction. These baroreceptor reflex mechanisms may be less responsive in the elderly and those with diabetes.

Stimulation of certain areas within the central nervous system (e.g., nucleus tractus solitarius, vagal nuclei, vasomotor center, area postrema) can either increase or decrease BP. For example, α_2-adrenergic stimulation within the central nervous system decreases BP through an inhibitory effect on the vasomotor center. However, angiotensin II increases sympathetic outflow from the vasomotor center, which increases BP.

The purpose of these neuronal mechanisms is to regulate BP and maintain homeostasis. Pathologic disturbances in any of the four major components (autonomic nerve fibers, adrenergic receptors, baroreceptors, central nervous system) could chronically elevate BP. These systems are physiologically interrelated. A defect in one component may alter normal function in another. Therefore, cumulative abnormalities may explain the development of essential hypertension.

Peripheral Autoregulatory Components

Abnormalities in renal or tissue autoregulatory systems could cause hypertension. It is possible that a renal defect in sodium excretion may develop, which can then cause resetting of tissue autoregulatory processes resulting in a higher BP. The kidney usually maintains a normal BP through a volume–pressure adaptive mechanism. When BP drops, the kidneys respond by increasing retention of sodium and water, which leads to plasma volume expansion that increases BP. Conversely, when BP rises above normal, renal sodium and water excretion are increased to reduce plasma volume and CO.

Local autoregulatory processes maintain adequate tissue oxygenation. When tissue oxygen demand is normal to low, the local arteriolar bed remains relatively vasoconstricted. However, increase in metabolic demand triggers arteriolar vasodilation that lowers peripheral vascular resistance (PVR) and increases blood flow and oxygen delivery.

Intrinsic defects in renal adaptive mechanisms could lead to plasma volume expansion and increased blood flow to peripheral tissues, even when BP is normal. Local tissue autoregulatory processes that vasoconstrict would then be activated to offset the increased blood flow. This effect would result in increased PVR and, if sustained, would also result in thickening of the arteriolar walls. This pathophysiologic component is plausible because increased TPR is a common underlying finding in patients with essential hypertension.

Vascular Endothelial Mechanisms

Vascular endothelium and smooth muscle play important roles in regulating blood vessel tone and BP. These regulating functions are mediated by vasoactive substances that are synthesized by endothelial cells. It has been postulated that a deficiency in local synthesis of vasodilating substances (e.g., prostacyclin and bradykinin) or excess vasoconstricting substances (e.g., angiotensin II and endothelin I) contribute to essential hypertension, atherosclerosis, and other CV diseases.

Nitric oxide is produced in the endothelium, relaxes the vascular epithelium, and is a very potent vasodilator. The nitric oxide system is an important regulator of arterial BP. Patients with hypertension may have an intrinsic nitric oxide deficiency, resulting in inadequate vasodilation.

Electrolytes

Epidemiologic and clinical data have associated excess sodium intake with hypertension. Population-based studies indicate that high-sodium diets are associated with a high prevalence of stroke and hypertension. Conversely, low-sodium diets are associated with a lower prevalence of hypertension. Clinical studies have shown that dietary sodium restriction lowers BP in many (but not all) patients with elevated BP. The exact mechanisms by which excess sodium leads to hypertension are not known.

Altered calcium homeostasis also may play an important role in the pathogenesis of hypertension. A lack of dietary calcium hypothetically can disturb the balance between intracellular and extracellular calcium, resulting in an increased intracellular calcium concentration. This imbalance can alter vascular smooth muscle function by increasing PVR. Some studies have shown that dietary calcium supplementation results in a modest BP reduction for patients with hypertension.

The role of potassium fluctuations is also inadequately understood. Potassium depletion may increase PVR, but the clinical significance of small serum potassium concentration changes is unclear. Furthermore, data demonstrating reduced CV risk with dietary potassium supplementation are very limited.

CLINICAL PRESENTATION

The clinical presentation of hypertension is described in Box 3-1.

Diagnostic Considerations

3 Hypertension is called the *silent killer* because most patients do not have symptoms. The primary physical finding is elevated BP. The diagnosis of hypertension cannot be made based on one elevated BP measurement. The average of two or more measurements taken during two or more clinical encounters is required to diagnose hypertension.[1] This BP average should be used to establish a diagnosis, and then classify the stage of hypertension using Table 3-3.

Measuring BP

The measurement of BP is a common routine medical screening tool that should be conducted at every healthcare encounter.[1]

Cuff Measurement Using Sphygmomanometry The most common procedure to measure BP in clinical practice is the indirect measurement of BP using sphygmomanometry.[13] The appropriate procedure to indirectly measure BP using sphygmomanometry has been described by the AHA.[13] It is imperative that the measurement equipment (inflation cuff, stethoscope, and manometer) meet certain national standards to ensure maximum quality and precision with measurement.

The AHA stepwise technique is recommended:

1. Patients should ideally refrain from nicotine and caffeine ingestion for 30 minutes and sit with lower back supported in a chair. Bare arm should be supported and resting near heart level. Feet should be flat on the floor (with legs not crossed). The measurement environment should be relatively quiet and provide privacy. Measuring BP in a position other than seated (supine or standing position) may be required under special circumstances (e.g., suspected orthostatic hypotension, or dehydration).
2. Measurement should begin only after a 5-minute period of rest.
3. A properly sized cuff (pediatric, small, regular, large, or extra large) should be used. The inflatable rubber bladder should be at least 80% and a width that is at least 40% of arm circumference.
4. The palpatory method should be used to estimate the SBP:
   a. Place the cuff on the upper arm 2 to 3 cm above the antecubital fossa and attach it to the manometer (either a mercury or an aneroid).
   b. Close the inflation valve and inflate the cuff to 70 mm Hg.
   c. Palpate the radial pulse with the index and middle fingers of the opposite hand.
   d. Inflate further in increments of 10 mm Hg until the radial pulse is no longer palpated.
   e. Note the pressure at which the radial pulse is no longer palpated; this is the estimated SBP.
   f. Release the pressure in the cuff by opening the valve.
5. The bell (not the diaphragm) of the stethoscope should be placed on the skin of the antecubital fossa, directly over

BOX 3-1 CLINICAL PRESENTATION Hypertension

General: The patient may appear healthy or may have the presence of additional CV risk factors:

- Age (≥55 years for men, ≥65 years for women)
- Diabetes mellitus
- Dyslipidemia
- Albuminuria
- Family history of premature CV disease
- Obesity (body mass index [BMI] ≥30 kg/m^2)
- Physical inactivity
- Tobacco use

Symptoms: Usually none related to elevated BP.

Signs: Previous BP values in either the prehypertension or the hypertension category.

Routine laboratory tests: Blood urea nitrogen (BUN)/serum creatinine, fasting lipid panel, fasting blood glucose, serum electrolytes (sodium, potassium), hemoglobin and hematocrit, and spot urine albumin-to-creatinine ratio. The patient may have normal values and still have hypertension. However, some may have abnormal values that are consistent with either additional CV risk factors or hypertension-related damage.

Other tests: 12-Lead electrocardiogram, estimated glomerular filtration rate (GFR; using modification of diet in renal disease [MDRD] equation).

Hypertension-related target-organ damage: The patient may have a previous medical history or diagnostic findings that indicate the presence of hypertension-related target-organ damage:

- Brain (stroke, transient ischemic attack, dementia)
- Eyes (retinopathy)
- Heart (left ventricular hypertrophy [LVH], angina, prior MI, prior coronary revascularization, heart failure)
- Kidney chronic kidney disease (CKD)
- Peripheral vasculature (peripheral arterial disease [PAD])

where the brachial artery is palpated. The stethoscope earpieces should be inserted appropriately. The valve should be closed with the cuff, and then inflated to 30 mm Hg above the estimated SBP from the palpatory method. The valve should be slightly opened to slowly release pressure at a rate of 2 to 3 mm Hg/s.

6. The clinician should listen for Korotkoff sounds with the stethoscope. The first phase of Korotkoff sounds is the initial presence of clear tapping sounds. Note the pressure at the first recognition of these sounds. This is the SBP. As pressure deflates, note the pressure when all sounds disappear, right at the last sound. This is the DBP.
7. Measurements should be rounded to the nearest 2 mm Hg.
8. A second measurement should be obtained after at least 1 minute. If these values differ by more than 5 mm Hg, additional measurements should be obtained.
9. Neither the patient nor the observer should talk during measurement.
10. When first establishing care with a patient, BP should be measured in both arms. If consistent interarm differences exist, the arm with the higher value should be used.

Inaccuracies with indirect measurements result from inherent biologic variability of BP, inaccuracies related to suboptimal technique, and the white coat effect.[13] Variations in BP occur with environmental temperature, the time of day and year, meals, physical activity, posture, alcohol, nicotine, and emotions. In the clinic setting, standard BP measurement procedures (e.g., appropriate rest period, correct technique, minimal number of measurements) are often not followed, which results in poor estimation of true BP. It is recommended that the stethoscope bell, rather than the diaphragm, be used for measurement, although some studies suggest little difference between two.[13]

Approximately 15% to 20% of patients have *white coat hypertension*, where BP values rise in a clinical setting but return to normal in nonclinical environments using home or ambulatory BP (ABP) measurements.[13] Interestingly, the rise in BP dissipates gradually over several hours after leaving the clinical setting. It may or may not be precipitated by other stresses in the patient's daily life. This is in contrast to *masked hypertension*, where a decrease in BP occurs in the clinical setting.[14] With masked hypertension, home BP is hypertensive, while the in-office BP is normotensive or substantially lower than that at home. This situation may lead to undertreatment or lack of treatment for hypertension. Moreover, patients with either white coat or masked hypertension have a high risk of progressing to develop sustained hypertension, which can result in a higher risk of CV events compared with normotensive patients.[15]

Pseudohypertension is a falsely elevated BP measurement. It may be seen in the elderly, those with long-standing diabetes, or those with CKD due to rigid, calcified brachial arteries.[13] In these patients, the true arterial BP when measured directly with intraarterial measurement (the most accurate measurement of BP) is much lower than that measured using the indirect cuff method. The Osler's maneuver can be used to test for pseudohypertension. In this maneuver, the BP cuff is inflated above peak SBP. If the radial artery remains palpable, the patient has a positive Osler's sign (rigid artery), which may indicate pseudohypertension.

Elderly patients with a wide pulse pressure may have an auscultatory gap that can lead to underestimated SBP or overestimated DBP measurements.[13] In this situation, as the cuff pressure falls from the true SBP value, the Korotkoff sound may disappear (indicating a false DBP measurement), reappear (a false SBP measurement), and then disappear again at the true DBP value. When an auscultatory gap is present, Korotkoff sounds are usually heard when pressure in the cuff first starts to decrease after inflation. This may be eliminated by raising the arm overhead by 30 seconds before bringing it to the proper position and inflating the cuff. This maneuver decreases the intravascular volume and improves inflow thereby allowing Korotkoff sounds to be heard.[13]

Ambulatory and Self-BP Monitoring Ambulatory BP (ABP) monitoring using an automated device can document BP at frequent time intervals (e.g., every 15 to 30 minutes) throughout a 24-hour period.[13] ABP values are usually lower than clinic-measured values. The definition of hypertension for ABP is ≥135/85 mm Hg during the day, ≥120/75 mm Hg nighttime (or asleep), and ≥130/80 mm Hg over 24 hours.[13] For self BP monitoring, a BP ≥135/85 mm Hg is considered hypertensive. Self-BP measurements are collected by patients, preferably in the morning, using home monitoring devices.

Neither ABP nor self-BP monitoring is needed for the routine diagnosis of hypertension according to JNC7 guidelines; however, these modalities can enhance the ability to identify patients with white coat and masked hypertension.[14] ABP and self-BP measurements may also be useful in evaluating and optimizing BP control for patients on antihypertensive drug therapy.[14,16] ABP monitoring may be helpful for patients with apparent drug resistance, hypotensive symptoms while on antihypertensive therapy, episodic hypertension (e.g., white coat hypertension), autonomic dysfunction, and in identifying "nondippers" whose BP does not decrease by >10% during sleep and who may portend increased risk of BP-related complications.[1,13]

Limitations of ABP and self-BP measurements may prohibit routine use of such technology. These include complexity of use, costs, and lack of prospective outcome data describing normal ranges for these measurements. Although self-monitoring of BP at home is less complicated and less costly than ambulatory monitoring, patients may omit or fabricate readings, or have poor technique (e.g., not resting for adequate period of time, improper placement, wrong cuff size).

Clinical Evaluation

Frequently, the only sign of essential hypertension is elevated BP. The rest of the physical examination may be completely normal. However, a complete medical evaluation (a comprehensive medical history, physical examination, and laboratory and/or diagnostic tests) is recommended after diagnosis to (a) identify secondary causes, (b) identify other CV risk factors or comorbid conditions that may define prognosis and/or guide therapy, and (c) assess for the presence or absence of hypertension-associated target-organ damage.[1] All patients with hypertension should have the tests described in Box 3-1 measured prior to initiating therapy.[1] For patients without a history of coronary artery disease, noncoronary atherosclerotic vascular disease, left ventricular dysfunction, or diabetes, it is also important to estimate future risk of CV disease. The 10-year risk of fatal coronary heart disease or nonfatal MI can be estimated using Framingham risk scoring (*http://www.nhlbi.nih.gov/guidelines/cholesterol/risk_tbl.htm*).[2]

Secondary Causes

The most common secondary causes of hypertension are listed in Table 3-1. A complete medical evaluation should provide clues for identifying secondary hypertension.

Patients with secondary hypertension might have signs or symptoms suggestive of the underlying disorder. Patients with pheochromocytoma may have a history of paroxysmal headaches, sweating, tachycardia, and palpitations. Over half of these patients suffer from episodes of orthostatic hypotension. In primary hyperaldosteronism symptoms related to hypokalemia usually include muscle cramps and muscle weakness. Patients with Cushing's syndrome may complain of weight gain, polyuria, edema, menstrual irregularities, recurrent acne, or muscular weakness and have several classic physical features (e.g., moon face, buffalo hump, hirsutism). Patients with coarctation of the aorta may have higher BP in the arms than in legs and diminished or even absent femoral pulses. Patients with renal artery stenosis may have an abdominal systolic–diastolic bruit.

Routine laboratory tests may also help identify secondary hypertension. Baseline hypokalemia may suggest mineralocorticoid-induced hypertension. Protein, red blood cells, and casts in the urine may indicate renovascular disease. Some laboratory tests are used specifically to diagnose secondary hypertension. These include plasma norepinephrine and urinary metanephrine for pheochromocytoma, plasma and urinary aldosterone concentrations for primary hyperaldosteronism, and plasma renin activity, captopril stimulation test, renal vein renin, and renal artery angiography for renovascular disease.

Certain drugs and other products can result in drug-induced hypertension (see Table 3-1). For some patients, the addition of these agents can be the cause of elevated BP or can exacerbate underlying hypertension. Identifying a temporal relationship between starting the suspected agent and developing elevated BP is most suggestive of drug-induced BP elevation.

Natural Course of Disease

Essential hypertension is usually preceded by elevated BP values that are in the prehypertension category. BP values may fluctuate between elevated and normal levels for an extended period of time. As the disease progresses, PVR increases, and BP elevation becomes chronic.

Hypertension-Associated Target-Organ Damage

Target-organ damage (see Box 3-1) can develop as a complication of hypertension. CV events (e.g., MI, cerebrovascular accidents, kidney failure) are clinical end points of hypertension-associated target-organ damage and are the primary causes of CV morbidity and mortality for patients with hypertension. The probability of CV events and CV morbidity and mortality in patients with hypertension is directly correlated with the severity of BP elevation.

Hypertension accelerates atherosclerosis and stimulates left ventricular and vascular dysfunction. These pathologic changes are thought to be secondary to both a chronic pressure overload and a variety of nonhemodynamic stimuli. Several nonhemodynamic disturbances have been implicated in these effects (e.g., the adrenergic system, RAAS, increased synthesis and secretion of endothelin I, and a decreased production of prostacyclin and nitric oxide). Atherosclerosis in hypertension is accompanied by proliferation of smooth muscle cells, lipid infiltration into the vascular endothelium, and enhancement of vascular calcium accumulation.

Cerebrovascular disease is a consequence of hypertension. A neurologic assessment can detect either gross neurologic deficits or a slight hemiparesis with some incoordination and hyperreflexia that are indicative of cerebrovascular disease. Stroke can result from lacunar infarcts caused by thrombotic occlusion of small vessels or intracerebral hemorrhage resulting from ruptured microaneurysms. Transient ischemic attacks secondary to atherosclerotic disease in the carotid arteries can also happen in patients with hypertension.

Retinopathies can occur in hypertension and may manifest as a variety of different findings. A funduscopic examination can detect hypertensive retinopathy, and the result can be categorized according to the Keith-Wagener-Barker retinopathy classification. Retinopathy manifests as arteriolar narrowing, focal arteriolar constrictions, arteriovenous crossing changes (nicking), retinal hemorrhages and exudates, and disk edema. Accelerated arteriosclerosis, a long-term consequence of essential hypertension, can cause nonspecific changes such as increased light reflex, increased tortuosity of vessels, and arteriovenous nicking. Focal arteriolar narrowing, retinal infarcts, and flame-shaped hemorrhages usually are suggestive of accelerated or malignant phase of hypertension. Papilledema is swelling of the optic disk caused by a breakdown in autoregulation of capillary blood flow in the presence of high pressure. It is usually only present in hypertensive emergencies.

Heart disease is the most well-identified form of target-organ damage. A thorough cardiac and pulmonary examination can identify cardiopulmonary abnormalities. Clinical manifestations include LVH, coronary heart disease (angina, prior MI, and prior coronary revascularization), and heart failure. These complications may lead to cardiac arrhythmias, angina, MI, and sudden death. Coronary disease (also called *coronary heart disease*) and associated CV events are the most common causes of death in patients with hypertension.

The kidney damage caused by hypertension is characterized pathologically by hyaline arteriosclerosis, hyperplastic arteriosclerosis, arteriolar hypertrophy, fibrinoid necrosis, and atheroma of the major renal arteries. Glomerular hyperfiltration and intraglomerular hypertension are early stages of hypertensive nephropathy. Albuminuria is followed by a gradual decline in renal function. The primary renal complication in hypertension is nephrosclerosis, which is secondary to arteriosclerosis. Atheromatous disease of a major renal artery may give rise to renal artery stenosis. Although overt kidney failure is an uncommon complication of essential hypertension, it is an important cause of end-stage kidney disease, especially in African Americans, Hispanics, and Native Americans.

The peripheral vasculature is a target organ. Physical examination of the vascular system can detect evidence of atherosclerosis, which may present as arterial bruits (aortic, abdominal, or peripheral), distended veins, diminished or absent peripheral arterial pulses, or lower extremity edema. PAD is a clinical condition that can result from atherosclerosis, which is accelerated in hypertension. Other CV risk factors (e.g., smoking) can increase the likelihood of PAD as well as all other forms of target-organ damage.

TREATMENT

Desired Outcomes

Overall Goal of Treatment

4 The overall goal of treating hypertension is to reduce hypertension-associated morbidity and mortality.[1] This morbidity and mortality is related to hypertension-associated target-organ damage (e.g., CV events, cerebrovascular events, heart failure, kidney disease). Reducing CV risk is the primary purpose of hypertension therapy and the specific choice of drug therapy should be determined by evidence demonstrating such CV risk reduction.

Surrogate Targets—Blood Pressure Goals

5 Treating patients with hypertension to achieve a desired target BP value is simply a surrogate goal of therapy. Reducing BP to goal does not guarantee prevention of hypertension-associated target-organ damage, but is associated with a lower risk of hypertension-associated target-organ damage.[1] Targeting a goal BP value is a tool that clinicians use to evaluate response to therapy. It is the primary method used to determine the need for titration and regimen modification.

The JNC7 guidelines recommend BP goals for the management of hypertension (Box 3-2). A goal BP of <140/90 mm Hg is recommended for most patients for general prevention of CV events or

BOX 3-2 Goal BP Values Recommended by the JNC7 in 2003, American Diabetes Association, and KDIGO

JNC7

- <140/90 mm Hg for most patients

American Diabetes Association (2013)

- <140/80 mm Hg for patients with diabetes.
- SBP goal of <130 mm Hg may be appropriate for certain individuals (e.g., younger patients) if achieved without undue treatment burden.

KDIGO (2012)

- <130/80 mm Hg only for patients with CKD (nondialysis) who have persistent urine albumin excretion of >30 mg per 24 hours (or equivalent)

CV disease (e.g., coronary artery disease).[1] The JNC7, published in 2003, recommends a lower BP goal of <130/80 mm Hg for patients with diabetes or significant CKD. However, data supporting that this goal provides better reductions in CV events than a goal of <140/90 mm Hg are lacking. In 2013 the American Diabetes Association changed their recommended goal BP in patients with diabetes to <140/80 mm Hg.[17] This was a significant change from their long-standing recommendation of <130/80 mm Hg. They do recommend that a SBP goal of <130 mm Hg may be appropriate for certain individuals (e.g., younger patients) if achieved without undue treatment burden, but the recommendation for most patients with diabetes is <140/80 mm Hg. Similarly, the Kidney Disease Improving Global Outcomes (KDIGO) guidelines recommend a BP goal of 140/90 mm Hg for patients with hypertension and CKD (nondialysis), with a lower BP goal of <130/80 mm Hg only for those patients who have persistent albuminuria (>30 mg urine albumin excretion per 24 hours or equivalent).[18,19]

Until a new clinical guideline based on the NHLBI evidentiary review is published, clinicians should use the most recent recommended BP goals from these consensus statements of <140/90 mm Hg for most patients, <140/80 mm Hg for patients with diabetes, and <130/80 mm Hg for patients with persistent increased urinary albumin excretion (see Box 3-2).

Evidence Supporting <140/90 mm Hg in Most Patients Lower goal DBP values have been evaluated prospectively in the Hypertension Optimal Treatment (HOT) study.[20] In this study, over 18,700 patients were randomized to target DBP values of ≤90, ≤85, or ≤80 mm Hg. Although the actual DBP values achieved were 85.2, 83.2, and 81.1 mm Hg, respectively, there were no significant differences in risk of major CV events when the three treatment groups were compared with each other among the total population. This lack of a benefit in reducing risk of CV events is consistent with findings from a 2009 Cochrane Collaboration systematic review that included seven clinical trials that evaluated different goal DBP values in hypertension.[21] When the relationship between actual BP values and risk of CV events was evaluated, there was a trend that lower was better. The risk of major CV events was the lowest with a BP of 139/83 mm Hg, and lowest risk of stroke was with a BP of 142/80 mm Hg.

A major limitation of the HOT study and the 2009 Cochrane Collaboration review is the use of DBP goal values. SBP is more directly correlated to CV risk than DBP in most patients with hypertension, especially those above the age of 50. Therefore, data from the HOT study cannot answer this question. It is important to note that no J-curve relationship was seen. The *J-curve hypothesis* suggests that lowering BP too much might increase the risk of CV events.[22] This theoretical hypothesis was described many years ago and was originally suggested in observational studies. Therefore, it remains an unproven hypothesis.

Limited data suggest lower is better when SBP goal values are targeted. The Cardio-Sys trial was a small open-label study in 1,111 patients with hypertension and without a history of diabetes.[23] These patients had additional CV risk factors and roughly reflect a population with a Framingham risk score of 10% or greater. Patients were randomized to SBP goals of <140 mm Hg or <130 mm Hg. After a median of 2 years, the incidence of LVH was lower in the group randomized to a SBP goal of <130 mm Hg. Interestingly, the incidence of CV events, which was a secondary end point, was also significantly lower in the <130 mm Hg group. These data suggest that the optional lower BP goals may be better. However, LVH is only a surrogate end point for CV events, and the open-label nature of this study limits broad application to patient care.

Clinical **Controversy...**

How low to go in most patients?

A standard BP goal of <140/90 mm Hg is recommended for most patients with hypertension. Lower goals are recommended in specific patient populations (e.g., diabetes, CKD with persistent albuminuria). However, some clinicians believe that lower BP goals are better, even for patients who do not have one of the aforementioned higher-risk conditions. One ongoing trial sponsored by the NHLBI, the Systolic Pressure Intervention Trial (SPRINT), is a prospective randomized trial that is evaluating standard BP goals with lower BP goals for patients without a history of diabetes or a history of stroke. Once this trial is completed, hopefully the controversy of how low to go in most patients will be resolved.

Evidence Supporting Lower BP Goals in Diabetes A BP goal of <130/80 mm Hg was historically recommended for patients with diabetes for many years, by multiple organizations.[1,2] The primary evidence supporting this recommendation was from the HOT study, where the only subgroup to show a lower risk of major CV events in the <80 mm Hg group versus the <90 mm Hg group was in patients with diabetes ($n = 1{,}501$).

The NHLBI-sponsored Action to Control Cardiovascular Risk in Diabetes Blood Pressure (ACCORD-BP) study questioned the benefit of lower BP goals for patients with diabetes.[24]

The ACCORD-BP was an open-label study that randomized 4,733 patients with type 2 diabetes to intensive therapy targeting a SBP of <120 mm Hg, or to standard therapy targeting a SBP <140 mm Hg for a mean followup of 4.7 years. After 1 year, an average of 3.4 medications was needed in the intensive therapy group to attain a mean SBP of 119.3 mm Hg, compared with an average of 2.1 medications in the standard therapy group to attain a mean SBP of 133.5 mm Hg. This difference was generally maintained throughout the study duration. However, there was no significant difference in the annual rate of the primary end point (nonfatal MI, nonfatal stroke, or CV death) between the two groups. The annual incidence of the secondary end point of stroke was lower with the intensive therapy group versus the standard therapy group, and this was the only prespecified end point that was different between the two groups.

Despite consensus guidelines historically recommending a BP goal of <130/80 mm Hg for patients with diabetes, evidence supporting this approach over a standard goal of <140/90 mm Hg is marginal, and comes at the cost of increased side effects (e.g., hypotension, hyperkalemia, bradycardia). While the ACCORD-BP provided additional evidence regarding BP goals for patients with diabetes, these data do not provide all of the clinical answers that are needed. The ACCORD-BP was open label, and those in the standard group (SBP <140 mm Hg) actually had SBP values that were closer to 130 mm Hg than to 140 mm Hg. Based on these data, in 2013 American Diabetes Association changed their recommendation to a goal BP of <140/80 mm Hg for most patients with hypertension and diabetes.[17] The KDIGO guidelines recommend a BP goal of <140/90 mm Hg for patients with hypertension and CKD (non-dialysis) and a BP goal of <130/80 mm Hg only for those patients who have persistently increased urine albumin excretion.[18]

Avoiding Clinical Inertia

Although hypertension is one of the most common medical conditions, BP control rates are poor. *Clinical inertia* in hypertension has been defined as an office visit at which no therapeutic move was made to lower BP in a patient with uncontrolled hypertension.[25] Clinical inertia is not the entire reason why many patients with hypertension do not achieve goal BP values. However, it is certainly a major reason that can be remedied simply through more aggressive treatment with drug therapy. This can involve initiating, titrating, or changing drug therapy.

General Approach to Treatment

Most patients should be placed on both lifestyle modifications and drug therapy concurrently after a diagnosis of hypertension is made. Lifestyle modification alone is appropriate for most patients with prehypertension. However, lifestyle modifications alone may not be adequate for patients with hypertension and either additional CV risk factors or hypertension-associated target-organ damage.

6 The choice of initial drug therapy depends on the degree of BP elevation and presence of compelling indications (discussed in the Pharmacotherapy section below). Most patients with stage 1 hypertension should be initially treated with a first-line antihypertensive drug or the combination of two agents. Combination drug therapy is recommended for patients with more severe BP elevation (stage 2 hypertension), using preferably two first-line antihypertensive drugs. This general approach is outlined in Figure 3-2. There are six compelling indications where specific antihypertensive drug classes have evidence showing unique benefits in patients with hypertension and the listed compelling indication (Fig. 3-3).

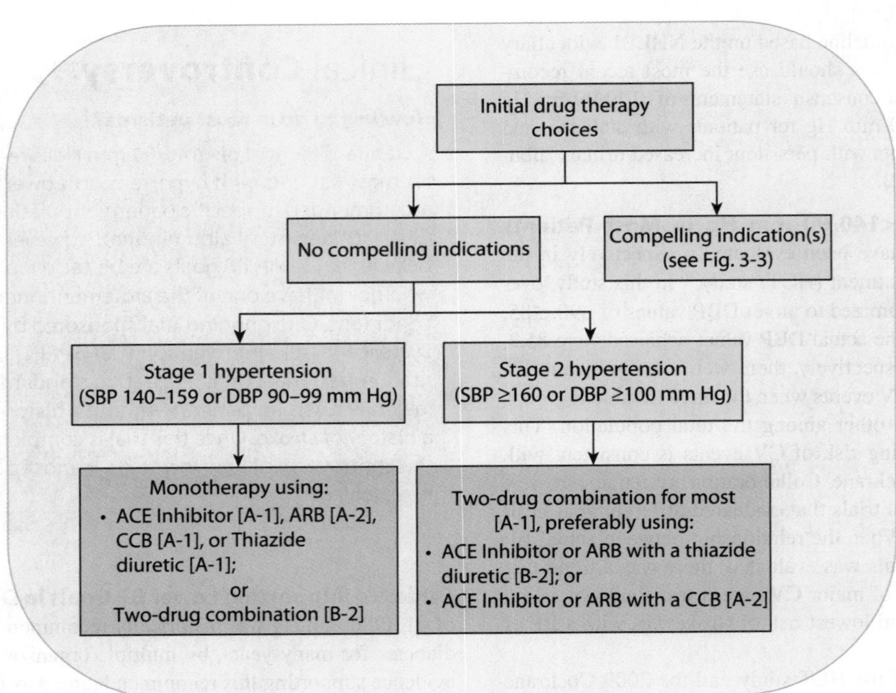

FIGURE 3-2 Algorithm for treatment of hypertension. Drug therapy recommendations are graded with strength of recommendation and quality of evidence in brackets. Strength of recommendations: A, B, and C are good, moderate, and poor evidence to support recommendation, respectively. Quality of evidence: (1) evidence from more than one properly randomized controlled trial; (2) evidence from at least one well-designed clinical trial with randomization, from cohort or case-controlled studies, or dramatic results from uncontrolled experiments or subgroup analyses; (3) evidence from opinions of respected authorities, based on clinical experience, descriptive studies, or reports of expert communities.

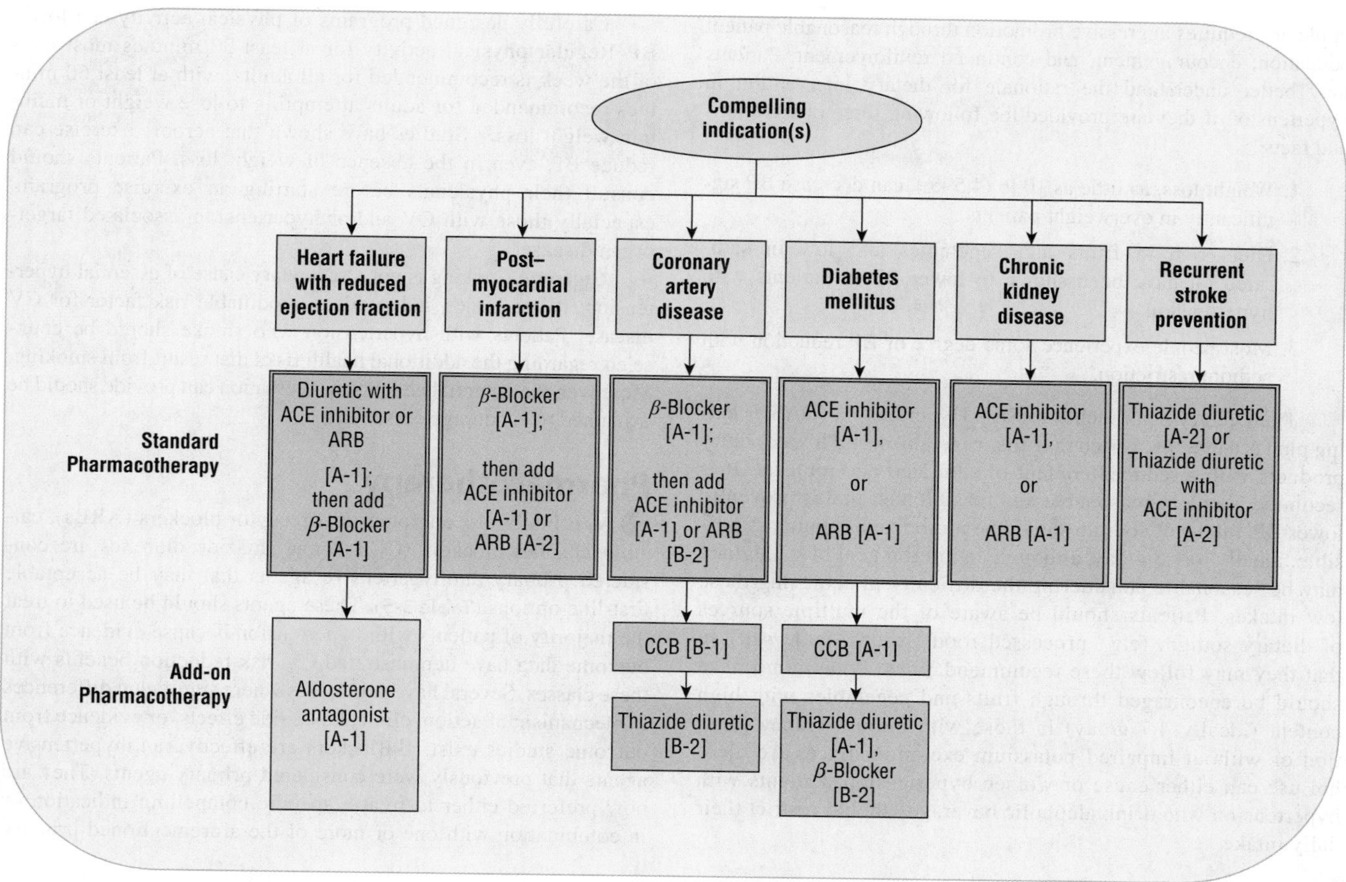

FIGURE 3-3 Compelling indications for individual drug classes. Compelling indications for specific drugs are evidenced-based recommendations from outcome studies or existing clinical guidelines. The order of drug therapies serves as a general guidance that should be balanced with clinical judgment and patient response; however, standard pharmacotherapy should be considered first-line recommendations, preferably in the order depicted. Then add-on pharmacotherapy recommendations are intended to further reduce risk of cardiovascular events when additional pharmacotherapy is needed to lower blood pressure to goal values. Blood pressure control should be managed concurrently with the compelling indication. Drug therapy recommendations are graded with strength of recommendation and quality of evidence in brackets. Strength of recommendations: A, B, and C are good, moderate, and poor evidence to support recommendation, respectively. Quality of evidence: (1) evidence from more than one properly randomized controlled trial; (2) evidence from at least one well-designed clinical trial with randomization, from cohort or case-controlled analytic studies or multiple time series, or dramatic results from uncontrolled experiments or subgroup analyses; (3) evidence from opinions of respected authorities, based on clinical experience, descriptive studies, or reports of expert communities.

Nonpharmacologic Therapy

7 All patients with prehypertension and hypertension should be prescribed lifestyle modifications. Recommended modifications that have been shown to lower BP are listed in Table 3-4.[1,26] They can provide small to moderate reductions in SBP. Aside from lowering BP in patients with known hypertension, lifestyle modification can decrease the progression to hypertension in patients with prehypertension BP values.[26]

A sensible dietary program is one that is designed to reduce weight gradually (for overweight and obese patients) and one that restricts sodium intake with only moderate alcohol consumption. Successful implementation of dietary lifestyle modifications by

TABLE 3-4 Lifestyle Modifications to Prevent and Manage Hypertension

Modification	Recommendation	Approximate Systolic Blood Pressure Reduction (mm Hg)[a]
Weight loss	Maintain normal body weight (body mass index, 18.5–24.9 kg/m^2)	5–20 per 10-kg weight loss
DASH-type dietary patterns	Consume a diet rich in fruits, vegetables, and low-fat dairy products with a reduced content of saturated and total fat	8–14
Reduced salt intake	Reduce daily dietary sodium intake as much as possible, ideally to ≈65 mmol/day (1.5 g/day sodium, or 3.8 g/day sodium chloride)	2–8
Physical activity	Regular aerobic physical activity (at least 30 min/day, most days of the week)	4–9
Moderation of alcohol intake	Limit consumption to ≤2 drink equivalents per day in men and ≤1 drink equivalent per day in women and lighter-weight persons[b]	2–4

[a]Effects of implementing these modifications are time- and dose-dependent and could be greater for some patients.
[b]One drink equivalent is equal to 1.5 oz (~45 mL) of 80-proof distilled spirits (e.g., whiskey), a 5 oz (~150 mL) glass of wine (12%), or 12 oz (~350 mL) of beer.

clinicians requires aggressive promotion through reasonable patient education, encouragement, and continued reinforcement. Patients may better understand the rationale for dietary intervention in hypertension if they are provided the following three observations and facts[26]:

1. Weight loss, as little as 10 lb (4.5 kg), can decrease BP significantly in overweight patients.
2. Diets rich in fruits and vegetables and low in saturated fat have been shown to lower BP in patients with hypertension.
3. Most people experience some degree of BP reduction with sodium restriction.

The Dietary Approaches to Stop Hypertension (DASH) eating plan is a diet that is rich in fruits, vegetables, and low-fat dairy products with a reduced content of saturated and total fat. It is recommended as a reasonable and feasible diet that is proven to lower BP. Intake of sodium should be minimized as much as possible, ideally to 1.5 g/day, although an interim goal of <2.3 g/day may be reasonable considering the difficulty in achieving these low intakes. Patients should be aware of the multiple sources of dietary sodium (e.g., processed foods, soups, table salt) so that they may follow these recommendations. Potassium intake should be encouraged through fruits and vegetables with high content (ideally 4.7 g/day) in those with normal kidney function or without impaired potassium excretion. Excessive alcohol use can either cause or worsen hypertension. Patients with hypertension who drink alcoholic beverages should restrict their daily intake.

Carefully designed programs of physical activity can lower BP. Regular physical activity for at least 30 minutes most days of the week is recommended for all adults, with at least 60 minutes recommended for adults attempting to lose weight or maintain weight loss.[27] Studies have shown that aerobic exercise can reduce BP, even in the absence of weight loss. Patients should consult their physicians before starting an exercise program, especially those with CV and/or hypertension-associated target-organ disease.

Cigarette smoking is not a secondary cause of essential hypertension; it is a major, independent, modifiable risk factor for CV disease. Patients with hypertension who smoke should be counseled regarding the additional health risks that result from smoking. Moreover, the potential benefits that cessation can provide should be explained to encourage cessation.

Pharmacotherapy

8 ACE inhibitors, angiotensin II receptor blockers (ARBs), calcium channel blockers (CCBs), and thiazide diuretics are considered primary antihypertensive agents that may be acceptable first-line options (Table 3-5). These agents should be used to treat the majority of patients with hypertension because evidence from outcome data have demonstrated CV risk reduction benefits with these classes. Several have subclasses where significant differences in mechanism of action, clinical use, side effects, or evidence from outcome studies exist. β-Blockers are effective antihypertensive agents that previously were considered primary agents. They are now preferred either to treat a specific compelling indication or in combination with one or more of the aforementioned primary

TABLE 3-5 First-Line and Other Common Antihypertensive Agents

Class	Subclass	Drug (Brand Name)	Usual Dose Range (mg/day)	Daily Frequency	Comments
ACE inhibitors		Benazepril (Lotensin)	10–40	1 or 2	May cause hyperkalemia in patients with chronic kidney disease or in those receiving a potassium-sparing diuretic, aldosterone antagonist, ARB, or direct renin inhibitor; can cause acute kidney failure in patients with severe bilateral renal artery stenosis or severe stenosis in artery to solitary kidney; do not use in pregnancy or in patients with a history of angioedema; starting dose should be reduced 50% in patients who are on a diuretic, are volume depleted, or are very elderly due to risks of hypotension
		Captopril (Capoten)	12.5–150	2 or 3	
		Enalapril (Vasotec)	5–40	1 or 2	
		Fosinopril (Monopril)	10–40	1	
		Lisinopril (Prinivil, Zestril)	10–40	1	
		Moexipril (Univasc)	7.5–30	1 or 2	
		Perindopril (Aceon)	4–16	1	
		Quinapril (Accupril)	10–80	1 or 2	
		Ramipril (Altace)	2.5–10	1 or 2	
		Trandolapril (Mavik)	1–4	1	
ARBs		Azilsartan (Edarbi)	40–80	1	May cause hyperkalemia in patients with chronic kidney disease or in those receiving a potassium-sparing diuretic, aldosterone antagonist, ACE inhibitor, or direct renin inhibitor; can cause acute kidney failure in patients with severe bilateral renal artery stenosis or severe stenosis in artery to solitary kidney; do not cause a dry cough like ACE inhibitors may; do not use in pregnancy; starting dose should be reduced 50% in patients who are on a diuretic, are volume depleted, or are very elderly due to risks of hypotension
		Candesartan (Atacand)	8–32	1 or 2	
		Eprosartan (Teveten)	600–800	1 or 2	
		Irbesartan (Avapro)	150–300	1	
		Losartan (Cozaar)	50–100	1 or 2	
		Olmesartan (Benicar)	20–40	1	
		Telmisartan (Micardis)	20–80	1	
		Valsartan (Diovan)	80–320	1	
Calcium channel blockers	Dihydropyridines	Amlodipine (Norvasc)	2.5–10	1	Short-acting dihydropyridines should be avoided, especially immediate-release nifedipine and nicardipine; dihydropyridines are more potent peripheral vasodilators than nondihydropyridines and may cause more reflex sympathetic discharge (tachycardia), dizziness, headache, flushing, and peripheral edema; have additional benefits in Raynaud's syndrome
		Felodipine (Plendil)	5–20	1	
		Isradipine (DynaCirc)	5–10	2	
		Isradipine SR (DynaCirc SR)	5–20	1	
		Nicardipine sustained release (Cardene SR)	60–120	2	
		Nifedipine long-acting (Adalat CC, Nifedical XL, Procardia XL)	30–90	1	
		Nisoldipine (Sular)	10–40	1	

(continued)

TABLE 3-5 First-Line and Other Common Antihypertensive Agents (*Continued*)

Class	Subclass	Drug (Brand Name)	Usual Dose Range (mg/day)	Daily Frequency	Comments
	Nondihydropyridines	Diltiazem sustained release (Cardizem SR)	180–360	2	Extended-release products are preferred for hypertension; these agents reduce heart rate; may produce heart block, especially in combination with β-blockers; these products are not AB rated as interchangeable on an equipotent milligram-per-milligram basis due to different release mechanisms and different bioavailability parameters; Cardizem LA, Covera-HS, and Verelan PM have delayed drug release for several hours after dosing, when dosed in the evening can provide chronotherapeutic drug delivery starting shortly before patients awake from sleep; nondihydropyridines have additional benefits in patients with atrial tachyarrhythmia
		Diltiazem sustained release (Cardizem CD, Cartia XT, Dilacor XR, Diltia XT, Tiazac, Taztia XT)	120–480	1	
		Diltiazem extended release (Cardizem LA)	120–540	1 (morning or evening)	
		Verapamil sustained release (Calan SR, Isoptin SR, Verelan)	180–480	1 or 2	
		Verapamil controlled onset, extended release (Covera-HS)	180–420	1 (in the evening)	
		Verapamil chronotherapeutic oral drug absorption system (Verelan PM)	100–400	1 (in the evening)	
Diuretics	Thiazides	Chlorthalidone (Hygroton)	12.5–25	1	Hydrochlorothiazide is a "thiazide-type" diuretic; chlorthalidone, indapamide, and metolazone are "thiazide-like" diuretics. Dose in the morning to avoid nocturnal diuresis; thiazides are more effective antihypertensives than loop diuretics in most patients; use usual doses to avoid adverse metabolic effects; hydrochlorothiazide, chlorthalidone, and indapamide are preferred; chlorthalidone is approximately 1.5 times as potent as hydrochlorothiazide; have additional benefits in osteoporosis; use with caution in patients with a history of gout
		Hydrochlorothiazide (Esidrix, HydroDiuril, Microzide, Oretic)	12.5–50	1	
		Indapamide (Lozol)	1.25–2.5	1	
		Metolazone (Zaroxolyn)	2.5–10	1	
	Loops	Bumetanide (Bumex)	0.5–4	2	Dose in the morning and late afternoon (when twice daily) to avoid nocturnal diuresis; higher doses may be needed for patients with severely decreased glomerular filtration rate or heart failure; preferred over thiazides in patient with concomitant renal dysfunction and resistant hypertension
		Furosemide (Lasix)	20–80	2	
		Torsemide (Demadex)	5–10	1	
	Potassium sparing	Amiloride (Midamor)	5–10	1 or 2	Weak diuretics that are generally used in combination with thiazide diuretics to minimize hypokalemia; do not significantly lower BP unless used with a thiazide diuretic; should generally be reserved for patients experiencing diuretic-induced hypokalemia; avoid in patients with chronic kidney disease (estimated creatinine clearance <30 mL/min [<0.5 mL/s]); may cause hyperkalemia, especially in combination with an ACE inhibitor, ARB, direct renin inhibitor, or potassium supplements
		Amiloride/hydrochlorothiazide (Moduretic)	5–10/50–100	1	
		Triamterene (Dyrenium)	50–100	1 or 2	
		Triamterene/hydrochlorothiazide (Dyazide)	37.5–75/25–50	1	
	Aldosterone antagonists	Eplerenone (Inspra)	50–100	1 or 2	Dose in the morning and late afternoon (when twice daily) to avoid nocturnal diuresis; eplerenone contraindicated in patients with an estimated creatinine clearance <50 mL/min (<0.83 mL/s), elevated serum creatinine (>1.8 mg/dL [159 µmol/L] in women, >2 mg/dL [177 µmol/L] in men), and type 2 diabetes with microalbuminuria; spironolactone often used as add-on therapy in resistant hypertension; avoid spironolactone in patients with chronic kidney disease (estimated creatinine clearance <30 mL/min [<0.5 mL/s]); may cause hyperkalemia, especially in combination with an ACE inhibitor, ARB, direct renin inhibitor, or potassium supplements
		Spironolactone (Aldactone)	25–50	1 or 2	
		Spironolactone/hydrochlorothiazide (Aldactazide)	25–50/25–50	1	
β-Blockers	Cardioselective	Atenolol (Tenormin)	25–100	1	Abrupt discontinuation may cause rebound hypertension; inhibit β_1-receptors at low to moderate dose, higher doses also block β_2-receptors; may exacerbate asthma when selectivity is lost; have additional benefits in patients with atrial tachyarrhythmia or preoperative hypertension
		Betaxolol (Kerlone)	5–20	1	
		Bisoprolol (Zebeta)	2.5–10	1	
		Metoprolol tartrate (Lopressor)	100–400	2	
		Metoprolol succinate extended release (Toprol XL)	50–200	1	

(*continued*)

TABLE 3-5 First-Line and Other Common Antihypertensive Agents (*Continued*)

Class	Subclass	Drug (Brand Name)	Usual Dose Range (mg/day)	Daily Frequency	Comments
	Nonselective	Nadolol (Corgard) Propranolol (Inderal) Propranolol long acting (Inderal LA, InnoPran XL) Timolol (Blocadren)	40–120 160–480 80–320 10–40	1 2 1 1	Abrupt discontinuation may cause rebound hypertension; inhibit β_1- and β_2-receptors at all doses; can exacerbate asthma; have additional benefits in patients with essential tremor, migraine headache, portal hypertension, thyrotoxicosis
	Intrinsic sympathomimetic activity	Acebutolol (Sectral) Carteolol (Cartrol) Penbutolol (Levatol) Pindolol (Visken)	200–800 2.5–10 10–40 10–60	2 1 1 2	Abrupt discontinuation may cause rebound hypertension; partially stimulate β-receptors while blocking against additional stimulation; no clear advantage for these agents; contraindicated in patients post–myocardial infarction
	Mixed α- and β-blockers	Carvedilol (Coreg) Carvedilol phosphate (Coreg CR) Labetalol (Normodyne, Trandate)	12.5–50 20–80 200–800	2 1 2	Abrupt discontinuation may cause rebound hypertension; additional α-blockade produces vasodilation and more orthostatic hypotension
	Cardioselective and vasodilatory	Nebivolol (Bystolic)	5–20	1	Abrupt discontinuation may cause rebound hypertension; additional vasodilation does not result in more orthostatic hypotension

antihypertensive agents for patients without a compelling indication. Other antihypertensive drug classes are considered alternative drug classes that may be used in select patients after first-line agents (Table 3-6).

Thiazide Diuretics as Historical First-Line Agents

Landmark placebo-controlled clinical trials demonstrate that thiazide diuretic therapy irrefutably reduces risk of CV morbidity and mortality.[28] The Systolic Hypertension in the Elderly Program (SHEP),[8] Swedish Trial in Old Patients with Hypertension (STOP-Hypertension),[9] and Medical Research Council (MRC)[10] studies showed significant reductions in stroke, MI, all-cause CV disease, and mortality with thiazide diuretic–based therapy versus placebo. These trials allowed for β-blockers as add-on therapy for BP control. Newer agents (e.g., ACE inhibitors, ARBs, and CCBs) were not available at the time of these studies. However, subsequent clinical trials have compared these newer antihypertensive agents with thiazide diuretics.[29–34] These data show similar effects, but most trials used a prospective open-label, blinded end point (PROBE) study methodology that is not double-blinded and limited their ability to prove equivalence of newer drugs to diuretics. Other prospective trials have compared different primary antihypertensive agents with each other.[35,36] Although these studies used head-to-head comparisons, they did not use a thiazide diuretic as their comparator treatment.

The Antihypertensive and Lipid Lowering Treatment to Prevent Heart Attack Trial (ALLHAT) The results of the ALLHAT were the deciding evidence that the JNC7 used to justify thiazide diuretics as first-line therapy.[32] It was designed to test the hypothesis that newer antihypertensive agents (an α-blocker, ACE inhibitor, or dihydropyridine CCB) would be superior to thiazide diuretic–based therapy. The primary objective was to compare the combined end point of fatal CHD and nonfatal MI. Other hypertension-related complications (e.g., heart failure, stroke) were evaluated as secondary end points. This was the largest prospective

TABLE 3-6 Alternative Antihypertensive Agents

Class	Drug (Brand Name)	Usual Dose Range (mg/day)	Daily Frequency	Comments
α_1-Blockers	Doxazosin (Cardura) Prazosin (Minipress) Terazosin (Hytrin)	1–8 2–20 1–20	1 2 or 3 1 or 2	Give first dose at bedtime; patients should rise from sitting or laying down slowly to minimize risk of orthostatic hypotension; additional benefits in men with benign prostatic hyperplasia
Direct renin inhibitor	Aliskiren (Tekturna)	150–300	1	May cause hyperkalemia in patients with chronic kidney disease and diabetes or in those receiving a potassium-sparing diuretic, aldosterone antagonist, ACE inhibitor, or ARB; may cause acute kidney failure in patients with severe bilateral renal artery stenosis or severe stenosis in artery to solitary kidney; do not use in pregnancy
Central α_2-agonists	Clonidine (Catapres) Clonidine patch (Catapres-TTS) Methyldopa (Aldomet)	0.1–0.8 0.1–0.3 250–1,000	2 1 weekly 2	Abrupt discontinuation may cause rebound hypertension; most effective if used with a diuretic to diminish fluid retention; clonidine patch is replaced once per week
Peripheral adrenergic antagonist	Reserpine (generic only)	0.05–0.25	1	Used in many of the landmark clinical trials; should be used with a diuretic to diminish fluid retention
Direct arterial vasodilators	Minoxidil (Loniten) Hydralazine (Apresoline)	10–40 20–100	1 or 2 2 to 4	Should be used with diuretic and β-blocker to diminish fluid retention and reflex tachycardia

hypertension trial ever conducted and included 42,418 patients aged 55 and older with hypertension and one additional CV risk factor. This double-blind trial randomized patients to chlorthalidone-, amlodipine-, doxazosin-, or lisinopril-based therapy for a mean of 4.9 years.

The doxazosin arm was terminated early when a significantly higher risk of heart failure versus chlorthalidone was observed.[37] The other arms were continued as scheduled and no significant differences in the primary end point was seen between the chlorthalidone and lisinopril or amlodipine treatment groups. However, chlorthalidone had statistically fewer secondary end points than amlodipine (heart failure) and lisinopril (combined CV disease, heart failure, and stroke). The study conclusions were that chlorthalidone-based therapy was superior in preventing one or more major forms of CV disease and was less expensive than amlodipine- or lisinopril-based therapy.

ALLHAT was designed as a superiority study with the hypothesis that amlodipine, doxazosin, and lisinopril would be better than chlorthalidone.[38] It did not prove this hypothesis because the primary end point was no different between chlorthalidone, amlodipine, and lisinopril. Many subgroup analyses of specific populations (e.g., black patients, CKD, diabetes) from the ALLHAT have been conducted to assess response in certain unique patient populations.[39–41] Surprisingly, none of these analyses demonstrated superior CV event reductions with lisinopril or amlodipine versus chlorthalidone. Overall, thiazide diuretics remain unsurpassed in their ability to reduce CV morbidity and mortality in most patients.

JNC7 guidelines (from 2003) recommend thiazide diuretics as a first-line therapy option for most patients, and are consistent with the historical treatment of hypertension.[1] The AHA 2007 guidelines clearly identify thiazide diuretics as a first-line therapy option, comparable to an ACE inhibitor, ARB, or CCB for first-line therapy. Contrary to the historical preference to use a thiazide diuretic as the preferred first-line agent for treating most patients with hypertension, they are simply one of four first-line drug therapy options. Figure 3-2 displays the algorithm for the treatment of hypertension and highlights that four drug classes are considered first-line agents for patients without a compelling indication for a specific drug class.

Clinical **Controversy. . .**

Is chlorthalidone superior to hydrochlorothiazide?

Chlorthalidone (thiazide-like) undisputedly reduces CV morbidity and mortality. It was used in the most influential landmark long-term placebo-controlled trials in hypertension, and is almost twice as potent in lowering BP on a milligram-per-milligram basis as hydrochlorothiazide, which has not been as extensively studied in major long-term hypertension clinical trials. In clinical practice, it is well accepted that CV benefits in hypertension apply to all thiazide diuretics, and benefits are considered a class effect. However, it is not definitively known if the clinical benefits of reducing CV morbidity and mortality that have been proven with chlorthalidone can be extrapolated to hydrochlorothiazide.

ACE Inhibitors, ARBs, and CCBs as First-Line Agents

Clinical trial data cumulatively demonstrate that ACE inhibitor–, CCB-, or ARB-based antihypertensive therapy reduces CV events. These agents may be used for patients without compelling indications as a first-line therapy. The Blood Pressure Lowering Treatment Trialists' Collaboration has evaluated the incidence of major CV events and death among different antihypertensive drug classes from 29 major randomized trials in 162,341 patients.[42] In placebo-controlled trials, the incidences of major CV events were significantly lower with ACE inhibitor– and CCB-based regimens versus placebo. Although there were differences in the incidences of certain CV events in some comparisons (e.g., stroke was lower with diuretic or CCB-based regiments versus ACE inhibitor–based regimens), there were no differences in total major CV events when ACE inhibitors, CCBs, or diuretics were compared with each other. In studies evaluating ARB-based therapy to control regimens, the incidence of major CV events was lower with ARB-based therapy. However, the control regimens used in these comparisons included both active antihypertensive drug therapies and placebo.

Data from meta-analyses may not be as influential as data from well-designed, prospective, randomized controlled trials (e.g., the ALLHAT). However, they provide clinically useful data that support using ACE inhibitor–, CCB-, or ARB-based treatment for hypertension as first-line antihypertensive agents. Clinicians can use meta-analyses data as supporting evidence when selecting a first-line antihypertensive regimen for hypertension in most patients.

Other major consensus guidelines recommend multiple first-line options for treating hypertension in most patients. The 2013 European Society of Hypertension/European Society of Cardiology guidelines and the 2011 UK's National Institute for Health and the Clinical Excellence guidelines list more than one drug therapy option as an acceptable first-line treatment approach.[43,44] The European Society of Hypertension/European Society of Cardiology guidelines are founded on the principle that CV risk reduction is a function of BP control that is largely independent of specific antihypertensives.[43] The UK guidelines stratify patients based on age and race; they recommend an ACE inhibitor or ARB first line for patients under the age of 55, and a CCB first line for patients age 55 or older or for black patients.[44]

9 β-Blockers Versus First-Line Agents Clinical trial data cumulatively suggest that β-blockers may not reduce CV events to the extent that ACE inhibitors, ARBs, CCBs, or thiazide diuretics do. These data are from three meta-analyses of clinical trials evaluating β-blocker–based therapy for hypertension.[45–48] Overall, these analyses demonstrated fewer reductions in CV events with β-blocker–based antihypertensive therapy compared mostly with ACE inhibitor– and CCB-based therapy. Although comparative data with ARB-based therapy are more limited, a similar trend was observed.

Meta-analyses data evaluating β-blockers and their ability to reduce CV events have limitations. Most studies that were included used atenolol as the β-blocker studied. Therefore, it is possible that atenolol is the only β-blocker that reduces CV events less than the other primary antihypertensive drug classes. However, consensus guidelines do extrapolate these findings to the β-blocker drug class in general.[2] In the absence of a compelling indication, the 2011 UK guidelines recommend a β-blocker as fourth-line therapy, only after other primary antihypertensive agents (e.g., ACE inhibitor or ARB, CCB, thiazide diuretic) have been used.[44] These findings also call in question the validity of results from prominent prospective, controlled clinical trials evaluating antihypertensive drug therapy that use β-blocker–based therapy, especially atenolol, as the primary comparator.[31,36] Of note, these studies used once-daily atenolol, which may be inadequate based on the shorter half-life of this agent.

β-Blocker therapy for patients without compelling indications still has a role in the management of hypertension. It is important for clinicians to remember that β-blocker–based antihypertensive therapy does not increase risk of CV events; β-blocker–based therapy reduces risk of CV events compared with no antihypertensive therapy. Using a β-blocker as a primary antihypertensive agent is optimal when an ACE inhibitor, ARB, CCB, or thiazide diuretic cannot be used as the primary agent. β-Blockers still have an important add-on role after first-line agents to reduce BP in patients with hypertension but without compelling indications.

Clinical **Controversy. . .**

Is atenolol the reason that β-blockers should not be used first-line?

Many of the clinical trials included in the meta-analyses that suggest β-blocker–based therapy may not reduce CV events as well as these other agents used atenolol dosed once daily. Atenolol has a half-life of 6 to 7 hours and is nearly always dosed once daily, while immediate-release forms of carvedilol and metoprolol have half-lives of 6 to 10 and 3 to 7 hours, respectively, and are always dosed at least twice daily. Therefore, it is possible that these findings might only apply to atenolol and also that these findings may be a result of using atenolol once daily instead of twice daily.

Patients with Compelling Indications

⑩ The JNC7 report identifies six compelling indications.[1] Compelling indications represent specific comorbid conditions where evidence from clinical trials supports using specific antihypertensive classes to treat both the compelling indication and hypertension. Drug therapy recommendations typically consist of combination drug therapies (see Fig. 3-3). Data from these clinical trials have demonstrated reduction in CV morbidity and/or mortality that justify use for patients with hypertension and with such a compelling indication. Some compelling indications include recommendations that are provided by other national treatment guidelines, or from newer clinical trials, which are complementary to the JNC7 guidelines.

Heart Failure with Reduced Ejection Fraction Five drug classes are listed as compelling indications for heart failure with reduced ejection fraction (HFrEF), also known as systolic heart failure or left ventricular dysfunction.[49] The primary physiologic abnormality in this compelling indication is decreased CO resulting from a decrease left ventricular ejection fraction. An evidence-based pharmacotherapy regimen for HFrEF, sometimes called *standard pharmacotherapy*, consists of three to four drugs: an ACE inhibitor or ARB plus diuretic therapy, followed by the addition of an appropriate β-blocker, and possibly an aldosterone receptor antagonist.

Evidence from clinical trials shows that ACE inhibitors significantly modify disease progression by reducing morbidity and mortality. Although HFrEF was the primary disease in these studies, ACE inhibitor therapy will also control BP in patients with systolic heart failure and hypertension. ARBs are acceptable as an alternative therapy for patients who cannot tolerate ACE inhibitors based on data from the Candesartan in Heart Failure—Assessment of Reduction in Mortality and Morbidity (CHARM) studies.[50] An ACE inhibitor or ARB should be started with low doses for patients with HFrEF, especially those in acute exacerbation. Heart failure induces a compensatory high-renin condition, and starting ACE inhibitors or ARBs under these conditions can cause a pronounced first-dose effect and possible orthostatic hypotension.

Diuretics are also a part of standard pharmacotherapy primarily to control symptoms. They provide symptomatic relief of edema by inducing diuresis. Loop diuretics are often needed, especially for patients with more advanced heart failure. However, some patients with well-controlled heart failure and without significant CKD may be managed with a thiazide diuretic.

β-Blocker therapy is appropriate to further modify disease in HFrEF and is a component of standard therapy for these patients. For patients on an initial regimen of diuretics and ACE inhibitors, β-blockers have been shown to reduce CV morbidity and mortality.[51,52] It is of paramount importance that β-blockers be dosed appropriately due to the risk of inducing an acute exacerbation of heart failure. They must be started in very low doses, doses much lower than that used to treat hypertension, and titrated slowly to high doses based on tolerability. Bisoprolol, carvedilol, and sustained-release metoprolol succinate are the only β-blockers proven to be beneficial in HFrEF.

After implementation of a standard three-drug regimen (diuretic, ACE inhibitor or ARB, and β-blocker), other agents may be added to further reduce CV morbidity and mortality, and reduce BP if needed. The addition of an aldosterone antagonist can reduce CV morbidity and mortality in HFrEF.[53,54] Spironolactone has been studied in severe HFrEF and has shown benefit in addition to diuretic and ACE inhibitor therapy.[53] Eplerenone has been studied in patients with symptomatic HFrEF within 3 to 14 days after an acute MI in addition to a standard three-drug regimen and in patients with mild left ventricular dysfunction.[54,55] Spironolactone and eplerenone are similar in their ability to lower risk of CV events in HFrEF.[56] For patients self-described as African Americans, the combination of a fixed dose of isosorbide dinitrate and hydralazine to standard three-drug regimen is recommended as an option to improve CV outcomes.[49]

Post-MI β-Blockers (those without intrinsic sympathomimetic activity [ISA]) and ACE inhibitor or ARB therapy are recommended in the AHA/American College of Cardiology Foundation and JNC7 guidelines.[1,2,57] β-Blockers decrease cardiac adrenergic stimulation and have been shown in clinical trials to reduce the risk of a subsequent MI or sudden cardiac death. ACE inhibitors have been shown to improve cardiac remodeling and cardiac function and to reduce CV events post-MI. These two drug classes, with β-blockers first, are considered the first drugs of choice for patients who have experienced an MI. One study, the Valsartan in Acute MI (VALIANT) trial, demonstrated that ARB therapy is similar to ACE inhibitor therapy for patients post-MI with heart failure and/or left ventricular systolic dysfunction.[58]

Coronary Artery Disease Chronic stable angina and acute coronary syndrome (unstable angina and acute MI) are forms of coronary artery disease (aka ischemic heart disease).[57,59] These are the most common forms of hypertension-associated target-organ disease. This compelling indication is also referred to as high coronary disease risk and high CV disease risk in the JNC7.[1] This compelling indication does not refer to patients without established CV disease (primary prevention patients) even if they have very high Framingham risk score (e.g., >20% over 10 years). β-Blocker therapy has been considered a standard of care for treating patients with coronary artery disease and hypertension. β-Blockers are first-line therapy in chronic stable angina and have the ability to reduce BP and improve ischemic symptoms by decreasing myocardial oxygen consumption and demand. β-Blocker therapy seems to be most effective in reducing the risk of CV events in patients with recent MI and/or ischemic symptoms. However, recent evidence indicates that the long-term risk of CV events and mortality may not be reduced with β-blocker in patients with very stable coronary artery disease (i.e., do not have ischemic symptoms or have a distant history of MI).[60]

Long-acting CCBs may considered alternatives to β-blockers (the nondihydropyridine CCBs diltiazem and verapamil) or as add-on therapy (dihydropyridine CCBs) in chronic stable angina for patients with ischemic symptoms.[59] The International Verapamil–Trandolapril Study (INVEST) demonstrated no difference in CV risk reduction when β-blocker–based therapy was compared with nondihydropyridine CCB-based therapy in this population.[61] Nonetheless, the preponderance of data is with β-blockers and they remain the therapy of choice.[1,57,59]

For acute coronary syndromes (ST-elevation MI and unstable angina/non–ST-segment MI), first-line therapy should consist of a β-blocker and ACE inhibitor.[62,63] An ARB is a reasonable alternative to an ACE inhibitor. This regimen will lower BP, control acute ischemia, and reduce CV risk.

CCBs (especially nondihydropyridine CCBs) and β-blockers provide antiischemic effects; they lower BP and reduce myocardial oxygen demand in patients with hypertension and coronary artery disease. However, cardiac stimulation may occur with dihydropyridine CCBs (particularly immediate release formulations) or β-blockers with ISA, making these agents less desirable. Therefore, β-blockers with ISA should be avoided. Nondihydropyridine CCBs should be used as alternatives to β-blockers, and dihydropyridines should be add-on therapy to β-blockers.

Once ischemic symptoms are controlled with β-blocker and/or CCB therapy, other antihypertensive drugs can be added to provide additional CV risk reduction. Clinical trials have demonstrated that the addition of an ACE inhibitor further reduces CV events in patients with chronic stable angina.[64] ARBs may provide similar benefits but have not been as extensively studied as ACE inhibitors.[64] Therefore, in coronary artery disease, ARBs are generally considered an alternative to ACE inhibitor therapy. Thiazide diuretics can be added thereafter to provide additional BP lowering and to further reduce CV risk; they do not provide antiischemic effects.

Diabetes Mellitus The primary cause of mortality in diabetes is CV disease, and hypertension management is a very important risk reduction strategy.[1,17] Five antihypertensive agents have evidence supporting their compelling indications in diabetes (see Fig. 3-3). All of these agents have been shown to reduce CV events in patients with diabetes. However, risk reduction may not be equal when comparing these agents.

11 All patients with diabetes and hypertension should ideally be treated with an ACE inhibitor or an ARB.[17] Pharmacologically, both of these agents should provide nephroprotection due to vasodilation in the efferent arteriole of the kidney. Moreover, ACE inhibitors have overwhelming data demonstrating CV risk reduction in patients with established forms of heart disease. Evidence from clinical studies have demonstrated reductions in both CV risk (mostly with ACE inhibitors) and reduction in risk of progressive kidney dysfunction (mostly with ARBs) in patients with diabetes.[17] There is debate surrounding which agent is better because data support both drug classes. Nonetheless, either drug class should be used to control BP as one of the drugs in the antihypertensive regimen for patients with diabetes, and multiple agents are often needed to attain goal BP values.

CCBs are the most appropriate add-on agents for BP control for patients with diabetes. Data indicate that these are the most optimal second agent added to either an ACE inhibitor or an ARB. Specifically, in the cohort of patients with diabetes from the Avoiding Cardiovascular Events Through Combination Therapy in Patients Living with Systolic Hypertension (ACCOMPLISH) trial, the combination of an ACE inhibitor with a CCB was better at reducing CV events than the combination of an ACE inhibitor with a thiazide.[65] The ACCOMPLISH trial is discussed later in this chapter.

A thiazide diuretic is recommended as an add-on agent to lower BP and provide additional CV risk reduction. A subgroup analysis of patients with diabetes from the ALLHAT trial showed no difference in long-term risk of CV events in the chlorthalidone and lisinopril treatment groups.[40] Therefore, some argue that thiazide diuretics, used in low doses, are equally effective for patients with hypertension and diabetes. Nonetheless, the entire body of evidence evaluating pharmacotherapy for patients with hypertension and diabetes supports an ACE inhibitor or ARB first line.[1,17,18,66]

β-Blockers, similar to CCBs, are useful add-on agents for BP control for patients with diabetes. These agents should also be used to treat another compelling indication (e.g., post-MI). β-Blockers (especially nonselective agents) can possibly mask the signs and symptoms of hypoglycemia in patients with tightly controlled diabetes because most of the symptoms of hypoglycemia (e.g., tremor, tachycardia, and palpitations) are mediated through the sympathetic nervous system. Sweating, a cholinergically mediated symptom of hypoglycemia, should still occur during a hypoglycemic episode despite β-blocker therapy. Patients may also have a delay in hypoglycemia recovery time because compensatory recovery mechanisms need the catecholamine inputs that are antagonized by β-blocker therapy. Finally, unopposed α-receptor stimulation during the acute hypoglycemic recovery phase (due to endogenous epinephrine release intended to reverse hypoglycemia) may result in acutely elevated BP due to vasoconstriction. Despite these potential problems, β-blockers can be safely used for patients with diabetes.

Based on the weight of all evidence, ACE inhibitors or ARBs are preferred first-line agents for controlling hypertension in diabetes. The need for combination therapy should be anticipated, and a CCB should be the second agent added. Thiazide diuretics, and even β-blockers, are useful evidence-based agents in this population, but are considered add-on therapies to the aforementioned agents.

Chronic Kidney Disease Patients with hypertension may develop damage to either the renal tissue (parenchyma) or the renal arteries.[19] CKD initially presents as moderately increased albuminuria (urine albumin-to-creatinine ratio 30 to 299 mg/g [3.4 to 33.8 mg/mmol] on a spot urine sample or ≥30 mg albumin in a 24-hour urine collection) that can progress to overt kidney failure. The rate of kidney function deterioration is accelerated when both hypertension and diabetes are present. Once patients have an estimated GFR <60 mL/min/1.73 m^2 or albuminuria, they have significant CKD and risk of CV disease and progression to severe CKD increases.[1] BP control can slow the decline in kidney function.

In addition to lowering BP, ACE inhibitors and ARBs reduce intraglomerular pressure, which can theoretically provide additional benefits by further reducing the decline in kidney function. ACE inhibitors and ARBs have been shown to reduce progression of CKD in diabetes[17,18] and in those without diabetes.[19,67] It is difficult to differentiate whether the kidney protection benefits are from RAAS blockade versus BP lowering. A meta-analysis failed to demonstrate any unique long-term kidney protective effects of RAAS-blocking drugs compared with other antihypertensive drugs.[68] Moreover, a subgroup analysis of patients from the ALLHAT stratified by different baseline GFR values also did not show a difference in long-term outcomes with chlorthalidone versus lisinopril.[39] Nonetheless, consensus guidelines recommend either an ACE inhibitor or an ARB as first-line therapy to control BP and preserve kidney function in CKD, and patients with urine albumin excretion >30 to 300 mg per 24 hours (or equivalent) should be treated to a goal BP of 130/80 mm Hg.

Patients may experience a rapid and profound drop in BP or acute kidney failure when given an ACE inhibitor or ARB. The potential to produce acute kidney failure is particularly problematic in patients with bilateral renal artery stenosis or a solitary functioning kidney with stenosis. Patients with renal artery stenosis are usually older, and the condition is more common in patients with diabetes or those who smoke. Patients with renal artery stenosis do not always have evidence of kidney disease unless sophisticated tests are performed. Starting with low dosages and evaluating serum creatinine soon after starting the drug can minimize this risk.

Recurrent Stroke Prevention Ischemic stroke (not hemorrhagic stroke) and transient ischemic attack are considered a form of hypertension-associated target-organ damage.[69] Attaining goal BP values in patients who have experienced an ischemic stroke is considered a primary modality to reduce risk of a second stroke. A thiazide diuretic, either in combination with an ACE inhibitor or as monotherapy, is considered an evidence-based antihypertensive regimen for patients with a history of stroke or transient ischemic attack.[1,69,70] ARBs have also been studied in this population.[71,72] Antihypertensive drug therapy should only be implemented after patients have stabilized following an acute cerebrovascular event.

Alternative Drug Treatments

It is necessary to use other agents such as a direct renin inhibitor, α-blockers, central α_2-agonists, adrenergic inhibitors, and arterial vasodilators in some patients. Although these agents are effective in lowering BP, they do not have compelling outcome data showing reduced morbidity and mortality in hypertension. Moreover, there is a much greater incidence of adverse effects with some of these agents (i.e., α-blockers, central α_2-agonists, and arterial vasodilators) than with first-line agents. They are generally reserved for patients with resistant hypertension or as add-on therapy with multiple other primary antihypertensive agents.

Special Populations Selection of drug therapy should follow the guidelines provided by established guidelines, which are summarized in Figures 3-2 and 3-3.[1] These should be maintained as the guiding principles of drug therapy. However, there are some patient populations where the approach to drug therapy may be slightly different, or utilize recommended agents using tailored dosing strategies. In some cases, this is because other agents have unique properties that benefit a coexisting condition, but may not be based on evidence from outcome studies in hypertension.

Hypertension in Older People Hypertension often presents as isolated systolic hypertension in the elderly.[73] Epidemiologic data indicate that CV morbidity and mortality are more directly correlated to SBP than to DBP for patients aged 50 and older, so this population is at high risk for hypertension-related target-organ damage.[1] Although several placebo-controlled trials have specifically demonstrated risk reduction in this form of hypertension, many older people with hypertension are either not treated, or treated but not controlled.

The SHEP was a landmark double-blind, placebo-controlled trial that evaluated chlorthalidone-based treatment (with atenolol or reserpine as add-on therapy) for isolated systolic hypertension.[8] A 36% reduction in total stroke, a 27% reduction in coronary artery disease, and 55% reduction in heart failure were demonstrated versus placebo. The Systolic Hypertension in Europe (Syst-Eur) trial was another placebo-controlled trial that evaluated treatment with a long-acting dihydropyridine CCB.[11] Treatment resulted in a 42% reduction in stroke, 26% reduction in coronary artery disease, and 29% reduction in heart failure. These data clearly demonstrate reductions in CV morbidity and mortality in older patients with isolated systolic hypertension, especially with thiazide diuretics and long-acting dihydropyridine CCBs.

The very elderly population (i.e., ≥80 years of age) were underrepresented in the SHEP and Syst-Eur studies. Historically, this population often was not treated to goal either because of a fear of side effects or because of limited data demonstrating benefit. However, the Hypertension in the Very Elderly Trial (HYVET) provided definitive evidence that antihypertensive drug therapy provides significant clinical benefits in the very elderly.[74] The HYVET was a prospective controlled clinical trial that randomized patients 80 years and older with hypertension to placebo or antihypertensive drug therapy. It was stopped early after a median of only 1.8 years because the incidence of death was 21% higher in placebo-treated patients. Based on these results, hypertension should be treated in the very elderly. This is also recommended by the AHA in a 2011 consensus statement on hypertension in the elderly.[73]

Thiazide diuretics or β-blockers have been compared with either ACE inhibitors or CCBs in elderly patients with either systolic hypertension, diastolic hypertension, or both in the Swedish Trial in Old Patients with Hypertension-2 (STOP-2) study.[75] In this trial no significant differences were seen between conventional drugs and either ACE inhibitors or CCBs. However, there were significantly fewer MIs and cases of heart failure in the ACE inhibitor group compared with the CCB group. These data suggest that overall treatment may be more important than specific antihypertensive agents in this population.

Elderly patients are more sensitive to volume depletion and sympathetic inhibition than younger patients. This may lead to orthostatic hypotension (see next section). In the elderly, this can increase the risk of falls due to the associated dizziness. Centrally acting agents and α_1-blockers should generally be avoided or used with caution in the elderly because they are frequently associated with dizziness and orthostatic hypotension. Diuretics, ACE inhibitors, and ARBs provide significant benefits and can safely be used in the elderly, but smaller-than-usual initial doses must be used for initial therapy.

The JNC7 and 2007 AHA goal BP recommendations are independent of age.[1,2] However, the AHA published an expert consensus on hypertension in the elderly in 2011.[73] Although age-adjusted goals are generally not recommended, for patients aged 80 years and older, a SBP of 140 to 145 mm Hg is recommended as appropriate for patients who do not tolerate treatment with a goal SBP of <140 mm Hg. The treatment of hypertension in older patients should follow the same principles that are outlined for general care of hypertension. However, initial drug doses may be lower, and dosage titrations over a longer period of time are usually needed to minimize the risk of hypotension.

Clinical **Controversy...**

How aggressively should BP be lowered in the very elderly?

It has been advocated for several years to target standard BP goals in the elderly population, regardless of age. This is a well-accepted standard of care for patients with hypertension who continue to have elevated BP as they age, meaning that a patient with a history of hypertension should not have his or her BP goal adjusted just because he or she has become older. However, for patients who initially develop hypertension when they are very elderly, it is less clear what their BP goal should be. The HYVET trial established that treating hypertension in patients aged 80 years or older reduces mortality, but the treatment goal in that population was <150/80 mm Hg with a mean SBP and DBP achieved of 145 and 79 mm Hg, respectively, at 2 years.

⓬ **Patients at Risk for Orthostatic Hypotension** *Orthostatic hypotension* is a significant drop in BP when standing and can be associated with dizziness and/or fainting. It is defined as a SBP decrease of >20 mm Hg or DBP decrease of >10 mm Hg when changing from supine to standing.[1] The risk of orthostatic hypotension is increased in older patients (especially those with isolated systolic hypotension) and those with diabetes, severe volume depletion, baroreflex dysfunction, autonomic insufficiency, and on concomittant venodilators (α-blockers, mixed α-/β-blockers, nitrates, and phosphodiesterase inhibitors). For patients with these risks factors, antihypertensive agents should be started in low doses, especially diuretics, ACE inhibitors, and ARBs.

Hypertension in Children and Adolescents Detecting hypertension in children requires special attention to BP measurement, which is defined as SBP and/or DBP that is >95th percentile for sex, age, and height on at least 3 occasions.[76] BP between the 90th and 95th percentile, or >120/80 mm Hg in adolescents, is considered prehypertension. Hypertensive children often have a family history of high BP, and many are overweight predisposing them to insulin resistance and associated CV disease. Unlike hypertension in adults, secondary hypertension is more common in children and adolescents. An appropriate workup for secondary causes is required if elevated BP is identified. Kidney disease (e.g., pyelonephritis, glomerulonephritis) is the most common cause of secondary hypertension in children. Coarctation of the aorta can also produce secondary hypertension. Medical or surgical management of the underlying disorder usually normalizes BP.

Nonpharmacologic treatment, particularly weight loss in those overweight, is the cornerstone of therapy for essential hypertension in children.[76] The goal is to reduce the BP to <95th percentile for sex, age, and height, or <90th percentile if concurrent conditions such as CKD, diabetes, or target-organ damage are present. ACE inhibitors, ARBs, β-blockers, CCBs, and thiazide diuretics are all acceptable choices in children and have data supporting their use. ACE inhibitors, ARBs, and direct renin inhibitors are contraindicated in sexually active girls due to potential teratogenic effect. As with adults, selection of initial agents should be based on the presence of compelling indications or concurrent conditions that may warrant their use (e.g., ACE inhibitor or ARB for those with diabetes or CKD).

Pregnancy Hypertension during pregnancy is a major cause of maternal and neonatal morbidity and mortality.[1,77] Hypertension during pregnancy is categorized as preeclampsia, eclampsia, gestational, chronic, and superimposition of preeclampsia on chronic hypertension. *Preeclampsia*, defined as an elevated BP >140/90 mm Hg that appears after 20 weeks' gestation accompanied by new-onset proteinuria (≥300 mg/24 hours), can lead to life-threatening complications for both mother and fetus. Eclampsia, the onset of convulsions in preeclampsia, is a medical emergency. *Gestational hypertension* is defined as new-onset hypertension arising after midpregnancy in the absence of proteinuria, and chronic hypertension is elevated BP that is noted before the pregnancy began. It is controversial whether treating elevated BP for patients with chronic hypertension in pregnancy is beneficial. However, women with chronic hypertension prior to pregnancy are at increased risk of a number of complications including superimposed preeclampsia, preterm delivery, fetal growth restriction or demise, placental abruption, heart failure, and acute kidney failure.[77]

Definitive treatment of preeclampsia is delivery. Delivery is indicated if pending or frank eclampsia is present. Otherwise, management consists of restricting activity, bedrest, and close monitoring. Salt restriction, or any other measures that contract blood volume, should not be employed. Antihypertensive agents are used prior to induction of labor if DBP is greater than 105 mm Hg with a target DBP of 95 to 105 mm Hg. IV hydralazine is most commonly used, and IV labetalol is also effective. Immediate-release oral nifedipine has been used in the past, but it is not approved by the FDA for hypertension, and untoward fetal and maternal effects (hypotension with fetal distress) have been reported.

TABLE 3-7 Treatment of Chronic Hypertension in Pregnancy

Drug/Class	Comments
Methyldopa	Preferred agent based on long-term followup data supporting safety; traditional drug of choice
β-Blockers	Generally safe, but intrauterine growth retardation reported (mostly with atenolol)
Labetalol	Increasingly preferred over methyldopa because of fewer side effects
Clonidine	Limited data available; used mainly in third trimester
CCBs	Limited data available; no increase in major teratogenicity with exposure (except immediate-release oral nifedipine should not be used)
Diuretics	Not first-line agents but probably safe in low doses if started prior to conception for essential hypertension
ACE inhibitors, ARBs, direct renin inhibitors	Contraindicated; major teratogenicity reported with exposure (fetal toxicity and death)

Many agents can be used to treat chronic hypertension in pregnancy (Table 3-7). Unfortunately, there is little consensus and few data regarding the most appropriate therapy in pregnancy. Methyldopa is still considered the drug of choice.[1] It is viewed as very safe based on long-term followup data (7.5 years) that have not demonstrated adverse effects on childhood development. β-Blockers (other than atenolol), labetalol, and CCBs are also reasonable alternatives. ACE inhibitors and ARBs are known teratogens and are absolutely contraindicated.[78]

African Americans Hypertension affects African American patients at a disproportionately higher rate, and hypertension-related target-organ damage is more prevalent than in other populations.[1,79] Reasons for these differences are not fully understood, but may be related to differences in electrolyte homeostasis, GFR, sodium excretion and transport mechanisms, plasma renin activity, and BP response to plasma volume expansion.

African Americans have an increased need for combination therapy to attain and maintain BP goals.[79] The International Society on Hypertension in Blacks consensus statement recommendations aggressively promote combination therapy. They recommend starting with two drugs for patients with SBP values ≥15 mm Hg from goal. This aggressive approach is reasonable considering that overall goal BP attainment rates are low in African Americans.

BP-lowering effects of antihypertensive classes vary in African Americans, primarily when used as monotherapy. Thiazide diuretics and CCBs are most effective at lowering BP in African Americans. When either of these two classes (especially thiazide diuretics) are used in combination with a β-blocker, ACE inhibitor, or ARB (which are three classes known to be less effective at lowering BP in African Americans), antihypertensive response is significantly increased. This may be due to the low-renin pattern of hypertension in African Americans, which can result in less BP lowering with β-blockers, ACE inhibitors, or ARBs when used as monotherapy compared with white patients. Interestingly, African Americans have a higher risk of angioedema and cough from ACE inhibitors compared with whites.[79]

Despite potential differences in antihypertensive effects, drug therapy selection should be based on evidence, no different from what is recommended for the hypertensive population in general. Drug therapies should be used if a compelling indication is present, even if the antihypertensive effect may not be as great as with another drug class (e.g., a β-blocker is first line for BP control in an African American patient who is post-MI).

Other Concomitant Conditions

Most patients with hypertension have some other coexisting conditions that may influence selection or utilization of drug therapy. The influence of concomitant conditions should only be complementary to, and never in replacement of, drug therapy choices indicated by compelling indications. Under some circumstances, these considerations are helpful in deciding on a particular antihypertensive agent when more than one antihypertensive class is recommended to treat a compelling indication. In some cases, an agent should be avoided because it may aggravate a concomitant disorder. In other cases, an antihypertensive can be used to treat hypertension, a compelling indication, and another concomitant condition. These are briefly summarized in Table 3-5.

Pulmonary Disease and Peripheral Arterial Disease β-Blockers, especially nonselective agents, have been generally avoided for patients with hypertension and reactive airway disease (asthma or chronic obstructive pulmonary disease [COPD] with a reversible obstructive component) due to a fear of inducing bronchospasm.[80] This precaution is more of a myth than a fact. Data suggest that cardioselective β-blockers can safely be used in patients with asthma or COPD.[81] Therefore, cardioselective β-blockers should be used to treat a compelling indication (i.e., post-MI, coronary disease, or heart failure) for patients with reactive airway disease.

PAD is considered a noncoronary form of atherosclerotic vascular disease and is a coronary artery disease risk equivalent.[57,80] β-Blockers can theoretically be problematic for patients with PAD due to possible decreased peripheral blood flow secondary to unopposed stimulation of α_1-receptors that results in vasoconstriction. If problematic, this can be mitigated by using a β-blocker that also has α_1-blocking properties (e.g., carvedilol). However, β-blockers are not contraindicated in PAD and have not been shown to adversely affect walking capacity.[82]

Metabolic Syndrome Metabolic syndrome is a cluster of multiple cardiometabolic risk factors.[12] It has been most recently defined as the presence of three of the following five criteria: abdominal obesity (based on waist circumference measurements), elevated triglycerides, low HDL cholesterol, elevated BP (≥130/≥85 mm Hg or receiving drug treatment for high BP), and elevated fasting blood glucose.[12]

Despite the debate regarding whether or not metabolic syndrome is a true "disease" or rather simply a cluster of risk factors, it is widely accepted that patients with metabolic syndrome have increased risk of developing CV disease and/or type 2 diabetes. Using an ACE inhibitor or ARB is associated with the lowest rate of developing new-onset diabetes in patients with hypertension.[83] However, studies specifically evaluating the most effective antihypertensive regimen for patients with metabolic syndrome have not been done. In addition, an ALLHAT subgroup analysis of patients with impaired fasting glucose showed that CV events were reduced more with chlorthalidone compared with lisinopril.[40] Thus, thiazide diuretics can be used first line for patients with metabolic syndrome, similar to ACE inhibitors, ARBs, or CCBs, but treated patients will have a higher risk of developing elevated fasting glucose.

Erectile Dysfunction Most antihypertensive agents have been associated with erectile dysfunction in men.[84] However, it is not clear if erectile dysfunction associated with antihypertensive treatment is solely a result of drug therapy or rather a symptom of underlying vascular disease. β-Blockers have traditionally been labeled as agents that significantly cause sexual dysfunction, and many practitioners have avoided prescribing them as a result. However, data supporting this notion are limited. A systematic review of 15 studies involving 35,000 patients assessing β-blocker use for MI, heart failure, and hypertension found only a very slight increased risk for erectile dysfunction.[85] In addition, prospective long-term data from the Treatment of Mild Hypertension Study (TOMHS) and the Veterans Administration Cooperative trial show no difference in the incidence of erectile dysfunction between diuretics and β-blockers versus ACE inhibitors and CCBs.[86,87] Centrally acting agents are associated with higher rates of sexual dysfunction and should be avoided in men with erectile dysfunction.

Hypertensive men frequently have atherosclerotic vascular disease, which frequently results in erectile dysfunction. Therefore, erectile dysfunction is associated with chronic arterial changes resulting from elevated BP, and lack of control may increase the risk of erectile dysfunction. These changes are even more pronounced in hypertensive men with diabetes.

Individual Antihypertensive Agents

ACE Inhibitors ACE inhibitors are a first-line therapy option in most patients with hypertension.[1,2,6] The ALLHAT demonstrated less heart failure and stroke with chlorthalidone versus lisinopril.[31] However, another outcome study has demonstrated similar, if not better, outcomes with ACE inhibitors versus hydrochlorothiazide.[34] It is possible that the different thiazide diuretics have different abilities to reduce hypertension-associated target-organ damage. Nonetheless, most clinicians will agree that if ACE inhibitors are not the first agent used in most patients with hypertension, they should be the second agent used.

ACE facilitates production of angiotensin II that has a major role in arterial BP regulation as depicted in Figure 3-1. ACE is distributed in many tissues and is present in several different cell types, but its principal location is in endothelial cells. Therefore, the major site for angiotensin II production is in the blood vessels, not the kidney. ACE inhibitors block the ACE, thus inhibiting conversion of angiotensin I to angiotensin II. Angiotensin II is a potent vasoconstrictor that stimulates aldosterone secretion, causing an increase in sodium and water reabsorption with accompanying potassium loss. By blocking the ACE, vasodilation and a decrease in aldosterone occur.

ACE inhibitors also block degradation of bradykinin and stimulate the synthesis of other vasodilating substances (prostaglandin E_2 and prostacyclin). The observation that ACE inhibitors lower BP in patients with normal plasma renin activity suggests that bradykinin and perhaps tissue production of ACE are important in hypertension. Increased bradykinin enhances the BP-lowering effects of ACE inhibitors, but also is responsible for the side effect of dry cough. ACE inhibitors effectively prevent or regress LVH by reducing direct stimulation by angiotensin II on myocardial cells.

There are many evidence-based uses for ACE inhibitors (see Fig. 3-3). ACE inhibitors reduce CV morbidity and mortality in patients with HFrEF,[49] and decrease progression of CKD.[66] They should be first line as disease-modifying therapy in all of these patients unless absolutely contraindicated. ACE inhibitors (or ARBs in certain patients) are first line for patients with diabetes and hypertension because of demonstrated CV disease and kidney benefits. A regimen including an ACE inhibitor with a thiazide diuretic is considered first line in recurrent stroke prevention based on proven benefits from the PROGRESS trial showing reduced risk of secondary stroke.[33] In combination with β-blocker therapy, evidence shows that ACE inhibitors further reduce CV risk in coronary disease and in patients post-MI.[57,59,62,63] These benefits of ACE inhibitors occur in patients with atherosclerotic vascular disease even in the absence of left ventricular dysfunction and have the potential to reduce the development of new-onset type 2 diabetes.[88]

Most ACE inhibitors can be dosed once daily in hypertension (Table 3-5). In some patients, especially when higher doses are used, twice-daily dosing is needed to maintain 24-hour effects with enalapril, benazepril, moexipril, quinapril, and ramipril.

ACE inhibitors are well tolerated,[89] but are not absent of side effects. They decrease aldosterone and can increase potassium serum concentrations. While this increase is usually small, hyperkalemia is possible. Patients with CKD or those on concomitant potassium supplements, potassium-sparing diuretics, ARBs, or a direct renin inhibitor are at risk for hyperkalemia. Judicious monitoring of serum potassium and creatinine values within 4 weeks of starting or increasing the dose of an ACE inhibitor can often identify these abnormalities early before they evolve into serious adverse events.

The most worrisome adverse effect of ACE inhibitor therapy is acute kidney failure. This serious adverse effect is rare, occurring in less than 1% of patients. Preexisting kidney disease increases the risk of this side effect. Bilateral renal artery stenosis or unilateral stenosis of a solitary functioning kidney renders patients dependent on the vasoconstrictive effect of angiotensin II on the efferent arteriole of the kidney, thus explaining why these patients are particularly susceptible to acute kidney failure from ACE inhibitors. Slow titration of the ACE inhibitor dose and judicious kidney function monitoring can minimize risk and allow for early detection of those with renal artery stenosis.

It is important to note that GFR does decrease somewhat in patients when started on ACE inhibitors or ARBs.[90] This is attributed to the inhibition of angiotensin II vasoconstriction on the efferent arteriole. This decrease in GFR often increases serum creatinine, and small increases should be anticipated when monitoring patients on ACE inhibitors. Either modest elevations of ≤35% (for baseline creatinine values ≤3 mg/dL [265 μmol/L]) or absolute increases <1 mg/dL (88 μmol/L) do not warrant changes. If larger increases occur, ACE inhibitor therapy should be stopped or the dose reduced.

Angioedema is a serious potential complication of ACE inhibitor therapy. It occurs in <1% of the population, and it is more likely in African Americans and smokers. Symptoms include lip and tongue swelling and possibly difficulty breathing. Drug withdrawal is appropriate for treating patients with angioedema. However, angioedema associated with laryngeal edema and/or pulmonary symptoms occasionally occurs and requires additional treatment with epinephrine, corticosteroids, antihistamines, and/or emergent intubations to support respiration. A history of angioedema, even if not from an ACE inhibitor, precludes use of another ACE inhibitor (it is a contraindication). Cross-reactivity between ACE inhibitors and ARBs does not appear to be a significant concern. The Telmisartan Randomized Assessment Study in ACE-Intolerant Subjects with Cardiovascular Disease (TRANSCEND) trial enrolled 75 patients with a history of ACE inhibitor–induced angioedema, and randomized these patients to either placebo or ARB therapy.[91] There were no cases of repeat angioedema among these patients. These data suggest the cross-reactivity is very low. Hence, an ARB can be used in a patient with a history of ACE inhibitor–induced angioedema when it is needed. However, clinicians should monitor for repeat occurrences, since idiopathic angioedema may still occur.

A persistent dry cough develops in up to 20% of patients treated with an ACE inhibitor. It is pharmacologically explained by the inhibition of bradykinin breakdown. This cough does not cause respiratory illness but is annoying to patients and can compromise adherence. It should be clearly differentiated from a wet cough due to pulmonary edema, which may be a sign of uncontrolled heart failure versus an ACE inhibitor–induced cough.

ACE inhibitors, as well as ARBs and direct renin inhibitors, are absolutely contraindicated in pregnancy.[1,78] Female patients of childbearing age should be counseled regarding effective forms of birth control as ACE inhibitors have been associated with major congenital malformations when exposed in the first trimester and fetopathy (group of conditions that includes renal failure, renal dysplasia, hypotension, oligohydramnios, pulmonary hypotension, hypocalvaria, and death) has occurred when exposed in the second and third trimesters.[78] Similar to diuretics, ACE inhibitors can increase lithium serum concentrations in patients on lithium therapy. Concurrent use of an ACE with a potassium-sparing diuretic (including aldosterone antagonists), potassium supplements, an ARB, or a direct renin inhibitor may result in hyperkalemia.

Starting doses of ACE inhibitors should be low, with even lower doses for patients at risk for orthostatic hypotension or severe renal dysfunction (e.g., elderly, CKD). Acute hypotension may occur at the onset of ACE inhibitor therapy. Patients who are sodium or volume depleted, in a heart failure exacerbation, very elderly, or on concurrent vasodilators or diuretics are at high risk for this effect. It is important to start with half the normal dose of an ACE inhibitor for all patients with these risk factors and to use slow dose titration.

ARBs Angiotensin II is generated by two enzymatic pathways: the RAAS, which involves ACE, and an alternative pathway that uses other enzymes such as chymase (aka "tissue ACE"). ACE inhibitors inhibit only the effects of angiotensin II produced through the RAAS, whereas ARBs inhibit angiotensin II from all pathways. It is unclear how these differences affect tissue concentrations of ACE. ACE inhibitors only partially block the effects of angiotensin II, although the clinical significance of this is not known.

ARBs directly block the AT_1 receptor that mediates the known effects of angiotensin II in humans: vasoconstriction, aldosterone release, sympathetic activation, antidiuretic hormone release, and constriction of the efferent arterioles of the glomerulus. They do not block the AT_2 receptor. Therefore, beneficial effects of AT_2 receptor stimulation (vasodilation, tissue repair, and inhibition of cell growth) remain intact when ARBs are used. Unlike ACE inhibitors, ARBs do not block the breakdown of bradykinin. Therefore, some of the beneficial effects of bradykinin, such as vasodilation, regression of myocyte hypertrophy and fibrosis, and increased levels of tissue plasminogen activator, are not present with ARB therapy.

ARB therapy has been directly compared with ACE inhibitor therapy in the management of hypertension.[92] The Ongoing Telmisartan Alone and in Combination with Ramipril Global End Point Trial (ON-TARGET) was a double-blind trial that randomized 25,620 patients with hypertension to ACE inhibitor–based therapy, ARB-based therapy, or the combination of an ACE inhibitor with an ARB. The primary end point was a composite end point of CV death or hospitalization for heart failure. After a median followup of 56 months, there was no difference in the primary end point between any of the three treatment groups. Therefore, these data establish that the CV event–lowering benefits of ARB therapy are similar to ACE inhibitor therapy in hypertension. Moreover, the combination of an ACE inhibitor with an ARB had no additional CV event lowering but was associated with a higher risk of side effects (renal dysfunction, hypotension). Therefore, there is no reason to use an ACE inhibitor with an ARB for the management of hypertension.

For patients with certain compelling indications, ARBs have outcome data showing long-term reductions in progression of target-organ damage. For patients with type 2 diabetes and nephropathy, progression of nephropathy has been shown to be significantly reduced with ARB therapy.[17] Some benefits appear to be independent of BP lowering, suggesting that the pharmacologic effects of ARBs on the efferent arteriole may result in attenuated progression of kidney disease. For patients with HFrEF, the CHARM study showed that ARB therapy reduces risk of hospitalization for heart failure when used as an alternative therapy in ACE-intolerant patients.[50]

ARBs have been compared head-to-head with CCBs. The Morbidity and Mortality After Stroke: Eprosartan Versus Nitrendipine in Secondary Prevention (MOSES) trial demonstrated that eprosartan reduced the occurrence of recurrent stroke greater than nitrendipine in patients with a past medical history of cerebrovascular disease.[71] Using nitrendipine was a reasonable comparator because the Syst-Eur had already demonstrated that nitrendipine reduces the occurrence of CV events, particularly stroke, in older patients with isolated systolic hypertension compared with placebo.[11] These data support the common notion that ARBs may have cerebroprotective effects that may explain CV event reductions.[93] Another outcome study, the Valsartan Antihypertensive Long-Term Use Evaluation (VALUE) trial, showed that valsartan-based therapy is equivalent to amlodipine-based therapy for the primary composite outcome of first CV event in patients with hypertension and additional CV risk factors.[35] However, occurrence of certain components of the primary end point (stroke and MI) and new-onset type 2 diabetes was lower in the valsartan group. Although patients treated with amlodipine had slightly lower mean BP values than valsartan-treated patients, there was no difference in the primary end point.

The addition of low doses of a CCB or thiazide diuretic to an ARB significantly increases antihypertensive efficacy. Similar to ACE inhibitors, most ARBs have long enough half-lives to allow for once-daily dosing. However, candesartan, eprosartan, losartan, and valsartan have the shortest half-lives and may require twice-daily dosing for sustained BP lowering.

ARBs have the lowest incidence of side effects compared with other antihypertensive agents.[89] Because they do not affect bradykinin, they do not illicit a dry cough like ACE inhibitors. While these drugs have been referred to as "ACE inhibitors without the cough," pharmacologic differences highlight that they could have very different effects on vascular smooth muscle and myocardial tissue that can correlate to different effects on target-organ damage and CV risk reduction when compared with ACE inhibitors. Data from the Randomized Olmesartan and Diabetes Microalbuminuria Prevention (ROADMAP) trial have demonstrated that ARB therapy delays the onset of albuminuria in patients with type 2 diabetes.[94] Regardless, their first-line role for patients with type 2 diabetic nephropathy is well established, and they also are very reasonable alternatives for patients requiring an ACE inhibitor but who experience an intolerable cough.

Like ACE inhibitors, ARBs may cause renal insufficiency, hyperkalemia, and orthostatic hypotension. The same precautions that apply to ACE inhibitors for patients with suspected bilateral renal artery stenosis, those on drugs that can raise potassium, and those on drugs that increase risk of hypotension apply to ARBs. As discussed in ACE Inhibitors, ARBs, and CCBs as First-Line Agents above, patients with a history of ACE inhibitor angioedema can be treated with an ARB when needed.[91] ARBs should not be used in pregnancy.

CCBs CCBs, both dihydropyridine CCBs and nondihydropyridine CCBs, are first-line therapy options and are very effective antihypertensive agents.[1,2] They also have compelling indications in coronary artery disease and in diabetes. However, with these compelling indications, they are in addition to, or instead of, other first-line antihypertensive drug classes.

Contraction of cardiac and smooth muscle cells requires an increase in free intracellular calcium concentrations from the extracellular fluid. When cardiac or vascular smooth muscle is stimulated, voltage-sensitive channels in the cell membrane are opened, allowing calcium to enter the cells. The influx of extracellular calcium into the cell releases stored calcium from the sarcoplasmic reticulum. As intracellular free calcium concentration increases, it binds to a protein, calmodulin, which then activates myosin kinase enabling myosin to interact with actin to induce contraction. CCBs work by inhibiting influx of calcium across the cell membrane. There are two types of voltage-gated calcium channels: a high-voltage channel (L-type) and a low-voltage channel (T-type). Currently available CCBs only block the L-type channel, which leads to coronary and peripheral vasodilation.

The two subclasses of CCBs, dihydropyridines and nondihydropyridines (see Table 3-5), are pharmacologically very different from each other. Antihypertensive effectiveness is similar with both subclasses, but they differ somewhat in other pharmacodynamic effects. Nondihydropyridines (verapamil and diltiazem) decrease heart rate and slow atrioventricular nodal conduction. Similar to β-blockers, these drugs may also treat supraventricular tachyarrhythmias (e.g., atrial fibrillation). Verapamil produces negative inotropic and chronotropic effects that are responsible for its propensity to precipitate or cause systolic heart failure in high-risk patients. Diltiazem also has these effects but to a lesser extent than verapamil. All CCBs (except amlodipine and felodipine) have negative inotropic effects. Dihydropyridines may cause a baroreceptor-mediated reflex tachycardia because of their potent peripheral vasodilating effects. This effect appears to be more pronounced with the first-generation dihydropyridines (e.g., nifedipine) and is significantly diminished with the newer agents (e.g., amlodipine) and when given in sustained-release dosage forms. Dihydropyridines do not alter conduction through the atrioventricular node and thus are not effective agents in supraventricular tachyarrhythmias.

Dihydropyridine CCBs CCBs, both dihydropyridines and nondihydropyridines, are as effective at lowering CV events as other first-line agents in most patients with hypertension. The dihydropyridine CCBs have been extensively studied. In ALLHAT there was no difference in the primary outcome between chlorthalidone and amlodipine, and only the secondary outcome of heart failure was higher with amlodipine.[32] A subgroup analysis of ALLHAT directly compared amlodipine with lisinopril and demonstrated that there was no difference in the primary outcome.[95] However, amlodipine was superior to lisinopril for BP control in blacks, and for stroke reduction in blacks and in women. There was a lower risk of heart failure in the lisinopril group. As discussed previously, the VALUE study also showed no difference between valsartan and amlodipine in the primary outcome of first CV event in high-risk patients.[35]

Dihydropyridine CCBs are very effective in older patients with isolated systolic hypertension. The placebo-controlled Syst-Eur trial demonstrated that a long-acting dihydropyridine CCB reduced the risk of CV events markedly in isolated systolic hypertension.[11] A long-acting dihydropyridine CCB should be strongly considered as preferred add-on therapy when a thiazide diuretic is not controlling BP in a patient with isolated systolic hypertension and no other compelling indications.

Among dihydropyridines, short-acting nifedipine may rarely cause an increase in the frequency, intensity, and duration of angina in association with acute hypotension. This effect is most likely due to a reflex sympathetic stimulation and is likely obviated by using sustained-release formulations of nifedipine. For this reason, all other dihydropyridines have an intrinsically long half-life or are sustained-release formulations. Immediate-release nifedipine has been associated with an increased incidence of adverse CV effects, is not approved for treatment of hypertension, and should not be used to treat hypertension. Other side effects with dihydropyridines include dizziness, flushing, headache, gingival hyperplasia, peripheral edema, mood changes, and various GI complaints. Side effects due to vasodilation such as dizziness, flushing, headache, and peripheral edema occur more frequently with all dihydropyridines than with the nondihydropyridines (i.e., verapamil, diltiazem) because they are less potent vasodilators.

Nondihydropyridine CCBs Diltiazem and verapamil can cause cardiac conduction abnormalities such as bradycardia or atrioventricular block. These problems occur mostly with high doses or when used for patients with preexisting abnormalities in the cardiac conduction system. Heart failure has been reported in otherwise healthy patients due to negative inotropic effects. Both drugs can cause anorexia, nausea, peripheral edema, and hypotension. Verapamil causes constipation in about 7% of patients. This side effect also occurs with diltiazem, but to a lesser extent.

Verapamil and to a lesser extent diltiazem can cause drug interactions due to their ability to inhibit the cytochrome P450 3A4 isoenzyme system. This inhibition can increase serum concentrations of other drugs that are metabolized by this isoenzyme system (e.g., cyclosporine, digoxin, lovastatin, simvastatin, tacrolimus, theophylline). Verapamil and diltiazem should be given very cautiously with a β-blocker because there is an increased risk of heart block with these combinations. When a CCB is needed in combination with a β-blocker for BP lowering, a dihydropyridine should be selected because it will not increase risk of heart block. The hepatic metabolism of CCBs, especially felodipine, nicardipine, nifedipine, and nisoldipine, may be inhibited by ingesting large quantities of grapefruit juice (e.g., ≥1 qt daily).

Many different formulations of verapamil and diltiazem are currently available (see Table 3-5). Although certain sustained-release verapamil and diltiazem products contain the same active drug (e.g., Calan SR and Verelan), they are usually not AB rated by the FDA as interchangeable on a milligram-per-milligram basis due to different biopharmaceutical release mechanisms. However, the clinical significance of these differences is likely negligible.

Two sustained-release verapamil products (Covera-HS and Verelan PM) and one diltiazem product (Cardizem LA) are chronotherapeutically designed to target the circadian BP rhythm. These agents are primarily dosed in the evening (with the exception of Cardizem LA, which may be dosed in the morning or evening) so that drug is released during the early morning hours when BP first starts to increase. The rationale behind chronotherapy in hypertension is that blunting the early morning BP surge may result in greater reductions in CV events than conventional dosing of regular antihypertensive products in the morning. However, evidence from the Controlled Onset Verapamil Investigation of Cardiovascular End-Points (CONVINCE) trial showed that chronotherapeutic verapamil was similar to, but not better than, a thiazide diuretic–β-blocker–based regimen with respect to CV events.[30]

Diuretics There are four subclasses of diuretics that are used in the treatment of hypertension: thiazide diuretics, loops, potassium-sparing agents, and aldosterone antagonists (see Table 3-5).[96] Thiazide diuretics are the preferred type of diuretic for most patients with hypertension.[1,2] The best available evidence justifying this recommendation is from the ALLHAT.[32] Moreover, when combination therapy is needed in hypertension to control BP, a thiazide diuretic as an add-on agent, but not necessarily the second agent, is very effective in lowering BP.[1,97]

Loops are more potent agents for inducing diuresis, but they are not ideal antihypertensive agents unless relief of edema is also needed. In general, loops are often preferred over a thiazide diuretic for hypertension in patients with CKD when estimated GFR is <30 mL/min/1.73 m^2.[96] However, many patients with an estimated GFR of <30 mL/min/1.73 m^2 but not on dialysis will still have antihypertensive effects with thiazide diuretics.[98] This is especially true with chlorthalidone.[96]

Potassium-sparing diuretics are very weak antihypertensive agents when used alone and provide minimal additive effect when used in combination with a thiazide or loop diuretic. Their primary use is in combination with another diuretic to counteract the potassium-wasting properties of the other diuretic agent. Aldosterone antagonists (spironolactone and eplerenone) may be technically considered potassium-sparing agents but are more potent as antihypertensives. However, they are viewed as an independent class due to evidence supporting compelling indications.

The exact hypotensive mechanism of action of diuretics is not known, but has been well hypothesized. The drop in BP seen when diuretics are first started is caused by an initial diuresis. Diuresis causes reductions in plasma and stroke volume, which decreases CO and BP. This initial drop in CO causes a compensatory increase in PVR. With chronic diuretic therapy, extracellular fluid and plasma volume return to near pretreatment values. However, PVR decreases to values that are lower than the pretreatment baseline. This reduction in PVR is responsible for chronic antihypertensive effects.

Thiazide diuretics have additional actions that may further explain their antihypertensive effects. They mobilize sodium and water from arteriolar walls. This effect would lessen the amount of physical encroachment on the lumen of the vessel created by excessive accumulation of intracellular fluid. As the diameter of the lumen relaxes and increases, there is less resistance to the flow of blood and PVR further drops. High dietary sodium intake can blunt this effect and a low salt intake can enhance this effect. Thiazide diuretics are also postulated to cause direct relaxation of vascular smooth muscle.

Diuretics should ideally be dosed in the morning if given once daily and in the morning and late afternoon when dosed twice daily to minimize risk of nocturnal diuresis. However, with chronic use, thiazide diuretics, potassium-sparing diuretics, and aldosterone antagonists rarely cause a pronounced diuresis.

The major pharmacokinetic differences between the various thiazide diuretics are serum half-life and duration of diuretic effect. The clinical relevance of these differences is unknown because the serum half-life of most antihypertensive agents does not correlate with the hypotensive duration of action. Moreover, diuretics lower BP primarily through extrarenal mechanisms. Hydrochlorothiazide and particularly chlorthalidone are the two most frequently used thiazide diuretics in landmark clinical trials that have demonstrated reduced morbidity and mortality. Hydrochlorothiazide is considered a "thiazide-type" diuretic while chlorthalidone is a "thiazide-like" diuretic. These agents are not equipotent on a milligram-per-milligram basis; chlorthalidone is 1.5 to 2 times more potent than hydrochlorothiazide.[96] This has been attributed to a longer half-life (45 to 60 hours vs. 8 to 15 hours) and longer duration of effect (48 to 72 hours vs. 16 to 24 hours) with chlorthalidone.

Diuretics are very effective in lowering BP when used in combination with most other antihypertensives. This additive response is explained by two independent pharmacodynamic effects. First, when two drugs cause the same overall pharmacologic effect (BP lowering) through different mechanisms of action, their combination usually results in an additive or synergistic effect. This is especially relevant when a β-blocker or ACE inhibitor is indicated in an African American, but does not elicit sufficient antihypertensive effect. Adding a diuretic in this situation can often significantly lower BP. Second, a compensatory increase in sodium and fluid retention may be seen with antihypertensive agents. This problem is counteracted with the concurrent use of a diuretic.

Side effects of thiazide diuretics include hypokalemia, hypomagnesemia, hypercalcemia, hyperuricemia, hyperglycemia, dyslipidemia, and sexual dysfunction. Many of these side effects were identified when high doses of thiazides were used in the past (e.g., hydrochlorothiazide 100 to 200 mg/day). Current guidelines recommend limiting the dose of hydrochlorothiazide or chlorthalidone to 12.5 to 25 mg/day, which markedly reduces the risk for most metabolic side effects. However, the most effective antihypertensive dose of hydrochlorothiazide is 50 mg daily, although many clinicians are dissuaded from this higher dose due to potential higher risk of hypokalemia.[99] Loop diuretics may cause the same side effects, although the effect on serum lipids and glucose is not as significant, hypokalemia is more pronounced, and hypocalcemia may occur.

Hypokalemia and hypomagnesemia may cause muscle fatigue or cramps. However, serious cardiac arrhythmias can occur in patients with severe hypokalemia and hypomagnesemia. Patients at greatest risk for this are patients with LVH, coronary disease, post-MI, a history of arrhythmia, or those concurrently receiving digoxin. Low-dose therapy (i.e., 25 mg hydrochlorothiazide or 12.5 mg chlorthalidone daily) causes small electrolyte disturbances. However, the most effective doses of these two thiazide diuretics are hydrochlorothiazide 50 mg daily and chlorthalidone 25 mg daily. Efforts should be made to keep potassium in the therapeutic range by careful monitoring, especially if these higher doses are used.

Diuretic-induced hyperuricemia can precipitate gout. This side effect may be especially problematic for patients with a previous history of gout and is more common with thiazide diuretics. However, acute gout is unlikely in patients with no previous history of gout. If gout does occur in a patient who requires diuretic therapy, allopurinol can be given to prevent gout and will not compromise the antihypertensive effects of the diuretic. High doses of thiazide and loop diuretics may increase fasting glucose and serum cholesterol values. These effects, however, usually are transient and often inconsequential.[100]

Potassium-sparing diuretics can cause hyperkalemia, especially in patients with CKD or diabetes and in patients receiving concurrent treatment with an ACE inhibitor, ARB, direct renin inhibitor, or potassium supplements. Hyperkalemia is especially problematic for the newest aldosterone antagonist eplerenone. This agent is a very selective aldosterone antagonist, and its propensity to cause hyperkalemia is greater than with the other potassium-sparing agents and even spironolactone. Due to this increased risk of hyperkalemia, eplerenone is contraindicated for patients with impaired kidney function or type 2 diabetes with proteinuria (see Table 3-5). While spironolactone may cause gynecomastia in up to 10% of patients, this occurs rarely with eplerenone.

Diuretics can be used safely with most other agents. However, concurrent administration with lithium may result in increased lithium serum concentrations and can predispose patients to lithium toxicity.

β-Blockers β-Blockers have been used in several large outcome trials in hypertension. However, in most of these trials, a thiazide diuretic was the primary agent with a β-blocker added on for additional BP lowering. Moreover, as previously discussed, for patients with hypertension but without compelling indications, other primary agents (ACE inhibitors, ARBs, CCBs, thiazide diuretics) should be used as the initial first-line agent before β-blockers. While this may be surprising to experienced clinicians, this recommendation is consistent with the 2007 AHA guidelines and the 2011 UK's National Institute for Health and the Clinical Excellence guidelines.[2,44] It is based on meta-analyses that suggest β-blocker–based therapy may not reduce CV events as well as these other agents when used as the initial drug to treat patients with hypertension and without a compelling indication for a β-blocker.[45–48]

β-Blockers are only considered appropriate first-line agents to treat specific compelling indications (post-MI, coronary artery disease). They are also evidenced-based as additional therapy for other compelling indications (HFrEF and diabetes). Numerous trials have shown a reduced risk of CV events when β-blockers are used following an MI, during an acute coronary syndrome, or in patients with chronic stable angina with ischemic symptoms. Although once contraindicated in heart failure, studies have shown that bisoprolol, carvedilol, and metoprolol succinate reduce mortality in patients with HFrEF who are treated with a diuretic and ACE inhibitor.

Several mechanisms of action have been proposed for β-blockers, but none of them alone has been shown to be consistently associated with a reduction in arterial BP. β-Blockers have negative chronotropic and inotropic effects that reduce CO, which explains some of the antihypertensive effect. However, CO falls equally for patients treated with β-blockers regardless of BP lowering. Additionally, β-blockers with ISA do not reduce CO, yet they lower BP and decrease peripheral resistance.

β-Adrenoceptors are also located on the surface membranes of juxtaglomerular cells, and β-blockers inhibit these receptors and thus the release of renin. However, there is a weak association between plasma renin and antihypertensive efficacy of β-blocker therapy. Some patients with low plasma renin concentrations do respond to β-blockers. Therefore, additional mechanisms likely also account for the antihypertensive effect of β-blockers. However, the ability of β-blockers to reduce plasma renin and thus angiotensin II concentrations may play a major role in their ability to reduce CV risk.

There are important pharmacodynamic and pharmacokinetic differences among β-blockers, but all agents provide a similar degree of BP lowering. There are three pharmacodynamic properties of the β-blockers that differentiate this class: cardioselectivity, ISA, and membrane-stabilizing effects. β-Blockers that possess a greater affinity for β_1-receptors than for β_2-receptors are *cardioselective*.

β_1-Adrenoceptors and β_2-adrenoceptors are distributed throughout the body, but they concentrate differently in certain organs and tissues. There is a preponderance of β_1-receptors in the heart and kidney, and a preponderance of β_2-receptors in the lungs, liver, pancreas, and arteriolar smooth muscle. β_1-Receptor stimulation increases heart rate, contractility, and renin release. β_2-Receptor stimulation results in bronchodilation and vasodilation. Cardioselective β-blockers are not likely to provoke bronchospasm and vasoconstriction. Insulin secretion and glycogenolysis are mediated by β_2-receptors. Blocking β_2-receptors may reduce these processes and cause hyperglycemia or blunt recovery from hypoglycemia.

Cardioselective β-blockers (e.g., atenolol, bisoprolol, metoprolol, nebivolol) have clinically significant advantages over nonselective β-blockers (e.g., propranolol, nadolol), and are preferred when using a β-blocker to treat hypertension. Cardioselective agents are safer than nonselective agents for patients with asthma or diabetes who have a compelling indication for a β-blocker. However, cardioselectivity is a dose-dependent phenomenon; at higher doses, cardioselective agents lose their relative selectivity for β_1-receptors and block β_2-receptors as effectively as they block β_1-receptors. The dose at which cardioselectivity is lost varies from patient to patient.

Some β-blockers (e.g., acebutolol, pindolol) have ISA and act as partial β-receptor agonists. When they bind to the β-receptor, they stimulate it, but far less than a pure β-agonist. If sympathetic tone is low, as it is during resting states, β-receptors are partially stimulated by ISA β-blockers. Therefore, resting heart rate, CO, and peripheral blood flow are not reduced when these types of β-blockers are used. Theoretically, ISA agents would appear to have advantages over β-blockers in certain patients with heart failure or sinus bradycardia. Unfortunately, they do not appear to reduce CV events as well as other β-blockers. In fact, they may increase CV risk post-MI or in those with coronary artery disease. Thus, agents with ISA are rarely needed.

All β-blockers exert a *membrane-stabilizing action* on cardiac cells when large doses are given. This activity is needed when β-blockers are used as an antiarrhythmic agent.

Pharmacokinetic differences among β-blockers relate to first-pass metabolism, route of elimination, degree lipophilicity, and serum half-lives. Propranolol and metoprolol undergo extensive first-pass metabolism, so the dose needed to attain β-blockade with either drug varies from patient to patient. Atenolol and nadolol are renally excreted. The dose of these agents may need to be reduced for patients with moderate-to-severe CKD.

β-Blockers, especially those with high lipophilic properties, penetrate the central nervous system and may cause other effects.

Propranolol is the most lipophilic drug and atenolol is the least lipophilic. Therefore, higher brain concentrations of propranolol compared with atenolol are seen after equivalent doses are given. It is thought that higher lipophilicity is associated with more central nervous system side effects (dizziness, drowsiness). However, the lipophilic properties can provide better effects for non-CV conditions such as migraine headache prevention, essential tremor, and thyrotoxicosis. BP lowering is equal among β-blockers regardless of lipophilicity.

Most side effects of β-blockers are an extension of their ability to antagonize β-adrenoceptors. β-Blockade in the myocardium can be associated with bradycardia, atrioventricular conduction abnormalities (e.g., second- or third-degree heart block), and the development of acute heart failure. The decrease in heart rate may actually benefit certain patients with atrial arrhythmias (atrial fibrillation, atrial flutter) and hypertension by both providing rate control and BP lowering. β-Blockers usually only produce heart failure if they are used in high initial doses for patients with preexisting left ventricular dysfunction or if started in these patients during an acute heart failure exacerbation. Blocking β_2-receptors in arteriolar smooth muscle may cause cold extremities and may aggravate intermittent claudication or Raynaud's phenomenon as a result of decreased peripheral blood flow. In addition, there is an increase of sympathetic tone during periods of hypoglycemia in patients with diabetes that may result in a significant increase in BP because of unopposed α-receptor–mediated vasoconstriction.

Abrupt cessation of β-blocker therapy can produce unstable angina, MI, or even death in patients with coronary disease. Abrupt cessation may also lead to rebound hypertension (a sudden increase in BP to or above pretreatment values). To avoid this, β-blockers should always be tapered gradually over 1 to 2 weeks before eventually discontinuing the drug. This acute withdrawal syndrome is believed to be secondary to progression of underlying coronary disease, hypersensitivity of β-adrenergic receptors due to upregulation, and increased physical activity after withdrawal of a drug that decreases myocardial oxygen requirements. For patients without coronary disease, abrupt discontinuation may present as tachycardia, sweating, and generalized malaise in addition to increased BP.

Like diuretics, β-blockers have been shown to increase serum cholesterol and glucose values, but these effects are transient and of little clinical significance. For patients with diabetes, the reduction in CV events was as great with β-blockers as with an ACE inhibitor in the United Kingdom Prospective Diabetes Study (UKPDS)[101] and far superior to placebo in the SHEP trial.[8] In the Glycemic Effects in Diabetes Mellitus: Carvedilol–Metoprolol Comparison in Hypertensives (GEMINI) trial, patients with diabetes and hypertension who were randomized to metoprolol had an increase in hemoglobin A1C values, while patients randomized to carvedilol did not.[102] This suggests that mixed α- and β-blocking effects of carvedilol may be preferential to metoprolol for patients with uncontrolled diabetes. However, differences in hemoglobin A1C values were small. Nebivolol is considered a third-generation β-blocker. Similar to carvedilol and labetalol, this β-blocker results in vasodilation. However, carvedilol and labetalol cause vasodilation because of their ability to block α_1-receptors, while nebivolol causes vasodilation through release of nitric oxide. The long-term clinical benefits of the nitric oxide effects seen with nebivolol are currently unknown, but this might explain a lower risk of β-blocker–associated fatigue, erectile dysfunction, and metabolic side effects (e.g., hyperglycemia) with this agent.

13 Alternative Agents The primary role of an alternative antihypertensive agent is to provide additional BP lowering in patients who are already treated with antihypertensive agents from a drug class proven to reduce hypertension-associated CV events (ACE inhibitors, ARBs, CCBs, diuretics, and/or β-blockers).

α_1-Blockers Prazosin, terazosin, and doxazosin are selective α_1-receptor blockers.[37] They work in the peripheral vasculature and inhibit the uptake of catecholamines in smooth muscle cells resulting in vasodilation and BP lowering.

Doxazosin was one of the original treatment arms of the ALLHAT. However, it was stopped prematurely when statistically more secondary end points of stroke, heart failure, and CV events were seen with doxazosin compared with chlorthalidone.[37] There were no differences in the primary end point of fatal coronary heart disease and nonfatal MI. These data suggest that thiazide diuretics are superior to α_1-blockers in preventing CV events in patients with hypertension. Therefore, α_1-blockers are alternative agents that should be used in combination with first-line antihypertensive agents.

α_1-Blockers can provide symptomatic benefits in men with benign prostatic hypertrophy. These agents block postsynaptic α_1-adrenergic receptors located on the prostate capsule, causing relaxation and decreased resistance to urinary outflow. However, when used to lower BP, they should only be in addition to other first-line antihypertensive agents.

A potentially severe side effect of α_1-blockers is a "first-dose" phenomenon that is characterized by transient dizziness or faintness, palpitations, and even syncope within 1 to 3 hours of the first dose. This adverse reaction can also happen after dose increases. These episodes are accompanied by orthostatic hypotension and can be obviated by taking the first dose and subsequent first increased doses at bedtime. Because orthostatic hypotension and dizziness may persist with chronic administration, these agents should be used very cautiously in elderly patients. Even though antihypertensive effects are achieved through a peripheral α_1-receptor antagonism, these agents cross the blood–brain barrier and may cause central nervous system side effects such as lassitude, vivid dreams, and depression. α_1-Blockers also may cause priapism. Sodium and water retention can occur with higher doses, and sometimes even with chronic administration of low doses. Therefore, these agents are most effective when given in combination with a diuretic to maintain antihypertensive efficacy and minimize potential edema.

Aliskiren Aliskiren is the only agent that is a direct renin inhibitor. This drug blocks the RAAS at its point of activation, which results in reduced plasma renin activity and BP lowering. It has a 24-hour half-life, is primarily eliminated through biliary excretion unchanged, and provides 24-hour antihypertensive effects with once-daily dosing.

The exact role of this drug class in the management of hypertension is unclear. Aliskiren is approved as monotherapy or in combination therapy. However, because of the lack of long-term studies evaluating CV event reduction and significant drug cost compared with older generic agents with outcome data, it should clearly be used as an alternative therapy for the treatment of hypertension. Moreover, aliskiren is considered a RAAS blocker. Therefore, it should not be used in combination with an ACE inhibitor or an ARB because of a higher risk of adverse effects without providing additional reduction in CV events.[103]

Many of the cautions and adverse effects seen with ACE inhibitors and ARBs apply to direct renin inhibitors (e.g., aliskiren). Aliskiren should never be used in pregnancy due to the known teratogenic effects of using other drugs that block the RAAS system. Angioedema has also been reported for patients treated with aliskiren. Increases in serum creatinine and serum potassium values have been observed. The mechanisms of these adverse effects are likely similar to those with ACE inhibitors and ARBs. It is reasonable to utilize similar monitoring strategies by measuring serum creatinine and serum potassium in patients treated with aliskiren.

Central α_2-Agonists Clonidine, guanabenz, guanfacine, and methyldopa lower BP primarily by stimulating α_2-adrenergic receptors in the brain. This stimulation reduces sympathetic outflow from the vasomotor center in the brain and increases vagal tone. It is also believed that peripheral stimulation of presynaptic α_2-receptors may further reduce sympathetic tone. Reduced sympathetic activity together with enhanced parasympathetic activity can decrease heart rate, CO, TPR, plasma renin activity, and baroreceptor reflexes. Clonidine is often used in resistant hypertension, and methyldopa is a first-line agent for pregnancy-induced hypertension.

Chronic use of centrally acting α_2-agonists results in sodium and water retention, which is most prominent with methyldopa. Low doses of clonidine (and guanfacine or guanabenz) can be used to treat hypertension without the addition of a diuretic. However, methyldopa should be given in combination with a diuretic to avoid the blunting of antihypertensive effect that happens with prolonged use when used to treat chronic hypertension (not necessary in pregnancy-induced hypertension). Sedation and dry mouth are common anticholinergic side effects that typically improve with chronic use of low doses, but they are more troublesome in the elderly. As with other centrally acting antihypertensives, depression can occur, especially with high doses. The incidence of orthostatic hypotension and dizziness is higher than with other antihypertensive agents, so they should be used very cautiously in the elderly. Lastly, clonidine has a relatively high incidence of anticholinergic side effects (sedation, dry mouth, constipation, urinary retention, and blurred vision). Thus, it should generally be avoided for chronic antihypertensive therapy in the elderly.

Abrupt cessation of central α_2-agonists may lead to rebound hypertension. This effect is thought to be secondary to a compensatory increase in norepinephrine release after abrupt discontinuation. In addition, other effects such as nervousness, agitation, headache, and tremor can also occur, which may be exacerbated by concomitant β-blocker use, particularly with clonidine. Thus, if clonidine is to be discontinued, it should be tapered. For patients who are receiving concomitant β-blocker therapy, the β-blocker should be gradually discontinued first several days before gradual discontinuation of clonidine.

Methyldopa can cause hepatitis or hemolytic anemia, although this is rare. Transient elevations in serum hepatic transaminases are occasionally seen with methyldopa therapy but are clinically irrelevant unless they are greater than three times the upper limit or normal. Methyldopa should be quickly discontinued if persistent increases in serum hepatic transaminases or alkaline phosphatase are detected because this may indicate the onset of fulminant life-threatening hepatitis. A Coombs-positive hemolytic anemia occurs in <1% of patients receiving methyldopa, although 20% exhibit a positive direct Coombs test without anemia. For these reasons, methyldopa has limited use in routine management of hypertension, except in pregnancy.

Reserpine Reserpine lowers BP by depleting norepinephrine from sympathetic nerve endings and blocking transport of norepinephrine into its storage granules. Norepinephrine release into the synapse following nerve stimulation is reduced and results in reduced sympathetic tone, PVR, and BP. Reserpine also depletes catecholamines in the brain and the myocardium, which may lead to sedation, depression, and decreased CO.

Reserpine has a slow onset of action and long half-life that allows for once-daily dosing. However, it may take 2 to 6 weeks before the maximal antihypertensive effect is seen. Because reserpine can cause significant sodium and water retention, it should be given in combination with a diuretic (preferably a thiazide). Reserpine's strong inhibition of sympathetic activity results in increased parasympathetic activity. This effect explains why side effects such as nasal stuffiness, increased gastric acid secretion, diarrhea, and bradycardia can occur. Depression has been reported, which is a consequence of central nervous system depletion of catecholamines and serotonin. The initial reports of depression with reserpine were in the 1950s and are not consistent with current definitions of depression. Regardless, reserpine-induced depression is dose related. Moreover, very high doses (above 1 mg daily) were frequently used in the 1950s, resulting in more depression. When reserpine is dosed between 0.05 and 0.25 mg daily (recommended doses), the rate of depression is equal to that seen with β-blockers, diuretics, or placebo.[8]

Reserpine was used as a third-line agent in many of the landmark clinical trials that have documented the benefit in treating hypertension, including the Veterans Administration Cooperative trials and the SHEP trial.[8] An analysis of the SHEP data found that reserpine was very well tolerated and that the combination of a thiazide diuretic and reserpine is very effective at lowering BP.

Direct Arterial Vasodilators Hydralazine and minoxidil directly relax arteriolar smooth muscle resulting in vasodilation and BP lowering. They exert little to no venous vasodilation. Both agents cause potent reductions in perfusion pressure that activates the baroreceptor reflexes. Activation of baroreceptors results in a compensatory increase in sympathetic outflow, which leads to an increase in heart rate, CO, and renin release. Consequently, tachyphylaxis can develop resulting in a loss of hypotensive effect with continued use. This compensatory baroreceptor response can be counteracted by concurrent use of a β-blocker.

All patients receiving hydralazine or minoxidil long-term for hypertension should first receive both a diuretic and a β-blocker. Direct arterial vasodilators can precipitate angina in patients with underlying coronary disease unless the baroreceptor reflex mechanism is completely blocked with a β-blocker. Nondihydropyridine CCBs can be used as an alternative to β-blockers in these patients, but a β-blocker is preferred. The side effect of sodium and water retention is significant but is minimized by using a diuretic concomitantly.

One side effect unique to hydralazine is a dose-dependent drug-induced lupus-like syndrome. Hydralazine is eliminated by hepatic *N*-acetyltransferase. This enzyme displays genetic polymorphism, and "slow acetylators" are especially prone to develop drug-induced lupus with hydralazine. This syndrome is more common in women and is reversible on discontinuation. Drug-induced lupus may be avoided by using less than 200 mg of hydralazine daily. Because of side effects, hydralazine has limited clinical use for chronic management of hypertension. However, it is especially useful for patients with severe CKD and in kidney failure on hemodialysis. Hydralazine, when used in combination with isosorbide dinitrate, has been shown to reduce the risk of CV events in black patients with HFrEF when added to a standard regimen of a diuretic, ACE inhibitor or ARB, and appropriate β-blocker therapy.[104]

Minoxidil is a more potent vasodilator than hydralazine. Therefore, the compensatory increases in heart rate, CO, renin release, and sodium retention are even more dramatic. Sodium and water retention can be so severe with minoxidil that heart failure can be precipitated. It is even more important to coadminister a β-blocker and a diuretic with minoxidil. A loop diuretic is often more effective than a thiazide in patients treated with minoxidil. A troublesome side effect of minoxidil is hypertrichosis (hirsutism), presenting as increased hair growth on the face, arms, back, and chest. This usually ceases when the drug is discontinued. Other minoxidil side effects include pericardial effusion and a nonspecific T-wave change on the electrocardiogram. Minoxidil is reserved for very-difficult-to-control hypertension and for patients requiring hydralazine that experience drug-induced lupus.

Pharmacoeconomic Considerations

The cost of effectively treating hypertension is substantial. It is projected that the direct costs of treating hypertension will rise from \$91.4 billion in 2015 to \$200.3 billion in 2030.[105] However, these costs are offset by savings that would be realized by reducing CV morbidity and mortality. Cost related to treating target-organ damage (e.g., MI, end-stage kidney failure) can drastically increase healthcare costs.

Antihypertensive drug costs are a major portion of the total cost of hypertensive care. First-line drug classes (i.e., ACE inhibitors, ARBs, CCBs, and diuretics) are predominantly generic.[1,2] Using these agents to treat hypertension results in lower drug acquisition costs. There are even multiple generic fixed-dose combinations of these agents. A comparative analysis of 133,624 patients with hypertension aged 65 and older from a state prescription drug assistance program demonstrated that 40% of patients were prescribed pharmacotherapy that was not necessarily according to JNC7 guideline recommendations.[106] If these 40% had drug therapy modifications made to follow evidence-based treatment, a reduction in costs of $11.6 million would have been realized in the 2001 calendar year based on discounted prices. This was projected to increase to $20.5 million using usual Medicaid pricing limits.

It is crucial to identify ways to control the cost of care without increasing the morbidity and mortality associated with uncontrolled hypertension. Using evidence-based pharmacotherapy will save costs. ACE inhibitors, ARBs, CCBs, and diuretics are first-line treatment options in most patients without compelling indications and most are very inexpensive. Just utilizing generic agents, either as monotherapy or in combination, is appropriate under most circumstances in hypertension management. Brand name drugs should also be used when needed. However, considerations to implement once-daily options and even fixed-dose combination options that are economical should be considered.

Team-Based Collaborative Care

Team-based care for patients with hypertension is a proven strategy that improves goal BP attainment rates.[107,108] These patient care models are interprofessional and utilize physicians, pharmacists, nurses, and other healthcare professionals. With the advent of healthcare reform, such approaches to chronic diseases are being viewed as high-quality and cost-effective improvement modalities. Within these models, pharmacists have been proven to be an effective component of team-based models both in ambulatory clinic settings[107] and in community pharmacist settings.[109] In addition to optimizing selection and implementation of antihypertensive drug therapy, clinical interventions by pharmacists have been proven to reduce the risk of adverse drug events and medication errors in ambulatory patients with CV disease.[110]

EVALUATION OF THERAPEUTIC OUTCOMES

Monitoring the Pharmacotherapy Plan

Routine ongoing monitoring to assess disease progression, the desired effects of antihypertensive therapy (efficacy, including BP goal attainment), and undesired adverse side effects (toxicity) is needed in all patients treated with antihypertensive drug therapy.

Disease Progression

Patients should be monitored for signs and symptoms of progressive hypertension-associated target-organ disease. A careful history for ischemic chest pain (or pressure), palpitations, dizziness, dyspnea, orthopnea, headache, sudden change in vision, one-sided weakness, slurred speech, and loss of balance should be taken to assess the presence of CV and cerebrovascular hypertensive complications. Other clinical monitoring parameters that may be used to assess target-organ disease include funduscopic changes on eye exam, LVH on electrocardiogram, proteinuria, and changes in kidney function. These parameters should be monitored periodically because any sign of deterioration requires immediate assessment and followup.

Efficacy

The most important strategy to prevent CV morbidity and mortality in hypertension is BP control to goal values (see Box 3-2). Routine goal BP values should be attained in elderly patients and in those with isolated systolic hypertension, but actual BP lowering can occur at a gradual pace over a period of several months to avoid orthostatic hypotension. Modifying other CV risk factors (e.g., smoking, dyslipidemia, and diabetes) is also important.

Clinic-based BP monitoring remains the standard for managing hypertension. BP response should be evaluated 2 to 4 weeks after initiating or making changes in therapy. With some agents, monitoring BP 4 to 6 weeks later may better represent steady-state BP values (e.g., thiazide diuretics, reserpine). Once goal BP values are attained, assuming no signs or symptoms of acute target-organ disease are present, BP monitoring can be done every 3 to 6 months. More frequent evaluations are required for patients with a history of poor control, nonadherence, progressive target-organ damage, or symptoms of adverse drug effects.

Self-measurements of BP or automated ABP monitoring can be useful clinically to establish effective 24-hour control. This type of monitoring may become the standard of care in the future because evolving data have demonstrated significant benefits of using these types of measurements to both diagnose hypertension[111,112] and optimize the use of antihypertensive drug therapy.[16] Currently, ABP monitoring is used in select situations such as suspected white coat hypertension.[14] If patients are measuring their BP at home, it is important that they measure during the early morning hours for most days and then at different times of the day on alternative days of the week. It is also of paramount importance that clinicians remember self-BP and ABP measurements are lower than clinic BP measurements.[14] Goal BP values should be lowered accordingly when clinicians use self-BP or ABP measurements to monitor and/or adjust antihypertensive pharmacotherapy.

Toxicity

Patients should be monitored routinely for adverse drug effects. The most common side effects associated with each class of antihypertensive agents were discussed in Individual Antihypertensive Agents above, and laboratory parameters for primary agents are listed in Table 3-8. Laboratory monitoring should typically occur 2 to 4 weeks after starting a new agent or dose increase, and then every 6 to 12 months in stable patients. Additional monitoring may be needed for other concomitant diseases if present (e.g., diabetes, dyslipidemia, gout). Moreover, patients treated with an aldosterone antagonist (eplerenone or spironolactone) should have potassium

TABLE 3-8 Select Monitoring for Antihypertensive Pharmacotherapy

Class	Parameters
Aldosterone antagonists	Blood pressure; BUN/serum creatinine; serum potassium
ACE inhibitors	Blood pressure; BUN/serum creatinine; serum potassium
ARBs	Blood pressure; BUN/serum creatinine; serum potassium
Calcium channel blockers	Blood pressure; heart rate
Diuretics	Blood pressure; BUN/serum creatinine; serum electrolytes (potassium, magnesium, sodium); uric acid (for thiazides)
β-Blockers	Blood pressure; heart rate

concentrations and kidney function assessed within 3 days of initiation and again at 1 week to detect potential hyperkalemia. The occurrence of an adverse drug event may require dosage reduction or substitution with an alternative antihypertensive agent.

Adherence and Persistence

Nonadherence and lack of persistence with hypertension treatment is a major problem in the United States and is associated with significant increases in costs due to development of complications. Since hypertension is a relatively asymptomatic disease, poor adherence is frequent, particularly in patients newly treated. It has been estimated that up to 50% of patients with newly diagnosed hypertension are continuing treatment at 1 year.[113] It has also been demonstrated that long-term risk of CV events is significantly reduced when newly diagnosed patients are adherent with their antihypertensive drug therapy.[114] Therefore, it is imperative to assess patient adherence on a regular basis.

The American Society of Hypertension has outlined four global practical considerations and recommendations for adherence in patients with hypertension.[115] These include: (a) focus on clinical outcomes (e.g., following national guidelines, simplifying drug regimens, encouraging self-monitoring of BP), (b) empowering informed activated patients (e.g., problem-solving and behavior change interventions, urge the use of pill boxes, help patients develop a system for refilling prescriptions), (c) implement a team approach (e.g., implementing collaborative models of care, using office practice policies and procedures to improve BP control), and (d) advocating for health policy reform (e.g., elevate medication adherence as a critical healthcare issue, structure/finance healthcare that stimulates behavioral aspects).

Identification of nonadherence should be followed up with appropriate patient education, counseling, and intervention. Once-daily regimens are preferred in most patients to improve adherence. Although some may believe that aggressive treatment may negatively impact quality of life and thus adherence, several studies have found that most patients actually feel better once their BP is controlled. Patients on antihypertensive therapy should be questioned periodically about changes in their general health perception, energy level, physical functioning, and overall satisfaction with treatment. Lifestyle modifications should always be recommended to provide additional BP lowering and other potential health benefits. Persistence with lifestyle modifications should be continually encouraged for patients engaging in such endeavors.

Combination Therapy

(14) Initial therapy with a combination of two drugs is highly recommended for patients with stage 2 hypertension and is an option for treating patients with stage 1 hypertension.[116] Using a fixed-dose combination product is an option for these types of patients and has been shown to improve adherence.[117] Initial two-drug combination therapy may also be appropriate for patients with multiple compelling indications for different antihypertensive agents. Moreover, combination therapy is often needed to control BP in patients who are already on drug therapy and most patients require two or more agents.[1,43,116]

The Avoiding Cardiovascular Events Through Combination Therapy for Patients Living with Systolic Hypertension Trial

Long-term safety and efficacy of initial two-drug therapy for hypertension has been evaluated in the ACCOMPLISH trial.[118] This was a prospective, randomized, double-blind trial in 11,506 patients with hypertension and other CV risk factors. All of these patients either had stage 2 hypertension or were on antihypertensive drug therapy on enrollment. Patients were randomized to receive either benazepril-with-hydrochlorothiazide or benazepril-with-amlodipine as initial drug therapy. Treatment was titrated to a goal BP of <140/90 mm Hg for most patients and <130/80 mm Hg for patients with diabetes or CKD.

The trial was terminated early after a mean of 36 months because the incidence of CV events was 20% lower in the benazepril-with-amlodipine group compared with the benazepril-with-hydrochlorothiazide group. What is most important for clinical practice is that this trial established that initial two-drug therapy, as is recommended in JNC and AHA guidelines, was safe and highly effective in lowering BP. Mean BP measurements were 132/73 and 133/74 mm Hg in the benazepril-with-amlodipine and the benazepril-with-hydrochlorothiazide groups, respectively. However, rates of attaining a BP of <140/90 mm Hg were 75.4% and 72.4% (benazepril-with-amlodipine and benazepril-with-hydrochlorothiazide, respectively). These goal attainment rates are higher than in any other long-term prospective study and are higher than what is seen in clinical practice.

The ACCOMPLISH trial established initial two-drug antihypertensive therapy as an evidence-based strategy to treat hypertension. Clinicians should consider this study as positive justification for implementing initial two-drug therapy antihypertensive regimens in appropriate patients.

Clinical **Controversy...**

Why is the most effective two-drug combination for reducing CV events not as frequently used as other combinations?

The ACCOMPLISH trial demonstrated that the combination of an ACE inhibitor with a dihydropyridine CCB was more effective in reducing risk of CV events than the combination of an ACE inhibitor with a thiazide diuretic. However, thiazide diuretics are very effective at lowering BP, especially when used in combination with other agents, and hydrochlorothiazide is easily available in many fixed-dose combination products. Therefore, the most ideal two-drug combination for the treatment of hypertension in the absence of compelling indications is an ACE inhibitor (an ARB is a reasonable alternative) with a dihydropyridine CCB. However, because of traditional habits and common availability of combination products, many clinicians use an ACE inhibitor with hydrochlorothiazide.

Optimal Use of Combination Therapy

Clinicians should anticipate the need for combination drugs to control BP in most patients. Using low-dose combinations also provides greater reductions in BP compared with high doses of single agents, with fewer drug-related side effects.[89] Contrary to popular myth, appropriately increasing the number of antihypertensive medications to attain goal BP values does not increase the risk of adverse effects.[119] The American Society of Hypertension has recommended three categories of combination therapy (see Box 3-3).[116] Preferred combinations are ideal for lowering BP, have complementary mechanisms of action, and use first-line drugs that have been shown to lower risk of CV events. Acceptable combinations may not provide all of the benefits that preferred combinations do, and may have additive side effect profiles. Less effective combinations are limited in their overall benefits, and should only be used when absolutely necessary.

Some combinations are not effective long-term in treating hypertension. As previously discussed, the ON-TARGET demonstrated that the use of an ACE inhibitor with an ARB in the

BOX 3-3 Recommendations for Combination Therapy

Preferred

- ACE inhibitor/CCB
- ARB/CCB
- ACE inhibitor/diuretic
- ARB/diuretic

Acceptable

- β-Blocker/diuretic
- CCB (dihydropyridine)/β-blocker
- CCB/diuretic
- Renin inhibitor/diuretic
- Thiazide diuretics/potassium-sparing diuretics

Less Effective

- ACE inhibitor/β-blocker
- ARB/β-blocker
- CCB (nondihydropyridine)/β-blocker
- Centrally acting agent/β-blocker

management of hypertension results in no additional reduction in incidence of CV events.[92] Moreover, this combination results in a higher risk of adverse events. These same effects are seen when aliskiren is used in combination with an ARB.[103] These combinations (using two RAAS blockers together) should not be used for the purpose of managing hypertension. Other combinations such as a thiazide diuretic with a potassium-sparing agent, both of which appear to have overlapping mechanisms of action, should be implemented primarily to minimize side effects. The combination of two CCBs, a dihydropyridine with a nondihydropyridine, might provide additional BP lowering[120,121] but has limited use in the routine management of most patients with hypertension. Under no circumstance should two drugs from the same exact class of medications (e.g., two β-blockers, two ACE inhibitors) be used to treat hypertension.

Fixed-Dose Combination Products Many fixed-dose combination products are commercially available, and some are generic (see Table 3-9). Most of these products contain a thiazide diuretic and have multiple dose strengths available. Individual

TABLE 3-9 Fixed-Dose Combination Products

Combination	Drugs (Brand Name)	Strengths (mg/mg)	Daily Frequency
ACE inhibitor with CCB	Amlodipine/benazepril (Lotrel)	2.5/10, 5/10, 10/20	1
	Enalapril/felodipine (Lexxel)	5/5	1
	Trandolapril/verapamil (Tarka)	2/180, 1/240, 2/240, 4/240	1 or 2
ARB with CCB	Amlodipine/olmesartan (Azor)	5/20, 10/20, 5/40, 10/40	1
	Telmisartan/amlodipine (Twynsta)	40/5, 40/10, 80/5, 80/10	1
	Valsartan/amlodipine (Exforge)	5/160, 10/160, 5/320, 10/320	1
ACE inhibitor with a thiazide diuretic	Benazepril/hydrochlorothiazide (Lotensin HCT)	5/6.25, 10/12.5, 20/12.5, 20/25	1
	Captopril/hydrochlorothiazide (Capozide)	25/15, 25/25, 50/15, 50/25	1 to 3
	Enalapril/hydrochlorothiazide (Vaseretic)	5/12.5, 10/25	1
	Lisinopril/hydrochlorothiazide (Prinizide, Zestoretic)	10/12.5, 20/12.5, 20/25	1
	Moexipril/hydrochlorothiazide (Uniretic)	7.5/12.5, 15/25	1 or 2
	Quinapril/hydrochlorothiazide (Accuretic)	10/12.5, 20/12.5, 20/25	1
ARB with a thiazide diuretic	Azilsartan/chlorthalidone (Edarbyclor)	40/12.5, 40/25	1
	Candesartan/hydrochlorothiazide (Atacand HCT)	16/12.5, 32/12.5	1
	Eprosartan/hydrochlorothiazide (Teveten HCT)	600/12.5, 600/25	1
	Irbesartan/hydrochlorothiazide (Avalide)	75/12.5, 150/12.5, 300/12.5	1
	Losartan/hydrochlorothiazide (Hyzaar)	50/12.5, 100/25	1
	Olmesartan/hydrochlorothiazide (Benicar HCT)	20/12.5, 40/12.5, 40/25	1
	Telmisartan/hydrochlorothiazide (Micardis HCT)	40/12.5, 80/12.5	1
	Valsartan/hydrochlorothiazide (Diovan HCT)	80/12.5, 160/12.5	1
β-Blocker with a thiazide diuretic	Atenolol/chlorthalidone (Tenoretic)	50/25, 100/25	1
	Bisoprolol/hydrochlorothiazide (Ziac)	2.5/6.25, 5/6.25, 10/6.25	1
	Propranolol/hydrochlorothiazide (Inderide)	40/25, 80/25	2
	Propranolol LA/hydrochlorothiazide (Inderide LA)	80/50, 120/50, 160/50	1
	Metoprolol/hydrochlorothiazide (Lopressor HCT)	50/25, 100/25	1 or 2
	Nadolol/bendroflumethiazide (Corzide)	40/5, 80/5	1
	Timolol/hydrochlorothiazide (Timolide)	10/25	1 or 2
Direct renin inhibitor with thiazide diuretic	Aliskiren/hydrochlorothiazide (Tekturna HCT)	150/12.5, 150/25, 300/12.5, 300/25	1
Direct renin inhibitor with CCB	Aliskiren/amlodipine (Tekamlo)	100/5, 150/10, 300/5, 300/10	1
ARB with CCB with a thiazide diuretic	Amlodipine/valsartan/hydrochlorothiazide (Exforge HCT)	5/160/12.5, 5/160/25, 10/160/12.5, 10/160/25, 10/320/25	1
	Olmesartan/amlodipine/hydrochlorothiazide (Tribenzor)	20/5/12.5, 40/5/12.5, 40/5/25, 40/10/12.5, 40/10/25	1
Direct renin inhibitor with CCB with a thiazide diuretic	Aliskiren/amlodipine/hydrochlorothiazide (Tekamlo)	150/5/12.5, 300/5/12.5, 300/5/25, 300/10/12.5, 300/10/25	1

dose titration is more complicated with fixed-dose combination products, but this strategy can reduce the number of daily tablets/capsules and can simplify regimens to improve adherence by decreasing pill burden.[116,117] This alone may increase the likelihood of achieving or maintaining goal BP values. Depending on the product, some may be less expensive to patients and to health systems. Nonadherence rates are 24% lower when fixed-dose combination products are used to treat hypertension compared with using free drug components (separate pills) to treat hypertension.[117]

Resistant Hypertension

⓯ Resistant hypertension is defined as patients who are uncontrolled (failure to achieve goal BP of <140/90 mm Hg, or lower when indicated) with the use of three or more drugs.[122] Ideally, these should be patients who are adhering to full doses of an appropriate three-drug regimen that includes a diuretic.[1] This also includes patients who are controlled but require the use of four or more medications.[122] Patients with newly diagnosed hypertension or who are not receiving drug therapy should not be considered to have resistant hypertension.[123] Difficult-to-control hypertension is persistently elevated BP despite treatment with two or three drugs that does not meet the criteria for resistant hypertension (e.g., maximum doses that include a diuretic).

Several causes of resistant hypertension are listed in Table 3-10. Volume overload is a common cause, thus highlighting the importance of diuretic therapy in the management of hypertension. Pseudoresistance should also be ruled out by assuring adherence with prescribed therapy and possibly use of home BP measurements (by using a self-monitoring device or 24-hour ABP monitor).[122] Patients should be closely evaluated to see if any of these causes can be reversed.

Treatment of patients with resistant hypertension should ultimately follow the principle of drug therapy selection from the JNC and AHA guidelines. Compelling indications, if present, should guide selection assuming these patients are on a diuretic. However, there are treatment philosophies that are germane to the management of resistant hypertension: (a) assuring adequate diuretic therapy, (b) appropriate use of combination therapies, and (c) using alternative antihypertensive agents when needed.

Assuring Appropriate Diuretic Therapy

Diuretics have a large role in the pharmacotherapy of resistant hypertension. Thiazide diuretics are the mainstay of treatment, but chlorthalidone (thiazide-like) should be preferentially used instead of hydrochlorothiazide, especially for patients with resistant hypertension, because it is more potent on a milligram-per-milligram basis.[96,122] Clinicians should identify that chlorthalidone therapy, like all thiazide diuretics, has dose-dependent metabolic side effects (hypokalemia and hyperglycemia) and that appropriate monitoring should be implemented. An aldosterone antagonist (e.g., spironolactone) is also very effective as an add-on agent.[122] Evolving data indicate that many patients with resistant hypertension have some degree of underlying hyperaldosteronism, emphasizing the role of adding an aldosterone antagonist. Clinicians should consider using a loop diuretic, even in place of a thiazide diuretic, for patients with resistant hypertension who have very compromised kidney function (estimated GFR <30 mL/min/1.73 m^2). Torsemide can be dosed once daily while furosemide must be dosed twice daily or three times daily.

TABLE 3-10 Causes of Resistant Hypertension

Improper BP measurement
Volume overload: • Excess sodium intake • Volume retention from kidney disease • Inadequate diuretic therapy
Drug induced or other causes: • Nonadherence • Inadequate doses • Agents listed in Table 3-1
Associated conditions: • Obesity, excess alcohol intake
Secondary hypertension

Hypertensive Urgencies and Emergencies

Both hypertensive urgencies and emergencies are characterized by the presence of very elevated BP, typically >180/120 mm Hg.[1,6] However, the need for urgent or emergent antihypertensive therapy must be determined based on the presence of acute or immediately progressing target-organ injury, not elevated BP alone. Urgencies are not associated with acute or immediately progressing target-organ injury, while emergencies are. Examples of acute target-organ injury include encephalopathy, intracranial hemorrhage, acute left ventricular failure with pulmonary edema, dissecting aortic aneurysm, unstable angina, and eclampsia or severe hypertension during pregnancy.

Hypertensive Urgency

⓰ A common error with hypertensive urgency is overly aggressive antihypertensive therapy. This treatment has likely been perpetrated by the classification terminology "urgency." Hypertensive urgencies are ideally managed by adjusting maintenance therapy, by adding a new antihypertensive, and/or by increasing the dose of a present medication. This is the preferred approach to these patients as it provides a more gradual reduction in BP. Very rapid reductions in BP to goal values should be discouraged due to potential risks. Because autoregulation of blood flow in patients with hypertension occurs at a much higher range of pressure than in normotensive persons, the inherent risks of reducing BP too precipitously include cerebrovascular accidents, MI, and acute kidney failure. Hypertensive urgency requires BP reductions with oral antihypertensive agents to stage 1 values over a period of several hours to several days. All patients with hypertensive urgency should be reevaluated within and no later than 7 days (preferably after 1 to 3 days).

Acute administration of a short-acting oral antihypertensive (e.g., captopril, clonidine, or labetalol) followed by careful observation for several hours to assure a gradual reduction in BP is an option for hypertensive urgency. However, there are no data supporting this approach as being absolutely needed. Oral captopril is one of the agents of choice and can be used in doses of 25 to 50 mg at 1- to 2-hour intervals. The onset of action of oral captopril is 15 to 30 minutes, and a marked fall in BP is unlikely to occur if no hypotensive response is observed within 30 to 60 minutes. For patients with hypertensive rebound following withdrawal of clonidine, 0.2 mg can be given initially, followed by 0.2 mg hourly until the DBP falls below 110 mm Hg or a total of 0.7 mg clonidine has been administered. A single dose may be all that is necessary. Labetalol can be given in a dose of 200 to 400 mg, followed by additional doses every 2 to 3 hours.

Oral or sublingual immediate-release nifedipine has been used for acute BP lowering in the past but is potentially dangerous. This approach produces a rapid reduction in BP. Immediate-release nifedipine should never be used for hypertensive urgencies due to risk of causing severe adverse events such as MIs and strokes.[124]

TABLE 3-11 Parenteral Antihypertensive Agents for Hypertensive Emergency

Drug	Dose	Onset (minutes)	Duration (minutes)	Adverse Effects	Special Indications
Clevidipine	1–2 mg/h (32 mg/h maximum)	2–4	5–15	Headache, nausea, tachycardia, hypertriglyceridemia	Most hypertensive emergencies except acute heart failure; caution with coronary ischemia; contraindicated in soy or egg allergy, defective lipid metabolism, and severe aortic stenosis
Enalaprilat	1.25–5 mg IV every 6 hours	15–30	360–720	Precipitous fall in pressure in high-renin states; variable response	Acute left ventricular failure; avoid in acute myocardial infarction, eclampsia
Esmolol hydrochloride	250–500 mcg/kg/min IV bolus, and then 50–100 mcg/kg/min IV infusion; may repeat bolus after 5 minutes or increase infusion to 300 mcg/min	1–2	10–20	Hypotension, nausea, asthma, first-degree heart block, heart failure	Aortic dissection; perioperative; avoid in patients already on β-blocker, bradycardic, or decompensated heart failure
Fenoldopam mesylate	0.1–0.3 mcg/kg/min IV infusion	<5	30	Tachycardia, headache, nausea, flushing	Most hypertensive emergencies; caution with glaucoma
Hydralazine hydrochloride	12–20 mg IV 10–50 mg intramuscular	10–20 20–30	60–240 240–360	Tachycardia, flushing, headache vomiting, aggravation of angina	Eclampsia
Labetalol hydrochloride	20–80 mg IV bolus every 10 minutes; 0.5–2 mg/min IV infusion	5–10	180–360	Vomiting, scalp tingling, bronchoconstriction, dizziness, nausea, heart block, orthostatic hypotension	Most hypertensive emergencies except acute heart failure or heart block
Nicardipine hydrochloride	5–15 mg/h IV	5–10	15–30, may exceed 240	Tachycardia, headache, flushing, local phlebitis	Most hypertensive emergencies except acute heart failure; caution with coronary ischemia
Nitroglycerin	5–100 mcg/min IV infusion	2–5	5–10	Headache, vomiting, methemoglobinemia, tolerance with prolonged use	Coronary ischemia
Sodium nitroprusside	0.25–10 mcg/kg/min IV infusion (requires special delivery system)	Immediate	1–2	Nausea, vomiting, muscle twitching, sweating, thiocyanate and cyanide intoxication	Most hypertensive emergencies; caution with high intracranial pressure, azotemia, or in chronic kidney disease

Hypertensive Emergency

Hypertensive emergencies are those rare situations that require immediate BP reduction to limit new or progressing target-organ damage (see Classification under Arterial BP above). Hypertensive emergencies require parenteral therapy, at least initially, with one of the agents listed in Table 3-11. The goal in hypertensive emergencies is not to lower BP to <140/90 mm Hg; rather, the initial target is a reduction in MAP of up to 25% within minutes to hours. If the patient is then stable, DBP can be reduced to 100–110 mm Hg within the next 2 to 6 hours. Precipitous drops in BP may lead to end-organ ischemia or infarction. If patients tolerate this reduction well, additional gradual reductions toward goal BP values can be attempted after 24 to 48 hours. The exception to this guideline is for patients with an acute ischemic stroke where maintaining an elevated BP is needed for a longer period of time.

The clinical situation should dictate which IV medication is used to treat hypertensive emergencies. Regardless, therapy should be provided in a hospital or emergency room setting with intraarticular BP monitoring. Table 3-11 lists special indications for agents that can be used.

Nitroprusside is widely considered the agent of choice for most cases, but it can be problematic for patients with CKD. It is a direct-acting vasodilator that decreases PVR but does not increase CO unless left ventricular failure is present. Nitroprusside can be given to treat most hypertensive emergencies, but in aortic dissection, propranolol should be given first to prevent reflex sympathetic activation. Nitroprusside is metabolized to cyanide and then to thiocyanate, which is eliminated by the kidneys. Therefore, serum thiocyanate levels should be monitored when infusions are continued longer than 72 hours. Nitroprusside should be discontinued if the concentration exceeds 12 mg/dL (~2 mmol/L). The risk of thiocyanate accumulation and toxicity is increased for patients with impaired kidney function.

IV nitroglycerin dilates both arterioles and venous capacitance vessels, thereby reducing both cardiac afterload and cardiac preload, which can decrease myocardial oxygen demand. It also dilates collateral coronary blood vessels and improves perfusion to ischemic myocardium. These properties make IV nitroglycerin ideal for the management of hypertensive emergency in the presence of myocardial ischemia. IV nitroglycerin is associated with tolerance when used over 24 to 48 hours and can cause severe headache.

Fenoldopam, nicardipine, and clevidipine are newer and more expensive agents. Fenoldopam is a dopamine-1 agonist. It can improve renal blood flow and may be especially useful for patients with kidney insufficiency. Nicardipine and clevidipine are dihydropyridine CCBs that provide arterial vasodilation and can treat cardiac ischemia similar to nitroglycerin, but they may provide more predictable reductions in BP.

The hypotensive response of hydralazine is less predictable than with other parenteral agents. Therefore, its major role is in the treatment of eclampsia or hypertensive encephalopathy associated with renal insufficiency.

CONCLUSIONS

Hypertension is a very common medical condition in the United States. Treatment of patients with hypertension should include both lifestyle modifications and pharmacotherapy. Evidence from outcome-based clinical trials have definitively demonstrated that treating hypertension reduces the risk of CV events and subsequently reduces morbidity and mortality. Moreover, evidence evaluating individual drug classes has resulted in an evidence-based approach to selecting pharmacotherapy in an individual patient ACE inhibitors, ARBs, CCBs, and thiazide diuretics are all first-line agents. Data suggest that using a β-blocker as the primary agent to treat patients with hypertension, without the presence of a compelling indication, may not be as beneficial in reducing risk of CV events compared with ACE inhibitor–, ARB-, CCB-, or thiazide diuretic–based therapy. Therefore, they are not first-line therapy options unless an appropriate compelling indication is present.

Patients should be treated to a goal BP value. In addition to selecting the most appropriate agent, attaining a goal BP is also of paramount importance to ensure maximum reduction in risk for CV events is provided. A BP goal of <140/90 mm Hg is recommended for most patients with hypertension and some patients are candidates for lower goal values. Most patients with hypertension require more than one drug to attain goal BP values; therefore, combination therapy should be anticipated.

Optimizing hypertension management can be achieved many ways. Team-based approaches to implement care and attain goal BP values are effective. Judicious use of cost-effective treatments and fixed-dose combination products should always be considered to improve sustainability of treatment. Lastly, interventions to reinforce adherence and lifestyle modifications also are highly recommended in the comprehensive management of hypertension.

ABBREVIATIONS

ABP	ambulatory blood pressure
ACCOMPLISH	Avoiding Cardiovascular Events Through Combination Therapy in Patients Living with Systolic Hypertension
ACCORD-BP	Action to Control Cardiovascular Risk in Diabetes Blood Pressure
ACE	angiotensin-converting enzyme
AHA	American Heart Association
ALLHAT	Antihypertensive and Lipid Lowering Treatment to Prevent Heart Attack Trial
ARB	angiotensin II receptor blocker
AT_1	angiotensin II type 1
AT_2	angiotensin II type 2
BP	blood pressure
BUN	blood urea nitrogen
CCB	calcium channel blocker
CHARM	Candesartan in Heart Failure—Assessment of Reduction in Mortality and Morbidity
CKD	chronic kidney disease
CO	cardiac output
CONVINCE	Controlled Onset Verapamil Investigation of Cardiovascular End-Points
COPD	chronic obstructive pulmonary disease
CV	cardiovascular
DASH	Dietary Approaches to Stop Hypertension
DBP	diastolic blood pressure
GEMINI	Glycemic Effects in Diabetes Mellitus: Carvedilol–Metoprolol Comparison in Hypertensives
GFR	glomerular filtration rate
HOT	Hypertension Optimal Treatment
HFrEF	Heart Failure with reduced Ejection Fraction
HYVET	Hypertension in the Very Elderly Trial
INVEST	International Verapamil–Trandolapril Study
ISA	intrinsic sympathomimetic activity
JNC7	Seventh Report of the Joint National Committee on Prevention, Detection, Evaluation, and Treatment of High Blood Pressure
KDIGO	Kidney Disease Improving Global Outcomes
LVH	left ventricular hypertrophy
MAP	mean arterial pressure
MDRD	modification of diet in renal disease
MI	myocardial infarction
MOSES	Morbidity and Mortality After Stroke: Eprosartan Versus Nitrendipine in Secondary Prevention
MRC	Medical Research Council
NHLBI	National Heart, Lung, and Blood Institute
ON-TARGET	Ongoing Telmisartan Alone and in Combination with Ramipril Global End Point Trial
PAD	peripheral arterial disease
PROBE	prospective open-label, blinded end point
PVR	peripheral vascular resistance
RAAS	renin–angiotensin–aldosterone system
ROADMAP	Randomized Olmesartan and Diabetes Microalbuminuria Prevention
SBP	systolic blood pressure
SHEP	Systolic Hypertension in the Elderly Program
SPRINT	Systolic Pressure Intervention Trial
STOP-2	Swedish Trial in Old Patients with Hypertension-2
STOP-Hypertension	Swedish Trial in Old Patients with Hypertension
Syst-Eur	Systolic Hypertension in Europe
TOMHS	Treatment of Mild Hypertension Study
TPR	total peripheral resistance
TRANSCEND	Telmisartan Randomized Assessment Study in ACE-Intolerant Subjects with Cardiovascular Disease
UKPDS	United Kingdom Prospective Diabetes Study
VALIANT	Valsartan in Acute MI
VALUE	Valsartan Antihypertensive Long-Term Use Evaluation

REFERENCES

1. Chobanian AV, Bakris GL, Black HR, et al. Seventh report of the Joint National Committee on Prevention, Detection, Evaluation, and Treatment of High Blood Pressure. Hypertension 2003;42:1206–1252.
2. Rosendorff C, Black HR, Cannon CP, et al. Treatment of hypertension in the prevention and management of ischemic heart disease: A scientific statement from the American Heart

Association Council for High Blood Pressure Research and the Councils on Clinical Cardiology and Epidemiology and Prevention. Circulation 2007;115:2761–2788.

3. Go AS, Mozaffarian D, Roger VL, et al. Heart disease and stroke statistics—2013 update: A report from the American Heart Association. Circulation 2013;127:e6–e245.
4. Staessen JA, Wang J, Bianchi G, Birkenhager WH. Essential hypertension. Lancet 2003;361:1629–1641.
5. Saseen JJ. Hypertension. In: Tisdale JE, Miller DA, eds. Drug-Induced Diseases: Prevention, Detection, and Management, 2nd ed. Bethesda: American Society of Health-Systems Pharmacists, Inc, 2010:516–528 [chapter 27].
6. Kaplan NM. Kaplan's Clinical Hypertension, 9th ed. Philadelphia, PA: Lippincott Williams & Wilkins, 2006:1–518.
7. MacMahon S, Peto R, Cutler J, et al. Blood pressure, stroke, and coronary heart disease. Part 1, prolonged differences in blood pressure: Prospective observational studies corrected for the regression dilution bias. Lancet 1990;335:765–774.
8. SHEP Cooperative Research Group. Prevention of stroke by antihypertensive drug treatment in older persons with isolated systolic hypertension. Final results of the Systolic Hypertension in the Elderly Program (SHEP). JAMA 1991; 265:3255–3264.
9. Dahlof B, Lindholm LH, Hansson L, Schersten B, Ekbom T, Wester PO. Morbidity and mortality in the Swedish Trial in Old Patients with Hypertension (STOP-Hypertension). Lancet 1991;338:1281–1285.
10. MRC Working Party. Medical Research Council trial of treatment of hypertension in older adults: Principal results. BMJ 1992;304:405–412.
11. Staessen JA, Fagard R, Thijs L, et al. Randomised double-blind comparison of placebo and active treatment for older patients with isolated systolic hypertension. The Systolic Hypertension in Europe (Syst-Eur) Trial Investigators. Lancet 1997;350:757–764.
12. Alberti KG, Eckel RH, Grundy SM, et al. Harmonizing the metabolic syndrome: A joint interim statement of the International Diabetes Federation Task Force on Epidemiology and Prevention; National Heart, Lung, and Blood Institute; American Heart Association; World Heart Federation; International Atherosclerosis Society; and International Association for the Study of Obesity. Circulation 2009;120:1640–1645.
13. Pickering TG, Hall JE, Appel LJ, et al. Recommendations for blood pressure measurement in humans and experimental animals: Part 1: Blood pressure measurement in humans: A statement for professionals from the Subcommittee of Professional and Public Education of the American Heart Association Council on High Blood Pressure Research. Circulation 2005;111:697–716.
14. Pickering TG, White WB. ASH position paper: Home and ambulatory blood pressure monitoring. When and how to use self (home) and ambulatory blood pressure monitoring. J Clin Hypertens (Greenwich) 2008;10:850–855.
15. Mancia G, Bombelli M, Facchetti R, et al. Long-term risk of sustained hypertension in white-coat or masked hypertension. Hypertension 2009;54:226–232.
16. Agarwal R, Bills JE, Hecht TJ, Light RP. Role of home blood pressure monitoring in overcoming therapeutic inertia and improving hypertension control: A systematic review and meta-analysis. Hypertension 2011;57:29–38.
17. American Diabetes Association. Standards of medical care in diabetes—2013. Diabetes Care 2013;36(Suppl 1):S11–S66.
18. Kidney Disease Improving Global Outcomes. Chapter 4: Blood pressure management in CKD ND patients with diabetes mellitus. Kidney Int Suppl 2012;2:363–369.
19. Kidney Disease Improving Global Outcomes. Chapter 3: Blood pressure management in CKD ND patients without diabetes mellitus. Kidney Int Suppl 2012;2:357–362.
20. Hansson L, Zanchetti A, Carruthers SG, et al. Effects of intensive blood-pressure lowering and low-dose aspirin in patients with hypertension: Principal results of the Hypertension Optimal Treatment (HOT) randomised trial. HOT Study Group. Lancet 1998;351:1755–1762.
21. Arguedas JA, Perez MI, Wright JM. Treatment blood pressure targets for hypertension. Cochrane Database Syst Rev 2009:CD004349.
22. Farnett L, Mulrow CD, Linn WD, Lucey CR, Tuley MR. The J-curve phenomenon and the treatment of hypertension. Is there a point beyond which pressure reduction is dangerous? JAMA 1991;265:489–495.
23. Verdecchia P, Staessen JA, Angeli F, et al. Usual versus tight control of systolic blood pressure in non-diabetic patients with hypertension (Cardio-Sis): An open-label randomised trial. Lancet 2009;374:525–533.
24. Cushman WC, Evans GW, Byington RP, et al. Effects of intensive blood-pressure control in type 2 diabetes mellitus. N Engl J Med 2010;362:1575–1585.
25. O'Connor PJ. Overcome clinical inertia to control systolic blood pressure. Arch Intern Med 2003;163:2677–2678.
26. Appel LJ, Brands MW, Daniels SR, Karanja N, Elmer PJ, Sacks FM. Dietary approaches to prevent and treat hypertension: A scientific statement from the American Heart Association. Hypertension 2006;47:296–308.
27. Lichtenstein AH, Appel LJ, Brands M, et al. Diet and lifestyle recommendations revision 2006: A scientific statement from the American Heart Association Nutrition Committee. Circulation 2006;114:82–96.
28. Moser M, Feig PU. Fifty years of thiazide diuretic therapy for hypertension. Arch Intern Med 2009;169: 1851–1856.
29. Saseen JJ, MacLaughlin EJ, Westfall JM. Treatment of uncomplicated hypertension: Are ACE inhibitors and calcium channel blockers as effective as diuretics and beta-blockers? J Am Board Fam Pract 2003;16:156–164.
30. Black HR, Elliott WJ, Grandits G, et al. Principal results of the Controlled Onset Verapamil Investigation of Cardiovascular End Points (CONVINCE) trial. JAMA 2003;289:2073–2082.
31. Dahlof B, Devereux RB, Kjeldsen SE, et al. Cardiovascular morbidity and mortality in the Losartan Intervention For Endpoint reduction in hypertension study (LIFE): A randomised trial against atenolol. Lancet 2002;359: 995–1003.
32. ALLHAT Officers and Coordinators for the ALLHAT Collaborative Research Group. Major outcomes in high-risk hypertensive patients randomized to angiotensin-converting enzyme inhibitor or calcium channel blocker vs diuretic: The Antihypertensive and Lipid-Lowering Treatment to Prevent Heart Attack Trial (ALLHAT). JAMA 2002;288:2981–2997.
33. PROGRESS Collaborative Group. Randomised trial of a perindopril-based blood-pressure-lowering regimen among 6,105 individuals with previous stroke or transient ischaemic attack. Lancet 2001;358:1033–1041.
34. Wing LM, Reid CM, Ryan P, et al. A comparison of outcomes with angiotensin-converting-enzyme inhibitors and diuretics for hypertension in the elderly. N Engl J Med 2003;348:583–592.
35. Julius S, Kjeldsen SE, Weber M, et al. Outcomes in hypertensive patients at high cardiovascular risk treated with regimens based on valsartan or amlodipine: The VALUE randomised trial. Lancet 2004;363:2022–2031.

36. Dahlof B, Sever PS, Poulter NR, et al. Prevention of cardiovascular events with an antihypertensive regimen of amlodipine adding perindopril as required versus atenolol adding bendroflumethiazide as required, in the Anglo-Scandinavian Cardiac Outcomes Trial-Blood Pressure Lowering Arm (ASCOT-BPLA): A multicentre randomised controlled trial. Lancet 2005;366:895–906.
37. Antihypertensive and Lipid-Lowering Treatment to Prevent Heart Attack Trial Collaborative Research Group. Diuretic versus alpha-blocker as first-step antihypertensive therapy: Final results from the Antihypertensive and Lipid-Lowering Treatment to Prevent Heart Attack Trial (ALLHAT). Hypertension 2003;42:239–246.
38. Davis BR, Cutler JA, Gordon DJ, et al. Rationale and design for the Antihypertensive and Lipid Lowering Treatment to Prevent Heart Attack Trial (ALLHAT). ALLHAT Research Group. Am J Hypertens 1996;9:342–360.
39. Rahman M, Pressel S, Davis BR, et al. Renal outcomes in high-risk hypertensive patients treated with an angiotensin-converting enzyme inhibitor or a calcium channel blocker vs a diuretic: A report from the Antihypertensive and Lipid-Lowering Treatment to Prevent Heart Attack Trial (ALLHAT). Arch Intern Med 2005;165:936–946.
40. Whelton PK, Barzilay J, Cushman WC, et al. Clinical outcomes in antihypertensive treatment of type 2 diabetes, impaired fasting glucose concentration, and normoglycemia: Antihypertensive and Lipid-Lowering Treatment to Prevent Heart Attack Trial (ALLHAT). Arch Intern Med 2005;165:1401–1409.
41. Wright JT Jr, Dunn JK, Cutler JA, et al. Outcomes in hypertensive black and nonblack patients treated with chlorthalidone, amlodipine, and lisinopril. JAMA 2005;293:1595–1608.
42. Turnbull F. Effects of different blood-pressure-lowering regimens on major cardiovascular events: Results of prospectively-designed overviews of randomised trials. Lancet 2003;362:1527–1535.
43. Mancia G, Fagard R, Narkiewicz K, et al. 2013 ESH/ESC Guidelines for the management of arterial hypertension: The Task Force for the management of arterial hypertension of the European Society of Hypertension (ESH) and of the European Society of Cardiology (ESC). J Hypertens 2013;31(7):1281–1357.
44. National Clinical Guideline Centre. Hypertension—The Clinical Management of Primary Hypertension in Adults. Clinical Guideline 127: Methods, Evidence, and Recommendations. London: The Royal College of Physicians; August 2011.
45. Carlberg B, Samuelsson O, Lindholm LH. Atenolol in hypertension: Is it a wise choice? Lancet 2004;364:1684–1689.
46. Lindholm LH, Carlberg B, Samuelsson O. Should beta blockers remain first choice in the treatment of primary hypertension? A meta-analysis. Lancet 2005;366:1545–1553.
47. Khan N, McAlister FA. Re-examining the efficacy of beta-blockers for the treatment of hypertension: A meta-analysis. CMAJ 2006;174:1737–1742.
48. Wiysonge C, Bradley H, Mayosi B, et al. Beta-blockers for hypertension. Cochrane Database Syst Rev 2007:CD002003.
49. Hunt SA, Abraham WT, Chin MH, et al. 2009 focused update incorporated into the ACC/AHA 2005 guidelines for the diagnosis and management of heart failure in adults: A report of the American College of Cardiology Foundation/American Heart Association Task Force on Practice Guidelines: Developed in collaboration with the International Society for Heart and Lung Transplantation. Circulation 2009;119:e391–e479.
50. Granger CB, McMurray JJ, Yusuf S, et al. Effects of candesartan in patients with chronic heart failure and reduced left-ventricular systolic function intolerant to angiotensin-converting-enzyme inhibitors: The CHARM-Alternative trial. Lancet 2003;362:772–776.
51. Effect of metoprolol CR/XL in chronic heart failure: Metoprolol CR/XL Randomised Intervention Trial in Congestive Heart Failure (MERIT-HF). Lancet 1999;353:2001–2007.
52. Packer M, Coats AJ, Fowler MB, et al. Effect of carvedilol on survival in severe chronic heart failure. N Engl J Med 2001;344:1651–1658.
53. Pitt B, Zannad F, Remme WJ, et al. The effect of spironolactone on morbidity and mortality in patients with severe heart failure. Randomized Aldactone Evaluation Study Investigators. N Engl J Med 1999;341:709–717.
54. Pitt B, Remme W, Zannad F, et al. Eplerenone, a selective aldosterone blocker, in patients with left ventricular dysfunction after myocardial infarction. N Engl J Med 2003;348:1309–1321.
55. Zannad F, McMurray JJ, Krum H, et al. Eplerenone in patients with systolic heart failure and mild symptoms. N Engl J Med 2011;364:11–21.
56. Chatterjee S, Moeller C, Shah N, et al. Eplerenone is not superior to older and less expensive aldosterone antagonists. Am J Med 2012;125:817–825.
57. Smith SC Jr, Benjamin EJ, Bonow RO, et al. AHA/ACCF secondary prevention and risk reduction therapy for patients with coronary and other atherosclerotic vascular disease: 2011 update: A guideline from the American Heart Association and American College of Cardiology Foundation. Circulation 2011;124:2458–2473.
58. Pfeffer MA, McMurray JJ, Velazquez EJ, et al. Valsartan, captopril, or both in myocardial infarction complicated by heart failure, left ventricular dysfunction, or both. N Engl J Med 2003;349:1893–1906.
59. Fihn SD, Gardin JM, Abrams J, et al. 2012 ACCF/AHA/ACP/AATS/PCNA/SCAI/STS guideline for the diagnosis and management of patients with stable ischemic heart disease: A report of the American College of Cardiology Foundation/American Heart Association Task Force on Practice Guidelines, and the American College of Physicians, American Association for Thoracic Surgery, Preventive Cardiovascular Nurses Association, Society for Cardiovascular Angiography and Interventions, and Society of Thoracic Surgeons. Circulation 2012;126:e354–e471.
60. Bangalore S, Steg G, Deedwania P, et al. Beta-blocker use and clinical outcomes in stable outpatients with and without coronary artery disease. JAMA 2012;308:1340–1349.
61. Pepine CJ, Handberg EM, Cooper-DeHoff RM, et al. A calcium antagonist vs a non-calcium antagonist hypertension treatment strategy for patients with coronary artery disease. The International Verapamil–Trandolapril Study (INVEST): A randomized controlled trial. JAMA 2003;290:2805–2816.
62. Jneid H, Anderson JL, Wright RS, et al. 2012 ACCF/AHA focused update of the guideline for the management of patients with unstable angina/non-ST-elevation myocardial infarction (updating the 2007 guideline and replacing the 2011 focused update): A report of the American College of Cardiology Foundation/American Heart Association Task Force on Practice Guidelines. Circulation 2012;126:875–910.
63. O'Gara PT, Kushner FG, Ascheim DD, et al. 2013 ACCF/AHA guideline for the management of ST-elevation myocardial infarction: A report of the American College

of Cardiology Foundation/American Heart Association Task Force on Practice Guidelines. J Am Coll Cardiol 2013;61:e78–e140.
64. Baker WL, Coleman CI, Kluger J, et al. Systematic review: Comparative effectiveness of angiotensin-converting enzyme inhibitors or angiotensin II-receptor blockers for ischemic heart disease. Ann Intern Med 2009;151:861–871.
65. Weber MA, Bakris GL, Jamerson K, et al. Cardiovascular events during differing hypertension therapies in patients with diabetes. J Am Coll Cardiol 2010;56:77–85.
66. Bakris GL, Sowers JR. ASH position paper: Treatment of hypertension in patients with diabetes—An update. J Clin Hypertens (Greenwich) 2008;10:707–713 [discussion 714–715].
67. Wright JT Jr, Bakris G, Greene T, et al. Effect of blood pressure lowering and antihypertensive drug class on progression of hypertensive kidney disease: Results from the AASK trial. JAMA 2002;288:2421–2431.
68. Casas JP, Chua W, Loukogeorgakis S, et al. Effect of inhibitors of the renin–angiotensin system and other antihypertensive drugs on renal outcomes: Systematic review and meta-analysis. Lancet 2005;366:2026–2033.
69. Furie KL, Kasner SE, Adams RJ, et al. Guidelines for the prevention of stroke in patients with stroke or transient ischemic attack: A guideline for healthcare professionals from the American Heart Association/American Stroke Association. Stroke 2011;42:227–276.
70. Rashid P, Leonardi-Bee J, Bath P. Blood pressure reduction and secondary prevention of stroke and other vascular events: A systematic review. Stroke 2003;34:2741–2748.
71. Schrader J, Luders S, Kulschewski A, et al. Morbidity and Mortality After Stroke, Eprosartan Compared with Nitrendipine for Secondary Prevention: Principal results of a prospective randomized controlled study (MOSES). Stroke 2005;36:1218–1226.
72. Yusuf S, Diener HC, Sacco RL, et al. Telmisartan to prevent recurrent stroke and cardiovascular events. N Engl J Med 2008;359:1225–1237.
73. Aronow WS, Fleg JL, Pepine CJ, et al. ACCF/AHA 2011 expert consensus document on hypertension in the elderly: A report of the American College of Cardiology Foundation Task Force on Clinical Expert Consensus Documents. Circulation 2011;123:2434–2506.
74. Beckett NS, Peters R, Fletcher AE, et al. Treatment of hypertension in patients 80 years of age or older. N Engl J Med 2008;358:1887–1898.
75. Hansson L, Lindholm LH, Ekbom T, et al. Randomised trial of old and new antihypertensive drugs in elderly patients: Cardiovascular mortality and morbidity the Swedish Trial in Old Patients with Hypertension-2 study. Lancet 1999;354:1751–1756.
76. National High Blood Pressure Education Program Working Group on High Blood Pressure in Children and Adolescents. The fourth report on the diagnosis, evaluation, and treatment of high blood pressure in children and adolescents. Pediatrics 2004;114:555–576.
77. Roberts JM, Pearson G, Cutler J, Lindheimer M. Summary of the NHLBI Working Group on Research on Hypertension During Pregnancy. Hypertension 2003;41:437–445.
78. Cooper WO, Hernandez-Diaz S, Arbogast PG, et al. Major congenital malformations after first-trimester exposure to ACE inhibitors. N Engl J Med 2006;354:2443–2451.
79. Flack JM, Sica DA, Bakris G, et al. Management of high blood pressure in blacks: An update of the International Society on Hypertension in Blacks consensus statement. Hypertension 2010;56:780–800.
80. Rooke TW, Hirsch AT, Misra S, et al. 2011 ACCF/AHA focused update of the guideline for the management of patients with peripheral artery disease (updating the 2005 guideline): A report of the American College of Cardiology Foundation/American Heart Association Task Force on Practice Guidelines. Circulation 2011;124:2020–2045.
81. Salpeter SR, Ormiston TM, Salpeter EE. Cardioselective beta-blockers in patients with reactive airway disease: A meta-analysis. Ann Intern Med 2002;137:715–725.
82. Paravastu SC, Mendonca D, Da Silva A. Beta blockers for peripheral arterial disease. Cochrane Database Syst Rev 2008:CD005508.
83. Elliott WJ, Meyer PM. Incident diabetes in clinical trials of antihypertensive drugs: A network meta-analysis. Lancet 2007;369:201–207.
84. Barksdale JD, Gardner SF. The impact of first-line antihypertensive drugs on erectile dysfunction. Pharmacotherapy 1999;19:573–581.
85. Ko DT, Hebert PR, Coffey CS, Sedrakyan A, Curtis JP, Krumholz HM. Beta-blocker therapy and symptoms of depression, fatigue, and sexual dysfunction. JAMA 2002;288:351–357.
86. Materson BJ, Reda DJ, Cushman WC, et al. Single-drug therapy for hypertension in men. A comparison of six antihypertensive agents with placebo. The Department of Veterans Affairs Cooperative Study Group on Antihypertensive Agents. N Engl J Med 1993;328:914–921.
87. Grimm RH Jr, Grandits GA, Prineas RJ, et al. Long-term effects on sexual function of five antihypertensive drugs and nutritional hygienic treatment in hypertensive men and women. Treatment of Mild Hypertension Study (TOMHS). Hypertension 1997;29:8–14.
88. Dagenais GR, Pogue J, Fox K, Simoons ML, Yusuf S. Angiotensin-converting-enzyme inhibitors in stable vascular disease without left ventricular systolic dysfunction or heart failure: A combined analysis of three trials. Lancet 2006;368:581–588.
89. Law MR, Wald NJ, Morris JK, Jordan RE. Value of low dose combination treatment with blood pressure lowering drugs: Analysis of 354 randomised trials. BMJ 2003;326:1427.
90. Bakris GL, Weir MR. Angiotensin-converting enzyme inhibitor-associated elevations in serum creatinine: Is this a cause for concern? Arch Intern Med 2000;160:685–693.
91. Yusuf S, Teo K, Anderson C, et al. Effects of the angiotensin-receptor blocker telmisartan on cardiovascular events in high-risk patients intolerant to angiotensin-converting enzyme inhibitors: A randomised controlled trial. Lancet 2008;372:1174–1183.
92. Yusuf S, Teo KK, Pogue J, et al. Telmisartan, ramipril, or both in patients at high risk for vascular events. N Engl J Med 2008;358:1547–1559.
93. Fournier A, Messerli FH, Achard JM, Fernandez L. Cerebroprotection mediated by angiotensin II: A hypothesis supported by recent randomized clinical trials. J Am Coll Cardiol 2004;43:1343–1347.
94. Haller H, Ito S, Izzo JL Jr, et al. Olmesartan for the delay or prevention of microalbuminuria in type 2 diabetes. N Engl J Med 2011;364:907–917.
95. Leenen FH, Nwachuku CE, Black HR, et al. Clinical events in high-risk hypertensive patients randomly assigned to calcium channel blocker versus angiotensin-converting enzyme inhibitor in the antihypertensive and lipid-lowering treatment to prevent heart attack trial. Hypertension 2006;48:374–384.
96. Ernst ME, Moser M. Use of diuretics in patients with hypertension. N Engl J Med 2009;361:2153–2164.

97. Chen JM, Heran BS, Wright JM. Blood pressure lowering efficacy of diuretics as second-line therapy for primary hypertension. Cochrane Database Syst Rev 2009:CD007187.
98. Dussol B, Moussi-Frances J, Morange S, Somma-Delpero C, Mundler O, Berland Y. A randomized trial of furosemide vs hydrochlorothiazide in patients with chronic renal failure and hypertension. Nephrol Dial Transplant 2005;20:349–353.
99. Messerli FH, Makani H, Benjo A, Romero J, Alviar C, Bangalore S. Antihypertensive efficacy of hydrochlorothiazide as evaluated by ambulatory blood pressure monitoring: A meta-analysis of randomized trials. J Am Coll Cardiol 2011;57:590–600.
100. Grimm RH Jr, Flack JM, Grandits GA, et al. Long-term effects on plasma lipids of diet and drugs to treat hypertension. Treatment of Mild Hypertension Study (TOMHS) Research Group. JAMA 1996;275:1549–1556.
101. UK Prospective Diabetes Study Group. Efficacy of atenolol and captopril in reducing risk of macrovascular and microvascular complications in type 2 diabetes: UKPDS 39. BMJ 1998;317:713–720.
102. Bakris GL, Fonseca V, Katholi RE, et al. Metabolic effects of carvedilol vs metoprolol in patients with type 2 diabetes mellitus and hypertension: A randomized controlled trial. JAMA 2004;292:2227–2236.
103. Parving HH, Brenner BM, McMurray JJ, et al. Cardiorenal end points in a trial of aliskiren for type 2 diabetes. N Engl J Med 2012;367:2204–2213.
104. Taylor AL, Ziesche S, Yancy C, et al. Combination of isosorbide dinitrate and hydralazine in blacks with heart failure. N Engl J Med 2004;351:2049–2057.
105. Heidenreich PA, Trogdon JG, Khavjou OA, et al. Forecasting the future of cardiovascular disease in the United States: A policy statement from the American Heart Association. Circulation 2011;123:933–944.
106. Fischer MA, Avorn J. Economic implications of evidence-based prescribing on hypertension: Can better care cost less? JAMA 2004;291:1850–1856.
107. Carter BL, Ardery G, Dawson JD, et al. Physician and pharmacist collaboration to improve blood pressure control. Arch Intern Med 2009;169:1996–2002.
108. Carter BL, Rogers M, Daly J, Zheng S, James PA. The potency of team-based care interventions for hypertension: A meta-analysis. Arch Intern Med 2009;169:1748–1755.
109. McLean DL, McAlister FA, Johnson JA, et al. A randomized trial of the effect of community pharmacist and nurse care on improving blood pressure management in patients with diabetes mellitus: Study of cardiovascular risk intervention by pharmacists-hypertension (SCRIP-HTN). Arch Intern Med 2008;168:2355–2361.
110. Murray MD, Ritchey ME, Wu J, Tu W. Effect of a pharmacist on adverse drug events and medication errors in outpatients with cardiovascular disease. Arch Intern Med 2009;169:757–763.
111. Lovibond K, Jowett S, Barton P, et al. Cost-effectiveness of options for the diagnosis of high blood pressure in primary care: A modelling study. Lancet 2011;378:1219–1230.
112. Hodgkinson J, Mant J, Martin U, et al. Relative effectiveness of clinic and home blood pressure monitoring compared with ambulatory blood pressure monitoring in diagnosis of hypertension: Systematic review. BMJ 2011;342:d3621.
113. Degli Esposti L, Valpiani G. Pharmacoeconomic burden of undertreating hypertension. Pharmacoeconomics 2004; 22:907–928.
114. Mazzaglia G, Ambrosioni E, Alacqua M, et al. Adherence to antihypertensive medications and cardiovascular morbidity among newly diagnosed hypertensive patients. Circulation 2009;120:1598–1605.
115. Hill MN, Miller NH, Degeest S, et al. Adherence and persistence with taking medication to control high blood pressure. J Am Soc Hypertens 2011;5:56–63.
116. Gradman AH, Basile JN, Carter BL, Bakris GL. Combination therapy in hypertension. J Am Soc Hypertens 2010;4:42–50.
117. Bangalore S, Kamalakkannan G, Parkar S, Messerli FH. Fixed-dose combinations improve medication compliance: A meta-analysis. Am J Med 2007;120:713–719.
118. Jamerson K, Weber MA, Bakris GL, et al. Benazepril plus amlodipine or hydrochlorothiazide for hypertension in high-risk patients. N Engl J Med 2008;359:2417–2428.
119. Weber CA, Leloux MR, Carter BL, Farris KB, Xu Y. Reduction in adverse symptoms as blood pressure becomes controlled. Pharmacotherapy 2008;28:1104–1114.
120. Saseen JJ, Carter BL, Brown TE, Elliott WJ, Black HR. Comparison of nifedipine alone and with diltiazem or verapamil in hypertension. Hypertension 1996;28:109–114.
121. Saseen JJ, Carter BL. Dual calcium-channel blocker therapy in the treatment of hypertension. Ann Pharmacother 1996;30:802–810.
122. Calhoun DA, Jones D, Textor S, et al. Resistant hypertension: Diagnosis, evaluation, and treatment: A scientific statement from the American Heart Association Professional Education Committee of the Council for High Blood Pressure Research. Circulation 2008;117:e510–e526.
123. Moser M, Cushman W, Handler J. Resistant or difficult-to-treat hypertension. J Clin Hypertens (Greenwich) 2006;8: 434–440.
124. Grossman E, Messerli FH, Grodzicki T, Kowey P. Should a moratorium be placed on sublingual nifedipine capsules given for hypertensive emergencies and pseudoemergencies? JAMA 1996;276:1328–1331.

4

Chronic Heart Failure

Robert B. Parker, Jean M. Nappi, and Larisa H. Cavallari

KEY CONCEPTS

1. Heart failure (HF) is a progressive clinical syndrome that can result from any changes in cardiac structure or function that impair the ability of the ventricle to fill with or eject blood. HF may be caused by an abnormality in systolic function, diastolic function, or both. The leading causes of HF are coronary artery disease and hypertension. The primary manifestations of the syndrome are dyspnea, fatigue, and fluid retention.

2. In response to a decrease in cardiac output, a number of compensatory responses are activated in an attempt to maintain adequate cardiac output, including activation of the sympathetic nervous system (SNS) and the renin–angiotensin–aldosterone system (RAAS), resulting in vasoconstriction and sodium and water retention as well as ventricular hypertrophy/remodeling. These compensatory mechanisms are responsible for the symptoms of HF and contribute to disease progression.

3. Our current understanding of HF pathophysiology is best described by the neurohormonal model. Activation of endogenous neurohormones including norepinephrine, angiotensin II, aldosterone, vasopressin, and numerous proinflammatory cytokines plays an important role in ventricular remodeling and the subsequent progression of HF. Importantly, pharmacotherapy targeted at antagonizing this neurohormonal activation has slowed the progression of HF and improved survival.

4. Most patients with symptomatic systolic heart failure (SHF) should be routinely treated with an angiotensin-converting enzyme (ACE) inhibitor, a β-blocker, and a diuretic. The benefits of these medications on slowing HF progression, reducing morbidity and mortality, and/or improving symptoms are clearly established. Patients should be treated with a diuretic if there is evidence of fluid retention. Treatment with digoxin may also be considered to improve symptoms and reduce hospitalizations.

5. In patients with SHF, ACE inhibitors improve survival, slow disease progression, reduce hospitalizations, and improve quality of life. The doses for these agents should be targeted at those shown in clinical trials to improve survival. When ACE inhibitors are contraindicated or not tolerated, an angiotensin II receptor blocker or the combination of hydralazine and isosorbide dinitrate is a reasonable alternative. Patients with asymptomatic left ventricular dysfunction and/or a previous myocardial infarction (MI) (Stage B of the American College of Cardiology [ACC]/American Heart Association [AHA] classification scheme) should also receive ACE inhibitors, with the goal of preventing symptomatic HF and reducing mortality.

6. The β-blockers carvedilol, metoprolol succinate, and bisoprolol have been shown to prolong survival, decrease hospitalizations and need for transplantation, and cause "reverse remodeling" of the left ventricle. These agents are recommended for all patients with a reduced left ventricular ejection fraction. Therapy must be instituted at low doses, with slow upward titration to the target dose.

7. Although chronic diuretic therapy frequently is used in HF patients, it is not mandatory. Diuretic therapy along with sodium restriction is required only in those patients with peripheral edema and/or pulmonary congestion. Many patients will need continued diuretic therapy to maintain euvolemia after fluid overload is resolved.

8. Digoxin does not improve survival in patients with SHF but does provide symptomatic benefits. Digoxin doses should be adjusted to achieve plasma concentrations of 0.5 to 1 ng/mL (0.6 to 1.3 nmol/L); higher plasma concentrations are not associated with additional benefits but may be associated with increased risk of toxicity.

9. Aldosterone antagonists, also known as mineralocorticoid receptor antagonists, reduce mortality in patients with SHF and New York Heart Association (NYHA) class II to IV symptoms and thus should be strongly considered in these patients provided that potassium and renal function can be carefully monitored. Aldosterone antagonists should also be considered soon after MI in patients with left ventricular dysfunction and either HF or diabetes.

10. The combination of hydralazine and nitrates improves the composite end point of mortality, hospitalizations for HF, and quality of life in African Americans receiving standard therapy. Current guidelines recommend the addition of hydralazine and nitrates to self-described African Americans with moderate to severe symptoms despite therapy with ACE inhibitors, diuretics, and β-blockers. This combination is also reasonable to consider in all patients who continue to have symptoms despite optimized therapy with an ACE inhibitor (or angiotensin receptor blocker [ARB]) and β-blocker. Hydralazine and a nitrate might be reasonable in patients unable to tolerate either an ACE inhibitor or ARB because of renal insufficiency, hyperkalemia, or possibly hypotension.

11. Treatment of HF with a preserved ejection fraction should be targeted at symptom reduction, causal clinical disease, and underlying basic mechanisms. Patients with HF and a preserved EF may be treated differently than those with systolic dysfunction.

INTRODUCTION

❶ ❷ Heart failure (HF) is a progressive clinical syndrome that can result from any abnormality in cardiac structure or function that impairs the ability of the ventricle to fill with or eject blood.[1] HF may be caused by an abnormality in systolic function, diastolic function, or both. Making the distinction is important because the prevalence, prognosis, and treatment of HF may be quite different depending on whether the predominant mechanism causing the symptoms is systolic or diastolic dysfunction. HF is the final common pathway for numerous cardiac disorders including those affecting the pericardium, heart valves, and myocardium. Diseases that adversely affect ventricular diastole (filling), ventricular systole (contraction), or both can lead to HF. For many years it was believed that reduced myocardial contractility, or systolic dysfunction (i.e., reduced left ventricular ejection fraction [LVEF]), was the sole disturbance in cardiac function responsible for HF. However, it is now recognized that large numbers of patients with the HF syndrome have relatively normal systolic function (i.e., normal LVEF). This is now referred to as HF with preserved LVEF (HFpEF) and is believed to be primarily due to diastolic dysfunction of the heart.[1] Recent estimates suggest approximately 50% of patients with HF have preserved LVEF with disturbances in relaxation (lusitropic) properties of the heart, or diastolic dysfunction.[2] However, regardless of the etiology of HF, the underlying pathophysiologic process and principal clinical manifestations (fatigue, dyspnea, and often volume overload) are similar and appear to be independent of the initial cause. Historically, this disorder was commonly referred to as *congestive HF*; the preferred nomenclature is now *HF* since a patient may have the clinical syndrome of HF without having symptoms of congestion. This chapter will focus on treatment of patients with chronic HF from reduced as well as preserved LVEF. Chapter 5 will discuss the treatment of acute decompensated HF.[2]

EPIDEMIOLOGY

HF is an epidemic public health problem in the United States.[3] Nearly 6 million Americans have HF with an additional 670,000 cases diagnosed each year.[3] Unlike most other cardiovascular diseases, the incidence and prevalence of HF are increasing and are expected to continue to increase over the next few decades as the population ages. A large majority of patients with HF are elderly, with multiple comorbid conditions that influence morbidity and mortality.[3] Improved survival after myocardial infarction (MI) is thought to be a likely contributor to the increased incidence and prevalence of HF.[4] Annual hospital discharges for HF now total over 1 million, although recent data suggest hospitalization rates are declining in the Medicare population.[4] However, HF remains the most common hospital discharge diagnosis in individuals over age 65.[3] The disorder also has a tremendous economic impact, with this expected to increase markedly as the baby-boom generation ages. Current estimates suggest annual expenditures for HF of approximately $39 billion, with the majority of these costs spent on hospitalized patients.[5] Thus, HF is a major medical problem, with substantial economic impact that is expected to become even more significant as the population ages.

Despite prodigious advances in our understanding of the etiology, pathophysiology, and pharmacotherapy of HF, the prognosis for patients with this disorder remains grim. Although the mortality rates have declined over the last 50 years, the overall 5-year survival remains approximately 50% for all patients with a diagnosis of HF, with mortality increasing with symptom severity.[3,4,6] Death is classified as sudden in about 40% of patients, implicating serious ventricular arrhythmias as the underlying cause.[1] Factors affecting the prognosis of patients with HF include, but are not limited to, age, gender, LVEF, renal function, natriuretic peptide plasma concentrations, diabetes, extent of underlying coronary artery disease, blood pressure (BP), HF etiology, and drug or device therapy. Recent models incorporating these and other factors enable clinicians to develop reliable estimates of an individual patient's prognosis.[5,6]

ETIOLOGY

❶ ❷ HF can result from any disorder that affects the ability of the heart to contract (systolic function) and/or relax (diastolic dysfunction); common causes of HF are shown in Table 4-1.[7] HF with reduced systolic function (i.e., reduced LVEF) is the classic, more familiar form of the disorder, but current estimates suggest up to 50% of patients with HF have preserved left ventricular systolic function with presumed diastolic dysfunction.[2,8] In contrast to systolic heart failure (SHF) that is usually caused by previous MI, patients with preserved LVEF typically are elderly, female, and obese, and have hypertension (HTN), atrial fibrillation, or diabetes.[8] Recent data indicate that survival is similar in patients with impaired or preserved LVEF.[8]

❶ Coronary artery disease is the most common cause of SHF, accounting for nearly 70% of cases.[8,9] MI leads to reduction in muscle mass due to death of affected myocardial cells. The degree to which contractility is impaired depends on the size of the infarction. To attempt to maintain cardiac output (CO), the surviving myocardium undergoes a compensatory remodeling, thus beginning the maladaptive process that initiates the HF syndrome and leads to further injury to the heart. This is discussed in greater detail in Pathophysiology below. Myocardial ischemia and infarction also affect the diastolic properties of the heart by increasing ventricular stiffness and slowing ventricular relaxation. Thus, MI frequently results in systolic and diastolic dysfunction.

Impaired systolic function is a cardinal feature of dilated cardiomyopathies. Although the cause of reduced contractility frequently is unknown, abnormalities such as interstitial fibrosis, cellular infiltrates, cellular hypertrophy, and myocardial cell degeneration are seen commonly on histologic examination. Inherited forms of dilated as well as hypertrophic cardiomyopathies may also occur.[9,10]

Pressure or volume overload causes ventricular hypertrophy, which attempts to return contractility to a near-normal state. If the pressure or volume overload persists, the remodeling process results in alterations in the geometry of the hypertrophied myocardial cells

TABLE 4-1 Causes of Heart Failure

Systolic dysfunction (decreased contractility)
- Reduction in muscle mass (e.g., myocardial infarction)
- Dilated cardiomyopathies
- Ventricular hypertrophy
  - Pressure overload (e.g., systemic or pulmonary hypertension, aortic or pulmonic valve stenosis)
  - Volume overload (e.g., valvular regurgitation, shunts, high-output states)

Diastolic dysfunction (restriction in ventricular filling)
- Increased ventricular stiffness
  - Ventricular hypertrophy (e.g., hypertrophic cardiomyopathy, other examples above)
  - Infiltrative myocardial diseases (e.g., amyloidosis, sarcoidosis, endomyocardial fibrosis)
  - Myocardial ischemia and infarction
- Mitral or tricuspid valve stenosis
- Pericardial disease (e.g., pericarditis, pericardial tamponade)

Data from Mann DL. Management of heart failure patients with reduced ejection fraction. In: Bonow RO, Mann DL, Zipes DP, Libby P, eds. Braunwald's Heart Disease: A Textbook of Cardiovascular Medicine, 9th ed. Philadelphia, PA: Elsevier, 2012:543–569.

and is accompanied by increased collagen deposition in the extracellular matrix. Thus, both systolic and diastolic functions may be impaired.[7] Examples of pressure overload include systemic or pulmonary HTN and aortic or pulmonic valve stenosis.

HTN remains an important cause and/or contributor to HF in many patients, particularly women, the elderly, and African Americans.[1,8] The role of HTN should not be underestimated because HTN is an important risk factor for ischemic heart disease and thus is also present in a high percentage of the patients with this disorder. HF is a largely preventable disorder such that appropriate management of lifestyle risk factors (e.g., HTN, coronary heart disease, smoking, obesity, physical activity, diabetes, etc.) is key to minimize the risk of HF development.

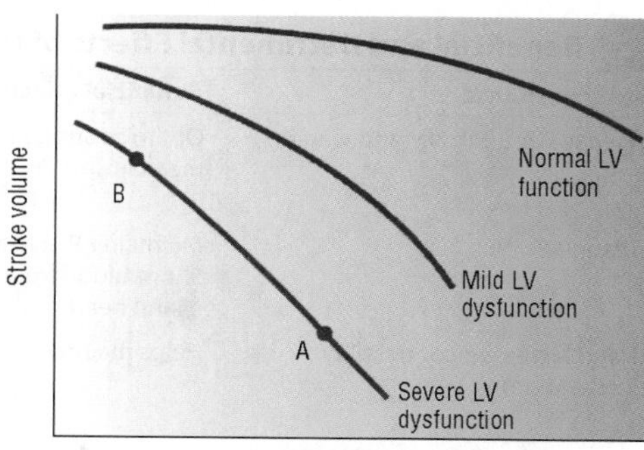

FIGURE 4-1 Relationship between stroke volume and systemic vascular resistance. In an individual with normal left ventricular (LV) function, increasing systemic vascular resistance has little effect on stroke volume. As the extent of LV dysfunction increases, the negative, inverse relationship between stroke volume and systemic vascular resistance becomes more important (B to A).

PATHOPHYSIOLOGY

Normal Cardiac Function

To understand the pathophysiologic processes in HF, a basic understanding of normal cardiac function is necessary. *CO* is defined as the volume of blood ejected per unit time (L/min) and is the product of heart rate (HR) and stroke volume (SV):

$$CO = HR \times SV$$

The relationship between CO and mean arterial pressure (MAP) is:

$$MAP = CO \times \text{systemic vascular resistance (SVR)}$$

HR is controlled by the autonomic nervous system. SV, or the volume of blood ejected during systole, depends on preload, afterload, and contractility.[7] As defined by the Frank-Starling mechanism, the ability of the heart to alter the force of contraction depends on changes in preload. As myocardial sarcomere length is stretched, the number of cross-bridges between thick and thin myofilaments increases, resulting in an increase in the force of contraction. The length of the sarcomere is determined primarily by the volume of blood in the ventricle; therefore, left ventricular end-diastolic volume (LVEDV) is the primary determinant of preload. In normal hearts, the preload response is the primary compensatory mechanism such that a small increase in end-diastolic volume results in a large increase in CO. Because of the relationship between pressure and volume in the heart, left ventricular end-diastolic pressure (LVEDP) is often used in the clinical setting to estimate preload. The hemodynamic measurement used to clinically estimate LVEDP is the pulmonary capillary wedge pressure (PCWP), also known as the pulmonary artery occlusion pressure (PAOP). Afterload is a more complex physiologic concept that can be viewed pragmatically as the sum of forces preventing active forward ejection of blood by the ventricle. Major components of afterload are ejection impedance, wall tension, and regional wall geometry. In patients with left ventricular systolic dysfunction, an inverse relationship exists between afterload (estimated clinically by SVR) and SV such that increasing afterload causes a decrease in SV (Fig. 4-1). Contractility is the intrinsic property of cardiac muscle describing fiber shortening and tension development.

HF with a preserved ejection fraction can be defined as a condition in which myocardial relaxation and filling are impaired and incomplete. The ventricle is unable to accept an adequate volume of blood from the venous system, does not fill at low pressure, and/or is unable to maintain normal SV. In its most severe form, HFpEF results in overt symptoms of HF. In modest HFpEF, symptoms of dyspnea and fatigue occur only during stress or activity, when HR and end-diastolic volume increase. In its mildest form, HFpEF can be manifested as a slow or delayed pattern of relaxation and filling with little or no elevation in diastolic pressure and few or no cardiac symptoms. The congestive symptoms that occur with HFpEF are a manifestation of increased pulmonary venous pressures. HFpEF is caused by impaired myocardial relaxation and/or increased diastolic stiffness. When HF is caused by a predominant abnormality in diastolic function, the ventricular chamber is not enlarged, and EF may be normal or even elevated.[2,11] Figure 4-2 shows the pressure–volume relationship in a patient with normal versus abnormal diastolic function. Changes in the myocardium are associated with a shift upward and to the left of the pressure–volume curve, so that for any increase in LV volume, diastolic pressure rises to a much greater level than normally would occur. Clinically, patients present with reduced exercise tolerance and dyspnea when they have elevated LV diastolic pressures. Patients with HFpEF have a predominant abnormality in diastolic function, whereas patients with SHF have a predominant abnormality in systolic function of the LV.

Recent data suggest that HFpEF may also be associated with abnormalities in endothelial and ventricular reserve function. During physical exertion, CO increases through integrated enhancements in venous return, contractility, HR, and peripheral vasodilation. The vasodilation that normally occurs during exercise is impaired in HFpEF. Pulmonary HTN is also a common finding. Abnormalities in each of these components of normal exercise reserve function have been identified in HFpEF and all may contribute to pathophysiology in individual patients.[2]

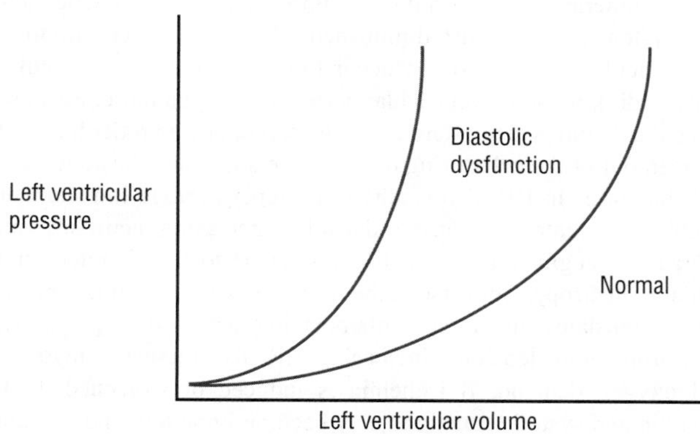

FIGURE 4-2 Diastolic pressure–volume relationship in a normal patient (*right trace*) and a patient with diastolic dysfunction (*left trace*).

TABLE 4-2 Beneficial and Detrimental Effects of the Compensatory Responses in Heart Failure

Compensatory Response	Beneficial Effects of Compensation	Detrimental Effects of Compensation
Increased preload (through Na^+ and water retention)	Optimize stroke volume via Frank-Starling mechanism	Pulmonary and systemic congestion and edema formation Increased MVO_2
Vasoconstriction	Maintain BP in face of reduced CO Shunt blood from nonessential organs to brain and heart	Increased MVO_2 Increased afterload decreases stroke volume and further activates the compensatory responses
Tachycardia and increased contractility (due to SNS activation)	Helps maintain CO	Increased MVO_2 Shortened diastolic filling time β_1-Receptor downregulation, decreased receptor sensitivity Precipitation of ventricular arrhythmias Increased risk of myocardial cell
Ventricular hypertrophy and remodeling	Helps maintain CO Reduces myocardial wall stress Decreases MVO_2	Diastolic dysfunction Systolic dysfunction Increased risk of myocardial cell death Increased risk of myocardial ischemia Increased arrhythmia risk Fibrosis

SNS, sympathetic nervous system; BP, blood pressure; MVO_2, myocardial oxygen demand; CO, cardiac output.

Compensatory Mechanisms in Heart Failure

2 HF is a progressive disorder initiated by any event that impairs the ability of the heart to contract and/or relax resulting in a decrease in CO. The index event may have an acute onset, as with MI, or the onset may be slow, as with long-standing HTN. Regardless of the index event, the decrease in CO results in activation of compensatory responses to maintain the circulation.[7,10,12] These compensatory responses include: (a) tachycardia and increased contractility through sympathetic nervous system (SNS) activation, (b) the Frank-Starling mechanism, whereby an increase in preload results in an increase in SV, (c) vasoconstriction, and (d) ventricular hypertrophy and remodeling. Compensatory responses evolved to provide short-term support to maintain circulatory homeostasis after acute reductions in BP or renal perfusion. However, the persistent decline in CO in HF results in long-term activation of these compensatory responses resulting in the complex functional, structural, biochemical, and molecular changes important for the development and progression of HF. The beneficial and detrimental effects of these compensatory responses are described below and are summarized in Table 4-2.

Tachycardia and Increased Contractility

The increase in HR and contractility that rapidly occurs in response to a drop in CO is primarily due to release of norepinephrine (NE) from adrenergic nerve terminals, although parasympathetic nervous system activity is also diminished.[12] Loss of atrial contribution to ventricular filling also can occur (atrial fibrillation, ventricular tachycardia), reducing ventricular performance even more. Because ionized calcium is sequestered into the sarcoplasmic reticulum and pumped out of the cell during diastole, the shortened diastolic time with increases in HR also results in a higher average intracellular calcium concentration during diastole, increasing actin–myosin interaction, augmenting the active resistance to fibril stretch, and reducing lusitropy. Conversely, the higher average calcium concentration translates into greater filament interaction during systole, generating more tension.[7] Increasing HR also increases myocardial oxygen demand. If ischemia is induced or worsened, both diastolic and systolic functions may become impaired, and SV can drop precipitously. In addition, polymorphisms in genes coding for adrenergic receptors (e.g., β_1- and α_{2c}-receptors) and their signaling pathways may affect the risk for development of HF and alter the response to endogenous NE.[13]

Fluid Retention and Increased Preload

Augmentation of preload is another compensatory response that is rapidly activated in response to decreased CO. Renal perfusion in HF is reduced due to both depressed CO and redistribution of blood away from nonvital organs. The kidney interprets the reduced perfusion as an ineffective blood volume, resulting in activation of the renin–angiotensin–aldosterone system (RAAS) in an attempt to maintain BP and increase renal sodium and water retention. Reduced renal perfusion and increased sympathetic tone also stimulate renin release from juxtaglomerular cells in the kidney. As shown in Figure 4-3, renin is responsible for conversion of angiotensinogen to angiotensin I. Angiotensin I is converted to angiotensin II by angiotensin-converting enzyme (ACE). Angiotensin II may also be generated via non–ACE-dependent pathways. Angiotensin II stimulates aldosterone release from the adrenal gland, thereby providing an additional mechanism for renal sodium and water retention. As intravascular volume increases secondary to sodium and water retention, left ventricular volume and pressure (preload) increase, sarcomeres are stretched, and the force of contraction is enhanced.[7] While the preload response is the primary compensatory mechanism in normal hearts, the chronically failing heart usually has exhausted its preload reserve.[7] As shown in Figure 4-4, increases in preload will increase SV only to a certain point. Once the flat portion of the curve is reached, further increases in preload will only lead to pulmonary or systemic congestion, a detrimental result.[7] Figure 4-4 also shows that the curve is flatter in patients with left ventricular dysfunction. Consequently, a given increase in preload in a patient with HF will produce a smaller increment in SV than in an individual with normal ventricular function.

Vasoconstriction and Increased Afterload

Vasoconstriction occurs in patients with HF to help redistribute blood flow away from nonessential organs to coronary and cerebral circulations to support BP, which may be reduced secondary to a decrease in CO (MAP = CO × SVR).[7] A number of neurohormones likely contribute to the vasoconstriction, including NE, angiotensin II, endothelin-1 (ET-1), neuropeptide Y, urotensin II, and arginine vasopressin (AVP).[7] Vasoconstriction impedes forward ejection of blood from the ventricle, further depressing CO and heightening the compensatory responses. The failing ventricle is exquisitely sensitive to changes in afterload (Fig. 4-1). Thus, increases in afterload often potentiate a vicious cycle of continued worsening and downward spiraling of the HF state.

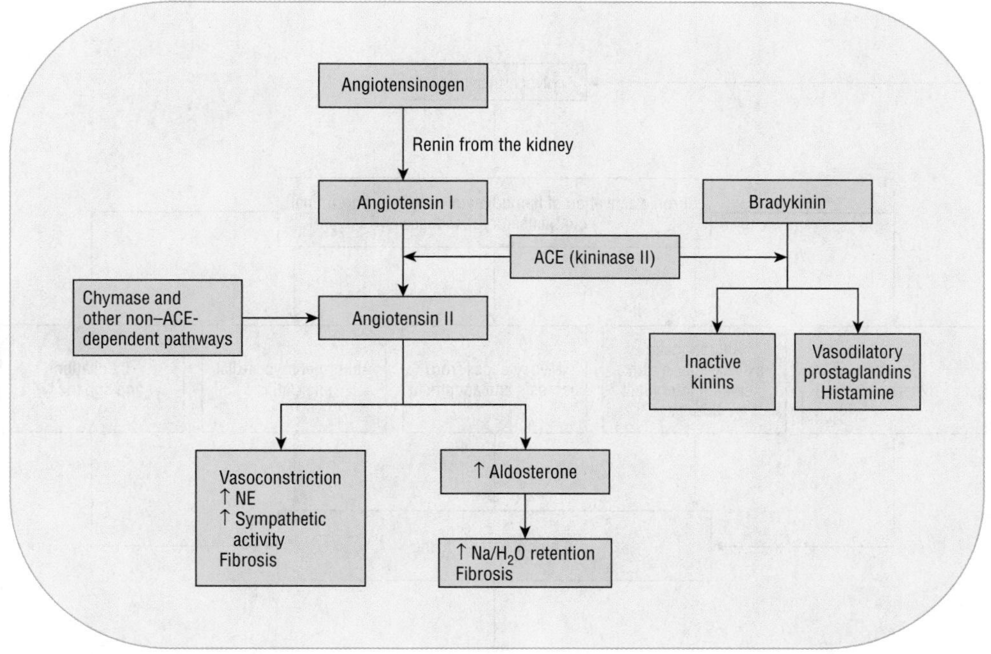

FIGURE 4-3 Physiology of the renin–angiotensin–aldosterone system. Renin produces angiotensin I from angiotensinogen. Angiotensin I is cleaved to angiotensin II by angiotensin-converting enzyme (ACE). Angiotensin II has a number of physiologic actions that are detrimental in heart failure. Note that angiotensin II can be produced in a number of tissues, including the heart, independent of ACE activity. ACE is also responsible for the breakdown of bradykinin. Inhibition of ACE results in accumulation of bradykinin that, in turn, enhances the production of vasodilatory prostaglandins.

Ventricular Hypertrophy and Remodeling

3 While the signs and symptoms of HF are closely associated with the items described above, the progression of HF appears to be independent of the patient's hemodynamic status. It is now recognized that left ventricular hypertrophy and remodeling are key components in the pathogenesis of progressive myocardial failure.[7] *Ventricular hypertrophy* is a term used to describe an increase in ventricular muscle mass. *Cardiac or ventricular remodeling* is a broader term describing changes in both myocardial cells and extracellular matrix that result in changes in the size, shape, structure, and function of the heart. These progressive changes in ventricular structure and function ultimately result in a change in shape of the left ventricle from an ellipse to a sphere. This change in ventricular size and shape serves to further depress the mechanical performance of the heart, increases regurgitant flow through the mitral valve, and, in turn, fuels the continued progression of remodeling. Ventricular hypertrophy and remodeling can occur in association with any condition that causes myocardial injury. The onset of the remodeling process precedes the development of HF symptoms.

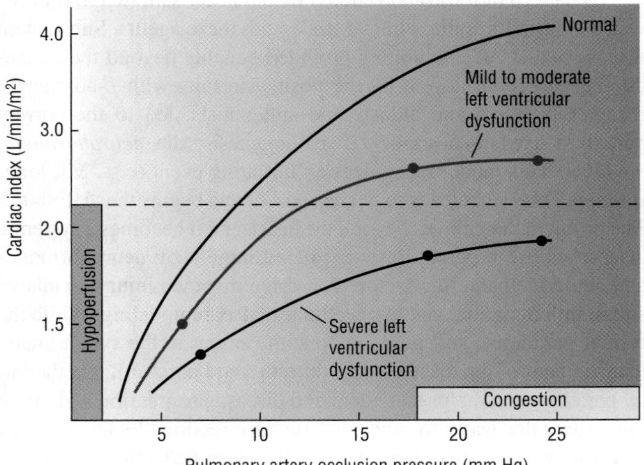

FIGURE 4-4 Relationship between cardiac output (shown as cardiac index which is CO/BSA) and preload (shown as pulmonary artery occlusion pressure).

Cardiac remodeling is a complex process that affects the heart at the molecular and cellular levels. Key elements in the process are shown in Figure 4-5. Collectively, these events result in progressive changes in myocardial structure and function such as cardiac hypertrophy, myocyte loss, and alterations in the extracellular matrix. The progression of the remodeling process leads to reductions in myocardial systolic and/or diastolic function that, in turn, results in further myocardial injury, perpetuating the remodeling process and the decline in left ventricular performance. Angiotensin II, NE, ET, aldosterone, vasopressin, and numerous inflammatory cytokines, as well as substances under investigation, that are activated both systemically and locally in the heart and vasculature play an important role in initiating the signal transduction cascade responsible for ventricular remodeling. Although these mediators produce harmful effects on the heart, their increased circulating and tissue concentrations are also toxic to other organs and serve as an important reminder that HF is a systemic as well as a cardiac disorder.[12]

Pressure overload (and probably hormonal activation) associated with HTN produces a concentric hypertrophy (increase in the ventricular wall thickness without chamber enlargement). Conversely, eccentric left ventricular hypertrophy (myocyte lengthening with increased chamber size with minimal increase in wall thickness) characterizes the hypertrophy seen in patients with systolic

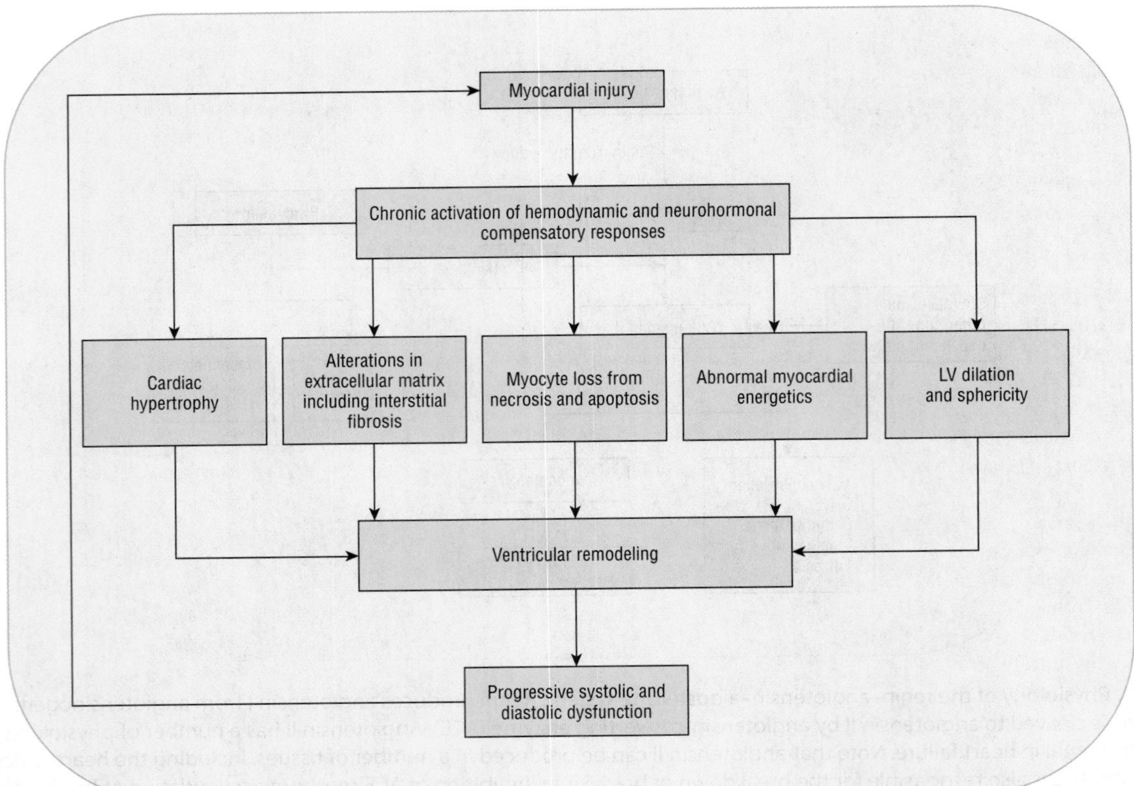

FIGURE 4-5 Key components of the pathophysiology of cardiac remodeling. Myocardial injury (e.g., myocardial infarction) results in the activation of a number of hemodynamic and neurohormonal compensatory responses in an attempt to maintain circulatory homeostasis. Chronic activation of the neurohormonal systems results in a cascade of events that affect the myocardium at the molecular and cellular levels. These events lead to the changes in ventricular size, shape, structure, and function known as ventricular remodeling. The alterations in ventricular function result in further deterioration in cardiac systolic and diastolic functions that further promotes the remodeling process.

dysfunction or previous MI. As the myocytes undergo change, so do various components of the extracellular matrix. For example, collagen degradation may lead to myocyte slippage, fibroblast proliferation, and increased fibrillar collagen synthesis, resulting in fibrosis and stiffening of the entire myocardium. Thus, a number of important ventricular changes that occur with remodeling include alterations in the geometry of the heart from an elliptical to a spherical shape, increases in ventricular mass (from myocyte hypertrophy), and changes in ventricular composition (especially the extracellular matrix) and volumes, all of which contribute to the impaired cardiac function. If the event producing cardiac injury is acute (e.g., MI), the ventricular remodeling process begins immediately. However, it is the progressive nature of this process that results in continual worsening of the HF state, and thus is now the major focus for identification of therapeutic targets. In fact, HF pharmacotherapy associated with decreased mortality, and/or slowing the progression of the disease, produces these effects largely by slowing or reversing ventricular remodeling, a process often referred to as *reverse remodeling*.

The Neurohormonal Model of Heart Failure and Therapeutic Insights It Provides

❷ ❸ Over the years, several different paradigms have guided our understanding of the pathophysiology and treatment of HF.[7] The early paradigm is often called the *cardiorenal model*, where the problem was viewed as excess sodium and water retention, and diuretic therapy was the main therapeutic approach. Next, the *cardiocirculatory model* focused on impaired CO (viewed as being due to both reduced pumping capacity of the heart and systemic vasoconstriction). Treatment strategies here focused on positive inotropes and, later, vasodilators, as the primary therapies to overcome reduced CO. While the therapeutic approaches associated with these paradigms provided some symptomatic benefits, they did little to slow progression of the disease. In fact, the detrimental effects of positive inotropic drugs on survival highlighted the inadequacy of the cardiocirculatory model to explain the progressive nature of HF.

Balanced (arterial and venous) vasodilation with ACE inhibitors was the basis for initial clinical trials with these agents. Subsequent discovery that ACE inhibitors provided benefits beyond their vasodilating effects, followed by the positive results with β-adrenergic receptor blockers and aldosterone antagonists, led to the current paradigm used to describe HF pathogenesis: the *neurohormonal model*.[7,14] This model recognizes an initiating event (e.g., MI, longstanding HTN) that leads to decreased CO and begins the "HF state." The problem then moves beyond the heart, and it becomes a systemic disease whose progression is mediated largely by neurohormones and autocrine/paracrine factors that drive myocyte injury, oxidative stress, inflammation, and extracellular matrix remodeling. While the former paradigms still guide us to some extent in the symptomatic management of the disease (e.g., diuretics and digoxin), it is the latter paradigm that helps us understand disease progression and, more important, the ways to slow disease progression. In the sections that follow, key neurohormones and autocrine/paracrine factors, sometimes now collectively termed biomarkers, are described with respect to their role in HF and its progression. The benefits of current and investigational drug therapies can be better understood through a solid understanding of the neurohormones they regulate/affect.

Although the neurohormonal model provides a logical framework for our current understanding of HF progression and the role of various medications in attenuating this progression, it must be emphasized that this model does not completely explain HF progression. For example, drug therapies that target the neurohormonal perturbations in HF usually only slow the progressive nature of the disorder rather than completely stop it. Ongoing research will likely identify additional targets for drug therapy.

Angiotensin II

Of the neurohormones and autocrine/paracrine factors that play an important role in SHF pathophysiology, angiotensin II is probably the best understood.[7,15] Although circulating angiotensin II produced from ACE activity is the most familiar route for generation of angiotensin II, recent evidence indicates that this hormone is synthesized directly in the myocardium through non–ACE-dependent pathways that also contribute to HF pathophysiology.

Angiotensin II has multiple actions that contribute to its detrimental effects in HF. It is a potent vasoconstrictor mediated by binding to the angiotensin type 1 (AT1) receptor in the vasculature and it also causes release of AVP and ET-1. Angiotensin II facilitates release of NE from adrenergic nerve terminals, heightening SNS activation. It promotes sodium retention through direct effects on the renal tubules and by stimulating aldosterone release. Its vasoconstriction of the efferent glomerular arteriole helps to maintain renal perfusion pressure in patients with severe HF or impaired renal function. Finally, angiotensin II, and many of the neurohormones released in response to angiotensin II, plays a central role in stimulating ventricular hypertrophy, remodeling, myocyte apoptosis, oxidative stress, inflammation, and alterations in the myocardial extracellular matrix. Clinical data suggest that attenuating angiotensin II–mediated effects contributes substantially to the benefits of ACE inhibitor–treated and angiotensin receptor blocker (ARB)–treated patients with SHF.[15,16] The favorable effects of ACE inhibitors and ARBs on hemodynamics, symptoms, hospitalizations, quality of life, and survival highlight the importance of angiotensin II in the pathophysiology of this disorder.

Norepinephrine

As described earlier in this chapter, NE plays a central role in the tachycardia, vasoconstriction, and increased contractility and plasma renin activity in HF.[12] Plasma NE concentrations are elevated in correlation with the degree of HF, and patients with the highest plasma NE concentrations have the poorest prognosis.[7,17] Excessive SNS activation causes downregulation of β_1-receptors, with a subsequent loss of sensitivity to receptor stimulation. Excess catecholamines increase the risk of arrhythmias and can cause myocardial cell loss by stimulating both necrosis and apoptosis. Finally, NE contributes to ventricular hypertrophy and remodeling. The detrimental effects of SNS activation are further highlighted by the clinical trials of chronic therapy with β-agonists, phosphodiesterase inhibitors, or other drugs that cause SNS activation, since these agents are uniformly associated with increased mortality. Conversely, β-blockers, ACE inhibitors, and digoxin all help to decrease SNS activation, through various mechanisms, and are beneficial in HF. Thus, it is clear that NE plays a critical role in the pathophysiology of the HF state.

Aldosterone

Aldosterone-mediated sodium retention and its key role in volume overload and edema have long been recognized as important components of the HF syndrome.[18] Circulating aldosterone is increased in HF due to stimulation of its synthesis and release from the adrenal cortex by angiotensin II and due to decreased hepatic clearance from reduced hepatic perfusion. Recent studies demonstrate direct effects of aldosterone on the heart that may be even more important than sodium retention in HF pathophysiology. Chief among these is the ability of aldosterone to produce interstitial cardiac fibrosis through increased collagen deposition in the extracellular matrix of the heart. By increasing the stiffness of the myocardium, cardiac fibrosis may decrease systolic function and impair diastolic function. Current research shows that extra-adrenal production of aldosterone in the heart, kidneys, and vascular smooth muscle also contributes to the progressive nature of HF through target organ fibrosis and vascular remodeling. Induction of a systemic proinflammatory state, increased oxidative stress, wasting of soft tissues and bone, secondary hyperparathyroidism, and mineral/micronutrient dyshomeostasis are other important pathologic actions of aldosterone that directly contribute to ventricular remodeling and HF progression.[19] Aldosterone also may increase the risk of ventricular arrhythmias through a number of mechanisms, including creation of reentrant circuits as a result of fibrosis, inhibition of cardiac NE reuptake, depletion of intracellular potassium and magnesium, and impairment of parasympathetic traffic. Other detrimental effects of aldosterone include insulin resistance and endothelial and baroreceptor dysfunction. Clinical trials with the aldosterone antagonists spironolactone[20] and eplerenone[21,22] showing significant reductions in morbidity and mortality in patients with HF provide compelling evidence of the important role of aldosterone in the initiation and progression of this syndrome.

Natriuretic Peptides

The natriuretic peptide family has three members, atrial natriuretic peptide (ANP), B-type natriuretic peptide (BNP), and C-type natriuretic peptide (CNP).[22] Of these, BNP is the one that is most useful in the diagnosis and management of HF.[23,24] BNP is synthesized and released from the ventricle in response to pressure or volume overload. BNP plasma concentrations are elevated in patients with HF functioning to increase natriuresis and diuresis and attenuate activation of the RAAS and SNS.

The development of easily performed commercial assays for BNP and the related biologically inactive peptide, NT-proBNP, resulted in widespread interest in the role of these peptides as a biomarker for prognostic, diagnostic, and therapeutic use. In patients with chronic HF, the degree of elevation in BNP levels is closely associated with increased mortality, risk of sudden death, symptoms, and hospital readmission.[23,24] Accurate diagnosis of acute decompensated HF in acute care settings is often difficult since many of the symptoms (e.g., dyspnea) mimic those of other disorders such as pulmonary disease or obesity. The most well-established clinical application of BNP testing is in the urgent care setting where the BNP or NT-proBNP assay is useful when combined with clinical evaluation for differentiating dyspnea secondary to either SHF or HFpEF from other causes. The Breathing Not Properly study evaluated 452 patients with echocardiography within 30 days of an emergency department visit. Of the 452 patients, 165 (36.5%) had EF >45% (mean EF 59%).[25] In the patients with preserved EF who had been admitted to the hospital for dyspnea, BNP levels were significantly lower than those found in patients with SHF (413 pg/mL vs. 821 pg/mL [119 pmol/L vs. 237 pmol/L]). However, there was considerable overlap in the BNP levels in patients with HFpEF compared with those in patients without HF, making BNP levels less useful. Furthermore, the sensitivity, specificity, and predictive accuracy of BNP levels in HFpEF are limited in part because BNP is altered by age, adiposity, gender, and other factors. Similar findings have been documented with NT-proBNP. In a study of 68 symptomatic patients with isolated HFpEF (EF >50%), NT-proBNP was significantly increased in patients with isolated HFpEF and correlated with disease severity. Compared with conventional echocardiography, Doppler imaging, and heart catheterization, NT-proBNP exhibited the best negative predictive value for detection of HFpEF.[26]

Much interest has focused on the benefits of serial measurement of BNP as a target to guide drug therapy, primarily diuretics. Recent studies evaluating this approach have not shown consistent improvement in long-term outcomes compared with standard medical therapy.[23,24] As a result, current guidelines do not support the routine use of serial measurement of BNP in the management of chronic HF.[1,27]

Arginine Vasopressin

AVP is a pituitary peptide hormone that regulates renal water excretion and plasma osmolality.[7,14] Plasma concentrations of AVP are elevated in patients with HF, supporting its role in the pathophysiology of this disorder. The physiologic effects of AVP are mediated through the V_{1a}, V_{1b}, and V_2 receptors. Stimulation of these receptors by increased circulating AVP results in several maladaptive responses including: (a) increased renal free water reabsorption in the face of plasma hypoosmolality resulting in volume overload and hyponatremia; (b) increased arterial vasoconstriction that contributes to reduced CO; and (c) stimulation of remodeling by cardiac hypertrophy and extracellular matrix collagen deposition.

Given the importance of AVP in HF, recent efforts have focused on the development of AVP antagonist drugs for treatment of acute and chronic HF. By blocking the AVP receptor, these agents primarily increase free water excretion (i.e., an "aquaretic" effect). Although clinical trials with tolvaptan demonstrate improvements in acute symptoms and increases in serum sodium and urine output without affecting HR, BP, renal function, or other electrolytes, no improvements in morbidity and mortality were seen.[28]

Other Circulating Biomarkers

The role of other biomarkers in HF pathogenesis, risk stratification, and identification of patients at risk for developing HF, and as potential therapeutic targets is an area of extensive ongoing research.[13,14,23] Many of these biomarkers (e.g., ET, C-reactive protein and other inflammatory cytokines, copeptin, procalcitonin) are involved in inflammation, oxidative stress, extracellular matrix remodeling, myocyte injury and stress, and kidney injury that drive the systemic response to the failing left ventricle. It is hoped that data from investigations will lead to improved understanding of disease pathophysiology, prognosis, and targets for therapy.

Factors Precipitating/Exacerbating Heart Failure

Although significant advancements have been made in treatment, symptom exacerbation, to the point that hospitalization is required, is a common and growing problem in patients with chronic HF. Hospitalization for HF exacerbation consumes large amounts of healthcare dollars and significantly impairs the patient's quality of life; thus, there is great interest in identifying and then remedying factors that increase the risk of decompensation. Appropriate therapy can often maintain patients in a "compensated" state, indicating that they are relatively symptom-free. However, there are many aggravating or precipitating factors that may cause a previously compensated patient to develop worsened symptoms necessitating hospitalization. Often, these precipitating factors are reversible or treatable, such that a thorough evaluation for their presence is imperative.

Cardiac events are a frequent cause of worsening HF.[1,29] Myocardial ischemia and infarction are potentially reversible causes that must be carefully considered since nearly 70% of HF patients have coronary artery disease. Revascularization should be considered in appropriate patients. Atrial fibrillation occurs in up to 10% to 50% of patients with HF and is associated with increased morbidity and mortality.[30,31] It can exacerbate HF through rapid ventricular response and loss of atrial contribution to ventricular filling. Conversely, HF can precipitate atrial fibrillation by increasing atrial distension from ventricular volume overload. Control of ventricular response, maintenance of sinus rhythm in appropriate patients, and prevention of thromboembolism are important elements in the treatment of HF patients with atrial fibrillation. Uncontrolled HTN is also an important contributing factor and should be treated according to current guidelines.[30,31]

Noncardiac events are also associated with HF decompensation. Pulmonary infections frequently cause worsening HF. Many of these events would be preventable with more widespread use of the pneumococcal and influenza vaccines. Pulmonary embolus, diabetes, worsening renal function, hypothyroidism, and hyperthyroidism should also be considered.

Nonadherence with prescribed HF medications or with dietary recommendations (e.g., sodium intake and fluid restriction) is also a common cause of HF exacerbation.[29,32] Recent estimates indicate that nonadherence is an important contributor to poor outcomes and that socioeconomically disadvantaged patients appear to be disproportionately affected.

A number of drugs can precipitate or exacerbate HF by one or more of the following mechanisms: (a) negative inotropic effects; (b) direct cardiotoxicity; or (c) increased sodium and/or water retention (Table 4-3).[33] The resulting symptoms are typically those associated with volume overload, but in more severe cases hypoperfusion may also be present. Nonsteroidal antiinflammatory drugs (NSAIDs) are increasingly recognized for their ability to exacerbate HF and increase risk of hospitalization and mortality through volume retention, decreased renal function, and increased BP.[33]

What should be evident is that many of the precipitating factors are preventable, particularly through appropriate healthcare

TABLE 4-3 Drugs That May Precipitate or Exacerbate Heart Failure

Negative inotropic effect
Antiarrhythmics (e.g., disopyramide, flecainide, and propafenone)
β-Blockers (e.g., propranolol, metoprolol, carvedilol)
Calcium channel blockers (e.g., verapamil, diltiazem)
Itraconazole
Cardiotoxic
Doxorubicin
Epirubicin
Daunomycin
Cyclophosphamide
Trastuzumab
Bevacizumab
Mitoxantrone
Ifosfamide
Mitomycin
Lapatinib
Sunitinib
Imatinib
Ethanol
Amphetamines (e.g., cocaine, methamphetamine)
Sodium and water retention
NSAIDs
Cyclooxygenase-2 (COX-2) inhibitors
Rosiglitazone and pioglitazone
Glucocorticoids
Androgens and estrogens
Salicylates (high dose)
Sodium-containing drugs (e.g., carbenicillin disodium, ticarcillin disodium)
Uncertain mechanism
Infliximab
Etanercept
Dronedarone

professional intervention. Specifically, patient education and counseling by a pharmacist should be able to identify and address inadequate HF therapy, identify medication nonadherence, and administration of drugs or the presence of drug–drug interactions that may worsen HF (Table 4-3). A careful medication history is an important aspect of evaluating the cause(s) of HF exacerbation. Discontinuation of medications known to exacerbate HF may help prevent hospitalizations. Use of medications such as antiarrhythmic agents, particularly disopyramide, dronedarone, and flecainide, and nondihydropyridine calcium channel blockers are important precipitants of exacerbations. The widespread use of NSAIDs, particularly the nonprescription ones that many patients perceive as having a low risk of adverse effects, is also problematic and should be discouraged. The thiazolidinedione (TZD) hypoglycemic drugs, rosiglitazone and pioglitazone, cause fluid retention and weight gain that may exacerbate HF. Current guidelines indicate these agents should not be used in patients with New York Heart Association (NYHA) class III or IV HF.[1] Thus, many of the factors precipitating HF exacerbations (nonadherence, inadequate/inappropriate drug therapy, uncontrolled HTN, etc.) are amenable to pharmacist intervention. Thus, the value of the pharmacist's role in careful and repeated education of patients and monitoring of the drug regimen should not be underestimated.[34,35] Attention to these factors may make an important contribution to reducing the risk of hospitalization and improving the patient's quality of life.

CLINICAL PRESENTATION

Signs and Symptoms

❷ The primary manifestations of HF are dyspnea and fatigue, which lead to exercise intolerance, and fluid overload, which can result in peripheral edema and pulmonary congestion.[1,33,36] The presence of these signs and symptoms may vary considerably from patient to patient such that some patients have dyspnea but no signs of fluid retention, whereas others may have marked volume overload with few complaints of dyspnea or fatigue. However, many patients have both dyspnea and volume overload. Clinicians should remember that symptom severity often does not correlate with the degree of LV dysfunction. Patients with a low LVEF (less than 20% to 25%) may be asymptomatic, whereas those with preserved LVEF may have significant symptoms. It is also important to note that symptoms can vary considerably over time in a given patient, even in the absence of changes in ventricular function or medications.

Pulmonary congestion arises as the left ventricle fails and is unable to accept and eject the increased blood volume that is delivered to it or if pulmonary pressures are elevated due to a stiff, nondistensible ventricle. Consequently, pulmonary venous and capillary pressures rise, leading to interstitial and bronchial edema, increased airway resistance, and dyspnea. The associated signs and symptoms may include (a) dyspnea (with or without exertion), (b) orthopnea, (c) paroxysmal nocturnal dyspnea (PND), and (d) pulmonary edema. Exertional dyspnea occurs when there is a reduction in the level of exertion that causes breathlessness. This is typically described as more breathlessness than was associated previously with a specific activity (e.g., vacuuming, stair climbing). As HF progresses, many patients eventually have dyspnea at rest.

Orthopnea is dyspnea that occurs with assumption of the supine position. It occurs within minutes of recumbency and is due to reduced pooling of blood in the lower extremities and abdomen. Orthopnea is relieved almost immediately by sitting upright and typically is prevented by elevating the head with pillows. An increase in the number of pillows required to prevent orthopnea (e.g., a change from "two-pillow" to "three-pillow" orthopnea) suggests worsening HF. Attacks of PND typically occur after 2 to 4 hours of sleep; the patient awakens from sleep with a sense of suffocation. The attacks are due to severe pulmonary and bronchial congestion, leading to shortness of breath, cough, and wheezing. The reasons these attacks occur at night are unclear but may include (a) reduced pooling of blood in the lower extremities and abdomen (as with orthopnea), (b) slow resorption of interstitial fluid from sites of dependent edema, (c) normal reduction in sympathetic activity that occurs with sleep (e.g., less support for the failing ventricle), and (d) normal depression in respiratory drive that occurs with sleep.

Rales (crackling sounds heard on auscultation) are present in the lung bases due to transudation of fluid into alveoli. The rales typically are bibasilar, but if heard unilaterally, they are usually right-sided. Rales are not present in most patients with chronic HF even though there is volume overload. This is thought to be due to a compensatory increase in lymphatic drainage. Detection of rales is usually indicative of a rapid onset of worsening HF rather than the amount of excess fluid volume. A third heart sound, or S_3 gallop, is heard frequently in patients with left ventricular failure and may be due to elevated atrial pressure and altered distensibility of the ventricle.

Pulmonary edema is the most severe form of pulmonary congestion, and is caused by accumulation of fluid in the interstitial spaces and alveoli. In HF patients, it is the result of increased pulmonary venous pressure. The patient experiences extreme breathlessness and anxiety and may cough pink, frothy sputum. Pulmonary edema can be terrifying for the patient, causing a feeling of suffocation or drowning. Patients with pulmonary edema may also report any of the above-mentioned signs or symptoms of pulmonary congestion.

Systemic congestion is associated with a number of signs and symptoms. Jugular venous distension (JVD) is the simplest and most reliable sign of fluid overload. Examination of the right internal jugular vein with the patient at a 45° angle is the preferred method for assessing JVD. The presence of JVD more than 4 cm above the sternal angle suggests systemic venous congestion. In patients with mild systemic congestion, JVD may be absent at rest, but application of pressure to the abdomen will cause an elevation of JVD (hepatojugular reflux).

Peripheral edema is a cardinal finding in HF. Edema usually occurs in dependent parts of the body, and thus is seen as ankle or pedal edema in ambulatory patients, although it may be manifested as sacral edema in bedridden patients. Adults typically have a 10-lb (4.5-kg) fluid weight gain before trace peripheral edema is evident; therefore, patients with acute decompensated HF may have no clinical evidence of systemic congestion except weight gain. Body weight is thus the best short-term end point for evaluating fluid status. Nonfluid weight gain and loss of muscle mass due to cardiac cachexia are potential confounders for long-term use of weight as a marker for fluid status. Hepatomegaly and ascites are other signs of systemic congestion.

Patients with HF may exhibit signs and symptoms of low CO alone or in addition to volume overload. The primary complaint associated with hypoperfusion is fatigue. Poor appetite or early satiety may be due to limited perfusion of the GI tract. Conversely, patients with such GI complaints may simply be experiencing gut edema. Subjective measures of low CO include worsening renal function, cool extremities, altered mental status, resting tachycardia, and narrow pulse pressure.

Diagnosis

No single test is available to confirm the diagnosis of HF—it is a clinical syndrome associated with specific signs and symptoms.[1,27,36] Because HF can be caused or worsened by multiple cardiac and noncardiac disorders, many of which may be treatable or reversible, accurate diagnosis is essential for development of therapeutic strategies. HF is often initially suspected in a patient based on his or her symptoms. However, signs and symptoms lack sensitivity for

CLINICAL PRESENTATION Heart Failure

General

- Patient presentation may range from asymptomatic to cardiogenic shock

Symptoms

- Dyspnea, particularly on exertion
- Orthopnea
- Paroxysmal nocturnal dyspnea
- Exercise intolerance
- Tachypnea
- Cough
- Fatigue
- Nocturia
- Hemoptysis
- Abdominal pain
- Anorexia
- Nausea
- Bloating
- Poor appetite, early satiety
- Ascites
- Mental status changes
- Weight gain or loss

Signs

- Pulmonary rales
- Pulmonary edema
- S_3 gallop
- Cool extremities
- Pleural effusion
- Cheyne-Stokes respiration
- Tachycardia
- Narrow pulse pressure
- Cardiomegaly
- Peripheral edema
- Jugular venous distention
- Hepatojugular reflux
- Hepatomegaly
- Venous stasis changes
- Lateral displacement of apical impulse

Laboratory Tests

- BNP >100 pg/mL (>29 pmol/L)
- NT-proBNP >300 pg/mL (>35 pmol/L)
- Electrocardiogram may be normal or it could show numerous abnormalities including acute ST-T wave changes from myocardial ischemia, atrial fibrillation, bradycardia, left ventricular hypertrophy
- Serum creatinine: it may be increased due to hypoperfusion. Preexisting renal dysfunction can contribute to volume overload
- Complete blood count useful to determine if heart failure due to reduced oxygen-carrying capacity
- Chest x-ray: useful for detection of cardiac enlargement, pulmonary edema, and pleural effusions
- Echocardiogram: used to assess LV size, valve function, pericardial effusion, wall motion abnormalities, and ejection fraction
- Hyponatremia: serum sodium <130 mEq/L (<130 mmol/L) is associated with reduced survival and may indicate worsening volume overload and/or disease progression

diagnosing HF since they are frequently found with many other disorders. Even in patients with known HF, there is poor correlation between the presence or severity of symptoms and the hemodynamic abnormality. With few exceptions, HFpEF cannot be distinguished from SHF on the basis of the history, physical examination, chest x-ray, and ECG alone. The frequency with which patients have symptoms and signs of HF on physical examination or chest x-ray is not dependent on whether they have SHF or HFpEF.[37] Patients with HFpEF are often elderly, hypertensive women.[37]

A complete history and physical examination targeted at identifying cardiac or noncardiac disorders or behaviors that may cause or hasten HF development or progression are essential in the initial patient evaluation. However, the physical examination cannot distinguish between HF due to decreased systolic function and that due to preserved systolic function. A careful medication history should also be obtained with a focus on use of ethanol, tobacco, illicit drugs (e.g., cocaine or methamphetamine), vitamins and supplements (including herbal or "natural" supplements), NSAIDs, and antineoplastic agents (anthracyclines, cyclophosphamide, trastuzumab, imatinib).

Particular attention should be paid to cardiovascular risk factors and to other disorders that can cause or exacerbate HF such as HTN, diabetes, atrial fibrillation, dyslipidemia, tobacco use, sleep-disordered breathing, and thyroid disease. Since coronary artery disease is the cause of HF in many patients, evaluation of the possibility of coronary disease is essential, especially in men. If coronary artery disease is detected, appropriate revascularization procedures may then be considered. The patient's volume status should be documented by assessing the body weight, JVD, and presence or absence of pulmonary congestion and peripheral edema. Laboratory testing may assist in identification of disorders that cause or worsen HF. The initial evaluation should include a complete blood count, serum electrolytes (including calcium and magnesium), assessment of renal and hepatic function, urinalysis, lipid profile, hemoglobin A1C, thyroid function tests, chest x-ray, and 12-lead ECG. There are no specific ECG abnormalities associated with HF, but findings may help detect coronary artery disease or conduction abnormalities that could affect prognosis and guide treatment decisions. Measurement of BNP or NT-proBNP may also assist in differentiating dyspnea caused by HF from other causes.

Although the history, physical examination, and laboratory tests provide important insight into the underlying cause of HF, the echocardiogram is the single most useful test in the evaluation of the patient. The echocardiogram is used to assess abnormalities in cardiac structure and function and should include evaluation of the pericardium, myocardium, and heart valves, and quantification of the LVEF to determine if systolic or diastolic dysfunction is present.

TREATMENT OF CHRONIC HEART FAILURE

Desired Outcomes

The goals of therapy in management of chronic HF are to improve the patient's quality of life, relieve or reduce symptoms, prevent or minimize hospitalizations for exacerbations of HF, slow progression of the disease process, and prolong survival. Pharmacotherapy plays a key role in achieving these goals.[1] In addition, identification of risk factors for HF development and recognition of its progressive nature have led to increased emphasis on preventing the development of this disorder. With this in mind, the American College of Cardiology (ACC)/American Heart Association (AHA) guidelines for the evaluation and management of chronic HF utilize a staging system that not only recognizes the evolution and progression of the disorder but also emphasizes risk factor modification and preventive treatment strategies (Fig. 4-6).[1] The four stages of this system differ from the NYHA functional classification (Table 4-4) with which most clinicians are familiar. The NYHA system is primarily intended to classify symptoms according to the clinician's subjective evaluation and does not recognize preventive measures or the progression of the disorder. A patient's symptoms can change frequently over a short period of time due to changes in medications, diet, intercurrent illnesses, etc. For example, a patient with ACC/AHA Stage C HF with NYHA class IV symptoms such as marked volume overload could rapidly improve to class I to II with aggressive diuretic therapy. Despite these limitations, this system can be useful for monitoring patients and is widely used in HF studies. In contrast, and consistent with the progressive nature of HF, a patient's ACC/AHA HF stage could not improve (e.g., go from Stage C to Stage B) even though the patient's symptoms could fluctuate from NYHA class IV to I. In addition, the ACC/AHA staging system provides a more comprehensive framework for evaluation, prevention, and treatment of HF.

The general principles used to guide the treatment of SHF are based on numerous large, randomized, double-blind, multicenter trials. Until recently, no such randomized trials had been performed in patients with HFpEF. Consequently, the guidelines for the management of HFpEF are based primarily on clinical investigations in relatively small groups of patients, clinical experience, and concepts based on the knowledge and understanding of the pathophysiology of the disease process. The treatment regimen outlined in Table 4-5 applies to patients with HFpEF who have clear manifestations of congestion either at rest or with exertion. Whether treatment of asymptomatic diastolic dysfunction confers any benefit has not been demonstrated.

TABLE 4-4 New York Heart Association Functional Classification

Functional class	
I	Patients with cardiac disease but without limitations of physical activity. Ordinary physical activity does not cause undue fatigue, dyspnea, or palpitation
II	Patients with cardiac disease that results in slight limitations of physical activity. Ordinary physical activity results in fatigue, palpitation, dyspnea, or angina
III	Patients with cardiac disease that results in marked limitation of physical activity. Although patients are comfortable at rest, less than ordinary activity will lead to symptoms
IV	Patients with cardiac disease that results in an inability to carry on physical activity without discomfort. Symptoms of congestive heart failure are present even at rest. With any physical activity, increased discomfort is experienced

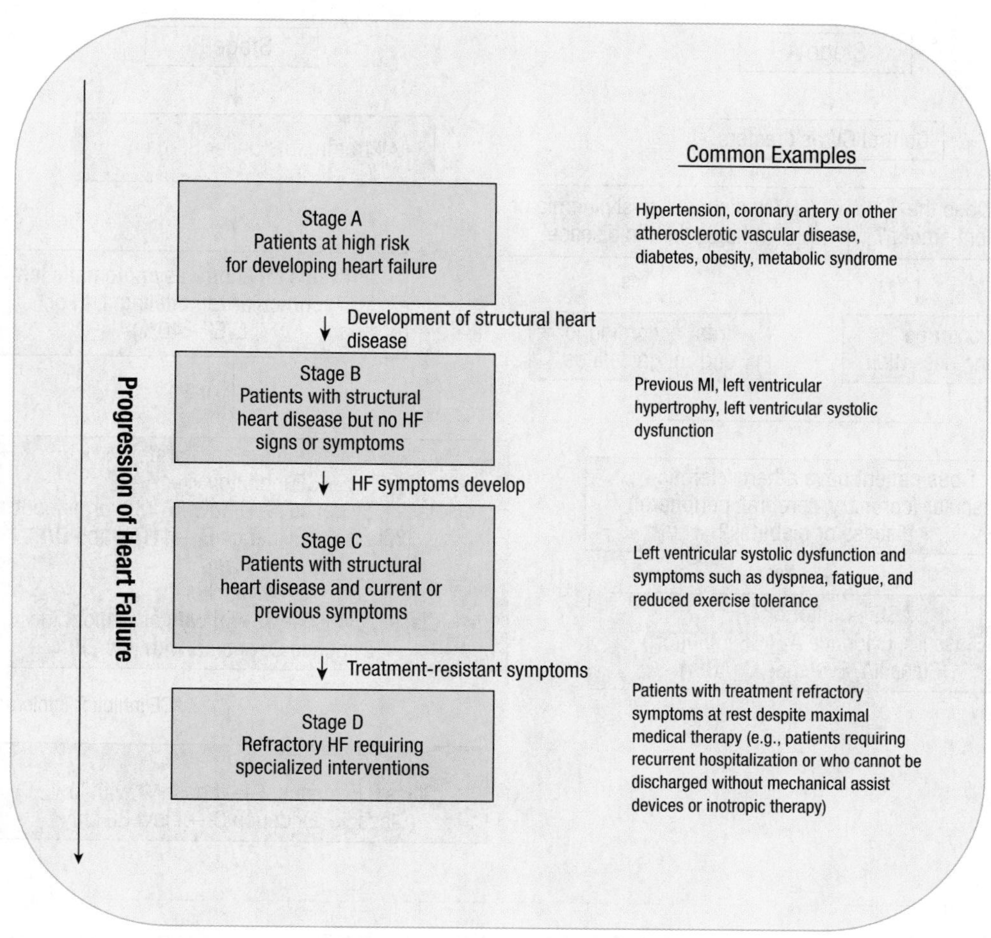

FIGURE 4-6 ACC/AHA heart failure staging system. *(Adapted with permission from Hunt SA, Abraham WT, Chin MH, et al. Circulation 2009; 119:e391–e479.)*

TABLE 4-5 Targeted Approach to Treatment of HFpEF

	Rationale	Agent
Symptom-Targeted Treatment		
Decrease pulmonary venous pressure	Reduce left ventricular volume	Diuretics, nitrates, salt restriction
Decrease myocardial oxygen consumption	Reduce heart rate Control blood pressure	β-Blockers, diltiazem, verapamil ACE inhibitors, angiotensin receptor blockers, calcium channel blockers
Maintain atrial contraction	Restore and/or maintain sinus rhythm	Cardioversion of atrial fibrillation
Improve exercise tolerance	As above	Use positive inotropic agents with caution
Disease-Targeted Treatment		
Prevent/treat myocardial ischemia		β-Blockers, diltiazem, verapamil, nitrates
Prevent/regress ventricular hypertrophy		Antihypertensive therapy
Mechanism-Targeted Treatment		
Modify myocardial and extramyocardial mechanisms		Possibly ACE inhibitors or angiotensin receptor blockers, diuretics, spironolactone
Modify intracellular and extracellular mechanisms		Possibly ACE inhibitors or angiotensin receptor blockers, spironolactone

ACE, angiotensin-converting enzyme; HFpEF, heart failure with preserved ejection fraction.

General Measures

The complexity of the HF syndrome necessitates a comprehensive approach to management that includes accurate diagnosis, identification and treatment of risk factors, elimination or minimization of precipitating factors, appropriate pharmacologic and nonpharmacologic therapy, and close monitoring and followup.

The first step in management of chronic HF is to determine the etiology (see Table 4-1) and/or any precipitating factors. Appropriate treatment of underlying disorders (e.g., hyperthyroidism, valvular heart disease) may obviate the need for specific HF treatment. Revascularization or antiischemic therapy in patients with coronary disease may reduce HF symptoms. Drugs that aggravate HF (see Table 4-3) should be discontinued if possible.

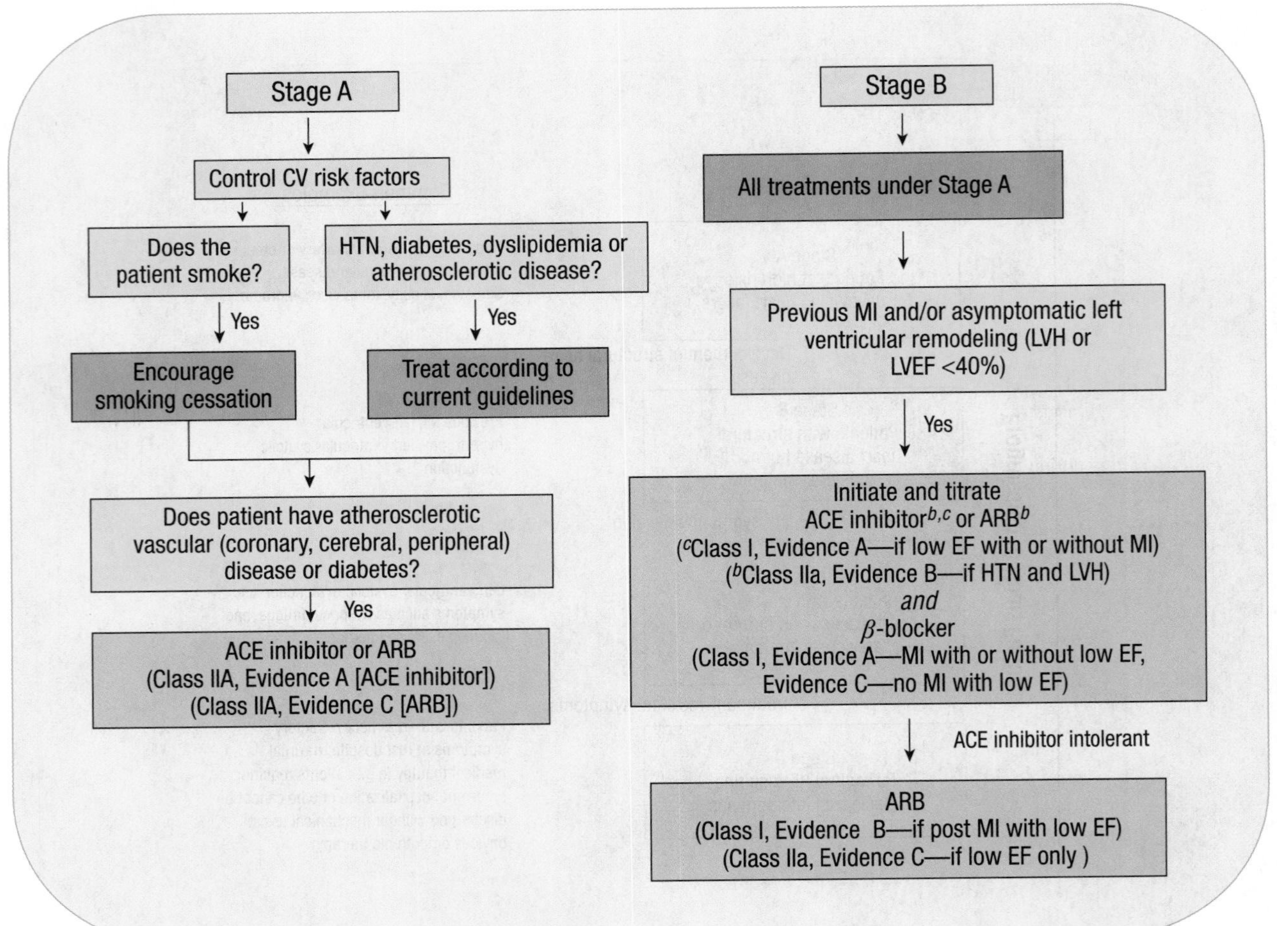

FIGURE 4-7 Treatment algorithm for patients with ACC/AHA Stage A and B heart failure. *(Adapted with permission from Hunt SA, Abraham WT, Chin MH, et al. Circulation 2009; 119:e391–e479.)*

Restriction of physical activity reduces cardiac workload and is recommended for virtually all patients with acute congestive symptoms. However, once the patient's symptoms have stabilized and excess fluid is removed, restrictions on physical activity are discouraged.[38] Exercise training may improve quality of life and yield trends toward reduced hospitalizations and death from cardiovascular causes.[34,38] Current guidelines support exercise training programs in stable patients to improve clinical status.[1]

Because a major compensatory response in HF is sodium and water retention, restriction of dietary sodium and fluid intake is an important lifestyle intervention. Mild (<3 g/day) to moderate (<2 g/day) sodium restriction, in conjunction with daily measurement of weight, should be implemented to minimize volume retention and allow use of lower and safer diuretic doses. The typical American diet contains 8 to 10 g of sodium per day, so most patients would need to reduce their intake by over 50%. Patients should avoid adding salt to prepared foods and eliminate foods high in sodium (e.g., salt-cured meats, salted snack foods, pickles, soups, delicatessen meats, and processed foods). In patients with hyponatremia (serum Na <130 mEq/L [<130 mmol/L]) or those with persistent volume retention despite high diuretic doses and sodium restriction, daily fluid intake should be limited to 2 L/day from all sources. However, both sodium and fluid restriction must be done with care in patients with HFpEF. Excessive restriction can lead to hypotension, low-output state, and/or renal insufficiency. Daily weights may help to assess volume status. Dietary and lifestyle factors that decrease the risk of development of CAD and HTN should be encouraged.[1] Although guidelines recommend reducing sodium intake in patients with HF, proven benefits of such restriction on clinical outcomes are lacking.[39] In fact, there is concern among some clinicians about the increased RAAS activity that results from sodium restriction.[39]

Other important general measures include patient and family counseling on the signs and symptoms of HF, detailed written instructions on the importance of appropriate medication use and compliance, activity level, diet, discharge medications, weight monitoring, continuity of care, and the need for close monitoring and followup to reinforce compliance and minimize the risk of HF exacerbations and subsequent hospitalization. These activities are now referred to as self-care and constitute an important means to improve such important outcomes as hospitalization and quality of life.[40]

General Approach to Treatment

4 The ACC/AHA treatment guidelines are organized around the four identified stages of HF, and the treatment recommendations are summarized in Figures 4-7 and 4-8.[1] Clinicians are reminded that,

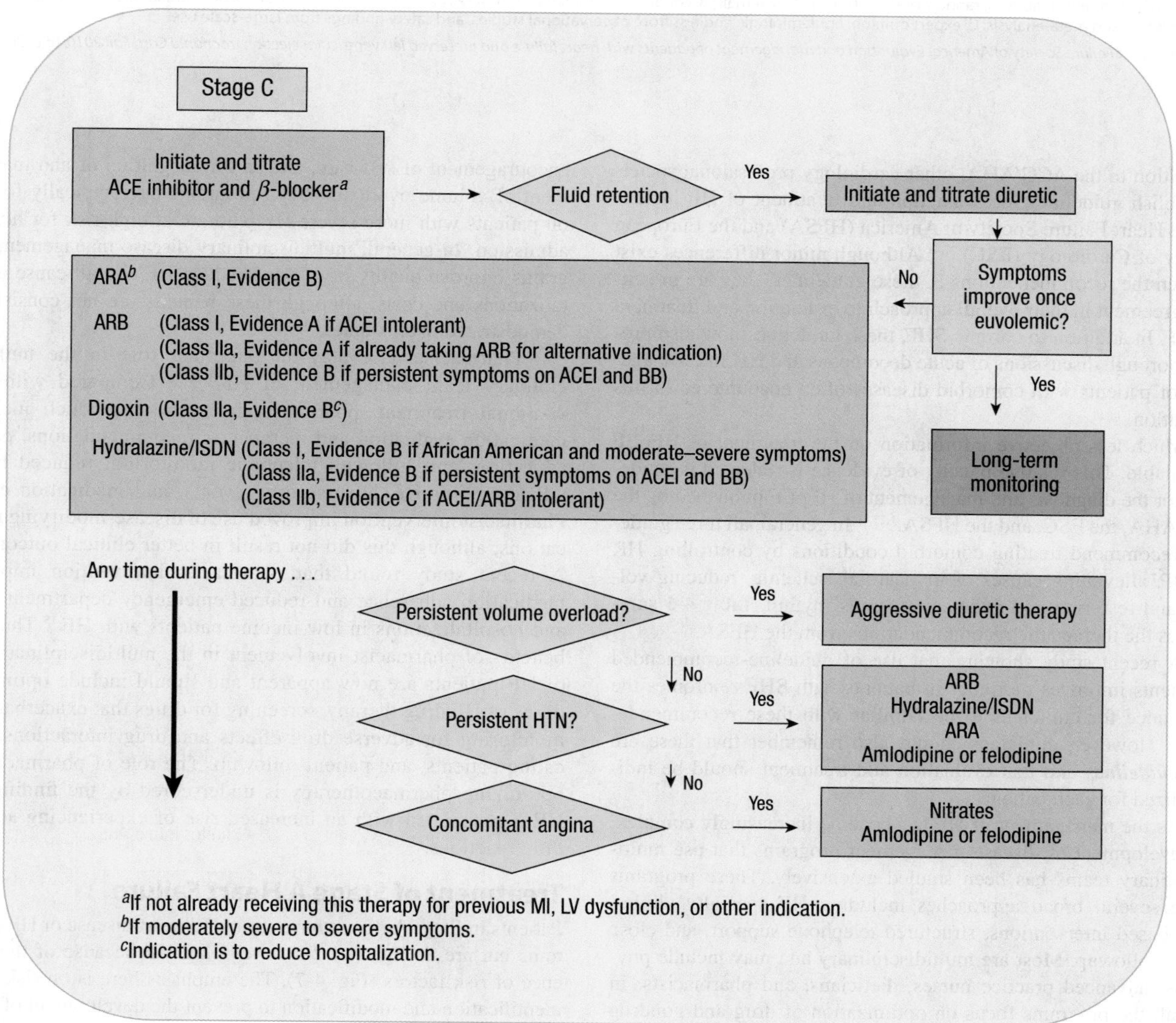

FIGURE 4-8 Treatment algorithm for patients with ACC/AHA Stage C heart failure. *(Adapted with permission from Hunt SA, Abraham WT, Chin MH, et al. Circulation 2009; 119:e391–e479.)*

TABLE 4-6 Evidence-Based Pharmacotherapy for Heart Failure with Preserved Ejection Fraction

Recommendations	Recommendation Grade[a]
Diuretics	
• A loop or a thiazide diuretic should be considered for patients with volume overload. However, with more severe volume overload or inadequate response to a thiazide, a loop diuretic should be implemented. Caution is warranted not to lower preload excessively, which may reduce stroke volume and cardiac output	C
ACE Inhibitors	
• ACE inhibitors may be considered in all patients	C
• ACE inhibitors should be considered in all patients who have symptomatic atherosclerotic cardiovascular disease or diabetes and one additional risk factor	C
Angiotensin Receptor Blockers	
• Angiotensin receptor blockers may be considered in all patients	C
• In patients who are intolerant of ACE inhibitors, an angiotensin receptor blocker can be considered an alternative	C
β-Blockers	
• β-Blockers should be considered in patients with one or more of the following conditions:	
Myocardial infarction	A
Hypertension	B
Atrial fibrillation requiring ventricular rate control	B
Calcium Channel Blockers	
• In patients with atrial fibrillation warranting ventricular rate control who either are intolerant to or have not responded to a β-blocker, diltiazem or verapamil should be considered	C
• A nondihydropyridine or dihydropyridine calcium channel blocker can be considered for symptom-limiting angina	A
• A nondihydropyridine or dihydropyridine calcium channel blocker can be considered for hypertension	C

ACE, angiotensin-converting enzyme.

[a]Strength of recommendations: A, randomized controlled clinical trials; B, cohort and case control studies based on observations from observational studies or registries, post hoc, subgroup, and meta-analysis; C, expert opinion, epidemiologic findings from observational studies, and safety findings from large-scale use.

Data from Heart Failure Society of America. Evaluation and management of patients with heart failure and preserved left ventricular ejection fraction. J Card Fail 2010;16:e126–e133.

in addition to the ACC/AHA, other cardiology professional societies publish guidelines for evaluation and treatment of HF including the Heart Failure Society of America (HFSA) and the European Society of Cardiology (ESC).[27,41] Although minor differences exist between the recommendations in these guidelines, they are in general agreement in their overall approach to evaluation and treatment of SHF. In addition to chronic SHF, these guidelines now also provide thorough discussions of acute decompensated HF and management of patients with comorbid diseases often encountered in this population.

Much less objective information on the treatment of HFpEF is available. This relative paucity of evidence is reflected in guidelines for the diagnosis and management of HFpEF published by the ACC/AHA, the ESC, and the HFSA.[1,27,41] In general, all three guidelines recommend treating comorbid conditions by controlling HR and BP, alleviating causes of myocardial ischemia, reducing volume, and restoring and maintaining sinus rhythm. Table 4-6 summarizes the therapeutic recommendations from the HFSA.

A recent study showing that use of guideline-recommended treatments improves mortality in patients with SHF reinforces the importance for clinicians to be familiar with these recommendations.[42] However, clinicians should also remember that these are only *guidelines* and that evaluation and treatment should be individualized for each patient.

As the management of HF has become increasingly complex, the development of disease management programs that use multidisciplinary teams has been studied extensively. These programs utilize several broad approaches including HF specialty clinics, home-based interventions, structured telephone support, and close patient followup. Most are multidisciplinary and may include physicians, advanced practice nurses, dieticians, and pharmacists. In general, the programs focus on optimization of drug and nondrug therapy, patient and family education and counseling, exercise and dietary advice, intense followup by telephone or home visits, improving adherence to medications and lifestyle recommendations, encouragement of self-care, and early recognition of and management of volume overload.[1] Such programs have typically focused on patients with more severe HF who are at high risk for hospital admission. In general, multidisciplinary disease management programs improve quality of life and reduce HF and all-cause hospitalizations and costs, although these benefits are not consistently demonstrated in all studies.[43,44]

Pharmacists can play an important role in the multidisciplinary team management of HF.[34,35,45] Compared with conventional treatment, pharmacist interventions, which included medication evaluation and therapeutic recommendations, patient education, and followup telephone monitoring, reduced hospitalizations for HF, adverse drug events, and medication errors. Pharmacist intervention improved use of disease-modifying medications, although this did not result in better clinical outcomes.[46] A recent study found that pharmacist intervention improved medication adherence and reduced emergency department visits and hospitalizations in low-income patients with HF.[45] Thus, the benefits of pharmacist involvement in the multidisciplinary care of HF patients are now apparent and should include optimizing doses of HF drug therapy, screening for drugs that exacerbate HF, monitoring for adverse drug effects and drug interactions, educating patients, and patient followup. The role of pharmacists in optimizing pharmacotherapy is underscored by the finding that HF is associated with an increased risk of experiencing adverse drug reactions.[47]

Treatment of Stage A Heart Failure

Patients in Stage A do not have structural heart disease or HF symptoms but are at high risk for developing HF because of the presence of risk factors (Fig. 4-7). The emphasis here is on risk factor identification and modification to prevent the development of structural heart disease and subsequent HF. Commonly encountered risk factors include HTN, dyslipidemia, diabetes, obesity, metabolic syndrome, smoking, and coronary artery disease. Although each of these disorders individually increases risk, they frequently coexist in many patients and act synergistically to foster the development of HF. Effective control of both systolic and diastolic BPs reduces the risk of developing HF by approximately 50%; thus, current HTN treatment guidelines should be followed.[1] Diabetes dramatically increases the risk of developing HF and adversely affects the prognosis of patients with known HF. Appropriate diabetic control is important to minimize the risk of end-organ damage but has not been shown to affect the risk of developing HF. Appropriate management of coronary disease and its associated risk factors is also important.[39,48] Although treatment must be individualized, ACE inhibitors or ARBs are recommended for HF prevention in patients with multiple vascular risk factors.[1]

Treatment of Stage B Heart Failure

Patients in Stage B have structural heart disease, but do not have HF symptoms (Fig. 4-7). This group includes patients with left ventricular hypertrophy, recent or remote MI, valvular disease, or reduced LVEF (less than 40%). These individuals are at risk for developing HF, and treatment is targeted at minimizing additional injury and preventing or slowing the remodeling process. In addition to the treatment measures outlined in Stage A, ACE inhibitors and β-blockers are important components of therapy. Patients with a previous MI should receive both ACE inhibitors and β-blockers, regardless of the LVEF.[1] Similarly, patients with a reduced LVEF and no symptoms should also receive both these agents, whether or not they have had an MI.[1] ARBs are an effective alternative in patients intolerant to ACE inhibitors.[1]

Treatment of Stage C Heart Failure

4 5 6 7 8 9 10 Patients with structural heart disease and previous or current HF symptoms are classified in Stage C (Fig. 4-8). In addition to treatments in Stages A and B, most patients in Stage C should be routinely treated with three medications: a diuretic, an ACE inhibitor, and a β-blocker (see Drug Therapies for Routine Use in Patients with Stage C Systolic Heart Failure below). The benefits of these medications on slowing HF progression, reducing morbidity and mortality, and improving symptoms are clearly established. Aldosterone receptor antagonists, ARBs, digoxin, and hydralazine–isosorbide dinitrate (ISDN) are also useful in selected patients. Nonpharmacologic therapy with devices such as an implantable cardioverter-defibrillator (ICD) or cardiac resynchronization therapy (CRT) with a biventricular pacemaker is also indicated in certain patients in Stage C (see Nonpharmacologic Therapy below). Other general measures noted earlier are also important as is careful followup and patient education to reinforce dietary and medication compliance to prevent clinical deterioration and reduce hospitalization.[1,40]

Dozens of trials evaluated pharmacotherapy in patients with SHF, but few focused on patients with HFpEF. In fact, most published HF studies specifically excluded patients with preserved EF. The results of large clinical trials for treatment of HFpEF as well as important ongoing studies are summarized in Table 4-7. The hope is that these studies will provide the future basis for evidence-based treatment for HFpEF.

Treatment of Stage D Heart Failure

Stage D HF includes patients with refractory symptoms at rest despite maximal medical therapy and those patients who undergo recurrent hospitalizations or cannot be discharged from the hospital without special interventions. These individuals have the most advanced form of HF and should be referred to HF management programs so that specialized therapies including mechanical circulatory support, continuous IV positive inotropic therapy, and cardiac transplantation can be considered in addition to standard treatments outlined in Stages A to C.[1] Discussions with the patient and family members regarding prognosis, patient priorities for minimizing symptoms versus prolonging survival, options for additional treatments, and end-of-life care should be started.[1,53] A scientific statement from the AHA on decision making in advanced HF is an excellent resource on these issues.[54]

Management of volume status can be challenging in these patients. Restriction of sodium and fluid intake may be beneficial. High doses of diuretics, combination therapy with a loop and thiazide diuretic, or mechanical methods of fluid removal such as ultrafiltration may be required. Patients in Stage D may be less tolerant to ACE inhibitors (hypotension, worsening renal insufficiency) and β-blockers (worsening HF) as high levels of neurohormonal activation maintain circulatory homeostasis. Initiation of therapy with low doses, slow upward dose titration, and close monitoring for signs and symptoms of intolerance are essential in this group of patients. The approach to treatment of patients with Stage D HF is discussed in more detail in Chapter 5.

Nonpharmacologic Therapy

Sudden cardiac death, primarily due to ventricular tachycardia and fibrillation, is responsible for 40% to 50% of the mortality in patients with HF. In general, patients in the earlier stages with milder symptoms are more likely to die from sudden death, whereas death from pump failure is more frequent in those with advanced HF. Many of these patients have complex and frequent ventricular ectopy, although it remains unknown whether these ectopic beats contribute to the risk of malignant arrhythmias or merely serve as markers for individuals at higher risk for sudden death. Drugs that attenuate disease progression such as β-blockers and aldosterone antagonists reduce the risk of sudden death. However, although class I antiarrhythmic agents can suppress ventricular ectopy, empiric treatment with them adversely affects survival.[55]

Implantation of an ICD is an effective primary prevention for reducing the risk of mortality from sudden death.[1] In patients with NYHA class II or III symptoms and LVEF ≤35%, the ICD was superior to amiodarone or placebo for reducing mortality.[56] Importantly, this study also found that amiodarone was no more effective than placebo. Thus, this drug, because of its multiple adverse effects, drug interactions, and lack of effect on mortality, should not be used for primary prevention of sudden death. However, because of the neutral effects of amiodarone on survival, it is often used in HF patients with symptomatic atrial fibrillation to maintain sinus rhythm and/or to prevent ICD discharges. The ACC/AHA guidelines recommend the ICD for both primary and secondary prevention to improve survival in patients with current or previous HF symptoms and reduced LVEF.[1] A thorough review of ICD therapy can be found in Chapter 8.

The use of CRT improves a number of important end points in selected patients with chronic SHF.[57,58] Delayed electrical activation of the left ventricle, characterized on the ECG by a QRS duration that exceeds 120 milliseconds, occurs in approximately one third of patients with moderate to severe SHF. Since the left and right ventricles normally activate simultaneously, this delay results in asynchronous contraction of the ventricles, which contributes to the hemodynamic abnormalities of HF. Implantation of a specialized biventricular pacemaker to restore synchronous activation of the ventricles improves ventricular contraction and hemodynamics. Use of CRT is associated with improvements in exercise capacity, NYHA classification, quality of life, hemodynamic function, hospitalizations, and mortality.[57,58] The ACC/AHA guidelines recommend CRT in NYHA class III to IV patients receiving optimal medical therapy and with a QRS duration ≥120 milliseconds and LVEF ≤35%.[1] However, trials published since the last guideline update show impressive benefits in patients with less severe symptoms (NYHA class I to III) and that this earlier use of CRT is associated

TABLE 4-7 Completed and Ongoing Large Clinical Trials for HFpEF

Trial (No. of Patients)	Treatment	Inclusion Criteria	Primary End Point	Results
DIG Ancillary Study[110] (*n* = 988)	Digoxin versus placebo for a mean of 37 months. Patients received ACE inhibitor (86%) and diuretics (85%)	EF >45%, NYHA II–IV, normal sinus rhythm	Composite of HF hospitalization or HF mortality	No significant difference was found in the primary end point between treatment groups (HR = 0.82, *P* = 0.136). Digoxin had no effect on all-cause mortality or cause-specific mortality or on all-cause or CV hospitalization. Compared with placebo, digoxin use was associated with a trend toward a reduction in HF hospitalizations (HR = 0.79, *P* = 0.094) and an increase in unstable angina admissions (HR = 1.37, *P* = 0.061)
CHARM-Preserved[96] (*n* = 3,023)	Candesartan versus placebo for a mean of 36.6 months. Patients continued their background HF medications: ACE inhibitor (19%), β-blocker (55%), diuretics (75%), spironolactone (11%)	EF >40%, NYHA II–IV, ≥1 hospitalization for CV reason	Composite of CV mortality or HF hospitalization	No significant difference was found in the primary end point between treatment groups (adjusted HR = 0.86, *P* = 0.051) or in CV deaths (adjusted HR = 0.95, *P* = 0.635). Compared with placebo, candesartan use was associated with fewer HF admissions (*P* = 0.047), lower incidence of new diabetes (HR = 0.60, *P* = 0.005), and a reduction in the composite of CV death, hospitalization for HF, MI, and stroke (adjusted HR = 0.86, *P* = 0.037)
PEP-CHF[49] (*n* = 850)	Perindopril versus placebo for a mean of 2.1 years	Clinical criteria for HF, EF ≥40%, age ≥70 years	Composite of total mortality and HF hospitalization	At 1 year and at study completion, no significant difference was found in the primary end point between treatment groups (HR = 0.69, *P* = 0.055; HR = 0.70, *P* = 0.545). In a subgroup analysis, patients ≤75 years of age (HR = 0.29, *P* = 0.035) and with a history of MI (HR = 0.38, *P* = 0.004) showed a reduction in the primary end point. Compared with placebo, perindopril use at 1 year was associated with fewer unplanned hospital admissions (HR = 0.63, *P* = 0.033), greater improvements in exercise tolerance (*P* = 0.011), and improvement in NYHA class (*P* = 0.030)
I-Preserve[97] (*n* = 4,128)	Irbesartan versus placebo for 2 years. ACE inhibitor can be used for any indication other than HTN	Clinical criteria for HF or hospitalized within 6 months for HF, age ≥60 years, NYHA II–IV, EF ≥45%	Composite of all-cause mortality or CV hospitalization	No significant difference was found in the primary end point between treatment groups (HR = 0.95, *P* = 0.35), overall death rates (HR = 1, *P* = 0.98), or CV hospitalization rate (HR = 0.95, *P* = 0.44)
J-DHF[50] (*n* = 800)	Carvedilol versus placebo for 2 years	Clinical criteria for HF, EF >40%	Composite of CV mortality and unplanned HF hospitalization	Expected to be completed in 2010
SENIORS[51] (*n* = 2,111)	Nebivolol versus placebo for 21 months	Clinical criteria for HF with either documented heart failure hospitalization with 1 year or documented EF ≤35% within 6 months, age ≥70 years	All-cause mortality or cardiovascular hospitalization	In the study, 1,359 patients (64%) had an EF ≤35% (mean 28.7%), and 752 (36%) had an EF >35% (mean 49.2%). In patients with EF >35%, the HR for nebivolol versus placebo for the primary end point was 0.81 (*P* = 0.104). No significant difference existed between groups (EF ≤35% vs. EF >35%, *P* = 0.720)
TOPCAT[52] (*n* = 4,500)	Spironolactone versus placebo for 2 years	Clinical criteria for HF, age ≥50 years, EF ≥45%, ≥1 hospitalization for HF, controlled SBP	CV mortality, aborted cardiac arrest, HF hospitalization	Expected to be completed in 2012

ACE, angiotensin-converting enzyme; CHARM, Candesartan in Heart Failure: Assessment of Reduction in Mortality and Morbidity; CV, cardiovascular; DIG, Digitalis Investigation Group.

with reverse remodeling.[46,57,59] It is likely that these findings will be incorporated into the next guideline revision. Combined CRT and ICD devices are available and can be used if the patient meets the indications for both devices.

Pharmacologic Therapy

11 With a few notable exceptions, many of the drugs used to treat SHF are the same as those for treatment of HFpEF. However, the rationale for their use, the pathophysiologic process that is being altered by the drug, and the dosing regimen may be entirely different depending on whether the patient has SHF or HFpEF. For example, β-blockers are recommended for the treatment of both SHF and HFpEF. In HFpEF, however, β-blockers are used to decrease HR, increase diastolic duration, and modify the hemodynamic response to exercise. In SHF, β-blockers are used in the long term to increase the inotropic state and modify LV remodeling. Diuretics also are used in the treatment of both SHF and HFpEF. However, the doses of diuretics used to treat HFpEF are, in general, much smaller than those used to treat SHF. Antagonists of the RAAS are useful in lowering BP and reducing LVH. Some drugs, however, are used to treat either SHF or HFpEF, but not both. Calcium channel blockers such as diltiazem, nifedipine, and verapamil have little utility in the treatment of SHF. In contrast, each of these drugs has been proposed as being useful in the treatment of HFpEF.

Drug Therapies for Routine Use in Patients with Stage C Systolic Heart Failure

❹ ❺ ❻ ❼ A treatment algorithm for management of patients with Stage C SHF is shown in Figure 4-8. In general, these patients should receive combined therapy with an ACE inhibitor or ARB (if ACE inhibitor intolerant) and a β-blocker, plus a diuretic if there is evidence of fluid retention. An aldosterone receptor antagonist should also be considered in selected patients.[1] Initiation of digoxin therapy can be considered at any time for symptom reduction, to decrease hospitalizations, or slow ventricular response in patients with concomitant atrial fibrillation.[1] Drug dosing and monitoring are summarized in Tables 4-8 and 4-9.

Diuretics ❼ The compensatory mechanisms in HF stimulate excessive sodium and water retention, often leading to pulmonary and systemic congestion.[60,61] Diuretic therapy, in addition to sodium restriction, is recommended in all patients with clinical evidence of fluid retention. Once fluid overload has been resolved, many patients require chronic diuretic therapy to maintain euvolemia. Among the drugs used to manage HF, diuretics are the most rapid in producing symptomatic benefits. However, diuretics do not prolong survival or (with the possible exception of torsemide) alter disease progression, and therefore are not considered mandatory therapy. Thus, patients who do not have fluid retention would not require diuretic therapy.

The primary goal of diuretic therapy is to reduce symptoms associated with fluid retention, improve exercise tolerance and quality of life, and reduce hospitalizations from HF. Diuretics accomplish this by decreasing pulmonary and peripheral edema through reduction of preload. Although preload is a determinant of CO, the Frank-Starling curve (see Fig. 4-4) shows that patients with congestive symptoms have reached the flat portion of the curve. A reduction in preload improves symptoms but has little effect on the patient's SV or CO until the steep portion of the curve is reached. However, diuretic therapy must be used judiciously because overdiuresis can lead to a reduction in CO, renal perfusion, and symptoms of volume depletion.

Diuretic therapy is usually initiated in low doses in the outpatient setting, with dosage adjustments based on symptom assessment and daily body weight. Change in body weight is a sensitive marker of fluid retention or loss, and it is recommended that patients monitor their status by taking daily morning body weights. Patients who gain 1 lb/day for several consecutive days or 3 to 5 lb (1.4 to 2.3 kg) in a week should contact their healthcare provider for instructions (which often will be to increase the diuretic dose temporarily). Such action often will allow patients to prevent a decompensation that requires hospitalization. One study demonstrated a significant reduction in emergency department visits with a protocol that directed patients to self-adjust their diuretic dose based on changes in HF symptoms and daily body weight.[62] Hypotension or worsening renal function (e.g., increases in serum creatinine) may be indicative of volume depletion and necessitates a reduction in the diuretic dose. Assessing volume status is particularly important before ACE inhibitor or β-blocker initiation or dose uptitration as overdiuresis may predispose patients to hypotension and other adverse effects with increases in ACE inhibitor or β-blocker doses.

⓫ In patients with HFpEF, diuretic treatment should be initiated at low doses in order to avoid hypotension and fatigue. Hypotension can be a significant problem in the treatment of HFpEF because these patients have a very steep LV diastolic pressure–volume curve such that a small change in volume causes a large change in filling pressure and CO. After the acute treatment of HFpEF has been completed, long-term treatment should include small to moderate oral doses of diuretics (furosemide 20 to 40 mg/day, chlorthalidone 25 to 100 mg, or hydrochlorothiazide 12.5 to 25 mg/day).

Thiazide Diuretics Thiazide diuretics such as hydrochlorothiazide block sodium reabsorption in the distal convoluted tubule (approximately 5% to 8% of filtered sodium). The thiazides therefore are relatively weak diuretics and infrequently are used alone in HF. However, thiazides or the thiazide-like diuretic metolazone can be used in combination with loop diuretics to promote a very effective diuresis. In addition, thiazide diuretics may be preferred in patients with only mild fluid retention and elevated BP because of their more persistent antihypertensive effects compared with loop diuretics.

Loop Diuretics Loop diuretics are usually necessary to restore and maintain euvolemia in HF. They act by inhibiting a Na–K–2Cl transporter in the thick ascending limb of the loop of Henle, where 20% to 25% of filtered sodium normally is reabsorbed. Because loop diuretics are highly bound to plasma proteins, they are not highly filtered at the glomerulus. They reach the tubular lumen by active transport via the organic acid transport pathway. Competitors for this pathway (probenecid or organic by-products of uremia) can inhibit delivery of loop diuretics to their site of action and decrease effectiveness. Loop diuretics also induce a prostaglandin-mediated increase in renal blood flow, which contributes to their natriuretic effect. Coadministration of NSAIDs blocks this prostaglandin-mediated effect and can diminish diuretic efficacy. Excessive dietary sodium intake may also reduce the efficacy of loop diuretics. Unlike thiazides, loop diuretics maintain their effectiveness in the presence of impaired renal function, although higher doses may be necessary to obtain adequate delivery of the drug to the site of action.

ACE Inhibitors ❺ ACE inhibitors are the cornerstone of pharmacotherapy for patients with SHF. By blocking the conversion of angiotensin I to angiotensin II by ACE, the production of angiotensin II and, in turn, aldosterone is decreased, but not completely eliminated.[16] This decrease in angiotensin II and aldosterone attenuates many of the deleterious effects of these neurohormones that drive HF progression including ventricular remodeling, myocardial fibrosis, myocyte apoptosis, cardiac hypertrophy, NE release, vasoconstriction, and sodium and water retention.[16] The endogenous vasodilator bradykinin, which is inactivated by ACE, is also increased by ACE inhibitors along with the release of vasodilatory prostaglandins and histamine.[16] The precise contribution of the effects of ACE inhibitors on bradykinin and vasodilatory prostaglandins is unclear. However, the persistence of clinical benefits with ACE inhibitors despite the fact that angiotensin II and aldosterone levels return to pretreatment levels in some patients suggests this is a potentially important effect.[16]

Numerous placebo-controlled clinical trials involving over 7,000 patients with reduced LVEF have documented the favorable effects of ACE inhibitor therapy on symptoms, NYHA functional classification, clinical status, hospitalizations, exercise tolerance, and quality of life.[16] When compared with placebo, patients treated with ACE inhibitors have fewer treatment failures, hospitalizations, and increases in diuretic dosages.[16] More importantly, ACE inhibitors improve survival by 20% to 30% compared with placebo and these benefits are maintained for years with continued therapy.[16] ACE inhibitors also reduce the combined risk of death or hospitalization, slow the progression of HF, and reduce the rate of reinfarction.[16] The benefits of ACE inhibitor therapy are independent of the etiology of HF (ischemic vs. nonischemic) and are observed in patients with mild, moderate, or severe symptoms.

ACE inhibitors also prevent the development of HF and reduce cardiovascular risk. Enalapril decreases the risk of hospitalization for worsening HF and reduces the composite end point of death and HF hospitalization in patients with asymptomatic left ventricular dysfunction.[63] In patients with established atherosclerotic vascular disease (e.g., coronary, cerebral, or peripheral

TABLE 4-8 Drug Dosing Table

Drug	Brand Name	Initial Dose	Usual Range	Special Population Dose	Comments
Loop Diuretics					
Furosemide	Lasix®	20–40 mg once or twice daily	20–160 mg once or twice daily	Cl_{cr} 20–50 mL/min (0.33–0.83 mL/s): 160 mg once or twice daily Cl_{cr} <20 mL/min (<0.33 mL/s): 400 mg daily	Single doses exceeding those listed are unlikely to elicit additional response
Bumetanide	Bumex®	0.5–1 mg once or twice daily	1–2 mg once or twice daily	Cl_{cr} 20–50 mL/min (0.33–0.83 mL/s): 2 mg once or twice daily Cl_{cr} <20 mL/min (<0.33 mL/s): 8–10 mg daily	Single doses exceeding those listed are unlikely to elicit additional response
Torsemide	Demadex®	10–20 mg once daily	10–80 mg once daily	Cl_{cr} 20–50 mL/min (0.33–0.83 mL/s): 40 mg once daily Cl_{cr} <20 mL/min (<0.33 mL/s): 200 mg daily	Single doses exceeding those listed are unlikely to elicit additional response
ACE Inhibitors					
Captopril	Capoten®	6.25 mg three times daily	50 mg three times daily[a]		
Enalapril	Vasotec®	2.5 mg twice daily	10–20 mg twice daily[a]		
Lisinopril	Zestril®, Prinivil®	2.5–5 mg once daily	20–40 mg once daily[a]		
Quinapril	Accupril®	5 mg twice daily	20–40 mg twice daily		
Ramipril	Altace®	1.25–2.5 mg	5 mg twice daily[a]		
Fosinopril	Monopril®	5–10 mg once daily	40 mg once daily		Undergoes both hepatic and renal elimination
Trandolapril	Mavik®	0.5–1 mg once daily	4 mg once daily[a]		Undergoes both hepatic and renal elimination
Perindopril	Aceon®	2 mg once daily	8–16 mg once daily		Undergoes both hepatic and renal elimination
Angiotensin Receptor Blockers					
Candesartan	Atacand®	4 mg once daily	32 mg once daily[a]		
Valsartan	Diovan®	20–40 mg twice daily	160 mg twice daily[a]		
Losartan	Cozaar®	25–50 mg once daily	150 mg once daily[a]		
***β*-Blockers**					
Bisoprolol	Zebeta®	1.25 mg once daily	10 mg once daily[a]		
Carvedilol	Coreg®	3.125 mg twice daily	25 mg twice daily[a]	Target dose for patients weighing >85 kg is 50 mg twice daily	Should be taken with food
Carvedilol phosphate	Coreg CR®	10 mg once daily	80 mg once daily		Should be taken with food
Metoprolol succinate CR/XL	Toprol-XL®	12.5–25 mg once daily	200 mg once daily[a]		
Aldosterone Antagonists					
Spironolactone	Aldactone®	12.5–25 mg once daily	25–50 mg once daily[a]		
Eplerenone	Inspra®	25 mg once daily	50 mg once daily[a]		
Other					
Hydralazine–isosorbide dinitrate	BiDil®	Hydralazine 37.5 mg three times daily Isosorbide dinitrate 20 mg three times daily	Hydralazine 75 mg three times daily[a] Isosorbide dinitrate 40 mg three times daily[a]		Indicated in conjunction with standard heart failure therapy to improve survival and reduce hospitalizations in self-identified black patients
Digoxin	Lanoxin®	0.125–0.25 mg once daily	0.125–0.25 mg once daily	Reduce dose in elderly and patients with impaired renal function	Target plasma concentration range is 0.5–1 ng/mL (0.6–1.3 nmol/L). Does not improve survival in patients with systolic heart failure

Cl_{cr}, creatinine clearance.

[a]Regimens proven in large clinical trials to reduce mortality.

Adapted from references 1 and 60.

TABLE 4-9 Drug Monitoring

Drug Class	Adverse Effect	Monitoring Parameters	Comments
ACE inhibitors	Angioedema, cough, hyperkalemia, hypotension, renal dysfunction	BP, electrolytes, BUN, and creatinine	Contraindicated in patients with bilateral renal artery stenosis, history of angioedema, or pregnancy. Assess BP, BUN, creatinine, and electrolytes at baseline and 1–2 weeks after initiation or increase in dose. Goal is target dose from clinical trials or highest tolerated
ARBs	Hyperkalemia, hypotension, renal dysfunction	BP, electrolytes, BUN, and creatinine	Contraindicated in patients with bilateral renal artery stenosis or pregnancy. Assess BP, BUN, creatinine, and electrolytes at baseline and 1–2 weeks after initiation or increase in dose. Use with caution in patients with a history of ACE inhibitor–associated angioedema. Goal is target dose from clinical trials or highest tolerated
Aldosterone antagonists	Gynecomastia/breast tenderness/ menstrual irregularities (spironolactone), hyperkalemia	BP, electrolytes, BUN, and creatinine	Assess BP, BUN, creatinine, and electrolytes at baseline. Check potassium 3 days and 1 week after initiation and then monthly for the first 3 months. Change to eplerenone if gynecomastia develops with spironolactone
β-Blockers	Bradycardia, heart block, bronchospasm, hypotension, worsening HF	BP, HR, ECG, signs and symptoms of worsening HF, blood glucose	Start with low dose and titrate upward no more often than every 2 weeks as tolerated based on BP, HR, and symptoms. Goal is target dose from clinical trials or highest tolerated. Patients may feel worse before they feel better
Digoxin	GI and CNS adverse effects, bradyarrhythmias and tachyarrhythmias See Table 4-11	Electrolytes, BUN, creatinine, ECG, serum digoxin concentration	Target serum digoxin concentration 0.5–1 ng/mL (0.6–1.3 nmol/L)
Diuretics	Hypovolemia, hypotension, hyponatremia, hypokalemia, hypomagnesemia, hyperuricemia, renal dysfunction, thirst	BP, electrolytes, BUN, creatinine, glucose, uric acid, changes in weight, JVD	Dose should be adjusted based on volume status, renal function, electrolytes, and BP. Reassess these parameters 1–2 weeks after dose changes. Goal is lowest dose that maintains euvolemia
Hydralazine	Hypotension, headache, rash, arthralgia, lupus, tachycardia	BP, HR	
Nitrates	Hypotension, headache, light-headedness	BP, HR	

circulations) and normal LVEF, ACE inhibitors reduce the development of new-onset HF and diabetes, cardiovascular death, overall mortality, MI, and stroke.[64]

The most common cause of SHF is ischemic heart disease, where MI results in loss of myocytes, followed by ventricular dilation and remodeling. Captopril, ramipril, and trandolapril all benefit post-MI patients whether therapy is initiated early or late after the infarct.[16] Collectively, these studies indicate that ACE inhibitors administered after MI improve overall survival, decrease development of severe HF, and reduce reinfarction and HF hospitalization rates.[16] The effects are most pronounced in higher-risk patients, such as those with symptomatic HF or reduced LVEF, with 20% to 30% reductions in mortality reported in these patients.[16] Post-MI patients without HF symptoms or decreases in LVEF (Stage B) should also receive ACE inhibitors to prevent the development of HF and to reduce mortality.[1,16]

The use of ACE inhibitors in patients with chronic kidney disease is particularly relevant since it is present in 25% to 50% of HF patients and is associated with an increased risk of mortality.[65] In spite of the perceived risks, ACE inhibitors are effective in patients with chronic kidney disease.[66,67] Since many patients have concomitant disorders (e.g., diabetes, HTN, previous MI) that also may be favorably affected by ACE inhibitors, chronic kidney disease should not be an absolute contraindication to ACE inhibitor use in patients with left ventricular dysfunction. However, these patients should be monitored carefully for the development of worsening renal function and/or hyperkalemia with special attention to risk factors associated with this complication of ACE inhibitor therapy.[1]

An important practical consideration is determining the proper dose of an ACE inhibitor. Despite the overwhelming benefit demonstrated with these agents, they remain underused and underdosed.[68,69] Also, for patients receiving an ACE inhibitor at hospital discharge, use significantly decreases over time and patients not prescribed ACE inhibitors at discharge were unlikely to have therapy initiated in the outpatient setting.[68,69] Common reasons cited for underuse or underdosing are concerns about safety and adverse reactions to ACE inhibitors, especially in patients with chronic kidney disease or hypotension. Clinical trials establishing the efficacy of these agents titrated drug doses to a predetermined target rather than according to therapeutic response. Although data on the dose-dependent effects of ACE inhibitors in patients with HF are limited, higher doses may reduce the risk of hospitalization, but not mortality, compared with lower doses.[70] In many positive trials of other HF therapies (e.g., β-blockers, aldosterone antagonists), intermediate ACE inhibitor doses were generally used as background therapy. These results emphasize that clinicians should attempt to use ACE inhibitor doses proven beneficial in clinical trials, but if these doses are not tolerated, lower doses can be used with the knowledge that it is unlikely there are differences in mortality between the high and low doses. Also, initiation of β-blocker therapy should not be delayed until target ACE inhibitor doses are achieved since the addition of a β-blocker is proven to reduce mortality, whereas that is not the case with increasing ACE inhibitor doses.

In summary, the evidence that ACE inhibitors improve symptoms, slow disease progression, and decrease mortality in patients with HF and reduced LVEF (Stage C) is unequivocal. As a result, current guidelines indicate these patients should receive ACE inhibitors, unless contraindications are present.[1] The clear benefit of ACE inhibitors is also evident by the selection of these agents as a key performance measure by the Joint Commission and Centers for Medicare and Medicaid Services (CMS). This measure states that patients with left ventricular systolic dysfunction discharged from the hospital should receive ACE inhibitors unless there is documentation in the medical record of an absolute contraindication or drug intolerance.

β-Blockers 6 There is overwhelming evidence from multiple randomized, placebo-controlled clinical trials that β-blockers reduce morbidity and mortality in patients with SHF. As such, the ACC/AHA guidelines on the management of HF recommend that β-blockers should be used in all stable patients with HF and a reduced left ventricular EF in the absence of contraindications or a clear history of β-blocker intolerance.[1] Patients should receive a β-blocker even if their symptoms are mild or well controlled with diuretic and ACE inhibitor therapy. Importantly, it is not essential that ACE inhibitor doses be optimized before a β-blocker is started because the addition of a β-blocker is likely to be of greater benefit than an increase in ACE inhibitor dose.[1] β-Blockers are also recommended for asymptomatic patients with a reduced left ventricular EF (Stage B) to decrease the risk of progression to HF.

β-Blockers have been studied in over 20,000 patients with SHF in placebo-controlled trials. Three β-blockers have been shown to significantly reduce mortality compared with placebo: carvedilol, metoprolol succinate (CR/XL), and bisoprolol. Each was studied in a large population with the primary end point of mortality. Carvedilol was the first β-blocker shown to improve survival in HF. In the U.S. Carvedilol Heart Failure Study, 1,094 patients were randomized to carvedilol or placebo in addition to standard therapy, including an ACE inhibitor, digoxin, and diuretic.[71] The study was stopped early because of a 65% reduction in the risk of death with carvedilol. Nearly 4,000 patients were randomized to metoprolol succinate (Toprol-XL®) or placebo in the Metoprolol CR/XL Randomised Intervention Trial in Congestive Heart Failure (MERIT-HF), the largest β-blocker mortality trial to date.[72] This trial was also stopped early because of a significant survival benefit with β-blockade. Specifically, metoprolol was associated with a 34% reduction in total mortality, a 41% reduction in sudden death, and a 49% reduction in death from worsening HF. Bisoprolol was studied in over 2,600 patients enrolled in the Cardiac Insufficiency Bisoprolol Study II (CIBIS II).[73] The study was also stopped prematurely because of a 34% reduction in total mortality with bisoprolol compared with placebo. Bisoprolol was also associated with a 44% reduction in sudden death and a 26% reduction in death due to worsening HF. Multiple post hoc subgroup analyses of data from the MERIT-HF and CIBIS II trials suggest that the benefits of β-blockade occur regardless of HF etiology or disease severity.

The majority of participants in MERIT-HF and CIBIS II had either NYHA class II or class III SHF. The efficacy and safety of β-blockers in patients with class IV HF were examined in the Carvedilol, Prospective, Randomized, Cumulative Survival (COPERNICUS) trial.[74] This trial randomized nearly 2,300 clinically stable patients who had symptoms at rest or with minimal exertion to carvedilol or placebo. Like the other studies, COPERNICUS was stopped prematurely after carvedilol produced a 35% relative reduction in mortality. Carvedilol was well tolerated in this population, with fewer participants receiving carvedilol compared with placebo requiring permanent discontinuation of study medication.

Data supporting the use of β-blockers in asymptomatic patients with left ventricular systolic dysfunction (Stage B) come from a study of carvedilol in post-MI patients with a decreased left ventricular EF.[75] While the primary end point of all-cause mortality or hospital admission for cardiovascular problems was similar in the carvedilol and placebo groups, carvedilol significantly reduced all-cause mortality alone compared with placebo. Cardiovascular mortality and nonfatal MI were also lower among carvedilol-treated patients.

In addition to improving survival, β-blockers have been shown to improve multiple other end points. All the large clinical trials demonstrated 15% to 20% reductions in all-cause hospitalization and 25% to 35% reductions in hospitalizations for worsening HF with β-blocker therapy.[73,76,77] Studies have also shown consistent improvements in left ventricular systolic function with β-blockers, with increases in LVEF of 5 to 10 units (e.g., from an EF of 20% to 25% or 30%) after several weeks to months of therapy. β-Blockers have also been shown to decrease ventricular mass, improve the sphericity of the ventricle, and reduce systolic and diastolic volumes (left ventricular end-systolic volume and LVEDV).[78,79] These effects are often collectively called *reverse remodeling*, referring to the fact that they return the heart toward more normal size, shape, and function.

The effects of β-blockers on symptoms and exercise tolerance varied among studies. Many studies showed improvements in NYHA functional class, patient symptom scores or quality-of-life assessments (such as the Minnesota Living with Heart Failure Questionnaire), and exercise performance, as assessed by the 6-minute walk test.[76–78] Other investigators found significant reductions in mortality with β-blockers but no significant improvement in symptoms.[80] As such, it is important to educate patients that β-blocker therapy is expected to positively influence disease progression and survival even if there is little to no symptomatic improvement.

Most participants in β-blocker trials were on ACE inhibitors at baseline since the benefits of ACE inhibitors were proven prior to β-blocker trials. Whether the strategy of starting a β-blocker prior to an ACE inhibitor is safe and effective was addressed in CIBIS III, in which patients with mild to moderate symptoms were randomized to initial therapy with either bisoprolol or enalapril.[81] Rates of death or hospitalization were similar with the two strategies. However, the trial failed to satisfy the prespecified statistical criterion for noninferiority of initial therapy with a β-blocker compared with an ACE inhibitor. In the absence of more compelling evidence, ACE inhibitors should be started first in most patients. Initiating a β-blocker first may be advantageous for patients with evidence of excessive SNS activity (e.g., tachycardia) and may also be appropriate for patients whose renal function or potassium concentrations preclude starting an ACE inhibitor (or ARB) at that time. However, the risk for decompensation during β-blocker initiation may be greater in the absence of preexisting ACE inhibitor therapy, and careful monitoring is essential.

β-Blockers antagonize the detrimental effects of the SNS described earlier in the chapter. To this end, potential mechanisms to explain the favorable effects of β-blockers in HF include antiarrhythmic effects, attenuating or reversing ventricular remodeling, decreasing myocyte death from catecholamine-induced necrosis or apoptosis, preventing fetal gene expression, improving left ventricular systolic function, decreasing HR and ventricular wall stress thereby reducing myocardial oxygen demand, and inhibiting plasma renin release.[1]

Components that are critical for successful β-blocker therapy include appropriate patient selection, drug initiation and titration, and patient education. β-Blockers should be initiated in stable patients who have no or minimal evidence of fluid overload.[1] While β-blockers are typically started in the outpatient setting, there are data indicating that initiation of a β-blocker prior to discharge in patients who are hospitalized for decompensated HF increases β-blocker usage compared with outpatient initiation without increasing the risk of serious adverse effects.[82] However, β-blockers should not be started in patients who are hospitalized in the intensive care unit or recently required IV inotropic support. In unstable patients, other HF therapy should be optimized and then β-blocker therapy reevaluated once stability is achieved.

Initiation of a β-blocker at normal doses in patients with HF may lead to symptomatic worsening or acute decompensation owing to the drug's negative inotropic effect. For this reason, β-blockers are listed as drugs that may exacerbate or worsen HF (see Table 4-3). To minimize the likelihood for acute decompensation, β-blockers should be started in very low doses with slow upward dose titration. β-Blocker doses should be doubled no more often than every 2 weeks, as tolerated, until the target or maximally tolerated dose is reached. According to current guidelines, target doses are those associated with reductions in mortality in placebo-controlled clinical trials.[1] The starting and target doses achieved in clinical trials are described in Table 4-8. Data with both metoprolol and carvedilol suggest that HR may serve as a guide to the degree of β-blockade and that lower β-blocker doses might be considered reasonable if the reduction in HR indicates a good response to β-blocker therapy.[83] In fact, it remains uncertain whether β-blocker dose or the degree of HR reduction is the optimal end point to guide dose titration and predict survival.

A recent meta-analysis of 23 randomized trials involving over 19,000 patients receiving β-blockers for HF compared HR reduction and β-blocker dose as predictors of survival.[83] Overall, β-blocker treatment was associated with a 24% mortality reduction. However, trials with the largest decrease in HR (median 15 beats per minute) reported a 36% reduction in mortality, whereas trials with the smallest HR reduction (median 8 beats/min) showed only a 9% mortality reduction. Greater magnitude of HR reduction was significantly associated with greater improvement in survival. On the other hand, no relationship between β-blocker dose and magnitude of mortality decrease was found. The results from this study suggest that the degree of β-blocker–mediated reduction in resting HR, but not β-blocker dose, is associated with the magnitude of improved survival. However, the analysis is limited by its retrospective design, inability to account for other factors affecting HR (e.g., vagal activity, β-receptor pharmacogenomics), and reliance on resting HR as a surrogate marker for extent of β-blockade. Although resting HR is routinely used clinically to evaluate extent of β-blockade, it is not as accurate as inhibition of exercise HR. Whether magnitude of resting HR reduction or achievement of clinical trial doses is the optimal surrogate marker for improved outcomes with β-blockers in HF remains uncertain and may only be definitively determined by prospective trials.

Of note, the smallest commercially available tablet of bisoprolol is a scored 5-mg tablet. Since the recommended starting dose of 1.25 mg/day is not readily available, bisoprolol is the least commonly used of the three agents and, in fact, is not approved by the FDA for use in HF. Thus, therapy is generally limited to either carvedilol or metoprolol succinate, and there is no compelling evidence that one drug is superior to the other. A controlled-release formulation of carvedilol (carvedilol CR) that allows once-daily dosing is available, and pharmacokinetic studies demonstrate similar degrees of drug exposure with the controlled- and immediate-release formations of the drug.[84]

Good communication between the patient and healthcare provider(s) is particularly important for successful therapy. Patients should understand that dose uptitration is a long, gradual process and that achieving the target dose is important to maximize the benefits of therapy. Patients should also be aware that response to therapy may be delayed and that HF symptoms may actually worsen during the initiation period. In the event of worsening symptoms, patients who understand the potential benefits of long-term β-blocker therapy may be more likely to continue treatment.

In summary, the data provide clear evidence that β-blockers slow disease progression, decrease hospitalizations, and improve survival in SHF. β-Blockers have also been shown to improve quality of life in many patients with HF, although this is not a universal finding. Based on these data, β-blockers are recommended as standard therapy for all patients with SHF, regardless of the severity of their symptoms. Clinical trial experience shows that target β-blocker doses can be achieved in the majority of patients provided that appropriate initiation, titration, and education are implemented.

11 In patients with HFpEF, β-blockers may help to lower and maintain low pulmonary venous pressures by decreasing HR and increasing the duration of diastole. Tachycardia is poorly tolerated in patients with HFpEF for several reasons. First, rapid HRs cause an increase in myocardial oxygen demand and a decrease in coronary perfusion time. This can promote ischemia even in the absence of epicardial CAD. Second, incomplete relaxation between cardiac cycles may result in an increase in diastolic pressure relative to volume. Third, a rapid rate reduces diastolic filling time and ventricular filling.[85] Thus, many clinicians use β-blockers (and nondihydropyridine calcium channel blockers) to prevent excessive tachycardia and produce a relative bradycardia in patients with diastolic dysfunction. However, excessive bradycardia can result in a fall of CO despite an increase in LV filling.[2] Such considerations underscore the need for individualizing therapeutic interventions that affect HR. In general, it is not necessary to start at an extremely low dose and titrate the β-blocker in a slow, progressive fashion in HFpEF as it is in SHF. However, because patients tend to be older, have numerous comorbidities, and take many concomitant medications, it is prudent to start with a moderate dose of β-blockers. A randomized, multicenter, open-label trial is ongoing to examine the effects of β-blocker therapy on clinical outcomes in patients with HF and a preserved left ventricular EF.[86]

Drug Therapies to Consider for Selected Patients

Angiotensin II Receptor Blockers 5 The crucial role of the RAAS in HF development and progression is well established as are the benefits of inhibiting this system with ACE inhibitors. ACE inhibitors decrease angiotensin II production in the short term, but these agents do not completely suppress generation of this hormone. With chronic administration of ACE inhibitors, *ACE escape*, characterized by increases in circulating angiotensin II and aldosterone, often occurs.[7,16] In addition, angiotensin II can be formed in a number of tissues, including the heart, through non–ACE-dependent pathways (e.g., chymase, cathepsin, and kallikrein).[7,16] Therefore, blockade of the detrimental effects of angiotensin II by ACE inhibition is incomplete. By blocking the angiotensin II receptor subtype, AT_1, ARBs attenuate the deleterious effects of angiotensin II on ventricular remodeling, regardless of the site of origin of the hormone. Since ARBs do not inhibit the ACE enzyme, these agents do not affect bradykinin, which is linked to ACE inhibitor cough. Because bradykinin-related adverse effects of ACE inhibitors such as angioedema and cough lead to drug discontinuation in some patients, the potential for an ARB to produce similar clinical benefits with fewer side effects is of great interest.

Although a number of ARBs are currently available, the primary clinical trials supporting the use of these agents in SHF used either valsartan or candesartan.[80] The addition of valsartan to standard background HF therapy did not improve mortality but did reduce hospitalizations due to HF.[87] In post-MI patients, valsartan was noninferior to captopril for reducing mortality and the combination of valsartan and captopril only increased the risk of adverse effects and did not improve survival compared with monotherapy with either agent.[88] Based on these findings, valsartan is now approved for use in patients with NYHA class II to IV HF as well as post-MI patients with left ventricular dysfunction.

The Candesartan in Heart Failure: Assessment of Reduction in Mortality and Morbidity (CHARM) trials were designed as three studies to evaluate candesartan in patients with symptomatic HF.[89] Both the CHARM-Added (patients receiving background ACE inhibitor therapy)[90] and CHARM-Alternative (patients intolerant of ACE inhibitor therapy)[91] trials found significant reductions in the primary end point of CV death or hospitalization for HF in patients receiving candesartan, although the benefit was modest in CHARM-Added (17% reduction). Overall, candesartan was well tolerated but its use was associated with an increased risk of hypotension, hyperkalemia, and renal dysfunction. On the basis of these results, candesartan is now approved for use in symptomatic

HF in patients with LVEF ≤40% to reduce cardiovascular death and reduce HF hospitalizations.

The effect of high-dose compared with low-dose losartan treatment was evaluated in the Heart Failure Endpoint Evaluation of Angiotensin II Antagonist Losartan (HEAAL) study.[92] Over 3,800 patients receiving standard background HF treatment who were intolerant to ACE inhibitors with a LVEF ≤40% and NYHA class II to IV symptoms were randomly assigned to losartan 50 or 150 mg daily. The higher losartan dose was associated with significant reductions (~10%) in the primary end point of death or hospital admission for HF. Significant increases in renal insufficiency, hyperkalemia, and hypotension were also associated with the higher dose, but the development of these adverse effects did not result in increased rates of drug discontinuation. The benefits of higher ARB doses were also seen in a recent registry-based study comparing the effects of losartan and candesartan on mortality in patients with SHF.[93] Overall, there were no differences in mortality in patients treated with losartan compared with that in patients treated with candesartan. However, in patients receiving low doses of losartan (12.5 to 50 mg daily), mortality was higher than in the candesartan group. High-dose losartan (100 mg daily) was equivalent to higher doses of candesartan. High-dose candesartan was superior to lower doses. These findings point out the importance of titrating the doses of these medications to the targets achieved in clinical trials.

Although ACE inhibitors remain first-line therapy in patients with Stage C SHF, the current guidelines recommend the use of ARBs in patients who are unable to tolerate (usually due to cough) ACE inhibitors.[1,27,41] Caution should be exercised when ARBs are used in patients with angioedema from ACE inhibitors as some cross-reactivity is reported.[94] ARBs are not an alternative in patients with hypotension, hyperkalemia, or renal insufficiency secondary to ACE inhibitors because they are as likely to cause these adverse effects. Also, the combined use of ACE inhibitors, ARBs, and aldosterone antagonists is not recommended because of the increased risk of renal dysfunction and hyperkalemia.[1] The specific drugs and doses proven to be effective in clinical trials should be used (Table 4-8).

Combination therapy with an ACEI inhibitor and an ARB remains controversial. The CHARM-Added trial found the addition of candesartan to ACE inhibitor and β-blocker therapy produced incremental reductions in cardiovascular death and hospitalizations for HF, but did not improve overall survival.[90] In contrast, neither the VALIANT nor the Val-HeFT trials found additional benefit from the addition of valsartan to ACE inhibitor treatment.[87,88] Moreover, a recent meta-analysis showed that combination therapy is associated with increased risk of medication discontinuation due to adverse effects, hyperkalemia, renal insufficiency, and hypotension.[95] Collectively, these results suggest the addition of an ARB to optimal HF therapy (ACE inhibitors, β-blockers, diuretics, etc.) offers, at best, marginal benefits with increased risk of adverse effects. The ACC/AHA guidelines recommend the addition of an ARB can be considered in patients who remain symptomatic despite receiving conventional HF pharmacotherapy. Some clinicians suggest that the addition of an aldosterone antagonist to ACE inhibitor and β-blocker therapy in patients with persistent symptoms is preferred over an ARB. Unlike ARBs, combination aldosterone antagonist and ACE inhibitor therapy improves survival in patients with NYHA class II–IV HF (RALES and EMPHASIS trial) and in post-MI patients with LV systolic dysfunction (EPHESUS trial), supports this approach.[20–22]

11 The role of ARBs in the treatment of HFpEF is less clear. The CHARM-Preserved trial was the first large prospective study to demonstrate some benefit (reduction in hospitalizations for HF) of an ARB in patients with HFpEF receiving standard background treatment, although no improvement in cardiovascular death was observed.[96] Adverse effects of candesartan in this study were frequent; 22% of candesartan-treated patients discontinued therapy because of hypotension, increased serum creatinine, or hyperkalemia. In the Irbesartan in Heart Failure with Preserved EF (I-PRESERVE) trial, irbesartan was compared with placebo in over 4,000 patients with symptoms of HF and a LVEF of at least 45% (0.45).[97] There was no significant difference between irbesartan and placebo with regard to death or hospitalization for cardiovascular causes. No benefit was seen in quality-of-life measures. There was a high discontinuation rate of the study drug in this trial (33%), as well as a high rate of postrandomization initiation of ACE inhibitors (20%) and spironolactone (10%), which may have contributed to the outcome in this trial.

Aldosterone Antagonists **9** Spironolactone and eplerenone are aldosterone antagonists that work by blocking the mineralocorticoid receptor, the target site for aldosterone, and, thus, they are also referred to as mineralocorticoid receptor antagonists. In the kidney, aldosterone antagonists inhibit sodium reabsorption and potassium excretion. While the diuretic effects with low doses of aldosterone antagonists are minimal, the potassium-sparing effects can have significant consequences as discussed below. In the heart, aldosterone antagonists inhibit cardiac extracellular matrix and collagen deposition, thereby attenuating cardiac fibrosis and ventricular remodeling.[98] Aldosterone antagonists also attenuate the systemic proinflammatory state, atherogenesis, and oxidative stress caused by aldosterone. In addition, there is evidence that aldosterone antagonists may attenuate aldosterone-induced calcium excretion and reductions in bone mineral density and protect against fractures in HF.[99] While spironolactone historically has been viewed as a diuretic, this is believed to contribute little to its benefits in HF, in part, because the doses used have minimal diuretic effect.[20] Thus, as with ACE inhibitors and β-blockers, the data on aldosterone antagonists also support the neurohormonal model of HF.

Three large, randomized controlled trials have evaluated low-dose aldosterone antagonism in patients with either HF or post-MI and left ventricular dysfunction. All three trials excluded patients with significant renal dysfunction (e.g., serum creatinine above 2.5 mg/dL [221 μmol/L]) and elevated serum potassium (e.g., above 5 mEq/L [5 mmol/L]) at baseline.

The RALES randomized over 1,600 patients with current or recent NYHA class IV HF to aldosterone blockade with spironolactone 25 mg/day or placebo.[20] Patients were also treated with standard therapy, usually including an ACE inhibitor, loop diuretic, and digoxin. Those with a serum creatinine concentration above 2.5 mg/dL (221 μmol/L) or a serum potassium concentration above 5 mEq/L (5 mmol/L) were excluded. The study was stopped prematurely after an average followup of 24 months because of a significant 30% reduction in the primary end point of total mortality with spironolactone. Spironolactone reduced mortality due to both progressive HF and sudden cardiac death. It also produced a 35% reduction in hospitalizations for worsening HF and significant symptomatic improvement, as assessed by changes in NYHA functional class. The low dose of spironolactone was well tolerated in RALES. The most common adverse effect was gynecomastia, which occurred in 10% of men on spironolactone compared with 1% of men on placebo, and led to treatment discontinuation in 2% of patients. There were statistically (but not clinically) significant increases in serum creatinine (by 0.05 to 0.10 mg/dL [4 to 9 μmol/L]) and potassium concentrations (by 0.30 mEq/L [0.30 mmol/L]) with spironolactone. The incidence of serious hyperkalemia (>6 mEq/L [>6 mmol/L]) was minimal and did not differ between spironolactone- and placebo-treated groups.

The EPHESUS trial evaluated the effect of selective antagonism of the mineralocorticoid receptor with eplerenone in patients with left ventricular dysfunction after MI.[21] To be eligible for study participation, patients had to have evidence of either HF or diabetes. Over 6,600 patients were randomized within 3 to 14 days of MI to eplerenone, titrated to 50 mg/day, or placebo in addition to standard therapy, which usually included an ACE inhibitor, β-blocker, aspirin, and diuretics. Treatment with eplerenone was associated with a significant 15% relative reduction in the risk for death from any cause and a 15% reduction in the risk of hospitalization from HF. Serious hyperkalemia occurred in 5.5% of eplerenone-treated patients and 3.9% of placebo-treated patients.

Most recently, the EMPHASIS-HF trial demonstrated significant improvements in clinical outcomes with aldosterone antagonism in mild HF.[22] Over 2,700 patients with NYHA class II HF and a LVEF of 35% or less were randomized to eplerenone up to 50 mg/day (mean dose of 39 mg/day) or placebo, in addition to receiving treatment with an ACE inhibitor or ARB and β-blocker. Eligible patients were hospitalized for a cardiovascular reason within 6 months of study entry or had a plasma BNP of at least 250 pg/mL (72 pmol/L) or an N-terminal proBNP of at least 500 pg/mL (59 pmol/L) in men and 750 pg/mL (89 pmol/L) in women. The trial was stopped prematurely after a median followup of 21 months because of a significant benefit with eplerenone. Eplerenone treatment reduced the primary end point of cardiovascular death or HF hospitalization by 37%, all-cause and cardiovascular mortality by 24%, and hospitalization for HF by 42%. A post hoc analysis of the data also showed a reduction in the incidence of new-onset atrial fibrillation or flutter with eplerenone. The rate of serum potassium greater than 5.5 mEq/L (5.5 mmol/L) was 11.8% in the eplerenone group and 7.2% with placebo.

Current guidelines recommend adding a low-dose aldosterone antagonist to standard therapy to improve symptoms, reduce the risk of HF hospitalization, and increase survival in select patients provided that potassium and renal function can be carefully monitored.[1] Based on the clinical trial data low-dose aldosterone antagonists are appropriate for two groups of patients: those with mild to moderately severe SHF (NYHA class II to IV) who are receiving standard therapy and those with left ventricular dysfunction and either acute HF or diabetes early after MI.[1,98] An aldosterone antagonist may be preferred over an ARB in patients with persisting symptoms despite ACE inhibitor and β-blocker therapy provided that serum potassium and renal function are acceptable.[98] For patients who fall outside the populations studied in these clinical trials, there are no clear guidelines on aldosterone antagonist use. Trials to address the efficacy of aldosterone antagonism in patients with preserved left ventricular systolic function are ongoing.

Despite the clear benefits of aldosterone antagonists in patients with mild to severe SHF, registry data show that only one third of patients meeting guideline criteria for an aldosterone antagonist actually receive one.[100] The low use of aldosterone antagonists is likely due in large part to safety concerns. The clinical trial data suggest that aldosterone antagonists in HF are associated with minimal risk when used appropriately (e.g., in those with adequate renal function and with close laboratory monitoring). However, shortly after publication of RALES, an observational study of approximately 1.3 million elderly patients in the Ontario Drug Benefit Program found that the increase in the spironolactone prescription rate following the publication of RALES was accompanied by nearly threefold increases in the rate of hospital admissions and the rate of death related to hyperkalemia.[101] In addition, small case series showed that 25% to 35% of patients treated outside the controlled clinical trial setting developed hyperkalemia (>5 mEq/L [>5 mmol/L]) and that 10% to 12% developed serious hyperkalemia.[102,103]

Potential factors contributing to the high incidence of hyperkalemia in clinical practice include the initiation of aldosterone antagonists in patients with impaired renal function or high potassium concentrations and the failure to decrease or stop potassium supplements when starting aldosterone antagonists. Other risk factors for hyperkalemia include diabetes, inadequate laboratory monitoring, and concomitant use of both ACE inhibitors and ARBs or NSAIDs. The ACC/AHA recently recommended strategies to minimize the risk for hyperkalemia with aldosterone antagonists in HF.[1] These strategies are summarized in Table 4-10. Chief among these recommendations is to avoid aldosterone antagonists in patients with renal dysfunction or elevated serum potassium. It is important to emphasize here that serum creatinine may overestimate renal function in the elderly and in patients with decreased muscle mass, in whom creatinine clearance should serve as a guide for the appropriateness of aldosterone antagonist therapy. The risk for hyperkalemia is dose dependent, and the morbidity and mortality reductions with aldosterone antagonists in clinical trials occurred at low doses (i.e., spironolactone 25 mg/day and eplerenone 50 mg/day). Therefore, the doses of aldosterone antagonists should be limited to those associated with beneficial effects in order to decrease the risk for hyperkalemia. Spironolactone also interacts with androgen and progesterone receptors, which may lead to gynecomastia, impotence, and menstrual irregularities in some patients. Such adverse effects are less frequent with eplerenone owing to its low affinity for the progesterone and androgen receptors.

Only 10% of RALES participants were taking β-blockers at baseline since the benefits of β-blockers in HF were not appreciated fully at the time the trial began.[20] β-Blockers inhibit plasma renin release and may provide additional suppression of the RAAS when used with ACE inhibitors. Thus, there has been some speculation about whether spironolactone will provide further benefit in patients receiving both ACE inhibitors and β-blockers. However, data from EPHESUS and EMPHASIS provide some clarity to this issue, since the majority of EPHESUS participants were on β-blockers at baseline, and the trial still demonstrated significant reductions in mortality with the addition of eplerenone.[21,22]

TABLE 4-10 Recommended Strategies for Reducing the Risk for Hyperkalemia with Aldosterone Antagonists

- Avoid starting aldosterone antagonists in patients with any of the following:
  - Serum creatinine concentration >2 mg/dL (>177 μmol/L) in women or >2.5 mg/dL (221 μmol/L) in men or a creatinine clearance <30 mL/min (<0.5 mL/s)
  - Recent worsening of renal function
  - Serum potassium concentration ≥5 mEq/L (≥5 mmol/L)
  - History of severe hyperkalemia
- Start with low doses (12.5 mg/day for spironolactone and 25 mg/day for eplerenone) especially in the elderly and in those with diabetes or a creatinine clearance <50 mL/min (<0.83 mL/s)
- Decrease or discontinue potassium supplements when starting an aldosterone antagonist
- Avoid concomitant use of NSAIDs or COX-2 inhibitors
- Avoid concomitant use of high-dose ACE inhibitors or ARBs
- Avoid triple therapy with an ACE inhibitor, ARB, and aldosterone antagonist
- Monitor serum potassium concentrations and renal function within 3 days and 1 week after the initiation or dose titration of an aldosterone antagonist or any other medication that could affect potassium homeostasis. Thereafter, potassium concentrations and renal function should be monitored monthly for the first 3 months, and then every 3 months
- If potassium exceeds 5.5 mEq/L (5.5 mmol/L) at any point during therapy, discontinue any potassium supplementation or, in the absence of potassium supplements, reduce or stop aldosterone antagonist therapy
- Counsel patients to:
  - Limit intake of high potassium–containing foods and salt substitutes
  - Avoid the use of nonprescription NSAIDs
  - Temporarily discontinue aldosterone antagonist therapy if diarrhea develops or diuretic therapy is interrupted

Adapted with permission from Hunt SA, Abraham WT, Chin MH, et al. Circulation 2009; 119:e391–e479.

Digoxin 8 In 1785, William Withering was the first to report extensively on the use of foxglove or *Digitalis purpurea* for the treatment of dropsy (i.e., edema). Although digitalis glycosides have been in clinical use for more than 200 years, not until the 1920s were they clearly demonstrated to have a positive inotropic effect on the heart. Furthermore, it was not until the late 1980s that clinical trials were conducted to critically evaluate the role of digoxin in the therapy of chronic HF. The view of digoxin has also shifted over the past decade. While it was historically considered useful in HF because of its positive inotropic effects, it now seems clear that its real benefits in HF are related to its neurohormonal modulating activity.[104,105]

The efficacy of digoxin in patients with SHF and supraventricular tachyarrhythmias such as atrial fibrillation is well established and widely accepted. Its role in HF patients with normal sinus rhythm has been considerably more controversial. Clinical trials have also shown that digoxin improves cardiac function, quality of life, exercise tolerance, and HF symptoms in patients with SHF and normal sinus rhythm.[106–108] However, these studies involved small numbers of patients followed for short time periods. Although these trials demonstrated hemodynamic and symptomatic improvement in HF patients receiving digoxin, an unresolved issue was the unknown effect of digoxin on mortality. This was of particular concern given the increased mortality seen with other positive inotropic drugs, and finally led to the Digitalis Investigation Group (DIG) trial to determine the effects of digoxin on survival in patients with HF in sinus rhythm.[109]

The DIG trial was a double-blind, randomized, placebo-controlled trial with the primary end point of all-cause mortality.[109] Patients (n = 6,800) with HF symptoms and a LVEF of 45% or less were eligible for the main DIG trial and were randomized to receive digoxin or placebo for a mean followup period of 37 months. Most patients received background therapy with diuretics and ACE inhibitors. Digoxin serum concentrations of 0.5 to 2 ng/mL (0.6 to 2.6 nmol/L) were targeted, with a mean serum digoxin concentration (SDC) of 0.8 ng/mL (1 nmol/L) achieved at 12 months. No significant differences in all-cause mortality were found between patients receiving digoxin and placebo. A trend toward lower mortality due to worsening HF was observed in the digoxin group, although this was offset by a trend toward an increased mortality from other cardiovascular causes (presumably arrhythmias) in patients receiving digoxin. Importantly, digoxin reduced hospitalizations for worsening HF by 28% compared with placebo (P <0.001). Therefore, DIG is the first trial to show that a positive inotropic agent does not increase mortality and actually decreases morbidity in patients with SHF. On the other hand, among an additional 988 patients with a LVEF greater than 45% (diastolic dysfunction) who were enrolled in an ancillary DIG trial, there was no apparent benefit of digoxin on hospitalizations or mortality during the 37-month followup period.[110]

The PROVED and RADIANCE trials investigated the effect of digoxin withdrawal in patients with chronic HF and normal sinus rhythm and further defined the role of digoxin in this setting.[107,108] Both of these trials were short-term (12-week), prospective, randomized, and placebo-controlled and were conducted prior to the use of β-blockers. Together, data from these trials suggested that digoxin produces important symptomatic benefits and that digoxin withdrawal results in worsening HF, decreased exercise capacity, and a reduction in ejection fraction. A post hoc analysis of the DIG trial data supports findings that discontinuation of digoxin may be detrimental. Specifically, among patients treated with digoxin prior to enrollment in the DIG trial, those assigned to the placebo arm (i.e., those discontinuing digoxin therapy) had an increased risk of all-cause hospitalization and HF-related hospitalization compared with patients assigned to the digoxin arm (i.e., those continuing digoxin therapy).[111]

Retrospective analyses of the combined PROVED/RADIANCE database[112] and the DIG trial database[113] suggest that the clinical benefits of digoxin are achieved at lower SDCs, with no additional benefit with higher concentrations. In particular, analysis of digoxin-treated patients in the PROVED and RADIANCE trials showed similar clinical outcomes among those with a SDC between 0.5 and 0.9 ng/mL (between 0.6 and 1.2 nmol/L) as those with higher serum concentrations.[112] While the DIG trial showed no reduction in mortality in the study population overall, a comprehensive analysis of the DIG trial database found that lower SDCs were associated with decreased mortality, whereas higher concentrations were not.[113] Specifically, compared with placebo, SDCs of 0.5 to 0.9 ng/mL (0.6 to 1.2 nmol/L) 1 month after digoxin initiation were associated with lower mortality, all-cause hospitalizations, and HF hospitalizations. Serum concentrations greater than or equal to 1 ng/mL (1.3 nmol/L) were associated with lower HF hospitalizations with no effect on mortality. A digoxin dose of 0.125 mg daily or less was predictive of SDCs of 0.4 to 0.9 ng/mL (0.5 to 1.2 nmol/L). While an initial, well-publicized study suggested that digoxin might be harmful in women,[114] subsequent analyses show no increased risks with digoxin in women, particularly with SDCs less than 1 ng/mL (1.3 nmol/L).[113,115]

Based on the available data, for most patients, the target SDC should be 0.5 to 1 ng/mL (0.6 to 1.3 nmol/L). This more conservative target would also be expected to decrease the risk of adverse effects from digoxin toxicity. In fact, recent assessment of the rate of digoxin toxicity has suggested a significant decline in the overall incidence.[116] In most patients with normal renal function, this serum concentration range can be achieved with a daily dose of 0.125 mg. Patients with decreased renal function, the elderly, or those receiving interacting drugs (e.g., amiodarone) should receive 0.125 mg daily or every other day. Routine measuring of SDCs is not necessary in the absence of suspected digoxin toxicity, worsening renal function, institution of an interacting drug, or other conditions that may significantly affect SDC. In patients with atrial fibrillation and a rapid ventricular response, the historic practice of increasing digoxin doses (and concentrations) until rate control is achieved is no longer recommended. Digoxin alone is often ineffective to control ventricular response in patients with atrial fibrillation and increasing the dose only increases the risk of toxicity. Digoxin combined with a β-blocker or amiodarone is superior to either agent alone for controlling ventricular response in patients with atrial fibrillation and HF.[1] Therefore, target SDCs are the same regardless of whether the patient is in sinus rhythm or atrial fibrillation. Several equations and nomograms have been proposed to estimate digoxin maintenance doses based on estimated renal function for a particular patient and population pharmacokinetic parameters. These methods are extensively reviewed elsewhere.[117] More recently, based on post hoc analyses from the DIG, PROVED, and RADIANCE trials, investigators developed a digoxin dosing nomogram that targets a lower digoxin plasma concentration.[118] In the absence of supraventricular tachyarrhythmias, a loading dose is not indicated because digoxin is a mild inotropic agent that will produce gradual effects over several hours, even after loading.

The DIG trial was conducted prior to the proven benefits and widespread use of β-blockers in HF, and, thus, some have called for a reexamination of digoxin in the context of contemporary HF therapy.[119] Based on the available data, digoxin's place in the pharmacotherapy of chronic SHF can be summarized for two patient groups. In patients with HF and supraventricular tachyarrhythmias such as atrial fibrillation, it should be considered early in therapy to help control ventricular response rate. For patients in normal sinus rhythm, although digoxin does not improve survival, its effects on symptom reduction and clinical outcomes are evident in patients with mild to severe HF with reduced systolic function. And thus, it should be used in conjunction with other standard HF therapies including diuretics, ACE inhibitors, and β-blockers in patients with symptomatic HF to reduce hospitalizations.[1,27] In the absence of digoxin toxicity or serious adverse effects, digoxin should be continued in most patients. Digoxin withdrawal may be considered for asymptomatic patients who have significant improvement in systolic function with optimal ACE inhibitor and β-blocker treatment.[120]

Nitrates and Hydralazine 10 Nitrates and hydralazine were originally combined in the treatment of SHF because of their complementary hemodynamic actions. Nitrates, by serving as nitric oxide donors, activate guanylate cyclase to increase cyclic guanosine monophosphate (cGMP) in vascular smooth muscle resulting in venodilation and decreased preload. Hydralazine is a direct-acting arterial vasodilator causing a decrease in SVR and resultant increases in SV and CO (see Fig. 4-1). However, recent evidence suggests that the beneficial effects of hydralazine and nitrates extend beyond their hemodynamic actions and interfere with the biochemical processes driving HF progression.[121]

The efficacy of the combination of hydralazine and ISDN has been evaluated in three large, randomized clinical trials. The first trial predated the use of ACE inhibitors and β-blockers and found that the combination of hydralazine 75 mg and ISDN 40 mg, each given four times daily, reduced mortality compared with placebo in patients receiving diuretics and digoxin.[122] A subsequent trial comparing the combination with an ACE inhibitor demonstrated greater mortality reduction with the ACE inhibitor.[123] Post hoc analysis of these trials suggested that the combination of hydralazine and ISDN was particularly effective in African Americans, and led to examining the efficacy of adding the combination to standard therapy in this group.[121]

The African-American Heart Failure Trial (A-HeFT) randomized 1,050 self-identified African Americans with NYHA class III or IV SHF receiving standard therapy to hydralazine plus ISDN or placebo.[124] The trial used a fixed-dose combination product, BiDil®, which contains hydralazine 37.5 mg and ISDN 20 mg. Therapy was initiated as a single tablet given three times daily, and then titrated to two tablets three times daily if tolerated. The trial was terminated early because of a significant 43% reduction in all-cause mortality in patients receiving hydralazine/ISDN compared with placebo. The primary composite end point of mortality, hospitalizations for HF, and quality of life was also significantly improved with the combination product. Based on these results, BiDil® was approved by the FDA to treat HF exclusively in African Americans.

The mechanism for the beneficial effects of hydralazine/ISDN remains uncertain but is most likely related to normalization of the increased oxidative stress and reduced nitric oxide signaling that contributes to HF progression. By serving as a nitric oxide donor, nitrates increase nitric oxide bioavailability and hydralazine reduces oxidative stress.[121,123] Nitric oxide attenuates myocardial remodeling and may play a protective role in HF. African Americans may have less nitric oxide availability compared with non–African Americans, and, thus, may derive particular benefit from therapy that enhances nitric oxide bioavailability. Whether the benefits of adding hydralazine/ISDN to standard therapy extend to non–African Americans remains to be prospectively evaluated.

Guidelines recommend the addition of hydralazine and nitrates to self-described African Americans with SHF and moderate to severe symptoms despite therapy with ACE inhibitors, diuretics, and β-blockers.[1,27] This combination is also reasonable to consider in all patients who continue to have symptoms despite optimized therapy with an ACE inhibitor (or ARB) and β-blocker.[1,27] For patients unable to tolerate an ACE inhibitor because of cough, an ARB is recommended as the first-line alternative.[1] Hydralazine and a nitrate might be reasonable in patients unable to tolerate either an ACE inhibitor or ARB because of renal insufficiency, hyperkalemia, or possibly hypotension.[1]

Despite the demonstrated benefits from hydralazine/ISDN, this therapy is significantly underused.[121] There are several potential obstacles that may explain this low rate of use. The first is the need for frequent dosing, with the fixed-dose combination administered three times daily. Second, adverse effects are common with hydralazine/ISDN, with nearly 30% of patients reporting dizziness, as well as headache and GI distress occurring more frequently with this combination compared with placebo in clinical trials.[122,124] A third potential obstacle is the high cost of the BiDil® fixed-dose combination product compared with that of the individual generic drugs purchased separately. Because of the high cost, many clinicians use generic hydralazine and ISDN as separate agents, rather than the combination product. Although the generic and brand name products are not bioequivalent as determined in healthy volunteer studies, it is unknown if these pharmacokinetic differences impact clinical outcomes.[121]

Calcium Channel Blockers 11 Calcium channel blockers can provide symptom-targeted treatment in patients with HFpEF by decreasing HR and increasing exercise tolerance. They can also provide disease-targeted therapy by treating HTN and coronary artery disease. However, the beneficial effect of these agents on exercise tolerance is not always paralleled by improved LV diastolic function or increased relaxation rate. Nonetheless, a number of small clinical trials have shown that the use of these agents results in both short- and long-term improvement in exercise capacity in patients with HFpEF.[27]

Of the calcium channel blockers, the nondihydropyridines (verapamil and diltiazem) are the most effective because they lower HR in addition to lowering BP.[125] Sustained-release nifedipine, because of its strong vasodilator properties, tends to cause hypotension, reflex tachycardia, and peripheral edema. These characteristics make it less useful in HFpEF. Amlodipine may be effective because it reduces BP. Initial doses are verapamil 120 to 240 mg/day, diltiazem 90 to 120 mg/day, and amlodipine 2.5 mg/day.

Heart block is a contraindication for the nondihydropyridines. The most common adverse effects are bradycardia and heart block (for the nondihydropyridines). Peripheral edema and headache also are common. Nondihydropyridines exacerbate the bradycardic effects of β-blockers, and verapamil raises digoxin serum concentrations by 70%. Diltiazem increases cyclosporine, tacrolimus, and sirolimus serum concentrations. Generic formulations, but not necessarily generic equivalents to the original brand names, are available for some of the calcium channel blockers.

Treatment of Concomitant Disorders

HF is often accompanied by other disorders whose natural history or therapy may affect morbidity, mortality, and treatment approach. Optimal management of these concomitant disorders in the context of the patient's HF is an important consideration in the overall care of the patient.

Hypertension Although ischemic heart disease has replaced HTN as the most common cause of HF, still nearly two thirds of patients with HF have current or a previous history of HTN.[1] HTN can contribute directly to the development of both SHF and HFpEF as well as indirectly by increasing the risk of coronary artery disease. Effective treatment of HTN reduces the risk of developing HF, especially in patients with diabetes.[1] Pharmacotherapy of HTN in patients with SHF should initially involve agents that can treat both disorders such as ACE inhibitors, β-blockers, and diuretics. Target levels of BP should be consistent with current guidelines.[1,27,48] If control of HTN is not achieved after optimizing treatment with these agents, the addition of an ARB, aldosterone antagonist, ISDN/hydralazine, or a second-generation calcium channel blocker such as amlodipine (or possibly felodipine) should be considered. Medications that should be avoided in patients with SHF include the calcium channel blockers with negative inotropic effects (e.g., verapamil, diltiazem) and direct-acting vasodilators (e.g., minoxidil) that cause sodium retention.

In patients with HFpEF, both verapamil and diltiazem can be safely used. However, clinicians should remember that HFpEF is associated with HTN and aging, making it a common diagnosis in elderly women. Because these women often are frail and have low muscle mass, their creatinine clearance and renal function may be compromised. Special care must be taken when selecting and titrating doses of drugs such as diuretics, ACE inhibitors, and ARBs and close attention paid to monitoring serum creatinine and electrolytes.

Angina Coronary artery disease is the most common etiology of SHF. Appropriate management of coronary disease and its risk factors is thus an important strategy for the prevention and treatment of HF. Coronary revascularization should be strongly considered in patients with both HF and angina.[1] Pharmacotherapy of angina in patients with HF should utilize drugs that can successfully treat both disorders. Nitrates and β-blockers are effective antianginals and are the preferred agents for patients with both disorders since they may improve hemodynamics and clinical outcomes.[1] It should be noted that the antianginal effectiveness of these agents may be significantly limited if fluid retention is not controlled with diuretics. Similar to their use in HTN, both amlodipine and felodipine appear to be safe to use in this setting. Optimization of other treatments for secondary prevention of coronary and other atherosclerotic vascular disease should also be considered.[48] Two large trials found that despite significant reductions in LDL cholesterol, rosuvastatin did not improve outcomes including mortality, nonfatal MI, nonfatal stroke, or hospital admission for cardiovascular causes in patients with SHF.[126,127] Therefore, the current data do not support the routine use of statins in SHF, although the precise role of these agents remains controversial.

Atrial Fibrillation Atrial fibrillation is the most frequently encountered arrhythmia and it is commonly found in patients with HF, affecting 10% to 50% of patients with the prevalence increasing in parallel to the severity of HF.[30] The high incidence of atrial fibrillation in these patients is not surprising since each disorder predisposes to the other and they share many risk factors including coronary artery disease, diabetes, obesity, and HTN. The presence of atrial fibrillation in patients with HF is associated with a worse long-term prognosis.[1,30] Detrimental effects of these disorders include increased risk of thromboembolism secondary to stasis of blood in the atria, a reduction in CO due to loss of the atrial contribution to ventricular filling, and hemodynamic compromise from the rapid ventricular response.[30] Moreover, HF exacerbations and atrial fibrillation are closely linked and it is often difficult to determine which disorder caused the other. For example, worsening HF results in volume overload, which, in turn, causes atrial distension and increases the risk of atrial fibrillation. Similarly, atrial fibrillation with a rapid ventricular response can reduce CO and lead to HF exacerbation. Thus, optimal management according to established guidelines is required with careful attention paid to control of ventricular response and anticoagulation for stroke prevention (see Chap. 8).[128]

Digoxin is frequently used to slow ventricular response in patients with HF and atrial fibrillation. However, it is more effective at rest than with exercise and it does not affect the progression of HF. β-Blockers are more effective than digoxin and have the added benefits of improving morbidity and mortality in patients with SHF. Combination therapy with digoxin and a β-blocker may be more effective for rate control than either agent used alone. Calcium channel blockers with negative inotropic effects such as verapamil or diltiazem should be avoided. Amiodarone is a reasonable alternative for rate control in those patients not responding to digoxin and/or β-blockers or with contraindications to these agents.[128] Appropriate selection of antithrombotic therapy for stroke prevention that takes into consideration the presence of risk factors for thromboembolism in an individual patient is also required.[126,128]

Because of the close association between atrial fibrillation, HF exacerbations, and hospitalizations, restoration and maintenance of sinus rhythm (i.e., rhythm control) is often attempted instead of the rate control approach. Although initial trials such as AFFIRM showed no differences in outcomes between the rhythm and rate control approaches, less than 10% of the patients in this study had left ventricular dysfunction.[129] The Atrial Fibrillation and Congestive Heart Failure (AF-CHF) trial prospectively compared the rhythm and rate control approaches in nearly 1,400 patients with symptomatic HF and LVEF ≤35%.[130] Rhythm control was primarily achieved with amiodarone, whereas a β-blocker and digoxin were used for rate control. Compared with rate control, there were no improvements in mortality, stroke, death from cardiovascular causes, or HF hospitalizations in the rhythm control arm. Therefore, overall rhythm control appears to offer no specific advantages over rate control in this population and can be reserved for patients in whom the rate cannot be controlled or who remain symptomatic. In general, amiodarone is the preferred agent if the rhythm control approach is taken. Although it has many noncardiac toxicities, amiodarone does not have cardiodepressant or significant proarrhythmic effects and appears to be safe in HF. Dofetilide also appears to be safe and effective in this population.[30,128] Class I antiarrhythmics should be avoided.[30,128]

Diabetes Diabetes is a common comorbid condition in patients with HF, with current estimates indicating it is present in approximately one third of HF patients.[131] As an important risk factor for coronary artery disease, diabetes directly contributes to the development of HF. Importantly though, diabetes is also a risk factor for HF, particularly in women, independent of coronary artery disease or HTN.[131] Diabetes is associated with more rapid HF progression and is a significant predictor of mortality in patients with HF.[131]

Pharmacotherapy of diabetes in patients with HF should be targeted to control hyperglycemia according to current guidelines, although this approach is not proven to reduce the risk of HF development.[1] The optimal approach to the treatment of diabetes in this population remains uncertain as most clinical trials of diabetes medications excluded patients with moderate to severe HF. Some medications used to treat diabetes can have important adverse effects in patients with HF. Because the TZDs (pioglitazone and rosiglitazone) are associated with fluid retention, these medications should not be used in patients with NYHA class III or IV HF and used cautiously in patients with NYHA class I or II symptoms with close observation needed to detect weight gain, edema formation, or HF exacerbation. TZDs should be discontinued in patients developing symptoms related to volume overload. Use of metformin in patients with HF has been contraindicated because of the purported risk of lactic acidosis. However, the product labeling was recently revised removing this contraindication, although a warning still remains specifically in patients with hypoperfusion and hypoxemia. A growing number of observational reports demonstrate that not only is metformin safe in HF, but it is also associated with improved morbidity and mortality.[132,133] However, no prospective data on metformin's safety and efficacy in HF are available, so careful monitoring of volume status and renal function is needed when this medication is used in these patients.[131]

Drug Class Information

Diuretics 7 Loop diuretics, as described earlier, represent the typical diuretic therapy for patients with HF due to their potency and, as such, are the only diuretics discussed here.[55,60] There are currently three loop diuretics available that are used routinely: furosemide, bumetanide, and torsemide. They share many similarities in their pharmacodynamics, with their differences being largely pharmacokinetic in nature. Relevant information on the loop diuretics is shown in Tables 4-8 and 4-9. Following oral administration, the peak effect with all the agents occurs in 30 to 90 minutes, with duration of 2 to 3 hours (slightly longer for torsemide). Following IV administration, the diuretic effect begins within minutes. All three drugs are highly (>95%) bound to serum albumin and enter the nephron by active secretion in the proximal tubule. The magnitude of effect is determined by the peak concentration achieved in the nephron, and there is a threshold concentration that must be achieved before any diuresis is seen.

The biggest difference between the agents is bioavailability. Bioavailability of bumetanide and torsemide is essentially complete (80% to 100%), whereas furosemide bioavailability exhibits marked intrapatient and interpatient variability. Furosemide bioavailability ranges from 10% to 100%, with an average of 50%. Thus, if bioequivalent IV and oral doses are desired, oral furosemide doses should be approximately double that of the IV dose, whereas IV and oral doses are the same for torsemide and bumetanide. Coadministration of furosemide and bumetanide with food can decrease bioavailability significantly, whereas food has no effect on bioavailability of torsemide. The intraabdominal congestion that can occur in HF also may slow the rate (and thus decrease the peak concentration) of furosemide, which can reduce the diuretic's efficacy. Thus, furosemide is most problematic with respect to rate and extent of absorption and the factors that influence it, whereas torsemide has the least variable bioavailability.

Recent data suggest that these differences in bioavailability and variability may have clinical implications. For example, several studies have suggested that torsemide is absorbed reliably and is associated with better outcomes than the more variably absorbed furosemide.[134,135] Torsemide is preferred in patients with persistent fluid retention despite high doses of other loop diuretics. And while the costs of torsemide exceed those of furosemide, pharmacoeconomic analyses suggest that the costs of care are similar or less with torsemide.[135] These data require confirmation in controlled, double-blind clinical trials but provide preliminary evidence that the more reliably absorbed loop diuretics may be superior to furosemide.

HF is one of the disease states in which the maximal response to loop diuretics is reduced. This is believed to result from a decrease in the rate of diuretic absorption and/or increased proximal or distal tubule reabsorption of sodium, possibly due to increased activity of the Na–K–2Cl transporter.[61] As a consequence, loop diuretics exhibit a ceiling effect in HF, meaning that once the ceiling dose is reached, no additional diuretic response is achieved by increasing the dose. Thus, when this dose is reached, additional diuresis can be achieved by giving the drug more often (twice daily or occasionally three times daily) or by giving combination diuretic therapy. Multiple daily dosing achieves a more sustained diuresis throughout the day. When dosed two or three times daily, the first dose is usually given first thing in the morning and the final dose in late afternoon/early evening. The appropriate chronic dose of a loop diuretic is that which maintains the patient at a stable dry weight without symptoms of dyspnea. Ranges of doses of loop diuretics and recommended ceiling doses are shown in Table 4-8.

Diuretics cause a variety of metabolic abnormalities, with severity related to the potency of the diuretic. The reader is referred to Chapter 3 for a detailed discussion on the adverse effects of diuretic therapy. Hypokalemia is the most common metabolic disturbance with thiazide and loop diuretics, which in HF patients may be exacerbated by hyperaldosteronism. Hypokalemia increases the risk for ventricular arrhythmias in HF and is especially worrisome in patients receiving digoxin. It is often accompanied by hypomagnesemia. Since adequate magnesium is necessary for entry of potassium into the cell, co-supplementation with both magnesium and potassium may be necessary to correct the hypokalemia. Concomitant ACE inhibitor (or ARB) and/or aldosterone antagonist therapy may help to minimize diuretic-induced hypokalemia because these drugs tend to increase serum potassium concentration through their inhibitory effect on aldosterone secretion. Nonetheless, the serum potassium concentration should be monitored closely in HF patients and supplemented appropriately when needed. In addition to metabolic abnormalities, a recent post hoc analysis of the DIG trial suggested that chronic diuretic use was associated with increased risk of mortality and hospitalization.[136] These findings must be interpreted with caution because this trial was not designed to evaluate outcomes associated with diuretic therapy. However, they do serve to remind clinicians of the importance of appropriate patient selection and monitoring when using diuretic therapy.

ACE Inhibitors ❺ A number of ACE inhibitors are currently available; those commonly used in the treatment of patients with HF are summarized in Table 4-8. Although ACE inhibitors vary in their chemical structure (e.g., sulfhydryl vs. non–sulfhydryl-containing agents) and tissue affinity, the major differences in the ACE inhibitors are not in these pharmacologic properties but in their pharmacokinetic properties.[16] To date all ACE inhibitors studied improve symptoms and mortality in SHF.[16] However, it seems most prudent to use those agents documented to reduce morbidity and mortality because the dose required for these end points has been determined.[1]

To minimize the risk of hypotension and renal insufficiency, ACE inhibitor therapy should be started with low doses followed by gradual titration as tolerated to the target doses.[1] Asymptomatic hypotension should not be considered a contraindication to starting therapy with an ACE inhibitor, although initiation or dose increases in patients with systolic BPs less than 90 to 100 mm Hg should be done cautiously. Renal function and serum potassium should be evaluated at baseline and within 1 to 2 weeks after therapy is started with subsequent periodic assessments. In the outpatient setting, clinicians should wait at least 2 weeks between dose increases and renal function and potassium should be checked 1 to 2 weeks after each increase. After titration of the drug to the target dose, most patients tolerate chronic therapy with few complications. Although symptoms may improve within a few days of initiating therapy, it may take weeks to months before the full benefits are apparent. Even if symptoms do not improve, long-term ACE inhibitor therapy should be continued to reduce the risk of mortality and hospitalization. Careful attention to appropriate doses of diuretics is important since fluid overload may blunt the beneficial effects of ACE inhibitors and overdiuresis increases the risk of hypotension and renal insufficiency.

Since ACE inhibitors were the first agents to show improvements in survival and were frequently used as background therapy in clinical trials of other medications, they are often used as the initial therapy in patients with HF. Traditionally, after titration of the ACE inhibitor dose, the addition of β-blockers was then considered. As a result, the expected ACE inhibitor–mediated decrease in BP prevented some clinicians from starting β-blocker therapy. However, initiation of β-blocker therapy should not be delayed while the ACE inhibitor is titrated to the target dose since low–intermediate ACE inhibitor doses are equally effective as higher doses for improving symptoms and survival.[1,70] Also, in β-blocker clinical trials, most patients were receiving background therapy with low–intermediate ACE inhibitor doses. Thus, in most patients, ACE inhibitors should be the initial therapy but it is important to remember that even a small dose of ACE inhibitor is better than no ACE inhibitor and that the greatest benefit is seen when these agents are combined with a β-blocker.

Because of the high prevalence of coronary artery disease in patients with HF, aspirin is frequently coadministered with

ACE inhibitors. Whether aspirin may attenuate the hemodynamic and mortality benefits of ACE inhibitors remains controversial. The postulated mechanism of this interaction involves opposing effects on synthesis of vasodilatory prostaglandins. The ACE inhibitor–mediated increase in bradykinin increases the synthesis of vasodilatory prostaglandins that have favorable hemodynamic benefits in HF. Because of aspirin's effect on prostaglandin synthesis, this potentially beneficial action of ACE inhibitors may be attenuated. However, in contrast with studies that showed an ACE inhibitor–aspirin interaction, other investigators have found no interaction, even in patients without coronary artery disease or with impaired renal function.[137] It is currently recommended that the decision to use each of these medications be made based on whether an individual patient has indications for each drug.[1,27] Aspirin doses of 160 mg/day or less should be considered. In the absence of atherosclerotic vascular disease, aspirin therapy is not recommended.[27]

Adverse Effects The primary adverse effects of ACE inhibitors are secondary to their major pharmacologic effects of suppressing angiotensin II and increasing bradykinin. The most common adverse effects with these agents are hypotension and functional renal insufficiency resulting from the drug-related reductions in angiotensin II. ACE inhibitors reduce BP in nearly all patients, with hypotension becoming problematic when symptoms such as dizziness, light-headedness, blurred vision, presyncope, or syncope are observed. Hypotension occurs most frequently soon after therapy is started or after an increase in dose, although it may occur at any time during treatment. Risk factors for hypotension include hyponatremia (serum sodium <130 mEq/L [<130 mmol/L]), hypovolemia, and overdiuresis.[1] The risk of hypotension may be minimized by initiating therapy with lower ACE inhibitor doses and/or temporarily withholding or reducing the dose of diuretic, and liberalizing salt and fluid intake.[1] An often overlooked solution to hypotension is to space the administration times of vasoactive medications (e.g., diuretics and β-blockers) throughout the day so that these medications are not all administered at or near the same time. Also, if the patient is receiving other vasodilating drugs (e.g., nitrates, amlodipine), the need for these medications or at least the feasibility of dose reduction should be considered. Many patients who experience symptomatic hypotension early in therapy are still good candidates for long-term treatment if risk factors for low BP are addressed.

Functional renal insufficiency causes increases in serum creatinine and blood urea nitrogen (BUN). As CO and renal blood flow decline, renal perfusion is maintained by the vasoconstrictor effect of angiotensin II on the efferent arteriole. Patients most dependent on this system for maintenance of renal perfusion (and therefore most likely to develop functional renal insufficiency with ACE inhibitors) are those with severe HF, hypotension, hyponatremia, volume depletion, bilateral renal artery stenosis, and concomitant use of NSAIDs.[138] Sodium depletion, usually secondary to diuretic therapy, is the most important factor in the development of functional renal insufficiency with ACE inhibitor therapy. Renal insufficiency therefore can be minimized in many cases by reduction in diuretic dosage or liberalization of sodium intake. Increases in serum creatinine of 10% to 20% from baseline are commonly observed after initiation of ACE inhibitor therapy. In some patients, the serum creatinine will return to baseline levels without a reduction in ACE inhibitor dose.[138] Increases in serum creatinine of >0.5 mg/dL if the baseline creatinine is <2 mg/dL or of >1 mg/dL if the creatinine is >2 mg/dL should prompt clinicians to reduce the dose of ACE inhibitors or reconsider ACE therapy and evaluate potential causes for the abrupt decline in renal function.[138] The safety and efficacy of ACE inhibitors in patients with baseline serum creatinine >2.5 mg/dL (>221 μmol/L) is uncertain as these patients were usually excluded from clinical trials. Caution should also be exercised when using ACE inhibitors in such patients. Since renal dysfunction with ACE inhibitors is secondary to alterations in renal hemodynamics, it is almost always reversible on discontinuation of the drug.[138]

Careful dose titration can minimize the risks of hypotension and transient worsening of renal function. Thus, usual initial doses should be about one fourth the final target dose with slow upward dose titration based on BP and serum creatinine. In certain patients, especially those hospitalized patients who seem at high risk for hypotension or worsening of renal function, it also may be advisable to initiate therapy with a short-acting agent such as captopril. This will help minimize the duration of these adverse effects should they occur. Once stabilized on captopril, the patient can then be switched to an agent given once daily.

Hyperkalemia with ACE inhibitor therapy can occur and is due to the reduced feedback of angiotensin II to stimulate aldosterone release. Hyperkalemia is most likely to occur in patients with renal insufficiency and in those taking concomitant potassium supplements, potassium-containing salt substitutes, or potassium-sparing diuretic therapy (including an aldosterone antagonist), especially if they have diabetes.[138] The more widespread use of aldosterone antagonists (e.g., spironolactone) in patients with HF may increase the risk of hyperkalemia.[101]

ACE inhibitors are also associated with other important adverse effects. A dry, hacking cough is the most common reason for discontinuation of ACE inhibitors, and this adverse effect occurs with a similar frequency with all the agents.[1] The incidence of cough is reported to range from 5% to 10%, but a recent report suggests cough occurs significantly more often (up to 15% of patients) than what is reported in the product labeling.[139] The cough is usually nonproductive, occurs within the first few months of therapy, resolves within 1 to 2 weeks of drug discontinuation, and reappears with rechallenge. Cough occurs in up to 40% of patients with HF, independent of ACE inhibitor use; therefore, it is important to rule out other potential causes of cough, such as pulmonary congestion. Because cough is a bradykinin-mediated effect, replacement of ACE inhibitor therapy with an ARB would be reasonable in those patients who cannot tolerate the cough. Angioedema is a rare, occurring in less than 1% of patients receiving an ACE inhibitor, but potentially life-threatening complication that may also be due to bradykinin accumulation. It occurs more frequently in African Americans, women, and patients with HF than in other populations.[140,141] Approximately 50% of patients develop angioedema within the first 90 days of therapy, but it can occur years after treatment was started.[140] Use of ACE inhibitors is contraindicated in patients with a history of angioedema. Extreme caution should be exercised if ARBs are used as an alternative therapy in patients with ACE inhibitor–induced angioedema, as cross-reactivity is reported.[1,91,141] ACE inhibitors are contraindicated during the second and third trimesters of pregnancy due to the increased risk of fetal renal failure, intrauterine growth retardation, and other congenital defects. A recent analysis using a Medicaid database of nearly 30,000 patients suggests that first-trimester use of ACE inhibitors should also be avoided as the risk of major congenital defects was increased 2.7-fold in infants exposed to these agents during the first trimester.[142]

Angiotensin II Receptor Blockers **5** Although ACE inhibitors remain the agents of first choice to treat Stage C SHF, ARBs are now the recommended alternatives in patients who are unable to tolerate an ACE inhibitor.[1] Although numerous ARBs are currently available, only three agents, candesartan, valsartan, and losartan, are recommended in the treatment guidelines.[1,27] The efficacy of these agents is supported by clinical trial data that document a target dose associated with improved survival and other important outcomes in patients with decreased LVEF.[87–89,91,92] ARBs are also alternatives to ACE inhibitors in patients with Stage A or B HF.[1]

The clinical use of ARBs is also similar to that of ACE inhibitors. Therapy should be initiated at low doses and then titrated to target doses (Table 4-8).[1] BP, renal function, and serum potassium should be evaluated within 1 to 2 weeks after initiation of therapy and after increases in dose and these end points used to guide subsequent dose changes. It is not necessary to reach target doses before adding a β-blocker, although incremental benefits may be associated with higher doses of ARBs.[86]

Adverse Effects The ARBs have a low incidence of adverse effects. Since they do not affect bradykinin, they are not associated with cough and have a lower risk of angioedema than ACE inhibitors.[141] However, because of reports of recurrences of angioedema after ARB administration to patients with a history of ACE inhibitor–related angioedema, ARBs should be used with extreme caution in any patient with a history of angioedema as cross-reactivity may occur in 2% to 17% of patients.[91,94,143]

The major adverse effects are related to suppression of the RAAS. The incidence and risk factors for developing hypotension, decreases in renal function, and hyperkalemia with the ARBs are similar to those with ACE inhibitors.[1,137] Thus, ARBs are not alternatives in patients who develop these complications from ACE inhibitors. Careful monitoring is required when an ARB is used with another inhibitor of the RAAS (e.g., ACE inhibitor or aldosterone antagonist) as this combination increases the risk of these adverse effects. Similar to the ACE inhibitors, the ARBs are contraindicated in the second and third trimesters of pregnancy and should be avoided in the first trimester because of increased risk of fetal/neonatal morbidity and mortality. Neither candesartan nor valsartan is metabolized by the cytochrome P450 system, so no pharmacokinetic drug–drug interactions with these agents are expected.

β-Blockers 6 Metoprolol succinate, carvedilol, and bisoprolol are the only β-blockers shown to reduce mortality in large trials in patients with SHF. Metoprolol and bisoprolol selectively block the β_1-receptor, while carvedilol blocks the β_1-, β_2-, and α_1-receptors and also possesses antioxidant effects. While there is no clear evidence that these pharmacologic differences result in differences in efficacy among agents, they may aid in selection of a specific agent. For example, carvedilol is expected to have greater antihypertensive effects than the other agents because of its α-receptor blocking properties and may be preferred in patients with poorly controlled BP. Conversely, metoprolol or bisoprolol may be preferred in patients with low BP or dizziness and in patients with significant airway disease. Bisoprolol is eliminated approximately 50% by the kidneys, whereas metoprolol and carvedilol are essentially completely metabolized and undergo extensive hepatic first-pass metabolism.

There is fairly strong evidence that benefits of β-blockers in SHF are not a class effect. Specifically, in a study powered for mortality reduction, there was no difference in survival between the nonselective β-blocker bucindolol and placebo.[144] While there has been considerable debate over why bucindolol failed to provide a survival benefit, it may be related to the drug's ancillary properties or differences among β-blocker trials in the characteristics of study participants. Additional data suggest that bucindolol's effects on survival might be genotype specific, as described in Personalized Pharmacotherapy below. In the absence of bucindolol's approval for HF, β-blocker use should be confined to one of the agents with proven survival benefits, especially given the diversity among β-blockers in their receptor sensitivities and ancillary properties.

There has been much debate over whether one β-blocker is superior to another. Specifically, it has been hypothesized that nonselective blockade with carvedilol might produce greater benefits than β_1-selective blockade. This hypothesis is based on observations that the β_1-receptor is downregulated, and the β_2- and α_1-receptors account for a larger proportion of total cardiac adrenergic receptors in the failing heart. Only one trial with a mortality end point has provided a head-to-head comparison of carvedilol and a β_1-selective blocker. The Carvedilol Or Metoprolol European Trial (COMET) compared carvedilol 25 mg twice daily and immediate-release metoprolol 50 mg twice daily and found a significant 17% lower mortality rate in patients treated with carvedilol.[145] However, concerns regarding the formulation and dose of metoprolol used in COMET limit the conclusions that can be drawn from these findings. Specifically, the study used the immediate-release formulation of metoprolol (metoprolol tartrate), not the sustained-release formation (metoprolol succinate) shown to reduce mortality. The efficacy of the immediate-release formulation in reducing mortality in HF has not been proven. Metoprolol succinate provides more consistent plasma concentrations over a 24-hour period and appears to provide more favorable effects on HR variability, autonomic balance, and BP, suggesting that this formulation might be superior to immediate-release metoprolol.[146] The target dose of metoprolol also differed between COMET and MERIT-HF. The target dose in COMET was 100 mg/day (50 mg twice daily), whereas the target dose of metoprolol in MERIT-HF was 200 mg/day. Many question whether the degree of β-blockade achieved in COMET with immediate-release metoprolol 50 mg twice daily is comparable to that achieved with metoprolol succinate 200 mg/day in MERIT-HF or carvedilol 25 mg twice daily in COMET. Thus, the debate over β-blocker superiority continues, and while some clinicians would argue superiority of carvedilol, it seems clear that what is most important is that one of the three β-blockers proven to reduce mortality is used.

Adverse Effects Possible adverse effects with β-blocker use in HF include bradycardia or heart block, hypotension, fatigue, impaired glycemic control in diabetic patients, bronchospasm in patients with asthma, and worsening HF. Clinicians should monitor vital signs and carefully assess for signs and symptoms of worsening HF during β-blocker initiation and uptitration. Hypotension is more common with carvedilol due to its α_1-receptor blocking properties. Bradycardia and hypotension generally are asymptomatic and require no intervention; however, β-blocker dose reduction is warranted in symptomatic patients. Fatigue usually resolves after several weeks of therapy, but sometimes requires dose reduction. In diabetic patients, β-blockers may worsen glucose tolerance and can mask the tachycardia and tremor (but not sweating) that accompany hypoglycemia. In addition, nonselective agents such as carvedilol may prolong insulin-induced hypoglycemia and slow recovery from a hypoglycemic episode. Despite this, there is evidence that carvedilol produces better glycemic control in diabetic patients compared with immediate-release metoprolol and may improve insulin sensitivity.[147] Furthermore, post hoc analysis of HF trials shows that β-blockers are well tolerated and significantly reduce morbidity and mortality in patients with diabetes and SHF.[148] Thus, while β-blockers should be used cautiously in patients with recurrent hypoglycemia, concerns of masking symptoms of hypoglycemia or worsening glycemic control should not preclude β-blocker use in patients with diabetes. Patients with diabetes should be warned of these potential adverse effects, and blood glucose monitored with initiation, adjustment, and discontinuation of β-blocker therapy. Adjustment of hypoglycemic therapy may be necessary with concomitant β-blocker use in diabetics.

Uptitration should be avoided if the patient experiences signs of worsening HF, including volume overload and poor perfusion. Fluid overload may be asymptomatic and manifest solely as an increase in body weight. Mild fluid overload may be managed by intensifying diuretic therapy. Once the patient has been stabilized, dose titration may continue as tolerated until the target or highest tolerated dose is reached. Despite their negative inotropic effects, continuing β-blocker therapy during hospitalization for acute decompensated HF appears to neither worsen symptoms nor delay clinical improvement. In fact, β-blocker withdrawal may increase the risk for mortality after hospital discharge.[149,150] Further, stopping β-blocker therapy during acute decompensation may lead to lower chronic β-blocker use due to failure to reinstitute β-blocker therapy once the patient has stabilized.[150,151] Guidelines recommend continuing β-blocker therapy during hospitalization for HF whenever possible.[1,27]

Absolute contraindications to β-blocker use include uncontrolled bronchospastic disease, symptomatic bradycardia, advanced heart block without a pacemaker, and acute decompensated HF. However, β-blockers may be tried with caution in patients with asymptomatic bradycardia, COPD, or well-controlled asthma. Particular caution is warranted in patients with marked bradycardia (<55 beats/min) or hypotension (systolic BP <80 mm Hg).

Digoxin Digoxin exerts its positive inotropic effect by binding to sodium- and potassium-activated adenosine triphosphatase (Na,K-ATPase or sodium pump). Inhibition of Na,K-ATPase decreases outward transport of sodium and leads to increased intracellular sodium concentrations. Higher intracellular sodium concentrations favor calcium entry and reduce calcium extrusion from the cell through effects on the sodium–calcium exchanger. The result is increased storage of intracellular calcium in the sarcoplasmic reticulum and, with each action potential, a greater release of calcium to activate contractile elements. Digoxin also has beneficial neurohormonal actions. These effects occur at low plasma concentrations, where little inotropic effect is seen, and are independent of inotropic activity. Unlike other positive inotropes that increase intracellular cyclic adenosine monophosphate (cAMP), digoxin attenuates the excessive SNS activation present in HF patients. Although the precise mechanism is unknown, a digoxin-mediated reduction in central sympathetic outflow and improvement in impaired baroreceptor function appear to play an important role. Because mortality and progression of HF are linked to the extent of SNS activation, these sympathoinhibitory effects may be an important component of the clinical response to the drug. Chronic HF is also marked by autonomic dysfunction, most notably suppression of the parasympathetic (vagal) system. Digoxin increases parasympathetic activity in HF patients and leads to a decrease in HR, thus enhancing diastolic filling. The vagal effects also result in slowed conduction and prolongation of AV node refractoriness, thus slowing the ventricular response in patients with atrial fibrillation. Because atrial fibrillation is a common complication of HF, the combined positive inotropic, neurohormonal, and negative chronotropic effects of digoxin can be particularly beneficial for such patients. The overall response to digoxin is usually an increase in cardiac index and a decrease in PCWP with relatively little change in arterial BP.[106,120]

Pharmacokinetics Numerous studies of digoxin pharmacokinetics have been published and are summarized in Table 4-11. Digoxin has a large volume of distribution and is extensively bound to various tissues, most notably to Na,K-ATPase in skeletal and cardiac muscles. Because it does not distribute appreciably to body fat, loading doses of digoxin (when necessary) should be calculated based on estimates of lean body weight. There is a long "distribution phase" after administration of oral or IV digoxin, resulting in a lag time before maximum pharmacologic response is observed (see Table 4-11). Transiently elevated SDCs during the distribution phase are not associated with increased therapeutic or adverse effects, although they can mislead the clinician who is unaware of the timing of blood sampling relative to the previous digoxin dose. Consequently, blood samples for measurement of SDCs should be collected at least 6 hours and preferably 12 hours or more after the last dose.

TABLE 4-11 Clinical Pharmacokinetics of Digoxin

Oral bioavailability	
Tablets	0.5–0.9 (0.65)[a]
Elixir	0.75–0.85 (0.80)
Capsules	0.9–1.0 (0.95)
Onset of action	
Oral	1.5–6 hours
IV	15–30 minutes
Peak effect	
Oral	4–6 hours
IV	1.5–4 hours
Terminal half-life	
Normal renal function	36 hours
Anuric patients	5 days
Volume of distribution at steady state	7.3 L/kg
Fraction unbound in plasma	0.75–0.80
Fraction excreted unchanged in urine	0.65–0.70

[a]Range and mean value in parentheses.

Data from Schentag JJ, Bang AJ, Kozinski-Tober JL. In: Burton ME, Shaw LM, Schentag JJ, Evans WE, eds. Applied Pharmacokinetics and Pharmacodynamics: Principles of Therapeutic Drug Monitoring, 4th ed. Baltimore, MD: Lippincott Williams and Wilkins, 2006:410–439.

In patients with normal renal function, 60% to 80% of a dose of digoxin is eliminated unchanged in urine via glomerular filtration and tubular secretion. The terminal half-life of digoxin is approximately 1.5 days in subjects with normal renal function but approximately 5 days in anuric patients (see Table 4-11). Recent evidence indicates that the drug efflux transporter P-glycoprotein (P-gp) plays an important role in the bioavailability, renal and nonrenal clearance, and drug interactions with digoxin. Clinically important pharmacokinetic/pharmacodynamic drug interactions are summarized in Table 4-12. An extensive review of the pharmacokinetics and pharmacodynamics of digoxin is available.[117]

Adverse Effects Digoxin can produce a variety of cardiac and noncardiac adverse effects, but it is usually well tolerated by most patients (Table 4-13).[105,120] Noncardiac adverse effects frequently involve the CNS or GI systems but also may be nonspecific (e.g., fatigue or weakness). Cardiac manifestations include numerous different arrhythmias caused by the drug's multiple electrophysiologic effects (Table 4-13). Cardiac arrhythmias may be the first evidence of toxicity in a patient (before any noncardiac symptoms occur). Rhythm disturbances are of particular concern because patients with chronic HF are already at increased risk for sudden cardiac death, presumably due to ventricular arrhythmias. Patients at increased risk of toxicity include those with impaired renal function, decreased lean body mass, the elderly, and those taking interacting drugs. Hypokalemia, hypomagnesemia, and hypercalcemia will predispose patients to cardiac manifestations of digoxin toxicity. Thus, concomitant therapy with diuretics may lead to electrolyte abnormalities and increase the likelihood of cardiac arrhythmias. Similarly, hypothyroidism, myocardial ischemia, and acidosis will also increase the risk of cardiac adverse effects. Although digoxin toxicity is commonly associated with plasma concentrations greater than 2 ng/mL (2.6 nmol/L), clinicians should remember that digoxin toxicity is based on the presence of symptoms rather than a specific plasma concentration.[117] Usual treatment of digoxin toxicity includes drug withdrawal or dose reduction and treatment of cardiac arrhythmias and electrolyte abnormalities. In patients with life-threatening digoxin toxicity, purified digoxin-specific Fab antibody fragments should be administered. SDCs will not be reliable until the antidote has been eliminated from the body.[120]

TABLE 4-12 Selected Digoxin Drug Interactions

Drugs	Mechanism/Effect	Suggested Clinical Management
Amiodarone, dronedarone	Inhibits P-glycoprotein resulting in decrease in renal and nonrenal clearance; can increase SDC by 70–100%	Monitor SDC and adverse effects; anticipate the need to reduce the dose by 50%
Antacids	Concurrent administration may decrease digoxin bioavailability by 20–35%	Space doses at least 2 hours apart or avoid concurrent use if possible
Cholestyramine, colestipol	Bind digoxin in gut and decrease bioavailability 20–35%; may also decrease enterohepatic recycling	Space doses at least 2 hours apart or avoid concurrent use if possible
Diuretics	Thiazides or loop diuretics may cause hypokalemia and hypomagnesemia, thereby increasing the risk of digitalis toxicity	Monitor and replace electrolytes if necessary
Erythromycin, clarithromycin, tetracycline	Alter gut bacterial flora; bioavailability and SDC increase 40–100% in about 10% of patients who extensively metabolize digoxin in the gut, may also be due to inhibition of P-glycoprotein by macrolides	Monitor SDC and anticipate the need to reduce the dose; avoid concurrent use if possible
Ketoconazole, itraconazole	Decrease in renal and nonrenal clearance by inhibition of P-glycoprotein; SDC may increase by 50–100%	Monitor SDC and anticipate the need to reduce the dose by 50%
Kaolin–pectin	Large dose (30–60 mL) may decrease digoxin bioavailability by about 60%	Space doses at least 2 hours apart or avoid concurrent use if possible
Metoclopramide	Increase in gut mobility may decrease bioavailability of slow dissolving tablets; unknown significance	Effect is minimized by administration of digoxin capsules
Neomycin, sulfasalazine	Decrease in bioavailability by 20–25%	Space doses at least 2 hours apart or avoid concurrent use if possible
Propafenone	Decrease in renal clearance; SDC may increase 30–40%	Monitor SDC and anticipate the need to reduce the dose
Quinidine	Inhibits P-glycoprotein resulting in decrease in renal and nonrenal clearance; also displacement of digoxin from tissue binding sites with decrease in the volume of distribution; SDC generally increases about twofold	Monitor SDC and adverse effects; anticipate the need to reduce dose by 50%
Spironolactone	Decrease in renal and nonrenal clearance; also interference with some digoxin assays thus increasing apparent SDC	Monitor SDC and anticipate the need to reduce dose; check assay for interference
Verapamil	Inhibits P-glycoprotein resulting in decrease in renal and nonrenal clearance; SDC may increase 70–100%	Monitor SDC and anticipate the need to reduce the dose by 50%; consider using another calcium channel blocker

SDC, serum digoxin concentration.

Personalized Pharmacotherapy

Pharmacogenetics holds promise for future personalized HF therapy. Most HF pharmacogenetic research has focused on genetic association responses to β-blockers. For example, there is evidence that the β_1-adrenergic receptor (ADRB1) Arg389Gly polymorphism is associated with improvement in left ventricular EF with β-blockers.[152] Further, the Arg389Gly variant was associated with clinical outcomes with bucindolol, the only β-blocker among those studied in large, randomized, multicenter HF trials that did not significantly improve outcomes.[144] The trial with bucindolol was unique in that it included a large number of African American patients. A subgroup analysis showed survival improvement with bucindolol in whites, but not African Americans. African Americans have a higher frequency of the ADRB1 389Gly allele and the α_{2c}-adrenergic receptor (ADRA2C) Del322–325 variant, both of which are associated with a lack of improvement in HF outcomes with bucindolol.[153,154] In contrast, the wild-type ADRB1 and ADRA2C genotypes, which occur more often among whites, were associated with a reduced risk for hospitalization and death with bucindolol. The manufacturer of bucindolol sought FDA approval of the drug for patients with the more favorable response genotype; however, their initial efforts have been unsuccessful.

Both metoprolol and carvedilol are also substrates for the cytochrome P450 2D6 enzyme, which is known to be polymorphic. A total of 7% of the white population and 1% to 2% of the Asian American and African American populations who are CYP2D6 poor metabolizers would be expected to have higher plasma concentrations than anticipated at the usual doses of carvedilol and metoprolol. However, given that β-blockers have a wide therapeutic index, it is unclear whether CYP2D6 phenotype significantly impacts hemodynamic and clinical effects.

There is also preliminary evidence of genetic determinants of outcomes with hydralazine/ISDN. Specifically, the endothelial nitric oxide synthase-3 (NOS3) Glu298Asp polymorphism was associated with the effects of hydralazine/ISDN on the composite end point of survival, hospitalization, and quality of life, with greater improvement with the Glu298Glu genotype.[155] A separate analysis focused on the gene for corin, a protein expressed in cardiomyocytes that

TABLE 4-13 Signs and Symptoms of Digoxin Toxicity

Noncardiac (mostly CNS) adverse effects

Anorexia, nausea, vomiting, abdominal pain
Visual disturbances
Halos, photophobia, problems with color perception (i.e., red-green or yellow-green vision), scotomata
Fatigue, weakness, dizziness, headache, neuralgia, confusion, delirium, psychosis

Cardiac adverse effects[a,b]

Ventricular arrhythmias
Premature ventricular depolarizations, bigeminy, trigeminy, ventricular tachycardia, ventricular fibrillation
Atrioventricular (A-V) block
First degree, second degree (Mobitz type I), third degree
A-V junctional escape rhythms, junctional tachycardia
Atrial arrhythmias with slowed A-V conduction or A-V block particularly paroxysmal atrial tachycardia with A-V block
Sinus bradycardia

[a]Some adverse effects may be difficult to distinguish from the signs/symptoms of heart failure.
[b]Digoxin toxicity has been associated with almost every known rhythm abnormality (only the more common manifestations are listed).

Data from reference 105.

cleaves pro-ANP and proBNP into active natriuretic peptides. The corin Gln568Pro variant leads to a dysfunctional protein and was associated with an increased risk for death or HF hospitalization in the A-HeFT population.[156] However, no detrimental effect of the 568Pro variant was observed among patients treated with hydralazine/ISDN, suggesting that the drug combination attenuates the adverse consequences of the 568Pro allele. Both the NOS3 Glu-298Glu genotype and corin 568Pro variant occur predominately in persons of African descent, potentially explaining why hydralazine/ISDN is especially effective in African Americans.

Clinical **Controversy...**

1. Treatment guidelines for SHF recommend that the dose of β-blockers be titrated to those achieved in the clinical efficacy trials. Attainment of these doses is not possible in some patients because of bradycardia, hypotension, or other β-blocker adverse effects. Thus, it is uncertain if these lower doses provide the same benefits as seen when target doses are achieved. Observational data suggest HR reduction may be a more sensitive therapeutic end point than dose as an indicator for the benefits of β-blockers.
2. Patients with SHF and sinus rhythm are at increased risk for stroke and other thromboembolic complications. The optimal approach to antithrombotic therapy (warfarin, aspirin, or no therapy) in these patients remains uncertain. A recent clinical trial showed no difference between warfarin and aspirin for preventing stroke (ischemic or hemorrhagic) or death. The risk of bleeding was higher in patients receiving warfarin compared with that in patients receiving aspirin. The optimal approach to preventing thromboembolic events in these patients remains to be determined.

EVALUATION OF THERAPEUTIC OUTCOMES

Although mortality is an important end point, it does not give a complete measure of the overall impact of this disorder because many patients are hospitalized repeatedly for HF exacerbations and continue to survive, albeit with a significantly reduced quality of life. Thus, some of the more important therapeutic outcomes in HF management, such as prolonged survival or prevention or slowing of the progression of HF, cannot be quantified in an individual patient. However, after appropriate diagnostic evaluation to determine the etiology of HF, ongoing clinical assessment of patients typically focuses on evaluation of three general areas: (a) functional capacity, (b) volume status, and (c) laboratory monitoring.

The evaluation of functional capacity should focus on the presence and severity of symptoms the patient experiences during activities of daily living and how his or her symptoms affect these activities. Questions directed toward the patient's ability to perform specific activities may be more informative than general questions about what symptoms the patient may be experiencing. For example, patients should be asked if they can exercise, climb stairs, get dressed without stopping, check the mail, go shopping, or clean the house. Another important component of assessment of functional capacity is to ask patients what activities they would like to do but are now unable to perform.

Assessment of volume status is a vital component of the ongoing care of patients with HF. This evaluation provides the clinician important information about the adequacy of diuretic therapy. Since the cardinal signs and symptoms of HF are caused by excess fluid retention, the efficacy of diuretic treatment is readily evaluated by the disappearance of these signs and symptoms. The physical examination is the primary method for the evaluation of fluid retention, and specific attention should be focused on the patient's body weight, extent of JVD, presence of hepatojugular reflux, presence

TABLE 4-14 ACC/AHA Clinical Performance Measures for Adults with Systolic Heart Failure

Performance Measure	Recommendation
Inpatient Measures	
Evaluation of left ventricular systolic function[a]	Echocardiogram with Doppler flow studies is the most useful test as it enables clinicians to determine the presence of pericardial, myocardial, or valvular abnormalities. Patients with LVEF <40% should be considered for specific therapy (e.g., ACE inhibitors, β-blockers). *Class I recommendation, Level of Evidence C*
ACE inhibitors or ARBs for patients with left ventricular systolic dysfunction[a]	Patients with a LVEF <40% or moderate or severe systolic dysfunction should receive an ACE inhibitor or ARB unless contraindications are present or there is a history of intolerance to both drugs. ACE inhibitors: *Class I recommendation, Level of Evidence A*. ARBs: *Class I, Level of Evidence A*
β-Blocker therapy for patients with left ventricular systolic dysfunction	All patients with stable heart failure and LVEF 40% should receive treatment with one of the three β-blockers proven to reduce mortality unless contraindicated. *Class I recommendation, Level of Evidence A*
Postdischarge followup appointment	At the time of hospital discharge, patients should receive an appointment for a followup visit to occur within 7–10 days of discharge
Outpatient Measures	
Evaluation of left ventricular systolic function	Echocardiogram with Doppler flow studies is the most useful test as it enables clinicians to determine the presence of pericardial, myocardial, or valvular abnormalities. Patients with LVEF <40% should be considered for specific therapy (e.g., ACE inhibitors, β-blockers). *Class I recommendation, Level of Evidence C*
Symptom and activity assessment	Both initial and ongoing quantitative assessment of symptom type, severity, duration, and their impact on the patient's functional capacity should be performed. This can be accomplished using the NYHA functional classification or other established evaluation instruments (e.g., Minnesota Living with Heart Failure Questionnaire). *Class I recommendation, Level of Evidence C*
β-Blocker therapy for patients with left ventricular systolic dysfunction	All patients with stable heart failure and decreased LVEF should receive treatment with one of the three β-blockers proven to reduce mortality unless contraindicated. *Class I recommendation, Level of Evidence A*
ACE inhibitors or ARBs for patients with left ventricular systolic dysfunction	Patients with a LVEF <40% or moderate or severe systolic dysfunction should receive an ACE inhibitor or ARB unless contraindications are present or there is a history of intolerance to both drugs. ACE inhibitors: *Class I recommendation, Level of Evidence A*. ARBs: *Class 1, Level of Evidence A*

[a]Also Center for Medicare and Medicaid Services (CMS) and Joint Commission Core Measures

Adapted from reference 158.

and severity of pulmonary congestion, and peripheral edema. Specifically, in a patient with pulmonary congestion, monitoring is indicated for resolution of rales and pulmonary edema and improvement or resolution of DOE, orthopnea, and PND. For patients with systemic congestion, a decrease or disappearance of peripheral edema, JVD, and hepatojugular reflux is sought. Other therapeutic outcomes include an improvement in exercise tolerance and fatigue, decreased nocturia, and a decrease in HR. Clinicians also will want to monitor BP and ensure that the patient does not develop symptomatic hypotension as a result of drug therapy. Body weight is a sensitive short-term marker of fluid loss or retention, and patients should be counseled to weigh themselves daily, reporting changes to their healthcare provider so that adjustments can be made in diuretic doses. Patients and healthcare providers should be aware that HF progression may be slowed even though symptoms have not resolved.

Routine monitoring of serum electrolytes and renal function is required in patients with HF. Assessment of serum potassium and magnesium is especially important because hypokalemia and hypomagnesemia are common adverse effects of diuretic therapy and are associated with an increased risk of arrhythmias and digoxin toxicity (hypokalemia). Serum potassium monitoring is also required because of the risk of hyperkalemia associated with ACE inhibitors, ARBs, and aldosterone antagonists. A serum potassium ≥4 mEq/L (≥4 mmol/L) should be maintained with some evidence suggesting it should be ≥4.5 mEq/L (≥4.5 mmol/L).[157] Assessment of renal function (BUN and serum creatinine) is also an important end point for monitoring diuretic and ACE inhibitor therapy. Common causes of worsening renal function in patients with HF include overdiuresis, adverse effects of ACE inhibitor or ARB therapy, and hypoperfusion.

Most of these therapeutic end points are incorporated into the ACC/AHA performance measures outlined in Table 4-14.[158]

ABBREVIATIONS

ACC	American College of Cardiology
ACE	angiotensin-converting enzyme
AF-CHF	Atrial Fibrillation and Congestive Heart Failure
AHA	American Heart Association
A-HeFT	African-American Heart Failure Trial
ANP	atrial natriuretic peptide
ARB	angiotensin receptor blocker
AT1	angiotensin type 1
AVP	arginine vasopressin
BNP	B-type natriuretic peptide
BP	blood pressure
BUN	blood urea nitrogen
cAMP	cyclic adenosine monophosphate
cGMP	cyclic guanosine monophosphate
CHARM	Candesartan in Heart Failure: Assessment of Reduction in Mortality and Morbidity
CIBIS II	Cardiac Insufficiency Bisoprolol Study II
CMS	Centers for Medicare and Medicaid Services
CNP	C-type natriuretic peptide
CO	cardiac output
COMET	Carvedilol Or Metoprolol European Trial
COPERNICUS	Carvedilol, Prospective, Randomized, Cumulative Survival
CRT	cardiac resynchronization therapy
DIG	Digitalis Investigation Group
ESC	European Society of Cardiology
ET	endothelin
HEAAL	Heart Failure Endpoint Evaluation of Angiotensin II Antagonist Losartan
HF	heart failure
HFpEF	heart failure with preserved ejection fraction
HFSA	Heart Failure Society of America
HR	heart rate
HTN	hypertension
ICD	implantable cardioverter-defibrillator
I-PRESERVE	Irbesartan in Heart Failure with Preserved EF
ISDN	isosorbide dinitrate
JVD	jugular venous distension
LVEDP	left ventricular end-diastolic pressure
LVEDV	left ventricular end-diastolic volume
LVEF	left ventricular ejection fraction
MAP	mean arterial pressure
MERIT-HF	Metoprolol CR/XL Randomised Intervention Trial in Congestive Heart Failure
MI	myocardial infarction
NE	norepinephrine
NOS3	nitric oxide synthase-3
NSAID	nonsteroidal antiinflammatory drug
NYHA	New York Heart Association
PAOP	pulmonary artery occlusion pressure
PCWP	pulmonary capillary wedge pressure
P-gp	P-glycoprotein
PND	paroxysmal nocturnal dyspnea
RAAS	renin–angiotensin–aldosterone system
RALES	Randomized Aldactone Evaluation Study
SDC	serum digoxin concentration
SHF	systolic heart failure
SNS	sympathetic nervous system
SV	stroke volume
SVR	systemic vascular resistance
TZD	thiazolidinedione

REFERENCES

1. Hunt SA, Abraham WT, Chin MH, et al. 2009 focused update incorporated into the ACC/AHA 2005 guidelines for the diagnosis and management of heart failure in adults: A report of the American College of Cardiology Foundation/American Heart Association Task Force on Practice Guidelines: Developed in collaboration with the International Society for Heart and Lung Transplantation. Circulation 2009;119:e391–e479.
2. Borlaug BA, Paulus WJ. Heart failure with preserved ejection fraction: Pathophysiology, diagnosis, and treatment. Eur Heart J 2011;32:670–679.
3. Roger VL, Go AS, Lloyd-Jones DM, et al. Heart disease and stroke statistics—2012 update: A report from the American Heart Association. Circulation 2012;125:e2–e220.
4. Chen J, Normand SL, Wang Y, Krumholz HM. National and regional trends in heart failure hospitalization and mortality rates for Medicare beneficiaries, 1998–2008. JAMA 2011;306:1669–1678.
5. Agarwal SK, Chambless LE, Ballantyne CM, et al. Prediction of incident heart failure in general practice: The Atherosclerosis Risk in Communities (ARIC) Study. Circ Heart Fail 2012;5:422–429.
6. Kalogeropoulos A, Psaty BM, Vasan RS, et al. Validation of the health ABC heart failure model for incident heart failure risk prediction: The Cardiovascular Health Study. Circ Heart Fail 2010;3:495–502.
7. Mann DL. Pathophysiology of heart failure. In: Bonow RO, Mann DL, Zipes DP, Libby P, eds. Braunwald's Heart Disease: A Textbook of Cardiovascular Medicine, 9th ed. Philadelphia, PA: Elsevier, 2012:487–504.

8. Maeder MT, Kaye DM. Heart failure with normal left ventricular ejection fraction. J Am Coll Cardiol 2009;53: 905–918.
9. McMurray JJ. Clinical practice. Systolic heart failure. N Engl J Med 2010;362:228–238.
10. Watkins H, Ashrafian H, Redwood C. Inherited cardiomyopathies. N Engl J Med 2011;364:1643–1656.
11. Leite-Moreira AF. Current perspectives in diastolic dysfunction and diastolic heart failure. Heart 2006;92:712–718.
12. Floras JS. Sympathetic nervous system activation in human heart failure: Clinical implications of an updated model. J Am Coll Cardiol 2009;54:375–385.
13. Johnson JA, Liggett SB. Cardiovascular pharmacogenomics of adrenergic receptor signaling: Clinical implications and future directions. Clin Pharmacol Ther 2011;89:366–378.
14. Braunwald E. Biomarkers in heart failure. N Engl J Med 2008;358:2148–2159.
15. McMurray JJ. CONSENSUS to EMPHASIS: The overwhelming evidence which makes blockade of the renin–angiotensin–aldosterone system the cornerstone of therapy for systolic heart failure. Eur J Heart Fail 2011; 13:929–936.
16. Wong J, Patel RA, Kowey PR. The clinical use of angiotensin-converting enzyme inhibitors. Prog Cardiovasc Dis 2004;47:116–130.
17. Triposkiadis F, Karayannis G, Giamouzis G, Skoularigis J, Louridas G, Butler J. The sympathetic nervous system in heart failure physiology, pathophysiology, and clinical implications. J Am Coll Cardiol 2009;54:1747–1762.
18. Weber KT. The proinflammatory heart failure phenotype: A case of integrative physiology. Am J Med Sci 2005;330: 219–226.
19. Weber KT, Weglicki WB, Simpson RU. Macro- and micronutrient dyshomeostasis in the adverse structural remodelling of myocardium. Cardiovasc Res 2009;81: 500–508.
20. Pitt B, Zannad F, Remme WJ, et al. The effect of spironolactone on morbidity and mortality in patients with severe heart failure. Randomized Aldactone Evaluation Study Investigators. N Engl J Med 1999;341:709–717.
21. Pitt B, Remme W, Zannad F, et al. Eplerenone, a selective aldosterone blocker, in patients with left ventricular dysfunction after myocardial infarction. N Engl J Med 2003;348:1309–1321.
22. Zannad F, McMurray JJ, Krum H, et al. Eplerenone in patients with systolic heart failure and mild symptoms. N Engl J Med 2011;364:11–21.
23. Maisel AS, Choudhary R. Biomarkers in acute heart failure—State of the art. Nat Rev Cardiol 2012;9:478–490.
24. Maisel AS, Daniels LB. Breathing not properly 10 years later: What we have learned and what we still need to learn. J Am Coll Cardiol 2012;60:277–282.
25. Maisel AS, McCord J, Nowak RM, et al. Bedside B-type natriuretic peptide in the emergency diagnosis of heart failure with reduced or preserved ejection fraction. Results from the Breathing Not Properly Multinational Study. J Am Coll Cardiol 2003;41:2010–2017.
26. Tschope C, Kasner M, Westermann D, Gaub R, Poller WC, Schultheiss HP. The role of NT-proBNP in the diagnostics of isolated diastolic dysfunction: Correlation with echocardiographic and invasive measurements. Eur Heart J 2005;26:2277–2284.
27. Lindenfeld J, Albert NM, Boehmer JP, et al. HFSA 2010 comprehensive heart failure practice guideline. J Card Fail 2010;16:e1–e194.
28. Reilly T, Schork MR. Vasopressin antagonists: Pharmacotherapy for the treatment of heart failure. Ann Pharmacother 2010;44:680–687.
29. Fonarow GC, Abraham WT, Albert NM, et al. Factors identified as precipitating hospital admissions for heart failure and clinical outcomes: Findings from OPTIMIZE-HF. Arch Intern Med 2008;168:847–854.
30. Anter E, Jessup M, Callans DJ. Atrial fibrillation and heart failure: Treatment considerations for a dual epidemic. Circulation 2009;119:2516–2525.
31. Mountantonakis SE, Grau-Sepulveda MV, Bhatt DL, Hernandez AF, Peterson ED, Fonarow GC. Presence of atrial fibrillation is independently associated with adverse outcomes in patients hospitalized with heart failure: An analysis of get with the guidelines-heart failure. Circ Heart Fail 2012;5:191–201.
32. Molloy GJ, O'Carroll RE, Witham MD, McMurdo ME. Interventions to enhance adherence to medications in patients with heart failure: A systematic review. Circ Heart Fail 2012;5:126–133.
33. Maxwell CB, Jenkins AT. Drug-induced heart failure. Am J Health Syst Pharm 2011;68:1791–1804.
34. Koshman SL, Charrois TL, Simpson SH, McAlister FA, Tsuyuki RT. Pharmacist care of patients with heart failure: A systematic review of randomized trials. Arch Intern Med 2008;168:687–694.
35. Murray MD, Ritchey ME, Wu J, Tu W. Effect of a pharmacist on adverse drug events and medication errors in outpatients with cardiovascular disease. Arch Intern Med 2009;169:757–763.
36. Greenberg B, Kahn A. Clinical assessment of heart failure. In: Bonow RO, Mann DL, Zipes DP, Libby P, eds. Braunwald's Heart Disease: A Textbook of Cardiovascular Medicine, 8th ed. Philadelphia, PA: Elsevier, 2012: 505–516.
37. Borlaug BA, Redfield MM. Diastolic and systolic heart failure are distinct phenotypes within the heart failure spectrum. Circulation 2011;123:2006–2013 [discussion 14].
38. Downing J, Balady GJ. The role of exercise training in heart failure. J Am Coll Cardiol 2011;58:561–569.
39. Gupta D, Georgiopoulou VV, Kalogeropoulos AP, et al. Dietary sodium intake in heart failure. Circulation 2012; 126:479–485.
40. Riegel B, Moser DK, Anker SD, et al. State of the science: Promoting self-care in persons with heart failure: A scientific statement from the American Heart Association. Circulation 2009;120:1141–1163.
41. McMurray JJ, Adamopoulos S, Anker SD, et al. ESC guidelines for the diagnosis and treatment of acute and chronic heart failure 2012: The Task Force for the Diagnosis and Treatment of Acute and Chronic Heart Failure 2012 of the European Society of Cardiology. Developed in collaboration with the Heart Failure Association (HFA) of the ESC. Eur Heart J 2012;33:1787–1847.
42. Fonarow GC, Albert NM, Curtis AB, et al. Incremental reduction in risk of death associated with use of guideline-recommended therapies in patient with heart failure: A nested case–control analysis of IMPROVE-HF. J Am Heart Assoc 2012;1:16–26.
43. Holland R, Battersby J, Harvey I, Lenaghan E, Smith J, Hay L. Systematic review of multidisciplinary interventions in heart failure. Heart 2005;91:899–906.
44. Clark AM, Savard LA, Thompson DR. What is the strength of evidence for heart failure disease-management programs? J Am Coll Cardiol 2009;54:397–401.

45. Murray M, Young J, Hoke S, et al. Pharmacist intervention to improve medication adherence in heart failure. A randomized trial. Ann Intern Med 2007;146:714–725.
46. Lowrie R, Mair FS, Greenlaw N, et al. Pharmacist intervention in primary care to improve outcomes in patients with left ventricular systolic dysfunction. Eur Heart J 2012; 33:314–324.
47. Catananti C, Liperoti R, Settanni S, et al. Heart failure and adverse drug reactions among hospitalized older adults. Clin Pharmacol Ther 2009;86:307–310.
48. Smith SC Jr, Benjamin EJ, Bonow RO, et al. AHA/ACCF secondary prevention and risk reduction therapy for patients with coronary and other atherosclerotic vascular disease: 2011 update: A guideline from the American Heart Association and American College of Cardiology Foundation. Circulation 2011;124:2458–2473.
49. Cleland JG, Tendera M, Adamus J, Freemantle N, Polonski L, Taylor J. The perindopril in elderly people with chronic heart failure (PEP-CHF) study. Eur Heart J 2006;27:2338–2345.
50. Hori M, Kitabatake A, Tsutsui H, et al. Rationale and design of a randomized trial to assess the effects of beta-blocker in diastolic heart failure; Japanese Diastolic Heart Failure Study (J-DHF). J Card Fail 2005;11:542–547.
51. van Veldhuisen DJ, Cohen-Solal A, Bohm M, et al. Beta-blockade with nebivolol in elderly heart failure patients with impaired and preserved left ventricular ejection fraction: Data From SENIORS (Study of Effects of Nebivolol Intervention on Outcomes and Rehospitalization in Seniors With Heart Failure). J Am Coll Cardiol 2009; 53:2150–2158.
52. Massie BM, Fabi MR. Clinical trials in diastolic heart failure. Prog Cardiovasc Dis 2005;47:389–395.
53. Goodlin SJ. Palliative care in congestive heart failure. J Am Coll Cardiol 2009;54:386–396.
54. Allen LA, Stevenson LW, Grady KL, et al. Decision making in advanced heart failure: A scientific statement from the American Heart Association. Circulation 2012;125:1928–1952.
55. Echt DS, Liebson PR, Mitchell LB, et al. Mortality and morbidity in patients receiving encainide, flecainide, or placebo. The Cardiac Arrhythmia Suppression Trial. N Engl J Med 1991;324:781–788.
56. Bardy GH, Lee KL, Mark DB, et al. Amiodarone or an implantable cardioverter-defibrillator for congestive heart failure. N Engl J Med 2005;352:225–237.
57. Adabag S, Roukoz H, Anand IS, Moss AJ. Cardiac resynchronization therapy in patients with minimal heart failure: A systematic review and meta-analysis. J Am Coll Cardiol 2011;58:935–941.
58. Holzmeister J, Leclercq C. Implantable cardioverter defibrillators and cardiac resynchronisation therapy. Lancet 2011;378:722–730.
59. Tang AS, Wells GA, Talajic M, et al. Cardiac-resynchronization therapy for mild-to-moderate heart failure. N Engl J Med 2010; 363:2385–2395.
60. Brater DC. Pharmacology of diuretics. Am J Med Sci 2000; 319:38–50.
61. Shankar SS, Brater DC. Loop diuretics: From the Na–K–2Cl transporter to clinical use. Am J Physiol Renal Physiol 2003;284:F11–F21.
62. Prasun MA, Kocheril AG, Klass PH, Dunlap SH, Piano MR. The effects of a sliding scale diuretic titration protocol in patients with heart failure. J Cardiovasc Nurs 2005;20: 62–70.
63. Dries DL, Strong MH, Cooper RS, Drazner MH. Efficacy of angiotensin-converting enzyme inhibition in reducing progression from asymptomatic left ventricular dysfunction to symptomatic heart failure in black and white patients. J Am Coll Cardiol 2002;40:311–317.
64. Dagenais GR, Pogue J, Fox K, Simoons ML, Yusuf S. Angiotensin-converting-enzyme inhibitors in stable vascular disease without left ventricular systolic dysfunction or heart failure: A combined analysis of three trials. Lancet 2006;368:581–588.
65. Zamora E, Lupon J, Vila J, et al. Estimated glomerular filtration rate and prognosis in heart failure: Value of the Modification of Diet in Renal Disease Study-4, chronic kidney disease epidemiology collaboration, and cockroft-gault formulas. J Am Coll Cardiol 2012;59:1709–1715.
66. Berger AK, Duval S, Manske C, et al. Angiotensin-converting enzyme inhibitors and angiotensin receptor blockers in patients with congestive heart failure and chronic kidney disease. Am Heart J 2007;153:1064–1073.
67. Ahmed A, Fonarow GC, Zhang Y, et al. Renin–angiotensin inhibition in systolic heart failure and chronic kidney disease. Am J Med 2012;125:399–410.
68. Rodgers JE, Stough WG. Underutilization of evidence-based therapies in heart failure: The pharmacist's role. Pharmacotherapy 2007;27:18S–28S.
69. Gheorghiade M, Albert NM, Curtis AB, et al. Medication dosing in outpatients with heart failure after implementation of a practice-based performance improvement intervention: Findings from IMPROVE HF. Congest Heart Fail 2012; 18:9–17.
70. Packer M, Poole-Wilson PA, Armstrong PW, et al. Comparative effects of low and high doses of the angiotensin-converting enzyme inhibitor, lisinopril, on morbidity and mortality in chronic heart failure. ATLAS Study Group. Circulation 1999;100:2312–2318.
71. Packer M, Bristow MR, Cohn JN, et al. The effect of carvedilol on morbidity and mortality in patients with chronic heart failure. U.S. Carvedilol Heart Failure Study Group. N Engl J Med 1996;334:1349–1355.
72. Effect of metoprolol CR/XL in chronic heart failure: Metoprolol CR/XL Randomised Intervention Trial in Congestive Heart Failure (MERIT-HF). Lancet 1999;353:2001–2007.
73. The Cardiac Insufficiency Bisoprolol Study II (CIBIS-II): A randomised trial. Lancet 1999;353:9–13.
74. Packer M, Coats AJ, Fowler MB, et al. Effect of carvedilol on survival in severe chronic heart failure. N Engl J Med 2001;344:1651–1658.
75. Dargie HJ. Effect of carvedilol on outcome after myocardial infarction in patients with left-ventricular dysfunction: The CAPRICORN randomised trial. Lancet 2001;357: 1385–1390.
76. Packer M, Fowler MB, Roecker EB, et al. Effect of carvedilol on the morbidity of patients with severe chronic heart failure: Results of the carvedilol prospective randomized cumulative survival (COPERNICUS) study. Circulation 2002;106:2194–2199.
77. Hjalmarson A, Goldstein S, Fagerberg B, et al. Effects of controlled-release metoprolol on total mortality, hospitalizations, and well-being in patients with heart failure: The Metoprolol CR/XL Randomized Intervention Trial in congestive heart failure (MERIT-HF). MERIT-HF Study Group. JAMA 2000;283:1295–1302.
78. Kukin ML, Kalman J, Charney RH, et al. Prospective, randomized comparison of effect of long-term treatment with metoprolol or carvedilol on symptoms, exercise, ejection fraction, and oxidative stress in heart failure. Circulation 1999;99:2645–2651.

79. Metra M, Nodari S, Parrinello G, Giubbini R, Manca C, Dei Cas L. Marked improvement in left ventricular ejection fraction during long-term beta-blockade in patients with chronic heart failure: Clinical correlates and prognostic significance. Am Heart J 2003;145:292–299.
80. Bristow MR, Gilbert EM, Abraham WT, et al. Carvedilol produces dose-related improvements in left ventricular function and survival in subjects with chronic heart failure. MOCHA Investigators. Circulation 1996;94:2807–2816.
81. Willenheimer R, van Veldhuisen DJ, Silke B, et al. Effect on survival and hospitalization of initiating treatment for chronic heart failure with bisoprolol followed by enalapril, as compared with the opposite sequence: Results of the randomized Cardiac Insufficiency Bisoprolol Study (CIBIS) III. Circulation 2005;112:2426–2435.
82. Gattis WA, O'Connor CM, Gallup DS, Hasselblad V, Gheorghiade M. Predischarge initiation of carvedilol in patients hospitalized for decompensated heart failure: Results of the Initiation Management Predischarge: Process for Assessment of Carvedilol Therapy in Heart Failure (IMPACT-HF) trial. J Am Coll Cardiol 2004;43:1534–1541.
83. McAlister FA, Wiebe N, Ezekowitz JA, Leung AA, Armstrong PW. Meta-analysis: Beta-blocker dose, heart rate reduction, and death in patients with heart failure. Ann Intern Med 2009;150:784–794.
84. Packer M. Controlled-release carvedilol: A concluding perspective. Am J Cardiol 2006;98:67–69.
85. Zile MR. Diastolic heart failure. Diagnosis, prognosis, treatment. Minerva Cardioangiol 2003;51:131–142.
86. Zhou J, Shi H, Zhang J, Lu Y, Fu M, Ge J. Rationale and design of the beta-blocker in heart failure with normal left ventricular ejection fraction (beta-PRESERVE) study. Eur J Heart Fail 2010;12:181–185.
87. Cohn JN, Tognoni G. A randomized trial of the angiotensin-receptor blocker valsartan in chronic heart failure. N Engl J Med 2001;345:1667–1675.
88. Pfeffer MA, McMurray JJ, Velazquez EJ, et al. Valsartan, captopril, or both in myocardial infarction complicated by heart failure, left ventricular dysfunction, or both. N Engl J Med 2003;349:1893–1906.
89. Pfeffer MA, Swedberg K, Granger CB, et al. Effects of candesartan on mortality and morbidity in patients with chronic heart failure: The CHARM-Overall programme. Lancet 2003;362:759–766.
90. McMurray JJ, Ostergren J, Swedberg K, et al. Effects of candesartan in patients with chronic heart failure and reduced left-ventricular systolic function taking angiotensin-converting-enzyme inhibitors: The CHARM-Added trial. Lancet 2003;362:767–771.
91. Granger CB, McMurray JJ, Yusuf S, et al. Effects of candesartan in patients with chronic heart failure and reduced left-ventricular systolic function intolerant to angiotensin-converting-enzyme inhibitors: The CHARM-Alternative trial. Lancet 2003;362:772–776.
92. Konstam MA, Neaton JD, Dickstein K, et al. Effects of high-dose versus low-dose losartan on clinical outcomes in patients with heart failure (HEAAL study): A randomised, double-blind trial. Lancet 2009;374:1840–1848.
93. Svanstrom H, Pasternak B, Hviid A. Association of treatment with losartan vs candesartan and mortality among patients with heart failure. JAMA 2012;307:1506–1512.
94. Haymore BR, Yoon J, Mikita CP, Klote MM, DeZee KJ. Risk of angioedema with angiotensin receptor blockers in patients with prior angioedema associated with angiotensin-converting enzyme inhibitors: A meta-analysis. Ann Allergy Asthma Immunol 2008;101:495–499.
95. Phillips CO, Kashani A, Ko DK, Francis G, Krumholz HM. Adverse effects of combination angiotensin II receptor blockers plus angiotensin-converting enzyme inhibitors for left ventricular dysfunction: A quantitative review of data from randomized clinical trials. Arch Intern Med 2007;167:1930–1936.
96. Yusuf S, Pfeffer MA, Swedberg K, et al. Effects of candesartan in patients with chronic heart failure and preserved left-ventricular ejection fraction: The CHARM-Preserved Trial. Lancet 2003;362:777–781.
97. Massie BM, Carson PE, McMurray JJ, et al. Irbesartan in patients with heart failure and preserved ejection fraction. N Engl J Med 2008;359:2456–2467.
98. Butler J, Ezekowitz JA, Collins SP, et al. Update on aldosterone antagonists use in heart failure with reduced left ventricular ejection fraction Heart Failure Society of America Guidelines Committee. J Card Fail 2012;18: 265–281.
99. Carbone LD, Cross JD, Raza SH, et al. Fracture risk in men with congestive heart failure risk reduction with spironolactone. J Am Coll Cardiol 2008;52:135–138.
100. Albert NM, Yancy CW, Liang L, et al. Use of aldosterone antagonists in heart failure. JAMA 2009;302:1658–1665.
101. Juurlink DN, Mamdani MM, Lee DS, et al. Rates of hyperkalemia after publication of the Randomized Aldactone Evaluation Study. N Engl J Med 2004;351:543–551.
102. Bozkurt B, Agoston I, Knowlton AA. Complications of inappropriate use of spironolactone in heart failure: When an old medicine spirals out of new guidelines. J Am Coll Cardiol 2003;41:211–214.
103. Svensson M, Gustafsson F, Galatius S, Hildebrandt PR, Atar D. How prevalent is hyperkalemia and renal dysfunction during treatment with spironolactone in patients with congestive heart failure? J Card Fail 2004;10:297–303.
104. Terra SG, Washam JB, Dunham GD, Gattis WA. Therapeutic range of digoxin's efficacy in heart failure: What is the evidence? Pharmacotherapy 1999;19:1123–1126.
105. Eichhorn EJ, Gheorghiade M. Digoxin. Prog Cardiovasc Dis 2002;44:251–266.
106. Gheorghiade M, Adams KF Jr, Colucci WS. Digoxin in the management of cardiovascular disorders. Circulation 2004;109:2959–2964.
107. Packer M, Gheorghiade M, Young JB, et al. Withdrawal of digoxin from patients with chronic heart failure treated with angiotensin-converting-enzyme inhibitors. RADIANCE Study. N Engl J Med 1993;329:1–7.
108. Uretsky B, Young JB, Shahidi FE, et al. Randomized study assessing the effect of digoxin withdrawal in patients with mild to moderate chronic congestive heart failure: Results of the PROVED trial. J Am Coll Cardiol 1993;22:955–962.
109. The Digitalis Investigation Group. The effect of digoxin on mortality and morbidity in patients with heart failure. N Engl J Med 1997;336:525–533.
110. Ahmed A, Rich MW, Fleg JL, et al. Effects of digoxin on morbidity and mortality in diastolic heart failure: The ancillary digitalis investigation group trial. Circulation 2006;114:397–403.
111. Ahmed A, Gambassi G, Weaver MT, Young JB, Wehrmacher WH, Rich MW. Effects of discontinuation of digoxin versus continuation at low serum digoxin concentrations in chronic heart failure. Am J Cardiol 2007;100:280–284.
112. Adams KF Jr, Gheorghiade M, Uretsky BF, Patterson JH, Schwartz TA, Young JB. Clinical benefits of low serum digoxin concentrations in heart failure. J Am Coll Cardiol 2002;39:946–953.

113. Ahmed A, Rich MW, Love TE, et al. Digoxin and reduction in mortality and hospitalization in heart failure: A comprehensive post hoc analysis of the DIG trial. Eur Heart J 2006;27:178–186.
114. Rathore SS, Wang Y, Krumholz HM. Sex-based differences in the effect of digoxin for the treatment of heart failure. N Engl J Med 2002;347:1403–1411.
115. Adams KF Jr, Patterson JH, Gattis WA, et al. Relationship of serum digoxin concentration to mortality and morbidity in women in the digitalis investigation group trial: A retrospective analysis. J Am Coll Cardiol 2005;46:497–504.
116. Bauman JL, Didomenico RJ, Galanter WL. Mechanisms, manifestations, and management of digoxin toxicity in the modern era. Am J Cardiovasc Drugs 2006;6:77–86.
117. Schentag J, Bang A, Kozinski-Tober J. Digoxin. In: Burton M, Shaw L, Schentag J, Evans W, eds. Applied Pharmacokinetics and Pharmacodynamics, 4th ed. Baltimore: Lippincott Williams & Wilkins, 2006:411–439.
118. Bauman JL, DiDomenico RJ, Viana M, Fitch M. A method of determining the dose of digoxin for heart failure in the modern era. Arch Intern Med 2006;166:2539–2545.
119. Butler J, Anand IS, Kuskowski MA, Rector T, Carson P, Cohn JN. Digoxin use and heart failure outcomes: Results from the Valsartan Heart Failure Trial (Val-HeFT). Congest Heart Fail 2010;16:191–195.
120. Gheorghiade M, van Veldhuisen DJ, Colucci WS. Contemporary use of digoxin in the management of cardiovascular disorders. Circulation 2006;113:2556–2564.
121. Cole RT, Kalogeropoulos AP, Georgiopoulou VV, et al. Hydralazine and isosorbide dinitrate in heart failure: Historical perspective, mechanisms, and future directions. Circulation 2011;123:2414–2422.
122. Cohn JN, Archibald DG, Ziesche S, et al. Effect of vasodilator therapy on mortality in chronic congestive heart failure. Results of a Veterans Administration Cooperative Study. N Engl J Med 1986;314:1547–1552.
123. Cohn JN, Johnson G, Ziesche S, et al. A comparison of enalapril with hydralazine–isosorbide dinitrate in the treatment of chronic congestive heart failure. N Engl J Med 1991;325:303–310.
124. Taylor AL, Ziesche S, Yancy C, et al. Combination of isosorbide dinitrate and hydralazine in blacks with heart failure. N Engl J Med 2004;351:2049–2057.
125. Chinnaiyan KM, Alexander D, Maddens M, McCullough PA. Curriculum in cardiology: Integrated diagnosis and management of diastolic heart failure. Am Heart J 2007;153:189–200.
126. Kjekshus J, Apetrei E, Barrios V, et al. Rosuvastatin in older patients with systolic heart failure. N Engl J Med 2007;357:2248–2261.
127. Tavazzi L, Maggioni AP, Marchioli R, et al. Effect of rosuvastatin in patients with chronic heart failure (the GISSI-HF trial): A randomised, double-blind, placebo-controlled trial. Lancet 2008;372:1231–1239.
128. Fuster V, Ryden LE, Cannom DS, et al. 2011 ACCF/AHA/HRS focused updates incorporated into the ACC/AHA/ESC 2006 guidelines for the management of patients with atrial fibrillation: A report of the American College of Cardiology Foundation/American Heart Association Task Force on practice guidelines. Circulation 2011;123:e269–e367.
129. Wyse DG, Waldo AL, DiMarco JP, et al. A comparison of rate control and rhythm control in patients with atrial fibrillation. N Engl J Med 2002;347:1825–1833.
130. Roy D, Talajic M, Nattel S, et al. Rhythm control versus rate control for atrial fibrillation and heart failure. N Engl J Med 2008;358:2667–2677.
131. Choy CK, Rodgers JE, Nappi JM, Haines ST. Type 2 diabetes mellitus and heart failure. Pharmacotherapy 2008;28:170–192.
132. Aguilar D, Chan W, Bozkurt B, Ramasubbu K, Deswal A. Metformin use and mortality in ambulatory patients with diabetes and heart failure. Circ Heart Fail 2011;4:53–58.
133. Shah DD, Fonarow GC, Horwich TB. Metformin therapy and outcomes in patients with advanced systolic heart failure and diabetes. J Card Fail 2010;16:200–206.
134. Murray MD, Deer MM, Ferguson JA, et al. Open-label randomized trial of torsemide compared with furosemide therapy for patients with heart failure. Am J Med 2001;111:513–520.
135. Young M, Plosker GL. Torasemide: A pharmacoeconomic review of its use in chronic heart failure. Pharmacoeconomics 2001;19:679–703.
136. Ahmed A, Husain A, Love TE, et al. Heart failure, chronic diuretic use, and increase in mortality and hospitalization: An observational study using propensity score methods. Eur Heart J 2006;27:1431–1439.
137. Masoudi FA, Wolfe P, Havranek EP, Rathore SS, Foody JM, Krumholz HM. Aspirin use in older patients with heart failure and coronary artery disease: National prescription patterns and relationship with outcomes. J Am Coll Cardiol 2005;46:955–962.
138. Schoolwerth AC, Sica DA, Ballermann BJ, Wilcox CS. Renal considerations in angiotensin converting enzyme inhibitor therapy: A statement for healthcare professionals from the Council on the Kidney in Cardiovascular Disease and the Council for High Blood Pressure Research of the American Heart Association. Circulation 2001;104:1985–1991.
139. Bangalore S, Kumar S, Messerli FH. Angiotensin-converting enzyme inhibitor associated cough: Deceptive information from the Physicians' Desk Reference. Am J Med 2010;123:1016–1030.
140. Miller DR, Oliveria SA, Berlowitz DR, Fincke BG, Stang P, Lillienfeld DE. Angioedema incidence in US veterans initiating angiotensin-converting enzyme inhibitors. Hypertension 2008;51:1624–1630.
141. Makani H, Messerli FH, Romero J, et al. Meta-analysis of randomized trials of angioedema as an adverse event of renin–angiotensin system inhibitors. Am J Cardiol 2012;110:383–391.
142. Cooper WO, Hernandez-Diaz S, Arbogast PG, et al. Major congenital malformations after first-trimester exposure to ACE inhibitors. N Engl J Med 2006;354:2443–2451.
143. Cicardi M, Zingale LC, Bergamaschini L, Agostoni A. Angioedema associated with angiotensin-converting enzyme inhibitor use: Outcome after switching to a different treatment. Arch Intern Med 2004;164:910–913.
144. The Beta-Blocker Evaluation of Survival Trial Investigators. A trial of the beta-blocker bucindolol in patients with advanced chronic heart failure. N Engl J Med 2001;344:1659–1667.
145. Poole-Wilson PA, Swedberg K, Cleland JG, et al. Comparison of carvedilol and metoprolol on clinical outcomes in patients with chronic heart failure in the Carvedilol Or Metoprolol European Trial (COMET): Randomised controlled trial. Lancet 2003;362:7–13.
146. Aquilante CL, Terra SG, Schofield RS, et al. Sustained restoration of autonomic balance with long- but not short-acting metoprolol in patients with heart failure. J Card Fail 2006;12:171–176.
147. Bakris GL, Fonseca V, Katholi RE, et al. Metabolic effects of carvedilol vs metoprolol in patients with type 2 diabetes mellitus and hypertension: A randomized controlled trial. JAMA 2004;292:2227–2236.

148. Deedwania PC, Giles TD, Klibaner M, et al. Efficacy, safety and tolerability of metoprolol CR/XL in patients with diabetes and chronic heart failure: Experiences from MERIT-HF. Am Heart J 2005;149:159–167.
149. Metra M, Torp-Pedersen C, Cleland JG, et al. Should beta-blocker therapy be reduced or withdrawn after an episode of decompensated heart failure? Results from COMET. Eur J Heart Fail 2007;9:901–909.
150. Fonarow GC, Abraham WT, Albert NM, et al. Influence of beta-blocker continuation or withdrawal on outcomes in patients hospitalized with heart failure: Findings from the OPTIMIZE-HF program. J Am Coll Cardiol 2008;52:190–199.
151. Jondeau G, Neuder Y, Eicher JC, et al. B-CONVINCED: Beta-blocker CONtinuation Vs. INterruption in patients with Congestive heart failure hospitalizED for a decompensation episode. Eur Heart J 2009;30:2186–2192.
152. Davis HM, Johnson JA. Heart failure pharmacogenetics: Past, present, and future. Curr Cardiol Rep 2011;13:175–184.
153. Bristow MR, Murphy GA, Krause-Steinrauf H, et al. An alpha2C-adrenergic receptor polymorphism alters the norepinephrine-lowering effects and therapeutic response of the beta-blocker bucindolol in chronic heart failure. Circ Heart Fail 2010;3:21–28.
154. Liggett SB, Mialet-Perez J, Thaneemit-Chen S, et al. A polymorphism within a conserved beta(1)-adrenergic receptor motif alters cardiac function and beta-blocker response in human heart failure. Proc Natl Acad Sci U S A 2006;103:11288–11293.
155. McNamara DM, Tam SW, Sabolinski ML, et al. Endothelial nitric oxide synthase (NOS3) polymorphisms in African Americans with heart failure: Results from the A-HeFT trial. J Card Fail 2009;15:191–198.
156. Rame JE, Tam SW, McNamara D, et al. Dysfunctional corin i555(p568) allele is associated with impaired brain natriuretic peptide processing and adverse outcomes in blacks with systolic heart failure: Results from the Genetic Risk Assessment in Heart Failure substudy. Circ Heart Fail 2009;2:541–548.
157. Macdonald JE, Struthers AD. What is the optimal serum potassium level in cardiovascular patients? J Am Coll Cardiol 2004;43:155–161.
158. Bonow RO, Ganiats TG, Beam CT, et al. ACCF/AHA/AMA-PCPI 2011 performance measures for adults with heart failure: A report of the American College of Cardiology Foundation/American Heart Association Task Force on Performance Measures and the American Medical Association-Physician Consortium for Performance Improvement. J Am Coll Cardiol 2012;59:1812–1832.

Acute Decompensated Heart Failure

Jo E. Rodgers and Brent N. Reed

5

KEY CONCEPTS

1. Unlike chronic heart failure therapies whose primary role is to improve survival, treatment goals for acute decompensated heart failure (ADHF) are directed toward relief of congestive symptoms, restoration of systemic oxygen transport and tissue perfusion through improved myocardial contractility, and minimization of further cardiac damage and other adverse effects.
2. Maximizing oral chronic heart failure therapy may assist with optimizing cardiac output and relieving congestion.
3. Patients presenting to the hospital with ADHF can be categorized into four subsets based upon fluid status (euvolemic or "dry" vs. fluid overloaded or "wet") and cardiac function (adequate cardiac output or "warm" vs. hypoperfusion or "cold"). Therefore, patients are either warm and dry, warm and wet, cold and dry, or cold and wet.
4. While invasive hemodynamic monitoring using a PA catheter does not alter outcomes in a broad population of ADHF patients, it is indicated in those who are refractory to initial therapy, whose volume status is unclear, or who have clinically significant hypotension (i.e., systolic blood pressure less than 80 mm Hg) or worsening renal function despite therapy.
5. Key hemodynamic parameters to monitor with a PA catheter include pulmonary capillary wedge pressure (PCWP; reflecting fluid status or "preload"), cardiac output or cardiac index (CI; reflecting the innate contractility of the heart), and systemic vascular resistance (reflecting vascular tone or "afterload"). While a normal PCWP (6 to 12 mm Hg) is desirable in healthy patients, higher filling pressures (15 to 18 mm Hg) are often necessary in patients with heart failure.
6. Three major therapeutic categories exist for the management of ADHF including diuretics, inotropes, and vasodilators. No therapy studied to date has conclusively been shown to decrease mortality and several may potentially worsen outcomes.
7. IV loop diuretics are considered first-line therapy for the management of ADHF associated with fluid overload nonresponsive to orally administered diuretics. While a variety of therapeutic options may be considered for refractory fluid overload, a recent clinical trial demonstrated no difference in outcomes between bolus and continuous administration of IV diuretics; however, administering high-dose IV diuretic (2.5-times the previous oral regimen) is associated with greater fluid removal rate. If patients continue to be refractory to, or experience worsening renal function with diuretic therapy, vasodilatory and inotropic therapy may be indicated. Placement of a pulmonary artery (PA) catheter may be helpful in guiding therapy in such patients.
8. IV inotropes are recommended for symptom relief or end-organ dysfunction in patients with left ventricular dysfunction and low cardiac output. Such therapy may be especially useful in patients with low systolic blood pressure (less than 90 mm Hg) or symptomatic hypotension in the setting of adequate filling pressures. Inotropic therapy may also be considered in patients who do not tolerate or respond to IV vasodilators or in patients with worsening renal function, but should be avoided in patients with reduced left heart filling pressures. Patients receiving these agents should be monitored continuously for arrhythmias.
9. Given the potential risks associated with inotropic therapy, vasodilators should be considered prior to their use.
10. IV vasodilators may be added to diuretics for rapid symptom resolution, especially in patients with acute pulmonary edema or severe hypertension. Such therapy may also be considered in patients who fail to respond to aggressive treatment with diuretics. Vasodilators should be avoided in patients with symptomatic hypotension and frequent blood pressure monitoring is necessary to ensure their safe use. In addition, these agents should not be used in patients with reduced left heart filling pressures. If patients fail to respond to IV diuretics or vasodilators or experience worsening renal function, IV inotropic therapy should be considered.
11. Vasopressin antagonists provide a new therapeutic option for managing hyponatremia in patients with euvolemic or hypervolemic hyponatremia. Tolvaptan is the only vasopressin antagonist indicated for hyponatremia associated with heart failure. Despite being an oral agent, tolvaptan should only be initiated in the hospital setting to allow for monitoring of volume status and serum sodium concentrations, as rapid correction of serum sodium may result in adverse neurological sequalae.
12. Given extended wait times for patients on the cardiac transplantation list, implantation of a ventricular assist device may be considered for those in whom extended time to identify a suitable donor is anticipated (i.e., "bridge" to transplant) or in whom transplantation is not an option (i.e., "destination" therapy).

INTRODUCTION

As discussed in the Systolic and Diastolic Heart Failure chapter (Chap. 4), the number of patients with heart failure (HF) is substantial and continues to increase. Despite survival from HF having improved over time, the 5-year mortality rate remains 50%. In addition, the growing number of patients with this disorder and the progressive nature of the disease have led to substantial increases in hospitalizations for HF. In addition, an estimated 5.1 million U.S. adults over 20 years of age have HF; it is estimated that by 2030, an additional 3 million people will have HF, representing a 25% increase in prevalence from 2013 estimates. At 40 years of age, the lifetime risk for developing HF is one in five in both men and women. Recent data indicate that over 1 million patients are hospitalized for HF annually, resulting in significant morbidity, mortality, and consumption of large quantities of healthcare resources.[1,2] Hospital admission for HF is associated with an increased risk of subsequent hospitalization and decreased survival.[3] The economic impact of heart failure is considerable with costs driven primarily by inpatient care.[2]

A number of terms have been used to characterize patients with worsening heart failure requiring hospitalization. Patients with persistent symptoms or *refractory* heart failure requiring specialized interventions despite optimal oral therapies are classified as Stage D in the American College of Cardiology/American Heart Association (ACC/AHA) classification scheme.[4–6] These patients typically fall into the category of New York Heart Association (NYHA) class III or IV. Specialized interventions may include the addition of select medications beyond standard therapy or consideration for various surgical options. The terms *acute decompensated heart failure* (ADHF) or *exacerbation of heart failure* refer to those patients with new or worsening signs or symptoms (often as a result of volume overload and/or hypoperfusion) requiring additional medical care such as emergency department visits and hospitalizations. The term *acute* heart failure may be misleading as it more often refers to the patient with a sudden onset of signs or symptoms in the setting of previously normal cardiac function. This chapter will focus on the management of patients with ADHF. Clinical syndromes within decompensated heart failure include pulmonary or systemic volume overload, low cardiac output, and acute pulmonary edema. Clinicians should recognize that patients may present with impaired or preserved left ventricular systolic function and a variety of etiologies may be responsible for the primary disease process. The clinical course of heart failure manifests as periods of relative stability with an increasing frequency in episodes of decompensation as the underlying disease progresses.[7]

Despite the considerable morbidity and mortality associated with ADHF, the first randomized placebo-controlled trials in this patient population were published in 2002.[8,9] In addition, it was not until 2005 that guidelines specifically addressing ADHF were promulgated. The Heart Failure Society of America (HFSA) and the ACC/AHA guidelines address the management of ADHF; however, the HFSA guidelines are more detailed and will be the focus of the remainder of this chapter.[4,6,10]

PATHOPHYSIOLOGY AND CLINICAL PRESENTATION

Patients requiring intensive therapy for ADHF may have a variety of underlying etiologies and clinical presentations.[10] Patients with worsening chronic heart failure comprise approximately 70% of heart failure hospitalizations. These patients can become refractory to oral therapies and decompensate following even a relatively mild insult (e.g., dietary indiscretion, nonsteroidal antiinflammatory drug use), medication noncompliance, or a concurrent noncardiac illness (e.g., infection). New or worsening cardiac processes, such as myocardial infarction, atrial fibrillation, hypertensive urgency/emergency, myocarditis, or acute valvular insufficiency may also result in decompensation in an otherwise stable patient. Secondly, de novo heart failure may occur when left ventricular dysfunction results from a large myocardial infarction or sudden elevation in blood pressure; such cases represent approximately 25% of admissions. A third group of patients with severe left ventricular systolic dysfunction associated with progressive worsening of cardiac output and refractoriness to therapy represents about 5% of heart failure admissions.[11] Additional insight into the clinical characteristics of patients presenting unexpectedly with ADHF indicates that a high percentage have hypertension and preserved left ventricular systolic function.[12]

Several studies have provided a better understanding of the prognostic factors associated with ADHF. Data from the Acute Decompensated Heart Failure National Registry (ADHERE), an archive of hospitalized patients with a primary diagnosis of ADHF, found blood urea nitrogen (BUN) greater than or equal to 43 mg/dL (15.4 mmol/L) to be the best individual predictor of in-hospital mortality, followed by systolic blood pressure less than 115 mm Hg and serum creatinine greater than or equal to 2.75 mg/dL (243 μmol/L). Using these three parameters, patients may be identified as low, intermediate, high, and very high risk with in-hospital mortalities of 2%, 6%, 13%, and 20%, respectively.[13] Hyponatremia, elevations in troponin I, ischemic etiology, and poor functional capacity are also negative prognostic factors.[11] Importantly, patients who survive a hospitalization for ADHF remain at high risk for rehospitalization or death. Data from the Organized Program to Initiate Lifesaving Treatment in Hospitalized Patients with Heart Failure (OPTIMIZE-HF) Registry, another archive of ADHF patients, indicated overall mortality and rehospitalization rates of 8.6% and 29.6%, respectively, at 60 to 90 days postdischarge.[14] In patients who survive a hospitalization for ADHF, low blood pressure and poor renal function are also negative prognostic markers for subsequent readmission or death.[14] However, use of standard heart failure therapies at discharge as well as coronary angiography or implantable cardioverter-defibrillator placement during hospitalization are associated with improved prognosis,[14] suggesting that optimal management of these patients during their hospitalization can yield beneficial effects on subsequent prognosis.

GENERAL APPROACH TO TREATMENT

❶ The overall goals of therapy in ADHF are to provide symptomatic relief while optimizing volume status and low cardiac output so that a patient can be discharged in a stable compensated state on oral drug therapy. Although diuretic, vasodilator, and positive inotropic therapy can be very effective at achieving these goals, their efficacy must be balanced against the potential for serious toxicity. Thus, another important goal is to minimize the risks associated with these therapies including renal dysfunction, myocardial injury, electrolyte depletion, hypotension, and arrhythmias.

In addition, all patients should be evaluated for potential etiologies contributing to decompensation as well as other precipitating factors, including atrial fibrillation and other arrhythmias, worsening hypertension, myocardial ischemia or infarction, anemia, hypothyroidism or hyperthyroidism, or other causes. Medications (including noncardiac medications) that may worsen cardiac function should also be considered as precipitating or contributing factors. Patients who may benefit from coronary revascularization should also be identified. Prior to discharge, optimization of chronic oral therapy and patient education are critical to preventing future hospitalizations. When available and appropriate, patients should be referred to a heart failure disease management program.[10]

A careful history and physical examination are key components in the diagnosis of ADHF. The history should focus on the potential etiologies of heart failure, the presence of any precipitating factors, onset, duration, and severity of symptoms, and a careful medication history. Current guidelines recommend making the diagnosis of ADHF based primarily on signs and symptoms.[10] The more common presentation of ADHF is severe fluid overload, and orthopnea is the symptom that best correlates with elevated pulmonary pressures.[15] Important elements of the physical examination include assessment of vital signs and weight, cardiac auscultation for heart sounds and murmurs, pulmonary auscultation for rales, and evaluation for the presence of peripheral edema. Jugular venous pressure is the most reliable indicator of volume status and should be carefully evaluated on admission and closely followed during hospitalization as an indicator of the efficacy of diuretic therapy.[15] An S3 gallop, suggestive of increased volume in the left ventricle, has high diagnostic specificity for heart failure decompensation.[16] Other physical findings such as pulmonary crackles and lower extremity edema have low specificity and sensitivity for the diagnosis of ADHF. The development of a bedside assay for plasma B-type natriuretic peptide (BNP) has focused considerable attention on the use of natriuretic peptide levels as an aid in the diagnosis of suspected heart failure.[17] Plasma BNP and N-terminal pro-BNP concentrations are positively correlated with the degree of left ventricular dysfunction and heart failure, and these assays are now frequently used in acute care settings to assist in the differential diagnosis of dyspnea (heart failure vs. asthma, chronic obstructive pulmonary disease, or infection). A low BNP concentration, often defined as less than 100 pg/mL (ng/L; 29 pmol/L), has a 96% predictive value for excluding heart failure as the underlying etiology of a patient presenting with dyspnea. In addition, an elevated BNP concentration prior to discharge is associated with an increased risk of poor long-term outcomes. However, some limitations exist with the use of BNP. For example, any disease process that increases right heart pressures will elevate BNP, including pulmonary emboli, chronic obstructive lung disease, and primary pulmonary hypertension. In addition, BNP concentrations may be mildly increased with advanced age, female gender, and renal dysfunction, and lower in the setting of obesity.[15] Although ongoing research will better characterize the role of BNP in the diagnosis and treatment of heart failure, current guidelines recommend obtaining a BNP concentration in conjunction with assessing signs and symptoms when the diagnosis of ADHF is uncertain.[10]

Hospitalization for ADHF *is recommended* or *should be considered* depending on patient presentation (Table 5-1). Most patients do not require admission to an intensive care unit and may be admitted to a monitored unit or general medical floor. If a patient experiences hemodynamic instability necessitating frequent monitoring of vital signs, invasive hemodynamic monitoring, or rapid titration of IV medications (with concurrent monitoring), admission to an intensive care unit may be required to assure safe and effective outcomes.

2 The first step in the management of ADHF is to ascertain that optimal treatment with oral medications has been achieved.[10] If fluid retention is evident on physical examination, aggressive diuresis should be pursued. Although increasing the dose of oral diuretic therapy may be effective in some cases, the use of IV diuretics is often necessary. Every effort should be made to optimize standard heart failure therapy including an ACE inhibitor and *β*-blocker. *β*-blocker therapy should generally be continued during a hospitalization unless recent dose initiation or uptitration was responsible for decompensation. In such cases, *β*-blocker therapy may be temporarily held or dose-reduced. Otherwise, discontinuation of *β*-blockers is discouraged as it has been associated with worse outcomes in patients in ADHF.[18,19] Appropriateness of initiating *β*-blockers prior to discharge will be discussed later in this chapter.

Discontinuation of ACE inhibitor or *β*-blocker therapy may be necessary in the setting of cardiogenic shock or symptomatic hypotension. Certain therapies may also need to be temporarily held in the setting of renal dysfunction, especially in the setting of oliguria or hyperkalemia (e.g., ACE inhibitor, angiotensin receptor blocker, aldosterone antagonist) or elevated serum digoxin concentrations. Therapies that can cause worsening renal function (e.g., ACE inhibitor) should only be initiatied or uptitrated cautiously during aggressive fluid removal with IV diuretic therapy. In addition, serum potassium concentrations should be monitored closely as IV diuretic therapy is transitioned to oral diuretic therapy, especially if an aldosterone antagonist was initiated during the hospital stay; this ensures such therapy can be tolerated on the oral diuretic dose prescribed at discharge. Most patients may continue to receive digoxin at low doses targeting a trough serum concentration of 0.5 to 1 ng/mL (0.6 to 1.3 nmol/L).[10] Discontinuation of digoxin is generally discouraged as an association between withdrawal of therapy and worsening HF has been well-documented.[20,21] Digoxin should only be discontinued if serum concentrations cannot be maintained in a desirable range.

Two general approaches exist for maximizing therapy in the ADHF patient. One is to use simple clinical parameters (e.g., signs and symptoms, blood pressure, renal function) and the other is to combine these parameters with invasive hemodynamic monitoring. In all ADHF patients, close monitoring is essential for ensuring an optimal response to therapy while avoiding adverse effects (summarized in Table 5-2). Daily monitoring to assess the efficacy of drug therapy should include weight, strict fluid intake and output, and heart failure signs and symptoms. Foley catheter placement is not recommended unless close monitoring of urine output is not otherwise possible. As safety endpoints, monitoring for electrolyte depletion, symptomatic hypotension, and renal dysfunction should

TABLE 5-1 Recommendations for Hospitalizing Patients Presenting with ADHF

Recommendation	Clinical Circumstances
Hospitalization recommended	Evidence of severely decompensated HF, including: • Hypotension • Worsening renal function • Altered mentation
	Dyspnea at rest • Typically reflected by resting tachypnea • Less commonly reflected by oxygen saturation <90% (<0.90)
	Hemodyamically significant arrhythmia • Including new onset of rapid atrial fibrillation
	Acute coronary syndromes
Hospitalization should be considered	Worsened congestion • Even without dyspnea • Typically reflected by a weight gain of ≥5 kg
	Signs and symptoms of pulmonary or systemic congestion • Even in the absence of weight gain
	Major electrolyte disturbance
	Associated comorbid conditions • Pneumonia • Pulmonary embolus • Diabetic ketoacidosis • Symptoms suggestive of transient ischemic accident or stroke
	Repeated implantable cardioverter-defibrillator firings
	Previously undiagnosed HF with signs and symptoms of systemic or pulmonary congestion

Data from Lindenfield J, et al. HFSA 2010 Comprehensive Heart Failure Practice Guidelines. J Card Fail 2010; 12:e134–e156.

TABLE 5-2 Monitoring Recommendations for Patients Hospitalized with ADHF

Value	Frequency	Specifics
Weight	At least daily	Determine after voiding in the morning Account for possible increased food intake due to improved appetite
Fluid intake/output	At least daily	
Vital signs	More than daily	Orthostatic blood pressure if indicated
Signs	At least daily	Edema, acites, pulmonary rales, hepatomegaly, increased jugular venous pressure, hepatojugular reflux, liver tenderness
Symptoms	At least daily	Orthopnea, paroxysmal nocturnal dyspnea, nocturnal cough, dyspnea, fatigue, lightheadedness
Electrolytes	At least daily	Potassium, sodium
Renal function	At least daily	Blood urea nitrogen, serum creatinine

Data from Lindenfield J, et al. HFSA 2010 comprehensive heart failure practice guidelines. J Card Fail 2010;12:e134–e156.

be assessed frequently. While many of the above parameters may be monitored daily, some will need to be monitored more frequently as dictated by patient clinical status. Vital signs should be assessed multiple times throughout the day at a frequency that is appropriate for the patient's degree of stability. Orthostatic blood pressure should be assessed at least once daily.[10]

PRINCIPLES OF THERAPY BASED ON CLINICAL PRESENTATION

3 Appropriate medical management of ADHF is guided by determining whether the patient has signs and symptoms of fluid overload ("wet" heart failure) or low cardiac output ("cold" heart failure).[15,22] As previously discussed, most patients present with *fluid overload* (or the "wet" profile). Symptoms consistent with pulmonary congestion include orthopnea and dyspnea with minimal exertion and those of systemic congestion include GI discomfort, ascites, and peripheral edema. Patients with no or minimal fluid overload (or the "dry" category of ADHF) may have symptoms that are more difficult to distinguish. Such patients may present with a syndrome of *low cardiac output* ("cold" heart failure) which is characterized principally by extreme fatigue as well as poor appetite, nausea, and early satiety, although GI symptoms may be a sign of congestion rather than low cardiac output to the GI tract. Patients with "cold" heart failure frequently exhibit worsening renal function and a decline in serum sodium concentrations, which, as previously discussed, are both associated with poor prognosis.

Many patients will present with signs and symptoms of both wet and cold types of ADHF. In these patients, low-output symptoms may not be obvious until congestion is optimally treated.

PRINCIPLES OF THERAPY BASED ON HEMODYNAMIC SUBSETS

Patients with ADHF may have critically reduced cardiac output, usually with low arterial blood pressure and systemic hypoperfusion resulting in organ system dysfunction (i.e., cardiogenic shock). They may also have pulmonary edema with hypoxemia, respiratory acidosis, and markedly increased work of breathing. With cardiopulmonary support, response to interventions should be assessed promptly to allow for timely adjustments in treatment. Since cardiopulmonary support must be instituted and adjusted rapidly, immediate assessment of each intervention limits risks and allows for more prompt adjustments in therapy. Continuous monitoring of ECG, continuous pulse oximetry, urine flow, and automated blood pressure recordings are standards of care for critically ill patients with cardiopulmonary decompensation. Peripheral or femoral arterial catheters may be utilized for continuous and accurate assessment of arterial pressure.

Hemodynamic Monitoring

4 The role of invasive hemodynamic monitoring in patients with ADHF remains controversial. In a clinical trial assessing the routine use of this strategy, PA catheter placement had no impact on survival after hospital discharge, although patients with a clear indication for its use were excluded.[23] Based on these results, the routine use of invasive monitoring is not currently recommended. However, invasive monitoring often provides essential information for adjusting drug therapy in patients with a confusing or complicated clinical picture and during dose titration of rapidly acting medications. Therefore, invasive monitoring should be considered in patients who are refractory to initial therapy, those in whom volume status is unclear, or those who have clinically significant hypotension (e.g., systolic blood pressure less than 80 mm Hg) or worsening renal function despite therapy. In addition, documentation of an adequate hemodynamic response to inotropic therapy is often necessary prior to committing patients to chronic outpatient inotropic therapy.[10] Finally, assessment of hemodynamic parameters is required to document adequate reversal of pulmonary hypertension prior to cardiac transplantation.[15]

5 Invasive hemodynamic monitoring is usually performed with a flow-directed PA catheter (also known as Swan-Ganz catheter) placed percutaneously through a central vein and advanced through the right side of the heart and into the PA. Inflation of a balloon proximal to the end port allows the catheter to "wedge," yielding the PA occlusion pressure, which estimates the pulmonary venous (left atrial) pressure and, in the absence of intracardiac shunt, mitral valve disease or pulmonary disease, the left ventricular end-diastolic pressure. While the term *pulmonary artery occlusion pressure* has previously been used to describe the filling pressure of the heart, the term *pulmonary capillary wedge pressure* (PCWP) is used more commonly in clinical practice and will be used henceforth. The PCWP is a useful marker of volume status; an elevated PCWP indicates fluid overload while a reduced PCWP indicates dehydration or inadequate filling pressures. Cardiac output may also be measured and represents the volume of blood being pumped by the heart (in particular by the left ventricle) in a minute. The cardiac index (CI) normalizes the cardiac output for body surface area, thus allowing measurements of heart performance to be made without being influenced by body size. Systemic vascular resistance is calculated using cardiac output and thus is inversely related to cardiac output. Mixed venous oxygen saturation represents the end result of both oxygen delivery and consumption at the tissue level.

Systemic vascular resistance (also referred to as total peripheral resistance) reflects the "afterload" or resistance applied to the left ventricle, which represents the force impeding ejection of blood from the left ventricle. Vasoconstriction (i.e., decrease in blood vessel diameter) increases vascular resistance, whereas vasodilation decreases it. An elevated systemic vascular resistance is common in untreated heart failure and is generally responsive to oral or IV arterial vasodilators. Conversely, a reduction in resistance is consistent with vasodilatory shock (e.g., sepsis) and is routinely managed with

TABLE 5-3 Hemodynamic Monitoring: Normal Values

Central venous (right atrial) pressure, mean, CVP	<5 mm Hg
Right ventricular pressure (systolic/diastolic)	25/10 mm Hg
Pulmonary artery pressure (systolic/diastolic), PAS/PAD	25/10 mm Hg
Pulmonary arterial pressure, mean, PAP	<18 mm Hg
Pulmonary capillary wedge pressure, mean, PCWP	<12 mm Hg
Systemic arterial pressure (systolic/diastolic), SBP/DBP	120/80 mm Hg
Mean arterial pressure, MAP = (DBP + (1/3(SBP – DBP))	90–110 mm Hg
Cardiac output, CO	4–6 L/min (0.067–0.1 L/s)
Cardiac index, CI = CO/BSA	2.8–4.2 L/min/m^2 (0.047–0.07 L/s/m^2)
Systemic vascular resistance, SVR = (MAP – CVP) × 80)/(CO)	900–1400 dyne s cm^{-5} (90–140 MPa s/m^3)
Pulmonary vascular resistance, PVR = ((PAP– CVP) × 80)/(CO)	150–250 dyne s cm^{-5} (15–25 MPa s/m^3)
Arterial oxygen content	20 mL/dL (200 mL/L)
Mixed venous oxygen content	15 mL/dL (15 mL/L)

BSA, body surface area.

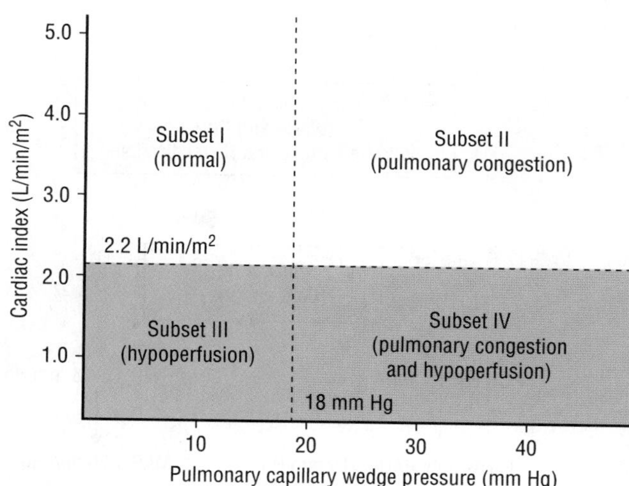

FIGURE 5-1 Hemodynamic subsets of heart failure based on cardiac index and pulmonary artery occlusion pressure. Cardiac index is expressed in conventional units of mL/min/m^2, and can be converted to SI units of mL/s/m^2 by multiplying by 0.0167. *(Forrester JS, Diamond G, Chatterjee K, et al. Medical Therapy of Acute Myocardial Infarction by Application of Hemodynamic Subsets. N Engl J Med 1976;295:1356–1362. Copyright © 1976 Massachusetts Medical Society. All rights reserved.)*

IV vasopressor therapy. In lieu of inotropic therapy, arterial vasodilators are the therapy of choice to reduce elevated systemic vascular resistance in ADHF.

Resistance present in the vasculature of the lungs is known as the pulmonary vascular resistance, and represents the impedance of blood flow from the right ventricle to the pulmonary circulation. Pulmonary hypertension and pulmonary edema are two common causes of elevated pulmonary vascular resistance. Patients with pulmonary hypertension must have proven reversibility in elevated pulmonary pressures prior to being listed for heart transplantation. If these pressures are irreversible, isolated right ventricular failure is likely to occur immediately following heart transplantation. Just as systemic resistance is calculated using mean arterial pressure, pulmonary vascular resistance is calculated using mean PA pressure, which incorporates the PA systolic and diastolic pressures. The PA diastolic pressure may be useful if the PA catheter fails to wedge (making it impossible to obtain PCWP). If PCWP and PA diastolic pressure correlate prior to the failure to wedge, then PA diastolic pressure can be followed as a surrogate marker of fluid status. Normal values for hemodynamic parameters are listed in Table 5-3.

In addition to understanding the initial clinical presentation, invasive hemodynamic monitoring assists with the classification of patients into specific subsets and subsequent selection of appropriate medical therapy. These *hemodynamic subsets* were first proposed for patients with left ventricular dysfunction following an acute myocardial infarction but also are applicable to patients with acute or severe heart failure from other causes (Fig. 5-1).[24] This classification scheme has four subsets and is based on a CI above or below 2.2 L/min/m^2 (0.037 L/s/m^2) and a PCWP above or below 18 mm Hg. A treatment algorithm, based on hemodynamic subsets, is provided in Figure 5-2. In addition to utilizing the above profiles or categories to stratify patients with ADHF, these four hemodynamic profiles are also predictive of clinical outcomes. Patients in the wet-warm and wet-cold profiles have a twofold and 2.5-fold greater risk of death at 1 year, respectively, compared to dry-warm patients.[15] Patients may experience compromised CI in the setting of significant fluid overload, which may improve as diuresis occurs. The underlying mechanism for how increasing fluid overload further worsens cardiac function is not clearly understood and is depicted in Figure 5-3.

Subset I

Patients in hemodynamic subset I have a CI and PCWP within generally acceptable ranges and have the lowest mortality of any subset. These patients do not need immediate specific interventions other than maximizing oral therapy and monitoring. Patients with significant left ventricular dysfunction may still present in subset I because normal compensatory mechanisms and/or appropriate drug therapy may at least partially correct an otherwise abnormal hemodynamic profile.

Subset II

As shown in Figure 5-1, patients in subset II have an adequate CI but a PCWP greater than 18 mm Hg. These patients are likely to have congestion (i.e., "wet" heart failure) secondary to increased hydrostatic pressure in the pulmonary and systemic circulation but no evidence of peripheral hypoperfusion. The primary goal of therapy in these patients is to reduce congestion by lowering PCWP without reductions in cardiac output, increases in heart rate, or further neurohormonal activation. Therefore, it is critically important that PCWP not be decreased excessively. Although the normal range of PCWP is 5 to 12 mm Hg for individuals without cardiac dysfunction, higher pressures (i.e., 15 to 18 mm Hg) are often necessary in patients with heart failure in order to optimize CI. Generally, the PCWP can be lowered to 15 to 18 mm Hg with relatively little decrease in cardiac output because the Frank-Starling curve is flatter at higher PCWP values in patients with heart failure (depicted in Figure 5-3). Cardiac output also declines when the PCWP desired in a heart failure patient (i.e., PCWP 15 to 18 mm Hg) is exceeded. This phenomenon may explain why patients may experience enhanced diuresis and improved renal function when the PCWP range of 15 to 18 mm Hg is achieved in a heart failure patient with fluid overload. IV administration of agents that reduce preload (i.e., loop diuretics, nitroglycerin, or nesiritide) are the most appropriate acute therapy to achieve the therapeutic goal for patients in subset II. Despite a very rapid onset with diuretic therapy, the time required for significant improvement in oxygenation with IV loop diuretics may take several hours in select patients. Thus, IV venodilators such as nitroglycerin and nesiritide may be utilized for rapid venodilation, which can acutely aid in improving hypoxia (Fig. 5-2).[9]

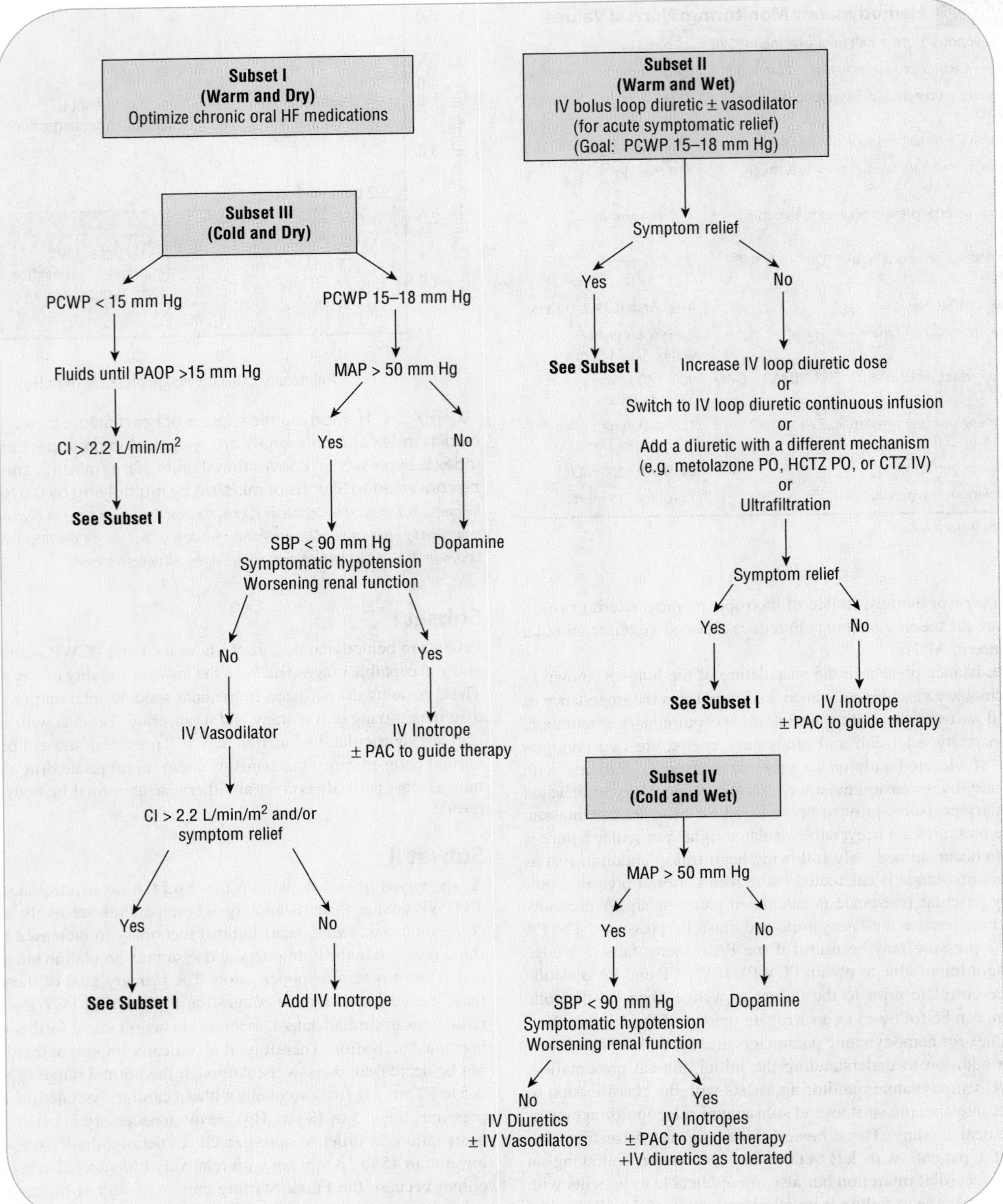

FIGURE 5-2 General treatment algorithm for ADHF based on clinical presentation. IV vasodilators that may be used include nitroglycerin, nesiritide, or nitroprusside. Metolazone or spironolactone may be added if the patient fails to respond to loop diuretics and a second diuretic is required. IV inotropes that may be used include dobutamine or milrinone. (CI, cardiac index; CTZ, chlorothiazide; HCTZ, hydrochlorothiazide; HF, heart failure; MAP, mean arterial pressure; PAC, pulmonary artery catheter; PCWP, pulmonary capillary wedge pressure; PO, by mouth; SBP, systolic blood pressure.) *Adapted from HFSA 2010 Comprehensive Heart Failure Practice Guideline. J Cardiac Fail 2010;16:e1–e2.*

Current guidelines recommend loop diuretics as first-line therapy for patients with fluid overload and that such agents typically be administered IV.[10] The rate of diuresis should achieve a desirable volume status without causing a rapid reduction in intravascular volume, which may result in symptomatic hypotension or renal dysfunction. Electrolyte depletion should be monitored closely especially when high doses or combination diuretic therapy is utilized. In addition to sodium restriction (less than 2 g daily), supplemental oxygen should be administered as needed for hypoxemia. In patients with moderate hyponatremia (less than 130 mEq/L

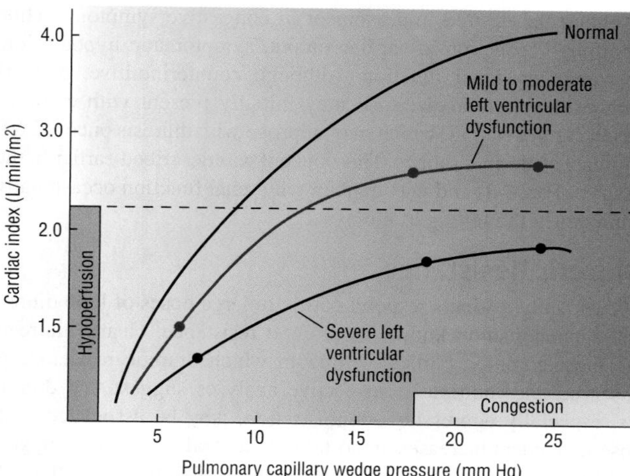

FIGURE 5-3 Relationship between cardiac output (shown as cardiac index which is CO/BSA) and preload (shown as pulmonary capillary wedge pressure). Cardiac index is expressed in conventional units of mL/min/m^2, and can be converted to SI units of mL/s/m^2 by multiplying by 0.0167.

[130 mmol/L]), fluid restriction (less than 2 L daily) should be considered, and in patients with worsening or severe hyponatremia (less than 125 mEq/L [125 mmol/L]), stricter fluid restriction may be necessary.[10] The arginine vasopressin (AVP) antagonists are a new class of agents indicated for the management of euvolemic or hypervolemic hyponatremia in a variety of disease states including heart failure.[25] Currently available vasopressin antagonists are discussed in greater detail later in this chapter.

IV vasodilators may be added to diuretics for rapid symptom resolution, especially in patients with acute pulmonary edema or severe hypertension. Such therapy may also be considered in patients who fail to respond to aggressive treatment with diuretics. Vasodilators should be avoided in patients with symptomatic hypotension, and frequent blood pressure monitoring is necessary to ensure their safe use. In addition, these agents should not be used in patients with reduced left heart filling pressures. If symptomatic hypotension occurs with vasodilator therapy, the dose should be reduced or the agent discontinued. If patients fail to respond to the above therapies or experience worsening renal function, IV inotropic therapy should be considered.[10]

Subset III

Patients in hemodynamic subset III have a CI of less than 2.2 L/min/m^2 but without an abnormal elevation in PCWP (Fig. 5-1). These patients usually present without evidence of congestion, but low cardiac output results in signs and symptoms of peripheral hypoperfusion (i.e., decreased urine output, weakness, peripheral vasoconstriction, weak pulses). The mortality rate of subset III patients is reportedly higher than that of patients without hypoperfusion.[24] Although the treatment goal is to alleviate signs and symptoms of hypoperfusion by increasing CI and perfusion to essential organs, therapy may differ based on initial presentation. If the PCWP is significantly below 15 mm Hg, IV fluids should be administered to provide a more optimal left ventricular filling pressure (i.e., 15 to 18 mm Hg), consequently improving CI (Fig. 5-2). Alternatively, diuretic therapy should be held and fluid restriction liberalized. When only mild left ventricular dysfunction is present, IV fluid administration may be all that is necessary to achieve a CI above 2.2 L/min/m^2 (0.037 L/s/m^2). However, many patients will have significant left ventricular dysfunction and depressed Frank-Starling relationship despite adequate filling pressures. In such patients, IV administration of positive inotropic agents (e.g., dobutamine, milrinone) and/or arterial vasodilators (e.g., nitroprusside or nesiritide) may be necessary to achieve an adequate CI (Fig. 5-2). Some positive inotropic medications also have arterial vasodilating activity (see specific drug classes that follow).

Current guidelines recommend IV inotropes for symptom relief or end-organ dysfunction in patients with left ventricular dysfunction and low cardiac output syndrome.[10] Such therapy may be especially useful in patients with low systolic blood pressure (less than 90 mm Hg) or symptomatic hypotension in the setting of adequate filling pressures. As previously discussed (see Subset II), inotropic therapy may be considered in patients who do not tolerate or respond to IV vasodilators or in patients with worsening renal function. As with vasodilators, inotrope administration requires frequent blood pressure monitoring as well as continuous monitoring for arrhythmias. If arrhythmias occur, dose reduction or discontinuation of inotropic therapy should be performed. As with vasodilators, these agents should be avoided in patients with low left heart filling pressures. Given the potential risks associated with inotropic therapy, vasodilators should be considered prior to using inotropes.[10]

In general, inotropic therapy should not be used routinely in the ADHF population. Instead, they should be reserved for the purpose of increasing cardiac output in the specific patients described above. These agents may also be used to "bridge" patients to heart transplantation or a left ventricular assist device, or as palliative therapy to improve functional status and quality of life in patients who are not candidates for these definitive therapies.[10]

Subset IV

Patients with a CI of less than 2.2 L/min/m^2 (0.037 L/s/m^2) and a PCWP higher than 18 mm Hg are in hemodynamic subset IV (Fig. 5-1). This subset is characterized by the worst prognosis of the four and represents the most common hemodynamic profile for patients with end-stage heart failure. Given the severity of systolic failure, such patients cannot maintain an adequate CI despite elevated left ventricular filling pressure and increased myocardial fiber stretch. Patients in subset IV will present with signs and symptoms of both congestion and hypoperfusion. Treatment goals for these patients include the alleviation of signs and symptoms by increasing CI above 2.2 L/min/m^2 (0.037 L/s/m^2) and reducing PCWP to 15 to 18 mm Hg while maintaining an adequate mean arterial pressure. As a consequence, therapy will involve a combination of agents used in Subsets II and III in order to achieve these goals (i.e., combination of diuretic plus positive inotrope). These targets may be difficult to achieve and often necessitate careful monitoring and individualization of drug therapy. Nitroprusside may be a particularly useful agent in this setting because of its mixed arterial-venous vasodilating effects. However, in the presence of significant hypotension and low mean arterial pressures, inotropic agents with vasopressor activity (e.g., dopamine) may be required initially to achieve an adequate end-organ perfusion pressure and can then be combined, if necessary, with diuretics and/or therapies to obtain the desired hemodynamic effects and clinical response (Fig. 5-2).

PHARMACOLOGIC THERAPY OF ACUTE DECOMPENSATED HEART FAILURE

6 Unfortunately, drug therapies utilized in the management of ADHF have not improved substantially in the last decade due primarily to a dearth of clinical trial data in this population. The agents used to treat patients with ADHF rarely, if ever, produce a single cardiovascular action. Even when intended for a specific purpose (e.g., positive inotropic effects), other cardiovascular effects (tachycardia,

TABLE 5-4 Usual Hemodynamic Effects of IV Agents Commonly Used for Treatment of Advanced or Decompensated Heart Failure[a]

Drug	Dose	HR	MAP	PCWP	CO	SVR
Dopamine	0.5–3 mcg/kg/min	0	0	0	0/+	–
	3–10 mcg/kg/min	+	+	0	+	0
	10–20 mcg/kg/min	+	+	+	+	+
Dobutamine	2.5–20 mcg/kg/min	0/+	0	–	+	–
Milrinone	0.1–0.75 mcg/kg/min	0/+	0/–	–	+	–
Nitroprusside	0.25–3 mcg/kg/min	0/+	0/–	–	+	–
Nitroglycerin	5–200 mcg/min	0/+	0/–	–	0/+	0/–
Furosemide	20–80 mg IVB (<0.4 mg/min)[b] Two to three times/day or 0.1 mg/kg/h CI	0	0/–	–	0	0
Enalaprilat	1.25–2.5 mg q 6–8 h	0	0/–	–	+	–
Nesiritide	2 mcg/kg IVB; 0.01 mcg/kg/min	0	0/–	–	+	–

+, increase; –, decrease; 0, no change; HR, heart rate; MAP, mean arterial pressure; PCWP, pulmonary capillary wedge pressure; CI, continuous infusion; CO, cardiac output; IVB, IV bolus; SVR, systemic vascular resistance.

[a]See the text for a more detailed description of the interpatient variability in response.
[b]IV bolus administered <0.4 mg/min.

vasodilation, or vasoconstriction) may either add to the therapeutic effect of the drug, or cause adverse effects that negate or even outweigh its intended therapeutic benefit. How an individual patient will respond to an intervention is often difficult to anticipate. For this reason, hemodynamic monitoring is often useful, and many drugs are considered first-line therapy due in part to their short half-lives and ease of titration. The description of expected drug actions outlined below should be viewed as a general guide to the clinician and patients should be continually reassessed for desired therapeutic outcomes. Table 5-4 contains a summary of the expected hemodynamic effects of the various drugs discussed below.

Diuretics

7 IV loop diuretics, including furosemide, bumetanide, and torsemide, are used commonly in the management of ADHF, with furosemide being the most widely studied and used in this setting.[26–29] Bolus administration of diuretics reduces preload within 5 to 15 minutes by functional venodilation and later (>20 minutes) via sodium and water excretion, thereby improving pulmonary congestion. However, an acute reduction in venous return may severely compromise effective preload in patients with significant diastolic dysfunction, intravascular depletion, or those in whom CI is significantly dependent on adequate filling pressure (i.e., preload-dependent). This reduction in preload may result in reflex elevation of renin, norepinephrine, and AVP and the expected consequences of arteriolar and coronary vasoconstriction, tachycardia, and increased myocardial oxygen consumption. Unlike arterial vasodilators and positive inotropic agents, diuretics do not cause an upward shift in the Frank–Starling curve or significantly increase CI in most patients (Table 5-4 and Fig. 5-3). In fact, excessive preload reduction, specifically diuresis to a PCWP of less than 15 mm Hg, can lead to a decline in cardiac output (Fig. 5-3). Furthermore, intravascular volume depletion may occur in the setting of rapid diuresis despite relative overload of total body fluid, and thus, daily diuresis goals must be highly individualized. Most patients tolerate a 2 L/day net negative diuresis. However, some end-stage patients, especially those who are malnourished due to early satiety, will only tolerate 1 L/day net negative diuresis. Thus, diuretics must be used judiciously to obtain the desired improvement in congestive symptoms while avoiding a reduction in cardiac output, symptomatic hypotension, or worsening renal function. Although counterintuitive, patients with excessive fluid overload may initially present with compromised cardiac output, which may improve with diuresis once PCWP approaches desired ranges. This concept was described earlier in the chapter (Fig. 5-3) and may explain why renal function occasionally improves in the setting of diuresis.

Diuretic Resistance

Occasionally, patients respond poorly to large doses of loop diuretics, a phenomenon known as diuretic resistance. Heart failure is the most common clinical setting in which diuretic resistance is observed and multiple retrospective analyses suggest that diuretics, especially aggressive administration, may be associated with dose-dependent increases in mortality.[30] Several studies also suggest that high doses are associated with renal dysfunction in ADHF,[29,31] which only further exacerbates diuretic resistance. Thus, the need for increased exposure to diuretics in the setting of resistance is concerning.

The mechanisms responsible for diuretic resistance in patients with heart failure are thought to be both pharmacokinetic and pharmacodynamic.[32] The oral bioavailability of furosemide is relatively normal in heart failure patients, but the rate of absorption is prolonged approximately twofold and peak concentrations are reduced by approximately 50%. Because loop diuretics have a sigmoidal-shaped concentration–response curve, prolonged absorption may result in concentrations that fail to reach the threshold necessary for producing effective diuresis. Resistance is also observed with IV administration, suggesting an equally important pharmacodynamic contribution to this phenomenon. The decreased responsiveness in patients with heart failure may be explained in part by the high concentrations of sodium reaching the distal tubule as a result of blocked sodium reabsorption in the loop of Henle. As a consequence, the distal tubule undergoes hypertrophy, which enhances its ability to reabsorb sodium. Additionally, neurohormonal activation, low cardiac output, reduced renal perfusion, and decreased drug delivery to the kidney may also contribute to resistance.

Several strategies may be employed to overcome diuretic resistance. Current guidelines support one of three pharmacologic options in patients who do not initially respond to diuretic therapy.[10] First, higher doses of loop diuretics may be administered to achieve concentrations near the top of the concentration–response curve. Although higher doses produce greater diuresis, these effects are not associated with improved long-term outcomes and must be weighed against the risk of worsening renal function.[33] A second approach for overcoming diuretic resistance is the use of a continuous IV infusion, although this strategy has produced mixed results in clinical trials. Initial studies of continuous-infusion furosemide suggest a greater natriuretic effect with no difference in metabolic adverse effects when compared to the same total daily dose given by IV bolus.[28,34,35] In another comparison of 56 patients with decompensated heart failure, use of a continuous furosemide infusion was associated with greater total urine output and shorter length of stay compared to IV bolus therapy, although net urine output and mean weight loss were unchanged.[36] In the largest investigation to date, 308 patients with decompensated heart failure were randomized to a four-way comparison of low- and high-dose furosemide administered as a continuous infusion or intermittent IV bolus every 12 hours; although differences were observed in the comparison of low and high-dose furosemide, no differences in relief of symptoms, urine output, weight loss, or long-term outcomes were observed when administration by continuous infusion or intermittent IV bolus were compared.[33]

A third strategy for overcoming diuretic resistance is to add a second diuretic with a different mechanism of action. Combining a loop diuretic with a distal tubule blocker such as oral metolazone, oral hydrochlorothiazide (HCTZ), or IV chlorothiazide can produce a synergistic diuretic effect. Inhibition of sodium reabsorption in the loop of Henle increases sodium delivery to (and reabsorption in) the distal convoluted tubule, which can be subsequently blocked by a thiazide-type diuretic. Thus, when thiazide-type diuretics are added to a loop diuretic, they inhibit more than the usual 5% to 8% of filtered sodium, resulting in synergistic natriuresis. The combination of a loop and thiazide diuretic should generally be reserved for hospitalized patients, as profound diuresis with severe electrolyte and volume depletion may occur. If used in the outpatient setting, very low doses or only occasional administration of a thiazide-type diuretic should be recommended. Patients should also receive close follow-up (e.g., weight, vital signs, serum potassium, dizziness) to avoid serious adverse events.

Nonpharmacologic strategies for managing diuretic resistance include additional sodium and fluid restriction (i.e., less than 1 g and less than 1 L per day, respectively) and ultrafiltration, a strategy discussed in further detail later in this chapter.

Poor response to diuretic therapy may also result from worsening renal perfusion in the setting of low cardiac output. Thus, the use of positive inotropes or arterial vasodilators may improve diuresis by improving central hemodynamics. However, given the adverse effects of inotropic therapy, this option is generally reserved for patients not responding to all other therapies or those with evidence of low cardiac output. Administration of low doses of dopamine (i.e., 2 to 5 mcg/kg/min) to enhance diuresis was once common practice, but evidence to support its use remains controversial, as most studies indicate minimal if any improvement in diuresis.[37] In a recent investigation comparing a high-dose furosemide infusion (20 mg/h) to the combination of a low-dose furosemide infusion (5 mg/h) and a dopamine infusion at 5 mcg/kg/h, reduced rates of worsening renal function were observed in the combination group despite similar rates of diuresis; however, because the trial did not include a group randomized to low-dose furosemide alone, it is not clear that these differences can be attributed to the addition of dopamine.[38] Additionally, at an infusion rate of 5 mcg/kg/min, dopamine exerts positive inotropic effects, thus it may not provide any advantages over a traditional inotrope when used in this setting.

Positive Inotropic Agents

8 9 The two positive inotropic agents currently approved for the management of ADHF are dobutamine and milrinone.[39,40] Although both drugs increase intracellular concentrations of cyclic adenosine monophosphate (cAMP), the two do so by slightly different mechanisms. Dobutamine activates adenylate cyclase through direct stimulation of β-adrenergic receptors, thus catalyzing the conversion of adenosine triphosphate to cAMP, while milrinone reduces degradation of cAMP by inhibiting phosphodiesterase. Increased intracellular cAMP enhances phospholipase (and subsequently phosphorylase) activity, increasing the rate and extent of calcium influx during systole and enhancing contractility. Additionally, cAMP enhances reuptake of calcium by the sarcoplasmic reticulum during diastole, improving active relaxation.

Digoxin has a limited role in hemodynamically unstable patients due to its limited inotropic effect. In patients who take digoxin as chronic therapy, discontinuation or dose-adjustment during an acute decompensation is generally unnecessary unless changes in renal function increase the risk of toxicity. As discussed previously in this chapter, discontinuation should be discouraged given the potential for digoxin withdrawal unless there is a concern for toxicity.[20,21]

Differences in the pharmacologic effects of dobutamine and milrinone may confer advantages or disadvantages in a given patient. Therefore, clinical considerations for their use in the management of ADHF will be reviewed in the sections to follow.

TABLE 5-5 Relative Effects of Adrenergic Drugs on Receptors

Drug	α_1	β_1	β_2	Dopamine
Dopamine[a]	++++	++++	++	++
Epinephrine	++++	++++	++	0
Norepinephrine	++++	++++	0	0
Phenylephrine	++++	0	0	0
Dobutamine	+	++++	++	0
Isoproterenol	0	++++	++++	0

[a]See the text for a more detailed description of the dose-dependent hemodynamic effects.

Dobutamine

The receptor activities of dobutamine and other adrenergic agonists are summarized in Table 5-5. Dobutamine, a synthetic catecholamine, is a β_1- and β_2-receptor agonist with some α_1-agonist effects. Unlike dopamine, dobutamine does not result in the release of norephinephrine from nerve terminals. Consequently, the positive inotropic effects of dobutamine are attributed to its effects on β_1-receptors. Stimulation of cardiac β_1-receptors by dobutamine does not generally produce a significant change in heart rate, thus explaining its more modest chronotropic effects compared with dopamine. Modest peripheral β_2-receptor-mediated vasodilation tends to offset minor α_1-receptor-mediated vasoconstriction with dobutamine. In addition, the increase in cardiac output often results in a reflexive decline in systemic vascular resistance. The net hemodynamic effect of dobutamine is usually vasodilation, which results from its effects on adrenergic receptors as well as reflex-mediated actions in vascular tissue.

The effects of dobutamine are observed within minutes but its peak effects may take up to 10 minutes to occur given an elimination half-life of 2 minutes. Initial doses of 2.5 to 5 mcg/kg/min may be increased progressively to 20 mcg/kg/min based on clinical and hemodynamic responses. Cardiac index is increased due to inotropic stimulation, arterial vasodilation, and a variable increase in heart rate. Because of offsetting changes in arteriolar resistance and CI, dobutamine usually causes relatively little change in mean arterial pressure, unlike the more consistent increases observed with dopamine. The vasodilating action of dobutamine usually reduces PCWP, making it particularly useful in the presence of low CI and an elevated left ventricular filling pressure; conversely, these effects may be detrimental in the presence of a reduced filling pressure. Although its impact on heart rate is variable, the major adverse effects of dobutamine are tachycardia and ventricular arrhythmias. Potentially detrimental increases in oxygen consumption have also been observed. While concerns exist regarding the attenuation of dobutamine's effects during prolonged administration, some effect is likely retained, requiring that the dose of dobutamine be slowly tapered rather than abruptly discontinued.

Milrinone

Milrinone is a bipyridine derivative that inhibits phosphodiesterase III, an enzyme responsible for the breakdown of cAMP to AMP. Milrinone has supplanted the use of its prototype amrinone due to less frequent occurrence of thrombocytopenia. Because both positive inotropic and vasodilating effects contribute to its therapeutic effects in ADHF, milrinone is often referred to as an *inodilator.* The relative balance of these pharmacologic effects may vary with dose and underlying cardiovascular pathology.

During IV administration, milrinone produces an increase in stroke volume (and, therefore, cardiac output) with minimal change in heart rate (Table 5-4). Despite an increase in CI, mean arterial pressure may remain constant due to a concomitant decrease in arteriolar resistance. However, the vasodilating effects of milrinone may predominate, leading to a decrease in blood pressure and reflex tachycardia. Like dobutamine, milrinone lowers PCWP by venodilation and thus is particularly useful in patients with a low CI and an elevated left ventricular filling pressure. Such a reduction in preload, however, can be hazardous for patients without excessive filling pressure (especially those with subset III heart failure), thus blunting the improvement in cardiac output produced by the positive inotropic and arterial dilating actions of milrinone. Furthermore, milrinone should be used cautiously in severely hypotensive patients because it does not increase, and may even decrease, arterial blood pressure. Comparisons between dobutamine and milrinone indicate that the two agents generally produce similar hemodynamic effects, although dobutamine is usually associated with more pronounced increases in heart rate.

Milrinone has a longer elimination half-life than other vasoactive agents. In healthy subjects, the half-life of milrinone is about 1 hour but may be as long as 3 hours in patients with ADHF. The long elimination half-life of milrinone presents several disadvantages in this patient population, including the need for a loading dose in order to obtain a prompt initial response, the inability to perform minute-to-minute titrations based on hemodynamic changes, and persistence of adverse effects (e.g., arrhythmias or hypotension) following drug discontinuation. The usual loading dose for milrinone is 50 mcg/kg administered over 10 minutes, although this practice is uncommon due to an increased risk of hypotension. Most patients are started on a maintenance infusion of 0.1 to 0.3 mcg/kg/min (up to 0.75 mcg/kg/min), although lower initial doses may be considered. Milrinone is excreted unchanged in the urine, and thus, its infusion rate should be decreased by 50% to 70% in patients with significant renal impairment.

The most notable adverse effects associated with milrinone are arrhythmia, hypotension, and thrombocytopenia. While the incidence of thrombocytopenia with milrinone is rare, patients should still have platelet counts measured before and during therapy.

The combination of dobutamine and milrinone is likely to produce additive effects on CI and PCWP, suggesting this regimen as an option in patients who have dose-limiting adverse effects with either drug class. However, whether this combination provides a therapeutic advantage over the combined use of a positive inotrope and a traditional vasodilator (e.g., nitroprusside) is unclear.

Although not supported by evidence from clinical trials, many patients without signs or symptoms of hypoperfusion receive inotropic therapy in an effort to improve hemodynamics and thus shorten length of hospitalization and improve clinical outcomes. In one randomized trial designed to evaluate this strategy, no difference in length of stay was observed when 949 patients with ADHF were randomized to either a 48-hour infusion of milrinone or placebo.[8] Adverse events were more common in the milrinone group, including sustained hypotension requiring intervention (10.7% vs. 3.2%; $P < 0.001$) and new onset of atrial fibrillation or flutter (4.6% vs. 1.5%; $P = 0.004$).

Recently, data from the ADHERE Registry (n = 15,230) has been used to compare in-hospital mortality among patients receiving IV nitroglycerin, nesiritide, milrinone, or dobutamine.[41] After adjusting for baseline parameters known to predict in-hospital mortality, both dobutamine- and milrinone-treated patients experienced higher in-hospital mortality compared to those receiving either nitroglycerin or nesiritide ($P < 0.005$). In-hospital mortality was higher among patients receiving dobutamine compared to milrinone ($P = 0.027$), and no difference in in-hospital mortality was observed between nitroglycerin- and nesiritide-treated patients ($P = 0.58$).

Results from these studies add to the growing concern regarding the use of inotropic drugs in patients with ADHF and strongly suggest that they not be routinely used for the treatment of heart failure exacerbations. However, clinicians should be aware that inotropic therapy may be needed in select patients, such as those with low cardiac output states, end-organ hypoperfusion, or cardiogenic shock.[10] Dobutamine should be considered when a significant decrease in mean arterial pressure might further compromise hemodynamic function, as this effect is more common with the initiation of milrinone. Selection of an inotropic drug should also take into account whether patients are receiving chronic β-blocker therapy and whether a β_1-selective agent (e.g., metoprolol succinate) or mixed α,β-blocking agent (e.g., carvedilol) is used. Generally, milrinone should be considered for patients who are receiving chronic β-blocker therapy because its inotropic effects do not involve stimulation of β-receptors. Continued β-blocker therapy may even augment the hemodynamic effects of milrinone, a phenomenon observed in studies with the structurally similar phosphodiesterase inhibitor enoximone.[42] The hemodynamic effects of dobutamine may persist in the presence of β_1-selective agents as a result of β-receptor upregulation or selective activation of β_2-receptors by dobutamine. However, these effects are not observed in the presence of carvedilol, which may inhibit the hemodynamic benefits of dobutamine entirely.[42]

In some patients, dose reduction or discontinuation of positive inotropic therapy results in acute decompensation, requiring the placement of an indwelling IV catheter for continuous outpatient therapy. This approach may be used to "bridge" patients awaiting cardiac transplantation or left ventricular assist device placement, or to facilitate the discharge of patients who are not transplant candidates but who cannot be weaned from inotrope therapy. In this latter group, the use of outpatient intropic therapy is palliative and should only be considered after multiple unsuccessful attempts to maximize oral therapy and discontinue IV inotrope therapy. Although this strategy may be effective for symptom palliation, the risk of mortality is likely increased. In contrast, the use of regularly scheduled intermittent inotropic infusions is not recommended in current guidelines.[10]

Dopamine

Although dopamine should generally be avoided in the treatment of ADHF, a clinical scenario where its pharmacologic actions may be preferable to dobutamine or milrinone is in patients with marked systemic hypotension or cardiogenic shock in the face of elevated ventricular filling pressures, where dopamine in doses greater than 5 mcg/kg/min may be necessary to raise central aortic pressure. Although this strategy is common in clinical practice, minimal data exist to support its use.

Dopamine is an endogenous precursor of norepinephrine and exerts its effects by directly stimulating adrenergic receptors as well as causing release of norepinephrine from adrenergic nerve terminals. Dopamine produces dose-dependent hemodynamic effects as a result of its relative affinity for α_1-, β_1-, β_2-, and D_1- (vascular dopaminergic) receptors (see Table 5-4).

The positive inotropic effects of dopamine are mediated primarily by β_1-receptors and become more prominent at doses of 2 to 5 mcg/kg/min. Cardiac index is increased because of an increase in stroke volume and a variable increase in heart rate, which is also partially dose-dependent. Minimal changes in systemic vascular resistance occur, presumably because neither vasodilation (D_1- and β_2-receptor-mediated) nor vasoconstriction (α_1-receptor-mediated) predominates. However, at doses between 5 and 10 mcg/kg/min, chronotropic and α_1-receptor-mediated vasoconstricting effects become more prominent. Mean arterial pressure is usually raised as a result of increases in both CI and systemic vascular resistance (Table 5-4). The vasoconstricting effects of higher doses may limit improvements in CI by increasing afterload and PCWP, thus complicating the management of patients with preexisting high afterload.

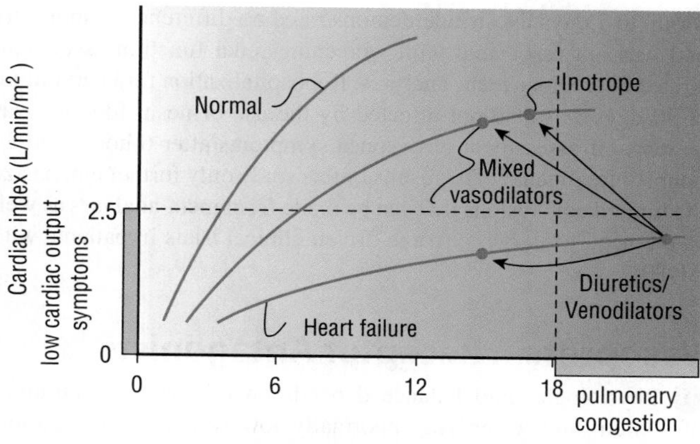

FIGURE 5-4 Relationship between stroke volume and systemic vascular resistance. In an individual with normal left ventricular function, increasing systemic vascular resistance has little effect on stroke volume. As the extent of left ventricular dysfunction increases, the negative, inverse relationship between stroke volume and systemic vascular resistance becomes more important. Cardiac index is expressed in conventional units of mL/min/m^2, and can be converted to SI units of mL/s/m^2 by multiplying by 0.0167.

In such patients, alternative agents (e.g., dobutamine, milrinone) or the addition of diuretics and/or vasodilators may be necessary.

Dopamine, particularly at higher doses, may also alter several parameters that increase myocardial oxygen demand (e.g., increased heart rate, contractility, and systolic pressure) and potentially decrease myocardial blood flow (e.g., coronary vasoconstriction and increased wall tension), which may worsen ischemia in patients with coronary artery disease. As with dobutamine and milrinone, arrhythmogenesis is also more common at higher dopamine doses.

Vasodilators

10 Activation of the sympathetic nervous system, renin–angiotensin–aldosterone system, and other neurohormonal mediators are characteristic features of both acute and chronic heart failure.[29,43] Peripheral vasoconstriction and increased systemic vascular resistance often results, leading to a severe decline in stroke volume and thus cardiac output (Fig. 5-4).

Vasodilators are commonly classified by their most prominent site of action (i.e., arterial or venous circulation). Arterial vasodilators act as impedance-reducing agents, reducing afterload and causing a reflexive increase in cardiac output. Venodilators act as preload reducers by increasing venous capacitance, thus reducing symptoms of pulmonary congestion in patients with high cardiac filling pressures. Mixed vasodilators act on both resistance and capacitance vessels, reducing congestive symptoms while increasing cardiac output. The most commonly used IV vasodilators in decompensated heart failure are nitroprusside, nitroglycerin, and nesiritide.

Nitroprusside

Sodium nitroprusside increases synthesis of nitric oxide in vascular smooth muscle, resulting in balanced arterial and venous vasodilation. As a result, nitroprusside increases CI and decreases venous pressure to a degree similar to dobutamine and milrinone, despite having no direct inotropic activity (Table 5-4); however, greater decreases in PCWP, systemic vascular resistance, and blood pressure are generally observed. Mean arterial pressure may remain fairly constant but often decreases depending on the relative increase in cardiac output and reduction in arteriolar tone. Hypotension is an important dose-limiting effect of nitroprusside; thus, it is used primarily in patients with significantly elevated systemic vascular resistance and often requires invasive hemodynamic monitoring.

Patients with normal left ventricular function do not experience an increase in stroke volume when systemic vascular resistance falls because the normal ventricle is fairly insensitive to small changes in afterload. Consequently, these patients may experience a significant decrease in blood pressure in response to arterial vasodilators. These differences explain why nitroprusside is a potent antihypertensive agent in patients without heart failure but causes less hypotension and reflex tachycardia in the presence of left ventricular dysfunction. Nonetheless, even a modest increase in heart rate can have adverse consequences in patients with underlying ischemic heart disease and/or resting tachycardia, thus necessitating close monitoring during therapy.

Nitroprusside is an effective strategy for the short-term management of patients with severe heart failure across a variety of settings (e.g., acute MI, valvular regurgitation, after coronary bypass surgery, decompensated chronic heart failure). Generally, nitroprusside does not worsen, and may even improve, the balance between myocardial oxygen demand and supply by lowering both left ventricular wall tension (thus reducing oxygen demand) and end-diastolic pressure (thereby increasing subendocardial blood flow). However, an excessive decrease in systemic arterial pressure may reduce coronary perfusion and worsen ischemia, leading to an increased risk of coronary steal.

Nitroprusside has a rapid onset of action but its effects last less than 10 minutes, necessitating its administration by continuous IV infusion. However, this method of administration allows precise dose-titration based on clinical and hemodynamic response. As with other vasodilators used in heart failure, nitroprusside should be initiated at low doses (0.1 to 0.2 mcg/kg/min) to avoid excessive hypotension and increased by small increments (0.1 to 0.2 mcg/kg/min) every 5 to 10 minutes as needed and tolerated. Effective doses usually range from 0.5 to 3 mcg/kg/min. A rebound phenomenon, which may be due to reflex neurohormonal activation during nitroprusside therapy, has been reported following abrupt withdrawal in patients with heart failure. Therefore, nitroprusside should be tapered slowly when transitioning patients to oral therapies. If renal perfusion pressure is compromised by nitroprusside administration, salt and water retention may contribute to volume expansion and tachyphylaxis, although this is typically only observed in patients with chronic hypertension, baseline azotemia, or when augmentation of cardiac output during therapy is minimal. Additionally, nitroprusside can cause cyanide and thiocyanate toxicity, but these effects are unlikely when doses less than 3 mcg/kg/min are administered for less than 3 days, except in patients with significant renal impairment (i.e., serum creatinine concentration greater than 3 mg/dL [265 μmol/L]). Nitroprusside should be avoided in the presence of elevated intracranial pressure because it may worsen cerebral edema in this setting. Given the potent pulmonary vasodilatory effects of nitroprusside as well as its short half-life, this agent is frequently used to determine reversibility of pulmonary hypertension in patients being evaluated for heart transplantation.

Unfortunately, no prospective randomized controlled trials have evaluated the use of nitroprusside in patients with ADHF. However, in one of the many retrospective studies in this population, patients with a reduced CI (i.e., less than or equal to 2 L/min/m^2 [0.033 L/s/m^2]) treated with nitroprusside (n = 78) experienced a reduction in all-cause mortality (P = 0.005) compared to patients who did not receive nitroprusside (n = 97). At baseline, patients receiving nitroprusside tended to have higher MAP, increased intracardiac filling pressures, and lower CI, but the observed improvements in mortality remained even after including only those patients who had initial MAP ≤85 mm Hg (P = 0.0001).[44]

Nitroglycerin

IV nitroglycerin is often the preferred agent for preload reduction in patients with ADHF, especially those with evidence of pulmonary congestion. Because of its short half-life, IV nitroglycerin is administered by continuous infusion. Its major hemodynamic effects are reductions in preload and PCWP via functional venodilation and mild arterial vasodilation that is particularly evident in patients with heart failure and elevated systemic vascular resistance (SVR) or when given in doses approaching 200 mcg/min (Table 5-4). In higher doses, nitroglycerin displays potent coronary vasodilating properties and thus beneficial effects on myocardial oxygen demand and supply, making it the vasodilator of choice for patients with severe heart failure and ischemic heart disease.

Nitroglycerin should be initiated at a dose of 5 to 10 mcg/min (0.1 mcg/kg/min) and increased every 5 to 10 minutes as necessary and tolerated. Hypotension and an excessive decrease in PCWP are important dose-limiting side effects. Maintenance doses usually vary from 35 to 200 mcg/min (0.5 to 3 mcg/kg/min). While tolerance to the hemodynamic effects of nitroglycerin may develop over 12 to 72 hours of continuous administration, some patients experience a sustained response. Like nitroprusside, nitroglycerin should not be used in the presence of elevated intracranial pressure because it may worsen cerebral edema in this setting.

In contrast to nitroprusside, one prospective randomized controlled trial has evaluated nitroglycerin in patients with ADHF. This study compared nitroglycerin to placebo as well as nesiritide and will be discussed in the following section.[9]

Nesiritide

Nesiritide is a recombinant form of BNP, which is secreted by the ventricular myocardium in response to volume overload. Exogenous administration of nesiritide mimics the vasodilatory and natriuretic actions of BNP by stimulating natriuretic peptide receptor A, which leads to increased levels of cGMP in target tissues. Nesiritide produces dose-dependent venous and arterial vasodilation; increases cardiac output, natriuresis, and diuresis; and decreases cardiac filling pressures and activation of the sympathetic nervous system and renin-angiotensin-aldosterone system. In contrast to nitroglycerin or dobutamine, tolerance does not develop to the pharmacologic actions of nesiritide. It also does not affect cAMP or β-receptors, mechanisms that are thought to contribute to the myocardial toxicity associated with the positive inotropic agents, including their proarrhythmic effects. Nesiritide is eliminated by several pathways including natriuretic peptide receptor C located on target tissues, proteolytic cleavage by neutral endopeptidase, and renal filtration. At 18 minutes, its elimination half-life is considerably longer than that of other IV vasoactive agents.

The precise role of nesiritide in the pharmacotherapy of ADHF remains controversial. Some of this controversy centers on the marginal lack of improvement in clinical outcomes with nesiritide compared to other IV vasodilators as well as its significantly greater costs (~$450 for a 24-hour nesiritide infusion compared to $10 to $15 for nitroglycerin). In a randomized, double-blind trial comparing nesiritide to nitroglycerin or placebo in patients with ADHF and dyspnea, nesiritide improved the incidence of dyspnea at 3 hours when compared to placebo but failed to demonstrate a significant difference compared to nitroglycerin.[9] In the subset of patients who received PA catheterization (permitted at the discretion of the investigators), nesiritide reduced PCWP at 3 hours when compared to both placebo and nitroglycerin. Two meta-analyses suggested an increased risk of negative outcomes with nesiritide including an increased risk of worsening renal function and an increased risk in mortality.[45–47] In a trial designed to address these concerns, 7,141 patients hospitalized for ADHF were randomized to receive nesiritide at 0.01 μg/kg/min (with an optional 2 μg/kg IV bolus) or placebo for up to 7 days. Nesiritide demonstrated no difference in mortality and was not associated with worsening renal function as demonstrated in previous meta-analyses. Rehospitalization for heart failure at 30 days was also not affected by the use of nesiritide, nor was patient self-assessment of dyspnea symptoms after 6 hours and 24 hours of treatment.[33] The results of this study only further emphasize the limited conclusions that can be made from meta-analyses as well as the need for large outcome-driven clinical trials in patients with ADHF.

Vasopressin Receptor Antagonists

11 Physiologic fluid balance depends on relative concentrations of sodium and water. An abnormally low sodium concentration, or *hyponatremia*, is commonly defined as less than 125 mEq/L (125 mmol/L) and can be classified as hypovolemic, euvolemic (urine sodium less than 30 mEq/L [30 mmol/L]), or hypervolemic (urine sodium greater than 30 mEq/L [30 mmol/L]) in nature. Diuretic administration may result in hypovolemic hyponatremia, excessive water consumption may result in euvolemic hyponatremia, and heart failure may be associated with hypervolemic hyponatremia. Other causes of hyponatremia include syndrome of inappropriate diuretic hormone (SIADH), cirrhosis with ascites, and medications.[48]

Hyponatremia is often characterized by inappropriately elevated concentrations of AVP, or antidiuretic hormone. In the setting of heart failure, reduced cardiac output leads to excess stimulation of arterial baroreceptors, which in turn enhances AVP secretion and consequently, net water retention. While the prevalence of hyponatremia in patients with heart failure varies by definition, as many as one in five patients hospitalized for acute heart failure presents with serum sodium concentrations less than 136 mEq/L (136 mmol/L).[49] Furthermore, the presence of hyponatremia has been associated with increased mortality in this population.[50]

While many cases of hyponatremia are mild, asymptomatic, and self-limited, prompt diagnosis and management is critical for the less common but life-threatening presentation, which may include lethargy, confusion, respiratory arrest, cerebral edema, seizures, coma, or death. Treatment is specific to the underlying etiology, as well as duration and severity of symptoms. Strategies for managing hyponatremia include removal of the underlying cause, fluid restriction, isotonic or hypertonic saline administration, or administration of diuretics, vasopressin antagonists, or other therapies. Importantly, while neurological sequalae may occur if treatment is not initiated promptly, overly rapid correction of hyponatremia (greater than 12 mEq/L [12 mmol/L] per 24 hours) may be just as detrimental.[51]

The two currently available vasopressin receptor antagonists, tolvaptan and conivaptan, inhibit one or two AVP receptors, V_{1A} or V_2.[52] Stimulation of V_{1A} receptors, which are present in vascular smooth muscle and myocardium, results in vasoconstriction as well as myocyte hypertrophy, coronary vasoconstriction, and positive inotropic effects. V_2 receptors are located in the renal tubules where they regulate water reabsorption. Tolvaptan selectively binds to and inhibits the V_2 receptor, whereas conivaptan nonselectively inhibits both V_{1A} and V_2 receptors. Tolvaptan is orally bioavailable and indicated for the management of hypervolemic and euvolemic hyponatremia in patients with SIADH, cirrhosis, or heart failure. Tolvaptan is typically initiated at 15 mg daily and then titrated to 30 mg or 60 mg as needed for resolution of hyponatremia. Importantly, tolvaptan is a substrate of cytochrome P450 3A4 and is contraindicated with potent inhibitors of this enzyme. Conivaptan is an IV agent indicated for hypervolemic and euvolemic hyponatremia resulting from a variety of causes; however, because it is not indicated in patients with heart failure, conivaptan will not be discussed in further detail here. Patients receiving vasopressin antagonists must be monitored closely to avoid an overly rapid rise in serum sodium, which may result in hypotension or hypovolemia, requiring that therapy be discontinued. Therapy may be restarted at a lower dose if hyponatremia recurs or persists and/or adverse effects resolve.[53]

The role of vasopressin antagonists in the long-term management of heart failure remains unclear at this time. In two trials of patients with euvolemic or hypervolemic hyponatremia (one-third of whom had heart failure as the underlying etiology of hyponatermia), tolvaptan effectively increased serum sodium at 4 and 30 days, although hyponatremia recurred in the week following discontinuation.[54] In a larger trial comprised entirely of hospitalized patients with NYHA class III to IV heart failure, tolvaptan was again associated with significant improvement in hyponatremia compared to placebo.[55,56] Additionally, patients receiving tolvaptan experienced an improvement in diuresis and symptoms of congestion. Unfortunately, the study failed to demonstrate an improvement in global clinical status at discharge or a reduction in 2-year all-cause mortality, cardiovascular mortality, or heart failure rehospitalization.

Overall, tolvaptan is well tolerated; common side effects include dry mouth, thirst, urinary frequency, constipation, and hyperglycemia. While tolvaptan is orally available, therapy in clinical trials was initiated in the inpatient setting, where serum sodium and volume status could be closely monitored. Because of the adverse consequences of rapid changes in serum sodium concentrations or fluid balance, caution should be exerted when initiating therapy.

MECHANICAL CIRCULATORY SUPPORT

Intraaortic Balloon Pump

The intraaortic balloon pump (IABP) is a type of mechanical circulatory assistance device occasionally employed in patients with advanced heart failure who do not respond adequately to drug therapy, such as those with intractable myocardial ischemia or cardiogenic shock.[57] The IABP consists of a polyethylene balloon mounted on a catheter that is usually inserted percutaneously into the femoral artery and advanced into the descending thoracic aorta. During counterpulsation, the balloon is synchronized with the ECG so that it inflates during diastole and displaces blood to the proximal aorta, thus increasing diastolic pressure and coronary perfusion. The balloon deflates just prior to the opening of the aortic valve during systole, which causes a sudden "vacuum-like" decrease in aortic pressure, allowing the left ventricle to pump against reduced arterial impedance. IABP support results in increased CI, coronary artery perfusion, and myocardial oxygen supply accompanied by decreased myocardial oxygen demand. Thus, it may be particularly useful for the short-term support of patients with myocardial ischemia complicated by cardiogenic shock, although it has not been shown to improve mortality in this setting.[58] The IABP is also used in hemodynamically unstable patients who are unresponsive to inotropic therapy, where it may serve as a bridge to a surgical device or transplantation. IV vasodilators and inotropic agents are generally used in conjunction with the IABP to maximize its hemodynamic and clinical benefits.

Ventricular Assist Devices

Ventricular assist devices (VAD) provide mechanical circulatory support by assisting and, in some cases, replacing the pumping functions of the right and/or left ventricles.[59] A left ventricular assist device (LVAD) removes blood directly from the left ventricle or left atrium and pumps it to the aorta, while a right VAD removes blood directly from the right ventricle or right atrium and pumps it to the PA. An RVAD may be used alone or in conjunction with an LVAD; this latter configuration is known as a biventricular assist device (BiVAD).

12 A number of VADs are currently available or under investigation. These devices may be used in the short term (days to weeks) for temporary stabilization while a patient awaits an intervention to correct the underlying cause of cardiac dysfunction, or they may be surgically implanted for the long term (months to years) as a bridge to heart transplantation. More recently, permanent device implantation (known as "destination therapy") has become an option for patients who are not heart transplant candidates. While an RVAD (used alone or in combination with an LVAD) is primarily reserved for acute hemodynamic support, an LVAD may be considered for both short- and long-term use.

Short-term VAD use is indicated in patients requiring acute hemodynamic support during high-risk invasive procedures (e.g., percutaneous coronary intervention, coronary artery bypass graft surgery, valve repair or replacement), postoperative cardiac dysfunction, or cardiogenic shock, often in the setting of cardiac surgery. Several device types may be employed in the short-term setting, including implantable, extracorporeal (e.g., AB5000, Abiomed, Danvers, MA), and percutaneous models (e.g., Impella, Abiomed, Danvers, MA).

Intermediate-term and long-term devices may serve as a bridge to heart transplantation or in the case of the latter type, destination therapy for patients who are not transplant candidates. In one of the first pivotal trials assessing LVAD implantation, 129 patients who were ineligible for heart transplantation were randomized to the HeartMate XVE (Thoratec Corp., Pleasanton, CA) or optimal medical therapy. Although overall survival was low in both groups, LVAD patients experienced improved 1- and 2-year survival (52% vs. 25% and 23% vs. 8%, respectively, $P = 0.009$).[60] In a trial evaluating the Novacor LVAD (WorldHeart, Ottawa, Canada) in an inotrope-dependent population, 1-year survival was improved in the LVAD arm (21% vs. 11% in medically treated patients, $P = 0.02$), but overall outcomes were inferior to those observed with the HeartMate XVE. Notably, some patients in the trial evaluating the Novacor device were more critically ill and would have been considered too high risk for the HeartMate XVE.[61] While previous devices employed a pulsatile flow mechanism, newer-generation devices such as the HeartMate II LVAD (Thoratec Corp., Pleasanton, CA) utilize continuous axial flow, which allows them to be smaller in size and less subject to deterioration over time. When compared to the HeartMate XVE, the HeartMate II LVAD improved the rate of survival free from stroke and device failure at 2 years (46% vs. 11%, $P < 0.001$) and actuarial survival rates at 2 years (58% vs. 24%, $P = 0.008$).

Complications of LVAD implantation include bleeding, air embolism, right ventricular failure, as well as those associated with any major surgical procedure, including infection. In addition, the devices can cause hemolysis, thrombosis, renal and hepatic dysfunction, and arrhythmias. Device malfunction may also occur, but as LVAD technology advances, many complications are unrelated to the device itself, further emphasizing the role of appropriate candidate selection and identifying the optimal window for LVAD implantation.

Controversy exists regarding the cost of such procedures given the already significant economic impact of heart failure on the healthcare system.[62] Although only a small number of patients have been studied, recent research suggests that prolonged unloading of the left ventricle with an LVAD in combination with drug therapy can produce sustained recovery in LV function and amelioration of symptoms.[63] Furthermore, more recent data suggest that patients referred for LVAD prior to the development of major complications of heart failure experience improved survival.[64]

For complete heart replacement therapy, total artificial heart systems continue to be investigated; however, embolic complications as well as the large size of the currently available systems limit their widespread use. Percutaneously inserted catheter-based LVADs are a more recent advancement. These small pumps may offer an advantage as they avoid the need for open-heart surgery; however, this technology is still in developmental stages.

Ultrafiltration

Renal impairment is common among patients with ADHF, and advanced forms may warrant the use of renal replacement therapy (e.g., hemodialysis). Ultrafiltration has emerged as another strategy for rapid fluid removal, where salt and water may be eliminated at rates of up to 500 mL/h. Ultrafiltration reduces PCWP and increases diuresis without adversely affecting hemodynamics (i.e., blood pressure, heart rate) or renal function, and is thought to be safer than diuretic therapy because fluid removal is isotonic. Potential candidates for ultrafiltration include patients demonstrating diuretic resistance, renal impairment following diuretic administration, or continued renal impairment despite inotropic therapy. Complications of ultrafiltration include those associated with central venous access (e.g., infection), rapid volume removal, and intravascular depletion, although electrolyte depletion is generally less significant compared to other treatment modalities.

Small studies suggest that ultrafiltration represents an effective strategy for fluid removal in heart failure patients and that early initiation prior to IV diuretics reduces hospital length of stay and readmission rates. In a study comparing early ultrafiltration to IV diuretics in patients with ADHF and evidence of fluid overload, ultrafiltration resulted in greater weight loss at 48 hours (5 kg vs. 3.1 kg) as well as net fluid loss (4.6 L vs. 3.3 L), although no differences in dyspnea scores were observed.[65] Several additional endpoints were improved among patients in the ultrafiltration group, including the incidence and duration of rehospitalization and incidence of unscheduled office or emergency department visits at 90 days. Although these results are promising, larger studies are necessary to determine the role of ultrafiltration in the management of ADHF.

HEART TRANSPLANTATION

Orthotopic heart transplantation remains the optimal management strategy for patients with chronic, irreversible NYHA class IV heart failure, as 10-year survival rates approach 50% among well-selected transplant recipients.[66] Unfortunately, the shortage of acceptable donor hearts has led to long waiting times and many patients succumb to their disease prior to transplantation. Another significant percentage of patients are deemed ineligible for transplantation because of age, concurrent illnesses, psychosocial factors, or other reasons. The shortage of donor hearts has prompted the development of new surgical strategies, including ventricular aneurysm resection, mitral valve repair, and myocardial cell transplantation, which have resulted in variable degrees of symptomatic improvement. Further development of these and other techniques may offer additional options in patients who are not considered candidates for transplantation.

EVALUATION OF THERAPEUTIC OUTCOMES

Assessment of therapeutic outcomes in patients with ADHF can be separated into two general categories: initial improvement of physiologic parameters and safe discharge from the hospital following transition to chronic oral medications. Both goals are equally important because hemodynamic improvement alone is not associated with prolonged symptom improvement or enhanced survival.

Initial stabilization requires an adequate arterial oxygen saturation, CI, and blood pressure necessary to maintain end-organ perfusion. Functional end-organ perfusion may be assessed by the presence of an appropriate mental status, renal function sufficient to prevent metabolic complications, hepatic function adequate to maintain synthetic and excretory functions, stable heart rate and rhythm (i.e., predominately sinus rhythm, rate-stabilized atrial fibrillation or flutter, or paced rhythm), absence of ongoing myocardial ischemia, skeletal muscle and skin blood flow sufficient to prevent ischemic injury, and normal arterial pH (7.34 to 7.47) and serum lactate concentration. Although these goals are most often achieved with a CI greater than 2.2 L/min/m^2 (0.037 L/s/m^2), mean arterial blood pressure greater than 60 mm Hg, and PCWP greater than 15 mm Hg, these absolute values are highly variable and depend on chronicity of illness, efficacy of chronic compensatory mechanisms, previous chronic therapy, and concurrent illnesses.

Discharge from the hospital requires maintaining the preceding parameters in the absence of ongoing IV therapy, mechanical circulatory support, or positive-pressure ventilation. Some patients may achieve this goal with markedly lower blood pressure or higher filling pressure than previously suggested; hence numerical goals cannot always be substituted for clinical status. Nonpharmacologic strategies aimed at the precipitants of a heart failure exacerbation include permanent pacing, chronic resynchronization therapy (i.e., biventricular pacing) with or without an implantable cardioverter-defibrillator, coronary angioplasty or valvuloplasty, pericardial drainage, cardiac surgery (coronary bypass, valve replacement or reconstruction, closure of intracardiac shunts), or cardiac transplantation to achieve initial stabilization, definitive therapy, or both.

PREPARATION FOR HOSPITAL DISCHARGE

All factors contributing to a heart failure decompensation should be addressed prior to discharge. Patients should be near or at optimal fluid status and transitioned from IV to oral diuretic therapy. Other chronic drug therapy should be optimized and appropriate follow-up clinic appointments scheduled. Typically, patients should be seen in clinic within 7 to 10 days of discharge. Both patients and their families should also receive appropriate education (see details below). For patients with recurrent hospital admissions, additional discharge criteria should be considered (Table 5-6).[10]

TABLE 5-6 Discharge Criteria for Patients with HF

Recommended for all HF patients	• Exacerbating factors addressed • Near optimal volume status observed • Transition from IV to oral diuretic successfully completed • Patient and family education completed, including clear discharge instructions • LVEF documented • Smoking cessation counseling initiated • Near optimal pharmacologic therapy achieved, including ACE inhibitor and β-blocker (for patients with reduced LVEF), or intolerance documented • Follow-up clinic visit scheduled, usually within 7–10 days
Should be considered for patients with advanced HF or recurrent admissions for HF	• Oral medication regimen stable for 24 hours • No IV vasodilator or inotropic agent for 24 hours • Ambulation before discharge to assess functional capacity after therapy • Plans for postdischarge management (scale present in home, visiting nurse or telephone follow-up generally no longer than 3 days after discharge) • Referral for disease management, if available

HF, heart failure; LVEF, left ventricular ejection fraction.

Data from Lindenfield J, et al. HFSA 2010 comprehensive heart failure practice guidelines. J Cardiac Fail 2010;12:e134–e156.

Patient education is essential in the discharge process and should involve input from a variety of disciplines, including dietitians, pharmacists, and other healthcare providers. Teaching should promote self-care by emphasizing specific positive and negative behaviors. By understanding key concepts of heart failure and its management, patient self-care should improve and future hospitalizations may be avoided.[10]

While all patients are likely to benefit from education, those with more severe symptoms (NYHA class III or IV) require the most comprehensive counseling. During the acute hospitalization, providers should educate on the most essential topics; this information should be reinforced and supplemented in the clinic setting within a couple of weeks after discharge. Recently hospitalized patients should also be considered for referral to a disease management program.

In end-stage disease, quality of life and prognosis should be discussed with patients and caregivers, and if possible, while the patient is still able to participate in the decision-making process. End-of-life care should be considered in patients with persistent symptoms at rest despite multiple attempts to optimize therapy, especially those with frequent hospitalizations, limited quality of life, dependence on intermittent or continuous IV therapy, or for those who might benefit from assist devices as destination therapy. In such cases, inactivation of an implantable cardioverter-defibrillator should be discussed and patients may be considered for a palliative care approach or hospice services.[10] As clinical status deteriorates and medical therapies become ineffective, healthcare providers should transition from focusing on mortality reduction to palliation of symptoms.[67]

PHARMACOECONOMIC CONSIDERATIONS

Heart failure imposes a tremendous economic burden on the healthcare system. Admission rates continue to grow and heart failure has become the most common reason for hospitalization among patients over the age of 65. Heart failure is also associated with unacceptably high readmission rates during the first 3 to 6 months after discharge. Current estimates of the costs of heart failure treatment in the United States approach $32 billion for 2013, with the greatest expense attributed to hospitalization. In addition, it is estimated that the total cost of HF will increase almost 120% to $70 billion by 2030.[1] The prevalence of heart failure and its associated costs are expected to increase as the population ages, especially as a result of improved survival from ischemic heart disease. Consequently, approaches aimed at improving the quality and cost-effectiveness of care for these patients may have a significant impact on healthcare costs.

Disease management programs have recently emerged as a novel approach for coordinating the increasingly complex management of heart failure. These programs utilize several approaches, including heart failure specialty clinics and/or home-based interventions. Most programs are multidisciplinary in nature and may include physicians, advanced practice nurses, dieticians, and pharmacists. Shown to reduce mortality, hospitalizations, and healthcare costs[68], this team-based approach allows providers to address a variety of issues, including optimization of drug and nondrug therapy; provide patient and family education, exercise and dietary advice, and intense follow-up by telephone or home visits; and monitoring and management of signs and symptoms of decompensation.

Pharmacists play an important role in the multidisciplinary management of heart failure and impact care in a number of ways, including optimization of doses of heart failure drug therapy, screening for drugs that exacerbate heart failure, monitoring for adverse drug effects and drug interactions, educating patients, and patient follow-up.[69,70] Compared to conventional care, these interventions have been shown to reduce hospitalizations for heart failure and improve adherence to guideline-recommended therapy. Additionally, a recent study found that pharmacist intervention also improved medication adherence and reduced emergency department visits and hospitalizations in low-income patients with heart failure.[71] Taken together, the results of these studies demonstrate the impact pharmacists can have on both patient outcomes and the cost-effectiveness of care.

FUTURE THERAPIES

Over the past decade, a number of large, international phase III development programs have failed to demonstrate a significant benefit in ADHF, including studies of the endothelin receptor antagonist tezosentan, calcium sensitizer levosimendan, vasopressin receptor antagonist tolvaptan, and adenosine A-1 receptor antagonist rolofylline. Potential explanations for the lack of positive findings include patient heterogeneity, limited understanding of underlying pathophysiology, improvements in background therapy, and limitations of study design including patient selection, timing and duration of intervention, and defined endpoints.[72] A number of investigations are currently underway to address these shortcomings as well as identify new and novel treatment strategies for patients with ADHF. Three pharmacologic therapies currently being investigated in patients with ADHF include serelaxin, omecamtiv mecarbil, and aliskiren.

Serelaxin is a novel recombinant form of human relaxin 2, a hormone that modulates the cardiovascular response during pregnancy (e.g., vasodilation, augmented renal function) as well as other important hemodynamic and neurohormonal effects.[73] A large randomized controlled trial is currently underway to assess the impact of serelaxin on shortness of breath and all-cause mortality in patients with ADHF and systolic blood pressure >125 mm Hg.[74] Preliminary results indicate a reduction in all-cause mortality among patients randomized to serelaxin compared to placebo.[75]

Omecamtiv mecarbil is a cardiac-specific activator of myosin, a motor protein responsible for cardiac contraction. Omecamtiv mecarbil activates myocardial ATPase, which improves energy utilization and enhances myosin cross-bridge formation and duration. It also increases the rate of phosphate release from myosin, thereby accelerating the rate-determining step of the cross-bridge cycle. As a result, omecamtiv mecarbil improves myocardial efficiency by increasing the duration of systolic ejection (and thus, stroke volume) without consuming additional energy or oxygen and without altering intracellular calcium levels.[76] Although omecamtiv mecarbil improves cardiac performance in the short term, its long-term effects have yet to be studied. An investigation of its role in patients with ADHF and left ventricular dysfunction is currently underway.[77,78]

Aliskiren is a direct renin inhibitor with favorable neurohormonal and hemodynamic effects that may be beneficial in patients with both chronic heart failure and ADHF. Given the neurohormonal abnormalities often present in patients with ADHF, the addition of aliskiren to standard therapy may reduce postdischarge mortality and rehospitalization. A trial evaluating these endpoints among patients with ADHF is currently underway.

Other therapies currently being investigated in ADHF include: nitroxyl, a reduced form of nitric oxide with arterial and venodilatory properties as well as positive inotropic and lusitropic properties; cenderitide (CD-NP), a chimeric protein that causes cGMP-mediated venodilation and aldosterone blockade; cinaciguat, a novel vasodilator that activates soluble guanylyl cyclase, leading to increased cGMP and subsequent venous and arterial vasodilation as well as reduced cell proliferation; clevidipine, a novel calcium channel blocker that selectively dilates arteries with no significant effect on myocardial contractility; and istaroxime, which inhibits sodium–potassium ATP activity and stimulates sarcoplasmic reticulum calcium adenosine triphosphatase isoform 2a (SERCA2a), thereby increasing lusitropy and inotropy.[79] Additional studies currently underway include investigations of novel biomarkers in determining diagnosis, prognosis, and optimal management of ADHF; renal optimization strategies such as low-dose nesiritide and low-dose dopamine; mechanical support devices; and various interdisciplinary models of care.

CLINICAL CONTROVERSIES

1. The optimal pharmacotherapy for patients with ADHF who are refractory to diuretic therapy has been clarified by investigations showing minimal to no difference between administration by IV bolus or continuous infusion. Higher doses (i.e., 2.5-times the previous oral dose) of IV diuretic are more effective than lower doses (i.e., equivalent to previous oral dose) but may also result in greater rates of renal dysfunction. The following controversies remain unaddressed by the current literature: the role of adding a diurectic with an alternative mechanism of action, which alternative diuretic should be added (e.g., metolazone, HCTZ, other), and the role of ultrafiltration.
2. The role of nesiritide in ADHF has also been clarified. After two meta-analyses suggested that its use was associated with worsening renal function and increased mortality, a recent investigation found that nesiritide neither improved nor worsened outcomes in ADHF. However, the efficacy and safety of other vasodilators have not been well established and the use of positive inotropes has been associated with poor outcomes.
3. Clinicians continue to struggle with avoiding cardiorenal syndrome while trying to manage ADHF patients. Novel therapies or therapeutic strategies to address cardiorenal syndrome continue to evolve. Evolving data regarding the role of LVADs as a bridge to transplantation or destination therapy provide further support for the use of these therapeutic modalities. Additional data are warranted to further define the most optimal candidates, timelines for implantation, and how to best minimize complications associated with these devices.

ABBREVIATIONS

ACC	American College of Cardiology
ACE	angiotensin-converting enzyme
AHA	American Heart Association
ANP	atrial natriuretic peptide
AVP	arginine vasopressin
BNP	B-type natriuretic peptide
cAMP	cyclic adenosine monophosphate
CI	cardiac index
CO	cardiac output
HFSA	Heart Failure Society of America
IABP	intraaortic balloon pump
LVAD	left ventricular assist device
NYHA	New York Heart Association
PCWP	pulmonary capillary wedge pressure
SVR	systemic vascular resistance
VAD	ventricular assist device

REFERENCES

1. Go AS, Mozaffarian D, Roger VL, et al. Heart Disease and Stroke Statistics—2013 Update: A Report From the American Heart Association. Circulation 2013;127:e6–e245. doi: 10.1161/CIR.0b013e31828124ad.
2. Roger VL, Go AS, Lloyd-Jones DM, et al. Heart disease and stroke statistics—2012 update: A report from the American Heart Association. Circulation 2012;125(1):e2–e220. doi: 10.1161/CIR.0b013e31823ac046.
3. Mehra MR. Optimizing outcomes in the patient with acute decompensated heart failure. Am Heart J 2006;151(3):571–579.
4. Hunt SA, Abraham WT, Chin MH, et al. 2009 focused update incorporated into the ACC/AHA 2005 Guidelines for the Diagnosis and Management of Heart Failure in Adults: A report of the American College of Cardiology Foundation/American Heart Association Task Force on Practice Guidelines: Developed in collaboration with the International Society for Heart and Lung Transplantation. Circulation 2009;119(14):e391–479. doi: 10.1161/circulationaha.109.192065
5. Hunt SA, Abraham WT, Chin MH, et al. ACC/AHA 2005 Guideline Update for the Diagnosis and Management of Chronic Heart Failure in the Adult: A report of the American College of Cardiology/American Heart Association Task Force on Practice Guidelines (Writing Committee to Update the 2001 Guidelines for the Evaluation and Management of Heart Failure): Developed in collaboration with the American College of Chest Physicians and the International Society for Heart and Lung Transplantation: Endorsed by the Heart Rhythm Society. Circulation 2005;112(12):e154–e235.
6. Jessup M, Abraham WT, Casey DE, et al. 2009 focused update: ACCF/AHA Guidelines for the Diagnosis and Management of Heart Failure in Adults: A report of the American College of Cardiology Foundation/American Heart Association Task Force on Practice Guidelines: Developed in collaboration with the International Society for Heart and Lung Transplantation. Circulation 2009;119(14):1977–2016.
7. Felker GM, Adams KF Jr, Konstam MA, O'Connor CM, Gheorghiade M. The problem of decompensated heart failure: Nomenclature, classification, and risk stratification. Am Heart J 2003;145(2 Suppl):S18–S25.
8. Cuffe MS, Califf RM, Adams KF, et al. Short-term intravenous milrinone for acute exacerbation of chronic heart failure: A randomized controlled trial. JAMA 2002;287(12):1541–1547.
9. The VMAC Investigators. Intravenous nesiritide vs nitroglycerin for treatment of decompensated congestive heart failure: A randomized controlled trial. JAMA 2002;287(12):1531–1540.
10. Lindenfeld J, Albert NM, Boehmer JP, et al. HFSA 2010 Comprehensive Heart Failure Practice Guideline. J Card Fail 2010;16(6):e1–e194. doi: 10.1016/j.cardfail.2010.04.004
11. Gheorghiade M, Zannad F, Sopko G, et al. Acute heart failure syndromes: Current state and framework for future research. Circulation 2005;112(25):3958–3968.
12. Adams KFJr, Fonarow GC, Emerman CL, et al. Characteristics and outcomes of patients hospitalized for heart failure in the United States: Rationale, design, and preliminary observations from the first 100,000 cases in the Acute Decompensated Heart Failure National Registry (ADHERE). Am Heart J 2005;149(2):209–216.
13. Fonarow GC, Adams KF Jr, Abraham WT, Yancy CW, Boscardin WJ. Risk stratification for in-hospital mortality in acutely decompensated heart failure: Classification and regression tree analysis. JAMA 2005;293(5):572–580.

14. O'Connor CM, Abraham WT, Albert NM, et al. Predictors of mortality after discharge in patients hospitalized with heart failure: An analysis from the Organized Program to Initiate Lifesaving Treatment in Hospitalized Patients with Heart Failure (OPTIMIZE-HF). Am Heart J 2008;156(4):662–673.
15. Nohria A, Mielniczuk LM, Stevenson LW. Evaluation and monitoring of patients with acute heart failure syndromes. Am J Cardiol 2005;96(6A):32G–40G.
16. Adams KF, Lindenfeld J, Arnold JMO, et al. HFSA 2006 Comprehensive Heart Failure Practice Guideline: Section 7: Heart failure in patients with left ventricular systolic dysfunction. J Card Fail 2006;12(1):e38–e57.
17. Maisel A, Mueller C, Adams K Jr, et al. State of the art: Using natriuretic peptide levels in clinical practice. Eur J Heart Fail 2008;10(9):824–839.
18. Fonarow GC, Abraham WT, Albert NM, et al. Influence of beta-blocker continuation or withdrawal on outcomes in patients hospitalized with heart failure: Findings from the OPTIMIZE-HF program. J Am Coll Cardiol 2008;52(3):190–199. doi: 10.1016/j.jacc.2008.03.048
19. Jondeau G, Neuder Y, Eicher JC, et al. B-CONVINCED: Beta-blocker continuation Vs. interruption in patients with congestive heart failure hospitalized for a decompensation episode. Eur Heart J 2009;30(18):2186–2192. doi: 10.1093/eurheartj/ehp323
20. Packer M, Gheorghiade M, Young JB, et al. Withdrawal of digoxin from patients with chronic heart failure treated with angiotensin-converting-enzyme inhibitors. RADIANCE Study. N Engl J Med 1993;329(1):1–7. doi: 10.1056/nejm199307013290101
21. Uretsky B, Young JB, Shahidi FE, et al. Randomized study assessing the effect of digoxin withdrawal in patients with mild to moderate chronic congestive heart failure: Results of the PROVED trial. J Am Coll Cardiol 1993;22:955–962.
22. Nohria A, Lewis E, Stevenson LW. Medical management of advanced heart failure. JAMA 2002;287(5):628–640.
23. Binanay C, Califf RM, Hasselblad V, et al. Evaluation study of congestive heart failure and pulmonary artery catheterization effectiveness: The ESCAPE trial. JAMA 2005;294(13):1625–1633.
24. Forrester JS, Diamond G, Chatterjee K, Swan HJC. Medical therapy of acute myocardial infarction by application of hemodynamic subsets. N Engl J Med 1976;295:1356–1362.
25. Finley JJ 4th, Konstam MA, Udelson JE. Arginine vasopressin antagonists for the treatment of heart failure and hyponatremia. Circulation 2008;118(4):410–421.
26. Brater DC. Pharmacology of diuretics. Am J Med Sci 2000;319(1):38–50.
27. Brater DC. Diuretic therapy in congestive heart failure. CHF 2000;6:197–210.
28. Iyengar S, Abraham WT. Diuretics for the treatment of acute decompensated heart failure. Heart Fail Rev 2007;12(2):125–130.
29. Stough WG, O'Connor CM, Gheorghiade M. Overview of current noninodilator therapies for acute heart failure syndromes. Am J Cardiol 2005;96(6A):41G–46G.
30. Eshaghian S, Horwich TB, Fonarow GC. Relation of loop diuretic dose to mortality in advanced heart failure. Am J Cardiol 2006;97(12):1759–1764.
31. Butler J, Forman DE, Abraham WT, et al. Relationship between heart failure treatment and development of worsening renal function among hospitalized patients. Am Heart J 2004;147(2):331–338.
32. Cleland JG, Coletta A, Witte K. Practical applications of intravenous diuretic therapy in decompensated heart failure. Am J Med 2006;119(12 Suppl 1):S26–36.
33. Felker GM, Lee KL, Bull DA, et al. Diuretic strategies in patients with acute decompensated heart failure. N Engl J Med 2011;364(9):797–805. doi: 10.1056/NEJMoa1005419
34. Adams KF, Lindenfeld J, Arnold JMO, et al. HFSA 2006 Comprehensive Heart Failure Practice Guideline: Section 12: Evaluation and management of patients with acute decompensated heart failure. J Card Fail 2006;12(1):e86–e103.
35. Dormans TP, van Meyel JJ, Gerlag PG, Tan Y, Russel FG, Smits P. Diuretic efficacy of high dose furosemide in severe heart failure: Bolus injection versus continuous infusion. J Am Coll Cardiol 1996;28(2):376–382.
36. Thomson MR, Nappi JM, Dunn SP, et al. Continuous versus intermittent infusion furosemide in acute decompensated heart failure. J Card Fail 2010;16(3):188–193.
37. Vargo DL, Brater DC, Rudy DW, Swan SK. Dopamine does not enhance furosemide-induced natriuresis in patients with congestive heart failure. J Am Soc Nephrol 1996;7(7):1032–1037.
38. Giamouzis G, Butler J, Starling RC, et al. Impact of dopamine infusion on renal function in hospitalized heart failure patients: Results of the dopamine in acute decompensated heart failure (DAD-HF) trial. J Card Fail 2010;16(12):922–930. doi: 10.1016/j.cardfail.2010.07.246
39. Bayram M, De Luca L, Massie MB, Gheorghiade M. Reassessment of dobutamine, dopamine, and milrinone in the management of acute heart failure syndromes. Am J Cardiol 2005;96(6A):47G–58G.
40. Lehtonen LA, Antila S, Pentikainen PJ. Pharmacokinetics and pharmacodynamics of intravenous inotropic agents. Clin Pharmacokinet 2004;43(3):187–203.
41. Abraham WT, Adams KF, Fonarow GC, et al. In-hospital mortality in patients with acute decompensated heart failure requiring intravenous vasoactive medications: An analysis from the Acute Decompensated Heart Failure National Registry (ADHERE). J Am Coll Cardiol 2005;46(1):57–64.
42. Metra M, Nodari S, D'Aloia A, et al. Beta-blocker therapy influences the hemodynamic response to inotropic agents in patients with heart failure: A randomized comparison of dobutamine and enoximone before and after chronic treatment with metoprolol or carvedilol. J Am Coll Cardiol 2002;40(7):1248–1258.
43. Dorsch MP, Rodgers JE. Nesiritide: Harmful or harmless? Pharmacotherapy 2006;26(10):1465–1478.
44. Mullens W, Abrahams Z, Francis GS, et al. Sodium nitroprusside for advanced low-output heart failure. J Am Coll Cardiol 2008;52(3):200–207. doi: 10.1016/j.jacc.2008.02.083
45. Aaronson KD, Sackner-Bernstein J. Risk of death associated with nesiritide in patients with acutely decompensated heart failure. JAMA 2006;296(12):1465–1466. doi: 10.1001/jama.296.12.1465
46. Sackner-Bernstein JD, Kowalski M, Fox M, Aaronson K. Short-term risk of death after treatment with nesiritide for decompensated heart failure: A pooled analysis of randomized controlled trials. JAMA 2005;293(15):1900–1905.
47. Sackner-Bernstein JD, Skopicki HA, Aaronson KD. Risk of worsening renal function with nesiritide in patients with acutely decompensated heart failure. Circulation 2005;111(12):1487–1491.
48. Reynolds RM, Padfield PL, Seckl JR. Disorders of sodium balance. BMJ 2006;332(7543):702–705.
49. Gheorghiade M, Gattis WA, O'Connor CM, et al. Effects of tolvaptan, a vasopressin antagonist, in patients hospitalized

with worsening heart failure: A randomized controlled trial. JAMA 2004;291(16):1963–1971.

50. Lee WH, Packer M. Prognostic importance of serum sodium concentration and its modification by converting-enzyme inhibition in patients with severe chronic heart failure. Circulation 1986;73(2):257–267.
51. Adrogue HJ, Madias NE. Hyponatremia. N Engl J Med 2000;342(21):1581–1589.
52. Lee CR, Watkins ML, Patterson JH, et al. Vasopressin: A new target for the treatment of heart failure. Am Heart J 2003;146(1):9–18.
53. Tolvaptan (Samsca™) package insert. Rockville, MD: Otsuka America Pharmaceutical, Inc., May 2009.
54. Schrier RW, Gross P, Gheorghiade M, et al. Tolvaptan, a selective oral vasopressin V2-receptor antagonist, for hyponatremia. N Engl J Med 2006;355(20):2099–2112.
55. Gheorghiade M, Konstam MA, Burnett JC Jr, et al. Short-term clinical effects of tolvaptan, an oral vasopressin antagonist, in patients hospitalized for heart failure: The EVEREST Clinical Status Trials. JAMA 2007;297(12):1332–1343.
56. Konstam MA, Gheorghiade M, Burnett JC Jr, et al. Effects of oral tolvaptan in patients hospitalized for worsening heart failure: The EVEREST outcome trial. JAMA 2007;297(12):1319–1331.
57. Boehmer JP, Popjes E. Cardiac failure: Mechanical support strategies. Crit Care Med 2006;34(9 Suppl):S268–S277.
58. Thiele H, Zeymer U, Neumann FJ, et al. Intraaortic balloon support for myocardial infarction with cardiogenic shock. N Engl J Med 2012;367(14):1287–1296. doi: 10.1056/NEJMoa1208410
59. Lietz K, Miller LW. Destination therapy: Current results and future promise. Semin Thorac Cardiovasc Surg 2008;20(3):225–233.
60. Rose EA, Gelijns AC, Moskowitz AJ, et al. Long-term mechanical left ventricular assistance for end-stage heart failure. N Engl J Med 2001;345(20):1435–1443.
61. Rogers JG, Butler J, Lansman SL, et al. Chronic mechanical circulatory support for inotrope-dependent heart failure patients who are not transplant candidates: Results of the INTREPID Trial. J Am Coll Cardiol 2007;50(8):741–747.
62. Russo MJ, Gelijns AC, Stevenson LW, et al. The cost of medical management in advanced heart failure during the final two years of life. J Card Fail 2008;14(8):651–658.
63. Birks EJ, Tansley PD, Hardy J, et al. Left ventricular assist device and drug therapy for the reversal of heart failure. N Engl J Med 2006;355(18):1873–1884.
64. Lietz K, Long JW, Kfoury AG, et al. Outcomes of left ventricular assist device implantation as destination therapy in the post-REMATCH era: Implications for patient selection. Circulation 2007;116(5):497–505.
65. Costanzo MR, Guglin ME, Saltzberg MT, et al. Ultrafiltration versus intravenous diuretics for patients hospitalized for acute decompensated heart failure. J Am Coll Cardiol 2007;49(6):675–683.
66. Taylor DO, Edwards LB, Boucek MM, et al. Registry of the International Society for Heart and Lung Transplantation: Twenty-third official adult heart transplantation report—2006. J Heart Lung Transplant 2006;25(8):869–879.
67. Hauptman PJ, Havranek EP. Integrating palliative care into heart failure care. Arch Intern Med 2005;165(4):374–378.
68. Holland R, Battersby J, Harvey I, Lenaghan E, Smith J, Hay L. Systematic review of multidisciplinary interventions in heart failure. Heart 2005;91(7):899–906.
69. Gattis WA, Hasselblad V, Whellan DJ, O'Connor CM. Reduction in heart failure events by the addition of a clinical pharmacist to the heart failure management team. Arch Int Med 1999;159:1939–1945.
70. Whellan DJ, Gaulden L, Gattis WA, et al. The benefit of implementing a heart failure disease management program. Arch Intern Med 2001;161(18):2223–2228.
71. Murray MD, Young J, Hoke S, et al. Pharmacist intervention to improve medication adherence in heart failure. A randomized trial. Ann Intern Med 2007;146:714–725.
72. Felker GM, Pang PS, Adams KF, et al. Clinical trials of pharmacological therapies in acute heart failure syndromes: Lessons learned and directions forward. Circ Heart Fail 2010;3(2):314–325. doi: 10.1161/circheartfailure.109.893222
73. Teichman SL, Unemori E, Teerlink JR, Cotter G, Metra M. Relaxin: Review of biology and potential role in treating heart failure. Curr Heart Fail Rep 2010;7(2):75–82. doi: 10.1007/s11897-010-0010-z
74. Ponikowski P, Metra M, Teerlink JR, et al. Design of the RELAXin in acute heart failure study. Am Heart J 2012;163(2):149–155 e141. doi: 10.1016/j.ahj.2011.10.009
75. Teerlink JR, Metra M, Felker GM, et al. Relaxin for the treatment of patients with acute heart failure (Pre-RELAX-AHF): A multicentre, randomised, placebo-controlled, parallel-group, dose-finding phase IIb study. Lancet 2009;373(9673):1429–1439. doi: 10.1016/s0140-6736(09)60622-x
76. Malik FI, Hartman JJ, Elias KA, et al. Cardiac myosin activation: A potential therapeutic approach for systolic heart failure. Science 2011;331(6023):1439–1443. doi: 10.1126/science.1200113
77. Cleland JG, Teerlink JR, Senior R, et al. The effects of the cardiac myosin activator, omecamtiv mecarbil, on cardiac function in systolic heart failure: A double-blind, placebo-controlled, crossover, dose-ranging phase 2 trial. Lancet 2011;378(9792):676–683. doi: 10.1016/s0140–6736(11)61126–4
78. Teerlink JR, Clarke CP, Saikali KG, et al. Dose-dependent augmentation of cardiac systolic function with the selective cardiac myosin activator, omecamtiv mecarbil: A first-in-man study. Lancet 2011;378(9792):667–675. doi: 10.1016/s0140-6736(11)61219-1
79. Majure DT, Teerlink JR. Update on the management of acute decompensated heart failure. Curr Treat Options Cardiovasc Med. 2011;13(6):570–585. doi: 10.1007/s11936-011-0149-2

Ischemic Heart Disease

Robert L. Talbert

6

KEY CONCEPTS

1. Ischemic heart disease (IHD) is primarily caused by coronary atherosclerotic plaque formation that leads to an imbalance between oxygen supply and demand resulting in myocardial ischemia.
2. Chest pain is the cardinal symptom of myocardial ischemia due to coronary artery disease (CAD).
3. Risk factor identification and modification are important interventions for individual patients with known or suspected IHD and as a population-based policy to reduce the impact of this disease.
4. Major risk factors that can be altered include dyslipidemia (high total and low-density lipoprotein [LDL] cholesterol, low HDL cholesterol, and high triglycerides), smoking, glycemic control in diabetes mellitus, hypertension, and adoption of therapeutic lifestyle changes (exercise, weight reduction, and reduced cholesterol and fat in the diet). Reduction in inflammation may also play an important role.
5. Most patients with CAD should receive antiplatelet therapy. Chronic stable angina should be managed initially with β-blockers because they provide better symptomatic control at least as well as nitrates or calcium channel blockers and decrease the risk of recurrent myocardial infarction (MI) and CAD mortality.
6. Nitroglycerin and other nitrate products are useful for prophylaxis of angina when patients are undertaking activities known to provoke angina; however, when angina is occurring on a regular, routine basis, chronic prophylactic therapy should be instituted.
7. Although calcium channel blockers are effective as monotherapy, they are generally used in combination with β-blockers or as monotherapy if patients are intolerant of β-blockers; most patients with moderate-to-severe angina will require two drugs to control their symptoms. Ranolazine is a second-line drug to be used with β-blockers and certain calcium channel blockers.
8. Pharmacologic management is as effective as revascularization (percutaneous transluminal coronary angioplasty [PTCA], coronary artery bypass grafting [CABG], etc.) if one or two vessels are involved and there are no differences in survival, recurrent MI, or other measures of effectiveness.
9. Multivessel involvement, especially if the patient has left main CAD or left main equivalent disease, or two- to three-vessel involvement with significant left ventricular dysfunction is best managed with revascularization. With improvements in stent technology, more patients are eligible for this approach compared with CABG.
10. PTCA and CABG produce similar results overall, but certain patient subsets (e.g., diabetics) should have CABG done.
11. The clinical performance measures for chronic stable CAD recommended by the American College of Cardiology and the American Heart Association include blood pressure measurement, lipid profile, symptom and activity assessment, smoking cessation, antiplatelet therapy, drug therapy for lowering LDL cholesterol, β-blocker therapy for prior MI, ACE inhibitor therapy, and screening for diabetes.

INTRODUCTION

Atherosclerosis of the epicardial vessels leading to coronary heart disease (CHD) is the main etiology of ischemic heart disease (IHD). This process begins early in life, often not being clinically manifest until the middle-aged years and beyond. IHD may present as an acute coronary syndrome (ACS includes unstable angina, non–ST-segment elevation myocardial infarction [MI] or ST-segment elevation MI—see Chap. 7), chronic stable exertional angina pectoris, and ischemia without clinical symptoms. Coronary artery vasospasm (variant or Prinzmetal's angina) produces similar symptoms but is not due to atherosclerosis. Microvascular angina that is myocardial ischemia without occlusive CHD is seen more commonly in women than in men. Other manifestations of atherosclerosis include heart failure, arrhythmias, cerebrovascular disease (stroke), and peripheral vascular disease. The American Heart Association (AHA), the American College of Cardiology, and the European Society of Cardiology have published management guidelines for stable and unstable angina.[1,2]

EPIDEMIOLOGY

The AHA estimates that 83,000,000 American adults have one or more types of cardiovascular disease (CVD) based on data from 2007 to 2010.[3] Nearly 2,300 Americans die of CVD each day, or an average of 1 death every 38 seconds. In 2009, the death rates from CVD were 387 (per 100,000) for black males, 281.4 for white males, 269.9 for black females, and 190.4 for white females.[3] Mortality data for 2010 show that CVD accounted for 34.3% of 2,468,435 deaths in 2009 or 1 of every ~4 deaths in the United States. Men die earlier from IHD and AMI than women, and aging of both sexes is associated with a higher incidence of these afflictions. The disparity in mortality from IHD between men and women decreases with aging, being about four to five times more common in men from the age of the mid-30s to a preponderance of female deaths in the very elderly.

The syndrome of angina pectoris is reported to occur with an average annual incidence rate (number of new cases per time period/total number of persons in the population for the same time period) of about 1.5% (range 0.1 to 5/1,000) depending on the patient's age, gender, and risk factor profile.[4] The estimated prevalence of angina in 2010 was 7,800,000 (3.2% of the population), and the incidence of stable angina was 500,000.[3] The presenting manifestation in women is more commonly angina, whereas men more frequently have MI as the initial event. Estimates of the incidence and prevalence of angina are not entirely accurate due to waxing and waning of symptoms; angina may disappear in up to 30% of patients with angina that is less severe and of recent onset.

Data from the Framingham study show that the prevalence in a 1970 cohort followed for 10 years was about 1.5% for women and 4.3% for men aged 50 to 59 years at inception.[4] The annual rates of new episodes of angina range from 28.3 to 33 per 1,000 population for non-black men, 22.4 to 39.5 for black men, 14.1 to 22.9 for non-black women, and 15.3 to 35.9 for black women in the age range of 65 to 84 years or older.[5] AHA estimates that the prevalence of angina was 10.2 million in 2006.[5] Between 1980 and 2002, death rates due to CHD among men and women ≥65 years of age fell by 52% in men and 49% in women.[5] The risk of developing IHD is not the same worldwide. Countries such as Japan and France are on the low end of the spectrum, whereas Finland, Northern Ireland, Scotland, and South Africa have very high rates of IHD.[6,7]

Angina may be classified according to symptom severity, disability induced, or a specific activity scale (Tables 6-1 and 6-2). The Specific Activity Scale developed by Goldman et al.[8] may be preferable because it has been shown to be equal to or better than the New York Heart Association (NYHA) or Canadian Cardiovascular Society functional classifications for reproducibility and provides better agreement with exercise treadmill testing.

TABLE 6-1 Criteria for Determination of the Specific Activity Scale Functional Class

	Any Yes	No
1. Can you walk down a flight of steps without stopping (4.5–5.2 MET)?	Go to 2	Go to 4
2. Can you carry anything up a flight of eight steps without stopping (5–5.5 MET)? Or can you: a. Have sexual intercourse without stopping (5–5.2 MET)? b. Garden, rake, weed (5.6 MET)? c. Roller skate, dance foxtrot (5–6 MET)? d. Walk at a 4-mph (6.5 km/h) rate on level ground (5–6 MET)?	Go to 3	Class III
3. Can you carry at least 24 lb (10.9 kg) up eight steps (10 MET)? Or can you: a. Carry objects that weigh at least 80 lb (36.4 kg) (18 MET)? b. Do outdoor work, shovel snow, spade soil (7 MET)? c. Do recreational activities such as skiing, basketball, touch football, squash, handball (7–10 MET)? d. Jog/walk 5 mph (8 km/h) (9 MET)?	Class I	Class II
4. Can you shower without stopping (3.6–4.2 MET)? Or can you: a. Strip and make bed (3.9–5 MET)? b. Mop floors (4.2 MET)? c. Hang washed clothes (4.4 MET)? d. Clean windows (3.7 MET)? e. Walk 2.5 mph (4 km/h) (3–3.5 MET)? f. Bowl (3–4.4 MET)? g. Play golf, walk and carry clubs (4.5 MET)? h. Push a power lawnmower (4 MET)?	Class III	Go to 5
5. Can you dress without stopping because of symptoms (2–2.3 MET)?	Class III	Class IV

MET, metabolic equivalents of activity.

From reference 8, with permission.

TABLE 6-2 Grading of Angina Pectoris by the Canadian Cardiovascular Society Classification System

Class	Description of Stage
Class I	Ordinary physical activity does not cause angina, such as walking and climbing stairs. Angina occurs with strenuous, rapid, or prolonged exertion at work or recreation
Class II	Slight limitation or ordinary activity. Angina occurs on walking or climbing stairs rapidly, on walking uphill, on walking or stair climbing after meals, in cold, in wind, under emotional stress, or only during the few hours after wakening. Walking more than two blocks on the level and climbing more than one flight of ordinary stairs at a normal pace and in normal condition
Class III	Marked limitations of ordinary physical activity. Angina occurs on walking one to two blocks on the level and climbing one flight of stairs in normal conditions and at a normal pace
Class IV	Inability to carry on any physical activity without discomfort—anginal symptoms may be present at rest

From Campeau L. Grading of angina [letter]. Circulation 1976;54:522–523, with permission.

An important determinate of outcome for the angina patient is the number of vessels obstructed. Twelve-year survival from the Coronary Artery Surgery Study (CASS) for patients with zero-, one-, two-, and three-vessel disease was 88%, 74%, 59%, and 40%, respectively.[9] Other factors that increase the risk of death in medically managed patients include the presence of heart failure (or markers such as poor ventricular wall motion and low ejection fraction), smoking, left main or left main equivalent coronary artery disease (CAD), diabetes, or prior MI. Twelve-year survival for patients with at least one diseased vessel and ejection fractions in the ranges of ≥50% (≥0.50), 35% to 49% (0.35 to 0.49), and 0% to 34% (0 to 0.34) is 73%, 54%, and 21%, respectively. Of particular note, patients with left main CAD (or left main equivalent) are at extremely high risk and constitute a unique group for therapeutic consideration.[10] In the CASS, at 15 years of follow-up, 37% of the surgery group and 27% of the medical group are surviving; median survival is 13.3 years versus 6.7 years, respectively ($P < 0.0001$). It is important to realize that these surgery studies are nearly 20 years old and event rates are now likely lower. Technology advances in coronary artery stent development may now allow more patients to be treated with primary percutaneous intervention (PCI) rather than coronary artery bypass grafting (CABG).[11] Indeed, current guidelines provide similar recommendations for PCI and CABG in certain patients.[12] If systolic function was normal, then median survival and percent surviving were not different between the surgery and medical groups (median survival of about 15 years). Patients screened but not randomized to CASS had similar survival rates, suggesting that results from randomized patients may be applicable to more generalized populations as a measure of external reliability.

ETIOLOGY AND PATHOPHYSIOLOGY

The pathophysiology that underlies this disease process is dynamic, evolutionary, and complex. An understanding of the determinants of myocardial oxygen demand (MVO_2), regulation of coronary blood flow, the effects of ischemia on the mechanical and metabolic function of the myocardium, and how ischemia is recognized is important to understand the rationale for the selection and use of pharmacotherapy for IHD.

1 Ischemia may be defined as lack of oxygen and decreased or no blood flow in the myocardium. In contrast, anoxia, defined as

the absence of oxygen to the myocardium, results in continued perfusion with washout of acid by-products of glycolysis, thereby preserving the mechanical and metabolic status of the heart to a greater extent than does ischemia for short periods of time.

Determinants of Oxygen Demand (MVO_2)

The major determinants of MVO_2 are (a) heart rate (HR), (b) contractility, and (c) intramyocardial wall tension during systole. Overall, intramyocardial wall tension is thought to be the most important among these three factors. As the consequences of IHD are a result of increased demand in the face of a fixed supply of oxygen in most situations, alterations in MVO_2 are critically important in producing ischemia and for interventions intended to alleviate ischemia. MVO_2 cannot be directly measured in patients; however, an indirect assessment that correlates reasonably well with MVO_2 as determined in experimental animal models is the tension–time index (TTI). This is a measure of the area under the curve of the left ventricular (LV) pressure curve. Tension in the ventricle wall is a function of the radius of the LV and intraventricular pressure. These factors are related through Laplace's law, which states that wall stress is related directly to the product of intraventricular pressure and internal radius and inversely to wall thickness multiplied by a factor of two. Increasing systemic blood pressure or ventricular dilation would increase wall tension and oxygen demand, whereas ventricular hypertrophy would tend to minimize increasing MVO_2. Clinical application of these principles has led to the use of the double product (DP), which is HR multiplied by systolic blood pressure (SBP) (DP = HR × SBP). Although this is a clinically useful indirect estimate of MVO_2, it does not consider changes in contractility (an independent variable), and because only changes in pressure are considered with the DP, volume loading of the LV and increased MVO_2 related to ventricular dilation are underestimated.

Regulation of Coronary Blood Flow

Coronary blood flow is influenced by multiple factors; however, the caliber of the resistance vessels delivering blood to the myocardium and MVO_2 are the prime determinants in the occurrence of ischemia. The anatomy of the vascular bed will affect oxygen supply and, subsequently, myocardial metabolism and mechanical function.

Anatomic Factors

The normal coronary system consists of large epicardial or surface vessels (R1) that normally offer little intrinsic resistance to myocardial flow and intramyocardial arteries and arterioles (R2), which branch into a dense capillary network (about 4,000 capillaries/mm^2) to supply basal blood flow of 60 to 90 mL/min per 100 g of myocardium. R1 and R2 are in series and total resistance is the algebraic sum; however, under normal circumstances, the resistance in R2 is much greater. Myocardial blood flow is inversely related to arteriolar resistance and directly related to the coronary driving pressure. The arterioles dynamically alter their intrinsic tone in response to demands for oxygen and other factors, and as a result, myocardial oxygen delivery and MVO_2 are tightly coupled in a rapidly responsive system.

Atherosclerotic lesions encroaching on the luminal cross-sectional area of the larger epicardial vessels (R1) transform the relationships among R1, R2, and blood flow. As resistance increases in R1 owing to occlusion, R2 can vasodilate to maintain coronary blood flow. This response is inadequate with greater degrees of obstruction, and the coronary flow reserve afforded by R2 vasodilation is insufficient to meet oxygen demand (also referred to as autoregulation). The extent of functional obstruction is important in the limitation of coronary blood flow, and the presence of relatively severe stenosis (>70%) may provoke ischemia and symptoms at rest, whereas less severe stenosis may allow a reserve of coronary blood flow for exertion.[13]

The diameter of the lesion impeding blood flow through a vessel is important, but other factors such as length of the lesion and the influence of pressure drop across an area of stenosis also affect coronary blood flow and function of the collateral circulation. Resistance to flow in a vessel is directly related to length of the obstructing lesion, but resistance is inversely related to the diameter of the vessel to the fourth power. Diameter is, therefore, much more important. As blood flows across a stenotic lesion, the pressure drops (energy losses) due to friction between blood and the lesion and due to the abrupt turbulent expansion as blood emerges from the stenosis. This pressure drop is dynamic and directly related to flow giving rise to a resistance that is not fixed, but rather fluctuates, as flow is changed. This relationship can dramatically affect collateral blood flow and its response to exercise, resulting in what has been called *coronary steal*. A similar situation may also occur when the epicardial or subepicardial vessels steal blood flow from the endocardium in the presence of a stenotic lesion.

Large and small coronary arteries may undergo dynamic changes in coronary vascular resistance and coronary blood flow. Dynamic coronary obstruction can occur in normal vessels and vessels with stenosis in which vasomotion or spasm may be superimposed on a fixed stenosis. Although it is possible that these changes may be active in small coronary arteries, it is also possible that the observed changes may reflect collapse owing to poststenotic intraluminal pressure drop or increased intramyocardial compressive forces associated with inadequate ventricular relaxation.

Collateral blood flow exists to a certain extent from birth as native collaterals, but persisting ischemia may promote collateral growth as developed collaterals. These two types of collaterals differ in anatomy and in their ability to regulate coronary blood flow. Collateral development is dependent on the severity of obstruction, the presence of various growth factors (basic fibroblast growth factor [β-FGF] and vascular endothelial growth factor [VEGF]), endogenous vasodilators (e.g., nitrous oxide, prostacyclin), hormones such as estrogen, and potentially exercise. Collateral development is highly species dependent and this should be considered when reading experimental literature. A recently developed technique called fractional flow reserve (FFR) allows for the measurement of coronary blood flow in the area of stenosis to assess the physiologic significance of stenosis (see Chap. 1 for details).

Metabolic Regulation

Coronary blood flow is closely tied to oxygen needs of the heart. Changes in oxygen balance lead to very rapid changes in coronary blood flow. Although a number of mediators may contribute to these changes, the most important ones are likely to be adenosine, other nucleotides, nitric oxide, prostaglandins, CO_2, and H^+. Adenosine, which is formed from adenosine triphosphate (ATP) and adenosine monophosphate (AMP) under conditions of ischemia and stress, is a potent vasodilator that links decreased perfusion to metabolically induced vasodilation or *reactive hyperemia*. The synthesis and release of adenosine into coronary sinus venous effluent occurs within seconds after coronary artery occlusion, and about 30% of the hyperemic response can be blocked by metabolic blockers of adenosine. Coronary reactivity can be used to detect individuals at risk for future events.[14]

Endothelial Control of Coronary Vascular Tone

The vascular endothelium, a single-cell tissue with an enormous surface area separating the blood from vascular smooth muscle of the artery wall, is capable of a broad range of metabolic functions. The endothelium functions as a protective surface for the artery wall, and as long as it remains intact and functional, it promotes vascular smooth muscle relaxation and inhibits thrombogenesis and atherosclerotic plaque formation; damaged endothelium reacts to numerous stimuli with vasoconstriction, thrombosis, and plaque formation. The vascular endothelium of the coronary arteries synthesizes large molecules such as fibronectin, interleukin-1, tissue plasminogen activator, and various growth factors. Small molecules that are also produced include prostacyclin, platelet-activating factor, endothelin-1, and endothelium-derived relaxing factor (EDRF) that is now characterized as nitric oxide. EDRF is synthesized from L-arginine via nitric oxide synthase and released by shear force on the endothelium as well as through interaction with many biochemical stimuli such as acetylcholine, histamine, arginine, catecholamines, arachidonic acid, ADP, endothelin-1, bradykinin, serotonin, and thrombin. Nitric oxide then causes relaxation of the underlying smooth muscle and may be thought of as a paracrine homeopathic defense mechanism against noxious stimuli. Denudation or loss of the vascular endothelium results in loss of EDRF and this protective mechanism. Loss of the endothelial cell layer and function may occur secondary to physical disruption (percutaneous transluminal coronary angioplasty [PTCA]), factors impinging from the vascular side (cyanide from smoke), or disruption of the intimal–medial layers (oxidized low-density lipoprotein [LDL]). Impaired endothelial function may be related to the development of premature atherosclerosis based on recent family studies. Endothelial function may be improved with angiotensin-converting enzyme inhibitors (ACEIs), statins, and exercise.[15]

Factors Extrinsic to the Vascular Bed

Blood flow to the coronary arteries arises from orifices located immediately distal to the aorta valve. Perfusion pressure is equal to the difference between the aortic pressure at an instantaneous point in time and the intramyocardial pressure. Coronary vascular resistance is influenced by phasic systolic compression of the vascular bed. The driving force for perfusion is, therefore, not constant throughout the cardiac cycle. Opening of the aortic valve may also lead to a Venturi effect, which can slightly decrease perfusion pressure. If perfusion pressure is elevated for a period of time, coronary vascular resistance declines and blood flow increases; however, continued perfusion pressure increases lead, within limits, to a return of coronary blood flow back toward baseline levels through autoregulation.

Alterations in intramyocardial wall tension throughout the cardiac cycle will also impose significant changes in coronary blood flow. Diastole is the period during which coronary artery filling can occur due to these pressure differences and little or no coronary blood flow occurs to the left ventricle during systole. The extent of pressure development in the ventricle and HR have a major effect on the development of wall tension, time for diastolic coronary artery filling, and MVO_2.

Under normal conditions, the average global distribution of blood flow between the epicardial and endocardial layer is about 1:1 at rest and remains approximately even during exercise secondary to autoregulatory changes. Regional disparity of blood flow distribution does exist normally, and these disparities are magnified in the presence of diseased coronary arteries and with increased cardiac work as the vasodilator reserve in the resistance vessels of the subendocardium layers is exhausted. Factors that favor a reduction in subendocardial blood flow include decreased perfusion pressure due to decreased diastolic blood pressure or coronary artery obstruction by atherosclerotic plaques with or without vasomotion, abbreviation of diastole (increased HR), and increased intraventricular diastolic pressure (e.g., valvular obstruction to flow).

Extravascular resistance may decrease coronary blood flow, primarily during systole. This effect is much more pronounced in the LV compared with that in the right ventricle (RV). When the effect of increased contractility is separated from the effect of ventricular pressure, about 75% of extravascular resistance is accounted for by passive stretch in equilibrium with ventricular pressure, whereas only 25% results from active myocardial contraction.

Factors Intrinsic to the Vascular Bed

Metabolic factors, myogenic responses, neural reflexes, and humoral substances within the vascular bed of the coronary circulation function in an orchestrated fashion to maintain relative consistency in blood flow to the myocardium in the face of imposed changes in perfusion pressures. Autoregulation, mediated primarily through the effects of myogenic responses and metabolic factors, is thought to be responsible for maintaining regional blood flow in a narrow range while systemic pressure varies over a range of approximately 50 to 150 mm Hg.

Myogenic control (also known as the Bayliss effect) of coronary artery tone occurs when the vessel is stretched secondary to an increase in pressure and contracts to return blood flow to normal. It is thought that the myogenic response to stretching in coronary arteries is a modest one and that metabolic factors such as nitric oxide play a much larger role in autoregulation.

There are three well-studied metabolic factors that have the ability to modify coronary artery resistance and blood flow at the local level. Basal coronary blood flow meets oxygen demands of 8 to 10 mL/min per 100 g of myocardium with essentially complete extraction of oxygen from the blood. As cardiac output or mean arterial blood pressure increases, the increased demand for oxygen is met by increasing blood flow because little additional oxygen is available from hemoglobin. Decreased oxygen availability causes vasodilation of vascular smooth muscle and relaxation of precapillary sphincters, which increase tissue oxygen and help maintain blood flow on a regional basis.

At perfusion pressures below 60 mm Hg, as the coronary arteries are maximally dilated and the buffering effect of autoregulation has reached its capacity, further reduction in coronary blood flow will decrease perfusion pressure and tissue oxygenation. It is thought that autoregulation works more efficiently in the epicardial layers than in subendocardial layers, and this may contribute to coronary steal.

Neural components that participate in the regulation of coronary blood flow include the sympathetic nervous system, the parasympathetic nervous system, coronary reflexes, and, possibly, central control of coronary blood flow. Within the sympathetic system, stimulation of the stellate ganglion elicits coronary vasodilation, which is associated with tachycardia and enhanced contractility. This indirect coronary vasodilation is secondary to increased MVO_2 related to increased HR, contractility, and aortic pressure and occurs following stellate stimulation. The direct effect of the sympathetic system is α_1-mediated vasoconstriction at rest and during exercise. Other receptor types, α_2 and β_1, have little influence on tone, whereas β_2 stimulation produces a modest vasodilatory effect. Although coronary atherosclerosis may decrease blood flow secondary to obstruction, severe coronary atherosclerosis and obstruction may also increase the sensitivity of coronary arteries to the effects of β_1 stimulation and vasoconstriction.

Vagal stimulation within the parasympathetic system produces a small to moderate increase in coronary blood flow, which involves the coronary efferent and afferent parasympathetic components (Bezold–Jarisch reflex). Indirectly, vasoconstriction may result, with vagal stimulation as the result of bradycardia and decreased contractility reducing MVO_2.

Coronary reflexes have an undetermined role in the regulation of coronary blood flow. Based on experimental data, coronary reflexes that may be important include the baroreceptor, the chemoreceptor, Bezold–Jarisch reflex, and the pulmonary inhalation reflex.

FACTORS LIMITING CORONARY PERFUSION

During exercise and pacing, as MVO_2 increases, coronary vascular resistance can be reduced to about 25% of basal values, which results in a fourfold to fivefold increase in coronary blood flow. The cross-sectional area can be reduced by about 80% prior to any mechanical or biochemical changes in the myocardium, reflecting a margin of safety for coronary blood flow. The extent of cross-sectional obstruction, the length of the lesion, lesion composition, and the geometry of the obstructing lesion can each affect flow across coronary arteries with atherosclerosis. Bernoulli's theorem states that the pressure drop across a lesion is directly related to the length of the lesion and inversely related to the radius of the lesion to the fourth power; critical stenosis occurs when the obstructing lesion encroaches on the luminal diameter and exceeds 70%. Lesions creating obstruction of 50% to 70% may reduce blood flow; however, these obstructions are not consistent and vasospasm and thrombosis superimposed on a *noncritical* lesion may lead to clinical events such as MI.[14] If the lesion enlarges from 80% to 90%, resistance in that vessel is tripled. Coronary reserve is diminished at about 85% obstruction owing to vasoconstriction. Exaggerated responsiveness can be seen when coronary stenosis reaches this critical level and the role of vasoactive substances such as prostaglandins, thromboxanes, and serotonin may play more of a role in the regulation of coronary vascular tone and thrombosis.

Little reserve exists for coronary blood flow and a relatively small reduction of 10% to 20% results in decreased myocardial fiber shortening as the first evidence for abnormal function. The subendocardial layers are affected to a greater extent than the epicardium by ischemia, considering changes in fiber shortening, arteriovenous (AV) difference in oxygen saturation, and lactate production. A reduction of 80% gives rise to akinesis and a 95% reduction of coronary blood flow produces dyskinesis during contraction of the ventricles. Although these abnormalities of contraction are associated with transient impaired function, depletion of high-energy phosphate compounds and ultrastructural changes may last for days even after transient ischemia; this has been referred to as *stunned myocardium*. Chronic hypoperfusion may lead to *hibernation*, in which ventricular function is impaired over longer time intervals. Hibernating myocardium can be differentiated from necrosis with various techniques (see Chap. 1) and revascularization of hibernating myocardium is useful in improving ventricular function. Regional loss of contractility may impose a burden on the remaining myocardial tissue, resulting in heart failure, increased MVO_2, and rapid depletion of blood flow reserve. Consequently, zones of tissue with marginal blood flow may develop in a lateral or transmural fashion; such development puts this tissue at risk for more severe damage if the ischemic episode persists or becomes more severe. Nonischemic areas of myocardium may compensate for the severely ischemic and border zones of ischemia by developing more tension than usual in an attempt to maintain cardiac output. At the cellular level, ischemia and the attendant acidosis are thought to alter calcium release from storage sites such as the sarcolemma and the sarcoplasmic reticulum as well as inhibit the binding of calcium to troponin, thereby impairing the association of actin and myosin. The clinical correlates of these cellular biochemical events leading to the development of LV or RV dysfunction include an S3, dyspnea, orthopnea, tachycardia, fluctuating blood pressure, transient murmurs, and mitral or tricuspid regurgitation.

CLINICAL PRESENTATION AND DIAGNOSIS

General

- Many episodes of ischemia do not cause symptoms of angina (silent ischemia).
- Patients often have a reproducible pattern of pain or other symptoms that appear after specific amount of exertion.
- Increased frequency, severity, duration, or symptoms at rest suggest an unstable angina pattern and the patient should seek help immediately.

Symptoms

- **2** Sensation of pressure or burning over the sternum or near it, often but not always radiating to the left jaw, shoulder, and arm; also chest tightness and shortness of breath.
- Pain usually lasts from 0.5 to 30 minutes often with a visceral quality (deep location).
- Precipitating factors include exercise, cold environment, walking after a meal, emotional upset, fright, anger, and coitus.
- Relief occurs with rest and nitroglycerin.

Signs

- Abnormal precordial (over the heart) systolic bulge
- Abnormal heart sounds

Laboratory Tests

- Typically no laboratory tests are abnormal; however, if the patient has intermediate- to high-risk features for unstable angina, electrocardiographic changes and serum troponin, or creatine kinase may become abnormal (Table 6-3).
- Patients are likely to have laboratory test abnormalities for the risk factors for IHD such as elevated total and LDL cholesterol, low HDL cholesterol, impaired fasting glucose or elevated glucose, high blood pressure, elevated C-reactive protein, and abnormal renal function. Hemoglobin should be checked to make sure the patient is not anemic.

Other Diagnostic Tests (see Chap. 1)

- A resting electrocardiogram followed by an exercise tolerance test is usually the first test done in stable patients. A chest x-ray should be done if the patient has heart failure symptoms. Cardiac imaging using radioisotopes to detect ischemic myocardium and measure ventricular function is commonly done when revascularization is being considered. Echocardiography may also be used to assess ventricular wall motion at rest or during stress. Cardiac catheterization and coronary arteriography are used to determine coronary artery anatomy and if the patient would benefit from angioplasty, coronary artery bypass surgery, or other revascularization procedures. Coronary artery calcium (CAC) may be useful in detecting early disease (see Chap. 1).

TABLE 6-3 Short-Term Risk of Death or Nonfatal Myocardial Infarction in Patients with Unstable Angina

Feature	High Risk (At Least One of the Following Features must be Present)	Intermediate Risk (No High-Risk Feature but must have One of the Following)	Low Risk (No High- or Intermediate-Risk Feature but may have Any of the Following)
History	Accelerating tempo of ischemic symptoms in preceding 48 hours	Prior MI, peripheral or cerebrovascular disease, or CABG, prior aspirin use	
Character of pain	Prolonged ongoing (>20 minutes), rest pain	Prolonged (>20 minutes), rest angina, now resolved, with moderate or high likelihood of CAD	New-onset CCS Class III or IV angina in the past 2 weeks without prolonged (>20 minutes) rest pain but with moderate or high likelihood of CAD
Clinical findings	Pulmonary edema, most likely caused by ischemia New or worsening MR murmur S_3 or new/worsening rales Hypotension, bradycardia, tachycardia Age >75 years		
ECG	Angina at rest with transient ST-segment changes >0.05 mV	T-wave inversions >0.2 mV	Normal or unchanged ECG during an episode of chest discomfort
	Bundle-branch block, new or presumed new	Pathologic Q waves	
Cardiac markers	Markedly elevated (e.g., TnT or TnI >0.1 ng/mL [>0.1 mcg/L])	Slightly elevated (e.g., TnT >0.01 but <0.1 ng/mL [>0.01 but <0.1 mcg/L])	Normal

CABG, coronary artery bypass grafting; CAD, coronary artery disease; CCS, Canadian Cardiovascular Society; ECG, electrocardiogram; MI, myocardial infarction; MR, mitral regurgitation; TnI, troponin; TnT, troponin T.

Calcium accumulation and overload secondary to ischemia impairs ventricular relaxation as well as contraction. This is apparently a result of impaired calcium uptake after systole from the myofilaments, leading to a less negative decline of the pressure in the ventricle over time. Impaired relaxation is associated with enhanced diastolic stiffness, decreased rate of wall thinning, and slowed pressure decay, producing an upward shift in the ventricular pressure–volume relationship; put more simply, MVO_2 is likely to be increased secondary to increased wall tension. Impairment of both diastolic and systolic function leads to elevation of the filling pressure of the left ventricle.

Important aspects of the clinical history for chest pain for patients with angina include the nature or quality of the pain, precipitating factors, duration, pain radiation, and the response to nitroglycerin or rest. Because there can be considerable variation in the manifestations of angina, it is more accurate to refer to these symptoms as an anginal syndrome. For some patients with significant coronary disease, their presenting symptoms may differ from the classical symptoms, yet the symptoms are due to ischemic pain, and these are often referred to as anginal equivalents. Obtaining an accurate and detailed family history is useful in placing symptoms in perspective. Significant positive information includes premature CHD (<55 years in men and <65 years in women) manifested as fatal and nonfatal MI, stroke, peripheral vascular disease, as well as other risk factors such as hypertension, smoking, familial lipid disorders, and diabetes mellitus (considered to be a risk equivalent). Typical pain radiation patterns include anterior chest pain (96%), left upper arm pain (83.7%), left lower arm pain (29.3%), and neck pain at some time (22%). Pain from other areas is less common. Ischemia detected by ECG monitoring is more likely to be detected in the morning hours (6 AM to 12 noon) than other periods throughout the day. Patients suffering from variant or Prinzmetal's angina secondary to coronary spasm are more likely to experience pain at rest and in the early morning hours. Prinzmetal's anginal pain is not usually brought on by exertion or emotional stress nor relieved by rest, and the ECG pattern is that of current injury with ST elevation rather than depression. Typical pain that occurs in nonocclusive CAD is referred to as microvascular angina.

It is also important to differentiate the pattern of pain for stable angina from that of unstable angina. Unstable angina may be stratified into categories of risk ranging from high to low (Table 6-3).[16] Ischemia may also be painless or *silent* in 60% to 100% of patients depending on the series cited and the patient population.[17] In patients with myocardial ischemia, approximately 70% of the episodes of documented ischemia are painless as determined by ambulatory ECG monitoring, and the ST-segment changes associated with these episodes can be ST elevation or depression. The mechanism of silent ischemia is unclear, but studies have shown that patients not experiencing pain have altered pain perception, with the threshold and tolerance for pain being higher than that of patients who have pain more frequently. Although patients with diabetes tend to have more extensive and microvascular coronary disease than those without diabetes and may suffer from autonomic neuropathy, asymptomatic ischemia is not more prevalent based on the Asymptomatic Cardiac Ischemia Pilot (ACIP) study.[18]

Lastly, it should be recognized that the threshold for pain due to exertion is fixed in some patients and variable in others and that the amount of exercise or stress necessary to provoke symptoms can change over time. A fixed threshold for the induction of pain or ECG evidence of ischemia means these indicators of ischemia occur at the same, or nearly so, double rate–pressure product (SBP × HR). This is apparently due to at least two factors. Over long periods of time atherosclerosis may progress, leading to more severe stenosis, reduced oxygen supply, and less of an increase in demand to precipitate ischemic symptoms. Once stenotic lesions reach a critical level of about 80% or greater, vasomotion, vasospasm, and thrombotic occlusion become significant factors impairing blood flow to the myocardium. Consequently, anatomic considerations and vasoactive substances may interact to provide an environment amenable to changing thresholds for the production of angina.

There appears to be little relationship between the historical features of angina and the severity or extent of coronary artery vessel involvement. Therefore, one may speculate that severe symptoms might be associated with multivessel disease, but no predictive markers exist on a routine basis.

Chest pain may resemble pain arising from a variety of noncardiac sources and the differential diagnosis of anginal pain from other etiologies may be quite difficult based on history alone. Table 6-4 outlines other common problems that may be present with episodic chest pain. Although much less common, nonatherosclerotic etiologies of CAD do exist and should be excluded with appropriate tests. The clinical classification of chest pain encompasses typical angina including (a) substernal chest pain with a characteristic quality and duration that is (b) provoked by exertion or emotional stress and (c)

TABLE 6-4 Differential Diagnosis of Episodic Chest Pain Resembling Angina Pectoris

	Duration	Quality	Provocation	Relief	Location	Comment
Effort angina	5–15 minutes	Visceral (pressure)	During effort or emotion	Rest, NTG	Substernal, radiates	First episode vivid
Rest angina	5–15 minutes	Visceral (pressure)	Spontaneous (with exercise?)	NTG	Substernal, radiates	Often nocturnal
Mitral prolapse	Minutes to hours	Superficial (rarely visceral)	Spontaneous (no pattern)	Time	Left anterior	No pattern, variable
Esophageal reflux	10 minutes to 1 hour	Visceral	Spontaneous, cold liquids, exercise, lying down	Foods, antacids, H_2 blockers, proton pump inhibitors, NTG	Substernal, radiates	Mimics angina
Peptic ulcer	Hours	Visceral, burning	Lack of food, "acid" foods	Foods, antacids, H_2 blockers, proton pump inhibitors	Epigastric, substernal	
Biliary disease	Hours	Visceral (wax and wane)	Spontaneous, food	Time, analgesia	Epigastric, radiates	Colic
Cervical disk	Variable (gradually subsides)	Superficial	Spontaneous, food	Time, analgesia	Arm, neck	Not relieved by rest
Hyperventilation	2–3 minutes	Visceral	Emotion, tachypnea	Stimulus removed	Substernal	Facial paraesthesia
Musculoskeletal	Variable	Superficial	Movement, palpation	Time, analgesia	Multiple	Tenderness
Pulmonary	30 minutes	Visceral (pressure)	Often spontaneous	Rest, time bronchodilator	Substernal	Dyspneic

NTG, nitroglycerin.

relieved by rest or nitroglycerin; atypical angina (meets two of the characteristics for typical angina); and noncardiac chest pain (meets ≤1 of the typical angina characteristics).[19,20]

There are few signs apparent on physical examination to indicate the presence of CAD and usually only the cardiovascular system reveals any useful information. Elevated HR or blood pressure can yield an increased DP and may be associated with angina, and it would be important to correct extreme tachycardia or hypertension if present. Other noncardiac physical findings that suggest that significant CVD may be associated with angina include abdominal aortic aneurysms or peripheral vascular disease. Cardiac examination findings in CAD are noted in Table 6-5. During an angina attack these findings may appear or become more prominent, making them more valuable if present.

In addition to screening for CVD risk factors, other recommended tests include hemoglobin, fasting glucose, fasting lipoprotein panel, resting ECG, and chest x-ray in patients with signs or symptoms of heart failure, valvular heart disease, pericardial disease, or aortic dissection/aneurysm.[20] Hemoglobin is assessed to insure adequate oxygen-carrying capacity. Fasting glucose determinations to exclude diabetes and glucose monitoring for concurrent diabetes should be performed routinely. Lipids are assessed total, LDL, and HDL cholesterol and triglycerides (see Chap. 11).[21] Other risk factors that may be important for some patients include high-sensitivity C-reactive protein, homocysteine level, evidence of chlamydia infection, and elevations in lipoprotein(a), fibrinogen, and plasminogen activator inhibitor.[22] Cardiac enzymes should all be normal in stable angina. Troponin T or I, myoglobin, or creatinine phosphokinase-MB isoform may be elevated in patients with unstable angina, and interventions such as anticoagulation or antiplatelet therapy have been shown to reduce cardiac end points when these markers for injury are elevated (Table 6-3).[23]

Patients presenting with chest pain are stratified into chronic stable angina or having features of intermediate- or high-risk unstable angina (Table 6-3). These features include rest pain lasting >20 minutes, age >65 years, ST- and T-wave changes, and pulmonary edema. Patients with ACS (unstable angina, non–ST-segment elevation AMI, and ST-segment elevation AMI) are managed differently than those with chronic stable angina. For more details on the management of ACS, please refer to Chapter 7.

TABLE 6-5 Cardiac Exam Findings in Coronary Artery Disease

Cardiac Finding	Clinical Significance
Common[a]	
Decreased intensity of S_1	Decrease in left ventricular contractility
S_4 (atrial gallop)	Reduced ventricular compliance
Infrequent[a]	
S_3 (ventricular gallop)	Increased left ventricular diastolic pressure, with or without clinical CHF
Apical systolic murmur	Papillary muscle dysfunction
Abnormal precordial systolic bulge	Left ventricular wall motion abnormality
Rare	
Paradoxical splitting of S_2	Left ventricular wall motion abnormality
Diastolic murmur	Coronary artery stenosis

CHF, congestive heart failure; S_1, first heart sound; S_2, second heart sound; S_3, third heart sound; S_4, fourth heart sound.

[a]Frequency typically increases in patients with angina or those who have suffered a prior myocardial infarction.

Courtesy of Dr. Emily Gordon, University Hospital Pharmacy Service.

Diagnostic Tests

See also Chapter 1 and Figure 6-1.

TREATMENT

Desired Outcome

Important goals in the treatment of IHD are to minimize the likelihood of death and maximize health and function. Objectives of management include:

1. Reduce premature CVD.
2. Prevent complications of IHD, for example, MI.
3. Maintain or restore activity, functional capacity, and quality of life.
4. Completely or nearly completely eliminate ischemic symptoms.

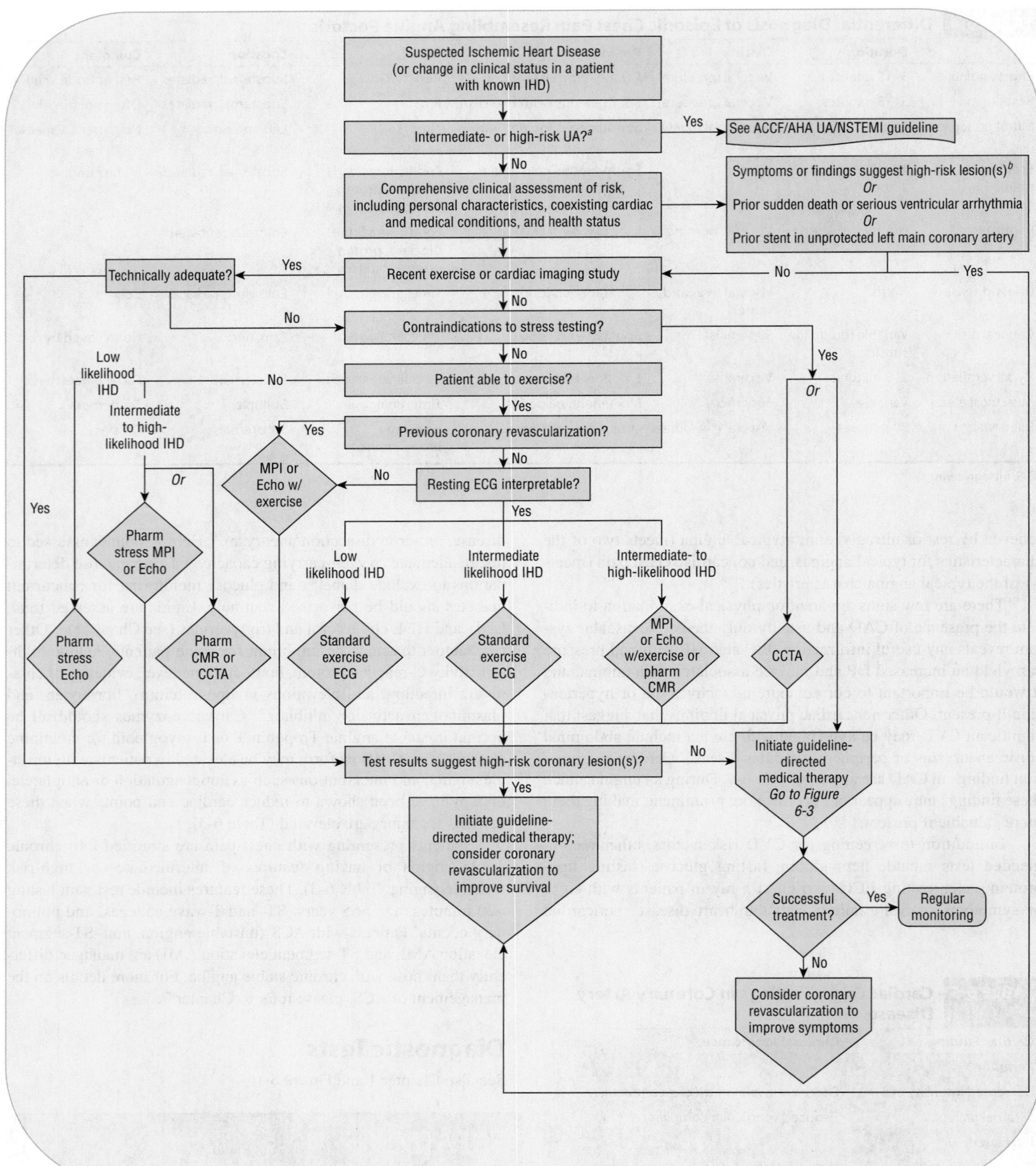

FIGURE 6-1 Diagnosis of patients with suspected ischemic heart disease. Colors correspond to the class of recommendations in the ACCF/AHA Table 6-13. The algorithms do not represent a comprehensive list of recommendations (see text for all recommendations). [a]See Table 6-3 for short-term risk of death or nonfatal MI in patients with UA/NSTEMI. [b]CCTA is reasonable only for patients with intermediate probability of IHD. (CCTA, computed coronary tomography angiography; CMR, cardiac magnetic resonance; ECG, electrocardiogram; Echo, echocardiography; IHD, ischemic heart disease; MI, myocardial infarction; MPI, myocardial perfusion imaging; Pharm, pharmacological; UA/NSTEMI, unstable angina/non–ST-elevation myocardial infarction.)

5. Minimize costs of heat care by avoiding unnecessary testing and treatment, preventing hospitalizations, and avoiding complications of testing.
6. Since there is little evidence that revascularization procedures such as angioplasty and coronary artery bypass surgery extend life, the primary focus should be on altering the underlying and ongoing process of atherosclerosis through risk factor modification while providing symptomatic relief through the use of β-blockers, calcium channel blockers, nitrates, and ranolazine for anginal symptoms.

Risk Factor Modification

3 Primary prevention of IHD through the identification and modification of risk factors prior to the initial morbid event would be the optimal management approach and should result in a significant impact on the prevalence of IHD. However, early recognition of some risk factors may not be possible in all cases, and in others, the patient may not be willing to undertake intervention until overt evidence of coronary disease is apparent. Secondary intervention continues to be more commonly pursued by both healthcare professionals and patients, and it is important to recognize this type of intervention as effective in reducing subsequent morbidity and mortality. The presence of risk factors in individual patients plays a major role in determining the occurrence and severity of IHD.[24,25] Risk factors are additive in nature and can be classified as alterable or unalterable (see Table 11-7). Unalterable risk factors include gender; age; family history or genetic composition; environmental influences such as climate, air pollution, and trace metal composition of drinking water; and, to some extent, diabetes mellitus. Improved glycemic control reduces the microvascular complications of diabetes mellitus (see Chap. 57); however, with publication of the ACCORD trial strict control of glucose did not improve the primary outcome.[2,26] 4 Risk factors that can be altered include smoking, hypertension, dyslipidemia, obesity, sedentary lifestyle, hyperuricemia, psychosocial factors such as stress and type A behavior patterns, and the use of certain drugs that may be detrimental including progestins, corticosteroids, and calcineurin inhibitors.

Cigarette smoking is common. The Centers for Disease Control and Prevention estimates that ~42 million people are current smokers (23.1% men; 16.7% women) in this country, and the risk for CHD is increased by about 1.8 in active smokers and by about 1.3 for passive or environmental smoke exposure.[3,5] Each year 443,000 Americans die from smoking-related illnesses and 142,000 of the deaths are attributable to CVD.[5] Risk due to smoking is related to the number of cigarettes smoked per day and the duration of smoking. Passive smoking in angina pectoris patients has been shown to decrease exercise time.[6] Pipe and cigar smokers are at increased risk compared with nonsmokers, but their risk is somewhat less than that of cigarette smokers.[27] The direct effects of cigarette smoke that are detrimental to patients with angina include (a) elevated HR and blood pressure from nicotine, which increases MVO_2, and impaired myocardial oxygen delivery due to carboxyhemoglobin generation from carbon monoxide inhalation in smoke; (b) the negative inotropic effect of carboxyhemoglobin; (c) increased platelet adhesiveness and promotion of aggregation resulting in thrombotic tendencies due to nicotine and carboxyhemoglobin; (d) lowered threshold for ventricular fibrillation during ischemia due to carboxyhemoglobin; and (e) impaired endothelial function owing to smoking.[31] Similar changes have been noted for marihuana smoking as well. Smoking also accelerates the risk for MI, sudden death, cerebrovascular disease, peripheral vascular disease, and hypertension, and it reduces high-density lipoprotein concentrations. Clearly, primary prevention is needed for this risk factor and much of the education effort to discourage initiation of smoking should be targeted for teenagers. Techniques for cessation of smoking that may be useful include aversive conditioning, group programs, self-help programs, hypnosis, *cold turkey*, and the use of nicotine substitutes (lobeline) or other sources of nicotine replacement products for short-term substitution during withdrawal syndrome. The antidepressant sustained-release buproprion has been shown to be more effective than placebo and best used with smoking cessation counseling. Varenicline, a partial agonist selective for the $\alpha_4\beta_2$ nicotinic acetylcholine receptor subtype, has been shown to improve cessation rates as well.[28,29] It may be more cost-effective than other interventions for smoking cessation.[30] Cessation of smoking reduces the incidence of coronary events to about 15% to 25% of that associated with continued smoking and these benefits are noted within 2 years of cessation.[31] A public ordinance reducing exposure to secondhand smoke was associated with a decrease in AMI hospitalizations in Pueblo, Colorado, by 27% in 2 years.[32]

Hypertension, whether labile or fixed, borderline or definite, casual or basal, systolic or diastolic, at any age regardless of gender, is the most common and a powerful contributor to atherosclerotic coronary vascular disease.[33] Morbidity and mortality increase progressively with the degree of blood pressure elevation of either systolic or diastolic pressure and pulse pressure, and no discernible critical value exists (see Chap. 3). Numerous trials have documented the reduction in risk associated with blood pressure lowering; however, most of these studies show that mortality and morbidity reduction is a result of fewer strokes and less renal failure and heart failure. The reduction in CHD end points is significant but not as dramatic. The reasons for this are unclear but perhaps relate to the multifactorial etiology of IHD. Recent guideline changes from the AHA recommend goal blood pressure of <130/80 mm Hg for patients with stable angina, unstable angina, non–ST-segment MI, and ST-segment MI and <120/80 mm Hg in patients with LV dysfunction.[33]

Hypercholesterolemia is a significant cardiovascular risk factor, and risk is directly related to the degree of cholesterol elevation.[24,25] As with hypertension, there is no critical value that defines risk, but rather risk is incrementally related to the degree of elevation and the presence of other risk factors (see Chap. 11 for a detailed discussion). A fasting lipoprotein panel should be obtained in all patients with known CAD. The goals for total, LDL, and HDL cholesterol and triglycerides are discussed in Chapter 11. All patients should undertake therapeutic lifestyle changes. Reductions in LDL cholesterol for primary prevention and secondary intervention have been shown to reduce total and CAD mortality and stroke as well as the need for interventions such as PTCA and CABG. Supplemental vitamin E or other antioxidants reduce the susceptibility of LDL cholesterol to oxidation but clinical trial data have failed to show any benefit with supplementation.[34]

Overweight and obesity, defined as a body mass index (BMI, weight in kilograms divided by height in meters squared) of ≥25 and ≥30 kg/m², respectively, are estimated to occur in 68.2% and 34.6% of the U.S. population. BMI is associated with an increased mortality ratio compared with individuals of normal body weight, and the objective for patients with IHD is to maintain or reduce to a normal body weight.[3,5] This may be accomplished through dietary modification, exercise, pharmacologic therapy, or surgical therapy. Frequently associated with obesity is a sedentary lifestyle, and inactivity may contribute to higher blood pressure, elevated blood lipid levels, and insulin resistance associated with glucose intolerance in diabetics (insulin resistance or metabolic syndrome). Exercise to the level of about 300 kcal (1,256 kJ) three times a week is useful in improving maximal oxygen uptake, improving cardiorespiratory efficiency, promoting collateral artery formation, and promoting potential alterations in the risk of ventricular fibrillation, coronary thrombosis, and improved tolerance to stress. Epidemiologic studies have found that mortality is directly related to resting HR and a low HR difference between resting and maximal exercise HR, and inversely related to exercise HR. A regular exercise program has been shown to reduce all-cause and cardiac mortality.[35,36]

Competitiveness, intense striving for achievement, easily provoked hostility, a sense of urgency about doing things quickly and being punctual, impatience, abrupt and rapid speech and gestures, and concentration on self-selected goals to the point of not perceiving and attending to other aspects of the environment are traits that characterize the behavioral pattern known as the type A or coronary prone personality. Although the issue is somewhat controversial, type A individuals may have increased cardiovascular risk with risk ratios ranging from insignificant to three times that of a matched population. Psychological stress and type D personality have been associated with adverse cardiac prognosis, but little is known about their relative effect on the pathogenesis of CHD. "Type D" refers to the tendency to experience negative emotions and to inhibit the expression of these emotions in social interactions. The mechanism by which personality affects the cardiovascular system is not understood, but may reflect the activity of the sympathetic system and enhanced responsiveness of other stress hormones when compared with non–type A personalities.

Alcohol ingestion in small to moderate amounts (<40 g/day of pure ethanol) reduces the risk of CHD; however, consumption of large amounts (>50 g/day) or binge drinking of alcohol is associated with increased mortality from stroke, cancer, vehicular accidents, and cirrhosis.[37,38] There appears to be a differential effect depending on race with an inverse relationship between ethanol consumption in whites but a direct relationship between consumption and CAD risk in blacks. The mechanisms for the presumed protective effects of alcohol are not known but the effects may be related to increased high-density lipoprotein levels, impaired platelet function, or associations between the amount of alcohol ingested and personality type. Long-term follow-up studies of alcohol ingestion have found that the beneficial effects on MI are small compared with the overall effects on mortality.[39] Whatever the relationship, it is well to remember that alcohol drinking is implicated in over 40% of all fatal automobile accidents and consumption of alcohol predisposes to hepatic cirrhosis, the sixth to seventh most common cause of death in middle age in the United States. With this in mind, it seems illogical to suggest alcohol ingestion as a prophylactic measure for coronary disease but rather advise moderation of alcohol consumption, if it is the preference of the individual.

Thiazide diuretics have been shown to elevate serum cholesterol and triglyceride levels, whereas β-blockers tend to lower HDL and raise LDL slightly; however, a direct association between these drugs and cardiovascular risk is tenuous and based on aggregating results rather than randomized clinical trials. Conjugated equine estrogen alone or in combination with progestin lowers LDL and raises HDL; unfortunately, the HERS trial showed no benefit of hormone replacement therapy for secondary intervention and increased risk for thromboembolism.[40] In secondary intervention, HRT or estrogen alone in women after hysterectomy found that hormonal therapy health risks exceeded benefits as well.[41,42] Unopposed estrogen is the optimal regimen for elevation of HDL, but the high rate of endometrial hyperplasia restricts use to women without a uterus. In women with a uterus, estrogen with cyclic medroxyprogesterone has the most favorable effect on HDL and no excess risk of endometrial hyperplasia. Use of oral contraceptives in women who smoke and are over the age of 35 years increases the risk of MI, stroke, and venous thromboembolism by threefold or higher. Alternative forms of contraception and cessation of smoking should be promoted in these patients. The risk for nonsmoking oral contraceptive users under the age of 35 is very small. The relative risk of breast cancer is increased, but in the absence of risk factors for breast cancer, the relative risk is approximately 1.3 (30% increase). Coffee consumption has also been linked to CHD and caffeine does transiently elevate blood pressure; however, the overall risk, if any, appears to be low and may be related to genetic makeup (CYP1A2 mutation).[43,44] Although thiazide diuretics and β-blockers (nonselective without intrinsic sympathomimetic activity) may elevate both cholesterol and triglycerides by approximately 10% to 20%, and these effects may be detrimental, no objective evidence exists from prospective well-controlled studies to support avoiding these drugs at this time. This controversy is most pertinent in the treatment of mild hypertension and it is discussed in greater detail in Chapter 3.

TREATMENT

Stable Ischemic Heart Disease

Table 6-6 contains evidence grading recommendations.

The guidelines for the management of stable IHD place a strong emphasis on patient education. Class I recommendations include education on the importance of medication adherence, modification of risk, a comprehensive review of all therapeutic options, appropriate levels of exercise, introduction to self-monitoring skills, and recognition of worsening symptoms and steps to take appropriate action if symptoms are changing.[12] Patients should be educated about adherence to a diet that is low in saturated fat, cholesterol, and *trans* fat; high in fresh fruits, whole grains, and vegetables; and reduced in sodium intake (Class IIa). Comprehensive behavioral approaches for the management of stress and depression and evolution and treatment of major depressive disorder are recommended as well (Class IIa, B, C).

Guideline-directed medical therapy (GDMT) provides guidance for risk factor modification in stable IHD. Lifestyle modifications including daily physical activity and weight management are strongly recommended (Class I, B) as well as dietary therapy including reduced saturated fat intake (7% of total calories), *trans* fat (<1% of total calories), and cholesterol <200 mg/day (Class I, B). In addition to therapeutic lifestyle changes a moderate or high dose of statin therapy is recommended in the absence of contraindications or adverse effects (Class I, A). Patients not tolerating a statin may be given a bile acid sequestrant, niacin, or both (Class IIa, B). The use

TABLE 6-6 The American College of Cardiology and American Heart Association Evidence Grading System

Recommendation Class		Level of Evidence	
I	Conditions for which there is evidence or general agreement that a given procedure or treatment is useful and effective	A	Data derived from multiple randomized clinical trials with large numbers of patients
II	Conditions for which there is conflicting evidence or a divergence of opinion that the usefulness/efficacy of a given procedure or treatment is useful and effective	B	Data derived from a limited number of randomized trials with small numbers of patients, careful analyses of nonrandomized studies, or observational registries
IIa	Weight of evidence/opinion is in favor or usefulness/efficacy	C	Expert consensus was the primary basis for the recommendation
IIb	Usefulness/efficacy is less well established by evidence/opinion		
III	Conditions for which there is evidence or general agreement that a given procedure or treatment is not useful/effective and in some cases may be harmful		

TABLE 6-7 Indications for Individual Drug Classes in SIHD

Indication	Diuretic	BB	ACEI	ARB	CCB	AA
Heart failure	X	X	X	X		X
LV dysfunction	X	X	X	X		X
Post-MI		X	X	X		X
Angina		X			X	
Diabetes		X	X	X		
CKD			X	X		

AA, aldosterone inhibitor; ACEI, angiotensin-converting enzyme inhibitor, ARB, angiotensin receptor blocker; BB, β-blocker; CCB, calcium channel blocker; CKD, chronic kidney disease; LV, left ventricular; SIHD, stable ischemic heart disease.

of niacin has become controversial and more detail can be found in Chapter 11. Under GDMT blood pressure management includes the lifestyle changes described above (Class I, B) with a target blood pressure of 140/90 mm Hg or less in addition to lifestyle modifications (Class I, A). Selection of a particular blood pressure–lowering agent should be based on specific patient characteristics and may include ACEI and/or β-blockers with the addition of other drugs such as thiazide diuretics or calcium channel blockers to achieve a goal blood pressure of <140/90 mm Hg (Class I, B). See Table 6-7 for indications for individual drug classes.

The goals for diabetes management take into consideration the duration of diabetes and life expectancy. Patients with a short duration of diabetes and long life expectancy have a goal of hemoglobin A1c of ≤7% (≤53 mmol/mol Hb) (Class IIa, B); a goal of 7% to 9% (53 to 75 mmol/mol Hb) is reasonable for certain patients based on age, history of hypoglycemia, presence of microvascular or macrovascular complications, or presence of coexisting medical conditions (Class IIa, C). Pharmacotherapy interventions to achieve the target A1c might be reasonable (Class IIb, A). Therapy with rosiglitazone should not be initiated in patients with SIHD (Class III, C). Another controversy now exists concerning how low to go with A1c. Recent trials described in Chapter 57 point out that lower may not be better.

Physical activity is recommended in all patients with a goal of 30 to 60 minutes of moderate-intensity aerobic activity at least 5 days and preferably 7 days/wk (Class I, B). Risk assessment with a physical activity history and/or an exercise test is recommended to guide prognosis and prescription (Class I, B). Cardiac rehabilitation and physician-directed, home-based programs are recommended for at-risk patient at first diagnosis (Class I, A). Resistance training is also considered to be reasonable at least 2 days/wk (Class IIa, C).

BMI should be assessed at every visit and the goal is to achieve a BMI of 18.5 to 24.9 kg/m^2 with a waist circumference of less than 102 cm in men and 88 cm in women (Class I, C). Smoking cessation and avoidance of exposure to environmental tobacco smoke should be encouraged for all patients with follow-up and referral to special programs to aid in cessation through counseling and pharmacologic interventions. The generally accepted approach is the ask, advise, assess, assist, arrange, and avoid approach (Class I, B). See Chapter 16 for more details concerning smoking cessation.

1. *Ask* each patient about tobacco use at every visit.
2. *Advise* each smoker to quit.
3. *Assess* each smoker's willingness to make a quit attempt.
4. *Assist* each smoker in making a quit attempt by offering medication and referral for counseling.
5. *Arrange* for follow-up.
6. *Avoid* exposure to environmental tobacco smoke.

It is reasonable to consider screening SIHD patients for depression and to refer or treat when indicated (Class IIa, B). Treatment of depression has not been shown to improve CVD outcomes but might be reasonable for its other clinical benefits (Class IIb, C). Alcohol consumption in patients with SIHD should not exceed 4 oz (120 mL) of wine, 12 oz (360 mL) of beer, or 1 oz (30 mL) of spirits a day (Class IIa, C). Patients with SIHD should avoid exposure to increased air pollution to reduce the risk of cardiovascular events (Class IIa, C).

Recommendations for Medical Therapy to Prevent MI and Death

Antiplatelet therapy with aspirin 75 to 162 mg day daily should be continued indefinitely in the absence of contraindications (Class I, A). Clopidogrel is a reasonable alterative when aspirin is contraindicated (Class I, A). Treatment with aspirin 65 to 162 mg daily and clopidogrel 75 mg daily might be reasonable in certain high-risk patients with SIHD (Class IIb, B). The major metabolic pathway for activation of clopidogrel is cytochrome (CYP) P450 2C19, and approximately 30% of whites and African Americans have reduced-function alleles and cannot fully activate clopidogrel, resulting in higher cardiovascular event rates. Asian populations have reduced-function alleles in as many as 60% of individuals. There has been concern over interactions with drugs that can inhibit 2C19 (such as omeprazole), but the clinical significance of these interactions remains uncertain. In certain situations such as placement of drug-eluting stents (DES) and certain valvular disorders this combination may be appropriate. Dipyridamole is not recommended as antiplatelet therapy for patients with SIHD (Class III, B).

β-Blocker therapy should be started and continued for 3 years in all patients with normal LV function after MI or an acute coronary syndrome (Class I, A). Patients with a reduced ejection fraction (≤40% [≤0.40]) with heart failure or prior MI should be started on β-blocker therapy unless contraindicated. Only carvedilol, metoprolol succinate, and bisoprolol have been shown to reduce the risk of death in heart failure patients (Class I, A). β-Blockers should be considered as chronic therapy for all other patients with coronary or other vascular disease (Class IIb, C).

ACEI should be used in all patients with SIHD who also have hypertension, diabetes mellitus, LV ejection fraction (≤40% [≤0.40]), or chronic kidney disease unless contraindicated (Class I, A). ARBs are recommended for patients who cannot tolerate ACEI (Class I, A). ACEIs are reasonable in patients with both SIHD and other vascular disease (Class IIa, B). In a similar vein, ARBs can be substituted for ACEI intolerance (Class IIa, C). Annual influenza vaccine is recommended for patients with SIHD (Class I, B).

Class III recommendations, that is, no benefit, include a number of interventions. Estrogen therapy is not recommended in postmenopausal women with SIHD with the intent of reducing CV risk or improving outcomes (Class III, A). Vitamins C and E and β-carotene supplementation are not recommended since there is no evidence that CV risk is reduced (Class III, A). The use of folate or vitamins B_6 and B_{12} and chelation therapy is not recommended due to the lack of evidence for effectively reducing CVD risk (Class III, A, C). Garlic, coenzyme Q10, selenium, or chromium is not recommended with the intent of reducing CVD risk in patient with SIHD (Class III, C).

Recommendations for Medical Therapy for the Relief of Symptoms

All of the following are Class I recommendations:

1. β-Blockers should be prescribed as initial therapy for relief of symptoms in patients with SIHD (LOE: B).
2. Calcium channel blockers or long-acting nitrates should be prescribed for the relief of symptoms when β-blockers are contraindicated or cause unacceptable adverse effects (LOE: B).

3. Calcium channel blockers or long-acting nitrates, in combination with β-blockers, should be prescribed for relief of symptoms when initial treatment with β-blockers is unsuccessful (LOE: B).
4. Sublingual (SL) nitroglycerin or nitroglycerin spray is recommended for immediate relief of angina in patients with SIHD (LOE: B) 6.

Class IIa recommendations include recommending the use of diltiazem or verapamil instead of a β-blocker as initial therapy for relief of symptoms is reasonable in SIHD (LOE: B). Ranolazine can be useful when prescribed as a substitute for β-blockers when β-blockers cause unacceptable adverse effects or are ineffective or contraindicated (LOE: B). Ranolazine in combination with β-blockers can be used for symptom relief when initial therapy with β-blockers is not successful in SIHD (LOE: A).

There are several interesting agents for the management of SIHD that are not available in the United States. Nicorandil activates ATP-sensitive potassium channels and promotes systemic venous and coronary vasodilation. The efficacy is considered to be similar to oral nitrates, calcium channel blockers, and β-blockers.[45] Ivabradine is an inhibitor of the *If* current of pacemaker cells reducing HR, prolonging diastole, and improving oxygen balance.[46] Trimetazidine improves the cellular tolerance to ischemia by inhibiting fatty acid metabolism and stimulating glucose metabolism.[47]

Alternative Therapies for Relief of Symptoms in Patients with Refractory Angina

Class IIb recommendations include enhanced external counterpulsation (LOE: B), spinal cord stimulation (LOE: C), and transmyocardial revascularization (LOE: B). None of these modalities are in common use in the United States. Acupuncture should not be used to improve symptoms or reduce risk of CVD in SIHD (Class III, C).

Recommendations for revascularization to improve survival and to improve symptoms can be found in Tables 6-8 and 6-9.[12] Generally speaking, the changes from previous guidelines are more use of PCI in more complex cases. This assumes that the patient has anatomy that can be addressed with PCI and that the SYNTAX (Synergy between Percutaneous Coronary Intervention with TAXUS and Cardiac Surgery) score is ≤22 that represents a high likelihood of a good long-term outcome. Early trials of CABG versus medical therapy found that survival was improved with CABG; however, many of these trials are more than 2 decades old and medical therapy has improved.[9,10] In the Clinical Outcomes Utilizing Revascularization and Aggressive Drug Evaluation (COURAGE) trial optimal medical therapy was as good as revascularization with the exception of certain subgroups such as patients with diabetes.[26,48] In the COURAGE trial the 4.6-year cumulative primary-event rates (death from any cause and nonfatal MI) were 19% in the PCI group and 18.5% in the medical-therapy group (hazard ratio for the PCI group, 1.05; 95% confidence interval [CI], 0.87 to 1.27; $P = 0.62$).[48,49] Medicine, Angioplasty, or Surgery Study (MASS II) found medical therapy was associated with an incidence of long-term events and rate of additional revascularization similar to those for PCI. CABG was superior to medical therapy in terms of the primary end points, reaching a significant 44% reduction in primary end points at the 5-year follow-up of patients with stable multivessel CAD.[50] Addition information is provided later in Revascularization below.

After assessing and manipulating the alterable risk factors as discussed previously, the next intervention that could be undertaken is the institution of a regular exercise program. Training is possible in many patients with angina and the observed benefits include decreased HR and SBP as well as increased ejection fraction and duration of exercise. Although the mechanism of these effects has been debated, improved overall cardiovascular and muscular condition is probably the most important. Improved production of nitric oxide and coronary vasomotion may account partially for the beneficial effects of exercise. The intensity of exercise influences training and more vigorous programs provide better overall results.[35,36] Obviously, an exercise program should be undertaken with caution and in a graded fashion with adequate supervision.

5 Chronic prophylactic therapy for patients with more than one angina episode per day may also be instituted with β-adrenergic blocking agents, and in many instances, β-blockers may be preferable because of less frequent dosing and other properties inherent in β-blockade (e.g., potential cardioprotective effects, antiarrhythmic effects, lack of tolerance, and antihypertensive effects), as well as their antianginal effects and documented protective effects in post-MI patients.[19,51] β-Blockers may also slow the progression of plaque volume.[52] Patients who continue to smoke have reduced antianginal efficacy of β-blockers. This may be due to enhanced hepatic metabolism of drugs that are eliminated through this route or related to the effects of smoking on MVO_2 and oxygenation.[53] The one characteristic that is relevant is the duration of effect on the DP. β-Blockers with longer half-lives (e.g., nadolol) are more likely to affect the DP for a longer period of time and require fewer doses per day. The choice of β-blocker for angina rests on choosing the appropriate dose to achieve the goals outlined for HR and DP, and choosing an agent that is well tolerated by individual patients and cost. Selective use may incorporate ancillary properties, but these are secondary considerations in overall drug product selection. Patients most likely to respond well to β-blockade are those who have a high resting HR and those having a relatively fixed anginal threshold. In other words, their symptoms appear at the same level of exercise or workload on a consistent basis. Symptoms appearing with variable workloads suggest fluctuations in myocardial oxygen supply, perhaps due to coronary artery vasomotion, and these patients are more likely to respond to calcium channel antagonists.

6 Nitrate therapy should be the first step in managing acute attacks for patients with chronic stable angina if the attacks are infrequent (i.e., a few times per month) or for prophylaxis of symptoms when undertaking activities known to precipitate attacks. In general, if angina occurs no more often than once every few days, then SL nitroglycerin tablets or spray or buccal products may be sufficient to allow the patient to maintain an adequate lifestyle. For episodes of *first-effort* angina occurring in a predictable fashion, nitroglycerin may be used in a prophylactic manner with the patient taking 0.3 to 0.4 mg SL about 5 minutes prior to the anticipated time of activity. Nitroglycerin spray may be useful when inadequate saliva is produced to rapidly dissolve SL nitroglycerin or if a patient has difficulty opening the container. Most patients have a response that lasts about 30 minutes or so, but this is subject to interindividual variability. When angina occurs more frequently than once a day, a chronic prophylactic regimen using β-blockers as the first line of therapy should be considered (see Fig. 6-2 for the SIHD algorithm). Chronic prophylactic therapy with long-acting forms of nitroglycerin (oral or transdermal), isosorbide dinitrate (ISDN), 5-mononitrate, and pentaerythritol trinitrate may be effective; however, the development of tolerance is a major limiting step in their continued effectiveness. Since long-acting nitrates are not as effective as β-blockers and do not have beneficial effects, monotherapy with nitrates should not be first-line therapy unless β-blockers and calcium channel blockers are contraindicated or not tolerated. As described previously, providing a nitrate-free interval of 8 hours/day or longer appears to be the most promising approach to maintaining the efficacy of chronic nitrate therapy. Recent investigations into the mechanisms of nitrate tolerance in normal volunteers have shown that treatment with isosorbide mononitrate (ISMN) for 7 days resulted in not only tolerance but also endothelial dysfunction that is thought to be due to reactive oxygen species generated during bioactivation of high-potency nitrates.[54,55] Chronic nitrate use may be associated with ACS presentation changes with a preponderance of unstable angina and NSTEMI over STEMI.[56]

TABLE 6-8 Revascularization to Improve Survival Compared with Medical Therapy

Anatomic Setting	COR	LOE
UPLM or complex CAD		
CABG and PCI	I—Heart team approach recommended	C
CABG and PCI	IIa—Calculation of STS and SYNTAX scores	B
UPLM[a]		
CABG	I	B
PCI	IIa—For SIHD when both of the following are present: • Anatomic conditions associated with a low risk of PCI procedural complications and a high likelihood of good long-term outcome (e.g., a low SYNTAX score of ≤22, ostial or trunk left main CAD) • Clinical characteristics that predict a significantly increased risk of adverse surgical outcomes (e.g., STS-predicted risk of operative mortality ≥5%)	B
	IIa—For UA/NSTEMI if not a CABG candidate	B
	IIa—For STEMI when distal coronary flow is TIMI flow grade <3 and PCI can be performed more rapidly and safely than CABG	C
	IIb—For SIHD when *both* of the following are present: • Anatomic conditions associated with a low to intermediate risk of PCI procedural complications and an intermediate to high likelihood of good long-term outcome (e.g., low–intermediate SYNTAX score of <33, bifurcation left main CAD) • Clinical characteristics that predict an increased risk of adverse surgical outcomes (e.g., moderate–severe COPD, disability from prior stroke, or prior cardiac surgery; STS-predicted operative mortality >2%)	B
	III: Harm—For SIHD in patients (vs. performing CABG) Anatomy for PCI and who are good candidates for CABG	B
Three-vessel disease with or without proximal LAD artery disease[a]	I	B
CABG	IIa—It is reasonable to choose CABG over PCI in patients with complex three-vessel CAD (e.g., SYNTAX score >22) who are good candidates for CABG	B
PCI	IIb—Of uncertain benefit	B
Two-vessel disease with proximal LAD artery disease[a]		
CABG	I	B
PCI	IIb—Of uncertain benefit	B
Two-vessel disease without proximal LAD artery disease[a]		
CABG	IIa—With extensive ischemia	B
	IIb—Of uncertain benefit without extensive ischemia	C
PCI	IIb—Of uncertain benefit	B
One-vessel proximal LAD artery disease[a]		
CABG	IIa—With LIMA for long-term benefit	B
PCI	IIb—Of uncertain benefit	B
One-vessel disease without proximal LAD artery involvement		
CABG	III: Harm	B
PCI	III: Harm	B
LV dysfunction		
CABG	IIa—EF 35–50%	B
CABG	IIb—EF <35% without significant left main CAD	B
PCI	Insufficient data	
Survivors of sudden cardiac death with presumed ischemia-mediated VT		
CABG	I	B
PCI	I	C
No anatomic or physiologic criteria for revascularization		
CABG	III: Harm	B
PCI	III: Harm	B

CABG, coronary artery bypass graft; CAD, coronary artery disease; COPD, chronic obstructive pulmonary disease; COR, class of recommendation; EF, ejection fraction; LAD, left anterior descending; LIMA, left internal mammary artery; LOE, level of evidence; LV, left ventricular; PCI, percutaneous coronary intervention; SIHD, stable ischemic heart disease; STEMI, ST-elevation myocardial infarction; STS, Society of Thoracic Surgeons; SYNTAX, Synergy between Percutaneous Coronary Intervention with TAXUS and Cardiac Surgery; TIMI, Thrombolysis in Myocardial Infarction; UA/NSTEMI, unstable angina/non–ST-elevation myocardial infarction; UPLM, unprotected left main disease; VT, ventricular tachycardia.

[a]In patients with multivessel disease who have diabetes mellitus, it is reasonable to choose CABG (with LIMA) over PCI (Class IIa; LOE: B).

TABLE 6-9 Revascularization to Improve Symptoms with Significant Anatomic (≥50% Left Main or ≥70% Non–Left Main CAD) or Physiologic (FFR ≤0.80) Coronary Artery Stenoses

Clinical Setting	COR	LOE
≥1 significant stenosis amenable to revascularization and unacceptable angina despite GDMT	1—CABG	A
	1—PCI	
≥1 significant stenosis and unacceptable angina in whom GDMT cannot be implemented because of medication contraindications, adverse effects, or patient preferences	IIa—CABG	C
	IIa—PCI	C
Previous CABG with ≥1 significant stenosis associated with ischemia and unacceptable angina despite GMDT	IIa—PCI	C
	IIb—CABG	C
Complex three-vessel CAD (e.g., SYNTAX score >22) with or without involvement of the proximal LAD artery and a good candidate for CABG	IIa—CABG preferred over PCI	B
Viable ischemic myocardium that is perfused by coronary arteries that are not amenable to grafting	IIb—TMR as an adjunct to CABG	B
No anatomic or physiologic criteria for revascularization	III: Harm—CABG	C
	III: Harm—PCI	C

CABG indicated coronary artery bypass graft; CAD, coronary artery disease; COR, class of recommendation; FFR, fractional flow reserve; GDMT, guideline-directed medical therapy; LOE, level of evidence; N/A, not available; PCI, percutaneous coronary intervention; SYNTAX, Synergy between Percutaneous Coronary Intervention with TAXUS and Cardiac Surgery; and TMR, transmyocardial revascularization.

Oral administration of nitrates is susceptible to a saturable first-pass effect; therefore, larger doses can produce a measurable hemodynamic effect and dose titration should be based on these changes in the DP. There are few well-controlled studies comparing oral or SL nitrate efficacy, and the choice among these products should be based on familiarity with the preparation, cost, and patient acceptance.

7 Calcium channel antagonists have the potential advantage of improving coronary blood flow through coronary artery vasodilation as well as decreasing MVO_2 and may be used instead of β-blockers for chronic prophylactic therapy; however, in chronic stable angina comparative trials of long-acting calcium channel blockers with β-blockers do not show significant differences in response.[57,58] They

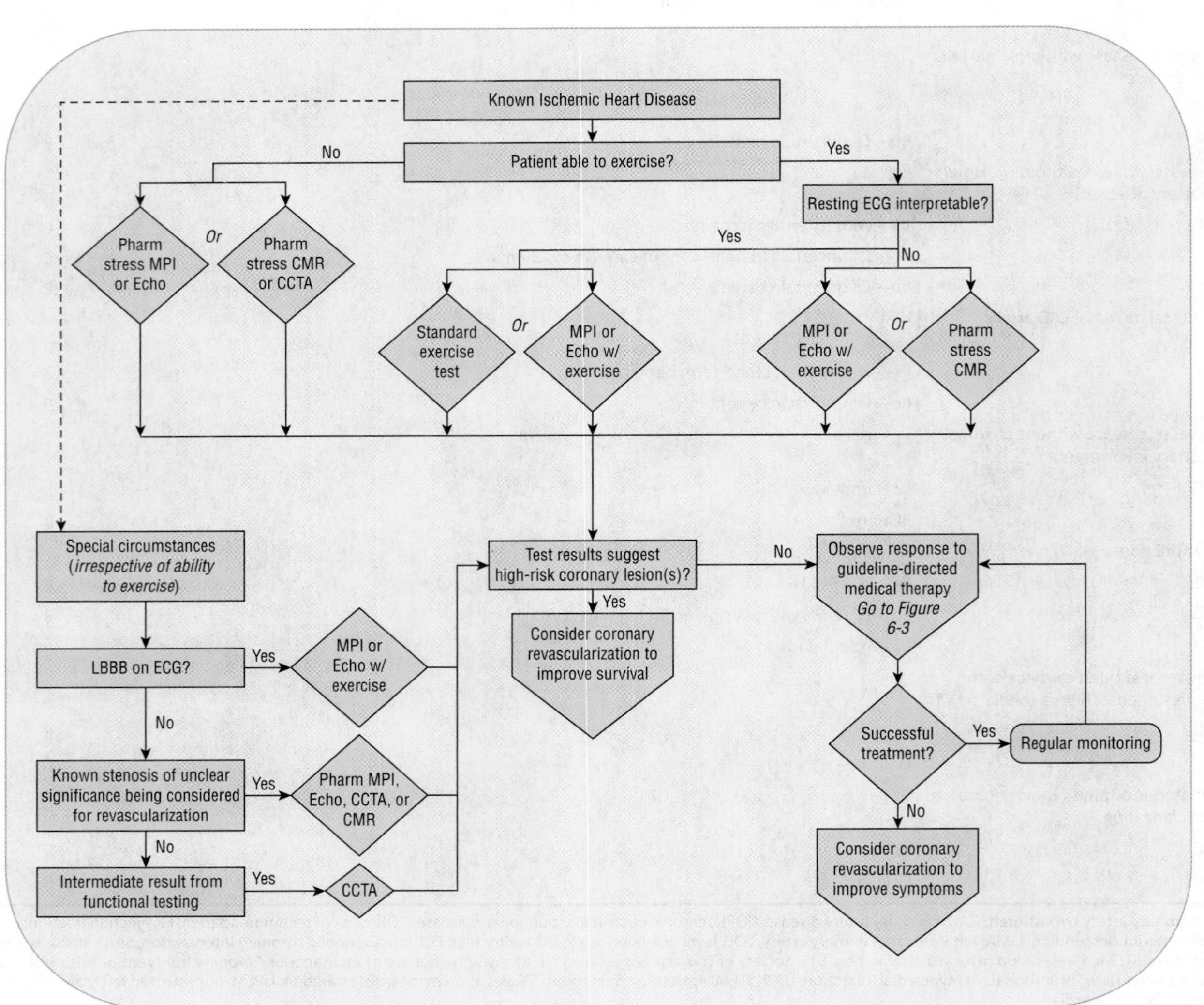

FIGURE 6-2 Algorithm for risk assessment in patients with SIHD.

are as effective as β-blockers and are most useful in patients who have a variable threshold for exertional angina. Calcium antagonists may provide better skeletal muscle oxygenation, resulting in decreased fatigue and better exercise tolerance. Additionally, if contraindications exist to β-blocker therapy, calcium antagonists can be safely used in many patients. The available calcium channel blockers appear to have similar efficacy in the management of chronic stable angina. Differences in their electrophysiology, peripheral and central hemodynamic effects, and adverse effect profiles are useful in selecting the appropriate agent. Patients with conduction abnormalities and moderate to severe LV dysfunction (ejection fraction <35% [<0.35]) should not be treated with verapamil or diltiazem, whereas amlodipine may be safely used in many of these patients. Diltiazem has significant effects on the AV node and can produce heart block in patients with preexisting conduction disease or when other drugs, such as digoxin or β-blockers, with effects on conduction are used concurrently. Nifedipine may cause excessive HR elevation, especially if the patient is not receiving a β-blocker, and this may offset the beneficial effect it has on MVO_2. Gingival hyperplasia has also been reported with nifedipine, and some dental authorities say this may be seen in as many as 20% of patients on nifedipine. Case–control studies with calcium blockers suggest an increased risk for MI and cancer.[59,60] The relationship to cancer appears to be weak to nonexistent, whereas the risk for MI is probably real and related to the type of drug used and relationship to recent MI. Immediate-release formulations of calcium blockers can activate the sympathetic nervous system and, in patients with recent MI or significant coronary disease, may induce ischemia. This effect has not been shown for longer-acting products. The hemodynamic effect of calcium antagonists is complementary to β-blockade, and, consequently, combination therapy is rational, but clinical trial data do not support the notion that combination therapy is always more effective.[57,61]

Nonpharmacologic Therapy 8

Revascularization The decision to undertake PCI or CABG for revascularization is based on the extent of coronary disease (number of vessels and location/amount of stenosis) and ventricular function. The recommended mode of coronary revascularization is outlined in Table 6-8.[62,63]

The largest randomized trial of PCI versus CABG is the Bypass Angioplasty Revascularization (BARI) trial conducted in 1,829 patients with two- or three-vessel disease; 64% of these patients had an admitting diagnosis of UA and 19% were diabetic.[64] The 10-year survival was 71% for PTCA and 73.5% for CABG ($P = 0.18$). At 10 years, the PTCA group had substantially higher subsequent revascularization rates than the CABG group (76.8% vs. 20.3%, $P < 0.001$), but angina rates for the two groups were similar. In the subgroup of patients with no treated diabetes, survival rates were nearly identical by randomization (PTCA 77% vs. CABG 77.3%, $P = 0.59$).[65] Insulin-requiring diabetics and chronic kidney disease seem to be at the highest risk and CABG is the revascularization procedure of choice for this population.[49] In a large observational study by Hannan et al., patients with proximal LAD lesions and multivessel disease had higher survival rates with CABG than with PTCA.[64,66,67] High-risk patients who should be considered for CABG over PCI are those with LV systolic dysfunction, patients with diabetes, and those with two-vessel disease with severe proximal LAD involvement or severe three-vessel or left main disease[62] (Table 6-8). Angina with Extremely Serious Operative Mortality (AWESOME) found that patients who were older than 70 years of age support the trial conclusions that either bypass or PCI effectively relieves medically refractory ischemia among high-risk unstable angina patients whose age was greater than 70 years.[68]

PCI has been used successfully in the management of unstable angina.[69] PTCA involves the insertion of a guidewire and inflatable balloon into the affected coronary artery and enlarging the lumen of the artery by stretching the vessel wall. This frequently causes atheroma plaque fracture by stretching inelastic components and denudation of the endothelium resulting in loss of nitric oxide and other vasodilators and exposure of plaque contents to the vascular compartment. Consequently, immediate vascular recoil, platelet adhesion and aggregation, mural thrombus formation, smooth muscle proliferation, and synthesis of extracellular matrix may give rise to acute occlusion and early or late restenosis.[70–72] The presence of coronary artery spasm and intraluminal thrombus, common occurrences in unstable angina, increases the hazard of these complications. The advent of combination therapy with ASA, UFH, or LMWH and IIb/IIIa receptor antagonists and coronary artery stents has dramatically reduced the occurrence of early reocclusion and late restenosis.[73,74] Patients best suited for PTCA are those with recent onset of worsening of angina without a long history of symptoms. Angiographic characteristics associated with these clinical findings that allow the greatest probability of success for PTCA are severe, discrete, proximal lesions found in a large epicardial vessel subtending a moderate or large area of viable myocardium and have high risk. Patients with focal saphenous vein graft lesions who are poor candidates for reoperation have a Class IIa recommendation for PCI. Class IIb indications include patients with one or more lesions to be dilated in vessels subtending a less than moderate area of viable myocardium and patients with multivessel disease and proximal LAD lesions, diabetes, or abnormal LV function.[63] Previously, candidates for PTCA must also be suited for CABG because a small percentage of procedures results in emergency CABG. Improvements in PCI and stent technology have led to some institutions performing procedures without surgical backup.[75] Success of PCI may be defined as angiographic success (TIMI 3 flow and <20% residual stenosis), procedural success (lack of in-hospital clinical complications), and clinical success (anatomic and procedural success with relief of ischemic pain for at least 6 months). In trials of invasive versus conservative strategies (medical management) using PCI, death or MI is less frequent in some trials but not all.[48,76,77] Numerous studies support the use of IIb/IIIa receptor antagonists in addition to ASA and UFH or LMWH and, as described previously, abciximab was superior to tirofiban in the only comparative study available.[78,79] The initial success rate for PTCA in unstable angina is ~80% to 90%, but these patients are at risk for more complications than are those with stable angina because of the underlying pathophysiology.

In the event of prolonged chest pain and ischemic ECG changes unrelieved by nitrate therapy or calcium channel antagonists, one may assume total occlusion of a coronary vessel and steps should be taken to restore blood flow with either PCI or CABG.

Coronary Artery Bypass Grafting Following the introduction of saphenous vein graft replacement for the severely occluded coronary arteries by Favorolo and Garrett in 1967, CABG became an accepted and commonly used approach for the management of IHD.[80] The objectives in performing CABG are twofold: (a) reduce the number of symptomatic anginal attacks not controlled with medical management or PCI and improve the lifestyle of the patient and (b) reduce the mortality associated with CAD. Surgery is effective in providing pain relief in large numbers of patients, with about 70% to 95% being pain-free at 1 year and 46% to 55% being pain-free at 5 years. This compares favorably with medical management, with which only about 30% are free of symptoms at 5 years. Mortality at 10 years from the largest published studies is 26.4% with CABG and 30.5% with medical management ($P = 0.03$), but there are significant differences based on subgroup analysis (e.g., left main disease vs. one-vessel disease without a proximal LAD lesion).[80] The second objective is met in certain patients and this has been addressed in three large, well-controlled trials of bypass surgery. These three studies, the Veterans Administration (VA), European Cooperative

Surgery Study (ECSS), and the CASS, are not directly comparable because the inclusion and exclusion criteria for entry into each study were different and patients were followed for different periods of time. They have also been criticized for not being representative of the population that may be candidates for surgery, lacking women or late-middle-aged or elderly patients, and crossover of medically managed patients to the surgical group. A major change in medical practice that influences the interpretation of these older studies is the common procedure of stent placement at the time of angioplasty.[11,81,83] There are about 20 different types of stents available and their use is associated with greater luminal diameter after angioplasty, fewer acute reocclusions, and less restenosis after stent placement.[84] Consequently, the validity of generalizing the results from these studies to routine practice has been questioned, but these studies are useful for providing a basis for decisions concerning surgery. Current Class I recommendations for CABG in asymptomatic or mild angina patient include significant (>50%) left main coronary artery stenosis, left main equivalent (≥70% stenosis of the proximal LAD and proximal left circumflex artery), and three-vessel disease, especially in patients with LV ejection fraction <50% (<0.50).[80] Class IIa recommendations for CABG are proximal LAD stenosis with one- or two-vessel disease and Class IIb one- or two-vessel disease not involving the proximal LAD. In stable angina, Class I recommendations are the same as for mild angina with the following additions: one- or two-vessel disease without significant proximal LAD stenosis, but with a large area of viable myocardium and high-risk criteria in noninvasive testing; disabling angina despite maximal medical therapy, when surgery can be performed with acceptable risk. Class IIb recommendations in stable angina include proximal LAD stenosis with one-vessel disease and one- or two-vessel disease without significant proximal LAD stenosis but with a moderate area of viable myocardium and ischemia on noninvasive testing. The indications for CABG in UA/NSTEMI are described previously. In ST-segment MI CABG is indicated for ongoing ischemia/infarction not responsive to maximal medical therapy (Class IIb).

In patients with poor LV function CABG is indicated for the same indications as in mild angina for Class I. Class IIa recommendations include poor LV function with significant viable, noncontracting, revascularizable myocardium without any of the aforementioned anatomic patterns (e.g., left main disease). CABG is useful in patients with life-threatening ventricular arrhythmia in the presence of left main disease and three-vessel disease (Class I) and in bypassable one- or two-vessel disease causing life-threatening ventricular arrhythmias and proximal LAD disease with one- or two-vessel disease (Class IIa).

CABG may also be used for patients who have failed PTCA if there is ongoing ischemia or threatened occlusion with significant myocardium at risk and in patients with hemodynamic compromise (Class I). Class IIa recommendations for failed PTCA include a foreign body in a crucial anatomic position and hemodynamic compromise in patient with impairment of the coagulation system and without a previous sternotomy. CABG may be repeated in patients with a previous CABG if disabling angina exists despite maximal noninvasive therapy (Class I) and if a large area of myocardium is threatened and is subtended by bypassable distal vessels (Class IIa).

The need for nitrates and β-blockers is clearly reduced by surgery, with only 30% of CABG patients requiring chronic medication, whereas 70% of their medical counterparts received anginal drugs. Employment status after surgery has been shown in CASS to be more dependent on the pretreatment status than an effect induced by the treatment arm, and about 70% of patients are employed before and after surgery. Recent follow-up analyses of these studies suggest that patients who have diabetes or peripheral vascular disease, who are African Americans, or who continued to smoke are at high risk for CAD events, and diabetics, in particular, are more likely to have a better outcome with CABG than with PTCA.[64,76] The overall benefit noted after CABG is similar in men and women, and elderly patients appear to have outcomes similar to younger patients.

Operative mortality is reported to range from 1% to 3% and is related to the number of vessels involved and preoperative ventricular function. Patients in CASS with one-, two-, or three-vessel disease had operative mortalities of 1.4%, 2.1%, and 2.8%, respectively. The relationship to LV ejection fraction follows a similar trend with ejection fractions of greater than 50% (0.50), 20% to 40% (0.20 to 0.40), and less than 20% (0.20) having operative mortality rates of 1.9%, 4.4%, and 6.7%, respectively. Perioperative infarction averages 5% depending on the sensitivity of the method for assessment, and the occurrence of an infarct reduces long-term survival. Neurologic dysfunction is relatively common postoperatively in CABG patients (~6%), but many of the deficits are clinically insignificant and resolve with time. Fatal brain damage occurs in 0.3% to 0.7%, stroke in about 5%, and ophthalmologic defects occur in 25%, but only 3% have clinically apparent field defects. Peripheral nerve lesions (12%) and brachial plexopathy (7%) are also reported to occur. Other complications include constrictive pericarditis (0.2%), cellulitis at the site of vein graft, and mediastinal infections (1% to 4%).

Graft patency influences the success for symptom control, and survival and the mechanism for early graft occlusion is probably different from that associated with late closure. Early occlusion is related to platelet adhesion and aggregation, whereas late occlusion may be related to endothelial proliferation and progression of atherosclerosis. Patency of grafts early on after the CABG is reported to range from 88% to 97% in at least one graft and 58% to 81% in all grafts at 1 year. Long-term patency based on the CASS Montreal Heart Institute experience suggests that 60% to 67% of all grafts remain patent at 5 to 11 years. Antiplatelet therapy has been demonstrated to improve early and late patency rates and should probably be used in all patients who do not have any contraindications.[78,79,82] Aspirin with or without other antiplatelet agents reduces the late development of vein graft occlusions. At the current time, prasugrel, a new antiplatelet drug, is only indicated for patients with ACS who are going to undergo PCI.[83] Late graft closure is related to elevated lipid levels and the progression of atherosclerosis in the grafted vessels as well as the native circulation. Elevation of very-low-density lipoprotein (VLDL), LDL, and LDL apolipoprotein B is correlated to disease progression and graft closure. Aggressive lipid lowering can stabilize the progression of CAD and may induce regression in selected coronary artery segments within a patient following CABG. Cessation of smoking is an important preoperative and postoperative objective as well as in the management of other coronary risk factors (e.g., hypertension) and institution of a supervised, daily exercise program is recommended. Internal mammary artery grafts should be used for revascularizing the left anterior descending artery system when possible owing to better graft survival and clinical outcomes.

Valvular heart disease can coexist with CHD, although this is relatively uncommon with rheumatic valve disease, usually the mitral valve, and more common with aortic stenosis and regurgitation. Angina may occur in 35% to 65% of patients with aortic stenosis or regurgitation, and, if severe, may be the cause of angina in the absence of CAD. Patients being evaluated for possible CABG should also be evaluated for valvular disease to determine if valve replacement needs to be performed along with bypass grafting.

Percutaneous Transluminal Coronary Angioplasty Since the introduction into clinical cardiology of PTCA by Gruentzig in 1977, this procedure has gained rapid acceptance as a safe and effective means of managing CAD.[69] It is estimated that more than 750,000 PCI procedures are done each year in this country and 525,000 of them are PTCA. The proposed mechanisms of reduced stenosis with PTCA include (a) compression and redistribution of the atherosclerotic plaque; (b) embolization of plaque contents;

(c) aneurysm formation; and (d) disruption of the plaque and arterial wall with distortion and tearing of the intima and media, which leads to denudation of the endothelium, platelet adhesion and aggregation, thrombus formation, and smooth muscle proliferation. Of these mechanisms, the last one is felt to be the most important, but the others may contribute to opening of the lesions in some situations.

9 The indications for PTCA have been provided by the ACC/AHA and now span single-vessel or multivessel disease as well as asymptomatic and symptomatic patients (see Table 6-9).[69] In addition to providing recommendations for which type of patients are appropriate for PTCA, the guidelines also provide recommendations for the volume of procedures, the use of intravascular ultrasound, and surgery backup when PTCA is being considered. 10 PTCA generally is not useful if only a small area of viable myocardium is at risk, when ischemia cannot be demonstrated, when borderline (<50%) stenosis or lesions are difficult to dilate, or when patients are at high risk for morbidity or mortality or both (e.g., left main or equivalent disease or three-vessel disease). PTCA alone or when used in conjunction or sequentially with thrombolysis for acute MI is discussed in Chapter 7. Stent placement accompanies balloon angioplasty in about 80% of cases in the United States. The current recommendations for PCI are provided in Table 6-10 based on class of angina.

Assessment of outcome with PCI can be based on several angiographic, procedural, and clinical outcomes as discussed previously. The success of PCI is dependent on the experience of the operator (high volume, better outcome), on complicating factors for the patient (including the number of vessels to be dilated), and on technical advances in the equipment used (e.g., steerable and low-profile catheters). The acute success rate for opening of uncomplicated stenotic lesions ranges from 96% to 99% with the combined balloon/device/pharmacologic approach in experienced hands, and angina is decreased or eliminated in about 80% of cases. The success rate for totally occluded lesions is somewhat less (~65%). Mortality at 1 year is 1% and 2.5% for single-vessel disease and multiple-vessel involvement, respectively, reflecting the good prognosis associated with this degree of CAD. At 10 years, survival is 95% and 81% for single and multiple disease, respectively.[69] Most patients remain event-free (no death, MI, or CABG) for an extended period. Symptomatic status, as measured by the NYHA classification, is improved in many patients. Restenosis is noted in 32% to 40% after balloon angioplasty at 6 months, and half of these patients will have symptoms associated with restenosis.[69] A few late restenotic events occur, but most restenosis occurs within the first 6 months. Anatomic factors that predict restenosis include lesions >20 mm in length, excessive tortuosity of the proximal segment, extremely angulated segments (>90°), total occlusions >3 months old and/or bridging collaterals, and inability to protect major side branches and degenerated vein grafts with friable lesions. Clinical factors that predict worse outcome include diabetes, advanced age, female gender, unstable angina, heart failure, and multivessel disease. A four-variable scoring system that predicts cardiovascular collapse for failed PTCA includes percentage of myocardium at risk (e.g., >50% viable myocardium at risk and LV ejection fraction <25% [<0.25]), preangioplasty percent diameter stenosis, multivessel CAD, and diffuse disease in the dilated segment or a high myocardial jeopardy score.[69] Strut thickness of the stent influences restenosis as well and thicker struts are associated with angiographic and clinical restenosis.[84,85] With the development of DES, early reocclusion has been reduced dramatically but late in-stent thrombosis has been a problem. As stent technology has evolved, due to better polymers, better strut design, and better antiproliferative agents (e.g., everolimus), stent thrombosis has dropped to as low as 0.3%, MI to 1.9%, and target lesion revascularization to 2.5%.[84]

The overall complication rate ranges from 2% to 21% depending on the lesion type. Coronary occlusion, dissection, or spasm occurs in 4% to 8% of patients, whereas ST-segment elevation MI occurs in 1.6% to 4.8%.[69] Prolonged angina and ventricular tachycardia or fibrillation occurs in 6.9% and 2.3%, respectively. In-hospital mortality ranges from 0.7% to 2.5% overall and high-risk events for mortality included ventricular arrhythmias and MI. The frequency of urgent CABG because of complications ranges from 0.4% to 5.8%.[69]

Current AHA/ACC recommendations for antithrombotic therapy in PCI are outlined in Table 6-10.[69,82] Antiplatelet therapy with ASA 80 to 325 mg/day given at least 2 hours prior to angioplasty is currently recommended. If patients are sensitive to ASA, clopidogrel or prasugrel is an acceptable alternative. In elective settings, clopidogrel should be started at least 72 hours in advance of the procedure to allow for maximal antiplatelet effects. Alternatively, a loading dose of clopidogrel (300 to 600 mg) or prasugrel 60 mg may be given to achieve a more rapid antiplatelet effect.[86–88] The combination of ASA plus clopidogrel or prasugrel is currently recommended for patients undergoing angioplasty and stenting and this combination is safer and superior to antiplatelet therapy plus anticoagulation with warfarin-like drugs.[82] Follow-up for up to 4 years from the Intracoronary Stenting and Antithrombotic Regimen (ISAR) trial shows that the benefit of combined antiplatelet therapy evident after 30 days is maintained after 4 years.[89] Aspirin is an incomplete inhibitor of platelet aggregation and combination therapy of ASA plus a GP IIb/IIIa receptor antagonist for PCI has shown a relative risk reduction of 37.5% for death and nonfatal MI at 30 days favoring GP IIb/IIIa receptor antagonists over placebo (absolute rates of 5.5% vs. 8.9% based on PCI trials of EPIC, IMPACT-II, EPILOG, CAPTURE, RESTORE, and EPISTENT).[69] As discussed in Revascularization above, high-risk patients and those having a stent placed are most likely to benefit from GP IIb/IIIa receptor antagonist use. Patients presenting with elevated cardiac biomarkers are also more likely to receive benefit from GP IIb/IIIa receptor antagonists than patients with normal levels of biomarkers.[90] In the only comparative trial (TARGET), abciximab was superior to tirofiban.[91]

During PTCA patients are usually heparinized to prevent immediate thrombus formation at the site of arterial injury and on coronary guidewires and catheters; anticoagulation is continued for up to 24 hours. The intensity of anticoagulation is monitored using the activated clotting time (ACT) and the targeted range for ACT is 250 to 300 seconds (HemoTec device) in the absence of GP IIb/IIIa receptor antagonist use.[69] When GP IIb/IIIa receptor antagonists are not used, UFH is given as an IV bolus of 70 to 100 international units/kg to achieve a target ACT of 200 seconds. The loading dose is lowered to 50 to 70 international units/kg when GP IIb/IIIa receptor antagonists are given. Target ACT for eptifibatide and tirofiban is <300 seconds during angioplasty; postprocedural UFH infusions are not recommended during GP IIb/IIIa receptor antagonist therapy. Mechanisms that result in restenosis include acute lumen loss owing to *recoil*, mural thrombosis formation, and smooth muscle cell proliferation with synthesis of extracellular matrix.[71] Approaches to prevent restenosis may be aimed at altering the underlying mechanisms. Recoil and loss of luminal diameter may be reduced by the use of stent placement; however, this beneficial effect is offset by an increased number of vascular complications. Cracking of the plaque leads to severe damage to the arterial wall, exposure of collagen, and endothelial dysfunction. These factors promote mural thrombi, and the propensity for thrombus formation is related, in part, to the composition of the plaque as well as the depth of injury. Combination therapy with ASA, heparin, and IIb/IIIa receptor antagonists is recommended to minimize acute occlusion and numerous clinical trials document the efficacy of this combined approach.[69,79,92] Bivalirudin is a specific and reversible direct thrombin inhibitor that is indicated for use as an anticoagulant in patients with unstable angina undergoing PTCA. Based on the REPLACE-2 and ACUITY studies, bivalirudin is comparable to heparin in preventing thrombosis and may

TABLE 6-10 Pharmacologic Management of Percutaneous Coronary Intervention

Recommendation	Comments
Antiplatelet and antithrombotic adjunctive therapies for PCI—oral antiplatelet therapy	
Class I	
1. Patients already taking daily chronic aspirin therapy should take 75–325 mg of aspirin before the PCI procedure is performed (*Level of Evidence: A*)	A daily dose of 75 mg of aspirin has been shown to result in improved cardiovascular outcomes similar to daily doses of 325 mg but with fewer bleeding complications
2. Patients not already taking daily chronic aspirin therapy should be given 300–325 mg of aspirin at least 2 hours and preferably 24 hours before the PCI procedure is performed (*Level of Evidence: C*)	Higher doses of aspirin are recommended for patients not already taking aspirin therapy immediately before PCI procedures
3. After the PCI procedure, in patients with no aspirin resistance, allergy, or increased risk of bleeding, aspirin 325 mg daily should be given for at least 1 month after bare-metal stent implantation, 3 months after sirolimus-eluting stent implantation, and 6 months after paclitaxel-eluting stent implantation, after which daily chronic aspirin use should be continued indefinitely at a dose of 75–162 mg (*Level of Evidence: B*)	The doses and duration of aspirin therapy recommended herein and derived from those used for U.S. Food and Drug Administration approval of the specific stent types noted in the recommendation. Daily chronic aspirin therapy is based on recommendations in the *ACC/AHA Guidelines for the Management of Patients with ST-Elevation Myocardial Infarction* and evidence indicating that aspiring therapy in dosages as low as 75 mg/day yields outcomes similar to those achieved with 325 mg/day but with fewer side effects
4. A loading dose of clopidogrel should be administered before PCI is performed (*Level of Evidence: A*). An oral loading dose of 300 mg, administered at least 6 hours before the procedure, has the best established evidence of efficacy (*Level of Evidence: B*)	Clopidogrel is an important adjunctive therapy for patients undergoing PCI with stent placement. The best evidence of efficacy exists for 300 mg given at lest 6 hours before PCI is performed
5. In patients who have undergone PCI, clopidogrel 75 mg daily should be given for at least 1 month after bare-metal stent implantation (unless the patient is at increased risk for bleeding; then it should be given for a minimum of 2 weeks), 3 months after sirolimus stent implantation, and 6 months after paclitaxel stent implantation, and ideally up to 12 months in patients who are not at high risk of bleeding (*Level of Evidence: B*)	Clopidogrel therapy in the dosage of 75 mg daily should be given after stent placement to all patients. The duration of therapy varies for each stent and is based on data from clinical trials used for U.S. Food and Drug Administration approval of that stent
Class IIa	
1. If clopidogrel is given at the time of procedure, supplementation with GP IIb/IIIa receptor antagonists can be beneficial to facilitate earlier platelet inhibition than with clopidogrel alone (*Level of Evidence: B*)	When clopidogrel is given at the time of a PCI procedure, supplementation with glycoprotein IIb/IIIa receptor antagonists can be beneficial, especially among high-risk patients
2. For patients with an absolute contraindication to aspirin, it is reasonable to give a 300-mg loading dose of clopidogrel, administered at least 6 hours before PCI, and/or GP IIb/IIIa antagonists, administered at the time of PCI (*Level of Evidence: C*)	A significant number of patients will have resistance to aspirin. The strongest evidence for clopidogrel benefit exists for doses of 300 mg given at least 6 hours before the procedure
3. When a loading dose of clopidogrel is administered, a regimen of greater than 300 mg is reasonable to achieve higher levels of antiplatelet activity more rapidly, but the efficacy and safety compared with a 300-mg loading dose are less established (*Level of Evidence: C*)	Many patients receive clopidogrel therapy at the time of PCI in dosages greater than 600 mg. Although more pronounced inhibition of platelet function has been demonstrated for doses of clopidogrel greater than 300 mg, the safety of these higher doses and their benefits on clinical outcome are not fully established
4. It is reasonable that patients undergoing brachytherapy be given daily clopidogrel 75 mg indefinitely and daily aspirin 75–325 mg indefinitely unless there is significant risk for bleeding (*Level of Evidence: C*)	Subacute or later thrombosis has been observed in patients undergoing brachytherapy, and for this reason long-term antiplatelet therapy is recommended
Class IIb	
In patients in whom subacute thrombosis may be catastrophic or lethal (unprotected left main, bifurcating left main, or last patent coronary vessel), platelet aggregation studies may be considered and the dose of clopidogrel increased to 150 mg/day if less than 50% inhibition of platelet aggregation is demonstrated (*Level of Evidence: C*)	Clopidogrel resistance is a significant problem, and owing to its contribution to catastrophic clinical outcomes, the Writing Committee recommends studies be performed with increases in clopidogrel dose being recommended for use in those with higher-risk lesions
Glycoprotein IIb/IIIa inhibitors	
Class I	
In patients with UA/NSTEMI undergoing PCI without clopidogrel administration, a C IIb/IIIa inhibitor (abciximab, eptifibatide, or tirofiban) should be administered (*Level of Evidence: A*). It is acceptable to administer the GP IIb/IIIa inhibitor before performance of the diagnostic angiogram ("upstream treatment") or just before PCI ("in-lab treatment")	This recommendation and phrasing are compatible with the *ACC/AHA 2002 Guideline Update for the Management of Patients with Unstable Angina and Non-ST-Segment Myocardial Infarction* and current evidence from randomized clinical trials. The benefits of GP IIb/IIa inhibition are especially efficacious when clopidogrel is not given
Class IIa	
1. In patients with UA/NSTEMI undergoing PCI with clopidogrel administration, it is reasonable to administer a GP IIb/IIIa inhibitor (abciximab, eptifibatide, or tirofiban) (*Level of Evidence: B*) It is acceptable to administer the GP IIb/IIIa inhibitor before performance of the diagnostic angiogram ("upstream treatment") or just before PCI ("in-lab treatment")	
2. In patients with STEMI undergoing PCI, it is reasonable to administer abciximab as early as possible (*Level of Evidence: B*)	Recommendation has been added for consistency with the *ACC/AHA Guidelines for the Management of Patients with ST-Elevation Myocardial Infarction*
3. In patients undergoing elective PCI with stent placement, it is reasonable to administer a GP IIb/IIIa inhibitor (abciximab, eptifibatide, or tirofiban) (*Level of Evidence: B*)	Phrasing has been changed to reflect current terminology, especially in a high-risk patient

(*continued*)

TABLE 6-10 Pharmacologic Management of Percutaneous Coronary Intervention (*Continued*)

Class IIb	
In patients with STEMI undergoing PCI, treatment with eptifibatide or tirofiban may be considered (*Level of Evidence: C*)	Recommendation has been added for consistency with the *ACC/AHA Guidelines for the Management of Patients with ST-Elevation Myocardial Infarction*
Antithrombotic therapy	
Unfractionated heparin, low-molecular-weight heparin, and bivalirudin	
Class I	
1. Unfractionated heparin should be administered to patients undergoing PCI (*Level of Evidence: C*)	Phrasing has been changed to reflect current terminology
2. For patients with heparin-induced thrombocytopenia, it is recommended that bivalirudin or argatroban be used to replace heparin (*Level of Evidence: B*)	Bivalirudin and argatroban are established therapies in place of heparin among patients with heparin-induced thrombocytopenia
Class IIa	
1. It is reasonable to use bivalirudin as an alternative to unfractionated heparin and glycoprotein IIb/IIIa antagonists in low-risk patients undergoing elective PCI (*Level of Evidence: B*)	New recommendation is based on data from a clinical trial (REPLACE-2) indicating bivalirudin is an acceptable alternative to heparin and GP IIb/IIIa antagonists in low-risk patients undergoing PCI
2. Low-molecular-weight heparin is a reasonable alternative to unfractionated heparin in patients with UA/NSTEMI undergoing PCI (*Level of Evidence: B*)	Recommendation from the *ACC/AHA 2002 Guideline Update for the Management of Patients with Unstable Angina and Non–ST-Segment Myocardial Infarction* has been approved by this Writing Committee and included in these guidelines for consistency
Class IIb	
Low-molecular-weight heparin may be considered as an alternative to unfractionated heparin in patients with STEMI undergoing PCI (*Level of Evidence: B*)	Recommendation from the *ACC/AHA Guidelines for the Management of Patients with ST-Elevation Myocardial Infarction* has been approved by this Writing Committee and included in these guidelines for consistency

GP, glycoprotein; NSTEMI, non–ST-segment elevation myocardial infarction; PCI, percutaneous coronary intervention; STEMI, ST-segment elevation myocardial infarction; UA, unstable angina.

From Smith SC Jr, Feldman TE, Hirshfeld JW Jr, et al. ACC/AHA/SCAI 2005 guideline update for percutaneous coronary intervention—Summary article: A report of the American College of Cardiology/American Heart Association Task Force on Practice Guidelines (ACC/AHA/SCAI Writing Committee to Update the 2001 Guidelines for Percutaneous Coronary Intervention). Circulation 2006;113:156–175.

be associated with less bleeding.[93,94] A more complete discussion of antithrombotic therapy can be found in Chapter 7.

When medical therapy, PTCA, and CABG have been compared, low-risk patients with single-vessel CAD and normal LV function had greater alleviation of symptoms with PTCA than with medical treatment; mortality rates and rates of MI were unchanged. In high-risk patients (risk was defined by severity of ischemia, number of diseased vessels, and presence of LV dysfunction), improvement of survival was greater with CABG than with medical therapy. In moderate-risk patients with multivessel CAD (most had two-vessel disease and normal LV function), PTCA and CABG produced equivalent mortality rates and rates of MI.

The development of DES has changed the natural course of stent thrombosis when compared with bare-metal stents (BMS) that have existed for a longer period of time. Currently there are three types of DES available (sirolimus [Cypher™], paclitaxel [Taxus™], and everolimus [Zortress™]). Soon after the introduction of BMS, it became apparent that early stent thrombosis (≤30 days) was an uncommon but serious complication of therapy.[71,84,85,95] Stent thrombosis is an infrequent but severe complication of both BMS and DES, but there is no apparent difference in overall stent thrombosis frequency at 4 years of follow-up, although the time course appears to be different. There is a relative numeric excess of stent thrombosis late after DES implantation; however, no differences in death or death and infarction have been observed. Target lesion revascularization is needed less often with DES compared with BMS. Implantation of DES stents outside of approved indications and lack of proper positioning of the stent are related to the occurrence of late stent thrombosis. Longer-term follow-up with larger subsets of patients (i.e., lesion number, type, and location and patient comorbidities) is needed to fully understand this issue and the evolution of newer platforms for drug delivery will likely alter the natural history of DES stent thrombosis.[96] A very important consideration is the use of combination antiplatelet therapy (aspirin + clopidogrel or prasugrel) for at least a year following implantation.[78,79,82] Patients who are unable to activate clopidogrel due to a reduced-function allele for CYP2C19 may be treated with 150 mg/day rather than 75 mg/day or switched to prasugrel.[97] Drugs that inhibit CYP2C19 should probably be avoided, although there is conflicting evidence in the literature.[98–100]

Pharmacologic Therapy

Historically, about 30% of anginal syndrome symptoms have responded regardless of which therapy was instituted. These observations stem from two problems inherent in clinical trials undertaken to assess the efficacy of any therapy for angina: (a) adequate trial design incorporating appropriate controls and washout periods, and (b) assessment of treatment effects using objective measures of efficacy including improvement in exercise performance, resting and ambulatory ECG improvement in ischemic changes, or other objective tests to address other aspects of myocardial function or metabolism. The use of pain episode frequency and nitroglycerin consumption is subjective, and their use as sole measures of efficacy should be avoided. Objective assessment using ETT has shown that placebo does not provide improvement in patients with exertional angina, substantiating this as a valid means to assess efficacy.

β-Adrenergic Blocking Agents Decreased HR, decreased contractility, and a slight to moderate decrease in blood pressure with β-adrenergic receptor antagonism reduce MVO_2.[101,102] The predominant receptor type in the heart is the β_1-receptor, and competitive blockade minimizes the influence of endogenous catecholamines on the chronotropic and inotropic state of the myocardium. These beneficial effects may be countered to some degree with increased ventricular volume and ejection time seen with β-blockade; however, the overall effect of β-blockers in patients with effort-induced angina is a reduction in oxygen demand (Table 6-11). The β-blockers do not improve oxygen supply, and in certain instances, unopposed α-adrenergic stimulation following the use of β-blockers may lead to coronary vasoconstriction. For patients with chronic exertional

TABLE 6-11 Effect of Drug Therapy on Myocardial Oxygen Demand[a]

			LV Wall Tension	
	Heart Rate	Myocardial Contractility	Systolic Pressure	LV Volume
Nitrates	⇓	0	⇓	⇓⇓
β-Blockers	⇓⇓	⇓	⇓	⇓
Nifedipine	⇓	0 or ⇓	0 or ⇓	0 or ⇓
Verapamil	⇓	⇓	⇓	0 or ⇓
Diltiazem	⇓⇓	0 or ⇓	⇓	0 or ⇓

LV, left ventricular.

[a]Calcium channel antagonists and nitrates also may increase myocardial oxygen supply through coronary vasodilation. Diastolic function also may be improved with verapamil, nifedipine, and, perhaps, diltiazem. These effects may vary from those indicated in the table depending on individual patient baseline hemodynamics.

stable angina, β-blockers improve symptoms about 80% of the time and objective measures of efficacy demonstrate improved exercise duration and delay in the time at which ST-segment changes and initial or limiting symptoms occur. β-Blockers do not alter the rate–pressure product (DP) for maximal exercise, therefore substantiating reduced demand rather than improved supply as the major consequence of their actions. Reflex tachycardia from nitrate therapy can be blunted with β-blocker therapy, making this a common and useful combination. Although β-blockade may decrease exercise capacity in healthy individuals or in patients with hypertension, it may allow angina patients previously limited by symptoms to perform more exercise and ultimately improve overall cardiovascular performance through a training effect. Ideal candidates for β-blockers include patients in whom physical activity figures prominently in their anginal attacks, those who have coexistent hypertension, those with a history of supraventricular arrhythmias or post-MI angina, and those who have a component of anxiety associated with angina.[3] β-Blockers may also be safely used in angina and heart failure as described in Chapter 4. Pertinent pharmacokinetics for the β-blockers includes half-life and route elimination, which are reviewed in Chapter 3. Drugs with longer half-lives need to be dosed less frequently than ones with shorter half-lives; however, disparity exists between half-life and duration of action for several β-blockers (e.g., metoprolol) and this may reflect attenuation of the central nervous system–mediated effects on the sympathetic system as well as the direct effects of this category on HR and contractility. Renal and hepatic dysfunction can affect the disposition of β-blockers, but these agents are dosed to effect, either hemodynamic or symptomatic, and route of elimination is not a major consideration in drug selection.

Guidelines for the use of β-blockers in treating angina include the objective of lowering resting HR to 50 to 60 beats/min and limiting maximal exercise HR to about 100 beats/min or less. It has also been suggested that exercise HR should be no more than about 20 beats/min or a 10% increment over resting HR with modest exercise. Because β-blockade is competitive and circulating catecholamine concentrations vary depending on the intensity of exercise and other factors, and cholinergic tone may be important in controlling HR in some patients, these guidelines are general in nature. These effects are generally dose and plasma concentration related, and for propranolol, plasma concentrations of 30 ng/mL (30 mcg/L; 115 nmol/L) are needed for a 25% reduction of anginal frequency. Initial doses of β-blockers should be at the lower end of the usual dosing range and titrated to response as indicated above.

There is little evidence to suggest superiority of any β-blocker; however, the duration of β-blockade is dependent partially on the half-life of the agent used, and those with longer half-lives may be dosed less frequently. Of note, propranolol may be dosed twice a day in most patients with angina and the efficacy is similar to that seen with more frequent dosing. The ancillary property of membrane-stabilizing activity is irrelevant in the treatment of angina, and intrinsic sympathomimetic activity appears to be detrimental in rest or severe angina because the reduction in HR would be minimized, therefore limiting a reduction in MVO_2. Cardioselective β-blockers may be used in some patients to minimize adverse effects such as bronchospasm in asthma, intermittent claudication, and sexual dysfunction. A common misunderstanding is that β-blockers are not well tolerated in peripheral arterial disease, but, in fact, their use is associated with a reduction in death and improved quality of life.[103] It should be remembered that cardioselectivity is a relative property and the use of larger doses (e.g., metoprolol 200 mg/day) is associated with the loss of selectivity and with adverse effects. Post–acute-MI patients with angina are particularly good candidates for β-blockade both because anginal symptoms may be treated as well as reducing the risk of post-MI reinfarction and because mortality has been demonstrated with timolol, propranolol, and metoprolol (see Chap. 4). Combined β-blockade (nonselective) and α-blockade with labetalol may be useful in some patients with marginal LV reserve, and fewer deleterious effects on coronary blood flow are seen when compared with other β-blockers.

Extension of pharmacologic effect is the underlying reason for many of the adverse effects seen with β-blockade. Hypotension, decompensated heart failure, bradycardia and heart block, bronchospasm, and altered glucose metabolism are directly related to β-adrenoreceptor antagonism. Patients with preexisting LV systolic and decompensated heart failure and the use of other negative inotropic agents are most prone to developing overt heart failure, and in the absence of these, heart failure is uncommon (less than 5%). Other drugs that depress conduction are additive to β-blockade, and intrinsic conduction system disease predisposes the patient to conduction abnormalities. Altered glucose metabolism is most likely to be seen in insulin-dependent diabetics, and β-blockade obscures the symptoms of hypoglycemia except for sweating. β-Blockers may also aggravate the lipid abnormalities seen in patients with diabetes; however, these changes are dose related, are more common with normal baseline lipids than dyslipidemia, and may be of short-term significance only. One of the more common reasons for discontinuation of β-blocker therapy is related to central nervous system adverse effects of fatigue, malaise, and depression. Cognition changes seen with β-blockers are usually minimal and comparable to other categories of drugs based on studies done in hypertension.[104] Abrupt withdrawal of β-blocker therapy in patients with angina has been associated with increased severity and number of pain episodes and MI. The mechanism of this effect is unknown but may be related to increased receptor sensitivity or disease progression during therapy, which becomes apparent following discontinuation of β-blockade. In any event, tapering of β-blocker therapy over about 2 days should minimize the risk of withdrawal reactions for those patients in whom therapy is being discontinued.

β-Adrenoreceptor blockade is effective in chronic exertional angina as monotherapy and in combination with nitrates and/or calcium channel antagonists. β-Blockers should be the first-line drug in chronic angina requiring daily maintenance therapy because β-blockers are more effective in reducing episodes of silent ischemia, reducing early morning peak of ischemic activity, and improving mortality after Q-wave MI than nitrates or calcium channel blockers (Fig. 6-3).[1] If β-blockers are ineffective or not tolerated, then monotherapy with a calcium channel blocker or combination therapy if monotherapy is ineffective for either alone may be instituted. Patients with severe angina, rest angina, or variant angina (i.e., a component of coronary artery spasm) may be better treated with calcium channel blockers or long-acting nitrates.

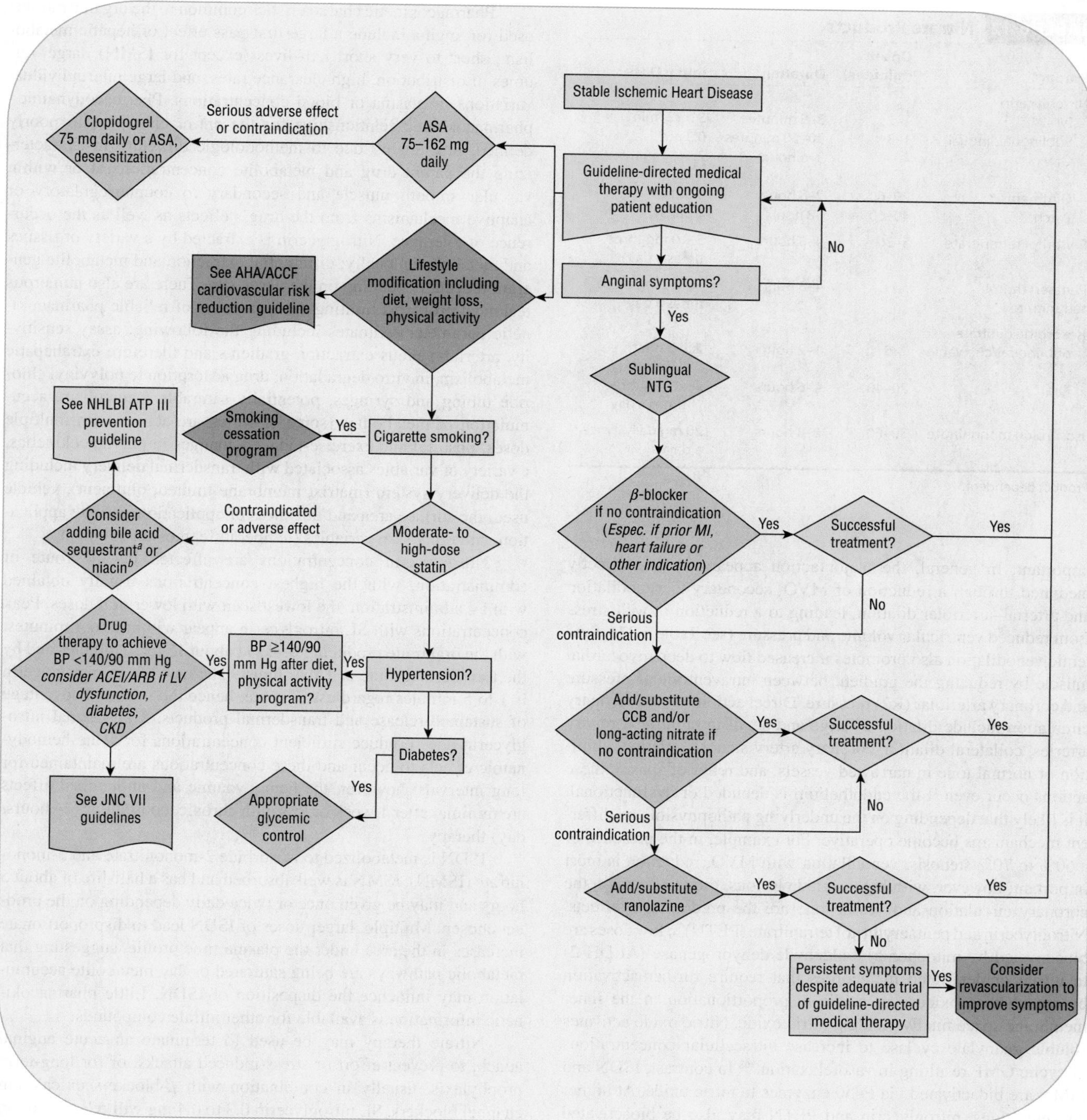

FIGURE 6-3 Algorithm for guideline-directed medical therapy for patients with SIHD. Colors correspond to the class of recommendations in the ACCF/AHA Table 6-13. The algorithms do not represent a comprehensive list of recommendations (see text for all recommendations). [a]The use of bile acid sequestrant is relatively contraindicated when triglycerides are 200 mg/dL and is contraindicated when triglycerides are 500 mg/dL. [b]Dietary supplement niacin must not be used as a substitute for prescription niacin. (ACCF, American College of Cardiology Foundation; ACEI, angiotensin-converting enzyme inhibitor; AHA, American Heart Association; ARB, angiotensin receptor blocker; ASA, aspirin; ATP III, Adult Treatment Panel 3; BP, blood pressure; CCB, calcium channel blocker; CKD, chronic kidney disease; HDL-C, high-density lipoprotein cholesterol; JNC VII, Seventh Report of the Joint National Committee on Prevention, Detection, Evaluation, and Treatment of High Blood Pressure; LDL-C, low-density lipoprotein cholesterol; LV, left ventricular; MI, myocardial infarction; NHLBI, National Heart, Lung, and Blood Institute; NTG, nitroglycerin.)

Nitrates Nitroglycerin has a well-documented role in the alleviation of acute anginal attacks when used as rapidly absorbed and readily available preparations by the oral and IV routes (see Table 6-12 and Fig. 6-3).[105] SL, buccal, or spray products are the products of choice for this indication. Prevention of symptoms may be accomplished by the prophylactic use of oral or transdermal products; however, recent concern has been expressed over the long-term efficacy of many of these preparations and the development of tolerance.[106–108]

Nitrates have multiple potential mechanisms of action, and for a given patient it is not always clear which of these is most

TABLE 6-12 Nitrate Products

Product	Onset (minutes)	Duration	Initial Dose
Nitroglycerin			
IV	1–2	3–5 minutes	5 mcg/min
Sublingual/lingual	1–3	30–60 minutes	0.3 mg
Oral	40	3–6 hours	2.5–9 mg three times a day
Ointment	20–60	2–8 hours	0.5–1 in
Patch	40–60	>8 hours	1 patch
Erythritol tetranitrate	5–30	4–6 hours	5–10 mg three times a day
Pentaerythritol tetranitrate	30	4–8 hours	10–20 mg three times a day
Isosorbide dinitrate			
Sublingual/chewable	2–5	1–2 hours	2.5–5 mg three times a day
Oral	20–40	4–6 hours	5–20 mg three times a day
Isosorbide mononitrate	30–60	6–8 hours	20 mg daily, twice a day[a]

[a]Product dependent.

important. In general, the major action appears to be indirectly mediated through a reduction of MVO_2 secondary to venodilation and arterial–arteriolar dilation, leading to a reduction in wall stress from reduced ventricular volume and pressure (see Table 6-11). Systemic venodilation also promotes increased flow to deep myocardial muscle by reducing the gradient between intraventricular pressure and coronary arteriolar (R2) pressure. Direct actions on the coronary circulation include dilation of large and small intramural coronary arteries, collateral dilation, coronary artery stenosis dilation, abolition of normal tone in narrowed vessels, and relief of spasm; these actions occur even if the endothelium is denuded or dysfunctional. It is likely that depending on the underlying pathophysiology, different mechanisms become operative. For example, in the presence of a 60% to 70% stenosis, venodilation with MVO_2 reduction is most important; however, with higher-grade lesions, direct effects on the coronary circulation and vessel tone are the predominant effects. Nitroglycerin and pentaerythritol tetranitrate (PETN) in low doses are bioactivated by mitochondrial aldehyde dehydrogenase (ALDH-2) to nitrite or denitrated metabolites that require further activation by cytochrome oxidase or acidic disproportionation in the inner membrane space finally yielding nitric oxide. Nitric oxide activates soluble guanylate cyclase to increase intracellular concentrations of cyclic GMP resulting in vasorelaxation.[108] In contrast, ISDN and ISMN are bioactivated via P450 enzymes to nitric oxide. At higher concentrations, nitroglycerin and PETN may also be bioactivated to nitric oxide via P450 enzymes. Increased cyclic GMP induces a sequence of protein phosphorylation associated with reduced intracellular calcium release from the sarcoplasmic reticulum or reduced permeability to extracellular calcium and, consequently, smooth muscle relaxation. Oxidative stress within the mitochondria causes inactivation of ALDH-2 leading to impaired bioactivation of nitroglycerin during prolonged treatment.[109] Thomas et al. performed a study in normal volunteers to evaluate the effect of ISMN 120 mg/day given for 7 days on endothelial function. They found that ISMN impaired endothelial function suggesting a role for oxygen free radicals and nitrate-induced abnormalities in endothelial-dependent vasomotor responses that were reversed with a vitamin C infusion of 24 mg/min given for 15 minutes.[106] Furthermore, ISDN has been shown to impair flow-mediated dilation and carotid intimal–medial thickness after 3 months of treatment.[110] These deleterious changes in endothelial function, intima–media thickness, and the occurrence of tolerance suggest that the role of nitrates in IHD may be changing.

Pharmacokinetic characteristics common to the organic nitrates used for angina include a large first-pass effect of hepatic metabolism, short to very short half-lives (except for ISMN), large volumes of distribution, high clearance rates, and large interindividual variations in plasma or blood concentrations. Pharmacodynamic–pharmacokinetic relationships for the entire class remain poorly defined, presumably due to methodologic difficulty in characterizing the parent drug and metabolite concentrations at or within vascular smooth muscle and secondary to counterregulatory or adaptive mechanisms from the drug's effects as well as the occurrence of tolerance. Nitroglycerin is extracted by a variety of tissues and metabolized locally; differential extraction and metabolite generation occur depending on the tissue site. There are also numerous technical problems limiting the generation of reliable pharmacokinetic parameter estimates including the following: assay sensitivity, arterial–venous extraction gradients and therefore extrahepatic metabolism, in vitro degradation, drug adsorption to polyvinyl chloride tubing and syringes, potentially saturable metabolism, accumulation of metabolites (some of which are active) with multiple doses, postural and exercise-induced changes in pharmacokinetics, a variety of variables associated with transdermal delivery including the delivery system (matrix, membrane-limited, ointment), vehicle used, the surface area and thickness of application, the site application, and other skin variables (temperature, moisture content).

Nitroglycerin concentrations are affected by the route of administration, with the highest concentrations usually obtained with IV administration, the lowest seen with lower oral doses. Peak concentrations with SL nitroglycerin appear within 2 to 4 minutes, with the oral route producing peaks at about 15 to 30 minutes and by the transdermal route at 1 to 2 hours. The half-life of nitroglycerin is 1 to 5 minutes regardless of route, hence the potential advantage of sustained-release and transdermal products. Transdermal nitroglycerin does produce sufficient concentrations for acute hemodynamic effects to occur and these concentrations are maintained for long intervals; however, the hemodynamic and antianginal effects are minimal after 1 week or less with chronic, continuous (24 hours/day) therapy.

ISDN is metabolized to isosorbide 2-mononitrate and 5-mononitrate (ISMN). ISMN is well absorbed and has a half-life of about 5 hours and may be given once or twice daily depending on the product chosen. Multiple, larger doses of ISDN lead to disproportionate increases in the area under the plasma time profile, suggesting that metabolic pathways are being saturated or that metabolite accumulation may influence the disposition of ISDN. Little pharmacokinetic information is available for other nitrate compounds.

Nitrate therapy may be used to terminate an acute anginal attack, to prevent effort or stress-induced attacks, or for long-term prophylaxis, usually in combination with β-blockers or calcium channel blockers. SL nitroglycerin 0.3 to 0.4 mg will relieve pain in about 75% of patients within 3 minutes, with another 15% becoming pain-free in 5 to 15 minutes. Pain persisting beyond about 20 to 30 minutes following the use of two or three nitroglycerin tablets is suggestive of ACS and the patient should be instructed to seek emergency aid. Patients should be instructed to keep nitroglycerin in the original, tightly closed glass container and to avoid mixing with other medication, because mixing may increase nitroglycerin adsorption and vaporization. Additional counseling should include the facts that nitroglycerin is not an analgesic but rather it partially corrects the underlying problem and that repeated use is not harmful or addicting. Patients should also be aware that enhanced venous pooling in the sitting or standing positions may improve the effect as well as the symptoms of postural hypotension, and that inadequate saliva may slow or prevent tablet disintegration and dissolution. An acceptable albeit expensive alternative is lingual spray, which may be more convenient and has a shelf life of 3 years compared with 6 months or so for some forms of nitroglycerin tablets.

Chewable, oral, and transdermal products are acceptable for the long-term prophylaxis of angina; however, considerable controversy surrounds their use and it appears that the development of tolerance or adaptive mechanisms limits the efficacy of all chronic nitrate therapies regardless of route. Dosing of the longer-acting preparations should be adjusted to provide a hemodynamic response, and as an example, this may require doses of oral ISDN ranging from 10 to 60 mg as often as every 3 to 4 hours owing to tolerance or first-pass metabolism, and similar large doses are required for other products. Nitroglycerin ointment has a duration of up to 6 hours, but it is difficult to apply in a cosmetically acceptable fashion over a consistent surface area, and response varies depending on the epidermal thickness, vascularity, and amount of hair. Percutaneous adsorption of nitroglycerin ointment may occur unintentionally if someone other than the patient applies the ointment, and limiting exposure through the use of gloves or some other means is advisable. Peripheral edema may also impair the response to nitroglycerin because venodilation cannot increase capacitance to a maximum and pooling may be reduced. Transdermal patch delivery systems were approved on the basis of sustained and equivalent plasma concentrations to other forms of therapy. Trials required by the Food and Drug Administration using transdermal patches as a continuous 24-hour delivery system revealed a lack of efficacy for improved exercise tolerance. Subsequently, large, randomized, double-blind, placebo-controlled trials of intermittent (10 to 12 hours on; 12 to 14 hours off) transdermal nitroglycerin therapy in chronic stable angina demonstrated modest but significant improvement in exercise time after 4 weeks for the highest doses at 8 to 12 hours after patch placement.[111] Subjective assessment methods for nitrate effects include reduction in the number of painful episodes and the amount of nitroglycerin consumed. Objective assessment includes the resolution of ECG changes at rest, during exercise, or with ambulatory ECG monitoring. Because nitrates work primarily through a reduction in MVO_2, the DP can be used to optimize the dose of SL and oral nitrate products. It is important to realize that reflex tachycardia may offset the beneficial reduction in SBP and calculation of the observed changes is necessary. The DP is best assessed in the sitting position and at intervals of 5 to 10 and 30 to 60 minutes following SL and oral therapy, respectively. Owing to the placebo effect, unpredictable and variable course of angina, numerous pharmacologic effects of nitroglycerin, diurnal variation in pain patterns, stringent investigative protocols, and interindividual sensitivity to nitroglycerin, assessment with transdermal and sustained-release products is difficult. ETT provides valuable information concerning efficacy and mechanism of action for nitrates, but its use is usually reserved for clinical investigation rather than for routine patient care. Most ETT studies have shown nitrates to delay the onset of ischemia (ST-segment changes or initial chest discomfort) at submaximal exercise, but the threshold for maximal exercise is unaltered, suggesting a reduction in oxygen demand rather than an improved oxygen supply. More sophisticated studies of myocardial function such as wall motion abnormalities and myocardial metabolism could be used to document efficacy; however, these studies are generally only for investigative purposes.

Adverse effects of nitrates are related most commonly to an extension of their pharmacologic effects and include postural hypotension with associated central nervous system symptoms, headaches and flushing secondary to vasodilation, and occasional nausea from smooth muscle relaxation. If hypotension is excessive, coronary and cerebral filling may be compromised leading to MI and stroke. While reflex tachycardia is most common, bradycardia with nitroglycerin has been reported. Other noncardiovascular adverse effects include rash with all products but particularly with transdermal nitroglycerin, the production of methemoglobinemia with high doses given for extended periods, and measurable concentrations of ethanol (intoxication has been reported) and propylene glycol (found in the diluent) with IV nitroglycerin.

Tolerance with nitrate therapy was first described in 1867 with the initial experience using amyl nitrate for angina and later widely recognized in munitions workers who underwent withdrawal reactions during periods of absence from exposure. Tolerance to nitrates is associated with a reduction in tissue cyclic GMP, which results from decreased production (guanylate cyclase) and increased breakdown via cyclic GMP-phosphodiesterase and increased superoxide levels. One proposed mechanism for the lack of cyclic GMP is lack of conversion of organic nitrates to nitric oxide as described previously.[105]

Most of the published information is from controlled trials examining nitrate tolerance that have been done with either ISDN or transdermal nitroglycerin, and these studies demonstrate the development of tolerance within as little as 24 hours of therapy. While the onset of tolerance is rapid, the offset may be just as rapid, and one alternative dosing strategy to circumvent or minimize tolerance is to provide a daily nitrate-free interval of 6 to 8 hours. Studies with a variety of nitrate preparations and dosing schedules demonstrate that this approach is useful and the nitrate-free interval should be a minimum of 8 hours and perhaps 12 hours for even better effects.[105] Another concern for intermittent transdermal nitrate therapy is the occurrence of rebound ischemia during the nitrate-free interval. Freedman et al. found more silent ischemia during the patch-free interval during a randomized, double-blind, placebo-controlled trial than during the placebo patch phase, although others have not noted this effect.[112] ISDN, for example, should not be used more often than three times per day if tolerance is to be avoided. Interestingly, hemodynamic tolerance does not always coincide with antianginal efficacy, but this is not well studied.

Nitrates may be combined with other drugs for anginal therapy including β-adrenergic blocking agents and calcium channel antagonists. These combinations are usually instituted for chronic prophylactic therapy based on complementary or offsetting mechanisms of action (Table 6-12). Combination therapy is generally used in patients with more frequent or symptoms not responding to β-blockers alone (nitrates plus β-blockers or calcium blockers), in patients intolerant of β-blockers or calcium channel blockers, and in patients having an element of vasospasm leading to decreased supply (nitrates plus calcium blockers).[113] Modulation of calcium entry into vascular smooth muscle and myocardium as well as a variety of other tissues is the principal action of the calcium antagonists. The cellular mechanism of these drugs is not completely understood and it differs among the available classes of the phenylalkylamines (verapamil-like), dihydropyridines (nifedipine-like), benzothiazepines (diltiazem-like), bepridil, and a recent class referred to as T-channel blockers. Receptor-operated channels stimulated by norepinephrine and other neurotransmitters, and potential-dependent channels activated by membrane depolarization, control the entry of calcium, and consequently the cytosolic concentration of calcium responsible for activation of actin–myosin complex leading to contraction of vascular smooth muscle and myocardium. In the myocardium, calcium entry triggers the release of intracellular stores of calcium to increase cytosolic calcium, whereas in smooth muscle calcium derived from the extracellular fluid may do this directly. Binding proteins within the cell, calmodulin and troponin, after binding with calcium, participate in phosphorylation reactions leading to contraction. Decreased calcium availability, through the actions of calcium antagonists, inhibits these reactions. Direct actions of the calcium antagonists include vasodilation of systemic arterioles and coronary arteries, leading to a reduction of arterial pressure and coronary vascular resistance as well as depression of the myocardial contractility and conduction velocity of the sinoatrial and atrioventricular nodes (see Chap. 8). Reflex β-adrenergic stimulation overcomes much of the negative inotropic effect, and depression of contractility becomes clinically apparent only in the presence of LV dysfunction and when other negative inotropic drugs are used concurrently. Verapamil and diltiazem cause less peripheral vasodilation than nifedipine, and, consequently, the risk of myocardial depression is greater with these two agents. Conduction through the AV node is predictably depressed with verapamil and diltiazem, and they must be used with caution in patients with preexisting conduction abnormalities or in the presence of other drugs with negative chronotropic properties. MVO_2 is reduced with all of the calcium channel antagonists because of reduced wall tension secondary to reduced arterial pressure and, to a minor extent, depressed contractility (Table 6-11). HR changes are dependent on the drug used and the state of the conduction system. Nifedipine generally increases HR or causes no change, whereas either no change or decreased HR is seen with verapamil and diltiazem because of the interaction of these direct and indirect effects. In contrast to the β-blockers, calcium channel antagonists have the potential to improve coronary blood flow through areas of fixed coronary obstruction and by inhibiting coronary artery vasomotion and vasospasm. Beneficial redistribution of blood flow from well-perfused myocardium to ischemic areas and from epicardium to endocardium may also contribute to improvement in ischemic symptoms. Overall, the benefit provided by calcium channel antagonists is related to reduced MVO_2 rather than improved oxygen supply based on lack of alteration in the rate pressure product at maximal exercise in most studies performed to date. However, as CAD progresses and vasospasm becomes superimposed on critical stenotic lesions, improved oxygen supply through coronary vasodilation may become more important.

Absorption of the calcium channel antagonists is characterized by excellent absorption and large, variable first-pass metabolism resulting in oral bioavailability ranging from about 20% to 50% or greater for diltiazem, nicardipine, nifedipine, verapamil, felodipine, and isradipine. Amlodipine has a range of bioavailability of ~60% to 80%. Saturation of this effect may occur with verapamil and diltiazem, resulting in greater amounts of drug being absorbed with chronic dosing. Nifedipine may have slow or fast absorption patterns, and the ingestion of food delays and impairs its absorption as well as potential enhanced absorption in elderly patients. This variability in absorption produces fluctuation in the hemodynamic response with nifedipine. SL nifedipine is frequently used to provide a more rapid response; however, the rationale for this application is suspect because little nifedipine is absorbed from the buccal mucosa and the swallowed drug is responsible for the observed plasma concentrations. Absorption of verapamil in sustained-release products may be influenced by food, and when used in the fasted state, dose dumping may occur, resulting in high peak concentrations with some products. The approved sustained-release products for nifedipine, verapamil, and diltiazem are approved primarily for the treatment of hypertension (see Chap. 3). The presence of severe liver disease (e.g., alcoholic liver disease with cirrhosis) has been shown to reduce the first-pass metabolism of verapamil, and this shunting of drug around the liver gives rise to higher plasma concentrations and lower dose requirements in these patients. Interestingly, this effect appears to be stereoselective for the more active isomer of verapamil. Verapamil may also reduce liver blood flow; however, evidence for this reduction is based primarily on animal experiments. Few data are available regarding the influence of liver disease on the kinetics of calcium blockers; however, these drugs undergo extensive hepatic metabolism with little unchanged drug being renally excreted, and liver disease can be expected to alter the pharmacokinetics. Nifedipine has no active metabolites, whereas norverapamil possesses 20% or less activity of the parent compound. Desacetyldiltiazem has not been studied in humans, but canine studies suggest its potency ranges from 100% to 40% of the parent compound for various cardiovascular effects; the clinical importance of these observations remains to be determined. With chronic dosing of verapamil and diltiazem, apparent saturation of metabolism occurs, producing higher plasma concentrations of each drug than those seen with single-dose administration. Consequently, the elimination half-life for verapamil is prolonged, and less frequent dosing intervals may be used in some patients. The elimination half-life for diltiazem is also somewhat prolonged and the half-life of desacetyldiltiazem is longer than that of the parent drug, but it is not clear if less frequent dosing may be used. Bepridil also undergoes hepatic elimination and an active metabolite, 4-hydroxyphenyl bepridil, is produced; the parent compound has a long half-life of 30 to 40 hours. Nifedipine does not accumulate with chronic dosing; however, it is eliminated via oxidative pathways that may be polymorphic, and slow and fast metabolizers have been described for nifedipine. Most of the calcium channel blockers are eliminated via CYP3A4 and other CYP isoenzymes and many inhibit CYP3A4 activity as well. Renal insufficiency has little or no effect on the pharmacokinetics of these three drugs. Although disease alterations in kinetics have been described, the most important quantitative alteration is the influence of liver disease on bioavailability and elimination that reduce the clearance of verapamil and diltiazem, and dosing in this population should be done with caution. Altered protein binding due to renal disease, decreased protein concentration, or increased α_1-acid glycoprotein has been noted, but the clinical import of these changes is unknown.

Good candidates for calcium channel blockers in angina include patients with contraindications or intolerance of β-blockers, coexisting conduction system disease (except for verapamil and diltiazem), patients with Prinzmetal's angina (vasospastic or variable threshold angina), the presence of peripheral vascular disease, severe ventricular dysfunction (amlodipine is probably calcium channel blocker of choice and others need to be used with caution if the ejection fraction is <40% [<0.40]), and concurrent hypertension.

Ranolazine is a new drug for angina that has a unique mechanism of action unlike any other drugs used to alter the relationship between oxygen supply and demand. It reduces calcium overload in the ischemic myocyte through inhibition of the late sodium current (I_{Na}). Myocardial ischemia produces a cascade of complex ionic exchanges that can result in intracellular acidosis, excess cytosolic Ca^{2+}, myocardial cellular dysfunction, and, if sustained, cell injury and death. Activation of the ATP-dependent K^+ current during ischemia results in a strong efflux of K^+ ions from myocytes. Sodium channels are activated on depolarization, leading to a rapid influx of sodium into the cells. The inactivation of I_{Na} has a fast component lasting a few milliseconds and a slowly inactivating component that can last hundreds of milliseconds.[114] Ranolazine is a relatively selective inhibitor for late I_{Na}. In isolated ventricular myocytes in which the late I_{Na} was pathologically augmented, ranolazine prevented or reversed the induced mechanical dysfunction, as well as ameliorated abnormalities of ventricular repolarization. Ranolazine does not affect HR, inotropic state, or hemodynamic state or increase coronary blood flow.

Ranolazine is extensively metabolized via CYP450 3A and potent inhibitors of 3A increase the plasma concentration by a factor of about three. Ketoconazole, diltiazem, and verapamil should not be coadministered with ranolazine. Absorption from the gut is quite variable and the apparent half-life is 7 hours. Steady state is reached 3 days of twice-daily dosing. Ranolazine is indicated for the treatment of chronic angina and because it prolongs the QT interval, it should be reserved for patients who have not achieved an adequate response with other antianginal agents. Contraindications include preexisting QT interval prolongation, hepatic impairment, concurrent QT interval prolonging drugs, and moderately potent to potent concurrent 3A inhibitors. QT prolongation occurs in a dose-dependent fashion with ranolazine with an average increase of 6 milliseconds, but 5% of the population has QTc prolongation of 15 milliseconds. Baseline and follow-up ECGs should be obtained to evaluate effects of the QT interval. In controlled trials, the most common adverse reactions are dizziness, headache, constipation, and nausea. Ranolazine should be started at 500 mg twice daily and increased to 1,000 mg twice daily as needed based on symptoms.[115]

Based on randomized, placebo-controlled trials, the improvement in exercise time is a modest increase of 15 to about 45 seconds compared with placebo.[116–118] In a large ACS trial, ranolazine reduced recurrent ischemia but did not improve the primary efficacy end point of the composite of cardiovascular death, MI, or recurrent ischemia.[119] Ranolazine may have antiarrhythmic effects as assessed by continuous ECG monitoring of patients in the first week after admission for acute coronary syndrome.[120] In a trial of non–ST-elevation acute coronary syndrome, ranolazine, compared with placebo, was not associated with increased risk for sudden cardiac death in patients with prolonged QTc.[121] It may also be cost-effective in patients not controlled well on otherwise optimal medical therapy.[122]

Coronary Artery Spasm and Variant Angina Pectoris (Prinzmetal's Angina)

Prinzmetal, in his original description of variant angina pectoris, noted the waxing and waning course of this syndrome associated with ST-segment elevation and most commonly resolves without progression to MI. Patients who develop variant angina are usually younger and have fewer coronary risk factors but more commonly smoke than patients with chronic stable angina. Hyperventilation, exercise, and exposure to cold may precipitate variant angina attacks or there may be no apparent precipitating cause. The onset of chest discomfort is usually in the early morning hours. The exact cause of variant angina is not well understood, but may be an imbalance between endothelium-produced vasodilator factors (prostacyclin, nitric oxide) and vasoconstrictor factors (e.g., endothelin, angiotensin II) as well as an imbalance of autonomic control characterized by parasympathetic dominance or inflammation may also play a role.[123,124] More recently there have been a number of potential common adrenoreceptor polymorphisms that may predispose patients to developing vasospasm.[118,119,125] Another possible explanation is a recently discovered genetic mutation. The eNOS T-786C mutation appears to be a reversible etiology of Prinzmetal's variant angina in white Americans whose angina might be ameliorated by L-arginine.[126]

The diagnosis of variant angina is based on ST-segment elevation during transient chest discomfort (usually at rest) that resolves when the chest discomfort diminishes in patients who have normal or nonobstructive coronary lesions. In the absence of ST-segment elevation, provocative test using ergonovine, acetylcholine, or methacholine may be used to precipitate coronary artery spasm, ST-segment elevation, and typical symptoms. Nitrates and calcium antagonists should be withdrawn prior to provocative testing. Provocative testing should not be used in patients with high-grade lesions. Hyperventilation may also be used to provoke spasm and patients who have a positive hyperventilation test are more likely to have higher frequency of attacks, multivessel disease, and a high degree of AV block or ventricular tachycardia.

Optimization of therapy includes dose titration using sufficiently high doses to obtain clinical efficacy without unacceptable adverse effects in individual patients. All patients should be treated for acute attacks and maintained on prophylactic treatment for 6 to 12 months following the initial episode. The occurrence of serious arrhythmias during attacks is associated with a greater risk of sudden death, and these patients should be treated more aggressively and for prolonged periods. For patients without arrhythmias who become asymptomatic and remain so for several months after treatment has been instituted, withdrawal of therapy may be safe after first ascertaining that disease activity is quiescent. Aggravating factors such as alcohol or cocaine use or cigarette smoking should be eliminated when instituting treatment.

Nitrates have been the mainstay of therapy for the acute attacks of variant angina and coronary artery spasm for many years. Most patients respond rapidly to SL nitroglycerin or ISDN; however, IV and intracoronary nitroglycerin may be very useful for patients not responding to SL preparations. In particular, vasospasm provoked by ergonovine may require intracoronary nitroglycerin. Although studies with nitrates generally show them to be efficacious, high doses are often required and it is unclear if they reduce mortality. Because calcium antagonists may be more effective, have few serious adverse effects in effective doses, and can be given less frequently than nitrates, some consider them the agents of choice for variant angina.

Nifedipine, verapamil, and diltiazem are all equally effective as single agents for the initial management of variant angina and coronary artery spasm. Dose titration is important to maximize the response with calcium antagonists. Comparative trials are few in number and do not reveal significant differences among these three drugs for variant angina. Patients unresponsive to calcium antagonists alone may have nitrates added. Combination therapy with nifedipine–diltiazem or nifedipine–verapamil has been reported useful for patients unresponsive to single-drug regimens. This is probably rational because, at the cellular level, the drugs have different receptors, but the combination of verapamil–diltiazem should be used cautiously owing to their potential additive effects on contractility and conduction.

β-Adrenergic blockade has little or no role in the management of variant angina according to most authorities.[127] Although not all studies report increased painful episodes of variant angina with the addition of β-blockers, they may induce coronary vasoconstriction and prolong ischemia, as documented by continuous ECG monitoring. Other approaches to therapy attempting to modify sympathetic/parasympathetic tone include α-antagonists, anticholinergics, plexectomy, surgical interruption of the sympathetic innervation of the heart, thromboxane receptor antagonism, prostacyclin, lipoxygenase inhibition, and ticlopidine, but these drugs or procedures do not occupy a major place in therapy at the present time. One interesting case report found that the likely cause of MI was coronary artery spasm in a woman with migraine headaches because of the possible increased serotonergic activity secondary to concomitant use of zolmitriptan and citalopram.[128]

Silent Ischemia

The objective in the treatment of silent myocardial ischemia is to reduce the total number of ischemic episodes, both symptomatic and asymptomatic, regardless of the direction of ST-segment shift.[17] The incidence of silent ischemia in the general, asymptomatic population is not known.[129–132] Significant day-to-day variability in the number of episodes, the duration of ischemia, and the amount of ST-segment deviation complicate both the understanding of this process and the utility of various therapeutic interventions. Silent ischemia in patients with known CAD is common (~80% of all ischemic episodes) and associated with the extent of disease as well as a high risk for MI and sudden death when compared with symptomatic episodes of ischemia. Although the underlying mechanisms for silent ischemia are continuing to be defined, increased physical activity, activation of the sympathetic nervous system, increased cortisol secretion, increased coronary artery tone, and enhanced platelet aggregation due to endothelia dysfunction leading to intermittent coronary obstruction may be additive in lowering the threshold for ischemia. Platelet aggregability is increased in the morning hours (7 to 11 AM), corresponding to circadian rhythms noted for the peak frequency of ischemia, acute MI, and sudden death. Silent ischemia is associated with ST-segment elevation or depression and frequently occurs without antecedent changes in HR or blood pressure, suggesting that this form of ischemia is a result of primary reduction in oxygen supply. Silent ischemia is classified into Class I, patients who do not experience angina at any time, and Class II, patients who have both asymptomatic and symptomatic ischemia. Patients with silent ischemia have a defective warning system for angina pain that may encourage excessive myocardial demand. Regardless of the exact mechanism, there is increasing concern that painless ischemia carries considerable risk for myocardial perfusion defects, detrimental hemodynamic changes, arrhythmogenesis, and sudden death.[129] Silent ischemia is associated with reduced survival and increased need for PTCA and CABG as well as increased risk of AMI.[133] Because it is apparently very common in some settings, major emphasis should be placed on its management. A consensus has not been reached for the most appropriate method of detecting and quantifying the magnitude of silent ischemia; however, ambulatory electrocardiogram monitoring is felt by many to be the most useful tool at the present time.

The initial step in management is to modify the major risk factors for IHD, hypertension, hypercholesterolemia, and smoking, and data from the Multiple Risk Factor Intervention Trial (MRFIT) show these interventions to be useful in patients with silent ischemia. In a subset of the study population who had abnormal baseline exercise ECG responses, the special intervention group had a 57% reduction in CHD death (22.2/1,000 vs. 51.8/1,000) and a reduction in sudden death resulting from cessation of smoking and lowering of blood pressure and cholesterol when compared with the usual-care group.

ACIP, a randomized trial of medical therapy versus revascularization (PTCA or CABG), at the 2-year follow-up demonstrates that total mortality was 6.6% in the angina-guided strategy (i.e., therapy based on symptoms), 4.4% in the ischemia-guided strategy (based on ECG changes), and 1.1% in the revascularization strategy ($P < 0.02$). The rate of death or MI was 12.1% in the angina-guided strategy, 8.8% in the ischemia-guided strategy, and 4.7% in the revascularization strategy ($P < 0.04$).[133] The rate of death, MI, or recurrent cardiac hospitalization was 41.8% in the angina-guided strategy, 38.5% in the ischemia-guided strategy, and 23.1% in the revascularization strategy ($P < 0.001$). Post-MI patients and those with a high level of sympathetic nervous system activity are perhaps the best candidates for β-blocker therapy.

Calcium channel antagonists alone and in combination have been shown to be effective in reducing symptomatic and asymptomatic ischemia; however, they do not interrupt the diurnal surge in ischemia observed on ambulatory monitoring and, in general, they are somewhat less effective than β-blockers for silent ischemia.[130,131] Nifedipine in particular seems to provide less protection and provides wide fluctuations in response with approximate reductions in the number of episodes ranging from 0% to 93% and in duration from 23% to 65% unless combined with β-blockers. Fewer studies are available with other calcium blockers and comparative trials are uncommon. Earlier studies have shown that combination therapy with calcium and β-blockers provides a better response than calcium blockers and nitrates or monotherapy.[132,133]

A randomized, unblinded, controlled trial (Swiss Interventional Study on Silent Ischemia Type II [SWISSI II]) of PCI in patients with silent ischemia after AMI found that PCI compared with antiischemic drug therapy reduced the long-term risk of major cardiac events with better preservation of ventricular function than with medical therapy.[134,135]

PHARMACOECONOMIC CONSIDERATIONS

Pharmacoeconomic studies have been performed primarily in patients with acute coronary syndromes and only with low-molecular-weight heparins, glycoprotein IIb/IIIa receptor antagonists, and statins.[136] Most of the studies on LMWHs have been cost-minimization analyses and have focused on enoxaparin sodium, because this is the only LMWH proven to be superior to UFH. Several analyses show that, compared with UFH plus aspirin, enoxaparin sodium provides cost savings during both hospitalization (30 days) and 1-year follow-up. These cost savings are mainly attributable to fewer cardiac interventions, shorter hospital stays, and lower administrative costs. Indeed, the clinical and economic advantages of enoxaparin sodium have led to its recommendation in recent guidelines as the antithrombotic agent of choice for CAD. Most of the economic analyses of GP IIb/IIIa inhibitors have been cost-effectiveness analyses.[137] Such analyses indicate that the high acquisition costs of these drugs may be at least partially offset by reductions in other costs if a noninvasive approach to risk stratification is used. Furthermore, use of GP IIb/IIIa inhibitors appears to give favorable cost-effectiveness ratios compared with other accepted therapies, such as fibrin-specific thrombolytic therapy, in the cardiovascular field, particularly in high-risk patients and those undergoing percutaneous coronary intervention. However, more comprehensive economic data on the GP IIb/IIIa inhibitors are needed. Bivalirudin combined with provisional glycoprotein IIb/IIIa inhibitors appears to be an acceptable alternative to the standard of care and is superior to UFH alone in PCI and is considered to be cost-effective.[138]

Atorvastatin when used in ACS has been shown to reduce events and this offsets the upfront acquisition costs.[139] The total expected cost was (British) £784.05 per patient in the placebo cohort and £851.59 per patient in the atorvastatin cohort, resulting in an incremental cost of £67.54 per patient in the atorvastatin group. The cost per event avoided was £1,762.04. One third of the cost of atorvastatin treatment was offset within 16 weeks by the cost savings resulting from the reduction in the number of events in the atorvastatin cohort compared with the placebo cohort. Other analyses of statins have found this class to be cost-effective especially in patients at higher risk.[139]

Aspirin and clopidogrel have been evaluated for secondary prevention of CHD and while aspirin is very cost-effective, clopidogrel is only cost-effective for patients who cannot take aspirin.

Clinical **Controversy. . .**

Once patients with angina develop symptoms sufficient for pharmacologic therapy on a daily basis, the initial prophylactic therapy recommended is a β-blocker. There is a paucity of comparative, long-term clinical trials of β-blockade versus calcium channel blockers to determine which is superior for survival benefit. β-Blockers are recommended first-line therapy because of their efficacy in post-MI patients and favorable adverse effect profile.

Recent developments in the understanding of bioactivation of organic nitrates have given rise to concern over endothelial dysfunction induced by nitrates when administered long term. Not all nitrate products are activated via the same mechanisms and this may impact how effective individual drugs are in long-term treatment.

In stable CAD, medical management has been reported for outcomes similar to revascularization and these findings may have a significant impact on how healthcare resources are utilized in the future.

EVALUATION OF THERAPEUTIC OUTCOMES

Improved symptoms of angina, improved cardiac performance, and improvement in risk factors may all be used to assess the outcome of treatment of IHD and angina. Symptomatic improvement in

TABLE 6-13 American College of Cardiology, American Heart Association, and Physician Consortium for Performance Improvement Chronic Stable Coronary Artery Disease Core Physician Performance Measurement Set[a]

	Clinical Recommendations
Blood pressure measurement	A blood pressure ready is recommended at every visit. Recommended blood pressure management targets are ≤130 mm Hg systolic (*Class I Recommendation, Level A Evidence*) and ≤85 mm Hg diastolic in patient with CAD coexisting condition (e.g., diabetes, heart failure, or renal failure) and <140/90 mm Hg in patient with CAD and no coexisting condition
Lipid profile	A lipid profile is recommended and should include total cholesterol, high-density lipoprotein cholesterol (HDL-C), low-density lipoprotein cholesterol (LDL-C), and triglycerides (*Class I Recommendation, Level C Evidence*)
Symptom and activity assessment	Regular assessment of patients' anginal symptoms and levels of activity is recommended (serves as a basis for treatment modification)
Smoking cessation	Smoking status should be determined and smoking cessation counseling and interventions are recommended (*Class I Recommendation, Level B Evidence*)
Antiplatelet therapy[d] *Denominator exclusion* Documentation of medical reason(s)[b] for not prescribing antiplatelet therapy; documentation of patient reason(s)[c] for not prescribing antiplatelet therapy	Routine use of aspirin is recommended in the absence of contraindications. If contraindications exist, other antiplatelet therapies may be substituted (*Class I Recommendation, Level A Evidence*)
Drug therapy for lowering LDL-cholesterol *Denominator exclusion* Documentation that a statin was not indicated[e]; documentation of medical reason(s)[b] for not prescribing a statin; documentation of patient reason(s)[c] for not prescribing statin	The LDL-C treatment goal is <100 mg/dL (<2.59 mmol/L). Persons with established coronary heart disease (CHD) who have a baseline LDL-C ≥130 mg/dL (≥3.36 mmol/L) should be started on a cholesterol-lowering drug simultaneously with therapeutic lifestyle changes and control of nonlipid risk factors (*Class I Recommendation, Level A Evidence*)
β-Blocker therapy—prior myocardial infarction (MI) *Denominator inclusion* Prior MI *Denominator exclusion* Documentation that a β-blocker was not indicated; documentation of medical reason(s)[b] for not prescribing a β-blocker; documentation of patient reason(s)[c] for not prescribing a β-blocker	β-Blocker therapy is recommended for all patients with prior MI in the absence of contraindications (*Class I Recommendation, Level A Evidence*)
ACE inhibitor therapy *Denominator inclusion* Patient with CAD who also has diabetes and/or left ventricular systolic dysfunction (LVSD) (left ventricular ejection fraction [LVEF] <40% [<0.40] or moderately or severely depressed left ventricular systolic function) *Denominator exclusion* Documentation that ACE inhibitor was not indicated (e.g., patients on angiotensin receptor blockers [ARB]); documentation of medical reason(s)[b] for not prescribing ACE inhibitor; documentation of patient reason(s)[c] for not prescribing ACE inhibitor	ACE inhibitor use is recommended in all patients with CAD who also have diabetes and/or LVSD (*Class I Recommendation, Level A Evidence*) ACE inhibitor use is also recommended in patients with CAD or other vascular disease (*Class IIa Recommendation, Level B Evidence*)
Screening for diabetes[f,g] *Denominator exclusion* Patients with documented diabetes	Screening for diabetes is recommended in patients who are considered high risk (e.g., CAD) (*Class I Recommendation, Level A Evidence*)

ACE, angiotensin-converting enzyme; CAD, coronary artery disease.

[a]Refers to all patients diagnosed with CAD.
[b]Medical reasons for not prescribing *antiplatelet therapy* (aspirin, clopidogrel, or combination of aspirin and dipyridamole): active bleeding in the previous 6 months with required hospitalization and/or transfusion(s), patient on other antiplatelet therapy, etc. Medical reasons for not prescribing a *statin*: clinical judgment, documented LDL-C <130 mg/dL (<3.36 mmol/L), etc. Medical reasons for not prescribing a *β-blocker*: bradycardia (defined as heart rate <50 beats/min without β-blocker therapy), history of Class IV (congestive) heart failure, history of second- or third-degree atrioventricular block without permanent pacemaker, etc. Medical reasons for not prescribing *ACE inhibitor (ACEI)*: allergy, angioedema caused by ACEI, anuric rental failure caused by ACEI, pregnancy, moderate or severe aortic stenosis, etc.
[c]Patient reasons for not prescribing antiplatelet therapy, statin, β-blocker, or ACEI: economic, social, and/or religious, etc.
[d]Antiplatelet therapy may include aspirin, clopidogrel, or combination of aspirin and dipyridamole.
[e]Not indicated for a stat refers to LDL-C <100 mg/dL (<2.59 mmol/L).
[f]Test measure.
[g]Screening for diabetes is usually done by fasting blood glucose or 2-hour glucose tolerance testing. Clinical recommendations indicate screening should be considered at 3-year intervals.

exercise capacity (longer duration) or fewer symptoms at the same level of exercise is subjective evidence that therapy is working. Once patients have been optimized on medical therapy, symptoms should improve over 2 to 4 weeks and remain stable until their disease progresses. There are several instruments (e.g., Seattle Angina Questionnaire, Specific Activity Scale [Table 6-1], Canadian Classification System [Table 6-2]) that could be used to improve the reproducibility of symptom assessment.[2] If the patient is doing well, then no other assessment may be necessary. Objective assessment is obtained through increase in exercise duration on ETT and the absence of ischemic changes on ECG or deleterious hemodynamic changes. Echocardiography and cardiac imaging may also be used; however, due to their expense, they are only used if a patient is not doing well to determine if revascularization or other measures should be undertaken. Coronary angiography may be used to assess the extent of stenosis or restenosis after angioplasty or CABG. (11) The performance measurement set recommended by the ACC/AHA is provided in Table 6-13.

ABBREVIATIONS

ACEI	angiotensin-converting enzyme inhibitor
ACIP	Asymptomatic Cardiac Ischemia Pilot
ACT	activated clotting time
AHA	American Heart Association
ALDH-2	aldehyde dehydrogenase
AMP	adenosine monophosphate
ATP	adenosine triphosphate
AV	arteriovenous
AWESOME	Angina with Extremely Serious Operative Mortality
BARI	Bypass Angioplasty Revascularization
BMI	body mass index
BMS	bare-metal stent
CABG	coronary artery bypass grafting
CAC	coronary artery calcium
CAD	coronary artery disease
CASS	Coronary Artery Surgery Study
CHD	coronary heart disease
CI	confidence interval
COURAGE	Clinical Outcomes Utilizing Revascularization and Aggressive Drug Evaluation
CVD	cardiovascular disease
CYP	cytochrome
DES	drug-eluting stent
DP	double product
ECSS	European Cooperative Surgery Study
EDRF	endothelium-derived relaxing factor
FFR	fractional flow reserve
β-FGF	fibroblast growth factor
GDMT	guideline-directed medical therapy
HR	heart rate
IHD	ischemic heart disease
ISAR	Intracoronary Stenting and Antithrombotic Regimen
ISDN	isosorbide dinitrate
ISMN	isosorbide mononitrate
LDL	low-density lipoprotein
LV	left ventricular
MASS II	Medicine, Angioplasty, or Surgery Study
MI	myocardial infarction
MRFIT	Multiple Risk Factor Intervention Trial
MVO_2	myocardial oxygen demand
NYHA	New York Heart Association
PCI	percutaneous intervention
PETN	pentaerythritol tetranitrate
PTCA	percutaneous transluminal coronary angioplasty
RV	right ventricle
SBP	systolic blood pressure
SL	sublingual
SWISSI II	Swiss Interventional Study on Silent Ischemia Type II
SYNTAX	Synergy between Percutaneous Coronary Intervention with TAXUS and Cardiac Surgery
TTI	tension–time index
VA	Veterans Administration
VEGF	vascular endothelial growth factor
VLDL	very-low-density lipoprotein

REFERENCES

1. Fox K, Garcia MA, Ardissino D, et al. Guidelines on the management of stable angina pectoris: Executive summary: The Task Force on the Management of Stable Angina Pectoris of the European Society of Cardiology. Eur Heart J 2006;27:1341–1381.
2. Fihn SD, Gardin JM, Abrams J, et al. 2012 ACCF/AHA/ACP/AATS/PCNA/SCAI/STS guideline for the diagnosis and management of patients with stable ischemic heart disease: A report of the American College of Cardiology Foundation/American Heart Association Task Force on Practice Guidelines, and the American College of Physicians, American Association for Thoracic Surgery, Preventive Cardiovascular Nurses Association, Society for Cardiovascular Angiography and Interventions, and Society of Thoracic Surgeons. J Am Coll Cardiol 2012;60:e44–e164.
3. Go AS, Mozaffarian D, Roger VL, et al. Heart disease and stroke statistics—2013 update: A report from the American Heart Association. Circulation 2013;127:e6–e245.
4. Sytkowski PA, D'Agostino RB, Belanger A, Kannel WB. Sex and time trends in cardiovascular disease incidence and mortality: The Framingham Heart Study, 1950-1989. Am J Epidemiol 1996;143:338–350.
5. Lloyd-Jones D, Adams RJ, Brown TM, et al. Heart disease and stroke statistics—2010 update: A report from the American Heart Association. Circulation 2010;121:e46–e215.
6. Menotti A, Keys A, Blackburn H, et al. Comparison of multivariate predictive power of major risk factors for coronary heart diseases in different countries: Results from eight nations of the Seven Countries Study, 25-year follow-up. J Cardiovasc Risk 1996;3:69–75.
7. Keys A. Mediterranean diet and public health: Personal reflections. Am J Clin Nutr 1995;61:1321S–1323S.
8. Goldman L, Hashimoto B, Cook EF, Loscalzo A. Comparative reproducibility and validity of systems for assessing cardiovascular functional class: Advantages of a new specific activity scale. Circulation 1981;64:1227–1234.
9. Emond M, Mock MB, Davis KB, et al. Long-term survival of medically treated patients in the Coronary Artery Surgery Study (CASS) Registry. Circulation 1994;90:2645–2657.
10. Caracciolo EA, Davis KB, Sopko G, et al. Comparison of surgical and medical group survival in patients with left main coronary artery disease. Long-term CASS experience. Circulation 1995;91:2325–2334.
11. Park SJ, Park DW. Percutaneous coronary intervention with stent implantation versus coronary artery bypass surgery for treatment of left main coronary artery disease: Is it time to change guidelines? Circ Cardiovasc Interv 2009;2:59–68.
12. Fihn SD, Gardin JM, Abrams J, et al. 2012 ACCF/AHA/ACP/AATS/PCNA/SCAI/STS guideline for the diagnosis and management of patients with stable ischemic heart disease: Executive summary: A report of the American College of Cardiology Foundation/American Heart Association Task Force on Practice Guidelines, and the American College of Physicians, American Association for Thoracic Surgery, Preventive Cardiovascular Nurses Association, Society for Cardiovascular Angiography and Interventions, and Society of Thoracic Surgeons. Circulation 2012;126:3097–3137.
13. Epstein SE, Cannon RO 3rd, Talbot TL. Hemodynamic principles in the control of coronary blood flow. Am J Cardiol 1985;56:4E–10E.
14. von Mering GO, Arant CB, Wessel TR, et al. Abnormal coronary vasomotion as a prognostic indicator of cardiovascular events in women: Results from the National Heart, Lung, and Blood Institute-Sponsored Women's Ischemia Syndrome Evaluation (WISE). Circulation 2004;109:722–725.
15. Ferrari R, Fox K. Insight into the mode of action of ACE inhibition in coronary artery disease: The ultimate 'EUROPA' story. Drugs 2009;69:265–277.

16. Anderson JL, Adams CD, Antman EM, et al. ACC/AHA 2007 guidelines for the management of patients with unstable angina/non ST-elevation myocardial infarction: A report of the American College of Cardiology/American Heart Association Task Force on Practice Guidelines (Writing Committee to Revise the 2002 Guidelines for the Management of Patients with Unstable Angina/Non ST-Elevation Myocardial Infarction): Developed in collaboration with the American College of Emergency Physicians, the Society for Cardiovascular Angiography and Interventions, and the Society of Thoracic Surgeons: Endorsed by the American Association of Cardiovascular and Pulmonary Rehabilitation and the Society for Academic Emergency Medicine. Circulation 2007;116:e148–e304.
17. Cohn PF. A new look at benefits of drug therapy in silent myocardial ischaemia. Eur Heart J 2007;28:2053–2054.
18. Caracciolo EA, Chaitman BR, Forman SA, et al. Diabetics with coronary disease have a prevalence of asymptomatic ischemia during exercise treadmill testing and ambulatory ischemia monitoring similar to that of nondiabetic patients. An ACIP database study. ACIP Investigators. Asymptomatic Cardiac Ischemia Pilot Investigators. Circulation 1996;93:2097–2105.
19. Fraker TD Jr, Fihn SD, Gibbons RJ, et al. 2007 chronic angina focused update of the ACC/AHA 2002 guidelines for the management of patients with chronic stable angina: A report of the American College of Cardiology/American Heart Association Task Force on Practice Guidelines Writing Group to develop the focused update of the 2002 guidelines for the management of patients with chronic stable angina. J Am Coll Cardiol 2007;50:2264–2274.
20. Gibbons RJ, Abrams J, Chatterjee K, et al. ACC/AHA 2002 guideline update for the management of patients with chronic stable angina—Summary article: A report of the American College of Cardiology/American Heart Association Task Force on Practice Guidelines (Committee on the Management of Patients with Chronic Stable Angina). J Am Coll Cardiol 2003;41:159–168.
21. Panel E. Summary of the second report of the National Cholesterol Education Program (NCEP) Expert Panel on Detection, Evaluation, and Treatment of High Blood Cholesterol in Adults (Adult Treatment Panel II). JAMA 1993;269:3015–3023.
22. Glynn RJ, Koenig W, Nordestgaard BG, Shepherd J, Ridker PM. Rosuvastatin for primary prevention in older persons with elevated C-reactive protein and low to average low-density lipoprotein cholesterol levels: Exploratory analysis of a randomized trial. Ann Intern Med 2010;152:488–496, W174.
23. Crowe E, Lovibond K, Gray H, Henderson R, Krause T, Camm J. Early management of unstable angina and non-ST segment elevation myocardial infarction: Summary of NICE guidance. BMJ 2010;340:c1134.
24. Panel E. Executive summary of the third report of the National Cholesterol Education Program (NCEP) Expert Panel on Detection, Evaluation, and Treatment of High Blood Cholesterol in Adults (Adult Treatment Panel III). JAMA 2001;285:2486–2497.
25. Grundy SM, Cleeman JI, Merz CN, et al. Implications of recent clinical trials for the National Cholesterol Education Program Adult Treatment Panel III guidelines. J Am Coll Cardiol 2004;44:720–732.
26. Group BDS, Frye RL, August P, et al. A randomized trial of therapies for type 2 diabetes and coronary artery disease. N Engl J Med 2009;360:2503–2515.
27. Wald NJ, Watt HC. Prospective study of effect of switching from cigarettes to pipes or cigars on mortality from three smoking related diseases. BMJ 1997;314:1860–1863.
28. Rigotti NA, Pipe AL, Benowitz NL, Arteaga C, Garza D, Tonstad S. Efficacy and safety of varenicline for smoking cessation in patients with cardiovascular disease: A randomized trial. Circulation 2010;121:221–229.
29. Swan GE, McClure JB, Jack LM, et al. Behavioral counseling and varenicline treatment for smoking cessation. Am J Prev Med 2010;38:482–490.
30. Keating GM, Lyseng-Williamson KA. Varenicline: A pharmacoeconomic review of its use as an aid to smoking cessation. Pharmacoeconomics 2010;28:231–254.
31. Russell LB, Carson JL, Taylor WC, Milan E, Dey A, Jagannathan R. Modeling all-cause mortality: Projections of the impact of smoking cessation based on the NHEFS. NHANES I Epidemiologic Follow-Up Study. Am J Public Health 1998;88:630–636.
32. Bartecchi C, Alsever RN, Nevin-Woods C, et al. Reduction in the incidence of acute myocardial infarction associated with a citywide smoking ordinance. Circulation 2006;114:1490–1496.
33. Rosendorff C. Hypertension and coronary artery disease: A summary of the American Heart Association scientific statement. J Clin Hypertens (Greenwich) 2007;9:790–795.
34. Bjelakovic G, Nikolova D, Gluud LL, Simonetti RG, Gluud C. Antioxidant supplements for prevention of mortality in healthy participants and patients with various diseases. Cochrane Database Syst Rev 2012;3:CD007176.
35. Haskell WL, Lee IM, Pate RR, et al. Physical activity and public health: Updated recommendation for adults from the American College of Sports Medicine and the American Heart Association. Circulation 2007;116:1081–1093.
36. Williams MA, Haskell WL, Ades PA, et al. Resistance exercise in individuals with and without cardiovascular disease: 2007 update: A scientific statement from the American Heart Association Council on Clinical Cardiology and Council on Nutrition, Physical Activity, and Metabolism. Circulation 2007;116:572–584.
37. Fuchs FD, Chambless LE, Folsom AR, et al. Association between alcoholic beverage consumption and incidence of coronary heart disease in whites and blacks: The Atherosclerosis Risk in Communities Study. Am J Epidemiol 2004;160:466–474.
38. Britton A, Marmot MG, Shipley MJ. How does variability in alcohol consumption over time affect the relationship with mortality and coronary heart disease? Addiction 2010;105:639–645.
39. Romelsjo A, Allebeck P, Andreasson S, Leifman A. Alcohol, mortality and cardiovascular events in a 35 year follow-up of a nationwide representative cohort of 50,000 Swedish conscripts up to age 55. Alcohol Alcohol 2012;47:322–327.
40. Hulley S, Grady D, Bush T, et al. Randomized trial of estrogen plus progestin for secondary prevention of coronary heart disease in postmenopausal women. Heart and Estrogen/progestin Replacement Study (HERS) Research Group. JAMA 1998;280:605–613.
41. Rossouw JE, Cushman M, Greenland P, et al. Inflammatory, lipid, thrombotic, and genetic markers of coronary heart disease risk in the women's health initiative trials of hormone therapy. Arch Intern Med 2008;168:2245–2253.
42. Marjoribanks J, Farquhar C, Roberts H, Lethaby A. Long term hormone therapy for perimenopausal and postmenopausal women. Cochrane Database Syst Rev 2012;7:CD004143.

43. El-Sohemy A, Cornelis MC, Kabagambe EK, Campos H. Coffee, CYP1A2 genotype and risk of myocardial infarction. Genes Nutr 2007;2:155–156.
44. Celik T, Iyisoy A, Amasyali B. The effects of coffee intake on coronary heart disease: Ongoing controversy. Int J Cardiol 2010;144:118.
45. Group IS. Effect of nicorandil on coronary events in patients with stable angina: The Impact of Nicorandil in Angina (IONA) randomised trial. Lancet 2002;359:1269–1275.
46. Fox K, Ford I, Steg PG, Tendera M, Ferrari R, BEAUTIFUL Investigators. Ivabradine for patients with stable coronary artery disease and left-ventricular systolic dysfunction (BEAUTIFUL): A randomised, double-blind, placebo-controlled trial. Lancet 2008;372:807–816.
47. Kantor PF, Lucien A, Kozak R, Lopaschuk GD. The antianginal drug trimetazidine shifts cardiac energy metabolism from fatty acid oxidation to glucose oxidation by inhibiting mitochondrial long-chain 3-ketoacyl coenzyme A thiolase. Circ Res 2000;86:580–588.
48. Boden WE, O'Rourke RA, Teo KK, et al. Optimal medical therapy with or without PCI for stable coronary disease. N Engl J Med 2007;356:1503–1516.
49. Maron DJ, Boden WE, O'Rourke RA, et al. Intensive multifactorial intervention for stable coronary artery disease: Optimal medical therapy in the COURAGE (Clinical Outcomes Utilizing Revascularization and Aggressive Drug Evaluation) trial. J Am Coll Cardiol 2010;55:1348–1358.
50. Hueb W, Lopes NH, Gersh BJ, et al. Five-year follow-up of the Medicine, Angioplasty, or Surgery Study (MASS II): A randomized controlled clinical trial of 3 therapeutic strategies for multivessel coronary artery disease. Circulation 2007;115:1082–1089.
51. Gibbons RJ, Abrams J, Chatterjee K, et al. ACC/AHA 2002 guideline update for the management of patients with chronic stable angina—Summary article: A report of the American College of Cardiology/American Heart Association Task Force on Practice Guidelines (Committee on the Management of Patients with Chronic Stable Angina). Circulation 2003;107:149–158.
52. Sipahi I, Tuzcu EM, Wolski KE, et al. Beta-blockers and progression of coronary atherosclerosis: Pooled analysis of 4 intravascular ultrasonography trials. Ann Intern Med 2007;147:10–18.
53. Kroon LA. Drug interactions with smoking. Am J Health Syst Pharm 2007;64:1917–1921.
54. Munzel T, Daiber A, Mulsch A. Explaining the phenomenon of nitrate tolerance. Circ Res 2005;97:618–628.
55. Daiber A, Munzel T. Characterization of the antioxidant properties of pentaerithrityl tetranitrate (PETN)-induction of the intrinsic antioxidative system heme oxygenase-1 (HO-1). Methods Mol Biol 2010;594:311–326.
56. Ambrosio G, Del Pinto M, Tritto I, et al. Chronic nitrate therapy is associated with different presentation and evolution of acute coronary syndromes: Insights from 52,693 patients in the Global Registry of Acute Coronary Events. Eur Heart J 2009;31:430–438.
57. Pehrsson SK, Ringqvist I, Ekdahl S, Karlson BW, Ulvenstam G, Persson S. Monotherapy with amlodipine or atenolol versus their combination in stable angina pectoris. Clin Cardiol 2000;23:763–770.
58. Verdecchia P, Reboldi G, Angeli F, et al. Angiotensin-converting enzyme inhibitors and calcium channel blockers for coronary heart disease and stroke prevention. Hypertension 2005;46:386–392.
59. Opie LH, Yusuf S, Kubler W. Current status of safety and efficacy of calcium channel blockers in cardiovascular diseases: A critical analysis based on 100 studies. Prog Cardiovasc Dis 2000;43:171–196.
60. Howes LG, Edwards CT. Calcium antagonists and cancer. Is there really a link? Drug Saf 1998;18:1–7.
61. Knight CJ, Fox KM. Amlodipine versus diltiazem as additional antianginal treatment to atenolol. Centralised European Studies in Angina Research (CESAR) Investigators. Am J Cardiol 1998;81:133–136.
62. Braunwald E, Antman EM, Beasley JW, et al. ACC/AHA guideline update for the management of patients with unstable angina and non-ST-segment elevation myocardial infarction—2002: Summary article: A report of the American College of Cardiology/American Heart Association Task Force on Practice Guidelines (Committee on the Management of Patients with Unstable Angina). Circulation 2002;106:1893–1900.
63. King SB 3rd, Smith SC Jr, Hirshfeld JW Jr, et al. 2007 focused update of the ACC/AHA/SCAI 2005 guideline update for percutaneous coronary intervention: A report of the American College of Cardiology/American Heart Association Task Force on Practice Guidelines: 2007 Writing Group to Review New Evidence and Update the ACC/AHA/SCAI 2005 Guideline Update for Percutaneous Coronary Intervention, Writing on Behalf of the 2005 Writing Committee. Circulation 2008;117:261–295.
64. Sobel BE. Coronary revascularization in patients with type 2 diabetes and results of the BARI 2D trial. Coron Artery Dis 2010;21:189–198.
65. BARI Investigators. The final 10-year follow-up results from the BARI randomized trial. J Am Coll Cardiol 2007;49:1600–1606.
66. Hannan EL, Racz MJ, Gold J, et al. Adherence of catheterization laboratory cardiologists to American College of Cardiology/American Heart Association guidelines for percutaneous coronary interventions and coronary artery bypass graft surgery: What happens in actual practice? Circulation 2010;121:267–275.
67. Simoons ML, Windecker S. Controversies in cardiovascular medicine: Chronic stable coronary artery disease: Drugs vs. revascularization. Eur Heart J 2010;31:530–541.
68. Ramanathan KB, Weiman DS, Sacks J, et al. Percutaneous intervention versus coronary bypass surgery for patients older than 70 years of age with high-risk unstable angina. Ann Thorac Surg 2005;80:1340–1346.
69. Smith SC Jr, Feldman TE, Hirshfeld JW Jr, et al. ACC/AHA/SCAI 2005 guideline update for percutaneous coronary intervention: A report of the American College of Cardiology/American Heart Association Task Force on Practice Guidelines (ACC/AHA/SCAI Writing Committee to Update 2001 Guidelines for Percutaneous Coronary Intervention). Circulation 2006;113:e166–e286.
70. Rathore S, Kinoshita Y, Terashima M, et al. A comparison of clinical presentations, angiographic patterns and outcomes of in-stent restenosis between bare metal stents and drug eluting stents. EuroIntervention 2010;5:841–846.
71. Lemesle G, Maluenda G, Collins SD, Waksman R. Drug-eluting stents: Issues of late stent thrombosis. Cardiol Clin 2010;28:97–105.
72. Onuma Y, Serruys PW, Kukreja N, et al. Randomized comparison of everolimus- and paclitaxel-eluting stents: Pooled analysis of the 2-year clinical follow-up from the SPIRIT II and III trials. Eur Heart J 2010;31:1071–1078.

73. Coons JC, Battistone S. 2007 guideline update for unstable angina/non-ST-segment elevation myocardial infarction: Focus on antiplatelet and anticoagulant therapies. Ann Pharmacother 2008;42:989–1001.
74. Vermeer NS, Bajorek BV. Utilization of evidence-based therapy for the secondary prevention of acute coronary syndromes in Australian practice. J Clin Pharm Ther 2008;33:591–601.
75. Tebbe U, Hochadel M, Bramlage P, et al. In-hospital outcomes after elective and non-elective percutaneous coronary interventions in hospitals with and without on-site cardiac surgery backup. Clin Res Cardiol 2009;98:701–707.
76. Chaitman BR, Hardison RM, Adler D, et al. The Bypass Angioplasty Revascularization Investigation 2 Diabetes randomized trial of different treatment strategies in type 2 diabetes mellitus with stable ischemic heart disease: Impact of treatment strategy on cardiac mortality and myocardial infarction. Circulation 2009;120:2529–2540.
77. Curzen NP. Is there evidence for prognostic benefit following PCI in stable patients? COURAGE and its implications: An interventionalist's view. Heart 2009;96:103–105.
78. Bottorff MB, Nutescu EA, Spinler S. Antiplatelet therapy in patients with unstable angina and non-ST-segment-elevation myocardial infarction: Findings from the CRUSADE national quality improvement initiative. Pharmacotherapy 2007;27:1145–1162.
79. Levine GN, Berger PB, Cohen DJ, et al. Newer pharmacotherapy in patients undergoing percutaneous coronary interventions: A guide for pharmacists and other health care professionals. Pharmacotherapy 2006;26:1537–1556.
80. Eagle KA, Guyton RA, Davidoff R, et al. ACC/AHA 2004 guideline update for coronary artery bypass graft surgery: A report of the American College of Cardiology/American Heart Association Task Force on Practice Guidelines (Committee to Update the 1999 Guidelines for Coronary Artery Bypass Graft Surgery). Circulation 2004;110:e340–e437.
81. King SB 3rd, Marshall JJ, Tummala PE. Revascularization for coronary artery disease: Stents versus bypass surgery. Annu Rev Med 2009;61:199–213.
82. Spinler SA. Managing acute coronary syndrome: Evidence-based approaches. Am J Health Syst Pharm 2007;64:S14–S24.
83. Toth PP. The potential role of prasugrel in secondary prevention of ischemic events in patients with acute coronary syndromes. Postgrad Med 2009;121:59–72.
84. Lange RA, Hillis LD. Second-generation drug-eluting coronary stents. N Engl J Med 2010;362:1728–1730.
85. Doostzadeh J, Clark LN, Bezenek S, Pierson W, Sood PR, Sudhir K. Recent progress in percutaneous coronary intervention: Evolution of the drug-eluting stents, focus on the XIENCE V drug-eluting stent. Coron Artery Dis 2010;21:46–56.
86. Bertrand ME, Rupprecht HJ, Urban P, Gershlick AH. Double-blind study of the safety of clopidogrel with and without a loading dose in combination with aspirin compared with ticlopidine in combination with aspirin after coronary stenting: The clopidogrel aspirin stent international cooperative study (CLASSICS). Circulation 2000;102:624–629.
87. Wiviott SD, Braunwald E, McCabe CH, et al. Prasugrel versus clopidogrel in patients with acute coronary syndromes. N Engl J Med 2007;357:2001–2015.
88. Mahoney EM, Wang K, Arnold SV, et al. Cost-effectiveness of prasugrel versus clopidogrel in patients with acute coronary syndromes and planned percutaneous coronary intervention: Results from the trial to assess improvement in therapeutic outcomes by optimizing platelet inhibition with Prasugrel-Thrombolysis in Myocardial Infarction TRITON-TIMI 38. Circulation 2010;121:71–79.
89. Schuhlen H, Kastrati A, Pache J, Dirschinger J, Schomig A. Sustained benefit over four years from an initial combined antiplatelet regimen after coronary stent placement in the ISAR trial. Intracoronary Stenting and Antithrombotic Regimen. Am J Cardiol 2001;87:397–400.
90. Takakuwa KM, Ou FS, Peterson ED, et al. The usage patterns of cardiac bedside markers employing point-of-care testing for troponin in non-ST-segment elevation acute coronary syndrome: Results from CRUSADE. Clin Cardiol 2009;32:498–505.
91. Topol EJ, Moliterno DJ, Herrmann HC, et al. Comparison of two platelet glycoprotein IIb/IIIa inhibitors, tirofiban and abciximab, for the prevention of ischemic events with percutaneous coronary revascularization. N Engl J Med 2001;344:1888–1894.
92. Spinler SA, Rees C. Review of prasugrel for the secondary prevention of atherothrombosis. J Manag Care Pharm 2009;15:383–395.
93. Stone GW, Ware JH, Bertrand ME, et al. Antithrombotic strategies in patients with acute coronary syndromes undergoing early invasive management: One-year results from the ACUITY trial. JAMA 2007;298:2497–2506.
94. Lincoff AM, Kleiman NS, Kereiakes DJ, et al. Long-term efficacy of bivalirudin and provisional glycoprotein IIb/IIIa blockade vs heparin and planned glycoprotein IIb/IIIa blockade during percutaneous coronary revascularization: REPLACE-2 randomized trial. JAMA 2004;292:696–703.
95. Canan T, Lee MS. Drug-eluting stent fracture: Incidence, contributing factors, and clinical implications. Catheter Cardiovasc Interv 2010;75:237–245.
96. Stone GW, Rizvi A, Newman W, et al. Everolimus-eluting versus paclitaxel-eluting stents in coronary artery disease. N Engl J Med 2010;362:1663–1674.
97. Mega JL, Close SL, Wiviott SD, et al. Cytochrome p-450 polymorphisms and response to clopidogrel. N Engl J Med 2009;360:354–362.
98. Ray WA, Murray KT, Griffin MR, et al. Outcomes with concurrent use of clopidogrel and proton-pump inhibitors: A cohort study. Ann Intern Med 2010;152:337–345.
99. Zairis MN, Tsiaousis GZ, Patsourakos NG, et al. The impact of treatment with omeprazole on the effectiveness of clopidogrel drug therapy during the first year after successful coronary stenting. Can J Cardiol 2010;26:e54–e57.
100. Juurlink DN, Gomes T, Ko DT, et al. A population-based study of the drug interaction between proton pump inhibitors and clopidogrel. CMAJ 2009;180:713–718.
101. Hall SL, Lorenc T. Secondary prevention of coronary artery disease. Am Fam Physician 2010;81:289–296.
102. Messerli FH, Bangalore S, Yao SS, Steinberg JS. Cardioprotection with beta-blockers: Myths, facts and Pascal's wager. J Intern Med 2009;266:232–241.
103. Feringa HH, van Waning VH, Bax JJ, et al. Cardioprotective medication is associated with improved survival in patients with peripheral arterial disease. J Am Coll Cardiol 2006;47:1182–1187.
104. Prince MJ, Bird AS, Blizard RA, Mann AH. Is the cognitive function of older patients affected by antihypertensive treatment? Results from 54 months of the Medical Research

Council's trial of hypertension in older adults. BMJ 1996;312:801–805.
105. Abrams J, Thadani U. Therapy of stable angina pectoris: The uncomplicated patient. Circulation 2005;112:e255–e259.
106. Thomas GR, DiFabio JM, Gori T, Parker JD. Once daily therapy with isosorbide-5-mononitrate causes endothelial dysfunction in humans: Evidence of a free-radical-mediated mechanism. J Am Coll Cardiol 2007;49:1289–1295.
107. Schuhmacher S, Wenzel P, Schulz E, et al. Pentaerythritol tetranitrate improves angiotensin II-induced vascular dysfunction via induction of heme oxygenase-1. Hypertension 2010;55:897–904.
108. Daiber A, Oelze M, Wenzel P, et al. Nitrate tolerance as a model of vascular dysfunction: Roles for mitochondrial aldehyde dehydrogenase and mitochondrial oxidative stress. Pharmacol Rep 2009;61:33–48.
109. Gori T, Daiber A, Di Stolfo G, et al. Nitroglycerine causes mitochondrial reactive oxygen species production: In vitro mechanistic insights. Can J Cardiol 2007;23:990–992.
110. Sekiya M, Sato M, Funada J, Ohtani T, Akutsu H, Watanabe K. Effects of the long-term administration of nicorandil on vascular endothelial function and the progression of arteriosclerosis. J Cardiovasc Pharmacol 2005;46:63–67.
111. Parker JO, Amies MH, Hawkinson RW, et al. Intermittent transdermal nitroglycerin therapy in angina pectoris. Clinically effective without tolerance or rebound. Minitran Efficacy Study Group. Circulation 1995;91:1368–1374.
112. Freedman SB, Daxini BV, Noyce D, Kelly DT. Intermittent transdermal nitrates do not improve ischemia in patients taking beta-blockers or calcium antagonists: Potential role of rebound ischemia during the nitrate-free period. J Am Coll Cardiol 1995;25:349–355.
113. Ajani AE, Yan BP. The mystery of coronary artery spasm. Heart Lung Circ 2007;16:10–15.
114. Reffelmann T, Kloner RA. Ranolazine: An anti-anginal drug with further therapeutic potential. Expert Rev Cardiovasc Ther 2010;8:319–329.
115. Fernandez SF, Tandar A, Boden WE. Emerging medical treatment for angina pectoris. Expert Opin Emerg Drugs 2010;15:283–298.
116. Chaitman BR. Efficacy and safety of a metabolic modulator drug in chronic stable angina: Review of evidence from clinical trials. J Cardiovasc Pharmacol Ther 2004;9(Suppl 1):S47–S64.
117. Chaitman BR, Skettino SL, Parker JO, et al. Anti-ischemic effects and long-term survival during ranolazine monotherapy in patients with chronic severe angina. J Am Coll Cardiol 2004;43:1375–1382.
118. Chaitman BR, Pepine CJ, Parker JO, et al. Effects of ranolazine with atenolol, amlodipine, or diltiazem on exercise tolerance and angina frequency in patients with severe chronic angina: A randomized controlled trial. JAMA 2004;291:309–316.
119. Morrow DA, Scirica BM, Karwatowska-Prokopczuk E, et al. Effects of ranolazine on recurrent cardiovascular events in patients with non-ST-elevation acute coronary syndromes: The MERLIN-TIMI 36 randomized trial. JAMA 2007;297:1775–1783.
120. Scirica BM, Morrow DA, Hod H, et al. Effect of ranolazine, an antianginal agent with novel electrophysiological properties, on the incidence of arrhythmias in patients with non ST-segment elevation acute coronary syndrome: Results from the Metabolic Efficiency with Ranolazine for Less Ischemia in Non ST-Elevation Acute Coronary Syndrome Thrombolysis in Myocardial Infarction 36 (MERLIN-TIMI 36) randomized controlled trial. Circulation 2007;116:1647–1652.
121. Karwatowska-Prokopczuk E, Wang W, Cheng ML, Zeng D, Schwartz PJ, Belardinelli L. The risk of sudden cardiac death in patients with non-ST elevation acute coronary syndrome and prolonged QTc interval: Effect of ranolazine. Europace 2013;15:429–436.
122. Phelps CE, Buysman EK, Gomez Rey G. Costs and clinical outcomes associated with use of ranolazine for treatment of angina. Clin Ther 2012;34:1395–1407.e4.
123. Sakata K, Miura F, Sugino H, et al. Assessment of regional sympathetic nerve activity in vasospastic angina: Analysis of iodine 123-labeled metaiodobenzylguanidine scintigraphy. Am Heart J 1997;133:484–489.
124. Hung MJ, Cherng WJ, Yang NI, Cheng CW, Li LF. Relation of high-sensitivity C-reactive protein level with coronary vasospastic angina pectoris in patients without hemodynamically significant coronary artery disease. Am J Cardiol 2005;96:1484–1490.
125. Park JS, Zhang SY, Jo SH, et al. Common adrenergic receptor polymorphisms as novel risk factors for vasospastic angina. Am Heart J 2006;151:864–869.
126. Glueck CJ, Munjal J, Khan A, Umar M, Wang P. Endothelial nitric oxide synthase T-786C mutation, a reversible etiology of Prinzmetal's angina pectoris. Am J Cardiol 2010;105:792–796.
127. Lanza GA, Pedrotti P, Pasceri V, Lucente M, Crea F, Maseri A. Autonomic changes associated with spontaneous coronary spasm in patients with variant angina. J Am Coll Cardiol 1996;28:1249–1256.
128. Acikel S, Dogan M, Sari M, Kilic H, Akdemir R. Prinzmetal-variant angina in a patient using zolmitriptan and citalopram. Am J Emerg Med 2010;28:257.e3–257.e6.
129. Schoenenberger AW, Kobza R, Jamshidi P, et al. Sudden cardiac death in patients with silent myocardial ischemia after myocardial infarction (from the Swiss Interventional Study on Silent Ischemia Type II [SWISSI II]). Am J Cardiol 2009;104:158–163.
130. Singh N, Mironov D, Goodman S, Morgan CD, Langer A. Treatment of silent ischemia in unstable angina: A randomized comparison of sustained-release verapamil versus metoprolol. Clin Cardiol 1995;18:653–658.
131. Dwivedi SK, Saran RK, Mittal S, Gupta R, Narain VS, Puri VK. Silent ischemic interval on exercise test is a predictor of response to drug therapy: A randomized crossover trial of metoprolol versus diltiazem in stable angina. Clin Cardiol 2001;24:45–49.
132. Pratt CM, McMahon RP, Goldstein S, et al. Comparison of subgroups assigned to medical regimens used to suppress cardiac ischemia (the Asymptomatic Cardiac Ischemia Pilot [ACIP] Study). Am J Cardiol 1996;77:1302–1309.
133. Davies RF, Goldberg AD, Forman S, et al. Asymptomatic Cardiac Ischemia Pilot (ACIP) study two-year follow-up: Outcomes of patients randomized to initial strategies of medical therapy versus revascularization. Circulation 1997;95:2037–2043.
134. Erne P, Schoenenberger AW, Burckhardt D, et al. Effects of percutaneous coronary interventions in silent ischemia after myocardial infarction: The SWISSI II randomized controlled trial. JAMA 2007;297:1985–1991.
135. Erne P, Schoenenberger AW, Zuber M, et al. Effects of anti-ischaemic drug therapy in silent myocardial ischaemia type I: The Swiss Interventional Study on Silent Ischaemia type I (SWISSI I): A randomized, controlled pilot study. Eur Heart J 2007;28:2110–2117.

136. Bosanquet N, Jonsson B, Fox KA. Costs and cost effectiveness of low molecular weight heparins and platelet glycoprotein IIb/IIIa inhibitors: In the management of acute coronary syndromes. Pharmacoeconomics 2003;21:1135–1152.

137. Plosker GL, Ibbotson T. Eptifibatide: A pharmacoeconomic review of its use in percutaneous coronary intervention and acute coronary syndromes. Pharmacoeconomics 2003;21:885–912.

138. Caron MF, McKendall GR. Bivalirudin in percutaneous coronary intervention. Am J Health Syst Pharm 2003;60:1841–1849.

139. Hay JW, Yu WM, Ashraf T. Pharmacoeconomics of lipid-lowering agents for primary and secondary prevention of coronary artery disease. Pharmacoeconomics 1999;15:47–74.

7 Acute Coronary Syndromes

Sarah A. Spinler and Simon de Denus

KEY CONCEPTS

1. The cause of an acute coronary syndrome (ACS) is the rupture of an atherosclerotic plaque with subsequent platelet adherence, activation, and aggregation, and the activation of the clotting cascade. Ultimately, a clot forms composed of fibrin and platelets.
2. The American College of Cardiology Foundation (ACCF), American Heart Association (AHA), and Society for Cardiovascular Angiography and Interventions (SCAI) recommend strategies, or guidelines, for ACS patient care for ST-segment elevation (STE) myocardial infarction (MI) and non–ST-segment elevation (NSTE) ACS, including guidelines for patients undergoing percutaneous coronary intervention (PCI).
3. Patients with ischemic chest discomfort and suspected ACS are risk-stratified based on a 12-lead electrocardiogram (ECG), past medical history, and results of the troponin and creatine kinase (CK)–myocardial band (MB) tests. The diagnosis of MI is confirmed based on the results of the CK-MB and troponin biochemical marker tests.
4. Early reperfusion therapy with primary PCI of the infarct artery is the recommended therapy for patients presenting with STE MI within 12 hours of symptom onset.
5. The most recent PCI ACCF/AHA/SCAI clinical practice guidelines recommend coronary angiography with either PCI or coronary artery bypass graft (CABG) surgery revascularization as an early treatment (early invasive strategy) for patients with NSTE ACS at an elevated risk for death or MI, including those with a high risk score or patients with refractory angina, acute heart failure, other symptoms of cardiogenic shock, or arrhythmias.
6. In addition to reperfusion therapy, other early pharmacotherapy that all patients with STE MI and without contraindications should receive within the first day of hospitalization, and preferably in the emergency department, are intranasal oxygen (if oxygen saturation is low), sublingual (SL) nitroglycerin (NTG), aspirin (ASA), a $P2Y_{12}$ inhibitor (clopidogrel, prasugrel, or ticagrelor depending on reperfusion strategy), and anticoagulation with bivalirudin, unfractionated heparin (UFH), enoxaparin, (agent dependent on reperfusion strategy), or fondaparinux. A glycoprotein (GP) IIb/IIIa inhibitor should be administered if UFH is selected as the anticoagulant for patients undergoing primary PCI. A statin should be administered prior to PCI. IV *β*-blockers and IV NTG should be given in selected patients. Oral *β*-blockers should be initiated within the first day in patients without contraindications.
7. In the absence of contraindications, all patients with NSTE ACS should be treated in the emergency department with intranasal oxygen (if oxygen saturation is low), SL NTG, ASA, and an anticoagulant (UFH, enoxaparin, fondaparinux, or bivalirudin). High-risk patients should proceed to early angiography, and may receive a GP IIb/IIIa inhibitor. A $P2Y_{12}$ inhibitor (selection of agent and timing of initiation dependent on selection of an interventional approach involving PCI or CABG surgery vs. a noninterventional approach with medical management alone) should be administered to all patients. A statin should be administered prior to PCI. IV *β*-blockers and IV NTG should be given in selected patients. Oral *β*-blockers should be initiated within the first day in patients without contraindications.
8. Secondary prevention guidelines from the ACCF/AHA suggest that following MI from either STE MI or NSTE ACS, all patients, in the absence of contraindications, should receive indefinite treatment with ASA, a *β*-blocker, a statin, and an angiotensin-converting enzyme (ACE) inhibitor for secondary prevention of death, stroke, or recurrent infarction. The goal low-density lipoprotein cholesterol is less than 100 mg/dL (2.59 mmol/L) and ideally less than 70 mg/dL (1.81 mmol/L). A $P2Y_{12}$ inhibitor should be continued for at least 12 months for patients undergoing PCI and for patients with NSTE ACS receiving a medical management strategy of treatment. Clopidogrel should be continued for at least 14 days in patients with STE MI in patients not undergoing PCI. An angiotensin II receptor blocker and a mineralocorticoid receptor antagonist should be given to selected patients. For all patients with ACS, treatment and control of modifiable risk factors such as hypertension (HTN), dyslipidemia, obesity, smoking, and diabetes mellitus are essential.
9. To determine the efficacy of nonpharmacologic treatments and pharmacotherapy, monitor patients for relief of ischemic discomfort, return of ECG changes to baseline, and absence or resolution of heart failure signs and symptoms. The most common adverse effects from pharmacotherapy of ACS are bleeding and hypotension.

INTRODUCTION

Cardiovascular disease (CVD) is the leading cause of death in the United States and one of the major causes of death worldwide. *Acute coronary syndromes* (ACSs), including unstable angina (UA) and myocardial *infarction* (MI), are a form of coronary heart disease (CHD) that comprises the most common cause of CVD death.[1] (1) The cause of an ACS is primarily the rupture of an atherosclerotic plaque with subsequent platelet adherence, activation, and aggregation, and the activation of the clotting cascade. Ultimately, a clot forms composed of fibrin and platelets. 2 The American Heart Association (AHA) and the American College of Cardiology Foundation (ACCF) recommend strategies, or guidelines, for ACS patient care for *ST-segment elevation* (STE) *and non–ST-segment elevation* (NSTE) ACS. In collaboration with the Society for Cardiovascular Angiography and Interventions (SCAI), the ACCF and AHA issue joint guidelines for *percutaneous coronary intervention* (PCI), including PCI in the setting of ACS. These practice guidelines are based on a review of available clinical evidence, have graded recommendations based on evidence and expert opinion, and are updated periodically. These guidelines form the cornerstone for quality care of the ACS patient.[2–7]

EPIDEMIOLOGY

Each year, more than 1.1 million Americans will experience an ACS, and 150,000 die of an MI.[1] In the United States, more than 7 million living persons have survived an MI.[1]

CVDs are the leading cause of hospitalization in the United States, resulting in about 6.2 million hospital discharges per year. Each year, there are more than 1.3 million MIs, and one in six deaths is secondary to CHD.[1]

The proportion of patients with MI presenting with STE MI compared with those presenting with NSTE MI decreased from approximately 80% in the early 1990s to between 25% and 30% currently.[1] This may be secondary to the use of the more sensitive biomarker troponin (increasing the diagnosis of MI in the NSTE ACS group), greater use of antecedent revascularization procedures, decreased reinfarction from enhanced medical therapy after an initial event, or prevention of progression of UA to MI through more effective anticoagulant and antiplatelet therapy.

According to data from the National Registry of Myocardial Infarction, in-hospital mortality has decreased by more than 20% during the last 20 years. Improvements in care that may have contributed to this mortality reduction include greater use of guideline-recommended drugs (e.g., aspirin [ASA], *β*-blockers, angiotensin-converting enzyme [ACE] inhibitors and angiotensin receptor blockers [ARBs], statins, clopidogrel), reductions in the door-to-needle time for administering fibrinolytics and in the corresponding first medical contact time to primary PCI, treatments for heart failure (HF), and increased use of early coronary angiography and PCI for high-risk patients with NSTE ACS.[1]

In patients with STE MI, in-hospital death rates are approximately 3% in patients receiving primary PCI, 7% for patients who are treated with fibrinolytics, and 16% for patients who do not receive reperfusion therapy. In patients with NSTE MI, in-hospital mortality is less than 5%. At 6 months and 1 year, mortality and reinfarction rates are similar between STE and NSTE MI.[1] Other than persistent ST-segment changes and troponin, other predictors of in-hospital mortality include older age, elevated serum creatinine (SCr), tachycardia, and HF.[1,2,8] One-year mortality following STE MI ranges from 7% to 18%.[2]

CHD is the leading cause of premature, chronic disability in the United States. The risks of CHD events, such as death, recurrent MI, and stroke, are higher for patients with established CHD and a history of MI than for patients with no known CHD. The cost of CHD is high, with estimated direct and indirect costs of more than $195 billion.[1] The estimated cost of hospitalization for MI is $14,000, and the median length of hospital stay is 3.2 days.[1,2] Risk-standardized hospital mortality for MI and 30-day hospital readmission rates following MI and PCI are quality performance measures and Outcome of Care Measures that are publically reportable by the Center for Medicare and Medicaid Services.[6] The Patient Protection and Affordable Care Act of 2010 links quality performance measures to hospital reimbursement.

ETIOLOGY

Endothelial dysfunction, inflammation, and the formation of fatty streaks contribute to the formation of atherosclerotic coronary artery plaques, the underlying cause of coronary artery disease (CAD).[7] 1 The predominant cause of ACS in more than 90% of patients is atheromatous plaque rupture, fissuring, or erosion of an unstable atherosclerotic plaque that occludes less than 50% of the coronary lumen prior to the event, rather than a more stable 70% to 90% stenosis of the coronary artery.[9] Stable stenoses are characteristic of stable angina.

PATHOPHYSIOLOGY

Spectrum of ACSs

ACSs include all clinical syndromes compatible with acute MI resulting from an imbalance between myocardial oxygen demand and supply. In contrast to stable angina, an ACS results primarily from diminished myocardial blood flow secondary to an occlusive or partially occlusive coronary artery thrombus. ACSs are classified according to electrocardiogram (ECG) changes into STE MI or NSTE ACS (NSTE MI and UA) (Fig. 7-1).[10] An STE MI occurs when symptoms of myocardial ischemia occur in conjunction with new STE with subsequent release of biomarkers of myocardial necrosis, mainly *troponins T* or *I*, but also *creatine kinase* (CK)–*myocardial band* (MB).[2] 2 An STE MI, formerly known as Q-wave or transmural MI, typically results in an injury that transects the thickness of the myocardial wall. Following an STE MI, pathologic Q waves are frequently seen on the ECG, indicating transmural MI, whereas such an ECG manifestation is seen less commonly in patients with NSTE MI.[3] NSTE MI, formerly known as non–Q-wave or nontransmural MI, is limited to the subendocardial myocardium. Patients in this case do not usually develop a pathologic Q wave on the ECG. Moreover, an NSTE MI is smaller and not as extensive as an STE MI. NSTE MI differs from UA in that ischemia is severe enough to produce myocardial necrosis resulting in the release of a detectable amount of biomarkers, mainly *troponins T* or *I*, but also *CK MB*, from the necrotic myocytes in the bloodstream. The clinical significance of serum markers will be discussed in greater detail in later sections of this chapter.

Plaque Rupture and Clot Formation

Following plaque rupture, a clot (a partially or completely occlusive thrombus) forms on top of the ruptured plaque. The thrombogenic contents of the plaque are exposed to blood elements. Exposure of collagen and tissue factor induces platelet adhesion and activation, which promote the release of platelet-derived vasoactive substances including adenosine diphosphate (ADP) and thromboxane A_2 (TXA_2).[7] These produce vasoconstriction and potentiate platelet activation. Furthermore, during platelet activation, a change in the conformation in the glycoprotein (GP) IIb/IIIa surface receptors of platelets occurs that cross-links platelets to each other through fibrinogen bridges. This is considered the final common pathway of platelet aggregation. Inclusion of platelets gives the clot a white appearance. Simultaneously, the extrinsic coagulation cascade pathway is activated as a result of exposure of blood components to the thrombogenic lipid core and disrupted endothelium, which are rich in tissue factor. This leads to the production of thrombin (factor IIa), which converts fibrinogen to fibrin through enzymatic activity. Fibrin stabilizes the clot and traps red blood cells, which gives the clot a red appearance. Therefore, the clot is composed of cross-linked platelets and fibrin strands.[9,11]

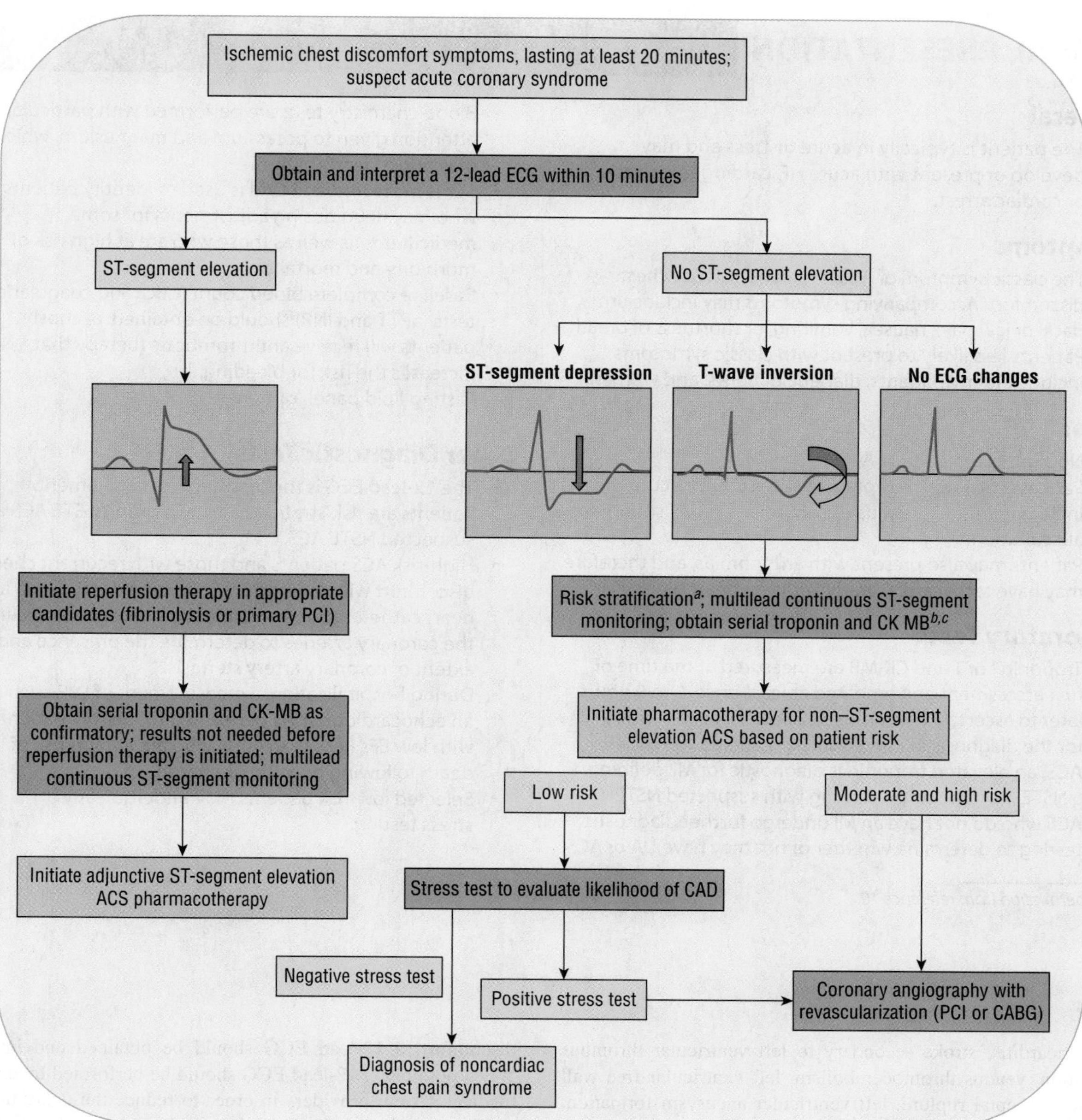

FIGURE 7-1 Evaluation of the acute coronary syndrome patient. [a]*As described in Table 7-1.* [b]"Positive": Above the myocardial infarction decision limit. [c]"Negative": Below the myocardial infarction decision limit. (ACS, acute coronary syndrome; CABG, coronary artery bypass graft; CAD, coronary artery disease; CK-MB, creatine kinase myocardial band; ECG, electrocardiogram; PCI, percutaneous coronary intervention.) *(Modified with permission from Spinler SA. Evolution of antithrombotic therapy used in acute coronary syndromes. In: Richardson MM, Chant C, Cheng JWM, et al., eds. Pharmacotherapy Self-Assessment Program. Book 1: Cardiology, 7th ed. Lenexa, KS: American College of Clinical Pharmacy, 2010.)*

Ventricular Remodeling Following an Acute MI

Ventricular remodeling is a process that occurs in several cardiovascular (CV) conditions including HF and following an MI. It is characterized by left ventricular dilation and reduced pumping function of the left ventricle, leading to cardiac failure.[12] Because HF represents one of the principal causes of mortality and morbidity following an MI, preventing ventricular remodeling is an important therapeutic goal.

ACE inhibitors, ARBs, β-blockers, and mineralocorticoid receptor antagonists (MRAs) are all agents that slow down or reverse ventricular remodeling through inhibition of the renin–angiotensin–aldosterone system and/or through improvement in hemodynamics (decreasing preload or afterload).[12] These agents also improve survival and will be discussed in more detail in subsequent sections of this chapter.

Complications

This chapter focuses on management of the uncomplicated ACS patient. However, it is important for clinicians to recognize complications of MI, because MI is associated with increased mortality. The most serious complication of MI is cardiogenic shock, occurring in approximately 5% to 6% of hospitalized patients presenting with STE MI.[13] Mortality complicated by cardiogenic shock with MI is high, approaching 60%.[14] Other complications that may result from MI are HF, valvular dysfunction, bradycardia, heart

CLINICAL PRESENTATION Diagnosis of ACSs

General

- The patient is typically in acute distress and may develop or present with acute HF, cardiogenic shock, or cardiac arrest.

Symptoms

- The classic symptom of ACS is midline anterior chest discomfort. Accompanying symptoms may include arm, back, or jaw pain, nausea, vomiting, or shortness of breath.
- Patients less likely to present with classic symptoms include elderly patients, diabetic patients, and women.

Signs

- No signs are classic for ACS.
- Patients with ACS may present with signs of acute HF including jugular venous distention and an S_3 sound on auscultation.
- Patients may also present with arrhythmias, and therefore may have tachycardia, bradycardia, or heart block.

Laboratory Tests

- Troponin I or T and CK-MB are measured at the time of first assessment and repeated at least once, 6 to 9 hours later to ascertain heart muscle damage, confirmatory for the diagnosis of infarction. For patients with NSTE ACS, an elevated troponin is diagnostic for MI, defining a NSTE MI. Patients presenting with suspected NSTE ACS who do not have an MI undergo further diagnostic testing to determine whether or not they have UA or ACS.
- Blood chemistry tests are performed with particular attention given to potassium and magnesium, which may affect heart rhythm.
- SCr is measured and CrCl is used to identify patients who may need dosing adjustments for some medications as well as those who are at high risk of morbidity and mortality.
- Baseline complete blood count (CBC) and coagulation tests (aPTT and INR) should be obtained, as most patients will receive antithrombotic therapy that increases the risk for bleeding.
- Fasting lipid panel (optional).

Other Diagnostic Tests

- The 12-lead ECG is the first step in management. Patients are risk-stratified into two groups: STE ACS and suspected NSTE ACS.
- High-risk ACS patients and those with recurrent chest discomfort will undergo coronary angiography via a left heart catheterization and injection of contrast dye into the coronary arteries to determine the presence and extent of coronary artery stenosis.
- During hospitalization, a measurement of LVF, such as an echocardiogram, is performed to identify patients with low EFs (less than 40%) who are at high risk of death following hospital discharge.
- Selected low-risk patients may undergo early stress testing.

With permission from reference 10.

block, pericarditis, stroke secondary to left ventricular thrombus embolization, venous thromboembolism, left ventricular free wall or ventricular septal rupture, left ventricular aneurysm formation, and ventricular and atrial tachyarrhythmias.[2] In fact, more than one quarter of MI patients die, presumably from ventricular fibrillation, prior to reaching the hospital.[1]

Symptoms and Physical Examination Findings

The classic symptom of an ACS is midline anterior anginal chest discomfort, most often occurring when an individual is at rest, as a severe new onset, or as an increasing angina that is at least 20 minutes in duration. The chest discomfort may radiate to the shoulder, down the left arm, and to the back or to the jaw. Associated symptoms that may accompany the chest discomfort include nausea, vomiting, diaphoresis, or shortness of breath. Although similar to stable angina, the duration may be longer and the intensity greater. All healthcare professionals should review these warning symptoms with patients at high risk for CHD. On physical examination, no specific features are indicative of ACS.

Twelve-Lead ECG

There are key features of a 12-lead ECG that identify and risk-stratify a patient with an ACS. Within 10 minutes of presentation to an emergency department with symptoms of ischemic chest discomfort, a 12-lead ECG should be obtained and interpreted. When possible, a 12-lead ECG should be performed by emergency medical system providers in order to reduce the delay until myocardial reperfusion. If available, a prior 12-lead ECG should be reviewed to identify whether or not the findings on the current ECG are new or old, with new findings being more indicative of an ACS. Key findings on review of a 12-lead ECG that indicate myocardial ischemia or infarction are STE, ST-segment depression, and T-wave inversion (Fig. 7-1).[10] ST-segment and/or T-wave changes in certain groupings of leads help to identify the location of the coronary artery that is the cause of the ischemia or infarction. In addition, the appearance of a new left bundle-branch block accompanied by chest discomfort is highly specific for acute MI. About one half of patients diagnosed with MI present with STE on their ECG, with the remainder having ST-segment depression, T-wave inversion, or, in some instances, no ECG changes. Some parts of the heart are more "electrically silent" than others, and myocardial ischemia may not be detected on a surface ECG. Therefore, it is important to review findings from the ECG in conjunction with biochemical markers of myocardial necrosis, such as troponin I or T, and other risk factors for CHD to determine the patient's risk for experiencing a new MI or having other complications.

Biochemical Markers/Cardiac Enzymes

Biochemical markers of myocardial cell death are important for confirming the diagnosis of MI. The diagnosis of acute MI is confirmed when the following conditions are met in a clinical setting consistent with myocardial ischemia: "Detection of a rise and/or fall of cardiac biomarkers (cardiac troponin preferred) with at least one value above the 99th percentile of the upper reference limit with at least one of the following: (a) symptoms of ischemia; (b) new or presumed new significant ST-segment–T wave changes or new left bundle-branch block; (c) development of pathologic Q waves; or (d) imaging evidence of new loss of viable myocardium or new regional wall motion abnormality."[15] Typically, a blood sample is obtained once in the emergency department, and then 6 to 9 hours later, and in patients at a high suspicion of MI but in whom previous measurements did not reveal elevations in biomarkers, 12 to 24 hours after. A single measurement of a biochemical marker is not adequate to exclude a diagnosis of MI, as up to 15% of values that were initially below the level of detection (a "negative" test) rise to the level of detection (a "positive" test) in subsequent hours. While troponins and CK-MB appear in the blood within 6 hours of infarction, troponins stay elevated for up to 10 days while CK-MB returns to normal values within 48 hours. Hence, traditionally, CK-MB was used to detect reinfarction. However, more recent data have suggested that troponins provide similar information to CK-MB in such a situation that has led to the use of troponins in this setting as well. Current guidelines suggest that, in patients in whom a recurrent MI is suspected, a cardiac biomarker should be immediately measured, followed by a second measurement 3 to 6 hours later. A recurrent MI is diagnosed when there is an increase of at least 20% in the second measurement of the biomarker, if this value exceeds the 99th percentile of the upper reference limit.[15]

Risk Stratification

Patient symptoms, past medical history, ECG, and biomarkers, particularly cardiac troponins, are utilized to stratify patients into low, medium, or high risk of death, MI, or likelihood of failing pharmacotherapy and needing urgent coronary angiography and PCI (Table 7-1).[3,5,16] ❸ Initial treatment according to risk stratification is depicted in Figure 7-1.[2–5,8,10] Patients with STE MI are at the highest risk of death. Initial treatment of STE MI should proceed without evaluation of the troponins because these patients have a greater than 97% chance of having an MI subsequently diagnosed with biochemical markers. The ACCF/AHA define a target time to initiate reperfusion treatment as within 30 minutes of hospital presentation for fibrinolytics (e.g., streptokinase, alteplase, reteplase, and tenecteplase) and within 90 minutes or less from first medical contact for primary PCI.[2,5] The sooner the infarct-related coronary artery is opened for these patients, the lower their mortality and the greater the amount of myocardium that is preserved.[17,18] Although all patients should be evaluated for reperfusion therapy, not all patients may be eligible. Indications and contraindications for fibrinolytic therapy are described in Treatment below. Less than 25% of hospitals in the United States are equipped to perform primary PCI. If patients are not eligible for reperfusion therapy, additional pharmacotherapy for STE patients should be initiated in the emergency department and the patient transferred to a coronary intensive care unit. The typical length of stay for a patient with uncomplicated STE MI is less than 4 days.[19]

Risk stratification of the patient with NSTE ACS is more complex because in-hospital outcomes for this group of patients vary with reported rates of death of 0% to 12%, reinfarction rates of 0% to 3%, and recurrent severe ischemia rates of 5% to 20%.[17] Not all patients presenting with suspected NSTE ACS will even have CAD. Some will eventually be diagnosed with nonischemic chest discomfort. In general, among NSTE patients, those with ST-segment depression (Fig. 7-1) and/or elevated biomarkers are at higher risk of death or recurrent infarction.

TABLE 7-1 Risk Stratification for Acute Coronary Syndromes (ACS)[3,4,16,23,24]

TIMI risk score for NSTE ACS

One point is assigned for each of the seven medical history and clinical presentation findings. The point total is calculated and the patient is assigned a risk for experiencing the composite end point of death, myocardial infarction, or urgent need for revascularization as follows:

- Age 65 years or older
- Three or more CHD risk factors: smoking, hypercholesterolemia, hypertension, diabetes mellitus, family history of premature CHD death/events
- Known CAD (50% or greater stenosis of at least one major coronary artery on coronary angiogram)
- Aspirin use within the last 7 days
- Two or more episodes of chest discomfort within the last 24 hours
- ST-segment depression 0.5 mm or greater
- Positive biochemical marker for infarction

High Risk	Medium Risk	Low Risk
TIMI Risk Score	TIMI Risk Score	TIMI Risk Score
5–7 points	3–4 points	0–2 points

TIMI Risk Score	Mortality, MI, or Severe Recurrent Ischemic Requiring Urgent Target Vessel Revascularization
0/1	4.7%
2	8.3%
3	13.2%
4	19.9%
5	26.2%
6/7	40.9%

GRACE risk factors for increased mortality and the composite of death or MI in ACS

- Signs and symptoms of heart failure
- Low systolic blood pressure
- Elevated heart rate
- Older age
- Elevated serum creatinine
- Baseline risk factors on clinical evaluation: cardiac arrest at admission, ST-segment deviation, elevated troponin
- A high-risk patient is defined as a GRACE risk score of >140 points

CAD, coronary artery disease; CHD, coronary heart disease; GRACE, Global Registry of Acute Coronary Events; MI, myocardial infarction; NSTE, non–ST-segment elevation; TIMI, thrombolysis in myocardial infarction.

An on-line calculator for the GRACE Risk Model is available at Grace Risk Model Calculator, http://www.outcomes-umassmed.org/GRACE/acs_risk/acs_risk_content.html.

Reproduced with permission from Spinler SA. Evolution of antithrombotic therapy used in acute coronary syndromes. In: Richardson MM, Chessman KH, Chant C, et al., eds. Pharmacotherapy Assessment Program. Book 1: Cardiology, 7th ed. Lenexa, KS: American College of Clinical Pharmacy, 2010:97–124. With permission from Spinler SA, de Denus S. Acute coronary syndromes. In: DiPiro JT, Talbert RL, Yee GC, et al., eds. Pharmacotherapy: A Pathophysiologic Approach, 8th ed. New York, NY: McGraw-Hill, 201:246.

TREATMENT

Desired Outcomes

Short-term desired outcomes in a patient with ACS are: (a) early restoration of blood flow to the infarct-related artery to prevent infarct expansion (in the case of MI) or prevent complete occlusion and MI (in UA); (b) prevention of death and other MI complications; (c) prevention of coronary artery reocclusion; and as evidence of restoration of coronary artery blood flow; (d) relief of ischemic chest discomfort; and (e) resolution of ST-segment and T-wave changes on the ECG.

Long-term desired outcomes are control of CV risk factors, prevention of additional CV events, including reinfarction, stroke, and HF, and improvement in quality of life.

General Approach to Treatment

Selecting evidence-based therapies described in the ACCF/AHA guidelines for patients without contraindications results in lower mortality.[20–22] General treatment measures for all STE MI and high- and intermediate-risk NSTE ACS patients include admission to hospital, oxygen administration (if oxygen saturation is low, less than 90%), continuous multilead ST-segment monitoring for arrhythmias and ischemia, frequent measurement of vital signs, bedrest for 12 hours in hemodynamically stable patients, avoidance of the Valsalva maneuver (prescribe stool softeners routinely), and pain relief (Figs. 7-2 and 7-3).[2–4,8,10,16]

Because risk varies and resources are limited, it is important to triage and treat patients according to their risk category. Initial approaches to treatment of STE MI and NSTE ACS patients are outlined in Figures 7-2 and 7-3. Patients with STE are at high risk of death, and efforts to reestablish coronary perfusion, as well as adjunctive pharmacotherapy, should be initiated immediately.

Features identifying low-, moderate-, and high-risk NSTE ACS patients are described in Table 7-1.[16,23,24]

Nonpharmacologic Therapy

Primary PCI for STE MIs

Early reperfusion therapy with primary PCI of the infarct artery within 90 minutes of first medical contact is the reperfusion treatment of choice for patients presenting with STE MI who present within 12 hours of symptom onset[2] (4) (Fig. 7-2). First, emergency medical services are activated for a patient complaining of ischemic symptoms. Paramedics arrive to care for the patient out of the hospital and they perform a 12-lead ECG that demonstrates STE. Sometimes, the 12-lead ECG is transmitted electronically or via telephone to an emergency department where a physician reviews the ECG and may "activate" the cardiac catheterization medical team to alert them that a patient with STE MI will be arriving at the hospital

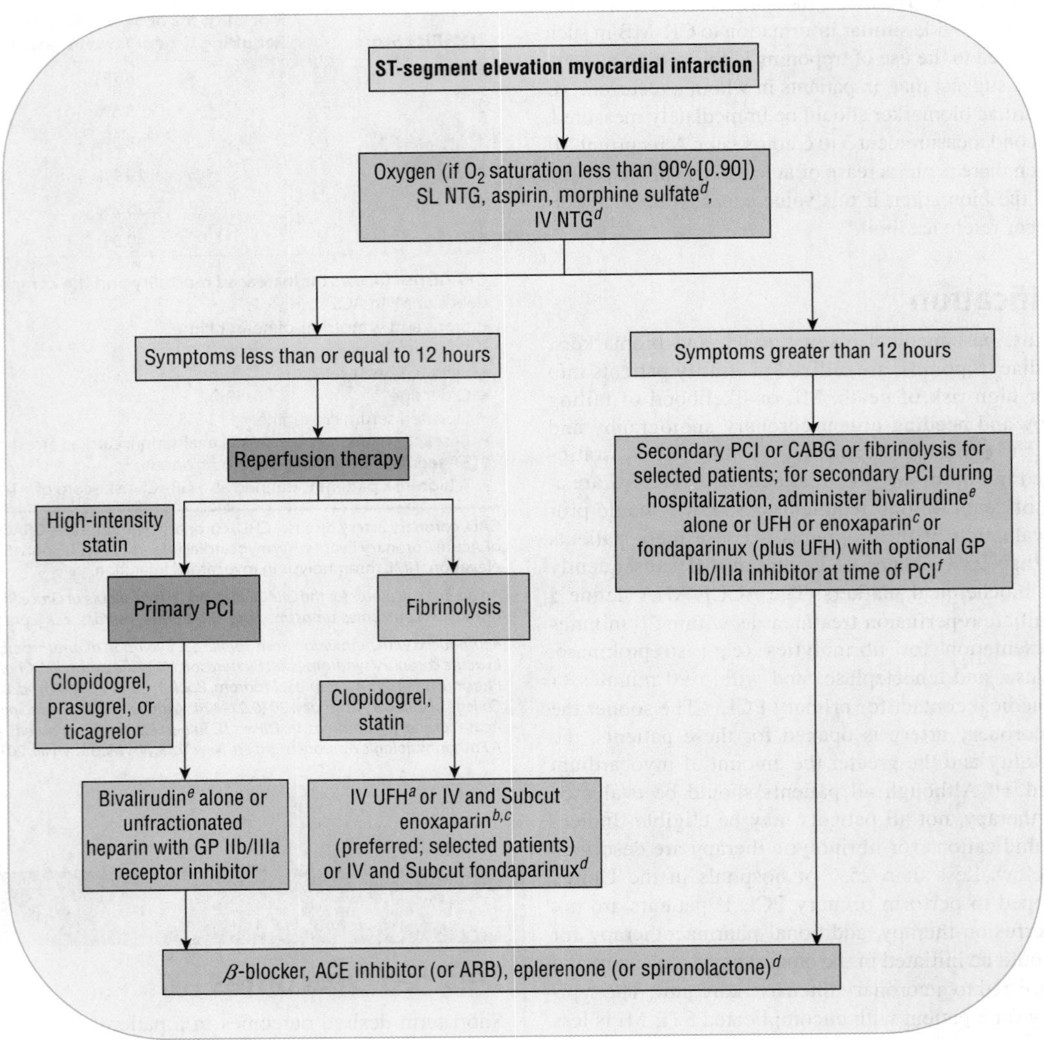

FIGURE 7-2 Initial pharmacotherapy for ST-segment elevation myocardial infarction. [a]For at least 48 hours. [b]See Table 7-2 for dosing and specific types of patients who should not receive enoxaparin. [c]For the duration of hospitalization, up to 8 days. [d]For selected patients, see Table 7-2. [e]If pretreated with UFH, stop UFH infusion for 30 minutes prior to administration of bivalirudin (bolus plus infusion). [f]Increased risk of major bleeding and intracranial hemorrhage if a GP IIb/IIIa inhibitor is added to an anticoagulant for PCI following fibrinolysis, especially in the elderly; weight risk versus benefit. (ACE, angiotensin-converting enzyme; ARB, angiotensin receptor blocker; CABG, coronary artery bypass graft; GP, glycoprotein; NTG, nitroglycerin; PCI, percutaneous coronary intervention; Subcut, subcutaneous; SL, sublingual; UFH, unfractionated heparin.) *(Modified with permission from Spinler SA. Evolution of antithrombotic therapy used in acute coronary syndromes. In: Richardson MM, Chant C, Cheng JWM, et al., eds. Pharmacotherapy Self-Assessment Program. Book 1: Cardiology, 7th ed. Lenexa, KS: American College of Clinical Pharmacy, 2010.)*

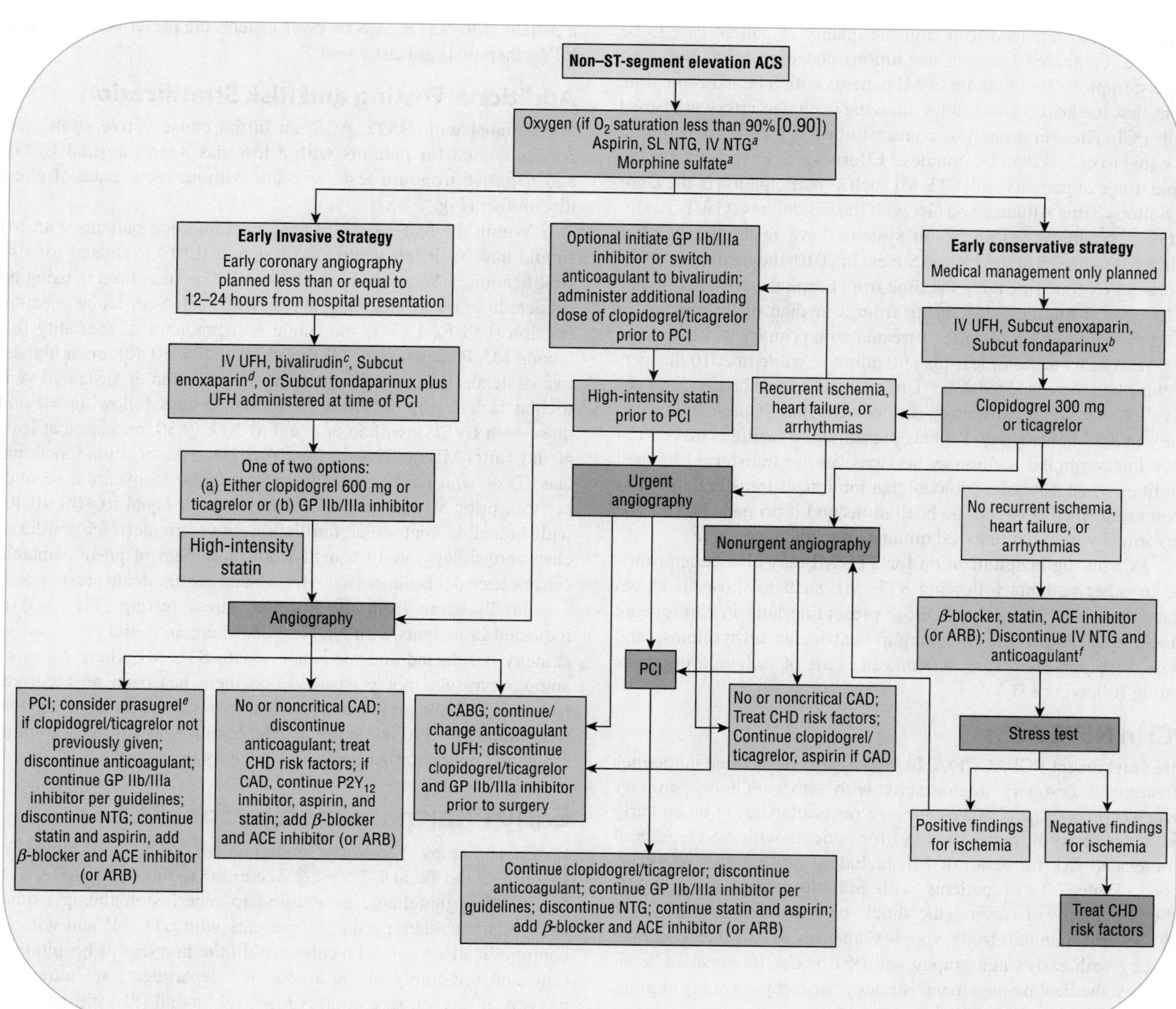

FIGURE 7-3 Initial pharmacotherapy for non–ST-segment elevation ACS. [a]For selected patients, see Table 7-2. [b]Preferred in patients at high risk for bleeding. [c]If pretreated with UFH, stop UFH infusion for 30 minutes prior to administration of bivalirudin bolus plus infusion. [d]May require IV supplemental dose of enoxaparin; see Table 7-2. [e]Do not use if prior history of stroke/transient ischemic attack (TIA), age older than 75 years, or body weight less than or equal to 60 kg. [f]Subcut enoxaparin or UFH can be continued at a lower dose for venous thromboembolism prophylaxis. (ACE, angiotensin-converting enzyme; ACS, acute coronary syndrome; ARB, angiotensin receptor blocker; CABG, coronary artery bypass graft; CAD, coronary artery disease; CHD, coronary heart disease; GP, glycoprotein; NTG, nitroglycerin; PCI, percutaneous coronary intervention; Subcut, subcutaneous; SL, sublingual; UFH, unfractionated heparin.)
(Modified with permission from reference 16.)

shortly. The patient is transported to the emergency department. For primary PCI, the patient is taken from the emergency department to the cardiac catheterization laboratory and undergoes coronary angiography with either balloon angioplasty or placement of a bare metal or drug-eluting intracoronary stent in the artery associated with the infarct. In order to meet the quality of care metric of less than 90 minutes from first medical contact to primary PCI, many transitions of care occur and care coordination between paramedics, emergency department staff, and cardiac catheterization is vital. Every minute delay results in additional myocardial cell damage that may be irreversible.

About 62% of patients with STE MI are treated with primary PCI; 18% are treated with fibrinolytics. Results from a meta-analysis of trials comparing fibrinolysis with primary PCI indicate a lower mortality rate with primary PCI.[25] One reason for the superiority of primary PCI compared with fibrinolysis is that more than 90% of occluded infarct-related coronary arteries are opened with primary PCI compared with fewer than 60% of coronary arteries opened with currently available fibrinolytics.[2] In addition, intracranial hemorrhage (ICH) and major bleeding risks from primary PCI are lower than the risks of severe bleeding events following fibrinolysis. An invasive strategy of primary PCI is generally preferred in patients presenting to institutions with skilled interventional cardiologists and a catheterization laboratory immediately available, patients in cardiogenic shock, those with contraindications to fibrinolytics, and those with continuing symptoms 12 to 24 hours after symptom onset.[2]

A quality performance measure (quality performance measures are measures of quality healthcare developed from practice guidelines and intended to permit the quality of patient care to be assessed, compared between institutions and over time, and, ultimately, improved) in the care of MI patients with STE MI is the time from first medical contact to the time the occluded artery is opened with PCI. This "first medical contact-to-primary PCI" time should be equal to or less than 90 minutes.[2] Efforts to improve system-wide rapid triage of patients with STE MI such as participation in the Door to Balloon Time Alliance and Get with the Guidelines (GWTG) educational programs within health systems have resulted in shorter primary PCI times in the United States. In 2010, the median door-to-primary PCI time (meaning the time from hospital arrival to primary PCI) was 64 minutes, decreasing from a median of 96 minutes in 2005.[26] In 2005, 44% of patients treated with primary PCI had door-to-primary PCI times of less than 90 minutes, while in 2010 this percentage had increased to 94%.[26] Unfortunately, most hospitals do not have interventional cardiology services capable of performing primary PCI 24 hours a day. Patients presenting to facilities that do not have interventional cardiology services can be transferred to such facilities when a transfer protocol that minimizes transfer delays has been established between the institutions and if primary PCI can be performed within the first 120 minutes of medical contact.[2]

PCI during hospitalization for STE MI may also be appropriate in other patients following STE MI, such as those in whom fibrinolysis is not successful, those presenting later in cardiogenic shock, those with life-threatening ventricular arrhythmias, and those with persistent rest ischemia or signs of ischemia on stress testing following MI.[2]

PCI in NSTE ACSs

The most recent PCI ACCF/AHA/SCAI clinical practice guidelines recommend coronary angiography with either PCI or *coronary artery bypass graft* (CABG) *surgery* revascularization as an early treatment (early invasive strategy) for patients with NSTE ACS at an elevated risk for death or MI, including those with a high risk score (Table 7-1) or patients with refractory angina, acute HF, other symptoms of cardiogenic shock, or arrhythmias (Fig. 7-3).[5,8] **5** Several clinical trials support an "invasive" interventional strategy with early angiography and PCI or CABG versus a "conservative medical management" strategy, whereby coronary angiography with revascularization is reserved for patients with symptoms refractory to pharmacotherapy and patients with signs of ischemia on stress testing.[5,27] An early invasive approach results in a lower rate of refractory angina during hospital admission and over the first year, as well as a lower frequency of MI at 5 years, but an increased frequency of minor bleeding related to the procedure.[27] An early invasive strategy is also less costly than the conservative medical stabilization approach.[28] Mortality is not reduced by an early invasive approach in patients with NSTE ACS.[27]

All patients undergoing PCI should receive low-dose ASA therapy indefinitely. A $P2Y_{12}$ inhibitor antiplatelet (clopidogrel, prasugrel, or ticagrelor) should be administered concomitantly with ASA for at least 12 months following PCI for a patient with ACS (Table 7-2).[2,5] Earlier discontinuation of the $P2Y_{12}$ inhibitor should be considered if the risk of bleeding outweighs the anticipated benefit in reduction in risk of death, MI, or stroke as well as stent thrombosis.[2,5] A longer duration of $P2Y_{12}$ inhibitor therapy may be considered for patients receiving a drug-eluting stent, as the risk of stent thrombosis is greater on cessation of dual antiplatelet therapy.[2,5] Drug-eluting stents reduce the rate of smooth muscle cell growth causing stent restenosis. However, there is a delay in endothelial cell regrowth at the site of the stent that places the patient at higher risk of thrombotic events following PCI. Therefore, dual antiplatelet therapy is indicated for a longer period of time following PCI with a drug-eluting stent. Trials are ongoing evaluating the need for an extended duration in patients without ACS undergoing PCI (greater than 12 months) of $P2Y_{12}$ inhibitor therapy following PCI. Regardless of whether or not a patient with NSTE ACS receives a stent, the preferred duration of $P2Y_{12}$ therapy is at least a year.[2,5]

Additional Testing and Risk Stratification

For patients with NSTE ACS, an initial conservative strategy is recommended for patients with a low risk score, normal ECGs, and negative troponin tests who are without recurrence of chest discomfort (Fig. 7-3).[3,4]

Within the first 3 days of hospital admission patients with MI should have their left ventricular function (LVF) evaluated for risk stratification.[2] The most common way LVF is measured is using an echocardiogram to calculate the patient's left ventricular ejection fraction (LVEF). LVF is the single best predictor of mortality following MI. Patients with LVEFs less than 40% (0.40) are at highest risk of death. Patients with ventricular fibrillation or sustained ventricular tachycardia occurring more than 2 days following MI and those with LVEF less than or equal to 30% (0.30, measured at least 40 days after MI) (and have a New York Heart Association functional class I) or who have nonsustained ventricular tachycardia secondary to a prior MI and a LVEF of less than or equal to 40% (0.40) with inducible ventricular fibrillation or ventricular tachycardia at electrophysiology study benefit from placement of an implantable cardioverter-defibrillator (ICD) for sudden cardiac death prevention.[29]

Predischarge from the hospital, stress testing (Fig. 7-3) is indicated in patients with NSTE ACS where an initial conservative strategy is selected and for patients with STE MI where coronary angiography was not performed and there has been no recurrent ischemia.[2–4] Following the stress test, patients deemed not at low risk should undergo left heart catheterization with coronary angiography and revascularization as indicated by the results.[3]

Early Pharmacotherapy for STE MIs

Pharmacotherapy for early treatment of ACS is outlined in Figure 7-2 and Table 7-2.[2–5,8] **6** According to the ACCF/AHA STE MI practice guidelines, in addition to reperfusion therapy, other early pharmacotherapy that all patients with STE MI and without contraindications should receive within the first day of hospitalization, and preferably in the emergency department, are intranasal oxygen (if oxygen saturation is low), sublingual (SL) nitroglycerin (NTG), ASA, a $P2Y_{12}$ inhibitor (clopidogrel, prasugrel, or ticagrelor depending on reperfusion strategy), and anticoagulation with bivalirudin, unfractionated heparin (UFH), enoxaparin, or fondaparinux (agent dependent on reperfusion strategy; see Table 7-2). A GP IIb/IIIa inhibitor should be administered with UFH for patients undergoing primary PCI. IV β-blockers and IV NTG should be given in selected patients. Oral β-blockers should be initiated within the first day in patients without cardiogenic shock.[2–4,8] Morphine is administered to patients with refractory angina as an analgesic and a venodilator that lowers preload. These agents should be administered early while the patient is still in the emergency department. An ACE inhibitor is recommended to be administered within the first 24 hours in patients with STE MI who have either an anterior wall MI or an LVEF less than or equal to 40% (0.40) and no contraindications. Dosing and contraindications for SL and IV NTG, ASA, clopidogrel, β-blockers, ACE inhibitors, anticoagulants, and fibrinolytics are listed in Table 7-2.[2–5,8]

Fibrinolytic Therapy

Administration of a fibrinolytic agent is indicated in patients with STE MI who present to the hospital within 12 hours of the onset of chest discomfort, have at least a 1 mm STE in two or more contiguous ECG leads, and are not able to undergo primary PCI within 120 minutes of medical contact.[2] The mortality benefit of fibrinolysis is highest with early administration and diminishes after 12 hours.[30] The use of fibrinolytics between 12 and 24 hours after symptom

TABLE 7-2 Evidence-Based Pharmacotherapy for ST-Segment Elevation Myocardial Infarction and Non–ST-Segment Elevation Acute Coronary Syndrome[2–5,8]

Drug	Brand Name	Clinical Condition and ACCF/AHA/SCAI Guideline Recommendation[a]	Contraindications[b]	Initial or Starting Dose	Usual Range or Maintenance Dose	Special Population Doses	Comments
Aspirin	Aspirin	STE MI, class I recommendation for all patients NSTE ACS, class I recommendation for all patients	Hypersensitivity, active bleeding, severe bleeding risk	160–325 mg orally once on hospital day 1	75–325 mg orally once daily starting hospital day 2, 81 mg preferred, and continued indefinitely in all patients		Limit dose to less than 100 mg orally daily if using ticagrelor Doses of 81 mg daily orally preferred following PCI in combination with a $P2Y_{12}$ inhibitor
Clopidogrel	Plavix	NSTE ACS, class I recommendation added to aspirin STE MI, class I recommendation added to aspirin PCI in STE and NSTE ACS, class I recommendation In patients with aspirin allergy, class I recommendation	Hypersensitivity, active bleeding, severe bleeding risk	300 mg (class I recommendation) to 600 mg (class IIa recommendation) oral loading dose on hospital day 1 followed by a maintenance dose of 75 mg orally daily starting on hospital day 2 in patients with NSTE ACS 300 mg oral loading dose followed by 75 mg orally daily in patients receiving a fibrinolytic or in patients with a STE MI who do not receive reperfusion therapy, avoid loading dose in patients aged 75 years or more 600 mg (class I recommendation) oral loading dose before or when primary PCI performed (unless within 24 hours of fibrinolytic therapy, a dose of 300 mg orally should be given)	75 mg orally once daily		Discontinue at least 5 days before CABG surgery if bleeding risk outweighs benefit (class I recommendation). Discontinue at least 24 hour before urgent on-pump CABG Administer indefinitely in patients with aspirin allergy (class I recommendation) Continue for at least 12 months (class I recommendation) and possibly beyond 12 months (class IIb recommendation) in patients with ACS managed with PCI/stent In patients with NSTE ACS treated medically, administer for 1 month and ideally for 1 year (class I recommendation) In patients receiving a fibrinolytic or who do not receive reperfusion therapy, administer for at least 14 days (class I recommendation) and up to 1 year (class IIa recommendation) Genetic testing might be considered to identify patients at high risk of poor response (class IIb recommendation). In these patients, an alternative $P2Y_{12}$ inhibitor might be considered (class IIb recommendation). The routine use of genetic testing is not recommended (class III recommendation)
Prasugrel	Effient	PCI in STE and NSTE ACS, added to aspirin, class I recommendation	Active bleeding, prior stroke or TIA	60 mg oral loading dose followed by 10 mg orally once daily for patients weighing 60 kg (132 lb) or more	10 mg once daily	60 mg oral loading dose followed by 5 mg once daily in patients weighing less than 60 kg (132 lb)	Initiate in patients with known coronary artery anatomy only (i.e., following coronary angiograph) so as to avoid use in patients needing CABG surgery (class I recommendation) Give no later than 1 hour after PCI Patients who have a history of prior stroke or TIA, are 75 years of age or more, and weigh less than 60 kg (132 lb) have higher risk of bleeding and no added benefit compared with clopidogrel Discontinue at least 7 days prior to CABG surgery if bleeding risk outweighs benefit (class I recommendation) Continue for at least 12 months (class I recommendation) and possibly beyond 12 months (class IIb recommendation) in patients with ACS managed with PCI/stent

(continued)

TABLE 7-2 Evidence-Based Pharmacotherapy for ST-Segment Elevation Myocardial Infarction and Non–ST-Segment Elevation Acute Coronary Syndrome[2–5,8] *(Continued)*

Drug	Brand Name	Clinical Condition and ACCF/AHA/SCAI Guideline Recommendation[a]	Contraindications[b]	Initial or Starting Dose	Usual Range or Maintenance Dose	Special Population Doses	Comments
Ticagrelor	Brilinta	PCI in STE and NSTE ACS, added to aspirin, class I recommendation NSTE ACS, conservative approach, added to aspirin, class I recommendation	Active bleeding, history of intracranial hemorrhage	180 mg (class I recommendation) oral loading dose in patients undergoing PCI, followed by 90 mg orally twice daily	90 mg twice daily		Patients with bradycardia were excluded from clinical trials Current data are too limited to recommend use in patients with STE MI not undergoing primary PCI Discontinue at least 5 days prior to CABG surgery if bleeding risk outweighs benefit (class I recommendation). Discontinue at least 24 hour before urgent on-pump CABG Continue for at least 12 months (class I recommendation) and possibly beyond 12 months (class IIb recommendation) in patients with ACS managed with PCI/stent
Unfractionated heparin		STE MI, class I recommendation in patients undergoing PCI and for those patients treated with fibrinolytics, class IIa recommendation for patients not treated with fibrinolytic therapy NSTE ACS, class I recommendation in combination with antiplatelet therapy for conservative or invasive approach PCI	Active bleeding, history of heparin-induced thrombocytopenia, severe bleeding risk, recent stroke	For STE MI with fibrinolytics, administer 60 units/kg IV bolus (maximum 4,000 units) heparin followed by a constant IV infusion at 12 units/kg/h (maximum 1,000 units/h) For STE MI primary PCI, administer 50–70 units/kg IV bolus if a GP IIb/IIIa inhibitor planned; 70–100 units/kg IV bolus if no GP IIb/IIIa inhibitor planned and supplement with IV bolus doses to maintain target ACT For NSTE ACS, administer 60 units/kg IV bolus (maximum 4,000 units) followed by a constant IV infusion at 1 (maximum 1,000 units/h)			Titrated to ACT of 250–300 seconds (HemoTec device) or 300–350 seconds (Hemochron device) for primary PCI without a GP IIb/IIIa inhibitor and 200–250 seconds in patients given a concomitant GP IIb/IIIa inhibitor The first aPTT should be measured at 4–6 hours for NSTE ACS and STE ACS in patients *not* treated with fibrinolytics or undergoing primary PCI The first aPTT should be measured at 3 hours in patients with STE ACS who are treated with fibrinolytics Continue for 48 hours or until the end of PCI

Enoxaparin	Lovenox	STE MI class I recommendation in patients receiving fibrinolytics and class IIa for patients not undergoing reperfusion therapy NSTE ACS, class I recommendation in combination with aspirin for conservative or invasive approach For PCI, class IIb recommendation as an alternative to UFH in patients with NSTE ACS For primary PCI in STE MI, class IIb recommendation as an alternative to UFH	Active bleeding, history of heparin-induced thrombocytopenia, severe bleeding risk, recent stroke, avoid enoxaparin if CrCl is less than 15 mL/min (less than 0.25 mL/s), avoid if CABG surgery planned	Enoxaparin 1 mg/kg SC every 12 hours for patients with NSTE ACS (CrCl greater than or equal to 30 mL/min) (greater than or equal to 0.50 mL/s) For all patients undergoing PCI following initiation of SC enoxaparin for NSTE ACS, a supplemental 0.3 mg/kg IV dose of enoxaparin should be administered at the time of PCI if the last dose of SC enoxaparin was given 8–12 hours prior to PCI or who received less than two therapeutic SC doses For patients with STE MI receiving fibrinolytics: Age less than 75 years: administer enoxaparin 30 mg IV bolus followed immediately by 1 mg/kg SC every 12 hours (first two doses administer maximum of 100 mg for patients weighing more than 100 kg). Wait 15 minutes between the IV bolus and the SC injection		Enoxaparin 1 mg/kg SC every 24 hours (CrCl 15–29 mL/min) for NSTE or STE MI For patients with STE MI receiving fibrinolytics: Age greater than or equal to 75 years: administer enoxaparin 0.75 mg/kg SC every 12 hours (first two doses administer maximum of 75 mg for patients weighing more than 75 kg)	Continue until end of PCI or throughout hospitalization or up to 8 days Discontinue at least 12–24 hours prior to CABG surgery
Bivalirudin	Angiomax	NSTE ACS class I recommendation for invasive strategy (PCI) PCI in STE MI (Class I recommendation)	Active bleeding, severe bleeding risk	Administer 0.75 mg/kg IV bolus followed by 1.75 mg/kg/h infusion		Dosage adjustment for renal failure: none required in the HORIZONS-AMI trial, but clinical guidelines recommend reducing infusion to 1 mg/kg/h if CrCl less than 30 mL/min	If prior UFH given, discontinue UFH and wait 30 minutes before initiating bivalirudin Discontinue at end of PCI or continue at 0.25 mg/kg/h if prolonged anticoagulation necessary Lower bleeding rates are mitigated when administered with a glycoprotein IIb/IIIa inhibitor Clopidogrel should be administered at least 6 hours before if a glycoprotein IIb/IIIa inhibitor is not used Discontinue at least 3 hours prior to CABG surgery
Fondaparinux	Arixtra	STE MI class I recommendation receiving fibrinolytics and IIa for patients not undergoing reperfusion therapy NSTE ACS class I recommendation for invasive or conservative approach Class III recommendation (i.e., avoid) as sole agent (without UFH) in PCI	Active bleeding, severe bleeding risk, SCr greater than or equal to 3 mg/dL (≥265 μmol/L) or CrCl less than 30 mL/min (less than 0.50 mL/s)	For STE MI, 2.5 mg IV bolus followed by 2.5 mg SC once daily starting on hospital day 2 For NSTE ACS, 2.5 mg SC once daily	2.5 mg SC once daily. Continue until hospital discharge or up to 8 days	Use with caution if CrCl 30–50 mL/min	For PCI, give additional heparin: 85 units/kg IV without a GP IIb/IIIa inhibitor and 60 units/kg IV with a GP IIb/IIIa inhibitor Continue until the end of PCI (used with UFH which is also discontinued), throughout hospitalization (without UFH), or up to 8 days (without UFH) Discontinue at least 24 hours prior to CABG surgery

(continued)

TABLE 7-2 Evidence-Based Pharmacotherapy for ST-Segment Elevation Myocardial Infarction and Non–ST-Segment Elevation Acute Coronary Syndrome[2–5,8] (*Continued*)

Drug	Brand Name	Clinical Condition and ACCF/AHA/SCAI Guideline Recommendation[a]	Contraindications[b]	Initial or Starting Dose	Usual Range or Maintenance Dose	Special Population Doses	Comments
Fibrinolytic therapy Alteplase Reteplase Tenecteplase	 Activase Retavase TNKase	STE MI, class I recommendation for patients presenting within 12 hours following the onset of symptoms, class IIa in patients presenting between 12 and 24 hours following the onset of symptoms with continuing signs of ischemia NSTE ACS, class III recommendation (avoid use)	See Table 7-3	Alteplase: 15 mg IV bolus followed by 0.75 mg/kg IV over 30 minutes (maximum 50 mg) followed by 0.5 mg/kg (maximum 35 mg) over 60 minutes (maximum dose = 100 mg) Reteplase: 10 units IV × 2, 30 minutes apart Tenecteplase: • Less than 60 kg (less than 132 lb) = 30 mg IV bolus • 60–69.9 kg (132–153 lb) = 35 mg IV bolus • 70–80 kg (154–76 lb) = 40 mg IV bolus			
Glycoprotein IIb/IIIareceptor inhibitors Abciximab Eptifibatide Tirofiban	 Reopro Integrilin Aggrastat	NSTE ACS PCI, class I recommendation for abciximab, high-bolus dose tirofiban or double-bolus eptifibatide at the time of PCI in high-risk patients already receiving aspirin and not pretreated with a $P2Y_{12}$ inhibitor and not receiving bivalirudin as the anticoagulant; class IIa at the time of PCI for high-risk patients already receiving aspirin and pretreated with a $P2Y_{12}$ inhibitor; class IIb for upstream use in high-risk patients already receiving aspirin and pretreated with a $P2Y_{12}$ inhibitor and not receiving bivalirudin as the anticoagulant; class I for upstream use in addition to aspirin without $P2Y_{12}$ inhibitor pretreatment for moderate- to high-risk patients	Active bleeding, thrombocytopenia, prior stroke, renal dialysis (eptifibatide)	Abciximab: 0.25 mg/kg IV bolus followed by 0.125 mcg/kg/min (maximum 10 mcg/min) for 12 hours (the bolus dose may be administered IC) Eptifibatide: 180 mcg/kg IV bolus × 2 (maximum 22.6 mg), 10 minutes apart followed by an infusion of 2 mcg/kg/min (maximum 15 mg/h) for 18–24 hours after PCI Tirofiban: 25 mcg/kg IV bolus, and then 0.15 mcg/kg/min up to 18–24 hours after PCI		Abciximab: no adjustment required in the presence of renal dysfunction Eptifibatide: reduce maintenance infusion to 1 mcg/kg/min for CrCl less than 50 mL/min; contraindicated if patient dependent on dialysis Tirofiban: reduce maintenance infusion by 50% for CrCl less than 30 mL/min	

		NSTE ACS for patients not undergoing PCI (conservative medical management), class IIb recommendation STE MI primary PCI, class IIa recommendation for abciximab, high-bolus dose tirofiban or double-bolus eptifibatide in patients receiving UFH					
High-intensity statins Atorvastatin Rosuvastatin	Lipitor Crestor	STE MI Class I recommendation STE MI or NSTE ACS Class IIa recommendation for administration prior to PCI	GI upset, myalgia, myopathy (rare), persistent elevations in LFTs, cognitive impairment (rare), increases in blood glucose and HbA1c levels	Atorvastatin 80 mg orally once daily Rosuvastatin 20 mg orally once daily	Atorvastatin: 10–80 mg orally once daily Rosuvastatin: 5–40 mg once daily		Initiate prior to PCI to reduce incidence of periprocedural MI
Nitroglycerin		STE MI and NSTE ACS, class I recommendation in patients with ongoing ischemic discomfort, control of hypertension or management of pulmonary congestion	Hypotension, sildenafil or vardenafil within 24 hours or tadalafil within 48 hours	0.4 mg SL, repeated every 5 minutes × 3 doses 5–10 mcg/min IV infusion	Titrate up to 75–100 mcg/min until relief of symptoms or limiting side effects (headache) with a systolic blood pressure less than 90 mm Hg or more than 30% below starting mean arterial pressure levels if significant hypertension is present (generally accepted maximum dose: 400 mcg/min)		Topical patches or oral nitrates are acceptable alternatives for patients without ongoing or refractory symptoms Continue IV infusion for 24–48 hours
β-Blockers[c] Metoprolol Propranolol Atenolol	Lopressor Inderal, Inderal LA Tenormin	STE MI and NSTE ACS, class I recommendation for oral β-blockers in all patients without contraindications in the first 24 hours, class IIa for IV β-blockers in hypertensive patients or patients with ongoing ischemia	PR ECG segment greater than 0.24 seconds, two-degree or three-degree atrioventricular heart block Heart rate less than 60 beats/min	Metoprolol: 5 mg slow IV push (over 1–2 minutes), repeated every 5 minutes for a total of 15 mg followed in 1–2 hours by 25–50 mg by mouth every 6 hours; if a very conservative regimen is desired, initial doses can be reduced to 1–2 mg	Metoprolol: 50–100 mg twice daily Propranolol: 180–240 mg in three or four divided doses Atenolol: 50–100 mg once daily	In patients with kidney dysfunction, metoprolol should be preferred over atenolol	Target resting heart rate of 50–60 beats/min Initiation of oral therapy without initial IV therapy preferred. Continue oral β-blocker for at least 3 years in patients without LV dysfunction and indefinitely in patients with LV dysfunction

(continued)

TABLE 7-2 Evidence-Based Pharmacotherapy for ST-Segment Elevation Myocardial Infarction and Non–ST-Segment Elevation Acute Coronary Syndrome[2–5,8] (*Continued*)

Drug	Brand Name	Clinical Condition and ACCF/AHA/SCAI Guideline Recommendation[a]	Contraindications[b]	Initial or Starting Dose	Usual Range or Maintenance Dose	Special Population Doses	Comments
			Systolic blood pressure less than 90 mm Hg, shock, left ventricular failure with congestive heart failure, severe reactive airway disease	Propranolol: 0.5–1 mg IV dose followed in 1–2 hours by 40–80 mg by mouth every 6–8 hours Atenolol: 5 mg IV dose followed in 5 minutes by a second 5 mg IV dose for a total of 10 mg followed in 1–2 hours by 50–100 mg by mouth once daily			
Calcium channel blockers Diltiazem Verapamil Amlodipine	 Cardizem Isoptin Norvasc	STE MI class IIa recommendation and NSTE ACS class I recommendation for patients with ongoing ischemia who are already taking adequate doses of nitrates and β-blockers or in patients with contraindications to or intolerance to β-blockers (diltiazem or verapamil preferred during initial presentation) NSTE ACS, class IIb recommendation for diltiazem for patients with AMI	For all: hypotension For diltiazem and verapamil: PR ECG segment greater than 0.24 second, second- or third-degree atrioventricular heart, pulse rate less than 60 beats/min	Diltiazem: 120 mg sustained release orally once daily Verapamil: 180 mg sustained release orally once daily Amlodipine: 5 mg orally once daily	Diltiazem: 120–360 mg sustained release orally once daily Verapamil: 180–480 mg sustained release orally once daily Amlodipine: 5–10 mg orally once daily		Continue indefinitely if contraindication to oral β-blocker persists
ACE inhibitors Captopril Enalapril Lisinopril Ramipril Trandolapril	 Capoten Vasotec Prinivil, Zestril Altace Mavik	NSTE ACS and STE MI, class I recommendation for patients with heart failure, LV dysfunction and EF less than or equal to 40%, type 2 diabetes mellitus, or CKD in the absence of contraindications Consider in all patients with CAD (class I recommendation, class IIa in low-risk patients) Indicated indefinitely for all patients with EF less than 40% (class I recommendation)	Hypotension, history of intolerance to an ACE inhibitor, bilateral renal artery stenosis, serum potassium greater than 5.5 mEq/L (greater than 5.5 mmol/L), acute renal failure, pregnancy	Captopril: 6.25–12.5 mg three times daily orally Enalapril: 2.5–5 mg twice daily orally Lisinopril: 2.5–5 mg once daily orally Ramipril: 1.25–2.5 mg once or twice daily orally Trandolapril 1 mg once daily orally	Target dose Captopril: 50 mg three times daily Enalapril: 10 twice daily orally Lisinopril: 10–20 mg once daily orally (20–40 mg in HF) Ramipril: 5 mg twice daily or 10 mg once daily orally Trandolapril: 4 mg once daily orally	In the presence of renal dysfunction, initiate a low dose	In patients with HF, ramipril should be given twice daily Continue all ACE inhibitors indefinitely Monitor serum creatinine and potassium carefully (see Table 7-5)

Angiotensin receptor blockers Candesartan Valsartan Losartan	 Atacand Diovan Cozaar	NSTE MI and STE MI, class I recommendation in patients with clinical signs of heart failure or left ventricular EF less than 40% and intolerant of an ACE inhibitor, class IIa recommendation in patients with clinical signs of heart failure or EF less than 40% and no documentation of ACE inhibitor intolerance. Class I recommendation in other ACE inhibitor–intolerant patients with hypertension	Hypotension, bilateral renal artery stenosis, serum potassium greater than 5.5 mEq/L (greater than 5.5 mmol/L), acute renal failure, pregnancy	Candesartan: 4–8 mg once daily orally Valsartan: 40 mg twice daily orally Losartan: 12.5–25 mg once daily orally	Target dose Candesartan: 32 once daily orally Valsartan: 160 twice daily orally Losartan: 150 once daily orally	In the presence of renal dysfunction, start at a low dose	Continue indefinitely Monitor serum creatinine and potassium carefully (see Table 7-5)
Mineralocorticoid receptor antagonists Eplerenone Spironolactone	 Inspra Aldactone	NSTE MI and STE MI class I recommendation in patients with LV EF less than or equal to 40% and either diabetes mellitus or heart failure symptoms who are already receiving an ACE inhibitor	Hypotension, hyperkalemia, serum potassium greater than 5 mEq/L, SCr greater than 2.5 mg/dL (221 μmol/L) and/or CrCl less than 30 mL/min (less than 0.50 mL/s)	Eplerenone: 25 mg once daily orally Spironolactone 12.5 mg once daily orally	Target dose Eplerenone: 50 mg once daily orally Spironolactone 25–50 mg once daily orally		Continue indefinitely Monitor serum creatinine and potassium carefully (see Table 7-5)
Morphine sulfate		STE and NSTE ACS, class I recommendation for patients whose symptoms are not relieved after three serial SL nitroglycerin tablets or whose symptoms recur with adequate antiischemic therapy	Hypotension, respiratory depression, confusion, obtundation	2–4 mg IV bolus dose May be repeated every 5–15 minutes as needed to relieve symptoms and maintain patient comfort			

ACCF, American College of Cardiology Foundation; ACE, angiotensin-converting enzyme; ACS, acute coronary syndrome; ACT, activated clotting time; AHA, American Heart Association; AMI, acute myocardial infarction; aPTT, activated partial thromboplastin time; CABG, coronary artery bypass graft; CAD, coronary artery disease; CKD, chronic kidney disease; CrCl, creatinine clearance; ECG, electrocardiogram; EF, ejection fraction; GP, glycoprotein; HORIZONS-AMI, Harmonizing Outcomes with Revascularization and Stents in Acute Myocardial Infarction; IC, intracoronary; LFTs, liver function tests; LV, left ventricular; MI, myocardial infarction; NSTE, non–ST-segment elevation; PCI, percutaneous coronary intervention; SC, subcutaneous; SCAI, Society for Cardiac Angiography and Interventions; SCr, serum creatinine; SL, sublingual; STE, ST-segment elevation; TIA, transient ischemic attack.

[a]Class I recommendations are those where the benefits greatly exceed risks and the treatment should be administered. Class IIa recommendations are those where the benefit exceeds risks and it is reasonable to administer the treatment. Class IIb recommendations are those where the benefit is equal to or greater than risks and the treatment may be considered. Class III recommendations are those where the treatment may be harmful.
[b]Allergy or prior intolerance contraindication for all categories of drugs listed in this chart.
[c]Choice of the specific agent is not as important as ensuring that appropriate candidates receive this therapy. If there are concerns about patient intolerance due to existing pulmonary disease, especially asthma, selection should favor a short-acting agent, such as metoprolol, or the ultrashort-acting agent, esmolol. Mild wheezing or a history of chronic obstructive pulmonary disease should prompt a trial of a short-acting agent at a reduced dose (e.g., 2.5 mg IV metoprolol, 12.5 mg oral metoprolol, or 25 mcg/kg/min esmolol as initial doses) rather than complete avoidance of β-blocker therapy.

TABLE 7-3 Indications and Contraindications to Fibrinolytic Therapy Per ACC/AHA Guidelines for Management of Patients with ST-Segment Elevation Myocardial Infarction[2]

Indications

1. Ischemic chest discomfort at least 20 minutes in duration but 12 hours or less since symptom onset, **and** ST-segment elevation of at least 1 mm in height in two or more contiguous leads, or new or presumed new left bundle-branch block
2. Ongoing ischemic chest discomfort at least 20 minutes in duration but 12–24 hours since symptom onset, **and** ST-segment elevation of at least 1 mm in height in two or more contiguous leads

Absolute contraindications

- Active internal bleeding (not including menses)
- Previous intracranial hemorrhage at any time; ischemic stroke within 3 months (except ischemic stroke within 4.5 hours)
- Known intracranial neoplasm (primary or metastatic)
- Known structural vascular lesion (e.g., arteriovenous malformation)
- Suspected aortic dissection
- Significant closed head or facial trauma within 3 months
- Intracranial or intraspinal surgery within 2 months
- For streptokinase, prior streptokinase treatment within the previous 6 months

ACC, American College of Cardiology; AHA, American Heart Association.

onset should be limited to patients with ongoing ischemia. Fibrinolytic therapy is preferred over primary PCI where there is no cardiac catheterization laboratory or there would be a delay in "door-to-primary PCI" of more than 90 minutes (of first medical contact) within the institution or 120 minutes (of first medical contact) if the patient is transferred. Indications and contraindications for fibrinolysis are listed in Table 7-3.[2] It is not necessary to obtain the results of biochemical markers before initiating fibrinolytic therapy. Because administration of fibrinolytics results in clot lysis, patients who are at high risk of major bleeding (including ICH) presenting with an absolute contraindication should not receive fibrinolytic therapy, as primary PCI is preferred. In patients who have a contraindication to fibrinolytics and PCI, or who do not have access to a facility that can perform PCIs, treatment with an anticoagulant (other than UFH) for up to 8 days can be administered.

A fibrin-specific agent, such as alteplase, reteplase, or tenecteplase, is preferred over a non–fibrin-specific agent such as streptokinase.[2] Fibrin-specific fibrinolytics open a greater percentage of infarcted arteries. Two trials compared alteplase with reteplase and alteplase with tenecteplase and found similar mortality between agents.[31,32] Therefore, alteplase, reteplase, and tenecteplase are acceptable as first-line agents. ICH and major bleeding are the most serious side effects of fibrinolytic agents. The risk of ICH is higher with fibrin-specific agents than with streptokinase.[17] However, the risk of systemic bleeding other than ICH is higher with streptokinase than with other more fibrin-specific agents and was higher with alteplase versus tenecteplase in one study.[17,30–32]

As mentioned previously, less than 20% of patients with STE MI receive fibrinolysis compared with more than 60% receiving primary PCI. However, 17% of eligible patients receive neither primary PCI nor fibrinolysis despite being eligible. The primary reason for lack of reperfusion therapy is that most patients present more than 12 hours after the time of symptom onset. The percentage of eligible patients who receive reperfusion therapy is a quality performance measure of care in patients with MI.[33] The "door-to-needle time," the time from hospital presentation to start of fibrinolytic therapy, is another quality performance measure.[33] The ACCF/AHA guidelines recommend a "door-to-needle time" of less than 30 minutes from the time of hospital presentation until start of fibrinolytic therapy.[8] The median administration time in the United States in 2006 was 29 minutes, with only 50% of patients meeting the quality performance target of less than 30 minutes.[34] All hospitals should have protocols addressing fibrinolysis eligibility, dosing, and monitoring.

Aspirin

ASA is the preferred antiplatelet agent in the treatment of all ACSs.[2–5,8] ASA administration to all patients who do not have contraindications to ASA therapy within 24 hours before or after hospital arrival is a quality performance measure for MI.[33] The antiplatelet effects of ASA are mediated by inhibiting the synthesis of TXA_2 through an irreversible inhibition of platelet cyclooxygenase-1. In patients undergoing PCI, ASA prevents acute thrombotic occlusion during the procedure. In patients receiving fibrinolytics, ASA reduces mortality, and its effects are additive to fibrinolysis alone.[2,8,35] Additionally, in patients undergoing PCI, ASA, in addition to a $P2Y_{12}$ inhibitor, reduces the risk of stent thrombosis.[5]

In patients experiencing an ACS, an initial dose equal to or greater than 160 mg nonenteric ASA is necessary to achieve a rapid platelet inhibition.[36,37] Current guidelines for STE MI recommend an initial ASA dose of 162 to 325 mg (Table 7-2).[2] This first dose can be chewed in order to achieve high blood concentrations and platelet inhibition rapidly. Preferably, patients undergoing PCI not previously taking ASA should receive 325 mg nonenteric-coated ASA.[5] The notion of chewing ASA came from the use of an enteric-coated formulation of ASA in the Second International Study of Infarct Survival (ISIS-2) trial in order to break the enteric coating to ensure more rapid effect.[35] Current data suggest that although an initial dose of 162 to 325 mg is required, long-term therapy with doses of 75 to 150 mg daily is as effective as higher doses, and therefore a daily maintenance dose of 75 to 162 mg is recommended in most patients to inhibit the 10% of the total platelet pool that is regenerated daily.[37,38] In a large (n = 25,086) randomized trial, high-dose ASA, 300 to 325 mg daily, had similar frequency of CV death, MI, or stroke as well as major bleeding compared with low-dose ASA in the first 30 days following ACS presentation.[39,40] Minor bleeding and GI bleeding were less frequent with low-dose ASA. In this trial, patients undergoing PCI during hospitalization had a lower frequency of death, MI, or stroke, but major bleeding was increased with high-dose ASA.[43] Post hoc analysis from the Harmonizing Outcomes with Revascularization and Stents in Acute Myocardial Infarction (HORIZONS-AMI) trial compared outcomes in patients treated with ASA doses of less than or equal to 200 mg with doses of greater than 200 mg daily and found that higher doses were a predictor of major bleeding but demonstrated similar 3-year risk of CV events.[41] In the Study of Platelet Inhibition and Patient Outcomes (PLATO), a randomized, double-blind clinical trial comparing ticagrelor with clopidogrel in patients receiving ASA, a post hoc analysis suggested that maintenance doses of ASA above 100 mg daily reduced the effectiveness of ticagrelor.[42] Because of increased bleeding risk in patients receiving ASA plus a $P2Y_{12}$ inhibitor compared with ASA alone, low-dose ASA (81 mg daily) is preferred following PCI.[5,43] Low-dose ASA should be continued indefinitely.[43]

Nonsteroidal antiinflammatory agents other than ASA, as well as cyclooxygenase-2 (COX-2) selective antiinflammatory agents, should be discontinued at the time of STE MI secondary to increased risk of death, reinfarction, HF, and myocardial rupture.[8]

The most frequent side effects of ASA are dyspepsia and nausea. Patients should be counseled about the risk of bleeding, especially GI bleeding, with ASA.

Platelet $P2Y_{12}$ Inhibitors

Clopidogrel, prasugrel, and ticagrelor block a subtype of ADP receptor, the $P2Y_{12}$ receptor, on platelets, preventing the binding of ADP to the receptor and subsequent expression of platelet GP IIb/IIIa receptors, reducing platelet activation and aggregation. Both clopidogrel and prasugrel are thienopyridines and prodrugs that are

TABLE 7-4 Pharmacokinetics of Clopidogrel, Prasugrel, and Ticagrelor[44–46]

	Clopidogrel	Prasugrel	Ticagrelor
Pharmacologic class	Thienopyridine	Thienopyridine	Cyclopentyl-triazolo-pyrimidine
ADP receptor binding	Irreversible	Irreversible	Reversible
Absorption and metabolism	Prodrug Inactive metabolite SR266334 Active metabolite R-130946 Metabolism to R-130946 is primarily by CYP2C19, 3A4, 2B6, and 1A2, with lesser contributions from CYP2C9 Exposure to the active metabolite is affected by CYP2C19 and possibly ATP-binding cassette B1 (ABCB1) transporter (also called P-glycoprotein) polymorphism Rapid conversion of the parent drug to active metabolite (mean time to peak plasma concentration of active metabolite approximately 1 hour)	Prodrug Active metabolite R-138727 Metabolism to R-138727 is primarily via CYP3A4 and CYP2B6 Exposure to the active metabolite is not affected by CYP2C19 and 2C9 polymorphism Rapid conversion of the parent drug to active metabolite (median time to peak plasma concentration of active metabolite approximately 30 minutes)	Active moiety, bioavailability 36% Active metabolite AR-C124910XX ~30–40% activity of parent compound Metabolism is primarily via CYP3A4/5 Exposure to the active metabolite is not affected by CYP2C19 and 2C9 polymorphism Rapid conversion of the parent drug to active metabolite (median time to peak plasma concentration of active metabolite 2.5 hours)
Food effect	According to one report in healthy volunteers, bioavailability of inactive metabolite concentrations unaffected by food; one report in healthy volunteers of clopidogrel demonstrated t_{max} delayed by 1.5 hours, C_{max} increased sixfold, and bioavailability increased ninefold	Fasting administration preferred; C_{max} is reduced by 49% and t_{max} delayed 0.5–1.5 hours when administered with high-fat, high-calorie meal, although AUC is unaffected	May be taken with or without food; no effect on C_{max} and 21% increase in AUC when administered with high-fat, high-calorie meal. Decrease in C_{max} by 22% and no effect on AUC of active metabolite when administered with high-fat, high-calorie meal
Disposition	Linear pharmacokinetics at doses of 50–150 mg	Linear pharmacokinetics at doses up to 75 mg	Linear pharmacokinetics at doses up to 600 mg daily
Elimination	Elimination half-life of active metabolite is approximately 30 minutes after a 75 mg dose Excretion is 50% urinary and 46% fecal	Median elimination half-life of the active metabolite approximately 7.4 hours Excretion is primarily urinary (approximately 70%); fecal excretion less than 30%	Median elimination half-life of the parent compound is approximately 7 hours and that of active metabolite approximately 9 hours Excretion is primarily metabolism (84%); fecal excretion 58%, urinary excretion 26%
Labeled drug interactions and suggested management of interaction	Enhanced bleeding with NSAIDs: avoid use Enhanced bleeding with warfarin: monitor carefully for bleeding; target INR to 2–2.5 for most indications Avoid use with moderate or strong CYP2C19 inhibitors (e.g., omeprazole, esomeprazole, chloramphenicol, cimetidine, efavirenz, etravirine, felbamate, fluoxetine, fluconazole, fluvoxamine, isoniazid, oxcarbazine, ketoconazole, voriconazole); select alternative noninteracting $P2Y_{12}$ inhibitor or alternative noninteracting drug	Enhanced bleeding with warfarin and NSAIDs: avoid use	Enhanced bleeding with warfarin and NSAIDs Use aspirin doses less than or equal to 100 mg daily Avoid use with strong CYP3A inhibitors (atazanavir, clarithromycin, indinavir, itraconazole, nefazodone, nelfinavir, ketoconazole, ritonavir, saquinavir, telithromycin, voriconazole) Avoid use with potent CYP3A inducers (carbamazepine, dexamethasone, phenobarbital, phenytoin, rifampin) Avoid simvastatin and lovastatin doses greater than 40 mg daily (ticagrelor inhibits CYP3A4 and increases statin concentration) Monitor digoxin serum concentrations with any change in ticagrelor dose (ticagrelor inhibits P-glycoprotein)

ADP, adenosine diphosphate; ATP, adenosine triphosphate; AUC, area under the curve; CYP, cytochrome P450; INR, international normalized ratio; NSAIDs, nonsteroidal antiinflammatory drugs.

converted to an active metabolite by a variety of cytochrome P450 (CYP) isoenzymes (Table 7-4).[44–46]

Both of these agents bind irreversibly to $P2Y_{12}$ receptor. Ticagrelor, which is not a thienopyridine, is a reversible, noncompetitive $P2Y_{12}$ receptor inhibitor. Ticagrelor parent compound has antiplatelet effects and is also metabolized primarily by CYP3A to an active metabolite producing its antiplatelet effects.

Both prasugrel and ticagrelor are more potent ADP inhibitors than clopidogrel. Prasugrel has the fewest significant drug–drug interactions. The production of clopidogrel's active metabolite and consequently its antiplatelet effect is reduced by moderate and strong inhibitors of CYP2C19, while ticagrelor's concentration is reduced by strong inhibitors of CYP3A. Labeled drug interactions are described in Table 7-4. A more detailed discussion of the interaction between clopidogrel and proton pump inhibitors may be found in Chapter 6.

A considerable amount of data support that genetic variations in the gene coding for *CYP2C19* significantly modulate the antiplatelet effects of clopidogrel. Specifically, carriers of reduced-function allele (i.e., *2 or *3) are not able to convert clopidogrel to its active metabolite in comparison to carriers of the wild-type allele. This results in decreased antiplatelet effects,[47] as well as higher rates of CV events, especially stent thrombosis and MI around the time of PCI.[48] Prasugrel is not as dependent on *CYP2C19* genotype for its conversion to the active metabolite and has a lower frequency of poor antiplatelet responsiveness.[49] Moreover, current data suggest that the benefit of prasugrel compared with clopidogrel may only be apparent in carriers of these reduced-function alleles,[49] whereas the benefits of ticagrelor over clopidogrel may be unrelated to *CYP2C19*.[50] Hence, ticagrelor or prasugrel may be considered preferred agents in carriers of *CYP2C19* reduced-function alleles.

Although the product labeling for clopidogrel suggests that genetic testing and alternative therapy should be selected for patients who are *CYP2C19* poor metabolizers,[44] the most recent clinical practice guidelines of the ACCF/AHA/SCAI have not endorsed routine genotyping to guide the prescription of $P2Y_{12}$ inhibitors because no prospective randomized clinical study has demonstrated the benefit of such a genotype-based prescribing approach.[5]

Administration of a $P2Y_{12}$ receptor inhibitor, in addition to ASA, is recommended for all patients with STE MI.[2,8] For STE MI undergoing primary PCI, clopidogrel, prasugrel, or ticagrelor, in addition to ASA, should be administered to prevent subacute stent thrombosis and longer-term CV events (Table 7-2).[2,5] Although not FDA approved, a clopidogrel loading dose of 600 mg is recommended over administration of 300 mg for patients undergoing PCI.[5] A systematic review and meta-analysis of randomized and nonrandomized trials in more than 25,000 patients demonstrated a reduction in CV ischemic events with a loading dose of 600 mg compared with 300 mg in patients undergoing PCI.[51]

In the most recent ACCF/AHA/SCAI PCI practice guidelines, no preference is given for one agent over the other. Nevertheless, clinical trials comparing these agents have highlighted distinct clinical differences between these antiplatelet agents.

A large randomized, double-blind study demonstrated that, compared with clopidogrel, the addition of prasugrel to ASA for patients undergoing PCI in the setting of STE MI or NSTE ACS significantly reduced risk of CV death or MI by 19% (9.9% vs. 12.1%), as well as MI and stent thrombosis, but increased the risk of major bleeding (not ICH) by 32% (2.4% vs. 1.8%).[52] Patients with a history of prior stroke or transient ischemic attack (TIA) had an increased risk of ICH and no net clinical benefit from prasugrel, and the product label lists prior stroke or TIA as a contraindication to prasugrel.[45,52] Patients older than 75 years and those weighing less than 60 kg (132 lb) are at increased risk of bleeding with prasugrel compared with clopidogrel.[52] Two subgroups of patients do not have an increased bleeding risk with prasugrel compared with clopidogrel and have even greater benefit, namely, patients undergoing primary PCI for STE MI and patients with a history of diabetes mellitus (DM).[53,54]

PLATO compared ticagrelor with clopidogrel in patients receiving ASA and presenting with either STE MI or NSTE ACS and undergoing an intended interventional management strategy with PCI or conservative noninterventional management strategy with medical therapy alone. In this trial, ticagrelor significantly reduced the rate of the CV death, MI, stroke, and stent thrombosis compared with clopidogrel.[55] Although no increase in study-defined major bleeding was noted with ticagrelor, the frequency of non-CABG major bleeding was increased compared with clopidogrel. As with the prasugrel trial described, several subgroups of patients enrolled in this trial had particular benefit with ticagrelor, including those with an intended invasive approach, those with an intended noninvasive approach, patients with STE MI primary PCI, and patients with DM.[56–59] Therefore, both of the more potent $P2Y_{12}$ inhibitors are more efficacious than clopidogrel but may also be associated with an increased risk of bleeding. No large randomized trial has directly compared ticagrelor and prasugrel. Figure 7-4 outlines the role of the newer $P2Y_{12}$ inhibitors in ACS compared with clopidogrel.[60]

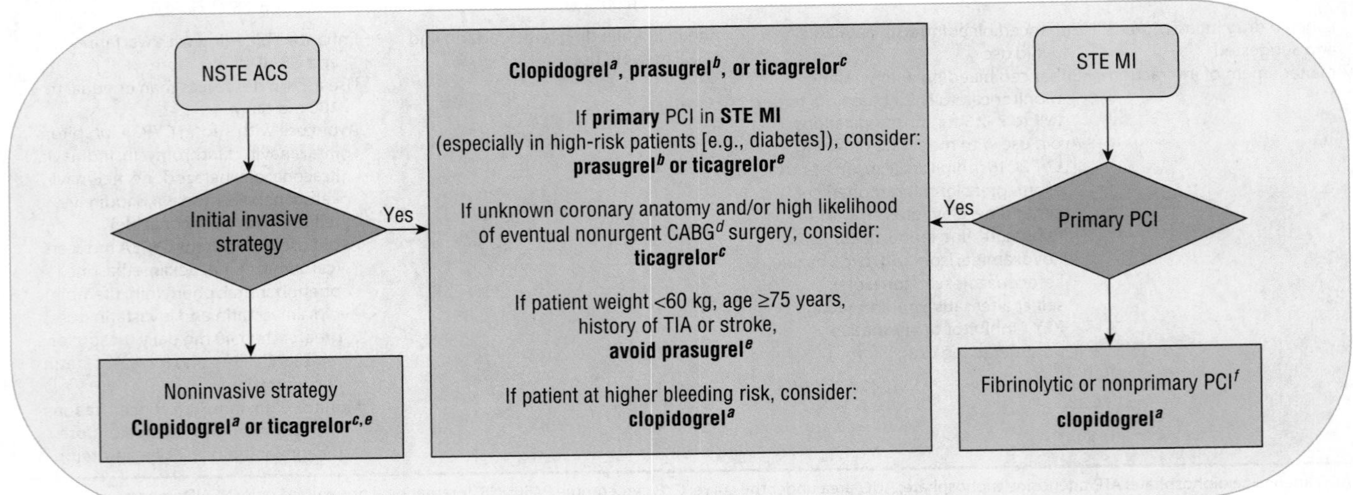

FIGURE 7-4 Proposed use of $P2Y_{12}$ inhibitors. [a]Do not use clopidogrel in patients with active pathologic bleeding; consider alternative $P2Y_{12}$ receptor inhibitor if documented clopidogrel ineffectiveness (e.g., poor metabolism, stent thrombosis during clopidogrel therapy) or drug–drug interactions (e.g., avoid moderate and strong CYP2C19 inhibitors); clopidogrel should be held for at least 5 days before CABG surgery, if the surgery can be delayed. [b]Do not use prasugrel in patients with active pathologic bleeding or a history of transient ischemic attack or stroke; if a patient subsequently goes on to receive CABG surgery, the drug should be held for at least 7 days if the surgery can be delayed. [c]Do not use ticagrelor in patients with active pathologic bleeding or a history of intracranial hemorrhage, or in patients planned to undergo urgent CABG surgery; concomitant maintenance aspirin dose above 100 mg should be avoided; dose of ticagrelor should be held for 5 days before CABG surgery, if the surgery can be delayed; when selecting this agent, consider patient compliance (dosed twice daily), unique adverse effects (e.g., dyspnea), and potential drug–drug interactions (e.g., avoid strong CYP3A inhibitors/inducers). [d]Prior to diagnostic angiography, it is difficult to determine the likelihood that an individual patient will receive CABG surgery; notable variables that predict this occurrence include previous CABG, male gender, previous heart failure, presence of diabetes, and previous percutaneous coronary intervention, among others. [e]Recommendation based on subgroup analysis. [f]At this time, there are insufficient data to support ticagrelor or prasugrel in the "fibrinolytic or nonprimary PCI" patient group. (ACS, acute coronary syndrome; CABG, coronary artery bypass graft; MI, myocardial infarction; NSTE, non–ST-segment elevation; PCI, percutaneous coronary intervention; STE, ST-segment elevation; TIA, transient ischemic attack.) *(Adapted from Crouch MA, Colucci VJ, Howard PA, Spinler SA. P2Y12 receptor inhibitors: Integrating ticagrelor into management of acute coronary syndrome. Ann Pharmacother 2011;45:1151–1156. Reprinted by Permission of SAGE Publications.)*

The recommended duration of $P2Y_{12}$ inhibitors for a patient undergoing PCI for ACS, either STE MI or NSTE ACS, is at least 12 months for patients receiving either a bare metal or a drug-eluting stent.[2,5] The benefit of prolonging treatment beyond 12 months is uncertain.[2,5] Nonadherence to $P2Y_{12}$ inhibitors is a major risk factor for stent thrombosis, and hence the likelihood of adherence to dual antiplatelet therapy (ASA and a $P2Y_{12}$ inhibitor) should be assessed prior to angiography.[5] The use of a bare metal stent over a drug-eluting stent should be considered in patients who are anticipated to be nonadherent to 12 months of dual antiplatelet therapy.[5]

To minimize the risk of CV events, elective noncardiac surgery should be delayed to more than 4 to 6 weeks after angioplasty or bare metal stent implantation, or 12 months after drug-eluting stent implantation if the discontinuation of the $P2Y_{12}$ inhibitor is required.[5] If CABG surgery is planned, clopidogrel and ticagrelor should be withheld preferably for 5 days, and prasugrel at least 7 days, to reduce the risk of postoperative bleeding, unless the need for revascularization outweighs the bleeding risk.[2]

Although a variety of blood tests can assess functional platelet aggregation inhibition to $P2Y_{12}$ inhibitors, especially clopidogrel, there is no one gold standard test. Moreover, despite using a higher maintenance dose of clopidogrel (150 mg daily) in patients with a high level of on-treatment platelet aggregation (low platelet aggregation inhibition) that resulted in improved platelet aggregation inhibition, dosing of clopidogrel via platelet aggregation testing does not result in improved clinical outcomes.[61] Therefore, the most recent PCI practice guidelines (2011) do not recommend routine platelet aggregation testing to determine $P2Y_{12}$ inhibitor strategy.[5]

The most frequent side effects of clopidogrel and prasugrel are nausea, vomiting, and diarrhea, which occur in approximately 2% to 5% of patients.[44,45] Rarely, thrombotic thrombocytopenic purpura (TTP) has been reported with clopidogrel.[44] In addition to nausea (4%) and diarrhea (3%), use of ticagrelor is associated with dyspnea (14%) and, rarely, ventricular pauses and bradyarrhythmias. Patients at risk of bradycardia were excluded from PLATO.[46] Small nonclinically significant increases in SCr and serum uric acid have also been reported with ticagrelor.[46]

In patients receiving fibrinolysis, early therapy with clopidogrel 75 mg once daily administered during hospitalization and up to 28 days (mean: 14 days) in patients with STE MI reduced mortality and reinfarction in patients treated with fibrinolytics without increasing the risk of major bleeding.[8,62,63] In adult patients younger than 75 years of age receiving fibrinolytics, the first dose of clopidogrel can be a 300 mg loading dose.[8,63] Although prasugrel and ticagrelor have been studied in the setting of PCI, no studies have evaluated their use when added to both ASA and a fibrinolytic.

Clopidogrel is currently the ACCF/AHA guideline–preferred $P2Y_{12}$ inhibitor added to ASA and should be continued for at least 14 days (and up to 1 year) for patients presenting with STE MI who do not undergo reperfusion therapy with either primary PCI or fibrinolysis.[2,62] However, recent subgroup analysis from PLATO suggests that ticagrelor may also be an option in medically managed patients with ACS not receiving fibrinolysis because the frequency of CV death, MI, or stroke as well as mortality was lower in ticagrelor-treated patients compared with those receiving clopidogrel (Fig. 7-4).[56,60] Ticagrelor use was not associated with a higher bleeding rate compared with clopidogrel.[56]

Clinical **Controversy. . .**

PERSONALIZED MEDICINE OF $P2Y_{12}$ INHIBITORS

In the last decade, a significant amount of information has been published with regard to the association of genetic factors with the antiplatelet response to clopidogrel.[47,64,65] Specifically, a great amount of evidence indicates that patients carrying a reduced or loss-of-function allele of the gene coding for *CYP2C19*, one of the isoenzymes implicated in the conversion of clopidogrel to its active metabolite, have a higher risk of CV events following an ACS, particularly those undergoing PCI. These data do not extend to other populations of patients receiving clopidogrel. Nevertheless, despite these extensive data, the most recent AHA/ACCF guideline does not endorse routine genotyping in patients receiving an ADP $P2Y_{12}$ inhibitor.[7] On the other hand, guidelines from the Clinical Pharmacogenetics Implementation Consortium (CPIC) recommend the use of genotyping in all patients with an ACS or undergoing PCI for whom clopidogrel is being prescribed.[66] The guideline specifically stressed that clopidogrel should not be given to intermediate or poor metabolizers (those carrying one or two *CYP2C19*2* alleles) and should be replaced by an alternative such as prasugrel. These inconsistencies between two professional organizations reflect differences in their level of evidence to evaluate the data. The AHA/ACCF guideline is primarily based on results from large, randomized controlled trials demonstrating a superiority of an approach before it can be strongly endorsed, whereas CPIC focused more on consistent results from well-designed clinical studies to give strong recommendations.

In the past, pharmacogenetic testing often involved lengthy waits for results to become available and thus lacked utility for clinical decision making at the time a patient was experiencing an ACS event. More recently, a simple rapid point-of-care assay demonstrated 100% sensitivity and 99% specificity for identifying patients with the *CYP2C19*2* allele demonstrating high on-treatment platelet reactivity.[65] This test utilizes a buccal swab and takes no longer than 8 minutes for results to become available. A recent randomized controlled study using this rapid pharmacogenetic assay suggested that a genotype-guided approach may be useful to select between antiplatelet agents, but was limited by a small sample size, and the use of surrogate CV end points.[65] Many have argued that the level of evidence to use these pharmacogenomic markers in clinical practice constitutes genetic exceptionalism as the level of evidence required to use these markers in clinical practice to guide therapy is considerably higher than the data used to adjust medication doses based on renal function or drug–drug interactions, for example.[67,68]

Glycoprotein IIb/IIIa Receptor Inhibitors

GP IIb/IIIa receptor inhibitors block the final common pathway of platelet aggregation, namely, cross-linking of platelets by fibrinogen bridges between the GP IIb and IIIa receptors on the platelet surface. In patients with STE MI undergoing primary PCI who are treated with UFH, abciximab (IV or intracoronary administration), eptifibatide, or tirofiban may be administered.[5] Routine use of a GP IIb/IIIa receptor inhibitor is not recommended in patients who have received fibrinolytics or in those receiving bivalirudin secondary to increased bleeding risk. GP IIb/IIIa inhibitors should not be administered for medical management of the patient with STE MI who will not be undergoing PCI.[2,8] A meta-analysis of STE MI primary PCI trials demonstrated no reduction in mortality or 30-day reinfarction but increased risk of major bleeding with GP IIb/IIIa inhibitors compared with control.[69] Although there are more clinical trial data with abciximab for primary PCI compared with the small-molecule GP IIb/IIIa inhibitors eptifibatide and tirofiban, the small-molecule agents are used more commonly in clinical practice. A meta-analysis found no difference in efficacy and safety between abciximab and the small-molecule GP IIb/IIIa inhibitors.[70]

Dosing and contraindications for GP IIb/IIIa inhibitors are described in Table 7-2. Bleeding is the most significant adverse effect associated with administration of GP IIb/IIIa inhibitors. GP IIb/IIIa inhibitors should not be administered to patients with a prior history of hemorrhagic stroke or recent ischemic stroke. The risk of bleeding is increased in patients with chronic kidney disease. Eptifibatide is contraindicated in patients dependent on dialysis and requires a reduced infusion dose in patients with creatinine clearance (CrCl) less than 50 mL/min (0.83 mL/s).[71] The STE MI PCI guideline–recommended dosing for tirofiban is not a FDA-approved regimen but one that has been studied in more contemporary clinical trials.[5,72] The dose of tirofiban should be halved in patients with CrCl less than 30 mL/min (0.50 mL/s).[73] No dosage adjustment for renal function is necessary for abciximab. An immune-mediated thrombocytopenia occurs in approximately 5% of patients with abciximab and less than 1% of patients receiving eptifibatide or tirofiban.[74]

Anticoagulants

Options for anticoagulant therapy for patients with STE MI are outlined in Figure 7-2 and Table 7-2.[2,5] For patients undergoing primary PCI, either UFH or bivalirudin is preferred, whereas for fibrinolysis, UFH, enoxaparin, or fondaparinux may be administered.[2] For patients undergoing PCI, anticoagulation is discontinued immediately following the PCI procedures. In patients receiving an anticoagulant plus a fibrinolytic, UFH is continued for a minimum of 48 hours and if either enoxaparin or fondaparinux is selected, those agents are continued for the duration of hospitalization, up to 8 days.[8] In patients who do not undergo reperfusion therapy, it is reasonable to administer anticoagulant therapy for up to 48 hours for UFH or for the duration of hospitalization for enoxaparin or fondaparinux.[2]

UFH has been the traditional anticoagulant administered to patients with STE MI to prevent reocclusion of an infarct artery for more than 50 years. The results of a meta-analysis of more than 7,500 patients suggest that low-molecular-weight heparins (LMWHs) reduce both mortality and reinfarction compared with placebo in patients treated with fibrinolytics and ASA.[75] In a randomized open-label clinical trial of primary PCI for STE MI, bivalirudin, a direct thrombin inhibitor, significantly reduced the frequency of CV mortality by 45% (2.9% vs. 5.1%) and all-cause mortality by 25% (5.9% vs. 7.7%) at 3 years of followup while lowering the risk of in-hospital major bleeding events by 40% (4.9% vs. 8.3%) compared with UFH plus a GP IIb/IIIa inhibitor (abciximab, eptifibatide, or tirofiban).[76,77] Therefore, bivalirudin has similar or greater efficacy but better safety than UFH in the setting of primary PCI.

In patients with STE MI treated with fibrinolytics, enoxaparin, administered for a median of 7 days, has shown a reduction in the risk of death or nonfatal MI but increased bleeding risk compared with UFH administered for a median of 2 days in a large randomized clinical trial.[78] Enoxaparin dosing is adjusted for body weight and renal function, and when administered in combination with fibrinolysis, it has special dosing requirements for older patients and those weighing more than 100 kg (Table 7-2).

Besides bleeding, the most serious adverse effect of UFH and enoxaparin is *heparin-induced thrombocytopenia*. ACS registry data indicate, however, that the frequency of heparin-induced thrombocytopenia is rare (less than 0.5%).[79] Bivalirudin would be a preferred anticoagulant for patients with a history of heparin-induced thrombocytopenia undergoing PCI.[2,5]

β-Blockers

A β-blocker should be administered early in the care of patients with STE MI and continued indefinitely. In ACS, the benefit of β-blockers results mainly from the competitive blockade of β_1-adrenergic receptors located on the myocardium. β_1-Blockade produces a reduction in heart rate (HR), myocardial contractility, and blood pressure (BP), decreasing myocardial oxygen demand. In addition, the reduction in HR increases diastolic time, thus improving ventricular filling and coronary artery perfusion. As a result of these effects, β-blockers reduce the risk for recurrent ischemia, infarct size, risk of reinfarction, and occurrence of ventricular arrhythmias in the hours and days following MI.

Landmark clinical trials have established the role of early β-blocker therapy in reducing MI mortality. Most of these trials were performed in the 1970s and 1980s before routine use of early reperfusion therapy.[80,81] However, data regarding the acute benefit of β-blockers in MI in the reperfusion era are derived mainly from a single large clinical trial that suggests that although initiating IV followed by oral β-blockers early in the course of STE MI was associated with a lower risk of reinfarction or ventricular fibrillation, there may be an early risk of cardiogenic shock, especially in patients presenting with pulmonary congestion or systolic BP less than 120 mm Hg.[82] Therefore, initiation of β-blockers, particularly when administered IV, should be limited to patients who present with hypertension (HTN) and/or have ongoing signs of myocardial ischemia and do not demonstrate any signs or symptoms of acute HF.[2] Careful assessment for signs of hypotension and HF should be performed following β-blocker initiation and prior to any dose titration. Patients already taking β-blockers can continue taking them.[8] The Joint Commission and Centers for Medicare & Medicaid Services retired the "Beta Blocker at Hospital Arrival" (acute myocardial infarction [AMI]-6 Core Measure) in 2009 and is no longer requiring hospital reporting of this measure.[83]

The most serious side effects of β-blocker administration early in ACSs are hypotension, acute HF, bradycardia, and heart block. Although initial acute administration of β-blockers is not appropriate for patients who present with acute HF, initiation of β-blockers may be attempted before hospital discharge in most patients following treatment of acute HF. β-Blockers should be continued for at least 3 years in patients with normal LV function and indefinitely in patients with LV systolic dysfunction and an LVEF less than or equal to 40% (0.40).[43]

Statins

A high-intensity statin (either atorvastatin 80 mg or rosuvastatin 40 mg) should be administered to all patients prior to PCI (regardless of prior lipid-lowering therapy) to reduce the frequency of periprocedural MI (a Type IVa MI) following PCI.[5,15]

Nitrates

One SL NTG tablet should be administered every 5 minutes for up to three doses in order to relieve myocardial ischemia. If patients have been previously prescribed SL NTG and ischemic chest discomfort persists for more than 5 minutes after the first dose, the patient should be instructed to contact emergency medical services before self-administering subsequent doses to activate emergency care sooner. IV NTG should then be initiated in all patients with an ACS who have persistent ischemia, HF, or uncontrolled high BP in the absence of contraindications.[2] IV NTG should be continued for approximately 24 hours after ischemia is relieved (Table 7-2). Nitrates promote the release of nitric oxide from the endothelium, which results in venous and arterial vasodilation. Venodilation lowers preload and myocardial oxygen demand. Arterial vasodilation may lower BP, thus reducing myocardial oxygen demand. Arterial vasodilation also relieves coronary artery vasospasm, dilating coronary arteries to improve myocardial blood flow and oxygenation. Although used to treat ACS, nitrates have been suggested to play a limited role in the treatment of ACS patients because two large randomized clinical trials failed to show a mortality benefit for IV nitrate therapy followed by oral nitrate therapy in acute MI.[84,85] The most significant adverse effects of nitrates are tachycardia, flushing, headache, and hypotension. Nitrate administration is contraindicated in patients who have received oral phosphodiesterase-5 inhibitors, such as sildenafil and vardenafil, within the last 24 hours, and tadalafil within the last 48 hours.[2]

Calcium Channel Blockers

Calcium channel blockers in the setting of STE MI are used for relief of ischemic symptoms in patients who have certain contraindications to β-blockers. Current data suggest little benefit on clinical outcomes beyond symptom relief for calcium channel blockers in the setting of ACS.[2] Therefore, calcium channel blockers should be avoided in the acute management of all ACSs unless there is a clear symptomatic need or a contraindication to β-blockers. Agent selection is based on presenting HR and LVF. Administration of an agent that lowers HRs, either diltiazem or verapamil, is preferred unless the patient has LV systolic dysfunction, bradycardia, or heart block, and then either amlodipine or felodipine is preferred.[8] Nifedipine should be avoided because it has demonstrated reflex sympathetic activation, tachycardia, and worsened myocardial ischemia.[2] Dosing and contraindications are described in Table 7-2.

Early Pharmacotherapy for NSTE ACSs

In general, early pharmacotherapy of NSTE ACS (Fig. 7-3) is similar to that of STE MI. In the absence of contraindications, all patients with NSTE ACS should be treated in the emergency department with intranasal oxygen (if oxygen saturation is low), SL NTG, ASA, and an anticoagulant: UFH, enoxaparin, fondaparinux, or bivalirudin. High-risk patients should proceed to early angiography and may receive a GP IIb/IIIa inhibitor (optional with either UFH or enoxaparin but should be avoided with bivalirudin). **7** A $P2Y_{12}$ inhibitor (selection of agent and timing of initiation dependent on selection of an interventional approach involving PCI or CABG surgery vs. a noninterventional approach with medical management alone) should be administered to all patients. IV β-blockers and IV NTG should be given in selected patients. Oral β-blockers should be initiated within the first 24 hours in patients without cardiogenic shock.[2–4] Morphine is also administered to patients with refractory angina as described previously. These agents should be administered early while the patient is still in the emergency department. Fibrinolytic therapy is never administered. Dosing and contraindications for SL and IV NTG (for selected patients), ASA, $P2Y_{12}$ inhibitors, β-blockers, and anticoagulants are listed in Table 7-2.

Fibrinolytic Therapy

Fibrinolytic therapy is not indicated in any patient with NSTE ACS because increased mortality has been reported with fibrinolytics compared with controls in clinical trials in which fibrinolytics have been administered to patients with NSTE ACS (patients with normal or ST-segment depression ECGs).[4]

Aspirin

ASA reduces the risk of death or developing MI by about 50% (compared with no antiplatelet therapy) in patients with NSTE ACS.[38] Therefore, ASA remains the cornerstone of early treatment for all ACS. Dosing of ASA for NSTE ACS is the same as that for STE MI (Table 7-2). Low-dose ASA is continued indefinitely.

Anticoagulants

The choice of anticoagulant for a patient with NSTE ACS is guided by risk stratification and initial treatment strategy, either an early invasive approach with early coronary angiography and PCI or an early conservative strategy with angiography in selected patients guided by relief of symptoms and stress testing (Fig. 7-3). For patients treated by an early invasive strategy, UFH, enoxaparin, or bivalirudin should be administered.[4,5] In a large open-label randomized clinical trial evaluating bivalirudin versus UFH or enoxaparin plus a GP IIb/IIIa inhibitor (abciximab, eptifibatide, or tirofiban) in moderate- and high-risk patients with NSTE ACS undergoing an early invasive strategy, bivalirudin demonstrated similar efficacy in preventing CV ischemic events but a lower bleeding rate.[86] Similarly, in a smaller randomized trial specifically comparing abciximab plus UFH with bivalirudin for patients with NSTE MI undergoing PCI, bivalirudin demonstrated no differences in clinical outcomes but a lower bleeding risk.[87]

In patients in whom an initial conservative strategy is planned (i.e., they are not anticipated to receive coronary angiography and revascularization), enoxaparin, UFH, or low-dose fondaparinux is recommended.[3,4] UFH and LMWH when added to ASA reduce the frequency of death or MI in patients presenting with NSTE ACS compared with control/placebo in patients primarily managed with a conservative strategy.[88,89] Compared with enoxaparin, fondaparinux showed similar ischemic outcomes with a lower bleeding rate in a large randomized trial of patients with NSTE ACS primarily managed with a conservative strategy.[90] If fondaparinux is chosen for a patient initially receiving a conservative strategy who subsequently undergoes angiography and PCI, it should be administered in combination with UFH (and not as the sole anticoagulant) because the dose of fondaparinux studied appears too low to prevent thrombotic events during PCI.[5] Neither fondaparinux nor bivalirudin is FDA approved for NSTE ACS despite being recommended by the ACCF/AHA NSTE ACS guidelines. Bivalirudin has not been studied for initial therapy in patients intended to receive a conservative management strategy. Guideline-recommended dosing and contraindications are described in Table 7-2.

Therapy should be continued for up at least 48 hours for UFH, until the patient is discharged from the hospital (or 8 days, whichever is shorter) for either enoxaparin or fondaparinux, or until the end of PCI or angiography procedure (or up to 72 hours following PCI for bivalirudin).[4,5] UFH is the preferred anticoagulant following angiography in patients subsequently undergoing CABG during the same hospitalization because it has a short duration of action following discontinuation when the patient is proceeding to surgery.[2,4] Because enoxaparin is eliminated renally and patients with renal insufficiency generally have been excluded from clinical trials, some practice protocols recommend UFH for patients with CrCl rates of less than 30 mL/min (0.50 mL/s) based on total patient body weight using the Cockroft-Gault equation.[3] Although recommendations for dosing adjustment of enoxaparin in patients with CrCl between 10 and 30 mL/min (0.27 and 0.50 mL/s) are listed in the product manufacturer's label, the safety and efficacy of enoxaparin in this patient population remain vastly understudied. Administration of enoxaparin should be avoided in dialysis patients with ACS. It is unclear whether or not bivalirudin requires dose adjustment for patients with significant renal dysfunction. Although bivalirudin is eliminated renally, the duration of infusion in recent trials has been short (several hours only), and therefore the actual need for dosing adjustment is unlikely. Practice guidelines recommend manufacturer's suggested dosing adjustment for patients with chronic kidney disease.[5] Patients with SCr greater than 3 mg/dL (265 μmol/L) were excluded from ACS trials with fondaparinux, and the product label states that fondaparinux is contraindicated in patients with CrCl less than 30 mL/min (0.50 mL/s) and in patients weighing less than 50 kg (110 lb).

UFH is monitored and the dose adjusted to a target activated partial thromboplastin time (aPTT), whereas enoxaparin is administered by a fixed actual body weight–based dose without routine monitoring of anti–factor Xa levels. Some experts recommend anti–factor Xa monitoring for LMWHs in patients with renal impairment during prolonged courses of administration of more than several days. No monitoring of coagulation is recommended for bivalirudin and fondaparinux.

$P2Y_{12}$ Inhibitors

Figure 7-4 delineates the role of different $P2Y_{12}$ inhibitors in ACS. For patients with NSTE ACS where an initial invasive management strategy is selected, two initial options for dual antiplatelet therapy are described by the practice guidelines depending on choice of $P2Y_{12}$ inhibitor. In addition to ASA administered either prehospital or in the emergency department, either of the following is recommended:

1. Early use of clopidogrel or ticagrelor (in the emergency department)[4]
2. Double-bolus dose eptifibatide plus an eptifibatide infusion or high-dose tirofiban bolus plus infusion administered at the time of PCI.[4] (Bivalirudin should not be administered as the anticoagulant in this option.)[4]

Subsequent antiplatelet therapy following PCI is selected based on the coronary anatomy at the time of angiography. For patients undergoing PCI initially treated with regimen 1 above, a GP IIb/IIIa inhibitor (abciximab, eptifibatide, or high-dose tirofiban) can be added, and then clopidogrel or ticagrelor continued with low-dose ASA. For patients undergoing PCI initially treated with option 2, clopidogrel, prasugrel, or ticagrelor can be selected following PCI (within 1 hour following PCI) and the $P2Y_{12}$ inhibitor continued with low-dose ASA. In a subgroup of patients undergoing PCI enrolled in a large clinical trial evaluating clopidogrel versus placebo added to ASA in patients with NSTE ACS, clopidogrel reduced the frequency of death or MI by 30%.[91] In the large pivotal trials of prasugrel versus clopidogrel and ticagrelor versus clopidogrel (PLATO), no added benefit of the newer $P2Y_{12}$ inhibitors was observed in the subgroup of patients with NSTE ACS undergoing PCI.[52,55] Following PCI in ACS, dual oral antiplatelet therapy is continued for at least 12 months.[2,5]

For patients receiving an initial conservative treatment strategy, the 2012 ACCF/AHA NSTE ACS guidelines recommend early administration of either clopidogrel or ticagrelor in addition to ASA.[4] The subgroup of medically managed patients in a large trial of clopidogrel in patients with NSTE ACS demonstrated a 20% reduction in the risk of CV death, MI, or stroke compared with ASA alone, a benefit similar to that seen in patients undergoing PCI.[92] Ticagrelor is an alternative in medically managed patients as described in the section Early Pharmacotherapy for STE MIs above.[56,60] Dual antiplatelet therapy is continued for at least 12 months.[5]

Specific dosing and contraindications of the $P2Y_{12}$ inhibitors are described in Table 7-2.

Glycoprotein IIb/IIIa Receptor Inhibitors

The role of GP IIb/IIIa inhibitors in NSTE ACS is diminishing as $P2Y_{12}$ inhibitors are used earlier in therapy, and bivalirudin is selected more commonly as the anticoagulant in patients receiving an early intervention approach. See $P2Y_{12}$ Inhibitors above, which includes the selection and timing of GP IIb/IIIa inhibitors in patients with NSTE ACS undergoing PCI.[4,5] Routine administration of eptifibatide (added to ASA and clopidogrel) prior to angiography and PCI (i.e., "upstream" use) in NSTE ACS does not reduce ischemic events and increases bleeding risk compared to placebo.[93] Therefore, the two antiplatelet initial therapy options, described in the previous section, are preferred.[4,5]

For low-risk patients where a conservative management strategy is selected, there is no role for routine GP IIb/IIIa inhibitors as the bleeding risk exceeds the benefit.[4] For patients in whom an initial conservative strategy was selected but who experience recurrent ischemia (chest discomfort and ECG changes), HF, or arrhythmias after initial medical therapy necessitating a change in strategy to angiography and revascularization, a GP IIb/IIIa inhibitor may be added to ASA and clopidogrel prior to the angiogram.[4,93]

Doses and contraindications to GP IIb/IIIa receptor inhibitors are described in Table 7-2.

Nitrates

SL NTG followed by IV NTG should be administered to patients with NSTE ACS and ongoing ischemia, HF, or uncontrolled high BP (Table 7-2). The mechanism of action, dosing, contraindications, and adverse effects are the same as those described in Early Pharmacotherapy for STE MIs above. IV NTG is typically continued for approximately 24 hours following ischemia relief.

β-Blockers

The use of β-blockers in NSTE ACS is similar to that in STE MI in that oral β-blockers should be initiated within 24 hours of hospital admission to all patients in the absence of contraindications. Benefits of β-blockers in this patient group are assumed to be similar to those seen in patients with STE MI. β-Blockers are continued indefinitely in patients with LVEF less than or equal to 40% (0.40) and for at least 3 years in patients with normal LV function.[43]

Calcium Channel Blockers

As described in the previous section, calcium channel blockers should not be administered to most patients with ACS. Their role is a second-line treatment for patients with certain contraindications to β-blockers and those with continued ischemia despite β-blocker and nitrate therapy. Agent selection for NSTE ACS is identical to that for STE MI with either diltiazem or verapamil preferred unless the patient has LV systolic dysfunction, bradycardia, or heart block, and then either amlodipine or felodipine is preferred. Nifedipine is contraindicated.[4]

Secondary Prevention Following MI

The long-term goals following MI are to (a) control modifiable CHD risk factors; (b) prevent the development of systolic HF; (c) prevent recurrent MI and stroke; (d) prevent death, including sudden cardiac death; and (e) prevent stent thrombosis following PCI. Pharmacotherapy, which has been proven to decrease mortality, HF, reinfarction or stroke, and stent thrombosis, should be initiated prior to hospital discharge for secondary prevention. Secondary prevention guidelines from the ACCF/AHA suggest that following MI, from either STE MI or NSTE ACS, all patients, in the absence of contraindications, should receive indefinite treatment with ASA, an ACE inhibitor, and a "high-intensity" statin for secondary prevention of death, stroke, or recurrent infarction.[43] (8) A β-blocker should be continued for at least 3 years in patients without HF or an ejection fraction (EF) of less than or equal to 40% (0.40) and indefinitely in patients with LV systolic dysfunction or HF symptoms.[43] A $P2Y_{12}$ inhibitor should be continued for at least 12 months for patients undergoing PCI and for patients with NSTE ACS receiving a medical management strategy of treatment.[2,5] Clopidogrel should be continued for at least 14 days in patients with STE MI not undergoing PCI.[8] An ARB and a MRA should be given to selected patients as discussed in greater detail later in the chapter.[2,43] For all patients with ACS, treatment and control of modifiable risk factors such as HTN, dyslipidemia, obesity, smoking, and DM are essential.[43] Dosing and contraindications are described in detail in Table 7-2. Benefits and adverse effects of long-term treatment with these medications are discussed in more detail later. Use of ICDs for the prevention of sudden cardiac death following MI in patients with diminished LVF and nonsustained ventricular arrhythmias is discussed in more detail in Chapter 8.

Aspirin

ASA decreases the risk of death, recurrent infarction, and stroke following MI. All patients should receive ASA indefinitely; those patients with a contraindication to ASA should receive clopidogrel.[43] The risk of major bleeding from chronic ASA therapy is approximately 2% and is dose related. Higher doses of ASA, 160 to 325 mg, are not more effective than ASA doses of 75 to 81 mg but have higher rates of bleeding.[94] Even in the setting of PCI, low-dose ASA (75 to 100 mg daily) was found to be equally safe and efficacious compared with higher doses of ASA (300 to 325 mg daily) in a prespecified subgroup analysis of 30-day outcomes in a large randomized, double-blind clinical trial of patients with ACS who underwent PCI.[42] (All patients received an initial dose on presentation to hospital of at least 300 mg.) Therefore, chronic doses of ASA should not exceed 81 mg.[2,5,43]

$P2Y_{12}$ Inhibitors

For patients with either STE MI or NSTE ACS, clopidogrel decreases the risk of CV events and stent thrombosis compared with placebo. Compared with clopidogrel, either prasugrel or ticagrelor lowers the risk of CV death, MI, or stroke by an additional 20% to 30% depending on the patient population studied. The frequency of stent thrombosis following PCI is also lower with prasugrel or ticagrelor compared with clopidogrel. However, the rate of non-CABG surgery-associated bleeding is higher with both prasugrel and ticagrelor compared with clopidogrel. For all patients with ACS, a $P2Y_{12}$ inhibitor should be continued for at least 1 year.[2–5,8] The ACCF/AHA/SCAI PCI guidelines recommend that for patients with ACS, a $P2Y_{12}$ inhibitor (clopidogrel, prasugrel, or ticagrelor) should be continued for at least 1 year following PCI.[5] For medically managed patients with STE MI, clopidogrel should be continued for at least 14 days and up to 1 year.[8] For medically managed NSTE ACS patients, clopidogrel or ticagrelor should be continued for up to 1 year.[4]

The combination of clopidogrel and ASA increases the risk of major bleeding by approximately 50% and minor bleeding by approximately 40% but not fatal bleeding compared with single agent alone.[95] Compared with clopidogrel, ticagrelor increased the risk of major bleeding not related to CABG surgery by 18% in a large randomized comparative trial of patients presenting with ACS and undergoing either PCI or medical management while prasugrel increased major bleeding by 33% compared with clopidogrel in a pivotal trial of patients with ACS undergoing PCI.[52,55] Oral antiplatelet agents are the third leading cause of adverse drug reaction–associated hospital admissions after emergency department visits among senior citizens.[96] Therefore, patients should be counseled on the risks and sites of potential bleeding and should be told to seek medical care immediately if significant bleeding is noticed. Lower-weight patients (less than or equal to 60 kg) and elderly patients are at higher risk of bleeding with prasugrel or ticagrelor compared with clopidogrel.[97,98] Prasugrel is contraindicated in patients with a prior history of stroke as the risk of ICH is increased with prasugrel compared with clopidogrel.[52,98]

Clinical **Controversy...**

TRIPLE ORAL ANTITHROMBOTIC THERAPY

Patients with ACS undergoing PCI and intracoronary stent placement with either a bare metal stent or a drug-eluting stent are managed with dual antiplatelet therapy that reduces stent thrombosis risk and reinfarction risk.[5] But what antithrombotic therapy is best for patients with a chronic or new indication for longer-term anticoagulant therapy following hospital discharge such as atrial fibrillation, the presence of a mechanical heart valve, venous thromboembolism, or left ventricular thrombus?

Which combination of antithrombotic agents is best to maximize efficacy while decreasing bleeding risk? A meta-analysis of nonrandomized controlled clinical trials suggests a significant reduction in all-cause mortality at a cost of increased major bleeding with triple antithrombotic therapy (ASA, clopidogrel, and an oral vitamin K antagonist) compared with dual antiplatelet therapy alone (ASA plus clopidogrel).[99] Current practice guidelines, a North American consensus statement, recommend triple antithrombotic therapy (warfarin, low-dose ASA, and clopidogrel) for 1 to 6 months for patients following PCI with a bare metal stent placement and between 6 and 12 months for patients following PCI with a drug-eluting stent placement, depending on bleeding risk. Thereafter, a single antiplatelet agent, either clopidogrel or low-dose ASA, is recommended in addition to warfarin.[100]

Only one randomized trial, the *W*hat is the *O*ptimal Antiplatelet and Anticoagulant Therapy in Patients with Oral Anticoagulation and Coronary *St*enting (WOEST) trial, has been published.[101] In this open-label study, patients undergoing PCI who were chronically treated with an oral vitamin K antagonist were randomized to receive clopidogrel alone or clopidogrel plus low-dose ASA 80 to 100 mg/day. The target international normalized ratio (INR) of anticoagulation was that recommended based on the indication. At 1-year followup, the primary end point, any bleeding episode was increased more than twofold in patients randomized to triple therapy compared with clopidogrel plus anticoagulation (44.4% vs. 19.4%, $P < 0.0001$). GI bleeding was the most common type of bleeding and was increased threefold by ASA (2.9% in patients receiving anticoagulation plus clopidogrel vs. 8.8% in patients receiving triple therapy). Therefore, consideration should be given to stopping ASA in patients receiving triple therapy as is an option in the practice guidelines recommended above.

The manufacturers of prasugrel and ticagrelor recommend against combining those $P2Y_{12}$ inhibitors with an oral anticoagulant due to a lack of data as well as clinical experience. Therefore, when triple therapy is needed, clopidogrel should be selected as the $P2Y_{12}$ inhibitor. Also, both rivaroxaban and apixaban have increased bleeding risk, including increased ICH risk when combined with ASA plus clopidogrel in patients with ACS, and there is no information on long-term treatment with dabigatran, ASA, and clopidogrel, and therefore warfarin should be selected as the anticoagulant of choice when triple antithrombotic therapy is needed.[102,103] While both the North American Consensus Document and the ACCF/AHA practice guidelines recommend a tighter warfarin INR range goal of 2 to 2.5 in patients receiving triple antithrombotic therapy, no clinical trial has prospectively tested this more stringent goal.[2,100]

In summary, triple antithrombotic therapy, when needed, should consist of warfarin (INR target 2 to 2.5), low-dose ASA 81 mg orally daily, and clopidogrel 75 mg orally daily. The anticoagulant should be discontinued if possible (such as in 3 to 6 months post-MI in patients at risk of left ventricular thrombus but without actual thrombi present), and then either clopidogrel or preferably ASA, discontinued after at least 1 month in a patient with a bare metal stent and after at least 6 months in a patient with a drug-eluting stent. Concomitant use of a proton pump inhibitor is recommended in patients receiving triple therapy undergoing PCI.[5]

β-Blockers, Nitrates, and Calcium Channel Blockers

Current treatment guidelines recommend that following an ACS, patients should receive a *β*-blocker for at least 3 years following MI in the absence of left ventricular dysfunction and regardless of whether they have residual symptoms of angina or not.[2,43] Patients with or without HF and LVEF less than or equal to 40% should receive a *β*-blocker indefinitely. Overwhelming data support the use of *β*-blockers in patients with a previous MI.[104] Currently, there are no data to support the superiority of one *β*-blocker over another in the absence of HF.

Although *β*-blockers should be avoided in patients with decompensated HF from left ventricular systolic dysfunction complicating an MI, clinical trial data suggest it is safe to initiate *β*-blockers prior to hospital discharge in these patients once HF symptoms have resolved.[105] These patients may actually benefit more than those without left ventricular dysfunction.[106] In patients who cannot tolerate or have a contraindication to a *β*-blocker, a calcium channel blocker can be used to prevent anginal symptoms but should not be used routinely in the absence of such symptoms.[2,4,107]

Finally, all patients should be prescribed short-acting, SL NTG or lingual NTG spray to relieve any anginal symptoms when necessary and instructed on its use.[107] Chronic long-acting nitrate therapy has not been shown to reduce CHD events following MI. Therefore, IV NTG is not routinely followed by chronic, long-acting oral nitrate therapy in ACS patients who have undergone revascularization, unless the patient has chronic stable angina or significant coronary stenoses that were not revascularized.[107]

ACE Inhibitors and ARBs

ACE inhibitors should be initiated in all patients following MI to reduce mortality, decrease reinfarction, and prevent the development of HF.[2–5,8,43] The benefit of ACE inhibitors in patients with MI most likely comes from their ability to prevent cardiac remodeling. The largest reduction in mortality is observed in patients with left ventricular dysfunction (low LVEF) or HF symptoms. Early initiation (within 24 hours) of an *oral* ACE inhibitor appears to be crucial during an acute MI because 40% of the 30-day survival benefit is observed during the first day, 45% from days 2 to 7, and approximately 15% from days 8 to 30.[108] However, current data do not support the early administration of IV ACE inhibitors in patients experiencing an MI because mortality may be increased.[109] Administration of ACE inhibitors should be continued indefinitely. Hypotension should be avoided because coronary artery filling may be compromised. Additional trials suggest that most patients with CAD, not just ACS or HF patients, benefit from ACE inhibitors. Therefore, ACE inhibitors should be considered in all patients following an ACS in the absence of a contraindication.

Many patients cannot tolerate chronic ACE inhibitor therapy secondary to adverse effects. The ARBs, candesartan, valsartan, and losartan, have been documented in trials to improve clinical outcomes in patients with HF.[110,111] Therefore, either an ACE inhibitor or candesartan, valsartan, or losartan is an acceptable choice for chronic therapy for patients who have a low LVEF and HF following MI. Besides hypotension, the most frequent adverse reaction to an ACE inhibitor is cough, which may occur in up to 30% of patients. Patients with an ACE inhibitor cough and either clinical signs of HF or LVEF less than 40% (0.40) may be prescribed an ARB.[43] Other, less common but more serious adverse effects to ACE inhibitors and ARBs include acute renal failure, hyperkalemia, and angioedema.

Mineralocorticoid Receptor Antagonists

To reduce mortality, administration of a MRA, either eplerenone or spironolactone, should be considered within the first 7 days following MI in all patients who are already receiving an ACE inhibitor (or ARB) and a *β*-blocker and have an LVEF of equal to or less than 40% (0.40) and either HF symptoms or DM.[2,43] Aldosterone plays an important role in HF and in MI because it promotes vascular and myocardial fibrosis, endothelial dysfunction, HTN, left ventricular hypertrophy, sodium retention, potassium and magnesium loss, and arrhythmias. MRAs have been shown in experimental and human studies to attenuate these adverse effects.[112] Spironolactone decreases all-cause mortality in patients with stable, severe HF.[113]

Eplerenone, like spironolactone, is an aldosterone antagonist that blocks the mineralocorticoid receptor. In contrast to spironolactone, eplerenone has no effect on the progesterone or androgen receptor, thereby minimizing the risk of gynecomastia, sexual dysfunction, and menstrual irregularities. In a large clinical trial,[114] eplerenone significantly reduced mortality as well as hospitalization for HF in post-MI patients with an LVEF less than 40% (0.40) and symptoms of HF at any time during hospitalization. Eplerenone has also been demonstrated to reduce mortality in patients with mild systolic HF.[115] The risk of hyperkalemia, however, was increased in both these studies. Patients with a SCr greater than 2.5 mg/dL (221 μmol/L) or CrCl less than 30 mL/min or serum potassium concentration of greater than 5 mmol/L (5 mEq/L) should not receive an MRA. Currently, there are no data to support that the more selective, more expensive eplerenone is superior to, or should be preferred to, the less expensive generic spironolactone unless a patient has experienced gynecomastia, breast pain, or impotence while receiving spironolactone.

Lipid-Lowering Agents

Following MI, statins reduce total mortality, CV mortality, and stroke. According to the National Cholesterol Education Program (NCEP) Adult Treatment Panel and the AHA secondary prevention of MI guidelines, all patients with CAD should receive dietary counseling and a statin in order to reach a low-density lipoprotein (LDL) cholesterol of less than 100 mg/dL (2.59 mmol/L) at a dose to reduce LDL cholesterol by 30%.[43,116] Results from landmark clinical trials have unequivocally demonstrated the value of statins in secondary prevention following MI. A meta-analysis of randomized controlled clinical trials in almost 18,000 patients with recent ACS (less than 14 days) found that statin therapy reduces mortality by 19%, with benefits observed after approximately 4 months of treatment.[117] Although the primary effect of statins is to decrease LDL cholesterol, statins are believed to produce many non–lipid-lowering or "pleiotropic" effects such as antiinflammatory and antithrombotic properties. Additional recommendations from the NCEP and AHA give an optional LDL cholesterol goal of less than 70 mg/dL (1.81 mmol/L).[118] The current evidence indicates that higher-dose statin therapy, such as atorvastatin 40 to 80 mg daily and rosuvastatin 10 to 20 mg daily, produces greater reduction in CV events such as MI, ischemic stroke, and revascularization than less intensive statin regimens (such as simvastatin 20 to 40 mg daily).[119] Moreover, the administration of high-dose statins prior to PCI reduces the risk of periprocedural MI and, hence, statins should be initiated as early as possible in ACS.[2,5]

Whether or not additional therapies such as ezetimibe, a fibrate derivative, niacin, or fish oil should be added to a statin in patients with an elevated non–high-density lipoprotein (non-HDL) cholesterol level or LDL cholesterol level despite maximally tolerated statin therapy or maximally dosed statin remains controversial as the benefits of this management strategy remain largely unproven.[43,120] In a large randomized trial of men with established CAD and low levels of HDL cholesterol, the use of gemfibrozil (600 mg twice daily, alone and not added to a statin) significantly decreased the risk of nonfatal MI or death from coronary causes.[121] Studies with fenofibrate and niacin have produced less definitive results.[122,123]

Other Modifiable Risk Factors

Smoking cessation, managing HTN, weight loss, exercise, and tight glucose control for patients with DM, in addition to treatment of dyslipidemia, are important treatments for secondary prevention of CHD events.[43] Referral to a comprehensive CV risk reduction program for cardiac rehabilitation is recommended.[43] The use of nicotine patches or gum, or of bupropion alone or in combination with nicotine patches, should be considered in appropriate patients.[8,43] HTN should be strictly controlled according to published guidelines.[43] Patients who are overweight should be educated on the importance of regular exercise, healthy eating habits, and reaching and maintaining an ideal weight. Moderate-intensity aerobic exercise for at least 30 minutes, 7 days/wk (minimum 5 days/wk) is recommended.[43] The goal body mass index is less than 25 kg/m^2. Finally, because patients with DM have up to a fourfold increased mortality risk compared with patients without DM, the importance of blood glucose control, as well as other CHD risk factor modifications, cannot be overstated.[43]

OUTCOME EVALUATION

To determine the efficacy of nonpharmacologic therapy and pharmacotherapy for both STE and NSTE ACS, monitor patients for: (a) relief of ischemic discomfort; (b) return of ECG changes to baseline; and (c) absence or resolution of HF signs and symptoms.

Monitoring parameters for recognition and prevention of adverse effects from ACS pharmacotherapy are described in Table 7-5. (9) In general, the most common adverse reactions from

TABLE 7-5 Therapeutic Drug Monitoring for Adverse Effects of Pharmacotherapy for Acute Coronary Syndromes

Drug	Adverse Effects	Monitoring
Aspirin	Dyspepsia, bleeding, gastritis	Clinical signs of bleeding,[a] GI upset; baseline CBC and platelet count; CBC platelet count every 6 months
Clopidogrel and prasugrel	Bleeding, diarrhea, rash, TTP (rare)	Clinical signs of bleeding[a]; baseline CBC and platelet count; CBC and platelet count every 6 months following hospital discharge
Ticagrelor	Bleeding, dyspnea, diarrhea, rash, elevated SCr, elevated serum uric acid	Clinical signs of bleeding[a]; baseline CBC and platelet count; CBC and platelet count every 6 months following hospital discharge
Unfractionated heparin	Bleeding, heparin-induced thrombocytopenia	Clinical signs of bleeding[a]; baseline aPTT, INR, CBC, and platelet count; aPTT every 6 hours until target, and then every 24 hours; daily CBC; platelet count every 2–3 days from days 4 to 14 until heparin is stopped (minimum, preferably every day)
Enoxaparin	Bleeding, heparin-induced thrombocytopenia	Clinical signs of bleeding[a]; baseline SCr, aPTT, INR, CBC, and platelet count; daily CBC, no routine platelet count monitoring unless recent UFH (less than 100 days), and then baseline and within 24 hours; daily CBC and SCr
Fondaparinux	Bleeding	Clinical signs of bleeding[a]; baseline SCr, aPTT, INR, CBC, and platelet count; daily CBC and SCr
Bivalirudin	Bleeding	Clinical signs of bleeding[a]; baseline SCr, aPTT, INR, CBC, and platelet count
Fibrinolytics	Bleeding, especially intracranial hemorrhage	Clinical signs of bleeding[a]; baseline aPTT, INR, CBC, and platelet count; mental status every 2 hours for signs of intracranial hemorrhage; daily CBC
Glycoprotein IIb/IIIa receptor inhibitors	Bleeding, acute profound thrombocytopenia	Clinical signs of bleeding[a]; baseline SCr (for eptifibatide and tirofiban), CBC, and platelet count; platelet count at 4 hours after initiation; daily CBC (and SCr for eptifibatide and tirofiban)
IV nitrates	Hypotension, flushing, headache, tachycardia	BP and HR every 2 hours
β-Blockers	Hypotension, bradycardia, heart block, bronchospasm, acute heart failure, fatigue, depression, sexual dysfunction	BP, RR, HR, 12-lead ECG, and clinical signs of heart failure every 5 minutes during bolus IV dosing; BP, RR, HR, and clinical signs of heart failure every shift during oral administration during hospitalization, and then BP and HR every 6 months following hospital discharge
Diltiazem and verapamil	Hypotension, bradycardia, heart block, heart failure, gingival hyperplasia	BP and HR every shift during oral administration during hospitalization, and then every 6 months following hospital discharge; dental examination and teeth cleaning every 6 months
Amlodipine	Hypotension, dependent peripheral edema, gingival hyperplasia	BP every shift during oral administration during hospitalization, and then every 6 months following hospital discharge; dental examination and teeth cleaning every 6 months
Angiotensin-converting enzyme (ACE) inhibitors and angiotensin receptor blockers (ARBs)	Hypotension, cough (with ACE inhibitors), hyperkalemia, prerenal azotemia, acute renal failure, angioedema (ACE inhibitors more so than ARBs)	BP every 4 hours × 3 for first dose, then every shift during oral administration during hospitalization, and then once every 6 months following hospital discharge; baseline SCr and potassium; daily SCr and potassium while hospitalized, and then every 6 months (or 1–2 weeks after each outpatient dose titration); closer monitoring required in selected patients using spironolactone or eplerenone or if renal insufficiency; counsel patient on throat, tongue, and facial swelling
Mineralocorticoid receptor antagonists	Hypotension, hyperkalemia, increased SCr	BP and HR every shift during oral administration during hospitalization, and then once every 6 months; baseline SCr and serum potassium concentration; SCr and potassium at 48 hours, at 7 days, then monthly for 3 months, and then every 3 months thereafter following hospital discharge
Morphine	Hypotension, respiratory depression	BP and RR 5 minutes after each bolus dose
Statins	GI upset, myopathy, hepatotoxicity	Liver function tests at baseline; counsel patient on myalgia; consider creatinine kinase at baseline if adding a fibrate or niacin

ACE, angiotensin-converting enzyme; aPTT, activated partial thromboplastin time; BP, blood pressure; CBC, complete blood count; ECG, electrocardiogram; HR, heart rate; INR, international normalized ratio; RR, respiratory rate; SCr, serum creatinine, TTP, thrombotic thrombocytopenic purpura.

[a]Clinical signs of bleeding include bloody stools, melena, hematuria, hematemesis, bruising, and oozing from arterial or venous puncture sites.

TABLE 7-6 Process of Care Quality Performance Measures for Myocardial Infarction[33,83]

- Median time to initial ECG (desired is less than or equal to 10 minutes)[a]
- Aspirin at hospital arrival[a,b]
- Fibrinolytic medication within 30 minutes of hospital arrival for STE MI ("door-to-needle" time)[a,b]
- Median time to fibrinolysis[a]
- PCI received within 90 minutes of hospital arrival for STE MI[a,b]
- Median time to transfer to another facility for PCI ("door-in to door-out time" desired is less than or equal to 30 minutes)[a,b]
- Percentage of eligible patients with STE MI receiving reperfusion therapy with either fibrinolytics or PCI[b]
- Aspirin at hospital discharge[a,b]
- ACE inhibitor or ARB for systolic dysfunction at hospital discharge[a,b]
- *β*-Blocker at hospital discharge[a,b]
- Smoking cessation advice/counseling[a,b]
- Statin at hospital discharge[b]
- Evaluation of LV function[b]
- Cardiac rehabilitation referral[b]

ACE, angiotensin-converting enzyme; ARB, angiotensin receptor blocker; ECG, electrocardiogram; LV, left ventricular; MI, myocardial infarction; PCI, percutaneous coronary intervention; STE, ST-segment elevation.

[a]2010 Center for Medicare and Medicaid Services process of care measures for myocardial infarction.
[b]American Heart Association 2008 myocardial infarction performance measure.

ACS therapies are hypotension and bleeding. To treat for bleeding and hypotension, discontinue the offending agent(s) until symptoms resolve. Severe bleeding resulting in hypotension secondary to hypovolemia may require blood transfusion.

Because poor medication adherence of secondary prevention medications following MI leads to worsened CV outcomes, patients should receive medication counseling (including counseling prior to hospital discharge) and be monitored for medication persistence.[2,5,124] Counseling should include assessment of health literacy level, assessment of barriers to adherence, assessment of access to medications, written and verbal instructions about the purpose of each medication, changes to previous medication regimen, optimal time to take each medication, new allergies or medication intolerances, need for timely prescription fill after discharge, anticipated duration of therapy, consequences of nonadherence, common and/or serious adverse reactions that may develop, drug–drug and drug–food interactions, and an assessment of instruction understanding.

Process of care quality performance measures for MI endorsed by the AHA and Centers for Medicare and Medicaid Services is described in Table 7-6.[33,83]

ABBREVIATIONS

ACCF	American College of Cardiology Foundation
ACE	angiotensin-converting enzyme
ACS	acute coronary syndrome
ADP	adenosine diphosphate
AHA	American Heart Association
AMI	acute myocardial infarction
aPTT	activated partial thromboplastin time
ARB	angiotensin receptor blocker
ASA	aspirin
BP	blood pressure
CABG	coronary artery bypass graft
CAD	coronary artery disease
CBC	complete blood count
CHD	coronary heart disease
CK	creatine kinase
COX-2	cyclooxygenase-2
CPIC	Clinical Pharmacogenetics Implementation Consortium
CrCl	creatinine clearance
CV	cardiovascular
CVD	cardiovascular disease
CYP	cytochrome P450
DM	diabetes mellitus
ECG	electrocardiogram
EF	ejection fraction
GP	glycoprotein
GWTG	Get with the Guidelines
HDL	high-density lipoprotein
HF	heart failure
HORIZONS-AMI	Harmonizing Outcomes with Revascularization and Stents in Acute Myocardial Infarction
HR	heart rate
HTN	hypertension
ICD	implantable cardioverter-defibrillator
ICH	intracranial hemorrhage
INR	international normalized ratio
ISIS-2	Second International Study of Infarct Survival
LDL	low-density lipoprotein
LMWH	low-molecular-weight heparin
LVEF	left ventricular ejection fraction
LVF	left ventricular function
MB	myocardial band
MI	myocardial infarction
MRA	mineralocorticoid receptor antagonist
NCEP	National Cholesterol Education Program
NSTE	non–ST-segment elevation
NTG	nitroglycerin
PCI	percutaneous coronary intervention
PLATO	Study of Platelet Inhibition and Patient Outcomes
SCAI	Society for Cardiovascular Angiography and Interventions
SCr	serum creatinine
SL	sublingual
STE	ST-segment elevation
TIA	transient ischemic attack
TTP	thrombotic thrombocytopenic purpura
TXA_2	thromboxane A_2
UA	unstable angina
UFH	unfractionated heparin
WOEST	What is the *O*ptimal Antiplat*e*let and Anticoagulant Therapy in Patients with Oral Anticoagulation and Coronary *St*enting

REFERENCES

1. Go AS, Mozaffarian D, Roger VL. Heart disease and stroke statistics—2013 update: A report from the American Heart Association. Circulation 2013;127:e6–e245.
2. O'Gara PT, Kushner FG, Ascheim DD, et al. 2013 ACCF/AHA guideline for the management of ST-elevation myocardial infarction: A report of the American College of Cardiology Foundation/American Heart Association Task Force on Practice Guidelines. J Am Coll Cardiol 2013;61:e78–e140.
3. Anderson JL, Adams CD, Antman AM, et al. ACC/AHA 2007 guidelines for the management of patients with unstable angina/non ST-elevation myocardial infarction: A report of the American College of Cardiology/American Heart Association Task Force on Practice Guidelines (Writing Committee to Revise the 2002 Guidelines for the

Management of Patients with Unstable Angina/Non ST-Elevation Myocardial Infarction): Developed in collaboration with the American College of Emergency Physicians, the Society for Cardiovascular Angiography and Interventions, and the Society of Thoracic Surgeons: Endorsed by the American Association of Cardiovascular and Pulmonary Rehabilitation and the Society for Academic Emergency Medicine [Erratum. Circulation 2008;117(9):e180]. Circulation 2007;116:e148–e304.

4. Jneid H, Andersen JL, Wright RS, et al. 2012 ACCF/AHA focused update of the guideline for the management of patients with unstable angina/non–ST-elevation myocardial infarction (updating the 2007 guideline and replacing the 2011 focused update): A report of the American College of Cardiology Foundation/American Heart Association Task Force on Practice Guidelines. Circulation 2012;126: 875–910.
5. Levine GN, Bates ER, Blankeship JC, et al. 2011 ACCF/AHA/SCAI guideline for percutaneous coronary intervention: A report of the American College of Cardiology Foundation/American Heart Association Task Force on Practice Guidelines and the Society for Cardiovascular Angiography and Interventions. J Am Coll Cardiol 2011;58:e44–e122.
6. U.S. Department of Health & Human Services. Calculation of 30-Day Risk Standardized Mortality Rates and Rates of Readmission. *http://www.cms.gov/Medicare/Quality-Initiatives-Patient-Assessment-Instruments/HospitalQualityInits/OutcomeMeasures.html.*
7. Borissoff JI, Spronk HMH, ten Cate H. The hemostatis system as a modulator of atherosclerosis. N Engl J Med 2011;364:746–760.
8. Antman EM, Hand M, Armstrong PW, et al. 2007 focused update of the ACCF/AHA 2004 guidelines for the management of patients with ST-elevation myocardial infarction: A report of the American College of Cardiology/American Heart Association Task Force on Practice Guidelines: Developed in collaboration with the Canadian Cardiovascular Society endorsed by the American Academy of Family Physicians: 2007 Writing Group to Review New Evidence and Update the ACC/AHA 2004 Guidelines for the Management of Patients with ST-Elevation Myocardial Infarction, Writing on Behalf of the 2004 Writing Committee. Circulation 2008;117:296–329.
9. Fuster V, Moreno PR, Fayad ZA, et al. Atherothrombosis and high-risk plaque: Part I: Evolving concepts. J Am Coll Cardiol 2005;46:937–954.
10. Spinler SA. Acute coronary syndromes. In: Dunsworth TS, Richardson MM, Cheng JWM, et al., eds. Pharmacotherapy Self-Assessment Program, Book 1: Cardiology, 6th ed. Kansas City: American College of Clinical Pharmacy, 2007:59–83.
11. Ruberg FL, Leopold JA, Loscalzo J. Atherothrombosis: Plaque instability and thrombogenesis. Prog Cardiovasc Dis 2003;44:381–394.
12. Gajarsa JJ, Kloner RA. Left ventricular remodeling in the post-infarction heart: A review of cellular, molecular mechanisms, and therapeutic modalities. Heart Fail Rev 2011;16:13–21.
13. Goodman SG, Huang W, Yan AT, et al. The expanded Global Registry of Acute Coronary Events: Baseline characteristics, management practices and outcomes of patients with acute coronary syndromes. Am Heart J 2009;158:193–205.e5.
14. Fox KAA, Steg PG, Eagle KA, et al. Decline in rates of death and heart failure in acute coronary syndromes, 1999-2006. JAMA 2007;297:1892–1900.
15. Thygesen K, Alpert JS, Jaffe AS, et al. Third universal definition of myocardial infarction. J Am Coll Cardiol 2012;60:1581–1598.
16. Spinler SA, de Denus S. Acute coronary syndromes. In: Chisholm-Burns M, Wells BG, Schwinghammer TL, Malone PM, Kolesar JM, DiPiro JT, eds. Pharmacotherapy Principles and Practice, 3rd ed. New York: McGraw-Hill, 2013:133–167.
17. Fibrinolytic Therapy Trialists' (FTT) Collaborative Group. Indications for fibrinolytic therapy in suspected myocardial infarction: Collaborative overview of early mortality and major morbidity results from all randomized trials of more than 1,000 patients. Lancet 1994;343:311–322.
18. Berger P, Ellis SG, Holmes DR Jr, et al. Relationship between delay in performing direct coronary angioplasty and early clinical outcome in patients with acute myocardial infarction: Results from the Global Use of Strategies to Open Occluded Arteries in Acute Coronary Syndromes (GUSTO-IIb) trial. Circulation 1999;100:14–20.
19. Steg PG, Goldberg RJ, Gore JM, et al. Baseline characteristics, management practices, and in-hospital outcomes of patients hospitalized with acute coronary syndromes in the Global Registry of Acute Coronary Events (GRACE). Am J Cardiol 2002;90:358–363.
20. Peterson ED, Roe MT, Muglund J, et al. Association between hospital process performance and outcomes among patients with acute coronary syndromes. JAMA 2006;295:1912–1920.
21. Eagle KA, Montoye CK, Riba AL, et al. Guideline-based standardized care is associated with substantially lower mortality in Medicare patients with acute myocardial infarction: The American College of Cardiology's Guidelines Applied in Practice (GAP) Projects in Michigan. J Am Coll Cardiol 2005;46:1242–1248.
22. Heidenreich PA, Lewis WR, LaBresh KA, et al. Hospital performance recognition with the Get with the Guidelines Program and mortality for acute myocardial infarction and heart failure. Am Heart J 2009;158:546–553.
23. Antman EM, Cohen M, Bernink PJ, et al. The TIMI risk score for unstable angina/non-ST-segment-elevation MI: A method for prognostication and therapeutic decision-making. JAMA 2000;284:835–842.
24. Pieper KS, Gore JM, FitzGerald G, et al. Validity of a risk-prediction tool for hospital mortality: The Global Registry of Acute Coronary Events. Am Heart J 2009;157:1097–1105.
25. Huynh T, Perron S, O'Loughlin J, et al. Comparison of primary percutaneous coronary intervention and fibrinolytic therapy in ST-segment-elevation myocardial infarction: Bayesian hierarchical meta-analyses of randomized controlled trials and observational studies. Circulation 2009;119:3101–3109.
26. Krumholz HM, Herrin J, Miller LE, et al. Improvements in door-to-balloon time in the United States, 2005 to 2010. Circulation 2011;124:1038–1045.
27. Hoenig MR, Aroney CN, Scott IA. Early invasive versus conservative strategies for unstable angina and non-ST elevation myocardial infarction in the stent era. Cochrane Database Syst Rev 2010;(3):CD004815.
28. Mahoney M, Jurkovitz CT, Chu H, et al. Cost and cost-effectiveness of an early invasive vs conservative strategy for the treatment of unstable angina and non-ST-segment elevation myocardial infarction. JAMA 2002;288:1851–1858.
29. Epstein AE, DiMarco JP, Ellenbogen KA, et al. ACCF/AHA/HRS focused update incorporated into the ACCF/AHA/HRS 2008 guidelines for device-based therapy of cardiac rhythm abnormalities: A report of the American College of

Cardiology Foundation/American Heart Association Task Force on Practice Guidelines and the Heart Rhythm Society. J Am Coll Cardiol 2013;31:e6–e75.

30. Effectiveness of intravenous thrombolytic treatment in acute myocardial infarction. Gruppo Italiano per lo Studio della Streptochinasi nell'Infarto MiCardico (GISSA). Lancet 1986;1:397–402.
31. The Global Use of Strategies to Open Occluded Coronary Arteries (GUSTO III) Investigators. A comparison of reteplase with alteplase for acute myocardial infarction. N Engl J Med 1997;337:1118–1123.
32. Assessment of the Safety and Efficacy of a New Thrombolytic (ASSENT-2) Investigators. Single-bolus tenecteplase compared with front-loaded alteplase in acute myocardial infarction: The ASSENT-2 double-blind randomized trial. Lancet 2000;354:716–722.
33. Krumholz HM, Anderson JL, Bachelder BL, et al. ACC/AHA 2008 performance measures for adults with ST-elevation and non-ST-elevation myocardial infarction: A report of the American College of Cardiology/American Heart Association Task Force on Performance Measures (Writing Committee to Develop Performance Measures for ST-Elevation and Non-ST-Elevation Myocardial Infarction) developed in collaboration with the American Academy of Family Physicians and American College of Emergency Physicians endorsed by the American Association of Cardiovascular and Pulmonary Rehabilitation, Society for Cardiovascular Angiography and Interventions, and Society of Hospital Medicine. J Am Coll Cardiol 2008;52:2046–2099.
34. Gibson CM, Pride YB, Frederick PD, et al. Trends in reperfusion strategies, door-to-needle and door-to-balloon times, and in-hospital mortality among patients with ST-segment elevation myocardial infarction enrolled in the National Registry of Myocardial Infarction from 1990 to 2006. Am Heart J 2008;156:1035–1044.
35. ISIS-2 (Second International Study of Infarct Survival) Collaborative Group. Randomised trial of intravenous streptokinase, oral aspirin, both, or neither among 17,187 cases of suspected acute myocardial infarction: ISIS-2. Lancet 1988;2:349–360.
36. Awtry EH, Loscalzo J. Aspirin. Circulation 2000;101: 1206–1218.
37. Campbell CL, Smyth S, Montalescot G, et al. Aspirin dose for the prevention of cardiovascular disease. JAMA 2007;297:2018–2024.
38. Antiplatelet Trialists' Collaboration. Collaborative meta-analysis of randomised trials of antiplatelet therapy for prevention of death, myocardial infarction, and stroke in high risk patients. BMJ 2002;324:71–86.
39. CURRENT-OASIS 7 Investigators, Mehta SR, Bassand JP, et al. Dose comparisons of clopidogrel and aspirin in acute coronary syndromes [Erratum. N Engl J Med 2010;363:1585]. N Engl J Med 2010;363:930–942.
40. Mehta SR, Tanguay JF, Eikelboom JW, et al. Double-dose versus standard-dose clopidogrel and high-dose versus low-dose aspirin in individuals undergoing percutaneous coronary intervention for acute coronary syndromes (CURRENT-OASIS 7): A randomised factorial trial. Lancet 2010;376:1233–1243.
41. Yu J, Mehran R, Dangas GD, et al. Safety and efficacy of high- versus low-dose aspirin after primary percutaneous coronary intervention in ST-segment elevation myocardial infarction: The HORIZONS-AMI (Harmonizing Outcomes with Revascularization and Stents in Acute Myocardial Infarction) trial. JACC Cardiovasc Interv 2012;5:1231–1238.
42. Smith SC, Benjamin EJ, Bonow RO, et al. AHA/ACCF secondary prevention and risk reduction therapy for patients with coronary and other atherosclerotic vascular disease: 2011 update: A guideline from the American Heart Association and American College of Cardiology Foundation endorsed by the World Heart Federation and the Preventive Cardiovascular Nurses Association. J Am Coll Cardiol 2011;58:2432–2446.
43. Mahaffey KW, Wojdyla DM, Carroll K, et al. Ticagrelor compared with clopidogrel by geographic region in the Platelet Inhibition and Patient Outcomes (PLATO) trial. Circulation 2011;124:544–554.
44. Plavix (clopidogrel bisulphate tablets). Bristol-Myers Squibb/Sanofi Pharmaceuticals Partnership [prescribing information], December 2011.
45. Eli Lilly and Company. Effient (prasugrel tablets). Daiichi Sankyo Inc and Eli Lilly and Company [prescribing information], November 30, 2012.
46. AstraZeneca. Brilinta (ticagrelor tablets) [prescribing information], January 24, 2013.
47. Mega JL Close SL, Wiviott SD, et al. Cytochrome P450 polymorphisms and response to clopidogrel. N Engl J Med 2009;360:354–362.
48. Sofi F, Giusti B, Marcucci R, et al. Cytochrome P450 2C19*2 polymorphism and cardiovascular recurrences in patients taking clopidogrel: A meta-analysis. Pharmacogenomics J 2011;11:199–206.
49. Mega JL, Close SL, Wiviott SD, et al. Cytochrome P450 genetic polymorphisms and the response to prasugrel: Relationship to pharmacokinetic, pharmacodynamic, and clinical outcomes. Circulation 2009;119:2553–2560.
50. Wallentin L, James S, Storey RF, et al. Effect of CYP2C19 and ABCB1 single nucleotide polymorphisms on outcomes of treatment with ticagrelor versus clopidogrel for acute coronary syndromes: A genetic substudy of the PLATO trial. Lancet 2010;376:1320–1328.
51. Siller-Matula JM, Huber K, Christ G. Impact of clopidogrel loading dose on clinical outcome in patients undergoing percutaneous coronary intervention: A systematic review and meta-analysis. Heart 2011;97:98–105.
52. Wiviott SD, Braunwald E, McCabe CH, et al. Prasugrel versus clopidogrel in patients with acute coronary syndromes. N Engl J Med 2007;357;2001–2015.
53. Montalescot G, Wiviott SD, Braunwald E, et al. Prasugrel compared with clopidogrel in patients undergoing percutaneous coronary intervention for ST-elevation myocardial infarction (TRITON-TIMI 38): Double-blind, randomised controlled trial. Lancet 2009;373:723–731.
54. Wiviott SD, Braunwald E, Angiolillo DJ, et al. Greater clinical benefit of more intensive oral antiplatelet therapy with prasugrel in patients with diabetes mellitus in the trial to assess improvement in therapeutic outcomes by optimizing platelet inhibition with prasugrel-Thrombolysis in Myocardial Infarction 38. Circulation 2008;118:1626–1636.
55. Wallentin L, Becker RC, Budaj A, et al. Ticagrelor versus clopidogrel in patients with acute coronary syndromes. N Engl J Med 2009;361:1045–1057.
56. James SK, Roe MT, Cannon CP, et al. Ticagrelor versus clopidogrel in patients with acute coronary syndromes intended for non-invasive management: Substudy from prospective randomised PLATelet inhibition and patient Outcomes (PLATO) trial. BMJ 2011;342:d3527.
57. James S, Angiolillo DJ, Cornel JH, et al.; PLATO Study Group. Ticagrelor vs. clopidogrel in patients with acute coronary syndromes and diabetes: A substudy from the PLATelet inhibition and patient Outcomes (PLATO) trial. Eur Heart J 2010;31:3006–3016.

58. Steg PG, James S, Harrington RA, et al.; PLATO Study Group. Ticagrelor versus clopidogrel in patients with ST-elevation acute coronary syndromes intended for reperfusion with primary percutaneous coronary intervention: A Platelet Inhibition and Patient Outcomes (PLATO) trial subgroup analysis. Circulation 2010;122:2131–2141.
59. Cannon CP, Harrington RA, James S, et al. Comparison of ticagrelor with clopidogrel in patients with a planned invasive strategy for acute coronary syndromes (PLATO): A randomised double-blind study. Lancet 2010;375:283–293.
60. Crouch MA, Colucci VJ, Howard PA, Spinler SA. $P2Y_{12}$ receptor inhibitors: Integrating ticagrelor into the management of acute coronary syndrome. Ann Pharmacother 2011;45:1151–1156.
61. Price MJ, Berger PB, Teirstein PS, et al. Standard- vs high-dose clopidogrel based on platelet function testing after percutaneous coronary intervention: The GRAVITAS randomized trial [Erratum. JAMA 2011;305;2174]. JAMA 2011;305:1097–1105.
62. Chen ZM, Jiang XL, Chen YP, et al. Addition of clopidogrel to aspirin in 45,852 patients with acute myocardial infarction: Randomised placebo-controlled trial. Lancet 2005;366:1607–1621.
63. Sabatine MS, Cannon CP, Gibson CM, et al. Addition of clopidogrel to aspirin and fibrinolytic therapy for myocardial infarction with ST-segment elevation. N Engl J Med 2005;352:1179–1189.
64. Simon T, Verstuyft C, Mary-Krause M, et al. Genetic determinants of response to clopidogrel and cardiovascular events. N Engl J Med 2009;360:363–375.
65. Roberts JD, Wells GA, Le May MR, et al. Point-of-care genetic testing for personalisation of antiplatelet treatment (RAPID GENE): A prospective, randomised, proof-of-concept trial. Lancet 2012;379:1705–1711.
66. Scott SA, Sangkuhl K, Gardner EE, et al. Clinical Pharmacogenetics Implementation Consortium guidelines for cytochrome P450-2C19 (CYP2C19) genotype and clopidogrel therapy. Clin Pharmacol Ther 2011;90:328–332.
67. Relling MV, Altman RB, Goetz MP, Evans WE. Clinical implementation of pharmacogenomics: Overcoming genetic exceptionalism. Lancet Oncol 2010;11:507–509.
68. de Denus S, Letarte N, Hurlimann T, et al. An evaluation of pharmacists' expectations towards pharmacogenomics. Pharmacogenomics 2013;14:165–175.
69. De Luca G, Navarese E, Marino P. Risk profile and benefits from Gp IIb–IIIa inhibitors among patients with ST-segment elevation myocardial infarction treated with primary angioplasty: A meta-regression analysis of randomized trials. Eur Heart J 2009;30:2705–2713.
70. Gurm HS, Tamhane U, Meier P, et al. A comparison of abciximab and small-molecule glycoprotein IIb/IIIa inhibitors in patients undergoing primary percutaneous coronary intervention: A meta-analysis of contemporary randomized controlled trials. Circ Cardiovasc Interv 2009;2:230–236.
71. Merck and Co. Inc. Integrilin (eptifibatide) injection [prescribing information], March 2011.
72. Juwana YB, Suryapranata H, Ottervanger JP, van't Hof AW. Tirofiban for myocardial infarction. Expert Opin Pharmacother 2010;11:861–866.
73. Medicure Pharma Inc. Aggrastat (tirofiban HCl) injection premixed [prescribing information], May 2012.
74. Dasgupta H, Blankenship JC, Wood C, et al. Thrombocytopenia complicating treatment with intravenous glycoprotein IIb/IIIa receptor inhibitors: A pooled analysis. Am Heart J 2000;140:206–211.
75. Eikelboom JW, Quinlan DJ, Mehta SR, et al. Unfractionated and low-molecular-weight heparin as adjuncts to thrombolysis in aspirin-treated patients with ST-elevation acute myocardial infarction: A meta-analysis of the randomized trials. Circulation 2005;112:3855–3867.
76. Stone GW, Witzenbichler B, Guagliumi G, et al. Bivalirudin during primary PCI in acute myocardial infarction. N Engl J Med 2008;358:2218–2230.
77. Stone GW, Witzenbichler B, Guagliumi G, et al. Heparin plus a glycoprotein IIb/IIIa inhibitor versus bivalirudin monotherapy and paclitaxel-eluting stents versus bare-metal stents in acute myocardial infarction (HORIZONS-AMI): Final 3-year results from a multicentre, randomised controlled trial. Lancet 2011;377:2193–2204.
78. Antman EM, Morrow DA, McCabe CH, et al. Enoxaparin versus unfractionated heparin with fibrinolysis for ST-elevation myocardial infarction. N Engl J Med 2006;354: 1477–1488.
79. Gore JM, Spencer FA, Gurfinkel EP, et al. Thrombocytopenia in patients with an acute coronary syndrome (from the Global Registry of Acute Coronary Events [GRACE]). Am J Cardiol 2009;103(2):175–180.
80. First International Study of Infarct Survival Collaborative Group. Randomised trial of intravenous atenolol among 16,027 cases of suspected acute myocardial infarction: ISIS-1. Lancet 1986;2:57–661.
81. Metoprolol in acute myocardial infarction (MIAMI). A randomised placebo-controlled international trial. Eur Heart J 1985;6:199–226.
82. COMMIT (Clopidogrel and Metoprolol in Myocardial Infarction Trial [Collaborative Group]). Early intravenous then oral metoprolol in 45,852 patients with acute myocardial infarction: Randomised placebo-controlled trial. Lancet 2005;366:1622–1632.
83. U.S. Department of Health & Human Services. Centers for Medicare & Medicaid Services. Office of Clinical Standards & Quality. Fact Sheet. *http://www.cms.gov/Medicare/Quality-Initiatives-Patient-Assessment-Instruments/HospitalQualityInits/downloads/HospitalAMI-6FactSheet.pdf*.
84. Gruppo Italioano per Lo Studio della Sopravivenza Nell'infarcto Myiocardio. GISSI-3: Effects of lisinopril and transdermal glyceryl trinitrate singly and together on 6-week mortality and ventricular function after acute myocardial infarction. Lancet 1994;343:1115–1122.
85. ISIS-4 (Fourth International Study of Infarct Survival [Collaborative Group]). ISIS-4: A randomised factorial trial assessing early oral captopril, oral mononitrate, and intravenous magnesium sulphate in 58,050 patients with suspected acute myocardial infarction. Lancet 1995;345:669–685.
86. Stone GW, McLaurin BT, Cox DA, et al. Bivalirudin for patients with acute coronary syndromes. N Engl J Med 2006;355:2203–2216.
87. Kastrati A, Neumann FJ, Schulz S, et al. Abciximab and heparin versus bivalirudin for non-ST-elevation myocardial infarction. N Engl J Med 2011;365:1980–1989.
88. Oler A, Whooley MA, Oler J, Grady D. Adding heparin to aspirin reduces the incidence of myocardial infarction and death in patients with unstable angina: A meta-analysis. JAMA 1996;276:811–815.
89. Fragmin During Instability in Coronary Artery Disease Study Group. Low-molecular-weight heparin during instability in coronary artery disease. Lancet 1996;347:561–568.

90. Yusuf S, Mehta SR, Chrolavicius S, et al. Effects of fondaparinux on mortality and reinfarction in patients with acute ST-segment elevation myocardial infarction: The OASIS-6 randomized trial. JAMA 2006;295:1519–1530.
91. Mehta SR, Yusuf S, Peters RJG, et al. Effects of pretreatment with clopidogrel and aspirin followed by long-term therapy in patients undergoing percutaneous coronary intervention: The PCI-CURE study. Lancet 2001;358:527–533.
92. Yusuf S, Zhao F, Meta SR, et al. Effects of clopidogrel in addition to aspirin in patients with acute coronary syndromes without ST-segment elevation. N Engl J Med 2001;345; 494–502.
93. Giugliano RP, White JA, Bode C, et al. Early versus delayed, provisional eptifibatide in acute coronary syndromes. N Engl J Med 2009;360:2176–2190.
94. Serebruany VL, Malinin AI, Sane DC, et al. The risk of bleeding complications with antiplatelet agents: A meta-analysis of 338,191 patients enrolled in 50 randomized controlled trials. Am J Cardiol 2005;95:1218–1222.
95. Serebruany VL, Malinin AI, Ferguson JJ, et al. Bleeding risks of combination vs. single antiplatelet therapy: A meta-analysis of 18 randomized trials comprising 129,314 patients. Fundam Clin Pharmacol 2008;22:315–321.
96. Budnitz DS, Lovegrove MC, Shehab N, Richards CL. Emergency hospitalizations for adverse drug events in older Americans. N Engl J Med 2011;365(21):2002–2012.
97. Becker RC, Bassan JP, Budaj A, et al. Bleeding complications with the P2Y12 receptor antagonists clopidogrel and ticagrelor in the PLATelet inhibition and patient outcome trial. Eur Heart J 2011;32:2933–2944.
98. Wiviott SD, Desai N, Murphy SA, et al. Efficacy and safety of intensive antiplatelet therapy with prasugrel from TRITON-TIMI 38 in a core clinical cohort defined by worldwide regulatory agencies. Am J Cardiol 2011;108: 905–911.
99. Zhao HJ, Zheng ZR, Wang ZH, et al. "Triple therapy" rather than "triple threat": A meta-analysis of the two antithrombotic regimens after stent implantation in patients receiving long-term oral anticoagulant treatment. Chest 2011;139:260–270.
100. Faxon DP, Eikelboom JW, Berger PB, et al. Antithrombotic therapy in patients with atrial fibrillation undergoing coronary stenting: A North American perspective: Executive summary. Circ Cardiovasc Interv 2011;4:522–534.
101. Dewilde WJM, Oirbans T, Verheugt FWA, Kelder JC, et al. Use of clopidogrel with or without aspirin in patients taking oral anticoagulant therapy and undergoing percutaneous coronary intervention: An open-label, randomised controlled trial. Lancet 2013;381:1107–1115 [Epub February 13, 2013].
102. Alexander JH, Lopes RD, James S, et al. Apixaban with antiplatelet therapy after acute coronary syndrome. N Engl J Med 2011;365:699–708.
103. Mega JL, Braunwald E, Wiviott SD, et al. Rivaroxaban in patients with a recent acute coronary syndrome. N Engl J Med 2012;366:9–19.
104. Freemantle N, Cleland J, Young P, et al. β-Blockade after myocardial infarction: Systematic review and meta regression analysis. Br Med J 1999;318:1730–1737.
105. Houghton T, Freemantle N, Cleland JG, et al. Are beta-blockers effective in patients who develop heart failure soon after myocardial infarction? A meta-regression analysis of randomised trials. Eur J Heart Fail 2000;2:333–340.
106. Dargie HJ. Effect of carvedilol on outcome after myocardial infarction in patients with left-ventricular dysfunction: The CAPRICORN randomised trial. Lancet 2001;357: 1385–1390.
107. Fihn SD, Gardin JM, Abrams J, et al. 2012 ACCF/AHA/ACP/AATS/PCNA/SCAI/STS guideline for the diagnosis and management of patients with stable ischemic heart disease: A report of the American College of Cardiology Foundation/American Heart Association Task Force on Practice Guidelines, and the American College of Physicians, American Association for Thoracic Surgery, Preventive Cardiovascular Nurses Association, Society for Cardiovascular Angiography and Interventions, and Society of Thoracic Surgeons. Circulation 2012;126:e354–e471.
108. ACE Inhibitor Myocardial Infarction Collaborative Group. Indications for ACE inhibitors in the early treatment of acute myocardial infarction: Systematic overview of individual data from 100,000 patients in randomized trials. Circulation 1998;97:2202–2212.
109. Swedberg K, Held P, Kjekshus J, et al. Effects of the early administration of enalapril on mortality in patients with acute myocardial infarction: Results of the Cooperative New Scandinavian Enalapril Survival Study II (CONSENSUS II). N Engl J Med 1992;327:678–684.
110. Pfeffer MA, McMurray JJV, Velazquez EJ, et al. Valsartan, captopril, or both in myocardial infarction complicated by heart failure, left ventricular dysfunction, or both. N Engl J Med 2003;349:1893–1906.
111. Granger CB, McMurray JV, Yusuf S, et al. Effects of candesartan in patients with chronic heart failure and reduced left-ventricular systolic function intolerant to angiotensin-converting-enzyme inhibitors: The CHARM-Alternative trial. Lancet 2004;362:772–776.
112. Makkar KM, Sanoski CA, Spinler SA. The role of angiotensin-converting enzyme inhibitors, angiotensin receptor blockers and aldosterone antagonists in the prevention of atrial and ventricular arrhythmias. Pharmacotherapy 2009;29:31–48.
113. Pitt B, Zannad F, Remme WJ, et al., for the Randomized Aldactone Evaluation Study Investigators. The effect of spironolactone on morbidity and mortality in patients with severe heart failure. N Engl J Med 1999;341:709–717.
114. Pitt B, Remme W, Zannad F, et al. Eplerenone, a selective aldosterone blocker in patients with left ventricular dysfunction after myocardial infarction. N Engl J Med 2003;348:1309–1321.
115. Zannad F, McMurray JJ, Krum H, et al. Eplerenone in patients with systolic heart failure and mild symptoms. N Engl J Med 2011;364:11–21.
116. Expert Panel on Detection, Evaluation, and Treatment of High Blood Cholesterol in Adults. Executive summary of the third report of the National Cholesterol Education Program (NCEP) Expert Panel on Detection, Evaluation, and Treatment of High Blood Cholesterol in Adults (Adult Treatment Panel III). JAMA 2001;285:2486–2497.
117. Hulten E, Jackson JL, Douglas K, et al. The effect of early, intensive statin therapy on acute coronary syndrome: A meta-analysis of randomized controlled trials. Arch Intern Med 2006;166:1814–1821.
118. Grundy SM, Cleeman JI, Merz CN, et al. Coordinating Committee of the National Cholesterol Education Program, endorsed by the National Heart, Lung, and Blood Institute, American College of Cardiology Foundation, and American Heart Association. Implications of recent clinical trials for the National Cholesterol Education Program Adult Treatment Panel III guidelines. Circulation 2004;110:227–239.
119. Cholesterol Treatment Trialists' (CTT) Collaboration, Baigent C, Blackwell L. Efficacy and safety of more intensive lowering of LDL cholesterol: A meta-analysis of data from 170,000 participants in 26 randomised trials. Lancet 2010;376:1670–1681.

120. Hayward RA, Krumholz HM. Three reasons to abandon low-density lipoprotein targets; an open letter to the Adult Treatment Panel IV of the National Institutes of Health. Circ Cardiovasc Qual Outcomes 2012;5:2–5.
121. Rubins HB, Robins SJ, Collins D, et al. Gemfibrozil for the secondary prevention of coronary heart disease in men with low levels of high-density lipoprotein cholesterol. Veterans Affairs High-Density Lipoprotein Cholesterol Intervention Trial Study Group. N Engl J Med 1999;341:410–418.
122. The ACCORD Study Group. Effects of combination lipid therapy in type 2 diabetes mellitus. N Engl J Med 2010;362:1563–1564.
123. The AIM-HIGH Investigators. Niacin in patients with low HDL cholesterol levels receiving intensive statin therapy. N Engl J Med 2011;365:2255–2267.
124. Ho PM, Spertus JA, Masoudi FA, et al. Impact of medication therapy discontinuation on mortality after myocardial infarction. Arch Intern Med 2006;166:1842–1847.

8

The Arrhythmias

Cynthia A. Sanoski and Jerry L. Bauman

KEY CONCEPTS

1. The use of antiarrhythmic drugs (AADs) in the United States has declined because of major trials that show increased mortality with their use in several clinical situations, the realization of proarrhythmia as a significant side effect, and the advancing technology of nonpharmacologic therapies such as ablation and the implantable cardioverter-defibrillator (ICD).
2. AADs frequently cause side effects and are complex in their pharmacokinetic characteristics. Close monitoring is required of all of these drugs to assess for adverse effects as well as potential drug interactions.
3. The most commonly prescribed AAD is now amiodarone. This drug is effective in terminating and preventing a wide variety of symptomatic supraventricular and ventricular arrhythmias. However, because this AAD is plagued by frequent side effects, it requires close monitoring. The most concerning toxicity is pulmonary fibrosis; side effect profiles of the IV (acute, short-term) and oral (chronic, long-term) forms of amiodarone differ substantially.
4. In patients with atrial fibrillation (AF), therapy is traditionally aimed at controlling ventricular rate (digoxin, nondihydropyridine calcium channel blockers, β-blockers), preventing thromboembolic complications (warfarin, aspirin), and restoring and maintaining sinus rhythm (AADs, direct current cardioversion). Studies show there is no need to aggressively pursue strategies to maintain sinus rhythm (i.e., long-term AAD therapy); rate control alone (leaving the patient in AF) is often sufficient in patients who can tolerate it. Nonetheless, chronic AAD therapy may still be needed in patients who continue to have symptoms despite adequate ventricular rate control.
5. Paroxysmal supraventricular tachycardia is usually a result of reentry in or proximal to the atrioventricular (AV) node or AV reentry incorporating an extranodal pathway; common tachycardias can be terminated acutely with AV nodal blocking drugs such as adenosine, and recurrences can be prevented by ablation with radio-frequency current.
6. Patients with Wolff-Parkinson-White (WPW) syndrome may have several different tachycardias that are acutely treated by different strategies: orthodromic reentry (adenosine), antidromic reentry (adenosine or procainamide), and AF (procainamide or amiodarone). AV nodal blocking drugs are contraindicated in patients with WPW syndrome and AF.
7. Because of the results of the Cardiac Arrhythmia Suppression Trial and other trials, AADs (with the exception of β-blockers) should not be routinely used in patients with prior myocardial infarction (MI) or left ventricular (LV) dysfunction and minor ventricular rhythm disturbances (e.g., premature ventricular complexes).
8. Patients with hemodynamically significant ventricular tachycardia (VT) or ventricular fibrillation not associated with an acute MI who are successfully resuscitated (electrical cardioversion, vasopressors, amiodarone) are at high risk for sudden cardiac death (SCD) and should receive an ICD ("secondary prevention").
9. Implantation of an ICD should be considered for the primary prevention of SCD in certain high-risk patient populations. High-risk patients include those with a history of MI and LV dysfunction (regardless of whether they have inducible sustained ventricular arrhythmias), as well as those with New York Heart Association class II or III heart failure as a result of either ischemic or nonischemic causes.
10. Life-threatening ventricular proarrhythmia generally takes two forms: sinusoidal or incessant monomorphic VT (class Ic AADs) and torsade de pointes (class Ia or III AADs and many other noncardiac drugs).

The heart has two basic properties, namely, an electrical property and a mechanical property. The synchronous interaction between these two properties is complex, precise, and relatively enduring. The study of the electrical properties of the heart has grown at a steady rate, interrupted by periodic salvos of scientific breakthroughs. Einthoven's pioneering work allowed graphic electrical tracings of cardiac rhythm and probably represents the first of these breakthroughs. This discovery of the surface electrocardiogram (ECG) has remained the cornerstone of diagnostic tools for cardiac rhythm disturbances. Since then, intracardiac recordings and programmed cardiac stimulation have advanced our understanding of arrhythmias, and microelectrode, voltage clamping, and patch clamping techniques have allowed considerable insight into the electrophysiologic actions and mechanisms of antiarrhythmic drugs (AADs). Certainly, the new era of molecular biology and mapping of the human genome promises even greater insights into mechanisms (and potential therapies) of arrhythmias. Noteworthy in this regard is the discovery of genetic abnormalities in the ion channels that control electrical repolarization (heritable long QT syndrome) or depolarization (Brugada syndrome).

The clinical use of drug therapy started with the use of digitalis and then quinidine. A surge of new agents followed somewhat later in the 1980s. A theme of drug discovery during this decade was initially to find orally absorbed lidocaine congeners (such as mexiletine and tocainide); later, the emphasis was on drugs with extremely potent effects on conduction (i.e., flecainide-like agents). The most recent focus of investigational AADs is the potassium channel blockers, with dronedarone being the most recently approved AAD in the United States in nearly a decade. Previously, there was some expectation that advances in AAD discovery would lead to a highly effective and nontoxic agent that would be effective for a majority of patients (i.e., the so-called magic bullet). Instead, significant problems with drug toxicity and proarrhythmia have resulted in a decline in the overall volume of AAD usage in the United States since 1989. 1 The other phenomenon that has significantly contributed to the decline in AAD utilization is the development of extremely effective nonpharmacologic therapies. Technical advances have made it possible to permanently interrupt reentry circuits with radiofrequency ablation, which renders long-term AAD use unnecessary in certain arrhythmias. Furthermore, the impressive survival data associated with the use of implantable cardioverter-defibrillators (ICDs) for the primary and secondary prevention of sudden cardiac death (SCD) have led most clinicians to choose "device" therapy as the first-line treatment for patients who are at high risk for life-threatening ventricular arrhythmias. Both of these nonpharmacologic therapies have become increasingly popular for the management of arrhythmias so that the potential proarrhythmic effects and organ toxicities associated with AADs can be avoided.

This chapter reviews the principles involved in both normal and abnormal cardiac conduction and addresses the pathophysiology and treatment of the more commonly encountered arrhythmias. Certainly, many volumes of complete text could be (and have been) devoted to basic and clinical electrophysiology. Consequently, this chapter briefly addresses those principles necessary for clinicians.

ARRHYTHMOGENESIS

Normal Conduction

Electrical activity is initiated by the sinoatrial (SA) node and moves through cardiac tissue by a tree-like conduction network. The SA node initiates cardiac rhythm under normal circumstances because this tissue possesses the highest degree of automaticity or rate of spontaneous impulse generation. The degree of automaticity of the SA node is largely influenced by the autonomic nervous system in that both cholinergic and sympathetic innervations control the sinus rate. Most tissues within the conduction system also possess varying degrees of inherent automatic properties. However, the rates of spontaneous impulse generation of these tissues are less than that of the SA node. Thus, these latent automatic pacemakers are continuously overdriven by impulses arising from the SA node (primary pacemaker) and do not become clinically apparent.

From the SA node, electrical activity moves in a wave front through an atrial specialized conducting system and eventually gains entrance to the ventricle via the atrioventricular (AV) node and a large bundle of conducting tissue referred to as the bundle of His. Aside from this AV node–bundle of His pathway, a fibrous AV ring that will not permit electrical stimulation separates the atria and ventricles. The conducting tissues bridging the atria and ventricles are referred to as the junctional areas. Again, this area of tissue (junction) is largely influenced by autonomic input and possesses a relatively high degree of inherent automaticity (about 40 beats/min, less than that of the SA node). From the bundle of His, the cardiac conduction system bifurcates into several (usually three) bundle branches: one right bundle and two left bundles. These bundle branches further arborize into a conduction network referred to as the Purkinje system. The conduction system as a whole innervates the mechanical myocardium and serves to initiate excitation–contraction coupling and the contractile process. After a cell or group of cells within the heart is electrically stimulated, a brief period of time follows in which those cells cannot again be excited. This time period is referred to as the refractory period. As the electrical wave front moves down the conduction system, the impulse eventually encounters tissue refractory to stimulation (recently excited) and subsequently dies out. The SA node subsequently recovers, fires spontaneously, and begins the process again.

Prior to cellular excitation, an electrical gradient exists between the inside and the outside of the cell membrane. At this time, the cell is polarized. In atrial and ventricular conducting tissues, the intracellular space is approximately 80 to 90 mV negative with respect to the extracellular environment. The electrical gradient just prior to excitation is referred to as the resting membrane potential (RMP) and is the result of differences in ion concentrations between the inside and the outside of the cell. At RMP, the cell is polarized primarily by the action of active membrane ion pumps, the most notable of these being the sodium–potassium pump. For example, this specific pump (in addition to other systems) attempts to maintain the intracellular sodium concentration at 5 to 15 mEq/L and the extracellular sodium concentration at 135 to 142 mEq/L, and the intracellular potassium concentration at 135 to 140 mEq/L and the extracellular potassium concentration at 3 to 5 mEq/L. The RMP can be calculated by using the Nernst equation:

$$\text{RMP} = 61.5 \log\left(\frac{[\text{K}^+]\text{ outside}}{[\text{K}^+]\text{ inside}}\right)$$

Electrical stimulation (or depolarization) of the cell will result in changes in membrane potential over time or a characteristic action potential curve (Fig. 8-1). The action potential curve results from the transmembrane movement of specific ions and is divided into different phases. Phase 0 or initial, rapid depolarization of atrial and ventricular tissues is caused by an abrupt increase in the permeability of the membrane to sodium influx. This rapid depolarization more than equilibrates (overshoots) the electrical potential, resulting in a brief initial repolarization or phase 1. Phase 1 (initial repolarization) is caused by a transient and active potassium efflux (i.e., the I_{Kto} current). Calcium begins to move into the intracellular space at about −60 mV (during phase 0), causing a slower depolarization. Calcium influx continues throughout phase 2 of the action potential (plateau phase) and is balanced to some degree by potassium efflux. Calcium entrance (only through L channels in myocardial tissue) distinguishes cardiac conducting cells from nerve tissue and provides the critical ionic link to excitation–contraction coupling and the mechanical properties of the heart as a pump. The membrane remains permeable to potassium efflux during phase 3, resulting in cellular repolarization. Phase 4 of the action potential is the gradual depolarization of the cell and is related to a constant sodium leak into the intracellular space balanced by a decreasing (over time) efflux of potassium. The slope of phase 4 depolarization determines, in large part, the automatic properties of the cell. As the cell is slowly depolarized during phase 4, an abrupt increase in sodium permeability occurs, allowing the rapid cellular depolarization of phase 0. The juncture of phase 4 and phase 0 where rapid sodium influx is initiated is referred to as the threshold potential of the cell. The level of threshold potential also regulates the degree of cellular automaticity.

Not all cells in the cardiac conduction system rely on sodium influx for initial depolarization. Some tissues depolarize in response to a slower inward ionic current caused by calcium influx. These "calcium-dependent" tissues are found primarily in the SA and AV nodes (both L and T channels) and possess distinct conduction properties in comparison to "sodium-dependent" fibers. Calcium-dependent cells generally have a less negative RMP (−40 to −60 mV) and a slower conduction velocity. Furthermore, in calcium-dependent tissues, recovery of excitability outlasts full repolarization, whereas in sodium-dependent tissues, recovery is prompt after repolarization. These two types of electrical fibers also differ dramatically in how drugs modify their conduction properties.

Ion conductance across the lipid bilayer of the cell membrane occurs via the formation of membrane pores or "channels" (Fig. 8-2). Selective ion channels probably form in response to specific electrical potential differences between the inside and the outside of the

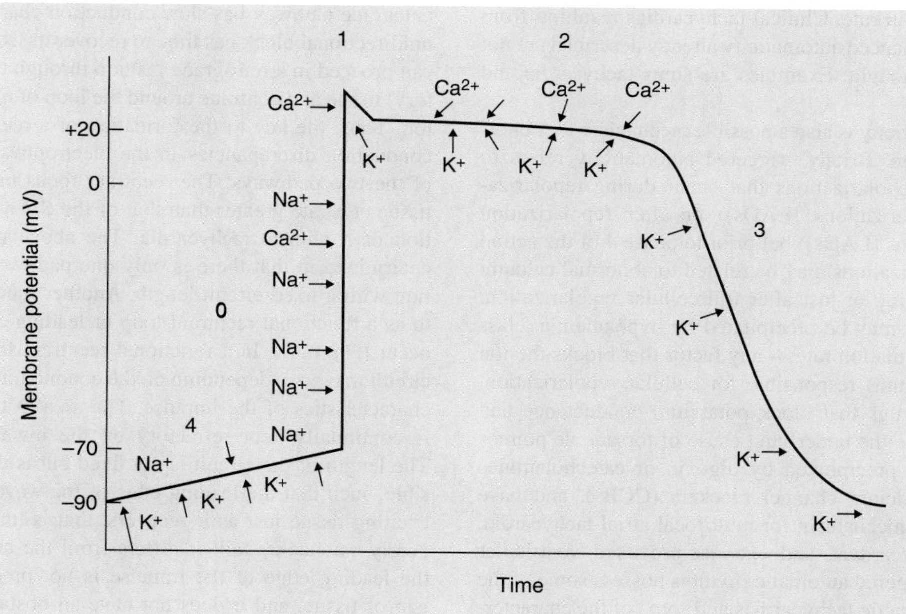

FIGURE 8-1 Purkinje fiber action potential showing specific ion flux responsible for the change in membrane potential. Ions outside of the line (e.g., sodium) move from the extracellular space to the intracellular space and ions on the inside of the line (e.g., potassium) move from the inside of the cell to the outside.

cell (voltage dependence). The membrane itself is composed of both organized and disorganized lipids and phospholipids in a dynamic sol-gel matrix. During ion flux and electrical excitation, changes in this sol-gel equilibrium occur and permit the formation of activated ion channels. Besides channel formation and membrane composition, intrachannel proteins or phospholipids, referred to as gates, also regulate the transmembrane movement of ions. These gates are thought to be positioned strategically within the channel to modulate ion flow (Fig. 8-2). Each ion channel conceptually has two types of gates: an activation gate and an inactivation gate. The activation gate opens during depolarization to allow the ion current to enter or exit from the cell, and the inactivation gate later closes to stop ion movement. When the cell is in a rested state, the activation gates are closed and the inactivation gates are open. The activation gates then open to allow ion movement through the channel, and the inactivation gates later close to stop ion conductance. Thus, the cell cycles between three states: resting, activated or open, and inactivated or closed. Activation of SA and AV nodal tissue is dependent on a slow depolarizing current through calcium channels and gates, whereas the activation of atrial and ventricular tissues is dependent on a rapid depolarizing current through sodium channels and gates.

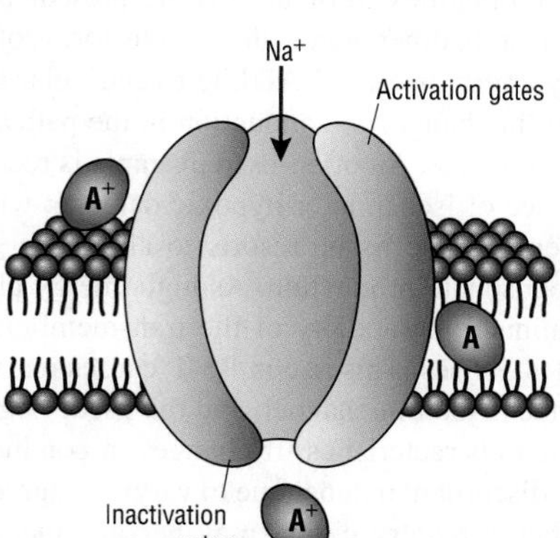

FIGURE 8-2 Lipid bilayer, sodium channel, and possible sites of action of the class I AADs (*A*). Class I AADs may theoretically inhibit sodium influx at an extracellular, intramembrane, or intracellular receptor site. However, all approved agents appear to block sodium conductance at a single receptor site by gaining entrance to the interior of the channel from an intracellular route. Active ionized drugs block the channel predominantly during the activated or inactivated state and bind and unbind with specific time constants (described as fast on–off, slow on–off, and intermediate). (AADs, antiarrhythmic drugs.)

Abnormal Conduction

The mechanisms of tachyarrhythmias have been classically divided into two general categories: those resulting from an abnormality in impulse generation or "automatic" tachycardias and those resulting from an abnormality in impulse conduction or "reentrant" tachycardias.

Automatic tachycardias depend on spontaneous impulse generation in latent pacemakers and may be a result of several different mechanisms. Drugs, such as digoxin or catecholamines, and conditions, such as hypoxia, electrolyte abnormalities (e.g., hypokalemia), and fiber stretch (cardiac dilation), may lead to an increased slope of phase 4 depolarization in cardiac tissues other than the SA node. These factors that experimentally lead to abnormal automaticity are also known to be arrhythmogenic in clinical situations. The increased slope of phase 4 causes heightened automaticity of these tissues and competition with the SA node for dominance of cardiac rhythm. If the rate of spontaneous impulse generation of the abnormally automatic tissue exceeds that of the SA node, then an automatic tachycardia may result. Automatic tachycardias have the following characteristics: (a) the onset of the tachycardia is unrelated to an initiating event such as a premature beat; (b) the initiating beat is usually identical to subsequent beats of the tachycardia; (c) the tachycardia cannot be initiated by programmed cardiac stimulation; and (d) the onset of the tachycardia is usually preceded by a gradual acceleration in rate and termination is usually preceded by a gradual deceleration in rate. Clinical tachycardias resulting from the classic forms of enhanced automaticity already described are not as common as once thought. Examples are sinus tachycardia and junctional tachycardia.

Triggered automaticity is also a possible mechanism for abnormal impulse generation. Briefly, triggered automaticity refers to transient membrane depolarizations that occur during repolarization (early afterdepolarizations [EADs]) or after repolarization (late afterdepolarizations [LADs]) but prior to phase 4 of the action potential. Afterdepolarizations may be related to abnormal calcium and sodium influx during or just after full cellular repolarization. Experimentally, EADs may be precipitated by hypokalemia, class Ia AADs, or slow stimulation rates—any factor that blocks the ion channels (e.g., potassium) responsible for cellular repolarization. EADs provoked by drugs that block potassium conductance and delay repolarization are the underlying cause of torsade de pointes (TdP). LADs may be precipitated by digoxin or catecholamines and suppressed by calcium channel blockers (CCBs), and have been suggested as the mechanism for multifocal atrial tachycardia, digoxin-induced tachycardias, and exercise-provoked ventricular tachycardia (VT). Triggered automatic rhythms possess some of the characteristics of automatic tachycardias and some of the characteristics of reentrant tachycardias (description follows).

Reentry is a concept that involves indefinite propagation of the impulse and continued activation of previously refractory tissue. There are three conduction requirements for the formation of a viable reentrant focus: 1) two pathways for impulse conduction, 2) an area of unidirectional block (prolonged refractoriness) in one of these pathways, and 3) slow conduction in the other pathway (Fig. 8-3). Usually, a critically timed premature beat initiates reentry. This premature impulse enters both conduction pathways but encounters refractory tissue in one of the pathways at the area of unidirectional block. The impulse dies out because the tissue is still refractory from the previous (sinus) impulse. Although it fails to propagate in one pathway, the impulse may still proceed in a forward direction (antegrade) through the other pathway because of this pathway's relatively shorter refractory period. The impulse may then proceed through a loop of tissue and "reenter" the area of unidirectional block in a backward direction (retrograde). Because the

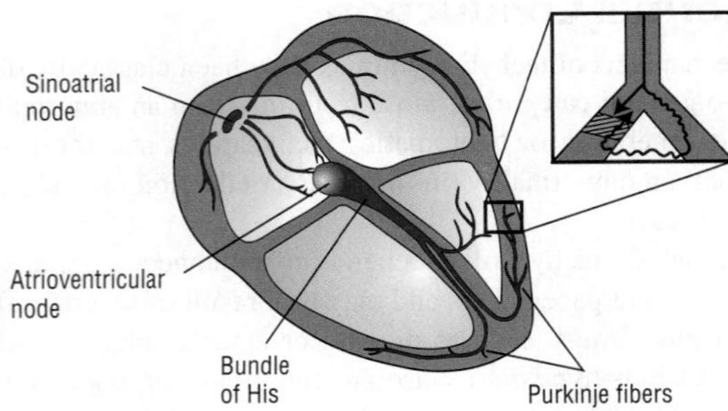

FIGURE 8-3 Conduction system of the heart. The magnified portion shows a bifurcation of a Purkinje fiber traditionally explained as the etiology of reentrant VT. A premature impulse travels to the fiber, damaged by heart disease or ischemia. It encounters a zone of prolonged refractoriness (area of unidirectional block; *cross-hatched area*) but fails to propagate because it remains refractory to stimulation from the previous impulse. However, the impulse may slowly travel (*squiggly line*) through the other portion of the Purkinje twig and will "reenter" the cross-hatched area if the refractory period is concluded and it is now excitable. Thus, the premature impulse never meets refractory tissue; circus movement ensues. If this site stimulates the surrounding ventricle repetitively, clinical reentrant VT results. (VT, ventricular tachycardia.)

antegrade pathway has slow conduction characteristics, the area of unidirectional block has time to recover its excitability. The impulse can proceed in a retrograde fashion through this (previously refractory) tissue and continue around the loop of tissue in a circular fashion. Thus, the key to the formation of a reentrant focus is crucial conduction discrepancies in the electrophysiologic characteristics of the two pathways. The reentrant focus may excite surrounding tissue at a rate greater than that of the SA node, leading to formation of a clinical tachycardia. The above model is anatomically determined in that there is only one pathway for impulse conduction with a fixed circuit length. Another model of reentry, referred to as a functional reentrant loop or leading circle model, may also occur (Fig. 8-4).[1] In a functional reentrant focus, the length of the circuit may vary depending on the conduction velocity and recovery characteristics of the impulse. The area in the middle of the loop is continually kept refractory by the inwardly moving impulse. The length of the circuit is not fixed but is the smallest circle possible, such that the leading edge of the wave front is continuously exciting tissue just as it recovers, that is, the head of the impulse nearly catches its tail. It differs from the anatomic model in that the leading edge of the impulse is not preceded by an excitable gap of tissue, and it does not have an obstacle in the middle or a fixed anatomic circuit. Clinically, many reentrant foci probably have both anatomic and functional characteristics. In the figure 8 model, a zone of unidirectional block is present, allowing for two impulse loops that join and reenter the area of block in a retrograde fashion to form a pretzel-shaped reentrant circuit. This model combines functional characteristics with an excitable gap. All of these theoretical models require a critical balance of refractoriness and conduction velocity within the circuit and as such have helped to explain the effects of drugs on terminating, modifying, and causing cardiac rhythm disturbances.

What causes reentry to become clinically manifest? Reentrant foci may occur at any level of the conduction system: within the branches of the specialized atrial conduction system, within the Purkinje network, and even within portions of the SA and AV nodes. The anatomy of the Purkinje system appears to provide a suitable substrate for the formation of microreentrant loops and is often used as a model to facilitate the understanding of reentry concepts (Fig. 8-4). Of course, because reentry does not usually occur in normal, healthy conduction tissue, various forms of heart disease or conduction abnormalities must usually be present before reentry becomes manifest. In other words, the various forms of heart disease (e.g., coronary artery disease [CAD], left ventricular [LV] dysfunction) can result in changes in conduction in the pathways of a suitable reentrant substrate. An often-used example is reentry occurring as a consequence of ischemic or hypoxic damage: with inadequate cellular oxygen, cardiac tissue resorts to anaerobic glycolysis for adenosine triphosphate production. As high-energy phosphate concentration diminish, the activity of the transmembrane ion pumps declines and RMP rises. This rise in RMP causes inactivation in the voltage-dependent sodium channel, and the tissue begins to assume slow conduction characteristics. If changes in conduction parameters occur in a discordant manner due to varying degrees of ischemia or hypoxia, then a reentry circuit may become manifest. Furthermore, an ischemic, dying cell liberates intracellular potassium, which also causes a rise in RMP. In other cases, reentry may occur as a consequence of anatomic or functional variants in the normal conduction system. For instance, patients may possess two (instead of one) conduction pathways near or within the AV node, or have an anomalous extranodal AV pathway that possesses different electrophysiologic characteristics from the normal AV nodal pathway. Reentry in these cases may occur within the AV node or encompass both atrial and ventricular tissues. Reentrant tachycardias have the following characteristics: (a) the onset of the tachycardia is usually related to an initiating event (i.e., premature beat); (b) the initiating

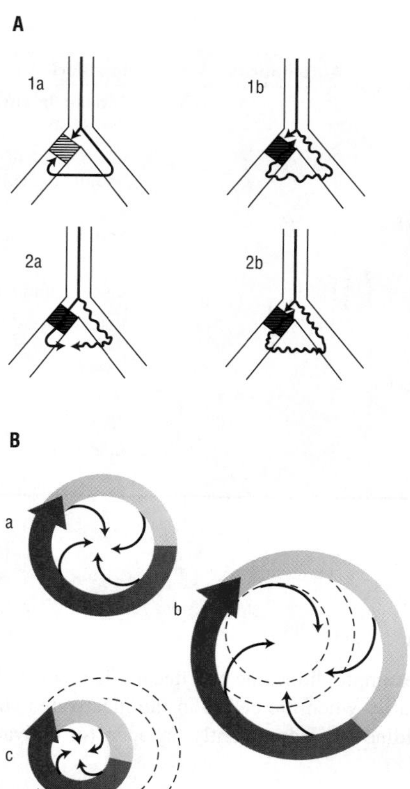

FIGURE 8-4 *A.* Possible mechanism of proarrhythmia in the anatomic model of reentry. *1a.* Nonviable reentrant loop due to bidirectional block (*shaded area*). *1b.* Instance where a drug slows conduction velocity without significantly prolonging the refractory period. The impulse is now able to reenter the area of unidirectional block (*shaded area*) because slowed conduction through the contralateral limb allows recovery of the block. A new reentrant tachycardia may result. *2a.* Nonviable reentrant loop due to a lack of a unidirectional block. *2b.* Instance where a drug prolongs the refractory period without significantly slowing conduction velocity. The impulse moving antegrade meets refractory tissue (*shaded area*) allowing for unidirectional block. A new reentrant tachycardia may result. *B.* Mechanism of reentry and proarrhythmia. *a.* Functionally determined (*leading circle*) reentrant circuit. This model should be contrasted with anatomic reentry; here the circuit is not fixed (it does not necessarily move around an anatomic obstacle) and there is no excitable gap. All tissue inside is held continuously refractory. *b.* Instance where a drug prolongs the refractory period without significantly slowing conduction velocity. The tachycardia may terminate or slow in rate as shown as a consequence of a greater circuit length. The *dashed lines* represent the original reentrant circuit prior to drug treatment. *c.* Instance where a drug slows conduction velocity without significantly prolonging the refractory period (i.e., class Ic *antiarrhythmic drugs*) and accelerates the tachycardia. The tachycardia rate may increase (proarrhythmia) as shown as a consequence of a shorter circuit length. The dashed lines represent the original reentrant circuit prior to drug treatment. *(Reproduced with permission from McCollam PL, Parker RB, Beckman KJ, et al. Proarrhythmia: A paradoxic response to antiarrhythmic agents. Pharmacotherapy 1989;9:146.)*

beat is usually different in morphology from subsequent beats of the tachycardia; (c) the initiation of the tachycardia is usually possible with programmed cardiac stimulation; and (d) the initiation and termination of the tachycardia is usually abrupt without an acceleration or deceleration phase. There are many examples of reentrant tachycardias, including atrial fibrillation (AF), atrial flutter, AV nodal or AV reentrant tachycardia, and recurrent VT.

ANTIARRHYTHMIC DRUGS

In a theoretical sense, drugs may have antiarrhythmic activity by directly altering conduction in several ways. First, a drug may depress the automatic properties of abnormal pacemaker cells. A drug may do this by decreasing the slope of phase 4 depolarization and/or by elevating threshold potential. If the rate of spontaneous impulse generation of the abnormally automatic foci becomes less than that of the SA node, normal cardiac rhythm can be restored. Second, drugs may alter the conduction characteristics of the pathways of a reentrant loop.[1,2] A drug may facilitate conduction (shorten refractoriness) in the area of unidirectional block, allowing antegrade conduction to proceed. On the other hand, a drug may further depress conduction (prolong refractoriness) either in the area of unidirectional block or in the pathway with slowed conduction and a relatively shorter refractory period. If refractoriness is prolonged in the area of unidirectional block, retrograde propagation of the impulse is not permitted, causing a "bidirectional" block. In the anatomic model, if refractoriness is prolonged in the pathway with slow conduction, antegrade conduction of the impulse is not permitted. In either case, drugs that reduce the discordance and cause uniformity in conduction properties of the two pathways may suppress the reentrant substrate. In the functionally determined model, if refractoriness is prolonged without significantly slowing conduction velocity, the tachycardia may terminate or slow in rate as a consequence of a greater circuit length (Fig. 8-4). There are other theoretical ways to stop reentry: a drug may eliminate the critically timed premature impulse that triggers reentry, a drug may slow conduction velocity to such an extent that conduction is extinguished, or a drug may reverse the underlying form of heart disease that was responsible for the conduction abnormalities that led to the arrhythmia (i.e., "reverse remodeling").

AADs have specific electrophysiologic actions that alter cardiac conduction in patients with or without heart disease. These actions form the basis of grouping AADs into specific categories based on their electrophysiologic actions in vitro. Vaughan Williams proposed the most frequently used classification system (Table 8-1).[2] This classification has been criticized for the following reasons: (a) it is incomplete and does not allow for the classification of drugs such as digoxin or adenosine; (b) it is not pure, and many agents have properties of more than one class of drugs; (c) it does not incorporate drug characteristics such as mechanisms of tachycardia termination/prevention, clinical indications, or side effects; and (d) drugs become "labeled" within a class, although they may be distinct in many regards.[3] These criticisms formed the basis for an attempt to reclassify AADs based on a variety of basic and clinical characteristics (called the Sicilian Gambit[3]). Nonetheless, the Vaughan Williams classification remains the most frequently used despite many proposed modifications and alternative systems.

The class Ia AADs, quinidine, procainamide, and disopyramide, slow conduction velocity, prolong refractoriness, and decrease the automatic properties of sodium-dependent (normal and diseased) conduction tissue. Although class Ia AADs are primarily considered sodium channel blockers, their electrophysiologic actions can also be attributed to blockade of potassium channels. In reentrant tachycardias, these drugs generally depress conduction and prolong refractoriness, theoretically transforming the area of unidirectional block into a bidirectional block. Clinically, class Ia drugs are broad-spectrum AADs that are effective for both supraventricular and ventricular arrhythmias. Procainamide is only available in the IV formulation as all of its oral formulations have been discontinued.

TABLE 8-1 Classification of Antiarrhythmic Drugs

Class	Drug	Conduction Velocity[a]	Refractory Period	Automaticity	Ion Block
Ia	Quinidine Procainamide Disopyramide	↓	↑	↓	Sodium (intermediate) Potassium
Ib	Lidocaine Mexiletine	0/↓	↓	↓	Sodium (fast on–off)
Ic	Flecainide Propafenone[b]	↓↓	0	↓	Sodium (slow on–off)
II[c]	β-Blockers	↓	↑	↓	Calcium (indirect)
III	Amiodarone[d] Dofetilide Dronedarone[d] Sotalol[b] Ibutilide	0	↑↑	0	Potassium
IV[c]	Verapamil Diltiazem	↓	↑	↓	Calcium

[a]Variables for normal tissue models in ventricular tissue.
[b]Also has β-blocking actions.
[c]Variables for sinoatrial (SA) and atrioventricular (AV) nodal tissue only.
[d]Also has sodium, calcium, and β-blocking actions; see Table 8-2 (for amiodarone).

The class Ib AADs, lidocaine, mexiletine, and phenytoin, were historically categorized separately from quinidine-like drugs. This was a result of early work demonstrating that lidocaine had distinctly different electrophysiologic actions. In normal tissue models, lidocaine generally facilitates actions on cardiac conduction by shortening refractoriness and having little effect on conduction velocity. Thus, it was postulated that these agents could improve antegrade conduction, eliminating the area of unidirectional block. Of course, arrhythmias do not usually arise from normal tissue, leading investigators to study the actions of lidocaine and phenytoin in ischemic and hypoxic tissue models. Interestingly, studies have shown these drugs to possess class Ia quinidine-like properties in diseased tissues. Therefore, it is probable that lidocaine acts in a similar fashion to the class Ia AADs (i.e., prolongs refractoriness in diseased ischemic tissues leading to bidirectional block in a reentrant circuit). Lidocaine and similar agents have accentuated effects in ischemic tissue caused by the local acidosis and potassium shifts that occur during cellular hypoxia. Changes in pH alter the time that local anesthetics occupy the sodium channel receptor, thereby affecting the agent's electrophysiologic actions. In addition, the intracellular acidosis that ensues as a consequence of ischemia could cause lidocaine to become "trapped" within the cell, allowing increased access to the receptor. The class Ib AADs are considerably more effective in ventricular arrhythmias than supraventricular arrhythmias. As a group, these drugs are relatively weak sodium channel antagonists (at normal stimulation rates).

The class Ic AADs, propafenone and flecainide, are extremely potent sodium channel blockers, profoundly slowing conduction velocity while leaving refractoriness relatively unaltered. The class Ic AADs theoretically eliminate reentry by slowing conduction to a point where the impulse is extinguished and cannot propagate further. Although the class Ic AADs are effective for both ventricular and supraventricular arrhythmias, their use for ventricular arrhythmias has been limited by the risk of proarrhythmia.

Class I AADs are grouped together because of their common action in blocking sodium conductance. The receptor site for these AADs is probably inside the sodium channel so that, in effect, the drug plugs the pore. The AAD may gain access to the receptor either via the intracellular space through the membrane lipid bilayer or directly through the channel. Several principles are inherent in antiarrhythmic sodium channel receptor theories[4]:

1. Class I AADs have predominant affinity for a particular state of the channel (e.g., during activation or inactivation). For example, lidocaine and flecainide block sodium current primarily when the cell is in the inactivated state, whereas quinidine is predominantly an open (or activated)-channel blocker.
2. Class I AADs have specific binding and unbinding characteristics to the receptor. For example, lidocaine binds to and dissociates from the channel receptor quickly ("fast on–off") but flecainide has very "slow on–off" properties. This explains why flecainide has such potent effects on slowing ventricular conduction, whereas lidocaine has little effect on normal tissue (at normal heart rates). In general, the class Ic AADs are "slow on–off," the class Ib AADs are "fast on–off," and the class Ia AADs are intermediate in their binding kinetics.
3. Class I AADs possess rate dependence (i.e., sodium channel blockade and slowed conduction are greatest at fast heart rates and least during bradycardia). For "slow on–off" drugs, sodium channel blockade is evident at normal rates (60 to 100 beats/min), but for "fast on–off" agents, slowed conduction is only apparent at fast heart rates.
4. Class I AADs (except phenytoin) are weak bases with a pK_a >7 and block the sodium channel in their ionized form. Consequently, pH will alter these actions: acidosis accentuates and alkalosis diminishes sodium channel blockade.
5. Class I AADs appear to share a single receptor site in the sodium channel. It should be noted, however, that a number of class I AADs have other electrophysiologic properties. For instance, quinidine has potent potassium channel blocking activity (manifests predominantly at low concentrations) as does *N*-acetylprocainamide (manifests predominantly at high concentrations), the primary metabolite of procainamide. Additionally propafenone has β-blocking actions.

These principles are important in understanding additive drug combinations (e.g., quinidine and mexiletine), antagonistic combinations (e.g., flecainide and lidocaine), and potential antidotes to excess sodium channel blockade (sodium bicarbonate). They also explain a number of clinical observations, such as why lidocaine-like drugs are relatively ineffective for supraventricular tachycardia. The class Ib AADs are "fast on–off," inactivated sodium channel blockers; atrial cells, however, have a very brief inactivated phase relative to ventricular tissue.

The β-blockers are classified as class II AADs. For the most part, the clinically relevant acute antiarrhythmic mechanisms of the β-blockers result from their antiadrenergic actions. Because the SA and AV nodes are heavily influenced by adrenergic innervation, β-blockers would be most useful in tachycardias in which these nodal tissues are abnormally automatic or are a portion of a reentrant loop. These drugs are also helpful in slowing ventricular response in atrial arrhythmias (e.g., AF) by their effects on the AV node. Furthermore, some tachycardias are exercise-related or precipitated by states of high sympathetic tone (perhaps through triggered activity), and β-blockers may be useful in these instances. β-Adrenergic stimulation results in increased conduction velocity, shortened refractoriness, and increased automaticity of the nodal tissues; β-blockers will antagonize these effects. In the nodal tissues, β-blockers interfere with calcium entry into the cell by altering catecholamine-dependent channel integrity and gating kinetics. In sodium-dependent atrial and ventricular tissues, β-blockers shorten repolarization somewhat but otherwise have little direct effect. The antiarrhythmic properties of β-blockers observed with long-term, chronic therapy in patients with heart disease are less well understood. Although it is clear that β-blockers decrease the likelihood of SCD (presumably arrhythmic death) after myocardial infarction (MI), the mechanism for this benefit remains unclear but may relate to the complex interplay of changes in sympathetic tone, damaged myocardium, and ventricular conduction. In patients with heart failure (HF), drugs such as β-blockers, angiotensin-converting enzyme inhibitors, and angiotensin II receptor blockers may prevent arrhythmias such as AF by attenuating the structural and/or electrical remodeling process in the myocardium.[5,6]

The class III AADs include those agents that specifically prolong refractoriness in atrial and ventricular tissues. This class includes amiodarone, dronedarone, sotalol, ibutilide, and dofetilide; these drugs share the common effect of delaying repolarization by blocking potassium channels. Amiodarone and sotalol are effective in most supraventricular and ventricular arrhythmias. Amiodarone displays electrophysiologic characteristics of all four Vaughan Williams classes; it is a sodium channel blocker with relatively "fast on–off" kinetics, has nonselective β-blocking actions, blocks potassium channels, and also has a small degree of calcium channel blocking activity (Table 8-2). At normal heart rates and with chronic use, its predominant effect is to prolong repolarization. With IV administration, its onset is relatively quick (unlike the oral form) and β-blockade predominates initially. Theoretically, amiodarone, like class I AADs, may interrupt the reentrant substrate by transforming an area of unidirectional block into an area of bidirectional block. However, electrophysiologic studies using programmed cardiac stimulation imply that amiodarone may leave the reentrant loop intact. The impressive effectiveness of amiodarone coupled with its low proarrhythmic potential has challenged the notion that selective ion channel blockade by AADs is preferable. Sotalol is a potent inhibitor of outward potassium movement during repolarization and also possesses nonselective β-blocking actions. Unlike amiodarone and sotalol, dronedarone, ibutilide, and dofetilide are only approved for the treatment of supraventricular arrhythmias. Both ibutilide (only available IV) and dofetilide (only available orally) can be used for the acute conversion of AF or atrial flutter to SR. Dofetilide can also be used to maintain SR in patients with AF or atrial flutter of longer than 1 week's duration who have been converted to sinus rhythm (SR). Dronedarone is approved to reduce the risk of cardiovascular hospitalization in patients with a history of paroxysmal or persistent AF. Although structurally related to amiodarone, dronedarone's structure has been modified through the addition of a methylsulfonyl group and the removal of iodine. Dronedarone is also similar to amiodarone in exhibiting electrophysiologic characteristics of all four Vaughan Williams classes (sodium channel blocker with relatively "fast on–off" kinetics, nonselective β-blocker, potassium channel blocker, and calcium channel antagonist).

There are a number of different potassium channels that function during normal conduction; all approved class III AADs inhibit the delayed rectifier current (I_K) responsible for phase 2 and phase 3 repolarization. Subcurrents make up I_K: an ultrarapid component (I_{Kur}), a rapid component (I_{Kr}), and the slow component (I_{Ks}). *N*-Acetylprocainamide, sotalol, ibutilide, and dofetilide selectively block I_{Kr}, whereas amiodarone and dronedarone block both I_{Kr} and I_{Ks}. New drugs that selectively block I_{Kur} (found predominantly in the atrium but not ventricle) are being investigated for supraventricular arrhythmias. The clinical relevance of selectively blocking components of the delayed rectifier current remains to be determined. Potassium channel blockers (particularly those with selective I_{Kr} blocking properties) display "reverse use dependence" (i.e., their effects on repolarization are greatest at low heart rates). Sotalol and drugs like it also appear to be much more effective in preventing ventricular fibrillation (VF) (in dog models) than the traditional sodium channel blockers. They also decrease defibrillation threshold in contrast to class I AADs, which tend to increase this parameter. This feature could be important in patients with ICDs, as concurrent therapy with class I AADs may require more energy for successful cardioversion or may render the ICD ineffective in terminating the ventricular arrhythmia. The Achilles' heel of all class III AADs is an extension of their underlying ionic mechanism (i.e., by blocking potassium channels and delaying repolarization, they may also cause proarrhythmia in the form of TdP by provoking EADs).

The nondihydropyridine (non-DHP) CCBs, verapamil and diltiazem, are categorized as class IV AADs. At least two types of calcium channels are operative in SA and AV nodal tissues: an L-type channel and a T-type channel. Both L-type channel blockers (verapamil and diltiazem) and selective T-type channel blockers (mibefradil was previously approved but withdrawn from the market) will slow conduction, prolong refractoriness, and decrease automaticity (e.g., due to EADs or LADs) of the calcium-dependent tissue in the

TABLE 8-2 Time Course and Electrophysiologic Effects of Amiodarone

				IV		Oral	
Class	Mechanism	EP	ECG	Minutes–Hours	Hours–Days	Days–Weeks	Weeks–Months
Class I	Na^+ block	↑ HV	↑ QRS	0	+	+	++
Class II	β-block	↑ AH	↑ PR ↓ HR	++	++	++	++
Class III	K^+ block	↑ VERP ↑ AERP	↑ QT	0	+	++	++++
Class IV	Ca^{2+} block[a]	↑ AH	↑ PR	+	+	+	+

AERP, atrial effective refractory period; AH, atria–His interval; ECG, electrocardiographic effects; EP, electrophysiologic actions; HR, heart rate; HV, His–ventricle interval; VERP, ventricular effective refractory period.

[a]Rate-dependent.

SA and AV nodes. Therefore, these agents are effective in automatic or reentrant tachycardias, which arise from or use the SA or AV nodes. In supraventricular arrhythmias (e.g., AF), these drugs can slow ventricular response by slowing AV nodal conduction. Furthermore, because calcium entry seems to be integral to exercise-related tachycardias and/or tachycardias caused by some forms of triggered automaticity, these agents may be effective in the treatment of these types of arrhythmias. The DHP CCBs (e.g., nifedipine) do not have significant antiarrhythmic activity because a reflex increase in sympathetic tone caused by vasodilation counteracts their direct negative dromotropic action.

All AADs currently available have an impressive side effect profile (Table 8-3). A considerable percentage of patients cannot tolerate long-term therapy with these drugs and will have to discontinue therapy because of side effects. ❷ Flecainide, propafenone, and disopyramide may precipitate congestive HF in a significant number of patients with underlying LV systolic dysfunction; consequently, these drugs should be avoided in this patient population.[7] The class Ib AAD, mexiletine, causes neurologic and/or gastrointestinal (GI) toxicity in a high percentage of patients. One of the most frightening side effects related to AADs is the aggravation of underlying ventricular arrhythmias or the precipitation of new (and life-threatening) ventricular arrhythmias.[8]

Amiodarone has assumed a prominent place in the treatment of both chronic and acute supraventricular and ventricular arrhythmias and is now the most commonly prescribed AAD.[9] Once considered a drug of last resort, it is now the first AAD considered in many arrhythmias. Yet amiodarone is a peculiar and complex drug, displaying unusual pharmacologic effects, pharmacokinetics, dosing regimens, and multiorgan side effects. Amiodarone has an extremely long elimination half-life (greater than 50 days) and large volume of distribution; consequently, its onset of action with the oral form is delayed (days to weeks) despite the use of a loading regimen, and its effects persist for a long period (months) after discontinuation. Amiodarone is a substrate of the cytochrome P450 (CYP) 3A4 isoenzyme, a moderate inhibitor of many CYP isoenzymes (e.g., CYP2C9, CYP2D6, CYP3A4), and a P-glycoprotein inhibitor, all of which can result in the potential for numerous drug interactions. Amiodarone interacts with digoxin and warfarin and can significantly increase plasma concentrations of both drugs. By inhibiting P-glycoprotein, amiodarone can increase digoxin concentrations by approximately twofold; therefore, the digoxin dose should be empirically reduced by 50% when amiodarone is initiated. When amiodarone and warfarin are initiated concurrently, warfarin should be started at a dose of 2.5 mg daily. When amiodarone is initiated in a patient already receiving warfarin, the warfarin dose should be reduced by approximately 30%.[10] Acute administration of amiodarone is usually well tolerated by patients, but severe organ toxicities may result with chronic use. Severe bradycardia (sometimes requiring pacing to allow the patient to remain on amiodarone), hyperthyroidism, hypothyroidism, peripheral neuropathy, GI discomfort, photosensitivity, and a blue-gray skin discoloration on exposed areas are common. Fulminant hepatitis (uncommon) and pulmonary fibrosis (5% to 10% of patients) have caused death.[11,12] Although amiodarone can cause corneal microdeposits (usually do not affect vision) in virtually every patient, it has also been associated with the development of optic neuropathy/neuritis, which can lead to blindness. All of these side effects mandate close and continued monitoring (liver enzymes, thyroid function tests, eye examinations, chest radiographs, pulmonary function tests) and have led to a proliferation of "amiodarone clinics" designed just for patients receiving this drug on a chronic basis (Table 8-4). ❸[13,14]

The modifications to dronedarone's chemical structure may confer an improved safety profile when compared with amiodarone. With the addition of a methylsulfonyl group and the deletion of the iodine moiety, dronedarone is less lipophilic than amiodarone; consequently, dronedarone is supposed to be less likely to accumulate in tissues and cause various organ toxicities. Dronedarone also has a considerably shorter half-life (~24 hours) when compared with amiodarone, which allows for steady state to be achieved in 5 to 7 days, without the need for using loading doses. Like amiodarone, dronedarone is a substrate of the CYP3A isoenzyme and a moderate inhibitor of the CYP2D6 and CYP3A isoenzymes. Its use with potent CYP3A4 inhibitors or inducers should be avoided. Dronedarone may increase plasma concentrations of (*S*)-warfarin; therefore, the international normalized ratio (INR) should be closely monitored with concurrent use of these drugs. Dronedarone also inhibits P-glycoprotein and can increase digoxin concentrations by about 2.5-fold. Consequently, when concomitantly using dronedarone and digoxin, the digoxin dose should be empirically reduced by 50%. Additionally, dronedarone can increase dabigatran and rivaroxaban concentrations in patients with renal impairment. To minimize the risk of bleeding when concomitantly using dronedarone and dabigatran in this patient population, the dose of dabigatran should be reduced to 75 mg twice daily in those with moderate renal impairment (creatinine clearance [CrCl] 30 to 50 mL/min). The concomitant use of dronedarone and dabigatran should be avoided in patients with severe renal impairment (CrCl 15 to 30 mL/min). Rivaroxaban should only be used if the benefit outweighs the risk in patients receiving dronedarone who have a CrCl of 15 to 50 mL/min.

Table 8-5 summarizes the pharmacokinetics of the AADs and Table 8-6 lists recommended dosages of the oral dosage forms.

TABLE 8-3 Side Effects of Antiarrhythmic Drugs

Drug	Side effects
Disopyramide	Anticholinergic symptoms (dry mouth, urinary retention, constipation, blurred vision), nausea, anorexia, TdP, HF, conduction disturbances, ventricular arrhythmias
Procainamide[a]	Hypotension, TdP, worsening HF, conduction disturbances, ventricular arrhythmias
Quinidine	Cinchonism, diarrhea, abdominal cramps, nausea, vomiting, hypotension, TdP, worsening HF, conduction disturbances, ventricular arrhythmias, fever, hepatitis, thrombocytopenia, hemolytic anemia
Lidocaine	Dizziness, sedation, slurred speech, blurred vision, paresthesia, muscle twitching, confusion, nausea, vomiting, seizures, psychosis, sinus arrest, conduction disturbances
Mexiletine	Dizziness, sedation, anxiety, confusion, paresthesia, tremor, ataxia, blurred vision, nausea, vomiting, anorexia, conduction disturbances, ventricular arrhythmias
Flecainide	Blurred vision, dizziness, dyspnea, headache, tremor, nausea, worsening HF, conduction disturbances, ventricular arrhythmias
Propafenone	Dizziness, fatigue, bronchospasm, headache, taste disturbances, nausea, vomiting, bradycardia or AV block, worsening HF, ventricular arrhythmias
Amiodarone	Tremor, ataxia, paresthesia, insomnia, corneal microdeposits, optic neuropathy/neuritis, nausea, vomiting, anorexia, constipation, TdP (<1%), bradycardia or AV block (IV and oral use), pulmonary fibrosis, liver function test abnormalities, hepatitis, hypothyroidism, hyperthyroidism, photosensitivity, blue-gray skin discoloration, hypotension (IV use), phlebitis (IV use)
Dofetilide	Headache, dizziness, TdP
Dronedarone	Nausea, vomiting, diarrhea, serum creatinine elevations, bradycardia, worsening HF, liver toxicity, pulmonary fibrosis, TdP (<1%)
Ibutilide	Headache, TdP, hypotension
Sotalol	Dizziness, weakness, fatigue, nausea, vomiting, diarrhea, bradycardia or AV block, TdP, bronchospasm, worsening HF

AV, atrioventricular; HF, heart failure; TdP, torsade de pointes.

[a]Side effects listed are for the IV formulation only; oral formulations are no longer available.

TABLE 8-4 Amiodarone Monitoring

Side Effect	Monitoring Recommendations	Management of Side Effect
Pulmonary fibrosis	Chest radiograph (baseline, and then every 12 months) Pulmonary function tests (if symptoms develop)	Discontinue amiodarone immediately; initiate corticosteroid therapy
Hypothyroidism	TFTs (baseline, and then every 6 months)	Thyroid hormone supplementation (e.g., levothyroxine)
Hyperthyroidism	TFTs (baseline, and then every 6 months)	Antithyroid drugs (e.g., methimazole)
Optic neuritis/ neuropathy	Ophthalmologic examination (baseline [only if significant visual abnormalities present], and then if symptoms develop)	Discontinue amiodarone immediately
Corneal microdeposits	Slit-lamp examination (routine monitoring not necessary)	No treatment necessary
Hepatotoxicity	LFTs (baseline, and then every 6 months)	Lower the dose or discontinue amiodarone if LFTs >3× the upper limit of normal
Bradycardia/heart block	ECG (baseline, and then every 3–6 months)	Lower the dose, if possible, or discontinue amiodarone if severe
Tremor, ataxia, peripheral neuropathy	History/physical examination (each office visit)	Lower the dose, if possible, or discontinue amiodarone if severe
Photosensitivity/blue-gray skin discoloration	History/physical examination (each office visit)	Advise patients to wear sunblock while outdoors

ECG, electrocardiogram; LFTs, liver function tests, TFTs, thyroid function tests.

TABLE 8-5 Pharmacokinetics of Antiarrhythmic Drugs

Drug	Oral Bioavailability (%)	Primary Route of Elimination[a]	Substrate[b]	Inhibitor[b]	V_{Dss} (L/kg)	Protein Binding (%)	$t_{1/2}$[c]	Therapeutic Range (mg/L)
Disopyramide	70–95	H/R	CYP3A4 (M)	—	0.8–2	50–80	4–8 hours	2–6 (6–18 μmol/L)
Procainamide	—	H/R	NAT CYP2D6 (M)	—	1.5–3	10–20	5–6 hours (SAs) 2–3 hours (FAs)	4–15 (17–64 μmol/L)
Quinidine	70–80	H	CYP3A4 (M) CYP2C9	CYP2D6 (S) CYP3A4 (S) CYP2C9 P-GP	2–3.5	80–90	5–9 hours	2–6 (6–18 μmol/L)
Lidocaine	—	H	CYP3A4 (M) CYP2D6 (M) CYP1A2 CYP2C9	CYP1A2 (S) CYP2D6 CYP2D6	1–2	65–75	1–3 hours	1.5–5 (6.4–21.3 μmol/L)
Mexiletine	80–95	H	CYP2D6 (M) CYP1A2 (M)	CYP1A2 (S)	5–12	60–75	12–20 hours (PMs) 7–11 hours (EMs)	0.8–2 (4.5–11.1 μmol/L)
Flecainide	90–95	H/R	CYP2D6 (M) CYP1A2	CYP2D6	8–10	35–45	14–20 hours (PMs) 10–14 hours (EMs)	0.2–1 (0.5–2.4 μmol/L)
Propafenone[d]	11–39	H	CYP2D6 (M) CYP1A2 CYP2D6	CYP1A2 CYP2D6	2.5–4	85–95	10–25 hours (PMs) 3–7 hours (EMs)	—
Amiodarone	22–88	H	CYP3A4 (M) CYP1A2 CYP2C19 CYP2D6	CYP2C9 CYP2D6 CYP3A4 CYP1A2 CYP2C19 P-GP	70–150	95–99	15–100 days	1–2.5 (1.6–3.9 μmol/L)
Dofetilide	85–95	R/H	CYP3A4	—	2.5–3.5	60–70	6–10 hours	—
Dronedarone	4 (fasting) 15 (with food)	H	CYP3A4	CYP2D6 CYP3A4	20	>98	13–19	—
Ibutilide	—	H	—	—	6–12	40–50	3–6 hours	—
Sotalol	90–95	R	—	—	1.2–2.4	30–40	10–20 hours	—
Diltiazem	35–50	H	CYP3A4 (M) CYP2C9 CYP2D6	CYP3A4 CYP2C9 CYP2D6 P-GP	3–5	70–85	4–10 hours	—
Verapamil	20–40	H	CYP3A4 (M) CYP1A2 CYP2C9	CYP3A4 CYP1A2 CYP2C9 CYP2D6 P-GP	1.5–5	95–99	4–12 hours	—

[a]H, hepatic; R, renal.
[b]CYP, cytochrome P450 isoenzyme; M, major; NAT, *N*-acetyltransferase; P-GP, P-glycoprotein; S, strong.
[c]EMs, extensive metabolizers; FAs, fast acetylators; PMs, poor metabolizers; SAs, slow acetylators.
[d]Variables for parent compound (not 5-OH-propafenone).

TABLE 8-6 Typical Maintenance Doses of Oral Antiarrhythmic Drugs

Drug	Dose	Dose Adjusted
Disopyramide	100–150 mg q 6 h 200–300 mg q 12 h (SR form)	HEP, REN
Quinidine	200–300 mg sulfate salt q 6 h 324–648 gluconate salt q 8–12 h	HEP
Mexiletine	200–300 mg q 8 h	HEP
Flecainide	50–200 mg q 12 h	HEP, REN
Propafenone	150–300 mg q 8 h 225–425 mg q 12 h (SR form)	HEP
Amiodarone	400 mg two to three times daily until 10 g total, and then 200–400 mg daily[a]	
Dofetilide	500 mcg q 12 h	REN[b]
Dronedarone	400 mg twice daily (with meals)[c]	
Sotalol	80–160 mg q 12 h	REN[d]

HEP, hepatic disease; REN, renal dysfunction; SR, sustained release.

[a]Usual maintenance dose for atrial fibrillation is 200 mg/day (may further decrease dose to 100 mg/day with long-term use if patient clinically stable in order to decrease risk of toxicity); usual maintenance dose for ventricular arrhythmias is 300–400 mg/day.

[b]Dose should be based on creatinine clearance; should not be used when creatinine clearance <20 mL/min.

[c]Should not be used in severe hepatic impairment.

[d]Should not be used for atrial fibrillation when creatinine clearance <40 mL/min.

Table 8-7 lists the dosing recommendations for the IV forms of various AADs.

SUPRAVENTRICULAR ARRHYTHMIAS

The common supraventricular tachycardias that often require drug treatment are: (a) AF or atrial flutter, (b) paroxysmal supraventricular tachycardia (PSVT), and (c) automatic atrial tachycardias. Other common supraventricular arrhythmias that usually do not require drug therapy include premature atrial complexes, wandering atrial pacemaker, sinus arrhythmia, and sinus tachycardia. As an example, premature atrial complexes rarely cause symptoms and never cause hemodynamic compromise; therefore, drug therapy is usually not indicated. Likewise, sinus tachycardia is usually the result of underlying metabolic or hemodynamic disorders (e.g., infection, dehydration, hypotension), and therapy should be directed at the underlying cause, not the tachycardia per se. Of course, there are exceptions to these suggestions. For example, sinus tachycardia may be deleterious in patients after cardiac surgery or MI. Therefore, AADs, such as β-blockers, may be indicated in these situations. Stated in another way, although many arrhythmias generally do not require therapy, clinical judgment and patient-specific variables play an important role in this decision. AF, atrial flutter, and PSVT tend to be the most common supraventricular arrhythmias seen in clinical practice; therefore, this discussion will focus only on these arrhythmias.

Atrial Fibrillation and Atrial Flutter

Mechanisms and Background

AF continues to be the most common sustained arrhythmia encountered in clinical practice, affecting between 2.7 and 6.1 million Americans.[15] In the general population, the overall prevalence of AF is 0.4% to 1%, and this increases with age (e.g., approximately an 8% prevalence in patients >80 years old).[16] The prevalence of AF also appears to increase as patients develop more severe HF, increasing from 4% in asymptomatic New York Heart Association (NYHA) class I patients to 50% in patients with NYHA class IV HF.[17] With the aging population, improved survival in patients with HF, CAD, and hypertension, and the increased frequency of surgical procedures being performed, it is expected that the prevalence of AF will dramatically increase to an estimated 12 to 15 million by the year 2050.[17] Based on data derived from the Framingham study cohort, the general lifetime risk for AF in men and women at least 40 years of age is estimated to be 1 in 4.[18]

AF and atrial flutter may present as a chronic, established tachycardia, an acute tachycardia, or a self-terminating, paroxysmal form. The following semantics and definitions are sometimes used specifically for AF[16,19]: acute AF (onset within 48 hours), paroxysmal AF (terminates spontaneously in <7 days), recurrent AF (two or more episodes), persistent AF (duration >7 days and does not terminate spontaneously), and permanent AF (does not terminate with attempts at pharmacologic or electrical cardioversion). AF is characterized by extremely rapid (atrial rate of 400 to 600 beats/min) and disorganized atrial activation. With this disorganized atrial activity, there is a loss of the contribution of synchronized atrial contraction

TABLE 8-7 IV Antiarrhythmic Dosing

Drug	Clinical Situation	Dose
Amiodarone	Pulseless VT/VF	300 mg IV/IO push (can give additional 150 mg IV/IO push if persistent VT/VF), followed by infusion of 1 mg/min for 6 hours, and then 0.5 mg/min
	Stable VT (with a pulse)	150 mg IV over 10 minutes, followed by infusion of 1 mg/min for 6 hours, and then 0.5 mg/min
	AF (termination)	5 mg/kg IV over 30 minutes, followed by infusion of 1 mg/min for 6 hours, and then 0.5 mg/min
Diltiazem	PSVT; AF (rate control)	0.25 mg/kg IV over 2 minutes (may repeat with 0.35 mg/kg IV over 2 minutes), followed by infusion of 5–15 mg/h
Ibutilide	AF (termination)	1 mg IV over 10 minutes (may repeat if needed)
Lidocaine	Pulseless VT/VF	1–1.5 mg/kg IV/IO push (can give additional 0.5–0.75 mg/kg IV/IO push every 5–10 minutes if persistent VT/VF [maximum cumulative dose = 3 mg/kg]), followed by infusion of 1–4 mg/min (1–2 mg/min if liver disease or HF)
	Stable VT (with a pulse)	1–1.5 mg/kg IV push (can give additional 0.5–0.75 mg/kg IV push every 5–10 minutes if persistent VT [maximum cumulative dose = 3 mg/kg]), followed by infusion of 1–4 mg/min (1–2 mg/min if liver disease or HF)
Procainamide	AF (termination); stable VT (with a pulse)	15–18 mg/kg IV over 60 minutes, followed by infusion of 1–4 mg/min
Verapamil	PSVT; AF (rate control)	2.5–5 mg IV over 2 minutes (may repeat up to maximum cumulative dose of 20 mg); can follow with infusion of 2.5–10 mg/h

AF, atrial fibrillation; HF, heart failure; IO, intraosseous; PSVT, paroxysmal supraventricular tachycardia; VF, ventricular fibrillation; VT, ventricular tachycardia.

CLINICAL PRESENTATION Supraventricular Tachycardias

Atrial Fibrillation/Flutter

General

- These arrhythmias are usually not directly life-threatening and do not generally cause hemodynamic collapse or syncope; 1:1 atrial flutter (ventricular response ~300 beats/min) is an exception. Also, patients with underlying forms of heart disease who are heavily reliant on atrial contraction to maintain adequate cardiac output (e.g., mitral stenosis, obstructive cardiomyopathy) display more severe symptoms of AF or atrial flutter.

Symptoms

- Most often, patients complain of rapid heart rate/palpitations and/or worsening symptoms of HF (shortness of breath, fatigue). Medical emergencies are severe HF (i.e., pulmonary edema, hypotension) or AF occurring in the setting of acute MI.

Diagnostic tests/signs (ECG; see text for details)

- AF is an irregularly irregular supraventricular rhythm with no discernible, consistent atrial activity (P waves). Ventricular rate is usually 120 to 180 beats/min and the pulse is irregular. Atrial flutter is (usually) a regular supraventricular rhythm with characteristic flutter waves (or sawtooth pattern) reflecting more organized atrial activity. Commonly, the ventricular rate is in factors of 300 beats/min (e.g., 150, 100, or 75 beats/min).

Paroxysmal Supraventricular Tachycardia Caused by Reentry

General

- This arrhythmia can be transient, resulting in little, if any, symptoms.

Symptoms

- Patients frequently complain of intermittent episodes of rapid heart rate/palpitations that abruptly start and stop, usually without provocation (but occasionally as a result of exercise). Severe symptoms include syncope. Often (in particular, those with AV nodal reentry), patients complain of a chest pressure or neck sensation. This is caused by simultaneous AV contraction with the right atrium contracting against a closed tricuspid valve. Life-threatening symptoms (syncope, hemodynamic collapse) are associated with an extremely rapid heart rate (e.g., >200 beats/min) and AF associated with an accessory AV pathway.

Diagnostic tests/signs (ECG; see text for details)

- Most commonly, PSVT is a rapid, narrow QRS tachycardia (regular in rhythm) that starts and stops abruptly. Atrial activity, although present, is difficult to ascertain on surface ECG because P waves are "buried" in the QRS or T wave.

(atrial kick) to forward cardiac output. Supraventricular impulses penetrate the AV conduction system in variable degrees resulting in an irregular activation of the ventricles and an irregularly irregular pulse. The AV junction will not conduct most of the supraventricular impulses, causing the ventricular response to be considerably slower (120 to 180 beats/min) than the atrial rate. It is sometimes stated that "AF begets AF," that is, the arrhythmia tends to perpetuate itself. Long episodes are more difficult to terminate perhaps because of tachycardia-induced changes in atrial function (mechanical and/or electrical "remodeling").

Atrial flutter occurs less frequently than AF but is similar in its precipitating factors, consequences, and drug therapy approach. This arrhythmia is characterized by rapid (atrial rate of 270 to 330 beats/min) but regular atrial activation. The slower and regular electrical activity results in a regular ventricular response that is in approximate factors of 300 beats/min (i.e., 1:1 AV conduction = ventricular rate of 300 beats/min; 2:1 AV conduction = ventricular rate of 150 beats/min; 3:1 AV conduction = ventricular rate of 100 beats/min). Atrial flutter may occur in two distinct forms (type I and type II). Type I flutter is the more common classic form with atrial rates of approximately 300 beats/min and the typical "sawtooth" pattern of atrial activation as shown by the surface ECG. Type II flutter tends to be faster, being somewhat of a hybrid between classic atrial flutter and AF. Although the ventricular response usually has a regular pattern with this arrhythmia, atrial flutter with varying degrees of AV block or that occur with episodes of AF ("fib-flutter") can cause an irregular ventricular rate.

It is generally accepted that the predominant mechanism of AF and atrial flutter is reentry. AF appears to result from multiple atrial reentrant loops (or wavelets), whereas atrial flutter is caused by a single, dominant, reentrant substrate (counterclockwise circus movement in the right atrium around the tricuspid annulus). AF or atrial flutter usually occurs in association with various forms of structural heart disease (SHD) that cause atrial distension, including myocardial ischemia or infarction, hypertensive heart disease, valvular disorders such as mitral stenosis or mitral insufficiency, congenital abnormalities such as septal defects, dilated or hypertrophic cardiomyopathy, and obesity. Disorders that cause right atrial stretch and are associated with AF or atrial flutter include acute pulmonary embolus and chronic lung disease resulting in pulmonary hypertension and cor pulmonale. AF may also occur in association with states of high adrenergic tone such as thyrotoxicosis, surgery, alcohol withdrawal, sepsis, and excessive physical exertion. AF that develops in the absence of clinical, electrocardiographic, radiographic, and echocardiographic evidence of SHD is defined as lone AF. Other states in which patients are predisposed to episodes of AF are the presence of an anomalous AV pathway (i.e., Kent's bundle) and sinus node dysfunction (i.e., sick sinus syndrome).

Patients with AF or atrial flutter may experience the entire range of symptoms associated with other supraventricular tachycardias, although syncope as a presenting symptom is uncommon. Because atrial kick is lost with the onset of AF, patients with LV systolic or diastolic dysfunction may develop worsening signs and symptoms of HF as they often depend on the contribution of their atrial kick to maintain an adequate cardiac output. Thromboembolic events, resulting from atrial stasis and poorly adherent mural thrombi, are an additional complication of AF. Of course, the most devastating complication in this regard is the occurrence of an embolic stroke. The average rate of ischemic stroke in patients with AF who are not receiving antithrombotic therapy is approximately 5% per year.[20,21] Stroke can precede the onset of documented AF, probably as a result of undetected paroxysms prior to the onset of established AF. The risk of stroke significantly increases with age, with the annual attributable risk increasing from 1.5% in individuals 50 to 59 years of age to almost 24% in those 80 to 89 years of age.[20] Patients with concomitant AF and rheumatic heart disease are at particularly high risk for stroke, with their risk being increased 17-fold compared with patients in SR.[20] Other risk factors for stroke identified from recent trials are previous ischemic stroke, transient ischemic attack, or other systemic embolic event; age >75 years; moderate or severe LV systolic dysfunction and/or congestive HF; hypertension; and diabetes.[20] The risk of stroke in patients with only atrial flutter has been traditionally believed to be low, prompting some to recommend only aspirin for prevention of thromboembolism in this particular patient population. However, because patients with atrial flutter may also intermittently have episodes of AF, this patient population may also be at risk for a thromboembolic event. Although the role of antithrombotic therapy in patients with atrial flutter has not been adequately studied in clinical trials, the most recent guidelines suggest that the same risk stratification scheme and antithrombotic recommendations used in patients with AF should also be applied to those with atrial flutter.[20]

Management

The traditional approach to the treatment of AF can be organized into several sequential goals. First, evaluate the need for acute treatment (usually administering drugs that slow ventricular rate). Next, contemplate methods to restore SR, taking into consideration the risks (e.g., thromboembolism). Lastly, consider ways to prevent the long-term complications of AF such as arrhythmia recurrence and thromboembolism. ❹ One of the biggest controversies in the management of AF is whether restoring and maintaining SR is a desirable goal for all patients. A review of the management of AF and atrial flutter, including a discussion of this controversy, follows, organized according to the goals already outlined. Figure 8-5 shows an algorithm for the management of AF and atrial flutter. In addition, Table 8-8 summarizes the recommendations for pharmacologically controlling ventricular rate and restoring and maintaining SR from the most recent AF guidelines developed by the American College of Cardiology (ACC)/American Heart Association (AHA)/ European Society of Cardiology (ESC).[16,22]

Acute Treatment First, consider the patient with new-onset, symptomatic AF or atrial flutter. Although uncommon, patients may present with signs and/or symptoms of hemodynamic instability (e.g., severe hypotension, angina, or pulmonary edema), which qualifies as a medical emergency. In these situations, direct current cardioversion (DCC) is indicated as first-line therapy in an attempt to immediately restore SR (without regard to the risk of thromboembolism). Atrial flutter often requires relatively low energy levels of countershock (i.e., 50 J), whereas AF often requires higher energy levels (i.e., greater than 200 J).

If patients are hemodynamically stable, there is no emergent need to restore SR. Instead, the focus should be directed toward controlling the patient's ventricular rate. Achieving adequate ventricular rate control should be a treatment goal for all patients with AF. To achieve this goal, drugs that slow conduction and increase refractoriness in the AV node (e.g., β-blockers, non-DHP CCBs, or digoxin) should be used as initial therapy. Although loading doses of digoxin have been historically recommended as first-line treatment to slow ventricular rate, use of this drug for this purpose, especially in patients with normal LV systolic function (left ventricular ejection fraction [LVEF] >40%), has declined.[9] In this patient population, IV β-blocker (propranolol, metoprolol, esmolol), diltiazem, or verapamil is preferred. A few of the potential reasons for the declining use of digoxin in this patient population are its relatively slow onset and its inability to control the ventricular rate during exercise. Although an initial decrease in the ventricular rate can sometimes be observed within 1 hour of IV administration of digoxin, full control (heart rate <80 beats/min at rest and <100 beats/min during exercise) is usually not achieved for 24 to 48 hours. In addition, digoxin tends to be ineffective for controlling ventricular rate under conditions of increased sympathetic tone (i.e., surgery, thyrotoxicosis) because it slows AV nodal conduction primarily through vagotonic mechanisms. In contrast, IV β-blockers and non-DHP CCBs have a relatively quick onset and can effectively control the ventricular rate at rest and during exercise. β-Blockers are also effective for controlling ventricular rate under conditions of increased sympathetic tone.

Based on the most recent guidelines for the treatment of AF, the selection of a drug to control ventricular rate in the acute setting should be primarily based on the patient's LV function.[16] In patients with normal LV function (LVEF >40%), IV β-blocker, diltiazem, or verapamil is recommended as first-line therapy to control ventricular rate.[16] All of these drugs have proven efficacy in controlling the ventricular rate in patients with AF. Propranolol and metoprolol can be administered as intermittent IV boluses, whereas esmolol (because of its very short half-life of 5 to 10 minutes) must be administered as a series of loading doses followed by a continuous infusion. Likewise, because control of ventricular rate can be transient with a single bolus, verapamil or diltiazem can be given as an initial IV bolus followed by a continuous infusion.[23] These continuous infusions can be adjusted in monitored settings to the desired ventricular response (e.g., acutely <100 beats/min). In situations where AF or atrial flutter is precipitated by states of increased sympathetic tone (i.e., surgery, thyrotoxicosis), IV β-blockers can be highly effective and should be considered first.

In patients with LV dysfunction (LVEF ≤40%), both IV diltiazem and verapamil should be avoided because of their potent negative inotropic effects. IV β-blockers should be used with caution in this patient population and should be avoided if patients are in the midst of an episode of decompensated HF. In those patients who are having an exacerbation of HF symptoms, IV administration of either digoxin or amiodarone should be used as first-line therapy to achieve ventricular rate control.[16] IV amiodarone can also be used in patients who are refractory to or have contraindications to β-blockers, non-DHP CCBs, and digoxin.[16] However, clinicians should be aware that the use of amiodarone for controlling ventricular rate may also stimulate the conversion of AF to SR and place the patient at risk for a thromboembolic event, especially if the AF has persisted for at least 48 hours or is of unknown duration.

Patients may present with a slow ventricular response (in the absence of AV nodal blocking drugs) and thus do not require therapy with β-blockers, non-DHP CCBs, or digoxin. This type of presentation should alert the clinician to the possibility of preexisting SA or AV nodal conduction disease such as sick sinus syndrome. In these patients, DCC should not be attempted without a temporary pacemaker in place.

Restoration of Sinus Rhythm? After treatment with AV nodal blocking drugs and a subsequent decrease in the ventricular rate, the patient should be evaluated for the possibility of restoring SR if AF persists. Within the context of this evaluation, several factors should be considered. First, many patients spontaneously convert to SR without intervention, obviating the need for therapy to achieve

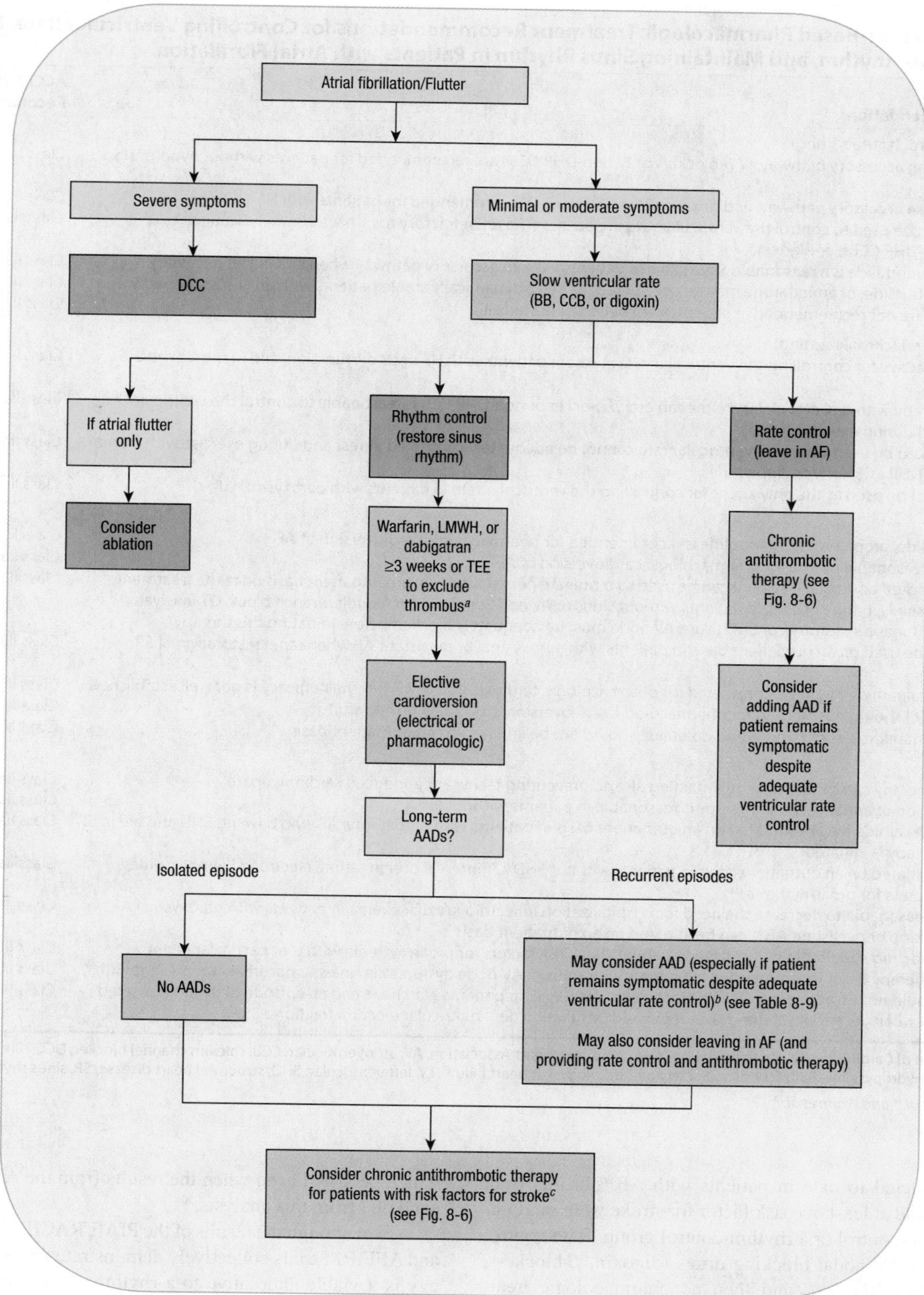

FIGURE 8-5 Algorithm for the treatment of AF and atrial flutter. [a]If AF <48 hours, anticoagulation prior to cardioversion is unnecessary; may consider TEE if patient has risk factors for stroke. [b]Ablation may be considered for patients who fail or do not tolerate ≥1 AAD. [c]Chronic antithrombotic therapy should be considered in all patients with AF and risk factors for stroke regardless of whether or not they remain in sinus rhythm. (AAD, antiarrhythmic drug; AF, atrial fibrillation; BB, β-blocker; CCB, calcium channel blocker [i.e., verapamil or diltiazem]; DCC, direct current cardioversion; LMWH, low-molecular-weight heparin; TEE, transesophageal echocardiogram.)

this goal. For instance, AF occurs frequently as a complication of cardiac surgery and often spontaneously reverts to SR without therapy. Second, restoring SR is not a necessary or realistic goal in some patients. The results of six landmark clinical trials (Pharmacological Intervention in Atrial Fibrillation [PIAF], Rate Control Versus Electrical Cardioversion for Persistent Atrial Fibrillation [RACE], Atrial Fibrillation Follow-Up Investigation of Rhythm Management [AFFIRM], Strategies of Treatment of Atrial Fibrillation [STAF], How to Treat Chronic Atrial Fibrillation [HOT-CAFE], and Atrial Fibrillation and Congestive Heart Failure [AF-CHF]) have shed significant light on the comparative efficacy of rate-control (controlling ventricular rate; patient remains in AF) and rhythm-control (restoring and maintaining SR) treatment strategies in patients with AF.[24–29] The AFFIRM trial is the largest rate-control versus rhythm-control

TABLE 8-8 Evidence-Based Pharmacologic Treatment Recommendations for Controlling Ventricular Rate, Restoring Sinus Rhythm, and Maintaining Sinus Rhythm in Patients with Atrial Fibrillation

Treatment Recommendations	ACC/AHA/ESC Guideline Recommendation
Ventricular rate control (acute setting)	
In the absence of an accessory pathway, IV β-blockers or IV non-DHP CCBs are recommended for patients without hypotension or HF	Class I
In the absence of an accessory pathway, IV digoxin or IV amiodarone is recommended for patients with HF	Class I
IV amiodarone can be used to control the ventricular rate in patients who are refractory to or have contraindications to IV β-blockers, non-DHP CCBs, or digoxin	Class IIa
IV procainamide or ibutilide is a reasonable alternative in patients with an accessory pathway when DCC is not necessary	Class IIa
IV procainamide, ibutilide, or amiodarone may be considered for hemodynamically stable patients with an accessory pathway	Class IIb
IV non-DHP CCBs are not recommended in patients with decompensated HF	Class III
Ventricular rate control (chronic setting)	
Oral digoxin is effective for controlling the ventricular rate at rest in patients with HF or LV dysfunction, and in those who are sedentary	Class I
Combination therapy with oral digoxin and either an oral β-blocker or non-DHP CCB is reasonable to control the ventricular rate both at rest and during exercise	Class IIa
Oral amiodarone can be used when the ventricular rate cannot be adequately controlled at rest and during exercise with an oral β-blocker, non-DHP CCB, and/or digoxin	Class IIb
Digoxin should not be used as the only agent for controlling the ventricular rate in patients with paroxysmal AF	Class III
Restoration of SR	
Flecainide, dofetilide, propafenone, or ibutilide is recommended for pharmacologic cardioversion of AF	Class I
Amiodarone is a reasonable option for pharmacologic cardioversion of AF	Class IIa
The "pill-in-the-pocket" approach (see text) can be used to terminate persistent AF on an outpatient basis once the treatment has been used safely in the hospital, in patients without sinus or AV node dysfunction, bundle-branch block, QT interval prolongation, Brugada syndrome, or SHD (*Note*: AV node must be adequately blocked before initiating this therapy)	Class IIa
Amiodarone can be used on an outpatient basis in patients with paroxysmal or persistent AF when rapid restoration of SR is not necessary	Class IIa
Quinidine or procainamide might be considered for pharmacologic cardioversion of AF, but their efficacy is not well established	Class IIb
Digoxin and sotalol should not be used for pharmacologic cardioversion of AF (may be harmful)	Class III
Quinidine, procainamide, disopyramide, and dofetilide should not be initiated on an outpatient basis	Class III
Maintenance of SR	
Antiarrhythmic therapy can be useful for maintaining SR and preventing tachycardia-induced cardiomyopathy	Class IIa
Outpatient initiation of antiarrhythmic therapy is reasonable in patients without SHD	Class IIa
Propafenone or flecainide may be initiated on an outpatient basis in patients with paroxysmal AF who have no SHD and are in SR at the time therapy is initiated	Class IIa
Sotalol may be initiated on an outpatient basis in patients without SHD, QT interval prolongation, electrolyte abnormalities, or other risk factors for proarrhythmia	Class IIa
Dronedarone is reasonable to decrease the need for hospitalization for cardiovascular events in patients with paroxysmal AF or after conversion of persistent AF. It can be initiated on an outpatient basis	Class IIa
An antiarrhythmic drug should not be used when patients have risk factors for proarrhythmia with that particular agent	Class III
Antiarrhythmic therapy is not recommended in patients with sinus or AV node dysfunction unless a pacemaker is present	Class III
Dronedarone should not be administered to patients with class IV HF or patients who have had an episode of decompensated HF in the last 4 weeks, especially if they have depressed LV function (left ventricular ejection fraction ≤35%)	Class III

ACC, American College of Cardiology; AF, atrial fibrillation; AHA, American Heart Association; AV, atrioventricular; CCB, calcium channel blocker; DCC, direct current cardioversion; DHP, dihydropyridine; ESC, European Society of Cardiology; HF, heart failure; LV, left ventricular; SHD, structural heart disease, SR, sinus rhythm.

Adapted from Fuster et al.[16] and Wann et al.[22]

study to be conducted to date in patients with AF.[26] In this trial, patients with AF and at least one risk factor for stroke were randomized to either a rate-control or a rhythm-control group. Rate-control treatment involved AV nodal blocking drugs (digoxin, β-blockers, and/or non-DHP CCBs) first, and then nonpharmacologic treatment (AV nodal ablation with pacemaker implantation), if necessary. All patients in this group were anticoagulated with warfarin to achieve an INR of 2 to 3. In the rhythm-control group, class I or III AADs were used to maintain SR. The choice of AAD therapy was left up to each patient's physician; however, by the end of the trial, more than 60% of patients had received at least one trial of amiodarone and approximately 40% of patients had received at least one trial of sotalol. In this group, anticoagulation was encouraged but could be discontinued if SR had been maintained for at least 4 weeks. After a mean follow-up period of 3.5 years, overall mortality was not statistically different between the two strategies but tended ($P = 0.08$) to be higher in the rhythm-control group. The results of the PIAF, RACE, STAF, and HOT-CAFE trials were consistent with those of the AFFIRM trial.[24,25,27,28] In addition, a meta-analysis of the data from all of these trials demonstrated no significant difference in overall mortality between rate-control and rhythm-control strategies, which persisted even when the results from the AFFIRM trial were excluded from this analysis.[30]

Even though the results of the PIAF, RACE, STAF, HOT-CAFE, and AFFIRM trials collectively demonstrate that a rate-control strategy is a viable alternative to a rhythm-control strategy in patients with persistent AF, a significant limitation of these results is that they cannot be applied to patients with HF because only a small proportion of patients enrolled in these trials had LV systolic dysfunction. The AF-CHF trial was conducted to specifically evaluate the safety and efficacy of rate-control and rhythm-control strategies in patients with systolic HF.[29] In this trial, patients with an LVEF ≤35%, a history of HF (defined as NYHA class II to IV HF within the last 6 months, NYHA class I HF with a hospitalization for HF during the previous 6 months, or an LVEF ≤25%), and a history of AF were randomized to either a rate-control or a rhythm-control group. Rate-control treatment involved concomitant therapy with a β-blocker and digoxin first, and then nonpharmacologic treatment (AV nodal ablation with pacemaker implantation), if necessary. In the rhythm-control group, amiodarone was the preferred AAD, whereas sotalol and dofetilide were considered alternatives (most of the patients ultimately received amiodarone). If patients in this group did not convert to SR within 6 weeks, electrical cardioversion was performed. Anticoagulation was recommended for all patients in both treatment groups. After a mean follow-up period of 37 months, no significant difference was observed between the treatment groups with regard to the primary end point of death from cardiovascular causes. Patients in the rhythm-control group tended to have more hospitalizations, primarily due to repeated cardioversions and adjustment of AAD therapy, compared with patients in the rate-control group; however, this difference was not statistically significant ($P = 0.06$). It is important to note that the results of this trial should not be applied to patients with HF and preserved LV function (i.e., diastolic HF). Nevertheless, the results of this trial are generally consistent with those of the PIAF, RACE, AFFIRM, STAF, and HOT-CAFE trials and suggest that a rhythm-control strategy does not confer any advantage over a rate-control strategy in patients with AF and systolic HF.

Clearly, these important findings temper the old approach of aggressively attempting to maintain SR. Because a rhythm-control strategy does not offer any significant advantage over a rate-control strategy in the management of patients with persistent or recurrent AF (including those with concomitant HF), it is acceptable to allow patients to remain in AF, while being chronically treated not only with AV nodal blocking drugs to achieve adequate ventricular rate control but also with appropriate antithrombotic therapy to prevent thromboembolic complications. ❹ The important question with this rate-control approach is: What defines "adequate" ventricular rate control? While adequate ventricular rate control was previously considered to be achieving a heart rate <80 beats/min at rest and <100 beats/min during exercise, evidence from the RACE II trial has suggested that selecting a more lenient rate-control strategy (resting heart rate <110 beats/min) may be a reasonable approach for certain patients with AF.[31] In this trial, a lenient rate-control strategy (resting heart rate <110 beats/min) was considered to be noninferior to a strict heart rate-control strategy (resting heart rate <80 beats/min and heart rate during moderate exercise <110 beats/min) with regard to the primary end point of cardiovascular death, hospitalization for HF, stroke, systemic embolism, bleeding, and life-threatening arrhythmic events. According to the most recent treatment guidelines for AF, this lenient rate-control strategy is recommended for those patients with persistent AF who have no or acceptable symptoms and stable LV function (LVEF >40%).[22] In patients with LV systolic dysfunction (LVEF ≤40%), a stricter rate-control approach (resting heart rate <80 beats/min) should be considered to minimize the potential harmful effects of a rapid heart rate response on ventricular function.

As in the acute setting, the selection of an AV nodal blocking drug to control ventricular rate in the chronic setting should be primarily based on the patient's LV function.[16] In patients with normal LV function (LVEF >40%), an oral β-blocker, diltiazem, or verapamil is preferred over digoxin because of their relatively quick onset and maintained efficacy during exercise. When adequate ventricular rate control cannot be achieved with one of these drugs, the addition of digoxin may result in an additive lowering of the heart rate. Verapamil and diltiazem should not be used in patients with LV dysfunction (LVEF ≤40%). Instead, β-blockers (i.e., metoprolol succinate, carvedilol, or bisoprolol) and digoxin are preferred in these patients, as these drugs are also concomitantly used to treat chronic HF. Specifically, in patients with NYHA class II or III HF, β-blockers should be considered over digoxin because of their survival benefits in patients with LV systolic dysfunction. If patients are having an episode of decompensated HF (NYHA class IV), digoxin is preferred as first-line therapy to achieve ventricular rate control because of the potential for worsening HF symptoms with the initiation and subsequent titration of β-blocker therapy. If adequate ventricular rate control during rest and exercise cannot be achieved with β-blockers, non-DHP CCBs, and/or digoxin in patients with normal or depressed LV function, oral amiodarone can be used as alternative therapy to control the heart rate.[16]

Because a rate-control strategy is now considered a reasonable initial approach for the chronic management of AF, the question that remains to be answered is, "In which patients should restoration of SR be considered?" Electrical or pharmacologic cardioversion should be considered for those patients with AF who remain symptomatic despite having adequate ventricular rate control or for those patients in whom adequate ventricular rate control cannot be achieved. In addition, a rhythm-control strategy may be considered in patients who are experiencing their first episode of AF if they are likely to convert to and remain in SR. Chronic AAD therapy is usually not needed in the latter population since the AF is often self-limiting.

In those patients in whom it is decided to restore SR, one must consider that this very act (regardless of whether an electrical or pharmacologic method is chosen) places the patient at risk for a thromboembolic event. The reason for this heightened risk is that the return of SR restores effective contraction in the atria, which may dislodge poorly adherent thrombi. Administering antithrombotic therapy prior to cardioversion not only prevents clot growth and the formation of new thrombi but also allows existing thrombi to become organized and well adherent to the atrial wall. It is a generally accepted principle that the risk of thrombus formation and a subsequent embolic event increases if the duration of the AF exceeds 48 hours. Therefore, it is vital for clinicians to estimate the duration of the patient's AF, so that appropriate antithrombotic therapy can be administered prior to cardioversion if needed.

According to the most recent guidelines on antithrombotic and thrombolytic therapy developed by the American College of Chest Physicians (ACCP), patients with AF lasting at least 48 hours or an unknown duration should be given therapeutic anticoagulation with warfarin (INR target range 2 to 3), a low-molecular-weight heparin (subcutaneously at treatment doses), or dabigatran for 3 weeks before cardioversion.[20] If the 3 weeks of therapeutic warfarin, low-molecular-weight heparin, or dabigatran therapy is not feasible, patients may alternatively undergo transesophageal echocardiography (TEE) to provide guidance regarding the need for antithrombotic therapy prior to cardioversion. If no thrombus is noted on TEE, these patients can be cardioverted without the mandatory 3 weeks of warfarin, low-molecular-weight heparin, or dabigatran pretreatment. In these patients, anticoagulation therapy with either IV unfractionated heparin or a low-molecular-weight heparin (subcutaneously at treatment doses) should be administered during the TEE and cardioversion procedure to prevent the formation of thrombi during the pericardioversion and postcardioversion periods. Cardioversion should then be performed within 24 hours of the TEE. Alternatively, warfarin therapy (INR target range of 2 to 3) may be used for at least 5 days prior to the TEE and cardioversion. If cardioversion is successful, therapeutic anticoagulation with either warfarin (INR target range of 2 to 3) or dabigatran should be continued for at least 4 weeks, regardless of the patient's baseline risk of stroke. The reason for continuing anticoagulation for this additional 4-week time period is that after restoration of SR, full atrial contraction does not occur immediately. Rather, it returns gradually to a maximum contractile force over a 3- to 4-week period. Decisions regarding long-term antithrombotic therapy after this 4-week time period should be primarily based on the patient's risk for stroke and not on whether he or she is in SR. If a thrombus is seen on TEE, cardioversion should not be performed and the patient should be anticoagulated indefinitely. If cardioversion is considered in these patients at a later time, a TEE should again be performed. Overall, the use of a TEE-guided approach to cardioversion in patients with AF has been compared with the conventional 3 weeks of anticoagulation before cardioversion in a large, multicenter, randomized trial.[32] In this trial, the incidence of thromboembolic events was not different between the two strategies, but bleeding episodes were higher in the group that received 3 weeks of warfarin therapy before cardioversion. Patients in the TEE strategy group had a higher success rate of achieving SR, probably because it is more difficult to terminate AF the longer a patient remains in this arrhythmia.

In patients with AF that is less than 48 hours in duration, anticoagulation prior to cardioversion is unnecessary because there has not been sufficient time to form atrial thrombi.[20] However, it is recommended that these patients should receive either IV unfractionated heparin or a low-molecular-weight heparin (subcutaneously at treatment doses) at presentation prior to and when proceeding to cardioversion. If these patients have risk factors for stroke, a TEE could alternatively be performed prior to cardioversion to exclude the presence of thrombus. If cardioversion is successful, therapeutic anticoagulation with either warfarin (INR target range 2 to 3) or dabigatran should be continued for at least 4 weeks, regardless of the patient's baseline risk of stroke. Decisions regarding long-term antithrombotic therapy after this 4-week time period should be primarily based on the patient's risk for stroke and not on whether he or she is in SR.

After prior anticoagulation or TEE, the process of restoring SR can be considered. There are two methods of restoring SR in patients with AF or atrial flutter: pharmacologic cardioversion and DCC. The decision to use either of these methods is generally a matter of clinical preference. The disadvantages of pharmacologic cardioversion are the risk of significant side effects (e.g., drug-induced TdP),[33] the potential for drug–drug interactions (e.g., digoxin–amiodarone), and the lower efficacy of AADs when compared with DCC. The advantages of DCC are that it is quick and more often successful (80% to 90% success rate). The disadvantages of DCC are the need for prior sedation/anesthesia and a risk (albeit small) of serious complications such as sinus arrest or ventricular arrhythmias.

Nonetheless, despite the relatively high success rate associated with DCC, clinicians often elect to use AADs first, and then resort to DCC in the event that these drugs fail. Pharmacologic cardioversion appears to be most effective when initiated within 7 days after the onset of AF.[16] According to the most recent treatment guidelines for AF, there is relatively strong evidence for efficacy of the class III pure I_K blockers (ibutilide and dofetilide), the class Ic AADs (e.g., flecainide and propafenone), and amiodarone (oral or IV) within this time frame.[16] Class Ia AADs have limited efficacy or have not been adequately studied in this setting. Sotalol is not effective for cardioversion of paroxysmal or persistent AF. Single, oral loading doses of propafenone (600 mg) and flecainide (300 mg) are effective compared with placebo for conversion of recent-onset AF and have been incorporated into the "pill-in-the-pocket" approach endorsed by the treatment guidelines.[16,34] With this method, outpatient, patient-controlled self-administration of a single, oral loading dose of either flecainide or propafenone can be a relatively safe and effective approach for the termination of recent-onset AF in a selected patient population that does not have sinus or AV node dysfunction, bundle-branch block, QT interval prolongation, Brugada syndrome, or SHD.[35] In addition, this treatment regimen should only be considered in patients who have previously been successfully cardioverted with these drugs on an inpatient basis. In patients with AF that is longer than 7 days in duration, only dofetilide, amiodarone, and ibutilide have proven efficacy for cardioversion.[16] The class Ia and Ic AADs have limited efficacy or have been inadequately studied in this setting.

Overall, when considering pharmacologic cardioversion, the selection of an AAD should be based on whether the patient has SHD (e.g., LV dysfunction, CAD, valvular heart disease, LV hypertrophy).[16] In the absence of any type of SHD, the use of a single, oral loading dose of flecainide or propafenone is a reasonable approach for cardioversion. Ibutilide can also be used as an alternative in this patient population; however, use of this agent is restricted to a monitored setting in the hospital because it requires QT interval monitoring. In patients with underlying SHD, flecainide, propafenone, and ibutilide should be avoided because of the increased risk of proarrhythmia; amiodarone or dofetilide should be used instead. Although amiodarone can be administered safely on an outpatient basis because of its low proarrhythmic potential, dofetilide therapy can only be initiated in the hospital (for QT interval monitoring). Additionally, it should be remembered that a patient's ventricular rate should be adequately controlled with AV nodal blocking drugs prior to administering a class Ic (or Ia) AAD for cardioversion. The class Ia and Ic AADs may paradoxically increase ventricular response. Traditionally, this observation has been attributed to the vagolytic action of these drugs despite the fact that only disopyramide displays significant anticholinergic side effects. Therefore, a more likely alternative explanation exists: all of these drugs slow atrial conduction, decreasing the number of impulses reaching the AV node; as a result, the AV node paradoxically allows more impulses to gain entrance to the ventricular conduction system, thereby increasing ventricular rate.

Long-Term Complications There are two forms of therapy that the clinician must consider in each patient with AF: long-term antithrombotic therapy to prevent stroke and long-term AADs to prevent recurrences of AF. Consider the issue of antithrombotic therapy first. Historically, warfarin has been the standard of care for stroke prevention in patients considered to be moderate or high risk for stroke. However, while warfarin is undoubtedly effective in preventing strokes in patients with AF, its use can be associated with a number of potential limitations, including a narrow therapeutic window, requirement for INR monitoring, food and drug interactions, and pharmacogenetic influences. Therefore, researchers have long been searching for an antithrombotic therapy that could be used as an alternative or even as a replacement for warfarin in patients with AF. Over the past few years, several oral antithrombotic therapies have been approved by the Food and Drug Administration for stroke prevention in patients with AF. These oral anticoagulant drugs include the direct thrombin inhibitor, dabigatran, and the factor Xa inhibitors, rivaroxaban and apixaban.

When initiating chronic antithrombotic therapy in patients with AF, assessing the patient's risk for stroke becomes important for selecting the most appropriate regimen. Based on the most recent ACCP guidelines, the CHADS2 index continues to be recommended for stroke risk stratification in patients with AF.[20] With this risk index, patients with AF are given two points if they have a history of a previous stroke or transient ischemic attack, and one point each for being ≥75 years old, having hypertension, having diabetes, or having congestive HF (CHADS2 is an acronym for each of these risk factors). The points are added up and the total score is then used to determine the most appropriate antithrombotic therapy for the patient (Fig. 8-6). Patients with a CHADS2 score of ≥2, 1, or 0 are considered to be at high risk, intermediate risk, and low risk for stroke, respectively. Based on the most recent ACCP guidelines, oral anticoagulant therapy is preferred over aspirin or aspirin plus clopidogrel therapy in patients who are at either high or intermediate risk for stroke. With regard to selection of an oral anticoagulant in both high-risk and intermediate-risk patients with AF, the updated ACCP guidelines suggest that dabigatran should be used rather than warfarin (INR target range 2 to 3). Either no antithrombotic therapy or aspirin is recommended for patients who are at low risk for stroke; however, no therapy is preferred in these patients. If the decision is made to initiate antithrombotic therapy in these low-risk patients, aspirin (75 to 325 mg/day) can be used.

The efficacy and safety of dabigatran were compared with those of warfarin in patients with AF in the Randomized Evaluation of Long-Term Anticoagulation Therapy (RE-LY) trial.[36] In this study, patients were randomized to receive dabigatran 110 mg twice daily, dabigatran 150 mg twice daily or adjusted-dose warfarin. The median follow-up period was 2 years. For the primary end point of

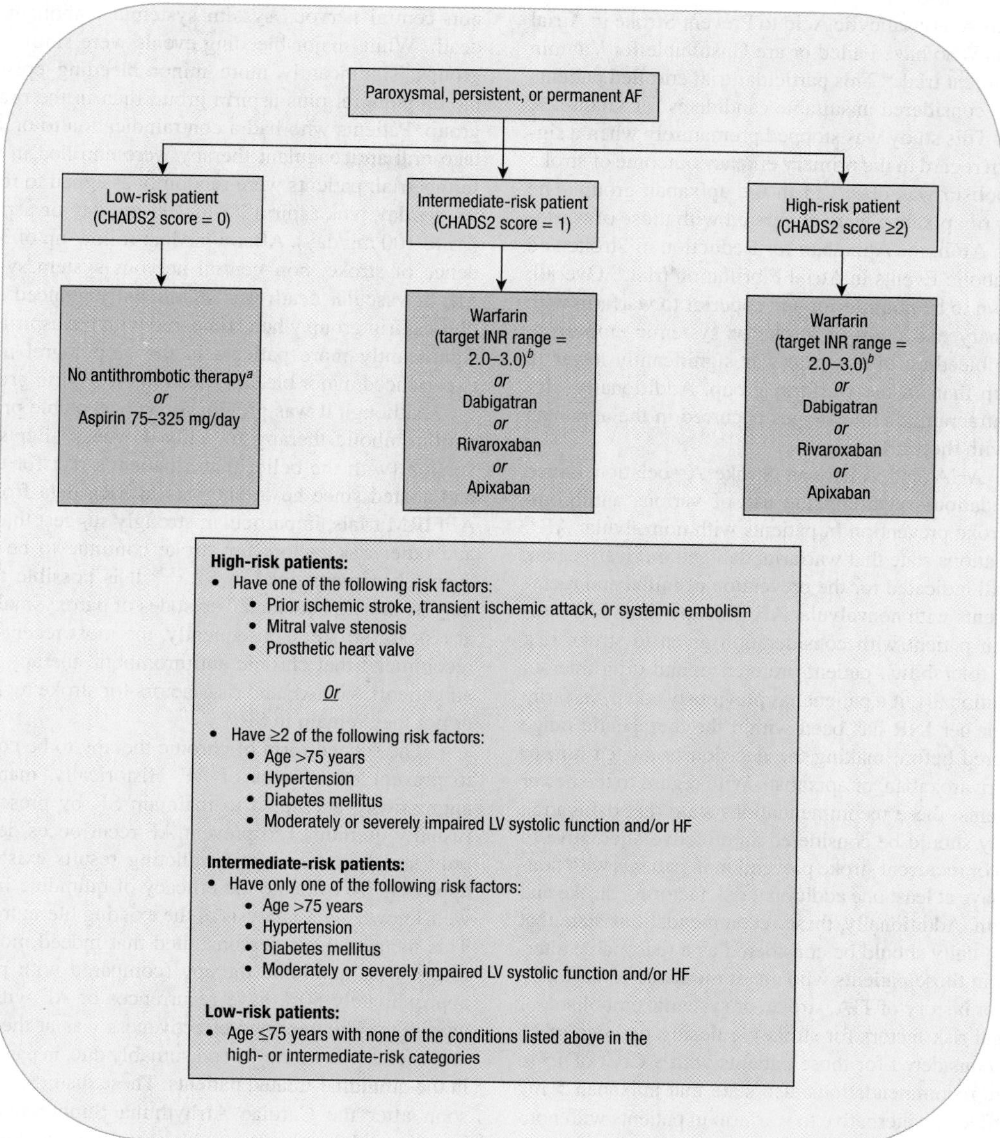

FIGURE 8-6 Algorithm for the prevention of thromboembolism in paroxysmal, persistent, or permanent AF. [a]No antithrombotic therapy preferred for low-risk patients. [b]The target INR for patients with prosthetic heart valves should be based on the type of valve that is present. (AF, atrial fibrillation; HF, heart failure; INR, international normalized ratio; LV, left ventricular.)

stroke or systemic embolism, both dabigatran groups were shown to be noninferior to warfarin. However, superiority was also assessed and the dabigatran 150-mg group was shown to be superior to warfarin in reducing this end point. The rate of major bleeding was similar between the dabigatran 150-mg and warfarin groups, while the rate of major bleeding was significantly lower in the dabigatran 110-mg group than in the warfarin group. The rate of intracranial hemorrhage was significantly lower in both dabigatran groups than in the warfarin group. Even though the 110- and 150-mg dosing regimens of dabigatran were evaluated in this trial, only the 150-mg dose was approved by the Food and Drug Administration. A lower 75-mg dose was also approved for patients with a CrCl of 15 to 30 mL/min, even though this dose has not been evaluated in a randomized, prospective clinical trial in patients with AF; this dose has only pharmacokinetic data to support its use.[37] It is important to note that the RE-LY trial excluded patients with a CrCl <30 mL/min. Therefore, the most recent ACCP guidelines made the evidence-based decision to recommend that dabigatran be contraindicated in patients with a CrCl <30 mL/min. Dabigatran is also contraindicated in patients with mechanical heart valves. The use of dabigatran is also not recommended in patients with bioprosthetic heart valves since the safety and efficacy of this antithrombotic have not been evaluated in this population. Patients with hemodynamically significant valvular disease or advanced liver disease are also not appropriate candidates for dabigatran therapy.[38]

The efficacy and safety of rivaroxaban were compared with those of warfarin in patients with AF in the Rivaroxaban Once Daily Oral Direct Factor Xa Inhibition Compared with Vitamin K Antagonism for Prevention of Stroke and Embolism Trial in Atrial Fibrillation.[39] In this study, patients were randomized to receive rivaroxaban 20 mg daily or adjusted-dose warfarin. The median follow-up period was 1.9 years. For the primary end point of stroke or systemic embolism, rivaroxaban was shown to be noninferior to warfarin. The rate of major and nonmajor clinically relevant bleeding was similar between the rivaroxaban and warfarin groups. Significantly fewer intracranial hemorrhages occurred in the rivaroxaban group compared with the warfarin group.

The efficacy and safety of the other factor Xa inhibitor, apixaban, were compared with those of aspirin in patients with AF in the Apixaban Versus Acetylsalicylic Acid to Prevent Stroke in Atrial Fibrillation Patients Who have Failed or are Unsuitable for Vitamin K Antagonist Treatment trial.[40] This particular trial enrolled patients who failed or were considered unsuitable candidates for vitamin K antagonist therapy. This study was stopped prematurely when a significant benefit with regard to the primary efficacy outcome of stroke and systemic embolism was observed in the apixaban group. The efficacy and safety of apixaban were compared with those of warfarin in patients with AF in the Apixaban for Reduction in Stroke and Other Thromboembolic Events in Atrial Fibrillation trial.[41] Overall, apixaban was shown to be noninferior and superior to warfarin with regard to the primary end point of stroke or systemic embolism. The rate of major bleeding in this trial was significantly lower in the apixaban group than in the warfarin group. Additionally, significantly fewer intracranial hemorrhages occurred in the apixaban group compared with the warfarin group.

Recently, the AHA and American Stroke Association issued revised recommendations regarding the use of various antithrombotic agents for stroke prevention in patients with nonvalvular AF.[42] These recommendations state that warfarin, dabigatran, rivaroxaban, and apixaban are all indicated for the prevention of initial and recurrent strokes in patients with nonvalvular AF. Therapy should be individualized for each patient with consideration given to stroke risk factors, drug cost, tolerability, patient preference, and drug interaction potential. Additionally, if a patient has previously taken warfarin, the time that his or her INR has been within the therapeutic range should be considered before making the decision to switch him or her to dabigatran, rivaroxaban, or apixaban. With regard to the newer antithrombotic agents, these recommendations state that dabigatran 150 mg twice daily should be considered an effective alternative to warfarin for initial or recurrent stroke prevention in patients with nonvalvular AF who have at least one additional risk factor for stroke and a CrCl >30 mL/min. Additionally, these recommendations state that rivaroxaban 20 mg daily should be considered as a reasonable alternative to warfarin in those patients who are at moderate-to-high risk of stroke (e.g., prior history of TIA, stroke, or systemic embolism, or at least 2 additional risk factors for stroke); a dosing regimen of 15 mg daily may be considered for those patients with a CrCl of 15 to 50 mL/min. These recommendations also state that apixaban 5 mg twice daily is an effective alternative to warfarin in patients with nonvalvular AF who have at least one risk factor for stroke; a dosing regimen of 2.5 mg twice daily may be considered for those patients with at least two of the following: age ≥80 years, weight ≤60 kg, or serum creatinine ≥1.5 mg/dL (133 μmol/L). Apixaban 5 mg twice daily is also considered an effective alternative to aspirin in those patients with nonvalvular AF who have at least one risk factor for stroke and are considered unsuitable candidates for warfarin; a similar dosage adjustment can be made based on the age, weight, and renal function criteria listed above.

Based on the most recent ACCP guidelines, dual antiplatelet therapy with aspirin plus clopidogrel is recommended over aspirin monotherapy for patients who are at high or intermediate risk for stroke and are not candidates for oral anticoagulant therapy for reasons other than bleeding (i.e., patient preference, unable to adhere to monitoring or dosing regimen requirements).[20] These recommendations are based on the results of the Atrial Fibrillation Clopidogrel Trial with Irbesartan for Prevention of Vascular Events (ACTIVE) W and ACTIVE A.[43,44] Both of these trials evaluated the efficacy and safety of this combination therapy in patients with AF and at least one risk factor for stroke. In the ACTIVE W, patients were randomized to receive oral anticoagulation therapy (with the vitamin K antagonist used in the investigator's country) titrated to achieve a target INR of 2 to 3 or clopidogrel 75 mg/day plus aspirin 75 to 100 mg/day.[43] This trial was prematurely discontinued when the oral anticoagulation therapy was found to be superior to the combination antiplatelet regimen in reducing the occurrence of stroke, non–central nervous system systemic embolism, MI, or vascular death. While major bleeding events were similar between the two groups, significantly more minor bleeding episodes occurred in the clopidogrel plus aspirin group than in the oral anticoagulation group. Patients who had a contraindication to or were unwilling to take oral anticoagulant therapy were enrolled in the ACTIVE A.[44] In this trial, patients were randomly assigned to receive clopidogrel 75 mg/day plus aspirin 75 to 100 mg/day or aspirin monotherapy (75 to 100 mg/day). After a median follow-up of 3.6 years, the incidence of stroke, non–central nervous system systemic embolism, MI, or vascular death was significantly reduced in the clopidogrel plus aspirin group when compared with the aspirin group. However, significantly more patients in the clopidogrel plus aspirin group experienced major bleeding than in the aspirin group.

Although it was previously an acceptable practice to continue antithrombotic therapy for only 4 weeks after successful cardioversion (with the belief that a patient's risk for thromboembolism had abated since he or she was in SR), data from the RACE and AFFIRM trials, in particular, strongly suggest that patients with AF and other risk factors for stroke continue to be at risk for stroke even when maintained in SR.[25,26] It is possible that these patients may be having undetected episodes of paroxysmal AF, placing them at risk for stroke. Consequently, the most recent ACCP guidelines recommend that chronic antithrombotic therapy be considered for all patients with AF and risk factors for stroke regardless of whether or not they remain in SR.[20]

The second form of chronic therapy to be considered is AADs to prevent recurrences of AF. Historically, many clinicians have aggressively attempted to maintain SR by prescribing oral AADs (usually quinidine) to prevent AF recurrences despite the fact that only small studies with conflicting results existed evaluating this approach. To evaluate the efficacy of quinidine in preventing AF, a well-known meta-analysis of the existing literature was completed.[45] This meta-analysis demonstrated that indeed more patients remain in SR with quinidine therapy (compared with placebo); however, approximately 50% have recurrences of AF within a year despite quinidine. This reported effectiveness was at the cost of an associated increase in mortality (presumably due, in part, to proarrhythmia) in the quinidine-treated patients. These disturbing results (published soon after the Cardiac Arrhythmia Suppression Trial [CAST][46]) became widely quoted and highly visible, making clinicians question the wisdom of long-term prevention of recurrences of AF with AADs. These results coupled with the findings of the PIAF, RACE, AFFIRM, STAF, HOT-CAFE, and AF-CHF trials question the need to use AADs to prevent AF recurrences.[24–29] In fact, based on the results of these landmark trials, the use of AADs to maintain SR may be more reasonable to consider in patients who remain symptomatic despite having adequate ventricular rate control or for those patients in whom adequate ventricular rate control cannot be achieved.

According to the most recent treatment guidelines for AF, the class Ic or III AADs are reasonable to consider to maintain patients in SR (Table 8-9).[16] The role of the class Ia AADs for maintenance of SR has been deemphasized throughout these guidelines as they are considered less effective or incompletely studied compared with the class Ic and III AADs. Realistically, however, these drugs can still be considered as last-line therapy in select patients. Interestingly, a systematic review of AADs for the maintenance of SR after cardioversion in patients with AF demonstrated that AF recurrences were significantly reduced with the use of class Ia, Ic, and III AADs; however, mortality was significantly increased with the class Ia drugs, in particular.[47]

The class Ic AADs, flecainide and propafenone, are effective for maintaining SR. However, because of the increased risk for proarrhythmia, these drugs should be avoided in patients with SHD.

Although all of the oral class III AADs have demonstrated efficacy in preventing AF recurrences, amiodarone is clearly the most

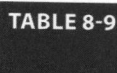

TABLE 8-9 Guidelines for Selecting Antiarrhythmic Drug Therapy for Maintenance of Sinus Rhythm in Patients with Recurrent Paroxysmal or Recurrent Persistent Atrial Fibrillation

No structural heart disease[a] (absence of heart failure, coronary artery disease, significant LVH, and valvular disease)
First line: dronedarone, flecainide, propafenone, or sotalol
Second line: amiodarone or dofetilide (catheter ablation could also be considered as an alternative to antiarrhythmic therapy)

Heart failure[a]
First line: amiodarone or dofetilide
Second line: catheter ablation

Coronary artery disease[a]
First line: dofetilide, dronedarone,[b] or sotalol[b]
Second line: amiodarone (catheter ablation could also be considered as an alternative to antiarrhythmic therapy)

Hypertension[a]
Presence of significant LVH:
First line: amiodarone
Second line: catheter ablation
Absence of significant LVH:
First line: dronedarone, flecainide, propafenone, or sotalol
Second line: amiodarone or dofetilide (catheter ablation could also be considered as an alternative to antiarrhythmic therapy)

LVH, left ventricular hypertrophy.

[a]Drugs are listed alphabetically and not in order of suggested use.
[b]Should only be used in this situation if the patient has normal left ventricular systolic function.

effective agent and is now the most frequently used AAD despite its potential for causing significant organ toxicity.[9] The superiority of amiodarone over other AADs for maintaining patients in SR has been demonstrated in a number of clinical trials. In the Canadian Trial of Atrial Fibrillation, amiodarone was significantly more effective than sotalol or propafenone in maintaining SR in patients with persistent or paroxysmal AF.[48] Furthermore, in a substudy of the AFFIRM trial, amiodarone appeared to be the most effective AAD in maintaining SR of those used in the study.[49] In the Sotalol Amiodarone Atrial Fibrillation Efficacy Trial, amiodarone and sotalol were equally effective at converting AF to SR.[50] However, amiodarone was significantly more effective than sotalol at maintaining SR in all patient subgroups, except for those with CAD where the efficacy of these two drugs was comparable.

Although sotalol is not effective for conversion of AF, it is an effective drug for maintaining SR. Sotalol appears to be at least as effective as quinidine or propafenone in preventing recurrences of AF.[48,51] However, treatment with either quinidine or sotalol is associated with a similar incidence of TdP. Because this form of proarrhythmia primarily occurs with higher doses of sotalol (quinidine usually causes TdP at low or therapeutic concentrations), it may be more easily predicted and therefore avoided. Nonetheless, sotalol may be similar to quinidine in increasing mortality in patients with AF; however, this finding requires further study.[52]

Dofetilide is effective in preventing recurrences of AF[53] but has not been directly compared with either amiodarone or sotalol. In a large, multicenter trial,[54] dofetilide was more effective than placebo in maintaining SR (approximately 35% to 50% at 1 year). The efficacy of dofetilide for the maintenance of SR has also specifically been demonstrated in patients with LV systolic dysfunction.[53] Like sotalol and quinidine, dofetilide also has significant potential to cause TdP (in a dose-related fashion).

The safety and efficacy of dronedarone for the treatment of AF and atrial flutter have been evaluated in several clinical trials. In the European Trial in Atrial Fibrillation or Flutter Patients Receiving Dronedarone for the Maintenance of Sinus Rhythm and the American–Australian–African Trial with Dronedarone in Atrial Fibrillation or Flutter Patients for the Maintenance of Sinus Rhythm, which were similar in design, dronedarone was more effective than placebo in maintaining SR in patients with paroxysmal or persistent AF or atrial flutter.[55] In another trial, the use of dronedarone in patients with persistent or paroxysmal AF or atrial flutter was associated with significantly fewer hospitalizations due to cardiovascular events or death when compared with placebo.[56] The safety and efficacy of dronedarone were also evaluated in a trial that included patients with NYHA class III or IV HF and an LVEF of 35% or less.[57] This trial was prematurely terminated because all-cause mortality (primarily due to worsening HF) was significantly higher in the dronedarone group when compared with the placebo group. Consequently, based on these findings, dronedarone is contraindicated in and has received a black box warning for patients with advanced HF (NYHA class IV or NYHA class II or III with a recent hospitalization for decompensated HF). The efficacy and safety of dronedarone in patients with AF have been compared with those of amiodarone.[58] In this trial, dronedarone was shown to be significantly less effective than amiodarone in reducing AF recurrences; however, tolerability was significantly better in the dronedarone group than in the amiodarone group as evidenced by higher rates of premature drug discontinuation and adverse events in the amiodarone group. Most recently, a trial that enrolled patients with permanent AF and risk factors for major vascular events was terminated prematurely after significantly more patients in the dronedarone group died (primarily from cardiovascular causes), were hospitalized for HF, and suffered a stroke when compared with the placebo group.[59] Based on the results of this trial, dronedarone is contraindicated in and has received a boxed warning for patients with permanent AF.

Overall, the selection of an AAD to maintain SR should be primarily based on whether the patient has SHD.[16,22] However, other factors, including renal and hepatic function, concomitant disease states and drugs, and the AAD's side effect profile, also need to be considered. For those patients with no underlying SHD, dronedarone, flecainide, propafenone, or sotalol should be considered initially because these drugs have the most optimal long-term safety profile in this setting. However, amiodarone or dofetilide could be used as alternative therapy if the patient fails or does not tolerate one of these initial AADs. In the presence of SHD, flecainide and propafenone should be avoided because of the risk of proarrhythmia. If LV systolic dysfunction is present (LVEF ≤40%), amiodarone should be considered the AAD of choice. Dofetilide can be used as an alternative if patients develop intolerable side effects with amiodarone. At this time, only amiodarone and dofetilide have been shown to be mortality-neutral in patients with AF and HF. Both dronedarone and sotalol should be avoided in patients with LV systolic dysfunction because of the risk for increased mortality (dronedarone) or worsening HF (sotalol). In patients with CAD, dofetilide, dronedarone, or sotalol can be used initially. Again, dronedarone and sotalol should not be used in patients with LV systolic dysfunction. Amiodarone could be used as an alternative therapy if the patient fails or does not tolerate one of these initial AADs. The presence of LV hypertrophy may predispose the myocardium to proarrhythmic events. Because of its low proarrhythmic potential, amiodarone should be considered first-line AAD therapy in these patients.

Nonpharmacologic forms of therapy, designed to maintain SR, are becoming increasingly popular treatment options for patients with AF or atrial flutter. For patients who have "pure" (i.e., not associated with concurrent AF) type I atrial flutter, ablation of the reentrant substrate with radiofrequency current is highly effective (~90%)[60] and can be considered first-line treatment of atrial flutter to prevent recurrences.[61] Catheter ablation for patients with AF is much more technically difficult for a variety of reasons, including the lack of a single, identifiable, and ablatable reentrant focus (as in atrial flutter). Nonetheless, progress has been made in this area. Patients with AF have been found to have arrhythmogenic foci that occur in atrial tissue near and within the pulmonary veins. During the ablation procedure, radiofrequency energy can be delivered to these areas in an attempt to abolish the foci. Historically, this procedure was often considered last-line therapy for patients who had failed all AADs, including amiodarone. However, in some of the recent trials, the use of catheter ablation in patients with AF has been associated with a significant reduction in recurrent episodes of AF and an improvement in quality of life when compared with AAD therapy.[62–64] There is even some evidence[65,66] to suggest that this procedure may be superior to AADs as first-line therapy of symptomatic AF. According to the most recent guidelines, for those patients with symptomatic episodes of AF who fail or do not tolerate at least one class I or III AAD, catheter ablation is recommended for those with paroxysmal AF, reasonable for those with persistent AF, and may be considered for those with long-standing persistent AF.[67] For those patients with symptomatic episodes of AF who have not yet received treatment with a class I or III AAD, catheter ablation is reasonable for those with paroxysmal AF and may be considered for persistent or long-standing persistent AF. This procedure is not without its risks, as major complications, such as pulmonary vein stenosis, thromboembolic events, cardiac tamponade, and new atrial flutter, have been reported in 4.5% of patients.[68]

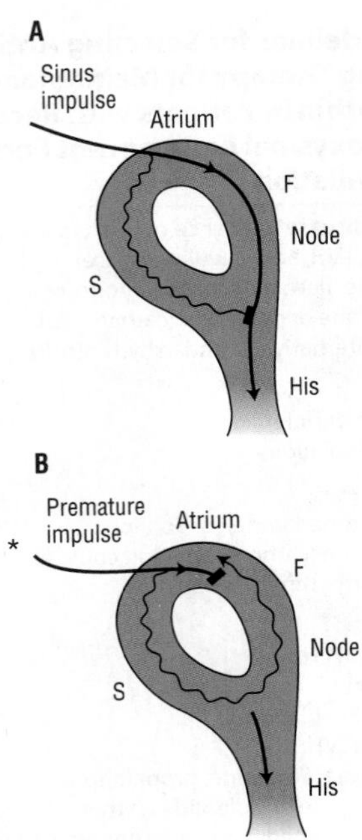

FIGURE 8-7 Reentry mechanism of dual AV nodal pathway PSVT. *A.* Sinus rhythm: the impulse travels from the atrium through the fast pathway (*F*) and then to the His-Purkinje system (*His*). The impulse also travels through the slow pathway (*S*) but is stopped when refractory tissue is encountered. *B.* Dual AV nodal reentry: a critically timed premature impulse (*) is stopped in the fast pathway (because of prolonged refractoriness) but is able to travel antegrade down the slow pathway and retrograde through the fast pathway. (AV, atrioventricular; PSVT, paroxysmal supraventricular tachycardia.)

Paroxysmal Supraventricular Tachycardia Caused by Reentry

PSVT arising by reentrant mechanisms includes those arrhythmias caused by AV nodal reentry, AV reentry incorporating an anomalous AV pathway, SA nodal reentry, and intraatrial reentry. AV nodal reentry and AV reentry are by far the most common of these tachycardias. 5

Mechanisms

The underlying substrate of AV nodal reentry is the functional division of the AV node into two (or more) longitudinal conduction pathways or "dual" AV nodal pathways.[69] It is now clear that there are not two distinct anatomic pathways inside the AV node itself; rather, it is likely that a fan-like network of perinodal fibers inserts into the AV node and represents the second pathway. The pathways possess key differences in conduction characteristics: one is a fast-conducting pathway with a relatively long refractory period (fast pathway) and the other is a slower-conducting pathway with a shorter refractory period (slow pathway). The presence of dual pathways does not necessarily imply that the patient will have clinical PSVT. In fact, it is estimated that between 10% and 50% of patients have discernible dual pathways, but the incidence of PSVT is considerably lower.[69] Sustenance of the tachycardia depends on the critical electrophysiologic discrepancies and the ability of one pathway (usually the slow) to allow repetitive antegrade conduction, and the ability of the other pathway (usually the fast) to allow repetitive retrograde conduction. During SR, a patient with dual pathways conducts supraventricular impulses antegrade through both pathways. Electrical activity reaches the distal common pathway at the level of or above the His bundle and continues to depolarize the ventricles in an antegrade direction. Conduction proceeds via the two pathways but reaches the distal common pathway first through the fast AV nodal route (Fig. 8-7). For this reason, a short PR interval is sometimes observed during SR.

PSVT caused by AV nodal reentry may occur by the following sequence of events. The occurrence of an appropriately timed premature impulse penetrates the AV node but is blocked in the fast pathway that is still refractory from the previous beat. However, the slow pathway, which has a shorter refractory period, permits antegrade conduction of the premature impulse. By the time the impulse has reached the distal common pathway, the fast pathway has recovered its excitability and now will permit retrograde conduction. The impulse reaches the common proximal pathway, preceded by an excitable gap of tissue, and reenters the slow pathway. A reentrant circuit that does not require atrial or ventricular tissue is completed within the AV node, and a tachycardia is thereby initiated (Fig. 8-7). The common form of this tachycardia uses the slow pathway for antegrade conduction and the fast pathway for retrograde conduction; an uncommon form exists in which the reentrant impulse travels in the opposite direction.

AV reentrant tachycardia depends on the presence of an anomalous, or accessory, extranodal pathway that bypasses the normal AV conduction pathway. Several different types of accessory pathways have been described, depending on the specific anatomic areas they connect (e.g., AV bundles or nodoventricular tracts); some are also referred to as eponyms, such as the Kent's bundle. A Kent's bundle is an extranodal AV connection that is associated with Wolff-Parkinson-White (WPW) syndrome. During SR (Fig. 8-8), patients with WPW syndrome depolarize the ventricles simultaneously through both AV pathways (AV nodal pathway and the Kent's bundle), creating a fusion pattern on the early portion of the QRS complex (delta wave). The degree of ventricular "preexcitation" depends on the contribution of antegrade ventricular activation through the accessory pathway. Patients may have an accessory pathway that is not evident on ECG, which is referred to as a "concealed" Kent's bundle. These concealed accessory pathways are often incapable of antegrade conduction and can only accept electrical stimulation in a retrograde fashion. The electrocardiographic expression of preexcitation (delta wave) depends on the location of the accessory pathway, the distance from the wave front of sinus activation, and the conduction characteristics of the various structures involved.

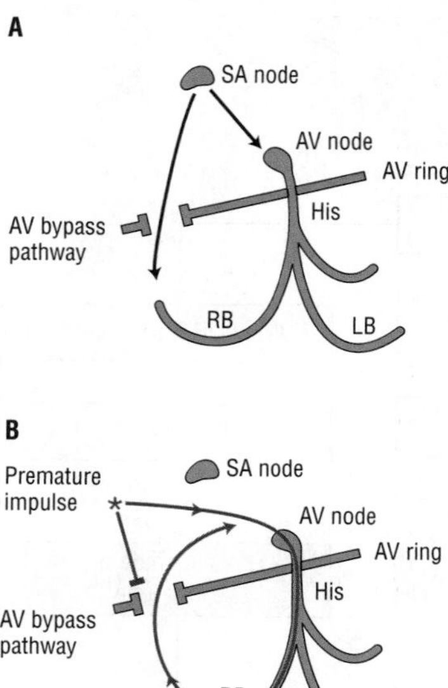

FIGURE 8-8 Reentry mechanism for AV accessory pathway PSVT in Wolff-Parkinson-White syndrome. *A.* Sinus rhythm: the impulse travels from the atrium to the ventricle by two pathways—the AV node and an accessory bypass pathway. *B.* AV reentry: a critically timed premature impulse (*) is stopped in the Kent's bundle (because of prolonged refractoriness) but travels antegrade through the AV node and retrograde through the Kent's bundle. (AV, atrioventricular; His, His-Purkinje system; LB, left bundle branch; PSVT, paroxysmal supraventricular tachycardia; RB, right bundle branch; SA, sinoatrial.)

It should be noted that (similar to patients with dual AV nodal pathways) not all patients with preexcitation with an accessory AV pathway are capable of having clinical PSVT.

Patients with an accessory AV pathway may have three forms of supraventricular tachycardia: orthodromic reentry, antidromic reentry, and/or AF or atrial flutter. AV reentrant PSVT usually occurs by the following sequence of events. Analogous to AV nodal reentry, two pathways (the normal AV nodal pathway and the accessory AV pathway) exist that have different electrophysiologic characteristics. The AV nodal pathway usually has a relatively slower conduction velocity and shorter refractory period, and the accessory pathway has a faster conduction velocity and a longer refractory period. A critically timed premature impulse may be blocked in the accessory pathway because this area is still refractory from the previous sinus beat. However, the AV nodal pathway, with a relatively shorter refractory period, may accept antegrade conduction of the premature impulse. Meanwhile, the accessory pathway may recover its excitability and now allow retrograde conduction. A macroreentrant tachycardia is thereby initiated in which the antegrade pathway is the AV nodal pathway, the distal common pathway is the ventricle, the retrograde pathway is the accessory pathway, and the proximal common pathway is the atrium (Fig. 8-8). This sequence of events (down the AV node, up the Kent's bundle), termed *orthodromic PSVT*, is the common variety of reentry in patients with an accessory AV pathway, resulting in a narrow QRS tachycardia. In the uncommon variety, conduction proceeds in the opposite direction (down the Kent's bundle, up the AV node), resulting in a wide QRS tachycardia, which is termed *antidromic PSVT*. Patients with WPW syndrome can have a third type of tachycardia, namely, AF. The occurrence of AF in the setting of an accessory AV pathway (i.e., WPW syndrome) can be extremely serious. As AF is an extremely rapid atrial tachycardia, conduction can proceed down the accessory AV pathway, resulting in a very fast ventricular response or even VF. Unlike the AV nodal pathway, the refractory period of the accessory bundle shortens in response to rapid stimulation rates.

Sinus node reentry and intraatrial reentry occur less commonly and are not as well described as AV nodal reentry and AV reentry. Aside from a characteristic abrupt onset and termination, coupled with subtle changes in P-wave morphology, these tachycardias can be difficult to diagnose. Electrophysiologic studies may be necessary to determine the ultimate mechanism of the PSVT.

Management

Both pharmacologic and nonpharmacologic methods have been used to treat patients with PSVT. Drugs used in the treatment of PSVT can be divided into three broad categories: (a) those that directly or indirectly increase vagal tone to the AV node (e.g., digoxin); (b) those that depress conduction through slow, calcium-dependent tissue (e.g., adenosine, β-blockers, and non-DHP CCBs); and (c) those that depress conduction through fast, sodium-dependent tissue (e.g., quinidine, procainamide, disopyramide, and flecainide). Drugs within these categories alter the electrophysiologic characteristics of the reentrant substrate so that PSVT cannot be sustained. In PSVT caused by AV nodal reentry, class I AADs, such as flecainide, act primarily on the retrograde fast pathway. Digoxin and β-blockers may work on either the retrograde fast or the antegrade slow pathway. Verapamil, diltiazem, and adenosine prolong conduction time and increase refractoriness, primarily in the slow antegrade pathway of the reentrant loop. In PSVT caused by AV reentry incorporating an extranodal pathway, class I AADs increase refractoriness in the fast accessory pathway or within the His-Purkinje system. β-Blockers, digoxin, adenosine, and verapamil all act by their effects on the AV nodal (antegrade, slow) portion of the reentrant circuit. Regardless of the mechanism, treatment measures are directed first at terminating an acute episode of PSVT and then at preventing symptomatic recurrences of the arrhythmia.

For those patients with PSVT who present with severe symptoms (i.e., syncope, near syncope, angina, or severe HF), synchronized DCC is the treatment of choice. Even at low energy levels (such as 25 J), DCC is almost always effective in quickly restoring SR and correcting symptomatic hypotension. Patients with only mild-to-moderate symptoms usually do not require DCC, and nonpharmacologic measures that increase vagal tone to the AV node can be used initially. Vagal techniques, such as unilateral carotid sinus massage, Valsalva maneuver, ice water facial immersion, or induced retching, are often successful in terminating PSVT, although carotid massage and Valsalva maneuver are the simplest, least obtrusive, and most frequently used of these techniques.

In the event that vagal maneuvers fail (approximately 80% of acute episodes) in those patients with tolerable symptoms, drug therapy is the next option. Figure 8-9 shows a therapeutic approach to the acute treatment of the different forms of reentrant PSVT. 6 This approach is based on analysis of the electrocardiographic characteristics of the rhythm because PSVT is not always discernible from other arrhythmias, and some forms of PSVT require different treatment. In patients with a narrow QRS, regular arrhythmia (AV nodal reentry or orthodromic AV reentry), IV verapamil (5 to 10 mg), IV diltiazem (15 to 25 mg), and adenosine (6 to 12 mg) are all equally efficacious. Approximately 80% to 90% of PSVT episodes will revert to SR within 5 minutes of these drug therapies.[70] The most recent guidelines for cardiopulmonary resuscitation (CPR) and emergency cardiovascular care (ECC) from the AHA,[71] and practice guidelines from the ACC/AHA/ESC,[61] promote adenosine as the drug of first choice in patients with PSVT. 5 These recommendations are particularly important when treating a patient who presents with a wide QRS, regular tachycardia that may be VT or PSVT

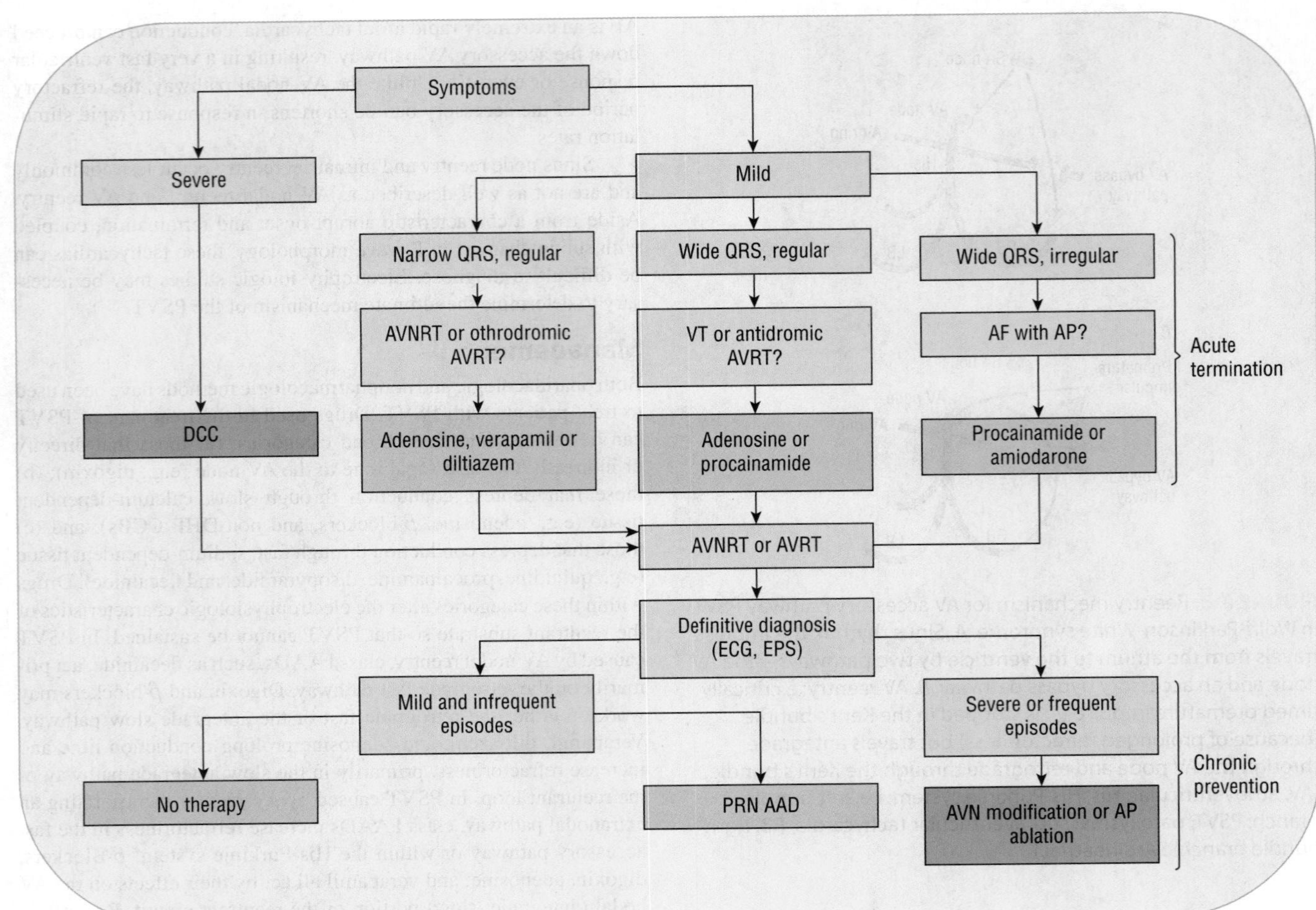

FIGURE 8-9 Algorithm for the treatment of acute (*top portion*) PSVT and chronic prevention of recurrences (*bottom portion*). *Note*: For empiric bridge therapy prior to radiofrequency ablation procedures, CCBs (or other AV nodal blockers) should not be used if the patient has AV reentry with an accessory pathway. (AAD, antiarrhythmic drug; AF, atrial fibrillation; AP, accessory pathway; AV, atrioventricular; AVN, atrioventricular nodal; AVNRT, atrioventricular nodal reentrant tachycardia; AVRT, atrioventricular reentrant tachycardia; CCBs, calcium channel blockers; DCC, direct current cardioversion; ECG, electrocardiogram; EPS, electrophysiologic studies; PRN, as needed; PSVT, paroxysmal supraventricular tachycardia; VT, ventricular tachycardia.)

(antidromic AV reentry or as a result of aberrancy). Because of its ultrashort duration of action (seconds), adenosine will not cause the severe and prolonged hemodynamic compromise seen in patients with VT who were mistakenly treated with verapamil and suffered from its negative inotropic effects and vasodilator properties.[72] If, in fact, the arrhythmia is PSVT, adenosine will likely terminate it. An alternative treatment for this type of patient is IV procainamide, which works on the fast, sodium-dependent extranodal pathway and is also effective for VT. Likewise, IV procainamide, or perhaps IV amiodarone (particularly in patients with LV dysfunction) should be used for the patient who presents with a wide QRS, irregular arrhythmia that is hemodynamically stable.[71] This rhythm could represent AF with rapid ventricular activation occurring primarily through an extranodal pathway. Administration of IV verapamil, diltiazem, digoxin, or adenosine to these patients may result in a paradoxical increase in ventricular response, causing severe symptoms requiring cardioversion. Consequently, these drugs are considered contraindicated in this specific setting.

Once the acute episode of PSVT is terminated, a decision on long-term preventive therapy must follow. Most patients require long-term therapy; preventive treatment is indicated if (a) frequent episodes occur that necessitate therapeutic intervention (i.e., emergency department visits or interference with the patient's lifestyle) or (b) infrequent but severely symptomatic symptoms occur. For those patients in whom a preventive treatment is deemed necessary, two methods of management have been used: preventive drug therapy and ablation.

AADs are no longer the treatment of choice to prevent recurrences of reentrant PSVT for the following reasons: (a) lifelong treatment is necessary in these generally young, but otherwise healthy, individuals; (b) there are few, if any, large controlled or comparative trials to assist the clinician in rationally choosing effective agents; and (c) most importantly, other nonpharmacologic treatments are clearly more effective. Nevertheless, drug therapy may occasionally be necessary in some patients, particularly those with mild symptoms and infrequent recurrences. A trial-and-error approach may be used, complemented by the use of ambulatory electrocardiographic recordings (Holter) or telephonic transmissions of cardiac rhythm (event monitors) to objectively document the efficacy or failure of the chosen drug regimen. Drugs known to be effective in preventing recurrences of PSVT are the AV nodal blocking drugs (digoxin, β-blockers, non-DHP CCBs, and combinations of these agents) and the class Ic AADs (flecainide, propafenone). Drugs such as quinidine, disopyramide, amiodarone, and dofetilide, although effective

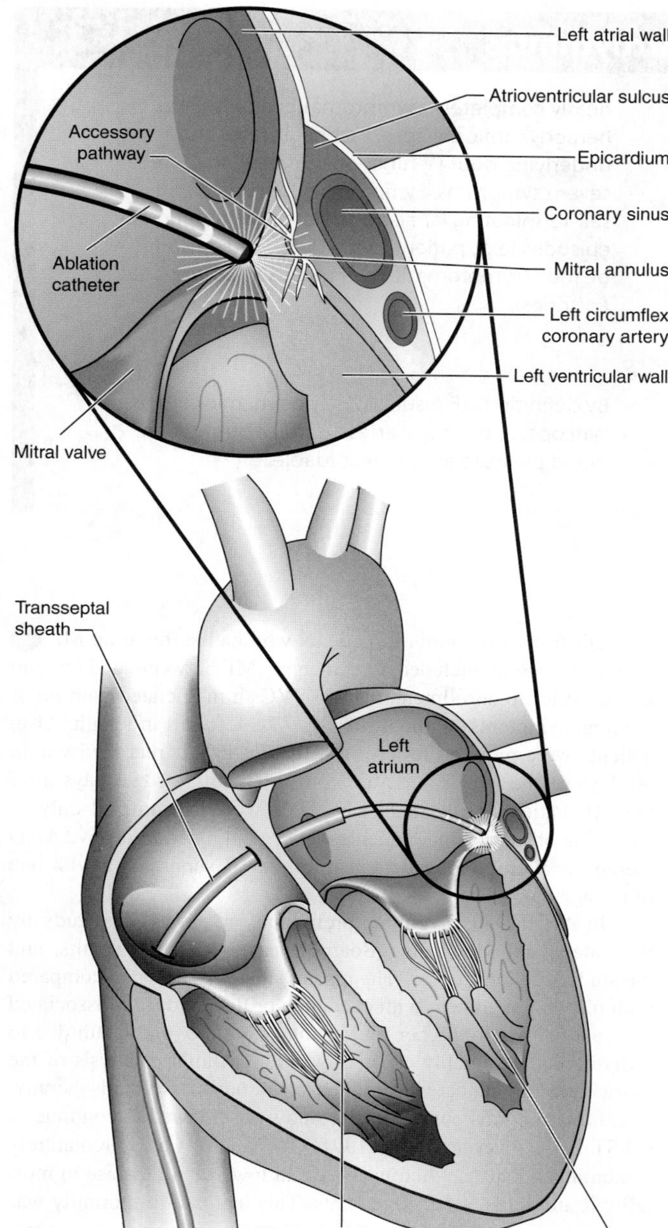

FIGURE 8-10 Drawing showing catheter placement for radiofrequency ablation of a left lateral free wall accessory pathway. Here, a venous (atrial) transseptal puncture to gain access to the Kent's bundle is shown; a retrograde arterial approach has also been used. *(Data from Lerman BB, Basson CT. High risk patients with ventricular preexcitation: A pendulum in motion. N Engl J Med 2003;349:1787–1789. Copyright © 2003 Massachusetts Medical Society. All rights reserved.)*

in some patients, should be discouraged because of the risk of toxicity with long-term treatment.

Transcutaneous catheter ablation using radiofrequency current on the PSVT substrate has dramatically altered the traditional treatment of these patients (Fig. 8-10). 5 Radiofrequency energy delivered through a transvenous or arterial catheter causes small, discrete lesions through thermal energy. During invasive electrophysiologic studies, portions of the reentrant circuit can be located (or mapped) by the use of a number of catheters. Once this is completed, radiofrequency energy is applied, creating thermal injury in the tissue necessary for reentry. In this way, the substrate for reentry is destroyed, "curing" the patient of recurrent episodes of PSVT and obviating the need for chronic drug therapy. Complications, although unusual, include tamponade, pericarditis, valvular insufficiency, and AV block. Radiofrequency ablation is highly effective, preventing the recurrences of PSVT in 85% to 98% of patients.[73,74] The procedure was originally used in patients with WPW syndrome.[73] In these patients, the extranodal pathway is most often located at the left lateral free wall of the left ventricle (Fig. 8-10). After the pathway is located, the catheter is put as close to the site as possible, and radiofrequency current is applied to make small burns in the tissue. Ablation of the extranodal connection occurs promptly, and evidence of preexcitation (delta waves) disappears. Thereafter, a similar approach was developed for patients with AV nodal reentry, placing the catheter in the coronary sinus, proximal to the AV node.[74] The preferred method in these individuals is to apply small amounts of radiofrequency current to the slow pathway of the reentrant circuit in order to modify its properties enough so that PSVT cannot recur.

It has been suggested that *all* patients with symptomatic PSVT undergo radiofrequency catheter ablation.[75] This is because the procedure is highly effective and curative, rarely results in complications, and obviates the need for chronic AAD therapy. In other words, radiofrequency catheter ablation should be considered in *any* patient who would previously be considered for chronic AAD treatment. Radiofrequency ablation is also a cost-effective approach (in the long term) because, if effective, the costs of drugs and repeated hospital visits are avoided. In one cost-effectiveness analysis, radiofrequency ablation improved quality of life and reduced lifetime medical expenditures by nearly $30,000 compared with chronic drug treatment.[76]

VENTRICULAR ARRHYTHMIAS

The common ventricular arrhythmias include (a) premature ventricular complexes (PVCs), (b) VT, and (c) VF. These arrhythmias may result in a wide variety of symptoms. PVCs often cause no symptoms or only mild palpitations. VT may be a life-threatening situation associated with hemodynamic collapse or may be totally asymptomatic. VF, by definition, is an acute medical emergency necessitating CPR.

Premature Ventricular Complexes and Prevention of Sudden Cardiac Death

PVCs are very common ventricular rhythm disturbances that occur in patients with or without SHD. Experimental models show that PVCs may be elicited by abnormal automaticity, triggered activity, or reentrant mechanisms. It is well known that PVCs are commonly observed in apparently healthy individuals; in these patients, the PVCs seem to have little, if any, prognostic significance. PVCs occur more frequently and in more complex forms in patients with SHD than in healthy individuals. The prognostic meaning of PVCs has been well studied in patients with MI (acute or remote) with several consistent themes. Patients with some forms of PVCs are at higher risk for SCD than if they did not have these minor rhythm disturbances. SCD can be defined as unexpected death occurring in a patient within 1 hour of experiencing symptoms. Studies of patients who experienced SCD (and happened to be wearing an electrocardiographic monitor at the time) often demonstrate the cause to be VF preceded by a short run of VT and frequent PVCs.[77]

Significance

Historically, investigators promoted the concept that patients in the acute phase of MI may have types of PVCs that are predictive of VF and SCD. These types of PVCs were referred to as "warning arrhythmias" and included frequent ventricular ectopy (more than

CLINICAL PRESENTATION Ventricular Arrhythmias

PVCs

- PVCs are non–life-threatening and usually asymptomatic. Occasionally, patients will complain of palpitations or uncomfortable heartbeats. Since the PVC, by definition, occurs early and the ventricle contracts when it is incompletely filled, patients do not feel the PVC. Rather, the next beat (after the PVC and a compensatory pause) is usually responsible for the patient's symptoms.

VT

- The symptoms of VT (monomorphic VT or TdP), if prolonged (i.e., sustained), can vary from nearly completely asymptomatic to pulseless, hemodynamic collapse. Fast heart rates and underlying poor LV function will result in more severe symptoms. Symptoms of nonsustained, self-terminating VT also correlate with duration of episodes (e.g., patients with 15-second episodes will be more symptomatic than those with three-beat episodes).

VF

- By definition, VF results in hemodynamic collapse, syncope, and cardiac arrest. Cardiac output and blood pressure are not recordable.

5 beats/min), multiform configuration (different morphology), couplets (two in a row), and R-on-T phenomenon (PVCs occurring during the repolarization phase of the preceding sinus beat in the vulnerable period of ventricular recovery). However, as a result of using continuous electrocardiographic monitoring techniques, it has become apparent that almost all patients have warning arrhythmias in the acute MI setting. In those patients who experience VF, warning arrhythmias are no more common than in those without VF. Consequently, warning arrhythmias observed during acute MI are neither sensitive nor specific for determining which patients will have VF. Thus, there is little need to direct drug therapy specifically at PVC suppression in these particular patients. Studies show that effective prevention of VF in the acute MI setting may be achieved without the abolition of PVCs.

Conversely, data strongly imply that PVCs documented in the convalescence period of MI do carry important long-term prognostic significance.[78] PVCs occurring after an MI seem to be a risk factor for patient death that is independent of the degree of LV dysfunction or the extent of coronary atherosclerosis. Ruberman et al.[78] employed a simple classification of PVCs: simple or benign (infrequent and monomorphic) versus "complex" (≥5 PVCs/min, couplets, R-on-T beats, and multiform). These investigators found that the presence of complex (but not simple) ventricular ectopy in the setting of CAD was associated with a higher incidence of overall mortality and cardiac death.

Because PVCs without associated SHD, in apparently healthy individuals, carry little or no risk, drug therapy is unnecessary. However, because of the prognostic significance of complex PVCs in patients with SHD, the use of AAD therapy to suppress them has been controversial. Historically, many supported the aggressive use of AAD therapy to suppress PVCs, based on the underlying premise of eliminating a risk factor for SCD in patients with CAD (namely, the presence of complex PVCs). However, others favored a more conservative approach and disregarded the use of AAD therapy in the absence of significant symptoms. An important study, the CAST,[46] abruptly put an end to this debate in noteworthy fashion; its results are reviewed in the following section because of its great historical significance and lingering impact.

The Cardiac Arrhythmia Suppression Trial

The CAST[46,79] was initiated by the National Institutes of Health in 1987 to determine if suppression of ventricular ectopy with encainide, flecainide, or moricizine could decrease the incidence of death from arrhythmia in patients who had suffered an MI. 7 Entrance criteria included documented MI between 6 days and 2 years prior to enrollment, and ≥6 PVCs/h (associated with no or minimal symptoms) without runs of VT >15 beats in length. Also, patients were required to have an LVEF ≤55% if recruited within 90 days of the MI or an LVEF ≤40% if recruited ≥90 days after the MI. Patients with an LVEF <30% were randomized only to encainide or moricizine. Patients were randomized to receive AAD therapy or placebo after demonstrating PVC suppression with one of the agents.

In April 1989, a routine, preliminary review of the study by the Safety and Monitoring Board revealed alarming results, and the study was interrupted. The results showed that when compared with placebo, treatment with encainide or flecainide was associated with a significantly higher rate of total mortality and death due to arrhythmia, presumably caused by proarrhythmia. Analysis of the moricizine arm indicated neither harm nor benefit from this therapy; therefore, only this portion of the study was allowed to continue as CAST II.[79] However, in July 1991, CAST II was also prematurely discontinued because there was a trend toward an increase in mortality in moricizine-treated patients. This increase in mortality was primarily observed during the initiation of moricizine (dose titration phase) but not during the chronic treatment phase. The overall results of the two CASTs conclusively prove that the use of AAD therapy (beyond the general use of β-blockers) to suppress PVCs in patients after an MI does not improve survival and is most likely detrimental.

Even though the CAST was conducted more than 2 decades ago, it is considered one of the most important trials ever undertaken and has had a tremendous influence on the overall approach to the treatment of arrhythmias, as well as a far-reaching impact on AAD development. The results of the CAST have clearly had a negative influence on the long-term use of all AADs, causing a broad skepticism in the risk-versus-benefit analysis of this class of drugs. Consequently, pharmaceutical companies have shifted their drug discovery and investigative efforts away from potent sodium channel blockers. The findings of the CAST have also provided additional fuel for the pursuit of nonpharmacologic therapies for arrhythmias, such as ablation and implantable devices.

Despite the discouraging results of the CAST, post-MI patients with complex ventricular ectopy remain at risk for death. Other drugs, besides the class Ic AADs, have been studied in this patient population, including sotalol. Sotalol is marketed as a racemic mixture of a D and L isomers: both are class III potassium channel blockers but the L isomer has β-blocking actions. Chronic therapy with D-sotalol was studied in patients with a remote MI complicated by complex ectopy in the Survival with Oral D-Sotalol trial.[80] In this trial, D-sotalol treatment was not designed to cause PVC suppression (unlike the CAST), yet (like the CAST) the trial was halted prematurely because of excessive mortality in the treatment arm. Again, the presumed reason for this observation was D-sotalol–related proarrhythmia. Currently, only two AADs have been shown *not* to increase mortality in post-MI patients with long-term use: amiodarone and dofetilide. A number of trials[81,82] have shown amiodarone to decrease the incidence of sudden (or arrhythmic) death, but not total mortality, in post-MI patients with complex ventricular ectopy. A meta-analysis of all trials (6,553 combined patients) demonstrated a reduction in total mortality (by 13%) with long-term amiodarone therapy.[83] It is unclear if these findings can be attributed to one of amiodarone's electrophysiologic properties (e.g., β-blocking) or a combination of its complex pharmacologic effects on conduction. It is noteworthy to mention that in two major studies, patients treated with amiodarone and a β-blocker generally did better than when no β-blocker was used.[81,82] Clearly, because of its impressive side effect profile and its inability to improve survival, amiodarone should not routinely be recommended in patients with heart disease such as remote MI and complex PVCs. Two randomized controlled trials[84,85] have also shown that chronic therapy with dofetilide has no effect on overall mortality in post-MI patients with LV dysfunction.

How should the clinician approach the patient with documented asymptomatic PVCs? Clearly, attempts to suppress asymptomatic PVCs should *not* be made with any AAD. Indeed, those patients who are at risk for arrhythmic death (recent MI, LV dysfunction, complex PVCs) should also *not* be routinely given *any* class I or III AAD.[86] If these patients have symptomatic PVCs, chronic drug therapy should be limited to the use of β-blockers. The use of β-blockers in post-MI patients is associated with a decrease in the incidence of total mortality and SCD, especially in the presence of LV dysfunction. β-Blockers can also be used in patients without underlying SHD to suppress symptomatic PVCs. 7

Ventricular Tachycardia

Mechanisms and Types of VT

VT is a wide QRS tachycardia that may acutely occur as a result of metabolic abnormalities, ischemia, or drug toxicity, or chronically recur as a paroxysmal form. On ECG, VT may appear as either repetitive monomorphic or polymorphic ventricular complexes. The definition of VT is three or more consecutive PVCs occurring at a rate >100 beats/min. An acute episode of VT may be precipitated by severe electrolyte abnormalities (hypokalemia or hypomagnesemia), hypoxia, or digoxin toxicity, or (most commonly) may occur during an acute MI or ischemia complicated by HF. In these cases, correction of the underlying precipitating factors will usually prevent further recurrences of VT. As an example, if VT occurs during the first 24 hours of an acute MI, it will probably not reappear on a chronic basis after the infarcted area has been reperfused or healed with scar formation. This form of acute VT may be caused by a transient reentrant mechanism within temporarily ischemic or dying ventricular tissue. In contrast, some patients have a chronic recurrent form of VT that is almost always associated with some type of underlying SHD. Common examples are paroxysmal VT associated with idiopathic dilated cardiomyopathy or remote MI with an LV aneurysm. In chronic, recurrent VT, microreentry within the distal Purkinje network is presumed to be responsible for the underlying substrate in a large majority of patients (Fig. 8-3). Theoretically, electrophysiologic discrepancies occur as a result of structural damage and heart disease within the ventricular conducting system. The reentrant circuit may possess both anatomically determined and functional properties coursing through normal tissue, damaged (but not dead) tissue, and islands of necrosed tissue. In a minority of patients, macroreentrant circuits may be responsible for recurrent VT, including reentry incorporating the bundle branches.

Patients with acute VT associated with a precipitating factor often suffer severe symptoms, requiring immediate treatment measures. Chronic recurrent VT may also cause severe hemodynamic compromise but may also be associated with only mild symptoms that are generally well tolerated. Sustained VT is that which requires therapeutic intervention to restore a stable rhythm or persists for a relatively long time (usually >30 seconds). Nonsustained VT is that which self-terminates after a brief duration (usually <30 seconds). If the patient has VT more frequently than SR (i.e., VT is the dominant rhythm), this is referred to as incessant VT. In monomorphic VT, the QRS complexes are similar in morphologic characteristics from beat to beat. In polymorphic VT, the QRS complexes vary in shape and/or size between beats. A characteristic type of polymorphic VT, in which the QRS complexes appear to undulate around a central axis and that is associated with evidence of delayed ventricular repolarization (long QT interval or prominent U waves), is referred to as TdP.

Most but not all forms of recurrent VT occur in patients with extensive SHD. VT occurring in a patient without SHD is sometimes referred to as idiopathic VT and may take several forms.[87–89] Fascicular VT arises from a fascicle of the left bundle branch (usually posterior) and is usually not associated with severe underlying SHD. In distinct contrast to the common form of recurrent VT associated with extensive SHD, non-DHP CCBs (but not adenosine) are effective in terminating an acute episode of fascicular VT. Ventricular outflow tract VT (usually originating from the right ventricular outflow tract) originates from near the pulmonic valve (or uncommonly the aortic valve or LV outflow tract) and also occurs in patients with normal LV function without discernible SHD.[89] Unlike other forms of VT, right ventricular outflow tract VT often terminates with adenosine and may be prevented with β-blockers and/or non-DHP CCBs.

Some unusual forms of VT are congenital or heritable (Table 8-10). TdP can be associated with heritable defects in the flux of ions that govern ventricular repolarization. Although multiple syndromes and genetic mutations have been described, the more

TABLE 8-10 Heritable Polymorphic Ventricular Tachycardia

Syndrome	Channel Defect	Mutant Gene	Characteristics	Treatment
$LQTS_1$	$\downarrow I_{Ks}$	KVLQT1	SCD/TdP with exercise	BB/ICD
$LQTS_2$	$\downarrow I_{Kr}$	HERG	SCD/TdP with arousal	BB/ICD
$LQTS_3$	$\uparrow I^+_{Na}$ during plateau/ repolarization	SCN5A	SCD/TdP at rest/ sleep	Flecainide/ mexiletine/ ICD
Brugada	$\downarrow I^+_{Na}$	SCN5A	SCD/PMVT or VF at rest/sleep in Asian males	ICD/ quinidine

BB, β-blocker; ICD, implantable cardioverter-defibrillator; LQTS, long QT syndrome; PMVT, polymorphic ventricular tachycardia; SCD, sudden death; TdP, torsade de pointes; VF, ventricular fibrillation.

Note: LQTS can be provoked by potassium channel blockers (e.g., quinidine, sotalol), and Brugada syndrome can be provoked by potent sodium channel blockers (e.g., cocaine, flecainide). $LQTS_3$ and Brugada syndrome may coexist.

common examples are long QT syndrome 1 (depressed I_{Ks}), long QT syndrome 2 (depressed I_{Kr}), and long QT syndrome 3 (enhanced inward sodium ion flux during repolarization).[90,91] Polymorphic VT (without a long QT interval) or VF may also occur as a result of a heritable defect in the sodium channel. This is the case in Brugada syndrome, which is described as a typical ECG pattern (ST-segment elevation in leads V_1 to V_3) in SR that is associated with SCD, and commonly occurs in males of Asian descent.[92]

Management

Consider the patient with the more common form of sustained monomorphic VT (i.e., those with SHD, usually ischemic in nature). Like other rapid tachycardias, the initial management of an acute episode of VT (with a pulse) requires a quick assessment of the patient's status and symptoms. If severe symptoms are present (i.e., severe hypotension, angina, pulmonary edema), synchronized DCC should be delivered immediately to attempt to restore SR. An investigation should be made into possible precipitating factors, and these should be corrected if possible. The diagnosis of acute MI should always be entertained. If the episode of VT is thought to be an isolated electrical event associated with a transient initiating factor (such as acute myocardial ischemia or digoxin toxicity), there is no need for long-term AAD therapy once the precipitating factors are corrected (e.g., an MI has been reperfused and healed and the patient is stable). Nevertheless, the patient should be monitored closely for possible recurrences of VT.

Patients presenting with an acute episode of VT (with a pulse) associated with only mild symptoms can be initially treated with AADs. The reader is referred to the most recent AHA guidelines for CPR and ECC.[71] IV procainamide, amiodarone, or sotalol can be considered in this situation. Lidocaine can be considered as an alternative. In one small study, procainamide was shown to be superior to lidocaine in terminating VT.[93] Synchronized DCC should be delivered if the patient's status deteriorates, VT degenerates to VF (would be unsynchronized in this situation), or drug therapy fails.

Once an acute episode of sustained VT has been successfully terminated by electrical or pharmacologic means and an acute MI has been ruled out, the possibility of a patient having recurrent episodes of VT should be considered. Evidence for the possibility of VT recurrence can often be gleaned from invasive electrophysiologic studies using programmed ventricular stimulation. Because these patients are at extremely high risk for death, trial-and-error attempts to find effective therapy are unwarranted. To gain some objective evidence of a response to a specific AAD regimen, serial testing of these drugs using the following two surrogate end points has been used: (a) inability to induce sustained VT with programmed extrastimuli by invasive electrophysiologic studies and (b) suppression of ventricular ectopic beats by serial 24-hour continuous electrocardiographic (Holter) monitoring. These two strategies have been compared[94,95] but largely abandoned for several reasons. First, the yield for finding an effective AAD is low. For instance, sustained monomorphic VT can be rendered noninducible or nonsustained by programmed stimulation protocols in only 20% to 25% of patients. Therefore, the clinician frequently must search for other therapeutic options or settle for other treatment end points such as slower and more tolerable inducible VT. Second, amiodarone is clearly the most effective (approximately 50% effective after 2 years) AAD in patients with recurrent VT; however, electrophysiologic drug testing does not necessarily predict the clinical efficacy of amiodarone. Patients may have continued inducibility of VT on amiodarone despite long-term success. Indeed, empiric amiodarone has been compared with therapy (with other AADs) guided by electrophysiologic testing in patients at high risk for recurrent VT.[96] In this trial, amiodarone therapy without invasive testing was superior in preventing SCD and recurrences of severe ventricular arrhythmias at all time points. Third, the recurrence rate of life-threatening VT is high (20% to 50% per year depending on the AAD chosen), regardless of the method of acute drug testing. Fourth, as referred to previously, there is a substantial side effect profile of the class I and III AADs. Lastly, and perhaps most importantly, is the impressive demonstrated effectiveness of nonpharmacologic approaches to the treatment of recurrent VT/VF.[97] For instance, some forms of recurrent VT are amenable to catheter ablation therapy using radiofrequency current. This approach is highly effective (approximately 90%) in idiopathic VT (right ventricular outflow tract or fascicular VT), but less so in recurrent VT associated with a cardiomyopathic process or remote MI with LV aneurysm. In the latter patients, ablation is usually regarded as second-line therapy after other methods have failed. Additionally, numerous trials have established the ICD as a superior treatment over AAD therapy not only for the prevention of SCD in patients who have been resuscitated from an episode of cardiac arrest or had sustained VT ("secondary prevention") but also for the prevention of an initial episode of SCD in certain high-risk patient populations ("primary prevention").

The Implantable Cardioverter-Defibrillator The introduction of and advances in the ICD (Fig. 8-11) have obviated the need to rely solely on the use of AADs to prevent episodes of life-threatening ventricular arrhythmias.[98] 8 Numerous advancements in device technology have allowed the ICD to become smaller, less invasive to implant, and programmable with advanced functions. Early ICDs required a thoracotomy to place the generator in the abdomen, whereas with the newer, smaller models, the leads are implanted transvenously with the generator placed into the pectoral region in a manner similar to cardiac pacemakers. Modern ICDs now employ a "tiered-therapy approach," meaning that overdrive pacing (i.e., antitachycardia pacing) can be attempted first to terminate the tachyarrhythmia (no painful shock delivered), followed by low-energy cardioversion, and, finally, by high-energy defibrillation

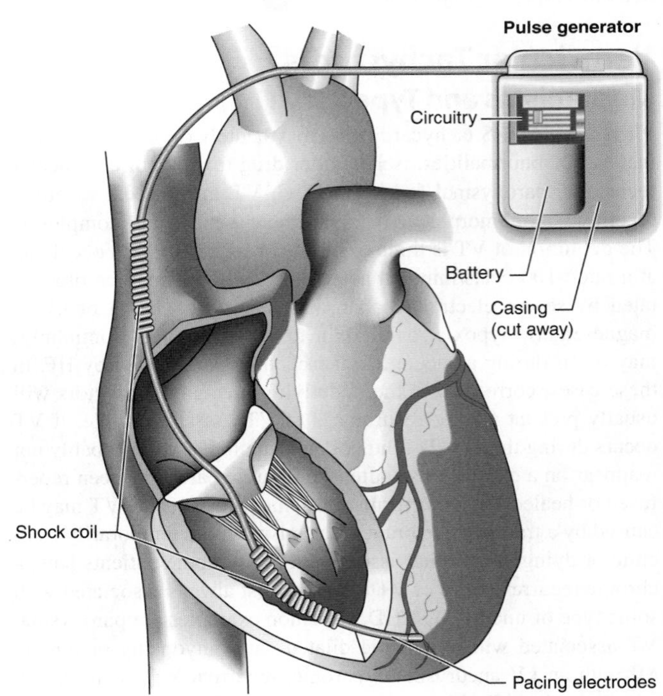

FIGURE 8-11 Drawing showing implantable cardioverter-defibrillator. *(Data from reference 98. Copyright © 2003 Massachusetts Medical Society. All rights reserved.)*

shocks. In addition, backup antibradycardia pacing and extended battery lives have made these newer devices much more attractive. All models store recordings during delivery of pacing shocks, which is extremely important in discerning appropriate shocks (i.e., delivers shock for serious ventricular arrhythmia) from inappropriate shocks (i.e., delivers shock for AF with rapid ventricular rate) and in documenting true recurrences of the patient's tachycardia.

Although the ICD is a highly effective method for preventing SCD due to recurrent VT or VF, several problems remain. First, the device itself, the implantation procedure, electrophysiologic studies, hospitalization, and physician fees are costly. Given that the indications for receiving an ICD have significantly expanded over the past several years, the total cost associated with the implantation of this device is likely to place a great burden on the healthcare system. Second, many patients (as high as 70% of patients) with ICDs end up receiving concomitant AAD therapy (usually amiodarone or sotalol).[99,100] AADs can be initiated in these patients for a number of reasons, including (a) decreasing the frequency of VT/VF episodes to subsequently reduce the frequency of appropriate shocks; (b) reducing the rate of VT so that it can be terminated with antitachycardia pacing; and (c) decreasing episodes of concomitant supraventricular arrhythmias (e.g., AF, atrial flutter) that may trigger inappropriate shocks. As a result of these potential benefits, the concomitant use of AADs can minimize patient discomfort and prolong the battery life of the ICD. The decision to initiate concomitant AAD therapy should be individualized, with treatment usually being reserved for those with frequent shocks because of VT or AF. If AADs are added to ICD therapy, one should note that many of these drugs alter defibrillation thresholds; consequently, the device may need to be reprogrammed to account for this alteration.[101]

Secondary Prevention of Sudden Cardiac Death The results of three trials, the Antiarrhythmics Versus Implantable Defibrillators (AVID), Cardiac Arrest Study Hamburg (CASH), and Canadian Implantable Defibrillator Study (CIDS), definitively support the ICD as first-line therapy for the secondary prevention of SCD.[102–104] Of these, the AVID trial was the largest, randomizing more than 1,000 patients with resuscitated VF, sustained VT with syncope, or hemodynamically significant sustained VT (with LVEF ≤40%) to either an ICD or AADs (~95% received amiodarone at discharge).[102] The trial was stopped early because of a demonstrated superiority of the ICD; patients in the ICD group had a better overall survival when compared with those in the AAD group (75% vs. 64%, respectively, at 3 years). Although they were smaller trials, both CASH and CIDS demonstrated the efficacy of an ICD compared with amiodarone in patients with a history of sustained VT or VF, with the ICD reducing overall mortality by 20% to 25%.[103,104] Overall, the results of these three trials provide strong support for the aggressive use of the ICD in patients who are at high risk for recurrent, life-threatening ventricular arrhythmias.

Primary Prevention of Sudden Cardiac Death One of the patient populations that appears to be at high risk for a first episode of SCD includes those with a prior MI, LV dysfunction, and nonsustained VT. The use of AADs to prevent SCD in this high-risk group has been significantly limited by the results of the CAST and other similar trials that have collectively demonstrated that these drugs may actually increase the risk of mortality in these patients. As a result of these trials, clinicians have sought a more clearly defined strategy for risk stratification in these patients before initiating drug therapy.

Traditionally, there are three strategies to approach the treatment of nonsustained VT: (a) conservative (i.e., no AAD treatment beyond β-blockers); (b) empiric amiodarone; and (c) aggressive (i.e., electrophysiologic studies with possible insertion of an ICD) (Fig. 8-12). 9 A number of early studies[105,106] suggested that tests such as electrophysiologic studies could be used to determine long-term risk in patients with nonsustained VT. For instance, Wilber et al.[105] demonstrated that post-MI patients with nonsustained VT and inducible sustained VT after programmed stimulation were at increased risk for subsequent VT/VF or SCD compared with those in whom sustained VT could not be induced. These data provided the basis for the Multicenter Automatic Defibrillator Implantation Trial (MADIT) and the Multicenter Unsustained Tachycardia Trial (MUSTT).[107,108] The MADIT was the first of these trials to be conducted to evaluate the efficacy of ICD therapy in this high-risk patient population. Specifically, this trial randomized patients with a previous MI, LVEF ≤36%, asymptomatic nonsustained VT, and inducible VT that was not suppressed with the use of IV procainamide to receive an ICD or conventional medical therapy (74% received amiodarone).[107] This trial was terminated prematurely after a significant survival benefit was detected in the ICD group. The findings of the MADIT were subsequently supported by those of the MUSTT. In the MUSTT, patients with a history of MI, LVEF ≤40%, asymptomatic nonsustained VT, and inducible sustained VT were randomized to a conservative approach (no AAD therapy beyond β-blockers) or electrophysiologically guided therapy (AADs and/or ICD).[108] The results showed that the conservative approach had a significantly higher event rate (cardiac arrest or death from arrhythmia). However, when the results of the electrophysiologically guided group were further stratified, those receiving only AADs (no ICD) were no different in terms of outcomes than those who received no treatment. In other words, only those treated with an ICD had a significantly lower event rate and greater survival. One problem with the MUSTT, however, is that, because the trial was initiated in 1989, nearly 50% of patients received class I AADs or drugs that are now known not to improve survival in patients with CAD, LV dysfunction, and ventricular arrhythmias; only 10% of patients received the most effective agent in this setting, amiodarone. Based on the results of the MADIT and MUSTT, it is reasonable for patients with CAD, LV dysfunction, and nonsustained VT to undergo electrophysiologic testing.[109] If these patients do not have inducible sustained VT/VF, chronic AAD therapy is unnecessary; however, if these patients do have inducible sustained VT/VF, implantation of an ICD is warranted.

Although the MADIT and MUSTT provide clinicians with important information regarding risk stratification, both of these trials targeted patients who had a history of nonsustained VT. The results of two landmark trials, the MADIT II and Sudden Cardiac Death in Heart Failure Trial (SCD-HeFT), have provided clinicians with additional information regarding the treatment of other groups of high-risk patients who have no prior history of ventricular arrhythmia (Fig. 8-13).[110,111] In the MADIT II, patients with a prior MI and LVEF ≤30% were randomized to receive either an ICD or a conventional therapy (routine post-MI and HF therapy).[110] Neither a history of ventricular arrhythmia nor electrophysiologic testing was required for inclusion in this study. Patients in the ICD group experienced a significant reduction in mortality when compared with the conventional therapy group; the reduction in mortality in the ICD group was primarily due to a reduction in arrhythmic death. Whereas the MADIT, MUSTT, and MADIT II limited enrollment to patients with ischemic cardiomyopathy, the SCD-HeFT is the largest trial, to date, to evaluate the efficacy of an ICD in a nonischemic HF population. In this trial, patients with NYHA class II or III HF (of either ischemic or nonischemic etiology) and LVEF ≤35% were randomized to receive placebo, amiodarone, or an ICD.[111] All patients were treated with appropriate HF therapies, as indicated. Implantation of an ICD resulted in a significantly lower mortality rate compared with treatment with either placebo or amiodarone (there was no difference between placebo and amiodarone). The survival benefits of the ICD were observed regardless of the etiology of the HF.

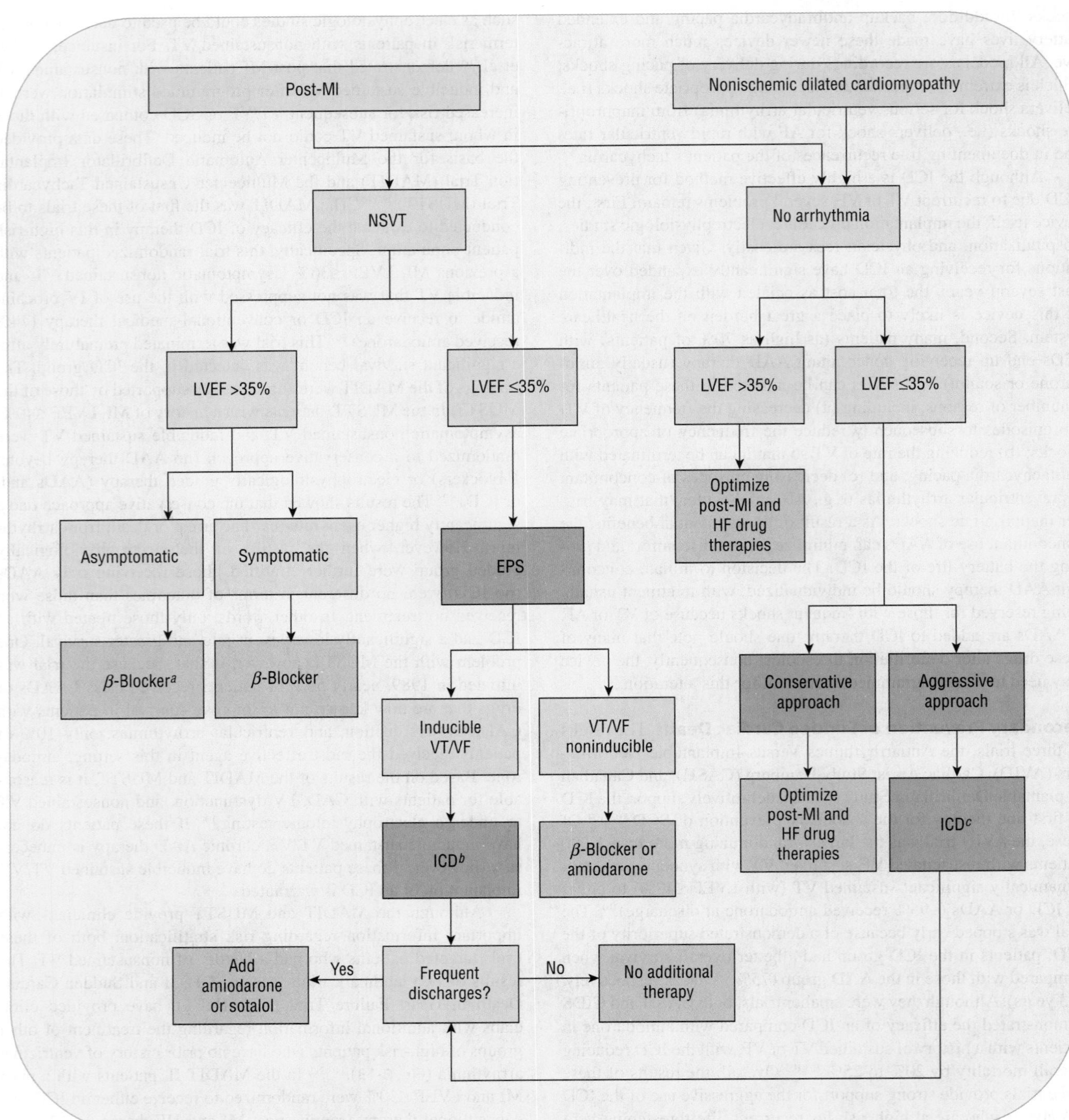

FIGURE 8-12 Algorithm for the primary prevention of SCD in patients with a history of MI or with a nonischemic dilated cardiomyopathy. [a]In these patients, the β-blocker is being used to reduce post-MI mortality. [b]Patients should be >40 days post-MI prior to insertion of the ICD. [c]Patients with an ischemic cardiomyopathy should be >40 days post-MI prior to insertion of the ICD. (EPS, electrophysiologic study; HF, heart failure; ICD, implantable cardioverter-defibrillator; LVEF, left ventricular ejection fraction; MI, myocardial infarction; NSVT, nonsustained VT; SCD, sudden cardiac death; VF, ventricular fibrillation; VT, ventricular tachycardia.)

Overall, as the ICD trials have evolved over the past decade, the indications for implanting these devices have significantly expanded (Table 8-11).[112] Based on the results of the MUSTT, MADIT, MADIT II, and SCD-HeFT, many patients will be eligible for an ICD. 9 In fact, just based on the results of the MADIT II and SCD-HeFT alone, it was estimated that an additional 500,000 Medicare beneficiaries would qualify for implantation of an ICD for primary prevention of SCD.

Ventricular Proarrhythmia

All AADs have the potential to aggravate existing arrhythmias or to cause new arrhythmias. It is believed that AADs may cause proarrhythmia in nearly 30% of patients.[8] Many definitions for proarrhythmia have been proposed; however, in the simplest terms, it indicates the development of a significant new arrhythmia (such as VT, VF, or TdP) or worsening of an existing arrhythmia (episodes

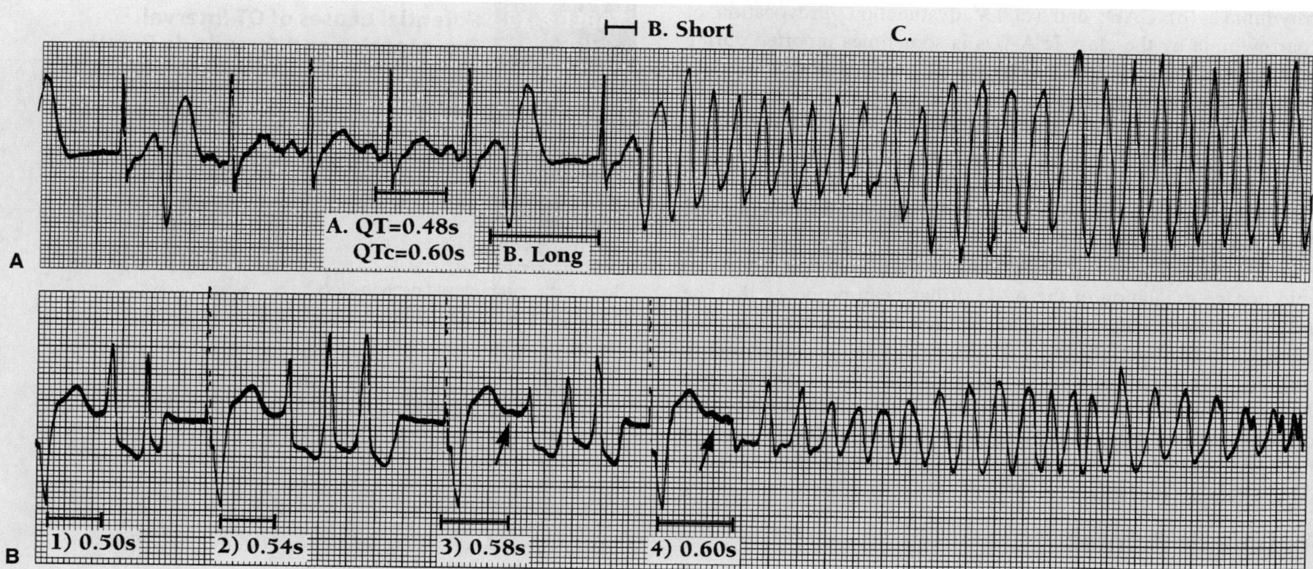

FIGURE 8-13 Torsade de pointes caused by quinidine. Note the presence of a couplet and two triplets following each extra systolic pause. The pause gets progressively longer until it is long enough to result in an episode of sustained torsade de pointes. Also, as the pause lengthens, discernible U waves (labeled ↑) (EADs?) begin to appear. The amplitude of the U wave is somewhat greater with the longest pause. *(Reproduced with permission from Bauman JL. Drug safety: Cardiac arrhythmias. Antihistamine update symposium. Hosp Med 1995;31:24.)*

are longer, faster, or more frequent). As with all arrhythmias, the consequences of proarrhythmia are varied. Some patients who develop proarrhythmia may be totally asymptomatic, others may notice a worsening of symptoms, and some may die suddenly. The development of proarrhythmia results from the same mechanisms that cause arrhythmias in general (e.g., quinidine-induced TdP due to EADs) or from an alteration in the underlying substrate due to the AAD (e.g., development of an accelerated tachycardia caused by flecainide, which decreases conduction velocity without significantly altering the refractory period).[8] The diagnosis of proarrhythmia is sometimes difficult to make because of the variable nature of the underlying arrhythmias. However, in all cases, the AAD should be discontinued if proarrhythmia is detected or suspected.

Incessant Monomorphic VT

The prototypical form of proarrhythmia caused by the class Ic AADs is a rapid, sustained, monomorphic VT with a characteristic sinusoidal QRS pattern that is often resistant to resuscitation with cardioversion or overdrive pacing. **10** It is sometimes referred to as sinusoidal or incessant VT and is the result of excessive sodium channel blockade and slowed conduction. Sinusoidal VT caused by the class Ic AADs was thought to occur within the first several days of drug initiation; however, the results of the CAST indicate that the risk for this type of proarrhythmia may exist as long as the AAD is continued. Factors that can predispose a patient to this form of proarrhythmia include: (a) the presence of underlying ventricular

TABLE 8-11 Current Indications for ICD Implantation

Indications	ACC/AHA/HRS Guideline Recommendation
Secondary Prevention	
An ICD is *indicated* in the following individuals:	
Patients who survived an episode of cardiac arrest due to VF or have hemodynamically unstable sustained VT, not due to a reversible cause	Class I, LOE A
Patients with structural heart disease who develop spontaneous sustained VT that is either hemodynamically stable or unstable	Class I, LOE B
Patients with unexplained syncope who have hemodynamically unstable sustained VT or VF induced by EPS	Class I, LOE B
An ICD is *considered reasonable* in the following individuals:	
Patients with unexplained syncope who have significant LV dysfunction and nonischemic dilated cardiomyopathy	Class IIa, LOE C
Patients with sustained VT and normal or near-normal LV function	Class IIa, LOE C
Primary Prevention	
An ICD is *indicated* in the following individuals:	
Patients with a prior MI (occurring >40 days before ICD implantation) and LVEF ≤30% who are in NYHA FC I	Class I, LOE A
Patients with an LVEF ≤35% due to a prior MI (occurring >40 days before ICD implantation) who are in NYHA FC II or III	Class I, LOE A
Patients with nonsustained VT due to prior MI, an LVEF ≤40%, and inducible, sustained VT or VF at EPS	Class I, LOE B
Patients with nonischemic dilated cardiomyopathy and an LVEF ≤35% who are in NYHA FC II or III	Class I, LOE B
An ICD is *considered reasonable* in patients who are not hospitalized and are awaiting cardiac transplantation	Class IIa, LOE C
An ICD *may be considered* in patients with nonischemic dilated cardiomyopathy and an LVEF ≤35% who are in NYHA FC I	Class IIb, LOE C

ACC, American College of Cardiology; AHA, American Heart Association; EPS, electrophysiologic study; FC, functional class; HRS, Heart Rhythm Society; ICD, implantable cardioverter-defibrillator; LV, left ventricular; LVEF, left ventricular ejection fraction; MI, myocardial infarction; NYHA, New York Heart Association; VF, ventricular fibrillation; VT, ventricular tachycardia.

arrhythmias; (b) CAD; and (c) LV dysfunction. Provocation of proarrhythmia by the class Ic AADs is sometimes reported during exercise, which is most likely a result of augmented slowed conduction at rapid heart rates (i.e., rate-dependent sodium blockade). The incidence of proarrhythmia caused by class Ic AADs is greatest in patients with all three of the above risk factors (approximately 10% to 20%) and extremely uncommon in those without these risk factors, such as patients with supraventricular tachycardias and normal LV function. Other factors that have a less well-defined association with proarrhythmia are elevated AAD serum concentrations and rapid dosage escalation of the AAD. It has been proposed that the presence of underlying ventricular conduction delays may also pose a risk for proarrhythmia. As mentioned earlier, incessant monomorphic VT is often resistant to resuscitation; however, some have had success with lidocaine ("fast on–off" AAD, which successfully competes with a "slow on–off" agent such as flecainide for sodium channel receptor) or sodium bicarbonate (reverses the excessive sodium channel blockade).

Torsade de Pointes

As defined previously, TdP is a rapid form of polymorphic VT (Fig. 8-13) that is associated with evidence of delayed ventricular repolarization (long QT interval or prominent U waves) on ECG. It is important to note that most forms of polymorphic VT occurring in the setting of a normal QT interval are similar to monomorphic VT in terms of etiology and treatment strategies (thus, a long QT interval is crucial to the diagnosis of TdP). Much has been learned about the underlying etiology of TdP. Basic defects (genetic, drugs, or diseases) that delay repolarization by influencing ion movement (usually by blocking potassium efflux) provoke EADs preferentially in cells deep in the heart muscle (termed *M cells*), which, in turn, trigger reentry and TdP. Drugs that cause TdP usually delay ventricular repolarization in an inhomogeneous way (termed *dispersion of refractoriness*), which facilitates the formation of multiple reentrant loops in the ventricle.[113] TdP may occur in association with hereditary syndromes or as an acquired form (i.e., a result of drugs or diseases). The underlying etiology in both cases is delayed ventricular repolarization due to blockade of potassium conductance. It is possible, however, that some individuals have a partially expressed form of these congenital syndromes but never suffer TdP unless some other external factor (e.g., drugs, diseases, electrolyte disturbances, abrupt heart rate changes) further delays ventricular repolarization. Specifically, acquired forms of TdP are associated with electrolyte disturbances (hypokalemia or hypomagnesemia), subarachnoid hemorrhage, myocarditis, liquid protein diets, arsenic poisoning, severe hypothyroidism, or, most commonly, drug therapy (notably phenothiazines, antibiotics, antihistamines, antidepressants, and AADs) (Table 8-12). 10

The class Ia AADs (especially quinidine) and class III I_{Kr} blockers are most notorious for precipitating TdP; the class Ib and Ic AADs rarely, if ever, cause TdP as they do not appreciably delay repolarization. Most AADs with I_{Kr} blocking activity cause TdP in approximately 2% to 4% of patients, with the exceptions being amiodarone and dronedarone (<1%). Risk factors and associated features of drug-induced TdP have been identified and can be summarized as follows[33,114]: (a) high dosages or plasma concentrations of the offending drug ("dose-related") (except for quinidine-induced TdP, which tends to occur more frequently at low-to-therapeutic plasma concentrations); (b) concurrent SHD (e.g., CAD, HF, and/or LV hypertrophy); (c) evidence of mild delayed repolarization (prolonged QT interval) at baseline; (d) evidence of a prolonged QT interval shortly after initiation of the offending drug; (e) concomitant electrolyte disturbances such as hypokalemia or hypomagnesemia; (f) female gender; and (g) a characteristic long–short initiating sequence (so-called "pause dependence") of the episode of TdP (Fig. 8-13). However, none of these associations are absolute

TABLE 8-12 Potential Causes of QT Interval Prolongation and Torsade de Pointes

Conditions
Congenital long QT syndromes
Myocarditis
Myocardial ischemia/infarction
Heart failure
Severe bradycardia (<50 beats/min)
Hypokalemia
Severe hypothermia
Hypomagnesemia
Severe starvation/liquid protein diets
Subarachnoid hemorrhage
Drugs
Antiarrhythmic drugs
Quinidine
Procainamide (also *N*-acetylprocainamide)
Disopyramide
Amiodarone (<1%)
Dofetilide
Dronedarone (<1%)
Sotalol
Ibutilide
Psychotropics
Phenothiazines (e.g., thioridazine, chlorpromazine)
Tricyclic and tetracyclic antidepressants
Haloperidol/droperidol
Pimozide
Atypical antipsychotics (e.g., quetiapine, ziprasidone)
Toxins
Organophosphate insecticides
Arsenic
Antibiotics
Pentamidine
Macrolides
Trimethoprim–sulfamethoxazole
Fluoroquinolones (levofloxacin, moxifloxacin, gemifloxacin)
Voriconazole
Pain
Methadone
Miscellaneous
Liquid protein diets[a]
Corticosteroids[a]
Diuretics[a]
Quinine
Ondansetron (IV)
Chloroquine
Tacrolimus

[a]More than likely a result of severe electrolyte imbalance.

Note: For a complete list, see *www.qtdrugs.org*.

prerequisites to the development of drug-induced TdP. For instance, although TdP is usually documented early in the course of quinidine therapy, patients may develop this arrhythmia during chronic treatment.[115] The reason for quinidine's relatively unique propensity for causing TdP at relatively low dosages and plasma concentrations requires explanation. Quinidine's ability to block I_{Kr} is clinically manifest at low plasma concentrations; at higher plasma concentrations, its sodium channel blocking properties predominate. Other drugs that block I_{Kr} usually do so in a concentration-dependent fashion. The observation that most patients who suffer drug-induced TdP have evidence of mildly delayed repolarization (long QT intervals) even before they are prescribed the offending drug has stimulated a search for a potential genetically linked risk. Indeed, it appears that at least some patients with acquired drug-induced TdP possess mutations of genes that encode for I_{Kr} or I_{Ks}.[114]

The common underlying electrophysiologic cause of TdP is a delay in ventricular repolarization (provoking EADs), which usually results from inhibition (drug-induced or genetic) of I_K current and manifests as QT interval prolongation on the ECG. Therefore, the extent of QT interval prolongation has been used as a measurement of risk of TdP; however, considerable controversy exists regarding this practice. Amiodarone, for example, commonly causes significant QT prolongation but is a relatively infrequent cause of TdP. Nonetheless, the QT interval should be measured and monitored in all patients prescribed drugs that have a high potential for causing TdP (Table 8-12). Patients with a baseline QT_c interval (QT interval corrected for heart rate, which can be calculated using Bazett's formula: $QT_c = QT\ measured / \sqrt{R\text{–}R\ interval}$) > 450 milliseconds should not be given drugs that have a high potential for causing TdP; an increase in the QT_c interval to ≥560 milliseconds after the initiation of the drug is an indication to discontinue the agent or, at least, to reduce its dosage and carefully observe and monitor.

Drug-induced TdP has become an extremely visible hazard plaguing new drugs, sometimes resulting in public health disasters. For instance, several drugs (cisapride, astemizole, levomethadyl, grepafloxacin, sparfloxacin, terfenadine, and high-dose [32 mg] IV ondansetron) have been withdrawn from the market in the United States because of their significant potential for causing TdP. One of the most visible and striking examples of drug withdrawal due to TdP occurred with the popular nonsedating antihistamine, terfenadine. Terfenadine is a potent I_{Kr} blocker but is rapidly metabolized by CYP3A4 to an active moiety (fexofenadine) that is not associated with delayed repolarization. Consequently, in the presence of drugs that block the CYP3A4 isoenzyme (e.g., ketoconazole, erythromycin, diltiazem), accumulation of the parent compound, terfenadine, causes clinically significant blockade of I_{Kr} that could result in TdP and even death.[116] Because of experiences like this, all new drug entities under investigation are screened for their ability to block I_K and cause significant QT prolongation.

Acute treatment of TdP is different than treatment for the more common acute monomorphic VT. For an acute episode of TdP, most patients will require and respond to DCC. However, TdP tends to be paroxysmal in nature and often will rapidly recur after DCC. Therefore, after the initial restoration of a stable rhythm, therapy designed to prevent recurrences of TdP should be instituted. AADs that further prolong repolarization such as IV procainamide are absolutely contraindicated. Lidocaine is usually ineffective. Although there are no true efficacy trials, IV magnesium sulfate, by suppressing EADs, is considered the drug of choice in preventing recurrences of TdP.[117] If IV magnesium sulfate is ineffective, treatment strategies designed to increase heart rate, shorten ventricular repolarization, and prevent the pause dependency should be initiated. Either temporary transvenous pacing (105 to 120 beats/min) or pharmacologic pacing (isoproterenol or epinephrine infusion) can be initiated for this purpose. All drugs that prolong the QT interval should be discontinued, and exacerbating factors (e.g., hypokalemia or hypomagnesemia) should be corrected.

Ventricular Fibrillation

Background and Prevention

VF is electrical anarchy of the ventricle resulting in no cardiac output and cardiovascular collapse. Death will ensue rapidly if effective treatment measures are not taken. Patients who die abruptly (within 1 hour of initial symptoms) and unexpectedly (i.e., "sudden death") usually have VF recorded at the time of death.[118] SCD accounts for about 310,000 deaths per year in the United States.[15] It occurs most commonly in patients with CAD and those with LV dysfunction; it occurs less commonly in those with WPW syndrome or mitral valve prolapse, and occasionally in those without associated heart disease (e.g., Brugada syndrome). Patients who have SCD (not associated with acute MI) but survive because of appropriate CPR and defibrillation (where warranted) often have inducible sustained VT and/or VF during electrophysiologic studies. These individuals are at high risk for the recurrence of VT and/or VF.

In contrast, patients who have VF associated with acute MI (i.e., within the first 24 hours after symptoms) usually have little risk of recurrence. Of all patients who die as a result of an acute MI, approximately 50% die suddenly prior to hospitalization. VF associated with acute MI can be subdivided into two types: primary VF and complicated or secondary VF. Primary VF occurs in an uncomplicated MI not associated with HF; secondary VF occurs in an MI complicated by HF. The time course, incidence, mechanisms, treatment, and complications of these two forms of VF are different. For example, approximately 2% to 6% of patients with acute MI suffer primary VF within 24 hours of chest pain, but the risk of VF declines rapidly over time and is nearly zero after the initial 24-hour period. Complicated or secondary VF does not follow such a predictable time course and may occur in the late infarction period. The premise of prophylactic AADs administered to all patients with uncomplicated MI is based on (a) the inability to predict which patients are at risk for primary VF and (b) the predictable time course of primary VF (in contrast to complicated VF). Of the prophylactic therapies used, lidocaine has been the most widely debated and studied. Lie et al.[119] performed the classic study showing the effectiveness of lidocaine in preventing primary VF. Although lidocaine significantly reduced the incidence of VF compared with placebo, there was no significant difference in mortality due to VF between the groups. These results, along with the effectiveness of rapidly instituted defibrillation in modern coronary care units with sophisticated monitoring techniques, have caused most to reject the notion of prophylactic lidocaine administration for all patients with uncomplicated MI. In support of this, two meta-analyses[120,121] concluded against the routine use of prophylactic lidocaine because of a possible increase in mortality in lidocaine-treated patients[120] as well as the declining incidence of primary VF documented in recent years (probably a result of the more aggressive and rapid use of β-blockers, thrombolytics, and percutaneous intervention for the treatment of acute coronary syndromes).[121]

Acute Management

A patient with pulseless VT or VF should be managed according to the most recent AHA guidelines for CPR and ECC.[71] A detailed discussion regarding the acute management of pulseless VT/VF can be found in Chapter 2.

BRADYARRHYTHMIAS

The previous sections reviewed the pathophysiology and treatment of tachyarrhythmias, and this section serves to briefly consider the bradyarrhythmias. For the most part, the symptoms of bradyarrhythmias result from a decline in cardiac output. Because cardiac output decreases as heart rate decreases (to a point), patients with bradyarrhythmias may experience symptoms in association with hypotension, such as dizziness, syncope, fatigue, and confusion. If LV dysfunction exists, patients may experience worsening HF symptoms. Except in the case of recurrent syncope, symptoms associated with bradyarrhythmias are often subtle and nonspecific.

Sinus Bradycardia

Sinus bradyarrhythmias (heart rate <60 beats/min) are a common finding, especially in young, athletically active individuals, and usually are neither symptomatic nor in need of therapeutic intervention. On the other hand, some patients, particularly the elderly, have sinus node dysfunction. This may be the result of underlying SHD and the normal aging process that attenuate SA nodal function over time. Sick sinus syndrome refers to this process resulting in symptomatic sinus bradycardia and/or periods of sinus arrest.[122] Sinus node dysfunction is usually reflective of diffuse conduction disease, and accompanying AV block is relatively common. Furthermore, symptomatic bradyarrhythmias may be accompanied by alternating periods of paroxysmal tachycardias such as AF. In this instance, AF sometimes presents with a rather slow ventricular response (in the absence of AV nodal blocking drugs) because of diffuse conduction disease. The occurrence of alternating bradyarrhythmias and tachyarrhythmias is referred to as the tachy-brady syndrome. The occurrence of paroxysmal AF in a patient with sinus node dysfunction may be a result of underlying SHD with atrial dysfunction or atrial escape in response to reduced sinus node automaticity. In fact, because the rate of impulse generation by the sinus node is generally depressed or may fail altogether, other automatic pacemakers within the conduction system may "rescue" the sinus node. These rescue rhythms often present as paroxysmal atrial rhythms (e.g., AF) or as a junctional escape rhythm.

The treatment of sinus node dysfunction involves the elimination of symptomatic bradycardia and potentially managing alternating tachycardias such as AF. In general, the long-term therapy of choice is a permanent ventricular pacemaker. Dual-chamber, rate-adaptive chronic pacing clearly improves symptoms and overall quality of life and decreases the incidence of paroxysmal AF and systemic embolism.[122] Drugs commonly employed to treat supraventricular tachycardias should be used with caution, if at all, in the absence of a functioning pacemaker. AADs prescribed to prevent AF recurrences may also suppress the escape or rescue rhythms that appear in severe sinus bradycardia or sinus arrest. Consequently, these drugs may transform an asymptomatic patient with bradycardia into a symptomatic one. The addition of class I AADs can also affect pacemaker threshold and result in loss of capture if the pacemaker is not appropriately interrogated and adjusted. Other drugs that depress SA or AV nodal function, such as β-blockers and non-DHP CCBs, may also significantly exacerbate bradycardia. Even drugs with indirect sympatholytic actions, such as methyldopa and clonidine, may worsen sinus node dysfunction. The use of digoxin in these patients is controversial; however, in most cases, it can be used safely.

Other Causes

Another reason for paroxysmal bradycardia and sinus arrest that is not directly due to sinus node dysfunction is carotid sinus hypersensitivity.[123,124] Again, this syndrome occurs commonly in the elderly with underlying SHD, and may precipitate falls and hip fractures. Symptoms occur when the carotid sinus is stimulated, resulting in an accentuated baroreceptor reflex. Often, however, symptoms are not well correlated with the obvious physical manipulation of the carotid sinus (in the lateral neck region). Patients may experience intermittent episodes of dizziness or syncope because of sinus arrest caused by increased vagal tone and sympathetic withdrawal (the cardioinhibitory type), a drop in systemic blood pressure caused by sympathetic withdrawal (the vasodepressor type), or both (mixed cardioinhibitory and vasodepressor types). The diagnosis can be confirmed by performing carotid sinus massage with ECG and blood pressure monitoring in controlled conditions. Symptomatic carotid sinus hypersensitivity should also be treated with permanent pacemaker therapy.[123] However, some patients, particularly those with a significant vasodepressor component, still experience syncope or dizziness. The choice of definitive drug therapy in this situation is marred by the lack of controlled trials, although α-adrenergic stimulants such as midodrine are often tried in addition to the pacemaker.[124]

Vasovagal syndrome, by causing bradycardia, sinus arrest, and/or hypotension, is the cause of syncope in many patients who present with recurrent fainting of unknown origin.[125–127] By history, many individuals can recount rare instances of fainting spells at times of duress or fear. These are most often caused by vasovagal syncope. However, some have extremely frequent, unexpected syncopal episodes that interfere with the patient's quality of life and cause physical danger (sometimes referred to as neurocardiogenic syncope syndrome or malignant vasovagal syndrome). Vasovagal syncope is presumed to be a neurally mediated, paradoxical reaction involving stimulation of cardiac mechanoreceptors (i.e., Bezold-Jarisch reflex). Forceful contraction of the ventricle (e.g., as with adrenergic stimulation) coupled with low ventricular volumes (e.g., with upright posture or dehydration) provides a powerful stimulus for cardiac mechanoreceptors. Syncope results from the spontaneous development of transient hypotension (sympathetic withdrawal) and bradycardia (vagotonia). However, the true mechanism of vasovagal syncope remains to be definitively determined. For instance, patients with denervated hearts (e.g., heart transplant recipients) can still experience this form of syncope. This observation has led some to question the ultimate role of the Bezold-Jarisch reflex in these patients. Regardless, patients believed to have frequent episodes of vasovagal syncope have been evaluated and diagnosed using the upright body-tilt test,[128] a potent stimulus for the development of vasovagal symptoms. Although commonly used, the sensitivity and reproducibility of this test have been questioned.[129]

Traditionally, β-blockers, such as metoprolol, were frequently chosen as the drugs of choice in preventing episodes of vasovagal syncope. Although these drugs may seem inappropriate to treat a syndrome resulting from vasodilation and bradycardia, the therapeutic approach is designed to block an inappropriate vasovagal reaction (i.e., they inhibit the sympathetic surge that causes forceful ventricular contraction and precedes the onset of hypotension and bradycardia). To most clinicians' surprise, most controlled trials of the use of β-blockers in patients with severe vasovagal syncope have shown no effect compared with placebo in preventing syncopal episodes.[130] Some trials have suggested that β-blockers are more effective and should be used in older patients (>40 years of age) with vasovagal syncope rather than the relatively young.[131] Other drugs that have been used successfully (with or without β-blockers) include mineralocorticoids as volume expanders (fludrocortisone), anticholinergic drugs (scopolamine patches, disopyramide), α-adrenergic agonists (midodrine), adenosine analogs (theophylline, dipyridamole), and selective serotonin receptor antagonists (sertraline, paroxetine).[132] Permanent pacing has been used with some success but should be reserved for drug-refractory patients.[126,127] Because of the questionable effectiveness of β-blockers and the paucity of controlled or comparative trials, there is not a true drug of choice for severe vasovagal syncope, and clinicians are left with choosing agents and judging clinical effectiveness in individual patients on a case-by-case basis.

Atrioventricular Block

Conduction delay or block may occur in any area of the AV conduction system: the AV node, the His bundle, or the bundle branches. AV block is usually categorized into three different types based on ECG findings (Table 8-13). First-degree AV block is 1:1 AV conduction with a prolonged PR interval. Second-degree AV block is divided into two forms: Mobitz I AV block (Wenckebach periodicity) is less than 1:1 AV conduction with progressively lengthening PR intervals until a ventricular complex is dropped; Mobitz II AV block is intermittently dropped ventricular beats in a random fashion without

TABLE 8-13 Forms of Atrioventricular Block

Type	Criteria	Site of Block
First-degree block	Prolonged PR interval (>0.2 second); 1:1 AV conduction	Usually AVN
Second-degree block		
Mobitz I	Progressive PR prolongation until QRS is dropped; <1:1 AV conduction	AVN
Mobitz II	Random nonconducted beats (absence of QRS); <1:1 AV conduction	Below AVN
Third-degree block	AV dissociation; absence of AV conduction	AVN or below

AV, atrioventricular; AVN, atrioventricular node.

progressive PR lengthening. Third-degree AV block is complete heart block where AV conduction is totally absent (AV dissociation). First-degree AV block usually represents prolonged conduction in the AV node. Mobitz I, second-degree AV block is also usually caused by prolonged conduction in the AV node. Indeed, Wenckebach periodicity is a normal AV nodal response to rapid supraventricular stimulation or high vagal tone. In contrast, Mobitz II, second-degree AV block is usually caused by conduction disease below the AV node (i.e., His bundle). Third-degree AV block may be caused by disease at any level of the AV conduction system: complete AV nodal block, His bundle block, or trifascicular block. In this situation, the ventricle beats independently of the atria (AV dissociation), and the rate of ventricular activation and QRS configuration are determined by the site of the AV block. The usual degree of automaticity of ventricular pacemakers progressively declines as the site of impulse generation moves down the ventricular conduction system. Therefore, the ventricular escape rate in cases of trifascicular block will be significantly less than complete AV nodal block. Consequently, trifascicular block is a much more dangerous form of AV block. For instance, complete AV block at the level of the AV node usually results in the ventricular rhythm being controlled by the stable AV junctional pacemaker (rate ~40 beats/min). In contrast, in complete AV block due to trifascicular or His bundle block, a much less reliable pacemaker with slower rates below the site of block controls ventricular rhythm.

AV block may be found in patients without underlying SHD such as trained athletes or during sleep when vagal tone is high. Also, AV block may be transient where the underlying etiology is reversible such as in myocarditis, myocardial ischemia, after cardiovascular surgery, or during drug therapy. β-Blockers, digoxin, or non-DHP CCBs may cause AV block, primarily in the AV nodal area. Class I AADs may exacerbate conduction delays below the level of the AV node (sodium-dependent tissue). In other cases, AV block may be irreversible, such as that caused by acute MI, rare degenerative diseases, primary myocardial disease, or congenital heart disease.

If patients with Mobitz II AV block or third-degree AV block develop signs or symptoms of poor perfusion (e.g., altered mental status, chest pain, hypotension, shock), IV atropine (0.5 mg given every 3 to 5 minutes, up to 3 mg total dose) should be administered.[71] If these patients do not respond to atropine, transcutaneous pacing can be initiated. Sympathomimetic infusions such as epinephrine (2 to 10 mcg/min) or dopamine (2 to 10 mcg/kg/min) can also be used in the event of atropine failure and are particularly effective in sinus bradycardia/arrest and AV nodal block. An isoproterenol infusion (2 to 10 mcg/min) may be considered if the patient does not respond to dopamine or epinephrine; however, this drug should be used with caution because of its vasodilating properties and ability to increase myocardial oxygen consumption (particularly during active MI). As would be expected, these drugs usually do not help when the site of AV block is below the AV node (e.g., Mobitz II or trifascicular AV block) because their primary mechanism is to accelerate conduction through the AV node. If patients with bradycardia or AV block present with signs and symptoms of adequate perfusion, no acute therapy other than close observation is recommended.

Patients with chronic symptomatic AV block should be treated with the insertion of a permanent pacemaker. Patients without symptoms can sometimes be followed closely without the need for a pacemaker. The reader is referred for more detail to the national consensus guidelines for pacemaker implantation.[112,133] Patients with acute MI and evidence of new AV block or conduction disturbances will often require the insertion of a temporary transvenous pacemaker. AV block more commonly occurs as a complication of inferior wall MIs because of high vagal innervation at this site, and the coronary blood flow to the nodal areas usually supplies the inferior wall. However, the AV block may only be transient, obviating the need for permanent pacing.

EVALUATION OF THERAPEUTIC AND ECONOMIC OUTCOMES

Generally, patients who suffer from tachyarrhythmias can be monitored for one or several possible therapeutic outcomes. Obviously, the presence or recurrence of any arrhythmia can be documented by electrocardiographic means (e.g., surface ECG, Holter monitor, or event monitor). Furthermore, patients may experience a decrease in blood pressure that may result in symptoms ranging from light-headedness to abrupt syncope, depending on the rate of the arrhythmia and the status of the underlying heart disease. For some patients, the potential alteration in hemodynamics may result in death if the arrhythmia is not detected and treated immediately. Besides these clinical outcomes, many patients with tachyarrhythmias experience alterations in quality of life as a result of recurrent symptoms of the arrhythmia or from side effects of therapy. And, finally, there are the economic considerations of medical or surgical intervention, continued medical care, and chronic drug or nonpharmacologic treatment.[134,135] Most of the studies are limited to the use of nonpharmacologic therapies such as the ICD or radiofrequency ablation.[76,136] Because that technology is rapidly evolving, what is not very cost-effective now may indeed be cost-effective in the next several years. For example, original cost-effectiveness analysis of the ICD showed it to be highly sensitive to the life of the generator, yet newer-generation devices have made significant advances not only in their size but also in their battery life. More recent data on the effect of the ICD on mortality coupled with the declining costs of an ICD imply that the device is indeed cost-effective in certain subsets of patients, which is similar to well-proven drug therapies used for other disorders.[136] Other nonpharmacologic treatments, such as radiofrequency ablation for PSVT, not only improve quality of life but also save money on medical expenditures compared with chronic drug therapy.[76]

There are some therapeutic outcomes that are unique to certain arrhythmias. For instance, patients with AF or atrial flutter need to be monitored for thromboembolism and for complications of antithrombotic therapy (bleeding, drug interactions). However, the most important monitoring parameters for most patients fall into the following categories: (a) mortality (total and arrhythmic); (b) arrhythmia recurrence (duration, frequency, symptoms); (c) hemodynamic consequences (heart rate, blood pressure, symptoms); and (d) treatment complications (side effects or need for alternative or additional drugs, devices, surgery) (Table 8-14). When evaluating the arrhythmia literature, care should be taken to consider

TABLE 8-14 Arrhythmia Outcomes

Mortality
Total, all-cause
Arrhythmic death (i.e., sudden cardiac death)
Recurrences documented by electrocardiogram
Time to recurrence
Frequency of recurrences
Tolerance
Symptoms
Blood pressure
Rate of tachycardia
Surrogate markers of efficacy such as:
Number of premature ventricular complexes per day
Inducibility of tachycardia with programmed stimulation
Necessity of nondrug interventions (e.g., ICD)
ICD shocks
Side effects of drugs/treatment complications
Quality of life
Economics
Outcomes specific to tachycardia (e.g., systemic embolism in atrial fibrillation)

ICD, implantable cardioverter-defibrillator.

real outcomes. For example, total mortality is more meaningful than SCD rates; it is possible an intervention prevents arrhythmic death but patients die from other causes, leaving all-cause mortality unaltered. Likewise, surrogate markers of drug efficacy (e.g., noninducible tachycardia, suppression of minor arrhythmias) should be judged with a degree of skepticism. One should ask: Did the treatment make patients live longer (reduce mortality)? Did the treatment make them feel better (improve humanistic outcomes or quality of life)? Was the treatment economically worth it (cost-effective)?

ABBREVIATIONS

AAD	antiarrhythmic drug
ACC	American College of Cardiology
ACCP	American College of Chest Physicians
ACTIVE	Atrial Fibrillation Clopidogrel Trial with Irbesartan for Prevention of Vascular Events
AF	atrial fibrillation
AF-CHF	Atrial Fibrillation and Congestive Heart Failure
AFFIRM	Atrial Fibrillation Follow-Up Investigation of Rhythm Management
AHA	American Heart Association
AV	atrioventricular
AVID	Antiarrhythmics Versus Implantable Defibrillators
CAD	coronary artery disease
CASH	Cardiac Arrest Study Hamburg
CAST	Cardiac Arrhythmia Suppression Trial
CCB	calcium channel blocker
CIDS	Canadian Implantable Defibrillator Study
CPR	cardiopulmonary resuscitation
CrCl	creatinine clearance
CYP	cytochrome P450
DCC	direct current cardioversion
DHP	dihydropyridine
EAD	early afterdepolarization
ECC	emergency cardiovascular care
ECG	electrocardiogram
ESC	European Society of Cardiology
HF	heart failure
HOT-CAFE	How to Treat Chronic Atrial Fibrillation
ICD	implantable cardioverter-defibrillator
INR	international normalized ratio
LAD	late afterdepolarization
LV	left ventricular
LVEF	left ventricular ejection fraction
MADIT	Multicenter Automatic Defibrillator Implantation Trial
MI	myocardial infarction
MUSTT	Multicenter Unsustained Tachycardia Trial
NYHA	New York Heart Association
PIAF	Pharmacological Intervention in Atrial Fibrillation
PSVT	paroxysmal supraventricular tachycardia
PVC	premature ventricular complex
RACE	Rate Control Versus Electrical Cardioversion for Persistent Atrial Fibrillation
RE-LY	Randomized Evaluation of Long-Term Anticoagulation Therapy
RMP	resting membrane potential
SA	sinoatrial
SCD	sudden cardiac death
SCD-HeFT	Sudden Cardiac Death in Heart Failure Trial
SHD	structural heart disease
SR	sinus rhythm
STAF	Strategies of Treatment of Atrial Fibrillation
TdP	torsade de pointes
TEE	transesophageal echocardiography
VF	ventricular fibrillation
VT	ventricular tachycardia
WPW	Wolff-Parkinson-White

REFERENCES

1. Alice MA, Bonke FIM, Schopman FJG. Circus movement in rabbit atrial muscle as a mechanism of tachycardia III. The "leading circle" concept: A new model of circus movement in cardiac tissue without the involvement of an anatomic obstacle. Circ Res 1977;41:9–18.
2. Vaughan Williams EM. A classification of antiarrhythmic actions reassessed after a decade of new drugs. J Clin Pharmacol 1984;24:129–147.
3. Working Group on Arrhythmias of the European Society of Cardiology. The Sicilian Gambit: A new approach to the classification of antiarrhythmic drugs based upon their actions on arrhythmogenic mechanisms. Circulation 1991;84:1831–1851.
4. Hondeghem LM, Katzung BG. Antiarrhythmic agents: The modulated receptor mechanism of action of sodium and calcium channel-blocking drugs. Annu Rev Pharmacol Toxicol 1984;24:387–423.
5. Nasr IR, Bouzamondo A, Hulot JS, et al. Prevention of atrial fibrillation onset by beta-blocker treatment in heart failure: A meta-analysis. Eur Heart J 2007;28:457–462.
6. Makkar KM, Sanoski CA, Spinler SA. Role of angiotensin-converting enzyme inhibitors, angiotensin II receptor blockers, and aldosterone antagonists in the prevention of atrial and ventricular arrhythmias. Pharmacotherapy 2009;29:31–48.
7. Podrid PJ, Schoeneburger A, Lown B. Congestive heart failure caused by oral disopyramide. N Engl J Med 1980;302:614–617.
8. Podrid PJ. Proarrhythmia, a serious complication of antiarrhythmic drugs. Curr Cardiol Rep 1999;1:289–296.
9. Fang MC, Stafford RS, Ruskin JN, et al. National trends in antiarrhythmic and antithrombotic medication use in atrial fibrillation. Arch Intern Med 2004;164:55–60.
10. Sanoski CA, Bauman JL. Clinical observations with the amiodarone/warfarin interaction: Dosing relationships with long-term therapy. Chest 2002;121:19–23.
11. Camus P, Martin WJ, Rosenow EC. Amiodarone pulmonary toxicity. Clin Chest Med 2004;25:65–75.
12. Babatin M, Lee SS, Pollak PT. Amiodarone hepatotoxicity. Curr Vasc Pharmacol 2008;6:228–236.
13. Sanoski C, Schoen MD, Gonzalez RD, et al. Rationale, development and outcomes of a multidisciplinary clinic for patients receiving chronic oral amiodarone. Pharmacotherapy 1998;18:1465–1515.
14. Goldschlager N, Epstein AE, Naccarelli GV, et al. A practical guide for clinicians who treat patients with amiodarone: 2007. Heart Rhythm 2007;4:1250–1259.
15. Go AS, Mozaffarian D, Roger VL, et al. Heart disease and stroke statistics 2013 update: A report from the American Heart Association. Circulation 2013;127:e6–e245.
16. Fuster V, Rydén LE, Cannom DS, et al. ACC/AHA/ESC 2006 guidelines for the management of patients with atrial fibrillation: A report of the American College of Cardiology/American Heart Association Task Force on Practice Guidelines and the European Society of Cardiology Committee for Practice Guidelines (Writing Committee to Revise the 2001 Guidelines for the Management of Patients

with Atrial Fibrillation). J Am Coll Cardiol 2006;48: e149–e246.

17. Miyasaka Y, Barnes ME, Gersh BJ, et al. Secular trends in incidence of atrial fibrillation in Olmsted County, Minnesota, 1980 to 2000, and implications on the projections for future prevalence. Circulation 2006;114:119–125.
18. Lloyd-Jones DM, Wang TJ, Leip EP, et al. Lifetime risk for developing atrial fibrillation: The Framingham Heart Study. Circulation 2004;110:1042–1046.
19. Levy S, Camm AJ, Saksena S, et al. International consensus on nomenclature and classification of atrial fibrillation. A collaborative project of the Working Group on Arrhythmias and the Working Group on Cardiac Pacing of the European Society of Cardiology and the North American Society of Pacing and Electrophysiology. Europace 2003;5:119–122.
20. You JJ, Singer DE, Howard PA, et al. Antithrombotic therapy for atrial fibrillation: Antithrombotic Therapy and Prevention of Thrombosis, 9th ed: American College of Chest Physicians Evidence-Based Clinical Practice Guidelines. Chest 2012;141:e531S–e575S.
21. Atrial Fibrillation Investigators. Risk factors for stroke and efficacy of antithrombotic therapy in atrial fibrillation: Analysis of pooled data from five randomized controlled trials. Arch Intern Med 1994;154:1449–1457.
22. Wann LS, Curtis AB, January CT, et al. 2011 ACCF/AHA/HRS focused update on the management of patients with atrial fibrillation (updating the 2006 guideline): A report of the American College of Cardiology Foundation/American Heart Association Task Force on Practice Guidelines. Circulation 2011;123:104–123.
23. Phillips BG, Gandhi AJ, Sanoski CA, et al. Comparison of intravenous diltiazem and verapamil for the acute treatment of atrial fibrillation and flutter. Pharmacotherapy 1997;17:1238–1245.
24. Hohnloser SH, Kuck KH, Lilienthal J. Rhythm or rate control in atrial fibrillation—Pharmacological Intervention in Atrial Fibrillation (PIAF): A randomised trial. Lancet 2000;356:1789–1794.
25. Van Gelder IC, Hagens VE, Bosker HA, et al. The Rate Control Versus Electrical Cardioversion for Persistent Atrial Fibrillation Study Group. A comparison of rate control and rhythm control in patients with recurrent persistent atrial fibrillation. N Engl J Med 2002;347:1834–1840.
26. The Atrial Fibrillation Follow-Up Investigation of Rhythm Management (AFFIRM) Investigators. A comparison of rate control and rhythm control in patients with atrial fibrillation. N Engl J Med 2002;347:1825–1833.
27. Carlsson J, Miketic S, Windeler J, et al. Randomized trial of rate-control versus rhythm-control in persistent atrial fibrillation: The Strategies of Treatment of Atrial Fibrillation (STAF) study. J Am Coll Cardiol 2003;41:1690–1696.
28. Opolski G, Torbicki A, Kosior DA, et al. Rate control vs rhythm control in patients with nonvalvular persistent atrial fibrillation: The results of the Polish How to Treat Chronic Atrial Fibrillation (HOT CAFE) Study. Chest 2004;126: 476–486.
29. Roy D, Talajic M, Nattel S, et al. Rhythm control versus rate control for atrial fibrillation and heart failure. N Engl J Med 2008;358:2667–2677.
30. de Denus S, Sanoski CA, Carlsson J, Opolski G, Spinler SA. Rate vs rhythm control in patients with atrial fibrillation: A meta-analysis. Arch Intern Med 2005;165:258–262.
31. Van Gelder IC, Groenveld HF, Crijns HJ, et al. Lenient versus strict rate control in patients with atrial fibrillation. N Engl J Med 2010;362:1363–1373.
32. Klein AL, Grimm RA, Murray D, et al. Use of transesophageal echocardiography to guide cardioversion in patients with atrial fibrillation. N Engl J Med 2001;344: 1411–1420.
33. Bauman JL, Bauernfeind RA, Hoff JV, et al. Torsade de pointes due to quinidine: Observations in 31 patients. Am Heart J 1984;107:425–430.
34. Slavik RS, Tisdale JE, Borzak S. Pharmacologic conversion of atrial fibrillation: A systematic review of available evidence. Prog Cardiovasc Dis 2001;44:121–152.
35. Alboni P, Botto GL, Baldi N, et al. Outpatient treatment of recent-onset atrial fibrillation with the "pill-in-the-pocket" approach. N Engl J Med 2004;351:2384–2391.
36. Connolly SJ, Ezekowitz MD, Yusuf S, et al. Dabigatran versus warfarin in patients with atrial fibrillation. N Engl J Med 2009;361:1139–1151.
37. Liesenfeld KH, Lehr T, Dansirikul C, et al. Population pharmacokinetic analysis of the oral thrombin inhibitor dabigatran etexilate in patients with non-valvular atrial fibrillation from the RE-LY trial. J Thromb Haemost 2011;9:2168–2175.
38. Wann LS, Curtis AB, Ellenbogen KA, et al. 2011 ACCF/AHA/HRS focused update on the management of patients with atrial fibrillation (update on dabigatran): A report of the American College of Cardiology Foundation/American Heart Association Task Force on Practice Guidelines. Circulation 2011;123:1144–1150.
39. Patel MR, Mahaffey KW, Garg J, et al. Rivaroxaban versus warfarin in nonvalvular atrial fibrillation. N Engl J Med 2011;365:883–891.
40. Connolly SJ, Eikelboom J, Joyner C, et al. Apixaban in patients with atrial fibrillation. N Engl J Med 2011;364: 806–817.
41. Granger CB, Alexander JH, McMurray JJ, et al. Apixaban versus warfarin in patients with atrial fibrillation. N Engl J Med 2011;365:981–992.
42. Furie KL, Goldstein LB, Albers GW, et al. Oral antithrombotic agents for the prevention of stroke in nonvalvular atrial fibrillation: A science advisory for healthcare professionals from the American Heart Association/American Stroke Association. Stroke 2012;43: 3442–3453.
43. Connolly SJ, Pogue J, Hart R, et al. Clopidogrel plus aspirin versus oral anticoagulation for atrial fibrillation in the Atrial fibrillation Clopidogrel Trial with Irbesartan for prevention of Vascular Events (ACTIVE W): A randomised controlled trial. Lancet 2006;367:1903–1912.
44. The ACTIVE Investigators. Effect of clopidogrel added to aspirin in patients with atrial fibrillation. N Engl J Med 2009;360:2066–2078.
45. Coplen SE, Antman EM, Berlin JA, et al. Efficacy and safety of quinidine therapy for maintenance of sinus rhythm after cardioversion: A meta-analysis of randomized control trials. Circulation 1990;82:1106–1116.
46. Echt DS, Liebson PR, Mitchell B, et al. Mortality and morbidity in patients receiving encainide, flecainide, or placebo. The Cardiac Arrhythmia Suppression Trial. N Engl J Med 1991;324:781–788.
47. Lafuente-LaFuente C, Mouly S, Longás-Tejero MA, et al. Antiarrhythmic drugs for maintaining sinus rhythm after cardioversion of atrial fibrillation. Arch Intern Med 2006;166:719–728.
48. Roy D, Talajic M, Dorian P, et al. Amiodarone to prevent recurrence of atrial fibrillation. Canadian Trial of Atrial Fibrillation Investigators. N Engl J Med 2000;324: 913–920.

49. AFFIRM First Antiarrhythmic Drug Substudy Investigators. Maintenance of sinus rhythm in patients with atrial fibrillation: An AFFIRM substudy of the first antiarrhythmic drug. J Am Coll Cardiol 2003;42:20–29.
50. Singh BN, Singh SN, Reda DJ, et al. Amiodarone versus sotalol for atrial fibrillation. N Engl J Med 2005;352: 1861–1872.
51. Juul-Moller S, Edvardsson N, Rehnqvist-Ahlberg N. Sotalol versus quinidine for the maintenance of sinus rhythm after direct current conversion of atrial fibrillation. Circulation 1990;82:1932–1939.
52. Southworth MR, Zarembski D, Viana M, Bauman JL. Comparison of sotalol versus quinidine for maintenance of normal sinus rhythm in patients with chronic atrial fibrillation. Am J Cardiol 1999;83:1629–1632.
53. Pedersen OD, Bagger H, Keller N, et al. Efficacy of dofetilide in the treatment of atrial fibrillation-flutter in patients with reduced left ventricular function, a Danish Investigation of Arrhythmia and Mortality on Dofetilide (DIAMOND) Substudy. Circulation 2001;104:292–296.
54. Singh S, Zoble RG, Yellen L, et al. Efficacy and safety of oral dofetilide in converting and maintaining sinus rhythm in patients with chronic atrial fibrillation or atrial flutter. The Symptomatic Atrial Fibrillation Investigative Research on Dofetilide (SAFIRE-D) Study. Circulation 2000;102: 2385–2390.
55. Singh BN, Connolly SJ, Crijns HJGM, et al. Dronedarone for maintenance of sinus rhythm in atrial fibrillation or flutter. N Engl J Med 2007;357:987–999.
56. Hohnloser SH, Crijns HJGM, van Eickels M, et al. Effect of dronedarone on cardiovascular events in atrial fibrillation. N Engl J Med 2009;360:668–678.
57. Køber L, Torp-Pedersen C, McMurray JJV, et al. Increased mortality after dronedarone therapy for severe heart failure. N Engl J Med 2008;358:2678–2687.
58. Le Heuzey JY, De Ferrari GM, Radzik D, et al. A short-term, randomized, double-blind, parallel-group study to evaluate the efficacy and safety of dronedarone versus amiodarone in patients with persistent atrial fibrillation: The DIONYSOS study. J Cardiovasc Electrophysiol 2010;21:597–605.
59. Connolly SJ, Camm AJ, Halperin JL, et al. Dronedarone in high-risk permanent atrial fibrillation. N Engl J Med 2011;365:2268–2276.
60. Spector P, Reynolds MR, Calkins H, et al. Meta-analysis of ablation of atrial flutter and supraventricular tachycardia. Am J Cardiol 2009;104:671–677.
61. Blomstrom-Lundgrist C, Scheimanman MM, Aliot EM, et al. ACC/AHA/ESC guidelines for the management of patients with supraventricular arrhythmias. A report of the American College of Cardiology/American Heart Association Task Force and the European Society of Cardiology Committee for Practice Guidelines. J Am Coll Cardiol 2003;42: 1493–1531.
62. Pappone C, Augello G, Sala S, et al. A randomized trial of circumferential pulmonary vein ablation versus antiarrhythmic drug therapy in paroxysmal atrial fibrillation: The APAF Study. J Am Coll Cardiol 2006;48:2340–2347.
63. Oral H, Pappone C, Chugh A, et al. Circumferential pulmonary-vein ablation for chronic atrial fibrillation. N Engl J Med 2006;354:934–941.
64. Wilber DJ, Pappone C, Neuzil P, et al. Comparison of antiarrhythmic drug therapy and radiofrequency catheter ablation in patients with paroxysmal atrial fibrillation: A randomized controlled trial. JAMA 2010;303:333–340.
65. Wazni OM, Marrouche NF, Martin DO, et al. Radiofrequency ablation vs antiarrhythmic drugs as first-line treatment of symptomatic atrial fibrillation: A randomized trial. JAMA 2005;293:2634–2640.
66. Jaïs P, Cauchemez B, Macle L, et al. Catheter ablation versus antiarrhythmic drugs for atrial fibrillation: The A4 study. Circulation 2008;118:2498–2505.
67. Calkins H, Kuck KH, Cappato R, et al. 2012 HRS/EHRA/ ECAS expert consensus statement on catheter and surgical ablation of atrial fibrillation: Recommendations for patient selection, procedural techniques, patient management and follow-up, definitions, endpoints, and research trial design. Heart Rhythm 2012;9:632–696.
68. Cappato R, Calkins H, Chen SA, et al. Updated worldwide survey on the methods, efficacy, and safety of catheter ablation for human atrial fibrillation. Circ Arrhythm Electrophysiol 2010;3:32–38.
69. Sung RJ, Lauer MR, Chun H. Atrioventricular node reentry: Current concepts and new perspectives. Pacing Clin Electrophysiol 1994;17:1413–1430.
70. DiMarco JP, Miles W, Akhtar M, et al. Adenosine for paroxysmal supraventricular tachycardia: Dose ranging and comparison with verapamil. Assessment in placebo-controlled, multicenter trials. Ann Intern Med 1990;1113:104–110.
71. 2010 American Heart Association guidelines for cardiopulmonary resuscitation and emergency cardiovascular care science. Circulation 2010;122:5640–5933.
72. Rankin AC, McGovern BA. Adenosine or verapamil for the acute treatment of supraventricular tachycardia? Ann Intern Med 1991;114:513–515.
73. Jackman WM, Wang Z, Friday KJ, et al. Catheter ablation of accessory atrioventricular pathways (Wolff-Parkinson-White syndrome) by radiofrequency current. N Engl J Med 1991;324:1605–1611.
74. Jackman WM, Beckman KJ, McClelland JH, et al. Treatment of supraventricular tachycardia due to atrioventricular nodal reentry by radiofrequency catheter ablation of slow pathway conduction. N Engl J Med 1992;327:313–318.
75. Scheinman MM. Radiofrequency catheter ablation for patients with supraventricular tachycardia. Pacing Clin Electrophysiol 1993;16:671–679.
76. Cheng CH, Sanders GD, Hlatky MA, et al. Cost effectiveness of radio-frequency ablation for supraventricular tachycardia. Ann Intern Med 2000;133:864–876.
77. Bayes deLuna A, Coumel P, LeClercq IF. Ambulatory sudden cardiac death: Mechanisms of production of fatal arrhythmia on the basis of data from 157 cases. Am Heart J 1989;117:151–159.
78. Ruberman W, Weinblatt E, Goldberg JD, et al. Ventricular premature beats and mortality after myocardial infarction. N Engl J Med 1977;297:750–757.
79. The Cardiac Arrhythmia Suppression Trial II Investigators. Effect of the antiarrhythmic agent moricizine on survival after myocardial infarction. N Engl J Med 1992;327: 227–233.
80. Waldo AL, Camm AJ, deRuyter H, et al. Effect of *d*-sotalol on mortality in patients with left ventricular dysfunction and remote myocardial infarction. Lancet 1996;348:7–12.
81. Julian DG, Camm AJ, Frangin G, et al. Randomized trial of effect of amiodarone on mortality in patients with left ventricular dysfunction after recent myocardial infarction: EMIAT. Lancet 1997;349:667–674.
82. Cairns JA, Connolly SJ, Roberts R, et al. Randomized trial of outcome after myocardial infarction in patients with frequent or repetitive ventricular premature depolarizations: CAMIAT. Lancet 1997;349:675–682.
83. Amiodarone Trials Meta-Analysis Investigators. Effect of prophylactic amiodarone on mortality after acute myocardial

infarction and in congestive heart failure: Meta-analysis of individual data from 6,500 patients in randomized trials. Lancet 1997;350:1417–1424.

84. Torp-Pederson C, Moller M, Bloch-Thomsen PE, et al. Dofetilide in patients with congestive heart failure and left ventricular dysfunction. N Engl J Med 1999;341:857–865.
85. Kober L, Block-Thomsen PE, Moller M, et al. Effect of dofetilide in patients with recent myocardial infarction and left ventricular dysfunction: A randomized trial. Lancet 2000;356:2052–2058.
86. Hilleman DE, Bauman JL. Role of antiarrhythmic therapy in patients at risk for sudden cardiac death: An evidence-based review. Pharmacotherapy 2001;21:556–575.
87. Edhouse J, Morris F. Broad complex tachycardia—Part I. BMJ 2002;312:719–722.
88. Edhouse J, Morris F. Broad complex tachycardia—Part II. BMJ 2002;324:776–779.
89. Cole CR, Marrouche NF, Natale A. Evaluation and management of ventricular outflow tract tachycardias. Card Electrophysiol Rev 2002;6:442–447.
90. Modell SM, Lehmann MH. The long QT syndrome family of cardiac ion channelopathies: A HuGE review. Genet Med 2006;8:143–155.
91. Keating MT, Sanguinetti MC. Molecular and cellular mechanisms of cardiac arrhythmias. Cell 2001;104:569–580.
92. Antzelevitch C, Brugada P, Brugada J, et al. Brugada syndrome: 1992–2002: A historical perspective. J Am Coll Cardiol 2003;41:1665–1671.
93. Gorgels A, van den Dool A, Hofs A, et al. Comparison of procainamide and lidocaine in terminating sustained monomorphic ventricular tachycardia. Am J Cardiol 1996;78:43–46.
94. Mason JW, Electrophysiologic Study Versus Electrocardiographic Monitoring Investigators. A comparison of electrophysiologic testing with Holter monitoring to predict antiarrhythmic drug efficacy for ventricular tachyarrhythmias. N Engl J Med 1993;329: 445–451.
95. Mason JW, Electrophysiologic Study Versus Electrocardiographic Monitoring Investigators. A comparison of seven antiarrhythmic drugs in patients with ventricular tachyarrhythmias. N Engl J Med 1993;329: 452–458.
96. The Cascade Investigators. Randomized antiarrhythmic drug therapy in survivors of cardiac arrest (the CASCADE Study). Am J Cardiol 1993;72:280–287.
97. Aliot EM, Stevenson WG, Almendral-Garrote JM, et al. EHRA/HRS expert consensus on catheter ablation of ventricular arrhythmias: Developed in a partnership with the European Heart Rhythm Association (EHRA), a registered branch of the European Society of Cardiology (ESC), and the Heart Rhythm Society (HRS); in collaboration with the American College of Cardiology (ACC) and the American Heart Association (AHA). Europace 2009;11:771–817.
98. DiMarco JP. Implantable cardioverter-defibrillators. N Engl J Med 2003;349:1836–1847.
99. Pacifico A, Hohnloser SH, Williams JH, et al. Prevention of implantable-defibrillator shocks by treatment with sotalol. N Engl J Med 1999;340:1855–1862.
100. Connolly SJ, Dorian P, Roberts RS, et al. Comparison of beta-blockers, amiodarone plus beta-blockers, or sotalol for prevention of shocks from implantable cardioverter defibrillators: The OPTIC Study: A randomized trial. JAMA 2006;295:165–171.
101. Dopp AL, Miller JM, Tisdale JE. Effects of drugs on defibrillation capacity. Drugs 2008;68:607–630.
102. The AVID Investigators. A comparison of antiarrhythmic-drug therapy with implantable defibrillators in patients resuscitated from near-fatal ventricular arrhythmias. N Engl J Med 1997;337:1576–1583.
103. Connolly SJ, Gene M, Roberts TS, et al. Cardiac Implantable Defibrillator Study (CIDS): A randomized trial of the implantable cardioverter-defibrillator against amiodarone. Circulation 2000;101:1297–1302.
104. Kuck KH, Cappato R, Siebels J, et al. Randomized comparison of antiarrhythmic drug therapy with implantable defibrillators in patients resuscitated from cardiac arrest: The Cardiac Arrest Study Hamburg (CASH). Circulation 2000;102:748–754.
105. Wilber DJ, Olshansky B, Moran JF, et al. Electrophysiological testing and nonsustained VT. Use and limitations in patients with coronary artery disease and impaired ventricular function. Circulation 1990;82:350–358.
106. Buxton AE, Leek KL, DiCarlo L, et al. Electrophysiologic testing to identify patients with coronary artery disease who are at risk for sudden death. Multicenter Unsustained Tachycardia Trial. N Engl J Med 2000;342:1937–1945.
107. Moss AJ, Hall WJ, Cannom DS, et al. Improved survival with an implanted defibrillator in patients with coronary disease at high risk for ventricular arrhythmia. N Engl J Med 1996;335:1933–1940.
108. Buxton AE, Lee KL, Fisher JD, et al. A randomized study of the prevention of sudden death in patients with coronary artery disease. N Engl J Med 1999;341:1882–1890.
109. Zipes DP, Camm AJ, Borggrefe M, et al. ACC/AHA/ESC 2006 guidelines for management of patients with ventricular arrhythmias and the prevention of sudden cardiac death—Executive summary: A report of the American College of Cardiology/American Heart Association Task Force and the European Society of Cardiology Committee for Practice Guidelines (Writing Committee to Develop Guidelines for Management of Patients with Ventricular Arrhythmias and the Prevention of Sudden Cardiac Death). Circulation 2006;114:1–45.
110. Moss AJ, Zareba W, Hall WJ, et al. Prophylactic implantation of a defibrillator in patients with myocardial infarction and reduced ejection fraction. N Engl J Med 2002;346:877–883.
111. Bardy GH, Lee KL, Mark DB, et al. Amiodarone or an implantable cardioverter-defibrillator for congestive heart failure. N Engl J Med 2005;352:225–237.
112. Epstein AE, DiMarco JP, Ellenbogen KA, et al. ACC/AHA/HRS 2008 guidelines for device-based therapy of cardiac rhythm abnormalities: A report of the American College of Cardiology/American Heart Association Task Force on Practice Guidelines (Writing Committee to Revise the ACC/AHA/NASPE 2002 Guideline Update for Implantation of Cardiac Pacemakers and Antiarrhythmia Devices). J Am Coll Cardiol 2008;51:e1–e62.
113. Antzelevitch C. Heterogeneity of cellular repolarization in LQTS: The role of M cells. Eur Heart J 2001;3:K2–K16.
114. Roden DM. Long QT syndrome: Reduced repolarization reserve and the genetic link. J Intern Med 2006;259:59–69.
115. Oberg KC, O'Toole MF, Gallastegui JL, Bauman JL. "Late" proarrhythmia due to quinidine. Am J Cardiol 1994;74: 192–194.
116. Bauman JL. The role of pharmacokinetics, drug interactions and pharmacogenetics in the acquired long QT syndrome. Eur Heart J 2001;3:K93–K100.
117. Tzivoni D, Banai S, Schuger C, et al. Treatment of torsade de pointes with magnesium sulfate. Circulation 1987;77: 392–397.

118. Koplan BA, Stevenson WG. Ventricular tachycardia and sudden cardiac death. Mayo Clin Proc 2009;84:289–297.
119. Lie KI, Wellens HJJ, Van Capelle FJ. Lidocaine in the prevention of primary ventricular fibrillation. N Engl J Med 1974;291:1324–1326.
120. MacMahon S, Collin R, Peto R, et al. Effects of prophylactic lidocaine in suspected acute myocardial infarction: An overview of results from the randomized controlled trials. JAMA 1988;260:1910–1916.
121. Antman EM, Berlin JA. Declining incidence of ventricular fibrillation in myocardial infarction: Implications for the prophylactic use of lidocaine. Circulation 1992;86:764–773.
122. Moya A, Sutton R, Ammirati F, et al. Guidelines for the diagnosis and management of syncope (version 2009). Eur Heart J 2009;30:2631–2671.
123. Sugrue DD, Gersh BJ, Holmes DR, et al. Symptomatic "isolated" carotid sinus hypersensitivity: Natural history and results of treatment with anticholinergic drugs or pacemaker. J Am Coll Cardiol 1986;7:158–162.
124. Seifer C. Carotid sinus syndrome. Prog Cardiol Clin 2013;31: 111–121.
125. Zagga M, Massumi A. Neurally mediated syncope. Tex Heart Inst J 2000;27:268–272.
126. Grubb BP. Neurocardiogenic syncope and related disorders of orthostatic intolerance. Circulation 2005;111:2997–3006.
127. Grubb BP. Neurocardiogenic syncope. N Engl J Med 2005;352:1004–1010.
128. Milstein S, Reyes WJ, Benditt DG. Upright body tilt for evaluation of patients with recurrent, unexplained syncope. Pacing Clin Electrophysiol 1989;12:117–124.
129. Almquist A, Goldenberg I, Milstein S. Provocation of bradycardia and hypotension by isoproterenol and upright posture in patients with unexplained syncope. N Engl J Med 1990;320:346–351.
130. Brignole M. Randomized clinical trials of neurally mediated syncope. J Cardiovasc Electrophysiol 2003;14(Suppl): S64–S69.
131. Sheldon R, Connolly S, Rose S, for the POST Investigators. Prevention of Syncope Trial (POST). A randomized, placebo-controlled study of metoprolol in the prevention of vasovagal syncope. Circulation 2006;113:1164–1170.
132. Armaganijan L, Morillo CA. Treatment of vasovagal syncope: An update. Curr Treat Options Cardiovasc Med 2010;12:472–488.
133. Tracy CM, Epstein AE, Darbar D, et al. 2012 ACCF/AHA/HRS focused updated of the 2008 guidelines for device-based therapy of cardiac rhythm abnormalities: A report of the American College of Cardiology Foundation/American Heart Association Task Force on Practice Guidelines. J Am Coll Cardiol 2012;60:1297–1313.
134. Kupersmith J, Holmes-Novner M, Hogan A, et al. Cost-effectiveness analysis in heart disease, I: General principles. Prog Cardiovasc Dis 1994;37:161–184.
135. Kupersmith J, Holmes-Novner M, Hogan A, et al. Cost-effectiveness analysis in heart disease, III: Ischemia, congestive heart failure, and arrhythmias. Prog Cardiovasc Dis 1995;37:307–346.
136. Sanders GD, Hlatky MA, Owens DK. Cost-effectiveness of implantable cardioverter-defibrillators. N Engl J Med 2005;353:1471–1480.

9

Venous Thromboembolism

Daniel M. Witt and Nathan P. Clark

KEY CONCEPTS

1. The risk of venous thromboembolism (VTE) is related to several easily identifiable factors, including age, major surgery (particularly orthopedic procedures of the lower extremities), previous VTE, trauma, malignancy, prolonged immobility or limb paralysis, and hypercoagulable states.
2. The diagnosis of VTE should be confirmed by objective testing.
3. At the time of hospital admission, all patients should receive prophylaxis against VTE that corresponds to their level of risk. Prophylaxis should be continued throughout the period of risk.
4. In the absence of contraindications, the treatment of VTE should initially include a rapid-acting anticoagulant (e.g., unfractionated heparin, low-molecular-weight heparin, fondaparinux, or rivaroxaban). If the patient is transitioned to warfarin therapy, the rapid-acting anticoagulant should be overlapped with warfarin for at least 5 days and until the patient's international normalized ratio is greater than 2.
5. Most patients with an uncomplicated deep vein thrombosis (DVT), with or without pulmonary embolism (PE), can be safely treated as an outpatient.
6. Emerging anticoagulants such as rivaroxaban may mark a significant advancement in the treatment of VTE.
7. Anticoagulant therapies require meticulous and systematic monitoring as well as ongoing patient education.
8. Bleeding is the most common adverse effect associated with anticoagulant drugs. A patient's risk of major hemorrhage is related to the intensity and stability of therapy, concurrent drug use, history of prior bleeding, prior history of stroke, renal or hepatic impairment, thrombocytopenia, recent surgery or trauma, and increasing age.
9. Anticoagulation therapies for VTE should be continued for a minimum of 3 months. The duration of anticoagulation therapy should be based on the patient's risks of VTE recurrence and major bleeding, and preference regarding continued treatment.

INTRODUCTION

Venous thromboembolism (VTE) is a potentially fatal disorder and a significant health problem in our aging society.[1] Although young, otherwise healthy adults can have VTE, it most frequently occurs in patients who are hospitalized, undergo major surgery, are immobile for a lengthy period of time, or have a hypercoagulable disorder. VTE is manifested as deep vein thrombosis (DVT) and/or pulmonary embolism (PE) and results from clot formation within the venous circulation, most commonly the legs, but clots can also form in the arms, and in the mesenteric and cerebral veins (Fig. 9-1).[1] DVT is rarely fatal, but death from PE can occur within minutes after symptom onset, before effective treatment can be given. Beyond the symptoms produced by the acute event, the complications of VTE, such as the postthrombotic syndrome and chronic thromboembolic pulmonary hypertension (CTPH), also cause substantial disability and suffering.[1]

Anticoagulant drugs used in the prevention and treatment of VTE require precise dosing and meticulous monitoring.[2,3] Systematic approaches to anticoagulant therapy management substantially reduce the risks, but bleeding remains an all too common and serious complication of administering anticoagulant drugs. Consequently, preventing VTE in at-risk patients is paramount to improving outcomes.[4–6] When there is a suspicion of VTE, the rapid and accurate diagnosis of the disorder is critical to making appropriate treatment decisions.[7] The optimal use of anticoagulant drugs requires an in-depth knowledge of their pharmacology and pharmacokinetic properties, and a comprehensive approach to patient management.[2,3]

EPIDEMIOLOGY

The true incidence of VTE in the general population is unknown because a substantial portion of patients have clinically silent disease. The annual incidence of symptomatic objectively diagnosed VTE is estimated at 2 to 3 per 1,000, increasing with age from 0.1 per 1,000 in adolescence to 8 per 1,000 in those over 80 years.[8] The incidence of VTE in specific high-risk patient populations has been extensively studied.[4–6] Patients sustaining multiple traumas or having orthopedic procedures involving the lower extremities are at particularly high risk as are those with a prior history of VTE and/or who have metastatic cancer. Likewise, the incidence of VTE after a myocardial infarction, stroke, and spinal cord injury is high. Several disorders of hypercoagulability have also been linked to a high lifetime incidence of VTE.[4–6]

ETIOLOGY

1 A number of factors increase the risk of developing VTE (Table 9-1). The majority of these risk factors can be easily identified in clinical practice. Stasis of blood favors clotting in part through reduced clearance of activated clotting factors from sites of clot formation.[9] The rate of blood flow in the venous circulation, particularly in the deep veins of the lower extremities, is relatively slow. Contraction of the calf and thigh muscles works with valves in the deep veins of the leg to facilitate the flow of blood back to the heart and lungs; thus, damage to the venous valves and periods of

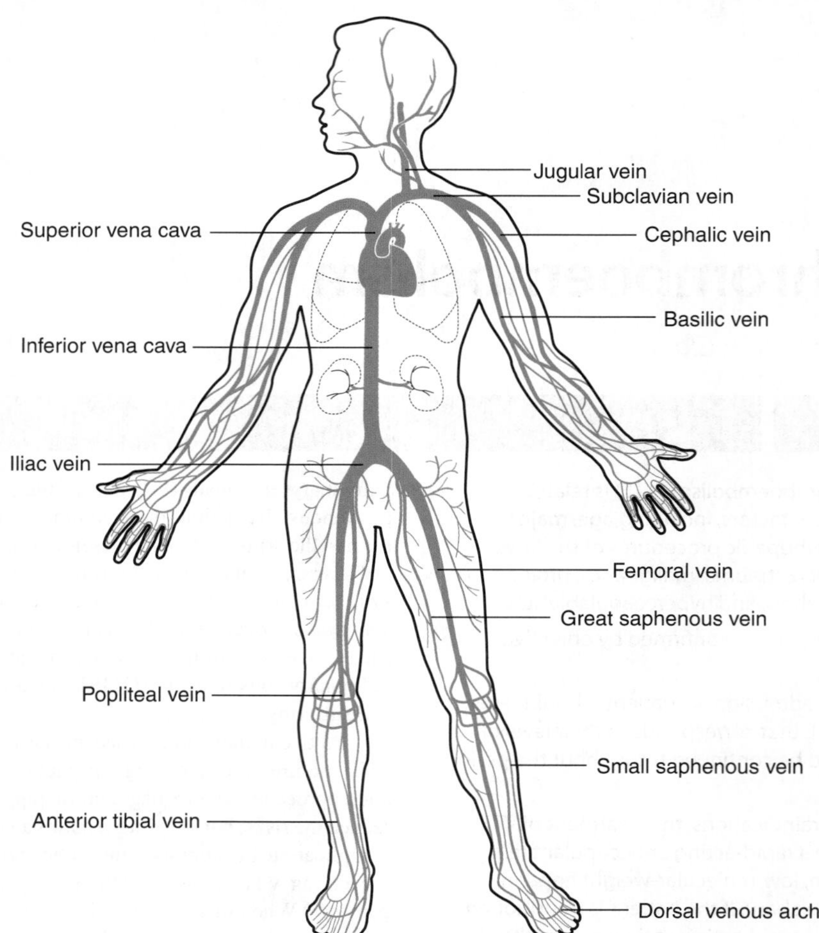

FIGURE 9-1 Venous circulation.

prolonged immobility result in venous stasis.[8] Vessel obstruction, from either external compression or a thrombus, also promotes clot propagation. Reduced venous blood flow explains, at least in part, why numerous medical conditions and surgical procedures are associated with an increased risk of VTE (Table 9-1). Increased blood viscosity, seen in myeloproliferative disorders such as polycythemia vera, may also contribute to thrombus formation.[8]

A growing list of inherited and acquired diseases has been linked to hypercoagulability (see Table 9-1). Activated protein C (aPC) resistance is the most common genetic disorder of hypercoagulability (prevalence rate of 2% to 7% in whites) accounting for many cases of DVT in unselected patients.[10] Most aPC resistance results from a mutation on factor V that renders it resistant to degradation by aPC.[10] This mutation is known as factor V Leiden, named after the city of Leiden, Holland, where the defect was first described. The prothrombin G20210A mutation is the second most frequent genetic risk factor, occurring in about 2% to 4% of whites and imparting about a threefold increased risk of VTE.[10] This mutation increases circulating prothrombin, but the degree of VTE risk does not rise proportionally. Enhanced thrombin generation has been observed, but the mechanism whereby this disorder increases VTE risk is not completely understood.[11] Although the rarity (present in <1% of the population) of inherited deficiencies of the natural anticoagulants protein C, protein S, and antithrombin precludes accurate quantification of their effect on the risk of initial VTE, many experts believe the lifetime risk is high.[12] Conversely, excessively high concentrations of factors VIII, IX, and XI or fibrinogen also increase the risk of VTE.[13] Given the prevalence of these inherited abnormalities in the general population, some patients have multiple genetic defects that have additive effects in terms of increasing the lifetime thrombotic risk.[13]

Acquired disorders of hypercoagulability may result from malignancy, the presence of antiphospholipid antibodies, and estrogen use.[13] The strong link between cancer and thrombosis has long been recognized.[14] Tumor cells secrete a number of procoagulant substances that activate the coagulation cascade. Furthermore, patients with cancer often have suppressed levels of endogenous anticoagulants (protein C, protein S, and antithrombin). It has been postulated that cancer cells use thrombotic mechanisms to recruit a blood supply (angiogenesis), metastasize, and create barriers against host defense mechanisms.[15] Antiphospholipid antibodies are a heterogeneous group of antibodies targeting proteins that bind phospholipids.[11] These include antibodies that prolong phospholipid-based clotting assays, known as lupus anticoagulants, as well as anticardiolipin and β_2-glycoprotein (β_2-gp) I antibodies. Antiphospholipid antibodies are found in up to 5% of normal healthy populations but are more common in patients with autoimmune disorders such as systemic lupus erythematosus and inflammatory bowel disease.[16] Transient and low titers of these antibodies are common and do not present a risk for thrombosis. A diagnosis of antiphospholipid antibody syndrome requires the presence of moderate- or high-titer antibodies or lupus anticoagulants measured at least 12 weeks apart in a patient with a history of arterial or venous thrombosis or recurrent miscarriage.[17] The precise mechanism by which antiphospholipid antibodies provoke thrombosis remains to be definitively determined. Contributing factors include complement activation, inhibition of proteins C and fibrinolysis, platelet activation, and increased tissue factor expression.[16] Estrogen-containing contraception,

TABLE 9-1 Risk Factors for Venous Thromboembolism

Risk Factor	Comments/Examples
Age	Annual incidence increases from 10 per 100,000 in adolescence to 1 per 100 in old age
History of VTE	Strongest known risk factor for recurrence, risk is highest during the first 6 months after VTE
Venous stasis	Acute medical illness requiring hospitalization Surgery (especially general anesthesia >30 minutes) Paralysis (e.g., status post stroke, spinal cord injury) Immobility (e.g., plaster casts, status post stroke or spinal cord injury) Polycythemia vera Obesity Varicose veins
Vascular injury	Major orthopedic surgery (e.g., knee or hip replacement) Trauma (especially fractures of the pelvis, hip, or leg) Indwelling venous catheters
Hypercoagulable states	Malignancy, diagnosed or occult Factor V Leiden Prothrombin (G20210A) gene mutation Protein C deficiency Protein S deficiency Antithrombin deficiency Factor VIII excess (>90th percentile) Factor XI excess (>90th percentile) Antiphospholipid antibodies Lupus anticoagulant Anticardiolipin antibodies Anti–β_2-glycoprotein I antibodies Dysfibrinogenemia Hyperhomocysteinemia Plasminogen activator inhibitor-1 excess Inflammatory bowel disease Nephrotic syndrome Paroxysmal nocturnal hemoglobinuria Pregnancy/postpartum
Drug therapy	Estrogen-containing contraception Estrogen replacement therapy Selective estrogen receptor modulators (e.g., tamoxifen, raloxifene) Cancer therapy Heparin-induced thrombocytopenia

VTE, venous thromboembolism.

From Rosendaal et al.,[18] Kahn et al.,[6] Gould et al.,[5] Falck-Ytter et al.,[4] and Giannakopoulos et al.[16]

estrogen replacement therapy, and the selective estrogen receptor modulators are all linked to venous thrombosis.[18] Estrogens increase serum clotting factor concentrations and induce aPC resistance. Women with underlying hypercoagulability are at particularly high risk of developing venous thrombosis while taking estrogens.[18]

In many cases, VTE is the result of converging combinations of inherited and acquired thrombotic risk factors. Thus, many individuals with congenital hypercoagulable conditions experience a first VTE only after being placed in situations of high risk for thrombosis such as orthopedic surgery, immobilization, the use of estrogen-containing oral contraceptives, or pregnancy.[19]

PATHOPHYSIOLOGY

The arrest of bleeding following vascular injury is an amazingly complex process that is essential to life (Fig. 9-2). In the late 1800s, Dr. Rudolf Virchow, a German pathologist, recognized the role played by blood vessels, circulating elements in the blood, and the speed of blood flow in the regulation of clot formation.[20] As described previously, alterations in any one of these elements, known today as Virchow's triad, may lead to pathologic clot formation. Through the years various descriptive models of blood clot formation have been proposed and continuously refined based on new information and fresh thinking derived from increasingly sophisticated experimental methodology. Still many questions remain and a complete understanding of in vivo thrombus formation remains incomplete.[21]

Hemostasis is the complex process responsible for maintaining the integrity of the pressurized circulatory system following damage to blood vessels.[22] Hemostatic clots remain localized to the vessel wall and do not greatly impair blood flow in the vessel. In contrast, thrombotic clots such as those causing VTE result in impairment of blood flow and even complete occlusion of the vessel. Under normal circumstances, endothelial cells forming the intima of vessels maintain blood flow by physically separating extravascular collagen and tissue factor from platelets and clotting factors (namely, activated factor VII [VIIa]), respectively, thus preventing activation of hemostasis. Vascular injury allows key components of the coagulation process to seal the breach through the interaction of activated platelets recruited to the site of injury and the clotting factor cascade initiated by tissue factor and culminating in the formation of thrombin and ultimately fibrin clot (see Fig. 9-2).[22] In contrast to physiologic hemostasis, pathologic venous thrombosis often occurs in the absence of gross vein wall disruption and may be triggered by circulating microparticles bearing tissue factor rather than the tissue factor expressed in the vessel wall. Venous clots often occur in areas of disturbed blood flow (e.g., valve cusps in the deep veins of the legs) and are mainly composed of fibrin with platelets and trapped red blood cells.[21] Platelet thrombus and fibrin clot formation overlap temporally and occur nearly simultaneously,[21] but are discussed separately below for simplicity.

Platelet Pathway

Platelets become actively involved in thrombus formation via two distinct pathways acting in parallel or separately. In one pathway, exposure of circulating blood to subendothelial collagen following vascular injury initiates platelet activation; in the other pathway platelets are activated by thrombin generated by tissue factor derived from the vessel wall or present in flowing blood.[22] Various adhesion proteins (e.g., von Willebrand factor, fibrinogen) appear to play critical roles in platelet–vessel wall interactions.[21] A platelet thrombus develops as activated platelets recruit unstimulated platelets, some of which are also activated while others remain loosely associated but do not undergo activation and may ultimately break away from the growing thrombus.[22] Activation causes platelet α and dense granules to release their cargo of components such as adenosine diphosphate (ADP) and calcium ions that are critical for sustaining further thrombus formation into the environment surrounding the developing clot.[22] Activated platelets accumulating in the thrombus also express P-selectin, an adhesion molecule that facilitates capture of blood-borne microparticles bearing tissue factor. Accumulation of tissue factor in the platelet thrombus is important as tissue factor is the primary initiator of fibrin clot formation via the coagulation cascade (Fig. 9-3).[22]

Tissue Factor Pathway

The tissue factor pathway triggers coagulation by generating a small (picomolar) amount of thrombin. Before this small amount of thrombin is generated, the tissue factor pathway proceeds inefficiently through factor IX or X because factors VIII and V, the circulating procofactors required in the tenase and prothrombinase complexes, are not yet available in their most active cofactor form (Fig. 9-4). However, once formed, this small amount of thrombin converts factors VIII and V to their active cofactor forms, factors

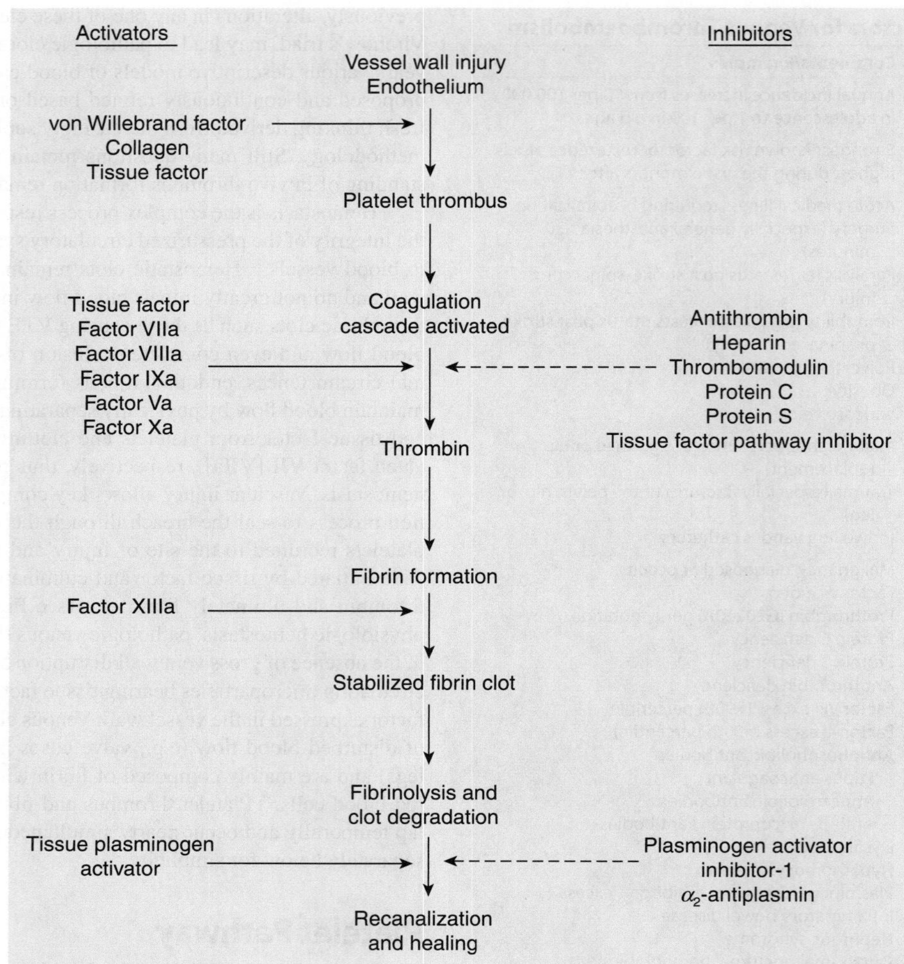

FIGURE 9-2 Overview of hemostasis.

VIIIa and Va, respectively.[22] The tenase and prothrombinase complexes now efficiently proceed to generate a large burst of thrombin. Even though the tissue factor pathway is rapidly downregulated, or inhibited, by the action of tissue factor pathway inhibitor, thrombin generation proceeds without replenishing active tissue factor.[22]

Fibrin Thrombus Formation

The final step in thrombus formation is the thrombin-mediated conversion of fibrinogen to form fibrin monomers. As fibrin monomers reach a critical concentration, they begin to precipitate and polymerize to form fibrin strands. Factor XIIIa, which is also activated by the action of thrombin, covalently bonds these strands to one another (Fig. 9-4) to form an extensive meshwork that surrounds and encases the aggregated platelet thrombus and red blood cells to form a stabilized clot that seals the site of vascular injury and prevents blood loss.[23] Coagulation reactions are eventually terminated when this expanding meshwork of platelets and fibrin "paves over" the initiation site and additional activated factors are unable to diffuse through the overlying layer of clot.[24]

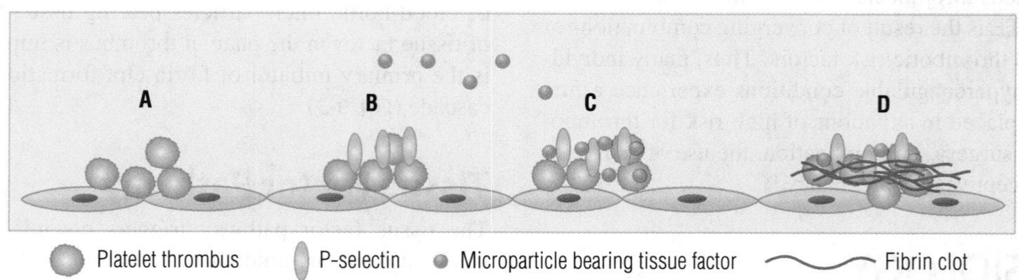

FIGURE 9-3 Model of pathologic thrombus formation: (*A*) activated platelets adhere to vascular endothelium; (*B*) activated platelets express P-selectin; (*C*) pathologic microparticles express active tissue factor and are present at a high concentration in the circulation—these microparticles accumulate, perhaps by binding to activated platelets expressing P-selectin; (*D*) tissue factor can lead to thrombin generation, and thrombin generation leads to platelet thrombus formation and fibrin generation. *(Adapted from Furie and Furie.[22])*

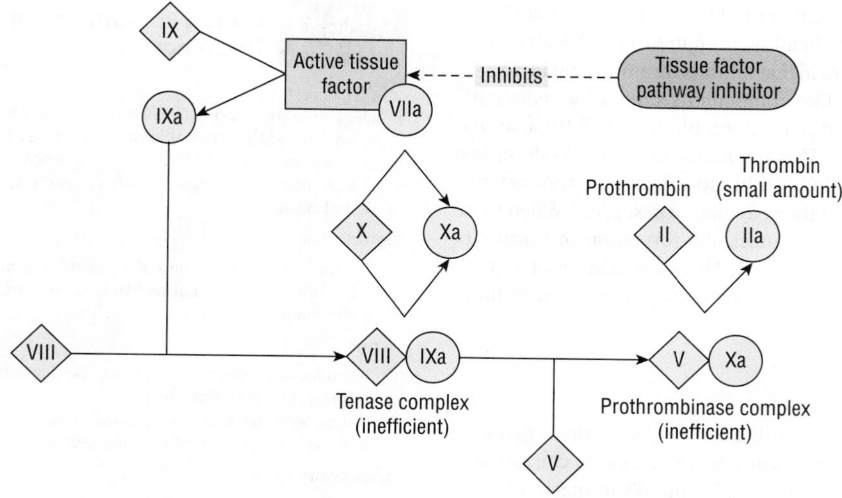

A

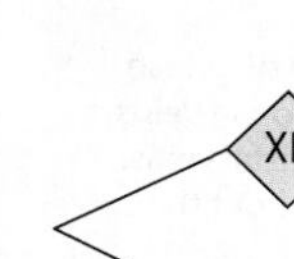

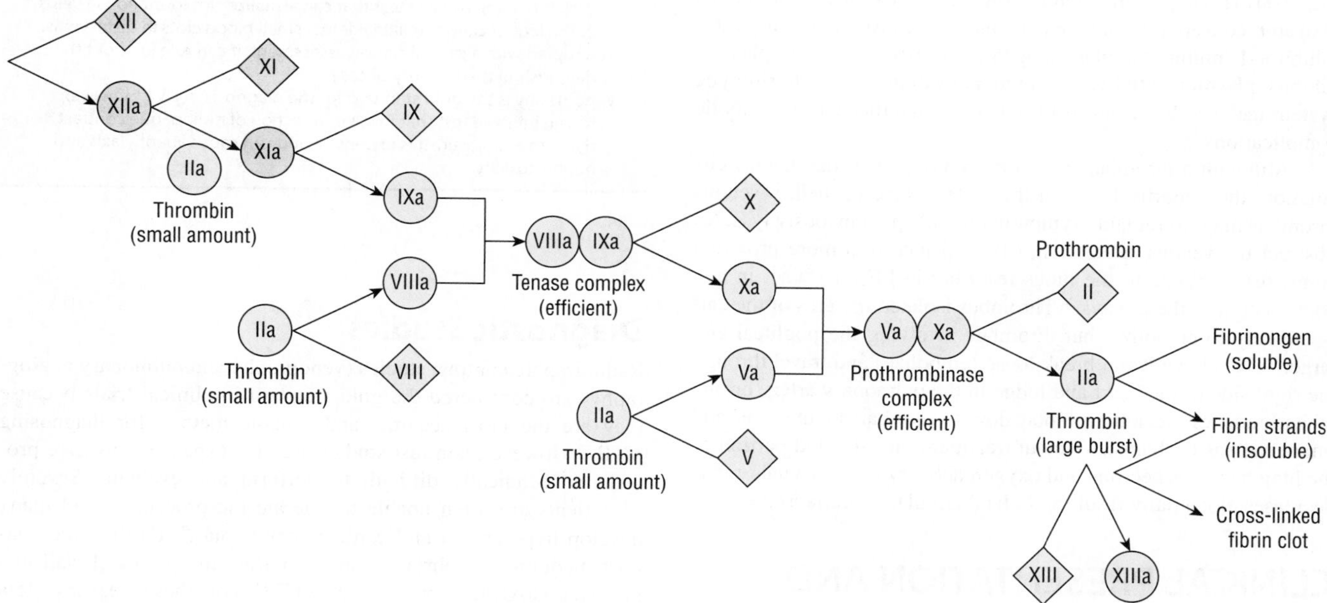

B

FIGURE 9-4 Coagulation cascade: (*A*) During the initiation phase the tissue factor–factor VIIa complex triggers blood coagulation by generating small amounts of thrombin. The tissue factor–factor VIIa complex activates factors IX and X. Factor IXa binds to factor VIII to form a tenase complex that inefficiently activates factor X to form factor Xa. Factor Xa, generated by the tissue factor–factor VIIa complex or the inefficient tenase complex, binds factor V on membrane surfaces to form a prothrombinase complex that inefficiently converts prothrombin to thrombin. The initiation phase is quickly downregulated by tissue factor pathway inhibitor. (*B*) During the amplification phase, the small amount of thrombin generated during initiation activates factors VIII and V, leading to a large burst of thrombin via highly efficient tenase and prothrombinase complexes. Thrombin converts fibrinogen to fibrin that forms strands that ultimately create an intricate web that traps red blood cells, platelets, and other cells to form a fibrin clot. Thrombin also activates factor XIII that cross-links fibrin to form a stabilized clot. *(Adapted from Furie and Furie.[22])*

Endogenous Control of Thrombus Formation

Normally, a number of tempering mechanisms control coagulation (see Fig. 9-2).[24] Without effective self-regulation, the coagulation cascade would continue unabated causing vascular occlusion at the site of injury. The intact endothelium adjacent to the damaged tissue actively secretes several antithrombotic substances.[9] As its name implies, thrombomodulin modulates thrombin activity by converting protein C to its active form (aPC). When joined with its cofactor protein S, aPC enzymatically inactivates factors Va and VIIIa regulating the functionality of the prothrombinase and tenase complexes, respectively.[9] The physiologic role of aPC is to prevent coagulation reactions from spreading to healthy, uninjured vessel walls. Antithrombin is a circulating protein that inhibits thrombin and factor Xa. Heparan sulfate, a heparin-like compound secreted by endothelial cells, exponentially accelerates antithrombin activity.[9] By a similar mechanism, heparin cofactor II also inhibits thrombin. As described previously, tissue factor pathway inhibitor plays an important role by regulating the initiation of the coagulation cascade.[22] When these self-regulatory mechanisms are intact, the formation of fibrin clot is limited to the zone of tissue injury. However, disruptions in the system, previously described hypercoagulable states, often result in pathologic thrombosis.[19]

Fibrinolysis

The fibrinolytic system is responsible for the dissolution of formed blood clots.[25] An inactive proenzyme, plasminogen, is converted to an active enzyme, plasmin, that degrades the fibrin mesh into soluble end products collectively known as fibrin degradation products including D-dimer.[25] The fibrinolytic system is also under the control of a series of stimulatory and inhibitory substances (see Fig. 9-2). Tissue plasminogen activator and urokinase plasminogen activator convert plasminogen to plasmin. Plasminogen activator inhibitor-1 inhibits the plasminogen activators, and α_2-antiplasmin inhibits plasmin activity. Impaired activation of the fibrinolytic system has also been linked to hypercoagulability and thrombotic complications.[25]

Although a thrombus can form in any part of the venous circulation, the majority begin in the leg(s). Once formed, a venous thrombus may (a) remain asymptomatic, (b) spontaneously lyse, (c) obstruct the venous circulation, (d) propagate into more proximal veins, (e) embolize to the lungs resulting in PE, or (f) act in any combination of these ways.[26] Thrombus isolated in veins of the calf is unlikely to embolize, but thrombus involving the popliteal and larger veins above it can break loose (embolize) and travel through the right side of the heart and lodge in the pulmonary artery or one of its branches, occluding blood flow to that part of the lung and impairing gas exchange. Without treatment, the affected portion of the lung becomes necrotic and oxygen delivery to other vital organs decreases, potentially resulting in fatal circulatory collapse.[27]

CLINICAL PRESENTATION AND DIAGNOSIS

Clinical Presentation

2 The symptoms of DVT or PE (Tables 9-2 and 9-3) are nonspecific and objective tests are required to confirm or exclude the diagnosis.[28] Patients with DVT frequently present with unilateral leg pain and swelling. Postthrombotic syndrome, a long-term complication of DVT caused by damage to the venous valves, may also result in chronic lower extremity swelling, pain, tenderness, skin discoloration, and, in the most severe cases, ulceration.[7] PE typically presents with chest pain, shortness of breath, tachypnea, and tachycardia. PE is a life-threatening condition that may result in cardiopulmonary collapse.[29]

Given that VTE can be debilitating or fatal, it is important to treat it quickly and aggressively.[7] Conversely, because major bleeding induced by antithrombotic drugs can be equally harmful, it is important to avoid treatment when the diagnosis is not a reasonable certainty.[28] Assessment of the patient's status should focus on the search for risk factors in the patient's medical history (see Table 9-1). Even in the presence of mild, seemingly inconsequential symptoms, VTE should be strongly suspected in those with multiple risk factors.

TABLE 9-2 Clinical Presentation of Deep Vein Thrombosis

General

Deep vein thrombosis (DVT) most commonly develops in patients with identifiable risk factors (see Table 9-1) during or following a period of acute illness or hospitalization. Many have asymptomatic disease. Patients may die suddenly of pulmonary embolism

Symptoms

The patient may complain of leg swelling, pain, or warmth. Symptoms are nonspecific and objective testing must be performed to establish the diagnosis

Signs

The patient's superficial veins may be dilated and a "palpable cord" may be felt in the affected leg

The patient may experience pain in back of the knee when the examiner dorsiflexes the foot of the affected leg (known as Homan's sign)

Laboratory tests

Serum concentration of D-dimer, a by-product of fibrin degradation, is nearly always elevated

Diagnostic tests

Compression ultrasound is the most commonly used test to diagnose DVT. It is a noninvasive test that can visualize clot formation in veins of the legs. It cannot reliably detect small blood clots in distal veins. Coupled with a careful clinical assessment, it can rule in or out the diagnosis in the majority of cases

Venography is the gold standard for the diagnosis of DVT. However, it is an invasive test that involves injection of radiopaque contrast dye into a foot vein. It is expensive and can cause anaphylaxis and nephrotoxicity

Diagnostic Studies

Radiographic contrast studies (venography and pulmonary angiography) are considered the gold standard in clinical trials because they are the most accurate and reliable method for diagnosing VTE.[28] However, contrast studies are also expensive invasive procedures technically difficult to perform and evaluate. Severely ill patients are often unable to tolerate the procedure, and many develop hypotension and cardiac arrhythmias.[28] Further, the contrast medium is nephrotoxic and irritating to the vessel wall and may paradoxically precipitate VTE.[28] For these reasons, less invasive tests, such as compression ultrasound (CUS), computed tomography (CT) scans, and the ventilation–perfusion (V/Q) scan, are used in clinical practice for the initial evaluation of patients with suspected VTE.

D-Dimer

D-dimer is a degradation product of fibrin clot and levels of D-dimer are usually significantly elevated in patients with acute thrombosis.[28] Although D-dimer is a very sensitive marker of clot formation, it is not sufficiently specific. A variety of conditions are associated with D-dimer elevations, including recent surgery or trauma, pregnancy, increasing age, and cancer; therefore, a positive D-dimer test is not conclusive evidence of VTE diagnosis. A wide variety of D-dimer assays of varying sensitivities for VTE are available. Enzyme-linked immunosorbent assays (ELISAs) and enzyme-linked immunofluorescence assays, along with the latex immunoturbidimetric assays, are generally termed "highly sensitive," whereas the whole blood D-dimer assay is considered "moderately sensitive."[28] Appropriate use of D-dimer should include initial risk stratification via a validated clinical assessment model.[28]

TABLE 9-3 Clinical Presentation of Pulmonary Embolism

General

Pulmonary embolism (PE) most commonly develops in patients with risk factors for venous thromboembolism (see Table 9-1) during or following a hospitalization. Although many patients develop a symptomatic deep vein thrombosis prior to developing a PE, some do not. Patients may die suddenly from cardiogenic shock and circulatory collapse before effective treatment can be initiated

Symptoms

The patient may complain of cough, chest pain, chest tightness, shortness of breath, or palpitation. The patient may spit or cough up blood (hemoptysis). When PE is massive, the patient may complain of dizziness or light-headedness. Symptoms may be confused with myocardial infarction, requiring objective testing to establish the diagnosis

Signs

The patient may have tachypnea (increased respiratory rate) and tachycardia (increased heart rate). The patient may appear diaphoretic (sweaty). The patient's neck veins may be distended. In massive PE, the patient may appear cyanotic and become hypotensive. In such cases, oxygen saturation by pulse oximetry or arterial blood gas will likely indicate that the patient is hypoxic. In the worse cases, the patient may go into cardiogenic shock and die within minutes

Laboratory tests

Serum concentration of D-dimer, a by-product of fibrin degradation, is nearly always elevated

Diagnostic tests

Computerized tomography (CT) scan is the most commonly used test to diagnose PE, but some centers still use the ventilation–perfusion (V/Q) scan. Spiral CT scans can detect emboli in the pulmonary arteries. A V/Q scan measures the distribution of blood and air flow in the lungs. When there is a large mismatch between blood and air flow in one area of the lung, there is a high probability that the patient has a PE

Pulmonary angiography is the gold standard for the diagnosis of PE. However, it is an invasive test that involves injection of radiopaque contrast dye into the pulmonary artery. The test is expensive and associated with a significant risk of mortality

TABLE 9-4 Clinical Assessment Models for Deep Vein Thrombosis and Pulmonary Embolism

Clinical Feature	Score
Pretest probability of deep vein thrombosis[a]	
Tenderness along entire deep vein system	1
Swelling of the entire leg	1
Greater than 3 cm difference in calf circumference	1
Pitting edema	1
Collateral superficial veins	1
Risk factors present	
Active cancer	1
Prolonged immobility or paralysis	1
Recent surgery or major medical illness	1
Alternative diagnosis likely (ruptured Baker's cyst, rheumatoid arthritis, superficial thrombophlebitis, or infective cellulitis)	−2
Pretest probability of pulmonary embolism[b]	
Deep vein thrombosis suspected	
Clinical features of deep vein thrombosis	3
Recent prolonged immobility or surgery	1.5
Active cancer	1
History of deep vein thrombosis or pulmonary embolism	1.5
Hemoptysis	1
Resting heart rate >100 beats/min	1.5
No alternative explanation for acute shortness of breath or chest pain	3

[a]Score: ≥3, high probability; 1–2, moderate probability; ≤0, low probability.
[b]Score: ≥6, high probability; 2–6, moderate probability; ≤1.5, low probability.

From Bauersachs.[30]

Risk Stratification

Clinical assessment significantly improves the diagnostic accuracy of noninvasive tests such as CUS, CT scanning, and D-dimer. Simple assessment checklists can be used to determine if a patient has a high, moderate, or low probability of DVT or PE (Table 9-4).[30] Patients with a high pretest probability of VTE have a greater than 50% chance of having VTE, compared with only 5% of those with low pretest probability.[31] Patients with a low pretest probability of VTE should receive testing with a moderate or highly sensitive D-dimer, if available.[28] If the D-dimer result is normal, VTE is ruled out. Patients with a moderate pretest probability should receive either highly sensitive D-dimer or CUS. CUS may be performed proximally (i.e., above the knee) or throughout the entire leg. A normal full leg ultrasound or highly sensitive D-dimer rules out VTE. A normal proximal ultrasound should be repeated in 1 week or paired with D-dimer testing to rule out VTE. All patients with high pretest probability of VTE should receive either proximal or full leg CUS. A normal full leg ultrasound rules out VTE, whereas a normal proximal ultrasound requires additional testing with highly sensitive D-dimer, full leg ultrasound, or repeat proximal ultrasound surveillance in 1 week.[28] Patients with CUS indicating proximal DVT should receive treatment, regardless of pretest probability. Evidence of calf vein DVT after full leg ultrasound may be managed by anticoagulation or further ultrasound surveillance to assess for propagation into the proximal deep veins of the leg.[7,28]

PREVENTION AND TREATMENT OF VENOUS THROMBOEMBOLISM

General Approach to the Prevention of Venous Thromboembolism

Given that VTE is potentially fatal and costly to treat, strategies to prevent DVT in at-risk populations positively impact patient outcomes.[32] Relying on the early diagnosis and treatment of VTE is unacceptable because some patients will die before treatment can be initiated. Effective prophylaxis can reduce the risk of fatal PE in high-risk surgical and medical populations, whereas early ambulation is often sufficient for those at low risk of VTE.[33] Educational programs and clinical decision support systems have been shown to improve the appropriate use of VTE prevention methods.[34]

3 The most authoritative and well-recognized evidence-based guidelines for the prevention and treatment of VTE are the *Antithrombotic Therapy and Prevention of Thrombosis, 9th ed: Evidence-Based Clinical Practice Guidelines* published by the American College of Chest Physicians (AT9). The AT9 attempt to balance concerns regarding the competing risks of symptomatic VTE and bleeding in their recommendations for thromboprophylaxis.[33] Compared with previous guideline editions, the AT9 have critically evaluated the relevance of surrogate end points, such as venographically detected asymptomatic DVT, and based current recommendations mainly on the risk of symptomatic VTE (Table 9-5).[33] An effective VTE prophylaxis program should identify and determine each patient's level of risk for VTE and bleeding, and select and implement regimens that optimally balance these risks in a cost-effective manner. Several pharmacologic and mechanical methods

TABLE 9-5 Guidelines for the Prevention of Venous Thromboembolism

Medical illness

For acutely ill hospitalized medical patients at increased risk of thrombosis, thromboprophylaxis with low-molecular-weight heparin (LMWH), low-dose unfractionated heparin (LDUH) twice or three times daily, or fondaparinux is recommended (Grade 1B)[a]

For acutely ill hospitalized medical patients at low risk of thrombosis, use of pharmacologic prophylaxis or mechanical prophylaxis is not recommended (Grade 1B)

For acutely ill hospitalized medical patients who are bleeding or at high risk for bleeding, anticoagulant thromboprophylaxis is not recommended (Grade 1B)

For acutely ill hospitalized medical patients at increased risk of thrombosis who are bleeding or at high risk for major bleeding, optimal use of mechanical thromboprophylaxis with graduated compression stockings or intermittent pneumatic compression (IPC) is suggested (Grade 2C). When bleeding risk decreases, and if venous thromboembolism (VTE) risk persists, substitution of pharmacologic thromboprophylaxis for mechanical thromboprophylaxis is suggested (Grade 2B)

In critically ill patients, routine ultrasound screening for deep vein thrombosis (DVT) is not recommended (Grade 2C)

For critically ill patients, thromboprophylaxis with LMWH or LDUH is suggested over no prophylaxis (Grade 2C)

For critically ill patients who are bleeding, or are at high risk for major bleeding, mechanical thromboprophylaxis with graduated compression stockings or IPC is suggested (Grade 2C). When bleeding risk decreases, substitution of pharmacologic thromboprophylaxis for mechanical thromboprophylaxis is suggested (Grade 2C)

In outpatients with cancer who have no additional risk factors for VTE, routine prophylaxis is not recommended with LMWH or LDUH (Grade 2B) or warfarin (Grade 1B)

Routine thromboprophylaxis is not recommended for chronically immobilized persons residing at home or at a nursing home (Grade 2C)

For long-distance travelers at increased risk of VTE (including previous VTE, recent surgery or trauma, active malignancy, pregnancy, estrogen use, advanced age, limited mobility, severe obesity, or known thrombophilia disorder), frequent ambulation, calf muscle exercise, sitting in an aisle seat or below-the-knee graduated compression stockings providing 15–30 mm Hg (2–4 kPa) pressure at the ankle are suggested (Grade 2C)

In persons with thrombophilia but no previous history of VTE, the long-term daily use of mechanical or pharmacologic thromboprophylaxis to prevent VTE is not recommended (Grade 1C)

Surgical populations excluding orthopedics

For general and abdominal–pelvic surgery patients at very low risk for VTE, no specific pharmacologic (Grade 1B) or mechanical (Grade 2C) prophylaxis other than early ambulation is recommended

For patients at low risk of VTE after abdominal–pelvic surgery or cardiac surgery with an uncomplicated course, mechanical prophylaxis, preferably with IPC, over no prophylaxis is suggested (Grade 2C)

For patients at moderate VTE risk after general, abdominal–pelvic, or thoracic surgery, or cardiac surgery with a prolonged course not at high risk for major bleeding complications, LMWH or LDUH (Grade 2B), or mechanical prophylaxis, preferably with IPC (Grade 2C), is suggested over no prophylaxis

For patients at moderate risk for VTE after general, abdominal–pelvic surgery, thoracic surgery, or cardiac surgery who are at high risk for major bleeding complications or those in whom the consequences of bleeding are thought to be particularly severe, mechanical prophylaxis, preferably with IPC, is suggested over no prophylaxis (Grade 2C)

For patients at high risk for VTE after general, abdominal–pelvic, and thoracic surgery who are not at high risk for major bleeding complications, pharmacologic prophylaxis with LMWH (Grade 1B) or LDUH (Grade 1B) is suggested over no prophylaxis. Combination with graduated compression stockings or IPC is also suggested (Grade 2C)

For high-VTE-risk general, abdominal–pelvic, and thoracic surgery patients who are at high risk for major bleeding complications or those in whom the consequences of bleeding are thought to be particularly severe, the use of mechanical prophylaxis, preferably with IPC, is suggested over no prophylaxis until the risk of bleeding diminishes and pharmacologic prophylaxis may be initiated (Grade 2C)

For high-VTE-risk patients undergoing abdominal or pelvic surgery for cancer who are not otherwise at high risk for major bleeding complications, extended-duration pharmacologic prophylaxis (4 weeks) with LMWH is recommended over shorter-duration prophylaxis (Grade 1B)

For general and abdominal–pelvic surgery patients at high risk for VTE in whom both LMWH and LDUH are contraindicated or unavailable and who are not at high risk for major bleeding complications, low-dose aspirin (Grade 2C), fondaparinux (Grade 2C), or mechanical prophylaxis, preferably with IPC (Grade 2C), is suggested over no prophylaxis

For general and abdominal–pelvic surgery patients, an inferior vena cava (IVC) filter is not recommended for primary VTE prevention (Grade 2C)

Orthopedic surgery

In patients undergoing total hip arthroplasty (THA) or total knee arthroplasty (TKA), use of one of the following for a minimum of 10–14 days is recommended: LMWH, fondaparinux, apixaban, dabigatran, rivaroxaban, LDUH, adjusted-dose warfarin, aspirin (all Grade 1B), or IPC (Grade 1C)

In patients undergoing hip fracture surgery (HFS), use of one of the following is recommended: antithrombotic prophylaxis for a minimum of 10–14 days, LMWH, fondaparinux, LDUH, adjusted-dose warfarin, aspirin (all Grade 1B), or IPC (Grade 1C)

For patients undergoing major orthopedic surgery (THA, TKA, HFS) and receiving LMWH as thromboprophylaxis, starting either 12 hours or more preoperatively or 12 hours or more postoperatively is recommended over starting within 4 hours or less preoperatively or 4 hours or less postoperatively (Grade 1B)

In patients undergoing THA, TKA, or HFS, irrespective of the concomitant use of IPC or length of treatment, the use of LMWH is suggested over other recommended alternatives, including fondaparinux, apixaban, dabigatran, rivaroxaban, LDUH (all Grade 2B), adjusted-dose warfarin, or aspirin (all Grade 2C)

For patients undergoing major orthopedic surgery, extending thromboprophylaxis in the outpatient period for up to 35 days from the day of surgery is suggested (Grade 2B)

In patients undergoing major orthopedic surgery, dual prophylaxis with an antithrombotic agent and IPC is suggested during the hospital stay (Grade 2C)

In patients undergoing major orthopedic surgery who decline injections or IPC, apixaban or dabigatran (alternatively rivaroxaban or adjusted-dose warfarin) is recommended over alternative forms of prophylaxis (all Grade 1B)

For primary prevention of VTE after major orthopedic surgery, no thromboprophylaxis is suggested over placement of an IVC filter in patients with an increased bleeding risk or contraindications to both pharmacologic and mechanical thromboprophylaxis (Grade 2C)

The use of screening compression ultrasound in asymptomatic patients following major orthopedic surgery is not recommended (Grade 1B)

No prophylaxis is suggested rather than pharmacologic thromboprophylaxis in patients with isolated lower leg injuries requiring leg immobilization (Grade 2C)

For patients undergoing knee arthroscopy without a history of prior VTE, no thromboprophylaxis is suggested (Grade 2B)

[a]Recommendations are graded as strong (Grade 1) or weak (Grade 2) based on high-quality (Grade A), moderate-quality (Grade B), or weak-quality (Grade C) evidence.

From Kahn et al.,[6] Gould et al.,[5] and Falck-Ytter et al.[4]

are effective for preventing VTE, and these can be used alone or in combination.[4–6] Mechanical methods improve venous blood flow, whereas drug therapy inhibits clotting factor activity or production. Despite ongoing efforts to minimize hospital-acquired VTE, up to one third of hospitalized patients at high risk of VTE without contraindications to anticoagulant therapy still do not receive appropriate prophylaxis.[35]

Clinical **Controversy...**

In the United States interest in VTE prevention peaked after the 2008 decision by the Centers for Medicare and Medicaid Services to withhold a portion of reimbursement to hospitals for patients in whom VTE complicated hip or knee replacement surgery. These so-called "never events" proved controversial because VTE occurs even among carefully selected populations receiving adequate prophylaxis in clinical trials, and many orthopedic surgeons believe overzealous use of anticoagulants increases the risk for postoperative bleeding complications.[36]

General Approach to the Treatment of Venous Thromboembolism

❹ Anticoagulation therapies remain the mainstay of treatment for VTE. DVT and PE are manifestations of the same disease process and are treated similarly.[7] Before prescribing a full course of anticoagulation therapy for the treatment of VTE, it is imperative to establish an accurate diagnosis, thus preventing unnecessary risk of bleeding and expense to the patient (Fig. 9-5).[7] Patients with high probability of VTE may need parenteral anticoagulation therapy while awaiting the results of diagnostic testing, whereas patients with intermediate probability may need parenteral anticoagulation only if diagnostic testing will be delayed more than 4 hours.[7] The acute phase of VTE treatment (~7 days) requires rapidly acting anticoagulants such as unfractionated heparin (UFH), low-molecular-weight heparin (LMWH), fondaparinux, or rivaroxaban to prevent thrombus extension and embolization. The early maintenance phase (7 days to 3 months) consists of continued therapeutic anticoagulation aimed at reducing the risk of long-term sequelae such as the postthrombotic syndrome and CTPH by allowing formed clot to be slowly dissolved by endogenous thrombolytic processes. Anticoagulation therapy extending beyond 3 months is aimed at long-term secondary prevention of recurrent VTE.[1,7] Anticoagulation therapy is usually initiated with an injectable anticoagulant and then transitioned to warfarin maintenance therapy (Table 9-6 and Fig. 9-5). A simpler single-drug approach using orally administered rivaroxaban has now been shown to be noninferior to this standard approach for VTE treatment for appropriately selected patients.[37,38]

Determining the optimal duration of anticoagulation involves weighing the risk of recurrent VTE against the risk of bleeding associated with anticoagulation therapy and determining patient preference regarding treatment duration (see Evaluation of Therapeutic Outcomes below). When bleeding risk outweighs VTE recurrence risk or if the informed patient's preference is to stop treatment, anticoagulation therapy should be discontinued.[7] In life- or limb-threatening circumstances, elimination of the obstructing thrombus may be warranted and the use of thrombolysis or thrombectomy can be considered.[7] Insertion of a removable filter in the inferior vena cava (IVC) is also an option in those with contraindications to anticoagulation therapy or in whom anticoagulant therapy has failed.[7]

❺ Once the diagnosis of VTE has been objectively confirmed (see Clinical Presentation and Diagnosis above), anticoagulant therapy with UFH, LMWH, fondaparinux, or rivaroxaban should be instituted as soon as possible. Evidence indicates that currently available injectable anticoagulants can be administered in the outpatient setting in most patients with DVT and in carefully selected hemodynamically stable patients with PE (see Table 9-6).[1] The decision to initiate therapy on an outpatient basis should be based on institutional resources and patient-specific variables (Table 9-7).[39]

NONPHARMACOLOGIC THERAPY

Mechanical Prevention and Treatment Strategies

Graduated compression stockings and intermittent pneumatic compression (IPC) devices improve venous blood flow and reduce the risk of VTE. These methods do not increase the risk of bleeding, which makes them attractive for postoperative VTE prophylaxis. However, they are not risk free as skin breakdown and ulceration can occur.[6]

Graduated compression stockings have failed to reliably demonstrate a reduction in VTE in medically ill patients.[6] However, they reduce the incidence of VTE (including asymptomatic and distal DVT) by approximately 65% when used after orthopedic surgery, cardiac surgery, gynecologic surgery, or neurosurgery.[5] Compression stockings work by increasing the velocity of venous blood flow through the application of graded pressure, with the greatest amount applied at the ankle. This treatment option is inexpensive and safe, and an excellent choice when pharmacologic intervention is either contraindicated or difficult to adequately monitor.[6] When combined with pharmacologic interventions, graduated compression stockings have an additive effect. However, they can be uncomfortable and some patients are unable to wear them because of the size or shape of their legs and adverse skin reactions.[6]

IPC devices utilize sequential inflation of a series of cuffs wrapped around the patient's legs to increase the velocity of blood flow.[6] The cuffs use graded pressure and inflate in 1- to 2-minute continuous cycles from the ankles to the thighs. IPC reduces the risk of VTE by more than 60% following general surgery, neurosurgery, and orthopedic surgery.[5] Although IPC is well tolerated and safe to use in patients who have contraindications to pharmacologic therapies, it does have drawbacks. There is some theoretical concern that external compression may dislodge a previously formed clot, IPC is more expensive and cumbersome to use than graduated compression stockings, and some patients have difficulty sleeping and getting in and out of bed while wearing the devices.[4] For optimal effectiveness, IPCs should be worn at least 18 hours/day. Battery-operated units facilitate mobility and monitoring. Like graduated compression stockings, IPCs can be used in combination with pharmacologic strategies.[4]

IVC filters can provide short-term protection against PE in very-high-risk patients by blocking embolization of thrombus formed below the filter.[5] Percutaneous insertion of an IVC filter is a minimally invasive procedure performed using fluoroscopic imaging to verify placement. Despite the widespread use of IVC filters, only limited data support effectiveness and long-term safety in the setting of VTE prevention. Nonrandomized data suggest IVC filters reduce the short-term risk of PE but are associated with complications including DVT, filter migration, IVC occlusion, and insertion site thrombosis.[5] IVC filters should be reserved for patients at highest risk for VTE in whom other prophylactic strategies cannot be used.

IVC filters also have a limited role in the management of acute VTE when anticoagulants are ineffective or unsafe, including in (a) patients with an absolute contraindication to anticoagulation therapy because of active bleeding or anticipated bleeding from a

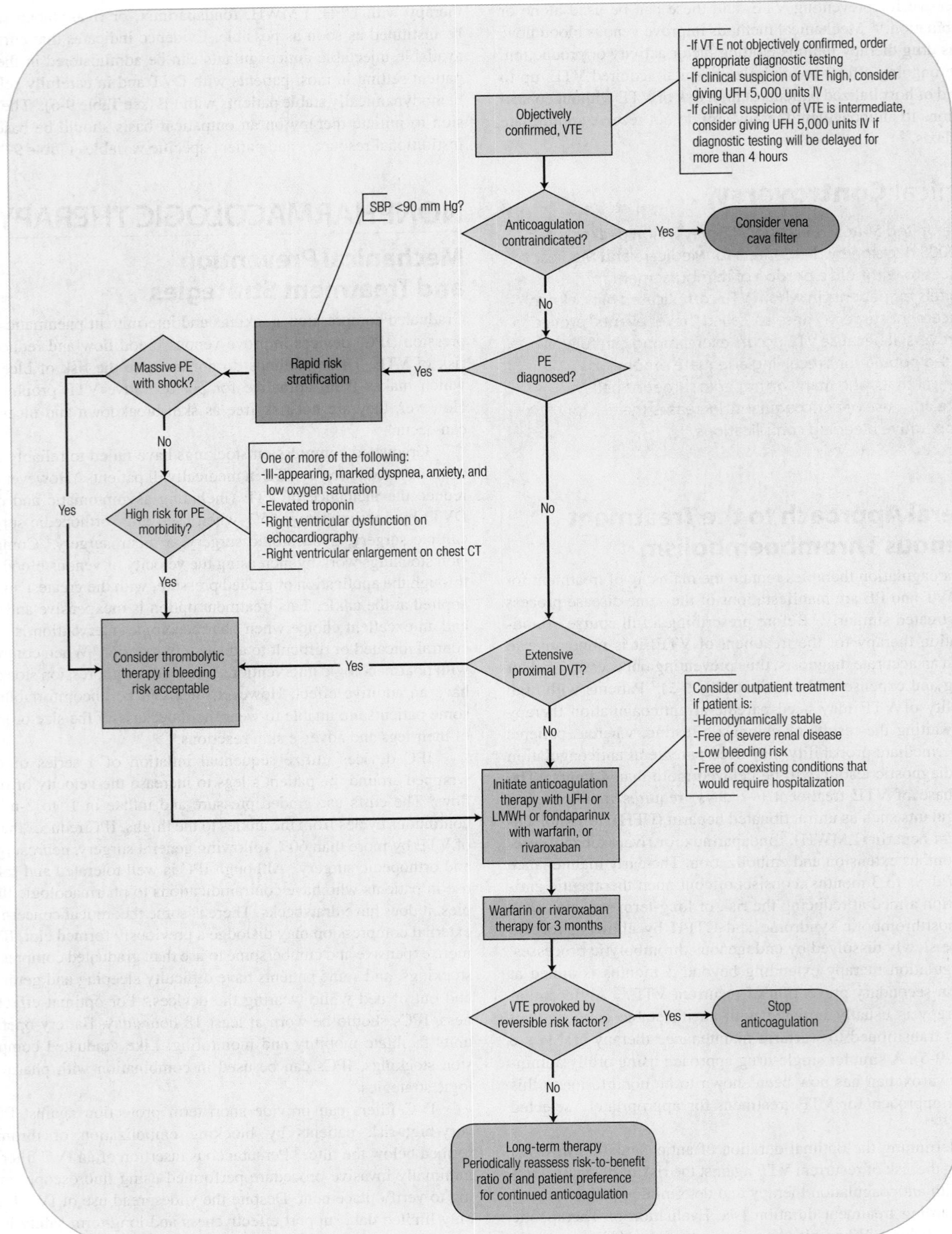

FIGURE 9-5 Treatment of venous thromboembolism (VTE). (DVT, deep vein thrombosis; LMWH, low-molecular-weight heparin; PE, pulmonary embolism; SBP, systolic blood pressure; UFH, unfractionated heparin.)

TABLE 9-6 Guidelines for the Treatment of Venous Thromboembolism

Deep vein thrombosis (DVT) and pulmonary embolism (PE)

In patients with acute DVT of the leg or PE treated with warfarin therapy, initial treatment with LMWH, fondaparinux, IV UFH, or SC UFH is recommended (Grade 1B)[a]

In patients with acute DVT of the leg or PE, early initiation of warfarin (e.g., same day as parenteral therapy is started) over delayed initiation, and continuation of parenteral anticoagulation for a minimum of 5 days and until the international normalized ratio (INR) is 2 or above for at least 24 hours are recommended (Grade 1B)

In patients with acute DVT of the leg or PE, LMWH or fondaparinux is suggested over IV UFH (Grade 2C [2B for fondaparinux in PE]) and over SC UFH (Grade 2B for LMWH; Grade 2C for fondaparinux)

In patients with proximal DVT of the leg or PE provoked by surgery, treatment with anticoagulation for 3 months is recommended over treatment of a shorter period (Grade 1B), treatment of a longer time-limited period (e.g., 6 or 12 months) (Grade 1B), or extended therapy (Grade 1B regardless of bleeding risk)

In patients with proximal DVT of the leg or PE provoked by a nonsurgical transient risk factor, treatment with anticoagulation for 3 months is recommended over treatment of a shorter period (Grade 1B), treatment of a longer time-limited period (e.g., 6 or 12 months) (Grade 1B), and extended therapy if there is a high bleeding risk (Grade 1B); anticoagulation for 3 months is suggested over extended therapy if there is a low or moderate bleeding risk (Grade 2B)

In patients with a first unprovoked DVT of the leg or PE, treatment with anticoagulation for at least 3 months is recommended over treatment of a shorter duration (Grade 1B); after 3 months of treatment, the risk-to-benefit ratio of extended therapy should be evaluated; for patients with low or moderate bleeding risk, extended anticoagulant therapy is suggested over 3 months of therapy (Grade 2B); for patients with high bleeding risk, 3 months of anticoagulant therapy is recommended over extended therapy (Grade 1B)

In patients with recurrent unprovoked VTE, extended anticoagulant therapy is recommended over 3 months of therapy in those with low bleeding risk (Grade 1B), and suggested in those with moderate bleeding risk (Grade 2B); in patients with high bleeding risk, 3 months of therapy is suggested over extended therapy (Grade 2B)

In all patients who receive extended anticoagulant therapy, the continuing use of treatment should be reassessed at periodic intervals (e.g., annually)

In patients with DVT of the leg or PE who are treated with warfarin, a therapeutic INR range of 2–3 (target INR of 2.5) is recommended for all treatment durations (Grade 1B)

In patients with DVT of the leg or PE and no cancer, warfarin therapy is suggested over LMWH for long-term therapy (Grade 2C); for patients with DVT or PE and no cancer who are not treated with warfarin therapy, LMWH is suggested over dabigatran or rivaroxaban for long-term therapy (Grade 2C)

In patients with DVT of the leg or PE and cancer, LMWH is suggested over warfarin therapy (Grade 2B); in patients with DVT or PE and cancer who are not treated with LMWH, warfarin is suggested over dabigatran or rivaroxaban for long-term therapy (Grade 2B)

In patients with DVT of the leg or PE who receive extended therapy, treatment with the same anticoagulant chosen for the first 3 months is suggested (Grade 2C)

In patients with acute DVT of the leg or PE, the use of an inferior vena cava (IVC) filter in addition to anticoagulants is not recommended (Grade 1B) unless anticoagulation therapy is contraindicated (Grade 1B); a conventional course of anticoagulant therapy is suggested if the risk of bleeding resolves (Grade 2B)

In patients who are incidentally found to have asymptomatic DVT of the leg or PE, the same initial and long-term anticoagulation as for comparable patients with symptomatic DVT of PE is suggested (Grade 2B)

DVT specific

In patients with acute DVT of the leg and whose home circumstances are adequate, initial treatment at home is recommended over treatment in hospital (Grade 1B)

In patients with acute DVT of the leg, early ambulation is suggested over initial bedrest (Grade 2C)

In patients with acute symptomatic DVT of the leg, the use of graduated compression stockings is suggested to reduce the risk of postthrombotic syndrome (Grade 2B)

PE specific

In patients with low-risk PE and whose home circumstances are adequate, early discharge is suggested over standard discharge (e.g., after first 5 days of treatment) (Grade 2B)

In patients with acute PE associated with hypotension (e.g., systolic BP <90 mm Hg) who do not have a high bleeding risk, systemically administered thrombolytic therapy is suggested (Grade 2C)

In selected patients with acute PE not associated with hypotension and with a low bleeding risk whose initial clinical presentation, or clinical course after starting anticoagulant therapy, suggests a high risk of developing hypotension, administration of thrombolytic therapy is suggested (Grade 2C)

In patients with acute PE, when a thrombolytic agent is used, short infusion times (e.g., a 2-hour infusion) are suggested over prolonged infusion times (e.g., a 24-hour infusion) (Grade 2C); thrombolytic administration through a peripheral vein is suggested over a pulmonary artery catheter (Grade 2C)

In patients with acute PE associated with hypotension and who have contraindications to thrombolysis, failed thrombolysis, or shock that is likely to cause death before systemic thrombolysis can take effect (e.g., within hours), catheter-assisted thrombus removal is suggested over no such intervention if appropriate expertise and resources are available (Grade 2C); surgical pulmonary embolectomy is suggested over no such intervention if catheter-assisted embolectomy fails provided surgical expertise and resources are available (Grade 2C)

In patients with chronic thromboembolic pulmonary hypertension (CTPH), extended anticoagulation is recommended over stopping therapy (Grade 1B); in selected patients with CTPH, such as those with central disease under the care of an experienced thromboendarterectomy team, pulmonary thromboendarterectomy is suggested (Grade 2C)

Upper extremity DVT

In patients with acute upper extremity DVT (UEDVT) involving the axillary or more proximal veins, acute treatment with parenteral anticoagulation (LMWH, fondaparinux, IV UFH, or SC UFH) is recommended over no such acute treatment (Grade 1B); LMWH or fondaparinux is suggested over IV UFH (Grade 2C) and over SC UFH (Grade 2B); anticoagulant therapy alone is suggested over thrombolysis (Grade 2C)

In patients with UEDVT who undergo thrombolysis, the same intensity and duration of anticoagulant therapy as in similar patients who do not undergo thrombolysis is recommended (Grade 1B)

In most patients with UEDVT associated with a central venous catheter, not removing the catheter is suggested if it is functional and there is an ongoing need for the catheter (Grade 2C)

In patients with UEDVT involving the axillary or more proximal veins, a minimum duration of anticoagulation of 3 months is suggested over a shorter period (Grade 2B); in patients who have UEDVT that is not associated with a central venous catheter or with cancer, 3 months of anticoagulation is recommended over a longer duration of therapy (Grade 1B); in patients who have UEDVT that is associated with a central venous catheter that is not removed, anticoagulation that continues as long as the central venous catheter remains is recommended over stopping after 3 months of treatment in patients with cancer (Grade 1C), and is suggested in patients with no cancer (Grade 2C)

[a]Recommendations are graded as strong (Grade 1) or weak (Grade 2) based on high-quality (Grade A), moderate-quality (Grade B), or weak-quality (Grade C) evidence.

From Kearon et al.[7]

TABLE 9-7 Outpatient Treatment Protocol for Deep Venous Thrombosis

Target population	Inclusion/exclusion criteria for outpatient venous thromboembolism (VTE) treatment
Inclusion	Patients with objectively diagnosed VTE
Relative exclusion	Patients with clinical evidence of pulmonary embolus or suspected embolism who are hemodynamically stable
Exclusion	Arterial thromboembolism or patients who are currently receiving dialysis, actively bleeding, have had recent (within 2 weeks) major surgery/trauma, or have other severe uncompensated comorbid conditions

Recommended procedure: may vary depending on the patient's clinical condition

A. Confirm diagnosis of VTE by objective testing
  1. Venous ultrasonogram
  2. Ventilation–perfusion (V/Q) scan
  3. Computed tomography (CT) scan

B. Day 1
  1. Baseline laboratory evaluation
    a. Prothrombin time (PT) and calculated international normalized ratio (INR)
    b. Activated partial thromboplastin time (aPTT)
    c. Serum creatinine (Scr)
    d. Complete blood count (CBC) with platelets
  2. Medication
    a. Low-molecular-weight heparin (LMWH) or fondaparinux injections
      i. Enoxaparin 1 mg/kg subcutaneously (SC) q 12 h or
      ii. Enoxaparin 1.5 mg/kg SC q 24 h (not recommended for patients with cancer or for obese patients)
      iii. Dalteparin 100 units/kg SC q 12 h or
      iv. Dalteparin 200 units/kg SC q 24 h or
      v. Tinzaparin 175 units/kg SC q 24 h or
      vi. Fondaparinux 7.5 mg SC q 24 h (5 mg if <50 kg and 10 mg if >100 kg)
    b. Warfarin sodium 5–10 mg orally every evening
    c. Pain medication if necessary (avoid nonsteroidal antiinflammatory drugs [NSAIDs])
  3. Patient education
    a. Clinical pharmacy/nursing
      i. Educate patient regarding the importance of proper monitoring of anticoagulation therapy and indications for additional medical evaluation; document activities in the medical record
      ii. Teach patient how to self-administer LMWH/fondaparinux (if patient or family member unwilling or unable to self-administer injection, visiting nurse services should be arranged); initial injection should be administered in the medical office or hospital
      iii. Instruct patient regarding local therapy: elevation of affected extremity, localized heat, antiembolic exercises (flexion–extension of ankle for lower extremity VTE, or hand squeezing–relaxation for upper extremity VTE)
    b. Pharmacy operations
      i. Provide backup for clinical pharmacy/nursing; reinforce patient education regarding indication, use, monitoring, side effects, and drug interactions with antithrombotic therapy
      ii. Repackage LMWH syringes (if indicated) in patient-specific doses and dispense 5–7 days of therapy
      iii. Screen patient's pharmacy profile for potential drug–drug interactions with anticoagulation therapy
    c. Anticoagulation service enrollment

C. Day 2
  1. Laboratory evaluation: not required on day 2 of therapy
  2. Medications: continue LMWH/fondaparinux and warfarin as directed
  3. Anticoagulation service
    a. Contact patient and evaluate for symptoms of pulmonary embolism (PE), clot extension, and/or bleeding
    b. Arrange for visiting nursing service if family or family member is having difficulty with outpatient therapy
    c. Continue reduced activity as long as pain persists (when possible, elevate extremity); increase activity as tolerated
    d. Document activities in medical record

D. Day 3
  1. Laboratory evaluation: check INR
  2. Medications: continue LMWH/fondaparinux and warfarin directed
  3. Anticoagulation service
    a. Contact patient and evaluate for symptoms of PE, clot extension, and/or bleeding
    b. Interpret results of INR and adjust dose of warfarin to achieve a target INR of 2.5
    c. Patient activity: continue reduced activity as long as pain persists (when possible, elevate extremity); increase activity as tolerated
    d. Document activities in medical record

E. Day 4
  1. Laboratory evaluation: check INR
  2. Medications: continue LMWH/fondaparinux and warfarin as directed
  3. Anticoagulation service
    a. Contact patient and evaluate for symptoms of PE, clot extensions, and/or bleeding
    b. Interpret results of INR and adjust dose of warfarin to achieve a target INR of 2.5
    c. Patient activity: no restrictions; if pain increases, contact anticoagulation service or provider
    d. Document activities in medical record

F. Day 5
  1. Laboratory evaluation: check INR and CBC with platelets
  2. Medications: continue LMWH/fondaparinux if indicated and warfarin as directed
  3. Anticoagulation service
    a. Contact patient and evaluate for symptoms of PE, clot extension, and/or bleeding
    b. Interpret results of INR and adjust dose of warfarin to achieve a target INR of 2.5
    c. Patient activity: no restriction; if pain increases, contact primary care provider
    d. Document activities in medical record

preexisting lesion; (b) patients with massive PE who survive but in whom recurrent embolism might be fatal; (c) patients who have recurrent VTE despite adequate anticoagulation therapy; and (d) demonstration of large free-floating clot loosely attached to the wall of the IVC.[40] IVC filters reduce the risk of PE in the short term, but also appear to increase the long-term risk for recurrent DVT presumably as a consequence of the accumulation of thrombus on the filter, which may partially occlude the vena cava, resulting in venous stasis.[40] Retrievable filters that can be removed after the period of greatest risk for PE or after a transient bleeding risk has resolved have been developed and suggested for use in patients with transient contraindications to anticoagulation therapy. In reality most (65% in one report) "retrievable" filters are not removed.[40] When an IVC filter is inserted as an alternative to anticoagulation, the AT9 suggest a conventional course of anticoagulant therapy once the risk of bleeding resolves.[7]

Ancillary Therapy

In addition to anticoagulant therapy for patients with proximal DVT, wearing graduated compression stockings can reduce the risk of developing the postthrombotic syndrome by 50%.[7] To be effective, graduated compression stockings must fit properly and provide adequate pressure at the ankle (30 to 40 mm Hg; 4 to 5.3 kPa).[7] Discomfort and unflattering appearance are barriers to adherence with compression stockings, particularly during the hot summer months. However, consistent daily use should be encouraged for at least 2 years after DVT or longer if symptoms of postthrombotic syndrome persist.[7]

Strict bedrest was traditionally recommended following acute DVT based on the assumption that leg movement would dislodge the clot, resulting in PE. However, ambulation in conjunction with graduated compression stockings results in faster reduction in pain and swelling with no apparent increase in the rate of embolization. Early ambulation and continued high activity level also reduce the likelihood of postthrombotic syndrome.[7] Patients should be encouraged to ambulate as much as their symptoms permit. If pain and swelling increase with ambulation, the patient should be instructed to lie down and elevate the affected leg until symptoms subside.

PHARMACOLOGIC STRATEGIES FOR VTE PREVENTION

Pharmacologic options for preventing VTE have been extensively evaluated in randomized clinical trials (see Table 9-5). Appropriately selected drug therapies can significantly reduce the incidence of VTE following hip and knee replacement, hip fracture repair, general surgery, myocardial infarction, ischemic stroke, and in appropriately selected hospitalized medical patients.[4–6] The optimal agent and dose to use for VTE prevention must be based on the patient's level of risk for thrombosis and bleeding complications, as well as cost and availability.

Medical Patients

Several risk assessment models have been developed to identify hospitalized and critically ill patients at high risk of VTE who would realize the greatest benefit from thromboprophylaxis. The Padua Prediction Score is a prospectively validated VTE risk assessment tool for hospitalized medical patients.[6] For this tool, 3 points each are assigned for active cancer, previous VTE, reduced mobility, and thrombophilia; 2 points are assigned for trauma and/or surgery within the last month; and 1 point each is assigned for age ≥70 years, heart and/or respiratory failure, acute myocardial infarction or ischemic stroke, acute infection and/or rheumatologic disorder, body mass index ≥30 kg/m^2, or ongoing hormonal treatment. Among high-risk patients (score ≥4 points) not receiving prophylaxis, VTE occurred in 11% within 90 days compared with just 0.3% of low-risk patients.[6]

Recommendations for preventing VTE during medical illness are summarized in Table 9-5. Compared with placebo, low-dose unfractionated heparin (LDUH), LMWH, and fondaparinux all reduce the risk of symptomatic VTE and fatal PE among high-risk medical patients.[6] Hospitalized and acutely ill medical patients at high risk of VTE and low risk of bleeding should receive pharmacologic prophylaxis with LDUH, LMWH, or fondaparinux for the duration of hospitalization or until fully ambulatory. Routine use of pharmacologic prophylaxis is not warranted in low-VTE-risk populations. In medical patients at high risk of bleeding who also require VTE prophylaxis, mechanical prophylaxis may be preferred over anticoagulation therapy.[6] The AT9 guidelines suggest that mechanical prophylaxis may be preferred in patients with any of the following bleeding risk factors: active gastric or duodenal ulcer, history of bleeding within 90 days, or platelet count <50 × 10^9/L.[6] Mechanical prophylaxis should also be considered if more than one of the following are present: Age 85 years or more, hepatic failure, renal failure (creatinine clearance <30 mL/min), admission to intensive care or cardiac care units, central venous catheter, rheumatic disease, active cancer, or male sex.[6]

Nonorthopedic Surgery Patients

Patient risk for VTE after general surgery can be estimated using the Caprini score.[5] This extensive risk assessment tool awards 1, 2, 3, or 5 points to patient-specific risk factors (e.g., age, BMI, VTE history) and procedure-related risk factors including minor or major surgery, laparoscopic or open procedures, and elective arthroplasty. Once all risk factor points are summed, VTE risk is categorized as very low (0 to 1 point), low (2 points), moderate (3 to 4 points), or high (≥5 points).[5] Estimating bleeding risk associated with surgery is challenging due to wide variety of surgery types, the effect of surgical technique, and the lack of a validated clinical predication rule. Table 9-5 summarizes the AT9 recommendation for preventing VTE following nonorthopedic surgery. In general, patients at high risk of VTE but at low risk of bleeding should receive prophylaxis with LDUH or LMWH in addition to graduated compression stockings or IPC. Patients at high risk of bleeding should receive IPC if the risk of VTE is moderate or high.[5]

Orthopedic Surgery

Total joint arthroplasty is associated with a very high risk of postoperative VTE. Recommended pharmacologic agents for the prevention of VTE following joint replacement surgery include aspirin, adjusted-dose warfarin, UFH, LMWH, fondaparinux, dabigatran, apixaban, and rivaroxaban for a minimum duration of 10 days postsurgery.[4] Head-to-head trials of these agents fail to reliably demonstrate differences in clinically relevant outcomes such as symptomatic VTE, fatal PE, major hemorrhage, and surgical site complications.[4] The endorsement of aspirin for VTE prevention in the AT9 is a major departure from previous guidelines that actually recommended against aspirin use in this setting.[4,41] The change in recommendation reflects recognition by AT9 panelists that previous recommendations did not reflect actual clinical practice due to overreliance on surrogate end points such as asymptomatic DVT detected via screening venography.[33]

The AT9 cite extensive clinical experience and similar or superior properties compared with other pharmacologic options as reasons for suggesting LMWH as preferred over other agents after total joint arthroplasty despite a lack of convincing evidence of superior efficacy or safety compared with older, less costly agents.[4] The risk of bleeding associated with LMWH use following orthopedic surgery relates closely to the timing of thromboprophylaxis initiation. Administration of LMWH within 2 hours preoperatively or postoperatively increases the risk of bleeding up to fivefold compared with starting 12 hours after surgery.[4]

Warfarin remains among the most commonly prescribed agents for VTE prevention after total joint arthroplasty offering some advantages over LMWH, including low acquisition cost and oral administration.[42] Warfarin's delayed onset of anticoagulant effect confers both a potential advantage (reduced immediate risk of postoperative bleeding) and a disadvantage (increased risk of early VTE). Previous American College of Chest Physician's guidelines recommended a goal international normalized ratio (INR) range of 2 to 3 following orthopedic surgery while American Academy of Orthopaedic Surgery (AAOS) guidelines recommended an INR target of 2 or "one which appropriately balances the risk of PE and bleeding."[41,43] The AT9 now simply recommend "dose-adjusted warfarin" without specific guidance on target INR, and the AAOS guidelines also no longer recommend a specific INR target.[4,43] Many orthopedic surgeons prefer low-intensity warfarin (e.g., INR 1.5 to 2.5) due to perceived lower risk of postoperative bleeding.[42] Regardless of INR target, warfarin use following orthopedic surgery requires a well-coordinated monitoring system and timely INR testing.[44] Arranging INR testing for patients following joint replacement surgery can be challenging due to limited patient mobility often requiring arrangement of home phlebotomy or use of point-of-care INR monitoring devices that erodes the cost advantage of warfarin.

Rivaroxaban, apixaban, and dabigatran offer the convenience of oral administration and fixed dosing without the need for routine coagulation testing. Clinical trials of these agents have demonstrated safety and efficacy similar to enoxaparin after total joint replacement, but they have not been studied after hip fracture surgery.[4] The AT9 express a preference for apixaban or dabigatran (alternatively warfarin or rivaroxaban) in patients unwilling to use injections of LMWH, but neither dabigatran nor apixaban is FDA approved for VTE prevention after total joint arthroplasty.[4] Postmarketing studies are needed to provide real-world context in a variety of patient populations to the favorable results of initial clinical trials for these new anticoagulants.

Duration of Therapy

The optimal duration of VTE prophylaxis following surgery is not well established.[41] Prophylaxis should be given throughout the period of increased VTE risk. For general surgical procedures and medical conditions, once the patient is able to ambulate regularly and other risk factors are no longer present, prophylaxis can be discontinued.[5,6] Because of the relatively high incidence of VTE in the first month following hospital discharge among patients who have undergone a lower extremity orthopedic procedure, extended prophylaxis following hospital discharge appears to be beneficial.[4] Most clinical trials support the use of antithrombotic therapy for 21 to 35 days following total hip replacement and hip fracture repair surgeries.[4]

Pharmacoeconomic Considerations in VTE Prevention

The acquisition costs of graduated compression stockings, UFH, and warfarin are considerably less than those of LMWH, fondaparinux, rivaroxaban, and dabigatran. However, the drug acquisition cost is relatively small when compared with the overall cost of care.[32] Economic analyses must take into account therapeutic efficacy, duration of use, complications, and monitoring costs.[45]

The determination of the cost-effectiveness of VTE prophylaxis is based on the premise that a reduction in future VTE events will reduce overall healthcare costs.[32] The cost of providing VTE prophylaxis for 1,000 patients declines as the incidence of VTE in a given population increases. Compared with no prophylaxis, prophylaxis with UFH or LMWH in immobilized medically ill patients appears to be cost-effective, with incremental costs ranging from \$65 to \$2,534 per quality-adjusted life-year.[6] Studies of nonorthopedic surgical populations suggest that use of graduated compression stockings, IPCs, LMWH, and LDUH is more cost-effective than no prophylaxis.[5] Pharmacologic prophylaxis in high-risk surgical and orthopedic populations is likely to be cost-effective compared with no prophylaxis given the high risk for postoperative VTE. In this population a systematic review showed that fondaparinux was more cost-effective than LMWH, and that warfarin and LMWH were similarly cost-effective.[46] The availability of generic enoxaparin may alter these findings. Extended prophylaxis is cost-effective after total hip arthroplasty, but the results of cost analysis after total knee arthroplasty are inconclusive.[46]

PHARMACOLOGIC STRATEGIES FOR VTE TREATMENT

Unfractionated Heparin

The parenteral administration of UFH is preferred for acute VTE treatment in patients with severe renal insufficiency (creatinine clearance <30 mL/min [<0.5 mL/s]).[7] UFH may be administered subcutaneously (SC) with or without coagulation monitoring or by continuous IV infusion (see Table 9-8). Because the anticoagulant response to UFH is highly variable, it is standard practice to adjust the dose based on the results of coagulation tests. When UFH is administered by IV infusion, the activated partial thromboplastin time (aPTT) is generally used to monitor the anticoagulant effect, although aPTT response varies between laboratories using different reagents and instruments and methods for improving interlaboratory agreement (e.g., standardization of aPTT ratios by reference to anti-Xa levels) have had limited success.[3] For these reasons, the therapeutic aPTT range at each institution should be adapted to the responsiveness of the reagent and instrument used.[3] Either weight-based dosing (see Table 9-8) or fixed dosing (e.g., 5,000 unit bolus

TABLE 9-8 Weight-Based[a] Dosing for Unfractionated Heparin Administered by Continuous IV Infusion

Indication	Initial Loading Dose	Initial Infusion Rate
Deep venous thrombosis/ pulmonary embolism	80–100 units/kg Maximum = 10,000 units	17–20 units/kg/h Maximum = 2,300 units/h
Activated Partial Thromboplastin Time (seconds)	**Maintenance Infusion Rate** *Dose Adjustment*	
<37 (or anti–factor Xa <0.20 unit/mL [<0.20 kU/L])	80 units/kg bolus, and then increase infusion by 4 units/kg/h	
37–47 (or anti–factor Xa 0.20–0.29 unit/mL [0.20–0.29 kU/L])	40 units/kg bolus, and then increase infusion by 2 units/kg/h	
48–71 (or anti–factor Xa 0.30–0.70 unit/mL [0.30–0.70 kU/L])	No change	
72–93 (or anti–factor Xa 0.71–1 unit/mL [0.71–1 kU/L])	Decrease infusion by 1–2 units/kg/h	
>93 (or anti–factor Xa >1 unit/mL [>1 kU/L])	Hold infusion for 1 hour, and then decrease by 3 units/kg/h	

[a]Use actual body weight for all calculations. Adjusted body weight may be used for obese patients (>130% of ideal body weight).

Adapted from Garcia et al.[3]

followed by 1,000 units/h continuous infusion) of UFH produces similar clinical outcomes.[44] However, failure to give a sufficient IV UFH dose has been shown to increase the risk of VTE recurrence not only during initial treatment but also during long-term therapy.[3] IV UFH requires hospitalization with frequent aPTT monitoring and dose adjustment. Inpatient anticoagulation management services have been shown to improve patient care by increasing the proportion of aPTT values in the therapeutic range, reducing the length of hospital stay, and lowering total hospital costs when compared with usual care.[47] However, some patients still fail to achieve an adequate response to UFH therapy.[3] Consequently, traditional IV UFH in the acute treatment of VTE has largely been replaced by LMWH or fondaparinux. However, as clearance of LMWH, fondaparinux, and the new oral anticoagulants is dependent in some degree on renal function, UFH will continue to have a role for acute VTE treatment in patients with creatinine clearance <30 mL/min (<0.5 mL/s).[7]

If a sufficient dose of UFH is administered SC, aPTT-guided dose titration may be unnecessary. Weight-based LMWH compared with weight-based UFH (initial dose 333 units/kg SC followed by 250 units/kg twice daily) without coagulation monitoring for the treatment of acute VTE revealed no difference in recurrent VTE, major bleeding, or death during followup. Both groups received warfarin therapy overlapped for at least 5 days and continued after LMWH or UFH was discontinued.[48] UFH administered in this manner may be a less costly option for treatment of acute VTE in appropriately selected patients. For patients weighing more than 80 kg, injection volume may be problematic.

Low-Molecular-Weight Heparin

Because of improved pharmacokinetic and pharmacodynamic profiles as well as ease of use, the LMWHs have largely replaced UFH for the treatment of VTE. LMWH given SC in fixed, weight-based doses (see Table 9-9) is at least as effective as UFH given IV for the treatment of VTE.[3] There appears to be similar efficacy and safety with inpatient or outpatient LMWH administration, once- or twice-daily dosing regimens, and use of different LMWH preparations. A preference for once-daily LMWH administration is suggested by the AT9, provided the once-daily regimen uses the same daily LMWH dose as the twice-daily regimen (i.e., the once-daily injection contains double the dose of each twice-daily injection).[7]

Given the predictable response and the reduced need for laboratory monitoring with LMWH, stable patients with DVT who have normal vital signs, low bleeding risk, and no other comorbid conditions requiring hospitalization can be discharged early or treated entirely on an outpatient basis (see Table 9-7).[7] In one survey, 91% of patients who received outpatient DVT treatment indicated a high degree of satisfaction.[39]

Patients presenting with PE and no evidence of hemodynamic instability are at low risk of subsequent morbidity and mortality. Evidence suggests that patients with submassive PE who are hemodynamically stable can be managed safely as outpatients with LMWH or fondaparinux.[1,7] However, hemodynamically unstable patients with PE should generally be admitted for anticoagulation therapy initiation. Rapidly reversible UFH is preferred if thrombolytic therapy or embolectomy is anticipated.[49]

TABLE 9-9 FDA-Approved Venous Thromboembolism Indications and Doses for Low-Molecular-Weight Heparins

Indications	Enoxaparin	Dalteparin	Tinzaparin
Hip replacement surgery (prophylaxis)	30 mg SC q 12 h initiated 12–24 hours after surgery *Or* 40 mg SC q 24 h initiated 12 hours prior to surgery Extended prophylaxis may be given for up to 3 weeks	Postoperative start: 2,500 units SC given 4–8 hours after surgery, and then 5,000 international units SC q 24 h *Or* Preoperative start (evening before surgery): 5,000 units SC 10–14 hours before surgery, then 5,000 units given 4–8 hours after surgery, and then 5,000 units SC q 24 h *Or* Preoperative start (day of surgery): 2,500 units SC within 2 hours of surgery, then 2,500 units given 4–8 hours after surgery, and then 5,000 units SC q 24 h	
Knee replacement surgery (prophylaxis)	30 mg SC q 12 h initiated 12–24 hours after surgery		
Abdominal surgery (prophylaxis)	40 mg SC q 24 h initiated 2 hours prior to surgery	2,500 units SC q 24 h initiated 1–2 hours prior to surgery Patients with malignancy: 5,000 units SC the evening prior to surgery, and then 5,000 units SC q 24 h *Or* 2,500 units SC 1–2 hours prior to surgery, and then 2,500 units 12 hours after surgery followed by 5,000 units SC q 24 h	
Acute medical illness (prophylaxis)	40 mg SC q 24 h	5,000 units SC q 24 h	
Deep vein thrombosis treatment (with or without pulmonary embolism)	1 mg/kg SC q 12 h *Or* 1.5 mg/kg SC q 24 h		175 units/kg SC q 24 h
Venous thromboembolism treatment in patients with cancer		200 units/kg SC q 24 h for 30 days, followed by 150 units SC q 24 h (total daily dose should not exceed 18,000 units)	

TABLE 9-10 Patient Education for Outpatient Venous Thromboembolism Therapy

General information regarding VTE and the goals of treatment
- Anticoagulant medications (injections and warfarin tablets) have been prescribed to prevent your blood clot from growing larger so that the body can begin to dissolve the clot
- Your body may be able to completely dissolve the clot, but in some cases the clot never goes completely away; even with adequate anticoagulation therapy, some people will have chronic pain and swelling in the affected limb; people who have had one clot are at increased risk of having future clots
- Warfarin tablets take several days to begin to work; LMWH or fondaparinux injections work right away, so at first LMWH or fondaparinux injections and warfarin tablets are used together
- When the warfarin has become effective, you will be able to stop the LMWH or fondaparinux injections; you will continue to take warfarin tablets for 3 months or longer to prevent blood clots from returning
- It is important for you to administer your LMWH or fondaparinux and warfarin exactly as directed

Subcutaneous injection technique
- You must learn to give yourself an injection of LMWH or fondaparinux under the skin; alternatively, you may have a family member or visiting nurse give it to you
- If your LMWH or fondaparinux syringes were filled by the manufacturer, they can be stored at room temperature; if your syringes were filled by the pharmacy, they should be stored in the refrigerator; if you were instructed to fill your own syringes, you should prepare the syringe immediately prior to injecting its contents
- If you see a bubble in the syringe, do not try to get it out; you may accidentally squirt out part of your dose
- Choose an injection site on your abdomen; clean the area with alcohol, and then position an uncapped syringe at a 90° angle; pinch the skin, stick the needle in as far as it will go, and gently but firmly push the plunger down; this will inject the medicine into the skin; when all the medication has been injected, remove the needle and dispose of it in an appropriate container
- You will likely experience a burning sensation when the medication is injected; this will go away after a few minutes
- Rotate injection sites from side to side; do not inject into the same site more than once; avoid the area around your navel; do not inject into any bruises

Blood test monitoring
- Regular blood tests are required to make sure your medication is working properly
- The prothrombin time tells how quickly your blood forms a clot; it is used to tell how well warfarin is working
- The INR is a way to standardize the prothrombin time between laboratories; your goal INR range is between 2 and 3; if your INR is less than 2, you are at higher risk for clotting; if your INR is greater than 3, you are at higher risk for bleeding; your dose of warfarin will be adjusted based on the results of this test
- You need to have a complete blood count test both before you begin therapy and after you have been on LMWH or fondaparinux for about 5 days; this will help detect internal bleeding and the occurrence of a rare side effect of heparin therapy that can decrease an element of your blood called platelets

Warfarin information
- Each strength of warfarin has a unique color; each time you refill your prescription, make sure your new tablets are the same color as the ones you have been taking; if not, ask your pharmacist why
- Warfarin should be taken at approximately the same time each day
- The most common and serious side effect of warfarin is bleeding; you should be careful to avoid situations or activities that increase your risk of injury; apply direct pressure to control bleeding from superficial cuts
- Warfarin has many drug interactions; always check with your provider before taking any new medications (including nonprescription medications and dietary supplements)
- Foods rich in vitamin K (green leafy vegetables, etc.) may interfere with warfarin; do not avoid foods rich in vitamin K, but try to maintain consistent dietary habits
- Alcohol can increase your risk for bleeding and interfere with warfarin therapy; drink alcohol in moderation (one to two drinks per day); avoid binge drinking

Contact your provider if you experience
- Persistent bleeding from a cut or scrape
- Blood in your urine
- Blood in your stool
- Persistent nose bleeding
- Increased swelling or pain in your affected extremity

Go to the emergency department if you experience
- Shortness of breath
- Chest pain
- Coughing up blood
- Black tarry-appearing stool
- Severe headache of sudden onset
- Slurred speech

INR, international normalized ratio; LMWH, low-molecular-weight heparin.

Not all patients are appropriate candidates for outpatient VTE treatment. At a minimum, patients must be reliable or have adequate caregiver support and be willing and active participants in the outpatient management of VTE.[39] Table 9-10 summarizes important aspects of patient education for outpatient VTE treatment. Patients who are unable to manage or who decline home treatment should be admitted to the hospital. These patients may subsequently opt for early discharge on LMWH. Daily patient contact either in person or via telephone is essential to identify potential complications and to address questions and concerns promptly. During daily contacts patients must be asked about symptoms that may indicate bleeding, thrombus extension, and PE.[39] Once acute treatment with LMWH has been transitioned to long-term warfarin therapy (usually after about 5 to 10 days) and the warfarin dose stabilizes, patient contacts can occur less frequently.

Fondaparinux

Fondaparinux has been shown to be a safe and effective alternative to LMWH for the treatment of acute VTE.[7] It is dosed once daily via weight-based SC injection as follows: 5 mg if <50 kg, 7.5 mg if 50 to 100 kg, and 10 mg if >100 kg.[50] Compared with weight-based LMWH dosing, this flexible dosing scheme may be particularly useful with very obese patients. Careful attention should be paid to renal function when fondaparinux is used to treat VTE as the drug is contraindicated if creatinine clearance is <30 mL/min (<0.5 mL/s).[50]

Warfarin

Warfarin monotherapy is an unacceptable choice for the acute treatment of VTE because it does not produce a rapid anticoagulation effect and is associated with high incidence of recurrent thromboembolism.

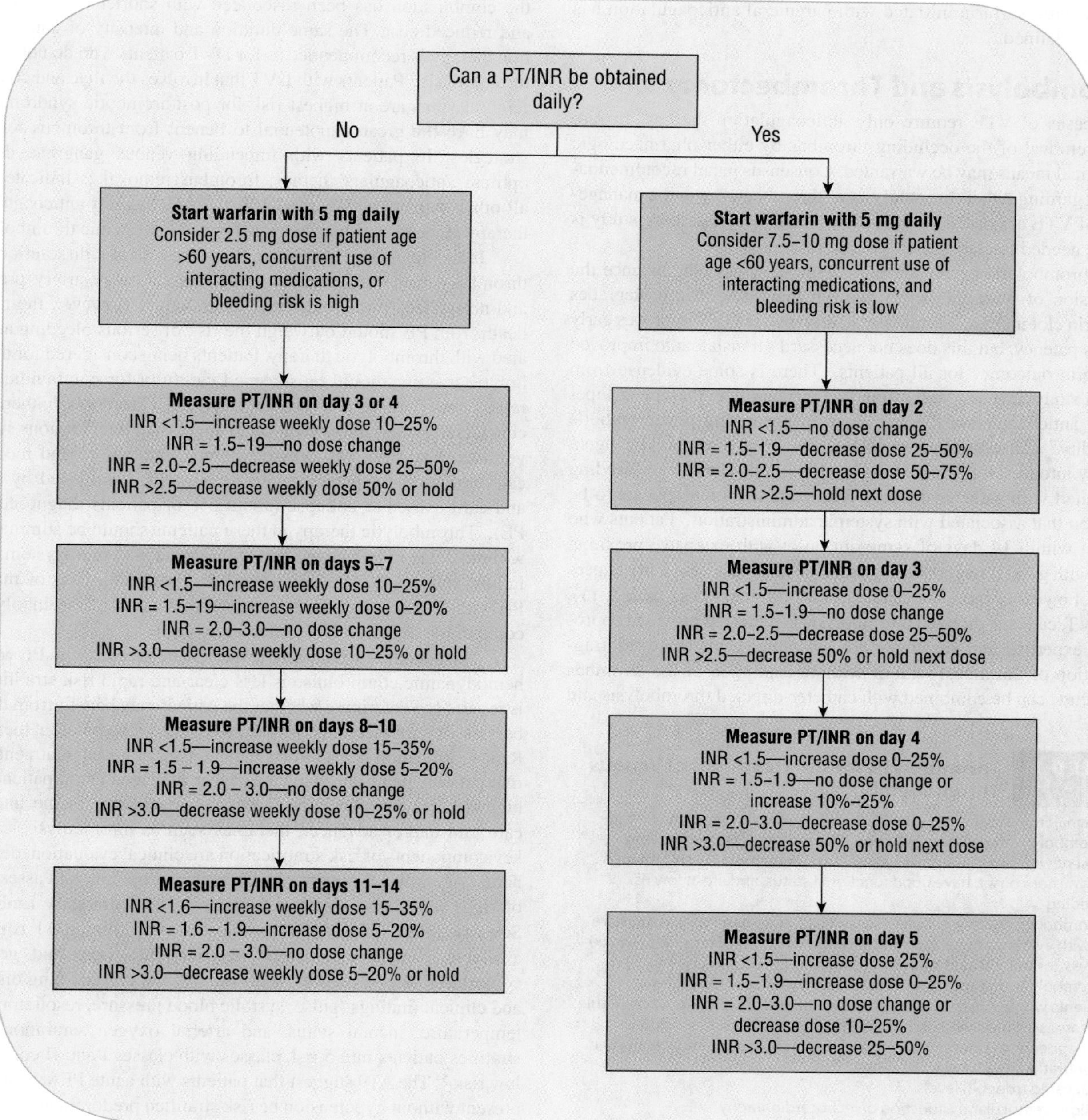

FIGURE 9-6 Initiation of warfarin therapy. (INR, international normalized ratio; PT, prothrombin time.)

However, warfarin is very effective in the long-term management of VTE and should be started concurrently with rapid-acting injectable anticoagulant therapy.[7] The rapid-acting injectable anticoagulant should overlap with warfarin therapy for at least 5 days and until an INR ≥2 has been achieved for at least 24 hours.[7] The initial dose of warfarin should be 5 to 10 mg for most patients (see Fig. 9-6) and periodically adjusted to achieve and maintain an INR between 2 and 3. For patients sufficiently healthy to be treated as outpatients, the AT9 suggest initiating warfarin therapy with 10 mg daily for the first 2 days followed by dosing based on INR measurements rather than starting with the estimated daily maintenance dose.[44]

Pharmacoeconomic Considerations in VTE Treatment

Hospitalization is the main cost driver in the management of VTE. Although the drug acquisition costs for the LMWHs and fondaparinux are substantially higher than those for UFH, avoiding hospitalization dramatically decreases the overall costs of DVT treatment.[51] Cost-effectiveness analyses using decision modeling suggest that the treatment of DVT with LMWHs is more cost-effective than the treatment with UFH in both inpatient and outpatient settings.[52] Based on this decision model, LMWH will reduce overall healthcare cost if as few as 8% of patients are treated entirely on an outpatients basis or 13% of patients are discharged from hospital early.

Despite the substantial cost savings stemming from outpatient DVT treatment from the perspective of the insurer, the reality is that some patients are unable to afford LMWH or fondaparinux prescriptions. Fixed-dose UFH as described previously may provide a lower-cost option for the outpatient treatment of VTE for selected patients who otherwise might not have been able to afford it.[48] A generic formulation of enoxaparin is now available in the United States. The cost-effectiveness of rivaroxaban or dabigatran (discussed below) compared with that of standard anticoagulation therapy with warfarin initiated with parenteral anticoagulation has yet to be defined.

Thrombolysis and Thrombectomy

Most cases of VTE require only anticoagulation therapy. In rare cases removal of the occluding thrombus by either pharmacologic or surgical means may be warranted. Consensus panel recommendations regarding either thrombolysis or thrombectomy in the management of VTE are based on low-quality evidence, and more study is clearly needed to clarify their precise role.[7]

Thrombolytic agents are proteolytic enzymes that enhance the conversion of plasminogen to plasmin that subsequently degrades the fibrin clot matrix.[7] Thrombolytic therapy for DVT improves early venous patency, but this does not necessarily translate into improved long-term outcomes for all patients.[7] There is some evidence from pooled study analyses suggesting that thrombolytic therapy is superior to anticoagulation therapy alone in preventing postthrombotic morbidity.[7] Catheter-directed instillation of a thrombolytic agent directly into the clot is increasingly being used. The risk of bleeding associated with catheter-directed drug administration appears to be less than that associated with systemic administration.[7] Patients who present within 14 days of symptom onset with extensive proximal DVT, with good functional status, low bleeding risk, and a life expectancy of a year or more are candidates for thrombolysis (Table 9-11). For DVT, catheter-directed thrombolysis is preferred provided appropriate expertise and resources are available. Catheter-based fragmentation of thrombus, with or without aspiration of the thrombus fragments, can be combined with catheter-directed thrombolysis and the combination has been associated with shorter treatment times and reduced cost. The same duration and intensity of anticoagulation therapy is recommended as for DVT patients who do not receive thrombolysis.[7] Patients with DVT that involves the iliac and common femoral veins are at highest risk for postthrombotic syndrome and may have the greatest potential to benefit from thrombus removal strategies. In patients with impending venous gangrene despite optimal anticoagulant therapy, thrombus removal is indicated; for all other patients with acute DVT, the AT9 suggest anticoagulation therapy alone over either catheter-directed or systemic thrombolysis.[7]

In the management of acute PE successful clot dissolution with thrombolytic therapy reduces elevated pulmonary artery pressure and normalizes right ventricular dysfunction. However, the risk of death from PE should outweigh the risk of serious bleeding associated with thrombolytic therapy. Patients being considered for thrombolytic therapy should be screened carefully for contraindications relating to bleeding risk (see Table 9-11).[7] Thrombolytic therapy is considered necessary in addition to aggressive interventions such as volume expansion, vasopressor therapy, intubation, and mechanical ventilation for patients with massive PE manifested by shock and cardiovascular collapse (about 5% of patients diagnosed with PE).[7] Thrombolytic therapy in these patients should be administered without delay to reduce the risk of progression to multisystem organ failure and death. While lifesaving in the acute phase of massive PE with hypotension, the hemodynamic benefit of thrombolysis is comparable to that of UFH after a few days.[53]

The benefit of thrombolytic therapy in patients with PE without hemodynamic compromise is less clear and rapid risk stratification is required to determine whether the patient may benefit from thrombolysis or embolectomy in addition to anticoagulation therapy.[49] Risk stratification helps inform the intensity of initial treatment, low-risk patients being discharged early or managed as outpatients and high-risk patients receiving intensive surveillance in the intensive care unit and/or advanced therapies such as thrombolysis.[54] Three key components of risk stratification are clinical evaluation, determination of cardiac biomarker levels such as troponin, and assessment of right ventricular size and function.[7] The Pulmonary Embolism Severity Index (PESI) is a prognostic tool utilizing 11 routinely available clinical parameters: demographics (age and gender), comorbid illnesses (cancer, heart failure, and chronic lung disease), and clinical findings (pulse, systolic blood pressure, respiratory rate, temperature, mental status, and arterial oxygen saturation), that stratifies patients into 5 risk classes with classes I and II considered low risk.[54] The AT9 suggest that patients with acute PE who initially present without hypotension be risk stratified predominantly by clinical signs indicating instability including a decrease in systolic blood pressure that still remains >90 mm Hg, tachycardia, elevated jugular venous pressure, clinical evidence of poor tissue perfusion, hypoxemia, and failure to improve on anticoagulant therapy.[7] Patients with one or more of these clinical features are at high risk for PE-related morbidity and mortality and may benefit from thrombolytic therapy, provided bleeding risk is acceptable, even in the absence of hemodynamic compromise (see Table 9-11).[7] The optimal role of thrombolysis in the management of PE requires further study.

In rare circumstances surgical thrombectomy for extensive ileofemoral DVT may be necessary, but catheter-directed thrombolysis is preferred if bleeding risk is acceptable.[7] For treatment of acute PE, catheter-based embolectomy might be particularly suitable for patients who have contraindications to thrombolytic therapy, have failed thrombolytic therapy, or in whom death is likely before onset of thrombolysis. In the absence of contraindications, catheter-based embolectomy in PE is usually combined with thrombolytic therapy unless bleeding risk is high.[7] Surgical embolectomy is reserved for massive PE and hemodynamic instability when thrombolysis is contraindicated and for when thrombolysis has failed clinically or will not have sufficient time to take effect.[7] In cases of chronic PE—where

TABLE 9-11 Thrombolysis for the Treatment of Venous Thromboembolism

- The majority of patients with VTE do not require thrombolytic therapy
- Thrombolytic therapy for DVT should be reserved for patients who present with extensive proximal DVT (e.g., ileofemoral) within 14 days of symptom onset, have good functional status, and are at low risk of bleeding
- Thrombolytic therapy should be administered to patients with massive PE with evidence of hemodynamic compromise (hypotension or shock) unless contraindicated by bleeding risk
- Thrombolytic therapy should be considered for selected high-risk patients without hypotension provided the risk of bleeding is acceptable
- Factors associated with high risk for adverse PE outcomes include:
  - Ill-appearing patients with marked dyspnea, anxiety, and low oxygen saturation
  - Elevated troponin levels
  - Right ventricular dysfunction on echocardiography
  - Right ventricular enlargement on chest CT
- Factors that increase the risk of bleeding must be evaluated before thrombolytic therapy is initiated (i.e., recent surgery, trauma or internal bleeding, uncontrolled hypertension, recent stroke or intracranial hemorrhage)
- Baseline labs should include CBC and blood typing in case transfusion is needed
- Alteplase 100 mg infused via peripheral vein over 2 hours is the most commonly used thrombolytic for patients with PE
- Before thrombolytic therapy for PE, IV UFH should be administered in full therapeutic doses
- During thrombolytic therapy it is acceptable to either continue or suspend IV UFH (suspending UFH is the most common practice in the United States)
- aPTT should be measured following the completion of thrombolytic therapy
  - If aPTT is <80 seconds, UFH infusion should be started and adjusted to maintain aPTT in therapeutic range
  - If aPTT is >80 seconds, measure every 2–4 hours and start UFH infusion when aPTT is <80 seconds
- Avoid phlebotomy, arterial puncture, and other invasive procedures during thrombolytic therapy to minimize the risk of bleeding

aPTT, activated partial thromboplastin time; CBC, complete blood cell count; DVT, deep vein thrombosis; PE, pulmonary embolism; UFH, unfractionated heparin.

From Kearon et al.[7] and Goldhaber.[49]

persistent emboli produce CTPH, hypoxemia, and right-sided heart failure—surgical pulmonary thromboendarterectomy offers greater benefit than anticoagulants and may be the treatment of choice if performed by an experienced surgical team. A permanent IVC filter is usually inserted before or during the procedure and these patients need long-term warfarin therapy targeted to an INR of 2 to 3.[7]

Alternative Drug Treatments

Rivaroxaban

6 A randomized, open-label, controlled noninferiority trial has demonstrated that oral rivaroxaban alone is noninferior to traditional therapy with warfarin (targeted INR 2 to 3) overlapped with enoxaparin at initiation for both acute DVT and PE with similar rates of recurrent VTE and clinically relevant bleeding.[37,38] Bleeding meeting the prespecified definition of major was lower with rivaroxaban in the PE trial, but not in the DVT trial. Rivaroxaban was administered in a fixed dose of 15 mg twice daily for 3 weeks followed by 20 mg once daily for at least 3 months without routine coagulation monitoring. Patients with creatinine clearance <30 mL/min (<0.5 mL/s) or cancer and those requiring thrombolytic therapy were excluded from study participation and should probably not be treated with rivaroxaban until additional information is available. Replacing the effective but cumbersome combination of LMWH or fondaparinux and warfarin with a single-drug regimen holds promise for simplifying the treatment of VTE; however, the higher acquisition cost of rivaroxaban and lack of an effective reversal agent will be of concern to some patients and clinicians.

Clinical **Controversy...**

Results of recent randomized clinical trials in patients with acute VTE indicate that initiation of anticoagulation with a single oral anticoagulant, rivaroxaban that does not require routine therapeutic monitoring, produced efficacy and safety outcomes that were noninferior to standard therapy.[37,38] These findings highlight the potential of rivaroxaban to greatly simplify the management of VTE. The lack of a reliable rivaroxaban reversal agent and limited experience managing rivaroxaban-associated bleeding will be concerning to some clinicians and patients. The cost-effectiveness of rivaroxaban for treatment of venous thrombosis also remains to be defined and assessing outcomes outside of carefully controlled clinical trials in real-world patient populations is needed.

Dabigatran

Oral dabigatran 150 mg twice daily was compared with warfarin (targeted INR 2 to 3) in a randomized, double-blind, noninferiority trial involving patients with acute VTE.[55] Both treatment groups were initially given parenteral anticoagulation therapy (UFH or LMWH). The primary outcome was the 6-month incidence of recurrent symptomatic VTE and related deaths, and the main safety end point was bleeding events. The results indicated that fixed dose of dabigatran was as effective as and had a safety profile that is similar to that of warfarin, and did not require laboratory monitoring. Patients with hemodynamically unstable PE or creatinine clearance <30 mL/min (<0.5 mL/s) were excluded as were those at high risk for bleeding. The requirement for parenteral anticoagulation at initiation of dabigatran therapy is a disadvantage compared with VTE treatment using rivaroxaban.

Apixaban

Oral apixaban administered as 10 mg twice daily for 7 days followed by 5 mg twice daily for 6 months is being compared with warfarin (targeted INR 2 to 3) with initial enoxaparin coverage in an ongoing double-blind, randomized clinical trial with results expected sometime in 2013.

Treatment of Venous Thromboembolism in Special Populations

Pregnancy

The use of anticoagulation therapy for the treatment and prevention of DVT or PE during pregnancy is common.[17] UFH and LMWH are preferred during pregnancy (Table 9-12) as they do not cross the placenta and evidence suggests they are safe for the fetus.[17] Warfarin crosses the placenta and can result in fetal bleeding, central nervous system abnormalities, and embryopathy and should not be used for treatment

TABLE 9-12 Unfractionated and Low-Molecular-Weight Heparin Use During Pregnancy

Acute treatment[a]	LMWH • Enoxaparin 1 mg/kg SC q 12 h or 1.5 mg/kg q 24 h *Or* • Dalteparin 100 units/kg SC q 12 h *Or* • Tinzaparin 175 units/kg SC q 24 h *Or* UFH • Initiate using weight-based IV therapy and adjust dose to achieve therapeutic anti-Xa level for at least 5 days • Transition to SC adjusted-dose UFH administered q 8–12 h with mid-interval anti-Xa activity in the therapeutic range[b]
Long-term treatment[c]	LMWH Maintain initial LMWH dose regimen throughout pregnancy *Or* Alter LMWH dose in proportion to any weight change (usually gain) *Or* Obtain monthly anti-Xa level measurements 4–6 hours after morning dose and adjust LMWH dose based on anti-Xa level (target = 0.5–1.2 units/mL [0.5–1.2 kU/L] if twice-daily dosing; 1–2 units/mL [1–2 kU/L] if once-daily dosing) *Or* UFH Obtain anti-Xa level at the midpoint of the dosing interval and adjust UFH dose to achieve an anti-Xa level of 0.3–0.7 unit/mL [0.3–0.7 kU/L]
Issues at time of delivery	Elective induction of labor • Discontinue UFH or LMWH 24 hours prior to induction • Initiate therapeutic doses of UFH by IV infusion and discontinue 4–6 hours prior to expected time of delivery if risk of recurrent VTE is deemed high Spontaneous labor • For LMWH, if there is a reasonable expectation that significant anticoagulant effect will be present at time of delivery: (a) epidural should be avoided and (b) reversal with protamine sulfate may be considered • For UFH, monitor the aPTT and reverse with protamine sulfate if aPTT is prolonged near the time of delivery Postpartum • Commence UFH or LMWH as soon as safely possible (usually 12 hours following delivery) • Concurrently initiate warfarin therapy and discontinue UFH or LMWH when the INR is 2 or greater • Continue anticoagulants for at least 4 weeks following delivery • Warfarin can be safely used by women who are breast-feeding

aPTT, activated partial thromboplastin time; INR, international normalized ratio; LMWH, low-molecular-weight heparin; SC, subcutaneously; UFH, unfractionated heparin; VTE, venous thromboembolism.

[a]Twice-daily LMWH preferred during pregnancy due to increased clearance.
[b]Anti-Xa monitoring preferred as the relationship between aPTT and heparin levels differs in pregnant compared with nonpregnant patients.
[c]As pregnancy progresses the volume of distribution of LMWH changes, glomerular filtration rate increases, and most women gain weight.

From Bates et al.[17] and Ginsberg and Bates.[56]

of VTE during pregnancy.[17] Women of childbearing age taking warfarin must be counseled regarding the fetal risks and effective contraception should be used. Dabigatran, rivaroxaban, and apixaban should be avoided in pregnancy until more information regarding safety is available.[57–59] Fondaparinux, rivaroxaban, dabigatran, and apixaban have not been formally evaluated in pregnant patients.[2,3]

All pregnant women with a history of VTE should receive VTE prophylaxis for 6 weeks after delivery. Antenatal prophylaxis may also be indicated depending on other risk factors, such as history of multiple VTE, VTE associated with pregnancy or estrogen therapy, or known thrombophilia. Anticoagulation for acute VTE during pregnancy should continue for at least 6 weeks postpartum and for a minimum total duration of 3 months.[28] Warfarin, UFH, and LMWH are safe for use during breast-feeding.[60]

Pediatric Patients

Although seen far more frequently in adults, VTE in pediatric patients is increasing secondary to prematurity, cancer, trauma, surgery, congenital heart disease, and systemic lupus erythematosus. Pediatric patients often develop DVTs associated with indwelling central venous catheters. In contrast to adults, pediatric patients rarely develop idiopathic VTE.[61] While recommendations for anticoagulant therapy in pediatric patients are largely extrapolated from recommendations in adults, there are likely important pharmacokinetic and pharmacodynamic differences that should be taken into consideration. The majority of literature supporting pediatric recommendations is derived from uncontrolled studies, case reports, or in vitro experiments. When possible, a pediatric hematologist with experience managing VTE should manage pediatric patients.[61]

Anticoagulation with UFH and warfarin remains the most frequently used approach for the treatment of VTE in pediatric patients. The recommended target aPTT and INR ranges as well as the duration of therapy are extrapolated from clinical trials in adults. Recent data suggest that extrapolating aPTT range from adults to pediatric patients is unlikely to be valid. However, in the absence of supporting clinical data, extrapolation of the adult aPTT range to pediatric patients remains necessary.[61] The recommended initial bolus dose of UFH is 75 to 100 units/kg given IV over 10 minutes followed by a maintenance infusion of 28 units/kg/h for infants 2 to 12 months of age and 20 units/kg/h for children aged 1 year or older.[61] Subsequent infusion rate adjustments should be made every 4 to 6 hours to maintain the aPTT within the institution-specific therapeutic range. The usual warfarin starting dose is 0.2 mg/kg with a maximum of 10 mg. Infants require higher doses of warfarin per kilogram to maintain a target INR of 2 to 3 compared with teenagers and adults (mean dose 0.33 mg/kg, 0.09 mg/g, and 0.04 to 0.08 mg/kg, respectively).[61] The INR target range for VTE treatment in children is 2 to 3. Frequent INR monitoring and warfarin dose adjustments are typically required. When compared with adults, only 10% to 20% of pediatric patients can be safely monitored once monthly.[61] Obtaining coagulation monitoring tests in pediatric patients is problematic because many have poor or nonexistent venous access. To address this problem, many clinicians recommend using finger-stick blood samples with a portable point-of-care monitor.[61] Despite need for daily injections, LMWH is an attractive alternative in pediatric patients due to low drug interaction potential and less frequent laboratory testing. Enoxaparin, dalteparin, and tinzaparin have been evaluated in pediatric patients. Most experts recommend that anti-Xa activity be monitored and the dose adjusted to maintain anti–factor Xa levels between 0.5 and 1 unit/mL (0.5 and 1 kU/L) 4 to 6 hours following SC injection. Compared with adults, children younger than 2 to 3 months of age or who weigh less than 5 kg have higher per-kilogram dose requirements to achieve a "therapeutic" response. The dose of LMWH for older children is generally similar to the weight-adjusted doses used in adults.[61] Warfarin can be initiated concurrently with UFH or LMWH therapy. Therapy should be overlapped for a minimum of 5 days and until the INR is therapeutic. Warfarin should be continued for at least 3 months for provoked VTE and 6 months for idiopathic VTE.[61] Thrombolysis and thrombectomy have been successfully employed in pediatric patients, but published data are very limited—routine use is not recommended.[61]

Patients with Cancer

VTE is a frequent complication of cancer. Furthermore, compared with patients without cancer, the natural history of VTE in patients with cancer is different having threefold higher rates of recurrent VTE and bleeding and more resistance to standard warfarin-based therapy.[7,14] Warfarin therapy in cancer patients is often complicated by drug interactions (e.g., chemotherapy and antibiotics) and the need to frequently interrupt therapy for invasive procedures (e.g., thoracentesis, percutaneous biopsies, and abdominal paracentesis). Maintaining stable INR control is more difficult in this patient population because of nausea, anorexia, and vomiting.[7]

Randomized trials provide evidence that long-term LMWH monotherapy for VTE in patients with cancer significantly decreases the rate of recurrent VTE without increasing bleeding risks compared with traditional warfarin-based therapy.[7,14] Despite recommendations from AT9, the American Society of Clinical Oncology, and the National Comprehensive Cancer Network that patients with cancer should be given LMWH monotherapy for the long-term treatment of VTE, most patients with cancer-related VTE continue to receive warfarin-based therapy.[62] The reasons for this phenomenon are unclear, but possible explanations might be patient preference for oral therapy over daily injections, and/or the higher cost of LMWH. Pooled analysis of clinical trials demonstrates no survival advantage of LMWH monotherapy compared with traditional therapy with warfarin.[7] Advantages of LMWH over warfarin for VTE treatment in cancer are expected to be greatest in those with one or more of the following: metastatic disease, treatment with aggressive chemotherapy, extensive VTE at presentation, liver dysfunction, poor or unstable nutritional status, or desire to avoid frequent blood draws for coagulation monitoring.[7]

For patients with VTE and cancer who do receive LMWH, therapy should continue for at least the first 3 to 6 months of long-term treatment, at which time further LMWH can be considered or warfarin therapy can be substituted. Anticoagulation therapy should continue for as long as the cancer is "active" and while the patient is receiving antitumor therapy.[7] A risk-to-benefit assessment should be performed on a regular basis and the overall clinical status of the patient should be considered, along with the risk for bleeding, quality of life, and life expectancy.[7] Because so few patients with cancer-related VTE were included in rivaroxaban and dabigatran clinical trials, an assessment of whether these anticoagulants are appropriate alternatives to warfarin or LMWH for VTE treatment in this patient population is not possible until additional information becomes available.[7]

Clinical **Controversy. . .**

Most VTE in patients with cancer occurs in the outpatient setting. Several recent randomized clinical trials evaluated the utility of thromboprophylaxis for patients with solid tumors receiving systemic chemotherapy.[14] While these studies demonstrate that outpatient thromboprophylaxis is feasible, safe, and effective, the rates of VTE in the placebo arms of the trials argue against a broad application of prophylaxis for cancer patients. How to prospectively identify cancer patients at sufficiently high VTE risk to justify the use of thromboprophylaxis is being actively studied, but is currently poorly understood.

Patients with Renal Insufficiency

Patients with acute or chronic renal compromise often require anticoagulation for concomitant risk or treatment of thromboembolic disorders. With the exception of warfarin, most anticoagulants have at least some dependency on renal elimination. Accumulation of drug is possible during treatment with LMWH, fondaparinux, dabigatran, rivaroxaban, and apixaban.[2,3] In addition, patients with chronic kidney disease are at increased risk of bleeding, independent of drug clearance.[63]

LMWHs are primarily reliant on renal elimination and should be used with caution in patients with severe renal impairment.[64] Enoxaparin has specific labeling for patients with creatinine clearance <30 mL/min (<0.5 mL/s), but supporting evidence is limited to pharmacokinetic modeling analyses and bleeding and thromboembolic outcomes in this patient population are not well defined.[65] UFH is preferred for acute VTE treatment when creatinine clearance is <30 mL/min (<0.5 mL/s).[7]

Dabigatran, rivaroxaban, and apixaban each relies on renal elimination and requires dose adjustment at varying degrees of renal impairment.[57–59] Use of these anticoagulants in patients with creatinine clearance <30 mL/min (<0.5 mL/s) should be avoided.

7 8 PHARMACOLOGIC AGENTS USED IN THE PREVENTION AND TREATMENT OF VENOUS THROMBOEMBOLISM

Unfractionated Heparin

UFH has been used for the prevention and treatment of thrombosis for decades. Commercially available UFH preparations are derived from bovine lung or porcine intestinal mucosa. Although some differences exist between the two sources, no differences in antithrombotic activity have been demonstrated.[3]

Pharmacology

UFH is a heterogeneous mixture of sulfated mucopolysaccharides of variable lengths and pharmacologic properties (Table 9-13).[3] Each heparin molecule is composed of repetitive units of D-glycosamine and uronic acid. The anticoagulant profile and clearance of each UFH molecule varies based on its length. Smaller chains are cleared less rapidly than their longer counterparts.[3]

The anticoagulant effect of UFH is mediated through a specific pentasaccharide sequence on the heparin molecule that binds to antithrombin, provoking a conformational change (Fig. 9-7). Only one third of the UFH molecules possess the unique pentasaccharide sequence with affinity for antithrombin.[3] The UFH–antithrombin complex is 100 to 1,000 times more potent as an anticoagulant compared with antithrombin alone. Antithrombin inhibits the activity of several clotting factors including IXa, Xa, XIIa, and thrombin. Through its action on thrombin, the UFH–antithrombin complex also inhibits the thrombin-induced activation of factors V and VIII.[3] UFH prevents the growth and propagation of formed thrombus and allows endogenous thrombolytic systems to degrade the clot.

Factors IIa (thrombin) and Xa are most sensitive to inhibition by the UFH–antithrombin complex. To inactivate thrombin, the heparin molecule must form a ternary complex bridging between antithrombin and thrombin (see Fig. 9-7).[3] Only molecules that contain more than 18 saccharides are able to bind to both antithrombin and thrombin simultaneously. Smaller heparin molecules cannot facilitate the interaction between antithrombin and thrombin. In contrast, the inactivation of factor Xa does not require UFH to form a bridge with antithrombin, but requires only UFH binding to antithrombin via the specific pentasaccharide sequence. UFH molecules with as few as five saccharide units are able to catalyze the inhibition of factor Xa. After it has produced its effect UFH uncouples from antithrombin and quickly recouples with another antithrombin molecule.[3] Because of its relatively large size, the UFH–antithrombin complex is incapable of inactivating thrombin or factor Xa within a formed clot or bound to surfaces. At high doses, UFH also binds to

TABLE 9-13 Comparison of the Chemical and Pharmacokinetic Properties of Antithrombotic Drugs Used for Venous Thrombosis

Agent	FDA Approved	Method of Preparation	Mean Molecular Weight (d)	Plasma Half-Life	Anti-Xa: Anti-IIa Activity	Bioavailability
Unfractionated heparin	Yes	Extracted from porcine gut mucosa or beef lung	≈15,000	30–90 minutes (dose dependent)	1:1	SC: 30–70% (dose dependent)
Low-molecular-weight heparins						
Dalteparin (Fragmin)	Yes	Nitrous acid depolymerization	≈6,000	119–139 minutes	2.7:1	SC: 87%
Enoxaparin (Lovenox)	Yes	Benzoylation and alkaline depolymerization	≈4,200	129–180 minutes	3.8:1	SC: 92%
Tinzaparin (Innohep)	Yes	Heparinase digestion	≈4,500	111–234 minutes	2.8:1	SC: 90%
Anti–factor Xa inhibitors						
Fondaparinux (Arixtra)	Yes	Synthetic	1,728	15–18 hours	100% anti-Xa	SC: 100%
Rivaroxaban (Xarelto)	Yes (VTE prophylaxis and atrial fibrillation)	Synthetic	NA	7–11 hours	100% anti-Xa	po: 80–100%
Apixaban (Eliquis)	No	Synthetic	460	9–14 hours	100% anti-Xa	po: 50%
Direct thrombin inhibitors						
Dabigatran (Pradaxa)	Yes (for atrial fibrillation)	Synthetic	471	14 hours	100% anti-IIa	Oral: 7%
Vitamin K antagonists						
Warfarin (Coumadin)	Yes	Synthetic	330	40 hours	1:1	Oral: 90–100%

NA, not available; SC, subcutaneous.

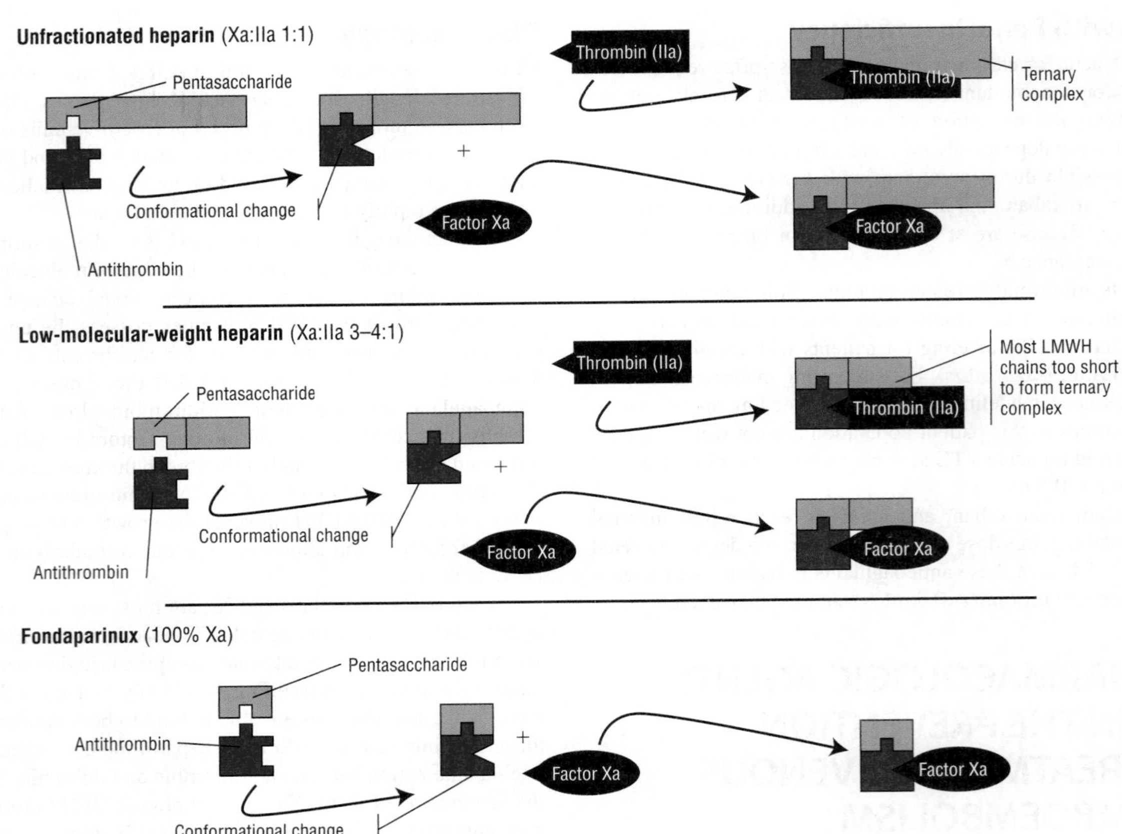

FIGURE 9-7 Pharmacologic activity of unfractionated heparin, low-molecular-weight heparins (LMWHs), and fondaparinux.

heparin cofactor II, further inhibiting the activity of thrombin.[3] UFH increases the release of tissue factor pathway inhibitor from vascular endothelium, augmenting its inhibitory effect on factor Xa. UFH, especially high-molecular-weight fractions, also binds to platelets and inhibits platelet aggregation.[3]

Pharmacokinetics

UFH is not reliably absorbed when taken orally as a result of its large molecular size and anionic structure. The bioavailability and biologic activity of UFH is limited by its propensity to bind to plasma proteins, platelet factor-4 (PF-4), macrophages, fibrinogen, lipoproteins, and endothelial cells. This may explain the substantial interpatient and intrapatient variability observed in the anticoagulation response to UFH.[3]

The SC bioavailability of UFH is dose dependent and ranges from 30% at low doses to as much as 70% at high doses. The onset of anticoagulant effect is usually evident 1 to 2 hours after SC injection and peaks at 3 hours.[3] When UFH is administered via the IV route, a continuous infusion is preferable.[7] Intramuscular administration is discouraged because of the risk of large hematoma formation.

UFH has a dose-dependent half-life of approximately 30 to 90 minutes, but may be prolonged to as much as 150 minutes when given in high doses.[3] There are two primary mechanisms for the elimination of UFH. One is a rapid, but saturable zero-order process involving enzymatic inactivation of heparin molecules bound to endothelial cells and macrophages.[3] The other mechanism is renal elimination via a slower, nonsaturable first-order process. With typical therapeutic regimens, a combination of the two mechanisms eliminates UFH with the saturable mechanism predominating.[3]

Dose and Administration

The dose of UFH is expressed in units of activity. For the prevention of VTE, UFH is given by SC injection in the abdominal fat layer. The typical dose for prophylaxis is 5,000 units every 8 to 12 hours. When immediate and full anticoagulation is required, an IV bolus dose followed by a continuous infusion is preferred (Table 9-8).[3] SC UFH (initial dose of 333 units/kg followed by 250 units/kg every 12 hours) also provides adequate therapeutic anticoagulation for the treatment of acute VTE.[48]

Therapeutic Monitoring

7 Administration of UFH requires close monitoring because of the unpredictable anticoagulant patient response.[3] The aPTT is the most widely used test to determine the degree of therapeutic anticoagulation and, although most experts advocate using the aPTT to monitor UFH provided that institution-specific therapeutic ranges are defined, the use of aPTT has several limitations as discussed previously. The aPTT should be measured prior to the initiation of therapy to determine the patient's baseline. With IV infusion, the aPTT response to UFH therapy should be measured 6 hours after initiation or a dose change; this is usually sufficient time to reach steady state. Promptly adjust the dose of UFH based on patient response and the institution-specific aPTT therapeutic range.[3]

Adverse Effects

8 Bleeding is the primary adverse effect associated with all anticoagulant drugs (Table 9-14).[63] Low-dose SC UFH is associated with a minimal risk of major bleeding, while the rates of major bleeding for patients receiving full therapeutic doses of UFH range from 0% to 2%.[63]

TABLE 9-14 Risk Factors for Major Bleeding While Taking Anticoagulation Therapy

Anticoagulation intensity
Initiation of therapy (first few days and weeks)
Unstable anticoagulation response
Age >65 years
Concurrent antiplatelet therapy
Concurrent nonsteroidal antiinflammatory drug use
History of GI bleeding
Recent surgery or trauma
High risk for fall/trauma
Heavy alcohol use
Renal failure
Cerebrovascular disease
Malignancy

From Schulman et al.[63]

Heparin-induced thrombocytopenia (HIT) is a rare drug-induced immunologic reaction requiring immediate intervention.[66] The most common complication of HIT is VTE; arterial thromboembolic events occur less frequently. Approximately 5% to 10% of patients with HIT die, usually as a result of thrombotic complications.[66] Thrombocytopenia (defined as a platelet count <150 × 10³/mm³ [<150 × 10⁹/L]) is the most common clinical manifestation of HIT and occurs in up to 95% of patients with confirmed HIT if a proportional fall in platelet count of 30% to 50% even though the count stays above 150 × 10³/mm³ (150 × 10⁹/L) is included in the definition.[66] The characteristic onset of falling platelet count in HIT is 5 to 10 days after initiation of UFH (day 0 being the first day of UFH), particularly when administered perioperatively.[66] Thrombocytopenia alone is not sufficient for diagnosing HIT; serologic confirmation of heparin antibodies using an assay available only in a few specialty laboratories is required.[66] Falsely diagnosing HIT can have serious consequences including unnecessary anxiety, unnecessary withdrawal of UFH, and the use of alternative anticoagulants with higher bleeding risk. One decision analysis found that strict adherence to platelet monitoring for HIT could, at best, prevent one thrombosis per 1,000 patients screened at the cost of one major bleeding event.[66] For these reasons, AT9 suggest monitoring platelet counts every 2 to 3 days from day 4 to 14 of UFH only in populations where the expected risk of HIT exceeds 1%.[66] The use of a clinical prediction rule, such as the 4 Ts score (*t*hrombocytopenia, *t*iming of platelet count fall or thrombosis, *t*hrombosis, o*t*her explanation for thrombocytopenia), can improve the predictive value of platelet count monitoring and heparin antibody testing (Table 9-15).[66,67] While a low 4 Ts score identifies patients with low probability of HIT (0% to 3%), a substantial proportion of patients with a high 4 Ts score do not have HIT either (24% to 61%).[66] A prospective trial is needed to definitively determine the role of the 4 Ts score in HIT surveillance and management. A 4 Ts score should be calculated when HIT is suspected in patients receiving heparin (UFH or LMWH). If the 4 Ts score is low, no further workup is needed, whereas if the 4 Ts score is moderate or high, further workup of HIT including serologic testing should be undertaken.[68] All heparin should be discontinued if new thrombosis occurs in the setting of falling platelets in conjunction with a moderate or high 4 Ts score. Alternative anticoagulation should then be initiated with a parenteral direct thrombin inhibitor.[66]

Long-term UFH has been reported to cause alopecia, priapism, and suppressed aldosterone synthesis with subsequent hyperkalemia.[3] The use of UFH in doses ≥20,000 units/day for more than 6 months, especially during pregnancy, is associated with significant bone loss and may lead to osteoporosis.[3] Few drug interactions are reported with UFH, but concurrent use with other anticoagulant, thrombolytic, and antiplatelet agents increases the risk of bleeding.[3]

Management of Bleeding

Hemorrhage can occur at any site in patients receiving UFH and close monitoring for signs and symptoms of bleeding is crucial.[3,63] When major bleeding occurs, UFH should be immediately discontinued and the underlying source of bleeding identified and treated. IV protamine sulfate in a dose of 1 mg per 100 units of UFH up to a maximum of 50 mg can be administered via slow IV infusion to reverse the anticoagulant effects of UFH.[3] Protamine sulfate neutralizes UFH in 5 minutes, and its effect persists for 2 hours. Multiple doses or prolonged infusion of protamine sulfate may be necessary if hemorrhage continues.[3]

Low-Molecular-Weight Heparin

LMWH fragments produced by either chemical or enzymatic depolymerization of UFH (see Table 9-13) are heterogeneous mixtures of sulfated glycosaminoglycans with approximately one third the molecular weight of UFH.[3] LMWH has a similar mechanism of action as UFH, but with reduced inhibitory activity against thrombin relative to factor Xa, less affinity for plasma proteins, and longer duration of activity.[3] Advantages of LMWH over UFH include (a) predictable anticoagulation dose response, (b) improved SC bioavailability, (c) dose-independent clearance, (d) longer biologic half-life, (e) lower incidence of thrombocytopenia, and (f) reduced need for routine laboratory monitoring.[3] Currently three LMWH

TABLE 9-15 The 4 Ts Probability Score for Heparin-Induced Thrombocytopenia

Category	2 Points	1 Point	0 Point
Thrombocytopenia	Platelet count falls >50% from baseline and nadir is ≥20 × 10³/mm³ (≥20 × 10⁹/L)	Platelet count falls 30% to 50% from baseline or platelet nadir is 10 × 10³/mm³ to 19 × 10³/mm³ (10 × 10⁹/L to 19 × 10⁹/L)	Platelet count fall <30% from baseline or platelet nadir is <10 × 10³/mm³ (<10 × 10⁹/L)
Timing of platelet count fall	Clear onset between 5 and 10 days of heparin exposure or platelet fall ≤1 day with history of heparin exposure in previous 30 days	Fall in platelet counts consistent with onset between days 5 and 10 but timing is not clear *or* onset after day 10 *or* fall in platelets ≤1 day with history of heparin exposure in previous 30–100 days	Platelet counts fall <4 days without history of recent heparin exposure
Thrombosis or other sequelae	New thrombosis, skin necrosis, or acute systematic reaction after heparin exposure	Progressive/recurrent thrombosis or unconfirmed but clinically suspected thrombosis	No thrombosis or thrombosis preceding heparin exposure only
Other causes of thrombocytopenia	None apparent	Possible other causes present	Probable other causes present

The 4 Ts score is determined by summing the values for each category. Scores: <4, low; 4–5, intermediate; >5, high.

Adapted from Crowther et al.[67]

products are available in the United States (see Table 9-13) with only enoxaparin being available in a generic formulation. The FDA-approved indications and doses relating to VTE for the LMWHs are product specific (Table 9-9).

Pharmacology

LMWH prevents the growth and propagation of formed thrombi by enhancing and accelerating the activity of antithrombin through binding to a specific pentasaccharide sequence present on about one third of LMWH molecules.[3] The principal difference in the pharmacologic activity of LMWH and UFH is their relative inhibition of factor Xa and thrombin. Because of smaller chain lengths, LMWH has limited activity against thrombin (see Fig. 9-7). The ratio of anti–factor Xa-to-IIa activity varies between 4:1 and 2:1. By comparison, UFH has an anti–factor Xa-to-IIa activity ratio of 1:1.[3]

Pharmacokinetics

Compared with UFH, LMWH has a more predictable anticoagulation response. The improved pharmacokinetic profile of LMWH is the result of reduced binding to proteins and cells.[3] The bioavailability of LMWH is about 90% when administered SC. The SC bioavailability of the available LMWH products differs only slightly. The peak anticoagulation effect is seen in 3 to 5 hours.[3] The predominant mode of elimination for LMWH is renal. Consequently, their biologic half-life may be prolonged in patients with renal impairment.[3] The plasma half-life of LMWH preparations is 3 to 6 hours. The clearance of LMWH is independent of dose.[3]

Dosing and Administration

LMWH is given in fixed or weight-based doses based on the product and indication (see Table 9-9). Doses should be based on actual body weight and studies in obese patients indicate that full weight-based doses do not lead to elevated LMWH concentrations when compared with normal subjects; consequently, dose capping is not recommended.[64] The dose for enoxaparin is expressed in milligrams, whereas dalteparin and tinzaparin are expressed in units of anti–factor Xa activity. LMWH is given by SC injection as described in Table 9-10.

The dosing interval for LMWH is every 12 or 24 hours depending on the indication and product. For VTE treatment, AT9 suggest once- over twice-daily LMWH administration provided the approved once-daily regimen contains double the dose of each twice-daily injection.[7] Given that the elimination half-life of LMWH is prolonged in patients with severe renal impairment, unadjusted therapeutic doses may lead to a significant accumulation in these patients.[3] The enoxaparin dose should be reduced and the dosing interval extended to once daily in patients with creatinine clearance <30 mL/min (<0.5 mL/s).[65] The pharmacokinetics of dalteparin and tinzaparin is less well characterized in patients with renal insufficiency, but some studies suggest that there is a lower degree of accumulation with tinzaparin.[3] Data on the use of LMWH in patients with end-stage renal disease receiving hemodialysis are very limited; thus, UFH is preferred for these patients.[3] Given that few published data are available regarding the use of LMWH in the setting of renal insufficiency, some experts recommend measuring anti–factor Xa activity if therapy is continued for more than a few days.[3] When given in prophylactic doses, LMWH has not been shown to increase the risk of bleeding complications, irrespective of the degree of renal function impairment. For patients with creatinine clearance <30 mL/min (<0.5 mL/s) who require VTE prophylaxis, enoxaparin 30 mg once daily is recommended, but dosing recommendations are not available in the setting of renal insufficiency for dalteparin or tinzaparin.[3]

Therapeutic Monitoring

Because LMWH anticoagulant response is predictable when given SC, routine laboratory monitoring is unnecessary.[3] Prior to initiation of LMWH, a baseline complete blood cell count with platelet count, and serum creatinine should be obtained. The complete blood cell count can be checked every 5 to 10 days during the first 2 weeks of LMWH therapy and every 2 to 4 weeks thereafter to monitor for occult bleeding. If neuraxial anesthesia has been used, patients should be closely monitored for signs and symptoms of neurologic impairment.[65]

Measurement of anti–factor Xa activity is the most widely used method to monitor LMWH in clinical practice. Routine anti–factor Xa activity measurement is unnecessary in patients whose condition is stable and uncomplicated.[3] Although very limited data support the use of laboratory monitoring to guide LMWH therapy, measuring anti–factor Xa activity may be helpful in patients who have significant renal impairment (e.g., creatinine clearance <30 mL/min [<0.5 mL/s]), weigh less than 50 kg, are morbidly obese, or require prolonged therapy (e.g., longer than 14 days). Periodic anti–factor Xa activity monitoring may also be useful in women treated with LMWH during pregnancy because of changing pharmacokinetic variables (e.g., volume of distribution and renal function).[3]

When anti–factor Xa activity is used to monitor LMWH therapy, the sample should be drawn after steady state has been achieved (after the second or third dose) and approximately 4 hours after the SC injection, during the peak period of anti–factor Xa activity.[3] The therapeutic range for anti–factor Xa activity is not well defined and has not been clearly correlated with efficacy or the risk of bleeding. For the treatment of VTE, an acceptable target range for the peak anti-Xa level for twice-daily enoxaparin dosing is 0.6 to 1 unit/mL (0.6 to 1 kU/L). For once-daily dosing likely peak targets are >1 unit/mL (>1 kU/L) for enoxaparin, 0.85 unit/mL (0.85 kU/L) for tinzaparin, and 1.05 units/mL (1.05 kU/L) for dalteparin.[3]

Adverse Effects

As with other anticoagulants, bleeding is the most common adverse effect of LMWH therapy.[63] The frequency of major bleeding is purported to be less with LMWH than with UFH, but this has not been consistently demonstrated in clinical trials.[63] Although there is no proven method for reversing LMWH anticoagulation if major bleeding does occur, IV protamine sulfate can be administered. However, because of limited binding to the shorter LMWH chains, protamine sulfate neutralizes only around 60% to 75% of LMWH anticoagulant activity.[3] The recommended dose of protamine sulfate is 1/1 mg of enoxaparin or 1 mg/100 anti–factor Xa units of dalteparin or tinzaparin administered in the previous 8 hours. A second protamine sulfate dose of 0.5/1 mg or 100 anti–factor Xa units can be given if bleeding continues. Smaller doses of protamine sulfate can be used if the LMWH dose was given in the previous 8 to 12 hours. The use of protamine sulfate is not recommended if LMWH was administered more than 12 hours earlier.[3]

Although thrombocytopenia can occur with the use of LMWH, the incidence of HIT is three times lower than that observed with UFH, perhaps due to the reduced propensity of LMWH to bind to platelets.[3] Because LMWH exhibits nearly 100% cross-reactivity with heparin antibodies in vitro, LMWH should be avoided in patients with an established diagnosis or history of HIT.[3] The risk of osteoporosis appears to be lower with LMWH than with UFH, but both agents have the potential to produce osteopenia.[3]

Fondaparinux

Fondaparinux, also known as pentasaccharide, is a synthetic molecule consisting of the five critical saccharide units that bind specifically, but reversibly, to antithrombin (see Fig. 9-7). Unlike UFH or LMWH, fondaparinux selectively inhibits factor Xa activity.[3]

Pharmacology

Similar to UFH and LMWH, fondaparinux prevents thrombus generation and clot formation by indirectly inhibiting factor Xa activity through its interaction with antithrombin. Fondaparinux is not destroyed during this process and is released to bind many other antithrombin molecules.[3]

Pharmacokinetics

Fondaparinux is rapidly and completely absorbed following SC administration (absolute bioavailability 100%). Peak plasma concentrations are achieved in approximately 2 hours after a single dose and 3 hours with repeated once-daily dosing. At therapeutic concentrations, fondaparinux is highly and specifically bound to antithrombin. It does not bind to red blood cells or other plasma proteins including albumin, gp, platelets, or PF-4.[3] Fondaparinux is primarily eliminated unchanged in the urine and is contraindicated in patients with creatinine clearance <30 mL/min (<0.5 mL/s). The terminal elimination half-life is 17 to 21 hours.[3] The anticoagulant effect of fondaparinux persists for 2 to 4 days following discontinuation of the drug in patients with normal renal function. Fondaparinux has no known pharmacokinetic drug interactions. However, concurrent use with other drugs with anticoagulant, fibrinolytic, or antiplatelet activity increases the risk of hemorrhage.[50]

Dosing and Administration

Fondaparinux is FDA approved for the prevention of VTE following orthopedic (hip fracture, hip and knee replacement) or abdominal surgery and for the treatment of DVT and PE (in conjunction with warfarin).[50] In the setting of VTE prevention, the dose of fondaparinux is 2.5 mg injected SC once daily starting 6 to 8 hours following surgery if hemostasis has been established. It is important to avoid initiating fondaparinux too soon because there is a significant relationship between the timing of the first dose and the risk of major bleeding complications.[3] Patients who weigh less than 50 kg should not be given fondaparinux for VTE prophylaxis.[50] The usual duration of therapy is 5 to 9 days, but may be given as extended prophylaxis following hospital discharge for up to 35 days.[4] For the treatment of DVT or PE, the dose of fondaparinux is 5 mg for patients up to 50 kg, 7.5 mg for 50 to 100 kg, and 10 mg for patients >100 kg.[50]

Therapeutic Monitoring

A complete blood cell count should be measured at baseline and monitored periodically to detect the possibility of occult bleeding.[50] Baseline kidney function should be determined as fondaparinux is contraindicated when creatinine clearance is <30 mL/min (<0.5 mL/s). Signs and symptoms of bleeding should be monitored daily, particularly in patients with a baseline creatinine clearance between 30 and 50 mL/min (0.5 and 0.83 mL/s). If neuraxial anesthesia has been used, patients should be closely monitored for signs and symptoms of neurologic impairment.[50]

Fondaparinux does not alter coagulation tests such as the aPTT and prothrombin time (PT). The role of anti–factor Xa monitoring during fondaparinux is not well defined. Patients receiving fondaparinux therapy do not require routine coagulation testing.[50]

Adverse Effects

The primary adverse effect associated with fondaparinux therapy is bleeding.[50] Similar to UFH and LMWH, fondaparinux should be used with extreme caution in patients with neuraxial anesthesia or following a spinal puncture because of the risk for spinal or epidural hematoma formation.[50] Some case reports have documented successful treatment of HIT with fondaparinux, while others have implicated fondaparinux as a cause of HIT.[69] A specific antidote to reverse the antithrombotic activity of fondaparinux is not currently available; if uncontrollable bleeding occurs during fondaparinux therapy, factor VIIa may be effective.[3]

Direct Anti-Xa Inhibitors

The introduction of LMWH and fondaparinux transformed the initial treatment of VTE from a purely inpatient endeavor to one where the majority of patients can be treated as outpatients. However, the need for daily SC injections is a significant barrier for some patients.[38] Warfarin therapy is notoriously unpredictable and labor intensive, and can be stressful for patients and anticoagulation providers. These shortcomings in available anticoagulants have driven the search for replacements with rapid onset of effect that can be administered orally without the need for anticoagulant monitoring. Two such agents that target factor Xa are rivaroxaban and apixaban. Neither of these agents has been FDA approved for use in VTE treatment in the United States, but rivaroxaban has been approved for prevention of VTE following hip or knee replacement surgery.[59]

Pharmacology and Pharmacokinetics

Rivaroxaban and apixaban are potent and selective inhibitors of both free and clot-bound factor Xa that do not require antithrombin to exert their anticoagulant effect.[2] Both drugs have good oral bioavailability (80% and 50% for rivaroxaban and apixaban, respectively) and reach peak plasma concentrations in about 3 hours. The terminal half-life is 5 to 9 hours for rivaroxaban and 9 to 14 hours for apixaban.[2] Both drugs are excreted in the urine and feces and are metabolized by CYP3A4 (among others) and cytochrome P450 (CYP)–independent mechanisms. Rivaroxaban is a substrate of CYP3A4/5, CYP2J2, and the P-gp and ATP-binding cassette G2 (ABCG2) transporters. Inhibitors and inducers of these CYP450 enzymes or transporters (e.g., P-gp) may result in changes in rivaroxaban exposure.[59] Both drugs should be used with caution in patients with renal dysfunction.[2]

Dosing and Administration

The dose of rivaroxaban for prevention of VTE following elective hip or knee replacement surgery is 10 mg orally once daily with or without food. Rivaroxaban should be initiated at least 6 to 10 hours after surgery once hemostasis has been established and continued for 12 days (knee replacement) or 35 days (hip replacement).[59] The dose used in clinical trials for VTE treatment was 15 mg orally twice daily for 3 weeks, and then 20 mg once daily thereafter.[37,38] When rivaroxaban doses of 20 mg are taken by patients with atrial fibrillation, administration with food is recommended.[59] Apixaban is not approved for use in the United States, but European prescribing information lists the recommended dose following elective hip or knee replacement surgery at 2.5 mg orally twice daily with or without food starting 12 to 24 hours after surgery and continuing for 10 to 14 days (knee replacement) or 32 to 38 days (hip replacement).[57]

Therapeutic Monitoring

Because of predictable pharmacokinetics, rivaroxaban and apixaban do not require routine laboratory monitoring or dose adjustments. In rare situations (e.g., overdose, bleeding, assessment of compliance, prior to an invasive procedure, drug interactions, or assessment of drug accumulation in renal or hepatic impairment) the ability to measure coagulation using a quantitative assay might be valuable.[2] However, there are currently no validated laboratory tests that can be recommended to monitor rivaroxaban or apixaban or any recommendations for dose adjustments based on observed test results.[2] Periodic assessment of renal function is important during long-term therapy with rivaroxaban or apixaban, especially for patients with creatinine clearance <50 mL/min (<0.83 mL/s). These drugs should not be used in patients with creatinine clearance less than 15 mL/min (0.25 mL/s) (apixaban) or 30 mL/min (0.5 mL/s) (rivaroxaban).[57,59] Patients should be observed closely and promptly evaluated for any signs or symptoms of blood loss.

Adverse Effects

Bleeding is the most common adverse effect associated with rivaroxaban and apixaban therapy.[57,59] Managing bleeding associated with rivaroxaban and apixaban is complicated by the lack of a specific reversal agent.[2] Patients presenting with significant bleeding during rivaroxaban or apixaban therapy should receive routine usual supportive care (fluid resuscitation, blood transfusion, maintenance of renal function, bleeding source identification, and surgical intervention if needed), and discontinuation of anticoagulation therapy.[70] Because rivaroxaban and apixaban have relatively short half-lives, these measures may control bleeding in many patients, especially those with normal renal function.[70] Activated charcoal may provide some benefit if drug intake occurred within a couple of hours of presentation, but hemodialysis is not expected to be effective for rivaroxaban and apixaban as they are both highly protein bound; fresh-frozen plasma (FFP) is also unlikely to provide clinical benefit.[70] It is unclear whether factor VIIa administration will be useful for emergent reversal of rivaroxaban or apixaban and its use has been associated with increased risk of arterial thrombosis in nonhemophiliac patients.[70] In dire circumstances, the use of nonactivated four-factor prothrombin complex concentrates (PCCs) may be reasonable based on a small study in normal volunteers receiving rivaroxaban.[70] However, it is important to note that there have been no studies evaluating the effect of PCCs in bleeding humans receiving rivaroxaban or apixaban, and four-factor PCCS are currently unavailable in the United States.[70] The most frequent nonbleeding adverse events in clinical trials of rivaroxaban and apixaban were nausea, vomiting, and constipation.[2]

Use in Special Populations

There are no adequate or well-controlled studies of rivaroxaban or apixaban in pregnant women, and use is not recommended in this patient population. It is not known if rivaroxaban is excreted in human milk and breast-feeding is not recommended in women taking either rivaroxaban or apixaban.[57,59] Oral administration and no need for routine coagulation monitoring make rivaroxaban and apixaban attractive alternatives in pediatric patients; however, safety and effectiveness in this population have not been established.[57,59]

Dabigatran

Dabigatran is a selective, reversible, direct thrombin inhibitor given as an orally absorbable prodrug dabigatran etexilate. Dosing schedules are 150 and 220 mg once daily when used to prevent VTE (starting with a half dose given soon after surgery) and 150 mg twice daily with therapeutic LMWH for the first 5 days for treatment of VTE.[2] Available data suggest that dabigatran is at least as effective and safe as LMWH in the prevention of VTE after major orthopedic surgery and it has been approved in Canada and Europe for VTE prevention after hip and knee replacement surgery, but is not yet approved for this indication in the United States, although it is on the market for stroke prevention in patients with nonvalvular atrial fibrillation.[58] The need for concurrent administration with LMWH at the initiation makes dabigatran a less attractive alternative compared with rivaroxaban for treatment of VTE.

Warfarin

Warfarin is currently the anticoagulant of choice for long-term or extended anticoagulation. Because of its narrow therapeutic index, predisposition to drug and food interactions, and propensity to cause bleeding, warfarin requires continuous patient monitoring and education to achieve optimal outcomes.[2]

Pharmacology

Warfarin exerts its anticoagulation effect by inhibiting the enzymes responsible for the cyclic interconversion of vitamin K in the liver.[2] Reduced vitamin K is a cofactor required for the carboxylation of the vitamin K–dependent coagulation proteins, namely, prothrombin, VII, IX, and X, as well as the endogenous anticoagulant proteins C and S. Carboxylation of the N-terminal region of these proteins in the liver is required for biologic activity. By inhibiting the supply of vitamin K to serve as a cofactor in the production of these proteins, warfarin results in the production of partially carboxylated and decarboxylated coagulation proteins with reduced activity.[2] Warfarin has no direct effect on previously circulating clotting factors or previously formed thrombus. The time required for warfarin to achieve its pharmacologic effect is dependent on the elimination half-lives of the coagulation proteins that vary between 4 and 6 hours for factor VII and 42 and 72 hours for prothrombin.[2] Given that prothrombin has a 2- to 3-day half-life, antithrombotic effect is not achieved for at least 6 days after the initiation of warfarin therapy. By suppressing the production of fully functional clotting factors, warfarin prevents the initial formation and propagation of thrombus.[2]

Pharmacokinetics

Commercially available warfarin is a racemic mixture of *R* and *S* isomers. The *S* isomer is 2.7 to 3.8 times more potent than the *R* isomer.[2] Warfarin is rapidly and extensively absorbed from the GI tract and reaches peak plasma concentration within 4 hours with a bioavailability of greater than 90% following oral administration. Warfarin is 99% bound to plasma proteins.[71] It undergoes stereoselective metabolism via CYP1A2, 2C9, 2C19, 2C8, 2C18, and 3A4 isoenzymes in the liver, with 2C9 being the main enzyme to modulate in vivo anticoagulant activity.[71] Pharmacokinetic parameters of warfarin, particularly hepatic metabolism, vary substantially between individuals leading to large interpatient differences in dose requirements. Genetic variations in the 2C9 isoenzyme and vitamin K epoxide reductase (VKOR) have been shown to correlate with warfarin dose requirements.[2] Given the relatively greater potency of *S*-warfarin, coadministration of drugs that induce or inhibit the CYP2C isoenzymes is more likely to cause clinically significant interactions.[2] These and other pharmacokinetic variations in warfarin metabolism likely explain the large interpatient dose–response seen with warfarin in clinical practice.

Dosing and Administration

The dose of warfarin is patient specific based on the desired intensity of anticoagulation and the patient's individual response.[2] There is tremendous interpatient variability with regard to the pharmacodynamic response and pharmacokinetic disposition of warfarin. In addition, there can be significant intrapatient variability in these parameters over time. Therefore, the dose of warfarin must be based on continual clinical and laboratory monitoring.[2]

Although the average weekly dose of warfarin is between 25 and 55 mg, some patient-related variables are associated with lower than usual dose requirement including advanced age (>65 years), elevated baseline INR, poor nutritional status, liver disease, hyperthyroidism, genetic polymorphisms in CYP2C9 and VKOR (see Personalized Pharmacotherapy below), and concurrent use of medications known to enhance the effect of warfarin.[2] Prior to initiating therapy, the clinician should screen for the presence of contraindications to anticoagulation therapy and risk factors for major bleeding (see Table 9-14). It is important to collect a complete medication history, including the use of herbal and nutritional products (Tables 9-16 and 9-17).

For most patients, initiating therapy with 5 to 10 mg daily and adjusting the dose based on the INR response will produce therapeutic INRs in 4 to 5 days (Fig. 9-6). Lower starting doses may be acceptable based on patient-related factors such as advanced age, malnutrition, liver disease, or heart failure. Starting doses >10 mg should be avoided.[2] Warfarin therapy can be safely initiated on an

TABLE 9-16 Warfarin Dietary Supplements Interactions Involving Cytochrome P450 Metabolism

Dietary Supplement	Mechanism
Bergamottin (component of grapefruit juice)	2C9 inhibitor
Bishop's weed (bergapten)	3A4 inhibitor
Bitter orange	3A4 inhibitor
Cat's claw	3A4 inhibitor
Chrysin	1A2 inhibitor
Cranberry	2C9 inhibitor
Devil's claw	2C9 inhibitor
Dehydroepiandrosterone (DHEA)	3A4 inhibitor
Diindolylmethane	1A2 inducer
Echinacea	3A4 inhibitor
Eucalyptus	3A4, 2C9, 2C19, 1A2 inhibitor
Feverfew	1A2, 2C9, 2C19, 3A4 inhibitor
Fo-ti	1A2, 2C9, 2C19, 3A4 inhibitor
Garlic	2C9, 2C19, and 3A4 inhibitor
Ginseng	CYP P450 inducer
Goldenseal	3A4 inhibitor
Guggul	3A4 inducer
Grape	1A2 inducer
Grapefruit juice	1A2, 2A6, and 3A4 inhibitor
Indole-3-carbinol	1A2 inducer
Ipriflavone	2C9, 1A2 inhibitor
Kava	1A2, 2C9, 2C19, 2D6, 3A4 inhibitor
Licorice	3A4 inhibitor
Lime	3A4 inhibitor
Limonene	2C9, 2C19 substrate, and 2C9 inducer
Lycium (Chinese wolfberry)	2C9 inhibitor
Milk thistle	2C9 and 3A4 inhibitor
Peppermint	1A2, 2C9, 2C19, 3A4 inhibitor
Red clover	1A2, 2C9, 2C19, 3A4 inhibitor
Resveratrol	1A, 2E1, 3A4 inhibitor
St. John's wort	1A2, 2C9, 3A4 inducer
Sulforaphane	1A2 inhibitor
Valerian	3A4 inhibitor
Wild cherry	3A4 inhibitor

From Nutescu et al.[72]

outpatient basis; the response to therapy should be measured every 1 to 3 days until stabilized. For patients with acute venous thrombosis, UFH, LMWH, or fondaparinux should be overlapped with warfarin therapy for at least 5 days regardless of whether the target INR has been achieved earlier.[2,7]

When adjusting the dose of warfarin, allow sufficient time for changes in the INR to occur. In general, maintenance dose changes should not be made more frequently than every 3 days. Doses should be adjusted by reducing or increasing the weekly dose by 5% to 25%. The full effect of dose changes may not become evident for 5 to 7 days. During maintenance therapy, patients should not have followup INR tests sooner than anticipated changes are likely to occur.[2]

Therapeutic Monitoring

Warfarin requires frequent laboratory monitoring to ensure optimal therapeutic outcomes and minimize bleeding complications. The PT has been used for decades to monitor the anticoagulation effects of warfarin. The PT measures the biologic activity of factors II, VII, and X and correlates well to warfarin's anticoagulation effect. The test is performed by measuring the time required for clot formation after adding calcium and thromboplastin to citrated plasma.[2] The PT is problematic to interpret because of the variable sensitivity of commercially available thromboplastin reagents. With a given blood sample, thromboplastins of differing sensitivity will produce substantially different results some of which could lead to inappropriate dosing decisions. The World Health Organization (WHO) addressed the need for standardization in the late 1970s by developing a reference thromboplastin and recommending the use of the INR to monitor warfarin therapy. The INR corrects for differences in thromboplastin reagents through the following formula:

$$\text{INR} = \left(\frac{\text{PT}^{\text{patient}}}{\text{PT}^{\text{control}}}\right)^{\text{ISI}}$$

The International Sensitivity Index (ISI) is a measure of thromboplastin responsiveness compared with the WHO reference standard.[2] Each thromboplastin reagent manufactured has an ISI value that should be used to calculate the INR. Although the INR system has a number of potential problems, it is currently the best means available to interpret the PT and the preferred method for monitoring warfarin therapy.[2]

The recommended target INR and associated goal range is based on the therapeutic indication. For most indications including treatment of VTE, the target INR is 2.5 with an acceptable range of 2 to 3.[2] A baseline INR and complete blood cell count should be obtained prior to initiating warfarin therapy. In patients with an acute thromboembolic event, an INR should be measured minimally every 3 days during the first week of therapy (daily INRs are common in hospitalized patients). Once the patient's dose–response is established, an INR should be determined every 7 to 14 days until it stabilizes and optimally every 4 to 12 weeks thereafter.[44,73]

At each encounter and especially when the INR is not in range, patients on warfarin therapy should be meticulously questioned regarding their medication use and symptoms related to bleeding and thromboembolic complications. Any changes in medications, including changes in dose as well as nonprescription drug and dietary supplement use, should be carefully explored (see Tables 9-16 and 9-17). If the INR is outside the therapeutic range, dietary intake of vitamin K–rich foods should also be evaluated (Table 9-18).

Anticoagulation therapy management services can optimize the care of patients who take warfarin therapy by providing structured care, comprehensive patient education, and evaluation of outcomes.[75] When anticoagulation management services are not available, individual clinicians should strive to implement a similar structured care process.[44]

Portable finger-stick INR devices are available for monitoring warfarin therapy. These devices permit clinicians to do "real-time" therapeutic drug monitoring, and enable patients to engage in self-testing and/or management at home.[44] Self-monitoring, in its simplest form, requires the patient to report his or her test results to a healthcare professional who continues to make warfarin dosing decisions. Highly motivated and sophisticated patients can be trained to manage themselves, independently altering the dose of warfarin therapy based on their INR results. Patients who engage in INR self-monitoring and warfarin self-management report high levels of satisfaction with care and maintain the INR within the therapeutic range slightly more frequently than those managed by "usual care."[44] However, home INR testing and self-management is clearly not for everyone; these modalities require careful patient selection and considerable patient education.[44] Finger-stick INR devices are relatively expensive, but some patients may qualify for limited coverage of the monitor and testing strips.

Adverse Effects

Warfarin's primary adverse effect is bleeding ranging from mild to life-threatening and can occur at any site in the body.[2] Although warfarin is not believed to cause bleeding per se, it can "unmask" bleeding from an existing lesion or enable massive bleeding from an ordinarily minor source. The GI tract and the nose are among the most frequent sites of bleeding, and intracranial hemorrhage is the most serious and feared complication related to warfarin therapy, often resulting in permanent disability or death.[2]

There are no universally accepted criteria for defining a bleeding event as major or minor. The International Society for

TABLE 9-17 Dietary Supplements that can Affect Platelet Function and Anticoagulation Status

Agent	Mechanism	Comments
Bladderwrack	Has anticoagulant effects	Increased risk of bleeding or bruising
Boldo	Constituents may have antiplatelet effects	Increased risk of bleeding or bruising
Bromelain	Decreased platelet aggregation	Increased risk of bleeding or bruising
Burdock	Decreased platelet aggregation by inhibiting platelet activation factor	Increased risk of bleeding or bruising
Caffeine	May have antiplatelet activity; not reported in humans	Increased risk of bleeding or bruising; found in black tea, green tea, guarana, mate, oolong tea
Clove	Eugenol has antiplatelet activity	Increased risk of bleeding or bruising
Cod liver oil	May inhibit platelet aggregation	Increased risk of bleeding or bruising; avoid concomitant use
Coltsfoot	May inhibit platelet aggregation	Increased risk of bleeding or bruising; avoid concomitant use
Danshen	Decreased platelet aggregation; may also have antithrombotic effects	Increased risk of bleeding or bruising; avoid concomitant use
Dong quai	May inhibit platelet aggregation	Increased risk of bleeding or bruising
Fenugreek	Constituents may have antiplatelet effects; concentration may not be clinically significant	Increased risk of bleeding or bruising
Fish oil	Has antiplatelet effects	Increased risk of bleeding or bruising
Flax seed	Decreased platelet aggregation and increased bleeding time	Increased risk of bleeding or bruising
γ-Linolenic acid (GLA)	Has anticoagulant effects	Increased risk of bleeding or bruising; found in borage and evening primrose oil
Garlic	Has anticoagulant effects and may inhibit platelet aggregation	Increased risk of bleeding or bruising
Ginger	Inhibits thromboxane synthetase and decreases platelet aggregation	Increased risk of bleeding or bruising
Ginkgo	Decreased platelet aggregation; ginkgolide B, a component of ginkgo, is a potent inhibitor of PAF	Increased risk of bleeding or bruising
Ginseng, panax	Components may decrease platelet aggregation through PAF antagonism; not shown in humans	Increased risk of bleeding or bruising; use with caution until more is known.
Ginseng, Siberian	A component, dihydroxybenzoic acid, may inhibit platelet aggregation	Increased risk of bleeding or bruising
Melatonin	Unknown; might increase the anticoagulant or antiplatelet effect; decreased prothrombin activity observed	Increased risk of bleeding or bruising
Nattokinase	Has thrombolytic activity	Increased risk of bleeding or bruising
Onion	Decreased platelet aggregation	Increased risk of bleeding or bruising
Pantethine	Decreased platelet aggregation	Increased risk of bleeding or bruising
Policosanol	Inhibits platelet aggregation	Increased risk of bleeding or bruising
Poplar	Contains salicylates and may cause decreased platelet aggregation	Increased risk of bleeding or bruising
Resveratrol	Has antiplatelet effects	Increased risk of bleeding or bruising
Sea buckthorn	Inhibits platelet aggregation	Increased risk of bleeding or bruising
Turmeric	Decreased platelet aggregation; has antiplatelet effects	Increased risk of bleeding or bruising
Vinpocetine	Has antiplatelet effects	Increased risk of bleeding or bruising
Vitamin E	Inhibits platelet aggregation and antagonizes the effects of vitamin K–dependent clotting factors	Dose dependent and significant with doses greater than 800 units/day; advise patients to avoid high doses of vitamin E; increased risk of bleeding or bruising
Willow bark	Decreased platelet aggregation; has antiplatelet effects but less than aspirin	Increased risk of bleeding or bruising

PAF, platelet activating factor.

From Nutescu et al.[72]

Thrombosis and Haemostasis defines major bleeding as fatal bleeding, any bleeding into a critical anatomic space (e.g., intracranial bleeding, hemarthrosis, or intraocular bleeding), bleeding that requires transfusion of 2 or more units of whole blood or red cells, or bleeding that leads to a greater than 2 g/dL (20 g/L; 1.2 mmol/L) drop in hemoglobin concentration.[76] Bleeding that does not meet the criteria for a major hemorrhage is generally considered to be a minor. Minor bleeding is common during warfarin therapy even in the most expertly managed patients.

Several risk factors for bleeding while taking anticoagulation therapy have been identified (see Table 9-14).[63] Intensity of anticoagulation therapy appears to be the most powerful risk factor with the likelihood of bleeding rising steeply as the INR increases above 5.[2] The risk of hemorrhage is greatest during the first few weeks of therapy; however, bleeding can occur at any time and the cumulative incidence steadily increases over time.[2]

Other adverse effects associated with warfarin are uncommon, but can be serious.[2] The "purple toe syndrome," manifested as a purplish discoloration of the toes, is reported in a very small percentage of patients receiving warfarin. The etiology of this unusual phenomenon is unknown, but is thought to be the result of cholesterol microembolization into the arterial circulation of the toes.[2]

TABLE 9-18 Vitamin K Content of Select Foods[a]

Very High (>200 mcg)	High (100–200 mcg)	Medium (50–100 mcg)	Low (<50 mcg)
Brussel sprouts	Basil	Apple, green	Apple, red
Chickpea	Broccoli	Asparagus	Avocado
Collard greens	Chive	Cabbage	Beans
Coriander	Coleslaw	Cauliflower	Breads, grains
Endive	Cucumber (with peel)	Mayonnaise	Carrot
Kale	Canola oil	Nuts, pistachio	Cereal
Lettuce, red leaf	Green onion/scallion	Squash, summer	Celery
Parsley	Lettuce, butterhead		Coffee
Spinach	Mustard greens		Corn
Swiss chard	Soybean oil		Cucumber (without peel)
Tea, green			Dairy products
Tea, black			Eggs
Turnip greens			Fruit (varies)
Watercress			Lettuce, iceberg
			Meats, fish, poultry
			Pasta
			Peanuts
			Peas
			Potato
			Rice
			Tomato

[a]Approximate amount of vitamin K per 100 g (3.5 oz) serving.

From Booth and Centurelli.[74]

Warfarin-induced skin necrosis is an uncommon but very serious dermatologic reaction that usually manifests in the first week of therapy as a painful maculopapular rash and ecchymosis or purpura that subsequently progresses to necrotic gangrene. It most frequently appears in areas of the body rich in SC fat, such as the breasts, thighs, buttocks, and abdomen.[2] The pathogenesis of warfarin-induced skin necrosis is not clearly understood, but patients with protein C or S deficiency appear to be at greater risk.[2] If the diagnosis of skin necrosis is suspected, warfarin therapy should be immediately discontinued, FFP and vitamin K administered, and full-dose UFH or LMWH therapy initiated. Restart warfarin therapy with extreme caution if at all in patients with a history of skin necrosis using small doses and gradual titration under the coverage of full-dose UFH or LMWH until therapeutic INR has been achieved.[2]

Management of Bleeding and Excessive Anticoagulation

The AT9 offer suggestions for the management of patients with an elevated INR.[44] When the INR is >4.5 without evidence of bleeding, the INR can be lowered by withholding warfarin, adjusting the dose of warfarin, and providing some dose of vitamin K to shorten the time to return to normal INR. Although vitamin K can be administered parenterally or orally, in the absence of major bleeding, the oral route is preferred. If the INR is between 4.5 and 10 and no bleeding is present, AT9 suggest against the routine use of vitamin K as it has not been shown to affect the risk of developing subsequent bleeding or thromboembolism compared with simply withholding warfarin alone. For INRs >10 without evidence of bleeding 2.5 mg of oral vitamin K is suggested.[44] Vitamin K should be used with caution in patients at high risk of recurrent thromboembolism because of the possibility of INR overcorrection. Conversely, simply withholding warfarin therapy may not lower a high INR quickly enough in patients at high risk for developing bleeding complications. Most patients with asymptomatic INR elevations can be safely managed by withholding warfarin alone. Patients with warfarin-associated major bleeding require supportive care as described previously, and in addition the AT9 suggest rapid reversal of anticoagulation with four-factor PCCs rather than FFP, but acknowledge that four-factor PCCs are currently not available in the United States. The guidelines further suggest that in addition to repletion of coagulation factors (via PCCs or FFP), 5 to 10 mg of vitamin K should be administered via slow IV injection.[44]

Drug–Drug and Drug–Food Interactions

The pharmacokinetic and pharmacodynamic properties of warfarin, coupled with its narrow therapeutic index, predispose this agent to numerous clinically important food and drug interactions.[77] Vitamin K can reverse warfarin's pharmacologic activity, and many foods contain sufficient vitamin K to reduce the anticoagulation effect of warfarin if a patient consumes them in large portions or repetitively within a short period of time.[2] Patients should be instructed to maintain a relatively consistent intake of vitamin K–rich foods. It is important to stress consistency rather than abstinence as patients with the highest daily intake of vitamin K have been shown to have more stable INR control.[78]

Pharmacokinetic drug interactions with warfarin are primarily a result of alterations in hepatic metabolism. Drugs that inhibit or induce the CYP2C9, CYP1A2, and CYP3A4 isoenzymes have the greatest potential to significantly alter the response to warfarin therapy.[2] Drugs that alter hemostasis, platelet function, or the clearance of clotting factors (e.g., thyroid hormone replacement) can alter the response to warfarin therapy or increase the risk of bleeding by pharmacodynamic mechanisms.[77] Clinicians should advise patients on warfarin therapy to seek information about potential interactions with warfarin whenever they start to take a new drug product, dietary supplement, or herbal product, whether it is prescribed or nonprescribed. If there is a known drug interaction or doubt about its

TABLE 9-19 General Approach to Periprocedural Anticoagulation Therapy Management

Days Relative to Procedure	Anticoagulation Management
−7 to −10	Assess thrombosis and bleeding risk
	Determine if bridging anticoagulation with LMWH is appropriate
	Obtain baseline INR
−7	Stop aspirin or other antiplatelet therapy if necessary
−5 or −4	Stop warfarin[a]
−3 or −2	Start LMWH[b]
−1	Give last dose of LMWH 24 hours before procedure[c]
	Verify attainment of preprocedure INR goal
0 = procedure	Resume warfarin[d] at usual maintenance dose on evening after procedure
+1	Resume LMWH[e]
	Resume aspirin or other antiplatelet therapy once hemostasis secured
>+6	Stop LMWH once INR is therapeutic

INR, international normalized ratio; LMWH, low-molecular-weight heparin.

[a]Warfarin stopped on day −5 or −4 if baseline INR 2–3 or day −6 if baseline INR is 2.5–3.5.

[b]LMWH is initiated approximately 72 hours prior to the procedure.

[c]Give only the morning dose of twice-daily therapeutic-dose LMWH and reduce by 50% the total dose of once-daily therapeutic-dose LMWH.

[d]Some clinicians instruct patients to take "booster" doses (e.g., 150% of usual dose) for 1–2 days when resuming warfarin therapy.

[e]Resume therapeutic-dose LMWH approximately 24 hours after (e.g., the day after) the procedure for minor surgical or other invasive procedures; for major surgery or high bleeding risk procedures wait 48–72 hours after the procedure and when hemostasis is secured before resuming therapeutic-dose LMWH, *or* administer prophylactic-dose LMWH when hemostasis is secured, *or* avoid LMWH completely.

From Douketis et al.[79]

potential to alter the response to warfarin, more frequent INR testing following the initiation of the new agent is prudent.[77]

Use in Special Populations

Patients scheduled to undergo invasive procedures often require temporary discontinuation of warfarin therapy.[79] The decision to withhold warfarin therapy should be based on the type of surgical procedure being performed and the patient's risk of bleeding and thromboembolism. Warfarin therapy should generally not be discontinued in patients undergoing minimally invasive procedures such as dental work, cataract surgery, or minor dermatologic procedures.[79] If the bleeding risk from the procedure is considerable, warfarin should be stopped 4 to 5 days prior to the procedure in order to allow the INR to return to near-normal values. Patients at high risk of thromboembolism (i.e., DVT or PE in the previous month) should be given so-called bridge therapy with UFH or a LMWH before and/or after the procedure (Table 9-19).[79]

PERSONALIZED PHARMACOTHERAPY

Warfarin Pharmacogenomics

At the initiation of warfarin therapy, it is difficult to predict the specific dose that an individual will require. Warfarin dosing algorithms that incorporate pharmacogenetic information regarding CYP2C9 and VKOR polymorphisms are currently being evaluated. However, the clinical utility and cost-effectiveness of using pharmacogenetic information to guide warfarin initiation remains unproven and AT9 suggest against routine use.[44]

EVALUATION OF THERAPEUTIC OUTCOMES

9 The appropriate initial duration of warfarin therapy to effectively treat an acute first episode of VTE for all patients is 3 months.[7] Three months of therapeutic anticoagulation therapy reduces the risk of recurrent VTE to as low as can be achieved by a time-limited duration of therapy. To prevent new episodes of VTE that are not directly related to the preceding episode, continued warfarin therapy is required.[1] Individually tailoring warfarin maintenance duration therapy past 3 months requires careful consideration of the circumstances surrounding the initial thromboembolic event, the presence of ongoing thromboembolic risk factors and the risk of bleeding, and patient preference.[7]

The most important considerations in determining the risk of recurrent VTE once anticoagulation therapy is stopped is whether the initial thrombotic event was associated with a major transient or reversible risk factor (e.g., surgery, plaster cast immobilization of a leg, or hospitalization in the month prior to VTE) and the presence of active cancer.[7] The estimated cumulative risk of recurrent VTE after stopping anticoagulant therapy for VTE provoked by surgery is 1% after 1 year and 3% after 5 years, and that for VTE provoked by a nonsurgical reversible risk factor is 5% after 1 year and 15% after 5 years. Three months of anticoagulation therapy is recommended in these situations.[7] Patients with a first unprovoked (idiopathic) VTE have a recurrence risk of approximately 10% in the first year and approximately 30% and 50% over 5 and 10 years, respectively. These patients should be considered for extended warfarin therapy when feasible.[7] Extended in this context refers to warfarin that is continued beyond 3 months without a scheduled stop date, but which may be stopped because of a subsequent increase in the risk of bleeding or change in patient preference for anticoagulation.[7] Anticoagulant treatment is rarely stopped in patients with VTE and active cancer because of a high risk for recurrence.[7] Factors that may lead to the decision to stop warfarin therapy after 3 months include noncompliance with therapy, initial clot even though idiopathic was isolated in calf veins, or a moderate to high risk of bleeding.[7]

Clinically important risk factors for bleeding include age >75 years, previous noncardioembolic stroke, history of GI bleeding, renal or hepatic impairment, anemia, thrombocytopenia, concurrent antiplatelet use (avoid if possible), noncompliance, poor anticoagulant control, serious acute or chronic illness, and the presence of a structural lesion (e.g., tumor, recent surgery) expected to be associated with bleeding. Presence of one to two bleeding risk factors suggests moderate bleeding risk while three or more risk factors suggest a high bleeding risk.[80] For patients with second episode of idiopathic VTE, extended anticoagulation is recommended.[7]

Various secondary strategies aimed at identifying patients at very low risk of recurrence after a first idiopathic VTE are being evaluated in clinical trials. Safe withdrawal of warfarin therapy may be possible if reliable identification of these patients proves possible. Estimating an individual patient's risk of recurrent VTE using a variety of interacting clinical, laboratory, and radiologic findings can be accomplished with increasing precision.[53] Some factors that may predict lower risk of recurrence include female gender, low D-dimer levels 1 month after stopping warfarin therapy, absence of residual clot on ultrasound, absence of hereditary and acquired thrombophilia, and absence of the postthrombotic syndrome. Risk assessment derived from combining several independent risk factors for recurrence has also been investigated.[7] Further validation is needed before any one factor or prediction rule using a combination of factors can justify routinely stopping warfarin after 3 months of therapy. The decision to continue extended warfarin therapy should be reassessed periodically. Patients should be involved in any decision to continue anticoagulation therapy with consideration given to the patient's long-term prognosis, risk of bleeding, ability to adhere to anticoagulation therapy instructions, financial resources, lifestyle, and quality of life.[7] Although warfarin targeted to an INR of 2 to 3 is very effective at preventing recurrence while patients are receiving therapy, when it is stopped, there is a similar risk of recurrence whether patients have been treated for 3 months or longer. The same is true for other anticoagulants used for extended therapy (e.g., LMWH, rivaroxaban).[7]

Increasingly, patients with VTE are being tested for hereditary and acquired hypercoagulable states (thrombophilia). The available evidence does not support an association between genetically transmitted thrombophilia and a higher chance of recurrent VTE.[13] Despite a lack of convincing evidence, most experts recommend indefinite anticoagulation for individuals with the antiphospholipid antibody syndrome, homozygotes for the factor V Leiden mutation, and heterozygotes with both the factor V Leiden and prothrombin 20210 gene mutations.

NATIONAL QUALITY INITIATIVES

Even though several clinical interventions are known to be effective in preventing and treating VTE, adherence with various consensus guidelines regarding thromboprophylaxis remains alarmingly low.[81] Although preventing VTE is a significant patient safety issue, there is little public awareness of the life-threatening nature of DVT and PE. A survey conducted on behalf of the American Public Health Association suggests that 75% of Americans have little or no awareness of DVT, and less than one half of respondents could identify any risk factors associated with its development.[82] Recognizing the lack of public awareness, several organizations have focused on increasing consumer knowledge of the risks, signs, and symptoms of VTE through increased media visibility.

Given the number and variety of clinical conditions or circumstances that place individuals at risk for VTE, improvements in VTE prevention and care have the potential to benefit many patients. Over the past decade, the focus on quality healthcare has been emphasized by the call to accountability through the Joint Commission's Agenda for Change, the Institute of Medicine's report on medical errors, the National Quality Forum's (NQF's) endorsed safe practices, the Leapfrog Group, and the demand for value by healthcare consumers (Table 9-20).[83,84] The NQF has developed national consensus standards for VTE prevention and treatment that will be applicable to a variety of healthcare settings.[84] The outcomes of this effort will provide a framework for measuring the effective screening, prevention, and treatment of VTE. NQF's recommendations include developing organizational policies that address staff education, treatment protocols, and adherence measurements to improve VTE prevention in the hospital. The ultimate goal of the NQF consensus standards is to facilitate early promulgation of VTE policies, risk assessment, prophylaxis, diagnosis, and treatment services as well as patient education and organizational accountability. To that end, the Joint Commission has developed performance measures to enforce the NQF's recommendations.[83] Four major domains have been identified: risk assessment, prevention, diagnosis, and treatment. Six measures have been selected for implementation as core VTE quality measures. It is expected that compliance and reporting on these measures eventually will be tied to payment from governmental entities such as Medicare and Medicaid (Table 9-21).

Hopefully, through the concerted efforts of government and accrediting agencies working with hospitals and other healthcare institutions, the incidence of DVT and PE will begin to fall. Systematic approaches to this problem are needed at every level, starting with increased public and health practitioner awareness, continuing with the uniform use of effective prophylactic strategies in patients at risk, and concluding with greater accountability with precise quality measurements.

TABLE 9-20 Organizations Monitoring Quality Care

The Joint Commission
www.jointcommission.org
A not-for-profit healthcare accreditation organization that issues performance-based standards and assesses organizational compliance to improve patient safety and quality of care

Leapfrog Group
www.leapfroggroup.org
An initiative of healthcare purchasing organizations seeking improvements in safety, quality, and affordability of healthcare, with funding from the Business Roundtable, Robert Wood Johnson Foundation, and member organizations

National Quality Forum
www.qualityforum.org
A not-for-profit that develops and implements national strategies for healthcare quality measurement and reporting

TABLE 9-21 The Joint Commission's Proposed Performance Measures for the Prevention and Treatment of Venous Thrombosis

Number	Description of Proposed Performance Measure
1	Documentation of venous thromboembolism risk assessment/ prophylaxis within 24 hours of hospital admission
2	Documentation of venous thromboembolism risk assessment/ prophylaxis within 24 hours of transfer to intensive care unit
3	Venous thromboembolism patients with overlap of parenteral and warfarin anticoagulation therapy
4	Venous thromboembolism patients receiving unfractionated heparin by nomogram/protocol and with platelet count monitoring
5	Venous thromboembolism discharge instructions
6	Incidence of potentially preventable hospital-acquired venous thromboembolism

From the Joint Commission.[83]

ABBREVIATIONS

AAOS	American Academy of Orthopaedic Surgery
ABCG2	ATP-binding cassette G2
ADP	adenosine diphosphate
aPC	activated protein C
aPTT	activated partial thromboplastin time
AT9	*Antithrombotic Therapy and Prevention of Thrombosis, 9th ed: Evidence-Based Clinical Practice Guidelines* published by the American College of Chest Physicians
CT	computed tomography
CTPH	chronic thromboembolic pulmonary hypertension
CUS	compression ultrasound
CYP	cytochrome P450
DVT	deep vein thrombosis
ELISA	enzyme-linked immunosorbent assay
FFP	fresh-frozen plasma
gp	glycoprotein
HIT	heparin-induced thrombocytopenia
INR	international normalized ratio
IPC	intermittent pneumatic compression
ISI	International Sensitivity Index
IVC	inferior vena cava
LDUH	low-dose unfractionated heparin
LMWH	low-molecular-weight heparin
NQF	National Quality Forum
PCCs	prothrombin complex concentrates

PE	pulmonary embolism
PESI	Pulmonary Embolism Severity Index
PF-4	platelet factor-4
PT	prothrombin time
SC	subcutaneous
UFH	unfractionated heparin
V/Q	ventilation–perfusion
VIIa	activated factor VII
VKOR	vitamin K epoxide reductase
VTE	venous thromboembolism
WHO	World Health Organization

REFERENCES

1. Goldhaber SZ, Bounameaux H. Pulmonary embolism and deep vein thrombosis. Lancet 2012;379(9828):1835–1846.
2. Ageno W, Gallus AS, Wittkowsky A, Crowther M, Hylek EM, Palareti G. Oral anticoagulant therapy: Antithrombotic Therapy and Prevention of Thrombosis, 9th ed: American College of Chest Physicians Evidence-Based Clinical Practice Guidelines. Chest 2012;141(2 Suppl):e44S–e88S.
3. Garcia DA, Baglin TP, Weitz JI, Samama MM. Parenteral anticoagulants: Antithrombotic Therapy and Prevention of Thrombosis, 9th ed: American College of Chest Physicians Evidence-Based Clinical Practice Guidelines. Chest 2012;141(2 Suppl):e24S–e43S.
4. Falck-Ytter Y, Francis CW, Johanson NA, et al. Prevention of VTE in orthopedic surgery patients: Antithrombotic Therapy and Prevention of Thrombosis, 9th ed: American College of Chest Physicians Evidence-Based Clinical Practice Guidelines. Chest 2012;141(2 Suppl):e278S–e325S.
5. Gould MK, Garcia DA, Wren SM, et al. Prevention of VTE in nonorthopedic surgical patients: Antithrombotic Therapy and Prevention of Thrombosis, 9th ed: American College of Chest Physicians Evidence-Based Clinical Practice Guidelines. Chest 2012;141(2 Suppl):e227S–e277S.
6. Kahn SR, Lim W, Dunn AS, et al. Prevention of VTE in nonsurgical patients: Antithrombotic Therapy and Prevention of Thrombosis, 9th ed: American College of Chest Physicians Evidence-Based Clinical Practice Guidelines. Chest 2012;141(2 Suppl):e195S–e226S.
7. Kearon C, Akl EA, Comerota AJ, et al. Antithrombotic therapy for VTE disease: Antithrombotic Therapy and Prevention of Thrombosis, 9th ed: American College of Chest Physicians Evidence-Based Clinical Practice Guidelines. Chest 2012;141(2 Suppl):e419S–e494S.
8. Reitsma PH, Versteeg HH, Middeldorp S. Mechanistic view of risk factors for venous thromboembolism. Arterioscler Thromb Vasc Biol 2012;32(3):563–568.
9. Turpie AG, Esmon C. Venous and arterial thrombosis—Pathogenesis and the rationale for anticoagulation. Thromb Haemost 2011;105(4):586–596.
10. Margaglione M, Grandone E. Population genetics of venous thromboembolism. A narrative review. Thromb Haemost 2011;105(2):221–231.
11. Anderson JA, Weitz JI. Hypercoagulable states. Crit Care Clin 2011;27(4):933–952, vii.
12. Dalen JE. Should patients with venous thromboembolism be screened for thrombophilia? Am J Med 2008;121(6):458–463.
13. Rosendaal FR, Reitsma PH. Genetics of venous thrombosis. J Thromb Haemost 2009;7(Suppl 1):301–304.
14. Khorana AA. Cancer and coagulation. Am J Hematol 2012;87(Suppl 1):S82–S87.
15. Buller HR, van Doormaal FF, van Sluis GL, Kamphuisen PW. Cancer and thrombosis: From molecular mechanisms to clinical presentations. J Thromb Haemost 2007;5(Suppl 1):246–254.
16. Giannakopoulos B, Passam F, Rahgozar S, Krilis SA. Current concepts on the pathogenesis of the antiphospholipid syndrome. Blood 2007;109(2):422–430.
17. Bates SM, Greer IA, Middeldorp S, Veenstra DL, Prabulos AM, Vandvik PO. VTE, thrombophilia, antithrombotic therapy, and pregnancy: Antithrombotic Therapy and Prevention of Thrombosis, 9th ed: American College of Chest Physicians Evidence-Based Clinical Practice Guidelines. Chest 2012;141(2 Suppl):e691S–e736S.
18. Rosendaal FR, Helmerhorst FM, Vandenbroucke JP. Female hormones and thrombosis. Arterioscler Thromb Vasc Biol 2002;22(2):201–210.
19. Crowther MA, Kelton JG. Congenital thrombophilic states associated with venous thrombosis: A qualitative overview and proposed classification system. Ann Intern Med 2003;138(2):128–134.
20. Dahlback B. Advances in understanding pathogenic mechanisms of thrombophilic disorders. Blood 2008;112(1):19–27.
21. Furie B, Furie BC. Thrombus formation in vivo. J Clin Invest 2005;115(12):3355–3362.
22. Furie B, Furie BC. Mechanisms of thrombus formation. N Engl J Med 2008;359(9):938–949.
23. Crawley JT, Zanardelli S, Chion CK, Lane DA. The central role of thrombin in hemostasis. J Thromb Haemost 2007;5(Suppl 1):95–101.
24. Monroe DM, Hoffman M. What does it take to make the perfect clot? Arterioscler Thromb Vasc Biol 2006;26(1):41–48.
25. Rijken DC, Lijnen HR. New insights into the molecular mechanisms of the fibrinolytic system. J Thromb Haemost 2009;7(1):4–13.
26. Kearon C. Natural history of venous thromboembolism. Circulation 2003;107(23 Suppl 1):I22–I30.
27. Pruitt B, Lawson R. What you need to know about venous thromboembolism. Nursing 2009;39(4):22–27.
28. Bates SM, Jaeschke R, Stevens SM, et al. Diagnosis of DVT: Antithrombotic Therapy and Prevention of Thrombosis, 9th ed: American College of Chest Physicians Evidence-Based Clinical Practice Guidelines. Chest 2012;141 (2 Suppl):e351S–e418S.
29. Tapson VF. Acute pulmonary embolism. N Engl J Med 2008;358(10):1037–1052.
30. Bauersachs RM. Clinical presentation of deep vein thrombosis and pulmonary embolism. Best Pract Res Clin Haematol 2012;25(3):243–251.
31. Righini M, Perrier A, De Moerloose P, Bounameaux H. D-dimer for venous thromboembolism diagnosis: 20 years later. J Thromb Haemost 2008;6(7):1059–1071.
32. Mahan CE, Holdsworth MT, Welch SM, Borrego M, Spyropoulos AC. Deep-vein thrombosis: A United States cost model for a preventable and costly adverse event. Thromb Haemost 2011;106(3):405–415.
33. Guyatt GH, Eikelboom JW, Gould MK, et al. Approach to outcome measurement in the prevention of thrombosis in surgical and medical patients: Antithrombotic Therapy and Prevention of Thrombosis, 9th ed: American College of Chest Physicians Evidence-Based Clinical Practice Guidelines. Chest 2012;141(2 Suppl):e185S–e194S.
34. Gray J, Razmus I. Improving venous thromboembolism prevention processes and outcomes at a community hospital. Jt Comm J Qual Patient Saf 2012;38(2):61–66.

35. Schiro TA, Sakowski J, Romanelli RJ, et al. Improving adherence to best-practice guidelines for venous thromboembolism risk assessment and prevention. Am J Health Syst Pharm 2011;68(22):2184–2189.
36. Streiff MB, Haut ER. The CMS ruling on venous thromboembolism after total knee or hip arthroplasty: Weighing risks and benefits. JAMA 2009;301(10): 1063–1065.
37. Bauersachs R, Berkowitz SD, Brenner B, et al. Oral rivaroxaban for symptomatic venous thromboembolism. N Engl J Med 2010;363(26):2499–2510.
38. Buller HR, Prins MH, Lensin AW, et al. Oral rivaroxaban for the treatment of symptomatic pulmonary embolism. N Engl J Med 2012;366(14):1287–1297.
39. ASHP Therapeutic Position Statement on the Use of Low-Molecular-Weight Heparins for Adult Outpatient Treatment of Acute Deep-Vein Thrombosis. Am J Health Syst Pharm 2004;61(18):1950–1955.
40. Anderson RC, Bussey HI. Retrievable and permanent inferior vena cava filters: Selected considerations. Pharmacotherapy 2006;26(11):1595–1600.
41. Geerts WH, Bergqvist D, Pineo GF, et al. Prevention of venous thromboembolism: American College of Chest Physicians Evidence-Based Clinical Practice Guidelines (8th Edition). Chest 2008;133(6 Suppl):381S–453S.
42. Anderson FA Jr, Huang W, Friedman RJ, Kwong LM, Lieberman JR, Pellegrini VD Jr. Prevention of venous thromboembolism after hip or knee arthroplasty: Findings from a 2008 survey of US orthopedic surgeons. J Arthroplasty 2012;27(5):659–666.
43. Mont MA, Jacobs JJ. AAOS clinical practice guideline: Preventing venous thromboembolic disease in patients undergoing elective hip and knee arthroplasty. J Am Acad Orthop Surg 2011;19(12):777–778.
44. Holbrook A, Schulman S, Witt DM, et al. Evidence-based management of anticoagulant therapy: Antithrombotic Therapy and Prevention of Thrombosis, 9th ed: American College of Chest Physicians Evidence-Based Clinical Practice Guidelines. Chest 2012;141(2 Suppl):e152S–e184S.
45. Matchar DB, Mark DB. Strategies for incorporating resource allocation and economic considerations: American College of Chest Physicians Evidence-Based Clinical Practice Guidelines (8th Edition). Chest 2008;133(6 Suppl): 132S–140S.
46. Kapoor A, Chuang W, Radhakrishnan N, et al. Cost effectiveness of venous thromboembolism pharmacological prophylaxis in total hip and knee replacement: A systematic review. Pharmacoeconomics 2010;28(7):521–538.
47. Mamdani MM, Racine E, McCreadie S, et al. Clinical and economic effectiveness of an inpatient anticoagulation service. Pharmacotherapy 1999;19(9):1064–1074.
48. Kearon C, Ginsberg JS, Julian JA, et al. Comparison of fixed-dose weight-adjusted unfractionated heparin and low-molecular-weight heparin for acute treatment of venous thromboembolism. JAMA 2006;296(8):935–942.
49. Goldhaber SZ. Advanced treatment strategies for acute pulmonary embolism, including thrombolysis and embolectomy. J Thromb Haemost 2009;7(Suppl 1):322–327.
50. Arixtra Prescribing Information. GlaxoSmithKline. September 2012, http://us.gsk.com/products/assets/us_arixtra.pdf.
51. Tillman DJ, Charland SL, Witt DM. Effectiveness and economic impact associated with a program for outpatient management of acute deep vein thrombosis in a group model health maintenance organization. Arch Intern Med 2000;160(19):2926–2932.
52. Gould MK, Dembitzer AD, Sanders GD, Garber AM. Low-molecular-weight heparins compared with unfractionated heparin for treatment of acute deep venous thrombosis. A cost-effectiveness analysis. Ann Intern Med 1999;130(10):789–799.
53. Baglin T. What happens after venous thromboembolism? J Thromb Haemost 2009;7(Suppl 1):287–290.
54. Aujesky D, Hughes R, Jimenez D. Short-term prognosis of pulmonary embolism. J Thromb Haemost 2009;7(Suppl 1): 318–321.
55. Schulman S, Kearon C, Kakkar AK, et al. Dabigatran versus warfarin in the treatment of acute venous thromboembolism. N Engl J Med 2009;361(24):2342–2352.
56. Ginsberg JS, Bates SM. Management of venous thromboembolism during pregnancy. J Thromb Haemost 2003;1(7):1435–1442.
57. Eliquis Prescribing Information. Bristol-Myers Squibb/Pfizer. September 2012, http://www.eliquis.eu/pdf/UK%20PI%20October%202011.pdf.
58. Pradaxa Prescribing Information. Boehringer-Ingelheim. September 2012, http://bidocs.boehringer-ingelheim.com/BIWebAccess/ViewServlet.ser?docBase=renetnt&folderPath=/Prescribing%20Information/PIs/Pradaxa/Pradaxa.pdf.
59. Xarelto Prescribing Information. Janssen Pharmaceuticals Inc. September 2012, http://www.xareltohcp.com/sites/default/files/pdf/xarelto_0.pdf#zoom=100/.
60. Stone SE, Morris TA. Pulmonary embolism and pregnancy. Crit Care Clin 2004;20(4):661–677, ix.
61. Monagle P, Chan AK, Goldenberg NA, et al. Antithrombotic therapy in neonates and children: Antithrombotic Therapy and Prevention of Thrombosis, 9th ed: American College of Chest Physicians Evidence-Based Clinical Practice Guidelines. Chest 2012;141(2 Suppl):e737S–e801S.
62. Delate T, Witt DM, Ritzwoller D, et al. Outpatient use of low molecular weight heparin monotherapy for first-line treatment of venous thromboembolism in advanced cancer. Oncologist 2012;17(3):419–427.
63. Schulman S, Beyth RJ, Kearon C, Levine MN. Hemorrhagic complications of anticoagulant and thrombolytic treatment: American College of Chest Physicians Evidence-Based Clinical Practice Guidelines (8th Edition). Chest 2008;133 (6 Suppl):257S–298S.
64. Clark NP. Low-molecular-weight heparin use in the obese, elderly, and in renal insufficiency. Thromb Res 2008;123(Suppl 1):S58–S61.
65. Lovenox Prescribing Information. Sanofi-Aventis Pharmaceuticals. September 2012, http://products.sanofi-aventis.us/lovenox/lovenox.html.
66. Linkins LA, Dans AL, Moores LK, et al. Treatment and prevention of heparin-induced thrombocytopenia: Antithrombotic Therapy and Prevention of Thrombosis, 9th ed: American College of Chest Physicians Evidence-Based Clinical Practice Guidelines. Chest 2012;141(2 Suppl):e495S–e530S.
67. Crowther MA, Cook DJ, Albert M, et al. The 4Ts scoring system for heparin-induced thrombocytopenia in medical-surgical intensive care unit patients. J Crit Care 2010;25(2):287–293.
68. Cuker A, Gimotty PA, Crowther MA, Warkentin TE. Predictive value of the 4Ts scoring system for heparin-induced thrombocytopenia: A systematic review and meta-analysis. Blood 2012;120(5):4160–4167.
69. Blackmer AB, Oertel MD, Valgus JM. Fondaparinux and the management of heparin-induced thrombocytopenia: The journey continues. Ann Pharmacother 2009;43(10): 1636–1646.

70. Kaatz S, Kouides PA, Garcia DA, et al. Guidance on the emergent reversal of oral thrombin and factor Xa inhibitors. Am J Hematol 2012;87(Suppl 1):S141–S145.
71. Coumadin Prescribing Information. Bristol-Myers Squibb. September 2012, http://packageinserts.bms.com/pi/pi_coumadin.pdf.
72. Nutescu EA, Shapiro NL, Ibrahim S, West P. Warfarin and its interactions with foods, herbs and other dietary supplements. Expert Opin Drug Saf 2006;5(3):433–451.
73. Rose AJ, Ozonoff A, Berlowitz DR, Ash AS, Reisman JI, Hylek EM. Reexamining the recommended follow-up interval after obtaining an in-range international normalized ratio value: Results from the Veterans Affairs study to improve anticoagulation. Chest 2011;140(2):359–365.
74. Booth SL, Centurelli MA. Vitamin K: A practical guide to the dietary management of patients on warfarin. Nutr Rev 1999;57(9 Pt 1):288–296.
75. Garcia DA, Witt DM, Hylek E, et al. Delivery of optimized anticoagulant therapy: Consensus statement from the Anticoagulation Forum. Ann Pharmacother 2008;42(7):979–988.
76. Seto AC, Kenyon K, Wittkowsky AK. Discrepancies in identification of major bleeding events in patients taking warfarin. Pharmacotherapy 2008;28(9):1098–1103.
77. Holbrook AM, Pereira JA, Labiris R, et al. Systematic overview of warfarin and its drug and food interactions. Arch Intern Med 2005;165(10):1095–1106.
78. Schurgers LJ, Shearer MJ, Hamulyak K, Stocklin E, Vermeer C. Effect of vitamin K intake on the stability of oral anticoagulant treatment: Dose–response relationships in healthy subjects. Blood 2004;104(9):2682–2689.
79. Douketis JD, Spyropoulos AC, Spencer FA, et al. Perioperative management of antithrombotic therapy: Antithrombotic Therapy and Prevention of Thrombosis, 9th ed: American College of Chest Physicians Evidence-Based Clinical Practice Guidelines. Chest 2012;141 (2 Suppl): e326S–e350S.
80. Kearon C. Balancing risks and benefits of extended anticoagulant therapy for idiopathic venous thrombosis. J Thromb Haemost 2009;7(Suppl 1):296–300.
81. Herner SJ, Paulson DC, Delate T, Witt DM, Vondracek TG. Evaluation of venous thromboembolism risk following hospitalization. J Thromb Thrombolysis 2011;32(1):32–39.
82. American Public Health Association. Deep-Vein Thrombosis: Advancing Awareness to Protect Patient Lives. White Paper, Public Health Leadership Conference on Deep-Vein Thrombosis. September 2009, http://www.apha.org/NR/rdonlyres/A209F84A-7C0E-4761-9ECF-61D22E1E11F7/0/DVT_White_Paper.pdf.
83. The Joint Commission. National Consensus Standards on the Prevention and Care of Venous Thromboembolism. September 2009, http://www.jointcommission.org/PerformanceMeasurement/PerformanceMeasurement/VTE.htm.
84. The National Quality Forum. Establishing a Patient-Centered National Action Plan for Deep Vein Thrombosis Prevention, Treatment, and Research. Conference Proceedings. Washington, DC: National Quality Forum, 2007.

10

Stroke

Susan C. Fagan and David C. Hess

KEY CONCEPTS

1. Stroke can be either ischemic (87%) or hemorrhagic (13%) and the two types are treated differently.
2. Transient ischemic attacks (TIAs) require urgent intervention to reduce the risk of stroke, which is known to be highest in the first few days after TIA.
3. Carotid endarterectomy should be performed in ischemic stroke patients with 70% to 99% stenosis of the ipsilateral carotid artery, provided that it is done in an experienced center.
4. Carotid stenting is an option for stroke patients eligible for carotid endarterectomy, especially in patients less than 70 years of age.
5. Early reperfusion (<4.5 hours from onset) with tissue plasminogen activator (tPA) has been shown to reduce the ultimate disability due to ischemic stroke.
6. Antiplatelet therapy is the cornerstone of antithrombotic therapy for the secondary prevention of noncardioembolic ischemic stroke.
7. Oral anticoagulation is recommended for the secondary prevention of cardioembolic stroke in moderate- to high-risk patients.
8. Blood pressure lowering is effective in both the primary and secondary prevention of both ischemic and hemorrhagic stroke regardless of blood pressure.
9. Blood pressure lowering in the acute ischemic stroke period (first 7 days) may result in decreased cerebral blood flow and worsened symptoms.
10. Statin therapy is recommended for all ischemic stroke patients, regardless of baseline cholesterol, to reduce stroke recurrence.

(1) Stroke is the leading cause of disability among adults and the fourth leading cause of death in the United States, behind cardiovascular disease, cancer, and chronic lower respiratory diseases.[1] Despite a 30% reduction in stroke mortality between 1995 and 2005, stroke occurs in the United States at a rate of almost 800,000 per year and resulted in 133,750,000 deaths in 2008.[1,2] Aggressive efforts to organize stroke care at the local and regional levels and increased utilization of evidence-based recommendations and national guidelines may have contributed to the improved outcomes.

EPIDEMIOLOGY

There are currently 6.5 million stroke survivors in the United States, and stroke is the leading cause of adult disability.[2] Of those free of the diagnosis of stroke or transient ischemic attack (TIA), however, almost 20% of individuals over the age of 45 years reported at least one stroke symptom,[3] suggesting rampant underdiagnosing. Owing in part to the need for expensive posthospitalization rehabilitation and nursing home care, the annual cost of stroke in the United States is estimated to be $69 billion.[2] Current projections are that death caused by stroke will increase exponentially in the next 30 years owing to aging of the population and our inability to control risk factors.[4]

African Americans have stroke rates that are twice those of whites, and the difference is exaggerated at younger ages.[2] In addition, geographic disparity in stroke incidence exists, such that many states in the southeastern United States have stroke mortality rates 40% higher than the national average.[2]

Etiology

(2) Stroke can be either ischemic or hemorrhagic (87% and 13%, respectively, of all strokes in the 2012 American Heart Association [AHA] report).[2] Hemorrhagic strokes include subarachnoid hemorrhage (SAH), intracerebral hemorrhage (ICH), and subdural hematomas. SAH occurs when blood enters the subarachnoid space (where cerebrospinal fluid is housed) owing to trauma, rupture of an intracranial aneurysm, or rupture of an arteriovenous malformation (AVM). By contrast, ICH occurs when a blood vessel ruptures within the brain parenchyma itself, resulting in the formation of a hematoma. These types of hemorrhages very often are associated with uncontrolled high blood pressure and sometimes antithrombotic or thrombolytic therapy. Subdural hematomas refer to collections of blood below the dura (covering of the brain), and they are caused most often by trauma. Hemorrhagic stroke, although less common, is significantly more lethal than ischemic stroke, with 30-day case-fatality rates that are two to six times higher.[5,6]

Ischemic strokes are caused either by local thrombus formation or by embolic phenomena, resulting in occlusion of a cerebral artery. Atherosclerosis, particularly of the cerebral vasculature, is a causative factor in most cases of ischemic stroke, although 30% are cryptogenic. Emboli can arise from either intracranial or extracranial arteries (including the aortic arch) or, as is the case in 20% of all ischemic strokes, the heart. Cardiogenic embolism is presumed to have occurred if the patient has concomitant atrial fibrillation, valvular heart disease, or any other condition of the heart that can lead to clot formation.[7] Distinguishing between cardiogenic embolism and other causes of ischemic stroke is important in determining long-term pharmacotherapy in a given patient.

Risk Factors

Risk factors for stroke can be subdivided into nonmodifiable, modifiable, and potentially modifiable. In addition, risk factors can be

TABLE 10-1 Risk Factors for Ischemic Stroke

Nonmodifiable risk factors or risk markers
Age
Sex
Low birth weight
Race
Family history of stroke/TIA
Modifiable, well documented
Cigarette smoking
Hypertension
Diabetes
High total cholesterol
Low HDL cholesterol
Atrial fibrillation
Sickle cell disease
Postmenopausal hormone therapy
Oral contraceptive use
High-sodium/low-potassium diet
Obesity
Physical inactivity
Other cardiac diseases (coronary heart disease, heart failure, PAD)
Potentially modifiable, less well documented
Migraine with aura
Metabolic syndrome
Drug and alcohol abuse
Hemostatic and inflammatory factors
Homocysteinemia
Sleep-disordered breathing
Periodontal disease
Infectious diseases (chlamydia, *Cytomegalovirus*, *Helicobacter pylori*)

Reproduced from reference 8.

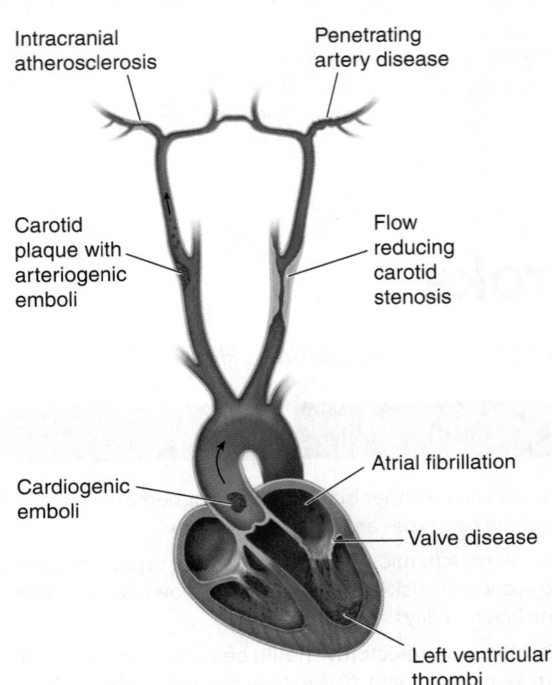

FIGURE 10-1 Pathophysiology of ischemic stroke. Diagram illustrating the three major mechanisms underlying ischemic stroke including occlusion of an intracranial vessel by an embolus that arises from a distant site (e.g., cardiogenic embolus), in situ thrombosis of an intracranial vessel, typically affecting the small penetrating arteries, and hypoperfusion caused by flow-limiting stenosis of a major extracranial artery. *(Reproduced with permission from Longo DL, Fauci AS, Kasper DL, et al. Harrison's Principals and Practice of Internal Medicine, 18th ed. New York: McGraw-Hill, 2012.)*

either well documented or less well documented.[8] The main risk factors of stroke are listed in Table 10-1. Recommendations for risk factor reduction aggressively target the modifiable, well-documented risk factors, even in individuals with nonmodifiable risk.[8] The nonmodifiable risk factors are age, race, sex, low birth weight, and family history. An individual's risk of having a stroke increases substantially as he or she ages, with a doubling of risk for each decade older than 55 years of age. African Americans, Asian-Pacific Islanders, and Hispanics experience higher death rates than their white counterparts.[2] Men are at a higher risk of stroke than women when matched for age, but women who suffer from a stroke are more likely to die from it.[2]

The most common modifiable, well-documented risk factors for stroke include hypertension, cigarette smoking, diabetes, atrial fibrillation, and dyslipidemia. The treatment of hypertension, beginning in the mid-20th century, is thought to be primarily responsible for the drastic reduction in stroke death rates between 1950 and 1980 in the United States.[4] A second very important risk factor for stroke is cardiac disease. Patients with coronary artery disease, congestive heart failure, left ventricular hypertrophy, and especially atrial fibrillation are at increased risk of stroke.[8] In fact, the presence of atrial fibrillation is one of the most potent risk factors for ischemic stroke, with stroke rates from 5% to 20% per year depending on the patient's comorbid conditions.[9] Other known risk factors for atherosclerosis are also known to place patients at risk of stroke. Diabetes mellitus, dyslipidemia, and cigarette smoking are known atherogenic states that lead to cerebrovascular disease and ischemic stroke.[9]

PATHOPHYSIOLOGY

Ischemic Stroke

Ischemic stroke results from an occlusion of a cerebral artery, leading to a reduction in cerebral blood flow. The pathophysiologic mechanisms of ischemic stroke are given in Figure 10-1. Normal cerebral blood flow averages 50 mL/100 g per minute, and this is maintained over a wide range of blood pressures (mean arterial pressures of 50 to 150 mm Hg) by a process called *cerebral autoregulation*. Cerebral blood vessels dilate and constrict in response to changes in blood pressure, but this process can be impaired by atherosclerosis, chronic hypertension, and acute injury, such as stroke. Arterial occlusion leads to severe reductions in cerebral blood flow leading to *infarction*. Tissue that is ischemic but maintains membrane integrity is referred to as the ischemic *penumbra* because it usually surrounds the infarct core. This penumbra is potentially salvageable through therapeutic intervention.

Reduction in the provision of nutrients to the ischemic cell eventually leads to depletion of the high-energy phosphates (e.g., adenosine triphosphate [ATP]) and accumulation of extracellular potassium, intracellular sodium, and water, leading to cell swelling and eventual lysis. The increase in intracellular calcium that follows results in the activation of lipases, proteases, and endonucleases and the release of free fatty acids from membrane phospholipids. In addition, there is a release of excitatory amino acids, such as glutamate and aspartate, that perpetuates the neuronal damage and the accumulation of free fatty acids, including arachidonic acid, and results in the formation of prostaglandins, leukotrienes, and free radicals. In ischemia, the magnitude of free radical production overwhelms normal scavenging systems, leaving these reactive molecules to attack cell membranes and contribute to the mounting intracellular acidosis. All these events occur within 2 to 3 hours of the onset of ischemia and contribute to the ultimate cell death.[10]

Later targets for intervention in the pathophysiologic process involved after cerebral ischemia include inflammation and apoptosis, or programmed cell death, occurring many hours after the acute insult and can interfere with recovery and repair of brain tissue.[10]

Hemorrhagic Stroke

The pathophysiology of hemorrhagic stroke is not as well studied as that of ischemic stroke. However, it is known that the presence of blood in the brain parenchyma causes damage to the surrounding tissue through the mechanical effect it produces (mass effect) and the neurotoxicity of the blood components and their degradation products.[5,6] Approximately 30% of ICHs continue to enlarge over the first 24 hours, most within 4 hours, and clot volume is the most important predictor of outcome, regardless of location.[11,12] Hemorrhage volumes >60 mL are associated with 71% to 93% mortality at 30 days.[5,6] Much of the early mortality of hemorrhagic stroke (up to 50% at 30 days) is caused by the abrupt increase in intracranial pressure that can lead to herniation and death.[1] There is also evidence to support that both early and late edema contributes to worsened outcome after ICH.[6]

CLINICAL PRESENTATION (INCLUDING DIAGNOSTIC CONSIDERATIONS)

Stroke is a term used to describe an abrupt-onset focal neurologic deficit that lasts at least 24 hours and is of presumed vascular origin. A TIA is the same but lasts less than 24 hours and usually less than 30 minutes. The abrupt onset and the duration of the symptoms are determined through the history. The use of sensitive imaging techniques (magnetic resonance imaging [MRI] with diffusion-weighted imaging [DWI]) has revealed that symptoms lasting more than 1 hour and less than 24 hours are associated with infarction, making TIA and minor stroke clinically indistinguishable. The location of the CNS injury and its reference to a specific arterial distribution in the brain are determined through the neurologic examination and confirmed by imaging studies such as computed tomography (CT) scanning and MRI. The main arterial supply to the cerebral hemispheres is illustrated in Figure 10-2. Further diagnostic tests are performed to identify the cause of the patient's stroke and to design appropriate therapeutic strategies to prevent further events.[13]

CLINICAL PRESENTATION Stroke

General

- The patient may not be able to reliably report the history owing to cognitive or language deficits. A reliable history may have to come from a family member or another witness

Symptoms

- The patient may complain of weakness on one side of the body, inability to speak, loss of vision, vertigo, or falling. Ischemic stroke is not usually painful, but patients may complain of headache, and with hemorrhagic stroke, it can be very severe

Signs

- Patients usually have multiple signs of neurologic dysfunction, and the specific deficits are determined by the area of the brain involved
- Hemiparesis or monoparesis occurs commonly, as does a hemisensory deficit
- Patients with vertigo and double vision are likely to have posterior circulation involvement
- Aphasia is seen commonly in patients with anterior circulation strokes
- Patients may also suffer from dysarthria, visual field defects, and altered levels of consciousness

Laboratory Tests

- Tests for hypercoagulable states (protein C deficiency, antiphospholipid antibody) should be done only when the cause of the stroke cannot be determined based on the presence of well-known risk factors for stroke. Protein C, protein S, and antithrombin III are best measured in the "steady state," not in the acute stage. Antiphospholipid antibodies as measured by anticardiolipin antibodies, β_2-glycoprotein I, and lupus anticoagulant screen are of higher yield than protein C, protein S, and antithrombin III but should be reserved for patients who are young (<50 years of age), have had multiple venous/arterial thrombotic events, or have livedo reticularis (a skin rash)

Other Diagnostic Tests

- CT scan of the head will reveal an area of hyperintensity (white) in the area of hemorrhage and will be normal or hypointense (dark) in the area of infarction. The CT scan may take 24 hours (and rarely longer) to reveal the area of infarction
- MRI of the head will reveal areas of ischemia with higher resolution and earlier than the CT scan. Diffusion-weighted imaging (DWI) will reveal an evolving infarct within minutes
- Carotid Doppler (CD) studies will determine whether the patient has a high degree of stenosis in the carotid arteries supplying blood to the brain (extracranial disease)
- An electrocardiogram (ECG) will determine whether the patient has atrial fibrillation, a potent etiologic factor for stroke
- Transthoracic echocardiography (TTE) will determine whether valve abnormalities or wall-motion abnormalities are sources of emboli to the brain. A "bubble test" can be done to look for an intraatrial shunt indicating an atrial septal defect or a patent foramen ovale
- Transesophageal echocardiography (TEE) is a more sensitive test for thrombus in the left atrium. It is effective at examining the aortic arch for atheroma, a potential source of emboli
- Transcranial Doppler (TCD) will determine whether the patient is likely to have intracranial stenosis (e.g., middle cerebral artery stenosis)

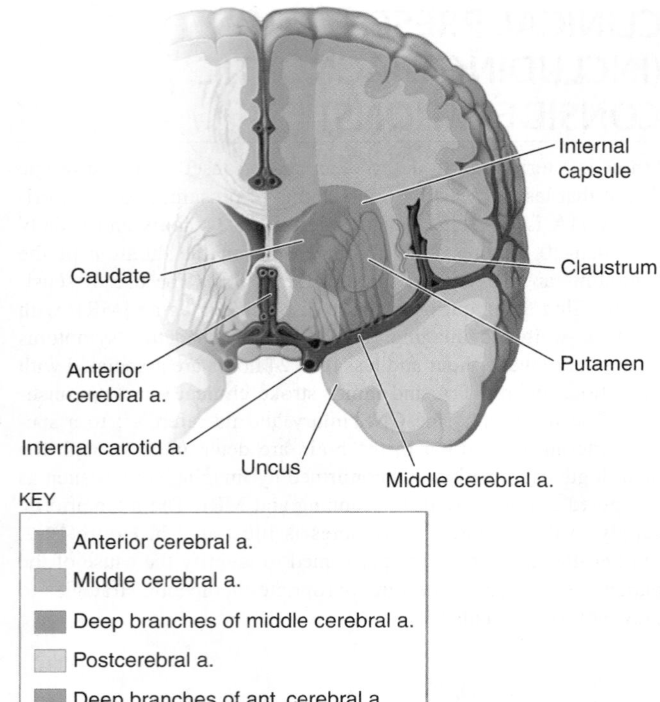

FIGURE 10-2 Diagram of a cerebral hemisphere in coronal section showing the territories of the major cerebral vessels branching from the internal carotid arteries. *(Reproduced with permission from Longo DL, Fauci AS, Kasper DL, et al. Harrison's Principals and Practice of Internal Medicine, 18th ed. New York: McGraw-Hill, 2012.)*

TREATMENT
Stroke

Desired Outcomes

The goals of treatment of acute stroke are to (a) reduce the ongoing neurologic injury and decrease mortality and long-term disability, (b) prevent complications secondary to immobility and neurologic dysfunction, and (c) prevent stroke recurrence.[14] Primary prevention of stroke is reviewed elsewhere.[8]

General Approach to Treatment

The initial approach to the patient with a presumed acute stroke is to ensure that the patient is supported from a respiratory and cardiac standpoint and to quickly determine whether the lesion is ischemic or hemorrhagic, based on a CT scan. Ischemic stroke patients presenting within hours of the onset of their symptoms should be evaluated for reperfusion therapy. **3** TIAs also require urgent intervention to reduce the risk of stroke, which is known to be highest in the first few days after TIA.[15] According to the American Stroke Association guidelines, patients with elevated blood pressure should remain untreated unless their blood pressure exceeds 220/120 mm Hg, or they have evidence of aortic dissection, acute myocardial infarction (AMI), pulmonary edema, or hypertensive encephalopathy. However, this level of blood pressure may be too high, and a number of clinical trials are currently testing more aggressive treatment of hypertension in the acute setting. If blood pressure is treated, short-acting parenteral agents, such as labetalol and nicardipine, or nitroprusside, are favored. Current recommendations regarding management of arterial hypertension in stroke patients are given in Table 10-2.[14] In patients with SAH, if an aneurysm is found by angiography, endovascular coiling or clipping via a craniotomy should be performed to reduce the risk of rebleeding.[16] In ICH, patients may require external ventricular drainage (EVD) if there is intraventricular blood and evolving hydrocephalus (enlargement of the ventricles). Once the patient is out of the hyperacute phase, attention is placed on preventing worsening, minimizing complications, and instituting appropriate secondary prevention strategies. The acute phase of the stroke includes the first week after the event.[14]

TABLE 10-2 Blood Pressure Treatment Guidelines in Acute Ischemic Stroke Patients

Treatment	Received tPA	Did Not Receive tPA
None	<180/105	<220/120
Labetalol IV[a] or nicardipine IV[b]	180–230/105–120	>220/121–140
Nitroprusside[c]	Diastolic >140	Diastolic >140

tPA, tissue plasminogen activator.

[a]Labetalol IV: 10–20 mg, doubled every 10–20 minutes, to a maximum of 300 mg. Also can use an infusion of 2–8 mg/min.

[b]Nicardipine IV: infusion starting at 5 mg/h up to 15 mg/h.

[c]Nitroprusside IV: infusion starting at 0.5 mcg/kg/min, with continuous arterial blood pressure monitoring.

Reproduced from reference 14. Source: American Heart Association, Inc.

Nonpharmacologic Therapy

Ischemic Stroke Surgical interventions in the acute ischemic stroke patient are limited. In less than 10% of patients with a large infarction in the middle cerebral artery territory, decompressive surgery to reduce intracranial pressure has been shown to significantly reduce mortality. However, the surgery must be performed within 48 hours of stroke onset to significantly improve functional outcome and this is at the cost of an increased number of surviving patients with severe disability.[17] In cases of significant swelling associated with a cerebellar infarction, surgical decompression can be lifesaving. Beyond surgical intervention, however, the use of an organized, multidisciplinary approach to stroke care that includes early rehabilitation has been shown to be very effective in reducing the ultimate disability owing to ischemic stroke. In fact, the use of "stroke units" has been associated with outcomes similar to those achieved with early thrombolysis when compared with usual care.[14]

4 In secondary prevention, carotid endarterectomy of an ulcerated and/or stenotic carotid artery is a very effective way to reduce stroke incidence and recurrence in appropriate patients and in centers where the operative morbidity and mortality are low. In fact, in ischemic stroke patients with 70% to 99% stenosis of an ipsilateral internal carotid artery, recurrent stroke risk can be reduced by up to 48% compared with medical therapy alone when combined with aspirin 325 mg daily.[18] In patients less than 70 years of age, carotid stenting is a less invasive alternative and can be effective in reducing recurrent stroke risk.[19] However, in patients with intracranial stenosis, aggressive medical management was shown to be superior to stenting in reducing recurrent stroke.[20]

Hemorrhagic Stroke In patients with SAH owing to a ruptured intracranial aneurysm, in AVMs, surgical intervention to either clip or ablate the offending vascular abnormality substantially reduces mortality owing to rebleeding.[16] In the case of primary ICH, surgical evacuation appears to be of benefit if undertaken within 8 hours of onset and in patients with intermediate hemorrhage volumes (20 to 50 mL).[12] Insertion of an EVD for hydrocephalus and subsequent monitoring of intracranial pressure are done commonly and are the least invasive of the procedures done in these patients.

Pharmacologic Therapy

Ischemic Stroke

Drug Treatments of First Choice: Published Guidelines The Stroke Council of the American Stroke Association and the American College of Chest Physicians have created and published guidelines that address the management of acute ischemic stroke.[7,14] For acute treatment, the only two pharmacologic agents with class I recommendations are IV tissue plasminogen activator (tPA) within 4.5 hours of onset and aspirin within 48 hours of onset.[7,14]

5 Early reperfusion (<4.5 hours from onset) with IV tPA has been shown to reduce the ultimate disability caused by ischemic stroke.[21,22] Caution must be exercised when using this therapy, and adherence to a strict protocol is essential to achieving positive outcomes.[14] The essentials of the treatment protocol can be summarized as (a) stroke team activation, (b) treatment as early as possible within 4.5 hours of onset, (c) CT scan to rule out hemorrhage, (d) meeting inclusion and exclusion criteria (Table 10-3), (e) administration of tPA 0.9 mg/kg over 1 hour, with 10% given as initial bolus over 1 minute, (f) avoidance of antithrombotic (anticoagulant or antiplatelet) therapy for 24 hours, and (g) close patient monitoring for elevated blood pressure, response, and hemorrhage.[14]

TABLE 10-3 Inclusion and Exclusion Criteria for Alteplase Use in Acute Ischemic Stroke[14,21,22]

Inclusion criteria (all YES boxes must be checked before treatment)

YES

- ☐ Age 18 years or older
- ☐ Clinical diagnosis of ischemic stroke causing a measurable neurologic deficit
- ☐ Time of symptom onset well established to be less than 4.5 hours before treatment would begin

Exclusion criteria (all NO boxes must be checked before treatment)

NO

- ☐ Evidence of intracranial hemorrhage on noncontrast head CT
- ☐ Only minor or rapidly improving stroke symptoms
- ☐ High clinical suspicion of subarachnoid hemorrhage even with normal CT
- ☐ Active internal bleeding (e.g., GI/GU bleeding within 21 days)
- ☐ Known bleeding diathesis, including but not limited to platelet count <100,000/mm^3 (<100 × 10^{12}/L)
- ☐ Patient has received heparin within 48 hours and had an elevated APTT
- ☐ Recent use of anticoagulant (e.g., warfarin) and elevated PT (>15 seconds)/INR
- ☐ Intracranial surgery, serious head trauma, or previous stroke within 3 months
- ☐ Major surgery or serious trauma within 14 days
- ☐ Recent arterial puncture at noncompressible site
- ☐ Lumbar puncture within 7 days
- ☐ History of intracranial hemorrhage, arteriovenous malformation, or aneurysm
- ☐ Witnessed seizure at stroke onset
- ☐ Recent acute myocardial infarction
- ☐ SBP >185 mm Hg or DBP >110 mm Hg at time of treatment

Additional exclusion criteria if within 3–4.5 hours of onset:

- ☐ Age greater than 80 years
- ☐ Current treatment with oral anticoagulants
- ☐ NIH Stroke Scale Score >25 (severe stroke)
- ☐ History of both stroke and diabetes

APTT, activated partial thromboplastin time; CT, computed tomography; DBP, diastolic blood pressure; GU, genitourinary; INR, international normalized ratio; PT, prothrombin time; SBP, systolic blood pressure.

Early aspirin therapy has also been shown to reduce long-term death and disability[23,24] but should never be given within 24 hours of the administration of tPA because it can increase the risk of bleeding in such patients.[14]

Antiplatelet therapy is the cornerstone of antithrombotic therapy for the secondary prevention of ischemic stroke and should be used in noncardioembolic strokes. Acetylsalicylic acid (ASA), clopidogrel, and extended-release dipyridamole plus aspirin (ERDP-ASA) are considered first-line antiplatelet agents.[25] Cilostazol is also a recommended first-line antiplatelet agent, but its use has been limited by a lack of data in other than Asian populations.[7]

In patients with atrial fibrillation and a presumed cardiac source of embolism, oral anticoagulation is recommended for secondary stroke prevention.[7,25] The choice of other oral anticoagulants (e.g., dabigatran) over vitamin K antagonism (warfarin) may be recommended in some patients.[7] Other pharmacotherapy recommended for secondary prevention of stroke includes blood pressure lowering and statin therapy. Current recommendations regarding the acute treatment and secondary prevention of stroke are given in Table 10-4.

General Information Regarding Safety and Efficacy (Including Pivotal Clinical Trials)

tPA The effectiveness of IV tPA in the treatment of ischemic stroke was first demonstrated in the National Institute of Neurologic Disorders and Stroke (NINDS) Recombinant Tissue-Type

TABLE 10-4 Recommendations for Pharmacotherapy of Ischemic Stroke

	Recommendation	Evidence[a]
Acute treatment	tPA 0.9 mg/kg IV[7,14] (maximum 90 mg) over 1 hour in selected patients within 3 hours of onset	IA
	tPA 0.9 mg/kg IV[7] (maximum 90 mg) over 1 hour between 3 and 4.5 hours of onset	1B
	ASA 160–325 mg daily[14] started within 48 hours of onset	IA
Secondary prevention		
Noncardioembolic	Antiplatelet therapy	IA
	Aspirin 50–325 mg daily[25]	IA
	Clopidogrel 75 mg daily[25]	IIa B
	Aspirin 25 mg + extended-release dipyridamole	
	200 mg twice daily[25]	IB
Cardioembolic (especially atrial fibrillation)	VKA (INR = 2.5)[25]	IA
	Dabigatran 150 mg twice daily[7]	2B
Atherosclerosis	Intense statin therapy[25]	IB
	50% reduction in LDL or ≤70 mg/dL (≤1.81 mmol/L)[7]	IIa B
All	BP reduction[25]	IA

ASA, acetylsalicylic acid; INR, international normalized ratio; tPA, tissue plasminogen activator; VKA, vitamin K antagonist.

[a]Classes: I, evidence or general agreement about usefulness and effectiveness; II, conflicting evidence about the usefulness; IIa, weight of evidence in favor of the treatment; IIb, usefulness less well established; III, not useful and maybe harmful. Levels of evidence: A, multiple randomized clinical trials; B, a single randomized trial or nonrandomized studies; C, expert opinion or case studies.[25] (Level 1A in reference 7, recommendation with high-quality evidence; 2B, suggested with moderate-quality evidence.)

Data from Lansberg et al.,[7] Jauch et al.,[14] and Furie et al.[25]

Plasminogen Activator (rtPA) Stroke Trial, published in 1995.[21] In 624 patients treated in equal numbers with either tPA 0.9 mg/kg IV or placebo within 3 hours of the onset of their neurologic symptoms, 39% of the treated patients achieved an "excellent outcome" at 3 months compared with 26% of the placebo patients. An "excellent outcome" was defined as minimal or no disability by several different neurologic scales. This beneficial effect was reported despite a 10-fold increase in the risk of symptomatic ICH in the tPA-treated patients (0.6% vs. 6.4%). Overall mortality was not significantly different between the two groups (17% with tPA and 21% with placebo). Patients with very severe symptoms at baseline (National Institutes of Health Stroke Scale [NIHSS] >20) and early ischemic changes on CT scan were shown to be at highest risk for the development of symptomatic intracranial hemorrhage. Even in patients at highest risk for bleeding, however, those receiving tPA had better outcomes at 90 days than those who received placebo.[21]

Thirteen years after the NINDS trial, the European Cooperative Acute Stroke Study (ECASS) III demonstrated that, even when administered between 3 and 4.5 hours after the onset of symptoms, ischemic stroke patients benefit from tPA when compared with placebo (52.4% vs. 45.2% excellent outcome; $P = 0.04$).[22] The benefit was less than that reported with earlier treatment but the rate of excess hemorrhage was similar, leading to a change in AHA guidelines to recommend extension of the window.[25] An important caveat was that the exclusion criteria for later treatment are more strict and are given in Table 10-3. The International Stroke Trial (IST)-3 reported subsequently, in a large group of 3,035 patients treated within 6 hours of ischemic stroke onset, that even patients outside the rigid criteria set forth by both the NINDS and ECASS III trials may experience improved functional outcome.[26] These investigators advocate that patients over the age of 80, presenting outside the 3-hour treatment window, may benefit from a personalized assessment of risk and benefit prior to excluding them from thrombolytic therapy.

ASA The use of early ASA to reduce long-term death and disability owing to ischemic stroke is supported by two large randomized clinical trials. In the IST,[24] aspirin 300 mg/day significantly reduced stroke recurrence within the first 2 weeks without effect on early mortality, resulting in a significant decrease in death and dependency at 6 months. In the Chinese Acute Stroke Trial (CAST),[23] aspirin 160 mg/day reduced the risk of recurrence and death in the first 28 days, but long-term death and disability were not different than with placebo. In both trials, a small but significant increase in hemorrhagic transformation of the infarction was demonstrated. Overall, the beneficial effects of early aspirin have been embraced and adopted into clinical guidelines.

Antiplatelet Agents All patients who have had an acute ischemic stroke or TIA should receive long-term antithrombotic therapy for secondary prevention.[25] ❻ In patients with noncardioembolic stroke, this will be some form of antiplatelet therapy. In a comprehensive meta analysis, the overall benefit of antiplatelet therapy in patients with atherothrombotic disorders was estimated to be 22%.[27] ASA is the best studied of the available agents but published literature has supported the use of clopidogrel, the combination product extended-release dipyridamole plus acetylsalicylic acid (ERDP-ASA), and cilostazol as additional first-line agents in secondary stroke prevention.[7,25]

The efficacy of clopidogrel as an antiplatelet agent in atherothrombotic disorders was demonstrated in the Clopidogrel versus Aspirin in Patients at Risk of Ischemic Events (CAPRIE) trial.[28] In this study of more than 19,000 patients with a history of myocardial infarction (MI), stroke, or peripheral arterial disease (PAD), clopidogrel 75 mg/day was compared with ASA 325 mg/day for its ability to decrease MI, stroke, or cardiovascular death. In the final analysis, clopidogrel was slightly (8% relative risk reduction [RRR]) more effective than ASA ($P = 0.043$) and had a similar incidence of adverse effects. It is not associated with the blood dyscrasias (neutropenia) common with its congener, ticlopidine, and is used widely in patients with atherosclerosis.

In the European Stroke Prevention Study 2 (ESPS-2), ASA 25 mg and ERDP 200 mg twice daily were compared alone and in combination with placebo for their ability to reduce recurrent stroke over a 2-year period.[29] In a total of more than 6,600 patients, all three treatment groups were shown to be superior to placebo—ASA alone (18% RRR), ERDP alone (16% RRR), and the combination (37% RRR). In addition, the combination demonstrated a significant advantage over the ASA-alone group (23% RRR; $P = 0.006$) and the ERDP-alone group (24% RRR; $P = 0.002$). Headache resulting in discontinuation occurred in approximately 15% of the ERDP groups (four times more common than in the placebo group), and the ASA-treated patients, even at the low dose of 50 mg/day, experienced significantly more bleeding than the other groups. The European/Australasian Stroke Prevention in Reversible Ischemia Trial (ESPRIT) confirmed the results of ESPS-2, in that the combination of dipyridamole (83% extended release) and ASA (30 to 325 mg daily) was more effective than ASA alone in reducing recurrent stroke.[30] Headache was again an important cause of discontinuation in the ESPRIT trial. In a large, multinational trial (Prevention Regimen for Effectively Avoiding Second Strokes [PRoFESS]) comparing ERDP-ASA with clopidogrel, the risk of recurrent stroke was similar for the two antiplatelet agents, but clopidogrel was better tolerated with less bleeding and headache.[31]

Cilostazol is an antiplatelet agent mostly used in the treatment of intermittent claudication. However, in a systematic assessment of two separate large randomized trials in Asian patients, cilostazol significantly reduced the risk of recurrent vascular events (RR 0.72) and hemorrhagic stroke (RR 0.26), compared with ASA.[32] Despite the fact that cilostazol caused less bleeding events than ASA, there were more overall minor adverse events, including headache (21.3% vs. 13.9%) and GI disturbance (9.66% vs. 5.02%).

Oral Anticoagulants ❼ Oral anticoagulation is the treatment of choice for the prevention of stroke in patients with atrial fibrillation.[7,25] In patients with atrial fibrillation and a recent history of stroke or TIA, the risk of recurrence places these patients in one of the highest risk categories known. In the European Atrial Fibrillation Trial (EAFT), 669 patients with nonvalvular atrial fibrillation (NVAF) and a prior stroke or TIA were randomized to warfarin (international normalized ratio [INR] = 2.5 to 4), ASA 300 mg/day, or placebo. Patients in the placebo group experienced stroke, MI, or vascular death at a rate of 17% per year compared with 8% per year in the warfarin group and 15% per year in the ASA group. This represents a 53% reduction in risk with anticoagulation.[33] Subsequent studies in the primary prevention of stroke in patients with NVAF have demonstrated that targeting an INR of 2.5 prevents stroke with the lowest bleeding risk (Stroke Prevention in Atrial Fibrillation [SPAF III]); therefore, a target INR of 2.5 is recommended in the secondary prevention of stroke.[7,25] Newer oral anticoagulants including dabigatran (direct thrombin inhibitor), rivaroxaban, and apixaban (direct factor Xa inhibitors) have significant advantages over warfarin in terms of ease of dosing and less food and drug interactions. In addition, in the prevention of stroke in selected patients with atrial fibrillation, all three agents have been shown to be as effective as, and in some cases, superior to, warfarin in reducing recurrent events and intracranial hemorrhage.[34,35] For the secondary prevention of stroke in patients with atrial fibrillation, dabigatran 150 mg twice daily is recommended as either a first-line agent (ACCP) or one of several first-line oral anticoagulants.[7,25] Use of warfarin in the secondary prevention of noncardioembolic stroke was addressed in the Warfarin Aspirin Recurrent Stroke Study.[36] In 2,206 patients with recent stroke, warfarin (INR = 1.4 to 2.8) was not superior to ASA 325 mg/day in the prevention of recurrent events. Further data from the Warfarin–Aspirin in Intracranial Disease (WASID) trial demonstrated that ASA therapy was as effective as and safer than warfarin in patients with intracranial stenosis.[37] These studies led most clinicians to abandon the practice of using warfarin in all but patients with cardioembolic sources of emboli, mainly atrial fibrillation.

Blood Pressure Lowering **8** Elevated blood pressure is very common in ischemic stroke patients, and treatment of hypertension in these patients is associated with a decreased risk of stroke recurrence.[38] In the Perindopril pROtection aGainst REcurrent Stroke Study (PROGRESS), a multinational stroke population (40% Asian) was randomized to receive either blood pressure lowering with the angiotensin-converting enzyme (ACE) inhibitor perindopril (with or without the thiazide diuretic indapamide) or placebo.[38] Treated patients achieved an overall 9 mm Hg systolic and 4 mm Hg diastolic blood pressure reduction, and this was associated with a 28% reduction in stroke recurrence. In the patients who received the combination treatment (clinician's discretion), the average blood pressure lowering achieved was 12 mm Hg systolic and 5 mm Hg diastolic, and this was associated with an even larger reduction in stroke recurrence (43%). Similar results were achieved in patients with and without hypertension. AHA/ASA guidelines recommend reduction of blood pressure in patients with stroke or TIA.[25] **9** Early blood pressure lowering can worsen symptoms, however; therefore, recommendations are limited to patients outside of the acute stroke period (first 7 days).[25]

Statins **10** The statins have been shown to reduce the risk of stroke by approximately 30% in patients with coronary artery disease and elevated plasma lipids.[39] The Stroke Prevention by Aggressive Reduction in Cholesterol (SPARCL) study demonstrated that atorvastatin 80 mg daily reduced the risk of recurrent stroke by 16% and coronary events by 42% in patients with no cardiac history. Although the high-dose statin caused an increase in liver enzymes, there was no increase in myopathy.[40] It is now recommended that ischemic stroke patients, regardless of baseline cholesterol, be treated with high-intensity statin therapy to achieve a reduction of low-density lipoprotein (LDL) of at least 50% for secondary stroke prevention.[25]

Heparin for Prophylaxis of Deep Vein Thrombosis (DVT) The use of low-molecular-weight heparins or low-dose subcutaneous unfractionated heparin (5,000 units three times daily) can be recommended for the prevention of DVT in hospitalized patients with decreased mobility owing to their stroke and should be used in all but the most minor strokes.[11]

Alternative Drug Treatments

ASA Plus Clopidogrel In the Management of ATherothrombosis with Clopidogrel in High-risk patients (MATCH) study, clopidogrel in combination with ASA 75 mg daily was no better than clopidogrel alone in secondary stroke prevention.[41] Also, when clopidogrel was used with ASA, the risk of life-threatening bleeding increased from 1.3% to 2.6%.[41] Again, in the Stroke Prevention in Subcortical Stroke (SPS)-3 trial of patients with recent minor strokes, the arm of the trial studying the combination of clopidogrel and ASA was stopped early due to excess mortality due to bleeding in this group.[42] However, the combination has been studied in patients with acute coronary syndromes and patients undergoing percutaneous coronary interventions and shown to be significantly more effective than ASA alone in reducing MI, stroke, and cardiovascular death.[43,44] Also, in patients with high-grade intracranial stenosis, short-term (3-month) use of the combination of clopidogrel and ASA was associated with better-than-expected outcome in the aggressive medical therapy group.[20] This combination should only be used in selected patients with a recent MI history or intracranial stenosis and only with ultra–low-dose ASA to minimize bleeding risk.[45]

Heparins The use of full-dose unfractionated heparin in the acute stroke period has never been proven to positively affect stroke outcome, and it significantly increases the risk of ICH.[7,14] Trials of low-molecular-weight heparins or heparinoids have been largely negative and do not support their routine use in stroke patients.[46–48] Other potential but unproven uses for treatment doses of either unfractionated or low-molecular-weight heparins include bridge therapy in patients being initiated on warfarin, carotid dissection, or continuous worsening of ischemia despite adequate antiplatelet therapy.[7]

Drug Class Information

ASA ASA exerts its antiplatelet effect by irreversibly inhibiting cyclooxygenase, which, in platelets, prevents conversion of arachidonic acid to thromboxane A_2 (TXA_2), which is a powerful vasoconstrictor and stimulator of platelet aggregation. Platelets remain impaired for their life span (5 to 7 days) after exposure to aspirin. ASA also inhibits prostacyclin (PGI_2) activity in the smooth muscle of vascular walls. PGI_2 inhibits platelet aggregation, and the vascular endothelium can synthesize PGI_2 such that the platelet antiaggregating effect is maintained.[7] There is probably a point at which lower doses of ASA do not completely block TXA_2, and recent studies indicate that the lowest effective dose may be in the range of 50 mg/day.[49] Upper GI discomfort and bleeding are the most common adverse effects of ASA and have been shown to be dose related. The highest rates of GI bleeding (5%) have been reported in patients receiving 1,200 mg/day as compared with rates of 2% in patients taking the more commonly prescribed 300 mg/day. Upper GI symptoms are much more common than frank bleeding, however, with 40% of patients affected at 1,200 mg/day and 25% at 300 mg/day.[50] In the ESPS-2 study, even 50 mg/day of ASA was associated with a twofold increase in bleeding over the placebo group.[29]

The onset of the antiplatelet effect of ASA is less than 60 minutes.[51] It has been reported, however, that some patients either have or develop "aspirin resistance" and can require higher doses to achieve the desired antiplatelet effect.[52] Despite this, routine testing for ASA resistance is not recommended. It was observed that administration of ibuprofen prior to the administration of a daily aspirin dose inhibits the ASA from binding irreversibly to the cyclooxygenase and can decrease its antiplatelet effect.[53] Current recommendations are to administer ASA at least 2 hours before ibuprofen or to wait at least 4 hours after an ibuprofen dose.

Clopidogrel Clopidogrel has a unique platelet antiaggregatory effect in that it is an inhibitor of the adenosine diphosphate (ADP) pathway of platelet aggregation and inhibits known stimuli to platelet aggregation.[7,28] This effect causes an alteration of the platelet membrane and interference with the membrane–fibrinogenic interaction leading to a blocking of the platelet glycoprotein IIb/IIIa receptor. A time lag of 3 to 7 days before the antiplatelet effect is maximal should be expected. The tolerability of clopidogrel 75 mg/day is at least as good as medium-dose (325 mg/day) ASA, and there is less GI bleeding.[28] Clopidogrel is associated with an increased risk of diarrhea and rash, but discontinuation rates owing to adverse effects are similar to those with ASA 325 mg/day (5.3% and 6%, respectively).[28] There is no excess neutropenia in patients taking clopidogrel, and rates of thrombotic thrombocytopenic purpura probably are no greater than background rate.

Extended-Release Dipyridamole Plus ASA Early studies of the role of dipyridamole in stroke prevention failed to show a benefit over that realized by ASA alone. Dipyridamole in high doses is thought to inhibit platelet aggregation by inhibiting phosphodiesterase, leading to accumulation of cyclic adenosine monophosphate (cAMP) and cyclic guanosine monophosphate (cGMP) intracellularly, which prevent platelet activation. In addition, dipyridamole also enhances the antithrombotic potential of the vascular wall.[54] The ESPS-2 demonstrated the efficacy of high-dose ERDP alone and in combination with ASA in secondary stroke prevention.[29] The extended-release formulation of dipyridamole is important in that it allows twice-daily administration and higher doses to be tolerated in patients. The use of immediate-release generic dipyridamole in combination with regular ASA, in order to reduce costs, is unproven and should be discouraged.

In the ESPS-2, 25% of the patients who received combination dipyridamole and ASA discontinued the therapy early, and the rate of discontinuation owing to headache was more than three times as common (10%) as in the aspirin-alone group (3%).[29] Even when patients were carefully educated and coached in the PRoFESS trial, discontinuation due to headache was six times higher in the ERDP-ASA group (5.9% vs. 0.9%).[31]

Investigational Strategies

Reperfusion Various investigations aimed at opening the occluded cerebral artery and preserving its patency are under way in acute ischemic stroke patients.[55] Strategies being tried include longer-acting fibrinolytic agents, intraarterial fibrinolysis with tPA and other agents, and endovascular clot removal using mechanical and laser-guided approaches. Although the endovascular devices are used extensively in some centers, expert guidelines recommend against their routine use.[7] In addition, investigators are trying to identify, using sensitive MRI techniques, which patients benefit from reperfusion at time points outside the approved time window. Undoubtedly, efforts to reperfuse the ischemic brain will continue to be explored, so more patients will be eligible for this therapy.

Neuroprotection and Neurorestoration Although many different neuroprotective agents have been studied in clinical trials of acute ischemic stroke, all have been unsuccessful.[55] Magnesium and albumin are still under investigation, but the drug development pipeline for acute neuroprotection is essentially nonexistent. However, hope exists that clinicians will be able to enhance the reparative process of the brain (neurorestoration) through targeted neurorehabilitation, growth factor enhancement, and the use of neural and cell transplantation.[55]

A promising nonpharmacologic strategy that has been shown to provide neuroprotection in patients has been hypothermia.[56] There remains uncertainty on the best way to optimize the mechanism of cooling the ischemic brain (intravascular coils vs. surface cooling) and rewarming the patient after hypothermia.

Hemorrhagic Stroke

There are currently no standard pharmacologic strategies for treating ICH.[11] Medical guidelines for the management of blood pressure, raised intracranial pressure, and other medical complications of ICH are those required for the management of any acutely ill patient in a neurointensive care unit.[11] When ICH occurs in a patient on oral anticoagulants, reversal of anticoagulation to prevent expansion and allow surgical intervention is recommended. The methods recommended to achieve reversal include IV vitamin K, fresh-frozen plasma (FFP), and hemostatic agents (factor VIIa and prothrombin complex concentrate [PCC]).[11] The optimal approach, particularly in patients on the newer oral anticoagulants, is yet to be determined.

SAH owing to aneurysm rupture is associated with a high incidence of delayed cerebral ischemia (DCI) in the 2 weeks following the bleeding episode. Vasospasm of the cerebral vasculature is thought to be responsible for DCI and occurs between 4 and 21 days after the bleed, peaking at days 5 to 9.[16] The calcium channel blocker nimodipine (60 mg every 4 hours for 21 days), along with maintenance of intravascular volume with pressor therapy, is recommended to reduce the incidence and severity of neurologic deficits owing to DCI.[16]

PERSONALIZED PHARMACOTHERAPY

Clopidogrel is a thienopyridine prodrug and needs to be biotransformed by the liver to an active metabolite. Evidence suggests that the antiplatelet effects of clopidogrel can be diminished in patients with reduced-function cytochrome P450 2C19 (CYP2C19)[57] or in those receiving agents that inhibit hepatic metabolism.[58] In patients receiving clopidogrel after stent placement, reduced-function CYP2C19 is associated with an increase in recurrent vascular events.[58] Although high doses of the lipophilic statins atorvastatin and simvastatin can diminish the effectiveness of clopidogrel to inhibit platelet aggregation in vitro, there does not appear to be any adverse effect on atherothrombotic event rates.[59] In contrast, in a retrospective analysis of 8,205 patients, concomitant proton pump inhibitor and clopidogrel treatment was associated with increased adverse vascular outcomes after acute coronary syndromes.[57] Careful consideration should be given to using clopidogrel in patients with reduced ability to biotransform the agent to its active metabolite.

The availability of genetic testing to identify patients with altered sensitivity to warfarin has led to questions regarding the ability of the tests to improve patient care. Polymorphisms in CYP2C9 and vitamin K epoxide reductase complex subunit 1 (VKORC1) contribute to the variability in warfarin response, but it is unclear whether knowledge of these genetic variations will improve dosing accuracy and reduce adverse events.[60] Clinical trial evidence is needed prior to instituting these tests in stroke patients who are candidates for warfarin therapy.

EVALUATION OF THERAPEUTIC OUTCOMES

Monitoring of the Pharmaceutical Care Plan

Patients with acute stroke should be monitored intensely for the development of neurologic worsening (recurrence or extension), complications (thromboembolism or infection), or adverse effects from pharmacologic or nonpharmacologic interventions. The most common reasons for deterioration in a stroke patient are (a) extension of the original lesion—ischemic or hemorrhagic—in the brain, (b) development of cerebral edema and raised intracranial pressure, (c) hypertensive emergency, (d) infection (urinary and respiratory most common), (e) venous thromboembolism (DVT and pulmonary embolism), (f) electrolyte abnormalities and cardiac rhythm disturbances (can be associated with brain injury), and (g) recurrent stroke.

TABLE 10-5 Monitoring Stroke Therapy

Drug	Adverse Effect	Monitoring Parameters	Comments
tPA	Bleeding	Neurologic exam	Every 15 minutes × 1 hour; every 0.5 hour × 6 hours; every 1 hour × 17 hours; every shift after
ASA	Bleeding		Daily
Clopidogrel	Bleeding		Daily
ERDP-ASA	Headache, bleeding		Daily
Warfarin	Bleeding	INR, Hb/Hct	Daily
Dabigatran	Bleeding		Daily

ERDP-ASA, extended-release dipyridamole plus aspirin; Hb/Hct, hemoglobin/hematocrit.

The approach to monitoring drug therapy in the hospitalized stroke patient is summarized in Table 10-5. The plan should be customized for individual patients based on their comorbidities and ongoing disease processes.

Clinical **Controversy...**

Rapid reversal of the INR with hemostatic agents in patients with oral anticoagulant–associated intracranial hemorrhage may reduce the risk of extension of the lesion but also carries a risk of thromboembolic events. The correct approach to management of this adverse effect of anticoagulant therapy is unknown.

Aggressive BP lowering in patients with intracranial hemorrhage may reduce the risk of hemorrhage extension. Although this practice may be safe, it is unclear whether it can improve outcome.

ABBREVIATIONS

ACE	angiotensin-converting enzyme
ADP	adenosine diphosphate
AHA	American Heart Association
AMI	acute myocardial infarction
ASA	acetylsalicylic acid
ATP	adenosine triphosphate
AVM	arteriovenous malformation
cAMP	cyclic adenosine monophosphate
CAPRIE	Clopidogrel versus Aspirin in Patients at Risk of Ischemic Events
CAST	Chinese Acute Stroke Trial
CD	carotid Doppler
cGMP	cyclic guanosine monophosphate
CT scan	computed tomographic scan
CYP2C19	cytochrome P450 2C19
DCI	delayed cerebral ischemia
DVT	deep vein thrombosis
DWI	diffusion-weighted imaging
EAFT	European Atrial Fibrillation Trial
ECASS	European Cooperative Acute Stroke Study
ECG	electrocardiogram
ERDP	extended-release dipyridamole
ESPRIT	European/Australasian Stroke Prevention in Reversible Ischemia Trial
ESPS-2	European Stroke Prevention Study 2
EVD	external ventricular drainage
FFP	fresh-frozen plasma
ICH	intracerebral hemorrhage
INR	international normalized ratio
IST	International Stroke Trial
LDL	low-density lipoprotein
MATCH	Management of ATherothrombosis with Clopidogrel in High-risk patients
MI	myocardial infarction
MRI	magnetic resonance imaging
NIHSS	National Institutes of Health Stroke Scale
NINDS	National Institute of Neurologic Disorders and Stroke
NVAF	nonvalvular atrial fibrillation
PAD	peripheral arterial disease
PCC	prothrombin complex concentrate
PGI_2	prostacyclin
PRoFESS	Perindopril pROtection aGainst REcurrent Stroke Study
PROGRESS	Perindopril pROtection aGainst REcurrent Stroke Study
RRR	relative risk reduction
rtPA	recombinant tissue-type plasminogen activator
SAH	subarachnoid hemorrhage
SPAF III	Stroke Prevention in Atrial Fibrillation
SPARCL	Stroke Prevention by Aggressive Reduction in Cholesterol
SPS	Stroke Prevention in Subcortical Stroke
TCD	transcranial Doppler
TEE	transesophageal echocardiography
TIA	transient ischemic attack
tPA	tissue plasminogen activator
TTE	transthoracic echocardiography
TXA_2	thromboxane A_2
VKORC1	vitamin K epoxide reductase complex subunit 1
WASID	Warfarin–Aspirin in Intracranial Disease

REFERENCES

1. National Center for Health Statistics. Centers for Disease Control and Prevention. Life expectancy declines slightly according to latest CDC deaths report. Press Release. Atlanta, GA: US Department of Health and Human Services, December 9, 2010.
2. Roger VL, Go AS, Lloyd-Jones DM, et al. Heart disease and stroke statistics—2012 update: A report from the American Heart Association. Circulation 2012;125:e2–e220.
3. Howard VJ, McClure LA, Meschia JF, Pulley L, Orr SC, Friday GH. High prevalence of stroke symptoms among persons without a diagnosis of stroke or transient ischemic attack in a general population: The Reasons for Geographic and Racial Differences in Stroke (REGARDS) Study. Arch Int Med 2006;166:1952–1958.
4. Elkins JS, Johnston SC. Thirty-year projections for deaths from ischemic stroke in the United States. Stroke 2003;34:2109–2113.
5. Juvela S, Kase CS. Advances in intracerebral hemorrhage management. Stroke 2006;37:301–304.
6. Qureshi AI, Mendelow AD, Hanley DF. Intracerebral hemorrhage. Lancet 2009;373:1632–1644.
7. Lansberg MG, O'Donnell MJ, Khatri P, et al. Antithrombotic and thrombolytic therapy for ischemic stroke: Antithrombotic therapy and prevention of thrombosis, 9th ed: American College of Chest Physicians evidence-based clinical practice guidelines. Chest 2012;141:e601S–e636S.

8. Goldstein LB, Bushnell CD, Adams R, et al. Guidelines for the primary prevention of ischemic stroke. A guideline for healthcare professionals from the American Heart Association/American Stroke Association. Stroke 2011; 42:517–584.
9. Wolf PA. Fifty years at Framingham: Contributions to stroke epidemiology. Adv Neurol 2003;92:165–172.
10. Xing C, Arai K, Lo EH, Hommel M. Pathophysiologic cascades in ischemic stroke. Int J Stroke 2012;7:378–385.
11. Morganstern LB, Hemphill JC, Anderson C, et al. Guidelines for the management of spontaneous intracerebral hemorrhage. A guideline for healthcare professionals from the American Heart Association/American Stroke Association. Stroke 2010;41:2108–2129.
12. Gregson BA, Broderick JP, Auer LM, et al. Individual patient data subgroup meta analysis of surgery for spontaneous supratentorial intracerebral hemorrhage. Stroke 2012;43:1496–1504.
13. Smith WS, English JD, Johnston SC. Cerebrovascular diseases. In: Longo DL, Fauci AS, Kasper DL, et al., eds. Harrison's Principles of Internal Medicine, 18th ed. New York: McGraw-Hill, 2012:3270–3299.
14. Jauch EC, Saver JL, Adams HP, et al. Guidelines for the early management of patients with ischemic stroke: A guideline for healthcare professionals from the American Heart Association/American Stroke Association. Stroke 2013;44:870–947.
15. Johnston SC, Nguyen-Huynh MN, Schwartz ME, et al. National Stroke Association guidelines for the management of transient ischemic attacks. Ann Neurol 2006;60(3):301–313.
16. Connolly ES, Rabinstein AA, Carhuapoma JR, et al. Guidelines for the management of aneurysmal subarachnoid hemorrhage. A guideline for healthcare professionals from the American Heart Association/American Stroke Association. Stroke 2012;43:1711–1737.
17. Vahedi K, Hofmeijer J, Juettler E, et al. Early decompressive surgery in malignant infarction of the middle cerebral artery: A pooled analysis of three randomized controlled trials. Lancet Neurol 2007;6:215–222.
18. Cina CA, Clase CM, Haynes RB. Carotid endarterectomy for symptomatic carotid stenosis [Cochrane review on CD-ROM]. In: The Cochrane Library, Issue 1. Oxford: Update Software, 2001.
19. Brott TG, Hobson RW, Howard G, et al. Stenting versus endarterectomy for treatment of carotid artery stenosis. N Engl J Med 2010;363:11–23.
20. Chimowitz MI, Lynn MJ, Derdeyn CP, et al. Stenting versus aggressive medical therapy for intracranial arterial stenosis. N Engl J Med 2011;365:993–1003.
21. The National Institute of Neurological Disorders and Stroke rt-PA Stroke Study Group. Tissue plasminogen activator for acute ischemic stroke. N Engl J Med 1995;333:1581–1587.
22. Hacke W, Kaste M, Bluhmki E, et al. Thrombolysis with alteplase 3 to 4.5 hours after acute ischemic stroke. N Engl J Med 2008;359:1317–1329.
23. Chinese Acute Stroke Trial (CAST) Collaborative Group. CAST: A randomized, placebo-controlled trial of early aspirin use in 20,000 patients with acute ischemic stroke. Lancet 1997;349:1641–1649.
24. International Stroke Trial Collaborative Group. The International Stroke Trial (IST): A randomized trial of aspirin, subcutaneous heparin, both, or neither among 19,435 patients with acute ischemic stroke. Lancet 1997; 349:1560–1581.
25. Furie KL, Kasner SE, Adams RJ, et al. Guidelines for prevention of stroke in patients with stroke or transient ischemic attack. A statement for healthcare professionals from the American Heart Association/American Stroke Association. Stroke 2011;42(1):227–276.
26. The IST-3 Collaborative Group. The benefits and harms of intravenous thrombolysis with recombinant tissue plasminogen activator within 6 h of acute ischaemic stroke (the third international stroke trial [IST-3]): A randomized controlled trial. Lancet 2012;379:2352–2363 [Epub ahead of print]. doi:10.1016/50140-6736(12)60768-5.
27. Antithrombotic Trialists' Collaboration. Collaborative meta analysis of randomized trials of antiplatelet therapy for prevention of death, myocardial infarction, and stroke in high risk patients. BMJ 2002;324:71–86.
28. CAPRIE Steering Committee. A randomized, blinded trial of clopidogrel versus aspirin in patients at risk of ischaemic events (CAPRIE). Lancet 1995;348:1329–1339.
29. Diener HC, Cunha L, Forbes C, et al. European Stroke Prevention Study 2: Dipyridamole and acetylsalicylic acid in the secondary prevention of stroke. J Neurol Sci 1996;143:1–13.
30. ESPRIT Study Group. Aspirin plus dipyridamole versus aspirin alone after cerebral ischaemia of arterial origin (ESPRIT): Randomized controlled trial. Lancet 2006;367:1665–1673.
31. Sacco RL, Diener HC, Yusuf S, et al. Aspirin and extended-release dipyridamole versus clopidogrel for recurrent stroke. N Engl J Med 2008;359:1238–1251.
32. Kamal AK, Naqvi I, Husain MR, Khealani BA. Cilostazol versus aspirin for secondary prevention of vascular events after stroke of arterial origin. Cochrane Database Syst Rev 2011;(1):CD008076. doi:10.1002/14651858.CD008076.pub2.
33. European Atrial Fibrillation Trial Study Group. Secondary prevention in nonrheumatic atrial fibrillation after transient ischaemic attack or minor stroke. Lancet 1993;342:1255–1262.
34. Katsnelson M, Sacco RL, Moscucci M. Progress for stroke prevention with atrial fibrillation. Emergence of alternative oral anticoagulants. Stroke 2012;43:1179–1185.
35. Connolly SJ, Ezekowitz MD, Yusuf S, et al. Dabigatran versus warfarin in patients with atrial fibrillation. N Engl J Med 2009;361(12):1139–1151.
36. Mohr JP, Thompson JLP, Lazar RM, et al. A comparison of warfarin and aspirin for the prevention of recurrent ischemic stroke. N Engl J Med 2001;345:1444–1451.
37. Chimowitz MI, Lynn MJ, Howlett-Smith H, et al. Comparison of warfarin and aspirin for symptomatic intracranial arterial stenosis. N Engl J Med 2005;352:1305–1316.
38. PROGRESS Collaborative Group. Randomized trial of perindopril-based blood-pressure-lowering regimen among 6105 individuals with previous stroke or transient ischaemic attack. Lancet 2001;358:1033–1041.
39. Hebert PR, Gaziano JM, Chan KS, Hennekens CH. Cholesterol lowering with statin drugs, risk of stroke, and total mortality: An overview of randomized trials. JAMA 1997;278:313–321.
40. The Stroke Prevention by Aggressive Reduction in Cholesterol Levels (SPARCL) Investigators. High-dose atorvastatin after stroke or transient ischemic attack. N Engl J Med 2006;355:549–559.
41. Diener HC, Bogousslavsky J, Brass LM, et al. Aspirin and clopidogrel compared with clopidogrel alone after recent ischemic stroke or transient ischaemic attack in high-risk patients (MATCH): Randomized, double-blind, placebo-controlled trial. Lancet 2004;364:331–337.
42. The SPS3 Investigators. Effects of clopidogrel added to aspirin in patients with recent lacunar stroke. N Engl J Med 2012;367:817–825.

43. Yusuf S, Zhao F, Mehta SR, et al. Effects of clopidogrel in addition to aspirin in patients with acute coronary syndromes without ST-segment elevation. N Engl J Med 2001;54: 1022–1028.
44. Steinhubl SR, Berger PB, Mann JT, et al. Early and sustained dual oral antiplatelet therapy following percutaneous coronary intervention: A randomized, controlled trial. JAMA 2002;288:2411–2420.
45. Peters RJG, Mehta SR, Fox KAA, et al. Effects of aspirin dose when used alone or in combination with clopidogrel in patients with acute coronary syndromes: Observations from the clopidogrel in unstable angina to prevent recurrent events (CURE) study. Circulation 2003;108:1682–1687.
46. The Publications Committee for the Trial of ORG 10172 in Acute Stroke Treatment (TOAST) Investigators. Low-molecular-weight heparinoid, ORG 10172 (danaparoid), and outcome after acute ischemic stroke: A randomized, controlled trial. JAMA 1998;279:1265–1272.
47. Bath PM, Lidenstrom E, Boysen G, et al. Tinzaparin in acute ischaemic stroke (TAIST): A randomized, aspirin-controlled trial. Lancet 2001;358:702–710.
48. Berge E, Abdelnoor M, Nakstad PH, et al. Low-molecular-weight heparin versus aspirin in patients with acute ischaemic stroke and atrial fibrillation: A double-blind, randomised study. HAEST Study Group. Heparin in Acute Embolic Stroke Trial. Lancet 2000;355:1205–1210.
49. Food and Drug Administration. FDA Approves New Prescribed Uses for Aspirin. FDA Talk Paper T98-76. 1998, *www.fda.gov/bbs/topics/ANSWERS/ANS00919.html*.
50. Farrell B, Godwin J, Richards S, Warlow C. The United Kingdom transient ischaemic attack (UK-TIA) aspirin trial: Final results. J Neurol Neurosurg Psychiatry 1991;54: 1044–1054.
51. Serebruany VL, Malinin AI, Sane DC. Rapid platelet inhibition after a single capsule of Aggrenox: Challenging a conventional full-dose aspirin antiplatelet advantage? Am J Hematol 2003;72:280–281.
52. Eikelboom JW, Hankey GJ. Aspirin resistance: A new independent predictor of vascular events? J Am Coll Cardiol 2003;41:966–968.
53. Catella-Lawson F, Reilly MP, Kapoor SC, et al. Cyclooxygenase inhibitors and the antiplatelet effects of aspirin. N Engl J Med 2001;345:1809–1817.
54. Eisert WG. Near-field amplification of antithrombotic effects of dipyridamole through vessel wall cells. Neurology 2001; 57(Suppl 2):S20–S23.
55. Sahota P, Savitz SI. Investigational therapies for ischemic stroke. Neurotherapeutics 2011;8:434–451.
56. Ginsberg MD. Current status of neuroprotection for cerebral ischemia: Synoptic overview. Stroke 2009;40(Suppl 1): S111–S114.
57. Ho PM, Maddox TM, Wang L, et al. Risk of adverse outcomes associated with concomitant use of clopidogrel and proton pump inhibitors following acute coronary syndrome. JAMA 2009;301:937–944.
58. Mega JL, Close SL, Wiviott SD, et al. Cytochrome P-450 polymorphisms and response to clopidogrel. N Engl J Med 2009;360:354–362.
59. Saw J, Steinhubl SR, Berger PB, et al. Lack of adverse clopidogrel atorvastatin clinical interaction from secondary analysis of a randomized, placebo-controlled clopidogrel trial. Circulation 2003;108:921–924.
60. Cavallari LH, Shin J, Perera MA. Role of pharmacogenomics in the management of traditional and novel oral anticoagulants. Pharmacotherapy 2011;31:1192–1207.

11

Hyperlipidemia

Robert L. Talbert

KEY CONCEPTS

1. Hypercholesterolemia, elevated low-density lipoprotein, and low high-density lipoprotein (HDL) are unequivocally linked to increased risk for coronary heart disease (CHD) and cerebrovascular morbidity and mortality; low-density lipoprotein (LDL) is the primary target.
2. Multiple genetic abnormalities and environmental factors are involved in clinical lipid abnormalities and routinely used clinical laboratory measurements do not define the underlying abnormalities.
3. Initial therapy for any lipoprotein disorder is therapeutic lifestyle changes with restricted intake of total and saturated fat and cholesterol and a modest increase in polyunsaturated fat intake along with a program of regular exercise and weight reduction if needed.
4. If therapy is insufficient after therapeutic lifestyle changes, lipid-lowering agents should be chosen based on the specific lipoprotein disorder presentation and the severity of the lipid abnormality.
5. Considering compliance, adverse effects, and effectiveness, statins are the drugs of choice for patients with hypercholesterolemia because they are the most potent form of monotherapy and are cost-effective in patients with known coronary artery disease (CAD) or multiple risk factors and in high-risk primary prevention patients.
6. Patients not responding to statin monotherapy may be treated with combination therapy for hypercholesterolemia, but should be monitored closely because of an increased risk for adverse effects and drug interactions.
7. Hypertriglyceridemia usually responds well to niacin, gemfibrozil, and fenofibrate; high-dose niacin should be used cautiously in diabetics because of worsening glycemic control. Statins lower triglycerides to a variable extent depending on baseline triglyceride concentration and statin potency.
8. Low HDL-C is addressed with lifestyle modifications such as smoking cessation and increased exercise; niacin and gemfibrozil and fenofibrate can significantly increase HDL-C as well.
9. Lipid-lowering therapy is generally considered to be cost-effective, particularly in secondary intervention and high-risk patients.
10. Reductions in elevated total cholesterol and LDL-C reduce CHD mortality and total mortality; increasing HDL may reduce CHD events as well. Aggressive treatment of hypercholesterolemia results in fewer patients progressing to myocardial infarction, angina, and stroke, and reduces the need for interventions such as coronary artery bypass graft and percutaneous transluminal coronary angioplasty.
11. Lomitapide and mipomersen have been recently approved for the treatment of homozygous familial hypercholesterolemia. Both have novel mechanisms of action to lower total and LDL cholesterol.

Cholesterol, triglycerides, and phospholipids are the major lipids in the body and they are transported as complexes of lipid and proteins known as lipoproteins. Plasma lipoproteins are spherical particles with surfaces that consist largely of phospholipid, free cholesterol, and protein, and cores that consist mostly of triglyceride and cholesterol ester (Fig. 11-1). The three major classes of lipoproteins found in serum are low-density lipoproteins (LDL), high-density lipoproteins (HDL), and very-low-density lipoproteins (VLDL). VLDL is carried in the circulation as triglyceride and can be estimated by dividing the triglyceride concentration by 5 if the triglyceride concentration is below 250 mg/dL (2.83 mmol/L). Intermediate-density lipoprotein (IDL) resides between VLDL and LDL and is included in the LDL measurement in routine clinical measurement. Abnormalities of plasma lipoproteins can result in a predisposition to coronary, cerebrovascular, and peripheral vascular arterial disease and constitute one of the major risk factors for coronary heart disease (CHD). Accumulating evidence over the past decades had linked elevated total and LDL cholesterol and reduced HDL to the development of CHD. Premature coronary atherosclerosis, leading to the manifestations of ischemic heart disease (IHD; see Chap. 6), is the most common and significant consequence of dyslipidemia. The National Cholesterol Education Program (NCEP) Adult Treatment Panel III (ATP III) published its third report summarizing these data and giving recommendations for the management of hypercholesterolemia in adults.[1,2] This report and the later update modify earlier recommendations and provide a new way of risk stratifying patients based on multiple risk factors, the presence of diabetes, and the metabolic syndrome. The American Heart Association (AHA) also provides guidelines for primary and secondary prevention of CHD.[3–5]

Total cholesterol and LDL-C increase throughout life in men and women, representing an atherogenic pattern characteristic of Westernized society diets.[6] Based on estimates from the AHA, 43.4% or 98.9 million American adults over age 20 years have total cholesterol levels of 200 mg/dL (5.17 mmol/L) or higher.[7] More than half of individuals at borderline high risk remain unaware that they have hypercholesterolemia and fewer than half of highest-risk persons (those with symptomatic CHD) are receiving lipid-lowering treatment. About one-third of treated patients are achieving their LDL goal; fewer than 20% of CHD patients are at their LDL goal.[8,9] Changes in the NCEP guidelines have increased the number of persons eligible for therapeutic lifestyle changes (TLCs) or lipid-lowering therapy by millions. NCEP estimates that only 26% of

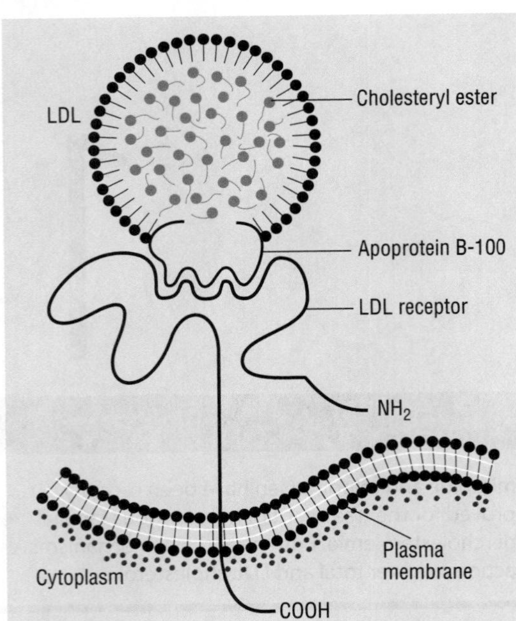

FIGURE 11-1 Diagrammatic representation of the structure of lowdensity lipoprotein (LDL), the LDL receptor, and the binding of LDL to the receptor via apolipoprotein B-100. *(From Ganong WF. Review of Medical Physiology, 22nd ed. New York: McGraw-Hill, 2005:303.)*

patients have an optimal LDL-C (<100 mg/dL [<2.59 mmol/L]) and that large numbers of patients are either untreated or undertreated.[1] Unfortunately, those patients at highest risk are less likely to be treated to desirable levels of LDL.[10] Although these numbers seem staggering in their enormity, substantial progress has been made, and the number of Americans with a desirable blood cholesterol level (<200 mg/dL [<5.17 mmol/L]) has risen to 49% from 45% from the earlier survey (1976 to 1980), while the average total cholesterol in this country has fallen from 220 mg/dL (5.69 mmol/L) in 1960 to 195 mg/dL for men and 201 mg/dL for women.[7] Patients who are at risk but who have not yet experienced their first cardiovascular or cerebrovascular event (e.g., myocardial infarction [MI]) are termed primary prevention, whereas those with manifest vascular disease are termed secondary intervention.

1 Data from the Framingham study and from other studies demonstrate that the risk for developing cardiovascular disease is related to the degree of total cholesterol and LDL elevation in a graded, continuous fashion.[11] Hypercholesterolemia is additive to the other nonlipid risk factors for CHD, including cigarette smoking, hypertension, diabetes, low HDL levels, and electrocardiographic abnormalities. The presence of established CHD or prior MI increases the risk of MI five to seven times that seen in men or women without CHD, and LDL is a significant predictor of subsequent morbidity and mortality. About 50% of all MIs and at least 70% of CHD deaths occur in patients with known CHD, and these patients should therefore be a target for screening, identification, and treatment. Unfortunately, the identification of patients at high risk because of hypercholesterolemia or other lipid disorders is too frequently overlooked, because blood lipid levels are not always evaluated in this population even after an event such as MI.

A comparison of the United States to other countries shows similar relationships between total cholesterol and LDL, and an inverse relationship with HDL to coronary artery disease (CAD) mortality.[11] On a positive note, the U.S. mortality rate is midway among the countries studied, and this country has had the greatest decline in CAD mortality (35% to 40%) in men and women over the past 10 years as compared with other countries. A decline in the prevalence of hypercholesterolemia in certain segments of the U.S. population parallels these trends in mortality.[1] LDL and the ratio of LDL to HDL have also been used to assess risk, but their use adds little information to total cholesterol alone unless HDL is abnormally high or low. McQueen et al. found that the ratio of apolipoprotein (Apo) B to ApoA-I was more predictive and consistent across gender and ethnic groups.[12] HDL transports cholesterol from lipid-laden foam cells to the liver. HDL has been shown to be protective for the occurrence of CHD, and an inverse relationship exists between CHD and HDL levels.[13] Recent clinical trials attempting to raise HDL have failed to demonstrate clinically meaningful reductions in cardiovascular end points challenging the importance of increasing HDL fractions and ApoA-I.[14]

VLDL, the major lipoprotein associated with triglycerides, is enriched with cholesterol esters, and is smaller, denser, and more atherogenic than less dense VLDL. Routine measurement of triglycerides cannot distinguish between the types of VLDL present in plasma. Elevation of triglyceride-rich lipoproteins is associated with low HDL, and this ratio predicts increased risk. The 8-year followup of the Copenhagen male study found a clear gradient of risk of IHD with increasing triglyceride levels within each level of HDL cholesterol. When compared with the lowest tertile of triglyceride concentrations, the highest tertile had 2.2 relative risk for IHD and the relationship extended across all concentrations of HDL.[15] The Helsinki Heart Study shows that hypertriglyceridemia and low HDL are associated with obesity (body mass index [BMI] >26 kg/m^2), smoking, sedentary lifestyle, blood pressure of ≥140/90 mm Hg, and blood glucose above 79 mg/dL (4.4 mmol/L), and that the benefit of gemfibrozil (risk reduction 68%, P <0.03) was largely confined to overweight subjects.[16] Hypertriglyceridemia in certain instances—for example, diabetes mellitus, nephrotic syndrome, and chronic renal disease, and perhaps in women—is associated with increased cardiovascular risk. This is thought to be a consequence of the presence of atherogenic lipoproteins and of hypertriglyceridemia being a marker for them, as triglycerides are usually not independently predictive for CHD.[17]

LIPOPROTEIN METABOLISM AND TRANSPORT

Cholesterol and triglycerides, as the major plasma lipids, are essential substrates for cell membrane formation and hormone synthesis, and provide a source of free fatty acids.[18] Dyslipidemia may be defined as an elevation in total cholesterol, elevation in LDL cholesterol, elevation in triglycerides or low HDL cholesterol concentration, or some combination of these abnormalities. Lipids, being water immiscible, are not present in free form in the plasma, but rather circulate as lipoproteins. Hyperlipoproteinemia describes an increased concentration of the lipoprotein macromolecules that transport lipids in the plasma. The density of plasma lipoproteins is determined by their relative content of protein and lipid. Density, composition, size, and electrophoretic mobility divide lipoproteins into four classes (Table 11-1).

LDL has been further divided into LDL$_1$, or IDL (density 1.006 to 1.019 g/mL), and LDL$_2$ (1.019 to 1.063 g/mL). LDL$_2$ is the major LDL component in plasma and it carries 60% to 70% of the total serum cholesterol. HDL has been subfractionated into HDL$_2$ (density 1.063 to 1.125 g/mL) and HDL$_3$ (1.125 to 1.21 g/mL). Fluctuations in HDL are usually caused by alterations in the levels of HDL$_2$. HDL normally carries about 20% to 30% of the total cholesterol. VLDL has also been subdivided into three classes, and it carries about 10% to 15% of serum cholesterol and most of the triglycerides in the fasting state. VLDL is the precursor for LDL, and VLDL

TABLE 11-1 Composition of Lipoprotein Isolated from Normal Subjects

Lipoprotein Class[a]	Density Range (g/mL)	Diameter (nm)	Composition (Weight %) Cholesterol				
			Protein	Triglyceride	Free	Ester	Phospholipid
Chylomicrons	<0.94	75–1,200	1–2	80–95	1–3	2–4	3–9
VLDL	0.94–1.006	30–80	6–10	55–80	4–8	16–22	10–20
LDL	1.006–1.063	18–25	18–22	5–15	6–8	45–50	18–24
HDL	1.063–1.21	5–12	45–55	5–10	3–5	15–20	20–30

[a]VLDL denotes very-low-density lipoprotein, LDL low-density lipoprotein, and HDL high-density lipoprotein.

remnants may also be atherogenic. Table 11-2 shows the characteristics of the protein constituent of lipoproteins known as Apos. The structure of LDL, the LDL receptor (LDL-R), and the binding of the LDL to the receptor via ApoB-100 are shown in Figure 11-1.

Chylomicrons, large triglyceride-rich particles containing Apos B-48, B-100, and E, are formed from dietary fat solubilized by bile salts in intestinal mucosal cells. Chylomicrons are normally not present in the plasma after a fast of 12 to 14 hours and are catabolized by lipoprotein lipase (LPL), which is activated by ApoC-II and in the vascular endothelium and hepatic lipase to form chylomicron remnants. The remnants that contain ApoE (Fig. 11-2) are taken up by the "remnant receptor," which may be an LDL-R-related protein, in the liver. Free cholesterol is liberated intracellularly after attachment to the remnant receptor. Chylomicrons also function to deliver dietary triglyceride to skeletal muscle and adipose tissue. During the catabolism of nascent chylomicrons to remnants, triglyceride is converted to free fatty acids and Apos A-I, A-II, A-IV (free in plasma), C-I, C-II, and C-III, and phospholipids are transferred to HDL. Apos E and C-II are transferred to chylomicrons from HDL and eventually back through these metabolic events. Hepatic VLDL synthesis is regulated in part by diet and hormones, and is inhibited by uptake of chylomicron remnants in the liver. VLDL is secreted from the liver and serially converted via LPL to IDL, and, finally, to LDL. VLDL receptors are found in adipose tissue and muscle, and bear close homology to the structure of LDL-Rs.

LDL, the major cholesterol transport lipoprotein and having virtually only ApoB-100, is mostly derived from VLDL catabolism and cellular synthesis. When fasting and on low-fat intake in normal subjects, most cholesterol is synthesized and used in the extrahepatic organs, while most of the cholesterol carried by LDL is taken up by the liver for catabolism. In patients with homozygous familial hypercholesterolemia, enhanced synthesis of LDL may occur, because LDL clearance is reduced as a consequence of the lack of LDL-Rs. LDL is catabolized through interaction of cell surface receptors found on liver, adrenal, and peripheral cells (including fibroblasts and smooth muscle cells). These cells recognize ApoB-100 on LDL, and after binding to a receptor on the cell membrane, LDL is internalized and degraded. In the normal fasting state, approximately 70% of LDL is cleared through receptor-dependent mechanism, although this is highly dependent on the availability and type of saturated and monounsaturated or polyunsaturated fat from dietary sources. Ingestion of cholesterol and saturated fatty acids such as C12:0, C14:0, and C16:0 is associated with reduction in LDL-R activity, increased

TABLE 11-2 Characteristics and Functions of Apolipoproteins

Apolipoprotein	Lipoprotein Density Class	Approximate Plasma Concentration (mg/dL [g/L])	Approximate Molecular Weight (kDa)	Reported Functions	Major Site of Synthesis
A-I	Chylomicrons, HDL	120 (1.2)	28	Cofactor with LCAT, structural protein on HDL, ligand for HDL receptor	Liver, intestine
A-II	Chylomicrons, HDL	35 (0.35)	17	Structural protein for HDL, ligand for HDL receptor	Liver
A-IV	Chylomicrons, 1.21B	15 (0.15)	46	Possibly facilitates transfer of other Apos between HDL and chylomicrons	Intestine
ApoLp(a)	LDL, HDL	10 (0.10)	500	Bound to B-100, high homology with plasminogen, may prevent LDL uptake by B, E receptor	Liver
B-100	VLDL, LDL, IDL	100 (1)	540	Necessary for assembly and secretion of VLDL from the liver, structural protein of VLDL, IDL, LDL, ligand for LDL receptor	Liver
B-48	Chylomicrons	Trace	264	Necessary for assembly and secretion of chylomicrons from the small intestine	Intestine
C-I	Chylomicrons, VLDL, HDL	7 (0.07)	6.6	Cofactor with LCAT; may inhibit hepatic uptake of chylomicron and VLDL remnants	Liver
C-II	Chylomicrons, VLDL, HDL	4 (0.04)	8.9	Activator of LPL	Liver
C-III	Chylomicrons, VLDL, HDL	13 (0.13)	8.8	Inhibitor with LPL; may inhibit hepatic uptake of chylomicron and VLDL remnants	Liver
D	HDL	6 (0.06)	32	?	?
E2-E4	Chylomicrons, VLDL, HDL	5 (0.05)	34	Ligand for several lipoproteins to LDL receptor, LRP, and possibly a separate hepatic ApoE receptor	Liver

IDL, intermediate-density lipoprotein; LCAT, lecithin-cholesterol acyltransferase; LRP, LDL receptor–related protein. Other abbreviations are in Table 11-1.

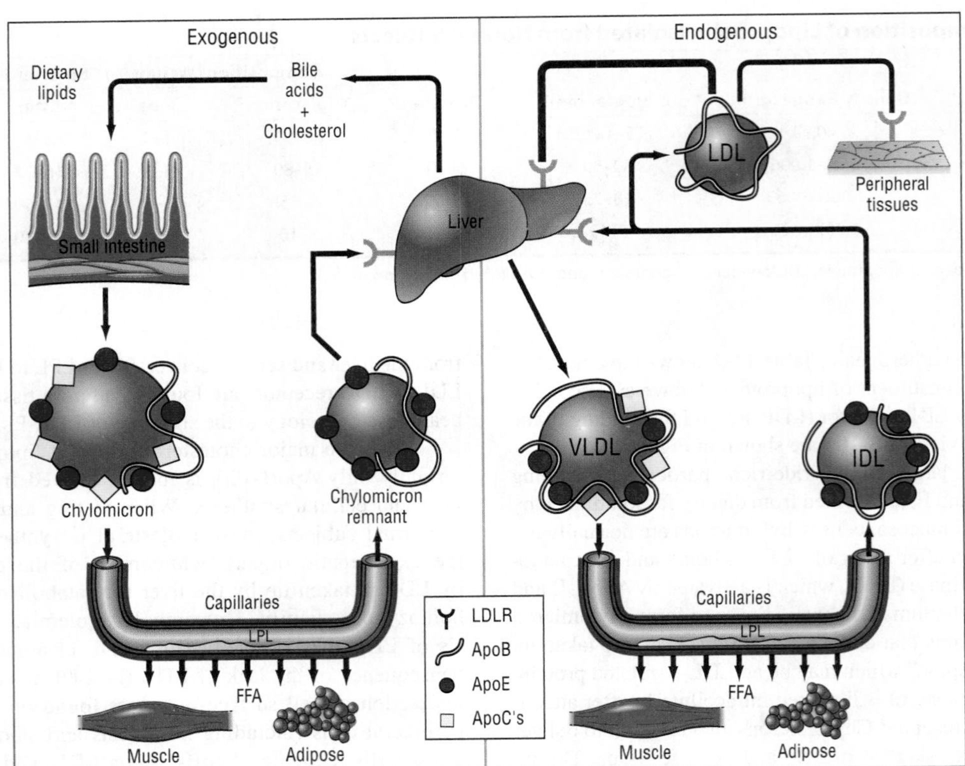

FIGURE 11-2 Simplified diagram of lipoprotein systems for transporting lipids in humans. In the exogenous system, chylomicrons rich in triglycerides of dietary origin are converted to chylomicron remnants rich in cholesteryl esters by the action of lipoprotein lipase (LPL). In the endogenous system, very-low-density lipoproteins (VLDL) rich in triglycerides are secreted by the liver and converted to intermediate-density lipoproteins (LDL) and then to low-density lipoproteins (LDL) rich in cholesteryl esters. Some of the LDLs enter the subendothelial space of arteries, are oxidized, and then are taken up by macrophages, which become foam cells. The letters on the chylomicrons, chylomicron remnants, VLDL, IDL, and LDL identify the primary apoproteins (ApoB, ApoC, ApoE) found in them. (LDLR, low-density lipoprotein receptor.) *(From Kasper DL, Braunwald E, Fauci AS, et al., eds. Harrison's Principles of Internal Medicine, 16th ed. New York, McGraw-Hill, 2005, p. 2289.)*

LDL production rate, and elevation in LDL plasma concentration. Receptor-independent mechanisms are also involved to a lesser extent in the catabolism of LDL, and these receptors are present in many tissues but are most active in animals in the adrenals and ovary. Increased intracellular cholesterol resulting from LDL catabolism inhibits the activity of 3-hydroxy-3-methylglutaryl coenzyme A reductase (HMG-CoA reductase), the rate-limiting enzyme for intracellular cholesterol biosynthesis (Fig. 11-3). Additional consequences of increased intracellular cholesterol include reduced synthesis of LDL-R, which limits subsequent cholesterol uptake from the plasma, and accelerated activity of acyl-coenzyme A-to-cholesterol acyltransferase (ACAT) to facilitate cholesterol storage within cells. LDL cholesterol may also be excreted into bile and become part of the enterohepatic pool or may be lost in the stool. Lp(a) is a cholesterol-rich lipoprotein similar to LDL in composition and density and with close homology to fibrinogen; it is reported to be an important independent risk factor for the development of premature cardiovascular disease.

Nascent HDL is derived from liver and gut synthesis primarily in the form of ApoA-I phospholipid disks.[13] Esterification of free cholesterol in nascent HDL and from peripheral tissues to cholesteryl esters by lecithin-cholesterol acyltransferase (LCAT) results in the production of HDL_3. Further addition of tissue cholesterol to HDL_3 results in the formation of HDL_2. HDL_2 can also be formed from remodeling of chylomicrons and VLDL catabolism. It may be converted back to HDL_3 by the action of hepatic lipase and by the transfer of cholesteryl esters to the liver, LDL, and VLDL. ApoA-I production is increased by estrogens, leading to higher HDL levels in women and in individuals receiving estrogen. Transfer of excess cholesterol from peripheral tissues by HDL is called *reverse cholesterol transport*. Putative HDL receptors in peripheral cells facilitate the uptake of cholesterol by HDL, which transfers cholesterol to either VLDL and LDL or the liver for secretion into bile or conversion into bile acids. These processes serve to rid peripheral tissue (e.g., coronary arteries) of excessive amounts of cholesterol, and account for some of the protective effects noted with increasing HDL in women and other factors that elevate HDL levels. Variants of the cholesterol ester transfer protein (CETP) have been demonstrated in humans, and the B1B1 genotype is associated with lower HDL and progression of coronary atherosclerosis. Inhibition of CETP leads to elevations in HDL; unfortunately when CETP inhibitors were tested in clinical trials, they did not induce regression of atherosclerotic plaque and were associated with higher blood pressure and CHD events.[19–22] The effect of CETP inhibition on blood pressure and HDL is discordant with some of these agents.[23]

The "response-to-injury" hypothesis states that risk factors such as oxidized LDL, mechanical injury to the endothelium (e.g., percutaneous transluminal angioplasty), excessive homocysteine, immunologic attack, or infection-induced (e.g., *Chlamydia*, herpes simplex virus-1) changes in endothelial and intimal function lead to endothelial dysfunction and a series of cellular interactions that culminate in atherosclerosis. C-reactive protein (CRP) is an acute phase reactant and a marker for inflammation; it may be useful in identifying patients at risk for developing CAD.[24] The transcription factor Kruppel-like factor 2 (KLF2) may be induced by statins in

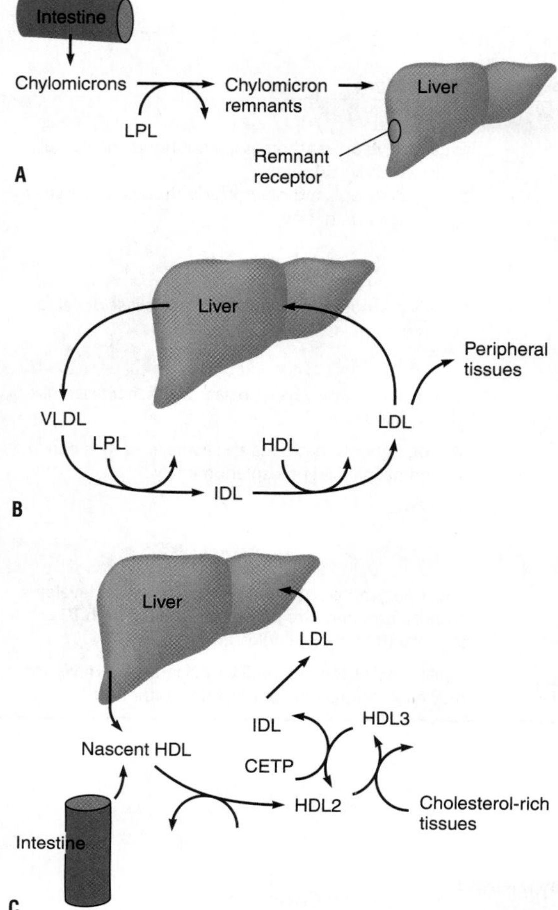

FIGURE 11-3 Biosynthetic pathway for cholesterol. The rate-limiting enzyme in this pathway is 3-hydroxy-3-methylglutaryl coenzyme A reductase (HMG-CoA reductase). (CETP, cholesterol ester transfer protein; HDL, high-density lipoprotein; IDL, intermediate-density lipoprotein; LDL, low-density lipoprotein; LPL, lipoprotein lipase; VLDL, very-low-density lipoprotein.) *A.* Exogenous pathway; *B.* Endogenous pathway; *C.* Reverse cholesterol transport. *(Modified from Breslow JL. Genetic basis of lipoprotein disorders. J Clin Invest 1989;84:373.)*

liver sinusoidal endothelial cells (SEC), orchestrating an efficient vasoprotective response. Upregulation of hepatic endothelial KLF2-derived transcriptional programs by statins confers vasoprotection and stellate cell deactivation, reinforcing the therapeutic potential of these drugs for liver diseases that course with endothelial dysfunction.

The eventual outcomes of this atherogenic cascade are clinical events such as angina, MI, arrhythmias, stroke, peripheral arterial disease, abdominal aortic aneurysm, and sudden death. Atherosclerotic lesions are thought to arise from transport and retention of plasma LDL cholesterol through the endothelial cell layer into the extracellular matrix of the subendothelial space. Once in the artery wall, LDL is chemically modified through oxidation and nonenzymatic glycation. Mildly oxidized LDL then recruits monocytes into the artery wall, which become transformed into macrophages. Macrophages have tremendous potential for accelerating LDL oxidation and ApoB accumulation, and altering the receptor-mediated uptake of LDL into the artery wall from the usual LDL-R to a "scavenger receptor" not regulated by cell content of cholesterol. Oxidized LDL increases plasminogen inhibitor levels (promotion of coagulation), induces the expression of endothelin (vasoconstrictive substance), inhibits the expression of nitric oxide (a vasodilator and platelet inhibitor), and is toxic to macrophages if highly oxidized. As oxidation of biologically active lipids proceeds, other lipids such as lysophosphatidylcholine, hydroperoxides, aldehydic breakdown products of fatty acids, and oxysterol are formed, which continue the reaction within the tissue. These events lead to a massive accumulation of cholesterol. The cholesterol-laden macrophages become foam cells; foam cells are the earliest recognized cells of the arterial fatty streak.

Oxidized LDL provokes an inflammatory response, which is mediated by a number of chemoattractants and cytokines. Examples of each that appear to be involved at different stages of lesion development include monocyte chemoattractant protein 1 (MCP-1), monocyte colony-stimulating factor (M-CSF), *gro*, vascular cell adhesion molecule (VCAM-1), E-selectin (ELAM-1), intercellular adhesion molecule (ICAM-1), platelet-derived growth factor (PDGF), vascular endothelial growth factor (VEGF), transforming growth factors (TGF-α and TGF-β), interleukin-1 (IL-1) and interleukin-6 (IL-6), and the ratio of interleukin-10 (IL-10) and interleukin-12 (IL-12). It appears that some of these factors (e.g., MCP-1 and M-CSF) participate early in the process of monocyte–macrophage attachment and transmigration across the endothelium, whereas others (PDGF and VCAM-1) promote later lesion growth.[25] The extent of oxidation and the inflammatory response is under genetic control of a major gene termed *Ath*-1 based on murine model studies. The process of aging may lead to lipoproteins that are more susceptible to oxidation and have longer resident time in the vascular compartment. Two proteins associated with HDL—ApoJ and paraoxonase (PON)—appear to play an important role to minimize the oxidation of LDL-C.[26] Increased recognition of the role of these growth-regulatory molecules provides the possibility of future directions for antagonists to regulatory molecules such as PDGF, TGF-β, and the interleukins. Repeated injury and repair within an atherosclerotic plaque eventually lead to a fibrous cap protecting the underlying core of lipids, collagen, calcium, and inflammatory cells such as T lymphocytes. Maintenance of the fibrous plaque is critical to prevent plaque rupture and subsequent coronary thrombosis.[27] An imbalance between plaque synthesis and degradation may lead to a weakened or vulnerable plaque prone to rupture. The fibrous cap may become weakened through decreased synthesis of the extracellular matrix or increased degradation of the matrix. The cytokine interferon-γ, produced by T lymphocytes, inhibits the ability of smooth muscle cells to synthesize collagen, a structurally important component of the fibrous cap. A family of enzymes known as matrix metalloproteinases can degrade all major constituents of the vascular extracellular matrix: collagen, elastin, and proteoglycans.[28]

2 Lipoprotein disorders are classified into six categories, which are commonly used for phenotypical description of dyslipidemia (Table 11-3). Specific genetic defects with disrupted protein, cell, and organ function give rise to several disorders within each

TABLE 11-3 Fredrickson-Levy-Lees Classification of Hyperlipoproteinemia

Type	Lipoprotein Elevation
I	Chylomicrons
IIa	LDL
IIb	LDL + VLDL
III	IDL (LDL_1)
IV	VLDL
V	VLDL + chylomicrons

IDL, intermediate-density lipoprotein; LDL, low-density lipoprotein; VLDL, very-low-density lipoprotein.

TABLE 11-4 Lipoprotein Disorders

Lipid Phenotype	Plasma Lipid Levels (mg/dL [mmol/L])	Lipoproteins Elevated	Lipoproteins Phenotype	Clinical Signs
Isolated Hypercholesterolemia				
Familial hypercholesterolemia	Heterozygotes TC = 275–500 (7.1–12.9)	LDL	IIa	Usually develop xanthomas in adulthood and vascular disease at 30–50 years
	Homozygotes TC >500 (>12.9)	LDL	IIa	Usually develop xanthomas in adulthood and vascular disease in childhood
Familial defective ApoB-100	Heterozygotes TC = 275–500 (7.1–12.9)	LDL	IIa	
Polygenic hypercholesterolemia	TC = 250–350 (6.5–9)	LDL	IIa	Usually asymptomatic until vascular disease develops; no xanthomas
Isolated Hypertriglyceridemia				
Familial hypertriglyceridemia	TG = 250–750 (2.8–8.5)	VLDL	IV	Asymptomatic; may be associated with increased risk of vascular disease
Familial LPL deficiency	TG >750 (>8.5)	Chylomicrons, VLDL	I, V	May be asymptomatic; may be associated with pancreatitits, abdominal pain, hepatosplenomegaly
Familial ApoC-II deficiency	TG >750 (>8.5)	Chylomicrons, VLDL	I, V	As above
Hypertriglyceridemia and Hypercholesterolemia				
Combined hyperlipidemia	TG = 250–750 (2.8–8.5); TC = 250–500 (6.5–12.9)	VLDL, LDL	IIb	Usually asymptomatic until vascular disease develops; familial form may also present as isolated high TG or an isolated high LDL cholesterol
Dysbetalipoproteinemia	TG = 250–750 (2.8–8.5); TC = 250–500 (6.5–12.9)	VLDL, IDL; LDL normal	III	Usually asymptomatic until vascular disease develops; may have palmar or tuboeruptive xanthomas

LPL, lipoprotein lipase; TC, total cholesterol; TG, triglycerides. Other abbreviations as in Table 11-1.

family of lipoproteins (Table 11-4). In other words, an elevated cholesterol level does not necessarily equate with familial hypercholesterolemia or type IIa, as cholesterol may also be elevated in other lipoprotein disorders and the lipoprotein pattern does not describe the underlying genetic defect. The preceding discussion has focused on primary or genetic dyslipoproteinemia; it should be remembered that secondary forms exist and that several drugs may also elevate lipid levels (Table 11-5). These secondary forms of hyperlipidemia should be initially managed by correcting the underlying abnormality, including modification of drug therapy when appropriate.

Familial hypercholesterolemia is characterized by (a) a selective elevation in the plasma level of LDL; (b) deposition of LDL-derived cholesterol in tendons (xanthomas) and arteries (atheromas); and (c) inheritance as an autosomal dominant trait with homozygotes more severely affected than heterozygotes. Homozygotes (prevalence 1 in 1,000,000) have severe hypercholesterolemia (650 to 1,000 mg/dL [16.8 to 25.9 mmol/L]), with the early appearance of cutaneous xanthomas and fatal CHD generally before the age of 20. The primary defect in familial hypercholesterolemia is the inability to bind LDL to the LDL-R or, rarely, a defect of internalizing the LDL-R complex into the cell after normal binding. Homozygotes have essentially no functional LDL-Rs. This leads to lack of LDL degradation by cells and unregulated biosynthesis of cholesterol, with total cholesterol and LDL-C being inversely proportional to the deficit in LDL-Rs. Heterozygotes have only about one half of the normal number of LDL-Rs, total cholesterol levels in the range of 300 to 600 mg/dL (7.76 to 15.52 mmol/L), and cardiovascular events beginning in the third and fourth decades of life.

Familial LPL deficiency is a rare, autosomal recessive trait characterized by a massive accumulation of chylomicrons and corresponding increase in plasma triglycerides or a type I lipoprotein pattern. VLDL concentration is normal. The presenting manifestations include repeated attacks of pancreatitis and abdominal pain, eruptive cutaneous xanthomatosis, and hepatosplenomegaly beginning in childhood. Symptom severity is proportional to dietary fat

TABLE 11-5 Secondary Causes of Lipoprotein Abnormalities

Hypercholesterolemia	Hypothyroidism Obstructive liver disease Nephrotic syndrome Anorexia nervosa Acute intermittent porphyria Drugs: progestins, thiazide diuretics, glucocorticoids, β-blockers, isotretinoin, protease inhibitors, cyclosporine, mirtazapine, sirolimus
Hypertriglyceridemia	Obesity Diabetes mellitus Lipodystrophy Glycogen storage disease Ileal bypass surgery Sepsis Pregnancy Acute hepatitis Systemic lupus erythematosus Monoclonal gammopathy: multiple myeloma, lymphoma Drugs: alcohol, estrogens, isotretinoin, β-blockers, glucocorticoids, bile acid resins, thiazides, asparaginase, interferons, azole antifungals, mirtazapine, anabolic steroids, sirolimus, bexarotene
Hypocholesterolemia	Malnutrition Malabsorption Myeloproliferative diseases Chronic infectious diseases: AIDS, tuberculosis Monoclonal gammopathy Chronic liver disease
Low HDL	Malnutrition Obesity Drugs: non-ISA β-blockers, anabolic steroids, probucol, isotretinoin, progestins

CLINICAL PRESENTATION

General

- Most patients are asymptomatic for many years prior to clinically evident disease.
- Patients with the metabolic syndrome may have three or more of the following: abdominal obesity, atherogenic dyslipidemia, raised blood pressure, insulin resistance ± glucose intolerance, prothrombotic state, or proinflammatory state.

Symptoms

- None to chest pain, palpitations, sweating, anxiety, shortness of breath, loss of consciousness or difficulty with speech or movement, abdominal pain, and sudden death.

Signs

- None to abdominal pain, pancreatitis, eruptive xanthomas, peripheral polyneuropathy, high blood pressure, BMI >30 kg/m^2, or waist size >40 in (102 cm) in men (35 in [89 cm] in women).

Laboratory Tests

- Elevations in total cholesterol, LDL, triglycerides, ApoB, and CRP.
- Low HDL.

Other Diagnostic Tests

- Lipoprotein(a), and small, dense LDL (pattern B), HDL subclassification, ApoE isoforms, ApoA-I, fibrinogen, folate, and lipoprotein-associated phospholipase A_2.
- Various screening tests for manifestations of vascular disease (ankle-brachial index, exercise testing, magnetic resonance imaging) and diabetes (fasting glucose, oral glucose tolerance test, hemoglobin A_{1c}).

intake, and consequently to the elevation of chylomicrons. LPL is normally released from vascular endothelium or by heparin and hydrolyzes chylomicrons and VLDL (see Fig. 11-2). Diagnosis is based on low or absent enzyme activity with normal human plasma or ApoC-II, a cofactor of the enzyme. Accelerated atherosclerosis is not associated with this disease. Abdominal pain, pancreatitis, eruptive xanthomas, and peripheral polyneuropathy characterize type V (VLDL and chylomicrons). Symptoms may occur in childhood, but usually the disorder is expressed at a later age. The risk of atherosclerosis is increased with this disorder. These patients are commonly obese, hyperuricemic, and diabetic, and alcohol intake, exogenous estrogens, and renal insufficiency tend to be exacerbating factors.

Patients with familial type III hyperlipoproteinemia (also called dysbetalipoproteinemia, broadband, or β-VLDL) develop the following clinical features after 20 years of age: xanthoma striata palmaris (yellow discolorations of the palmar and digital creases), tuberous or tuberoeruptive xanthomas (bulbous cutaneous xanthomas), and severe atherosclerosis involving the coronary arteries, internal carotids, and abdominal aorta. A defective structure of ApoE does not allow normal hepatic surface receptor binding of remnant particles derived from chylomicrons and VLDL (known as IDL); aggravating factors such as obesity, diabetes, or pregnancy may promote overproduction of ApoB–containing lipoproteins. Although homozygosity for the defective allele (E_2/E_2) is common (1 in 100), only 1 in 10,000 expresses the full-blown picture, and interaction with other genetic or environmental factors, or both, is needed to produce clinical disease.

Familial combined hyperlipidemia is characterized by elevations in total cholesterol, triglycerides, decreased HDL, increased ApoB, and small, dense LDL.[29] It is associated with premature CHD and may be difficult to diagnose since the lipid levels do not consistently display the same pattern.

Type IV hyperlipoproteinemia is common and occurs in adulthood primarily in patients who are obese, diabetic, and hyperuricemic and do not have xanthomas. It may be secondary to alcohol ingestion and can be aggravated by stress, progestins, oral contraceptives, thiazides, or β-blockers. Two genetic patterns occur in type IV hyperlipoproteinemia: familial hypertriglyceridemia, which does not carry a great risk for premature CAD, and familial combined hyperlipidemia, which is associated with increased risk of cardiovascular disease.

Rare forms of lipoprotein disorders may include hypobetalipoproteinemia, abetalipoproteinemia, Tangier disease, LCAT deficiency (fish-eye disease), cerebrotendinous xanthomatosis (CTX), and sitosterolemia. Most of these rare lipoprotein disorders do not result in premature atherosclerosis, with the exceptions of familial LCAT deficiency, CTX, and sitosterolemia with xanthomatosis. Their treatment consists of dietary restriction of plant sterols (sitosterolemia with xanthomatosis), chenodeoxycholic acid (CTX), or, potentially, blood transfusion (LCAT deficiency).

PATIENT EVALUATION

A fasting lipoprotein profile including total cholesterol, LDL-C, HDL-C, and triglycerides should be measured in all adults 20 years of age or older at least once every 5 years.[1] If the profile is obtained in the nonfasted state, only total cholesterol and HDL-C will be usable because LDL-C is usually a calculated value; if total cholesterol is ≥200 mg/dL (≥5.17 mmol/L), or if HDL-C is <40 mg/dL (<1.03 mmol/L), a followup fasting lipoprotein profile should be obtained. After a lipid abnormality is confirmed (Table 11-6), major components of the evaluation are the history (including age, gender, and, if female, menstrual and hormone replacement status), physical examination, and laboratory investigations. A complete history and physical examination should assess (a) presence or absence of cardiovascular risk factors (Table 11-7) or definite cardiovascular disease in the individual; (b) family history of premature cardiovascular disease or lipid disorders; (c) presence or absence of secondary causes of lipid abnormalities, including concurrent medications (see Table 11-5); and (d) presence or absence of xanthomas or abdominal pain, or history of pancreatitis, renal or liver disease, peripheral vascular disease, abdominal aortic aneurysm, or cerebral vascular disease (carotid bruits, stroke, or transient ischemic attack [TIA]). An important change in the ATP III guidelines is that diabetes mellitus is regarded as a CHD risk equivalent.[1] The presence of diabetes in patients without known CHD is associated with the same

TABLE 11-6 Classification of Total, LDL, and HDL Cholesterol, and Triglycerides

Total Cholesterol	
<200 mg/dL (<5.17 mmol/L)	Desirable
200–239 mg/dL (5.17–6.20 mmol/L)	Borderline high
≥240 mg/dL (≥6.21 mmol/L)	High
LDL Cholesterol	
<100 mg/dL (<2.59 mmol/L)	Optimal
100–129 mg/dL (2.59–3.35 mmol/L)	Near or above optimal
130–159 mg/dL (3.36–4.13 mmol/L)	Borderline high
160–189 mg/dL (4.14–4.90 mmol/L)	High
≥190 mg/dL (≥4.91 mmol/L)	Very high
HDL Cholesterol	
<40 mg/dL (<1.03 mmol/L)	Low
≥60 mg/dL (≥1.55 mmol/L)	High
Triglycerides	
<150 mg/dL (<1.70 mmol/L)	Normal
150–199 mg/dL (1.70–2.25 mmol/L)	Borderline high
200–499 mg/dL (2.26–5.64 mmol/L)	High
≥500 mg/dL (≥5.65 mmol/L)	Very high

HDL, high-density lipoproteins; LDL, low-density lipoproteins.

level of risk as in patients without diabetes but having confirmed CHD.[30,31] ATP III identifies four categories of risk that modify the goals and modalities of LDL-lowering therapy (Table 11-8).[2] The highest category is known CHD or CHD risk equivalents, which is defined as the risk for major coronary events equal to or greater than established CHD, that is, >20% per 10 years (2% per year). The next category is moderately high risk consisting of patients with multiple (2+) risk factors in which 10-year risk for CHD is 10% to 20%. Moderate risk is defined as ≥2 risk factors and a 10-year risk of ≤10%. The lowest risk category is persons with zero to one risk factor. Risk is estimated from Framingham risk scores.[32] Risk is estimated based on the patient's age, LDL-C or total cholesterol level, blood pressure, the presence of diabetes, and smoking status (Table 11-7). This approach for a single patient is referred to as case finding or patient-based approach, whereas large-scale screening and recommendations for the general populace, healthcare providers, and the food industry are called a population-based approach.

Measurement of plasma cholesterol (which is about 3% lower than serum determinations), triglyceride, and HDL-C levels after a 12-hour or longer fast is important, as triglycerides may be elevated in nonfasted individuals; total cholesterol is only modestly affected by fasting. Analytic and biologic variability can have a major impact on the measurement and interpretation of cholesterol (or any other laboratory test). Analytic variability can be minimized through the use of adequate quality control procedures, including internal training, routine calibration and monitoring, and external proficiency testing. Even with these measures, the coefficient of variability in the best procedures can acceptably be up to 5%, and when combined with average biologic variability, total variability may be as high as about 22%. Analytic variability with desktop equipment generally is greater in the finger-stick capillary blood methods, usually yielding measurements less than those from a clinical laboratory, and this technology should be considered for use only as a screening method. Reliance on desktop methods can result in misclassification of 7% to 14% of patients if capillary blood is used. Two determinations, 1 to 8 weeks apart, with the patient on a stable diet and weight, and in the absence of acute illness, are recommended to minimize variability and to obtain a reliable baseline.[1] If the total cholesterol is greater than 200 mg/dL (5.17 mmol/L), a second determination is recommended, and if the values are more than 30 mg/dL (0.78 mmol/L) apart, the average of three values should be used. Familiarity with the method and quality control procedures employed by local laboratories is essential for interpretation of reported values. If the physical examination and history are insufficient to diagnose a familial disorder, then agarose-gel lipoprotein electrophoresis is useful to determine which class of lipoproteins is affected. If the triglyceride levels are below 400 mg/dL (4.52 mmol/L) and neither type III hyperlipidemia nor chylomicrons are detected by electrophoresis, then one can calculate VLDL and LDL concentrations: VLDL = triglyceride/5; LDL = total cholesterol − (VLDL − HDL).

Because total cholesterol is composed of cholesterol derived from LDL, VLDL, and HDL, determination of HDL is useful when total plasma cholesterol is elevated. HDL may be elevated by moderate alcohol ingestion (less than two drinks per day), physical exercise, smoking cessation, weight loss, oral contraceptives, phenytoin, and terbutaline. Smoking, obesity, a sedentary lifestyle, and drugs such as β-blockers lower HDL. Only exercise and smoking cessation could be recommended as interventions for low HDL concentrations. Niacin and gemfibrozil also increase HDL concentrations.

The range of lipid concentrations represents a population mean plus or minus two standard deviations and does not define the risk of disease. Reference values for plasma total, LDL, and HDL cholesterol concentrations for men and women, as well as various ethnic groups, are available from the NHANES III.[6] Cholesterol and triglycerides increase throughout life until about the fifth decade for men and the sixth decade for women. Past these ages, total cholesterol and LDL plateau and fall slightly. HDL tends to fall slightly with time and more rapidly after menopause in women. Institution of a population-based approach for cholesterol reduction should shift the entire curve to the left, and the potential reduction in cardiovascular mortality would be proportional to mean reductions at any cholesterol concentration.

Based on a careful review of the experimental pathologic, genetic, and epidemiologic evidence relating to the relationship between blood cholesterol levels and CHD, the ATP III of the NCEP recommends that a fasting lipoprotein profile and risk factor assessment be used in the initial classification of adults.[1,33] If total cholesterol is less than 200 mg/dL (5.17 mmol/L), then the patient has a *desirable blood cholesterol level* (Table 11-6). Cholesterol levels between 200 and 239 mg/dL (5.17 and 6.18 mmol/L) are classified as *borderline high blood cholesterol levels*, and assessment of risk factors (Table 11-7) is needed to more clearly define disease risk. Blood cholesterol levels of 240 mg/dL (6.21 mmol/L) and above are classified as *high blood cholesterol levels*. Clinicians are awaiting the publication of ATP IV and it is anticipated that these categories of lipoproteins may be revised downward. If the total cholesterol is below 200 mg/dL (5.17 mmol/L) and the HDL is above 40 mg/dL (1.03 mmol/L), no further followup is recommended for patients without known CHD and who have fewer than two risk factors. In patients with evidence of CHD or other clinical atherosclerotic disease, the LDL goal is less than 100 mg/dL (2.59 mmol/L) and most patients will require diet and/or drug intervention. In patients with

TABLE 11-7 Major Risk Factors (Exclusive of LDL Cholesterol) that Modify LDL Goals[a]

Age: men: ≥45 years; women: ≥55 years or premature menopause without estrogen replacement therapy, family history of premature CHD (definite myocardial infarction or sudden death before 55 years of age in father or other male first-degree relative, or before 65 years of age in mother or other female first-degree relative)
Cigarette smoking
Hypertension (≥140/90 mm Hg or on antihypertensive medication)
Low HDL cholesterol (<40 mg/dL [<1.03 mmol/L])[b]

[a]Diabetes is regarded as a coronary heart disease (CHD) risk equivalent; LDL indicates low-density lipoprotein; HDL indicates high-density lipoprotein.
[b]HDL cholesterol (≥60 mg/dL [≥1.55 mmol/L]) counts as a "negative" risk factor; its presence removes one risk factor from the total count.

TABLE 11-8 LDL Cholesterol Goals and Cut Points for Therapeutic Lifestyle Changes (TLCs) and Drug Therapy in Different Risk Categories[a]

Risk Category	LDL Goal (mg/dL [mmol/L])	LDL Level at which to Initiate TLC (mg/dL [mmol/L])	LDL Level at which to Consider Drug Therapy (mg/dL [mmol/L])
High risk: CHD or CHD risk equivalents (10-year risk >20%)	<100 (<2.59) (optional goal: <70 [<1.81])	≥100 (≥2.59)	≥100 (≥2.59) (<100 mg/dL [<2.59]; consider drug options)[b]
Moderately high risk: 2+ risk factors (10-year risk >10–20%)	<130 (<3.36)	≥130 (≥3.36)	≥130 (≥3.36) (100–129 [2.59–3.35]: consider drug options)
Moderate risk: 2+ risk factors (10-year risk <10%)	<130 (<3.36)	≥130 (≥3.36)	≥160 (≥4.14)
Lower risk: 0–1 risk factor[c]	<160 (<4.14)	≥160 (≥4.14)	≥190 (≥4.91) (160–189 [4.14–4.90]: LDL-lowering drug optional)

[a]LDL indicates low-density lipoprotein; CHD, coronary heart disease.
[b]Some authorities recommend use of LDL-lowering drugs in this category if an LDL cholesterol level of <100 mg/dL (<2.59 mmol/L) cannot be achieved by TLC. Others prefer use of drugs that primarily modify triglycerides and HDL, for example, nicotinic acid or fibrates. Clinical judgment also may call for deferring drug therapy in this subcategory.
[c]Almost all people with zero to one risk factor have a 10-year risk <10%; thus, 10-year risk assessment in people with zero to one risk factor is not necessary.

very high risk (known CHD and multiple risk factors) the LDL goal may be set at <70 mg/dL (<1.81 mmol/L) based on evidence from newer studies.[33] Decisions regarding classification and management are based on the LDL-C levels as outlined in Table 11-8. An increasing number of persons have the metabolic syndrome that is characterized by abdominal obesity, atherogenic dyslipidemia (elevated triglycerides, small LDL particles, low HDL-C), raised blood pressure, insulin resistance (with or without glucose intolerance), and prothrombotic and proinflammatory states. ATP III recognizes the metabolic syndrome as a secondary target of risk reduction therapy after LDL-C has been addressed and if the metabolic syndrome is present, the patient is considered to have a CHD risk equivalent. Other lipid targets include non-HDL goals for patients with triglycerides >200 mg/dL (>2.26 mmol/L). Non-HDL is calculated by subtracting HDL from total cholesterol and the targets are 30 mg/dL (0.78 mmol/L) greater than LDL for each risk stratum. Non-HDL takes into consideration atherogenic particles such as remnant lipoproteins and IDL that are not measured in routine clinical laboratory testing.[34] HDL raising has potential benefit, but no specific goals are set in the current guidelines and the evidence is modest to support aggressively increasing HDL levels.[35]

The Expert Panel on Children and Adolescents of the NCEP recommends screening in higher-risk children (positive family history or parental high blood cholesterol, ≥240 mg/dL [≥6.21 mmol/L]).[36] The American Academy of Pediatrics categorizes total and LDL cholesterol into acceptable (<75th percentile; total cholesterol <170 mg/dL [<4.40 mmol/L]), borderline (75th to 95th percentile; total cholesterol 170 to 199 mg/dL [4.40 to 5.15 mmol/L], LDL cholesterol 110 to 129 mg/dL [2.84 to 3.34 mmol/L]), and elevated (>95th percentile; total cholesterol >200 mg/dL [>5.17 mmol/L], LDL cholesterol >130 mg/dL [>3.36 mmol/L]).[36] The rationale, in part, for this approach is based on the recognition that atherosclerosis begins in the childhood and adolescent years as documented in the pathobiologic determinants of atherosclerosis in youth (PDAY) and the Bogalusa studies.[37] Similarly, if children with high blood lipids or lipoprotein levels are identified, and the levels in the parents are unknown, the parents should be screened as well, as they are likely to be at high risk. Racial and gender differences do exist in the determination of lipoprotein fractions, and these factors should be considered in screening. Use of the serum cholesterol level alone may be of insufficient specificity or sensitivity, depending on the cut points used in screening, and other discretionary factors, such as hypertension, smoking, obesity, high-fat diet, and use of cholesterol-raising medication, may be needed to correctly identify children at risk. Presently, children over the age of 10 years are candidates for drug therapy if a trial of diet (6 months to 1 year) proves to be inadequate and LDL-C remains above 190 mg/dL (4.91 mmol/L), or above 160 mg/dL (4.14 mmol/L) if two or more risk factors or CHD are present in the child or adolescent, or if there is a history of premature CHD. In children with diabetes mellitus, pharmacologic treatment should be considered when LDL cholesterol is ≥130 mg/dL (≥3.36 mmol/L).[36] The Dietary Intervention Study in Children (DISC) in pubertal children found that a fat-restricted diet modestly lowered LDL-C and maintained psychological well-being and dietary changes are acceptable to children.[38,39] Although bile acid sequestrants have been the recommended drugs for this population, clinical trials demonstrate that statin therapy is effective and well tolerated in pediatric populations.[40,41] The long-term consequences of drug therapy in this population are unknown. In special instances, familial hypercholesterolemia (particularly the homozygous form), or the existence of CHD or two or more risk factors in the child, would prompt the earlier institution of drug therapy after a trial of dietary intervention.

TREATMENT

Desired Outcomes

The goals of therapy expressed as LDL-C levels and the level of initiation of TLC and drug therapy are provided in Tables 11-8 and 11-9 for adults and children, respectively. While these goals are surrogate end points, the primary reason to institute TLC and drug therapy is to reduce the risk first or recurrent events such as MI, angina, heart failure, ischemic stroke, or other forms of peripheral arterial disease such as carotid stenosis or abdominal aortic aneurysm.

General Approach

Establishing targeted changes and outcomes with consistent reinforcement of goals and measures at followup visits to attain goals is important to reduce barriers for optimizing TLC and pharmacologic

TABLE 11-9 Cut Points for Total Cholesterol and LDL Concentrations in Children and Adolescents

Category	Percentile	Total Cholesterol (mg/dL [mmol/L])	LDL Cholesterol (mg/dL [mmol/L])
Acceptable	<75th	<170 (<4.40)	<110 (<2.84)
Borderline	75th to 95th	170–199 (4.40–5.16)	110–129 (2.84–3.35)
Elevated	>95th	>200 (>5.17)	>130 (>3.36)

Data from reference 36.

therapy.[1] 3 TLC should be implemented in all patients prior to considering drug therapy. The components of TLC include reduced intakes of saturated fats and cholesterol, dietary options to reduce LDL such as plant stanols and sterols and increased soluble fiber intake, weight reduction, and increased physical activity. In general, physical activity of moderate intensity 30 minutes/day for most days of the week should be encouraged.[42,43] Patients with known CAD or at high risk should be evaluated before undertaking vigorous exercise. Weight and BMI should be determined at each visit and lifestyle patterns to induce a weight loss of 10% should be discussed in persons who are overweight. All patients should also be counseled to stop smoking and to meet the Joint National Committee VII guidelines for control of hypertension.

Nonpharmacologic Therapy

Individualized diet counseling that provides acceptable substitutions for unhealthy foods and ongoing reinforcement by a registered dietitian are necessary for maximal effect. The objectives of dietary therapy are to progressively decrease the intake of total fat, saturated fatty acids (i.e., saturated fat), and cholesterol, and to achieve a desirable body weight. Typical American diets now include 13% to 20% of total calories from saturated fat and a cholesterol intake of 350 to 450 mg/day, both in excess of a "heart-healthy" diet for normal Americans, let alone patients with a lipid disorder. Excessive dietary intake of cholesterol and saturated fatty acids lead to decreased hepatic clearance of LDL and deposition of LDL and oxidized LDL in peripheral tissues. The targeted saturated fatty acids have carbon chain lengths of 12 (lauric acid), 14 (myristic acid), and 16 (palmitic acid). The rationale for using a nutritionally balanced low-fat, low-cholesterol diet for the treatment of hypercholesterolemia is based on the following principles: (a) it represents a reasonable extension of the diet recommended for the general public; (b) it progressively decreases the major cholesterol-raising constituent of the diet; (c) it precludes large intakes of polyunsaturated fats; and (d) it facilitates weight reduction by removing foods of high caloric density.[44–47]

Dietary expertise in providing a wide range of options and suggestions in preparation of food can make the difference between a good and an inadequate response to diet. Information concerning eating out in a healthy fashion and advice for shopping are also important factors for success in diet therapy. An example is being aware of products with misleading labels such as coffee creamers that state they contain "no cholesterol," when they may contain hydrogenated (saturated) fats or oils (e.g., palmitic acid, palm kernel oil, or coconut oil), which makes them undesirable because of their saturated fat content. Variations in polyunsaturated and saturated fat and cholesterol intake influence the LDL concentration, but the amount of cholesterol has been found to have a greater effect than the proportion of polyunsaturated or saturated fat. There were also racial differences in elevation of LDL with high saturated fat diets being greater in whites than in other racial groups. The isomeric form of fatty acids is also important.[44] Fatty acids with the *cis* configuration are the preferred substrate for the ACAT reaction and significantly increase hepatic LDL-R clearance while reducing LDL cholesterol production rate. The *trans* isomeric form cannot be used by ACAT and is biologically inactive with no effect on LDL concentration.

Ideally, therapeutic TLC including reduced intake of saturated fats and cholesterol, increased stanol/sterol and fiber intake, weight reduction, and increased physical activity should be used to attain lower LDL-C and to achieve reductions in CHD risk (Table 11-10). TLC may obviate the need for drug therapy, augment LDL-lowering drug therapy, and allow for lower doses. Weight control plus increased physical activity reduces risk beyond LDL cholesterol lowering, is the primary management approach for the metabolic syndrome, and raises HDL and reduces non-HDL cholesterol.[48,49] Many persons should be given a 3-month trial (two visits spaced 6 weeks apart) of dietary therapy and TLC before advancing to drug therapy unless patients are at very high risk (severe hypercholesterolemia, known CHD, CHD risk equivalents, multiple risk factors, strong family history). Although changes in blood lipid levels may change before 3 months, adoption of a different eating pattern may require a longer period of time. It is important to involve all family members, especially if the patient is not the primary person preparing food. Both the NCEP and AHA have excellent Internet-based resources to aid patients in altering their diet in a culturally sensitive manner (*http://www.americanheart.org/presenter.jhtml?identifier=1200009*; *http://www.nhlbi.nih.gov/health/index.htm*). If all of the recommended dietary changes from NCEP, the estimated reduction, on average, in LDL would range from 20% to 30%.[1] Adherence to diet and interindividual variability in macronutrient intake would obviously influence the eventual LDL level achieved. Based on the NHANES data, less than one half of the patients who should be instructed on heart-healthy diet receive any dietary instructions.

TABLE 11-10 Macronutrient Recommendations for the TLC Diet

Component[a]	Recommended Intake
Total fat	25–35% of total calories
Saturated fat	Less than 7% of total calories
Polyunsaturated fat	Up to 10% of total calories
Monounsaturated fat	Up to 20% of total calories
Carbohydrates[b]	50–60% of total calories
Cholesterol	<200 mg/day
Dietary fiber	20–30 g/day
Plant sterols	2 g/day
Protein	Approximately 15% of total calories
Total calories	To achieve and maintain desirable body weight

[a]Calories from alcohol not included.
[b]Carbohydrates should derive from foods rich in complex carbohydrates such as whole grains, fruits, and vegetables.

Other dietary interventions or diet supplements may be useful in certain patients with lipid disorders. Increased intake of soluble fiber in the form of oat bran, pectins, certain gums, and psyllium products can result in useful adjunctive reductions in total and LDL cholesterol, but these dietary alterations or supplements should not be substituted for more active forms of treatment. Total daily fiber intake should be about 20 to 30 g/day, with about 25% or 6 g/day being soluble fiber.[1] Studies with psyllium seed in doses of 10 to 15 g/day show reductions in total and LDL cholesterol ranging from about 5% to 20%.[50,51] They have little or no effect on HDL-C or triglyceride concentrations. These products may also be useful in managing constipation associated with the bile acid sequestrants. Psyllium binds cholesterol in the gut and also reduces hepatic production and clearance. Fish oil supplementation provides an increased amount of the omega-3 polyunsaturated fatty acids such as eicosapentaenoic acid and docosahexaenoic acid. In epidemiologic studies, ingestion of large amounts of cold water, oily fish is associated with a reduction in CHD risk, but it is unclear whether the same advantage is conferred with commercially prepared fish oil products. Each 20 g/day ingestion of fish lowers CHD risk by 7% and eating fish once weekly or more should reduce CHD mortality.[52] Fish oil supplementation has a fairly large effect in reducing triglycerides and VLDL-C, but it either has no effect on total and LDL cholesterol or may cause elevations in these fractions. Other actions of fish oil may account for their protective effects. These effects include quantitative and qualitative alterations in the synthesis of prostanoid substances, changes in immune function and cellular proliferation, and potential antioxidative actions.[53] Responses noted with fish oil are further discussed in Pharmacologic Therapy below.[54]

Fat substitutes such as olestra (Olean, sucrose polyester, Procter and Gamble), a mixture of hexa-, hepta-, and octa-esters formed from the reaction of sucrose with long-chain fatty acids, are approved by the FDA as a nondigestible, nonabsorable, noncaloric fat substitute for snack foods. Olestra is heat stable, an advantage over several other fat substitutes, enabling it to be used in the preparation of fried and baked foods. It is similar in composition to triglycerides, but olestra is not hydrolyzed in the GI tract by pancreatic lipase, and, consequently, is not taken up by the intestinal mucosa. The principal adverse effects associated with olestra use are bloating, flatulence, diarrhea, and "anal leakage." Because of the ability of olestra to solubilize lipophilic substances, there has been concern over potential drug interactions in which lipophilic drugs (e.g., cyclosporin, or colchicine) or vitamins (vitamins A, D, E, and K) are solubilized in olestra and excreted in the feces.

Recent studies have demonstrated the LDL-lowering effect of plant sterols, which are isolated from soybean and tall pine-tree oils. Ingestion of 2 to 3 g/day will reduce LDL by 6% to 15%.[1] Plant sterols can be esterified to unsaturated fatty acids (creating sterol esters) to increase lipid solubility. Hydrogenating sterols produces plant stanols and, with esterification, stanol esters. The efficacy of plant sterols and plant stanols is considered to be comparable. Because lipids are needed to solubilize stanol/sterol esters, they are usually available in commercial margarines. The presence of plant stanols/sterols is listed on the food label. When margarine products are used, persons must be advised to adjust caloric intake to account for the calories contained in the products. Benecol® (McNeil), as an example, is a butter-like spread that contains a plant stanol ester, an ingredient that can lower cholesterol and that is derived from plant stanols found naturally in small amounts in foods such as wheat, rye, and corn.[55] In August 2007, the FDA issued a warning about the consumption of red yeast rice and red yeast rice/policosanol-containing products. These products contained lovastatin that could interact with other drugs and would have the same toxicity of statins but would not be recognized by the consumer and the reduction in LDL is minimal.[56]

Drug therapy is indicated following an adequate trial of TLC changes as outlined in Tables 11-8 and 11-9.

Pharmacologic Therapy

There are now numerous randomized, double-blinded clinical trials demonstrating that reduction of LDL reduces CHD event rates in primary prevention, secondary intervention, and angiographic trials.[57] Generally speaking, for every 1% reduction in LDL, there is a 1% reduction in CHD event rates.[1] However, if treatment extends beyond the typical duration of a clinical trial (2 to 5 years), the accumulated benefit could be greater. Elevations of HDL of 1% result in approximately 2% reduction in CHD events.[13,58] Of interest, angiographic trials, which typically cause small changes in luminal diameter (e.g., about a 0.04-mm difference in change between placebo and active treatment), result in fewer clinical events such as MI or the need for revascularization. This unexpected finding suggests that plaque size and luminal encroachment by plaque may be less important than the effects that cholesterol lowering may have on the activity in the plaque and endothelial dysfunction. These studies provide a strong rationale for attempting to lower plasma cholesterol and LDL in patients with hypercholesterolemia.

4 Although many efficacious lipid-lowering drugs exist, none is effective in all lipoprotein disorders, and all such agents are associated with some adverse effects.[59] Lipid-lowering drugs can be broadly divided into agents that decrease the synthesis of VLDL and LDL, agents that enhance VLDL clearance, agents that enhance LDL catabolism, agents that decrease cholesterol absorption, agents that elevate HDL, or some combination of these characteristics (Table 11-11). Table 11-12 lists recommended drugs of choice for

TABLE 11-11 Effects of Drug Therapy on Lipids and Lipoproteins

Drug	Mechanism of Action	Effects on Lipids	Effects on Lipoproteins	Comment
Cholestyramine, colestipol, and colesevelam	↑ LDL catabolism ↓ cholesterol absorption	↓ cholesterol	↓ LDL ↑ VLDL	Problem with compliance; bind many coadministered acidic drugs
Niacin	↓ LDL and VLDL ↓ synthesis	↓ triglyceride and ↓ cholesterol	↓ VLDL, ↓ LDL, ↑ HDL	Problems with patient acceptance; good in combination with bile acid resins; extended-release niacin causes less flushing and is less hepatotoxic than sustained release
Gemfibrozil, fenofibrate, clofibrate	↑ VLDL clearance ↓ VLDL synthesis	↓ triglyceride and cholesterol	↓ VLDL, ↓ LDL, ↑ HDL	Clofibrate causes cholesterol gall stones; modest LDL lowering; raises HDL; gemfibrozil inhibits glucuronidation of simvastatin, lovastatin, and atorvastatin
Lovastatin, pravastatin, simvastatin, fluvastatin, atorvastatin, rosuvastatin	↑ LDL catabolism; inhibit LDL synthesis	↓ cholesterol	↓ LDL	Highly effective in heterozygous familial hypercholesterolemia and in combination with other agents
Ezetimibe	Blocks cholesterol absorption across the intestinal border	↓ cholesterol	↓ LDL	Few adverse effects; effects additive to other drugs
Mipomersen	Inhibitor of apolipoprotein B-100	↓ cholesterol, LDL, non-HDL	↓ LDL, non-HDL	Increase in transaminases, risk of hepatosteatosis and hepatotoxicity; must be given by SQ injection. Only indicated for familial hypercholesterolemia. To be used along with other lipid-lowering therapies (statins)
Lomitapide	Microsomal triglyceride transfer protein inhibitor	↓ cholesterol	↓ LDL, non-HDL	Hepatotoxicity must be monitored via Juxtapid Risk Evaluation and Mitigation Strategy program. Only indicated for familial hypercholesterolemia. To be used along with other lipid-lowering therapies (statins)

TABLE 11-12 Lipoprotein Phenotype and Recommended Drug Treatment

Lipoprotein Type	Drug of Choice	Combination Therapy
I	Not indicated	—
IIa	Statins	Niacin or BAR
	Cholestyramine or colestipol	Statins or niacin
	Niacin	Statins or BAR
		Ezetimibe
		Mipomersen, lomitapide[a]
IIb	Statins	BAR or fibrates or niacin
	Fibrates	Statins or niacin or BAR[b]
	Niacin	Statins or fibrates
		Ezetimibe
III	Fibrates	Statins or niacin
	Niacin	Statins or fibrates
		Ezetimibe
IV	Fibrates	Niacin
	Niacin	Fibrates
V	Fibrates	Niacin
	Niacin	Fish oils

BAR, bile acid resins; fibrates include gemfibrozil or fenofibrate.

[a]Mipomersen and lomitapide are used in combinations with other lipid-lowering therapy, in particular, statins.

[b]BARs are not used as first-line therapy if triglycerides are elevated at baseline since hypertriglyceridemia may worsen with BAR alone.

each lipoprotein phenotype and alternate agents. Table 11-13 lists available products and their doses.

Treatment of type I hyperlipoproteinemia is directed toward reduction of chylomicrons derived from dietary fat with the subsequent reduction in plasma triglycerides. Total daily fat intake should be no more than 10 to 25 g/day, or approximately 15% of total calories. Secondary causes of hypertriglyceridemia (see Table 11-5) should be excluded or, if present, the underlying disorder should be treated appropriately. Type V hyperlipoproteinemia also requires a stringent restriction of the fat component of dietary intake; in addition, drug therapy is indicated, as outlined in Table 11-12, if the response to diet alone is inadequate. Medium-chain triglycerides, which are absorbed without chylomicron formation, may be used as a dietary supplement for caloric intake if needed for types I and V. Hepatic fibrosis has been reported with medium-chain triglycerides. Omega-3 fatty acids may be useful in LPL deficiency in some patients. In patients with ApoC-II deficiency, infusion of plasma may normalize plasma triglyceride levels.

Primary hypercholesterolemia (familial hypercholesterolemia, familial combined hyperlipidemia, type IIa hyperlipoproteinemia) is treated with the bile acid resins or sequestrants (BARs, colestipol, cholestyramine, and colesevelam), HMG Co-A reductase inhibitors (statins), niacin, or ezetimibe. 5 Of these choices, statins are first choice because they are the most potent LDL-lowering agents. Statins interrupt the conversion of HMG-CoA to mevalonate, the rate-limiting step in de novo cholesterol biosynthesis, by inhibiting HMG-CoA reductase (see Fig. 11-3). Currently available products include lovastatin, pravastatin, simvastatin, fluvastatin, atorvastatin, and pitvastatin.[60] Rosuvastatin is the most potent statin currently on the market. Table 11-14 lists the pharmacokinetic properties of the statins.[61] The plasma half-lives for all the statins are reported to be short except for atorvastatin and rosuvastatin, and this may account for their potency. In CURVES, the largest head-to-head comparison of statins, atorvastatin was found to be the most potent drug for lowering total cholesterol and LDL-C, with reductions in LDL-C of 38%, 46%, 51%, and 54% for the 10-, 20-, 40-, and 80-mg doses, respectively.[62] Metabolic studies with statins in normal volunteers and patients with hypercholesterolemia suggest reduced synthesis of LDL-C, as well as enhanced catabolism of LDL mediated through LDL-Rs, as the principal mechanisms for lipid-lowering effects. Total and LDL cholesterol are reduced in a dose-related fashion by 30% or more on average when added to dietary therapy, with the effects being more pronounced in nonfamilial than in familial hypercholesterolemia. 6 Combination therapy with bile acid sequestrants and lovastatin is rational as LDL-R numbers are increased, leading to greater degradation of LDL-C; intracellular synthesis of cholesterol is inhibited, and enterohepatic recycling of bile acids is interrupted. Combination therapy with a statin plus ezetimibe is also so rational since ezetimibe inhibits cholesterol absorption across the gut border and adds 12% to 20% further reduction when combined to a statin or other drugs.[63] However, the combination of a statin and ezetimibe has not been shown to affect surrogate end points such as carotid intimal medial thickness (CIMT) even with further reduction in LDL cholesterol.[64] Elevation of serum transaminase levels (primarily alanine aminotransferase) to greater than three times the upper limit of normal occurs in approximately 1.3% of patients on moderate to high doses of statins and serious muscle toxicity occurs in <0.6% of patients.[65] Meta-analysis of placebo-controlled studies with statins demonstrates a low risk of abnormal ALT or CK and a low risk of myopathy without or with rhabdomyolysis.[66] Lens opacities have been reported with lovastatin; however, in the age groups studied, these abnormalities are common and tend to wax and wane with time irrespective of drug therapy, and no statistical association is known to exist. As a category of monotherapy, the HMG-CoA reductase inhibitors are the most potent total and LDL cholesterol–lowering agents and among the best tolerated.[65,66] In an analysis of more than 75,000 patients allocated to statins in clinical trials, Alsheikh-Ali et al. found that risk of statin-associated elevated liver enzymes or rhabdomyolysis is not related to the magnitude of LDL-C lowering. A highly significant inverse relationship between achieved LDL-C levels and rates of newly diagnosed cancer was observed ($R^2 = 0.43$, $P = 0.009$).[67] The WHO Foundation Collaborating Centre for International Drug Monitoring has issued a report suggesting that a rare relationship may exist between statin use and the onset of upper motor neuron diseases such as amyotrophic lateral sclerosis, but this association remains uncertain.[68] Statin use is associated with a small risk of diabetes (9%).[69] There are numerous pharmacokinetic and pharmacodynamic differences among statins and patients that give rise to variable response to therapy.[70]

The primary action of BAR is to bind bile acids in the intestinal lumen, with a concurrent interruption of enterohepatic circulation of bile acids and a markedly increased excretion of acidic steroids in the feces. This decreases the bile acid pool size and stimulates hepatic synthesis of bile acids from cholesterol. Depletion of the hepatic pool of cholesterol results in an increase in cholesterol biosynthesis and an increase in the number of LDL-Rs on the hepatocyte membrane. The increased number of receptors stimulates an enhanced rate of catabolism from plasma and lowers LDL levels. CETP, which is correlated with total and LDL cholesterol concentrations, is also reduced by BAR, perhaps by interfering with hepatic microsomal cholesterol content, but this effect is not as great as with statins.[71] Patients with homozygous familial hypercholesterolemia genetically lack the ability to increase synthesis of LDL-Rs and BARs are generally ineffective. The increase in hepatic cholesterol biosynthesis may be paralleled by increased hepatic VLDL production and, consequently, BARs may aggravate hypertriglyceridemia in patients with combined hyperlipidemia. GI complaints of constipation, bloating, epigastric fullness, nausea, and flatulence are most commonly reported.[1] With intensive education, patients can learn to tolerate resins on a long-term basis as evidenced by adherence in clinical trials to active drug regimens, but in routine clinical practice 40% or more of patients will discontinue therapy within 1 year; however, with pharmacists' interventions, adherence rates can be improved.[72,73] These adverse effects can be managed by increasing

TABLE 11-13 Comparison of Drugs Used in the Treatment of Hyperlipidemia

Drug	Manufacturer	Dosage Forms	Usual Daily Dose	Maximum Daily Dose
Cholestyramine (Questran)	BMS	Bulk powder/4-g packets	8 g three times a day	32 g
Cholestyramine (Questran Light)	BMS	Bulk powder/4-g packets		
Cholestyramine (Cholybar)	Parke-Davis	4-g resin per bar		
Colestipol hydrochloride (Colestid)	Upjohn	Bulk powder/5-g packets	10 g twice daily	30 g
Colesevelam (Welchol)	Sankyo	625 mg tablets	1,875 mg twice daily	4,375 mg
Niacin	Various	50-, 100-, 250-, and 500-mg tablets; 125-, 250-, and 500-mg capsules	2 g three times a day	9 g
Extended-release niacin (Niaspan)	Kos	500-, 750-, and 1,000-mg tablets	500 mg	2,000 mg
Extended-release niacin + lovastatin (Advicor)[a]	Kos	Niacin/lovastatin 500-/20-mg tablets Niacin/lovastatin 750-/20-mg tablets Niacin/lovastatin 1,000-/20-mg tablets	Niacin/lovastatin 500/20 mg	Niacin/lovastatin 1,000/20 mg
Fenofibrate (Tricor and others)	Abbott, various	67-, 134-, and 200-mg capsules (micronized); 54- and 160-mg tablets; 40- and 120-mg tablets; 50- and 160-mg tablets	54 or 67 mg	201 mg
Gemfibrozil (Lopid)	Parke-Davis	300-mg capsules	600 mg twice daily	1.5 g
Lovastatin (Mevacor)	MSD	20- and 40-mg tablets	20–40 mg	80 mg
Pravastatin (Pravachol)	Bristol-Myers Squibb	10- and 20-mg tablets	10–20 mg	40 mg
Simvastatin (Zocor)	MSD	5-, 10-, 20-, 40-, and 80-mg tablets	10–20 mg	80 mg
Atorvastatin (Lipitor)	Pfizer	10-mg tablets	10 mg	80 mg
Rosuvastatin (Crestor)	Astra-Zeneca	5- and 10-mg tablets	5 mg	40 mg
Pitavastatin (Livalo)	Kowa	1-, 2-, and 4-mg tablets	2 mg	4 mg
Ezetimibe (Zetia)	MSD	10-mg tablet	10 mg	10 mg
Atorvastatin/amlodipine (Caduet)	Pfizer	Atorvastatin/amlodipine 10/5 mg Atorvastatin/amlodipine 20/5 mg Atorvastatin/amlodipine 40/5 mg Atorvastatin/amlodipine 80/5 mg Atorvastatin/amlodipine 10/10 mg Atorvastatin/amlodipine 20/10 mg Atorvastatin/amlodipine 40/10 mg Atorvastatin/amlodipine 80/10 mg	Atovastatin/amlodipine 10/5 mg	Atovastatin/amlodipine 80/10 mg
Pravastatin/aspirin (Pravigard PAC)	BMS	Pravastatin/aspirin 20/81 mg Pravastatin/aspirin 20/325 mg Pravastatin/aspirin 40/81 mg Pravastatin/aspirin 40/325 mg Pravastatin/aspirin 80/81 mg Pravastatin/aspirin 80/325 mg		
Simvastatin/ezetimibe (Vytorin)	Merck/Schering-Plough	Simvastatin/ezetimibe 10/10 mg Simvastatin/ezetimibe 20/10 mg Simvastatin/ezetimibe 40/10 mg	Simvastatin/ezetimibe 20/10 mg	Simvastatin/ezetimibe 40/10 mg
Omega-3 acid ethyl esters (Lovaza)	Reliant	Eicosapentaenoic acid (EPA) 465 mg, docosahexaenoic acid (DHA) 375 mg	Four 1 g capsules daily or two 1 g capsules twice daily	Four 1 g capsules daily or two 1 g capsules twice daily
Lomitapide	Aegerion	5-, 10-, and 20-mg capsules	5 mg daily increasing at 2-week intervals to response or maximum dose; dose 2 hours after evening meal	60 mg daily
Mipomersen	Genzyme	200 mg/mL for SQ injection	200 mg SQ once weekly	200 mg SQ once weekly

Probucol is no longer on the market in the United States; gemfibrozil, fenofibrate, atorvastatin, and lovastatin are available as generic products.

BMS, Bristol-Myers Squibb; MSD, Merck Sharp & Dohme; SQ, subcutaneously.

[a]The manufacturer does not recommend use of the fixed combination as initial therapy of primary hypercholesterolemia or mixed dyslipidemia. It is specifically indicated in patients receiving lovastatin alone plus diet who require an additional reduction in triglyceride levels or increase in HDL cholesterol levels; it is also indicated in those treated with niacin alone who require additional decreases in LDL cholesterol. Lomitapide and mipomersen can be hepatotoxic and close monitoring is recommended for both.

TABLE 11-14 Pharmacokinetics of the Statins

Parameter	Lovastatin	Simvastatin	Pravastatin	Fluvastatin	Atorvastatin	Rosuvastatin	Pitavastatin
Isoenzyme	3A4	3A4	None	2C9	3A4	2C9/2C19	UGT1A3/UGT2B7
Lipophilic	Yes	Yes	No	Yes	Yes	No	Yes
Protein binding (%)	>95	95–98	~50	>90	96	88	99
Active metabolites	Yes	Yes	No	No	Yes	Yes	No
Elimination half-life (hours)	3	2	1.8	1.2	7–14	13–20	12

Isoenzyme refers to the specific isoenzyme in the cytochrome P450 system that is responsible for the metabolism of each drug. Pharmacokinetic parameters in this table are based on studies and reviews presented in the literature.

the fluid intake, modifying the diet to increase bulk, and using stool softeners. The other major limiting complaint is the gritty texture and bulk; these problems may be minimized by mixing the powder with orange drink or juice. Tablet forms of bile acid sequestrants should help in improving compliance with this form of therapy, whereas the bar does not improve compliance.[74] Other potential adverse effects include impaired absorption of fat-soluble vitamins A, D, E, and K; hypernatremia and hyperchloremia; GI obstruction; and reduced bioavailability of acidic drugs such as coumarin anticoagulants, nicotinic acid, thyroxine, acetaminophen, hydrocortisone, hydrochlorothiazide, loperamide, and possibly iron. Hyperchloremic metabolic acidosis, hypernatremia, and GI obstruction have been reported almost exclusively in children, and malabsorption of fat-soluble vitamins is probably most common with high doses (e.g., 30 g/day of cholestyramine) of the BARs. Drug interactions may be avoided by alternating administration times with an interval of 6 hours or greater between the BAR and other drugs. Colestipol and cholestyramine have comparable side effects; however, colestipol may have better palatability because it is odorless and tasteless. Colesevelam is the newest BAR and total and LDL-C reduction is dose related. The adverse effects are qualitatively similar to the older BAR but may occur less often. Because of adverse effects occurring commonly with BAR at higher doses, BARs are increasingly used in combination with other drugs, as low doses are tolerated well and they work in a complementary fashion with other agents.

Niacin (nicotinic acid) may also be used in primary hypercholesterolemia in combination with bile acid sequestrants or as monotherapy for this disorder and others (Table 11-12). Niacin reduces the hepatic synthesis of VLDL, which, in turn, leads to a reduction in the synthesis of LDL. Factors responsible for decreased production of VLDL include inhibition of lipolysis with a decrease in free fatty acids in plasma, decreased hepatic esterification of triglycerides, and a possible direct effect on the hepatic production of ApoB.[75] The complementary action of niacin and bile acid sequestrants to increase catabolism and decrease synthesis of LDL may account for the additive effects of this combination in hyperlipidemia. Niacin also increases HDL by reducing its catabolism. It selectively decreases hepatic removal of HDL ApoA-I but not removal of cholesterol esters, thereby increasing the capacity of retained ApoA-I to augment reverse cholesterol transport in isolated hepatic cells. The principal use of niacin is for mixed hyperlipemia or as a second-line agent in combination therapy for hypercholesterolemia. It is also considered to be the first-line agent or an alternative for the treatment of hypertriglyceridemia and diabetic dyslipidemia.[76,77] There are numerous smaller trials suggesting that lower doses of niacin may be combined with statins or gemfibrozil to minimize adverse effects and maximize response. One meta-analysis showed that combination therapy was no more effective than high-dose statin therapy.[78] These combinations require careful monitoring because interactions do occur.

Niacin has many adverse drug reactions that occur commonly; fortunately, most of the symptoms and biochemical abnormalities seen do not require discontinuation of therapy. Cutaneous flushing and itching appear to be prostaglandin mediated and can be reduced by aspirin 325 mg given shortly before niacin ingestion.[1,79] Flushing seems to be related to rising plasma concentrations of niacin; taking the dose with meals and slowly titrating the dose upward may minimize these effects. Laropiprant is a selective antagonist of the prostaglandin D(2) receptor subtype 1 (DP1), which may mediate niacin-induced vasodilation. Coadministration of laropiprant 30, 100, and 300 mg with extended-release (ER) niacin significantly lowered flushing symptom scores (by approximately 50% or more) and also significantly reduced malar skin blood flow measured by laser Doppler perfusion imaging.[80,81] GI intolerance and flushing are common problems. Acanthosis nigricans, a darkening of the skin in skinfold areas and an external marker of insulin resistance, may be seen with high doses of niacin. Sustained-release products may minimize these complaints in some patients, but controlled trials with regular-release products do not demonstrate much of a difference between sustained- and regular-release products. The only legend form of niacin, Niaspan® (Abbott), is an ER form of niacin with pharmacokinetics intermediate between instant and sustained-release products that are sold as food supplements rather than legend products. In controlled trials, Niaspan® is reported to have fewer dermatologic reactions and has a low risk for hepatotoxicity. When combined with statins, this combination produces large reductions in LDL and increases in HDL.[82] Potentially important laboratory abnormalities occurring with niacin therapy include elevated liver function tests, hyperuricemia, and hyperglycemia. Recent experience with niacin in diabetes suggests that some diabetic patients do not have worsened glycemic control with dose titration and sustained-release products.[83] BMI and fasting plasma glucose predict loss of blood glucose control.[84] With less than 3 g/day, the degree of liver function test elevation is generally not marked and often transient, and a temporary reduction in dosage frequently corrects the problem. Niacin-associated hepatitis is more common with sustained-release preparations, and their use should be restricted to patients intolerant of regular-release products.[83,85] Sustained-release products are often more expensive and given the lack of data for reduced adverse effects and increased incidence of hepatitis, regular-release products should always be used first. Preexisting gout and diabetes may be exacerbated by niacin; these patients should be monitored more closely and their medication titrated appropriately. Patients with well-controlled type 2 diabetes mellitus do not have significant changes in glycemic control with niacin at doses of 2 g/day or less.[85] Niacin is contraindicated in patients with active liver disease. Dry eyes and other ophthalmologic complaints are also occasionally noted. Concomitant alcohol and hot drinks may magnify flushing and pruritus with niacin and they should be avoided at the time of ingestion. Nicotinamide should not be used in the treatment of hyperlipidemia, as it does not effectively lower cholesterol or triglyceride levels.

Combined hyperlipoproteinemia (type IIb) may be treated with statins, niacin, or gemfibrozil combinations to lower LDL cholesterol without elevating VLDL and triglycerides. Niacin is the most effective agent and may be combined with a bile acid sequestrant. BARs alone in this disorder may elevate VLDL and triglycerides, and their use as single agents for treating combined hyperlipoproteinemia should be avoided. Fibric acid (gemfibrozil, fenofibrate) monotherapy is effective in reducing VLDL, but a reciprocal rise in LDL may occur, and total cholesterol values may remain relatively unchanged. Gemfibrozil reduces the synthesis of VLDL and, to a lesser extent, ApoB, with a concurrent increase in the rate of removal of triglyceride-rich lipoproteins from plasma. Plasma HDL concentrations may rise 10% to 15% or more with fibrates. Fenofibrate may have fewer drug interactions than gemfibrozil, but fenofibrate has been reported to worsen renal function.[86] Ezetimibe could also be used in combination therapy in type IIb. GI complaints with fibric acid derivatives occur in 3% to 5% of patients, rash in 2% of patients, dizziness in 2.4% of patients, and transient elevations in transaminase levels and alkaline phosphatase in 4.5% and 1.3% of patients, respectively.[87] Gemfibrozil and probably fenofibrate may enhance the formation of gallstones associated with an increase in the lithogenic index; however, the rate is low (0.5% to 7%) and similar to that seen with placebo in the Helsinki Heart Study.[87] Fibric acid derivatives may potentiate the effects of oral anticoagulants and international normalized ratio (INR) should be monitored very closely with this combination.

Type III hyperlipoproteinemia may be treated with fibric acid derivatives or niacin. Although fibric acid derivatives have been suggested as the drugs of choice for this disorder, given the lack of data supporting its efficacy in altering cardiovascular mortality in the major studies on hypercholesterolemia, and numerous, well-documented, and serious adverse effects, it is reasonable to consider niacin. Gemfibrozil increases the activity of LPL and reduces to a lesser extent the synthesis or secretion of VLDL from the liver into the plasma. A myositis syndrome of myalgia, weakness, stiffness, malaise, and elevations in creatinine phosphokinase and aspartate aminotransaminase is seen with the fibric acid derivatives, and it seems to be more common in patients with renal insufficiency.[87] Enhanced hypoglycemic effects are reported to occur when fibric acid derivatives are given to patients on sulfonylurea compounds, but the mechanisms for these interactions are not well understood.

Two fibric acid derivatives (gemfibrozil and fenofibrate) are approved in the United States. Both reduce LDL-C by 20% to 25% in heterozygous familial hypercholesterolemia. The response of LDL-C, HDL-C, and triglycerides to this category of drug is very dependent on the specific lipoprotein type (e.g., type IIa vs. IIb) and the baseline triglyceride concentration.[88]

As a potential alternative therapy, for this phenotype, numerous epidemiologic and normal volunteer studies have found that diets high in omega-3 polyunsaturated fatty acids (from fish oil), mostly commonly eicosapentaenoic acid, reduce cholesterol, triglycerides, LDL-C, and VLDL-C, and may elevate HDL-C.[54] The effects of fish oil on lipoprotein metabolism are mediated through a reduction in VLDL production and suppression of VLDL ApoB. In patients with hypertriglyceridemia, either phenotypes type IIb or type V, a diet high in omega-3 fatty acids given for 4 weeks reduced cholesterol 27% and 45%, and triglyceride 64% and 79%, in the type IIb and type V patients, respectively.[52] A diet high in eicosapentaenoic acid given to hyperlipidemic hemodialysis patients resulted in significant decreases in cholesterol and triglycerides for as long as 13 weeks. Fish oil supplementation may be most useful in patients with hypertriglyceridemia; however, its role in treatment is not well defined. Potential complications of fish oil supplementation, such as thrombocytopenia and bleeding disorders, have been noted, especially with high doses (eicosapentaenoic acid 15 to 30 g/day), and well-controlled trials are needed to determine if fish oils are safe and effective before their use may be broadly recommended. Based a recent meta-analysis, fish consumption lowers the risk of CHD, but nutraceuticals have not been adequately tested.[52] Recently, a prescription form of concentrated fish oil, Lovaza®, has become available.[54] This product lowers triglycerides by 14% to 30% and raises HDL by about 10% depending on baseline values. Another fish oil derivative product being considered by the FDA, Epanova contains EPA and DHA in their free fatty acid form at a total concentration of 50% to 60% EPA and 15% to 25% DHA along with other potentially active omega-3 fatty acids stored in a patent-protected capsule with a patent-protected coating designed to maximize bioavailability and tolerability.

Combination drug therapy may be considered after adequate trials of monotherapy and for patients documented compliant to the prescribed regimen. Two or three lipoprotein profiles at 6-week intervals should confirm lack of response prior to initiation of combination therapy. Cholestyramine may be added in patients with fasting hypertriglyceridemia, but it should not be used as the initial drug, because triglycerides are likely to increase. Contraindications to and drug interactions with combined therapy should be carefully screened, as well as consideration of the extra cost of drug product and monitoring that may be required. In general, a statin and a BAR or niacin with a BAR provide the greatest reduction in total and LDL cholesterol. Regimens intended to increase HDL levels should include either gemfibrozil or niacin, and it should be remembered that statins combined with either of these drugs may result in a greater incidence of hepatotoxicity or myositis. This is particularly important for statins that are eliminated via cytochrome 3A4 or through glucuronidation.[61] Familial combined hyperlipidemia may respond better to a fibric acid and a statin than to a fibric acid and a BAR.[89]

Severe forms of hypercholesterolemia—such as familial hypercholesterolemia, familial defective ApoB-100, severe polygenic hypercholesterolemia, familial combined hyperlipidemia, and familial dysbetalipoproteinemia (type III)—may require more intensive therapy. In particular, familial hypercholesterolemia patients often require combination therapy (two or three drugs) and are managed with surgical therapy (partial ileal bypass), plasmapheresis (LDL-apheresis), and liver transplantation (to replace LDL-Rs).

Hypertriglyceridemia

It is important to remember that lipoprotein pattern types I, III, IV, and V are associated with hypertriglyceridemia, and that these primary lipoprotein disorders and underlying diseases should be excluded prior to implementing therapy (see Table 11-5). In a national survey, approximately one-third of participants tested had a triglyceride concentration exceeding 150 mg/dL (1.70 mmol/L).[90] A positive family history of CHD is important in identifying patients at risk for premature atherosclerosis.[17,91] If a patient with CHD has elevated triglycerides, the associated abnormality is probably a contributing factor to CHD and should be treated.[33]

High serum triglycerides (see Tables 11-6 and 11-12) should be treated by achieving desirable body weight, consumption of a low saturated fat and cholesterol diet, regular exercise, smoking cessation, and restriction of alcohol (in selected patients). ATP III identifies the sum of LDL and VLDL (termed *non-HDC* [total cholesterol − HDL]) as a secondary target of therapy in persons with high triglycerides (≥200 mg/dL [≥2.26 mmol/L]).[1,33] This approach is used when triglycerides exceed 200 mg/dL (2.26 mmol/L) and accounts for atherogenic particles carried in VLDL and remnant particles. The goal for non-HDL in persons with high serum triglycerides can be set at 30 mg/dL (0.78 mmol/L) higher than that for LDL on the premise that a VLDL level ≤30 mg/dL (≤0.78 mmol/L) is normal. **7** In patients with borderline high triglycerides but with accompanying risk factors of established CHD disease, family history of premature CHD, concomitant LDL elevation or low HDL, and genetic forms of hypertriglyceridemia associated with CHD (familial dysbetalipoproteinemia, familial combined hyperlipidemia), drug therapy with niacin should be considered. Niacin may be used cautiously in diabetics based on the results of the ADMIT trial, which found triglycerides were reduced by 23%, HDL-C increased by 29%, only a slight increase in glucose (mean 8.7 mg/dL [0.5 mmol/L]), and no change in hemoglobin A_{1c}.[92] Elevated BMI and plasma glucose predict loss of glycemic control.[84] Alternative therapies include gemfibrozil or fenofibrate, statins, and fish oil.[17,93,94] Fibrates may increase LDL, and their use in borderline high triglyceridemia requires careful monitoring to detect this deleterious change in lipid profile. Statins may also be used, because they provide modest reductions in triglycerides and modest elevations in HDL. Higher doses of statins may reduce HDL as well as LDL and triglycerides with amount of reduction related to the baseline concentration and dose.[17,94] The goal of therapy in this situation is to lower triglycerides and VLDL particles that may be atherogenic, increase HDL, and reduce LDL.

Very high triglycerides are associated with pancreatitis and other consequences of the chylomicron syndrome. At this level of elevation of triglycerides, a genetic form of hypertriglyceridemia often coexists with other causes of elevated triglycerides such as diabetes. Dietary fat restriction (10% to 20% of calories as fat), weight loss, alcohol restriction, and treatment of the coexisting disorder are the basic elements of management. Drugs useful in hypertriglyceridemia include gemfibrozil or fenofibrate, niacin, and higher-potency statins (atorvastatin, rosuvastatin, pitvastatin, and simvastatin). Gemfibrozil and fenofibrate are the preferred drugs in diabetics because of the effect of niacin on glycemic control unless the newer ER forms are used. Fenofibrate may be preferred in combination with statin therapy since it does not impair glucuronidation and minimizes potential drug interactions. Success in treatment is defined as a reduction in triglycerides below 500 mg/dL (5.65 mmol/L).[1]

Low HDL Cholesterol

Low HDL is a strong independent risk predictor of CHD. ATP III redefined low HDL-C as <40 mg/dL (<1.03 mmol/L), but specified no goal for HDL-C raising.[1] Low HDL may be a consequence of insulin resistance, physical inactivity, type 2 diabetes, cigarette smoking, very high carbohydrate intake, and certain drugs (see Table 11-5). 8 In low HDL the primary target remains LDL according to ATP III, but emphasis shifts to weight reduction, increased physical activity, and smoking cessation, and, if drug therapy is required, to fibric acid derivatives and niacin. Niacin has the potential for the greatest increase in HDL and the effect is more pronounced with regular or immediate-release forms than with sustained-release forms.[95]

Diabetic Dyslipidemia

Diabetic dyslipidemia is characterized by hypertriglyceridemia, low HDL, and LDL that is minimally elevated. Small, dense LDL (pattern B) in diabetes is more atherogenic than larger, more buoyant forms of LDL (pattern A); routine lipoprotein profiles do not differentiate between pattern A and pattern B.[96–98] Diabetes in ATP III is a CHD risk equivalent and the primary target is LDL with a goal of treatment being to lower LDL-C <100 mg/dL (<2.59 mmol/L).[1] When LDL is >130 mg/dL (>3.36 mmol/L), most patients will require simultaneous TLCs and drug therapy. When LDL-C is between 100 and 129 mg/dL (2.59 and 3.34 mmol/L), intensifying glycemic control, adding drugs for the atherogenic dyslipidemia (fibric acid derivatives, niacin), and intensifying LDL-C–lowering therapy are options. Because the primary target is LDL-C in diabetic dyslipidemia, statins are considered by many to be initial drugs of choice.[1,33] The relative risk reduction for CHD in diabetics versus nondiabetics is greater in the West of Scotland (37% vs. 20%),[99] AFCAPS/TexCAPS (43% vs. 36%),[100] CARE (25% vs. 23%),[101] and 4S (55% vs. 32%) trials.[102] All statins are fairly comparable in triglyceride lowering and because statins differ in potency for LDL reduction, a ratio of LDL reduction to triglyceride reduction can be applied. Statin therapy may protect against the development of diabetes.[30] The most recent trial to evaluate the benefit of LDL lowering in type 2 diabetes mellitus is the Collaborative Atorvastatin Diabetes Study (CARDS).[103] This was a randomized, double-blind, placebo-controlled comparison of atorvastatin 10 mg/day versus placebo in 2,838 diabetics to reduce first CHD events. Baseline LDL was 118 mg/dL (3.05 mmol/L) and with atorvastatin LDL fell by 46 mg/dL (1.19 mmol/L). The primary end point, a composite of acute CHD death, nonfatal MI, hospitalized unstable angina, resuscitated cardiac arrest, coronary revascularization, or stroke, was reduced by 37%. This study suggests that all diabetics should have an LDL much lower than 100 mg/dL (2.59 mmol/L) and these results are consistent with the Heart Protection Study analysis of diabetic patients.[104]

Fenofibrate, according to the DIAS trial, reduced the angiographic progression of CAD in type 2 diabetes.[105] Fewer CHD events were seen with fenofibrate compared with placebo, but the difference was not significant. Fibric acids principally lower VLDL and triglycerides while increasing HDL with only modest lowering of total and LDL cholesterol; on occasion, fibric acid derivatives may increase LDL levels. Fibric acid derivatives tend to improve glucose tolerance, in contrast to niacin; the greatest effect has been seen with bezafibrate. The Helsinki Heart Study found gemfibrozil to be most effective in diabetic dyslipidemia.[106] Although the effect of statins on triglycerides and HDL abnormalities commonly seen in diabetes is less than with fibric acids, the subgroup analyses cited earlier suggest that they reduce CHD risk significantly. In the Action to Control Cardiovascular Risk in Diabetes (ACCORD) the combination of a statin and fenofibrate in patients with type 2 diabetes did not reduce the rate of fatal cardiovascular events, nonfatal MI, or nonfatal stroke compared with simvastatin alone.[107] Cholestyramine in diabetic patients may result in lower LDL levels, but VLDL and triglyceride levels, which are commonly elevated in diabetes, may be further increased in this population. Resins may aggravate constipation, which is common in diabetics. As demonstrated in the ADMIT and ADVENT trials, immediate-release and ER niacin are very effective in raising HDL and lowering triglycerides and LDL.[92,108]

Special Considerations

Elderly

Hypercholesterolemia is an independent risk factor for CHD in the elderly (>65 years old), as it is in the younger patient. The attributable risk, which is the difference in absolute rates of CHD between segments of the population with higher or lower serum cholesterol levels, increases with age. Older patients potentially benefit to a greater extent from cholesterol lowering than younger populations. Data from studies of elderly men in a variety of settings are consistent with a relative risk of at least 1.5 in the highest compared with the lowest quartile of cholesterol levels and a relative risk reduction of 22% for heart-related mortality.[109–111] Treatment of hypercholesterolemia in the elderly may bring about a comparable reduction in absolute risk to that obtained in younger persons.[1] Subgroup analyses of the West of Scotland (primary) and 4S (secondary) intervention studies show that elderly patients have lower CHD risk reduction (relative risk reduction of 27% and 29%, respectively) as compared with younger patients (relative risk reduction of 40% and 39%, respectively).[99,112] The Framingham study suggests that elderly women are at higher risk because of high blood cholesterol levels, but no other large studies included women, and their risks or benefits from cholesterol reduction are not well defined. Primary prevention in younger patients requires about 2 years before reduction in CHD risk is apparent, and this lag time should be taken into consideration in patient selection for therapy. Nonlipid CHD risk factors do not decline in relative risk with aging, and aggressive management of the modifiable nonlipid risk factors is important in the older patient. High-risk elderly patients are less likely to be prescribed statins and their potent benefits are not realized.[113] Because most women with CHD are elderly and also at risk for osteoporosis, they are logical candidates for diet therapy with consideration of calcium intake consistent with osteoporosis prevention, exercise, and perhaps estrogen replacement therapy. Recent evidence suggests that statins may reduce the risk of osteoporosis; however, there are conflicting data from various studies.[114]

Drug therapy in principle differs little from younger patients, and older patients respond to lipid-lowering drugs as well as younger patients.[115,116] Based on the Heart Protection Study with more elderly patients than any other trial, simvastatin 40 mg/day produced the CHD event rate reduction in patients over 70 years of age as in younger patients.[117] The gain in life expectancy may be small depending on the age at the start of treatment and the magnitude of cholesterol reduction. Changes in body composition, renal function, and other physiologic changes of aging may make older patients more susceptible to adverse effects of lipid-lowering drug therapy. In particular, older patients are more likely to have constipation (BARs), skin and eye changes (niacin), gout (niacin), gallstones (fibric acid derivatives), and bone/joint disorders (fibric acid derivatives, statins). Therapy should be started with lower doses and titrated up slowly to minimize adverse effects.

Women

Cholesterol is an important determinant of CHD in women, but the relationship is not as strong as that seen in men. HDL may be a more important predictor of disease in women.[4] LDL and HDL genetic regulation in women and men does not appear to be different. Based on the Nurses' Health Study, obesity is an important determinant of CHD in women, with the relative risk being 3.3 in the highest Quetelet's index (weight in kilograms divided by the square of the height in meters) as compared with the lowest category (i.e., <21 vs. ≥29); low HDL levels usually accompany obesity.[118] No major differences exist in the influence of exercise, alcohol ingestion, and smoking on lipid levels between men and women. Women in the highest tertile of cholesterol appear to be more responsive to dietary therapy than those in the lower tertiles, and more responsive than formulas based on men predict.

Based on the HERS[119] and WHI trials,[120–122] recently published national guidelines recommended similar types of lifestyle and risk factor goals and interventions as recommended by NCEP for the entire population.[4] Hormone therapy may continue to have a role for postmenopausal symptoms; however, a notable exception is hormone replacement therapy and heart protection. Combined estrogen plus progestin hormone therapy should not be initiated to prevent CVD in postmenopausal women. Combined estrogen plus progestin hormone therapy should not be continued to prevent CVD in postmenopausal women. Other forms of menopausal hormone therapy (e.g., unopposed estrogen) should not be initiated or continued to prevent CVD in postmenopausal women pending the results of ongoing trials. Results of the WISDOM trial confirm lack of benefit as seen in HERS and WHI.[123] In a recent post hoc analysis of the WHI, women who initiated hormone therapy closer to menopause tended to have reduced CHD risk compared with the increase in CHD risk among women more distant from menopause, but this trend did not meet statistical significance.[120] Based on the Justification for the Use of Statins in Prevention: An Intervention Trial Evaluating Rosuvastatin (JUPITER), women experience the same benefit of LDL cholesterol lowering as men with rosuvastatin.[124]

Cholesterol and triglyceride levels rise progressively throughout pregnancy, with an average increment in cholesterol of 30 to 40 mg/dL (0.78 to 1.03 mmol/L) occurring around the 36th to 39th weeks. Triglyceride levels may go up by as much as 150 mg/dL (1.70 mmol/L). Drug therapy is neither instituted nor usually continued during pregnancy. If the patient is very high risk, a BAR may be considered since there is no systemic drug exposure.[1] Statins are category X and are contraindicated. Ezetimibe might be an alternative since it is a category C drug (animal studies have shown that the drug exerts teratogenic or embryocidal effects, and there are no adequate, well-controlled studies in pregnant women, or no studies are available in either animals or pregnant women), but no data are available in humans. Dietary therapy is the mainstay of treatment, with emphasis on maintaining a nutritionally balanced diet as per the needs of pregnancy.

Children

Drug therapy in children is not recommended until the age of 8 years or older, and the guidelines for institution of therapy and the goals of therapy are different from those in adults (see Table 11-9).[125] Younger children are generally managed with TLCs until after the age of 2 years.[1,47] Although bile acid sequestrants have been recommended in the past as first-line therapy, there is now evidence that statins are safe and effective in children and provide greater lipid lowering than BAR.[126–129] Severe forms of hypercholesterolemia (e.g., familial hypercholesterolemia) may require more aggressive treatment.

Concurrent Disease States

Nephrotic syndrome, end-stage renal disease, and hypertension compound the risk of dyslipidemia and may present difficult-to-treat lipid abnormalities. Abnormalities of lipoprotein metabolism in the nephrotic syndrome include elevated total and LDL cholesterol, Lp(a), VLDL, and triglycerides. The Apo C-III-to-C-II ratio is elevated, consistent with greater LPL inhibitor activity, and the extent of hypoalbuminemia is correlated with dyslipidemia. The basic abnormality appears to be one of overproduction of LDL-ApoB from VLDL, rather than reduced clearance of LDL-C and related proteins. Protein restriction and a "vegan" diet correct lipid abnormalities to some extent. Statins have been shown to be effective in reducing elevated total and LDL cholesterol in the nephrotic syndrome, although the levels do not usually return to normal.[130] Fibric acid derivatives and statins reduce small, dense LDL-C by different mechanisms, suggesting a potential role for combination therapy to optimize lowering of small, dense LDL-C and remnant lipoproteins. Statins appear to be safe and effective for lowering LDL cholesterol in renal insufficiency, but they may not affect CHD end points.[131,132]

Renal insufficiency without proteinuria leads to hypertriglyceridemia, slightly elevated total and LDL cholesterol (particularly with chronic ambulatory peritoneal dialysis), and low HDL levels (especially during hemodialysis). These abnormalities are thought to be caused by a deficiency in ApoC-II, perhaps as a result of sustained use of heparin during hemodialysis and depletion of LPL, carbohydrate-induced obesity and hypertriglyceridemia, loss of carnitine during hemodialysis, use of acetate buffer (acetate is a precursor to fatty acid synthesis) during hemodialysis, and decreased LCAT activity during hemodialysis. Dialysis does not correct the lipid abnormalities. Renal transplantation may correct lipid abnormalities in some patients; however, in others, the use of transplantation-related medications such as corticosteroids, cyclosporine, and certain antihypertensive agents (see Chaps. 3 and 70) may aggravate the lipid abnormalities. Cyclosporine interferes with the metabolism of statins metabolized by cytochrome P450 3A4 (Table 11-14), and patients need to be observed closely for myositis and worsening renal function. Of interest, correction of lipid abnormalities may improve renal hemodynamics. Pravastatin and fluvastatin may be safer than other statins, but this needs to be validated in larger, long-term trials. Diet will modify lipoprotein levels and polyunsaturated fatty acids may have a role in impeding the progression of renal disease as well as the cardiovascular complications. Bile acid sequestrants do not correct the lipid abnormalities seen in renal insufficiency. Lovastatin or its active metabolite may accumulate in renal insufficiency, and lower doses of reductase inhibitors should be used to avoid adverse effects. Gemfibrozil may be used with caution as its pharmacokinetics is unchanged and it lowers triglycerides and increases HDL.[133] Statins (simvastatin, lovastatin, and atorvastatin) and fibric acid derivatives may increase the risk of severe myopathy, and attention to symptoms of myositis is needed. Niacin may also be useful in nondiabetic patients with renal insufficiency.

Hypertensive patients have a greater-than-expected prevalence of high blood cholesterol levels and, conversely, patients with hypercholesterolemia have a higher-than-expected prevalence of hypertension caused by the metabolic syndrome. Recommendations for the management of hypertension in patients with hypercholesterolemia include avoiding the use of drugs that elevate cholesterol such as diuretics and β-blockers and using agents that either are lipid neutral or may reduce cholesterol slightly (see Chap. 3).[1] Bile acid sequestrants may bind to thiazide diuretics and some β-blockers, and may interfere with their absorption; reaction may be avoided by giving the antihypertensive 1 hour before or 4 hours after the resin. Niacin may magnify the hypotensive effects of vasodilators.

Pharmacoeconomic Considerations

9 The clinical benefits of lipid-lowering therapy for primary and secondary interventions are now well established based on the results of studies showing a reduction in CHD morbidity and mortality.[134–136] The balance of benefits and costs has been examined in a few studies. The cost per year of life saved has been estimated to range from less than $10,000 to over $1 million depending on the presence or absence of CHD, age of the patient, baseline total or LDL-C level and reduction in cholesterol, and number of risk factors present. In general, intervention in patients with known CHD, those who have CHD risk equivalents, or those with a 10-year risk of 10% to 20% is cost-effective with statin therapy, while other types of therapy may be cost-effective if certain assumptions concerning compliance, efficacy, and so forth are met. The range for secondary intervention based on the 4S study is $3,800 for a 70-year-old man with a high cholesterol level to $27,400 per year of life gained for a middle-aged woman with an average cholesterol level.[137] In contrast, primary prevention in men based on the West of Scotland trial averages about $35,000 per year of life gained.[138] These studies demonstrate that primary and secondary interventions are well within the accepted boundary of less than $50,000 for a medical intervention to be considered cost-effective. Based on the specific lipoprotein phenotype, fibric acid derivatives, niacin, or combination therapy of statins plus BAR may be cost-effective. Cost-effectiveness is maximized by treating high-risk patients and those with established CHD.

Specialty lipid clinics have become increasingly popular and many use pharmacists to provide direct patient care in this setting. An interesting recent analysis shows that a specialty clinic may be more expensive ($659 ± $43 vs. $477 ± $42 per patient, P <0.001) than usual care. However, the overall cost-effectiveness is improved when expressed as program costs per unit (mmol/L) reduction in the LDL-C, a measure of cost-effectiveness that was significantly lower for specialized care ($758 ± $58 vs. $1,058 ± $70, P = 0.002) because more patients achieve their targeted goal.[139] Project ImPACT demonstrated that pharmacists, working collaborative with patients and physicians, can improve persistence and compliance and that nearly two-thirds of patients achieved their NCEP lipid goal.[140] Other programs show similar trends.[73,141,142]

Other Therapies

Partial ileal bypass has been used in severe heterozygous and homozygous familial hypercholesterolemia; however, it is ineffective in the latter case. Ileal bypass removes the site of bile acid reabsorption, depleting the bile acid pool and increasing the catabolism of cholesterol. A randomized trial of diet versus surgery, Program on the Surgical Control of the Hyperlipidemias (POSCH), reported that total and LDL cholesterol were decreased (23.3% and 37.7%, respectively) and HDL increased (4.3%) in patients who had undergone ileal bypass for hypercholesterolemia.[143] Overall death was delayed by nearly 3 years (P = 0.032) and CHD mortality was delayed by nearly 4 years (P = 0.046) by surgery, as compared with the control group. Revascularization procedures were delayed by an average of 7 years (P <0.001). Postsurgery diarrhea was more common in the surgical group, as was the rate of kidney stones (4% vs. 0.4%), gallstones (10% vs. 2%), and bowel obstruction (13.5% vs. 3.6%).

Portacaval shunts have been used to decrease the formation of LDL-C and reductions of 10% to 20% have been reported. Plasma exchange combined with niacin was found to reduce plasma cholesterol levels by about 50% in homozygous familial hypercholesterolemia over 5 years, and coronary atherosclerosis did not progress as documented by angiography. LDL-apheresis, selective removal of LDL-C via a filtering system, plus statin therapy is effective in LDL-C and appears to affect the progression of vascular disease. LDL-apheresis may be combined with statin therapy for greater effect. Combined liver and heart transplantation in homozygous familial hypercholesterolemia reduces total and LDL cholesterol concentrations from about 1,100 and 900 mg/dL (28.45 and 23.27 mmol/L) to about 300 and 185 mg/dL (7.76 and 4.78 mmol/L), prior to and after surgery, respectively. Liver transplantation replaced the missing LDL-Rs, enhanced catabolism, and reduced lipoprotein synthesis in this patient.

Summary of Major Studies

10 Primary and secondary prevention diet and drug trials have been performed to determine whether lowering of cholesterol will prevent CHD; Tables 11-15 and 11-16 summarize these trials. A number of earlier angiographic studies demonstrated that cholesterol reduction leads to regression of atherosclerosis and plaque stabilization.

TABLE 11-15 Primary Prevention Trials with Lipid-Lowering Drugs

Trial	F/U (years)	*N*	Treatment	Control Events (%)	Treatment Events (%)	*P*-Value	RRR	ARR (%)	NNT
AFCAPS/TexCAPS	5	6,605	Lovastatin 20–40 mg	5.5	3.5	<0.001	36.4%	2.0	50
Helsinki	5	4,081	Gemfibrozil 1,200 mg	4.1	2.7	<0.02	34%	1.4	71
LRC-CPPT	7.4	3,806	Cholestyramine 24 g	9.8	8.1	<0.05	17.3%	1.7	59
Oslo	5	1,232	Diet + smoking cessation	4.2	2.5	0.03	40.5%	1.7	59
WOSCOPS	4.9	6,595	Pravastatin 40 mg	7.8	5.5	<0.001	29.5%	2.3	43
ALLHAT	4.8	10,355	Usual care Pravastatin 40 mg	10.4	9.3	0.16	9%	1.1	91
WHI	5.2	16,608	Usual care Diet, CEE 0.625 mg + MPA 2.5 mg	1.5	1.9	0.05	1.29[a]	0.4	200[b]
WHI	5.2	16,608	Usual care Diet, CEE 0.625 mg	3.7	3.3	NS	9%	0.4	250
CARDS	4	2,838	Atorvastatin 10 mg	9	5.8	0.001	37%	3.2	32
JUPITER	1.9	17,802	Rosuvastatin 20 mg	2.82	1.59	0.00001	44%	1.2	82

AFCAPS/TexCAPS, Air Force/Texas Coronary Atherosclerosis Prevention Study[100]; ALLHAT, Antihypertensive and Lipid-Lowering Treatment to Prevent Heart Attack Trial (approximately 13–15% of patients had a history of coronary heart disease [CHD]; events are CHD events only); ARR, absolute risk reduction; CARDS, Collaborative Atorvastatin Diabetes Study (presented at the 2004 American Diabetes Association meeting); CEE, conjugated equine estrogen; Helsinki, the Helsinki Heart Study (Frick et al., 1987); JUPITER, Justification for the Use of Statins in Prevention (Ridker, 2008); LRC-CPPT, the Lipid Research Clinics Coronary Primary Prevention Trial (Insull et al., 1984); MPA, medroxyprogesterone acetate; NNT, number needed to treat; Oslo, the Oslo Study (Hjermann et al., 1988); RRR, relative risk reduction; WHI, Women's Health Initiative; WOSCOPS, the West of Scotland Coronary Prevention Study.[99]

[a]The risk of CHD was increased by 29%.

[b]Number needed to harm since CEE + MPA was worse than placebo.

TABLE 11-16 Secondary Prevention Trials with Lipid-Lowering Drugs

Trial	F/U (years)	N	Treatment	Control Events	Treatment Events	P-Value	RRR (%)	ARR	NNT
VA-HIT	5.1	2,531	Gemfibrozil 1,200 mg	23.7%	17.3%	0.006	22	4.4%	23
AVERT	1.5	341	Atorvastatin 80 mg	21%	13%	0.048	38	8%	12
CARE	5	4,159	Pravastatin 40 mg	13.2%	10.2%	0.003	22.7	3%	33
CDP	5	8,341	Niacin 3 g + clofibrate 1.8 g	20.9%	20.6%	NS	1.4	0.3%	333
HERS	4.1	2,673	Estrogen 0.625 mg + progestin 2.5 mg	12.7%	12.5%	0.91	1.6	0.2%	500
LIPID	7.4	3,806	Pravastatin 40 mg	9.8%	8.1%	<0.05	17.3	1.7%	59
4S	5	4,444	Simvastatin 20 mg	11.5%	8.2%	0.0003	28.7	3.3%	30
WHO	5.3	15,745	Clofibrate 1.6 g	3.9%	3.1%	<0.005	20.5	0.8%	125
BIP	6.2	3,090	Placebo Bezafibrate 400 mg	15%	13.6%	0.26	9.3	1.4%	72
TIMI-22	2	4,162	Pravastatin 40 mg Atorvastatin 80 mg	26.3% (P)	22.4% (A)	0.005	16	3.9%	26
HPS	5	20,536	Simvastatin 40 mg	14.7%	12.9%	0.003	13	1.8%	56
MIRACL		3,086	Atorvastatin 80 mg	17.4%	14.8%	0.048	16	2.6%	39
PROSPER	3	5,804	Pravastatin 40 mg	16.2%	14.1%	0.014	24	2.1%	48
SPARCL	4	4,731	Atorvastatin 80 mg	13.1	11.2	0.03	16	2.2	46
TNT	4.9	10,001	Atorvastatin 10 mg versus 80 mg	10.9	8.7	<0.001	22	2.2	46
ACCORD	4.7	5,518	Fenofibrate 160 mg	2.4%	2.2%	0.32	8	0.2%	500
AIM-HIGH	2	3,414	Niacin 1,500–2,000 mg + simvastatin	16.2%	16.4	0.80	−0.2	+1.2%	NA
HPS 2-THRIVE	3.9	25,673	Niacin 2 g + laropiprant	13.7%	13.2%	0.29	4.9	0.5%	200

ACCORD, Action to Control Cardiovascular Risk in Diabetes (Accord Study Group, 2010); AIM-HIGH, Low HDL/High Triglycerides: Impact on Global Health Outcomes (AIM-HIGH Investigators); ARR, absolute risk reduction; AVERT, Atorvastatin Versus Revascularization Treatments; BIP, Bezafibrate Infarction Prevention; CARE, Cholesterol and Recurrent Events (Melendez et al., 1996); CDP, Coronary Drug Project (Berge et al., 1975); HERS, Heart and Estrogen Replacement Study[119]; HPS, Heart Protection Study, results expressed as all-cause mortality (HPS Collaborative Group, 2002); HPS2-THRIVE, Heart Protection Study—Treatment of HDL to Reduce the Incidence of Vascular Events; LIPID, Long-Term Intervention with Pravastatin in Ischaemic Disease Study (MacMahon et al., 1995); MIRACL, Myocardial Ischemia Reduction with Aggressive Cholesterol Lowering (Schwartz et al., 2001); NNT, number needed to treat; PROSPER, PROspective Study of Pravastatin in the Elderly at Risk[151]; RRR, relative risk reduction; 4S, Scandinavian Simvastatin Survival Study (Pederson et al., 1994); SPARCL, Stroke Prevention by Aggressive Reduction in Cholesterol Levels (SPARCL Investigators, 2006); TIMI-22, Thrombolysis in Myocardial Infarction 22 study, also known as the PROVE-IT trial[152]; TNT, Treatment to New Targets[153]; VA-HIT, Veterans Administration High-Density Lipoprotein Cholesterol (HDL-C) Intervention Trial; WHO, World Health Organization (Committee of Principal Investigators, 1978).

Most of the primary and secondary studies were double blinded, randomized, and placebo controlled, lasting for 5 years or longer, and most had sufficient patient numbers to be meaningful. Exceptions to these qualifications were seen in the early studies such as the Newcastle and Edinburgh trials, which were small and generally did not show much benefit, and the Coronary Drug Project (CDP) using dextrothyroxine, which was terminated early due to adverse effects on CHD mortality. The Helsinki Heart Study, using gemfibrozil, resulted in a reduction in nonfatal MI, which was the primary contributor to reduced CHD incidence (Table 11-15).[16]

Total and LDL cholesterol were reduced an average of 13.4% and 20.3%, respectively, by cholestyramine in the LRC-CPPT, and the reduction of lipid levels was related to the amount of drug ingested (e.g., one to two packets, 5.4% reduction in total cholesterol, vs. five or more packets, 19% reduction).[144] The prescribed dose of cholestyramine was 24 g, or six packets, per day. The cholestyramine group experienced a 19% reduction in risk (P <0.05) of the primary end point—definite CHD death and/or definite nonfatal MI—reflecting a 24% reduction in definite CHD death and a 19% reduction in nonfatal MI. Other end points were reduced by 25%, 20%, and 21% for new positive exercise tests, angina, and coronary bypass surgery, respectively. Death from all causes was not significantly reduced by cholestyramine secondary to more accidents and violence in this group. The mean falls in total and LDL cholesterol in the cholestyramine group were 8% and 12% relative to levels in placebo-treated men, providing evidence that for every 1% reduction in cholesterol, a 2% decline in CHD mortality can be realized.

AFCAPS/TexCAPS, a primary prevention trial conducted in 6,605 men and women aged 57 to 63 years with average total cholesterol and LDL (<221 and <150 mg/dL [<5.72 and <3.88 mmol/L], respectively) who were treated with lovastatin 20 to 40 mg/day for 5.2 years, a 37% reduction (P <0.001) was shown in the risk for first acute major coronary event (fatal or nonfatal MI, unstable angina, or sudden cardiac death).[100] The need for revascularization procedures was also reduced by 33% (P <0.001). The implications of this trial are enormous; potentially millions of "normal" people could benefit from lipid lowering with statins based on these results. The number of patients who need to be treated (NNT, Table 11-15) for primary prevention ranges from 43 in the West of Scotland trial to 71 in the Helsinki Heart Study. This range is within the typical boundary used for treatment decisions and described previously; cost-effectiveness is achieved routinely in patients with moderate to high risk. The Antihypertensive and Lipid-Lowering Treatment to Prevent Heart Attack Trial (ALLHAT-LLT) tested pravastatin 40 mg/day versus placebo in hypertensive patients with at least one CHD risk factor. Pravastatin did not reduce either all-cause mortality or CHD significantly when compared with usual care in older participants with well-controlled hypertension and moderately elevated LDL-C. The results may be due to the modest differential in total cholesterol (9.6%) and LDL-C (16.7%) between pravastatin and usual care compared with prior statin trials supporting cardiovascular disease prevention.[145] The Women's Health Initiative trial proved to be disappointing with no beneficial effects on CHD event reduction in the hormone replacement arm (conjugated equine estrogens [CEE] + medroxyprogesterone) or the CEE alone arm compared with placebo.[119,121] Women did experience greater risk for thromboembolism, a slight increase in breast cancer, and a reduced risk of hip fracture. Consequently, hormone replacement therapy can no longer be recommended for cardiovascular protection.[4] Publication of the recent WISDOM trial found that when combined hormone therapy (N = 2,196) was compared with placebo (N = 2,189), there was a significant increase in the number of major cardiovascular events (7 vs. 0, P = 0.016) and venous thromboembolism (22 vs. 3, hazard ratio 7.36 [95% CI 2.20 to 24.60]) confirming the findings of HERS and WHI. There were no statistically significant differences in numbers of breast or other cancers' cerebrovascular events, fractures, and overall death.[123]

Niacin in the CDP significantly reduced definite, nonfatal MI as compared with placebo (10.1% vs. 13.9%), whereas clofibrate did not reduce death from any cause or nonfatal or fatal MI at the 5-year followup period.[146]

One of the most important studies published in the last few years is the 4S trial, a secondary intervention trial in a large number of patients.[147] Simvastatin, 20 to 40 mg/day, reduced LDL cholesterol by 35% and reduced the risk of death from any cause by 30%. Coronary deaths were also reduced with simvastatin (relative risk, 0.58; confidence interval, 0.46 to 0.73). Therapy was also shown to be effective in women (18% to 19% of patients enrolled) and in the elderly (≥60 years). Indeed, the relative risk of death or major coronary event was reduced to a greater extent in the elderly than in younger patients. Death from noncardiovascular causes was similar for simvastatin and placebo (2.1% and 2.2%, respectively). The survival curves for simvastatin and placebo began to separate at 1 year and became more divergent with additional followup. The 4S study clearly demonstrates the benefit in cholesterol lowering and placates long-held fears of death from non-CHD causes. The Long-Term Intervention with Pravastatin in Ischemic Disease (LIPID) study (N = 7,498 men and 1,516 women) has investigated the effect of pravastatin on CHD mortality in patients with prior MI or unstable angina and mean cholesterol level of 219 mg/dL (5.66 mmol/L) over 6 years.[148] Pravastatin reduced the risk of CHD mortality by 24% (8.3% vs. 6.4%, $P = 0.0004$) and total mortality by 23% (14.1% vs. 11%, $P = 0.00002$); stroke was also reduced by 20% (4.3% vs. 3.5%, $P = 0.22$), and there was reduction in the need for coronary artery bypass graft (11.3% vs. 8.9%, $P = 0.0001$) or percutaneous transluminal coronary angioplasty (5.3% vs. 4.4%, $P = 0.04$).

The Veterans Administration High-Density Lipoprotein Intervention Trial (VA-HIT) was a double-blind trial that compared gemfibrozil (1,200 mg/day) with placebo in 2,531 men with CHD, an HDL cholesterol level of ≤40 mg/dL (≤1.03 mmol/L), and an LDL cholesterol level of ≤140 mg/dL (≤3.62 mmol/L).[149] The primary study outcome was nonfatal MI or death from coronary causes. The median followup was 5.1 years. At 1 year, the mean HDL cholesterol level was 6% higher, the mean triglyceride level was 31% lower, and the mean total cholesterol level was 4% lower in the gemfibrozil group than in the placebo group. LDL cholesterol levels did not differ significantly between the groups. A primary event occurred in 21.7% of the patients assigned to placebo and in 17.3% of the patients assigned to gemfibrozil. The overall reduction in the risk of an event was 4.4 percentage points, and the reduction in relative risk was 22% ($P = 0.006$). This trial presents the strongest evidence to date that raising HDL-C and lowering triglycerides reduce risk for CHD.

The Atorvastatin Versus Revascularization Treatments (AVERT) study compared atorvastatin 80 mg/day with percutaneous transluminal coronary angioplasty.[150] The followup period was 18 months. Of the patients who received aggressive lipid-lowering treatment with atorvastatin, 13% had ischemic events, as compared with 21% of the patients who underwent angioplasty. The incidence of ischemic events was thus 36% lower in the atorvastatin group over an 18-month period ($P = 0.048$, which was not statistically significant after adjustment for interim analyses). This reduction in events was because of a smaller number of angioplasty procedures, coronary artery bypass operations, and hospitalizations for worsening angina (the most common end point). As compared with the patients who were treated with angioplasty and usual care, the patients who received atorvastatin had a significantly longer time to the first ischemic event ($P = 0.03$). In low-risk patients with stable CAD, aggressive lipid-lowering therapy is at least as effective as angioplasty and usual care in reducing the incidence of ischemic events.

Pravastatin in the elderly individuals at risk for vascular disease (PROSPER) studied men and women in the age range of 70 to 82 years and found that pravastatin 40 mg/day reduced CHD events by 24% with no effect on cognitive function.[151] A more recent trial, TIMI-22 (also known as Pravastatin or Atorvastatin Evaluation and Infection Therapy [PROVE-IT]) enrolled 4,162 patients who had been hospitalized for an acute coronary syndrome within the preceding 10 days and compared 40 mg of pravastatin daily (standard therapy) with 80 mg of atorvastatin daily (intensive therapy).[152] An intensive lipid-lowering statin regimen with atorvastatin 80 mg/day provided greater protection against death or major cardiovascular events than does a standard regimen. This study clearly points to "lower is better" for LDL concentration and will likely lead to revision in guideline goals to lower LDL levels. The Treatment to New Targets (TNT) assessed the efficacy and safety of lowering LDL cholesterol levels below 100 mg/dL (2.6 mmol/L) in patients with stable CHD.[153,154] Intensive lipid-lowering therapy with 80 mg of atorvastatin per day in patients with stable CHD provides significant clinical benefit beyond that afforded by treatment with 10 mg of atorvastatin per day providing further evidence that intensive lipid lowering brings greater benefits.

Statins reduce the incidence of strokes among patients at increased risk for cardiovascular disease; whether they reduce the risk of stroke after a recent stroke or TIA was addressed by Stroke Prevention by Aggressive Reduction in Cholesterol Levels (SPARCL).[155] During a median followup of 4.9 years, 265 patients (11.2%) receiving atorvastatin 80 mg/day and 311 patients (13.1%) receiving placebo had a fatal or nonfatal stroke (5-year absolute reduction in risk, 2.2%; adjusted hazard ratio, 0.84; 95% confidence interval, 0.71 to 0.99; $P = 0.03$; unadjusted $P = 0.05$).[155] JUPITER randomized healthy patients to rosuvastatin on placebo and, on the basis of elevated CRP, found a 55% reduction in vascular events (event rate 1.11 vs. 0.51 per 100 person-years; hazard ratio 0.45, $P < 0.0001$).[24]

Recent clinical trials attempting to increase HDL-C have been disappointing and one was stopped early due to futility.[156] Neither the AIM-HIGH nor HPS2-THRIVE trial demonstrated a reduction in cardiovascular end points.[14] Both trials included background therapy with statins ± ezetimibe and the changes in HDL-C were somewhat smaller than expected. Some have suggested that extensive prior treatment may have depleted the lipid core making plaque less susceptible to rupture leading to clinical events.

Clinical **Controversy. . .**

The CETP inhibitor torcetrapib was associated with a substantial increase in HDL cholesterol and decrease in LDL cholesterol. It was also associated with an increase in blood pressure, and there was no significant decrease in the progression of coronary atherosclerosis. The lack of efficacy may be related to the mechanism of action of this drug class or to molecule-specific adverse effects. Other means of raising HDL cholesterol (HDL mimetics, which include ApoA-I mutants and peptide mimetics of ApoA-I, and HDL Milano A, a synthetic form of HDL) still hold hope of HDL modification leading a reduction in clinical events.

The enzyme ACAT esterifies cholesterol in a variety of tissues. In some animal models, ACAT inhibitors have antiatherosclerotic effects. Unfortunately, when tested in clinical trials, ACAT inhibition is not an effective strategy for limiting atherosclerosis and may promote atherogenesis.[157]

With the failure of AIM-HIGH and HPS2-THRIVE, the HDL hypothesis, raising HDL-C lowers cardiovascular risk, may be called into question. Others argue that trial design limited the outcome in these studies and a true test of the HDL-C hypothesis remains to be completed.

Statins differ in their pharmacokinetic properties and in pleiotropic effects (i.e., non–lipid lowering). The contribution of lipid lowering alone (a class effect) versus other effects (antiinflammatory, antithrombotic, etc.) continues to create controversy.

Proteinuria has been associated with high-dose rosuvastatin therapy (40 mg/day), but a review of a clinical trial database revealed an increase in eGFR for rosuvastatin-treated patients was consistent across all major demographic and clinical subgroups of interest, including patients with baseline proteinuria, baseline eGFR <60 mL/min/1.73 m^2 (<0.58 mL/s/m^2), and in patients with hypertension and/or diabetes.[158]

11 Mipomersen is an oligonucleotide inhibitor of ApoB-100 synthesis indicated as an adjunct to lipid-lowering medications and diet to reduce LDL cholesterol, ApoB, total cholesterol, and non-HDL cholesterol in patients with homozygous familial hypercholesterolemia. The average reduction in LDL cholesterol is ~25% with the most common adverse events being injection site pain (~10%).[159] Lomitapide oral capsule is a microsomal triglyceride transfer protein (MTP) inhibitor. Inhibiting MTP reduces the level of cholesterol that the liver and intestines assemble and secrete into the circulation.[160] The average decrease in LDL cholesterol beyond baseline is ~40%. Hepatic steatosis associated with lomitapide may be a risk factor for progressive liver disease including steatohepatitis and cirrhosis. GI complaints and mild to moderate elevations in liver enzymes have been reported with both drugs.

The role of nontraditional risk factors (hsCRP, homocysteine, etc.) is continuing to be clarified and may lead to recommendations for the use of these tests in patient evaluation.

EVALUATION OF THERAPEUTIC OUTCOMES

Short-term evaluation of therapy for hyperlipidemia is based on response to diet and drug treatment as measured in the clinical laboratory by total cholesterol, LDL cholesterol, HDL cholesterol, and triglycerides for patients being treated for primary intervention, as well as on response to secondary intervention. The interval for followup is dependent on the severity of illness, and patients with known CAD or multiple risk factors should be monitored more closely. Less commonly used laboratory measurements include CRP, homocysteine, ApoB, and Lp(a) levels. Because many patients being treated for primary hyperlipidemia have no symptoms and may not have any clinical manifestations of a genetic lipid disorder such as xanthomas or eruptions, monitoring and outcome are solely laboratory based. In patients treated for secondary intervention, symptoms of atherosclerotic cardiovascular disease, such as angina or intermittent claudication, may improve over months to years. If patients have xanthomas or other external manifestations of hyperlipidemia, these lesions should regress with therapy. Lipid measurements should be obtained in the fasted state to minimize interference from chylomicrons, and once the patient is stable, monitoring is needed at intervals of 6 months to 1 year. The goals for LDL and HDL cholesterol are provided in Tables 11-8 and 11-9.

Patients with multiple risk factors and established CHD should also be monitored and evaluated for progress in managing their other risk factors such as hypertension, smoking cessation, exercise and weight control, and glycemic control if diabetic. The goals are to maintain a blood pressure of below 130/80 mm Hg or less (presence of diabetes or renal insufficiency), stop smoking, maintain an ideal body weight, exercise for at least 20 minutes three or more times per week, and keep plasma glucose below 100 mg/dL (5.6 mmol/L) (threshold for glucose intolerance). Invasive evaluation, such as cardiac catheterization, is useful in patients with established CHD and is typically used for planning revascularization rather than monitoring of lipid-lowering therapy.

Evaluation of dietary therapy is part of the outcome evaluation for treating hyperlipidemia and the assistance of a dietitian is recommended. Use of diet diaries and recall survey instruments enables information about diet to be collected in a systematic fashion and may improve patient adherence to dietary recommendations. Patients on resin therapy should have a FLP panel checked every 4 to 8 weeks until a stable dose; triglycerides should be checked at stable dose to insure they have not increased. Niacin requires baseline liver function tests, uric acid, and glucose; repeat tests are appropriate at doses of 1,000 to 1,500 mg/day. Symptoms of myopathy or diabetes-like symptoms should be investigated and may require CK or glucose determinations; more frequent monitoring in diabetics may be necessary. A FLP 4 to 8 weeks after the initial dose or dose changes with statins is appropriate. Liver function tests should be obtained at baseline and periodically thereafter based on package insert information; recognized experts believe that monitoring for hepatotoxicity and myopathy should be symptom triggered.[59,66] Ezetimibe requires little specific monitoring; however, with the publication of the SEAS trial, there is concern over the increased risk of cancer.[161] Other studies underway will clarify this issue.

ABBREVIATIONS

ACAT	acyl-coenzyme A-to-cholesterol acyltransferase
ACCORD	Action to Control Cardiovascular Risk in Diabetes
AHA	American Heart Association
ALLHAT-LLT	Antihypertensive and Lipid-Lowering Treatment to Prevent Heart Attack Trial
Apo	apolipoprotein
ATP III	Adult Treatment Panel III
AVERT	Atorvastatin Versus Revascularization Treatments
BAR	bile acid resin
BMI	body mass index
CAD	coronary artery disease
CARDS	Collaborative Atorvastatin Diabetes Study
CDP	Coronary Drug Project
CEE	conjugated equine estrogens
CETP	cholesterol ester transfer protein
CHD	coronary heart disease
CIMT	carotid intimal medial thickness
CRP	C-reactive protein
CTX	cerebrotendinous xanthomatosis
DISC	Dietary Intervention Study in Children
DP1	D(2) receptor subtype 1
ER	extended release
HDL	high-density lipoprotein
HMG-CoA reductase	3-hydroxy-3-methylglutaryl coenzyme A reductase
ICAM-1	intercellular adhesion molecule
IDL	intermediate-density lipoprotein
IHD	ischemic heart disease
IL-1	interleukin-1
IL-6	interleukin-6
IL-10	interleukin-10
IL-12	interleukin-12
INR	international normalized ratio

JUPITER	Justification for the Use of Statins in Prevention: An Intervention Trial Evaluating Rosuvastatin
KLF2	Kruppel-like factor 2
LCAT	lecithin-cholesterol acyltransferase
LDL	low-density lipoprotein
LDL-R	LDL receptor
LIPID	Long-Term Intervention with Pravastatin in Ischemic Disease
LPL	lipoprotein lipase
M-CSF	monocyte colony-stimulating factor
MCP-1	monocyte chemoattractant protein 1
MI	myocardial infarction
MTP	microsomal triglyceride transfer protein
NCEP	National Cholesterol Education Program
NNT	number of patients who need to be treated
PDAY	pathobiologic determinants of atherosclerosis in youth
PDGF	platelet-derived growth factor
PON	paraoxonase
POSCH	Program on the Surgical Control of the Hyperlipidemias
PROVE-IT	Pravastatin or Atorvastatin Evaluation and Infection Therapy
SEC	sinusoidal endothelial cells
SPARCL	Stroke Prevention by Aggressive Reduction in Cholesterol Levels
TIA	transient ischemic attack
TLC	therapeutic lifestyle change
TNT	Treatment to New Targets
VA-HIT	Veterans Administration High-Density Lipoprotein Intervention Trial
VCAM-1	vascular cell adhesion molecule
VEGF	vascular endothelial growth factor
VLDL	very-low-density lipoprotein

REFERENCES

1. Expert Panel on Detection, Evaluation, and Treatment of High Blood Cholesterol in Adults. Executive summary of the third report of the National Cholesterol Education Program (NCEP) Expert Panel on Detection, Evaluation, and Treatment of High Blood Cholesterol in Adults (Adult Treatment Panel III). JAMA 2001;285:2486–2497.
2. Grundy SM, Cleeman JI, Merz CN, et al. Implications of recent clinical trials for the National Cholesterol Education Program Adult Treatment Panel III guidelines [erratum appears in Circulation 2004;110(6):763]. Circulation 2004;110:227–239.
3. Smith SC Jr, Allen J, Blair SN, et al. AHA/ACC guidelines for secondary prevention for patients with coronary and other atherosclerotic vascular disease: 2006 update: Endorsed by the National Heart, Lung, and Blood Institute [erratum appears in Circulation 2006;113(22):e847]. Circulation 2006;113:2363–2372.
4. Mosca L, Banka CL, Benjamin EJ, et al. Evidence-based guidelines for cardiovascular disease prevention in women: 2007 update. Circulation 2007;115:1481–1501.
5. Fletcher B, Berra K, Ades P, et al. Managing abnormal blood lipids: A collaborative approach. Circulation 2005;112: 3184–3209.
6. Ford ES, Mokdad AH, Giles WH, Mensah GA. Serum total cholesterol concentrations and awareness, treatment, and control of hypercholesterolemia among US adults: Findings from the National Health and Nutrition Examination Survey, 1999 to 2000 [see comment]. Circulation 2003;107: 2185–2189.
7. Go AS, Mozaffarian D, Roger VL, et al. Heart disease and stroke statistics—2013 update: A report from the American Heart Association. Circulation 2013;127:e6–e245.
8. Arnett DK, Jacobs DR Jr, Luepker RV, Blackburn H, Armstrong C, Claas SA. Twenty-year trends in serum cholesterol, hypercholesterolemia, and cholesterol medication use: The Minnesota Heart Survey, 1980-1982 to 2000-2002. Circulation 2005;112:3884–3891.
9. Lloyd-Jones D, Adams RJ, Brown TM, et al. Executive summary: Heart disease and stroke statistics—2010 update: A report from the American Heart Association. Circulation 2010;121:948–954.
10. Foley KA, Denke MA, Kamal-Bahl S, et al. The impact of physician attitudes and beliefs on treatment decisions: Lipid therapy in high-risk patients. Med Care 2006;44:421–428.
11. Menotti A, Lanti M, Nedeljkovic S, Nissinen A, Kafatos A, Kromhout D. The relationship of age, blood pressure, serum cholesterol and smoking habits with the risk of typical and atypical coronary heart disease death in the European cohorts of the Seven Countries Study. Int J Cardiol 2006;106: 157–163.
12. McQueen MJ, Hawken S, Wang X, et al. Lipids, lipoproteins, and apolipoproteins as risk markers of myocardial infarction in 52 countries (the INTERHEART study): A case–control study. Lancet 2008;372:224–233.
13. Rader DJ. Mechanisms of disease: HDL metabolism as a target for novel therapies. Nat Clin Pract Cardiovasc Med 2007;4:102–109.
14. AIM-HIGH Investigators, Boden WE, Probstfield JL, et al. Niacin in patients with low HDL cholesterol levels receiving intensive statin therapy. N Engl J Med 2011;365:2255–2267.
15. Jeppesen J, Hein HO, Suadicani P, Gyntelberg F. Triglyceride concentration and ischemic heart disease: An eight-year follow-up in the Copenhagen Male Study. Circulation 1998;97:1029–1036.
16. Huttunen JK, Manninen V, Manttari M, et al. The Helsinki Heart Study: Central findings and clinical implications. Ann Med 1991;23:155–159.
17. Yuan G, Al-Shali KZ, Hegele RA. Hypertriglyceridemia: Its etiology, effects and treatment. CMAJ 2007;176:1113–1120.
18. Ganong WF. Pathophysiology of Disease: An Introduction to Clinical Medicine, 5th ed. New York: McGraw Hill, 2006.
19. Nissen SE, Tardif JC, Nicholls SJ, et al. Effect of torcetrapib on the progression of coronary atherosclerosis [see comment]. N Engl J Med 2007;356:1304–1316.
20. Libby P, Aikawa M, Jain MK. Vascular endothelium and atherosclerosis. Handb Exp Pharmacol 2006;176:285–306.
21. Miller DT, Ridker PM, Libby P, Kwiatkowski DJ. Atherosclerosis: The path from genomics to therapeutics. J Am Coll Cardiol 2007;49:1589–1599.
22. Schwartz GG, Olsson AG, Abt M, et al. Effects of dalcetrapib in patients with a recent acute coronary syndrome. N Engl J Med 2012;367:2089–2099.
23. Sofat R, Hingorani AD, Smeeth L, et al. Separating the mechanism-based and off-target actions of cholesteryl ester transfer protein inhibitors with CETP gene polymorphisms. Circulation 2010;121:52–62.
24. Ridker PM, Danielson E, Fonseca FA, et al. Reduction in C-reactive protein and LDL cholesterol and cardiovascular event rates after initiation of rosuvastatin: A prospective study of the JUPITER trial. Lancet 2009;373:1175–1182.
25. Eagle KA, Ginsburg GS, Musunuru K, et al. Identifying patients at high risk of a cardiovascular event in the near future: Current status and future directions: Report of a

National Heart, Lung, and Blood Institute working group. Circulation 2010;121:1447–1454.
26. Kujiraoka T, Hattori H, Miwa Y, et al. Serum apolipoprotein j in health, coronary heart disease and type 2 diabetes mellitus. J Atheroscler Thromb 2006;13:314–322.
27. Libby P. How our growing understanding of inflammation has reshaped the way we think of disease and drug development. Clin Pharmacol Ther 2010;87:389–391.
28. Huang CY, Wu TC, Lin WT, et al. Effects of simvastatin withdrawal on serum matrix metalloproteinases in hypercholesterolaemic patients. Eur J Clin Invest 2006;36:76–84.
29. Suviolahti E, Lilja HE, Pajukanta P. Unraveling the complex genetics of familial combined hyperlipidemia. Ann Med 2006;38:337–351.
30. Buse JB, Ginsberg HN, Bakris GL, et al. Primary prevention of cardiovascular diseases in people with diabetes mellitus: A scientific statement from the American Heart Association and the American Diabetes Association. Diabetes Care 2007;30:162–172.
31. Grundy SM, Cleeman JI, Daniels SR, et al. Diagnosis and management of the metabolic syndrome: An American Heart Association/National Heart, Lung, and Blood Institute scientific statement [erratum appears in Circulation 2005;112(17):e297]. Circulation 2005;112:2735–2752.
32. Grundy SM, Pasternak R, Greenland P, Smith S Jr, Fuster V. AHA/ACC scientific statement: Assessment of cardiovascular risk by use of multiple-risk-factor assessment equations: A statement for healthcare professionals from the American Heart Association and the American College of Cardiology. J Am Coll Cardiol 1999;34:1348–1359.
33. Grundy SM, Cleeman JI, Merz CN, et al. A summary of implications of recent clinical trials for the National Cholesterol Education Program Adult Treatment Panel III guidelines. Arterioscler Thromb Vasc Biol 2004;24: 1329–1330.
34. Grundy SM, Cleeman JI, Merz CN, et al. Implications of recent clinical trials for the National Cholesterol Education Program Adult Treatment Panel III guidelines. J Am Coll Cardiol 2004;44:720–732.
35. Singh IM, Shishehbor MH, Ansell BJ. High density lipoprotein as a therapeutic target. A systematic review. JAMA 2007;298:786–798.
36. Daniels SR, Greer FR, Committee on Nutrition. Lipid screening and cardiovascular health in childhood. Pediatrics 2008;122:198–208.
37. Strong JP, Malcom GT, Oalmann MC, Wissler RW. The PDAY Study: Natural history, risk factors, and pathobiology. Pathobiological Determinants of Atherosclerosis in Youth. Ann N Y Acad Sci 1997;811:226–235 [discussion 35–37].
38. Lauer RM, Obarzanek E, Hunsberger SA, et al. Efficacy and safety of lowering dietary intake of total fat, saturated fat, and cholesterol in children with elevated LDL cholesterol: The Dietary Intervention Study in Children. Am J Clin Nutr 2000;72:1332S–1342S.
39. Van Horn L, Obarzanek E, Friedman LA, Gernhofer N, Barton B. Children's adaptations to a fat-reduced diet: The Dietary Intervention Study in Children (DISC). Pediatrics 2005;115:1723–1733.
40. Iughetti L, Predieri B, Balli F, Calandra S. Rational approach to the treatment for heterozygous familial hypercholesterolemia in childhood and adolescence: A review. J Endocrinol Invest 2007;30:700–719.
41. Wierzbicki AS, Viljoen A. Hyperlipidaemia in paediatric patients: The role of lipid-lowering therapy in clinical practice. Drug Saf 2010;33:115–125.
42. Trejo-Gutierrez JF, Fletcher G. Impact of exercise on blood lipids and lipoproteins. J Clin Lipidol 2007;1: 175–181.
43. Williams MA, Haskell WL, Ades PA, et al. Resistance exercise in individuals with and without cardiovascular disease: 2007 update: A scientific statement from the American Heart Association Council on Clinical Cardiology and Council on Nutrition, Physical Activity, and Metabolism. Circulation 2007;116:572–584.
44. Eckel RH, Borra S, Lichtenstein AH, Yin-Piazza SY, Trans Fat Conference Planning Group. Understanding the complexity of trans fatty acid reduction in the American diet: American Heart Association Trans Fat Conference 2006: Report of the Trans Fat Conference Planning Group. Circulation 2007;115:2231–2246.
45. American Heart Association Nutrition Committee, Lichtenstein AH, Appel LJ, et al. Diet and lifestyle recommendations revision 2006: A scientific statement from the American Heart Association Nutrition Committee [erratum appears in Circulation 2006;114(1):e27]. Circulation 2006;114:82–96.
46. Sacks FM, Lichtenstein A, Van Horn L, et al. Soy protein, isoflavones, and cardiovascular health: An American Heart Association Science Advisory for professionals from the Nutrition Committee. Circulation 2006;113:1034–1044.
47. Gidding SS, Dennison BA, Birch LL, et al. Dietary recommendations for children and adolescents: A guide for practitioners: Consensus statement from the American Heart Association [erratum appears in Circulation 2005;112(15):2375]. Circulation 2005;112:2061–2075.
48. Grundy SM, Cleeman JI, Daniels SR, et al. Diagnosis and management of the metabolic syndrome: An American Heart Association/National Heart, Lung, and Blood Institute scientific statement. Curr Opin Cardiol 2006;21:1–6.
49. Assmann G, Guerra R, Fox G, et al. Harmonizing the definition of the metabolic syndrome: Comparison of the criteria of the Adult Treatment Panel III and the International Diabetes Federation in United States American and European populations. Am J Cardiol 2007;99:541–548.
50. Shrestha S, Volek JS, Udani J, et al. A combination therapy including psyllium and plant sterols lowers LDL cholesterol by modifying lipoprotein metabolism in hypercholesterolemic individuals. J Nutr 2006;136: 2492–2497.
51. Petchetti L, Frishman WH, Petrillo R, Raju K. Nutriceuticals in cardiovascular disease: Psyllium. Cardiol Rev 2007;15:116–122.
52. He K, Song Y, Davigius ML, et al. Accumulated evidence on fish consumption and coronary heart disease mortality: A meta-analysis of cohort studies. Circulation 2004;109:2705–2711.
53. von Schacky C, Harris WS. Cardiovascular benefits of omega-3 fatty acids. Cardiovasc Res 2007;73:310–315.
54. McKenney JM, Sica D. Role of prescription omega-3 fatty acids in the treatment of hypertriglyceridemia. Pharmacotherapy 2007;27:715–728.
55. Bhattacharya S. Therapy and clinical trials: Plant sterols and stanols in management of hypercholesterolemia: Where are we now? Curr Opin Lipidol 2006;17:98–100.
56. Berthold HK, Unverdorben S, Degenhardt R, Bulitta M, Gouni-Berthold I. Effect of policosanol on lipid levels among patients with hypercholesterolemia or combined hyperlipidemia: A randomized controlled trial. JAMA 2006;295:2262–2269.
57. Baigent C, Keech A, Kearney PM, et al. Efficacy and safety of cholesterol-lowering treatment: Prospective meta-analysis

of data from 90,056 participants in 14 randomised trials of statins. Lancet 2005;366:1267–1278.

58. Link JJ, Rohatgi A, de Lemos JA. HDL cholesterol: Physiology, pathophysiology, and management. Curr Probl Cardiol 2007;32:268–314.
59. McKenney JM. Introduction. Report of the National Lipid Association's Safety Task Force: The nonstatins. Am J Cardiol 2007;99:1C–58C.
60. Wensel TM, Waldrop BA, Wensel B. Pitavastatin: A new HMG-CoA reductase inhibitor. Ann Pharmacother 2010;44:507–514.
61. Shitara Y, Sugiyama Y. Pharmacokinetic and pharmacodynamic alterations of 3-hydroxy-3-methylglutaryl coenzyme A (HMG-CoA) reductase inhibitors: Drug–drug interactions and interindividual differences in transporter and metabolic enzyme functions. Pharmacol Ther 2006;112: 71–105.
62. Jones P, Kafonek S, Laurora I, Hunninghake D. Comparative dose efficacy study of atorvastatin versus simvastatin, pravastatin, lovastatin, and fluvastatin in patients with hypercholesterolemia (the CURVES Study). Am J Cardiol 1998;81:582–587.
63. Robinson JG, Davidson MH. Combination therapy with ezetimibe and simvastatin to achieve aggressive LDL reduction. Expert Rev Cardiovasc Ther 2006;4:461–476.
64. Nissen SE. ENHANCE and ACCORD: Controversy over surrogate end points. Curr Cardiol Rep 2008;10:159–161.
65. Davidson MH, Robinson JG. Safety of aggressive lipid management. J Am Coll Cardiol 2007;49:1753–1762.
66. McKenney JM, Davidson MH, Jacobson TA, Guyton JR, National Lipid Association Statin Safety Assessment Task Force. Final conclusions and recommendations of the National Lipid Association Statin Safety Assessment Task Force. Am J Cardiol 2006;97:17.
67. Alsheikh-Ali AA, Maddukuri PV, Han H, Karas RH. Effect of the magnitude of lipid lowering on risk of elevated liver enzymes, rhabdomyolysis, and cancer: Insights from large randomized statin trials. J Am Coll Cardiol 2007;50: 409–418.
68. Edwards IR, Star K, Kiuru A. Statins, neuromuscular degenerative disease and an amyotrophic lateral sclerosis-like syndrome: An analysis of individual case safety reports from vigibase. Drug Saf 2007;30:515–525.
69. Sattar N, Preiss D, Murray HM, et al. Statins and risk of incident diabetes: A collaborative meta-analysis of randomised statin trials. Lancet 2010;375:735–742.
70. Mangravite LM, Thorn CF, Krauss RM. Clinical implications of pharmacogenomics of statin treatment. Pharmacogenomics J 2006;6:360–374.
71. McPherson R. Comparative effects of simvastatin and cholestyramine on plasma lipoproteins and CETP in humans. Can J Clin Pharmacol 1999;6:85–90.
72. Tsuyuki RT, Bungard RJ. Poor adherence with hypolipidemic drugs: A lost opportunity. Pharmacotherapy 2001;21:576–582.
73. Tsuyuki RT, Olson KL, Dubyk AM, Schindel TJ, Johnson JA. Effect of community pharmacist intervention on cholesterol levels in patients at high risk of cardiovascular events: The Second Study of Cardiovascular Risk Intervention by Pharmacists (SCRIP-plus). Am J Med 2004;116:130–133.
74. McCrindle BW, O'Neill MB, Cullen-Dean G, Helden E. Acceptability and compliance with two forms of cholestyramine in the treatment of hypercholesterolemia in children: A randomized, crossover trial. J Pediatr 1997;130:266–273.
75. Zhang Y, Schmidt RJ, Foxworthy P, et al. Niacin mediates lipolysis in adipose tissue through its G-protein coupled receptor HM74A. Biochem Biophys Res Commun 2005;334:729–732.
76. Carlson LA. Nicotinic acid: The broad-spectrum lipid drug. A 50th anniversary review. J Intern Med 2005;258: 94–114.
77. Shepherd J, Betteridge J, Van Gaal L, European Consensus Panel. Nicotinic acid in the management of dyslipidaemia associated with diabetes and metabolic syndrome: A position paper developed by a European Consensus Panel. Curr Med Res Opin 2005;21:665–682.
78. Sharma M, Ansari MT, Abou-Setta AM, et al. Systematic review: Comparative effectiveness and harms of combination therapy and monotherapy for dyslipidemia. Ann Intern Med 2009;151:622–630.
79. Stern RH. The role of nicotinic acid metabolites in flushing and hepatoxicity. J Clin Lipidol 2007;1:191–193.
80. Lai E, De Lepeleire I, Crumley TM, et al. Suppression of niacin-induced vasodilation with an antagonist to prostaglandin D2 receptor subtype 1. Clin Pharmacol Ther 2007;81:849–857.
81. Maccubbin D, Koren MJ, Davidson M, et al. Flushing profile of extended-release niacin/laropiprant versus gradually titrated niacin extended-release in patients with dyslipidemia with and without ischemic cardiovascular disease. Am J Cardiol 2009;104:74–81.
82. McKenney JM, Jones PH, Bays HE, et al. Comparative effects on lipid levels of combination therapy with a statin and extended-release niacin or ezetimibe versus a statin alone (the COMPELL study). Atherosclerosis 2007;192:432–437.
83. McKenney J. Niacin for dyslipidemia: Considerations in product selection. Am J Health Syst Pharm 2003;60: 995–1005.
84. Libby A, Meier J, Lopez J, Swislocki AL, Siegel D. The effect of body mass index on fasting blood glucose and development of diabetes mellitus after initiation of extended-release niacin. Metab Syndr Relat Disord 2010;8:79–84.
85. Guyton JR, Bays HE. Safety considerations with niacin therapy [see comment]. Am J Cardiol 2007;99:19.
86. Forsblom C, Hiukka A, Leinonen ES, Sundvall J, Groop PH, Taskinen MR. Effects of long-term fenofibrate treatment on markers of renal function in type 2 diabetes: The FIELD Helsinki substudy. Diabetes Care 2010;33:215–220.
87. Davidson MH, Armani A, McKenney JM, Jacobson TA. Safety considerations with fibrate therapy. Am J Cardiol 2007;99:19.
88. Sveger T, Flodmark CE, Nordborg K, Nilsson-Ehle P, Borgfors N. Hereditary dyslipidaemias and combined risk factors in children with a family history of premature coronary artery disease. Arch Dis Child 2000;82: 292–296.
89. Grundy SM, Vega GL, Yuan Z, Battisti WP, Brady WE, Palmisano J. Effectiveness and tolerability of simvastatin plus fenofibrate for combined hyperlipidemia (the SAFARI trial) [erratum appears in Am J Cardiol 2006;98(3): 427–428]. Am J Cardiol 2005;95:462–468.
90. Ford ES, Li C, Zhao G, Pearson WS, Mokdad AH. Hypertriglyceridemia and its pharmacologic treatment among US adults. Arch Intern Med 2009;169:572–578.
91. Capell WH, Eckel RH. Treatment of hypertriglyceridemia. Curr Diab Rep 2006;6:230–240.
92. Elam MB, Hunninghake DB, Davis KB, et al. Effect of niacin on lipid and lipoprotein levels and glycemic control

in patients with diabetes and peripheral arterial disease: The ADMIT study: A randomized trial. Arterial Disease Multiple Intervention Trial. JAMA 2000;284:1263–1270.

93. McKenney JM, Sica D. Prescription omega-3 fatty acids for the treatment of hypertriglyceridemia. Am J Health Syst Pharm 2007;64:595–605.
94. Oh RC, Lanier JB. Management of hypertriglyceridemia. Am Fam Physician 2007;75:1365–1371.
95. McKenney J. New perspectives on the use of niacin in the treatment of lipid disorders. Arch Intern Med 2004;164: 697–705.
96. Gadi R, Samaha FF. Dyslipidemia in type 2 diabetes mellitus. Curr Diab Rep 2007;7:228–234.
97. Tan KC. Management of dyslipidemia in the metabolic syndrome. Cardiovasc Hematol Disord Drug Targets 2007;7:99–108.
98. Garg A, Simha V. Update on dyslipidemia. J Clin Endocrinol Metab 2007;92:1581–1589.
99. Shepherd J, Cobbe SM, Ford I, et al. Prevention of coronary heart disease with pravastatin in men with hypercholesterolemia. West of Scotland Coronary Prevention Study Group. N Engl J Med 1995;333:1301–1307.
100. Downs JR, Clearfield M, Weis S, et al. Primary prevention of acute coronary events with lovastatin in men and women with average cholesterol levels: Results of AFCAPS/ TexCAPS. JAMA 1998;279:1615–1622.
101. Sacks FM, Pfeffer MA, Moye LA, et al. The effect of pravastatin on coronary events after myocardial infarction in patients with average cholesterol levels. N Engl J Med 1996;335:1001–1009.
102. Anonymous. Design and baseline results of the Scandinavian Simvastatin Survival Study of patients with stable angina and/or previous myocardial infarction. Am J Cardiol 1993;71:393–400.
103. Colhoun HM, Betteridge DJ, Durrington PN, et al. Primary prevention of cardiovascular disease with atorvastatin in type 2 diabetes in the Collaborative Atorvastatin Diabetes Study (CARDS): Multicentre randomised placebo-controlled trial [see comment]. Lancet 2004;364:685–696.
104. Collins R, Armitage J, Parish S, Sleight P, Peto R, Heart Protection Study Collaborative Group. Effects of cholesterol-lowering with simvastatin on stroke and other major vascular events in 20536 people with cerebrovascular disease or other high-risk conditions [see comment]. Lancet 2004;363:757–767.
105. Anonymous. Effect of fenofibrate on progression of coronary-artery disease in type 2 diabetes: The Diabetes Atherosclerosis Intervention Study, a randomised study. Lancet 2001;357:905–910.
106. Backes JM, Gibson CA, Ruisinger JF, Moriarty PM. Fibrates: What have we learned in the past 40 years? Pharmacotherapy 2007;27:412–424.
107. ACCORD Study Group, Ginsberg HN, Elam MB, et al. Effects of combination lipid therapy in type 2 diabetes mellitus. N Engl J Med 2010;362:1563–1574.
108. Grundy SM, Vega GL, McGovern ME, et al. Efficacy, safety, and tolerability of once-daily niacin for the treatment of dyslipidemia associated with type 2 diabetes: Results of the assessment of diabetes control and evaluation of the efficacy of Niaspan trial [see comment]. Arch Intern Med 2002;162:1568–1576.
109. Davidson MH, Kurlandsky SB, Kleinpell RM, Maki KC. Lipid management and the elderly. Prev Cardiol 2003;6: 128–133.
110. Mazza A, Tikhonoff V, Schiavon L, Casiglia E. Triglycerides + high-density-lipoprotein-cholesterol dyslipidaemia, a coronary risk factor in elderly women: The CArdiovascular STudy in the ELderly. Intern Med J 2005;35:604–610.
111. Afilalo J, Duque G, Steele R, Jukema JW, de Craen AJ, Eisenberg MJ. Statins for secondary prevention in elderly patients: A hierarchical Bayesian meta-analysis. J Am Coll Cardiol 2008;51:37–45.
112. Anonymous. Randomised trial of cholesterol lowering in 4444 patients with coronary heart disease: The Scandinavian Simvastatin Survival Study (4S). Lancet 1994;344: 1383–1389.
113. Berger AK, Duval SJ, Armstrong C, Jacobs DR Jr, Luepker RV. Contemporary diagnosis and management of hypercholesterolemia in elderly acute myocardial infarction patients: A population-based study [see comment]. Am J Geriatr Cardiol 2007;16:15–23.
114. Hatzigeorgiou C, Jackson JL. Hydroxymethylglutaryl-coenzyme A reductase inhibitors and osteoporosis: A meta-analysis. Osteoporos Int 2005;16:990–998.
115. Blue Cross Blue Shield Association, Technology Evaluation Center. Special report: The efficacy and safety of statins in the elderly. Technol Eval Cent Assess Program Exec Summ 2007;21:1–3.
116. Anonymous. Pravastatin benefits elderly patients: Results of PROSPER study. Cardiovasc J S Afr 2003;14:48.
117. Heart Protection Study Collaborative Group. MRC/ BHF Heart Protection Study of cholesterol lowering with simvastatin in 20,536 high-risk individuals: A randomised placebo-controlled trial [see comment] [summary for patients in Curr Cardiol Rep 2002;4(6):486–487]. Lancet 2002;360:7–22.
118. Abate N. Obesity and cardiovascular disease. Pathogenetic role of the metabolic syndrome and therapeutic implications. J Diabetes Complications 2000;14:154–174.
119. Hulley S, Grady D, Bush T, et al. Randomized trial of estrogen plus progestin for secondary prevention of coronary heart disease in postmenopausal women. Heart and Estrogen/ progestin Replacement Study (HERS) Research Group. JAMA 1998;280:605–613.
120. Rossouw JE, Prentice RL, Manson JE, et al. Postmenopausal hormone therapy and risk of cardiovascular disease by age and years since menopause. JAMA 2007;297: 1465–1477.
121. Anderson GL, Limacher M, Assaf AR, et al. Effects of conjugated equine estrogen in postmenopausal women with hysterectomy: The Women's Health Initiative randomized controlled trial [see comment]. JAMA 2004;291: 1701–1712.
122. Wassertheil-Smoller S, Hendrix SL, Limacher M, et al. Effect of estrogen plus progestin on stroke in postmenopausal women: The Women's Health Initiative: A randomized trial [see comment]. JAMA 2003;289: 2673–2684.
123. Vickers MR, MacLennan AH, Lawton B, et al. Main morbidities recorded in the women's international study of long duration oestrogen after menopause (WISDOM): A randomised controlled trial of hormone replacement therapy in postmenopausal women. BMJ 2007;335:239. doi:10.1136/ bmj.39266.425069.AD.
124. Mora S, Glynn RJ, Hsia J, MacFadyen JG, Genest J, Ridker PM. Statins for the primary prevention of cardiovascular events in women with elevated high-sensitivity C-reactive protein or dyslipidemia: Results from the Justification for the Use of Statins in Prevention: An Intervention Trial Evaluating Rosuvastatin (JUPITER) and meta-analysis of women from primary prevention trials. Circulation 2010;121:1069–1077.

125. Davis V, Schatz D, Winter W. Pediatric lipid disorders in clinical practice. eMedicine 2006, *http://www.emedicine.com/ped/topic2787.htm*.
126. Clauss SB, Holmes KW, Hopkins P, et al. Efficacy and safety of lovastatin therapy in adolescent girls with heterozygous familial hypercholesterolemia. Pediatrics 2005;116:682–688.
127. Wiegman A, Hutten BA, de Groot E, et al. Efficacy and safety of statin therapy in children with familial hypercholesterolemia: A randomized controlled trial [see comment]. JAMA 2004;292:331–337.
128. de Jongh S, Ose L, Szamosi T, et al. Efficacy and safety of statin therapy in children with familial hypercholesterolemia: A randomized, double-blind, placebo-controlled trial with simvastatin. Circulation 2002;106:2231–2237.
129. O'Gorman CS, Higgins MF, O'Neill MB. Systematic review and metaanalysis of statins for heterozygous familial hypercholesterolemia in children: Evaluation of cholesterol changes and side effects. Pediatr Cardiol 2009;30:482–489.
130. Toto RD, Grundy SM, Vega GL. Pravastatin treatment of very low density, intermediate density and low density lipoproteins in hypercholesterolemia and combined hyperlipidemia secondary to the nephrotic syndrome. Am J Nephrol 2000;20:12–17.
131. Fellstrom BC, Jardine AG, Schmieder RE, et al. Rosuvastatin and cardiovascular events in patients undergoing hemodialysis. N Engl J Med 2009;360:1395–1407.
132. Baber U, Toto RD, de Lemos JA. Statins and cardiovascular risk reduction in patients with chronic kidney disease and end-stage renal failure. Am Heart J 2007;153:471–477.
133. Samuelsson O, Attman PO, Knight-Gibson C, et al. Effect of gemfibrozil on lipoprotein abnormalities in chronic renal insufficiency: A controlled study in human chronic renal disease. Nephron 1997;75:286–294.
134. Peterson AM, McGhan WF. Pharmacoeconomic impact of non-compliance with statins. Pharmacoeconomics 2005;23:13–25.
135. Tarraga-Lopez PJ, Celada-Rodriguez A, Cerdan-Oliver M, et al. A pharmacoeconomic evaluation of statins in the treatment of hypercholesterolaemia in the primary care setting in Spain [erratum appears in Pharmacoeconomics 2006;24(1):106]. Pharmacoeconomics 2005;23:275–287.
136. Cziraky MJ, Watson KE, Talbert RL. Targeting low HDL-cholesterol to decrease residual cardiovascular risk in the managed care setting. J Manag Care Pharm 2009;14:S3–S28.
137. Johannesson M, Jonsson B, Kjekshus J, Olsson AG, Pedersen TR, Wedel H. Cost effectiveness of simvastatin treatment to lower cholesterol levels in patients with coronary heart disease. Scandinavian Simvastatin Survival Study Group. N Engl J Med 1997;336:332–336.
138. Caro J, Klittich W, McGuire A, et al. The West of Scotland coronary prevention study: Economic benefit analysis of primary prevention with pravastatin. BMJ 1997;315:1577–1582.
139. Schectman G, Wolff N, Byrd JC, Hiatt JG, Hartz A. Physician extenders for cost-effective management of hypercholesterolemia. J Gen Intern Med 1996;11:277–286.
140. Bluml BM, McKenney JM, Cziraky MJ. Pharmaceutical care services and results in project ImPACT: Hyperlipidemia [see comment]. J Am Pharm Assoc 2000;40:157–165.
141. Charrois TL, Johnson JA, Blitz S, Tsuyuki RT. Relationship between number, timing, and type of pharmacist interventions and patient outcomes. Am J Health Syst Pharm 2005;62:1798–1801.
142. Yamada C, Johnson JA, Robertson P, Pearson G, Tsuyuki RT. Long-term impact of a community pharmacist intervention on cholesterol levels in patients at high risk for cardiovascular events: Extended follow-up of the second study of cardiovascular risk intervention by pharmacists (SCRIP-plus). Pharmacotherapy 2005;25:110–115.
143. Buchwald H, Campos CT, Boen JR, Nguyen PA, Williams SE. Disease-free intervals after partial ileal bypass in patients with coronary heart disease and hypercholesterolemia: Report from the Program on the Surgical Control of the Hyperlipidemias (POSCH). J Am Coll Cardiol 1995;26:351–357.
144. Anonymous. The Lipid Research Clinics Coronary Primary Prevention Trial results. I. Reduction in incidence of coronary heart disease. JAMA 1984;251:351–364.
145. ALLHAT Officers and Coordinators for the ALLHAT Collaborative Research Group, The Antihypertensive and Lipid-Lowering Treatment to Prevent Heart Attack Trial. Major outcomes in moderately hypercholesterolemic, hypertensive patients randomized to pravastatin vs usual care: The Antihypertensive and Lipid-Lowering Treatment to Prevent Heart Attack Trial (ALLHAT-LLT) [see comment]. JAMA 2002;288:2998–3007.
146. Canner PL, Berge KG, Wenger NK, et al. Fifteen year mortality in Coronary Drug Project patients: Long-term benefit with niacin. J Am Coll Cardiol 1986;8:1245–1255.
147. Strandberg TE, Pyorala K, Cook TJ, et al. Mortality and incidence of cancer during 10-year follow-up of the Scandinavian Simvastatin Survival Study (4S). Lancet 2004;364:771–777.
148. Tonkin AM, Colquhoun D, Emberson J, et al. Effects of pravastatin in 3260 patients with unstable angina: Results from the LIPID study. Lancet 2000;356:1871–1875.
149. Rubins HB, Robins SJ, Collins D. The Veterans Affairs High-Density Lipoprotein Intervention Trial: Baseline characteristics of normocholesterolemic men with coronary artery disease and low levels of high-density lipoprotein cholesterol. Veterans Affairs Cooperative Studies Program High-Density Lipoprotein Intervention Trial Study Group. Am J Cardiol 1996;78:572–575.
150. Pitt B, Waters D, Brown WV, et al. Aggressive lipid-lowering therapy compared with angioplasty in stable coronary artery disease. Atorvastatin versus Revascularization Treatment Investigators. N Engl J Med 1999;341:70–76.
151. Shepherd J, Blauw GJ, Murphy MB, et al. Pravastatin in elderly individuals at risk of vascular disease (PROSPER): A randomised controlled trial. Lancet 2002;360:1623–1630.
152. Cannon CP, Braunwald E, McCabe CH, et al. Intensive versus moderate lipid lowering with statins after acute coronary syndromes [see comment] [erratum appears in N Engl J Med 2006;354(7):778]. N Engl J Med 2004;350:1495–1504.
153. LaRosa JC, Grundy SM, Waters DD, et al. Intensive lipid lowering with atorvastatin in patients with stable coronary disease. N Engl J Med 2005;352:1425–1435.
154. Waters DD, LaRosa JC, Barter P, et al. Effects of high-dose atorvastatin on cerebrovascular events in patients with stable coronary disease in the TNT (treating to new targets) study. J Am Coll Cardiol 2006;48:1793–1799.
155. Amarenco P, Bogousslavsky J, Callahan A 3rd, et al. High-dose atorvastatin after stroke or transient ischemic attack. N Engl J Med 2006;355:549–559.

156. HPS2-THRIVE Collaborative Group. HPS2-THRIVE randomized placebo-controlled trial in 25 673 high-risk patients of ER niacin/laropiprant: Trial design, pre-specified muscle and liver outcomes, and reasons for stopping study treatment. Eur Heart J 2013;34:1279–1291.
157. Nissen SE, Tuzcu EM, Brewer HB, et al. Effect of ACAT inhibition on the progression of coronary atherosclerosis [see comment] [erratum appears in N Engl J Med 2006;355(6):638]. N Engl J Med 2006;354:1253–1263.
158. Vidt DG, Harris S, McTaggart F, Ditmarsch M, Sager PT, Sorof JM. Effect of short-term rosuvastatin treatment on estimated glomerular filtration rate. Am J Cardiol 2006;97:1602–1606.
159. Raal FJ, Santos RD, Blom DJ, et al. Mipomersen, an apolipoprotein B synthesis inhibitor, for lowering of LDL cholesterol concentrations in patients with homozygous familial hypercholesterolaemia: A randomised, double-blind, placebo-controlled trial. Lancet 2010;375: 998–1006.
160. Cuchel M, Meagher EA, du Toit Theron H, et al. Efficacy and safety of a microsomal triglyceride transfer protein inhibitor in patients with homozygous familial hypercholesterolaemia: A single-arm, open-label, phase 3 study. Lancet 2013;381:40–46.
161. Pedersen TR. Lipid-lowering drugs and risk for cancer. Curr Atheroscler Rep 2009;11:350–357.

Peripheral Arterial Disease

Barbara J. Hoeben and Robert L. Talbert

12

KEY CONCEPTS

1. The prevalence of peripheral arterial disease is dependent on age and the presence of traditional risk factors for cardiovascular disease and many patients are undiagnosed; undiagnosed patients have substantial risk for coronary and cerebrovascular events.
2. The clinical presentation of peripheral arterial disease is variable and includes a range of symptoms. The two most common characteristics of peripheral arterial disease are intermittent claudication and pain at rest in the lower extremities.
3. The ankle-brachial index (ABI) is a simple, noninvasive, quantitative test that has been proven to be a highly sensitive and specific tool in the diagnosis of peripheral arterial disease.
4. As with any atherosclerotic condition, several risk factors play an important role in the morbidity and mortality of peripheral vascular disease. Many of these risk factors are modifiable with the help of various nonpharmacologic and pharmacologic interventions.
5. Nonpharmacologic interventions such as smoking cessation and walking exercise programs have the ability to positively impact several of the pathophysiologic abnormalities present in patients with peripheral arterial disease.
6. Data proving that antiplatelet therapies can prevent or delay the progression of peripheral arterial disease are currently unavailable. However, aspirin therapy has repeatedly been proven to significantly reduce serious vascular events in these "high-risk" patients and, in the absence of contraindications, is highly recommended.
7. After appropriate exercise therapy and therapeutic lifestyle changes have been implemented, patients who continue to experience severe intermittent claudication may benefit from additional pharmacologic therapy with cilostazol.

Peripheral arterial disease (PAD), the most common form of peripheral vascular disease, is a manifestation of progressive narrowing of arteries due to atherosclerosis.[1] PAD is associated with elevated risk of cardiovascular disease (CVD) morbidity and mortality, even in the absence of prior history of acute myocardial infarction (AMI), stroke, or other manifestations of CVD.[2] Patients with PAD have approximately the same relative risk of death from CVD as do patients with a history of coronary or cerebrovascular disease, and PAD should be considered a surrogate marker of subclinical coronary artery disease (CAD) and other vascular territories.[1] The treatment of PAD focuses on decreasing the functional impairment caused by symptoms of intermittent claudication (IC) through nonpharmacologic and pharmacologic therapy and by minimizing the impact of other cardiovascular risk factors.[1]

EPIDEMIOLOGY

1 PAD should be defined with the ankle-brachial index (ABI) and compatible signs and symptoms. The normal range is 1 to 1.40 and ABI ≤0.90 in either leg or >1.40 representing noncompressible arteries. The National Health and Nutrition Examination Survey (NHANES) found a 4.6% prevalence of PAD among adults aged 40 years and older in the United States.[1] The prevalence of PAD is highly dependent on age, being infrequent in younger individuals and common in older individuals (Fig. 12-1). In age- and gender-adjusted logistic regression analyses, black race/ethnicity (odds ratio [OR] 2.83), current smoking (OR 4.46), diabetes (OR 2.71), hypertension (HTN; OR 1.75), hypercholesterolemia (OR 1.68), and impaired renal function (estimated glomerular filtration rate less than 60 mL/min/1.73 m^2) (OR 2) were associated with more prevalent PAD.[1,6] Individuals with PAD are also more likely to have a self-reported history of any CAD or CVD but, interestingly, no association with elevated body mass index. The reported relative risk of death from CVD in patients with PAD is reported to range from 2 to 5.1 in patients with or without CVD and 2.9 to 5.7 in patients with known CVD.[3] CVD accounts for 75% of all deaths in patients with PAD.[4] The risk of death is approximately the same in men and women and is elevated even in asymptomatic patients. Annual mortality is 25% in patients with critical leg ischemia who have the lowest ABI values.[5]

More than ~8.5 million (estimated range 4 to 7 million) adults aged 40 years have PAD. Ninety-five percent of individuals with PAD have at least one cardiovascular risk factor; the majority of patients have multiple risk factors for CVD.[6] Based on the PAD Awareness, Risk, and Treatment: New Resources for Survival (PARTNERS) program, the prevalence of PAD in primary care practices is high, yet physician awareness of the PAD diagnosis is relatively low.[7] In this cross-sectional study, PAD was detected in 29% of 6,979 patients. Eighty-three percent of the patients were aware of their diagnosis, but only 49% of their patients' physicians were aware. The reason for this observation is that patient self-report of symptoms and the use of questionnaires to detect PAD are not sufficiently sensitive and specific to reproducibly diagnose PAD and the cardinal symptom of PAD—IC—is present in the minority of patients (1% to 27%, typically ~10%).[1,3,8] A simple ABI measurement will identify a large number of patients with previously unrecognized PAD. Atherosclerosis risk factors were very prevalent in PAD patients, but these patients received less intensive treatment for lipid disorders and HTN and were prescribed antiplatelet therapy less frequently than were patients with CVD. These results demonstrate that underdiagnosis of PAD in primary care practice may be a barrier to effective secondary prevention of the high ischemic cardiovascular risk associated with PAD.[7] Because of the systemic nature of atherosclerosis and the

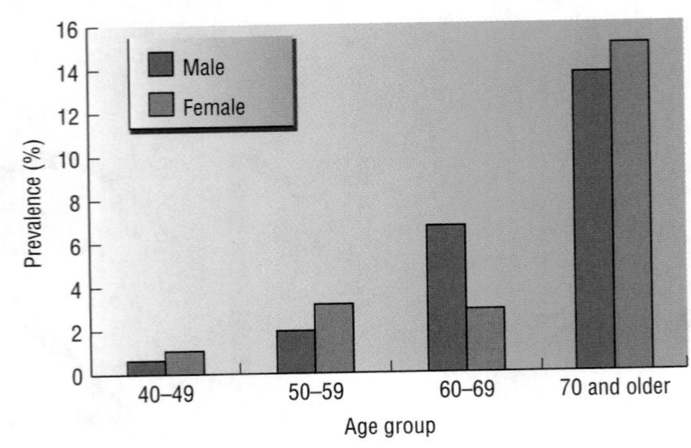

FIGURE 12-1 Prevalence of peripheral arterial disease by age and gender.

TABLE 12-1 Clinical Presentation

General

- Patients with PAD are likely to be 40 years of age and older with hypertension, hypercholesterolemia, diabetes, impaired renal function, a history of coronary artery disease or cardiovascular disease, and/or a history of smoking

Signs and symptoms

- The clinical presentation of PAD is variable and includes symptoms ranging from no symptoms at all (typically early in the disease) to pain and discomfort
- The two most common characteristics of PAD are intermittent claudication and pain at rest in the lower extremities
- Intermittent claudication is generally regarded as the primary indicator in PAD. It has been described as fatigue, discomfort, cramping, pain, or numbness in the affected extremities (typically the buttock, thigh, or calf) during exercise and resolves within a few minutes with rest
- Physical examination may reveal nonspecific signs of decreased blood flow to the extremities (e.g., cool skin temperature, thickened toenails, lack of hair on the calf, feet, and/or toes)

Laboratory tests

- None specific to PAD

Other diagnostic tests

- The ankle-brachial index (ABI) is a simple, noninvasive, quantitative test that has been proven to be a highly sensitive and specific (≥90%) tool in the diagnosis of PAD

PAD; peripheral arterial disease.

Data from references 6, 9, 12–24.

high risk of ischemic events, patients with PAD should be considered for secondary prevention strategies including aggressive risk factor modification and antiplatelet drug therapy.[3,8]

ETIOLOGY AND PATHOPHYSIOLOGY

PAD is most commonly a manifestation of systemic atherosclerosis in which the arterial lumen of the lower extremities becomes progressively occluded by atherosclerotic plaque.[4,8] The major risk factors for the development of atherosclerosis are older age (greater than 40 years), cigarette smoking, diabetes mellitus, hypercholesterolemia, HTN, and hyperhomocysteinemia.[3,4,9] The arteries most commonly involved, in order of occurrence, are the femoropopliteal-tibial, aortoiliac, carotid and vertebral, splenic and renal, and brachiocephalic.[10] Familial hypercholesterolemia (FH) leading to hypercholesterolemia and elevated low-density lipoprotein (LDL) levels are associated with accelerated development of atherosclerosis earlier and with more severe symptoms (e.g., IC) and abnormal blood flow studies compared with controls.[10,11] Intima–media thickness can be used as a surrogate phenotype for cardiovascular risk in FH and carotid and/or femoral artery atherosclerosis results in increased intima–media thickness and it is correlated to cardiovascular risk in FH patients compared with normolipidemic individuals.

CLINICAL PRESENTATION AND DIAGNOSIS

2 The clinical presentation of PAD is variable, ranging from no symptoms at all (typically early in the disease) to pain and discomfort (Table 12-1). This finding was illustrated in a study by Wang et al.,[12] who attempted to aid the diagnosis of PAD by using defined categories of exertional leg pain in patients with and without PAD. They determined that not one of the five categories of leg pain (no pain, pain on exertion and rest, noncalf pain, atypical calf pain, and classic claudication) was sufficiently sensitive or specific to enable a link to a PAD diagnosis. The two most common characteristics of PAD are IC and pain at rest in the lower extremities.[11,12,25] IC is generally regarded as the primary indicator of PAD. It is described as reproducible fatigue, discomfort, cramping, pain, or numbness in the affected extremities (typically the buttock, thigh, or calf) during exercise and is resolved within a few minutes with rest.[11,13–15,25,26] Symptoms of IC occur during exercise as the increase in blood flow is limited by occlusive atherosclerotic lesions in the peripheral arteries leading to an inability for oxygen supply to meet the demands of increased metabolic demand by the muscles.[26] Resting pain typically occurs later in the disease when the blood supply is not adequate to perfuse the extremity (critical limb ischemia). This most often can be felt at night in the feet (typically the toes or heel) while the patient is lying in bed.[11,12,25] Although IC is the primary indicator of PAD, it alone cannot be used to diagnose PAD. Unfortunately only ~10% of patients present with classical IC.[8] As explained by the Inter-Society Consensus for the Management of Peripheral Arterial Disease (TransAtlantic Inter-Society Consensus [TASC] II),[26] patients with PAD may not have symptoms of IC because they may have a sedentary lifestyle or some other condition that may be limiting the ability to exercise.

As with any good medical encounter, a detailed patient history of symptoms and atherosclerosis risk factors (e.g., smoking, HTN, hyperlipidemia, and diabetes) can be helpful in the diagnosis of PAD. Unfortunately, as illustrated by the PARTNERS program, providers who rely on a history alone will miss approximately 85% to 90% of patients with PAD.[16] Therefore, examination of the patient is vital to proper diagnosis. Requesting that the patient remove socks and shoes may reveal nonspecific signs of decreased blood flow to the extremities (e.g., cool skin temperature, shiny skin, thickened toenails, lack of hair on the calf, feet, and/or toes) or, in severe cases, visible sores or ulcers that are slow to heal and may even be black in appearance.[11,12,16,17,25]

An important criterion for the accurate diagnosis of PAD is the exclusion of other conditions that possess similar signs and symptoms. Differential diagnosis should rule out other neurologic conditions (e.g., peripheral neuropathy), inflammatory conditions (e.g., arthritis), and vascular conditions (e.g., deep venous thrombosis or venous congestion) that may mimic PAD.[11,15,18]

3 The ABI is a simple, noninvasive, quantitative test that has been proven to be a highly sensitive and specific (≥90%) tool in the diagnosis of PAD.[13,19,27] For measurement of the ABI, the patient lies in the supine position as the systolic blood pressure is measured at the brachial arteries on both arms and the dorsalis pedis and posterior tibial arteries of the legs with a standard sphygmomanometer and a continuous-wave Doppler device. The pressures obtained at the dorsalis pedis and posterior tibial arteries are averaged and divided by the mean measurement taken at the left and right brachial arteries.[3,16,20,26,28] An ABI of 1 to 1.40 is considered normal while a measurement under 0.9 is consistent with PAD. ABI from 0.7 to 0.9 correlates with mild PAD, 0.4 to 0.7 indicates moderate disease, and under 0.4 denotes severe PAD.[4,14,20] An ABI of >1.40 is consistent with noncompressible arteries. In addition to providing diagnostic information, the ABI measurement has been shown to be a strong predictor of future cardiovascular events associated with PAD.[21,29] The ABI can also be useful after a test of exercise tolerance (e.g., 5 minutes on a treadmill or 30 to 50 repetitions of heel raises). Patients with PAD will demonstrate a significant drop in the ABI after exercise, but their pain will be normal or unchanged. ABI can rule out PAD and suggest alternate diagnoses.[4,14,16,26] ABI can be considered as a useful tool in diagnosing both symptomatic and nonsymptomatic patients at high risk of PAD.[7,30]

Other noninvasive tools are available for the diagnosis of PAD. One study has suggested a calculation that takes into consideration the patient's history of AMI and the number of auscultated and palpated posterior tibial arteries.[31,32] Magnetic resonance angiography (MRA) can be used to examine the presence and location of significant stenosis, or lack thereof, and is a reasonable option in patients who are being considered for surgical revascularization.[33] Similarly, computed tomographic angiography (CTA) can be used to determine the presence of significant stenosis and soft-tissue diagnostic information that may be associated with PAD (e.g., aneurysms).[33,34] However, as ABI is a sufficient means of diagnosis, arteriography is not necessary or encouraged.[15,25,27]

TREATMENT
Peripheral Arterial Disease

Goals of Treatment

PAD is the result of atherosclerotic plaque formation in the arteries that results in decreased blood flow to the legs. Several of the treatment goals for these patients involve the reduction of confounding variables that attribute to the disease process, progress, and eventual outcome. Specific goals should include increasing maximal walking distance, duration, and pain-free walking, improving control of comorbid conditions contributing to the morbidity of the condition (e.g., HTN, hyperlipidemia, and diabetes), improvement in overall quality of life, and reduction in cardiovascular complications and death.

General Approach to Treatment

4 As with any atherosclerotic condition, several risk factors play an important role in the morbidity and mortality of PAD. Many of these risk factors are modifiable with the help of various nonpharmacologic and pharmacologic interventions.

Nonpharmacologic Therapy

Smoking Cessation

5 Not only cigarette smoking increases the risk of developing PAD and other cardiovascular disorders, but also the duration and quantity smoked can negatively impact disease progression (e.g., increase the risk of amputation) and increase mortality.[3,18,21,26,29,35–38] As a result, providers must advise patients to quit and should offer nonpharmacologic and pharmacologic means to aid the patient in that goal. Individual or group behavior modification therapy with or without the addition of certain antidepressants (e.g., bupropion), varenicline, or nicotine replacement therapy (e.g., gum or patches) has been proven effective in numerous studies. Varenicline has demonstrated superior quit rates compared with nicotine replacement therapy and bupropion.[8] Other forms of tobacco use should be discouraged as well. Reassessment of smoking status and progress encouragement at each encounter can help to reemphasize to the patient the vital importance of this lifestyle change.

Exercise

5 Walking exercise programs for patients with PAD have been proven to result in an increase in walking duration and distance, an increase in pain-free walking, and a delayed onset of claudication by 179%.[9,17,18,35,36,39–48] Walking, or any aerobic exercise program conducted under the supervision of a healthcare provider, has the ability to positively impact several of the pathophysiologic abnormalities present in patients with PAD. Benefits of exercise programs include improving diabetes and lipid management, reducing weight, improving blood viscosity and flow, and reducing blood pressure.[49] Walking distance can also be used as a prognostic tool for future outcomes in patients with normal and impaired ABIs. A recent study by de Liefde et al.[50] examined patients with normal ABI (≥0.90) and impaired ABI (<0.90) in relation to walking distance. It was demonstrated that walking impairment in conjunction with impaired ABI was associated with higher cardiovascular events, including death. Other studies have likewise observed a link between impaired exercise/walking distance and negative long-term outcomes in patients with PAD.[51,52]

The American College of Cardiology/American Heart Association (ACC/AHA) Guidelines for the Management of PAD recommend supervised exercise training for patients with IC, for a minimum of 30 to 45 minutes, to be performed at least three times per week for a minimum of 12 weeks.[33] During exercise sessions, walking should be performed at a speed and grade of incline to produce the symptoms of IC within 3 to 5 minutes. The patient should stop walking when the symptoms become moderate in intensity, wait for the symptoms to resolve, and then resume walking, thus repeating the cycle for the duration of the session.[26] A prospective, observational study performed by Gardner et al. concluded that PAD patients with higher physical activity (as measured with a vertical accelerometer) have reduced mortality and cardiovascular events compared with those with low physical activity, regardless of confounders.[45] Exercise treadmill walking testing should be repeated at regular intervals (e.g., quarterly to biannually) to assess improvement or decline in walking duration and distance, as well as the time to pain onset while performing this activity. The type of aerobic activity recommended, as well as the duration and frequency of the activity, should be individually designed on a patient-to-patient basis.

Surgical Interventions

Various surgical procedures are available for patients with severe, debilitating claudication who have attempted, and failed, other means of nonpharmacologic and pharmacologic therapy. The TASC document on PAD provides clear recommendations for invasive therapy.[27] First, there must be a lack of adequate response to exercise therapy and risk factor modification. Second, the patient must have severe disability from IC resulting in impairment of daily activities. Third, there must be a thorough evaluation of the risks versus benefits of an invasive intervention including probability of success, the anticipated future course of the disease if an intervention is not performed, as well as an evaluation of concomitant disease states.[27] The decision to attempt percutaneous revascularization is often made with the guidance of diagnostic angiography. Angiography can help to identify the location and size of lesions and provide valuable information as to the likelihood of success with surgical revascularization.[27]

Percutaneous transluminal angioplasty (PTA) is an example of an invasive treatment for PAD. A randomized controlled clinical trial performed by Whyman et al.[53] determined that in a 2-year post intervention, PTA outcomes on maximum walking distance and ABI were not significantly different than in patients who had only received daily low-dose aspirin (acetylsalicylic acid [ASA]; $P > 0.05$). Nevertheless, patients who had received PTA had significantly fewer occluded arteries ($P = 0.003$), but the true clinical significance of this finding was not able to be realized in the time allotted for the study. PTA typically is reserved for patients whose lifestyle and/or job performance are compromised secondary to claudication despite adequate pharmacologic interventions and exercise.[9,37] Another consideration for balloon angioplasty is life expectancy. PTA is preferred over surgery if life expectancy is <2 years.[8]

Stent placement in PAD patients has also been an area of study and controversy. A meta-analysis examining the use of stent placement versus PTA for the treatment of aortoiliac occlusive disease determined that, although stent placement and PTA yielded similar complication and mortality rates, posttreatment ABI was more improved with stents (0.87 with PTA and 0.76 with stents, $P < 0.03$) and the risk of long-term failure was 39% less with stent placement.[54] However, other studies have not demonstrated improvement in patency rates in peripheral arteries versus PTA alone.[13,55] The TASC document provides specific recommendations for PTA, with or without stenting, depending on how diffuse the disease process is, the number and size of the lesions, and the location of the lesions.[27]

For patients with severe IC resulting in critical leg ischemia, physicians may need to discuss alternate surgical interventions including aortofemoral bypass, femoral popliteal bypass, or even amputation.[13,14,39]

Pharmacologic Therapy

Hypertension

HTN is a major risk factor for PAD and can lead to AMI, stroke, heart failure (HF), and death.[56] Current guidelines recommend the treatment goal for blood pressure in patients with PAD to mirror those in patients with documented CVD, 130/85 mm Hg.[38,56] Although the Heart Outcomes Prevention Evaluation (HOPE)[57] study demonstrated that angiotensin-converting enzyme (ACE) inhibitors reduced not only blood pressure but also other cardiovascular events (e.g., AMI, stroke, and death) in high-risk patients, including those with PAD, no specific class of antihypertensives is recommended over another for the treatment of HTN in patients with PAD. Therefore, selection of drug therapy for HTN should be made in accordance with the seventh report of the Joint National Committee on Prevention, Detection, Evaluation, and Treatment of High Blood Pressure (JNC VII)[56] on the basis of comorbid disease states, drug costs and availability, drug allergies, or other possible limiting factors. For example, patients with concomitant Raynaud's phenomenon may benefit from calcium channel blockers while patients with documented CAD may receive a dual benefit by the selection of a β-blocker.[38,56,58] Hesitation to use β-blockers in patients with PAD without harm was recently supported with the publication of a review of six randomized controlled trials by Paravastu et al.[59] The review concluded that there was no evidence of harm in the use of these agents in patients with PAD; however, β-blockers should be used with caution in patients with critical leg ischemia where acute lowering of blood pressure is contraindicated.[59] In 2012, Tseng et al. described a relationship between ACE insertion/deletion polymorphisms with the DD genotype carrying greatest risk for cardiovascular outcomes.[60] It is not known if ACE inhibitors would lead to greater risk reduction. Dosing, monitoring guidelines, and contraindications for specific agents used in the treatment of HTN may be found in Chapter 3.[61]

Hyperlipidemia

Although it has been shown that a reduction in lipid levels can reduce the progression of PAD and the severity of claudication, the current recommendations for the management of hyperlipidemia in PAD are based on only a few small studies and sub-hoc analyses from larger trials.[3,38,62–64] The Expert Panel on Detection, Evaluation, and Treatment of High Blood Cholesterol in Adults (Adult Treatment Panel III, or ATP III) considers PAD to be in the category of highest risk, or a coronary heart disease (CHD) risk equivalent. Therefore, it was recommended by the Expert Panel that levels of LDL be maintained at <100 mg/dL (<2.59 mmol/L) and non–high-density lipoprotein (non-HDL) levels (total cholesterol – HDL cholesterol) at <130 mg/dL (<3.36 mmol/L).[62] Results of clinical trials conducted since the time of this recommendation, specifically the Heart Protection Study (HPS)[64] and the Pravastatin or Atorvastatin Evaluation and Infection—Thrombolysis in Myocardial Infarction (PROVE IT)[65] trial, have led many clinical experts to now recommend an LDL goal of <70 mg/dL (<1.81 mmol/L) for additional retardation of atherosclerotic plaque formation in persons considered to be at very high risk, including patients with PAD.[13] Regardless of the goal LDL chosen, initiation of patient therapeutic lifestyle changes (TLC; e.g., reduction in saturated fat, weight reduction, and increased physical activity) is vital to achieving these recommendations.[10,62] Unfortunately, in many cases, TLC alone will not achieve the desired goals.

Several options are available for the initiation of drug therapy for LDL lowering in patients with PAD. Statins, bile acid sequestrants, and nicotinic acid are all effective treatment options. However, in most cases, statins are the preferred starting agent in this patient population.[16,39,62,64] As proven in the HPS, simvastatin not only demonstrated potent action in reducing LDL but also provided a significant reduction in cardiovascular events overall (e.g., AMI, stroke, and death).[64] If an increase in HDL levels is also necessary, niacin should be considered alone or in combination with a statin without the fear of worsening glucose metabolism, as previously believed.[3,14,28,58,66] Niacin has not been shown to be effective in increasing exercise time when compared with dietary intervention.[67] Dosing, monitoring guidelines, and contraindications for specific agents may be found in Chapter 11.

Diabetes Mellitus

A meta-analysis of over 95,000 diabetic patients provided additional support for the accepted premise that glycemic control serves as a risk factor for CVD.[68] The analysis demonstrated an increasing risk of death from cardiovascular events as blood glucose concentrations increased, with the same relationship observed even at levels below the threshold of clinically defined diabetes mellitus. This relationship is just one illustration of the criticality of good glycemic control. Due to the high prevalence of PAD among diabetic patients, the American Diabetes Association recommends ABI screening for PAD in all diabetics older than 50 years.[69] Due to the presence of peripheral neuropathy, patients with diabetes may be less likely to experience or report symptoms of PAD and the first sign may be as drastic as the appearance of a gangrenous foot ulcer. Therefore, although there is currently a lack of randomized controlled studies illustrating that the degree of glycemic control is predictive of the extent of PAD present, it is widely recommended that all patients with concomitant diabetes and PAD maintain good glycemic control, as evidenced by a hemoglobin A-1c level of <7% (<0.07; <53 mmol/mol Hb).[3,27,28,38,40,69,70] This recommendation is supported by a prospective cohort study of 1,894 diabetic patients, which demonstrated that patients with poor glucose control (A-1c >7.5% [>0.075; >58 mmol/mol Hb]) were five times more likely to develop IC and also to be hospitalized for PAD compared with those with a hemoglobin A-1c <6% (<0.06; <42 mmol/mol Hb).[71] Despite this, a study

TABLE 12-2 Pharmacotherapy Options for Patients with Peripheral Arterial Disease

Agent	Daily Dose (Oral)	Mechanism of Action (MOA)	Side Effects	Contraindications	Level of Evidence[a]
Aspirin	81–325 mg	Irreversibly inhibits prostaglandin cyclooxygenase in platelets, prevents formation of thromboxane A_2	GI upset and/or bleeding	Active bleeding; hemophilia; thrombocytopenia	With coronary or cerebrovascular (Grade 1A), without (Grade 1C+)
Dipyridamole ER (Aggrenox)	400 mg (+ aspirin 50 mg)	May act by inhibiting platelet aggregation (complete MOA unknown)	Angina; dyspnea; hypotension; headache; dizziness	Active bleeding; CAD ("coronary steal syndrome")	Recommendation for use not specified in report
Cilostazol (Pletal)[b]	100 mg twice daily	Phosphodiesterase inhibitor, suppresses platelet aggregation; direct artery vasodilator	Fever: infection; tachycardia	All CHF patients (decreased survival)	With IC (Grade 2A)
Clopidogrel (Plavix)	75 mg	Inhibits binding of ADP analogues to its platelet receptor causing irreversible inhibition of platelets	Chest pain; purpura generalized pain; rash	Active pathologic bleeding (e.g., peptic ulcer, intracranial hemorrhage)	Recommend clopidogrel over no antiplatelet therapy (Grade 1C+)
Pentoxifylline (Trental)	1.2 g	Alters RBC flexibility; decreases platelet adhesion; reduces blood viscosity; decreases fibrinogen concentration	Dyspnea; nausea; vomiting; headache; dizziness	Recent retinal or cerebral hemorrhage; active bleeding	Not recommended in patients with IC (Grade 1B)
Ticlopidine (Ticlid)	500 mg	Inhibits binding of ADP analogues to its platelet receptor causing irreversible inhibition of platelets	Leukopenia; rash; thrombocytopenia; neutropenia; agranulocytosis; aplastic anemia	Active bleeding; hemophilia; thrombocytopenia	Clopidogrel recommended over ticlopidine (Grade 1C+)

ADP, adenosine 5′-diphosphate; CAD, coronary artery disease; CHF, congestive heart failure; ER, extended release; IC, intermittent claudication; RBC, red blood cell.
[a]Grades of recommendation for antithrombotic and thrombolytic therapy are part of the Seventh ACCP Conference on Antithrombotic and Thrombolytic Therapy.[73]
[b]Cilostazol should be used in combination with antiplatelet therapy.
Data from references 15, 21, 28, 74–82.

by Rehring et al.[72] of 365 patients with known PAD and concomitant diabetes showed that only 45.8% of these patients had a hemoglobin A-1c <7% (<0.07; <53 mmol/mol Hb). Oral antidiabetic agents, insulin regimens, as well as other pharmacologic and nonpharmacologic strategies to reduce the risk of complications associated with diabetes mellitus are discussed at length in Chapter 57.

Antiplatelet Drug Therapy

See Table 12-2.

Aspirin

6 By far, the most compelling evidence for the use of any pharmacologic agent in PAD can be found for ASA. The Antithrombotic Trialists' Collaboration (ATC) conducted a meta-analysis of 195 randomized trials, composed of over 135,000 patients at high risk for occlusive arterial disease, and concluded that low-dose ASA (75 to 160 mg) and medium-dose ASA (160 to 325 mg/day) lead to a significant reduction in serious vascular events (12%) in "high-risk" patients, such as those with PAD.[74] The ATC also noted in this analysis that the risk of major extracranial bleed was similar between the low-dose and medium-dose regimens.

Tran and Anand[83] conducted a systematic review of the literature in an effort to summarize the best evidence for oral antiplatelet therapy in patients with cerebrovascular disease, CAD, and PAD. This review included 111 trials (42 of which included patients with PAD, n = 9,214) and concluded that patients with PAD should use ASA (160 to 325 mg/day) or clopidogrel (75 mg/day) when ASA is not tolerated or contraindicated.[83] This is in concordance with the recommendations of the Ninth American College of Chest Physicians (ACCP) Conference on Antithrombotic and Thrombolytic Therapy that recommends lifelong ASA (75 to 325 mg/day) over clopidogrel and ticlopidine, and no antithrombotic therapy in patients with PAD.[75,84] Unfortunately, no data are currently available from large, clinical, randomized trials that ASA, or any other antiplatelet therapies, can actually prevent or delay the progression of PAD.[75]

Aspirin + Dipyridamole Extended Release (Aggrenox)

The ATC also examined the use of dipyridamole extended release (Aggrenox) in combination with ASA in "high-risk" patients, such as those with PAD. The meta-analysis of 25 trials (which included more than 10,000 patients) concluded that the addition of dipyridamole to ASA led to an additional reduction in serious vascular events over ASA alone (6%); however, this reduction was unable to reach statistical significance (P = 0.32).[74,83] It should also be taken into consideration that most of the reduction in nonfatal stroke in this analysis came from one trial, and these data are not replicated in the other studies.[74,85] The addition of dipyridamole to ASA may cause an increased risk of bleeding and GI side effects when compared with placebo and should not be used with CAD.[85]

Clopidogrel (Plavix)

The ATC meta-analysis also reviewed the effectiveness of clopidogrel (Plavix) 75 mg/day in "high-risk" patients, including those with PAD. The ATC concluded that although clopidogrel was able to reduce serious vascular events by 10%, this was significantly less than the reduction seen with ASA (12%, P = 0.03) described previously.[74] Included in this meta-analysis was the report from the Clopidogrel versus ASA in Patients at Risk of Ischemic Events (CAPRIE)[76] trial that had concluded that clopidogrel (75 mg daily) was more effective than ASA (325 mg daily) in preventing vascular events in "high-risk" patients. In comparison to the ASA therapy, the clopidogrel regimen resulted in an overall reduction in ischemic stroke, MI, or vascular death from 5.83% to 5.32% (P = 0.043). This difference was even more pronounced in the subgroup analysis of PAD patients, in which clopidogrel therapy led to a significant reduction of 4.86% versus 3.71% in the ASA group ($P = 0.0028$).[21,33,76] Although a generic clopidogrel product is now available, it remains significantly more expensive than ASA therapy, not only in drug costs but also due to the fact that clopidogrel remains a by-prescription-only medication and, thus, requires a physician visit to obtain a prescription for the medication. For all these reasons, the current recommendations list clopidogrel as a first-line agent, but only in cases where ASA therapy is either not tolerated or contraindicated.[74]

Ticlopidine (Ticlid)

Although ticlopidine has the same mechanism of action as clopidogrel and possesses a similar molecular structure, the results of clinical trials among the two agents are strikingly different.[15] The Swedish Ticlopidine Multicenter Study (STIMS)[86] had determined that ticlopidine therapy (500 mg/day) was able to reduce total mortality in comparison to placebo in patients with IC ($P = 0.015$).[15,86,87] However, the once promising results seen with ticlopidine therapy have now been overshadowed by the severe hematologic side effects unique to this agent. Ticlopidine has a "black box" warning from the FDA warning providers that use of this agent can cause neutropenia/agranulocytosis, thrombotic thrombocytopenic purpura, and aplastic anemia.[77] Other agents, namely, clopidogrel, are now used instead of ticlopidine.[3,28,40]

Intermittent Claudication

See Table 12-2.

Cilostazol (Pletal)

7 In a head-to-head, randomized, placebo-controlled study in 698 patients with moderate-to-severe claudication, Dawson et al.[88] assigned patients to cilostazol (100 mg twice a day), pentoxifylline (400 mg three times a day), or placebo in an effort to improve maximal walking distance. After 24 weeks, the cilostazol group demonstrated a 54% mean increase in distance versus pentoxifylline that demonstrated only a 30% mean increase ($P < 0.001$).[88] Similarly, a meta-analysis of eight randomized, double-blind, placebo-controlled, parallel-design trials supported this conclusion with a reported increase in maximal walking distance and pain-free walking distance with cilostazol at doses of 50 and 100 mg twice daily ($P < 0.05$ for all) over placebo.[89] Regrettably, improvement in walking distance has appeared to come with a price (in addition to the high drug cost); cilostazol has a "black box" warning from the FDA warning providers not to use this medication in patients with PAD and coexisting HF.[78] However, the Seventh ACCP Conference on Antithrombotic and Thrombolytic Therapy does suggest the use of this agent in patients with PAD who are not candidates for surgical interventions to improve severe IC that persists even after implementation of appropriate exercise therapy and TLC.[75]

Pentoxifylline (Trental)

Unlike cilostazol, pentoxifylline has produced less promising results in clinical trials, as illustrated by the randomized, placebo-controlled trial by Dawson et al.[88] Not only did cilostazol outperform pentoxifylline in improvement in walking distance, but also the improvement seen with pentoxifylline was no different from placebo ($P = 0.82$).[88] This nonsignificant improvement in walking distance has been observed in other studies as well.[3,90] Meanwhile, other meta-analyses of pentoxifylline in comparison to placebo for the improvement of maximal walking distance have shown some minimal improvement over placebo, but the average effects were relatively small.[3,91–94] For these reasons, the Seventh ACCP Conference on Antithrombotic and Thrombolytic Therapy does not recommend the use of this agent.[75]

EVALUATION OF THERAPEUTIC OUTCOMES

It is vital that the patient be counseled on the evaluation measures that will be used to monitor the outcomes of therapeutic interventions for PAD. Various laboratory measurements will assess patient progress in glycemic control (e.g., hemoglobin A-1c) and lipid management (e.g., total cholesterol, LDL, HDL, and non-HDL cholesterol), while blood pressure checks in the clinic and patient home blood pressure monitoring can assess the effectiveness of antihypertensive therapy. Repeat exercise treadmill walking testing should be repeated at regular intervals (e.g., quarterly to biannually) to assess improvement or decline in walking duration and distance, as well as the time to pain onset while performing this activity. Repeat ABI measurements should be assessed at each patient visit to determine if there has been stabilization or progression of the disease process. Most importantly to many patients, simple concern and questioning about improvements to their daily quality of life will highlight your concern for their well-being and aid in an overall picture of the patient's general state of health.

ABBREVIATIONS

ABI	ankle-brachial index
ACC	American College of Cardiology
ACCP	American College of Chest Physicians
ACE	angiotensin-converting enzyme
AHA	American Heart Association
AMI	acute myocardial infarction
ASA	aspirin (acetylsalicylic acid)
ATC	Antithrombotic Trialists' Collaboration
ATP III	Adult Treatment Panel III (Expert Panel on Detection, Evaluation, and Treatment of High Blood Cholesterol in Adults)
CAD	coronary artery disease
CAPRIE	Clopidogrel versus ASA in Patients at Risk of Ischemic Events
CHD	coronary heart disease
CTA	computed tomographic angiography
CVD	cardiovascular disease
FH	familial hypercholesterolemia
HDL	high-density lipoprotein
HF	heart failure
HOPE	Heart Outcomes Prevention Evaluation
HPS	Heart Protection Study
HTN	hypertension
IC	intermittent claudication
JNC VII	seventh report of the Joint National Committee on Prevention, Detection, Evaluation, and Treatment of High Blood Pressure
LDL	low-density lipoprotein
MRA	magnetic resonance angiography
NHANES	National Health and Nutrition Examination Survey
OR	odds ratio
PAD	peripheral arterial disease
PARTNERS	PAD Awareness, Risk, and Treatment: New Resources for Survival
PROVE IT	Pravastatin or Atorvastatin Evaluation and Infection—Thrombolysis in Myocardial Infarction
PTA	percutaneous transluminal angioplasty
STIMS	Swedish Ticlopidine Multicenter Study
TASC	TransAtlantic Inter-Society Consensus
TLC	therapeutic lifestyle changes

REFERENCES

1. Go AS, Mozaffarian D, Roger VL, et al. AHA statistical update. Heart disease and stroke statistics—2013 update. Circulation 2013;127:e1–e203.
2. Coutinho T, Rooke TW, Kullo IJ. Arterial dysfunction and functional performance in patients with peripheral artery disease: A review. Vasc Med 2011;16:203–211.
3. Hiatt WR. Medical treatment of peripheral arterial disease and claudication. N Engl J Med 2001;344:1608–1621.
4. Mohler ER 3rd. Peripheral arterial disease. Identification and implications. Arch Intern Med 2003;163:2306–2314.
5. Dormandy JA, Murray GD. The fate of the claudicant—A prospective study of 1969 claudicants. Eur J Vasc Surg 1991;5:131–133.
6. Selvin E, Erlinger TP. Prevalence of and risk factors for peripheral arterial disease in the United States. Results from the National Health and Nutrition Examination Survey, 1999-2000. Circulation 2004;110:738–743.
7. Hirsch AT, Hiatt WR, PARTNERS Steering Committee. PAD awareness, risk, and treatment: New resources for survival—The USA PARTNERS program. Vasc Med 2001;6:9–12.
8. Rooke TW, Hirsch AT, Misra S, et al. 2011 ACCF/AHA focused update of the guideline for the management of patients with peripheral artery disease (updating the 2005 guideline). Vasc Med 2011;16:452–476.
9. White C. Intermittent claudication. N Engl J Med 2007; 356:1241–1250.
10. Grundy S, Cleeman J, Merz CB, et al. Implications of recent clinical trials for the National Cholesterol Education Program Adult Treatment Panel III guidelines. Circulation 2004;110:227–239.
11. Hutter C, Austin M, Humphries S. Familial hypercholesterolemia, peripheral arterial disease, and stroke: A HuGE minireview. Am J Epidemiol 2004;160:430–435.
12. Wang JC, Criqui MH, Denenberg JO, McDermott MM, Golomb BA, Fronek A. Exertional leg pain in patients with and without peripheral arterial disease. Circulation 2005;112:3501–3508.
13. Hirsch AT, Haskal ZJ, Hertzer NR, et al. ACC/AHA 2005 practice guidelines for the management of patients with peripheral arterial disease (lower extremity, renal, mesenteric, and abdominal aortic): A collaborative report from the American Association for Vascular Surgery/Society for Vascular Surgery, Society for Cardiovascular Angiography and Interventions, Society for Vascular Medicine and Biology, Society of Interventional Radiology, and the ACC/AHA Task Force on Practice Guidelines (Writing Committee to Develop Guidelines for the Management of Patients with Peripheral Arterial Disease): Endorsed by the American Association of Cardiovascular and Pulmonary Rehabilitation; National Heart, Lung, and Blood Institute; Society for Vascular Nursing; TransAtlantic Inter-Society Consensus; and Vascular Disease Foundation. Circulation 2006;113:e463–e654.
14. Hiatt W, Nehler MR, eds. Peripheral Arterial Disease, 4th ed. New York: Spring-Verlag, 2003.
15. Hiatt WR. Preventing atherothrombotic events in peripheral arterial disease: The use of antiplatelet therapy. J Intern Med 2002;251:193–206.
16. Hirsch AT, Criqui MH, Treat-Jacobson D, et al. Peripheral arterial disease detection, awareness, and treatment in primary care. JAMA 2001;286:1317–1324.
17. Dormandy JA, Rutherford RB. Management of peripheral arterial disease (PAD). TASC Working Group. TransAtlantic Inter-Society Consensus (TASC). J Vasc Surg 2000;31:S1–S296.
18. Carman TL, Fernandez BB Jr. A primary care approach to the patient with claudication. Am Fam Physician 2000;61:1027–1032, 1034.
19. Schmieder FA, Comerota AJ. Intermittent claudication: Magnitude of the problem, patient evaluation, and therapeutic strategies. Am J Cardiol 2001;87:3D–13D.
20. Sontheimer DL. Peripheral vascular disease: Diagnosis and treatment. Am Fam Physician 2006;73:1971–1976.
21. Aronow WS. Management of peripheral arterial disease of the lower extremities in elderly patients. J Gerontol A Biol Sci Med Sci 2004;59:172–177.
22. O'Hare AM, Glidden DV, Fox CS, Hsu CY. High prevalence of peripheral arterial disease in persons with renal insufficiency: Results from the National Health and Nutrition Examination Survey 1999-2000. Circulation 2004;109:320–323.
23. Criqui MH. Systemic atherosclerosis risk and the mandate for intervention in atherosclerotic peripheral arterial disease. Am J Cardiol 2001;88:43J–47J.
24. Mannava K, Money SR. Current management of peripheral arterial occlusive disease: A review of pharmacologic agents and other interventions. Am J Cardiovasc Drugs 2007;7:59–66.
25. Jackson M, Clagett G. Antithrombotic therapy in peripheral arterial occlusive disease. Chest 2001;119:283S–299S.
26. Norgren L, Hiatt W, Dormandy J, Nehler MR, Harris KA, Fowkes FG. Inter-Society Consensus for the Management of Peripheral Arterial Disease (TASC II). J Vasc Surg 2007; 45(Suppl S):S5–S67.
27. TransAtlantic Inter-Society Consensus (TASC) Working Group. Management of peripheral arterial disease (PAD). TransAtlantic Inter-Society Consensus (TASC). Section B: Intermittent claudication. Eur J Vasc Endovasc Surg 2000;19: S47–S114.
28. Gey DC, Lesho EP, Manngold J. Management of peripheral arterial disease. Am Fam Physician 2004;69:525–532.
29. Doobay AV, Anand SS. Sensitivity and specificity of the ankle-brachial index to predict future cardiovascular outcomes: A systematic review. Arterioscler Thromb Vasc Biol 2005;25:1463–1479.
30. Mourad JJ, Cacoub PP, Collet JP, et al. Screening of unrecognized peripheral arterial disease (PAD) using ankle-brachial index in high cardiovascular risk patients free from symptomatic PAD. J Vasc Surg 2009;50:572–580. doi:10.1016/j.jvs.2009.04.055.
31. McDermott MM, Greenland P, Liu K, et al. The ankle brachial index is associated with leg function and physical activity: The Walking and Leg Circulation Study. Ann Intern Med 2002;136:873–883.
32. McDermott MM, Criqui MH, Liu K, et al. Lower ankle/brachial index, as calculated by averaging the dorsalis pedis and posterior tibial arterial pressures, and association with leg functioning in peripheral arterial disease. J Vasc Surg 2000;32:1164–1171.
33. Belch JJ, Topol EJ, Agnelli G, et al. Critical issues in peripheral arterial disease detection and management: A call to action. Arch Intern Med 2003;163:884–892.
34. Met R, Bipat S, Legemate DA, Reekers JA, Koelemay MJW. Diagnostic performance of computed tomography angiography in peripheral arterial disease: A systematic review and meta-analysis. JAMA 2009;301:415–424.
35. Farkouh ME. Improving the clinical examination for a low ankle-brachial index. Int J Angiol 2002;11:41–45.
36. Khan NA, Rahim SA, Anand SS, Simel DL, Panju A. Does the clinical examination predict lower extremity peripheral arterial disease? JAMA 2006;295:536–546.

37. Hirsch AT, Haskal ZJ, Hertzer NR, et al. ACC/AHA guidelines for the management of patients with peripheral arterial disease (lower extremity, renal, mesenteric, and abdominal aortic): Executive summary: A collaborative report from the American Association for Vascular Surgery/Society for Vascular Surgery, Society for Vascular Medicine and Biology, Society of Interventional Radiology, and the ACC/AHA Task Force on Practice Guidelines (Writing Committee to Develop Guidelines for the Management of Patients with Peripheral Arterial Disease [Lower Extremity, Renal, Mesenteric, and Abdominal Aortic]). J Am Coll Cardiol 2006;46:1239–1312.
38. Hiatt WR. Pharmacologic therapy for peripheral arterial disease and claudication. J Vasc Surg 2002;36:1283–1291.
39. Burns P, Gough S, Bradbury AW. Management of peripheral arterial disease in primary care. BMJ 2003;326:584–588.
40. Regensteiner JG, Hiatt WR. Current medical therapies for patients with peripheral arterial disease: A critical review. Am J Med 2002;112:49–57.
41. Kannel WB, Shurtleff D. National Heart and Lung Institute, National Institutes of Health. The Framingham Study: Cigarettes and the development of intermittent claudication. Geriatrics 1973;28:61–68.
42. Tierney S, Fennessy F, Hayes DB. ABC of arterial and vascular disease: Secondary prevention of peripheral vascular disease. BMJ 2000;320:1262–1265.
43. Gardner AW, Katzel LI, Sorkin JD, Goldberg AP. Effects of long-term exercise rehabilitation on claudication distances in patients with peripheral arterial disease: A randomized controlled trial. J Cardiopulm Rehabil 2002;22:192–198.
44. Langbein WE, Collins EG, Orebaugh C, et al. Increasing exercise tolerance of persons limited by claudication pain using polestriding. J Vasc Surg 2002;35:887–893.
45. Gardner AW, Katzel LI, Sorkin JD, et al. Exercise rehabilitation improves functional outcomes and peripheral circulation in patients with intermittent claudication: A randomized controlled trial. J Am Geriatr Soc 2001;49:755–762.
46. Falcone RA, Hirsch AT, Regensteiner JG, et al. Peripheral arterial disease rehabilitation: A review. J Cardiopulm Rehabil 2003;23:170–175.
47. Tan KH, De Cossart L, Edwards PR. Exercise training and peripheral vascular disease. Br J Surg 2000;87:553–562.
48. Garg PK, Tian L, Criqui MH, et al. Physical activity during daily life and mortality in patients with peripheral arterial disease. Circulation 2006;114:242–248.
49. Stewart KJ, Hiatt WR, Regensteiner JG, Hirsch AT. Exercise training for claudication. N Engl J Med 2002; 347:1941–1951.
50. de Liefde II, Hoeks SE, van Gestel YR, et al. The prognostic value of impaired walking distance on long-term outcome in patients with known or suspected peripheral arterial disease. Eur J Vasc Endovasc Surg 2009;38:482–487. doi:10.1016/j.ejvs.2009.02.022.
51. McDermott MM, Tian L, Liu K, Guralnik JM, Ferrucci L, Tan J. Prognostic value of functional performance for mortality in patients with peripheral artery disease. J Am Coll Cardiol 2008;51:1482–1489.
52. Schiano V, Brevetti G, Sirico G, Silvestro A, Giugliano G, Chiariello M. Functional status measured by walking impairment questionnaire and cardiovascular risk prediction in peripheral arterial disease: Results of the peripheral arteriopathy and cardiovascular events (PACE) study. Vasc Med 2006;11:147–154.
53. Whyman MR, Fowkes FG, Kerracher EM, et al. Is intermittent claudication improved by percutaneous transluminal angioplasty? A randomized controlled trial. J Vasc Surg 1997;26:551–557.
54. Bosch J, Hunink M. Meta-analysis of the results of percutaneous transluminal angioplasty and stent placement for aortoiliac occlusive disease [Erratum. Radiology 1997;205(2):584]. Radiology 1997;204:87–96.
55. Bradbury AW, Adam DJ, Bell J, et al. Bypass versus Angioplasty in Severe Ischaemia of the Leg (BASIL) trial: Analysis of amputation free and overall survival by treatment received. J Vasc Surg 2010;51:18S–31S.
56. Chobanian AV, Bakris GL, Black HR, et al. The seventh report of the Joint National Committee on Prevention, Detection, Evaluation, and Treatment of High Blood Pressure: The JNC 7 report. JAMA 2003;289:2560–2571.
57. The Heart Outcomes Prevention Evaluation Study Investigators. Effects of an angiotensin-converting-enzyme inhibitor, ramipril, on cardiovascular events in high-risk patients. N Engl J Med 2000;342:145–153.
58. McDermott MM. Peripheral arterial disease: Epidemiology and drug therapy. Am J Geriatr Cardiol 2002;11:258–266.
59. Paravastu SCV, Mendonca DA, de Silva A. Beta blockers for peripheral arterial disease. Eur J Endovasc Surg 2009; 38:66–70.
60. Tseng CH, Tseng FH, Chong CK, Tseng CP, Cheng JC. Angiotensin-converting enzyme genotype and peripheral arterial disease in diabetic patients. Exp Diabetes Res 2012; 2012:698695.
61. Aggarwal S, Loomba RS, Arora R. Preventive aspects in peripheral artery disease. Ther Adv Cardiovasc Dis 2012;6:53–70.
62. Expert Panel on Detection, Evaluation, and Treatment of High Blood Cholesterol in Adults. Executive summary of the third report of the National Cholesterol Education Program (NCEP) Expert Panel on Detection, Evaluation, and Treatment of High Blood Cholesterol in Adults (Adult Treatment Panel III). JAMA 2001;285:2486–2497.
63. Leng GC, Price JF, Jepson RG. Lipid-lowering for lower limb atherosclerosis. Cochrane Database Syst Rev 2000;(2):CD000123.
64. Heart Protection Study Collaborative Group. MRC/BHF Heart Protection Study of cholesterol lowering with simvastatin in 20536 high-risk individuals: A randomised placebo-controlled trial. Lancet 2002;360:7–22.
65. Cannon CP, Braunwald E, McCabe CH, et al. Intensive versus moderate lipid lowering with statins after acute coronary syndromes. N Engl J Med 2004;350:1495–1504.
66. Elam MB, Hunninghake DB, Davis KB, et al. Effect of niacin on lipid and lipoprotein levels and glycemic control in patients with diabetes and peripheral arterial disease: The ADMIT study: A randomized trial. JAMA 2000;284:1263–1270.
67. National Cholesterol Education Program Expert Panel on Detection, Evaluation, and Treatment of High Blood Cholesterol in Adults. Third report of the National Cholesterol Education Program (NCEP) Expert Panel on Detection, Evaluation, and Treatment of High Blood Cholesterol in Adults (Adult Treatment Panel III) final report. Circulation 2002;106:3143–3421.
68. Coutinho M, Gerstein H, Wang Y, Yusuf S. The relationship between glucose and incident cardiovascular events. A metaregression analysis of published data from 20 studies of 95,783 individuals followed for 12.4 years. Diabetes Care 1999;22:233–240.
69. American Diabetes Association. Peripheral arterial disease in people with diabetes. Diabetes Care 2003;26:3333–3341.
70. Creager MA, Luscher TF, Cosentino F, Beckman JA. Diabetes and vascular disease: Pathophysiology, clinical consequences, and medical therapy: Part I. Circulation 2003;108:1527–1532.

71. Selvin E, Wattanakit K, Steffes MW, Coresh J, Sharrett AR. HbA1c and peripheral arterial disease in diabetes: The atherosclerosis risk in communities study. Diabetes Care 2006;29:877–882.
72. Rehring TF, Sandhoff BG, Stolcpart RS, Merenich JA, Hollis HW Jr. Atherosclerotic risk factor control in patients with peripheral arterial disease. J Vasc Surg 2005;41:816–822.
73. Guyatt G, Schunemann HJ, Cook D, Jaeschke R, Pauker S. Applying the grades of recommendation for antithrombotic and thrombolytic therapy: The seventh ACCP conference on antithrombotic and thrombolytic therapy. Chest 2004;126: 179S–187S.
74. Antithrombotic Trialists' Collaboration. Collaborative meta-analysis of randomised trials of antiplatelet therapy for prevention of death, myocardial infarction, and stroke in high risk patients. BMJ 2002;324:71–86.
75. Clagett GP, Sobel M, Jackson MR, Lip GYH, Tangelder M, Verhaeghe R. Antithrombotic therapy in peripheral arterial occlusive disease: The seventh ACCP conference on antithrombotic and thrombolytic therapy. Chest 2004; 126:609S–626S.
76. CAPRIE Steering Committee. A randomised, blinded, trial of clopidogrel versus aspirin in patients at risk of ischaemic events (CAPRIE). CAPRIE Steering Committee. Lancet 1996;348:1329–1339.
77. Ticlid—Ticlopidine hydrochloride. Roche Laboratories Inc; December 2005.
78. Cilostazol—"C" Monographs. DrugPoints. July 15, 2009 ed. Thomson Healthcare; 2009.
79. Plavix—Clopidogrel Bisulfate. Bristol-Myers Squibb/Sanofi Pharmaceuticals Partnership; May 2009.
80. Aspirin—"A" Monographs. DrugPoints. August 3, 2009 ed. Thomson Healthcare; 2009.
81. Dipyridamole—"D" Monographs. DrugPoints. July 15, 2009 ed. Thomson Healthcare; 2009.
82. Pentoxifylline—"P" Monographs. DrugPoints. July 15, 2009 ed. Thomson Healthcare; 2009.
83. Tran H, Anand SS. Oral antiplatelet therapy in cerebrovascular disease, coronary artery disease, and peripheral arterial disease. JAMA 2004;292:1867–1874.
84. Eikelboloom JW, Hirsh J, Spencer FA, Baglin TP, Weitz JI. Antiplatelet drugs: Antithrombotic Therapy and Prevention of Thrombosis, 9th ed: American College of Chest Physicians Evidence-Based Clinical Practice Guidelines. Chest 2012;141:e89S–e119S.
85. Diener HC, Cunha L, Forbes C, Sivenius J, Smets P, Lowenthal A. European Stroke Prevention Study 2. Dipyridamole and acetylsalicylic acid in the secondary prevention of stroke. J Neurol Sci 1996;143:1–13.
86. Janzon L. The STIMS trial: The ticlopidine experience and its clinical applications. Swedish Ticlopidine Multicenter Study. Vasc Med 1996;1:141–143.
87. Janzon L, Bergqvist D, Boberg J, et al. Prevention of myocardial infarction and stroke in patients with intermittent claudication; effects of ticlopidine. Results from STIMS, the Swedish Ticlopidine Multicentre Study [Erratum. J Intern Med 1990;228(6):659]. J Intern Med 1990;227:301–308.
88. Dawson DL, Cutler BS, Hiatt WR, et al. A comparison of cilostazol and pentoxifylline for treating intermittent claudication. Am J Med 2000;109:523–530.
89. Thompson PD, Zimet R, Forbes WP, Zhang P. Meta-analysis of results from eight randomized, placebo-controlled trials on the effect of cilostazol on patients with intermittent claudication. Am J Cardiol 2002;90:1314–1319.
90. Lindgarde F, Jelnes R, Bjorkman H, et al. Conservative drug treatment in patients with moderately severe chronic occlusive peripheral arterial disease. Scandinavian Study Group. Circulation 1989;80:1549–1556.
91. Girolami B, Bernardi E, Prins MH, et al. Treatment of intermittent claudication with physical training, smoking cessation, pentoxifylline, or nafronyl: A meta-analysis [see comment]. Arch Intern Med 1999;159:337–345.
92. Radack K, Wyderski RJ. Conservative management of intermittent claudication. Ann Intern Med 1990;113:135–146.
93. Ernst E. Pentoxifylline for intermittent claudication. A critical review. Angiology 1994;45:339–345.
94. Hood SC, Moher D, Barber GG. Management of intermittent claudication with pentoxifylline: Meta-analysis of randomized controlled trials. CMAJ 1996;155:1053–1059.

Use of Vasopressors and Inotropes in the Pharmacotherapy of Shock

Robert Maclaren and Joseph F. Dasta

13

KEY CONCEPTS

1. Continuous hemodynamic monitoring with an arterial catheter or a central venous catheter capable of measuring mixed venous oxygen saturation (Svo_2) or central venous oxygen saturation ($Scvo_2$) should be used early and throughout the course of septic shock to assess intravascular fluid status and ventricular filling pressures, determine cardiac output (CO), and monitor arterial and venous oxygenation. They can be used for monitoring the response to drug therapy and guiding dosage titration.
2. Early goal-directed therapy with aggressive fluid resuscitation in the emergency department within the first 6 hours of presentation improves survival of patients with sepsis and septic shock.
3. Lactate production is increased under anaerobic conditions. Elevated serum lactate concentrations represent global perfusion abnormalities. Lactate clearance may be used to assess repayment of oxygen to the tissues. GI tonometry and sublingual capnometry represent methods of assessing regional perfusion but are used infrequently.
4. Derangements in adrenergic receptor sensitivity or activity frequently result in resistance to catecholamine vasopressor and inotropic therapy in critically ill patients. These changes may be a function of endogenous catecholamine concentrations, dosage/duration of exposure to and type of exogenously administered vasopressors, stage of septic shock, preexisting illness, and other factors.
5. In refractory septic shock, rational use of vasopressor or inotropic agents should be guided by receptor activity, pharmacologic and pharmacokinetic characteristics, and regional and systemic hemodynamic effects of the drug and should be tailored to the patient's physiologic needs. Pharmacologically sound combinations of vasopressor and/or inotrope agents should be initiated early to optimize and facilitate rapid response.
6. Goals of therapy with vasopressors and inotropes should be predetermined and should optimize global and regional perfusion parameters (e.g., cardiac, renal, mesenteric, and periphery) to normalize cellular metabolism. This can be accomplished by continuous or intermittent measurements. Targeted goals should be central venous pressure (CVP) of 8 to 12 mm Hg (up to 15 mm Hg in mechanically ventilated patients, patients with preexisting left ventricular dysfunction, or patients with abdominal distension), mean arterial pressure (MAP) ≥65 mm Hg, Svo_2 ≥65% or $Scvo_2$ ≥70%, and lactate clearance of ≥20%.
7. Dose titration and monitoring of vasopressor and inotropic therapy should be guided by the "best clinical response" while observing for and minimizing evidence of myocardial ischemia (e.g., tachydysrhythmias, electrocardiographic changes, troponin elevation), renal (decreased glomerular filtration rate and/or urine production), splanchnic/gastric (low intramucosal pH, bowel ischemia), or peripheral (cold extremities) hypoperfusion, and worsening of partial pressure of arterial oxygen (Pao_2), pulmonary artery occlusive pressure (PAOP), and other hemodynamic variables.
8. Much higher dosages of all vasopressors and inotropes than traditionally recommended are required to improve hemodynamic and oxygen-transport variables in patients with septic shock. Arbitrarily targeting vasopressor and inotrope therapy to supranormal values of global oxygen-transport variables cannot be recommended because of the lack of clear benefit and possible increased morbidity.
9. First-line therapy of septic shock is aggressive volume resuscitation with crystalloid or colloid types of fluids. Norepinephrine is the preferred initial vasopressor agent for hemodynamic support. Norepinephrine achieves greater hemodynamic response than dopamine and is less likely to cause tachydysrhythmias and a decrease in splanchnic oxygen utilization. Dopamine is also limited by its inability to adequately increase CO and complications of increased PAOP and decreased splanchnic oxygen use. Low-dose dopamine should not be used to prevent renal failure.
10. Phenylephrine may be a particularly useful alternative in patients who cannot tolerate tachycardia or tachydysrhythmia associated with the use of other agents. Its effects on cardiac performance and splanchnic oxygen utilization are variable.
11. Epinephrine is an effective initial agent and as an add-on agent. It is particularly useful in the young, in patients with otherwise healthy myocardium, and potentially in patients when used early in the course of treatment. However, because epinephrine causes a significant increase in lactate and worsening of splanchnic oxygen utilization, it is not the agent of first choice in patients with septic shock and is reserved as adjunctive therapy when other vasopressors do not adequately increase MAP. It should be used cautiously in patients with a history of coronary artery disease or underlying cardiac disturbances.
12. Dobutamine may be used as adjunctive therapy for its inotropic effect. It enhances CO and may increase Svo_2/$Scvo_2$. Concurrent vasopressor therapy is needed because dobutamine causes vasodilation. Dobutamine therapy may be limited by tachycardia and dysrhythmias.

13 Therapy with vasopressors and inotropes is continued until the myocardial depression and vascular hyporesponsiveness of septic shock improve, usually measured in hours to days. Discontinuation of vasopressor or inotropic therapy should be executed slowly; therapy should be "weaned" to avoid a precipitous worsening in regional and systemic hemodynamics.

14 Vasopressin produces vasoconstriction independent of adrenergic receptors and reduces the dosages of catecholamine vasopressors. Replacement dosages of vasopressin (0.01 to 0.04 units/min) can be considered in patients with septic shock refractory to catecholamine vasopressors despite adequate fluid resuscitation. Dosage rates should not be titrated upward. Vasopressin may enhance urine production but it may worsen splanchnic and peripheral perfusion. Given the current data, corticosteroids can be administered to patients with septic shock refractory to vasopressors or when adrenal insufficiency is suspected. Side effects of short-term corticosteroids are minimal.

Shock is an acute, generalized state of inadequate perfusion of critical organs that can produce serious pathophysiologic consequences, including death, when therapy is not optimal. Shock is defined as systolic blood pressure <90 mm Hg or reduction of at least 40 mm Hg from baseline with perfusion abnormalities despite adequate fluid resuscitation.[1] Previously, mortality from septic or cardiogenic shock exceeded 70% but now ranges between 20% and 40%.[2–5] This chapter reviews the theory and current status of hemodynamic monitoring and presents an update on the optimal use of inotropes and vasopressor drugs in shock states, specifically septic shock.[6–15]

The general goal of therapy during resuscitation from shock is to achieve and maintain mean arterial pressure (MAP) above 65 mm Hg while ensuring adequate perfusion to the critical organs.[6–15] Hemodynamic and perfusion monitoring can be categorized into two broad areas: global versus regional monitoring. Global parameters, such as systemic blood pressure, oxygen tension, and lactate, assess perfusion and oxygen utilization of the entire body. Regional monitoring techniques, such as tonometry or cardiac function, focus on oxygen delivery and subsequent changes in metabolism of individual organs and tissues. Patients in shock generally have several modes of monitoring so therapies are based on all gathered information and correlating with the patient's clinical response. Normal values for commonly monitored parameters are listed in Table 13-1. Evidence-based goals of therapy are listed in Table 13-2.[6–21] The adequacy of regional perfusion can be assessed by indices of specific organ perfusion.[6,15–21] These measurements include coagulation abnormalities (disseminated intravascular coagulation), altered renal function with reduced urine production or increased serum concentrations of blood urea nitrogen and creatinine, altered hepatic parenchymal function with increased serum concentrations of transaminases and bilirubin, altered GI perfusion manifested by ileus and diminished bowel sounds, cool extremities, cardiac ischemia with elevated troponin concentrations and electrocardiographic changes, and altered sensorium. Although none of these indices alone is a reliable indicator of adequate resuscitation, they offer immediate detection and may be prognostic of recovery when combined and defined at the level of organ function. As a result, these indices are frequently used as surrogate endpoints for the goals of resuscitation.[22] While it is assumed that normalization of these parameters infers benefit, the clinician must first treat the patient clinically rather than relying solely on data from continuous monitoring to guide therapy.[22]

TABLE 13-1 Hemodynamic and Oxygen-Transport Monitoring Parameters

Parameter	Normal Value[a]
Blood pressure (systolic/diastolic)	100–130/70–85 mm Hg
Mean arterial pressure (MAP)	80–100 mm Hg
Pulmonary artery pressure (PAP)	25/10 mm Hg
Mean pulmonary artery pressure (MPAP)	12–15 mm Hg
Central venous pressure (CVP)	8–12 mm Hg
Pulmonary artery occlusive pressure (PAOP)	12–15 mm Hg
Heart rate (HR)	60–80 beats/min
Cardiac output (CO)	4–7 L/min
Cardiac index (CI)	2.8–3.6 L/min/m²
Stroke volume index (SVI)	30–50 mL/m²
Systemic vascular resistance index (SVRI)	1,300–2,100 dyne • s/m² • cm⁵
Pulmonary vascular resistance index (PVRI)	45–225 dyne • s/m² • cm⁵
Arterial oxygen saturation (Sao_2)	97% (range, 95–100%)
Mixed venous oxygen saturation (Svo_2)	70–75%
Arterial oxygen content (Cao_2)	20.1 vol% (range, 19–21)
Venous oxygen content (Cvo_2)	15.5 vol% (range, 11.5–16.5)
Oxygen content difference ($C[a-v]O_2$)	5 vol% (range, 4–6)
Oxygen consumption index (VO_2)	131 mL/min/m² (range, 100–180)
Oxygen delivery index (Do_2)	578 mL/min/m² (range, 370–730)
Oxygen extraction ratio (O_2ER)	25% (range, 22–30)
Intramucosal pH (pHi)	7.40 (range, 7.35–7.45)
Index (I)	Parameter indexed to body surface area

[a]Normal values may not be the same as values needed to optimize the management of a critically ill patient.

GLOBAL PERFUSION MONITORING

Arterial Blood Pressure Measurement

MAP is the product of cardiac output (CO) and systemic vascular resistance (SVR). Conditions that may lower blood pressure through diminished CO in critically ill patients include cardiac failure (etiology may be myocardial infarction, arrhythmia, acute heart failure, or valvular disease) and hypovolemia (etiology may be hemorrhage, intractable diarrhea, or heat stroke). Vasodilatory conditions such as sepsis, anaphylaxis, pancreatitis, acute hepatic failure, or neurotrauma, lower blood pressure by reducing SVR. Arterial blood pressure is the commonly used end point of therapy; however, restoration of adequate perfusion pressure is the primary criterion of effectiveness.[6–21] Profound hypotension (MAP <60 mm Hg) is associated with pressure-dependent decreases in coronary, cerebral, and renal blood flow and may rapidly produce myocardial, cerebral, and renal ischemia. Therefore, a goal MAP of 65 mm Hg is often targeted for shock to maintain perfusion.

Arterial blood pressure can be determined by noninvasive and invasive methods. All noninvasive blood pressure monitoring techniques depend on the use of an occluding cuff. Systolic and diastolic blood pressures are further determined by oscillometry, auscultation, palpation (systolic pressure only), or Doppler technique (systolic pressures are most reliable). Oscillometry is the only noninvasive method used in the intensive care unit (ICU) to measure MAP because the data are valid during low-flow states and the method provides automatic cycling and serial

TABLE 13-2 Evidence-Based Treatment Recommendations for Management of Severe Sepsis or Septic Shock

Recommendations	Grade
Crystalloids are the initial fluid resuscitation of severe sepsis	1B
Albumin is additional therapy after substantial amounts of crystalloid have been used in the initial resuscitation regimen of severe sepsis and septic shock	2C
Hydroxyethyl starches with molecular weights exceeding 200 Da or molar substitution exceeding 0.4 should not be used	1B
Initial fluid challenge in patients with sepsis-induced tissue hypoperfusion and suspicion of hypovolemia should be initiated with ≥1,000 mL of crystalloid to achieve a minimum of 30 mL/kg of crystalloid in the first 4–6 hours of resuscitation. More rapid fluid administration and greater amounts of fluid may be needed in some patients	1B
An incremental fluid challenge technique of fluid boluses should be applied wherein fluid administration is continued until hemodynamic improvement, either based on dynamic (e.g., pulse pressure, stroke volume variation) or static (arterial pressure, heart rate) variables	1C
Resuscitation of patients with sepsis-induced shock, defined as tissue hypoperfusion (hypotension persisting after fluid challenge or blood lactate ≥4 mmol/L) should be protocolized. This protocol should be initiated as soon as hypoperfusion is recognized and should not be delayed pending ICU admission. The goal of initial resuscitation of sepsis-induced hypotension during the initial 6 hours should include all of the following: (a) CVP 8–12 mm Hg,[a] (b) MAP ≥65 mm Hg, (c) urine production ≥0.5 mL/kg/h, and (d) Svo_2 ≥65% or $Scvo_2$ ≥70%	1C
Resuscitation should target normal lactate concentrations in patients with elevated lactate levels as a marker of tissue hypoperfusion	2C
If Svo_2 ≤65% or $Scvo_2$ ≤70% persists during the initial 6 hours of resuscitation of severe sepsis or shock despite fluid resuscitation to CVP target, then transfusion of packed red blood cells to achieve a hematocrit of 30% and/or the administration of dobutamine at ≤20 mcg/kg/min should be used to achieve Svo_2 ≥65% or $Scvo_2$ ≥70%	No consensus
Use vasopressors to initially target MAP ≥65 mm Hg	1C
Norepinephrine is the initial vasopressor of choice	1B
Epinephrine (added or substituted) should be used when an additional agent is needed to maintain adequate blood pressure	2B
Dopamine should be used as an alternative vasopressor agent to norepinephrine in highly select patients with low CO and/or low heart rate and at very low risk of arrhythmias	2C
Dobutamine infusion should be administered or added to vasopressor therapy in the presence of (a) myocardial dysfunction as suggested by elevated filling pressures and low CO or (b) ongoing signs of hypoperfusion despite achieving adequate intravascular volume and adequate MAP	1C
Vasopressin 0.03 U/min may be added to norepinephrine with the intent of raising MAP or decreasing norepinephrine dosage	2A
Do not use corticosteroid in adult septic shock patients if adequate fluid resuscitation and vasopressor therapy is able to restore hemodynamic stability. If hemodynamic stability is not achieved, hydrocortisone at daily doses of 200 mg by continuous IV infusion may be administered	2C
ACTH stimulation test should not be used to identify the subset of adult patients with septic shock who should receive hydrocortisone	2B
Hydrocortisone is the preferred corticosteroid	2B
Hydrocortisone alone instead of hydrocortisone plus fludrocortisone should be used	1B
Corticosteroid therapy may be weaned once vasopressors are no longer required	2D
Do not use corticosteroids to treat sepsis in the absence of shock unless the patient's endocrine or corticosteroid history warrants it	1D

ACTH, adrenocorticotropic hormone; CO, cardiac output; CVP, central venous pressure; MAP, mean arterial pressure; $Scvo_2$, central-venous oxygen saturation; Svo_2, mixed venous oxygen saturation. *Level of recommendations*: 1, a strong recommendation indicating that the intervention's desirable effects clearly outweigh its undesirable effects; 2, a suggestion indicating that the tradeoff between desirable and undesirable effects is less clear. *Quality of evidence*: A, supported by a randomized control trial; B, supported by a downgraded randomized control trial or upgraded observational studies; C, supported by observational studies; D, supported by case series or expert opinion.

[a]A higher target CVP of 12 to 15 mm Hg may be required in the presence of mechanical ventilation or preexisting left ventricular dysfunction or abdominal distension.

Based on data from references 6–15.

measurements (every 1 to 3 minutes) that do not require operator intervention, a key component in ICU monitoring. The oscillometry method operates by sensing arterial blood pressure changes, or oscillations, against an inflated cuff. Rapid changes in oscillation amplitude correspond to systolic and diastolic pressure. The use of narrow cuffs or cuffs applied too loosely can result in falsely high readings, whereas wide cuffs may produce falsely low readings. Fingertip devices offer another avenue for continuous indirect blood pressure measurement, but their accuracy in ICU patients may be significantly diminished by concurrent administration of vasoactive drugs.

1 The use of invasive arterial catheters makes possible the continuous measurement of MAP as well as procurement of blood samples for laboratory testing. The radial artery is the most commonly used vessel, but the dorsalis pedis, femoral, brachial, and axillary arteries and the umbilical artery in the newborn also can be accessed. This method of blood pressure monitoring is the standard technique used in the ICU against which all other methods are compared. Major complications of peripheral artery catheterization include infection and distal ischemia. Acute distal ischemia and catheter-related bacteremia occur in <1% of catheter insertions. This translates to 2.9% of bloodstream infections per 1,000 catheter-days.[23] Ischemia is most common in patients with multiple or prolonged arterial cannulations, hypertension, or vasopressor therapy.[8] Invasive techniques are labor intensive, require aseptic techniques, and offer potential sources of equipment errors, such as length and quality of tubing, air bubbles, stopcocks, thrombus formation, tube kinking, and transducer placement. Hypertension, advanced age, and atherosclerosis also may affect the accuracy of invasive blood pressure readings.

Central Venous Catheter

1 The central venous catheter is used to measure the central venous pressure (CVP), to obtain venous samples for laboratory testing, and to administer drugs or fluids directly to the central circulation. A triple-lumen catheter frequently is used, whereby drugs with known incompatibility can be administered. Blood volume, venous wall compliance, right-sided cardiac function, intraabdominal and intrathoracic pressures, and vasopressor therapy affect

CVP. The CVP is not a reliable estimate of blood volume but can be used to qualitatively assess blood volume changes in patients during the early phases of fluid resuscitation.[24,25] The goal of fluid administration is to maintain the CVP at 8 to 12 mm Hg, but values of 15 mm Hg may be targeted in mechanically ventilated patients or patients with abdominal distension or preexisting ventricular dysfunction.[24,25] Sustained elevated pressures may be indicative of fluid overloading. Few data support the use of continuous CVP monitoring in the ICU. However, CVP monitoring of fluid therapy during resuscitation of septic shock is associated with reduced mortality.[6–8,24,25]

Pulmonary Artery Catheter

Pulmonary artery catheterization provides multiple cardiovascular parameters, including CVP, pulmonary artery pressure, pulmonary artery occlusive pressures (PAOP, commonly called the "wedge pressure"), CO, SVR, and the mixed-venous oxygen saturation (Svo_2).[26] Ideally, the pulmonary artery catheter should be positioned fluoroscopically; however, satisfactory placement also may be obtained by observing pulmonary artery pressure readings and electrocardiographic waveforms during catheter advancement. Proper positioning, or wedging, in the lower lung (zone 3) is essential to measure PAOP and to prevent distal pulmonary artery collapse. Inflation of the balloon at the catheter tip occludes the pulmonary artery, isolates the distal catheter tip from the right side of the heart, and allows the user to measure the PAOP, an approximate measure of the left ventricular end-diastolic volume and a major determinant of left ventricular preload. Poor wedging may be caused by catheter migration, patient movement, mechanical ventilation, or eccentric balloon inflation. Pulmonary artery catheters equipped with a distal thermistor also allow measurement of CO by thermodilution. Rapid injection of cold saline or dextrose solutions via the right atrial port allows complete mixing of blood with the injectate, and the resulting change in blood temperature is measured in the pulmonary artery. From the temperature change, the patient's CO can be calculated. Newer pulmonary artery catheters contain a temperature coil or filament that intermittently warms the blood in the right ventricle for near-continuous CO measurement. Significant tricuspid regurgitation, an intracardiac shunt, the respiratory phase, and significant positive end-expiratory pressure decrease the validity of CO measurements. The most common complications of pulmonary artery catheterization include mural thrombus formation (14% to 91%), transient ventricular tachydysrhythmias (11% to 63%), pulmonary infarction (1% to 7%), pulmonary artery rupture (0.06% to 2.0%), and sepsis (0.3% to 0.5%).[27,28] Most pulmonary artery catheters are heparin bonded which requires consideration in patients with unexplained thrombocytopenia. The relative risk (RR) of infection is 2.6 per 1,000 patient-days, similar to the risk with central venous catheters of 2.3 per 1,000 patient-days.[27,28] Controversy surrounds the utility and safety of the pulmonary artery catheter, including issues surrounding correct placement and impact of the device on patient outcome. Recent studies failed to demonstrate beneficial outcomes with the use of the pulmonary artery catheter.[29] The most recent guidelines suggest careful evaluation of the indications and the risk of placing a pulmonary artery catheter for resuscitation of critically ill patients.[30]

The optimal PAOP needs to be individualized for each patient. Administering a fluid bolus followed by simultaneous PAOP and CO measurements with the goal of increasing the PAOP until CO does not change can be accomplished and is based on Starling's law of the heart. However, clinical experience suggests that most patients have an optimal response to PAOP values in the range from 12 to 15 mm Hg. Limited data are available comparing the use of CVP and PAOP for guiding therapy in patients with shock. The results of recent studies of critically ill patients suggest CVP and PAOP are equivalent in terms of clinical outcomes, including mortality.[31] Therefore, a pulmonary artery catheter should be inserted when hemodynamic data are needed that cannot be obtained from a central venous catheter or when the validity of measurements from the central venous catheter is questionable.

Other methods used to assess CO include carbon dioxide (CO_2) partial rebreathing, esophageal Doppler, and transpulmonary (ultrasound) indicator dilution.[15–22] The CO_2 partial rebreathing technique compares end-tidal CO_2 partial pressure obtained during a nonrebreathing period with that obtained during a subsequent rebreathing period. The ratio of change in end-tidal CO_2 and CO_2 elimination estimates CO but must be corrected for blood shunting. Poor to acceptable agreement exists between this method and the thermodilution method of assessing CO in critically ill patients. In addition, low minute ventilation, a high shunt fraction, or a high CO produce inaccurate results. The esophageal Doppler technique measures flow velocity in the descending aorta by means of a Doppler transducer. CO is calculated based on the diameter of the aorta, the distribution of CO to the aorta, and the flow velocity of blood in the aorta. The CO reported by this method correlates with therapeutic interventions and demonstrates excellent agreement with the pulmonary artery catheter. Unfortunately, this method is technologically difficult and may not produce reliable measurements over time. The transpulmonary (ultrasound) indicator dilution method is functionally similar to the pulmonary artery catheter in that it employs thermodilution to calculate CO but it uses a central venous catheter rather than introducing a catheter into the pulmonary artery. This method of measuring CO correlates well with the values obtained from the pulmonary artery catheter and may display less respiratory phase variations. It also may estimate global end diastolic volume but other hemodynamic variables are not readily obtained.

Oxygen Tension and Saturation Monitoring

Partial pressure of arterial oxygen (Pao_2) and arterial oxygen saturation (Sao_2) can be assessed subjectively by assessing capillary refill or invasively by obtaining an arterial blood sample. Arterial blood gases measured by conventional arterial sampling are considered standard, but their accuracy and usefulness are affected by poor sampling techniques, transportation and analysis delays, analyzer accuracy, sample cellular metabolism, and inability to trend results. Indwelling fiberoptic and electrochemical systems that allow continuous monitoring and trend analyses of blood pH, Pao_2, and partial pressure of arterial carbon dioxide ($Paco_2$) while decreasing patient blood loss from less frequent sampling are in development. Mixed-venous oxygen saturation (Svo_2) and central-venous oxygen saturation ($Scvo_2$) reflect oxygen delivery (Do_2, or Do_2I, indexed to body surface area) with low values indicative of inadequate tissue perfusion that may occur during the early stages of septic shock, cardiogenic shock, or hypovolemic shock. Both measurements depend on CO, oxygen demand, hemoglobin, and Sao_2.

Svo_2 is measured in patients using a pulmonary artery catheter. Initially, critically ill septic patients may present with a low Svo_2 value (<65%), indicating high extraction of oxygen by tissues or lack of adequate Do_2 to tissues. In patients with sepsis and other conditions who present with a low Svo_2 value, rapid intervention should be undertaken to increase Do_2 to tissues, with the goal of obtaining Svo_2 ≥65%.[24,32] The length of time Svo_2 is <65% is associated with mortality.[24] As sepsis worsens, however, Svo_2 may be ≥65%. This occurs because extraction of oxygen in the arteriolar beds is hampered and is indicative of poor outcome.

❶ $Scvo_2$ is a less invasive measure of venous oxygen saturation because the catheter is placed at the junction of the inferior and superior venae cavae rather than at the pulmonary artery.[18–21] It is as accurate as Svo_2 but provides slightly higher normal values. Concentrations of $Scvo_2$ <70% reliably indicate inadequate oxygenation in shock states and detect subclinical ("cryptic") shock much earlier than hypotension. Targeting fluid and hemodynamic resuscitation to achieve $Scvo_2$ ≥70% is a sensitive indicator and measure of the extent of global tissue hypoxia, a determinant of the adequacy of hemodynamic resuscitation, and is associated with improved survival in patients with sepsis and septic shock.[15–21,24,32]

Oxygen Delivery and Consumption

Tissue oxygen debt is indicative of organ damage in critical illness. In normal individuals, oxygen consumption (Vo_2 or Vo_2I [oxygen consumption index], indexed to body surface area) depends on Do_2 (or Do_2I) up to a certain critical level (Vo_2 flow dependency). At this point, tissue oxygen requirements apparently are satisfied and further increases in Do_2 will not alter Vo_2 (Vo_2 flow independency). The point that Vo_2 becomes dependent on Do_2 represents a pathologic transition from aerobic to anaerobic cellular metabolism and lactate production.[21,24,33,34] Although animal models of sepsis substantiate this relationship, studies in critically ill humans show a continuous, pathologic dependence relationship of Vo_2 with Do_2.[21,24,33,34] The Vo_2/Do_2 ratio, or oxygen extraction ratio (O_2ER), can be used to assess adequacy of perfusion and metabolic response.[21,24,33,34] Maintaining the O_2ER at <25% without a changing Vo_2 may be helpful in maintaining or improving the body's reserve in meeting the oxygen demands. However, low Vo_2 and O_2ER values are indicative of poor oxygen utilization and lead to greater mortality. Patients who are able to increase Vo_2 when Do_2 is increased show improved survival. This finding became the basis for targeting supranormal Do_2 and Vo_2 values in the treatment of ICU patients in the 1970s and 1980s. However, a meta-analysis of randomized clinical trials involving 1,016 adult ICU patients failed to show that achievement of this goal improved mortality.[35] This may have been due in part to the heterogeneous nature of the ICU patients studied and therapies provided, lack of study blinding, crossover patients (control patients who achieve supranormal Do_2 and Vo_2 values by themselves), or lack of adequate control of cointerventions. The debate continues in more homogeneous patient populations. For example, in high-risk surgical patients, supranormal Do_2 values decrease mortality except in the subgroup of patients exceeding 75 years of age in whom achieving Do_2I >600 mL/m²/min shows mixed mortality results.[35] Of note, the systematic assessment of Do_2 and Vo_2 dependence is rarely done in practice but the concepts are frequently applied indirectly.

A review of alternative potential mechanisms of beneficial effect of supranormal Do_2 suggests that catecholamines exert antiinflammatory actions by modulating cytokine response.[6–15] In general, catecholamines inhibit the production of inflammatory cytokines (e.g., interleukin [IL]-6, tumor necrosis factor [TNF]-α) and may enhance synthesis of antiinflammatory cytokines (e.g., IL-4 and IL-10). The actions of epinephrine on these cytokines are blocked by propranolol and thus are mediated by adrenergic β-receptors.

Another issue with therapy directed to achieve supranormal oxygen transport values is that the apparent linear relationship between Do_2 and Vo_2 has been questioned because both share variables, and this *mathematical coupling* can produce artifactual relationships between variables.[21,24,33,34] The Do_2 and Vo_2 indexed parameters are calculated as follows:

$$Do_2 = CI \times Cao_2$$

$$Vo_2 = CI \times (Cao_2 - Cvo_2)$$

where CI is the cardiac index, Cao_2 is the arterial oxygen content determined by hemoglobin concentration and Sao_2, and Cvo_2 is the mixed venous oxygen content determined by hemoglobin concentration and Svo_2.

However, variable relationships between Do_2 and Vo_2 are observed when Vo_2 is measured independently by indirect calorimetry. Therefore, a linear relationship between Do_2 and Vo_2 may be the result of mathematical coupling or flow-dependent Vo_2. Currently available data do not support the concept that patient outcome or survival is improved by treatment measures directed toward achieving supranormal Do_2 and Vo_2 values.[35] In fact, a consensus conference concluded that although pulmonary artery catheterization is useful for guiding therapy, routinely increasing cardiac index to predetermined supranormal values does not improve outcome.[7] Furthermore, achievement of a supranormal Do_2 does not ensure parallel improvements in regional organ blood flow and oxygenation. One approach that may decrease the effect of mathematical coupling and provide individualized therapy may lie in titrated therapy, with sequential measurements of Do_2 and Vo_2 to achieve Vo_2 flow independency along with normalization of blood lactate and hemodynamic parameters.

❷ The most recent data regarding goal-directed therapy in the hemodynamic support of sepsis relates to the importance of achieving predetermined parameters early in the management of sepsis.[36] In a meta-analysis of early (defined as 8 to 12 hours postoperatively or before the development of organ failure) versus late (defined as after the onset of organ failure) resuscitative efforts targeting supranormal oxygen-transport variables, early goal-directed therapy reduced mortality and the development of organ failure in patients who were more severely ill when therapeutic interventions produced differences in Do_2.[36] Survival outcome was not improved significantly in less severely ill patients (control group mortality <15% and normal Do_2 values as goals) or when therapy did not improve Do_2.

❷ ❻ The rapid initiation of therapy to optimize the components of Do_2 (CO, hemoglobin, and Sao_2) improves survival. In a prospective, randomized controlled trial, Rivers et al. demonstrated a significant reduction in mortality (30.5% vs. 46.5%; $P < 0.001$) in patients with severe sepsis and septic shock randomized to receive therapy based on goal-directed hemodynamic end points that were achieved within 6 hours of hospital presentation.[32] They used a strategy of serial administering (a) fluids rapidly to achieve CVP 8 to 12 mm Hg, (b) vasopressor agents to achieve MAP at least 65 mm Hg, (c) red blood cell transfusion to maintain hematocrit ≥30%, and (d) dobutamine to achieve $Scvo_2$ ≥70%. During the 6-hour window, the goal-directed therapy group received substantially more fluid, blood transfusions, and dobutamine administration but required less vasopressor and ventilator support later. This approach demonstrates the benefits of initiating therapy early in the course of sepsis and directs therapy toward clearly defined goals of optimizing Do_2 in a consistent manner. The results of several evaluations of protocols or order sets designed to achieve the hemodynamic end points of early goal-directed therapy show that implementation is easily accomplished, cost is reduced, and patient outcomes, including survival, are improved.[37–43] A meta-analysis of nine studies showed reduced mortality when quantitative resuscitation goals are used to guide therapy (odds ratio [OR] 0.64; 95% confidence interval [CI]: 0.43 to 0.96; $P = 0.03$).[43] Therefore, healthcare facilities should implement strategies to achieve early goal-directed therapy using the predefined hemodynamic variables of the study by Rivers et al.[32]

Clinical Controversy...

GOALS OF EARLY GOAL-DIRECTED THERAPY

The results of studies cannot delineate which end point or combination of end points was most beneficial with respect to early goal-directed therapy. These studies also offer limited information about specific interventions to achieve the predefined goals. In addition, whether these goals must be maintained after resuscitation is unknown. Several studies are ongoing to address some of these issues. Current practice should rapidly target all the parameters of early goal-directed therapy by employing a protocol.

Blood Lactate

3 Lactate is a metabolic product of pyruvate. Its production is increased under anaerobic conditions when Vo_2 exceeds Do_2, such as may occur during shock.[21,24,33,34] Blood lactate concentrations are used as a diagnostic and prognostic tool in sepsis; they also are used to measure the repayment of oxygen debt to tissues.[15–21] Several studies have demonstrated risk stratification of mortality rates based on initial lactate concentrations.[44,45] Serial lactate concentrations may show better correlation with outcome than oxygen transport parameters and may be superior to hemodynamic markers in determining adequacy of restoration of systemic oxygenation. Continuously elevated concentrations are predictive of morbidity and mortality. Maintaining lactate elimination (commonly termed "clearance") of 10% for 6 hours during initial resuscitation produces similar survival outcomes as achieving $Scvo_2 \geq 70\%$.[46] The utility of blood lactate measurements in guiding therapy was recently demonstrated in a study of 348 septic patients that showed targeting a 20% lactate reduction during the first 2 hours of resuscitation reduced hospital mortality compared to conventional assessment methods (hazard ratio [HR], 0.61; 95% CI: 0.43 to 0.87; $P = 0.006$).[47]

Several caveats guide the use of lactate concentrations in septic patients. First, lactate may accumulate in patients with other conditions, such as significant hepatic dysfunction or acute respiratory distress syndrome, who are not in shock. Second, both well-perfused and poorly perfused tissues contribute to arterial and mixed venous lactate concentrations and therefore are not reflective of regional perfusion. Third, elevated lactate concentrations may result from cellular metabolic failure rather than global hypoperfusion in shock.

Clinical Controversy...

Svo_2 or $Scvo_2$ versus lactate

The goal of resuscitation is to reverse tissue hypoxia by facilitating Do_2. Both Svo_2 OR $Scvo_2$ and lactate clearance measure global tissue perfusion. Limited data are available comparing the use of Svo_2 or $Scvo_2$ and lactate clearance for guiding therapy in patients with shock. The results of a recent study of critically ill septic patients suggest that they are equivalent in terms of clinical outcomes, including mortality.[47] The decision to use one parameter over the other will depend on clinician preference and patient characteristics.

REGIONAL PERFUSION MONITORING

GI Tonometry

Blood pressures, CO, blood lactate, and global oxygen homeostasis parameters do not offer information about the function of individual organs. Organ-specific hypoxia may be evident by coagulopathy as indicated by thrombocytopenia (platelet count <100,000/L and/or prolonged clotting times [international normalized ratio >1.5 or activated partial thromboplastin time at least 1.5-fold the upper limit of normal]), impaired renal function with urine production <0.5 mL/kg/h and/or increased serum concentrations of blood urea nitrogen and creatinine, altered hepatic function with substantially increased serum concentrations of transaminases and bilirubin, altered GI perfusion manifested by ileus and diminished bowel sounds, cardiac ischemia with elevated troponin levels and electrocardiogram changes, and altered sensorium.[6,22] Objective measurement of regional perfusion to detect inadequate tissue oxygenation has focused on the mesenteric/splanchnic circulation, which is sensitive to changes in blood flow and oxygenation for several reasons.[15–20,34,48] Normally, most blood flow to the gut mucosa is redistributed toward the serosa and muscularis. Second, the gut may have a higher critical Do_2 threshold than other organs. Third, the tip of the villus has a countercurrent oxygen-exchange mechanism, rendering it highly sensitive to alterations in regional blood flow and oxygenation.

3 Gastric tonometry measures gut luminal partial pressure of carbon dioxide (Pco_2) at equilibrium by placing a saline- or air-filled gas-permeable balloon in the gastric lumen. Assuming that carbon dioxide (Co_2) permeates freely among tissues and that the arterial bicarbonate (HCO_3^-) concentration is equal to that of the gut mucosa, the intramucosal pH (pHi) may be calculated using the Henderson–Hasselbalch equation:

$$pHi = 6.1 \log (HCO_3^-)\ 0.03 \times Pco_2$$

Increases in mucosal Pco_2 and calculated decreases in pHi are associated with mucosal hypoperfusion and perhaps increased mortality.[15–20,34,48] Calculation of pHi can be confounded by increases in luminal Pco_2, such as may occur when buffering antacids are used. Histamine$_2$-receptor antagonists or proton pump inhibitors can be used instead. The presence of respiratory acid–base disorders; systemic bicarbonate administration; arterial blood gas measurement errors; or enteral feeding products, blood, or stool in the gut may confound pHi determinations. As a result, the change in gastric mucosal Pco_2 may be more accurate than pHi. Furthermore, because mucosal Pco_2 is influenced by arterial Pco_2, the mucosal–arterial Pco_2 difference (Pco_2 gap) likely is the optimal measurement.[15–20,34,48] Gastric tonometry can be performed using either a saline- or air-filled balloon. The time delay (30 minutes) associated with equilibration of saline inside the balloon makes this method impractical for monitoring of resuscitation and inconvenient for routine bedside monitoring. An air-filled balloon requires a shorter equilibrium time, is simpler to use, and is equally accurate. However, the clinical utility of gastric tonometry remains uncertain. Clinical trials of pHi-directed therapy do not show that it aids resuscitation when other goals are concomitantly targeted. Gastric tonometry, in general, inconsistently predicts mortality.

3 Evidence suggests that the most proximal part of the GI tract, the sublingual mucosa, may be an acceptable location for monitoring regional perfusion and Pco_2.[15–20,34,48] Unlike GI circulation, limited intra- and interpatient variability exists in the microvasculature and only few arterioles are available for assessment. Sublingual capnometry is noninvasive, is not technically complex, and provides results within minutes. The device consists of a disposable sublingual carbon dioxide pressure ($Pslco_2$) sensor, a fiberoptic cable that connects the disposable sensor to a blood gas analyzer, and a blood gas monitoring instrument. Small studies of critically ill patients with and without sepsis and septic shock show that the $Pslco_2$ and the sublingual-to-arterial Pco_2 gap correlate better with the enhancement of Do_2 with dobutamine than the mucosal Pco_2 and the mucosal-to-arterial Pco_2 gap.[15–20,34,48] The initial sublingual-to-arterial

P_{CO_2} gap is a better predictor of mortality. These pilot studies must be expanded before this technology becomes part of routine practice, but it offers the possibility of noninvasive measurement of regional perfusion. Of note, some institutions have incorporated the P_{slCO_2} into their algorithms of early goal-directed therapy in an effort to provide additional information about the effectiveness of therapies during resuscitation.

Myocardial Dysfunction

1 Although loss of vascular tone is the hallmark of septic shock, myocardial dysfunction characterized by transient impairment of contractility is a recognized complication.[5,49] The range of left ventricular ejection fraction (LVEF) upon presentation is wide, but approximately 35% of patients with septic shock have left ventricular hypokinesis (mean ejection fraction 38% ± 17%) and low CO.[5,49] Because LVEF also is affected by preload and afterload, the low SVR of septic shock may mask depressed myocardial contractility that may be revealed upon restoration of MAP by administration of fluid and vasopressors. Therefore, CO may not reflect the extent of myocardial dysfunction. While it requires technical and interpretive training, echocardiography is a relatively simple method of assessing cardiac function and ventricular response to therapies.[50] It can assess chamber size, ventricular contractility, valve function, blood flow, and CO. Patients with tissue hypoxia or a hypercontractile left ventricle may benefit from fluid administration or vasopressor therapy; whereas, patients with poor left ventricular function may require inotropic intervention. Like sublingual capnometry, some institutions use echocardiography to direct resuscitation therapies.

Cardiac troponin release in septic patients occurs in the absence of flow-limiting disease, likely due to a loss in membrane integrity with subsequent leakage or microvascular thrombosis. Elevation of cardiac troponin concentrations in patients with sepsis indicates left ventricular dysfunction and portends a poor prognosis.[49–51] Troponin concentrations also correlate with the duration of hypotension and the intensity of vasopressor therapy. Early recognition of myocardial dysfunction is crucial for administration of appropriate therapy. In the absence of other mechanisms for assessing cardiac function, echocardiographic findings and troponin concentrations may help guide and monitor therapy. Whereas cardiac troponins may be integrated into the monitoring of myocardial dysfunction to identify patients requiring aggressive therapy, natriuretic peptides show variable correlation with LVEF and should not be routinely monitored.[49–51]

VASOPRESSORS AND INOTROPES

6 Vasopressors and inotropes in patients with septic shock are required when volume resuscitation fails to maintain adequate blood pressure (MAP ≥65 mm Hg) and organs and tissues remain hypoperfused despite optimizing CVP to 8 to 12 mm Hg or PAOP to 12 to 15 mm Hg.[6] However, vasopressors may be needed temporarily to treat life-threatening hypotension when filling pressures are inadequate despite aggressive fluid resuscitation. Inotropes are frequently used to optimize cardiac function in cases of cardiogenic shock. The clinician must decide on the choice of agent, therapeutic end points, and safe and effective doses of vasopressors and inotropes to be used. This section reviews adrenergic receptor pharmacology, exogenous catecholamine use, and alterations in receptor function in critically ill patients. It also provides guidelines for the clinical use of adrenergic agents, optimization of pharmacotherapeutic outcomes, and minimization of adverse effects in critically ill patients with septic shock. Therapies of hypovolemic shock and cardiogenic shock are discussed in other chapters.

Of note, agents other than catecholamines have been used as inotropes and vasopressors in shock states. They include phosphodiesterase III inhibitors, naloxone, nitric oxide (NO) synthase (NOS) inhibitors, and calcium sensitizers. This chapter focuses on catecholamines. Vasopressin and corticosteroids, as they relate to septic shock, also are emphasized because they have pharmacologic interactions with catecholamines, possess hemodynamic effects, and are frequently used.

Catecholamine Receptor Pharmacology

5 Comparative receptor activities of endogenous and exogenously administered catecholamines are summarized in Table 13-3.[6–15,52–54] Endogenous catecholamines are responsible for regulation of

TABLE 13-3 Adrenergic, Dopaminergic, and Vasopressin Receptor Pharmacology, and Organ Distribution

Effector Organ	Receptor Subtype	Physiologic Response
Heart		
Sinoatrial node	β_1, β_2	Increased heart rate
Atria	β_1, β_2	Increased contractility Increased conduction velocity
Atrioventricular node	β_1, β_2	Increased automaticity Increased conduction velocity
His-Purkinje system	β_1, β_2	Increased automaticity Increased conduction velocity
Ventricles	β_1, β_2	Increased contractility Increased conduction velocity Increased automaticity Increased rate idioventricular pacemaker cells
Arterioles		
Coronary	$\alpha_1, \alpha_2, V_1; \beta_2, D_1, V_2$ (via NO)	Constriction; dilation
Skin and mucosa	α_1, α_2, V_1	Constriction
Skeletal muscle	$\alpha_1, V_1; \beta_2$	Constriction; dilation
Cerebral	$\alpha_1, V_1; V_2$ (via NO)	Constriction (slight); dilation
Pulmonary	$\alpha_1; \beta_2, V_2$ (via NO)	Constriction; dilation
Abdominal viscera (mesentery)	$\alpha_1, V_1; \beta_2, D_1$	Constriction; dilation
Renal	$\alpha_1, \alpha_2, V_1; \beta_1, \beta_2, D_1$	Constriction; dilation
Veins (systemic)	$\alpha_1, \alpha_2; \beta_2$	Constriction; dilation
Lungs		
Tracheal/bronchial smooth muscle	β_2	Relaxation
Bronchial glands	$\alpha_1; \beta_2$	Decreased; increased secretion
Stomach		
Motility and tone	$\alpha_1, \alpha_2, \beta_1, \beta_2$	Decreased (usually)
Sphincter	α_1	Contraction (usually)
Secretions	α_2	Inhibition
Intestine		
Motility and tone	$\alpha_1, \alpha_2, \beta_1, \beta_2; V_1$	Decreased (usually); increased?
Sphincters	α_1	Contraction
Secretions	α_2	Inhibition
Kidney		
Renin secretion	$\alpha_1; \beta_1$	Decreased; increased
Reabsorption of water	V_2	Increased
Skeletal muscle	β_2	Increased contractility, glyconeogenesis, K^+ uptake
Liver	α_1, β_2	Glycogenolysis and gluconeogenesis
Fat cells	$\alpha_1, \beta_1, \beta_2$	Lipolysis (thermogenesis)

D, dopamine; NO, nitric oxide; V, vasopressin.

Based on data from references 6–15, 52, 53.

vascular and bronchiolar smooth muscle tone and myocardial contractility. These effects are mediated by sympathetic adrenergic receptors of the autonomic nervous system located in the vasculature, myocardium, and bronchioles. Postsynaptic adrenoceptors are located at or near the synaptic junction. These receptors can be activated by naturally circulating or exogenous catecholamines (e.g., norepinephrine, epinephrine, and phenylephrine), whereas presynaptic adrenoceptors are stimulated by locally released neurotransmitters (e.g., norepinephrine) and are controlled by a negative feedback mechanism.

The signal transduction pathways associated with catecholamine and vasopressin-induced effects in the heart and blood vessels are illustrated in Figure 13-1.[6–15,52–54] Agonists of β-adrenoceptors and dopamine (D_1) receptors stimulate adenylate cyclase by a G-protein (G_s)-dependent mechanism (Fig. 13-1, top). Adenylate cyclase generates cyclic adenosine monophosphate (cAMP) from adenosine triphosphate (ATP). cAMP-dependent protein kinase A, which is activated by elevations in intracellular cAMP, phosphorylates target proteins to modify cellular function. Through these mechanisms, β_1-adrenoceptor activation exerts positive inotropic and chronotropic effects in the heart, and β_2-adrenoceptor and D_1-receptor activation induces vascular smooth muscle relaxation. Agonists of α_1-adrenoceptors stimulate phospholipase C-β (PLC-β) through a G-protein (G_q)-dependent process (Fig. 13-1, bottom). PLC-β produces inositol trisphosphate and diacylglycerol from cell membrane phosphatidylinositol bisphosphate. Diacylglycerol activates protein kinase C, an enzyme that phosphorylates several key proteins (e.g., extracellular signal-regulated kinases, c-Jun NH2-terminal kinases, and mitogen-activated protein kinases) that modify cellular function (e.g., hypertrophy). Inositol trisphosphate elicits the release of calcium from intracellular stores, such as the sarcoplasmic reticulum. Calcium forms a complex with calmodulin, which then activates calcium–calmodulin-dependent protein kinases (CaMK). CaMKs phosphorylate target proteins to alter cellular function. Myosin light-chain kinase is an example of a CaMK. Its action

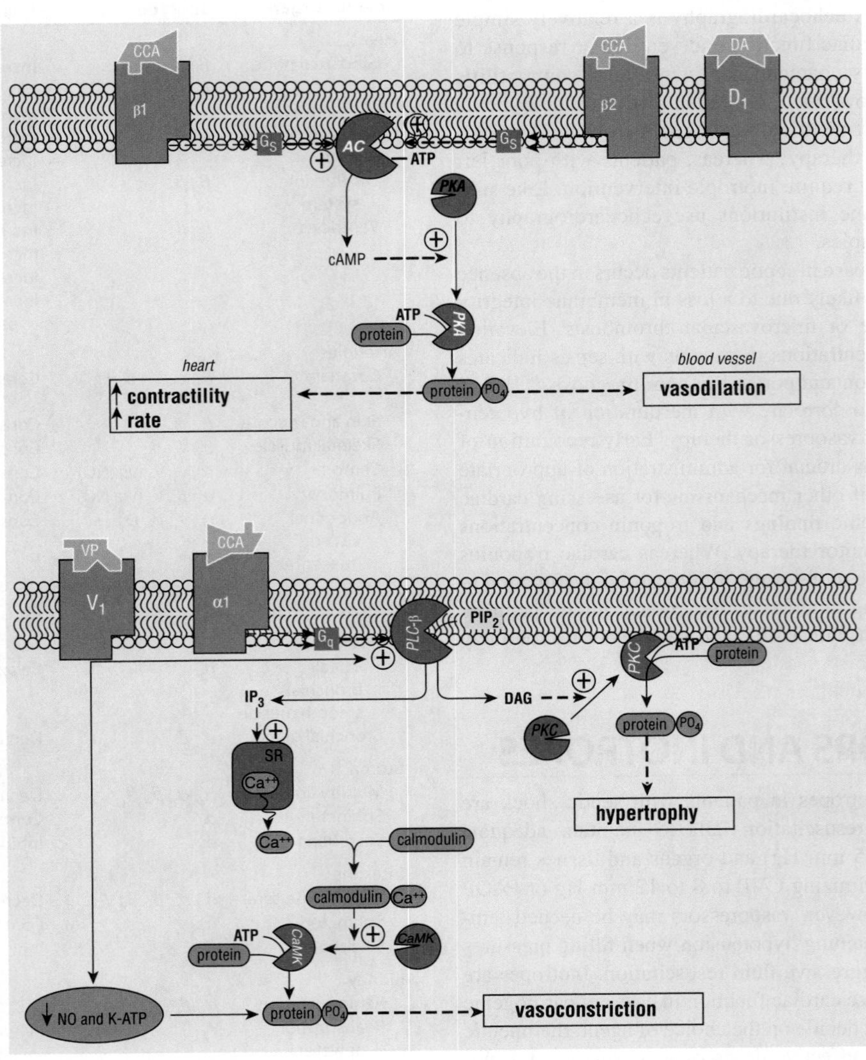

FIGURE 13-1 Signal transduction pathways in heart and blood vessels. *Top*: Catecholamine (CCA)-induced effects mediated in heart (β_1) or vascular smooth muscle (β_2, D_1). (AC, adenylate cyclase; ATP, adenosine triphosphate; cAMP, cyclic adenosine monophosphate; PKA, cAMP-dependent protein kinase; +, stimulation.) *Bottom*: CCA (α_1) and vasopressin (VP)-induced actions in vascular smooth muscle. (Ca^{++}, calcium ion; CaMK, calcium/calmodulin-dependent protein kinase; DAG, diacylglycerol; IP_3, inositol trisphosphate; NO, nitric oxide; PIP_2, phosphatidylinositol bisphosphate; PKC, protein kinase C; PLC-β, phospholipase C-β; SR, sarcoplasmic reticulum.) These pathways have been extensively simplified, and denoted cellular effects represent one of many produced. *(Figure based on data from references 6–15, 52–54.)*

of phosphorylating myosin light chain leads to vascular smooth muscle contraction.

The normal heart contains primarily postsynaptic β_1-receptors, which when stimulated cause increased rate and force of contraction. This effect is mediated by activation of adenylate cyclase and subsequent generation and accumulation of cAMP. Stimulation of postsynaptic cardiac α_1-receptors causes a significant increase in contractility without an increase in rate, an effect mediated by PLC rather than adenylate cyclase. The increased contractility is more pronounced at lower heart rates and has a slower onset and longer duration in comparison with β_1-mediated inotropic response. Presynaptic α_2-adrenoceptors also are found in the heart and appear to be activated by norepinephrine released by the sympathetic nerve itself. Their activation inhibits further norepinephrine release from the nerve terminal.

Both presynaptic and postsynaptic adrenoceptors are present in the vasculature. Postsynaptic α_1- and α_2-receptors mediate vasoconstriction, whereas postsynaptic β_2-receptors induce vasodilation. Presynaptic α_2-receptors inhibit norepinephrine release in the vasculature, also promoting vasodilation. Presynaptic β_1-adrenoceptors promote neurotransmitter release. Stimulation of peripheral D_1-receptors produces renal, coronary, and mesenteric vasodilation and a natriuretic response. Stimulation of D_2-receptors inhibits norepinephrine release from sympathetic nerve endings, sequesters prolactin and aldosterone, and may induce nausea and vomiting. D_1- and D_2-receptor stimulation also suppresses peristalsis and may precipitate ileus.

5 Vasopressin-induced vasoconstriction occurs through a variety of direct and indirect mechanisms.[52,53] Stimulation of vascular vasopressin $(V)_1$ receptors causes vasoconstriction by receptor-coupled activation of PLC and calcium release from intracellular stores via secondary messengers similar to α_1-adrenergic stimulation (Fig. 13-1, bottom). Vasopressin also directly inhibits vascular potassium-sensitive ATP channels to produce vasoconstriction (Fig. 13-1, bottom). V_1-receptor stimulation inhibits the actions of IL-1β and thereby facilitates vasoconstriction. Vasopressin also increases the activity of adrenergic receptors. The greatest vasoconstriction occurs in the skin and soft tissue, skeletal muscle, fat tissue, pancreas, and thyroid gland. In contrast, vasopressin causes vasodilation in the cerebral, pulmonary, coronary, and selected renal vascular beds by enhancing endothelial NO release through V_1-receptor stimulation in these tissues.[52–54] Vasopressin has minimal to no inotropic or chronotropic effects.

V_2 receptors located in the kidneys are responsible for the antidiuretic properties of vasopressin.[52–54] Stimulation of V_2 receptors facilitates integration of aquaporins into the luminal cell membrane of distal tubules and collecting duct capillaries to increase permeability and thus retain intravascular volume. However, vasopressin stimulation of V_1 receptors causes vasoconstriction of efferent arterioles and relative vasodilation of afferent arterioles to increase glomerular perfusion pressure and filtration rate to enhance urine production.

Vasopressin rapidly increases serum cortisol concentration by stimulating V_3 receptors in the pituitary gland to enhance the release of adrenocorticotropic hormone (ACTH).[52–54] Cortisol helps regulate the proinflammatory state associated with sepsis and increases blood pressure through several mechanisms, including inhibition of inducible nitric oxide synthase (iNOS) to reduce NO production, reversal of adrenergic receptor desensitization, and increased intravascular volume through retention of sodium and water.

Altered Adrenoceptor Function: Implications for Critically Ill Patients

4 Most of the work describing receptor function and associated clinical pharmacology has been performed in either animal models or human volunteers. In critically ill septic patients, derangements in adrenergic receptor activity may result in resistance to exogenously administered catecholamine.[6–15,52,53] This "desensitization" frequently is characterized by myocardial and vascular hyporesponsiveness to high dosages of inotropes and vasopressor agents. Prolonged exposure of vascular endothelial tissue to vasopressor drugs (α-adrenergic agonists) or endogenous catecholamines may promote additional receptor downregulation. Increased endogenous catecholamine concentrations have been reported in endotoxemic and other critically ill patients, suggesting an acquired adrenergic receptor defect and desensitization of adrenergic receptors and alteration in voltage-sensitive calcium channels. The problem in critically ill patients may be related to decreased receptor activity or density. However, in patients with septic shock, catecholamine concentrations are even higher, so abnormalities in adrenergic receptor function are greater, with associated reductions in the concentrations of intracellular signal transduction mediators. The worsened receptor abnormality may be explained by defects distal to the receptor site, such as uncoupling of adrenergic receptors from adenylate cyclase or PLC, or dysfunction in the regulatory G-protein unit of signal transduction pathways.

In addition to catecholamines, circulating inflammatory cytokines may be partly responsible for distal alterations.[52,53] Macrophage-derived IL-1 and TNF-α produce impaired coupling of β-adrenoceptors to adenylate cyclase. Patients with septic shock exhibit impaired β-adrenergic receptor stimulation of cAMP associated with myocardial hyporesponsiveness to various vasopressors and inotropes. However, increased chronotropic sensitivity to β-adrenergic stimulation with hypersensitivity of the adenylate cyclase system to isoproterenol stimulation also has been reported in animal models of bacteremia and endotoxemia. In the presence of intrinsic myocardial dysfunction and increased metabolic demands, this dysfunctional adrenergic system is incapable of mobilizing functional cardiac reserve to maintain adequate myocardial performance.[49,52,53]

IL-1 and TNF-α suppress gene expression of α_1-adrenoceptors, resulting in fewer receptor proteins. Overproduction of NO by iNOS directly contributes to vasodilation by cyclic guanosine monophosphate-mediated smooth muscle relaxation. NO indirectly produces vasodilation by combining with superoxide to form peroxynitrite, a highly toxic reactive species that causes endothelial dysfunction, uncoupling of α_1-adrenoceptors to PLC, and deactivation of catecholamines. The result of sepsis-induced inflammation is a system that promotes adrenergic receptor dysfunction to accentuate vasodilation and shock.[6–15,49,52,53]

5 Functional α_1-adrenergic receptor changes occur at various stages of sepsis; thus, adrenoceptor sensitivity may be time dependent during progression of sepsis to septic shock. The findings are not always consistent in various animal models of sepsis and in critically ill septic patients. Time-dependent alterations in the production of NO, a potent vasodilator, may explain the apparent differences in vascular reactivity to phenylephrine during the phases of endotoxemia. This finding suggests that the clinical response to vasopressors and possibly inotropic agents is variable during the stages of hemodynamic, myocardial, and peripheral vascular derangements of septic shock. β-adrenergic receptor changes are present within 24 to 48 hours of septic shock. In summary, α- and β-adrenergic receptor derangements may vary among patients and during each bacteremic insult; therefore, doses of catecholamines vary among patients and during the insult.[6–15,52,53] For these reasons, these drugs should be dosed to clinical end points and not to arbitrary maximal doses. High dosages are frequently required.

Relative Deficiencies of Vasopressin and Cortisol

14 Endogenous arginine vasopressin, a peptide hormone also known as antidiuretic hormone, is important for osmoregulation

under normal physiologic conditions. Vasopressin is produced in the hypothalamus, stored in the posterior pituitary, and released from magnocellular neurons of the hypothalamus.[54] Increased serum osmolality and hypovolemia are the major stimuli for vasopressin release.[54] Other stimuli commonly associated with shock are dopamine, histamine, angiotensin II, prostaglandins, pain, hypoxia, acidosis, hypotension, hypercarbia, and α_1-adrenergic receptor stimulation. Vasopressin release is inhibited by NO, natriuretic peptides, γ-aminobutyric acid, β-adrenergic receptor stimulation, and α_2-adrenergic receptor stimulation.[54]

Normal serum vasopressin concentrations are <4 pg/mL.[54] Serum vasopressin concentrations are elevated with hypotension. Vasopressin response in septic shock is biphasic. During the first 8 hours of septic shock requiring catecholamine adrenergic therapy, serum concentrations of vasopressin are appropriately high to help maintain blood pressure and organ perfusion. Thereafter, serum vasopressin concentrations decline dramatically over the next 96 hours to physiologically normal but inappropriately low values, resulting in a state of "relative deficiency." In contrast, serum vasopressin concentrations remain elevated in patients with cardiogenic shock. Administration of vasopressin at 0.01 to 0.06 units/min produces concentrations similar to those observed in early septic shock and other hypotensive states; however, vasopressin concentrations do not correlate with blood pressure.[54] Administration of vasopressin improves arterial pressure while minimizing the dose of catecholamine vasopressors.[54]

The mechanism of vasopressin insufficiency in septic shock is not well understood. Neurohypophyseal stores in the posterior lobe of the pituitary gland are depleted during septic shock, likely as a result of excessive and continuous baroreceptor stimulation that eventually exhausts the limited vasopressin secretory stores. In addition, secretion of vasopressin is inhibited by enhanced endothelial production of NO, high circulating concentrations of adrenergic agonists (both endogenous and exogenous), and tonic inhibition by stretch receptors in response to volume replacement and mechanical ventilation.[54]

14 As with vasopressin, during sepsis a state of "relative adrenal insufficiency" is produced by continuous activation of the hypothalamic–pituitary–adrenal axis by IL-1, IL-6, and TNF-α that causes depletion of cortisol in the adrenal glands.[55] Administration of corticosteroids improves arterial pressure while minimizing the dose of catecholamine vasopressors.[56,57] Current proposed mechanisms of the vasoconstrictor effect of corticosteroids include increasing the number and stimulating the function of α_1- and β-adrenergic receptors and attenuating the production of inflammatory mediators responsible for vasodilation.

The use of corticosteroids for treatment of septic shock has been a topic of controversy for many years. Meta-analyses of early studies of steroids in patients with sepsis demonstrated a lack of benefit and potential harm in sepsis and septic shock.[56,57] Interest in corticosteroid use is renewed because of the increased awareness of adrenocortical insufficiency in critically ill patients with septic shock.[55] Relative adrenal insufficiency has been defined as a random cortisol concentration <10 mcg/dL (278 nmol/L) or an increase of <9 mcg/dL (250 nmol/L) following a dose of synthetic ACTH irrespective of the initial serum cortisol concentration.[58] Although absolute insufficiency is rare, relative adrenocortical insufficiency is present in 50% to 70% of patients with septic shock and is associated with a poor outcome.[59–62]

An elevated random cortisol concentration (>34 mcg/dL) is an independent predictor of mortality.[58] Mortality is further increased if ACTH response is <9 mcg/dL, suggesting that the risk of mortality is greatest in situations of adrenal gland "fatigue" (i.e., degree of stress is not matched by sufficient cortisol production by the adrenal glands despite operating at maximal functional capacity).

Clinical Pharmacology of Vasopressors and Inotropes

5 14 The receptor selectivity of clinically used, catecholamine-based vasopressors and inotropes and hemodynamic effects are listed in Table 13-4.[6–15,52–54,63,64] In general, these drugs are fast acting, with short durations of action. As such, these drugs are given as continuous infusions and titrated rapidly to predetermined effects.[6] Vasopressin is administered as a replacement dosage of 0.01 to 0.04 units/min and should not be titrated.[54] Careful monitoring and calculation of infusion rates are advised for all vasopressors because dosing adjustments are made frequently, and varying admixtures and concentrations are used in volume-restricted patients.

TABLE 13-4 Receptor Pharmacology and Adverse Events of Selected Inotropic and Vasopressor Agents Used in Septic Shock[a]

Agent (Adverse Events)	α_1	α_2	β_1	β_2	D	V_1	V_2
Dobutamine (0.5–4 mg/mL D_5W or NS)	Tachycardia, dysrhythmias, hypotension						
2–10 mcg/kg/min	+	0	++++	++	0	0	0
>10–20 mcg/kg/min	++	0	++++	+++	0	0	0
Dopamine (0.8–3.2 mg/mL D_5W or NS)	Tachycardia, dysrhythmias, decreased Pao_2, mesenteric hypoperfusion, GI motility inhibition, T-cell inhibition						
1–3 mcg/kg/min	0	0	+	0	++++	0	0
3–10 mcg/kg/min	0/+	0	++++	+	++++	0	0
>10–20 mcg/kg/min	+++	0	++++	+	0	0	0
Epinephrine (0.008–0.016 mg/mL D_5W or NS)	Tachycardia, dysrhythmias, decreased Pao_2, mesenteric hypoperfusion, increased lactate, hyperglycemia, immunomodulation						
0.01–0.05 mcg/kg/min	++	++	++++	+++	0	0	0
0.05–3 mcg/kg/min	++++	++++	+++	+	0	0	0
Norepinephrine (0.016–0.064 mg/mL D_5W)	Mixed effects on myocardial performance and mesenteric perfusion, peripheral ischemia						
0.02–3 mcg/kg/min	+++	+++	+++	+/++	0	0	0
Phenylephrine (0.1–0.4 mg/mL D_5W or NS)	Mixed effects on myocardial performance, peripheral ischemia						
0.5–9 mcg/kg/min	+++	+	+	0	0	0	0
Vasopressin (0.8 units/mL D_5W or NS)	Mixed effects on myocardial performance, mesenteric hypoperfusion, peripheral ischemia, hyponatremia, thrombocytopenia						
0.01–0.04 units/min	0	0	0	0	0	+++	+++

D, dopamine; D_5W, dextrose 5% in water; NS, normal saline; Pao_2, arterial oxygen pressure; V, vasopressin.

[a]Activity ranges from no activity (0) to maximal (++++) activity.

Based on data from references 6–15, 52–54, 63, and 64.

9 Norepinephrine is a combined α- and β-agonist that produces vasoconstriction primarily via its more prominent α-effects on all vascular beds, thus increasing SVR.[6–15,52,53,63,64] Norepinephrine administration generally produces either no change or some increase in CO. Norepinephrine is considered the first-line option for initial vasopressor therapy of septic shock.[6]

10 Phenylephrine is a pure α_1-agonist and increases blood pressure through vasoconstriction.[6–15,52,53,63,64] Given the presence of cardiac α_1-receptors, phenylephrine also may increase contractility and CO although no change or a slight reduction in CO is often observed. It is a therapeutic option in hypotensive patients experiencing a tachyarrhythmia when a vasopressor with minimal to no β_1-agonist activity is indicated.[6]

11 Epinephrine exerts combined α- and β-agonist effects.[6–15,52,53,63,64] At the high epinephrine infusion rates used for patients with septic shock, predominantly α-adrenergic effects are observed, and SVR and MAP are increased. While epinephrine traditionally has been reserved as the vasopressor of last resort due to peripheral vasoconstriction, particularly in the splanchnic and renal beds, it is considered second-line therapy according to the current guidelines.[6] It is widely used in other countries where other agents may not be readily available or are relatively expensive.

9 Dopamine has been described as having dose-related receptor activity at D_1-, D_2-, β_1-, and α_1-receptors (Table 13-4).[6–15,52,53,63,64] This dose–response relationship has not been confirmed in critically ill patients. In patients with septic shock, great overlap of hemodynamic effects occur, even at dosages as low as 3 mcg/kg/min. Tachydysrhythmias are common due to the release of endogenous norepinephrine by dopamine entering the sympathetic nerve terminal. For this reason, it is no longer considered first-line therapy for septic shock.[6] Dopamine may increase PAOP through pulmonary vasoconstriction. This drug also may depress ventilation and worsen hypoxemia in patients dependent on the hypoxic ventilatory drive.

12 Dobutamine, a synthetic catecholamine, is primarily a selective β_1-agonist with mild β_2- and vascular α_1-activity, resulting in strong positive inotropic activity without concomitant vasoconstriction.[6–15,52,53,63,64] In comparison with dopamine, dobutamine produces a larger increase in CO and is less arrhythmogenic. α_1-Adrenoceptors in the heart are directly stimulated by the (–) isomer of dobutamine, but β_1 and β_2 activity resides in the (+) isomer. The strong inotropic action of dobutamine is a function of its structure, the additive effect of cardiac α_1- and β_1-agonist activity, and a relatively weak chronotropic effect limited to the (+) isomer action on the β-receptors. Clinically, β_2-induced vasodilation and the increased myocardial contractility with subsequent reflex reduction in sympathetic tone lead to a decrease in SVR. Dobutamine is used optimally for patients in low CO states with high filling pressures (e.g., CI <3 L/min/m^2, left ventricular dysfunction demonstrated with echocardiography, or $Scvo_2$ <70%) or in those in cardiogenic shock; however, vasopressors may be needed to counteract arterial vasodilation.[6,32]

14 Unlike adrenergic receptor agonists, the vasoconstrictive effects of vasopressin are preserved during hypoxia and severe acidosis. Initiating vasopressin at ≤0.04 units/min in patients with septic shock increases SVR and arterial blood pressure to reduce the dose requirements of catecholamine adrenergic agents.[54,63–66] These effects are rapid and sustained. Organ-specific vasodilation reduces pulmonary artery pressure and may preserve cardiac and renal function. It may enhance urine production, likely due to increased glomerular filtration rate.[54,67] At dosages exceeding 0.04 units/min, however, vasopressin is associated with ischemia of the mesenteric mucosa, skin, and myocardium. Limiting the dosage to a maximum of 0.04 units/min may minimize the development of these adverse effects. At present, vasopressin is not recommended as a replacement for norepinephrine in patients with septic shock but may be considered as adjunctive therapy in patients who are refractory to catecholamine vasopressors despite adequate fluid resuscitation.[6] If used, vasopressin should be administered at dosages not exceeding 0.04 units/min.[6,54,65]

Desired Outcomes and Clinical Application

Resuscitation Goals of Septic Shock

6 7 9 Initial hemodynamic therapy for septic shock is the administration of IV fluid (30 mL/kg of crystalloid fluid), with the goal of attaining CVP of 8 to 12 mm Hg or 15 mm Hg in mechanically ventilated patients or patients with abdominal distension or preexisting ventricular dysfunction.[6–15] Crystalloid fluids (e.g., normal saline, Ringer lactate) and colloid fluids (e.g., albumin, hydroxyethyl starch, dextran products, blood products) are considered equivalent for shock resuscitation.[6,68–70] Crystalloid fluids are generally preferred unless patients are at risk for adverse events from redistribution of IV fluids to extravascular tissues and/or are fluid restricted (e.g., patients with renal dysfunction, decompensated heart failure, ascites compromising diaphragmatic function).[6] Recent data suggest hydroxyethyl starch may increase the risk of acute renal dysfunction in a dose-dependent manner and possibly enhance mortality.[71,72] Its use warrants extreme caution and consideration of a dose threshold.

8 Norepinephrine is the preferred initial vasopressor agent in septic shock not responding to fluid administration.[6] Other agents include phenylephrine, epinephrine, dopamine, and dobutamine. Optimizing MAP to 65 mm Hg as the goal of vasopressor therapy does not uniformly correlate with decreased mortality in patients with septic shock but global perfusion may be improved.[15–21] Historically, significant concerns about the adverse effects of vasopressors limited their use. The past focus of achieving supranormal oxygen-transport variables also yielded poor results in patients with septic shock.[35] In fact, normalization of systemic Do_2 and Vo_2, whether spontaneously or with intervention, is associated with improved outcome and is not dependent on administration of vasopressor agents.[35] Part of the inability to detect an improvement with vasopressor or inotropic therapies may result from the limited ability to quantify regional tissue perfusion. However, use of early goal-directed therapy to MAP ≥65 mm Hg and $Scvo_2$ ≥70% reduces mortality in patients with sepsis and septic shock.[32]

6 7 9 10 11 12 13 Dosage titration and monitoring of vasopressor and inotropic therapy should be guided by the "best clinical response," the goals of early goal-directed therapy, and lactate clearance.[6–21,32] Norepinephrine is considered the agent of choice as initial vasopressor therapy.[6] Epinephrine may be added in cases where suboptimal hemodynamic response is obtained from to norepinephrine.[6] Phenylephrine may be tried as the initial vasopressor in cases of severe tachydysrhythmias.[6] Dobutamine is used in states of low CO states despite adequate fluid resuscitation pressures (e.g., CI <3 L/min/m^2, left ventricular dysfunction demonstrated with echocardiography, or $Scvo_2$ <70%). Low dosage rates are initiated and titrated rapidly (usually every 5 to 15 minutes) to clinical response. Clinically effective dosing of vasopressors and inotropes in septic shock often requires doses much higher than recommended by most references.[6–21] These large infusion rates must be tempered with the development of adverse effects. The goal is to use the lowest effective infusion rate while minimizing evidence of myocardial ischemia (e.g., tachydysrhythmias, electrocardiographic changes, troponin elevations), renal (decreased glomerular filtration rate and/or urine output), splanchnic/gastric (low pHi, bowel ischemia), or peripheral (cold extremities) hypoperfusion, and worsening Pao_2, PAOP, and other hemodynamic variables.

14 Vasopressin may be considered as adjunctive therapy in patients who are refractory to catecholamine vasopressors despite adequate fluid resuscitation.[6] Dosages of ≤0.04 units/min increase

SVR and arterial blood pressure to reduce the dose requirements of catecholamine adrenergic agents.[54,63–66]

13 Therapy with catecholamine vasopressors and inotropes is continued until myocardial depression and vascular hyporesponsiveness (i.e., blood pressure) of septic shock improve, usually measured in hours to days.[6] Discontinuation of vasopressor or inotropic therapy should be executed slowly; therapy should be "weaned" to avoid a precipitous worsening in regional and systemic hemodynamics. Careful monitoring of global and regional end points also should be geared toward discontinuation of vasopressors and inotropes as soon as the patient is hemodynamically stable. This requires constant observation. Because vasopressors and inotropes often are started while the patient is not yet optimally volume resuscitated, clinicians should reevaluate intravascular volume status continuously so that the patient can be weaned from the vasopressor as soon as possible. Dosage rates should be titrated carefully downward approximately every 10 minutes to determine if the patient can tolerate gradual withdrawal and eventual discontinuation of the vasopressor and/or inotrope. Discontinuation of agents may occur only minutes to hours after their initiation, or it may take days to weeks. Septic shock requiring vasopressor and/or inotropic support usually resolves within several days to 1 week.

Comparative Studies of Catecholamine Vasopressors

7 9 The results of several observational and randomized studies support norepinephrine as the first-line vasopressor for septic shock.[6] A recent meta-analysis of 11 trials ($N = 2768$) showed dopamine was associated with increased risk of death (RR, 1.23; 95% CI: 1.05 to 1.43; $P < 0.01$) compared to norepinephrine.[63] Tachydysrhythmias were more common with dopamine (RR, 2.34; 95% CI: 1.46 to 3.77; $P = 0.001$). The results of two recent studies contribute to the majority of data. The first randomized 1,679 patients with shock unresponsive to volume resuscitation to norepinephrine or dopamine and found similar 28-day mortality rates (48.5% vs. 52.5% of patients; $P = 0.10$) although death from refractory shock tended to occur less frequently with norepinephrine (41% vs. 46%; $P = 0.05$).[73] The mortality rate was significantly lower in the subgroup of 280 patients with cardiogenic shock that received norepinephrine ($P = 0.03$). Overall, patients receiving norepinephrine had fewer arrhythmic events (12.4% vs. 24.2%; $P < 0.001$) despite using dobutamine more frequently, had more vasopressor-free days, and were less likely to require open-label vasopressor support (20% vs. 26%; $P < 0.001$). Limitations of this landmark study include combining heterogeneous shock etiologies (cardiogenic, septic, hypovolemic, and other), the use of a relatively conservative definition of "shock unresponsive to fluid administration" (only 1 L of crystalloid or 0.5 L of colloid), the use of open-label norepinephrine in patients with inadequate hemodynamic response to study drug regimens, and the lack of standardization of other shock therapies that affect hemodynamic variables (e.g., corticosteroids, vasopressin, dobutamine, additional fluid administration). Another recent study randomized 252 septic shock patients found statistically similar 28-day mortality rates between norepinephrine and dopamine (43% vs. 50%; $P = 0.282$).[74] Similar to the aforementioned study, arrhythmic events were less likely to occur with norepinephrine (5.3% vs. 23.3%; $P < 0.0001$).

7 9 11 Two randomized, double-blind studies compared epinephrine with norepinephrine in 330 and 280 patients with septic shock, respectively.[75,76] Both studies found similar 28-day mortality rates with epinephrine and norepinephrine (40% vs. 31%; $P = 0.31$; and 22.5% vs. 26.1%; $P = 0.48$). Time to hemodynamic recovery and vasopressor withdrawal were also similar between agents in both studies. One study found more events of tachydysrhythmias with epinephrine leading to study discontinuation.[75] Both studies also showed that epinephrine was associated with lower arterial pH values and higher serum lactate concentrations over the first days of therapy, possibly demonstrating deleterious circulation, exaggerated glycolysis, or mobilization of lactate with epinephrine. These findings support the use of epinephrine in septic shock but it is considered second-line therapy due to its association with impaired lactate clearance.[6]

Vasopressin

14 Small studies of septic shock patients demonstrate that initial therapy with vasopressin achieves blood pressure control as effectively as traditional catecholamine vasopressors but the response is delayed.[54] Therefore, vasopressin therapy should not be initiated as first-line therapy. Several small studies showed that adjunctive vasopressin therapy reduces the dose requirements of catecholamine vasopressors and maintains blood pressure to expedite the discontinuation of catecholamine vasopressors.[54] A recent meta-analysis of 10 trials ($N = 1{,}134$) confirmed a negative correlation between vasopressin and norepinephrine dosages.[66] Some studies document enhancement of urine production.[54,67] The results of a randomized, double-blind study of 776 patients with septic shock requiring catecholamine vasopressors showed that 28-day mortality rates were similar when vasopressin 0.01 to 0.03 units/min or norepinephrine 5 to 15 mcg/min was added to traditional catecholamine therapy (35.4% vs. 39.3%; $P = 0.26$).[65] A trend toward reduced 28-day mortality favored vasopressin in the subset of patients categorized as having less severe septic shock defined by a baseline norepinephrine requirement of <15 mcg/min (26.5% vs. 35.7%; $P = 0.05$). This trend was evident when sepsis severity was defined by lactate quartiles or number of organ failures, suggesting that adjunctive vasopressin may be most beneficial when it is started prior to escalation of therapy with catecholamine vasopressors. Post hoc analyses demonstrated greatest benefit with early vasopressin treatment relative to the onset of shock. The adverse event profiles were similar between groups. Of note, vasopressin therapy expedited the discontinuation of catecholamine vasopressors in all patients and helped preserve renal function in patients with acutely declining urine production as defined by the injury (doubling of serum creatinine concentration, glomerular filtration rate reduced by half, or urine production less than 0.5 mL/kg/h) category of Risk, Injury, Failure, loss, End-stage renal disease (RIFLE).[67] Whereas V_2 stimulation promotes water retention from the distal tubules and collecting ducts, V_1 receptors cause vasoconstriction of efferent arterioles and relative vasodilation of afferent arterioles to increase glomerular perfusion pressure and filtration rate, enhancing urine production. In the studies reporting benefit on renal function, the maximum dosage used was 0.08 units/min.[54] Use of vasopressin for preventing dose escalation of adrenergic agents should be considered, but the risks must be weighed prior to initiating therapy. At present, vasopressin should not be used for the sole purpose of improving or maintaining renal function.[6]

Clinical **Controversy...**

Epinephrine or vasopressin

Current guidelines suggest epinephrine or vasopressin may be added to norepinephrine but do not delineate which agent is preferred or when this should occur with respect to resuscitation goals.[6] Adding epinephrine may worsen lactate clearance while adding vasopressin may enhance the occurrence of ischemic events to digits. Both agents may worsen splanchnic circulation.

Corticosteroids

14 Since two meta-analyses reported in 1995 increased mortality with corticosteroids,[56,57] several randomized controlled trials

of low-dose corticosteroids in vasopressor-dependent septic shock patients have been published.[58–62] These studies use moderate physiologic dosages (200 to 300 mg/day) of hydrocortisone. A meta-analysis of five studies ($N = 465$) showed that steroid therapy was associated with an overall improvement in the survival rate (RR, 1.23; 95% CI: 1.01 to 1.50; $P = 0.036$) and shock reversal (RR, 1.71; 95% CI: 1.29 to 2.26; $P < 0.001$).[59] These effects were beneficial in both responders and nonresponders to ACTH stimulation testing. These studies also showed that low-dose corticosteroid administration improves hemodynamics and reduces the duration of vasopressor support. All of these studies differ from earlier studies in that steroids were administered at lower total doses (hydrocortisone equivalents: 1,209 mg vs. 23,975 mg; $P = 0.01$) starting later in septic shock (23 hours vs. <2 hours; $P = 0.02$) for longer courses (6 days vs. 1 day; $P = 0.01$) to patients with higher control group mortality rates (mean, 57% vs. 34%; $P = 0.06$) who were more likely to be vasopressor dependent (100% vs. 65%; $P = 0.03$). The relationship between corticosteroid dose and survival was linear, with survival benefit at low doses ($P = 0.02$). Another meta-analysis of 17 trials ($N = 2,138$) found similar results with long-term administration of corticosteroids associated with lower mortality in hospital (RR, 0.83; 95% CI: 0.68 to 1; $P = 0.05$) and at 28 days (RR, 0.84; 95% CI: 0.71 to 1; $P = 0.05$), reduced ICU stay by 4.49 days (95% CI: −7.04 to −1.95; $P < 0.001$), and greater shock reversal at 28 days (RR, 1.12; 95% CI, 1.02 to 1.23; $P = 0.02$).[60] The rates of GI bleeding, super infections, and neuromuscular weakness were similar.

14 The results of these meta-analyses are heavily driven by data supplied by two, somewhat discordant, studies.[61,62] The first randomized 300 patients with septic shock within 8 hours of hypotension to placebo or a daily combination of hydrocortisone 50 mg IV every 6 hours and fludrocortisone 0.05 mg enterally for 7 days.[61] Similar to the meta-analyses, use of hydrocortisone reduced 28-day mortality (OR, 0.65; 95% CI: 0.39 to 1.07; $P = 0.09$), but all the benefit was seen in patients with adrenal insufficiency (OR, 0.54; 95% CI: 0.31 to 0.97; $P = 0.04$). The placebo group was more likely to continually require vasopressor therapy (HR, 1.54; 95% CI: 1.10 to 12.16; $P = 0.01$), but differences between groups were exhibited only in patients with adrenal insufficiency (HR, 1.91; 95% CI: 1.29 to 2.84; $P = 0.001$). Approximately 77% of patients were deemed adrenally insufficient. The second study randomized 499 of 800 intended subjects with severe sepsis or shock within 72 hours of presentation to placebo or hydrocortisone 50 mg IV every 6 hours for 5 days followed by a 6-day taper.[62] Mortality rates were similar between groups (32% vs. 34%), irrespective of adrenal function. Median time to shock reversal was shorter in patients receiving corticosteroid therapy (3.3 vs. 5.8 days; $P < 0.001$), again irrespective of adrenal function. Reversal of organ dysfunction was also expedited with corticosteroid therapy. Unlike the previous study, however, only 47% of patients demonstrated adrenal insufficiency likely reflective of the entry criteria and lower overall mortality rate of the study population.

Clinical **Controversy...**

Corticosteroid therapy

Current guidelines do not suggest assessing adrenal function to determine the need for corticosteroid therapy.[6] Instead, they recommend initiating corticosteroids when hemodynamic goals are not achieved with fluid resuscitation or vasopressor therapy. This is controversial given the limitations and differences between studies and the difficulty of determining the adequate achievement of hemodynamic goals in patients requiring vasopressor therapy.

14 A post hoc analysis of the large vasopressin study revealed a significant interaction between vasopressin and corticosteroids.[77] In patients receiving vasopressin therapy, concurrent corticosteroid administration increased vasopressin concentrations by 33% to 67% over the initial 24 hours compared with patients only receiving vasopressin. The addition of corticosteroids to vasopressin was associated with reduced mortality compared with concurrent administration of corticosteroids and norepinephrine (35.9% vs. 44.7%; $P = 0.03$). In the absence of corticosteroid therapy, however, mortality was greater with vasopressin therapy compared with norepinephrine (33.7% vs. 21.3%; $P = 0.06$). Similar results were reported in a retrospective, matched assessment that found lower 7-day mortality was associated with combination therapy compared with vasopressin alone (19.1% vs. 52.4%; $P = 0.02$).[78] This interaction warrants further investigation in studies.

Hemodynamic Considerations and Adverse Effects

5 7 9 10 11 Catecholamine vasopressors may result in adverse peripheral vasoconstrictive, metabolic, and dysrhythmogenic effects that limit or outweigh their positive effects on the central circulation.[6–15,52,53] Table 13-4 lists potential adverse effects of commonly used vasopressors and inotropes.[6–15,52,53] Excessive peripheral vasoconstriction may cause ischemia or necrosis of already poorly perfused tissues such as the skin and the mesenteric and splanchnic circulations. Some of these profound vasoconstrictive effects have been compounded by the concurrent use of other vasopressor agents in patients with septic shock who are significantly hypovolemic. These agents may be used in the context of late septic shock, where hypotension is refractory to less selective vasoconstrictors (e.g., dopamine) such that very large doses of norepinephrine or epinephrine or phenylephrine are required but provide little or no benefit. Myocardial ischemia and dysrhythmias may occur in patients with coronary artery disease, atherosclerosis, cardiomyopathies, left ventricular hypertrophy, congestive heart failure, or underlying dysrhythmias because of their inability to tolerate β_1 cardiac stimulation that mediates increases in CO. However, the effect usually is opposite in healthy myocardium and in young patients. β_1 cardiac stimulation is well tolerated, ventricular filling pressures decrease, and CO and Do_2 increase, with a resulting increase in peripheral perfusion. The dysrhythmogenic potential of the catecholamine vasopressors includes a variety of resulting atrial and ventricular arrhythmias. Norepinephrine, phenylephrine, and especially epinephrine can produce lactic acidosis secondary to excessive constriction in peripheral arterioles or enhanced glycogenolysis, or as a result of mobilization of lactate from peripheral tissues as a result of improved oxygenation. Sympathomimetic vasopressors also have been found to possess immunomodulatory actions, primarily mediated by β_2-adrenergic actions (e.g., epinephrine) because almost all immune cells express this receptor. The actions include down regulating the expression of proinflammatory cytokines such as TNF-α by neutrophils, suppression of oxygen free radical production from neutrophils, and direct proapoptotic effects. Dopamine suppresses prolactin secretion from the anterior pituitary gland, which may lead to reduced T-cell responsiveness. These effects may be either beneficial or deleterious by dampening harmful effects of oxygen free radical-mediated tissue injury or by reducing neutrophilic defense against bacteria.

Vasopressor catecholamines have the potential to cause extravasation-associated tissue damage if infusions infiltrate during peripheral administration. In the event of infiltration, an α-receptor antagonist such as phentolamine (10 mg in 10 mL saline) should be injected intradermally to reverse local vasoconstriction, with administration of vasopressor drugs into a large central vein.

Norepinephrine

7 8 9 13 Norepinephrine is the first-line therapy for septic shock as it effectively increases MAP.[6–15,52,53,73–76] It has combined strong α_1-activity and less potent β_1-agonist effects while maintaining weak vasodilatory effects of β_2-receptor stimulation.[6–19,49,50,68–76] Several studies have demonstrated improved MAP and mortality in ICU patients with severe hypotension treated with norepinephrine either as first-line therapy or after therapeutic failure with fluid resuscitation treatment.[63,73–76]

Norepinephrine infusions are initiated at 0.05 to 0.1 mcg/kg/min and rapidly titrated to preset goals of MAP (usually at least 65 mm Hg), improvement in peripheral perfusion (to restore urine production or decrease blood lactate), and/or achievement of desired oxygen-transport variables while not compromising the cardiac index. Norepinephrine 0.01 to 2 mcg/kg/min reliably and predictably improves hemodynamic parameters to "normal" values in most patients with septic shock. As with other vasopressors, norepinephrine dosages exceeding those recommended by most references frequently are needed in critically ill patients with septic shock to achieve predetermined goals. A significant increase in MAP generally is caused by an increase in SVR. Heart rate generally does not increase significantly with norepinephrine because of diminished stimulation of cardiac β_1-receptors in septic shock and reflex bradycardia from increased SVR.[6–15,52,53,73–76] Increasing norepinephrine doses to maintain higher MAPs may increase heart rates, cardiac index, Do_2, and cutaneous blood flow but these results are inconsistent. Older patients may benefit from the combined α- and β-adrenergic effects of norepinephrine given the higher incidence of coronary disease and compromised ventricles in this patient population. By virtue of restored MAP and hence coronary perfusion, cardiac index is increased in older patients, whereas in younger patients with less coronary artery disease and a higher cardiac index at baseline, norepinephrine acts primarily as a vasopressor. Norepinephrine does not influence PAOP.

The effect of norepinephrine on oxygen transport parameters is variable and depends on baseline values and concurrently administered vasoactive agents. In most studies of norepinephrine alone, either an increase or no change in Do_2 is seen with no change in O_2ER, particularly when Do_2 values were "supranormal" prior to therapy. Norepinephrine demonstrates either no effect or improvement in Pco_2 gap, pHi, or serum lactate concentrations. Splanchnic blood flow and fractional blood flow are higher with norepinephrine than either dopamine or epinephrine despite higher CO with the two latter agents.

Taken together, these data suggest that norepinephrine should be the primary vasopressor of choice in patients in septic shock because of its multiple benefits: (a) norepinephrine may decrease mortality in septic shock; (b) it reverses inappropriate vasodilation and low global oxygen extraction; (c) it attenuates myocardial depression at unchanged or increased CO and increased coronary blood flow; (d) it improves renal perfusion pressure and renal filtration; (e) it enhances splanchnic perfusion; and (f) it is less likely than other vasopressors to cause tachycardias and tachydysrhythmias.[6–15,52,53,73–76] The primary limitation to use is that norepinephrine is not available as premixed ready-to-use solutions so use requires preparation time.

Phenylephrine

7 8 10 13 Despite its purported use in refractory septic shock, little information is available regarding the clinical efficacy of phenylephrine. Nevertheless, it is an attractive agent for use in sepsis because of its selective α-agonism with primarily vascular effects.[6–15,52,53] As with other vasopressors, phenylephrine dosages required to achieve goals of therapy are significantly higher than dosages traditionally recommended for use.

Phenylephrine 0.5 to 9 mcg/kg/min, used alone or in combination with dobutamine or low doses of dopamine, improves blood pressure and myocardial performance in fluid-resuscitated septic patients. Incremental doses of phenylephrine result in linear dose-related increases in MAP, SVR, heart rate, and stroke index when administered alone as a single agent in stable, nonhypotensive but hyperdynamic, volume-resuscitated surgical ICU patients. In septic shock, phenylephrine does not impair the cardiac index, PAOP, or peripheral perfusion. In sepsis, phenylephrine improves MAP by increasing the cardiac index through enhanced venous return to the heart (increase in CVP and stroke index) and by acting as a positive inotrope. It improves myocardial performance in hyperdynamic, normotensive septic patients but worsens myocardial performance in cardiac controls. In cardiac patients, myocardial performance worsens as a result of a decrease in the cardiac index and an increase in SVR. Therefore, phenylephrine use warrants caution in septic shock patients with impaired myocardial performance.

In septic shock, phenylephrine appears to increase global tissue oxygen use, although data regarding the relationship of the oxygen-transport variables with increases in MAP and cardiac index are conflicting. Increases in Vo_2 appear to be dissociated from Do_2, representing an increase in O_2ER as the cardiac index remains unchanged. Increases in Vo_2 may result from redistribution of blood flow to previously underperfused areas, improving oxygen use as a result of changes in MAP and SVR. Evidence of globally improved peripheral tissue perfusion is observed as lactic acid concentration declines or remains unchanged and urine production increases significantly at increased or maximal Vo_2. An increased O_2ER may contribute to improved tissue response.

Few data regarding the effect of phenylephrine on regional hemodynamics and oxygen-transport variables are available. When phenylephrine replaced norepinephrine in patients with septic shock, phenylephrine selectively reduced splanchnic blood flow and thus splanchnic Do_2 and splanchnic lactate uptake rate without changing the overall splanchnic Vo_2. Concomitantly, pHi decreased and arterial lactate concentrations increased. Because all of these parameters normalized when norepinephrine was reinstated, these data suggest that exogenous β-adrenergic stimulation (norepinephrine) may determine hepatosplanchnic perfusion and oxygen availability but not utilization in septic shock. Phenylephrine and norepinephrine demonstrate similar hemodynamic profiles and indices of global and regional perfusion.[6–15]

The available data on hemodynamics, oxygen-transport variables, and mortality with phenylephrine in septic shock patients may not be generalizable because of the small numbers of patients evaluated. Adverse effects, such as tachydysrhythmias, are notably infrequent with phenylephrine, particularly when it is used as a single agent or at higher doses, because phenylephrine does not exert any activity on β_1-adrenergic receptors. Whether the beneficial effects can be sustained with longer administrations of phenylephrine is unclear. Phenylephrine may be a particularly useful alternative in patients who cannot tolerate tachycardia or tachydysrhythmias with use of dopamine or norepinephrine and in patients who are refractory to dopamine or norepinephrine (because of β-adrenergic receptor desensitization).[6] Its use in patients with myocardial dysfunction warrants further investigation. Like norepinephrine, it is not available as premixed ready-to-use solutions.

Epinephrine

7 8 11 13 Epinephrine is an acceptable choice for hemodynamic support of septic shock because of its combined vasoconstrictor and inotropic effects but it is associated with tachydysrhythmias and lactate elevation.[75,76] As a result, it is considered an alternative agent.[6] It is as effective as norepinephrine for blood pressure control. Epinephrine infusion rates of 0.04 to 1 mcg/kg/min alone increase

hemodynamic and oxygen-transport variables to "supranormal" values without adverse effects in septic patients without coronary artery disease. Large dosages (0.5 to 3 mcg/kg/min) often are required. Smaller dosages (0.10 to 0.50 mcg/kg/min) are effective when epinephrine is added to other vasopressors and inotropes. In addition, younger patients appear to respond better to epinephrine, possibly due to greater β-adrenergic reactivity.

Despite a linear dose–response curve with rapid improvement of hemodynamic variables and Do_2, epinephrine has deleterious effects on regional hemodynamics and oxygen utilization. Although Do_2 increases mainly as a function of increases in the cardiac index and a more variable increase in SVR, Vo_2 may not increase, and O_2ER may fall. A fall in pHi may be seen during epinephrine administration but the impairment in gastric mucosal perfusion can be counteracted in part by dobutamine. This may be explained by the vasodilatory effect of dobutamine on gastric mucosal microcirculation resulting in a redistribution of blood flow toward the mucosa. In contrast to other vasopressors, lactate concentrations frequently rise during epinephrine therapy resulting in variable arterial pH values. When compared with a combination of norepinephrine and dobutamine, epinephrine preferentially decreases splanchnic Do_2, worsens pHi, and increases systemic lactate concentration without increasing Vo_2. The effects of epinephrine on absolute and fractional splanchnic blood flow are more pronounced during severe shock. The increase in lactate may be a result of worsened Do_2 to the liver (and subsequent anaerobic metabolism) or to the hepatosplanchnic circulation, a direct increase in calorigenesis and breakdown of glycogen, or lactate mobilization. However, evidence suggests that epinephrine, in contrast to dopamine, increases the proportion of total CO delivered to the splanchnic circulation, although Vo_2 is not increased sufficiently. As a result, O_2ER values are usually lower with epinephrine than with other vasopressors but the concomitant administration of dobutamine helps maintain O_2ER. Of all the vasopressors, epinephrine exhibits the most pronounced capacity to induce hyperglycemia by increased gluconeogenesis and glycogenolysis with α-mediated suppression of insulin secretion.[52,53]

Despite the administration of high doses, epinephrine-associated clinically important dysrhythmias or cardiac ischemia occur at variable rates irrespective of age or underlying cardiac status.[6–15,52,53,75,76] Nevertheless, caution must be exercised before considering epinephrine for managing hypoperfusion in hypodynamic patients with coronary artery disease, in whom ischemia, chest pain, or myocardial infarction may result. Based on the current evidence, epinephrine should not be used as initial therapy in patients with septic shock refractory to fluid administration.[6] Although it effectively increases CO and Do_2, it has deleterious effects on the splanchnic circulation. If it is used as a second-line agent in septic shock, factors that may influence successful therapy with epinephrine include the time from onset of septic shock to effective therapy, the age of the population, and the selection of concurrent vasopressors and inotropes. Like norepinephrine and phenylephrine, it is not available as premixed ready-to-use solutions.

Dopamine

7 8 9 13 Dopamine is a natural precursor to norepinephrine and epinephrine and generally not as effective as these two agents for achieving goal MAP in patients with septic shock.[6–15,52,53,73,74] Most studies of patients with septic shock have shown that dopamine at dosages of 5 to 10 mcg/kg/min increase the cardiac index by improving contractility and heart rate, primarily from its β_1 effects. It increases MAP and SVR as a result of both increased CO and, at higher doses (>10 mcg/kg/min), its α_1 effects.

The clinical utility of dopamine as a vasopressor in the setting of septic shock is limited because large dosages are frequently necessary to maintain CO and MAP. At dosages exceeding 20 mcg/kg/min, further improvement in cardiac performance and regional hemodynamics is limited. Its clinical use frequently is hampered by tachycardia and tachydysrhythmias, which may lead to myocardial ischemia. Although tachydysrhythmias theoretically should not be expected to occur until administration of dopamine 5 to 10 mcg/kg/min, these β_1 effects are observed with dosages as low as 3 mcg/kg/min. They seem to be more prevalent in patients who are inadequately resuscitated (hypovolemic), in the elderly, in those with preexisting or concurrent cardiac ischemia or dysrhythmias, and in patients currently receiving other dysrhythmogenic agents, including vasopressors and inotropes.

Dopamine increases PAOP and pulmonary shunting to decrease Pao_2. The increase in PAOP may be due to changes in diastolic volumes from decreased cardiac compliance or increased venous return to the heart by α-adrenergic receptor-mediated venoconstriction. This may affect gas exchange and decrease Pao_2. The increase in pulmonary shunting also may result from acute enhancement of pulmonary blood flow to nonhomogeneous lung regions. Thus, dopamine should be used with caution in patients with elevated preload because the drug may worsen pulmonary edema. In the instance of high filling pressures, tachycardia, or tachydysrhythmias, dopamine should be replaced by another vasopressor and/or inotrope such as norepinephrine, dobutamine, phenylephrine, or epinephrine, depending on the desired effect.

The effect of dopamine on global oxygen-transport variables parallels the hemodynamic effects. Although dopamine improves global Do_2 in septic patients, it may compromise O_2ER in the splanchnic and mesenteric circulations by α_1-mediated vasoconstriction. Splanchnic blood flow and Do_2 increase with dopamine, but with no preferential increase in splanchnic perfusion as a fraction of CO and systemic increases in Do_2. Large doses of dopamine worsen pHi and the Pco_2 gap. This is reflected by a decrease or lack of change in regional Vo_2 and a decrease in tissue O_2ER. Dopamine at low or vasopressor dosages directly impedes gastric motility in critical illness and may aggravate gut ischemia in septic shock. Similar to high-dose administration, low-dose dopamine increases splanchnic blood flow but lowers splanchnic Vo_2 in sepsis. Therefore, dopamine at all dosages impairs hepatosplanchnic metabolism despite an increase in regional perfusion. Low dosages increase renal blood flow and glomerular filtration rate in studies of animals and healthy volunteers but did not demonstrate improved renal function in a randomized, placebo-controlled study of 328 critically ill patients with early renal dysfunction.[79] A meta-analysis of 61 trials ($N = 3359$) confirmed that low-dose dopamine fails to enhance renal function or survival in critically ill patients.[80]

While dopamine may improve hemodynamic function, the use of dopamine for septic shock is questionable because regional hemodynamics, oxygen-transport variables, and functional parameters of improved organ perfusion are not consistently enhanced in a sustained manner and may be negatively impaired.[6] The negative findings of low-dose dopamine use and the deleterious effects of inotropic and vasopressor dosages of dopamine on regional hemodynamics, oxygen transport, and functional performance of organ perfusion raise concern over whether dopamine should be considered in patients with severe sepsis or septic shock.[6,79] Unlike other vasopressor agents, however, dopamine is available as premixed ready-to-use solutions of various concentrations that can be stored in automated dispensing systems for rapid initiation.

Dobutamine

6 7 12 13 Dobutamine is an inotrope with vasodilatory properties (an "inodilator").[6–15,52,53] It is used for treatment of septic and cardiogenic shock to increase the cardiac index, typically by 25% to 50%.[6] In septic shock, LVEF and right ventricular function are depressed despite a high cardiac index, whereas ventricular volumes and compliance are increased. Stroke index is maintained by

an increased heart rate and ventricular dilation. In survivors, myocardial depression is reversible and normalizes 5 to 10 days after the onset of sepsis. Dobutamine increases stroke index, left ventricular stroke work index, and thus cardiac index and Do_2 without increasing PAOP.[6–15] The ability of dobutamine to enhance cardiac index and Do_2 during septic shock appears to be related to its chronotropic effect. However, dosage increments of dobutamine beyond 20 mcg/kg/min are limited by complications of tachycardia, ischemic changes on electrocardiogram, hypertension, and tachydysrhythmias despite the absence of preexisting cardiac abnormalities. The combination of dobutamine and norepinephrine results in a lower increase in heart rate compared with use of other vasopressors alone.

Increased cardiac performance measures in response to adjunctive dobutamine therapy are predictive of survival during sepsis. However, the achievement of supranormal oxygen transport values with dobutamine is of little value compared with treatment to normal values. In addition, administration of dobutamine to achieve these high values may increase the mortality rate and/or the incidence of adverse effects. Dobutamine increases Do_2 without affecting Vo_2, resulting in decreased O_2ER. Arterial lactate concentrations decrease significantly with norepinephrine and dobutamine compared with dopamine and epinephrine infusions.

Studies have focused on the effects of dobutamine on gastric mucosal flow and the splanchnic circulation. The addition of dobutamine to other vasopressors improves gastric mucosal perfusion without increasing the cardiac index. This is consistent with findings that dobutamine may improve pHi and mucosal perfusion in septic patients. The addition of dobutamine to norepinephrine or epinephrine treatment improves gastric mucosal perfusion as measured by improvements in pHi and Pco_2 gap. This effect may relate to blood flow redistribution toward gastric mucosa, due to either an increase in the fraction of CO distributed to the global hepatosplanchnic blood flow and/or a redistribution of blood flow within gastric wall layers toward the mucosa by "stealing" blood away from the muscularis potentially as a result of greater β_2-mediated vasodilation. Sublingual microcirculation improves after dobutamine is added to vasopressor-dependent septic shock patients in a manner unrelated to arterial pressure or cardiac index, suggesting that enhanced perfusion is the result of the "steal" phenomenon. Of note, gastric mucosal perfusion and tissue oxygen utilization are most improved with concurrent norepinephrine and dobutamine therapies compared with other vasopressor combinations at the same level of MAP.

Dobutamine should be started at dosages ranging from 2.5 to 5 mcg/kg/min. In the study of early goal-directed therapy, dobutamine was administered to 13.7% of patients within 6 hours of resuscitation to achieve $Scvo_2$ ≥70%.[32] Although a dose response may be seen, evidence now suggests that dosages >5 mcg/kg/min may provide limited beneficial effects on oxygen transport values and hemodynamics and may increase adverse cardiac effects. If given to patients who are intravascularly depleted, dobutamine will result in hypotension and a reflexive tachycardia. Pathophysiologic factors influence dosing requirements and pharmacokinetic parameters over the time course of the illness and the duration of the infusion. Decreases in Pao_2, as well as myocardial adverse effects such as tachycardia, ischemic changes on electrocardiogram, tachydysrhythmias, and hypotension are seen. Thus, infusion rates should be guided by clinical end points and Svo_2/$Scvo_2$ or lactate clearance. Dobutamine, like other inotropes, usually is given until improvement in myocardial function with resolution of the septic episode or dose-limiting side effects are observed. Dobutamine is available as premixed ready-to-use solutions.

Vasopressin

14 Studies involving vasopressin infusion for management of septic shock show rapid and sustained improvement in hemodynamic parameters.[54,65,66] These effects are evident with administration of dosages not exceeding 0.04 units/min. Administration of dosages >0.04 units/min are associated with negative changes in CO and mesenteric mucosal perfusion. The reduction in CO likely is the result of lowered stroke volume.[54] The studies that reported cardiac function indicate patients had adequate CO prior to initiating vasopressin therapy. Therefore, vasopressin use in septic shock patients with cardiac dysfunction warrants extreme caution. Cardiac ischemia appears to be a rare occurrence and may be related to administration of dosages ≥0.05 units/min.

Mesenteric ischemia associated with vasopressin may be clinically relevant. Increased hepatic transaminases and total bilirubin concentrations may occur with vasopressin therapy, suggesting impaired hepatic blood flow or a direct effect on excretory hepatic function.[54] Most studies have found that vasopressin at dosages of 0.04 to 1.8 units/min worsen pHi or Pco_2 gap when it is added to low or high doses of catecholamine vasopressors.[54] Mesenteric mucosal hypoperfusion may be expected with vasopressin because mesenteric vasoconstriction occurs at vasopressin serum concentrations as low as 10 pg/dL, and the effect is dose dependent. Of concern is the additive effective with norepinephrine despite substantially reduced dosages of norepinephrine when vasopressin is initiated. Although controversial, the degree of hypoperfusion with vasopressin may be greater than with norepinephrine alone unless the dose of norepinephrine is markedly increased to maintain adequate arterial blood pressure.

Vasopressin's strongest vasoconstrictive action occurs in the skin and soft tissues, skeletal muscles, and fat tissues.[54] As a result, ischemic skin lesions have been observed in several studies, with an occurrence rate as high as 30% after vasopressin was added to norepinephrine-resistant shock.[54,60] Although vasopressin may have deleterious effects on mesenteric and skin perfusion, studies report vasodilation of cerebral, pulmonary, coronary, and some renal vasculature beds. The clinical outcomes associated with selective vasodilation are not yet determined except for the possibility of enhanced urine production in patients not anuric at baseline.[67]

In order to minimize the potential for adverse events and maximize the beneficial effects, vasopressin should be used as add-on therapy to one or two catecholamine adrenergic agents rather than as first-line therapy or salvage therapy and dosages should be limited to 0.04 units/min.[6,54] The results of studies showed that vasopressin markedly reduced the requirements for adrenergic agents, but few studies demonstrated complete discontinuation of these therapies.[54,65,66] Therefore, vasopressin should be used only if response to one or two adrenergic agents is inadequate or as a method for reducing the dosage of these therapies.[6] Increased arterial pressure should be evident within the first hour of vasopressin therapy, at which time the dose(s) of adrenergic agent(s) should be reduced while maintaining goal MAP. This method should help limit the degree of ischemia.

Most studies evaluated vasopressin use for <48 hours, and several studies reported difficulty discontinuing vasopressin therapy. Whether additional benefits, deleterious effects, or tolerance is observed with longer infusions remains unclear. Long-term administration of vasopressin is associated with hyponatremia and thrombocytopenia. Because vasopressin is being used to replace a physiologic deficiency, it stands to reason that the requirement for vasopressin will subside with reversal of the septic process. Attempts to discontinue vasopressin should occur when the dosage(s) of adrenergic agent(s) has been minimized (e.g., dopamine ≤5 mcg/kg/min, norepinephrine ≤0.1 mcg/kg/min, phenylephrine ≤1 mcg/kg/min, and epinephrine ≤0.15 mcg/kg/min). At present, vasopressin should not be initiated as first-line therapy or added to existing therapy solely because a patient is septic. Vasopressin is not available as premixed ready-to-use solutions.

Corticosteroids

14 Corticosteroids can be initiated in cases of septic shock when adrenal insufficiency is suspected (e.g., patients receiving long-term corticosteroid therapy for other indications prior to the onset of shock), when vasopressor dosages are escalating, or when weaning of vasopressor therapy proves futile.[55–62] Assessment of adrenal function to guide therapy is no longer recommended.[6] Adverse events are few because corticosteroids are administered for a finite period of time, usually 7 days. Acutely, elevated serum concentrations of blood urea nitrogen, white blood cell count, and glucose occur. Although long-term administration of corticosteroids is associated with several chronic disease states, meta-analyses do not show an increase in adverse events, including GI hemorrhage (RR, 1.12; 95% CI: 0.81 to 1.53; $P = 0.5$), superinfections (RR, 1.01; 95% CI: 0.82 to 1.25; $P = 0.92$), and neuromuscular weakness (RR, 0.63; 95% CI: 0.12 to 3.35; $P = 0.58$).[59,60] Hyperglycemia (RR, 1.16; 95% CI: 1.07 to 1.25; $P < 0.001$) and hypernatremia (RR, 1.61; 95% CI: 1.26 to 2.06; $P < 0.001$) are associated with corticosteroid therapy.[59,60] Therefore, therapy of septic shock with corticosteroids improves hemodynamic variables and lowers catecholamine vasopressor dosages with minimal to no effect on patient safety.[6]

EXPERIMENTAL THERAPIES

Nitric Oxide Inhibitors

NO is a short-acting, potent vasodilator derived from enzymatic oxidation of arginine. Its production is under control of NOS. This enzyme is present (expressed) in two forms: a constitutive form (constitutive nitric oxide synthase [ecNOS]) and an inducible form (iNOS). Small amounts of NO normally are produced by the vascular endothelium under the control of ecNOS for physiologic control of vascular tone and blood flow distribution. Under pathophysiologic conditions such as stimulation by lipopolysaccharide or cytokines, iNOS becomes diffusely expressed, producing large amounts of NO. The latter has been implicated in the cardiovascular failure of septic shock.

Pharmacologic inhibition of NO production has been investigated as an adjunct to standard therapies of septic shock.[81] L-Arginine analogs such as monomethyl-L-arginine (L-NMMA) and L-arginine-methylester (L-NAME) are competitive inhibitors of NOS and have been shown to increase blood pressure, partially restore vascular reactivity, and reduce vasopressor use.[11] However, because these arginine analogs nonselectively block ecNOS and iNOS, their use has been associated with extensive vasoconstriction, decreased CO, and regional hypoperfusion, thus promoting organ failure and mortality.[82] Some *S*-substituted thiourea derivatives have demonstrated, both in vitro and in vivo (rodent), dose-dependent selectivity for iNOS inhibition, but the clinical application must be evaluated. Several phase I/IIa clinical trials of septic shock patients are underway.

Pyridoxalated hemoglobin polyoxyethylene is a scavenger of NO. A phase II study of 62 patients with vasodilatory shock requiring vasopressors showed that an infusion of 20 mg/kg/h for up to 100 hours rapidly increases blood pressure and shortens the duration of vasopressor therapy.[83] Additional studies are needed.

Methylene Blue

Methylene blue counteracts ecNOS, iNOS, and soluble guanylate cyclase to reduce serum concentrations of NO and cyclic guanosine monophosphate.[84] Despite these effects, methylene blue does not alter the expression of inflammatory cytokines. Clinically, methylene blue at dosages of 0.25 to 3 mg/kg/h increases SVR, MAP, myocardial contractility, and DO_2 in septic shock patients refractory to vasopressors while improving P_{CO_2} gap.[84] Dosages exceeding 3 mg/kg/h worsen splanchnic perfusion. It may increase pulmonary vascular resistance, potentially worsening oxygenation. Additional studies are needed before methylene blue can be recommended; at present, it has been used only for salvage therapy.

Terlipressin

Terlipressin, a prodrug that is converted into lysine vasopressin, has been used in septic shock patients and is available in other countries.[66,85] This drug has a half-life of 6 hours and acts via vascular V_1 receptors and renal tubular V_2 receptors. Terlipressin increases MAP to a greater extent than norepinephrine when it is used as the initial vasopressor in septic shock. Despite a decrease in CO, heart rate, and Do_2I, terlipressin increases gastric mesenteric perfusion, urine production, and creatinine clearance while reducing lactate concentration. Both terlipressin and vasopressin increase blood pressure and decrease heart rate to the same extent but terlipressin is associated with less supplemental norepinephrine usage and improved mesenteric perfusion.[66,85] These preliminary findings suggest that a clinical trial evaluating mortality as well as hemodynamic effects should be conducted.

Levosimendan

Levosimendan is a novel inotropic and vasodilator calcium-sensitizing drug.[86] In acute decompensated heart failure, it improves cardiac contractility by sensitizing troponin C to calcium. In septic shock patients with and without left ventricular dysfunction, levosimendan 0.1 to 0.2 mcg/kg/min decreases PAOP, increases LVEF and cardiac index, improves mesenteric and sublingual perfusion, and enhances urine production.[86] Levosimendan improves S_{CVO_2} to the same extent as dobutamine when it is used in early goal-directed therapy. Levosimendan is associated with declining serum lactate concentrations. While additional clinical trials of levosimendan in septic shock are needed, increased mortality was demonstrated in studies of acute decompensated heart failure.

Dopexamine and Isoproterenol

Dopexamine is a structural and synthetic analog of dopamine that exerts systemic vasodilation through stimulation of β_2-adrenoceptors and peripheral D_1 and D_2 receptors and weak inotropic properties through stimulation of β_1-adrenoceptors.[8–12,52,53] It has been used in patients with acute heart failure and septic shock. Similar to dobutamine, dopexamine is administered in combination with a vasopressor in septic shock. In small studies of septic shock, dopexamine produced a dose-related (range, 2 to 6 mcg/kg/min) increase in cardiac index, stroke volume, and heart rate, as well as a decrease in SVR over the course of 0.5 to 1 hour while the dosages of other vasopressors were kept constant. The increase in myocardial oxygen demand is less than with dopamine, but tachycardia and tachydysrhythmia may lead to myocardial ischemia, especially when ischemic heart disease is present. Global oxygen-transport variables are similar to those of dopamine: Do_2 increases but Vo_2 increases insufficiently, resulting in impaired O_2ER. The combined β_2-adrenoceptors and peripheral D_1 agonistic effects of dopexamine should improve distribution of blood flow. However, the results of studies of dopexamine use in septic shock failed to show preferential increase in splanchnic blood flow. In fact, gastric pHi was lowered. When administered over 7 days, dopexamine had no impact on renal function. Therefore, initial data do not support a role for dopexamine in improving regional hemodynamics and blood flow, but studies continue to investigate dopexamine as an alternative therapy for septic shock.

Isoproterenol is a synthetic catecholamine that stimulates only β_1- and β_2-adrenoceptors to produce vasodilatory and inotropic effects.[87] Although not thought of as a traditional agent for managing septic shock, isoproterenol has received attention because of the concepts of early goal-directed therapy.[32] The strong β-adrenergic effects of isoproterenol make it a potential alternative to dobutamine for optimizing Do_2 in patients with low Svo_2 despite use of other therapies (e.g., fluid resuscitation, vasopressors, red blood cell transfusion). In patients with septic shock and Svo_2 <70% despite volume administration, norepinephrine, and red blood cell transfusion, adding isoproterenol increases Svo_2, cardiac index, and stroke index while decreasing lactate concentration without increasing heart rate or causing myocardial ischemia. Although these results are intriguing, additional studies are needed to define the role of isoproterenol, especially considering that dobutamine has become standard therapy for early goal-directed therapy. At present, isoproterenol is an agent of last resort.

Other Therapies

As with vasopressin and cortisol, critical illness impairs hypothalamic–pituitary function, producing relative deficiencies of triiodothyronine (T_3) and thyroxine (T_4). This condition, referred to as *euthyroid sick syndrome*, may contribute to hypotension and mortality.[88,89] Concentrations of thyrotropin-releasing hormone and thyroid-stimulating hormone are inappropriately low. Measured concentrations of free T_3 and T_4 may be low or normal, but synthesis is consistently impaired. Only scant data regarding the replacement of these hormones in critically ill patients are available, and the results are variable, depending on the extent of additional hormone replacement (growth hormone, gonadotropin-releasing hormone, leptin, insulin, thyrotropin-releasing hormone, and thyroid-stimulating hormone). Given the data for replacing vasopressin and cortisol in septic shock, it is reasonable to assume that one day a "thyroid replacement" regimen will be offered as an adjunctive treatment to vasopressors.

GENERAL CONCLUSIONS AND RECOMMENDATIONS

Norepinephrine is the recommended first-line vasopressor for septic shock.[6] The choice of additional vasopressor or inotropic agents should be made according to the clinical needs of the patient and the data obtained from hemodynamic and perfusion monitoring.[6–15] Figure 13-2 presents an algorithm for the management of septic

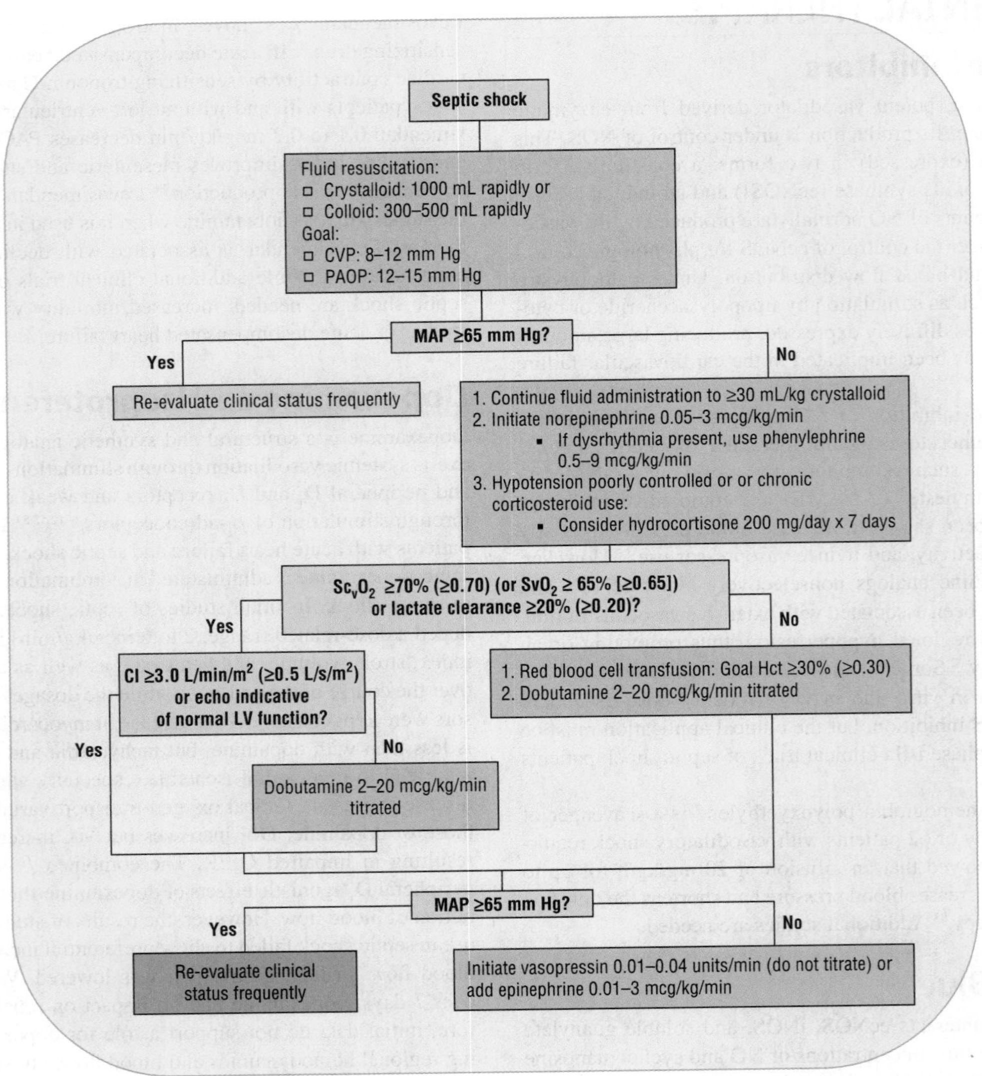

FIGURE 13-2 Algorithmic approach to resuscitative management of septic shock. The algorithmic approach is intended to be used in conjunction with clinical judgment, hemodynamic monitoring parameters, and therapy end points, as discussed in the text. (CI, cardiac index; CVP, central venous pressure; echo, echocardiography; Hct, hematocrit; MAP, mean arterial pressure; PAOP, pulmonary artery occlusive pressure; $Scvo_2$, central venous oxygen saturation; Svo_2, mixed venous oxygen saturation.) *(Figure based on data from references 6–15.)*

shock.[6–15] This algorithm suggests a stepwise approach of early goal-directed therapy to optimize Do_2, first with fluid resuscitation and using norepinephrine. Dobutamine is added for low CO states or to optimize $Svo_2/Scvo_2$ or lactate clearance. Occasionally, epinephrine and phenylephrine are used when necessary. Although this approach is empirical, it is used broadly in clinical practice and has been justified by the desire to avoid the adverse events associated with strong vasoconstriction. Developing a strategy to titrate therapy early in the course of illness to predetermined values reduces mortality. Goals of initial resuscitation should include fluids to achieve CVP 8 to 12 mm Hg, vasopressor agents to achieve MAP at least 65 mm Hg, red blood cell transfusion to maintain hematocrit ≥30%, and inotropic therapy to achieve $Scvo_2$ ≥70% or lactate clearance ≥20%.[6,32] For all catecholamine vasopressors, doses higher than recommended traditionally are required for goal-directed therapy to MAP and for normalization of oxygen-transport variables. Patients who develop supranormal Do_2 and Vo_2 values have lower mortality, but whether this effect is achieved intrinsically or with exogenous administration of vasopressors/inotropes appears inconsequential. Therefore, goal-directed therapy to supranormal oxygen-transport variables cannot be recommended because little or no benefit has been demonstrated. Further work is required to better elucidate the differential effects of vasopressors on regional hemodynamic and oxygen-transport values as measures of local tissue perfusion.

This algorithmic approach (Fig. 13-2) is consistent with the recommendations made in the Surviving Sepsis Campaign[6] and the American College of Critical Care Medicine's guidelines to the hemodynamic support of adult patients with sepsis (Table 13-2).[7] Personalized pharmacotherapy (Table 13-5) for hemodynamic support of shock may be rationale in certain situations but it is difficult to achieve because patient response is variable and the acute nature of emergent resuscitation often necessitates treatment before pharmacotherapy can be personalized. Although difficult to demonstrate, true differences in clinical outcomes as a result of differences in the pharmacologic activity of vasopressors and inotropes may exist. For example, evidence suggests that norepinephrine, when used appropriately with fluid replenishment, is safe and effective in treating septic shock; it decreases mortality, particularly when started early in the course of septic shock. It is effective in optimizing hemodynamic variables and improving systemic and regional (e.g., renal, gastric mucosal, and splanchnic) perfusion. Epinephrine causes a greater increase in the cardiac index and Do_2 and increases gastric mucosal flow but may not preserve splanchnic circulation adequately. It may cause increases in lactic acid. Epinephrine may be particularly useful when used earlier in the course of septic shock in young patients. Unlike epinephrine, dopamine does not increase the proportion of CO that preferentially goes to the splanchnic circulation. The ability of dopamine to increase CO by not more than 35% accompanied by a tachycardia or tachydysrhythmias limits its utility. Dopamine, as opposed to norepinephrine, has been shown to worsen splanchnic Vo_2 and O_2ER and is of limited value in improving urine production. The only benefit of dopamine is that it is readily available as a premixed solution. Low-dose dopamine has not been shown consistently to increase the glomerular filtration rate, does not prevent renal failure, and actually worsens splanchnic tissue oxygen utilization. Low-dose dopamine should not be used. Phenylephrine should be used when a pure vasoconstrictor is desired in patients who may not require or cannot tolerate the β-effects of other vasopressors or inotropes. In patients with a high filling pressure and hypotension, the combination of phenylephrine and dobutamine may be useful.

TABLE 13-5 Personalized Pharmacotherapy for Shock

Situational Considerations	Pharmacotherapy
Initial vasopressor of choice for resuscitation	Norepinephrine
Rapidly progressing shock requiring IMMEDIATE therapy	Dopamine
Presence of tachydysrhythmia	Phenylephrine
Healthy myocardium (e.g., young patients)	Epinephrine
Acutely declining renal function	Vasopressin
Myocardial dysfunction (elevated filling pressures and low CO)	Dobutamine
Hypoperfusion despite adequate intravascular volume (e.g., $Scvo_2$ <70% or Svo_2 <65% or lactate clearance <20%)	Dobutamine
MAP <65 mm Hg despite norepinephrine	Vasopressin or epinephrine
Vasopressor refractory shock	Corticosteroid

CO, cardiac output; MAP, mean arterial pressure; $Scvo_2$, central-venous oxygen saturation; Svo_2, mixed venous oxygen saturation.

Shortcomings of study methodology prevent the establishment of definitive conclusions. As a consequence, published guidelines for the management of severe sepsis and septic shock have many inconclusive recommendations (Table 13-2). Short infusions during studies may show differences that are not clinically significant after 24 hours, as demonstrated for epinephrine and dobutamine. Most studies comparatively evaluated vasopressors once patients were hemodynamically stable as the process of obtaining consent and randomization precluded the initiation of study drug during early resuscitation. Clinically, vasopressors and inotropes are used for hours to days. Possible confounding factors are the variable times at which studies are initiated with respect to the stage of sepsis or septic shock, the inherent differences in circulating catecholamine concentrations, changes in receptor activity, as well as differences in prestudy duration and type of exogenous catecholamine administration.

Initial studies with vasopressin suggest a potential role in the management of vasopressor-dependent septic shock patients. Vasopressin reduces the requirements of adrenergic agents while maintaining hemodynamic function. While it may enhance urine production, it is associated with mesenteric and peripheral ischemia. Therefore, vasopressin should be used only if response to one or two adrenergic agents is inadequate or as a method for reducing the dosage of these therapies. Close monitoring of ischemic events is needed. Data indicate that moderate doses of hydrocortisone (200 to 300 mg/day) administered over several days may reverse septic shock and dependency on vasopressor agents. Given the discrepancy of the current data, corticosteroids may be administered to patients with septic shock refractory to vasopressors or when adrenal insufficiency is suspected. Data on optimal dosage regimens and definitive outcomes still are needed.

Further pharmacotherapeutic and outcome studies are required to elucidate the place in therapy of individual vasopressors and inotropes or their combinations in the supportive care of patients with bacteremia or septic shock. As supportive therapy, it is imperative that primary therapy aimed at the source of (antimicrobials) and consequences of (anticytokines) infection be initiated quickly to afford the patient the best chance of survival. Once this goal is accomplished, we will need to direct our efforts to pharmacoeconomics and the cost-effectiveness of these therapies.

ABBREVIATIONS

ACTH	adrenocorticotropic hormone
ATP	adenosine triphosphate
CaMK	calcium–calmodulin-dependent protein kinase
cAMP	cyclic adenosine monophosphate
Cao_2	arterial oxygen content

CI confidence interval
CO cardiac output
CO_2 carbon dioxide
Cvo_2 venous oxygen content
CVP central venous pressure
Do_2 oxygen delivery
DO_2I oxygen delivery index
ecNOS constitutive nitric oxide synthase
HR hazard ratio
ICU intensive care unit
IL interleukin
iNOS inducible nitric oxide synthase
L-NAME L-arginine-methylester
L-NMMA monomethyl-L-arginine
LVEF left ventricular ejection fraction
MAP mean arterial pressure
NO nitric oxide
NOS nitric oxide synthase
O_2ER oxygen extraction ratio
OR odds ratio
$Paco_2$ arterial carbon dioxide pressure (tension)
Pao_2 arterial oxygen pressure (tension)
PAOP pulmonary artery occlusive pressure
Pco_2 gut luminal partial pressure of carbon dioxide
pHi intramucosal pH
PLC phospholipase
$Pslco_2$ sublingual carbon dioxide pressure
RR relative risk
Sao_2 arterial oxygen saturation
$Scvo_2$ central venous oxygen saturation
Svo_2 mixed venous oxygen saturation
SVR systemic vascular resistance
T_3 triiodothyronine
T_4 thyroxine
TNF tumor necrosis factor
Vo_2 oxygen consumption
Vo_2I oxygen consumption index

REFERENCES

1. Marik PE, Lipman J. The definition of septic shock: Implications for treatment. Crit Care Resusc 2007;9:101–103.
2. Vincent JL, Sakr Y, Sprung CL, et al. Sepsis in European intensive care unit: Results of the SOAP study. Crit Care Med 2006;34:344–353.
3. Sakr Y, Vincent JL, Roukonen E, et al. Sepsis and organ failure are major determinants of post-intensive care unit mortality. J Crit Care 2008;23:475–483.
4. Blanco J, Muriel-Bombin A, Sagredo V, et al. Incidence, organ dysfunction and mortality in severe sepsis: A Spanish multicentre study. Crit Care 2008;12:R158.
5. Patel AK, Hollenberg SM. Cardiovascular failure and cardiogenic shock. Semin Respir Crit Care Med 2011;32:598–606.
6. Dellinger RP, Levy MM, Carlet JM, et al. Surviving sepsis campaign: International guidelines for management of severe sepsis and septic shock: 2012. Crit Care Med 2013;41:580–637.
7. Hollenberg SM, Ahrens TS, Annane D, et al. Practice parameters for hemodynamic support of sepsis in adult patients in sepsis. Crit Care Med 2004;32:1928–1948.
8. Beale RJ, Hollenberg SM, Vincent JL, et al. Vasopressor and inotropic support in septic shock: An evidence-based review. Crit Care Med 2004;32(Suppl):S455–S465.
9. Hollenberg SM. Vasoactive drugs in circulatory shock. Am J Respir Crit Care Med 2011;183:847–855.
10. Bangash MN, Kong ML, Pearse RM. Use of inotropes and vasopressor agents in critically ill patients. Br J Pharmacol 2012;165:2015–2033.
11. Cinel I, Dellinger RP. Advances in the pathogenesis and management of sepsis. Curr Opin Infect Dis 2007;20:345–352.
12. Holmes CL, Walley KR. Vasoactive drugs for vasodilatory shock in ICU. Curr Opin Crit Care 2009;15:398–402.
13. Gullo A, Bianco N, Berlot G. Management of severe sepsis and septic shock: Challenges and recommendations. Crit Care Clin 2006;22:489–501.
14. Leone M, Martin C. Vasopressor use in septic shock: An update. Curr Opin Anesthesiol 2008;21:141–147.
15. Zanotti-Cavazzoni SL, Dellinger RP. Hemodynamic optimization of sepsis-induced tissue hypoperfusion. Crit Care 2006;10(Suppl 3):S2.
16. Pinsky MR. Hemodynamic evaluation and monitoring in the ICU. Chest 2007;132:2020–2029.
17. Marik PE, Baram M. Noninvasive hemodynamic monitoring in the intensive care unit. Crit Care Clin 2007;23:383–400.
18. Vincent JL, Rhodes A, Perel A, et al. Clinical review: Update on hemodynamic monitoring—A consensus of 16. Crit Care 2011;15:229.
19. Holley A, Lukin W, Paratz J, Hawkins T, Boots R, Lipman J. Review article: Part one: Goal-directed resuscitation—Which goals? Hemodynamic targets. Emerg Med Australas 2012;24:14–22.
20. Holley A, Lukin W, Paratz J, Hawkins T, Boots R, Lipman J. Review article: Part two: Goal-directed resuscitation—which goals? Perfusion targets. Emerg Med Australas 2012;24:127–135.
21. Nichols D, Nielsen ND. Oxygen delivery and consumption: A macrocirculatory perspective. Crit Care Clin 2010;26:239–253.
22. Levy MM, Macias WL, Vincent JL, et al. Early changes in organ function predict eventual survival in severe sepsis. Crit Care Med 2005;33:2194–2201.
23. O'Grady N, Alexander M, Dellinger E, et al. Guidelines for the prevention of intravascular catheter-related infections. Clin Infect Dis 2002;35:1281–1307.
24. Maddirala S, Khan A. Optimizing hemodynamic support in septic shock using central and mixed venous oxygen saturation. Crit Care Clin 2010;26:323–333.
25. Walley KR. Use of central venous oxygen saturation to guide therapy. Am J Respir Crit Care Med 2011;184:514–520.
26. Greenberg SB, Murphy GS, Vender JS. Current use of the pulmonary artery catheter. Curr Opin Crit Care 2009;15:249–253.
27. Bernard GR, Sopko G, Cerra F, et al. Pulmonary artery catheterization and clinical outcomes: National Heart, Lung, and Blood Institute and Food and Drug Administration Workshop Report. Consensus Statement. JAMA 2000;283:2568–2572.
28. Evans DC, Doraiswamy VA, Prosciak MP, et al. Complications associated with pulmonary artery catheters: A comprehensive clinical review. Scand J Surg 2009;98:199–208.
29. Harvey S, Young D, Brampton W, et al. Pulmonary artery catheter for adult patients in intensive care. Cochrane Database Syst Rev 2006;19:CD003408.
30. Practice Guidelines for Pulmonary Artery Catheterization: An updated report by the American Society of Anesthesiologists Task Force on Pulmonary Artery Catheterization. Anesthesiology 2003;99:988–1014.

31. The National Heart, Lung, and Blood Institute Acute Respiratory Distress Syndrome (ARDS) Clinical Trials Network. Pulmonary-artery central venous catheter to guide treatment of acute lung injury. N Engl J Med 2006;354:2213–2224.
32. Rivers E, Nguyen B, Havstad S, et al. Early goal-directed therapy in the treatment of severe sepsis and septic shock. N Engl J Med 2001;345:1368–1377.
33. Loiacono LA, Shapiro DS. Detection of hypoxia at the cellular level. Crit Care Clin 2010;26:409–421.
34. De Backer D, Ospina-Tascon G, Salgado D, Favory R, Creteur J, Vincent JL. Monitoring the microcirculation in the critically ill patients: Current methods and future approaches. Intensive Care Med 2010;36:1813–1825.
35. Heyland DK, Cook DJ, King D, et al. Maximizing oxygen delivery in critically ill patients: A methodologic appraisal of the evidence. Crit Care Med 1996;24:517–524.
36. Kern JW, Shoemaker WC. Meta-analysis of hemodynamic optimization in high-risk patients. Crit Care Med 2002;30:1686–1692.
37. Micek ST, Roubinian N, Heuring T, et al. Before–after study of a standardized hospital order set for the management of septic shock. Crit Care Med 2006;34:2707–2713.
38. Shorr AF, Micek ST, Jackson WL, et al. Economic implications of an evidence-based sepsis protocol: Can we improve outcomes and lower costs? Crit Care Med 2007;35:1257–1262.
39. Girardis P, Rinaldi L, Donno L, et al. Effects on management and outcome of severe sepsis and septic shock patients admitted to the intensive care unit after implementation of a sepsis program: A pilot study. Crit Care 2009;13:R143.
40. Shapiro NI, Howell MD, Talmor D, et al. Implementation and outcomes of the multiple urgent sepsis therapies (MUST) protocol. Crit Care Med 2006;34:1025–1032.
41. Suarez D, Ferrer R, Artigas A, et al. Cost-effectiveness of the Surviving Sepsis Campaign protocol for severe sepsis: A prospective nation-wide study in Spain. Intensive Care Med 2011;37:444–452.
42. Levy MM, Dellinger RP, Townsend SR, et al. The Surviving Sepsis Campaign: Results of an international guideline-based performance improvement program targeting severe sepsis. Crit Care Med 2010;38:367–374.
43. Jones AE, Brown MD, Trzeciak S. The effect of a quantitative resuscitation strategy on mortality in the patients with sepsis: A meta-analysis. Crit Care Med 2008;36: 2734–2739.
44. Okorie ON, Dellinger P. Lactate: Biomarker and potential therapeutic target. Crit Care Clin 2011;27:299–326.
45. Fuller BM, Dellinger RP. Lactate as a hemodynamic marker in the critically ill. Curr Opin Crit Care 2012;18:267–272.
46. Jones AE, Shapiro NI, Trzeciak S, et al. Lactate clearance vs. central venous oxygen saturation as goals on early sepsis therapy. A randomized clinical trial. JAMA 2010;303: 739–746.
47. Jansen TC, van Bommel J, Schoonderbeek J, et al. Early lactate-guided therapy in intensive care unit patients. A multicenter, open-label, randomised controlled trial. Am J Respir Crit Care Med 2010;182:752–761.
48. Boerma EC. The microcirculation as a clinical concept: Work in progress. Curr Opin Crit Care 2009;15:261–265.
49. Zanotti-Cavazzoni SL, Hollenberg SM. Cardiac dysfunction in severe sepsis and septic shock. Curr Opin Crit Care 2009;15:392–397.
50. Griffee MJ, Merkel MJ, Wei KS. The role of echocardiography in hemodynamic assessment of septic shock. Crit Care Clin 2010;26:365–382.
51. Ventetuolo CE, Levy MM. Cardiac biomarkers in critically ill. Crit Care Clin 2011;27:327–343.
52. Asfar P, Hauser B, Radermacher P, et al. Catecholamines and vasopressin during critical illness. Crit Care Clin 2006;22:131–149.
53. Boerma EC, Ince C. The role of vasoactive agents in the resuscitation of microvascular perfusion and tissue oxygenation in critically ill patients. Intensive Care Med 2010;36:2004–2018.
54. Russell JA. Bench-to-bedside review: Vasopressin in the management of septic shock. Crit Care 2011;15:226.
55. Marik PE, Pastores SM, Annane D, et al. Recommendations for the diagnosis and management of corticosteroid insufficiency in critically ill adult patients: Consensus statements from an international task force by the American College of Critical Care Medicine. Crit Care Med 2008;36:1937–1949.
56. Lefering LR, Neugebauer EAM. Steroids controversy in sepsis and septic shock: A meta-analysis. Crit Care Med 1995;23:1294–1303.
57. Cronin L, Cook DJ, Carlet J, et al. Corticosteroid treatment for sepsis: A critical appraisal and meta-analysis. Crit Care Med 1995;23:1430–1439.
58. Annane D, Sebille V, Troche G, et al. A 3-level prognostic classification in septic shock based on cortisol levels and cortisol response to corticotropin. JAMA 2000;283: 1038–1045.
59. Minneci PC, Deans KJ, Banks SM, et al. Meta-analysis: The effect of steroids on survival and shock during sepsis depends on the dose. Ann Intern Med 2004;141:47–56.
60. Annane D, Bellissant E, Bollaert PE, et al. Corticosteroids in the treatment of severe sepsis and septic shock in adults. JAMA 2009;301:2362–2375.
61. Annane D, Sébille V, Charpentier C, et al. Effect of treatment with low doses of hydrocortisone and fludrocortisone on mortality in patients with septic shock. JAMA 2002;288:862–871.
62. Sprung CL, Annane D, Keh D, et al. Hydrocortisone therapy for patients with septic shock. N Engl J Med 2008;358: 111–124.
63. De Backer D, Aldecoa C, Nimi H, Vincent JL. Dopamine versus norepinephrine in the treatment of septic shock: A meta-analysis. Crit Care Med 2012;40:725–730.
64. Havel C, Arrich J, Losert H, Gamper G, Mullner M, Herkner H. Vasopressors for hypotensive shock. Cochrane Database Syst Rev 2011;5:CD003709.
65. Russell JA, Walley KR, Singer J, et al. Vasopressin versus norepinephrine in patients with septic shock. N Engl J Med 2008;358:877–887.
66. Polito A, Parisini E, Ricci Z, Picardo S, Annane D. Vasopressin for treatment of vasodilatory shock: An ESICM systematic review and meta-analysis. Intensive Care Med 2012;38:9–19.
67. Gordon AC, Russell JA, Walley KR, et al. The effects of vasopressin on acute kidney injury in septic shock. Intensive Care Med 2010;36:83–91.
68. Finfer S, Bellomo R, McEvoy S, et al. A comparison of albumin and saline for fluid resuscitation in the intensive care unit. N Engl J Med 2004;350:2247–2256.
69. Perel P, Roberts I. Colloids versus crystalloids for fluid resuscitation in critically ill patients. Cochrane Database Syst Rev 2012;6:CD00056766.
70. Vincent JL, Gottin L. Type of fluid in severe sepsis and septic shock. Minerva Anesthesiol 2011;77:1190–1196.
71. Brunkhorst FM, Engel C, Bloos F, et al. Intensive insulin therapy and pentastarch resuscitation in severe sepsis. N Engl J Med 2008;358:125–139.

72. Perner A Hasse N, Guttormsen AB, et al. Hydroxyethyl starch 130/0.42 versus Ringer's acetate in severe sepsis. N Engl J Med 2012;367:124–134.
73. De Backer D, Biston P, Devriendt J, et al. Comparison of dopamine and norepinephrine in the treatment of shock. N Engl J Med 2010;362:779–789.
74. Patel GP, Grahe JS, Sperry M, et al. Efficacy and safety of dopamine versus norepinephrine in the management of septic shock. Shock 2010;33:375–380.
75. Myburgh JA, Higgins A, Jovanovska A, et al. A comparison of epinephrine and norepinephrine in critically ill patients. Intensive Care Med 2008;34:2226–2234.
76. Annane D, Vignon P, Renault A, et al. Norepinephrine plus dobutamine versus epinephrine alone for the management of septic shock: A randomised trial. Lancet 2007;370:678–684.
77. Russell JA, Walley KR, Gordon AC, et al. Interaction of vasopressin infusion, corticosteroid treatment, and mortality of septic shock. Crit Care Med 2009;37:811–818.
78. Bauer SR, Lam SW, Cha SS, et al. Effect of corticosteroids on arginine vasopressin-containing vasopressor therapy for septic shock: A case control study. J Crit Care 2008;23: 500–506.
79. Bellomo R, Chapman M, Finfer S, et al. Low-dose dopamine in patients with early renal dysfunction: A placebo-controlled randomized trial. Australian and New Zealand Intensive Care Society (ANZICS) Clinical Trials Group. Lancet 2000;356:2139–2143.
80. Friedrich JO, Adhikari N, Herridge MS, et al. Meta-analysis: Low-dose dopamine increases urine output but does not prevent renal dysfunction or death. Ann Intern Med 2005;142:510–524.
81. Suffredini AF, Munford RS. Novel therapies for septic shock over the past 4 decades. JAMA 2011;306:194–199.
82. Lopez A, Lorente JA, Steingrub J, et al. Multiple-center, randomized, placebo-controlled, double-blind study of the nitric oxide synthase inhibitor 546C88: Effect on survival in patients with septic shock. Crit Care Med 2004;32:21–30.
83. Kinasewitz GT. Privalle CT, Imm A, et al. Multicenter, randomized, placebo-controlled study of the nitric oxide scavenger pyridoxalated hemoglobin polyoxyethylene in distributive shock. Crit Care Med 2008;36:1999–2007.
84. Kwok ES, Howes D. Use of methylene blue in sepsis: A systematic review. J Intensive Care Med 2006;21:359–363.
85. Morelli A, Ertmer C, Peitropaoli P, et al. Terlipressin: A promising vasoactive agent in hemodynamic support of septic shock. Expert Opin Pharmacother 2009;10: 2569–2575.
86. Pinto BB, Rehberg S, Ertmer C, et al. Role of levosimendan in sepsis and septic shock. Curr Opin Anesthesiol 2008;21:168–177.
87. Leone M, Boyadjiev I, Boulos E, et al. A reappraisal of isoproterenol in goal-directed therapy of septic shock. Shock 2006;26:353–357.
88. De Groot LJ. Non-thyroidal illness syndrome is a manifestation of hypothalamic–pituitary dysfunction, and in view of current evidence, should be treated with appropriate replacement therapies. Crit Care Clin 2006;22:57–86.
89. Angelousi AG, Karageorgopoulos DE, Kapaskelis AM, Falagas ME. Association between thyroid function tests at baseline and the outcome of patients with sepsis or septic shock: A systematic review. Eur J Endocrinol 2011;164: 147–155.

14

Hypovolemic Shock

Brian L. Erstad

KEY CONCEPTS

1. Plasma does not have to be lost from the body for hypovolemic shock to occur.
2. Patients may die of hypovolemic shock despite having normal serum electrolyte concentrations.
3. Although the Starling's equation of fluid transport is useful for understanding the factors involved in fluid shifting between compartments, it is not a practical tool for use in the clinical setting.
4. Patients may have complications and death as a result of reperfusion injury as well as the initial insult.
5. The clinical presentation of patients with hypovolemic shock can vary substantially, depending on concomitant disease states, medications, and cause of hypovolemia.
6. The initial monitoring of a patient with suspected intravascular depletion always should include vital signs, urine output, mental status, and physical examination.
7. The need for IV (vs. oral) rehydration in children often is overestimated.
8. Crystalloid (sodium-containing) solutions should be used for most forms of circulatory insufficiency that are associated with hemodynamic instability.
9. Neither crystalloids nor colloids have the oxygen-carrying properties of red blood cells.
10. Vasoactive medications should not be considered for hypovolemic shock until fluid resuscitation has been optimized.

INTRODUCTION

This chapter discusses the assessment and management of hypovolemic shock. Neurogenic shock resulting from loss of sympathetic activity and anaphylactic shock resulting from increased vascular permeability often are considered separately from hypovolemic shock because fluid loss from the body is not necessary for their occurrence. Although these forms of shock are not discussed in detail, it is important to note that IV fluid administration (in conjunction with vasoactive medications) is a mainstay of therapy because circulating volume is decreased. In this regard, adequate fluid resuscitation to maintain circulating blood volume is a common principle in managing all forms of shock.

EPIDEMIOLOGY

Because shock is not a reportable category by state and federal agencies that track causes of death, the incidence is unknown. Estimates of deaths due to shock are complicated by differences in definitions and classification systems. Part of the problem is defining when progressive circulatory insufficiency results in the loss of normal compensatory responses by the body, which could reverse the processes leading to irreversible organ dysfunction. This loss of appropriate compensation varies from patient to patient and is not always readily apparent during the initial patient presentation. Therefore, forms of hypovolemic shock, such as hemorrhagic shock, are subsumed by more readily identifiable categories of death, such as accidental injuries and homicides. Crude and conservative estimates of death due to hypovolemic shock are available for some of its forms. More than 100,000 deaths each year in the United States are due to unintentional injuries that frequently involve bleeding,[1] and more than 600 deaths each year are due to natural heat-related illness.[2] The figures are much higher when considered on a global basis. For example, electrolyte depletion and dehydration due to diarrheal disease result in approximately 2 million deaths each year in children younger than 5 years.[3] The most liberal estimates of death include all causes of circulatory failure (i.e., the last stage of shock).

ETIOLOGY

1 Hypovolemic shock may result from blood loss (plasma and red blood cells) due to trauma, surgery, or internal hemorrhage or from plasma loss due to fluid sequestered within the body or lost from the body (Table 14-1). In some cases, such as in postoperative patients, a number of these problems occur at the same time. For example, a patient may have blood loss secondary to trauma or surgery, with additional fluid being third spaced (e.g., as tissue edema in the GI tract with a concomitant ileus) and lost through a high-output GI fistula postoperatively. As this example of third-spaced fluid indicates, fluid (i.e., plasma) does not have to be lost from the body for a person to develop hypovolemic shock, although the fistula output would clearly aggravate the situation. Approximately 10 L of fluid is secreted and reabsorbed daily in the GI tract; so, it is not surprising that volume loss could be substantial depending on the location of the fistula and function of the tract preceding the fistula.

Dehydration may result from primary water deficiency, usually because of decreased intake, but in some instances (e.g., diabetes insipidus) it may result from increased losses of water. With most forms of dehydration, such as those caused by diarrheal disease and heat-related illness, a combination of inadequate intake and higher than normal losses occurs. In general, the term *dehydration* implies primary intracellular water depletion, in contrast to *volume depletion*, which implies extracellular, and particularly intravascular, sodium and water loss. However, there is substantial overlap in the definitions and use of terms such as *dehydration* and *volume depletion* in the medical literature, so the reader must be cognizant of the intended meaning. In the case of primary water

TABLE 14-1 Causes of Hypovolemic Shock[a]

Decreased blood (plasma + red blood cells) volume
External: surgery or trauma
Internal (e.g., cerebral, chest, GI and other abdominal sources, long bone fractures, and retroperitoneum)
Decreased plasma volume
External: losses from urine, GI tract (e.g., vomiting, nasogastric suctioning, fistula, and diarrhea), lungs, or skin (including thermal injury)
Internal (decreased oncotic pressure or increased capillary permeability): fluid accumulation in bowel, peritoneal or pleural cavities

[a]Shock may result from various combinations of blood and plasma volume losses listed (i.e., causes are not mutually exclusive).

deficit, cell dehydration occurs. Initially, the patient may be thirsty and possibly have some mental status changes, such as confusion. If cellular dehydration occurs slowly, intracellular substances, referred to as *idiogenic osmoles*, develop that limit progressive complications (e.g., cerebral edema or coma). Death due to primary water deficit, if it occurs, is usually a result of delayed circulatory failure. With combined water and salt deficiencies, such as might occur with GI (e.g., diarrhea) and skin losses (e.g., heat stroke), interstitial and intravascular depletion is an early occurrence. Fortunately, dehydration is relatively easy to prevent with routine vigilance and water replacement compared with some of the other causes of shock.

PATHOPHYSIOLOGY

2 Hypovolemic shock often is described in terms of monitoring parameters such as lowered blood pressure, but patients with shock may die despite normal surrogate markers of circulatory insufficiency. Therefore, an appropriate definition should mention the underlying problem, which is inadequate tissue perfusion resulting from circulatory failure. In the case of hypovolemic shock, the cause of the altered perfusion is fluid (or volume) depletion resulting from trauma, surgery, thermal injury, or some form of dehydration. Figure 14-1 provides a simplified view of the pathophysiology of circulatory insufficiency assuming the acute insult causing the plasma volume depletion did not result in immediate patient death. Cell damage and death may occur from the primary insult or from reperfusion injury. The latter problem is associated most frequently with trauma and blood loss that cause a systemic inflammatory response syndrome (SIRS) with the release of a multitude of mediators of inflammation and injury that have complex interactions. Cells have varying responses to hypoxia, ranging from astrocytes that quit functioning almost immediately to other cells that may tolerate more prolonged periods of hypoperfusion. Left unmitigated, cell death occurs with prolonged injury and is usually heralded by acidosis, hypothermia, and coagulopathy—referred to as the lethal triad.

The body attempts to compensate for volume depletion beginning with autoregulatory changes involving smaller blood vessels. When the cause of circulatory insufficiency continues unabated, local mechanisms eventually fail to provide adequate compensation,

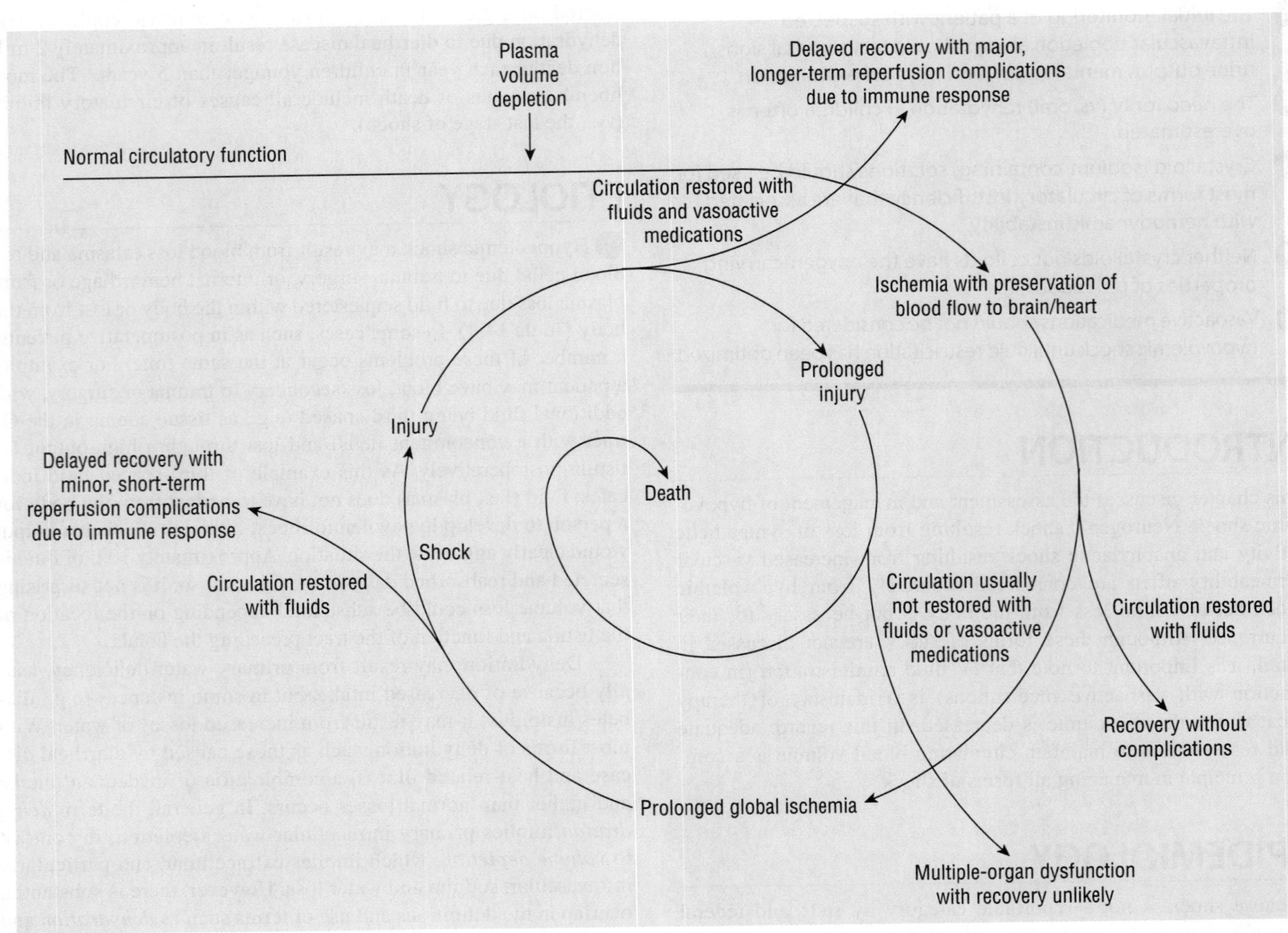

FIGURE 14-1 Pathophysiology of circulatory insufficiency and failure (shock).

and macrocirculatory changes ensue. The majority of blood volume is contained in venous capacitance vessels, with gravity being the major impedance to flow back to the heart. With increasing volume depletion, blood flow to the heart (preload) is decreased, with subsequent activation of baroreceptors and chemoreceptors leading to sympathetic discharge. Also, fluid shifting from the interstitial space to the intravascular space occurs through a phenomenon known as *transcapillary refill*, and hormones (e.g., adrenocorticotropic hormone, angiotensin, catecholamines, and vasopressin) that cause sodium and water retention by the kidneys are released. The phenomenon of transcapillary refill means that the body can have fluid losses exceeding normal plasma volume. These responses cause alterations in stroke volume, heart rate, and peripheral vascular resistance so that blood pressure and hence tissue perfusion can be maintained.

The microcirculatory changes associated with shock are complex and difficult to study. Although some mediators such as catecholamines, angiotensin II, arginine vasopressin, and endothelin-1 cause vasoconstriction, other mediators, such as adenosine and nitric oxide, yield vasodilation. These changes result in hypoperfusion or hyperperfusion, depending on the organs involved. As these microcirculatory changes fail to maintain adequate organ perfusion, more widespread sympathetic nervous system activation and vasoconstriction ensue. Even assuming general circulation is restored, capillaries may not function properly due to ongoing edema and ischemia. Failure to respond to sympathetic stimulation and fluid administration is indicative of the vasodilation that occurs in the final phase of circulatory failure leading to death.

The factors involved in fluid shifting between the intravascular and interstitial spaces are described by the modified Starling's equation:

$$J_V = K_{f,c}[(P_c - P_t) - [\sigma(\pi_c - \pi_t)]]$$

where J_V is the net transvascular flow rate (cannot be measured in the clinical setting), $K_{f,c}$ is the capillary filtration coefficient for fluids (cannot be measured in the clinical setting), P_c is the capillary hydrostatic pressure (indirectly estimated in the clinical setting, e.g., pulmonary artery occlusive pressure), P_t is the tissue hydrostatic pressure (cannot be measured in the clinical setting), σ is the reflection coefficient for proteins (cannot be measured in the clinical setting), π_c is the plasma colloid osmotic pressure (not usually measured in the clinical setting, but technology is available), and π_t is the tissue colloid osmotic pressure (cannot be measured in the clinical setting). The physiology of the parameters associated with the Starling equation continue to be elucidated. For example, the plasma colloid osmotic pressure is more appropriately referred to as the oncotic pressure within the endothelial surface layer and the tissue colloid osmotic pressure is more appropriately referred to as the oncotic pressure beneath the endothelial surface layer.

Proteins act as oncotic agents in each of these spaces to attract fluid, whereas hydrostatic forces push fluid into or out of the vessels. The equation has distinct permeability values for water and protein because each crosses the vascular membrane at a different rate. The values for the variables listed in the equation are not the same for capillaries in all parts of the body. For example, on a scale from 0 to 1 with 0 being free passage of protein and 1 being impermeable to protein, the typical value for the reflection coefficient in most capillaries is >0.9. However, in the pulmonary capillaries the value is closer to 0.7 and approaches 0 in inflammatory states associated with increased capillary permeability.[4] As the value approaches 0, the capillaries are freely permeable not only to the usual fluid and electrolytes but also to plasma proteins such as albumin. Because albumin accounts for approximately 80% of the plasma oncotic pressure, its free passage into the interstitial space effectively negates its intravascular oncotic benefit. 3 Although the Starling's equation is useful to practitioners in terms of understanding the factors involved in fluid shifting between compartments, the rate and direction of transvascular flow cannot be calculated accurately in the clinical setting because most factors cannot be measured directly and the values for the factors vary in different capillaries in the body.

The body's compensatory mechanisms may have beneficial and harmful consequences. For example, cardiac output can be increased substantially by increases in stroke volume or heart rate. Although this may be useful for providing blood flow to inadequately perfused tissues, it may cause large increases in oxygen consumption by the heart that could aggravate preexisting ischemia in patients with underlying coronary artery disease (CAD). Another example is the sympathetic nervous system–mediated vasoconstriction that causes blood to shift from the skin, skeletal muscle, and some internal organs such as the kidneys and GI tract to organs (e.g., heart and brain) that are less tolerant of inadequate flow. If the vasoconstriction continues unabated, the hypoperfused organs eventually become damaged. Figure 14-2 provides an overview of the compensatory changes that occur with a loss of circulating blood volume.

4 In addition to the more acute implications of hypovolemia and attendant complications, reperfusion damage is likely to occur, particularly after prolonged resuscitation attempts. In addition to edematous obstruction of capillaries and oxygen-free radical damage of cell membranes, a number of cellular (e.g., white blood cells and platelets) and humoral (e.g., procoagulants, anticoagulants, complement, and kinins) components are activated, causing the release of other inflammatory mediators. The resulting reperfusion injury may range from readily reversible organ dysfunction to multiple-organ failure and death. The lungs are frequently the first system affected either by excessive fluid resuscitation or by the mediators of secondary reperfusion injury. The latter form of injury often results in the acute respiratory distress syndrome that is defined by an arterial oxygen tension-to-fraction of inspired oxygen ratio of less than or equal to 300 (with additional subdivisions of mild, moderate, and severe) with bilateral lung opacities in the absence of hypervolemia.

Although the basic pathophysiology is similar for the various causes of hypovolemic shock, there are unique considerations relative to each. For example, whereas isolated head injuries associated with trauma typically do not result in substantial blood loss or shock, long bone or pelvic fractures may sequester several liters of blood. Patients with traumatic or thermal injuries, as well as postoperative patients, may have substantial fluid accumulation in sites where the fluid cannot be readily transferred back into blood vessels (i.e., third-spaced fluid) for maintaining pressure. With these types of injuries, prompt control of compressible bleeding sources with rapid patient transfer to the hospital for definitive treatment may preclude the cascade of events leading to shock. Indeed, with trauma patients, a "scoop and run" approach that places a priority on rapid transport to a hospital is used by most urban hospitals.

In the case of hemorrhagic shock, prompt attention must be given to cell as well as plasma losses. Red blood cells lost during the bleeding episode may lead to ischemic damage in vital organs. Packed red blood cell transfusions may be needed to increase the oxygen-carrying capacity of the blood because oxygen transport is a function not only of cardiac output but also of hemoglobin concentration and saturation and of hemoglobin affinity for oxygen. Once hemostasis has been achieved, a more restrictive transfusion strategy (i.e., transfusion if hemoglobin <7 g/dL [<70 g/L; 4.34 mmol/L]) is indicated for the majority of patients without severe cardiovascular disease (see Trauma/Perioperative Patients below).

Clotting factors and platelets are also lost in hemorrhage. The resulting bleeding problems may be aggravated by the dilutional effect of fluid resuscitation on clotting factor activity. Fresh-frozen plasma that contains necessary clotting factors and platelets is needed in massive blood loss to restore adequate coagulation. On the other hand, trauma patients are at increased risk for deep vein thrombosis and pulmonary embolism caused by multiple factors,

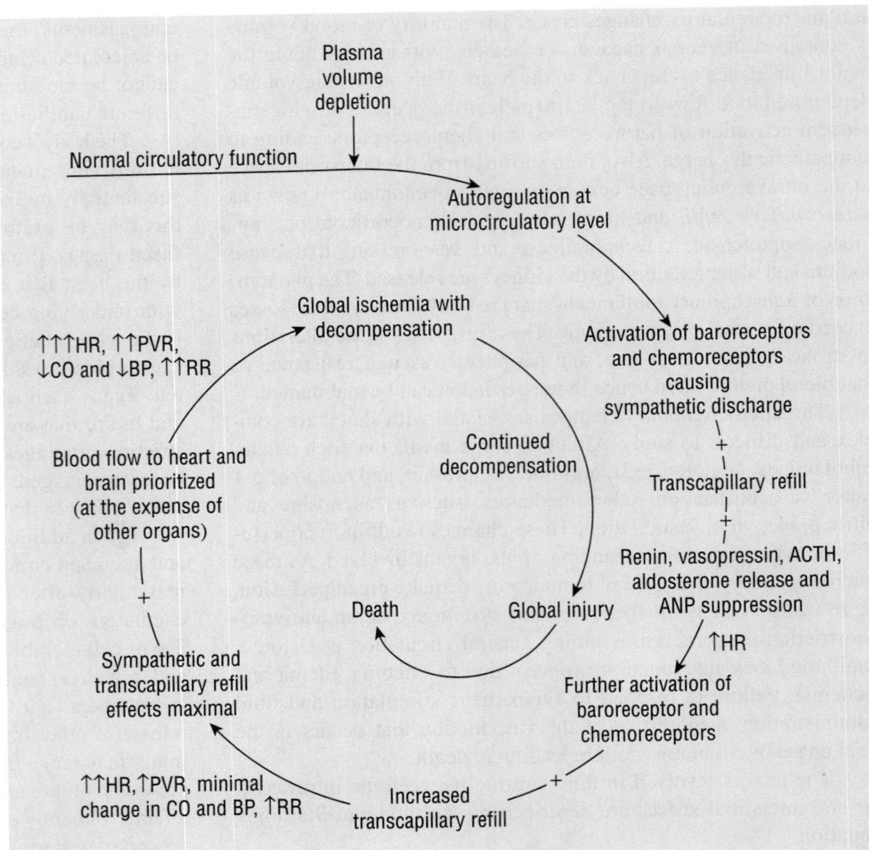

FIGURE 14-2 Activation of compensatory mechanisms with loss of circulatory volume. Certain stages may be absent, depending on a number of factors, such as age, preexisting disease states, and cause of circulatory insufficiency. (ACTH, adrenocorticotropin; ANP, atrial natriuretic peptide; BP, blood pressure; CO, cardiac output; HR, heart rate; PVR, peripheral vascular resistance; RR, respiratory rate.)

including vessel damage, abnormal blood flow patterns, and the hypercoagulable state associated with injury. Therefore, some form of venous thromboembolism prophylaxis usually is indicated in multiple-trauma patients or patients with severe single-system injuries (e.g., spinal cord damage) once hemostasis of major injury-related bleeding has been achieved.

The pathophysiology becomes more complicated if the severity of shock is sufficient to require patient admission to the intensive care unit (ICU) after initial resuscitation or surgery. Most patients admitted to the ICU have SIRS, which is the body's response to injury. This syndrome is defined by a number of hypermetabolic changes reflected in the patient's temperature, white blood cell count and differential, and respiratory and heart rates. The stress response involves complex interactions between the nervous system and immunomodulating substances and has similar (if not the same) harmful and helpful consequences described with reperfusion following shock. If the underlying problems are left untreated, the patient with SIRS may develop multiple-organ dysfunction syndrome (MODS) during the final stages of illness.

CLINICAL PRESENTATION

5 The initial presentation of patients with suspected volume depletion can vary markedly, depending on factors such as age, concomitant disease states and medications, and the etiology and rapidity of depletion (see Clinical Presentation of Hypovolemic Shock box). Intravascular depletion as a consequence of blood loss is signified by postural vital sign changes (i.e., changes in pulse and blood pressure between supine, sitting, and standing measurements), and such measurements should be performed unless the diagnosis is obvious, as in the case of bleeding associated with trauma. Early signs and symptoms of dehydration and intravascular depletion caused by GI or urinary losses often are relatively nonspecific. Plasma volume losses of <10 mL/kg of body weight usually are associated with minor signs and symptoms of distress. Larger losses are not likely to be well tolerated (Table 14-2), particularly in patients older than 65 years. An 18-year-old athlete and a 65-year-old sedentary individual are likely to have much different responses to a similar amount of fluid loss. The young patient may lose one-fourth of his or her circulating blood volume with minimal changes in arterial blood pressure and a relatively low heart rate. However, the elderly patient may have orthostatic changes in blood pressure that are not well tolerated by organs such as the kidneys. Unfortunately, this same elderly patient may not have common signs and symptoms of volume depletion, such as skin turgor changes or thirst, but instead may have more subtle changes (e.g., mental status alterations).

The diagnosis of dehydration and intravascular depletion in children is complicated by difficulties in obtaining an accurate history. However, some excellent resources are available for healthcare providers, such as the Centers for Disease Control and Prevention (CDC) guidelines (*www.cdc.gov*), which discuss the evaluation and management of diarrhea in patients of all ages. In younger children, parental observations are important for estimating fluid deficits and deciding whether hospitalization is necessary. Fortunately, prospective data suggest that parental histories are predictive of acidosis and the need for hospitalization.[5] **6** Regardless of patient age or preexisting conditions, the initial monitoring of a patient with suspected volume depletion should include the following noninvasive parameters: vital signs, urine output, mental status, and physical examination (Fig. 14-3). An increase in blood pressure with passive leg raising may also be useful for the assessment of suspected hypovolemia, but should not be used to guide responsiveness to fluid administration.

TABLE 14-2 Acute Circulatory Insufficiency: Initial Presentation and Therapy[a]

	Mild	Severe
Plasma/blood loss	Adult: 10 mL/kg Child: 20 mL/kg	Adult: 30 mL/kg Child: 35 mL/kg
Mental status/level of consciousness	None to small changes (e.g., anxious, irritable)	Marked changes (e.g., confusion to unconsciousness)
Vital signs/orthostatic changes	Minor changes	Marked changes
Therapy	20 mL/kg lactated Ringer's or normal saline IV[a] over 10–15 minutes Unlikely to need blood cell replacement even if hemorrhagic loss	Lactated Ringer's or normal saline IV as rapidly as possible until response in adult, and then decrease rate of infusion 20 mL/kg lactated Ringer's or normal saline IV in child (repeat quickly if minimal response); likely to need blood cell replacement and surgery if hemorrhagic

[a]Patients may have intermediate degrees of volume loss in addition to those listed, but the amount of loss often is difficult to quantify. The presentations may also vary greatly in patients with similar amounts of loss (young athlete vs. sedentary, elderly person). In patients particularly prone to complications associated with fluid overload, the fluid can be administered in multiple smaller boluses titrated to clinical response. See text for a more in-depth discussion of some of the guidelines in this table.

Although the presenting signs and symptoms of circulatory insufficiency are variable, patients usually have decreased blood pressure, increased heart and respiratory rates, and a normal or low–normal temperature (e.g., 36°C to 37°C [96.8°F to 98.6°F]) in the absence of infection, exposure to extremes of temperature, and medications that impair thermoregulation. As mentioned earlier, recordings of vital signs must be interpreted in light of known or suspected baseline conditions. For example, alcohol, β-blockers, diuretics, and medications with anticholinergic effects may impair thermoregulation. Medications such as β-blockers and calcium channel blockers may alter resting blood pressure and heart rate, as well as the subsequent response to therapeutic interventions.

Although a blood pressure reading of 110/70 mm Hg (systolic/diastolic) may be acceptable in many patients, it may be inadequate in a patient with preexisting hypertension who normally has a blood pressure of 170/105 mm Hg. At the other extreme, patients with very low blood pressure may have inaudible or inaccurate determinations with cuff (sphygmomanometric) measurements. Chapters 1 and 3 detail blood pressure measurement (e.g., cuff size, position). In this case, intraarterial monitoring is indicated. The respiratory rate may be elevated because of anxiety or as a compensatory mechanism for the metabolic acidosis caused by lactic acidosis associated with poor tissue perfusion.

Although the kidneys continually produce urine, the bladder stores the urine for intermittent elimination. For the initial diagnosis and management of acute circulatory insufficiency, a catheter can be inserted into the bladder for measuring urine output. In contrast to thirst, which is a relatively insensitive indicator of volume depletion, urine output is generally diminished with inadequate fluid administration and increases with appropriate resuscitation. This presumes, of course, that acute renal failure or medications such as diuretics are not altering the expected response. Adults should produce at least 0.5 to 1 mL/kg/h of urine, whereas children up to 12 years of age should produce at least 1 mL/kg/h (2 mL/kg/h if younger than 1 year).

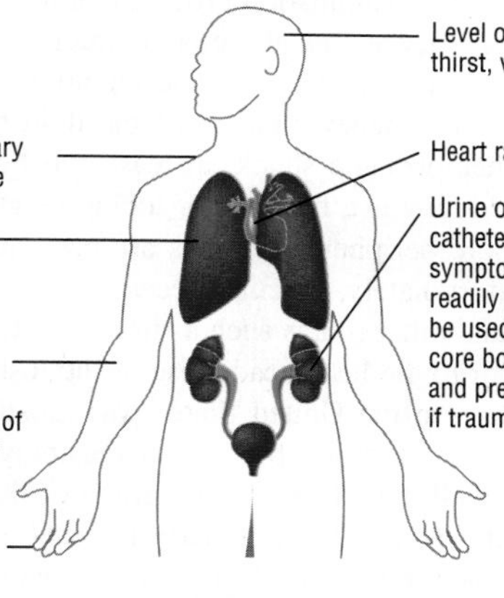

Mental status changes associated with volume depletion, if present, may range from subtle fluctuations in mood to unconsciousness. Although the latter finding typically is indicative of more severe depletion, less dramatic findings should not be interpreted as indicating mild fluid deficits. Losses of 3 to 4 L of plasma volume may be associated only with lassitude in an otherwise healthy adult patient. Similar interpretation difficulties must be considered when performing the initial physical examination. An orderly progression from warm, reddish skin with appropriate capillary refill (rapid return of blood flow to the extremity after removal of compression) to cold, cyanotic discoloration with impaired refill may not occur. Also, dry mucous membranes in elderly patients may be caused by mouth breathing or medications and not by fluid depletion.

FIGURE 14-3 Noninvasive assessment of circulatory insufficiency.

TREATMENT

Milder forms of volume depletion may be managed in outpatient settings. For example, supplemental fluids can be added to the usual estimated daily requirements of 30 to 35 mL/kg in patients older than 12 years with dehydration. Commercially available carbohydrate/electrolyte drinks generally are more palatable than water and may promote earlier recovery. The rationale for combining carbohydrates with sodium is based on the cotransport absorption mechanism in the intestinal tract. With diarrheal states in particular, sodium absorption is impaired. Because water follows sodium, the diarrhea is likely to continue despite oral crystalloid fluid administration until the intestinal pathology resolves. However, when dextrose and sodium are combined in 1:1 equimolar amounts, both are absorbed via the cotransport mechanism, which also allows for absorption of water. This concept forms the basis for the World Health Organization's (WHO's) oral rehydration solution, which contains 75 mmol/L of dextrose, 75 mmol/L of sodium, 20 mmol/L of potassium, 65 mmol/L of chloride, and 10 mmol/L of citrate for a total osmolarity of 245 mOsm/L.[3] Commercially available nonprescription rehydration drinks for children in the United States also have an osmolarity of approximately 250 mOsm/L but typically contain 50 mmol/L or less of sodium, and the dextrose-to-sodium ratio often is 3:1. How these differences between commercially available formulations and the WHO rehydration formula might affect hospitalization rates is unclear, but ad hoc attempts to alter the commercially available products to make them more

CLINICAL PRESENTATION Hypovolemic Shock

General

- The initial presentation of adult patients with suspected volume depletion could vary markedly, depending on factors such as age, concomitant disease states and medications, and the etiology and rapidity of depletion.
- Plasma volume losses of <10 mL/kg of body weight usually are associated with minor signs and symptoms of distress.

Symptoms

- Patients may present with thirst, nausea, anxiousness, weakness, light-headedness, and dizziness.
- Patients may report scanty urine output and dark yellow urine.

Signs

With more severe volume loss:

- Patients would have marked increases in heart rate (e.g., >120 beats/min) and respiratory rate (e.g., >30 breaths/min).
- Blood pressure would be decreased (e.g., systolic blood pressure <90 mm Hg).
- Mental status changes or unconsciousness may occur.
- Agitation may be present if the patient is conscious.
- Body temperature would be low or normal (e.g., 36°C to 37°C [96.8°F to 98.6°F]) in the absence of concomitant infection with cold extremities and decreased capillary refill on physical examination.

Laboratory Tests

- Sodium and chloride concentrations usually are high with acute depletion but may be low or normal depending on type of fluid intake.
- The ratio of blood urea nitrogen (BUN) to creatinine is likely to be elevated initially, but the creatinine level would increase as renal dysfunction occurs.
- Elevated base deficit and lactate concentrations in conjunction with decreased bicarbonate concentrations and pH due to metabolic acidosis.
- The complete blood count should be normal in the absence of concomitant disease states such as infection; in hemorrhagic shock, the red cell count, hemoglobin, and hematocrit would decrease over time, while the prothrombin time (PT) and international normalized ratio would increase.
- With more severe volume depletion, other organs may become dysfunctional, which may be reflected in laboratory testing (e.g., elevated transaminase levels with hepatic dysfunction).

Other Diagnostic Tests

- Urine output would be decreased to <0.5 to 1 mL/h.

consistent with the WHO formula may be dangerous and are not recommended.

Outpatient rehydration of children usually is recommended for those with uncomplicated (e.g., vomiting less than 48 hours) acute gastroenteritis and relatively mild dehydration after the exclusion of more severe illnesses such as bowel obstruction. (7) The need for IV rehydration often is overestimated. Randomized studies conducted in pediatric emergency departments have found oral or nasogastric rehydration to be at least as effective as IV rehydration using end points such as length of stay and need for hospital admission.[6,7] While dehydration is primarily a problem of intracellular fluid depletion, ongoing losses will result in extracellular fluid depletion as well. The remainder of this chapter will focus on more severe forms of volume depletion (i.e., hypovolemic shock) that are not amenable to oral rehydration.

Desired Outcomes

The desired outcomes of therapy for patients with hypovolemic shock are to reduce morbidity and mortality by preventing disease progression with subsequent organ damage and, to the extent possible, to reverse organ dysfunction that has already taken place.

Desired Outcome

Reduce morbidity and mortality by preventing disease progression with subsequent organ damage.

Desired Outcome

To the extent possible, reverse organ dysfunction that has already taken place.

General Approach to Treatment

Hospitalization is indicated for more severe forms of circulatory insufficiency. If access to the circulatory system for administration of fluids and medication is not obtained prior to hospitalization, this should be a priority. Venous access generally is obtained during the preliminary examination process that includes the ABCs of life support (i.e., airway, breathing, and circulation), assessment of vital signs and mental status, and determination of urine output after catheterization. Whenever large-volume fluid resuscitation is expected, as in hemorrhagic shock, at least two IV catheters are desirable. Because flow is a function of tubing length and catheter diameter, large-bore peripheral IV lines are preferred over longer central lines. Unfortunately, vascular access in some patients may be problematic, and other routes such as intraosseous infusion may be necessary. Prior to the last decade, use of intraosseous fluid and drug administration in the United States was mostly restricted to children with IV access issues, but it is increasingly being used in adult patients as well. One interesting method of fluid administration that has been investigated in elderly patients is subcutaneous infusion, or hypodermoclysis. With hypodermoclysis, common dextrose- and sodium-containing fluids typically given by the IV route are given by subcutaneous infusion at sites such as the upper arm, chest, abdomen, or thigh, depending on factors such as patient or provider preference. Hyaluronidase has been used as a spreading agent to facilitate fluid absorption by this route, but its benefit versus risk profile has yet to be clearly elucidated; in particular, allergic reactions with this agent have been a concern, although a recombinant form is now available that has the potential for fewer reactions compared with the older bovine-derived products. Hypodermoclysis is not used commonly in the United States, probably because of concerns of adverse effects that were found in early studies that used excessively hypotonic or hypertonic solutions, as well as issues related to reimbursement when considered in ambulatory, home, or palliative care settings. Although relatively high fluid administration rates have been achieved in some studies involving hypodermoclysis, this method of infusion should not be used in patients with more severe forms of dehydration or hypovolemia until additional supportive information from clinical trials is available. Although alternative methods of fluid administration, such as hypodermoclysis, are desirable, well-conducted trials are needed before such methods can be recommended for routine use.

After the immediate postresuscitation phase of the treatment of hypovolemic shock, proper attention must be paid to general supportive care measures that include appropriate assessment and management of pain, anxiety/agitation, and delirium. This is particularly true for patients who develop shock after trauma, surgery, or thermal injury and require admission to an ICU.

Nonpharmacologic Therapy

Nonpharmacologic therapy for shock is dependent on the inciting event, although the basic life support measures such as a secure airway with appropriate oxygenation apply to all patients. For patients with more severe traumatic injury, additional measures would include surgery, stabilization of fractures, control of blood loss by physical compression or surgical control, and prevention of heat loss since hypothermia may aggravate other problems such as bleeding. For patients with heat exposure, cooling measures are indicated. Patients with thermal injuries should have the wound sites covered with cool, moist sterile dressings until more definitive care can take place.

Pharmacologic Therapy

Since IV fluids are the primary therapy for hypovolemic shock, they will be considered as pharmacologic agents for this discussion.

Drug Treatments of First Choice

8 Dextrose-in-water solutions may be appropriate for uncomplicated dehydration caused by water deprivation, but isotonic crystalloid (sodium-containing) solutions should be used for forms of circulatory insufficiency that are associated with hemodynamic instability. In the latter situation, IV solutions with sodium concentrations approximating normal serum sodium values usually are indicated because they cause more expansion of the intravascular and interstitial spaces compared with dextrose solutions (Table 14-3). Lactated Ringer's and normal saline solutions are examples of such crystalloid solutions that frequently need to be administered in large volumes when given to patients with more severe forms of hypovolemia. A "large" amount of fluid does not mean a single bolus volume typically used as fluid challenge in a critically ill patient. An isolated bolus (e.g., 250 to 500 mL) in a young adult trauma patient is unlikely to cause a substantial change in blood pressure or acid–base balance.[8] Therefore, multiple fluid boluses usually are often needed in such patients to achieve hemodynamic stability in the perioperative period. On the other hand, overly aggressive fluid administration should be avoided, especially in patients with heart failure or impending pulmonary edema. In a randomized trial involving patients with acute lung injury and radiographic presence of pulmonary edema, a more conservative fluid management strategy led to significantly fewer ventilator-free days and days not spent in an ICU ($P < 0.001$).[9]

Published Guidelines or Treatment Protocols Recommendations for shock associated with trauma have been published as part of the Advanced Trauma Life Support (ATLS) course (http://www.facs.org/trauma/atls/).[10] In the past, the ATLS guidelines were derived more from consensus of expert participants than evidence, but this has changed in more recent revisions. Guidelines for prehospital fluid administration in patients with trauma have been published by the Eastern Association for the Surgery of Trauma (EAST).[11] Other evidence relative to fluid choice for resuscitation is available from systematic reviews,[12–14] a guideline for perioperative fluid resuscitation,[15] and a guideline pertaining to burn shock resuscitation.[16] Taken as a whole, the recommendations from all of these sources are consistent in that isotonic (or near isotonic) crystalloid solutions are the initial fluid of choice for resuscitation in hypovolemic shock (Table 14-4).

General Information Reporting Efficacy and Safety The choice between normal saline and lactated Ringer's solutions for

TABLE 14-3 Fluid Distribution and Major Indications[a]

Fluid	Intracellular	Interstitial	Intravascular	Major Indication
Normal saline or lactated Ringer's	None	750 mL	250 mL	Intravascular repletion in symptomatic patients
3% sodium chloride	→	750 mL+	250 mL+	Small amounts (e.g., 250 mL) by intermittent infusion have been used in conjunction with normal saline or lactated Ringer's for intravascular depletion in patients with head trauma
5% dextrose/0.45% sodium chloride	333 mL	500 mL	167 mL	Maintenance fluid in euvolemic or dehydrated (sodium and water loss) patients with mild signs/symptoms of volume depletion
5% dextrose	667 mL	250 mL	83 mL	Dehydration (primarily water loss) in patients with mild signs/symptoms of volume depletion
5% albumin	None	None	1,000 mL[b]	Intravascular repletion in symptomatic patients
25% albumin	→	→	1,000 mL+++[b]	Usually given by intermittent infusion of small volumes (e.g., 50–100 mL) or by continuous infusion titrated to response in hypovolemic patients with excess interstitial fluid accumulation

[a]Based on administration of 1 L of each solution *for comparative purposes only*. This amount of fluid, particularly for 3% saline and 25% albumin, would be inappropriate and likely harmful if given over a short period of time. Numbers are approximations and are likely not reflective of actual fluid distribution in critically ill patients; arrows indicate direction of fluid shift and plus signs indicate fluid pulled from other compartments.

[b]After distribution and attainment of steady-state conditions, 60% of albumin (and associated fluid) is in interstitial compartment and 40% is in intravascular compartment.

TABLE 14-4 Summary of Evidence for Choice of Plasma Expander for Hypovolemic Shock

Source	Type of Evidence	Recommendation/Conclusion
ATLS recommendations[10]	Evidence-based consensus recommendations of fluids in trauma patients with shock	Warmed isotonic crystalloid solutions such as normal saline or lactated Ringer's should be used (LOE3); hypertonic sodium chloride is an alternative with no mortality advantage (LOE4)
EAST guideline[11]	Evidence-based consensus recommendations for prehospital fluids in trauma patients	Insufficient data to recommend one fluid over another when comparing normal saline, lactated Ringer's, 3% sodium chloride, or 7.5% sodium chloride (level I)
Cochrane Collaboration[12]	Systematic review of colloids versus crystalloids in critically ill patients	No evidence that colloids reduce mortality compared with crystalloids in patients with trauma or burns, or after surgery; hydroxyethyl starch products may increase mortality
Cochrane Collaboration[13]	Systematic review of different colloids for fluid resuscitation	No evidence that one colloid is more effective than another in terms of efficacy or safety; could not exclude clinically important differences due to wide confidence intervals; did not include trials after December 1, 2011
Cochrane Collaboration[14]	Systematic review of albumin solutions versus no albumin or crystalloids for fluid resuscitation in critically ill patients	No evidence that albumin reduces mortality when compared with crystalloid solutions such as normal saline but cannot exclude benefit in specific subsets of critically ill patients
British consensus guidelines[15]	Guidelines for perioperative fluid prescribing	Balanced salt solutions such as lactated Ringer's are preferred over normal saline for crystalloid resuscitation unless hypochloremia is present (level 1b); balanced salt solutions or colloids until packed red blood cells are available for hypovolemia with blood loss (level 1b)
American Burn Association[16]	Guidelines for burn shock resuscitation that include fluid recommendations	Near isotonic crystalloid recommended for initial resuscitation (grade C); hypertonic sodium chloride reserved for clinicians experienced with use (grade B); addition of colloid after 12–24 hours postburn may decrease fluid requirements (grade A)

ATLS, Advanced Trauma Life Support; EAST, Eastern Association for the Surgery of Trauma; grade A, at least one large prospective trial with clear-cut results; grade B, several small prospective trials with similar results; grade C, single small prospective trial, retrospective studies, or expert opinion; level 1b, randomized controlled trial with narrow confidence interval, or quality cohort studies (specific definitions); level I, convincingly justifiable; LOE3, level of evidence based on case–control or retrospective cohort studies, or a systematic review with at least three studies; LOE4, level of evidence based on case series.

hypovolemia is largely based on clinician preference and adverse effect concerns (Table 14-5). Traditionally, lactated Ringer's solution has been recommended for patients with hemorrhage because it is unlikely to cause the hyperchloremic metabolic acidosis that is seen with infusions of large volumes of normal saline. More recently, concerns have been raised relative to the proinflammatory effects (e.g., neutrophil activation) of the D-isomer form of lactate that is contained along with the L-isomer in commercially available racemic isomer solutions. There are advocates for the use of lactated Ringer's solution containing only L-isomer lactate, particularly for more severe forms of hemorrhagic shock, since it avoids the proinflammatory effects of the racemic solution, while avoiding the hyperchloremia associated with normal saline.[17] Additionally, other substitutes for racemic lactate such as ketone or pyruvate have shown beneficial effects on neutrophil activation and gene expression in vitro and are the subject of ongoing studies.

TABLE 14-5 Adverse Effects of Plasma Expanders: Crystalloids

Normal saline
- Primarily extensions of pharmacologic actions (e.g., fluid overload, dilutional coagulopathy)
- Hyperchloremic metabolic acidosis (has 154 mEq/L [154 mmol/L] of chloride)
- Hypernatremia (has 154 mEq/L [154 mmol/L] of sodium)

Lactated Ringer's
- Primarily extensions of pharmacologic actions (e.g., fluid overload, dilutional coagulopathy)
- Hyponatremia (has 130 mEq/L [130 mmol/L] of sodium)
- Aggravation of preexisting hyperkalemia (has 4 mEq/L [4 mmol/L] of potassium)

Hypertonic saline
- Primarily extensions of pharmacologic actions (e.g., fluid overload, dilutional coagulopathy; intracellular volume depletion)
- Hypernatremia (has 513 mEq/L [513 mmol/L] of sodium)
- Hyperchloremia (has 513 mEq/L [513 mmol/L] of chloride)

Although lactated Ringer's solution does contain lactate, it does not cause substantial elevations in circulating lactate concentrations when used as a resuscitation solution.[18] Once adequate plasma volume has been restored by fluid administration, the body can readily clear the blood of the excess lactate that has accumulated from both anaerobic metabolism and lactated Ringer's solution. However, blood samples for lactate determinations drawn through catheters (arterial and venous) that have not been cleared appropriately may have spurious increases or decreases in lactate concentrations because of retained lactated Ringer's and nonlactated solutions (e.g., varying concentrations of dextrose-in-water or sodium chloride), respectively.[19] Therefore, blood samples for lactate concentration determinations should be drawn from a catheter that has been cleared adequately (e.g., 5 mL) of infusate after temporarily stopping the fluid infusion.

Alternative Drug Treatments

A number of pharmacologic therapies show promise in animal models of shock, but few demonstrate success in subsequent trials involving patients with shock. In large part this is a result of the lack of acceptable animal models of shock that mimic the pathophysiology of patients. In cases in which a relevant animal model is available, care must be taken when extrapolating the information to forms of shock other than the one under study. This may be the problem with naloxone, which has been shown to raise blood pressure in some studies of shock but not in others.

While research continues on medications that improve oxygen transport, optimize oxygen utilization, and reduce reactive oxygen species and reperfusion injuries, fluids remain the mainstay of therapy for shock. Hypertonic sodium chloride solutions have been used as an alternative to isotonic crystalloid solutions for hypovolemic shock in some studies. By causing redistribution (i.e., pulling fluid) from the intracellular space, hypertonic solutions cause rapid expansion of the intravascular compartment, which is essential for vital organ perfusion. In head-injured patients, it has been postulated that this redistribution should decrease intracranial pressure because the vessels of the brain are more impermeable to sodium ions than are vessels in other areas of the body. Additionally, hypertonic sodium chloride solutions have beneficial immunomodulating actions when compared with more isotonic solutions in experiments with animals, although these actions have not always translated into similar beneficial effects in patients.

From a safety standpoint, hypertonic sodium chloride is considered to be a high-risk concentrated electrolyte solution. Potential dosing and administration errors and related adverse events can occur when hypertonic sodium solution is ordered and administered by clinicians relatively unfamiliar with its use. Potential adverse events include cellular crenation and damage caused by the dramatic fluid shifts associated with hypernatremia, hyperchloremic metabolic acidosis from hyperchloremia, and peripheral vein destruction from high osmolality. The osmolarity of 3% sodium chloride is 1,026 mOsm/L. Although there are some notable exceptions (e.g., peripheral parenteral nutrition solutions often approach 1,000 mOsm/L), IV solutions with osmolarity values above 600 mOsm/L are usually recommended for administration by central lines. In the limited number of studies conducted in humans to date, adverse effects related to hypertonic sodium solutions have been uncommon and apparently of little clinical importance. Larger-molecular-weight solutions (i.e., >30,000 Da) known as *colloids* have been recommended in conjunction with or as replacements for crystalloid solutions, although their use is controversial. The major theoretical advantage of these compounds is their prolonged intravascular retention time compared with crystalloid solutions. In contrast to isotonic crystalloid solutions that have substantial interstitial distribution within minutes of IV administration, colloids remain in the intravascular space for hours or days, depending on factors such as capillary permeability. Examples of colloids used as plasma expanders in the United States include albumin, hydroxyethyl starch, and dextran. Albumin is known as a *monodisperse colloid* because all its molecules are of the same molecular size and weight (~67,000 Da), whereas hydroxyethyl starch and dextran solutions are *polydisperse compounds* with molecules of varying molecular size that are roughly proportional to molecular weight (weight-*averaged* molecular weights of 600,000 Da [range 450,000 to 800,000 Da] for 6% hetastarch in normal saline 450/0.75, 670,000 Da [range 450,000 to 800,000 Da] for 6% hetastarch in lactated electrolyte 670/0.75, 130,000 Da [range 110,000 to 150,000 Da] for 6% tetrastarch in normal saline 130/0.4, 40,000 Da [range 10,000 to 90,000 Da] for dextran 40, or 70,000 to 75,000 Da [range 20,000 to 200,000 Da] for dextran 70 or dextran 75, respectively). In light of these differences, colloid comparisons are based on weight-averaged ([number of molecules at each weight × particle weight]/total weight of all molecules) or number-averaged (arithmetic mean of all particles' weights) molecular weight.[20] The size and weight differences of the colloids have important implications for the distribution of the products because lower-molecular-weight substances are retained in the intravascular space for a shorter period of time as a result of more rapid leakage across the vessel membrane. The theoretical benefit common to all colloids is based on their increased molecular weight (average molecular weight in the case of hydroxyethyl starch and dextran) that corresponds to increased intravascular retention time in the absence of increased capillary permeability compared with crystalloids. Even in patients with intact capillary permeability, the colloid molecules eventually will leak through the membrane. In the case of albumin with a distribution half-life of 15 hours in normal subjects, approximately 60% of administered albumin molecules (and associated fluid) would be shifted to the interstitial space within 3 to 5 days of exogenous administration. In patients with altered permeability (e.g., acute respiratory distress syndrome), the leakage of albumin from the intravascular to the interstitial space may occur within hours, not days. The primary adverse effect concern of all colloids is fluid overload, which is an extension of their pharmacologic action. Another adverse effect of increasing concern is renal dysfunction that seems to be related to hyperoncotic (e.g., 25%) albumin and other starch and dextran products. The mechanism of this adverse effect may be related to alteration of normal glomerular oncotic pressure differences or formation of lesions in the kidney.[21]

Clinical **Controversy. . .**

There is no widespread agreement on the upper limit of osmolarity for hypertonic sodium solutions that are given by peripheral vein infusion.

Albumin is available in 5% and 25% concentrations. Plasma protein fraction has oncotic actions similar to a 5% albumin solution, which is not surprising because albumin is the predominant protein in this product. When given in equipotent amounts, albumin is much more costly than crystalloid solutions. Additionally, the 5% and 25% albumin solutions typically are priced such that no cost saving is associated with dilution of the 25% product to make a 5% concentration. In general, dilution should be avoided because of the possibility of preparation errors; cases of hemolysis and death have occurred when 25% albumin was inappropriately diluted with sterile water for injection, causing a dramatic lowering of effective osmolarity. The 5% albumin solution is relatively *iso-oncotic*, which means that it does not pull fluid into the compartment in which it is contained. In contrast, 25% albumin is referred to as *hyperoncotic* albumin because it tends to pull fluid into the compartment containing the albumin molecules. In general, the 5% albumin solution is used for hypovolemic states. The 25% solution should not be used for acute circulatory insufficiency unless it is used in combination with other fluids or it is being used in patients with excess total body water but intravascular depletion as a means of pulling fluid into the intravascular space. An example of the latter condition is cirrhosis with ascites in which total body water is substantially increased, but the patient is hypotensive as a consequence of lack of intravascular volume. To justify this use of hyperoncotic albumin from a cost-effectiveness standpoint presumes that there is evidence of adverse effects associated with the excess water (e.g., interstitial fluid accumulation in the lungs) and that the albumin remains in the intravascular space long enough to be of benefit. Albumin has a variety of functions beyond plasma expansion, such as binding properties, inflammatory gene modification, and antioxidant and free radical scavenging effects, which have been used to justify its administration instead of less expensive crystalloid or other colloid products. Although appealing theoretically, improved patient outcomes related to these properties have not been documented in adequately powered, randomized controlled trials. Additionally, the clinician must realize that the properties of commercially available albumin products are not biologically identical to those of native albumin. For example, denaturation of the products may lead to inefficient binding and decreased oncotic activity.

Hydroxyethyl starch products have been developed as synthetic alternatives to albumin that is derived through the fractionation of donated human blood. The various products are differentiated by two numbers, one for the average mean molecular weight and one for the degree of hydroxyethyl substitution of glucose. For example, hetastarch is expressed as 450/0.7 based on weight and substitution, respectively. Most of the trials comparing albumin with hydroxyethyl starch products for volume expansion were inadequately powered and found no significant differences in clinically important outcomes (e.g., mortality). Two large randomized trials have directly compared hydroxyethyl starch products with crystalloid solutions for intravascular expansion. Although these trials used newer, low-molecular-weight (140), low-substitution (0.4 or 0.42) starch products, hemostasis and renal function problems noted in older trials involving high-molecular-weight, high-substitution starch products were found, suggesting these are class adverse effects. One of these large trials (Scandinavian Starch for Severe Sepsis/Septic Shock, also known as the 6S trial) found significantly higher rates of renal replacement therapy, red blood cell transfusions, and 90-day mortality in patients receiving hydroxyethyl starch versus a Ringer's acetate solution.[22] The second trial (referred to as the CHEST trial) involved 7000 general intensive care unit patients, making it the largest randomized study to date involving a starch product. As in the other large trial, patients in the hydroxyethyl starch group required significantly more renal replacement therapy versus patients receiving normal saline, but the 90-day mortality rates were similar.[23] Possible explanations for the lack of a mortality difference include the relatively low overall mortality that might be related to the exclusion criteria (e.g., patients unlikely to survive), or to the use of normal saline as a control solution since saline has a high concentration of chloride ion and a low strong ion difference compared to plasma.

Hydroxyethyl starch may aggravate bleeding through mechanisms specific to this colloid (e.g., decreased factor VIII/von Willebrand factor). These mechanisms have not been well elucidated and often are difficult to distinguish from the dilutional effects on clotting factors caused by all plasma expanders; however, the risk of coagulopathy appears to be related to increasing doses and durations of administration.[22] Renal dysfunction associated with hydroxyethyl starch products may also be a function of dose and duration of administration. Regardless of potential mechanisms, the FDA considers the serious adverse effects of the hydroxyethyl starch products to be class effects that warrant changes to product labeling. The changes include a boxed warning that states these products are contraindicated in critically ill patients. Additional warnings have also been added about excessive bleeding when used in patients undergoing cardiopulmonary bypass. Hydroxyethyl starch may cause elevations in serum amylase concentrations but does not cause pancreatitis.

Clinical **Controversy...**

The mechanisms by which hydroxyethyl starch products cause bleeding and acute kidney injury have yet to be fully elucidated.

Dextran 40, dextran 70, and dextran 75 are available for use as plasma expanders in the United States. The numbers refer to the average molecular weight of the solutions. In general, dextran solutions are not used as often as albumin for plasma expansion because of a lack of adequately powered randomized trials, and because of concerns related to aggravation of bleeding (i.e., anticoagulant actions related to inhibiting stasis of microcirculation), acute kidney injury, and anaphylaxis that is more likely to occur with the higher-molecular-weight solutions. There are few comparative trials involving the dextran solutions, but the intravascular expansion within hours after infusion is approximately equal to the amount of dextran infused. Apart from the acute kidney injury and bleeding associated with starch and dextran products, adverse effects associated with colloids generally are extensions of their pharmacologic activity (Table 14-6).

From a historical perspective, the so-called crystalloid versus colloid debate was intensified when a meta-analysis by the well-respected Cochrane group found an overall increase in mortality associated with albumin using pooled results of randomized investigations.[24] The meta-analysis involved 30 randomized trials with 1,419 patients (relative risk of death with albumin vs. no administration or crystalloid administration, 1.68; 95% confidence interval [CI], 1.26 to 2.23). For hypovolemia (caused by blood loss in the majority of studies), the risk of death associated with albumin administration was not quite statistically significant (relative risk, 1.46; 95% CI, 0.97 to 2.22). With the notable exception of trauma patients, a subsequent and more comprehensive systematic review did not find increased mortality attributable to albumin.[25] Furthermore, a landmark investigation involving almost 7,000 critically ill patients (conducted after the previously mentioned meta-analyses) did not find statistically significant differences in 28-day mortality between patients resuscitated with either normal saline or 4% albumin.[26] As in the previous meta-analysis, there was a trend toward increased mortality in patients with trauma, which became statistically significant ($P = 0.003$) when analyzed at 24 months in a subset of patients with traumatic brain injury.[27] This multicenter, randomized, double-blind investigation, referred to as the Saline versus Albumin Fluid Evaluation (SAFE) study, involved a heterogeneous group of ICU patients and was not sufficiently powered to look at various subsets, so clinicians must be cautious when extrapolating the results to more specific patient populations. With this caution in mind, this trial provides strong evidence that crystalloid solutions should be considered first-line therapy in patients with hypovolemic shock.

TABLE 14-6 Adverse Effects of Plasma Expanders: Colloids

Albumin
Primarily extensions of pharmacologic actions (e.g., fluid overload; dilutional coagulopathy)
Amino acid profile and catabolism alterations (clinical significance?); potential protein overload if given with exogenous protein (e.g., parenteral nutrition)
Anaphylactoid/anaphylaxis reactions (life-threatening reactions rare; higher in patients with immunoglobulin A deficiency)
Infectious complications (all reported cases have been associated with improper handling by manufacturer or institution; no reported cases of human immunodeficiency virus or hepatitis transmission)
Interactions with medications and nutrients (clinical significance varies)
Metal loading, particularly aluminum (long-term administration in patients with renal failure)
Negative inotropic effect; reductions in ionized calcium concentrations (not well documented)
Pyrogenic reactions (not well documented)
Renal dysfunction with hyperoncotic albumin
Hydroxyethyl starch
Primarily extensions of pharmacologic actions (e.g., fluid overload, dilutional coagulopathy)
Bleeding; not recommended in critically ill patients or in patients with bleeding conditions such as subarachnoid hemorrhage
Macroamylase formation may cause elevation in blood amylase that leads to inaccurate diagnosis of pancreatitis
Anaphylactoid/anaphylaxis reactions
Pruritus (particularly when large amounts are given; may take months to resolve)
Renal dysfunction; not recommended in critically ill patients, patients at risk for renal dysfunction or patients with preexisting renal dysfunction
Dextrans
Primarily extensions of pharmacologic actions (e.g., fluid overload, dilutional coagulopathy)
Anaphylactoid/anaphylaxis reactions (increased incidence of anaphylaxis with increased molecular weight)
Bleeding (sometimes used for anticoagulant activity, so not recommended for patients with or at risk for bleeding)
Renal dysfunction

The colloids are expensive solutions. Therefore, it is difficult to justify the additional cost of colloidal products unless the benefit-to-risk ratio is substantially greater than that associated with inexpensive crystalloid solutions. This does not appear to be the case based on randomized controlled studies and meta-analyses comparing colloid and crystalloid solutions for acute circulatory insufficiency. While the use of albumin in specific patient populations (e.g., septic shock) is still debated, the documented adverse effect profile of hydroxyethyl starch products and the lack of adequately powered trials for dextran products renders them all unsuitable for use in critically ill patients including those with shock.

In contrast to other forms of shock such as anaphylactic or septic, medications are a distant alternative to the primary therapy for hypovolemic shock, fluids. In hypovolemic shock, peripheral resistance is high due to compensatory mechanisms aimed at maintaining tissue perfusion. Early or overzealous use of vasopressors in lieu of fluids may exacerbate this resistance to the point that flow is stopped. Therefore, vasoactive agents that dilate the peripheral vasculature such as dobutamine are preferred if the blood pressure is stable and high enough to tolerate the vasodilation. Vasopressors are only used as a temporizing measure or as a last resort when all other measures to maintain perfusion have been exhausted.[28] Because vasopressors have such a limited role in hypovolemic shock, there are very few studies that compare various agents. In one of the few studies that included patients with hypovolemic shock, norepinephrine and dopamine had similar effects on mortality, but dopamine was associated with more adverse effects, particularly atrial fibrillation.[29]

Special Populations

Trauma/Perioperative Patients

The need for immediate treatment of hemorrhagic circulatory insufficiency with plasma expanders (i.e., crystalloids or colloids) seems obvious, but no large, well-controlled trials conducted in humans have supported this practice. To the contrary, evidence suggests that fluid resuscitation beyond minimal levels (i.e., mean arterial pressure >60 mm Hg) is harmful in patients with penetrating abdominal trauma due to hemodilution and clot destabilization. One prospective study involving 598 adult patients with gunshot or stab wound injuries to the torso and systolic blood pressure measurements of 90 mm Hg or less found that delayed fluid resuscitation until operation was associated with increased survival and discharge from the hospital ($P = 0.04$).[30] Since concerns were expressed about the comparability of the immediate and delayed resuscitation groups, particularly because true randomization did not take place, a follow-up randomized trial was conducted to verify the findings. There were no differences in survival (four deaths in each group) in the second trial regardless of whether systolic blood pressure was titrated to >100 mm Hg or to 70 mm Hg.[31] Both studies were conducted in populated urban areas with approximately 2 hours from the time of injury to operation. Therefore, the results may not be applicable to rural areas with extended transport times. There also is a concern in applying the results of these investigations to patients with certain kinds of single-system injuries, particularly head trauma, where cerebral perfusion pressure is of primary importance. Although the applicability of these studies to other populations and settings is debatable, the *presumption* of benefits from immediate plasma expansion in all preoperative patients with circulatory insufficiency caused by hemorrhage is no longer valid. Instead, the initial priority should be surgical control of the bleeding source; until this is possible, fluids should be given in small aliquots to yield a palpable pulse and to maintain mean arterial pressures no more than 60 mm Hg and systolic pressures no more than 90 mm Hg based on accurate measurements (e.g., arterial monitoring).

Beneficial outcome data attributable to hypertonic solutions are lacking. Most of these studies were conducted in prehospital and emergency department settings using 250 mL of 7.5% sodium chloride with or without 6% dextran 70. For example, a double-blind, randomized controlled trial involving 229 patients with hypotension and severe brain injury demonstrated no significant differences in neurologic function at 6 months when 250 mL of 7.5% saline or lactated Ringer's solution was administered as part of a prehospital resuscitation regimen.[32] Part of the explanation for this finding may be related to supplemental crystalloid fluids that were given routinely to patients in both the treatment and control groups, which probably would increase the number of patients needed to demonstrate a statistically significant difference in mortality.

In order to address ongoing questions of efficacy, the National Heart, Lung, and Blood Institute evaluated hypertonic sodium chloride solutions with or without a colloid (i.e., 7.5% sodium chloride or 7.5% sodium chloride in 6% dextran 70) for prehospitalized trauma patients with shock and severe traumatic brain injury in two trials conducted by a network of sites known as the Resuscitation Outcomes Consortium (ROC). Both the parallel trials were stopped when it was determined that the hypertonic sodium chloride solutions were no better than normal saline and further enrollment would not change the 33 outcomes.[33,34] Therefore, normal saline is the fluid of choice since it is equal in efficacy with a lower risk of adverse effects compared with hypertonic solutions that are high-risk electrolyte solutions. Given their relatively poor intravascular expansion and association with poor outcome in animal models of closed head injury, hypotonic solutions should be avoided in this population.

In addition to crystalloid solutions, colloids have been used for plasma expansion in trauma patients with perioperative circulatory insufficiency. No large randomized studies have compared crystalloids and colloids for circulatory insufficiency in trauma patients. Until such studies are performed, there is no compelling reason to suspect that colloids have any substantial clinical benefits beyond crystalloids in these patients given the results of previous trials and systematic reviews performed in more general critical care populations. Further, bleeding and renal injury concerns for both starch and dextran products precludes their use in critically ill trauma patients.

The preceding discussion dealt primarily with acute circulatory insufficiency, but there are other considerations with regard to fluid replacement in other patients undergoing surgical procedures. Preoperative fluid deficits in patients undergoing minor procedures may be associated with increased perioperative morbidity, some of which (e.g., drowsiness, dizziness) may be reduced by appropriate fluid administration prior to surgery. However, care must be taken to avoid overhydration in the perioperative period because excess fluid will lead to weight gain and decreased pulmonary function. Some evidence suggests that fluid restriction on the day of surgery may reduce postoperative morbidity in patients undergoing major surgical procedures. In one randomized, multicenter trial, use of a restricted intraoperative and postoperative IV fluid protocol led to significantly fewer cardiopulmonary (7% vs. 24%; $P = 0.007$) and wound (16% vs. 31%; $P = 0.04$) complications.[35] As the preceding discussion indicates, the benefits and risks of fluid administration in the perioperative period are not just a function of too little or too much fluid but involve other patient- and procedure-related issues.

Another consideration in the patient with penetrating injuries or surgery is the potential need for blood product administration (Table 14-7) to replace oxygen-carrying and clotting functions. Although a small group of trauma patients respond to the initial fluid bolus and remain stable, most patients respond initially and then deteriorate. The latter patients, as well as patients undergoing blood loss associated with surgery, frequently need blood

TABLE 14-7 General Indications for Blood Products in Acute Circulatory Insufficiency Due to Hemorrhage[a]

Packed red blood cells	Increase oxygen-carrying capacity of blood: Usually indicated in patients with continued deterioration after volume replacement or obvious exsanguination; must be warmed, particularly when used in children
Fresh-frozen plasma	Replacement of clotting factors: Generally overused; indicated if ongoing hemorrhage in patients with PT/PTT >1.5 times normal, severe hepatic disease, or other bleeding diathesis
Platelets	Used for bleeding due to severe thrombocytopenia (i.e., platelet count <10,000/μL [<10 × 10^9/L]) or rapidly dropping platelet counts as would occur with massive bleeding
Other products	With the exception of recombinant activated factor VII, which is currently undergoing trials for use in life-threatening hemorrhage unresponsive to traditional blood product administration, components such as cryoprecipitate and factor VIII are generally not indicated in acute hemorrhage but rather are used after specific deficiencies are identified

[a]Although whole blood can be used for large-volume blood loss, most hospitals use component therapy, and use crystalloids or colloids for plasma expansion. PT, prothrombin time; PTT, partial thromboplastin time.

components such as packed red blood cells. **9** In the case of the latter component, red blood cells contain hemoglobin that delivers oxygen to tissues. Neither crystalloids nor colloids perform this function.

Administration of excessive blood products may be counterproductive. In the case of red blood cells, attempts to raise the hematocrit to high–normal or supranormal concentrations may decrease oxygen delivery by increasing blood viscosity. Additionally, there are immunomodulatory concerns with red blood cell administration. Although there is no optimal hematocrit value for all patients, a minimum hematocrit of 30% (0.30) (equivalent to a hemoglobin concentration of 10 g/dL [100 g/L; 6.21 mmol/L]) traditionally has been used as the threshold for transfusion, particularly in patients at risk for ischemia, such as those with CAD. Use of a more liberal transfusion strategy has been curtailed in many institutions with the publication of a randomized, multicenter trial involving critically ill patients that found 30-day mortality to be similar whether patients were transfused at a hemoglobin concentration less than 7 or 10 g/dL (70 to 100 g/L; 4.34 to 6.21 mmol/L) (18.7% vs. 23.3%, respectively; $P = 0.11$).[36] The mortality during hospitalization was significantly lower in the restrictive group (22.2% vs. 28.1%; $P = 0.05$). Although the investigators were cautious about extrapolating the results of this investigation to patients with myocardial ischemia, a subsequent study performed in patients undergoing cardiac surgery found similar results.[37] With the exception of the critically ill or perioperative patient with acute exsanguination, there is little justification for a liberal transfusion strategy based solely on hemoglobin concentrations.

Blood products have risks beyond immunomodulation. There is the rare but important risk of virus transmission (e.g., human immunodeficiency virus [HIV], hepatitis). Citrate that is added to stored blood to prevent coagulation may bind to calcium, resulting in hypocalcemia, although potassium and phosphate concentrations often are elevated in stored blood, particularly when hemolysis has occurred during storage. In patients receiving large amounts of blood, prophylactic calcium administration may be warranted until levels are available. Other issues that must be considered with blood product administration include monitoring for transfusion-related reactions and attention to appropriate warming, particularly when large volumes are given to pediatric patients, because hypothermia is associated with increased fluid requirements and mortality.

Since its commercial release in the United States, recombinant factor VIIa has been used for a variety of off-label uses related to trauma and bleeding. For example, in patients with massive blood loss a cocktail of cryoprecipitate, platelets, and recombinant factor VIIa has been suggested to rapidly attain hemostasis. These more severe forms of blood loss are a function of not only the type of injury but also factors such as medications (e.g., aspirin, Coumadin, clopidogrel, enoxaparin) and disease states that impair normal coagulation. Large well-controlled trials are needed to define the role of recombinant factor VIIa in clinical practice given its high cost and potential thromboembolic complications. Concerns with its use in trauma patients are issues related to appropriate dose, timing, and diminished effectiveness in patients with acidosis and severe hypothermia. Evidence of efficacy in a general trauma population that would offset these concerns is lacking. In the largest randomized controlled trial conducted to date that enrolled patients with penetrating and blunt trauma, factor VIIa did not decrease mortality compared with placebo when the trial was prematurely terminated due to futility.[38]

The periodic shortages, high costs, and adverse effect concerns related to blood products have prompted investigations of alternative "bloodless" strategies. In addition to the use of more restrictive transfusion thresholds, as mentioned previously, these strategies have included hemoglobin-based oxygen carriers and perfluorocarbon compounds to deliver oxygen to tissues. Other strategies have aimed at reducing blood loss through the use of improved procedural and surgical techniques, as well as the administration of hemostatic medications. The only hemostatic medication with a proven mortality benefit is the antifibrinolytic agent, tranexamic acid. The best evidence for efficacy was data from a multicenter trial involving more than 20,000 adult trauma patients with significant bleeding (or risk for significant bleeding) who were randomized to IV tranexamic acid (1 g over 10 minutes followed by 1 g over 8 hours by infusion) or matching placebo within 8 hours of injury.[39] There was a significant reduction in all-cause mortality with tranexamic acid compared with placebo (14.5% vs. 16%, $P = 0.0035$) with no increase in vascular or other adverse events. While additional data are still needed in specific subpopulations such as patients with traumatic brain injuries, this study is relatively unique in that an intervention apart from surgery and blood product administration was demonstrated to reduce mortality.

Patients with Thermal Injuries

There are a number of formulas for estimating fluid requirements in thermally injured patients, but there is little reason to choose one over another based on well-controlled studies. In general, the amount of loss corresponds to the size of the thermal injury. Guidelines recommend approximately 2 to 4 mL/kg of isotonic fluid (lactated Ringer's solution) for each percent burn can be used for calculating the expected fluid requirements for the first 24 hours after the burn.[16] For example, a 60-kg person with 30% body surface area (BSA) burns is expected to require 5,400 to 7,200 mL of fluid over the initial 24 hours. Regardless of the calculated deficit, fluids should be administered until adequate tissue perfusion has been documented (e.g., maintenance of urine output of 0.5 to 1 mL/kg in adults) or adverse effects (e.g., pulmonary edema) occur. Crystalloids are preferred as initial therapy for burn victims because there is no substantial evidence that colloids mobilize edematous fluid, and there is a theoretical concern that extravascular fluid accumulation might be prolonged by the oncotic actions of albumin and other colloid products that have leaked through vessel walls. Additionally, there is no evidence that colloids reduce mortality in patients with thermal injuries and there is a concern that hydroxyethyl starch and dextran products might even increase mortality through deleterious effects on coagulation and renal function. Some novel therapies for thermal resuscitation have been studied, although larger confirmatory trials are needed prior to use apart from research protocols. For example, in a prospective study involving patients with >30% BSA burns, antioxidant therapy with extremely high doses of IV vitamin C (66 mg/kg/h for 24 hours) reduced resuscitation fluid requirements and wound edema.[40] The proposed mechanism is reduction in free radical–induced increases in capillary permeability.

Personalized Pharmacotherapy

At this time there is little genetic/genomic information that is available to guide personalized pharmacotherapy in patients with hypovolemic shock. Further, as stressed throughout this chapter, fluids are by far the first choice of therapy in conjunction with other definitive interventions such as surgery for traumatic injuries. Nevertheless, there are individual factors that may influence the specific fluid being administered. For example, the lower chloride concentration in lactated Ringer's would usually make it preferred over normal saline in patients with a hyperchloremic metabolic acidosis, while the increased osmolarity of normal saline would usually make it preferred over lactated Ringer's in a patient with increased intracranial pressure.

Clinical Controversies

Some clinicians believe that hypertonic solutions should be used to lower intracranial pressure in patients with head injuries.

The appropriate use of invasive hemodynamic monitoring tools, such as right-sided heart catheterization in patients with hypovolemic shock, is controversial.

EVALUATION OF THERAPEUTIC OUTCOMES

Monitoring of the Pharmaceutical Care Plan

One form of monitoring that may take place in the emergency and operating rooms, as well as in the ICU, requires placement of a central venous pressure (CVP) line. Monitoring of CVP provides the clinician with a somewhat insensitive yet useful estimate of the relationship between increased right atrial pressure and cardiac output. A protocol that used a particular type of central catheter to perform continuous monitoring of central venous oxygen saturation in conjunction with so-called goal-directed therapy in the first 6 hours of patient arrival in an urban emergency department resulted in decreased mortality compared with standard monitoring (30.5% vs. 46.5%; $P = 0.009$).[41] However, the patients in this study had severe sepsis and septic shock, so the results might not be applicable to other forms of shock with different pathophysiologic considerations. For example, in hemorrhagic shock due to trauma, the most important intervention is surgical control of bleeding, and anything that delays this control is likely to increase, not decrease, mortality. Until additional studies have been performed, it would be premature to mandate goal-directed therapy with the associated central venous monitoring in patients with nonseptic forms of shock, particularly shock due to blood loss. In fact, so-called "upstream" measurements of perfusion such as CVP are not a useful guide for fluid management in hospitalized patients, and are being replaced by "downstream" markers such as urine output and lactate levels that are more likely to reflect end-organ dysfunction.[42] A more complete discussion of invasive and noninvasive hemodynamic monitoring is given in Chapter 1.

Clinical **Controversy...**

The most appropriate, cost-effective, and practical parameter(s) for monitoring adequacy of fluid resuscitation in shock is unresolved.

A number of laboratory tests are indicated for subacute monitoring of shock in the ICU setting. These include a renal battery for assessing possible electrolyte alterations and kidney perfusion (e.g., BUN and creatinine). Among other things, a complete blood count will enable assessment of possible infection (white blood cell count), oxygen-carrying capacity of the blood (hemoglobin, hematocrit), and ongoing bleeding (hemoglobin, hematocrit, and platelet count). The PT or international normalized ratio and partial thromboplastin time (PTT) will give an indication of the ability of the blood to clot because, in the case of hemorrhagic shock, clotting factors are lost and diluted. An increasing lactate concentration (arterial, mixed venous, or central venous), an increasing arterial base deficit, or a decreasing bicarbonate concentration are global markers indicative of inadequate perfusion leading to anaerobic metabolism with accumulation of lactic acid. Although the value of these surrogate markers for improving patient outcomes is more controversial, they are considered traditional end points of resuscitation in certain populations such as trauma patients. Other tests may be indicated if organ dysfunction is likely. For example, when blood flow to the liver is interrupted because of sustained hypotension, a condition known as *shock liver* may occur. In this condition, the levels of transaminases on a liver panel may be markedly elevated in the first couple of days after marked hypotension, although the concentrations should decrease over time. Along with laboratory testing, a more extensive history can be obtained during the subacute monitoring period.

The value of pulmonary artery catheters (also known as right-sided heart or Swan-Ganz catheters) has been debated hotly since their introduction. Such catheters are placed to obtain various oxygen-transport variables, some of which cannot be determined reliably from peripheral or other central vessels. The debate was intensified when early studies suggested improved outcomes when cardiac output and other oxygen-transport variables were raised to supranormal levels, the monitoring of which required placement of a pulmonary artery catheter. The controversy led to consensus conferences and workshops, the development of organizational guidelines, and the publication of a meta-analysis (which found a statistically significant reduction in *morbidity* using pulmonary artery catheters to guide therapy).[43] Ultimately, a large randomized controlled trial involving pulmonary artery catheters was conducted in high-risk surgical patients.[44] The trial involved 1,994 patients. The mortality was almost identical for the catheter and control groups (7.8% vs. 7.7%; 95% CI, 2.3 to 2.5). There were no episodes of pulmonary embolism in the catheter group and eight episodes in the control group ($P = 0.004$). This trial is important not only because of the implications for high-risk surgical patients but also because it allows for the conduct of future trials in other patient populations without some of the ethical issues raised about such trials in the past.

Part of the concern regarding pulmonary artery catheterization relates to interpretation of its results by inexperienced practitioners. Studies in Europe and the United States found that one of two physicians incorrectly interpreted a tracing from a pulmonary artery catheter.[45] This could explain some of the results of studies finding no benefits to pulmonary artery catheterization or, in some cases, worse outcomes in the pulmonary artery catheterization group by actions taken as a result of inaccurate measurements or misinterpretation of information obtained from the monitoring process.

Complications related to pulmonary artery catheter insertion, maintenance, and removal include damage to vessels and organs during insertion, arrhythmias, infections, and thromboembolic damage. To avoid the complications associated with pulmonary artery catheterization, other less invasive tools were developed to obtain similar information. For example, cardiac output determinations have been made by Doppler, bioimpedance, dye, and ionic dilution techniques, although such measurements would not provide other data that are obtained routinely with pulmonary artery catheters (e.g., left-sided heart filling pressure). Additionally, advances in pulmonary artery catheter technology that expand the information obtained from such monitoring (e.g., mixed venous oxyhemoglobin) are under investigation. However, given the lack of well-defined outcome data associated with pulmonary artery catheterization, its use is best reserved for complicated cases of shock not responding to conventional fluid and medication therapies.

Commonly measured and calculated hemodynamic and oxygen-transport indices associated with invasive monitoring are primarily global indicators of tissue perfusion. Attempts have been made to find regional and local indicators of hypoperfusion so that circulatory insufficiency could be treated before overt shock occurs. One focus of recent research has been monitoring modalities involving the GI tract. Although the literature is fairly consistent concerning low gastric intramucosal pH (pHi) values being predictive of death, pHi-guided therapy to decrease mortality has not been demonstrated.[46] Additionally, a number of technical considerations remain to be resolved when using pHi or, more recently, capnometry (luminal Pco_2 tonometry) for monitoring and therapy. Despite these concerns, measures of regional tissue oxygenation continue to be investigated through a variety of novel monitoring techniques.

In addition to regional monitoring of tissue perfusion, local methods of monitoring are being studied. For example, subcutaneous measurement of tissue oxygen pressure shows promise in preliminary investigations. Regional and local measurements likely will not replace more global indicators of perfusion; rather, the methods will complement each other.

Proper attention to monitoring of plasma volume must be continued into the intraoperative and postoperative periods. A number of neurohormonal changes take place that affect urine output, and patients may have substantial third spacing of fluid depending on the operation and preexisting conditions. Furthermore, postoperative patients are prone to hyponatremia from renal generation of electrolyte-free water and from antidiuretic hormone release. As in acute resuscitation, the administration of hypotonic solutions in the perioperative period does not prevent the decrease in extracellular volume that often occurs. Therefore, although excess fluid administration is to be avoided in the perioperative setting, isotonic crystalloid solutions should be used when fluids are indicated to prevent intravascular depletion and circulatory insufficiency. There is general agreement that the choice of crystalloid solution in the perioperative period should be either normal saline or a lactated Ringer's (or equivalent) solution. However, there is substantial debate as to which of these two solutions is preferable since comparative studies have involved small numbers of patients.

Of the randomized studies comparing albumin with crystalloid solutions in the perioperative period, the majority found no statistically significant differences between groups. Any significant differences found involved isolated hemodynamic or respiratory variables with no obvious clinical correlates (e.g., duration of mechanical ventilation). Therefore, albumin cannot be recommended for the prevention or initial treatment of circulatory insufficiency, although its use may be appropriate in patients who are not responding to crystalloids and are developing problems such as interstitial fluid accumulation.

In contrast to many other forms of shock, vasoactive medications are not indicated in the initial therapy of hypovolemic shock but rather play an adjunctive role in patients who continue to have circulatory insufficiency after fluids have been maximized and volume-overload concerns exist. In a multicenter cohort study of blunt-injured patients with hemorrhagic shock, the use of vasopressors within 12 hours of injury was associated with significantly higher mortality at 24 hours ($P = 0.001$).[47] With hypovolemia, the body's natural response is to increase cardiac output and to constrict blood vessels to maintain blood pressure. There is no evidence that vasoactive medications improve outcome in patients with hypovolemic shock assuming that fluid therapy is adequate. **10** However, once the cause of acute circulatory insufficiency has been stopped or treated and fluids have been optimized, some patients continue to have signs and symptoms of inadequate tissue perfusion. This may be caused by reperfusion injury. Although the search for a cryptogenic source (e.g., intraabdominal bleeding in a trauma patient) should continue, the clinician may need to administer vasoactive medications to improve perfusion.

Pressor agents such as norepinephrine and high-dose dopamine are to be avoided, if possible, because they may increase blood pressure at the expense of peripheral tissue ischemia. Some sources use stronger language and state that vasopressors are contraindicated in certain forms of shock (e.g., hemorrhagic). This does not help the clinician who is treating a patient with unstable blood pressure despite massive fluid replacement and increasing interstitial fluid accumulation. In such situations, inotropic agents such as dobutamine are preferred if blood pressure is adequate (e.g., systolic blood pressure ≥80 to 90 mm Hg) because they should not aggravate the existing vasoconstriction. The inotropic agents are justified by presumed inadequate cardiac output for the specific situation, although the measured values may be in the normal range.

When pressure cannot be maintained with inotropic agents or when inotropic agents with vasodilatory properties cannot be used because of inadequate blood pressure concerns, pressors may be required as a last resort. In general, the need for pressors is predictive of the development of MODS and increased length of hospital stay. Although the response to pressor agents may be variable in hypovolemic shock, there does not appear to be resistance as a consequence of altered receptor response, as is sometimes seen in patients with septic shock. Potent vasoconstrictors such as norepinephrine and phenylephrine should be given through central veins because of the possibility of extravasation and necrosis with peripheral administration.

In managing patients with hypovolemic shock, the clinician must be aware of potential adverse effects of medications being used for supportive care purposes. For example, some patients are particularly susceptible to the histamine release associated with morphine and may have substantial decreases in blood pressure. Sodium bicarbonate would seem to be a logical therapy in patients with shock who typically have a metabolic acidosis, but bicarbonate administration has not been shown to improve surrogate hemodynamic markers or patient outcomes and has known disadvantages such as the associated increase in arterial carbon dioxide levels and decrease in serum ionized calcium levels.[48] Propofol is commonly used for sedation in the ICU, but it may cause substantial decreases in blood pressure. The initial dose of propofol should be substantially reduced or avoided in patients with hemorrhagic shock who may not be fully resuscitated.

A number of interesting treatments for shock are under investigation, including autotransfusion for removing harmful cytokines from the body. Various alternatives to conventional blood components also are being studied, such as stroma-free hemoglobin and perfluorocarbon compounds, as virus-free alternatives to red blood cell transfusion. Hopefully, these methods will be useful adjuncts to adequate volume replacement, which is the primary therapeutic intervention in managing acute circulatory insufficiency as a result of volume depletion.

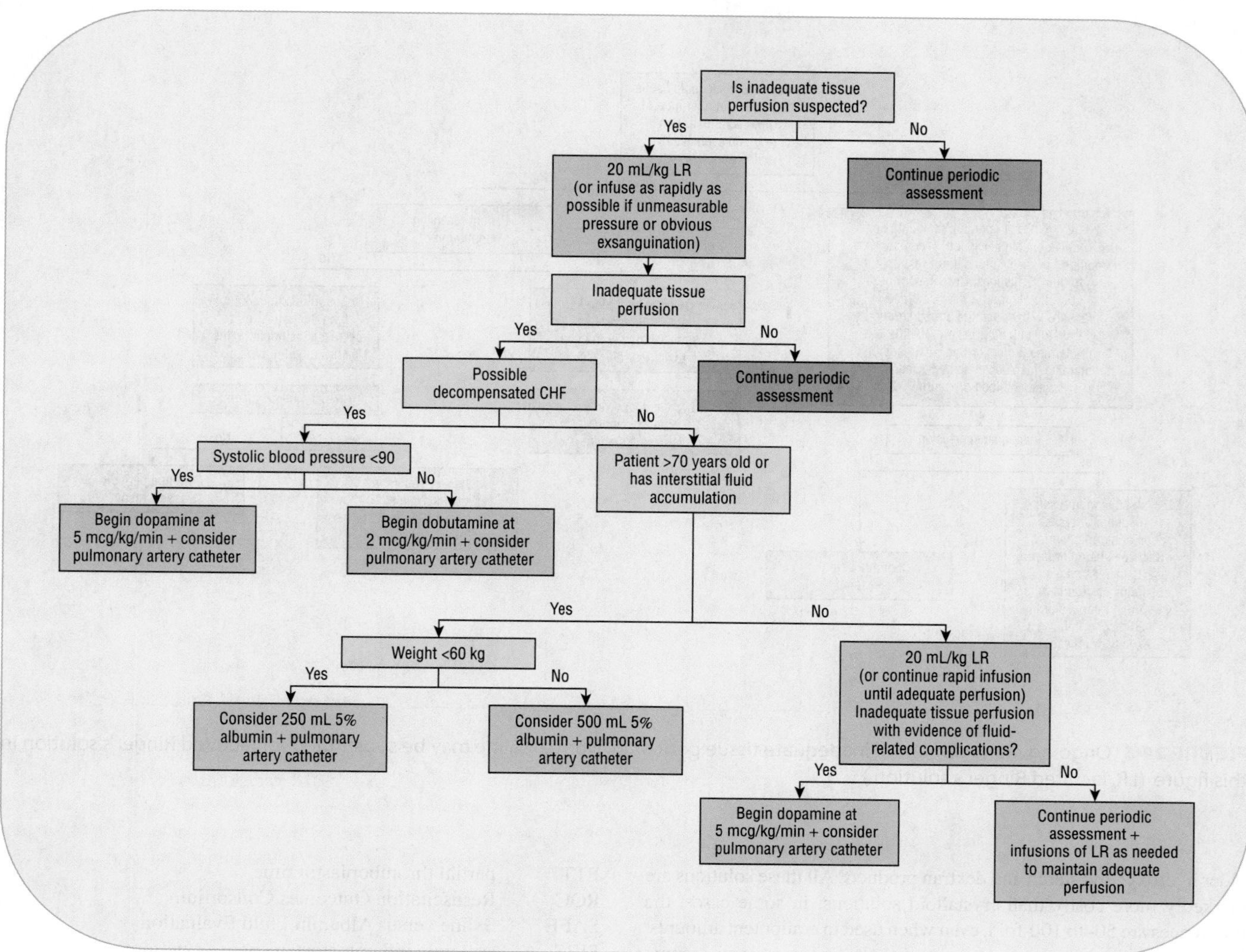

FIGURE 14-4 Hypovolemia protocol for adults. Normal saline may be used instead of lactated Ringer's solution. This protocol is not intended to replace or delay therapies such as surgical intervention or blood products for restoring oxygen-carrying capacity or hemostasis. For the resuscitation of patients with trauma prior to bleeding control, usually no more than 1 liter of crystalloid should be given initially in an attempt to use the minimal amount of fluid necessary to maintain perfusion and not exacerbate bleeding. If available, some measurements can be used in addition to those listed in the algorithm, such as mean arterial pressure or pulmonary artery catheter recordings. The latter can be used to assist in medication choices (e.g., agents with primary pressor effects may be desirable in patients with normal cardiac outputs, whereas dopamine or dobutamine may be indicated in patients with suboptimal cardiac outputs). Lower maximal doses of the medications in this algorithm should be considered when pulmonary artery catheterization is not available. See text for an in-depth discussion of these and other issues involved in this protocol. (CHF, congestive heart failure; LR, lactated Ringer's solution.)

CLINICAL BOTTOM LINE

Figure 14-4 is an algorithm that summarizes many of the treatment principles discussed in this chapter. The algorithm is an example of one approach to the adult patient presenting with hypovolemic shock. It presumes that initial rehydration attempts (i.e., outpatient or prehospital) were unsuccessful in restoring circulation. Obviously, modifications may be needed for patient-specific forms of hypovolemic shock. For example, in patients with severe traumatic brain injury albumin would be contraindicated as a plasma expander, while hypertonic sodium solution might be considered for its ability to lower elevated intracranial pressure without causing the diuresis associated with mannitol administration. Other limitations of the algorithm should be recognized, particularly the decisions to add or to substitute medication therapies when crystalloid solutions are not yielding desired results and when to perform pulmonary artery catheterization for more invasive monitoring. Medications become more important for the ongoing management of hypovolemic shock, but only when the patient is unresponsive to fluids (Fig. 14-5). Medications for more complicated cases of hemorrhagic shock should not detract from the primary effective resuscitative measure—surgical stabilization of bleeding.

The algorithm in Figure 14-4 attempts to incorporate economic considerations. The institutional cost of 1 L of most crystalloid solutions is less than $1. Assuming that such fluids are used, the associated costs of personnel and equipment then become the primary economic considerations in the resuscitation of patients with hypovolemic shock. However, as mentioned, many clinicians recommend that colloid plasma expanders (e.g., albumin, hydroxyethyl starch, or dextrans) be used to replace some or all of the standard crystalloid solutions. Although the costs of these solutions vary, depending on contractual arrangements, in general, albumin solutions are more expensive than

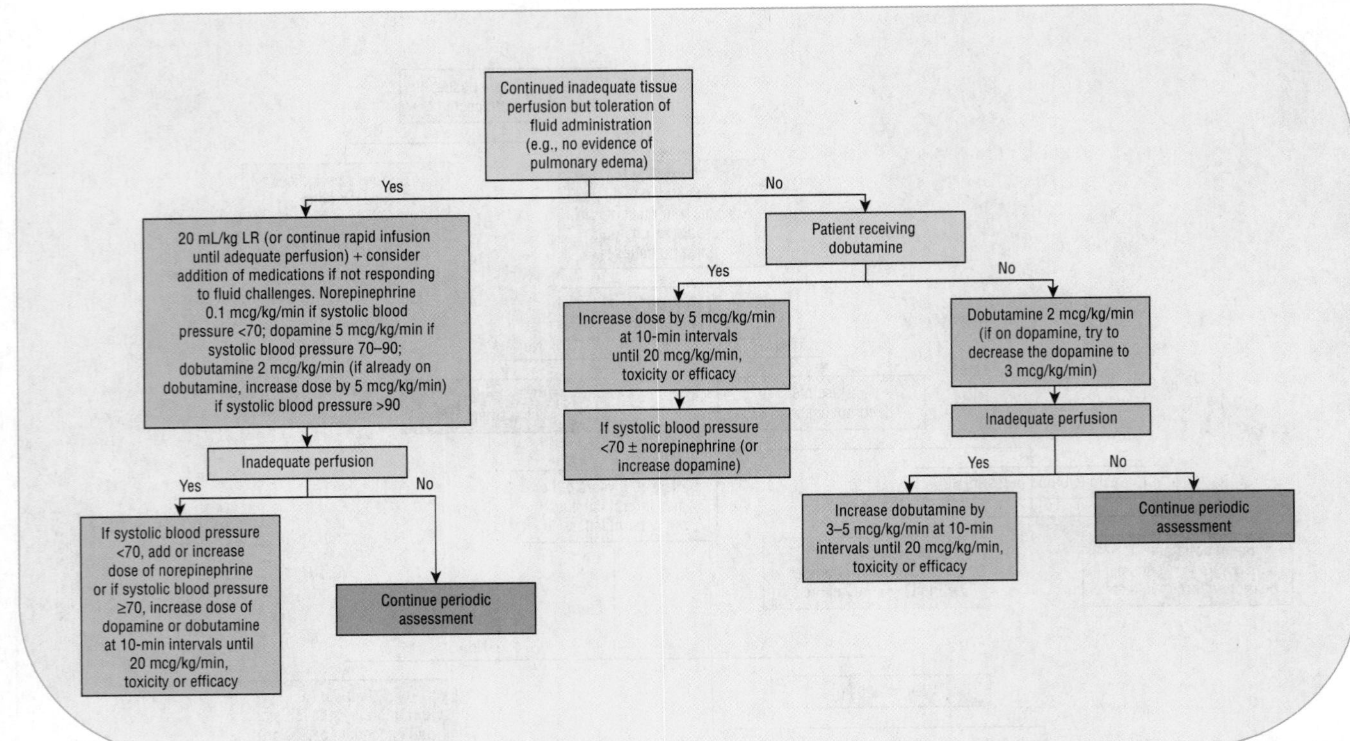

FIGURE 14-5 Ongoing management of inadequate tissue perfusion. Normal saline may be substituted for lactated Ringer's solution in this figure. (LR, lactated Ringer's solution.)

older hydroxyethyl starch and dextran products. All these solutions are markedly more costly than crystalloid solutions; in some cases, the differences are 50- to 100-fold, even when used in equipotent amounts. It is important to note that these cost minimization statements assume no differences in efficacy or toxicity between colloids and crystalloids when given in equipotent amounts. This is almost certainly not the case with respect to adverse effects of hydroxyethyl starch and dextran products. A cost-effectiveness analysis that takes into account adverse effects would be needed for the latter products and such an analysis would likely demonstrate they are not cost-effective versus crystalloids even if equipotent efficacy is presumed.

Because medications are not simply alternatives to crystalloids but rather are used when crystalloid therapy has been optimized, there is little reason to compare medication and fluid therapies from an economic perspective. Furthermore, there are no economic comparisons of the various inotropic and vasopressor medications used in the treatment of hypovolemic shock.

ABBREVIATIONS

ATLS	Advanced Trauma Life Support
BSA	body surface area
BUN	blood urea nitrogen
CAD	coronary artery disease
CDC	Centers for Disease Control and Prevention
CI	confidence interval
CVP	central venous pressure
EAST	Eastern Association for the Surgery of Trauma
HIV	human immunodeficiency virus
ICU	intensive care unit
MODS	multiple-organ dysfunction syndrome
pHi	gastric intramucosal pH
PT	prothrombin time
PTT	partial thromboplastin time
ROC	Resuscitation Outcomes Consortium
SAFE	Saline versus Albumin Fluid Evaluation
SIRS	systemic inflammatory response syndrome
WHO	World Health Organization

REFERENCES

1. Murphy SL, Xu J, Kochanek KD. Deaths: Preliminary Data for 2010. National Vital Statistics Reports, Vol. 60, No. 4. Hyattsville, MD: National Center for Health Statistics, 2012.
2. Anonymous. QuickStats: Number of Heat-Related Deaths,* by Sex—National Vital Statistics System, United States, 1999–2010. MMWR Morb Mortal Wkly Rep 2012;61(36):729.
3. Duggan C, Fontaine O, Pierce NF, et al. Scientific rationale for a change in the composition of oral rehydration solution. JAMA 2004;291:2628–2631.
4. Vercueil A, Grocott MPW, Mythen MG. Physiology, pharmacology, and rationale for colloid administration for the maintenance of effective hemodynamic stability in critically ill patients. Trans Med Rev 2005;19:93–109.
5. Porter SC, Fleisher GR, Kohane IS, Mandl KD. The value of parental report for diagnosis and management of dehydration in the emergency department. Ann Emerg Med 2003;41:196–205.
6. Spandorfer PR, Alessandrini EA, Joffe MD, et al. Oral versus intravenous rehydration of moderately dehydrated children: A randomized, controlled trial. Pediatrics 2005;115:295–301.
7. Atherly-John YC, Cunningham SJ, Crain EF. A randomized trial of oral vs intravenous rehydration in a pediatric emergency department. Arch Pediatr Adolesc Med 2002;156:1240–1243.
8. Axler OA, Tousiganant C, Thompson CR, et al. Small hemodynamic effect of typical rapid volume infusions in critically ill patients. Crit Care Med 1997;25:965–970.

9. The National Heart, Lung, and Blood Institute Acute Respiratory Distress Syndrome (ARDS) Clinical Trials Network. Comparison of two fluid-management strategies in acute lung injury. N Engl J Med 2006;354:2564–2575.
10. The ATLS Subcommittee, American College of Surgeons' Committee on Trauma, and the International ATLS working group. Advanced trauma life support (ATLS®): The ninth edition. J Trauma Acute Care Surg 2013;74:1363–1366.
11. Cotton BA, Jerome R, Collier BR, et al. Guidelines for prehospital fluid resuscitation in the injured patient. J Trauma 2009;67:389–402.
12. Perel P, Roberts I, Ker K. Colloids versus crystalloids for fluid resuscitation in critically ill patients. Cochrane Database Syst Rev 2013, Issue 2. Art. No.: CD000567. DOI: 10.1002/14651858.CD000567.pub6.
13. Bunn F, Trivedi D. Colloid solutions for fluid resuscitation. Cochrane Database Syst Rev 2012, Issue 7. Art. No.: CD001319. DOI: 10.1002/14651858.CD001319.pub5.
14. Roberts I, Blackhall K, Alderson P, Bunn F, Schierhout G. Human albumin solution for resuscitation and volume expansion in critically ill patients. Cochrane Database Syst Rev 2011, Issue 11. Art. No.: CD001208. DOI: 10.1002/14651858.CD001208.pub4.
15. Soni N. British consensus guidelines on intravenous fluid therapy for adult surgical patients—Cassandra's view. Anesthesia 2009;64:235–238.
16. Pham TN, Cancio LC, Gibran NS. American Burn Association practice guidelines burn shock resuscitation. J Burn Care Res 2008;29:257–266.
17. Alam HB, Rhee P. New developments in fluid resuscitation. Surg Clin North Am 2007;87:55–72.
18. Didwania A, Miller J, Kassel D, et al. Effect of intravenous lactated Ringer's solution infusion on the circulating lactate concentration: Results of a prospective, randomized, double-blind, placebo-controlled trial. Crit Care Med 1997;25:1851–1854.
19. Jackson EV, Wiese J, Sigal B, et al. Effects of crystalloid solutions on circulating lactate concentrations: 1. Implications for the proper handling of blood specimens obtained in critically ill patients. Crit Care Med 1996;24:1840–1846.
20. Grocott MPW, Mythen MG, Gan TJ. Perioperative fluid management and clinical outcomes in adults. Anesth Analg 2005;100:1093–1106.
21. Schortgen F, Giron E, Deye N, Brochard L. The risk associated with hyperoncotic colloids in patients with shock. Intensive Care Med 2008;34:2157–2168.
22. Perner A, Haase N, Guttormsen AB, et al. Hydroxyethyl starch 130/0.42 versus Ringer's acetate in severe sepsis. N Engl J Med 2012;367:124–134.
23. Myburgh JA, Finfer S, Bellomo R, et al. Hydroxyethyl starch or saline for fluid resuscitation in intensive care. N Engl J Med 2012;367:1901–1911.
24. Cochrane Injuries Group Albumin Reviewers. Human albumin administration in critically ill patients: Systematic review of randomized controlled trials. BMJ 1998;317:235–240.
25. Choi PTL, Yip G, Quinonez LG, Cook DJ. Crystalloids vs. colloids in fluid resuscitation: A systematic review. Crit Care Med 1999;27:200–210.
26. The SAFE Study Investigators. A comparison of albumin and saline for fluid resuscitation in the intensive care unit. N Engl J Med 2004;350:2247–2256.
27. The SAFE Study Investigators. Saline or albumin for fluid resuscitation in patients with traumatic brain injury. N Engl J Med 2007;357:874–884.
28. Hollenberg SM. Vasoactive drugs in circulatory shock. Am J Respir Crit Care Med 2011;183:847–855.
29. De Backer D, Biston P, Devriendt J, et al. Comparison of dopamine and norepinephrine in the treatment of shock. N Engl J Med 2010;362:779–789.
30. Bickell WH, Wall MJ, Pepe PE, et al. Immediate versus delayed fluid resuscitation for hypotensive patients with penetrating torso injuries. N Engl J Med 1994;331:1105–1109.
31. Dutton RP, Mackenzie CF, Scalea TM. Hypotensive resuscitation during active hemorrhage: Impact on in-hospital mortality. J Trauma 2002;52:1141–1146.
32. Cooper DJ, Myles PS, McDermott FT, et al. Prehospital hypertonic saline resuscitation of patients with hypotension and severe traumatic brain injury. JAMA 2004;291:1350–1357.
33. Bulger EM, May S, Brasel KJ, et al. Out-of-hospital hypertonic resuscitation following severe traumatic brain injury: a randomized controlled trial. JAMA 2010;304:1455–1464.
34. Bulger EM, May S, Kirby JD, et al. Out-of-hospital hypertonic resuscitation after traumatic hypovolemic shock: A randomized, placebo controlled trial. Ann Surg 2011;253:431–421.
35. Brandstrup B, Tonnesen H, Beier-Holgersen R, et al. Effects of intravenous fluid restriction on postoperative complications: Comparison of two perioperative fluid regimens. Ann Surg 2003;238:641–648.
36. Hebert PC, Wells G, Blajchman MA, et al. A multicenter, randomized, controlled clinical trial of transfusion requirements in critical care. N Engl J Med 1999;340:409–417.
37. Hajjar LA, Vincent JL, Galas FRBG, et al. Transfusion requirements after cardiac surgery: The TRACS randomized controlled trial. JAMA 2010;304:1559–1567.
38. Hauser CJ, Boffard K, Dutton R, et al. Results of the CONTROL trial: Efficacy and safety of recombinant activated factor VII in the management of refractory traumatic hemorrhage. J Trauma 2010;69:489–500.
39. CRASH-2 Trial Collaborators. Effects of tranexamic acid on death, vascular occlusive events, and blood transfusion in trauma patients with significant hemorrhage (CRASH-2): A randomised, placebo-controlled trial. Lancet 2010;376:23–32.
40. Tanaka J, Matsuda T, Miyagantani Y, et al. Reduction of resuscitation fluid volumes in severely burned patients using ascorbic acid administration. Arch Surg 2000;135:326–331.
41. Rivers E, Nguyen B, Havstad S, et al. Early goal-directed therapy in the treatment of severe sepsis and septic-shock. N Engl J Med 2001;345:1368–1377.
42. Marik PE, Baram M, Vahid B. Does central venous pressure predict fluid responsiveness? Chest 2008;134:172–178.
43. Ivanov R, Allen J, Calvin JE. The incidence of major morbidity in critically ill patients managed with pulmonary artery catheters: A meta-analysis. Crit Care Med 2000;28:615–619.
44. Sandham JD, Hull RD, Brant RF, et al. A randomized, controlled trial of the use of pulmonary-artery catheters in high-risk surgical patients. N Engl J Med 2003;348:5–14.
45. Ginosar Y, Thijs LG, Sprung CL. Raising the standard of hemodynamic monitoring: Targeting the practice or the practitioner? Crit Care Med 1997;25:209–211.
46. Gomersall CD, Joynt GM, Freebairn RC, et al. Resuscitation of critically ill patients based on the results of gastric tonometry: A prospective, randomized, controlled trial. Crit Care Med 2000;28:607–614.
47. Sperry JL, Minei JP, Frankel HL, et al. Early use of vasopressors after injury: Caution before constriction. J Trauma 2008;64:9–14.
48. Boyd JH, Walley KR. Is there a role for sodium bicarbonate in treating lactic acidosis from shock? Curr Opin Crit Care 2008;14:379–383.

15

Asthma

H. William Kelly and Christine A. Sorkness

KEY CONCEPTS

1. Asthma is a disease of increasing prevalence that is a result of genetic predisposition and environmental interactions; it is one of the most common chronic diseases of childhood.
2. Asthma is primarily a chronic inflammatory disease of the airways of the lung for which there is no known cure or primary prevention; the immunohistopathologic features include cell infiltration by neutrophils, eosinophils, T-helper type 2 lymphocytes, mast cells, and epithelial cells.
3. Asthma is characterized by either the intermittent or persistent presence of highly variable degrees of airflow obstruction from airway wall inflammation and bronchial smooth muscle constriction; in some patients, persistent changes in airway structure occur.
4. The inflammatory process in asthma is treated most effectively with corticosteroids, with the inhaled corticosteroids having the greatest efficacy and safety profile for long-term management.
5. Bronchial smooth muscle constriction is prevented or treated most effectively with inhaled β_2-adrenergic receptor agonists.
6. Variability in response to medications requires individualization of therapy within existing evidence-based guidelines for management. This is most evident in patients with severe asthma phenotypes.
7. Ongoing patient education, for a partnership in asthma care, is essential for optimal patient outcomes and includes trigger avoidance and self-management techniques.

Asthma has been known since antiquity, yet it is a disease that still defies precise definition. The word *asthma* is of Greek origin and means "panting." More than 2,000 years ago, Hippocrates used the word *asthma* to describe episodic shortness of breath; however, the first detailed clinical description of the asthmatic patient was made by Aretaeus in the second century.[1] The National Institutes of Health, National Asthma Education and Prevention Program (NAEPP) Expert Panel Report 3 (EPR3), has provided the following working definition of asthma[2]:

> Asthma is a chronic inflammatory disorder of the airways in which many cells and cellular elements play a role: in particular, mast cells, eosinophils, T-lymphocytes, macrophages, neutrophils, and epithelial cells. In susceptible individuals, this inflammation causes recurrent episodes of wheezing, breathlessness, chest tightness, and coughing, particularly at night or in the early morning. These episodes are usually associated with widespread but variable airflow obstruction that is often reversible either spontaneously or with treatment. The inflammation also causes an associated increase in the existing bronchial hyperresponsiveness (BHR) to a variety of stimuli. Reversibility of airflow limitation may be incomplete in some patients with asthma.

This definition encompasses the important heterogeneity of the clinical presentation of asthma by describing the scientific and clinically accepted characteristics of asthma.

EPIDEMIOLOGY

1 An estimated 25.7 million persons in the United States have asthma (about 8.4% of the population).[3] Asthma is the most common chronic disease among children in the United States, with approximately 7 million children affected. The prevalence rate is highest in children 0 to 17 years of age at 9.5%.[3] In the United States, as in other industrialized countries, the prevalence of asthma is increasing from 7.3% in 2001. Asthma prevalence is higher in persons with incomes below 100% of poverty level at 11.2% and in blacks 11.2% and multiple races 14.1%. Asthma accounts for 1.6% of all ambulatory care visits (10.6 million physician office visits and 1.2 million hospital outpatient visits) and resulted in 440,000 hospitalizations and 1.7 million emergency department (ED) visits in 2006 (both declined from peaks in the 1990s).[4] It is the third leading cause of preventable hospitalization in the United States; however, hospitalizations have decreased per 100 patients with asthma since 2001. Asthma accounts for more than 12.8 million missed school days per year.[4] In young children (0 to 10 years of age), the risk of asthma is greater in boys than in girls, becomes about equal during puberty, and then is greater in women than in men.[4]

Ethnic minorities continue to share the burden of asthma disproportionately. African Americans are two times as likely to be hospitalized and approximately two times more likely to die from asthma than whites.[3] Hispanics in general, with the exception of Puerto Ricans, at 16.1% prevalence have lower disease and hospitalization rates than African Americans or whites.

The estimated direct medical cost of asthma in the United States in 2007 was $14.7 billion.[4] The societal burden of asthma (indirect medical expenditures: loss of productivity and death) in the United States was $5 billion. Prescription drugs were the largest single direct medical expenditure at $6.2 billion; however, the combined costs of emergency care of acute asthma exacerbations make up 36% of direct medical costs.[4]

The natural history of asthma is still not well defined. Although asthma can occur at any time, it is principally a pediatric disease, with most patients being diagnosed by 5 years of age and up to 50% of children having symptoms by 2 years of age.[2] Between 30% and 70% of children with asthma will improve markedly or become symptom-free by early adulthood; chronic disease persists in about 30% to 40% of patients, and generally 20% or less develop severe chronic disease.[2] Predictors of persistent adult asthma include atopy, onset during school age, and presence of bronchial hyperresponsiveness (BHR).[2] Diminished lung growth may occur in some children (approximately 10%) with asthma.[2]

In adults, most longitudinal studies have suggested a more rapid rate of decline in lung function in asthmatics than in nonasthmatic normals, primarily reflected in forced expiratory volume in 1 second (FEV_1).[2] However, the annual decline in FEV_1 is less than in smokers or in patients with a diagnosis of emphysema. In general, individuals with less frequent asthma attacks and normal lung function on initial assessment have higher remission rates, whereas smokers have the lowest remission and highest relapse rates.[2] The level of BHR tends to predict the rate of decline in FEV_1, with a greater decline with high levels of BHR.[2] Thus, airway obstruction in asthma may become irreversible and also worsen over time owing to airway remodeling (see below).[2] However, most patients do not die from long-term progression of their disease and their life span is not different from the general population.[2]

As with prevalence and morbidity, mortality from acute exacerbations of asthma has been decreasing over the past 10 years, with a death rate of 0.14 per 1,000 persons with asthma reported in 2009.[3] Despite the relatively low number of asthma deaths, 80% to 90% are preventable.[2] Most deaths from asthma occur outside the hospital, and death is rare after hospitalization. The most common cause of death from asthma is inadequate assessment of the severity of airway obstruction by the patient or physician and inadequate therapy. The most common cause of death in hospitalized patients is also inadequate or inappropriate therapy. Thus, the key to prevention of death from asthma, as advocated by the U.S. NAEPP, is education.[2]

TABLE 15-1 List of Agents and Events Triggering Asthma

Respiratory infection
Respiratory syncytial virus (RSV), rhinovirus, influenza, parainfluenza, *Mycoplasma pneumonia*, *Chlamydia*
Allergens
Airborne pollens (grass, trees, weeds), house dust mites, animal dander, cockroaches, fungal spores
Environment
Cold air, fog, ozone, sulfur dioxide, nitrogen dioxide, tobacco smoke, wood smoke
Emotions
Anxiety, stress, laughter
Exercise
Particularly in cold, dry climate
Drugs/preservatives
Aspirin, NSAIDs (cyclooxygenase inhibitors), sulfites, benzalkonium chloride, nonselective β-blockers
Occupational stimuli
Bakers (flour dust); farmers (hay mold); spice and enzyme workers; printers (arabic gum); chemical workers (azo dyes, anthraquinone, ethylenediamine, toluene diisocyanates, polyvinyl chloride); plastics, rubber, and wood workers (formaldehyde, western cedar, dimethylethanolamine, anhydrides)

ETIOLOGY

1 Epidemiologic studies strongly support the concept of a genetic predisposition plus environmental interaction to the development of asthma, yet the picture remains complex and incomplete.[5] Genetic factors account for 60% to 80% of the susceptibility. Asthma represents a complex genetic disorder in that the asthma phenotype is likely a result of polygenic inheritance or different combinations of genes. Initial searches focused on establishing links between atopy (genetically determined state of hypersensitivity to environmental allergens) and asthma, but more recent genome-wide searches have found linkages with genes for metalloproteinases (e.g., *ADAM33*) and handling bacteria (*CHI3L1*).[5] Although genetic predisposition to atopy is a significant risk factor for developing asthma, not all atopic individuals develop asthma, nor do all patients with asthma exhibit atopy. Disparate phenotypes of asthma (progressive or remodeled vs. nonprogressive) are likely genetically determined.[5]

1 Environmental risk factors for the development of asthma include socioeconomic status, family size, exposure to secondhand tobacco smoke in infancy and in utero, allergen exposure, urbanization, respiratory syncytial virus (RSV) infection, and decreased exposure to common childhood infectious agents.[6,7] The "hygiene hypothesis" proposes that genetically susceptible individuals develop allergies and asthma by allowing the allergic immunologic system (T-helper cell type 2 [Th_2] lymphocytes) to develop instead of the system to fight infections (T-helper type 1 [Th_1] lymphocytes) and may explain the increase of asthma in developed countries.[6,7] The first 2 years of life appear to be most important for the exposures to produce an alteration in the immune response system.[6] The hygiene hypothesis is supported by studies demonstrating a lower risk for asthma in children who are exposed to high levels of bacteria or endotoxin, in those with a large number of older siblings, in those with early enrollment into child care, in those with exposure to cats and dogs early in life, or in those with exposure to fewer antibiotics.[5–7]

Risk factors for early (<3 years of age) recurrent wheezing associated with viral infections include low birth weight, male gender, and parental smoking. However, this early pattern is due to smaller airways, and these risk factors are not necessarily risk factors for asthma in later life.[6] Atopy is the predominant risk factor for children to have continued asthma.[6,7] Asthma can begin in adults later in life. Occupational asthma in previously healthy individuals emphasizes the effect of environment on the development of asthma.[8] The heterogeneity of the asthma phenotype appears most obvious when listing the diverse triggers of bronchospasm[2,6] (Table 15-1). The various triggers have relative degrees of importance from patient to patient. Environmental exposures are the most important precipitants of severe asthma exacerbations[9] (see Table 15-1). Epidemics of severe asthma in cities have followed exposures to high concentrations of aeroallergens.[9] Viral respiratory tract infections remain the single most significant precipitant of severe asthma in children and are an important trigger in adults as well.[10] Other possible factors include air pollution, sinusitis, food preservatives, and drugs.

PATHOPHYSIOLOGY

2 The major characteristics of asthma include a variable degree of airflow obstruction (related to bronchospasm, edema, and mucus hypersecretion), BHR, and airway inflammation (Fig. 15-1). To understand the pathogenetic mechanisms that underlie the many phenotypes of asthma, it is critical to identify factors that initiate,

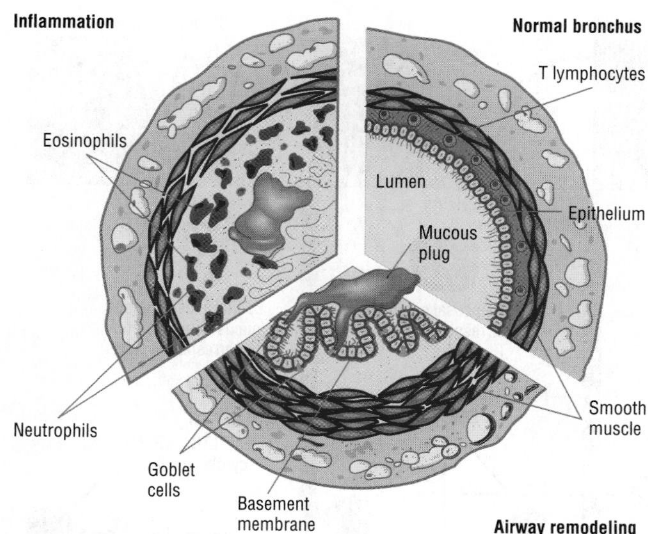

FIGURE 15-1 Representative illustration of the pathology found in the asthmatic bronchus compared with a normal bronchus (*upper right*). Each section demonstrates how the lumen is narrowed. Hypertrophy of the basement membrane, mucus plugging, smooth muscle hypertrophy, and constriction contribute (*lower section*). Inflammatory cells infiltrate, producing submucosal edema, and epithelial desquamation fills the airway lumen with cellular debris and exposes the airway smooth muscle to other mediators (*upper left*).

intensify, and modulate the inflammatory response of the airways and to determine how these processes produce the characteristic airway abnormalities.

Acute Inflammation

Inhaled allergen challenge models contribute most to our understanding of acute inflammation in asthma.[7] Inhaled allergen challenge in allergic patients leads to an early phase reaction that, in some cases, may be followed by a late-phase reaction. The activation of cells bearing allergen-specific immunoglobulin E (IgE) initiates the early phase reaction. It is characterized by the rapid activation of airway mast cells and macrophages leading to the rapid release of proinflammatory mediators such as histamine, eicosanoids, and reactive oxygen (O_2) species that induce contraction of airway smooth muscle, mucus secretion, and vasodilation.[7] The bronchial microcirculation has an essential role in this inflammatory process. Inflammatory mediators induce microvascular leakage with exudation of plasma in the airways.[7] Acute plasma protein leakage induces a thickened, engorged, and edematous airway wall and a consequent narrowing of the airway lumen. Plasma exudation may compromise epithelial integrity, and the presence of plasma in the lumen may reduce mucus clearance.[7] Plasma proteins also may promote the formation of exudative plugs mixed with mucus and inflammatory and epithelial cells. Together these effects contribute to airflow obstruction (Fig. 15-1).

The late-phase inflammatory reaction occurs 6 to 9 hours after allergen provocation and involves the recruitment and activation of eosinophils, $CD4^+$ thymically derived lymphocytes (T cells), basophils, neutrophils, and macrophages.[7] There is selective retention of airway T cells, the expression of adhesion molecules, and the release of selected proinflammatory mediators and cytokines involved in the recruitment and activation of inflammatory cells.[7] The activation of T cells after allergen challenge leads to the release of Th_2-like cytokines that may modulate the late-phase response.[7] The release of preformed cytokines by mast cells is the likely initial trigger for the early recruitment of inflammatory cells that then recruit and induce the more persistent involvement by T cells.[7] The enhancement of nonspecific BHR usually can be demonstrated after the late-phase reaction but not after the early phase reaction following allergen or occupational challenge.

Chronic Inflammation

Airway inflammation has been demonstrated in all forms of asthma, and an association between the extent of inflammation and the clinical severity of asthma has been demonstrated in selected studies.[7] It is accepted that both central and peripheral airways are inflamed.

In asthma, all cells of the airways are involved and become activated (Fig. 15-2). Included are eosinophils, T cells, mast cells, macrophages, epithelial cells, fibroblasts, and bronchial smooth muscle cells. These cells also regulate airway inflammation and initiate the process of remodeling by the release of cytokines and growth factors.[7,11]

Epithelial Cells

Bronchial epithelial cells participate in mucociliary clearance and removal of noxious agents; however, they also enhance inflammation by releasing eicosanoids, peptidases, matrix proteins, cytokines, chemokines, and nitric oxide (NO).[7,11] Epithelial cells can be activated by IgE-dependent mechanisms, viruses, pollutants, or histamine. In asthma, especially fatal asthma, extensive epithelial shedding occurs. The functional consequences of epithelial shedding may include heightened airway responsiveness, release of the chemokine eotaxin that attracts eosinophils, altered permeability of the airway mucosa, depletion of epithelial-derived relaxant factors, and loss of enzymes responsible for degrading proinflammatory neuropeptides. The integrity of airway epithelium may influence the sensitivity of the airways to various provocative stimuli. Epithelial cells also may be important in the regulation of airway remodeling and fibrosis.[7,11]

Eosinophils

Eosinophils play an effector role in asthma by releasing proinflammatory mediators, cytotoxic mediators, and cytokines.[7] Circulating eosinophils migrate to the airways by cell rolling, through interactions with selectins, and eventually adhere to the endothelium through the binding of integrins to adhesion proteins (vascular cell adhesion molecule 1 [VCAM-1] and intercellular adhesion molecule 1 [ICAM-1]). As eosinophils enter the matrix of the membrane, their survival is prolonged by interleukin 5 (IL-5) and granulocyte-macrophage colony-stimulating factor (GM-CSF). On activation, eosinophils release inflammatory mediators such as leukotrienes (LTs) and granule proteins to injure airway tissue.[7]

Lymphocytes

Mucosal biopsy specimens from patients with asthma contain lymphocytes, many of which express surface markers of inflammation. There are two types of T-helper $CD4^+$ cells. Th_1 cells produce IL-2 and interferon-γ (IFN-γ), both essential for cellular defense mechanisms. Th_2 cells produce cytokines (IL-4, -5, and -13) that mediate allergic inflammation. It is known that Th_1 cytokines inhibit the production of Th_2 cytokines, and vice versa. It is hypothesized that allergic asthmatic inflammation results from a Th_2-mediated mechanism (an imbalance between Th_1 and Th_2 cells).[7] However, more recently it has been observed that there exists a low Th_2 cytokine phenotype of asthma in adults that appears more resistant to usual therapies for asthma.[12]

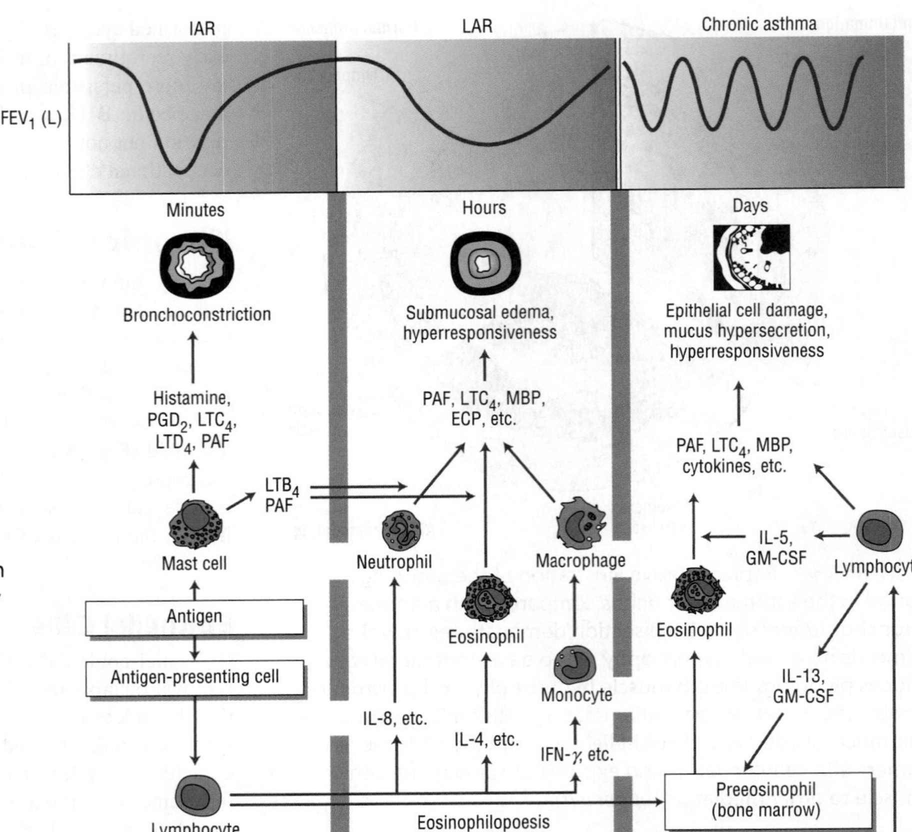

FIGURE 15-2 Diagrammatic presentation of the relationship between inflammatory cells, lipid and preformed mediators, inflammatory cytokines, and proposed pathogenesis and clinical presentation in asthma. See text for details. (GM-CSF, granulocyte-macrophage colony-stimulating factor; IL, interleukin; LT, leukotriene; MBP, major basic protein; PAF, platelet-activating factor; PG, prostaglandin.)

Th_1 and Th_2 Cell Imbalance

The T-cell population in the cord blood of newborn infants is skewed toward a Th_2 phenotype.[6,7] The extent of the imbalance between Th_1 and Th_2 cells (as indicated by diminished IFN-γ production) during the neonatal phase may predict the subsequent development of allergic disease, asthma, or both. It has been suggested that infants at high risk of asthma and allergies should be exposed to stimuli that upregulate Th_1-mediated responses in order to restore the balance during a critical time in the development of the immune system and the lungs.[6]

The basic premise of the hygiene hypothesis is that the newborn's immune system needs timely and appropriate environmental stimuli to create a balanced immune response. Factors that enhance Th_1-mediated responses include infection with *Mycobacterium tuberculosis*, measles virus, and hepatitis A virus; endotoxin exposure; increased exposure to infections through contact with older siblings; and daycare attendance during the first 6 months of life. Restoration of the balance between Th_1 and Th_2 cells may be impeded by frequent administration of oral antibiotics, with concomitant alterations in GI flora. Other factors favoring the Th_2 phenotype include residence in an industrialized country, urban environment exposure, diet, and sensitization to house dust mites and cockroaches.[6] Immune "imprinting" may begin in utero by transplacental transfer of allergens and cytokines.

Mast Cells

Mast cell degranulation is important in the initiation of immediate responses following exposure to allergens.[2] Mast cells reside throughout the walls of the respiratory tract, and increased numbers of these cells (threefold to fivefold) have been described in the airways of allergic asthmatics.[7] Once binding of allergen to cell-bound IgE occurs, mediators such as histamine; eosinophil and neutrophil chemotactic factors; LTs C_4, D_4, and E_4; prostaglandins; platelet-activating factor (PAF); and others are released from mast cells (see Fig. 15-2). Histologic examination has revealed decreased numbers of granulated mast cells in the airways of patients who have died from acute asthma attacks, suggesting that mast cell degranulation is a contributing factor. Sensitized mast cells are also activated by osmotic stimuli to account for exercise-induced bronchospasm (EIB).[13]

Alveolar Macrophages

The primary function of alveolar macrophages in the normal airway is to serve as "scavengers," engulfing and digesting bacteria and other foreign materials. Macrophages are found in large and small airways, ideally located for affecting the asthmatic response. A number of mediators produced and released by macrophages have been identified, including PAF, LTB_4, LTC_4, and LTD_4.[7] Additionally, alveolar macrophages are able to produce neutrophil chemotactic factor and eosinophil chemotactic factor, which in turn amplify the inflammatory process.

Neutrophils

The role of neutrophils in the pathogenesis of asthma remains somewhat unclear because they normally may be present in the airways and usually do not infiltrate tissues showing chronic allergic inflammation despite the potential to participate in late-phase inflammatory reactions. However, high numbers of neutrophils have been observed in the airways of patients who died from sudden-onset fatal asthma and in those with severe disease.[14] This suggests that neutrophils may play a pivotal role in the disease process, at least in some patients with long-standing or corticosteroid-resistant asthma.[14] The neutrophil also can be a source for a variety of mediators, including PAF, prostaglandins, thromboxanes, and LTs, that contribute to BHR and airway inflammation.[14]

Fibroblasts and Myofibroblasts

Fibroblasts are found frequently in connective tissue. Human lung fibroblasts may behave as inflammatory cells on activation by IL-4 and IL-13. The myofibroblast may contribute to the regulation of inflammation via the release of cytokines and to tissue remodeling. In asthma, myofibroblasts are increased in numbers beneath the reticular basement membrane, and there is an association between their numbers and the thickness of the reticular basement membrane.[7,11]

Inflammatory Mediators

Associated with asthma for many years, histamine is capable of inducing smooth muscle constriction and bronchospasm and is thought to play a role in mucosal edema and mucus secretion.[2] Lung mast cells are an important source of histamine. The release of histamine can be stimulated by exposure of the airways to a variety of factors, including physical stimuli (airway drying with exercise) and relevant allergens.[7] Histamine is involved in acute bronchospasm following allergen exposure; however, other mediators such as LTs are also involved.

Besides histamine release, mast cell degranulation releases ILs, proteases, and other enzymes that activate the production of other mediators of inflammation. Several classes of important mediators, including arachidonic acid and its metabolites (i.e., prostaglandins, LTs, and PAF), are derived from cell membrane phospholipids.

Once arachidonic acid is released, it can be metabolized by the enzyme cyclooxygenase to form prostaglandins. Prostaglandin D_2 is a potent bronchoconstricting agent; however, it is unlikely to produce sustained effects and its role in asthma remains to be determined. Similarly, prostaglandin $F_{2\alpha}$ is a potent bronchoconstrictor in patients with asthma and can enhance the effects of histamine.[2,7] However, its pathophysiologic role in asthma is unclear. Another cyclooxygenase product, prostacyclin (prostaglandin I_2), is known to be produced in the lung and may contribute to inflammation and edema owing to its effects as a vasodilator.

Thromboxane A_2 is produced by alveolar macrophages, fibroblasts, epithelial cells, neutrophils, and platelets within the lung.[7] It may have several effects, including bronchoconstriction, involvement in the late asthmatic response, and involvement in the development of airway inflammation and BHR.

The 5-lipoxygenase pathway of arachidonic acid metabolism is responsible for the production of the *cysteinyl LTs*.[7] LTC_4, LTD_4, and LTE_4 are released during inflammatory processes in the lung. LTs D_4 and E_4 share a common receptor (LTD_4 receptor) that, when stimulated, produces bronchospasm, mucus secretion, microvascular permeability, and airway edema, whereas LTB_4 is involved with granulocyte chemotaxis.

Thought to be produced by macrophages, eosinophils, and neutrophils within the lung, PAF is involved in the mediation of bronchospasm, sustained induction of BHR, edema formation, and chemotaxis of eosinophils.[7]

Adhesion Molecules

Adhesion molecules are glycoproteins that facilitate infiltration and migration of inflammatory cells to the site of inflammation. They have additional functions involved in the inflammatory process aside from promoting cell adhesion, including activation of cells and cell–cell communication, and promoting cellular migration and infiltration.[2] The many adhesion molecules are divided into families on the basis of their chemical structure. These families are the integrins, cadherins, immunoglobulin supergene family, selectins, vascular adressins, and carbohydrate ligands.[7] Those thought to be important in inflammation include the integrins, immunoglobulin supergene family, selectins, and carbohydrate ligands, including ICAM-1 and VCAM-1.[7] Adhesion molecules are found on a variety of cells, such as neutrophils, monocytes, lymphocytes, basophils, eosinophils, granulocytes, platelets, endothelial cells, and epithelial cells, and can be expressed or activated by the many inflammatory mediators present in asthma.[7]

Clinical Consequences of Chronic Inflammation

Chronic inflammation is associated with nonspecific BHR and increases the risk of asthma exacerbations. Exacerbations are characterized by increased symptoms and worsening airway obstruction over a period of days or even weeks, and rarely hours. Hyperresponsiveness of the airways to physical, chemical, and pharmacologic stimuli is a hallmark of asthma.[2] BHR also occurs in some patients with chronic bronchitis and allergic rhinitis.[2] Normal healthy subjects also may develop a transient BHR after viral respiratory infections or ozone exposure. However, the degree of BHR in patients with asthma is quantitatively greater than in other populations. Bronchial responsiveness of the general population fits a unimodal distribution that is skewed toward increased reactivity; individuals with clinical asthma represent the extreme end of this distribution. The degree of BHR within asthma correlates with its clinical course and medication requirement necessary to control symptoms.[2] Patients with mild symptoms or in remission demonstrate lower levels of BHR.

The current understanding is that the BHR seen in asthma is at least in part due to and correlative with the extent of airway inflammation.[2] Airway remodeling also correlates somewhat with BHR.[11]

Remodeling of the Airways

Acute inflammation is a beneficial, nonspecific response of tissues to injury and generally leads to repair and restoration of the normal structure and function. In contrast, asthma represents a chronic inflammatory process of the airways followed by healing that in some may result in altered structure referred to as *remodeling*.[11] Repair involves replacement of injured tissue by parenchymal cells of the same type and replacement by connective tissue and its maturation into scar tissue. In asthma, remodeling presents as extracellular matrix fibrosis, an increase in smooth muscle and mucus gland mass, and angiogenesis.[11]

The precise mechanisms of remodeling of the airways are under intense study. Airway remodeling is of concern because it may represent an irreversible process that can have more serious sequelae such as the development of chronic obstructive pulmonary disease (COPD).[2,11] Observations in children with asthma indicate that some loss of lung function may occur during the first 5 years of life.[6] Importantly, no current therapies have been shown to alter either early decreased lung growth or later progressive loss of lung function.

Mucus Production

The mucociliary system is the lung's primary defense mechanism against irritants and infectious agents. Mucus, composed of 95% water and 5% glycoproteins, is produced by bronchial epithelial glands and goblet cells.[7] The lining of the airways consists of a continuous aqueous layer controlled by active ion transport across the epithelium in which water moves toward the lumen along the concentration gradient. Catecholamines and vagal stimulation enhance the ion transport and fluid movement. Mucus transport depends on its viscoelastic properties. Mucus that is either too watery or too viscous will not be transported optimally. The exudative inflammatory process and sloughing of epithelial cells into the airway lumen impair mucociliary transport. The bronchial glands are increased in size and the goblet cells are increased in size and number in asthma. Expectorated mucus from patients with asthma tends to have a high viscosity. The mucus plugs in the airways of patients who died in status asthmaticus are tenacious and tend to be connected by mucous strands to the goblet cells. Asthmatic airways also may become plugged with casts consisting of epithelial and inflammatory cells. Although it is tempting to speculate that death from asthma attacks is a result of the mucus plugging resulting in irreversible obstruction, there is no direct evidence for this. Autopsies of asthmatics who died from other causes have shown similar pathology. In addition, some patients who have died of sudden severe asthma did not show the characteristic mucus plugging on necropsy.[7]

Airway Smooth Muscle

The smooth muscle of the airways does not form a uniform coat around the airways but is wrapped around in a connecting network best described as a spiral arrangement.[15] The muscle contraction displays a sphincteric action that is capable of completely occluding the airway lumen. The airway smooth muscle extends from the trachea through the respiratory bronchioles. When expressed as a percentage of wall thickness, the smooth muscle represents 5% of the large central airways and up to 20% of the wall thickness in the bronchioles. Total smooth muscle mass decreases rapidly past the terminal bronchioles to the alveoli, so the contribution of smooth muscle tone to airway diameter in this region is relatively small. In the large airways of asthmatics, smooth muscle may account for 11% of the wall thickness. It is possible that the increased smooth muscle mass of the asthmatic airways is important in magnifying and maintaining BHR in persistent disease. However, it appears that the hypertrophy and hyperplasia are secondary processes caused by chronic inflammation and are not the primary cause of BHR.[15]

Neural Control/Neurogenic Inflammation

The airway is innervated by parasympathetic, sympathetic, and nonadrenergic inhibitory nerves.[2] Parasympathetic innervation of the smooth muscle consists of efferent motor fibers in the vagus nerves and sensory afferent fibers in the vagus and other nerves.[15] The normal resting tone of human airway smooth muscle is maintained by vagal efferent activity. Maximum bronchoconstriction mediated by vagal stimulation occurs in the small bronchi and is absent in the small bronchioles. The nonmyelinated C fibers of the afferent system lie immediately beneath the tight junctions between epithelial cells lining the airway lumen.[15] These endings probably represent the irritant receptors of the airways. Stimulation of these irritant receptors by mechanical stimulation, chemical and particulate irritants, and pharmacologic agents such as histamine produces reflex bronchoconstriction.[7]

The nonadrenergic, noncholinergic (NANC) nervous system has been described in the trachea and bronchi. Substance P, neurokinin A, neurokinin B, and vasoactive intestinal peptide (VIP) are the best characterized neurotransmitters in the NANC nervous system.[7] VIP is an inhibitory neurotransmitter. Inflammatory cells in asthma can release peptidases that can degrade VIP, producing exaggerated reflex cholinergic bronchoconstriction. NANC excitatory neuropeptides such as substance P and neurokinin A are released by stimulation of C-fiber sensory nerve endings. The NANC system may play an important role in amplifying inflammation in asthma by releasing NO.

Nitric Oxide

NO is produced by cells within the respiratory tract. It has been thought to be a neurotransmitter of the NANC nervous system.[16] Endogenous NO is generated from the amino acid L-arginine (L-Arg) by the enzyme NO synthase.[16] There are three isoforms of NO synthase. One isoform is induced in response to proinflammatory cytokines, inducible NO synthase (iNOS), in airway epithelial cells and inflammatory cells of asthmatic airways.[16] NO produces smooth muscle relaxation in the vasculature and bronchials; however, it appears to amplify the inflammatory process and is unlikely to be of therapeutic benefit. Investigations measuring the fraction of exhaled NO (FeNO) concentrations have suggested that it may be a useful measure of ongoing lower airway inflammation in patients with asthma and for guiding asthma therapy.[16]

CLINICAL PRESENTATION

Chronic Asthma

❸ Classic asthma is characterized by episodic dyspnea associated with wheezing; however, the clinical presentation of asthma is as diverse as the number of triggering events (see Clinical Presentation: Chronic Ambulatory Asthma below). Although wheezing is the characteristic symptom of asthma, the medical literature is replete with the warning that "not all that wheezes is asthma."

CLINICAL PRESENTATION Chronic Ambulatory Asthma

General

- Asthma is a disease of exacerbation and remission, so the patient may not have any signs or symptoms at the time of examination.

Symptoms

- The patient may complain of episodes of dyspnea, chest tightness, coughing (particularly at night), wheezing, or a whistling sound when breathing. These often occur in association with exercise, but also occur spontaneously or in association with known allergens.

Signs

- Expiratory wheezing on auscultation, dry hacking cough, or signs of atopy (allergic rhinitis and/or eczema) may occur.

Laboratory

- Spirometry demonstrates obstruction (reduced FEV_1/forced vital capacity [FVC]) with reversibility following inhaled β_2-agonist administration (at least a 12% improvement in FEV_1).

Other Diagnostic Tests

- A fall in FEV_1 of at least 15% following 6 minutes of near maximal exercise. Elevated eosinophil count and IgE concentration in blood. Elevated FeNO (greater than 20 ppb in children less than 12 years of age and greater than 25 ppb in adults). Positive methacholine challenge (PC_{20} FEV_1 less than 12.5 mg/mL) or mannitol challenge (FEV_1 decrease of at least 15% from baseline after 635 mg or less).

TABLE 15-2 Sample Questions[a] for the Diagnosis and Initial Assessment of Asthma

A "yes" answer to any question suggests that an asthma diagnosis is likely.
In the last 12 months...

- Have you had a sudden severe episode or recurrent episodes of coughing, wheezing (high-pitched whistling sounds when breathing out), chest tightness, or shortness of breath?
- Have you had colds that "go to the chest" or take more than 10 days to get over?
- Have you had coughing, wheezing, or shortness of breath during a particular season or time of the year?
- Have you had coughing, wheezing, or shortness of breath in certain places or when exposed to certain things (e.g., animals, tobacco smoke, perfumes)?
- Have you used any medications that help you breathe better? How often?
- Are your symptoms relieved when the medications are used?

In the last 4 weeks, have you had coughing, wheezing, or shortness of breath...

- At night that has awakened you?
- On awakening?
- After running, moderate exercise, or other physical activity?

[a]These questions are recommended by the NAEPP but have not been formally validated.

A wheeze is a high-pitched, whistling sound created by turbulent airflow through an obstructed airway, so any condition that produces significant obstruction can result in wheezing as a symptom. In addition, "all of asthma does not wheeze" is an equally justifiable warning. Patients may present with a chronic persistent cough as their only symptom.[2]

There is no single diagnostic test for asthma. The diagnosis is based primarily on a good history[2] (Table 15-2). The patient may have a family history of allergy or asthma or have symptoms of allergic rhinitis.[2] Reversibility of airway obstruction following administration of a short-acting inhaled β_2-agonist provides confirmation but is not by itself diagnostic. Patients with normal values of spirometry can be challenged by exercise or substances that produce bronchoconstriction, such as methacholine or mannitol, to determine if they have BHR, but, again, positive challenges are not diagnostic. Newer tests of inflammation in the airways such as induced sputum eosinophil and/or neutrophil counts and FeNO measurements are consistent with but not diagnostic of asthma.

Asthma has a widely variable presentation from chronic daily symptoms to only intermittent symptoms. The intervals between symptoms can be days, weeks, months, or years. Asthma also can vary as to its severity, the intrinsic intensity of the disease process. Severity is most easily and directly measured in a patient who is not currently receiving asthma treatment. The NAEPP has provided a means of classifying asthma severity that is divided into two domains: impairment and risk.[2] This classification system is individualized for three age groups (0 to 4, 5 to 11, and ≥12 years) and summarized in Table 15-3. The intermittent and/or chronic nature of symptoms does not necessarily determine the severity of symptoms during exacerbations. Asthma severity is determined by lung function, symptoms, nighttime awakenings, and interference with normal activity prior to therapy. Patients can present with a range from intermittent symptoms that require no medications or only occasional use of short-acting inhaled β_2-agonists to severe persistent asthma symptoms despite treatment with multiple medications.

Acute Severe Asthma

Uncontrolled asthma, with its inherent variability, can progress to an acute state where inflammation, airway edema, excessive mucus accumulation, and severe bronchospasm result in a profound airway narrowing that is poorly responsive to usual bronchodilator therapy[2,9] (see Clinical Presentation: Acute Severe Asthma below). Although this progression is the most common scenario, some patients experience rapid-onset or hyperacute attacks.[2,9] Hyperacute attacks are associated with neutrophilic as opposed to eosinophilic infiltration and resolve rapidly with bronchodilator therapy, suggesting that smooth muscle spasm is the major pathogenic mechanism.[9,14] In most cases, ED visits for acute severe asthma represent the failure of an adequate therapeutic regimen to control persistent asthma. Underutilization of antiinflammatory drugs and excessive reliance on short-acting inhaled β_2-agonists are the major risk factors for severe exacerbations.[2] However, frequent exacerbations may represent a specific phenotype of asthma.[9] A blunted perception of airway obstruction may predispose certain individuals to fatal asthma attacks.[2]

CLINICAL PRESENTATION Acute Severe Asthma

General

- An episode can progress over several days or hours (usual scenario) or progresses rapidly over 1 to 2 hours.

Symptoms

- The patient is anxious in acute distress and complains of severe dyspnea, shortness of breath, chest tightness, or burning. The patient is only able to say a few words with each breath. Symptoms are unresponsive to usual measures (short-acting inhaled β_2-agonist administration).

Signs

- Signs include expiratory and inspiratory wheezing on auscultation (breath sounds may be diminished with very severe obstruction), dry hacking cough, tachypnea, tachycardia, pale or cyanotic skin, hyperinflated chest with intercostal and supraclavicular retractions, and hypoxic seizures if very severe.

Laboratory

- Peak expiratory flow [PEF] and/or FEV_1 less than 40% of normal predicted values. Decreased arterial O_2 (Pao_2), and O_2 saturations by pulse oximetry (SaO_2 less than 90% [0.90] on room air is severe). Decreased arterial or capillary CO_2 if mild, but in the normal range or increased in moderate to severe obstruction.

Other Diagnostic Tests

- Blood gases to assess metabolic acidosis (lactic acidosis) in severe obstruction. Complete blood count if there are signs of infection (fever and purulent sputum). Serum electrolytes as therapy with β_2-agonist and corticosteroids can lower serum potassium, magnesium, and phosphate, and increase glucose. Chest radiograph if signs of consolidation on auscultation.

TABLE 15-3 Classifying Asthma Severity for Patients Who Are Not Currently Taking Long-Term Control Medications

	Children 0–4 and 5–11 Years of Age				
			Persistent		
	Components	Intermittent	Mild	Moderate	Severe
Impairment	Symptoms	≤2 days/wk	>2 days/wk but not daily	Daily	Throughout the day
	Nighttime awakenings (0–4 years)	0	1–2 × month	3–4 × month	>1 × week
	5–11 years	≤2 × month	3–4 × month	>1 × week, but not nightly	Often 7 × week
	SABA use for Sx control	≤2 days/wk	>2 days/wk but not daily	Daily	Several times per day
	Interference with normal activity	None	Minor limitation	Some limitation	Extremely limited
	Lung function	FEV_1 >80%	FEV_1 >80%	FEV_1 60–80%	FEV_1 <60%
	5–11 years	FEV_1/FVC >85% (>0.85)	FEV_1/FVC >80% (>0.80)	FEV_1/FVC 75–80% (0.75–0.80)	FEV_1/FVC <75% (<0.75)
	Exacerbations	Intermittent	Persistent		
Risk	0–4 years	0–1/y	≥2 in 6 months or ≥4 wheezing episodes/1 year lasting >1 day		
	5–11 years	0–2/y	>2 in 1 year →		
	Recommended step for initiating treatment	Step 1	Step 2	Step 3 and consider short course of oral corticosteroids	
	Youths ≥12 Years of Age and Adults				
			Persistent		
	Components	Intermittent	Mild	Moderate	Severe
Impairment	Symptoms	≤2 days/wk	>2 days/wk but not daily	Daily	Throughout the day
	Nighttime awakenings	≤2 × month	3–4 × month	>1 × week, but not nightly	Often 7 × week
	SABA use for Sx control	≤2 days/wk	>2 days/wk, but not >1 × day	Daily	Several times per day
	Interference with normal activity	None	Minor limitation	Some limitation	Extremely limited
	Lung function[a]	FEV_1 >80% FEV_1/FVC normal	FEV_1 >80% FEV_1/FVC normal	FEV_1 60–80% FEV_1/FVC reduced 5% (0.05)	FEV_1 <60% FEV_1/FVC reduced >5% (>0.05)
	Exacerbations	Intermittent	Persistent		
Risk		0–2/y	>2 in 1 year →		
	Recommended step for initiating treatment	Step 1	Step 2	Step 3 and consider short course of oral corticosteroids	Step 4 or 5 course of oral corticosteroid

SABA, short-acting β-agonist.

[a]Normal FEV_1/FVC: 8–19 years 85% (0.85); 20–39 years 80% (0.80); 40–59 years 75% (0.75); 60–80 years 70% (0.70).

Exercise-Induced Bronchospasm

During vigorous exercise, pulmonary function measurements (FEV_1 and PEF) in patients with asthma increase during the first few minutes but then begin to decrease after 6 to 8 minutes (Fig. 15-3).[2] EIB is defined as a drop in FEV_1 of 15% or greater from baseline (pre-exercise value).[2] Most studies suggest that many patients with persistent asthma experience EIB.[2] The exact pathogenesis of EIB is unknown, but heat loss and/or water loss from the central airways appears to play an important role.[13] EIB is provoked more easily in cold, dry air; alternatively, warm, humid air can blunt or block it.[13] Studies have demonstrated increased plasma histamine, cysteinyl LTs, prostaglandins, and tryptase concentrations during EIB, suggesting a role for mast cell degranulation.[13] These findings have led to the development of inhaled mannitol, an osmotic agent, as an indirect pharmacologic bronchoprovocation test to assist in the diagnosis of asthma.[17]

A refractory period following EIB lasts up to 3 hours after exercise in some patients. During this period, repeat exercise of the same intensity produces either no decrease in pulmonary function or a drop of less than 50% of the initial response.[13] This refractory period is thought to be caused by an acute depletion of mast cell mediators and time required for their repletion. Patients with known refractoriness to exercise will still respond to

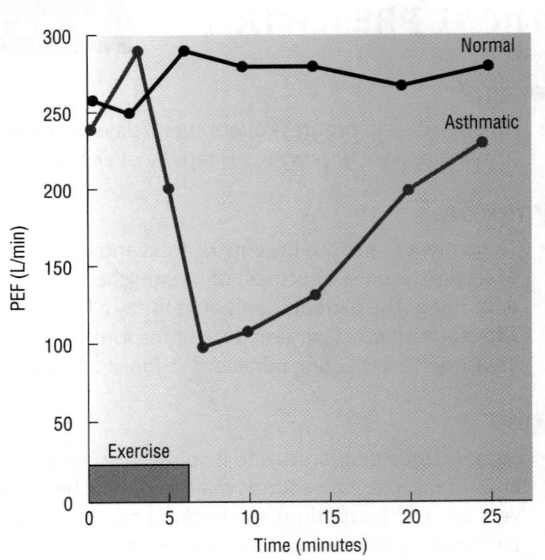

FIGURE 15-3 Typical responses to exercise in a normal subject and an asthmatic subject. Note the initial bronchodilation. (PEF, peak expiratory flow.)

histamine, so acute hyporesponsiveness of airway smooth muscle does not appear to be a factor.[13]

EIB is believed to be a reflection of increased BHR associated with asthma. A correlation, though not perfect, exists between EIB and reactivity to histamine, methacholine, and mannitol.[13,17] Other patient groups with BHR (e.g., after viral infection, cystic fibrosis, or allergic rhinitis) show bronchoconstriction after exercise to a lesser degree (5% to 10% drops) than patients with asthma (15% to 40% drops).[13] Patients will not always demonstrate the same sensitivity. During periods of remission, a decreased sensitivity to the same degree of exercise is often observed. Finally, a number of children and adults with EIB are otherwise normal, without symptoms or abnormal pulmonary function except in association with exercise.[2] Elite athletes have a higher prevalence of EIB than the general population.[13]

Nocturnal Asthma

3 Worsening of asthma during sleep is referred to as *nocturnal asthma*. Patients with nocturnal asthma exhibit significant falls in pulmonary function between bedtime and awakening.[2] Typically, their lung function reaches a nadir at 3 to 4 AM. Although the pathogenesis of this phenomenon is unknown, it has been associated with diurnal patterns of endogenous cortisol secretion and circulating epinephrine.[2] Direct evidence for an inflammatory component to nocturnal asthma includes increased circulating histamine and activated eosinophils and LT excretion at night associated with increased BHR to methacholine.[2]

Numerous other factors that may affect nocturnal worsening of asthma, including allergies and improper environmental control, gastroesophageal reflux, obstructive sleep apnea, and sinusitis, also must be considered when evaluating these patients.[2] Most experts consider nocturnal symptoms to be a sign of inadequately treated persistent asthma.[2] Awakening from nocturnal asthma is a sensitive indicator of both severity and inadequate control.[2]

FACTORS CONTRIBUTING TO ASTHMA SEVERITY

Viral Respiratory Infections

Viral respiratory infections are primarily responsible for exacerbations of asthma, particularly in children under age 10.[9,10] Infants are particularly susceptible to airway obstruction and wheezing with viral infections because of their small airways. The most common cause of exacerbations in both children and adults is the rhinovirus, which is the most frequent virus associated with the common cold and distributed worldwide.[10] Other viruses isolated include RSV, parainfluenza virus, adenoviruses, coronavirus, and influenza viruses. Certain viruses (RSV and parainfluenza virus) are capable of inducing specific IgE antibodies, and rhinovirus can activate eosinophils directly in asthmatics.[10] The increase in asthma symptoms and BHR that occurs may last for days or weeks following resolution of the symptoms of the viral infection. Evidence does not support a beneficial effect of influenza vaccine for preventing asthma exacerbations from subsequent influenza infections.[2]

Environmental and Occupational Factors

Agents and events and the mechanisms that are known to trigger asthma are listed in Table 15-1.[2] The general mechanisms are unknown but presumably are the result of epithelial damage and inflammation in the airway mucosa. Ozone and sulfur dioxide, common components of air pollution, have been used to induce BHR in animals. Exposure to 0.2 ppm ozone for 2 to 3 hours can induce bronchoconstriction and increase BHR in asthmatics.[2,8] Sulfur dioxide in the ambient atmosphere is highly irritating and presumably induces bronchoconstriction through mast cell or irritant-receptor involvement.[2] Asthma produced by repeated prolonged exposure to industrial inhalants is a significant health problem. It has been estimated that occupational asthma accounts for 2% of all asthmatic persons.[8] Persons with occupational asthma have the typical symptoms of asthma with cough, dyspnea, and wheeze. Typically, the symptoms are related to workplace exposure and improve on days off and during vacations.[8] In some instances, symptoms may persist even after termination of exposure.[8]

Stress, Depression, and Psychosocial Factors in Asthma

Observational studies demonstrate an association between increased stress and worsening asthma, but the role is not clearly defined.[2] Bronchoconstriction from psychological factors appears to be mediated primarily through excess parasympathetic input. Atropine has been shown to block experimental psychogenic bronchoconstriction. It is most important to emphasize to both patients and parents that asthma is not an emotional disease; however, coping skills may benefit the patient who becomes emotionally distraught during an asthma attack.

Rhinitis/Sinusitis

Disorders of the upper respiratory tract, particularly rhinitis and sinusitis, have been linked with asthma for many years. As many as 40% to 50% of asthmatics have abnormal sinus radiographs.[2] However, chronic sinusitis may just represent a nonbacterial coexisting condition with allergic asthmatics because the histologic changes in the paranasal sinuses are similar to those seen in the lung and nose.[2] Treatment of upper airway disease may optimize overall asthma control. The mechanism by which sinusitis aggravates asthma is unknown. The treatment of allergic rhinitis with intranasal corticosteroids and cromolyn but not antihistamines will reduce BHR in asthmatic patients.[2] It has been postulated that transport of mucus chemotactic factors and inflammatory mediators from nasal passages during allergic rhinitis into the lung may accentuate BHR.

Gastroesophageal Reflux Disease

Symptoms of gastroesophageal reflux disease (GERD) as well as asymptomatic reflux are common in both children and adults who have asthma.[2] Nocturnal asthma may be associated with nighttime reflux.[2] Reflux of acidic gastric contents into the esophagus is thought to initiate a vagally mediated reflex bronchoconstriction.[2] Also of concern is that most medications that decrease airway smooth muscle tone may have a relaxant effect on gastroesophageal sphincter tone. However, treatment of reflux in asthma patients has produced inconsistent results on asthma control.[2,18] The current recommendation is to initiate standard antireflux therapy in those patients exhibiting symptoms of reflux.[2]

Female Hormones and Asthma

Premenstrual worsening of asthma has been reported in as many as 30% to 40% of women in some studies, whereas worsening of pulmonary functions has been reported even in women not aware of worsening symptoms.[19] The pathophysiology is uncertain because estrogen replacement in postmenopausal women has been shown to worsen asthma, whereas estradiol and progesterone administration has been variably reported to improve or have no effect on asthma in women with premenstrual asthma.[19,20] Asthma symptoms may vary significantly during different stages of the menstrual cycle. The clinical significance of menstruation-related asthma is still unclear because some studies have reported that up to 50% of ED visits by women were premenstrual, whereas others have reported no association with menstrual phase.[19,20] In general, BHR and symptoms improve in asthmatic women during pregnancy.[2,19]

FOODS, DRUGS, AND ADDITIVES

Documentation in the literature of food allergens as triggers for asthma is not available.[2] However, additives, specifically sulfites used as preservatives, can trigger life-threatening asthma exacerbations. Beer, wine, dried fruit, and open salad bars, in particular, have high concentrations of metabisulfites.[2] Severe oral corticosteroid-dependent patients should be warned about ingesting foods processed with sulfites. Another additive producing bronchospasm is benzalkonium chloride, which is found as a preservative in some nebulizer solutions of antiasthmatic drugs.[21]

Aspirin and other nonsteroidal antiinflammatory drugs can precipitate an attack in up to 20% of adults and 5% of children with asthma.[22] The mechanism is related to cyclooxygenase inhibition, and 5-lipoxygenase inhibition can alter dose–response but not completely block the symptoms.[22] The prevalence increases with age and severity of asthma.[2] The greatest frequency occurs in severe corticosteroid-resistant asthmatics in their fourth and fifth decades who also have perennial rhinitis and nasal polyposis (presence of several polyps).[22] Other drugs that do not precipitate bronchospasm but that prevent its reversal are the nonselective β-blocking agents.[2]

Nutritional Factors

Epidemiologic data suggest that obesity increases the prevalence of asthma and may reduce asthma control.[23] Lung volume and tidal volume are reduced in obesity, promoting airway narrowing. Obesity also produces low-grade systemic inflammation that may act on the lung to worsen asthma.[23] The mechanism is likely the release of adipose-derived proinflammatory mediators such as IL-6, IL-10, eotaxin, tumor necrosis factor-α, transforming growth factors-β_1, C-reactive protein, leptin, and adiponectin or a result of common predisposing dietary factors. Although not all studies find relationship between body mass index and asthma control, management of asthma in obese patients should include weight loss measures.[24]

More recently it has been shown that children with vitamin D insufficiency are at greater risk of uncontrolled asthma (increased hospitalizations, BHR, and eosinophil counts).[25] Vitamin D helps regulate T cells and improves their secretion of antiinflammatory cytokines in response to corticosteroids.[25] Clinical trials defining the potential therapeutic role of vitamin D supplementation in asthma management are underway.

TREATMENT
Asthma

Aerosol Therapy for Asthma

4 5 Aerosol delivery of drugs for asthma has the advantage of being site specific and thus enhancing the therapeutic ratio.[2,26] Inhalation of short-acting β_2-agonists provides more rapid bronchodilation than either parenteral or oral administration, as well as the greatest degree of protection against EIB and other challenges.[2] Inhaled corticosteroids (ICSs) have been developed with rapid oral and systemic clearance to enhance lung activity and reduce systemic activity. Specific agents (e.g., cromolyn, formoterol, salmeterol, and ipratropium bromide) are only effective by inhalation.[2] Therefore, an understanding of aerosol drug delivery is essential to optimal asthma therapy. Table 15-4 lists the factors determining lung deposition of therapeutic aerosols.

TABLE 15-4 Factors Determining Lung Deposition of Aerosols

Device	Device Factors	Patient Factors
Metered-dose inhaler (MDI)	Canister held inverted Formulation (solution or suspension) Actuator cleanliness Addition of a spacer device	Inspiratory flow (slow, deep) Breath-holding Coordinating actuation with inhalation Priming and shaking the device
Dry powder inhaler (DPI)	Device cleanliness Resistance to inhalation Humidity	Inspiratory flow (deep, forceful) Tilting head back Maintaining parallel to ground once activated
Jet nebulizer (small volume)	Volume fill (3–6 mL) Gas flow (6–12 L/min) Dead space volume Open versus closed system Thumb-activating valve Mouthpiece versus face mask	Inspiratory flow (slow, deep) Breath-holding Tapping nebulizer
Ultrasonic nebulizer	Volume fill Not effective for suspensions Mouthpiece versus face mask	Inspiratory flow (slow, deep) Breath-holding Tapping nebulizer
Spacer device	Volume (≥650 mL) One-way valves Holding chamber versus open-ended Antistatic lining Mouthpiece versus face mask	Inspiratory flow (slow, deep) Time between actuation and inhalation (<5 seconds) Cleaning with detergent to reduce static Multiple actuations decrease delivery Coordination of actuation and inhalation for the simple open-tube spacers

Device Determinants of Delivery

Devices used to generate therapeutic aerosols include jet nebulizers, ultrasonic nebulizers, metered-dose inhalers (MDIs), and dry powder inhalers (DPIs). The single most important device factor determining the site of aerosol deposition is particle size.[26] Devices for delivering therapeutic aerosols generate particles with aerodynamic diameters from 0.5 to 35 μm.[26] Particles larger than 10 μm deposit in the oropharynx, particles between 5 and 10 μm deposit in the trachea and large bronchi, particles 1 to 5 μm in size reach the lower airways, and particles smaller than 0.5 μm act as a gas and are exhaled. In asthma, the airways, not the alveoli, are the target for delivery. Respirable particles are deposited in the airways by three mechanisms: (a) inertial impaction, (b) gravitational sedimentation, and (c) Brownian diffusion.[26] The first two mechanisms are the most important for therapeutic aerosols and probably are the only factors that can be manipulated by patients.

Each delivery device within a classification generates specific aerosol characteristics, so extrapolation of delivery data from one device cannot be applied to the other devices in the class. For instance, MDIs can deliver 15% to 50% of the actuated dose; DPIs, 10% to 30% of the labeled dose; and nebulizers, 2% to 15% of the starting dose.[26] MDIs and DPIs are portable and convenient, unlike jet nebulizers. Small portable ultrasonic nebulizers have also been developed. MDIs consist of a pressurized canister with a metering valve; the canister contains active drug, low-vapor-pressure propellants such as hydrofluoroalkane (HFA), cosolvents, and/or surfactants.[26] The international ban on the production and use of chlorofluorocarbon (CFC) propellant (due to their ozone layer–depleting properties) has resulted in no CFC-propelled MDIs available in the United States with the exception of pirbuterol Autohaler

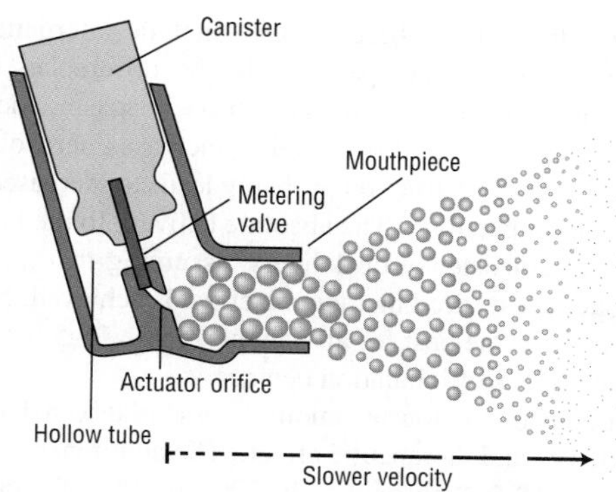

FIGURE 15-4 Illustration of a metered-dose inhaler demonstrating the particle size difference as the aerosol cloud extends outward.

until December 31, 2013. With any change in the components of an MDI, the FDA considers it to be a new drug that requires stability, safety, and efficacy studies prior to approval. The drug is either in solution or a suspended micronized powder. In order to disperse the suspension for accurate delivery, the canister must be shaken. The metering chamber measures a liquid volume, and, therefore, the device must be held with the valve stem downward so that the chamber is covered with liquid[26] (Fig. 15-4). When the canister is actuated, the device releases the propellant and drug in a forceful spray whose particles are large (mass median aerodynamic diameter [MMAD] = 45 μm)[26] (see Fig. 15-4). As evaporation occurs, the particle size is reduced to a final MMAD of 0.5 to 5.5 μm depending on the MDI. The aerosol cloud extends about 6 in beyond the MDI at the lowest MMAD.[26] Each MDI has different conditions for storage and durations to expiration, so the pharmacist must become familiar with and counsel the patient on these factors.

The breath-actuated MDI Autohaler is cocked with a lever to "load" the dose of medication, a baffle is opened by inspiratory pressure, and the dose is expelled from the canister metering chamber.[26] While the need for hand–lung coordination for proper actuation is reduced significantly with breath-actuated MDIs, these devices do not accommodate the use of a spacer device.

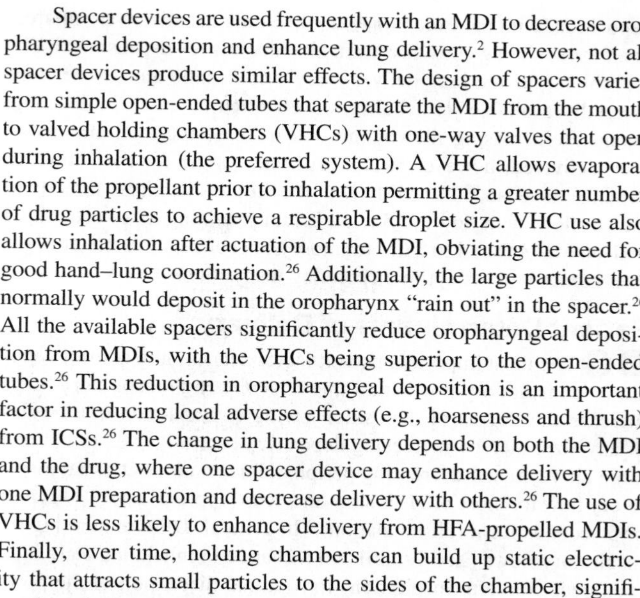

Spacer devices are used frequently with an MDI to decrease oropharyngeal deposition and enhance lung delivery.[2] However, not all spacer devices produce similar effects. The design of spacers varies from simple open-ended tubes that separate the MDI from the mouth to valved holding chambers (VHCs) with one-way valves that open during inhalation (the preferred system). A VHC allows evaporation of the propellant prior to inhalation permitting a greater number of drug particles to achieve a respirable droplet size. VHC use also allows inhalation after actuation of the MDI, obviating the need for good hand–lung coordination.[26] Additionally, the large particles that normally would deposit in the oropharynx "rain out" in the spacer.[26] All the available spacers significantly reduce oropharyngeal deposition from MDIs, with the VHCs being superior to the open-ended tubes.[26] This reduction in oropharyngeal deposition is an important factor in reducing local adverse effects (e.g., hoarseness and thrush) from ICSs.[26] The change in lung delivery depends on both the MDI and the drug, where one spacer device may enhance delivery with one MDI preparation and decrease delivery with others.[26] The use of VHCs is less likely to enhance delivery from HFA-propelled MDIs. Finally, over time, holding chambers can build up static electricity that attracts small particles to the sides of the chamber, significantly reducing aerosol availability. Some spacers should be washed weekly with household detergent with a single rinse and allowed to drip dry.[2] Other VHCs have been developed with antistatic materials.

Dry micronized powders can be inhaled directly into the lung. A number of DPIs are now available for use in the United States.[26] Currently, there are no generic DPIs as each drug plus device has its own patent. Each DPI has unique characteristics with advantages and disadvantages (Table 15-5). The primary advantage of DPIs is that they are breath actuated and require minimal hand–lung coordination, and it is thus easier to teach patients proper technique.[26] Some DPIs are more flow dependent than others.[26] Thus, similar to MDIs and spacers, delivery data from one DPI cannot be extrapolated to another.

Nebulizers come in two basic types, the jet nebulizer and the ultrasonic nebulizer. Jet nebulizers produce an aerosol from a liquid solution or suspension placed in a cup. A tube connected to a stream of compressed air or O_2 flows up through the bottom and draws the liquid up an adjacent open-ended tube.[26] The air and liquid strike a baffle, creating a droplet cloud that is then inhaled.[26] Ultrasonic nebulizers produce an aerosol by vibrating liquid lying above a transducer at speeds of about 1 mHz.[26] Both produce similar degrees of lung

TABLE 15-5 Characteristics of Various Inhalation Devices

Device	Drugs	Breath Activated	Dose Counter	Other Excipients	Disadvantages
MDI	All classes	No	No/yes	Propellants, surfactants, cosolvents	Requires coordination of actuation and inhalation. Large pharyngeal deposition. Difficult to teach
Autohaler MDI	Pirbuterol	Yes	No	CFC propellant, surfactant	Requires rapid inhalation to activate
MDI plus valved holding chamber	All classes	No	No		More expensive than MDI alone; less portable; some payers will not pay; inconsistent effect on delivery; nonstatic preferred
Jet nebulizers	All classes	No	—	Preservatives in some solutions	Significant interbrand variability; expensive and time consuming; less efficient than MDIs; contamination possible; preparations may be light and temperature sensitive (short shelf life)
Ulrasonic nebulizer	Cromolyn solution, short-acting β_2-agonist solutions	No	—	Preservatives in some solutions	Same as for jet nebulizers plus cannot be used for suspensions; battery operated are portable
Flexhaler	Budesonide	Yes	Yes	Lactose filler	Requires high inspiratory flow (60 L/min). Pharyngeal deposition Not approved for <6 years of age
Diskus	Fluticasone; salmeterol; fluticasone/salmeterol	Yes	Yes	Lactose filler	Not approved for <4 years of age Requires inspiratory flow of 30–60 L/min
Aerolizer	Formoterol	Yes	—	Lactose filler	Single-dose capsules. Not approved for <5 years of age Requires flow of 30–60 L/min
Twisthaler	Mometasone	Yes	Yes	Lactose filler	Not approved for <4 years of age

deposition, with the exception that ultrasonic nebulizers are ineffective for nebulizing currently available micronized suspensions.[26] The aerosol output and lung delivery vary significantly among the commercially available jet nebulizers even when operated in the same manner.[26] Increasing fill volume will increase the total amount of drug delivered; however, it also will take longer for the patient to nebulize the dose.[26] The MMAD of the droplets is related directly to the gas flow, with flows of 5 to 12 L/min providing an aerosol cloud with an MMAD of 4 to 8 μm for most jet nebulizers.[26] Each jet nebulizer comes with its optimal operating instructions.

Patient Determinants of Delivery

6 7 The most important patient factor determining aerosol deposition is inspiratory flow (see Table 15-4).[2,26] High inspiratory flows increase the degree of deposition owing to impaction of particles of any size, thereby increasing deposition centrally (i.e., throat and large airways) and decreasing peripheral deposition. Optimal inspiratory flow for most MDIs is slow and deep (approximately 30 L/min or 5 seconds for a full inhalation).[2] In general, DPIs require higher inspiratory flows (≥60 L/min) and a change in inhalation technique (i.e., deep, forceful inspiration) for optimal dispersion of the powder, which, in turn, increases the amount of drug delivered to the larger central airways.[26] However, this difference in delivery may not produce clinically significant differences.[26] Patients should be cautioned not to exhale into DPIs because this causes loss of dose and moistens the dry powder, causing aggregation into larger particles. Patient factors that cannot be controlled include interpatient variability in airway geometry (particularly the differences between children and adults)[26] and the effects of bronchospasm, edema, and mucus hypersecretion. Mild obstruction increases aerosol deposition; however, severe obstruction probably leads to increased central deposition from impaction.[26] The absolute delivery to the lung is not as important as consistency of delivery, assuming that a sufficient dose to produce the desired therapeutic effect is achieved. No single inhalation device is the best for all patients. Table 15-5 lists the differing characteristics of inhalation devices.

Appropriate inhalation technique is essential to achieve optimal drug delivery and therapeutic effect.[2] The components are illustrated in Figure 15-5. Approximately 50% to 80% of a dose from MDIs and DPIs impacts on the oropharynx and is then swallowed; the rest is either left in the device or exhaled.[26] It is important that actuation occurs during inhalation, although the time during inspiration is unimportant.[2,26] Although radiolabeled studies with MDIs indicate improved delivery by holding the actuator 2 to 3 cm in front of an open mouth to allow more evaporation and less impaction, physiologic studies with bronchodilators have failed to document an advantage for this method.[2,26] Many patients do not use their MDIs optimally, and patient instruction with demonstration is the most effective means of improving inhaler technique.[2,26] Even with instruction, up to 30% of patients, particularly young children and the elderly, cannot master the use of an MDI. For these patients, attachment of a VHC to the MDI or use of a breath-actuated MDI can

Steps for Using Your Inhaler

Please demonstrate your inhaler technique at every visit.

1. Remove the cap and hold inhaler upright.
2. Shake the inhaler.
3. Tilt your head back slightly and breathe out slowly.
4. Position the inhaler in one of the following ways (B is acceptable for those who have difficulty with A or C: C is required for breath-activated inhalers):

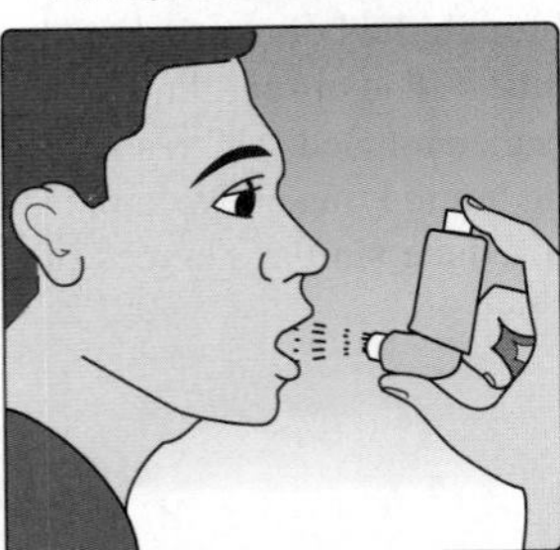

A Open mouth with inhaler 1 to 2 in away.

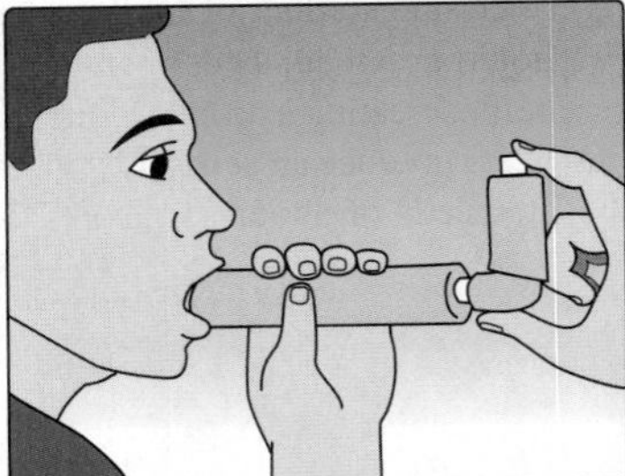

B Use spacer/holding chamber (which is recommended especially for young children and for people using corticosteroids).

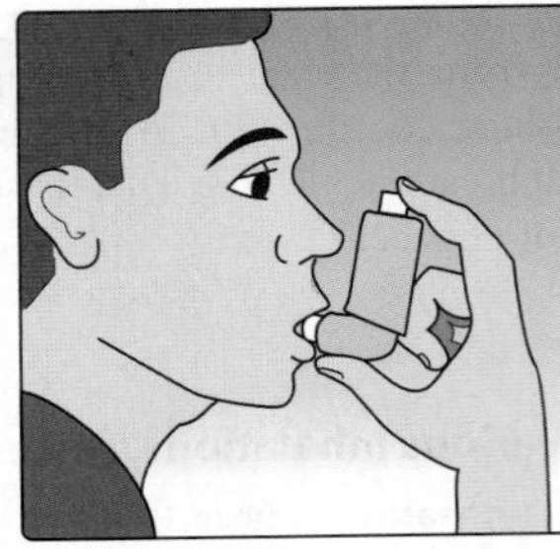

C In the mouth.

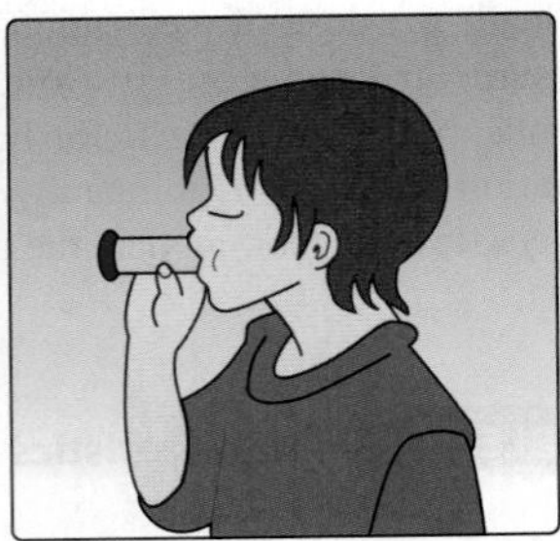

D NOTE: Inhaled dry powder capsules require a different inhalation technique. To use a dry powder inhaler, it is important to close the mouth tightly around the mouthpiece of the inhaler and to inhale rapidly.

5. Press down on the inhaler to release medication as you start to breathe in slowly.
6. Breathe in slowly (3–5 seconds).
7. Hold your breath for 10 seconds to allow the medicine to reach deeply into your lungs.
8. Repeat puff as directed. Waiting 1 minute between puffs may permit second puff to penetrate your lungs better.
9. Spacers/holding chambers are useful for all patients. They are particularly recommended for young children and older adults and for use with corticosteroids.

Avoid common inhaler mistakes. Follow these inhaler tips:

- Breathe out *before* pressing your inhaler.
- Inhale *slowly.*
- Breathe in through your mouth, not your nose.
- Press down on your inhaler at the *start* of inhalation (or within the first second of inhalation).
- Keep inhaling as you press down on inhaler.
- Press your inhaler only *once* while you are inhaling (one breath for each puff).
- Make sure you breathe in evenly and deeply.

NOTE: Other inhalers are becoming available in addition to those illustrated above. Different types of inhalers require different techniques.

FIGURE 15-5 Instructions for inhaler use from the adapted NAEPP Expert Panel Report 2. *http://www.nhlbi.nih.gov/guidelines/archives/epr-2/index.htm.*

improve efficacy significantly.[2,26] However, addition of a VHC offers no advantage in patients who can use an MDI optimally alone.[26] Mouth rinsing following treatment with MDI- and DPI-ICSs is important to minimize local adverse effects and oral absorption.[2,26]

Delivery from high-resistance DPIs is more flow dependent than from low-resistance DPIs. Thus, younger children and possibly elderly adults will have more variability in delivery from high-resistance devices.[26] Most children younger than 4 years of age cannot generate a sufficient inspiratory flow to use DPIs. Young children (<4 years) and infants generally require the use of a face mask attached to either an MDI plus VHC or nebulizer. The use of a face mask results in a reduction in lung delivery due to the portion of the aerosol inhaled nasally, so the doses of drugs used in these patients are often not decreased.

TREATMENT

Acute Severe Asthma

The primary goal is prevention of life-threatening asthma by early recognition of signs of deterioration and early intervention. As such, the principal goals of treatment include[2]:

1. Correction of significant hypoxemia
2. Rapid reversal of airflow obstruction
3. Reduction of the likelihood of relapse of the exacerbation or future recurrence of severe airflow obstruction
4. Development of a written asthma action plan in case of a further exacerbation

These goals are best achieved by early initiation or intensification of treatment and close monitoring of objective measures of oxygenation and lung function.[2] Early response to treatment as measured by the improvement in FEV_1 at 30 minutes following inhaled β_2-agonists is the best predictor of outcome.[2,27] Providing adequate O_2 supplementation to maintain O_2 saturations above 90% (0.90) (or >95% [0.95] in pregnant women and those who have coexistent heart disease) is essential. In children younger than 6 years of age, in whom lung function measures are difficult to obtain, a combination of objective (e.g., O_2 saturation, capillary CO_2, respiratory rate, and heart rate) and subjective measures may be used to assess severity.[2,28]

The primary therapy of acute exacerbations is pharmacologic, which includes short-acting inhaled β_2-agonists and, depending on the severity, systemic corticosteroids, inhaled ipratropium, and O_2 (Figs. 15-6 and 15-7).[2] It is important that therapy not be delayed, so the history and physical examination should be obtained while initial therapy is being provided. Patients at risk for life-threatening exacerbations require special attention. Risk factors include a history of previous severe asthma exacerbations (e.g., hospitalizations, intubations, or hypoxic seizures), difficulty

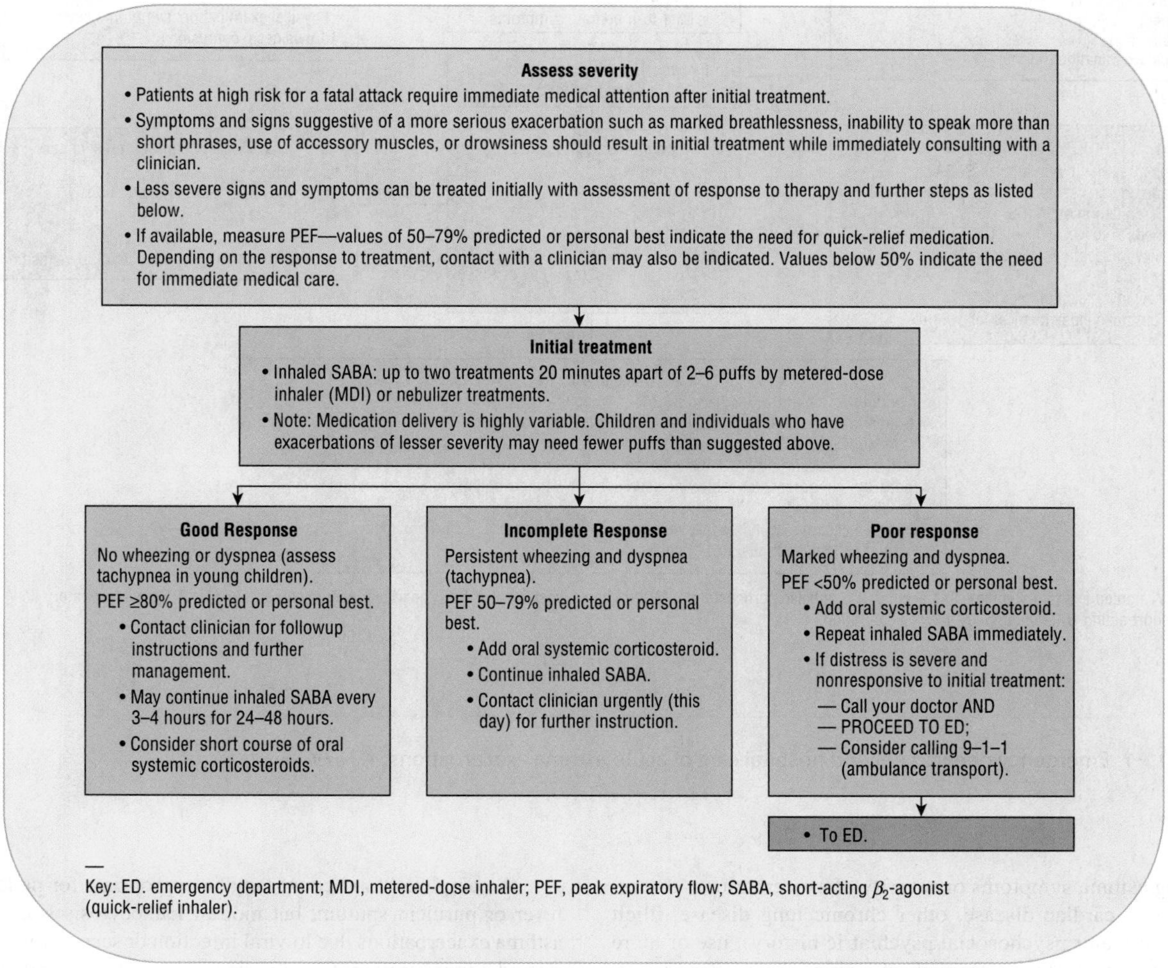

Assess severity

- Patients at high risk for a fatal attack require immediate medical attention after initial treatment.
- Symptoms and signs suggestive of a more serious exacerbation such as marked breathlessness, inability to speak more than short phrases, use of accessory muscles, or drowsiness should result in initial treatment while immediately consulting with a clinician.
- Less severe signs and symptoms can be treated initially with assessment of response to therapy and further steps as listed below.
- If available, measure PEF—values of 50–79% predicted or personal best indicate the need for quick-relief medication. Depending on the response to treatment, contact with a clinician may also be indicated. Values below 50% indicate the need for immediate medical care.

↓

Initial treatment

- Inhaled SABA: up to two treatments 20 minutes apart of 2–6 puffs by metered-dose inhaler (MDI) or nebulizer treatments.
- Note: Medication delivery is highly variable. Children and individuals who have exacerbations of lesser severity may need fewer puffs than suggested above.

↓

Good Response

No wheezing or dyspnea (assess tachypnea in young children).

PEF ≥80% predicted or personal best.

- Contact clinician for followup instructions and further management.
- May continue inhaled SABA every 3–4 hours for 24–48 hours.
- Consider short course of oral systemic corticosteroids.

Incomplete Response

Persistent wheezing and dyspnea (tachypnea).

PEF 50–79% predicted or personal best.

- Add oral systemic corticosteroid.
- Continue inhaled SABA.
- Contact clinician urgently (this day) for further instruction.

Poor response

Marked wheezing and dyspnea.

PEF <50% predicted or personal best.

- Add oral systemic corticosteroid.
- Repeat inhaled SABA immediately.
- If distress is severe and nonresponsive to initial treatment:
  - — Call your doctor AND
  - — PROCEED TO ED;
  - — Consider calling 9–1–1 (ambulance transport).

↓

- To ED.

Key: ED. emergency department; MDI, metered-dose inhaler; PEF, peak expiratory flow; SABA, short-acting β_2-agonist (quick-relief inhaler).

FIGURE 15-6 Home management of acute asthma exacerbation. Patients at risk for asthma-related death should receive immediate clinical attention after initial treatment. Additional therapy may be required. *(From reference 2.)*

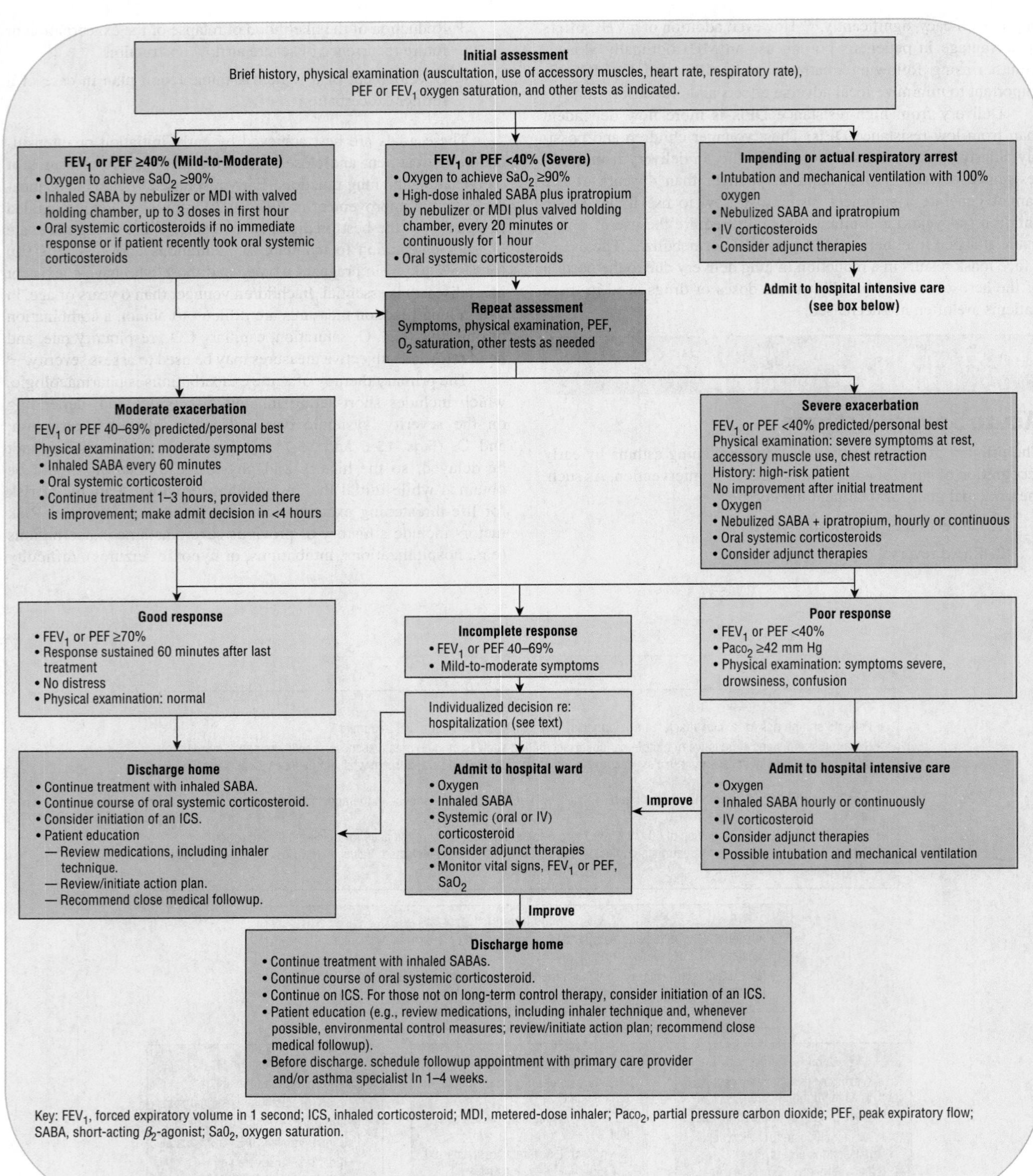

FIGURE 15-7 Emergency department and hospital care of acute asthma exacerbations. *(From reference 2.)*

perceiving asthma symptoms or severity of exacerbations, comorbidities (e.g., cardiac disease, other chronic lung disease, illicit drug use, or major psychosocial/psychiatric history), use of more than two canisters per month of short-acting inhaled β_2-agonists, and current intake of oral corticosteroids or recent withdrawal from oral corticosteroids.[2]

A complete blood count may be appropriate for patients with fever or purulent sputum, but modest leukocytosis is common in asthma exacerbations due to viral infection or secondary to corticosteroid administration. Chest radiography is not recommended for routine assessment but should be obtained for patients suspected of a complicating cardiopulmonary process or another pulmonary process (pneumothorax or pulmonary consolidation).[2] Serum electrolytes should be monitored if high-dose continuous inhaled or systemic β_2-agonists are to be used because they can produce transient decreases in potassium, magnesium, and phosphate.[2] Measurement of serum electrolytes is also prudent in patients who take diuretics regularly and in patients with coexistent cardiovascular disease. The combination of high-dose β_2-agonists and systemic corticosteroids occasionally may result in excessive elevations of glucose and lactic acid.[2]

Initial response should be achieved within minutes, and most patients experience significant improvement within the first 30 to 60 minutes of therapy, with most patients doubling their FEV_1 or PEF.[2] In patients ultimately admitted to the hospital, only a 10% to 20% improvement is seen within the first 2 hours. Hypoxemia, primarily a result of ventilation–perfusion mismatch, is immediately correctable by low-flow O_2.[2] While reversal of lung function into the normal range may take 12 to 24 hours, complete restoration takes much longer—up to 3 to 7 days.[2] A strategy to prevent recurrence includes systemic corticosteroids and symptom or PEF monitoring.[2] It is essential to provide the patient with a written self-management action plan for dealing with exacerbations. Patients at risk for severe exacerbations should be taught how to use a peak flow meter and monitor morning peak flows at home.[2] In young children, an increased respiratory rate, increased heart rate, and inability to speak more than one or two words between breaths are signs of severe obstruction.[2] O_2 saturations by pulse oximetry and peak flows should be measured in all patients not completely responding to initial intensive inhaled β_2-agonist therapy. Initially, on admission, the peak flows or clinical symptoms should be monitored every 2 to 4 hours. Prior to discharge from the ED or hospital, the patient should be given a sufficient supply of prednisone, taught the purpose of the medications and proper inhaler technique, and referred to followup asthma care within 1 to 4 weeks; initiation of ICSs should also be considered.[2]

7 Early recognition of deterioration and aggressive treatment are the keys to successful treatment of acute asthma exacerbations. Thus, patient and/or parent education, teaching self-management skills, and written action plans for early institution of therapy for acute exacerbations improve outcomes.[2] For more moderate to severe patients, this therapeutic plan also may include the availability of oral prednisone to begin at home.[2] Easy access by telephone to healthcare providers is also needed. Because of the rapid progression to severe asthma that can occur, patients and parents should be encouraged to communicate promptly with their asthma care provider during an exacerbation.

Figures 15-6 and 15-7 illustrate the recommended therapies for the treatment of acute asthma exacerbations in home and ED/hospital settings, respectively.[2] The dosages of the drugs for acute severe exacerbations are provided in Table 15-6.[2,6] Institutions should strongly consider developing critical pathways/treatment

TABLE 15-6 Dosages of Drugs of Acute Severe Exacerbations of Asthma in the Emergency Department or Hospital

Medications	Dosages		Comments
	≥12 Years Old	<12 Years Old	
Inhaled β-Agonists			
Albuterol nebulizer solution (5 mg/mL, 0.63 mg/3 mL, 1.25 mg/3 mL, 2.5 mg/3 mL)	2.5–5 mg every 20 minutes for three doses, and then 2.5–10 mg every 1–4 hours as needed, or 10–15 mg/h continuously	0.15 mg/kg (minimum dose 2.5 mg) every 20 minutes for three doses, and then 0.15–0.3 mg/kg up to 10 mg every 1–4 hours as needed, or 0.5 mg/kg/h by continuous nebulization	Only selective β_2-agonists are recommended. For optimal delivery, dilute aerosols to minimum of 4 mL at gas flow of 6–8 L/min. Use face mask if <4 years
Albuterol MDI (90 mcg/puff)	4–8 puffs every 30 minutes up to 4 hours, and then every 1–4 hours as needed	4–8 puffs every 20 minutes for three doses, and then every 1–4 hours as needed	In patients in severe distress, nebulization is preferred; use VHC-type spacer with face mask if <4 years old
Levalbuterol nebulizer solution (0.31 mg/3 mL, 0.63 mg/3 mL, 2.5 mg/1 mL, 1.25 mg/3 mL)	Give at one half the milligram dose of albuterol above	Give at one half the milligram dose of albuterol above	The single isomer of albuterol is twice as potent on a milligram basis
Levalbuterol MDI (45 mcg/puff)	See albuterol dose MOI dose	See albuterol dose MOI dose above	See albuterol MOI dose one half as potent as albuterol on a microgram basis
Pirbuterol MDI (200 mcg/puff)	See albuterol MOI dose above		Has not been studied in acute severe asthma
Systemic β-Agonists			
Epinephrine 1:1,000 (1 mg/mL)	0.3–0.5 mg every 20 minutes for three doses SQ	0.01 mg/kg up to 0.5 mg every 20 minutes for three doses SQ	No proven advantage of systemic therapy over aerosol
Terbutaline (1 mg/mL)	0.25 mg every 20 minutes for three doses SQ	0.01 mg/kg every 20 minutes for three doses, and then every 2–6 hours as needed SQ	Not recommended
Anticholinergics			
Ipratropium bromide nebulizer solution (0.25 mg/mL)	500 mcg every 30 minutes for three doses, and then every 2–4 hours as needed	250 mcg every 20 minutes for three doses, and then 250 mcg every 2–4 hours	May mix in same nebulizer with albuterol; do not use as first-line therapy; only add to β_2-agonist therapy
Ipratropium bromide MDI (18 mcg/puff)	8 puffs every 20 minutes as needed for up to 3 hours	4–8 puffs as needed every 2–4 hours	
Corticosteroids			
Prednisone, methylprednisolone, prednisolone	40–80 mg in one or two divided doses until PEF reaches 70% of personal best	1 mg/kg (maximum 60 mg/day) in two divided doses until PEF is 70% of normal predicted	For outpatient "burst" use 1–2 mg/kg/day, maximum 60 mg, for 3–10 days in children and 40–60 mg/day in one or two divided doses for 5–10 days in adults

Note: No advantage has been found for very-high-dose corticosteroids in acute severe asthma, nor is there any advantage for IV administration over oral therapy. The usual regimen is to continue the oral corticosteroid for duration of hospitalization. The final duration of therapy following a hospitalization or emergency department visit may be from 3 to 10 days. If patients are then started on ICSs, there is no need to taper the systemic corticosteroid dose. ICSs can be started at any time during the exacerbation.

From reference 2.

algorithms for their EDs because their implementation has been shown to improve outcomes and decrease the cost of care.[27] Finally, it is strongly recommended that an appointment with the patient's primary care provider be made within 1 week of the ED visit.[27]

Nonpharmacologic and Ancillary Therapy

Infants and young children may be mildly dehydrated owing to increased insensible loss, vomiting, and decreased intake.[2] Unless dehydration has occurred, increased fluid therapy is not indicated in acute asthma management because the capillary leak from cytokines and increased negative intrathoracic pressures may promote edema in the airways.[2] Correction of significant dehydration is always indicated, and the urine specific gravity may help to guide therapy in young children, in whom the state of hydration may be difficult to determine.[2] Chest physical therapy and mucolytics are not recommended in the therapy of acute asthma.[2] Sedatives should not be given because anxiety may be a sign of hypoxemia, which could be worsened by central nervous system depressants. Antibiotics also are not indicated routinely because viral respiratory tract infections are the primary cause of asthma exacerbations.[2] Antibiotics should be reserved for patients who have signs and symptoms of pneumonia (e.g., fever, pulmonary consolidation, and purulent sputum from polymorphonuclear leukocytes). *Mycoplasma* and *Chlamydia* are infrequent causes of severe asthma exacerbations but should be considered in patients with high O_2 requirements.[2,28]

Respiratory failure or impending respiratory failure as measured by rising $Paco_2$ (≥45 mm Hg [≥6 kPa]) or failure to correct hypoxemia with supplemental O_2 therapy is treated with intubation and mechanical ventilation.[27] In order to prevent barotrauma and pneumothoraces from excess positive pressure, it is recommended that controlled hypoventilation or permissive hypercapnia be used (correcting the hypoxemia, Pao_2 >60 mm Hg [>8 kPa], but allowing the $Paco_2$ to rise to the high 60 mm Hg [8 kPa] range).[27]

Pharmacotherapy

β_2-Agonists

4 The short-acting inhaled β_2-agonists are the most effective bronchodilators and the treatment of first choice for the management of acute severe asthma.[2,27] Up to 66% of adults presenting to an ED require only three doses of 2.5 mg nebulized albuterol to be discharged.[27] Most well-controlled clinical trials have demonstrated equal to greater efficacy and greater safety of aerosolized β_2-agonists over systemic administration regardless of the severity of obstruction.[2,27] Systemic adverse effects, hypokalemia, hyperglycemia, tachycardia, and cardiac dysrhythmias are more pronounced in patients receiving systemic β_2-agonist therapy. Children younger than 2 years of age achieve clinically significant responses from nebulized albuterol.[2] Effective doses of aerosolized β_2-agonists can be delivered successfully through mechanical ventilator circuits to infants, children, and adults in respiratory failure secondary to severe airway obstruction.[29]

Frequent administration of inhaled β_2-agonists (every 20 minutes or continuous nebulization) has been found to be superior to the same dosage administered at 1-hour intervals.[2] In the subset of more severely obstructed patients, continuous nebulization decreases the hospital admission rate, provides greater improvement in the FEV_1 and PEF, and reduces duration of hospitalization when compared with intermittent (hourly) nebulized albuterol in the same total dose.[2] Thus, continuous nebulization is recommended for patients having an unsatisfactory response (achieving less than 50% of normal FEV_1 or PEF) following the initial three doses (every 20 minutes) of aerosolized β_2-agonists and potentially for patients presenting initially with PEF or FEV_1 values of less than 30% of predicted normal.[2]

The doses of inhaled β_2-agonists for acute severe asthma exacerbations (see Table 15-6) have been derived empirically. The β_2-agonists follow a log-linear dose–response curve.[30] In addition, the dose–response curve is shifted to the right by more severe bronchospasm or by increased concentrations of bronchospastic mediators, which is characteristic of functional antagonists.[30] The ability to increase the dose of the short-acting aerosolized β_2-agonists by as much as 5- to 10-fold over doses producing adequate bronchodilation in chronic stable asthma is what contributes to their efficacy in reversing the bronchospasm of acute severe exacerbations. The nebulizer dose of inhaled β_2-agonists for children often is listed on a weight basis (milligrams per kilogram). However, a fixed minimal dose (2.5 mg albuterol or equivalent), as opposed to a weight-adjusted dose, is more appropriate in younger children because children younger than 5 years of age receive a lower lung dose.[2] Adults dosed on a weight basis demonstrate excessive cardiac stimulation, so they have fixed maximal doses[2] (see Table 15-6). Initial doses of inhaled β_2-agonists can produce vasodilation, worsening ventilation–perfusion mismatch, slightly lowering O_2 saturation or Pao_2.[27] High doses of inhaled β_2-agonists can produce a decrease in serum potassium concentration, an increase in heart rate, and an increase in serum glucose and lactic acid concentration.[28] However, both children and adults receiving continuously nebulized β_2-agonists have demonstrated decreased heart rates as their lung function improves.[2] Thus, an elevated heart rate is not an indication to use lower doses or to avoid using inhaled β_2-agonists.

The inhaled β_2-agonists produce similar efficacy whether delivered by MDI plus VHC or nebulization in treating acute severe exacerbations in the ED and hospital; thus, the choice depends on the experience and comfort of the treating clinicians.[2] The DPIs are currently not indicated for the treatment of acute severe asthma exacerbations due to the higher inspiratory flows required for adequate drug delivery.[2]

Corticosteroids

Systemic corticosteroids are indicated in all patients with acute severe asthma exacerbations not responding completely to initial inhaled β_2-agonist administration (every 20 minutes for three to four doses).[2] IV therapy offers no therapeutic advantage over oral administration.[2,31] This therapy usually is continued until hospital discharge. Tapering the systemic corticosteroid dose following discharge from the hospital appears unnecessary, provided that patients are prescribed ICSs for outpatient therapy.[31] Most patients achieve 70% of predicted normal FEV_1 within 48 hours and 80% of predicted by 6 days after plateauing by day 3. Thus, maintaining systemic corticosteroid courses for 10 to 14 days may be unnecessarily long in some patients. Indeed, many patients not admitted to the hospital respond to 3- to 5-day courses of systemic corticosteroids. Short courses of oral prednisone (3- to 10-day "bursts") have been effective in preventing hospitalizations in infants and young children.[2] It is recommended that a full dose of the corticosteroid be continued until the patient's peak flow reaches 70% of predicted normal or personal best.[2]

Multiple daily dosing of systemic corticosteroids for the initial therapy of acute asthma exacerbations appears warranted because receptor binding affinities of lung corticosteroid receptors are decreased in the face of airway inflammation.[31] However, patients with less severe exacerbations may be treated adequately with once-daily administration. High-dose and very-high-pulse-dose corticosteroid regimens have not been shown to enhance the outcomes in severe acute asthma but are associated with a higher likelihood of side effects.[31]

Studies of ICSs in acute exacerbations of asthma have provided conflicting results. Studies have demonstrated both greater and lesser efficacy than standard doses of oral corticosteroids.[28,31] Currently, there is insufficient evidence supporting efficacy in the ED setting, although continued research appears warranted.[28] There is evidence that prescribing ICSs on discharge from the ED reduces the risk of relapse.[31] This policy is rational because inflammation is the underlying cause of deterioration in most cases.[2]

Anticholinergics

Inhaled ipratropium bromide produces a further improvement in lung function of 10% to 15% over inhaled β_2-agonists alone. In children and adults, multiple-dose ipratropium bromide added to initial therapy reduces hospitalization rate in the subset of patients with a baseline FEV_1 of less than 30% of predicted.[32] Ipratropium bromide, a quaternary amine, is poorly absorbed and produces minimal or no systemic effects.[28] Care should be taken when administering ipratropium bromide by nebulizer. If a tight mask or mouthpiece is not used, the ipratropium bromide that deposits in the eyes may produce pupillary dilation and difficulty in accommodation.[2] Ipratropium bromide is not a vasodilator, so unlike β_2-agonists it will not worsen ventilation–perfusion mismatch.[32]

Alternative Therapies

The ED use of aminophylline, a moderate bronchodilator, for acute asthma has not been recommended for a number of years.[2] Aminophylline in adults and children hospitalized with acute asthma does not enhance improvement in lung function or reduce length of hospitalization but has increased the risk of adverse effects.[2] Adverse effects of theophylline include nausea and vomiting and potentiation of the cardiac effects of the inhaled β_2-agonists.

Magnesium sulfate is a moderately potent bronchodilator, producing relaxation of smooth muscle and central nervous system depression. The use of IV magnesium sulfate in patients presenting to the ED is controversial (see below).[28] The adverse effects of magnesium sulfate include hypotension, facial flushing, sweating, nausea, loss of deep tendon reflexes, and respiratory depression.[28] Helium is an inert gas of low density with no pharmacologic properties that can lower resistance to gas flow and increase ventilation because the low density decreases the pressure gradient needed to achieve a given level of turbulent flow, converting turbulent flow to laminar flow.[28] Helium is given as a mixture of helium and O_2 (heliox), usually 60% to 70% helium with 30% to 40% O_2.[33] Heliox has been effective in some but not all clinical trials.[33] Although heliox is free of adverse effects, its use is limited to patients with a low inspired O_2 requirement because the decrease in density generally is insignificant clinically with less than 60% helium.[28]

The inhalational anesthetics halothane, isoflurane, and enflurane all have been reported to have a positive effect in children and adults with acute severe asthma that is unresponsive to standard medical therapy.[2] The proposed mechanisms for inhalational anesthetics include direct action on bronchial smooth muscle, inhibition of airway reflexes, attenuation of histamine-induced bronchospasm, and interaction with β_2-adrenergic receptors.[2] Well-controlled trials with these agents have not been completed.[27] Potential adverse effects include myocardial depression, vasodilation, arrhythmias, and depression of mucociliary function.[27] In addition, the practical problem of delivery and scavenging these agents in the intensive care environment as opposed to the operating room is a concern. The use of volatile anesthetics cannot be recommended based on insufficient evidence of efficacy.

Ketamine has been recommended for rapid induction of anesthesia in patients with asthma who require intubation and mechanical ventilation.[2] Although anecdotal reports have suggested that ketamine is useful as a short-term adjunct in acute severe asthma, controlled trials have not provided evidence of efficacy. Ketamine has several significant adverse effects, including the anesthesia emergence reaction, which can alter mood and cause delirium. These emergence phenomena occur in at least 25% of patients over 16 years of age; the incidence seems to be much lower in younger patients.[2] Other risks include an increase in heart rate, arterial blood pressure, and cerebral blood flow because of its sympathetic effects.[27]

Special Populations

6 Infants and children younger than 4 years of age may be at greater risk of respiratory failure than older children and adults. Although treated with the same drugs, these younger children require the use of a face mask as opposed to a mouthpiece for delivery of aerosolized medication. Use of the face mask reduces delivery of drug to the lung by one half so that a minimal dose is recommended as opposed to a weight-adjusted dose.[26] The face mask should be sized appropriately and should fit snugly over the nose and mouth. Use of the "blow-by" method, where the respiratory therapist or parent places the mask or extension tubing near the child's nose and mouth, should be discouraged because holding the mask as few as 2 cm from the patient's face reduces lung delivery of the aerosol by 80%.[2,26]

Drug Class Information

Short-Acting β_2-Agonists

5 **6** The β_2-agonists are the most effective bronchodilators available. The β_2-adrenergic receptors are transmembrane proteins consisting of clusters of seven helices of amino acids that form the ligand-binding core.[30] The human β_2-adrenergic receptors are polymorphic in structure, with the most common polymorphisms in the amino terminus of the receptor at amino acid positions 16 (encoding either arginine [Arg] or glycine [Gly]) and 27 (encoding either glutamine [Gln] or glutamic acid [Glu]).[34] Some of the polymorphisms determine responsiveness to β_2-agonists, whereas others may act as disease modifiers (see below).[35] Stimulation of β_2-adrenergic receptor activates cytoplasmic G proteins, which in turn activate adenylyl cyclase to produce cyclic adenosine monophosphate (cAMP), generally thought to be responsible for the bulk of activity through activation of various proteins by cAMP-dependent protein kinase A (PKA).[30] This activation, in turn, decreases unbound intracellular calcium, producing smooth muscle relaxation, mast cell membrane stabilization, and skeletal muscle stimulation.[30] Despite the fact that β_2-agonists are potent inhibitors of mast cell degranulation in vitro, they do not inhibit the late asthmatic response to allergen challenge or the subsequent BHR.[2,30] Long-term administration of β_2-agonists does not reduce BHR, confirming a lack of significant antiinflammatory activity.[34] β_2-Adrenergic stimulation also activates Na^+-K^+-ATPase, produces gluconeogenesis, and enhances insulin secretion, resulting in a mild to moderate decrease in serum potassium concentration by driving potassium intracellularly.[30] The chronotropic response to β_2-agonists is mediated in part by baroreceptor reflex mechanisms as a result of the drop in blood pressure from vascular smooth muscle relaxation, as well as by direct stimulation of cardiac β_2-receptors and some β_1 stimulation at high concentrations.[30] Table 15-7 lists the pharmacologic effects of adrenergic receptor stimulation. Because β_1-receptor stimulation produces excessive cardiac stimulation, resulting in cardiac arrhythmias, and because the inotropic effect enhancing myocardial O_2 consumption leads to myocardial necrosis, there is no rationale for using non–β_2-selective agonists in the treatment of asthma.[2]

TABLE 15-7 Pharmacologic Responses to Sympathomimetic Agonists

Tissue	Receptor Type	Response
Airways	β_2	Smooth muscle relaxation (bronchodilation), increased ciliary beat, increased serous secretion, and inhibition of mast cell degranulation
	α	Smooth muscle contraction (bronchoconstriction?)
Heart	β_1	Inotropic and chronotropic
	β_2	Chronotropic
Vasculature	β_2	Vasodilation, decreased microvascular leakage
	α	Vasoconstriction
Skeletal	β_2	Increased neuromuscular transmission (tremor and increased strength of contraction)
Uterus	β_2	Relaxation (tocolysis)
Metabolic	α, β_1	Glycogenolysis, lipolysis
	β_2	Gluconeogenesis, hypokalemia, increased lactate production

Table 15-8 compares the various β-adrenergic agonists used in asthma in terms of selectivity, potency, oral activity, and duration of action. The β_2-agonists are functional or physiologic antagonists in that they relax airway smooth muscle regardless of the mechanism for constriction.[30] When administered in equipotent doses, all the short-acting drugs produce the same intensity of response; the only differences are in duration of action and cardiac toxicity.[2,30] The catecholamine derivatives all have the disadvantage of rapid inactivation of their 3,4-hydroxyl catechol group from catechol-*O*-methyltransferase located in the GI tract, rendering them orally inactive. In addition, catecholamines are taken up rapidly into tissues by secondary uptake mechanisms that limit their receptor occupancy and thus have a shorter duration of action.[30] All the β_2-agonists are more bronchoselective when administered by the aerosol route. Aerosol administration of the short-acting β_2-agonists provides more rapid response and greater protection against provocations that induce bronchospasm such as exercise and allergen challenges than does systemic administration.[2,30] Differences in myocardial effects are discernible between selective and nonselective agents even when administered as aerosols, particularly at the higher doses used for acute severe asthma. The β_2-agonists also differ in efficacy or ability to activate the β_2-adrenergic receptors. Full agonists include the catecholamines while the synthetic β_2-agonists all exhibit various levels of partial agonism in the following order of fuller agonism: formoterol > albuterol = terbutaline = pirbuterol > salmeterol.[30] Although partial agonists by definition cannot produce maximum dilation or protection as full agonists and can potentially block the effect of a full agonist, these differences have not been proven to be clinically significant.

All synthetic β_2-agonists are 1:1 racemic mixtures of two mirror images (enantiomers) owing to an asymmetric or chiral carbon.[30] Since most physiologic functions (receptor occupancy and activation and enzymatic metabolism) are stereoselective, the (*R*)-enantiomers of the β_2-agonists are the most pharmacologically active isomer.[30] While it was felt initially that the (*S*)-enantiomers were essentially inactive owing to the 100- to 1,000-fold potency difference between the enantiomers, studies in animal models and isolated in vitro tissue preparations have suggested that the (*S*)-enantiomer of albuterol may be proinflammatory and could induce BHR.[30] However, evidence that this occurs consistently in humans or is clinically relevant is lacking.[30] The pharmacokinetics are stereoselective as well, although not predictable. (*R*)-Albuterol is metabolized more rapidly than (*S*)-albuterol, which could lead to accumulation of (*S*)-albuterol with continued dosing.[30] On the other hand, (*S*)-terbutaline is eliminated more rapidly than (*R*)-terbutaline.[34]

Both the intensity and duration of response are dose dependent, and, more important, the dose–response relationship is dynamic.[30,34] At increasing levels of baseline bronchoconstriction (irrespective of the stimulus), the dose–response curve is shifted to the right, and the duration of bronchodilation is decreased.[30] This shift is reflected in the need for higher, more frequent doses in acute asthma exacerbations; the duration of protection against significant provocation is much less than the duration of bronchodilation in chronic stable asthma (see Table 15-8).[30,34]

Chronic administration of β_2-agonists leads to downregulation (decreased number of β_2-receptors) and a decreased binding affinity (desensitization) for these receptors.[30] Systemic corticosteroid therapy can both prevent and partially reverse this phenomenon.[2,30] However, the use of ICSs appears to have minimal ability to prevent tolerance to β_2-agonists.[30] Although in vitro differences in downregulation of the β_2-receptors exist (Gly-16 homozygotes >Arg-16 homozygotes), clinical desensitization is seen in all polymorphisms.[34] Tolerance primarily reduces duration of bronchodilation as opposed to peak response, although the latter can occur as well. A significantly greater tolerance develops in other tissues (e.g., lymphocytes and cardiac and skeletal muscle) compared with the lung, primarily as a result of the surplus β_2-receptors found in respiratory smooth muscle.[30] Tolerance to the extrapulmonary effects (cardiac stimulation and hypokalemia) may account for a lack of significant cardiac effects with retention of the bronchodilator response despite chronic inhaled β_2-agonist therapy, whereas tolerance to mast cell stabilization may be a drawback to chronic use.[30] Thus, chronic β_2-agonist administration produces a tolerance of minimal clinical significance that is overcome easily by increasing the dose or by administering corticosteroids.[2,30,34] Most of the tolerance occurs within a week of regular administration and does not worsen with continued administration. As would be expected from a receptor phenomenon, tolerance

TABLE 15-8 Relative Selectivity, Potency, and Duration of Action of the β-Adrenergic Agonists

Agent	Selectivity β_1	Selectivity β_2	Potency, β_2[b]	Duration of Action[a]: Bronchodilation (hours)	Duration of Action[a]: Protection (hours)[c]	Oral Activity
Isoproterenol	++++	++++	1	0.5–2	0.5–1	No
Albuterol	+	++++	2	4–8	2–4	Yes
Pirbuterol	+	++++	5	4–8	2–4	Yes
Terbutaline	+	++++	4	4–8	2–4	Yes
Formoterol	+	++++	0.12	≥12	6–12	Yes
Salmeterol	+	++++	0.5	≥12	6–12	No

[a]Median durations with the highest value after a single dose and lowest after chronic administration.
[b]Relative molar potency to isoproterenol: 15 = lowest potency.
[c]Protection refers to the prevention of bronchoconstriction induced by exercise or nonspecific bronchial challenges.

TABLE 15-9 Pharmacodynamic/Pharmacokinetic Comparison of the Corticosteroids

Systemic	Antiinflammatory Potency	Mineralocorticoid Potency	Duration of Biologic Activity (hours)	Elimination Half-Life (hours)
Hydrocortisone	1	1	8–12	1.5–2
Prednisone	4	0.8	12–36	2.5–3.5
Methylprednisolone	5	0.5	12–36	3.3
Dexamethasone	25	0	36–54	3.4–4
ICS	**Receptor Binding Affinity**	**Oral Bioavailability (%)**	**Systemic Clearance (L/h)**	**Half-Life (hours) (IV/Inhaled)**
BDP/BMP[a]	0.4/13.5	20/40	150/120	(0.5/2.7)/(UK/2.7)
BUD	9.4	11	84	2.8/2
CIC/des-CIC[a]	0.12/12	<1/<1	152/228	(0.36/3.4)/(0.5/4.8)
FLU	1.8	20	58	1.6/1.6
FP	18	≤1	66	7.8/14.4
MF	23[b]	<1	53	5.8/UK

Note: Receptor binding affinities are relative to dexamethasone equal to 1. BDP, beclomethasone dipropionate; BMP, beclomethasone 17-monopropionate; BUD, budesonide; CIC, ciclesonide; des-CIC, des-ciclesonide; FLU, flunisolide; FP, fluticasone propionate; MF, mometasone furoate; UK, unknown.

[a]BDP and CIC are prodrugs that are activated in the lung to their active metabolites BMP and des-CIC, respectively.
[b]MF studied in a different receptor system. Value estimated from relative values of BDP and FP in that system.

is a cross-tolerance to all β_2-agonists.[30] Regular use of short-acting inhaled β_2-agonists may produce slight worsening of asthma in a subset of patients, but it does not appear to occur in the entire population.[34] Regular treatment with short-acting β_2-agonists can increase BHR and in homozygous Arg-16 patients reduces morning PEF and increases exacerbations.[35] Regular treatment (four times daily) does not improve symptom control over as-needed use and is not indicated.[2] Regular treatment with the long-acting inhaled β_2-agonists (LABAs) is discussed in Chronic Asthma below.

In conclusion, the short-acting inhaled selective β_2-agonists are indicated for the as-needed treatment of intermittent episodes of bronchospasm. They are the first treatment of choice for acute severe asthma and EIB.[2,13] They inhibit EIB in a dose-dependent fashion and provide complete protection for a 2-hour period following inhalation with varying levels of patient-dependent protection over 4 hours.[13] Although the regular administration of β_2-agonists slightly decreases the protective effect, two inhalations prior to exercise still essentially block EIB completely (1% vs. 5% drop in FEV_1).[30]

Systemic Corticosteroids

4 The corticosteroids are the most effective antiinflammatories available to treat asthma.[2] Actions useful in treating asthma include (a) increasing the number of β_2-adrenergic receptors and improving the receptor responsiveness to β_2-adrenergic stimulation, (b) reducing mucus production and hypersecretion, (c) reducing BHR, and (d) reducing airway edema and exudation.[2,36] The glucocorticoid receptor is found in the cytoplasm of most body cells, explaining the multiple effects of systemic corticosteroids. There is no difference between glucocorticoid receptors found throughout the body; however, genetic differences between glucocorticoid receptors from different individuals may determine some of the variations in response.[35] The corticosteroids are lipophilic, readily cross the cell membrane, and combine with the glucocorticoid receptor. The activated complex then enters the nucleus, where it acts as a transcription factor leading to gene activation or suppression.[36] This leads to specific mRNA production, resulting in increased production of antiinflammatory mediators; suppression of several proinflammatory cytokines such as IL-1, GM-CSF, IL-4, IL-5, IL-6, and IL-8, reducing inflammatory cell activation, recruitment, and infiltration; and decreasing vascular permeability.[36] In addition, the activated glucocorticoid receptor complex can act directly with cytoplasmic transcription factors, nuclear factor-κB, and activating protein 1 to prevent the action of proinflammatory cytokines on the cell.[36]

Owing to the mechanism that modifies gene expression, the time required to see a particular effect depends on the time required for new protein synthesis, decreased formation of the particular mediator, and resolution of the inflammatory response.[36] Generally, the cellular and biochemical effects are immediate, but varying amounts of time are required to produce a clinical response. β_2-Receptor density increases within 4 hours of corticosteroid administration.[36] Improved responsiveness to β_2-agonists occurs within 2 hours.[36] In acute severe asthma, 4 to 12 hours may be required before any clinical response is noted.[31,36] Reversal of seasonally increased BHR requires at least 1 week of therapy.[36] The chronic use of corticosteroids does not induce a state of corticosteroid dependence, there is no evidence of tolerance produced by chronic administration.

The corticosteroids used in asthma are compared in Table 15-9.[36,37] Besides acute severe asthma, systemic corticosteroids are also recommended for the treatment of impending episodes of severe asthma unresponsive to bronchodilator therapy.[2,28] The effects of corticosteroids in asthma are dose and duration dependent. This pattern is true for the adverse effects as well (Table 15-10). The clinician must continually balance the toxicity of chronic systemic corticosteroid therapy with control of asthma symptoms. Because short-term (1 to 2 weeks) high-dose corticosteroids (1 to 2 mg/kg/day of prednisone) do not produce serious toxicities, the ideal use is to administer the systemic corticosteroids in a short "burst" and then to maintain the patient on appropriate long-term control therapy with ICSs (discussed below).[2,28] In general, therapy for more than 5 days at doses that exceed the usual physiologic endogenous cortisol production will cause temporary aberration in adrenal cortisol release.[36] However, this hypothalamic–pituitary–adrenal (HPA) axis suppression is short-lived (1 to 3 days)

TABLE 15-10 Adverse Effects of Chronic Systemic Glucocorticoid Administration

Hypothalamic–pituitary–adrenal suppression	Hypertension
Growth retardation	Skin striae
Skeletal muscle myopathy	Impaired wound healing
Osteoporosis/fractures	Inhibition of leukocyte and monocyte function
Aseptic necrosis of bone	Subcutaneous tissue atrophy
Pancreatitis	Glaucoma
Pseudotumor cerebri	Posterior subcapsular cataracts
Psychiatric disturbances	Moon facies
Sodium and water retention	Central redistribution of fat
Hypokalemia/hyperglycemia	

and readily reversible following short bursts (≤10 days) of pharmacologic doses.[36] A maximum number of short bursts that a patient can receive probably exists, after which chronic corticosteroid side effects occur. Adult patients receiving at least eight bursts (≥10 days each) have a similar decrease in trabecular bone density as patients on daily or alternate-day corticosteroids over 1 year.[36] Children who received four or more bursts per year of prednisone exhibited a subnormal response to hypoglycemic stress or adrenocorticotropic hormone (ACTH) administration.[36] Just two or more bursts per year increase the risk for osteopenia in children with concomitant vitamin D insufficiency.[38] Very short courses (3 to 5 days) have been effective in reducing hospitalization from acute exacerbations.[2] Use of the shorter-acting corticosteroids such as prednisone will produce less adrenal suppression than the longer-acting dexamethasone.[36]

Anticholinergics

The anticholinergic agents have a long history of use for asthma, but they do not have an FDA-labeled indication for asthma.[2] Anticholinergics are competitive inhibitors of muscarinic receptors.[39] Unlike β_2-agonists, they are not functional antagonists; they only reverse cholinergic-mediated bronchoconstriction. Normal bronchial tone is maintained through parasympathetic innervation of the airways via the vagus nerve.[39] A number of the triggers and mediators of asthma (i.e., histamine, prostaglandins, sulfur dioxide, exercise, and allergens) produce bronchoconstriction in part through vagal reflex mechanisms.[39] Studies consistently demonstrate that anticholinergics are effective bronchodilators in asthma, although not as effective as β_2-agonists. Anticholinergics attenuate but do not block allergen-induced asthma in a dose-dependent fashion and have no effect on BHR.[39] Anticholinergics attenuate but do not block EIB.[13]

Ipratropium bromide is a nonselective muscarinic receptor blocker, and blockade of inhibitory muscarinic receptors theoretically could result in an increased release of acetylcholine and overcome the block on the smooth muscle receptors (M_3).[39] Only the quaternary ammonium derivatives such as ipratropium bromide should be used because they have the advantage of poor absorption across mucosae and the blood–brain barrier. This attribute contributes to negligible systemic effects with a prolonged local effect (i.e., bronchodilation). In addition, the quaternary compounds do not appear to produce a decrease in mucociliary clearance.[39] Ipratropium bromide has a duration of action of 4 to 8 hours. Both intensity and duration of action are dose dependent. Tiotropium bromide, a long-acting inhaled anticholinergic with duration of 24 hours, is more selective for M_1 and M_3 receptors and less likely to affect the inhibitory M_2 receptors.[39] Time to reach maximum bronchodilation for ipratropium is considerably slower than for aerosolized short-acting β_2-agonists (30 to 60 minutes vs. 5 to 10 minutes). However, this difference is of little clinical consequence because some bronchodilation is seen within 30 seconds; 50% of maximum response occurs within 3 minutes.[39] Ipratropium bromide is only indicated as adjunctive therapy in acute severe asthma not completely responsive to β_2-agonists alone because it does not improve outcomes in chronic asthma.[2,31] Recent trials of tiotropium bromide in chronic asthma suggest that it may be as effective as LABAs added to ICSs and add additional control in severe asthma when added to ICS/LABA combinations.[40,41]

PHARMACOECONOMICS

ED visits for asthma exceed the number of hospitalizations by approximately four times, yet the annual expenditures for ED visits remain significantly less than that spent on in-patient hospital services for patients with acute severe asthma.[42] Thus, reducing the number of patients requiring hospitalizations is a primary goal of therapy. Since the primary drugs used to treat acute severe asthma are available generically, drug costs account for only a small portion of the overall costs of care. Few of these therapies have been evaluated formally for their pharmacoeconomic impact. One evaluation based on a meta-analysis of inhaled anticholinergics added to short-acting inhaled β_2-agonists in children with acute severe asthma suggested that this approach was cost-effective and would reduce overall costs by reducing hospitalizations.[32] In children with acute severe asthma admitted to an intensive care unit, the use of continuously nebulized albuterol resulted in a decreased cost of care compared with intermittent nebulization.[2]

Clinical **Controversy...**

Some clinicians believe that IV magnesium sulfate is effective for the treatment of acute severe asthma exacerbations unresponsive to standard doses of inhaled β_2-agonists in the ED. This belief is based on subset analyses of two studies showing that patients with the most severe obstruction following initial inhaled β_2-agonists demonstrated a reduction in hospitalizations with magnesium treatment compared with placebo.[2] However, the subset with severe obstruction is the one demonstrating an improved response to the addition of ipratropium bromide and continuous nebulization of inhaled β_2-agonists. In addition, a large, randomized trial failed to confirm a decrease in hospitalization even in the severe group.[28] The 2007 NAEPP guidelines state that magnesium can be considered for use in patients with severe episodes with a poor response to initial inhaled β_2-agonists.[2]

EVALUATION OF THERAPEUTIC OUTCOMES

Figures 15-6 and 15-7 provide the monitoring parameters for acute severe asthma. Lung function, either spirometric or peak flow measurements, should be monitored 5 to 10 minutes after each treatment.[2,28] O_2 saturations can be easily monitored continuously with pulse oximetry. For young children and infants, pulse oximetry, lung auscultation, and observation of the presence of supraclavicular retractions are useful.[2,27] The majority of patients will respond within the first hour of initial inhaled β_2-agonists regardless of history of pre-ED administration of drug.[27] Patients not achieving an initial response should be monitored every 0.5 to 1 hour. Depending on whether there is a standard ED or a special unit for acute severe asthma, the decision to admit to the hospital should be made within 4 to 6 hours of entry to the ED.[28] The mean duration of hospitalization following admission is 2 to 3 days. Frequency of monitoring depends on the severity of the exacerbation. With mild exacerbations, monitor lung function every 2 to 3 hours and with severe exacerbations every 0.5 to 1 hour.

TREATMENT

Chronic Asthma

The diagnosis of chronic asthma is made primarily by history and confirmatory spirometry (see Clinical Presentation above).[2] The NAEPP has provided a list of questions that would lead to the diagnosis of asthma[2] (see Table 15-2). In the older child and adult patient in whom spirometric evaluations can be performed, failure of pulmonary functions to improve acutely does not necessarily rule out asthma. Patients with long-standing disease or substantial inflammation may require an intensive, prolonged course of bronchodilators and glucocorticoids before reversibility is detected.[2] If baseline spirometry is normal, challenge testing with exercise, histamine, methacholine, or mannitol can be used to elicit BHR.[2] Patients with significant symptoms and/or an FEV_1 of less than 70% of predicted normal should not be challenged. Vocal cord dysfunction, particularly with exercise, may mimic asthma symptoms.[2] Studies for atopy such as serum IgE and sputum and blood eosinophil determinations are not necessary to make the diagnosis of asthma, but they may help differentiate asthma from chronic bronchitis in adults. Clinically, this distinction is often difficult to make. Some patients with chronic bronchitis may have a reversible component, and some patients with long-standing severe chronic asthma may have significant irreversible damage and obstruction. Very high peripheral blood eosinophil counts may point to the diagnosis of allergic bronchopulmonary aspergillosis (ABPA) or other hypereosinophilic syndromes.[2] Skin testing is of no value in diagnosing asthma but is useful in identifying triggers.[2] In small infants unable to perform spirometry, the diagnosis is more difficult. Hyperinflation may be demonstrated on the chest roentgenogram.[2] Radiologic examination is helpful in ruling out other causes of wheezing (e.g., foreign-body aspiration, parenchymal lung disease, cardiac disease, and congenital anomalies).[2] In place of pulmonary function measures, the parents should be given a diary card to record symptoms and precipitating events.

Desired Outcomes for the Long-Term Management of Asthma

The NAEPP has provided key points for managing asthma long term.[2] The desired outcomes for therapy to control asthma are outlined below:

Reducing impairment:

1. Prevent chronic and troublesome symptoms (e.g., coughing or breathlessness in the daytime, in the night, or after exertion).
2. Require infrequent use (≤2 days a week) of short-acting inhaled β_2-agonist for quick relief of symptoms[2] (not including prevention of EIB).
3. Maintain (near) normal pulmonary function.
4. Maintain normal activity levels (including exercise and other physical activity and attendance at work or school).
5. Meet patients' and families' expectations of and satisfaction with asthma care.

Reducing risk:

1. Prevent recurrent exacerbations of asthma and minimize the need for ED visits or hospitalizations.
2. Prevent loss of lung function; for children, prevent reduced lung growth.
3. Minimal or no adverse effects of therapy.

Nonpharmacologic Therapy

Although the mainstay of the management of asthma is pharmacologic therapy, it is likely to fail without concurrent attention to relevant environmental control and management of comorbid conditions. Figure 15-8 depicts the stepwise approach for managing asthma recommended in the 2007 update by the NAEPP.[2] Nonpharmacologic aspects of therapy are incorporated into the steps. The guidelines were designed to give primary healthcare providers a framework with which to develop the proper approach to the individualized therapy of patients. The heterogeneity of asthma demands an individualized approach to therapy with the basic goals of therapy as primary outcome measures.[2] The focus of therapy is the prevention and suppression of the underlying inflammation.[2] Thus, current therapeutic options in asthma consist of acute reliever medications used for acute symptoms and exacerbations and long-term control medications used for the prevention of symptoms and exacerbations and the suppression of inflammation and reduction of BHR.[2]

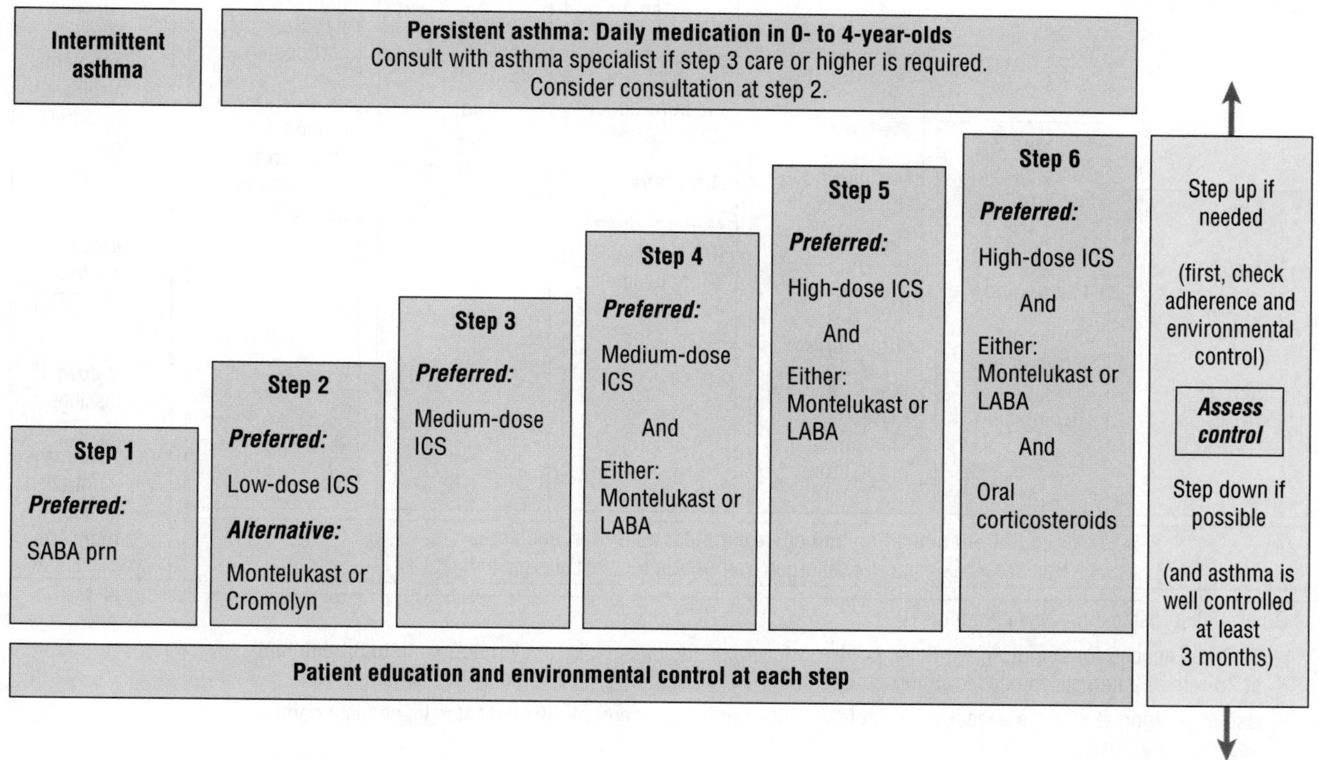

FIGURE 15-8 Stepwise approach for managing asthma in adults and children 0 to 4 and 5 to 11 years old. *(From reference 2.)*

Intermittent asthma	Persistent asthma: Daily medication in 5- to 11-year-olds Consult with asthma specialist if step 4 care or higher is required. Consider consultation at step 3.					
Step 1 ***Preferred:*** SABA prn	**Step 2** ***Preferred:*** Low-dose ICS ***Alternative:*** LTRA Cromolyn, Nedocromil, or Theophylline	**Step 3** ***Preferred:*** Medium-dose ICS Or Low-dose ICS + LABA, LTRA, or Theophylline	**Step 4** ***Preferred:*** Medium-dose ICS + LABA ***Alternative:*** Medium-dose ICS + either LTRA or Theophylline	**Step 5** ***Preferred:*** High-dose ICS + LABA ***Alternative:*** High-dose ICS + either LTRA or Theophylline	**Step 6** ***Preferred:*** High-dose ICS + LABA + oral corticosteroid ***Alternative:*** High-dose ICS + either LTRA or Theophylline + oral corticosteroid	Step up if needed (first, check adherence and environmental control and comorbid conditions) ***Assess control*** Step down if possible (and asthma is well controlled at least 3 months)
Patient education and environmental control at each step Steps 2–4: Consider SQ allergen immunotherapy for allergic patients						

Intermittent asthma	Persistent asthma: Daily medication in ≥12-year-olds and adults Consult with asthma specialist if step 4 care or higher is required. Consider consultation at step 3.					
Step 1 ***Preferred:*** SABA prn	**Step 2** ***Preferred:*** Low-dose ICS ***Alternative:*** Cromolyn, Nedocromil, LTRA, or Theophylline	**Step 3** ***Preferred:*** Medium-dose ICS Or Low-dose ICS + LABA ***Alternative:*** Low-dose ICS + LTRA, Theophylline, or Zileuton	**Step 4** ***Preferred:*** Medium-dose ICS + LABA ***Alternative:*** Medium-dose ICS + LTRA, Theophylline or Zileuton	**Step 5** ***Preferred:*** High-dose ICS + LABA And Consider Omalizumab for patients who have allergies	**Step 6** ***Preferred:*** High-dose ICS + LABA + oral corticosteroid And Consider Omalizumab for patients who have allergies	Step up if needed (first, check adherence and environmental control, and comorbid conditions) ***Assess control*** Step down if possible (and asthma is well controlled at least 3 months)
Patient education and environmental control at each step Steps 2–4: Consider SQ allergen immunotherapy for allergic patients						

Quick-Relief Medication for All Patients

- SABA as needed for symptoms. Intensity of treatment depends on severity of symptoms: up to 3 treatments at 20-minute intervals as needed. Short course of systemic oral corticosteroids may be needed.
- Use of β_2-agonist >2 days a week for symptom control (not prevention of EIB) indicates inadequate control and the need to step up treatment.

FIGURE 15-8 *(Continued)*

TABLE 15-11 Key Educational Messages for Patients

Basic facts about asthma
- The contrast between asthmatic and normal airways
- What happens to the airways in an asthma attack

Roles of medications
- How medications work
- Long-term control: medications that prevent symptoms, often by reducing inflammation
- Quick relief: short-acting bronchodilator relaxes muscles around airways
- Stress importance of long-term control medications and not to expect quick relief from them

Skills
- Inhaler use (patient demonstrate)
- Spacer and holding chamber use
- Use of the nebulizer
- Symptom monitoring, peak flow monitoring, and recognizing early signs of deterioration
- How to assess asthma control after therapy has begun

Environmental control measures
- Identifying and avoiding environmental precipitants or exposures, including tobacco smoke

When and how to adjust treatment
- Using written action plan
- Responding to changes in asthma control

7 The development of a partnership in care through patient education and the teaching of patient self-management skills should be the cornerstone of any treatment program.[2] There are a number of published self-management programs for children and adults available through local American Lung Association chapters, as well as asthma treatment centers, and nationally through the NAEPP and the Asthma and Allergy Foundation of America.[2] Asthma self-management programs have been shown to improve patient adherence to medication regimens, improve self-management skills, and improve use of healthcare services.[2,43,44] Table 15-11 lists the key educational messages recommended by the NAEPP.[2]

Self-management programs instruct patients in the pathogenesis of asthma and the appropriate use of their medications but focus principally on teaching patients to recognize triggers for their asthma and how to recognize early signs of deterioration.[43] Home PEF monitoring is part of some programs.[2] However, routine PEF monitoring in and of itself does not improve patient outcomes.[2]

The NAEPP advocates the use of PEF monitoring only for patients with severe persistent asthma who have difficulty perceiving airway obstruction.[2] It also has recommended a system based on a traffic light scenario (based on percentage of normal predicted values or personal best values): the green zone is equal to 80% to 100%, the yellow zone is equal to 50% to 79%, and the red zone is less than 50%. The yellow zone is cautionary and requires increasing as-needed bronchodilator use and possibly beginning prednisone if not improved, whereas the red zone warrants contacting the patient's healthcare provider.[2]

Patient education is essential before monitoring can be effective. It has proved successful regardless of the health professional who provided the information (physician, nurse, or pharmacist). The NAEPP advocates significant involvement of all points of patient care in the educational process.[2] The provision of written action plans enhances the success of education and is considered an essential component of care.[2] Samples of clinically tested written action plans are available from NAEPP guidelines and other sources.[2]

In patients with known allergic triggers for their asthma, allergen avoidance has resulted in an improvement in symptoms, a reduction in medication use, and a decrease in BHR.[2] A comprehensive approach to environmental control is advocated. For example, for patients with house dust mite allergy removing carpeting from bedrooms, washing sheets in hot water (>54.4°C [>130°F]) and using special dust-proof pillow and mattress covers can reduce symptoms and need for medications.[2] Obvious environmental triggers (e.g., animal dander, cockroaches), if the patient is sensitive, should be avoided. Evidence for home air-filtering systems and chemicals for killing house dust mites is limited.[2] Immunotherapy (allergy shots) with single antigens particularly has been beneficial and may be considered in patients with persistent asthma with documented sensitivity.[2] Immunotherapy with multiple antigens has been less effective.

Patients who smoke should be encouraged to stop. Parents of children with asthma should stop or at least not smoke around their children.[2]

Pharmacologic Therapy

The current NAEPP recommendations for therapy of persistent asthma are illustrated in Figure 15-8.[2] Therapy should be adjusted based on control status of the patient (refer to later section). Regardless of the long-term therapy, all patients need to have quick-relief medication in the form of short-acting inhaled β_2-agonists available for acute symptoms. The ICSs are considered the preferred long-term control therapy for persistent asthma in all patients due to their potency and consistent effectiveness.[2] Low- to medium-dose ICSs reduce BHR, improve lung function, and reduce severe exacerbations leading to ED visits and hospitalizations. They are more effective than cromolyn, theophylline, or the LT receptor antagonists.[2] In addition, the ICSs are the only therapy that reduces the risk of dying from asthma.[2] In the low to medium doses recommended by NAEPP guidelines (Table 15-12), ICSs are safe for long-term administration (see below).[2,45] They do not appear to reduce airway remodeling and loss of lung function found in some patients with persistent asthma. The ICSs do not enhance lung growth in children with asthma, prevent the development of asthma in high-risk infants, or induce remission of asthma as BHR and other measures of inflammation return to pretreatment levels on discontinuation of therapy.[46,47] The sensitivity and consequent clinical response to ICSs can vary among patients.[2]

Although studies of the alternative long-term control therapies (e.g., cromolyn, LT receptor antagonists, and theophylline) demonstrate improvement in symptoms, lung function, and as-needed, short-acting inhaled β_2-agonist use, they do not reduce BHR, suggesting minimal antiinflammatory activity.[2] The evidence suggests minimal to no differences in efficacy between these alternatives. Therefore, NAEPP lists them in alphabetical order to show no preference of one over the other.[2]

For those patients inadequately controlled on low-dose ICSs either an increased dose of the ICS or the combination of ICS and LABA is the next step to gain control of more moderate persistent asthma.[2] Alternatives could be the addition of LT modifiers or theophylline to ICSs.[2] The addition of theophylline or LT modifiers to ICSs is no more effective than doubling the dose of the ICS.[2] The combination of ICS/LABA is more effective at reducing severe asthma exacerbations than doubling the dose of ICS in moderate persistent asthma; increasing the dose of ICSs fourfold also will result in a significant reduction in exacerbations.[48,49] However, doses of ICSs in the high range significantly enhance the risk of toxicity.[37,45,46] Thus, high doses of ICSs plus LABA are reserved for patients with severe persistent asthma.[2]

Although the addition of a third controller medication is often used clinically in patients with severe persistent asthma uncontrolled on high-dose ICS/LABA, there are few studies evaluating this practice.[2] LT receptor antagonists or theophylline added to high-dose combination ICS/LABA do not improve outcomes.[2] Omalizumab, a recombinant anti-IgE, has demonstrated significant activity in these

TABLE 15-12 Available Inhaled Corticosteroid Products, Lung Delivery, and Comparative Daily Dosages

ICS	Product		Lung Delivery[a]
Beclomethasone dipropionate (BDP)	40 and 80 mcg/actuation HFA MDI, 120 actuations		55–60%
Budesonide (BUD)	90 or 180 mcg/dose DPI, Flexhaler, 200 doses 200 and 500 mcg ampules, 2 mL each		32% (15–30%) 5–8%
Ciclesonide (CIC)	80 or 160 mcg/actuation HFA MDI		50%
Flunisolide (FLU)	80 mcg/actuation HFA MDI, 120 actuations		68%
Fluticasone propionate (FP)	44, 110, and 220 mcg/actuation HFA MDI, 120 actuations 50, 100, and 250 mcg/dose DPI, Diskus, 60 doses		20% 15%
Mometasone furoate (MF)	110 and 220 mcg/dose DPI, Twisthaler, 14, 30, 60, and 120 doses		11%
	Comparative Daily Dosages (mcg) of Inhaled Corticosteroids		
	Low Daily Dose Child[a]/Adult	**Medium Daily Dose Child[a]/Adult**	**High Daily Dose Child[a]/Adult**
BDP HFA MDI	80–160/80–240	>160–320/>240–480	>320/>480
BUD DPI Nebules	180–360/180–540 500/UK	>360–720/>540–1,080 1,000/UK	>720/>1,080 2,000/UK
CIC HFA MDI	80–160/160–320	>160–320/>320–640	>320/>640
FLU HFA MDI	160/320	320/320–640	≥640/>640
FP HFA MDI DPIs	88–176/88–264 100–200/100–300	176–352/264–440 200–400/300–500	>352/>440 >400/>500
MF, DPI	110/220	220–440/440	>440/>440

[a]5–11 years of age, except for BUD Nebules, which is 2–11 years of age.

severe uncontrolled atopic patients.[2,50] More recently tiotropium bromide has shown promise as add-on to ICS/LABA combination but is not yet approved by the FDA for use in asthma.[41,51]

Special Populations

6 Children younger than 5 years of age have not been studied adequately. Thus, many of the recommendations in this age group are extrapolated from older children and adults.[2] The studies of ICSs in this younger group demonstrate improvement in symptoms, as-needed bronchodilator use, and exacerbations. The nebulized suspension of budesonide gained FDA approval from three pivotal efficacy and safety trials.[2] Recently, high-dose nebulized budesonide administered intermittently (1 mg twice a day for 7 days) at early signs of upper respiratory tract infections was as effective at preventing severe episodes of wheezing in infants 12 to 53 months of age with recurrent wheezing as low-dose (0.5 mg daily) continuous therapy.[52] The FDA approval for montelukast in children younger than age 6 was based on safety and pharmacokinetic studies establishing doses but not on efficacy, although improvement in symptoms and as-needed bronchodilators was noted.[2] Cromolyn nebulizer solution was approved down to age 2 years based on efficacy.[2] Theophylline has not been evaluated adequately, except for pharmacokinetics.[2] Combination therapy of any kind has not been studied sufficiently.[2]

The FDA approval of the fluticasone/salmeterol DPI 100/50 in patients 4 to 11 years of age was largely based on extrapolation of efficacy data from patients older than 12 years of age and by a single safety and efficacy study in children with asthma aged 4 to 11 years. In children 5 to 11 years old, the ICS/LABA combination has not yet been definitively shown to decrease exacerbations compared with medium-dose ICS, although impairment domains improved.[2] More recently, the addition of a LABA to low-dose ICS improved overall asthma control compared with either doubling the dose of ICS or the addition of montelukast in children 6 to 17 years old.[53]

The elderly are at highest risk from dying of asthma.[3] Owing to the increased risk of osteoporosis and cataracts in the elderly, patients requiring high doses of ICSs should have routine height measurements, bone mineral density determinations, and ophthalmic examinations.[2,54] Appropriate therapies for prevention of osteoporosis should be instituted.[2,54]

Asthma affects 7% of pregnant women, making it potentially the most common serious medical condition to complicate pregnancy.[19] Maternal asthma has been reported to increase the risk of perinatal mortality, preeclampsia, preterm birth, and low-birth-weight infants.[19] More severe asthma is associated with increased risks, whereas better-controlled asthma is associated with decreased risks. A systematic review of the evidence on the safety of asthma medications has concluded that it is safer for pregnant women with asthma to be treated with effective medications than for them to have exacerbations.[19] Proper monitoring and control of asthma should enable a woman with asthma to maintain a normal pregnancy with little or no risk to mother or her fetus. Regular visits are recommended and should include objective assessment of lung function and validated assessment of symptoms.

A stepwise approach to managing asthma during pregnancy and lactation has been published, with low-dose ICSs recommended as preferred treatment for mild persistent asthma with the addition of a LABA if not adequately controlled.[19] Budesonide is considered the preferred ICS to initiate because it has the greatest amount of safety data, and the data are reassuring.[19] Albuterol is considered the preferred rescue therapy.[19] Conditions that may aggravate asthma such as allergic rhinitis and sinusitis should be aggressively treated.[19]

Drug Class Information

Inhaled Corticosteroids

The mechanism of action of the corticosteroids has been reviewed (see above). The principal advantage of the ICSs is their high topical potency to reduce inflammation in the lung and low systemic activity.[37,46] The ICSs have high antiinflammatory potency, approximately 1,000-fold greater than endogenous cortisol, and differ from each other by as much as fourfold to sixfold.[37] However, potency differences, which are simply a measure of binding affinity to the receptor, can be overcome simply by giving different microgram dosages of drug. Aerosol delivery of the preparations is remarkably variable, ranging from 10% to 60% of the nominal dose (i.e., that dose which leaves an actuator for an MDI or, in the case of a DPI, that which is released on actuation of the inhaler).[26,37] Different devices for the same chemical entity may result in twofold differences in delivery, so that delivery method can make a significant difference in the relative comparable dose or therapeutic index.[2,37]

The ICSs, beclomethasone dipropionate, budesonide, ciclesonide, flunisolide, fluticasone propionate, and mometasone furoate, that are currently available for use are compared and listed in Table 15-12. The ICSs have pharmacokinetic differences that result in different topical/systemic activity.[37] Most evidence is consistent with log-linear dose–response curves for both indirect and direct responses.[46] The log-linear nature of the dose–response curve for ICS activity raises the issue of how much of a difference in dose (or lung delivery) or potency is detectable. The measures used to assess efficacy (lung function, BHR, symptoms, and as-needed short-acting inhaled β_2-agonist use) are downstream events from the antiinflammatory activity.[46] It takes a fourfold difference in potency or dose to detect clinically significant differences in efficacy.[49] The table of comparable ICS doses (see Table 15-12) is based on extensive clinical trial data.[2,37] Clinically comparable doses take into consideration drug potency differences as well as device delivery differences but not the potential for systemic activity.

Since the glucocorticoid receptors within the various tissues are the same, differences in the pharmacokinetic profile are required to produce differences in the topical/systemic effect ratio (therapeutic index).[37] Pharmacokinetic properties that enhance topical selectivity include rapid systemic clearance, poor oral bioavailability, and prolonged residence time in the lung.[37] Owing to their high lipophilicity, systemic clearance of the available ICSs is very rapid, approaching the rate of liver blood flow with the exception of ciclesonide, which is inactivated by blood esterases as well.[37] However, the ICSs differ markedly in their oral bioavailability, although they all undergo rather extensive first-pass metabolism to less active substances when absorbed[37] (see Table 15-9). The ICSs produce dose-dependent systemic effects, contributed by the orally absorbed fraction and the fraction absorbed from the lung[2,37,46] (Table 15-13). Essentially all the drug that reaches the lung is absorbed systemically; thus, a slow absorption from the lung results in an apparent long elimination half-life and enhances topical selectivity by lowering the systemic concentration.[37] Ciclesonide and beclomethasone dipropionate differ from the other ICSs in that the parent compounds are prodrugs that are metabolized in the lung to the active compounds desciclesonide and beclomethasone monopropionate.[37] The potential advantage of the drugs with low oral bioavailability is obviated by using a spacer device with the MDI for the drugs with higher oral bioavailability because appropriate spacers reduce the oral dose by 80%.[37] The use of VHCs also can increase systemic activity by increasing lung delivery of drugs not absorbed significantly orally.[37] If this increase in lung deposition is twofold or less, it will increase systemic activity without producing a clinically important increase in efficacy, thus decreasing the therapeutic index.[37] Mouth rinsing and spitting will also reduce the oral availability and are particularly useful for DPI devices.[2,37] Although ciclesonide and its active metabolite have rapid systemic clearance suggesting an improved therapeutic index, it has not yet been clearly established in clinical trials.[37]

TABLE 15-13 Effects of Inhaled Corticosteroids

Beneficial Effects	Potential Adverse Effects
Decrease eosinophil numbers	Growth retardation, skeletal muscle myopathy
Decrease mast cell numbers	Osteoporosis, fractures and aseptic necrosis of hip
Decrease T-lymphocyte cytokine production	Posterior subcapsular cataract formation and glaucoma
Inhibit transcription of inflammatory genes in airway epithelium	Adrenal axis suppression, immunosuppression
Reduce endothelial cell leak	Impaired wound healing, easy bruising, skin striae
Upregulate β_2-receptor production	Hyperglycemia/hypokalemia, hypertension
Reduce airway epithelial subbasement membrane thickening	Psychiatric disturbances

The response to ICSs is somewhat delayed. Most patients' symptoms will improve in the first 1 to 2 weeks of therapy and will reach maximum improvement in 4 to 8 weeks.[46] Improvement in baseline FEV_1 and PEF may require 3 to 6 weeks for maximum improvement, whereas improvement in BHR requires 2 to 3 weeks and approaches maximum in 1 to 3 months but may continue to improve over 1 year.[46] Most of the improvement in these parameters occurs at low to medium doses, and there is a large variability in response, with 10% of patients not demonstrating an improvement in either parameter.[46] Whether these nonresponders also show no improvement in rates of exacerbations is unknown. Significant decreases in FeNO occur within 1 to 2 days with maximum effect in 2 to 3 weeks.[16,46] Sensitivity to exercise challenge decreases after 4 weeks of therapy.[46] Although single doses do not inhibit the immediate asthmatic response to antigen challenge or exercise, continued therapy for 1 week partially suppresses the response. The two latter effects are likely due to a reduction in mucosal mast cells.[46]

Local adverse effects from ICSs include oropharyngeal candidiasis and dysphonia that are dose dependent. The dysphonia (reported in 5% to 20% of patients) appears to be due to a local corticosteroid-induced myopathy of the vocal cords.[2] The use of a spacer device with MDIs can decrease oropharyngeal deposition and thus decrease the incidence and severity of local side effects.[2,46] In infants who require ICS delivery through a face mask, the parent should clean the nasal–perioral area with a damp cloth following each treatment to prevent topical candidal infections.

Systemic adverse effects can occur with any of the ICSs given in a sufficiently high dose.[46] Long-term adverse effects of greatest concern include growth suppression in children, osteoporosis, cataracts, dermal thinning, and adrenal insufficiency and crisis.[45,46] Of these, only growth retardation occurs in low to medium doses. However, the growth reduction appears to be transient in that growth velocity is reduced in the first 6 months to 2 years of therapy and then returns to normal.[2,45] The effect is small (1 to 2 cm total) and not cumulative, but does persist into adulthood.[55] The suppression of the HPA axis and decreased bone mineralization are dose dependent and do not appear to be significant clinically except at high doses.[46] The risks therefore depend on the therapeutic index of each ICS and its delivery device. The effect of delivery device is illustrated by fluticasone propionate, which has both the greatest therapeutic index when administered by DPI and the lowest therapeutic index when administered by MDI plus VHC.[37] Many of the ICSs, including fluticasone propionate, budesonide, ciclesonide, and mometasone furoate, are metabolized in the GI tract and liver by CYP3A4 isoenzymes. Potent inhibitors of CYP3A4 such as ritonavir and ketoconazole have the potential for increasing systemic concentrations of these ICSs by increasing oral availability and decreasing systemic clearance.[37] Some cases of clinically significant Cushing's syndrome and secondary adrenal insufficiency have been reported.[37]

Most patients with moderate disease can be controlled with twice-daily dosing of most ICSs.[2,37] Twice-daily dosing produces less thrush than three- to four-times-daily dosing regimens. In milder asthma, once-daily dosing is often sufficient to maintain control.[37,46] Some of the newer products have gained once-daily dosing indications, particularly in mild asthma once initial control is established.[37] There is no specific pharmacologic or pharmacokinetic aspect of the current ICSs that allows for once-daily dosing because all the agents studied (both the older low-potency ICSs and newer high-potency ICSs) have been effective, provided that patients had relatively mild-to-moderate asthma.[37] More severe patients require multiple daily dosing. The inflammatory response of asthma has been shown to inhibit corticosteroid-receptor binding.[37] Once asthma is controlled, many patients are able to reduce the ICS dose and maintain control.[37,46] There has been a recent interest in using ICSs as needed or intermittently in patients with mild persistent asthma; however, the as-needed use has shown inconsistent results with better overall control from regular use.[56,57]

Long-Acting Inhaled β_2-Agonists

The two LABAs, formoterol and salmeterol, provide long-lasting bronchodilation (≥12 hours) when administered as aerosols[34] (see Table 15-8). Unlike the more water-soluble short-acting β_2-agonists, the long-acting agents are lipid soluble, readily partitioning into the outer phospholipid layer of the cell membrane.[34] More recently, indacaterol, a 24-hour LABA, was developed and approved for use in COPD.[58,59] However, due to concerns of safety of LABAs in asthma it has not yet been approved for asthma.[58] The LABAs are more β_2-selective than albuterol and more bronchoselective by virtue of their property of remaining in the lung tissue cell membrane, which produces its longer duration.[30] However, all LABAs will produce dose-dependent systemic β_2-agonist effects.[30,58]

The principal difference between formoterol and salmeterol is that formoterol has a more rapid onset of action. This is unlikely to produce a clinically significant advantage because both LABAs are recommended for chronic therapy only in combination with ICSs.[2] LABAs are available singly and as fixed-dose combinations with ICSs (see below). Neither has approved FDA labeling for acute relief of asthma, although formoterol has an onset of activity similar to albuterol. Patients need to be counseled to continue to use their short-acting inhaled β_2-agonists for acute exacerbations while receiving the LABA/ICS combination products.

The LABAs are preferred adjunctive therapy to ICSs in children 12 years and older and adults for step 3 and children 5 to 11 years of age for steps 4 and 5.[2] Combination treatment with ICS/LABA provides greater asthma control than increasing the dose of ICS alone, while at the same time reducing the frequency of mild and severe exacerbations.[48] Since they are devoid of antiinflammatory activity, LABAs should not be used as monotherapy for asthma. Patients treated with LABA monotherapy added to usual therapy are at an increased risk for severe, life-threatening exacerbations and asthma-related death.[60,61] This risk may be greater in African American patients. Whether this risk is obviated by concomitant ICS use is controversial at this time (see below).[61–63] A genotype stratified study failed to detect lung function deterioration or increased exacerbations in Arg-16 homozygotes receiving a LABA plus ICS.[64]

As with short-acting β_2-agonists, tolerance is produced with chronic administration of LABAs. Long-term trials have shown no diminution in bronchodilator response but a partial loss of the bronchoprotective effect against methacholine, histamine, and exercise challenge.[30] In particular, the duration of protection against EIB following a single dose of salmeterol is up to 9 hours but is reduced to less than 4 hours following regular treatment.[30] Following regular treatment with LABAs, decreased protection against nonspecific bronchoprovocation with methacholine also occurs, although they continue to provide greater protection than placebo.[30] Responsiveness to short-acting β_2-agonists has been reported to be slightly decreased but easily overcome by increasing the dose (by 1–2 puff) following chronic therapy with LABAs.[30]

There is ample evidence that the use of a LABA in combination with ICS therapy does not mask inflammation.[30] In children 4 to 11 years of age, LABAs added to ICS reduce impairment and improve asthma control but have yet to be adequately studied for reducing the risk domain of exacerbations over ICS alone.[30,53]

Methylxanthines

Methylxanthines have been used for asthma therapy for more than 50 years, but their use has declined markedly owing to the high risk of severe life-threatening toxicity and numerous drug interactions, as well as decreased efficacy compared with ICSs and LABAs. Theophylline, the primary methylxanthine of interest, is a moderately potent bronchodilator with mild antiinflammatory properties.[2] Like the β_2-agonists, the methylxanthines are functional antagonists of bronchospasm; however, their clinical utility is limited by their low therapeutic index.[2] Theophylline as a sustained-release product is the preferred oral preparation, whereas its complex with ethylenediamine (aminophylline) is the preferred injectable product owing to increased solubility.[2]

The mechanism by which theophylline produces bronchodilation appears to be through nonselective phosphodiesterase (PDE) inhibition–producing increased cAMP and cyclic guanosine monophosphate (cGMP) concentrations.[2] The PDE isoenzymes currently thought to be important for theophylline's clinical effects are isoenzymes III, predominant in airway smooth muscle, and IV, important in inflammatory cell regulation such as mast cells, neutrophils, eosinophils, and T lymphocytes.[2] Selective PDE isoenzyme IV inhibitors, however, have no significant effects in clinical asthma. Theophylline also activates histone deacetylase that is involved in the corticosteroid-induced decrease in proinflammatory gene expression.[65] It is a competitive antagonist of adenosine and stimulates endogenous catecholamine release, which are important determinants of toxic symptoms of excess theophylline.[2]

Theophylline has a log-linear dose–response curve.[66] Most chronic stable patients with asthma will obtain significant bronchodilation when the serum theophylline concentration reaches 5 mcg/mL (28 μmol/L), and most patients will have no toxic symptoms with serum concentrations of less than 15 mcg/mL (83 μmol/L).[2,66] The percentage of patients experiencing adverse effects increases sharply as concentrations exceed 15 mcg/mL (83 μmol/L). As with the β_2-agonists, the dose–response curves for smooth muscle relaxation by theophylline are dynamic and shifted to the right in the face of increasing contractile stimuli.[66] This property probably explains theophylline's relative lack of bronchodilatory effect in acute severe asthma.[2,66] The severity of theophylline's toxicity precludes even doubling the usual dosage. Toxicities include caffeine-like effects of nausea, vomiting, tachycardia, jitteriness, and difficulty sleeping to more severe toxicities such as cardiac tachyarrythmias and seizures. Death has occurred in children receiving their usual doses of theophylline during acute systemic viral illnesses.[66]

Routine monitoring of serum concentrations is essential for the safe and effective use of theophylline.[2] Theophylline is eliminated primarily by metabolism via the hepatic cytochrome P450 (CYP) mixed-function oxidase microsomal enzymes (primarily the CYP1A2 and CYP3A3 isozymes), with 10% or less excreted unchanged in the kidney.[2] Theophylline clearance is age dependent, with 1- to 9-year-olds having the highest systemic

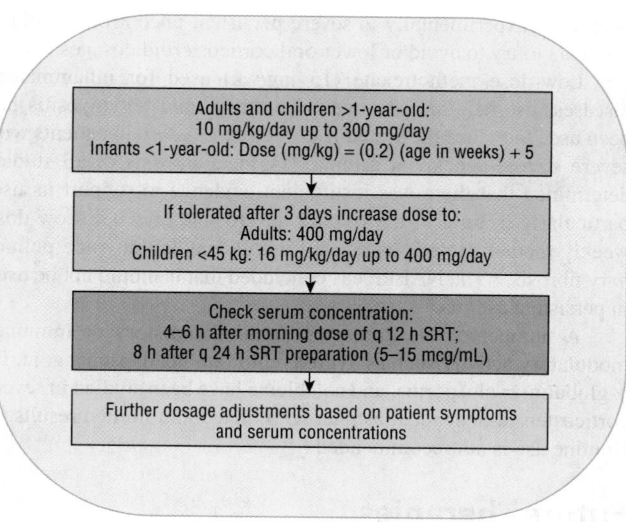

FIGURE 15-9 Algorithm for slow titration of theophylline dosage and guide for final dosage adjustment based on serum theophylline concentration measurement. For infants younger than 1 year of age, the initial daily dosage can be calculated by the following regression equation: Dose (mg/kg) = (0.2) (age in weeks) + 5. Whenever side effects occur, dosage should be reduced to a previously tolerated lower dose.

clearances and therefore requiring the largest dosages (on a weight basis). However, even within the same age groups, theophylline clearance can vary twofold to threefold.[2] Figure 15-9 outlines a dosing and monitoring schedule for theophylline. Factors affecting theophylline's hepatic metabolism are listed in Table 15-14.[2] Only drugs or diseases that produce a ≥20% inhibition or a ≥50% induction of theophylline metabolism are likely to result in clinically significant interactions.[66]

Sustained-release theophylline is less effective than ICSs and no more effective than oral sustained-release β_2-agonists, cromolyn, or LT antagonists.[2] The addition of theophylline to ICSs is similar to doubling the dose of the ICS and is overall less effective than the LABAs as adjunctive therapy.[2] The addition of theophylline to patients with poorly controlled asthma receiving ICS/LABA combination does not improve outcomes.[67]

TABLE 15-14 Factors Affecting Theophylline Clearance

Decreased Clearance	% Decrease	Increased Clearance	% Increase
Cimetidine	−25 to −60	Rifampin	+53
Macrolides: erythromycin, TAO, clarithromycin	−25 to −50	Carbamazepine Phenobarbital Phenytoin	+50 +34 +70
Allopurinol	−20	Charcoal-broiled meat	+30
Propranolol	−30		
Quinolones ciprofloxacin, enoxacin, perfloxacin	−20 to −50	High-protein diet Smoking	+25 +40
Interferon	−50	Sulfinpyrazone	+22
Thiabendazole	−65	Moricizine	+50
Ticlopidine	−25	Aminoglutethimide	+50
Zileuton	−35		
Systemic viral illness	−10 to −50		

Cromolyn Sodium

Cromolyn is classified as a mast cell stabilizer and inhibits the early and late asthmatic response to allergen challenge, as well as inhibiting EIB.[13,68] Long-term treatment produces minimal to no change in baseline BHR.[2] Cromolyn inhibits neurally mediated bronchoconstriction through C-fiber sensory nerve stimulation in the airways, although it does not have a bronchodilatory effect.[68]

Cromolyn is only effective by inhalation, and available as a nebulizer solution.[68] It is not bioavailable orally, but the portion of the dose that reaches the lung is absorbed completely.[68] Absorption from the airway is significantly slower than elimination (hours vs. minutes). The short duration in the lung likely limits its efficacy. Both the intensity and duration of protection against various challenges are dose dependent.[68]

Cromolyn is remarkably nontoxic. No evidence of mutagenesis or teratogenesis has been found. Cough and wheeze have been reported following inhalation.[2] Tolerance to cromolyn has not been demonstrated. It is not considered to be an ICS-sparing agent.

Cromolyn is no more or less effective than theophylline or the LT antagonists for persistent asthma.[2,66] It is not as effective as the ICSs for controlling persistent asthma.[66] Cromolyn is not as effective as the inhaled β_2-agonists for preventing EIB but can be used in conjunction for patients not responding completely to the inhaled β_2-agonists.[13]

Most patients will experience an improvement in 1 to 2 weeks, but it may take longer to achieve maximum benefit. Patients initially should receive cromolyn four times daily, and then only after stabilization of symptoms may the frequency be reduced to three times daily.

Leukotriene Modifiers

Two cysteinyl LT receptor antagonists (zafirlukast and montelukast) and one 5-lipoxygenase inhibitor (zileuton) are available in the United States.[69] In challenge studies, they reduce allergen-, exercise-, cold-air hyperventilation–, irritant-, and aspirin-induced asthma.[69] Clinical use of zileuton is limited due to the potential for elevated liver enzymes (especially in the first 3 months of therapy), and the potential inhibition of drugs metabolized by the CYP3A4 isoenzymes.[66,69] They are not preferred alternatives in mild persistent asthma nor as alternative add-on therapy for moderate persistent asthma (Fig. 15-8).[2]

These drugs improve pulmonary function tests (FEV_1 and PEF), decrease nocturnal awakenings and β_2-agonist use, and improve asthma symptoms.[69] A major advantage is that they are effective orally, and can be administered once or twice a day.[69] However, they are less effective in asthma than low doses of ICSs.[66,69] Although montelukast is approved for EIB in adults, it is significantly less effective than short-acting inhaled β_2-agonists. In adults with severe uncontrolled asthma they do not improve outcomes.[69] They are not as effective as LABAs when added to ICSs for moderate persistent asthma.[69] It is not yet possible to predict which patients respond best to LT modifiers, although there is some evidence that patients with aspirin-sensitive asthma do well, as predicted by studies showing increased cysteinyl LT production in these patients.[69] It is possible that genetic polymorphisms in the 5-lipoxygenase or LTC_4 synthase pathways or in cys-LT_1 receptors might predict better responders in the future.[69] Anti-LTs also have modest efficacy in allergic rhinitis.

In general, the LTD_4 receptor antagonists are well tolerated and do not appear to have serious class-specific effects.[2] An idiosyncratic syndrome similar to the Churg-Strauss syndrome, with marked circulating eosinophilia, heart failure, and associated eosinophilic vasculitis, has been reported in a small number of patients treated with zafirlukast and montelukast.[66] The majority of these patients had been receiving high-dose ICS or oral corticosteroids and were able to reduce the dose as a consequence of the LTD_4 receptor antagonists. It is unclear whether the increased reports are due to increased case findings among patients with asthma prescribed a new drug or whether the syndrome is related to corticosteroid dose reduction or an idiosyncratic effect of LT modifiers in general. Whatever the cause, it appears to be a rare syndrome, with an estimated incidence of fewer than 1 case per 15,000 to 20,000 patient-years of treatment.[66]

Reports of adverse neuropsychiatric events have caused the manufacturers of the LT inhibitors to revise their labeling. However, evidence for causality of suicidal thoughts and suicide is lacking.[70] Reports of fatal hepatic failure associated with zafirlukast have prompted a warning for patients to be made aware of signs and symptoms of hepatic dysfunction.[2]

Zileuton can be administered twice daily as controlled-release tablets.[2] Efficacy data are more limited, liver function monitoring is recommended, and drug interactions are reported with warfarin and theophylline.

Anti-IgE (Omalizumab)

Omalizumab is a recombinant anti-IgE antibody approved for the treatment of allergic asthma not well controlled on oral corticosteroids or ICSs.[71] It is a composite of 95% human and 5% antihuman murine IgE sequences. Omalizumab binds to the Fc portion of the IgE antibody preventing the binding of IgE to its high-affinity receptor (FcεRI) on mast cells and basophils. The decreased binding of IgE on the surface of mast cells leads to a decrease in the release of mediators in response to allergen exposure. Omalizumab also decreases FcεRI expression on basophils and airway submucosal mast cells over 8 to 12 weeks.[71]

Omalizumab is administered subcutaneously and has a slow absorption rate; peak serum concentration is achieved in 3 to 14 days.[71] Omalizumab is eliminated primarily through the reticuloendothelial system and has an elimination half-life of 17 to 22 days; serum free IgE levels return to previous level in about 3 weeks.[71] Omalizumab should be administered under medical observation with drugs for treating anaphylaxis available.

The dosage of omalizumab is determined by the patient's baseline total serum IgE level (international units per milliliter) and body weight (kilograms).[71] Doses range from 150 to 375 mg and are given at either 2- or 4-week intervals. No further adjustments for variations in total serum IgE are required, and patients receive a consistent dose for the duration of treatment.[71] Omalizumab is approved for patients greater than 12 years with allergic asthma.[71] Clinical trials in 5- to 12-year-olds are ongoing. Due to its significant cost, it is only indicated as step 5 or 6 care for patients who have allergies and severe persistent asthma that are inadequately controlled with the combination of high-dose ICS/LABA and at risk for severe exacerbations.[2,72] It is the only adjunctive therapy that has demonstrated improved outcomes in patients uncontrolled on ICS/LABA and has allowed oral corticosteroid reduction in a number of studies.[2,71] Omalizumab therapy is associated with a 0.2% rate of anaphylaxis prompting an FDA warning that patients should remain in the healthcare provider's office for a reasonable period of time past the injection as 70% of reactions occur within 2 hours. In addition, patients should be counseled on the signs and symptoms of anaphylaxis because some reactions have occurred up to 24 hours following an injection.[2,71]

Miscellaneous Therapies (Immunomodulators)

The following therapies have been loosely categorized by the NAEPP with omalizumab as immunomodulators because they either affect the immune system or have antiinflammatory properties. Many have been used experimentally in severe persistent uncontrolled asthma for years to try to avoid or lower oral corticosteroid dosages.

Low-dose methotrexate (15 mg/wk) used for inflammatory diseases, psoriatic and rheumatoid arthritis, and polymyositis has been used to reduce the systemic corticosteroid dose in patients with severe steroid-dependent asthma.[73] A meta-analysis of all studies determined that there was insufficient evidence to support its use, particularly in light of the risk for severe side effects.[73] Low-dose weekly methotrexate is associated with hepatotoxicity and pulmonary fibrosis.[73] The NAEPP has concluded that it should not be used in persistent asthma.[2]

A number of the drugs with antiinflammatory or immunomodulatory activity such as hydroxychloroquine, dapsone, gold, IV γ-globulin, cyclosporine, and colchicine have been studied in severe corticosteroid-dependent asthma with mixed and limited results.[2,74] Routine use is not recommended.[2]

Future Therapies

In addition to a number of once-daily ICSs and ICS/LABA combinations, agents that are now in development for asthma focus on the treatment of allergic inflammation.[75] Examples include inhibitors of eosinophilic inflammation, drugs that may inhibit allergen presentation, and inhibitors of Th_2 cells. Multiple cytokines have been implicated in allergic inflammation, and several possible inhibiting approaches are being explored. These range from drugs that inhibit cytokine synthesis (cyclosporin A and tacrolimus), humanized blocking antibodies to cytokines or their receptors, soluble receptors to mop up secreted cytokines, receptor antagonists, and drugs that block the signal-transduction pathways activated by cytokines.[75] Unfortunately specific anticytokine therapy against IL-5 and IL-4 has been disappointing to date.[75]

The FDA has approved Asthmatx, Inc's Alair Bronchial Thermoplasty System to treat severe asthma in adult patients. This is the first nondrug treatment for asthma. The Alair treatment (three sessions of 30 minutes each) is performed via a bronchoscope that is inserted into the lungs. A tip of a small catheter then expands to deliver thermal energy to reduce the presence of airway smooth muscle that narrows the airways.[76]

PHARMACOECONOMIC CONSIDERATIONS

Of the estimated $19.7 billion cost of asthma in the United States in 2004, direct medical expenditure accounted for $14.7 billion of the total, with emergency care (ED and in-patient hospital care) reaching $4.7 billion.[4] A cost-of-illness approach takes in all measurable costs; both indirect costs or costs to society and direct medical costs are considered.[77,78] Using this approach, indirect costs such as lost work and death accounted for 25% of total expenditures per patient. Although prescription drugs were the largest single direct medical expenditure at $6.7 billion,[4] an increase in these costs secondary to improved patient adherence could significantly reduce other costs due to missed school days and lost productivity secondary to asthma morbidity and mortality.

The medication cost increase over the past years resulted from an increase in prescribed medications, as well as an increase in unit cost per medication. The latter may improve in the next few years as a number of existing products go off patent and become generic. Asthma severity affects cost of care as studies from health maintenance organizations suggest that up to 45% of the cost of asthma is accrued by 10% of the patients, primarily as a result of emergency care.[78]

Numerous studies have demonstrated the cost-effectiveness of patient education programs for asthma, particularly those providing guided self-management.[2] Several studies have reported positive results from pharmacist interventions reducing overall cost of care.[2] Similar studies have demonstrated the cost-effectiveness of specialist care compared with generalist care. However, the results of these trials may be confounded by changes in prescribing as part of the overall program.[77] Indeed, use of ICSs reduces both morbidity, particularly hospitalizations, and mortality in asthma patients.[2,77]

The NAEPP recommendations provide numerous alternatives for long-term controllers in mild-to-moderate persistent asthma, and few studies have compared their relative cost-effectiveness. This comparison is important because outside the realm of randomized clinical trials that evaluate efficacy, other factors such as concern about adverse effects and adherence to therapy may alter the overall clinical effectiveness. Use of ICSs in children has produced a cost of $9.45 per symptom-free day gained and in adults $5 per symptom-free day.[2] Retrospective analyses of large managed-care-linked pharmacy claims and healthcare utilization databases have allowed direct comparisons of the various long-term controllers in a general population to assess clinical effectiveness and cost-effectiveness. While these studies have confirmed comparative randomized clinical trials showing ICSs to be significantly more cost-effective than LT antagonists, many have flaws, including the short duration of followup for a chronic illness such as asthma.[77]

Clinical **Controversy. . .**

The potential for chronic use of inhaled β_2-agonists to worsen asthma has been a concern for more than 40 years. A large multicenter clinical trial of the addition of LABA as monotherapy to patient's usual therapy produced a significant increased risk of death from asthma.[60] However, post hoc analysis from that study did not show an increased risk of death in those patients whose usual therapy included ICSs.[60] Other meta-analyses also failed to demonstrate an increased risk of death or hospitalizations from asthma in patients receiving ICS/LABA combination therapy.[61,62] However, the FDA's stance is that the number of patients in the trials was too low to detect rare events, so it has mandated the pharmaceutical companies to perform large clinical trials in both children and adults to determine whether ICSs protect against the risk of severe life-threatening asthma exacerbations in those on combination therapy.[63] Those studies are underway. The LABAs should be used only in combination with ICSs where the risk of severe life-threatening exacerbations has not been demonstrated.[61,62]

EVALUATION OF ASTHMA CONTROL

Control of asthma is defined as reducing both impairment and risk domains.[77] The stepwise approach to therapy should be used to achieve and maintain this control. The steps of care appropriate to the three age ranges of asthma have been outlined in Figure 15-8.[2] Depending on the severity of the patient's asthma, compromises from the ideal control are made, and the best possible outcome balancing disease control and possible adverse effects from the drugs is attempted. Regular followup contact is essential (at 1- to 6-month intervals, depending on control). A step-down in therapy can be considered, if well-controlled status has been achieved for at least 3 months.[2]

Components of control classification include symptoms, nighttime awakenings, interference with normal activities, pulmonary function, quality of life, exacerbations, medication adherence, treatment-related adverse effects, and satisfaction with care.[77] The categories of well controlled, not well controlled, and very poorly controlled are recommended. Validated questionnaires such as the Asthma Therapy Assessment Questionnaire (ATAQ), the Asthma Control Questionnaire (ACQ), and the Asthma Control Test (ACT) can be regularly administered.[77] The NAEPP minimally recommends spirometric tests at initial assessment, after treatment is initiated, and then every 1 to 2 years.[2] In moderate-to-severe persistent asthma, PEF monitoring is recommended. PEF monitoring should also be considered in patients who are poor symptom perceivers or those with a history of severe exacerbations.[2] Patients should also be asked about exercise tolerance. All patients on inhaled drugs should have their inhalation delivery technique evaluated periodically—monthly initially and then every 3 to 6 months. Before stepping up therapy, adherence, environmental control, and comorbid conditions should be reviewed.[2]

Following initiation of antiinflammatory therapy or an increase in dosage, most patients should begin experiencing a decrease in symptoms in 1 to 2 weeks and achieve maximum symptomatic improvement within 4 to 8 weeks. The use of higher ICS doses or more potent agents may accelerate the process. Improvement in FEV_1 and PEF should follow a similar time frame; however, a decrease in BHR, as measured by morning PEF, PEF variability, and exercise tolerance, may take longer and improve over 1 to 3 months.[2] Patients should be informed that following a viral respiratory infection, they may experience decreased exercise tolerance for up to 4 weeks.

Initial visits with the patient should focus on the patient's concerns, expectations, and goals of treatment. Basic education should focus on asthma as a chronic lung disease, the types of medications, and how they are to be used. Inhaler technique is taught, as is when to seek medical advice. Written action plans should be provided. Either peak flow–based or symptom-based self-monitoring can be effective, if taught and followed correctly.[2] The first followup visit should be in 2 to 6 weeks, to evaluate control. At that time, the educational messages of the first visit should be repeated, as well as review of the patient's current medications, adherence, and any difficulties related to the therapy.

CONCLUSION

Asthma is a complicated disease with a multitude of clinical presentations. The exact defect in asthma has not been defined, and it may be that asthma is a common presentation of a heterogeneous group of diseases. Asthma is defined and characterized by excessive reactivity of the bronchial tree to a wide variety of noxious stimuli. The reaction is characterized by bronchospasm, excessive mucus production, and inflammation. The central role of inflammation in inducing and maintaining BHR is now becoming widely appreciated. The goal of asthma therapy is to normalize, as much as possible, the patient's life and prevent chronic irreversible lung changes. Drugs are the mainstay of asthma management. The goal of drug therapy is to use the minimum amount of medications possible to completely control the disease. In persistent asthma, therapy should be aimed at both bronchospasm and inflammation in order to produce the best results. Patients should be followed and monitored diligently for toxicities. Although death from asthma is an uncommon event, the most common cause of death is underassessment of the severity of obstruction either by the patient or by the clinician; the next common cause is undertreatment. A cornerstone of any therapy is education and the realization that most asthma deaths are avoidable.

ABBREVIATIONS

ABPA	allergic bronchopulmonary aspergillosis
ACQ	Asthma Control Questionnaire
ACT	Asthma Control Test
ACTH	adrenocorticotropic hormone
Arg	arginine
ATAQ	Asthma Therapy Assessment Questionnaire
BHR	bronchial hyperresponsiveness
cAMP	cyclic adenosine monophosphate
CFC	chlorofluorocarbon
cGMP	cyclic guanosine monophosphate
COPD	chronic obstructive pulmonary disease
CYP	cytochrome P450
DPI	dry powder inhaler
ED	emergency department
EIB	exercise-induced bronchospasm
EPR3	Expert Panel Report 3
FeNO	fraction of exhaled nitric oxide
FEV_1	forced expiratory volume in 1 second
FVC	forced vital capacity
GERD	gastroesophageal reflux disease
Gln	glutamine
Glu	glutamic acid
Gly	glycine
GM-CSF	granulocyte-macrophage colony-stimulating factor
HFA	hydrofluoroalkane
HPA	hypothalamic–pituitary–adrenal
ICAM-1	intercellular adhesion molecule 1
ICS	inhaled corticosteroid
IFN-γ	interferon-γ
IgE	immunoglobulin E
IL	interleukin
iNOS	inducible nitric oxide synthase
LABA	long-acting inhaled β_2-agonist
LT	leukotriene
MDI	metered-dose inhaler
MMAD	mass median aerodynamic diameter
NAEPP	National Asthma Education and Prevention Program
NANC	nonadrenergic, noncholinergic
NO	nitric oxide
O_2	oxygen
PAF	platelet-activating factor
PDE	phosphodiesterase
PEF	peak expiratory flow
PKA	protein kinase A
RSV	respiratory syncytial virus
T cells	thymically derived lymphocytes
Th_1	type 1 T-helper
Th_2	T-helper cell type 2
VCAM-1	vascular cell adhesion molecule 1
VHC	valved holding chamber
VIP	vasoactive intestinal peptide

REFERENCES

1. Rosenblatt MB. History of bronchial asthma. In: Weiss EB, Segal MS, Stein M, eds. Bronchial Asthma: Mechanisms and Therapeutics, 2nd ed. Boston: Little, Brown, 1976:5–17.
2. National Institutes of Health, National Heart, Lung, and Blood Institute. National Asthma Education and Prevention Program. Full Report of the Expert Panel: Guidelines for the Diagnosis and Management of Asthma (EPR-3). July 2007, *http://www.nhlbi.nih.gov/guidelines/asthma*.
3. Akinbami LJ, Moorman JE, Bailey C, et al. Trends in asthma prevalence, health care use, and mortality in the United States, 2001-2010. NCHS Data Brief 2012;94:1–8.
4. American Lung Association. Trends in Asthma Morbidity and Mortality. American Lung Association Epidemiology & Statistics Unit Research and Program Services. January 2009, *http://www.lungusa.org*.
5. Melén E, Pershagen G. Pathophysiology of asthma: Lessons from genetic research with particular focus on severe asthma. J Intern Med 2012;272:108–120.
6. Gelfand EW. Pediatric asthma: A different disease. Proc Am Thorac Soc 2009;6:278–282.
7. Busse WW, Lemanske RF Jr. Asthma. N Engl J Med 2001;344:350–362.
8. Dykewicz MS. Occupational asthma: Current concepts in pathogenesis, diagnosis, and management. J Allergy Clin Immunol 2009;123:519–528.
9. Sears MR. Epidemiology of asthma exacerbations. J Allergy Clin Immunol 2008;122:662–668.
10. Busse WW, Lemanske RF Jr, Gern JE. Role of viral respiratory infections in asthma and asthma exacerbations. Lancet 2010;376(9743):826–834.
11. Fixman ED, Stewart A, Martin JG. Basic mechanisms of development of airway structural changes in asthma. Eur Respir J 2007;29:379–389.
12. Woodruff PG, Modrek B, Choy DF, et al. T-helper type 2-driven inflammation defines major subphenotypes of asthma. Am J Respir Crit Care Med 2009;180:388–395.
13. Weiler JM, Anderson SD, Randolph C, et al. Pathogenesis, prevalence, diagnosis, and management of exercise-induced bronchoconstriction: A practice parameter. Ann Allergy Asthma Immunol 2010;105(6 Suppl):S1–S47.
14. Fahy JV. Eosinophilic and neutrophilic inflammation in asthma: Insights from clinical studies. Proc Am Thorac Soc 2009;6:256–259.
15. An SS, Bai TR, Bates JHT, et al. Airway smooth muscle dynamics: A common pathway of airway obstruction in asthma. Eur Respir J 2007;29:834–860.
16. Kharitonov SA, Barnes PJ. Exhaled biomarkers. Chest 2006; 130:1541–1546.
17. Anderson SD, Charlton B, Weiler JM, et al. Comparison of mannitol and methacholine to predict exercise-induced bronchoconstriction and a clinical diagnosis of asthma. Respir Res 2009;10:4.
18. The American Lung Association Clinical Research Centers. Efficacy of esomeprazole for treatment of poorly controlled asthma. N Engl J Med 2009;360:1487–1499.
19. National Institutes of Health, National Heart, Lung and Blood Institute. NAEPP Expert Panel Report Managing Asthma During Pregnancy: Recommendations for Pharmacologic Treatment—Update 2004. NIH Publication No. 04-5246. Bethesda, MD: National Heart, Lung and Blood Institute, National Institutes of Health, March 2004.
20. Brenner BE, Holmes TM, Mazal B, Camargo CA Jr. Relation between phase of the menstrual cycle and asthma presentations in the emergency department. Thorax 2005;60: 806–809.
21. Beasley R, Burgess C, Holt S. Call for a worldwide withdrawal of benzalkonium chloride from nebulizer solutions. J Allergy Clin Immunol 2001;107:222–223.
22. Jenkins C, Costello J, Hodge L. Systematic review of the prevalence of aspirin induced asthma and its implications for clinical practice. BMJ 2004;328(7437):434.
23. Dixon AE, Holguin F, Sood A, et al. An official American Thoracic Society workshop report: Obesity and asthma. Proc Am Thorac Soc 2010;7(5):325–335.

24. Marcon A, Corsico A, Cazzoletti L, et al. Body mass index, weight gain, and other determinants of lung function decline in adult asthma. J Allergy Clin Immunol 2009;123: 1069–1074.
25. Brehm JM, Schuemann B, Fuhlbrigge AL, et al. Serum vitamin D levels and severe asthma exacerbations in the Childhood Asthma Management Program study. J Allergy Clin Immunol 2010;126:52–58.
26. Dolovich MB, Dhand R. Aerosol drug delivery: Developments in device design and clinical use. Lancet 2011;377(9770):1032–1045.
27. Schatz M, Kazzi AAN, Brenner B, et al. American Thoracic Society documents: Joint task force report: Supplemental recommendations for the management and follow-up of asthma exacerbations. Proc Am Thorac Soc 2009;6: 353–393.
28. Lazarus SC. Clinical practice. Emergency treatment of asthma. N Engl J Med 2010;363:755–764.
29. Dhand R. Aerosol delivery during mechanical ventilation: From basic techniques to new devices. J Aerosol Med Pulm Drug Deliv 2008;21:45–60.
30. Kelly HW. Risk versus benefit considerations for the beta(2)-agonists. Pharmacotherapy 2006;26:164S–174S.
31. Rowe BH, Edmonds ML, Spooner CH, Diner B, Camargo CA Jr. Corticosteroid therapy for acute asthma. Respir Med 2004;98:275–284.
32. Rodrigo GJ, Castro-Rodriguez JA. Anticholinergics in the treatment of children and adults with acute asthma: A systematic review with meta-analysis. Thorax 2005;60: 740–746.
33. Rodrigo G, Pollack C, Rodrigo C, Rowe BH. Heliox for nonintubated acute asthma patients. Cochrane Database Syst Rev 2006;(4):CD002884.
34. Kelly HW. What is new with the β_2 agonists: Issues in the management of asthma. Ann Pharmacother 2005;39: 931–938.
35. Tse SM, Tantisira K, Weiss ST. The pharmacogenetics and pharmacogenomics of asthma therapy. Pharmacogenomics J 2011;11:383–392.
36. Green RH, Wardlaw AJ. Systemic corticosteroids in asthma. In: Li JT, ed. Pharmacotherapy of Asthma. New York, NY: Taylor and Francis, 2006:233–262.
37. Kelly HW. Comparison of inhaled corticosteroids: An update. Ann Pharmacother 2009;43:519–527.
38. Tse SM, Kelly HW, Litonjua AA, et al. Corticosteroid use and bone mineral accretion in children with asthma: Effect modification by vitamin D. J Allergy Clin Immunol 2012;130:53–60.
39. Gross NJ. Anticholinergic bronchodilators. In: Li JT, ed. Pharmacotherapy of Asthma. New York, NY: Taylor and Francis, 2006:65–82.
40. Peters SP, Kunselman SJ, Icitovic N, et al. Tiotropium bromide step-up therapy for adults with uncontrolled asthma. N Engl J Med 2010;363:1715–1726.
41. Kerstjens HA, Disse B, Schröder-Babo W, et al. Tiotropium improves lung function in patients with severe uncontrolled asthma: A randomized controlled trial. J Allergy Clin Immunol 2011;128:308–314.
42. Rank MA, Liesinger JT, Ziegenfuss JY, et al. Asthma expenditures in the United States comparing 2004 to 2006 and 1996 to 1998. Am J Manag Care 2012;18:499–504.
43. Boyd M, Lasserson TJ, McKean MC, Gibson PG, Ducharme FM, Haby M. Interventions for educating children who are at risk of asthma-related emergency department attendance. Cochrane Database Syst Rev 2009;(2):CD001290.
44. Janson SL, McGrath KW, Covington JK, Cheng SC, Boushey HA. Individualized asthma self-management improves medication adherence and markers of asthma control. J Allergy Clin Immunol 2009;123:840–846.
45. Pedersen S. Clinical safety of inhaled corticosteroids for asthma in children: An update of long-term trials. Drug Saf 2006;29:599–612.
46. Masoli M, Shirtcliffe P, Weatherall M, Holt S, Beasley R. Inhaled corticosteroid therapy in the management of asthma in adults. In: Li JT, ed. Pharmacotherapy of Asthma. New York, NY: Taylor & Francis, 2006:83–115.
47. Strunk RC, Sternberg AL, Szefler SJ, et al. Long-term budesonide or nedocromil treatment, once discontinued, does not alter the course of mild to moderate asthma in children and adolescents. J Pediatr 2009;154:682–687.
48. Ducharme F, Ni Chroinin M, Greenstone I, Lasserson TJ. Addition of long-acting beta2-agonists to inhaled corticosteroids versus same dose inhaled corticosteroids for chronic asthma in adults and children. Cochrane Database Syst Rev 2010;(5):CD005535.
49. Kelly HW. Inhaled corticosteroid dosing: Double for nothing? J Allergy Clin Immunol 2011;128:278–281.
50. Casale TB, Stokes JR. Immunomodulators for allergic respiratory disorders. J Allergy Clin Immunol 2008;121: 288–296.
51. Kerstjens HA, Engel M, Dahl R, et al. Tiotropium in asthma poorly controlled with standard combination therapy. N Engl J Med 2012;367:1198–1207 [Epub ahead of print].
52. Zeiger RS, Mauger D, Bacharier LB, et al. Continuous or intermittent budesonide in preschool children with recurrent wheezing. N Engl J Med 2011;365:1990–2001.
53. Lemanske RF Jr, Mauger DT, Sorkness CA, et al. Step-up therapy for children with uncontrolled asthma receiving inhaled corticosteroids. N Engl J Med 2010;362:975–985.
54. Weldon D. The effects of corticosteroids on bone growth and bone density. Ann Allergy Asthma Immunol 2009;103:3–11.
55. Kelly HW, Sternberg AL, Lescher R, et al. Effect of inhaled glucocorticoids in childhood on adult height. N Engl J Med 2012;367:904–912.
56. Papi A, Canonica GW, Maestrelli P, et al. Rescue use of beclomethasone and albuterol in a single inhaler for mild asthma. N Engl J Med 2007;356(20):2040–2052.
57. Martinez FD, Chinchilli VM, Morgan WJ, et al. Use of beclomethasone dipropionate as rescue treatment for children with mild persistent asthma (TREXA): A randomised, double-blind, placebo-controlled trial. Lancet 2011;377(9766):650–657.
58. Chowdhury BA, Seymour SM, Michele TM, Durmowicz AG, Liu D, Rosebraugh CJ. The risks and benefits of indacaterol—The FDA's review. N Engl J Med 2011;365:2247–2249.
59. Ray SM, McMillen JC, Treadway SA, Helmer RS, Franks AS. Indacaterol: A novel long-acting β(2)-agonist. Pharmacotherapy 2012;32:456–474.
60. Nelson HS, Weiss ST, Bleecker ER, Yancey SW, Dorinsky PM. The Salmeterol Multicenter Asthma Research Trial: A comparison of usual pharmacotherapy for asthma or usual pharmacotherapy plus salmeterol. Chest 2006;129:15–26.
61. McMahon AW, Levenson MS, McEvoy BW, Mosholder AD, Murphy D. Age and risks of FDA-approved long-acting β_2-adrenergic receptor agonists. Pediatrics 2011;128: e1147–e1154.
62. Jaeschke R, O'Byrne PM, Mejza F, et al. The safety of long-acting beta-agonists among patients with asthma using inhaled corticosteroids: Systematic review and meta-analysis. Am J Respir Crit Care Med 2008;178:1009–1016.

63. Chowdhury BA, Seymour SM, Levenson MS. Assessing the safety of adding LABAs to inhaled corticosteroids for treating asthma. N Engl J Med 2011;364:2473–2475.
64. Wechsler ME, Kunselman SJ, Chinchilli VM, et al. Effect of β_2-adrenergic receptor polymorphism on response to longacting β_2 agonist in asthma (LARGE trial): A genotype-stratified, randomized, placebo-controlled, crossover trial. Lancet 2009;374:1754–1764.
65. Adcock IM, Barnes PJ. Molecular mechanisms of corticosteroid resistance. Chest 2008;134:394–401.
66. Kelly HW. Non-corticosteroid therapy for the long-term control of asthma. Expert Opin Pharmacother 2007;8: 2077–2087.
67. The American Lung Association Asthma Clinical Research Centers. Clinical trial of low-dose theophylline and montelukast in patients with poorly controlled asthma. Am J Respir Crit Care Med 2007;175:235–242.
68. Lowery M, Kelly KJ. Cromolyn and nedocromil. In: Li JT, ed. Pharmacotherapy of Asthma. New York, NY: Taylor & Francis, 2006:195–231.
69. O'Byrne PM, Gauvreau GM, Murphy DM. Efficacy of leukotriene receptor antagonists and synthesis inhibitors in asthma. J Allergy Clin Immunol 2009;124:397–403.
70. Manalai P, Woo JM, Postolache TT. Suicidality and montelukast. Expert Opin Drug Saf 2009;8:273–282.
71. Ledford DK. Omalizumab: Overview of pharmacology and efficacy in asthma. Expert Opin Biol Ther 2009;9:933–943.
72. Wu AC, Paltiel AD, Kuntz KM, et al. Cost-effectiveness of omalizumab in adults with severe asthma: Results from the Asthma Policy Model. J Allergy Clin Immunol 2007;120:1146–1152.
73. Davies H, Olson L, Gibson P. Methotrexate as a steroid sparing agent for asthma in adults. Cochrane Database Syst Rev 2000;(2):CD000391.
74. Dykewicz MS. Immunosuppressive and other alternate treatments for asthma. In: Li JT, ed. Pharmacotherapy of Asthma. New York, NY: Taylor & Francis, 2006: 299–317.
75. Barnes PJ. Drugs for asthma. Br J Pharmacol 2006; 147(Suppl 1):S297–S303.
76. Castro M, Rubin AS, Laviolette M, et al. Effectiveness and safety of bronchial thermoplasty in the treatment of severe asthma: A multicenter, randomized, double-blind, sham-controlled clinical trial. Am J Respir Crit Care Med 2010;181:116–124.
77. Reddel HK, Taylor DR, Bateman ED, et al. An official American Thoracic Society/European Respiratory Society statement: Asthma control and exacerbations: Standardizing endpoints for clinical asthma trials and clinical practice. Am J Respir Crit Care Med 2009;180: 59–99.
78. Campbell JD, Spackman DE, Sullivan SD. Health economics of asthma: Assessing the value of asthma interventions. Allergy 2008;63:1581–1592.

Chronic Obstructive Pulmonary Disease

16

Sharya V. Bourdet and Dennis M. Williams

KEY CONCEPTS

1. Chronic obstructive pulmonary disease (COPD) is a treatable and preventable disease characterized by progressive airflow limitation that is not fully reversible and is associated with an abnormal inflammatory response of the lungs to noxious particles or gases.
2. COPD is historically described as either *chronic bronchitis* or *emphysema*. Chronic bronchitis is defined in clinical terms, whereas emphysema is defined in terms of anatomic pathology. Because most patients exhibit some features of each disease, the appropriate emphasis of COPD pathophysiology is on small airway disease and parenchymal damage that contributes to chronic airflow limitation.
3. Mortality from COPD has increased steadily over the past three decades; it currently is the third leading cause of death in the United States.
4. The primary cause of COPD is cigarette smoking, implicated in 85% of diagnosed cases. Other risks include a genetic predisposition, environmental exposures (including occupational dusts and chemicals), and air pollution.
5. Smoking cessation, and avoidance of other known toxins causing COPD, are the only management strategies proven to slow the progression.
6. Oxygen therapy has been shown to reduce mortality in selected patients with COPD. Oxygen therapy is indicated for patients with a resting Pao_2 of less than 55 mm Hg or a Pao_2 of less than 60 mm Hg and evidence of right-sided heart failure, polycythemia, or impaired neurologic function.
7. Bronchodilators represent the mainstay of drug therapy for COPD. Pharmacotherapy is used to relieve patient symptoms and improve quality of life. Guidelines recommend short-acting bronchodilators as initial therapy for patients with mild or intermittent symptoms.
8. For the patient who experiences chronic symptoms, long-acting bronchodilators are appropriate. Either a β_2-agonist or an anticholinergic offers significant benefits. Combining long-acting bronchodilators is recommended if necessary, despite limited data.
9. The role of inhaled corticosteroid therapy in COPD is controversial. International guidelines suggest that patients with severe COPD and frequent exacerbations may benefit from inhaled corticosteroids.
10. Acute exacerbations of COPD have a significant impact on disease progression and mortality. Treatment of acute exacerbations includes intensification of bronchodilator therapy and a short course of systemic corticosteroids.
11. Antimicrobial therapy should be used during acute exacerbations of COPD if the patient exhibits at least two of the following: increased dyspnea, increased sputum volume, and increased sputum purulence.

1 Chronic obstructive pulmonary disease (COPD) is a common lung disease characterized by airflow limitation that is not fully reversible and is both chronic and progressive.[1] COPD is preventable and treatable and causes significant extrapulmonary effects that contribute to disease severity in a subset of patients. The prevalence and mortality of COPD have increased substantially over the past 2 decades. Currently, COPD is the third leading cause of death in the United States, with 6/3% of adults reporting a physician diagnosis of COPD.[2] By 2020, it is estimated that COPD will rank fifth in burden of disease and third as a cause of death throughout the world.

Although national guidelines for management have been available for over 2 decades, questions have been raised concerning their quality and supporting evidence. In order to standardize the care of patients with COPD and present evidence-based recommendations, the National Heart, Lung, and Blood Institute (NHLBI) and the World Health Organization (WHO) launched the Global Initiative for Chronic Obstructive Lung Disease (GOLD) in 2001. This report was most recently revised in December 2013.[1] The goals of the GOLD organization are to increase awareness of COPD and reduce morbidity and mortality associated with the disease. International guidelines have also been developed through a collaborative effort of the American College of Physicians (ACP), the American College of Chest Physicians (ACCP), the American Thoracic Society (ATS), and the European Respiratory Society (ERS) and are widely available.[3] These two guidelines are generally concordant in their recommendations.

COPD is differentiated from asthma in that the airflow limitation that is present is not fully reversible. In a subset of patients, it is fixed with minimal improvement in response to a bronchodilator or with optimal treatment. However, the natural course of the disease is quite variable among patients. The chronic and progressive nature of COPD is associated with an abnormal inflammatory response of the lungs to noxious particles or gases.[1] Nonetheless, COPD is preventable and treatable. In recent years, there has been an increased appreciation for the impact of the systemic consequences of chronic inflammatory diseases, including COPD, and for the impact of comorbidities in individual patients that can complicate COPD management.

For many years, clinicians and researchers have exhibited a nihilistic attitude toward the value of treatments for COPD. This was based on the paucity of effective therapies, the destructive nature of the condition, and the fact that the common etiology is cigarette smoking, a modifiable health risk. There is now a renewed interest in evaluating the value of treatments and prevention based on the availability of new therapeutic options for pharmacotherapy and guidelines based on evidence. The international guidelines emphasize the terms *preventable* and *treatable* to support a positive approach to managing the patient with COPD. Support is also reflected in the availability of research funding to improve understanding about this disease and its management. This includes NHLBI funding of Specialized Centers of Clinically Oriented Research (SCCOR) programs in COPD that have an objective to promote multidisciplinary research on clinically relevant questions enabling basic science findings to be more rapidly applied to clinical problems.[4]

2 The term *COPD* has historically been used to describe various pulmonary diseases with a fixed component of airflow limitation. The two principal conditions are chronic bronchitis and emphysema. Chronic bronchitis is associated with chronic or recurrent excessive mucus secretion into the bronchial tree with cough that is present on most days for at least 3 months of the year for at least 2 consecutive years in a patient in whom other causes of chronic cough have been excluded.[3] While chronic bronchitis is defined in clinical terms, emphysema is defined in terms of anatomic pathology. Emphysema historically was defined on histologic examination at autopsy. Because this histologic definition is of limited clinical value, emphysema also has been defined as abnormal permanent enlargement of the airspaces distal to the terminal bronchioles accompanied by destruction of their walls, yet without obvious fibrosis.[3]

Differentiating COPD as either chronic bronchitis or emphysema as descriptive subsets of COPD is no longer considered relevant. This is based on the observation that the majority of COPD is caused by a common risk factor (cigarette smoking) and most patients exhibit features of both chronic bronchitis and emphysema. Currently, emphasis is placed on the pathophysiologic features of small airways disease and parenchymal destruction as contributors to chronic airflow limitation. Most patients with COPD demonstrate features of both chronic bronchitis and emphysema. Chronic inflammation affects the integrity of the airways and causes damage and destruction of the parenchymal structures. The underlying problem is persistent exposure to noxious particles or gases that sustain the inflammatory response. The airways of both the lung and the parenchyma are susceptible to inflammation, and the result is the chronic airflow limitation that characterizes COPD (see Fig. 16-1).

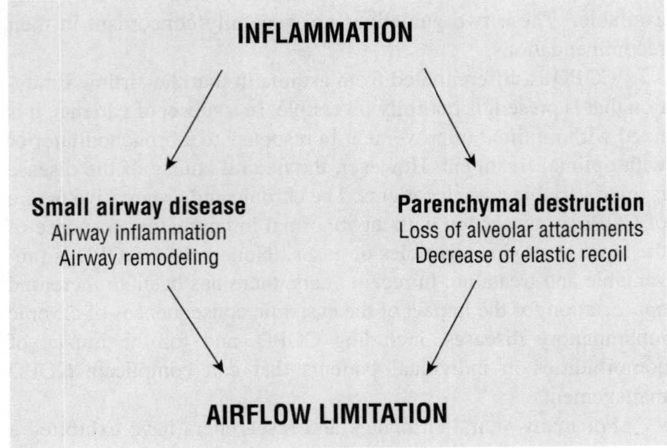

FIGURE 16-1 Mechanisms for developing chronic airflow limitation in COPD. *(From reference 1.)*

EPIDEMIOLOGY

The true prevalence of COPD is likely underreported in the United States. Data from the National Health Interview Survey in 2001 indicate that 12.1 million people over age 25 years have COPD.[5] Over 9 million of these individuals have chronic bronchitis; the remaining number have emphysema or a combination of both diseases. According to national surveys, the true prevalence of people with symptoms of chronic airflow obstruction may exceed 24 million.[6] The burden may be even greater because more than one third of adults in the United States reported respiratory complaints compatible with symptomatic COPD in some surveys.[7]

3 COPD is the fourth leading cause of death in the United States, exceeded only by cancer, heart disease, and cerebrovascular accidents. In 2005, COPD accounted for 126,005 deaths in the United States, representing 1 in every 20 deaths. Deaths attributed to COPD increased 8% from 2000 to 2005.[8] It is the only leading cause of death to increase over the past 30 years and is projected to be the third leading cause by 2020.[9] Overall, the mortality rate is higher in males; however, the female death rate has doubled over the past 25 years, and the number of female deaths exceeded male deaths in each year since 2000. The mortality rate is higher in whites compared with that in blacks.[9]

Cigarette smoking is the primary cause of COPD and, although the prevalence of cigarette smoking has declined compared with 1965, approximately 25% of individuals in the United States currently smoke. The trend of increasing COPD mortality likely reflects the long latency period between smoking exposure and complications associated with COPD.

The mortality of COPD is significant; however, morbidity associated with the disease also has a significant impact on patients, their families, and the healthcare system. COPD represents the second leading cause of disability in the United States. In the last 20 years, COPD has been responsible for nearly 50 million hospital visits nationwide.[10] In recent years, a diagnosis of COPD accounts for over 15 million physician office visits, 1.5 million emergency room visits, and 700,000 hospitalizations annually. A survey by the American Lung Association revealed that among COPD patients, 51% reported that their condition limits their ability to work, 70% were limited in normal physical activity, 56% were limited in performing household chores, and 50% reported that sleep was affected adversely.[11]

The economic impact of COPD continues to increase as well. It was estimated at $23 billion in 2000 and rose to $37.2 billion in 2004, including $20.9 billion in direct costs and $16.3 billion in indirect morbidity and mortality costs.[9,12] By 2020, COPD will be the fifth most burdensome disease, as measured by disability-adjusted life years lost due to illness. The cost of care for COPD patients is high compared with that for patients without the disease. There is a relationship among the severity of COPD, resources consumed, and the costs of care.[13]

ETIOLOGY

4 Cigarette smoking is the most common risk factor and accounts for 85% to 90% of cases of COPD.[1] Components of tobacco smoke activate inflammatory cells, which produce and release the inflammatory mediators characteristic of COPD. Smokers are 12 to 13 times more likely to die from COPD than nonsmokers.[14] Although the risk is lower in pipe and cigar smokers, it is still higher than in nonsmokers. Age of starting, total pack-years, and current smoking status are predictive of COPD mortality.

However, only 15% to 20% of all smokers go on to develop COPD, and not all smokers who have equivalent smoking histories develop the same degree of pulmonary impairment, suggesting

TABLE 16-1 Risk Factors for Development of Chronic Obstructive Pulmonary Disease (COPD)

Exposures	Host Factors
Environmental tobacco smoke	Genetic predisposition (AAT deficiency)
Occupational dusts and chemicals	Airway hyperresponsiveness
Air pollution	Impaired lung growth

that other host and environmental factors contribute to the degree of lung dysfunction. Nevertheless, the rate of loss of lung function is determined primarily by smoking status and history.[3] Children and spouses of smokers have increased risk of developing significant pulmonary dysfunction through passive smoking, also known as *environmental tobacco smoke* or *secondhand smoke*.

In addition to cigarette smoking, COPD is attributed to a combination of risk factors that results in lung injury and tissue destruction. Risk factors can be divided into host factors and environmental factors (Table 16-1), and, commonly, the interaction between these risks leads to expression of the disease. Host factors, such as genetic predisposition, may not be modifiable but are important for identifying patients at high risk of developing the disease.

Environmental factors, such as tobacco smoke and occupational dust and chemicals, are modifiable factors that, if avoided, may reduce the risk of disease development. Environmental exposures associated with COPD are particles that are inhaled by the individual, which result in inflammation and cell injury. Exposure to multiple environmental toxins increases the risk of COPD. Thus, the total burden of inhaled particles (e.g., cigarette smoke as well as occupational and environmental particles and pollutants) can play a significant role in the development of COPD. In such cases, it is helpful to assess an individual's total burden of inhaled particles. For example, an individual who smokes and works in a textile factory has a higher total burden of inhaled particles than an individual who smokes and has no occupational exposure.

In nonindustrialized countries, occupational exposures may be a more common risk than cigarette smoking. These exposures include dust and chemicals such as vapors, irritants, and fumes. Reduced lung function and deaths from COPD are higher for individuals who work in gold and coal mining, in the glass or ceramic industries with exposure to silica dust, and in jobs that expose them to cotton dust or grain dust, toluene diisocyanate, or asbestos. Other occupational risk factors include chronic exposure to open cooking or heating fires.

It is unclear whether air pollution alone is a significant risk factor for the development of COPD in smokers and nonsmokers with normal lung function. However, in individuals with existing pulmonary dysfunction, significant air pollution worsens symptoms. As evidence for this, emergency department visits are increased during higher-intensity periods of air pollution.

Individuals exposed to the same environmental risk factors do not have the same chance of developing COPD, suggesting that host factors play an important role in pathogenesis.[1,3] While many not-yet-identified genes may influence the risk of developing COPD, the best documented genetic factor is a hereditary deficiency of α_1-antitrypsin (AAT). AAT-associated emphysema is an example of a pure genetic disorder inherited in an autosomal recessive pattern. Inheritance is sometimes described as autosomal codominant by some researchers, because heterozygotes can also have decreased concentrations of AAT enzyme.[15] The consequences of AAT deficiency are discussed in the following section as protease–antiprotease imbalance. True AAT deficiency accounts for less than 1% of COPD cases.[3]

AAT is a 42 kDa plasma protein that is synthesized in hepatocytes. A primary role of AAT is to protect cells, especially those in the lung, from destruction by elastase released by neutrophils. In fact, AAT may be responsible for 90% of the inhibition of this destructive enzyme.[16] In individuals with the most common allele (M), plasma levels of AAT are approximately 20 to 50 μmol (100 to 350 mg/dL). The protective effect of AAT in the lungs is significantly diminished when plasma levels are less than 11 μmol (80 mg/dL).[16] AAT is an acute-phase reactant, and the serum concentration can be quite variable.

Several types of AAT deficiency have been identified and are due to mutations in the AAT gene. Two main gene variants, S and Z, have been identified. For patients who are homozygous with the S variant, AAT levels are at least 60% of those of normal individuals. These patients usually do not have an increased risk of COPD compared with normal individuals. Patients with homozygous Z deficiency (ZZ) represent 95% of clinical cases[15] and have AAT levels that are 10% of those of normal individuals, while patients with heterozygous Z variant (SZ) have levels closer to 40% of those of normal individuals. Homozygous Z patients have a higher risk of developing COPD compared with heterozygous Z patients. A history of cigarette smoking increases this risk. A small number of patients have a null phenotype and are at high risk for developing emphysema because they produce virtually no AAT.

Patients with AAT deficiency develop COPD at an early age (20 to 50 years) primarily owing to an accelerated decline in lung function. Compared with an average annual decline in forced expiratory volume in 1 second (FEV_1) of 25 mL/y in healthy nonsmokers, patients with homozygous Z deficiency have been reported to have declines of 54 mL/y for nonsmokers and 108 mL/y for current smokers. Effective diagnosis is dependent on clinical suspicion, diagnostic testing of serum concentrations, and genotype confirmation.[15] Patients developing COPD at an early age or those with a strong family history of COPD should be screened for AAT deficiency. If the concentration is low, genotype testing (DNA) should be performed.

Other genes have been implicated with increased risk of developing COPD, including chromosome 2q, transforming growth factor β_1, microsomal epoxide hydrolase 1, and tumor necrosis factor-α (TNF-α). However, there are no definite conclusions about an association other than AAT. One genetic factor that may reduce the risk of developing COPD is a polymorphism in the gene encoding for matrix metalloproteinase 12 (MMP12). A cohort of smokers with the polymorphism exhibited a lower risk for developing COPD (0.63).[17]

Two additional host factors that may influence the risk of COPD include airway hyperresponsiveness and lung growth. Individuals with airway hyperresponsiveness to various inhaled particles may have an accelerated decline in lung function compared with those without airway hyperresponsiveness. Additionally, individuals who do not attain maximal lung growth owing to low-birth-weight, prematurity at birth, or childhood illnesses may be at risk for COPD in the future.[1]

PATHOPHYSIOLOGY

COPD is characterized by chronic inflammatory changes that lead to destructive changes and the development of chronic airflow limitation. The inflammatory process is widespread and not only involves the airways but also extends to the pulmonary vasculature and lung parenchyma. The inflammation of COPD is often referred to as *neutrophilic* in nature, but macrophages and CD8+ lymphocytes also play major roles.[18–20] The inflammatory cells release a variety of chemical mediators, of which TNF-α, interleukin 8 (IL-8), and leukotriene B_4 (LTB_4) play major roles.[1,21] The actions of these cells and mediators are complementary and redundant, leading to the widespread destructive changes. The stimulus for activation of inflammatory cells and mediators is an exposure to noxious particles

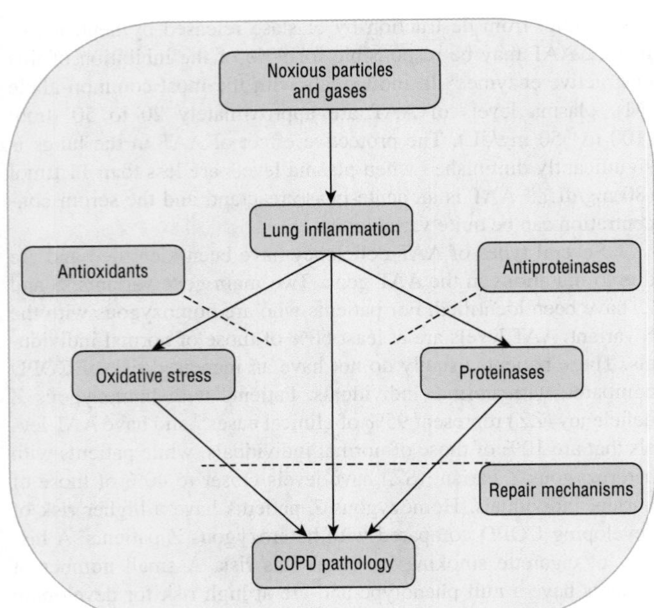

FIGURE 16-2 Pathogenesis of COPD.

and gas through inhalation. The most common etiologic factor is exposure to environmental tobacco smoke, although other chronic inhalational exposures can lead to similar inflammatory changes.

Other processes that have been proposed to play a major role in the pathogenesis of COPD include oxidative stress and an imbalance between aggressive and protective defense systems in the lungs (proteases and antiproteases).[18] These processes may be the result of ongoing inflammation or occur as a result of environmental pressures and exposures (Fig. 16-2).

An altered interaction between oxidants and antioxidants present in the airways is responsible for the increased oxidative stress present in COPD. Increases in markers (e.g., hydrogen peroxide and nitric oxide) of oxidants are seen in the epithelial lining fluid.[1] The increased oxidants generated by cigarette smoke react with and damage various proteins and lipids, leading to cell and tissue damage. Oxidants also promote inflammation directly and exacerbate the protease–antiprotease imbalance by inhibiting antiprotease activity.

The consequences of an imbalance between proteases and antiproteases in the lungs were described over 40 years ago when the hereditary deficiency of the protective antiprotease AAT was discovered to result in an increased risk of developing emphysema prematurely. This enzyme (AAT) is responsible for inhibiting several protease enzymes, including neutrophil elastase. In the presence of unopposed activity, elastase attacks elastin, a major component of alveolar walls.[1]

In the inherited form of emphysema, there is an absolute deficiency of AAT. In cigarette smoking–associated emphysema, the imbalance is likely associated with increased protease activity or reduced activity of antiproteases. Activated inflammatory cells release several proteases other than AAT, including cathepsins and metalloproteinases (MMPs). In addition, oxidative stress reduces antiprotease (or protective) activity.

It is helpful to differentiate inflammation occurring in COPD from that present in asthma because the response to antiinflammatory therapy differs. The inflammatory cells that predominate differ between the two conditions, with neutrophils playing a major role in COPD and eosinophils and mast cells in asthma. Mediators of inflammation also differ leukotriene B_4 (LTB_4), interleukin 8 (IL-8), and tumor necrosis factor alpha (TNF-α) predominating in COPD, compared with leukotriene D_4 (LTD_4), interleukin 4 (IL-4),

TABLE 16-2 Features of Inflammation in COPD Compared with Asthma

	COPD	Asthma
Cells	Neutrophils Large increase in macrophages Increase in CD8+ T lymphocytes	Eosinophils Small increase in macrophages Increase in CD4+ Th2 lymphocytes Activation of mast cells
Mediators	LTB_4 IL-8 TNF-α	LTD_4 IL-4, IL-5 (Plus many others)
Consequences	Squamous metaplasia of epithelium Parenchymal destruction Mucus metaplasia Glandular enlargement	Fragile epithelium Thickening of basement membrane Mucus metaplasia Glandular enlargement
Response to treatment	Glucocorticosteroids have variable effect.	Glucocorticosteroids inhibit inflammation.

and interleukin 5 (IL-5) among the numerous mediators modulating inflammation in asthma.[1] Characteristics of inflammation for the two diseases are summarized in Table 16-2.

Pathologic changes of COPD are widespread, affecting large and small airways, lung parenchyma, and the pulmonary vasculature.[1] An inflammatory exudate is often present that leads to an increase in the number and size of goblet cells and mucus glands. Mucus secretion is increased, and ciliary motility is impaired. There is also a thickening of smooth muscle and connective tissue in the airways. Inflammation is present in central and peripheral airways. The chronic inflammation results in a repeated injury and repair process that leads to scarring and fibrosis. Diffuse airway narrowing is present and is more prominent in smaller peripheral airways. The decrease in FEV_1 is attributed to the presence of inflammation in the airways, while the blood gas abnormalities result from impaired gas transfer due to parenchymal damage.

Parenchymal changes affect the gas-exchanging units of the lungs, including the alveoli and pulmonary capillaries. The distribution of destructive changes varies depending on the etiology. Most commonly, smoking-related disease results in centrilobular emphysema that primarily affects respiratory bronchioles. Panlobular emphysema is seen in AAT deficiency and extends to the alveolar ducts and sacs.

The vascular changes of COPD include a thickening of pulmonary vessels and often are present early in the disease. Increased pulmonary pressures early in the disease are due to hypoxic vasoconstriction of pulmonary arteries. If persistent, the presence of chronic inflammation may lead to endothelial dysfunction of the pulmonary arteries. Later, structural changes lead to an increase in pulmonary pressures, especially during exercise. In severe COPD, secondary pulmonary hypertension leads to the development of right-sided heart failure.

Mucus hypersecretion is present early in the course of the disease and is associated with an increased number and size of mucus-producing cells. The presence of chronic inflammation perpetuates the process, although the resulting airflow obstruction and chronic airflow limitation may be reversible or irreversible. The various causes of airflow obstruction are summarized in Table 16-3.

Thoracic overinflation is a relevant feature in the pathophysiology of COPD, because it is a central factor in causing dyspnea. Chronic airflow obstruction leads to air trapping, resulting in thoracic hyperinflation that can be detected on chest radiograph. This problem results in several dynamic changes in the chest, including

TABLE 16-3 Etiology of Airflow Limitation in COPD

Reversible
Presence of mucus and inflammatory cells and mediators in bronchial secretions
Bronchial smooth muscle contraction in peripheral and central airways
Dynamic hyperinflation during exercise
Irreversible
Fibrosis and narrowing of airways
Reduced elastic recoil with loss of alveolar surface area
Destruction of alveolar support with reduced patency of small airways

flattening of diaphragmatic muscles. Under normal circumstances, the diaphragms are dome-shaped muscles tethered at the base of the lungs. When the diaphragm contracts, the muscle becomes shorter and flatter, which creates the negative inspiratory force through which air flows into the lung during inspiration. In the presence of thoracic hyperinflation, the diaphragmatic muscle is placed at a disadvantage and is a less efficient muscle of ventilation. The increased work required by diaphragmatic contractions predisposes the patient to muscle fatigue, especially during periods of exacerbations.

The other consequence of thoracic hyperinflation is a change in lung volumes. For patients with COPD who exhibit thoracic hyperinflation, there is an increase in the functional residual capacity (FRC), which is the amount of air left in the lung after exhalation at rest. Therefore, these patients are breathing at higher lung volumes, which perturbs gas exchange. In addition, the increased FRC limits the inspiratory reserve capacity, which is the amount of air that the patient can inhale to fill the lungs. The increased FRC also limits the duration of inhalation time, and this has been associated with an increase in dyspnea complaints by patients.[22] Drug therapy for COPD, especially bronchodilators, can reduce thoracic hyperinflation by reducing airflow obstruction. This may partially explain the improvement in symptoms reported by patients with COPD despite minimal improvements in lung function with drug therapy.

Airflow limitation is assessed through spirometry, which represents the "gold standard" for diagnosing and monitoring COPD. The hallmark of COPD is a reduction in the ratio of FEV_1 to forced vital capacity (FVC) to less than 70%.[1,3] The FEV_1 generally is reduced, except in very mild disease, and the rate of FEV_1 decline is greater in COPD patients compared with that in normal subjects.

The impact of the numerous pathologic changes in the lung perturbs the normal gas-exchange and protective functions of the lung. Ultimately, these are exhibited through the common symptoms of COPD, including dyspnea and a chronic cough productive of sputum. As the disease progresses, abnormalities in gas exchange lead to hypoxemia and/or hypercapnia, although there often is not a strong relationship between pulmonary function and arterial blood gas (ABG) results.

Significant changes in ABGs usually are not present until the FEV_1 is less than 1 L.[1] In these patients, hypoxemia and hypercapnia can become chronic problems. Initially, when hypoxemia is present, it usually is associated with exercise. However, as the disease progresses, hypoxemia at rest develops. Patients with severe COPD can have a low arterial oxygen tension (pressure exerted by oxygen gas in arterial blood [Pa_{O_2}] = 45 to 60 mm Hg) and an elevated arterial carbon dioxide tension (pressure exerted by carbon dioxide gas in arterial blood [Pa_{CO_2}] = 50 to 60 mm Hg). The hypoxemia is attributed to hypoventilation ($\dot{V}$) of lung tissue relative to perfusion ($\dot{Q}$) of the area. This low $\dot{V}/\dot{Q}$ ratio will progress over a period of several years, resulting in a consistent decline in the Pa_{O_2}. Some COPD patients lose the ability to increase the rate or depth of respiration in response to persistent hypoxemia. Although this is not completely understood, the decreased ventilatory drive may be due to abnormal peripheral or central respiratory receptor responses. This relative hypoventilation subsequently leads to hypercapnia. In this case, the central respiratory response to a chronically increased Pa_{CO_2} can be blunted. These changes in Pa_{O_2} and Pa_{CO_2} are subtle and progress over a period of many years. As a result, the pH usually is nearly normal because the kidneys compensate by retaining bicarbonate. If acute respiratory distress develops, such as might be seen in pneumonia or a COPD exacerbation with impending respiratory failure, the Pa_{CO_2} may rise sharply, and the patient presents with an uncompensated respiratory acidosis.

The consequences of long-standing COPD and chronic hypoxemia include the development of secondary pulmonary hypertension that progresses slowly if appropriate treatment of COPD is not initiated. Pulmonary hypertension is the most common cardiovascular complication of COPD and can result in cor pulmonale, or right-sided heart failure.[23]

The elevated pulmonary artery pressures are attributed to vasoconstriction (in response to chronic hypoxemia), vascular remodeling, and loss of pulmonary capillary beds. If elevated pulmonary pressures are sustained, cor pulmonale can develop, characterized by hypertrophy of the right ventricle in response to increases in pulmonary vascular resistance.

The risks of cor pulmonale include venous stasis with the potential for thrombosis and pulmonary embolism. Another important systemic consequence of COPD is a loss of skeletal muscle mass and general decline in the overall health status.

While airway inflammation is prominent for patients with COPD, there is also evidence of systemic inflammation.[24] A consequence is widespread skeletal muscle dysfunction, especially in the leg muscles involved with ambulation.[25] The systemic manifestations can have devastating effects on overall health status and comorbidities. These include cardiovascular events associated with ischemia, cachexia, osteoporosis, anemia, and muscle wasting. There is some interest in the role of measuring C-reactive protein as a parameter to assess systemic inflammation and its impact on COPD severity; however, it is premature to recommend this strategy currently.[26]

PATHOPHYSIOLOGY OF EXACERBATION

The natural history of COPD is characterized by recurrent exacerbations associated with increased symptoms and a decline in overall health status. An exacerbation is defined as a change in the patient's baseline symptoms (dyspnea, cough, or sputum production) beyond day-to-day variability sufficient to warrant a change in management.[1,3] Exacerbations have a significant impact on the natural course of COPD and occur more frequently for patients with more severe chronic disease. Because many patients experience chronic symptoms, the diagnosis of an exacerbation is based, in part, on subjective measures and clinical judgment. Repeated exacerbations, especially those requiring hospitalization, are associated with an increased mortality risk.

There are limited data about pathology during exacerbations owing to the nature of the disease and the condition of patients. However, inflammatory mediators including neutrophils and eosinophils are increased in the sputum. Chronic airflow limitation is a feature of COPD and may not change remarkably even during an exacerbation.[1] The lung hyperinflation present in chronic COPD is worsened during an exacerbation, which contributes to worsening dyspnea and poor gas exchange.

The primary physiologic change is often a worsening of ABG results due to poor gas exchange and increased muscle fatigue. For a patient experiencing a severe exacerbation, profound hypoxemia and hypercapnia can be accompanied by respiratory acidosis and respiratory failure.

CLINICAL PRESENTATION

Symptoms
- Chronic cough
- Sputum production
- Dyspnea

Exposure to Risk Factors
- Tobacco smoke
- α_1-Antitrypsin deficiency
- Occupational hazards

Physical Examination
- Cyanosis of mucosal membranes
- Barrel chest
- Increased resting respiratory rate
- Shallow breathing
- Pursed lips during expiration
- Use of accessory respiratory muscles

Diagnostic Tests
- Spirometry with reversibility testing
- Radiograph of chest
- Arterial blood gas (not routine)

CLINICAL PRESENTATION

The diagnosis of COPD is made based on the patient's symptoms, including cough, sputum production, and dyspnea, and a history of exposure to risk factors such as tobacco smoke and occupational exposures. Patients may have these symptoms for several years before dyspnea develops and often will not seek medical attention until dyspnea is significant. A diagnosis of COPD should be considered for any patient, age 40 years or older, with persistent or progressive dyspnea, with chronic cough productive of sputum, and who exhibits an unusual or abnormal decline in activity, especially in the presence of positive cigarette smoke exposure. In addition, the presence of genetic factors, including AAT deficiency, and occupational exposures should be evaluated because approximately 15% of patients with COPD do not have a history of cigarette smoking.

The presence of airflow limitation should be confirmed with spirometry. Spirometry represents a comprehensive assessment of lung volumes and capacities. The hallmark of COPD is an FEV_1:FVC ratio of less than 70%, which indicates airway obstruction, and a postbronchodilator FEV_1 of less than 80% of predicted confirms the presence of airflow limitation that is not fully reversible.[1] There is an increased awareness that the use of a fixed ratio of less than 70% may be problematic because normal aging may affect this result; however, it continues to be the current standard. An improvement in FEV_1 of less than 12% following inhalation of a rapid-acting bronchodilator is considered to be evidence of irreversible airflow obstruction. Reversibility of airflow limitation is measured by a bronchodilator challenge, which is described in Table 16-4. The use of peak expiratory flow measurements is not adequate for the diagnosis of COPD owing to low specificity and the high degree of effort dependence; however, a low peak expiratory flow is consistent with COPD. A comprehensive discussion about spirometry can be found in Chapter 15.

Spirometry combined with a physical examination improves the diagnostic accuracy of COPD.[7] Spirometry also is useful to determine the severity of airflow limitation. Patients with all levels of severity of COPD exhibit the hallmark finding of airflow obstruction, that is, a reduction in the FEV_1:FVC ratio to less than 70%. FVC is the total amount of air exhaled after a maximal inhalation. Currently, the GOLD consensus guidelines suggest a four-grade classification of airflow limitation (see Table 16-5). Patients in GOLD 3 or 4 have the most significant airflow limitation and are at the highest risk for future exacerbations, while patients in GOLD 1 and 2 have less airflow limitation and are at lower risk for exacerbations.

Dyspnea is typically the most troublesome complaint for the patient with COPD and often is the stimulus for the patient seeking

TABLE 16-4 Procedures for Reversibility Testing

Preparation

Tests should be performed when patients are clinically stable and free from respiratory infection.

Patients should not have taken inhaled short-acting bronchodilators in the previous 6 hours, long-acting β-agonists in the previous 12 hours, or sustained-release theophylline in the previous 24 hours.

Spirometry

FEV_1 should be measured before bronchodilator is given.

Bronchodilators can be given by either metered-dose inhaler or nebulization.

Usual doses are 400 mcg of β-agonist, 80 mcg of anticholinergic, or the two combined.

FEV_1 should be measured again 30–45 minutes after bronchodilator is given.

Results

An increase in FEV_1 that is both greater than 200 mL and 12% above the prebronchodilator FEV_1 is considered significant.

TABLE 16-5 Classification of Severity of Airflow Obstruction (Based on Postbronchodilator FEV_1)

I: mild
$FEV_1/FVC < 70\%$
$FEV_1 \geq 80\%$
With or without symptoms

II: moderate
$FEV_1/FVC < 70\%$
$50\% < FEV_1 < 80\%$
With or without symptoms

III: severe
$FEV_1/FVC < 70\%$
$30\% < FEV_1 < 50\%$
With or without symptoms

IV: very severe
$FEV_1/FVC < 70\%$
$FEV_1 < 30\%$

From reference 1.

TABLE 16-6 Modified Medical Research Council (MRC) Dyspnea Scale

Grade 0	No dyspnea	Not troubled by breathlessness except with strenuous exercise
Grade 1	Slight dyspnea	Troubled by shortness of breath when hurrying on a level surface or walking up a slight hill
Grade 2	Moderate dyspnea	Walks slower than normal based on age on a level surface due to breathlessness or has to stop for breath when walking on level surface at own pace
Grade 3	Severe dyspnea	Stops for breath after walking 100 yards or after a few minutes on a level surface
Grade 4	Very severe dyspnea	Too breathless to leave the house or becomes breathless while dressing or undressing

From reference 2.

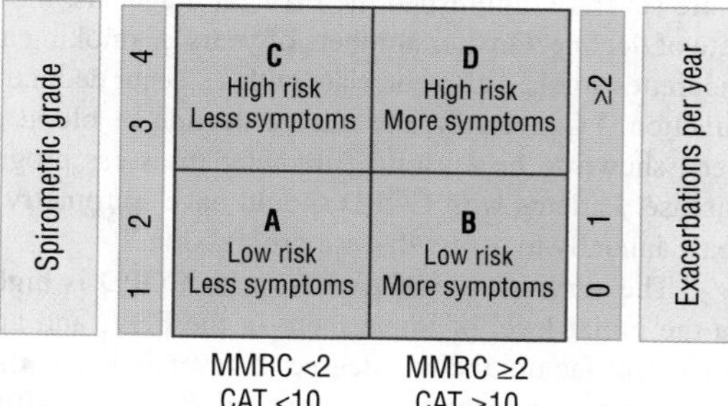

FIGURE 16-3 Groups of COPD classification.

medical attention. It can impair exercise performance and functional capacity and is frequently associated with depression and anxiety. Together, these have a significant effect on health-related quality of life.[22] As a subjective symptom, dyspnea is often difficult for the clinician to assess. Various tools are available to evaluate the severity of dyspnea. The modified Medical Research Council (mMRC) scale is commonly employed and categorizes dyspnea grades from 0 to 4 (see Table 16-6).[27] The effect of COPD on overall well-being can be assessed using the COPD Assessment Test (CAT), which includes eight statements about symptoms and activities. The patient scores each statement on a scale of 0 to 5 and the impact of COPD is assessed by the cumulative score (see Table 16-7).[28]

Previously, guidelines have defined disease severity solely by spirometry. Observations that patients with similar spirometric parameters exhibit variations in symptom severity and risk of adverse health events, such as exacerbations, have led to a revision in severity classification. In order to incorporate multiple factors that contribute to disease risk, the revised GOLD consensus guidelines recommend that three separate parameters be assessed when classifying disease severity. Parameters include an assessment of airflow limitation by spirometry, measurement of symptom severity, and an assessment of exacerbation frequency. Symptom assessment should be measured using either CAT or mMRC. Frequency of exacerbations can be assessed either by predicted risk of future exacerbations based on classification of airflow limitation or through a review of exacerbation history for the past 12 months. Patients with at least two exacerbations in the last 12 months would be considered high risk for future exacerbations. If both methods of exacerbation risk are assessed, the method with the highest risk result should be used to classify the patient (see Fig. 16-3).

While a physical examination is appropriate in the diagnosis and assessment of COPD, most patients who present in the milder stages of COPD will have a normal physical examination. In later stages of the disease, when airflow limitation is severe, patients may have cyanosis of mucosal membranes, development of "barrel chest" due to hyperinflation of the lungs, an increased respiratory rate and shallow breathing, and changes in breathing mechanics such as pursing of the lips to help with expiration or use of accessory respiratory muscles.

TABLE 16-7 Staging Acute Exacerbations of COPD[a]

Mild (type 1)	One cardinal symptom[a] plus at least one of the following: URTI[b] within 5 days, fever without other explanation, increased wheezing, increased cough, increase in respiratory or heart rate >20% above baseline
Moderate (type 2)	Two cardinal symptoms[a]
Severe (type 3)	Three cardinal symptoms[a]

[a]Cardinal symptoms include worsening of dyspnea, increase in sputum volume, and increase in sputum purulence.
[b]URTI, upper respiratory tract infection.

Classification Based on Severity

In 2011, the GOLD guidelines included a modified system for classifying COPD based on severity. As discussed above, the new system is based on numerous factors that have a significant impact on the patient, including the degree of airflow obstruction, the frequency and severity of symptoms, and the frequency of exacerbations (see Fig. 16-3). A patient can first be classified according to the severity of airflow obstruction into grades ranging from 1 to 4 (Table 16-5). Then the patient is placed into a group (A, B, C, or D) based on the impact of symptoms and the risk for future exacerbations. The extent of symptoms is assessed using a validated symptom assessment tool (e.g., the mMRC or the CAT). Finally, the risk for an exacerbation is based on previous exacerbations. A patient is categorized based on a history of less than two annual exacerbations, or two or more. This new classification system by group provides an appropriate emphasis for each of the parameters included (see Fig. 16-3). Another advantage is that classifying patients according to these groups informs treatment decisions.

Prognosis

For the patient with COPD, the combination of impaired lung function and recurrent exacerbations promotes a clinical scenario characterized by dyspnea, reduced exercise tolerance and physical activity, and deconditioning. These factors lead to disease progression, poor quality of life, possible disability, and premature mortality.[29] COPD is ultimately a fatal disease if it progresses and advanced directives and end-of-life care options are appropriate to consider. The primary causes of death of patients with COPD include respiratory failure, cardiovascular events or diseases, and lung cancer.[30]

The FEV_1 is the most important prognostic indicator for a patient with COPD. The average rate of decline of FEV_1 is the most useful objective measure to assess the course of COPD. The average rate of decline in FEV_1 for healthy, nonsmoking patients owing to age alone is 25 to 30 mL/y. The rate of decline for smokers is steeper, especially for heavy smokers compared with light smokers. The decline in pulmonary function is a steady curvilinear path. The more severely diminished the FEV_1 at diagnosis, the steeper is the rate of decline. Greater numbers of years of smoking and number of cigarettes smoked also correlate with a steeper decline in pulmonary function.[27] Conversely, the rate of decline of blood gases has not been shown to be a useful parameter to assess progression of the disease. Patients with COPD should have spirometry performed at least annually to assess disease progression.[31]

The survival rate of patients with COPD is highly correlated to the initial level of impairment in the FEV_1 and age. Other less important factors include degree of reversibility with bronchodilators, resting pulse, perceived physical disability, diffusing capacity for carbon monoxide (D_LCO), cor pulmonale, and blood gas abnormalities. A rapid decline in pulmonary function tests indicates a poor prognosis. Median survival is approximately 10 years when the FEV_1 is 1.4 L, 4 years when the FEV_1 is 1 L, and about 2 years when the FEV_1 is 0.5 L.

While ABG measurements are important, they do not carry the prognostic value of pulmonary function tests. Measurement of ABGs is more useful for patients with severe disease and is recommended for all patients with an FEV_1 of less than 40% of predicted or those with signs of respiratory failure or right-sided heart failure.[1]

Asthma is usually differentiated from COPD based on the patient's medical history, risk factors, and improvements on postbronchodilator spirometry; however, in some cases, asthma patients exhibit COPD-like features and COPD patients exhibit asthma-like features. It is also possible for the two conditions to coexist.

CLINICAL PRESENTATION OF COPD EXACERBATION

Because of the subjective nature of defining an exacerbation of COPD, the criteria used among clinicians vary widely; however, most rely on a change in one or more of the following clinical findings: worsening symptoms of dyspnea, increase in sputum volume, or increase in sputum purulence. Acute exacerbations have a significant impact of the economics of treating COPD as well, estimated at 35% to 45% of the total costs of the disease in some settings.[32]

A widely accepted definition of an exacerbation is that it is an event in the natural course of COPD that is characterized by a worsening in baseline dyspnea, cough, and/or sputum that is beyond the normal day-to-day variation, is acute in onset, and may warrant a change in regular medication. With an exacerbation, patients using rapid-acting bronchodilators may report an increase in the frequency of use. Exacerbations are commonly staged as mild, moderate, or severe according to the criteria summarized in Table 16-7.[33]

An important complication of a severe exacerbation is acute respiratory failure. In the emergency department or hospital, an ABG usually is obtained to assess the severity of an exacerbation. The diagnosis of acute respiratory failure in COPD is made based on an acute change in the ABGs. Defining acute respiratory failure as a Pao_2 of less than 50 mm Hg or a $Paco_2$ of greater than 50 mm Hg often may be incorrect and inadequate because these values may not represent a significant change from a patient's baseline values. A more precise definition is an acute drop in Pao_2 of 10 to 15 mm Hg or any acute increase in $Paco_2$ that decreases the serum pH to 7.3 or less. Additional acute clinical manifestations of respiratory failure include restlessness, confusion, tachycardia, diaphoresis, cyanosis, hypotension, irregular breathing, miosis, and unconsciousness.

Prognosis

COPD exacerbations are associated with significant morbidity and mortality. While mild exacerbations may be managed at home, mortality rates are higher for patients admitted to the hospital. In one study of patients hospitalized with COPD exacerbations, in-hospital mortality was 6% to 8%.[34] Many patients experiencing an exacerbation do not have a return to their baseline clinical status for several weeks, significantly affecting their quality of life. Additionally, as many as half the patients originally hospitalized for an exacerbation are readmitted within 6 months.[35]

There is good evidence that acute exacerbations of COPD have a tremendous impact on disease progression and ultimate mortality. For exacerbations requiring hospitalizations, mortality rates range from 22% to 43% after 1 year, and 36% to 49% in 2 years.[34,36,37]

TREATMENT
Chronic Obstructive Pulmonary Disease

Desired Outcome

Given the nature of COPD, a major focus in healthcare should be on prevention. However, for patients with a diagnosis of COPD, the primary goal is to prevent or minimize progression. Specific goals of management are listed in Table 16-8. The primary goal of pharmacotherapy has been relief of symptoms, including dyspnea. However, more recently there has been increased interest in the value of therapeutic interventions that reduce exacerbation frequency and severity, as well as reduce mortality. In fact, a reduction in exacerbation frequency is an important outcome measure to consider when evaluating the role and benefit of individual chronic therapies used in COPD management.

Optimally, these goals can be accomplished with minimal risks or side effects. The therapy of the patient with COPD is

CLINICAL PRESENTATION Features of COPD Exacerbation

Symptoms

- Increased sputum volume
- Acutely worsening dyspnea
- Chest tightness
- Presence of purulent sputum
- Increased need for bronchodilators
- Malaise, fatigue
- Decreased exercise tolerance

Physical Examination

- Fever
- Wheezing, decreased breath sounds

Diagnostic Tests

- Sputum sample for Gram stain and culture
- Chest radiograph to evaluate for new infiltrates

TABLE 16-8 Goals of COPD Management

Prevent disease progression
Relieve symptoms
Improve exercise tolerance
Improve overall health status
Prevent and treat exacerbations
Prevent and treat complications
Reduce morbidity and mortality

multifaceted and includes pharmacologic and nonpharmacologic strategies. Appropriate measures of effectiveness of the management plan include continued smoking cessation, symptom improvement, reduction in FEV_1 decline, reduction in the number of exacerbations, improvements in physical and psychological well-being, and reduction in mortality, hospitalizations, and days lost from work.

Unfortunately, most treatments for COPD have not been shown to improve survival or to slow the progressive decline in lung function. However, many therapies do improve pulmonary function and quality of life and reduce exacerbations and duration of hospitalization. Several disease-specific quality-of-life measures are available to assess the overall efficacies of therapies for COPD, including the CAT, Chronic Respiratory Questionnaire (CRQ), and the St. George's Respiratory Questionnaire (SGRQ). These questionnaires measure the impact of various therapies on such disease variables as severity of dyspnea and level of activity. They do not measure impact of therapies on survival. While early studies of COPD therapies focused primarily on improvements in pulmonary function measurements such as FEV_1, there is a trend toward greater use of these disease-specific quality-of-life measures to evaluate the benefits of therapy on larger clinical outcomes.

General Approach to Treatment

To be effective, the clinician should address four primary components of management: assess and monitor the condition, avoid or reduce exposure to risk factors, manage stable disease, and treat exacerbations. These components are addressed through a variety of nonpharmacologic and pharmacologic approaches.

Nonpharmacologic Therapy

Patients with COPD should receive education about their disease, treatment plans, and strategies to slow progression and prevent complications.[1] Advice and counseling about smoking cessation are essential, if applicable, and should be addressed for patients in all stages of the disease. Because the natural course of the disease leads to respiratory failure, the clinician should address end-of-life decisions and advanced directives prospectively with the patient and family.[38]

Smoking Cessation

5 Smoking cessation represents the single most important intervention in preventing the development, as well as the progression, of COPD. A primary component of COPD management is avoidance of or reduced exposure to risk factors. Exposure to environmental tobacco smoke is a major risk factor, and smoking cessation is the most effective strategy to reduce the risk of developing COPD and to slow or stop disease progression. The cost-effectiveness of smoking-cessation interventions compares favorably with interventions made for other major chronic diseases.[39] The importance of smoking cessation cannot be overemphasized. Smoking cessation leads to decreased symptomatology and slows the rate of decline of pulmonary function even after significant abnormalities in pulmonary function tests have been detected (FEV_1:FVC <60%).[31] As confirmed by the Lung Health Study, smoking cessation is the only intervention proven at this time to affect long-term decline in FEV_1 and slow the progression of COPD.[40] In this 5-year prospective trial, smokers with early COPD were randomly assigned to one of the following three groups: smoking-cessation intervention plus inhaled ipratropium three times a day, smoking-cessation intervention alone, or no intervention. During an 11-year followup, the rate of decline in FEV_1 among subjects who continued to smoke was more than twice the rate in sustained quitters. Smokers who underwent smoking-cessation intervention had fewer respiratory symptoms and a smaller annual decline in FEV_1 compared with smokers who had no intervention. However, this study also demonstrated the difficulty in achieving and sustaining successful smoking cessation.

Tobacco cessation has mortality benefits beyond those related to COPD. A followup analysis of the Lung Health Study data conducted more than 14 years later demonstrated an 18% reduction in all-cause mortality in patients who received the intervention compared with usual care.[41] Intervention patients had lower death rates due to coronary artery disease (the leading cause of mortality), cardiovascular diseases, and lung cancer, although all categories did not reach clinical significance.

Every clinician has a responsibility to assist smokers in smoking-cessation efforts. A clinical practice guideline for treating tobacco dependence from the U.S. Public Health Service (PHS) was updated in 2008.[42] The major findings and recommendations of that report are summarized in Table 16-9. An earlier report from the Surgeon General in 2004 on the health consequences of smoking broadened

TABLE 16-9 Key Guideline Recommendations Regarding Tobacco Use and Dependence[42]

Tobacco dependence is a chronic disease that often requires repeated intervention and multiple attempts to quit. Effective treatments are available that can significantly improve rates of long-term abstinence.
Clinicians and healthcare delivery systems should consistently identify and document tobacco use status and treat every tobacco user.
Tobacco-dependence treatments are effective over a broad range of populations. Clinicians should encourage every patient willing to make a quit attempt to use counseling treatments and medications recommended in the guideline.
Brief tobacco-dependence treatments are effective. Clinicians should offer every patient who uses tobacco at least these brief treatments.
Individual, group, and telephone counseling are effective, and their effectiveness increases with treatment intensity. Practical counseling (problem-solving and/ or skills training) and social support are especially effective and should be employed as a part of treatment.
There are numerous effective medications for tobacco dependence, and clinicians should encourage their use by patients during a quit attempt, except when medically contraindicated or with populations in which the evidence of effectiveness is insufficient (pregnancy, smokeless tobacco users, light smokers, and adolescents). Seven first-line medications (5 nicotine and 2 non-nicotine) consistently increase long-term abstinence rates. Clinicians should also consider the use of combinations as identified in the guideline.
Counseling and medication are effective when used by themselves for treating tobacco dependence. The combination of the two is more effective than either alone. Patients should be encouraged to use both counseling and medication.
Telephone quitline counseling is effective for diverse populations and offers the advantage of broad reach. Clinicians should ensure patient access to quitlines and promote quitline use.
For a tobacco user who is currently unwilling to make a quit attempt, clinicians should use motivational treatments that have been shown to be effective in increasing future quit attempts.
Tobacco-dependence treatments are both clinically effective and highly cost-effective relative to interventions for other clinical disorders. Providing coverage for these treatments increases quit rates. Insurers and purchasers should ensure that all insurance plans include the counseling and medications identified as effective in the guideline as covered benefits.

TABLE 16-10 Five-Step Strategy for Smoking-Cessation Program (5 A's)

Ask	Use systematic approach to identify all tobacco users.
Advise	Urge all tobacco users to quit.
Assess	Determine willingness to make a cessation attempt.
Assist	Provide support for the patient to quit smoking.
Arrange	Schedule follow-up and monitor for continued abstinence.

the scope of the detrimental effects of cigarette smoking, indicating that "Smoking harms nearly every organ of the body, causing many diseases and reducing the health of smokers in general."[14]

All clinicians should take an active role in assisting patients with tobacco dependence in order to reduce the burden on the individual, his or her family, and the healthcare system. It is estimated that over 75% of smokers want to quit and that one-third have made a serious effort. Yet complete and permanent tobacco cessation is difficult.[40] Counseling that is provided by clinicians is associated with greater success rates than self-initiated efforts.[42]

The PHS guidelines recommend that clinicians take a comprehensive approach to smoking-cessation counseling. Advice should be given to smokers even if they have no symptoms of smoking-related disease or if they are receiving care for reasons unrelated to smoking. Clinicians should be persistent in their efforts because relapse is common among smokers owing to the chronic nature of dependence. Brief interventions (3 minutes) of counseling are proven effective. However, it must be recognized that the patient must be ready to stop smoking because there are several stages of decision making. Based on this, a five-step intervention program is proposed (Table 16-10).

There is strong evidence to support the use of pharmacotherapy to assist in smoking cessation. In fact, it should be offered to most patients as part of a cessation attempt. In general, available therapies will double the effectiveness of a cessation effort. Agents that are considered first line are listed in Table 16-11. The usual duration of therapy is 8 to 12 weeks, although some individuals may require longer courses of treatment. Precautions to consider before using bupropion include a history of seizures or an eating disorder. Nicotine replacement therapies are contraindicated for patients with unstable coronary artery disease, active peptic ulcers, or recent myocardial infarction or stroke. Nicotine patch, bupropion, and the combination of bupropion and the nicotine patch were compared with placebo in a controlled trial.[43] The treatment groups that received bupropion had higher rates of smoking cessation than the groups that received placebo or the nicotine patch. The addition of the nicotine patch to bupropion slightly improved the smoking-cessation rate compared with bupropion monotherapy. Recently, a new agent became available to assist in tobacco cessation attempts. Varenicline is a nicotine acetylcholine receptor partial agonist that has shown benefit in tobacco cessation.[44] It relieves physical withdrawal symptoms and reduces the rewarding properties of nicotine. Nausea and headache are the most frequent complaints associated with varenicline. Currently, varenicline has not been studied in combination with other tobacco cessation therapies. Second-line agents are less effective or associated with greater side effects; however, they may be useful in selected clinical situations. These therapies include clonidine and nortriptyline, a tricyclic antidepressant.

Behavioral modification techniques or other forms of psychotherapy also may be helpful in assisting in smoking cessation. Programs that address the many issues associated with smoking (i.e., learned behaviors, environmental influences, and chemical dependence) using a team approach are more likely to be successful. The role of alternative medicine therapies in smoking cessation is controversial. Hypnosis may aid in improving abstinence rates when added to a smoking-cessation program but appears to give little benefit when used alone. Acupuncture has not been shown to contribute to smoking cessation and is not recommended.[3]

Other Environmental Triggers

Although cigarette smoke represents the overwhelming majority of risk for developing COPD, exposure to other environmental toxins also confers risks.[45,46] Exposures to occupational dusts and fumes have been implicated as a cause of COPD in 19% of smokers and 31% of nonsmokers with COPD in the United States. In the case of known environmental hazards, primary prevention is appropriate. Policies to limit airborne exposures in the workplace and outdoors, as well as education efforts of workers and policy makers, are recommended.

Pulmonary Rehabilitation

Exercise training is beneficial in the treatment of COPD to improve exercise tolerance and to reduce symptoms of dyspnea and fatigue.[1] Pulmonary rehabilitation programs are an integral component in the management of COPD and should include exercise training along with smoking cessation, breathing exercises, optimal medical treatment, psychosocial support, and health education. Pulmonary rehabilitation has no direct effect on lung function or gas exchange. Instead, it optimizes other body systems so that the impact of poor lung function is minimized. Exercise training reduces the CNS response to dyspnea, ameliorates anxiety and depression, reduces thoracic hyperinflation, and improves skeletal muscle function.[25] High-intensity training (70% maximal workload) is possible even in advanced COPD patients, and the level of intensity improves peripheral muscle and ventilatory function. Studies have demonstrated that pulmonary rehabilitation with exercise three to seven times per week can produce long-term improvement in activities of daily living, quality of life, exercise tolerance, and dyspnea for patients with moderate-to-severe COPD.[47] Improvements in dyspnea can be achieved without concomitant improvements in spirometry. While rehabilitation programs vary based on length of program, and exercise frequency and intensity, those with longer length and more frequent sessions have demonstrated the best clinical benefit.

Immunizations

Vaccines can be considered as pharmacologic agents; however, their role is described here in reducing risk factors for COPD

TABLE 16-11 First-Line Pharmacotherapies for Smoking Cessation

Agent	Usual Dose	Duration	Common Complaints
Bupropion SR	150 mg orally daily for 3 days, then twice daily	12 weeks, up to 6 months	Insomnia, dry mouth
Nicotine gum	2–4 mg gum prn, up to 24 pieces daily	12 weeks	Sore mouth, dyspepsia
Nicotine inhaler	6–16 cartridges daily	Up to 6 months	Sore mouth and throat
Nicotine nasal spray	8–40 doses daily	3–6 months	Nasal irritation
Nicotine patches	Various, 7–21 mg every 24 hours	Up to 8 weeks	Skin reaction, insomnia
Varenicline	0.5 mg daily for 3 days, then 0.5 mg twice daily for 4 days, then 1 mg twice daily	12 weeks	Nausea, sleep disturbances

exacerbations. Because influenza is a common complication in COPD that can lead to exacerbations and respiratory failure, an annual vaccination with the inactivated intramuscular influenza vaccine is recommended. Immunization against influenza can reduce serious illness and death by 50% in COPD patients.[48] Influenza vaccine should be administered in the fall of each year (October and November) during regular medical visits or at vaccination clinics. There are few contraindications to influenza vaccine except for a patient with a serious allergy to eggs. An oral antiinfluenza agent (oseltamivir) can be considered for patients with COPD during an outbreak for patients who have not been immunized; however, this therapy is less effective and causes more side effects.[49]

The polyvalent pneumococcal vaccine, usually administered one time, is widely recommended for people from 2 to 64 years of age who have chronic lung disease and for all people older than 65 years. Thus, COPD patients at any age are candidates for vaccination. Although evidence for the benefit of the pneumococcal vaccine in COPD is not strong, the argument for continued use is that the current vaccine provides coverage for 85% of pneumococcal strains causing invasive disease and the increasing rate of resistance of pneumococcus to selected antibiotics. Currently, administering the vaccine remains the standard of practice and is recommended by the Centers for Disease Control and Prevention and the American Lung Association. Repeated vaccination with the 23-valent product is not recommended for patients aged 2 to 64 years with chronic lung disease; however, revaccination is recommended for patients over 65 years of age if the first vaccination was more than 5 years earlier and the patient was younger than age 65. The GOLD guidelines recommend pneumococcal vaccine for all COPD patients 65 years and older and for patients less than 65 years only if the FEV_1 is less than 40% predicted.[50,51] In 2009, the CDC broadened their recommendations for the pneumococcal polysaccharide vaccine to include all persons aged 18 and over who smoke based on a higher risk of pneumococcal infection in these patients.

Long-Term Oxygen Therapy

6 The use of supplemental oxygen therapy increases survival in COPD patients with chronic hypoxemia. Although long-term oxygen has been used for many years for patients with advanced COPD, it was not until 1980 that data became available documenting its benefits. At that time, the Nocturnal Oxygen Therapy Trial Group published its data comparing nocturnal oxygen therapy (NOT), 12 hours/day, with continuous oxygen therapy (COT), average of 20 hours/day.[52] Among patients who were followed for at least 12 months, the results revealed a mortality rate in the NOT group that was nearly double that of the COT group (51% vs. 26%). Statistical estimates of the COT group suggest that COT may have added 3.25 years to a COPD patient's life. Additional data from the Nocturnal Oxygen Therapy Trial Group revealed that COT patients had fewer (but statistically insignificant) hospitalizations, improved quality of life and neuropsychological function, reduced hematocrit, and decreased pulmonary vascular resistance.[52]

The decline in mortality with oxygen therapy was further substantiated in 1981 in a study by the British Medical Research Council that compared 15 hours/day of oxygen versus no supplemental oxygen in COPD patients.[53] Patients receiving oxygen therapy for at least part of the day had lower rates of mortality than those not receiving oxygen. Long-term oxygen therapy provides even more benefit in terms of survival after at least 5 years of use, and it improves the quality of life of these patients by increasing walking distance and neuropsychological condition and reducing time spent in the hospital.[54] Before patients are considered for long-term oxygen therapy, they should be stabilized in the outpatient setting, and pharmacotherapy should be optimized. Once this is accomplished, long-term oxygen therapy should be instituted if either of the following two conditions is observed and documented twice in a 3-week period:

1. A resting Pao_2 of less than 55 mm Hg or SaO_2 less than 88% with or without hypercapnia
2. A resting Pao_2 between 55 and 60 mm Hg or SaO_2 less than 88% with evidence of right-sided heart failure, polycythemia, or pulmonary hypertension

The most practical means of administering long-term oxygen is with the nasal cannula, at 1 to 2 L/min, which provides 24% to 28% oxygen. The goal is to raise the Pao_2 above 60 mm Hg. Patient education about flow rates and avoidance of flames (i.e., smoking) is of the utmost importance.

There are three different ways to deliver oxygen, including (a) in liquid reservoirs, (b) compressed into a cylinder, and (c) via an oxygen concentrator. Although conventional liquid oxygen and compressed oxygen are quite bulky, smaller, portable tanks are available to permit greater patient mobility. Oxygen concentrator devices separate nitrogen from room air and concentrate oxygen. These are the most convenient and the least expensive method of oxygen delivery. Oxygen-conservation devices are available that allow oxygen to flow only during inspiration, making the supply last longer. These may be particularly useful to prolong the oxygen supply for mobile patients using portable cylinders. However, the devices are bulky and subject to failure.

Adjunctive Therapies

In addition to supplemental oxygen, adjunctive therapies to consider as part of a pulmonary rehabilitation program are psychoeducational care and nutritional support. Psychoeducational care (such as relaxation) has been associated with improvement in the functioning and well-being of adults with COPD.[1,3] The role of nutritional support for patients with COPD is controversial. Several studies have shown an association among malnutrition, low body mass index (BMI), and impaired pulmonary status among patients with COPD. However, a meta-analysis suggests that the effect of nutritional support on outcomes in COPD is small and not associated with improved anthropometric measures, lung function, or functional exercise capacity.[55]

Pharmacologic Therapy

Results from numerous recent clinical trials have improved insight and understanding about the respective roles of various medications used in chronic COPD management; yet, some controversies still exist related to both effectiveness and safety. In contrast to the survival benefit conferred by supplemental oxygen therapy, there is no medication available for the treatment of COPD that has been conclusively shown to modify the progressive decline in lung function or prolong survival.[1] There is limited evidence that chronic treatment with long-acting inhaled β-agonists, inhaled corticosteroids (ICs), or the combination can reduce the rate of decline in spirometry in a subset of patients with more severe disease.[56] Currently, the primary goal of pharmacotherapy is to control patient symptoms and reduce complications, including the frequency and severity of exacerbations and improving the overall health status and exercise tolerance of the patient.

International guidelines recommend a stepwise approach to the use of pharmacotherapy based on disease severity,[1,3] which is determined by the results of spirometry, nature of symptoms, and exacerbation rates. The impact of recurrent exacerbations on accelerating disease progression is increasingly recognized as an important factor to be considered. The primary goals of pharmacotherapy are to control symptoms (including dyspnea), reduce exacerbations, and improve exercise tolerance and health status. Currently, there is inadequate evidence to support the use of more aggressive pharmacotherapy early in the course of disease because of the lack of a disease-modifying benefit. Because of the progressive nature of COPD, pharmacotherapy tends to be chronic and cumulative and step-down approaches in stable patients are not successful. Patients exhibit variable responses to available therapies and the treatment approach should be individualized.

Pharmacotherapy of COPD typically involves the use of inhaled medications, requiring patient knowledge, understanding, and skills using the various inhalation devices. Several delivery devices are available (e.g., metered-dose inhalers [MDIs], dry powder inhalers [DPIs], nebulizers, and ancillary devices such as holding chambers), and the instructions about proper use vary. Comorbidities that are common for patients with COPD, including physical and mental conditions, can have a significant effect on the patient's ability to use the devices. Periodic and frequent reinforcement and observation by the clinician is required for the patient's benefit.

7 Pharmacotherapy focuses on the use of bronchodilators to control symptoms. Bronchodilators relax bronchial smooth muscle, improve lung emptying, reduce thoracic hyperinflation at rest and during exercise, and improve exercise tolerance.[1] These effects can be seen in the absence of objective improvements on spirometry. There are several classes of bronchodilators to choose from, and no single class has been proven to provide superior benefit over other available agents. The initial and subsequent choice of medications should be based on the specific clinical situation and patient characteristics. Medications can be used as needed or on a scheduled basis depending on the clinical situation, and additional therapies should be added in a stepwise manner depending on the response and severity of disease. Considerations should be given to individual patient response, tolerabililty, adherence, and economic factors. Recommendations for management of COPD have been proposed based on a combined assessment of airflow limitation, symptoms, and risk of exacerbations, according to the new classification system for disease severity (Fig. 16-4). This schema provides clearer guidance on management compared with previous recommendations, and also allows for the individualization of pharmacotherapy based on patient-specific factors of lung function, symptom frequency and severity, and exacerbation risk.

According to the guidelines, patients with intermittent symptoms and low risk for exacerbations (Group A) should be treated with short-acting bronchodilators as needed. When symptoms become more persistent (Group B), long-acting bronchodilators should be initiated. For patients at high risk for exacerbations (Groups C and D), ICs should be considered. Short-acting bronchodilators relieve symptoms and increase exercise tolerance. Long-acting bronchodilators relieve symptoms, reduce exacerbation frequency, and improve quality of life and health status. Patients have a variety of choices in using inhalational therapies, including MDIs, DPIs, or nebulizers. There is no clear advantage of one delivery method over another, and it is recommended that patient-specific factors and preferences should be considered in selecting the device.[57]

The benefit of individual therapies in reducing the severity and frequency of exacerbations has been a major focus for the past several years. Each of the agents typically used in the long-term treatment of COPD has been shown to reduce exacerbation frequency, and each does so to a similar degree. In a meta-analysis that included many clinical trials, it was reported that exacerbations were reduced by long-acting inhaled β_2-agonists (LABAs) (23%), tiotropium (29%), ICs (22%), and ICs plus LABAs (28%).[58] There were no significant differences between the agents. These exacerbation reduction rates are consistent with those seen in the large clinical trials for tiotropium (Understanding Potential Long-term Impacts on Function with Tiotropium [UPLIFT] and Towards a Revolution in COPD Health [TORCH] [ICs plus LABAs]).

Bronchodilators

Bronchodilator classes available for the treatment of COPD include β_2-agonists, anticholinergics, and methylxanthines. There is no clear benefit to one agent or class over others, although inhaled therapy generally is preferred. In general, it can be more difficult for patients with COPD to use inhalation devices effectively compared with other populations owing to advanced age and the presence of other comorbidities. Clinicians should advise, counsel, and observe patient technique with the devices frequently and consistently.

Bronchodilators generally work by reducing the tone of airway smooth muscle (relaxation), thus minimizing airflow limitation. For patients with COPD, the clinical benefits of bronchodilators include increased exercise capacity, decreased air trapping in the lungs, and relief of symptoms such as dyspnea. However, use of bronchodilators may not be associated with significant improvements in

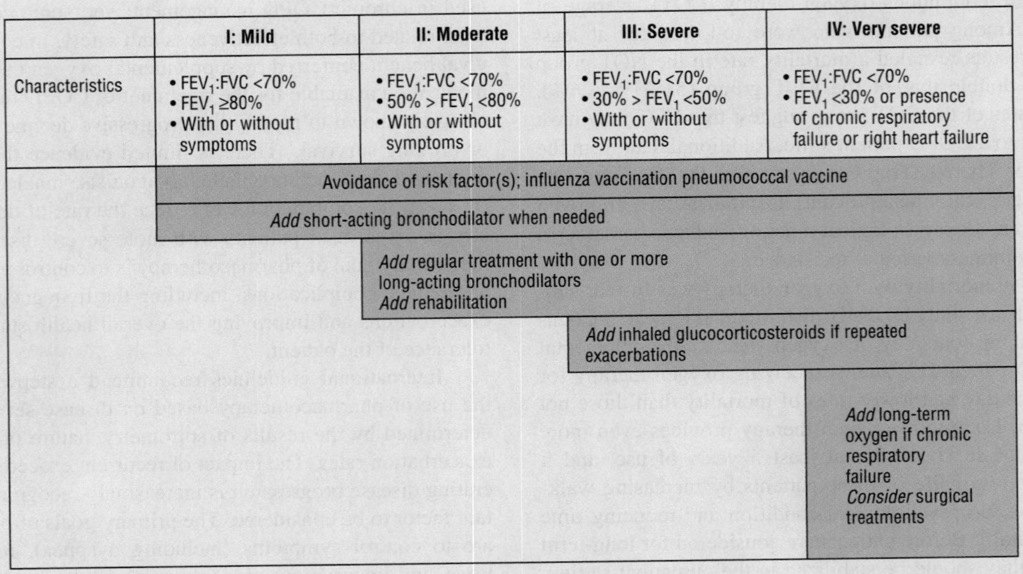

	I: Mild	II: Moderate	III: Severe	IV: Very severe
Characteristics	• FEV_1:FVC <70% • FEV_1 ≥80% • With or without symptoms	• FEV_1:FVC <70% • 50% > FEV_1 <80% • With or without symptoms	• FEV_1:FVC <70% • 30% > FEV_1 <50% • With or without symptoms	• FEV_1:FVC <70% • FEV_1 <30% or presence of chronic respiratory failure or right heart failure
	Avoidance of risk factor(s); influenza vaccination pneumococcal vaccine			
	Add short-acting bronchodilator when needed			
		Add regular treatment with one or more long-acting bronchodilators *Add* rehabilitation		
			Add inhaled glucocorticosteroids if repeated exacerbations	
				Add long-term oxygen if chronic respiratory failure *Consider* surgical treatments

FIGURE 16-4 Pharmacotherapy recommendations based on group classification.

pulmonary function measurements such as FEV_1. In clinical studies, regular use of a long-acting inhaled bronchodilator (LABA or anticholinergic) or ipratropium is associated with improved health status. Regular use of tiotropium also reduces exacerbation rates. In general, side effects of bronchodilator medications are related to their pharmacologic effects and are dose dependent. Because COPD patients are older and more likely to have comorbid conditions, the risk for side effects and drug interactions is higher compared with patients with asthma.

Short-Acting Bronchodilators The initial therapy for COPD patients who experience symptoms intermittently is short-acting bronchodilators. Among these agents, the choices are a short-acting β_2-agonist or an anticholinergic. Either class of agents has a relatively rapid onset of action, relieves symptoms, and improves exercise tolerance and lung function. In general, both classes are equally effective.

Short-Acting Sympathomimetics (β_2-Agonists) A number of sympathomimetic agents are available in the United States. They vary in selectivity, route of administration, and duration of action. In COPD management, sympathomimetic agents with β_2-selectivity, or β_2-agonists, should be used as bronchodilators. β_2-Agonists cause bronchodilation by stimulating the enzyme adenyl cyclase to increase the formation of cyclic adenosine monophosphate (cAMP). cAMP is responsible for mediating relaxation of bronchial smooth muscle, leading to bronchodilation. In addition, β_2-agonists may improve mucociliary clearance. Although shorter-acting and less selective β-agonists are still used widely (e.g., metaproterenol, isoetharine, isoproterenol, and epinephrine), they should not be used owing to their shorter duration of action and increased cardiostimulatory effects. Short-acting, selective β_2-agonists such as albuterol, levalbuterol, and pirbuterol are preferred for therapy.

Sympathomimetics are available in inhaled, oral, and parenteral dosage forms. The preferred route of administration is by inhalation. The use of oral and parenteral β-agonists in COPD is discouraged because they are no more effective than a properly used MDI or DPI, and the incidence of systemic adverse effects such as tachycardia and hand tremor is greater. Administration of β_2-agonists in the outpatient and emergency room settings via inhalers (MDIs or DPIs) is at least as effective as nebulization therapy and usually favored for reasons of cost and convenience.[57] Chapter 15 includes a complete description of the devices used for delivering aerosolized medication and a comparison of β_2-agonist therapies.

Albuterol is the most frequently used β_2-agonist. It is available as an oral and inhaled preparation. Albuterol is a racemic mixture of (*R*)-albuterol, which is responsible for the bronchodilator effect, and (*S*)-albuterol, which has no therapeutic effect. (*S*)-Albuterol is considered by some clinicians to be inert, whereas others believe that it may be implicated in worsening airway inflammation and antagonizing the response to (*R*)-albuterol. Levalbuterol is a single-isomer formulation of (*R*)-albuterol. A retrospective evaluation of levalbuterol versus albuterol use for patients with asthma and COPD concluded that levalbuterol offered significant advantages over albuterol for hospitalized patients.[59] Other clinicians feel that there are no significant differences between the products and that the use of levalbuterol is not justified owing to its higher acquisition cost.[60] The effects of a single dose of levalbuterol have been compared with those of albuterol and ipratropium plus albuterol for patients with COPD. No significant differences in pulmonary function improvements or adverse effects were noted.[61]

In COPD patients, β_2-agonists exert a rapid onset of effect, although the response generally is less than that seen in asthma. Short-acting inhaled β_2-agonists cause only a small improvement in FEV_1 acutely but may improve respiratory symptoms and exercise tolerance despite the small improvement in spirometric measurements.[62] Patients with COPD can use quick-onset β_2-agonists as needed for relief of symptoms or on a scheduled basis to prevent or reduce symptoms. The duration of action of short-acting β_2-agonists is 4 to 6 hours.

Inhaled β_2-agonists are generally well tolerated. They can cause sinus tachycardia and rhythm disturbances in predisposed patients, but these are rarely reported. Skeletal muscle tremors can occur initially but subside as tolerance develops.

Short-Acting Anticholinergics When given by inhalation, anticholinergics such as ipratropium or atropine produce bronchodilation by competitively inhibiting cholinergic receptors in bronchial smooth muscle. This activity blocks acetylcholine, with the net effect being a reduction in cyclic guanosine monophosphate (cGMP), which normally acts to constrict bronchial smooth muscle. Muscarinic receptors on airway smooth muscle include M_1, M_2, and M_3 subtypes. Activation of M_1 and M_3 receptors by acetylcholine results in bronchoconstriction; however, activation of M_2 receptors inhibits further acetylcholine release.

Ipratropium is the primary short-acting anticholinergic agent used for COPD in the United States. Atropine has a tertiary structure and is absorbed readily across the oral and respiratory mucosa, whereas ipratropium has a quaternary structure that is absorbed poorly. The lack of systemic absorption of ipratropium greatly diminishes the anticholinergic side effects such as blurred vision, urinary retention, nausea, and tachycardia associated with atropine. Ipratropium bromide is available as an MDI and a solution for inhalation. The MDI was recently reformulated with an HFA propellant and delivers 17 mcg per puff. Ipratropium is also available as an MDI in combination with albuterol and as a solution for nebulization at 200 mcg/mL. It provides a peak effect in 1.5 to 2 hours and has a duration of effect of 4 to 6 hours. Ipratropium has a slower onset of action and a more prolonged bronchodilator effect compared with standard β_2-agonists. Because of the slower onset of effect (15 to 20 minutes compared with 5 minutes for albuterol), it may be less suitable for as-needed use; however, it is often prescribed in that manner. The role of inhaled anticholinergics in COPD is well established.[63–65] However, results from the Lung Health Study showed that treatment with ipratropium did not affect the progressive decline in lung function.[40] Studies comparing ipratropium with inhaled β_2-agonists have generally reported similar improvements in pulmonary function. Others report a modest benefit with ipratropium, including a lower incidence of side effects such as tachycardia.[63,64]

Although the recommended dose of ipratropium is 2 puffs four times a day, there is evidence for a dose–response, so the dose can be titrated upward often to 24 puffs a day. Ipratropium has been shown to increase maximum exercise performance in stable COPD patients with doses of 8 to 12 puffs prior to exercise but not with doses of 4 puffs or less.[65,66] During sleep, ipratropium also has been shown to improve arterial oxygen saturation and sleep quality.[67] Ipratropium is well tolerated. The most frequent patient complaints are dry mouth, nausea, and an occasional metallic taste.

Clinicians differ about preference in choosing the initial short-acting bronchodilator therapy for the patient with COPD. Both a short-acting β_2-agonist and ipratropium represent reasonable choices for initial therapy.

8 Long-Acting Bronchodilators For patients with moderate-to-severe COPD who experience symptoms on a regular and consistent basis, or in whom short-acting therapies do not provide adequate relief, long-acting bronchodilator therapies are the recommended treatment. Long-acting inhaled bronchodilator therapy can be administered as an inhaled β_2-agonist (LABA) or an anticholinergic. Long-acting, inhaled bronchodilator therapy is more convenient and effective, compared with short-acting agents, for patients with chronic symptoms. There are superior outcomes in lung function as measured by spirometry, symptoms including dyspnea, and, importantly, reductions in exacerbation frequency and improved quality of life.

Long-Acting Inhaled β_2-Agonists LABAs offer the convenience and benefit of a long duration of action for patients with persistent symptoms. Most of the currently available agents, salmeterol, formoterol, and arformoterol, are dosed every 12 hours and provide sustained bronchodilation. An ultra-long-acting agent, indacaterol, requires only once-daily dosing and was recently approved in July 2011. Arformoterol, formoterol, and indacaterol have an onset of action similar to albuterol (less than 5 minutes), whereas salmeterol has a slower onset (15 to 20 minutes); however, none of these agents are recommended for acute relief of symptoms. There is no dose titration for any of these agents; the starting dose is the effective and recommended dose for all patients. The clinical benefits of LABAs compared with short-acting therapies include similar or superior improvements in lung function and symptoms, as well as reduced exacerbation rates in some studies.[68–71] The use of the long-acting agents should be considered for patients with frequent and persistent symptoms. When patients require short-acting β_2-agonists on a scheduled basis, LABAs are more convenient based on dosing frequency but are also more expensive. Salmeterol, indacaterol, and formoterol are available in dry powder inhalation devices, and formoterol and arformoterol as solutions for nebulization. LABAs are also useful to reduce nocturnal symptoms and improve quality of life. When compared with short-acting bronchodilators or theophylline, both salmeterol and formoterol improve lung function, symptoms, exacerbation frequency, and quality of life.[70] These benefits are apparent even for patients with poorly reversible lung function and are related to improvements in inspiratory capacity.[72] Both salmeterol and formoterol have been compared with ipratropium. In separate studies, each agent improved FEV_1 compared with ipratropium and, in addition, the LABA was more effective for other selected outcomes (e.g., prolonged time to exacerbation for salmeterol while formoterol reduced symptoms and rescue inhaler use).[73,74] Comparative data for indacaterol and other bronchodilators are limited. Available studies have demonstrated similar effects with indacaterol on FEV_1 and symptoms compared with other long-acting bronchodilators; however, the effect on other outcomes such as exacerbation frequency has not been evaluated.

Long-Acting Anticholinergics Tiotropium bromide, a long-acting quaternary anticholinergic agent, has been available in the United States since 2004. This agent blocks the effects of acetylcholine by binding to muscarinic receptors in airway smooth muscle and mucus glands, blocking the cholinergic effects of bronchoconstriction and mucus secretion. Tiotropium is more selective than ipratropium at blocking important muscarinic receptors. It dissociates slowly from M_1 and M_3 receptors, allowing prolonged bronchodilation. The dissociation from M_2 receptors is much faster, allowing inhibition of acetylcholine release. Binding studies of tiotropium in the human lung show that it is approximately 10-fold more potent than ipratropium and protects against cholinergic bronchoconstriction for greater than 24 hours.[75]

When inhaled, tiotropium is minimally absorbed into the systemic circulation and results in bronchodilation within 30 minutes, with a peak effect in 3 hours. Bronchodilation persists for at least 24 hours, allowing for a once-daily dosing. There is no titration of tiotropium dose; a regimen of 18 mcg inhaled once daily is recommended for all patients. In the United States, it is delivered via the HandiHaler, a single-load, dry powder, breath-actuated device. Because it acts locally, tiotropium is well tolerated, with the most common complaint being a dry mouth. Other anticholinergic side effects that are reported include constipation, urinary retention, tachycardia, blurred vision, and precipitation of narrow-angle glaucoma symptoms.

The benefits of tiotropium have been evaluated in numerous trials of patients with COPD. Similar to long-acting β-agonists, tiotropium improves lung function and dyspnea, exacerbation frequency, and health-related quality of life.[76] Benefits have been demonstrated compared with placebo[77] and with ipratropium.[78] Tiotropium therapy is associated with a decreased risk of exacerbations compared with placebo or ipratropium, and equal or superior efficacy compared with LABAs in various studies.[79] The tolerance that is demonstrated with chronic use of β-agonists does not occur with tiotropium therapy, as improvements in lung function are sustained with long-term therapy.[80]

As a long-acting bronchodilator, tiotropium is an option to consider in addition to LABAs for COPD management. Once-daily tiotropium has been compared with twice-daily salmeterol in two placebo-controlled trials of 6 months' duration. Tiotropium reduced asthma exacerbations and hospital admissions and improved quality of life, whereas both active treatments improved lung function and reduced dyspnea.[78] In another 6-month randomized controlled trial of patients with COPD, patients were randomized to receive tiotropium once daily by DPI, salmeterol twice daily by MDI, or placebo.[81] Patients receiving tiotropium had greater improvements in trough FEV_1 and dyspnea scores than those receiving salmeterol. Patients also were more likely to have improvements in quality-of-life indicators with tiotropium than with salmeterol. However, no differences in frequency of exacerbations were noted among the three groups.

The most notable study involving the use of tiotropium in recent years for patients with COPD was the UPLIFT trial.[82] This was a randomized, double-blind study of 4 years' duration. A total of 5,993 subjects received either tiotropium 18 mcg daily inhaled via a HandiHaler device or a matching placebo. All other COPD therapies were allowed except for other anticholinergic therapies (e.g., ipratropium). The mean postbronchodilator FEV_1 among subjects was 1.32 L, and the primary outcome was the rate of decline in FEV_1 on spirometry. The results showed that tiotropium treatment resulted in prebronchodilator FEV_1 improvement of 87 to 103 mL, and postbronchodilator improvement of 47 to 65 mL, both of which were statistically significant. However, the rate of decline in the mean FEV_1 result was not statistically significant between the groups. Tiotropium-treated subjects benefited from treatment as reflected in improved quality-of-life scores, reduced exacerbation rates, fewer hospitalizations, and instances of respiratory failure. Tiotropium was associated with a lower overall risk of mortality, including deaths from respiratory and cardiac causes.

The safety of tiotropium documented in the UPLIFT trial is reassuring. Recently, retrospective analysis have reported an increased risk of cardiovascular events associated with ipratropium[83] and tiotropium use.[84,85] However, the UPLIFT study, which was a prospective trial over 4 years, did not report an increased cardiovascular risk associated with tiotropium use.[82]

Recently, another long-acting agent has been approved. Aclidinium bromide is expected to have a similar role to tiotropium. In one clinical trial, aclidinium administered at 400 mcg twice daily provided similar improvements in spirometry and COPD symptom scores compared with tiotropium.[86]

Combination Anticholinergics and β-Agonists Combination regimens of bronchodilators are used often in the treatment of COPD, especially as the disease progresses and symptoms worsen over time. Combining bronchodilators with different mechanisms of action allows the lowest possible effective doses to be used and reduces potential adverse effects from individual agents.[1] Combinations of both short- and long-acting β_2-agonists with ipratropium have been shown to provide added symptomatic relief and improvements in pulmonary function.[86–88] A combination of albuterol and ipratropium (Combivent) is available as an MDI in the United States for chronic maintenance therapy of COPD. This product offers the obvious convenience of two classes of bronchodilators in a single inhaler.

Although clinical practice guidelines recommend that combinations of long-acting bronchodilators are appropriate for patients who do not receive adequate benefit from a single agent, data to support the use of these combinations have been lacking. These approaches have been the focus of more recent research. A recent Cochrane review evaluated five trials comparing combination long-acting bronchodilators (LABA plus tiotropium) versus tiotropium alone. Combination therapy resulted in significant improvement in FEV_1 and quality-of-life measures compared with tiotropium alone, although no difference was shown for frequency of exacerbations or symptom scores.[89] Future combination inhalation products may contain long-acting β_2-agonists with tiotropium to reduce the need for frequent dosing.

Methylxanthines Methylxanthines, including theophylline and aminophylline, have been available for the treatment of COPD for at least 5 decades and at one time were considered first-line therapy. However, with the availability of LABAs and inhaled anticholinergics, the role of methylxanthine therapy is significantly limited. Inhaled bronchodilator therapy is preferred for COPD. Because of the risk for drug interactions and the significant intrapatient and interpatient variability in dosage requirements, theophylline therapy generally is considered for patients who are intolerant or unable to use an inhaled bronchodilator. Theophylline is still an alternative to commonly used inhaled therapies partially due to the potential for multiple mechanisms (bronchodilation and antiinflammatory) and the possible benefit that systemic administration may exert on peripheral airways.[90]

The methylxanthines may produce bronchodilation through numerous mechanisms, including (a) inhibition of phosphodiesterase, thereby increasing cAMP levels, (b) inhibition of calcium ion influx into smooth muscle, (c) prostaglandin antagonism, (d) stimulation of endogenous catecholamines, (e) adenosine receptor antagonism, and (f) inhibition of release of mediators from mast cells and leukocytes.[91]

Chronic theophylline use for patients with COPD has been shown to exert improvements in lung function, including vital capacity (VC), FEV_1, minute ventilation, and gas exchange.[90] Subjectively, theophylline has been shown to reduce dyspnea, increase exercise tolerance, and improve respiratory drive in COPD patients.[90,91] Other nonpulmonary effects of theophylline that may contribute to improved overall functional capacity for patients with COPD include improved cardiac function and decreased pulmonary artery pressure.

Regular use of methylxanthines has not been shown to have either a beneficial or a detrimental effect on the progression of COPD. However, methylxanthines may be added to the treatment plan of patients who have not achieved an optimal clinical response to inhaled bronchodilators. Studies suggest that adding theophylline to a combination of albuterol and ipratropium provides added benefit for stable COPD patients, supporting the hypothesis that there is a synergistic bronchodilator effect.[92–94] The efficacy of combination therapy with salmeterol and theophylline for patients with COPD was reported to improve pulmonary function and reduce dyspnea better than either treatment alone.[95] Combination treatment also was associated with a reduced number of exacerbations only when compared with the theophylline group, suggesting that the salmeterol component was responsible for this beneficial effect.

As is the case with other bronchodilator therapy, parameters other than objective measurements, such as FEV_1, should be monitored to assess efficacy of theophylline in COPD. Subjective parameters, such as perceived improvements in symptoms of dyspnea and exercise tolerance, become increasingly important in assessing the acceptability of methylxanthines for COPD patients. Although objective improvement may be minimal, patients may experience an improvement in clinical symptoms, and thus benefit to the individual may be meaningful.

Although theophylline is available in a variety of oral dosage forms, sustained-release preparations are most appropriate for the long-term management of COPD. These products have the advantages of improving patient compliance and achieving more consistent serum concentrations over rapid-release theophylline and aminophylline preparations. However, caution must be used in switching from one sustained-release preparation to another because there are considerable variations in sustained-release characteristics.[91] Aside from IV aminophylline, there is no need to use any of the various salt forms of theophylline.

Therapy can be initiated at 200 mg twice daily and titrated upward every 3 to 5 days to the target dose. Most patients required daily doses of 400 to 900 mg. Dosage adjustments generally should be made based on serum concentration results. Traditionally, the therapeutic range of theophylline was identified as 10 to 20 mcg/mL; however, because of the frequency of dose-related side effects and the relatively minor benefit of higher concentrations, a more conservative therapeutic range of 8 to 15 mcg/mL often is targeted. This is especially preferable for the elderly. When concentrations are measured, trough measurements are most appropriate.

Once a dose is established, serum concentrations should be monitored once or twice a year unless the patient's disease worsens, medications that interfere with theophylline metabolism are added to therapy, or toxicity is suspected. The most common side effects of theophylline therapy are related to the GI system, the cardiovascular system, and the CNS. Side effects are dose related; however, there is overlap in side effects between the therapeutic and toxic ranges. Minor side effects include dyspepsia, nausea, vomiting, diarrhea, headache, dizziness, and tachycardia. More serious toxicities, especially at toxic concentrations, include arrhythmias and seizures.

Factors that decrease theophylline clearance and lead to reduced maintenance dose requirements include advanced age, bacterial or viral pneumonia, left or right ventricular failure, liver dysfunction, hypoxemia from acute decompensation, and use of drugs such as cimetidine, macrolides, and fluoroquinolone antibiotics. Factors that may enhance theophylline clearance and result in the need for higher maintenance doses include tobacco and marijuana smoking, hyperthyroidism, and the use of such drugs as phenytoin, phenobarbital, and rifampin.

In summary, there are decades of experience with theophylline and other methylxanthine products in the management of patients with COPD. However, inhalation therapy is currently preferred based on superior efficacy and safety, as well as ease of use by the clinician. Theophylline is a challenging medication to dose, monitor, and manage due to the significant intrapatient and interpatient variability in pharmacokinetics and the potential for drug interactions and toxicities.

Corticosteroids

9 Corticosteroid therapy has been studied and debated in COPD therapy for half a century; however, owing to the poor risk-to-benefit ratio, chronic systemic corticosteroid therapy should be avoided if possible.[1] Because of the potential role of inflammation in the pathogenesis of the disease, clinicians hoped that corticosteroids would be promising agents in COPD management. However, their use continues to be debated, especially in the management of stable COPD.

The antiinflammatory mechanisms whereby corticosteroids exert their beneficial effect in COPD include (a) reduction in capillary permeability to decrease mucus, (b) inhibition of release of proteolytic enzymes from leukocytes, and (c) inhibition of prostaglandins. Unfortunately, the clinical benefits of systemic corticosteroid therapy in the chronic management of COPD are often not evident, and the risk of toxicity is extensive and far-reaching. Currently, the appropriate situations to consider corticosteroids in COPD include (a) short-term systemic use for acute exacerbations and (b) inhalation therapy for chronic stable COPD.

The role of oral steroid use in chronic stable COPD patients was evaluated in a meta-analysis over a decade ago.[96] Investigators concluded that only a small fraction (10%) of COPD patients treated with steroids showed clinically significant improvement in baseline FEV_1 (increase of 20%) compared with those treated with placebo. While a small number of COPD patients are considered responders to oral steroids, many of these patients actually may have an asthmatic, or reversible, component to their disease. The best predictors for response to oral steroids are the presence of eosinophils on sputum examination (≥3%) and a significant response to sympathomimetics on pulmonary function tests.[97] Both the presence of eosinophils in sputum and the responsiveness to sympathomimetics suggest an asthmatic component to the disease process and thus may explain the clinical benefit seen with steroids.

Previously, a common clinical practice was to administer a short course (2 weeks) of oral corticosteroids as a trial to predict which patients would benefit from chronic oral or ICs. There is now sufficient evidence suggesting that this practice is not effective in predicting a long-term response to ICs and should not be recommended.[98]

Long-term adverse effects associated with systemic corticosteroid therapy include osteoporosis, muscular atrophy, thinning of the skin, development of cataracts, and adrenal suppression and insufficiency. The risks associated with long-term steroid therapy are much greater than the clinical benefits. If a decision to treat with long-term systemic corticosteroids is made, the lowest possible effective dose should be given once per day in the morning to minimize the risk of adrenal suppression. If therapy with oral agents is required, an alternate-day schedule should be used.

The use of chronic IC therapy has been of interest for the past decade. Their use has been common despite the lack of firm evidence about significant clinical benefit until recently. ICs have an improved risk-to-benefit ratio compared with systemic corticosteroid therapy. Using the model for asthma, it was hoped that the inhalation of potent corticosteroid would result in high local efficacy and limited systemic exposure and toxicity. In the latter part of the 1990s, several large international trials were initiated to evaluate the effect on ICs in COPD. Unfortunately, the results of these major clinical trials failed to demonstrate any benefit from chronic treatment with ICs in modifying long-term decline in lung function that is characteristic of COPD.[99] Therefore, the role of ICs in COPD continues to be debated in the literature, unlike in asthma, where their use is clearly advocated. Much of the debate centers on the appropriate outcome measures in this population of patients.

During the last decade, several studies of ICs in COPD were designed to detect a benefit on slowing the progressive loss of lung function, but the results were disappointing.[100–105] None of the large national or international trials were able to demonstrate a benefit of high-dose IC therapy on this primary outcome. However, ICs have been associated with other important benefits in some patients, including a decrease in exacerbation frequency and improvements in overall health status.[101,105,106] Clinicians continue to debate the most appropriate and relevant outcome measure to evaluate in COPD studies. A meta-analysis evaluating randomized clinical trials involving ICs for patients with COPD indicated that treatment was associated with a relative risk reduction in exacerbation frequency of 33%. The report indicated that 12 patients would require treatment for 20.8 months to prevent one exacerbation episode. The benefit was evident for patients with moderate-to-severe COPD.[107] This meta-analysis did not detect a mortality benefit.

Other investigators have reported a reduction in mortality for patients with COPD who were treated with ICs. In an epidemiologic study of a Canadian database, patient mortality 3 months to 1 year following a hospitalization for a COPD exacerbation was evaluated for patients who received ICs in the first 3 months compared with those who did not. For patients over 65 years of age, IC therapy reduced mortality by 25%. Much of the mortality reduction was reflected in deaths due to cardiovascular causes. Conversely, patients who received only bronchodilator therapy trended toward higher mortality rates, although this was not significant.[108] A pooled analysis of seven large trials also concluded that ICs reduced all-cause mortality in COPD patients.[109]

Currently, the recommended role of IC therapy is for patients with severe or very severe COPD and at high risk of exacerbation (Groups C and D) who are not controlled with inhaled bronchodilators. The initial hope that treatment with ICs would prevent or slow the progressive decline in FEV_1 remains unproven; however, it is often argued that additional important outcomes for patients with COPD include relief of symptoms, fewer and less severe exacerbations, and improved quality of life.[110] ICs do not prolong survival in COPD patients and there is good evidence to suggest that treatment with ICs increases the risk of pneumonia for patients with COPD.[111–113]

Although a dose–response relationship for ICs has not been demonstrated in COPD, the major clinical trials employed moderate to high doses for treatment. Side effects of ICs are relatively mild compared with the toxicity from systemic therapy. Hoarseness, sore throat, oral candidiasis, and skin bruising have been reported in the clinical trials. Severe side effects, such as adrenal suppression, osteoporosis, and cataract formation, have been reported less frequently than with systemic corticosteroids, but clinicians should monitor patients who are receiving high-dose chronic therapy.[114,115]

There is evidence supporting a dose relationship between IC use and the risk of fractures. In a cohort of over 1,600 subjects with a diagnosis of asthma or COPD (mean age 80 years), the risk of a fracture was 2.53 times higher (CI, 1.65 to 3.89) in those receiving a mean daily dose of IC of 601 mcg or greater.[116] However, the data are conflicting about this issue. A meta-analysis found no evidence supporting an increased risk of fractures or decreased bone mineral density with chronic IC use.[117] It appears prudent to suggest that, to minimize the risk of fracture, patients should be treated with the lowest effective dose of ICs.[118] It may also be helpful to recommend adequate intake of calcium and vitamin D and possibly periodic bone mineral density testing.

Combination Therapy: Bronchodilators and Inhaled Corticosteroids

Following the disappointing results of chronic IC studies and the progressive decline in lung function, investigators became interested in the combination of potent antiinflammatory therapies and long-acting bronchodilators. Subsequently, several studies have shown an additive benefit with long-acting bronchodilators.[119–122] In various studies, combination therapy with salmeterol plus fluticasone or formoterol plus budesonide was associated with greater improvements in clinical outcomes such as FEV_1, health status, and frequency of exacerbations compared with ICs or long-acting bronchodilators alone. The availability of combination inhalers (e.g., salmeterol plus fluticasone and budesonide plus formoterol) makes administration of both ICs and long-acting bronchodilators more convenient for patients and decreases the total number of inhalations needed daily. An IC combined with a long-acting β-agonist is superior to the individual components in reducing exacerbations, improving lung function and overall health status.[111] Therefore, there is growing evidence that IC and long-acting β-agonist combinations improve lung function, as well as reduce symptoms of dyspnea and exacerbation frequency.[121–123]

The combination of a long-acting β-agonist and IC has been compared with the long-acting β-agonist therapy alone. In a study involving nearly 1,000 patients with severe but stable COPD, subjects received either salmeterol 50 mcg/fluticasone 500 mcg twice daily or salmeterol 50 mcg twice daily for 44 weeks. Exacerbation frequency was significantly lower in the combination group (334 episodes vs. 464 episodes), which corresponded to a 35% reduction in the annualized rate. The time to the first exacerbation was also delayed with the combination therapy.[124] One finding of concern reported in this trial was the increased number of pneumonia cases for patients receiving combination therapy compared with salmeterol alone. There were 23 cases reported compared with 7 in the salmeterol group.[124] An increase in the risk for pneumonia was also reported in the TORCH study described below.[111]

The largest prospective study to date is referred to as the TORCH study.[111] This trial consisted of 6,112 patients who received one of four treatments for 3 years. Treatment groups were placebo, salmeterol 50 mcg twice daily, fluticasone 500 mcg twice daily, or the combination of salmeterol and fluticasone in a single inhaler. The primary outcome was death from any cause and secondary outcomes were exacerbation rates, lung function, and health status. None of the active treatments differed significantly from placebo, although the combination of salmeterol and fluticasone trended toward fewer deaths ($P = 0.052$). The combination also reduced exacerbation rates, and improved lung function and health status compared with the other treatments. Exacerbation rates were also significantly reduced with combination therapy compared with either single agent alone. Both treatment groups that included fluticasone had higher rates of pneumonia. Although this study did not reflect a mortality benefit, the authors indicated the risk of death was reduced by 17.5% with the combination and that the number needed to treat for 1 year to provide a benefit was 4.

In a post hoc analysis of this trial, both individual agents and the combination decreased the rate of spirometry decline in patients with an FEV_1 of less than 60% predicted.[56] While this observation is interesting, it is in contrast to previous randomized controlled studies that have not demonstrated an effect of pharmacotherapy on rate of disease progression.

In a head-to-head trial, a large study comparing a combination of salmeterol and fluticasone with tiotropium alone showed no difference in the exacerbation rates between the groups, although the combination therapy was associated with a higher study completion rate.[125]

Combinations of Long-Acting Bronchodilators Compared with Long-Acting Bronchodilators Plus Inhaled Corticosteroids The combination of salmeterol and tiotropium has also been evaluated in a short-term crossover study involving only 22 subjects who received salmeterol (50 mcg twice daily) plus fluticasone (500 mcg twice daily), fluticasone plus tiotropium (18 mcg once daily), or fluticasone, salmeterol, and tiotropium for 1 week. The triple combination provided a significant benefit of improved lung function compared with either of the dual treatments in subjects with moderate-to-severe COPD.[126] The benefit of triple therapy was evaluated in a 1-year randomized, double-blind, placebo-controlled study involving 449 subjects with moderate-to-severe COPD. Treatment consisted of tiotropium, tiotropium plus salmeterol, or tiotropium, salmeterol, and fluticasone.[127] There was no difference between treatments for the primary outcome of percentage of patients experiencing an exacerbation requiring systemic corticosteroids or antibiotics. The triple-drug regimen improved lung function, quality of life, and reduced hospitalization compared with tiotropium alone, while two-drug therapy did not offer any benefit in lung function improvement or hospitalization rates compared with the single agent. Another small study evaluated the addition of tiotropium for 1 month to a regimen of an IC and a long-acting β-agonist.[128] The addition of tiotropium improved lung function and quality-of-life scores, apparently by improving dynamics of lung capacity (inspiratory capacity). These effects were reversed when tiotropium therapy was discontinued. These data involving combinations of long-acting bronchodilators are limited and preliminary. More research is required and should include other outcome parameters including relief of symptoms, exacerbation rates, and quality of life. Larger sample sizes and longer durations will provide insight into the value of combinations.

A retrospective cohort study of 42,090 patients in the Veterans Affairs healthcare system evaluated outcomes for patients with COPD who received tiotropium as part of a COPD regimen compared with a cohort of COPD patients who did not receive the medication. Patients who received tiotropium with ICs plus a long-acting β-agonist exhibited a 40% reduction in mortality compared with patients treated with ICs plus a long-acting β-agonist alone (95% CI of 0.45 to 0.79). Triple therapy patients also significantly reduced exacerbations and hospitalization rates. However, this same study demonstrated that tiotropium combined with two other medications (various) increased mortality and morbidity risks.[83]

Phosphodiesterase Inhibitors

Phosphodiesterase 4 (PDE4) is the major phosphodiesterase found in airway smooth muscle cells and inflammatory cells and is responsible for degrading cAMP. Inhibition of PDE4 results in relaxation of airway smooth muscle cells and decreased activity of inflammatory cells and mediators such as TNF-α and IL-8. One PDE4 inhibitor, roflumilast, was approved in February 2011 to reduce the risk of exacerbations in patients with severe COPD. When either used as monotherapy or added to a maintenance regimen with other inhaled bronchodilators, roflumilast was associated with a modest increase in FEV_1 and reduction in rate of exacerbation by approximately 15%. Of note, patients in phase III trials evaluating roflumilast were not allowed to receive ICs as part of their maintenance regimen.

Roflumilast is dosed at 500 mcg orally once a day. Major adverse effects include weight loss and neuropsychiatric effects such as suicidal thoughts, insomnia, anxiety, and new or worsened depression. Weight loss may be of concern in patients with low BMI and drug discontinuation may be necessary if significant weight loss is observed. Both patients and family members should be counseled regarding the potential for mood and behavior changes and to alert healthcare providers if they occur.

Roflumilast is metabolized by CYP3A4 and 1A2 and coadministration with strong inducers of cytochrome P450 is not recommended due to potential for subtherapeutic plasma concentrations. Although there are no recommended dose adjustments, caution should also be used when administering roflumilast with strong inhibitors of cytochrome P450 due to potential for adverse effects.

Given the limited evidence demonstrating long-term clinical benefit and the lack of evidence for coadministration with ICs, the role of roflumilast in the management of COPD is not entirely clear. Current consensus guidelines recommend roflumilast for patients with severe or very severe COPD who are at high risk of exacerbation (Groups C and D) and are not controlled by inhaled bronchodilators. Roflumilast may also be considered for patients who are intolerant or unable to use inhaled bronchodilators or corticosteroids. Given that both theophylline and roflumilast have similar mechanisms of action through inhibition of phosphodiesterases, it is not recommended to use both together for the management of COPD.

α_1-Antitrypsin Replacement Therapy

For patients with inherited AAT deficiency–associated emphysema, treatment focuses on reduction of risk factors such as smoking, symptomatic treatment with bronchodilators, and augmentation therapy with replacement AAT. Based on knowledge about the relationship between serum concentrations of AAT and the risk of developing emphysema, the rationale for augmentation therapy is to maintain serum concentrations above the protective threshold throughout the dosing interval.[129] Indirect evidence of AAT activity in the interstitium of the lung has been demonstrated by measuring concentrations of the enzyme in epithelial lining fluid obtained during bronchoalveolar lavage. Augmentation therapy consists of weekly infusions of pooled human AAT to maintain AAT plasma levels over 10 μmol/L. Much of the data supporting the use of AAT replacement are based on evidence of biochemical efficacy (e.g., administering the product and demonstrating protective serum concentrations of AAT).

Clinical evidence for slowing lung function decline or improving outcomes with augmentation therapy is sparse. Stated challenges to performing randomized clinical trials include the large sample size and long duration of followup required, and the expense of conducting such a trial. One observational study followed patients in the National Registry of Severe AAT Deficiency over a period of several years and documented clinical outcomes. In this study, patients who received weekly augmentation therapy with purified AAT had slower declines in FEV_1 and decreased mortality compared with patients who never received augmentation therapy.[130] However, this was an observational study of patients, not a randomized, placebo-controlled trial, and so direct cause-and-effect relationships cannot be concluded. One randomized, placebo-controlled study of patients with severe AAT deficiency (ZZ phenotype) did show a significant reduction in lung tissue loss and destruction as measured by computed tomographic (CT) scan for patients receiving augmentation therapy.[131] Other measures of lung function and mortality were not recorded.

The recommended dosing regimen for replacement AAT is 60 mg/kg administered IV once a week at a rate of 0.08 mL/kg/min, adjusted to patient tolerance. It has been estimated that this form of augmentation therapy will cost over $54,000 annually.[132] In the absence of alternative treatments, it is difficult to assess the cost-effectiveness using conventional criteria. There have been repeated problems with supply of this biologic replacement therapy (derived from pooled blood donors) related to production difficulty and contamination issues. Currently, there are four products available (Prolastin-C [Talecris], Aralast-NP [Baxter], Zemaira [CSL Behring], and Glassia [Kamata]) that should minimize this problem in the future. Drug development research continues in the area of recombinant products and inhalational therapy.

The safety of AAT replacement therapy has been evaluated in two large observational studies. In the most recent study, 174 patients ($n = 747$) reported 720 adverse events, classified as severe in 8.8% of cases and moderate in 72.4% of cases.[133] Common complaints included headache, dizziness, nausea, dyspnea, and fever. The overall rate of adverse events was low (i.e., two events over 5 years).

TREATMENT
COPD Exacerbation

Desired Outcomes

10 The goals of therapy for patients experiencing exacerbations of COPD are (a) prevention of hospitalization or reduction in hospital stay, (b) prevention of acute respiratory failure and death, and (c) resolution of exacerbation symptoms and a return to baseline clinical status and quality of life.[134] Acute exacerbations can range from mild to severe. Factors that influence the severity, and subsequently the level of care required, include the severity of airflow limitation, presence of comorbidities, and the history of previous exacerbations. Table 16-12 includes factors that warrant treatment in the hospital.

Various therapeutic options for exacerbation management are summarized in Table 16-13. Pharmacotherapy consists of intensification of bronchodilator therapy and a short course of systemic corticosteroids. Antimicrobial therapy is indicated in the presence of selected symptoms. Since the frequency and severity of exacerbations are closely related to each patient's overall health status, all patients should receive optimal chronic treatment, including smoking cessation, appropriate pharmacologic therapy, and preventative therapy such as vaccinations.

TABLE 16-12 Factors Favoring Hospitalization for Treatment of COPD Exacerbation

Presence of high risk comorbidity (e.g., pneumonia, arrhythmia, CHF, diabetes, renal or hepatic failure)
Suboptimal response to outpatient management
Marked worsening of dyspnea
Inability to eat or sleep due to symptoms
Worsening hypoxemia or hypercapnia
Mental status changes
Lack of home support for care
Uncertain diagnosis

Nonpharmacologic Therapy

Controlled Oxygen Therapy

Oxygen therapy should be considered for any patient with hypoxemia during an exacerbation. Caution must be used, however, because many patients with COPD rely on mild hypoxemia to trigger their drive to breathe. In normal, healthy individuals, the drive to breathe is triggered by carbon dioxide accumulation. For patients with COPD who retain carbon dioxide as a result of their disease progression, hypoxemia rather than hypercapnia becomes the main trigger for their respiratory drive. Overly aggressive administration of oxygen to patients with chronic hypercapnia may result in respiratory depression and respiratory failure. Oxygen therapy should be used to achieve a Pao_2 of greater than 60 mm Hg or oxygen saturation of greater than 90%. However, an ABG should be obtained after oxygen initiation to monitor carbon dioxide retention owing to hypoventilation.

Noninvasive Mechanical Ventilation

Noninvasive positive-pressure ventilation (NPPV) provides ventilatory support with oxygen and pressurized airflow using a face or nasal mask with a tight seal but without endotracheal intubation. There have been numerous trials reporting the benefits of NPPV for patients with acute respiratory failure due to COPD exacerbations. In one meta-analysis

TABLE 16-13 Therapeutic Options for Acute Exacerbations of COPD

Therapy	Comments
Antibiotics	Recommended if two or more of the following are present: Increased dyspnea Increased sputum production Increased sputum purulence
Corticosteroids	Oral or IV therapy may be used. If IV is used, it should be changed to oral after improvement in pulmonary status. If continued longer than 14 days, then the dose should be tapered to avoid HPA Axis suppression.
Bronchodilators	MDIs and DPIs equal in efficacy to nebulization. β-Agonists also may increase mucociliary clearance. Long-acting β-agonists should not be used for quick relief of symptoms or on an as-needed basis.
Controlled oxygen therapy	Titrate oxygen to desired oxygen saturation (>90%). Monitor arterial blood gas for development of hypercapnia.
Noninvasive mechanical ventilation	Consider for patients with acute respiratory failure. Not appropriate for patients with altered mental status, severe acidosis, respiratory arrest, or cardiovascular instability.

of eight studies, NPPV was associated with lower mortality, lower intubation rates, shorter hospital stays, and greater improvements in serum pH in 1 hour compared with treatment with usual care alone.[135] The benefits seen with NPPV generally can be attributed to a reduction in the complications that often arise with invasive mechanical ventilation. Not all patients with COPD exacerbations are appropriate candidates for NPPV. Patients with altered mental status may not be able to protect their airway and thus may be at increased risk for aspiration. Patients with severe acidosis (pH <7.25), respiratory arrest, or cardiovascular instability should be not considered for NPPV. Patients failing a trial of NPPV or those considered poor candidates might be considered for intubation and mechanical ventilation.

Pharmacologic Therapy

Bronchodilators

During exacerbations, intensification of bronchodilator regimens is used commonly. The doses and frequency of bronchodilators are increased to provide symptomatic relief. Short-acting β_2-agonists are preferred owing to rapid onset of action. Anticholinergic agents may be added if symptoms persist despite increased doses of β_2-agonists. In fact, combinations of these agents are employed often, although data are lacking about the benefit versus higher doses of one agent. Bronchodilators may be administered via MDIs or nebulization with equal efficacy. Nebulization may be considered for patients with severe dyspnea who are unable to hold their breath after actuation of an MDI. Clinical evidence supporting the use of theophylline during exacerbations is lacking, and thus theophylline generally should be avoided. However, addition of one of these agents may be considered for patients not responding to other therapies. The risk of adverse effects such as cardiac arrhythmias should be considered and serum levels monitored closely.

Corticosteroids

Until recently, the literature supporting the use of corticosteroids in acute exacerbations of COPD was sparse. However, since 1996, five studies have been performed that document the value of systemic corticosteroids in exacerbations of COPD.[136–140] The Systemic Corticosteroids in Chronic Obstructive Pulmonary Disease Exacerbations (SCCOPE) trial evaluated three groups of patients hospitalized for exacerbations of COPD.[136] The first group received an 8-week course of corticosteroids given as methylprednisolone 125 mg IV every 6 hours for 72 hours, followed by once-daily oral prednisone (60 mg on days 4 to 7, 40 mg on days 8 to 11, 20 mg on days 12 to 43, 10 mg on days 44 to 50, and 5 mg on days 51 to 57). The second group received a 2-week course given as methylprednisolone 125 mg IV every 6 hours for 72 hours, followed by oral prednisone (60 mg on days 5 to 7, 40 mg on days 8 to 11, and 20 mg on days 12 to 15) and placebo on days 16 to 57. The third group received placebo for all 57 days of study. Rates of treatment failure and hospital stay were significantly higher in the placebo group than in either treatment group at 30 and 90 days. Groups randomized to corticosteroid treatment also had a significantly shorter length of hospital stay compared with the placebo group. The 8-week regimen was not found to be superior to the 2-week regimen. Significant treatment benefits were no longer evident at 6 months.

Davies et al.[137] evaluated the oral use of corticosteroids in hospitalized patients with acute exacerbations of COPD. Patients received either 30 mg/day oral prednisolone or placebo for 14 days. Patients who were treated with corticosteroids had a significantly more rapid improvement in FEV_1 and a shorter hospital stay than did patients who received placebo. There was no significant difference between groups at 6-week follow-up.

In total, results from these trials suggest that patients with acute exacerbations of COPD should receive a short course of IV or oral corticosteroids. However, because of the large variability in dosage ranges, the optimal dose and duration of corticosteroid treatment are not known. It appears that short courses (9 to 14 days) are as effective as longer courses and have a lower risk of associated adverse effects owing to less time of exposure. Several trials used high initial doses of steroids before tapering to a lower maintenance dose. Adverse effects such as hyperglycemia, insomnia, and hallucinations may occur at higher doses. Depending on the clinical status of the patient, treatment may be initiated at a lower dose or tapered more quickly if these effects occur. It appears that a regimen of prednisone 40 mg orally daily (or equivalent) for 10 to 14 days can be effective for most patients.[141] If steroid treatment is continued for greater than 2 weeks, a tapering oral schedule should be employed to avoid hypothalamic–pituitary–adrenal (HPA) axis suppression.

Recent data suggest that ICs may be beneficial for treating COPD exacerbations, although this is not the standard of care. In one study, inhaled budesonide, alone or combined with formoterol, was as effective as oral corticosteroids in treating COPD exacerbations.[142]

Antimicrobial Therapy

11 It is thought that most acute exacerbations of COPD are caused by viral or bacterial infections. However, as many as 30% of exacerbations are caused by unknown factors.[1] A meta-analysis of nine studies evaluating the effectiveness of antibiotics in treating exacerbations of COPD determined that patients receiving antibiotics had a greater improvement in peak expiratory flow rate than those who did not.[143]

This meta-analysis concluded that antibiotics are of most benefit and should be initiated if at least two of the following three symptoms are present: increased dyspnea, increased sputum volume, and increased sputum purulence. The utility of sputum Gram stain and culture is questionable because some patients have chronic bacterial colonization of the bronchial tree between exacerbations.

The emergence of drug-resistant organisms has mandated that antibiotic regimens be chosen judiciously. Selection of empirical antimicrobial therapy should be based on the most likely organism(s) thought to be responsible for the infection based on the individual patient profile. The most common organisms for any acute exacerbation of COPD are *Haemophilus influenzae*, *Moraxella catarrhalis*, *Streptococcus pneumoniae*, and *Haemophilus parainfluenzae*. More virulent bacteria may be present for patients with more complicated acute exacerbations of COPD, including drug-resistant pneumococci, β-lactamase–producing *H. influenzae* and *M. catarrhalis*, and enteric gram-negative organisms, including *Pseudomonas aeruginosa*. Table 16-14 summarizes recommended antimicrobial therapy for exacerbations of COPD and the most common organisms based on patient presentation.[144]

Therapy with antibiotics generally should be continued for at least 7 to 10 days. Studies evaluating shorter treatment courses (usually 5 days) with the fluoroquinolones, second- and third-generation cephalosporins, and macrolide antimicrobials have demonstrated comparable efficacy with the longer treatment regimens.[145] If the patient deteriorates or does not improve as anticipated, hospitalization may be necessary, and more aggressive attempts should be made to identify potential pathogens responsible for the exacerbation.

COPD patients are at increased risk for pulmonary embolism during severe exacerbations requiring hospitalizations. An increased awareness of this risk and appropriate preventative measures are warranted.[146]

Complications

Cor Pulmonale

Cor pulmonale is right-sided heart failure secondary to pulmonary hypertension. Long-term oxygen therapy and diuretics have been the mainstays of therapy for cor pulmonale. Increasing the Pao_2 above 60 mm Hg with supplemental oxygen therapy decreases pulmonary hypertension and thus decreases the force against which the

TABLE 16-14 Recommended Antimicrobial Therapy in Acute Exacerbations of COPD

Patient Characteristics	Likely Pathogens	Recommended Therapy
Uncomplicated exacerbations <4 exacerbations per year No comorbid illness FEV_1 >50% of predicted	*S. pneumoniae* *H. influenzae* *M. catarrhalis* *H. parainfluenzae* Resistance uncommon	Macrolide (azithromycin, clarithromycin) Second- or third-generation cephalosporin Doxycycline Therapies not recommended[a]: TMP/SMX, amoxicillin, first-generation cephalosporins, and erythromycin
Complicated exacerbations: Age ≥65 and >4 exacerbations per year FEV_1 <50% but >35% of predicted	As above plus drug-resistant pneumococci, β-lactamase–producing *H. influenzae* and *M. catarrhalis*	Amoxicillin/clavulanate Fluoroquinolone with enhanced pneumococcal activity (levofloxacin, gemifloxacin, moxifloxacin)
Complicated exacerbations with risk of *P. aeruginosa* Chronic bronchial sepsis[b] Need for chronic corticosteroid therapy Resident of nursing home with <4 exacerbations per year FEV_1 <35% of predicted	Some enteric gram-negatives As above plus *P. aeruginosa*	Fluoroquinolone with enhanced pneumococcal and *P. aeruginosa* activity (levofloxacin) IV therapy if required: β-lactamase resistant penicillin with antipseudomonal activity 3rd- or 4th-generation cephalosporin with antipseudomonal activity

[a]TMP/SMX should not be used due to increasing pneumococcal resistance; amoxicillin and first-generation cephalosporins are not recommended due to β-lactamase susceptibility; and erythromycin is not recommended due to insufficient activity against *H. influenzae*.
[b]In sepsis, double antipseudomonal coverage should be considered (e.g., addition of aminoglycoside).

right ventricle has to work. While diuretics may help decrease fluid overload, caution should be used because patients with significant right-sided heart failure are highly dependent on preload for cardiac output. Therefore, the decision to use diuretics must be based on a risk-to-benefit ratio. Digitalis glycosides have no role in the treatment of cor pulmonale.

Other pharmacologic agents that have been investigated to treat cor pulmonale include hydralazine, calcium channel blockers, angiotensin-converting enzyme inhibitors, and angiotensin II antagonists. However, there is insufficient evidence to offer guidelines for the role of these agents in COPD patients with cor pulmonale.

Polycythemia

Polycythemia secondary to chronic hypoxemia in COPD patients can be improved by either oxygen therapy or periodic phlebotomy if oxygen therapy alone is not sufficient. COT was shown by the Nocturnal Oxygen Therapy Trial Group to reduce hematocrit values in treated patients.[31] Acute phlebotomy is indicated if the hematocrit is above 55% to 60% and the patient is experiencing CNS effects suggestive of sludging from high blood viscosity. Long-term oxygen then can be used to maintain a lower hematocrit.

Other Pharmacologic Considerations

A number of other treatments have been explored over the years. Among these therapies, either there is insufficient evidence to warrant recommending their use or they have been proven to not be beneficial in the management of COPD. A brief summary is provided because the clinician likely will encounter patients who are receiving or inquire about these treatments.

Suppressive Antimicrobial Agents

Because COPD patients often are colonized with bacteria and experience recurrent exacerbations of their condition, a common practice employed in the past has been the use of low-dose antimicrobial therapy as preventative or prophylaxis against these acute exacerbations. However, clinical studies over the past 40 years have failed to demonstrate any significant benefit from this practice.[1]

In certain pulmonary conditions such as cystic fibrosis and bronchiectasis, chronic therapy with macrolide antibiotics, specifically azithromycin, has shown clinical benefit based on its proposed antiinflammatory properties and is used in clinical practice. A recent study evaluated the effect of chronic azithromycin in patients with COPD. Patients were randomized to azithromycin (250 mg orally daily) or placebo in addition to maintenance therapy for COPD and were followed for 1 year.[147] Chronic azithromycin was associated with a lower rate of exacerbations and improved quality-of-life scores; however, more patients in the azithromycin group reported hearing deficits (25% vs. 20% in the placebo group). Therapy with azithromycin was also associated with a higher rate of colonization with macrolide-resistant bacteria during the study period. Of note, patients were carefully screened for hearing impairment and risk factors for QT prolongation prior to entering the study and were excluded if either was present.

In May 2012, a retrospective, observational study reported an increase in cardiac events with short courses of azithromycin and the FDA has since updated the product labeling to include a precaution about QT prolongation.[148] Given the limited evidence for long-term treatment (beyond 1 year) with azithromycin, it would be prudent to wait for more long-term safety data before routinely recommending this therapy for patients with COPD who are at risk for exacerbations. Clinicians may choose to consider azithromycin for individual patients at high risk for exacerbations after weighing the risks and benefits of therapy.

Expectorants and Mucolytics

Adequate water intake generally is acceptable to maintain hydration and assist in the removal of airway sections. Beyond this, the regular use of mucolytics or expectorants for COPD patients has no proven benefit. This includes the use of saturated solutions of potassium iodide, ammonium chloride, acetylcysteine, and guaifenesin. In 2011, the FDA announced its intention to remove various unapproved cough and cold preparations (including several containing guaifenesin) from the market due to safety and efficacy concerns. Two formulations are currently approved by the FDA (Humibid and Mucinex); however, data are lacking on their benefit.

Narcotics

Systemic (oral and parenteral) opioids, especially morphine, can relieve dyspnea for patients with end-stage COPD. Nebulized therapy is sometimes used in clinical practice, although data about clinical benefit are lacking.[149] Opioids should be used carefully, if at all, to avoid adverse effects on ventilatory drive.

Respiratory Stimulants

There is no role for respiratory stimulants in the long-term management of COPD.[1] Agents that have shown some utility in the acute setting include almitrine and doxapram. However, almitrine is available only in Europe, and its usefulness is limited by neurotoxicity. Doxapram is available for IV use only and may be no better than intermittent NPPV.

Secondary pulmonary hypertension is a feature of severe COPD. This has prompted interest about the potential role of agents used to treat primary pulmonary hypertension. However, the use of an endothelin receptor antagonist (bosentan) failed to improve exercise tolerance and worsened hypoxemia in one trial.[150] Investigations with sildenafil, a phosphodiesterase type 5 (PDE5) inhibitor, have been conflicting in uncontrolled clinical trials. Due to concerns that PDE5 inhibitors may worsen gas exchange in patients with COPD, they are not recommended outside of clinical trials.

Surgical Intervention

Various surgical options have been employed in the management of COPD. These include bullectomy, lung volume reduction surgery (LVRS), and lung transplantation. Bullectomy has been performed for many years and may be useful when large bullae (>1 cm) are noted on computerized axial tomography (CT or CAT) scan. The presence of bullae may contribute to complaints of dyspnea, and their removal can improve lung function and reduce symptoms, although there is no evidence of a mortality benefit.

Because of the prevalence of COPD, it is the most frequent indication for lung transplantation. Transplantation is considered when predicted survival is less than 2 years, FEV_1 is <25% predicted, and hypoxemia, hypercapnia, and pulmonary hypertension exist despite medical management.[3] Experience to date shows 2-year survival of 65% to 90%, and 5-year survival of 41% to 53%.

Recent trials have evaluated the effect of bilateral LVRS for management of severe COPD. Short-term trials comparing the effects of pulmonary rehabilitation plus LVRS with pulmonary rehabilitation alone reported that the combination of treatments resulted in greater improvements in lung function, gas exchange, and quality of life at 3 months. Only recently have data evaluating the long-term effect of LVRS compared with pulmonary rehabilitation been published. The National Emphysema Treatment Trial (NETT), a prospective, randomized trial evaluating the long-term effects of LVRS plus pulmonary rehabilitation compared with pulmonary rehabilitation alone, followed 1,218 patients for 3 years.[151] The primary end points for the study were mortality and maximal exercise capacity 2 years after randomization. Secondary end points included pulmonary function, distance walked in 6 minutes, and quality-of-life measurements. At an interim analysis, patients with an FEV_1 of less than 20% of predicted or a carbon monoxide diffusing capacity of less than 20% of predicted were noted to be at high risk of death after surgery and subsequently were excluded from the study. Results of the study showed no mortality benefit with LVRS compared with pulmonary rehabilitation alone. Patients undergoing surgery had improved exercise capacity, lung function, and quality of life at 2 years, but these patients also had a higher risk of short-term morbidity and mortality associated with the surgery. A subgroup analysis of the study noted that patients with predominately upper-lobe emphysema and low exercise capacity undergoing surgery had lower mortality rates at 2 years compared with patients treated with medical therapy alone. Because of the costs and risks associated with LVRS, more studies are needed to better determine the ideal surgical candidates and identify subgroups of patients that would benefit most from surgery. The long-term benefits of LVRS are exhibited as improved oxygenation and decreased requirements for supplemental oxygen during treadmill walking as well as self-reported oxygen requirements for up to 24 months after the procedure.[152]

Dietary Supplements

There has been increasing interest in the role of antioxidants, including vitamins E and C and β-carotene, in reducing the frequency of exacerbations. It is postulated that they may be beneficial in COPD as a result of an imbalance between oxidants and antioxidants that has been considered in the pathogenesis of smoking-induced lung disease. However, there is no good evidence that antioxidant therapies improve COPD symptoms or slow disease progression. Nutritional supplements, including creatine, have not proven beneficial to improve the benefit of pulmonary rehabilitation programs.[153]

Investigational Therapies

Based on the knowledge about the importance of neutrophilic inflammation in COPD and potential therapeutic benefit of inhibition of neutrophil activity, a number of antiinflammatory compounds are being explored. Specifically, agents inhibiting LTB_4, neutrophil elastase, and phosphodiesterases currently are being evaluated. To date, studies evaluating leukotriene-modifying therapies have been disappointing. Further studies are needed to evaluate the clinical benefit of such inhibitors for patients with COPD.

Neutrophil elastase is implicated in the induction of bronchial disease, causing structural changes in lungs, impairment of mucociliary clearance, and impairment of host defenses. Protease inhibitors, namely, inhibitors of neutrophil elastase, are being investigated currently for the treatment of COPD.

Results have been disappointing in evaluating the benefit of infliximab, a TNF-α-blocker, in treating COPD. A total of 234 patients with moderate-to-severe COPD received either infliximab 3 or 5 mg/kg or placebo at baseline, 2, 6, 12, 18, and 24 weeks. Subjects completed a quality-of-life questionnaire (CRQ) during treatment and out to 44 weeks. There were no differences on the CRQ or on any secondary end points including lung function, exercise capacity, or exacerbation rates. The discontinuation rate due to adverse events was high (20% to 27%) in the active treatment group.[154]

PHARMACOECONOMIC CONSIDERATIONS

The overall cost of therapy is an important consideration in contemporary medical practice. Meaningful cost analysis goes beyond the cost of the medication itself and incorporates the impact of a given therapeutic agent on overall healthcare cost. Because of the relative lack of benefit among objective outcome measures in COPD clinical trials, pharmacoeconomic studies can be useful in decision making about pharmacotherapy options. Pharmacoeconomic analyses in COPD, although limited, are available regarding antibiotic use in acute exacerbations and some therapies for management of chronic stable COPD.

The costs of managing an acute exacerbation of COPD in the ambulatory setting were evaluated in over 2,400 patients. Subjects were followed for 1 month following the diagnosis of the exacerbation. The overall relapse rate was 21%, with 31% and 16% of subjects requiring care in the emergency department and hospital, respectively. The overall costs for exacerbation treatment averaged $159, with 58% attributed to hospitalization.[155] These authors concluded that a significant cost saving would result from improving the successful ambulatory management of acute exacerbations.

Grossman et al. conducted a trial investigating the use of aggressive antimicrobial therapy (ciprofloxacin) compared with usual antibiotic therapy (defined as any nonquinolone) in the treatment of acute exacerbations of COPD.[156] Overall, the results indicated no preference for either treatment arm. However, for patients who were categorized as high risk (severe underlying lung disease, more than four exacerbations per year, duration of bronchitis greater than 10 years, elderly, significant comorbid illness), the use of aggressive antibiotic therapy was associated with improved clinical outcome, higher quality of life, and fewer costs. The results of this study are consistent with Table 16-14, which suggests that higher-risk patients are likely to have more resistant strains of organisms and thus require more aggressive antimicrobial treatment.

Few data are available about the cost-effectiveness of educational programs for patients with COPD. In an outpatient clinic, patients attending one 4-hour group session, followed by one to two individual sessions with a clinician, reported improved outcomes, and costs were reduced in an evaluation 12 months later.[157] Additional research is needed regarding the best model for education and also the specific self-management strategies to teach.

Friedman et al. conducted a post hoc pharmacoeconomic evaluation of two multicenter, randomized trials comparing the combination of ipratropium and albuterol with both drugs used as monotherapy.[158] Patients who received a combination of ipratropium and albuterol had lower rates of exacerbations, lower overall treatment costs, and improved cost-effectiveness compared with either drug used alone. With the introduction of new bronchodilator therapies and with no clearly consistent advantage of one class of agents over another, pharmacoeconomic analyses may be useful for clinicians in determining the most appropriate therapy for their patients.

Clinical **Controversy. . .**

In the United States, all products containing a LABA agent, either alone or in combination with ICs, include a black box warning about an increased risk of severe asthma attacks or death associated with their use. This caution applies to patients with asthma, and it is strongly recommended that LABAs use should always be in conjunction with another controller therapy (e.g., ICs) and that use should be limited in duration. This concern only applies to patients with asthma and is not relevant concerning the use of LABA therapy for COPD patients.

A combination product of a long-acting inhaled β-agonist (salmeterol) and an inhaled corticosteroid agent (fluticasone) is one of the most commonly prescribed medications for lung disease, including COPD. However, in expert guidelines, ICs are indicated only for patients with more severe disease who experience frequent exacerbations. Many patients now receiving therapy with the combination inhaler may be candidates for bronchodilator therapy alone, although the benefit of ICs continues to be a focus of clinical research, including the potential for a mortality benefit.

The role of systemic corticosteroids for acute exacerbations of COPD has been clarified in recent years. However, the appropriate dosage regimen is not well established. Regimens range from initial high doses (methylprednisolone 125 mg every 6 hours) to more conservative dosing (prednisone 40–60 mg/day). Consensus guidelines indicate that bronchodilator therapy is the focus of pharmacotherapy for COPD. However, there is no clear choice for the initial agent. For patients with daily but not persistent symptoms, either ipratropium or albuterol offers advantages as initial therapy. Both also have limitations if chosen as the initial therapy.

International guidelines recommend long-acting bronchodilator therapy for patients with moderate to very severe disease or when symptoms are not adequately managed with short-acting agents or as-needed therapy. When response to a single long-acting bronchodilator is not optimal, guidelines recommend the use of combinations. However, data are lacking presently about the therapeutic benefit of combinations of long-acting bronchodilators, and this approach is associated with substantial costs.

EVALUATION OF THERAPEUTIC OUTCOMES

To evaluate therapeutic outcomes of COPD effectively, the practitioner must first delineate between chronic stable COPD and acute exacerbations. In chronic stable COPD, pulmonary function tests should be assessed periodically and with any therapy addition, change in dose, or deletion of therapy. Because objective improvements often are minimal, subjective assessments are important. Other outcome parameters are commonly evaluated, including dyspnea score, quality-of-life assessments, and exacerbation rates, including visits to the emergency department or hospitalization. In acute exacerbations of COPD, white blood cell count, vital signs, chest x-ray, and changes in frequency of dyspnea, sputum volume, and sputum purulence should be assessed at the onset and throughout treatment of an exacerbation. In more severe exacerbations, ABGs and oxygen saturation also should be monitored. As with any drug therapy, patient adherence to therapeutic regimens, side effects, potential drug interactions, and subjective measures of quality of life also must be evaluated.

To date, there is no evidence that any of the available pharmacotherapies for COPD impact disease progression. Removal of the primary causative factor for COPD (e.g., cessation of cigarette smoking) does improve survival, as does supplemental oxygen therapy in a subset of patients with COPD. The most pertinent clinical outcomes that have emerged from clinical trials over the past decade are symptom improvement and reductions in exacerbation frequency. While it is important to continue to explore strategies to improve survival, consideration should be given to these two relevant and important outcome measures when initiating, continuing, and monitoring therapy. Because of the tremendous impact of exacerbations on disease progression, a reduction in exacerbation frequency may be predicted to show a benefit; however, this has not been proven.

END-OF-LIFE CARE

Based on the natural course of COPD, characterized by the progressive decline in lung function and development of complications, consideration should be given to end-of-life decisions and advanced directives.[159] Factors associated with expected mortality within 1 year have been identified. These include older age, diagnosis of depression, declining overall health status, hypercapnia, an FEV_1 of less than 30% predicted, ability to walk only a few steps without resting, more than one emergent hospitalization in the past year, and the presence of comorbidities, including congestive heart failure. An effective strategy to discuss end-of-life care involves the patient's participation in identifying advanced directives. Patients should be assured that symptoms, including pain, will be managed and their dignity will be preserved. Specific issues that should be addressed include location and provider for terminal care, desires to use or withhold mechanical ventilation, and involvement of other family members in decisions on behalf of the patient.

ABBREVIATIONS

AAT	α_1-antitrypsin
ABG	arterial blood gas
ACCP	American College of Chest Physicians
ACP	American College of Physicians
ATS	American Thoracic Society
BMI	body mass index
cAMP	cyclic adenosine monophosphate
CAT	COPD Assessment Test
cGMP	cyclic guanosine monophosphate
COPD	chronic obstructive pulmonary disease
COT	continuous oxygen therapy
CRQ	Chronic Respiratory Questionnaire
CT	computed tomographic
D_LCO	diffusing capacity for carbon monoxide
DPI	dry powder inhaler
ERS	European Respiratory Society
FEV_1	forced expiratory volume in 1 second
FRC	functional residual capacity
FVC	forced vital capacity
GOLD	Global Initiative for Chronic Obstructive Lung Disease
HPA	hypothalamic–pituitary–adrenal
IC	inhaled corticosteroid
IL-8	interleukin 8
LABA	long-acting inhaled β_2-agonist
LTB_4	leukotriene B_4
LVRS	lung volume reduction surgery
MDI	metered-dose inhaler
MMP12	matrix metalloproteinase 12
mMRC	modified Medical Research Council
NETT	National Emphysema Treatment Trial
NHLBI	National Heart, Lung, and Blood Institute
NOT	nocturnal oxygen therapy
NPPV	noninvasive positive-pressure ventilation
$Paco_2$	pressure exerted by carbon dioxide gas in arterial blood
Pao_2	pressure exerted by oxygen gas in arterial blood
PDE4	phosphodiesterase 4
PDE5	phosphodiesterase type 5
PHS	Public Health Service
SCCOPE	Systemic Corticosteroids in Chronic Obstructive Pulmonary Disease Exacerbations
SCCOR	Specialized Centers of Clinically Oriented Research
SGRQ	St. George's Respiratory Questionnaire
TNF-α	tumor necrosis factor-α
TORCH	Towards a Revolution in COPD Health
UPLIFT	Understanding Potential Long-Term Impacts on Function with Tiotropium
VC	vital capacity
WHO	World Health Organization

REFERENCES

1. Global Initiative for Chronic Obstructive Lung Disease. Global Strategy for the Diagnosis, Management, and Prevention of Chronic Obstructive Pulmonary Disease (GOLD). 2013, *http://www.goldcopd.com/*.
2. Centers for Disease Control and Prevention. Chronic obstructive pulmonary disease among adults—United States, 2011. MMWR 2012;61(46):938–943.
3. Qaseem A, Wilt TJ, Weinberger SE, et al. Diagnosis and management of stable COPD: A clinical practice guideline update from the American College of Physicians, the American College of Chest Physicians, the American Thoracic Society, and the European Respiratory Society. Ann Intern Med 2011;155:179–191.
4. National Institutes of Health. Specialized Centers of Clinically Oriented Research (SCCOR) in Chronic Obstructive Pulmonary Disease (COPD). RFA Number: REA-HL-05-008. Bethesda, MD: National Institutes of Health, August 2004.
5. National Center for Health Statistics. National Health Interview Survey. Hyattsville, MD: U.S. Department of Health and Human Services, CDC, NCHS, 2001, *www.cdc.gov/nchs/nhis.htm*.
6. Mannino DM, Homa DM, Akinbami LJ, Ford ES, Redd SC. Chronic obstructive pulmonary disease surveillance—United States, 1971–2000. MMWR Surveill Summ 2002;51:1–16.
7. Wilt TJ, Niewoehner D, Kim C, et al. Use of Spirometry for Case Finding, Diagnosis, and Management of Chronic Obstructive Pulmonary Disease (COPD). Evidence Report #121. AHRQ Publication 05-E017–1. Rockville, MD: Agency for Healthcare Research and Quality, August 2005.
8. Centers for Disease Control and Prevention. Deaths from chronic obstructive pulmonary disease—United States, 2000–2005. MMWR Morb Mortal Wkly Rep 2008;57: 1229–1232.
9. Chronic Obstructive Pulmonary Disease: Data Fact Sheet. NIH Publication 03-5529. Bethesda, MD: U.S. Department of Health and Human Services, National Institutes of Health, NHLBI, March 2003.
10. Holguin F, Folch E, Redd SC, Mannino DM. Comorbidity and mortality in COPD-related hospitalizations in the United States, 1979–2001. Chest 2005;128:2005–2011.
11. Chronic Obstructive Pulmonary Disease (COPD) Fact Sheet. Washington, DC: American Lung Association, February 2010, *www.lungusa.org/lung-disease/COPD/resources/fact-figures/COPD-Fact-Sheet.html*.
12. National Institutes of Health. NHLBI Morbidity & Mortality: 2004 Chart Book on Cardiovascular, Lung, and Blood Diseases. Washington, DC: U.S. Department of Health and Human Services, May 2004, *http://www.nhlbi.nih.gov/resources/docs/cht-book.htm*.
13. Jansson SA, Andersson F, Borg S, Ericsson A, Jonsson E, Lundback B. Costs of COPD in Sweden according to disease severity. Chest 2002;122:1994–2002.
14. U.S. Department of Health and Human Services. The Health Consequences of Smoking: A Report of the Surgeon General. Washington, DC: U.S. Department of Health and Human Services, 2004.
15. Sandford AJ, Silverman EK. Chronic obstructive pulmonary disease. 1: Susceptibility factors for COPD the genotype–environment interaction. Thorax 2002;57:736–741.
16. Carrel RW, Lomas DA. Alpha-1 antitrypsin deficiency: A model for conformational diseases. N Engl J Med 2002;346:45–53.
17. Hunninghake GM, Cho MH, Tesfaigzi Y, et al. MMP12, lung function, and COPD in high-risk populations. N Engl J Med 2009;361:2599–2608.
18. Barnes PJ. Chronic obstructive pulmonary disease. N Engl J Med 2000;343:269–280.
19. Stockley RA. Neutrophils and the pathogenesis of COPD. Chest 2002;121:151S–155S.
20. Hogg JC. Pathophysiology of airflow limitation in chronic obstructive pulmonary disease. Lancet 2004;364: 709–721.
21. Hill AT, Bayley D, Stockely RA. The interrelationship of sputum inflammatory markers in patients with chronic bronchitis. Am J Respir Crit Care Med 1999;160:893–898.

22. Ries AL. Impact of chronic obstructive pulmonary disease on quality of life: The role of dyspnea. Am J Med 2006;119:S12–S20.
23. MacNee W. Pathophysiology of cor pulmonale in chronic obstructive pulmonary disease. Part 2. Am J Respir Crit Care Med 1994;150:1158–1168.
24. Sin DD, Man SF. Why are patients with chronic obstructive pulmonary disease at increased risk of cardiovascular disease? The potential role of systemic inflammation in chronic obstructive pulmonary disease. Circulation 2003;107:1514–1519.
25. Casaburi R, ZuWallack R. Pulmonary rehabilitation for management of chronic obstructive pulmonary disease. N Engl J Med 2009;360:1329–1335.
26. Rodriguez-Roisin R. Toward a consensus definition for COPD exacerbations. Chest 2000;117(Suppl 2):398S–401S.
27. Ferris BG. Epidemiology standardization project (American Thoracic Society). Am Rev Respir Dis 1978;118:1–120.
28. Jones PW, Harding G, Berry P, Wiklund L, Chen W-H, Kline Leidy N. Development and first validation of the COPD Assessment Test. Eur Respir J 2009;34:648–665.
29. Anzueto A. Clinical course of chronic obstructive pulmonary disease: Review of therapeutic interventions. Am J Med 2006;119:S46–S53.
30. Mannino DM, Doherty DE, Buist S. Global initiative on obstructive lung disease (GOLD) classification of lung disease and mortality: Findings from the atherosclerosis risk in communities (ARIC) study. Respir Med 2006;100: 115–122.
31. Celli BR. The importance of spirometry in COPD and asthma. Chest 2000;117:15S–19S.
32. Andersson F, Borg S, Janson S-A, et al. The costs of exacerbations in chronic obstructive pulmonary disease (COPD). Respir Med 2002;96:700–708.
33. Anthonisen NR, Manfreda J, Warren CPW, et al. Antibiotic therapy in exacerbations of chronic obstructive pulmonary disease. Ann Intern Med 1987;106:196–204.
34. Groenewegen KH, Schols AMW, Wouters EFM. Mortality and mortality-related factors after hospitalization for acute exacerbation of COPD. Chest 2003;124:459–467.
35. Bach PB, Brown C, Gelfand SE, McCrory DC. Management of acute exacerbations of chronic obstructive pulmonary disease: A summary and appraisal of published evidence. Ann Intern Med 2001;134:600–620.
36. Almagro P, Calbo E, Ochoa de Echaguen A, et al. Mortality after hospitalization for COPD. Chest 2002;121:1441–1448.
37. Anzueto A. Impact of exacerbations on COPD. Eur Respir Rev 2010;19(116):113–118.
38. Heffner JE, Fahy B, Hilling L, Barbieri C. Outcomes of advanced directive education of pulmonary rehabilitation patients. Am J Respir Crit Care Med 1997;155:1055–1059.
39. Parrott S, Godfrey C, Raw M, et al. Guidance for commissioners on the cost-effectiveness of smoking cessation interventions. Health International Authority. Thorax 1998;53(Suppl 5):S1–S38.
40. Anthonisen NR, Connett JE, Kiley JP, et al. Effects of smoking intervention and the use of an inhaled anticholinergic bronchodilator on the rate of decline in FEV_1: The Lung Health Study. JAMA 1994;272: 1497–1505.
41. Anthonisen NR, Skeans MA, Wise RA, Manfreda J, Kanner RE, Connett JE. The effects of a smoking cessation intervention on 14.5 year mortality: A randomized clinical trial. Ann Intern Med 2005;142:233–239.
42. Fiore MC, Jaén CR, Baker TB, et al. Treating Tobacco Use and Dependence: 2008 Update. Clinical Practice Guideline. Public Health Service. Rockville, MD: U.S. Department of Health and Human Services, May 2008, *www.surgeongeneral.gov/tobacco*.
43. Jorenby DE, Leischow SJ, Nides MA, et al. A controlled trial of sustained-release bupropion, a nicotine patch, or both for smoking cessation. N Engl J Med 1999;340:685–691.
44. Tonstad S, Tonnesen P, Hajek P, et al. Effect of maintenance therapy with varenicline on smoking cessation: A randomized controlled trial. JAMA 2006;296:64–71.
45. Celli BR, Halbert RJ, Nordyke RJ, Schan B. Airway obstruction in never smokers: Results from the Third National Health and Nutrition Examination Survey. Am J Med 2005;118:1364–1372.
46. Oroczo-Levi M, Garcia-Aymerich J, Villar J, Ramirez-Samiento A, Anto JM, Gea J. Wood smoke exposure and risk of chronic obstructive pulmonary disease. Eur Respir J 2006;27:542–546.
47. American Thoracic Society/European Respiratory Society. Statement on pulmonary rehabilitation. Am J Respir Crit Care Med 2006;173:1390–1413.
48. Nichol KL, Margolis KL, Wourenma J, Von Sternberg T. The efficacy and cost effectiveness of vaccination against influenza among elderly persons living in the community. N Engl J Med 1994;331:778–784.
49. Advisory Committee on Immunization Practices, Smith NM, Bresee JS, et al. Prevention and control of influenza: Recommendations of the Advisory Committee on Immunization Practices (ACIP). MMWR Recomm Rep 2006;55:1–42.
50. Jackson LA, Neuzil KM, Yu O, et al. Effectiveness of pneumococcal polysaccharide vaccine in older adults. N Engl J Med 2003;348:1747–1755.
51. Alfageme I, Vazquez R, Reyes N, et al. Clinical efficacy of anti-pneumococcal vaccination in patients with COPD. Thorax 2006;61:189–195.
52. Nocturnal Oxygen Therapy Trial Group. Continuous or nocturnal oxygen therapy in hypoxemic chronic obstructive lung disease. Ann Intern Med 1980;93:391–398.
53. Medical Research Council Working Party. Long-term domiciliary oxygen therapy in chronic hypoxic cor pulmonale complicating chronic bronchitis and emphysema. Lancet 1981;1:681–685.
54. O'Donohue WJ. Home oxygen therapy. Med Clin North Am 1996;80:611–622.
55. Ferreira IM, Brooks D, Lacasse Y, et al. Nutritional support for individuals with COPD: A meta-analysis. Chest 2000;117:672–678.
56. Celli BR, Thomas NE, Anderson JA, et al. Effect of pharmacotherapy on rate of decline of lung function in chronic obstructive pulmonary disease: Results from the TORCH study. Am J Respir Crit Care Med 2008;178: 332–338.
57. Dolovich MB, Ahrens RC, Hess DR, et al. Device selection and outcomes of aerosol therapy: Evidence-based guidelines. Chest 2005;127:335–371.
58. Puhan MA, Bachmann LM, Kleijnen J, ter Riet G, Kessels AG. Inhaled drugs to reduce exacerbations in patients with chronic obstructive pulmonary disease: A network meta-analysis. BMC Med 2009;7:2.
59. Truitt T, Witko J, Halpern M. Levalbuterol compared to racemic albuterol: Efficacy and outcomes in patients hospitalized with COPD or asthma. Chest 2003;123: 128–135.
60. Asmus MJ, Hendeles L. Levalbuterol nebulizer solution: Is it worth five times the cost of albuterol? Pharmacotherapy 2000;20:123–129.

61. Datta D, Vitale A, Lahiri B, ZuWallack R. An evaluation of nebulized levalbuterol in stable COPD. Chest 2003;124: 844–849.
62. O'Donnel DE, Lam M, Webb KA. Measurement of symptoms, lung hyperinflation, and endurance during exercise in chronic obstructive pulmonary disease. Am J Respir Crit Care Med 1998;158:1557–1565.
63. Friedman M. A multicenter study of nebulized bronchodilator solutions in chronic obstructive pulmonary disease. Am J Med 1996;100(Suppl 1A):30S–39S.
64. Wiggins J. The role of anticholinergics in "stable" chronic obstructive pulmonary disease: Unanswered questions. Respiration 1994;61:303–304.
65. Ikeda A, Nishimura K, Koyama H, et al. Dose–response study of ipratropium bromide aerosol on maximum exercise performance in stable patients with chronic obstructive pulmonary disease. Thorax 1996;51:48–53.
66. Tsukino M, Nishimura K, Ikeda A, et al. Effects of theophylline and ipratropium bromide on exercise performance in patients with stable chronic obstructive pulmonary disease. Thorax 1998;53:269–273.
67. Martin RJ, Bartelson BL, Smith P, et al. Effect of ipratropium bromide treatment on oxygen saturation and sleep quality in COPD. Chest 1999;115:1338–1345.
68. Mahler DA, Donohue JF, Barbee RA, et al. Efficacy of salmeterol xinafoate in the treatment of COPD. Chest 1999;115:957–965.
69. Rennard SI, Anderson W, ZuWallack R, et al. Use of a long-acting β_2-agonist, salmeterol xinafoate, in patients with chronic obstructive pulmonary disease. Am J Respir Crit Care Med 2001;163:1087–1092.
70. van Noord JA, Smeets JJ, Raaijmakers JA, Bommer AM, Maesen FP. Salmeterol versus formoterol in patients with moderately severe asthma: Onset and duration of action. Eur Respir J 1996;9:1684–1688.
71. Dougherty JA, Didur BL, Aboussouan LS. Long-acting inhaled beta2 agonists for stable COPD. Ann Pharmacother 2003;37:1247–1255.
72. Bouros D, Kottakis J, LeGros V, Overend T, Della Cioppa G, Siafakas N. Effects of formoterol and salmeterol on resting inspiratory capacity in COPD patients with poor FEV_1 reversibility. Curr Med Res Opin 2004;20: 581–586.
73. Rennard, SI, Anderson W, ZuWallack R, et al. Use of a long-acting inhaled beta2 adrenergic agonist, salmeterol xinafoate, in patients with chronic obstructive pulmonary disease. Am J Respir Crit Care Med 2001;163:1087–1092.
74. Dahl R, Greefhorst LA, Nowak D, et al. Inhaled formoterol dry powder versus ipratropium bromide in chronic obstructive pulmonary disease. Am J Respir Crit Care Med 2001;164:778–784.
75. Barnes PJ. The pharmacological properties of tiotropium. Chest 2000;117:63S–66S.
76. Casaburi R, Mayler DA, Jones PW, et al. A long-term evaluation of once daily inhaled ipratropium in chronic obstructive pulmonary disease. Eur Respir J 2002;19: 217–224.
77. Brusasco V, Hodder R, Miravitlles M, Korducki L, Towse L, Kesten S. Health outcomes following treatment for six months with once daily tiotropium compared with twice daily salmeterol in patients with COPD. Thorax 2003;58:399–404.
78. Vincken W, van Noord JA, Greefhorst AP, et al. Improved health outcomes in patients with COPD during one year treatment with tiotropium. Eur Respir J 2002;19: 209–216.
79. Barr RG, Bourbeau J, Camargo CA Jr, Ram FSF. Tiotropium for stable chronic obstructive pulmonary disease: A meta-analysis. Thorax 2006;61:854–862.
80. Anzueto A, Tashkin D, Menjoge S, Kesten S. One year analysis of longitudinal changes in spirometry in patients with COPD receiving tiotropium. Pulm Pharmacol Ther 2005;18:75–81.
81. Donohue JF, van Noord JA, Bateman ED, et al. A 6-month placebo-controlled study comparing lung function and health status changes in COPD patients treated with tiotropium or salmeterol. Chest 2002;122:47–55.
82. Tashkin DP, Celli B, Senn S, et al. A 4 year trial of tiotropium in chronic obstructive pulmonary disease. N Engl J Med 2008;359:1543–1554.
83. Lee TA, Pickard S, Au DH, Bartle B, Weiss KB. Risk for death associated with medications for recently diagnosed chronic obstructive pulmonary disease. Ann Intern Med 2008;149:380–390.
84. Lee TA, Wilke C, Joo M, et al. Outcomes associated with tiotropium use in patients with chronic obstructive pulmonary disease. Arch Intern Med 2009;169:1403–1410.
85. Celli B, Decramer M, Leimer I, Vogel U, Kesten S, Tashkin DP. Cardiovascular safety of tiotropium in patients with COPD. Chest 2010;137:2–30.
86. Fuhr R, Magnussen H, Sarem K, et al. Efficacy of aclidinium bromide 400 μg twice daily compared with placebo and tiotropium in patients with moderate to severe COPD. Chest 2012;141(3):745–752.
87. Combivent Inhalation Aerosol Study Group. In chronic obstructive pulmonary disease, a combination of ipratropium and albuterol is more effective than either agent alone. Chest 1994;105:1411–1419.
88. D'Urzo AD, De Salvo MC, Ramirez-Rivera A, et al. In patients with COPD, treatment with a combination of formoterol and ipratropium is more effective than a combination of salbutamol and ipratropium. Chest 2001;119:1347–1356.
89. Karner C, Cates CJ. Long-acting $beta_2$-agonist in addition to tiotropium versus either tiotropium alone or long-acting $beta_2$-agonist alone for chronic obstructive pulmonary disease. Cochrane Database Syst Rev 2012; 4:CD008989.
90. Barnes PJ. Theophylline in chronic obstructive pulmonary disease: New horizons. Proc Am Thorac Soc 2005;2: 334–339.
91. Barnes PJ. Theophylline: New perspectives for an old drug. Am J Respir Crit Care Med 2003;167:813–818.
92. Man GC, Chapman KR, Ali SH, Darke AC. Sleep quality and nocturnal respiratory function with once-daily theophylline (Uniphyl) and inhaled salbutamol in patients with COPD. Chest 1996;110:648–653.
93. Nishimura K, Koyama H, Ikeda A, et al. The additive effect of theophylline on a high-dose combination of inhaled salbutamol and ipratropium bromide in stable COPD. Chest 1995;107:718–723.
94. Karpel JP, Kotch A, Zinny M, et al. A comparison of inhaled ipratropium, oral theophylline plus inhaled beta agonist, and the combination of all three in patients with COPD. Chest 1994;105:1089–1094.
95. ZuWallack RL, Mahler DA, Reilly D, et al. Salmeterol plus theophylline combination therapy in the treatment of COPD. Chest 2001;119:1661–1670.
96. Callahan CM, Dittus RS, Katz BP. Oral corticosteroid therapy for patients with stable chronic obstructive pulmonary disease: A meta-analysis. Ann Intern Med 1991;114:216–223.

97. Pizzichini E, Pizzichini MM, Gibson P, et al. Sputum eosinophilia predicts benefit from prednisone in smokers with chronic obstructive bronchitis. Am J Respir Crit Care Med 1998;158:1511–1517.
98. Senderovitz T, Vestbo J, Frandsen J, et al. Steroid reversibility test followed by inhaled budesonide or placebo in outpatients with stable chronic obstructive pulmonary disease. The Danish Society of Respiratory Medicine. Respir Med 1999;93:715–718.
99. Pauwels RA, Claes-Goran L, Latinen LA, et al. Long-term treatment with inhaled budesonide in persons with mild chronic obstructive pulmonary disease who continue smoking. N Engl J Med 1999;340:1948–1953.
100. Vestbo J, Sorenson T, Lange P, et al. Long-term effect of inhaled budesonide in mild and moderate chronic obstructive pulmonary disease: A randomized, controlled trial. Lancet 1999;353:1819–1823.
101. Burge PS, Calverley PM, Jones PW, et al. Randomised, double-blind, placebo-controlled study of fluticasone propionate in patients with moderate to severe chronic obstructive pulmonary disease: The ISOLDE trial. Br Med J 2000;320:1297–1303.
102. Nishimura K, Koyama H, Ikeda A, et al. The effect of high-dose inhaled beclomethasone dipropionate in patients with stable COPD. Chest 1999;115:31–37.
103. Weir DC, Bale GA, Bright P, Sherwood Burge P. A double-blind placebo-controlled study of the effect of inhaled beclomethasone dipropionate for 2 years in patients with nonasthmatic chronic obstructive pulmonary disease. Clin Exp Allergy 1999;29(Suppl 2):125–128.
104. Paggiaro PL, Dahle R, Bakran I, et al. Multicentre, randomized, placebo-controlled trial of inhaled fluticasone propionate in patients with chronic obstructive pulmonary disease. International COPD Study Group. Lancet 1998;351:773–780.
105. The Lung Health Study Research Group. Effect of inhaled triamcinolone on the decline in pulmonary function in chronic obstructive pulmonary disease. N Engl J Med 2000;343:1902–1909.
106. Sutherland ER, Allmers H, Ayas NT, Venn AJ, Martin RJ. Inhaled corticosteroids reduce the progression of airflow limitation in chronic obstructive pulmonary disease: A meta-analysis. Thorax 2003;58:937–941.
107. Gartlehner G, Hansen RA, Carson SS, Lohr KN. Efficacy and safety of inhaled corticosteroids in patients with COPD: A systematic review and meta-analysis of health outcomes. Ann Fam Med 2006;4:253–262.
108. Macie C, Wooldrage K, Manfreda J, Anthonisen NR. Inhaled corticosteroids and mortality in COPD. Chest 2006;130: 640–646.
109. Sin DD, Wu L, Anderson JA, et al. Inhaled corticosteroids and mortality in chronic obstructive pulmonary disease. Thorax 2005;60:992–997.
110. Mapel DW, Hurley JS, Roblin D, et al. Survival of COPD patients using inhaled corticosteroids and long-acting beta agonists. Respir Med 2006;100:595–609.
111. Calverley PMA, Anderson JA, Celli B, et al. Salmeterol and fluticasone propionate and survival in chronic obstructive pulmonary disease. N Engl J Med 2007;356:775–789.
112. Drummond MB, Dasenbrook EC, Pitz MW, Murphy DJ, Fan E. Inhaled corticosteroids in patients with stable chronic obstructive pulmonary disease: A systematic review and meta-analysis. JAMA 2008;300:2407–2416.
113. Singh S, Amin AV, Loke YK. Long-term use of inhaled corticosteroids and the risk of pneumonia in chronic obstructive pulmonary disease: A meta-analysis. Arch Intern Med 2009;169:219–229.
114. Lipworth BJ. Systemic adverse effects of inhaled corticosteroid therapy: A systematic review and meta-analysis. Arch Intern Med 1999;159:941–955.
115. van Grunsven PM, van Schayck CP, Derenne JP, et al. Long-term effects of inhaled corticosteroids in chronic obstructive pulmonary disease: A meta-analysis. Thorax 1999;54:7–14.
116. Hubbard R, Tatterfield A, Smith C, et al. Use of inhaled corticosteroids and the risk of fracture. Chest 2006;130:1082–1088.
117. Jones A, Fay JK, Burr M, Stone M, Hood K, Roberts G. Inhaled corticosteroid effects on bone metabolism in asthma and mild chronic obstructive pulmonary disease. Cochrane Database Syst Rev 2002;(1):CD003537.
118. Decramer M, Ferguson G. Clinical safety of long acting beta2 agonists and inhaled corticosteroid combination therapy in COPD. COPD 2006;3:163–171.
119. Calverly P, Pauwels R, Vestbo J, et al. Combined salmeterol and fluticasone in the treatment of chronic obstructive pulmonary disease: A randomized, controlled trial. Lancet 2003;361:449–456.
120. Szafranski W, Cukier A, Ramirez A, et al. Efficacy and safety of budesonide/formoterol in the management of chronic obstructive pulmonary disease. Eur Respir J 2003;21:74–81.
121. Mahler DA, Wire P, Horstman D, et al. Effectiveness of fluticasone propionate and salmeterol combination delivered via the Diskus device in the treatment of chronic obstructive pulmonary disease. Am J Respir Crit Care Med 2002;166:1084–1091.
122. Hanania NA, Darken P, Horstman D, et al. Efficacy and safety of fluticasone propionate (250 mcg) and salmeterol (50 mcg) combined in the Diskus inhaler for the treatment of COPD. Chest 2003;124:834–843.
123. Calverley PM, Boonsawat W, Cseke Z, Zhong N, Peterson S, Olsson H. Maintenance therapy with budesonide and formoterol in chronic obstructive pulmonary disease. Eur Respir J 2003;22:912–919.
124. Kardos P, Wencker M, Glaab T, Vogelmeier C. Impact of salmeterol/fluticasone propionate versus salmeterol on exacerbations in severe chronic obstructive pulmonary disease. Am J Respir Crit Care Med 2007;175:144–149.
125. Wedzicha JA, Calverley PM, Seemungal TA, et al. The prevention of chronic obstructive pulmonary disease exacerbations by salmeterol/fluticasone propionate or tiotropium bromide. Am J Respir Crit Care Med 2008;177:19–26.
126. Baloria VA, Vialrino PC. Bronchodilator efficacy of combined salmeterol and tiotropium in patients with chronic obstructive pulmonary disease. Arch Bronchopneumol 2005;41:130–134.
127. Aaron SD, Vandemheen KL, Fergusson D, et al. Tiotropium in combination with placebo, salmeterol or fluticasone–salmeterol for treatment of chronic obstructive pulmonary disease. Ann Intern Med 2007;146:545–555.
128. Perng DW, Wu CC, Su KC, Lee YC, Perng RP, Tao CW. Additive benefits of tiotropium in COPD patients treated with long-acting beta2 agonists and corticosteroids. Respirology 2006;11:598–602.
129. Juvelekian GS, Stoller JK. Augmentation therapy for alpha1 antitrypsin deficiency. Drugs 2004;64:1743–1756.
130. Alpha-1-Antitrypsin Deficiency Registry Study Group. Survival and FEV_1 decline in individuals with severe deficiency of alpha-1-antitrypsin. Am J Respir Crit Care Med 1998;158:49–59.
131. Dirksen A, Dijkman JH, Madsen F, et al. A randomized clinical trial of alpha-1-antitrypsin augmentation therapy. Am J Respir Crit Care Med 1999;160:1468–1472.

132. Gildea TR, Shermock KM, Singer ME, et al. Cost-effectiveness analysis of augmentation therapy for severe alpha1 antitrypsin deficiency. Am J Respir Crit Care Med 2003;167:1387–1392.
133. Stoller JK, Fallat R, Schluchter MD, et al. Augmentation therapy with alpha1 antitrypsin: Patterns of use and adverse events. Chest 2003;123:1425–1434.
134. Quon BS, Gan WQ, Sin DD. Contemporary management of acute exacerbations of COPD: A systematic review and metaanalysis Chest 2008;133:756–766.
135. Lightowler JV, Wedzicha JA, Elliott MW, et al. Noninvasive positive pressure ventilation to treat respiratory failure resulting from exacerbations of chronic obstructive pulmonary disease: Cochrane systemic review and meta-analysis. Br Med J 2003;326:185–189.
136. Niewoehner DE, Erbland ML, Deupree RH, et al. Effect of systemic glucocorticoids on exacerbations of chronic obstructive pulmonary disease. Department of Veterans Affairs Cooperative Study Group. N Engl J Med 1999;340:1941–1947.
137. Davies L, Angus RM, Calverley PMA. Oral corticosteroids in patients admitted to hospital with exacerbations of chronic obstructive pulmonary disease: A prospective, randomised, controlled trial. Lancet 1999;354:456–460.
138. Thompson WH, Nielson CP, Carvalho P, et al. Controlled trial of oral prednisone in outpatients with acute COPD exacerbation. Am J Respir Crit Care Med 1996;154:407–412.
139. Sayiner A, Aytemur ZA, Cirit M, et al. Systemic glucocorticoids in severe exacerbations of COPD. Chest 2001;119:726–730.
140. Aaron SD, Vandemheen KL, Hebert P, et al. Outpatient oral prednisone after emergency treatment of chronic obstructive pulmonary disease. N Engl J Med 2003;348:2618–2625.
141. Vondracek SF, Hemstreet BA. Is there an optimal corticosteroid regimen for the management of an acute exacerbation of chronic obstructive pulmonary disease? Pharmacotherapy 2006;26:522–532.
142. Stallberg B, Selroos O, Vogelmeier C, Andersson E, Ekstrom T, Larsson K. Budesonide/formoterol as effective as prednisolone plus formoterol in acute exacerbations of COPD: A double blind, randomized, non-inferiority, parallel group, multicenter study. Respir Res 2009;10:11.
143. Saint S, Bent S, Vittinghoff E, Grady D. Antibiotics in chronic obstructive pulmonary disease exacerbations: A meta-analysis. JAMA 1995;273:957–960.
144. Niederman MS. Antibiotic therapy for exacerbations of chronic bronchitis. Semin Respir Infect 2000;15:59–70.
145. Chodosh S, DeAbate C, Haverstock D, Aneiro L, Church D. Short-course moxifloxacin therapy for treatment of acute bacterial exacerbations of chronic bronchitis. Respir Med 2000;94:18–27.
146. Rizkallah J, Man SF, Sin DD. Prevalence of pulmonary embolism in acute exacerbations of COPD: A systematic review and metaanalysis. Chest 2009;135:786–793.
147. Albert RK, Connett J, Bailey WD, et al. Azithromycin for prevention of exacerbation in COPD. N Engl J Med 2011;365:689–698.
148. Ray WA, Murray KT, Hall K, et al. Azithromycin and the risk of cardiovascular death. N Engl J Med 2012;366: 1881–1890.
149. Jenning AL, Davies AN, Higgins JP, Gibbs JS, Broadley KE. A systematic review of the use of opioids in the management of dyspnea. Thorax 2002;57:939–944.
150. Stolz D, Linka A, Di Valentino M, Meyer A, Brutsche M, Tamm M. A randomized, controlled trial of bosentan in severe COPD. Eur Respir J 2008;32:619–628.
151. Fishman A, Martinez F, Naunheim K, et al. A randomized trial comparing lung-volume-reduction surgery with medical therapy for severe emphysema. N Engl J Med 2003;348:2059–2073.
152. Snyder ML, Goss CH, Neradilek B, et al. National Emphysema Treatment Trial Research Group. Changes in arterial oxygenation and self-reported oxygen use after lung volume reduction surgery. Am J Respir Crit Care Med 2008;178:339–345.
153. Deacon SJ, Vincent EE, Greenhaff PL, et al. Randomized controlled trial of dietary creatine as an adjunct therapy to physical training in chronic obstructive pulmonary disease. Am J Respir Crit Care Med 2008;178:233–239.
154. Rennard SI, Fogarty C, Kelsen S, et al. The safety and efficacy of infliximab in moderate to severe chronic obstructive pulmonary disease. Am J Respir Crit Care Med 2007;175:926–934.
155. Miravitlles M, Murio C, Guerrero T, Gisbert R. Pharmacoeconomic evaluation of acute exacerbations of chronic bronchitis and COPD. Chest 2002;121: 1449–1455.
156. Grossman RF, Mukerjee J, Vaughan D, et al. A one-year community-based health economic study of ciprofloxacin versus usual antibiotic treatment in acute exacerbations of chronic bronchitis. Chest 1998;113: 131–141.
157. Gallefoss F. The effects of patient education in COPD in a 1-year follow-up randomized, controlled trial. Patient Educ Couns 2004;52:259–266.
158. Friedman M, Serby CW, Menjoge SS, et al. Pharmacoeconomic evaluation of a combination of ipratropium plus albuterol compared with ipratropium alone and albuterol alone in COPD. Chest 1999;115: 635–641.
159. Hansen-Flashen J. Chronic obstructive pulmonary disease: The last year of life. Respir Care 2004;49:90–97.

17

Pulmonary Arterial Hypertension

Rebecca L. Attridge, Rebecca Moote, and Deborah J. Levine

KEY CONCEPTS

1. Pulmonary arterial hypertension (PAH) is defined as a mean pulmonary artery pressure (mPAP) ≥25 mm Hg at rest with a pulmonary wedge pressure (also known as pulmonary artery occlusion pressure) or left ventricular end-diastolic pressure (LVEDP) ≤15 mm Hg measured by right cardiac catheterization.
2. Diagnosis of PAH is growing due to increased awareness and knowledge of the disease state, leading to earlier and improved evaluation and identification.
3. Regardless of the etiology, be it unknown or related to an associated medical condition, subgroups of PAH are based on similar clinical and pathologic physiology.
4. The underlying cause of PAH is a complicated amalgam of endothelial cell dysfunction, a procoagulant state, platelet activation, vasoconstriction, loss of relaxing factors, cellular proliferation, hypertrophy, fibrosis, and inflammation.
5. Patients with PAH present with exertional dyspnea, fatigue, weakness, and exertion intolerance. As the disease progresses, symptoms of right heart dysfunction and failure, such as dyspnea at rest, lower extremity edema, chest pain, and syncope, are seen.
6. The only way to make a definitive diagnosis of PAH is by right heart catheterization. The right heart catheterization provides important prognostic information and can be used to assess pulmonary vasoreactivity prior to initiating therapy.
7. The goals of treatment are to alleviate symptoms, improve the quality of life, slow the progression of the disease, and improve survival.
8. A general goal of PAH treatment is to correct the imbalance between vasoconstriction and vasodilation and prevent adverse thrombotic events to improve oxygenation and quality of life.
9. Nonpharmacologic therapy is frequently used to address comorbid conditions that often accompany PAH.
10. Conventional therapy of PAH includes oral anticoagulants, diuretics, oxygen, and digoxin.
11. Prostacyclin analogs such as epoprostenol, treprostinil, and iloprost induce potent vasodilation of pulmonary vascular beds.
12. Endothelin receptor antagonists, bosentan and ambrisentan, improve exercise capacity, hemodynamics, and functional class in PAH.
13. Phosphodiesterase-5 inhibitors, including sildenafil and tadalafil, are potent and highly specific drugs that have been shown to reduce mPAP and improve functional class.
14. Combination therapy in PAH may address more than one mechanism causing this disease. Combination therapy in clinical trials has provided additional benefit, but more studies are needed.

Pulmonary hypertension is a term describing a group of conditions relating to elevated blood pressure measured within the pulmonary artery. Pulmonary hypertension is not a specific diagnosis; rather it is a complex group of disorders relating to the pulmonary circulation. Pulmonary hypertension is classified into five groups according to the World Health Organization (WHO; see Table 17-1).[1] Pulmonary arterial hypertension (PAH) or Group 1 pulmonary hypertension is a progressive disease characterized by an elevation in pulmonary arterial pressure and pulmonary vascular resistance. **1** PAH may be defined as a mean pulmonary artery pressure (mPAP) ≥25 mm Hg at rest, with a pulmonary wedge pressure (also known as a pulmonary artery occlusion pressure or left ventricular end-diastolic pressure [LVEDP]) ≤15 mm Hg measured by cardiac catheterization.[2]

PAH may occur in the setting of underlying medical conditions or as an idiopathic disease (idiopathic PAH [IPAH]). Historically, medical treatment of PAH has been limited due to lack of effective, targeted therapy. Without medical therapy, IPAH portends a poor prognosis (median survival 2.8 years) after diagnosis.[3] Prior to the availability of disease-specific therapy for IPAH, survival rates for 1, 3, and 5 years were 68%, 48%, and 34%, respectively.[4] Since the approval of epoprostenol in 1995, a number of new therapeutic options have been developed. In a recent epidemiologic study, survival rates for 1, 2, and 3 years in patients on targeted therapy were 83%, 67%, and 58%, respectively.[5]

EPIDEMIOLOGY

The prevalence of PAH is estimated to be 15 to 50 patients per million individuals. Unfortunately, only 15,000 to 20,000 of the afflicted patients have an established diagnosis of PAH and are currently receiving treatment. In a French registry study of more than 600 patient with PAH, Humbert found that the most common cause of PAH was IPAH (approximately 40%), followed by PAH associated with connective tissue diseases (15.3%), congenital heart disease (11.3%), portal hypertension (10.4%), and familial PAH (FPAH) (3.9%).[6] **2** However, diagnosis of PAH is growing due to increased awareness and knowledge of the disease state, leading to earlier and improved evaluation and identification.

TABLE 17-1 World Health Organization Classification of Pulmonary Hypertension

Group 1—Pulmonary Arterial Hypertension (PAH)
1.1. Idiopathic (IPAH)
1.2. Heritable
1.2.1. BMPR2
1.2.2. ALK-1, endoglin (with or without hereditary hemorrhagic telangiectasia)
1.2.3. Unknown
1.3. Drug and toxin induced
1.4. Associated with (APAH)
1.4.1. Connective tissue diseases
1.4.2. HIV infection
1.4.3. Portal hypertension
1.4.4. Congenital heart diseases
1.4.5. Schistosomiasis
1.4.6. Chronic hemolytic anemia
1.5. Persistent pulmonary hypertension of the newborn
1.6. Pulmonary venoocclusive disease (PVOD) and/or pulmonary capillary hemangiomatosis (PCH)
Group 2—Pulmonary Hypertension Owing to Left Heart Disease
2.1. Systolic dysfunction
2.2. Diastolic dysfunction
2.3. Valvular disease
Group 3—Pulmonary Hypertension Owing to Lung Diseases and/or Hypoxemia
3.1. Chronic obstructive pulmonary disease
3.2. Interstitial lung disease
3.3. Other pulmonary diseases with mixed restrictive and obstructive pattern
3.4. Sleep-disordered breathing
3.5. Alveolar hypoventilation disorders
3.6. Chronic exposure to high altitude
3.7. Developmental abnormalities
Group 4—Chronic Thromboembolic Pulmonary Hypertension (CTEPH)
Group 5—Pulmonary Hypertension with Unclear Multifactorial Mechanisms
5.1. Hematologic disorders: myeloproliferative disorders, splenectomy
5.2. Systemic disorders: sarcoidosis, pulmonary Langerhans' cell histiocytosis, lymphangioleiomyomatosis, neurofibromatosis, vasculitis
5.3. Metabolic disorders: glycogen storage disease, Gaucher's disease, thyroid disorders
5.4. Others: tumoral obstruction, fibrosing mediastinitis, chronic renal failure on dialysis

ALK-1, activin receptor-like kinase type-1; BMPR2, bone morphogenetic protein receptor 2; HIV, human immunodeficiency virus.

Data from reference 11.

ETIOLOGY

PAH most often originates with a predisposing state and one or more inciting factors that could be genetic or environmental exposures.[7] Once a permissive environment exists, multiple mechanisms can be activated leading to vascular constriction, cellular proliferation, and a prothrombotic state resulting in PAH and its sequelae.[8] PAH can be associated with numerous conditions as well as being an idiopathic condition (IPAH). The incidence of IPAH is estimated to be 5 to 6 per 1 million in North America and Europe, with a marked female predominance (male-to-female ratio, 1:1.7), and mean age at time of recognition is approximately 37 years, although there is considerable variation.[8,9] Although uncommon in the United States, the commonest form of PAH worldwide is schistosomiasis followed by congenital heart disease and pulmonary hypertension of early childhood.[10] Rheumatologic diseases such as scleroderma, systemic lupus erythematosus, rheumatoid arthritis, and myositis are also associated with development of PAH. Patients with scleroderma who develop PAH, estimated between 7% and 12% of patients, have markedly worse outcomes in comparison to other PAH subgroups. Patients with human immunodeficiency virus (HIV) infection can develop PAH with a prevalence of 0.5%. In patients with liver disease, portal hypertension may cause concurrent pulmonary hypertension in an estimated 2% to 6% of patients.[11] Multiple drugs and toxins have been associated with PAH but those that definitively precipitate PAH include anorexigens such as aminorex, fenfluramine, and dexfenfluramine.[10,12] Other drugs considered to be likely or possible causative agents for PAH include amphetamines, L-tryptophan, cocaine, and certain chemotherapeutic agents (mitomycin C, carmustine, etoposide, cyclophosphamide, bleomycin).[9] Heritable PAH (HPAH) includes both IPAH with germline mutations and familial cases without an identified mutation. Germline mutations seen in PAH include bone morphogenetic protein receptor 2 (BMPR2) and activin receptor-like kinase 1 (ALK-1). Genetic testing for these mutations may be offered and professional genetic counseling should be provided.[11]

PATHOPHYSIOLOGY

❸ Regardless of etiology, all subgroups of PAH are based on similar clinical and pathologic physiology. ❹ The pathobiology of PAH involves several key biologic events, including endothelial cell dysfunction, a procoagulant state, platelet activation, constricting factors, loss of relaxing factors, cellular proliferation, hypertrophy, fibrosis, and inflammation—all combining to produce progressive and deleterious vascular remodeling (Fig. 17-1).[13,14] Multiple genetic mutations are known to contribute to the pathophysiology of PAH, including BMPR2, ALK-1, nitric oxide synthase (ec-NOS), carbamoyl-phosphate synthase gene, and 5-hydroxytryptamine (serotonin [5-HT]) transporter (5-HTT).[13,15] A mutation of BMPR2 receptor is an aberration of signal transduction in the pulmonary vascular smooth muscle cell that is postulated to alter apoptosis favoring cellular proliferation. ALK-1 is part of the transforming growth factor-β superfamily and is seen in hereditary hemorrhagic telangiectasia and PAH.[16] 5-HTT is associated with pulmonary artery smooth muscle proliferation and is present in IPAH in the homozygous form in 65% of patients.[17] Dysregulation of 5-HT synthesis mediated via tryptophan hydroxylases is closely linked to the hypoxic PAH phenotype in mice and may contribute to PAH development.[18]

Molecular, cellular, and genetic mechanisms are mediated by a variety of biologically active compounds, including prostacyclin (PGI_2), endothelin-1 (ET-1), nitric oxide (NO), and 5-HT. PGI_2 is a vasodilatory and antiproliferative substance that is produced by the endothelial cells, and the synthesis of PGI_2 and its circulating levels are reduced in PAH. Furthermore, thromboxane, a vasoconstrictor, is increased in PAH. ET-1 is produced in the endothelium, and it possesses potent vasoconstrictor and mitogenic effects. ET-1 levels are increased in PAH and clearance is reduced. ET-1 acts via the endothelin receptors (ET_A and ET_B) to promote vascular smooth muscle proliferation and vasoconstriction.[14,19] Plasma levels of ET-1 are correlated with severity of PAH and prognosis.[20] NO is produced in the endothelium via NO synthase and leads to vasodilation and opening of cell membrane potassium channels to allow potassium ion efflux, membrane depolarization, and calcium channel inhibition. Voltage-dependent potassium channels are inhibited by a number of stimuli that promote PAH, including hypoxia and fenfluramine, resulting in

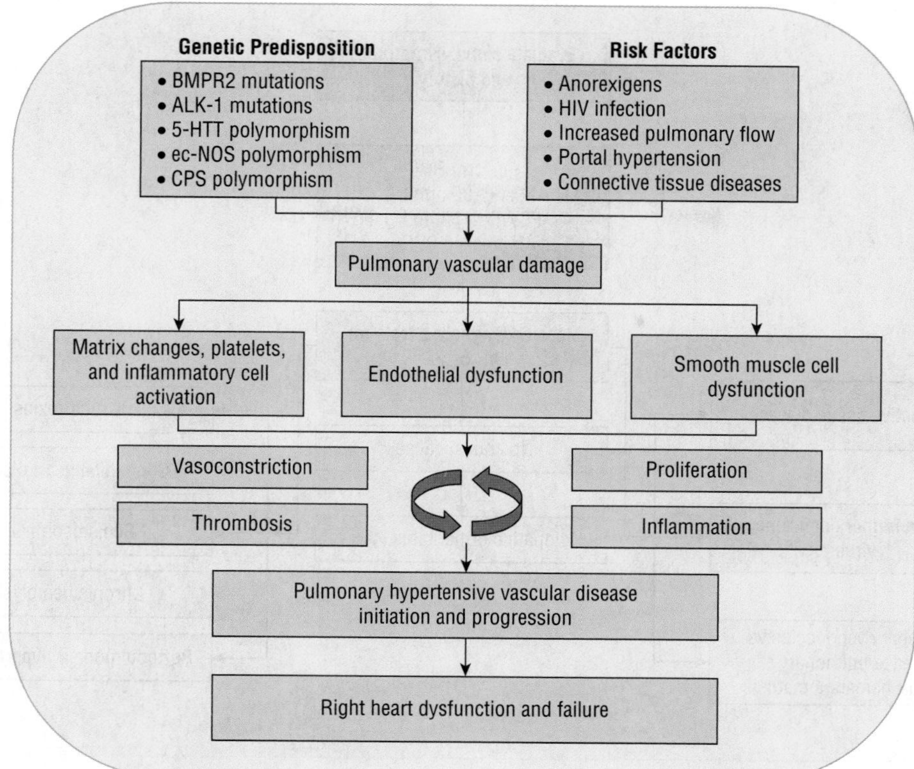

FIGURE 17-1 Pulmonary arterial hypertension; potential pathogenetic and pathobiologic mechanisms. (ALK-1, activin receptor-like kinase 1 gene; BMPR2, bone morphogenetic protein receptor 2 gene; CPS, carbamoyl-phosphate synthase gene; ec-NOS, nitric oxide synthase gene; 5-HTT, serotonin transporter gene; HIV, human immunodeficiency virus.) *(Reproduced with permission from reference 30.)*

downregulated potassium channels in patients with PAH. Entering calcium is a signal for release of sarcoplasmic calcium and activation of the contractile apparatus. NO promotes vasodilation through calcium channel inhibition. In PAH there is evidence of decreased NO synthase expression, leading to vasoconstriction and cell proliferation.[21] Elevated 5-HT has been observed and vasoconstriction mediated via the increased expression of the 5-HT_{1B} receptor is seen in PAH.[8]

Autoantibodies, proinflammatory cytokines, and inflammatory infiltrates may also participate in the pathogenesis of PAH. Coagulation is disordered in PAH as evidenced by increased levels of von Willebrand factor, plasma fibrinopeptide A, plasminogen activator inhibitor-1, 5-HT, and thromboxane. Furthermore, tissue plasminogen activator, thrombomodulin, NO, and PGI_2 are decreased, leading to an imbalance favoring thrombosis. Endothelial dysfunction is the common denominator of mechanisms for PAH, and a variety of injuries, such as shear stress, inflammation, toxins, and hypoxia, are thought to be involved.[10,13]

5 The signs and symptoms of PAH are highly variable depending on the stage of the disease and comorbidities (Table 17-2). Symptoms may include exertional dyspnea, fatigue, and weakness. As the disease progresses, patients may experience dyspnea at rest, chest pain, presyncope, syncope, lower extremity edema, and abdominal bloating and distension. On physical exam, patients with PAH may have an accentuated component of S_2 audible at the apex of the heart, midsystolic ejection murmur, palpable left parasternal lift, right ventricular S_4 gallop, and a prominent "a" wave.[10] Hepatojugular reflux, a diastolic murmur of pulmonary regurgitation, and a systolic murmur of tricuspid regurgitation may be present in advanced disease.[9]

Several comorbidities and environmental factors play a role in the development of PAH and must be evaluated when establishing an initial diagnosis of PAH (Fig. 17-2). In patients with a clinical suspicion of PAH, Doppler echocardiography should be performed as a noninvasive screening test that can detect increased pulmonary pressures, although this study cannot be used to definitively diagnose PAH.[22] Echocardiography can also be used to assess treatment interventions and to follow disease progression.[10] **6** However, right heart catheterization is the definitive study to

TABLE 17-2 World Health Organization Functional Classification of Pulmonary Arterial Hypertension (PAH)

Class	Description
I	Patients with PAH in whom there is no limitation of usual physical activity; ordinary physical activity does not cause increased dyspnea, fatigue, chest pain, or presyncope
II	Patients with PAH who have mild limitation of physical activity. There is no discomfort at rest, but normal physical activity causes increased dyspnea, fatigue, chest pain, or presyncope
III	Patients with PAH who have marked limitation of physical activity. There is no discomfort at rest, but less than normal physical activity causes increased dyspnea, fatigue, chest pain, or presyncope
IV	Patients with PAH who are unable to perform any physical activity at rest and who may have signs of right ventricular failure. Dyspnea and/or fatigue may be present at rest, and symptoms are increased by almost any physical activity

Data from reference 3.

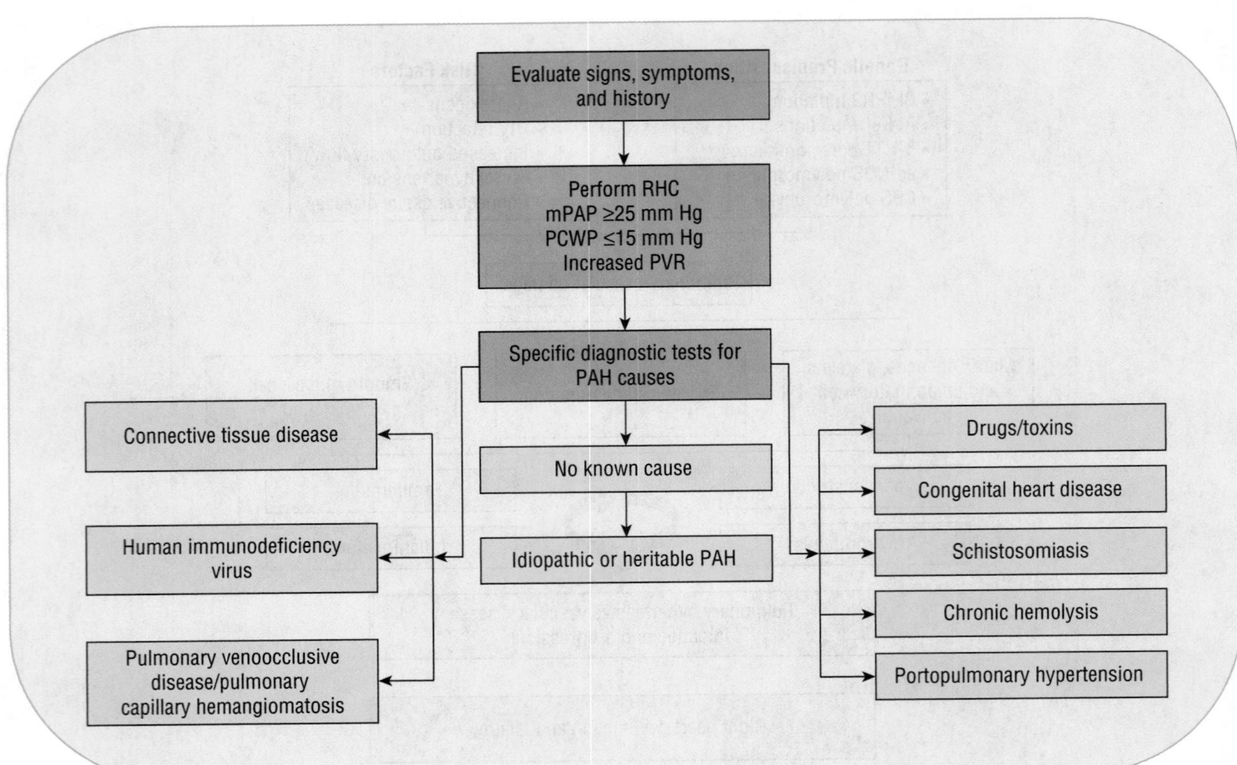

FIGURE 17-2 Evaluation of causes of PAH. *(Adapted from Galiè N, Hoeper MM, Humbert M, et al. Guidelines for the diagnosis and treatment of pulmonary hypertension: The Task Force for the Diagnosis and Treatment of Pulmonary Hypertension of the European Society of Cardiology (ESC) and the European Respiratory Society (ERS), endorsed by the International Society of Heart and Lung Transplantation (ISHLT). Eur Heart J 2009;30:2493–2537.)*

use in diagnosis of PAH and when patients are worsening clinically.[15] Right heart catheterization provides important prognostic information and can be used to assess pulmonary vasoreactivity with the administration of fast-acting, short-duration vasodilators to determine the extent of vascular smooth muscle constriction and vasodilator response to calcium channel blockers (CCBs; strength of recommendation: A for IPAH; E/C for associated pulmonary arterial hypertension [APAH]).[9] Table 17-3 lists the grading criteria for recommendations, and Table 17-4 lists commonly used agents and their dosages. The consensus definition of a positive response is defined as a reduction of mPAP by at least 10 mm Hg to a value of 40 mm Hg or less.[23] Patients with an acute response (approximately 13% on initial testing) are most likely to have a beneficial hemodynamic and clinical response. These patients may be able to be treated with CCBs. However, about half of these patients lose an acute vasodilator response when tested 1 year later.[24] Therefore, even this small group of patients who may be treated with CCBs must be followed closely for safety and efficacy. If the patient loses the acute vasodilator response, he or she needs to be switched to different PAH therapy. Patients who have a negative response on initial vasodilator testing are not candidates for treatment with CCBs.[9,25]

Because PAH commonly occurs in the setting of connective tissue disease, serologic markers should be obtained to confirm or exclude these diagnoses.[9,26] Liver function tests (LFTs) should also be evaluated due to the increased risk for PAH in patients with cirrhosis and portal hypertension. HIV is associated with an increased prevalence of PAH, and HIV testing should be done as part of the initial PAH workup.[9] Chronic thromboembolic pulmonary hypertension (CTEPH) should be evaluated with ventilation–perfusion lung scans and/or pulmonary angiography. Pulmonary function testing and arterial blood oxygenation should be evaluated. The diffusing capacity of carbon monoxide may be particularly helpful in systemic sclerosis and PAH.[10] In

TABLE 17-3 Relationship of Strength of Recommendation Scale to Quality of Evidence and Net Benefit

	Net Benefit					
Quality of Evidence	Substantial	Intermediate	Small/Weak	None	Conflicting	Negative
Good	A	A	B	D	I	D
Fair	A	B	C	D	I	D
Low	B	C	C	I	I	D
Expert opinion	E/A	E/B	E/C	I	I	E/D

A, strong recommendation; B, moderate recommendation; C, weak recommendation; D, negative recommendation; I, inconclusive (no recommendation possible); E/A, strong recommendation based on expert opinion only; E/B, moderate recommendation based on expert opinion only; E/C, weak recommendation based on expert opinion only; E/D, negative recommendation based on expert opinion only.

Data from reference 1.

CLINICAL PRESENTATION Pulmonary Arterial Hypertension

Symptoms

- Exertional dyspnea
- Fatigue
- Weakness
- Exertional chest pain
- Complaints of general exertion intolerance
- Dyspnea at rest as disease progresses
- Syncope
- Lower extremity edema

Symptoms of Related Conditions

- Paroxysmal nocturnal dyspnea as a result of left-sided heart disease
- Raynaud's phenomenon, arthralgia, or swollen hands and other symptoms of connective tissue disease
- Orthopnea
- A history of snoring as reported by the patient's partner may be a consequence of sleep-disordered breathing and can be associated with PAH

Symptoms of Disease Progression

- Leg swelling
- Abdominal bloating and distension
- Anorexia
- More profound fatigue
  May develop as right ventricular dysfunction and triscuspid valve regurgitation evolve

Signs

- Accentuated component of S_2 audible at the apex of the heart
- Early systolic ejection click
- Midsystolic ejection murmur
- Palpable left parasternal lift
- Right ventricular S_4 gallop
- Prominent "a" wave

Signs of Advanced Disease

- Diastolic murmur of pulmonary regurgitation
- Holosystolic murmur of tricuspid regurgitation
- Hepatojugular reflux
- A pulsatile liver
- Right ventricular S_3 gallop
- Marked distension of jugular veins
- Peripheral edema
- Hypotension
- Cool extremities suggesting markedly reduced cardiac output and peripheral vasoconstriction
- Diminished pulse pressure
- Cyanosis (suggests right-to-left shunting)
- Digital clubbing
- Rales
- Dullness
- Decreased breath sounds
- Accessory muscle use
- Wheezing
- Prolonged exhalation
- Peripheral venous insufficiency (suggests venous thrombosis or pulmonary thrombotic disease)

Diagnostic Tests

- Electrocardiogram for chamber enlargement
- Chest radiography to detect enlarged pulmonary arteries
- Doppler echocardiography to evaluate right ventricular/right atrial morphology and calculate right ventricular pressure and pulmonary arterial systolic pressure
- Magnetic resonance imaging may be used to exclude other diagnoses and evaluate right heart morphology
- Pulmonary function testing and arterial blood oxygenation
- Ventilation–perfusion scanning
- Computed tomography or magnetic resonance imaging can be used to exclude other diagnoses
- Right heart catheterization may be used to confirm the presence of PAH and to guide therapy
- Tests for connective disease or other risk factors

patients with PAH, serial determinations of functional class, exercise capacity (assessed by the 6-minute walk distance), and serial biomarkers provide benchmarks for disease severity, response to therapy, and progression.[9,26]

TABLE 17-4 Agents for Vasodilator Testing in Pulmonary Arterial Hypertension

	NO	Epoprostenol	Adenosine
Route	Inhaled	IV	IV
Dose range	10–80 ppm	2–10 ng/kg/min	50–250 mcg/kg/min
Dosing increments	10–80 ppm for 5 minutes	2 ng/kg/min every 15 minutes	50 mcg/kg/min every 2 minutes
Common side effects	None	Headache, flushing, nausea	Chest tightness, dyspnea

NO, nitric oxide.

Data from reference 33.

TREATMENT

Pulmonary Arterial Hypertension

Desired Outcomes

7 The goals of treatment are alleviation of symptoms, improvement in the quality of life, prevention of disease progression, and improvement in survival.[1,9] While the first two outcomes are obtainable based on data from randomized trials, controversy exists over improvement in survival with current treatment regimens. Meta-analyses are conflicting; a 2007 meta-analysis of 16 trials demonstrated no mortality benefit in functional classes III/IV while a later 2009 study of 21 trials (6 of which were not included in the 2007 study) in predominately functional class III patients showed a 43% reduction in mortality.[27] Unfortunately, overall mortality remained high.[28] In addition, individual trials also show survival benefit, at least in the short term (i.e., 3 years).[29]

General Approach to Treatment

Treatment of PAH may be categorized into nonpharmacologic, pharmacologic, and surgical interventions. **8** The principal endothelial abnormalities that are current pharmacologic therapeutic targets include (a) supplementing endogenous vasodilators, (b) inhibiting endogenous vasoconstrictors, and (c) reducing endothelial platelet interaction and limiting thrombosis. Nonpharmacologic therapy can be quite broad and should be used when clinically appropriate. Surgical therapy is indicated in certain situations and includes atrial septostomy, pulmonary thromboendarterectomy for CTEPH, and lung or heart–lung transplantation (for disease that is not responsive to medical therapy).[1]

Nonpharmacologic Therapy

9 Nonpharmacologic therapy is frequently used to address comorbid conditions that often accompany PAH. Patients with PAH should be counseled on several important points. Pregnancy should be avoided due to high morbidity and mortality rates in females with PAH during pregnancy and in the postpartum course.[3] Immunization against influenza and pneumococcal disease should be provided.[9] Hypoxemia may aggravate vasoconstriction in patients with PAH; therefore, PAH patients may require supplemental oxygen, particularly when using air travel.[30] Patients should adhere to a low-sodium diet to avoid fluid retention predisposing to right heart failure.[31] Cardiopulmonary rehabilitation improves functional status and is safe and important for patients with PAH.[32]

Pharmacologic Therapy

The number of potential therapies for PAH has expanded dramatically in the last decade. In addition to adjunctive background therapy, multiple drugs have been developed specifically for treatment of PAH. Figure 17-3 illustrates the current recommended treatment algorithm based on the most recent guidelines.[1,3]

Conventional Pharmacologic Treatment **10** Conventional therapy includes oral anticoagulants, diuretics, oxygen, and digoxin.[26] Anticoagulation with warfarin may be considered in

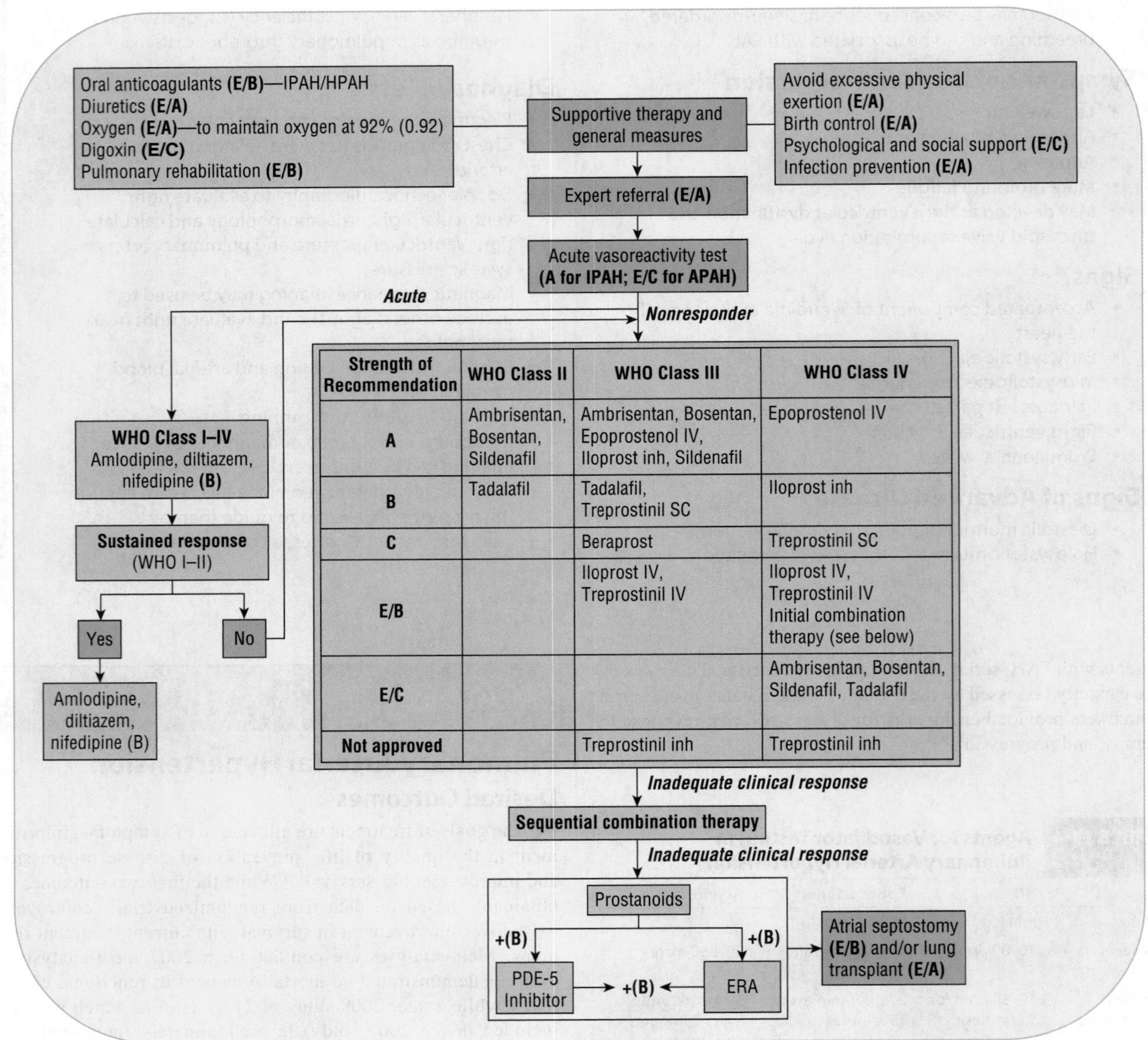

FIGURE 17-3 Treatment algorithm for pulmonary arterial hypertension (PAH). Designators (A), (B), (C), (D), (E/A), (E/B), and (E/C) are defined in Table 17-3. (APAH, associated pulmonary arterial hypertension; CCB, calcium channel blocker; FC, functional class; HPAH, heritable pulmonary arterial hypertension; IPAH, idiopathic pulmonary arterial hypertension.) *(Data from reference 1.)*

patients with PAH, particularly if they have IPAH. The rationale for oral anticoagulants is based on the presence of traditional risk factors for venous thromboembolism, such as heart failure and sedentary lifestyle, as well as on the demonstration of thrombotic predisposition and thrombotic changes in the pulmonary microcirculation. The target international normalized ratio (INR) in most centers is 1.5 to 2.5.[10,23] Anticoagulation is recommended for patients with IPAH (strength of recommendation: E/B).[1,9]

Loop diuretics such as furosemide are helpful adjunctive therapy in patients with decompensated right heart failure and associated findings of increased central venous pressure, abdominal organ congestion, peripheral edema, and ascites.[9] Appropriate diuretic therapy in right heart failure provides symptomatic and clinical benefits in patients with PAH (strength of recommendation: E/A).[9] Patients should be maintained at as close to a euvolemic state as possible.

Oxygen therapy with a goal oxygen saturation greater than 90% (0.90) may be beneficial in some patients, although there are no data regarding the long-term effects of oxygen treatment in PAH (strength of recommendation: E/A).[9] Oxygen treatment is controversial in patients with PAH associated with shunts (i.e., Eisenmenger's syndrome).

Digoxin may be used for patients with PAH with right heart failure as adjunctive therapy along with diuretics to control symptoms (strength of recommendation: E/C).[9] There are no long-term trials and benefit is uncertain. Optimal plasma concentrations are unknown; however, in light of recent trials of digoxin in left systolic dysfunction, the typical target concentration is between 0.5 and 0.8 ng/mL (0.64 and 1 nmol/L). Patients on digoxin should receive periodic monitoring of potassium.

Specific Pharmacologic Therapy In recent years, there has been a surge in availability of drug therapy for the treatment of PAH. Figure 17-4 illustrates the timeline of drug approval over the past few decades.

Synthetic Prostacyclin and Prostacyclin Analogs **11** PGI_2 is produced predominantly by endothelial cells, and it induces potent vasodilation of all vascular beds. It is also a potent inhibitor of platelet aggregation and possesses cytoprotective and antiproliferative activities. PGI_2 synthase expression is reduced in pulmonary arteries, and urinary excretion of PGI_2 metabolites is reduced in PAH. Epoprostenol is a synthetic analog of PGI_2 and has a short half-life of 3 to 5 minutes; consequently, it must be given by continuous IV infusion. Initiation of epoprostenol should be done in a hospital setting at low doses ranging from 2 to 4 ng/kg/min and increased at a rate limited by side effects (flushing, headache, diarrhea, jaw pain, backache, abdominal cramping, foot/leg pain, and hypotension). The two available products, Flolan® (now available generic) and Veletri®, have unique stability and reconstitution parameters; both pharmacists and patients should be aware of the differences and follow the manufacturer recommendations. Because of the short half-life of the drug, it is recommended that the patient have a backup supply of the drug and infusion pump.[23] Because the drug must be administered by continuous infusion with a central venous catheter and pump, infection, catheter obstruction, and sepsis are potential complications. A Centers for Disease Control and Prevention study found that bloodstream infections occurred with epoprostenol and treprostinil in the range of 0.3 to 2.1 per 1,000 medicine days (approximately 1 infection every 3 years) when these drugs are given by the IV route. The target dose for the first 2 to 4 weeks is around 10 to 15 ng/kg/min, and periodic dose increases are then required to maximize efficacy. Optimal doses are variable but are in the range of 25 to 40 ng/kg/min.[30,33] Observational series have documented an improvement in survival in patients with IPAH compared with either historical control or predicted survival based on the National Institutes of Health Registry equation.[33–35] Based on current guidelines, epoprostenol is indicated for WHO functional class III and IV (strength of recommendation: A).[1]

Treprostinil (Remodulin) is a stable analog of PGI_2 given for subcutaneous (SC) or IV infusion approved for functional classes II, III, and IV.[33] The major advantages of treprostinil over epoprostenol include ease of use and increased safety due to a longer half-life, lowering the risk of rebound effects that may happen with drug interruption.[19] Treprostinil has been shown to improve 6-minute walk distance and hemodynamics with outcomes that are similar to epoprostenol.[36,37] In clinical trials, the greatest exercise improvement was observed in patients who were more compromised at baseline and in patients who could tolerate doses in the upper quartile (>13.8 ng/kg/min). The initial dose for treprostinil is 1.25 ng/kg/min by either the SC or the IV route. If not tolerated, the dose should be reduced to 0.625 ng/kg/min and retitration attempted at 4 weeks. If transitioning from epoprostenol to treprostinil, start with 10% of the epoprostenol dose. Dose may be increased by 1.25 ng/kg/min but no more than 2.5 ng/kg/min per week. Infusion site pain is common with the SC route, leading to discontinuation of the treatment in 8% of patients and limiting dose increase in other patients.[30] Patients unable to tolerate SC can be transitioned to IV treprostinil.[23] Other side effects are similar to epoprostenol. Based

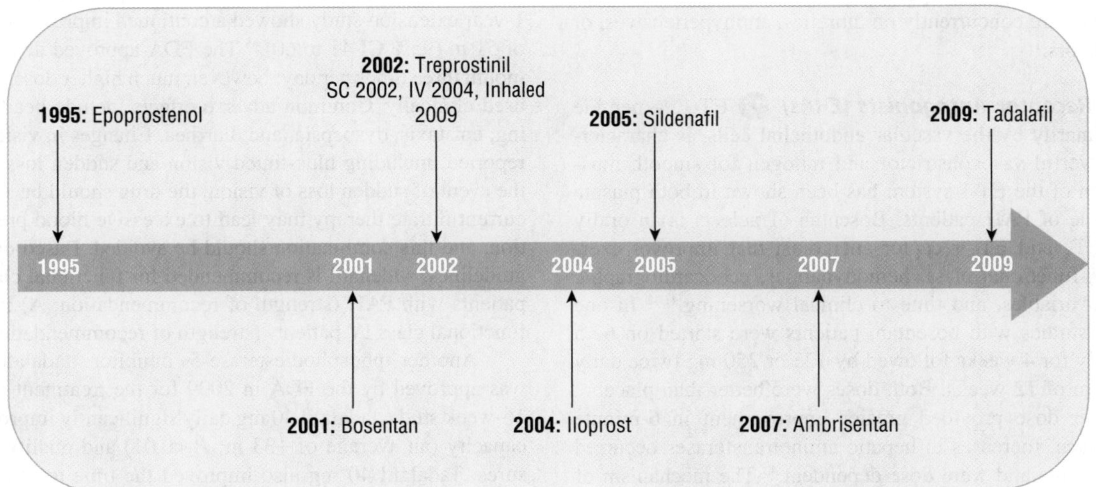

FIGURE 17-4 Timeline of pulmonary arterial hypertension (PAH) medication approvals. Epoprostenol: 1995; treprostinil: SC 2002, IV 2004, inhaled 2009; iloprost: 2004; bosentan: 2001; ambrisentan: 2007; sildenafil: 2005; tadalafil: 2009.

on international guidelines, treprostinil is recommended for functional class III (SC administration—strength of recommendation: B; IV administration—strength of recommendation: E/B), and functional class IV (SC administration—strength of recommendation: C; IV administration—strength of recommendation: E/B).[1]

In an effort to prevent complications and use of pumps and central venous catheters for PGI_2 analog administration, aerosolized formulations were developed. The first approved formulation, iloprost (Ilomedin, Ventavis), is a PGI_2 analog that is given by inhalation using a dosing system provided by the manufacturer (ADD system) with the initial inhaled dose being 2.5 mcg six to nine times per day up to every 2 hours during waking hours. The dose should be titrated and maintained at 5 mcg/dose if tolerated. In a 3-month, randomized, double-blind, placebo-controlled trial, iloprost via inhalation provided at least a 10% improvement in 6-minute walking distance and improvement in functional class.[38] Inhaled iloprost can be cumbersome to use as each inhalation dose can take 4 to 10 minutes to administer. Patients should also be instructed to have a backup supply as iloprost has a short half-life, similar to epoprostenol.[23] Adverse effects are similar to other PGI_2 analogs with the exception of infectious complications related to catheter use for drug delivery. Inhaled iloprost is indicated for functional class III (strength of recommendation: A) and functional class IV (strength of recommendation: B), although many clinicians prefer using the IV or SC route in patients with more severe disease.[1]

The second aerosolized formulation, inhaled treprostinil (Tyvaso), was approved by the FDA in July 2009 to improve exercise capacity in functional class III patients. In a randomized, double-blind, 12-week trial, patients receiving inhaled treprostinil experienced a 20-m improvement in 6-minute walk distance compared with those on placebo (P <0.0006). All patients included in the trial were concurrently receiving bosentan or sildenafil for at least 3 months.[39] An open-label extension of the trial found that inhaled treprostinil provided sustained benefit and was safe and efficacious over a 2-year period.[40] The approved dosing of inhaled treprostinil is three breaths (18 mcg each) four times daily during waking hours. The dose may be titrated based on patient tolerance at 1- to 2-week intervals to maximum dose of nine breaths four times daily. Inhaled treprostinil requires less time to administer, but the formulation is more complicated to prepare than inhaled iloprost.[23] While inhaled treprostinil avoids the infusion-related complications of the other PGI_2 analogs, use is cautioned in patients with acute pulmonary infections or underlying lung disease. The most common adverse effects seen in clinical trials include throat irritation, cough, headache, nausea, dizziness, and flushing. Inhaled treprostinil may also cause systemic hypotension, and patients should be monitored carefully if they are concurrently on diuretics, antihypertensives, or other vasodilators.[1]

Endothelin Receptor Antagonists (ERAs) **12** ET-1, a peptide produced primarily by the vascular endothelial cells, is characterized as a powerful vasoconstrictor and mitogen for smooth muscle. Activation of the ET-1 system has been shown in both plasma and lung tissue of PAH patients. Bosentan (Tracleer) is an orally active dual ET_A and ET_B receptor antagonist that improves exercise capacity, functional class, hemodynamics, echocardiographic and Doppler variables, and time to clinical worsening.[41,42] In one of the larger studies with bosentan, patients were started on 62.5 mg twice daily for 4 weeks followed by 125 or 250 mg twice daily for a minimum of 12 weeks. Both doses were better than placebo, and the higher dose provided greater improvement in 6-minute walking distance. Increases in hepatic aminotransferases occurred in 11% of patients and were dose dependent.[42] The mechanism of increased liver enzymes is thought to be competition by bosentan and its metabolites with the biliary excretion of bile salts, resulting in retention of bile salts that can be cytotoxic to hepatocytes. Because of this toxicity, bosentan is only available through a distribution program, the Tracleer Access Program.[23] Bosentan should be started at 62.5 mg twice daily in adults and adolescents for 4 weeks. After 4 weeks of therapy, the dose should be increased to 125 mg twice daily. If LFTs are confirmed to be in the range of three to five times the upper limit of normal, reduce the daily dose or interrupt treatment. If LFTs return to pretreatment levels, bosentan may be continued or reintroduced if indicated. LFTs should be monitored at baseline and monthly thereafter, and monthly pregnancy testing is required in females (category X). Complete blood count should be monitored every 3 months as bosentan has been associated with anemia. Bosentan is indicated for WHO functional class II and III (strength of recommendation: A) as well as functional class IV (strength of recommendation: E/C).[1]

Ambrisentan (Letairis) is a once-daily selective ET_A receptor antagonist that improves exercise capacity and hemodynamics and delays clinical worsening in PAH.[43,44] Two large (n = 202 and 192) trials recently evaluated the efficacy of ambrisentan compared with placebo. In 12 weeks, both studies demonstrated a significant improvement in functional capacity at doses of 2.5, 5, and 10 mg daily (range of 31 to 59 m). However, greater response was seen with increased doses. All doses were well tolerated, with no patients on therapy experiencing an increase in LFTs >3 times the upper limit of normal. Similar to bosentan, ambrisentan is category X for pregnancy; the distribution program for ambrisentan is referred to as Letairis Education and Access Program (LEAP).[23] Unlike bosentan, liver toxicity occurs very rarely with ambrisentan (0.8% in 12-week trials and 2.8% for up to 1 year).[33] Common side effects include peripheral edema, nasal congestion, flushing, and palpitations. Treatment should be initiated with 5 mg once daily and increased to 10 mg once daily if required. Ambrisentan is recommended for WHO functional class II and III (strength of recommendation: A) and may be used for WHO functional class IV (strength of recommendation: E/C).[1]

Phosphodiesterase Inhibitors There are two phosphodiesterase-5 inhibitors available for the treatment of PAH—sildenafil (Revatio) and tadalafil (Adcirca). **13** Sildenafil is a potent and highly specific phosphodiesterase-5 inhibitor that is approved for erectile dysfunction but also has been shown to reduce mPAP and improve functional class. Sildenafil exerts its pharmacologic effect by increasing the intracellular concentration of cyclic guanosine monophosphate, leading to vasorelaxation and antiproliferative effects on vascular smooth muscle cells. In a double-blind, placebo-controlled trial, sildenafil with conventional therapy significantly improved 6MWD and hemodynamic parameters at 12 weeks compared with placebo. A 1-year extension study showed a continued improvement in 6MWD of 51 m (95% CI 41 to 60).[45] The FDA-approved dose is 20 mg by mouth three times per day; however, much higher doses are routinely used clinically. Common adverse effects include headaches, flushing, epistaxis, dyspepsia, and diarrhea. Changes in vision have been reported, including blue-tinted vision and sudden loss of vision. In the event of sudden loss of vision, the drug should be stopped. Concurrent nitrate therapy may lead to excessive blood pressure reduction, and this combination should be avoided. Based on the current guidelines, sildenafil is recommended for functional class II and III patients with PAH (strength of recommendation: A) in addition to functional class IV patients (strength of recommendation: E/C).[1]

Another phosphodiesterase-5 inhibitor, tadalafil (Adcirca), was approved by the FDA in 2009 for the treatment of PAH. In a 16-week study, tadalafil 40 mg daily significantly improved exercise capacity (an average of +33 m; P <0.01) and quality of life measures. Tadalafil 40 mg also improved the time to clinical worsening (P = 0.041), which has not been demonstrated with sildenafil. Fifty-three percent of patients in this study were also on background bosentan therapy. Treatment-naïve patients demonstrated not only

TABLE 17-5 Drug Dosing Table

Drug	Brand Name	Initial Dose	Usual Range	Special Population Dose	Other
Synthetic Prostacyclin and Prostacyclin Analogs					
Epoprostenol	Flolan®	Starting dose 2–4 ng/kg/min IV	Titrate up to 20–40 ng/kg/min		
Treprostinil (IV or SC)	Remodulin®	Initially 1.25 ng/kg/min continuous subcutaneous or IV infusion	Decrease to 0.625 ng/kg/min if not tolerated Increase by no more than 1.25 ng/kg/min weekly for the first 4 weeks of therapy and no more than 2.5 ng/kg/min weekly for the duration of therapy		
Treprostinil (inhaled)	Tyvaso®	Initially three breaths (18 mcg) via oral inhalation four times daily during waking hours (approximately 4 hours apart)	Reduce to one to two breaths if three breaths not tolerated; increase to three breaths when tolerance improves Goal maintenance dose is nine breaths (54 mcg) per treatment four times daily; titrate by increasing three breaths at 1- to 2-week intervals as tolerated		
Iloprost	Ventavis®	Initially 2.5 mcg inhaled six to nine times daily (dosing at ≥2-hour intervals while awake)	Titrate to 5 mcg per dose with a maximum daily dose of 45 mcg		
Endothelin Receptor Antagonists					
Bosentan	Tracleer®	Initially 62.5 mg orally twice daily for 4 weeks	Increase to 125 mg orally twice daily		Available through Tracleer Access Program
Ambrisentan	Letairis®	Initial dose 5 mg orally daily	Titrate to maximum dose of 10 mg daily		Available through Letairis Education and Access Program
Phosphodiesterase Inhibitors					
Sildenafil	Revatio®	Initial dose 20 mg orally three times daily, taken at least 4–6 hours apart	Maximum FDA-approved dose is 20 mg orally three times a day; higher doses frequently used clinically		
Tadalafil	Adcirca®	40 mg orally once daily, with or without food	40 mg orally once daily		Not recommended to divide the dose

greater improvement in exercise capacity than those on bosentan therapy (+44 m vs. 23 m) but also greater improvement on all secondary outcomes. One possible explanation is decreased tadalafil levels as bosentan is a potent CYP450 3A4 inducer. Higher doses of tadalafil may be required in patients on concurrent bosentan therapy.[46] The most commonly reported adverse events were headache, myalgia, and flushing. The recommended dose is 40 mg by mouth once a day.[46] Concurrent use with nitrate therapy should also be avoided with tadalafil. Current guidelines indicate tadalafil for functional class II and III (strength of recommendation: B) and functional class IV (strength of recommendation: E/C).[1]

Calcium Channel Blockers **14** Since such a small number of patients have a positive response to acute vasodilator testing, CCBs are rarely used in the management of PAH. Approximately 13% of patients with IPAH will demonstrate an acute vasodilator response and may be initiated on CCB therapy; however, the number responding to long-term therapy is low (7%).[24] CCBs should not be used in the absence of demonstrated acute vasoreactivity.[1] The preferred drugs are dihydropyridine CCBs as they lack the negative inotropic effects seen with verapamil. Diltiazem may be used in patients with tachycardia to slow heart rate through atrioventricular node blockade. If left ventricular systolic dysfunction is present, diltiazem and verapamil should not be used. Assessment of CCB therapy should occur soon after initiation, and if improvement in functional class to class I or II is not seen, additional or alternative PAH therapy must be initiated. In acute responders, CCBs may be used in WHO functional classes I to IV (strength of recommendation: B).[1] The doses of these drugs are relatively high—that is, up to 120 to 240 mg/day for nifedipine and 240 to 720 mg/day for diltiazem—however, initial doses should be much lower and titrated upward to response.[30]

Combination Therapy **14** Combination therapy is an attractive option to address the multiple pathophysiologic mechanisms in PAH, resulting in improvement in hemodynamics, symptoms, and exercise capacity. Unfortunately, use of combination therapy has not been shown to decrease mortality, admission for worsening PAH, lung transplantation, or escalation of PAH therapy.[44] Combination therapy can be pursued by the simultaneous initiation of two (or more) treatments or by the addition of a second (or third) agent if previous treatment has been insufficient. Potential indications for combination therapy include signs of right heart failure, 6-minute walk distance <380 m, and persistent functional class III or IV symptoms despite active treatment. ERAs plus PDE-5 inhibitors, PDE-5 inhibitors with PGI_2 analogs, ERAs with PGI_2 analogs, and all three classes used in combination have all shown improved functional outcomes.[41,42,47–49] Sequential combination therapy is recommended for patients with inadequate clinical response to monotherapy; combinations of prostanoids, phosphodiesterase-5 inhibitors, and endothelin antagonists may be used (strength of recommendation: B).[1] Initial combination therapy may be necessary in WHO functional class IV patients (strength of recommendation: E/C).[1] More specific information concerning individual drugs used for PAH is shown in Tables 17-5 to 17-7.

TABLE 17-6 Desired Treatment Outcomes

Parameter	Frequency
Six-minute walk distance	Every 3–6 months
Functional class	Every 3 months
Echocardiography	Center dependent
Right heart catheterization	Center dependent

TABLE 17-7 Drug Monitoring Information

Drug	ADR	Monitoring Parameter	Comments
Synthetic Prostacyclin and Prostacyclin Analogs			
Epoprostenol	Pain (chest and jaw), flushing, headache	Titrate to balance efficacy and adverse effect	Occurs with dose titration
	GI (nausea, vomiting, diarrhea, anorexia)		
	Hypotension	Blood pressure	Occurs with dose titration; additive hypotensive effects with monoamine oxidase inhibitors
	Thrombocytopenia	Platelets	Monitor with concurrent anticoagulants
Treprostinil (IV or SC)	SC site pain See epoprostenol		
Treprostinil (inhaled)	Cough and sore throat		
Iloprost			
Endothelin Receptor Antagonists			
Bosentan	Hepatotoxicity	Monthly liver function tests required	Black box warning for liver injury
	Anemia	Hemoglobin	
	Edema	Edema on physical exam	
Ambrisentan	Anemia	Hemoglobin	
	Edema	Edema on physical exam	
Phosphodiesterase-5 Inhibitors			
Sildenafil	Headache		
	Nasal congestion		
	Hypotension	Blood pressure	Concurrent use with nitrates potentiates effects
	Visual changes	Consider baseline exam; repeat exam if visual changes occur	
Tadalafil	See sildenafil		

Evaluation of Therapeutic Outcomes

Response to treatment in PAH can be objectively measured by the 6-minute walk distance, echocardiography to assess pulmonary pressures, and right heart catheterization as the gold standard to assess ventricular function and pulmonary pressures (see Table 17-6). The WHO functional classification system is clinically useful, but correlations to hemodynamics may be imprecise. Other outcomes that are useful in clinical trials include hospitalization for exacerbations of PAH and the development of complications and death.

CONCLUSIONS

Significant advances have been made in elucidating the pathogenesis of PAH as well as in the evaluation and treatment of these patients over the past 2 decades. With approved targeted therapies such as ERAs, phosphodiesterase-5 inhibitors, and PGI_2 analogs, clinical improvement is possible in most patients, leading to a better quality of life and delay of disease progression. Patient education is important to improve acceptance of this disease and referral to specialty care centers may provide the best outcomes.

ABBREVIATIONS

ALK-1	activin receptor-like kinase 1
APAH	associated pulmonary arterial hypertension
BMPR2	bone morphogenetic protein receptor 2
CCB	calcium channel blocker
CTEPH	chronic thromboembolic pulmonary hypertension
ec-NOS	nitric oxide synthase
ERA	endothelin receptor antagonist
ET-1	endothelin-1
FPAH	familial pulmonary arterial hypertension
5-HT	serotonin
5-HTT	5-hydroxytryptamine transporter
HIV	human immunodeficiency virus
HPAH	heritable pulmonary arterial hypertension
INR	international normalized ratio
IPAH	idiopathic pulmonary arterial hypertension
LEAP	Letairis Education and Access Program
LFT	liver function test
LVEDP	left ventricular end-diastolic pressure
mPAP	mean pulmonary artery pressure
NO	nitric oxide
PAH	pulmonary arterial hypertension
PGI_2	prostacyclin
SC	subcutaneous
WHO	World Health Organization

REFERENCES

1. Barst RJ, Gibbs JSR, Ghofrani HA, et al. Updated evidence-based treatment algorithm in pulmonary arterial hypertension. J Am Coll Cardiol 2009;54:S78–S84.
2. Gladwin MT, Ghofrani HA. Update on pulmonary hypertension 2009. Am J Respir Crit Care Med 2010; 181:1020–1026.
3. Badesch DB, Abman SH, Simonneau G, Rubin LJ, McLaughlin VV. Medical therapy for pulmonary arterial hypertension: Updated ACCP evidence-based clinical practice guidelines. Chest 2007;131:1917–1928.
4. D'Alonzo GE. Survival in patients with primary pulmonary hypertension. Results from a national prospective registry. Ann Intern Med 1991;115:343–349.

5. Humbert M, Sitbon O, Chaouat A, et al. Survival in patients with idiopathic, familial, and anorexigen-associated pulmonary arterial hypertension in the modern management era. Circulation 2010;122:156–163.
6. Humbert M. Pulmonary arterial hypertension in France: Results from a national registry. Am J Respir Crit Care Med 2006;173:1023–1030.
7. Yuan JXJ. Pathogenesis of pulmonary arterial hypertension: The need for multiple hits. Circulation 2005;111:534–538.
8. McLaughlin VV, McGoon MD. Pulmonary arterial hypertension. Circulation 2006;114:1417–1431.
9. McLaughlin VV, Archer SL, Badesch DB, et al. ACCF/AHA 2009 expert consensus document on pulmonary hypertension: A report of the American College of Cardiology Foundation Task Force on Expert Consensus Documents and the American Heart Association: Developed in collaboration with the American College of Chest Physicians, American Thoracic Society, Inc., and the Pulmonary Hypertension Association. Circulation 2009;119:2250–2294.
10. Chin KM. Pulmonary arterial hypertension. J Am Coll Cardiol 2008;51:1527–1538.
11. Simonneau G, Robbins IM, Beghetti M, et al. The 4th World Health Symposium. Updated clinical classification of pulmonary hypertension. J Am Coll Cardiol 2009; 54(Suppl S):S43–S54.
12. Humbert M, McLaughlin VV. The 4th World Symposium on Pulmonary Hypertension. Introduction. J Am Coll Cardiol 2009;54:S1–S2.
13. Schermuly RT, Ghofrani HA, Wilkins MR, Grimminger F. Mechanisms of disease: Pulmonary arterial hypertension. Nat Rev Cardiol 2011;8:443–455.
14. Olsson KM, Hoeper MM. Novel approaches to the pharmacotherapy of pulmonary arterial hypertension. Drug Discov Today 2009;14:284–290.
15. Humbert M. Update in pulmonary hypertension 2008. Am J Respir Crit Care Med 2009;179:650–656.
16. Trembath RC. Clinical and molecular genetic features of pulmonary hypertension in patients with hereditary hemorrhagic telangiectasia. N Engl J Med 2001;345:325–334.
17. Eddahibi S. Serotonin transporter overexpression is responsible for pulmonary artery smooth muscle hyperplasia in primary pulmonary hypertension. J Clin Invest 2001;108: 1141–1150.
18. Izikki M. Tryptophan hydroxylase 1 knockout and tryptophan hydroxylase 2 polymorphism: Effects on hypoxic pulmonary hypertension in mice. Am J Physiol Lung Cell Mol Physiol 2007;293:L1045–L1052.
19. Park MH. Advances in diagnosis and treatment in patients with pulmonary arterial hypertension. Catheter Cardiovasc Interv 2008;71:205–213.
20. Rubens C. Big endothelin-1 and endothelin-1 plasma levels are correlated with the severity of primary pulmonary hypertension. Chest 2001;120:1562–1569.
21. Giaid A. Reduced expression of endothelial nitric oxide synthase in the lungs of patients with pulmonary hypertension. N Engl J Med 1995;333:214–221.
22. Janda S, Shahidi N, Gin K, Swiston J. Diagnostic accuracy of echocardiography for pulmonary hypertension: A systematic review and meta-analysis. Heart 2011;97: 612–622.
23. Bishop BM, Mauro VF, Khouri SJ. Practical considerations for pharmacotherapy for pulmonary arterial hypertension. Pharmacotherapy 2012;32:838–855.
24. Sitbon O. Long-term response to calcium channel blockers in idiopathic pulmonary arterial hypertension. Circulation 2005;111:3105–3111.
25. O'Callaghan DS, Savale L, Montani D, et al. Treatment of pulmonary arterial hypertension with targeted therapies. Nat Rev Cardiol 2011;8:526–538.
26. Agarwal R, Gomberg-Maitland M. Current therapeutics and practical management strategies for pulmonary arterial hypertension. Am Heart J 2011;162:201–213.
27. Macchia A. A meta-analysis of trials of pulmonary hypertension: A clinical condition looking for drugs and research methodology. Am Heart J 2007;153:1037–1047.
28. Galie N, Manes A, Negro L, Palazzini M, Bacchi-Reggiani ML, Branzi A. A meta-analysis of randomized controlled trials in pulmonary arterial hypertension. Eur Heart J 2009; 30:394–403.
29. McLaughlin VV, Presberg KW, Doyle RL, et al. Prognosis of pulmonary arterial hypertension: ACCP evidence-based clinical practice guidelines. Chest 2004;126:78S–92S.
30. Galie N, Torbicki A, Barst R, et al. Guidelines on diagnosis and treatment of pulmonary arterial hypertension. The Task Force on Diagnosis and Treatment of Pulmonary Arterial Hypertension of the European Society of Cardiology. Eur Heart J 2004;25:2243–2278.
31. McGoon M, Gutterman D, Steen V, et al. Screening, early detection, and diagnosis of pulmonary arterial hypertension: ACCP evidence-based clinical practice guidelines. Chest 2004;126:14S–34S.
32. Uchi M. Feasibility of cardiopulmonary rehabilitation in patients with idiopathic pulmonary arterial hypertension treated with intravenous prostacyclin infusion therapy. J Cardiol 2005;46:183–193.
33. McLaughlin VV, Archer SL, Badesch DB, et al. ACCF/ AHA 2009 expert consensus document on pulmonary hypertension a report of the American College of Cardiology Foundation Task Force on Expert Consensus Documents and the American Heart Association developed in collaboration with the American College of Chest Physicians; American Thoracic Society, Inc.; and the Pulmonary Hypertension Association. J Am Coll Cardiol 2009;53:1573–1619.
34. Badesch DB, Tapson VF, McGoon MD, et al. Continuous intravenous epoprostenol for pulmonary hypertension due to the scleroderma spectrum of disease. A randomized, controlled trial. Ann Intern Med 2000;132:425–434.
35. Sitbon O. Long-term intravenous epoprostenol infusion in primary pulmonary hypertension: Prognostic factors and survival. J Am Coll Cardiol 2002;40:780–788.
36. Simonneau G. Continuous subcutaneous infusion of treprostinil, a prostacyclin analogue, in patients with pulmonary arterial hypertension: A double-blind, randomized, placebo-controlled trial. Am J Respir Crit Care Med 2002;165:800–804.
37. Gomberg-Maitland M, Tapson VF, Benza RL, et al. Transition from intravenous epoprostenol to intravenous treprostinil in pulmonary hypertension. Am J Respir Crit Care Med 2005;172:1586–1589.
38. Olschewski H. Inhaled iloprost for severe pulmonary hypertension. N Engl J Med 2002;347:322–329.
39. McLaughlin VV, Rubin LJ, Benza RL, et al. TRIUMPH I: Efficacy and safety of inhaled treprostinil sodium in patients with pulmonary arterial hypertension (PAH) [abstract]. Am J Respir Crit Care Med 2008;177:A965.
40. Benza RL, Rubin LJ, McLaughlin VV, et al. TRIUMPH I: Long-term safety and efficacy of inhaled treprostinil sodium in patients with pulmonary arterial hypertension (PAH)—Two year follow-up. Am J Respir Crit Care Med 2009;179:A1041.
41. Hoeper MM, Leuchte H, Halank M, et al. Combining inhaled iloprost with bosentan in patients with idiopathic pulmonary arterial hypertension. Eur Respir J 2006;28:691–694.

42. Humbert M, Barst RJ, Robbins IM, Channick RN, Galie N, Boonstra A. Combination of bosentan with epoprostenol in pulmonary arterial hypertension: BREATHE-2. Eur Respir J 2004;24:353–359.
43. Galie N. Ambrisentan therapy for pulmonary arterial hypertension. J Am Coll Cardiol 2005;46:529–535.
44. Barst RJ. A review of pulmonary arterial hypertension: Role of ambrisentan. Vasc Health Risk Manag 2007;3:11–22.
45. Galie N. Sildenafil citrate therapy for pulmonary arterial hypertension. N Engl J Med 2005;353:2148–2157.
46. Galie N, Brundage BH, Ghofrani HA, et al. Tadalafil therapy for pulmonary arterial hypertension. Circulation 2009;119: 2894–2903.
47. Abraham T, Wu G, Vastey F, Rapp J, Saad N, Balmir E. Role of combination therapy in the treatment of pulmonary arterial hypertension. Pharmacotherapy 2010;30: 390–404.
48. Ghofrani HA. Combination therapy with oral sildenafil and inhaled iloprost for severe pulmonary hypertension. Ann Intern Med 2002;136:515–522.
49. Simonneau G, Rubin LJ, Galiè N, et al. Addition of sildenafil to long-term intravenous epoprostenol therapy in patients with pulmonary arterial hypertension: A randomized trial. Ann Intern Med 2008;149:521–530.

18

Cystic Fibrosis

Chanin C. Wright and Yolanda Y. Vera

KEY CONCEPTS

1. Good nutrition with appropriate pancreatic enzyme and vitamin supplementation are essential in the management of cystic fibrosis (CF).
2. Airway clearance and antiinflammatory therapies are key components to improve pulmonary health in CF patients.
3. Antipseudomonal agents are the cornerstone of antibiotic therapy for chronic lung infections in the CF patient.
4. Altered pharmacokinetics of CF patients can impact the dosing and clearance of pharmacologic therapy.

"Woe to that child which when kissed on the forehead tastes salty. He is bewitched and soon must die." This European adage accurately describes the fate of an individual diagnosed with cystic fibrosis during ancient times.[1]

Cystic fibrosis (CF) is a disease state resulting from a dysfunction in the cystic fibrosis transmembrane conductance regulator (CFTR). It is the most common life-limiting disorder in the Caucasian population, with an incidence of 1 in 2000 to 4000 live births and a prevalence of 30,000 affected individuals in the United States.[2–7]

Currently with care, affected individuals have an expected life span of 36 years of age. Multiple organ systems are affected in CF individuals, especially, the lungs, the digestive system, and the reproductive organs. Mortality is most commonly due to chronic organ damage or resistant pulmonary infections.[8]

The pharmacist plays an essential role in the development and management of a pharmacotherapeutic care plan for the CF patient.

EPIDEMIOLOGY

Cystic fibrosis occurs in approximately 1 in 3,500 newborns. In the 1970s, patients only survived into their teen years. By 2006, progress in care had extended survival to 36 years. Institution of care at a young age impacts long-term survival; hence, timing of diagnosis and recognition of signs and symptoms are crucial.[2–7]

Although CF occurs in all ethnicities, other ethnicities besides the Caucasian population display lower frequencies: 1 in 9,200 Hispanic-Americans, 1 in 10,900 Native Americans, 1 in 15,000 African Americans, and 1 in 100,000 Asians. The carrier frequency is 1 in 28 North American white populations, 1 in 29 Ashkenazi Jews, and 1 in 60 African Americans.[2]

ETIOLOGY

The cause of CF is due to a mutation of the CFTR gene. Extensive genetic studies have increased awareness regarding the large spectrum of mutations in the CF population. Over 1,800 mutations have been identified due to the extensive collaboration of the CF Foundation with international researchers. The most common mutation identified in CF patients is ΔF508.[3]

CF is an autosomal recessive disease, in which one mutation present on each allele of the CFTR gene results in presentation of the disease. The presentation of a mutation on only one allele of the CFTR gene will prevent the full expression of CF. Genetic studies have increased the understanding of genotype–phenotype relationships. Various mutations on the CFTR gene can result in various pathologies such as primary lung disease to minor GI involvement.[3]

PATHOPHYSIOLOGY

In order to successfully treat CF, a good understanding of the disease's underlying mechanism of action is crucial. It is well established that gene mutations cause an abnormality in the cystic fibrosis transmembrane conductance regulator (CFTR). This initiates the sequence of events responsible for the manifestations of CF. Mucosal obstruction occurs in the distal airways of the lung and submucosal glands, which express the CFTR. The CFTR also performs numerous cellular functions, including the regulation of chloride transport across the cell membrane. Studies in genotype–phenotype relationships have shown that an abnormality on the CFTR contributes to the expression of other gene proteins involved with inflammatory responses, ion transport, and cell signaling. These various expressions result in differences in clinical severity among patients with the same mutations on the CFTR.[3,9–11]

Under normal conditions, the CFTR helps regulate ion transport and salt homeostasis in the sweat glands. Typically, the sodium ion is followed by the chloride ion, and is reabsorbed from the lumen by the CFTR and apical sodium channels. As a result of the CFTR's malfunction in CF patients, chloride fails to be reabsorbed, which impacts the sodium ion reabsorption as well. This failed process produces sweat that contains high levels of salt. The endpoint of this process is a highly negatively charged lumen, which leads to an increased salt content in the sweat gland. This is known as the transepithelial potential difference, which is two to three times greater in CF patients. These processes can lead to organ damage in the CF patient (Fig. 18-1).

There are several theories as to how mucosal obstruction occurs in the airways. One of these theories, known as the "low-volume model," explains that the pulmonary surface epithelium behaves the opposite of a sweat gland in CF patients. There is an increased absorption of sodium, chloride, and fluid, which causes dehydration of the airway surfaces and defective mucociliary transport. An alternative theory known as the "high-salt model" indicates that the

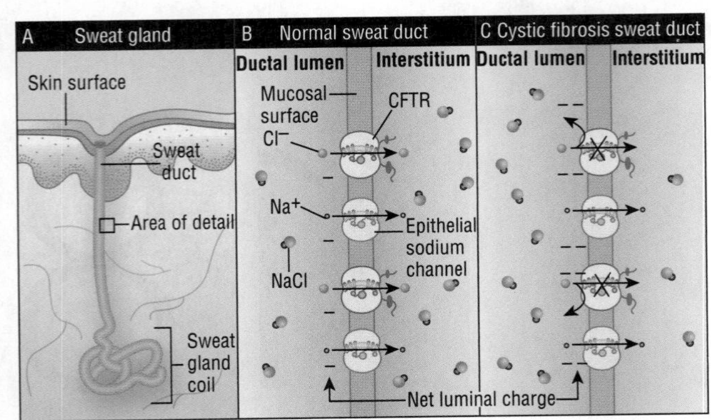

FIGURE 18-1 Mechanism of underlying elevated sodium chloride levels in the sweat of patients with cystic fibrosis (CF). Sweat ducts (Panel *A*) in patients with CF differ from those in people without the disease in the ability to reabsorb chloride before the emergence of sweat on the surface of the skin. A major pathway for Cl^- absorption is through CFTR, situated within luminal plasma membranes of cells lining the duct (i.e., on the apical, or mucosal, cell surface) (Panel *B*). Diminished chloride reabsorption in the setting of continued sodium uptake leads to an elevated transepithelial potential difference across the wall of the sweat duct, and the lumen becomes more negatively charged because of a failure to reabsorb chloride (Panel *C*). The result is that total sodium chloride flux is markedly decreased, leading to increased salt content. The thickness of the arrows corresponds to the degree of movement of ions. *(From Rowe SM, Miller S, Sorscher EJ. Cystic fibrosis. N Engl J Med 2005;352(19):1992–2001.)*

pulmonary surface epithelium behaves similarly to the sweat gland. A high salt content predisposes the CF patient to bacterial infections. Both theories agree that CF airways lack the ability to transport chloride through the CFTR.[9,12,13]

One of the common causes of morbidity and mortality in CF patients is mucosal obstruction of the exocrine glands. Mucosal obstruction causes the ducts to dilate, which results in the coating of lung surfaces by thick, viscous, neutrophil-dominated debris. These secretions initiate a cascade of events that lead to inflammation and formation of scar tissue in the lungs[14] (Fig. 18-2).

Other organ systems are impacted by the absence of CFTR activity as well. Ten percent of CF patients are born with meconium ileus, which is an intestinal obstruction that may be fatal if left untreated. Blockage of the pancreatic duct leads to complications such as chronic fibrosis and fatty replacement of the pancreatic gland. Bile duct obstruction causes cirrhosis of the liver, and male CF patients can experience infertility due to obstruction of the vas deferens in utero.[9]

CLINICAL PRESENTATION

In the classic presentation of CF, there are two mutations present (Table 18-1). The patients show signs and symptoms of chronic sinus and pulmonary infections, pancreatic insufficiency, and elevated sweat chloride levels. Patients with nonclassic CF have one mutation present, therefore retaining partial function of the CFTR and maintaining appropriate pancreatic function (Fig. 18-3).

Sinus and Pulmonary Presentation

Cystic fibrosis patients will usually experience chronic infections and frequently develop polyps in the sinus cavity. Daily symptomatology includes shortness of breath and cough, with sputum production. A common finding in radiology chest films is a flat diaphragm with an increased chest diameter and air trapping. Pulmonary function tests will reflect a decrease in FEV_1. Older patients will experience digital clubbing, a deformity of the fingers and fingernails often associated with chronic hypoxia.

Bacterial growth in the lungs will often drive CF patients to a state of exacerbation, resulting in increased cough, a reduction in pulmonary function, and increased sputum production with a change in color.

GI System Presentation

Most patients with nonclassic CF will maintain adequate pancreatic function. However in classic CF patients, steatorrhea, or greasy stools, is typically present that can lead to a failure to thrive, resulting in malnutrition. Infants and small children will show an increase in frequency of small stools. Newborns may present with meconium ileus, which is considered diagnostic of CF. Older patients may experience constipation, abdominal cramping, and flatulence. This presentation is due to the obstruction of the pancreatic ducts and intestinal tract and their inability to digest essential nutrients.

Pancreatic malfunction can also lead to an insulin deficiency, which is often a later finding detected by a loss in weight, an increase in blood glucose levels, and a failed oral glucose tolerance test (OGTT).

Reproductive Presentation

As patients reach adolescent and adult ages, tests may show azoospermia due to blockage of or the congenital bilateral absence of the vas deferens. Females may experience reduced fertility as cervical fluids have lower water content and decreased thinning during ovulation.[9,15,16]

DIAGNOSIS

As of 2010, all states were required to perform CF newborn screening.[17] The screening test checks for immunoreactive trypsinogen (IRT), a chemical produced by the pancreas. The IRT tends to be high in babies with CF. A second test may be done with a follow-up IRT test or a DNA test to look for a genetic mutation that causes CF. The CF newborn screening consists of a test called the quantitative pilocarpine iontophoresis sweat test (QPIT). The QPIT came about due to the risk of hyperpyrexia associated with older methods that utilized plastic body bags to make patients sweat. QPIT uses only a small area on the forearm, which is then stimulated to secrete sweat through the skin by iontophoresis of pilocarpine. Sweat from the

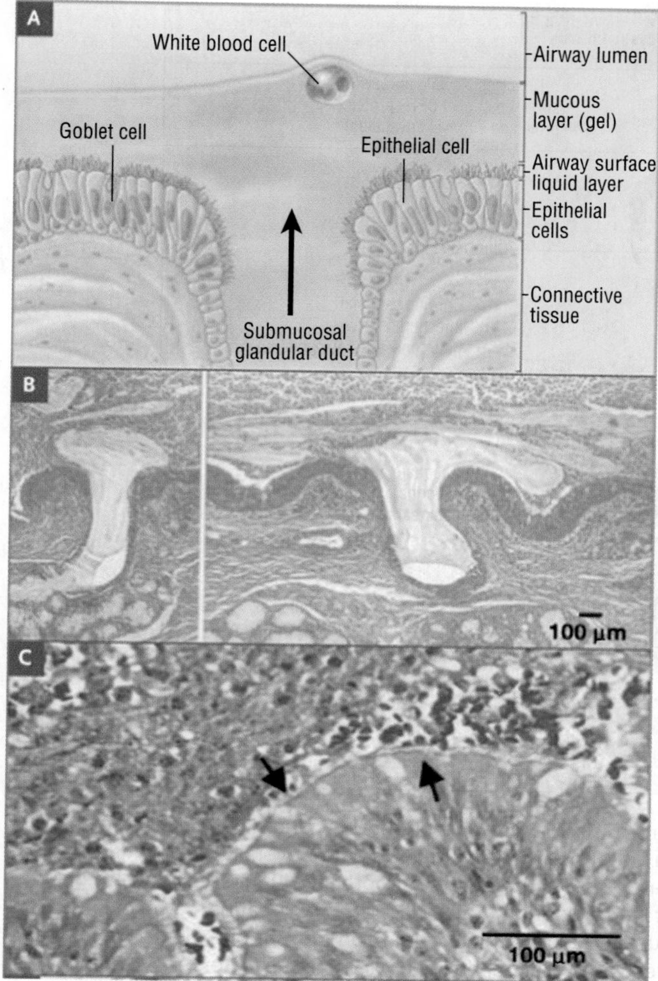

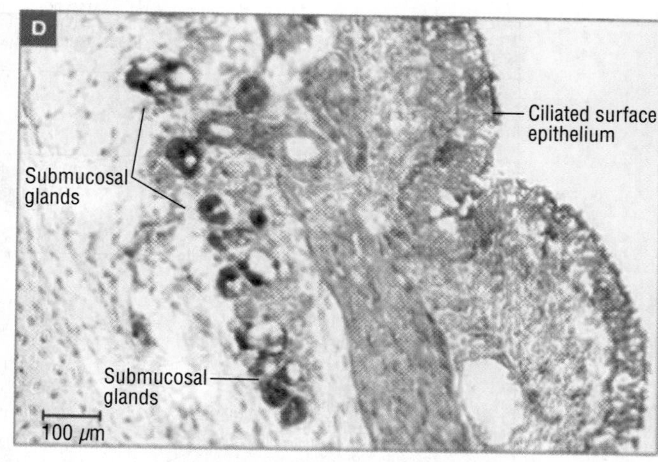

FIGURE 18-2 Extrusion of mucus secretion onto the epithelial surface of airways in cystic fibrosis. Panel *A* shows a schematic of the surface epithelium and supporting glandular structure of the human airway. In Panel *B*, the submucosal glands of a patient with CF are filled with mucus, and mucopurulent debris overlies the airway surfaces, essentially burying the epithelium. Panel *C* is a higher-magnification view of a mucus plug tightly adhering to the airway surface, with arrows indicating the interface between infected and inflamed secretions and the underlying epithelium to which the secretions adhere. (Both Panels *B* and *C* were stained with hematoxylin and eosin, with the colors modified to highlight structures.) Infected secretions obstruct airways and, over time, dramatically disrupt the normal architecture of the lung. In Panel *D*, CFTR is expressed in surface epithelium and serous cells at the base of submucosal glands in a porcine lung sample, as shown by the dark staining, signifying binding by CFTR antibodies to epithelial structures (aminoethylcarbazole detection of horseradish peroxidase with hematoxylin counterstain). *(From Rowe SM, Miller S, Sorscher EJ. Cystic fibrosis. N Engl J Med 2005;352(19):1992–2001.)*

stimulated area is then collected and analyzed for chloride content. Chloride concentrations are quantified as: normal: ≤39 mmol/L; intermediate: 40 to 59 mmol/L; and abnormal: ≥60 mmol/L. Values ≥60 mmol/L are consistently diagnostic of CF. It is suggested that samples from two sites will increase the reliability of the diagnosis[3,7] (Fig. 18-4).

DESIRED OUTCOMES

Pharmacists play a vital role in assisting patients to reach the following long- and short-term goals. Since CF affects multiple organ systems, there are several therapeutic goals that must be addressed for each system.[8]

TABLE 18-1 Cystic Fibrosis Foundation Diagnosis Criteria and Clinical Presentation

A. Meets one or more of the following clinical features associated with the CF phenotype plus:
- (a) Two CF mutations
- (b) Two positive QPIT results
- (c) An abnormal transepithelial potential difference value

B. The following are typical phenotypes associated with CF:
- (a) Chronic sinopulmonary disease
  - (i) Persistent colonization/infection with pathogens typical of CF lung disease
  - (ii) Endobronchial disease manifested by
    1. Cough and sputum production
    2. Wheeze and air trapping
    3. Radiographic abnormalities
    4. Evidence of obstruction on pulmonary function test
    5. Digital clubbing
  - (iii) Chronic sinus disease
    1. Nasal polyps
    2. Radiographic changes
- (b) GI/nutritional abnormalities
  - (i) Intestinal abnormalities
    1. Meconium ileus
    2. Exocrine pancreatic insufficiency
    3. Distal intestinal obstruction syndrome
    4. Rectal prolapse
    5. Recurrent pancreatitis
  - (ii) Chronic hepatobiliary disease manifested by clinical and/or laboratory evidence of
    1. Focal biliary cirrhosis
    2. Multilobar cirrhosis
  - (iii) Failure to thrive
  - (iv) Hypoproteinemia–edema
  - (v) Fat-soluble vitamin deficiencies
- (c) Obstructive azoospermia in males
- (d) Salt-loss syndromes
  - (i) Acute salt depletion
  - (ii) Chronic metabolic alkalosis
- (e) CF in a first-degree relative

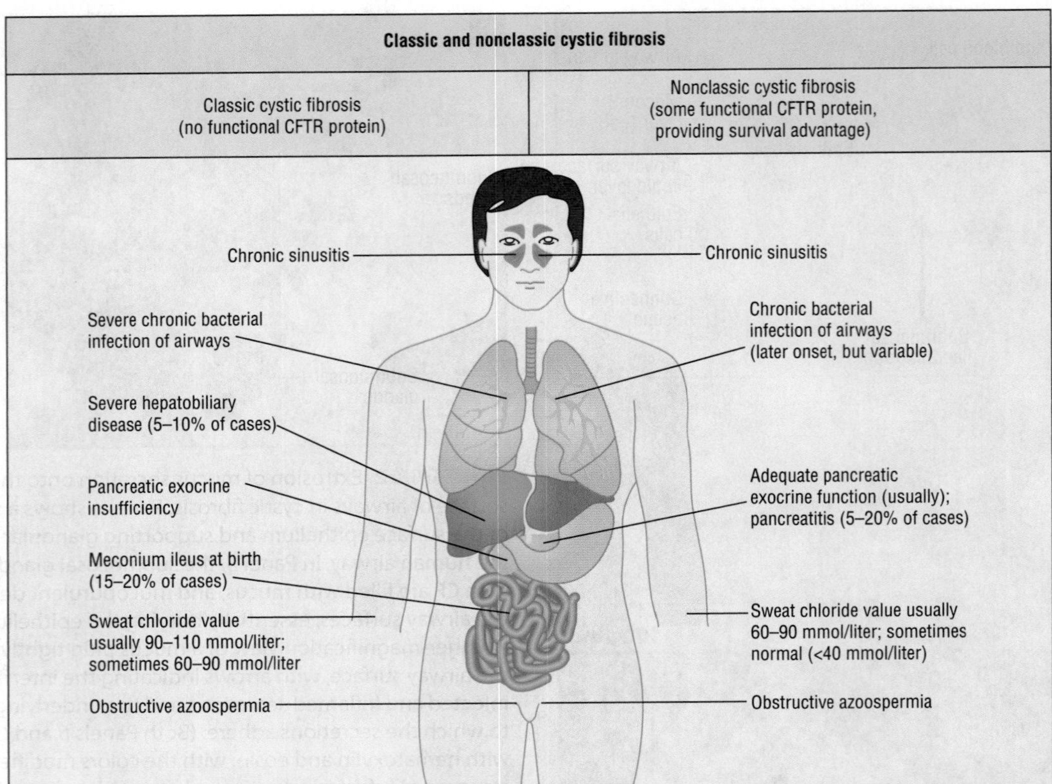

FIGURE 18-3 Classic and nonclassic cystic fibrosis (CF). The findings in classic CF are shown on the left-hand side, and those of nonclassic CF on the right-hand side. Patients with nonclassic CF have better nutritional status and better overall survival. Although the lung disease is variable, patients with nonclassic CF usually have late-onset or more slowly progressive lung disease. Sweat-gland function, as evidenced by the sweat chloride test, is abnormal but not to the extent noted in classic CF. Pancreatitis may occur in patients with nonclassic disease. However, chronic sinusitis and obstructive azoospermia occur in both groups of patients. On the basis of these findings, one can infer that mutations in *CTFR,* perhaps coupled with other genetic or environmental factors, may confer a predisposition to sinusitis, pancreatitis, or congenital bilateral absence of the vas deferens (azoospermia) in the general population. *(From Knowles MR, Durie PR. What is cystic fibrosis? N Engl J Med 2002;347(6):439–442.)*

Sinopulmonary

1. Prevent and treat sinusitis.
2. Increase FEV_1 and promote optimal pulmonary function tests and prevent pulmonary exacerbations.
   a. Promote effective airway clearance by providing counseling on the use of appropriate medications and chest physiotherapy.
   b. Prevent and treat colonization of the lungs with pathogens.
   c. Prevent and treat acute exacerbations.

GI

1. Control pancreatic insufficiency by providing adequate enzyme supplementation.
2. Optimize growth and nutritional status.
3. Promote healthy bowel habits.
4. Maintain normal fat-soluble vitamin levels.

Reproduction

1. Provide mutation analysis with appropriate genetic counseling at the time of diagnosis and periodically thereafter.

Psychosocial

1. Keep these patients living essentially normal lives by being active in school and the workplace.
2. Encourage compliance with pharmacological and nonpharmacological therapies in order to help prolong CF patient's lives.

NUTRITION

❶ In healthy individuals, the pancreas is vital to the absorption and digestion of essential nutrients for the body's growth and function. In pancreatic-insufficient CF individuals, the resulting inability to absorb these nutrients may lead to malnourishment. The focus of treatment lies in achieving and maintaining normal weight for adults and normal growth patterns for children. This is mostly achieved by managing GI and pulmonary symptoms, monitoring nutrient and energy intakes, and addressing psychosocial and financial issues. Numerous population-based studies have provided strong evidence to support optimization of nutritional status, due to its association with an improved pulmonary function. The CF Foundation recommends that both children and adults maintain normal nutritional status, due to its association with healthy pulmonary function, including a better FEV_1, and an increase in survival.

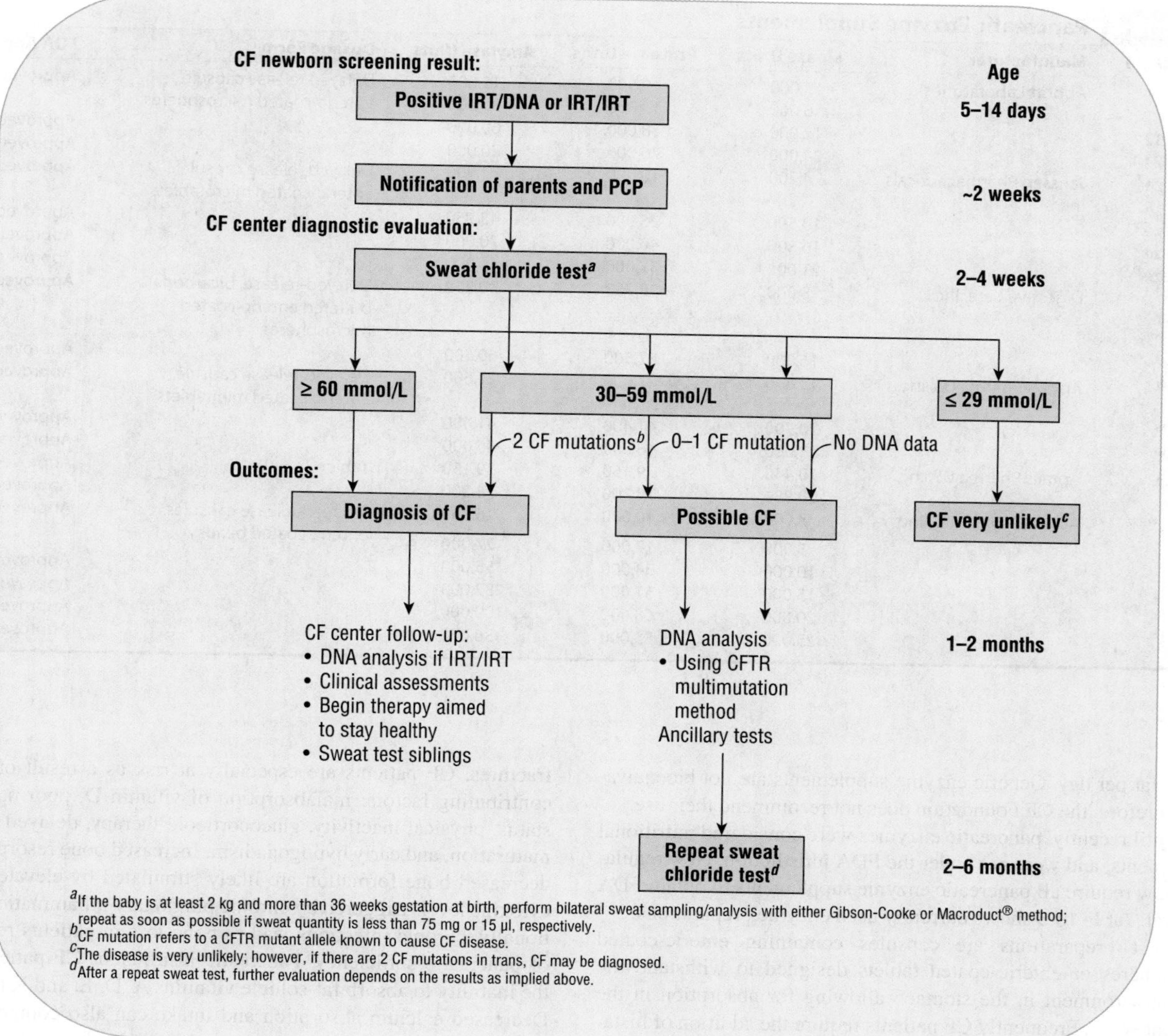

FIGURE 18-4 The CF diagnostic process for screened newborns. *(From Farrell PM, Rosenstein BJ, White TB, et al. Guidelines for the diagnosis of cystic fibrosis in newborns through older adults: Cystic Fibrosis Foundation Consensus Report. J Pediatr 2008;153(2):S4–S14.)*

To help meet this desired outcome, the CF Foundation recommends energy intakes greater than the standard for the general population to support weight gain and maintenance in children over 2 years and in adults. Trial evidence gathered from population-based studies has shown that energy intakes of 110% to 200% compared to the general health population intakes yield improved nutritional status in CF individuals. The CF Foundation has also established consensus-based assessment parameters to monitor nutritional status in CF individuals. These parameters and goals are listed in Table 18-2. In order to achieve these goals, pancreatic enzyme replacement therapy (PERT) is utilized to improve fat absorption due to pancreatic insufficiency. For patients who consistently fail to meet weight requirements, the clinician must consider the use of nutritional supplements that may be given orally or enterally via a percutaneous endoscopic gastrostomy (PEG) tube.

PERT has been proven both safe and efficacious in improving nutritional status in CF patients and is recommended in addition to adequate dietary intake. Consensus-based guidelines have established a dose of 500 to 2500 lipase units per kilogram (kg) of body weight per meal; or 10,000 units per kg per day; or 4,000 units per gram of

TABLE 18-2 Cystic Fibrosis Foundation Nutritional Assessment Parameters and Recommendations

- Age-appropriate BMI method should be utilized to assess weight and height
- Better FEV_1 status at about 80% (0.80) predicted or above was associated with BMI % at 50th percentile or higher
- For children and adolescents aged 2 to 20 years, the CF Foundation recommends that weight-for-stature assessment uses the BMI percentile method and that children and adolescents maintain a BMI at or above the 50th percentile
- For children diagnosed before age 2 years, the CF Foundation recommends that children reach a weight-for-length status of 50th percentile by age 2 years
- For adults aged 20 years and older, the CF Foundation recommends that weight-for-stature assessment use the BMI method and that women maintain a BMI ≥22, and men maintain a BMI ≥23
- For adults aged 20 years and older, the CF Foundation recommends that unintentional weight loss be avoided. When encountered in patient care, unintentional weight loss should be evaluated in the context of the patient's usual weight and health status

BMI, body mass index.

TABLE 18-3 Pancreatic Enzyme Supplements

Trade Name	Manufacturer	Lipase Units	Protease Units	Amylase Units	Dosage Form	FDA Approval
Creon	Abbott Laboratories	3,000	9,500	15,000	Delayed release capsule, enteric-coated microspheres	Approved
Creon®		6,000	19,000	30,000		
Creon® 12		12,000	38,000	60,000		Approved
Creon® 24		24,000	76,000	120,000		Approved
Pancreaze®	Janssen Pharmaceuticals, Inc.	4,200	10,000	17,500	Delayed release capsule, enteric-coated microtablets	Approved
Pancreaze®		10,500	25,000	43,750		Approved
Pancreaze®		16,800	40,000	70,000		Approved
Pancreaze®		21,000	37,000	61,000		Approved
Pertzye	Digestive Care, Inc.	8,000	28,750	30,250	Delayed-release, bicarbonate-buffered enteric-coated microspheres	Approved
Pertzye		16,000	57,500	60,500		Approved
Ultresa®	Aptalis Pharma US, Inc.	13,800	27,600	27,600	Delayed-release capsule, enteric-coated minitablets	Approved
Ultresa®		20,700	41,400	41,400		Approved
Ultresa®		23,000	46,000	46,000		Approved
Viokace	Aptalis Pharma US, Inc.	10,440	39,150	39,150	Tablet	Approved
Viokace		20,880	78,300	78,300		Approved
Zenpep®	Aptalis Pharma US, Inc.	3,000	10,000	16,000	Delayed-release capsules, enteric-coated beads	Approved
		5,000	17,000	27,000		
		10,000	34,000	55,000		Approved
		15,000	51,000	82,000		Approved
		20,000	68,000	109,000		Approved
		25,000	85,000	136,000		Approved

dietary fat per day. Generic enzyme supplements are not bioequivalent; therefore, the CF Foundation does not recommend their use.

Until recently, pancreatic enzymes were considered nutritional supplements, and were not under the FDA jurisdiction. New regulations now require all pancreatic enzyme supplements to obtain FDA approval. Table 18-3 shows currently used enzyme preparations.[18–39]

Most preparations are capsules containing enteric-coated microspheres or enteric-coated tablets designed to withstand the acidic environment in the stomach allowing for absorption in the small intestine. Frequently CF patients require the addition of histamine receptor antagonists or proton-pump inhibitors in order to create an alkaline environment in the intestine. Enteric-coated capsules should not be crushed but may be opened and mixed with nonalkaline food. However, if allowed to sit in food for a prolonged amount of time, the enteric coating will be lost and enzymes inactivated. Enzymes are administered prior to meals and snacks.[40]

Patients dosed beyond the recommended guidelines may develop fibrosing colonopathy, which leads to colonic strictures. This condition should be considered in individuals who have evidence of obstruction, bloody diarrhea, or ascites, as well as in patients who have a combination of abdominal pain, ongoing diarrhea, and/or poor weight gain. Risk factors for fibrosing colonopathy include: age <12 years; enzyme dosages >6,000 lipase units/kg/meal for more than 6 months; history of meconium ileus or distal intestinal obstruction syndrome (DIOS); history of any intestinal surgery; and inflammatory bowel disease.

Patients who experience fibrosing colonopathy are treated by reducing the dose of enzyme supplements, or with oral laxatives and/or enemas, all of which have been proven effective. More severe cases may require surgical intervention.[41]

BONE HEALTH AND VITAMIN SUPPLEMENTATION

Increased longevity in CF patients has revealed bone disease as an emerging complication. Many studies have observed that 50% to 75% of CF adults have low bone density and increased rates of fractures. CF patients are especially at risk as a result of several contributing factors: malabsorption of vitamin D, poor nutritional status, physical inactivity, glucocorticoid therapy, delayed pubertal maturation, and early hypogonadism. Increased bone resorption and decreased bone formation are likely stimulated by elevated serum cytokine levels triggered by chronic pulmonary inflammation. Additionally, chronic infections lead to bone loss in patients regardless of pancreatic sufficiency. Pancreatic insufficient CF patients have the inability to absorb fat-soluble vitamins A, D, E, and K (ADEK). Decreased calcium absorption and intake can also compound this problem. As bone disease progresses, this can lead to exclusion from lung transplantation, which is often a life-saving operation for individuals with CF.

Appropriate bone density monitoring for CF patients requires obtaining levels of fat-soluble vitamins yearly, as well as treatment with daily supplementation. Special multivitamin formulations contain high amounts of fat-soluble vitamins designed to deliver the appropriate doses required. Recommended vitamin D levels are a minimum of 30 ng/mL (75 nmol/L). Even with these precautions, adequate vitamin D levels may be difficult to maintain due to altered absorption, reduced fat mass, and minimal exposure to sun light. Medical management of CF patients can also contribute to bone disease by the administration of glucocorticoids, posttransplant immunosuppressant therapies, and antibiotic therapies that require protection from sunlight exposure.[42–51]

PULMONARY HEALTH AND TREATMENT

2 One of the fundamentals of pulmonary care in CF patients is airway clearance. CF patients, in general, have impaired mucociliary clearance that results in thick sputum, predisposing them to chronic infections and inflammation. Effective airway clearance involves the use of a bronchodilator, a mucolytic medication, and chest percussion. It is recommended that airway clearance therapy (ACT) be initiated within the first few months of life. Table 18-4 shows typical medications used in airway clearance.

TABLE 18-4 Airway Clearance Therapies

	Dose
Albuterol	2 puffs prior to therapy 2–4 times a day
HyperSal™ (hypertonic saline)	4 mL delivered via a nebulizer 2–4 times a day
Pulmozyme® (dornase alfa)	2.5 mg delivered via a nebulizer 1–2 times a day

Choosing a particular ACT routine for a patient is based on the patient's needs. There is no consensus on the optimal method of ACT. The regimen including duration or number of treatments per day may be changed in response to acute illness or exacerbations.

Chest percussion was originally performed by hand, with a cupped hand pounding on the chest that generates percussion or vibration. Currently, the most convenient method is the use of a percussion vest. Aerobic exercise is also effective and recommended for improved airway clearance.[52]

The recommended sequence of clearance therapy or "pulmonary toilet" regimen is as follows (note that these therapies are recommended for individuals ≥6 years of age and are administered concurrently with percussion therapy):

1. Bronchodilator: Albuterol is commonly used for this indication. It helps open up the airways and prevents bronchospasm.
2. Hypertonic saline (HyperSal®): It hydrates the airway mucus secretions and facilitates mucociliary function.
3. Dornase alfa (Pulmozyme®): Enzyme that cleaves extracellular DNA, which results in decreased viscosity of mucus.
4. Aerosolized antibiotics (i.e., Aztreonam [Cayston], tobramycin [TOBI®]): If this therapy is indicated based on severity of lung disease and sputum cultures, it is administered after the CF patient completes percussion therapy.

Bronchodilator therapy is recommended for patients ≥6 years of age who demonstrate bronchiole hyperresponsiveness or a bronchodilator response. Chronic use of bronchodilator therapy is recommended to improve lung function by enhancing mucociliary action.[53,54]

Inhaled hypertonic saline is a novel agent used for the treatment of CF. Based on the "low-volume model" theory, the use of hypertonic saline would restore airway hydration and enhance mucociliary function.[55] Hypertonic saline is recommended for patients ≥6 years of age. A study conducted in Australia showed that CF patients who surfed had better pulmonary outcomes than other patients who did not surf.[56] Researchers believed that the inhalation of ocean water helped to improve FEV_1 in CF patients that surfed. In this study, 24 patients were randomly assigned to receive a daily treatment of 7% hypertonic saline with or without pretreatment of a control. Clearance and pulmonary function were measured during a 14-day period. Results showed significant improvement in FEV_1 and FVC, as well as improvement of respiratory symptoms in hypertonic saline patients. The study also demonstrated that these patients were able to sustain mucus clearance for >8 hours. Other studies assessing the use of hypertonic saline have supported this study, showing an improvement in lung function and a 56% reduction in exacerbations.[53–57]

Dornase alfa (Pulmozyme®) is also recommended in all patients ≥6 years of age, and is strongly recommended in patients with moderate-to-severe lung disease, to improve lung function and reduce exacerbations. Three randomized controlled trials and a crossover trial involving 520 patients were conducted. Study results showed improvement in FEV_1 by 3.2% and a reduction in exacerbations.[53,58,59]

Antiinflammatory Therapies

Pulmonary inflammation begins early in life, as shown by the predominance of proinflammatory mediators that can be seen on bronchiolar lavage. A normal inflammatory response to bacteria becomes pathologic in CF patients who have both a prolonged and exaggerated reaction. Treatment of this inflammatory response is crucial to treating the CF patient.

Antiinflammatory therapies must address the neutrophil response and inhaled therapies will target the endobronchial location, which is the site of inflammation. Using medications that terminate the inflammatory process may be effective. Airway clearance and antibiotics will help control the inflammatory stimulation. Steroids and nonsteroidal antiinflammatory drugs (NSAIDs) are not widely used due to long-term safety concerns. High-dose ibuprofen (20 to 30 mg/kg of body weight twice daily) has proven efficacious in a study where patients showed less decline in pulmonary function when compared to patients given placebo. Patients on high dose ibuprofen were able to maintain weight and had less hospital admissions. The benefits of this regimen exceed the risks of GI complications and nephrotoxicity. Despite these outcomes, less than 10% of CF patients in the United States are on this regimen. The low number of patients utilizing this proven therapy may be related to the requirement to obtain a specific therapeutic level of ibuprofen, which in turn requires frequent blood draws for pharmacokinetic monitoring.[53,60–63]

Studies with macrolides have shown an inhibition of the neutrophil migration and a decrease in production of proinflammatory mediators. It is unclear at this point if the antiinflammatory effects of macrolides are a combination of antimicrobial and/or immunomodulatory mechanisms of action. A study conducted in Japan first demonstrated the benefit of macrolides against *Pseudomonas aeruginosa*. Four randomized controlled trials have since demonstrated this effect with azithromycin (250 to 500 mg) given three times weekly, which has led to increased nutritional status and decreased pulmonary infections. Other treatments are under investigation, but larger studies are needed before they become recommended therapies.[53,60,64,65]

Infectious Disease

3 Antibiotic therapy plays two integral roles in the treatment of CF patients: improving pulmonary function and preventing pulmonary failure. Oral, IV, and aerosolized antibiotic formulations are indicated and utilized in patients who experience acute pulmonary exacerbations, are chronically infected with *P. aeruginosa*, or require prevention of chronic *P. aeruginosa* infection. A major disadvantage of treatment in CF patients is that pathogens are not fully eradicated from the airways and will often develop resistance. Unfortunately, this limits antimicrobial selection, and can contribute to deterioration of pulmonary function (Table 18-5).

Early in life, patients will routinely be colonized with *S. aureus* and then later with *P. aeruginosa*. A 5 to 7 year study of cephalexin prophylaxis in young CF children showed decreased *S. aureus* colonization, however, there was an increase in frequency of *P. aeruginosa* infections. Ultimately, this study showed no significant improvement in health outcomes, therefore, prophylaxis for *S. aureus* colonization is not recommended.[66,67]

The finding of *P. aeruginosa* on sputum culture is a predictor of morbidity and mortality. There are relatively few antibiotics available for the treatment of *P. aeruginosa*. Antibiotics available include extended-spectrum penicillins, select cephalosporins, select carbapenems, aztreonam, quinolones, colistimethate, and aminoglycosides. The only two mechanisms of action represented in this group are cell wall destruction and inhibited cell wall synthesis by ribosomal attachment. Standard practice is to combine these two mechanisms

TABLE 18-5 Antimicrobial Agents Utilized in CF

Antibiotic Oral	Pediatric Dose (mg/kg/day)	Adult Dose	Frequency Range	Pathogens
Ciprofloxacin	40	750 mg	Q 12 H	*Pseudomonas, Alcaligenes*
Sulfamethoxazole/ Trimethoprim	15–20 mg of TMP	15–20 mg of TMP/kg/day	Q 6-8 H	*Staphylococcus* (MRSA, MSSA), *Burkholderia Stenotrophomonas, Alcaligenes*
Doxycycline	2–4	Max 200 mg/day	Q 12–24 H	*Stenotrophomonas, Staphylococcus*
IV				
Amikacin	22.5–30	15 mg/kg/day	Q 8 H	*Pseudomonas*
Aztreonam	200	2 g	Q 6–8 H	*Pseudomonas*
Cefepime	150	2 g	Q 8 H	*Pseudomonas*
Ceftazidime	150	2 g	Q 8 H	*Pseudomonas, Burkholderia, Alcaligenes*
Ciprofloxacin	30	400 mg	Q 8 H	*Pseudomonas, Alcaligenes*
Colistimethate	5–8	5–8 mg/kg/day	Q 8 H	*Pseudomonas*
Doxycycline	2–4	Max 200 mg/day	Q 12–24 H	*Stenotrophomonas, Staphylococcus*
Gentamicin	7.5–10	7.5–10 mg/kg/day	Q 6–8 H	*Pseudomonas*
Imipenem	60–100	2–4 g	Q 6 H	*Pseudomonas, Burkholderia, Alcaligenes*
Meropenem	30–50	1–2 g	Q 8 H	*Pseudomonas, Burkholderia, Alcaligenes*
Piperacillin–Tazobactam	300–400 (piperacillin component)	4.5 g	Q 4–6 H	*Pseudomonas, Alcaligenes, Staphylococcus MSSA*
Ticarcillin–Clavulanate	300–400 (ticarcillin component)	3.1 g	Q 4 H	*Pseudomonas, Alcaligenes Staphylococcus* (MSSA)
Tobramycin	7.5–10	7.5–10 mg/kg/day	Q6–8H	*Pseudomonas*
Vancomycin	60	15 mg/kg	Q 6–12 H	Staphylococcus (MRSA, MSSA)
Inhalation				
Tobramycin	60–600 mg/day	60–600 mg/day	Q 12 H	*Pseudomonas*
Colistimethate	75 mg/day	75 mg/day	Q 12 H	*Pseudomonas*
Aztreonam	225 mg/day	225 mg/day	Q 8 H	*Pseudomonas*

for the best bactericidal results. It is not unusual for patients to have multiple organisms growing in their sputum. The clinician can review the quantitative sputum culture for both the organisms present and the amount or colony forming units grown. By targeting the organisms with the most numerous organisms present and reviewing the susceptibility panels, the clinician can choose the most appropriate regimen. After years of drug exposure, older CF patients will exhibit multidrug-resistant *P. aeruginosa*. At this point, sputum cultures can be sent to specialized laboratories that will test combinations of antibiotics and report out any synergy results. Aerosolized antibiotics are directly deposited into the lung, providing concentrations that may overcome the standard measures of resistance.[68]

Other organisms that may be seen are *Alcaligenes, Stenotrophomonas, Mycobacteria, Aspergillus*, and *Burkholderia*. The importance of *Alcaligenes* as a pathogen is not well described. Originally only thought to have a prevalence of 2.7%, better lab testing and more studies have found infection rates closer to 8% in CF patients greater than 6 years old.[69–72] *Stenotrophomonas* is intrinsically multidrug resistant and pathogenic. A risk factor for acquiring this organism may be broad-spectrum antibiotic use (carbapenems and cephalosporins).[73,74] Quite often this bacteria is misidentified and confirmatory testing may show *Burkholderia*. Prevalence in American CF patients is reported to be 8.4%; however, some centers report incidence to be as high as 25%.[75–77] Treatment choice is trimethoprim–sulfamethoxazole or doxycycline. *Mycobacteria* have been reported with more frequency in the last 10 years. Species include *M. tuberculosis*, nontuberculosis *M. chelonei, M. fortuitum*, and *M. avium-intracellulare* (MAI). The impact of *Mycobacteria* in the CF patient is unclear. Caseating granulomas have been found in some patients with clinical disease while other patients with nontuberculous mycobacteria (NTM) have shown no adverse consequences.[78–81] *Aspergillus* species has a prevalence of 10% to 25% in American CF patients. During the TOBI® trials, patients treated with aerosolized tobramycin appeared to be more at risk for colonization with *Aspergillus* than the placebo group. Although *Aspergillus* does not directly inhibit lung function, it may cause allergic bronchopulmonary aspergillosis which is an immunologic-mediated response to the presence of *Aspergillus* in the lungs.[82,83] *Burkholderia cepacia* is now known to be a bacterial species called "genomovars." Currently, up to nine species have been identified.

The two typical antimicrobial choices to treat *B. cepacia* are ceftazidime and trimethoprim-sulfamethoxazole®. It is important to recognize the transmission of *B. cepacia* from patient to patient has been shown via droplet route and therefore proper infection control precautions should be taken.[84–86]

Although CF patients are not more susceptible to respiratory viral infections, the outcome of such illnesses may be more severe. Decline in pulmonary function can be directly related to the number of annual viral infections. Newborns diagnosed with CF should receive respiratory syncytial virus (RSV) prevention with Synagis®, a monoclonal antibody for the first 2 years of life. Synagis® is usually dosed at 15 mg/kg intramuscularly once a month during the RSV season. All CF patients who are 6 months of age or older should receive the annual influenza vaccine.[87–93]

Tobramycin (TOBI®) is recommended in all patients ≥6 years of age, and is strongly recommended in patients with moderate-to-severe lung disease and *Pseudomonas* present in sputum cultures. Aerosolized antibiotics deliver drug locally to the lung while decreasing the risk of systemic side effects. In 1998, the FDA approved TOBI® for treating bacterial lung infections in patients with CF. Routine monitoring of serum aminoglycoside levels is unnecessary in patients with normal renal function using approved doses. It is recommended that CF patients use a preservative-free formulation of aerosolized antibiotics to prevent occurrence of bronchospasm.[94]

Geller et al. describes the pharmacokinetics of inhaled TOBI®, specifically looking at sputum concentrations in CF patients receiving three cycles of routine TOBI® (i.e., 28 days on, 28 days off), 300 mg twice daily. The study followed 258 patients for 24 weeks, and showed that approximately 95% of patients achieved sputum concentrations of >25 times the minimum inhibitory concentration (MIC) of *Pseudomonas* isolates. This confirmed that inhaled TOBI® can be efficacious in helping prevent the progression of lung disease. At 25 times the MIC, tobramycin has a bactericidal effect.[95]

In 2010, the FDA approved a new inhaled antibiotic, Cayston®, for the treatment of *Pseudomonas*. This inhaled formulation of aztreonam is currently in Phase 3 clinical trials and has demonstrated improvement in respiratory symptoms and lung function in patients greater than 6 years of age. Cayston® has been compared to TOBI® in a head-to-head trial and met noninferiority and superiority endpoints. It will require an Altera nebulizer that can deliver the medication in 3 minutes. This in itself would increase compliance and have a positive impact on the quality of life in CF patients.[96]

Pharmacokinetics

❹ CF patients are unique in respect to a larger volume of distribution and a faster rate of clearance. With a larger volume of distribution, patients may require larger antibiotic doses. Dosing intervals become shorter because drugs are eliminated faster. Critically ill patients may vary from their baseline function and require closer monitoring. However, as patients age, they tend to approach normal population parameters. Therapeutic drug monitoring and necessary dosage and regimen adjustments are critical to the successful treatment of CF patients.

Once daily dosing of aminoglycosides is preferred for ease of home care administration, and may actually work well in this setting. However, given the possibility of a shortened half-life, each patient's unique pharmacokinetic parameters must be calculated to determine if once daily dosing is appropriate.[97,98]

REPRODUCTION

Fertility discussions with older CF patients may arise during clinic visits, and these conversations should include genetic counseling and options for contraception. Drug–drug interactions between oral contraceptive pills (OCPs) and antibiotics should be monitored. Studies have shown that OCP use in CF patients is safe and effective in comparison to other contraception methods. Patches may not reliably adhere to the skin as a result of increased sweat on the surface of the skin.

The issues surrounding the use of contraception among CF men are similar to those among the normal population. CF men should not assume they are infertile, and should adhere to using protective measures in order to prevent unwanted pregnancy and the spread of sexually transmitted diseases. Should a CF male with a nonfunctioning vas deferens desire to become a biological parent, microsurgical epididymal aspiration of spermatozoa with intracytoplasmic sperm injection into the oocyte can be performed.[16]

DIABETES

As CF patients live longer, glucose intolerance and cystic fibrosis related diabetes (CFRD) are common complications. Even though it shares features of type 1 and type 2 diabetes, CFRD is unique because it is influenced by factors specific to CF, including: insulin deficiency, undernutrition, chronic and acute infection, elevated energy expenditure, glucagon deficiency, malabsorption, abnormal intestinal transit time, and liver dysfunction.[99] In comparison to the general CF population, patients with CFRD show a higher mortality rate. In a study of 448 patients, 60% of non-CFRD population and 25% of the CFRD were alive at age 30. The average onset of CFRD is between 18 and 21 years, with a slight female predominance and is more commonly seen in CF gene mutation ΔF508.[99–104]

It is now recommended that at age 10 years and every year thereafter, CF patients be screened for CFRD. The OGTT should be used as the HbA1c is not a reliable indicator of diabetes in this population. During an acute illness, fasting glucose levels of ≥126 mg/dL (7.0 mmol/L) are diagnostic of CFRD. A mid- or postfeeding plasma glucose level of >200 mg/dL (>11.1 mmol/L) repeated on two separate days during continuous drip feedings may also be diagnostic of CFRD.[105]

A desired goal in this population is to control hyperglycemia and hypoglycemia in order to reduce acute and chronic diabetes complications. Because insulin deficiency is the hallmark of CFRD, insulin is the recommended medical treatment. Insulin regimens are individualized based on the patient's lifestyle and circumstances. Exercise is encouraged because it can improve peripheral insulin sensitivity and have beneficial effects in overall health, pulmonary function, and well-being.[100–103]

Oral antidiabetic agents have inconsistent results in the literature; therefore, support for their use in therapy for CFRD patients is not recommended. Medications that help improve insulin sensitivity do not address the primary problem of insulin deficiency in CF. Metformin's mechanism of action is to improve hepatic and peripheral insulin sensitivity; however, it is contraindicated in patients with hypoxia due to the risk of fatal lactic acidosis. Additionally, metformin's multiple GI effects include, anorexia, diarrhea, flatulence, and abdominal discomfort. Thiazolidinediones help to enhance peripheral insulin sensitivity, but there is serious potential for hepatic toxicity due to the underlying liver problems in CF patients. The use of acarbose is also discouraged due to its mechanism of action, which reduces postprandial glucose and insulin excursion by limiting intestinal absorption of glucose. This inhibits the energy absorption in malnourished individuals while causing diarrhea, anorexia, and abdominal discomfort. Sulfonylureas are being considered due to their ability to enhance insulin secretion by acting on a specific islet beta cell receptor; however, evidence has also shown that these agents bind and inhibit the CFTR. Use of sulfonylureas is not recommended at this time.[100,104]

SPECIAL POPULATIONS

Pregnancy

As women with CF live longer, more choose to become pregnant. CF women considering pregnancy and their partners should both undergo genetic counseling. CF women who become pregnant are considered a high-risk pregnancy; therefore, several considerations should be addressed at the onset of and during pregnancy. At the beginning, both current medications and medications that might be used to treat exacerbations need to be considered. Several of these medications are classified as category C and may pose a potential harm to the fetus. These patients should also be screened and treated accordingly for CFRD.

Several complications that will arise during CF pregnancy include increases in minute ventilation, increased oxygen uptake, increased blood volume, and cardiac output. In a woman with severe lung disease, these changes can cause right-sided heart failure.

Other pharmacotherapy issues that are seen in this population are altered pharmacokinetics and increased maintenance of nutritional and pulmonary health.

The addition of the fetus impacts the CF woman's health by placing a strain on a precariously balanced state of being. The CF woman who chooses to breastfeed must take into account the additional nutritional requirement of approximately 500 kcal/day (2,093 kJ/day).[16]

Pediatrics

Education of the parents is emphasized in this population, concerning administration of pancreatic enzymes and infant formula. Parents are also counseled to encourage their child to adhere with pulmonary health and nutritional health practices. As the child grows into adolescence, compliance becomes an issue. Peer pressure and social restraints may interfere with CF compliance and may influence the patients to disregard their personal well-being.

Transplant Patients

Lung transplantation has become an option with a 5-year survival rate of approximately 50%. Criteria for selection of transplant candidates include not only an FEV_1 of <30% (<0.30), but also gender, nutritional status, diabetic status, sputum microbiology, and number of pulmonary exacerbations. Factors affecting compliance to CF care and to immunosuppressant therapy may also be taken under consideration for candidacy.[16]

NEW THERAPIES

Antibiotic resistance is a common focus for new therapies, and quinolone inhaled formulations are currently being evaluated in phase 2 and 3 trials. Inhaled levofloxacin and ciprofloxacin will be used for treatment of *Pseudomonas* and other bacterial lung infections. Tobramycin inhaled powder (TIP®) has been approved in Canada and Chile. TIP® demonstrates an advantage over TOBI® due to its faster administration time. Arikase™, the liposomal amikacin formulation, penetrates into the lung surface and delivers a high concentration of drug to the site of infection and is currently in phase 3 trials.[108–110]

Bronchitol, an inhaled dry powder form of mannitol, is a new agent to help restore normal airway hydration by drawing water to the airway surface, which hydrates secretions to help improve airway clearance. Bronchitol has completed two large multinational phase 3 trials, has been approved for CF treatment in Australia, and will be submitted to the FDA in 2012.[111]

An exciting breakthrough in CF treatment focuses on treating the basic defect of the disease: CFTR dysfunction. Kalydeco™ (ivacaftor) was approved on January 31, 2012, for patients >6 years of age with the G551D mutation. Ivacaftor works by potentiating the activity of the CFTR protein so that the channels stay open longer on the cell surface. As a result, mucus is thinned by fluid movement into the airways making airway clearance easier for the patient.

In a randomized, double-blind, placebo-controlled trial evaluating ivacaftor in patients 12 years of age or older, ivacaftor met effectiveness endpoints. Researchers saw significant improvements in lung function, risk of pulmonary exacerbations, respiratory symptoms, and weight and sweat chloride concentrations. The change in baseline FEV_1 was greater than 10.6 percentage points (0.106) in comparison to placebo ($P < 0.001$) with an improvement in pulmonary function noted by 2 weeks and sustained through week 48. An average weight increase of 2.7kg was seen in the ivacaftor group versus placebo at the end of 48 weeks. No significant safety issues were noted in the study. Two other CFTR modulating agents are currently being evaluated: VX-809 and PTC 124 (ataluren). Clinical trials are currently evaluating the safety and efficacy of these agents.[112,113]

Clinical **Controversy...**

CF is a worldwide problem, with a variety of approaches toward treatment. Discussions regarding controversial methods are constantly being held while new therapies are tried. Due to the relatively small population of CF patients, any studies that are conducted are frequently small in number or do not accurately reflect this population. This makes it difficult to extrapolate and come to a consensus regarding therapy. Some of these controversies will be discussed.

The development of novel CFTR modulators brings the promise of improvement in quality and duration of life for the CF patient. It also brings the question of who will finance these expensive drugs. It is estimated that ivacaftor will cost hundreds of thousands of dollars per year. Even with support from insurance and pharmaceutical companies, these drugs are unaffordable for most families. Pharmacists could play an important role in assisting families to obtain financial assistance for these new agents.

Inhaled and/or oral *N*-acetylcysteine (NAC) is an antioxidant that may have some antiinflammatory effect. The CF Foundation does not recommend this therapy due to insufficient evidence; however, a few published studies have led some clinicians to utilize this therapy. To date, there is not enough information to identify an NAC dosing strategy that is tolerable.[52,59,104]

Bisphosphonate therapy is being added to bone health regimens in both adult and pediatric patients. Pediatric CF trials with these medications have not been conducted, although adult CF trials indicated potential value. CF children will develop bone disease that forces clinicians to decide whether to utilize this controversial therapy. In adult CF patients, there have been a few studies assessing the use of injectable bisphosphonate. The use of IV pamidronate showed significant gains in bone mineral density (BMD); however, there was a high incidence of adverse events, such as moderate-severe bone pain, fever, and phlebitis. Injectable formulations are useful to the CF population because they bypass the malabsorption issue. A once-a-week oral bisphosphonate trial is underway. There has been at least one promising adult study with oral alendronate; however, no study has been performed with risedronate.[42,49,50,105]

Colistimethate (Colistin®) is an antibiotic commonly used to treat pseudomonal infections. It is available in the injectable form that can be diluted and nebulized. Reports show a high incidence of bronchospasm and decline of FEV_1 in CF patients, especially in those with underlying reactive airway disease. Administration via inhalation can also be problematic due to low surface tension resulting in foaming of the solution. Thus, the recommended dose is questionable, due to variable drug delivery. However, for patients with multiple-drug-resistant pseudomonas, this may be the only alternative.[93,106,107]

SOCIAL

The social worker is an integral part of the CF team, due to the complex social issues that surround CF patients. Maintaining health insurance is a lifelong problem for CF patients. The inability to pay for CF meds may often influence compliance. Life insurance and homeowners insurance may never be obtainable. Maintaining employment is difficult because some employers may penalize for frequent hospitalizations. Thus, many CF patients have low-paying jobs without insurance coverage.

Building relationships and confiding in others about personal health issues can be intimidating and difficult for CF patients. Children do not have opportunities to engage in friendships with other CF children. Due to infection control guidelines, group settings are limited. Support groups, although available, are restricted to online discussions. The decision to marry and have children is complicated by an awareness of a shortened life span.[16]

SUMMARY

Multidisciplinary care for CF patients should involve pulmonologists, gastroenterologists, pharmacists, social workers, respiratory therapists, and dieticians. Complexity of care requires good communication within the CF team. Although IV antibiotics have historically been a mainstay of therapy, recent focus has shifted to optimizing nutrition status and promoting effective pulmonary clearance. New treatment modalities such as CFTR modulators will necessitate greater involvement by pharmacists. As patients live longer, more social issues arise and medical issues become more complex.

ABBREVIATIONS

ACT	airway clearance therapy
ADEK	fat-soluble vitamins A, D, E, K
BMD	bone mineral density
CF	cystic fibrosis
CFRD	cystic fibrosis related diabetes
CFTR	cystic fibrosis transmembrane conductance regulator
DIOS	distal intestinal obstruction syndrome
FEV_1	forced expiratory volume at 1 second
FVC	forced vital capacity
MIC	minimum inhibitory concentration
NAC	*N*-acetylcysteine
NTM	nontuberculous mycobacteria
OGTT	oral glucose tolerance test
OCP	oral contraceptive pills
PEG	percutaneous endoscopic gastrostomy
PERT	pancreatic enzyme replacement therapy
QPIT	quantitative pilocarpine iontophoresis test

REFERENCES

1. Quinton PM. Cystic fibrosis: Lessons from the sweat gland. Physiology 2007;22:212–225.
2. Moskowitz SM, Chmiel JF, Sternen DL, et al. Clinical practice and genetic counseling for cystic fibrosis and CFTR-related disorders. Genet Med 2008;10(12):851–866.
3. Farrell PM, Rosenstein BJ, White TB, et al. Guidelines for the diagnosis of cystic fibrosis in newborns through older adults: Cystic Fibrosis Foundation Consensus Report. J Pediatr 2008;153(2):S4–S14.
4. Sontag MK, Hammond KB, Zielenski J, et al. Two-tiered immunoreactive trypsinogen (IRT/IRT)-based newborn screening for cystic fibrosis in Colorado: Screening efficacy and diagnostic outcomes. J Pediatr 2005;147(Suppl): S83–S88.
5. Parad RB, Corneau AM. Newborn screening for cystic fibrosis. Pediatr Ann 2003;32:528–535.
6. Corneau AM, Parad RB, Dorkin HL, et al. Population-based newborn screening for genetic disorders when multiple mutations DNA testing is incorporated: A cystic fibrosis newborn screening model demonstrating increased sensitivity but more carrier detections. Pediatrics 2004;113: 1573–1581.
7. Cystic Fibrosis Foundation. Cystic Fibrosis Foundation Patient Registry, 2005 Annual Data Report to the Center Directors. Bethesda, MD: Cystic Fibrosis Foundation, 2006.
8. Cystic Fibrosis Foundation. Clinical Practice Guidelines for Cystic Fibrosis: Preventive and maintenance care for the patient with cystic fibrosis. May 2006;1–24. https://www.portcf.org/Resources/Consensus%20&%20Guidelines/Chapter%201.pdf.
9. Rowe SM, Miller S, Sorscher EJ. Cystic fibrosis. N Engl J Med 2005;352(19):1992–2001.
10. Groman JD, Karczeski B, Sheridan M, et al. Phenotypic and genetic characterization of patients with features of "nonclassic" forms of cystic fibrosis. J Pediatr 2005;146: 675–680.
11. Mickle JE, Cutting GR. Genotype–phenotype relationships in cystic fibrosis. Med Clin North Am 2000;84:597–607.
12. Mall M, Grubb BR, Harkema JR, et al. Increased airway epithelial Na+ absorption produces cystic fibrosis-like lung disease in mice. Nat Med 2004;10:487–493.
13. Smith JJ, Travis SM, Greenberg EP, et al. Cystic fibrosis airway epithelia fail to kill bacteria because of abnormal airway surface fluid. Cell 1996;85:229–236.
14. Engelhardt JF, Yankaskas JR, Ernst SA, et al. Submucosal glands are the predominant site of CFTR expression in the human bronchus. Nat Genet 1992;2:240–248.
15. Knowles MR, Durie PR. What is cystic fibrosis? N Engl J Med 2002;347(6):439–442.
16. Yankaskas JR, Marshall BC, Sufian B, et al. Cystic fibrosis adult care. Chest 2004;125:1S–39S.
17. Kerr M. Cystic fibrosis screening legislated for all newborns by 2010. Medscape Medical News. 2009 Medscape, LLC. July 15, 2009. *http://www.medscape.com/viewarticle/705589_print*.
18. Stallings VA, Stark LJ, Robinson KA, et al. Evidence-based practice recommendations for nutrition-related management of children and adults with cystic fibrosis and pancreatic insufficiency: Results of a systematic review. J Am Diet Assoc 2008;108(5):832–839.
19. Steinkamp G, Demmelmair H, Ruhl-Bagheri I, et al. Energy supplements rich in linoleic acid improve body weight and essential fatty acid status of cystic fibrosis patients. J Pediatr Gastroenterol Nutr 2000;31:418–423.
20. Richardson I, Nyulasi I, Cameron K, et al. Nutritional status of an adult cystic fibrosis population. Nutrition 2000;16: 255–259.
21. Stark LJ, Bowen AM, Tyc VL, et al. A behavioral approach to increasing calorie consumption in children with cystic fibrosis. J Pediatr Psychol 1990;15:309–326.
22. Stark LJ, Knapp LG, Bowen AM, et al. Increasing calorie consumption in children with cystic-fibrosis—Replication with 2-year follow-up. J Appl Behav Anal 1993;26:435–450.
23. Lloyd-Still JD, Smith AE, Wessel HU. Fat intake is low in cystic fibrosis despite unrestricted dietary practices. JPEN J Parenter Enteral Nutr 1989;13:296–298.
24. Luder E, Kattan M, Thornton JC, et al. Efficacy of a nonrestricted fat diet in patients with cystic fibrosis. Am J Dis Child 1989;143:458–464.
25. Shepherd RW, Holt TL, Cleghorn G, et al. Short-term nutritional supplementation during management of pulmonary exacerbations in cystic fibrosis: A controlled study, including effects of protein turnover. Am J Clin Nutr 1988;48:235–239.

26. Hanning RM, Blimkie CJR, Baror O, et al. Relationships among nutritional status and skeletal and respiratory muscle function in cystic fibrosis: Does early dietary supplementation make a difference? Am J Clin Nutr 1993;57:580–587.
27. Bentur L, Kalnins D, Levison H, et al. Dietary intakes of young children with cystic fibrosis: Is there a difference? J Pediatr Gastroenterol Nutr 1996;22:254–258.
28. Vaisman N, Clarke R, Pencharz PB. Nutritional rehabilitation increases resting energy expenditure without affecting protein turnover in patients with cystic fibrosis. J Pediatr Gastroenterol Nutr 1991;13:383–390.
29. Van Biervliet S, De Waele K, Van Winekel M, et al. Percutaneous endoscopic gastrostomy in cystic fibrosis: Patient acceptance and effect of overnight tube feeding on nutritional status. Acta Gastroenterol Belg 2004;67: 241–244.
30. Peterson ML, Jacobs DR Jr, Mills CE. Longitudinal changes in growth parameters are correlated with changes in pulmonary function in children with cystic fibrosis. Pediatrics 2003;112(3 Pt 1):588–592.
31. Konstan MW, Butler SM, Wohl ME, et al. Growth and nutritional indexes in early life predict pulmonary function in cystic fibrosis. J Pediatr 2003, 142:624–630.
32. Thomson MA, Quirk P, Swanson CE, et al. Nutritional growth-retardation is associated with defective lung growth in cystic-fibrosis: A preventable determinant of progressive pulmonary dysfunction. Nutrition 1995;11:350–354.
33. Walker SA, Gozal D. Pulmonary function correlates in the prediction of long-term weight gain in cystic fibrosis patients with gastrostomy tube feedings. J Pediatr Gastroenterol Nutr 1998;27:53–56.
34. Navarro J, Rainisio M, Harms HK, et al. Factors associated with poor pulmonary function: Cross-sectional analysis of data from the ERCF. European Epidemiologic Registry of Cystic Fibrosis. Eur Respir J 2001;18:298–305.
35. Oliver MR, Heine RG, Ng CH, et al. Factors affecting clinical outcomes in gastrostomy-fed children with cystic fibrosis. Pediatr Pulmonol 2004;37:324–329.
36. Smith DL, Clarke JM, Stableforth DE. A nocturnal nasogastric feeding programme in cystic fibrosis adults. J Hum Nutr Diet 1994;7:257–262.
37. Williams SG, Ashworth F, McAlweenie A, et al. Percutaneous endoscopic gastrostomy feeding in patients with cystic fibrosis. Gut 1999;44:87–90.
38. Steinkamp G, von der Hardt H. Improvement of nutritional status and lung function after long-term nocturnal gastrostomy feedings in cystic fibrosis. J Pediatr 1994;124:244–249.
39. FDA approves pancreatic enzyme replacement product for marketing in United States: Creon designed to help those with cystic fibrosis, others with exocrine pancreatic insufficiency. U.S. Food and Drug Administration. U.S. Department of Health & Human Services, 2009.
40. Cystic Fibrosis Foundation. Concepts in CF Care, Vol X, Section 1. Consensus Conferences. Bethesda, MD: Cystic Fibrosis Foundation, 2001.
41. Houwen RH, van der Doef HP, Sermer I, et al. Defining DIOS and constipation in cystic fibrosis with a multicentre study on the incidence, characteristics, and treatment of DIOS. J Pediatr Gastroenterol Nutr 2009;49(1):54–58.
42. Aris RM, Merkel PA, Bachrach LK, et al. Consensus statement: Guide to bone health and disease in cystic fibrosis. J Clin Endocrinol Metab 2005;90(3):1888–1896.
43. Elkin SL, Fairney A, Burnett S, et al. Vertebral deformities and low bone mineral density in adults with cystic fibrosis: A cross-sectional study. Osteoporos Int 2001;12:366–372.
44. Aris RM, Renner JB, Winders AD, et al. Increased rate of fractures and severe kyphosis: Sequelae of living to adulthood with cystic fibrosis. Ann Intern Med 1998;128:186–193.
45. Conway SP, Morton AM, Oldroyd B, et al. Osteoporosis and osteopenia in adults and adolescents with cystic fibrosis: Prevalence and associated factors. Thorax 2000;55: 798–804.
46. Borowitz D, Baker RD, Stallings V. Consensus report on nutrition for pediatric patients with cystic fibrosis. J Pediatr Gastroenterol Nutr 2002;35:246–259.
47. Wilson DC, Rashid M, Durie PR, et al. Treatment of vitamin K deficiency in cystic fibrosis: Effectiveness of a daily fat-soluble vitamin combination. J Pediatr 2001;138: 851–855.
48. Ontjes DA, Lark RK, Lester GE, et al. Vitamin D depletion and replacement in patients with cystic fibrosis. In: Norman A, Bouillon R, eds. Vitamin D Endocrine System: Structural, Biological, Genetic and Clinical Aspects. Riverside, CA: Thomasset, University of California, 2000:893–896.
49. Haworth CS, Selby PL, Adams JE, et al. Effect of intravenous pamidronate on bone mineral density in adults with cystic fibrosis. Thorax 2001;56:314–316.
50. Haworth CS, Selby PL, Webb AK, et al. Severe bone pain after intravenous pamidronate in adult patients with cystic fibrosis. Lancet 1998;86:1753–1754.
51. Tangpricha V, Kelly A, Stephenson A, et al. An update on the screening, diagnosis, management, and treatment of vitamin d deficiency in individuals with cystic fibrosis: Evidence-based recommendations from the Cystic Fibrosis Foundation. J Clin Endocrinol Metab 2012; 2011–3050.
52. Flume PA, Robinson KA, O'Sullivan BP, et al. Cystic fibrosis pulmonary guidelines: Airway clearance therapies. Respir Care 2009;54(4):522–537.
53. Flume PA, O'Sullivan BP, Robinson KA, et al. Cystic fibrosis pulmonary guidelines: Chronic medications for maintenance of lung health. Am J Respir Crit Care Med 2007;176:957–969.
54. Halfhide C, Evans HJ, Couriel J. Inhaled bronchodilators for cystic fibrosis. Cochrane Database Syst Rev 2008;4:CD003428.
55. Ratjen F. Restoring airway surface liquid in cystic fibrosis. N Engl J Med 2006;354(3):291–293.
56. Robinson M, Rose BR, et al. A controlled trial of long-term inhaled hypertonic saline in patients with cystic fibrosis. N Engl J Med 2006;354(3):229–240.
57. Ballmann M, von der Hart H. Hypertonic saline and recombinant human DNase: A randomised cross-over pilot study in patients with cystic fibrosis. J Cyst Fibros 2002;1: 35–37.
58. Quan JM, Tiddens HA, Sy JP, et al. A two-year randomized, placebo-controlled trial of dornase alfa in young patients with cystic fibrosis with mild lung function abnormalities. J Pediatr 2001;139(6):813–820.
59. Nasr SZ, Kuhns LR, Brown RW, et al. Use of computerized tomography and chest x-rays in evaluating efficacy of aerosolized recombinant human DNase in cystic fibrosis patients younger than age 5 years: A preliminary study. Pediatr Pulmonol 2001;31(5):377–382.
60. Nichols DP, Konstan MW, Chmiel JF. Anti-inflammatory therapies for cystic fibrosis-related lung disease. Clin Rev Allerg Immunol 2008;35(3):135–153.
61. Lands LC, Milner R, Cantin AM, et al. High-dose ibuprofen in cystic fibrosis: Canadian safety and effectiveness trial. J Pediatr 2007;151(3):249–254.

62. Konstan MW, Schluchter MD, Xue W, et al. Clinical use of ibuprofen is associated with slower FEV1 decline in children with cystic fibrosis. Am J Respir Crit Care Med 2007;176(11):1084–1089.
63. Konstan MW, Byard PJ, Hoppel CL, et al. Effect of high-dose ibuprofen in patients with cystic fibrosis. N Engl J Med 1995;332(13):848–854.
64. Saiman L, Marshall BC, Mayer-Hamblett N, et al. Azithromycin in patients with cystic fibrosis chronically infected with *Pseudomonas aeruginosa*: A randomized controlled trial. JAMA 2003;290(13):1749–1756.
65. Wolter J, Seeney S, Bell S, et al. Effect of long term treatment with azithromycin on disease parameters in cystic fibrosis: A randomised trial. Thorax 2002;57(3): 212–216.
66. Saiman L, Siegel J. Infection control recommendations for patients with cystic fibrosis: Microbiology, important pathogens, and infection control practices to prevent patient-to-patient transmissions. Infect Control Hosp Epidemiol 2003;24(5):S6–S52.
67. Stutman HR, Lieberman JM, Nussbaum E, et al. Antibiotic prophylaxis in infants and young children with cystic fibrosis: A randomized controlled trial. J Pediatr 2002;140:299–305.
68. Saiman L, Mehar F, Niu WW, et al. Antibiotic susceptibility of multiply resistant *Pseudomonas aeruginosa* isolated from patients with cystic fibrosis, including candidates for transplantation. Clin Infect Dis 1996;23:532–537.
69. Cystic Fibrosis Foundation. Patient Registry 1996. In: *Annual Report*. Bethesda, MD: Cystic Fibrosis Foundation, 1997.
70. Cystic Fibrosis Foundation. Patient Registry 1997. In: *Annual Report*. Bethesda, MD: Cystic Fibrosis Foundation, 1998.
71. Burns JL, Emerson J, Stapp JR, et al. Microbiology of sputum from patients at cystic fibrosis centers in the United States. Clin Infect Dis 1998;27:158–163.
72. Saiman L, Chen Y, Tabibi S, et al. Identification and antimicrobial susceptibility of *Alcaligenes xylosoxidans* isolated from patients with cystic fibrosis. J Clin Microbiol 2001;39:3942–3945.
73. Sattler C, Mason EJ, Kaplan S. Nonrespiratory *Stenotrophomonas maltophilia* infection at a children's hospital. Clin Infect Dis 2000;31:1321–1330.
74. Elting LS, Khardori N, Bodey GP, et al. Nosocomial infection caused by *Xanthomonas maltophilia*: A case–control study of predisposing factors. Infect Control Hosp Epidemiol 1990;11:134–138.
75. Burde DR, Noble MA, Campbell ME, et al. *Xanthomonas maltophilia* misidentified as *Pseudomonas cepacia* in cultures of sputum from patients with cystic fibrosis: A diagnostic pitfall with major clinical implications. Clin Infect Dis 1995;20:445–448.
76. Demko CA, Stern RC, Doershuk CF. *Stenotrophomonas maltophilia* in cystic fibrosis: Incidence and prevalence. Pediatr Pulmonol 1998;25:304–308.
77. Denton M, Todd NJ, Kerr KG, et al. Molecular epidemiology of *Stenotrophomonas maltophilia* isolated from clinical specimens from patients with cystic fibrosis and associated environmental samples. J Clin Microbiol 1998;36: 1953–1958.
78. Kilby JM, Gilligan PH, Yankaskas JR, et al. Nontuberculous mycobacteria in adult patients with cystic fibrosis. Chest 1992;102:70–75.
79. Torrens JK, Dawkins P, Conway SP, et al. Non-tuberculous mycobacteria in cystic fibrosis. Thorax 1998;53:182–185.
80. Tomashefski JF Jr, Stern RC, Demko CA, et al. Nontuberculous mycobacteria in cystic fibrosis. An autopsy study. Am J Respir Crit Care Med 1996;154:523–528.
81. Cullen AR, Cannon CL, Mark EJ, et al. *Mycobacterium abscessus* infection in cystic fibrosis. Colonization or infection? Am J Respir Crit Care Med 2003;167:828–834.
82. Equi A, Balfour-Lynn IM, Bush A, et al. Long term azithromycin in children with cystic fibrosis: A randomised, placebo-controlled crossover trial. Lancet 2002;360(9338)978–980
83. Bargon J, Dauletbaev N, Kohler B, et al. Prophylactic antibiotic therapy is associated with an increased prevalence of *Aspergillus* colonization in adult cystic fibrosis patients. Respir Med 1999;93:835–838.
84. Coenye T, Vandamme P, Govan JRW, et al. Taxonomy and identification of the *Burkholderia cepacia* complex. J Clin Microbiol 2001:3427–3436.
85. Humphreys H, Peckham D, Patel P, et al. Airborne dissemination of *Burkholderia* (*Pseudomonas*) *cepacia* from adult patients with cystic fibrosis. Thorax 1994;49:1157–1159.
86. McMeamin JD, Zaccone TM, Coenye T, et al. Misidentification of *Burkholderia cepacia* in US cystic fibrosis treatment centers: An analysis of 1,051 recent sputum isolates. Chest 2000;117:1661–1665.
87. Ramsey BW, Gore EJ, Smith AL, et al. The effect of respiratory viral infections on patients with cystic fibrosis. Am J Dis Child 1989;143:662–668.
88. Hiatt PW, Grace SC, Kozinetz CA, et al. Effects of viral lower respiratory tract infection on lung function in infants with cystic fibrosis. Pediatr 1999;103:619–626.
89. Abman SH, Ogle JW, Harbeck RJ, et al. Early bacteriologic, immunologic, and clinical courses of young infants with cystic fibrosis identified by neonatal screening. J Pediatr 1991;119:211–217.
90. Synagis (Palivizumab) package insert. MedImmune Incorporated. July 2008
91. Gruber WC, Campbell PW, Thompson JM, et al. Comparison of live attenuated and inactivated influenza vaccines in cystic fibrosis patients and their families: Results of a 3-year study. J Infect Dis 1994;169:241–247.
92. Gross PA, Denning CR, Gaerlan PF, et al. Annual influenza vaccination: Immune response in patients over 10 years. Vaccine 1996;14:1280–1284.
93. Grohskopf L, Uyeki T, Bresee J, et al. Prevention and control of influenza with vaccines: Recommendations of the Advisory Committee on Immunization Practices (ACIP)—United States, 2012–2013 Influenza Season. MMWR 2012; 61:613–618.
94. Fiel SB. Aerosolized antibiotics in cystic fibrosis: Current and future trends. Expert Rev Respir Med 2009 Medscape, LLC. July 15, 2009. *http://www.medscape.com/viewarticle/579507_print*
95. Geller, DE, Pitlick WH, Nardella PA. "Pharmacokinetics and bioavailability of aerosolized tobramycin in cystic fibrosis." Chest 2002: 22 (1):219–226.
96. Assael BM, Pressler T, Bilton D, et al. Inhaled aztreonam lysine vs. inhaled tobramycin in cystic fibrosis: A comparative efficacy trial. J Cyst Fibros 2012. doi:pii: S1569–1993(12)00136-1.10.1016/j.jcf.2012.07.006.
97. Yaffe S, Gerbracht LM, Mosovich LL, et al. Pharmacokinetics of methicillin in patients with cystic fibrosis. J Infect Dis 1977;135(5):828–831.
98. Powell SH, Thompson WL, Luthe MA, et al. Once-daily vs. continuous aminoglycoside dosing: Efficacy and toxicity in animal and clinical studies of gentamicin, netilmicin and tobramycin. J Infect Dis 1983;5:918–932.

99. Cystic Fibrosis Foundation. Diagnosis, Screening, and Management of Cystic Fibrosis Related Diabetes Mellitus. Consensus Conferences, Vol IX. Section II. Bethesda, MD: Cystic Fibrosis Foundation, 1999.
100. Rosenecker J, Eichler I, Kuhn L, et al. Genetic determination of diabetes mellitus in patients with cystic fibrosis. J Pediatr 1995;127:441–443.
101. Lanng S, Thorsteinsson B, Lund-Andersen C, et al. Diabetes mellitus in Danish CF patients: Prevalence and late diabetic complications. Acta Paediatr 1994;83:72–77.
102. Finkelstein SM, Wielinski CL, Elliott GR, et al. Diabetes mellitus associated with cystic fibrosis. J Pediatr 1988;112: 373–377.
103. Geffner ME, Lippe BM, Maclaren NK, et al. Role of autoimmunity in insulinopenia and carbohydrate derangements with cystic fibrosis. J Pediatr 1988;112:419–421.
104. Sheppard DJ, Welsh MJ. Effect on ATP-sensitive K+ channel regulators on cystic fibrosis transmembrance conductance regulator chloride currents. J Gen Physiol 1992;100:573–591.
105. Moran A, Brunzell C, Cohen RC, et al. Clinical care guidelines for cystic fibrosis-related diabetes. Diabetes Care 2010 ;33(12):2697–2708.
106. Trouvanziam R, Conrad CK, Bottiglieri T, et al. High-dose oral *N*-acetylcysteine, a glutathione prodrug, modulates inflammation in cystic fibrosis. Proc Natl Acad Sci USA 2006;103:4628–4633.
107. Aris RM, Lester GE, Camaniti M, et al. Alendronate for cystic fibrosis adults with low bone density: Results of a randomized, controlled trial. Am J Respir Crit Care Med 2006;169:77–82.
108. Rebelo K. ATS 2009: Inhalation powder tobramycin safe, effective to treat *Pseudomonas aeruginosa* in cystic fibrosis patients. Medscape Medical News. 2009 Medscape, LLC. July 15, 2009. *http://www.medscape.com/viewarticle/702973_print*
109. PARI's Altera Delivers Gilead's Cayston, approved by European Commission to treat cystic fibrosis. 2009 PARI Pharma. Sept 23, 2009. http://www.paripharma.com.
110. Cystic Fibrosis Foundation Website, 2013. Cystic Fibrosis Drug Pipeline: Arikace. http://www.cff.org/research/DrugDevelopmentPipeline/.
111. Cystic Fibrosis Foundation Website, 2013. Cystic Fibrosis Drug Pipeline: Bronchitol. http://www.cff.org/research/DrugDevelopmentPipeline/.
112. Ramsey BW, Davies J, McElvaney NG et al. A CFTR Potentiator in Patients with Cystic Fibrosis and the G551D Mutation. N Eng J Med 2011;365:1663–1672.
113. Accurso FJ, Rowe SM, Clancy JP, et al. Effect of VX-770 in persons with cystic fibrosis and the G551D-CFTR mutation. N Eng J Med 2010;363:1991–2003.

19 Gastroesophageal Reflux Disease

Dianne B. May and Satish SC Rao

KEY CONCEPTS

1. Gastroesophageal reflux disease (GERD) can be described on the basis of either esophageal symptoms or esophageal tissue injury. The common symptoms include heartburn, acid brash, regurgitation, chest pain, and dysphagia.
2. Endoscopy is commonly used to evaluate mucosal injury from GERD and to assess for the presence of Barrett's esophagus or other complications such as bleeding or stricture.
3. Ambulatory pH monitoring (with or without impedance monitoring) is useful for confirming acid or nonacid reflux in patients with persistent symptoms without evidence of mucosal damage or for patients with atypical symptoms such as hoarseness of voice, chest pain, persistent cough/throat clearing, or erosion of dental enamel; manometry is useful for patients who are candidates for antireflux surgery and for ensuring proper placement of pH probes.
4. The goals of GERD treatment are to alleviate symptoms, decrease the frequency of recurrent disease, promote healing of mucosal injury, and prevent complications.
5. GERD treatment is determined by disease severity and includes lifestyle changes and patient-directed therapy, pharmacologic treatment, and antireflux surgery.
6. Patients with typical GERD symptoms should be treated with lifestyle modifications as appropriate and a trial of empiric acid-suppression therapy. Those who do not respond to empiric therapy or who present with alarm symptoms such as dysphagia, weight loss, anemia, or GI bleeding should undergo endoscopy, or, less commonly, a barium swallow study.
7. Surgical intervention is a viable alternative treatment for select patients when long-term pharmacologic management is undesirable or when patients have refractory symptoms or complications.
8. Acid suppression is the mainstay of GERD treatment. Proton pump inhibitors provide the greatest symptom relief and the highest healing rates, especially for patients with erosive disease or moderate to severe symptoms or with complications.
9. Many patients with GERD will relapse if medication is withdrawn; so long-term maintenance treatment may be required. A proton pump inhibitor is the drug of choice for maintenance of patients with moderate to severe GERD. Both step-up and step-down therapies have been advocated.
10. Patient medication profiles should be reviewed for drugs that may aggravate GERD. Patients should be monitored for adverse drug reactions and potential drug–drug interactions.

Gastroesophageal reflux disease (GERD) is a common medical disorder. A consensus definition of GERD states it is "a condition that occurs when the refluxed stomach contents lead to troublesome symptoms and/or complications."[1] The key is that these troublesome symptoms adversely affect the well-being of the patient. Episodic heartburn that is not frequent enough or painful enough to be considered bothersome by the patient is not included in this definition of GERD.[1]

Esophageal GERD syndromes are classified as either symptom-based or tissue injury–based depending on how the patient presents.[1] Symptom-based esophageal GERD syndromes may exist with or without esophageal injury and most commonly present as heartburn, regurgitation, or dysphagia. Less commonly, odynophagia (painful swallowing) or hypersalivation may occur. Tissue injury–based syndromes may exist with or without symptoms. The spectrum of injury includes esophagitis (inflammation of the lining of the esophagus), Barrett's esophagus (when tissue lining the esophagus is replaced by tissue similar to the lining of the intestine), strictures, and esophageal adenocarcinoma.[2] Esophagitis occurs when the esophagus is repeatedly exposed to refluxed gastric contents for prolonged periods of time. This can progress to erosion of the squamous epithelium of the esophagus (erosive esophagitis). Complications of long-term reflux may include the development of strictures, Barrett's esophagus, or possibly adenocarcinoma of the esophagus.

Gastroesophageal reflux symptoms associated with disease processes in organs other than the esophagus are referred to as extraesophageal reflux syndromes. Patients with extraesophageal reflux syndromes may present with chest pain, hoarseness of voice, chronic cough/throat clearing, or asthma. An association between these syndromes and GERD should only be considered when they occur along with esophageal GERD syndrome because these extraesophageal symptoms are nonspecific and have many other causes.[1]

Many patients suffering from mild GERD do not go on to develop erosive esophagitis and are often managed with lifestyle changes, antacids, and nonprescription histamine-2 (H_2) receptor antagonists or nonprescription proton pump inhibitors. Those with more severe symptoms (with or without tissue injury) predictably follow a course of relapsing disease, requiring more intensive treatment with acid-suppression therapy followed by long-term maintenance therapy. Antireflux surgery offers an alternative for select patients in whom prolonged medical management is undesirable or who have refractory symptoms or complications.

EPIDEMIOLOGY

GERD occurs in people of all ages but is most common in those older than age 40 years. Although mortality is rare, GERD symptoms may have a significant impact on quality of life. The true prevalence of GERD is difficult to assess because many patients do not seek medical treatment, symptoms do not always correlate well with the severity of the disease, and there is no standardized definition or universal gold standard method for diagnosing the disease. However, 10% to 20% of adults in Western countries suffer from GERD symptoms on a weekly basis.[3]

The prevalence of GERD varies depending on the geographic region but appears highest in Western countries and is on the rise.[3]

Except during pregnancy, there does not appear to be a major difference in incidence between men and women. Although gender does not generally play a major role in the development of GERD, it is an important factor in the development of Barrett's esophagus. Alarmingly, adenocarcinoma of the esophagus has increased twofold to sixfold over the past two decades.[2] The relationship of adenocarcinoma to Barrett's esophagus, or even just long-standing GERD, which may be an independent risk factor for esophageal adenocarcinoma, remains to be clearly defined.

Other risk factors and comorbidities that may contribute to the development or worsening of GERD symptoms include family history, obesity, smoking, alcohol consumption, certain medications and foods, respiratory diseases, and reflux chest pain syndrome.

PATHOPHYSIOLOGY

The key factor in the development of GERD is the abnormal reflux of gastric contents from the stomach into the esophagus.[4] In some cases, gastroesophageal reflux is associated with defective lower esophageal sphincter (LES) pressure or function (see Fig. 19-1). Patients may have decreased gastroesophageal sphincter pressures related to (a) spontaneous transient LES relaxations, (b) transient increases in intraabdominal pressure, or (c) an atonic LES, all of which may lead to the development of gastroesophageal reflux. Problems with other normal mucosal defense mechanisms, such as abnormal esophageal anatomy, improper esophageal clearance of gastric fluids, reduced mucosal resistance to acid, delayed or ineffective gastric emptying, inadequate production of epidermal growth factor, and reduced salivary buffering of acid, may also contribute to the development of GERD. Substances that may promote esophageal damage on reflux into the esophagus include gastric acid, pepsin, bile acids, and pancreatic enzymes. Thus, the composition and volume of the refluxate, as well as duration of exposure, are important aggressive factors in determining the consequences of gastroesophageal reflux. Rational therapeutic regimens in the treatment of gastroesophageal reflux are designed to maximize normal mucosal defense mechanisms and attenuate the aggressive factors.

Lower Esophageal Sphincter Pressure

The LES is a specialized thickening of the smooth muscle lining of the distal esophagus with an elevated basal resting pressure. The sphincter is normally in a tonic, contracted state, preventing the reflux of gastric material from the stomach, but relaxes on swallowing to permit the passage of food into the stomach. Mechanisms by which defective LES pressure may cause gastroesophageal reflux are threefold. First, and probably most importantly, reflux may occur following spontaneous transient LES relaxations that are not associated with swallowing. Although the exact mechanism is unknown, esophageal distension, vomiting, belching, and retching cause relaxation of the LES. While not thought to contribute significantly to erosive esophagitis, these transient relaxations, which are normal postprandially, may play an important role in symptom-based esophageal reflux syndromes. Transient decreases in sphincter pressure are responsible for more than half of the reflux episodes in patients with GERD. The propensity to develop gastroesophageal reflux secondary to transient decreases in LES pressure is probably dependent on numerous factors, including the degree of sphincter relaxation, efficacy of esophageal clearance, patient position (more common in recumbent position), gastric volume, and intragastric pressure. Second, reflux may occur following transient increases in intraabdominal pressure (stress reflux). An increase in intraabdominal pressure such as that occurring during straining, bending over, coughing, eating, or a Valsalva maneuver may overcome a weak LES, and thus may lead to reflux. Third, the LES may be atonic, thus permitting free reflux as seen in patients with scleroderma. Although transient relaxations are more likely to occur when there is normal LES pressure, the latter two mechanisms are more likely to occur when the

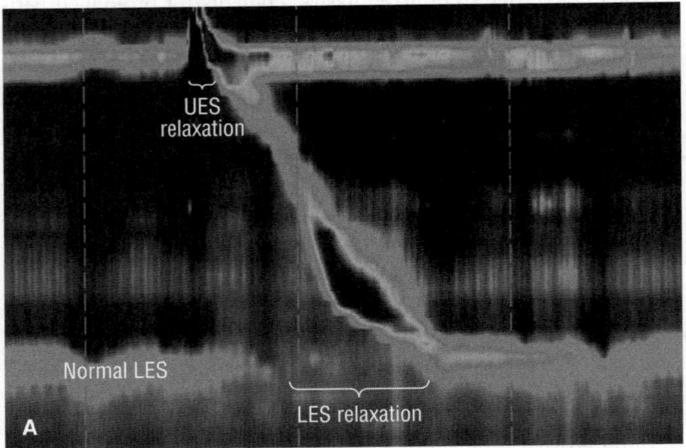

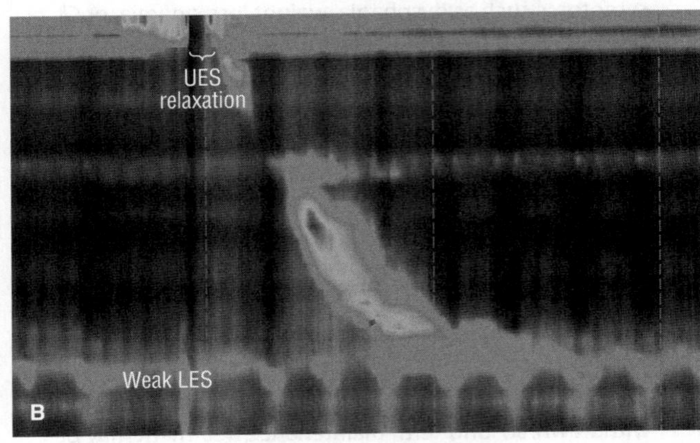

FIGURE 19-1 Comparison of a normal esophageal high-resolution manometry showing normal upper esophageal sphincter and lower esophageal sphincter (LES) resting pressure and relaxations with a water bolus (*A*), compared with that seen in a patient with GERD and a weak resting LES (*B*).

TABLE 19-1 Foods and Medications That May Worsen GERD Symptoms

Foods/Beverages	Medications
Decreased Lower Esophageal Sphincter Pressure	
Fatty meal	Anticholinergics
Carminatives (peppermint, spearmint)	Barbiturates
Chocolate	Caffeine
Coffee, cola, tea	Dihydropyridine calcium channel blockers
Garlic	Dopamine
Onions	Estrogen
Chili peppers	Nicotine
Alcohol (wine)	Nitrates
	Progesterone
	Tetracycline
	Theophylline
Direct Irritants to the Esophageal Mucosa	
Spicy foods	Aspirin
Orange juice	Bisphosphonates
Tomato juice	Nonsteroidal antiinflammatory drugs (NSAIDs)
Coffee	Iron
Tobacco	Quinidine
	Potassium chloride

LES pressure is decreased by such factors as fatty foods, gastric distension, smoking, or certain medications (see Table 19-1).[5] Various foods aggravate esophageal reflux by decreasing LES pressure or by precipitating symptomatic reflux by direct mucosal irritation (e.g., spicy foods, orange juice, tomato juice, and coffee). Pregnancy is a condition in which reflux is common. There are many postulated reasons for the increased incidence of heartburn during pregnancy, including hormonal effects on esophageal muscle, LES tone, and physical factors (increased intraabdominal pressure) resulting from an enlarging uterus. A decrease in LES pressure resulting from any of the previously mentioned causes is not always associated with gastroesophageal reflux. Likewise, individuals who experience decreases in sphincter pressures and subsequently reflux do not always develop GERD. The other natural defense mechanisms (anatomic factors, esophageal clearance, mucosal resistance, and other gastric factors) must be evoked to explain this phenomenon.

Anatomic Factors

Disruption of the normal anatomic barriers by a hiatal hernia (when a portion of the stomach protrudes through the diaphragm into the chest) was once thought to be a primary etiology of gastroesophageal reflux and esophagitis. Now it appears that a more important factor related to the presence or absence of symptoms in patients with hiatal hernia is the LES pressure. Patients with hypotensive LES pressures and large hiatal hernias are more likely to experience gastroesophageal reflux following abrupt increases in intraabdominal pressure compared with patients with a hypotensive LES and no hiatal hernia. Although anatomic factors are still considered significant by some, the diagnosis of hiatal hernia is currently considered a separate entity with which gastroesophageal reflux may simultaneously occur.

Esophageal Clearance

In many patients with GERD, the problem is not that they produce too much acid but that the acid produced ends up in the wrong place and spends too much time in contact with the esophageal mucosa. This is not surprising, because the symptoms and/or severity of damage produced by gastroesophageal reflux are partially dependent on the duration of contact between the gastric contents and the esophageal mucosa. This contact time is, in turn, dependent on the rate at which the esophagus clears the noxious material, as well as the frequency of reflux. The esophagus is cleared by primary peristalsis in response to swallowing, or by secondary peristalsis in response to esophageal distension and gravitational effects. Swallowing contributes to esophageal clearance by increasing salivary flow. Saliva contains bicarbonate that buffers the residual gastric material on the surface of the esophagus. The production of saliva decreases with increasing age, making it more difficult to maintain a neutral intraesophageal pH. Therefore, esophageal damage caused by reflux occurs more often in the elderly, and similarly, for patients with *Sjögren's syndrome* or *xerostomia*. In addition, swallowing is decreased during sleep, making nocturnal GERD a problem in many patients.

Mucosal Resistance

Within the esophageal mucosa and submucosa there are mucus-secreting glands that may contribute to the protection of the esophagus. Bicarbonate moving from the blood to the lumen can neutralize acidic refluxate in the esophagus. When the mucosa is repeatedly exposed to the refluxate in GERD, or if there is a defect in the normal mucosal defenses, hydrogen ions diffuse into the mucosa, leading to the cellular acidification and necrosis that ultimately cause esophagitis. In theory, mucosal resistance may be related not only to esophageal mucus but also to tight epithelial junctions, epithelial cell turnover, nitrogen balance, mucosal blood flow, tissue prostaglandins, and the acid–base status of the tissue. Saliva is also rich in epidermal growth factor, stimulating cell renewal.

Gastric Emptying

Delayed gastric emptying can contribute to gastroesophageal reflux. An increase in gastric volume may increase both the frequency of reflux and the amount of gastric fluid available to be refluxed. Gastric volume is related to the volume of material ingested, rate of gastric secretion, rate of gastric emptying, and amount and frequency of duodenal reflux into the stomach. Factors that increase gastric volume and/or decrease gastric emptying, such as smoking and high-fat meals, are often associated with gastroesophageal reflux. This partially explains the prevalence of postprandial gastroesophageal reflux. Fatty foods may increase postprandial gastroesophageal reflux by increasing gastric volume, delaying the gastric emptying rate, and decreasing the LES pressure. Patients with gastroesophageal reflux, particularly infants, may have a defect in gastric antral motility. The delay in emptying may promote regurgitation of feedings, which might, in turn, contribute to two common complications of GERD in infants (e.g., failure to thrive and pulmonary aspiration).[6]

Composition of Refluxate

The composition, pH, and volume of the refluxate are important aggressive factors in determining the consequences of gastroesophageal reflux. In animals, acid has two primary effects when it refluxes into the esophagus. First, if the pH of the refluxate is less than 2, esophagitis may develop secondary to protein denaturation. In addition, pepsinogen is activated to pepsin at this pH and may also cause esophagitis. Duodenogastric reflux esophagitis, or "alkaline esophagitis," refers to esophagitis induced by the reflux of bilious and pancreatic fluid. The term alkaline esophagitis may be a misnomer in that the refluxate may be either weakly alkaline or acidic in nature. An increase in gastric bile concentrations may be caused by duodenogastric reflux as a result of a generalized motility disorder, slower clearance of the refluxate, or after surgery.[7] Although bile acids have both a direct irritant effect on the esophageal mucosa and an indirect effect of increasing hydrogen ion permeability of the mucosa, symptoms are more often related to acid reflux than to bile reflux. Specifically, the percentage of time that the esophageal pH is <4 is greater for patients with severe disease as compared with that for patients with mild disease. Esophageal pH monitoring in conjunction with 24-hour bile monitoring has shown a higher incidence of Barrett's esophagus for patients who have both acid and alkaline reflux.[7] More study is needed to substantiate this finding. Nevertheless, the combination of acid, pepsin, and/or bile is a potent refluxate in producing esophageal damage.

Complications

Several complications may occur with gastroesophageal reflux, including esophagitis, esophageal strictures, Barrett's esophagus, and esophageal adenocarcinoma. Strictures are common in the distal esophagus and are generally 1 to 2 cm in length. The use of nonsteroidal antiinflammatory drugs or aspirin is an additional risk factor that may contribute to the development or worsening of GERD complications.[3] Although GERD may lead to esophageal bleeding, the blood loss is usually chronic and low grade in nature, but anemia may occur. In some patients, the reparative process leads to the replacement of the squamous epithelial lining of the esophagus by specialized columnar-type epithelium (Barrett's esophagus), which increases the incidence of esophageal strictures by as much as 30%. Barrett's esophagus is most prevalent in white males in Western countries. The risk of esophageal adenocarcinoma may be higher for patients with Barrett's esophagus as compared with that for the general population, although not as high as previously thought. The absolute annual risk of esophageal adenocarcinoma was 0.12% in those with Barrett's esophagus.[8] The pathophysiology of gastroesophageal reflux is a complex cyclic process. It is difficult, if not impossible, to determine which occurs first: gastroesophageal reflux leading to defective peristalsis with delayed clearing or an incompetent LES pressure leading to gastroesophageal reflux. Understanding the factors associated with the development of GERD provides insight into the treatment modalities currently used to manage patients suffering from this disease.

CLINICAL PRESENTATION

(1) GERD can be described on the basis of either esophageal symptoms or esophageal tissue injury. The severity of the symptoms of gastroesophageal reflux does not always correlate with the degree of esophageal tissue injury, but it does correlate with the duration of reflux. Patients with symptom-based esophageal syndromes may have symptoms as severe as those with esophageal tissue injury. It is important to distinguish GERD symptoms from those of other diseases, especially when chest pain or pulmonary symptoms are present.[9]

CLINICAL PRESENTATION GERD[2]

Symptom-based GERD Syndromes (With or Without Esophageal Tissue Injury)

Typical symptoms (may be aggravated by activities that worsen gastroesophageal reflux such as recumbent position, bending over, or eating a meal high in fat):

- Heartburn (hallmark symptom described as a substernal sensation of warmth or burning rising up from the abdomen that may radiate to the neck; may be waxing and waning in character)
- Acid brash (hypersalivation)
- Regurgitation/belching
- Chest pain (~50% with normal electrocardiogram have GERD)[9]

Alarm symptoms (these symptoms may be indicative of complications of GERD such as Barrett's esophagus, esophageal strictures, or esophageal adenocarcinoma and require further diagnostic evaluation):

- Dysphagia (common)
- Odynophagia
- Bleeding
- Weight loss

Tissue Injury–based GERD Syndromes (With or Without Esophageal Symptoms)

Symptoms (may present with alarm symptoms such as dysphagia, odynophagia, or unexplained weight loss):

- Esophagitis
- Strictures
- Barrett's esophagus
- Esophageal adenocarcinoma

Extraesophageal GERD Syndromes

Symptoms (these symptoms have an association with GERD, but causality should only be considered if a concomitant esophageal GERD syndrome is also present):

- Chronic cough
- Laryngitis
- Asthma (~50% with asthma have GERD)
- Dental enamel erosion

Diagnostic Tests for GERD

Clinical history:

- Generally sufficient to diagnose GERD in patients with typical symptoms

Endoscopy:

- Preferred for assessing for mucosal injury and to assess for other complications, such as bleeding or strictures. Biopsies are necessary to identify Barrett's esophagus, adenocarcinoma, and eosinophilic esophagitis (a nonacid-related esophageal disorder that generally does not respond well to proton pump inhibitor therapy).
- Noninflammatory GERD and major motor disorders may be missed by endoscopy.
- Absence of erosions does not definitively show symptoms are GERD related.

Ambulatory pH monitoring:

- Identifies patients with excessive esophageal acid exposure and helps determine if symptoms are acid related

(continued)

CLINICAL PRESENTATION GERD[2] *(continued)*

- Useful for patients not responding to acid-suppression therapy
- Documents the percentage of time the intraesophageal pH is <4 and determines the frequency and severity of reflux
- Measures only acid reflux (not nonacid reflux)

Combined impedance–pH monitoring:

- Measures both acid and nonacid reflux

Manometry/high-resolution esophageal pressure topography (HREPT):

- Useful in those who have failed twice-daily proton pump inhibitor therapy with normal endoscopic findings to identify motor disorders, to evaluate peristaltic function in those who are candidates for antireflux surgery, and to assure proper placement of pH probes (the recent advancement of the tubeless pH monitoring system using endoscopic landmarks for placement may negate the need for manometry for ensuring proper placement of esophageal pH probes)[1]

Impedance manometry:

- Evaluates bolus transit esophageal clearance/retention
- Evaluates LES and upper esophageal sphincter pressures and peristalsis

Empiric trial of a proton pump inhibitor as a diagnostic test for GERD:

- Less expensive and more convenient than ambulatory pH monitoring but lacks standardized dosing regimen and duration of the diagnostic trial

Barium radiography:

- Not routinely used to diagnose GERD because it lacks sensitivity and specificity; cannot identify Barrett's esophagus. Can detect hiatal hernia.

Diagnostic Tests

The most useful tool in the diagnosis of gastroesophageal reflux is the clinical history, including presenting symptoms and associated risk factors. Patients presenting with typical symptoms of reflux, such as heartburn or regurgitation, do not usually require invasive esophageal evaluation. These patients generally benefit from an initial empiric trial of acid-suppression therapy. A clinical diagnosis of GERD can be assumed in patients who respond to appropriate therapy.[4] Further diagnostic evaluation is useful to prevent misdiagnosis, identify complications, and assess treatment failures.[2] Diagnostic tests should be performed in those patients who do not respond to therapy and in those who present with alarm symptoms (e.g., dysphagia, odynophagia, weight loss), which may be more indicative of complicated disease.

Useful tests in diagnosing GERD include upper *endoscopy*, ambulatory pH monitoring test or impedance monitoring, and manometry. **2** Endoscopy is commonly used to evaluate mucosal injury from GERD and to assess other complications, such as bleeding or stricture. A camera-containing capsule swallowed by the patient offers the newest technology for visualizing the esophageal mucosa via endoscopy. The PillCam ESO is less invasive than traditional endoscopy and takes less than 15 minutes to perform in the clinician's office. Images of the esophagus are downloaded through sensors placed on the patient's chest that are connected to a data collector. The camera-containing capsule is later eliminated in the stool. The main disadvantage of the PillCam is that biopsies cannot be obtained. Of note, it is not recommended to use endoscopy as a "screening tool" for Barrett's esophagus and esophageal adenocarcinoma just because a patient has long-standing GERD.[1]

Clinical **Controversy...**

What constitutes refractory GERD is not well defined. Some consider failure to respond to twice-daily proton pump use to be the threshold for refractory GERD. Symptom indexes are available, but their interpretation is controversial.

Unfortunately, the presence or absence of mucosal damage does not prove the patient's symptoms are reflux related; for that, ambulatory pH monitoring is useful. **3** Ambulatory pH monitoring (with or without impedance monitoring) is useful for confirming acid or nonacid reflux in patients with persistent symptoms without evidence of mucosal damage or for patients with atypical symptoms such as hoarseness of voice, chest pain, persistent cough or throat clearing, or erosion of dental enamel. Ambulatory pH monitoring can be performed by passing a small pH probe transnasally and placing it approximately 5 cm above the LES. Patients are asked to keep a diary of symptoms that later are correlated with the pH measurement corresponding to the time the symptom was reported (see Fig. 19-2). Two developments related to ambulatory reflux monitoring include (a) the use of combined *impedance–pH monitoring* and (b) the use of a wireless method of pH monitoring.[4] Whereas ambulatory pH monitoring only measures acid reflux, combined impedance–pH monitoring measures both acid and nonacid reflux. The wireless pH monitoring involves attaching a radiotelemetry capsule to the esophageal mucosa. The advantages of this method are that a longer period of monitoring is possible (48 hours), it may demonstrate superior recording accuracy compared with some catheter designs, and it is more comfortable for the patient because a nasogastric tube is unnecessary.[1] Proton pump inhibitor therapy should be withheld for 7 days prior to performing ambulatory catheter pH, impedance–pH, or wireless pH monitoring when evaluating patients who have failed an initial empiric therapy and who have normal findings on endoscopy and manometry.[1] Manometry is also useful and can be performed before ambulatory pH/impedance testing. Reasons for choosing manometry are described in Clinical Presentation of GERD above.

TREATMENT

Therapeutic modalities used in the treatment of gastroesophageal reflux are targeted at reversing the various pathophysiologic abnormalities.

Desired Outcomes

4 The goals of treatment are to (a) alleviate or eliminate the patient's symptoms, (b) decrease the frequency or recurrence and duration of gastroesophageal reflux, (c) promote healing of the injured mucosa, and (d) prevent the development of complications. Therapy is directed at augmenting defense mechanisms that prevent reflux and/or decrease the aggressive factors that worsen reflux or

A

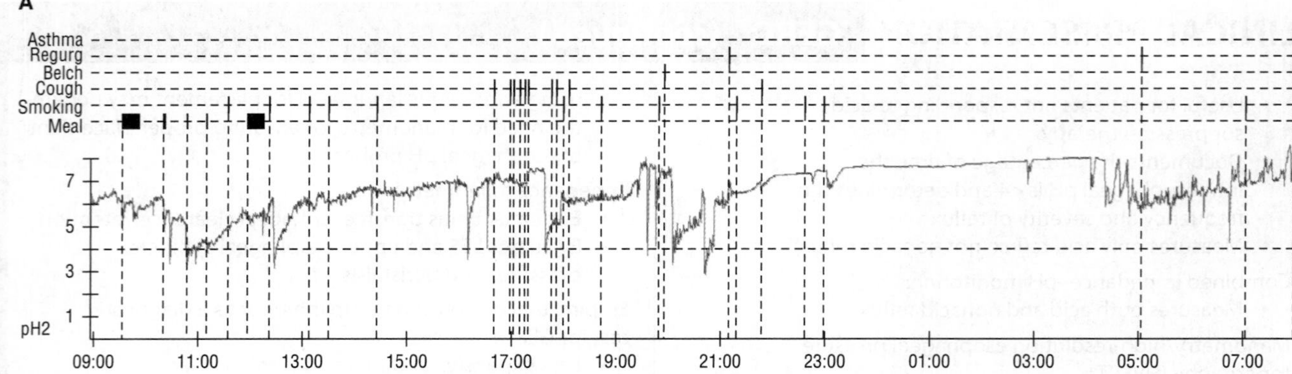

Normal 24 hour ambulatory esophageal pH test	Total	Normal	Upright	Normal	Supine	Normal
• Fraction time pH <4 (%)	1.9	<4.2	1.9	<6.3	0	<1.2
• Number of refluxes	81		81		0	
• Number of long refluxes (>5 minutes)	0		0		0	
• Duration of longest reflux (minutes)	2.3		2.3		0	
• Time pH <4 (minutes)	25.9		25.9		0	

B

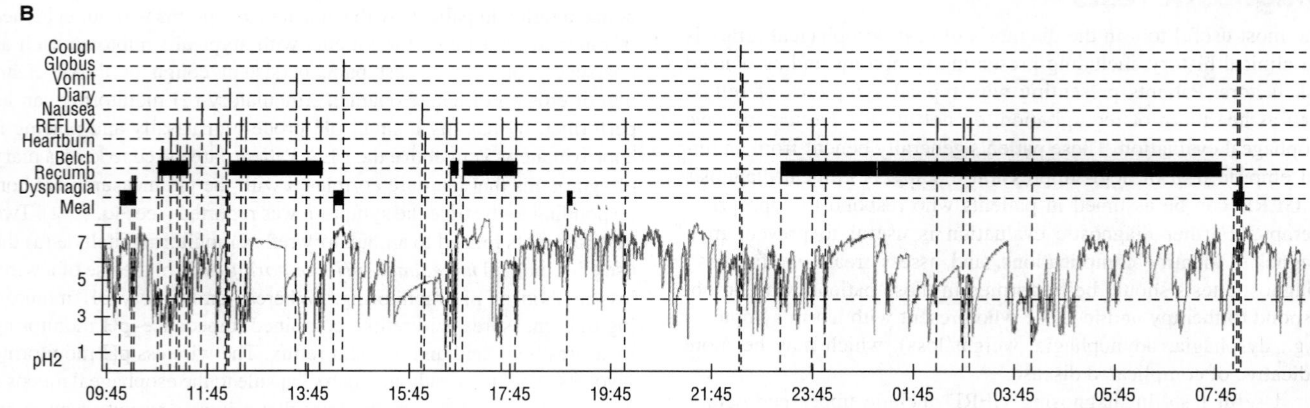

Abnormal 24-hour ambulatory esophageal pH test	Total	Normal	Upright	Normal	Supine	Normal
• Fraction time pH <4 (%)	16	<4.2	10.6	<6.3	20.6	<1.2
• Number of refluxes	332		143		189	
• Number of long refluxes (>5 minutes)	10		6		4	
• Duration of longest reflux (minutes)	7.9		7.1		7.9	
• Time pH <4 (minutes)	220.5		66.8		153.7	

FIGURE 19-2 Graphical representation of a normal 24-hour ambulatory esophageal pH test profile in a healthy subject and a table summarizing key results (*A*) compared with an abnormal 24-hour ambulatory esophageal pH test (*B*) showing significant acid reflux (multiple events of pH drop below 4) and abnormal 24-hour profile in the table.

mucosal damage (see Fig. 19-3). Therapy is directed at (a) decreasing the acidity of the refluxate, (b) decreasing the gastric volume available to be refluxed, (c) improving gastric emptying, (d) increasing LES pressure, (e) enhancing esophageal acid clearance, and (f) protecting the esophageal mucosa.

General Approach to Treatment

5 GERD treatment is determined by disease severity and includes: (a) lifestyle changes and patient-directed therapy with antacids, nonprescription H_2-receptor antagonists, and/or nonprescription proton pump inhibitors; (b) pharmacologic treatment with prescription-strength acid-suppression therapy; (c) and antireflux surgery (see Table 19-2). The initial therapeutic modality used is in part dependent on the patient's condition (frequency of symptoms, degree of esophagitis, and presence of complications) (see Table 19-3). Historically, a step-up approach was used, starting with noninvasive lifestyle modifications and patient-directed therapy and progressing to pharmacologic management or antireflux surgery. A step-down approach, starting with a proton pump inhibitor instead of an H_2-receptor antagonist and then stepping down to the lowest dose of acid suppression (either an H_2-receptor antagonist or proton pump inhibitor) needed to

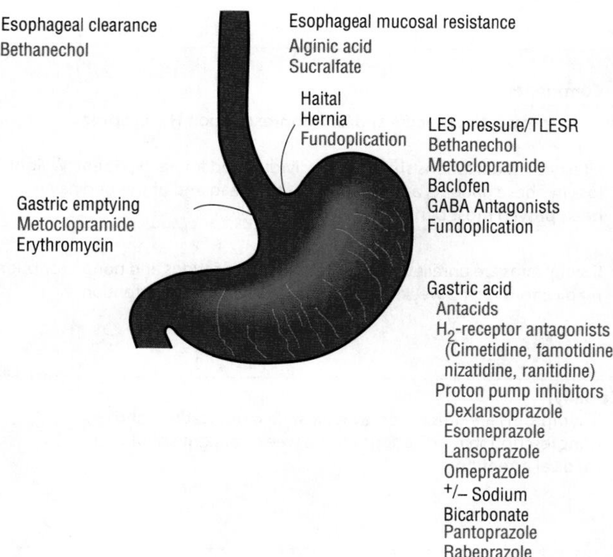

FIGURE 19-3 Therapeutic interventions in the management of gastroesophageal reflux disease. Pharmacologic interventions are targeted at improving defense mechanisms or decreasing aggressive factors. (LES, lower esophageal sphincter.)

control symptoms, has also been advocated. Neither the step-up nor the step-down approach has superior efficacy over the other. The clinician should determine the most appropriate approach for the individual patient. Every attempt should be made to aggressively control symptoms and to prevent relapses early in the course of the patient's disease in order to prevent the complications. For patients with moderate to severe GERD, especially those with erosive disease, starting with a proton pump inhibitor as initial therapy is advocated because of its superior efficacy over H_2-receptor antagonists.

While weight loss in obese patients and elevation of the head end of the bed are beneficial for most GERD patients, recommending all lifestyle modifications to all patients is not recommended.[1] Instead, education on lifestyle modifications should be tailored to the individual needs of the patient. Table 19-4 lists some of the lifestyle modifications that can be recommended.[4]

6 Initially, patients with typical GERD symptoms should be treated with lifestyle modifications and patient-directed therapy. Patients who do not respond to lifestyle modifications and patient-directed therapy after 2 weeks or those with alarm symptoms, such as dysphagia, should seek medical attention and are generally started on empiric therapy consisting of an acid-suppression agent. Those who do not respond to empiric therapy or who present with alarm symptoms should undergo endoscopy or, less commonly, a barium swallow study. Acid-suppression therapy with proton pump inhibitors or H_2-receptor antagonists is the mainstay of GERD treatment. Patients presenting with moderate to severe symptoms (with or without esophageal erosions) should be started on a proton pump inhibitor as initial therapy because it provides the most rapid symptomatic relief and healing in the highest percentage of patients.[4] H_2-receptor antagonists in divided doses are effective for patients with milder GERD symptoms. Standard H_2-receptor antagonist doses may be increased to two to four times the normal dose for patients who do not respond to standard doses. However, if this is necessary, it is more cost-effective and efficacious to switch to a proton pump inhibitor.

Promotility agents are not as effective as acid-suppression agents. Combining promotility agents with acid-suppression drugs offers only modest improvements in symptoms over standard doses of H_2-receptor antagonists and should not be routinely recommended. In addition, the availability of a promotility agent that has an acceptable adverse-effect profile is lacking. Mucosal protectants, such as sucralfate, have a limited role in the treatment of GERD.

TABLE 19-2 Evidence-Based Treatment Recommendations for GERD[2]

Recommendation	Level of Evidence[a]
Lifestyle modifications	
• Weight loss is recommended for overweight or obese patients with GERD	B
• Elevation of the head end of the bed is beneficial when troublesome	
Heartburn or regurgitation occurs when recumbent	
• Other lifestyle modifications should be tailored to the individual patient	
Acid-suppression therapy	
• Acid-suppression therapy is the preferred treatment for GERD	A
Proton pump inhibitors provide more rapid relief of symptoms and are more effective at healing the esophageal mucosa compared with H_2-receptor antagonists	
• Patients with esophageal syndromes not responding to once-daily proton pump inhibitor therapy should receive twice-daily proton pump inhibitor therapy. Endoscopy with biopsy is recommended for those not responding to twice-daily proton pump inhibitor therapy	B
• Patients with extraesophageal GERD syndrome (e.g., laryngitis, asthma) who also have a concomitant esophageal GERD syndrome should be treated with once- or twice-daily acid-suppression therapy. These patients may also require maintenance therapy	B
• Use of acid-suppression therapy in patients with extraesophageal GERD syndrome without concomitant esophageal GERD syndrome	D
• When symptomatic control is primary goal (no esophagitis present), short courses of as-needed acid-suppression therapy may be beneficial. Proton pump inhibitors are more effective than H_2-receptor antagonists	B
Promotility therapy	
• Metoclopramide is not recommended as monotherapy or as adjunctive therapy for patients with GERD	D
Maintenance therapy	
• Most patients with esophageal GERD syndromes will require continuous therapy to control symptoms and to prevent complications. Titrate down to the lowest effective dose	A
• Use of less than daily dosing as maintenance therapy in patients with GERD and previous erosive esophagitis	D
Surgery	
• Proton pump inhibitor therapy is preferred as initial therapy over antireflux surgery due to superior safety	A
• Antireflux surgery represents a viable alternative for patients with an established diagnosis of GERD who are responsive to, but intolerant of, acid-suppression therapy	A

[a]Level of evidence: A, strongly recommended based on good evidence that it improves outcomes; B, recommended based on fair evidence that it improves outcomes; D, recommended against based on fair evidence that it is ineffective or harm outweighs benefit.

Maintenance therapy is generally necessary to control symptoms and to prevent complications. For patients with more severe symptoms (with or without esophageal erosions) or for patients with other complications, maintenance therapy with a proton pump inhibitor is most effective. Routine use of combination therapy has no role in GERD maintenance therapy. In cases of refractory GERD, the diagnosis should be confirmed through further diagnostic tests before long-term, high-dose therapy or antireflux surgery is considered.[4]

Nonpharmacologic Therapy

Nonpharmacologic treatment of GERD includes lifestyle modifications and antireflux surgery, which may be viable maintenance modalities in select patients. Endoscopic therapies, such as

TABLE 19-3 Therapeutic Approach to GERD in Adults

Recommended Treatment Regimen	Brand Name	Dose	Comments
Intermittent, mild heartburn (individualized lifestyle modifications + patient-directed therapy with antacids and/or nonprescription H_2-receptor antagonists *or* nonprescription proton pump inhibitor)			
Individualized lifestyle modifications			Lifestyle modifications should be individualized for each patient. Weight loss in obese patients and elevation of the head end of the bed have been proven most beneficial
Patient-directed therapy with antacids			
Magnesium hydroxide/aluminum hydroxide	For example, Maalox®	30 mL as needed or after meals and at bedtime	If symptoms are unrelieved with lifestyle modifications and nonprescription medications after 2 weeks, patient should seek medical attention
Antacid/alginic acid	Gaviscon®	2 tablets or 15 mL after meals and at bedtime	
Calcium carbonate	Tums®	500 mg, 2–4 tablets as needed	
Patient-directed therapy with nonprescription H_2-receptor antagonists (up to twice daily)			
Cimetidine	Tagamet HB®	200 mg	If symptoms are unrelieved with lifestyle modifications and nonprescription medications after 2 weeks, patient should seek medical attention
Famotidine	Pepcid AC®	10 mg	
Nizatidine	Axid AR®	75 mg	
Ranitidine	Zantac 75®	75 mg	
Patient-directed therapy with nonprescription proton pump inhibitors (taken once daily)			
Omeprazole	Prilosec OTC®	20 mg	If symptoms are unrelieved with lifestyle modifications and nonprescription medications after 2 weeks, patient should seek medical attention
Omeprazole/sodium bicarbonate	Zegerid OTC®	20 mg/1,100 mg	
Lansoprazole	Prevacid® 24HR	15 mg	
Symptomatic relief of GERD (individualized lifestyle modifications + prescription-strength H_2-receptor antagonists *or* prescription-strength proton pump inhibitors)			
Individualized lifestyle modifications			Lifestyle modifications should be individualized for each patient. Weight loss in obese patients and elevation of the head end of the bed have been proven most beneficial
Prescription-strength H_2-receptor antagonists (for 6–12 weeks)			
Cimetidine	Tagamet®	400 mg twice daily	• For typical symptoms, treat empirically with prescription-strength acid-suppression therapy • Mild GERD can usually be treated effectively with H_2-receptor antagonists • If symptoms recur, consider maintenance therapy. Note: Most patients will require standard doses for maintenance therapy
Famotidine	Pepcid®	20 mg twice daily	
Nizatidine	Axid®	150 mg twice daily	
Ranitidine	Zantac®	150 mg twice daily	
Prescription-strength proton pump inhibitors (for 4–8 weeks)			
Dexlansoprazole	Dexilant®	30 mg once daily	• For typical symptoms, treat empirically with prescription-strength acid-suppression therapy • Patients with moderate to severe symptoms should receive a proton pump inhibitor as initial therapy • If symptoms recur, consider maintenance therapy. Note: Most patients will require standard doses for maintenance therapy
Esomeprazole	Nexium®	20 mg once daily	
Lansoprazole	Prevacid®	15–30 mg once daily	
Omeprazole	Prilosec®	20 mg once daily	
Omeprazole/sodium bicarbonate	Zegrid®	20 mg once daily	
Pantoprazole	Protonix®	20 mg once daily	
Rabeprazole	Aciphex®		
Healing of erosive esophagitis or treatment of patients with moderate to severe symptoms or complications (individualized lifestyle modifications + high-dose H_2-receptor antagonists *or* proton pump inhibitors *or* antireflux surgery)			
Individualized lifestyle modifications			Lifestyle modifications should be individualized for each patient. Weight loss in obese patients and elevation of the head end of the bed have been proven most beneficial
Proton pump inhibitors (up to twice daily for 4–16 weeks)			
Dexlansoprazole	Dexilant®	60 mg daily	• For atypical or alarm symptoms, obtain endoscopy with biopsy to evaluate mucosa • If symptoms are relieved, consider maintenance therapy. Proton pump inhibitors are the most effective maintenance therapy for patients with atypical symptoms, complications, and erosive disease. Start with twice-daily proton pump inhibitor therapy if reflux chest syndrome present • Patients not responding to pharmacologic therapy, including those with persistent atypical symptoms, should be evaluated via manometry and/or ambulatory reflux monitoring
Esomeprazole	Nexium®	20–40 mg daily	
Lansoprazole	Prevacid®	30 mg twice daily	
Omeprazole	Prilosec®	20 mg twice daily	
Rabeprazole	Aciphex®	20 mg twice daily	
Pantoprazole	Protonix®	40 mg twice daily	

(*continued*)

TABLE 19-3 Therapeutic Approach to GERD in Adults (*Continued*)

Recommended Treatment Regimen	Brand Name	Dose	Comments
High-dose H_2-receptor antagonists (up to twice daily for 8–12 weeks)			
Cimetidine	Tagamet®	400 mg four times daily or 800 mg twice daily	Note: If high-dose H_2-receptor antagonist needed, may consider using proton pump inhibitor to lower cost, increase convenience, and increase tolerability
Famotidine	Pepcid®	40 mg twice daily	
Nizatidine	Aciphex®	150 mg four times daily	
Ranitidine	Zantac®	150 mg four times daily	
Interventional therapy			
Antireflux surgery			

endoscopic sewing devices and endoluminal application of radiofrequency heat energy, have fallen out of favor and are not routinely recommended.

Lifestyle Modifications

The most common lifestyle modifications that a patient should be educated about include weight loss in obese patients and elevation of the head end of the bed, especially for those patients who have symptoms while in a recumbent position. Other lifestyle modifications should be individualized based on the patient's specific situation. These include consumption of smaller meals and not sleeping for at least 3 hours after eating, avoidance of foods or medications that exacerbate GERD, smoking cessation, avoidance of tight-fitting clothes, and avoidance of alcohol (see Table 19-4).

Obesity increases the risk of GERD, most likely through increased intraabdominal pressure and possibly by disruption of the esophagogastric junction.[10] A high-fat meal will decrease LES pressure for 2 hours or more postprandially. In contrast, a high-protein, low-fat meal will elevate LES pressure. Consequently, weight loss and a low-fat diet may help to improve GERD symptoms. Elevating the head end of the bed by approximately 6 to 8 in (15 to 20 cm) with a foam wedge under the mattress (not just elevating the head with pillows) decreases nocturnal esophageal acid contact time and should be recommended. Many foods may worsen the symptoms of GERD. Fats and chocolate can decrease LES pressure, whereas citrus juice, tomato juice, coffee, and pepper may irritate damaged endothelium.

Patient profiles should be evaluated to identify potential medications that may exacerbate GERD symptoms. Some medications decrease LES pressure, while other medications can act as direct contact irritants to the esophageal mucosa (Table 19-1). Proper patient education can help prevent dysphagia or esophageal ulceration. Patients should be closely monitored for worsening symptoms when any of these medications are started. If symptoms worsen, alternative therapies may be warranted. The clinician must weigh the risks and benefits of continuing a drug known to worsen GERD and esophagitis.

Smoking can cause *aerophagia*, which leads to increased belching and regurgitation. However, data are lacking to show that symptoms improve for patients who quit smoking. Nevertheless, patients with GERD should be encouraged to quit smoking. Alcohol, although not thought to play a role in severe disease, decreases LES pressure and may exacerbate symptoms such as heartburn.

Many patients are noncompliant with lifestyle modifications, and even those who do comply generally continue to have symptoms that require acid-suppression therapy. Nonetheless, it is important to regularly stress the potential benefits of lifestyle modifications that would benefit each individual patient.

TABLE 19-4 Nonpharmacologic Treatment of GERD with Lifestyle Modifications[4]

- Elevate the head end of the bed (increases esophageal clearance). Use 6- to 8-in (15–20 cm) blocks under the head side of the bed
- Weight reduction (reduces symptoms) in obese patients
- Avoid foods that may decrease lower esophageal sphincter pressure or increase transient lower esophageal sphincter relaxation (TLESR) (fats, chocolate, alcohol, peppermint, and spearmint)
- Include protein-rich meals in diet (augments lower esophageal sphincter pressure)
- Avoid foods that have a direct irritant effect on the esophageal mucosa (spicy foods, orange juice, tomato juice, and coffee)
- Behaviors that may reduce esophageal acid exposure:
  - Eat small meals and avoid sleeping immediately after meals (sleep after 3 hours if possible; decreases gastric volume)
  - Stop smoking (decreases spontaneous esophageal sphincter relaxation)
  - Avoid alcohol (increases amplitude of the lower esophageal sphincter, peristaltic waves, and frequency of contraction)
  - Avoid tight-fitting clothes
  - Always take drugs in the sitting upright or standing position and with plenty of liquid, especially for those that have a direct irritant effect on the esophageal mucosa (e.g., bisphosphonates, tetracyclines, quinidine, and potassium chloride, iron salts, aspirin, nonsteroidal antiinflammatory drugs)

Interventional Approaches

Interventional approaches include antireflux surgery and endoscopic therapies.

Antireflux Surgery 7 Surgical intervention is a viable alternative treatment for select patients when long-term pharmacologic management is undesirable or when patients have refractory symptoms or complications. The goal of antireflux surgery is to reestablish the antireflux barrier, to position the LES within the abdomen where it is under positive (intraabdominal) pressure, and to close any associated defect in the diaphragmatic hiatus by reinforcing the crural muscles. Antireflux surgery should be considered for patients (a) who fail to respond to pharmacologic treatment, (b) who opt for surgery despite successful treatment because of lifestyle considerations, including age, time, or expense of medications, (c) who have complications of GERD (e.g., Barrett's esophagus, strictures), or (d) who have atypical symptoms and reflux documented with ambulatory pH monitoring. The antireflux surgical procedure chosen depends on the surgeon's expertise and preference, as well as on anatomic considerations. In general, 90% of patients have symptom resolution following successful Nissen fundoplication. The major complications with antireflux surgery include gas bloat syndrome (inability to belch or vomit), dysphagia, vagal denervation, and splenic trauma. Antireflux surgery is superior to medical management with an H_2-receptor antagonist or a promotility agent. In a 7-year followup study of omeprazole compared with antireflux surgery for patients with esophagitis, symptoms (regurgitation and heartburn) were better controlled in the surgical group; however, treatment failures were also higher in the surgical group. In addition, more patients in the surgical group complained of complications, such as inability to belch, flatulence, and dysphagia.[11] Long-term effectiveness of antireflux surgery is uncertain.

Endoscopic Therapies Endoscopic approaches for the management of GERD have included endoscopic sewing devices and endoluminal application of radio-frequency heat energy resulting in tissue injury or nerve ablation (the Stretta procedure). Unfortunately, results from these endoscopic therapies have proven disappointing and are not routinely recommended. Currently in their infancy stages, natural orifice transluminal surgery and surgical techniques may evolve.

Pharmacologic Therapy

Pharmacologic treatment consists of (a) patient-directed therapy with nonprescription antacids, H_2-receptor antagonists, or proton pump inhibitors and (b) prescription-strength acid-suppression therapy or promotility medications.

Patient-Directed Therapy

Patient-directed therapy, where patients self-treat themselves with nonprescription medications, is appropriate for mild, intermittent symptoms. Patients with continuous symptoms lasting longer than 2 weeks should seek medical attention.

Antacids and Antacid–Alginic Acid Products Patients should be educated that antacids are an appropriate component of treating milder GERD symptoms, even though documentation of their efficacy in placebo-controlled clinical trials is lacking.[4] Although the literature is somewhat controversial on the superiority of antacids to placebo, clinicians and patients clearly consider antacids to be effective for immediate symptomatic relief, and antacids are often used concurrently with other acid-suppression therapies. Maintaining the intragastric pH >4 decreases the activation of pepsinogen to pepsin, a proteolytic enzyme. Also, neutralization of gastric fluid leads to increased LES pressure. Patients who require frequent use of antacids for chronic symptoms should be treated with prescription-strength acid-suppression therapy because their illness is considered more significant.

An antacid product combined with alginic acid is not a potent neutralizing agent and does not enhance LES pressure; however, it does form a highly viscous solution that floats on the surface of the gastric contents. This viscous solution is thought to serve as a protective barrier for the esophagus against reflux of gastric contents. It also reduces the frequency of the reflux episodes. The combination product may be superior to antacids alone in relieving the symptoms of GERD.[4] Efficacy data indicating endoscopic healing are lacking.

Antacid or antacid combination products interact with a variety of medications by altering gastric pH, increasing urinary pH, adsorbing medications to their surfaces, providing a physical barrier to absorption, or forming insoluble complexes with other medications. Antacids have clinically significant drug interactions with tetracycline, ferrous sulfate, isoniazid, quinidine, sulfonylureas, and quinolone antibiotics. Antacid–drug interactions are influenced by composition, dose, dosage schedule, and formulation of the antacid.

Dosage recommendations for antacids in the management of GERD are somewhat difficult to derive from the literature. Doses range from hourly to an as-needed basis (Table 19-3). In general, antacids have a short duration of action, which necessitates frequent administration throughout the day to provide continuous neutralization of acid. Taking antacids after meals can increase the duration of action from about 1 to 3 hours; however, nighttime acid suppression cannot be maintained with bedtime doses.

Nonprescription H_2-Receptor Antagonists and Proton Pump Inhibitors Nonprescription H_2-receptor antagonists (cimetidine, famotidine, nizatidine, and ranitidine) are effective in diminishing gastric acid secretion when taken prior to meals and decrease GERD symptoms associated with exercise. Antacids may have a slightly faster onset of action, while the H_2-receptor antagonists have a much longer duration of action compared with antacids.

The proton pump inhibitors omeprazole 20 mg (alone or combined with sodium bicarbonate) and lansoprazole 15 mg are available without a prescription for the short-term treatment of heartburn. Patients who do not respond to lifestyle modifications and patient-directed therapy after 2 weeks should be seen by their clinician.

Acid-Suppression Therapy

8 Acid suppression is the mainstay of GERD treatment. Proton pump inhibitors provide the greatest symptom relief and the highest healing rates, especially for patients with erosive disease or moderate to severe symptoms or with complications.

Proton Pump Inhibitors (Dexlansoprazole, Esomeprazole, Lansoprazole, Omeprazole, Pantoprazole, and Rabeprazole) Proton pump inhibitors are superior to H_2-receptor antagonists in treating patients with moderate to severe GERD and should be given empirically to those with troublesome symptoms. This includes not only patients with esophageal tissue injury (e.g., Barrett's esophagus, strictures, or esophagitis) but also patients with symptom-based GERD syndromes. Twice-daily proton pump inhibitor use is indicated in those not responding to a standard once-daily course of therapy. Further diagnostic evaluation is indicated for patients not responding to twice-daily proton pump inhibitor therapy.

Proton pump inhibitors block gastric acid secretion by inhibiting gastric H^+/K^+-adenosine triphosphatase in gastric parietal cells. This produces a profound, long-lasting antisecretory effect capable of maintaining the gastric pH >4, even during postprandial acid surges. A correlation exists between the percentage of time the gastric pH remains >4 during the 24-hour period and healing erosive esophagitis.

In general, healing rates at 4 and 8 weeks are similar among proton pump inhibitors. Symptomatic relief is seen in approximately 83% of patients with endoscopic evidence of injury after 8 weeks treated with a proton pump inhibitor, whereas the endoscopic healing rate at 8 weeks is 78%.[4]

Enteric infections, vitamin B_{12} deficiency, hypomagnesemia, and bone fractures are potential long-term adverse effects associated with proton pump inhibitors (Table 19-5).[1,12–18] It is becoming more apparent that overuse of proton pump inhibitors should be minimized as the clinical implications of chronic therapy are better elucidated.

Drug interactions with the proton pump inhibitors vary slightly with each agent. All proton pump inhibitors can decrease the absorption of drugs such as ketoconazole or itraconazole, which require an acidic environment to be absorbed. Pantoprazole is the least likely to have drug interactions because it undergoes cytosolic sulfotransferase metabolism instead of through the cytochrome P450 (CYP) enzyme system. While no interactions with lansoprazole, pantoprazole, or rabeprazole have been seen with CYP2C19 substrates such as diazepam, warfarin, and phenytoin, concerns have been raised regarding the concomitant use of proton pump inhibitors, particularly omeprazole, with clopidogrel since it is the strongest inhibitor of CYP2C19.[19,20] Clopidogrel, a prodrug, is converted to its active metabolite via the CYP2C19 and CYP3A4 enzymes. Inhibition of CYP2C19 by proton pump

TABLE 19-5 Drug Monitoring

Drug	Adverse Drug Reaction	Monitoring Parameter	Comments
Antacids			
• Magnesium hydroxide/aluminum hydroxide • Antacid/alginic acid • Calcium carbonate	• Diarrhea or constipation (depending on product) • Alterations in mineral metabolism • Acid–base disturbances	• Periodic calcium and phosphate levels in patients on chronic therapy	• Use caution with aluminum- and calcium-containing antacids in patients with renal impairment • Aluminum-containing antacids may bind to phosphate in the gut and lead to bone demineralization
H_2-Receptor Antagonists			
• Cimetidine • Famotidine • Nizatidine • Ranitidine	• Headache, somnolence, fatigue, dizziness, and either constipation or diarrhea	• Monitor for CNS effects, especially in the elderly	• May see increased CNS effects (rare) in those over 50 years of age or in those with renal or hepatic dysfunction
Proton Pump Inhibitors			
• Dexlansoprazole • Esomeprazole • Lansoprazole • Omeprazole • Omeprazole/sodium bicarbonate • Pantoprazole • Rabeprazole	*Most common adverse effects*: • Headache, dizziness, somnolence, diarrhea, constipation, flatulence, abdominal pain, and nausea *Other important adverse effects*: • Enteric infections (*C. difficile* infections) • Increased risk of pneumonia *Long-term adverse effects*: • Hypomagnesemia • Bone fractures • Vitamin B_{12} deficiency	• Number and type of diarrhea episodes • Periodic magnesium levels warranted in those on higher doses or who are on therapy for greater than 1 year • Routine bone density studies or calcium supplementation should only be considered if other risk factors for osteoporosis or bone fractures are present[1]	• Acid suppression may result in loss of host defense against ingested spores and bacteria permitting a higher burden of exposure. Recent meta-analysis showed 65% increase in *Clostridium difficile*–associated diarrhea among those on proton pump inhibitors[13] • Hypomagnesemia is uncommon but can be life-threatening • Data related to increased risk of bone fractures are conflicting. Prescription proton pump inhibitors carry an FDA advisory regarding fracture risk in patients on higher doses or those on therapy for greater than 1 year[15,16] • Proton pump inhibitors may inhibit secretion of intrinsic factor, which potentially can lead to vitamin B_{12} deficiency; this is not well documented in literature as a major concern

inhibitors, specifically omeprazole, may decrease the effectiveness of clopidogrel causing cardiovascular adverse events. Careful review of the risk-to-benefit profile regarding the use of proton pump inhibitors for patients on clopidogrel should be considered. Patients with upper GI bleeding or those with multiple risk factors for GI bleeding who require antiplatelet therapy would benefit from proton pump inhibitor therapy. Risk factors for GI bleeding include advanced age, use of anticoagulants, steroids or nonsteroidal anti-inflammatory drugs, presence of *Helicobacter pylori*, or previous history of bleeding or peptic ulcer disease complications.[21] Otherwise, using an alternative agent, such as an H_2-receptor antagonist, may be prudent in this patient population.

Esomeprazole does not appear to interact with warfarin or phenytoin, and an interaction with diazepam is generally not considered clinically relevant. Although generally not a problem, omeprazole has the potential to inhibit the metabolism of warfarin, diazepam, and phenytoin, and lansoprazole may decrease theophylline concentrations. Patients on potentially interacting drugs, such as warfarin, should be monitored closely for potential problems.

The proton pump inhibitors degrade in acidic environments and are therefore formulated in a delayed-release capsule or tablet formulation. Dexlansoprazole, esomeprazole, lansoprazole, and omeprazole contain enteric-coated (pH-sensitive) granules in a capsule form. Dexlansoprazole is unique in that the capsule is a dual delayed-release formulation, with the first release occurring 1 to 2 hours after the dose and the second release occurring 4 to 5 hours after the dose. The clinical significance of this dual release is to allow the drug to have a longer-lasting benefit, at least 16 to 18 hours. Patients taking pantoprazole or rabeprazole should be instructed not to crush, chew, or split the delayed-release tablets.

For patients who are unable to swallow the capsule or for pediatric patients, there are several alternative administration methods available. The contents of the delayed-release capsules can be mixed in applesauce or placed in orange juice. If a patient has a nasogastric tube, the contents of an omeprazole capsule can be mixed in 8.4% sodium bicarbonate solution. Esomeprazole granules can be dispersed in water. Esomeprazole, omeprazole, and pantoprazole are also available in a delayed-release oral suspension powder packet, and lansoprazole is available as a delayed-release, orally disintegrating tablet. Esomeprazole and pantoprazole are available in an IV formulation, which offers an alternative route of administration for patients who are unable to take an oral proton pump inhibitor. Importantly, the IV product is not more efficacious than oral proton pump inhibitors and is significantly more expensive. Careful patient selection is necessary to avoid the increased cost from the use of the IV product.

The newest dosage form of omeprazole is in a delayed-release tablet; it is also available in a combination product with sodium bicarbonate in an immediate-release capsule and oral suspension (Zegerid®). This is the first immediate-release proton pump inhibitor and it should be taken on an empty stomach at least 1 hour before a meal. Zegerid® offers an alternative to the delayed-release capsules, powder for suspension, or IV formulation in adult patients with a nasogastric tube.

Patients should be instructed to take their proton pump inhibitor in the morning, 15 to 30 minutes before breakfast or before their biggest meal of the day, to maximize efficacy, because these agents inhibit only actively secreting proton pumps. Dexlansoprazole can be taken without regards to meals. Patients with nocturnal symptoms may benefit from taking their proton pump inhibitor prior to the evening meal. If dosed twice daily, the second dose should be administered approximately 10 to 12 hours after the morning dose and prior to a meal or snack.

H_2-Receptor Antagonists (Cimetidine, Famotidine, Nizatidine, and Ranitidine) H_2-receptor antagonists in divided doses are effective in treating patients with mild to moderate GERD.[4] The majority of the trials assessing the efficacy of standard doses of H_2-receptor antagonists indicate that symptomatic improvement is achieved in an average of 60% of patients after 12 weeks of therapy.[4] However, endoscopic healing rates tend to be lower, an average of 50% of patients at 12 weeks.[4]

The efficacy of H_2-receptor antagonists in the management of GERD is extremely variable and is frequently lower than desired. Response to the H_2-receptor antagonists is dependent on the (a) severity of disease, (b) dosage regimen used, and (c) duration of therapy. These factors are important to keep in mind when comparing clinical trials and/or assessing a patient's response to therapy. The severity of esophagitis at baseline has a profound impact on the patient's response to H_2-receptor antagonists. For symptomatic relief of mild GERD, low-dose, nonprescription H_2-receptor antagonists or standard doses given twice daily may be beneficial. Patients who do not respond to standard doses may be hypersecreters of gastric acid and will require higher doses. Although higher doses of H_2-receptor antagonists may provide higher symptomatic and endoscopic healing rates, limited information exists regarding the safety of these regimens, and they can be less effective and more costly than once-daily proton pump inhibitors. Unlike duodenal ulcer disease, in which the duration of therapy is relatively short (e.g., 4 to 6 weeks), prolonged courses of H_2-receptor antagonists are frequently required in the treatment of GERD.

Because all of the H_2-receptor antagonists have similar efficacy, selection of the specific agent to use in the management of GERD should be based on factors such as differences in pharmacokinetics, safety profile, and cost. Patients should be monitored for the presence of adverse effects as well as potential drug interactions, especially when on cimetidine. Cimetidine may inhibit the metabolism of theophylline, warfarin, phenytoin, nifedipine, and propranolol, among others. An alternate H_2-receptor antagonist should be selected if the patient is on any of these medications.

Promotility Agents

Promotility agents may be useful as an adjunct to acid-suppression therapy for patients with a known motility defect (e.g., LES incompetence, decreased esophageal clearance, delayed gastric emptying). Unfortunately, all available promotility agents are fraught with undesirable side effects and are not generally as effective as acid-suppression therapy.

Metoclopramide Metoclopramide, a dopamine antagonist, increases LES pressure in a dose-related manner and accelerates gastric emptying in gastroesophageal reflux patients. However, it does not improve esophageal clearance. Metoclopramide provides symptomatic improvement for some patients with GERD; however, substantial data supporting endoscopic healing are lacking. In addition, metoclopramide's adverse-effect profile, including extrapyramidal effects, tardive dyskinesia, tachyphylaxis, and other CNS effects, limits its usefulness in treating many patients with GERD. The risk of adverse effects is much greater for elderly patients and for patients with renal dysfunction because the drug is primarily eliminated by the kidneys. Contraindications include Parkinson's disease, mechanical obstruction, concomitant use of other dopamine antagonists or anticholinergic agents, and pheochromocytoma.

Bethanechol Bethanechol, a promotility drug, has limited value in the treatment of GERD because of unwanted side effects, such as urinary retention, abdominal discomfort, nausea, and flushing. It is not routinely recommended for the treatment of GERD.

Other Promotility Drugs Under Investigation Other promotility drugs under investigation include itopride and baclofen. Because domperidone does not cross the blood–brain barrier, it does not cause the CNS effects seen with metoclopramide. However, it is not currently available in the United States. Baclofen, an gamma aminobutyric acid (GABA) receptor type B agonist, may decrease esophageal acid exposure and the number of reflux episodes by decreasing the number of transient relaxations of the LES. However, this agent has many side effects, limiting its usefulness in GERD. Other GABA type B agonists, as well as metabotropic glutamate type 5 (mGluR5) receptor antagonists, macrolide antibiotics, and cannabinoid agonists, are under development as potential prokinetic agents.[22]

Mucosal Protectants

Sucralfate, a nonabsorbable aluminum salt of sucrose octasulfate, has limited value in the treatment of GERD. It may not be useful in the routine treatment of acid reflux but can be quite useful in the management of radiation esophagitis and bile or nonacid reflux GERD.

Combination Therapy

Combination therapy with an acid-suppression agent and a promotility agent or a mucosal protectant agent would seem logical given the multifactorial nature of the disease, particularly in light of the disappointing results seen with many monotherapy regimens. However, data to support combination therapy are limited, and this approach should not routinely be recommended unless a patient has GERD plus motor dysfunction occurring. The effectiveness of the addition of an H_2-receptor antagonist at bedtime to proton pump inhibitor therapy for the treatment of nocturnal symptoms may decrease over time due to tachyphylaxis with H_2-receptor antagonists. Using the omeprazole–sodium bicarbonate immediate-release product in addition to once-daily proton pump inhibitors may offer an alternative for nocturnal GERD symptoms.

Maintenance Therapy

9 Many patients with GERD will relapse if medication is withdrawn; so long-term maintenance treatment may be required. A proton pump inhibitor is the drug of choice for maintenance of patients with moderate to severe GERD. Both step-up and step-down therapies have been advocated.

Although healing and/or symptomatic improvement may be achieved via many different therapeutic modalities, a large percentage of patients with gastroesophageal reflux will relapse following discontinuation of proton pump inhibitor or H_2-receptor antagonist therapy, especially those with more severe disease. Patients who have symptomatic relapse following discontinuation of therapy or lowering of drug doses, including patients with complications such as Barrett's esophagus, strictures, or esophagitis, should be considered for long-term maintenance therapy to prevent complications or worsening of esophageal function.[4] The goal of maintenance therapy is to improve quality of life by controlling the patient's symptoms and preventing complications. These goals cannot generally be achieved by decreasing the dose of the therapeutic modality used for initial healing or switching to a less potent acid-suppression agent. Most patients will require standard doses to prevent relapses. Patients should be counseled on the importance of complying with lifestyle changes and long-term maintenance therapy in order to prevent recurrence or worsening of disease.[4]

H_2-receptor antagonists may be effective maintenance therapy for patients with mild disease.[4] The proton pump inhibitors are the drugs of choice for maintenance treatment of moderate to severe esophagitis or symptoms. Low doses of a proton pump inhibitor or alternate-day dosing may be effective in some patients with mild symptoms, thereby allowing titration in some cases. "On-demand" maintenance therapy, by which patients take their proton pump inhibitor only when they have symptoms, may be effective for patients with endoscopy-negative GERD.[4] Although not well studied, many patients with only mild to moderate symptoms may decide on their own to take their medication this way for the financial benefit. However, patients with persistent symptoms and/or complications should be maintained on standard doses of proton pump inhibitors.

Long-term chronic use of proton pump inhibitor doses higher than standard treatment doses is not indicated unless the patient has complicated symptoms, has erosive esophagitis per endoscopy, or has had further diagnostic evaluation to determine the level of acid exposure. Metoclopramide is not approved for maintenance therapy, and its use is limited by adverse-effect profile. Antireflux surgery may also be considered a viable alternative to long-term drug therapy for maintenance of healing for patients who are candidates.

Maintenance Therapy with H_2-Receptor Antagonists The studies evaluating the efficacy of the H_2-receptor antagonists in maintaining GERD patients in remission have been disappointing. Currently, ranitidine 150 mg twice daily is the only H_2-receptor antagonist regimen that is FDA approved for maintenance of healing of erosive esophagitis.

Maintenance Therapy with Proton Pump Inhibitors Long-term use of the proton pump inhibitors is associated with adverse effects such as hypomagnesemia, enteric infections, and risk for bone fractures; however, there is no evidence of carcinoid tumors directly linked to their use. Prolonged hypergastrinemia leading to the development of colonic polyps, and potentially adenocarcinoma, was also a concern that has proven unfounded with long-term use. However, the role of *H. pylori* status for patients with GERD has been questioned. As a consequence of the controversy surrounding *H. pylori* and GERD, specific guidelines on how to handle patients who are *H. pylori* positive are lacking. Most clinicians would probably opt to eradicate *H. pylori* infections once detected. Further studies are needed to determine the role of *H. pylori* for patients with GERD.

Special Populations

There are several special populations that should be considered when discussing GERD, such as patients with atypical symptoms, pediatric patients, elderly patients, and patients with refractory symptoms.

Patients with Extraesophageal (Atypical) GERD

Patients presenting with atypical symptoms may require higher doses and longer treatment courses as compared with patients with typical symptoms. Patients with suspected reflux chest pain syndrome may benefit from an empiric course of twice-daily proton pump inhibitor therapy for 4 weeks once cardiac workup is known to be negative.[1] If symptoms continue, patients should be evaluated with manometry, ambulatory pH, or impedance–pH monitoring to rule out dysmotility or refractory symptoms.[1] Because there are many causes of asthma and laryngeal symptoms, a concomitant esophageal GERD syndrome must also be present to associate these symptoms with GERD. In practice, these patients may benefit from twice-daily proton pump inhibitor for 3 to 4 months even though evidence supporting this regimen is not well established.[1] This recommendation is based more on pH monitoring data showing normalization of gastric pH with twice-daily dosing.[1] For patients not responding to empiric therapy, pH monitoring may be beneficial in determining acid exposure as it relates to symptoms. The optimal dose of proton pump inhibition is not well defined. Maintenance therapy is generally indicated for patients who respond to the therapeutic trial or have endoscopic evidence of reflux. Antireflux surgery may be an option in select patients.

Pediatric Patients with GERD

Many infants have physiologic reflux with little or no clinical consequence. Uncomplicated gastroesophageal reflux usually manifests as regurgitation or "spitting up" and resolves without incident by 12 to 14 months of life.[6] It usually responds to supportive therapy, including dietary adjustments, postural management, and reassurance for the parents. Thickened feedings may be useful in milder cases. While this does not decrease the time the pH is <4, it may decrease the incidence of regurgitation.[6] Chronic vomiting associated with gastroesophageal reflux must be distinguished from other causes, such as neurologic, metabolic, eating, and rumination disorders. Smaller, more frequent feedings may be beneficial. In formula-fed infants, an extensively hydrolyzed protein may help identify milk protein sensitivity as the cause of unexplained vomiting and crying.[6] Developmental immaturity of the LES is one suspected cause of gastroesophageal reflux in infants.[6] Like adults, transient LES relaxations seem to be the most common cause of gastroesophageal reflux in children. Other causes include impaired luminal clearance of gastric acid, neurologic impairment, and type of infant formula. Complications, although rare, include distal esophagitis, failure to thrive, esophageal peptic strictures, Barrett's esophagus, and pulmonary disease. Further diagnostic evaluation is indicated in all who experience apnea or an apparent life-threatening event.

Clinical **Controversy...**

While the use of proton pump inhibitors in children has increased, there are little safety data in premature infants. Many feel that the proton pump inhibitors are overused in this population.

The benefits of using promotility medications, such as metoclopramide, erythromycin, bethanechol, and baclofen, are outweighed by the potential adverse effects that may occur and, therefore, cannot be routinely recommended.[6] Careful consideration should be made before medication is recommended, especially in children less than 1 year of age. Overprescribing of acid-suppression therapy may lead to increased risk of infection and other adverse effects in premature infants.[23,24] When medication is deemed necessary, ranitidine is commonly used at a dose of 2 to 4 mg/kg twice daily.[6] Tachyphylaxis may develop making the effectiveness of H_2-receptor antagonists less than optimal. The use of proton pump inhibitor use in children is increasing, especially in those with esophagitis. Most patients will respond to once-daily proton pump inhibitor dosing. Lansoprazole, esomeprazole, and omeprazole are indicated for treating symptomatic and erosive GERD for pediatric patients older than age 1 year. Lansoprazole 15 mg once daily is recommended for children who weigh 30 kg or less, and a dose of 30 mg once daily is recommended for those who weigh more than 30 kg. Esomeprazole may be dosed 10 to 20 mg daily for children 1 to 11 years old and 20 to 40 mg daily for children 12 to 17 years old. Omeprazole 5 mg daily may be used in children weighing between 5 and 10 kg, 10 mg for children weighing between 10 and 20 kg, and 20 mg daily for children weighing >20 kg. Omeprazole has been used off-label for children less than 1 year of age at a dose of 1 mg/kg/day. Long-term use of a proton pump inhibitor without a clear diagnosis of GERD is not recommended.[6]

Elderly Patients with GERD

Many elderly patients have decreased host defense mechanisms, such as saliva production. In addition, they have more comorbidities, medications, and physiologic changes that put them at higher risk. More aggressive therapy with a proton pump inhibitor may be warranted for patients older than 60 years of age with symptomatic GERD. Often these patients do not seek medical attention because they feel their symptoms are part of the normal aging process. They may also present with atypical symptoms such as chest pain, asthma, poor dentition, or jaw pain. Decreased GI motility is a common problem in elderly patients. Unfortunately, there are no good promotility agents available to these patients. Elderly patients are especially sensitive to the CNS effects of metoclopramide. They may also be sensitive to the CNS effects of H_2-receptor antagonists. Proton pump inhibitors appear to be the most useful treatment modality because they have superior efficacy and are dosed once daily, which is beneficial in all patients, but is especially beneficial in the elderly. Long-term risk of bone fractures may be of concern in this population. Patients at risk for bone fractures should be monitored appropriately.

Patients with Refractory GERD

What constitutes refractory GERD is not well defined. It should be considered in patients who have not responded to a standard course of twice-daily proton pump inhibitor therapy.[1] In this case, other causes for the patient's symptoms should be evaluated. The majority of patients with refractory symptoms experience nocturnal acid breakthrough. Other reasons for refractory symptoms may be related to compliance, timing of proton pump inhibitor, and drug metabolism differences in certain patients. Switching to another proton pump inhibitor may be effective for refractory symptoms in some patients. Manometry or ambulatory pH monitoring is useful for patients who are not responding to therapy with normal endoscopic findings. Adding an H_2-receptor antagonist at bedtime for nocturnal symptoms has been suggested; however, the effect may be short-lived. Antireflux surgery may also be considered in this patient population. Eosinophilic esophagitis or dysmotility syndromes may be causes of nonacid-related esophageal symptoms.[25]

PERSONALIZED PHARMACOTHERAPY

Significant liver impairment may result in a sevenfold to ninefold increase in area under the curve and increase half-life of proton pump inhibitors. While clear recommendations are not available, it may be prudent to consider a lower dose in this population.

The hepatic enzyme CYP2C19 is involved in the metabolism of many medications, including proton pump inhibitors, particularly omeprazole. Further evaluation is needed to determine the role of polymorphic gene variation in the hepatic activity of CYP2C19.

Drug interactions with omeprazole are of particular concern for patients who are considered "slow metabolizers" of omeprazole, which is more common in the Asian population but also found in approximately 3% of the white population. Unfortunately, it is unclear which patients have the polymorphic gene variation that makes them slow metabolizers. Like omeprazole, the metabolism of esomeprazole may also be altered for patients with this polymorphic gene variation.

EVALUATION OF THERAPEUTIC OUTCOMES

The long-term benefits of treatment are difficult to assess because of the limited information known about the epidemiology and natural history of GERD. Consequently, successful outcomes are generally measured in terms of three separate end points: (a) relieving symptoms, (b) healing the injured mucosa, and (c) preventing complications.

The short-term goal of therapy is to relieve symptoms such as heartburn and regurgitation to the point at which they do not impair the patient's quality of life. Patients should be educated regarding specific lifestyle modifications that are applicable to their individual situation including weight loss, raising the head end of the bed, smoking cessation, eating smaller meals, and avoiding eating prior to bedtime. Patients should also be instructed to avoid or limit foods that aggravate GERD symptoms, such as fat and chocolate. **10** In addition, patient medication profiles should be reviewed for drugs that may aggravate GERD. Patients should be monitored for adverse drug reactions. Table 19-5 reviews common adverse drug reactions and monitoring of medications used in GERD. Drug–drug interactions should also be assessed and these agents should be avoided if possible. Table 19-6 lists recommendations for providing pharmaceutical care to patients with GERD.

The frequency and severity of symptoms should be monitored, and patients should be counseled on symptoms that suggest the presence of complications requiring immediate medical attention, such as dysphagia or odynophagia. Patients should also be monitored for the presence of atypical symptoms such as laryngitis asthma or chest pain. These symptoms require further diagnostic evaluation. Long-term maintenance treatment is indicated for patients who have strictures because the strictures commonly recur if reflux esophagitis is not treated.

The second goal is to heal the injured mucosa. Again, individualized lifestyle modifications and the importance of complying with the therapeutic regimen chosen to heal the mucosa should be stressed. Patients should be educated about the risk of relapse and the need for long-term maintenance therapy to prevent recurrence or complications.

The final, long-term goal of therapy is to decrease the risk of complications (esophagitis, strictures, Barrett's esophagus, and esophageal adenocarcinoma). A small subset of patients may continue to fail treatment despite therapy with high doses of H_2-receptor antagonists or a proton pump inhibitor. Patients should be monitored for the presence of continual pain, dysphagia, or odynophagia.

TABLE 19-6 Recommendations for Providing Pharmaceutical Care to Patients with GERD

1. Assess the patient's symptoms to determine if patient-directed therapy is appropriate or whether patient should be evaluated by a clinician. Determine the type of symptoms, frequency, and exacerbating factors. Refer any patient with alarm or atypical symptoms to a clinician for further diagnostic workup
2. Obtain a thorough history of prescription, nonprescription, and natural drug product use
3. Counsel the patient on lifestyle modifications that will improve symptoms
4. Recommend appropriate drug therapy based on patient presentation
5. Develop a plan to assess effectiveness of acid-suppression therapy after an appropriate amount of time (8–16 weeks). Recommend alternative therapy if necessary
6. Assess improvement in quality-of-life measures such as physical, psychological, and social functioning and well-being
7. Evaluate patient for the presence of adverse drug reactions, allergies, and drug interactions
8. Stress the importance of compliance with the therapeutic regimen, including lifestyle modifications. Recommend a therapeutic regimen that is easy for the patient to accomplish
9. Provide patient education with regard to disease state, lifestyle modifications, and drug therapy. Patients should be counseled on:
   - What causes GERD and what things to avoid
   - When to take their medications
   - What potential adverse effects or drug interactions may occur
   - What alarm signs they should report to their clinician

ABBREVIATIONS

CYP	cytochrome P450
GABA	gamma aminobutyric acid
GERD	gastroesophageal reflux disease
H_2	histamine-2
HREPT	high-resolution esophageal pressure topography
LES	lower esophageal sphincter
mGluR5	metabotropic glutamate type 5

REFERENCES

1. The American Gastroenterological Association (AGA) Institute Medical Position Panel. American gastroenterological association medical position statement on the management of gastroesophageal reflux disease. Gastroenterology 2008;135:1383–1391.
2. Kahrilas PJ. Gastroesophageal reflux disease. N Engl J Med 2008;359:1700–1707.
3. Dent J, El-Serag HB, Wallander MA, Johansson S. Epidemiology of gastro-oesophageal reflux disease: A systematic review. Gut 2005;54:710–717.
4. DeVault KR, Castell DO. Updated guidelines for the diagnosis and treatment of gastroesophageal reflux disease. Am J Gastroenterol 2005;100:190–200.
5. DeVault KR. Review article: The role of acid suppression in patients with non-erosive reflux disease or functional heartburn. Aliment Pharmacol Ther 2006;23(Suppl 1):33–39.
6. Vandenplas Y, Rudolph CD, Di Lorenzo C, et al. Pediatric gastroesophageal reflux clinical practice guidelines: Joint recommendations of the North American Society for Pediatric Gastroenterology, Hepatology, and Nutrition (NASPGHAN) and the European Society for Pediatric Gastroenterology, Hepatology, and Nutrition (ESPGHAN). J Pediatr Gastroenterol Nutr 2009;49:498–547.
7. Hirano I. Review article: Modern technology in the diagnosis of gastrooesophageal reflux disease—Bilitec, intraluminal impedance and Bravo capsule pH monitoring. Aliment Pharmacol Ther 2006;23(Suppl 1):12–24.
8. Hvid-Jensen F, Pedersen L, Drewes AM, et al. Incidence of adenocarcinoma among patients with Barrett's esophagus. N Engl J Med 2011;365:1375–1383.
9. Liu JJ, Carr-Lock DL, Osterman MT, et al. Endoscopic treatment for atypical manifestations of gastroesophageal reflux disease. Am J Gastroenterol 2006;101:440–445.
10. Pandolfino JE, El-Serag HB, Zhang Q, et al. Obesity: A challenge to esophagogastric junction integrity. Gastroenterology 2006;130:639–649.
11. Lundell L, Miettinen P, Myrvold E, et al. Seven-year follow-up of a randomized clinical trial comparing proton-pump inhibition with surgical therapy for reflux oesophagitis. Br J Surg 2007;94:198–203.
12. Aseeri M, Schroeder T, Kramer J, Zackula R. Gastric acid suppression by proton pump inhibitors as a risk factor for *Clostridium difficile*-associated diarrhea in hospitalized patients. Am J Gastroenterol 2008;103:2308–2313.
13. Janarthanan S, Ditah I, Phil M, et al. *Clostridium difficile*-associated diarrhea and proton pump inhibitor therapy: A meta-analysis. Am J Gastroenterol 2012;107:1001–1010.
14. Thomson ABR, Sauve MD, Kassam N, Kamitakahara H. Safety of the long-term use of proton pump inhibitors. World J Gastroenterol 2010;16(19):2323–2330.
15. FDA Drug Safety Communication: Possible Increased Risk of Fractures of the Hip, Wrist, and Spine with the Use of Proton Pump Inhibitors. 2010, *www.fda.gov*.
16. FDA Drug Safety Communication: Possible Increased Risk of Fractures of the Hip, Wrist, and Spine with the Use of Proton Pump Inhibitors. Update. 2011, *www.fda.gov*.
17. Ngamruengphong S, Leontiadis GI, Radhi S, et al. Proton pump inhibitors and risk of fracture: A systematic review and meta-analysis of observational studies. Am J Gastroenterol 2011;106:1209–1218.
18. Corley DA, Kubo A, Zhao W, Quesenberry C. Proton pump inhibitors and histamine-2 receptor antagonists are associated with hip fractures among at-risk patients. Gastroenterology 2010;139:93–101.
19. Ho MP, Maddox TM, Wang L, et al. Risk of adverse outcomes associated with concomitant use of clopidogrel and proton pump inhibitors following acute coronary syndrome. JAMA 2009;301:937–944.
20. Laine L, Henneken SC. Proton pump inhibitor and clopidogrel interaction: Fact or fiction? Am J Gastroenterol 2010;105:34–41.
21. Abraham NS, Hlatky MA, Antman EM, et al. ACCF/ACG/AHA 2010 expert consensus document on the concomitant use of proton pump inhibitors and thienopyridines: A focused update of the ACCF/ACG/AHA 2008 expert consensus document on reducing the gastrointestinal risks of antiplatelet therapy and NSAID use: A report of the American College of Cardiology Foundation Task Force on Expert Consensus Documents. Circulation 2010;122: 2619–2633.
22. Kuo P, Holloway RH. Beyond acid suppression: New pharmacologic approaches for treatment of GERD. Curr Gastroenterol Rep 2010;12:175–180.
23. Hassall E. Over-prescription of acid-suppressing medications in infants: How it came about, why it's wrong, and what to do about it. J Pediatr 2012;160(2):193–198.
24. Terrin G, Passariello A, De Curtis M, et al. Ranitidine is associated with infections, necrotizing enterocolitis, and fatal outcome in newborns. Pediatrics 2012;129:e40–e45.
25. Dellon ES, Shaheen NJ. Persistent reflux symptoms in the proton pump inhibitor era: The changing face of gastroesophageal reflux disease. Gastroenterology 2010;139:7–13.

20

Peptic Ulcer Disease

Bryan L. Love and Matthew N. Thoma

KEY CONCEPTS

1. Patients with peptic ulcer disease (PUD) should reduce psychological stress, cigarette smoking, and nonsteroidal antiinflammatory drug (NSAID) use and avoid foods and beverages that exacerbate ulcer symptoms.
2. Eradication is recommended for all *Helicobacter pylori*–positive patients, especially those patients with an active ulcer, a documented history of a prior ulcer, or a history of ulcer-related complications.
3. The selection of an *H. pylori* eradication regimen should be based on efficacy, safety, antibiotic resistance, cost, and the likelihood of medication adherence. Treatment should be initiated with a proton pump inhibitor (PPI)–based three-drug regimen. If a second course of *H. pylori* therapy is required, the regimen should contain different antibiotics.
4. PPI cotherapy reduces the risk of NSAID-related gastric and duodenal ulcers and is at least as effective as recommended dosages of misoprostol and superior to the histamine-2 receptor antagonists (H_2RAs).
5. Standard PPI dosages and a nonselective NSAID are as effective as a selective cyclooxygenase-2 (COX-2) inhibitor in reducing the risk of NSAID-induced ulcers and upper GI complications.
6. Patients with PUD, especially those receiving *H. pylori* eradication or misoprostol cotherapy, require patient education regarding their disease and drug treatment to successfully achieve a positive therapeutic outcome.
7. The recommended treatment for severe peptic ulcer bleeding after appropriate endoscopic treatment is the IV administration of a PPI loading dose followed by a 72-hour continuous infusion with a goal of maintaining an intragastric pH of 6 or greater.
8. Critically ill patients at the highest risk of developing stress-related mucosal bleeding (SRMB) who require prophylactic drug therapy include those with respiratory failure on mechanical ventilation or those with coagulopathy.
9. There are limited data to support the selection of a PPI over an IV H_2RA for SRMB prophylaxis. The decision should be based on appropriate individual patient characteristics (e.g., nothing by mouth, presence of nasogastric tube, renal failure).

PEPTIC ULCER DISEASE

Acid-related diseases (gastritis, erosions, and peptic ulcer) of the upper GI tract require gastric acid for their formation.[1–3] Peptic ulcer disease (PUD) differs from gastritis and erosions in that ulcers typically extend deeper into the muscularis mucosa.[1] There are three common forms of peptic ulcers: *Helicobacter pylori* positive, nonsteroidal antiinflammatory drug (NSAID) induced, and stress ulcers (Table 20-1). The term *stress-related mucosal damage* (SRMD) is preferred to stress ulcer or stress gastritis, because the mucosal lesions range from superficial gastritis and erosions to deep ulcers.

H. pylori–positive and NSAID-induced ulcers are chronic peptic ulcers that differ in etiology, clinical presentation, and tendency to recur (see Table 20-1). These ulcers develop most often in the stomach and duodenum of ambulatory patients (Fig. 20-1). Occasionally, ulcers develop in the esophagus, jejunum, ileum, or colon. The natural course of chronic PUD is characterized by frequent ulcer recurrence. The most important factors that influence ulcer recurrence are *H. pylori* infection and NSAID use. Other factors include cigarette smoking, alcohol use, ulcer-related complications, gastric acid hypersecretion, and patient noncompliance. The cause of ulcer recurrence is most likely multifactorial.

Peptic ulcers are also associated with Zollinger-Ellison syndrome (ZES), radiation, chemotherapy, vascular insufficiency, and other chronic diseases (Table 20-2).[1,3] Although a strong association exists between chronic pulmonary diseases, chronic renal failure, and cirrhosis, the pathophysiologic mechanisms of these associations remain unclear.[1] In contrast, SRMD occurs primarily in the stomach in critically ill patients (see Table 20-1).[1]

This chapter focuses on chronic PUD associated with *H. pylori* and NSAIDs. A brief discussion of ZES and upper GI bleeding related to PUD and SRMD is included.

EPIDEMIOLOGY

The epidemiology of PUD is complicated and difficult to estimate given the variability in the prevalence of *H. pylori* infection, NSAID use, and cigarette smoking as well as the various methods used to detect ulcers, for example, endoscopy, radiology, symptoms, or complications.[1,4] The prevalence and incidence of PUD in the United States also reflects improvements in drug therapy, the dramatic shift to ambulatory management, and changes in the criteria and coding system for mortality and hospitalization data.[1] Recent trends suggest a shift from predominance in men to a similar occurrence in men and women with increasing rates of disease in older individuals and a decrease in the younger population.[1,4] Despite a modest decline in mortality, hospitalizations, and office visits, PUD remains one of the most common GI diseases, resulting in impaired quality of life, work loss, and high-cost medical care.

TABLE 20-1 Comparison of Common Forms of Peptic Ulcer

Characteristic	*H. pylori* Induced	NSAID Induced	SRMD
Condition	Chronic	Chronic	Acute
Site of damage	Duodenum > stomach	Stomach > duodenum	Stomach > duodenum
Intragastric pH	More dependent	Less dependent	Less dependent
Symptoms	Usually epigastric pain	Often asymptomatic	Asymptomatic
Ulcer depth	Superficial	Deep	Most superficial
GI bleeding	Less severe, single vessel	More severe, single vessel	More severe, superficial mucosal capillaries

NSAID, nonsteroidal antiinflammatory drug; SRMD, stress-related mucosal damage.

ETIOLOGY AND RISK FACTORS

Most peptic ulcers occur in the presence of acid and pepsin when *H. pylori*, NSAIDs, or other factors (see Table 20-2) disrupt the normal mucosal defense and healing mechanisms.[1] Hypersecretion of acid is the primary pathogenic mechanism in hypersecretory states such as ZES.[3] Benign gastric ulcers can occur anywhere in the stomach, although most are located on the lesser curvature, just distal to the junction of the antral and acid-secreting mucosa (see Fig. 20-1). Most duodenal ulcers occur in the first part of the duodenum (duodenal bulb).

H. pylori

H. pylori infection causes chronic gastritis in infected individuals and is causally linked to PUD, mucosa-associated lymphoid tissue (MALT) lymphoma, and gastric cancer (Fig. 20-2).[1,2,5–8] The majority of infected individuals remain asymptomatic, but 10% to 20% will develop PUD during their lifetime and about 1% will develop gastric cancer.[1,2,8] Host-specific cofactors and *H. pylori* strain variability play an important role in the pathogenesis of PUD and gastric cancer.[2,8] Although an association between *H. pylori* and PUD bleeding is less clear, there is evidence that eradication of *H. pylori* decreases recurrent bleeding.[5,9] No specific link has been established between *H. pylori* and dyspepsia, nonulcer dyspepsia (NUD), or gastroesophageal reflux disease (GERD).[5,9–11] However, some patients with dyspepsia and NUD may have symptom improvement from *H. pylori* eradication.[5,9] Although eradication of *H. pylori* may worsen GERD symptoms in some patients, eradication should not be withheld.[5,10] An association between *H. pylori* infection and iron deficiency anemia has been established, but cause and effect have not been proven, and whether *H. pylori* eradication is beneficial is uncertain.[5,11] There are insufficient data to support a link between

TABLE 20-2 Potential Causes of Peptic Ulcer

Common causes
- *Helicobacter pylori* infection
- Nonsteroidal antiinflammatory drugs
- Critical illness (stress-related mucosal damage)

Uncommon causes of chronic peptic ulcer
- Idiopathic (non–*H. pylori*, non-NSAID peptic ulcer)
- Hypersecretion of gastric acid (e.g., Zollinger-Ellison syndrome)
- Viral infections (e.g., cytomegalovirus)
- Vascular insufficiency (e.g., crack cocaine associated)
- Radiation therapy
- Chemotherapy (e.g., hepatic artery infusions)
- Infiltrating disease (e.g., Crohn's disease)

Diseases and medical conditions associated with chronic peptic ulcer
- Cirrhosis
- Chronic renal failure
- Chronic obstructive pulmonary disease
- Cardiovascular disease
- Organ transplantation

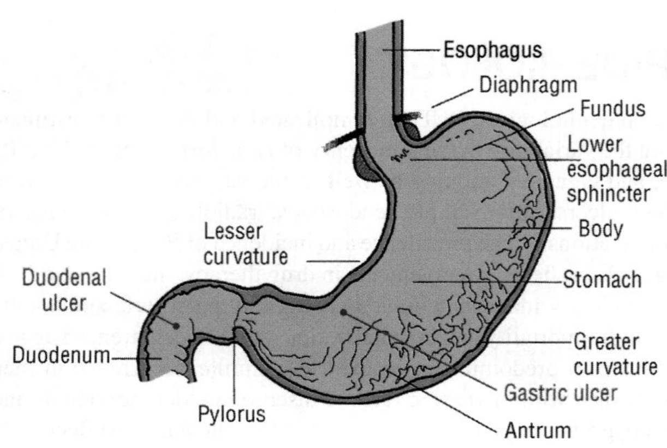

FIGURE 20-1 Anatomic structure of the stomach and duodenum and most common locations of gastric and duodenal ulcers.

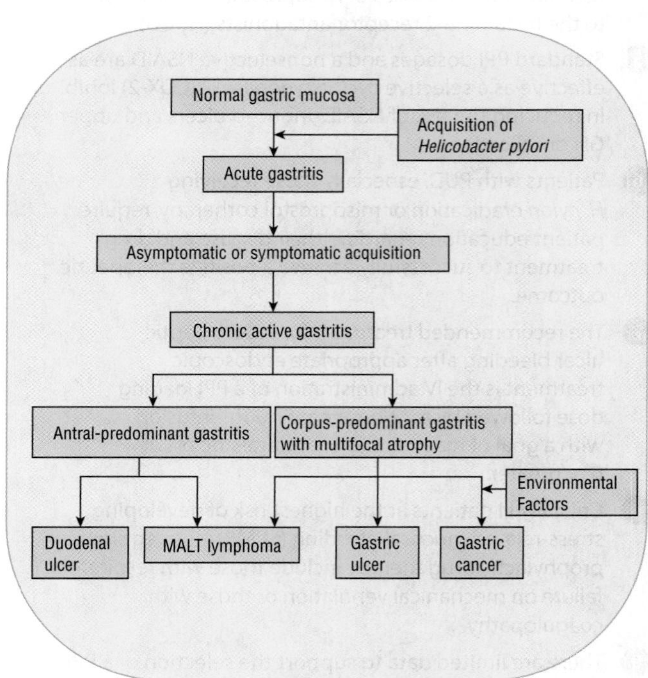

FIGURE 20-2 The natural history of *Helicobacter pylori* infection in the pathogenesis of gastric ulcer and duodenal ulcer, mucosa-associated lymphoid tissue (MALT) lymphoma, and gastric cancer.

TABLE 20-3 Selected Nonsteroidal Antiinflammatory Drugs (NSAIDs) and Cyclooxygenase-2 (COX-2) Inhibitors

Nonsalicylates[a]
- Nonselective (traditional) NSAIDs: indomethacin, piroxicam, ibuprofen, naproxen, sulindac, ketoprofen, ketorolac, flurbiprofen
- Partially selective NSAIDs: etodolac, nabumetone, meloxicam, diclofenac, celecoxib
- Selective COX-2 inhibitors: rofecoxib,[b] valdecoxib[b]

Salicylates
- Acetylated: aspirin
- Nonacetylated: salsalate, trisalicylate

[a]Based on COX-1-to-COX-2 selectivity ratio.
[b]Withdrawn from U.S. market.

H. pylori and extragastric manifestations including cardiovascular, hematologic, respiratory, hepatobiliary, and neurologic diseases.[5,11]

The prevalence of *H. pylori* varies by geographic location, socioeconomic conditions, ethnicity, and age. In developing countries, *H. pylori* prevalence is more common than in industrialized countries and correlates with lower socioeconomic levels.[2,5,6] The prevalence of *H. pylori* in the United States is 30% to 40% but is much higher in individuals over 60 years (50% to 60%) than in children under 12 years (10% to 15%) of age.[2,5] Although most individuals in the United States acquire *H. pylori* in childhood, the rate of acquisition in children is declining and most likely will continue to fall as a consequence of improved socioeconomic conditions.[2] Whites are infected with *H. pylori* less frequently than African Americans and Hispanic persons, but this is thought to be related to lower socioecomonic status and living conditions. Infection rates do not differ with gender or smoking status.

The most common route of *H. pylori* transmission is person to person by either gastro–oral (vomitus) or fecal–oral (diarrhea) contact that occurs primarily during childhood.[2] Members of the same household are likely to become infected when someone in the same household is infected.[2] *H. pylori* can also be transmitted by the use of inadequately sterilized endoscopes.

Nonsteroidal Antiinflammatory Drugs

NSAIDs (Table 20-3), including both prescription and nonprescription medications, are widely used in the United States, particularly in individuals over 60 years of age, to treat chronic pain and inflammation.[1] Low-dose aspirin is used for cardiovascular and cerebrovascular risk reduction.[1,12–14] There is overwhelming evidence linking chronic NSAID (including aspirin) use to a variety of upper GI tract injuries.[1,12–16] NSAIDs cause superficial (topical) mucosal damage consisting of petechiae (intramucosal hemorrhages) within minutes of ingestion, and progress to erosions with continued use.[1] These lesions typically heal within a few days and rarely cause ulcers or acute upper GI bleeding. Gastroduodenal ulcers develop in about 25% of chronic NSAID users with continued use.[12] Gastric ulcers are most common, occur primarily in the antrum, and are of greater concern because of their potential to cause ulcer-related upper GI complications (see Table 20-1). As many as 2% to 4% of patients with an NSAID ulcer will bleed or perforate.[12] Each year, NSAIDs account for at least 100,000 hospitalizations and between 7,000 and 10,000 deaths in the United States.[12] NSAID-induced ulcers occur less frequently in the esophagus, small bowel, and colon.[16,17] How NSAIDs damage the lower GI tract is unclear, but the enteropathy is associated with lower GI bleeding.

Table 20-4 lists the risk factors associated with NSAID-induced ulcers and upper GI complications. Combinations of factors confer an additive risk.[12–16,18] Advanced age is an independent risk factor, and the incidence of NSAID-induced ulcers increases linearly with

TABLE 20-4 Risk Factors Associated with Nonsteroidal Antiinflammatory Drug (NSAID)–Induced Ulcers and Upper GI Complications[a]

Age >65
Previous peptic ulcer
Previous ulcer-related upper GI complication
High-dose NSAIDs
Multiple NSAID use
Selection of NSAID (e.g., COX-1 vs. COX-2 inhibition)
NSAID-related dyspepsia
Aspirin (including cardioprotective dosages)
Concomitant use of
- NSAID plus low-dose aspirin
- Oral bisphosphonates (e.g., alendronate)
- Corticosteroids
- Anticoagulant or coagulopathy
- Antiplatelet drugs (e.g., clopidogrel)
- Selective serotonin reuptake inhibitor

Chronic debilitating disorders (e.g., cardiovascular disease, rheumatoid arthritis)
Helicobacter pylori infection
Cigarette smoking
Alcohol consumption

[a]Combinations of risk factors are additive.
Data from references 1, 12–15, 20, and 29.

the age of the patient.[1] The high incidence of ulcer complications in older individuals may be explained by age-related changes in gastric mucosal defense. The relative risk of NSAID complications is increased for patients with a previous peptic ulcer and may be as high as 14-fold in those with a history of an ulcer-related complication.[1,16] Although the risk of ulcer complications is greatest during the first few months after initiating continuous NSAID therapy, it does not vanish with long-term treatment.[12]

NSAID ulcers and related complications are dose dependent, but may occur with low doses of nonprescription NSAIDs and low cardioprotective dosages of aspirin (81 to 325 mg/day).[1,12–16] Factors such as NSAID potency, longer duration of effect, and a greater propensity to inhibit cyclooxygenase-1 (COX-1) versus cyclooxygenase-2 (COX-2) isoenzymes are associated with increased risk (see Table 20-3).[1,16,18,19] NSAID-related dyspepsia, in itself, does not correlate directly with mucosal injury or clinical events. However, new-onset dyspepsia, changes in severity, or dyspepsia not relieved by antiulcer medications may suggest an ulcer or ulcer complication.[1] Nonacetylated salicylates (e.g., salsalate) may be associated with decreased GI toxicity.[1] Buffered or enteric-coated aspirin confers no added protection from upper GI events.[13]

NSAID ulcer and GI complication risk are increased with the use of multiple NSAIDs or the concomitant use of low-dose aspirin, oral bisphosphonates, corticosteroids, anticoagulants, antiplatelet drugs, and selective serotonin reuptake inhibitors.[1,12–16,20] The risk of an ulcer-related GI complication is greater when an NSAID or COX-2 inhibitor (see Table 20-3) is coadministered with low-dose aspirin than when either drug is taken alone.[1,13,16] The NSAID may also reduce the antiplatelet effects of aspirin, although NSAIDs vary in their effects on platelet function.[13–15] Corticosteroids, when used alone, do not potentiate the risk of ulcer or complications, but the relative risk is increased twofold in corticosteroid users who are also taking concurrent NSAIDs.[1,16] The relative risk of GI bleeding increases up to 20-fold when NSAIDs are taken concomitantly with anticoagulants (e.g., warfarin) and up to 6-fold with the concurrent use of serotonin reuptake inhibitors.[16,17] When clopidogrel is taken in combination with aspirin, an NSAID, or an anticoagulant, the risk of GI bleeding is increased compared with when these agents are taken alone.[13,15,16] Even when prescribed as monotherapy, clopidogrel increases the risk of rebleeding for patients with a history of a bleeding ulcer.[13,15,16]

H. pylori and NSAIDs act independently to increase ulcer risk and ulcer-related bleeding and appear to have additive effects.[5,16] Thus, the incidence of peptic ulcer is higher in *H. pylori*–positive NSAID users. Whether *H. pylori* infection is actually a risk factor for NSAID ulcers remains controversial.[1,5,16] However, eradication is reported to reduce the incidence of peptic ulcer if undertaken prior to starting the NSAID but does not reduce the risk for patients who were previously taking an NSAID.[1,5,16]

Cigarette Smoking

Epidemiologic evidence links cigarette smoking to PUD, but it is uncertain whether smoking causes peptic ulcers.[1] Ulcer risk is proportional to the number of cigarettes smoked and is modest when fewer than 10 cigarettes are smoked per day. Cigarette smoking impairs ulcer healing, promotes ulcer recurrence, and increases ulcer risk.[1] The exact mechanism by which cigarette smoking contributes to PUD remains unclear. Possible mechanisms include mucosal ischemia, inhibition of pancreatic bicarbonate secretion, and increases in gastric acid secretion, but these effects are inconsistent. Whether nicotine or other components of smoke are responsible for these physiologic alterations is unknown.

Psychological Stress

The importance of psychological factors in the pathogenesis of PUD remains controversial.[1] Clinical observation suggests that ulcer patients are adversely affected by stressful life events. However, results from controlled trials are conflicting and have failed to document a cause-and-effect relationship.[1] Emotional stress may induce behavioral risks such as smoking and the use of NSAIDs or alter the inflammatory response or resistance to *H. pylori* infection. The role of stress and how it affects PUD is complex and probably multifactorial.

Dietary Factors

The role of diet and nutrition in PUD is uncertain.[1] Coffee, tea, carbonated beverages, beer, milk, and spices may cause dyspepsia but do not increase the risk for PUD. Beverage restrictions and bland diets do not alter the frequency of ulcer recurrence. Although caffeine is a gastric acid stimulant, constituents in decaffeinated coffee or tea, caffeine-free carbonated beverages, beer, and wine may also increase gastric acid secretion. In high concentrations, alcohol ingestion is associated with acute gastric mucosal damage and upper GI bleeding; however, there is insufficient evidence to confirm that alcohol causes ulcers.[1]

PATHOPHYSIOLOGY

A physiologic imbalance between aggressive (gastric acid and pepsin) and protective (mucosal defense and repair) factors remains an important issue in the pathophysiology of gastric and duodenal ulcers.[1,21] Gastric acid is secreted by the parietal cells, which contain receptors for histamine, gastrin, and acetylcholine.[21] Acid (as well as *H. pylori* infection and NSAID use) is an independent factor that contributes to the disruption of mucosal integrity.[1] Increased acid secretion has been observed for patients with duodenal ulcers and may be a consequence of *H. pylori* infection.[2,22] Patients with ZES (described in Zollinger-Ellison Syndrome below) have profound gastric acid hypersecretion resulting from a gastrin-producing tumor.[3] In contrast, patients with gastric ulcer usually have normal or reduced rates of acid secretion (hypochlorhydria).

Acid secretion is expressed as the amount of acid secreted under basal or fasting conditions, basal acid output (BAO); after maximal stimulation, maximal acid output (MAO); or in response to a meal.[21] Basal, maximal, and meal-stimulated acid secretion varies according to time of day and the individual's psychological state, age, gender, and health status. The BAO follows a circadian rhythm, with the highest acid secretion occurring at night and the lowest in the morning. An increase in the BAO:MAO ratio suggests a basal hypersecretory state such as ZES. A review of gastric acid secretion and its regulation can be found elsewhere.[21]

Pepsin is an important cofactor that plays a role in the proteolytic activity involved in ulcer formation.[21] Pepsinogen, the inactive precursor of pepsin, is secreted by the chief cells located in the gastric fundus (see Fig. 20-1). Pepsin is activated by acid pH (optimal pH of 1.8 to 3.5), reversibly inactivated at pH 4, and irreversibly destroyed at pH 7.

Mucosal defense and repair mechanisms (mucus and bicarbonate secretion, intrinsic epithelial cell defense, and mucosal blood flow) protect the gastroduodenal mucosa from noxious endogenous and exogenous substances.[1,21] The viscous nature and near-neutral pH of the mucus–bicarbonate barrier protect the stomach from the acidic contents in the gastric lumen. Mucosal repair after injury is related to epithelial cell restitution, growth, and regeneration. The maintenance of mucosal integrity and repair is mediated by the production of endogenous prostaglandins (PGs). The term *cytoprotection* is often used to describe this process, but *mucosal defense* and *mucosal protection* are more accurate terms, as PGs prevent deep mucosal injury and not superficial damage to individual cells. Gastric hyperemia and increased PG synthesis characterize adaptive cytoprotection, the short-term adaptation of mucosal cells to mild topical irritants. This phenomenon enables the stomach to initially withstand the damaging effects of irritants. Alterations in mucosal defense that are induced by *H. pylori* or NSAIDs are the most important cofactors in the formation of peptic ulcers.

H. pylori

H. pylori is a spiral-shaped, pH-sensitive, gram-negative, microaerophilic bacterium that resides between the mucus layer and surface epithelial cells in the stomach, or any location where gastric-type epithelium is found.[2,22] The combination of its spiral shape and flagellum permits it to move from the lumen of the stomach, where the pH is low, to the mucus layer, where the local pH is neutral. *H. pylori* produces large amounts of urease, which hydrolyzes urea in the gastric juice and converts it to ammonia and carbon dioxide.[2] The local buffering effect of ammonia creates a neutral microenvironment within and surrounding the bacterium, protecting it from the lethal effect of gastric acid. *H. pylori* also produces acid-inhibitory proteins, which allow it to adapt to the low-pH environment of the stomach.[2]

H. pylori binds to specific regions within the stomach. It attaches to gastric-type epithelium by adherence pedestals, which prevent the organism from being shed during cell turnover and mucus secretion.[2] Colonization of the antrum and corpus (body) of the stomach is associated with gastric ulcer and cancer.[1,2,22] Antral organisms colonize gastric metaplastic tissue (gastric tissue that develops in the duodenum secondary to changes in gastric acid or bicarbonate secretion) leading to duodenal ulcer (see Fig. 20-2).[1,2] Although *H. pylori* causes chronic gastric mucosal inflammation in all infected individuals, only a minority actually develop an ulcer or gastric cancer.[1,2,8] The difference in the diverse clinical outcomes is related to variations in bacterial pathogenicity and host susceptibility.[2,22]

Mucosal injury is produced by (a) elaborating bacterial enzymes (urease, lipases, and proteases), (b) adherence, and (c) *H. pylori* virulence factors.[2,22] Lipases and proteases degrade gastric mucus, ammonia produced by urease may be toxic to gastric epithelial cells, and bacterial adherence enhances the uptake of toxins into gastric epithelial cells. *H. pylori* induces gastric inflammation by altering the host inflammatory response and damaging epithelial cells directly by cell-mediated immune mechanisms or indirectly by activated neutrophils or macrophages attempting to phagocytose bacteria or bacterial products.[2,22] However, *H. pylori* strains are genetically diverse and account for differences in adaptation within the human host. Two of the most important are cytotoxin-associated gene protein (CagA) and vacuolating cytotoxin (VacA). About 60% of *H. pylori* strains in the United States possess CagA, but CagA-positive strains increase the risk for severe PUD, gastritis, and gastric cancer compared with CagA-negative strains.[2,22] The VacA gene codes for the VacA cytotoxin, a vacuolating toxin. Although VacA is present in most *H. pylori* strains, strains vary in cytotoxicity and increased risk for peptic ulcer and gastric cancer.[2,22] Host polymorphisms are important markers of disease susceptibility and may identify high-risk patients.[2,22] Polymorphisms of interleukin (IL)-1β and its receptor antagonist, as well as tumor necrosis factor-α (TNF-α) and IL-10, may be associated with increased gastric acid secretion and duodenal ulcer or acid suppression and gastric cancer.[2,22]

Nonsteroidal Antiinflammatory Drugs

NSAIDs, including aspirin (see Table 20-3), cause gastric mucosal damage by two important mechanisms: (a) direct or topical irritation of the gastric epithelium and (b) systemic inhibition of endogenous mucosal PG synthesis.[1,13] Although the onset of injury is initiated topically by the acidic properties of many of the NSAIDs, systemic inhibition of the protective PGs limits the ability of the mucosa to defend itself against injury and thus plays the predominant role in the development of gastric ulcer.[1,13]

Topical irritant properties are predominantly associated with acidic NSAIDs (e.g., aspirin) and their ability to decrease the hydrophobicity of the mucous gel layer in the gastric mucosa. Most nonaspirin NSAIDs have topical irritant effects, but aspirin is the most damaging. Although NSAID prodrugs, enteric-coated aspirin tablets, salicylate derivatives, and parenteral or rectal preparations are associated with less acute topical gastric mucosal injury, they can cause ulcers and related GI complications as a result of their systemic inhibition of endogenous PGs.[1]

Cyclooxygenase (COX) is the rate-limiting enzyme in the conversion of arachidonic acid to PGs and is inhibited by NSAIDs (Fig. 20-3). Two similar COX isoforms have been identified: COX-1 is found in most body tissue, including the stomach, kidney,

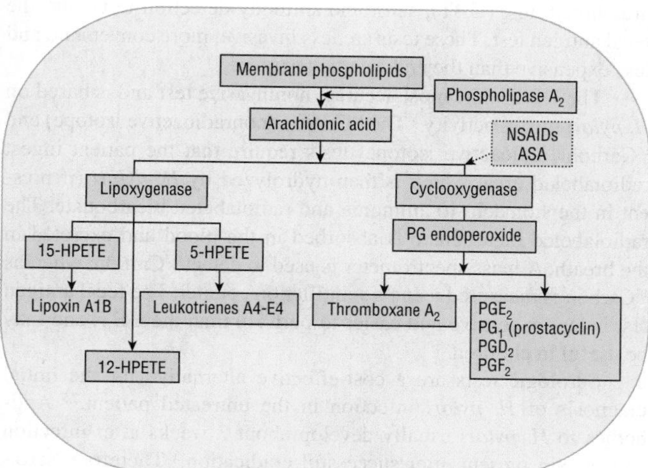

FIGURE 20-3 Metabolism of arachidonic acid after its release from membrane phospholipids. *Broken arrow* indicates inhibitory effects. (ASA, aspirin; HPETE, hydroperoxyeicosatetraenoic acid; NSAIDs, nonsteroidal antiinflammatory drugs; PG, prostaglandin.)

Cyclooxygenase

COX-1
Constitutively expressed

COX-2
Induced at inflammation site

Nonselective
NSAID/ASA

Selective
COX-2
inhibitor

Stomach
Kidney
Platelets
Intestinal endothelium

Macrophages
Leukocytes
Fibroblasts
Endothelial cells
Other

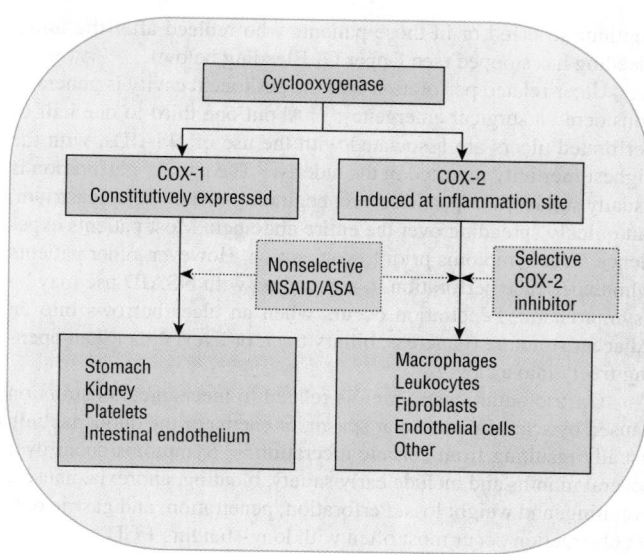

FIGURE 20-4 Tissue distribution and actions of cyclooxygenase (COX) isoenzymes. Nonselective nonsteroidal antiinflammatory drugs (NSAIDs) including aspirin (ASA) inhibit COX-1 and COX-2 to varying degrees; COX-2 inhibitors inhibit only COX-2. *Broken arrow* indicates inhibitory effects.

intestine, and platelets; COX-2 is undetectable in most tissues under normal physiologic conditions, but its expression can be induced during acute inflammation and arthritis (Fig. 20-4).[1,13] COX-1 produces protective PGs that regulate physiologic processes such as GI mucosal integrity, platelet homeostasis, and renal function. COX-2 is induced (unregulated) by inflammatory stimuli such as cytokines and produces PGs involved with inflammation, fever, and pain. It is also constitutionally expressed in organs such as the brain, kidney, and reproductive tract. Adverse effects (e.g., GI or renal toxicity) of NSAIDs are primarily associated with the inhibition of COX-1, whereas antiinflammatory actions result primarily from NSAID inhibition of COX-2.[1,13]

The COX-1-to-COX-2 inhibitory ratio determines the relative GI toxicity of a specific NSAID. Nonselective NSAIDs, including aspirin (see Table 20-3), inhibit both COX-1 and COX-2 to varying degrees and are associated with an increased propensity to cause gastric ulcers.[1,13] In contrast, the selective COX-2 inhibitors are associated with a reduction in ulcers and related GI complications, but the benefit of celecoxib is less than that of rofecoxib and valdecoxib (see Table 20-3). The addition of aspirin to a selective COX-2 inhibitor reduces its ulcer-sparing benefit and increases ulcer risk.[1,13] Aspirin and nonaspirin NSAIDs irreversibly inhibit platelet COX-1, resulting in decreased platelet aggregation and prolonged bleeding times, thereby increasing the potential for upper and lower GI bleeding.[1,13,15] Coadministration of selected NSAIDs may reduce the antiplatelet effects of aspirin.[13–15] Clopidogrel and other medications that impair angiogenesis do not cause ulcers, per se, but may impair healing of gastric erosions leading to ulceration.[13,15]

Complications

Upper GI bleeding, perforation, and obstruction occur with *H. pylori*–associated and NSAID-induced ulcers and constitute the most serious, life-threatening complication of chronic PUD.[1,23] Bleeding is caused by the erosion of an ulcer into an artery. It may be occult (hidden) and insidious or may present as melena (black-colored stools) or hematemesis (vomiting of blood). The use of NSAIDs (especially in older adults) is the most important risk factor for upper GI bleeding. Deaths occur primarily in patients who continue to bleed or in those patients who rebleed after the initial bleeding has stopped (see Upper GI Bleeding below).

Ulcer-related perforation into the peritoneal cavity is generally considered a surgical emergency.[1,23] About one third to one half of perforated ulcers are associated with the use of NSAIDs, with the highest mortality reported in the elderly.[23] The pain of perforation is usually sudden, sharp, and severe, beginning first in the epigastrium, but quickly spreading over the entire abdomen. Most patients experience ulcer symptoms prior to perforation. However, older patients who experience perforation in association with NSAID use may be asymptomatic. Penetration occurs when an ulcer burrows into an adjacent structure (pancreas, biliary tract, or liver) rather than opening freely into a cavity.

Gastric outlet obstruction is related to mechanical obstruction caused by scarring, muscular spasm, or edema of the duodenal bulb usually resulting from chronic ulceration.[1,23] Symptoms occur over several months and include early satiety, bloating, anorexia, nausea, vomiting, and weight loss. Perforation, penetration, and gastric outlet obstruction occur most often with long-standing PUD.

Treatment of PUD has improved so that even the most virulent ulcers can be managed with medication. Intractability to drug therapy is an infrequent manifestation of PUD and an infrequent indication for surgery.

CLINICAL PRESENTATION

The clinical presentation of PUD varies depending on the severity of epigastric pain and the presence of complications (Table 20-5).[1] Ulcer-related pain in duodenal ulcer often occurs 1 to 3 hours after meals and is usually relieved by food, but this is variable. In gastric ulcer, food may precipitate or accentuate ulcer pain. Antacids usually provide immediate pain relief in most ulcer patients. Pain usually diminishes or disappears during treatment; however, recurrence of epigastric pain after healing often suggests an unhealed or recurrent ulcer.

The presence or absence of epigastric pain does not define an ulcer.[1] Ulcer healing does not necessarily render the patient asymptomatic. Why symptoms remain is unclear, but it may relate to sensitization of afferent nerves in response to mucosal injury.[1] Conversely, the absence of pain does not preclude an ulcer diagnosis especially in the elderly who may present with a "silent" ulcer complication. The reasons for this are unclear, but may relate to differences in the way the elderly perceive pain or the analgesic effect of NSAIDs.

Dyspepsia in itself is of little clinical value when assessing subsets of patients who are most likely to have an ulcer. Patients taking NSAIDs often report dyspepsia, but dyspeptic symptoms do not directly correlate with an ulcer. Individuals with dyspeptic symptoms may have either uninvestigated (no upper endoscopy) or investigated (underwent upper endoscopy) dyspepsia. If an ulcer is not confirmed in a patient with ulcer-like symptoms at the time of endoscopy, the disorder is referred to as *NUD*.[9] Ulcer-like symptoms may occur in the absence of peptic ulceration in association with *H. pylori* gastritis or duodenitis. There is no one sign or symptom that differentiates between *H. pylori*–positive and NSAID-induced ulcer.

TABLE 20-5 Clinical Presentation of Peptic Ulcer Disease

General
- Mild epigastric pain or acute life-threatening upper GI complications

Symptoms
- Abdominal pain that is often epigastric and described as burning but may present as vague discomfort, abdominal fullness, or cramping
- A typical nocturnal pain that awakens the patient from sleep (especially between 12 and 3 AM)
- The severity of ulcer pain varies from patient to patient and may be seasonal, occurring more frequently in the spring or fall; episodes of discomfort usually occur in clusters, lasting up to a few weeks and followed by a pain-free period or remission lasting from weeks to years
- Changes in the character of the pain may suggest the presence of complications
- Heartburn, belching, and bloating often accompany the pain
- Nausea, vomiting, and anorexia are more common for patients with gastric ulcer than with duodenal ulcer but may also be signs of an ulcer-related complication

Signs
- Weight loss associated with nausea, vomiting, and anorexia
- Complications including ulcer bleeding, perforation, penetration, or obstruction

Laboratory tests
- Gastric acid secretory studies
- The hematocrit and hemoglobin are low with bleeding, and stool hemoccult tests are positive
- Tests for *Helicobacter pylori* (see Table 20-6)

Diagnostic tests
- Fiber-optic upper endoscopy (esophagogastroduodenoscopy) detects more than 90% of peptic ulcers and permits direct inspection, biopsy, visualization of superficial erosions, and sites of active bleeding
- Upper GI radiography with barium has been replaced with upper endoscopy as the diagnostic procedure of choice for suspected peptic ulcer

DIAGNOSIS

Routine laboratory tests are not helpful in establishing the diagnosis of PUD (see Table 20-5).[1]

Tests for *H. pylori*

The diagnosis of *H. pylori* infection can be made using endoscopic or nonendoscopic tests (Table 20-6).[2,5,24] The tests that require upper endoscopy are invasive, more expensive, and usually require a mucosal biopsy for histology, culture, or detection of urease activity. At least four tissue samples are taken from specific areas of the stomach, as patchy distribution of *H. pylori* infection can lead to false-negative results. Because certain medications may decrease the sensitivity of rapid urease test, antibiotics and bismuth salts should be withheld for 4 weeks and proton pump inhibitors (PPIs) for 1 to 2 weeks prior to endoscopic testing.[2,5] If the patient has been taking these medications, then a gastric biopsy for histology should be performed.[5]

Two types of nonendoscopic tests are available: tests that identify active infection and tests that detect antibodies (see Table 20-6). Antibody tests do not differentiate between active infection and previously eradicated *H. pylori*. The nonendoscopic tests include the urea breath test (UBT), serologic antibody detection tests, and the fecal antigen test. These tests are less invasive, more convenient, and less expensive than the endoscopic tests.[2,5,24]

The UBT is the most accurate noninvasive test and is based on *H. pylori* urease activity.[5] The ^{13}Carbon (nonradioactive isotope) and ^{14}Carbon (radioactive isotope) tests require that the patient ingest radiolabeled urea, which is then hydrolyzed by *H. pylori* (if present in the stomach) to ammonia and radiolabeled bicarbonate. The radiolabeled bicarbonate is absorbed in the blood and excreted in the breath. A mass spectrometer is used to detect ^{13}Carbon, whereas ^{14}Carbon is measured using a scintillation counter. The fecal antigen test is less expensive and easier to perform than the UBT, and may be useful in children.

Serologic tests are a cost-effective alternative for the initial diagnosis of *H. pylori* infection in the untreated patient.[2,5] Antibodies to *H. pylori* usually develop about 3 weeks after infection and remain present after successful eradication.[5] Therefore, serology should not be used to confirm *H. pylori* eradication.[2,5] Office-based tests are less expensive, widely available, and provide rapid results, but the results are less accurate and more variable than the laboratory-based tests. Salivary and urine antibody tests are under investigation.[2]

TABLE 20-6 Tests for Detection of *Helicobacter pylori*

Test	Description	Comments
Endoscopic Tests		
Histology	Microbiologic examination using various stains	Gold standard; >95% sensitive and specific; permits classification of gastritis; results are not immediate; not recommended for initial diagnosis; tests for active *H. pylori* infection
Culture	Culture of biopsy	Enables sensitivity testing to determine appropriate treatment or antibiotic resistance; 100% specific; results are not immediate; not recommended for initial diagnosis; used after failure of second-line treatment; tests for active *H. pylori* infection
Biopsy (rapid) urease	*H. pylori* urease generates ammonia, which causes a color change	Test of choice at endoscopy; >90% sensitive and specific; easily performed; rapid results (usually within 24 hours); tests for active *H. pylori* infection
Polymerase chain reaction	*H. pylori* DNA detected in gastric tissue	Test is highly specific and sensitive; high rate of false-positives and false-negatives; positive DNA does not directly equate top presence of the organism; considered a research technique
Nonendoscopic Tests		
Antibody detection (laboratory based)	Detects antibodies to *H. pylori* in serum using laboratory-based enzyme-linked immunosorbent assay (ELISA) tests and latex agglutination techniques	Quantitative; less sensitive and specific than endoscopic tests; more accurate than in office; unable to determine if antibody is related to active or cured infection; antibody titers vary markedly among individuals and take 6 months to 1 year to return to the uninfected range; not affected by PPIs or bismuth; antibiotics given for unrelated indications may cure the infection, but antibody test will remain positive
Antibody detection (can be performed in office or near patient)	Detects IgG antibodies to *H. pylori* in whole blood or finger stick	Qualitative; quick (within 15 minutes); unable to determine if antibody is related to active or cured infection; most patients remain seropositive for at least 6 months to 1 year after *H. pylori* eradication; not affected by PPIs, bismuth, or antibiotics
Urea breath test	*H. pylori* urease breaks down ingested labeled C-urea, patient exhales labeled CO_2	Tests for active *H. pylori* infection; 95% sensitive and specific; results take about 2 days; antibiotics, bismuth, PPIs, and H_2RAs may cause false-negative results; withhold PPIs or H_2RAs (1–2 weeks) and bismuth or antibiotics (4 weeks) prior to testing; recommended test to confirm posttreatment eradication of *H. pylori*
Fecal antigen	Identifies *H. pylori* antigen in stool by enzyme immunoassay using polyclonal anti–*H. pylori* antibody	Tests for active *H. pylori* infection; sensitivity and specificity comparable to urea breath test when used for initial diagnosis; antibiotics, bismuth, and PPIs may cause false-negative results, but to a lesser extent than with the urea breath test; may be used posttreatment to confirm eradication, but patients may have a reluctance to obtain stool samples

H_2RA, H_2-receptor antagonist; PPI, proton pump inhibitor.

Data from references 2, 5, and 25.

Testing for *H. pylori* is only recommended if eradication is planned. Serologic antibody testing is a reasonable choice if endoscopy is not planned. The diagnostic accuracy of *H. pylori* tests for patients with an active bleeding ulcer has been questioned because of the potential for false-negative results. However, endoscopic biopsy-based tests such as the rapid urease test have a high degree of specificity in these patients (see Peptic Ulcer–Related Bleeding below).[5]

Confirmation of eradication is indicated posttreatment of active ulcers, previous ulcers, MALT lymphoma, endoscopic resection of gastric cancer, and uninvestigated dyspepsia, but routine testing for all patients is neither cost-effective nor practical.[5] The decision to test posttreatment should be patient-specific and take into consideration the patient's diagnosis, age, and ulcer history. The UBT and fecal antigen are preferred nonendoscopic tests to confirm *H. pylori* eradication but must be delayed at least 4 weeks after the completion of treatment to avoid confusing bacterial suppression with eradication. The term *eradication* or *cure* is used when posttreatment tests conducted 4 weeks after the end of treatment do not detect the organism. Quantitative antibody tests are impractical for posttreatment as antibody titers remain elevated for long periods of time. A negative posttreatment antibody test, however, is considered reliable.

Imaging and Endoscopy

The diagnosis of PUD depends on visualizing the ulcer crater by either upper GI radiography or upper endoscopy (see Table 20-5).[1] In the past, radiography was the initial diagnostic procedure of choice because of its lower cost, greater availability, and greater safety. Today, upper endoscopy has replaced radiography because it provides a more accurate diagnosis and permits direct visualization of the ulcer.

CLINICAL COURSE AND PROGNOSIS

The natural history of PUD is characterized by periods of exacerbations and remissions.[1] Ulcer pain is usually recognizable and episodic, but symptoms are variable, especially in older adults and for patients taking NSAIDs. Antiulcer medications, including the histamine-2 receptor antagonists (H_2RAs), PPIs, and sucralfate, relieve symptoms, accelerate ulcer healing, and reduce the risk of ulcer recurrence, but they do not cure the disease. Both duodenal and gastric ulcers recur unless the underlying cause (*H. pylori* or NSAID) is removed. Successful *H. pylori* eradication markedly decreases ulcer recurrence and complications. Prophylactic cotherapy or a COX-2 inhibitor decreases the risk of upper GI events for patients who are taking NSAIDs. GI bleeding, perforation, and obstruction remain troublesome complications of chronic PUD. Mortality for patients with gastric ulcer is slightly higher than in duodenal ulcer and the general population. The development of gastric cancer in *H. pylori*–infected individuals is a slow process that occurs over 20 to 40 years and is associated with a lifetime risk of less than 1%.[2,8]

TREATMENT

Desired Outcome

The treatment of chronic PUD varies depending on the etiology of the ulcer (*H. pylori* or NSAID), whether the ulcer is initial or recurrent, and whether complications have occurred (Fig. 20-5). Overall treatment is aimed at relieving ulcer pain, healing the ulcer, preventing ulcer recurrence, and reducing ulcer-related complications. The goal of therapy for *H. pylori*–positive patients with an active ulcer, a previously documented ulcer, or a history of an ulcer-related complication is to eradicate *H. pylori*, heal the ulcer, and cure the disease. Successful eradication heals ulcers and reduces the risk of recurrence for most patients. The goal of therapy for a patient with an NSAID-induced ulcer is to heal the ulcer as rapidly as possible. Patients who are at high risk of developing NSAID ulcers should receive prophylactic cotherapy or be switched to a selective COX-2 inhibitor NSAID (if available) to reduce ulcer risk and related complications. When possible, the most cost-effective drug regimen should be used.

General Approach to Treatment

Antimicrobials such as clarithromycin, metronidazole, amoxicillin, bismuth salts, and antisecretory drugs (PPIs or H_2RAs) relieve ulcer symptoms, heal the ulcer, and eradicate *H. pylori* infection. PPIs are preferred to H_2RAs or sucralfate for healing *H. pylori*–negative NSAID-induced ulcers because they accelerate ulcer healing and provide more effective relief of symptoms. Treatment with a PPI should be extended from 4 to 8-12 weeks if the NSAID must be continued. A PPI-based *H. pylori* eradication regimen is recommended when the patient with an active ulcer is taking an NSAID and is *H. pylori* positive. Prophylactic cotherapy with either a PPI or misoprostol decreases ulcer risk and upper GI complications for patients taking nonselective NSAIDs. Selective COX-2 inhibitor NSAIDs (if available) may be used as an alternative to a nonselective NSAID, but their beneficial GI

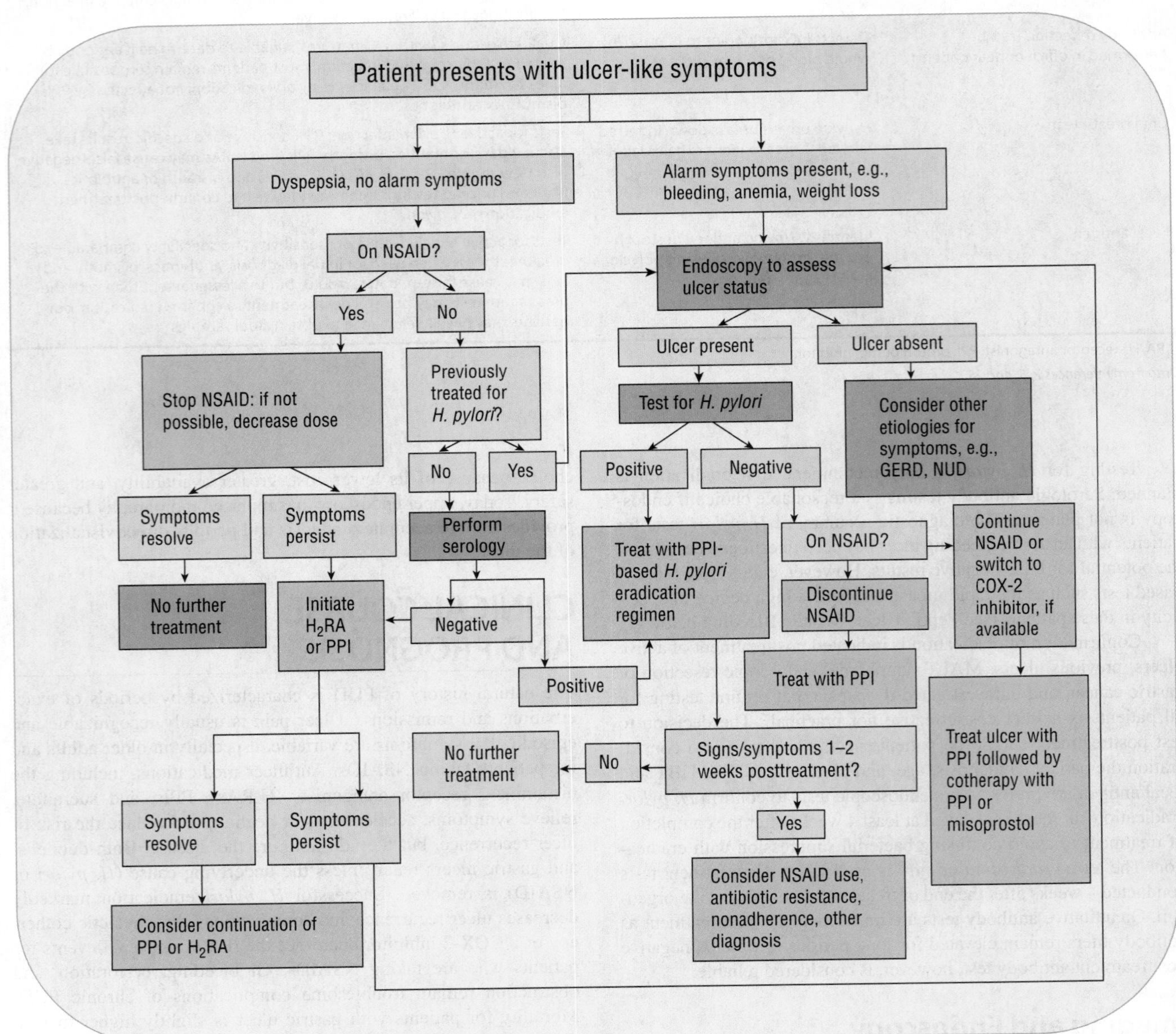

FIGURE 20-5 Algorithm. Guidelines for the evaluation and management of a patient who presents with dyspeptic or ulcer-like symptoms. (COX-2, cyclooxygenase-2; GERD, gastroesophageal reflux disease; H_2RA, H_2-receptor antagonist; NSAID, nonsteroidal antiinflammatory drug; NUD, nonulcer dyspepsia; PPI, proton pump inhibitor.)

effect when taken with low-dose aspirin is negated and their association with adverse cardiovascular effects reduces their usefulness.

Dietary modifications are important for patients who are unable to tolerate certain foods and beverages. Lifestyle modifications such as reducing stress and stopping cigarette smoking are encouraged. Surgery may be necessary for patients with ulcer-related complications.

Nonpharmacologic Therapy

1 Patients with PUD should eliminate or reduce psychological stress, cigarette smoking, and the use of NSAIDs (including aspirin). Although there is no "antiulcer diet," the patient should avoid foods and beverages (e.g., spicy foods, caffeine, and alcohol) that cause dyspepsia or that exacerbate ulcer symptoms. If possible, alternative agents such as acetaminophen or nonacetylated salicylate (e.g., salsalate) should be used for relief of pain. Elective surgery for PUD is rarely performed today because of highly effective medical management. A subset of patients, however, may require emergency surgery for bleeding, perforation, or obstruction. In the past, surgical procedures were performed for medical treatment failures and included vagotomy with pyloroplasty or vagotomy with antrectomy.[23] Vagotomy (truncal, selective, or parietal cell) inhibits vagal stimulation of gastric acid. A truncal or selective vagotomy frequently results in postoperative gastric dysfunction and requires a pyloroplasty or antrectomy to facilitate gastric drainage. When an antrectomy is performed, the remaining stomach is anastomosed with the duodenum (Billroth I) or with the jejunum (Billroth II). A vagotomy is unnecessary when an antrectomy is performed for gastric ulcer. Postoperative consequences include postvagotomy diarrhea, dumping syndrome, anemia, and recurrent ulceration.

Pharmacologic Therapy

Recommendations

2 Table 20-7 presents guidelines for the eradication of infection in *H. pylori*–positive individuals. Table 20-8 lists regimens used to eradicate *H. pylori* infection.

TABLE 20-7 Guidelines for the Eradication of *Helicobacter pylori* Infection

Indications for treatment of *H. pylori* infection

- Established indications for the treatment of *H. pylori* include gastric or duodenal ulcer, mucosa-associated lymphoid tissue (MALT) lymphoma, after endoscopic resection of gastric cancer, and uninvestigated dyspepsia
- Controversial indications for the treatment of *H. pylori* infection include nonulcer dyspepsia, gastroesophageal reflux disease, individuals taking nonsteroidal antiinflammatory drugs (NSAIDs), individuals at high risk for gastric cancer, and unexplained iron deficiency anemia

Initial treatment of *H. pylori* infection

- Use only those eradication regimens that are of proven effectiveness in the United States
- In the United States, first-line treatment should include a proton pump inhibitor (PPI), clarithromycin, and either amoxicillin or metronidazole (PPI-based triple therapy) for 10–14 days
- The PPI-based triple-therapy amoxicillin-containing regimen is preferred initially because bacterial resistance to amoxicillin is almost absent, it has fewer adverse effects, and it leaves metronidazole as a backup agent for second-line therapy
- In penicillin-allergic patients, metronidazole should be substituted for amoxicillin in the PPI-based triple-therapy regimen and yields similar results when combined with clarithromycin
- An alternate initial strategy includes a PPI or H_2RA, bismuth salt, tetracycline, and metronidazole (bismuth-based quadruple therapy) for 10–14 days
- Sequential therapy consisting of a PPI and amoxicillin for 5 days followed by a PPI, clarithromycin, and metronidazole for 5 days is an alternative to PPI-based triple therapy or PPI-based quadruple therapy, but requires further validation before it can be recommended as first-line therapy in the United States

Eradication of *H. pylori* after initial treatment failure

- Avoid antibiotics that have been used in previous eradication regimens
- Bismuth-based quadruple therapy with a bismuth salt, tetracycline, metronidazole, and a PPI or H_2RA for 10–14 days is an acceptable treatment regimen for persistent *H. pylori* infections
- PPI-based triple therapy with levofloxacin and amoxicillin for 10 days may be more effective and better tolerated than PPI-based quadruple therapy with a bismuth salt, tetracycline, and metronidazole, but it requires further validation in the United States

Data from references 5, 25–29.

TABLE 20-8 Drug Regimens Used to Eradicate *Helicobacter pylori*

Drug #1	Drug #2	Drug #3	Drug #4
Proton Pump Inhibitor–Based Triple Therapy[a]			
PPI once or twice daily[b]	Clarithromycin 500 mg twice daily	Amoxicillin 1 g twice daily *or* metronidazole 500 mg twice daily	
Bismuth-Based Quadruple Therapy[a]			
PPI or H_2RA once or twice daily[b,c]	Bismuth subsalicylate[d] 525 mg four times daily	Metronidazole 250–500 mg four times daily	Tetracycline 500 mg four times daily
Sequential Therapy[e]			
PPI once or twice daily on days 1–10[b]	Amoxicillin 1 g twice daily on days 1–5	Metronidazole 250–500 mg twice daily on days 6–10	Clarithromycin 250–500 mg twice daily on days 6–10
Second-Line (Salvage) Therapy for Persistent Infections			
PPI or H_2RA once or twice daily[b,c]	Bismuth subsalicylate[d] 525 mg four times daily	Metronidazole 250–500 mg four times daily	Tetracycline 500 mg four times daily
PPI once or twice daily[b,f]	Amoxicillin 1 g twice daily	Levofloxacin 250 mg twice daily	

H_2RA, H_2-receptor antagonist; PPI, proton pump inhibitor.

[a]Although treatment is minimally effective if used for 7 days, 10–14 days is recommended. The antisecretory drug may be continued beyond antimicrobial treatment for patients with a history of a complicated ulcer, for example, bleeding, or in heavy smokers.

[b]Standard PPI peptic ulcer healing dosages given once or twice daily.

[c]Standard H_2RA peptic ulcer healing dosages may be used in place of a PPI.

[d]Bismuth subcitrate potassium (biskalcitrate) 140 mg, as the bismuth salt, is contained in a prepackaged capsule (Pylera), along with metronidazole 125 mg and tetracycline 125 mg; three capsules are taken with each meal and at bedtime; a standard PPI dosage is added to the regimen and taken twice daily. All medications are taken for 10 days.

[e]Requires validation as first-line therapy in the United States.

[f]Requires validation as rescue therapy in the United States.

Data from references 5, 25–29.

TABLE 20-9 Drug Dosing Table

Drug	Brand Name	Initial Dose	Usual Range	Special Population Dose	Other
Proton Pump Inhibitors					
Omeprazole, sodium bicarbonate	Prilosec, Zegerid	40 mg daily	20–40 mg/day	Consider adjustment for hepatic disease	Pregnancy Category C
Lansoprazole	Prevacid, various	30 mg daily	15–30 mg/day	Consider adjustment for hepatic disease	Pregnancy Category B
Rabeprazole	Aciphex	20 mg daily	20–40 mg/day	Use with caution in severe hepatic disease	Pregnancy Category B
Pantoprazole	Pantoprazole, various	40 mg daily	40–80 mg/day	Consider adjustment for severe hepatic disease	Pregnancy Category B
Esomeprazole	Nexium	40 mg daily	20–40 mg/day	Limit dose to 20 mg/day in severe hepatic disease	Pregnancy Category B
Dexlansoprazole	Dexilant	30–60 mg daily	30–60 mg/day	Consider dose limit of 30 mg/day in moderate hepatic impairment, dose not established in severe hepatic disease	Pregnancy Category B
H_2-Receptor Antagonists					
Cimetidine	Tagamet, various	300 mg four times daily, 400 mg twice daily, or 800 mg at bedtime	800–1,600 mg/day in divided doses	Adjust dose for renal and severe hepatic impairment	Pregnancy Category B
Famotidine	Pepcid, various	20 mg twice daily, or 40 mg at bedtime	20–40 mg/day	Adjust dose for renal impairment	Pregnancy Category B
Nizatidine	Axid, various	150 mg twice daily, or 300 mg at bedtime	150–300 mg/day	Adjust dose for renal impairment	Pregnancy Category B
Ranitidine	Zantac, various	150 mg twice daily, or 300 mg at bedtime	150–300 mg/day	Adjust dose for renal impairment	Pregnancy Category B
Mucosal Protectants					
Sucralfate	Carafate, various	1 g four times daily, or 2 g twice daily	2–4 g/day		Aluminum may accumulate in renal failure, Pregnancy Category B
Misoprostol	Cytotec	100–200 mcg four times daily	400–800 mcg/day		Pregnancy Category X

Data from references 32, 70, and 72.

3 First-line therapy is usually initiated with a PPI-based three-drug regimen for 10 to 14 days. If a second course of treatment is required, the PPI-based three-drug regimen should contain different antibiotics or a four-drug regimen with a bismuth salt, metronidazole, tetracycline, and a PPI should be used.

Patients with NSAID-induced ulcers should be tested to determine their *H. pylori* status. If *H. pylori* positive, treatment should be initiated with a PPI-based three-drug regimen. If *H. pylori* negative, the NSAID should be discontinued, and the patient treated with a PPI, H_2RA, or sucralfate (see Table 20-9). If the NSAID is continued, treatment should be initiated with a PPI (if *H. pylori* negative) or with a PPI-based three-drug regimen (if *H. pylori* positive). Cotherapy with a PPI or misoprostol or switching to a selective COX-2 inhibitor (if available) is recommended for patients at risk of developing an ulcer-related complication.

Maintenance therapy with a PPI or H_2RA should be limited to high-risk patients with ulcer complications, patients who fail eradication, and those with *H. pylori*–negative ulcers. Treatment failure is associated with poor medication adherence, antimicrobial resistance, NSAID use, cigarette smoking, acid hypersecretion, or tolerance to the antisecretory effects of an H_2RA.

Treatment of *H. pylori*–Positive Ulcers

This chapter focuses on the eradication of *H. pylori* in adults.[25–29] A discussion of the treatment of *H. pylori* infection in children is found elsewhere.[30,31]

The treatment of *H. pylori*–positive PUD should be effective, well tolerated, easy to adhere to, and cost-effective. Historically, none of these factors have been addressed in a systematic way making it difficult to identify the best evidence-based treatment regimens.[1] Successful eradication depends on the drug regimen, resistance to the antibiotics used, duration of therapy, medication adherence, and genetic polymorphism.[25–29] *H. pylori* regimens should have eradication (cure) rates of at least 80% based on intention-to-treat analysis or at least 90% based on per-protocol analysis, and they should minimize the potential for antimicrobial resistance.[1,25,29] Not one antibiotic, bismuth salt, or antiulcer drug achieves this goal, but clarithromycin is the single most effective antibiotic. Two-drug regimens that combine a PPI and either amoxicillin or clarithromycin have yielded marginal and variable eradication rates in the United States and are not recommended.[1,5] In addition, the use of only one antibiotic is associated with a higher rate of antimicrobial resistance.

Drug regimens (see Table 20-8) that combine an antisecretory drug with two antibiotics (triple therapy) or with two antibiotics and a bismuth salt (quadruple therapy) usually increase eradication rates to acceptable levels and reduce the risk of antimicrobial resistance.[5,25–29] When selecting an initial eradication regimen, an antibiotic combination should be used that permits second-line treatment (if necessary) with different antibiotics. The antibiotics that have been most extensively studied and found to be effective in various combinations include clarithromycin, amoxicillin, metronidazole, and tetracycline.[1] Because of insufficient data, ampicillin should not be substituted for amoxicillin, doxycycline should not be substituted for tetracycline, and azithromycin or erythromycin should not be substituted for clarithromycin. Antisecretory drugs enhance antibiotic activity and stability by increasing intragastric pH and by decreasing intragastric volume thereby enhancing the topical antibiotic concentration.[27]

Proton Pump Inhibitor–Based Three-Drug Regimens

PPI-based triple therapy (see Table 20-8) is the initial treatment of choice for eradicating *H. pylori* (see Table 20-7).[5,25–29] The regimens that combine either clarithromycin and amoxicillin or clarithromycin and metronidazole are more effective than the amoxicillin–metronidazole regimen. In most cases, increasing the antibiotic dosage does not improve eradication rates. The clarithromycin–amoxicillin regimen is preferred initially (see Table 20-7), but metronidazole should be substituted for amoxicillin for penicillin-allergic patients unless alcohol is consumed.[5,25–27] Unfortunately, eradication rates for PPI-based triple therapy have declined substantially in recent years in North America and Europe due primarily to an increase in clarithromycin-resistant *H. pylori* strains (see Factors that Predict *H. pylori* Eradication Outcomes below).[5,25–27] Other antibiotics and antibiotic combinations have been investigated, but these regimens should not be used as initial treatment in the United States until well-designed trials confirm their effectiveness.[5,27]

The recommended duration of therapy in the United States is 10 to 14 days, but the 14-day regimen is preferred in light of the decreasing eradication rate with the PPI-based triple-therapy regimens containing clarithromycin.[5] Although a 7-day course has been approved by the FDA and is used in Europe, the longer treatment periods favor higher eradication rates and are less likely to be associated with antimicrobial resistance.[5,25–27]

Clinical **Controversy. . .**

Although clinical guidelines recommend a 10- or 14-day treatment course, some clinicians favor an initial 7-day *H. pylori* regimen. These clinicians believe that the shorter treatment period enhances the compliance of a complicated drug regimen.

The PPI is an integral part of the three-drug regimen and should be taken 30 to 60 minutes before a meal along with the two antibiotics (see Table 20-8).[5,32] Prolonged PPI treatment beyond 2 weeks after eradication is usually not necessary for ulcer healing. A single daily dose of a PPI may be less effective than a twice-daily dose.[33] Substitution of one PPI for another is acceptable and does not enhance or diminish *H. pylori* eradication.[32,34] An H_2RA should not be substituted for a PPI, as H_2RA is associated with lower eradication rates.[35,36] Pretreatment with a PPI does not influence *H. pylori* eradication.[37]

Bismuth-Based Four-Drug Regimens

Bismuth-based quadruple therapy (see Table 20-8) is recommended as an alternative first-line eradication therapy (see Table 20-7) for those allergic to penicillin.[5,25–29] Although this regimen may be used initially, it is often reserved as a second-line therapy after treatment failure with the PPI-based clarithromycin–amoxicillin regimen (see Eradication of *H. pylori* After Initial Treatment Failure below). Eradication rates for bismuth-based quadruple therapy (bismuth salicylate, metronidazole, tetracycline, and either a PPI or H_2RA) are similar to those achieved with PPI-based triple therapy.[5,27,38] Eradication rates are comparable when bismuth subcitrate potassium (biskalcitrate) is substituted for bismuth subsalicylate (see Table 20-8).[39] Substitution of clarithromycin 250 to 500 mg four times a day for tetracycline yields similar results but increases adverse effects. Bismuth salts have a topical antimicrobial effect.[1] The antisecretory drug hastens ulcer healing and relieves pain in patients with an active ulcer. All medications except the PPI should be taken with meals and at bedtime.

The original bismuth-based regimens contained an H_2RA in place of a PPI, but a meta-analysis indicated that quadruple therapy with a PPI provides greater efficacy and permits a shorter treatment duration (7 days) when compared with the H_2RA-based regimens (10 to 14 days).[40] However, a 10- to 14-day duration is recommended in the United States as it generally provides higher eradication rates.[5] When treating an active ulcer, the antisecretory drug is usually continued for 2 (PPI) to 4 (H_2RA) weeks after stopping bismuth and antibiotics.

Bismuth-based quadruple therapy is the treatment of choice when medication costs are of overriding importance. However, major concerns include a four-times-a-day dosing regimen (see Table 20-8), poor medication adherence, and frequent adverse effects. Although minor adverse effects are more common, the frequency of moderate or severe adverse effects is similar to those reported for the PPI-based triple therapy.[41]

Sequential Therapy Sequential therapy is a new form of eradication therapy whereby the antibiotics are administered in a sequence rather than all together.[5,26,29] The rationale for sequential therapy is to initially treat with antibiotics that rarely promote resistance (e.g., amoxicillin) to reduce the bacterial load and preexisting resistant organisms and then to follow with different antibiotics (e.g., clarithromycin and metronidazole) to kill the remaining organisms.[1] Treatment consists of a PPI and amoxicillin for 5 days followed by a PPI, clarithromycin, and tinidazole (or metronidazole) for an additional 5 days (see Table 20-8).[5,26,42] Although this regimen has achieved eradication rates that are superior to the PPI-based three-drug regimens containing clarithromycin,[42] the regimen requires a change in medication midtreatment, which may contribute to nonadherence.[43] The advantages of sequential therapy need to be confirmed in the United States before it can be recommended as a first-line *H. pylori* eradication therapy (see Table 20-7).[5,26,27]

Eradication of *H. pylori* After Initial Treatment Failure

H. pylori eradication is often more difficult after initial treatment fails and successful eradication after retreatment is extremely variable.[5,44] Treatment failures should be referred to a gastroenterologist for further diagnostic evaluation. Second-line (salvage) treatment should (a) use antibiotics that were not previously used during initial therapy; (b) use antibiotics that are not associated with resistance; (c) use a drug that has a topical effect such as bismuth; and (d) extend the duration of treatment to 14 days.[5,44,45] The most commonly used second-line therapy, after unsuccessful initial treatment with a PPI–amoxicillin–clarithromycin regimen, is a 14-day course of the PPI-based quadruple therapy (see Table 20-8).[5,26,27,45] A levofloxacin-containing regimen (see Table 20-8) may be an alternative second-line eradication regimen and may be better tolerated than PPI-based quadruple therapy (see Table 20-7).[46] Additionally, the levofloxacin regimen may serve as an alternative to PPI–clarithromycin–metronidazole usually recommended in penicillin-allergic patients.[47] However, concerns about using fluoroquinolones for *H. pylori* eradication are related to the development of resistance and adverse effects such as tendonitis and hepatotoxicity.[26] Other second-line regimens that include rifabutin and furazolidone are discussed elsewhere.[5,25–27]

Factors that *Predict H. pylori* Eradication Outcomes

Factors that predict *H. pylori* eradication outcomes include antibiotic resistance, poor medication adherence, short duration of therapy, CagA status, high bacterial load, low intragastric pH, and genetic polymorphism.[5,45,48–50] Medication adherence decreases with multiple medications, increased frequency of administration, intolerable adverse effects, and costly drug regimens. One meta-analysis reported that CYP2C19 polymorphism may alter the effect of PPIs on gastric acid secretion thereby influencing eradication outcomes.[49] Tolerability varies with different regimens.[1,5] Common adverse effects include nausea, vomiting, abdominal pain, diarrhea, and taste disturbances (metronidazole and clarithromycin). Adverse effects with metronidazole are dose related (especially when >1 g/day) and include a disulfiram-like reaction with alcohol. Tetracycline may cause photosensitivity and should not be used in children because of possible tooth discoloration. Bismuth salts may cause darkening of the stool and tongue. Antibiotic-associated diarrhea and *Clostridium difficile*–associated disease can occur. Oral thrush and vaginal candidiasis may also occur.

An important predictor of *H. pylori* eradication is the presence or absence of resistant microorganisms.[5,50–52] U.S. data from 1993 to 1999 report resistance rates among *H. pylori* strains for metronidazole (37%), clarithromycin (10%), and amoxicillin (1.4%).[51] Data from 1998 to 2002 reveal rates of 25% for metronidazole, 13% for clarithromycin, and 0.9% for amoxicillin.[52] In one study, the proportion of clarithromycin resistance increased with increasing courses of macrolide antibiotics, from 7% resistance with no prior exposure to 80% resistance with ≥5 courses of macrolides. It is possible that the increased rate of clarithromycin resistance partially explains the decrease in efficacy of clarithromycin-containing regimens. The clinical importance of metronidazole resistance remains uncertain, as resistance can be overcome by using higher dosages and combining metronidazole with other antibiotics.[5] Resistance to tetracycline and amoxicillin is uncommon.[5] Resistance to bismuth has not been reported. The role of antibiotic sensitivity testing prior to initiating *H. pylori* treatment has not been established.

Probiotics

Probiotics (e.g., strains of *Lactobacillus* and *Bifidobacterium*) and foodstuffs (e.g., cranberry juice and some milk proteins) with bioactive components have been used proactively to control *H. pylori* colonization in at-risk individuals and, when taken as a supplement to eradication therapy, may have a role in improving *H. pylori* eradication and reducing the adverse effects of PPI-based triple therapy.[53–55] However, the administration of probiotics alone does not eradicate *H. pylori* infection. In the future, the regular intake of probiotics may constitute a low-cost alternative for individuals who are at risk for *H. pylori* infection and, in combination with antibiotics, augment eradication rates. These preliminary data are encouraging and warrant more research in this area.

Treatment of NSAID-Induced Ulcers

Nonselective NSAIDs should be discontinued (when possible) on confirmation of an active ulcer. If the NSAID is stopped, most uncomplicated ulcers heal with standard regimens of an H_2RA, PPI, or sucralfate (see Table 20-9).[1,13,29] However, PPIs are usually preferred because they provide more rapid symptom relief and ulcer healing. If the NSAID is continued despite ulceration, consideration should be given to reducing the NSAID dose, switching to acetaminophen or a nonacetylated salicylate, or using a more selective COX-2 inhibitor (see Table 20-3). PPIs are the drugs of choice when the NSAID is continued, as potent acid suppression is required to accelerate ulcer healing.[1,13,29] If the ulcer is *H. pylori* positive, eradication should be initiated with a regimen that contains a PPI.[1,13,29]

Strategies to Reduce the Risk of NSAID Ulcer and GI Complications There are three therapeutic approaches to reducing the risk of NSAID ulcers and related upper GI complications (see Table 20-10). Medical cotherapy with either a PPI or misoprostol decreases ulcer risk and GI complications in high-risk patients.[12–14,16,19,29] The use of a selective COX-2 inhibitor instead of a nonselective NSAID also decreases risk of ulcers and upper GI events.[12–14,16,18,19,29] Unfortunately, these strategies do not completely eliminate ulcers and complications for patients at the "highest risk." When selecting a gastroprotective strategy, the GI benefits must be balanced against the cardiovascular risks associated with selective COX-2 inhibitor NSAIDs, nonselective NSAIDs, and concomitant antiplatelet therapy.[12–16] Strategies aimed at reducing the topical irritant effects of nonselective NSAIDs, for example, prodrugs, slow-release formulations, and enteric-coated products, do not prevent ulcers or GI complications.

Misoprostol Cotherapy Misoprostol, 200 mcg orally four times per day, reduces the risk of NSAID-induced gastric and duodenal ulcer, and related upper GI complications, but diarrhea and abdominal cramping limit its use.[12,16,56] Because a dosage of 200 mcg three times per day is comparable in efficacy to 800 mcg/day, the lower dosage should be considered for patients unable to tolerate the higher dose.[12,16] Reducing the misoprostol dosage to 400 mcg/day or less to minimize diarrhea compromises its gastroprotective effects. A fixed combination of misoprostol 200 mcg and diclofenac (50 or 75 mg) may enhance compliance, but the flexibility to individualize drug dosage is lost. A large clinical trial in rheumatoid arthritis patients provided the most compelling evidence that misoprostol reduces the risk of upper GI complications for high-risk patients.[57]

Proton Pump Inhibitor Cotherapy ❹ PPI cotherapy reduces NSAID-related gastric and duodenal ulcer risk and is better tolerated than misoprostol.[12–14,16,56] All PPIs are effective when used in standard dosages (see Table 20-9). Although head-to-head comparative trials are few, there are limited data to indicate that PPIs are superior to standard H_2RA dosages.[12,13,16] When lansoprazole (15 or 30 mg/day) was compared with misoprostol 800 mcg/day or placebo, both dosages of lansoprazole and misoprostol effectively

TABLE 20-10 Drug Monitoring Table

Drug	Adverse Drug Reaction	Monitoring Parameter	Comments
Proton pump inhibitors	Headache, N/V/D, flatulence Less common: thrombocytopenia, neutropenia, hypomagnesemia, hypocalcemia, liver function abnormalities, renal impairment	Baseline and periodic CBC, serum electrolytes, renal/liver function	Well tolerated; may be associated with increased risk of fractures, pneumonia, *Clostridium difficile* infection
Histamine-2 receptor antagonists	Headache, dizziness, diarrhea, somnolence, gynecomastia (cimetidine) Less common: thrombocytopenia, neutropenia, liver function abnormalities, renal impairment, pancreatitis	Baseline and periodic CBC, serum electrolytes, renal/liver function	
Sucralfate	Constipation		
Misoprostol	Diarrhea, abdominal pain, headache, nausea/vomiting, flatulence, dysmenorrhea, hypophosphatemia	Pregnancy test Serum phosphate	Avoid in pregnancy

Data from references 32, 70, 72, 85–93.

reduced ulcer recurrence, although the PPI was better tolerated.[58] A greater proportion of those in the misoprostol group reported treatment-related adverse events and withdrew early from the study. Results from observational studies and meta-analyses indicate the PPIs reduce the risk of NSAID-related ulcer bleeding.[12,16,19,59]

H_2-Receptor Antagonist Cotherapy Standard H_2RA dosages (e.g., famotidine 40 mg/day) are effective in reducing NSAID-related duodenal ulcer but not gastric ulcer (the most frequent type of ulcer associated with NSAIDs).[12,13,16] Higher dosages (e.g., famotidine 40 mg twice daily, ranitidine 300 mg twice daily) may reduce the risk of gastric and duodenal ulcer, but studies comparing double dosages with PPIs or misoprostol are not available.[12,13] One study suggests that famotidine 20 mg twice daily may be an alternative to PPIs for patients taking low cardioprotective dosages of aspirin, but additional studies are required to confirm these findings.[60] The H_2RAs are not recommended as prophylactic cotherapy because it is likely that they are not as effective as the PPIs or misoprostol in preventing NSAID-induced gastric ulcer and related GI complications.[16] An H_2RA, however, may be used to relieve NSAID-related dyspepsia.

Cyclooxygenase-2 Inhibitors Two large outcome trials have compared celecoxib[61] and rofecoxib[62] with nonselective NSAIDs. Patients in the Celecoxib Long-Term Arthritis Safety Study (CLASS) trial who were taking celecoxib and required cardioprotection (antiplatelet effects of aspirin) were permitted to take low-dose aspirin.[61] Although a 6-month analysis found a nonsignficant reduction in ulcer complications with celecoxib when compared with ibuprofen and diclofenac, results after 1 year found no difference between the groups. Today, celecoxib is not considered a selective COX-2 inhibitor (Table 20-3) by the FDA as it contains the same GI warnings as the nonselective and partially selective NSAIDs.[63] A post hoc analysis confirmed that any gastroprotective benefits of celecoxib were negated in aspirin users. Similar effects have been observed with rofecoxib. Additionally, an increased number of nonfatal myocardial infarctions and thrombotic stroke were observed in studies of rofecoxib leading to its withdrawal from the market.[64] Subsequently, valdecoxib was withdrawn from the market amid concerns about cardiovascular risk.

Cardiovascular safety was also evaluated in the CLASS trial, but serious cardiovascular thromboembolic events were no different between celecoxib and the comparative nonselective NSAIDs. In contrast, the results of a meta-analysis of randomized trials of COX-2 inhibitor NSAIDs reported a dose-dependent increase in cardiovascular events with all COX-2 inhibitor NSAIDs, including celecoxib.[65] Increased cardiovascular risk appears to be dependent on a number of factors including increased COX-2 selectivity, higher dosages, and a longer duration of treatment.[12,18,19] Thus, the lowest effective celecoxib dose should be used for the shortest duration of time. Dyspepsia and abdominal pain, fluid retention, hypertension, and renal toxicity are associated with the COX-2 inhibitors and nonselective NSAIDs.[1]

COX-2 Inhibitor Versus NSAID Plus PPI ❺ There are limited data that suggest that for high-risk, *H. pylori*–negative patients, a COX-2 inhibitor NSAID may be as beneficial as a nonselective NSAID plus a PPI in reducing NSAID-related ulcer complications.[12,18,19] However, neither the COX-2 inhibitor NSAID nor the NSAID plus a PPI will eliminate upper GI events for these patients. Combining a COX-2 inhibitor NSAID with a PPI may be considered for very high-risk patients, but this regimen is likely to be of modest benefit.[12,18]

GI and Cardiovascular Safety Issues

There is no difference in cardiovascular risk between the selective COX-2 inhibitor NSAIDs and the nonselective or partially selective NSAIDs, with the exception of naproxen.[12,18,65] Thus, individual patient risk factors for NSAID-related GI bleeding and cardiovascular events must be weighed when determining treatment (see Table 20-11). Naproxen is preferred compared with other nonselective NSAIDs and COX-2 inhibitors because of its comparative cardiovascular safety and not because of its GI safety profile. There is insufficient evidence regarding the preferred NSAID for patients also taking low-dose aspirin.[14] Clopidogrel should not be substituted for low-dose aspirin in order to reduce recurrent GI bleeding as it is inferior to a PPI plus low-dose aspirin.[13] Despite limited evidence to suggest an interaction via the hepatic cytochrome P450 (CYP450) pathway, combining a PPI and clopidogrel with or without low-dose aspirin results in less GI bleeding.[13] Ongoing studies for patients

TABLE 20-11 Guidelines for Reducing GI Risk for Patients Receiving Chronic NSAID Therapy

Cardiovascular Risk	No or Low GI Risk (No Risk Factors)	Moderate GI Risk (1–2 Risk Factors)	High GI Risk (>2 Risk Factors or Prior Ulcer or Ulcer-Related Complication)
GI Risk Factors (see Table 20-4)			
	Age <65 years)	Age ≥65 years High-dose NSAIDs Concomitant use of aspirin, corticosteroids, or anticoagulants	Age ≥65 years Concomitant use of aspirin corticosteroids, or anticoagulants Dual antiplatelet therapy
No or low CV risk (patient does not require low-dose aspirin)	Nonselective NSAID or partially selective NSAID (see Table 20-3)	Nonselective NSAID or partially selective NSAID + PPI or misoprostol Selective COX-2 inhibitor NSAID (if available)	Avoid NSAID or selective COX-2 inhibitor, if possible; use alternative therapy Nonselective NSAID or partially selective NSAID + PPI or misoprostol Selective COX-2 inhibitor NSAID (if available) + PPI or misoprostol
High CV risk (patient requires low-dose aspirin), no NSAID	No prophylaxis required	PPI or misoprostol	PPI or misoprostol
High CV risk (patient requires low-dose aspirin) and NSAID	Naproxen + PPI or misoprostol	Naproxen + PPI or misoprostol	Avoid NSAID or selective COX-2 inhibitor If antiinflammatory drug is needed and CV risk is >GI risk, use naproxen and aspirin + PPI or misoprostol If antiinflammatory drug and aspirin are needed and GI risk is >CV, use selective COX-2 inhibitor + PPI or misoprostol

COX-2, cyclooxygenase-2 inhibitor; CV, cardiovascular; NSAID, nonsteroidal antiinflammatory drug; PPI, proton pump inhibitor.

Data from references 12–15, 18, 19, and 59.

with cardiovascular disease should provide the necessary information to help resolve these issues. The lowest possible daily dose of a COX-2 inhibitor should be used as the cardiovascular risk may be dose dependent. However, no studies, to date, have evaluated the safety of low-dose COX-2 inhibitor NSAIDs for patients with or at risk for cardiovascular disease. In the future, there will be new formulations and classes of NSAIDs and COX-2 inhibitors with an improved GI and cardiovascular safety profile.[66] Until then patients who take NSAIDs or COX-2 inhibitors should be counseled about the signs and symptoms of upper GI bleeding and major cardiovascular events and what they should do if they occur.

Treatment of Non–*H. pylori*, Non-NSAID Ulcers

Very few individuals have non–*H. pylori*, non-NSAID (idiopathic) ulcers.[29,67,68] Patients should be double-checked to verify that they are *H. pylori* negative and that they are not taking ulcerogenic medications. Possible explanations for *non–H. pylori*, non-NSAID ulcers include gastric hypersecretion, gastric outlet obstruction, genetic predisposition, concomitant diseases (see Table 20-2), and heavy tobacco use. Treatment should be initiated with conventional ulcer healing therapy (see Table 20-9). Although standard H_2RA or sucralfate dosage regimens heal the majority of gastric and duodenal ulcers in 6 to 8 weeks, PPIs provide comparable ulcer healing rates in 4 weeks.[32] A higher daily dose or a longer treatment duration is sometimes needed to heal larger gastric ulcers. Antacids are not used as single agents to heal ulcers because of the high volume and frequent doses required. When conventional antiulcer therapy is discontinued after ulcer healing, most patients develop a recurrent ulcer within 1 year.[32] Maintenance therapy may be required to prevent ulcer recurrence.

Long-Term Maintenance of Ulcer Healing

Continuous antiulcer therapy is aimed at the long-term maintenance of ulcer healing and the prevention of ulcer-related complications. Because *H. pylori* eradication dramatically decreases ulcer recurrence, continuous maintenance therapy is primarily used to treat high-risk patients who failed *H. pylori* eradication, have a history of ulcer-related complications, have frequent recurrences of *H. pylori*–negative ulcers, and are heavy smokers or NSAID users. For most patients, standard maintenance dosages (see Table 20-9) are effective.[32]

Treatment of Refractory Ulcers

Ulcers are considered refractory to therapy when symptoms, ulcers, or both persist beyond 8 to 12 weeks despite conventional treatment or when several courses of *H. pylori* eradication fail.[1,45] Poor patient compliance, antimicrobial resistance, cigarette smoking, NSAID use, gastric acid hypersecretion, or tolerance to the antisecretory effects of an H_2RA (see Antiulcer Agents below) may contribute to refractory PUD. Patients with refractory ulcers should undergo upper endoscopy to confirm a nonhealing ulcer, exclude malignancy, and assess *H. pylori* status. *H. pylori*–positive patients should receive eradication therapy (see Treatment of *H. pylori*–Positive Ulcers above). In *H. pylori*–negative patients, higher PPI dosages (e.g., omeprazole 40 mg/day) heal the majority of ulcers. Continuous treatment with a PPI is often necessary to maintain healing, as refractory ulcers recur when therapy is discontinued or the dose is reduced. Switching from one PPI to another is not beneficial. Patients with refractory gastric ulcer may require surgery because of the possibility of malignancy.

Antiulcer Agents

Proton Pump Inhibitors The PPIs (omeprazole, esomeprazole, lansoprazole, dexlansoprazole, rabeprazole, and pantoprazole) dose-dependently inhibit basal and stimulated gastric acid secretion.[32] When PPI therapy is initiated, the degree of acid suppression increases over the first 3 to 4 days of therapy, as more proton pumps are inhibited.[32] Because PPIs inhibit only those proton pumps that are actively secreting acid, they are most effective when taken 30 to 60 minutes before meals.[32] The duration of acid suppression is a function of binding to the H^+/K^+-adenosine triphosphatase (ATPase) enzyme and is longer than their elimination half-lives.[32] Symptomatic acid rebound on withdrawal of a PPI has been reported in healthy volunteers after 8 weeks of treatment.[1,69]

Various PPI dosage forms and formulations exist (see Table 20-12) and include the delayed-release enteric-coated dosage

TABLE 20-12 Proton Pump Inhibitor Formulations and Options for Administration

	Omeprazole	Esomeprazole	Lansoprazole	Pantoprazole	Rabeprazole	Dexlansoprazole
Commercially available oral formulations						
Capsule	X[a]	X	X			X[b]
Tablet	X[c]			X	X	
Oral disintegrating tablet			X			
Packet for oral suspension	X[d]	X[d]				
Extemporaneous oral preparations						
Pellets from capsule in water		X				
Pellets from capsule in applesauce	X		X			X
Pellets from capsule in juice	X	X[e]	X			
Extemporaneous preparation of delayed-release PPI in bicarbonate (omeprazole-sodium bicarbonate)	X		X	X		
Parenteral formulations						
IV	Not available in the United States	X		X		

X, product is available.

[a]Omeprazole is available as delayed-release enteric-coated pellets in a capsule or as immediate-release capsule that contains 20 or 40 mg of omeprazole with 1,100 mg sodium bicarbonate (equivalent to 304 mg of sodium). Because 20 and 40 mg dosages contain the same amount of bicarbonate, two 20 mg capsules should not be substituted for the 40 mg immediate-release omeprazole-sodium bicarbonate capsule.

[b]Dexlansoprazole is available as a dual delayed-release formulation in capsules for oral administration. The capsule contains dexlansoprazole in a mixture of two types of enteric-coated granules with different pH-dependent dissolution profiles.

[c]Omeprazole oral tablets are available as 20 mg delayed-release nonprescription tablets.

[d]Omeprazole oral suspension is available as 20 or 40 mg omeprazole with 1,680 mg sodium bicarbonate (equivalent to 460 mg of sodium). Because 20 and 40 mg dosages contain the same amount of bicarbonate, two 20 mg packets should not be substituted for the 40 mg immediate-release omeprazole-bicarbonate packet.

[e]No published information; based on omeprazole data.

Data from references 32, 70, and 72.

forms that have pH-sensitive granules contained in gelatin capsules (omeprazole, esomeprazole, prescription and nonprescription lansoprazole, and dexlansoprazole), rapidly disintegrating tablets (lansoprazole), and delayed-release enteric-coated tablets (rabeprazole, pantoprazole, and nonprescription omeprazole).[32] The pH-sensitive enteric coating prevents degradation and premature protonation of the drug in stomach acid but dissolves at a higher pH in the duodenum where the drug is absorbed. Dexlansoprazole is formulated with a dual-release mechanism that results in inhibition of proton pumps that become activated after initial release of the medication.[70,71] Omeprazole is also available as an immediate-release formulation (oral suspension, oral capsule) containing sodium bicarbonate, which raises intragastric pH and protects omeprazole from acid degradation in the stomach thus permitting rapid absorption from the duodenum.[72] IV products available in the United States include pantoprazole and esomeprazole.

Five of the PPIs provide similar rates of ulcer healing (dexlansoprazole has not been labeled at this time for these indications), maintenance of ulcer healing, and symptom relief when used in recommended dosages (see Table 20-9). When higher dosages are indicated, the daily dose should be divided in order to obtain better 24-hour control of intragastric pH. A dosage reduction is unnecessary for patients with renal impairment or in older adults but should be considered in severe hepatic disease.[32] The short-term adverse effects of the PPIs are similar to those observed with the H_2RAs and include headache, nausea, and abdominal pain.[32] Because the immediate-release formulations contain sodium bicarbonate, they are contraindicated for patients with metabolic alkalosis and hypokalemia.[72] The sodium should also be taken into consideration for patients who are on sodium-restricted diets, for example, congestive heart failure.

Drug Interactions All PPIs increase intragastric pH and may alter the bioavailability of orally administered drugs, such as ketoconazole (weak bases) and digoxin, or pH-dependent dosage forms.[32,73] This interaction is especially important with atazanavir, a protease inhibitor. Concomitant use with a PPI can significantly reduce the oral bioavailability of atazanavir and potentially lead to therapeutic failure and viral resistance in patients infected with HIV.[74] Omeprazole and esomeprazole selectively inhibit the hepatic CYP2C19 pathway and may decrease the elimination of phenytoin, warfarin, diazepam, and carbamazepine.[32] The PPIs may increase the metabolic clearance and decrease the GI absorption of levothyroxine resulting in increased thyroid-stimulating hormone levels and a corresponding increase in the levothyroxine dose.[75] Clinically significant drug interactions with PPIs are rare and usually do not constitute a major clinical risk.[76,94]

Clinical **Controversy...**

Some clinicians believe that the antiplatelet effect of clopidogrel is attenuated by omeprazole resulting in an increased risk of adverse cardiac events when these medications are taken concomitantly. Strategies to avoid this interaction for patients at risk of NSAID-related GI events include switching omeprazole to another PPI or substituting an H_2RA for the PPI. Others believe that the use of a PPI (if indicated) and clopidogrel is not a safety concern and that it is not necessary to switch omeprazole to another PPI.

One of the most perplexing potential PPI drug interactions is with the antiplatelet drug clopidogrel. This interaction is especially important given recent consensus guidelines that recommend the use of a PPI for high-risk patients on antiplatelet therapies to prevent ulcers and related GI bleeding.[13] Clopidogrel, a prodrug, is converted to its active form through CYP2C19. PPIs may attenuate the antiplatelet effect of clopidogrel by inhibiting or competing for this metabolic pathway. FDA safety guidelines recommend that the coadministration of omeprazole, omeprazole/sodium bicarbonate, or esomeprazole with clopidogrel be avoided because they reduce the effectiveness of clopidogrel.[77–79] Details of new studies performed by the manufacturer and submitted to the FDA, as well as warnings regarding omeprazole, esomeprazole, and other interacting drugs (e.g., cimetidine), are contained in the clopidogrel package insert.[80] A reduced antiplatelet effect of clopidogrel may also result from genetic polymorphisms of the CYP2C19 pathway leading to decreased biotransformation of the drug to its active form.[81,82] Whether the use of other PPIs such as pantoprazole, lansoprazole, dexlansoprazole, and rabeprazole interacts with clopidogrel remains uncertain as the capacity to inhibit CYP2C19 varies among these PPIs.[83,84] While some reports suggest a "class effect" among the different PPIs, other pharmacodynamic studies suggest an interaction with omeprazole and esomeprazole but not with pantoprazole.[83,84] Because of the uncertainty of the effect of the PPI–clopidogrel interaction on clinical outcomes and the extent to which other PPIs may interact with clopidogrel, caution is warranted. The only randomized double-blind trial comparing clopidogrel with or without omeprazole yielded no apparent increase in cardiovascular events due to clopidogrel and omeprazole cotherapy; however, there was a significant reduction in the rate of upper GI bleeding. This trial has been criticized by many due to the low number of cardiovascular events, formulation of omeprazole used, and premature termination of the study due to loss of funding by the sponsor. Patients should have an acceptable indication for a PPI recognizing that risk versus benefit must be weighed on an individual basis. If a PPI is absolutely necessary with clopidogrel, many clinicians continue to avoid the use of omeprazole and esomeprazole.

Potential Risks and Long-Term Safety Issues Numerous potential risks and safety issues (see Table 20-13) have been associated with the long-term use of PPIs as a consequence of prolonged hypergastrinemia and chronic hypochlorhydria.[32,85–88] In most cases, causality is difficult to ascertain because of the study design, confounding variables, and subject selection. All of the PPIs dose-dependently increase serum gastrin concentrations twofold to fourfold as a function of their potent acid-inhibitory effect.[32,85] Fasting gastrin elevations are usually within the normal range and return to baseline within 1 month of discontinuing the drug. In humans, PPIs may lead to enterochromaffin-like (ECL) hyperplasia as a result of the hypergastrinemia, but there is no evidence that these changes result in dysplasia, carcinoid tumors, or gastric adenocarcinoma.[85,86]

TABLE 20-13 Potential Risks and Safety Issues Associated with the Proton Pump Inhibitors

Gastric cancers or malignancy
Carcinoid tumors
Atrophic gastritis
Adenocarcinoma
Bacterial overgrowth
Increase in *N*-nitroso compounds from ingested nitrates (carcinogenic)
Enteric infections (*Clostridium difficile, Salmonella typhimurium, and Campylobacter jejuni*)
Community-acquired pneumonia
Decreased nutrient absorption:
Iron
Calcium
Cyanocobalamin (vitamin B_{12})
Magnesium
Osteoporosis and related fractures

Data from references 32, 85–88.

Although long-term PPI therapy in *H. pylori*–positive individuals is associated with progressive atrophic gastritis, there are insufficient data to link chronic PPI use with gastric cancer in *H. pylori*–positive patients.[85,86] Despite theoretical and in vitro data, there is no evidence to support an association between PPIs and colonic polyps or colorectal cancer.[85,86] Bacterial overgrowth occurs in the stomach as a consequence of hypochlorhydria and may lead to carcinogenic *N*-nitroso compounds in animals but is unlikely to result in significant gastric nitrosation in humans.[85,88]

Chronic PPI therapy may be associated with an increased risk of infection and nutritional deficiences.[85–87] Gastric acid (low stomach pH) plays an important role in the defense against bacterial colonization of the stomach and in nutrient absorption. Acid suppression has been implicated as a risk factor for community-acquired pneumonia (CAP) and enteric infections (*C. difficile*, *Salmonella*, *Campylobacter*).[86] Three case-controlled studies demonstrate a higher adjusted relative risk of CAP for patients currently using PPIs compared with controls.[89–91] The results of these retrospectively designed studies, however, need to be interpreted cautiously because of the variability in the length of therapy for current PPI users and the inclusion of older (>60 years of age) patients with concomitant comorbidities. A systematic review of the literature has linked PPIs with various enteric infections, but the most convincing data were with *C. difficile*.[92] It is likely that sustained elevations in intragastric pH facilitate the survival of *C. difficile* spores. However, the magnitude of risk varies and causality is difficult to establish. The risk of various infections associated with PPI therapy cannot be firmly established until the results of large prospective studies are made available.

The absorption of vitamin B_{12}, dietary iron, and calcium requires an acidic environment and may be adversely affected by PPI-induced prolonged hypochlorhydria (see Table 20-10).[86] Although a few studies have investigated the long-term use of PPIs on vitamin B_{12} and iron absorption, the clinical importance of their effect on absorption has not been established, and monitoring of B_{12} and iron levels cannot be recommended.[86] However, adequate supplementation and monitoring should be considered in high-risk populations (e.g., older patients, vegetarians, alcoholism) who may be already depleted.[85,86] High PPI dosage and long-term therapy have been associated with an increased risk of hip, wrist, and spine fractures related to reduction in calcium absorption.[26,93] Although the results of the studies vary, the FDA has revised the warnings and precautions of prescription and nonprescription PPIs to reflect this potential risk.[93] Bone density tests for osteoporosis screening, calcium supplementation, or other precautions cannot be recommended solely based on chronic PPI therapy.[94] However, it is appropriate to screen and treat older patients for osteoporosis regardless of whether they are receiving long-term PPI therapy.

On the basis of numerous case reports of hypomagnesemia, the FDA has revised the warnings and precautions of prescription and nonprescription PPIs. Hypomagnesemia, both symptomatic and asymptomatic, has been reported with serious adverse events including tetany, arrhythmias, and seizures (see Table 20-10). In most cases it occurs in patients taking PPIs more than 1 year, but can occur with as little as 3 months of therapy.

H_2-Receptor Antagonists Ulcer healing is comparable among H_2RAs (cimetidine, famotidine, nizatidine, and ranitidine) with equipotent multiple daily doses or a single full dose given after dinner or at bedtime (see Table 20-9), but tolerance to their antisecretory effect may occur.[95] Twice-daily administration suppresses daytime acid and benefits patients with daytime ulcer pain. Cigarette smokers may require higher doses or a longer duration of treatment. H_2RAs are eliminated renally and therefore a dosage reduction is recommended for patients with moderate-to-severe renal failure.[96] The short- and long-term safety of all four H_2RAs is similar.[1] Thrombocytopenia, the most common hematologic adverse effect, is reversible and occurs with all four H_2RAs (see Table 20-10). However, the propensity for H_2RAs to cause thrombocytopenia is likely overestimated.[97] Cimetidine inhibits several CYP450 isoenzymes, resulting in numerous drug interactions (e.g., theophylline, lidocaine, phenytoin, warfarin, and clopidogrel).[77,96] Ranitidine has less potential for hepatic CYP450 drug interactions, while famotidine and nizatidine do not interact with drugs metabolized by the hepatic CYP450 pathway.[96] The H_2RAs decrease acid secretion and may alter the bioavailability of orally administered drugs, similar to that seen with the PPIs.

Sucralfate Sucralfate heals peptic ulcers, but is not widely used today for this indication.[1] Deterrents to its use include the requirement for multiple doses per day, large tablet size, and the need to separate the drug from meals and potentially interacting medications. Drug interactions can be minimized by giving the interacting drug at least 2 hours before sucralfate. Alternative therapy is warranted for patients taking oral fluoroquinolones. Constipation may be troublesome especially in older individuals. Seizures may occur in dialysis patients taking aluminum-containing antacids. Hypophosphatemia may develop with long-term treatment. Gastric bezoar formation has also been reported (see Table 20-10).

Prostaglandins Misoprostol, a synthetic PGE_1 analogue, moderately inhibits acid secretion and enhances mucosal defense.[1,98,99] Antisecretory effects are dose dependent over the range of 50 to 200 mcg; cytoprotective effects occur in humans at doses of greater than 200 mcg. Because protective effects occur at higher doses, it is difficult to establish the protective effect independent of the antisecretory action. A dose of 200 mcg four times daily or 400 mcg twice daily (although not recommended in the United States) heals duodenal ulcers and gastric ulcers comparable to standard H_2RA or sucralfate regimens. Diarrhea, the most troublesome adverse effect, is dose dependent and develops in 10% to 30% of patients.[1,98,99] Abdominal cramping, nausea, flatulence, and headache typically accompany the diarrhea. Taking the drug with or after meals and at bedtime may minimize the diarrhea (see Table 20-10). Misoprostol is contraindicated in pregnant women because it is uterotropic and produces uterine contractions that may endanger pregnancy.[98,99] If misoprostol is prescribed to women in their childbearing years, contraceptive measures must be confirmed and a negative serum pregnancy test should be documented within 2 weeks of initiating treatment (see Table 20-10). Patients should be counseled about the GI effects and the need to avoid magnesium antacids, as they may increase the propensity for GI adverse effects.

Bismuth Preparations Bismuth subsalicylate and bismuth subcitrate potassium (biskalcitrate) are the only available bismuth salts in the United States.[1,96] Possible ulcer healing mechanisms include an antibacterial effect, a local gastroprotective effect, and stimulation of endogenous PGs. Bismuth salts do not inhibit or neutralize acid. Bismuth subsalicylate is regarded as safe and has few adverse effects when taken in recommended dosages. Because renal insufficiency may decrease bismuth elimination, bismuth salts should be used with caution in older patients and in renal failure. Bismuth subsalicylate may cause salicylate sensitivity or bleeding disorders and should be used with caution for patients receiving concurrent salicylate therapy. Bismuth salts impart a black color to stool and possibly the tongue (liquid preparations). Long-term use of bismuth salts is not recommended due to the potential for bismuth toxicity.

Antacids Antacids neutralize gastric acid, inactivate pepsin, and bind bile salts.[96,98,99] Aluminum-containing antacids also suppress *H. pylori* and enhance mucosal defense. The GI adverse effects are most common and are dose dependent. Magnesium salts cause an osmotic diarrhea, whereas aluminum salts cause constipation. Diarrhea usually predominates with magnesium/aluminum preparations.

Aluminum-containing antacids (except aluminum phosphate) form insoluble salts with dietary phosphorus and interfere with phosphorus absorption. Hypophosphatemia occurs most often for patients with low dietary phosphate intake (e.g., malnutrition or alcoholism). Combined treatment with sucralfate may amplify the hypophosphatemia and aluminum toxicity.

Magnesium-containing antacids should not be used for patients with a creatinine clearance of less than 30 mL/min (0.5 mL/s) because magnesium excretion is impaired, which may lead to toxicity. Hypercalcemia may occur for patients with normal renal function taking more than 20 g/day of calcium carbonate and for patients with renal failure who are taking more than 4 g/day. The milk-alkali syndrome (hypercalcemia, alkalosis, renal stones, increased blood urea nitrogen, and increased serum creatinine concentration) occurs with high calcium intake for patients with systemic alkalosis produced by either ingestion of absorbable antacids (sodium bicarbonate) or prolonged vomiting. Antacids may alter the absorption and excretion of drugs when administered concomitantly.[96,98,99] Drug interactions may occur when antacids are administered with iron, warfarin, tetracycline, digoxin, quinidine, isoniazid, ketoconazole, or the fluoroquinolones. Most interactions can be avoided by separating the antacid from the oral drug by at least 2 hours.

PERSONALIZED PHARMACOTHERAPY

The metabolism of PPIs occurs primarily through CYP2C19 and polymorphisms of CPY2C19 result in significant differences in enzymatic activity (poor, intermediate, or rapid metabolizers). For example, approximately 85% of white and nearly 100% of Asian populations have polymorphisms resulting in poor metabolism of substrates for CYP2C19. Eradication response rates of *H. pylori* are influenced by pharmacogenomics, with poor metabolizers achieving 100% eradication, intermediate metabolizers achieving 60%, and rapid metabolizers achieving 30% eradication.[100] Prior knowledge of CYP2C19 genotype may help to optimize the PPI dose and interval to minimize therapeutic failure. Rapid metabolizers may need more frequent PPI dosing, up to four times daily, to ensure an optimal gastric pH. Further studies are required to determine if increased AUC achieved in poor metabolizers translates to an additional risk of adverse effects.[101] Pharmacologic properties such as bioavailability and plasma concentrations of individual PPIs differ between individuals, but it remains unclear whether these differences impact the efficacy of *H. pylori* eradication.

Patients with high BMI have reduced antibiotic concentration at the gastric mucosal level and may result in higher risk of treatment failure. Likewise, prior allergy information and history of antimicrobial use is important in tailoring a regimen for *H. pylori* eradication. Tailoring eradication therapy based on *H. pylori* clarithromycin sensitivities is gaining popularity as molecular diagnostic testing improves. In one study, eradication rates improved from 70% in the control group to 94.3% in the treatment arm by tailoring eradication therapy from detection of clarithromycin-resistant *H. pylori* in feces.[102]

Smoking is a risk factor for treatment failure or ulcer recurrence; therefore, patients should be encouraged to quit smoking.

EVALUATION OF THERAPEUTIC OUTCOMES

❻ Table 20-14 lists the recommendations for treating and monitoring patients with PUD. Relief of epigastric pain should be monitored throughout the course of treatment for patients with either

TABLE 20-14 Recommendations for Treating and Monitoring Patients with *Helicobacter pylori*–Associated and Nonsteroidal Antiinflammatory Drug (NSAID)–Induced Ulcers

H. pylori–associated ulcer

1. Recommend drug treatment as presented in the chapter text. See Tables 20-7 and 20-8
2. Assess patient allergies to determine if allergic to penicillin (or other antibiotics) so that drug regimens that contain penicillin (or other antibiotics) can be avoided. Avoid regimens that contain tetracycline in children
3. Assess patient use of alcohol or alcohol-containing products with metronidazole and oral birth control medications with antibiotics and counsel appropriately
4. Assess likelihood of nonadherence to the drug regimen as a cause of treatment failure
5. Recommend a different antibiotic combination if *H. pylori* eradication fails and a second treatment is planned
6. Inform the patient of change in stool color when bismuth salicylate is included in an *H. pylori* eradication regimen
7. Assess and monitor patients for potential adverse effects, especially those associated with metronidazole, clarithromycin, and amoxicillin
8. Assess and monitor patients for potential drug interactions, especially those receiving metronidazole, clarithromycin, or cimetidine
9. Monitor patients for salicylate toxicity, especially patients receiving cotherapy with other salicylates and anticoagulants and patients with renal failure
10. Monitor patients for persistent or recurrent symptoms within 14 days after completion of a course of *H. pylori* eradication therapy
11. Provide patient education to patients who are receiving *H. pylori* eradication therapy and include why antibiotic and antiulcer combinations are used; when and how to take medications; adverse effects; alarm symptoms; the importance of adherence to the entire course of drug treatment; and contact their healthcare provider if alarm symptoms develop (e.g., blood in the stools, black tarry stools, vomiting, severe abdominal pain), or if symptoms persist or return after *H. pylori* eradication

NSAID-induced ulcer

1. Recommend drug treatment as presented in the chapter text
2. Assess risk factors for NSAID-induced ulcers and ulcer-related complications and recommend appropriate strategies for reducing ulcer risk (see Table 20-11)
3. Weigh patient risk factors for NSAID-related GI bleeding and cardiovascular events when selecting a strategy to reduce ulcer risk
4. Recommend eradication treatment for *H. pylori*–positive patients taking NSAIDs
5. Monitor patients for signs and symptoms of NSAID-related upper GI complications
6. Assess and monitor patients for potential drug interactions and adverse effects (especially misoprostol)
7. Provide patient education to patients who are at risk of NSAID-induced ulcers or GI-related complications and include why cotherapy is used with nonselective NSAIDs, when and how to take medications, adverse effects, alarm symptoms, when to contact their healthcare provider, and the importance of adherence to drug treatment

H. pylori– or NSAID-related ulcers. Ulcer pain typically resolves in a few days when NSAIDs are discontinued and within 7 days on initiation of antiulcer therapy. Most patients with uncomplicated PUD will be symptom free after treatment with any one of the recommended antiulcer regimens. The persistence, or recurrence, of symptoms within 14 days after the end of treatment suggests failure of ulcer healing or *H. pylori* eradication or an alternative diagnosis such as GERD. Most patients with uncomplicated *H. pylori*–positive ulcers do not require confirmation of ulcer healing or *H. pylori* eradication. However, eradication should be confirmed after treatment in individuals who are at risk for complications, for example, individuals who had a prior bleeding ulcer. The UBT is the preferred test to confirm *H. pylori* eradication when endoscopy is not indicated. Medication adherence should be assessed for patients who fail therapy. Because a large number of at-risk patients treated with NSAIDs do not receive adequate prophylaxis for GI complications, therapeutic outcomes can be improved by advocating preventive strategies. Patients on NSAIDs should be closely monitored for signs or symptoms of bleeding, obstruction, penetration, or perforation. A followup endoscopy is justified for patients with frequent symptomatic recurrence, refractory disease, complications, or suspected hypersecretory states.

ZOLLINGER-ELLISON SYNDROME

ZES is characterized by gastric acid hypersecretion and recurrent peptic ulcers that result from a gastrin-producing tumor (gastrinoma).[21,45] In the United States, ZES accounts for 0.1% to 1% of patients with duodenal ulcer; however, this may be an underestimation of the true incidence because of the heterogeneity of clinical manifestations.[21] Gastrinomas are classified as those associated with multiple endocrine neoplasia type 1 (MEN 1) or sporadic tumors, which have a greater tendency to behave as malignant tumors. In more than 80% of cases, gastrinomas are localized in an area referred to as the *triangle of gastrinomas*, which includes the convergence of the cystic duct and the common bile duct, the junction of the second and third portions of the duodenum, and the junction of the head and body of the pancreas.[21] More than 50% of the gastrinomas are malignant, often with metastases to regional lymph nodes, liver, and bone.[21]

ZES is suspected for patients with multiple ulcers and recurrent or refractory PUD, often accompanied by esophagitis or ulcer complications.[21,45] Ulcers occur most often in the duodenum but may involve the stomach or jejunum. Diarrhea occurs in about 50% of patients, and results from high concentrations of acid that overwhelm the duodenum's buffering capacity and cause damage to the mucosa.[21] Intraluminal acid also causes steatorrhea by inactivating pancreatic lipase and precipitating bile acids. Vitamin B_{12} malabsorption may result from reduced intrinsic factor activity. The diagnosis is established when the serum gastrin is higher than 1,000 pg/mL (ng/L; 481 pmol/L) and the BAO ≥15 mEq/h (≥15 mmol/h) for patients with an intact stomach (BAO ≥5 mEq/h [≥5 mmol/h] for patients with previous gastric surgery) or when hypergastrinemia is associated with a gastric pH value of ≤2.[21] In situations in which the serum gastrin is between 100 and 1,000 pg/mL (ng/L; 48 and 481 pmol/L) and gastric pH is ≤2, a secretin or calcium proactive test is used to aid the diagnosis.[21] Identification of the location of the tumor with imaging techniques is essential, as early surgical resection prior to liver metastases is often curative.[21] The widespread use of PPIs, although effective in reducing symptoms, may mask the clinical presentation and PPI-related hypergastrinemia may further complicate the diagnosis.[21]

Treatment is based on the presence or absence of peptic ulcers, esophagitis, diarrhea, and a gastrinoma, which may be malignant. The PPIs are the oral drugs of choice for managing gastric acid hypersecretion. Treatment should be instituted with omeprazole 60 mg/day (or an equivalent dose of the available PPIs) and should be adjusted based on individual patient response.[21] Dividing the daily dose and giving the PPI every 8 to 12 hours is most effective in controlling acid output and relieving symptoms. The goal of therapy for uncomplicated patients is to maintain BAO between 1 and 10 mEq/h (1 and 10 mmol/h), in the hour preceding the next dose of the PPI. In complicated cases, such as patients with MEN 1, GERD, or those who are undergoing partial gastrectomy, the BAO should be maintained below 5 mEq/h (5 mmol/h). A gradual reduction in PPI dose is recommended after the adequate control of gastric acid hypersecretion is achieved. IV PPIs are used to suppress gastric acid secretion in patients who are unable to take oral PPIs. The somatostatin analogues, octreotide and lanreotide, directly inhibit the release of gastrin and gastric acid secretion and have been used with varying degrees of success.[21] However, these drugs are not considered first-line therapy as they are only available in the injectable form. Preliminary studies have found the long-acting depot formation of octreotide to be efficacious in the treatment of GI neuroendocrine tumors.[21] Patients with metastatic gastrinoma require tumor resection or treatment with chemotherapeutic agents.

UPPER GI BLEEDING

There are about 160 cases of upper GI bleeding per 100,000 adults annually in the United States.[103] Despite a decreased incidence of PUD and improvements in the management of upper GI bleeding, the mortality rate associated with acute hemorrhage remains between 5% and 15%.[103–105] Upper GI bleeding is categorized as variceal or nonvariceal bleeding. Two common types of nonvariceal bleeding are bleeding from chronic peptic ulcers and bleeding from SRMD (stress gastritis, stress ulcer, or stress erosions), both of which are acid peptic complications.[103–107] Upper GI bleeding associated with chronic PUD usually precedes hospital admission, whereas bleeding associated with SRMD develops in severely ill patients during hospitalization.[103,107]

The underlying pathophysiology of bleeding from a peptic ulcer or from SRMD is similar in that impaired mucosal defense in the presence of gastric acid and pepsin leads to mucosal damage. In chronic PUD, *H. pylori* infection and NSAID use are the most important etiologic factors, whereas the primary pathogenic factor of SRMD in critically ill patients is thought to be mucosal ischemia, which is a result of reduced gastric blood flow (decreased oxygen and nutrient delivery) resulting from splanchnic hypoperfusion.[1,103,107–109] Defense mechanisms are normally in place to protect the gastric mucosa against the damaging effects of gastric acid, pepsin, and bile (see Pathophysiology above). However, these defense mechanisms become diminished in the face of the overwhelming physiologic stress from critical illness and coupled with mucosal ischemia and subsequent reperfusion injury along with gastric acid result in the rapid development of mucosal lesions.[107,108] In contrast to chronic PUD, stress-related mucosal lesions are characteristically asymptomatic, numerous, located in the proximal stomach, and unlikely to perforate.[108] Bleeding from SRMD occurs from superficial mucosal capillaries, whereas bleeding associated with chronic PUD usually results from a single vessel.[108]

The mortality rate associated with clinically important stress-related mucosal bleeding (SRMB) is approximately 50% and is related to the underlying severity of disease and comorbidities in this patient population.[106,108,110] In contrast, the mortality associated with chronic PUD-related bleeding is approximately 10% but can increase dramatically in select patient populations.[104,111,112] Although the initial management of acute upper GI bleeding focuses on aggressive resuscitative measures and ensuring hemodynamic stability, the medical management of PUD-related bleeding and SRMB is distinctly different.[103,104,107,108]

Peptic Ulcer–Related Bleeding

The most common presenting signs and symptoms of PUD-related bleeding are hematemesis (vomiting up blood) or melena (dark, tarry stools) or possibly both. When evaluating patients with PUD-related bleeding, the degree of risk for adverse outcomes must be rapidly assessed in order to determine if the patient's condition constitutes a medical emergency.[103,104] Two risk stratification tools exist for early assessment and triage.[113,114] The Blatchford score is a newer risk stratification scale and is used to evaluate the need for urgent endoscopic intervention for patients presenting with PUD-related bleeding.[113] The scale values range from 0 to 23, with higher scores indicating higher risk. The most well-known scale, however, is the Rockall Score.[114] This validated risk assessment instrument is composed of two assessments: the clinical score, which is performed prior to endoscopy, and the endoscopic score. The use of these risk stratification tools can reduce the requirement of endoscopic procedures and lead to early discharge for low-risk patients while ensuring rapid intervention for patients at higher risk.[103] These data will also allow the pharmacist to make appropriate pharmacotherapy decisions based on the patient's assessed level of risk. When considering the risk of death due to PUD bleeding, the following patients generally have poorer prognoses and usually require more aggressive intervention including admission to an intensive care unit (ICU)[103,104,107,108]:

1. Older than 60 years of age
2. Comorbid conditions (e.g., ischemic heart disease, congestive heart failure, renal failure, hepatic failure, metastatic cancer)
3. High transfusion requirements
4. Ongoing blood loss
5. Presence of hypovolemic shock (i.e., tachycardia with a pulse of ≥100 beats/min, hypotension with a systolic blood pressure of <100 mm Hg with concomitant orthostatic changes, such as an increase in the heart rate of ≥20 beats/min or decrease in systolic blood pressure of ≥20 mm Hg on standing from a sitting position)
6. Prolonged prothrombin time (or increased international normalized ratio [INR])
7. Erratic mental status

Initial therapy for patients with defined hemostatic instability should focus on correcting fluid volume loss though appropriate volume resuscitative measures. This is usually accomplished with a continuous 0.9% sodium chloride infusion (or blood products if clinically indicated) through two large-bore peripheral IV catheters (i.e., 16 to 18 gauge).[103,105] The use of nasogastric (NG) tubes remains controversial but may aid in early assessment and gastric lavage.[103]

Diagnostic endoscopy is usually performed as early as possible (preferably within 24 hours of presentation) to identify the source of the bleeding, assess the potential risk for rebleeding, and, if appropriate, employ therapeutic interventions to promote hemostasis.[103,105] Several endoscopic treatment approaches (e.g., thermocoagulation, argon plasma coagulation therapy, injection sclerotherapy, hemoclipping, and ligation) can be used; however, to maximize the likelihood of positive outcomes, patients should be treated with a combination of at least two endoscopic modalities, such as thermocoagulation and injection of lesions with epinephrine.[103–105] The appearance of the ulcer at the time of endoscopy is a prognostic indicator for the risk of rebleeding.[103,105,111] Clean-based and flat spot (pigmented) ulcers are most commonly seen and are associated with a low risk of rebleeding (5% and 10%, respectively).[105,111] In most cases, patients with clean-based ulcers can be immediately discharged after endoscopy on antiulcer therapy (usually twice-daily PPI), while patients with flat spot ulcers may be admitted to the general hospital ward for a brief observation period. Patients with an adherent clot overlying the ulcer base are at intermediate risk of rebleeding (22%), and controversy exists as to the appropriate management of these patients.[105,111] Adherent clots can be removed, and then the lesion be reclassified based on what is observed following clot removal.[105,111] Patients with a visible vessel or active bleeding are at the highest risk of rebleeding (43% and 55%, respectively) and should be managed within an ICU for at least 24 hours and then monitored on a general medical/surgical service for an additional 48 hours (total of 72 hours), as rebleeding significantly increases mortality.[103,104,111]

7 Antisecretory therapy is often used as adjuvant therapy to endoscopic procedures to prevent PUD rebleeding in high-risk patients because acid impairs clot stability.[103] However, endoscopic hemostatic techniques remain the treatment of choice for patients with life-threatening bleeding, as this has been associated with better outcomes when compared with either placebo or pharmacotherapy alone.[103–105,110] H_2-receptor antagonists are ineffective in preventing PUD rebleeding because they do not achieve an intragastric pH of 6 (which is needed to promote hemostatis and clot stability) and tolerance to their antisecretory effect develops rapidly (especially with high-dose or IV therapy).[103–105,109,115,116] In contrast, PPIs reduce the incidence of rebleeding and need for surgery but have no significant impact on overall mortality.[103,104,115,116] Interestingly, subgroup analysis from two differing meta-analyses has suggested a mortality benefit with high-dose IV PPIs in a subpopulation of patients with the highest risk of rebleeding (i.e., nonbleeding visible vessel or active bleeding).[115,117]

The precise route (oral or IV) and the dose of PPI should be based on the clinical situation, risk of rebleeding, endoscopic identification of the lesion, and patient risk.[115,116] Because of the theoretical goal of maintaining intragastric pH values >6, and data from randomized controlled trials, practice guidelines recommend that high-dose continuous-infusion PPI (equivalent to omeprazole 80 mg given IV as a loading dose, followed by 8 mg/h continuous infusion for 72 hours) be used to reduce the risk of rebleeding in high-risk patients who have undergone endoscopy hemostasis.[103,104,115,116] Because IV omeprazole is not available in the United States and three small randomized controlled trials have not demonstrated any evidence of improved outcomes between the available IV PPIs and omeprazole, most clinicians consider IV pantoprazole and esomeprazole to be equivalent to IV omeprazole on a milligram-per-milligram basis. Thus, IV pantoprazole and esomeprazole can be interchanged as there is currently no evidence to suggest that one PPI is superior to another.[116,118] The administration of high-dose continuous-infusion PPIs given prior to endoscopy hastens resolution of bleeding stigmata.[119] However, PPI therapy is not a replacement for interventional endoscopy for patients who are at high risk of rebleeding, as data demonstrate that the combination of a high-dose PPI continuous IV infusion with therapeutic endoscopy is superior to either strategy alone.[116,120] High-dose oral PPI therapy (omeprazole 80 mg/day for 5 days) is also effective; however, concerns exist as to whether critically ill patients will absorb the medication.[110,115] The risk of rebleeding is greatest within the first 72 hours (especially the first 24 hours), and it is during this time that antisecretory therapy to prevent rebleeding in high-risk patients should be employed.[103,104] Patients should be transitioned to an oral PPI on completion of IV therapy. Somatostatin and octreotide have not demonstrated any significant benefit in treating nonvariceal bleeding and are not recommended at this time.[103,104]

Patients with upper GI bleeding should be tested for *H. pylori* at the time of endoscopy (see Tests for *H. pylori* above). However, the tests are associated with an increased rate of false-negatives when obtained during acute bleeding episodes.[121] If the initial results of the rapid urease test and/or histology are negative, a confirmatory test (^{14}C-UBT or serology) should be performed following the acute bleeding episode. There is no rationale for using IV therapy to eradicate *H. pylori*. Ulcer treatment, including *H. pylori* eradication, if appropriate, should be initiated after the acute bleeding episode has resolved (see Treatment of *H. pylori*–Positive Ulcers and Treatment of NSAID-Induced Ulcers above).

Stress-Related Mucosal Bleeding

Critically ill patients may develop SRMD leading to SRMB because of the homeostatic compromise that is associated with severe illness.[107,108] More than 75% (some studies suggesting up to 100%) of critically ill patients develop SRMD within the first 1 to 3 days of admission to an ICU, but the incidence of clinically important SRMB (defined as overt bleeding with concomitant hemodynamic instability and likely requirement for blood products) is 1% to 4%.[107–109] Clinically important bleeding increases the length of ICU stay by up to 11 days, results in excessive healthcare costs, and is associated with increased mortality.[107,108,122] Thus, attempts to prevent SRMB are warranted in high-risk patients. Prophylactic therapy to prevent bleeding is most effective if initiated early in the patient's course.

(8) Patients who are at risk for SRMB include those with respiratory failure (need for mechanical ventilation for longer than 48 hours), coagulopathy (INR >1.5, platelet count <50,000 mm^3 [$<50 \times 10^9$/L]), hypotension, sepsis, hepatic failure, acute renal failure, high-dose corticosteroid therapy (>250 mg/day hydrocortisone or equivalent), multiple trauma, severe burns (>35% of body surface area), head injury, traumatic spinal cord injury, major surgery, prolonged ICU admission (>7 days), or history of GI bleeding.[106–108,122] The relative importance of the various risk factors remains controversial, but most clinicians concur that patients with respiratory failure or coagulopathy should receive prophylaxis, as these two factors are independent risk factors for SRMB.[106,107] In the absence of these risk factors, some clinicians only administer prophylaxis to patients who have two of the aforementioned risk factors.[106] Since not all patients in a hospital or ICU are at increased risk of SRMB, a cost-effective approach should be developed to target prophylactic therapy at high-risk patients.

Clinical **Controversy. . .**

Some clinicians feel that SRMB prophylaxis is indicated for all critically ill patients given the associated mortality and increased length of stay for patients who develop this complication. Others adhere to clinical guidelines that suggest only high-risk patients such as those with respiratory failure requiring ventilation or patients with coagulopathy and perhaps those patients with two or more other risk factors will benefit from prophylaxis.

Prevention of SRMB includes resuscitative measures that restore mucosal blood and pharmacotherapy that either maintains an intragastric pH of >4 or provides gastric mucosal protection.[106–108] Although the benefits of enteral nutrition to patient outcome (e.g., improved nutritional status enhances mucosal integrity) are of overall clinical importance, its precise role as a sole modality to prevent SRMB remains controversial.[107,108] Therapeutic options for the prevention of SRMB include antacids (which are of historical interest, as they are no longer used because of cumbersome dosage schedules and side effects), antisecretory drugs (H_2RAs and PPIs), and sucralfate (mucosal protectant).[106–108,110,122]

Antisecretory therapy is generally preferred for SRMB prophylaxis for several reasons. First, a large landmark study demonstrated that IV ranitidine was superior to oral sucralfate in preventing SRMB.[123] Second, ranitidine did not increase the risk for nosocomial pneumonia, as the incidence of pneumonia was not different between the two treatment groups.[123] Third, although sucralfate is an evidence-based option, it is cumbersome, requiring multiple daily dosage administration (up to four times daily), which may occlude NG tubes, cause constipation, interact with several medications, and/or increase the potential for aluminum toxicity in patients with renal dysfunction. Finally, sucralfate does not have any appreciable effect on reducing intragastric pH. Although data published in 2004 indicated that H_2RAs were the most commonly prescribed antisecretory agents used to prevent SRMB,[124] PPIs have become the mainstay of therapy.[107] Regardless, numerous studies and years of experience support the use of H_2RAs, and they remain a recommended option for the prevention of SRMB.[106–108,124]

TABLE 20-15 Pharmacotherapy Options for Prophylaxis of Stress-Related Mucosal Bleeding

Drug and Route	Dosage
Parenteral H_2RAs	
Cimetidine	300 mg IV loading dose followed by 50 mg/h as a continuous infusion[a] or 300 mg IV every 6–8 hours
Ranitidine	6.25 mg/h as a continuous infusion or 50 mg IV every 6–8 hours
Famotidine	1.7 mg/h as a continuous infusion or 20 mg IV every 12 hours
Oral/NG Tube PPIs	
Omeprazole	20–40 mg orally/NG tube[b] every 12–24 hours
Omeprazole/bicarbonate powder for oral suspension	40 mg orally/NG tube to start, then followed by an additional 40 mg in 6–8 hours as a loading dose, and then 40 mg every 24 hours
Lansoprazole	30 mg orally/NG tube[b,c] every 12–24 hours
Pantoprazole	40 mg orally/NG tube[b] every 12 to 24 hours
Parenteral PPIs	
Pantoprazole	40–80 mg IV every 12–24 hours
Esomeprazole	40 mg IV every 12–24 hours

H_2RA, histamine-2 receptor antagonist; NG, nasogastric; PPI, proton pump inhibitor.

[a]Product is FDA approved for the prevention of stress-related mucosal bleeding.
[b]Administered as an extemporaneously compounded suspension made with sodium bicarbonate.
[c]Administered as a rapidly disintegrating tablet given orally or by NG tube dissolved in 10 mL of water.

Parenteral H_2RAs may be administered as either continuous infusions or intermittent bolus doses (see Table 20-15). Cimetidine, given as a continuous IV infusion, is the only FDA-labeled H_2RA for the prevention of SRMB. Despite evidence suggesting that continuous infusions of the H_2RAs are superior to intermittent dosing at maintaining an intragastric pH >4, there is no evidence to suggest better outcomes with respect to prevention of SRMB.[107] Thus, intermittent bolus doses of H_2RAs are used more commonly than continuous infusions.[108,110] Drug interactions are more common with cimetidine, and for this reason the other H_2RAs (famotidine, ranitidine) are used more frequently.[107] Adverse events associated with the use of H_2RAs for the critically ill patient include thrombocytopenia, mental status changes (more common in older patients or individuals with renal or hepatic compromise), and tachyphylaxis (especially with parenteral or high-dose therapy).[107] Given that the H_2RAs are renally eliminated, dosage reductions are recommended for patients with renal dysfunction.

The PPIs are more potent than H_2RAs in inhibiting acid secretion and, unlike H_2RAs, tolerance does not develop.[107,108,110,122] Although there are limited data assessing the efficacy of PPIs for the prevention of SRMB, recent reports suggest that PPIs may be used as alternatives to H_2RAs or sucralfate.[122,125,126] Initial open-label studies of PPIs for SRMB prophylaxis were performed with omeprazole compounded suspensions given as 40 mg for two doses on the first day, followed by 20 mg/day thereafter in critically ill or trauma patients requiring mechanical ventilation and the presence of at least one additional risk factor.[127,128] The results of these studies demonstrated significant pH control above 4 and no GI bleeding in either trial. Because of the small number of subjects, no firm clinical outcomes can be derived from these studies. Since then, numerous extemporaneously compounded sodium bicarbonate suspensions of PPIs (see Tables 20-12 and 20-15) have been used as cost-effective regimens for stress ulcer prophylaxis in patients with NG tubes.[107,110,122,129] In one study, immediate-release omeprazole–sodium bicarbonate suspension (40 mg × 2 doses, and then 40 mg/day) was more effective than continuous-infusion cimetidine in maintaining intragastric pH >4 in critically ill patients, but there was no difference in the incidence of clinically important SRMD between the two groups.[125] Based on meeting the prespecified criteria for noninferiority, immediate-release omeprazole gained FDA labeling for the prevention of SRMB.[125] In another trial of ICU patients requiring mechanical ventilation, patients were randomized to receive either lansoprazole 30 mg given as a rapidly disintegrating tablet mixed in 10 mL of water and administered via an NG tube or lansoprazole 30 mg given as an IV infusion (no longer available in the United States) once daily for 72 hours.[130] Enterally administered lansoprazole, despite having a lower bioavailability, resulted in superior intragastric pH control when compared with the IV-administered lansoprazole.

One of the most compelling dose-finding pilot studies to evaluate the use of IV PPIs for SRMB prophylaxis was performed in over 200 ICU patients examining five different dosing strategies of pantoprazole (40 mg given every 8 hours, every 12 hours, and every 24 hours or 80 mg given every 12 hours or every 24 hours) versus cimetidine given as a 300 mg IV bolus followed by a 50 mg/h continuous infusion.[126] Each regimen was given for at least 48 hours and for up to 7 days. The time the intragastric pH was ≥4 increased from day 1 to 2 in all the pantoprazole groups, whereas it actually decreased in the cimetidine group suggesting tachyphylaxis. No bleeding was identified in any of the treatment groups. The results suggest appropriate pH control can be obtained with doses of 80 mg given on day 1 and 40 mg given every 12 hours thereafter. The use of IV esomeprazole has also demonstrated efficacy in a small number of clinical studies.[107] Given the relatively limited data, the overall efficacy, optimal dosage, frequency, and route of administration for PPIs in the prevention of SRMB remain to be fully elucidated.[107,108] Based on the available evidence, several PPI dosing regimens for SRMB prophylaxis exist (see Table 20-15). Adverse events that have been described when the PPIs are used for this indication include an increased risk of enteric infections, including *C. difficile*–associated diarrhea and nosocomial pneumonia.[107]

9 When deciding on the most appropriate pharmacotherapy plan for the prevention of SRMB for a specific patient, the clinical presentation of the patient and medication costs should be used as a guide. Patients who can take oral medication or have a working NG tube in place may be placed on an oral or compounded PPI suspension as a cost-effective measure. For most patients who are not able to utilize one of these routes, an IV H_2RA is appropriate. However, if the patient has renal dysfunction, develops thrombocytopenia, or mental status changes while on an H_2RA, then an IV PPI may be the most appropriate prophylaxis option. Consideration should be given to both the patient's clinical condition and the most cost-effective option when developing protocols for preventing SRMB.

Improvement in the patient's overall medical condition (resolution of risk factors, discharge from the ICU, extubation, and oral intake) suggests that prophylactic therapy can be discontinued.[107] Too often the patient is continued on SRMB prophylaxis on transition to the general medical/surgical unit and is often discharged on oral PPI therapy without an appropriate indication.[87] This results in unnecessary costs for the patient and the healthcare system.[87] Pharmacists should identify patients in whom SRMB prophylaxis is no longer indicated.[107] If a patient develops clinically important bleeding, endoscopic evaluation of the GI tract is indicated along with aggressive antisecretory therapy (see Peptic Ulcer–Related Bleeding above).

ABBREVIATIONS

ATPase	adenosine triphosphatase
BAO	basal acid output
CAP	community-acquired pneumonia
CLASS	Celecoxib Long-Term Arthritis Safety Study
COX	cyclooxygenase
COX-1	cyclooxygenase-1
COX-2	cyclooxygenase-2
CYP450	cytochrome P450
ECL	enterochromaffin-like
GERD	gastroesophageal reflux disease
H_2RA	histamine-2 receptor antagonist
ICU	intensive care unit
IL	interleukin
INR	international normalized ratio
MALT	mucosa-associated lymphoid tissue
MAO	maximal acid output
MEN 1	multiple endocrine neoplasia type 1
NG	nasogastric
NSAID	nonsteroidal antiinflammatory drug
NUD	nonulcer dyspepsia
PG	prostaglandin
PPI	proton pump inhibitor
PUD	peptic ulcer disease
SRMB	stress-related mucosal bleeding
SRMD	stress-related mucosal damage
TNF-α	tumor necrosis factor-α
UBT	urea breath test
ZES	Zollinger-Ellison syndrome

REFERENCES

1. Soll AH, Graham DY. Peptic ulcer disease. In: Yamada T, Alpers DH, Kalloo KN, et al., eds. Textbook of Gastroenterology, 5th ed. Hoboken, NJ: Wiley-Blackwell, 2009:936–981.
2. Washington MK, Peek RM. Gastritis and gastropathy. In: Yamada T, Alpers DH, Kalloo KN, et al., eds. Textbook of Gastroenterology, 5th ed. Hoboken, NJ: Wiley-Blackwell, 2009:1005–1025.
3. Del Valle J. Zollinger-Ellison syndrome. In: Yamada T, Alpers DH, Kalloo KN, et al., eds. Textbook of Gastroenterology, 5th ed. Hoboken, NJ: Wiley-Blackwell, 2009:982–1004.
4. Everhart JE, Ruhl CE. Burden of digestive diseases in the United States part I: Overall and upper gastrointestinal diseases. Gastroenterology 2009;136:376–386.
5. Chey WD, Wong BCY, Practice Parameters Committee of American College of Gastroenterology. Guideline on the management of *Helicobacter pylori* infection. Am J Gastroenterol 2007;102:1–18.
6. Azevedo NF, Huntington J, Goodman KJ. The epidemiology of *Helicobacter pylori* and public health implications. Helicobacter 2009;14(Suppl 1):1–7.
7. Talley NJ, Fock KM, Moayyedi P. Gastric cancer consensus conference recommends *Helicobacter pylori* screening and treatment in asymptomatic persons from high-risk populations to prevent gastric cancer. Am J Gastroenterol 2008;103:510–514.
8. Leung WK, Ng EKW, Sung JJY. Tumors of the stomach. In: Yamada T, Alpers DH, Kalloo KN, et al., eds. Textbook of Gastroenterology, 5th ed. Hoboken, NJ: Wiley-Blackwell, 2009:1026–1053.
9. Talley NJ, Holtmann G. Approach to the patient with dyspepsia and related functional gastrointestinal complaints. In: Yamada T, Alpers DH, Kalloo KN, et al., eds. Principles of Clinical Gastroenterology, 1st ed. Hoboken, NJ: Wiley-Blackwell, 2008:38–61.
10. Furuta T, Delchier JC. *Helicobacter pylori* and non-malignant diseases. Helicobacter 2009;14(Suppl 1):29–35.

11. Pellicano R, Franceschi F, Saracco G, et al. *Helicobacters* and extragastric diseases. Helicobacter 2009;14(Suppl 1):58–68.
12. Lanza FL, Chan FKL, Quigley EMM, Practice Parameters Committee of the American College of Gastroenterology. Guidelines for prevention of NSAID-related ulcer complications. Am J Gastroenterol 2009;104:728–738.
13. Bhatt DL, Scheiman J, Abraham NS, et al. ACCF/ACG/AHA 2008 expert consensus document on reducing the gastrointestinal risks of antiplatelet therapy and NSAID use: A report of the American College of Cardiology Foundation Task Force on clinical expert consensus documents. Am J Gastroenterol 2008;103:2890–2907.
14. Chan FKL Abraham NS, Scheiman JM, Laine L. Management of patients on nonsteroidal anti-inflammatory drugs: A clinical practice recommendation from the First International Working Party on Gastrointestinal and Cardiovascular Effects of Nonsteroidal Anti-Inflammatory Drugs and Anti-Platelet Agents. Am J Gastroenterol 2008;103:2908–2918.
15. Cryer B. Management of patients with high gastrointestinal risk on antiplatelet therapy. Gastroenterol Clin North Am 2009;38:289–303.
16. Rostom A, Moayyedi P, Hunt R, Canadian Association of Gastroenterology Consensus Group. Canadian consensus guidelines on long-term nonsteroidal anti-inflammatory drug therapy and the need for gastroprotection: Benefits versus risks. Aliment Pharmacol Ther 2009;29:481–496.
17. Lanas A, Sopena F. Nonsteroidal anti-inflammatory drugs and lower gastrointestinal complication. Gastroenterol Clin North Am 2009;38:333–352.
18. Chan FKL. The David Y. Graham Lecture: Use of nonsteroidal antiinflammatory drugs in a COX-2 restricted environment. Am J Gastroenterol 2008;103:221–227.
19. Scheiman JM. Balancing risks and benefits of cyclooxygenase-2 selective nonsteroidal anti-inflammatory drugs. Gastroenterol Clin North Am 2009;38:305–314.
20. Loke YK, Trivedi AN, Singh S. Meta-analysis: Gastrointestinal bleeding due to interaction between selective serotonin uptake inhibitors and non-steroidal anti-inflammatory drugs. Aliment Pharmacol Ther 2008;27:31–40.
21. Del Valle J, Tedisco A. Gastric secretion. In: Yamada T, Alpers DH, Kalloo KN, et al., eds. Textbook of Gastroenterology, 5th ed. Hoboken, NJ: Wiley-Blackwell, 2009:284–329.
22. Costa AC, Figueiredo C, Touati E. Pathogenesis of *Helicobacter pylori* infection. Helicobacter 2009;14(Suppl 1): 15–20.
23. Glasglow RE, Mulvihill SJ. Surgery for peptic ulcer disease and postgastrectomy syndromes. In: Yamada T, Alpers DH, Kalloo KN, et al., eds. Textbook of Gastroenterology, 5th ed. Hoboken, NJ: Wiley-Blackwell, 2009:1054–1070.
24. Monteiro L, Oleastro M, Lehours P, Megraud F. Diagnosis of *Helicobacter pylori* infection. Helicobacter 2009;14(Suppl 1): 8–14.
25. Malfertheiner P, Megraud F, O'Morain C, et al. Current concepts in the management of *Helicobacter pylori* infection—The Maastricht III Consensus Report. Gut 2007;56:772–781.
26. O'Connor A, Gisbert J, O'Morain C. Treatment of *Helicobacter pylori* infection. Helicobacter 2009;14(Suppl 1):46–51.
27. Vakil N. *H. pylori* treatment: New wine in old bottles? Am J Gastroenterol 2009;104:26–30.
28. Rokkas P, Sechopoulos P, Robotis I, et al. Cumulative *H. pylori* eradication rates in clinical practice by adopting first and second-line regimens proposed by the Maastricht III Consensus and a third-line empirical regimen. Am J Gastroenterol 2009;104:21–25.
29. Malfertheiner P, Chan FKL, McColl KEL. Peptic ulcer disease. Lancet 2009;374:1449–1461.
30. Kindermann A, Lopes AI. *Helicobacter pylori* infection in pediatrics. Helicobacter 2009;14(Suppl 1):52–57.
31. Francavilla R, Lionetti E, Cavallo L. Sequential treatment for *Helicobacter pylori* eradication in children. Gut 2008;57:1178.
32. Boparai V, Rajagopalan J, Triadafilopoulos G. Guide to the use of proton pump inhibitors in adult patients. Drugs 2008;68:925–947.
33. Villoria A, Garcia P, Calvet X, et al. Meta-analysis: High-dose proton pump inhibitors vs. standard dose in triple therapy for *Helicobacter pylori* eradication. Aliment Pharmacol Ther 2008;28:868–877.
34. Vergara M, Vallve M, Gisbert JP, et al. Meta-analysis: Comparative efficacy of different proton-pump inhibitors in triple therapy for *Helicobacter pylori* eradication. Aliment Pharmacol Ther 2003;18:647–654.
35. Graham DY, Hammoud F, el-Zimaity HM, et al. Meta-analysis: Proton pump inhibitor or H_2-receptor antagonist for *Helicobacter pylori* eradication. Aliment Pharmacol Ther 2003;17:1229–1236.
36. Gisbert JP, Khorrami S, Calvet X, et al. Meta-analysis: Proton pump inhibitors vs. H_2-receptor antagonists—Their efficacy with antibiotics in *Helicobacter pylori* eradication. Aliment Pharmacol Ther 2003;18:757–766.
37. Janssen MJR, Laheij RJF, Boer WA, et al. Meta-analysis: The influence of pre-treatment with a proton pump inhibitor on *Helicobacter pylori* eradication. Aliment Pharmacol Ther 2005;21:341–345.
38. Luther J, Higgins PDR, Schoenfeld PS, et al. Empiric quadruple vs. triple therapy for primary treatment of *Helicobacter pylori* infection: Systematic review and meta-analysis of efficacy and tolerability. Am J Gastroenterol 2010;105:65–73.
39. Laine L, Hunt R, el-Zimaity H, et al. Bismuth-based quadruple therapy using a single capsule of bismuth biskalcitrate, metronidazole, and tetracycline given with omeprazole versus omeprazole, amoxicillin, and clarithromycin for eradication of *Helicobacter pylori* in duodenal ulcer patients: A prospective, randomized, multicenter, North American trial. Am J Gastroenterol 2003;98:562–567.
40. Fischbach LA, van Zanten S, Dickason J. Meta-analysis: The efficacy, adverse events, and adherence related to firstline anti-*Helicobacter pylori* quadruple therapies. Aliment Pharmacol Ther 2004;20:1071–1082.
41. Laine L. Is it time for quadruple therapy to be first line? Can J Gastroenterol 2003;17(Suppl B):33B–35B.
42. Jafri NS, Hornung CA, Howden CW. Meta-analysis: Sequential therapy appears superior to standard therapy for *Helicobacter pylori* infection in patients naive to treatment. Ann Intern Med 2008;148:1–9.
43. O'Morain CA, O'Connor JP. Is sequential therapy superior to standard triple therapy for the treatment of *Helicobacter pylori* infection? Nat Clin Pract Gastroenterol Hepatol 2009;6:8–9.
44. Megraud F, Lamouliatte H. Review article: The treatment of refractory *Helicobacter pylori* infection. Aliment Pharmacol Ther 2003;17:1333–1343.
45. Napolitano L. Refractory peptic ulcer disease. Gastroenterol Clin North Am 2009;38:267–288.
46. Saad RJ, Schoenfeld P, Kim HM, et al. Levofloxacin-based triple therapy versus bismuth-based quadruple therapy for persistent *Helicobacter pylori* infection: A meta-analysis. Am J Gastroenterol 2006;101:488–496.
47. Gisbert JP, Perez-Aisa A, Castro-Fernandez M, et al. *Helicobacter pylori* first-line treatment and rescue option

containing levofloxacin in patients allergic to penicillin. Dig Liver Dis 2010;42:287–290.

48. Suzuki T, Matsuo K, Sawaki A, et al. Systematic review and meta-analysis: Importance of CagA status for successful eradication of *Helicobacter pylori* infection. Aliment Pharmacol Ther 2006;24:273–280.
49. Padol S, Yuan Y, Thabane M, et al. The effect of CYP2C19 polymorphisms on *H. pylori* eradication rate in dual and triple first-line PPI therapies: A meta-analysis. Am J Gastroenterol 2006;101:1467–1475.
50. Fischbach L, Evans EL. Meta-analysis: The effect of antibiotic resistance status on the efficacy of triple and quadruple first-line therapies for *Helicobacter pylori*. Aliment Pharmacol Ther 2007;26:343–357.
51. Meyer JM, Silliman NP, Wang W, et al. Risk factors for *Helicobacter pylori* resistance in the United States: The surveillance of *H. pylori* antimicrobial resistance partnership (SHARP) study, 1993–1999. Ann Intern Med 2002;136:13–24.
52. Duck WM, Sobel J, Pruckler JM, et al. Antimicrobial resistance incidence and risk actors among *Helicobacter pylori*-infected persons in the United States. Emerg Infect Dis 2004;10:1088–1094.
53. Gotteland M, Brunser O, Cruchet S. Systematic review: Are probiotics useful in controlling gastric colonization by *Helicobacter pylori*. Aliment Pharmacol Ther 2006;23: 1077–1086.
54. Kim MN, Kim N, Lee SH, et al. The effects of probiotics on PPI-triple therapy for *Helicobacter pylori* eradication. Helicobacter 2008;13:261–268.
55. Scaccianoce G, Zullo A, Hassan C, et al. Triple therapies plus different probiotics for *Helicobacter pylori* eradication. Eur Rev Med Pharmacol Sci 2008;12:251–256.
56. Targownik LE, Metge CJ, Leung S, et al. The relative efficacies of gastroprotective strategies in chronic users of nonsteroidal anti-inflammatory drugs. Gastroenterology 2008;134:937–944.
57. Silverstein FE, Graham DY, Senior JR, et al. Misoprostol reduces serious gastrointestinal complications in patients with rheumatoid arthritis receiving nonsteroidal anti-inflammatory drugs: A randomized, double-blind, placebo-controlled trial. Ann Intern Med 1995;123:241–249.
58. Graham DY, Agrawal NM, Campbell DR, et al. Ulcer prevention in long-term users of nonsteroidal anti-inflammatory drugs: Results of a double-blind, randomized, multicenter, active- and placebo-controlled study of misoprostol vs lansoprazole. Arch Intern Med 2002;152:169–175.
59. Arora G, Singh G, Triadafilopoulos G. Proton pump inhibitors for gastroduodenal damage related to nonsteroidal antiinflammatory drugs or aspirin: Twelve important questions for clinical practice. Clin Gastroenterol Hepatol 2009;7:725–736.
60. Taha AT, McCloskey C, Prasad R, Bezlyak V. Famotidine for the prevention of peptic ulcers and oesophagitis in patients taking low-dose aspirin (FAMOUS): A phase III, randomised, double-blind, placebo-controlled trial. Lancet 2009;374:119–125.
61. Silverstein F, Faich G, Goldstein JL, et al. Gastrointestinal toxicity with celecoxib vs nonsteroidal antiinflammatory drugs for osteoarthritis and rheumatoid arthritis. The CLASS study: A randomized controlled trial. JAMA 2000;284:1247–1255.
62. Bombardier C, Laine L, Reicin A, et al. Comparison of upper intestinal toxicity of rofecoxib and naproxen in patients with rheumatoid arthritis. VIGOR Study Group. N Engl J Med 2000;343:1520–1528.
63. US Food and Drug Administration. Drug Information. COX-2 Selective and Non-Selective Non-Steroidal Anti-Inflammatory Drugs (NSAIDs). *http://www.fda.gov/cder/drug/infopage/cox2/default.htm*.
64. Bresalier RS, Sandler RS, Quan H, et al. Cardiovascular events associated with rofecoxib in colorectal adenoma chemoprevention trial. N Engl J Med 2005;352:1092–1102.
65. Kearney PM, Baigent C, Godwin J, et al. Do selective cyclooxygenase-2 inhibitors and traditional non-steroidal antiinflammatory drugs increase the risk of atherothrombosis? Meta-analysis of randomized trials. BMJ 2006;322:1302–1308.
66. Fiorucci S. Prevention of nonsteroidal anti-inflammatory drug-induced ulcer: Looking forward to the future. Gastroenterol Clin North Am 2009;38:315–322.
67. McColl KEL. How I manage *H. pylori*-negative, NSAID/aspirin-negative peptic ulcers. Am J Gastroenterol 2009;104:190–193.
68. Gisbert JP, Calvert X. *Helicobacter pylori*-negative duodenal ulcer disease. Aliment Pharmacol Ther 2009;30:791–815.
69. Reimer C, Sondergaard G, Hilsted L, et al. Proton-pump inhibitor therapy induces acid-related symptoms in healthy volunteers after withdrawal of therapy. Gastroenterology 2009;137:80–87.
70. Dexilant (dexlansoprazole) [package insert]. Deerfield, IL: Takeda Pharmaceuticals America Inc. *http://www.dexilant.com/PI.aspx*.
71. Metz DC, Valiky M, Dixit T, et al. Review article: Dual delayed release formulation of dexlansoprazole MR, a novel approach to overcome the limitations of conventional single release proton pump inhibitor therapy. Aliment Pharmacol Ther 2009;29:928–937.
72. Zegerid (omeprazole/sodium bicarbonate) [package insert]. San Diego, CA: Santarus Inc. *http://www.zegerid.com/assets/pdfs/prescribing_information.pdf*.
73. Lahner E, Annibale B, Fave GD. Systematic review: Impaired drug absorption related to the co-administration of antisecretory therapy. Aliment Pharmacol Ther 2009;29: 219–229.
74. Béïque L, Giguère P, la Porte C, Angel J. Interactions between protease inhibitors and acid-reducing agents: A systematic review. HIV Med 2007;8:335–345.
75. Sachmechi I, Reich DM, Aninyei M, et al. Effect of proton pump inhibitors on serum thyroid-stimulating hormone level in euthyroid patients treated with levothyroxine for hypothyroidism. Endocr Pract 2007;13:345–349.
76. Parikh N, Howden CW. The safety of drugs used in acid-related disorders and functional gastrointestinal disorders. Gastroenterol Clin North Am 2010;39:529–542.
77. U.S. Food and Drug Administration. Information for Healthcare Professionals: Update to the Labeling of Clopidogrel Bisulfate (Marketed as Plavix) to Alert Healthcare Professionals About a Drug Interaction with Omeprazole (Marketed as Prilosec and Prilosec OTC). *http://www.fda.gov/Drugs/DrugSafety/PostmarketDrugSafetyInformationforPatientsandProviders/DrugSafetyInformationforHeathcareProfessionals/ucm190787.htm*.
78. U.S. Food and Drug Administration. Public Health Advisory: Updated Information About a Drug Interaction Between Clopidogrel Bisulfate (Marketed as Plavix) and Omeprazole (Marketed as Prilosec and Prilosec OTC). 2009, *http://www.fda.gov/Drugs/DrugSafety/PublicHealthAdvisories/ucm190825.htm*.
79. U.S. Food and Drug Administration. Information for Healthcare Professionals: Update to the Labelling of Clopidogrel Bisulfate (Marketed as Plavix) to Alert Healthcare Practitioners About a Drug Interaction

with Omeprazole (Marketed as Prilosec and Prilosec OTC). *http://www.fda.gov/Drugs/DrugSafety/PostmarketDrugSafetyInformationforPatientsandProviders/DrugSafetyInformationforHeathcareProfessionals/ucm19078.htm.*

80. Plavix (clopidogrel bisulfate tablets). Bridgewater, NJ: Bristol-Myers Squibb/Sanofi Pharmaceuticals Partnership. Revised 2009, *http://products.sanofi-aventis.us/PLAVIX/plavix.pdf.*
81. Mega JL, Close SL, Wiviott SD, et al. Cytochrome P-450 polymorphisms and response to clopidogrel. N Engl J Med 2009;360:354–362.
82. Freedman JE, Hylek EM. Clopidogrel, genetics, and drug responsiveness. N Engl J Med 2009;360:411–413.
83. Last EJ, Sheehan AH. Review of recent evidence: Potential interaction between clopidogrel and proton pump inhibitors. Am J Health Syst Pharm 2009;66:2117–2122.
84. Norgard NB, Mathews KD, Wall GC. Drug–drug interaction between clopidogrel and proton pump inhibitors. Ann Pharmacother 2009;43:1266–1274.
85. Sheen E, Triadafilopoulos G. Adverse effects of long-term proton pump inhibitor therapy. Dig Dis Sci 2011;56: 931–950.
86. Ali T, Roberts DN, Tierney WM. Long-term safety concerns with proton pump inhibitors. Am J Med 2009;122:896–903.
87. Heidelbaugh JJ, Goldberg KL, Inadomi JM. Overutilization of proton pump inhibitors: A review of cost-effectiveness and risk. Am J Gastroenterol 2009;104(Suppl):S27–S32.
88. Williams C, McColl KE. Review article: Proton pump inhibitors and bacterial overgrowth. Aliment Pharmacol Ther 2006;23:3–10.
89. Laheij RJF, Sturkenboom MCJM, Hassing R-J, et al. Risk of community-acquired pneumonia and use of gastric acid-suppressive drugs. JAMA 2004;292:1955–1960.
90. Gulmez SE, Holm A, Frederiksen H, et al. Use of proton pump inhibitors and the risk of community-acquired pneumonia: A population-based case–control study. Arch Intern Med 2007;167:950–955.
91. Sarkar M, Hennessy S, Yang YX. Proton-pump inhibitor use and the risk of community-acquired pneumonia. Ann Intern Med 2008;149:391–398.
92. Leonard J, Marshall JK, Moayyedi P. Systematic review of the risk of enteric infection in patients taking acid suppression. Am J Gastroenterol 2007;102:2047–2056.
93. US Food and Drug Administration. FDA Safety Communication: Possible Increase Risk of Fractures of the Hip, Wrist and Spine with the Use of Proton Pump Inhibitors. *http://www.fda.gov/Drugs/DrugSafety/PostmarketDrugSafetyInformationforPatientsandProviders/ucm213206.htm.*
94. Kahrilas PJ, Shaheen NJ, Vaezi MF. American Gastroenterological Association Medical Position Statement on management of GERD. Gastroenterology 2008;135:1383–1391.
95. Furuta K, Adachi K, Komazawa Y, et al. Tolerance to H_2-receptor antagonist correlates well with the decline in efficacy against gastroesophageal reflux in patients with gastroesophageal reflux disease. J Gastroenterol Hepatol 2006;21:1581–1585.
96. Zweber A, Berardi RR. Heartburn and Dyspepsia. In: Berardi RR, Ferreri SP, Hume AL, et al., eds. Handbook of Nonprescription Drugs, 16th ed. Washington, DC: American Pharmaceutical Association, 2009:231–246.
97. Wade EE, Rebuck JA, Healey MA, Rogers FB. H_2 antagonist-induced thrombocytopenia: Is this a real phenomenon? Intensive Care Med 2002;28:459–465.
98. Chong YS, Su LL, Arulkumaran S. Misoprostol: A quarter century of use, abuse and creative misuse. Obstet Gynecol Surg 2004;59:128–140.
99. Maton PN, Burton ME. Antacids revisited: A review of their clinical pharmacology and recommended therapeutic use. Drugs 1999;57:855–870.
100. Kang JM, Kim N, Lee DH, et al. Effect of the CYP2C19 polymorphism on the eradication rate of *Helicobacter pylori* infection by 7-day triple therapy with regular proton-pump inhibitor dosage. J Gastroenterol Hepatol 2008;23:1287–1291.
101. Ma Q, Lu AYH. Pharmacogenetics, pharmacogenomics, and individualized medicine. Pharmacol Rev 2011;63:437–459.
102. Kawai T, Yamagishi T, Yagi K, et al. Tailored eradication therapy based on fecal *Helicobacter pylori* clarithromycin sensitivities. J Gastroenterol Hepatol 2008;23:S171–S174.
103. Gralnek IM, Barkun AN, Bardou M. Management of acute bleeding from a peptic ulcer. N Engl J Med 2008;359:928–937.
104. Barkun AN, Bardou M, Kuipers EJ, et al. International consensus recommendations on the management of patients with nonvariceal upper gastrointestinal bleeding. Ann Intern Med 2010;152:101–113.
105. Bjorkman DJ. Endoscopic diagnosis and treatment of nonvariceal upper gastrointestinal hemorrhage. In: Yamada T, Alpers DH, Kalloo KN, et al., eds. Textbook of Gastroenterology, 5th ed. Hoboken, NJ: Wiley-Blackwell, 2009:3018–3031.
106. American Society of Health-System Pharmacists therapeutic guidelines on stress ulcer prophylaxis. Am J Health Syst Pharm 1999;56:347–379.
107. Ali T, Harty RF. Stress-induced ulcer bleeding in critically ill patients. Gastroenterol Clin North Am 2009;38:245–265.
108. Stollman N, Metz DC. Pathophysiology and prophylaxis of stress ulcer in intensive care unit patients. J Crit Care 2005;20:35–45.
109. Laine L, Takeuchi K, Tarnawski A. Gastric mucosal defense and cytoprotection: Bench to bedside. Gastroenterology 2008;135:41–60.
110. Devlin JW, Welage LS, Olsen KM. Proton pump inhibitor formulary considerations in the acutely ill—Part 2: Clinical efficacy, safety, and economics. Ann Pharmacother 2005;39:1844–1851.
111. Elmunzer BJ, Inadomi JM, Elta GH. Risk stratification in upper gastrointestinal bleeding. J Clin Gastroenterol 2007;41:559–563.
112. Chiu PWY, Ng EKW. Predicting poor outcome from acute upper gastrointestinal hemorrhage. Gastroenterol Clin North Am 2009;38:215–230.
113. Blatchford O, Murray WR, Blatchford M. A risk score to predict need for treatment for upper-gastrointestinal haemorrhage. Lancet 2000;356:1318–1321.
114. Rockall TA, Logan RF, Devlin HB, et al. Risk assessment after acute upper gastrointestinal haemorrhage. Gut 1996;38:316–321.
115. Leontiadis GI, Sharma VK, Howden CW. Proton pump inhibitor therapy for peptic ulcer bleeding: Cochrane Collaboration meta-analysis of randomized controlled trials. Mayo Clin Proc 2007;82:286–296.
116. Leontiadis GI, Howden CW. The role of proton pump inhibitors in the management of upper gastrointestinal bleeding. Gastroenterol Clin North Am 2009;38:199–213.
117. Bardou M, Toubouti Y, Benhaberou-Brun D, et al. Meta-analysis: Proton-pump inhibitors in high-risk patients with acute peptic ulcer bleeding. Aliment Pharmacol Ther 2005;21:677–686.
118. Sung JYJ, Barkun A, Kuipers EJ, et al. Intravenous esomeprazole for prevention of recurrent peptic

ulcer bleeding: A randomized trial. Ann Intern Med 2009;150:455–464.

119. Lau JY, Leung WK, Wu JCY, et al. Omeprazole before endoscopy in patients with gastrointestinal bleeding. N Engl J Med 2007;356:1631–1640.

120. Sung JJ, Chan FK, Lau JY. The effect of endoscopic therapy in patients receiving omeprazole for bleeding ulcers with nonbleeding visible vessels or adherent clots. Ann Intern Med 2003;139:237–243.

121. Gisbert JP, Abraiira V. Accuracy of *Helicobacter pylori* diagnostic tests in patients with bleeding peptic ulcer: A systematic review and meta-analysis. Am J Gastroenterol 2006;101:848–863.

122. Jung R, MacLaren R. Proton-pump inhibitors for stress ulcer prophylaxis in critically ill patients. Ann Pharmacother 2002;36:1929–1937.

123. Cook D, Guyatt G, Marshall J, et al. A comparison of sucralfate and ranitidine for the prevention of upper gastrointestinal bleeding in patients requiring mechanical ventilation. N Engl J Med 1998;338:791–797.

124. Daley RJ, Rebuck JA, Welage LS, Rogers FB. Prevention of stress ulceration: Current trends in critical care. Crit Care Med 2004;32:2008–2013.

125. Conrad SA, Gabrielli A, Margolis B, et al. Randomized, double-blind comparison of immediate-release omeprazole oral suspension versus intravenous cimetidine for the prevention of upper gastrointestinal bleeding in critically ill patients. Crit Care Med 2005;33:760–765.

126. Somberg L, Morris J, Fantus R, et al. Intermittent intravenous pantoprazole and continuous cimetidine infusion: Effect on gastric pH control in critically ill patients at risk of developing stress-related mucosal disease. J Trauma 2008;64:1202–1210.

127. Phillips JO, Metzler MH, Palmirei MT, et al. A prospective study of simplified omeprazole suspension for the prophylaxis of stress-related mucosal damage. Crit Care Med 1996;24:1793–1800.

128. Lasky MR, Metzler MH, Phillips JO. A prospective study of omeprazole suspension to prevent clinically significant gastrointestinal bleeding from stress ulcers in mechanically ventilated trauma patients. J Trauma 1998;44:527–533.

129. Devlin JW, Welage LS, Olsen KM. Proton pump inhibitor formulary considerations in the acutely ill—Part 1: Pharmacology, pharmacodynamics and available formulations. Ann Pharmacother 2005;39:1667–1677.

130. Olsen KM, Devlin JW. Comparison of the enteral and intravenous lansoprazole pharmacodynamic responses in critically ill patients. Aliment Pharmacol Ther 2008;28: 326–333.

21 Inflammatory Bowel Disease

Brian A. Hemstreet

KEY CONCEPTS

1. The exact cause of inflammatory bowel disease (IBD) is unknown. Proposed causes include infectious, genetic, and environmental factors, as well as immune dysregulation.
2. Ulcerative colitis (UC) is confined to the rectum and colon, causes continuous lesions, and affects primarily the mucosa and the submucosa. Crohn's disease (CD) can involve any part of the GI tract, often causes discontinuous (skip) lesions, and is a transmural process that can result in fistulas, perforations, or strictures.
3. Common GI complications of IBD include rectal fissures, fistulas (CD), perirectal abscess (UC), toxic megacolon (UC), and colon cancer. Extraintestinal manifestations include hepatobiliary complications, arthritis, uveitis, skin lesions (including erythema nodosum and pyoderma gangrenosum), osteoporosis, anemia, and aphthous ulcerations of the mouth.
4. The severity of UC may be assessed by stool frequency, presence of blood in stool, fever, pulse, hemoglobin, erythrocyte sedimentation rate (ESR), C-reactive protein (CRP), abdominal tenderness, and radiologic or endoscopic findings. The severity of CD can be assessed using similar parameters, in addition to the CD Activity Index, which includes stool frequency, presence of blood in stool, endoscopic appearance, and physician's global assessment.
5. The goals of IBD treatment are resolution of acute inflammation and complications, alleviation of systemic manifestations, and maintenance of remission.
6. The first line of treatment for mild to moderate extensive UC consists of oral aminosalicylates with oral controlled release budesonide as an alternative. Mesalamine or steroid enemas or suppositories may be used for distal disease. Mesalamine is less effective for CD; however, certain delayed-release oral formulations of mesalamine may be used for Crohn's ileitis. Controlled-release budesonide is preferred as a first-line agent for CD confined to the terminal ileum and/or ascending colon.
7. Systemic corticosteroids are often required for acute UC or CD. The duration of steroid use should be minimized and the dose tapered gradually over 3 to 4 weeks.
8. Infliximab or adalimumab is a treatment option for patients with moderate to severe active UC and for those patients with UC who are corticosteroid dependent. Azathioprine or mercaptopurine may be used for maintenance of remission as an alternative to or in combination with infliximab for patients with UC who have failed aminosalicylates and for patients who are corticosteroid dependent.
9. IV continuous infusion of cyclosporine may be effective in treating severe colitis that is refractory to corticosteroids as an option to delay or prevent the need for surgery.
10. Aminosalicylates can prevent recurrence of acute UC in many patients, while steroids are ineffective for this purpose.
11. Other treatments for CD include infliximab, adalimumab, and certolizumab (for moderate to severe or fistulizing disease as both induction and maintenance therapies); methotrexate, azathioprine, or mercaptopurine (for inadequate response or to reduce steroid dosage and in combination with infliximab); metronidazole (for perineal or colonic disease); natalizumab (for patients failing tumor necrosis factor-α [TNF-α] antagonists); and cyclosporine (for refractory disease).

There are two forms of idiopathic inflammatory bowel disease (IBD): (a) ulcerative colitis (UC), a mucosal inflammatory condition confined to the rectum and colon, and (b) Crohn's disease (CD), a transmural inflammation of the GI tract that can affect any part, from the mouth to the anus.

EPIDEMIOLOGY

IBD is most prevalent in Western countries and in areas of northern latitude.[1] Rates of IBD are highest in North America, Northern Europe, and Great Britain.[1,2] The incidence of IBD is increasing worldwide.[2,3] CD has an incidence of 0.03 to 15.5 cases per 100,000 persons per year and a prevalence of 3.6 to 214 per 100,000 people per year.[1,2] The incidence of UC ranges from 1.2 to 20 cases per 100,000 persons per year with a prevalence of 7.6 to 246 per 100,000 persons per year.[1] Although most epidemiologic studies combine ulcerative proctitis with UC, 17% to 49% of cases are classified as proctitis.

Both sexes are affected somewhat equally with IBD, although 20% to 30% more women are affected with CD and slightly more males (60%) are affected with UC.[2] Both UC and CD have bimodal distributions in age of initial presentation. The peak incidence occurs in the second (CD) or third (UC) decade of life, with a second peak occurring between 60 and 70 years of age.[1–3] A higher incidence of IBD occurs in the Jewish population, while black and Asian populations have a relatively similar, and possibly lower, incidence of IBD.[2]

ETIOLOGY

1 The exact etiology of UC and CD is unknown; however, there are similar factors believed responsible for both conditions. The major theories behind the cause of IBD involve a combination of infectious, genetic, environmental, and immunologic factors. This may involve abnormal regulation of the innate immune response or

a reaction to various antigens.[4–6] The microflora of the GI tract may provide an environmental trigger to activate inflammation and are highly implicated in the development of IBD.[5,6]

Infectious Factors

Microorganisms are proposed to be a major factor in the initiation of inflammation in IBD. In general, there is thought to be shift toward the presence of more proinflammatory bacteria in the GI tract.[4] However, no one definitive infectious cause of IBD has been found. Patients with IBD have an increased density of intestinal microbiotica compared with those without IBD, including increased numbers of mucus, mucosal, and intraepithelial bacteria.[1,4] The development and composition of the intestinal microbiotica may be influenced by dietary factors.[5] The pathogenesis of IBD may involve a loss of tolerance toward normal GI bacterial flora.[1] Other supporting evidence for an infectious etiology are that colitis does not appear to occur in genetically altered germ-free animals, intestinal lesions in IBD predominate in areas of highest bacterial exposure, and differences are observed in the makeup of the resident luminal and mucosal bacterial flora in healthy subjects versus those with IBD.[7,8]

Microorganisms may play a key role in the development of IBD. Suspect infectious agents include viruses, protozoans, mycobacteria such as *Mycobacterium paratuberculosis* or *avium*, and other bacteria such as *Ruminococcus gnavus*, *Ruminococcus torques*, *Listeria monocytogenes*, *Chlamydia trachomatis*, and *Escherichia coli*.[4–9] Patients with CD typically have circulating antibodies to *Saccharomyces cerevisiae*, which demonstrates some immunologic response to intestinal organisms.[4] Bacterial gene products may promote alteration of the intestinal barrier while bacterial antigens or ligands may include and propagate the inflammatory response.[4,5,10]

Genetic Factors

Genetic factors play a significant role in the predisposition to IBD. Studies of monozygotic twins demonstrate a high concordance rate of IBD in both individuals (particularly CD).[1,11] First-degree relatives of patients with IBD may have up to a 20-fold increase in the risk of disease.[4] Several genetic markers and loci have been identified that occur more frequently in patients with IBD. Genes may not act independently, but rather function in an integrated manner. This is referred to as the "limited pathway model."[4] The nucleotide-binding oligomerization domain protein 2 (NOD2), a key component involved in pathogen recognition in the innate immune system, is the major contributor of genetic predisposition to CD.[11,12] Other genes involved in the innate immune system autophagy, such as ATG16L1 and IRGM, as well as genes involved in the interleukin (IL) biologic pathway such as polymorphisms of the IL-23 receptor IL-23R, and IL-12B, STAT3, and CCR6, are strongly associated with CD and possibly UC (IL23R).[1,11–13] The major genetic region for UC is on chromosome 6p21, in the major histocompatibility region, near human leukocyte antigen (HLA) class II genes.[11] Alterations in the genes encoding for IL-10 and the IL-10 receptor have been implicated in UC.[11,13] Other possible high-risk loci involved in epithelial barrier function such as ECM1, HNF4A, CDH1, and LAMB1, and Th1 and Th17, involved with helper T-cell types, are implicated in the pathophysiology of UC.[1]

Immunologic Mechanisms

The immune system plays a critical role in the pathogenesis of IBD. Potential immunologic mechanisms include both autoimmune and nonautoimmune phenomena. The innate immune system largely involves the intestinal wall epithelial barrier and its associated secretions in response to contact with organisms.[4] NOD proteins (for recognition of organisms) and toll-like membrane receptors (TLRs) are involved in intestinal surveillance and can lead to release of antibacterial peptides such as defensins, among other functions.[4] Reduction in defensin secretion by Paneth cells is thought to be one contributing factor in the loss of effective barrier function.[4,10] Consequently, the bowel wall in CD is infiltrated with lymphocytes, plasma cells, mast cells, macrophages, and neutrophils, often leading to formation of granulomas. Similar infiltration has been observed in the colonic mucosal layer in patients with UC. Given that inflammation is limited to the colon in UC, dysfunction of colonocytes is highly implicated.[1] The colonic mucosal layer in UC may be thinner and less effective in protecting the epithelial cells. This may be due to reduced mucin secretion secondary to defective goblet cell differentiation.[4,10,17] Autoimmune features may be directed against mucosal epithelial cells or against neutrophil cytoplasmic elements.

Antineutrophil cytoplasmic antibodies are found in a high percentage of patients with UC (70%) and less frequently in CD.[6,14] Circulating antibodies to goblet cells and anti-tropomysin are present in UC, although their contribution to the disease process is not fully elucidated.[10] Overproduction of circulating IgG1 antibodies in UC may react with epithelium in the eyes, skin, joints, and biliary tract.[1] Dysfunction or reduced expression of the peroxisome proliferator–activated receptor γ in colonocytes may play a role in this process.[1]

Dysregulation of cytokines is a key component of IBD. Specifically, Th_1 cytokine activity is excessive in CD and increased expression of interferon-γ in the intestinal mucosa and production of IL-12 production are features of the immune response in CD.[6,10] In contrast, Th_2 cytokine activity is excessive with UC.[1,14,15] This is mediated by excess production of IL-13, which contributes to epithelial cell dysfunction by enhancing natural killer T-cell cytotoxicity, and IL-5, which is involved with eosinophil recruitment and activation.[1,10,14] Upregulation of the IL-13 receptor-2α occurs as well.[1,10,14,15] Activated epithelial cells secrete a variety of substances involved in the recruitment of inflammatory cells. These include IL1β, epithelial neutrophil-activating peptide 78, IL-8, and monocyte chemoattractant protein 1.[1] Neutrophils produce proteolytic enzymes, such as matrix metalloproteinase-8 and neutrophil elastase, which further contribute to epithelial damage.[14]

Lastly, tumor necrosis factor-α (TNF-α) is a pivotal proinflammatory cytokine that is increased in the mucosa and intestinal lumen of patients with CD and UC. TNF-α can recruit inflammatory cells to inflamed tissues, activate coagulation, promote the formation of granulomas in patients with CD, and possibly modify epithelial cell apoptosis.[1,14,15]

Psychological Factors

Mental health changes, particularly stress, appear to possibly correlate with disease flares in IBD, but whether psychological factors are true etiologic factors in the pathophysiologic process is unclear.[16–18] Given the complex nature of the disease process and lack of standard measurement processes, documenting the effects of stress in IBD is difficult.[17] Some studies demonstrate that perceived stress and negative mood is significantly different between patients in remission and those experiencing a disease flare.[17,18] Mood-related components, such as anxiety and depression, may contribute to exacerbations of CD.[19] Approximately 50% of patients with IBD reported some type of significant stress during any 3-month period.[20] Additionally, subjects with IBD matched by sex, age, and geographic region to control subjects reported significantly worse psychological well-being and more distress compared with controls.[21] Stress-related interventions in another study did not appear to alter disease course for patients with IBD, but may result in improved quality of life (QOL).[22] While stress and psychological factors may not be a direct cause of IBD, they may significantly affect QOL. This is compounded by the fact that many patients are young at the time of diagnosis, and may require surgical intervention and temporary or permanent ostomy placement.[23]

Lifestyle, Dietary, and Drug-Related Causes

Several theories regarding dietary influence on the development of IBD have been proposed. Intake of refined sugars has been associated with development of CD, while increased protein intake has been associated with a higher risk of developing IBD.[13] Diet composition may directly influence the makeup of the gut microbiotica, possibly triggering IBD.[24,25] The "hygiene hypothesis" proposes that cleaner conditions in more industrialized countries expose patients to fewer microorganisms at an early age. The immune response to these organisms is altered when encountered later in life.[13,25] Diets low in fruits and vegetables and high in ω-6 polyunsaturated fats have been suggested to increase the risk of CD.[24] Changes in expression of the aryl hydrocarbon receptor, a transcription factor activated by dietary ligands and involved in the maintenance of the innate immune response, may increase development of IBD.[26]

Smoking plays an important but contrasting role in UC and CD. It appears to be protective for UC and is associated with fewer disease flare-ups and reduced disease severity. The risk of developing UC is increased for 2 to 3 years after smoking cessation in patients without IBD.[24] In contrast, smoking is associated with increased frequency and severity of CD, and appears to worsen ileal disease more than colonic.[24] Patients with CD who stop smoking have a disease severity that is similar to nonsmokers. Smoking cessation should be offered to all patients. There are data to support transdermal nicotine replacement as an adjunctive therapy in UC.[27]

Use of nonsteroidal antiinflammatory drugs (NSAIDs) may trigger disease occurrence or lead to disease flares.[24,28,29] Inhibition of prostaglandin production through cyclooxygenase inhibition may impair mucosal barrier protective mechanisms. Alteration in platelet function, release of inflammatory mediators, and alteration in the microvascular response to stress are other potential mechanisms of worsening of IBD. Cyclooxygenase-2 inhibitors and cyclooxygenase-1 inhibitors increase risk; however, it is unclear whether cyclooxygenase-2 inhibitors may be safer in select patients with IBD.[2] A large cohort study in U.S. women revealed an increase in risk of developing IBD with NSAID use; however, no association was found with use of aspirin.[28] Use of NSAIDs may be warranted in some patients with IBD, particularly those with arthritic symptoms, if the benefit outweighs the potential risk of disease flare.

An association with development of IBD following use of antibiotics has been found, but a direct causal relationship remains unclear.[24,29] Since antibiotics alter the intestinal flora, this appears to be a viable mechanism; however, delineating antibiotics as a causative factor is difficult given that symptoms may not manifest for several weeks to years following a treatment course. Furthermore, antibiotics may induce *Clostridium difficile* infection, which is a cause of colitis.[24,29] Patients presenting with severe diarrhea for whom a diagnosis of IBD is being entertained should be asked about recent antibiotic use.

Oral contraceptives and isotretinoin have been implicated in the development of IBD as well.[25,30]

PATHOPHYSIOLOGY

UC and CD differ in two general respects: the extent and distribution of inflammation within the GI tract and depth of involvement within the bowel wall. A small fraction of patients have features of both diseases. Confusion can occur, particularly when the inflammation is limited to the colon. For patients in whom it cannot be determined whether they have UC or CD, they are often classified as indeterminate colitis.[1] Table 21-1 compares pathologic and clinical findings of the two diseases.

TABLE 21-1 Comparison of the Clinical and Pathologic Features of Crohn Disease and Ulcerative Colitis

Feature	Crohn Disease	Ulcerative Colitis
Clinical		
Malaise, fever	Common	Uncommon
Rectal bleeding	Common	Common
Abdominal tenderness	Common	May be present
Abdominal mass	Common	Absent
Abdominal pain	Common	Unusual
Abdominal wall and internal fistulas	Common	Absent
Distribution	Discontinuous	Continuous
Aphthous or linear ulcers	Common	Rare
Pathologic		
Rectal involvement	Rare	Common
Ileal involvement	Very common	Rare
Strictures	Common	Rare
Fistulas	Common	Rare
Transmural involvement	Common	Rare
Crypt abscesses	Rare	Very common
Granulomas	Common	Rare
Linear clefts	Common	Rare
Cobblestone appearance	Common	Absent

Ulcerative Colitis

2 UC is confined to the rectum and colon and affects the mucosal and the submucosal layers. In some instances, a short segment of terminal ileum may be inflamed; this is referred to as *backwash ileitis*. Unlike CD, the deeper longitudinal muscular layers, serosa, and regional lymph nodes are not usually involved.[1] Fistula, perforation, or obstruction is uncommon because this is a superficial inflammation.

In UC abscess formation in the crypts of the mucosa occurs (crypts of Lieberkuhn) secondary to infiltration of lymphocytes, plasma cells, and granulocytes.[1] Crypt abscesses are usually visible only with microscopy but may be visible when coalescence results in ulceration. Reduced crypt density, distorted crypt architecture and atrophy, and depletion of goblet cells are typical findings.[1,31] Extension and coalescence of ulcers may surround areas of uninvolved mucosa, causing *pseudopolyp* formation. Mucosal damage and friability in UC can result in significant diarrhea and bleeding, although a small percentage of patients experience constipation.

3 Complications of UC may be local, including hemorrhoids, anal fissures, or perirectal abscesses, and are more likely to be present during active colitis. Extraintestinal manifestations (not directly associated with the colon) may occur and are discussed later.

A major complication is toxic megacolon, which is a segmental or total colonic distension of greater than 6 cm with acute colitis and signs of systemic toxicity.[1,32] It occurs in up to 7.9% of UC patients admitted to hospitals and results in death rates of up to 50%. With toxic megacolon, ulceration extends below the submucosa, sometimes reaching the serosa. Vasculitis, swelling of the vascular endothelium, and thrombosis of small arteries occur. Involvement of the muscularis propria causes loss of colonic tone, leading to dilation and potential perforation. Patients typically have a high fever, tachycardia, distended abdomen, and elevated white blood cell count, and a dilated colon is observed on x-ray.[7,31] Colonic perforation may occur with or without toxic megacolon and is a greater risk with the first episode. Another infrequent major complication is massive colonic hemorrhage. Colonic stricture, sometimes with clinical obstruction, may also complicate long-standing UC.

The risk of colonic dysplasia with transition to colorectal carcinoma (CRC) is fivefold greater for patients with chronic UC with colonic involvement compared with the general population.[33] Patients with ulcerative proctitis or proctosigmoiditis are generally not considered to be at increased risk.[33,34] The cumulative risk of developing CRC in patients with chronic UC may be as high as 20% to 30% at 30 years.[1] Risk factors for CRC include young age at onset (<50 years), severe inflammation, a positive family history, and presence of primary sclerosing cholangitis (PSC) or inflammatory polyps.[1,33,34] Screening colonoscopy with multiple biopsies should be performed at 8 years after onset of symptoms in patients with left-sided or extensive colitis, with subsequent screenings at 1 to 2 years if negative.[34] Patients with PSC should undergo yearly colonoscopy.[34]

Crohn's Disease

CD is characterized as a transmural inflammatory process. The terminal ileum is the most common site of the disorder, but it may occur in any part of the GI tract from mouth to anus.[35,36] Patients often have normal bowel separating segments of diseased bowel resulting in discontinuous disease. The mesentery first becomes thickened and edematous, and then fibrotic. Ulcers are typically deep and elongated and extend along the longitudinal axis of the bowel, at least into the submucosa. The "cobblestone" appearance of the bowel wall results from deep mucosal ulceration intermingled with nodular submucosal thickening.

Bowel wall injury is generally extensive and the intestinal lumen is often narrowed. Small bowel stricture and subsequent obstruction is a complication that may require surgery. Fistula formation is also common, occurring much more frequently than with UC, and is reported as a 20% to 40% lifetime risk in CD.[35] Fistulas often occur in highly inflamed areas, where loops of bowel become matted together by fibrous adhesions. Fistulas may connect a segment of the GI tract to skin (enterocutaneous), two segments of the GI tract (enteroenteric), or the intestinal tract with the bladder (enterovesicular) or vagina. Fistulae associated with CD frequently require surgical treatment.

Bleeding with CD is usually not as severe as with UC, although patients with CD may develop hypochromic anemia. The risk of carcinoma is increased but not as greatly as with UC.[34]

Nutritional deficiencies are common with CD.[37,38] Frequencies of various nutritional parameters are: weight loss, 40% to 80%, up to 90% reported in children at the time of diagnosis; growth failure in children, 15% to 88%; iron deficiency anemia, 39%; vitamin B_{12} deficiency, 18.4%; folate deficiency, 19%; hypoalbuminemia, 17% to 76%; hypokalemia, 33%; and osteomalacia, 36%. There are usually decreased fat stores and lean tissue. Growth failure in children may be associated with low zinc levels.

Extraintestinal Manifestations of IBD

Both forms of IBD are associated with development of symptoms and organ involvement outside of the GI tract referred to as extraintestinal manifestations.

Hepatobiliary Complications

Approximately 11% of patients with UC are reported to have hepatobiliary complications with overall frequencies ranging from 5% to 95% for patients with IBD.[1,39,40] Hepatic complications include fatty liver, pericholangitis, autoimmune hepatitis, and cirrhosis. Biliary complications include PSC, cholangiocarcinoma, and cholelithiasis.[1,20,39]

Fatty infiltration of the liver may result from malabsorption, protein-losing enteropathy, or corticosteroid use. Pericholangitis (acute inflammation surrounding the intrahepatic portal venules, bile ducts, and lymphatics) occurs in up to one third of UC patients. PSC is associated with progressive fibrosis of intrahepatic and extrahepatic bile ducts in 3% to 7% of patients with UC.[39] Cirrhosis may result from cholangitis or chronic active hepatitis. Often the severity of hepatic disease does not correlate with GI disease activity. Gallstones occur in 13% to 34% of patients with CD (particularly with terminal ileal disease) and are related to bile salt malabsorption.[39]

Joint Complications

Arthritis in IBD is typically asymmetric (unlike rheumatoid arthritis) and migratory, involving one or a few usually large joints. The severity parallels IBD disease activity.[1,39] Arthritis may be peripheral or axial in nature and includes sacroiliitis, ankylosing spondylitis, and IBD-associated spondyloarthropathy. Patients positive for HLA-B27 often exhibit axial arthropathy, such as ankylosing spondylitis. Rheumatoid factors are generally not detected and the arthritis is nondeforming and nondestructive. Patients may exhibit enthesopathy, tenosynovitis, or dactylitis.[39]

Ocular Complications

Ocular complications including iritis, uveitis, episcleritis, and conjunctivitis occur in up to 2% to 29% of patients with IBD.[1,39] Commonly reported symptoms with iritis and uveitis include blurred vision, eye pain, and photophobia. Episcleritis is associated with scleral injection, burning, and increased secretions. These complications may parallel the severity of intestinal disease, and recurrence after colectomy with UC is uncommon.

Dermatologic and Mucocutaneous Complications

Skin and mucosal lesions associated with IBD include erythema nodosum, pyoderma gangrenosum, aphthous ulceration, and Sweet's syndrome.[40] Raised, red, tender nodules on the tibial surfaces of the legs and arms that vary in size from 1 cm to several centimeters are manifestations of erythema nodosum, and may occur in 2% to 20% of patients with IBD.[40] These lesions are more commonly observed in CD patients and often correlate with disease severity.

Pyoderma gangrenosum occurs in 0.5% to 2% of patients with IBD and is characterized by discrete skin ulcerations that have a necrotic center and a violaceous color of the surrounding skin.[1,40] They can be seen on any part of the body but commonly occur on the lower extremities.

Oral lesions are found in 4% to 20% of patients with IBD.[35,40] The most common lesion seen with CD is aphthous stomatitis. The severity of these lesions tends to parallel the disease course. Sweet's syndrome, also known as acute febrile neutrophilic dermatosis, is characterized by tender erythematous skin lesions secondary to dermal neutrophil infiltration, and is often associated with fever and a distribution on the upper trunk, face, neck, and arms.[40]

Hematologic, Coagulation, and Metabolic Abnormalities

Patients with IBD may develop anemia, with a prevalence reported up to 74%.[1,40] The anemia may present as iron deficiency related to chronic blood loss, ongoing inflammation, malnutrition, hemolysis, or bone marrow suppression from drug treatment.[40] Alternatively, it may be more characteristic of anemia of chronic disease secondary to chronic inflammation and overproduction of cytokines. Patients with IBD are at a 1.5 to 3.6 times higher risk of venous thromboembolism (VTE) compared with the general population.[41] This is secondary to activation of the clotting cascade and platelet activation secondary to inflammation.[40,41] Occurrence of VTE is higher during disease flares and occurs more often in peripheral veins.[1,41] Patients should be considered for pharmacologic VTE prophylaxis when admitted to the hospital for a disease flare. Patients with IBD may be at increased risk for metabolic bone disease and development of osteoporosis. Osteomalacia is less common in IBD.[40,42] Bone disease may be related to a combination of nutritional deficiencies, especially calcium and vitamin D, chronic cytokine-related inflammatory effects on bone, disease-associated hypogonadism, and use of corticosteroids.[40,42]

CLINICAL PRESENTATION

The patterns of clinical presentation of IBD can vary widely. Patients may have a single acute episode that resolves and does not recur, but most patients experience acute flares with alternating periods of remission.

Ulcerative Colitis

There is a wide range of presentation in UC, ranging from mild abdominal cramping with frequent small-volume bowel movements to profuse diarrhea (Table 21-2). Most patients with UC experience intermittent bouts of illness after varying intervals of remission with symptoms. A small percentage of patients have continuous unremitting symptoms or a single acute attack with no subsequent symptoms.

4 While various disease classifications are available for UC, a standard disease severity scoring system is not universally accepted.[43] The arbitrary distinctions of mild, moderate, severe, and fulminant disease activity are generally used in treatment guideline recommendations, and are determined largely by clinical signs and symptoms[1,31,43]:

1. Mild: Fewer than four stools daily, with or without blood, with no systemic disturbance and a normal erythrocyte sedimentation rate (ESR)
2. Moderate: More than four stools per day but with minimal systemic disturbance
3. Severe: More than six stools per day with blood, with evidence of systemic disturbance as shown by fever, tachycardia, anemia, or ESR of greater than 30 mm/h (8.3 μm/s)
4. Fulminant: More than 10 bowel movements per day with continuous bleeding, toxicity, abdominal tenderness, requirement for transfusion, and colonic dilation

TABLE 21-2 Clinical Presentation of Ulcerative Colitis

Signs and symptoms
- Abdominal cramping
- Frequent bowel movements, often with blood in the stool
- Weight loss
- Fever and tachycardia in severe disease
- Blurred vision, eye pain, and photophobia with ocular involvement
- Arthritis
- Raised, red, tender nodules that vary in size from 1 cm to several centimeters

Physical examination
- Hemorrhoids, anal fissures, or perirectal abscesses may be present
- Iritis, uveitis, episcleritis, and conjunctivitis with ocular involvement
- Dermatologic findings with erythema nodosum, pyoderma gangrenosum, or aphthous ulceration

Laboratory tests
- Decreased hematocrit/hemoglobin
- Increased ESR or CRP
- Leukocytosis and hypoalbuminemia with severe disease
- (+) perinuclear antineutrophil cytoplasmic antibodies

With severe disease, the patient typically has profuse bloody diarrhea with a high fever, leukocytosis, and hypoalbuminemia. The patient may be dehydrated with tachycardia and hypotension. This presentation may have a sudden onset with rapid progression.

Determining disease extent, that is, which sections of the colon are involved, is important. This is accomplished via endoscopy. Patients with "distal" disease have inflammation limited to areas distal to the splenic flexure (also referred to as *left-sided* disease), while those with "extensive disease" have inflammation extending proximal to the splenic flexure.[1,31] Inflammation confined to the rectal area is referred to as *proctitis*, while disease involving the rectum and sigmoid colon is referred to as *proctosigmoiditis*.[29] Inflammation of the majority of the colon is called *pancolitis*.

The diagnosis of UC is made on clinical suspicion and confirmed by biopsy, stool examinations, sigmoidoscopy or colonoscopy, or barium radiographic contrast studies. The presence of extracolonic manifestations may also aid in establishing the diagnosis.[1,31,40]

Crohn's Disease

As with UC, the presentation of CD is highly variable. The time between the onset of complaints and the initial diagnosis may be as long as 3 years. The patient typically presents with diarrhea and abdominal pain. Hematochezia occurs in about one half of patients with colonic involvement and much less frequently when there is no colonic involvement. A patient may first present with a perirectal or perianal lesion (Table 21-3). The diagnosis should also be suspected in children with growth retardation, especially with abdominal complaints.

Much like UC, global classification guidelines for scoring severity of active CD are not available. For patients with luminal nonfistulizing CD, the Crohn's Disease Activity Index (CDAI) is used most often to gauge response to therapy and determine remission and is employed mostly in the research setting.[44] This score system ranges from 0 to 600, with score great than 150 defined as active disease. The Harvey Bradshaw Index (HBI) is another scoring system that is also used for CD, and tends to correlate well with the CDAI.[44] A decrease of 3 points in the HBI is defined as a clinical response in the with complete remission defined as a score of <4. Treatment guidelines use the presence of signs and symptoms as their marker for disease activity and severity.[35] Patients with mild to moderate CD are typically ambulatory and have no evidence of dehydration, systemic toxicity, loss of body weight, or abdominal tenderness, mass, or obstruction. Moderate to severe disease is considered in patients who fail to respond to treatment for mild to moderate disease or those with fever, weight loss, abdominal pain or tenderness, vomiting, intestinal obstruction, or significant anemia. Severe to fulminant CD is classified as the presence of persistent symptoms or evidence of systemic toxicity despite corticosteroid or biologic treatment or

TABLE 21-3 Clinical Presentation of Crohn Disease

Signs and symptoms
- Malaise and fever
- Abdominal pain
- Frequent bowel movements
- Hematochezia
- Fistula
- Weight loss and malnutrition
- Arthritis

Physical examination
- Abdominal mass and tenderness
- Perianal fissure or fistula

Laboratory tests
- Increased white blood cell count, ESR, and CRP
- (+) anti-*Saccharomyces cerevisiae* antibodies

presence of cachexia, rebound tenderness, intestinal obstruction, or abscess. Disease activity may be assessed and correlated by evaluation of serum C-reactive protein (CRP) concentrations.

The course of CD is characterized by periods of remission and exacerbation. Patients may be symptom-free for years, while others experience chronic symptoms in spite of medical therapy. As with UC, the diagnosis of CD involves a thorough evaluation using laboratory, endoscopic, and radiologic testing to detect the extent and characteristic features of the disease. Small bowel involvement, strictures detected on radiographs, and presence of fistulae are characteristic of CD.

TREATMENT

Desired Outcomes

5 The clinician must have a clear concept of realistic therapeutic goals for each patient with IBD. Goals may relate to resolution of acute inflammatory processes, resolution of complications (e.g., fistulae and abscesses), alleviation of extraintestinal manifestations, maintenance of remission, or surgical palliation or cure.

When determining goals of therapy and selecting therapeutic regimens, it is important to understand the natural history of IBD.[1,13,31,35] Some cases of acute UC are self-limited. With mild to moderate acute colitis without systemic symptoms, 20% of patients may experience spontaneous improvement in their disease within a few weeks; however, a small percentage of patients may go on to experience more serious disease. With severe colitis, improvement without treatment cannot be expected. The response to medical management of toxic megacolon is variable and emergent colectomy may be required. When remission of UC is achieved, it is likely to last at least 1 year with medical therapy; however, long-term sustained remission rates are typically less than 50%.[43] In the absence of medical therapy, one half to two thirds of patients relapse within 9 months.[31]

Approximately 20% of patients with CD will experience a relapse annually.[35] Sustained remission is impacted by response to treatment. Patients remaining in remission for 1 year have an 80% chance of remaining in remission the subsequent year, while 70% of patients will continue to have active disease in the year following a 12-month period in which they had active disease.[35] Thus, inducing and maintaining remission is an important aspect of treatment to improve outcomes and QOL and reduce complications. There has been recent interest in mucosal healing as a more objective end point or goal for the treatment of IBD.[45,46] Mucosal healing is accessed via endoscopy; however, there is not a universal scoring system that has been adopted for either CD or UC. The natural course of the disease may be altered and outcomes improved, such as sustained remission and reduced hospitalization, if mucosal healing is achieved.[45,46] Mucosal healing is directly related to the efficacy of drug therapies used in the treatment of IBD and may be used to determine the need for escalation or de-escalation of drug therapy.[45,46] At this time mucosal healing is a promising end point; however, as more studies incorporate this end point, it can be better determined if this is achievable in all patients, particularly those with CD whose disease typically penetrates below the mucosal layer.

General Approach to Treatment

6 Treatment of IBD centers on agents used to relieve the inflammatory process and induce disease remission. Aminosalicylates (ASAs), corticosteroids, antimicrobials, immunosuppressive, and biologic agents are commonly used to treat active disease and for some agents to maintain disease remission. The severity and extent of the disease should be taken into account, as this will often dictate the dose, route, frequency, and formulation of drug therapy that will be most effective. Patient preference for different drug formulations and cost of therapies should also be taken into account.

Surgical procedures are sometimes performed when active disease is inadequately controlled with drugs or when the required drug dosages pose an unacceptable risk of adverse effects. Nutritional considerations are also important because many patients may develop malnutrition. A variety of adjunctive therapies may be used to address complications or symptoms of IBD. For example, antidiarrheal agents such as loperamide may be used in some patients with relatively well-controlled disease, although these are generally to be avoided in active moderate to severe IBD because they may contribute to the development of toxic megacolon.

Nonpharmacologic Therapy

Nutritional Support

Proper nutritional support is an important aspect of the treatment of patients with IBD. Specific types of diets are not useful in alleviating the inflammatory conditions; however, patients with moderate to severe disease are often malnourished.[37,38,47] Malabsorption or maldigestion may occur secondary to the catabolic effects of the disease process. Elevated activity of IL-6 and TNF-α increases protein turnover, resulting in protein loss and muscle wasting.[38] Malabsorption and malnutrition may occur more often in the patient with CD with involvement of the small bowel, as this is where many nutrients are absorbed.[47] Protein–energy malnutrition and suboptimal weight is reported in up to 85% of patients with CD.[47] Patients who have undergone multiple small bowel resections may have reduction in the absorptive surface of the intestine (i.e., "short gut"). Maldigestion with accompanying diarrhea can also occur if there is a bile salt deficiency in the gut.

Many specific diets have been tried to improve nutritional status and symptoms in IBD, but none has gained widespread acceptance. On an individual patient basis, elimination of specific foods that appear to exacerbate symptoms can be tried; however, exclusion diets are generally not endorsed, even in the setting of severe disease.[48] If attempted, the elimination process must be conducted cautiously, as patients may exclude a wide range of nutritious products without adequate justification. Some patients with IBD may have lactase deficiency as well; therefore, diarrhea may be associated with intake of dairy products. For these patients, avoidance of dairy products or supplementation with lactase generally improves the patient's symptoms.[48] Patients with small bowel strictures due to CD should avoid excessive high-residue foods, such as citrus fruits and nuts, in order to prevent obstruction.

The nutritional needs of patients with IBD may be adequately addressed with use of enteral supplementation in acute or chronic situations.[37,38,47] Use of enteral nutrition has favorable effects on reducing inflammation and intestinal cytokine production.[47] This may lead to a greater chance of induction and maintenance of remission as well as facilitation of mucosal healing, particularly in patients with CD.[47] No specific enteral formula is recommended, so initiation of polymeric feeds may be tried first.[47] Monitoring for efficacy of the enteral feeding is similar to other patient populations receiving enteral nutrition.

Parenteral nutrition has a more limited role in CD or UC. It is generally reserved for patients with severe malnutrition or those who fail enteral therapy or have a contraindication to receiving enteral therapy, such as perforation, protracted vomiting, short-bowel syndrome, or severe intestinal stenosis.[47] Parenteral therapy is not preferred as primary therapy for IBD even in the setting of acute disease flares in hospitalized patients.[48] Home parenteral nutrition may be necessary for patients requiring long-term therapy, particularly those with short-bowel syndrome. Parenteral nutrition is more costly and is associated with more complications, such as serious infections, compared with enteral nutrition.

Given that the intestinal microbiotica may play a key role in IBD pathogenesis, probiotic administration as an adjunctive treatment of IBD has been explored. Postulated mechanisms for using probiotics in IBD include reestablishment of normal bacterial flora within the gut, reduction in bacterial adhesion and competition for nutrients with pathogenic bacteria, production of antibacterial substances, and promotion of favorable effects on the host immune response.[49–51] Probiotic preparations often contain various organisms such as nonpathogenic *E. coli Nissle*, bifidobacteria, lactobacilli, *Streptococcus thermophilus, or Saccharomyces boulardii.* Probiotics have demonstrated some effectiveness in inducing and maintaining remission in some trials for patients with UC; however, differences in methodology, probiotics used, and underlying treatments for IBD make comparison of trials difficult.[49–54] A formulation of *Bifidiobacterium*, lactobacilli, and streptococci (VSL #3) is marketed specifically for use in UC as an adjunctive therapy and for patients who have a surgically constructed ileal pouch anal anastomosis (IPAA) to prevent or treat pouchitis.[31,49–51] Use of probiotics as adjunctive agents to avoid stepping up drug therapy to potentially more toxic agents is another potential use.[49] Evidence of probiotic use in the induction and maintenance of CD is less compelling and has led to recommendations not supporting widespread use, but rather further investigation.[52–54] While probiotics are considered to be generally safe in patients with IBD, the added cost and requirement to often take multiple doses per day should also weigh into the decision to use them in IBD.

Surgery

Despite the availability of medications to treat IBD, many patients will often require surgery. Surgical procedures may involve resection of segments of intestine that are affected, as well as correction of complications (e.g., fistulas) or drainage of abscesses.

Rates of colectomy for UC are 5% to 30%.[1,31,55] Colectomy may be necessary when the patient has disease uncontrolled by maximum medical therapy or when there are complications of the disease such as colonic perforation, toxic megacolon, uncontrolled colonic hemorrhage, or colonic strictures.[1,31,55] Colectomy may be indicated for patients with long-standing disease (greater than 8 to 10 years), as a prophylactic measure against the development of CRC, and for patients with premalignant changes (severe dysplasia) on surveillance mucosal biopsies.[33,34,55] Proctocolectomy, after which the patient is left with a permanent ileostomy, is generally considered curative for UC; however, the decision to perform this should take into account the effects on the patient's QOL. Restorative proctocolectomy with construction of an IPAA is the most common surgical procedure performed in UC and is typically well tolerated with a reported failure rate of less than 10%.[55] Patients may develop inflammation of the IPAA, often referred to as pouchitis.[53] The risk from surgery for these patients is relatively low if the operations are performed on a nonemergent basis.

Indications for surgery with CD are not as well established as for UC. Surgery is usually reserved for patients with complications of the disease. A recognized problem with intestinal resection for CD is the high rate of recurrence. Surgery may be appropriate in well-selected patients who have severe or incapacitating disease or obstruction in spite of aggressive medical management. The surgical procedures performed most often include resections of the major intestinal areas of involvement. Patients who undergo multiple resections of the small intestine may develop malabsorption related to short-bowel syndrome. For some patients with severe rectal or perianal disease, particularly abscesses, diversion of the fecal stream is performed with a colostomy. Other indications for surgery include resection of strictures or performance of stricturoplasty, or presence of colon cancer, an inflammatory mass, intestinal perforation, or fistulas.[35]

Pharmacologic Therapy

Drug therapy plays an integral role in the treatment of IBD. None of the drugs used for IBD are curative; therefore, reasonable goals of drug therapy are resolution of acute disease symptoms and induction of remission. The major types of drug therapy used in IBD include ASAs, corticosteroids, immunosuppressive agents (azathioprine, mercaptopurine [MP], cyclosporine, and methotrexate), antimicrobials (metronidazole and ciprofloxacin), and agents to inhibit TNF-α (anti–TNF-α antibodies) or leukocyte adhesion and migration (natalizumab).

Sulfasalazine is the prototypical ASA, and is composed of a sulfonamide moiety (sulfapyridine) and mesalamine (5-aminosalicylate acid [5-ASA]) joined by a diazo bond in the same molecule.[55,56] Sulfasalazine has been used for years to treat IBD but was originally intended to treat arthritis. It is cleaved by gut bacteria in the colon to sulfapyridine (which is mostly absorbed and excreted in the urine) and mesalamine (which mostly remains in the colon and is excreted in stool).[54–56]

The active component of sulfasalazine is mesalamine, which exerts its effects locally in the GI tract; however, the mechanism of action is not completely understood. Beneficial effects of mesalamine may include scavenging of free radicals, inhibition of leukocyte motility, interference with TNF-α, transforming growth factor-β (TGF-β) and nuclear factor κB (NF-$\kappa\beta$), suppression of IL-1 production, and inhibition of leukotriene and prostaglandin production.[55–59]

Because the effectiveness of sulfasalazine is not related to the sulfapyridine component and since sulfapyridine is believed to be responsible for many of the adverse reactions to sulfasalazine, mesalamine can be administered alone. Given that mesalamine is rapidly and completely absorbed in the small intestine but poorly absorbed in the colon, drug formulations must be designed to deliver mesalamine to the affected areas in the GI while preventing premature absorption.[55–60] Mesalamine can be used topically as an enema, to treat left-sided disease, or as a suppository for treatment of proctitis (Fig. 21-1). In general, the use of topical mesalamine preparations such as enemas and suppositories is more effective than oral preparations.[60] Likewise, these therapies may be used concomitantly with the oral mesalamine preparations, which may result in additive efficacy in patients with UC.[61] Oral slow-release formulations will deliver mesalamine to the small intestine and/or colon based on the product design (Table 21-4). Slow-release oral formulations of mesalamine, such as Pentasa, release mesalamine from the duodenum to the ileum, with up to 59% of the drug passing into the colon.[57] Some dose forms (Asacol, Asacol HD, Delzicol) utilize a pH-dependent coating that releases in response to intestinal pH.[58] Another tablet formulation of mesalamine (Lialda) uses a pH-dependent coating that releases at a pH of 7, in combination with a polymeric matrix core, referred to as the Multi-MatriX (MMX) system, and releases drug evenly throughout the colon also allowing

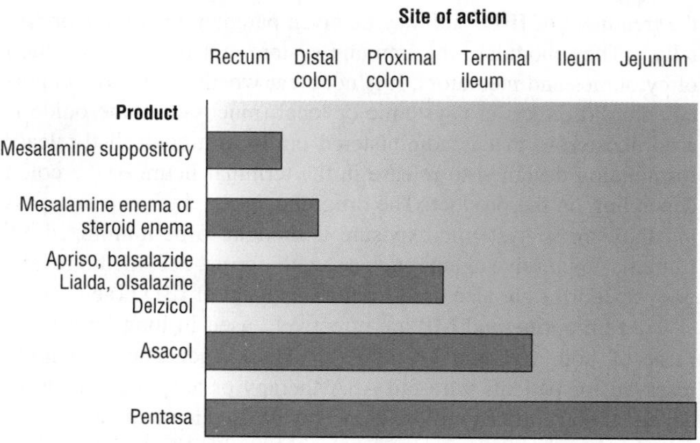

FIGURE 21-1 Site of activity of various agents used to treat inflammatory bowel disease.

TABLE 21-4 Agents for the Treatment of Inflammatory Bowel Disease

Drug	Brand Name	Initial Dose (g)	Usual Range
Sulfasalazine	Azulfidine	500 mg to 1 g	4–6 g/day
	Azulfidine EN	500 mg to 1 g	4–6 g/day
Mesalamine suppository	Rowasa	1 g	1 g daily to three times weekly
Mesalamine enema	Canasa	4 g	4 g daily to three times weekly
Mesalamine (oral)	Asacol	1.2 g/day	2.8–4.8 g/day
	Asacol HD	1.6 g/day	2.8–4.8 g/day
	Apriso	1.5 g/day	1.5 g/day once daily
	Lialda	1.2–2.4 g/day	1.2–4.8 g/day once daily
	Pentasa	2 g/day	2–4 g/day
	Delzicol	1.2 g/day	2.4–4.8 g/day
Olsalazine	Dipentum	1.5 g/day	1.5–3 g/day
Balsalazide	Colazal	2.25 g/day	2.25–6.75 g/day
Azathioprine	Imuran, Azasan	50–100 mg	1–2.5 mg/kg/day
Cyclosporine	Gengraf	2–4 mg/kg/day IV	2–4 mg/kg/day IV
	Neoral, Sandimmune	2–8 mg/kg/day oral	
Mercaptopurine	Purinethol	50–100 mg	1–2.5 mg/kg/day
Methotrexate	Trexall	15–25 mg IM weekly	15–25 mg IM weekly
Adalimumab	Humira	160 mg SC day 1	80 mg SC 2 (day 15), and then 40 mg every 2 weeks
Certolizumab	Cimzia	400 mg SC	400 mg SC weeks 2 and 4, and then 400 mg SC monthly
Infliximab	Remicade	5 mg/kg IV	5 mg/kg weeks 2 and 6, 5–10 mg/kg every 8 weeks
Natalizumab	Tysabri	300 mg IV	300 mg IV every 4 weeks
Budesonide	Enterocort EC Uceris	9 mg	6–9 mg daily

SC, subcutaneous; IM, intramuscular.

for once-daily dosing.[59] A capsule formulation of mesalamine (Apriso) utilizes enteric-coated mesalamine granules in a polymer matrix for delayed and extended delivery of mesalamine to the colon and also allows for once-daily dosing.[57,58] Use of once-daily oral mesalamine preparations may enhance adherence, which may help to prevent relapse.[57,59] Olsalazine is a dimer of two 5-ASA molecules linked by an azo bond. Mesalamine is released in the colon after colonic bacteria cleave the azo bond.[56] Balsalazide is a mesalamine prodrug that couples mesalamine with the inert carrier molecule 4-aminobenzoyl-β-alanine and is also enzymatically cleaved in the colon to release mesalamine.[56] The recommended daily doses of the oral mesalamine derivatives are intended to approximate the molar equivalent of mesalamine present in 4 g of sulfasalazine. Because the oral mesalamine formulations are delayed-release coated tablets or granules, they should not be crushed or chewed. Unlike sulfasalazine, all of these agents are safe to use for patients with sulfonamide allergies.

7 Corticosteroids are used to suppress acute inflammation in the treatment of IBD, and may be given parenterally, orally, or rectally.[62] They modulate the immune system and inhibit production of cytokines and mediators. It is not clear whether the most important steroid effects are systemic or local (mucosal). Budesonide is a corticosteroid that is administered orally in a controlled-release formulation designed to release in the terminal ileum or the colon depending on the product. The drug undergoes extensive first-pass metabolism; so systemic exposure is thought to be minimized.[36,62] Immunosuppressive agents such as azathioprine, MP, methotrexate, or cyclosporine are also used for the treatment of IBD (Table 21-4).

Azathioprine and MP are effectively used in long-term treatment of both CD and UC.[1,31,35,63–65] These agents are generally reserved for patients who fail ASA therapy or are refractory to or dependent on corticosteroids. They may be used in conjunction with mesalamine derivatives, corticosteroids, and TNF-α antagonists, and must be used for extended periods of time, ranging from a few weeks up to 12 months, before benefits may be observed.[63–65]

Cyclosporine has a short-term benefit in the treatment of acute, severe UC to avoid colectomy in patients failing corticosteroids.[1,13,31,48,66] It is used initially as a continuous IV infusion of 2 to 4 mg/kg daily.[48,67] Cyclosporine poses a risk of nephrotoxicity and neurotoxicity. Studies evaluating tacrolimus for the treatment of IBD suggest a potential role for use for patients with luminal or perianal CD; however, results have been variable with few data to support its routine use.[68] Methotrexate 15 to 25 mg given intramuscularly or subcutaneously once weekly is useful for treatment and maintenance of CD and may result in steroid-sparing effects, while data supporting use in UC are lacking.[13,35,44,63]

Clinical **Controversy...**

The treatment of CD has traditionally used a "step-up" approach, with use of ASAs and corticosteroids first, followed by azathioprine, MP, methotrexate, or biologic agents. Introducing immunosuppressants or biologic agents earlier in a "top-down" approach has gained interest.[36] Use of these agents earlier may significantly alter the disease course; however, these agents are costly and may be associated with significant toxicities. More studies are needed to define the role of the "top-down" approach before it is implemented in a wider range of patients.

Antimicrobial agents, particularly metronidazole and ciprofloxacin, are frequently used as adjunctive therapies in IBD. Metronidazole and ciprofloxacin, often given in combination, have demonstrated some value in both induction of remission and decrease in relapse rates in CD with some data supporting use in UC as well.[13,36,44,69] Antibiotics are often used in patients with perineal CD or when fistulas or abscesses are present.[5] Rifamycin antibiotics have demonstrated some efficacy in treatment of both UC and CD.[69]

Risks of long-term antibiotic use include the development of antibiotic resistance, predisposition to *C. difficile* infection, and adverse effects such as neurotoxicity secondary to metronidazole use.

Biologic agents that target TNF-α have become a key class of agents in the treatment and maintenance of IBD.[70–72] Infliximab is an IgG_1 chimeric monoclonal antibody that is administered IV and binds TNF-α and inhibits its inflammatory effects. In addition, it lyses activated T cells and macrophages and induces T-cell apoptosis.[72] Infliximab is useful for moderate to severe active CD and UC disease, as well as steroid-dependent or fistulizing disease, as both an induction and a maintenance therapy. Adalimumab is also an IgG1 antibody to TNF-α; however, this agent, unlike infliximab, is fully humanized and contains no murine sequences. Theoretically, the lack of a murine component in adalimumab reduces antibody development seen with use of infliximab. This agent is administered subcutaneously and is a treatment option for patients with moderate to severe active UC and CD and those previously treated with infliximab who have lost response. Certolizumab pegol is a humanized pegylated Fab fragment directed against TNF-α that is also administered subcutaneously. Both adalimumab and certolizumab inhibit soluble and membrane-bound TNF and can be used as both induction and maintenance therapies.[72]

Lastly, natalizumab is a novel biologic agent that inhibits leukocyte adhesion and migration by targeting the α_4 subunit of integrin.[71,72] This agent can be used in the treatment of CD for patients who are unresponsive to other therapies, including corticosteroids and TNF-α inhibitors.

Clinical **Controversy. . .**

Use of the combination of anti–TNF-α antagonists and immunosuppressants in patients with CD has gained interest based on recent data.[84] This combination appears to be more effective than azathioprine or infliximab alone. Despite this efficacy, controversy remains as to the level of immunosuppression that is needed versus the risk of potential toxicities, such as serious infections or lymphoma.[65] Likewise, the timing and approach to de-escalation of one or both therapies and which therapies should be stopped or reduced first remains an unclear area.[65,83]

Treatment of Ulcerative Colitis

Mild to Moderate Active Disease Most patients with mild to moderate active UC can be managed on an outpatient basis with oral and/or topical ASAs (Fig. 21-2; Table 21-5). For patients with extensive disease, oral sulfasalazine or an oral mesalamine derivative is preferred, with rates of induction of remission reported as 36% to 60% in 2 to 4 weeks after initiating therapy.[1,31,60,61,73,74] Topical mesalamine in an enema or suppository formulation is more effective than oral mesalamine or topical steroids for distal disease.[60,61] The combination of oral and topical mesalamine is more effective than either alone for patients with left-sided or extensive disease; however, patients may be less willing to use these formulations.[60,61] Usually 4 to 6 g/day of sulfasalazine given in four divided doses is required to suppress active inflammation.[31] There does not appear to be an increased rate of response with dosages over 6 g/day, although adverse effects typically increase.

Oral mesalamine derivatives (Table 21-2) are alternatives to sulfasalazine for treatment of mild to moderate UC with similar rates of efficacy. Mesalamine preparations are typically better tolerated than sulfasalazine and thus are often chosen preferentially as first-line therapies. Mesalamine suppositories will only reach to approximately 10 to 20 cm within the lower GI tract and thus are reserved for patients with proctitis.[1] Enemas will reach to the splenic flexure and can be used for left-sided disease.[60] The various oral mesalamine products generally have similar rates of efficacy and the effective daily dose range is 2.4 to 4.8 g/day. Doses greater than 2.4 g/day generally do not demonstrate significant additional benefit; however, patients with moderate disease may respond better to higher doses.[1,13,67,73] The choice of oral formulations may be dictated by patient-specific factors, such as use of a once-daily formulation to help improve patient adherence and reduce pill burden, or use of a generically available product in patients with limited financial resources.[56–59,75] Controlled release budesonide (Uceris) is an alternative for mild-moderate UC. Oral corticosteroids in doses of 40 to 60 mg/day prednisone equivalent can be used for patients with moderate extensive disease who are refractory to oral ASAs or require more rapid control of symptoms.[31,62] Topical corticosteroids, given as foams, enemas, and suppositories, while effective for patients with distal disease, are generally less effective than mesalamine but can be used for patients with tenesmus.[31]

Moderate to Severe Active Disease Patients with moderate to severe active disease require prompt initiation of therapies to quickly suppress inflammation. Systemic corticosteroids are used in the treatment of moderate to severe active UC regardless of disease location or in those patients who are unresponsive to maximal doses of oral and/or topical mesalamine derivatives.[21,31] Oral doses of 40 to 60 mg prednisone equivalent daily are recommended.[31]

Use of TNF-α inhibitors is an option for patients with moderate to severe disease who are unresponsive to ASAs, corticosteroids, or other immunosuppressive agents and is generally the next step in therapy. Infliximab has demonstrated rates of induction of remission of up to 65% using a 5 mg/kg three-dose induction regimen at day 0, 2 weeks, and 6 weeks.[1,13,74] Adalimumab has also demonstrated efficacy in moderate to severe UC with reported rates of remission as 16.5% to 18.5% at 8 weeks using a four-dose regimen of 160 mg on day 1, 80 mg 2 weeks later, and then 40 mg every other week starting 2 weeks later.[76,77]

Severe or Fulminant Disease Patients with uncontrolled severe colitis or those with incapacitating symptoms require hospitalization for effective management. Under these conditions, patients generally receive nothing by mouth to promote bowel rest. Medications are given by the parenteral route and oral sulfasalazine or mesalamine derivatives are not typically beneficial in this setting because of rapid elimination of these agents from the colon with diarrhea.

Systemic corticosteroids are used in the treatment of severe disease and may allow some patients to avoid colectomy. IV hydrocortisone 300 mg daily in three divided doses or methylprednisolone 60 mg once daily is considered a first-line agent.[31,67] Methylprednisolone is typically preferred due to its lesser mineralocorticoid effects. A trial of steroids is warranted in most patients before proceeding to colectomy, unless the condition is grave or rapidly deteriorating. The length of corticosteroid therapy before consideration of surgery is open to debate, with recommendations ranging from 3 to 7 days.[1,31,48] Steroids do increase surgical risk, particularly infectious, if an operation is required later.

8 Patients who are unresponsive to parenteral corticosteroids after 3 to 7 days have the option of receiving higher-potency agents such as cyclosporine or infliximab. Seventy-six percent to 85% of hospitalized patients who are unresponsive to corticosteroids will typically respond to IV cyclosporine.[66] A continuous IV infusion of cyclosporine 2 to 4 mg/kg/day is the typical dose range utilized and may delay the need for colectomy.[1,31,48,66,67] Persistent fever, tachycardia, elevated CRP, hypoalbuminemia, and deep colonic ulcerations may be predictors of failure to respond to cyclosporine.[31,66] Patients who are controlled on IV cyclosporine can then be switched to an oral cyclosporine (4 to 8 mg/kg/day) tapered regimen with transition to azathioprine or MP.[1,31,48,66,78] Infliximab is an alternative to cyclosporine at a dose of 5 mg/kg and has demonstrated similar results regarding delaying the need for colectomy for patients with severe disease unresponsive to

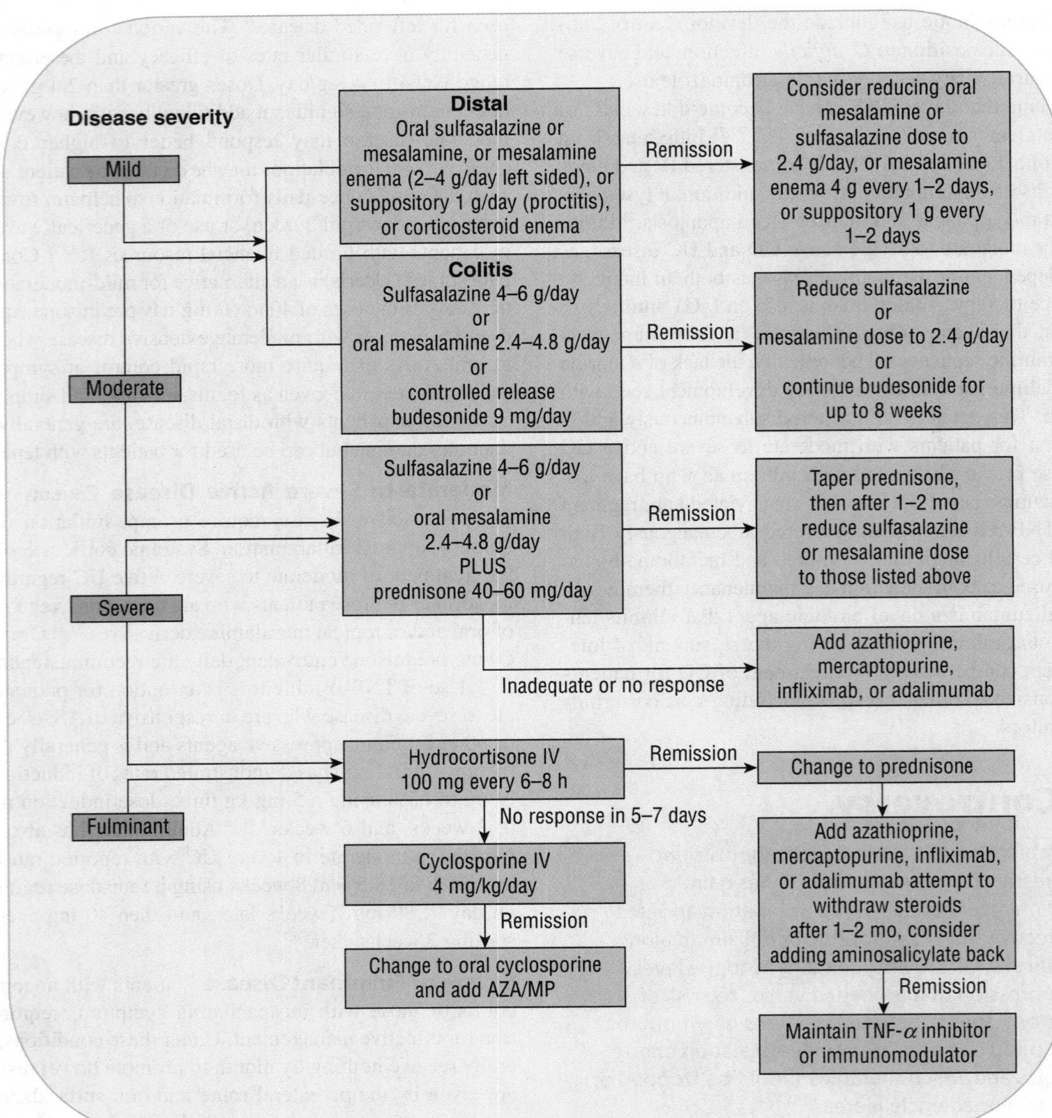

FIGURE 21-2 Treatment approaches for ulcerative colitis.

steroids.[1,48,66,67] Patients who respond to infliximab should be considered for additional doses at 2 and 6 weeks later.[48] The sequential use of cyclosporine and infliximab, or the drugs given in reverse order, is not recommended.[48] The adverse effects of both cyclosporine and infliximab are potentially serious and should be taken into consideration when using either therapy for patients with severe disease.[66,67]

Clinical **Controversy. . .**

For patients with severe or fulminant IBD that is unresponsive to corticosteroids, cyclosporine has traditionally been a last-line agent. The use of infliximab for this indication has recently gained interest. Both cyclosporine and infliximab appear to be similar in efficacy; however, data are variable and each may have its own role.[66] Each agent is associated with potentially serious adverse effects and the decision to use either should take into account each individual case. Few head-to-head trials exist, and more data are needed to determine if either agent should be preferred over the other.

Maintenance of Remission

9 After remission from active disease is achieved, the goal of therapy is to maintain remission. The major agents used for maintenance of remission are sulfasalazine and the newer mesalamine derivatives, infliximab and adalimumab, and azathioprine or MP.

Oral agents, including sulfasalazine, mesalamine, and balsalazide, are all effective options for maintenance therapy. The optimal dose to prevent relapse is 2 to 2.4 g/day of mesalamine equivalent, with rates of relapse over 6 to 12 months reported as 40%.[13,31,71,73,74] The newer mesalamine derivatives are generally better tolerated than sulfasalazine and are associated with fewer adverse effects often making them a preferred choice.[31,71] For patients with left-sided disease or proctitis, mesalamine enemas or suppositories are preferred.[60] The frequency of administration of topical agents may possibly be lessened to every third night over time.[29,39,60,70] The combination of topical and oral mesalamine is superior to either regimen alone for maintenance therapy.[60]

Corticosteroids do not have a role in the maintenance of remission with UC because they are ineffective and are associated with serious adverse effects with long-term use.[1,31] Steroids should be gradually withdrawn after 2 to 4 weeks after induction of remission.

TABLE 21-5 Levels of Evidence for Therapeutic Interventions in Inflammatory Bowel Disease

Interventions	Evidence Grades[a]
Ulcerative Colitis	
Mild to moderate active distal disease may be treated with oral aminosalicylates, topical mesalamine, or topical steroids	A
Combined oral and topical aminosalicylates are more effective than either is alone for mild to moderate active distal disease	A
Oral prednisone in doses of 40–60 mg/day or 1 mg/kg/day may be used in patients with mild to moderate distal disease unresponsive to oral or topical aminosalicylates	B
Sulfasalazine in doses of 4–6 g/day or an alternate aminosalicylate in doses of up to 4.8 g/day of the active 5-aminosalicylate moiety is effective for induction of mild to moderate extensive colitis	A
Infliximab and adalimumab are effective for moderate to severe disease in those patients not responding to corticosteroids or an immunosuppressive agent	A
Systemic corticosteroids are effective in moderate to severe active disease	A
Hospitalization for parenteral steroids is indicated for patients with severe disease or those failing to respond to oral steroids	A
Failure to demonstrate improvement following 3 days of parenteral steroids in patients with severe disease is an indication for cyclosporine or colectomy	1B
Sulfasalazine, mesalamine, or balsalazide is effective in maintenance of remission of distal disease; combining oral and topical mesalamine is more effective than is either alone	A
Sulfasalazine, olsalazine, mesalamine, and balsalazide are effective in preventing relapses in patients with mild to moderate extensive disease	A
Corticosteroids are not effective as maintenance treatment	A
Azathioprine, mercaptopurine, infliximab, and adalimumab are effective in lowering or eliminating corticosteroid use in corticosteroid-dependent patients	A
Azathioprine, mercaptopurine, or infliximab may be effective in patients with severe disease flares or those requiring retreatment with corticosteroids within 1 year	C
Oral cyclosporine is effective for patients with corticosteroid refractory disease but requires concomitant administration of azathioprine or mercaptopurine	C
Infliximab or adalimumab therapy is effective for maintenance if there is an initial response	A
Crohn Disease	
Oral aminosalicylates are effective for mild to moderate ileal, ileocolonic, or colonic active disease	D
Metronidazole may be effective in patients not responding to sulfasalazine	D
Ileal release budesonide is effective for mild to moderate ileal or right-sided colonic disease	A
Topical hydrocortisone is effective for distal colonic inflammation	A
Systemic corticosteroids are effective in moderate to severe active disease	A
Systemic corticosteroids are not effective for patients with perianal fistulas	C
Hospitalization for parenteral steroids is indicated for patients with severe disease or those failing to respond to oral steroids	A
Parenteral methotrexate is effective for induction of remission in patients with active disease and for reducing corticosteroid dependency	B
Infliximab, adalimumab, and certolizumab are effective for moderate to severe disease in those patients not responding to corticosteroids or an immunosuppressive agent	A
Infliximab and adalimumab are effective for those patients with fistulas who have not responded to antibiotics, immunosuppressive agents, or surgical drainage	A
High-dose oral cyclosporine (7.6 mg/kg) has short-term efficacy in patients with active disease	B
IV cyclosporine is effective for the treatment of fistulizing disease	B
Corticosteroids are not effective as maintenance treatment	A
Budesonide is effective as short-term maintenance therapy (3 months) but not long term	A
Azathioprine, mercaptopurine, infliximab, adalimumab, and certolizumab are effective in lowering or eliminating corticosteroid use in corticosteroid-dependent patients	A
Azathioprine or mercaptopurine is effective for maintenance of remission regardless of disease distribution	A
Azathioprine or mercaptopurine may be effective for treating perianal or enteric fistulae	C
Methotrexate maintenance therapy (15–25 mg IM weekly) is effective for patients whose active disease has responded to IM methotrexate	A
Methotrexate 25 mg IM for up to 16 weeks followed by 15 mg IM weekly is effective for patients with chronic active disease	A
Infliximab, adalimumab, and certolizumab therapy is effective for maintenance if there is an initial response	A

[a]A, homogenous evidence from multiple well-designed, randomized (therapeutic) or cohort (descriptive) controlled trials, each involving a number of participants to be of sufficient statistical power; B, evidence from at least one large well-designed clinical trial with or without randomization from cohort or case–control analytic studies or well-designed meta analysis; C, evidence based on clinical experience, descriptive studies, or reports of expert committees; D, not rated.

From references 31, 35, 48, and 82.

For patients who require chronic steroid use and are steroid dependent, there is a strong justification for use of alternative therapies. Azathioprine is effective in preventing relapse of UC for patients who fail ASAs or who are steroid dependent.[1,13,63,67] Approximately one third of patients will maintain remission on azathioprine; however, the onset of action is slow and 3 to 6 months may be required before beneficial effects are noted.[73] As mentioned earlier, azathioprine is also recommended for patients with severe UC who are transitioned to oral cyclosporine.[1,13,31,48,66,78]

The TNF-α inhibitors are options for maintenance in patients with moderate to severe UC following induction, and in those who are steroid dependent or have failed azathioprine. Despite their effectiveness in inducing remission, less than half of patients with UC will be able to maintain remission with a TNF-α inhibitor.[74] For patients who initially respond to infliximab, continued dosing of 5 mg/kg as maintenance therapy every 8 weeks can be used with a 10% colectomy rate reported at 54 weeks.[1,13,31,71,74] Adalimumab is an alternative to infliximab and has rates of remission at week 52 reported as 16% in patients failing corticosteroids or immunosuppressants.[77]

Crohn's Disease

Management of CD often proves more difficult than management of UC because of the greater complexity of presentation (Fig. 21-3; Table 21-3). There is a greater potential for reliance on drug therapy with CD because resection of involved areas of the GI tract may not be possible. Recurrence of CD is common following surgery with reported rates of endoscopic recurrence reported as up to 75% at 1 year.[79]

The drug treatment of CD involves many of the same agents used for UC. While the treatment strategy for CD has often followed

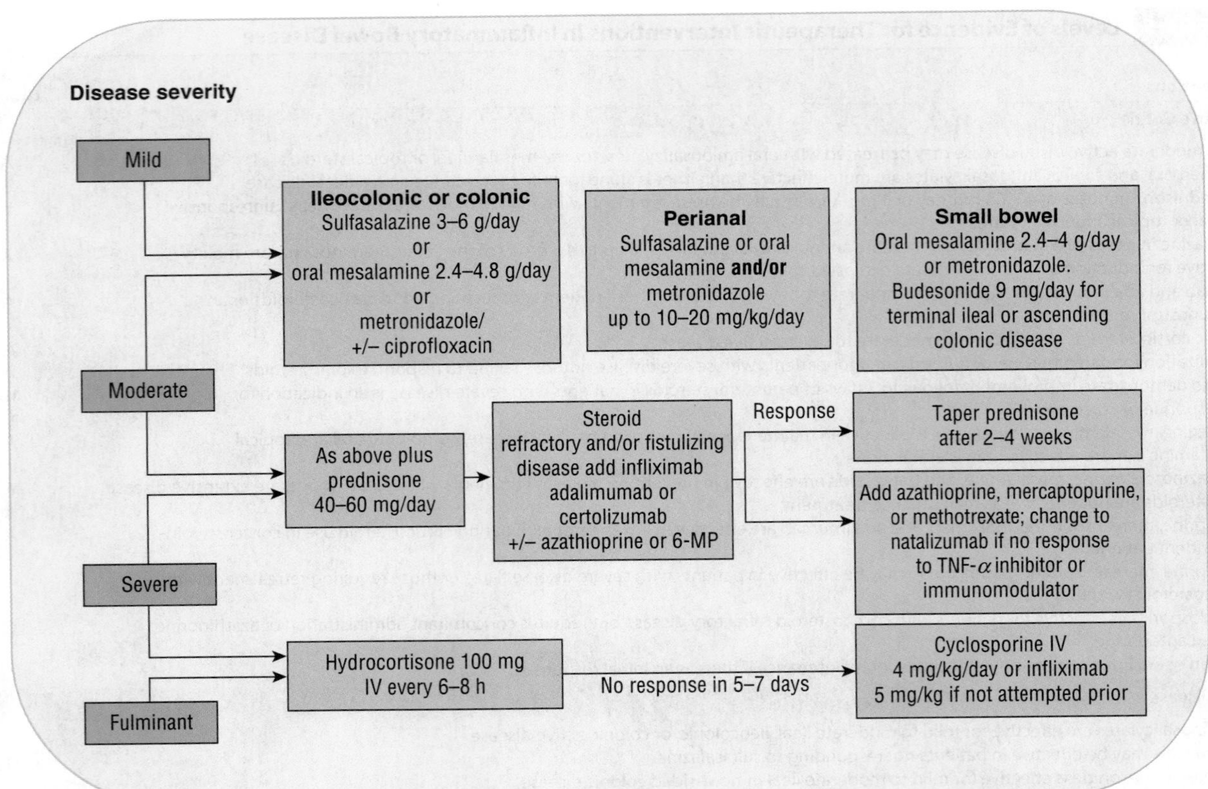

FIGURE 21-3 Treatment approaches for Crohn disease.

a similar "step-up" pattern as seen with UC, which involves initiating therapy with ASAs first, there has been interest in using higher-potency agents first, such as TNF-α inhibitors in a "top-down" approach in patients with severe disease.[36]

Mild to Moderate Active Crohn's Disease

While effective in UC, ASAs have not demonstrated significant efficacy in CD. Sulfasalazine is reported to have marginal efficacy when compared with placebo for patients with mild to moderate CD, while the newer mesalamine derivatives are generally considered to have minimal efficacy.[13,35,36,44,71,80] Despite limited and variable effectiveness, the mesalamine derivatives are often tried as an initial therapy for mild to moderate CD given their favorable adverse effect profile. Since CD often involves the small intestine, formulations such as Pentasa, which release in the small intestine, may be used.

Systemic corticosteroids are frequently used for the treatment of moderate to severe active CD; however, controlled-release budesonide (Entocort) at a dose of 9 mg daily is a viable first-line option for patients with mild to moderate ileal or right-sided (ascending colonic) disease.[13,13,35,36,44,62] This agent is superior to placebo and has demonstrated superiority to mesalamine with reported remission rates of up to 69% at 8 weeks.[13,41,71] Budesonide has a low systemic bioavailability, reported as 10%, so it has less potential for systemic adverse effects compared with conventional corticosteroids.[36]

Antibiotics may have some roles in the treatment of CD. Metronidazole, given orally as 10 to 20 mg/kg/day in divided doses, has demonstrated variable efficacy but may possibly be useful in some patients with CD, particularly for patients with colonic or ileocolonic involvement, those with perineal disease, or those who are unresponsive to sulfasalazine.[13,35,36,69] For patients with colonic or perineal disease, metronidazole can be added to a mesalamine product or steroids as adjunctive therapy when satisfactory control of CD is not gained with first-line agents, or in attempts to reduce steroid dosage.[36] Ciprofloxacin 1 g/day is another antibiotic used in CD, often in combination with metronidazole for patients with perianal disease or septic complications; however, results have been variable due to differences in study design and patient numbers.[35,41,44,69] Other antibiotics such as rifaximin and clofazimine have also been studied with variable efficacy reported.[44,69] While there has been some demonstrated efficacy with antibiotics in mild to moderate CD, they are generally not recommended as a first-line therapy.[35,36,44,69]

Moderate to Severe Active Crohn's Disease

Patients with moderate to severe active CD require rapid suppression of inflammation for symptom improvement and prevention of complications. Oral corticosteroids, such as prednisone 40 to 60 mg/day, are generally considered first-line therapies for moderate to severe active CD who are unresponsive to ASAs and are effective in inducing remission for up to 70% of patients.[13,36,62] Traditional oral systemic steroids have greater efficacy in inducing remission compared with budesonide in patients with moderate disease; however, the potential for adverse effects is greater.[62,71] Hospitalized patients with moderate to severe disease who are unable to tolerate oral therapy are candidates for administration of parenteral steroids, with methylprednisolone or hydrocortisone being first-line options.[36,48] Systemic steroids do not appear to be effective for treatment of perianal fistulas.[36,71]

⑩ Immunomodulators (azathioprine and MP) are not recommended to induce remission in moderate to severe CD; however, they are effective in maintaining steroid-induced remission and are generally limited to use for patients not achieving adequate response to standard medical therapy or in the setting of steroid dependency.[13,36,63] The usual doses of azathioprine are 2 to 3 mg/kg/day, and for MP 1 to 1.5 mg/kg/day.[71] Starting doses are typically 50 mg/day and increased at 2-week intervals.

Clinical response to MP may be related to whole-blood concentrations of the metabolite 6-thioguanine (6-TGN), while toxicity is correlated with concentrations of another metabolite, 6-methylmercaptopurine.[71]

11 Although mostly used in the setting of maintenance therapy as an alternative to azathioprine, methotrexate is another option for use as induction and/or maintenance therapy for patients with moderate to severe CD. Use of a weekly intramuscular or subcutaneous injection of 15 to 25 mg has demonstrated efficacy for induction of remission in CD and corticosteroid-sparing effects.[13,36,44,63]

The TNF-α inhibitors are effective agents in the management of CD. Collectively these agents have demonstrated rates of remission of 28% at 4 to 12 weeks versus 19% with placebo ($P < 0.001$).[70] Infliximab is a well-established treatment option for moderate to severe active CD for patients failing immunosuppressive therapy, in those who are corticosteroid dependent, and for treatment of fistulizing disease.[13,36,70,81,82] In large trials infliximab has resulted in remission in up to 46% of patients at 10 to 12 weeks.[13,70,81–83] Following the standard dose regimen of 5 mg/kg at 0, 2, and 6 weeks, 69% of patients with fistulizing disease responded with a 50% reduction in draining fistulae.[81–83] Data comparing infliximab with azathioprine and the combination of infliximab and azathioprine demonstrated significantly greater rates of remission of 57% at week 26 with the combination and infliximab alone (44%) compared with azathioprine alone (30%) in immunomodulator and biologic naive patients with CD.[84] Patients with CRP levels greater than 0.8 mg/dL (8 mg/L) and those with mucosal lesions responded better in both groups receiving infliximab. Earlier use of infliximab is efficacious, particularly in patients with luminal disease; however, this has also raised concerns regarding development of serious adverse effects such as infections and lymphoma.[64,80,85]

Adalimumab is another viable option for moderate to severe CD. It has the advantage of subcutaneous administration and may be considered as an alternate to infliximab as initial therapy or in those patients losing response to infliximab. Trials evaluating treatment with adalimumab for patients with moderate to severe active CD demonstrate rates of remission of approximately 25% at 4 weeks.[70] In patients who have lost response to infliximab, adalimumab use has resulted in rates of remission of 21% at 4 weeks.[72] Certolizumab has also demonstrated efficacy in moderate to severe CD with patients who have a baseline CRP of greater than 10 mg/dL (100 mg/L) exhibiting the best response rates, reported as 25% to 37% at 6 to 12 weeks.[70,83] Natalizumab is reserved for patients who do not respond to steroids or TNF-α inhibitors. Patients who initially responded to natalizumab treatment had rates of sustained response reported as 61% versus 28% for placebo at week 36.[71]

Severe/Fulminant Active Disease

Patients with severe or fulminant disease require prompt management in the inpatient setting and are often considered for surgical intervention. Parenteral corticosteroids at a dose equivalent of 40 to 60 mg prednisone should be instituted once the presence of abscess has been excluded.[36] Unresponsive cyclosporine has been tried at doses of 2 to 4 mg/h via IV infusion with reported in-hospital colectomy rates of 12.5%; however, despite these findings, there are few data to support its use in this setting.[13,86] It may also be effective as a last-line option for patients with severe fistulizing disease.[86]

Maintenance of Remission

Maintaining remission is typically more difficult with CD than with UC. There is minimal evidence that sulfasalazine and oral mesalamine derivatives are effective therapies for maintenance of CD following medically induced remission.[35,74] Despite these findings, an attempt to maintain remission with sulfasalazine or oral mesalamine following a medically induced remission may be carried out given the favorable side-effect profile and cost of these drugs compared with those of immunosuppressive and biologic agents. Mesalamine appears to have some efficacy in preventing postsurgical relapse following resection, with absolute risk reductions of approximately 14% for relapse in some studies, and can be considered in patients who do not qualify for or have a contraindication to immunosuppressive therapy.[79]

Systemic corticosteroids have no place in the prevention of recurrence of CD. These agents do not alter the long-term course of the disease and predispose patients to serious adverse effects with long-term use.[36] Budesonide has been studied at maintenance doses of 6 mg/day for up to 52 weeks with minimal efficacy in maintaining remission.[13,61,74] Despite this recommendation, use of budesonide as maintenance therapy for up to 1 year can be considered, particularly in patients who have become corticosteroid dependent, for whom switching to budesonide is an option.[13]

Azathioprine and MP are effective in maintaining remission in CD in up to 70% of patients, particularly in infliximab- or steroid-induced remission, and therefore these drugs are generally considered first-line agents.[36,74] Patients who may benefit from these agents include those with quiescent disease who are steroid dependent or refractory, postsurgical patients to prevent recurrence, those with frequent flares requiring steroid bursts, and those with perianal or enteric fistulas.[13,63,74] For patients who initially respond to methotrexate, continued dosing at 15 to 25 mg intramuscularly once weekly is also effective in maintaining remission in up to 66% of patients and may be considered as an alternative to azathioprine and MP.[13,63,74]

All of the currently approved TNF-α inhibitors are viable options for maintenance of remission in CD. Infliximab given at a dose of 5 mg/kg every 8 weeks is more effective than placebo in maintaining remission for patients who initially respond.[13] Reported rates of steroid-free remission at 48 to 52 weeks range from 12% to 16%[70,74,81] An increase in the dose to 10 mg/kg or shortening of the dosing interval to 6 weeks is possible if loss of efficacy over time is evident.[72] Additionally, infliximab is the effective maintenance therapy for fistulizing disease, and may be used in combination with azathioprine or MP.[81] Adalimumab is also a treatment option for maintenance therapy of CD. Following induction therapy, doses of 40 mg subcutaneously every other week have resulted in clinical remission rates of 40% to 47% after 20 to 30 weeks of therapy.[13,70,74] Certolizumab is effective for maintenance of CD, with remission rates for patients who initially responded reported as 48% at 20 to 30 weeks.[74] For patients treated with natalizumab who initially respond, maintenance therapy led to significant response rates of 40% at 60 weeks compared with 15% with placebo.[70]

Selected Complications

Toxic Megacolon

The treatment required for toxic megacolon includes general supportive, consideration for early surgical intervention, and drug therapy.[32,36] Perforation is reported in up to 36% of patients and can significantly worsen outcomes.[48] Aggressive fluid and electrolyte management is required for dehydration. Transfusion may be necessary if significant blood loss has occurred. Opiates and medications with anticholinergic properties should be discontinued because these agents enhance colonic dilation, thereby increasing the risk of bowel perforation.[48] Broad-spectrum antimicrobials that include coverage for gram-negative bacilli and intestinal anaerobes should be used as preemptive therapy in the event that perforation occurs.[32] If the patient is not receiving corticosteroids, then high-dose IV therapy should be administered to reduce acute inflammation. Emergent surgical intervention, mainly an abdominal colectomy with formation of an ileostomy, is an important consideration for patients with toxic megacolon and prevents death in some patients.[48]

Extraintestinal Manifestations

For some extraintestinal manifestations of IBD, specific therapies can be instituted, whereas for others the treatment that is used for the GI inflammatory process also addresses the systemic manifestations.

Anemia secondary to blood loss from the GI tract can be treated with oral ferrous sulfate. If the patient is unable to take oral medication and the patient's hematocrit is sufficiently low, blood transfusions or IV iron infusions may be required.[40] Anemia may also be related to malabsorption of vitamin B_{12} or folic acid, particularly for patients who have had ileal resection, so supplementation may be required. Screening for osteoporosis via dual x-ray absorptiometry is recommended for patients using steroids for >3 months, in postmenopausal females, patients of age over 60, and those who have sustained a low-stress fracture.[42] If the patient is deemed high risk for osteoporosis or exhibits a reduced serum vitamin D concentration, vitamin D and calcium should be instituted. If osteoporosis is present, then calcium, vitamin D, and a bisphosphonate or possibly teriparatide are recommended.[40,42] Corticosteroid use should be avoided or limited, and weight-bearing exercise initiated if possible.

There are no consistently recommended therapies for aphthous ulcers; however, topical viscous lidocaine may provide symptom relief while topical corticosteroids may promote healing.[40] Episcleritis or uveitis is often worse during exacerbations of the intestinal disease, and measures improving intestinal disease will improve these systemic manifestations. Cool compresses and topical corticosteroids may provide symptomatic relief, while TNF-α inhibitors when in use may also provide benefit.[40] For arthritis associated with IBD, aspirin or another NSAID may be beneficial, as are corticosteroids. However, NSAID use may exacerbate the underlying IBD and predispose patients to GI bleeding. Intraarticular corticosteroids may be tried to limit the adverse effects of systemically administered agents.[40] Skin manifestations often require local wound care and use of topical or systemic corticosteroids.[40] Anti–TNF-α therapies may also improve severe dermatologic manifestations. Although ursodiol may improve liver enzymes in patients with IBD-associated PSC, it has not been demonstrated to have favorable effects on outcomes.[39,40] Liver transplantation is being used more frequently for definitive treatment of PSC.

Special Considerations

Pregnancy and Breast-Feeding

The occurrence or consideration of pregnancy may cause significant concerns for the patient with IBD. Patients with IBD have similar infertility rates as the general female population. The rate of normal childbirth is similar to that for healthy populations.[87,88] Some studies have noted a greater risk of spontaneous abortion, low birth weight, caesarian section, or congenital abnormalities.[87] However, most patients can conceive normally and have a normal pregnancy.[87–91] There is a small risk of preterm labor or low-gestational-weight infants.[87,90,91] Preconception counseling is key for female patients with IBD who are considering becoming pregnant. This includes improving prepregnancy nutrition, implementing supplementation with folate, calcium, and vitamin D, ceasing alcohol and tobacco use, and inducing disease remission if possible.[87] Overall, pregnancy appears to have minimal effects on the course of IBD.[86–90] Likewise, IBD appears to have little effect on the course of pregnancy, particularly if the IBD is quiescent at the time of conception.[87,88,90] Patients who are pregnant experience IBD recurrence rates similar to those of nonpregnant females.[90] Patients are recommended to wait until their disease is in remission for 3 months prior to conceiving if possible.[86] Patients requiring colectomy for UC should preferentially receive rectal-sparing surgery if they are considering conceiving, followed by IPAA after delivery.[87]

Most classes of medications used in IBD are relatively safe in pregnancy. Sulfasalazine is generally well tolerated; however, it does interfere with folate absorption, so supplementation with folic acid 1 mg twice daily should be used during the pregnancy.[87,88] Sulfasalazine causes decreased sperm counts and reduced fertility in males. This effect is reversible on discontinuation of the drug, and it is not reported with mesalamine. Other ASAs can be used as well; however, there are concerns regarding the presence of dibutyl phthalate in the coating of Asacol.[87] Mesalamine preparations not containing dibutyl phthalate should be preferentially used. Steroids given systemically do not appear to be detrimental to the fetus, with the exception of dexamethasone.[87,90] Maternal cortisol is generally inactivated by placental 11β-hydroxysteroid dehydrogenase type 2; however, dexamethasone is not inactivated by this enzyme and may accumulate in fetal tissue. Therefore, dexamethasone should be avoided in pregnancy.[87] Immunosuppressive drugs (azathioprine and MP) may be associated with fetal deformities in humans and are classified as pregnancy category D; however, they have been used commonly in IBD without detriment for most patients.[87,90] Infliximab, adalimumab, and certolizumab are classified as pregnancy category B drugs and appear to be relatively safe for use in pregnant patients.[87–91] Use of infliximab should be restricted to the first and second trimesters if possible due to placental transfer of infliximab and the potential for neonatal adverse effects.[91] There is a similar concern with adalimumab, although this agent is more difficult to detect in the neonatal bloodstream. Consideration can be given to stopping it 8 to 10 weeks prior to delivery.[91] Natalizumab is a pregnancy category C drug and not much is known about its safety in pregnancy, and thus may be used if benefit is thought to outweigh risk.[91] Metronidazole may be used for short courses for treatment of trichomoniasis, but prolonged use should be avoided due to potential mutagenic effects.[90] Methotrexate should not be used during pregnancy, as it is a known abortifacient (category X).[87–91] Cyclosporine has been used in pregnant patients with success and therefore is an option for patients with severe disease.[87,90]

Use of agents in breast-feeding women is also a consideration. Sulfasalazine does pose a small risk of kernicterus, as levels of sulfapyridine in breast milk are low or undetectable, and thus monitoring for this symptom should be implemented.[87] Other mesalamine derivatives are considered safe in breast-feeding.[87,90] Corticosteroids can be detected in breast milk, with fetal levels approximately 10% to 12% of maternal levels.[88] However, breast-feeding is believed to be safe for the infant when doses of prednisone less than 40 mg are used.[88] Optimally mothers should wait at least 4 hours after an oral dose of systemic corticosteroids before breast-feeding to limit exposure to the child.[87,90] The anti–TNF-α agents are generally considered safe for use in breast-feeding and carry minimal risk of adverse effects.[88,91] Metronidazole and cyclosporine should not be given to nursing mothers because these agents are excreted into breast milk and may cause adverse effects.[87–90]

Adverse Drug Effects

Drug intolerance often limits the usefulness of agents used to treat IBD. In some cases, adverse effects can be significant and require discontinuation of the therapy. Knowledge of the common or important adverse reactions will assist in avoiding or minimizing their effects.

Compared with mesalamine, sulfasalazine is more often associated with adverse drug effects, and these effects may be classified as either dose related or idiosyncratic (Table 21-6).[55] The sulfapyridine portion of the sulfasalazine molecule is believed to be responsible

TABLE 21-6 Drug Monitoring Guidelines

Drug(s)	Adverse Drug Reaction	Monitoring Parameters	Comments
Sulfasalazine	Nausea, vomiting, headache	Folate, complete blood count	Increase the dose slowly, over 1–2 weeks
	Rash, anemia, pneumonitis	Liver function tests, Scr, BUN	
	Hepatotoxicity, nephritis		
	Thrombocytopenia, lymphoma		
Mesalamine	Nausea, vomiting, headache	GI disturbances	
Corticosteroids	Hyperglycemia, dyslipidemia	Blood pressure, fasting lipid panel	Avoid long-term use if possible or consider budesonide
	Osteoporosis, hypertension, acne	Glucose, vitamin D, bone density	
	Edema, infection, myopathy, psychosis		
Azathioprine/mercaptopurine	Bone marrow suppression, pancreatitis	Complete blood count	Check TMPT activity
	Liver dysfunction, rash, arthralgia	Scr, BUN, liver function tests, genotype/phenotype	
Methotrexate	Bone marrow suppression, pancreatitis	Complete blood count Scr, BUN	Check baseline pregnancy test
	Pneumonitis, pulmonary fibrosis, hepatitis	Liver function tests	Chest x-ray
Infliximab	Infusion-related reactions (infliximab), infection	Blood pressure/heart rate (infliximab)	Need negative PPD and viral serologies
Adalimumab	Heart failure, optic neuritis, demyelination, injection site reaction, signs of infection	Neurologic exam, mental status	
Certolizumab	Lymphoma	Trough concentrations (infliximab)	
Natalizumab	Infusion-related reactions	Brain MRI, mental status, progressive multifocal leukoencephalopathy	

for much of the sulfasalazine toxicity.[31] Dose-related side effects usually include GI disturbances such as nausea, vomiting, diarrhea, or anorexia but may also include headache and arthralgia. These adverse reactions tend to occur more commonly on initiation of therapy and decrease in frequency as therapy is continued. Approaches to the management of these adverse effects include discontinuing the agent for a short period and then reinstituting therapy at a reduced dosage with subsequent slower dose escalation, administration with food, or substituting another enteric-coated 5-ASA product. Folic acid absorption is impaired by sulfasalazine, which may lead to anemia, so oral folic acid supplementation should be administered.

Idiosyncratic effects commonly include rash, fever, or hepatotoxicity, as well as relatively uncommon but serious reactions such as bone marrow suppression, thrombocytopenia, pancreatitis, pneumonitis, interstitial nephritis, and hepatitis. For most patients with idiosyncratic reactions, sulfasalazine must be discontinued. In some patients who have experienced allergic reactions to sulfasalazine, a desensitization procedure can be instituted. By gradually increasing sulfasalazine dosage over weeks to months, patient tolerance has been improved.[31]

Oral mesalamine derivatives may impose a lower frequency of adverse effects as compared with sulfasalazine.[31,73] Up to 80% of patients who are intolerant to sulfasalazine will tolerate oral mesalamine derivatives.[31] The most commonly encountered adverse effects are nausea, vomiting, and headache.[73] However, olsalazine may cause watery diarrhea in up to 25% of patients, often requiring drug discontinuation.

There is a greater potential for adverse effects from corticosteroids when used for the treatment of IBD because there is often a requirement for use of high doses for extended periods of time. Adverse effects of corticosteroids include hyperglycemia, hypertension, osteoporosis, acne, fluid retention, electrolyte disturbances, myopathies, muscle wasting, increased appetite, psychosis, infection, and adrenocortical suppression.[31,62] To minimize corticosteroid effects, clinicians have used alternate-day steroid therapy; however, some patients do not do well clinically on the days when no steroid is given. For most patients a single daily corticosteroid dose suffices, and divided daily doses are unnecessary. Adrenal insufficiency after abrupt steroid withdrawal often necessitates gradual tapering of steroid therapy for patients using these agents daily for more than 2 to 3 weeks. Due to its lower bioavailability and lower potential for adverse effects, budesonide may be used as alternate steroid therapy in CD involving the ileum or right colon, or in UC, or may be substituted for prednisone in CD patients who are steroid dependent or require long-term therapy.[35,36]

Complete blood counts with differential should be monitored every 2 weeks while doses are being titrated. Azathioprine and MP may be associated with serious adverse effects such as lymphomas, pancreatitis, or nephrotoxicity.[31,36,65] Adverse events to thiopurines are typically divided into two groups, type A and type B.[92,93] Type A are dose related and include malaise, nausea, infectious complications, hepatitis, and myelosuppression. Type B reactions are considered idiosyncratic and include fever, rash, arthralgia, and pancreatitis (3% to 15% of patients).[92,93] Predisposition to development of these adverse effects may be related to polymorphisms in the enzyme thiopurine methyltransferase (TPMT), which is partially responsible for activation and metabolism of these drugs. Determination of TPMT activity is recommended prior to initiation of therapy to determine which patients require lower doses of these agents.[36,71] Alternatively, evaluating TPMT genotype or phenotype can also assist in assessing a patient's risk for toxicity.[63–65,71] Adjusting azathioprine and MP doses by measuring concentrations of metabolites, particularly 6-TGN, may be useful, with higher levels associated with greater remission rates.[63–65,67]

With the advent of coadministration of azathioprine with infliximab, development of hepatosplenic T-cell lymphoma (HSTCL) has become a concern. The overall impact of using both drugs together, the contribution of drug classes to the development of lymphoma, and the risk and effects of both drugs are unclear. Those most at risk appear to be younger male patients.[64,85,94] Methotrexate is associated with the development of nausea, vomiting, pulmonary fibrosis, pneumonitis, hepatotoxicity, anemia, and renal dysfunction, and is a known abortifacient. Patients should have baseline liver function tests, serum creatinine, BUN, complete blood count, and chest x-ray prior to use. Female patients should have a negative pregnancy test prior to use. Some patients may require supplementation with folic acid.

Most patients receiving metronidazole for CD tolerate the agent fairly well; however, mild adverse effects occur frequently. They commonly include nausea, metallic taste, urticaria, and glossitis.[32,35] More serious effects that occur with long-term use include development of paresthesias and reversible peripheral neuropathy. Other effects include a disulfiram-like reaction if alcohol is ingested in conjunction.

The TNF-α inhibitors may be associated with development of serious adverse effects and carry similar adverse effect profiles for the available agents. Patients who receive infliximab often develop antibodies to infliximab (ATIs), also referred to as antidrug antibodies (ADAs), which can result in increases in the occurrence of serious infusion-related reactions and loss of response to the drug. Up to 10% of patients per year require discontinuation of infliximab due to adverse effects and loss of efficacy related to development of ATIs.[71,81,95] Strategies to reduce ATI formation include administration of a second dose within 8 weeks of the first dose, concurrent administration of steroids (hydrocortisone 200 mg IV on the day of the infusion or oral prednisone the day prior), and use of concomitant immunosuppressive agents.[71,84] Loss of efficacy may be managed by a dose escalation to 10 mg/kg or reducing the dosing interval.[80,84] Delayed hypersensitivity reactions may also occur up to 14 days after administration, with 5 to 7 days being the most common time frame.[81,95] Due to administration via the subcutaneous route, adalimumab and certolizumab may be more associated with injection site reactions versus infusion-related reactions. Likewise, development of antibodies to adalimumab appears to be minimal due to its humanized structure.[81] Autoimmune phenomena, such as lupus and hemolytic anemia, may also occur during infliximab therapy but are uncommon, as are adverse neurologic events such as optic neuritis and demyelinating syndrome.[72,81,95] As mentioned earlier, risk of HSTCL may be increased with use of infliximab, particularly if used in combination with immunomodulators such as azathioprine. For these reasons patients with a history of demyelinating disease, optic neuritis, or lymphoma should avoid use of TNF-α antagonists.[95] Infliximab may also cause worsening of heart failure and thus is contraindicated for patients with New York Heart Association Class III or IV heart failure.[85] While the mechanism is unclear, it may relate in part to the cytoprotective effects of TNF on ischemic cardiac tissue, increases in production of nitric oxide and increased peripheral perfusion secondary to TNF, or TNF's role in cardiac remodeling and repair.[81]

All TNF-α inhibitors predispose patients to development of serious infections, including fungal, bacterial, and viral. Patients with clinically significant active infections should not receive TNF-α inhibitors. While the overall risk of hospitalization for serious infections may be less than previously suspected, development of infection remains a serious concern.[96] Reactivation of latent mycobacterial infections may occur because of the inhibition of TNF-protective mechanisms; therefore, patients should receive a tuberculin skin test (purified protein derivative [PPD] test) and a chest x-ray prior to initiating therapy to rule out undiagnosed tuberculosis.[81,95] Reactivation of hepatitis B may occur; thus, patients should also be screened for hepatitis B virus infection prior to initiating therapy. Patients should also be screened for hepatitis C infection, although it does not appear that use of TNF-α inhibitors is unsafe or significantly alters the disease course.[81] Lastly, use of natalizumab is associated with development of progressive multifocal leukoencephalopathy and is only available via the manufacturer's TOUCH prescribing program.[95] Patients receiving natalizumab should be monitored for development of adverse neurologic events and undergo MRI of the brain should development of progressive multifocal leukoencephalopathy be suspected.

PERSONALIZED PHARMACOTHERAPY

The approach to treatment of IBD should consider all aspects of each individual patient in order to maximize therapy, improve patient symptoms and QOL, and prevent complications. To ensure optimal drug therapy, an assessment of each patient's health literacy and potential barriers to understanding and adherence should be performed. Involving the patient in the care process will help to keep him or her engaged. For the drug classes that are used in the management of IBD, there are several aspects of individualization that may improve efficacy and safety. Since patients with IBD are often seen by GI specialists or surgeons, ensuring that each provider has a current, accurate, and complete medication list will help to prevent potential medication errors. Female patients of childbearing age should discuss with their providers their goals for becoming pregnant, as this may dictate the choice of drugs used.

For the ASAs picking the appropriate formulation and dose of drug for the disease severity and extent is key. Enemas and suppositories, while generally more effective than oral preparations, may not be as acceptable for use, particularly by younger patients. Therefore, individuating the patient's preference for a specific formulation should be taken into account when choosing ASA preparations.[57] Consideration can be given to the use of once-daily products if there is evidence that multiple-daily dosing is affecting patient adherence.[57–59] This must be weighed against the higher cost of these preparations. If expense is an issue, use of generically available agents may be preferred.

Patients receiving systemic corticosteroids for extended periods of time should be assessed for risk of bone loss and fracture and the need for vitamin D and calcium supplementation. In addition, a review of the patient's medical history should be performed to identify other conditions that may be worsened by corticosteroids, such as diabetes or hypertension. Adjustment of medications for these types of conditions may need to be made based on the dose and duration of corticosteroid use.

Patients in whom azathioprine or MP is being considered should undergo TPMT activity testing or have a genotype or phenotype test performed to determine if dose adjustments are required. Since the initial dosing of these agents is weight based, obtaining a current accurate weight for the patient is necessary as well. Obtaining a family history regarding lymphoproliferative disorders or lymphoma is important for determining if the potential risks outweigh the benefits of long-term use. For female patients in whom methotrexate is being considered, a pregnancy test should be obtained and the potential desire to become pregnant in the future should be discussed. Female patients of childbearing age opting to use methotrexate should have a safe and effective method of birth control available that is based on their preference.

For patients receiving TNF-α antagonists, baseline screening for latent infections should be performed. Obtaining an accurate weight will assist in the dosing of infliximab. Likewise use of infliximab requires administration in an observed infusion center or clinic. If patients are unable to afford to get to their appointment, use of a self-administered agent, such as adalimumab or certolizumab, may be preferred. If patients appear to be losing response to infliximab, evaluating for ATIs, if assays are available, in addition to evaluating serum trough concentrations may assist the clinician in determining if dose and frequency need to be altered. In vitro infliximab concentrations of 0.2 to 10 mcg/mL (mg/L) are shown to inhibit TNF-α activity, while the optimal in vivo concentration is not known.[72] Targeting trough concentrations of least 12 mcg/mL (mg/L) at 4 weeks is reasonable, as higher concentrations appear to improve disease activity and significantly reduce inflammatory markers such as CRP.[72] Patients who lose response may need to be switched to adalimumab or certolizumab.

From a health maintenance standpoint, patients should be evaluated for use of recommended vaccines; however, if patients are receiving immunosuppressants or biologic agents, the use of live or attenuated vaccines may be contraindicated. Patients who currently use tobacco should be encouraged to undergo tobacco cessation, as tobacco use will worsen CD. Since nicotine often improves symptoms in UC, it may be more difficult to cease tobacco use in this patient population. Choice of tobacco cessation products should also be based on current amount and patient preference. Nutritional status of patients should also be routinely assessed, and patient-specific diets or delivery, such as enteral or parenteral nutrition, should be implemented.

EVALUATION OF THERAPEUTIC OUTCOMES

The success of therapeutic regimens to treat IBD can be measured by patient-reported complaints, signs, and symptoms; by direct clinician examination (including endoscopy); by history and physical examination; by selected laboratory tests; and by QOL measures. Evaluation of IBD severity is difficult because much of the assessment is subjective. Disease rating scales, such as the CDAI or other indices, have been created to try and make disease assessment more objective. The CDAI is a commonly used scale for patients with nonfistulizing disease and for evaluation of patients during clinical trials.[44] The scale incorporates eight elements: (a) number of stools in the past 7 days, (b) sum of abdominal pain ratings from the past 7 days, (c) rating of general well-being in the past 7 days, (d) use of antidiarrheals, (e) body weight, (f) hematocrit, (g) finding of abdominal mass, and (h) a sum of extraintestinal symptoms present in the past week. Elements of this index provide a guide for those measures that may be useful in assessing the effectiveness of treatment regimens. A decrease in CDAI of 100 points is considered a clinically significant response, with a score of <150 considered to be disease remission.[44] A subsequent scale was developed specifically for perianal CD, known as the *Perianal CD Activity Index* (PDAI).[44] The PDAI includes five items: presence of discharge, pain, restriction of sexual activity, type of perianal disease, and degree of induration. The HBI may also be used in place of the CDAI.

Standardized assessment tools have also been constructed for UC.[43] Elements in these scales vary and include (a) stool frequency, (b) presence of blood in the stool, (c) mucosal appearance (from endoscopy), and (d) physician's global assessment based on physical examination, endoscopy, and laboratory data. While these tools are often used for assessment of patients in clinical trials, they are sometimes used in the clinical setting as well.

Additional studies that are often useful include direct endoscopic examination of affected areas and/or radiocontrast studies. As mentioned earlier, mucosal healing is being explored as a major end point for patients with luminal disease.[46] For patients with acute disease, assessment of fluid and electrolyte status is important, because these may be lost during diarrheal episodes. Other laboratory tests, such as serum albumin, transferrin, or other markers of visceral protein status as well as markers of inflammation such as ESR or CRP, may be used to monitor disease and drug therapy.

Assessment of the IBD patient must include consideration of adverse drug effects. Because many of the agents used have a relatively high probability of causing adverse effects, particularly corticosteroids and other immunosuppressive agents, patient assessment should include collection of history and physical and laboratory data that are necessary to prevent or recognize adverse drug effects.

Finally, a patient QOL assessment should be performed regularly.[43,44] Inquiry should be made regarding patient's general well-being, emotional function, and social function. Social function may include assessment of the ability to perform routine daily functions and to maintain occupational activities, sexual function, and recreation. The most common tool used to assess QOL is the Inflammatory Bowel Disease Questionnaire (IBDQ), a 32-item questionnaire that covers four disease dimensions: bowel function, emotional status, systemic symptoms, and social function. The IBDQ has shown good correlation with the CDAI.[44] The standard short form-36 is often used as a measure of QOL in IBD intervention trials.[43,44]

ABBREVIATIONS

ADA antidrug antibody
ASA aminosalicylate
ATI antibody to infliximab
CD Crohn's disease
CDAI Crohn's Disease Activity Index
CRC colorectal carcinoma
CRP C-reactive protein
ESR erythrocyte sedimentation rate
HBI Harvey Bradshaw Index
HLA human leukocyte antigen
HSTCL hepatosplenic T-cell lymphoma
IBD inflammatory bowel disease
IBDQ Inflammatory Bowel Disease Questionnaire
IL interleukin
IPAA ileal pouch anal anastomosis
MMX Multi-MatriX
MP mercaptopurine
NF-κB nuclear factor κB
NOD2 nucleotide-binding oligomerization domain protein 2
NSAID nonsteroidal antiinflammatory drug
PDAI Perianal Crohn's Disease Activity Index
PPD purified protein derivative
PSC primary sclerosing cholangitis
QOL quality of life
TGF-β transforming growth factor-β
TGN thioguanine
TLR toll-like membrane receptor
TNF-α tumor necrosis factor-α
TPMT thiopurine methyltransferase
UC ulcerative colitis
VTE venous thromboembolism

REFERENCES

1. Danese S, Fiocchi C. Ulcerative colitis. N Engl J Med 2011;356(18):1713–1725.
2. Cosnes J, Gower-Rousseau C, Seksik P, Cortot A. Epidemiology and natural history of inflammatory bowel diseases. Gastroenterology 2011;140:1786–1795.
3. Molodecky NA, Soon IS, Rabi DM, et al. Increasing incidence and prevalence of the inflammatory bowel diseases with time, based on systematic review. Gastroenterology 2012;142:46–54.
4. Gerseman M, Wehkamp J, Strange EF. Innate immune dysfunction in inflammatory bowel disease. J Intern Med 2012;271:421–428.
5. Scharl M, Rogler G. Inflammatory bowel disease pathogenesis: What is new? Curr Opin Gastroenterol 2012;28:301–309.
6. Nanau R, Neuman MG. Metabolome and inflammasome in inflammatory bowel disease. Transl Res 2012;160:1–28.

7. Seksik P, Sokol H, Lepage P, et al. Review article: The role of bacteria in onset and perpetuation of inflammatory bowel disease. Aliment Pharmacol Ther 2006;24(Suppl 3):11–18.
8. Gentschew L, Ferguson LR. Role of nutrition and microbiota in susceptibility to inflammatory bowel diseases. Mol Nutr Food Res 2012;56:524–535.
9. Lakatos PL, Fischer S, Lakatos L, et al. Current concept on the pathogenesis of inflammatory bowel disease-crosstalk between genetic and microbial factors: Pathogenic bacteria and altered bacterial sensing or changes in mucosal integrity take "toll". World J Gastroenterol 2006;12:1829–1841.
10. Murphy SF, Kwon JH, Boone DL. Novel players in inflammatory bowel disease pathogenesis. Curr Gastroenterol Rep 2012;14:146–152.
11. Cho JH, Brant SR. Recent insights into the genetics of inflammatory bowel disease. Gastroenterology 2011;140:1704–1712.
12. Neuman MG, Nanau R. Single nucleotide polymorphisms in inflammatory bowel disease. Transl Res 2012;160:45–64.
13. Talley NJ, Abreu MT, Achkar JP, et al. An evidence-based systematic review on medical therapies for inflammatory bowel disease. Am J Gastroenterol 2011;106:S2–S25.
14. Di Sabatino A, Biacnheri P, Rovedatti L, MacDonald TT, Corazza GR. Recent advances in understanding ulcerative colitis. Intern Emerg Med 2012;7:103–111.
15. Hamilton MJ, Snapper SB, Blumberg RS. Update on biologic pathways in inflammatory bowel disease and their therapeutic relevance. J Gastroenterol 2012;47:1–8.
16. Andrews JM, Holtmann G. Stress causes flares of IBD—Much evidence is enough? Nat Rev Gastroenterol Hepatol 2011;8:13–14.
17. Rampton DS. The influence of stress on the development and severity of immune mediated diseases. J Rheumatol 2011;38(Suppl 88):43–47.
18. Rampton DS. Does stress influence inflammatory bowel disease? The clinical data. Dig Dis 2009;27(Suppl 1):76–79.
19. Camara RJ, Schoepfer AM, Pittet V, Begre S, von Kanel R, Swiss Inflammatory Bowel Disease Cohort Study (SIBDCS) Group. Mood and nonmood components of perceived stress and exacerbation of Crohn's disease. Inflamm Bowel Dis 2011;17(11):2358–2365.
20. Singh S, Blanchard A, Walker JR, Graff LA, Miller N, Bernstein CN. Common symptoms and stressors among individuals with inflammatory bowel diseases. Clin Gastroenterol Hepatol 2011;9(9):769–775.
21. Graff LA, Walker JR, Clara I, Lix L, Miller N, Rogala L. Stress coping, distress, and health perceptions in inflammatory bowel disease and community controls. Am J Gastroenterol 2009;104(12):2959–2969.
22. Boye B, Lundin KE, Jantschek G, et al. INSPIRE study: Does stress management improve the course of inflammatory bowel disease and disease-specific quality of life in distressed patients with ulcerative colitis or Crohn's disease? A randomized controlled trial. Inflamm Bowel Dis 2011;17(9):1863–1873.
23. Savard J, Woodgate R. Young peoples' experience of living with ulcerative colitis and an ostomy. Gastroenterol Nurs 2009;32(1):33–41.
24. Neuman MG, Nanau RM. Inflammatory bowel disease: Role of diet, microbiota, life style. Transl Res 2012;160:29–44.
25. Albenberg LG, Lewis JD, Wu GD. Food and gut microbiotica in inflammatory bowel disease: A critical connection. Curr Opin Gastroenterol 2012;28:314–320.
26. Monteleone I, MacDonald TT, Pallone F, Monteleone G. The aryl hydrocarbon receptor in inflammatory bowel disease: Linking environment to disease pathogenesis. Curr Opin Gastroenterol 2012;28:310–313.
27. McGrath J, McDonald JWD, MacDonald JK. Transdermal nicotine for induction of remission in ulcerative colitis. Cochrane Database Syst Rev 2004;(4):CD004722. doi:10.1002/14651858.CD004722.pub2.
28. Ananthakrishnan AN, Higuchi LM, Huang ES, et al. Aspirin, nonsteroidal anti-inflammatory drug use, and risk for Crohn disease and ulcerative colitis. Ann Intern Med 2012;156:350–359.
29. Singh S, Graff LA, Bernstein CN. Do NSAIDs, antibiotics, infections, or stress trigger flares in IBD? Am J Gastroenterol 2009;104:1298–1313.
30. Crockett SD, Porter CQ, Martin CF, Sandler RS, Kappelman MD. Isotretinoin use and the risk of inflammatory bowel disease: A case–control study. Am J Gastroenterol 2010;105(9):1986–1993.
31. Kornbluth A, Sachar DB. Ulcerative practice guidelines in adults: American College of Gastroenterology, Practice Parameters Committee. Am J Gastroenterol 2010;105: 501–523.
32. Gan SI, Beck PL. A new look at toxic megacolon: An update and review of incidence, etiology, pathogenesis, and management. Am J Gastroenterol 2003;98:2363–2371.
33. Velayos F. Managing risks of neoplasia in inflammatory bowel disease. Curr Gastroenterol Rep 2012;14:174–180.
34. Farraye FA, Odze RD, Eaden J, Itzkowitz SH. AGA technical review on the diagnosis and management of colorectal neoplasia in inflammatory bowel disease. Gastroenterology 2010;138(2):746–774.
35. Lichtenstein GR, Hanauer SB, Sandborn WJ, The Practice Parameters Committee of the American College of Gastroenterology. Management of Crohn's disease in adults. Am J Gastroenterol 2009;104:465–483.
36. Buchner AM, Blonski W, Lichtenstein GR. Update on the management of Crohn's disease. Curr Gastroenterol Rep 2011;3:465–474.
37. Hartman C, Eliakim R, Shamir R. Nutritional status and nutritional therapy in inflammatory bowel diseases. World J Gastroenterol 2009;15:2570–2578.
38. Filippi J, Al-Jaouni R, Wiroth JB, et al. Nutritional deficiencies in patients with Crohn's disease in remission. Inflamm Bowel Dis 2006;12:185–191.
39. Navaneethan U, Shen B. Hepatopancreatobiliary manifestations and complications associated with inflammatory bowel disease. Inflamm Bowel Dis 2010;16(9):1598–1619.
40. Larsen S, Bendtzen K, Nielsen OH. Extraintestinal manifestations of inflammatory bowel disease: Epidemiology, diagnosis, and management. Ann Med 2010;42(2):97–114.
41. Murthy SK, Nguyen CG. Venous thromboembolism in inflammatory bowel disease: An epidemiological review. Am J Gastroenterol 2011;106:713–718.
42. American Gastroenterological Association medical position statement: Guidelines on osteoporosis in gastrointestinal diseases. Gastroenterology 2003;124:791–794.
43. Travis SPL, Higgins PDR, Orchard T, et al. Review article: Defining remission in ulcerative colitis. Aliment Pharmacol Ther 2011;34:113–124.
44. Cottone M, Renna S, Orlando A, Mocciaro F. Medical management of Crohn's disease. Expert Opin Pharmacother 2011;12(16):2505–2525.
45. Pineton de Chambrun G, Lemann M, Peyrin-Biroule L. Clinical implications of mucosal healing for the management of IBD. Nat Rev Gastroenterol Hepatol 2010;7:15–29.

46. Flynn A, Kane S. Mucosal healing in Crohn's disease and ulcerative colitis: What does it tell us? Curr Opin Gastroenterol 2011;27:342–345.
47. Forbes A, Goldesgeyme E, Paulon E. Nutrition in inflammatory bowel disease. J Parenter Enteral Nutr 2011;35:571–580.
48. Bitton A, Buie D, Enns R, et al. Treatment of hospitalized adult patients with severe ulcerative colitis: Toronto consensus statements. Am J Gastroenterol 2012;107:179–194.
49. Meijer BJ, Dieleman LA. Probiotics in the treatment of human inflammatory bowel diseases update 2011. J Clin Gastroenterol 2011;45:S139–S144.
50. Cain AM, Dowhower Karpa K. Clinical utility of probiotics in inflammatory bowel disease. Altern Ther Health Med 2011;17(l):72–79.
51. Jonkers D, Penders J, Masclee A, Pierik M. Probiotics in the management of inflammatory bowel disease: A systematic review of intervention studies in adult patients. Drugs 2012;72(6):803–823.
52. Rahimi R, Nikfar S, Rahimi F, et al. A meta-analysis on the efficacy of probiotics for maintenance of remission and prevention of clinical and endoscopic relapse in Crohn's disease. Dig Dis Sci 2008;53:2524–2531.
53. Prantera C, Scribano ML. Antibiotics and probiotics in inflammatory bowel disease: Why, when, and how. Curr Opin Gastroenterol 2009;25:329–333.
54. Butterworth AD, Thomas AG, Akobeng AK. Probiotics for induction of remission in Crohn's disease. Cochrane Database Syst Rev 2008;(3):CD006634. doi:10.1002/14651858.CD006634.pub2.
55. Biondi A, Zoccali M, Costa S, Troci A, Contessini-Avesani E, Fichera A. Surgical treatment of ulcerative colitis in the biologic therapy era. World J Gastroenterol 2012;18(16):1861–1870.
56. Campregher C, Gasche C. Aminosalicylates. Best Pract Res Clin Gastroenterol 2011;25:535–546.
57. Tindall WN. New approaches to adherence issues when dosing oral aminosalicylates in ulcerative colitis. Am J Health Syst Pharm 2009;66:451–457.
58. Oliveira L, Cohen RD. Maintaining remission in ulcerative colitis—Role of once daily extended-release mesalamine. Drug Des Dev Ther 2011;5:111–116.
59. Yang LPH, McCormack PL. MMX mesalamine: A review of its use in the management of mild to moderate ulcerative colitis. Drugs 2011;71(2):221–235.
60. Harris MS, Lichtenstein GR. Review article: Delivery and efficacy of topical 5-aminosalicylic acid (mesalazine) therapy in the treatment of ulcerative colitis. Aliment Pharmacol Ther 2011;33:996–1009.
61. Ford AC, Khan KJ, Achkar JP, Moayyedi P. Efficacy of oral vs. topical, or combined oral and topical 5-aminosalicylates, in ulcerative colitis: Systematic review and meta-analysis. Am J Gastroenterol 2012;107:167–176.
62. Ford AC, Bernstein CN, Khan KJ, et al. Glucocorticosteroid therapy in inflammatory bowel disease: Systematic review and meta-analysis. Am J Gastroenterol 2011;106:590–599.
63. Khan KJ, Dubinsky MC, Ford AC, Ullman TA, Talley NJ, Moayyedi P. Efficacy of immunosuppressive therapy for inflammatory bowel disease: A systematic review and meta-analysis. Am J Gastroenterol 2011;106:630–642.
64. Van Assche G, Vermeire S, Rutgeerts P. Immunosuppression in inflammatory bowel disease: Traditional, biological or both? Curr Opin Gastroenterol 2009;25:323–328.
65. Cohen BL, Torres J, Colombel JF. Immunosuppression in inflammatory bowel disease: How much is too much? Curr Opin Gastroenterol 2012;28:341–348.
66. Burger DC, Travis S. Colon salvage therapy for acute severe colitis: Cyclosporine or infliximab? Curr Opin Gastroenterol 2011;27:358–362.
67. Hoentjen F, Sakuraba A, Hanauer S. Update on the management of ulcerative colitis. Curr Gastroenterol Rep 2011;13:475–485.
68. McSharry K, Dalzell AM, Leiper K, El-Matary W. Systematic review: The role of tacrolimus in the management of Crohn's disease. Aliment Pharmacol Ther 2011;34:1282–1294.
69. Khan KJ, Ullman TA, Ford AC, et al. Antibiotic therapy in inflammatory bowel disease: A systematic review and meta-analysis. Am J Gastroenterol 2011;106:661–673.
70. Ford AC, Sandboarn WJ, Khan KJ, Hanauer SB, Talley NJ, Moayyedi P. Efficacy of biological therapies in inflammatory bowel disease: Systematic review and meta-analysis. Am J Gastroenterol 2011;106:644–659.
71. Blonski W, Buchner AM, Lichtenstein GR. Inflammatory bowel disease therapy: Current state-of-the-art. Curr Opin Gastroenterol 2011;27:346–357.
72. Yanai H, Hanauer SB. Assessing response and loss of response to biologic therapies in IBD. Am J Gastroenterol 2011;106:685–698.
73. Ford AC, Ackhar AC, Khan KJ, et al. Efficacy of 5-aminosalicylates in ulcerative colitis: Systematic review and meta-analysis. Am J Gastroenterol 2011;106: 601–616.
74. Peyrin-Biroulet L, Lémann M. Review article: Remission rates achievable by current therapies for inflammatory bowel disease. Aliment Pharmacol Ther 2011;33:870–879.
75. Zhu Y, Tang R, Zhao P, Zhu S, Li Y, Li J. Can oral 5-aminosalicylic acid be administered once daily in the treatment of mild-to-moderate ulcerative colitis? A meta-analysis of randomized-controlled trials. Eur J Gastroenterol Hepatol 2012;24:487–494.
76. Reinisch W, Sandborn WJ, Hommes DW, et al. Adalimumab for induction of clinical remission in moderately to severely active ulcerative colitis: Results of a randomised controlled trial. Gut 2011;60:780–787.
77. Sandborn WJ, van Assche G, Reinisch W, et al. Adalimumab induces and maintains clinical remission in patients with moderate-to-severe ulcerative colitis. Gastroenterology 2012;142(2):257–266.
78. Cheifetz AS, Stern J, Garud S, et al. Cyclosporine is safe and effective in patients with severe ulcerative colitis. J Clin Gastroenterol 2011;45:107–112.
79. Ford AC, Khan KK, Talley NJ, Moayyedi P. 5-Aminosalicylates prevent relapse of Crohn's disease after surgically induced remission: Systematic review and meta-analysis. Am J Gastroenterol 2011;106:413–420.
80. Ford AC, Kane SV, Khan KJ, Achkar AJ, Talley NJ, Marshall JK. Efficacy of 5-aminosalicylates in Crohn's disease: Systematic review and meta-analysis. Am J Gastroenterol 2011;106:617–629.
81. Danese S, Colombel JF, Reinisch W, Rutgeerts PJ. Review article: Infliximab for Crohn's disease treatment shifting therapeutic strategies after 10 years of clinical experience. Aliment Pharmacol Ther 2011;33:857–869.
82. Peyrin-Biroulet L, Deltenre P, de Suray N, et al. Efficacy and safety of tumor necrosis factor antagonists in Crohn's disease: Meta-analysis of placebo-controlled trials. Clin Gastroenterol Hepatol 2008;6:644–653.
83. D'Haens G, Panaccione R, Higgins PDR, et al. The London Position Statement of the World Congress of Gastroenterology on Biological Therapy for IBD with the European Crohn's and Colitis Organization: When to start,

when to stop, which drug to choose, and how to predict response? Am J Gastroenterol 2011;106:199–212.

84. Colombel J-F, Sandborn WJ, Reinisch W, et al. Infliximab, azathioprine, or combination therapy for Crohn's disease. N Engl J Med 2010;362:1383–1395.
85. Van Assche G, Lewis JD, Lichtenstein GR, Loft EV, Ouyang Q, Panes J. The London Position Statement of the World Congress of Gastroenterology on Biological Therapy for IBD with the European Crohn's and Colitis Organisation: Safety. Am J Gastroenterol 2011;106:1594–1602.
86. Lazarev M, Present DH, Lichtiger S, et al. The effect of intravenous cyclosporine on rates of colonic surgery in hospitalized patients with severe Crohn's colitis. J Clin Gastroenterol 2012;46(9):764–767.
87. Dubinsky M, Abraham B, Mahadevan U. Management of the pregnant IBD patient. Inflamm Bowel Dis 2008;14:1736–1750.
88. Habal FM, Huang VW. Review article: A decision-making algorithm for the management of pregnancy in the inflammatory bowel disease patient. Aliment Pharmacol Ther 2012;35:501–515.
89. Nasef NA, Ferguson LR. Inflammatory bowel disease and pregnancy: Overlapping pathways. Transl Res 2012;160:65–83.
90. Beaulieu DB, Kane S. Inflammatory bowel disease in pregnancy. Gastroenterol Clin North Am 2011;40:399–413.
91. van Mahade U, Cucchiara S, Hyams JS, et al. The London Position Statement of the World Congress of Gastroenterology on Biological Therapy for IBD with the European Crohn's and Colitis Organization: Pregnancy and pediatrics. Am J Gastroenterol 2011;106:214–223.
92. Derijks LJJ, Gilissen LPL, Hooymans PM, Hommes DW. Review article: Thiopurines in inflammatory bowel disease. Aliment Pharmacol Ther 2006;24:715–729.
93. Pascal Juillerat P, Pittet V, Felley C, et al. Drug safety in Crohn's disease. Digestion 2007;76:161–168.
94. Kotlyar DS, Osterman MT, Diamond RH, et al. A systematic review of factors that contribute to hepatosplenic T-cell lymphoma in patients with inflammatory bowel disease. Clin Gastroenterol Hepatol 2011;9:36–41.e1.
95. Connor V. Anti-TNF therapies: A comprehensive analysis of adverse effects associated with immunosuppression. Rheumatol Int 2011;31:327–337.
96. Grijalva CG, Chen L, Delzell E, et al. Initiation of tumor necrosis factor antagonists and the risk of hospitalization for infection in patients with autoimmune diseases. JAMA 2011;306(21):2331–2339.

22

Nausea and Vomiting

Cecily V. DiPiro and Robert J. Ignoffo

KEY CONCEPTS

1. Nausea and/or vomiting is often a part of the symptom complex for a variety of GI, cardiovascular, infectious, neurologic, metabolic, or psychogenic processes.
2. Nausea or vomiting is caused by a variety of medications or other noxious agents.
3. The overall goal of treatment should be to prevent or eliminate nausea and vomiting regardless of etiology.
4. Treatment options for nausea and vomiting include drug and nondrug modalities such as relaxation, biofeedback, and self-hypnosis.
5. The primary goal with chemotherapy-induced nausea and vomiting (CINV) is to prevent nausea and/or vomiting. Optimal control of acute nausea and vomiting positively impacts the incidence and control of delayed and anticipatory nausea and vomiting.
6. The emetic risk of the chemotherapeutic regimen is the primary factor to consider when selecting prophylactic antiemetics for CINV.
7. Patients at high risk of vomiting should receive prophylactic antiemetics for postoperative nausea and vomiting.
8. Patients undergoing radiation therapy to the upper abdomen or receiving total or hemibody irradiation should receive prophylactic antiemetics for radiation-induced nausea and vomiting.

Nausea and vomiting are common complaints from individuals of all ages. Management can be quite simple or detailed and complex, essentially innocuous or associated with therapy-induced adverse reactions. This chapter provides an overview of nausea and vomiting, two multifaceted problems.

Nausea is defined as the inclination to vomit or as a feeling in the throat or epigastric region alerting an individual that vomiting is imminent. Vomiting is defined as the ejection or expulsion of gastric contents through the mouth and is often a forceful event. Either condition may occur transiently with no other associated signs or symptoms; however, these conditions also may be only part of a more complex clinical presentation.

ETIOLOGY

❶ Nausea and vomiting may be associated with a variety of conditions, including GI, cardiovascular, infectious, neurologic, or metabolic disease processes. Nausea and vomiting may be a feature of such conditions as pregnancy, or may follow operative procedures or administration of certain medications, such as those used in cancer chemotherapy. Psychogenic etiologies of these symptoms may be present. Anticipatory etiologies may be involved, such as in patients who have previously received cytotoxic chemotherapy. Table 22-1 lists specific etiologies associated with nausea and vomiting.[1]

The etiology of nausea and vomiting may vary with the age of the patient. For example, vomiting in the newborn during the first day of life suggests upper digestive tract obstruction or an increase in intracranial pressure. ❷ Drug-induced nausea and vomiting are of particular concern, especially with the increasing number of patients receiving cytotoxic treatment. A four-level classification system defines the risk for emesis with agents used in oncology (Table 22-2).[2] Although some agents may have greater emetic risk than others, combinations of agents, high doses, clinical settings, psychological conditions, prior treatment experiences, and unusual stimulus of sight, smell, or taste may alter a patient's response to drug treatment. In this setting, nausea and vomiting may be unavoidable and some patients experience these problems so intensely that chemotherapy is postponed or discontinued.

PATHOPHYSIOLOGY

The three consecutive phases of emesis include nausea, retching, and vomiting. Nausea, the imminent need to vomit, is associated with gastric stasis and may be considered a separate and singular symptom. Retching is the labored movement of abdominal and thoracic muscles before vomiting. The final phase of emesis is vomiting, the forceful expulsion of gastric contents caused by GI retroperistalsis. The act of vomiting requires the coordinated contractions of the abdominal muscles, pylorus, and antrum, a raised gastric cardia, diminished lower esophageal sphincter pressure, and esophageal dilation.[1] Vomiting should not be confused with regurgitation, an act in which the gastric or esophageal contents rise to the pharynx but is not usually associated with forceful ejection seen with vomiting. Accompanying autonomic symptoms of pallor, tachycardia, and diaphoresis account for many of the distressing feelings associated with emesis.

Vomiting is triggered by afferent impulses to the vomiting center, a nucleus of cells in the medulla. Impulses are received from sensory centers, which include the chemoreceptor trigger zone (CTZ), cerebral cortex, and visceral afferents from the pharynx and GI tract. The vomiting center integrates the afferent impulses, resulting in efferent impulses to the salivation center, respiratory center, and the pharyngeal, GI, and abdominal muscles, leading to vomiting.

The CTZ, located in the area postrema of the fourth ventricle of the brain, is a major chemosensory organ for emesis and is usually

TABLE 22-1 Specific Etiologies of Nausea and Vomiting

GI mechanisms
Mechanical obstruction
Gastric outlet obstruction
Small bowel obstruction
Functional GI disorders
Gastroparesis
Nonulcer dyspepsia
Chronic intestinal pseudoobstruction
Irritable bowel syndrome
Organic GI disorders
Peptic ulcer disease
Pancreatitis
Pyelonephritis
Cholecystitis
Cholangitis
Hepatitis
Acute gastroenteritis
Viral
Bacterial
Cardiovascular diseases
Acute myocardial infarction
Congestive heart failure
Radio-frequency ablation
Neurologic processes
Increased intracranial pressure
Migraine headache
Vestibular disorders
Metabolic disorders
Diabetes mellitus (diabetic ketoacidosis)
Addison's disease
Renal disease (uremia)
Psychiatric causes
Psychogenic vomiting
Anxiety disorders
Anorexia nervosa
Therapy-induced causes
Cytotoxic chemotherapy
Radiation therapy
Theophylline preparations
Anticonvulsant preparations
Digitalis preparations
Opiates
Antibiotics
Volatile general anesthetics
Drug withdrawal
Opiates
Benzodiazepines
Miscellaneous causes
Pregnancy
Noxious odors
Operative procedures

Reprinted and adapted from reference 1.

associated with chemically induced vomiting. Because of its location, bloodborne and cerebrospinal fluid toxins have easy access to the CTZ. Cytotoxic agents primarily stimulate this area rather than the cerebral cortex and visceral afferents. Similarly, pregnancy-associated vomiting probably occurs through stimulation of the CTZ.

Numerous neurotransmitter receptors are located in the vomiting center, CTZ, and GI tract, including cholinergic, histaminic, dopaminergic, opiate, serotonergic, neurokinin (NK), and benzodiazepine receptors. Chemotherapeutic agents, their metabolites, or other emetic compounds theoretically trigger the process of emesis through stimulation of one or more of these receptors. Antiemetics have been developed to antagonize or block these emetogenic receptors.

CLINICAL PRESENTATION

Nausea and vomiting are commonly seen in many clinical situations. Patients may present in varying degrees of distress summarized in Table 22-3 as *simple* or *complex* in presentation.

TREATMENT

Desired Outcome

3 The overall goal of antiemetic therapy is to prevent or eliminate nausea and vomiting. This should be accomplished without adverse effects or with clinically acceptable adverse effects. Although this goal may be accomplished easily in patients with simple nausea and vomiting, patients with more complex problems require greater assistance. In addition to these clinical goals, appropriate cost issues should be considered, particularly in the management of chemotherapy-induced nausea and vomiting (CINV) and postoperative nausea and vomiting (PONV).

General Approach to Treatment

4 Treatment options include drug and nondrug modalities. Initially patients may choose to do nothing or to self-medicate with nonprescription drugs. As symptoms become worse or are associated with more serious medical problems, patients are more likely to benefit from prescription antiemetic drugs. When prescribed according to reliable clinical information, these agents often provide acceptable relief; however, some patients will never be totally free of symptoms. This lack of relief is most disabling when it is associated with an unresolved medical problem or when the necessary therapy for this condition is the cause of the nausea or vomiting, as in the case of patients who are receiving chemotherapy of moderate or high emetic risk.

Nonpharmacologic Management

Nonpharmacologic management of nausea and vomiting involves dietary, physical, or psychological strategies that are consistent with the etiology of nausea and vomiting. For patients with simple complaints, perhaps resulting from excessive or disagreeable food or beverage consumption, avoidance or moderation in dietary intake may be preferable. Patients suffering symptoms of systemic illness may improve dramatically as their underlying condition resolves. Finally, patients in whom these symptoms result from labyrinthine changes produced by motion may benefit quickly by assuming a stable physical position.

Nonpharmacologic interventions are classified as behavioral interventions and include relaxation, biofeedback, self-hypnosis, cognitive distraction, guided imagery, acupuncture, and systematic desensitization.[3,4] The reader is referred to references 5 to 7 for a more complete discussion on nonpharmacologic strategies.

Pharmacologic Therapy

4 Although many approaches to the treatment of nausea and vomiting have been suggested, antiemetic drugs (nonprescription and prescription) are most often recommended. These agents represent a variety of pharmacologic and chemical classes, as well as dosage regimens and routes of administration. With so many treatment possibilities available, factors that enable the clinician to discriminate among various choices include (a) the suspected etiology of the symptoms; (b) the frequency, duration, and severity of the episodes; (c) the ability of the patient to use oral, rectal, injectable, or transdermal medications; and (d) the success of previous

TABLE 22-2 Emetic Risk of Agents Used in Oncology

Emetic Risk (If No Prophylactic Medication Is Administered)	Cytotoxic Agent (in Alphabetical Order)
High (>90%)	Combination of either doxorubicin or epirubicin + cyclophosphamide
	Carmustine
	Cisplatin (>50 mg/m²)
	Cyclophosphamide (≥1,500 mg/m²)
	Dacarbazine
	Ifosfamide (>10 g/m²)
	Mechlorethamine
	Streptozotocin
Moderate (30–90%)	Aldesleukin (>12–15 million units/m²)
	Amifostine (>300 mg/m²)
	Arsenic trioxide
	Azacitidine
	Bendamustine
	Busulfan
	Carboplatin
	Cisplatin (<50 mg/m²)
	Clofarabine
	Cytarabine (>200 mg/m²)
	Cyclophosphamide (<1,500 mg/m²)
	Daunorubicin
	Dactinomycin
	Doxorubicin
	Epirubicin
	Idarubicin
	Ifosfamide
	Interferon alfa (10 million units/m²)
	Irinotecan
	Melphalan
	Methotrexate (>250 mg/m²)
	Oxaliplatin
	Procarbazine
	Temozolomide
Low (10–30%)	Cabazitaxel
	Capecitabine
	Cetuximab
	Cytarabine (≤200 mg/m²)
	Docetaxel
	Eribulin
	Erlotinib
	Etoposide
	Floxuridine
	Fluorouracil
	Gemcitabine
	Interferon alfa (<10 million units/m²)
	Ixabepilone
	Lapatinib
	Methotrexate (<250 mg/m²)
	Mitomycin
	Mitoxantrone
	Paclitaxel
	Paclitaxel albumin
	Pemetrexed
	Pentostatin
	Romidepsin
	Sorafenib
	Sunitinib
	Thiotepa
	Topotecan
	Trastuzumab
Minimal (<10%)	Alemtuzumab
	Asparaginase
	Bevacizumab
	Bleomycin
	Bortezomib
	Cladribine
	Cytarabine (<200 mg/m²)
	Decitabine
	Denileukin diftitox
	Dexrazoxane
	Fludarabine
	Ipilimumab
	Nelarabine
	Ofatumumab
	Panitumumab
	PEG-asparaginase
	Rituximab
	Temsirolimus
	Trastuzumab
	Valrubicin
	Vinblastine
	Vincristine
	Vinorelbine

Adapted from reference 30. Adapted with permission from reference 2.

TABLE 22-3 Clinical Presentation of Nausea and Vomiting

General
Depending on severity of symptoms, patients may present in mild to severe distress

Symptoms
Simple: Self-limiting, resolves spontaneously, and requires only symptomatic therapy
Complex: Not relieved after administration of antiemetics; progressive deterioration of patient secondary to fluid–electrolyte imbalances; usually associated with noxious agents or psychogenic events

Signs
Simple: Patient complaint of queasiness or discomfort
Complex: Weight loss; fever; abdominal pain

Laboratory tests
Simple: None
Complex: Serum electrolyte concentrations; upper/lower GI evaluation

Other information
Fluid input and output
Medication history
Recent history of behavioral or visual changes, headache, pain, or stress
Family history positive for psychogenic vomiting

antiemetic medications. Please see Table 22-4 for dosing information of commonly available antiemetic preparations.

The treatment of simple nausea and vomiting often involves self-care from a lengthy list of nonprescription products. Both nonprescription and prescription drugs useful in the treatment of simple nausea and vomiting are usually effective in small, infrequently administered doses associated with minimal side effects. Although suitable for occasional simple nausea and vomiting, nonprescription agents are often abandoned by the patient as symptoms continue or become progressively worse. As the patient's condition warrants, prescription medications may be chosen, either as single-agent therapy or in combination.

The management of complex nausea and vomiting, for example, in patients who are receiving cytotoxic chemotherapy, may require combination therapy. In combination regimens, the goal is to achieve symptomatic control through administration of agents with different pharmacologic mechanisms of action.

Antacids

Patients who are experiencing simple nausea and vomiting may use various antacids. In this setting, single or combination nonprescription antacid products, especially those containing magnesium

TABLE 22-4 Common Antiemetic Preparations and Adult Dosage Regimens

Drug	Adult Dosage Regimen	Dosage Form/Route	Availability	Adverse Drug Reactions	Monitoring Parameters	Comments
Antacids						
Antacids (various)	15–30 mL every 2–4 hours prn	Liquid/oral	OTC	Magnesium products: diarrhea Aluminum or calcium products: constipation	Assess for symptom relief	Useful with simple nausea/vomiting
Antihistaminic–Anticholinergic Agents						
Dimenhydrinate (Dramamine)	50–100 mg every 4–6 hours prn	Tab, chew tab, cap	OTC	Drowsiness, confusion, blurred vision, dry mouth, urinary retention	Assess for episodic relief of motion sickness or nausea/vomiting	Especially problematic in the elderly Increased risk of complications in patients with BPH, narrow angle glaucoma, or asthma
Diphenhydramine (Benadryl)	25–50 mg every 4–6 hours prn	Tab, cap, liquid	Rx/OTC	See above	See above	See above
	10–50 mg every 2–4 hours prn	IM, IV		See above	See above	See above
Hydroxyzine (Vistaril, Atarax)	25–100 mg every 4–6 hours prn	IM (unlabeled use)	Rx	See above	See above	See above
Meclizine (Bonine, Antivert)	12.5–25 mg 1 hour before travel; repeat every 12–24 hours prn	Tab, chew tab	Rx/OTC	See above	See above	See above
Scopolamine (Transderm Scop)	1.5 mg every 72 hours	Transdermal patch	Rx	See above	See above	See above
Trimethobenzamide (Tigan)	300 mg three to four times daily	Cap	Rx	See above	See above	See above
	200 mg three to four times daily	IM		See above	See above	See above
Benzodiazepines						
Alprazolam (Xanax)	0.5–2 mg three times daily prior to chemotherapy	Tab	Rx (C-IV)	Dizziness, sedation, appetite changes, memory impairment	Assess for episodes of ANV	Place in therapy: ANV
Lorazepam (Ativan)	0.5–2 mg on night before and morning of chemotherapy	Tab	Rx (C-IV)	See above	See above	See above
Butyrophenones						
Haloperidol (Haldol)	1–5 mg every 12 hours prn	Tab, liquid, IM, IV	Rx	Sedation, constipation, hypotension	Observe for additive sedation especially if used with narcotic analgesics	Place in therapy: palliative care
Droperidol (Inapsine)[a]	2.5 mg; additional 1.25 mg may be given	IM, IV	Rx	QT prolongation and/or torsade de pointes	12-Lead electrocardiogram prior to administration, followed by cardiac monitoring for 2–3 hours after administration	Limited use outside of clinical trials
Cannabinoids						
Dronabinol (Marinol)	5–15 mg/m^2 every 2–4 hours prn	Cap	Rx (C-III)	Euphoria, somnolence, xerostomia	Assess for symptom relief	May be useful with refractory CINV
Nabilone (Cesamet)	1–2 mg twice daily	Cap	Rx (C-II)	Somnolence, vertigo, xerostomia	See above	See above

Corticosteroids						
Dexamethasone	See Table 22-6 for CINV dosing and Table 22-8 for PONV dosing	Tab, IV	Rx	Insomnia, GI symptoms, agitation, appetite stimulation	Assess for efficacy as prophylactic agent: episodes of nausea/vomiting and hydration status	Useful as single-agent or combination therapy for prophylaxis of CINV and PONV
Histamine (H_2) Antagonists						
Cimetidine (Tagamet HB)	200 mg twice daily prn	Tab	OTC	Headache	Assess for symptom relief	Useful when nausea due to heartburn or GERD
Famotidine (Pepcid AC)	10 mg twice daily prn	Tab	OTC	Constipation, diarrhea	See above	See above
Nizatidine (Axid AR)	75 mg twice daily prn	Tab	OTC	Diarrhea, headache	See above	See above
Ranitidine (Zantac 75)	75 mg twice daily prn	Tab	OTC	Constipation, diarrhea	See above	See above
5-Hydroxytryptamine-3 Receptor Antagonists						
	See Table 22-6 for CINV dosing and Table 22-8 for PONV dosing	Tab, IV	Rx	Asthenia, constipation, headache	Assess for efficacy as prophylactic agent: episodes of nausea/vomiting and hydration status	Useful as single-agent or combination therapy for prophylaxis of CINV and PONV
Miscellaneous Agents						
Metoclopramide (Reglan)	10 mg four times daily	Tab	Rx	Asthenia, headache, somnolence	Assess for symptom relief	Prokinetic activity useful in diabetic gastroparesis
Olanzapine (Zyprexa)	2.5–5 mg twice daily	Tab	Rx	Sedation	Assess for decrease in episodes of nausea/vomiting	Use with caution in elderly. May be useful in breakthrough CINV
Phenothiazines						
Chlorpromazine (Thorazine)	10–25 mg every 4–6 hours prn	Tab, liquid	Rx	Constipation, dizziness, tachycardia, tardive dyskinesia	Assess for decrease in episodes of nausea/vomiting	Useful with simple nausea/vomiting
	25–50 mg every 4–6 hours prn	IM, IV		See above	See above	See above
Prochlorperazine (Compazine)	5–10 mg 3–4 times daily prn	Tab, liquid	Rx	Prolonged QT interval, sedation, tardive dyskinesia	Assess for decrease in episodes of nausea/vomiting	Useful with simple nausea/vomiting and for breakthrough CINV
	5–10 mg every 3–4 hours prn	IM		See above	See above	See above
	2.5–10 mg every 3–4 hours prn	IV	Rx	See above	See above	See above
	25 mg twice daily prn	Supp	Rx	See above	See above	See above
Promethazine (Phenergan)	12.5–25 mg every 4–6 hours prn	Tab, liquid, IM, IV, supp	Rx	Drowsiness, sedation	Assess for decreased nausea/vomiting episodes and improvement in hydration status	See above
Substance P/Neurokinin 1 Receptor Antagonist						
Aprepitant	See Table 22-6 for CINV dosing and Table 22-8 for PONV dosing	Cap, IV	Rx	Constipation, diarrhea, headache, hiccups	Assess for efficacy as prophylactic agent: episodes of nausea/vomiting and hydration status	Useful in combination therapy for prophylaxis of CINV and PONV

ANV, anticipatory nausea and vomiting; C-II, C-III, and C-IV, controlled substance schedule 2, 3, and 4, respectively; cap, capsule; chew tab, chewable tablet; CINV, chemotherapy-induced nausea and vomiting; GERD, gastroesophageal reflux disease; liquid, oral syrup, concentrate, or suspension; OTC, nonprescription; PONV, postoperative nausea and vomiting; Rx, prescription; supp, rectal suppository; tab, tablet.

[a]See text for current warnings.

hydroxide, aluminum hydroxide, and/or calcium carbonate, may provide sufficient relief, primarily through gastric acid neutralization.

Antihistamine–Anticholinergic Drugs

Antiemetic drugs from the antihistaminic–anticholinergic category appear to interrupt various visceral afferent pathways that stimulate nausea and vomiting. These drugs are often initiated as self-care by the patient for simple nausea or vomiting, especially associated with motion sickness.

Benzodiazepines

Since nausea and vomiting are often associated with chemotherapy, radiotherapy, and surgery, anticipatory anxiety may occur prior to these therapies and may exacerbate symptoms. Benzodiazepines may be useful in this setting.

Benzodiazepines are relatively weak antiemetics and are primarily used to prevent anxiety or anticipatory nausea and vomiting (ANV) in patients receiving highly emetogenic chemotherapy. They are also useful against akathisia associated with metoclopramide therapy. Both alprazolam and lorazepam are used as adjuncts to other antiemetics in patients treated with cisplatin-containing regimens. Alprazolam is usually given orally and has an onset of about 60 minutes, while lorazepam is given orally or sublingually, which has a more rapid onset.

Butyrophenones

Two butyrophenone compounds that have antiemetic activity are haloperidol and its congener droperidol; both block dopaminergic stimulation of the CTZ. Although each agent is effective in relieving nausea and vomiting, haloperidol is not considered first-line therapy for uncomplicated nausea and vomiting but has been used in palliative care situations.[8] The current labeling of droperidol recommends that all patients should undergo a 12-lead electrocardiogram prior to administration, followed by cardiac monitoring for 2 to 3 hours after administration because of the possibility of the development of potentially fatal QT prolongation and/or torsade de pointes.[9] The clinical use of droperidol has effectively ceased outside of clinical trials in anesthesia.

Cannabinoids

Cannabinoids have complex effects on the CNS and their effects at receptors in neural tissues may explain efficacy in CINV. Oral dronabinol and nabilone are therapeutic options when CINV is refractory to other antiemetics; they are not indicated as first-line agents.[10]

Corticosteroids

Corticosteroids have demonstrated antiemetic efficacy since the initial recognition that patients who received prednisone as part of their Hodgkin's disease protocol appeared to develop less nausea and vomiting than did those patients who were treated with protocols that excluded this agent. Methylprednisolone has also been used as a component of an antiemetic regimen, but the majority of trials have included dexamethasone. The site and mechanism of action of corticosteroids for CINV is unknown.

Dexamethasone is the most commonly used corticosteroid in the management of CINV and PONV, either as a single agent or in combination with 5-hydroxytryptamine-3 receptor antagonists (5-HT_3-RA). Dexamethasone is effective in the prevention of both cisplatin-induced acute emesis and delayed nausea and vomiting associated with CINV when used alone or in combination.[11–14] Corticosteroids affect almost every organ system. For patients with simple nausea and vomiting, steroids are not indicated and may be associated with unacceptable risks.

H_2-Receptor Antagonists

Histamine$_2$-receptor antagonists work by decreasing gastric acid production and are used to manage simple nausea and vomiting associated with heartburn or gastroesophageal reflux. Except for potential drug interactions with cimetidine, these agents cause few side effects when used for episodic relief.

5-Hydroxytryptamine-3 Receptor Antagonists

5-HT_3-RAs block presynaptic serotonin receptors on sensory vagal fibers in the gut wall, effectively blocking the acute phase of CINV. These agents do not completely block the acute phase of CINV and are less efficacious in preventing the delayed phase, but they are the standard of care in the management of CINV, PONV, and radiation-induced nausea and vomiting (RINV). Issues involved in the use of dolasetron, granisetron, ondansetron, and palonosetron are reviewed in detail in the sections that follow.

Metoclopramide

Metoclopramide, a procainamide congener, blocks dopaminergic receptors centrally in the CTZ. It increases lower esophageal sphincter tone, aids gastric emptying, and accelerates transit through the small bowel, possibly through the release of acetylcholine. The prokinetic activity of metoclopramide makes it useful in patients with nausea and vomiting associated with diabetic gastroparesis. The introduction of the 5-HT_3-RAs in the early 1990s supplanted the use of metoclopramide in CINV.

Olanzapine

Olanzapine is an antipsychotic that blocks several neurotransmitters including dopamine at D_2 and 5-HT_3-RA. Use of olanzapine, in combination with palonosetron and dexamethasone, effectively controlled acute and delayed CINV in patients receiving highly emetogenic chemotherapy as compared with aprepitant, palonosetron, and dexamethasone in a randomized, phase 3 clinical trial.[15] The National Comprehensive Cancer Network (NCCN) antiemesis practice guideline includes olanzapine as one of many options in patients who experience breakthrough nausea and/or vomiting following prophylaxis for CINV.[16] Sedation is the most common side effect with olanzapine; it should be used with caution in the elderly.

Phenothiazines

Phenothiazines have been the most widely prescribed antiemetic agents and appear to block dopamine receptors, most likely in the CTZ. They are marketed in an array of dosage forms, none of which appears to be more efficacious than another. These agents may be most practical for long-term treatment and are inexpensive in comparison with newer drugs. Rectal administration is a reasonable alternative in patients in whom oral or parenteral administration is not feasible.

Phenothiazines are most useful in adult patients with simple nausea and vomiting. IV prochlorperazine provided quicker and more complete relief with less drowsiness than IV promethazine in adult patients treated in an emergency department for nausea and vomiting associated with uncomplicated gastritis or gastroenteritis.[17]

Substance P/Neurokinin 1 Receptor Antagonists

Substance P is a peptide neurotransmitter in the NK family whose preferred receptor is the NK_1 receptor. The acute phase of CINV is believed to be mediated by both serotonin and substance P, whereas substance P is believed to be the primary mediator of the delayed phase. Aprepitant and fosaprepitant are the first substance P/NK_1 receptor antagonists in clinical use; at the time of this writing, casopitant is still in development.

The efficacy of aprepitant was demonstrated in patients receiving high-dose cisplatin-based chemotherapy[13,14] and in patients receiving doxorubicin and cyclophosphamide,[18] a regimen of moderate to high emetic risk. The three-drug regimen of aprepitant, dexamethasone, and ondansetron provided improved protection from vomiting for the 5 days after chemotherapy administration as compared with the combination of dexamethasone and ondansetron.

Aprepitant has the potential for numerous drug interactions because it is a substrate, moderate inhibitor, and an inducer of cytochrome isoenzyme CYP3A4 and an inducer of CYP2C9. It can increase serum concentrations of many drugs metabolized by CYP3A4, including docetaxel, paclitaxel, etoposide, irinotecan, ifosfamide, imatinib, vinorelbine, vincristine, and vinblastine. In clinical studies, aprepitant was concomitantly administered with etoposide, vinorelbine, or paclitaxel, with no adjustment in the doses of these agents to account for potential drug interactions. The efficacy of oral contraceptives may be reduced when given with aprepitant. Concomitant administration with warfarin may result in a clinically significant decrease in the international normalized ratio.[19] The dose of oral dexamethasone should be reduced 50% when coadministered with aprepitant, because of the 2.2-fold increase in observed area under the plasma-concentration-versus-time curve.[20] Aprepitant is not approved for use in children.

Fosaprepitant, an injectable form of aprepitant, has been approved by the FDA as an IV substitute for oral aprepitant on day 1 of the standard 3-day CINV prevention regimen, with oral aprepitant administered on days 2 and 3.[21]

TABLE 22-5 Nonchemotherapy Etiologies of Nausea and Vomiting in Cancer Patients

Fluid and electrolyte abnormalities
Hypercalcemia
Volume depletion
Water intoxication
Adrenocortical insufficiency
Drug induced
Opiates
Antibiotics
Antifungals
GI obstruction
Increased intracranial pressure
Peritonitis
Metastases
Brain
Meninges
Hepatic
Uremia
Infections (septicemia, local)
Radiation therapy

Data from reference 26.

CHEMOTHERAPY-INDUCED NAUSEA AND VOMITING

There are five categories of CINV: acute, delayed, anticipatory, breakthrough, and refractory. Nausea and vomiting that occurs within 24 hours of chemotherapy administration is defined as acute CINV, whereas when it starts more than 24 hours after chemotherapy administration, it is defined as delayed CINV.

Nausea or vomiting that occurs prior to receiving chemotherapy is termed ANV. ANV is believed to be a learned, conditioned, or psychological response that occurs in about 25% of patients by the fourth cycle of chemotherapy.[22] ANV triggers include tastes, odors, sights, or thoughts associated with chemotherapy. Risk factors associated with ANV include age under 50, nausea and/or vomiting after the previous chemotherapy session, anxiety, sweating and a feeling of warmth after the last chemotherapy cycle, and susceptibility to motion sickness.[23]

In the setting of optimal antiemetic prophylaxis and no prior emesis, reported chemotherapy-induced ANV is rare. Use of newer antiemetic regimens appears to have resulted in a decreased rate of ANV.[24]

Breakthrough nausea and vomiting is defined as emesis occurring despite prophylactic administration of antiemetics and requiring the use of rescue antiemetics. Historically, breakthrough emesis occurs in 10% to 40% treated with modern-day antiemetics.[25]

Refractory nausea and vomiting is evident when there is a poor response to multiple antiemetic regimens. In addition to the emetic risk of various cytotoxic regimens, other common etiologies have been proposed for the development of nausea and vomiting in cancer patients (Table 22-5).[26]

5 The primary goal for CINV is to *prevent* nausea and/or vomiting. Optimal control of acute nausea and vomiting is known to impact positively on the incidence and control of delayed nausea and vomiting and ANV.[25]

Clinical practice guidelines for the use of antiemetics in CINV have been published by the NCCN,[16] the Multinational Association of Supportive Care in Cancer/European Society of Oncology (MASCC/ESMO),[24] and the American Society of Clinical Oncology (ASCO).[27] The NCCN guidelines are updated annually, while the ASCO and ESMO guidelines appear to be updated less frequently. Despite the demonstrated improvement in outcomes with the use of these practice guidelines, they are underutilized by a high percentage of practitioners.[28] Furthermore, product availability and recommended doses are often institution-specific and may vary considerably from the doses listed in Table 22-6.

Principles of Antiemetic Use for CINV

ASCO, MASCC, and the NCCN consensus groups share several of the principles listed below that appear to be important for the effective prevention of CINV in adults[29,30]:

1. The primary goal of emesis prevention is no nausea and/or vomiting throughout the period of emetic risk.
2. The duration of emetic risk is 2 days for patients receiving moderately emetogenic chemotherapy and 3 days for highly emetogenic chemotherapy. Emetic prophylaxis should be provided through the entire period of risk.
3. **6** The selection of the antiemetic regimen should be based on the chemotherapy drug with highest emetogenicity (see Table 22-2). Prior emetic experience and patient-specific factors should also be considered.
4. When given in equipotent doses, oral and IV 5-HT_3-RAs are equivalent in efficacy.
5. The toxicities of antiemetics should be considered and managed appropriately.

Prophylaxis of Acute CINV

Each of the practice guidelines states that the most effective classes of drugs for the prevention of acute emesis are the 5-HT_3-RAs, NK_1 receptor antagonists, and glucocorticoids (especially dexamethasone). Treatment recommendations for the different categories of emesis are outlined in Table 22-6.

High Emetogenic Chemotherapy (HEC)

Patients receiving HEC should receive a three-drug antiemetic regimen given before the administration of chemotherapy (day 1) that

TABLE 22-6 Dosage Recommendations for CINV for Adult Patients

Emetic Risk	Prophylaxis of Acute Phase of CINV (One Dose Administered Prior to Chemotherapy)	Prophylaxis of Delayed Phase of CINV
High (including the AC regimen[a])	5-HT_3 receptor antagonists (5-HT_3-RA): Palonosetron 0.25 mg IV (preferred); Dolasetron 100 mg orally; Granisetron 2 mg orally or 1 mg IV or 0.01 mg/kg IV or 34.3 mg transdermal patch; Ondansetron 16–24 mg orally or 8–12 mg IV (maximum 32 mg)	
	And dexamethasone 12 mg orally or IV	Dexamethasone 8 mg orally twice daily on days 2–4
	And Aprepitant 125 mg orally	Aprepitant 80 mg orally on days 2 and 3 after chemotherapy
	Or Fosaprepitant 115 mg IV	
	±Lorazepam 0.5–2 mg po or IV or SL every 4–6 hours on days 1–4	
	±H_2 blocker or proton pump inhibitor	
Moderate	5-HT_3-RA:	
	Palonosetron 0.25 mg IV (preferred)	5-HT_3-RA: dolasetron 100 mg orally daily[b]
	Dolasetron 100 mg orally	
	Granisetron 2 mg orally or 1 mg IV or 0.01 mg/kg IV or 34.3 mg transdermal patch	Granisetron 1–2 mg orally daily[b]
	Ondansetron 16–24 mg orally or 8–12 mg IV (maximum 32 mg)	Ondansetron 8 mg orally daily or twice daily[b]
	And Dexamethasone 8–12 mg orally or IV	Dexamethasone 8 mg orally twice daily[b]
	And in select patients[c] aprepitant 125 mg orally	Aprepitant 80 mg orally on days 2 and 3 if used on day 1
	Or fosaprepitant 115 mg IV	
	±Lorazepam 0.5–2 mg po or IV or SL every 4–6 hours on days 1–4	
	±H_2 blocker or proton pump inhibitor	
Low	Dexamethasone 8–12 mg orally or IV	None
Minimal	None	None

Doses included in this table reflect the recommendations from published guidelines.[16,24,27] These doses may differ from manufacturer labeling; they reflect the consensus of the guideline participants. CINV, chemotherapy-induced nausea and vomiting.

[a]See reference 27.
[b]For 2–3 days following chemotherapy.
[c]Patients receiving other chemotherapies of moderate emetic risk, for example, carboplatin, cisplatin, doxorubicin, epirubicin, ifosfamide, irinotecan, or methotrexate.

includes a 5-HT_3-RA (e.g., dolasetron, granisetron, ondansetron, or palonosetron), dexamethasone, and an NK_1 receptor antagonist (e.g., aprepitant or fosaprepitant). Dexamethasone should be given on days 2 to 4 and aprepitant on days 2 and 3 to prevent delayed emesis.

Any of the 5-HT_3-RAs may be used on day 1. The ASCO and NCCN guidelines prefer IV palonosetron. The use of IV dolasetron is contraindicated because it has a higher association of prolonged QT_c interval. Granisetron transdermal patch should be applied 24 to 48 hours prior to chemotherapy (duration of effect is 7 days).

Clinical **Controversy...**

Is triple therapy necessary in all patients receiving HEC? The major guidelines all recommend that a combination of a corticosteroid, a 5-HT_3-RA, and aprepitant should be standard prophylaxis for HEC-associated vomiting. The data raise some doubt about whether all anthracycline and cyclophosphamide chemotherapy and dacarbazine regimens require an NK_1 receptor antagonist at least when palonosetron is used. Few studies have carefully evaluated the risk of emesis with any chemotherapy other than cisplatin or anthracycline and cyclophosphamide in women.[31]

Moderate Emetogenic Chemotherapy (MEC)

Patients receiving MEC should receive a two-drug antiemetic regimen containing a 5-HT_3-RA on day 1 and dexamethasone on days 1 to 3. Both ASCO and NCCN guidelines recommend palonosetron as the preferred 5-HT_3-RA for MEC. The exception to this is patients who are receiving combination chemotherapies with carboplatin, cisplatin, doxorubicin, epirubicin, ifosfamide, irinotecan, or methotrexate; these patients may be given the triple-drug combination described for regimens of high emetic risk.

For chemotherapy regimens that are of low emetic risk, dexamethasone or any of the following may be used: prochlorperazine, metoclopramide, and/or diphenhydramine, and/or lorazepam alone.[16]

Prophylaxis of Delayed CINV

Management of delayed CINV has historically challenged practitioners. The best strategy for preventing delayed CINV (nausea and/or vomiting occurring 24 or more hours after chemotherapy) is to control acute CINV and provide adequate prophylaxis for delayed CINV.[32] Aprepitant, dexamethasone, and metoclopramide are effective in preventing delayed CINV, whereas 5-HT_3-RAs are inconsistent. However, palonosetron controlled delayed emesis more effectively than granisetron, suggesting that another 5-HT_3-RA should not be prescribed as a rescue medication when palonosetron is given prophylactically for acute CINV.[33]

Patients receiving cisplatin and other HEC regimens are at highest risk for experiencing delayed CINV. The combination of aprepitant and dexamethasone on days 2 and 3 appears to be superior to the use of dexamethasone alone or ondansetron plus dexamethasone in preventing delayed emesis.[34] Use of aprepitant also decreased delayed CINV in patients receiving an anthracycline plus cyclophosphamide, as compared with twice-daily ondansetron (49% vs. 55%).[18] Fosaprepitant, a parenteral formulation of aprepitant, given on day 1 plus dexamethasone on days 1 to 4 was effective for prevention of both acute and delayed emesis from cisplatin therapy.[35] Current practice guidelines recommend administration of aprepitant and dexamethasone on days 2 and 3 and dexamethasone with or without lorazepam on day 4.[16,24]

The incidence of delayed CINV following MEC is less well defined. The NCCN recommends aprepitant or any of the following: dexamethasone, a 5-HT_3-RA, and/or lorazepam, and/or a histamine$_2$-blocker, or a proton pump inhibitor on days 2 and 3 for chemotherapy regimens that contain carboplatin, doxorubicin, epirubicin, ifosfamide, irinotecan, or methotrexate.[16] In contrast, the ASCO guidelines do not recommend aprepitant for MEC.[27]

Palonosetron protected more patients from delayed emesis than ondansetron, granisetron, or dolasetron in adult patients receiving MEC.[36–39] Although these studies showed that palonosetron is superior to other 5-HT_3-RAs, it is unclear whether these results would persist if an NK_1 antagonist were included in the combination. Palonosetron may also be better than ondansetron in patients receiving multiday chemotherapy, but a larger randomized, prospective trial is needed to substantiate this finding.[40]

Prophylaxis of Anticipatory Nausea and Vomiting

The 2009 update of the MASCC antiemetic guidelines for preventing ANV stated that although there was only a moderate level of *confidence*, there was a high level of *consensus* for using a benzodiazepine combined with standard antiemetics for preventing ANV.[22] Alprazolam or lorazepam given the night before and the morning of chemotherapy is recommended.

Treatment of Anticipatory Nausea and Vomiting

ANV is more difficult to control than acute or delayed CINV. A key principle in the treatment of ANV is that effective management of delayed CINV or ANV requires adequate control of acute CINV. The most effective treatment for prevention of ANV is to give optimal antiemetic prophylaxis with each cycle of chemotherapy.[41]

Treatment of Breakthrough CINV

A general principle in all patients receiving chemotherapy is to prescribe an antiemetic from a different pharmacologic class for rescue of breakthrough nausea and vomiting. Rescue medications used in adult patients include prochlorperazine, promethazine, lorazepam, metoclopramide, haloperidol, 5-HT_3-RAs, dexamethasone, cannabinoids, or olanzapine.[16,42]

Around-the-clock dosing of rescue antiemetics should be considered rather than as-needed administration. The choice of agent should be based on patient-specific factors, including potential adverse drug reactions and cost. Chlorpromazine, lorazepam, and dexamethasone are recommended for pediatric patients.[43]

Treatment of Refractory Nausea and Vomiting

The general approach to the management of refractory CINV is to upgrade the antiemetic strategy to the next level of prophylaxis or to add breakthrough antiemetics to the regimen.[44] Some patients will experience nausea and vomiting despite optimal acute and delayed prophylaxis and failure of rescue antiemetics. Addition of another agent from a different pharmacologic class is recommended and routes other than the oral route may be required.

Treatment of Multiday Chemotherapy

Chemotherapy regimens are occasionally administered over multiple days. The MASCC guidelines state that the combination of a 5-HT_3-RA plus daily dexamethasone is the standard.[24] For highly emetogenic regimens, dexamethasone should be administered daily on the days of chemotherapy. Dexamethasone should not be prescribed for patients receiving a corticosteroid in their chemotherapy regimen or with interferon alfa or interleukin-2.[30] The use of a 5-HT_3-RA daily or granisetron transdermal patch plus daily dexamethasone and either aprepitant has been recommended on days 1 to 3, or fosaprepitant on day 1.[36]

TABLE 22-7 Risk Factors for Postoperative Nausea and Vomiting (PONV)

Factors unrelated to anesthesia
History of motion sickness
Metabolic factors:
Uremia
Diabetes mellitus
Electrolyte disturbances
Patient-related factors
Age
Female gender (two to three times greater incidence of PONV vs. males)
Nonsmoker
History of PONV or motion sickness (threefold increase in incidence of PONV)
Hydration status
Factors related to anesthesia
Use of volatile anesthetics
Nitrous oxide
Use of opioids (intraoperative or postoperative)
Factors related to surgery
Operative site (higher incidence of PONV after eye, oral, plastic, ear, nose and throat, head and neck, gynecologic, obstetric, laparoscopic, and abdominal procedures)
Duration of surgery

Adapted from references 45 and 47.

POSTOPERATIVE NAUSEA AND VOMITING

PONV in adults occurs in 25% to 30% of patients and within 24 hours of undergoing anesthesia.[45] Patients with multiple risk factors are at highest risk for PONV (Table 22-7). Patients with zero or one of the four risk factors present in Table 22-7 are at lowest risk (10% to 20%) and those with three or four risk factors are at highest risk for PONV (60% to 80%). Moderate risk is defined by this model as the presence of two risk factors. Patients at low risk for PONV are unlikely to benefit from prophylaxis and may potentially experience adverse reactions from the medications. The use of a risk assessment tool can help identify patients most likely to benefit from prophylaxis.[46]

In addition to using prophylactic antiemetics in high-risk patients, other strategies include using regional rather than systemic anesthesia, propofol, and hydration, as well as avoiding nitrous oxide, volatile anesthetics, and opioids.

Prophylaxis of PONV

Adherence to consensus guidelines for prophylaxis and treatment of PONV decreases emetic episodes.[47,48] 7 Patients at highest risk of vomiting should receive two prophylactic antiemetics from different pharmacologic classes, while those at moderate risk should receive one or two drugs.[47,49] Optimal outcomes appear to be achieved when the drugs are administered at the end of the surgery. When the different combinations were compared, no differences were found between 5-HT_3-RA plus droperidol, 5-HT_3-RA plus dexamethasone, and droperidol plus dexamethasone.[50] However, QT prolongation and/or torsade de pointes has been reported in some cases, with some fatalities in patients receiving droperidol at doses at or below recommended doses. Droperidol should be avoided in patients who have a history of QT prolongation, are over 65 years old, or have a history of alcohol abuse, or when used concomitantly with benzodiazepines, volatile anesthetics, and IV opiates.[9] Optimal dosing of agents used in combination has not been determined.

Cyclizine, dexamethasone, dolasetron, droperidol, granisetron, metoclopramide, ondansetron, tropisetron, scopolamine, and palonosetron are as effective as placebo for the prophylaxis of PONV.[51–53]

TABLE 22-8 Recommended Prophylactic Doses of Selected Antiemetics for Postoperative Nausea and Vomiting in Adults and Postoperative Vomiting in Children

Drug	Adult Dose	Pediatric Dose (IV)	Timing of Dose[a]
Aprepitant[b]	40 mg orally	Not labeled for use in pediatrics	Within 3 hours prior to induction
Dexamethasone	4–5 mg IV	150 mcg/kg up to 5 mg	At induction
Dimenhydrinate	1 mg/kg IV	0.5 mg/kg up to 25 mg	Not specified
Dolasetron	12.5 mg IV	350 mcg/kg up to 12.5 mg	At end of surgery
Droperidol[c]	0.625–1.25 mg IV	10–15 mcg/kg up to 1.25 mg	At end of surgery
Granisetron	0.35–1.5 mg IV	40 mcg/kg up to 0.6 mg	At end of surgery
Haloperidol	0.5–2 mg (IM or IV)	[d]	Not specified
Ondansetron	4 mg IV	50–100 mcg/kg up to 4 mg	At end of surgery
Palonosetron[b]	0.075 mg IV	Not labeled for patients <18 years	At induction
Prochlorperazine	5–10 mg IM or IV	[d]	At end of surgery
Promethazine[c]	6.25–25 mg IV	[d]	At induction
Scopolamine	Transdermal patch	[d]	Prior evening or 4 hours before surgery
Tropisetron	2 mg IV	0.1 mg/kg up to 2 mg	At end of surgery

[a]Based on recommendations from consensus guidelines; may differ from manufacturer's recommendations.
[b]Labeled for use in PONV but not included in consensus guidelines.
[c]See FDA "black box" warning.
[d]Pediatric dosing not included in consensus guidelines.

From reference 47.

Acquisition cost may be the primary factor that determines drug selection of the 5-HT_3-RAs.[47] Dexamethasone is an effective, inexpensive prophylactic agent when administered either alone or in combination with other antiemetic drugs before the induction of anesthesia.[49,51] Table 22-8 summarizes the doses for prophylactic antiemetics from the consensus guidelines.[47]

Aprepitant was approved for the prevention of PONV given orally within 3 hours prior to induction of anesthesia.[19] Aprepitant is equivalent to ondansetron 4 mg IV in reducing the incidence of nausea and the need for rescue in the 24 hours after surgery, but was significantly better than ondansetron for preventing vomiting in the 24 and 48 hours after surgery.[54]

Clinical **Controversy. . .**

When should droperidol be used for prophylaxis of PONV? Several clinical practice guidelines include droperidol as a first-line agent in the prevention of nausea and vomiting in high-risk patients receiving preoperative anesthesia. The black box warning in the product information recommends that this drug be reserved for patients who cannot tolerate or do not respond to other agents. This has led to debate and controversy in the literature as to the role of droperidol for PONV.[55,56]

Treatment of PONV

Patients who experience PONV after receiving prophylactic treatment with a 5-HT_3-RA plus dexamethasone should be given rescue therapy from a different drug class such as a phenothiazine, metoclopramide, or droperidol.[47] Repeating the agent given for PONV prophylaxis within 6 hours of surgery is of no additional benefit.[57] Furthermore, a repeated dose of a 5-HT_3-RA is not effective in treatment of PONV.[58,59] An emetic episode occurring more than 6 hours postoperatively can be treated with any of the drugs used for prophylaxis except dexamethasone and transdermal scopolamine.[47]

If no prophylaxis was given initially, the recommended treatment is low-dose 5-HT_3-RA as follows: dolasetron 12.5 mg, granisetron 0.1 mg, ondansetron 1 mg, and tropisetron 0.5 mg. Alternative treatments for established PONV include dexamethasone 2 to 4 mg IV, droperidol 0.625 mg IV, or promethazine 6.25 to 12.5 mg IV.[60]

RADIATION-INDUCED NAUSEA AND VOMITING

Nausea and vomiting associated with radiation therapy (RT) is not well understood and often underestimated by radiation oncologists.[61] RINV is neither as predictable nor as severe as CINV, and many patients receiving RT will not experience nausea or vomiting. The incidence of RINV ranges from 50% to 80%, is site dependent, and can have a substantial impact on a patient's quality of life. Risk factors associated with the development of RINV include combination chemoradiotherapy, prior CINV, upper abdomen RT, and field size.[62]

Four radiotherapy-induced emesis risk groups have been defined by the Antiemetic Subcommittee of the MASCC and the ASCO antiemetic practice guidelines[24,27]:

1. Highest risk: Total-body or nodal irradiation (TBI/TNI)
2. Moderate risk: Upper body or abdomen and hemibody RT
3. Low risk: Cranial, craniospinal, head and neck, lower thorax, and pelvic RT
4. Minimal risk: Extremity or breast RT

Prophylaxis of RINV

8 Several randomized trials have demonstrated that prophylactic 5-HT_3-RA and dexamethasone are more effective than placebo,[62] which was confirmed by a recent meta-analysis.[63] In addition, 5-HT_3-RAs were more effective than placebo or non-5-HT_3-RAs (prochlorperazine or metoclopramide), even in patients undergoing TBI.[62]

ASCO, ESMO/MASCC, and NCCN recommend preventive therapy with a 5-HT_3-RA throughout RT and dexamethasone on fractions 1 to 5 in patients who are receiving TBI (high emetic risk).[16,27,61] Patients undergoing RT procedures with moderate emetic risk should receive a 5-HT$_3$-RA prior to each fraction and dexamethasone on fractions 1 to 5. Those receiving low emetic risk radiotherapy may be given a 5-HT$_3$-RA either throughout RT or as rescue. For minimal emetic risk a 5-HT$_3$-RA, metoclopramide, or prochlorperazine may be offered.

There has not been adequate study of prophylactic NK$_1$ antagonists, palonosetron, or transdermal granisetron in the setting of RINV.

DISORDERS OF BALANCE

Disorders of balance include vertigo, dizziness, and motion sickness. The etiology of these complaints may include diseases that are infectious, postinfectious, demyelinative, vascular, neoplastic, degenerative, traumatic, toxic, psychogenic, or idiopathic. Symptoms of imbalance perceived by the patient present a particular clinical challenge. Whether associated with a minor or complex disorder, motion sickness may be associated with nausea and vomiting.

Beneficial therapy for patients in this setting can most reliably be found among the antihistaminic–anticholinergic agents. However, the precise mechanisms of action of these agents are currently unknown. Neither the antihistaminic nor the anticholinergic potency appears to correlate well with the ability of these agents to prevent or treat the nausea and vomiting associated with motion sickness. When used for their depressant effects on labyrinth excitability, these agents produce variable efficacy and safety profiles. Oral regimens of antihistaminic–anticholinergic agents given one to several times each day may be effective, especially when the first dose is administered prior to motion.

Scopolamine is commonly used to prevent nausea or vomiting caused by motion. The usefulness of scopolamine in preventing motion sickness was enhanced with the development of the transdermal system (patch) that increased patient satisfaction and decreased untoward side effects. A review of 12 randomized controlled studies showed that scopolamine provided better protection from motion-induced sickness than did placebo, but was not superior to antihistamines and combinations of scopolamine and ephedrine.[64]

ANTIEMETIC USE DURING PREGNANCY

As many as 75% of pregnant women experience nausea and vomiting to some degree during the first trimester of pregnancy. The severity of the symptoms varies considerably, from mild nausea to incapacitating nausea and vomiting. The etiology of nausea and vomiting of pregnancy (NVP) is not well understood. Symptoms are self-limited for a majority of women, although approximately 1% to 3% develop hyperemesis gravidarum, a serious condition marked by severe physical symptoms and/or medical complications requiring hospitalization. In its most severe state, hyperemesis gravidarum may result in volume contraction, starvation, and electrolyte abnormalities.

Initial management of NVP often involves dietary changes and/or lifestyle modifications. Nonpharmacologic interventions including ginger and acupressure are not supported by high-quality consistent evidence.[65] Persistent nausea and/or vomiting leads to the consideration of drug therapy at a time when teratogenic potential of each agent must be considered.

Treatment recommendations for the management of NVP are available from the American College of Obstetricians and Gynecologists (ACOG).[66] A comprehensive review of treatment options for NVP was published.[67] Pyridoxine (10 to 25 mg one to four times daily), with or without doxylamine (12.5 to 20 mg one to four times daily), is recommended as first-line therapy.

Patients with persistent NVP or who show signs of dehydration should receive IV fluid replacement with thiamine. Ondansetron 2 to 8 mg orally/IV every 8 hours as needed may alleviate NVP, but IV ondansetron was no more effective than promethazine for treatment of severe NVP.[68] Corticosteroids should be reserved for patients with refractory NVP or hyperemesis gravidarum; methylprednisolone 16 mg orally/IV every 8 hours for 3 days followed by a 2-week taper is recommended. This regimen may be repeated if necessary, but treatment should not exceed a total of 6 weeks.

ANTIEMETIC USE IN CHILDREN

Chemotherapy-Induced Nausea and Vomiting

Updated practice guidelines recommend that a corticosteroid (such as dexamethasone) plus a 5-HT$_3$-RA be administered as prophylaxis of acute CINV to children receiving chemotherapy of high or moderate emetic risk.[69] Consensus guidelines suggest that there are no differences between 5-HT$_3$-RAs in safety or efficacy. One small, randomized, comparative study demonstrated that one dose of palonosetron 0.25 mg IV significantly reduced emesis and nausea in the first 3 days as compared with ondansetron (8 mg/m^2 IV every 8 hours while receiving chemotherapy) in children treated with moderately to highly emetogenic chemotherapy.[70] This study needs to be confirmed in a larger randomized trial.

One small study has evaluated the safety and efficacy of aprepitant in adolescents. Patients were randomized to dexamethasone and ondansetron with or without aprepitant, using the recommended oral adult 3-day regimen. The emetogenicity of the chemotherapy administered was not discussed. Patients in the aprepitant arm had higher complete response rates and a parallel pharmacokinetic study suggests that the adult dose regimen was appropriate for adolescents.[71]

Gastroenteritis

Nausea and vomiting associated with pediatric gastroenteritis is self-limited and improves with correction of dehydration. The majority of patients can be successfully treated with oral rehydration therapy (ORT). Use of phenothiazines, such as promethazine, has declined due to potential serious adverse events in children and adolescents, including death.[72] Administration of a single dose of ondansetron appears to decrease persistent vomiting as a barrier to ORT and decreases need for IV rehydration and hospital admission.[73–75]

PERSONALIZED PHARMACOTHERAPY

Antiemetics are 70% to 80% effective in the prevention of CINV. One potential factor that might explain less than optimal response is the variability in genetic enzymes responsible for the metabolism, transport, and receptor affinity of antiemetics.[76] The literature on the pharmacogenetics of antiemetic drugs is limited regarding the impact of the polymorphic variability in the multidrug resistance gene (MDR1), the 5-HT$_3$-RA A, B, and C receptor genes, and the CYP2D6 gene on the efficacy of the 5-HT$_3$-RAs. Individuals who are ultrametabolizers of the CYP2D6 enzymes generally respond poorly to 5-HT$_3$-RAs and dopamine D$_2$ receptor antagonists (prochloperazine and metoclopramide).[77] Variant genotypes in the 5-HT$_3$-RA C gene appear to invoke resistance to ondansetron and tropisetron and were associated with an increased risk of nausea and vomiting.[78] In another study, complete antiemetic control was greater in patients with the TT genotype of the MDR1 compared with that in patients with the TC or CC genotype.[79] Until there are confirmatory studies of these results, it is premature to utilize genomic analysis for personalized clinical decision making for use of 5-HT_3-RAs.

With regard to the effect of pharmacokinetics on drug efficacy in PONV, clinical studies suggest that palonosetron is more effective against delayed emesis than other 5-HT_3-RAs because of its higher receptor binding affinity and longer plasma elimination half-life.[80] However, these studies were not compared with dexamethasone as part of the regimen. Although all the 5-HT_3-RAs are hepatically metabolized and excreted in the urine, renal and hepatic dysfunction does not require dose adjustment.

EVALUATION OF EMETIC OUTCOMES

In assessing emetic outcomes, standardized monitoring criteria should include a subjective assessment and objectives parameters including:

1. Severity of nausea
2. Change in patient weight
3. Number of vomiting episodes each day
4. Estimated fluid loss
5. Acid–base balance
6. Serum sodium, potassium, and chloride concentrations
7. Serum BUN and creatinine concentrations
8. Daily urine volume and urine-specific gravity

Physical assessment should include evaluation of mucous membranes and skin turgor. For patients on chemotherapy, evaluation of emetic outcomes should occur after the administration of each chemotherapy cycle. Adherence to outpatient antiemetic regimens occurs in about 65% of patients. Delayed nausea and vomiting occurs in 15% to 40% of patients, depending on the emetic risk of the chemotherapy and the antiemetic regimen used for prophylaxis. Patients receiving high-risk regimens are most likely to report symptoms of nausea and vomiting on day 3 after chemotherapy.[81] Symptom management assessments should be performed on the third or fourth day after chemotherapy. Documentation of a nausea and/or vomiting event will assist the clinician in modifying the antiemetic regimen for the next cycle of chemotherapy.

In the postsurgical anesthesia setting, assessment of nausea and vomiting is important since they may lead to dehydration, decreased blood pressure, or cardiac arrhythmias. Other complications of PONV include suture line tension, wound dehiscence, and increased bleeding under surgical flaps.[82]

ABBREVIATIONS

ACOG	American College of Obstetricians and Gynecologists
ANV	anticipatory nausea and vomiting
ASCO	American Society of Clinical Oncology
CINV	chemotherapy-induced nausea and vomiting
CTZ	chemoreceptor trigger zone
ESMO	European Society of Oncology
HEC	high emetogenic chemotherapy
5-HT_3-RA	5-hydroxytryptamine-3 receptor antagonist
MASCC	Multinational Association of Supportive Care in Cancer
MDR1	multidrug resistance gene
MEC	moderate emetogenic chemotherapy
NCCN	National Comprehensive Cancer Network
NK_1	neurokinin 1
NVP	nausea and vomiting of pregnancy
ORT	oral rehydration therapy
PONV	postoperative nausea and vomiting
RINV	radiation-induced nausea and vomiting
RT	radiation therapy
TBI	total-body irradiation
TNI	total nodal irradiation

REFERENCES

1. Malagelada JR, Malagelada C. Nausea and vomiting. In: Feldman M, ed. Sleisenger and Fordtran's Gastrointestinal and Liver Disease: Pathophysiology/Diagnosis/Management. St. Louis, MO: Elsevier, 2010:197–209.
2. Grunberg SM, Osoba D, Hesketh PJ, et al. Evaluation of new antiemetic agents and definition of antineoplastic agent emetogenicity—An update. Support Care Cancer 2011;19(Suppl 10):S43–S47.
3. Mundy EA, DuHamel KN, Montgomery GH. The efficacy of behavioral interventions for cancer treatment-related side effects. Semin Clin Neuropsychiatr 2003;8:253–275.
4. Matteson S, Roscoe J, Hickok J, Morrow GR. The role of behavioral conditioning in the development of nausea. Am J Obstet Gynecol 2002;186:S239–S243.
5. Morrow GR, Carroll J, Ryan EP, et al. Behavioral interventions in treating anticipatory nausea and vomiting. J Natl Compr Canc Netw 2007;5:44–50.
6. Lee J, Dodd M, Dibble S, Abrams D. Review of acupressure studies for chemotherapy-induced nausea and vomiting control. J Pain Symptom Manage 2008;36:529–544.
7. Lotfi-Jam K, Carey M, Jefford M, et al. Nonpharmacologic strategies for managing common chemotherapy adverse effects: A systematic review. J Clin Oncol 2008;26:5 618–5629.
8. Perkins P, Dorman S. Haloperidol for the treatment of nausea and vomiting in palliative care patients. Cochrane Database Syst Rev 2009;(2):CD006271.
9. Inapsine (Droperidol). 2012, *http://www.fda.gov/Safety/MedWatch/SafetyInformation/SafetyAlertsforHumanMedicalProducts/ucm173778.htm*.
10. Todaro B. Cannabinoids in the treatment of chemotherapy-induced nausea and vomiting. J Natl Compr Canc Netw 2012;10:487–492.
11. Italian Group for Antiemetic Research. Double-blind, dose-finding study of four intravenous doses of dexamethasone in the prevention of cisplatin-induced acute emesis. J Clin Oncol 1998;16:2937–2942.
12. Ioannidis JT, Hesketh PJ, Lau J. Contribution of dexamethasone to control of chemotherapy-induced nausea and vomiting: A meta-analysis of randomized evidence. J Clin Oncol 2000;18:3409–3422.
13. Poli-Bigelli S, Rodrigues-Pereira J, Carides AD, et al. Addition of the neurokinin 1 receptor antagonist aprepitant to standard antiemetic therapy improves control of chemotherapy-induced nausea and vomiting. Results from a randomized, double-blind, placebo-controlled trial in Latin America. Cancer 2003;97:3090–3098.
14. Hesketh PJ, Grunbert SM, Gralla RJ, et al. The oral neurokinin-1 antagonist aprepitant for the prevention of chemotherapy-induced nausea and vomiting: A multinational, randomized, double-blind, placebo controlled trial in patients receiving high-dose cisplatin—

The Aprepitant Protocol 052 Study Group. J Clin Oncol 2003;21:4112–4119.

15. Navari RM, Gray SE, Kerr AC. Olanzapine versus aprepitant for the prevention of chemotherapy-induced nausea and vomiting: A randomized phase III trial. J Support Oncol 2011;9:188–195.
16. National Comprehensive Cancer Network. Clinical Practice Guidelines in Oncology. Antiemesis. Version 1. 2012, *http://www.nccn.org/professionals/physician_gls/PDF/antiemesis.pdf.*
17. Ernst A, Weiss SJ, Park S, et al. Prochlorperazine versus promethazine for uncomplicated nausea and vomiting in the emergency department: A randomized, double-blind clinical trial. Ann Emerg Med 2000;36:89–94.
18. Warr DG, Hesketh PJ, Gralla RJ, et al. Efficacy and tolerability of aprepitant for the prevention of chemotherapy-induced nausea and vomiting in patients with breast cancer after moderately emetogenic chemotherapy. J Clin Oncol 2005;23:2822–2830.
19. Merck & Co Inc. Prescribing Information. Emend (Aprepitant) Capsules. 2011, *http://www.merck.com/product/usa/pi_circulars/e/emend/emend_pi.pdf.*
20. McCrea JB, Majumdar AK, Goldberg MR, et al. Effects of the neurokinin-1 receptor antagonist aprepitant on the pharmacokinetics of dexamethasone and methylprednisolone. Clin Pharmacol Ther 2003;74:17–24.
21. Van Belle S, Cocquyt V. Fosaprepitant dimeglumine (MK-0517 or L-785,298), an intravenous neurokinin-1 antagonist for the prevention of chemotherapy induced nausea and vomiting. Expert Opin Pharmacother 2008;9:3261–3270.
22. Roscoe JA, Morrow GR, Aapro MS, et al. Anticipatory nausea and vomiting. Support Care Cancer 2011;19: 1533–1538.
23. Morrow GR, Roscoe JA, Kirshner JJ, et al. Anticipatory nausea and vomiting in the era of 5-HT3 antiemetics. Support Care Cancer 1998;6:244–247.
24. Roila F, Herrstedt J, Aapro M, et al. Guideline update for MASCC and ESMO in the prevention of chemotherapy- and radiotherapy-induced nausea and vomiting: Results of the third Perugia consensus conference. Ann Oncol 2010;21(Suppl 5):v232–v243.
25. Kris MG, Hesketh PJ, Herrstedt J, et al. Consensus proposals for the prevention of acute and delayed vomiting and nausea following high-emetic-risk chemotherapy. Support Care Cancer 2005;13:85–96.
26. Stephenson J, Davies A. An assessment of etiology-based guidelines for the management of nausea and vomiting in patients with advanced cancer. Support Care Cancer 2006;14:348–353.
27. Basch E, Prestrud AA, Hesketh PJ, et al. Antiemetics: American Society of Clinical Oncology clinic practice guideline update. J Clin Oncol 2011;29:4189–4198.
28. Grunberg SM, Deuson RR, Mavros P, et al. Incidence of chemotherapy-induced nausea and emesis after modern antiemetics. Cancer 2004;100:2261–2268.
29. Wickham R. Best practice management of CINV in oncology patients II. Antiemesis guidelines and rational for use. J Support Oncol 2010;8(2 Suppl 1):10–15.
30. Ettinger DS, Armstrong DK, Barbour S, et al. Antiemesis. Clinical practice guidelines in oncology. J Natl Compr Canc Netw 2012;10:456–485.
31. Warr D. Management of highly emetogenic chemotherapy. Curr Opin Oncol 2012;24:371–375.
32. Ihbe-Heffinger A, Ehlken B, Bernard R, et al. The impact of delayed chemotherapy-induced nausea and vomiting on patients, health resource utilization and costs in German cancer centers. Ann Oncol 2004;15:526–536.
33. Saito M, Aogi K, Sekine I, et al. Palonosetron plus dexamethasone versus granisetron plus dexamethasone for prevention of nausea and vomiting during chemotherapy: A double-blind, double-dummy, randomised, comparative phase III trial. Lancet Oncol 2009;10:115–124.
34. Schmoll HJ, Aapro MS, Poli-Bigelli S, et al. Comparison of an aprepitant regimen with a multiple-day ondansetron regimen, both with dexamethasone, for antiemetic efficacy in high-dose cisplatin treatment. Ann Oncol 2006;17: 1000–1006.
35. Grunberg SM, Chua D, Maru A, et al. Single-dose fosaprepitant for the prevention of chemotherapy-induced nausea and vomiting associated with a broad range of moderately emetogenic chemotherapies: A randomized, double-blind study protocol—EASE. J Clin Oncol 2011;29:1495–1501.
36. Hesketh P. Prevention and Treatment of Chemotherapy-Induced Emesis. UpToDate. 2012, *http://www.uptodate.com.*
37. Aapro MS, Grunberg SM, Manikhas GM, et al. A phase III, double-blind, randomized trial of palonosetron compared with ondansetron in preventing chemotherapy-induced nausea and vomiting following highly emetogenic chemotherapy. Ann Oncol 2006;17:1441–1449.
38. Eisenberg P, Figueroa-Vadillo J, Zamora R, et al. Improved prevention of moderately emetogenic chemotherapy-induced nausea and vomiting with palonosetron, a pharmacologically novel 5-HT3 receptor antagonist: Results of a phase III, single-dose trial versus dolasetron. Cancer 2003;98:2473–2482.
39. Gralla R, Lichinitser M, Van Der Vegt S, et al. Palonosetron improves prevention of chemotherapy-induced nausea and vomiting following moderately emetogenic chemotherapy: Results of a double-blind randomized phase III trial comparing single doses of palonosetron with ondansetron. Ann Oncol 2003;14:1570–1577.
40. Musso M, Scalone R, Bonanno V, et al. Palonosetron (Aloxi) and dexamethasone for the prevention of acute and delayed nausea and vomiting in patients receiving multiple-day chemotherapy. Support Care Cancer 2009;17:205–209.
41. Aapro MS, Molassiotis A, Olver I. Anticipatory nausea and vomiting. Support Care Cancer 2005;13:117–121.
42. Hawkins R, Grunberg S. Chemotherapy-induced nausea and vomiting: Challenges and opportunities for improved outcomes. Clin J Oncol Nurs 2009;13:54–64.
43. Dupuis LL, Nathan PC. Options for the prevention and management of acute chemotherapy-induced nausea and vomiting in children. Paediatr Drugs 2003;5:597–613.
44. Lohr L. Chemotherapy-induced nausea and vomiting. Cancer J 2008;14:85–93.
45. Kovac AL. Prevention and treatment of postoperative nausea and vomiting. Drugs 2000;59:213–243.
46. Kapoor R, Hola ET, Adamson RT, Mathis AS. Comparison of two instruments for assessing risk of postoperative nausea and vomiting. Am J Health Syst Pharm 2008;65:448–453.
47. Gan TJ, Meyer TA, Apfel CC, et al. Society for Ambulatory Anesthesia guidelines for the management of postoperative nausea and vomiting. Anesth Analg 2007;105:1615–1628.
48. White PF, O'Hara JF, Roberson CR, Wender RH, Candiotti KA, POST-OP Study Group. The impact of current antiemetic practices on patient outcomes: A prospective study on high-risk patients. Anesth Analg 2008;107: 452–458.
49. Apfel CA, Korttila K, Abdalla M, et al. A factorial trial of six interventions for the prevention of postoperative nausea and vomiting. N Engl J Med 2004;350:2441–2451.

50. Habib AS, El-Moalem HE, Gan TJ. The efficacy of the 5-HT3 receptor antagonists combined with droperidol for PONV prophylaxis is similar to their combination with dexamethasone. A meta-analysis of randomized controlled trials. Can J Anaesth 2004;51:311–319.
51. Carlisle JB, Stevenson CA. Drugs for preventing postoperative nausea and vomiting. Cochrane Database Syst Rev 2006;(3):CD004125.
52. Kranke P, Morin AM, Roewer N, Wulf H, Eberhart LH. Palonosetron 04–07 Study Group. A randomized, double-blind study to evaluate the efficacy and safety of three different doses of palonosetron versus placebo in preventing postoperative nausea and vomiting over a 72-hour period. Anesth Analg 2008;107:439–444.
53. Candiotti KA, Kovac AL, Melson TI, et al. The Palonosetron 04-06 Study Group. A randomized, double-blind study to evaluate the efficacy and safety of three different doses of palonosetron versus placebo for preventing postoperative and post-discharge nausea and vomiting. Anesth Analg 2008;107:445–451.
54. Gan TJ, Apfel C, Kovac A, et al. A randomized, double-blind comparison of the NK_1 antagonist, aprepitant versus ondansetron for the prevention of postoperative nausea and vomiting. Anesth Analg 2007;104:1082–1089.
55. Habib AS, Gan TJ. Pro: The Food and Drug Administration black box warning on droperidol is not justified. Anesth Analg 2008;106:1414–1417.
56. Ludwin DB, Shafer SL. Con: The black box warning on droperidol should not be removed (but should be clarified!). Anesth Analg 2008;106:1418–1420.
57. Kovac AL, O'Connor TA, Pearman MH, et al. Efficacy of repeat intravenous dosing of ondansetron in controlling postoperative nausea and vomiting: A randomized, double-blind, placebo-controlled multicenter trial. J Clin Anesth 1999;11:453–459.
58. Kreisler NS, Spiekermann BF, Ascari CM, et al. Small-dose droperidol effectively reduces nausea in a general surgical adult patient population. Anesth Analg 2000;91:1256–1261.
59. Candiotti KA, Nhuch F, Kamat A, et al. Granisetron versus ondansetron treatment for breakthrough postoperative nausea and vomiting after prophylactic ondansetron failure: A pilot study. Anesth Analg 2007;104:1370–1373.
60. Habib AS, Gan TJ. The effectiveness of rescue antiemetics after failure of prophylaxis with ondansetron or droperidol: A preliminary report. J Clin Anesth 2005;17:62–65.
61. Fever P, Maranzano E, Molassiotis A, et al. Radiotherapy-induced nausea and vomiting (RINV): MASCC/ESMO guideline for antiemetics in radiotherapy: Update 2009. Support Care Cancer 2011;19(Suppl 1):S5–S14.
62. Maranzano E, De Angelis V, Pergolizzi S, et al. A prospective observational trial on emesis in radiotherapy: Analysis of 1020 patients recruited in 45 Italian radiation oncology centres. Radiother Oncol 2010;94:36–41.
63. Salvo N, Doble B, Khan L, et al. Prophylaxis of radiation-induced nausea and vomiting using 5-hydroxytryptamine-3 serotonin receptor antagonists: A systematic review of randomized trials. Int J Radiat Oncol Biol Phys 2012;82:408–417.
64. Spinks AB, Wasiak J, Villaneuva EV, Bernath V. Scopolamine (hyoscine) for preventing and treating motion sickness. Cochrane Database Syst Rev 2011;(6):CD002851.
65. Matthews A, Dowswell T, Haas DM, et al. Interventions for nausea and vomiting in early pregnancy. Cochrane Database Syst Rev 2010;(9):CD007575.
66. Nausea and vomiting of pregnancy. ACOG Practice Bulletin no. 52. American College of Obstetricians and Gynecologists. Obstet Gynecol 2004;103:803–815.
67. Badell ML, Ramin SM, Smith JA. Treatment options for nausea and vomiting during pregnancy. Pharmacotherapy 2006;26:1273–1287.
68. Sullivan CA, Johnson CA, Roach H, et al. A pilot study of intravenous ondansetron for hyperemesis gravidarum. Am J Obstet Gynecol 1996;174:1565–1568.
69. Jordan K, Roila F, Molassiotis A, et al. Antiemetics in children receiving chemotherapy. MASCC/ESMO guideline update 2009. Support Care Cancer 2011;19(Suppl 1): S37–S42.
70. Sepulveda-Vildosola AC, Betanzos-Cabrera Y, Lastiri GG, et al. Palonosetron hydrochloride is an effective and safe option to prevent chemotherapy-induced nausea and vomiting in children. Arch Med Res 2008;39:601–606.
71. Gore L, Chawla S, Petrilli A, et al. Aprepitant in adolescent patients for prevention of chemotherapy-induced nausea and vomiting: A randomized, double-blind, placebo-controlled study of efficacy and tolerability. Pediatr Blood Cancer 2009;52:242–247.
72. Starke PR, Weaver J, Chowdhury BA. Boxed warning added to promethazine labeling for pediatric use. N Engl J Med 2005;352:2653.
73. Freedman SB, Adler M, Seshadri R, Powell EC. Oral ondansetron for gastroenteritis in a pediatric emergency department. N Engl J Med 2006;354:1698–1705.
74. Roslund G, Hepps TS, McQuillen KK. The role of oral ondansetron in children with vomiting as a result of acute gastritis/gastroenteritis who have failed oral rehydration therapy: A randomized controlled trial. Ann Emerg Med 2008;52:22–29.
75. Fedorowicz Z, Jagannath VA, Carter B. Antiemetics for reducing vomiting related to acute gastroenteritis in children and adolescents. Cochrane Database Syst Rev 2011;(9):CD005506.
76. Perwitasari DA, Gelderblom H, Atthobari J, et al. Anti-emetic drugs in oncology: Pharmacology and individualization by pharmacogenetics. Int J Clin Pharm 2011;33:33–43.
77. Kaiser R, Sezer O, Papies A, et al. Patient-tailored antiemetic treatment with 5-hydroxytryptamine type 3 receptor antagonists according to cytochrome P-450 2D6 genotypes. J Clin Oncol 2002;20:2805–2811.
78. Fasching PA, Kollmannsberger B, Strissel PL, et al. Polymorphisms in the novel serotonin receptor subunit gene HTR3C show different risks for acute chemotherapy-induced vomiting after anthracycline chemotherapy. J Cancer Res Clin Oncol 2008;134:1079–1086.
79. Babaoglu MO, Bayar B, Aynacioglu AS, et al. Association of the ABCB1 3435C>T polymorphism with antiemetic efficacy of 5-hydroxytryptamine type 3 antagonists. Clin Pharmacol Ther 2005;78:619–626.
80. Ho KY, Gan TJ. Pharmacology, pharmacogenetics, and clinical efficacy of 5-hydroxytryptamine type 3 receptor antagonists for postoperative nausea and vomiting. Curr Opin Anaesthesiol 2006;19:606–611.
81. Shih V, Wan HS, Chan A. Clinical predictors of chemotherapy-induced nausea and vomiting in breast cancer patients receiving adjuvant doxorubicin and cyclophosphamide. Ann Pharmacother 2009;43:444–452.
82. Gundzik K. Nausea and vomiting in the ambulatory surgical setting. Orthop Nurs 2008;27:182–188.

Diarrhea, Constipation, and Irritable Bowel Syndrome

23

Patricia H. Fabel and Kayce M. Shealy

KEY CONCEPTS

1. Diarrhea is caused by many viral and bacterial organisms. It is most often a minor discomfort, not life-threatening, and usually self-limited.
2. The four pathophysiologic mechanisms of diarrhea have been linked to the four broad diarrheal groups, which are secretory, osmotic, exudative, and altered intestinal transit. The three mechanisms by which absorption occurs from the intestines are active transport, diffusion, and solvent drag.
3. Management of diarrhea focuses on preventing excessive water and electrolyte losses, dietary care, relieving symptoms, treating curable causes, and treating secondary disorders.
4. Bismuth subsalicylate is marketed for indigestion, relieving abdominal cramps, and controlling diarrhea, including traveler's diarrhea, but may cause interactions with several components if given excessively.
5. Constipation is defined as difficult or infrequent passage of stool, at times associated with straining or a feeling of incomplete defecation.
6. Underlying causes of constipation should be identified when possible and corrective measures taken (e.g., alteration of diet or treatment of diseases such as hypothyroidism).
7. The foundation of treatment of constipation is dietary fiber or bulk-forming laxatives that provide 20 to 25 g/day of raw fiber.
8. Irritable bowel syndrome (IBS) is one of the most common GI disorders characterized by lower abdominal pain, disturbed defecation, and bloating. Many non-GI manifestations also exist with IBS. Visceral hypersensitivity is a major culprit in the pathophysiology of the disease.
9. Diarrhea-predominant IBS should be managed by dietary modification and drugs such as loperamide when diet changes alone are insufficient to promote control of symptoms.
10. Several drug classes are involved in the treatment of the pain associated with IBS including tricyclic compounds and the gut-selective calcium channel blockers.

DIARRHEA

Diarrhea is a troublesome discomfort that affects most individuals in the United States at some point in their lives and can be thought of as both a symptom and a sign. Usually diarrheal episodes begin abruptly and subside within 1 or 2 days without treatment. This chapter focuses primarily on noninfectious diarrhea, with only minor reference to infectious diarrhea (see Chap. 91 for a discussion of GI infections). Diarrhea is often a symptom of a systemic disease, and not all possible causes of diarrhea are discussed in this chapter. Acute diarrhea is commonly defined as <14 days' duration, persistent diarrhea as >14 days' duration, and chronic diarrhea as >30 days' duration.

To understand diarrhea, one must have a reasonable definition of the condition; unfortunately, the literature is extremely variable on this. Simply put, diarrhea is an increased frequency and decreased consistency of fecal discharge as compared with an individual's normal bowel pattern. Frequency and consistency are variable within and between individuals. For example, some individuals defecate as often as three times per day, whereas others defecate only two or three times per week. A Western diet usually produces a daily stool weighing between 100 and 300 g, depending on the amount of nonabsorbable materials (mainly carbohydrates) consumed. Patients with serious diarrhea may have a daily stool weight in excess of 300 g; however, a subset of patients experience frequent small, watery passages. Additionally, vegetable fiber-rich diets, such as those consumed in some Eastern cultures (e.g., those in Africa), produce stools weighing more than 300 g/day.

Diarrhea may be associated with a specific disease of the intestines or secondary to a disease outside the intestines. For instance, bacillary dysentery directly affects the gut, whereas diabetes mellitus causes neuropathic diarrheal episodes. Furthermore, diarrhea can be considered as acute or chronic disease. Infectious diarrhea is often acute; diabetic diarrhea is chronic. Congenital disorders in GI ion transport mechanisms are another cause of chronic diarrhea.[1] Whether acute or chronic, diarrhea has the same pathophysiologic causes that help in identification of specific treatments.

Epidemiology

The epidemiology of diarrhea varies in developed versus developing countries.[2] In the United States, diarrheal illnesses are usually not reported to the Centers for Disease Control and Prevention (CDC) unless associated with an outbreak or an unusual organism or condition. For example, the acquired immune deficiency syndrome (AIDS) has been identified with protracted diarrheal illness. Diarrhea is a major problem in daycare centers and nursing homes, probably because early childhood and senescence plus environmental conditions are risk factors. Although an exact epidemiologic profile in the United States is not available through the CDC or published literature, chronic diarrhea affects approximately 5% of the adult population and ranges from 3% to 20% in children worldwide.[3–5] In developing countries, diarrhea is a leading cause of illness and death in children, creating a tremendous economic strain on healthcare costs.

(1) Most cases of acute diarrhea are caused by infections with viruses, bacteria, or protozoa and are generally self-limited.[6] Although viruses are more commonly associated with acute

gastroenteritis, bacteria are responsible for more cases of acute diarrhea.

Evaluation of a noninfectious cause is considered if diarrhea persists and no infectious organism can be identified, or if the patient falls into a high-risk category for metabolic complications with persistent diarrhea. Common causative bacterial organisms include *Shigella*, *Salmonella*, *Campylobacter*, *Staphylococcus*, and *Escherichia coli*. Foodborne bacterial infection is a major concern, as several major food poisoning episodes have occurred that were traced to poor sanitary conditions in meat processing plants. Acute viral infections are attributed mostly to the Norwalk and rotavirus groups.

Physiology

In the fasting state, 9 L of fluid enters the proximal small intestine each day. Of this fluid, 2 L is ingested through diet, while the remainder consists of internal secretions. Because of meal content, duodenal chyme is usually hypertonic. When chyme reaches the ileum, the osmolality adjusts to that of plasma, with most dietary fat, carbohydrate, and protein being absorbed. The volume of ileal chyme decreases to about 1 L/day on entering the colon, which is further reduced by colonic absorption to 100 mL daily. If the small intestine water absorption capacity is exceeded, chyme overloads the colon, resulting in diarrhea. In humans, the colon absorptive capacity is about 5 L daily. Colonic fluid transport is critical to water and electrolyte balance.

Absorption from the intestines back into the blood occurs by three mechanisms: active transport, diffusion, and solvent drag. Active transport and diffusion are the mechanisms of sodium transport. Because of the high luminal sodium concentration (142 mEq/L [142 mmol/L]), sodium diffuses from the sodium-rich gut into epithelial cells, where it is actively pumped into the blood and exchanged with chloride to maintain an isoelectric condition across the epithelial membrane.

Hydrogen ions are transported by an indirect mechanism in the upper small intestine. As sodium is absorbed, hydrogen ions are secreted into the gut. Hydrogen ions then combine with bicarbonate ions to form carbonic acid, which then dissociates into carbon dioxide and water. Carbon dioxide readily diffuses into the blood for expiration through the lung. The water remains in the chyme.

Paracellular pathways are major routes of ion movement. As ions, monosaccharides, and amino acids are actively transported, an osmotic pressure is created, drawing water and electrolytes across the intestinal wall. This pathway accounts for significant amounts of ion transport, especially sodium. Sodium plays an important role in stimulating glucose absorption. Glucose and amino acids are actively transported into the blood via a sodium-dependent cotransport mechanism. Cotransport absorption mechanisms of glucose–sodium and amino acid–sodium are extremely important for treating diarrhea.

Gut motility influences absorption and secretion. The amount of time in which luminal content is in contact with the epithelium is under neural and hormonal control. Neurohormonal substances, such as angiotensin, vasopressin, glucocorticoid, aldosterone, and neurotransmitters, also regulate ion transport.

Pathophysiology

❷ Four general pathophysiologic mechanisms disrupt water and electrolyte balance, leading to diarrhea, and are the basis of diagnosis and therapy. These are (a) a change in active ion transport by either decreased sodium absorption or increased chloride secretion; (b) change in intestinal motility; (c) increase in luminal osmolarity; and (d) increase in tissue hydrostatic pressure. These mechanisms have been related to four broad clinical diarrheal groups: secretory, osmotic, exudative, and altered intestinal transit.

Secretory diarrhea occurs when a stimulating substance either increases secretion or decreases absorption of large amounts of water and electrolytes. Substances that cause excess secretion include vasoactive intestinal peptide (VIP) from a pancreatic tumor, unabsorbed dietary fat in steatorrhea, laxatives, hormones (such as secretion), bacterial toxins, and excessive bile salts. Many of these agents stimulate intracellular cyclic adenosine monophosphate and inhibit Na^+/K^+-adenosine triphosphatase (ATPase), leading to increased secretion. Also, many of these mediators inhibit ion absorption simultaneously. Secretory diarrhea is recognized by large stool volumes (>1 L/day) with normal ionic contents and osmolality approximately equal to plasma. Fasting does not alter the stool volume in these patients.

Poorly absorbed substances retain intestinal fluids, resulting in osmotic diarrhea. This process occurs with malabsorption syndromes, lactose intolerance, administration of divalent ions (e.g., magnesium-containing antacids), or consumption of poorly soluble carbohydrate (e.g., lactulose). As a poorly soluble solute is transported, the gut adjusts the osmolality to that of plasma; in so doing, water and electrolytes flux into the lumen. Clinically, osmotic diarrhea is distinguishable from other types, as it ceases if the patient resorts to a fasting state.

Inflammatory diseases of the GI tract discharge mucus, serum proteins, and blood into the gut. Sometimes bowel movements consist only of mucus, exudate, and blood. Exudative diarrhea affects other absorptive, secretory, or motility functions to account for the large stool volume associated with this disorder.

Altered intestinal motility produces diarrhea by three mechanisms: reduction of contact time in the small intestine, premature emptying of the colon, and bacterial overgrowth. Chyme must be exposed to intestinal epithelium for a sufficient time period to enable normal absorption and secretion processes to occur. If this contact time decreases, diarrhea results. Intestinal resection or bypass surgery and drugs (such as metoclopramide) cause this type of diarrhea. On the other hand, an increased time of exposure allows fecal bacteria overgrowth. A characteristic small intestine diarrheal pattern is rapid, small, coupling bursts of waves. These waves are inefficient, do not allow absorption, and rapidly dump chyme into the colon. Once in the colon, chyme exceeds the colonic capability to absorb water.

Etiologic Examination of the Stool

Stool characteristics are important in assessing the etiology of diarrhea. A description of the frequency, volume, consistency, and color provides diagnostic clues. For instance, diarrhea starting in the small intestine produces a copious, watery or fatty (greasy), and foul-smelling stool; contains undigested food particles; and is usually free from gross blood. Colonic diarrhea appears as small, pasty, and sometimes bloody or mucoid movements. Rectal tenesmus with flatus accompanies large intestinal diarrhea.

Clinical Presentation

Table 23-1 outlines the clinical presentation of diarrhea, and Table 23-2 shows common drug-induced causes of diarrhea. A medication history is extremely important in identifying drug-induced diarrhea. Many agents, including antibiotics and other drugs, cause diarrhea or, less commonly, pseudomembranous colitis. Self-inflicted laxative abuse for weight loss is popular.

Most acute diarrhea is self-limiting, subsiding within 72 hours. However, infants, young children, the elderly, and debilitated persons are at risk for morbid and mortal events in prolonged or voluminous diarrhea. These groups are at risk for water, electrolyte, and acid–base disturbances, and potentially cardiovascular collapse and death. The prognosis for chronic diarrhea depends on the cause; for example, diarrhea secondary to diabetes mellitus waxes and wanes throughout life.

TABLE 23-1 Clinical Presentation of Diarrhea

General
- Usually, acute diarrheal episodes subside within 72 hours of onset, whereas chronic diarrhea involves frequent attacks over extended time periods

Signs and symptoms
- Abrupt onset of nausea, vomiting, abdominal pain, headache, fever, chills, and malaise
- Bowel movements are frequent and never bloody, and diarrhea lasts 12–60 hours
- Intermittent periumbilical or lower right quadrant pain with cramps and audible bowel sounds is characteristic of small intestinal disease
- When pain is present in large intestinal diarrhea, it is a gripping, aching sensation with tenesmus (straining, ineffective, and painful stooling). Pain localizes to the hypogastric region, right or left lower quadrant, or sacral region
- In chronic diarrhea, a history of previous bouts, weight loss, anorexia, and chronic weakness are important findings

Physical examination
- Typically demonstrates hyperperistalsis with borborygmi and generalized or local tenderness

Laboratory tests
- Stool analysis studies include examination for microorganisms, blood, mucus, fat, osmolality, pH, electrolyte and mineral concentration, and cultures
- Stool test kits are useful for detecting GI viruses, particularly rotavirus
- Antibody serologic testing shows rising titers over a 3- to 6-day period, but this test is not practical and is nonspecific
- Occasionally, total daily stool volume is also determined
- Direct endoscopic visualization and biopsy of the colon may be undertaken to assess for the presence of conditions such as colitis or cancer
- Radiographic studies are helpful in neoplastic and inflammatory conditions

TABLE 23-2 Drugs Causing Diarrhea

Laxatives
Antacids containing magnesium
Antineoplastics
Auranofin (gold salt)
Antibiotics
- Clindamycin
- Tetracyclines
- Sulfonamides
- Any broad-spectrum antibiotic

Antihypertensives
- Reserpine
- Guanethidine
- Methyldopa
- Guanabenz
- Guanadrel
- Angiotensin-converting enzyme inhibitors

Cholinergics
- Bethanechol
- Neostigmine

Cardiac agents
- Quinidine
- Digitalis
- Digoxin

Nonsteroidal antiinflammatory drugs
Misoprostol
Colchicine
Proton pump inhibitors
H_2-receptor blockers

TREATMENT

Prevention

Acute viral diarrheal illness often occurs in daycare centers and nursing homes. Because person-to-person contact is the mechanism by which viral disease spreads, isolation techniques must be initiated. For bacterial, parasitic, and protozoal infections, strict food handling, sanitation, water, and other environmental hygiene practices can prevent transmission. If diarrhea is secondary to another illness, controlling the primary condition is necessary. Antibiotics and bismuth subsalicylate are advocated to prevent traveler's diarrhea, in conjunction with treatment of drinking water and caution with consumption of fresh vegetables.[7]

Desired Outcome

3 If prevention is unsuccessful and diarrhea occurs, therapeutic goals are to (a) manage the diet; (b) prevent excessive water, electrolyte, and acid–base disturbances; (c) provide symptomatic relief; (d) treat curable causes; and (e) manage secondary disorders causing diarrhea (Figs. 23-1 and 23-2).

Clinicians must clearly understand that diarrhea, like a cough, may be a body defense mechanism for ridding itself of harmful substances or pathogens. The correct therapeutic response is not necessarily to stop diarrhea at all costs.

Nonpharmacologic Management

Dietary management is a first priority in the treatment of diarrhea. Most clinicians recommend discontinuing consumption of solid foods and dairy products for 24 hours. However, fasting is of questionable value, as this treatment modality has not been extensively studied. In osmotic diarrhea, these maneuvers control the problem. If the mechanism is secretory, diarrhea persists. For patients who are experiencing nausea and/or vomiting, a mild, digestible, low-residue diet should be administered for 24 hours. If vomiting is present and uncontrollable with antiemetics (see Chap. 22), nothing is taken by mouth. As bowel movements decrease, a bland diet is begun.

Feeding should continue in children with acute bacterial diarrhea. Fed children have less morbidity and mortality, whether or not they receive oral rehydration fluids. Studies are not available in the elderly or in other high-risk groups to determine the value of continued feeding in bacterial diarrhea.

Water and Electrolytes

Rehydration and maintenance of water and electrolytes are primary treatment goals until the diarrheal episode ends. If the patient is volume depleted, rehydration should be directed at replacing water and electrolytes to normal body composition. Then water and electrolyte composition are maintained by replacing losses. Many patients will not develop volume depletion and therefore will only require maintenance fluid and electrolyte therapy. Parenteral and enteral routes may be used for supplying water and electrolytes. If vomiting and dehydration are not severe, enteral feeding is the less costly and preferred method. In the United States, many commercial oral rehydration preparations are available (Table 23-3).

Because of concerns about hypernatremia, physicians continue to hospitalize patients and use IV fluids to correct fluid and electrolyte deficits in severe dehydration. Oral solutions are strongly recommended.[8–10] In developing countries, the World Health Organization oral rehydration solution (WHO-ORS) saves the lives of millions of children annually.

During diarrhea, the small intestine retains its ability to actively transport monosaccharides such as glucose. Glucose actively carries sodium with water and other electrolytes. The WHO now recommends an ORS with a lower osmolarity, sodium content, and glucose load (see Table 23-3).[11] A separate oral supplement of zinc 20 mg daily for 14 days in addition to ORS significantly reduces the severity and duration of acute diarrhea in developing countries.[8,12]

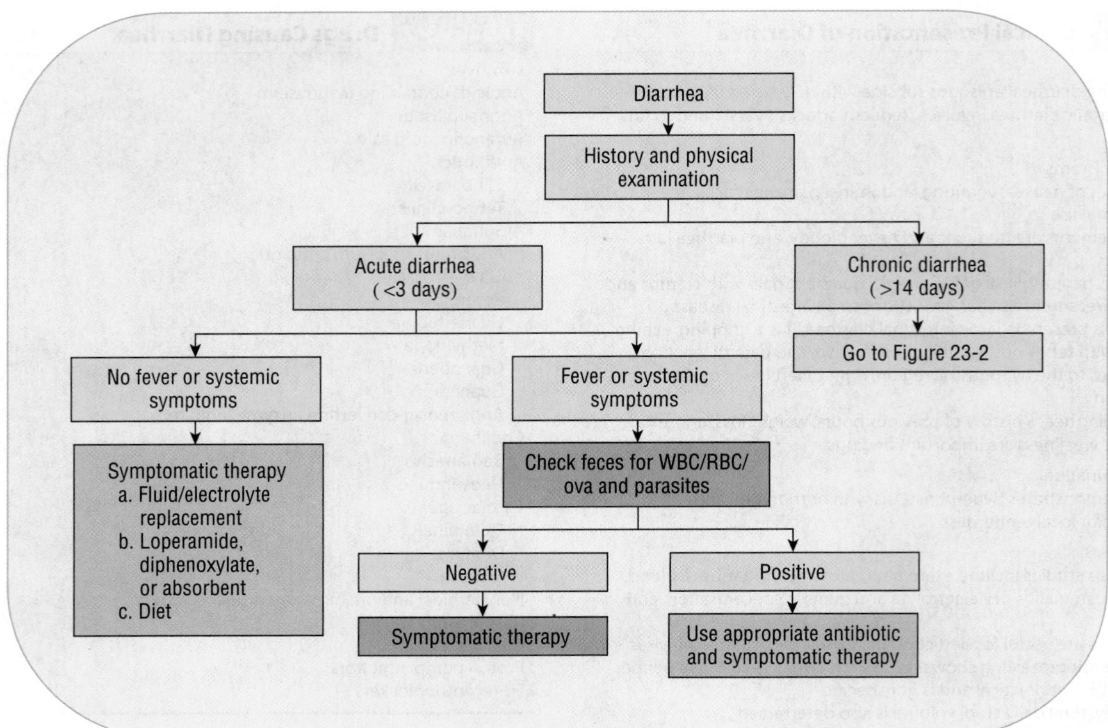

FIGURE 23-1 Recommendations for treating acute diarrhea. Follow the following steps: (a) Perform a complete history and physical examination. (b) Is the diarrhea acute or chronic? If chronic diarrhea, go to Figure 23-2. (c) If acute diarrhea, check for fever and/or systemic signs and symptoms (i.e., toxic patient). If systemic illness (fever, anorexia, or volume depletion), check for an infectious source. If positive for infectious diarrhea, use appropriate antibiotic/anthelmintic drug and symptomatic therapy. If negative for infectious cause, use only symptomatic treatment. (d) If no systemic findings, then use symptomatic therapy based on severity of volume depletion, oral or parenteral fluid/electrolytes, antidiarrheal agents (see Table 23-4), and diet. (RBC, red blood cells; WBC, white blood cells.)

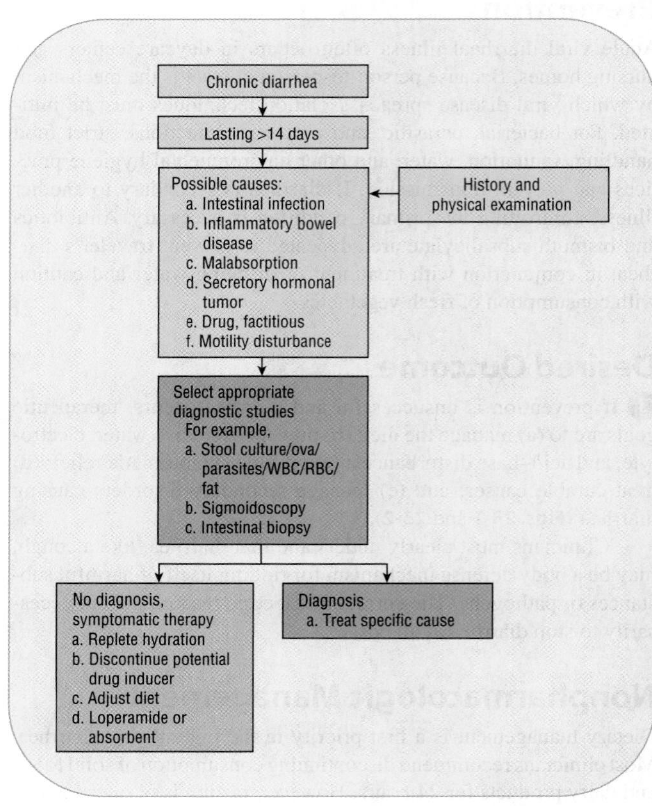

FIGURE 23-2 Recommendations for treating chronic diarrhea. Follow the following steps: (a) Perform a careful history and physical examination. (b) The possible causes of chronic diarrhea are many. These can be classified into intestinal infections (bacterial or protozoal), inflammatory disease (Crohn's disease or ulcerative colitis), malabsorption (lactose intolerance), secretory hormonal tumor (intestinal carcinoid tumor or vasoactive intestinal peptide-secreting tumor [VIPoma]), drug (antacid), factitious (laxative abuse), or motility disturbance (diabetes mellitus, irritable bowel syndrome, or hyperthyroidism). (c) If the diagnosis is uncertain, selected appropriate diagnostic studies should be ordered. (d) Once diagnosed, treatment is planned for the underlying cause with symptomatic antidiarrheal therapy. (e) If no specific cause can be identified, symptomatic therapy is prescribed. (RBC, red blood cells; WBC, white blood cells.)

TABLE 23-3 Oral Rehydration Solutions

	WHO-ORS[a]	Pedialyte[b] (Ross)	CeraLyte (Cera Products)	Enfalyte (Mead Johnson)
Osmolality (mOsm/kg or mmol/kg)	245	249	220	167
Carbohydrates[b] (g/L)	13.5	25	40[c]	30[c]
Calories (cal/L [J/L])	65 [272]	100 [418]	160 [670]	126 [527]
Electrolytes (mEq/L; mmol/L)				
Sodium	75	45	50–90	50
Potassium	20	20	20	25
Chloride	65	35	40–80	45
Citrate	—	30	30	34
Bicarbonate	30	—	—	—
Calcium	—	—	—	—
Magnesium	—	—	—	—
Sulfate	—	—	—	—
Phosphate	—	—	—	—

[a]World Health Organization reduced osmolarity oral rehydration solution.
[b]Carbohydrate is glucose.
[c]Rice syrup solids are carbohydrate source.

ORS is a lifesaving treatment for millions afflicted in developing countries. Acceptance in developed countries is less enthusiastic; however, the advantage of this product in reducing hospitalizations may prove its use as a cost-effective alternative, saving millions of dollars in healthcare expenditures.

Pharmacologic Therapy

Various drugs have been used to treat diarrheal attacks (Table 23-4), including antimotility agents, adsorbents, antisecretory compounds, antibiotics, enzymes, and intestinal microflora. Usually these drugs are not curative but palliative.

Opiates and Their Derivatives

Opiates and opioid derivatives (a) delay the transit of intraluminal contents or (b) increase gut capacity, prolonging contact and absorption. Enkephalins, which are endogenous opioid substances, regulate fluid movement across the mucosa by stimulating absorptive processes. Limitations to the use of opiates include an addiction potential (a real concern with long-term use) and worsening of diarrhea in selected infectious diarrhea.

Most opiates act through peripheral and central mechanisms with the exception of loperamide, which acts only peripherally. Loperamide is antisecretory; it inhibits the calcium-binding protein

TABLE 23-4 Selected Antidiarrheal Preparations

	Dose Form	Adult Dose
Antimotility		
Diphenoxylate	2.5 mg/tablet 2.5 mg/5 mL	5 mg four times daily; do not exceed 20 mg/day
Loperamide	2 mg/capsule 2 mg/capsule	Initially 4 mg, and then 2 mg after each loose stool; do not exceed 16 mg/day
Paregoric	2 mg/5 mL (morphine)	5–10 mL one to four times daily
Opium tincture	10 mg/mL (morphine)	0.6 mL four times daily
Difenoxin	1 mg/tablet	Two tablets, and then one tablet after each loose stool; up to eight tablets per day
Adsorbents		
Kaolin–pectin mixture	5.7 g kaolin + 130.2 mg pectin/30 mL	30–120 mL after each loose stool
Polycarbophil	500 mg/tablet	Chew 2 tablets four times daily or after each loose stool; do not exceed 12 tablets per day
Attapulgite	750 mg/15 mL 300 mg/7.5 mL 750 mg/tablet 600 mg/tablet 300 mg/tablet	1,200–1,500 mg after each loose bowel movement or every 2 hours; up to 9,000 mg/day
Antisecretory		
Bismuth subsalicylate	1,050 mg/30 mL 262 mg/15 mL 524 mg/15 mL 262 mg/tablet	Two tablets or 30 mL every 30 minutes to 1 hour as needed up to eight doses per day
Enzymes (lactase)	1,250 neutral lactase units/4 drops 3,300 FCC lactase units per tablet	Three to four drops taken with milk or dairy product
Bacterial replacement (*Lactobacillus acidophilus*, *Lactobacillus bulgaricus*)		Two tablets or one granule packet three to four times daily; give with milk, juice, or water
Octreotide	0.05 mg/mL 0.1 mg/mL 0.5 mg/mL	Initial: 50 mcg subcutaneously One to two times per day and titrate dose based on indication up to 600 mcg/day in two to four divided doses

calmodulin, controlling chloride secretion. Loperamide, available as 2 mg capsules or 1 mg/5 mL solution (both are nonprescription products), is suggested for managing acute and chronic diarrhea. The usual adult dose is initially 4 mg orally, followed by 2 mg after each loose stool, up to 16 mg/day. Used correctly, this agent has rare side effects, such as dizziness and constipation. If the diarrhea is concurrent with a high fever or bloody stool, the patient should be referred to a physician. Also, diarrhea lasting 48 hours beyond initiating loperamide warrants medical attention. Loperamide can also be used in traveler's diarrhea. It is comparable to bismuth subsalicylate for treatment of this disorder.[7]

Diphenoxylate is available as a 2.5 mg tablet and as a 2.5 mg/5 mL solution. A small amount of atropine (0.025 mg) is included in the product to discourage abuse. In adults, when taken as 2.5 to 5 mg three or four times daily, not to exceed a 20 mg total daily dose, diphenoxylate is rarely toxic. Some patients may complain of atropinism (blurred vision, dry mouth, and urinary hesitancy). Like loperamide, it should not be used in patients who are at risk of bacterial enteritis with *E. coli*, *Shigella*, or *Salmonella*.

Difenoxin, a diphenoxylate derivative also chemically related to meperidine, is also combined with atropine and has the same uses, precautions, and side effects. Marketed as a 1 mg tablet, the adult dosage is 2 mg initially, followed by 1 mg after each loose stool, not to exceed 8 mg/day.

Paregoric, camphorated tincture of opium, is marketed as a 2 mg/5 mL solution and is indicated for managing both acute and chronic diarrhea. It is not widely prescribed today because of its abuse potential.

Clinical **Controversy...**

Long-term use of oral opiates is not routinely recommended for several pharmacologic reasons. Some opioids such as morphine and codeine have the tendency to cause constipation by slowing down the peristaltic action of the bowels, which can also result in a functional ileus. This effect can be minimized by administering laxatives and/or stool softeners in patients who require long-term opiate therapy. Prokinetic agents may also be helpful in treating opiate-related constipation.

Adsorbents

Adsorbents are used for symptomatic relief. These products, many not requiring a prescription, are nontoxic, but their effectiveness remains unproven. Adsorbents are nonspecific in their action; they adsorb nutrients, toxins, drugs, and digestive juices. Polycarbophil absorbs 60 times its weight in water and can be used to treat both diarrhea and constipation. It is a nonprescription product and is sold as a 500 mg chewable tablet. This hydrophilic, nonabsorbable product is safe and may be taken four times daily, up to 6 g/day in adults. See Table 23-4 for selected antidiarrheal preparations.

Antisecretory Agents

Bismuth subsalicylate appears to have antisecretory, antiinflammatory, and antibacterial effects. As a nonprescription product, it is marketed for indigestion, relieving abdominal cramps, and controlling diarrhea, including traveler's diarrhea. Bismuth subsalicylate dosage strengths are a 262 mg chewable tablet, 262 mg/5 mL liquid, and 524 mg/15 mL liquid. The usual adult dose is two tablets or 30 mL every 30 minutes to 1 hour up to eight doses per day.

(4) Bismuth subsalicylate contains multiple components that might be toxic if given excessively to prevent or treat diarrhea. For instance, an active ingredient is salicylate, which may interact with anticoagulants or may produce salicylism (tinnitus, nausea, and vomiting). Bismuth reduces tetracycline absorption and may interfere with select GI radiographic studies. Patients may complain of a darkening of the tongue and stools with repeat administration. Salicylate can induce gout attacks in susceptible individuals.

Bismuth subsalicylate suspension has been evaluated in the treatment of secretory diarrhea of infectious etiology as well. In a dose of 30 mL every 30 minutes for eight doses, unformed stools decrease in the first 24 hours. Bismuth subsalicylate may also be effective in preventing traveler's diarrhea.

Octreotide, a synthetic octapeptide analog of endogenous somatostatin, is effective for the symptomatic treatment of carcinoid tumors and other peptide-secreting tumors, dumping syndrome, and chemotherapy-induced diarrhea.[13] It has had limited success in patients with AIDS-associated diarrhea and short-bowel syndrome, does not appear to have an advantage over various opiate derivatives in the treatment of chronic idiopathic diarrhea, and has the disadvantage of being administered by injection.[14] Metastatic intestinal carcinoid tumors secrete excessive amounts of vasoactive substances, including histamine, bradykinin, serotonin (5-HT), and prostaglandins. Primary carcinoid tumors occur throughout the GI tract, with most in the ileum. Predominant signs and symptoms experienced by patients with these tumors are attributable to excessive concentrations of 5-hydroxytryptophan and 5-HT. The totality of their clinical effects is termed the carcinoid syndrome. Some patients have a violent, watery diarrhea with abdominal cramping. Initially, diarrhea might be managed with various agents such as codeine, diphenoxylate, cyproheptadine, methysergide, phenoxybenzamine, or methyldopa. But octreotide is now considered first-line therapy for carcinoid syndrome.

Octreotide blocks the release of 5-HT and many other active peptides and has been effective in controlling diarrhea and flushing. It is reported to have direct inhibitory effects on intestinal secretion and stimulatory effects on intestinal absorption. Non–gastrin-secreting adenomas of the pancreas are tumors associated with profuse watery diarrhea. This condition has been referred to as Verner-Morrison syndrome, WDHA (watery diarrhea, hypokalemia, and achlorhydria) syndrome, pancreatic cholera, watery diarrhea syndrome, and vasoactive intestinal peptide-secreting tumor (VIPoma). Excessive secretion of VIP from a retroperitoneal or pancreatic tumor produces most of the clinical features. Surgical tumor dissection is the treatment of choice. In nonsurgical candidates, the profuse watery diarrhea and other symptoms commonly encountered are managed with octreotide.

The dose of octreotide varies with the indication, disease severity, and patient response.[13] For managing diarrhea and flushing associated with carcinoid tumors in adults, the initial dosage range is 100 to 600 mcg/day in two to four divided doses subcutaneously for 2 weeks. For controlling secretory diarrhea of VIPomas, the dosage range is 200 to 300 mcg/day in two to four divided doses for 2 weeks. Some patients may require higher doses for symptomatic control. Patients responding to these initial doses may be switched to Sandostatin LAR Depot, a long-acting octreotide formulation. This product consists of microspheres containing the drug. Initial doses consist of 20 mg given intramuscularly intragluteally at 4-week intervals for 2 months. It is recommended that during the first 2 weeks of therapy the short-acting formulation also be administered subcutaneously. At the end of 2 months, patients with good symptom control may have the dose reduced to 10 mg every 4 weeks, while those without sufficient symptom control may have the dose increased to 30 mg every 4 weeks. For patients experiencing recurrence of symptoms on the 10 mg dose, dosage adjustment to 20 mg should be made. It is not uncommon for patients with carcinoid tumors or VIPomas to experience periodic exacerbation of symptoms. Subcutaneous octreotide for several days should be reinstituted in these individuals. In so-called carcinoid crisis, octreotide is given as an IV infusion at 50 mcg/h for 8 to 24 hours.

Because octreotide inhibits many other GI hormones, it has a variety of intestinal side effects. With prolonged use, gallbladder and biliary tract complications such as cholelithiasis have been reported. Approximately 5% to 10% of patients complain of nausea, diarrhea, and abdominal pain. Local injection pain occurs with about an 8% incidence. With high doses, octreotide may reduce dietary fat absorption, leading to steatorrhea.

Two other somatostatin analogs, lanreotide and vapreotide, have been studied.[14,15] Lanreotide is approved for use in the United States for acromegaly. The starting dose is 90 mg subcutaneously every 4 weeks for 3 months, and then the dose is adjusted based on growth hormone and insulin-like growth factor levels.[16] Vapreotide is an orphan drug that is indicated for pancreatic and GI fistulas as well as esophageal variceal bleeding.

Miscellaneous Products

Probiotics are microorganisms that have been used for many years to replace colonic microflora. This supposedly restores normal intestinal function and suppresses the growth of pathogenic microorganisms. *Saccharomyces boulardii*, *Lactobacillus* GG, and *Lactobacillus acidophilus* decrease the duration of infectious and antibiotic-induced diarrhea in adults and children.[17] A combination probiotic product, VSL#3 (which contains multiple strains of lactobacilli and bifidobacteria) may have benefit in preventing radiation-induced diarrhea when given three times a day.[18] A meta-analysis suggests that probiotics may prevent antibiotic-associated diarrhea (AAD).[19] The dosage of probiotic preparations varies depending on the brand used. Intestinal flatus is the primary patient complaint experienced with this modality.

Anticholinergic drugs such as atropine block vagal tone and prolong gut transit time. Drugs with anticholinergic properties are present in many nonprescription products. Their value in controlling diarrhea is questionable and limited because of side effects. Angle-closure glaucoma, selected heart diseases, and obstructive uropathies are relative contraindications to the use of anticholinergic agents.

Lactase enzyme products are helpful for patients who are experiencing diarrhea secondary to lactose intolerance. Lactase is required for carbohydrate digestion. When a patient lacks this enzyme, eating dairy products causes an osmotic diarrhea. Several products are available for use each time a dairy product, especially milk or ice cream, is consumed.

Clinical **Controversy...**

The use of probiotics to treat and prevent AAD is controversial. A meta-analysis published in 2012 concluded that adjunctive probiotics significantly reduce the risk of acquiring AAD, but individual studies have been unclear as to whether there is any benefit. Additional studies are needed to compare different probiotic formulations, determine optimal dosing, and evaluate whether efficacy differs based on the antibiotic used. Additional safety data are also required before probiotics can be recommended routinely for this purpose.

Investigational Drugs

Several new classes of compounds are undergoing clinical trials for efficacy in acute diarrhea. Enkephalins are endogenous opiate compounds in the gut that have antisecretory and proabsorptive activity in the small intestine. They promote sodium and chloride reabsorption via stimulation of a nonadrenergic, noncholinergic neurotransmitter. Enkephalinase inhibitors are compounds that slow down the enzymatic (i.e., enkephalinase) breakdown of endogenous enkephalins found in the small intestines. They exert an antisecretory effect without affecting GI motility or CNS-related effects/side effects. One specific compound, originally called acetorphan but now referred to as racecadotril, has been extensively tested in humans and found to be equal to other opiate antidiarrheals such as loperamide, while causing less GI motility side effects such as abdominal bloating, pain, and constipation.[20–22] Racecadotril is currently licensed only in France and a few developing countries with a high incidence of childhood diarrhea.

Vaccines are a new therapeutic frontier in controlling infectious diarrheas, especially in developing countries.[23,24] An oral vaccine for cholera is licensed and available in other countries (Dukoral from SBL Vaccines) and appears to provide somewhat better immunity and has fewer adverse effects than the previously available parenteral vaccine. However, the CDC does not recommend cholera vaccines for most travelers, nor is the vaccine available in the United States.

Oral *Shigella* vaccine, although effective under field conditions, requires five weekly oral doses and repeat booster doses, thereby limiting its practicality for use in developing nations. With about 1,500 serotypes for *Salmonella*, a vaccine is not currently available for humans. There are two newer typhoid vaccine formulations, one a parenteral inactivated whole-cell vaccine and the other an oral live-attenuated (Ty21a) vaccine that is administered in four doses on days 1, 3, 5, and 7, to be completed at least 1 week before exposure. Two rotavirus vaccines have been shown to prevent gastroenteritis due to rotavirus infection in infants and children.[25] The pentavalent human-bovine reassortant vaccine (RotaTeq from Merck) is administered as a three-oral-dose sequence, and the monovalent human vaccine (Rotarix from GlaxoSmithKline) is administered as a two-oral-dose sequence. A rotavirus vaccine program has been formed to reduce child morbidity and mortality from diarrheal disease by accelerating the availability of rotavirus vaccines appropriate for use in developing countries.

Evaluation of Therapeutic Outcomes

Therapeutic outcomes are directed toward key symptoms, signs, and laboratory studies. Constitutional symptoms usually improve within 24 to 72 hours. Monitoring for changes in the frequency and character of bowel movements on a daily basis in conjunction with vital signs and improvement in appetite are of utmost importance. Also, the clinician needs to monitor body weight, serum osmolality, serum electrolytes, complete blood cell counts, urinalysis, and culture results (if appropriate).

Acute Diarrhea

Most patients with acute diarrhea experience mild to moderate distress. In the absence of moderate to severe dehydration, high fever, and blood or mucus in the stool, this illness is usually self-limiting within 3 to 7 days. Mild to moderate acute diarrhea is usually managed on an outpatient basis with oral rehydration, symptomatic treatment, and diet. Elderly persons with chronic illness as well as infants may require hospitalization for parenteral rehydration and close monitoring.

Severe Diarrhea

In the urgent/emergent situation, restoration of the patient's volume status is the most important outcome. Toxic patients (fever dehydration, hematochezia, or hypotension) require hospitalization, IV fluids and electrolyte administration, and empiric antibiotic therapy while awaiting culture and sensitivity results. With timely management, these patients usually recover within a few days.

CONSTIPATION

5 Constipation is a common complaint among the general population and accounts for many medical visits each year in the United States.[26] It is generally defined by the American Gastroenterology Association (AGA) as difficult or infrequent passage of stool, at times associated with straining or a feeling of incomplete defecation.[27]

Constipation may be further defined by quantitative or qualitative measures. For instance, physicians often use stool frequency to define constipation (most commonly fewer than three bowel movements per week); however, the "normal" frequency of bowel movement is not well established and can vary from person to person. Patients more often describe constipation in terms of symptoms or a combination of quantitative and qualitative descriptors that are difficult to quantify: bowel movement frequency, stool size or consistency (hard or lumpy stools), straining on defecation, inability to defecate at will, and symptoms such as sensation of incomplete evacuation. The condition is considered chronic if symptoms last for at least 3 months. Many people believe that daily bowel movements are required for normal health or that accumulation of toxic substances will occur with infrequent defecation. Inappropriate laxative use by the general public may result from these misconceptions.

Though often considered more of a minor uncomfortable or unpleasant problem, constipation can have serious consequences and be costly to the healthcare system. Costs for medical evaluation of constipation alone have been estimated at more than $2,500 per patient, and patients spend more than an estimated $800 million each year on nonprescription laxatives.[26,28]

Epidemiology

The prevalence of constipation depends on the definition used and whether the condition is self-reported or provider-diagnosed. A systematic review of 45 studies reported the prevalence of chronic constipation in adults (≥15 years old) worldwide to be 14%.[27] The highest incidence was found in South America (16%) and the lowest incidence in Southeast Asia. A review of the epidemiology of constipation in North America specifically found a prevalence for constipation up to 27%, with most reported estimates ranging from 12% to 19%.[29] Similarly, in a multinational survey of 13,879 adult participants from seven countries, the rate of self-reported constipation was 12.3% overall (range 5% to 18%).[29,30]

Constipation is more common in women (2.4-fold more likely) and the elderly.[27] Other factors associated with constipation in some reports include inactivity, lower socioeconomic class, lower income, non-white race, symptoms of depression, and history of physical or sexual abuse.

Pathophysiology

Constipation may be primary or secondary. Primary, or idiopathic, constipation occurs without an identifiable underlying cause, whereas secondary constipation may be the result of constipating drugs, lifestyle factors, or medical disorders (Table 23-5).[31] Primary constipation can be further divided into three categories—functional, slow transit, and outlet dysfunction, or disordered defecation. Functional constipation, often referred to as normal transit, is the most common type. These patients have normal GI motility and stool frequency but may experience difficulty evacuating, passage of hard stools, or bloating and abdominal discomfort. Slow transit constipation represents an abnormality of GI transit time that leads to infrequent defecation. Dysfunction of the pelvic floor muscles and/or anal sphincter is the most frequently encountered reason for disordered defecation. In patients with defecatory disorders, these muscles or sphincter contract during defecation instead of relax and impede evacuation of stool. It is common for patients to have and present with more than one type of constipation.

TABLE 23-5 Possible Causes of Constipation

Conditions	Possible Causes
GI disorders	Irritable bowel syndrome Diverticulitis Upper GI tract diseases Anal and rectal diseases Hemorrhoids Anal fissures Ulcerative proctitis Tumors Hernia Volvulus of the bowel Syphilis Tuberculosis Helminthic infections Lymphogranuloma venereum Hirschsprung's disease
Metabolic and endocrine disorders	Diabetes mellitus with neuropathy Hypothyroidism Panhypopituitarism Pheochromocytoma Hypercalcemia Enteric glucagon excess
Cardiac disorders	Heart failure
Pregnancy	Depressed gut motility Increased fluid absorption from colon Use of iron salts
Lifestyle factors	Dietary changes Inadequate fluid intake Low dietary fiber Decreased physical activity
Neurogenic causes	CNS diseases Trauma to the brain (particularly the medulla) Spinal cord injury CNS tumors Cerebrovascular accidents Parkinson's disease
Psychogenic causes	Ignoring or postponing urge to defecate Psychiatric diseases
Drug induced	See Table 23-6

Factors associated with the increased prevalence of constipation in the elderly include a higher number of daily medications, particularly anticholinergic agents, increased incidence of chronic comorbidities, and changes in mobility status.[28] Changes in diet such as decreased fluid and/or fiber intake, diminished physical activity, and institutionalization can lead to constipation. Physiologic changes such as mesenteric dysfunction and changes in anorectal function, including loss of rectal wall elasticity, are also thought to predispose elderly patients to constipation.

Drug-Induced Constipation

Use of drugs that inhibit the neurologic or muscular function of the GI tract, particularly the colon, may result in secondary constipation.[31] Medications that are commonly associated with causing constipation include opiates, anticholinergic agents, and certain antacids.[28] With most of the agents listed in Table 23-6, the inhibitory effects on bowel function may be dose dependent, with larger doses causing constipation more frequently.

Opiates have effects on all segments of the bowel, but effects are most pronounced on the colon.[27] The major mechanism by which opiates produce constipation has been proposed to be prolongation

TABLE 23-6 Drugs Causing Constipation

Analgesics
Inhibitors of prostaglandin synthesis
Opiates
Anticholinergics
Antihistamines
Antiparkinsonian agents (e.g., benztropine or trihexyphenidyl)
Phenothiazines
Tricyclic antidepressants
Antacids containing calcium carbonate or aluminum hydroxide
Barium sulfate
Calcium channel antagonists
Clonidine
Diuretics (non–potassium-sparing)
Ganglionic blockers
Iron preparations
Muscle blockers (D-tubocurarine, succinylcholine)
Nonsteroidal antiinflammatory agents
Polystyrene sodium sulfonate

of intestinal transit time by causing spastic, nonpropulsive contractions. An additional contributory mechanism may be an increase in electrolyte absorption.

While all opiate derivatives are associated with constipation, the degree of intestinal inhibitory effects seems to differ between agents. Orally administered opiates appear to have greater inhibitory effects than parenterally administered products. In some reports, transdermal fentanyl has been associated with less constipation than oral sustained-release morphine.[32]

Other medications may increase the risk of constipation by a variety of mechanisms. Anticholinergic agents decrease contractility of intestinal muscle while calcium channel blockers are thought to cause rectosigmoid dysfunction, leading to constipation. Nonsteroidal antiinflammatory drugs (NSAIDs) may lead to constipation due to their inhibition of prostaglandin synthesis.[28]

Clinical Presentation

A symptom-based system for classifying functional constipation (and other functional GI disorders) is often used to define constipation in clinical trials. The Rome criteria encompass both quantitative (frequency) and qualitative (stool consistency, etc.) symptoms associated with constipation.[33] Table 23-7 outlines general clinical presentation of patients with constipation. According to the Rome III criteria, patients should have at least 2 of the signs and symptoms listed in Table 23-7 apply to a minimum of 25% of bowel movements.

Evaluation of constipation should attempt to clarify the patient's specific symptoms (i.e., exactly what the patient means by constipation).[33] A complete and thorough history should be obtained from the patient, including frequency of bowel movements and duration of symptoms. Constipation occurring abruptly in an adult may indicate significant colon pathology such as malignancy. Constipation present since early infancy may be indicative of neurologic disorders. The patient should also be carefully questioned about usual diet and laxative regimens. Does the patient have a diet consistently deficient in high-fiber items and containing mainly high refined foods? What laxatives or cathartics has the patient used to attempt relief of constipation? The patient should be questioned about other concurrent medications, with interest focused on agents that might cause constipation.

Evaluation should also include perianal and anal examinations to identify fecal impaction or other anatomical obstructions that may be contributing to or causing constipation. General health status, signs of underlying medical illness (i.e., hypothyroidism),

TABLE 23-7 Clinical Presentation of Constipation

Signs and symptoms
- Infrequent bowel movements (less than 3 per week)
- Stools that are hard, small, or dry
- Difficulty or pain of defecation
- Feeling of abdominal discomfort or bloating, incomplete evacuation, etc.

Alarm signs and symptoms
- Hematochezia
- Melena
- Family history of colon cancer
- Family history of inflammatory bowel disease
- Anemia
- Weight loss
- Anorexia
- Nausea and vomiting
- Severe, persistent constipation that is refractory to treatment
- New-onset or worsening constipation in elderly without evidence of primary cause

Physical examination
- Perform rectal exam for presence of anatomical abnormalities (such as fistulas, fissures, hemorrhoids, rectal prolapse) or abnormalities of perianal descent
- Digital examination of rectum to check for fecal impaction, anal stricture, or rectal mass

Laboratory and other diagnostic tests
- No routine recommendations for lab testing—as indicated by clinical discretion
- In patients with signs and symptoms suggestive of organic disorder, specific testing may be performed (i.e., thyroid function tests, electrolytes, glucose, complete blood count) based on clinical presentation
- In patients with alarm signs and symptoms or when structural disease is a possibility, select appropriate diagnostic studies:
  1. Protoscopy
  2. Sigmoidoscopy
  3. Colonoscopy
  4. Barium enema

and psychological status (e.g., depression or other psychological illness) should also be assessed. Laboratory tests may be performed, particularly if the patient is presumed to suffer from secondary causes.

Specific attention should be given to identify any "alarm symptoms" that would warrant further diagnostic workup (see Table 23-7).[34] Patients with alarm symptoms, a family history of colon cancer, or those >50 years old with new symptoms may need further diagnostic evaluation.

TREATMENT

Desired Outcome

The major goals of treatment are to (a) relieve symptoms; (b) reestablish normal bowel habits; and (c) improve quality of life by minimizing adverse effects of treatment.

TABLE 23-8 Constipation Treatment Algorithm

Diagnosis
1. Treat specific cause
2. No underlying diagnosis, then choose symptomatic therapy
   A. Bulk-forming agents
   B. Dietary modification
   C. Alter lifestyle (exercise)
   D. Increase fluid intake
   E. Discontinue potential drug inducer

General Approach to Treatment

Table 23-8 presents a general treatment algorithm for the management of constipation.

6 Approaches to the treatment of constipation should begin with attempts to determine its cause. If an underlying disease is recognized as the cause of constipation, attempts should be made to correct it. GI malignancies may be removed via surgical resection. Endocrine and metabolic derangements should be corrected by the appropriate methods. For example, when hypothyroidism is the cause of constipation, cautious institution of thyroid replacement therapy is the most important treatment measure.

As discussed earlier, many drug substances may cause constipation. If a patient is consuming medications known to cause constipation, consideration should be given to alternative agents. If no reasonable alternatives exist to the medication thought to be responsible for constipation, consideration should be given to lowering the dose. If a patient must remain on constipating medications, then more attention must be given to general measures for prevention of constipation, as discussed in the next section.

The proper management of constipation will require a combination of nonpharmacologic and pharmacologic therapies. Laxative therapy is considered the preferred first line for the treatment of constipation, in addition to increasing dietary fiber. Patients are often encouraged to increase daily fluid intake and physical activity as well dedicate time to respond to the urge to defecate, although efficacy data are conflicting for these measures.[35]

Nonpharmacologic Therapy

Dietary Modification

The most important aspect of therapy for constipation for the majority of patients is dietary modification to increase the amount of fiber consumed. Fiber, the portion of vegetable matter not digested in the human GI tract, increases stool bulk, retention of stool water, and rate of transit of stool through the intestine. The result of fiber therapy is an increased frequency of defecation. Also, fiber decreases intraluminal pressures in the colon and rectum, which is thought to be beneficial for diverticular disease and for irritable bowel syndrome (IBS).

7 The specific physiologic effects of fiber are not well understood. Patients should be advised to gradually increase daily fiber intake to 20 to 25 g, through either dietary changes or fiber supplement products (see Bulk-Forming Agents below), a grade B recommendation from the American College of Gastroenterology.[36] Fruits, vegetables, and cereals typically have the highest fiber content. Bran, a by-product of milling of wheat, is often added to foods to increase fiber content and contains a high amount of soluble fiber, which may be extremely constipating in larger doses. Raw bran is generally 40% fiber. A small randomized controlled trial revealed that adding prunes (approximately 6 g fiber/day), or dried plums, to daily diet was more effective than adding psyllium (6 g fiber/day) in treating mild to moderate constipation.[37]

A trial of dietary modification with high-fiber content should be continued for at least 1 month before effects on bowel function are determined. Most patients begin to notice effects on bowel function 3 to 5 days after beginning a high-fiber diet, but some patients may require a considerably longer period of time. Patients should be cautioned that abdominal distension and flatulence may be particularly troublesome in the first few weeks of fiber therapy, particularly with high bran consumption. Gradually increasing dietary fiber over a few weeks to the goal of 20 to 25 g may help reduce some of the adverse abdominal effects. In most cases these problems resolve with continued use.

Surgery

In a small percentage of patients who present with complaints of constipation, surgical procedures are necessary because of the presence of colonic malignancies or GI obstruction from a number of other causes. Patients who have slow-transit-type primary constipation that is refractory to treatment are also surgical candidates.[35] Surgery may be required in some endocrine disorders that cause constipation, such as pheochromocytoma, which requires removal of a tumor. In each case, the involved segment of intestine may be resected or revised.

Biofeedback

Patients with constipation due to pelvic floor dysfunction/disordered defecation may have a less favorable response to fiber therapy than other constipation subtypes.[36] Many adult patients with functional defecatory disorders appear to benefit from pelvic floor retraining with biofeedback therapy. The goals of biofeedback are to improve pelvic floor relaxation to facilitate the passage of stool and the procedure is typically performed over 4- to 6-hour-long sessions. Success rates of 65% to 80% have been reported in controlled and uncontrolled studies, and improvement has been sustained for up to 1 year. The value of biofeedback in children with chronic constipation has not been well demonstrated.[3]

Electrical Stimulation

Sacral nerve stimulation is a minimally invasive technique that has been used for treatment of fecal incontinence and there are some reports of its use in severe refractory chronic constipation.[38] However, clinical data supporting the use of electrical stimulation for this purpose are limited and there are currently no recommendations for general practice.

Pharmacologic Therapy

Three general classes of laxatives are discussed in this section: (a) those causing softening of feces in 1 to 3 days; (b) those that result in soft or semifluid stool in 6 to 12 hours; and (c) those causing watery evacuation in 1 to 6 hours (Table 23-9). Other pharmacologic agents available for the treatment of constipation include a calcium channel activator, guanylate cyclase C agonist, and serotonergic agents.

Bulk-Forming Agents

Medicinal products, often called "bulk-forming agents," such as psyllium hydrophilic colloids, methylcellulose, or polycarbophil, have properties similar to those of dietary fiber and may be taken as tablets, powders, or granules.[28] These agents increase the water content of stool to increase stool bulk and weight and relieve the symptoms of constipation within 3 days of initiating therapy.

Bulk-forming laxatives have few adverse effects. The most common effects include flatulence, abdominal bloating, and distention. Rarely, these agents may lead to bowel obstruction. Patients should also be cautioned to consume sufficient fluid while supplementing with bulk-forming agents to avoid obstruction of the esophagus, stomach, small intestine, and colon.

Emollient Laxatives

Emollient laxatives, including docusate in its various salts, are surfactant agents that work by facilitating mixing of aqueous and fatty materials within the intestinal tract.[39] They may increase water and electrolyte secretion in the small and large bowel. Increased stool moisture content should lead to a softer, easier-to-pass stool. These products are generally given orally, although docusate potassium has also been used rectally. With these products, softening of stools occurs within 1 to 3 days of therapy.

TABLE 23-9 Dosage Recommendations for Laxatives and Cathartics

Agent	Recommended Dose
Agents that Cause Softening of Feces in 1–3 Days	
Bulk-forming agents/osmotic laxatives	
Methylcellulose	4–6 g/day
Polycarbophil	4–6 g/day
Psyllium	Varies with product
Polyethylene glycol 3350	17 g/dose
Emollients	
Docusate sodium	50–360 mg/day
Docusate calcium	50–360 mg/day
Docusate potassium	100–300 mg/day
Lactulose	15–30 mL orally
Sorbitol	30–50 g/day orally
Agents that Result in Soft or Semifluid Stool in 6–12 Hours	
Bisacodyl (oral)	5–15 mg orally
Senna	Dose varies with formulation
Magnesium sulfate (low dose)	<10 g orally
Agents that Cause Watery Evacuation in 1–6 Hours	
Magnesium citrate	18 g 300 mL water
Magnesium hydroxide	2.4–4.8 g orally
Magnesium sulfate (high dose)	10–30 g orally
Sodium phosphates	Varies with salt used
Bisacodyl	10 mg rectally
Polyethylene glycol–electrolyte preparations	4 L

Emollient laxatives are ineffective in treating constipation but are used mainly to prevent this condition. They may be helpful in situations in which straining at stool should be avoided, such as after recovery from myocardial infarction, with acute perianal disease, or after rectal surgery. It is unlikely that these agents would be effective in preventing constipation if major causative factors (e.g., heavy opiate use, uncorrected pathology, or inadequate dietary fiber) are not concurrently addressed. The use of mineral oil is generally not recommended due to safety concerns.

Although docusates are generally safe, a few adverse effects have been noted. They may increase the intestinal absorption of agents administered concurrently and alter toxic potential. Reports of increased fecal soiling associated with docusate use in elderly patients may limit their use in this population.[39]PEG solutions with electrolytes are used as bowel cleansing regimens prior to GI-related procedures.

Hyperosmolar Agents

Lactulose and Sorbitol Lactulose is a nonabsorbable disaccharide that is metabolized by colonic bacteria to low-molecular-weight acids, resulting in an osmotic effect whereby fluid is retained in the colon.[39] The fluid retained in the colon lowers the pH and increases colonic peristalsis within 2 to 3 days of use. Lactulose increases stool frequency and consistency in patients with chronic constipation (vs. placebo) and may be more effective than fiber alone. In comparison to polyethylene glycol (PEG), lactulose is slightly less effective in increasing stool frequency per week and patients are more likely to need additional products for constipation relief.[40] The most common adverse effects include flatulence, nausea, and abdominal discomfort or bloating—although lactulose can be useful in some patients. It may be justified as an alternative for acute constipation or in patients with an inadequate response to increased dietary fiber and bulking agents. In some patients with more complex disease or nonmodifiable risk factors for constipation (such as bedridden, elderly patients with chronic or debilitating illnesses and constipating medications), lactulose may be required on a more regular basis.[39] In addition to the adverse abdominal effects associated with lactulose, diarrhea and electrolyte imbalances can occasionally occur. Sorbitol, a monosaccharide, also exerts its effect by osmotic action and has been recommended as a cost-effective alternative to lactulose. It is as effective as lactulose but may cause less nausea and is much less expensive.

Polyethylene Glycol PEG is FDA-approved for treatment of constipation at low doses and is expected to produce a bowel movement in 1 to 3 days.[39,40] For this indication, PEG is administered in smaller volumes (10 to 30 or 17 to 34 g per 120 to 240 mL) usually once (or twice) daily. PEG is not absorbed systemically or metabolized by colonic bacteria, and therefore has a lower incidence of adverse effects compared with other osmotic laxatives. Daily use in low dose (17 g) may be safe and effective for up to 6 months.[41] PEG is a grade A recommendation from the American College of Gastroenterology for the treatment of chronic constipation and is available as a nonprescription drug.[34] The most common adverse effects are GI-related and include nausea, vomiting, flatulence, and abdominal cramping.[39] PEG solutions with electrolytes are used as bowel cleansing regimens prior to GI-related procedures.

Magnesium Salts Magnesium salts, including hydroxide, phosphate, and citrate, and sodium phosphate are categorized as saline cathartics.[39] These agents are frequently used as bowel preparations prior to diagnostic procedures such as colonoscopy.[31] Milk of magnesia (an 8% suspension of magnesium hydroxide), though, may be used occasionally to treat constipation in otherwise healthy adults, but efficacy data are limited. Saline cathartics should not be used on a routine basis. These agents may cause fluid and electrolyte depletion. Also, magnesium or sodium accumulation may occur in patients with renal dysfunction or congestive heart failure. These risks increase with long-term use.

Glycerin Glycerin is usually administered as a suppository and exerts its effect by osmotic action in the rectum. As with most agents given as suppositories, the onset of action is usually less than 30 minutes. Glycerin is considered a safe laxative, although it may occasionally cause rectal irritation. Its use is acceptable on an intermittent basis for constipation or fecal impaction, particularly in children.[42]

Stimulant Laxatives

Stimulant laxatives such as diphenylmethane (bisacodyl) and anthraquinone (senna and others) derivates primarily affect the colon.[39] These agents stimulate the mucosal nerve plexus of the colon and may also affect intestinal fluid secretion by altering fluid and electrolyte transport, and are expected to cause a bowel movement within 8 to 12 hours of administration. Stimulant laxatives may cause severe abdominal cramping and electrolyte imbalances, particularly with chronic use. Compared with placebo, bisacodyl is effective in treatment of constipation[43]; however, stimulant laxatives are not recommended as first-line treatment. These agents are typically reserved for intermittent use or in patients who fail to respond adequately to bulking and osmotic laxatives. Some patients, though, with severe chronic constipation and nonmodifiable risk factors may use these agents on a more regular basis.[28,34]

Lubiprostone

Lubiprostone is a chloride channel activator that acts locally in the gut to open chloride channels on the GI luminal epithelium, which, in turn, stimulates chloride-rich fluid secretion into the intestinal lumen. Increased intraluminal fluid secretion helps to soften stool and accelerate GI transit time.[27] Lubiprostone (Amitiza) is

FDA-approved for chronic idiopathic constipation in adults at a recommended dose of one 24 mg capsule twice daily with food as well as treatment of patients with constipation-predominant irritable bowel syndrome (IBS-C). Clinical trials have shown a significant increase in spontaneous bowel movements in patients treated with lubiprostone versus placebo as well as improvement in straining, stool consistency, and overall constipation severity.[44] Lubiprostone appears safe and effective for long-term treatment (up to 48 weeks). For most patients, bowel movements occur within 24 to 48 hours of lubiprostone administration. Common adverse effects include nausea, headache, and diarrhea and may be dose dependent.[31] Because of its high cost (especially relative to other available laxative agents) and lack of comparative data with other laxative therapies, lubiprostone is reserved for patients with chronic constipation who fail conventional first-line agents.

Linaclotide

Linaclotide (Linzess) is the newest agent approved for the treatment of constipation and IBS-C.[45] It is a synthetic 14-amino-acid peptide that binds to and activates the guanylate cyclase C receptor found on the intestinal epithelium. This increases intestinal fluid secretion and quickens intestinal motility. In two randomized controlled trials involving approximately 1,276 patients, linaclotide 145 and 290 mcg daily was more effective than placebo at increasing spontaneous bowel movements in patients with chronic constipation at 12 weeks.[46] Only the 145 mcg dose is approved for treatment of constipation due to the lack of improved efficacy with the higher dosing. Diarrhea was the most commonly reported adverse event in clinical trials, followed by flatulence and abdominal pain. Linaclotide should not be used in patients under the age of 18.[45]

Opioid Receptor Antagonists

Alvimopan (Entereg) is an oral GI-specific μ-opioid antagonist approved for short-term use in hospitalized patients to accelerate recovery of bowel function after large or small bowel resection.[47] It antagonizes the GI (peripheral) effects of opioids without affecting analgesia because it does not cross the blood–brain barrier. Alvimopan is only available through a special use program (ENTEREG access support and education [EASE]), which requires hospitals to register and meet all requirements before the drug can be administered. Additionally, alvimopan is contraindicated in patients receiving therapeutic doses of opioids for more than 7 consecutive days prior to surgery as they may be more sensitive to the drug's effects. Dosing for alvimopan is as follows: 12 mg capsule administered 30 minutes to 5 hours before surgery and then 12 mg twice daily for up to 7 days or until discharge (maximum of 15 doses).

Methylnaltrexone (Relistor) is μ-receptor antagonist approved for opioid-induced constipation in patients with advanced disease receiving palliative care or when response to laxative therapy has been insufficient.[47] This agent does not cross the blood–brain barrier or antagonize analgesia; it acts on peripheral μ-receptors to block unwanted opioid side effects such as constipation. It is administered at a weight-based dose as a subcutaneous injection, usually every other day (no more than once daily), and is contraindicated in patients with known or suspected GI obstruction.

Naltrexone and naloxone are also opioid antagonists. Although they do cross the blood–brain barrier and may potentially reverse CNS effects of opioids (respiratory depression and analgesia), use of naloxone for treatment of opioid-induced constipation may be effective when used in a prolonged-release formulation.[47]

Other Agents

Prucalopride is a selective 5-hydroxytryptamine-4 (5-HT_4) receptor agonist being developed for treatment of chronic constipation and IBS-C.[48] It demonstrates proenterokinetic effects (increased colonic motility and transit), specifically in the GI tract. Prucalopride, however, is more selective than the previously available serotonergic agonists cisapride and tegaserod with higher affinity for the 5-HT_4 receptor. Receptor selectivity is thought to improve the safety profile of prucalopride over cisapride and tegaserod, which were removed from the market due to concerns for adverse cardiovascular events. In clinical trials, prucalopride significantly increased the number of complete, spontaneous bowel movements in adults with chronic constipation. Constipation symptoms and quality of life were also improved with prucalopride. This agent has been safely tolerated in clinical trials with no adverse cardiovascular effects versus placebo (although data are limited) and is approved for use in Europe. Prucalopride has not yet been approved by the FDA.

Probiotics may be useful in the treatment of constipation. Five randomized controlled trials conducted in children and adults revealed that certain strains of probiotics increased weekly stool frequency.[49] However, these trials were small (370 patients total) and only slight improvement was realized (one additional stool per week). More studies are needed to strengthen evidence involving probiotics, but these may be an option for patients seeking alternative treatment.

Investigational drugs

Velusetrag and norcisapride are selective 5-HT_4 agonists that are currently being developed for chronic constipation.[28] Both agents appear to be effective and well tolerated in preliminary studies.

Prevention

For certain groups of patients, such as those recovering from myocardial infarction or rectal surgery, straining at defecation should be avoided. The basis of preventive therapy in these patients should be bulk-forming laxatives. Additionally, the use of docusate is popular, although its effectiveness is debated. In pregnant patients, constipation may result because of alterations in hormones or iron supplementation. As described earlier, bulk-forming laxatives and docusates should be the first line of prevention.

Evaluation of Therapeutic Outcomes

The ultimate goal of treatment for constipation is to prevent further episodes of constipation. Short-term goals include alleviation of acute constipation with relief from symptoms. For patients with chronic constipation, the goals include use of proper diet and decreased reliance on laxatives in addition to relief of symptoms for the patient so that quality of life is not diminished. Effective treatment of constipation requires the patient to become more knowledgeable about the causes of constipation, proper diet, and appropriate use of laxatives.

IRRITABLE BOWEL SYNDROME

IBS is a GI syndrome characterized by chronic abdominal pain and altered bowel habits in the absence of any organic cause. It is the most commonly diagnosed GI condition.

Epidemiology

The prevalence of IBS is approximately 10% to 15% based on North American and European population-based studies; however, there is a wide variation in prevalence by individual country.[50–53] IBS affects men and women, young patients, and the elderly with an overall 2:1 female predominance in North America.[52] However, younger patients and women are more likely to be diagnosed with IBS. Although only 15% of those affected actually seek medical attention, IBS is the cause of between 25% and 50% of all referrals to gastroenterologists.[50]

Pathophysiology

Although the exact pathophysiologic abnormalities with IBS are still being actively investigated, IBS likely results from altered somatovisceral and motor dysfunction of the intestine from a variety of causes. Abnormal CNS processing of afferent signals may lead to visceral hypersensitivity, with the specific nerve pathway affected determining the exact symptomatology expressed. This visceral hypersensitivity is a neuroenteric phenomenon that is independent of motility and psychological disturbances.[54] Factors known to contribute to these alterations include genetics, motility factors, inflammation, colonic infections, mechanical irritation to local nerves, stress, and other psychological factors.

Serotonin-Type Receptors

The enteric nervous system contains a significant percentage of the body's 5-HT.[55] Two types of 5-HT exist within the gut: serotonin type 3 (HT_3) and serotonin type 4 (HT_4), which are responsible for secretion, sensitization, and motility. There is an increase in the postprandial levels of 5-HT in those who suffer from diarrhea-predominant IBS when compared with nonsufferers.[55] Therefore, stimulation and antagonism of these 5-HT receptors have become a focused area for research on new drug therapies for both diarrhea- and constipation-predominant diseases.

Clinical Presentation

8 IBS presents as either diarrhea- or constipation-predominant disease and can be defined as lower abdominal pain, disturbed defecation (constipation, diarrhea, or an alternating pattern of both), and bloating in the absence of structural or biochemical factors that might explain these symptoms (Table 23-10). Because IBS can consist of a variable number of signs and symptoms, two diagnostic criteria "checklists" are commonly used to aid in the workup of a patient suspected of having IBS. The Manning criteria were first proposed in 1978, whereas the Rome criteria were initially proposed in 1999 and revised as recently as 2006 by an international working group in an effort to help standardize the diagnostic criteria used in clinical research protocols. Table 23-11 shows the symptom criteria for both of the Manning[56] and Rome III[33] symptom-based criteria.

Additional diagnostic steps that can be taken include sigmoidoscopy or colonoscopy, examination of the stool for occult blood and ova and parasites, complete blood cell count, erythrocyte sedimentation rate, and serum electrolytes. In some cases, radiographic imaging studies, such as computed tomography scans or barium swallows or enemas, may also be necessary if the findings of the foregoing assessment are not typical for IBS.[50]

TABLE 23-10 Clinical Presentation of Irritable Bowel Syndrome

Signs and symptoms
• Lower abdominal pain
• Abdominal bloating and distension
• Diarrhea symptoms, >3 stools/day
• Extreme urgency
• Passage of mucus
• Constipation symptoms, <3 stools/wk, straining, incomplete evacuation
• Psychological symptoms such as depression and anxiety
Non-GI symptoms
• Urinary symptoms
• Fatigue
• Dyspareunia
Other concurrent conditions
• Fibromyalgia
• Functional dyspepsia
• Chronic fatigue syndrome
Reduced health-related quality of life

TABLE 23-11 Symptom-Based Criteria for Irritable Bowel Syndrome

The Manning criteria[56]
Chronic or recurrent abdominal pain for at least 6 months and two or more of the following:
1. Abdominal pain relieved with defecation
2. Abdominal pain associated with more frequent stools
3. Abdominal pain associated with looser stools
4. Abdominal distension
5. Feeling of incomplete evacuation after defecation
6. Mucus in stools
Rome III diagnostic criteria for irritable bowel syndrome[33]
Recurrent abdominal pain or discomfort at least 3 days per month in the last 3 months associated with two or more of the following:
1. Relieved with defecation
2. Onset associated with a change in frequency of stool
3. Onset associated with a change in form (appearance) of stool

TREATMENT

General Approach to Treatment

The treatment approach to IBS is based on the predominant symptoms and their severity (Fig. 23-3). Milder, less frequent episodes can be managed with dietary restrictions and a higher-fiber diet, with addition of bulk-forming laxatives, if necessary. More persistent disease may require as-needed uses of various antispasmodic or antidiarrheal agents such as loperamide. Lastly, the most severe forms of this disease may call for pharmacologic agents directed specifically at the underlying neurohormonal imbalance, such as the 5-HT_4 agonists (e.g., tegaserod), or the 5-HT_3 receptor antagonists (e.g., alosetron).

Alosetron, a 5-HT_3 receptor antagonist, was withdrawn from the U.S. market in 2000 as a result of serious adverse effects, including severe constipation and ischemic colitis that did not appear in the initial clinical trials. It was reintroduced in 2002 and is now limited to an FDA-approved restricted-use program in lower initial doses, and requires extensive postmarketing surveillance. Results of these trials are necessary to definitively determine alosetron's true safety profile, especially with regard to its association with or causation of fatal ischemic colitis.

Constipation-Predominant Disease

In the constipation-predominant patient, dietary fiber may be beneficial. Patients should be instructed to begin with one tablespoonful of fiber with one meal daily and gradually increase the dose to include fiber with two and three meals a day until the desired outcome is achieved. End points that the patient should aim for include bulkier and more easily passed stools. For patients unable to tolerate dietary bran, bulking agents such as psyllium may be substituted.[57] Laxative use is not encouraged in these patients, and it should only be used in the smallest dose for the least amount of time in cases of severe constipation.

The 5-HT_4 partial agonist tegaserod was the first therapy approved by the FDA specifically for short-term, intermittent treatment of IBS-C.[58] tegaserod was suspended from marketing in early 2007 at the request of the FDA due to an analysis of clinical trial data

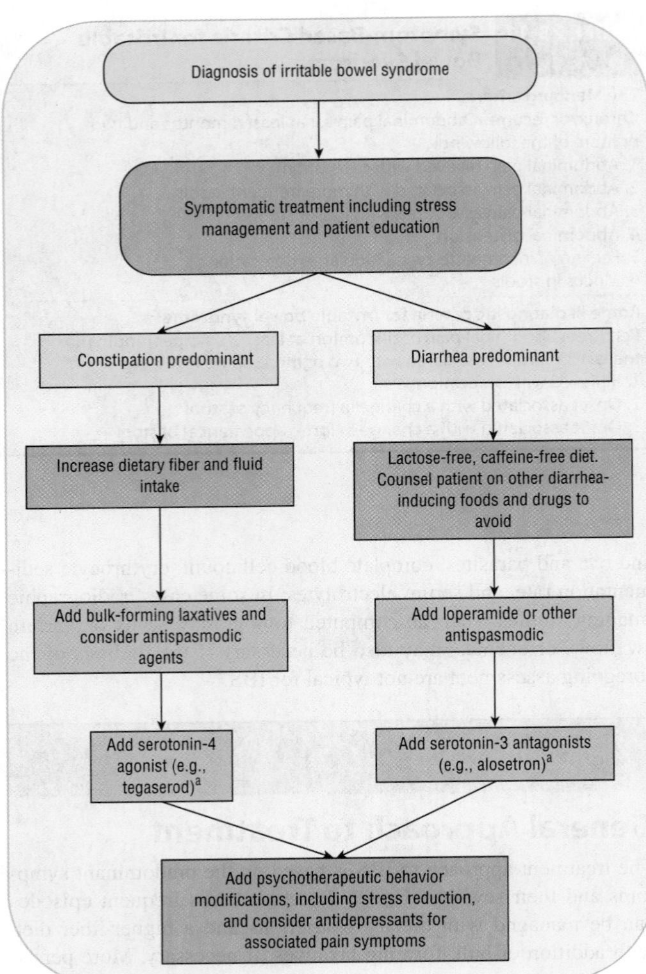

FIGURE 23-3 A general stepwise approach to the management of both constipation- and diarrhea-predominant irritable bowel syndrome. [a]Consider manufacturer-sponsored patient access program.

showing a small, yet significant, increase in ischemia events (MI, cerebrovascular accident [CVA], and unstable angina) in patients with preexisting cardiovascular disease and/or cardiovascular risk factors. In July 2007, the drug's manufacturer, Novartis, began a tegaserod (Zelnorm) restricted-access program for patients in the United States. Tegaserod is a 5-HT derivative that activates 5-HT_4 receptors on the neurons in the GI tract, increasing GI motility and decreasing visceral sensations. It is approved as 2 or 6 mg doses given twice daily 30 minutes prior to a meal with water for up to 12 weeks.[59] Stimulation of the 5-HT_4 receptors by tegaserod increases gastric secretions and promotes motility, with improvement in symptoms generally occurring within the first week of therapy. Currently this therapy is only approved for use in women; efficacy and safety in men have not been established because of inadequate numbers of men enrolled in clinical trials to date.[60] Diarrhea was the most common adverse effect, resulting in drug discontinuation in 1.6% of study subjects.

Diarrhea-Predominant Disease

9 For patients in whom diarrhea is the primary complaint, avoidance of certain food products may be necessary. Caffeine, alcohol, and artificial sweeteners (sorbitol, fructose, and mannitol) are known to irritate the gut and produce a laxative effect. Lactose intolerance should be considered in certain patients; however, the prevalence of this condition may be exaggerated.

Herbal medicines or teas often contain senna, which may produce diarrhea. In patients with disease persistence following dietary modification, loperamide may be used for episodic management of urgent diarrhea, or in situations in which the patient wishes to avoid the possibility of an acute onset of symptoms.[59] Loperamide decreases intestinal transit, enhances water and electrolyte absorption, and strengthens rectal sphincter tone. Some patients may require continuous therapy, and careful dosage titration can usually be undertaken to prevent the development of constipation.

Diarrhea-predominant IBS caused by excessive stimulation of the 5-HT_3 receptor can be relieved by the drug alosetron. Alosetron was the first effective treatment for diarrhea-predominant IBS.[55] However, in November 2000 it was voluntarily withdrawn from the market because of severe GI adverse effects, including 113 reported cases of serious constipation and 8 cases of possible ischemic colitis and death. This decision was met with a great public outcry, as many who had suffered for years had experienced relief for the first time. Because this drug was highly effective in many patients, the FDA approved restricted use of alosetron in June 2002. Alosetron is now available via an FDA-approved restricted-use program in conjunction with GlaxoSmithKline as detailed at http://www.lotronex.com. It is now indicated, in lower initial doses of 0.5 mg twice daily, for women with diarrhea-predominant symptoms of longer than 6 months' duration that are not relieved by conventional therapy. Healthcare providers must use extreme caution in therapy with this drug and must follow strict FDA-mandated guidelines.

Probiotics (see Diarrhea above) such as *Lactobacillus* and *Bifidobacterium* reduced IBS symptoms in several investigative trials.[17] Another 5-HT_3 antagonist, cilansetron, has demonstrated efficacy similar to that of alosetron in phase II trials and enrolled enough male patients to show benefit in males as well.[55]

Use of Antidepressants in Irritable Bowel Syndrome

Tricyclic antidepressants have shown some benefit in treatment of diarrhea-predominant IBS associated with moderate to severe abdominal pain, by modulating perception of visceral pain, altering GI transit time, and treating underlying comorbidities.[61,62] Selective 5-HT reuptake inhibitors are less well studied, with only one report with paroxetine showing some improvement in stool passage and "well-being" but no decrease in abdominal pain.[63–65]

Figure 23-3 shows a general stepwise approach to the management of both constipation and diarrhea-predominant IBS.

Pain in Irritable Bowel Syndrome

10 Some patients with IBS suffer significant pain associated with their disease. Data supporting the use of antispasmodic agents in these patients are conflicting.[50] A trial of low-dose antidepressant therapy is indicated, especially if pain is associated with eating. Both tricyclic antidepressants and 5-HT reuptake inhibitors produce analgesia and may relieve depressive symptoms if present. Preprandial doses of drugs containing anticholinergic properties may suppress pain (and/or diarrhea) associated with an overactive postprandial gastrocolonic response. Tricyclic antidepressants should be avoided in patients with pain and constipation. In addition, psychotherapy, including cognitive behavioral therapy, relaxation therapy, and hypnotherapy, has been shown to decrease IBS symptoms.[66]

Evaluation of Therapeutic Outcomes

IBS is usually classified as constipation-predominant, diarrhea-predominant, or IBS with abdominal pain and bloating. Therapeutic goals in IBS should focus on the patient's primary complaint. Dietary and drug therapy goals should focus on end-organ treatment to relieve abdominal pain (antispasmodic drugs) or disturbed bowel habits (antidiarrheals and bulk-forming agents). Additionally, severe symptoms from CNS dysregulation should be treated with antidepressants, psychotherapy, relaxation/stress management, cognitive behavior treatment, and/or hypnosis aimed at specific affective disorders.[50] Lastly, the 5-HT receptor agonists and antagonists can be used in carefully selected patients whose symptoms are not adequately controlled with other agents. The AGA recommends that patients with severe IBS consider psychological treatments such as psychotherapy, relaxation/stress management, and/or cognitive behavior treatment.

ABBREVIATIONS

AAD	antibiotic-associated diarrhea
AGA	American Gastroenterology Association
AIDS	acquired immune deficiency syndrome
ATPase	adenosine triphosphatase
CDC	Centers for Disease Control and Prevention
CVA	cerebrovascular accident
EASE	ENTEREG access support and education
5-HT	serotonin
HT_3	serotonin type 3
HT_4	serotonin type 4
5-HT_4	5-hydroxytryptamine-4
IBS	irritable bowel syndrome
IBS-C	constipation-predominant irritable bowel syndrome
NSAID	nonsteroidal antiinflammatory drug
ORS	oral rehydration solution
PEG	polyethylene glycol
VIP	vasoactive intestinal peptide
VIPoma	vasoactive intestinal peptide-secreting tumor
WDHA	watery diarrhea, hypokalemia, and achlorhydria
WHO	World Health Organization

REFERENCES

1. Sandle GI. Infective and inflammatory diarrhea: Mechanisms and opportunities for novel therapies. Curr Opin Pharmacol 2011;11(6):634–639.
2. World Gastroenterology Organisation. WGO Practice Guideline: Acute Diarrhea. 2008, *http://www.worldgastroenterology.org/global-guidelines.html*.
3. Sandler RS, Stewart WF, Liberman JN, Ricci JA, Zorich NL. Abdominal pain, bloating, and diarrhea in the United States: Prevalence and impact. Dig Dis Sci 2000;45(6):1166–1171.
4. Scallan E, Majowicz S, Hall G, et al. Prevalence of diarrhoea in the community in Australia, Canada, Ireland, and the United States. Int J Epidemiol 2005;34:454–460.
5. Jones T, McMillian M, Scallan E, et al. A population-based estimate of the substantial burden of diarrhoeal disease in the United States; FoodNet, 1996–2003. Epidemiol Infect 2007;135:293–301.
6. Musher DM, Musher BL. Contagious acute gastrointestinal infections. N Engl J Med 2004;351(23):2417–2427.
7. DuPont HL, Ericsson CD, Farthing MJG, et al. Expert review of the evidence base for self-therapy of travelers' diarrhea. J Travel Med 2009;16(3):161–171.
8. Bhatnagar S, Bhandari N, Mouli U, Bhan M. Consensus statement of IAP National Task Force: Status report on management of acute diarrhea. Indian Pediatr 2004;41:335–348.
9. Atia AN, Buchman AL. Oral rehydration solutions in non-cholera diarrhea: A review. Am J Gastroenterol 2009;104(10):2596–2604.
10. Fine KD, Schiller LR. AGA technical review on the evaluation and management of chronic diarrhea. Gastroenterology 1999;116(6):1464–1486.
11. World Health Organization. WHO/UNICEF Joint Statement: Clinical Management of Acute Diarrhea (WHO/FCH/CAH/04.7). Geneva, Switzerland: World Health Organization, 2004.
12. Bhandari N, Mazumder S, Taneja S, et al. Effectiveness of zinc supplementation plus oral rehydration salts compared with oral rehydration salts alone as a treatment for acute diarrhea in a primary care setting: A cluster randomized trial. Pediatrics 2008;121(5):e1279–e1285.
13. Harris AG, Odorisio TM, Woltering EA, et al. Consensus statement—Octreotide dose titration in secretory diarrhea—Diarrhea Management Consensus Development Panel. Dig Dis Sci 1995;40(7):1464–1473.
14. Schiller LR. Review article: Anti-diarrhoeal pharmacology and therapeutics. Aliment Pharmacol Ther 1995;9(2):87–106.
15. Ruszniewski P, Ducreux M, Chayvialle JA, et al. Treatment of the carcinoid syndrome with the longacting somatostatin analogue lanreotide: A prospective study in 39 patients. Gut 1996;39(2):279–283.
16. Lombardi G, Minuto F, Tamburrano G, et al. Efficacy of the new long-acting formulation of lanreotide (lanreotide Autogel) in somastatin analogue-naive patients with acromegaly. J Endocrinol Invest 2009;32(3):202–209.
17. Floch MH, Walker WA, Guandalini S, et al. Recommendations for probiotic use—2008. J Clin Gastroenterol 2008;42:S104–S108.
18. Delia P, Sansotta G, Donato V, et al. Use of probiotics for prevention of radiation-induced diarrhea. World J Gastroenterol 2007;13(6):912–915.
19. Hempel S, Newberry SJ, Maher AR, et al. Probiotics for the prevention and treatment of antibiotic-associated diarrhea. A systematic review and meta-analysis. JAMA 2012;307(18):1959–1969.
20. Gallelli L, Colosimo M, Tolotta G, et al. Prospective randomized double-blind trial of racecadotril compared with loperamide in elderly people with gastroenteritis living in nursing homes. Eur J Clin Pharmacol 2010;66(2):137–144.
21. Wang H, Shieh M, Liao K. A blind, randomized comparison of racecadotril and loperamide for stopping acute diarrhea in adults. World J Gastroenterol 2005;11(10):1540–1543.
22. Lehert P, Cheron G, Calatayud GA, et al. Racecadotril for childhood gastroenteritis: An individual patient data meta-analysis. Dig Liver Dis 2011;43(9):707–713.
23. Thompson RF, Bass DM, Hoffman SL. Travel vaccines. Infect Dis Clin North Am 1999;13(1):149–167.
24. Tacket CO, Kotloff KL, Losonsky G, et al. Volunteer studies investigating the safety and efficacy of live oral El Tor *Vibrio cholerae* 01 vaccine strain CVD 111. Am J Trop Med Hyg 1997;56(5):533–537.
25. CDC. Prevention of rotavirus gastroenteritis among infants and children: Recommendations of the Advisory Committee

on Immunization Practices (ACIP). MMWR 2009; 58(RR-2):1–26.
26. Choung RS, Locke GR, Rey E, et al. Factors associated with persistent and nonpersistent chronic constipation, over 20 years. Clin Gastroenterol Hepatol 2012;10:494–500.
27. Suares NC, Ford AC. Prevalence of, and risk factors for, chronic idiopathic constipation in the community: Systematic review and meta-analysis. Am J Gastroenterol 2011;106:1582–1591.
28. Gallegos-Orozco JF, Foxx-Orenstein AE, Sterler SM, Stoa JM. Chronic constipation in the elderly. Am J Gastroenterol 2012;107:18–25.
29. Higgins P, Johanson J. Epidemiology of constipation in North America: A systematic review. Am J Gastroenterol 2004;99(4):750–759.
30. Wald A, Scarpignato C, Mueller-Lissner S, et al. A multinational survey of prevalence and patterns of laxative use among adults with self-defined constipation. Aliment Pharmacol Ther 2008;28(7):917.
31. Foxx-Orenstein AE, McNally MA, Odunsi ST. Update on constipation: One treatment does not fit all. Cleve Clin J Med 2008;75(11):813–824.
32. Allan L, Richarz U, Simpson K, Slappendel R. Transdermal fentanyl versus sustained release oral morphine in strong-opioid naive patients with chronic low back pain. Spine 2005;30(22):2484–2490.
33. Longstreth G, Thompson W, Chey W, Houghton L, Mearin F, Spiller R. Functional bowel disorders. Gastroenterology 2006;130(5):1480–1491.
34. Brandt L, Prather C, Quigley E, Schiller L, Schoenfeld P, Talley N. Systematic review on the management of chronic constipation in North America. Am J Gastroenterol 2005;100:S5–S21.
35. Ternent CA, Bastawrous AL, Morin NA, et al. Practice parameters for the evaluation and management of constipation. Dis Colon Rectum 2007;50:2013–2022.
36. Schey R, Cromwell J, Rao SSC. Medical and surgical management of pelvic floor disorders affecting defecation. Am J Gastroenterol 2012;107:1624–1633. doi:10.1038/ajg.2012.247.
37. Attaluri A, Donahoe R, Valestin J, Brown K, Rao SSC. Randomised clinical trial: Dried plums (prunes) vs. psyllium for constipation. Aliment Pharmacol Ther 2011;33:822–828.
38. Ortiz H, de Miguel M, Rinaldi M, Oteiza F, Altomare DE. Functional outcome of sacral nerve stimulation in patients with severe constipation. Dis Colon Rectum 2012;55:876–880.
39. Gallagher PF, O'Mahony D, Quigley EM. Management of chronic constipation in the elderly. Drugs Aging 2008;25(10):807–821.
40. Lee-Robichaud H, Thomas K, Morgan J, Nelson RL. Lactulose versus polyethylene glycol for chronic constipation. Cochrane Database Syst Rev 2010;(7):CD007570. doi:10.1002/14651858.CD007570.pub2.
41. DiPalma JA, Cleveland MV, McGowan J, Herrar JL. A randomized, multicenter, placebo-controlled trial of polyethylene glycol laxative for chronic treatment of chronic constipation. Am J Gastroenterol 2007;102:1436–1441.
42. North American Society for Pediatric Gastroenterology, Hepatology, and Nutrition. Evaluation and treatment of constipation in infants and children: Recommendations from the North American Society of Pediatric Gastroenterology, Hepatology, and Nutrition. J Pediatr Gastroenterol Nutr 2006;43(3):e1–e13.
43. Ford AC, Suares NC. Effect of laxatives and pharmacological therapies in chronic idiopathic constipation: Systematic review and meta-analysis. Gut 2011;60:209–218.
44. Lembo AJ, Johanson JF, Parkman HP, Rao SS, Miner PB Jr, Ueno R. Long-term safety and effectiveness of lubiprostone, a calcium channel (ClC-2) activator, in patients with chronic idiopathic constipation. Dig Dis Sci 2011;56:2639–2645.
45. Food and Drug Administration (FDA). FDA approves Linzess to treat certain cases of irritable bowel syndrome and constipation [news release]. Silver Spring, MD: FDA, August 30, 2012.
46. Lembo AJ, Schneier AH, Shiff SJ, et al. Two randomized trials of linaclotide for chronic constipation. N Engl J Med 2011;365:527–536.
47. Camilleri M. Opioid-induced constipation: Challenges and therapeutic opportunities. Am J Gastroenterol 2011;106:835–842.
48. Camilleri M, Kerstens R, Rykx A, Vandeplassche L. A placebo-controlled trial of prucalopride for severe chronic constipation. N Engl J Med 2008;358(22):2344–2354.
49. Chmielewska A, Szajewska H. Systematic review of randomized controlled trials: Probiotics for functional constipation. World J Gastroenterol 2010;16(7):69–75.
50. Brandt L, Chey W, Foxx-Orenstein A, et al. An evidence-based position statement on the management of irritable bowel syndrome. Am J Gastroenterol 2009;104(S1):S1–S35.
51. Hungin A, Chang L, Locke G, Dennis E, Barghout V. Irritable bowel syndrome in the United States: Prevalence, symptom patterns and impact. Aliment Pharmacol Ther 2005;21(11):1365–1375.
52. Brandt L, Bjorkman D, Fennerty M, et al. Systematic review on the management of irritable bowel syndrome in North America. Am J Gastroenterol 2002;97(s11):S7–S26.
53. Hungin A, Whorwell P, Tack J, Mearin F. The prevalence, patterns and impact of irritable bowel syndrome: An international survey of 40,000 subjects. Aliment Pharmacol Ther 2003;17(5):643–650.
54. Gerson CD, Gerson M-J, Awad RA, et al. Irritable bowel syndrome: An international study of symptoms in eight countries. Eur J Gastroenterol Hepatol 2008;20(7):659–667.
55. Ford AC, Brandt LJ, Young C, et al. Efficacy of 5-Ht3 antagonists and 5-HT5 agonists in irritable bowel syndrome: A systematic review and meta-analysis. Am J Gastroenterol 2009;104:1831–1843.
56. Manning A, Thompson W, Heaton K, Morris A. Towards positive diagnosis of the irritable bowel. Br Med J 1978;2(6138):653–654.
57. Thompson WG. Irritable bowel syndrome: A management strategy. Best Pract Res Clin Gastroenterol 1999;13(3):453–460.
58. Camilleri M. Review article: Tegaserod. Aliment Pharmacol Ther 2001;15(3):277–289.
59. Tougas G, Snape WJ, Otten MH, et al. Long-term safety of tegaserod in patients with constipation-predominant irritable bowel syndrome. Aliment Pharmacol Ther 2002;16(10):1701–1708.
60. Muller-Lissner SA, Fumagalli I, Bardhan KD, et al. Tegaserod, a 5-HT4 receptor partial agonist, relieves symptoms in irritable bowel syndrome patients with abdominal pain, bloating and constipation. Aliment Pharmacol Ther 2001;15(10):1655–1666.
61. Rahimi R, Nikfar S, Rezaie A, Abdollahi M. Efficacy of tricyclic antidepressants in irritable bowel syndrome: A meta-analysis. World J Gastroenterol 2009;15(13):1548–1553.

62. Abdul-Baki S, El Hajj I, ElZahabi L, et al. A randomized controlled trial of imipramine in patients with irritable bowel syndrome. World J Gastroenterol 2009;15(29): 3636–3642.

63. Tabas G, Beaves M, Wang J, Friday P, Mardini H, Arnold G. Paroxetine to treat irritable bowel syndrome not responding to high-fiber diet: A double-blind, placebo-controlled trial. Am J Gastroenterol 2004;99(5):914–920.

64. Han C, Masand PS, Krulewicz S, et al. Childhood abuse and treatment response in patients with irritable bowel syndrome: A post-hoc analysis of a 12-week, randomized, double-blind, placebo-controlled trial of paroxetine controlled release. J Clin Pharm Ther 2009;34(1):79–88.

65. Masand PS, Pae C-U, Krulewicz S, et al. A double-blind, randomized, placebo-controlled trial of paroxetine controlled-release in irritable bowel syndrome. Psychosomatics 2009;50(1):78–86.

66. Heymann-Monnikes I, Arnold R, Florin I, Herda C, Melfsen S, Monnikes H. The combination of medical treatment plus multicomponent behavioral therapy is superior to medical treatment alone in the therapy of irritable bowel syndrome. Am J Gastroenterol 2000;95(4):981–994.

Portal Hypertension and Cirrhosis

Julie M. Sease

24

KEY CONCEPTS

1. Cirrhosis is a severe, chronic, irreversible disease associated with significant morbidity and mortality. However, the progression of cirrhosis secondary to alcohol abuse can be interrupted by abstinence. It is therefore imperative for the clinician to educate and support abstinence from alcohol as part of the overall treatment strategy of the underlying liver disease.
2. Patients with cirrhosis should receive endoscopic screening for varices, and certain patients with varices should receive primary prophylaxis with nonselective β-adrenergic blockade therapy to prevent variceal hemorrhage.
3. When nonselective β-adrenergic blocker therapy is used to prevent rebleeding, β-blocker therapy can be titrated to achieve a goal heart rate of 55 to 60 beats/min or the maximal tolerated dose.
4. Octreotide is the preferred vasoactive agent for the medical management of variceal bleeding. Endoscopy employing endoscopic band ligation is the primary therapeutic tool for the management of acute variceal bleeding.
5. The combination of spironolactone and furosemide is the recommended initial diuretic therapy for patients with ascites.
6. All patients who have survived an episode of spontaneous bacterial peritonitis should receive long-term antibiotic prophylaxis.
7. The mainstay of therapy of hepatic encephalopathy involves therapy to lower blood ammonia concentrations and includes diet therapy, lactulose, and antibiotics alone or in combination with lactulose.

Chronic liver injury causes damage to normal liver tissue resulting in the development of regenerative nodules surrounded by fibrous bands.[1] Cirrhosis is an advanced stage of liver fibrosis. The advanced fibrosis of cirrhosis leads to shunting of the portal and arterial blood supply directly into hepatic outflow through the central veins, and exchange between hepatic sinusoids and hepatocytes is compromised. Clinical consequences of cirrhosis include impaired hepatocyte function, the increased intrahepatic resistance of portal hypertension, and hepatocellular carcinoma. Circulatory irregularities such as splanchnic vasodilation, vasoconstriction and hypoperfusion of the kidneys, water and salt retention, and increased cardiac output also occur. The word *cirrhosis* is derived from the Greek *kirrhos*, meaning orange-yellow, and refers to the color of the cirrhotic liver as seen on autopsy or during surgery.[2]

(1) While cirrhosis has many causes (Table 24-1), in the Western world, excessive alcohol intake and hepatitis C are the most common causes.[1,3] This chapter elucidates the pathophysiology of cirrhosis and the resultant effects on human anatomy and physiology. Treatment strategies for managing the most commonly encountered clinical complications of cirrhosis are discussed.

EPIDEMIOLOGY

The exact prevalence of cirrhosis is unknown, but a reasonable estimate is that 1% of populations have histologically diagnosable cirrhosis.[1] Cirrhosis was responsible for over 31,000 deaths in America in 2010, and chronic liver disease continues to be ranked 12th among the leading causes of death in the United States.[4] Acute variceal bleeding and spontaneous bacterial peritonitis (SBP) are among the immediately life-threatening complications of cirrhosis. Associated conditions causing significant morbidity include ascites and hepatic encephalopathy (HE). Approximately 50% of patients with cirrhosis develop ascites during 10 years of observation and, within 2 years, nearly half of patients who develop ascites will die.[5]

PATHOPHYSIOLOGY OF CIRRHOSIS

Any discussion of cirrhosis must be based on a firm understanding of hepatic anatomy and vascular supply. Conceptually, the liver can be thought of as an elaborate blood filtration system receiving blood from the hepatic artery and the portal vein (Fig. 24-1), with

TABLE 24-1 Etiology of Cirrhosis

Chronic alcohol consumption
Chronic viral hepatitis (types B, C)
Metabolic liver disease
Hemochromatosis
Wilson's disease
α_1-Antitrypsin deficiency
Nonalcoholic steatohepatitis ("fatty liver")
Immunologic disease
Autoimmune hepatitis
Primary biliary cirrhosis
Vascular disease
Budd-Chiari
Cardiac failure
Drugs
Isoniazid, methyldopa, amiodarone, dronedarone, methotrexate, tamoxifen, retinol (vitamin A), propylthiouracil, didanosine

Data from references 1 and 3.

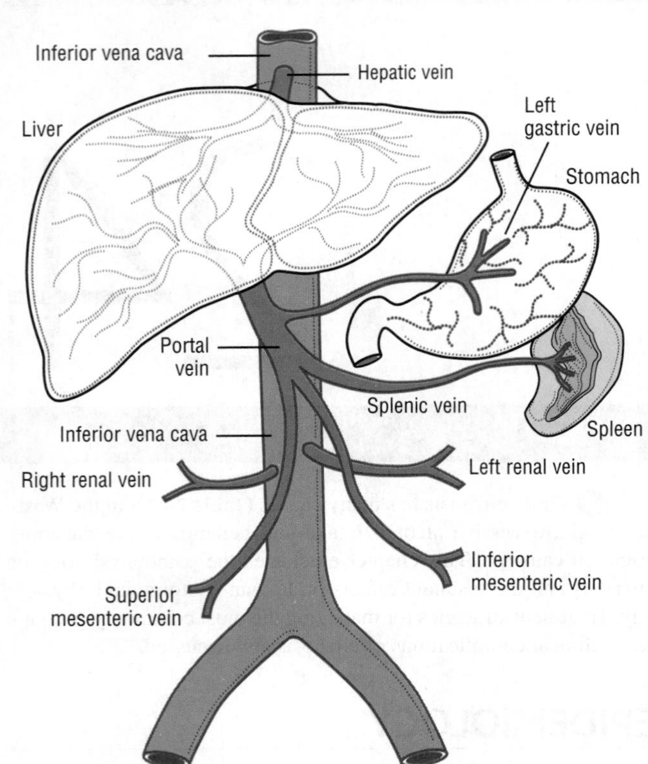

FIGURE 24-1 The portal venous system.

portal blood originating from the small intestines.[6] Blood enters the liver via the portal triad, which contains branches of the portal vein, hepatic artery, and bile ducts. It then drains through the sinusoidal spaces (also known as the space of Disse) of the hepatic lobule (Fig. 24-2), which are lined by the workhorses of the liver, the hepatocytes. Individual hepatocytes are arranged in plates that are one cell thick and organized around individual central veins. The six or more surfaces of each individual hepatocyte make contact with adjacent hepatocytes, border the bile canaliculi, or are exposed to the sinusoidal space. Filtered blood travels into the terminal hepatic venules, also called central veins, and then empties into larger hepatic veins and eventually into the inferior vena cava. Functional gradients of hepatocytes based on oxygen saturation have been reported. Hepatocytes closest to the portal triad, which contains the hepatic artery, have greater oxygen saturation than those hepatocytes nearer to the terminal hepatic venule. Blood flows past hepatocytes in zone one, then zone two, and finally zone three before entering the central vein. Hepatocytes in zone one are involved in gluconeogenesis, urea synthesis, and oxidative energy metabolism while those in zone three carry out the functions of glycolysis and lipogenesis.

Normally, hepatic stellate cells function to store vitamin A and help to maintain the normal matrix in the sinusoidal space.[7] During chronic liver disease, however, hepatic stellate cells undergo an "activation" process, which is the central event in the development of hepatic fibrosis. Activation causes stellate cells to lose vitamin A, become highly proliferative, and synthesize fibrotic scar tissue, which accumulates in the sinusoidal space. This leads to loss

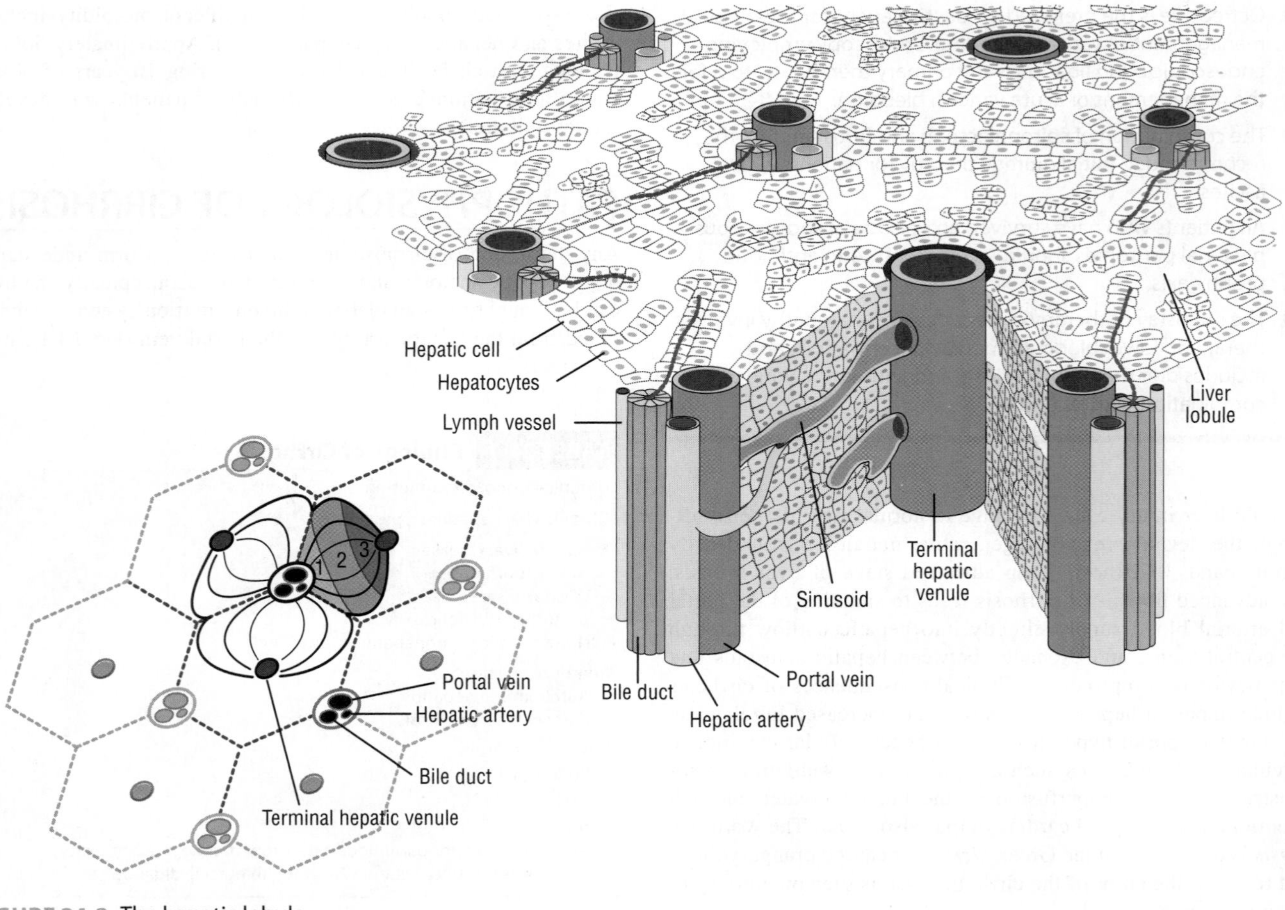

FIGURE 24-2 The hepatic lobule.

of hepatocyte microvilli, loss of sinusoidal endothelial fenestrae, deterioration of hepatocyte function, and, if fibrosis progresses, eventual cirrhosis.

Cirrhosis causes changes to the splanchnic vascular bed as well as the systemic circulation.[8] Splanchnic vasodilation, decreased responsiveness to vasoconstrictors, and the formation of new blood vessels contribute to an increased splanchnic blood flow, formation of gastroesophageal varices, and variceal bleeding. All of these components are part of the portal hypertensive syndrome. Portal hypertension is characterized by hypervolemia, increased cardiac index, hypotension, and decreased systemic vascular resistance. This is a so-called hyperkinetic syndrome that leads to a marked activation of neurohumoral vasoactive factors, a response that occurs in an effort to maintain the arterial blood pressure within normal limits. Activation of neurohumoral vasoactive factors is a main component in the pathophysiology of the ascites and renal dysfunction that often accompany chronic liver disease. Portal-systemic shunting may also occur and is involved in HE and other complications.

In summary, cirrhosis results from fibrotic changes within the hepatic sinusoids and results in changes in the levels of vasodilatory and vasoconstrictor mediators and an increase in blood flow to the splanchnic vasculature.

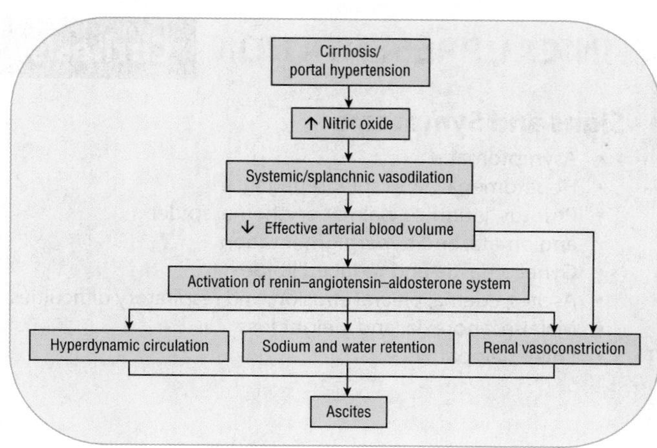

FIGURE 24-3 Pathogenesis of ascites.

ANATOMIC AND PHYSIOLOGIC EFFECTS OF CIRRHOSIS

Cirrhosis and the pathophysiologic abnormalities that cause it result in the commonly encountered problems of ascites, portal hypertension, esophageal varices, HE, and coagulation disorders. Other less commonly seen problems in patients with cirrhosis include hepatorenal syndrome, hepatopulmonary syndrome, and endocrine dysfunction. These are discussed in Management of Portal Hypertension and Variceal Bleeding below.

Ascites

Ascites is the accumulation of an excessive amount of fluid within the peritoneal cavity.[9] It is the most commonly occurring major complication of cirrhosis.[5] Approximately half of all cirrhotic patients develop ascites within 10 years of diagnosis. Several hypotheses have been offered to explain the mechanism for the development of ascites in decompensated cirrhosis.[9] Most acceptable theories state that ascites formation begins as a result of the development of sinusoidal hypertension and portal hypertension. Portal hypertension activates vasodilatory mechanisms that are mediated mostly by nitric oxide overproduction. This leads to splanchnic and peripheral arteriolar vasodilation and, in advanced disease, a drop in arterial pressure. Baroreceptor-mediated activation of the renin–angiotensin–aldosterone system, activation of the sympathetic nervous system, and release of antidiuretic hormone occur in response to the resulting arterial hypotension in an effort to restore normal blood pressure (Fig. 24-3). These changes cause renal sodium and water retention. Additionally, ongoing splanchnic vasodilation increases splanchnic lymph production beyond the capacity of the lymph transportation system. Leakage of lymphatic fluid into the peritoneal cavity occurs. Persistent renal sodium and water retention, increased splanchnic vascular permeability, and lymph leakage into the peritoneal cavity combine to create the sustained ascites formation of end-stage liver disease.

Portal Hypertension and Varices

Sinusoidal portal hypertension is most often caused by cirrhosis.[10] It is associated with acute variceal bleeding, a medical emergency that carries a mortality rate of 10% to 20% at 6 weeks, and is among the most severe complications of cirrhosis.[11] Portal hypertension is defined by the presence of a gradient of greater than 5 mm Hg between the portal and central venous pressures (see Fig. 24-1).[10] This gradient is called the hepatic venous pressure gradient (HVPG). Esophageal and gastric varices and variceal bleeding may arise after a HVPG pressure gradient of 10 mm Hg is reached.

Progression to bleeding can be predicted by Child-Pugh score, size of varices, and the presence of red wale markings on the varices. First variceal hemorrhage occurs at an annual rate of about 15% and carries a mortality of 7% to 15%. Rebleeding is common following initial hemorrhage with a median rate of 60% and carries a mortality rate as high as 33%. Prevention of bleeding is a major goal in the therapy of portal hypertension, and strategies include both pharmacologic and surgical approaches.

Hepatic Encephalopathy

HE is a metabolically induced functional disturbance of the brain that is potentially reversible.[12] Symptoms of HE are thought to result from an accumulation of gut-derived nitrogenous substances in the systemic circulation as a consequence of decreased hepatic functioning and shunting through portosystemic collaterals bypassing the liver.[13] Once these substances enter the CNS, they cause alterations of neurotransmission that affect consciousness and behavior. Ammonia is the most commonly cited culprit in the pathogenesis of HE, but glutamine, benzodiazepine receptor agonists, aromatic amino acids, and manganese are also potential causes.[12,13] Arterial ammonia levels are increased commonly in both acute and chronic liver diseases, but an established correlation between blood ammonia levels and mental status does not exist.[13] Despite this, interventions to lower blood ammonia levels remain the mainstay of treatment for HE.

HE is now categorized as type A, B, or C based on nomenclature developed by the 11th World Congress of Gastroenterology.[12] Type A is HE induced by acute liver failure, type B is due to portal-systemic bypass without associated intrinsic liver disease, and type C is HE that occurs in patients with cirrhosis. Minimal HE refers to cirrhotic patients who do not suffer clinically overt cognitive dysfunction but who are found to have cognitive impairment on psychological studies. The onset of HE in a patient with liver failure may be related to the presence of several known precipitating factors. In cases of HE associated with a precipitant, if that precipitant can be cured or discontinued, it may also be possible to discontinue treatment for HE. In many cases, no precipitant is found and, therefore, long-term treatment of HE may be required.

CLINICAL PRESENTATION Cirrhosis

Signs and Symptoms

- Asymptomatic
- Hepatomegaly and splenomegaly
- Pruritus, jaundice, palmar erythema, spider angiomata, and hyperpigmentation
- Gynecomastia and reduced libido
- Ascites, edema, pleural effusion, and respiratory difficulties
- Malaise, anorexia, and weight loss
- Encephalopathy

Laboratory Tests

- Hypoalbuminemia
- Elevated prothrombin time (PT)
- Thrombocytopenia
- Elevated alkaline phosphatase
- Elevated aspartate transaminase (AST), alanine transaminase (ALT), and γ-glutamyl transpeptidase (GGT)

Coagulation Defects

The liver synthesizes most of the proteins that are responsible for the maintenance of hemostasis (the balance between coagulation and anticoagulation).[14] Hepatocellular damage can lead to a disruption in hemostasis because of defects it may cause in the function of coagulation and fibrinolytic factors. These defects include a reduction in the synthesis of clotting factors, excessive fibrinolysis, disseminated intravascular coagulation, thrombocytopenia, and platelet dysfunction. Most coagulation factors are created in the liver, and the levels of these factors can be significantly reduced in chronic liver disease associated with extensive hepatocellular damage. Factor VII is the first factor to decrease as liver function declines due to its short half-life. A reduction in clotting factor VII is common in end-stage liver disease, affecting 60% of patients. Low factor VII activity is prognostic for reduced survival, and the prothrombin time (PT) is a standard component of the Child-Pugh scoring system. Accelerated intravascular coagulation and fibrinolysis can be detected in some patients with cirrhosis. The coexistence of sepsis, shock, surgery, trauma, or ascites may cause a progression from accelerated intravascular coagulation to disseminated intravascular coagulation. In patients with cirrhosis, disseminated intravascular coagulation involves increased release of procoagulants, impaired removal of activated coagulation factors and endotoxins produced by gut bacteria, and reduced synthesis of coagulation inhibitors. Both platelet number and function may also be affected in cirrhosis. Platelet numbers are reduced by multiple mechanisms, including splenomegaly due to portal hypertension and sequestration of platelets in the spleen, reduced hepatic production of thrombopoietin, bone marrow suppression, and increased platelet destruction. Mild to moderate thrombocytopenia occurs in 15% to 70% of patients with cirrhosis. The net effect of the coagulation disorders that occur in cirrhosis is the development of bleeding.

CLINICAL PRESENTATION

Cirrhotic patients may present in a variety of ways, from asymptomatic with abnormal radiographic or laboratory studies to decompensated with ascites, SBP, HE, or variceal bleeding.[15]

The approach to a patient with suspected liver disease begins with a thorough history and physical exam. Some presenting characteristics of patients with cirrhosis include anorexia, weight loss, weakness, fatigue, jaundice, pruritus, GI bleeding, coagulopathy, increasing abdominal girth with shifting flank dullness, mental status changes, and vascular spiders. Osteoporosis, as a result of vitamin D malabsorption and resultant calcium deficiency, can also occur.

A thorough history including risk factors that predispose patients to cirrhosis should be taken. Quantity and duration of alcohol intake should be determined. Risk factors for hepatitis B and C transmission should be inquired about. These include birthplace in endemic areas, sexual history, intranasal or IV drug use, body piercing or tattooing, and accidental contamination of body tissues or blood. Information concerning any history of transfusions, as well as any personal history of autoimmune or hepatic diseases, should be gathered. A family history should also be taken, looking especially for any family member with a prior history of autoimmune or hepatic diseases.

Laboratory Abnormalities

There are no laboratory or radiographic tests of hepatic function that can accurately diagnose cirrhosis. Despite this, liver function tests, a complete blood count with platelets, and a PT test should be performed if liver disease is suspected. Tests that measure the level of serum liver enzymes are usually referred to as liver function tests.[16] However, these tests actually reflect hepatocyte integrity or cholestasis, not liver function.

Routine liver tests include alkaline phosphatase, bilirubin, AST, ALT, and GGT. Additional markers of hepatic synthetic activity include albumin and PT. Liver function tests are often the first step in the evaluation of patients who present with symptoms or signs suggestive of cirrhosis.[15] The use of liver function tests in the diagnosis and management of cirrhosis is discussed in the following sections. It may be useful to group the tests into two broad categories: markers of hepatocyte integrity such as the transaminases and markers of liver function mass such as PT and albumin.[16]

Aminotransferases

The aminotransferases, AST and ALT, are enzymes that are highly concentrated in the liver. Liver injury, whether acute or chronic, results, at some point in the course of the disease, in increases in the serum concentrations of the aminotransferase enzymes. The degree of elevation, rate of rise, and nature of the course of alteration in aminotransferase serum levels are helpful in suggesting possible etiologies. Liver function tests will typically be elevated to the highest levels in acute viral, ischemic, or toxic liver injury. Chronic hepatitis and cirrhosis patients may present with elevated aminotransferase levels, but they may also present with aminotransferase levels within the normal reference range. The degree of aminotransferase level elevation is dependent on the course of the hepatic injury being experienced by the patients and also depends on when the enzyme levels are tested. In a landmark study by Cohen and Kaplan, alcoholic liver disease resulted in AST elevations of only six to seven times the upper limit of normal in 98% of patients.[17] The ratio of AST to ALT also provides information in patients with suspected alcoholic liver disease. Seventy percent of patients with alcoholic liver disease in the study by Cohen and Kaplan had ratios greater than 2, whereas 92% of patients had ratios greater than 1.

Alkaline Phosphatase and γ-Glutamyl Transpeptidase

Elevated serum levels of alkaline phosphatase and GGT occur in cases of liver injury with a cholestatic pattern and therefore accompany conditions such as primary biliary cirrhosis, primary sclerosing cholangitis, drug-induced cholestasis, bile duct obstruction, autoimmune cholestatic liver disease, and metastatic cancer of the liver.[16] Neither alkaline phosphatase nor GGT is found solely in the liver, and elevations in either of these biomarkers can occur in a variety of disease states affecting other bodily tissues. However, the combination of an elevation in alkaline phosphatase level with a concomitant elevation in GGT level increases clinical suspicion of hepatic etiology.

Child-Pugh Classification and Model for End-Stage Liver Disease Score

The Child-Pugh classification system has gained widespread acceptance as a means of quantifying the myriad effects of the cirrhotic process on the laboratory and clinical manifestations of this disease.[18] Recommended drug dosing adjustments for patients in liver failure, when available, are normally based on the Child-Pugh score. The newer Model for End-Stage Liver Disease (MELD) scoring system is now the accepted classification scheme used by the United Network for Organ Sharing in the allocation livers for transplantation.[19] The Child-Pugh classification system employs a combination of physical and laboratory findings (Table 24-2), whereas the MELD score calculation takes into account a patient's serum creatinine, bilirubin, international normalized ratio (INR), and etiology of liver disease, omitting the more subjective reports of ascites and encephalopathy used in the Child-Pugh system. The MELD scoring calculation* is as follows[20]:

$$\begin{aligned}\text{MELD score} = {} & 0.957 \times \log_e(\text{creatinine [mg/dL]}) \\ & + 0.378 \times \log_e(\text{bilirubin [mg/dL]}) \\ & + 1.120 \times \log_e(\text{INR}) + 0.643\end{aligned}$$

or using SI units*:

$$\begin{aligned}\text{MELD score} = {} & 0.957 \times \log_e(\text{creatinine [}\mu\text{mol/L]} \times 0.01131) \\ & + 0.378 \times \log_e(\text{bilirubin [}\mu\text{mol/L]} \times 0.05848) \\ & + 1.120 \times \log_e(\text{INR}) + 0.643\end{aligned}$$

These classification systems are important because they are used to assess and define the severity of the cirrhosis, and as a predictor for patient survival, surgical outcome, and risk of variceal bleeding.

Bilirubin

Bilirubin is the product of the breakdown of hemoglobin molecules in the reticuloendothelial system.[16] Elevations in serum conjugated bilirubin indicate that the liver has lost at least half of its excretory capacity and are usually a sign of liver disease. When found in conjunction with markedly elevated AST and ALT, conjugated hyperbilirubinemia indicates the possible presence of acute viral hepatitis, autoimmune hepatitis, toxic liver injury, or ischemic liver injury. Elevated conjugated bilirubin levels with concomitant increases in alkaline phosphatase and normal aminotransferase levels are a sign of cholestatic disease and possible cholestatic drug reactions. Causes of elevations in unconjugated bilirubin include hemolysis, Gilbert's syndrome, hematoma reabsorption, and ineffective erythropoiesis. Causes of conjugated hyperbilirubinemia include bile duct obstruction, hepatitis, cirrhosis, primary sclerosing cholangitis, primary biliary cirrhosis, total parenteral nutrition, drug toxins, and vanishing bile duct syndrome. When cirrhosis has been established, the degree of bilirubin elevation has prognostic significance and is used as a component of the Child-Pugh and MELD scoring systems for quantifying the degree of cirrhosis.[18,20]

Figure 24-4 describes a general algorithm for the interpretation of liver function tests. The algorithm first separates the tests into two categories based on the underlying pathology (pattern of elevations): obstructive (alkaline phosphatase, GGT, and bilirubin) versus hepatocellular (AST and ALT). If a hepatocellular pattern predominates, the magnitude of elevation provides diagnostic assistance. If the degree of elevation is greater than 10 times normal, the etiology is likely a result of drugs or other toxins, ischemia, or acute viral hepatitis.[16] Elevations less than 10 times normal have a broad differential. Unfortunately, most liver enzyme abnormalities will fall into a mixed pattern providing limited diagnostic assistance.

TABLE 24-2 Criteria and Scoring for the Child-Pugh Grading of Chronic Liver Disease

Score	1	2	3
Total bilirubin (mg/dL)	1–2 (17.1–34.2 μmol/L)	2–3 (34.2–51.3 μmol/L)	>3 (>51.3 μmol/L)
Albumin (g/dL)	>3.5 (>35 g/L)	2.8–3.5 (28–35 g/L)	<2.8 (<28 g/L)
Ascites	None	Mild	Moderate
Encephalopathy (grade)	None	1 and 2	3 and 4
Prothrombin time (seconds prolonged)	1–4	4–6	>6

Grade A, <7 points; grade B, 7–9 points; grade C, 10–15 points.
Data from reference 18.

Albumin and Coagulation Factors

Albumin and coagulation proteins are markers of hepatic synthetic activity and are therefore used to estimate the level of hepatic functioning in cirrhosis. Albumin and PT are used in the Child-Pugh

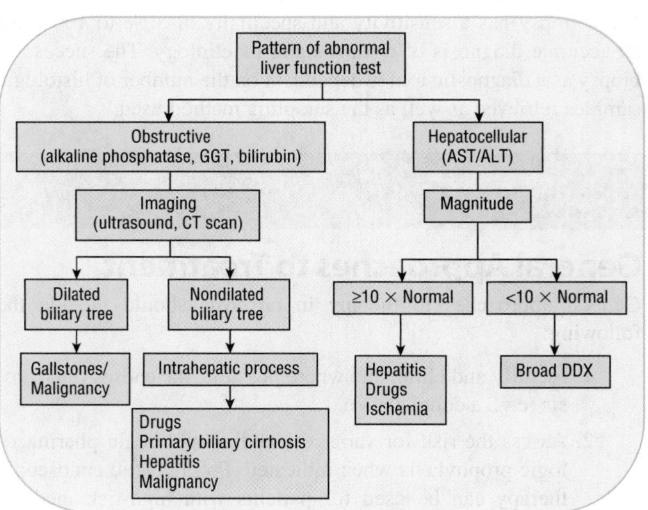

FIGURE 24-4 Interpretation of liver function tests. (DDX, differential diagnosis.)

*Multiply the score by 10 and round to the nearest whole number. (Laboratory values less than 1 are rounded up to 1 for the purposes of the MELD calculation.)

system for quantifying liver disease, and the INR is used in the MELD scoring system as a marker of coagulation.[18,20] Albumin levels can be affected by a number of factors, including malnutrition, malabsorption, and protein losses from renal and intestinal sources.[16]

Coagulation factors I, II, V, VII, VIII, IX, X, XI, XII, and XIII are synthesized in the liver.[14] Significantly reduced levels of coagulation factors II, V, VII, and XIII have been observed in patients with chronic liver disease resulting in PT prolongation and systemic bleeding unrelated to portal hypertension.

Thrombocytopenia

Thrombocytopenia (generally defined as a platelet count less than 150,000/mm^3 [150 × 10^9/L]) is a common feature of chronic liver disease found in 15% to 70% of cirrhotic patients depending on the stage of liver disease and definition of thrombocytopenia. The etiology of thrombocytopenia in liver disease is multifactorial, involving primarily splenomegaly due to portal hypertension with pooling of platelets in the spleen. A decrease in thrombopoietin due to decreased hepatic synthesis occurs as well as an immune-mediated destruction of platelets. Additionally, bone marrow suppression related to the hepatitis C virus or interferon antiviral treatment may exist and lead to thrombocytopenia associated with the cirrhotic process.

Endoscopic and Radiographic Abnormalities

While no radiographic test is considered a diagnostic standard for cirrhosis, radiographic studies may be used to detect ascites, hepatosplenomegaly, hepatic or portal vein thromboses, and hepatocellular carcinoma.[15] Ultrasonography, because it does not require radiation exposure or IV contrast and is relatively low cost, should be the first radiographic study in the evaluation of a patient with suspected cirrhosis. Hepatic nodularity, irregularity, increased echogenicity, and atrophy are all ultrasonographic findings indicative of cirrhosis. Ascites may also be detected on ultrasound. Computed tomography and magnetic resonance imaging can demonstrate liver nodularity as well as atrophic and hypertrophic changes. Ascites and varices may also be detected on computed tomography or magnetic resonance imaging scans. Portal vein patency can be assessed by computer tomography imaging.

Liver Biopsy

Liver biopsy should be considered after a thorough noninvasive workup has failed to confirm a diagnosis in suspected cirrhosis. Liver biopsy has a sensitivity and specificity of 80% to 100% for an accurate diagnosis of cirrhosis and its etiology. The success of biopsy as a diagnostic tool is dependent on the number of histologic samples retrieved as well as the sampling method used.

TREATMENT

General Approaches to Treatment

General approaches to therapy in cirrhosis should include the following:

1. Identify and eliminate, where possible, the causes of cirrhosis (e.g., alcohol abuse).
2. Assess the risk for variceal bleeding and begin pharmacologic prophylaxis when indicated. Prophylactic endoscopic therapy can be used for patients with high-risk medium and large varices as well as in patients with contraindications or intolerance to nonselective β-adrenergic blockers. Endoscopic therapy is also appropriate for patients suffering acute bleeding episodes. Variceal obliteration with endoscopic techniques in conjunction with pharmacologic intervention is the recommended treatment of choice in patients with acute bleeding.
3. Evaluate the patient for clinical signs of ascites and manage with pharmacologic therapy (e.g., diuretics) and paracentesis. Careful monitoring for SBP should be used in patients with ascites who undergo acute deterioration.
4. HE is a common complication of cirrhosis and requires clinical vigilance and treatment with dietary restriction, elimination of CNS depressants, and therapy to lower ammonia levels.
5. Frequent monitoring for signs of hepatorenal syndrome, pulmonary insufficiency, and endocrine dysfunction is necessary.

Desired Outcomes

The desired therapeutic outcomes can be viewed in two categories: *resolution of acute complications* such as tamponade of bleeding and resolution of hemodynamic instability for an episode of acute variceal hemorrhage and *prevention of complications* through lowering of portal pressure with medical therapy using β-adrenergic blocker therapy or supporting abstinence from alcohol. Treatment end points and desired therapeutic outcomes are presented for each of the recommended therapies discussed.

Management of Portal Hypertension and Variceal Bleeding

The management of varices involves three strategies: (a) primary prophylaxis (prevention of the first bleeding episode); (b) treatment of acute variceal hemorrhage; and (c) secondary prophylaxis (prevention of rebleeding in patients who have previously bled).[11]

Primary Prophylaxis

β-Adrenergic Blockade The mainstay of primary prophylaxis is the use of nonselective β-adrenergic blocking agents such as propranolol or nadolol.[10,11,21] These agents reduce portal pressure by reducing portal venous inflow via two mechanisms: a decrease in cardiac output through β_1-adrenergic blockade and a decrease in splanchnic blood flow through β_2-adrenergic blockade.[10]

Endoscopic Variceal Ligation (EVL) EVL is an endoscopic therapy that consists of placing rubber bands around varices until the varices are obliterated.[21]

Treatment Recommendations: Variceal Bleeding—Primary Prophylaxis

2 All patients with cirrhosis should be screened for varices on diagnosis.[10,11,21] β-Adrenergic blocker therapy is not indicated in patients without varices to prevent the formation of varices. Patients with small varices plus risk factors for variceal hemorrhage including red wale marks or Child-Pugh class C should receive prophylaxis therapy with a nonselective β-adrenergic blocker. β-Adrenergic blocker therapy is recommended preferentially to EVL in this situation due to the technical difficulty of EVL in the treatment of small varices. β-Adrenergic blocker therapy is not recommended for patients with small varices in the absence of risk factors as there is insufficient evidence to support this therapy to slow the growth of varices in this scenario. All patients found to have medium to large varices that have not bled should receive primary prophylaxis therapy with a nonselective β-adrenergic blocker or EVL. The choice of treatment should be based on a consideration of resources and expertise as well as patient preferences and characteristics with a particular emphasis on

side effects and contraindications.[11] If β-adrenergic blocker therapy is chosen, initiate therapy with oral propranolol 20 mg twice daily or nadolol 20 to 40 mg once daily and titrate every 2 to 3 days to maximal tolerated dose to heart rates of 55 to 60 beats/min.[10,21] Once a patient is started on nonselective β-adrenergic blocker therapy, it should be continued indefinitely. Following initiation and appropriate titration of the β-adrenergic blocker, further endoscopic surveillance is not needed. If EVL is chosen, it will be performed every 1 to 2 weeks until the obliteration of varices.[21] Followup surveillance will occur at 1 to 3 months and again every 6 to 12 months thereafter.

Patients with contraindications to therapy with nonselective β-adrenergic blockers (i.e., those with asthma, insulin-dependent diabetes with episodes of hypoglycemia, and peripheral vascular disease) or intolerance to β-adrenergic blockers should be considered for alternative prophylactic therapy with EVL.[22] Also, EVL may be considered as a possible first option for primary prophylaxis in patients with high-risk medium to large varices. Nitrates are no longer recommended as alternative therapy for primary prophylaxis against variceal bleeding in patients with intolerance to nonselective β-adrenergic blocker due to a potential for higher mortality with this therapy.[21] At this time, there is also insufficient evidence to support the use of other therapies and procedures (such as combination nonselective β-adrenergic blocker therapy with isosorbide mononitrate, combination nonselective β-adrenergic blocker therapy with spironolactone, combination nonselective β-adrenergic blocker therapy with EVL, shunt surgery, and endoscopic sclerotherapy) for primary prevention of variceal hemorrhage.

Acute Variceal Hemorrhage

Variceal hemorrhage is a medical emergency that carries a mortality rate of 15% to 20%, requires admission to an intensive care unit, and is one of the most feared complications of cirrhosis.[10,21] Treatment of acute variceal bleeding includes general stabilizing and assessment measures as well as specific measures to control the acute hemorrhage and prevent complications.

Initial treatment goals include (a) adequate blood volume resuscitation, (b) protection of airway from aspiration of blood, (c) correction of significant coagulopathy and/or thrombocytopenia with fresh-frozen plasma and platelets, (d) prophylaxis against SBP and other infections, (e) control of bleeding, (f) prevention of rebleeding, and (g) preservation of liver function.[22] Prompt stabilization of blood volume with a goal of maintaining hemodynamic stability and a hemoglobin of 8 g/dL (80 g/L; 4.97 mmol/L) should be undertaken. Volume should be expanded to maintain a systolic blood pressure of 90 to 100 mm Hg and a heart rate of less than 100 beats/min, but vigorous resuscitation with saline solution should generally be avoided because this may lead to recurrent variceal hemorrhage or accumulation of ascites and/or fluid at other anatomic sites.[21,22] Use of recombinant factor VIIa therapy is not recommended in cirrhotic patients with GI hemorrhage at this time. Airway management is critical in patients with variceal hemorrhage, especially those with concomitant HE or severe bleeding.[22] Elective or more emergent intubation may be required prior to diagnostic endoscopy. Combination pharmacologic therapy plus endoscopic therapy with preferably EVL, or sclerotherapy if EVL is not technically feasible, is considered the most rational approach to the treatment of acute variceal bleeding.[10,21]

Vasoactive drug therapy (usually octreotide) is routinely used early to stop or slow bleeding for patient management as soon as a diagnosis of variceal bleeding is suspected, and potentially even before endoscopy. Antibiotic therapy to prevent SBP and other infections, as well as to prevent rebleeding and decrease mortality, should be implemented. Figure 24-5 presents an algorithm for the management of variceal hemorrhage.

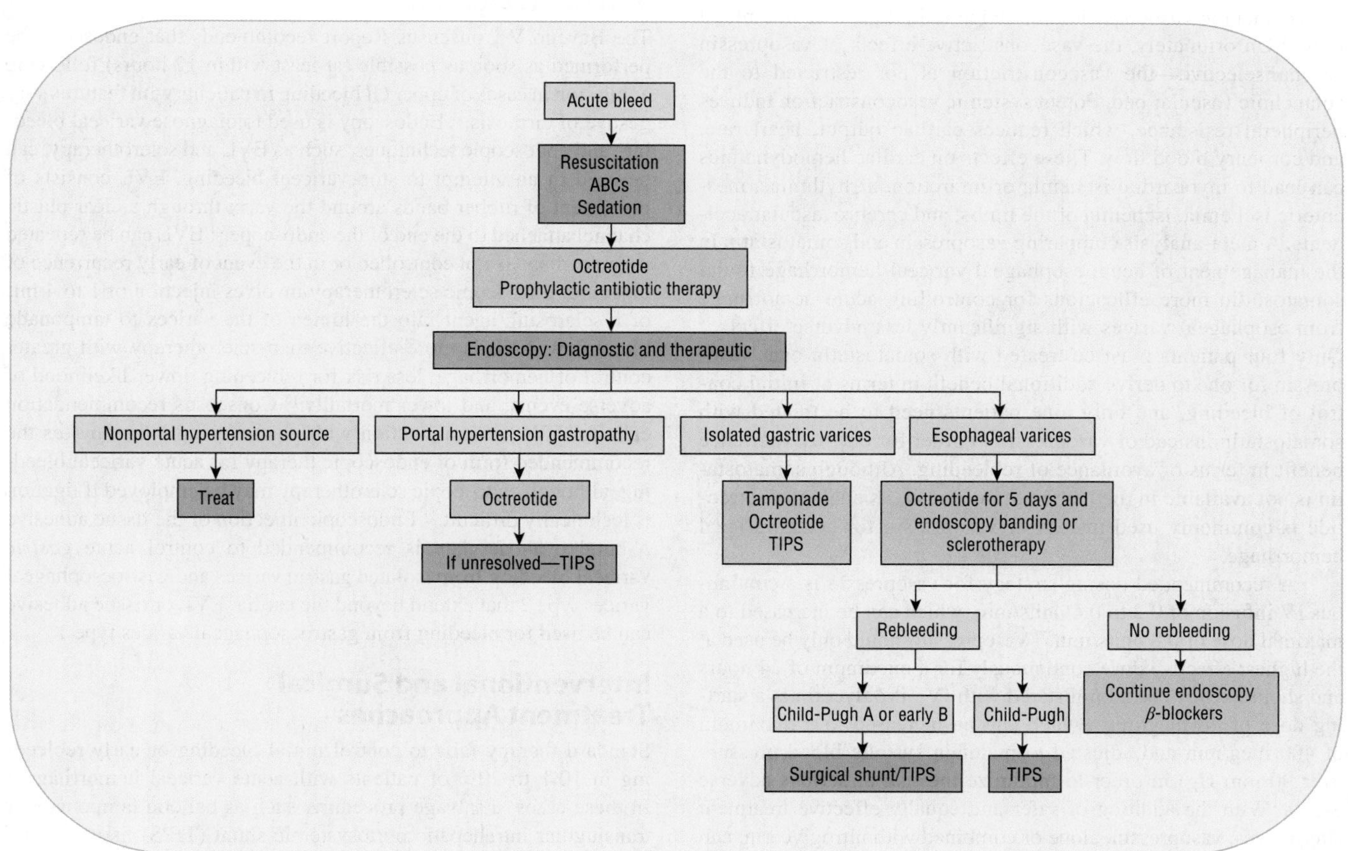

FIGURE 24-5 Management of acute variceal hemorrhage.

Drugs employed to manage acute variceal bleeding in the United States include (a) the somatostatin analogue octreotide and (b) vasopressin. These agents work as splanchnic vasoconstrictors, thus decreasing portal blood flow and pressure.[21] Agents available in other countries also include terlipressin, which is an analogue of vasopressin, and another somatostatin analogue, vapreotide.

Somatostatin and Octreotide

Somatostatin is a naturally occurring tetradecapeptide hormone, and octreotide is a synthetic octapeptide that shares a four–amino acid segment with somatostatin and has similar pharmacologic activity with greater potency and longer duration of action as compared with somatostatin.[23] Somatostatin and octreotide cause a reduction in portal pressure and port-collateral blood flow through inducing splanchnic vasoconstriction without causing the systemic effects associated with vasopressin.[22,23] The splanchnic vasoconstriction found with somatostatin and octreotide therapy is due to inhibition of the release of vasodilatory peptides such as glucagon; however, octreotide has a local vasoconstrictive effect confined to the splanchnic vasculature.[22] Somatostatin and somatostatin analogues are associated with fewer side effects as compared with vasopressin. The side effects of somatostatin therapy may include sinus bradycardia, hypertension, arrhythmia, and abdominal pain.[10] The currently recommended dosing of octreotide for variceal bleeding consists of an initial IV bolus of 50 mcg followed by a continuous IV infusion of 50 mcg/h. Because octreotide is safe for continuation for multiple days and because around half of early recurrent bleeding occurs within the first 3 to 5 days, guidelines suggest continuation of octreotide for 5 days after acute variceal bleeding.[11,21]

Vasopressin

Vasopressin (also known as antidiuretic hormone) is a potent, nonselective vasoconstrictor that reduces portal pressure by causing splanchnic vasoconstriction, which reduces splanchnic blood flow.[23] Unfortunately, the vasoconstrictive effects of vasopressin are nonselective—the vasoconstriction is not restricted to the splanchnic vascular bed. Potent systemic vasoconstriction induces peripheral resistance, which reduces cardiac output, heart rate, and coronary blood flow. These effects on cardiac hemodynamics can lead to myocardial ischemia or infarction, arrhythmias, mesenteric ischemia, ischemia of the limbs, and cerebrovascular accidents. A meta-analysis comparing vasopressin and somatostatin in the management of acute esophageal variceal hemorrhage found somatostatin more efficacious for controlling acute hemorrhage from esophageal varices with significantly less adverse effects.[24] Only four patients must be treated with somatostatin over vasopressin for one to derive additional benefit in terms of initial control of bleeding, and only nine patients need to be treated with somatostatin instead of vasopressin in order for one to experience benefit in terms of avoidance of rebleeding. Although somatostatin is not available in the United States today, its analogue octreotide is commonly used instead of vasopressin for acute variceal hemorrhage.

A recommended dosing strategy for vasopressin is a continuous IV infusion of 0.2 to 0.4 units/min, which can be increased to a maximal dose of 0.8 units/min.[22] Vasopressin should only be used at the highest effective dose continuously for a maximum of 24 hours and should always be administered with IV nitroglycerin at a starting dose of 40 mcg/min (which can be increased to a maximum of 400 mcg/min and adjusted to maintain systolic blood pressure over 90 mm Hg) in order to minimize the risk of serious adverse events. With the addition of safer and equally effective treatment alternatives, vasopressin, alone or combined with nitroglycerin, can no longer be recommended as first-line therapy for the management of variceal hemorrhage.[10,22] Terlipressin, a synthetic analogue of vasopressin, has fewer side effects and a longer duration of action than vasopressin. It reduces mortality in acute variceal hemorrhage, but is not currently available in the United States.[10]

Cirrhotic patients with active bleeding are at high risk of severe bacterial infections such as SBP.[22] Short-term prophylactic antibiotic therapy to reduce the risk of infection during episodes of bleeding not only reduces the likelihood of development of SBP and other infections but also reduces the incidence of rebleeding and increases short-term survival.[21] Prophylactic antibiotic therapy should be prescribed for all patients with cirrhosis and acute variceal bleeding.[22] A short course (7 days maximum) of oral norfloxacin 400 mg twice daily or IV ciprofloxacin when the oral route is not available is recommended. Alternatively, in patients with severe cirrhosis in areas with high quinolone resistance, IV ceftriaxone 1 g/day may be preferable.

Clinical **Controversy. . .**

Whether nonselective β-blocker or EVL is best for primary prophylaxis against variceal bleeding remains unsettled.[10] Some centers tend to perform EVL more readily in this indication. Others favor the more conservative approach of instituting a trial with nonselective β-blocker first, reserving EVL for patients unable to tolerate the β-blocker. Carvedilol is a nonselective β-blocker with α_1-adrenergic activity that shows promise for potentially being more effective than EVL in preventing first variceal hemorrhage. Further research is needed before carvedilol can be routinely recommended for this indication, however.

Endoscopic Interventions: Sclerotherapy and Band Ligation

The Baveno V Consensus Report recommends that endoscopy be performed as soon as possible (at least within 12 hours) following admission in cases of upper GI bleeding in patients with features suggestive of cirrhosis.[11] Endoscopy is used to diagnose variceal bleeding, and endoscopic techniques, such as EVL and sclerotherapy, can be used in an attempt to stop variceal bleeding. EVL consists of placement of rubber bands around the varix through a clear plastic channel attached to the end of the endoscope.[21] EVL can be repeated if hemorrhage is not controlled or in the event of early recurrence of bleeding. Endoscopic sclerotherapy involves injection of 1 to 4 mL of a sclerosing agent into the lumen of the varices to tamponade blood flow. EVL is more effective than sclerotherapy with greater control of hemorrhage, less risk for rebleeding, lower likelihood of adverse events, and lower mortality.[10] Consensus recommendation calls for EVL (in conjunction with pharmacologic therapy) as the recommended form of endoscopic therapy for acute variceal bleeding, although endoscopic sclerotherapy may be employed if ligation is technically difficult.[11] Endoscopic injection of the tissue adhesive *N*-butyl cyanoacrylate is recommended to control acute *gastric* variceal bleeding from isolated gastric varices and gastroesophageal varices type 2 that extend beyond the cardia. EVL or tissue adhesive can be used for bleeding from gastroesophageal varices type 1.

Interventional and Surgical Treatment Approaches

Standard therapy fails to control initial bleeding or early rebleeding in 10% to 20% of patients with acute variceal hemorrhage.[21] In these cases, a salvage procedure, such as balloon tamponade or transjugular intrahepatic portosystemic shunt (TIPS), is necessary. Balloon tamponade is effective in controlling variceal bleeding temporarily; however, rebleeding is common after balloon deflation,

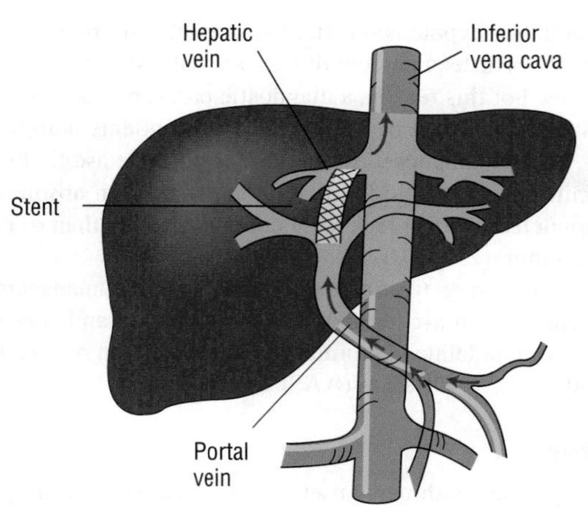

FIGURE 24-6 Transjugular intrahepatic portosystemic shunt (TIPS).

and complications result in mortality rates of up to 20% with balloon tamponade. Sengstaken-Blakemore tubes are recommended for use in esophageal variceal bleeding. Linton tubes are preferred for bleeding from fundal gastric varices. Balloon tamponade should be reserved as a temporizing measure until a more definitive treatment, such as TIPS, can be performed.

The TIPS procedure involves the placement of one or more stents between the hepatic vein and the portal vein (Fig. 24-6). TIPS (preferably with polytetrafluoroethylene-covered stents) is recommended for patients who fail to achieve hemostasis despite combined endoscopic and pharmacologic therapy.[11] TIPS provides an effective decompressive shunt without laparotomy and can be employed regardless of Child-Pugh score, unlike shunt surgery, which is restricted to Child-Pugh class A patients.[22] TIPS decreases the incidence of variceal rebleeding and decreases the incidence of deaths due to rebleeding.[25] There is a significantly increased rate of posttreatment encephalopathy found in TIPS-treated patients.

Treatment Recommendations: Variceal Hemorrhage

Patients require cautious resuscitation with colloids and blood products to correct intravascular losses and to reverse existing coagulopathies.[10,11,21,22] ❹ Drug therapy with octreotide should be initiated early to control bleeding and facilitate diagnostic and therapeutic endoscopy. Therapy is initiated with an IV bolus of 50 mcg and is followed by a continuous infusion of 50 mcg/h for 3 to 5 days.[21,22] Monitor patients for bradycardia, hypertension, arrhythmia, and abdominal pain.[10] Endoscopy is recommended in any patient with suspected upper GI bleeding due to ruptured varices.[10,11,21,22] EVL is the recommended form of endoscopic therapy, but endoscopic sclerotherapy may be employed if EVL is technically difficult. An additional endoscopic therapy option is injection of the tissue adhesive *N*-butyl cyanoacrylate for gastric varices.[11] Short-term antibiotic prophylaxis (maximum 7 days) is recommended.[11,22] Appropriate choices include norfloxacin 400 mg twice daily or IV ciprofloxacin if the oral route is unavailable.[22] In patients with advanced cirrhosis in areas of high quinolone resistance, IV ceftriaxone 1 g daily may be preferred. Surgical shunts and TIPS are employed as salvage therapy in patients who have failed repeated endoscopy and vasoactive drug therapy.[11]

Secondary Prophylaxis

Because rebleeding after initial control of variceal hemorrhage occurs in a median of 60% of patients and because rebleeding carries a mortality rate of 33%, it is inappropriate to simply observe patients for evidence of further bleeding.[10,22] Only patients who underwent shunt surgery or TIPS to control their initial acute bleeding require no further intervention as secondary prophylaxis. Patients who underwent one of these procedures to treat their initial bleeding should be referred for transplantation if they are a candidate. Candidates include those with a Child-Pugh score greater than or equal to 7 or MELD score greater than or equal to 15.[22] Combination therapy with β-adrenergic blockers and chronic EVL to eradicate varices is the best treatment option for secondary prophylaxis of variceal bleeding.[10,11,21,22] Secondary prophylaxis should be started once vasoactive drug therapy is discontinued and as soon as possible (as early as day 6) following the acute bleeding event.[10,11]

Drug Therapy

The combination of EVL and a nonselective β-adrenergic blocking agent provides the most rational approach for secondary prophylaxis because nonselective β-adrenergic blocking agents can protect against variceal rebleeding before variceal obliteration can be accomplished through EVL, and β-adrenergic blocking agents will also delay variceal recurrence.[21,22] The addition of isosorbide mononitrate to nonselective β-adrenergic blocker therapy reduces portal pressure more than β-adrenergic blocker alone, but there is no difference in the overall rate of rebleeding with this combination and side effects are more likely than with β-adrenergic blocker monotherapy (namely, headache and light-headedness).[26] Pharmacologic therapy (either isosorbide mononitrate plus nonselective β-adrenergic blocker therapy or β-adrenergic blocker therapy alone) plus EVL is associated with lower rebleeding rates than either pharmacologic or EVL therapy alone.[27,28]

The lowest rate of variceal rebleeding occurs in patients when pharmacologic therapy leads to a reduction in HVPG of greater than 20% of baseline or to a measurement less than 12 mm Hg.[10] Ideally, portal pressure monitoring would help to assess the response to nonselective β-adrenergic blocker therapy and identify responders from nonresponders earlier in the treatment course. In order to utilize the HVPG measurement for clinical decision making, the technique used to make this measurement would first have to be standardized.

Treatment Recommendations: Variceal Bleeding—Secondary Prophylaxis

The combination of EVL plus pharmacologic therapy to prevent rebleeding is currently considered the most rational therapeutic approach.[21,22] Pharmacologic therapy should be initiated with a nonselective β-blocker such as propranolol 20 mg twice daily or nadolol at a dose of 20 to 40 mg once daily.[21] ❸ β-Blocker therapy can be titrated to achieve a goal heart rate of 55 to 60 beats/min or the maximal tolerated dose. Monitor patients for evidence of heart failure, bronchospasm, and glucose intolerance, particularly hypoglycemia in patients with insulin-dependent diabetes. EVL should be conducted every 1 to 2 weeks until variceal obliteration, and then the patient should be followed by surveillance endoscopy in 1 to 3 months and then every 6 to 12 months. Combination therapy with nonselective β-blocker plus isosorbide mononitrate can be considered in patients who are unable to undergo EVL as well in patients who are hemodynamic nonresponders.[11] Patients who cannot tolerate or who fail pharmacologic and endoscopic interventions can be considered for TIPS or surgical shunting to prevent bleeding. A summary of evidence-based treatment recommendations regarding portal hypertension and variceal bleeding is found in Table 24-3.

Management of Ascites and Spontaneous Bacterial Peritonitis

Patients with cirrhosis experience overt fluid retention and ascites as liver disease progresses.[9] The classic physical exam findings of

TABLE 24-3 Evidence-Based Table of Selected Treatment Recommendations: Variceal Bleeding in Portal Hypertension

Recommendation	Grade
Prevention of variceal bleeding	
Nonselective β-blocker therapy should be initiated in:	
Patients with small varices and criteria for increased risk of hemorrhage	IIaC
Patients with medium/large varices without high risk of hemorrhage	IA
Endoscopic variceal ligation (EVL) should be offered to patients who have contraindications or intolerance to nonselective β-blockers	IA
EVL may be recommended for prevention in patients with medium/large varices at high risk of hemorrhage instead of nonselective β-blocker therapy	IA
Treatment of variceal bleeding	
Short-term antibiotic prophylaxis should be instituted on admission	IA
Vasoactive drugs should be started as soon as possible, prior to endoscopy, and maintained for 3–5 days	IA
Endoscopy should be performed within 12 hours to diagnose variceal bleeding and to treat bleeding with either sclerotherapy or EVL	IA
Secondary prophylaxis of variceal bleeding	
Nonselective β-blocker therapy plus EVL is the best therapeutic option for prevention of recurrent variceal bleeding	IA

Recommendation grading:
Class I—Conditions for which there is evidence and/or general agreement
Class II—Conditions for which there is conflicting evidence and/or a divergence of opinion
Class IIa—Weight of evidence/opinion is in favor of efficacy
Class IIb—Efficacy less well established
Class III—Conditions for which there is evidence and/or general agreement that treatment is not effective and/or potentially harmful
Level A—Data from multiple randomized trials or meta-analyses
Level B—Data derived from single randomized trial or nonrandomized studies
Level C—Only consensus opinion, case studies, or standard of care

Data from reference 22.

ascites are a bulging abdomen with shifting flank dullness.[5] The development of ascites in patients with cirrhosis is an indication of advanced liver disease and is a poor prognostic sign.[5,9] The principle therapeutic goals for patients with ascites are to control the ascites; to prevent or relieve ascites-related symptoms such as dyspnea, abdominal pain, and abdominal distention; and to prevent life-threatening complications such as SBP and the hepatorenal syndrome.[9] Treatment of ascites is expected to have little effect on survival, however.[21] Workup includes a history and physical exam, abdominal paracentesis and/or ultrasound, and ascitic fluid analysis.[5] The treatment of ascites is based on oral diuretics and is carried out in a slow, stepwise fashion.[21] Treatment of ascites should be initiated only in stable patients (e.g., those without ongoing variceal hemorrhage, bacterial infection, or renal dysfunction).

SBP is an infection of ascitic fluid that occurs in the absence of any evidence of an intraabdominal, surgically treatable source of infection.[5] It is a common complication that develops in 10% to 20% of patients hospitalized with severe liver disease, cirrhosis, and ascites.[21] The key mechanism behind the development of SBP is thought to be bacterial translocation.[29] Decreased motility of the GI tract with disturbances of the gut flora, changes in the structure of the GI tract, and reduced local and humoral immunity combine to lead to the free flow of microorganisms and endotoxins to the mesenteric lymph nodes. Most episodes of SBP are caused by *Escherichia coli*, *Klebsiella pneumonia*, and pneumococci.[5] Symptoms and signs of SBP include fever, abdominal pain, abdominal tenderness, rebound, encephalopathy, renal failure, acidosis, peripheral leukocytosis, and altered mental status.[5,29] Paralytic ileus, hypotension, and hypothermia are poor prognostic indicators.[29] Thirteen percent of patients with SBP present with no symptoms. For this reason, a diagnostic paracentesis with analysis of ascitic fluid should be performed in all patients admitted with ascites.[5] SBP is diagnosed when there is possible ascitic fluid bacterial culture and ascitic fluid cell counts show an absolute polymorphonuclear (PMN) leukocyte count of greater than or equal to 250 cells/mm^3 (250 × 10^6/L).

The following treatment guidelines for the management of adult patients with ascites and SBP were updated and approved by the Practice Guidelines Committee of the American Association for the Study of Liver Diseases (AASLD).

Ascites

In adult patients with new-onset ascites as determined by physical exam or radiographic studies, abdominal paracentesis should be performed, and ascitic fluid analysis should include a cell count with differential, ascitic fluid total protein, and a serum-ascites albumin gradient (SAAG). If infection is suspected, ascitic fluid cultures should be obtained at the time of the paracentesis. The SAAG can accurately determine whether ascites is a result of portal hypertension or another process. If the SAAG is greater than or equal to 1.1 g/dL (11 g/L), the patient almost certainly has portal hypertension. The treatment of ascites secondary to portal hypertension is relatively straightforward and includes abstinence from alcohol, sodium restriction, and diuretics.

❶ Abstinence from alcohol is an essential element of the overall treatment strategy. Abstinence from alcohol can result in improvement of the reversible component of alcoholic liver disease, resolution of ascites, or improved responsiveness of ascites to medical therapy. Patients with cirrhosis not caused by alcohol have less reversible liver disease, and, by the time ascites is present, these patients may be best managed with liver transplantation rather than protracted medical therapy.

Beyond avoidance of alcohol, the primary treatment of ascites due to portal hypertension and cirrhosis is salt restriction and oral diuretic therapy. Fluid loss and weight change depend directly on sodium balance in these patients. A goal of therapy is to increase urinary excretion of sodium to greater than 78 mmol/day. Evaluation of urinary sodium excretion, preferably utilizing a 24-hour urine collection, may be helpful, although this collection can be difficult. A random spot urine sodium concentration that is greater than the potassium concentration correlates very well with a 24-hour urinary sodium excretion over 78 mmol/day and is an easier test to complete. Severe hyponatremia, defined as serum sodium less than a threshold of 120 to 125 mEq/L (120 to 125 mmol/L), does warrant fluid restriction. However, rapid correction of asymptomatic hyponatremia is not recommended as patients with cirrhosis are usually asymptomatic until their serum sodium concentrations are less than 110 mEq/L (110 mmol/L) or unless the decline in serum sodium is rapid.

Diuretic Therapy The AASLD practice guidelines recommend that diuretic therapy be initiated with the combination of spironolactone and furosemide. At one time, spironolactone was commonly recommended for initial therapy as a single agent. However, due to the likelihood for development of drug-induced hyperkalemia with spironolactone when used as monotherapy, the drug is now recommended only for use as a lone diuretic agent in patients with minimal fluid overload. If tense ascites is present, paracentesis should be performed prior to institution of diuretic therapy and salt restriction. For patients who respond to diuretic therapy, this approach is preferred over the use of serial paracenteses. In patients with refractory ascites, serial paracenteses may be employed. Albumin infusion postparacentesis is controversial, but reasonable for extraction volumes exceeding 5 L. Laboratory tests for renal function and electrolytes need to be monitored during therapy. Referral for liver transplantation should be made in patients with refractory ascites. TIPS is a therapeutic modality for the treatment of refractory ascites that may be considered in appropriately selected patients. Peritoneovenous shunting may be considered in treatment refractory patients who are not candidates for paracenteses, transplant, or TIPS.

Spontaneous Bacterial Peritonitis

Relatively broad-spectrum antibiotic therapy that adequately covers the three most commonly encountered pathogens (*E. coli*, *K. pneumoniae*, and pneumococci) is warranted in patients with documented or suspected SBP.[5,21,29] Empiric therapy should not be delayed while awaiting culture results. In some patients, signs and symptoms of infection are present such as fever, abdominal pain, and unexplained encephalopathy at the bacterascites stage (i.e., signs and symptoms are present before the PMN count in the ascitic fluid is elevated).[5] In these patients, signs and symptoms of infection justify empiric antibiotic therapy until culture results are known, regardless of the PMN count in the ascitic fluid.

Cefotaxime 2 g every 8 hours, or a similar third-generation cephalosporin, is considered the drug of choice for SBP. A 5-day course of antibiotic therapy is as efficacious as 10 days of therapy. Ofloxacin 400 mg every 12 hours administered orally for an average of 8 days is an alternative for patients without vomiting, shock, significant HE, or serum creatinine over 3 mg/dL (265 μmol/L). IV ciprofloxacin offers another potential treatment alternative. Patients with SBP who previously received quinolone therapy as prophylaxis should be treated with an alternative agent since patients who have received quinolone therapy may become infected with quinolone-resistant flora.

Secondary bacterial peritonitis, ascitic fluid infection caused by a surgically treatable intraabdominal source, can masquerade as SBP. Free perforation should be considered when multiple or atypical organisms are cultured, a very high ascitic fluid PMN count is seen, or at least two of the following are seen on ascitic fluid analysis: total protein greater than 1 g/dL (10 g/L), lactate dehydrogenase greater than the upper limit of normal for serum, and glucose less than 50 mg/dL (2.8 mmol/L). A 48-hour followup PMN count that rises above pretreatment levels despite antibiotic treatment is indicative of secondary nonperforation peritonitis. Patients with free perforation or nonperforation secondary peritonitis should receive a third-generation cephalosporin plus anaerobic coverage in addition to undergoing laparotomy.

Treatment Recommendations: Ascites and Spontaneous Bacterial Peritonitis

Adult patients admitted to the hospital with new-onset ascites should have an abdominal paracentesis performed to establish the SAAG, the ascitic fluid cell count and differential, and the ascitic fluid total protein. If ascitic fluid infection is suspected, ascitic fluid should be cultured at the bedside. ❶ Patients who drink alcohol should be strongly discouraged from further alcohol use. ❺ Sodium restriction to 2,000 mg/day, together with spironolactone and furosemide, is the mainstay of therapy. Diuretic therapy should be initiated with single morning doses of spironolactone 100 mg and furosemide 40 mg administered orally. Titrate diuretic therapy every 3 to 5 days using the 100:40 mg dose ratio to attain adequate natriuresis and weight loss (reasonable daily weight loss goal is 0.5 kg). Maximum daily doses are 400 mg spironolactone and 160 mg furosemide. This combination ratio is used because it usually maintains normokalemia. Fluid restriction, unless the serum sodium is less than 120 to 125 mEq/L (120 to 125 mmol/L), and bedrest are not recommended. Utilize the random spot urine test to confirm a sodium concentration that is greater than the potassium concentration as this correlates very well with a 24-hour urinary sodium excretion over the goal of 78 mmol/day. Monitor serum potassium and renal function frequently. Avoid rapid correction of asymptomatic hyponatremia in patients with cirrhosis. If tense ascites is present, paracentesis should be performed prior to institution of diuretic therapy and salt restriction. For patients who respond to diuretic therapy, this approach is preferred over the use of serial paracenteses. Discontinue diuretic therapy in patients who experience uncontrolled or recurrent encephalopathy, severe hyponatremia (serum sodium less than 120 mEq/L [120 mmol/L]) despite fluid restriction, or renal insufficiency (serum creatinine greater than 2 mg/dL [177 μmol/L]). Serial paracenteses may be considered for patients with refractory ascites and albumin infusion of 6 to 8 g/L of fluid removed can be considered postparacentesis when paracentesis volumes exceed 5 L.

Patients with ascitic fluid PMN counts greater than or equal to 250 cells/mm^3 (250 × 10^6/L) should receive empiric antibiotic therapy with IV cefotaxime 2 g every 8 hours or a similar third-generation cephalosporin. Oral ofloxacin 400 mg twice daily may be an alternative option in patients without prior exposure to quinolones, vomiting, shock, severe encephalopathy, or serum creatinine over 3 mg/dL (265 μmol/L). Patients with ascitic fluid PMN counts less than 250 cells/mm^3 (250 × 10^6/L) but with signs and symptoms of infection (symptoms such as abdominal pain, abdominal tenderness, and fever) should also receive empiric antibiotic treatment. Patients with ascitic fluid PMN counts greater than or equal to 250 cells/mm^3 (250 × 10^6/L) and suspicion of SBP should also receive 1.5 g of albumin per kilogram body weight within 6 hours of detection and 1 g of albumin per kilogram body weight on day 3 if they also have a serum creatinine over 1 mg/dL (88 μmol/L), blood urea nitrogen over 30 mg/dL (10.7 mmol/L), or total bilirubin over 4 mg/dL (68.4 μmol/L).

❻ All patients who have survived an episode of SBP should receive long-term antibiotic prophylaxis with daily norfloxacin 400 mg or double strength trimethoprim–sulfamethoxazole. Long-term prophylaxis should also be considered for the prevention of SBP in patients with low-protein ascites (less than 1.5 g/dL [15 g/L]) who also have one of the following: serum creatinine greater than or equal to 1.2 mg/dL (106 μmol/L), blood urea nitrogen greater than or equal to 25 mg/dL (8.9 mmol/L), serum sodium less than or equal to 130 mEq/L (130 mmol/L), or Child-Pugh score of greater than or equal to 9 with bilirubin greater than or equal to 3 mg/dL (51.3 μmol/L). Short-term prophylaxis (7 days) is indicated in patients with cirrhosis and GI hemorrhage. A summary of evidence-based treatment recommendations regarding ascites and SBP is found in Table 24-4.

Management of Hepatic Encephalopathy

The clinical manifestations of HE vary widely.[30] Patients with minimal HE do not suffer from clinically overt cognitive dysfunction; nevertheless, it adversely affects their ability to function socially and perform in the workplace, and it may also affect their ability to drive safely.[31] Episodic HE refers to precipitated, spontaneous, or recurrent acute episodes of HE. *Recurrent HE* refers to two spontaneous or precipitated episodes of HE that occur within 1 year. Persistent HE refers to mild, severe, or treatment-dependent symptoms that are chronic in nature and negatively impact a patient's quality of life.

The prevalence of HE among cirrhotics is variable but may be found in up to 70% of patients. To determine the severity of HE, a grading system that relates neurologic and neuromuscular signs can be used (Table 24-5). The primary substances thought to be involved in the development of HE are ammonia, glutamate, manganese, and the γ-aminobutyric acid (GABA)-benzodiazepine receptor agonists.[30,31]

TABLE 24-4 Evidence-Based Table of Selected Treatment Recommendations: Ascites and Spontaneous Bacterial Peritonitis

Recommendation	Grade
Ascites	
Paracentesis should be performed in patients with apparent new-onset ascites	IC
Sodium restriction of 2,000 mg/day should be instituted as well as oral diuretic therapy with spironolactone and furosemide	IIaA
Diuretic-sensitive patients should be treated with sodium restriction and diuretics rather than serial paracentesis	IIaC
Refractory ascites	
Serial therapeutic paracenteses may be performed	IC
Postparacentesis albumin infusion of 6–8 g/L of fluid removed can be considered if more than 5 L is removed during paracentesis	IIaC
Treatment of SBP	
If ascitic fluid PMN counts are greater than 250 cells/mm^3 (250 × 10^6/L), empiric antibiotic therapy should be instituted (cefotaxime 2 g every 8 hours)	IA
If ascitic fluid PMN counts are less than 250 cells/mm^3 (250 × 10^6/L), but signs or symptoms of infection exist, empiric antibiotic therapy should be initiated while awaiting culture results	IB
Ofloxacin 400 mg twice daily may be substituted for cefotaxime in patients without vomiting, shock, grade II or higher encephalopathy, or serum creatinine greater than 3 mg/dL (265 μmol/L) and if there is no prior exposure to quinolones	IIaB
If ascitic fluid polymorphonuclear leukocyte counts are greater than 250 cells/mm^3 (250 × 10^6/L), clinical suspicion of SBP is present, and the patient has a serum creatinine greater than 1 mg/dL (88 μmol/L), blood urea nitrogen greater than 30 mg/dL (10.7 mmol/L), or total bilirubin over 4 mg/dL (68.4 μmol/L), 1.5 g/kg albumin should be infused within 6 hours of detection and 1 g/kg albumin infusion should also be given on day 3	IIaB
Prophylaxis against SBP	
Short-term antibiotic prophylaxis should be used for 7 days to prevent SBP in cirrhosis patients with GI hemorrhage	IA
Patients who survive an episode of SBP should receive long-term prophylaxis with either daily norfloxacin or trimethoprim–sulfamethoxazole	IA
Patients with low-protein ascites (less than 1.5 g/dL [15 g/L]) plus at least one of the following: serum creatinine greater than or equal to 1.2 mg/dL (106 μmol/L), blood urea nitrogen greater than or equal to 25 mg/dL (8.9 mmol/L), serum sodium less than or equal to 130 mEq/L (130 mmol/L), or Child-Pugh score of greater than or equal to 9 with bilirubin greater than or equal to 3 mg/dL (51.3 μmol/L) may also justifiably receive long-term norfloxacin or sulfamethoxazole/trimethoprim as prophylaxis	IB

Recommendation grading:
Class I—Conditions for which there is evidence and/or general agreement
Class II—Conditions for which there is conflicting evidence and/or a divergence of opinion
Class IIa—Weight of evidence/opinion is in favor of efficacy
Class IIb—Efficacy less well established
Class III—Conditions for which there is evidence and/or general agreement that treatment is not effective and/or potentially harmful
Level A—Data from multiple randomized trials or meta-analyses
Level B—Data derived from single randomized trial or nonrandomized studies
Level C—Only consensus opinion, case studies, or standard of care

Data from reference 5.

Episodic HE may develop in a clinically stable cirrhotic patient as the result of a precipitating event.[31] Table 24-6 lists the most commonly encountered precipitating factors and suggests general treatment alternatives. Table 24-7 describes the treatment goals for patients with HE and contrasts the differences between episodic and persistent HE. The general approach to the management of HE is to first identify and treat any precipitating factors, and, when associated with a precipitant, the clinical features of HE may resolve after the precipitating factor is treated or removed.[13,31]

Treatment approaches for episodic and persistent HE include (a) reducing ammonia blood concentrations by dietary restrictions and drug therapy aimed at inhibiting ammonia production or enhancing its removal and (b) inhibiting the GABA-benzodiazepine receptors.[13] Additionally, treatment for persistent HE should include avoidance and prevention of precipitating factors in an effort to avoid acute decompensation.

Hyperammonemia

7 Treatment interventions to reduce ammonia blood concentrations are recommended in patients with HE. Decreasing ammonia blood concentrations by reducing the nitrogenous load from the gut remains a mainstay of therapy for patients with HE. Treatment options most commonly used to decrease ammonia load from the gut include nutritional management, nonabsorbable disaccharides, and antibiotics.

TABLE 24-5 Grading System for Hepatic Encephalopathy

Grade	Level of Consciousness	Personality/Intellect	Neurologic Abnormalities
0	Normal	Normal	None
1	Inverted sleep patterns/restless	Mild confusion, euphoria or depression, decreased attention, irritable, slowing of ability to perform mental tasks	Slight tremor, apraxia, incoordination
2	Lethargic, drowsy, intermittent disorientation (usually for time)	Obvious personality changes, inappropriate behavior, gross deficits in ability to perform mental tasks	Asterixis, abnormal reflexes
3	Somnolent but arousable, markedly confused, disorientation to time and/or place, amnesia	Unable to perform mental tasks, occasional fits of rage, speech present but incomprehensible	Abnormal reflexes
4	Coma/unarousable	None	Decerebrate, Babinski sign present

Data from reference 31.

TABLE 24-6 Portosystemic Encephalopathy: Precipitating Factors and Therapy

Factor	Therapy Alternatives
GI bleeding	
Variceal	Band ligation/sclerotherapy Octreotide
Nonvariceal	Endoscopic therapy Proton pump inhibitors
Infection/sepsis	Antibiotics Paracentesis
Electrolyte abnormalities	Discontinue diuretics Fluid and electrolyte replacement
Sedative ingestion	Discontinue sedatives/tranquilizers Consider reversal (flumazenil/naloxone)
Dietary excesses	Limit daily protein Lactulose
Constipation	Cathartics Bowel cleansing/enema
Renal insufficiency	Discontinue diuretics Discontinue NSAIDs, nephrotoxic antibiotics Fluid resuscitation

Data from references 13, 30, and 31.

Guidelines for nutritional support of patients with liver disease have been published by the European Society for Parenteral and Enteral Nutrition.[32] Protein withdrawal is a cornerstone of treatment for patients during acute episodes of HE.[13] However, prolonged restriction can lead to malnutrition and poorer prognosis among HE patients. Therefore, once successful reversal of HE symptoms is achieved, protein is added back to the diet in combination with other therapies until a target of 1 to 1.5 g/kg/day is reached. Vegetable-source and dairy-source protein may be preferable to meat-source protein because the latter contains a higher calorie-to-nitrogen ratio. Also, the higher fiber content of vegetable protein lowers colonic pH, increasing catharsis. Most patients will tolerate at least 1 g/kg/day of standard proteins without becoming encephalopathic.[33] Branched-chain amino acid formulations may provide a better-tolerated source of protein in those patients with protein intolerance.[13] Bowel cleansing using cathartics or lactulose enemas (see following discussion) results in rapid removal of ammonia substrate from the colon and may be combined with dietary intervention to help the patient eliminate ammonia and tolerate dietary protein.

The use of lactulose, a nonabsorbable disaccharide, is standard therapy for both acute and chronic HE. Lactulose, when administered orally through ingestion or a nasogastric tube, passes through the GI tract and reaches the colon unchanged. It can also be administered by retention enema. Lactulose is metabolized by gut flora into acetic acid and lactic acid, which lower colonic pH and create a cathartic effect.

TABLE 24-7 Treatment Goals: Episodic and Persistent Hepatic Encephalopathy

Episodic HE	Persistent HE
Control precipitating factor	Reverse encephalopathy
Reverse encephalopathy	Avoid recurrence
Hospital/inpatient therapy	Home/outpatient therapy
Maintain fluid and hemodynamic support	Manage persistent neuropsychiatric abnormalities Manage chronic liver disease
Expect normal mentation after recovery	High prevalence of abnormal mentation after recovery

Lactulose administration lowers ammonia levels in the blood in several ways: (a) through creation of a laxative effect that reduces the time period available for ammonia absorption, (b) through leaching of ammonia from the circulation into the colon and increasing bacterial uptake of ammonia by colonic bacteria, and (c) through reducing ammonia production by the small intestine by interfering directly with the uptake of glutamine by the intestinal wall and its subsequent metabolism to ammonia.[34]

Clinical **Controversy. . .**

Whether lactulose retains benefit once antibiotic therapy is begun for recurrent HE has been an area of uncertainty.[12] This controversy stems from concern over whether or not antibiotic-altered gut flora is able to metabolize lactulose appropriately. Rifaximin has been established as the second-line agent of choice for patients with recurrent HE. A placebo-controlled trial examining rifaximin's effectiveness for maintaining remission in patients with a history of recurrent HE found significant improvement among patients allocated to receive rifaximin.[35] In this study, 90% of patients received concomitant lactulose therapy. Hence, at least in the case of rifaximin, it seems that continuing lactulose may be an appropriate therapeutic choice.

Inhibiting the activity of urease-producing bacteria by using neomycin or metronidazole can decrease production of ammonia.[13] Neomycin at doses of 3 to 6 g daily can be given for 1 to 2 weeks during an acute episode of HE. For persistent HE, a dose of 1 to 2 g daily could be used with periodic renal and annual auditory monitoring. Despite poor absorption, chronic use of neomycin can lead to irreversible ototoxicity, nephrotoxicity, and the possibility of staphylococcal superinfection. As such, neomycin should not be routinely recommended.[34] Metronidazole initiated at 250 mg twice daily may also produce a favorable clinical response in HE.[13] However, neurotoxicity caused by impaired hepatic clearance of the drug may be problematic. *Helicobacter pylori* eradication is not routinely recommended as a way to improve ammonia levels or symptoms of encephalopathy.

Rifaximin is a synthetic antibiotic structurally similar to rifamycin with a systemic absorption of only 0.4%.[34] It lowers blood ammonia levels and improves neuropsychiatric symptoms in HE. In a randomized, double-blind, placebo-controlled trial, patients in remission from recurrent HE were randomized to either rifaximin 550 mg twice daily or placebo for 6 months.[35] Rifaximin significantly reduced the risk of a recurrent episode of HE as well as hospitalization due to HE. Lactulose was used concomitantly in 90% of patients in this study. The incidence of adverse effects was similar between rifaximin and placebo with the most common serious adverse events reported being nausea and diarrhea.

Zinc is a cofactor of urea cycle enzymes and can be deficient in cirrhotic patients, especially in cases of malnourishment.[13] Zinc acetate 220 mg twice daily is recommended for patients with zinc deficiency.

Drugs Affecting Neurotransmission

The GABA-receptor complex is the primary inhibitory neural network within the CNS. An enhanced GABA-ergic tone and an increased amount of endogenous benzodiazepines may contribute to HE. Flumazenil 1 mg IV bolus may be considered for short-term therapy in refractory patients with suspected benzodiazepine intake, but cannot be recommended for routine clinical use.

Alterations of dopaminergic neurotransmission have also been thought to play a role in the symptoms of HE, particularly the extrapyramidal signs. Improvements of extrapyramidal symptoms have been reported with bromocriptine therapy. Bromocriptine 30 mg twice daily is indicated for chronic HE treatment in patients who are unresponsive to other therapies. Prolactin levels may become elevated during bromocriptine treatment.

Treatment Recommendations: Hepatic Encephalopathy

Treatment recommendations depend on the type of HE being managed: episodic HE, persistent HE, or minimal HE.[21] The general approach to the management of HE is first to identify patients with acute episodic HE and then to provide aggressive management of any precipitating events (see Table 24-7).[13] When the precipitating event has been discovered and appropriate therapy initiated, steps to rapidly reverse the encephalopathy should be implemented.

7 The mainstay of therapy of HE involves measures to lower blood ammonia concentrations and includes diet therapy, lactulose, and antibiotics alone or in combination with lactulose. Other commonly used adjunctive therapies include zinc replacement in patients with zinc deficiency, flumazenil, and possibly bromocriptine.

In patients with episodic HE, protein is withheld or limited while maintaining the total caloric intake until the clinical situation improves. Then dietary protein is titrated back up based on tolerance, increasing gradually to a total of 1 to 1.5 g/kg/day. Consider the substitution of meat-source protein with vegetable or dairy protein. Zinc acetate supplementation at a dose of 220 mg twice daily is recommended for long-term management in patients with cirrhosis who are zinc deficient.

In episodic HE, lactulose is initiated at a dose of 45 mL orally every hour (or by retention enema: 300 mL lactulose syrup in 1 L water held for 60 minutes) until catharsis begins. The dose is then decreased to 15 to 45 mL orally every 8 to 12 hours and titrated to produce two to three soft stools per day. The enema is retained for 1 hour with the patient in the Trendelenburg position. For chronic encephalopathy, dosing is the same except that the initial hourly administration is not required. Patients are maintained on this regimen to prevent recurrence of episodic HE. Monitor electrolytes periodically, follow patients for changes in mental status, and titrate to the number of stools as already described.

Rifaximin 550 mg twice daily plus lactulose has been proven superior to lactulose alone in patients with a history of recurrent HE.[35] Because of its more favorable adverse effect profile, rifaximin is now considered the next line of therapy for recurrent HE over either metronidazole or neomycin.[21]

Systemic Complications

In addition to the more common complications of chronic liver disease discussed earlier, other complications can occur, including hepatorenal syndrome, hepatopulmonary syndrome, coagulation disorders, and endocrine dysfunction.

Hepatorenal syndrome, which is a functional renal failure in the setting of cirrhosis, occurs in the absence of structural kidney damage.[36] It develops in patients with cirrhosis as a result of intense renal vasoconstriction, which results from extreme systemic vasodilation. The resultant reduction in blood supply to the kidneys causes avid sodium retention and oliguria. As liver disease progresses, systemic vasodilation worsens and, subsequently, increased renal vasoconstriction occurs and renal blood flow is further decreased. As this occurs, the heart's response becomes insufficient to maintain perfusion pressure, which the kidneys rely heavily on at this point to maintain adequate blood flow. Hepatorenal syndrome is common and develops in approximately 20% of hospitalized patients with cirrhosis.

Management of hepatorenal syndrome begins with a first step of discontinuing diuretics and any other medication that could potentially decrease effective blood volume and to expand the intravascular volume with IV albumin at a dose of 1 g/kg up to a maximum of 100 g.[21] Precipitating factors such as infection, fluid loss, and blood loss should be investigated and treated if found. Liver transplantation is the only definitive therapy for hepatorenal syndrome and the only therapy that will prolong survival. Therapies used to bridge patients until transplantation include arteriolar vasoconstrictor-based treatments with terlipressin or midodrine plus octreotide used in addition to IV albumin infusion as already discussed.

Hepatopulmonary syndrome affects somewhere between 5% and 32% of patients with cirrhosis.[37] This abnormality is characterized by a defect in arterial oxygenation, which is caused by the pulmonary vascular dilation that occurs in the presence of liver disease. Less commonly, pleural and pulmonary arteriovenous shunting can occur as well as portopulmonary venous anastomoses. These patients present with dyspnea on exertion, at rest, or both. Cirrhotic patients with these findings should be evaluated for hepatopulmonary syndrome, which is diagnosed based on the presence of arterial hypoxemia. Arterial hypoxemia is defined based on measurements of the partial pressure of oxygen that are performed with patients sitting and at rest. Testing for an increased alveolar–arterial oxygen gradient is also particularly important as this gradient can rise abnormally before the patient's partial pressure of oxygen measurement becomes abnormally low. Long-term management requires supportive therapy with supplemental oxygen. The prognosis for these patients is poor. Ultimately, liver transplantation offers the best chance for long-term recovery.

Correction of the coagulopathy is essential for patients actively bleeding. The pathophysiology of the coagulopathy is complex and involves impaired synthesis of clotting factors, excessive fibrinolysis, disseminated intravascular coagulation, thrombocytopenia, and platelet dysfunction. Acute therapy involves platelet transfusions for thrombocytopenia and fresh-frozen plasma for prolongation of the PT because of clotting factor deficiencies.[21]

The presence of cirrhosis can produce abnormal circulating levels of various hormones.[38] Hypogonadism, diabetes mellitus, osteoporosis, and thyroid disorders are among the endocrine disorders that may develop related to advanced liver disease. Erectile dysfunction related to hypogonadism can be treated with the administration of testosterone and the removal of causative factors such as alcohol.

Liver Transplantation

The complications seen in patients with chronic liver disease are essentially functional as a secondary effect of the circulatory and metabolic changes that accompany liver failure. Consequently, liver transplantation is the only treatment that can offer a cure for complications of end-stage cirrhosis.

PERSONALIZED PHARMACOTHERAPY

Cirrhosis modulates the behavior of drugs in the body by inducing kinetic alterations in drug absorption, distribution, and clearance.[39] Additionally, patients with cirrhosis may exhibit pharmacodynamic changes with increased sensitivity to the effects of certain drugs, namely, opiates, benzodiazepines, and nonsteroidal antiinflammatory drugs. These pharmacodynamic changes are separate and distinct from the enhancement of drug effects seen in cirrhosis patients as a result of pharmacokinetic changes. Hepatic drug clearance is primarily dependent on protein binding, hepatic blood flow,

TABLE 24-8 Drug Monitoring Guidelines

Drug	Adverse Drug Reaction	Monitoring Parameter	Comments
Nonselective β-adrenergic blocker	Heart failure, bronchospasm, glucose intolerance	BP, HR Goal HR: 55–60 beats/min or maximal tolerated dose	Nadolol or propranolol
Octreotide	Bradycardia, hypertension, arrhythmia, abdominal pain	BP, HR, EKG, abdominal pain	
Vasopressin	Myocardial ischemia/infarction, arrhythmia, mesenteric ischemia, ischemia of the limbs, cerebrovascular accident	EKG, distal pulses, symptoms of myocardial, mesenteric, or cerebrovascular ischemia/infarction	
Spironolactone/furosemide	Electrolyte disturbances, dehydration, renal insufficiency, hypotension	Serum electrolytes (especially potassium), SCr, blood urea nitrogen, BP Goal sodium excretion: >78 mmol/day	Spot urine sodium concentration greater than potassium concentration correlates well with daily sodium excretion >78 mmol/day
Lactulose	Electrolyte disturbances	Serum electrolytes Goal number of soft stools per day: 2–3	
Neomycin	Ototoxicity, nephrotoxicity	SCr, annual auditory monitoring	
Metronidazole	Neurotoxicity	Sensory and motor neuropathy	
Rifaximin	Nausea, diarrhea		

BP, blood pressure; HR, heart rate; beats/min, beats per minute; EKG, electrocardiogram; SCr, serum creatinine; mmol, millimole.

and metabolic enzyme activity. The pathophysiologic changes that occur in patients with cirrhosis, including reduced liver blood flow, intrahepatic and extrahepatic portal-systemic shunting, diminished metabolic and synthetic function, and capillarization of the sinusoids, can have a significant impact on each of these factors. The consequence of these changes is a reduction in intrinsic metabolic activity, a reduction in the delivery of blood to the liver that decreases clearance and prolongs half-life, and a reduction in the degree of protein binding that increases the fraction of unbound drug in the serum. Finally, patients with cirrhosis frequently accumulate large amounts of interstitial fluid resulting in substantial changes in the volume of distribution, which also prolongs drug half-life. These changes occur most commonly in combination in patients with cirrhosis and are dynamic throughout the disease course. The effect that these changes will have depends on the drug and the type of biotransformation that the drug undergoes.

Drugs with a high extraction ratio (high-extraction drugs) are dependent on blood flow for metabolism, and the rate of metabolism will be sensitive to changes in blood flow. Drugs with a low extraction ratio (low-extraction drugs) are dependent on intrinsic metabolic activity for metabolism, and the rate of metabolism will reflect changes in intrinsic clearance and protein binding. Furthermore, hepatic biotransformation involves two types of metabolic processes: phase I reactions and phase II reactions. Phase I reactions involve the cytochrome P450 system and include hydrolysis, oxidation, dealkylation, and reduction reactions. Phase II reactions involve conjugation of the drug with an endogenous molecule such as sulfate or an amino acid, rendering it more water soluble and enhancing its elimination. Drugs metabolized by phase I reactions, especially oxidation, tend to be significantly impaired in patients with cirrhosis, whereas drugs eliminated by conjugation are relatively unaffected.

The variability and complexity of the interaction between the extent and severity of liver disease and individual characteristics of the drug make it difficult to predict the degree of pharmacokinetic perturbation in an individual patient. Unfortunately, there are no sensitive and specific clinical or biochemical markers that allow us to quantify the extent of liver insufficiency or the degree of metabolic activity. In addition, renal insufficiency and alterations that commonly accompany cirrhosis further complicate empiric dosing recommendations in these patients. Dosing recommendations are most commonly nonspecific, with recommendations labeled for patients with mild to moderate liver impairment. Dosing information for patients with more severe liver impairment is not available. As a result, when patients with cirrhosis require therapy with drugs that undergo hepatic metabolism (e.g., benzodiazepines), monitoring response to therapy and anticipating drug accumulation and enhanced effects is essential. In the case of benzodiazepines, selection of an agent such as lorazepam, an intermediate-acting agent that is metabolized via conjugation and has no active metabolites, is easier to monitor than a drug such as diazepam, a long-acting benzodiazepine that is oxidized in the liver and has an active metabolite with a long half-life of its own.

EVALUATION OF THERAPEUTIC OUTCOMES

Table 24-8 summarizes the management approach for patients with cirrhosis and includes possible adverse drug effects. Cirrhosis is generally a chronic progressive disease that requires aggressive medical management to prevent or delay common complications. Table 24-8 also lists monitoring criteria that need to be carefully followed in order to achieve the maximum benefit from the medical therapies employed and prevent adverse effects. A therapeutic plan including therapeutic end points for each medical and diet therapy needs to be developed and discussed with the patient.

ABBREVIATIONS

AASLD	American Association for the Study of Liver Diseases
ALT	alanine transaminase
AST	aspartate transaminase
EVL	endoscopic variceal ligation
GABA	γ-aminobutyric acid
GGT	γ-glutamyl transpeptidase
HE	hepatic encephalopathy
HVPG	hepatic venous pressure gradient
INR	international normalized ratio
MELD	Model for End-Stage Liver Disease
PMN	polymorphonuclear
PT	prothrombin time
SAAG	serum-ascites albumin gradient
SBP	spontaneous bacterial peritonitis
TIPS	transjugular intrahepatic portosystemic shunt

REFERENCES

1. Schuppan D, Afdhal NH. Liver cirrhosis. Lancet 2008; 371(9615):838–851.
2. Guha IN, Iredale JP. Clinical and diagnostic aspects of cirrhosis. In: Rodés J, Benhamou J, Blei A, eds. Textbook of Hepatology: From Basic Science to Clinical Practice, 3rd ed. Malden, MA: Blackwell Publishing, 2007.
3. Abboud G, Kaplowitz N. Drug-induced liver injury. Drug Saf 2007;30(4):277–294.
4. Murphy SL, Xu J, Kochanek KD. Deaths: Preliminary data for 2010. Natl Vital Stat Rep 2012;60(4):1–52.
5. Runyon BA. Management of adult patients with ascites due to cirrhosis: An update. Hepatology 2009;49(6):2087–2107.
6. Khalili M, Liao CE, Nquyen T. Liver disease. In: McPhee SJ, Hammer GD, eds. Pathophysiology of Disease, 6th ed. New York: McGraw-Hill, 2010, *http://www.accessmedicine.com/content.aspx?aID=5369827* [chapter 14].
7. Friedman SL. Hepatic stellate cells: Protean, multifunctional, and enigmatic cells of the liver. Physiol Rev 2008;88: 125–172.
8. Bosch J, Berzigotti A, Garcia-Pagan JC, et al. The management of portal hypertension: Rational basis, available treatments and future options. J Hepatol 2008;48:S68–S92.
9. Kashani A, Landaverde C, Medici V, et al. Fluid retention in cirrhosis: Pathophysiology and management. Q J Med 2008;101:71–85.
10. Bari K, Garcia-Tsao G. Treatment of portal hypertension. World J Gastroenterol 2012;18(11):1166–1175.
11. de Franchis R. Evolving consensus in portal hypertension: Report of the Baveno V consensus workshop on methodology of diagnosis and therapy in portal hypertension. J Hepatol 2010;53(4):762–768.
12. Cash WJ, McConville P, McDermott E, McCormick PA, Callender ME, McDougall NI. Current concepts in the assessment and treatment of hepatic encephalopathy. Q J Med 2010;103:9–16.
13. Blei AT, Cordoba J, Practice Parameters Committee of the American College of Gastroenterology. Hepatic encephalopathy. Am J Gastroenterol 2001;96:1968–1976.
14. Peck-Radosavljevic M. Review article: Coagulation disorders in chronic liver disease. Aliment Pharmacol Ther 2007;26(Suppl 1):21–28.
15. Heidelbaugh JJ, Bruderly M. Cirrhosis and chronic liver failure, I: Diagnosis and evaluation. Am Fam Physician 2006;74:756–762, 781.
16. Giannini EG, Testa R, Savarino V. Liver enzyme alteration: A guide for clinicians. Can Med Assoc J 2005;172(3): 367–379.
17. Cohen JA, Kaplan MM. The SGOT/SGPT ratio—An indicator of alcoholic disease. Dig Dis Sci 1979;24:835–838.
18. Pugh RNH, Murray-Lyon IM, Dawson JL, et al. Transection of the oesophagus for bleeding oesophagus varices. Br J Surg 1973;60:646–649.
19. About the MELD/PELD Calculator, *http://optn.transplant.hrsa.gov/resources/MeldPeldCalculator.asp?index=97.*
20. MELD/PELD Calculator Documentation, *http://www.unos.org/docs/MELD_PELD_Calculator_Documentation.pdf.*
21. Garcia-Tsao G, Lim J, Members of the Veterans Affairs Hepatitis C Resource Center Program. Management and treatment of patients with cirrhosis and portal hypertension: Recommendations from the Department of Veterans Affairs Hepatitis C Resource Center Program and the National Hepatitis C Program. Am J Gastroenterol 2009;104: 1802–1829.
22. Garcia-Tsao G, Sanyal AJ, Grace ND, et al. Prevention and management of gastroesophageal varices and variceal hemorrhage in cirrhosis. Hepatology 2007;46(3):922–938.
23. de Franchis R. Somatostatin, somatostatin analogues and other vasoactive drugs in the treatment of bleeding oesophageal varices. Dig Liver Dis 2005;36(Suppl 1): S93–S100.
24. Imperiale TF, Teran JC, McCullough AJ. A meta-analysis of somatostatin versus vasopressin in the management of acute esophageal variceal hemorrhage. Gastroenterology 1995;109(4):1289–1294.
25. Zheng M, Chen Y, Bai J, et al. Transjugular intrahepatic portosystemic shunt versus endoscopic therapy in the secondary prophylaxis of variceal rebleeding in cirrhotic patients meta-analysis update. J Clin Gastroenterol 2008; 42(5):507–516.
26. Gluud LL, Langholz E, Drag A. Meta-analysis: Isosorbide-mononitrate alone or with either β-blockers or endoscopic therapy for the management of oesophageal varices. Aliment Pharmacol Ther 2010;32:859–871.
27. Garcia-Tsao G, Bosch J. Management of varices and variceal hemorrhage in cirrhosis. N Engl J Med 2010; 362:823–832.
28. Gonzalez R, Zamora J, Gomez-Camarero J, Molinero LM, Bañares R, Albillos A. Meta-analysis: Combination endoscopic and drug therapy to prevent variceal rebleeding in cirrhosis. Ann Intern Med 2008;149:109–122.
29. Koulaouzidis A, Bhat S, Saeed AA. Spontaneous bacterial peritonitis. World J Gastroenterol 2009;15(9):1042–1049.
30. Mas A. Hepatic encephalopathy: From pathophysiology to treatment. Digestion 2006;73(Suppl 1):86–93.
31. Stewart CA, Cerhan J. Hepatic encephalopathy: A dynamic or static condition. Metab Brain Dis 2005;20(3):193–204.
32. Plauth M, Cabré E, Kondrup J, et al. ESPEN guidelines on parenteral nutrition: Hepatology. Clin Nutr 2009;28(4): 436–444.
33. Charlton M. Branched-chain amino acid enriched supplements as therapy for liver disease. J Nutr 2006;136: 295S–298S.
34. Morgan MY, Blei A, Grüngreiff K, et al. The treatment of hepatic encephalopathy. Metab Brain Dis 2007;22: 389–405.
35. Bass NM, Mullen KD, Sanyal A, et al. Rifaximin treatment in hepatic encephalopathy. N Engl J Med 2010;362: 1071–1081.
36. Garcia-Tsao G, Parikh CR, Viola A. Acute kidney injury in cirrhosis. Hepatology 2008;48:2064–2077.
37. Rodriquez-Roisin R, Krowka MJ. Hepatopulmonary syndrome—A liver-induced lung vascular disorder. N Engl J Med 2008;358:2378–2387.
38. Minemura M, Tajri K, Shimizu Y. Systemic abnormalities in liver disease. World J Gastroenterol 2009;15(24):2960–2974.
39. Verbeeck RK. Pharmacokinetics and dosage adjustment in patients with hepatic dysfunction. Eur J Clin Pharmacol 2008;64:1147–1161.

25

Pancreatitis

Scott Bolesta and Patricia A. Montgomery

KEY CONCEPTS

ACUTE PANCREATITIS

1. Factors that can contribute to acute pancreatitis should be corrected, including discontinuation of medications that could be potential causes.
2. Patients with acute pancreatitis without the systemic inflammatory response syndrome should receive aggressive fluid replacement, but goal-directed therapy has not been defined.
3. Patients with severe acute pancreatitis and the systemic inflammatory response syndrome require early and aggressive IV fluid resuscitation and should be managed similarly to patients with sepsis.
4. Parenteral opioid analgesics are used to control abdominal pain associated with acute pancreatitis.
5. The only definitive indication for antibiotic use in acute pancreatitis is to treat known or suspected infection.

CHRONIC PANCREATITIS

6. Chronic pain, malabsorption with resultant steatorrhea, and diabetes mellitus are the hallmark complications and symptoms of chronic pancreatitis.
7. Pain from chronic pancreatitis can initially be treated with nonopioid analgesics, but opioids will eventually be required as the disease progresses.
8. Reduction in dietary fat intake and pancreatic enzyme supplementation are the primary treatments for malabsorption due to chronic pancreatitis.
9. Enteric-coated pancreatic enzyme supplements are the preferred dosage form in the treatment of malabsorption and steatorrhea due to chronic pancreatitis.
10. The addition of an antisecretory agent to pancreatic enzyme supplementation may increase the effectiveness of enzyme therapy for malabsorption and steatorrhea due to chronic pancreatitis.

Pancreatitis is inflammation of the pancreas with variable involvement of regional tissues or remote organ systems.[1,2] Acute pancreatitis is characterized by severe pain in the upper abdomen and elevations of pancreatic enzymes in the blood.[2] In the majority of patients, acute pancreatitis is a mild, self-limiting disease that resolves spontaneously without complications. Approximately 20% of adults with acute pancreatitis have a severe course, and 10% to 30% of those with severe acute pancreatitis die.[1,2] Severe pancreatitis with either organ failure or infected necrosis is associated with a mortality of approximately 30% and it increases when both are present.[3] Although exocrine and endocrine pancreatic functions may remain impaired for variable periods after an attack, acute pancreatitis usually does not progress to chronic pancreatitis.[4]

Chronic pancreatitis is characterized by long-standing inflammation that eventually leads to a loss of pancreatic exocrine and endocrine functions.[4–6] It is a progressive disease that often goes unnoticed for many years. Usually patients first present with complaints of chronic abdominal pain. Later in the disease process malabsorption with resultant steatorrhea occurs. This leads to malnutrition and weight loss. Finally, patients develop diabetes mellitus due to a loss of pancreatic endocrine function.[4,5]

EPIDEMIOLOGY

The prevalence of pancreatitis varies widely with geographic, etiologic (e.g., alcohol consumption), environmental, and genetic factors. Hospitalizations for acute pancreatitis have increased in the United States, most likely related to an increase in gallstones in association with obesity.[7] Admission rates for acute pancreatitis are approximately 40 per 100,000 per year in the United States.[7] Approximately 6 per 100,000 population will develop chronic pancreatitis with a peak incidence between ages 35 and 54 and about 85% of cases occurring in men.[6] However, this incidence may be underestimated due to diagnostic difficulties and various classification systems. Also, the prevalence of chronic pancreatitis varies widely based on geographic location.[4,6] Hospitalization for chronic pancreatitis has also doubled in the past decade with black patients being almost two to three times as likely to be hospitalized for chronic pancreatitis than for alcoholic cirrhosis.[6]

PANCREATIC EXOCRINE PHYSIOLOGY

The pancreas possesses both endocrine and exocrine functions. The islets of Langerhans, which contain the cells of the endocrine pancreas, secrete insulin, glucagon, somatostatin, and other polypeptide hormones. The exocrine pancreas is composed of acini and ductules that secrete about 2.5 L/day of isotonic fluid that contains water, electrolytes, and pancreatic enzymes necessary for digestion. Bicarbonate and other electrolytes are secreted primarily by the centroacinar (ductular) cells in order to neutralize gastric acid. Pancreatic juice is delivered to the duodenum via the pancreatic ducts (Fig. 25-1) where the alkaline secretion neutralizes gastric acid and provides an appropriate pH for maintaining the activity of pancreatic enzymes.[8]

The major pancreatic exocrine enzyme groups are as follows:

1. Amylolytic: amylase
2. Lipolytic: lipase, procolipase, prophospholipase A_2, and carboxylesterase

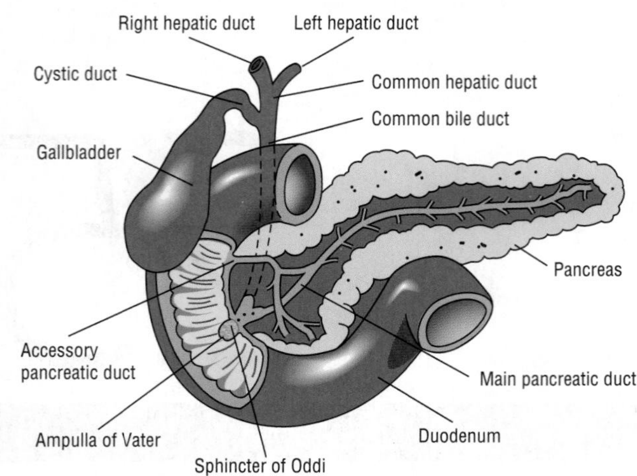

FIGURE 25-1 Anatomic structure of the pancreas and biliary tract.

3. Proteolytic: trypsinogen, chymotrypsinogen, procarboxypeptidase, and proelastase
4. Nucleolytic: ribonuclease and deoxyribonuclease
5. Other: trypsin inhibitor

Amylase is responsible for digestion of starches and glycogen through hydrolysis. The lipolytic enzymes break down triglycerides, cholesterol, and other fats in the digestive tract. Specifically, lipase hydrolyzes triglycerides into fatty acids and monoglycerides. Colipase and bile acids facilitate this process by allowing lipase to act on the hydrophobic surface of fat droplets in the mainly hydrophilic environment. Phospholipase A_2 and carboxylesterase continue to break down fatty acids, cholesterol, monoglycerides, and other products of fat digestion. Proteolytic enzymes digest proteins into oligopeptides and free amino acids, while nucleases break down nucleic acids.[8,9]

The production of proteolytic enzymes in the pancreas occurs in a manner that prevents self-digestion of the pancreas. These enzymes are synthesized within the acinar cells and secreted into the duodenum as zymogens (inactive enzymes). Enterokinase secreted by the duodenal mucosa converts trypsinogen to trypsin, which then activates all other proteolytic zymogens along with procolipase and prophospholipase A_2. Thus, two important mechanisms protect the pancreas from the potential degradative action of its own digestive enzymes. First, the synthesis of proteolytic enzymes as zymogens requires extrapancreatic activation by trypsin. Second, pancreatic juice contains a low concentration of trypsin inhibitor, which inactivates any autocatalytically formed trypsin within the pancreas. Proteolytic activity of trypsin in the intestinal lumen is not inhibited because the concentration of trypsin inhibitor is minimal. Lipase, amylase, ribonuclease, and deoxyribonuclease are secreted by the acinar cells in their active form.[8]

The regulation of exocrine pancreatic secretion is a complex interplay of neurohormonal feedback with three distinct phases. The first phase is the cephalic phase where the sight, smell, and taste of food produce pancreatic enzyme secretion through stimulus of the vagus nerve. Vasoactive intestinal peptide (VIP) and gastrin-releasing peptide (GRP) released from efferent vagus nerve terminals bind to receptors on the acinar cells stimulating enzyme release.[8] Water and bicarbonate are also released from ductal cells due to VIP stimulation. The gastric phase occurs due to gastric distension from food entering the stomach. This results primarily in secretion of digestive enzymes from the pancreas. Once chyme enters the duodenum, the intestinal phase begins. The chyme causes secretin to be released from the duodenal mucosa when its pH is less than 4.5. Secretin results in water and bicarbonate secretion from the pancreas, which is necessary since lipolytic enzymes are inactivated at a pH below 5.[9] Digestive enzymes are released from the pancreas due to the presence of fatty acids, peptides, amino acids, and glucose in the duodenum.[8]

The feedback mechanism for continued release of pancreatic enzymes involves the hormone cholecystokinin (CCK). When products of fat, protein, and starch digestion enter the upper small intestine, they stimulate release of CCK from I cells into the blood. Elevated levels of CCK in the serum activate a vagovagal reflex causing further release of VIP and GRP, leading to enhanced pancreatic enzyme secretion. Inhibition of this feedback loop is thought to be due to trypsin. After digestion is complete, unoccupied trypsin is thought to inhibit the release of CCK.[8] A more in-depth discussion of pancreatic physiology can be found elsewhere.[8]

ACUTE PANCREATITIS

Acute pancreatitis varies from mild to severe disease. The morphologic appearance of the pancreas and surrounding tissue ranges from interstitial edema and inflammatory cells (interstitial pancreatitis) to pancreatic and extrapancreatic necrosis (necrotizing pancreatitis). Necrotizing pancreatitis has a higher risk of infection, organ failure, and mortality.[10,11] The rupture of blood vessels within or around the pancreas can also lead to a collection of blood in the retroperitoneal space.

Etiology

Table 25-1 lists the etiologic risk factors associated with acute pancreatitis. Obstruction caused by gallstones is the most common cause of acute pancreatitis and alcohol abuse the second; together they account for 70% to 80% of all cases of acute pancreatitis.[6] Genetic and autoimmune causes of acute pancreatitis have been identified.[14] Most of the remaining cases are idiopathic.[2] Acute pancreatitis can occur as a result of an endoscopic retrograde cholangiopancreatography (ERCP) procedure and is more common following therapeutic ERCP than diagnostic, with overall rates of 1.6% to 5.4% and 0.4% to 5.4%, respectively. High-risk populations may have rates of acute pancreatitis as high as 15%.[15] Cigarette smoking appears to increase the risk of pancreatitis, especially in alcohol-related

TABLE 25-1 Etiologic Risk Factors Associated with Acute Pancreatitis

Structural	Gallstone disease, sphincter of Oddi dysfunction, pancreas divisum, pancreatic tumors
Toxins	Alcohol (ethanol) consumption, scorpion bite, organophosphate insecticides
Infectious	Bacterial, viral (including HIV and H1N1 influenza), parasitic
Metabolic	Hypertriglyceridemia, chronic hypercalcemia
Genetic	Cystic fibrosis, α_1-antitrypsin deficiency, hereditary (trypsinogen gene mutations)
Medications	See Table 25-2 for specific drugs
Iatrogenic	Abdominal surgery, ERCP
Kidney disease	Chronic kidney disease, dialysis-related
Trauma	Blunt abdominal trauma
Vascular	Vasculitis, atherosclerosis, cholesterol emboli, coronary artery bypass surgery
Other etiologies	Congenital, Crohn's disease, autoimmune, tropical, solid organ transplantation (e.g., liver, kidney, heart), refeeding syndrome
Idiopathic	Undetermined cause

HIV, human immunodeficiency virus; ERCP, endoscopic retrograde cholangiopancreatography.

From references 7, 10, 12, and 13.

disease.[16] Pregnancy is not considered a cause of acute pancreatitis; however, pregnant women develop pancreatitis as a result of a coincident process, most commonly cholelithiasis. In pediatric patients, the common etiologies are systemic illness, biliary disease, trauma, and medications.[17]

Medications

Drug-induced acute pancreatitis should be suspected when other causes have been excluded and there is a temporal relationship with the initiation of a medication that has been implicated as a cause. The percentage of acute pancreatitis cases caused by medications is reported to be 0.1 to 2.[18] Most information on drug-induced acute pancreatitis is obtained from case reports, which do not provide reliable information on incidence. The most convincing case reports involve recurrence on rechallenge; however, rechallenge is rare, occurring only when alternative therapy is not available. When evaluating case reports, clinicians should review data supporting the diagnosis of acute pancreatitis, attempts to rule out other causes, and the onset of acute pancreatitis in relation to drug therapy. Further complicating the evaluation of some reports is that certain patient populations may have an increased risk of pancreatitis.

Proton pump inhibitors and histamine$_2$-receptor antagonists may be initiated in response to early symptoms of unrecognized pancreatitis and may confound the association between the drug and the disease. However, a retrospective cohort study does not support an association between acute pancreatitis and proton pump inhibitors or histamine$_2$-receptor antagonists.[19] Medications that alter serum lipid concentrations, such as propofol and tamoxifen, are associated with pancreatitis from hyperlipidemia.[20,21] In contrast, a meta-analysis of lipid-lowering therapies found that statins were associated with a decreased number of acute pancreatitis cases.[22] Pancreatitis was not a stated end point of any of the trials included and there are numerous case reports of apparent drug-induced pancreatitis with statins. There is a higher incidence of drug-induced acute pancreatitis in U.S. patients with human immunodeficiency virus (HIV) treated with antiretroviral therapy.[23] However, there was no increase in acute pancreatitis associated with antiretroviral use in a well-controlled trial including data from 33,742 person-years.[24] Medications used in the treatment of inflammatory bowel disease and type II diabetes mellitus have also been associated with a higher incidence of drug-induced acute pancreatitis.[25,26] In addition, patients with diabetes mellitus may also have an inherent increased risk of acute pancreatitis. The commonly prescribed medication metformin is associated with acute pancreatitis at toxic serum concentrations.[27] There have also been case reports of acute pancreatitis in patients receiving some of the newer antihyperglycemic agents, including the dipeptidyl peptidase-4 (DPP-4) inhibitors, sitagliptin, linagliptin, and vildagliptin, and the glucagon-like peptide-1 (GLP-1) receptor agonists, exenatide and liraglutide.[18] Exenatide and liraglutide continue to account for a substantial percentage of drug-induced pancreatitis reported to the U.S. FDA.[28]

The onset of drug-induced pancreatitis after initiation of medications ranges from a few months to several years, with a median of 5 weeks; onset after rechallenge can occur within hours. The onset may differ according to the mechanism. Clinicians should be especially suspicious of drug-induced acute pancreatitis in high-risk patients, such as those receiving immunomodulating drugs or who have HIV infection, the elderly, or those with diabetes mellitus.[18]

Mechanisms of drug-induced pancreatitis are not clearly defined but may fall into several general categories, including direct toxic effects of the drug or its metabolites, hypersensitivity, drug-induced hypertriglyceridemia, and alterations of cellular function in the pancreas and pancreatic duct.[26] Once the process is initiated, disease severity is determined by the propagation of proinflammatory mediators. Although acute pancreatitis is an infrequent complication of drug therapy, it is prudent to withdraw medication when an association is suspected.

Numerous drugs are believed to cause acute pancreatitis, but ethical and practical considerations prevent rechallenge with suspected agents. Table 25-2 lists specific agents associated with acute pancreatitis based on known association. Class I (definite association) implies a temporal relationship of drug administration to abdominal pain and hyperamylasemia in at least 20 reported cases with at least one positive response to rechallenge with the offending

TABLE 25-2 Medications Associated with Acute Pancreatitis

Class I (Definite Association)	Class II (Probable Association)	Class III (Possible Association)	
5-Aminosalicylic acid	Acetaminophen	Aldesleukin	Indomethacin
Asparaginase	Carbamazepine	Amiodarone	Infliximab
Azathioprine	Cisplatin	Atorvastatin	Ketoprofen
Corticosteroids	Erythromycin	Bortezomib	Ketorolac
Cytarabine	Hydrochlorothiazide	Asparaginase	Lipid emulsion
Didanosine	Ifosfamide	Calcium	Lisinopril
Enalapril	Interferon α_{2b}	Capecitabine	Mefenamic acid
Estrogens	Lamivudine	Celecoxib	Metformin
Furosemide	Octreotide	Clozapine	Methyldopa
Mercaptopurine	Sitagliptin	Cholestyramine	Metolazone
Opiates		Cimetidine	Metronidazole
Pentamidine		Ciprofloxacin	Nitrofurantoin
Pentavalent antimonials		Clarithromycin	Omeprazole
Sulfasalazine		Clonidine	Ondansetron
Sulfamethoxazole and trimethoprim		Cyclosporine	Paclitaxel
Sulindac		Danazol	Pravastatin
Tamoxifen		Diazoxide	Propofol
Tetracycline		Etanercept	Propoxyphene
Valproic acid/salts		Ethacrynic acid	Rifampin
		Exenatide	Sertraline
		Famciclovir	Zalcitabine
		Glyburide	
		Gold therapy	
		Granisetron	
		Ibuprofen	
		Indinavir	

From references 18, 25, 29–32.

agent. Class II medications are implicated in more than 10, but less than 20, reported cases of acute pancreatitis and suggest a probable association. Class III includes medications with a possible association, defined as fewer than 10 published cases or unpublished reports in pharmaceutical or FDA files. Table 25-2 only includes selected class III medications. A comprehensive list of class III drugs can be found elsewhere.[33]

Pathophysiology

The pathophysiology of acute pancreatitis is based on events that initiate injury and secondary events that establish and perpetuate the injury (Fig. 25-2). Alcohol abuse and gallstones cause different initial insults to the pancreas. However, acute pancreatitis of any etiology has long been thought to result from the premature activation of trypsinogen to trypsin within the pancreas, leading to activation of other digestive enzymes and autodigestion of the gland.[2] The lysosomal proteinase, cathepsin B, and intracellular calcium may be involved in the activation of trypsinogen as well as decreased activity of trypsin inhibitor.[34] Genetic abnormalities in pathways that protect the pancreas from autodigestion also play a pathophysiologic role in the development of some forms of acute pancreatitis, and may be the differentiating factor in the minority of alcoholics who develop disease.[35]

In addition to increased production, activated enzymes are retained in the acinar cells in higher concentrations than normal.[36] Activated pancreatic enzymes released into the pancreas and surrounding tissues produce damage and necrosis to the pancreatic tissue, the surrounding fat, the vascular endothelium, and adjacent structures. Lipase damages the fat cells, producing noxious substances that cause further pancreatic and peripancreatic injury. The release of cytokines by acinar cells directly causes their injury and enhances the inflammatory response.[34] Injured acinar cells liberate chemoattractants that recruit neutrophils, macrophages, and other cells to the area of inflammation. These immune responses cause a systemic inflammatory response syndrome (SIRS). Vascular damage and ischemia causes the release of kinins, which makes capillary walls permeable and promotes tissue edema. The release of damaging oxygen-free radicals appears to correlate with the severity of pancreatic injury.[10] Finally, pancreatic infection may result from increased intestinal permeability and translocation of colonic bacteria.[35]

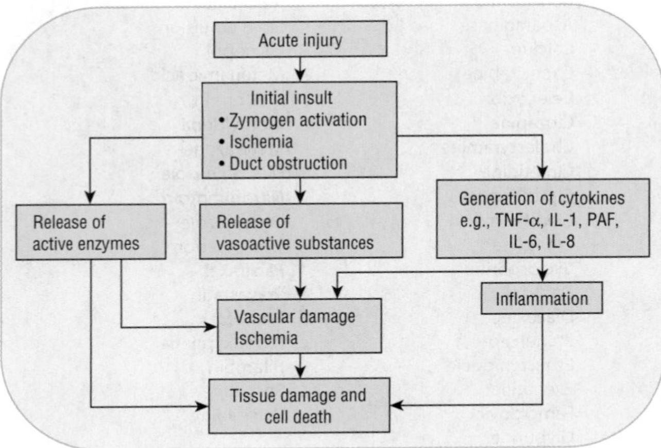

FIGURE 25-2 Pathophysiology of acute pancreatitis: initiating and secondary events. (IL-1β, interleukin-1β; IL-6, interleukin-6; IL-8, interleukin-8; PAF, platelet-activating factor; TNF-α, tumor necrosis factor-α.)

Complications

Early complications are a result of fluid losses and SIRS. Hypotension results from hypovolemia, hypoalbuminemia, the release of kinins, and sepsis. Even patients with mild disease have significant fluid losses. Renal complications are usually caused by hypovolemia. The most common systemic complication of acute pancreatitis is respiratory failure.[1] GI bleeding occurs secondary to numerous causes including rupture of a pseudocyst. Severe acute pancreatitis is also associated with confusion and coma.

Local complications—including acute fluid collection, pancreatic necrosis, infection, abscess (collection of pus in or adjacent to the pancreas), and pseudocyst—develop approximately 3 to 4 weeks after the initial attack. Pancreatic infections occur in 15% to 30% of those with pancreatic necrosis and are usually secondary infections of necrotic tissue.[7] Pancreatic ascites occurs when pancreatic secretions spread throughout the peritoneal cavity. Systemic complications include cardiovascular, renal, pulmonary, metabolic, hemorrhagic, and CNS abnormalities.[10] Long-term complications include glucose intolerance and recurrence of acute pancreatitis.[37]

Clinical Presentation

Signs and Symptoms

The clinical presentation of acute pancreatitis varies depending on the severity of the inflammatory process and whether damage is confined to the pancreas or involves local and systemic complications (Table 25-3).[7]

Diagnosis

Most guidelines agree that the diagnosis should be made within 48 hours based on characteristic abdominal pain and amylase, lipase, or both that are elevated to at least three times the upper limit of normal. Lipase is more sensitive and specific than amylase and is preferred. Contrast-enhanced computed tomography (CECT) of the abdomen may be used to confirm the diagnosis, including in patients with amylase or lipase that is not three times the upper limit of normal. Some guidelines consider ultrasonography to be an acceptable alternative to CECT.[1,10,41] However, it is best used to ascertain the presence of gallstones. The diagnosis of acute pancreatitis should also be considered when evaluating patients with SIRS (see Table 25-3).[10,41,42] For further information on laboratory tests and abdominal imaging, refer to Table 25-3.

Prediction of Disease Severity Prediction of severity of acute pancreatitis is useful for decisions involving the need for aggressive treatment, including admission to an intensive care unit. The risk for severe acute pancreatitis should be assessed on admission and on an ongoing basis.[10,11] Several scoring systems have been developed to assess the likelihood of severe disease (Table 25-4). However, development and validation of such systems remains an ongoing area of research. Scoring systems are developed based on retrospectively identified associations between clinical and laboratory findings and morbidity and mortality.[1,43,44] Many are too complicated for bedside use or rely on measurements that are not widely available. Some scoring systems have not been validated in prospective trials or have poor predictive ability.

The first scoring system developed for pancreatitis was the Ranson's criteria. It assesses 11 variables that must be monitored at the time of admission and during the initial 48 hours of hospitalization.[10] Severe acute pancreatitis is characterized by three or more criteria. While still used by many clinicians, the Ranson's score does not correlate well with disease severity. The Atlanta scoring system was developed based on consensus opinions; it consolidates clinical indicators, organ failure, and local complications to provide an ongoing assessment of disease severity.[7]

TABLE 25-3 Presentation and Diagnosis of Acute Pancreatitis

General

- The patient may have acute mild symptoms or present with a severe acute attack with life-threatening complications

Symptoms

- The patient may present initially with moderate abdominal discomfort to excruciating pain, nausea, shock, and respiratory distress
- Abdominal pain occurs in 95% of patients. The pain is usually epigastric and radiates to either of the upper quadrants or the back in two thirds of patients. In gallstone pancreatitis, the pain is typically sudden and quite severe and the intensity is often described as "knife-like" or "boring." The pain usually reaches its maximum intensity within 30 minutes and may persist for hours or days. Repositioning the patient relieves very little of the pain. In alcohol abuse and other cases, the onset of pain may be less abrupt and poorly localized. Pain may not be the dominant symptom if it is masked by multiorgan failure
- Nausea and vomiting occur in 85% of patients and usually follow the onset of abdominal pain. Vomiting does not provide relief of the abdominal pain

Signs

- Marked epigastric or diffuse tenderness on palpation with rebound tenderness and guarding in severe cases. The abdomen is often distended and tympanic, with bowel sounds decreased or absent in severe disease
- Vital signs may be normal, but hypotension, tachycardia, and low-grade fever are often observed, especially with widespread pancreatic inflammation and necrosis
- Dyspnea and tachypnea are often signs of acute respiratory complications. Jaundice and altered mental status may be present and have multiple causes. Other signs of alcoholic liver disease may be present in patients with alcoholic pancreatitis

Laboratory tests

- Leukocytosis is frequently present; hyperglycemia or hypoalbuminemia may be present. Liver transaminases, alkaline phosphatase, and bilirubin are usually elevated in gallstone pancreatitis and in patients with intrinsic liver disease. Elevated serum triglycerides may also be a possible etiology
- The hematocrit may be normal, but hemoconcentration results from multiple factors (e.g., vomiting). In patients with third-space fluid loss, hemoconcentration is present and a reasonably accurate marker of severe disease. A hematocrit concentration of greater than 47% (0.47) predicts severe acute pancreatitis and one of less than 44% (0.44) predicts mild disease. Further, failure to reverse hemoconcentration has been associated with pancreatic necrosis
- Blood urea nitrogen (BUN) that is elevated or rising over the first 24 hours has been associated with increased mortality
- The total serum calcium is usually normal initially, but hypocalcemia disproportionate to the hypoalbuminemia may develop. Marked hypocalcemia is an indication of severe necrosis and a poor prognostic sign
- The serum amylase concentration usually rises within 4–8 hours of the initial attack, peaks at 24 hours, and returns to normal over the next 8–14 days. Serum amylase concentrations greater than three times the upper limit of normal are highly suggestive of acute pancreatitis. Persistent elevations suggest extensive pancreatic necrosis and related complications. Normal concentrations may be observed if testing is delayed (i.e., amylase may have returned to normal) or in patients with hyperlipidemic pancreatitis (i.e., marked triglyceride elevations may interfere with amylase assay). In addition, many nonpancreatic diseases may be associated with hyperamylasemia, including salivary, kidney, hepatobiliary, metabolic, female reproductive tract, and neoplastic diseases
- Serum lipase is specific to the pancreas and concentrations are elevated and parallel the elevations in serum amylase. Levels remain elevated with pancreatic inflammation and return to normal when the inflammatory process resolves. Because of its longer half-life, elevations of serum lipase can be detected after the serum amylase has returned to normal
- Additional biomarkers: C-reactive protein (CRP) is a widely available test and levels greater than 150 mg/L at 48–72 hours predict severe acute pancreatitis with accuracy similar to that of APACHE II. Urinary trypsinogen activation peptide is specific for acute pancreatitis but not sensitive and not widely available. Procalcitonin has been studied for severity assessment as well as identification of patients with bacterial infection, but is not routinely utilized or widely available
- Thrombocytopenia and an increase in the international normalized ratio are seen in some patients with severe acute pancreatitis and associated liver disease

Abdominal imaging

- CECT is used to identify the cause of pancreatitis and confirm the diagnosis. It is less accurate for evaluating the gallbladder and biliary ducts. The test distinguishes interstitial from necrotizing pancreatitis, but does not distinguish between fat necrosis and acute fluid collection. Tests that are performed in the first few days may miss necrosis. A CECT performed too early may result in unnecessary exposure to risk and increased cost. Formal scoring systems may be used to evaluate the findings
- Magnetic resonance imaging is used to grade the severity of acute pancreatitis, identify biliary duct problems that are not seen on CT, or if there are contraindications to CECT. Patients over the age of 40 with pancreatitis of an unknown etiology should be evaluated for pancreatic malignancy with CT or endoscopic ultrasonography
- Ultrasonography of the abdomen is useful to determine pancreatic enlargement and peripancreatic fluid collections. It is also sensitive for detecting dilated biliary ducts and stones in the gallbladder

APACHE, Acute Physiology and Chronic Health Evaluation; CECT, contrast-enhanced computed tomography; CT, computed tomography.

From references 38–40.

The Acute Physiology and Chronic Health Evaluation II (APACHE II) system uses 12 indicators of physiologic and biochemical function, age, and previous health status to predict mortality in critically ill patients, but it is not specific to pancreatitis. The APACHE II score is calculated within the first 24 hours and is considered among the best predictors of severity on admission. A score greater than or equal to 8 points is associated with an increased risk of organ failure and mortality.[10] Other scoring systems include the Bedside Index of Severity in Acute Pancreatitis (BISAP), the Harmless Acute Pancreatitis Score (HAPS), and a computer-based tool using blood urea nitrogen (BUN), pleural effusion, and serum calcium. SIRS criteria alone are sensitive for predicting organ failure and death, but are not specific to severe acute pancreatitis.[1,44]

Clinical Course and Prognosis

The clinical course of acute pancreatitis varies from a mild transitory disorder to a severe necrotizing disease. Mild acute pancreatitis is self-limiting and subsides spontaneously within 3 to 5 days. Mortality is influenced by etiology, as idiopathic and postoperative acute pancreatitis have higher rates than gallstone- or alcohol-related disease. First and second occurrences also carry a higher mortality than subsequent episodes. Mortality increases with unfavorable early prognostic signs, local complications, and organ failure. Persistent organ failure is a greater risk than transient organ failure.[3] Severe pancreatitis with either organ failure or infected necrosis is associated with a mortality of approximately 30%, which increases when both are present.[3] Death during the first few days results from SIRS and multiorgan failure. When death occurs after this period, it is usually a result of infected necrosis, pancreatic abscess, and sepsis.[10]

TREATMENT
Acute Pancreatitis

Desired Outcome

Treatment of acute pancreatitis is aimed at relieving abdominal pain and nausea, replacing fluids, correcting electrolyte, glucose, and lipid abnormalities, minimizing systemic complications, and

TABLE 25-4 Prognostic Indicators for Severe Acute Pancreatitis

Prognostic Factor	Criterion
Ranson's criteria	
On admission	
Age (years)	>55
WBC (cells/mm³)	>16,000 (>16 × 10⁹/L)
Glucose (mg/dL)	>200 (>11.1 mmol/L)
LDH (international units/L)	>350 (>5.83 μkat/L)
AST (units/L)	>250 (>4.17 μkat/L)
Within 48 hours of admission	
Decrease in hematocrit (% points)	>10 (>0.10)
Increase in BUN (mg/dL)	>5 (>1.8 mmol/L)
Calcium (mg/dL)	<8 (<2 mmol/L)
PaO_2 (mm Hg)	<60 (<8 kPa)
Base deficit (mmol/L)	>4
Estimated fluid deficit (L)	>6
Atlanta criteria	
Unfavorable prognostic signs	
Ranson's criteria	≥3
APACHE II score	≥8
Organ failure (shock)	
Systolic blood pressure (mm Hg)	<90
Pulmonary insufficiency (PaO_2, mm Hg)	<60 (<8 kPa)
Kidney failure after hydration (serum creatinine [mg/dL])	>2 (177 μmol/L)
GI tract bleeding (mL in 24 hours)	>500
Systemic complications	
Disseminated intravascular coagulation	
Platelets (mm³)	≤100,000 (≤100 × 10⁹/L)
Fibrinogen (g/L)	<1
Fibrin-split products (mcg/mL or mg/L)	>80
Metabolic disturbance	
Calcium (mg/dL)	≤7.5 (≤1.88 mmol/L)
Local complications	
Pseudocyst	Present
Necrosis	Present
Abscess	Present

WBC, white blood cells; LDH, lactate dehydrogenase; AST, aspartate aminotransferase; BUN, blood urea nitrogen; PaO_2, partial pressure of arterial oxygen; APACHE, Acute Physiology and Chronic Health Evaluation.

From references 7, 10, 43, and 44.

preventing pancreatic necrosis and infection. Management varies depending on the severity of the attack (Fig. 25-3). Patients with mild acute pancreatitis respond very well to the initiation of supportive care and the reduction of pancreatic secretions. Patients with severe acute pancreatitis should be treated aggressively and monitored closely.

General Approach to Treatment

All patients with acute pancreatitis should receive supportive care, including IV fluid resuscitation, adequate nutrition, and effective relief of pain and nausea. The use of nasogastric aspiration offers no clear advantage in patients with mild acute pancreatitis, but it is beneficial in patients with profound pain, severe disease, paralytic ileus, and intractable vomiting.[10] Patients predicted to follow a severe course will require treatment of cardiovascular, respiratory, renal, and metabolic complications.[1] Aggressive fluid resuscitation is essential to correct intravascular volume depletion.[45] Patients with pancreatitis and SIRS should be treated according to SIRS guidelines. IV potassium, calcium, and magnesium are used to correct electrolyte deficiency states. Insulin is used to treat hyperglycemia. Local complications resolve as the inflammatory process subsides. However, patients with necrotizing pancreatitis may require antibiotics and surgical intervention.[10] Medications listed in Table 25-2 should be discontinued if possible (1).

Nonpharmacologic Therapy

Nonpharmacologic therapy includes ERCP for removal of any underlying biliary tract stones, surgery, and nutritional support. Surgery is indicated in patients with pancreatic pseudocyst or abscess or to drain the pancreatic bed if hemorrhagic or necrotic material is present. The need for admission to an intensive care unit should also be addressed. Advances in minimally invasive surgical techniques are changing practice with respect to timing and approach to managing infected necrotizing pancreatitis, and may help lower the risk of mortality in the most critical patients.[2,11,46,47]

Nutrition and Probiotics

Nutritional support plays an important role in the management of patients with mild or severe disease as acute pancreatitis creates a catabolic state that promotes nutritional depletion. This can impair recovery, increase the risk of complications, and prolong hospitalization.[48,49] Patients with mild acute pancreatitis can begin oral feeding when bowel sounds have returned and pain has resolved.[7] In severe or complicated disease, nutritional deficits develop rapidly and are complicated by tissue necrosis, organ failure, and surgery. Nutritional support should begin when it is anticipated that oral nutrition will be withheld for more than 1 week.[50] In the past, there was concern that enteral feeding stimulated pancreatic enzyme secretion and exacerbated the underlying disease. However, a Cochrane Collaboration review that included eight randomized controlled trials found that enteral nutrition results in decreased morality, multiple organ failure, and need for surgical intervention compared with parenteral nutrition.[50] Possible mechanisms for this include protection of the gut barrier and prevention of colonization with pathogenic bacteria, both of which may prevent translocation of bacteria and infection.[11] Therefore, the enteral route is preferred over the parenteral in patients with severe acute pancreatitis provided that it can be tolerated. Ongoing trials are addressing some remaining issues such as the optimal timing to initiate enteral feeding and the safety of the nasogastric route as compared with nasojejunal. If enteral feeding is not possible or if the patient is unable to obtain sufficient nutrients, total parenteral nutrition should be implemented before protein and calorie depletion become advanced. IV lipids should not be withheld unless the serum triglyceride concentration is greater than 500 mg/dL (5.65 mmol/L).[10]

Clinical trials do not support the use of probiotics in the treatment of acute pancreatitis as they have not shown a benefit. One prospective randomized trial in patients with predicted severe acute pancreatitis showed an increase in mortality with probiotics compared with placebo.[51]

Pharmacologic Therapy

Recommendations

Patients with acute pancreatitis often require IV antiemetics for nausea. Those with severe acute pancreatitis should be treated with antisecretory agents to prevent stress-related mucosal bleeding. Patients also require appropriate fluid resuscitation and pain management, but there is controversy surrounding both of these therapies. Octreotide has been studied as a specific therapy in severe acute pancreatitis, but its efficacy remains uncertain (see Fig. 25-3). Prophylactic antibiotics used to be widely used, but clinical trials have failed to identify a group of patients that benefit from this therapy.

Fluid Resuscitation

Vasodilation from the inflammatory response, vomiting, and nasogastric suction contribute to hypovolemia and fluid and electrolyte abnormalities, thus necessitating replacement. Evidence for the benefit of adequate fluid resuscitation comes from observational studies

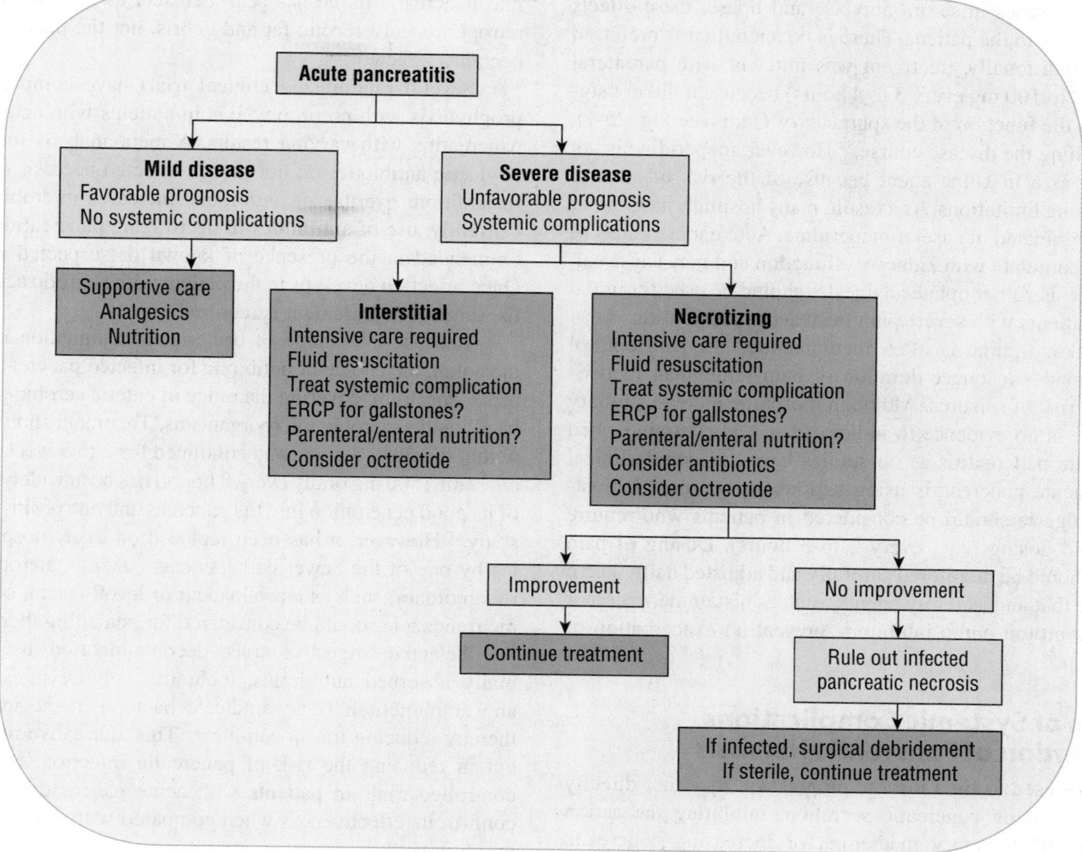

FIGURE 25-3 Algorithm of guidelines for evaluation and treatment of acute pancreatitis. (ERCP, endoscopic retrograde cholangiopancreatography.)

demonstrating an associated increase in morbidity and mortality with failure to improve laboratory indicators of hemoconcentration (i.e., hematocrit and BUN). There are no large randomized trials to provide specific recommendations. Guidelines call for rapid replacement of fluid, without details on rate or type of fluid ❷.

Observational studies have identified both benefit (decreased mortality and organ failure) and harm (abdominal compartment syndrome) associated with early aggressive fluid administration. Most studies have compared standard therapy with aggressive fluid therapy over the first 24 hours retrospectively. One trial found that administration during the first 24 hours of at least one third the cumulative volume given over the first 72 hours was associated with a decrease in mortality.[52] A similar trial found a decrease in SIRS, organ failure at 72 hours, and length of stay in patients who received more fluid during the first 24-hour period than subsequent 24-hour periods.[53] In contrast, another study found that patients who received more than 3.1 L of fluid during the first 24 hours had higher rates of persistent organ failure, respiratory failure, and renal failure than those who received smaller volumes.[54] In a prospective, randomized trial, goal-directed fluid replacement therapy of 3 mL/kg/h for the first 20 hours did not result in a reduction in SIRS or C-reactive protein (CRP).[55] Replacement at rates of 10 to 15 mL/kg/h was associated with more abdominal compartment syndrome, mechanical ventilation, and sepsis in the first 2 weeks following presentation than standard therapy in another trial.[56]

Interpretation of these trials is complicated by the likelihood that sicker patients were given larger volumes of fluid. Studies of fluid resuscitation in acute pancreatitis suggest that some patients may not require aggressive fluid resuscitation, while others may require gradual fluid administration. For example, those with reduced cardiac reserve may do better if fluid is replaced over 72 hours rather than 24 to 48 hours.[57]

In addition to questions about the rate and volume of fluid that should be administered to patients with acute pancreatitis, there is also debate regarding which fluid is most appropriate. A small randomized trial found that goal-directed resuscitation with lactated Ringer's produced a reduction in SIRS and CRP at 24 hours compared with normal saline.[55] The study protocol used aggressive replacement with a bolus of 20 mL/kg of lactated Ringer's followed by 150 to 300 mL/h for the first 24 hours. If patients responded to this therapy as assessed by BUN, the rate could be reduced to 2 mL/kg/h. Patients with SIRS or sepsis should be resuscitated according to sepsis guidelines ❸.[58]

Clinical **Controversy. . .**

Aggressive fluid resuscitation is generally recommended, but adequate studies on the volume and type of fluid have not been conducted. Excessive rates of administration have been associated with increased mortality in retrospective trials. Use of lactated Ringer's solution may be preferred over normal saline.

Relief of Abdominal Pain

Parenteral opioid analgesics are used to control abdominal pain associated with acute pancreatitis ❹. The most important factors to consider in selecting an analgesic are efficacy and safety. Although the administration of some opioids is associated with mild and transient increases in serum amylase and lipase, these effects are not deleterious to the patient. There is no agent that is preferred over others. Traditionally, treatment was initiated with parenteral meperidine (50 to 100 mg every 3 to 4 hours) because it did not significantly alter the function of the sphincter of Oddi (see Fig. 25-1), thereby worsening the disease course.[59] However, meperidine is not recommended as a first-line agent because of the risk of adverse effects and dosing limitations. As a result, many hospitals have either restricted or eliminated the use of meperidine. Active metabolites of meperidine accumulate with kidney dysfunction and may cause seizures or psychosis. Other opiate analgesics should be used for initial analgesia in patients with severe pain from acute pancreatitis.

Parenteral morphine is often recommended for pain control because it provides a longer duration of pain relief than meperidine with less risk of seizures. Although morphine increases biliary pressure, there is no evidence to indicate that it is contraindicated for use in acute pancreatitis as no studies have compared clinical outcomes of acute pancreatitis using various analgesics.[59] Patient-controlled analgesia should be considered in patients who require frequent opioid dosing (e.g., every 2 to 3 hours). Dosing of pain medications should be monitored carefully and adjusted daily. There is no evidence that antisecretory agents, such as histamine$_2$-receptor antagonists or proton pump inhibitors, prevent an exacerbation of abdominal pain.[60]

Limitation of Systemic Complications and Prevention of Pancreatic Necrosis

Agents may be used to limit disease progression by either directly or indirectly reducing pancreatic secretion, inhibiting the action of circulating inflammatory mediators, or increasing pancreatic microcirculation, but there is currently no specific therapy for acute pancreatitis. The use of parenteral histamine$_2$-receptor antagonists or proton pump inhibitors does not improve the overall outcome of patients with acute pancreatitis.[7] The platelet-activating factor inhibitor antagonist, lexipafant, was not effective in preventing organ failure in acute pancreatitis.[61] Clinical studies with protease inhibitors such as aprotinin, gabexate, and nafamostat have failed to show consistent benefit in acute pancreatitis, and their use is not supported by guidelines.[7,10,41,42,62] None of these agents is currently available in the United States. Somatostatin and its synthetic analog octreotide are potent inhibitors of pancreatic enzyme secretion and have been used to interrupt the inflammatory process. Several studies and a meta-analysis that evaluated the efficacy of somatostatin and octreotide suggest a slight trend toward benefit in patients with severe pancreatitis.[10,63] Limitations of these studies include small numbers of patients, no placebo, and inclusion of patients with mild disease. There are insufficient data to support the routine use of somatostatin or octreotide in the treatment of acute pancreatitis and guidelines do not recommend their use.[42]

Prevention of Infection

Prophylactic antibiotics do not offer any benefit in cases of mild acute pancreatitis or when there is no necrosis. Use of antibiotics in patients with severe acute pancreatic necrosis (with or without the presence of pancreatic necrosis), but without infection, is not currently supported by randomized controlled trials.

Antibiotic prophylaxis in early clinical trials showed no benefit, but these studies were limited due to inclusion of patients with a wide range of disease severity and insufficient enrollment of patients with severe necrotizing pancreatitis. In addition, they used ampicillin, which does not penetrate well into pancreatic tissue.[64] Imipenem–cilastatin, metronidazole, cefotaxime, piperacillin, mezlocillin, ofloxacin, and ciprofloxacin all achieve satisfactory bactericidal tissue concentrations, whereas aminoglycosides have poor penetration.[64–66] However, the importance of antibiotic penetration into pancreatic tissue has been debated, as it is the peripancreatic retroperitoneal necrotic fat and debris, not the pancreas itself, that becomes infected.

Several randomized clinical trials have compared antibiotic prophylaxis with no prophylaxis in patients with acute necrotizing pancreatitis with varying results. A meta-analysis found that prophylactic antibiotics do not reduce infected necrosis or mortality.[64] In addition, overuse of antibiotics increases microbial resistance. Currently, use of antibiotics in necrotizing pancreatitis is only recommended in the presence of known or suspected infection 5. Once infection develops in the patient with necrotic acute pancreatitis, surgical debridement is required.

Because the source of bacterial contamination is most likely the colon, the choice of antibiotic for infected pancreatitis should be broad-spectrum, covering the range of enteric aerobic gram-negative bacilli and anaerobic microorganisms. Treatment should be initiated within the first 48 hours and continued for 2 to 3 weeks. Imipenem–cilastatin (500 mg orally every 8 hours) has been widely used because of its good penetration into the pancreas and one positive prophylaxis study.[67] However, it has been replaced on many hospital formularies by one of the newer carbapenems (such as meropenem). Fluoroquinolones, such as ciprofloxacin or levofloxacin, combined with metronidazole should be considered for penicillin-allergic patients.[66]

Selective digestive tract decontamination uses oral minimally absorbed antibiotics, including polymyxin E, tobramycin, and amphotericin B, to eradicate bacteria in the intestinal flora, thereby reducing translocation.[66,68] This alternative may be of benefit in reducing the risk of pancreatic infection, but randomized controlled trials in patients with acute pancreatitis are needed to confirm its effectiveness when compared with parenteral antibiotic prophylaxis.[66]

Post-ERCP Pancreatitis

The clinical characteristics of post-ERCP pancreatitis are similar to those of acute pancreatitis from other causes. In most cases the disease course is mild and resolves in several days. Pretreatment with octreotide, corticosteroids, calcium channel blockers, allopurinol, natural β-carotene, and aprotinin has been disappointing.[69,70] Some benefit has been demonstrated with somatostatin, diclofenac suppositories, and gabexate.[71,72] Indomethacin suppositories decreased the incidence of post-ERCP pancreatitis by 46% in a population at increased risk.[73] This therapy was not associated with an increase in bleeding or renal failure. However, patients at increased risk for adverse effects from nonsteroidal antiinflammatory drugs (NSAIDs) were excluded. To date, there have not been any studies to evaluate the cost-effectiveness of prophylactic therapy.[74,75]

CHRONIC PANCREATITIS

Chronic pancreatitis results from long-standing pancreatic inflammation resulting in irreversible destruction of pancreatic tissue with fibrin deposition, leading to a loss of exocrine and endocrine functions.[4–6] It has four different stages beginning with a preclinical inflammatory stage where patients remain asymptomatic or have indistinguishable symptoms.[6] In the second stage patients present with acute attacks that often resemble those of acute pancreatitis. The third stage consists of episodes of intermittent or constant abdominal pain. Finally, in the burnout stage patients present with diminished or absent pain, but develop malabsorption syndrome due to loss of pancreatic exocrine function and diabetes mellitus from loss of endocrine function.

Etiology

Chronic alcohol consumption, especially heavy drinking, remains the leading cause of chronic pancreatitis in Western society,

TABLE 25-5 M-ANNHEIM Classification of Risk Factors for Chronic Pancreatitis

Pancreatitis with *M*ultiple risk factors	
*A*lcohol	Excessive consumption (>80 g/day) Increased consumption (20–80 g/day) Moderate consumption (<20 g/day)
*N*icotine	Quantitated in pack years for current smokers
*N*utritional factors	High-fat and -protein diet Hyperlipidemia (especially hypertriglyceridemia)
*H*ereditary factors	Hereditary pancreatitis Familial pancreatitis Early and late-onset idiopathic pancreatitis Tropical pancreatitis Possible gene mutations (e.g., *PRSS1*, *SPINK1*, and *CFTR*)
*E*fferent duct factors	Pancreas divisum Annular pancreas/congenital abnormalities Pancreatic duct obstruction Posttraumatic pancreatic duct scars Sphincter of Oddi dysfunction
*I*mmunologic factors	Autoimmune pancreatitis
*M*iscellaneous and rare factors	Hypercalcemia and hyperparathyroidism Chronic kidney disease Medications Toxins

PRSS1, cationic trypsinogen; *SPINK1*, serine protease inhibitor Kazal type 1; *CFTR*, cystic fibrosis transmembrane conductance regulator.

From reference 85.

accounting for approximately 70% to 80% of cases.[6,76] Generally, consumption of ≥150 g/day of alcohol for ≥15 years poses a significant risk of chronic pancreatitis.[77,78] Twenty percent of the remaining cases can be classified as idiopathic, while 10% are due to rare causes, such as autoimmune, hereditary, and tropical pancreatitis.[6,79] Various genetic alterations have also been associated with the occurrence of chronic pancreatitis, including mutations of the cationic trypsinogen (*PRSS1*), serine protease inhibitor Kazal type 1 (*SPINK1*), and the cystic fibrosis transmembrane conductance regulator (*CFTR*) genes.[77,79] There is also a demonstrated risk of chronic pancreatitis with cigarette smoking that appears to be dose-dependent and may contribute to mortality from chronic pancreatitis.[76,80–84] A proposed classification system called the M-ANNHEIM classification takes into account the various risk factors for chronic pancreatitis (Table 25-5).[85]

Pathophysiology

Although the exact mechanism for the pathogenesis of chronic pancreatitis is unknown, several theories have been proposed. The oxidative stress theory proposes that the pancreas is exposed to by-products of mixed-function oxidases that lead to an inflammatory reaction.[77,79] Increased activity of hepatic and pancreatic oxidases may be due to increased exposure to substrates (e.g., fat), inducers (e.g., alcohol), or other substances. A comparison of serum oxidative markers in chronic pancreatitis patients versus healthy volunteers supports this theory.[86] A toxic-metabolic theory focuses on alcohol as a primary causative agent where by-products of its metabolism in the pancreas lead to lipid accumulation in acinar cells and eventual fatty degeneration of the pancreas.[77] Ductal obstruction theories state that alcohol leads to obstruction of pancreatic ductals secondary to increased protein deposition and stone formation. This leads to scarring of ductal epithelial cells, which potentiates further obstruction and eventually results in acinar atrophy and fibrin deposition. The final major theory suggests that periductular necrosis from repeated episodes of acute pancreatitis eventually leads to ductal obstruction and stone formation with subsequent acinar atrophy and fibrosis.

Regardless of the pathophysiologic mechanism, several pieces of evidence now point to activation of pancreatic stellate cells as the cause of fibrin deposition in chronic pancreatitis. Various toxins, oxidative stress, and inflammatory mediators activate pancreatic stellate cells.[77,87] Cellular signaling pathways involved in this activation are modulated by hydroxymethylglutaryl-coenzyme A reductases and peroxisome proliferator–activated receptor-γ nuclear receptors.[88] As an example, exposure of the pancreas to alcohol and its metabolites leads to the production of various mediators and proinflammatory cytokines, especially tumor necrosis factor-α and interleukin-1 and -6.[87,88] These then activate pancreatic stellate cells that initiate fibrinogenesis. Other mediators generated by the stellate cells themselves perpetuate continued stellate cell activation.

The pathogenesis of pain in chronic pancreatitis has long been thought to be the result of increased pancreatic parenchymal pressure from obstruction, inflammation, and necrosis.[89,90] A neurogenic mechanism may also be responsible. Continued activation of trypsin not only damages afferent neurons but also has effects on sensory pain receptors within the pancreas.[89] Changes also occur within the CNS that further contribute to the neurogenic mechanism of pain.[89,91] This was demonstrated in a study that compared electroencephalogram recordings from chronic pancreatitis patients and healthy volunteers.[92] Therefore, compression of pancreatic nerve fibers after a meal along with continuous firing of peripheral and central neurons may explain the burning and shooting pain of chronic pancreatitis.[91]

Clinical Presentation

Chronic pain, malabsorption with resultant steatorrhea, and diabetes mellitus are the hallmark complications and symptoms of chronic pancreatitis 6. Although abdominal pain is the most common symptom at any stage, patients may present with various signs and symptoms depending on the stage of the disease. A more comprehensive list of the common signs and symptoms is presented in Table 25-6.

Diagnosis

The diagnosis of chronic pancreatitis is based primarily on presenting signs and symptoms in combination with either imaging or pancreatic function studies (Table 25-6). Although histology would be the best diagnostic test, it is difficult and risky to perform and is generally not recommended.[77] Therefore, testing usually begins with noninvasive and inexpensive studies such as serum trypsinogen, fecal elastase, mixed triglyceride breath test, and abdominal ultrasonography.[4,94,95] However, these tests are usually only useful in advanced disease.[4] Magnetic resonance cholangiopancreatography or computed tomography (CT) may be used next. The most sensitive studies are the secretin and CCK stimulation tests for exocrine pancreatic insufficiency.[5,77,79] Performing these studies is uncomfortable for patients and they are not widely available, so they are usually reserved to rule out chronic pancreatitis if imaging studies are nondiagnostic.[4,5] The gold standard invasive study is ERCP.[5,79] However, due to the risks associated with this procedure, endoscopic ultrasonography (EUS) has become an accepted alternative for the diagnosis of chronic pancreatitis.[5,79]

Clinical Course and Prognosis

The clinical course of chronic pancreatitis depends on the etiology. The median age at onset is as early as 10 years for hereditary chronic pancreatitis, whereas alcoholic and late-onset idiopathic chronic pancreatitis have median onsets of 36 and 62 years, respectively.[96] Exocrine insufficiency, which occurs when lipase secretion is less than 10% of normal,[4,79] develops about 5 years after diagnosis in alcoholic chronic pancreatitis and 22 years in hereditary chronic

TABLE 25-6 Signs, Symptoms and Diagnosis of Chronic Pancreatitis

Signs
- Malnutrition (especially in chronic alcoholism)
- Abdominal mass (may indicate a pancreatic pseudocyst)
- Jaundice may be seen
- Splenomegaly (rare)

Symptoms
- Abdominal pain
- Commonly in epigastric area
- May radiate to the back
- Described as deep and penetrating
- May be relieved by bending/leaning forward or bringing knees to the chest
- Often occurs with meals and at night
- May be associated with nausea and vomiting
- Steatorrhea
- Patients describe bulky or foul-smelling stools often with obvious oil droplets
- Usually have an average of three to four stools per day
- May be associated with deficiencies in fat-soluble vitamins
- Watery diarrhea, excess gas, and abdominal cramps are uncommon
- Pancreatic diabetes mellitus
- Diarrhea (associated with steatorrhea)
- Weight loss
- May be due to severe malabsorption or acute/chronic pain
- Substantial loss may be due to associated or unrelated malignancy
- Dyspepsia

Laboratory studies
- CBC to rule out infection (i.e., infected pseudocyst)
- Serum amylase and lipase
- Low specificity for chronic pancreatitis
- May be elevated in acute exacerbations
- Usually are normal or only slightly elevated
- Total bilirubin, alkaline phosphatase, and hepatic transaminases may be elevated with ductal obstruction
- Fasting serum glucose
- Pancreatic function tests
- Serum trypsinogen (<20 ng/mL [or mcg/L] is abnormal)
- Fecal elastase (<200 mcg/g of stool is abnormal)
- Fecal fat estimation (>7 g/day is abnormal; need to collect 72 hours of stool)
- Secretin stimulation (evaluates duodenal bicarbonate secretion)
- ^{13}C-mixed triglyceride breath test
- Serum albumin (may be low with malnutrition)
- Serum calcium (may be low with malnutrition)

Imaging studies
- Noninvasive
- Abdominal ultrasound
- Computed tomography (CT)
- Magnetic resonance cholangiopancreatography (MRCP)
- Invasive
- Endoscopic ultrasonography (EUS)
- Endoscopic retrograde cholangiopancreatography (ERCP)

CBC, complete blood count.

From references 4, 5, and 93.

pancreatitis. Diabetes mellitus has been shown to occur about 8 years after diagnosis of alcoholic chronic pancreatitis and up to 27 years after diagnosis of early onset idiopathic chronic pancreatitis. Resolution of pain from pancreatic burnout tends to coincide with exocrine insufficiency.

The life expectancy of patients with chronic pancreatitis is shorter than that of the general population. The 10-year survival rate is approximately 70%, while the 20-year rate is 45%.[6] However, death in patients with chronic pancreatitis most commonly results from cardiovascular disease, infection, or malignancy rather than from the disease itself.[6,96] One of the most significant complications of long-standing disease is pancreatic cancer. Patients with alcoholic chronic pancreatitis are 15 times as likely as the general population to develop pancreatic cancer, while 40% of those with hereditary chronic pancreatitis may be diagnosed.[6,79]

TREATMENT
Chronic Pancreatitis

Desired Outcome

The major goals in the treatment of uncomplicated chronic pancreatitis are relief of abdominal pain, treatment of the associated complications of malabsorption and diabetes mellitus, and improvement in quality of life. Secondary goals include treating associated disorders such as depression and malnutrition.

General Approach to Treatment

Treatment of chronic pancreatitis and its complications involves various nonpharmacologic and pharmacologic interventions. Lifestyle modifications should include abstinence from alcohol and smoking cessation.[5,79] Also, patients with steatorrhea may need to eat smaller, more frequent meals and reduce dietary fat intake.[4,5] The majority of patients require analgesics and pancreatic enzyme supplementation.[5,79] Pain can initially be controlled with medications, but may require more aggressive medical and surgical therapies as the disease progresses. Patients with malabsorption require pancreatic enzymes to reduce steatorrhea and maintain adequate nutrient absorption.[5,79] An antisecretory agent may be added to the regimen when enzymes alone provide an inadequate reduction in steatorrhea.[4,5,79]

Nonpharmacologic Therapy

In addition to medical management, the treatment of chronic pancreatitis includes both lifestyle and dietary modifications. Patients should be counseled to abstain from alcohol use, and smoking cessation should be advocated. It is unclear if cessation of alcohol use reduces pain in patients with alcoholic chronic pancreatitis, but its use hastens disease progression.[4] Smoking has been associated with an increased mortality in patients with chronic pancreatitis.[82] Patients with steatorrhea should be counseled to eat small and frequent meals.[97] A reduction in dietary fat is not needed routinely, but a decrease to 0.5 g/kg/day is recommended for those whose symptoms are uncontrolled with enzyme supplementation. Patients who do not consume adequate calories from their normal diet may be given whole protein or peptide-based oral nutritional supplements. Supplementation with medium-chain triglycerides, which do not require lipolysis, should be considered for patients with steatorrhea who are unable to gain weight. Complete enteral nutrition is recommended for patients who cannot consume adequate calories, have continued weight loss, experience complications, or require surgery. A jejunal feeding tube is the recommended route for administration of enteral nutrition in chronic pancreatitis patients; it increases patient weight and decreases abdominal pain and opioid use.[97]

Invasive procedures and surgery are primarily used to treat uncontrolled pain and the associated complications of chronic pancreatitis. Stents placed via ERCP may be used to treat pancreatic duct strictures in order to relieve parenchymal pressure and reduce pain.[90,98] Extracorporeal shock wave lithotripsy can be used to break up pancreatic stones with ultrasonic vibration prior to removal by ERCP.[90,98] However, combining these procedures to treat pain provides no additional benefit and increases cost.[99] Blockade of pain signals through the celiac plexus may be achieved utilizing EUS.[90,98,100,101] The various complications of chronic pancreatitis that can be treated endoscopically include common bile duct strictures, duodenal obstructions, and pancreatic pseudocysts.[98] Various surgical techniques including total pancreatectomy may also be used to relieve pain associated with chronic pancreatitis.[5,90,102] Surgery is more effective at relieving pain than endoscopic procedures, but

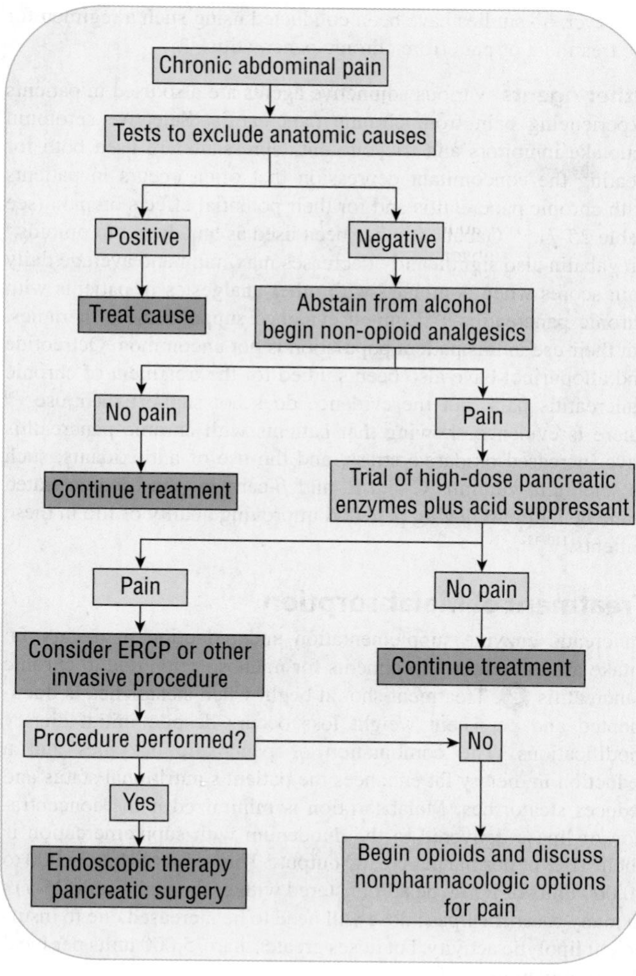

FIGURE 25-4 Algorithm for the treatment of abdominal pain in chronic pancreatitis. (ERCP, endoscopic retrograde cholangiopancreatography.)

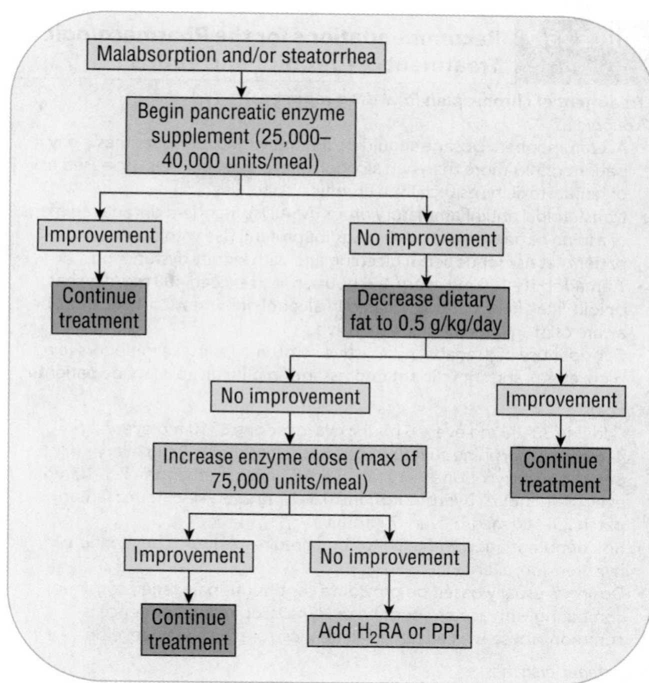

FIGURE 25-5 Algorithm for the treatment of malabsorption and steatorrhea in chronic pancreatitis. (H_2RA, histamine$_2$-receptor antagonist; PPI, proton pump inhibitor.)

these trials have a number of limitations.[103,104] Finally, total pancreatectomy with transplantation of pancreatic islet cells to reduce the need for exogenous insulin is a possible option for the treatment of pain due to chronic pancreatitis.[105,106]

Pharmacologic Therapy

General Recommendations

Pharmacologic therapy of chronic pancreatitis is aimed at controlling pain, treating malabsorption and associated steatorrhea, and controlling diabetes mellitus. Once other causes have been excluded, nonopioid analgesics should be tried initially for pain management (Fig. 25-4).[4,5] Patients unresponsive to nonopioid analgesics may be given a trial of pancreatic enzyme supplements prior to adding opioids.[4,90] If these measures fail, an oral opioid should be added to the drug regimen. Opioids administered by nonoral routes should be reserved for patients who cannot take oral medications or whose pain is unresponsive to oral opioids. Additional agents may be considered for added pain control and disorders associated with chronic pancreatitis.

Most patients with malabsorption will require a modification in diet along with pancreatic enzyme supplementation in order to achieve adequate nutritional status and reduction in steatorrhea (Fig. 25-5). An antisecretory agent should be added to the regimen when there is an inadequate response to enzyme therapy alone.[4] If these measures are ineffective, documentation of the diagnosis and exclusion of other diseases should be undertaken. Exogenous insulin is the primary pharmacologic agent used in the treatment of diabetes mellitus associated with chronic pancreatitis.[4] However, some patients may have favorable results with the use of oral agents for control of blood glucose.

Relief of Chronic Abdominal Pain

Analgesics Pain from chronic pancreatitis can initially be treated with nonopioid analgesics, but opioids will eventually be required as the disease progresses 7. Therapy should begin with acetaminophen or NSAIDs (Table 25-7).[4,5] Regimens should be individualized and should begin with the lowest effective dose. The dosage regimen should be maximized before adding or substituting agents. Analgesics should be scheduled around the clock rather than as needed in order to maximize efficacy. Also, scheduling short-acting analgesics prior to meals should help decrease postprandial pain. When nonopioid analgesics fail to control pain, low-potency opioids (e.g., hydrocodone) should be added to the regimen (see Table 25-7). Tramadol has also been used successfully to treat pain in patients with chronic pancreatitis, but at a higher dose than that approved in the United States.[4] Severe pain unresponsive to these therapies necessitates the use of opiate analgesics. Although opioids carry about a 10% to 30% risk of addiction in this population, their use should not be withheld.[4] Unless contraindicated, oral opioids should be used before parenteral, transdermal, or other dosage forms. Although oxycodone was found to relieve pain better than morphine in a study of simulated chronic pancreatitis pain, adequate trials comparing agents have not been conducted.[107] Therefore, the choice of agent should be based on cost, compliance, and avoidance of adverse drug events (e.g., allergic reactions).

Pancreatic Enzymes Although pancreatic enzymes are primarily used to treat malabsorption associated with chronic pancreatitis,

TABLE 25-7 Recommendations for the Pharmacologic Treatment of Chronic Pancreatitis

Treatment of chronic pain (oral drug regimens)

Nonopioids

- Acetaminophen: Dosage should be limited to 500 mg four times a day if patient drinks more than two alcoholic beverages per day; increased risk of hepatotoxicity, especially in chronic alcohol use
- Nonsteroidal antiinflammatory drugs (NSAIDs): Standard dosage regimens of aspirin or traditional NSAIDs (e.g., ibuprofen). Use with caution in patients at risk for upper GI bleeding and with kidney dysfunction
- Tramadol: 50–100 mg every 4–6 hours, not to exceed 400 mg/day; has opioid-like effect; contraindicated in alcohol or hypnotic intoxication; be aware of drug interactions; expensive
- Consider use of pregabalin, selective serotonin reuptake inhibitors (e.g., paroxetine), and tricyclic antidepressants in difficult-to-manage patients

Opioids

- Codeine 30–60 mg every 6 hours; hydrocodone 5–10 mg every 4–6 hours; morphine sulfate (extended-release) 30–60 mg every 8–12 hours; oxycodone 5–10 mg every 6 hours; methadone 2.5–10 mg every 8–12 hours; hydromorphone 0.5–1 mg every 4–6 hours; fentanyl patch 25–100 mcg/h every 72 hours
- Risk of potentiation with alcohol; impaired respiration; constipation; hypotension; allergy
- Dosing is usually based on providing continuous pain relief; consider combining with acetaminophen or NSAIDs; opioid dependence is common; abuse is a concern in alcoholics; tolerance may develop

Pancreatic enzymes

- Four to eight tablets/capsules of a preferred product (see Table 25-8) with each meal plus either a histamine$_2$-receptor antagonist or proton pump inhibitor; no clinical trials support such a regimen for pain management

Treatment of malabsorption and steatorrhea

- Start with pancreatic enzymes containing 25,000–40,000 USP units of lipase with each meal of a preferred product (see Table 25-8); administer dose during or just after meals
- Increase dose to a maximum of 75,000 USP units of lipase per meal
- Products containing enteric-coated microspheres or minimicrospheres may be more effective than other dose forms

Acid-suppression agents

- May improve efficacy of enzyme therapy for malabsorption and steatorrhea
- May allow a lower dose of enzyme supplements to be used

USP, United States Pharmacopeia.

From references 4, 5, 9, 90, 109, 113, 114, 116, and 117.

they are also used to treat pain from the disease. Relief of pain using pancreatic enzymes is thought to be due to their ability to break down CCK.[4,9,77,90] Normally, the release of CCK, which causes an increase in pancreatic secretion, is inhibited by trypsin. However, there is a decrease in the production of trypsin in patients with chronic pancreatitis. This leads to a loss of negative feedback on the release of CCK and thus an increase in pain due to unabated pancreatic secretion. The proteases in pancreatic enzyme supplements are thought to act as substitutes for endogenous trypsin, leading to a decrease in CCK release.

Despite this intuitive mechanism, mixed results have been found from trials investigating pancreatic enzyme supplements for the treatment of pain from chronic pancreatitis. This may be due to the differences between the various enzyme formulations used in the trials as well as the small number of subjects enrolled.[4,9,90] A Cochrane Collaborative review found no beneficial effect on pain relief.[108] However, trials that used non–enteric-coated enzyme formulations have demonstrated a benefit in the treatment of pain.[4,9,90] It is thought that enteric-coated formulations may not release enough proteases in the duodenum to inhibit CCK release. A trial of non–enteric-coated enzyme supplements may be used for patients with less advanced disease before more aggressive therapy was considered.[4,9] An alternative is to administer an enteric-coated product with an antisecretory agent in order to increase the amount of proteases available in the duodenum from these products (Table 25-7). However, no studies have been conducted using such a regimen for the treatment of pain from chronic pancreatitis.

Other Agents Various adjunctive agents are also used in patients experiencing pain from chronic pancreatitis. Selective serotonin reuptake inhibitors and tricyclic antidepressants are used both for treating the concomitant depression that often occurs in patients with chronic pancreatitis and for their potential effects on pain (see Table 25-7).[4,90] Gabapentin has been used as an adjunct to opioids.[4] Pregabalin also significantly decreases maximum and average daily pain scores when combined with other analgesics in patients with chronic pancreatitis.[109] Limited evidence supports these therapies, but their use in this patient population is not uncommon. Octreotide and allopurinol have also been studied for the treatment of chronic pancreatitis pain, but the evidence does not support their use.[4,90] There is evidence showing that patients with chronic pancreatitis have increased oxidative stress, and the use of antioxidants, such as selenium, vitamins C and E, and β-carotene, has demonstrated some benefit in relieving pain and improving quality of life in these patients.[110–112]

Treatment of Malabsorption

Pancreatic enzyme supplementation and reduction in dietary fat intake are the primary treatments for malabsorption due to chronic pancreatitis (8). Treatment should begin when steatorrhea is documented and persistent weight loss occurs despite initial dietary modifications. The combination of pancreatic enzymes and a reduction in dietary fat enhances the patient's nutritional status and reduces steatorrhea. Malabsorption is minimized if the concentration of lipase delivered to the duodenum with supplementation is about 10% of normal pancreatic output.[4] This requires that 25,000 to 40,000 units of lipase be administered with each meal (Table 25-7).[9] In many cases the lipase dose will need to be increased due to insufficient lipolytic activity, but doses greater than 75,000 units per meal are not recommended.

There is little evidence regarding the optimal dosage form and administration of pancreatic enzyme supplements. Most studies have compared them with placebo rather than other enzyme products, and used quantitation of fat absorption or elimination as a primary measure of efficacy rather than weight gain.[113] Although they have been shown to improve fat absorption, they may not completely eliminate steatorrhea.[113,114] However, they improve the quality of life of patients with chronic pancreatitis.[115] Since most exogenous lipase is rapidly and irreversibly destroyed at low intragastric pH, enteric-coated products are preferred for the treatment of malabsorption and steatorrhea (9). The enteric coating only dissolves at a pH greater than 5.5, which allows a sufficient quantity of enzymes to remain intact until dissolution of the coating in the duodenum.[9] However, enzymes must also be emptied from the stomach into the duodenum at the same rate and time as ingested food. The size of the enteric-coated enzyme preparation influences the rate of enzyme delivery to the duodenum.[4,9] Likewise, the administration time relevant to a meal influences the timing of enzyme delivery. Products that contain enzymes in small enteric-coated microspheres or minimicrospheres are often the best products because they are thought to mix effectively with chyme, thus leaving the stomach at a similar rate.[9] Also, the optimal administration time of enzymes containing minimicrospheres appears to be either with a meal or just after.[4,116]

Despite enzyme therapy, patients may continue to have steatorrhea and fail to gain sufficient weight. Compliance should be assessed in these patients as the number of capsules required with each meal can lead to noncompliance. Alternative products with higher lipase content can be tried in order to reduce the number of capsules needed. If this fails, the dose of lipase should be increased. Finally, addition of an antisecretory agent may be tried to increase the availability of active enzymes in the duodenum.[117]

TABLE 25-8 Commercially Available Pancreatic Enzyme (Pancrelipase) Preparations

Product	Enzyme Content Per Unit Dose (USP Units)		
	Lipase	Amylase	Protease
Tablets			
Viokace™ 10,440 lipase units	10,440	39,150	39,150
Viokace™ 20,880 lipase units	20,880	78,300	78,300
Enteric-coated beads			
Zenpep® 3,000 lipase units	3,000	16,000	10,000
Zenpep® 5,000 lipase units	5,000	27,000	17,000
Zenpep® 10,000 lipase units	10,000	55,000	34,000
Zenpep® 15,000 lipase units	15,000	82,000	51,000
Zenpep® 20,000 lipase units	20,000	109,000	68,000
Zenpep® 25,000 lipase units	25,000	136,000	85,000
Enteric-coated microspheres with bicarbonate buffer			
Pertzye™ 8,000 lipase units	8,000	30,250	28,750
Pertzye™ 16,000 lipase units	16,000	60,500	57,500
Enteric-coated minimicrospheres			
Creon® 3,000 lipase units	3,000	15,000	9,500
Creon® 6,000 lipase units	6,000	30,000	19,000
Creon® 12,000 lipase units	12,000	60,000	38,000
Creon® 24,000 lipase units	24,000	120,000	76,000
Enteric-coated minitablets/microtablets			
Pancreaze® 4,200 lipase units	4,200	17,500	10,000
Pancreaze® 10,500 lipase units	10,500	43,750	25,000
Pancreaze® 16,800 lipase units	16,800	70,000	40,000
Pancreaze® 21,000 lipase units	21,000	61,000	37,000
Ultresa™ 13,800 lipase units	13,800	27,600	27,600
Ultresa™ 20,700 lipase units	20,700	41,400	41,400
Ultresa™ 23,000 lipase units	23,000	46,000	46,000

USP, United States Pharmacopeia.

Pancreatic Enzyme Supplements Until recently none of the pancreatic enzyme supplements were approved by the FDA because they predated enactment of the Food, Drug, and Cosmetic Act of 1938. Since the FDA announced in 2004 that all products would have to seek approval, six products have been approved. Only two of these products are specifically approved for exocrine pancreatic insufficiency associated with chronic pancreatitis.[118,119] Dosage forms of approved products include regular-release tablets, enteric-coated beads, bicarbonate-buffered enteric-coated microspheres, enteric-coated minimicrospheres, and enteric-coated minitablets or microtablets encased in a cellulose or gelatin capsule (Table 25-8). Enzymes are easily administered to patients able to swallow the capsules or their contents. However, administration to patients with enteral feeding tubes presents a challenge. Products containing microspheres may be administered through feeding tubes in an applesauce or apple juice mixture.[9] Clinicians must be aware, however, that available products are not equivalent and should consider this before substituting products in patients who require administration through a nonoral route.

Adverse reactions from pancreatic enzyme supplements are generally benign. High doses can lead to nausea, diarrhea, and intestinal upset.[9] One of the more serious adverse effects of these products is fibrosing colonopathy. It occurs when the enzymes cause deposition of fibrin in the colon leading to colonic stricture. This reaction is uncommon and has been reported mostly in children with cystic fibrosis who received high doses of enzymes for prolonged periods.[9] Certain enteric coatings may specifically invoke this reaction. Another concern with pancreatic enzymes is the risk of possible viral infection due to contamination of these porcine-derived products.[120] Finally, pancreatic enzymes have been associated with deficiencies in fat-soluble vitamins, and appropriate monitoring and supplementation, especially of vitamin D, should be instituted.[4,79]

Clinical **Controversy...**

Since the evidence supporting the use of pancreatic enzyme supplements for treating pain associated with chronic pancreatitis is not overwhelming, clinicians debate over their use for this purpose. Often the decision to use enzyme supplements for the treatment of pain comes from clinical experience and the knowledge that their use carries minimal risk of adverse effects.

Adjuncts to Enzyme Therapy The addition of a histamine$_2$-receptor antagonist or proton pump inhibitor to pancreatic enzyme supplementation may increase the effectiveness of enzyme therapy for malabsorption and steatorrhea (10). The beneficial effects of these agents result from an increase in gastric and duodenal pH.[9,79] This is thought to result in an increase in the amount of active enzymes available in the duodenum. Traditionally, their use has been advocated with non–enteric-coated enzyme products.[4,9] In fact, the only non–enteric-coated formulation currently approved by the FDA is indicated for administration with a proton pump inhibitor.[119] However, evidence shows that their use in combination with enteric-coated preparations results in similar efficacy between standard and low-dose enzyme regimens.[117]

PERSONALIZED PHARMACOTHERAPY

Some cases of drug-induced pancreatitis are associated with elevated concentrations of the causative medications, and it is possible that genetic differences in drug metabolism contribute to this. A pharmacogenetic analysis was performed in one case of drug-induced pancreatitis that was associated with high concentrations of clozapine.[121] However, the patient was not found to have any genetic variants that would affect the metabolism of clozapine.

Although several genetic variations have been associated with the occurrence of chronic pancreatitis, variation in response to therapy related to these factors has not been studied. One cautionary note regarding pancreatic enzyme supplements is that they are all porcine-derived and thus contain purines. Therefore, they may increase uric acid levels and should be used cautiously in patients prone to the effects of hyperuricemia. This would include patients with a history of gout, impaired kidney function, and known hyperuricemia. One physiologic parameter affecting the efficacy of pancreatic enzyme supplements is GI transit. Non–enteric-coated formulations are preferred for patients with rapid gastrojejunal transit secondary to pancreatectomy associated with partial gastrectomy or vagotomy and gastroenteroscopy. These patients have hyposecretion of gastric acid and enteric-coated formulations would not be released early enough in the small intestine to confer a beneficial effect.[9]

EVALUATION OF THERAPEUTIC OUTCOMES

Acute Pancreatitis

Hydration status, serum electrolytes, pain control, and nutritional status should be assessed periodically in patients with mild acute pancreatitis, depending on the degree of abdominal pain and fluid loss. Patients with severe acute pancreatitis should receive intensive care and close monitoring of vital signs, fluid and electrolyte status, white blood cell count, blood glucose, lactate dehydrogenase, aspartate aminotransferase, serum albumin, hematocrit, BUN, serum creatinine, and international normalized ratio. Continuous hemodynamic and arterial blood gas monitoring is essential. Serum lipase, amylase, and bilirubin require less frequent monitoring. The patient should also be monitored for signs of infection, relief of abdominal pain, and adequate nutritional status. Severity of disease and patient response should be assessed using an evidence-based method, for example, APACHE II.

Chronic Pancreatitis

The severity and frequency of abdominal pain should be assessed periodically in patients with chronic pancreatitis using a standardized scale in order to determine the efficacy of pain therapy. Patients receiving opioids should be prescribed laxatives on an as-needed or scheduled basis and be monitored for constipation. Patients receiving pancreatic enzymes for malabsorption should have their weight and stool frequency and consistency monitored periodically. More objective assessments of fecal fat content, such as the ^{13}C-mixed triglyceride breath test, can be utilized, but are usually unnecessary and impractical in general clinical practice.[4,109,122] Blood glucose must be closely monitored in patients with diabetes mellitus, and those with long-standing disease should receive appropriate monitoring for nephropathy, retinopathy, and neuropathy.[4]

ABBREVIATIONS

APACHE	Acute Physiology and Chronic Health Evaluation
BISAP	Bedside Index of Severity in Acute Pancreatitis
BUN	blood urea nitrogen
CCK	cholecystokinin
CECT	contrast-enhanced computed tomography
CFTR	cystic fibrosis transmembrane conductance regulator gene
CRP	C-reactive protein
CT	computed tomography
DPP-4	dipeptidyl peptidase-4
ERCP	endoscopic retrograde cholangiopancreatography
EUS	endoscopic ultrasonography
GLP-1	glucagon-like peptide-1
GRP	gastrin-releasing peptide
HAPS	Harmless Acute Pancreatitis Score
HIV	human immunodeficiency virus
NSAID	nonsteroidal antiinflammatory drug
PRSS1	cationic trypsinogen gene
SIRS	systemic inflammatory response syndrome
SPINK1	serine protease inhibitor Kazal type 1 gene
VIP	vasoactive intestinal peptide

REFERENCES

1. Anand N, Park JH, Wu BU. Modern management of acute pancreatitis. Gastroenterol Clin North Am 2012;41(1):1–8.
2. Lippi G, Valentino M, Cervellin G. Laboratory diagnosis of acute pancreatitis: In search of the Holy Grail. Crit Rev Clin Lab Sci 2012;49(1):18–31.
3. Petrov MS, Shanbhag S, Chakraborty M, Phillips AR, Windsor JA. Organ failure and infection of pancreatic necrosis as determinants of mortality in patients with acute pancreatitis. Gastroenterology 2010;139(3):813–820.
4. Forsmark CE. Chronic pancreatitis. In: Feldman M, Friedman LS, Brandt LJ, eds. Sleisenger and Fordtran's Gastrointestinal and Liver Disease: Pathophysiology, Diagnosis, Management, 9th ed. Philadelphia: Saunders, 2010:985–1016.
5. Nair RJ, Lawler L, Miller MR. Chronic pancreatitis. Am Fam Physician 2007;76(11):1679–1688.
6. Spanier BW, Dijkgraaf MG, Bruno MJ. Epidemiology, aetiology and outcome of acute and chronic pancreatitis: An update. Best Pract Res Clin Gastroenterol 2008;22(1):45–63.
7. Lowenfels AB, Maisonneuve P, Sullivan T. The changing character of acute pancreatitis: Epidemiology, etiology, and prognosis. Curr Gastroenterol Rep 2009;11(2):97–103.
8. Pandol SJ. Pancreatic secretion. In: Feldman M, Friedman LS, Brandt LJ, eds. Sleisenger and Fordtran's Gastrointestinal and Liver Disease: Pathophysiology, Diagnosis, Management, 9th ed. Philadelphia: Saunders, 2010:921–930.
9. Ferrone M, Raimondo M, Scolapio JS. Pancreatic enzyme pharmacotherapy. Pharmacotherapy 2007;27(6):910–920.
10. Forsmark CE, Baillie J. AGA Institute technical review on acute pancreatitis. Gastroenterology 2007;132(5): 2022–2044.
11. Talukdar R, Swaroop VS. Early management of severe acute pancreatitis. Curr Gastroenterol Rep 2011;13(2):123–130.
12. Baran B, Karaca C, Soyer OM, et al. Acute pancreatitis associated with H1N1 influenza during 2009 pandemic: A case report. Clin Res Hepatol Gastroenterol 2012;36(4): e69–e70.
13. Lee JK, Enns R. Review of idiopathic pancreatitis. World J Gastroenterol 2007;13(47):6296–6313.
14. Finkelberg DL, Sahani D, Deshpande V, Brugge WR. Autoimmune pancreatitis. N Engl J Med 2006;355(25):2670–2676.
15. Feurer ME, Adler DG. Post-ERCP pancreatitis: Review of current preventive strategies. Curr Opin Gastroenterol 2012;28(3):280–286.
16. Morton C, Klatsky AL, Udaltsova N. Smoking, coffee, and pancreatitis. Am J Gastroenterol 2004;99(4):731–738.
17. Lowe ME, Greer JB. Pancreatitis in children and adolescents. Curr Gastroenterol Rep 2008;10(2):128–135.
18. Nitsche C, Maertin S, Scheiber J, Ritter CA, Lerch MM, Mayerle J. Drug-induced pancreatitis. Curr Gastroenterol Rep 2012;14(2):131–138.
19. Eland IA, Alvarez CH, Stricker BH, Rodriguez LA. The risk of acute pancreatitis associated with acid-suppressing drugs. Br J Clin Pharmacol 2000;49(5):473–478.
20. Lin HH, Hsu CH, Chao YC. Tamoxifen-induced severe acute pancreatitis: A case report. Dig Dis Sci 2004;49(6):997–999.
21. Devlin JW, Lau AK, Tanios MA. Propofol-associated hypertriglyceridemia and pancreatitis in the intensive care unit: An analysis of frequency and risk factors. Pharmacotherapy 2005;25(10):1348–1352.
22. Preiss D. Lipid-modifying therapies and risk of pancreatitis: A meta-analysis. JAMA. 2012;308(8):804–811.
23. Fessel J, Hurley LB. Incidence of pancreatitis in HIV-infected patients: Comment on findings in EuroSIDA cohort. AIDS 2008;22(1):145–147.
24. Smith CJ, Olsen CH, Mocroft A, et al. The role of antiretroviral therapy in the incidence of pancreatitis in HIV-positive individuals in the EuroSIDA study. AIDS 2008;22(1):47–56.
25. Dhir R, Brown DK, Olden KW. Drug-induced pancreatitis: A practical review. Drugs Today (Barc) 2007;43(7):499–507.
26. Balani AR, Grendell JH. Drug-induced pancreatitis: Incidence, management and prevention. Drug Saf 2008;31(10):823–837.
27. Mallick S. Metformin induced acute pancreatitis precipitated by renal failure. Postgrad Med J 2004;80(942):239–240.
28. Institute for Safe Medication Practices. QuarterWatch 2011 annual report: An estimated 2 to 4 million drug-induced

serious injuries in 2011. ISMP Medication Safety Alert! Acute Care 2012;17(11):1–3.
29. Knezevich E, Crnic T, Kershaw S, Drincic A. Liraglutide-associated acute pancreatitis. Am J Health Syst Pharm 2012;69(5):386–389.
30. Bain SC, Stephens JW. Exenatide and pancreatitis: An update. Expert Opin Drug Saf 2008;7(6):643–644.
31. Ahmad SR, Swann J. Exenatide and rare adverse events. N Engl J Med 2008;358(18):1970–1971.
32. U.S. Food and Drug Administration. Information for Healthcare Professionals—Acute Pancreatitis and Sitagliptin (Marketed as Januvia and Janumet). September 25, 2009, *http://www.fda.gov/Drugs/DrugSafety/PostmarketDrugSafetyInformationforPatientsandProviders/DrugSafetyInformationforHeathcareProfessionals/ucm183764.htm.*
33. Trivedi CD, Pitchumoni CS. Drug-induced pancreatitis: An update. J Clin Gastroenterol 2005;39(8):709–716.
34. Criddle DN, McLaughlin E, Murphy JA, Petersen OH, Sutton R. The pancreas misled: Signals to pancreatitis. Pancreatology 2007;7(5–6):436–446.
35. Vonlaufen A, Wilson JS, Apte MV. Molecular mechanisms of pancreatitis: Current opinion. J Gastroenterol Hepatol 2008;23(9):1339–1348.
36. Gorelick F. Pancreatic protease-activated receptors: Friend and foe. Gut 2007;56(7):901–902.
37. Sand J, Nordback I. Acute pancreatitis: Risk of recurrence and late consequences of the disease. Nat Rev Gastroenterol Hepatol 2009;6(8):470–477.
38. Balthazar EJ. Staging of acute pancreatitis. Radiol Clin North Am 2002;40(6):1199–1209.
39. Banks PA, Freeman ML. Practice guidelines in acute pancreatitis. Am J Gastroenterol 2006;101(10):2379–2400.
40. Mofidi R, Patil PV, Suttie SA, Parks RW. Risk assessment in acute pancreatitis. Br J Surg 2009;96(2):137–150.
41. Pezzilli R, Uomo G, Zerbi A, et al. Diagnosis and treatment of acute pancreatitis: The position statement of the Italian Association for the study of the pancreas. Dig Liver Dis 2008;40(10):803–808.
42. Working Party of the British Society of Gastroenterology, Association of Surgeons of Great Britain and Ireland, Pancreatic Society of Great Britain and Ireland, Association of Upper GI Surgeons of Great Britain and Ireland. UK guidelines for the management of acute pancreatitis. Gut 2005;54(Suppl 3):iii1–iii9.
43. Wu BU. Prognosis in acute pancreatitis. Can Med Assoc J 2011;183(6):673–677.
44. Vege SS, Gardner TB, Chari ST, et al. Low mortality and high morbidity in severe acute pancreatitis without organ failure: A case for revising the Atlanta classification to include "moderately severe acute pancreatitis". Am J Gastroenterol 2009;104(3):710–715.
45. Gardner TB, Vege SS, Pearson RK, Chari ST. Fluid resuscitation in acute pancreatitis. Clin Gastroenterol Hepatol 2008;6(10):1070–1076.
46. Bakker OJ, van Santvoort HC, van Brunschot S, et al. Endoscopic transgastric vs surgical necrosectomy for infected necrotizing pancreatitis. JAMA 2012;307(10):1053–1061.
47. Falor AE, de Virgilio C, Stabile BE, et al. Early laparoscopic cholecystectomy for mild gallstone pancreatitis: Time for a paradigm shift. Arch Surg 2012;1–5.
48. McClave SA, Chang WK, Dhaliwal R, Heyland DK. Nutrition support in acute pancreatitis: A systematic review of the literature. J Parenter Enteral Nutr 2006;30(2):143–156.
49. Meier RF, Beglinger C. Nutrition in pancreatic diseases. Best Pract Res Clin Gastroenterol 2006;20(3):507–529.
50. Al-Omran M, Albalawi ZH, Tashkandi MF, Al-Ansary LA. Enteral versus parenteral nutrition for acute pancreatitis. Cochrane Database Syst Rev 2010;(1):CD002837.
51. Besselink MG, van Santvoort HC, Buskens E, et al. Probiotic prophylaxis in predicted severe acute pancreatitis: A randomised, double-blind, placebo-controlled trial. Lancet 2008;371(9613):651–659.
52. Gardner TB, Vege SS, Chari ST, et al. Faster rate of initial fluid resuscitation in severe acute pancreatitis diminishes in-hospital mortality. Pancreatology 2009;9(6):770–776.
53. Warndorf MG, Kurtzman JT, Bartel MJ, et al. Early fluid resuscitation reduces morbidity among patients with acute pancreatitis. Clin Gastroenterol Hepatol 2011;9(8):705–709.
54. de-Madaria E, Soler-Sala G, Sanchez-Paya J, et al. Influence of fluid therapy on the prognosis of acute pancreatitis: A prospective cohort study. Am J Gastroenterol 2011;106(10):1843–1850.
55. Wu BU, Hwang JQ, Gardner TH, et al. Lactated Ringer's solution reduces systemic inflammation compared with saline in patients with acute pancreatitis. Clin Gastroenterol Hepatol 2011;9(8):710–717.
56. Mao EQ, Tang YQ, Fei J, et al. Fluid therapy for severe acute pancreatitis in acute response stage. Chin Med J (Engl) 2009;122(2):169–173.
57. Trikudanathan G, Navaneethan U, Vege SS. Current controversies in fluid resuscitation in acute pancreatitis: A systematic review. Pancreas 2012;41(6):827–834.
58. Nasr JY, Papachristou GI. Early fluid resuscitation in acute pancreatitis: A lot more than just fluids. Clin Gastroenterol Hepatol 2011;9(8):633–634.
59. Thompson DR. Narcotic analgesic effects on the sphincter of Oddi: A review of the data and therapeutic implications in treating pancreatitis. Am J Gastroenterol 2001;96(4):1266–1272.
60. Banks PA. Practice guidelines in acute pancreatitis. Am J Gastroenterol 1997;92(3):377–386.
61. Johnson CD, Kingsnorth AN, Imrie CW, et al. Double blind, randomised, placebo controlled study of a platelet activating factor antagonist, lexipafant, in the treatment and prevention of organ failure in predicted severe acute pancreatitis. Gut 2001;48(1):62–69.
62. Kitagawa M, Hayakawa T. Antiproteases in the treatment of acute pancreatitis. J Pancreas 2007;8(4 Suppl):518–525.
63. Andriulli A, Leandro G, Clemente R, et al. Meta-analysis of somatostatin, octreotide and gabexate mesilate in the therapy of acute pancreatitis. Aliment Pharmacol Ther 1998;12(3):237–245.
64. Bai Y, Gao J, Zou DW, Li ZS. Prophylactic antibiotics cannot reduce infected pancreatic necrosis and mortality in acute necrotizing pancreatitis: Evidence from a meta-analysis of randomized controlled trials. Am J Gastroenterol 2008;103(1):104–110.
65. Buchler M, Malfertheiner P, Friess H, et al. Human pancreatic tissue concentration of bactericidal antibiotics. Gastroenterology 1992;103(6):1902–1908.
66. Lankisch PG, Lerch MM. The role of antibiotic prophylaxis in the treatment of acute pancreatitis. J Clin Gastroenterol 2006;40(2):149–155.
67. Rokke O, Harbitz TB, Liljedal J, et al. Early treatment of severe pancreatitis with imipenem: A prospective randomized clinical trial. Scand J Gastroenterol 2007;42(6):771–776.
68. Luiten EJ, Bruining HA. Antimicrobial prophylaxis in acute pancreatitis: Selective decontamination versus antibiotics.

Baillieres Best Pract Res Clin Gastroenterol 1999;13(2): 317–330.
69. Poon RT, Fan ST. Antisecretory agents for prevention of post-ERCP pancreatitis: Rationale for use and clinical results. J Pancreas 2003;4(1):33–40.
70. Lavy A, Karban A, Suissa A, Yassin K, Hermesh I, Ben-Amotz A. Natural beta-carotene for the prevention of post-ERCP pancreatitis. Pancreas 2004;29(2):e45–e50.
71. Murray B, Carter R, Imrie C, Evans S, O'Suilleabhain C. Diclofenac reduces the incidence of acute pancreatitis after endoscopic retrograde cholangiopancreatography. Gastroenterology 2003;124(7):1786–1791.
72. Hoogerwerf WA. Pharmacological management of pancreatitis. Curr Opin Pharmacol 2005;5(6):578–582.
73. Elmunzer BJ, Scheiman JM, Lehman GA, et al. A randomized trial of rectal indomethacin to prevent post-ERCP pancreatitis. New Engl J Med 2012;366(15): 1414–1422.
74. Bai Y, Gao J, Zou DW, Li ZS. Prophylactic octreotide administration does not prevent post-endoscopic retrograde cholangiopancreatography pancreatitis: A meta-analysis of randomized controlled trials. Pancreas 2008;37(3): 241–246.
75. Zheng M, Chen Y, Bai J, Xin Y, Pan X, Zhao L. Meta-analysis of prophylactic allopurinol use in post-endoscopic retrograde cholangiopancreatography pancreatitis. Pancreas 2008;37(3):247–253.
76. Yadav D, Hawes RH, Brand RE, et al. Alcohol consumption, cigarette smoking, and the risk of recurrent acute and chronic pancreatitis. Arch Intern Med 2009;169(11):1035–1045.
77. Braganza JM, Lee SH, McCloy RF, McMahon MJ. Chronic pancreatitis. Lancet 2011;377(9772):1184–1197.
78. Balakrishnan V, Unnikrishnan AG, Thomas V, et al. Chronic pancreatitis. A prospective nationwide study of 1,086 subjects from India. J Pancreas 2008;9(5):593–600.
79. Tattersall SJ, Apte MV, Wilson JS. A fire inside: Current concepts in chronic pancreatitis. Intern Med J 2008;38(7):592–598.
80. Maisonneuve P, Lowenfels AB, Mullhaupt B, et al. Cigarette smoking accelerates progression of alcoholic chronic pancreatitis. Gut 2005;54(4):510–514.
81. Maisonneuve P, Frulloni L, Mullhaupt B, et al. Impact of smoking on patients with idiopathic chronic pancreatitis. Pancreas 2006;33(2):163–168.
82. Seicean A, Tantau M, Grigorescu M, Mocan T, Seicean R, Pop T. Mortality risk factors in chronic pancreatitis. J Gastrointestin Liver Dis 2006;15(1):21–26.
83. Tolstrup JS, Kristiansen L, Becker U, Gronbaek M. Smoking and risk of acute and chronic pancreatitis among women and men: A population-based cohort study. Arch Intern Med 2009;169(6):603–609.
84. Andriulli A, Botteri E, Almasio PL, Vantini I, Uomo G, Maisonneuve P. Smoking as a cofactor for causation of chronic pancreatitis: A meta-analysis. Pancreas 2010;39(8): 1205–1210.
85. Schneider A, Löhr JM, Singer MV. The M-ANNHEIM classification of chronic pancreatitis: Introduction of a unifying classification system based on a review of previous classifications of the disease. J Gastroenterol 2007;42(2): 101–119.
86. Verlaan M, Roelofs HM, van-Schaik A, et al. Assessment of oxidative stress in chronic pancreatitis patients. World J Gastroenterol 2006;12(35):5705–5710.
87. Talukdar R, Tandon RK. Pancreatic stellate cells: New target in the treatment of chronic pancreatitis. J Gastroenterol Hepatol 2008;23(1):34–41.
88. Talukdar R, Saikia N, Singal DK, Tandon R. Chronic pancreatitis: Evolving paradigms. Pancreatology 2006;6(5): 440–449.
89. Anaparthy R, Pasricha PJ. Pain and chronic pancreatitis: Is it the plumbing or the wiring? Curr Gastroenterol Rep 2008;10(2):101–106.
90. Gachago C, Draganov PV. Pain management in chronic pancreatitis. World J Gastroenterol 2008;14(20):3137–3148.
91. Drewes AM, Krarup AL, Detlefsen S, Malmstrom ML, Dimcevski G, Funch-Jensen P. Pain in chronic pancreatitis: The role of neuropathic pain mechanisms. Gut 2008;57(11): 1616–1627.
92. Drewes AM, Gratkowski M, Sami SA, Dimcevski G, Funch-Jensen P, Arendt-Nielsen L. Is the pain in chronic pancreatitis of neuropathic origin? Support from EEG studies during experimental pain. World J Gastroenterol 2008;14(25):4020–4027.
93. Chen WX, Zhang WF, Li B, et al. Clinical manifestations of patients with chronic pancreatitis. Hepatobiliary Pancreat Dis Int 2006;5(1):133–137.
94. Sun DY, Jiang YB, Rong L, Jin SJ, Xie WZ. Clinical application of 13C-Hiolein breath test in assessing pancreatic exocrine insufficiency. Hepatobiliary Pancreat Dis Int 2003; 2(3):449–452.
95. Conwell DL, Banks PA. Chronic pancreatitis. Curr Opin Gastroenterol 2008;24(5):586–590.
96. Mullhaupt B, Truninger K, Ammann R. Impact of etiology on the painful early stage of chronic pancreatitis: A long-term prospective study. Z Gastroenterol 2005;43(12):1293–1301.
97. Grant JP. Nutritional support in acute and chronic pancreatitis. Surg Clin North Am 2011;91(4):805–820.
98. Kowalczyk LM, Draganov PV. Endoscopic therapy for chronic pancreatitis: Technical success, clinical outcomes, and complications. Curr Gastroenterol Rep 2009;11(2): 111–118.
99. Dumonceau JM, Costamagna G, Tringali A, et al. Treatment for painful calcified chronic pancreatitis: Extracorporeal shock wave lithotripsy versus endoscopic treatment: A randomised controlled trial. Gut 2007;56(4):545–552.
100. Puli SR, Reddy JB, Bechtold ML, Antillon MR, Brugge WR. EUS-guided celiac plexus neurolysis for pain due to chronic pancreatitis or pancreatic cancer pain: A meta-analysis and systematic review. Dig Dis Sci 2009;54(11):2330–2337.
101. Kaufman M, Singh G, Das S, et al. Efficacy of endoscopic ultrasound-guided celiac plexus block and celiac plexus neurolysis for managing abdominal pain associated with chronic pancreatitis and pancreatic cancer. J Clin Gastroenterol 2010;44(2):127–134.
102. Deviere J, Bell RH Jr, Beger HG, Traverso LW. Treatment of chronic pancreatitis with endotherapy or surgery: Critical review of randomized control trials. J Gastrointest Surg 2008;12(4):640–644.
103. Cahen DL, Gouma DJ, Nio Y, et al. Endoscopic versus surgical drainage of the pancreatic duct in chronic pancreatitis. N Engl J Med 2007;356(7):676–684.
104. Ahmed AU, Pahlplatz JM, Nealon WH, van Goor H, Gooszen HG, Boermeester MA. Endoscopic or surgical intervention for painful obstructive chronic pancreatitis. Cochrane Database Syst Rev 2012;1:CD007884.
105. Garcea G, Weaver J, Phillips J, et al. Total pancreatectomy with and without islet cell transplantation for chronic pancreatitis: A series of 85 consecutive patients. Pancreas 2009;38(1):1–7.
106. Bramis K, Gordon-Weeks AN, Friend PJ, et al. Systematic review of total pancreatectomy and islet autotransplantation for chronic pancreatitis. Br J Surg 2012;99(6):761–766.

107. Staahl C, Dimcevski G, Andersen SD, et al. Differential effect of opioids in patients with chronic pancreatitis: An experimental pain study. Scand J Gastroenterol 2007;42(3): 383–390.
108. Shafiq N, Rana S, Bhasin D, et al. Pancreatic enzymes for chronic pancreatitis. Cochrane Database Syst Rev 2009;(4): CD006302.
109. Olesen SS, Bouwense SA, Wilder-Smith OH, van Goor H, Drewes AM. Pregabalin reduces pain in patients with chronic pancreatitis in a randomized, controlled trial. Gastroenterology 2011;141(2):536–543.
110. Bhardwaj P, Garg PK, Maulik SK, Saraya A, Tandon RK, Acharya SK. A randomized controlled trial of antioxidant supplementation for pain relief in patients with chronic pancreatitis. Gastroenterology 2009;136(1):149–159.
111. Shah NS, Makin AJ, Sheen AJ, Siriwardena AK. Quality of life assessment in patients with chronic pancreatitis receiving antioxidant therapy. World J Gastroenterol 2010;16(32): 4066–4071.
112. Grigsby B, Rodriguez-Rilo H, Khan K. Antioxidants and chronic pancreatitis: Theory of oxidative stress and trials of antioxidant therapy. Dig Dis Sci 2012;57(4):835–841.
113. Waljee AK, Dimagno MJ, Wu BU, Schoenfeld PS, Conwell DL. Systematic review: Pancreatic enzyme treatment of malabsorption associated with chronic pancreatitis. Aliment Pharmacol Ther 2009;29(3):235–246.
114. Safdi M, Bekal PK, Martin S, Saeed ZA, Burton F, Toskes PP. The effects of oral pancreatic enzymes (Creon 10 capsule) on steatorrhea: A multicenter, placebo-controlled, parallel group trial in subjects with chronic pancreatitis. Pancreas 2006;33(2):156–162.
115. Czako L, Takacs T, Hegyi P, et al. Quality of life assessment after pancreatic enzyme replacement therapy in chronic pancreatitis. Can J Gastroenterol 2003;17(10):597–603.
116. Dominguez-Munoz JE, Iglesias-Garcia J, Iglesias-Rey M, Figueiras A, Vilarino-Insua M. Effect of the administration schedule on the therapeutic efficacy of oral pancreatic enzyme supplements in patients with exocrine pancreatic insufficiency: A randomized, three-way crossover study. Aliment Pharmacol Ther 2005;21(8):993–1000.
117. Vecht J, Symersky T, Lamers CB, Masclee AA. Efficacy of lower than standard doses of pancreatic enzyme supplementation therapy during acid inhibition in patients with pancreatic exocrine insufficiency. J Clin Gastroenterol 2006;40(8):721–725.
118. Creon (pancrelipase) [package insert]. North Chicago, IL: Abbott Laboratories, 2011.
119. Viokace (pancrelipase) [package insert]. Birmingham, AL: Aptalis Pharma US Inc, 2012.
120. Traynor K. First FDA-approved pancrelipase product may mark new era for providers, patients. Am J Health Syst Pharm 2009;66(12):1066, 1068.
121. Sani G, Kotzalidis GD, Simonetti A, et al. Development of asymptomatic pancreatitis with paradoxically high serum clozapine levels in a patient with schizophrenia and the CYP1A2*1F/1F genotype. J Clin Psychopharmacol 2010;30(6):737–739.
122. Dominguez-Munoz JE, Iglesias-Garcia J, Vilarino-Insua M, Iglesias-Rey M. 13C-mixed triglyceride breath test to assess oral enzyme substitution therapy in patients with chronic pancreatitis. Clin Gastroenterol Hepatol 2007;5(4):484–488.

26

Viral Hepatitis

Paulina Deming

KEY CONCEPTS

1. Hepatitis A is transmitted via the fecal–oral route. Transmission is most likely to occur through travel to countries with high rates of hepatitis A, poor sanitation and hygiene, and overcrowded areas.
2. Hepatitis A causes an acute, self-limiting illness and does not lead to chronic infection. There are three stages of infection: incubation, acute hepatitis, and convalescence. Rarely, the infection progresses to liver failure.
3. Treatment of hepatitis A consists of supportive care. There is no role for antiviral agents in treatment.
4. Hepatitis B causes both acute and chronic infection. Infants and children are at high risk for chronic infection.
5. Several therapies are available for hepatitis B, including lamivudine, interferon-alfa, pegylated interferon-alfa, entecavir, adefovir, telbivudine, and tenofovir. Patient status, extent of disease, viral load, and viral resistance are all considered when deciding on treatment.
6. Chronic hepatitis B patients may require long-term therapy. Long-term therapy poses a challenge because of the potential for developing resistance. Resistance to lamivudine and telbivudine is most common, limiting the use of these treatments. Optimal treatment of resistant strains is unknown.
7. Prevention of hepatitis B infections focuses on immunization of all children and at-risk adults.
8. Hepatitis C is an insidious, blood-borne infection. Many people are unaware of their infection and risk significant morbidity and mortality.
9. Combination pegylated interferon and ribavirin therapy with either boceprevir or telaprevir is the treatment of choice for hepatitis C genotype 1 infections. Treatment duration varies depending on response, previous treatment history, and the presence of cirrhosis. For genotypes 2, 3, and 4 the treatment of choice includes pegylated interferon and ribavirin.
10. Boceprevir and telaprevir offer significant improvements in outcome for the treatment of hepatitis C genotype 1 infections but pose additional challenges and new concerns for multiple drug interactions.

The major hepatotrophic viruses responsible for viral hepatitis are hepatitis A, hepatitis B, hepatitis C, delta hepatitis, and hepatitis E. All share clinical, biochemical, immunoserologic, and histologic findings. Both hepatitides A and E are spread through fecal–oral contamination, whereas hepatitides B, C, and delta are transmitted parenterally. Infection with delta hepatitis requires coinfection with hepatitis B. Although the rates of acute infection have declined, viral hepatitis remains a major cause of morbidity and mortality with a significant impact on healthcare costs in the United States. Compared with human immunodeficiency virus (HIV), there are three to five times as many people infected with chronic viral hepatitis. In the United States, there is a general lack of knowledge among healthcare providers, social service providers, and the public regarding the risks of chronic hepatitis B and C infections.[1]

Unprecedented therapeutic advances have occurred with the treatment for hepatitis C with the approval of new agents, updated guidelines for care, and more novel therapies eagerly anticipated. For both hepatitides B and C, the challenge remains to increase awareness of the viral hepatic epidemic and to prevent the profound morbidity and mortality associated with chronic infection. This chapter focuses on hepatitides A, B, and C.

HEPATITIS A

Hepatitis A virus (HAV), or infectious hepatitis, is often a self-limiting and acute viral infection of the liver posing a health risk worldwide. The infection is rarely fatal. According to the Centers for Disease Control and Prevention (CDC), rates of reported cases of acute clinical hepatitis A infection in the United States continue to decline with 1,670 cases in 2010.[2] The significant declines in rates of acute HAV are associated with major vaccination campaigns that successfully reduced the incidence rate.

Epidemiology

Various patient groups are at increased risk for infection with HAV. Children pose a particular problem with the spread of the disease because they often remain clinically asymptomatic and are infectious for longer periods of time than adults. Traditionally, the most likely patient group affected is household or close personal contacts of an infected person. (1) Infection primarily occurs through the fecal–oral route, by person-to-person, or by ingestion of contaminated food or water. Incidentally, HAV's prevalence is linked to regions with low socioeconomic status and specifically to those with poor sanitary conditions and overcrowding. International travel and immigration also mitigate potential exposure to the virus.

International travel, in particular travel to HAV endemic areas, continues to be a major risk factor for HAV infection. Other identified risk factors include sexual and household contact with an HAV-infected person, men who have sex with men (MSM), and injection-drug users (IDUs).[2] Additional patient groups that are at risk include patients with chronic liver disease and persons working with nonhuman primates. In 2010, 75% of case reports of acute

HAV reported no identifiable risk factor.[2] Among MSMs, specific sexual practices may be associated with an increased risk for infection.[3] Foodborne outbreaks also occur. In general, mortality rates are low but highest among persons ≥75 years of age.[2]

Despite low endemic rates and successful vaccination programs in the United States, travel to HAV endemic areas is a recognized risk for acquiring acute HAV infections. According to the CDC, the majority of travel-related cases correspond to travel to Central and South America and Mexico.[2] Most Americans traveling to Mexico do not consider that country to be a risk in part because of Mexico's proximity to the United States. Moreover, most tourists falsely believe that higher-end resorts imply safety and that short visits to foreign countries are not associated with a risk for infection. Travel related to international adoptions can also be of risk. In 2009, HAV vaccination was recommended for household members and close personal contacts of newly adopted children from countries of high or intermediate HAV endemicity.[4]

Etiology

Hepatitis A is a RNA virus belonging to the genus *Hepatovirus* of the Picornaviridae family. Humans are the only known reservoir for the virus and transmission occurs primarily through the fecal–oral route.[6] The virus is stable in the environment for at least a month and requires heating foods to a minimum of 85°C (185°F) for 1 minute or disinfecting with a 1:100 dilution of sodium hypochlorite (bleach) in tap water for inactivation.[5,7]

Multiple genotypes of the virus exist and although the clinical implications of infection by particular type are unknown, types I and III are the most commonly identified in human outbreaks.[6]

Pathophysiology

HAV infection is usually acute, self-limiting, and confers lifelong immunity. HAV's life cycle in the human host classically begins with ingestion of the virus. Absorption in the stomach or small intestine allows entry into the circulation and uptake by the liver. Replication of the virus occurs within hepatocytes and GI epithelial cells. New virus particles are released into the blood and secreted into bile by the liver. The virus is then either reabsorbed to continue its cycle or excreted in the stool. The enterohepatic cycle will continue until interrupted by antibody neutralization.[6] The exact mechanism of replication and secretion is unknown; however, the initial viral expansion does not seem to be associated with hepatic injury as peak viral fecal excretion precedes clinical signs and symptoms of infection.[5]

Clinical Presentation

2 The incubation period of HAV is approximately 28 days, with a range of 15 to 50 days. Viremia occurs within 1 to 2 weeks of exposure as patients begin to shed the virus.[5] Table 26-1 summarizes the clinical features of acute hepatitis A. Peak fecal shedding of the virus precedes the onset of clinical symptoms and elevated liver enzymes. Acute hepatitis follows, beginning with the preicteric or prodromal period. The phase is marked by an abrupt onset of nonspecific symptoms, some very mild.[5] Other, more unusual symptoms include chills, myalgia, arthralgia, cough, constipation, diarrhea, pruritus, and urticaria. The phase generally lasts 2 months. There are no specific symptoms unique to HAV. Liver enzyme levels rise within the first weeks of infection, peaking approximately in the fourth week and normalizing by the eighth week. Conjugated bilirubinemia, clinically evident as dark urine, precedes the onset of the icteric period. GI symptoms may persist or subside during this time and some patients may have hepatomegaly. Duration of the icteric period varies and corresponds to disease duration. It averages between 7 and 30 days.[6]

TABLE 26-1 Clinical Presentation of Acute Hepatitis A

Signs and symptoms

- The preicteric phase brings nonspecific influenza-like symptoms consisting of anorexia, nausea, fatigue, and malaise
- Abrupt onset of anorexia, nausea, vomiting, malaise, fever, headache, and right upper quadrant abdominal pain with acute illness
- Icteric hepatitis is generally accompanied by dark urine, acholic (light-colored) stools, and worsening of systemic symptoms
- Pruritus is often a major complaint of icteric patients

Physical examination

- Icteric sclera, skin, and secretions
- Mild weight loss of 2–5 kg
- Hepatomegaly

Laboratory tests

- Positive-serum immunoglobulin M anti–hepatitis A virus
- Mild elevations of serum bilirubin, γ-globulin, and hepatic transaminase (alanine transaminase and aspartate transaminase) values to about twice normal in acute anicteric disease
- Elevations of alkaline phosphatase, γ-glutamyl transferase, and total bilirubin in patients with cholestatic illness

Symptoms and severity of HAV vary according to age. Children younger than 6 years of age typically are asymptomatic. Symptoms, if they do occur, do not include jaundice. In older children and adults, the majority of patients present with symptoms that last less than 2 months and 70% of adults experience jaundice. Peak viral shedding precedes the onset of GI symptoms in adults. In young children, shedding can occur for months following diagnosis.[5] Because children are often asymptomatic and will shed the virus for long periods of time, they can serve as a reservoir for the spread of HAV.

Serum HAV RNA is detectable approximately 2 weeks prior to the onset of symptoms or peak alanine aminotransferase (ALT) levels and can persist for an average of 79 days after the onset of symptoms. In some patients, serum HAV is detectable for more than a year.[11] The use of nucleic acid sequencing to detect HAV RNA is limited to research and instead immunoglobulin (Ig) M antibody to HAV (anti-HAV) is required for a diagnosis of acute infection in clinical settings. IgM anti-HAV is detectable 5 to 10 days prior to symptomatic HAV infections in the majority of patients. IgG anti-HAV replaces IgM and indicates host immunity following the acute phase of the infection.[7] FDA-approved assays for serologic testing detect IgM anti-HAV only and total anti-HAV (IgM and IgG anti-HAV). Patients who have detectable total anti-HAV with a negative IgM have resolved their infection. Patients who are successfully immunized or who receive Ig may have lower levels of total anti-HAV that are below the levels of detection of most commercial assays.[5,7] Concentrations of antibody often fall to 10 to 100 times lower than what would be expected after a natural course of infection. Although a positive anti-HAV result confirms protection, undetectable concentration of anti-HAV may not necessarily imply that protective levels were not achieved.[7]

HAV does not lead to chronic infections. Some patients may experience symptoms for up to 9 months. Rarely, patients experience complications from HAV, including relapsing hepatitis, cholestatic hepatitis, and fulminant hepatitis. Fatalities from HAV are generally rare, although more likely in patients older than age 50 years and in persons with preexisting liver disease.[7]

A diagnosis of HAV is based on clinical criteria of an acute onset of fatigue, abdominal pain, loss of appetite, intermittent nausea and vomiting, jaundice or elevated serum aminotransferase levels, and serologic testing for IgM anti-HAV. Serologic testing is necessary to differentiate the diagnosis from other types of hepatitis.

TREATMENT

Desired Outcome

3 The majority of people infected with HAV can be expected to fully recover without clinical sequelae.[6] Nearly all individuals will have clinical resolution within 6 months of the infection, and a majority will have done so by 2 months. Rarely, symptoms persist for longer or patients relapse. The ultimate goal of therapy is complete clinical resolution. Other goals include reducing complications from the infection, normalization of liver function, and reducing infectivity and transmission. Prevention of HAV infection is important because significant costs are accrued during acute HAV infections, from both direct costs of hospitalizations and indirect costs from loss of work days.

General Approach to Treatment

No specific treatment options exist for HAV infections. Instead, patients should receive general supportive care. Prevention and prophylaxis are key to managing the virus. The importance of good hand hygiene cannot be overemphasized in preventing disease transmission. Ig is used for preexposure and postexposure prophylaxis, and offers passive immunity. Active immunity is achieved through vaccination. Vaccines were approved for use in 1995 and implemented in the routine vaccination of children, as well as at-risk adults, to reduce the overall incidence of HAV.[7]

Prevaccination serologic testing to determine susceptibility is generally not recommended. In some cases, testing may be cost-effective if the cost of the test is less than that of the vaccine and if the person is from a moderate to high endemic area and likely to have prior immunity. Prevaccination serologic testing of children is not recommended. Similarly, because of high vaccine response, postvaccine serologic testing is not recommended.[7]

Prevention of Hepatitis A

HAV is easily preventable with vaccination. Because children often serve as reservoirs of the disease, vaccine programs have targeted children as the most effective means to control HAV. Two vaccines for HAV are available and are incorporated into the routine childhood vaccination schedule. In October 2005, the FDA reduced the minimum age for the vaccines to 12 months of age. In response, the Advisory Committee on Immunization Practices (ACIP) recommended expanding vaccine coverage to all children, including catch-up programs for children living in areas without existing vaccination programs. The new recommendations were enacted in the attempt to further reduce HAV incidence rates and possibly to eradicate the virus.[13] Following a CDC health advisory report of HAV infection from international adoptees, in 2009 ACIP updated its guidelines to include hepatitis A vaccination for previously unvaccinated persons anticipating close personal contact with international adoptees from a country of high or intermediate endemicity. Complete HAV vaccination recommendations are available from the CDC (Table 26-2).

Routine prevention of HAV transmission includes regular hand washing with soap and water after using the bathroom, changing a diaper, and before food preparation. For travelers to countries with high endemic rates of HAV, even short-term stays in urban and upscale resorts are not risk-free.[7] In particular, contaminated water and ice, fresh produce, and any uncooked foods pose a risk.[6]

Vaccines to Prevent Hepatitis A

The inactivated virus vaccines currently licensed in the United States are the single-antigen HAVRIX® and VAQTA® and the combination of HAV and hepatitis B virus (HBV) antigen vaccine TWINRIX®. Both single-antigen vaccines are available for pediatric and adult use while the TWINRIX is indicated for adults only (Table 26-3). The differences in the vaccines are in the use of a preservative and in expression of antigen content. VAQTA is formulated without a preservative and uses units of HAV antigen to express potency. HAVRIX and TWINRIX use 2-phenoxyphenol as a preservative and antigen content is expressed as enzyme-linked immunosorbent assay (ELISA) units.[7] Although high seroconversion rates of ≥94% are achieved with the first dose, VAQTA and HAVRIX recommend a booster shot to achieve the highest possible antibody titers. Although seroconversion exceeds 90% for HAV after the first dose of TWINRIX, the full three-dose series is required for maximal HBV seroconversion. An accelerated dosing schedule is available but requires a total of four doses for optimal response. The combined vaccine offers the advantage of immunization against both types of hepatitis in a single vaccine.

In situations of postexposure prophylaxis, either the vaccine or Ig can be used. The use of the vaccine is advantageous as vaccination confers the benefit of long-term immunity against HAV; however, experience in patients aged >40 years or with underlying medical conditions is limited.[8] Both vaccines may be given concomitantly with Ig and the two brands are interchangeable for booster shots.[7]

TABLE 26-2 Recommendations for Hepatitis A Virus (HAV) Vaccination

All children at 1 year of age
Children and adolescents aged 2–18 years who live in states or communities where routine hepatitis A vaccination has been implemented because of high disease incidence
Persons traveling to or working in countries that have high or intermediate endemicity of infection[a]
Men who have sex with men
Illegal drug users
Persons with occupational risk for infection (e.g., persons who work with HAV-infected primates or with HAV in a research laboratory)
Persons who have clotting factor disorders
Persons with chronic liver disease
All previously unvaccinated persons anticipating close personal contact (e.g., household contact or regular babysitter) with an international adoptee from a country of high or intermediate endemicity within the first 60 days following the arrival of the adoptee

[a]Travelers to Canada, Western Europe, Japan, Australia, or New Zealand are at no greater risk for infection than they are in the United States. All other travelers should be assessed for HAV risk.

From reference 8.

TABLE 26-3 Recommended Dosing of Hepatitis A Vaccines

Vaccine	Age (years)	Dose of Hepatitis A Antigen	No. of Doses	Schedule
HAVRIX	1–18	720 ELISA units	2	0, 6–12 months
	≥19	1,440 ELISA units	2	0, 6–12 months
VAQTA	1–18	25 units	2	0, 6–18 months
	≥19	50 units	2	0, 6–18 months
TWINRIX[a]	≥18	720 ELISA units	3	0, 1, 6 months
	≥18 (accelerated schedule)	720 ELISA units	4	0, 7 days, 21–30 days, +12 months

ELISA, enzyme-linked immunosorbent assay.

[a]Combination hepatitis A and B vaccine, also contains 20 mcg of hepatitis B surface antigen and requires a three-dose schedule.

From Centers for Disease Control and Prevention.[8]

Vaccine is recommended for international travel to areas of high or intermediate endemicity and can be given regardless of scheduled dates of departure. For older patients, immunocompromised, or any patients with chronic liver disease or any other chronic medical conditions traveling within 2 weeks, both Ig and vaccine are recommended.[8]

The most common side effects of the vaccines include soreness and warmth at the injection site, headache, malaise, and pain. More than 65 million doses of the vaccine have been administered and despite routine monitoring for adverse events, there are no data to suggest a greater incidence of serious adverse events among vaccinated people compared with nonvaccinated. The vaccine is considered safe.[7]

Immunoglobulin

Ig is used when preexposure or postexposure prophylaxis against HAV infection is needed in persons for whom vaccination is not an option. Vaccination is preferred for multiple reasons, including that it induces active immunity and therefore a longer time of protection against HAV than Ig. Ig is preferred for children <12 months of age and for postexposure prophylaxis in patients aged >60 years, patients with chronic liver disease, and persons allergic to any part of the vaccine. Among this patient population, Ig is preferred because it is effective and these populations are the most likely to experience fulminant hepatitis and mortality secondary to active HAV infections.

A sterile preparation of concentrated antibodies against HAV, Ig provides protection by passive transfer of antibody. Ig is most effective if given in the incubation period of the infection. Receipt of Ig within the first 2 weeks of infection will reduce infectivity and moderate the infection in 85% of patients. Patients who receive at least one dose of the HAV vaccine at least 1 month earlier do not need preexposure or postexposure prophylaxis with Ig.[7] Ig is available as both an IV and IM injection, but for HAV exposure, only the IM is used. If given to infants or pregnant women, the thimerosal-free formulation should be used.

Serious adverse events are rare. Anaphylaxis has been reported in patients with IgA deficiency. Patients who had an anaphylaxis reaction to Ig should not receive it. There is no contraindication for use in pregnancy or lactation.

Dosing of Ig is the same for adults and children. For postexposure prophylaxis and for short-term preexposure coverage of <3 months, a single dose of 0.02 mL/kg is given intramuscularly. For long-term preexposure prophylaxis of ≤5 months, a single dose of 0.06 mL/kg is used. Either the deltoid or gluteal muscle may be used. In children younger than 24 months of age, Ig can be given in the anterolateral thigh muscle.[7]

For people who were recently exposed to HAV and who had not been previously vaccinated, postexposure prophylaxis with vaccination is preferred for most patients. Ig prophylaxis is preferred in the following situations: patients are <12 months of age or >40 years of age, are immunocompromised, have chronic liver disease or have underlying medical conditions, or for whom vaccine is contraindicated.[8]

Ig can be given concomitantly with the HAV vaccine. Although the antibody titer will be lower than if the vaccine were administered alone, the response is still protective and coadministration should be considered for the advantages of long-term HAV protection. However, Ig can interfere with the response of other live, attenuated vaccines and should be delayed.

Personalized Pharmacotherapy

Vaccine efficacy may be reduced in certain patient populations. In HIV-infected patients, greater immunogenic response may correlate with higher baseline CD4 cell counts. Response to the HAV vaccine as determined by detection of anti-HAV after vaccination found that among HIV patients, patients with CD4 counts <200 cells/mm^3 (<200 × 10^6/L) at vaccination had a reduced response rate.[9]

HEPATITIS B

Hepatitis B is highly infectious, approximately 50 to 100 times more so than HIV.[10] Although a vaccine was made available in 1981, HBV has acutely infected more than 2 billion people globally, leading to chronic infection in more than 240 million people.[10] Chronic infection with HBV is a major public health issue as it serves as a reservoir for continued HBV transmission and poses a significant risk of death resulting from liver disease. More than 600,000 people per year die as a result of liver cirrhosis and hepatocellular carcinoma (HCC). In the United States, estimates of prevalence and incidence of viral hepatitis are difficult because there is no national chronic hepatitis surveillance program.[1]

Epidemiology

According to the World Health Organization (WHO), an estimated 2 billion people have been infected with HBV; only 12% of the global population lives in an area of low prevalence for hepatitis B, defined as an area where <2% of the population is hepatitis B surface antigen (HBsAg) positive.[10] Prevalence can vary regionally; however, areas commonly associated with high infectivity rates include sub-Saharan Africa, most of Asia, as well as the Amazon and southern parts of Eastern and Central Europe.[10] Areas of high prevalence, approximately 45% of the global population, are of special concern because most infections are of infants and children and >90% of cases lead to a chronic carrier state. Myths and misinformation about hepatitis B abound and can result in discrimination and social injustice.[1] There are approximately 1.4 million chronically infected HBV people in the United States. Rates of acute infection in the United States continue to decline and in 2010, an estimated 38,000 people developed new infections. In 2010, the highest incidence rate was among persons aged 30 to 39 years and among non-Hispanic blacks. Data from a limited chronic surveillance program indicate Asian/Pacific Islanders account for the highest proportion of chronic HBV infections.[2] Annually, 3,000 people die from chronic liver disease attributable to HBV.[1]

HBV is transmitted sexually, parenterally, and perinatally. In areas of high HBV prevalence, perinatal transmission from mother to infant at birth is most common, whereas in areas of intermediate prevalence, horizontal transmission from child to child is most common. Sexual contact, both homosexual and heterosexual, and injection-drug use are the predominant forms of transmission in low endemic countries such as the United States.[10] Concentration of HBV is high in blood, serum, and wound exudates of infected persons. Transmission occurs via blood-to-blood contact or semen or vaginal fluid of an infected person. The virus can be stable in the environment for at least 7 days and can cause infection during this time but is not spread via contaminated food or water and is not casually transmitted in the workplace.[10] In the United States in 2010, no risk factor could be identified for the majority of acute infections with HBV. Among patients with identifiable risk factors, the most common risk continues to be sexual contact, specifically multiple sexual partners, MSM, and sexual contact with a known HBV-positive person. Sexual contact was a consistent risk among all patients but especially among those aged 45 years or younger. Other known risk factors include IDU and household contact of HBV-positive person.[11]

The mode of transmission has clinical implications because chronic infections are associated with infection acquired in

PERSONS AT HIGH RISK FOR HBV: RECOMMENDED SCREENING

Individuals From the Following Areas	Other Groups
Asia	U.S.-born persons not vaccinated as infants whose parents were born in high HBV endemic regions
Africa	Household and sexual contacts of HBsAg positive patients
South Pacific Islands	Persons who have ever injected drugs
Middle East (except Cyprus and Israel)	Persons with multiple sexual partners of history of sexually transmitted disease
Malta	MSM
Spain	Inmates of correctional facilities
Arctic (indigenous populations of Alaska, Canada, Greenland)	Individuals with chronically elevated AST or ALT
South America: Ecuador, Guyana, Suriname, Venezuela, Amazon regions of Bolivia, Brazil, Colombia, Peru	Individuals with HIV or hepatitis C virus (HCV)
Eastern Europe (except Hungary)	Patients undergoing dialysis
Antigua and Barbuda, Dominica, Granada, Haiti, Jamaica, St. Kitts and Nevis, St. Lucia, Turks and Caicos	All pregnant women
	Persons requiring immunosuppressive therapy

Data from references 14 and 20.

younger patients, especially those infected perinatally and in early childhood.[10]

Clinical **Controversy. . .**

A total of 19 healthcare-associated HBV outbreaks have been identified and linked to lapses in infection control. Inappropriate use of glucose meters without cleaning and disinfection was the suspected mode of transmission in the majority of cases occurring in long-term care facilities.

Etiology

The HBV is a DNA virus that preferentially replicates within the liver.[12] There are at least 10 HBV genotypes (A to J) with distinct geographic and ethnic distribution (Table 26-4). Genotype prevalence may depend on mode of transmission as types B and C are found in areas where vertical transmission is the primary mode of infection.[13] Additionally, various subtypes of genotypes exist with varying clinical outcomes. Correlations between clinical outcomes and HBV genotypes suggest infections with genotype C are associated with more severe liver injury, including liver cirrhosis and progression to HCC. Noted limitations of studies are frequently small sample sizes and a predominance of research from Asia, primarily comparing genotypes B and C.[13] Nonetheless, risk of more severe liver fibrosis was significantly higher in HBV genotype A-, C-, and D-infected patients. Genotype B may be more benign because it is associated with faster seroconversion, although clinical studies suggest genotype A may have equivalent, if not higher, rates of seroconversion.[13] Patients with genotype C tend to have persistently higher viral DNA levels. Higher viral DNA levels are associated with increased incidence of cirrhosis and HCC. Resistance mutations may contribute to genotype virulence and hence impact severity of liver disease in infection.[13–15] Testing for HBV genotype is not currently recommended for clinical practice.[14]

TABLE 26-4 Worldwide Distribution of Hepatitis B Virus Genotypes

Genotype	Geographic Distribution
A	Northern/Central Europe, sub-Saharan Africa, Western Africa
B	East Asia, Japan, Alaska, Northern Canada, Greenland, Philippines, Vietnam, Indonesia, Taiwan, China
C	Taiwan, China, Korea, Southeast Asia, Australia, Philippines, Vietnam
D	Mediterranean region, Middle East, India, Africa
E	West Africa
F	Central and South America
G	France, Germany, United States
H	Central America
I	Vietnam, Laos
J	Japan

Data from reference 13.

Pathophysiology

On infection, replication of the virus begins by attachment of the virion to the hepatocyte cell surface receptors. The particles are transported to the nucleus where the DNA is converted into closed, circular DNA that serves as a template for pregenomic RNA. Viral RNA is then transcribed and transported back to the cytoplasm where it can alternatively serve as a reservoir for future viral templates or bud into the intracellular membrane with the viral envelope proteins and infect other cells.[13] The viral genome has four reading frames coding for various proteins and enzymes required for viral replication and spread. Several of these proteins are used diagnostically (Table 26-5). The HBsAg is the most abundant of the three surface antigens and is detectable at the onset of clinical symptoms. Its persistence past 6 months after initial detection corresponds to chronic infection and indicates an increased risk for cirrhosis, hepatic decompensation, and HCC. Development of antibody to HBsAg (anti-HBsAg) confers immunity to the virus and clearance of HBsAg is associated with favorable outcomes.[16] The precore polypeptide encodes for the secretory protein hepatitis B e antigen (HBeAg) and the hepatitis B core antigen (HBcAg) proteins. HBeAg is present in an acute infection and is replaced by antibodies (anti-HBeAg) once an infection is resolved. HBeAg was assumed to be a marker of viral replication and infectivity; however, it is now known that some viral mutants exist that are unable to have or have downregulated expression of HBeAg, although their ability to replicate is not affected.[14] HBeAg-negative mutants pose a particular clinical challenge because they are refractory to treatment. The HBcAg is a nucleocapsid protein that, when expressed on hepatocytes, promotes immune-mediated cell death. High levels of antibodies (IgM anti-HBcAg) are detectable during acute infections. Patients who respond to vaccine will have anti-HBsAg only.[7]

HBV itself does not seem to be pathogenic to cells; rather, it is thought that the immune response to the virus is cytotoxic to hepatocytes.[13] The immune response is critical to viral clearance. If the response is weak, chronic infection is likely. Liver injury is likely caused by secondary, nonspecific inflammation activated by the initial cytotoxic lymphocyte response and as an attempt by the immune system to clear the virus by destroying HBV antigen-presenting hepatocytes. Destruction of hepatocytes results in release of circulating, and hence increased, ALT levels.

Cirrhosis

Cirrhosis results as the liver attempts to regenerate while in an environment of persistent inflammation. Most patients with

TABLE 26-5 Interpretation of Serologic Tests in Hepatitis B Virus

Tests	Result	Interpretation
HBsAg Anti-HBc Anti-HBs	(–) (–) (–)	Susceptible
HBsAg Anti-HBc Anti-HBs	(–) (+) (+)	Immune because of natural infection
HBsAg Anti-HBc Anti-HBs	(–) (–) (+)	Immune because of vaccination (valid only if test performed 1–2 months after third vaccine dose)
HBsAg Anti-HBc IgM anti-HBc	(+) (+) (+)	Acute infection
HBsAg Anti-HBc IgM anti-HBc Anti-HBs	(+) (+) (–) (–)	Chronic infection
HBsAg Anti-HBc Anti-HBs	(–) (+) (–)	Four interpretations possible: 1. Recovery from acute infection 2. Distant immunity and test not sensitive enough to detect low level of HBs in serum 3. Susceptible with false-positive anti-HBc 4. May have undetectable level of HBsAg in serum and be chronically infected

HBc, hepatitis B core; HBs, hepatitis B surface; HBsAg, hepatitis B surface antigen; IgM, immunoglobulin M.

From Centers for Disease Control and Prevention. Hepatitis B Serology. http://www.cdc.gov/ncidod/diseases/hepatitis/b/Bserology.htm.

compensated cirrhosis either are asymptomatic or have mild symptoms of epigastric pain. During cirrhosis, the liver enters a cycle of ongoing liver damage, fibrosis, and attempts at regeneration. The classical appearance of a small and knobby liver reflects the irreversible effect of nodules of regenerating cells integrated with infiltrates of inflammation-induced fibrous tissue. Both viral and clinical factors affect the outcome of cirrhosis (Table 26-6). Cirrhosis develops at an annual incidence rate of 2.1% to 3.5%.[13] The development of cirrhosis is mostly insidious and patients can remain stable for years before disease progression. An estimated 20% of all chronic hepatitis B patients develop complications of hepatic insufficiency and portal hypertension as their compensated cirrhosis progresses to decompensated cirrhosis within a 5-year period.[14]

TABLE 26-6 Factors Associated with Hepatitis B Virus (HBV) Cirrhosis and Disease Progression

Persistence of HBV serum DNA
Infection with genotype C
Coinfection with HCV, delta hepatitis, or HIV
Age at diagnosis
Severity of liver disease at diagnosis
Male sex
Frequency of severe hepatic flares
Alcohol use
Laboratory/physical findings of abnormal liver function
Obesity and metabolic disorders
Smoking

HCV, hepatitis C virus; HIV, human immunodeficiency virus.

Data from references 13, 14, and 19.

Hepatocellular Carcinoma

HBV is a known risk factor for the development of HCC and in areas of high HBV endemicity, a major complication of the infection.[10] The development of HCC can be insidious, occurring in the absence of cirrhosis or in the presence of clinically silent, compensated cirrhosis. Many patients with HCC have no signs of cirrhosis.[14] The virus itself is not likely the causative agent of the cancer. In most cases, HCC develops after years of inflammatory processes provoked by ongoing HBV infection. Compared with HCV, however, HBV does seem to provoke a more direct carcinogenic effect as evidenced by its presence in less severe liver disease, and among patients with advanced HCC, HBV infection is associated with a worse survival rate.[17] Several factors influence the development of HCC, as well as predict survival (see Table 26-6). HCC is more prevalent in males; in older patients; in patients coinfected with HCV or delta hepatitis; and in patients with serologic markings of past or present HBV infection, preexisting cirrhosis, or continued alcohol ingestion. Risks for death and decompensation increase with underlying liver disease. Other host-specific or environmental factors may impact the course of liver disease. Persistently elevated HBV DNA levels (≥10,000 copies/mL [$\geq 10 \times 10^6$ copies/L]) predict HCC development, even after adjusting for sex, age, cigarette smoking, alcohol consumption, HBeAg status, ALT level, and liver cirrhosis.[18] Smoking is a risk factor among European and Asian patients.[19,20] HBeAg status is not a risk factor. In otherwise healthy patients without coinfection or who do not have HCC or decompensation at the time of seroclearance, HBsAg seroclearance does predict a favorable long-term outcome.[16]

Clinical Presentation

4 The clinical symptoms and course of an HBV infection are indistinguishable from other types of viral hepatitis. Several phases of an HBV infection exist and are dynamic.[15] During the initial or acute phase of an HBV infection in adults and older children, the HBV enters a 4- to 10-week incubation period, during which antibodies toward the HBV core are produced and the virus replicates profusely. Active viral replication results in high serum HBV DNA levels and HBeAg secretion. ALT levels may rise slightly, but most patients will remain asymptomatic. Symptoms, if they do occur, include fever, anorexia, nausea, vomiting, jaundice, dark urine, clay-colored or pale stools, and abdominal pain. Most neonates and children are anicteric and have no clinical symptoms; many adults are also asymptomatic.[10] HBsAg does not become detectable until after significant viremia. The initial phase is considered immunotolerant because no hepatic injury is sustained, as evidenced by generally normal ALT levels, and the virus replicates profusely. Patients are highly infectious during this time.[15] In perinatally acquired infections, and in young children, the phase can last for decades—until adulthood.[15] Infected children pose a particular risk because they are often asymptomatic, undiagnosed, and highly infectious.

The immunoactive phase marks a decrease in HBV DNA levels with ongoing secretion of HBeAg. Patients are symptomatic with intermittent flares of hepatitis and marked increases in ALT levels. More frequent flares are associated with disease progression and reflect host immune response against HBV-infected hepatocytes, increased cell death in an attempt to clear the virus.[13,19] The phase can last a few weeks in acute disease, and for years in patients with chronic disease. As the host immune system attempts to gain control of the infection by stopping active viral replication, serum HBV DNA levels drop to undetectable, ALT levels normalize, and liver necroinflammation resolves.[13]

If the infection is self-limiting, HBV DNA quickly subsides, HBeAg disappears within weeks, and HBsAg usually resolves within 4 months. The final phase is seroconversion and is defined by the replacement of HBeAg with anti-HBeAg. Factors favoring seroconversion include female sex, older age, biochemical activity, and genotype. Flares of hepatitis with ALT levels >5 times the upper limits of normal, compared with <5 times the upper limits of normal, correspond to increased immune system activity and precede seroconversion.

Chronic HBV

4 Patients who continue to have detectable HBsAg for more than 6 months have chronic HBV.[13] Table 26-7 lists the clinical features of chronic hepatitis B. The most predictive factor for developing a chronic infection is age. Perinatal infections almost always result in chronic infections because of immune tolerance to the virus. Risks of chronicity decline to a rate of 30% in infants and to less than 5% of acute adult infections.[14]

Chronic infections can be controlled in many cases, but cure is not possible because the HBV template is integrated into the host genome. In patients with recurring cycles of viral expression and host immune response, progressive liver damage ensues.[21] Patients can be divided into two types of chronic hepatitis B: those who are HBeAg positive and those who are HBeAg negative. The ability to express HBeAg by the virus differentiates the two types of chronic infection. Patients are considered to be in the "immune-tolerant" phase when HBeAg is positive, high serum HBV DNA levels are detected, and ALT levels are normal. Typically these patients were infected early in life and develop elevated ALT levels later in life. Spontaneous HBeAg clearance is possible and is associated with older age, higher ALT, and infection with HBV genotype B.[14]

Patients who are HBeAg negative can be further subdivided into the active or inactive carrier. HBeAg-negative chronic HBV patients who are active carriers have a worse clinical course with a very low rate of spontaneous remission. Patients may have long periods of disease remission, but recurring flares of hepatitis with increased frequency and severity can progress to cirrhosis and HCC. In contrast, HBeAg-negative chronic HBV patients who are inactive carriers have detectable HBsAg and anti-HBeAg, normal ALT, and either low or undetectable levels of HBV DNA. This patient population usually experiences a more benign course of disease, with the possibility of long-term remission, even seroconversion, although reactivation is possible with the progression to cirrhosis and HCC.

TABLE 26-7 Clinical Presentation of Chronic Hepatitis B[a]

Signs and symptoms

- Easy fatigability, anxiety, anorexia, and malaise
- Ascites, jaundice, variceal bleeding, and hepatic encephalopathy can manifest with liver decompensation
- Hepatic encephalopathy is associated with hyperexcitability, impaired mentation, confusion, obtundation, and eventually coma
- Vomiting and seizures

Physical examination

- Icteric sclera, skin, and secretions
- Decreased bowel sounds, increased abdominal girth, and detectable fluid wave
- Asterixis
- Spider angiomata

Laboratory tests

- Presence of hepatitis B surface antigen >6 months
- Intermittent elevations of hepatic transaminase (alanine transaminase and aspartate transaminase) and hepatitis B virus DNA >20,000 international units/mL (10^5 copies/mL) or >20 × 10^6/L (10^8 copies/L)
- Liver biopsies for pathologic classification as chronic persistent hepatitis, chronic active hepatitis, or cirrhosis

[a]Chronic hepatitis B can be present even without all the signs, symptoms, and physical examination findings listed being apparent.

Up to 20% of patients in the inactive carrier state may revert to detectable HBeAg, emphasizing the need for lifelong followup to confirm quiescence.[14]

Reactivation of hepatitis B, defined as the recurrence or abrupt rise in HBV replication by an increase in serum HBV DNA of at least 1 $\log_{10}$ and a marked increase in transaminase levels, can occur and is well described in the literature in patients receiving cancer chemotherapy, steroids, and other immunosuppressive agents.[22,23] Reactivation can occur in anyone with a prior or current HBV exposure, but patients who are HBsAg positive are most likely to experience a reactivation.[23] The causes of reactivation include spontaneous mutations of the virus that allow it to escape immune control, development of resistance to HBV drug therapy or the cessation of HBV therapy, or changes in immunity, such as those that occur in patients undergoing immunosuppressive therapies or coinfection with HIV.

The CDC recommends testing for hepatitis B for all patients who are to receive chemotherapy or other immunosuppressive agents.

HBV Mutations

6 Among the DNA viruses, HBV is notable for its significantly higher mutation rate.[24] Long-term therapy is problematic because of the high likelihood of developing viral resistance. One of the most common mutations consists of a nucleotide substitution either preventing or causing downregulation of the production of HBeAg. The mutation results in a chronic infection that may have a poorer long-term prognosis. Typically, the mutation emerges during the infection and represents a later stage in the course of chronic HBV infection with more advanced liver disease.

The selective pressures of the L-nucleoside analog antivirals, including lamivudine, cause the YMDD mutation. The mutation is associated with the active site of the DNA polymerase and causes an altered active site. The incidence of lamivudine resistance increases with each subsequent year of therapy and may be associated with a more severe disease progression.[14] An added risk of developing resistance is the retention of the mutation within the virus even 4 years after lamivudine therapy.[25] Cross-resistance of lamivudine-resistant mutants to telbivudine has been demonstrated and patients treated with lamivudine and telbivudine showed resistance mutations to both drugs. Telbivudine-specific resistance can also occur at rates lower than that seen in lamivudine.[26] Other mutations include resistance to adefovir and entecavir. Resistance to adefovir is associated with substitutions of aspargine by threonine (rtN236T) and substitution of alanine by valine or threonine (rtA181V/T), as well as other possible mutations to the HBV polymerase gene. The addition of lamivudine in adefovir resistance may overcome resistance, although the optimal management of either adefovir- or entecavir-resistant strains is not clear.[13–15,24]

Prevention of Hepatitis B

The development of the HBV vaccine represented the first vaccine against a major human cancer.[10] Despite the availability of the HBV vaccine in 1982, rates of HBV did not decline in the early 1980s. Initial declines in incidence were likely attributable to behavioral changes among high-risk groups as a result of the acquired immune deficiency syndrome (AIDS) epidemic. A 94% decline in rates between 1990 and 2004 was seen in children and adolescents, which began with the initiation of screening of pregnant women and subsequent immunizations of infants and recommendations set forth in the 1990s to immunize adolescents. Regulations enacted by Occupational Safety and Health Administration (OSHA) further reduced overall U.S. rates by 75%.[12]

7 Prophylaxis against HBV can be achieved by vaccination or by passive immunity in postexposure cases with hepatitis B Ig.

TABLE 26-8 Recommendations for Hepatitis B Virus (HBV) Vaccination

Infants
Adolescents including all previously unvaccinated children <19 years
All unvaccinated adults at risk for infection
All unvaccinated adults seeking vaccination (specific risk factor not required)
Men and women with a history of other sexually transmitted diseases and persons with a history of multiple sex partners (>1 partner/6 months)
Men who have sex with men
Current or recent injection-drug users
Household contacts and sex partners of persons with chronic hepatitis B infection and healthcare and public safety workers with exposure to blood in the workplace
Clients and staff of institutions for the developmentally disabled
International travelers to regions with high or intermediate levels (HBsAg prevalence ≥2%) of endemic HBV infection
Recipients of clotting factor concentrates
Sexually transmitted disease clinic patients
HIV patient/HIV-testing patients
Drug abuse treatment and prevention clinic patients
Correctional facilities inmates
Chronic dialysis/ESRD patients including predialysis, peritoneal dialysis, and home dialysis patients
Persons with chronic liver disease

ESRD, end-stage renal disease; HIV, human immunodeficiency virus.
From reference 11.

Vaccination is the most effective strategy to prevent infection and a comprehensive vaccination strategy has been implemented in the United States (Table 26-8). Vaccines use HBsAg for the antigen via recombinant DNA technology using yeast to prompt active immunity. More than 60 million adolescents and more than 40 million infants and children have received an HBV vaccine in the United States since 1982. The vaccine is considered safe. Since 2000, vaccines licensed in the United States contain either none or trace amounts of thimerosal as a preservative. Available vaccines include two single-antigen products and three combination products. The two single-antigen products are Recombivax HB and Engerix-B. TWINRIX is a combination vaccine for HAV and HBV in adults. Comvax and Pediarix are used for children and are used for HBV along with other scheduled vaccines.

Passive immunity in the form of anti-HBsAg offers temporary protection against HBV and is used in conjunction with the hepatitis B vaccine for postexposure prophylaxis.[12]

TREATMENT

Desired Outcome

HBV infections are not curable; rather, the goals of therapy are to suppress HBV replication and prevent disease progression to cirrhosis and HCC. The loss of HBsAg is becoming an increasingly more important goal in therapy.

General Approach to Treatment

5 Response to therapy is monitored by biochemical, histologic, and virologic response (Table 26-9).[14] Maintenance of viral suppression is defined as durability of response. In HBeAg-positive patients, successful therapy includes loss of HBeAg status and seroconversion to anti-HBeAg. Other serologic markers are typically not evaluated in clinical trials. Recommendations for treatment consider the patient's age, serum HBV DNA and ALT levels, as well as histologic evidence and clinical progression of disease (Fig. 26-1 and 26-2). Not all chronic HBV patients are candidates for treatment.

TABLE 26-9 Definitions of Response in HBV Therapy

Biochemical	Normalization of ALT
Histologic	Decrease in histology activity by at least 2 points as compared with baseline biopsy
Virologic	Undetectable HBV DNA and, in patients previously HBeAg positive, loss of HBeAg

In general, treatment is indicated if the risk of liver-related morbidity and mortality is within the foreseeable future and the likelihood for achieving sustained viral suppression is high.[14] Some patients may be best managed with periodic monitoring for disease progression because the chances for therapeutic response are unlikely and do not outweigh the risks and costs associated with treatment. The major organizations providing guidelines on the management of HBV infections are the American Association for the Study of Liver Diseases (AASLD), the European Association for the Study of Liver Disease, and the Asian Pacific Association for the Study of the Liver.[13–15]

Nonpharmacologic Therapy

All chronic HBV patients should be counseled on preventing disease transmission. Sexual and household contacts should be vaccinated. To minimize further liver damage, all chronic HBV patients should avoid alcohol and be immunized against HAV. No level of alcohol use has been established as safe.[14] Moreover, patients are encouraged to consult their medical provider before using any new medications, including herbals and nonprescription drugs.[12]

Herbal medicines are an intriguing option to many patients. Although some of the products may have some physiologic benefits, there are insufficient data and the methodologic qualities of the trials

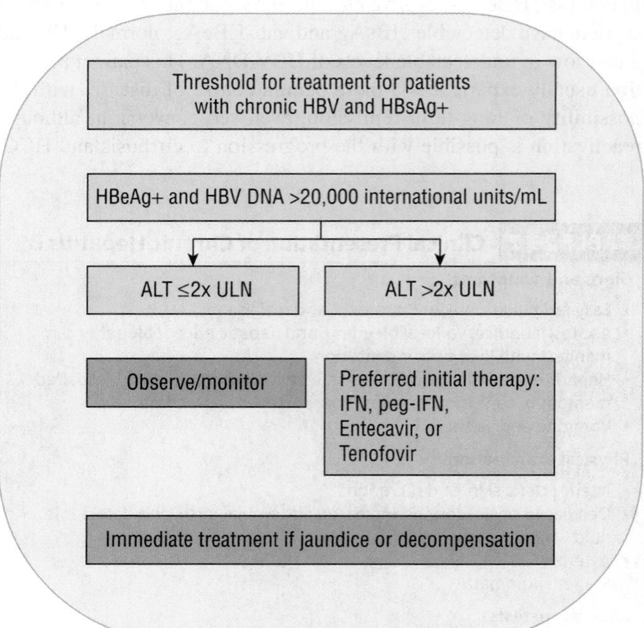

FIGURE 26-1 Suggested management algorithm for chronic hepatitis B virus infection based on the recommendations of the American Association for the Study of Liver Diseases. (ALT, alanine transaminases; HBeAg, hepatitis B e antigen; peg-IFN, pegylated interferon; HBV DNA concentration of >20,000 international units/mL is equivalent to >20 × 10[6] international units/L.) *(Adapted from reference 14.)*

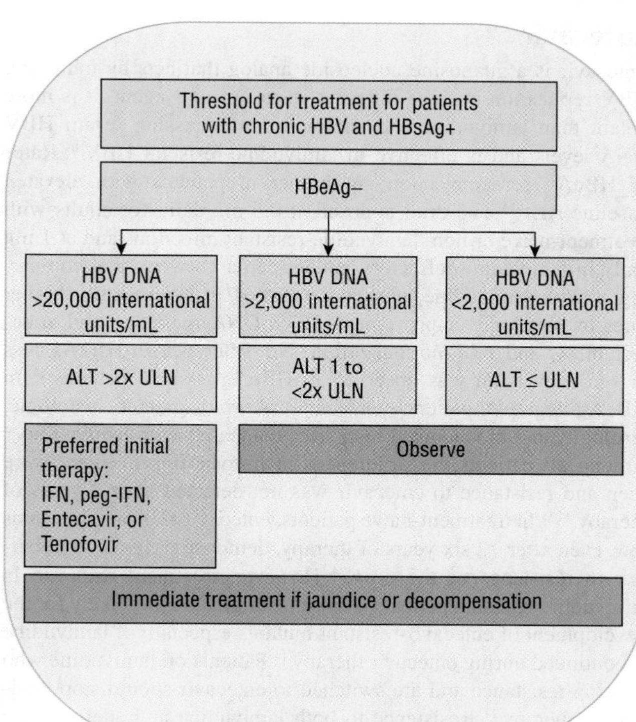

FIGURE 26-2 Suggested management algorithm based on the recommendations of the American Association for the Study of Liver Diseases for chronic hepatitis B virus–infected patients with cirrhosis. (HBV DNA concentrations of >20,000, >2,000, and ≤2,000 international units/mL are equivalent to $>20 \times 10^6$, $>2 \times 10^6$, and $\leq 2 \times 10^6$ international units/L, respectively.)
(Adapted from reference 14.)

evaluating the herbs are poor. Randomized, placebo-controlled studies and long-term followup data are lacking.[27]

Pharmacologic Therapy

5 Because hepatic damage is sustained by ongoing viral replication, drug therapy aims to suppress viral replication by either immunomodulating agents or antivirals—the nucleos(t)ide agents. In the United States, the immune-mediating agents approved as first-line therapy are interferon (IFN)-alfa and pegylated (peg) IFN-alfa. The antiviral agents lamivudine, telbivudine, adefovir, entecavir, and tenofovir are all approved as first-line therapy options for chronic HBV.[14] A major difference in therapy is duration of use: IFN-based therapies are typically administered for a predefined duration, whereas nucleos(t)ide analogs are used until a specific end point is achieved. For HBeAg-positive patients, treatment is recommended until HBeAg seroconversion and an undetectable HBV viral load are achieved and for 6 months of additional treatment. In HBeAg-negative patients, treatment should be continued until HBsAg clearance.[14]

Interferon

IFN-alfa therapy was the first approved therapy for treatment of HBV and improves long-term outcomes and survival. Acting as a host cytokine, it has antiviral, antiproliferative, and immunomodulatory effects in chronic HBV.[14] Several factors correlate with improved response to IFN therapy, including increased ALT and HBV DNA levels, high histologic activity score at biopsy, and being non-Asian. Asian patients tend to have more normal ALT levels in chronic infection, confounding the actual impact of ethnicity on infection.[14] The main mechanism of action of the IFNs is to enhance the host immune system to mount a defense against HBV.

TABLE 26-10 Recommendations for Hepatitis C Virus (HCV) Screening

Anyone born between 1945 and 1965
Current or past use of injection-drug use
Coinfection with HIV
Received blood transfusions or organ transplantations before 1992
Received clotting factors before 1987
Patients who have ever been on hemodialysis
Patients with unexplained elevated ALT levels or evidence of liver disease
Healthcare and public safety workers after a needle-stick or mucosal exposure to HCV-positive blood
Children born to HCV-positive mothers
Sexual partners of HCV-positive patients

ALT, alanine transaminase; HIV, human immunodeficiency virus.
Data from reference 62.

Patients who respond to IFN therapy tend to have a more durable response than that seen with lamivudine, likely as a consequence of IFN's stimulation of the immune response for seroconversion. Seroconversion rates range from 30% to 40% and are often permanent, although relapse is more likely in HBeAg-negative patients.[21,28] The duration of therapy is finite, although the optimal duration of treatment is unclear. Treatment for a minimum of 12 months is associated with greater sustained virologic response (SVR) rates than treatment for 4 to 6 months. Seroconversion can occur during or after therapy is complete. An extended treatment duration of 24 months may benefit the difficult-to-treat HBeAg-negative patient.[21] Conventional IFN therapy is plagued with numerous problems, including the inconvenience of thrice-weekly injections; however, standard IFN therapy has virtually been replaced by the use of peg-IFN because of the benefits in ease of administration, decreased side effect profile, and improvements in efficacy. Compared with conventional IFN, peg-IFN has a longer half-life enabling once-weekly injections. Studies comparing peg-IFN monotherapy with peg-IFN–lamivudine combination therapies suggest that combination therapy caused greater HBV DNA suppression than peg-IFN monotherapy; peg-IFN monotherapy better achieved HBeAg seroconversion than lamivudine monotherapy with no difference in combination therapy; and combination therapy resulted in less lamivudine resistance than lamivudine monotherapy. IFN-based therapies are still limited by multiple adverse effects (Table 26-10). The high risk of infection precludes use of IFN in decompensated cirrhotic patients.[14] In patients with compensated cirrhosis, IFN appears to be safe and effective, although it can provoke hepatic flares and precipitate hepatic decompensation.[14,21] Ongoing clinical trials are investigating the use of either sequential or combination therapy with peg-IFN and nucleos(t)ides. The optimal role of IFN-based therapies in HBV treatment is not defined.

Lamivudine

Lamivudine, a nucleoside analog, has antiviral activity against both HIV and HBV. It inhibits HBV DNA synthesis by being incorporated into growing DNA chains causing premature chain termination.[14] The optimal duration of treatment for HBV is unknown and can be limited by virologic breakthrough. In both HBeAg-positive and -negative patients, lamivudine at a 100 mg daily dose demonstrates profound viral suppression. HBV DNA serum levels are undetectable in 90% of lamivudine-treated patients after 4 weeks.[21] Normalization of ALT levels occurs gradually over 3 to 6 months in most patients. Additionally, fibrotic changes are reduced and may be reversed in some cases. Response to lamivudine is dependent on baseline ALT levels, with higher levels corresponding to greater likelihood of seroconversion. Seroconversion rates increase with duration of therapy and are at 50% by the fifth year of therapy.[14] The advantages of lamivudine-based therapy include its safety profile and patient tolerability and the convenience of an oral tablet. Moreover, lamivudine can safely be used in immunosuppressed and cirrhotic patients.[28] Patients who can maintain long-term viral suppression have reduced and possibly reversed cirrhotic changes. However, lamivudine therapy is not without problems. There is no clear duration of treatment and HBeAg-negative patients have a less than 20% viral suppression rate after 12 months of therapy. Serum HBV DNA levels return to baseline on cessation of therapy.[14] Seroconversion rates are less than 20% after 1 year of therapy and will relapse in up to 58% of patients. Relapse rates are highest among Asian patients.[28] Resistance is inevitable and can undermine the value of treatment. The emergence of resistant mutants increases with each subsequent year of therapy, with rates approaching 80% after 5 years of therapy, and is associated with returns of serum HBV DNA and elevated ALT levels.[24] Relapse is associated with reversion of histologic benefits.[14] Although seroconversion can occur even after the appearance of resistant mutants, the prognosis is poor for most patients who develop resistance.[21] In HBeAg-negative chronic hepatitis B, where therapy is long-term and the exact duration of therapy unknown, resistance is an especially daunting problem.[14] Given the availability of more potent antivirals and the low threshold for resistance with lamivudine, lamivudine is not recommended as first-line therapy for chronic HBV infections.

Patients on lamivudine therapy require monitoring for breakthrough infection. If patients have confirmed lamivudine-resistant mutations, therapy should be changed to include agents with activity against lamivudine-resistant HBV.[14]

Adefovir

Adefovir dipivoxil is an acyclic nucleotide analog of adenosine monophosphate. The drug acts by inhibiting HBV reverse transcriptase and DNA polymerase and is effective in both wild-type and lamivudine-resistant HBV. It is dosed at 10 mg daily for 1 year in adults, although the optimal duration of therapy is unknown.[14] A 48-week course of treatment is effective in improving histologic findings, reducing serum HBV DNA and ALT levels, and increasing HBeAg seroconversion in both HBeAg-negative and -positive patients.[29,30] The durability of the response is likely related to a long duration of treatment following seroconversion.[31] Further suppression of HBV DNA and ALT levels occurred in long-term therapy over 4 to 5 years with improved histologic findings.[32] In HBeAg-negative patients treated for 48 weeks, the benefits of therapy were lost within 4 weeks of stopping adefovir. In contrast, patients treated for 144 weeks maintained benefits throughout the treatment duration and saw continued improvement in fibrosis as the therapy continued. However, rates of seroconversion were low.[32] Adefovir is well tolerated at the 10 mg daily dose. Previous reports of nephrotoxicity were associated with clinical trials where adefovir was dosed at 30 mg/day. In patients treated chronically at a dose of 10 mg daily, the incidence of nephrotoxicity was the same as placebo. In patients treated with 10 mg/day for a subsequent 48 weeks, the incidence of serum creatinine abnormalities did not change from the first year of therapy.[32] Routine monitoring of serum creatinine is recommended every 3 months in patients at risk for renal insufficiency and in all patients treated for more than a year with adefovir.[14]

Resistance to adefovir has not been seen within the first year of therapy.[24] Resistant mutants have been identified and do respond to lamivudine therapy, although the full impact on clinical outcomes is not known.[14] The risk of adefovir resistance is higher among patients switched from lamivudine to adefovir rather than among those who received a combination therapy of lamivudine and adefovir.[33] To prevent adefovir resistance, lamivudine should be continued even in patients with lamivudine-resistant HBV, although the optimal duration for combination therapy is not known.[14] The optimal drug therapy in adefovir resistance is not known.[14]

Entecavir

Entecavir is a guanosine nucleoside analog that acts by inhibiting HBV replication at three different steps. An oral agent, it is more potent than lamivudine and adefovir in suppressing serum HBV DNA levels and is effective in lamivudine-resistant HBV.[14] Rates of HBeAg seroconversion are higher in patients with elevated baseline ALT.[14] The drug is dosed at 0.5 mg daily for adults with treatment-naïve or non–lamivudine-resistant infections and at 1 mg daily in lamivudine-refractory patients. In a 48-week trial comparing it with lamivudine, entecavir resulted in significantly higher rates of histologic improvement, HBV DNA reduction and undetectability, and ALT normalization. No difference in HBeAg loss or seroconversion was observed in HBeAg-positive patients.[34] In HBeAg-negative patients, entecavir showed greater histologic, virologic, and biochemical responses compared with lamivudine.[35] Among all patients, no differences in fibrosis improvement were seen and resistance to entecavir was not detected after 2 years of therapy.[34,35] In treatment-naïve patients, entecavir resistance remains low, even after 72 six years of therapy, demonstrating the high barrier to resistance of the drug.[24] However, treatment response in lamivudine-resistant patients is lower overall and more likely for the development of entecavir-resistant mutants especially if lamivudine is continued during entecavir therapy.[14] Patients on lamivudine who develop resistance and are switched to entecavir should stop lamivudine therapy.[14] Resistance to both lamivudine and adefovir is a risk factor for entecavir resistance.[36] In terms of safety, entecavir is comparable to lamivudine. Entecavir is considered to be a first-line agent for HBV therapy.

Telbivudine

Telbivudine is an HBV-specific nucleoside analog that acts as a competitive inhibitor of viral reverse transcriptase and DNA polymerase. The drug inhibits HBV DNA synthesis with no activity against other viruses or human polymerases.[26] Compared with lamivudine, telbivudine is a more potent suppressor of HBV DNA with greater median HBV DNA log reductions and more patients achieving undetectable viral loads.[26,37] More patients also experienced a normalization of ALT levels. Although more telbivudine-treated patients experienced seroconversion, the difference was not significant even at 2 years of therapy. Treatment failure, including an inability to suppress HBV DNA levels below 5 log, occurred significantly more often in lamivudine-treated patients than in telbivudine-treated ones.[37] However, similar to lamivudine, telbivudine has a high rate of mutations that limits its efficacy. During a 2-year evaluation, resistance increased substantially from year 1 at 5% to 25.1% in year 2 in HBeAg-positive patients and from 2.3% to 10.8% in HBeAg-negative patients.[37,38] Moreover, telbivudine-resistant mutations are cross-resistant with lamivudine. Telbivudine monotherapy is comparable with lamivudine in safety with few case reports of myopathy and elevations of creatinine kinase.[37,38] Overall, due to resistance concerns, telbivudine monotherapy has a limited role in the treatment of HBV.[14]

Tenofovir

Tenofovir is a nucleotide analog first approved for use in HIV and approved for HBV in 2008. It is available either as a single-agent oral tablet or as a combination therapy with emtricitabine. Tenofovir is similar to adefovir but without the nephrotoxicity seen with adefovir, permitting adult dosing to be 300 mg versus 10 mg of adefovir. The higher dosing strategy likely confers several advantages to tenofovir in comparison with adefovir. Among HBeAg-positive patients, more patients treated with tenofovir had undetectable HBV DNA, ALT normalization, and loss of HBsAg than the adefovir-treated group. Rates of histologic response and seroconversion were similar. Among HBeAg-negative patients, more patients treated with tenofovir had undetectable HBV DNA, but there was no difference in ALT normalization and histologic response, and no patients lost HBsAg.[39] In lamivudine-resistant chronic hepatitis B, tenofovir showed an earlier and greater suppression of HBV DNA than adefovir. In studies of treatment-naïve patients on tenofovir for up to 3 years, no resistant mutations were detected.[40] Additional data suggest sustained viral suppression with regression of fibrosis and no resistance in patients treated with tenofovir for 6 years.[41] Tenofovir can overcome adefovir treatment failure, but adefovir mutants persist, suggesting cross-resistance.[42] A study of 113 treatment-experienced patients who had previously failed nucleos(t)ide therapy and were started on tenofovir demonstrated viral suppression in 100% of patients without adefovir resistance and in 52% of patients with adefovir resistance.[43] The optimal management to prevent resistance is unknown at this time. Tenofovir is considered to be a first-line therapy in the treatment of HBV.[14]

Alternative Drug Treatments

Emtricitabine is a cytosine analog approved for use in HIV and with activity against HBV. It is currently not approved for HBV but has been used in combination with tenofovir. In a comparative study with placebo, emtricitabine showed a significant decrease in viral load to undetectable in 54% of patients, normalization of ALT levels in 65% of patients, and improvement in necroinflammatory score. However, seroconversion to anti-HBeAg and HBeAg loss did not differ between placebo and emtricitabine. Emtricitabine safety was comparable to placebo. At the end of the 48-week treatment, 20 emtricitabine-treated patients had YMDD or YMDD-related resistance mutations.[43] Emtricitabine is similar to lamivudine and thus induces similar mutations.[14]

Combination therapy has been proposed to increase drug effectiveness and to counter the issues of resistance. Potential disadvantages for combination therapy include costs, toxicity, and drug interactions. Currently no data exist that combination therapy of two antiviral agents improves effectiveness. Data for preventing resistance are mixed as complete suppression of resistance has not been achieved with combination therapy. Combination therapy with IFN and lamivudine creates less resistance than lamivudine monotherapy, but the combination did not change the posttherapy viral response in comparison to IFN monotherapy.[14] Switching to peg-IFN after entecavir therapy increased the rates of HBeAg seroconversion and HBsAg loss as compared with continuing entecavir therapy.[44] Adding adefovir to patients on lamivudine when HBV DNA levels began to increase better maintained normal ALT levels and suppressed HBV DNA than waiting to add adefovir until after ALT levels increased.[31] Adding adefovir to lamivudine when lamivudine resistance develops in HBeAg-negative patients was associated with improved ALT normalization and a lower likelihood for virologic breakthrough or development of adefovir resistance. Both groups had similar rates of virologic response.[33] In a comparison study of lamivudine monotherapy versus lamivudine–adefovir combination therapy in treatment-naïve patients, similar rates of seroconversion, HBV DNA suppression, and ALT normalization were observed. There was a lower rate of resistance in the combination therapy group at 15% versus 43% in the lamivudine monotherapy group.[45] Entecavir combined with tenofovir in HBeAg-positive patients resulted in greater viral suppression but only in patients with an initial baseline viral load of $\geq 10^8$ international units/mL ($\geq 10^{11}$ international units/L).[46] The AASLD recommends combination therapy with lamivudine or telbivudine plus adefovir, tenofovir, or entecavir for decompensated cirrhotic patients with chronic HBV regardless of HBV DNA levels or HBeAg status.[14] Moreover, current guidelines suggest combination therapy with two or more agents in patients who develop antiviral resistant HBV.[13–15]

Special Populations

Cirrhosis

The decision to treat cirrhotic patients depends on disease progression. Patients with decompensated cirrhosis require referral for liver transplant. Most recently updated guidelines suggest lamivudine, telbivudine, adefovir, tenofovir, and entecavir are possible agents for use in cirrhotic patients (see Fig. 26-2).[14]

Clinical **Controversy...**

Although previously published guidelines do not support the use of IFN in cirrhosis because of the potential for an IFN-induced hepatic flare progressing to decompensation, some experts suggest peg-IFN alfa-2a may be an option for some patients with compensated cirrhosis. Moreover, some experts argue that lamivudine, although indicated for use in cirrhosis, may cause clinical decompensation because of the drug's high risk for resistance and, hence, viral rebound triggering decompensation.

Coinfection with HCV

In patients coinfected with HCV, the clinical practice is to treat the more dominant form of the hepatitis virus. There are no current recommendations on management of HBV/HCV coinfection. Previously published recommendations suggested treating HCV according to published guidelines and to consider the addition of entecavir or adefovir if HBV DNA levels remained stable or rose.[14]

Coinfection with Hepatitis D

Patients coinfected with hepatitis D, which requires infection with hepatitis B, may be treated with high-dose IFN-alfa or peg-IFN.[14] There is an overall paucity of data on HBV–HDV coinfection treatment. Lamivudine has not been shown to be effective, neither has ribavirin, a drug used in combination therapy with IFN for HCV treatment.[47,48]

Coinfection with HIV

In HIV-coinfected patients, therapy should be tailored specifically to the patient. If the patient is being treated for HIV, certain regimens may be optimized to include drugs with efficacy against HBV, including tenofovir, emtricitabine, or lamivudine. If patients are on a stable regimen that does not include HBV-active drugs or are not considered for highly active antiretroviral therapy (HAART), peg-IFN or adefovir may be used.[14] Because of neutropenia associated with peg-IFN, patients considered for IFN therapy should have CD4 counts >500 cells/μL (>500 × 10^6/L). In patients being considered for HAART, combination therapy is recommended for HBV with either tenofovir and lamivudine or tenofovir and emtricitabine. Patients with confirmed lamivudine resistance should have tenofovir added to their regimens.[14]

Pediatrics

Although the majority of chronic HBV patients are adults, children may be treated. Lamivudine is indicated for children aged 2 years and older and IFN is approved for use in children aged 1 year and older. Entecavir is approved for adolescents aged 16 years and older and adefovir for children 12 years and older. Although peg-IFN-alfa does have indications for children 3 years and older, the approval is for the use in chronic hepatitis C infections.

Pregnant Females

Perinatal transmission of HBV is a major cause of chronic HBV globally. To prevent mother-to-child transmission, the use of lamivudine or telbivudine in the third trimester is recommended for women. Tenofovir is an alternative.[13]

Immunosuppressive or Cytotoxic Therapy

Patients who will undergo chemotherapy or immunosuppressive therapy should be assessed for risk of HBV. Prophylactic therapy is recommended prior to initiation of cancer chemotherapy or immunosuppressive therapy. Patients who have undetectable HBV DNA and who are expected to be on treatment for 1 year or less should be treated for 6 months after completion of chemotherapy or immunosuppressive therapy with either lamivudine or telbivudine. Tenofovir or entecavir should be used in patients where the duration of therapy is expected to be longer.[14]

Resistance Concerns

Current guidelines favor the use of potent agents with low rates of resistance. Resistance potential in HBV is evaluated by an antiviral agent's genetic barrier to resistance, or the number of primary mutations needed for antiviral drug resistance to occur. Other factors include cross-resistance and drug potency. Viral suppression is important because the HBV virus requires ongoing viral replication in the setting of antiviral drug pressure to mutate. HBV therapy can be cost prohibitive for many patients and can favor the use of lamivudine. Unfortunately lamivudine-based therapies are prone to resistance and may have long-term implications on viral activity, notably the concerns for development of vaccine-resistant mutants.[12,24]

Another major factor in resistance is patient adherence to therapy. Studies on adherence suggest suboptimal adherence is common with approximately 40% of patients missing doses.[49] Moreover, in patients experiencing virologic breakthrough, studies have shown that 40% of cases were not related to antiviral drug resistance, emphasizing the impact of medication adherence on viral suppression.[50]

PERSONALIZED PHARMACOTHERAPY

Vaccination for HBV is less effective than for HAV and requires multiple doses for improved response. Several host factors are implicated in a reduced response. Patients who are immunocompromised and patients on hemodialysis may require additional doses to induce antibody response. Some patients may require repeat vaccination.[51] Sleep deprivation may also contribute to decreased antibody response.[52]

The role of IFN sensitivity in treatment response is known for hepatitis C where allelic variants of interleukin 28B (IL28B) are strongly associated with spontaneous clearance and associated with responsiveness to treatment.[53] Currently, the role of IFN sensitivity is not well understood for hepatitis B.

HEPATITIS C

HCV is approximately 5 times as common as HIV and is responsible for an estimated 10,000 chronic liver disease–associated deaths per year.[1] More than 190,000 deaths from HCV-related disease are expected between 2010 and 2019, with projected costs exceeding $10 billion.[54] Most acute infections are asymptomatic and the course of the infection is insidious. As a result, many patients are not diagnosed until significant disease progression.

Epidemiology

8 HCV is the most common blood-borne pathogen. In the United States, approximately 3.2 million people are chronically infected with HCV.[1] An estimated 17,000 new HCV infections occurred in 2007; however, because of the clinically silent nature of acute infections and the 20- to 30-year disease progression to cirrhosis, it is the 200,000 patients infected per year in the late 1980s who contribute to today's HCV burden.[54] In 2007, the number of deaths attributable to HCV exceeded the number of deaths due to HIV.[55] The impact of undiagnosed and untreated HCV is expected to increase dramatically over the next 40 to 50 years with 1.76 million persons developing cirrhosis, 400,000 developing HCC, and 1 million persons dying from HCV-associated complications.[56] Considering that HCV infection is prevalent in high-risk populations such as prisoners, IDUs, and the homeless, and that this population is generally excluded from most surveys, the actual number of chronically infected people is significantly higher. Nearly 75% of infected people may not be identified.[1,54] The single largest risk factor for infection is injection-drug use. Some experts also consider other illicit drug use, for example, intranasal cocaine, as a risk factor because of the possible contamination of drug paraphernalia not limited to syringes and needles. Historically, blood transfusion posed a major risk for infection. Improved screening of blood in 1992 decreased the risk of transfusion-related HCV.[57] Currently both hemodialysis and transfusions represent less than 1% of risk factors in known HCV exposures.[4] Healthcare-associated transmission is rare; however, a much publicized outbreak linked to an endoscopy center in Nevada in 2007 prompted an examination of HCV outbreaks associated with healthcare. Since 1998, over 58,000 patients have been screened for possible exposure to HCV in nonhospital healthcare venues, including the Nevada incident. The identified risk in Nevada was unsafe injection practices.

Screening

Although acute HCV infections are often not recognized and many progress to chronic infections, routine screening for infection is not recommended. Various guidelines and position papers for the screening and treatment of chronic HCV infection exist. In 2012, the CDC released recommendations to perform a one-time screening of all patients born between 1945 and 1965. The recommendation was made due to the high rates of HCV in this birth cohort. The CDC estimates approximately 75% of adults with HCV were born in that age range. Screening is also warranted in patients who are at high risk for infection (Table 26-10). Although the risk of HCV in monogamous relationships is very low and barrier methods are not recommended, sexual partners are recommended to be tested for the sake of reassurance.[57] No specific sexual practices are associated with an increased risk of transmission.[58] Although sexual contact is considered an inefficient means of HCV transmission, multiple sexual partners and coinfection with sexually transmitted diseases, including HIV, increase the risk for HCV sexual transmission. The risk of infection from other needle-borne exposures, such as acupuncture, tattooing, and body piercing, is unclear and at this time not an indication for routine screening for HCV.[57]

Etiology

HCV is a single-stranded RNA virus of the family Flaviviridae notable for lacking a proofreading polymerase and enabling frequent viral mutations.[54] The virus replicates within hepatocytes and, like hepatitis B, is not directly cytopathic. HCV replicates copiously with an estimated serum half-life of 2 to 3 hours, posing an immense challenge for host immune control.

HCV is differentiated into six major genotypes, numbered 1 to 6. Genotypes are further classified into subtypes (a, b, c, etc.). The most widely distributed genotypes are 1 and 2, with genotype 1 the most common. In the United States, the majority of infections are caused by genotypes 1a and 1b, followed by genotypes 2 and 3. Although infection caused by any of the genotypes can lead to cirrhosis, end-stage liver disease (ESLD), or HCC, the significance of the infecting genotype is related to therapeutic response. Historically genotype 1 infections were least likely to respond to therapy, but with the release of protease inhibitor (PI) therapies, major advances in response are now possible. Genotypes 2 and 3 respond well to therapy; however, genotypes 4, 5, and 6 continue to pose a therapeutic challenge.

Pathophysiology

In the vast majority of cases, an acute HCV infection leads to chronic infection. The immune response in an acute HCV infection is mostly insufficient to eradicate the virus. The extent of hepatocyte apoptosis may correlate with the course of the disease. Liver damage and HCC are associated with high levels of hepatocyte apoptosis. Low levels of apoptosis are associated with viral persistence and may promote an environment conducive for other immune responses damaging to the liver. Although HCV infects less than 10% of hepatocytes, up to 20% of cells are activated for apoptosis.[59]

HCV poses a daunting challenge for immune control because of its rapid viral diversification. HCV genomic mutations are detectable within 1 year of infection. Resolved cases of HCV are defined by a vigorous T-cell response with highly active CD8 and persistent CD4 cell response. It is hypothesized that the CD8 activity mediates protective immunity but requires the aid of CD4 cells to maintain the response during viral mutations.[59]

Clinical Presentation

In an acute HCV infection, most patients are asymptomatic and undiagnosed. HCV RNA is detectable within 1 to 2 weeks of exposure and levels rise quickly during the initial weeks. The HCV RNA levels plateau at 10^5 to 10^7 international units/mL (10^8 to 10^{10} international units/L) and precede a peak in ALT levels and the onset of symptoms. Rising ALT levels indicate hepatic injury and cell necrosis and may exceed values 10 times the upper limits of normal. Although HCV RNA serum levels can show interpatient variability, the levels tend to be stable for the individual patient.[48] Typically, symptoms occur 7 weeks after the infection, with a range of 3 to 12 weeks. Approximately one-third of adults will experience some mild and nonspecific symptoms, including fatigue, anorexia, weakness, jaundice, abdominal pain, or dark urine.[54] Acute infections rarely progress to fulminant hepatitis, although the course can be severe and prolonged. If the infection is self-limiting, symptoms last several weeks as ALT and HCV RNA levels subside. Almost all patients, including immunosuppressed patients, will develop antibodies to HCV. Typically, antibodies are not detectable until either at the time of or shortly after the development of symptoms, limiting their usefulness in diagnosing an acute infection.

Up to 85% of acutely infected patients will go on to develop a chronic HCV infection, defined as persistently detectable HCV RNA for 6 months or more. HCV RNA levels and ALT levels can fluctuate and even have periods of undetectable HCV RNA and normal ALTs. Most patients will have few, if any, symptoms. The most common symptom is persistent fatigue. Additional symptoms include right upper quadrant pain, nausea, or poor appetite. On physical examination, hepatomegaly is usually present. With advanced disease, stigmata of liver disease are evident, such as spider nevi, splenomegaly, palmar erythema, testicular atrophy, and caput medusae. However, almost all patients with chronic HCV will have some degree of necroinflammatory disease on liver biopsy. Chronic inflammation of the liver from chronic HCV infection may result in fibrosis. Fibrosis is defined by altered hepatic perfusion creating a distorted structure and affecting normal function.[60] The speed of fibrosis progression can vary and is not necessarily predicative of cirrhosis development. An estimated 20% of chronic HCV patients will develop cirrhosis and half of those patients will progress to either decompensated cirrhosis or HCC. Historically, one-third of untreated patients may expect to develop cirrhosis within 20 years, while another third of patients may delay the onset of cirrhosis for 50 years or never develop it.

Viral load and genotypes other than genotype 3 are not factors for disease progression. Infection with genotype 3 may be associated with fibrosis progression.[60] The development of HCV cirrhosis poses a 30% risk over 10 years for the development of ESLD, as well as a 1% to 2% risk per year of developing HCC.[57] Progression to cirrhosis is the primary concern in patients infected with HCV for 2 decades or longer. Unfortunately, because acute infections are typically not recognized, the diagnosis of HCV is often not made until disease progression.

HCV is also rarely associated with extrahepatic manifestations. The most common is cryoglobulinemia, a local deposition of immune complexes that cause vasculitis. Typical manifestations involve the skin and internal organ damage, predominantly affecting the kidneys. Other, more rare symptoms include B-cell non-Hodgkin's lymphoma, Sjögren's syndrome, glomerulonephritis, arthritis, corneal ulcers, thyroid disease, neuropathies, and porphyria cutanea tarda.[61]

For many patients, a diagnosis of hepatitis C is incidental. Some patients are diagnosed after finding persistently abnormal transaminases. Unfortunately, those patients who present with symptoms typically have advanced disease. Due to the profound morbidity and mortality associated with HCV, the overall lack of awareness of the HCV epidemic, and the advances in treatment, the CDC recommends testing for HCV for anyone born between 1945 and 1965.[62] Early diagnosis and treatment can prevent liver damage, cirrhosis, HCC, and death. The U.S. Preventative Task Force opposed routine screening in previous reports but released a preliminary draft of recommendations for screening of HCV in high-risk individuals and for clinicians to consider birth cohort screening.[63]

TREATMENT

Desired Outcome

The primary goal of therapy is to eradicate HCV infection. Resolving the infection prevents the development of chronic HCV infection sequelae including death. Even patients who are unable to achieve cure may see histologic improvements with therapy.[57]

General Approach to Treatment

Treatment for HCV is necessary because nearly 85% of acutely infected patients develop chronic infections and are at risk of developing cirrhosis, ESLD, and HCC. Moreover, HCV infection is the most common indication for liver transplant. Treatment is indicated for patients previously untreated who have chronic HCV, circulating HCV RNA, increased ALT levels, evidence on biopsy of moderate-to-severe hepatic grade and stage, and compensated liver disease.[57] According to the AASLD, among chronic HCV patients, symptomatic cryoglobulinemia is an indication for HCV antiviral therapy irrespective of the stage of liver disease.[57] Therapy is not without risk, and in some cases may not be recommended, such as in patients with decompensated liver disease, a history of severe uncontrolled psychiatric disorder, and in patients with severe hematologic cytopenias.[57] Table 26-11 lists the contraindications to therapy.

Before therapy is initiated, quantitative HCV testing and genotyping are performed. A liver biopsy is also recommended.[57] Quantitative amplification assays for HCV RNA are performed in patients who are candidates for therapy to obtain baseline information on the viral load. A baseline HCV RNA level serves as a

TABLE 26-11 Contraindications to Hepatitis C Virus Combination Therapy

Autoimmune hepatitis
Patients aged 2 and under
Pregnant or unwilling to comply with contraception
Patients with untreated thyroid disease
Hypersensitivity to HCV medications
Patients with major, uncontrolled depression
Patients with severe concurrent medical disease
Patients with solid organ transplant including renal, heart, or lung

From reference 57.

prognostic indicator for response and is used to monitor virologic response once therapy is initiated. Genotyping is also necessary for treatment candidates because response to therapy and duration of therapy vary depending on the infecting genotype. Liver biopsy is used to determine histologic grade and stage and to guide therapy.[57] Because most chronic HCV patients are not diagnosed for years, a biopsy can provide clinical information on the extent of hepatic damage incurred since infection and offer baseline data to assess disease progression.[57] In some patients, liver biopsy may support a decision to delay treatment.

Adherence to therapy is a crucial component in response, especially among genotype 1–infected patients. Patients who take at least 80% of their medications for at least 80% of the treatment time are more likely to successfully respond to therapy.[64] Treatment response is monitored according to the following terminology:

1. *Rapid virologic response (RVR)*: undetectable viral load at week 4 of treatment
2. *Extended rapid virologic response (eRVR)*: undetectable viral load at weeks 4 and 12 of therapy; used to evaluate response with telaprevir-based treatment regimens
3. *Early virologic response (EVR)*: a ≥2-log reduction in viral load by the 12th week of treatment (partial EVR) or a patient with undetectable viral load by the 12th week of treatment (complete EVR)
4. *End-of-treatment response (ETR)*: undetectable viral load at the end of treatment
5. *SVR*: patient with no detectable viral load at the conclusion of therapy and 24 weeks later
6. *Early responder*: used with boceprevir-based treatment regimens, a patient who has an undetectable viral load at week 8 of treatment
7. *Late responder*: used with boceprevir-based treatment regimens, a patient who has an undetectable viral load at week 8 of treatment but subsequently an undetectable viral load at week 12 of treatment
8. *Relapser*: patient who achieves an ETR but who has a detectable viral load after treatment is completed; person who fails to achieve an SVR
9. *Partial responder*: a patient who achieves a ≥2 log drop in viral load but whose viral load never becomes undetectable
10. *Null responder*: patient who does not achieve a ≥2 log drop in viral load at week 12 of therapy
11. *IFN sensitivity*: refers to a >1 log decline after 4 weeks of peg-IFN and ribavirin lead in, as in boceprevir-based regimens; suggests a lower chance of resistance to treatment and an increased chance of successful therapy than in patients who experience a <1 log decline

Patients who achieve a RVR are highly likely to achieve cure; however, patients who do not achieve RVR should not be assumed to be nonresponsive. A negative RVR does not imply inability to achieve SVR; rather it indicates patients will require a full course of therapy and potentially an extended duration of therapy. Patients who experience a complete EVR are more likely to also have an SVR. Less than 3% of patients who fail to have an EVR can be expected to achieve an SVR.[57] Achieving a complete EVR is a better marker of SVR than achieving a partial EVR.

Nonpharmacologic Therapy

All chronic HCV patients should be vaccinated against hepatitides A and B. Lifestyle changes are an important factor in reducing health consequences in hepatitis C. Continued alcohol use is a known risk factor for disease progression and severity. There is no established lower limit of alcohol consumption at which disease progression is not seen. Obesity is also a factor and patients should be encouraged to eat a balanced diet and exercise regularly to maintain a normal weight. Progression of fibrotic changes is associated with obesity. Moreover, obesity and decreased insulin resistance contribute to decreased response to IFN. Smoking may also contribute to disease progression. Marijuana smoking, especially daily use, is a risk factor for progression of liver disease in patients with HCV.[65,66] Patients should be encouraged to maintain good overall health, stop smoking, and avoid alcohol and illicit drugs.[57] The use of herbal therapy is ineffective. Patients should consult with their physician prior to initiating any herbal therapies and minimize prescriptive drug use if possible.[57]

Pharmacologic Therapy

9 The treatment of chronic HCV was revolutionized with the approval of the PIs boceprevir and telaprevir in 2011 and marks the beginning of an era of direct-acting antiviral (DAA) agents in HCV therapy. The current standard of care for chronic HCV genotype 1 patients is a combination therapy of a once-weekly injection of peg-IFN, a daily oral dose of ribavirin, and either boceprevir or telaprevir. The PIs must be used in combination with peg-IFN and ribavirin to limit the development of resistance. Therapy is optimized with boceprevir and telaprevir dependent on viral response, the presence of cirrhosis, and previous treatment history. For all other genotypes, the standard of care remains peg-IFN and ribavirin. Table 26-12 lists current therapeutic regimens. For genotype 1, evaluation for RVR at 4 weeks is recommended as an indicator of the probability of achieving an SVR. Additionally, patients who are on treatment with boceprevir should be assessed for responsiveness to therapy at week 8, which corresponds to 4 weeks of boceprevir-based therapy after a 4-week lead in with peg-IFN and ribavirin. Treatment-naïve patients without cirrhosis on PI-based therapies may be treated for 24 weeks (telaprevir) or 28 weeks (boceprevir) if RVR is achieved. Patients who were previously treated, have cirrhosis, or who do not achieve RVR require longer durations of therapy.[67] Current guidelines suggest patients with genotypes 2 and 3 be treated for the full 24 weeks of therapy. Patients with genotype 4 require a minimum of 48 weeks of therapy.[57] A comparison of the use of the PIs in HCV management is found in Table 26-12.

TABLE 26-12 Recommended Hepatitis C Virus Treatment Algorithm

Genotype	Therapeutic Regimen	Duration[a]
1	Peg-IFN + ribavirin + boceprevir or telaprevir	Variable 24–48 weeks
2, 3, 4	Peg-IFN + ribavirin	24 weeks

[a]*Actual treatment duration may be different depending on virologic response.*

Clinical Controversy. . .

Although ribavirin is dosed by patient weight for genotype 1 infections, many clinicians will dose adjust based on clinical response (decline in hemoglobin).

Interferon

Historically, treatment of HCV involved the use of IFN-alfa. Although IFN monotherapy resulted in an SVR in less than 10% of patients, the response was durable. The addition of a peg moiety to IFN improved the pharmacokinetic profile of the drug to reduce injection frequency from three times to once a week, and doubled SVR rates. Two peg-IFNs are available, peg-IFN alfa-2a (Pegasys) and peg-IFN alfa-2b (Peg-Intron). Table 26-13 lists the differences between the two drugs. Achievement of SVR may be more likely in patients with an early and intense viral suppression. The current guidelines do not address which formulation of IFN should be preferentially used in HCV treatment.

Ribavirin

Ribavirin, a synthetic guanosine analog, is ineffective as a monotherapy for HCV and its exact mechanism of action is unknown. When added to IFN, ribavirin significantly increases SVR rates, especially among genotypes 2 and 3. Ribavirin is dosed based on weight for optimal response in genotype 1 and 4 infections. Although monotherapy with peg-IFN is an option for patients with contraindications to ribavirin, ribavirin is ineffective as monotherapy and should not be used alone.[57]

Protease Inhibitors: Boceprevir and Telaprevir

Boceprevir and telaprevir, both inhibitors of the NS3/4A serine protease, demonstrated profound HCV inhibition when combined with peg-IFN and ribavirin for genotype 1 infections. Their approval in 2011 changed the standard of care for the treatment of HCV genotype 1 infections to include either one of the agents in combination with peg-IFN and ribavirin (Table 26-14).[67] Neither boceprevir nor telaprevir should be used as monotherapy because each PI rapidly selects for HCV-resistant mutants. Similarly, neither PI should be dose adjusted during treatment. Both PIs have multiple drug interactions involving the cytochrome P450 (CYP) system (CYP2C, CYP3A4, or CYP1A).[67] The package insert lists known interactions; however, there are many unknown and theoretical interactions. Pharmacy can play an integral role in evaluating the potential for clinically significant drug interactions.

Boceprevir Boceprevir is used in therapy after an initial 4-week lead in with peg-IFN and ribavirin. The drug is dosed at 800 mg every 8 hours. The *SPRINT-2* trial of boceprevir with peg-IFN and ribavirin showed markedly improved SVR rates in treatment-naïve white patients as compared with peg-IFN and ribavirin (63% to 66% vs. 38%).[68] The study also demonstrated the efficacy of response-guided therapy (RGT) that allows patients to complete a total of 28 weeks of therapy if HCV viral load is undetectable at week 8 (corresponding to week 4 of boceprevir therapy) and at week 24. Patients with fibrosis and cirrhosis have lower SVR rates and benefit for longer durations of therapy; they are not candidates for RGT. Previously treated patients also benefit from retreatment with high SVR rates in prior relapsers (75%) and partial responders (52%) with 48 weeks of therapy. Null responders were not enrolled in the boceprevir trials but are likely to experience minimal benefit based on data from the telaprevir studies.[69,70] Given the toxicities and costs of therapy as well as concerns for resistance, futility rules for boceprevir exist that assess patient response at weeks 12 and 24 to identify patients who are likely experiencing viral rebound and are therefore unlikely to achieve SVR.[71]

TABLE 26-13 Pegylated Interferon Comparison

	Pegasys	Peg-Intron
Interferon	Alfa-2a	Alfa-2b
Indications	HBV, HCV	HCV
Peg moiety (weight)	Branched (40 kDa)	Linear (12 kDa)
Distribution	8–12 L; highest concentration in liver, spleen, kidneys	Body weight dependent: 1 L/kg; distributes throughout body
Metabolism	Liver	Liver
Excretion	Renal	Renal
Dosing	Fixed: 180 mcg/wk subcutaneously	Weight dependent: 1.5 mcg/kg/wk subcutaneously

HBV, hepatitis B virus; HCV, hepatitis C virus.

TABLE 26-14 Comparison of Protease Inhibitors in HCV Therapy

	Boceprevir	Telaprevir
Dose	800 mg every 8 hours with snack	750 mg every 8 hours with 20 g of fat
Initiation in treatment	Requires a 4-week lead in with peg-IFN and ribavirin before started on week 5 of therapy	Started with peg-IFN and ribavirin on day 1 of treatment
Duration of use	Variable—20–44 weeks depending on previous treatment history and virologic response at week 8; total duration of HCV therapy varies from 24 to 48 weeks	12 weeks total; total duration of HCV therapy can vary from 24 to 48 weeks

Telaprevir Telaprevir is used in the initial 12 weeks of treatment in conjunction with peg-IFN and ribavirin at a dose of 750 mg every 8 hours and must be taken with 20 g of fat for adequate absorption. The SVR rate in treatment-naïve patients was 75% as compared with 44% in patients treated with peg-IFN and ribavirin. Treatment-naïve patients who achieve an eRVR are treated for a duration of 24 weeks and can expect SVR rates of >80%.[72] Relapsers and partial responders also fared well when re-treated with a telaprevir-based regimen with SVR rates of 83% and 59%, respectively, when treated for a combined total of 48 weeks of therapy. The telaprevir trials did enroll previous null responders and the benefit of retreatment was significantly reduced with SVR rates at 29%.[73] Patients with fibrosis and cirrhosis should be treated for a total of 48 weeks of therapy.[67]

(10) Side effects of therapy are extensive and a major obstacle to successful patient completion of therapy (see Tables 26-15 and 26-16). The most common laboratory abnormalities are neutropenia, thrombocytopenia, and anemia. Ribavirin-induced hemolytic

TABLE 26-15 Common Side Effects of Therapy

Interferons	Ribavirin	Boceprevir	Telaprevir
• Flu-like symptoms: fever, headache, myalgia • Fatigue • Depression • Irritability • Insomnia • Vomiting • Anorexia • Cognitive dysfunction	• Rash • Fatigue • Nausea • Vomiting	• Fatigue • Nausea • Headache • Dysgeusia	• Rash • Anorectal symptoms (hemorrhoids, anal pruritus, anal discomfort)

TABLE 26-16 Common Laboratory Abnormalities of Therapy

Interferons	Ribavirin	Boceprevir	Telaprevir
• Neutropenia • Thrombocytopenia • Lymphopenia • Anemia • Autoimmune thyroiditis—hyper or hypo • Transaminitis	• Anemia	• Anemia • Neutropenia	• Anemia • Subclinical uric acid elevations • Transient elevations in bilirubin

anemia is an inevitable effect of therapy, although varying in severity among patients. Anemia results from ribavirin uptake into erythrocytes, inducing membrane damage and resulting in hemolysis. Patients may complain of fatigue as hemoglobin levels decrease even though dose reductions are not recommended until hemoglobin levels fall to 10 g/dL (100 g/L; 6.21 mmol/L). The mean decrease in hemoglobin is 3 g/dL (30 g/L; 1.86 g/L) in the initial weeks of therapy; thereafter, levels stabilize until discontinuation of therapy. Hemoglobin levels normalize once ribavirin is stopped. Ribavirin-induced anemia is exacerbated by PI therapy. Initial clinical experience with telaprevir included profound anemia requiring blood transfusion. IFN can cause bone marrow suppression, resulting in neutropenia and thrombocytopenia. Peg-IFNs are more likely to cause neutropenia than non–peg-IFN. Dose reductions are recommended for neutrophil counts <750 cells/mm^3 (<750 × 10^6/L); discontinuation is recommended at <500 cells/mm^3 (<500 × 10^6/L). Risk for infection is unclear. Neither nadir neutrophil counts nor total neutrophil decrease from baseline is related to infection. One study examined the risk for total, viral, fungal, and bacterial infections and concluded that neither dose reductions of IFN nor the addition of granulocyte-stimulating factor in HCV-treatment-induced neutropenia is warranted.[74]

Up to one-third of patients are expected to experience some degree of depression during treatment, partly because of IFN's interference with the serotonin pathways.[57] Although many patients can be managed with selective serotonin reuptake inhibitors, various degrees of counseling and psychiatric consultations may be necessary. Severe depression and suicidal behaviors are rare but documented. More common side effects include flu-like symptoms, which can be managed by acetaminophen or nonsteroidal inflammatory drugs. Rash is common; serious rashes and death have occurred with telaprevir.

Special Populations

Clinical trials are conducted with a patient population that generally does not reflect the patient spectrum encountered in clinical practice. There are no contraindications to the treatment of IDUs, prisoners, persons with substance abuse issues, or persons with psychiatric disorders. However, barriers exist that can prevent access to care. A multidisciplinary approach to HCV treatment that includes mental health and substance abuse professionals and pharmacy should be considered in providing care to special populations.[75]

Published recommendations for treatment in various populations are as follows.[57]

Patients with Normal ALTs The decision to treat patients with normal ALTs is somewhat controversial and made on an individual patient basis. Clinicians should consider the risks and benefits of therapy, including histologic data, genotype, likelihood for response, and other factors, such as patient willingness to undergo therapy. Successful treatment significantly improves patient quality of life and reduces fatigue.[76]

Patients with Decompensated Cirrhosis Patients with evidence of decompensation are candidates for liver transplantation. Therapy is generally not recommended unless administered by experienced clinicians. Serious adverse events including neutropenia and anemia are more likely in cirrhotics and may be managed through the use of growth factors.

Clinical **Controversy...**

In patients with advanced disease, a biopsy may be risky and offer no additional clinical information of whether to treat or not. Some clinicians believe that if therapy is to be initiated regardless, the liver biopsy offers no additional information.

Histologic improvement is not limited to patients who experience an SVR. Some clinicians believe IFN-based antiviral therapies, regardless of response, can decrease the incidence of HCC development.

Although ribavirin dosing is different for the treatment of genotype 1 depending on the formulation of peg-IFN, most clinicians will dose ribavirin according to patient weight, irrespective of the formulation.

Treatment-Experienced Patients The decision to re-treat genotype 1–infected patients should consider the previous response. Retreatment with a PI-based therapy is recommended in patients who had a virologic relapse or were partial responders with a previous course of therapy that included IFN, peg-IFN, and/or ribavirin. Patients with a prior null response to a previous course of therapy may be considered for retreatment.[67]

Accidental Needle-Stick Exposures Prophylactic treatment immediately following an accidental needle-stick exposure is not recommended for multiple reasons. Risk of transmission is considered low and among those infected, a percentage will successfully seroconvert and not require treatment. Because an initial delay in therapy does not increase the risk for developing a chronic infection, most experts wait 8 to 12 weeks before initiating treatment to allow for spontaneous remission. No formal guidelines exist as the optimal duration of treatment is unknown. Treatment is suggested for 12 to 24 weeks.

Injection-Drug Users Injection-drug use is a major factor in the cycle of HCV transmission. There are no recommendations against treatment for active IDUs, although ongoing drug abuse can create many complications and expert opinion dictates that the decision to treat be made on a case-by-case basis. Treatment is recommended for recovering drug users, including those in drug treatment programs, assuming patients are willing to comply with close monitoring and contraception requirements. Reinfection rates are low among IDUs who achieve SVR.[77] It is recommended that patients continue ongoing drug abuse and psychiatric counseling while on HCV therapy.

Alcoholism Because continued alcohol use affects disease progression and severity and thus response to therapy, the cessation of alcohol use during therapy is recommended. Moreover, a period of abstinence before initiation of therapy is also recommended.

End-Stage Renal Disease The role of chronic HCV treatment is not defined for patients with end-stage renal disease. Hemodialysis is a risk factor for acquiring HCV infection yet a contraindication for ribavirin use. Patients with mild renal insufficiency (GFR ≥60 mL/min [≥1 mL/s]) may be treated with combination peg-IFN and ribavirin. Monotherapy with IFN is an option in patients with renal insufficiency or with end-stage renal disease as ribavirin is contraindicated in these patients due to risks of ribavirin accumulation and severe hemolytic anemia. Peg-IFN can pose toxicity problems and requires careful monitoring.

HIV Coinfection Current guidelines do not recommend treatment for HIV–HCV coinfection with the PIs; however, trials are ongoing.[67] A large portion of HIV-infected patients who acquired the virus via injection-drug use will be coinfected with HCV. The PIs have multiple drug interactions, including with many of the drugs used in HAART. Treatment poses additional problems because of hepatotoxicity issues associated with HAART, hepatic complications from HIV-associated diseases, as well as flares in hepatitis as CD4 counts recover. Current guidelines recommend a 48-week course of therapy regardless of genotype with peg-IFN and ribavirin only. The prognosis for an SVR is worse than in patients infected with HCV only. In general, treatment is recommended and both HIV and HCV therapies can be coadministered with the exception of didanosine and zidovudine. The combination of ribavirin and didanosine can result in fatal lactic acidosis. Ribavirin causes hemolytic anemia and when combined with zidovudine can result in severe anemia.[78]

Children Currently therapy is indicated for children aged 2 years and older and consists of peg-IFN-alfa dosed at 60 mcg/m^2 weekly in combination with ribavirin 15 mg/kg daily for 48 weeks. Ribavirin is available in a liquid formulation. Pediatric patients tend to better tolerate therapy than adults. They should be evaluated as candidates for therapy similarly to the criteria for adults (Table 26-12).

African Americans Response rates of African Americans to HCV therapy are lower than rates observed with whites and non-Hispanic whites, and genetic mutations of HCV may partially explain the discrepancies. African Americans have higher rates of chronic HCV than non-Hispanic whites and Hispanics and have greater rates of baseline neutropenia. African Americans with HCV should be evaluated for treatment and treated according to current guidelines.

Prevention

No vaccine is available for HCV. It is unlikely that a vaccine will be developed in the near future because of the mutagenesis of the virus. Patients infected with HCV should be counseled on not being blood, organ, or semen donors. Although the likelihood of household transmission is small, patients should minimize risks by avoiding possible blood or mucus exposure, such as not sharing razors or toothbrushes and covering open wounds. Patients who continue to use illegal drugs should avoid sharing all drug paraphernalia, as risk of transmission is not limited to needles and syringes.

PERSONALIZED PHARMACOTHERAPY

It is currently not possible to definitively identify patients at risk for disease progression.[60] Several factors may correlate with a decreased risk for chronicity and include host, virus, and environmental factors. Important host factors that minimize the risk of developing chronic infection include being younger than 40 years old, female, non-black, not immunosuppressed, and with a symptomatic acute HCV infection. Being older than age 20 years at infection triples the risk for chronic HCV. Blacks, especially black men, are more likely to develop chronic infection and have lower treatment responses.[57] Becoming symptomatic and having jaundice is associated with a lower likelihood of chronic infection, perhaps correlating to a stronger immune response to the acute infection. Finally, immunosuppressed patients, such as those with HIV, are more prone to chronic infection, although they are not inherently unable to clear the infection.[57] Similarly, disease progression is associated with increased age, male sex, continued alcohol intake, obesity, and HIV coinfection. Diabetes, as well as steatosis, may also potentiate fibrosis progression.

Variation on a gene encoding for endogenous IFN, IL28, has been described that is associated with a difference in response to treatment and may explain differences in response between patients of African American and European ancestry.[53] Patients who have the CC genotype have higher rates of spontaneous clearance and higher rates of cure than patients who have IL genotype CT or TT.[53] The PI-based therapies demonstrated the ability to overcome differences in IL28 genotypes due to the potent antiviral effects of the PIs. Nonetheless, IL28 variants may affect decisions on choice and duration of therapy.[79]

Ribavirin-induced anemia can affect dosing strategies and is likely related to polymorphisms of the ITPA gene. The exact mechanism is not fully understood and the clinical relevance is not clear.[79]

ABBREVIATIONS

AASLD	American Association for the Study of Liver Diseases
ACIP	Advisory Committee on Immunization Practices
AIDS	acquired immune deficiency syndrome
ALT	alanine aminotransferase
Anti-HAV	antibody to hepatitis A virus
Anti-HBsAg	antibody to HBsAg
CDC	Centers for Disease Control and Prevention
CYP	cytochrome P450
DAA	direct-acting antiviral
ELISA	enzyme-linked immunosorbent assay
eRVR	extended rapid virologic response
ESLD	end-stage liver disease
ETR	end-of-treatment response
EVR	early virologic response
HAART	highly active antiretroviral therapy
HAV	hepatitis A virus
HBcAg	hepatitis B core antigen
HBeAg	hepatitis B e antigen
HBsAg	hepatitis B surface antigen
HBV	hepatitis B virus
HCC	hepatocellular carcinoma
HCV	hepatitis C virus
HIV	human immunodeficiency virus
IDU	injection-drug user
IFN	interferon
Ig	immunoglobulin
IL28B	interleukin 28B
MSM	men who have sex with men
OSHA	Occupational Safety and Health Administration
peg	pegylated
PI	protease inhibitor
RGT	response-guided therapy
RVR	rapid virologic response
SVR	sustained virologic response
WHO	World Health Organization

REFERENCES

1. IOM (Institute of Medicine). Hepatitis and Liver Cancer: A National Strategy for Prevention and Control of Hepatitis B and C. Washington, DC: The National Academic Press, 2010.
2. Centers for Disease Control and Prevention. Viral Hepatitis Statistics and Surveillance—United States. 2010, *http://www.cdc.gov/hepatitis/Statistics/2010Surveillance/Commentary.htm.*

3. Workowski KA, Berman S; Centers for Disease Control and Prevention (CDC). Sexually transmitted diseases treatment guidelines, 2010. MMWR Recomm Rep 2010;59(RR-12):1–110.
4. Centers for Disease Control and Prevention (CDC), Advisory Committee on Immunization Practices. Updated recommendations from the Advisory Committee on Immunization Practices (ACIP) for use of hepatitis A vaccine in close contacts of newly arriving international adoptees. MMWR Morb Mortal Wkly Rep 2009;58(36):1006–1007.
5. Nainan OV, Xia G, Vaughan G, Margolis HA. Diagnosis of hepatitis A virus infection: A molecular approach. Clin Microbiol Rev 2006;19:63–79.
6. Cuthbert JA. Hepatitis A. Old and new. Clin Microbiol Rev 2001;14:38–58.
7. Centers for Disease Control and Prevention. Prevention of hepatitis A through active or passive immunizations: Recommendations of the Advisory Committee on Immunization Practices (ACIP). MMWR Morb Mortal Wkly Rep 2006;55(RR07):1–23.
8. Advisory Committee on Immunization Practices (ACIP) Centers for Disease Control and Prevention (CDC). Update: Prevention of hepatitis A after exposure to hepatitis A virus and in international travelers. Updated recommendations of the Advisory Committee on Immunization Practices (ACIP). MMWR Morb Mortal Wkly Rep 2007;56(41):1080–1084.
9. Weissman S, Feucht C, Moore BA. Response to hepatitis A vaccine in HIV-positive patients. J Viral Hepat 2006;13:81–86.
10. World Health Organization. Hepatitis B. Fact Sheet No. 204. 2012, *http//www.who.int/mediacentre/factsheets/fs204/en/#*.
11. Weinbaum CM, Williams I, Mast EE, et al.; Centers for Disease Control and Prevention (CDC). Recommendations for identification and public health management of persons with chronic hepatitis B virus infection. MMWR Morb Mortal Wkly Rep 2008;57(RR-8):1–20.
12. Lapinski TW, Pogorzelska J, Flisiak R. HBV mutations and their clinical significance. Adv Med Sci 2012;57:18–22.
13. Liaw Y-F, Kao J-H, Piratvisuth T, et al. Asian-Pacific consensus statement on the management of chronic hepatitis B: A 2012 update. Hepat Int 2012;6:531–561.
14. Lok ASF, McMahon BJ. AASLD practice guidelines: Chronic hepatitis B: Update 2009. Hepatology 2009;50:661–662.
15. European Association for the Study of the Liver. EASL clinical practice guidelines: Management of chronic hepatitis B virus infection. J Hepatol 2012;57:167–185.
16. Arase Y, Ikeda K, Suzuki F, et al. Long-term outcome after hepatitis B surface antigen seroclearance in patients with chronic hepatitis B. Am J Med 2006;119:71.e9–71.e16.
17. Cantarini MC, Trevisani F, Morselli-Labate AM, et al. Effect of the etiology of viral cirrhosis on the survival of patients with hepatocellular carcinoma. Am J Gastroenterol 2006;101:91–98.
18. Chen CJ, Yang HI, Su J, et al. Risk of hepatocellular carcinoma across a biological gradient of serum hepatitis B virus DNA level. JAMA 2006;295:65–73.
19. Trichopoulos D, Bamia C, Lagiou P, et al. Hepatocellular carcinoma risk factors and disease burden in a European cohort: A nested case–control study. J Natl Cancer Inst 2011;103:1686–1695.
20. Koh WP, Robien K, Wang R, Govindarajan S, Yuan JM, Yu MC. Smoking as an independent risk factor for hepatocellular carcinoma: The Singapore Chinese Health Study. Br J Cancer 2011;105:1430–1435.
21. Farrell GC, Teoh NC. Management of chronic hepatitis B virus infection: A new era of disease control. Intern Med J 2006;36:100–113.
22. Manzano-Alonso ML, Castellano-Tortajada G. Reactivation of hepatitis B virus infection after cytotoxic chemotherapy or immunosuppressive therapy. World J Gastroenterol 2011;17:1531–1537.
23. Hwang JP, Vierling JM, Zelenetz AD, Lackey SC, Loomba R. Hepatitis B virus management to prevent reactivation after chemotherapy: A review. Support Care Cancer 2012;20:2999–3008.
24. Gish R, Jia J-D, Locarnini S, Zoulim F. Selection of chronic hepatitis B therapy with a high barrier to resistance. Lancet Infect Dis 2012;12:341–354.
25. Yim HJ, Hussain M, Liu Y, et al. Evolution of multi-drug resistant hepatitis B virus during sequential therapy. Hepatology 2006;44:703–712.
26. Kim JW, Park SH, Louie SG. Telbivudine: A novel nucleoside analog for chronic hepatitis B. Ann Pharmacother 2006;40:472–478.
27. Zhang L, Wang G, Hou W, Li P, Dulin A, Bonkovsky HL. Contemporary clinical research of traditional Chinese medicines for chronic hepatitis B in China: An analytical review. Hepatology 2010;51:690–698.
28. Craxi A, Antonucci G, Camma C. Treatment options in HBV. J Hepatol 2006;44(Suppl 1):s77–s83.
29. Marcellin P, Chang TT, Lim SG, et al. Adefovir dipivoxil for the treatment of hepatitis B e antigen-positive chronic hepatitis B. N Engl J Med 2003;348:808–816.
30. Hadziyannis SJ, Tassopoulos NC, Heathcote EJ, et al. Adefovir dipivoxil for the treatment of hepatitis B e antigen-negative chronic hepatitis B. N Engl J Med 2003;348:800–807.
31. Wu IC, Shiffman ML, Tong MJ, et al. Sustained hepatitis B e antigen seroconversion in patients with chronic hepatitis B after adefovir dipivoxil treatment: Analysis of precore and basal core promoter mutants. Clin Infect Dis 2008;47(10):1305–1311.
32. Hadziyannis SJ, Tassopoulos NC, Heathcote EJ, et al. Long-term therapy with adefovir dipivoxil for HBeAg-negative chronic hepatitis B. N Engl J Med 2005;352:2673–2681.
33. Vassiliadis TG, Giouleme O, Koumerkeridis G, et al. Adefovir plus lamivudine are more effective than adefovir alone in lamivudine-resistant HBeAg-chronic hepatitis B patients: A 4-year study. J Gastroenterol Hepatol 2010;25:54–60.
34. Chang TT, Gish RG, de Man R, et al. A comparison trial of entecavir and lamivudine for HBeAg-positive chronic hepatitis B. N Engl J Med 2006;354:1001–1010.
35. Lai CL, Shouval D, Lok AS, et al. Entecavir versus lamivudine for patients with HBeAg-negative chronic hepatitis B. N Engl J Med 2006;354:1011–1020.
36. Shim JH, Suh DJ, Kim KM, et al. Efficacy of entecavir in patients with chronic hepatitis B resistant to both lamivudine and adefovir or to lamivudine alone. Hepatology 2009;50:1064–1071.
37. Liaw YF, Gane E, Leung N, et al. 2-Year GLOBE trial results: Telbivudine is superior to lamivudine in patients with chronic hepatitis B. Gastroenterology 2009;136:486–495.
38. Lai CL, Gane E, Liaw YF, et al. Telbivudine versus lamivudine in patients with chronic hepatitis B. N Engl J Med 2007;357:2576–2588.
39. Marcellin P, Heathcote EJ, Buti M, et al. Tenofovir disoproxil fumarate versus adefovir dipivoxil for chronic hepatitis B. N Engl J Med 2008;359:2442–2455.
40. Heathcote EJ, Marcellin P, Buti M, et al. Three year efficacy and safety of tenofovir disoproxil fumarate treatment for chronic hepatitis B. Gastroenterology 2011;140:132–143.

41. Marcellin P, Buti M, Gane E, et al. Six years of treatment with tenofovir disoproxil fumarate for chronic hepatitis B virus infection is safe and well tolerated and associated with sustained virological, biochemical, and serological responses with no detectable resistance. In: Oral presentation at 63rd Annual Meeting of the American Association for the Study of Liver Disease; November 2012; Boston, MA.
42. Tan J, Degertekin B, Wong SN, et al. Tenofovir monotherapy is effective in hepatitis B patients with antiviral treatment failure to adefovir in the absence of adefovir-resistant mutants. J Hepatol 2008;48:391–398.
43. Lim SG, Ng TM, Kung N, et al. A double-blind placebo-controlled study of emtricitabine in chronic hepatitis B. Arch Intern Med 2006;166:49–56.
44. Ning Q, Han M, Sun Y, et al. New treatment strategy: Switching from long-term entecavir to peginterferon alfa-2a (40 kD) induces HBeAg seroconversion/HBsAg loss in patients with HBeAg-positive chronic hepatitis B (the OSST study). In: Oral presentation at 63rd Annual Meeting of the American Association for the Study of Liver Disease; November 2012; Boston, MA.
45. Sung JJY, Lai JY, Zeuzem S. Lamivudine compared with lamivudine and adefovir dipivoxil for the treatment of HBeAg-positive chronic hepatitis B. J Hepatol 2008;48:728–735.
46. Lok AS, Trinh H, Carosi G, et al. Efficacy of entecavir with or without tenofovir disoproxil fumarate for nucleos(t)ide-naïve patients with chronic hepatitis B. Gastroenterology 2012;143:619–628.
47. Niro G, Ciancio A, Gaeta GB, et al. Pegylated interferon alpha-2b as monotherapy or in combination with ribavirin in chronic hepatitis delta. Hepatology 2006;44:713–720.
48. Yurdaydin C, Bozkaya H, Onder FO, et al. Treatment of chronic delta hepatitis with lamivudine vs lamivudine + interferon vs interferon. J Viral Hepat 2008;15:314–321.
49. Giang L, Selinger CP, Lee AU. Evaluation of adherence to oral antiviral hepatitis B treatment using structured questionnaires. World J Hepatol 2012;4:43–49.
50. Hongthanakorn C, Chotiyaputta W, Oberhelman K, et al. Current nucleos(t)ide analogue therapy for chronic hepatitis B. Gut Liver 2011;5:278–287.
51. Mast EE, Weinbaum CM, Fiore AE, et al.; Advisory Committee on Immunization Practices (ACIP) Centers for Disease Control and Prevention (CDC). A comprehensive immunization strategy to eliminate transmission of hepatitis B virus infection in the United States. Recommendations of the Advisory Committee on Immunization Practices (ACIP) part II: Immunization of Adults. MMWR Recomm Rep 2006;55(RR-16):1–33.
52. Prather AA, Hall M, Fury JM, et al. Sleep and antibody response to hepatitis B vaccination. Sleep 2012;35:1063–1069.
53. Ge D, Fellay J, Thompson AJ, et al. Genetic variation in IL28B predicts hepatitis C treatment-induced viral clearance. Nature 2009;461:399–401.
54. McHutchison JG, Bacon BR. Chronic hepatitis C: An age wave of disease burden. Am J Manag Care 2005;11(Suppl 10):s286–s295.
55. Ly KN, Xing J, Klevens M, Jiles RB, Ward JW, Holmberg SD. The increasing burden of mortality from viral hepatitis in the United States between 1999 and 2007. Ann Internal Med 2012;156:271–278.
56. Rein DB, Wittenborn JS, Weinbaum CM, Sabin M, Smith BD, Lesesne SB. Forecasting the morbidity and mortality associated with prevalent cases of pre-cirrhotic chronic hepatitis C in the United States. Dig Liver Dis 2011;43: 66–72.
57. Ghany MG, Strader DB, Thomas DL, et al. American Association for the Study of Liver Diseases practice guidelines: Diagnosis, management, and treatment of hepatitis C. Hepatology 2009;49:1335–1374.
58. Terrault NA, Dodge JL, Murphy EL, et al. Sexual transmission of HCV among monogamous heterosexual couples: The HCV partners study. Hepatology 2013;57: 881–889. doi:10.1002/hep.26164 [Epub ahead of print].
59. Kanto T, Hayashi N. Immunopathogenesis of hepatitis C virus infection: Multifaceted strategies subverting innate and adaptive immunity. Intern Med 2006;45:183–191.
60. Massard J, Ratziu V, Thabut D, et al. Natural history and predictors of disease severity in chronic hepatitis C. J Hepatol 2006;44:s19–s24.
61. Mayo MJ. Extrahepatic manifestations of hepatitis C infection. Am J Med Sci 2002;325:135–148.
62. Smith BD, Morgan RL, Beckett GA, et al.; Centers for Disease Control and Prevention. Recommendations for the identification of chronic hepatitis C virus infection among persons born during 1945-1965. MMWR Recomm Rep 2012;61(RR-4):1–18.
63. U.S. Preventive Services Task Force. Screening for hepatitis C virus infection in adults: Recommendation statement. Ann Intern Med 2004;140:462–464.
64. McHutchison JG, Manns M, Patel K, et al. Adherence to combination therapy enhances sustained response in genotype-1 infected patients with chronic hepatitis C. Gastroenterology 2002;123:1061–1069.
65. Hezode C, Zafrani ES, Roudot-Thoraval F, et al. Daily cannabis use: A novel risk factor of steatosis severity in patients with chronic hepatitis C. Gastroenterology 2008;134:432–439.
66. Ishida JH, Peters MG, Jin C, et al. Influence of cannabis use on severity of hepatitis C disease. Clin Gastroenterol Hepatol 2008;6:69–75.
67. Ghany MG, Nelson DR, Strader DB, Thomas DI, Seeff LB. An update on treatment of genotype 1 chronic hepatitis C virus infection: 2011 practice guideline by the American Association for the Study of Liver Diseases. Hepatology 2011;54:1433–1444.
68. Poordad F, McCone J Jr, Bacon BR, et al.; for SPRINT-1 Investigators. Boceprevir for untreated chronic HCV genotype 1 infection. N Engl J Med 2011;364:1195–1206.
69. Bruno S, Vierling JM, Esteban R, et al. Efficacy and safety of boceprevir plus peginterferon–ribavirin in patients with HCV G1 infection and advanced fibrosis/cirrhosis. J Hepatol 2013;58:479–487. doi:10.1016/j.jhep.2012.11.020 [Epub ahead of print].
70. Bacon BR, Gordon SC, Lawitz E, et al. Boceprevir for previously treated chronic HCV genotype 1 infection. N Engl J Med 2011;364:1207–1217.
71. Jacobson IM, Marcellin P, Zeuzem S, et al. Refinement of stopping rules during treatment of hepatitis C genotype 1 infection with boceprevir and peginterferon/ribavirin. Hepatology 2012;56:567–575.
72. Jacobson IM, McHutchison JG, Dusheiko G, et al.; for ADVANCE Study Team. Telaprevir for previously untreated chronic hepatitis C virus infection. N Engl J Med 2011;364:2405–2416.
73. Zeuzem S, Andreone P, Pol S, et al. Telaprevir for retreatment of HCV infection. N Engl J Med 2011;364:2417–2428.
74. Cooper CL, Al-Bedwawi S, Lee C, Garber G. Rate of infectious complications during interferon-based therapy

for hepatitis C is not related to neutropenia. Clin Infect Dis 2006;42:1674–1678.

75. Arora S, Thornton K, Murata G, et al. Outcomes of treatment for hepatitis C virus infection by primary care providers. N Engl J Med 2011;364:2199–2207.
76. Arora S, O'Brien C, Zeuzem S, et al. Treatment of chronic hepatitis C patients with persistently normal alanine aminotransferase levels with the combination of peginterferon alpha-2a (40 kDa) plus ribavirin: Impact on health-related quality of life. J Gastroenterol Hepatol 2006;21:406–412.
77. Grebely J, Conway B, Raffa JD, et al. Hepatitis C virus reinfection in injection drug users. Hepatology 2006;44:1139–1145.
78. Soriano V, Puoti M, Sulkowski M, et al. Care of patients coinfected with HIV and hepatitis C virus: 2007 updated recommendations from the HCV-HIV International Panel. AIDS 2007;21:1073–1089.
79. Soriano V, Poveda E, Vispo E, et al. Pharmacogenetics of hepatitis C. J Antimicrob Chemother 2012;67:523–529.

Celiac Disease

Robert A. Mangione and Priti N. Patel

27

KEY CONCEPTS

1. Celiac disease is a chronic, small intestinal immune-mediated enteropathy caused by intolerance to gluten found in wheat, barley, rye, and other foods when a genetically predisposed person is exposed to the environmental trigger, gluten.
2. Celiac disease affects 1 in 100 to 120 adults and 1 in 80 to 300 children in the North American population and appears to be increasing in prevalence.
3. The integrity of the tissue junctions of the intestinal epithelium is compromised in patients with celiac disease; this enables gluten to reach the lamina propria. The presence of gluten in the lamina propria and an inherited combination of genes contribute to the heightened immune sensitivity to gluten that is found in patients with celiac disease.
4. The classic presenting symptom in adults is diarrhea, which may be accompanied by abdominal pain or discomfort; however, it is noteworthy that during the past decade diarrhea has been reported as the main presenting symptom of celiac disease in less than 50% of cases.
5. Dermatitis herpetiformis is a skin manifestation of small intestinal immune-mediated enteropathy caused by exposure to dietary gluten. All patients with celiac disease will not develop dermatitis herpetiformis; however, it is generally agreed that all patients with dermatitis herpetiformis also have celiac disease.
6. The frequency of diagnosis of patients with celiac disease has increased; however, the majority of patients with this condition remain undiagnosed.
7. A confirmed diagnosis of celiac disease requires both positive findings on duodenal biopsy and a positive response to a gluten-free diet. The most common serologic markers that are used for screening patients are serum anti–tissue transglutaminase antibodies and serum immunoglobulin A (IgA) endomysial antibodies.
8. Strict, lifelong adherence to a gluten-free diet is the only treatment for celiac disease that is currently available.
9. Clinicians must evaluate the patient with celiac disease for nutritional deficiencies (including folic acid, vitamin B_{12}, fat-soluble vitamins, iron, and calcium) due to malabsorption. Iron-deficiency anemia may be the only presenting sign of disease in patients without diarrhea.

1 Celiac disease is a small intestinal immune-mediated enteropathy caused by intolerance to ingested gluten, a storage protein found in wheat, barley, and rye. Genetic, environmental, and immune factors all play a role in the development of celiac disease. The mainstay of treatment of the disease is strict, lifelong adherence to a gluten-free diet.[1,2]

A disease resembling celiac disease was first described by a Greek physician in the second century AD.[3] In the mid-1900s, the connection between the ingestion of cereals and celiac disease was made. For many years, celiac disease was considered a disease of childhood with primarily GI symptoms. It is now recognized as a disease of all ages with varied presentation.

Celiac disease has also been known as celiac sprue, nontropical sprue, and gluten-sensitive enteropathy; however, these terms are currently not recommended. The disease is characterized by both GI and extraintestinal symptoms. Chronic inflammation caused by exposure to gluten leads to GI discomfort, nutrient malabsorption, and systemic complications. GI symptoms, including diarrhea, cramping, bloating, and flatulence, are the "classic" symptoms; however, a patient with celiac disease may initially present with a variety of extraintestinal symptoms. Patients with subclinical celiac disease have no or minimal symptoms but manifest mucosal damage on biopsy and have positive serologic testing. Patients with celiac disease classified as potential are asymptomatic patients who may show positive serology and have the human leukocyte antigen (HLA)-DQ2 and/or DQ8 haplotype, but have normal mucosa on biopsy.[1,4]

Adherence to a gluten-free diet is essential because it improves symptoms and prevents long-term complications of celiac disease, which include T-cell lymphomas, small bowel adenocarcinoma, and esophageal and oropharyngeal carcinomas.[5]

EPIDEMIOLOGY

2 Originally thought to be a pediatric disease, celiac disease is now being diagnosed in increasing numbers of adult and pediatric patients due to increased awareness and improved diagnostic techniques.[5] Celiac disease is common in Europe and North America. The prevalence of the disease is 1 in 100 to 120 adults in Western nations.[5,6] In children in the United States, the prevalence of the disease is 1 in 80 to 300 children.[7] Similar to other autoimmune diseases, the prevalence of celiac disease is higher in females than in males at rates ranging from 2:1 to 3:1.[8] In Finland and the United States, the prevalence of celiac disease has increased fourfold during the past 50 years. This finding has resulted from a true increase in the prevalence of the disease rather than simply an increase in the number of individuals who are diagnosed. While the reason for this increase is not known, it may be due to environmental factors such as the changing nature of gluten or other factors associated with diet.[9]

Celiac disease has been less well studied in other parts of the world. Previously believed to rarely occur in nonwhite populations, improved screening and diagnostic techniques now provide evidence that the prevalence of celiac disease in many non-Western nations is similar to that in Europe and North America.[10,11] In addition, in Asian countries where rice has traditionally been a staple, meals with rice are increasingly being replaced by a Western-style wheat-based diet. This transition in dietary preferences may lead to an increased prevalence of the disease in those populations.[12]

ETIOLOGY

Celiac disease is known to occur when a genetically predisposed person ingests gluten. Wheat gluten proteins exist in two fractions: gliadins and glutenins. Storage proteins similar to glutenins, called hordeins and secalins, are found in barley and rye, respectively. Table 27-1 refers to grains and other foods that do and do not contain gluten and related proteins. Ingestion of any of these proteins will lead to an autoimmune response in celiac disease patients.

TABLE 27-1 Grains and Other Foods that Do and Do Not Contain Gluten

Contain Gluten	Do Not Contain Gluten
Wheat	Amaranth
Barley	Buckwheat
Rye	Corn
Bran	Flax
Graham flour	Millet
Spelt	Potato flour
Wheat germ	Quinoa
Triticale	Rice
Oats[a]	Sorghum
	Soybeans
	Tapioca
	Teff

[a]Oats are in a different plant family, but they have also been regarded as problematic, although the ingestion of certified pure gluten-free oats appears to be safe in most patients with celiac disease.[6] Due to the continued difference of opinion regarding the safety of oats, patients are generally advised to discuss the risks and benefits associated with consuming oats with their healthcare provider before they include oats in their diet.

Clinical **Controversy...**

It is still a matter of controversy whether or not oats are safe for consumption by patients with celiac disease. Wheat, barley, and rye, which contain the disease-activating proteins gliadin, hordein, and secalin, respectively, are all derived from the Triticeae tribe of the grass (Gramineae) family. Oats, from the Aveneae tribe, are distantly related and therefore only contain few disease-activating proteins.[13] Another concern with oats is that they may be contaminated with gluten during the manufacturing process.[14] Gluten-free uncontaminated oats are now commercially available. Although a small number of individuals with celiac disease may not tolerate even pure, uncontaminated oats, clinical evidence has confirmed that the consumption of 50 to 70 g (1/2 to 3/4 cup [120 to 180 mL] dry certified gluten-free oats) is safe in adults with celiac disease.[14] It has raised concern that some celiac disease patients are found to have avenin-reactive T cells that can cause mucosal inflammation.[15] Investigators examined nine different cultivars of oats and found some to be more toxic than others regardless of their purity, leading them to conclude that some oats may trigger a greater immunologic response than others.[16] Although the consumption of limited quantities of oats is generally considered to be acceptable, clinical followup of celiac disease patients who consume oats is advisable even if these patients are maintaining a strict gluten-free diet.[14,15]

Genetic factors, in combination with exposure to gluten, are necessary for the development of celiac disease. A concordance rate of 85% in monozygotic twins has been reported, indicating that genetics play a large role in the disease, but other factors are likely also involved.[17,18]

Virtually all patients with celiac disease have variants of HLA-DQ2 or HLA-DQ8 molecules that are expressed on the surface of antigen-presenting cells.[19] Other non-HLA genes may also play a role in enhancing genetic susceptibility to celiac disease.[18]

Certain infectious agents and other compounds may contribute to the development of celiac disease. Both adenovirus and hepatitis C viruses are thought to act as triggers, whereas other agents, including *Campylobacter jejuni*, *Giardia lamblia*, rotavirus, and enterovirus infections, have been described in case reports as associated with celiac disease.[20] The biologic agent interferon-α has also been suggested to play a role in celiac disease development.[21]

In Sweden, increased rates of diagnosis of celiac disease in the mid-1980s corresponded to a change in infant feeding practices where mothers reduced breast-feeding and introduced cereal into babies' diets earlier than had been previously in practice. Based on this finding, prolonged breast-feeding with introduction of gluten-containing grains during breast-feeding may help avoid the development of celiac disease.[22]

PATHOPHYSIOLOGY

3 During normal digestion, peptides that remain from gastric or pancreatic digestion are broken down into amino acids, dipeptides, or tripeptides by the small intestinal brush-border membrane enzymes.[23] These GI proteases that are found in the intestinal lumen are one of the body's first defenses against potentially toxic dietary proteins.[6] The intestinal epithelium, with its intact intercellular tight junctions, functions as the primary barrier to the passage of macromolecules into the lamina propria. Gluten is unusually rich in the amino acids glutamine and proline, which enable part of the molecule to withstand the digestive processes. These peptides are kept within the GI tract and are primarily excreted before they can illicit an immune reaction. Small fractions of gluten do cross this important defense barrier in patients without celiac disease; however, the quantity of gluten that passes across the GI lining is generally insufficient to illicit a significant response from a normally functioning immune system.[24,25]

Events likely associated with the pathophysiology of celiac disease have been characterized as an interaction between gluten and immune, genetic, and environmental factors.[26] In celiac disease, the integrity of the tissue junctions of the intestinal epithelium is compromised, enabling gluten to reach the lamina propria through different routes. The presence of gluten in the lamina propria and an inherited combination of genes contribute to the heightened immune sensitivity to gluten found in patients with celiac disease (Table 27-2).[24,25] The notable immune response to gluten consists of both adaptive and innate immune responses that occur only in individuals who carry the HLA type DQ2 or in some populations DQ8.[27] The precise mechanism by which the immune

TABLE 27-2 Proposed Pathophysiology of Celiac Disease

- Enterocytes release the protein zonulin in response to the presence of indigestible fragments of gluten in the intestine
- Zonulin loosens the intercellular tight junctions
- Abundant quantities of gluten fragments cross the intestinal lining and accumulate under the enterocytes (epithelial cells)
- Gluten induces the enterocytes to secrete interleukin-15 (IL-15)
- IL-15 induces an immune response of intraepithelial lymphocytes against the enterocytes
- The damaged cells release the enzyme tissue transglutaminase (tTG), which modifies the gluten
- Antigen-presenting cells of the immune system join the modified gluten to human leukocyte antigen (HLA) molecules and display the resulting complexes to other immune cells (i.e., helper T cells)
- Helper T cells that recognize the complexes secrete molecules that attract other immune cells, which may result in damage to the enterocytes
- Helper T cells spur killer T cells that directly attack the enterocytes
- B cells release antibody molecules that are targeted to gluten and tTG (the role that these antibodies play remains to be further clarified; however, they may cause further damage when they contact their targets on or near the enterocytes)
- Enterocytes are disabled or killed

See reference 25.

system leads to damage of the intestinal lining of patients with celiac disease continues to be studied.

The primary toxic components of wheat gluten are a family of closely related proteins called gliadins.[23] The gliadin peptides induce changes in the epithelium through innate immunity and in the lamina propria through adaptive immunity.[18] Researchers have concluded that protected transport of gliadin peptides occurs in patients with celiac disease via a CD71-mediated transcytosis of immunoglobulin A (IgA)/gliadin peptides immune complexes from the lumen of the intestine to the lamina propria. In patients without celiac disease, the gliadin peptides are entirely degraded by lysosomal acid proteases during intestinal transcytosis. The abnormal expression of the IgA receptor CD71 at the apical side of the enterocytes that is found in celiac disease patients allows a protected retrotransport of serum immunoglobulin A (SIgA) gliadin immune complexes that could play an important role in triggering the immune activation that is characteristic of celiac disease. These researchers note that the normal function of SIgA (i.e., the containment of harmful antigens in the intestinal lumen) is deficient in celiac disease. They further state that the fate of the immune complexes once absorbed is unknown; however, the complexes may bind to IgA receptors that are present on local antigen-presenting cells and trigger the activation of local memory CD4+ T cells, which will perpetuate the inflammation.[28]

Tissue transglutaminase (tTG), a ubiquitous enzyme that catalyzes posttranslational modification of proteins and is released during inflammation, may play at least two crucial roles in celiac disease by serving as the main target autoantigen for antiendomysial enzymes and as a deaminating enzyme that raises the immunostimulatory effect of gluten. Expression and activity of tTG are raised in the mucosa of patients with celiac disease.[6] This enzyme, by deaminating glutamine to glutamic acid, makes the gliadin peptides become negatively charged and therefore more capable of fitting into pockets of the HLA-DQ2 (or HLA-DQ8) antigen-binding groove on the antigen-presenting cells.[6,26] Gliadin is presented to gliadin-reactive CD4+ T cells through a T-cell receptor, which then results in the production of cytokines that cause tissue damage. This then leads to villous atrophy, crypt hyperplasia, and the expansion of antibody-producing B cells found in celiac disease.[26]

CLINICAL PRESENTATION

❹ The recognition of celiac disease may be quite challenging due to the wide range of presenting symptoms, which includes patients who are asymptomatic.[6] Clinical manifestations of celiac disease also significantly vary according to age group (Table 27-3). Infants and young children generally experience diarrhea, abdominal distention, and failure to thrive. Vomiting, irritability, anorexia, and even constipation are also common in these young patients. Extraintestinal manifestations such as short stature, neurologic findings (e.g., peripheral neuropathy, ataxia, seizure, migraine, and dementia[30]), or anemia are often found in older children and adolescents. The classic presenting symptom in adults is diarrhea, which may be accompanied by abdominal pain or discomfort; however, it is noteworthy that during the past decade diarrhea has been reported as the main presenting symptom of celiac disease in less than 50% of cases. Adults may exhibit what are sometimes characterized as silent manifestations of this disease such as iron-deficiency anemia or osteoporosis. Less common but important presentations of celiac disease in adults include abdominal pain, constipation, weight loss, neurologic symptoms, dermatitis herpetiformis, hypoproteinemia, hypocalcemia, and elevated liver enzymes. Some adults may be diagnosed as a result of having an endoscopy performed in response to their complaints of symptoms associated with gastroesophageal reflux.[26] Prior to age 65 years, the disease is two to three times more common in adult women than in adult men.[6] Regrettably, patients with celiac disease often experience symptoms for a long period of time and may experience multiple hospitalizations and undergo surgical procedures before celiac disease is diagnosed.[26]

❺ Dermatitis herpetiformis is a skin manifestation of small intestinal immune-mediated enteropathy caused by the ingestion of gluten (Figs. 27-1 and 27-2).[1] It occurs in approximately 15% to 25% of patients with celiac disease.[31] This extremely pruritic, bullous skin rash is generally found on the elbows, knees, buttocks, and scalp but can occur anywhere on the body.[30,31] Although dermatitis herpetiformis is most frequently observed in patients who are 30 to 40 years of age, it can also be found in children and elderly patients.[32] Patients with dermatitis herpetiformis often do

TABLE 27-3 Selected Signs and Symptoms of Celiac Disease

Children	Adults
Symptoms • Fatigue • Bloating • Constipation • Abdominal pain • Chronic diarrhea • Irritability • Vomiting	Symptoms • Abdominal pain • Chronic diarrhea • Abdominal distension • Recurrent spontaneous abortion • Peripheral neuropathy • Depression • Fatigue/malaise • Ataxia
Signs • Muscle wasting • Failure to thrive/weight loss • Short stature • Delayed puberty • Osteopenia/osteoporosis • Hepatitis • Dental anomalies • Anemia	Signs • Weight loss • Infertility • Dermatitis herpetiformis • Hepatitis • Anemia • Aphthous ulcers • Alopecia • Malignancy • Seizures • Osteopenia/osteoporosis • Arthritis

See references 4 and 29.

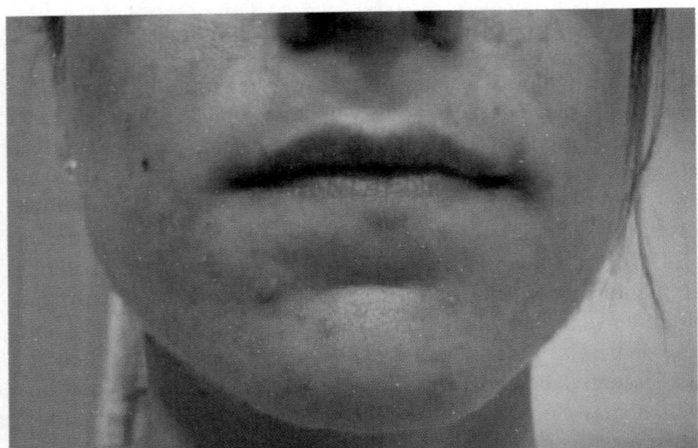

FIGURE 27-1 Photograph of dermatitis herpetiformis of the face. *(Copyright © American Pharmacists Association [APhA]. Reprinted by permission of APhA. Photographs provided by Peter H.R. Green, MD, Professor of Clinical Medicine, College of Physicians & Surgeons, Columbia University, New York.)*

not have the typical GI symptoms that are associated with celiac disease; however, they are at risk for developing intestinal damage.[33] Although dermatitis herpetiformis was once considered to be a skin disease that was often found in patients with celiac disease, researchers have also suggested that it is actually a cutaneous manifestation of the disease.[34] Although every patient with celiac disease does not develop dermatitis herpetiformis, it is generally agreed that every individual with dermatitis herpetiformis also has celiac disease.[33]

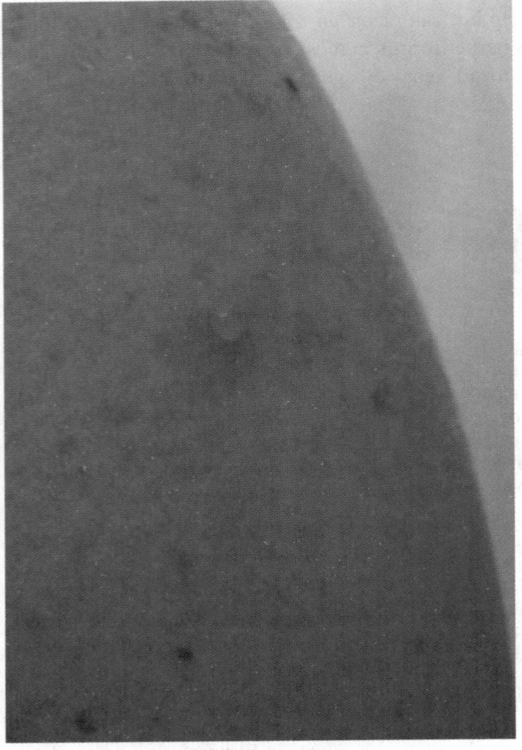

FIGURE 27-2 Photograph of bullous dermatitis herpetiformis. *(Copyright © American Pharmacists Association [APhA]. Reprinted by permission of APhA. Photographs provided by Peter H.R. Green, MD, Professor of Clinical Medicine, College of Physicians & Surgeons, Columbia University, New York.)*

TABLE 27-4 Selected Common Misdiagnoses

Irritable bowel syndrome
Viral gastroenteritis
Lactose intolerance
Amoebic/parasitic infection
Inflammatory bowel disease
Psychological dysfunction
Gallbladder disease
Chronic fatigue syndrome
Gastroesophageal reflux disease
Allergies
Ulcers
Cystic fibrosis
Colitis

See reference 33.

6 The diagnosis of celiac disease is based on clinical suspicion and confirmation with laboratory tests and duodenal biopsy.[35] When suspected, the diagnosis of celiac disease is easily established.[26] Although the frequency of diagnosis of patients with celiac disease has increased, the majority of patients (an estimated 97%) with this condition remain undiagnosed.[30] This is particularly concerning as undiagnosed celiac disease has been associated with a nearly fourfold increased risk of death compared with subjects without serologic evidence of disease.[36]

Perhaps the most important initial step in making this diagnosis is for healthcare providers to recognize its many and diverse possible symptoms.[37] Only 11% of celiac disease cases are diagnosed in a timely manner, with an average reported period of 5.8 to 11.7 years from the onset of symptoms to the diagnosis.[38] Clinicians can help reduce the time from the onset of symptoms to the diagnosis of celiac disease by being aware of the common diseases with which many celiac patients are misdiagnosed (Table 27-4). Although these disorders may be mistakenly diagnosed instead of celiac disease, they may also coexist with celiac disease.[38]

Clinicians should also note that individuals with certain disorders are more likely to have celiac disease than the general population. Examples include other autoimmune diseases, such as thyroid disease, diabetes mellitus (type 1), multiple sclerosis, myasthenia gravis, Raynaud's disease, rheumatoid arthritis, Addison's disease, chronic active hepatitis, cystic fibrosis, scleroderma, and Sjögren's syndrome; Down's syndrome; neurologic conditions such as ataxia, epilepsy, and cerebral calcifications; and primary biliary cirrhosis. Although patients with these disorders are more frequently found to have celiac disease than the general population, these associated conditions are not believed to cause celiac disease.[33]

7 Diagnostic testing for celiac disease must be performed while the patient continues to consume gluten.[39] A confirmed diagnosis of celiac disease requires both a positive finding on duodenal biopsy and a positive response to a gluten-free diet.[26] The identification of villous atrophy with small bowel endoscopy and biopsy is generally regarded as the diagnostic gold standard (although guidelines from the European Society of Paediatric Gastroenterology, Hepatology, and Nutrition suggest that a small intestinal biopsy may not be required in children with typical symptoms, titers of anti-tTG greater than 10 times the upper normal limit and predisposing HLA genotype).[2,40] Although villous atrophy is associated with celiac disease, clinicians must consider that this may also be found in other diseases, including giardiasis, autoimmune enteropathy, tuberculosis, Crohn's disease, intolerance to food other than gluten, intestinal lymphoma, and Zollinger-Ellison syndrome.[5,26]

Positive findings on biopsy include increased intraepithelial lymphocytes (i.e., >30/100 enterocytes), loss of nuclear polarity, change from columnar to cuboid cells, lamina propria cellular infiltration, crypt elongation and hyperplasia, increased crypt mitotic index, and progressive villous flattening or blunting.[40] The Marsh classification system is a standardized approach used by pathologists to describe the histologic changes seen in celiac disease. This classification includes ratings of Marsh I to IV with Marsh III being further subdivided into Marsh IIIa (partial villous atrophy), IIIb (subtotal villous atrophy), and IIIc (total villous atrophy). Most celiac disease patients (50% to 60%) are placed in one of the Marsh III categories.[41] Histologic findings lead to a presumptive diagnosis that is followed by placing the patient on a gluten-free diet. A definitive diagnosis can only be made after the patient's symptoms clearly improve while maintaining the special diet. A second biopsy to confirm histologic improvement is not required except in cases when the clinical symptoms of celiac disease were absent.[40] Some clinicians have suggested that a repeat biopsy after dietary intervention may have merit to demonstrate histologic improvement that will support the diagnosis, assess the patient's dietary compliance, and reassure the patient. A second biopsy can be useful for patients whose initial biopsy demonstrated ambiguous histologic changes, whose serology was negative or discrepant, or who continue to have symptoms after initiating the gluten-free diet.[6] Dermatitis herpetiformis is diagnosed by taking a small skin biopsy from normal skin that is next to the blister site.[33] The characteristic skin biopsy finding in this disorder is the deposition of IgA granules at the dermal–epidermal junction.[31] The 2004 National Institutes of Health (NIH) Consensus Development Conference on Celiac Disease reported that patients with skin biopsy–proven dermatitis herpetiformis generally are not required to have small bowel biopsies.[37]

Serologic test results provide clinicians with a useful noninvasive tool that helps to determine if symptomatic patients, or patients who are at risk for celiac disease, require a biopsy.[4,24,42] Available tests include those for antigliadin antibodies, connective tissue antibodies (antireticulum and antiendomysial antibodies), and antibodies against tTG.[26] The most common serologic markers that are used for screening patients are serum IgA endomysial antibodies and IgA tTG antibodies.[39] Both of these tests have over 90% sensitivity; therefore, a test for either marker is considered to be the best means of screening for celiac disease.[26] Antiendomysial antibody testing is operator dependent, rather time consuming, and more expensive than the test for IgA tTG antibodies, which is operator independent.[4] A rapid test for anti-tTG antibodies that only requires a sample of fingertip blood may be a convenient point-of-care test to aid with diagnosis and dietary monitoring.[26] Testing for gliadin antibodies is no longer utilized because of its low sensitivity and specificity for celiac disease.[35,39] Although serology is a good method to identify patients who will benefit from endoscopy and biopsy, negative serology should not preclude a biopsy examination in individuals for whom disease is suspected on clinical grounds.[5,6]

Genetic testing can be performed as a means of confirming the diagnosis of celiac disease or to determine which family members of a diagnosed patient may develop the disease (the prevalence of celiac disease has been reported to be 10% to 12% in first-degree relatives and is also higher than that found in the general population in second-degree relatives).[30] Patients and their family members can be tested for HLA-DQ2 and HLA-DQ8 as the HLA-DQ2 is found in up to 95% of celiac disease patients, with most other patients being HLA-DQ8 positive.[4,35] Although nearly all celiac disease patients carry one of these alleles, they are also found in 30% to 40% of the general population. Therefore, when these alleles are absent, it is extremely unlikely that the individual has celiac disease (i.e., the test has a high negative predictive value [NPV]).[37] A patient-administered saliva-based test for HLA-DQ2/DQ8 was released for direct sale to consumers.[43] It will be interesting to observe how the availability of this test will impact on the already rather strong interest of those patients who seek self-diagnostic methods.[44]

More accurate diagnostic measures will assist with the management and hopeful reduction of comorbid conditions (correcting deficiencies of iron, folic acid, vitamin B_{12}, fat-soluble vitamins; diagnosing and treating osteoporosis; etc.) and complications (a gluten-free diet may reduce the increased mortality related to risk of malignancy) that are associated with celiac disease.[39] Preventing additional comorbid conditions and/or celiac disease complications not only will improve the patient's quality of life but may also avoid the costs that are associated with treating these other disorders.

TREATMENT

Desired Outcome

Overall goals of treatment include relieving symptoms, healing the intestine, and reversing the consequences of malabsorption while enabling the patient to adhere to a healthy, interesting, and practical gluten-free diet.[27,45]

Nonpharmacologic

8 Table 27-5 presents a mnemonic that summarizes the major principles of the treatment of celiac disease. Strict lifelong adherence to a gluten-free diet is the only proven treatment for celiac disease.[6] Patients must recognize that adhering to a gluten-free diet includes not ingesting anything that contains gluten or has been contaminated with gluten. Wheat, barley, and rye must be avoided.[27] Although oats are in a different plant family, they have also been regarded to be problematic; however, the ingestion of certified pure gluten-free oats appears to be safe.[6] Due to the continued difference of opinion regarding the safety of oats, patients are generally advised to discuss the risks and benefits associated with consuming oats with their healthcare provider before they include oats in their diet. Patients must also commit to avoiding the ingestion of gluten found in nonfood items such as toothpaste, lip balm, lipstick, etc. A list of gluten-free grains can be found in Table 27-1.

Oral prescription drugs, nonprescription drugs, vitamin and mineral supplements, and health and beauty aids and cosmetics that have oral ingestion potential must not be overlooked as sources of gluten due to its presence in their formulation or due to contamination or contact.[46,47] Although clinicians have concluded that as little as 10 to 50 mg/day of gluten is the minimum dose required to produce measurable damage to the small intestinal mucosa, it is difficult to set a universal threshold given the individual variability among patients.[2,30,34,42]

The FDA's Office of Food Safety Center of Food Safety and Applied Nutrition determined, after an evaluation of all low-dose–response data available on the adverse health effects of gluten in celiac disease patients, the tolerable daily intake level for gluten in individuals with celiac disease to be 0.4 mg gluten/day for adverse morphologic effects and 0.015 mg gluten/day for adverse clinical effects.[48] These concerns regarding low-level exposure emphasize why healthcare providers must check to determine whether prescription drugs contain gluten in their formulation or have been contaminated with gluten before these drugs are provided to the patient

TABLE 27-5 Mnemonic for Celiac Disease

C	Consultation with a skilled dietician
E	Education about the disease
L	Lifelong adherence to a gluten-free diet
I	Identifying and treating nutritional deficiencies
A	Access to an advocacy group
C	Continuous long-term followup by a multidisciplinary team

See reference 37.

with celiac disease. Patients should also be assisted with determining whether nonprescription drugs and health and beauty aids are safe for their use.[49] Lack of reliable information may lead individuals with celiac disease to mistakenly assume that their prescription or nonprescription drugs contain gluten and therefore refuse to take newly recommended or prescribed medications, or stop taking previously prescribed and needed medications without conferring with their healthcare provider.[50] Although there are published lists of gluten-free drugs, it is often difficult to obtain information about the gluten content of medications.[51–53]

It is extremely important that patients become thoroughly knowledgeable about celiac disease. Although there are an increasing number of articles, reference materials, and other sources of information readily available to patients and their families, patients should still be advised to obtain advice and guidance from their healthcare providers. Consultations with a knowledgeable dietician will assist the patient to understand and effectively adhere to the gluten-free diet.[54]

9 Newly diagnosed patients should be evaluated for nutritional deficiencies associated with vitamin and mineral malabsorption. This assessment should include assuring that the patient does not have deficiencies of folic acid, vitamin B_{12}, fat-soluble vitamins, iron, and calcium.[26] Iron-deficiency anemia may be the only presenting sign of disease in patients without diarrhea.[55] Monitoring for potential nutritional deficiencies should also continue during subsequent followup visits.

Most adults with celiac disease are found to have some degree of bone loss; therefore, all patients must be screened for osteoporosis or osteopenia. A dual-energy x-ray absorptiometry (DEXA) scan is often performed to assist with this evaluation.[30,45] Supplementing a calcium-rich gluten-free diet with calcium, magnesium, and vitamin D may arrest or reverse celiac decrease–related bone loss. Although their use has not been extensively studied in patients with celiac disease, bisphosphonates, selective estrogen receptor modulators, anabolic agents, and other drugs have been prescribed for patients with bone disease.[27] Antiresorptive drugs have been utilized in some instances when patients do not adequately improve after at least 1 year of observing an appropriate diet and taking calcium supplements. These drugs have also been used sooner in patients with low bone mineral density and little or no intestinal malabsorptive problems. Clinicians must note that these drugs can cause serious adverse effects if they are administered before the intestine properly heals. Excessive dangerous drops in blood calcium can lead to cardiac dysrhythmias, muscle weakness, and seizures.[30]

Implementing a gluten-free diet presents some challenges. A dietician will be helpful, particularly when the patient is newly diagnosed. Patients are advised to initiate a complete gluten-free lifestyle immediately after diagnosis. Partial adherence to this diet is not adequate. In order to accomplish this objective, patients must be aware of what foods are gluten-free and when in doubt must know how to confirm whether a food contains gluten. Reading labels is extremely important; however, it may be difficult to identify hidden sources of gluten listed among the ingredients. Patients with celiac disease must also determine whether products were processed on equipment shared with wheat, barley, or rye. It may be necessary to call the manufacturers or check their website to obtain the needed information.[33]

Individuals with celiac disease must also be advised to maintain a gluten-free kitchen. A dedicated toaster, bread maker, waffle iron, and other appliances should be obtained for use in preparing gluten-free meals. Utensils and dishes must be carefully cleaned to avoid gluten contamination. Care must also be taken when dining in restaurants and homes of family and friends. The individuals who prepare and serve the food must be knowledgeable about gluten-free foods and food preparation.[30] Patients with celiac disease will often eat before leaving home and will bring gluten-free food with them when dining out.[33]

The economic burden associated with maintaining a gluten-free diet may present some challenges.[45,56,57] The relatively low availability and high cost of these foods contributes to the challenges associated with adhering to the required strict diet and may lead to varying degrees of noncompliance.[56,57] Patients also find that the extra cost associated with the special diet is not reimbursed by healthcare plans, and most policies do not pay for consultations with a dietician.[58] These challenges with compliance are particularly concerning as noncompliance with the gluten-free diet is associated with an increased mortality rate and compromised quality of life.[57] Patients are also encouraged to investigate their personal circumstances as to whether some of the costs of maintaining a gluten-free diet are eligible for approval as a tax deduction.[58]

Pharmacologic

Dietary avoidance of gluten remains the mainstay of treatment of celiac disease. Novel pharmacologic treatment modalities are under investigation. Most reports related to pharmacotherapy for celiac disease focus on the treatment of refractory disease.

In case reports, corticosteroids, azathioprine, cyclosporine, tacrolimus, infliximab, and alemtuzumab have been reported as effective treatments for refractory celiac disease.[59–62] Patients characterized to have refractory celiac disease have persistent or recurrent malabsorptive symptoms and signs with villous atrophy despite maintaining a gluten-free diet for more than 12 months.[1] Less than 5% of adult patients are found to have refractory celiac disease.[63]

Based on the pathophysiology of celiac disease, two categories of novel targets for the treatment of the disease have been identified: decreasing the antigenic load and modulation of the immune response.

Methods of decreasing the antigenic load include blocking the activity of tTG, GI destruction of proline peptides via enzyme therapy, blocking the binding of deaminated proteins to HLA-DQ2 and HLA-DQ8, detoxification of gluten peptides, and decreasing intestinal permeability in patients with celiac disease, in particular through inhibition of zonulin.[64–66] Investigational tTG inhibitors have been developed; however, their safety is questioned due to the presence of the enzyme throughout the body and its role in many functions necessary for homeostasis.[67] In the area of gluten detoxification, gluten proteins were developed in which the proline residues were replaced by azidoprolines; these azidoproline residues bound to HLA-DQ2 but did not stimulate an autoimmune response.[68] A zonulin inhibitor was shown to be well tolerated and effective in a small study and is currently being studied in larger populations.[67]

Means of modulating the immune response include the neutralization of inflammatory cytokines and regulation of T cells.[65] All of these methods are currently investigational but may offer hope in the future.

Clinical **Controversy...**

Changes in intestinal microflora have been linked with celiac disease.[69] One theory behind this link suggests that changes in the glycosylation in the mucous layer in the intestines can promote adhesion of harmful bacteria, leading to celiac disease. A second theory behind this link suggests that harmful bacteria are responsible for the changes in mucous layer glycosylation, which in turn promotes celiac disease. Among the strains of probiotics studied in in vitro and in animal studies for improving the bacterial flora in patients with celiac disease are *Bifidobacterium longum*, *B. bifidum*, *Lactobacillus paracasei*, *L. fermentun*, and *L. casei*. As of this writing, none have been proven to be beneficial in either preventing or treating celiac disease.

Evaluation of Therapeutic Outcomes

Clinical improvement will often be observed within days or weeks of instituting the required diet.[26] Although dermatitis herpetiformis is also treated with the prescribed diet, these cutaneous lesions may not completely resolve for 1 to 2 years after initiating strict dietary measures.[55]

Healthcare providers must also be mindful of conditions that are related to celiac disease and that are potential complications of the disease, including certain forms of cancer, neurologic manifestations, osteoporosis, depression, diabetes, infertility, as well as other autoimmune and related illnesses. Cancers that are of particular concern include thyroid cancer, adenocarcinoma of the small intestine, lymphoma (predominantly non-Hodgkin's lymphoma of any type), esophageal cancer, melanoma, and malignancies found in childhood.[31] Patients with celiac disease have also been found to have an increased risk of developing certain infectious diseases that include pneumococcal or staphylococcal sepsis and tuberculosis.[70] The immune system of celiac patients is not compromised as it is actually overactive. The risk of infections due to encapsulated organisms (pneumococcal pneumonia, meningococcal infections) arises from hyposplenism, which is common in active celiac disease. Therefore, patients over 50 years of age are advised to receive pneumococcal vaccine.[30] Annual influenza vaccine is advisable as this will reduce the incidence of secondary bacterial infections.[70]

Increased hazard ratios (HRs) for death were found in individuals with biopsy-verified celiac disease, inflammation, and potential celiac disease (the absolute risks were small). Individuals undergoing small-intestinal biopsy in childhood had increased HRs for death. These researchers concluded that the main causes of death in patients they studied were cardiovascular disease and malignancy.[71]

ABBREVIATIONS

DEXA	dual-energy x-ray absorptiometry
HLA	human leukocyte antigen
HR	hazard ratio
IgA	immunoglobulin A
NIH	National Institutes of Health
NPV	negative predictive value
SIgA	serum immunoglobulin A
tTG	tissue transglutaminase

REFERENCES

1. Ludvigsson JF, Leffler DA, Bai JC, et al. The Oslo definitions of celiac disease and related terms. Gut 2013;62:43–52.
2. Fasano A, Catassi C. Celiac disease. N Engl J Med 2012; 367(25):2419–2426.
3. Fasano A. Celiac disease: The past, the present, the future. Pediatrics 2001;107(4):768–777.
4. Jatla M, Pierly PA, Hlywiak K, et al. Overview of celiac disease: Differences between children and adults. Pract Gastroenterol 2008:18–34.
5. Gasbarrini G, Miele L, Malandrino N, et al. Celiac disease in the 21st century: Issues of under- and overdiagnosis. Int J Immunopathol Pharmacol 2009;22(1):1–7.
6. DiSabatino A, Corazza GR. Coeliac disease. Lancet 2009; 373:1480–1493.
7. Hill I, Dirks M, Liptak G, et al. Guideline for the diagnosis and treatment of celiac disease in children: Recommendations of the North American Society for Pediatric Gastroenterology, Hepatology and Nutrition. J Pediatr Gastroenterol Nutr 2005;40(1):1–19.
8. Green PHR, Stavropolous SN, Panagi SG, et al. Characteristics of adult celiac disease in the USA: Results of a national survey. Am J Gastroenterol 2001; 96:126–131.
9. Green PHR. Mortality in celiac disease, intestinal inflammation, and gluten sensitivity. JAMA 2009;302(11):1225–1226.
10. Malekzadeh R, Sachdev A, Ali AF. Coeliac disease in developing countries: Middle East, India, and North Africa. Best Pract Res Clin Gastroenterol 2005;19(3):351–358.
11. Cataldo F, Montalto G. Celiac disease in developing countries: A new and challenging public health problem. World J Gastroenterol 2007;13(15):2153–2159.
12. Cummins AG, Roberts-Thomson IC. Prevalence of celiac disease in the Asia-Pacific region. J Gastroenterol Hepatol 2009;24:1347–1351.
13. Kagnoff MF. Overview and pathogenesis of celiac disease. Gastroenterology 2005;128:S10–S18.
14. Rashid M, Butzner D, Burrows V, et al. Consumption of pure oats by individuals with celiac disease: A position statement by the Canadian Celiac Association. Can J Gastroenterol 2007;21:649–651.
15. Arentz-Hansen H, Fleckenstein B, Molberg O, et al. The molecular basis for oat intolerance in patients with celiac disease. PLoS Med 2004;1:84–92.
16. Comino I, Real A, de Lorenzo L, et al. Diversity in oat potential immunogenicity: Basis for the selection of oat varieties with no toxicity in coeliac disease. Gut 2011;60: 915–922.
17. Nistico L, Fagnani C, Coto I, et al. Concordance, disease progression, and heritability of coeliac disease in Italian twins. Gut 2006;55:803–808.
18. Wolters VM, Wijmenga C. Genetic background of celiac disease and its clinical implications. Am J Gastroenterol 2008;103(1):190–195.
19. AGA Institute. AGA Institute medical position statement on the diagnosis and management of celiac disease. Gastroenterology 2006;131(6):1977–1980.
20. Plot L, Amital H. Infectious associations of celiac disease. Autoimmun Rev 2009;8:316–319.
21. Cammarota G, Cuoco L, Cianci R, et al. Onset of coeliac disease during treatment with interferon for chronic hepatitis C. Lancet 2000;356;1494–1495.
22. Ivarsson A, Persson LA, Lystrom L, et al. Epidemic of coeliac disease in Swedish children. Acta Paediatr 2000;89(2):165–171.
23. Shan L, Molberg O, Parrot I, et al. Structural basis for gluten intolerance in celiac sprue. Science 2002;297:2275–2279.
24. Drago S, Di Pierro M, Catassi C, Fasano A. Recent developments in the pathogenesis, diagnosis and treatment of celiac disease. Expert Opin Ther Patents 2002;12:45–51.
25. Fasano A. Surprises from celiac disease. Sci Am 2009; 301:54–61.
26. Green PHR, Cellier C. Celiac disease. N Engl J Med 2007; 357:1731–1743.
27. See J, Murray JA. Gluten-free diet: The medical and nutrition management of celiac disease. Nutr Clin Pract 2006;21:1–15.
28. Heyman M, Menard S. Pathways of gliadin transport in celiac disease. Ann N Y Acad Sci 2009;1165:274–278.
29. Fasano A, Catassi C. Coeliac disease in children. Best Pract Res Clin Gastroenterol 2005;19:467–478.
30. Green PHR, Jones R. Celiac Disease: A Hidden Epidemic. New York: HarperCollins, 2010.
31. Murray JA. The widening spectrum of celiac disease. Am J Clin Nutr 1999;69:354–365.
32. Turchin I, Barankin B. Dermatitis herpetiformis and gluten-free diet. Dermatol Online J 2005;11:6.

33. Korn D. Wheat Free, Worry Free: The Art of Happy, Healthy Gluten-Free Living. Carlsbad, NY: Hay House, 2002.
34. Collin P, Reunala T. Recognition and management of the cutaneous manifestations of celiac disease: A guide for dermatologists. Am J Clin Dermatol 2003;4:13–20.
35. Harrison MS, Wehbi M, Obideen K. Celiac disease: More common than you think. Cleve Clin J Med 2007; 74:209–215.
36. Rubio-Tapia A, Kyle RA, Kaplan EL, et al. Increased prevalence and mortality in undiagnosed celiac disease. Gastroenterology 2009;137:88–93.
37. NIH consensus development conference on celiac disease. NIH Consens State Sci Statements 2004;21:1–23.
38. Thom S, Longo BM, Running A, Ashley J. Celiac disease: A guide to successful diagnosis and treatment. J Nurse Pract 2009;5:244–253.
39. Presutti RJ, Cangemi JR, Cassidy HD, Hill DA. Celiac disease. Am Fam Physician 2007;76:1795–1802.
40. Briani C, Samaroo D, Alaedini A. Celiac disease: From gluten to autoimmunity. Autoimmun Rev 2008;7:644–650.
41. Kupfer SS. Making sense of Marsh. In: Impact: A Publication of the University of Chicago Celiac Disease Center. Chicago, IL: University of Chicago Celiac Disease Center, Fall 2009;1–3.
42. Catassi C, Fabiani E, Iacono F, et al. A prospective, double-blind, placebo-controlled trial to establish a safe gluten threshold for patients with celiac disease. Am J Clin Nutr 2007;85:160–166.
43. Prometheus Launches MyCeliac ID, the First Do It Yourself, Saliva-Based Genetic Test Dedicated to Celiac Disease. *http://phx.corporate-ir.net/phoenix.zhtml?c=130685&p=irol-newsArticle&ID=1302745&highlight=*.
44. Copelton DA, Valle G. "You don't need a prescription to go gluten-free": The scientific self-diagnosis of celiac disease. Soc Sci Med 2009;69:623–631.
45. Lowell JP. The Gluten-Free Bible: The Thoroughly Indispensable Guide to Negotiating Life without Wheat. New York: Henry Holt and Company, 2005.
46. Hlywiak KH. Hidden sources of gluten. Pract Gastroenterol 2008;32:27–39.
47. Mangione RA, Patel PN. Caring for patients with celiac disease: The role of the pharmacist. J Am Pharm Assoc 2008;48(4):e125–e135.
48. Office of Food Safety Center of Food Safety and Applied Nutrition, Food and Drug Administration. Health Hazard Assessment for Gluten Exposure in Individuals with Celiac Disease: Determination of Tolerable Daily Intake Levels and Levels of Concern for Gluten. 2011, *http://www.fda.gov/downloads/food/scienceresearch/researchaccess/riskassessmentsafetyassessment/ucm264152.pdf*.
49. Mangione RA. Pharmacy care and celiac disease. Hosp Pharm 2009;44:373.
50. Esteban S, Podder N, Cruciani R. Celiac disease: Not all medications are contaminated with gliadin. J Pain Symptom Manage 2006;31:195–196.
51. Gluten-free drugs for celiac disease patients. Med Lett 2008;50:19–20.
52. King AR. The impact of celiac sprue on patients' medication choices. Hosp Pharm 2009;44:105–106.
53. Mangione RA, Patel PN, Shin E, et al. Determining the gluten content of over the counter drugs: Information for patients with celiac disease. J Am Pharm Assoc 2011;51: 734–737.
54. Bebb HR, Knight LT, Long RG. Long-term follow-up of coeliac disease: What do coeliac disease patients want? Aliment Pharmacol Ther 2006;23:827–831.
55. Rodrigo L. Celiac disease. World J Gastroenterol 2006;12: 6585–6593.
56. Lee A, Ng D, Zivin J, Green H. Economic burden of a gluten-free diet. J Hum Nutr Diet 2007;20:423–430.
57. Stevens L, Rashid M. Gluten-free and regular foods: A cost comparison. Can J Diet Pract Res 2008;69:147–150.
58. Alderman L. The expense of eating with celiac disease. New York Times August 15, 2009:B7.
59. al-Toma A, Verbeek WH, Mulder CJ. Update on the management of refractory coeliac disease. J Gastrointestin Liver Dis 2007;16(1):57–63.
60. Costantino G, della Torre A, Lo Presti MA, et al. Treatment of life-threatening type I refractory coeliac disease with long-term infliximab. Dig Liver Dis 2008;40:74–77.
61. Vivas S, Ruiz de Morales M, Ramos F, Suarez-Vilela D. Alemtuzumab for refractory celiac disease in a patient at risk for enteropathy-associated T-cell lymphoma. N Engl J Med 2006;354:2514–2515.
62. Verbeek WHM, Mulder CJJ, Zweegman S. Alemtuzumab for refractory celiac disease. N Engl J Med 2006;35(13): 1396–1397.
63. Mulder CJJ, Wahab PJ, Meijer JWR, Metselaar E. A pilot study of recombinant human interleukin-10 in adults with refractory coeliac disease. Eur J Gastroenterol Hepatol 2001;13:1183–1186.
64. Cerf-Nensussan N, Matysiak-Budnik T, Cellier C, Heyman M. Oral proteases: A new approach to managing coeliac disease. Gut 2007;56:157–160.
65. Gianfrani C, Auricchio S, Troncone R. Possible drug targets for celiac disease. Expert Opin Ther Targets 2006;10(4): 601–611.
66. Sollid LM, Khosla C. Future therapeutic options for celiac disease. Nat Clin Pract Gastroenterol Hepatol 2005;2(3): 140–147.
67. Sanz Y. Novel perspectives in celiac disease therapy. Mini Rev Med Chem 2009;9:359–367.
68. Sanz Y, De Pama G, Laparra M. Unraveling the ties between celiac disease and intestinal microbiota. Int Rev Immunol 2011;30(4):207–218.
69. Walters JRF, Bamford KB, Ghosh S. Coeliac disease and the risk of infections. Gut 2008;57:1034–1035.
70. Ludvigsson JF, Montgomery SM, Ekbom A, et al. Small-intestinal histopathology and mortality risk in celiac disease. JAMA 2009;302:1171–1178.
71. Picarelli A, Salvi I, Di Tola M, et al. Impact of gluten-free diet on quality of life in celiac disease patients. Dig Liver Dis 2009;41S:288.

28 Acute Kidney Injury

William Dager and Jenana Halilovic

KEY CONCEPTS

1. Three classification systems exist for staging severity of acute kidney injury (AKI): (a) Risk, Injury, Failure, Loss of Kidney Function, and End-Stage Kidney Disease (RIFLE), (b) Acute Kidney Injury Network (AKIN), and (c) Kidney Disease: Improving Global Outcomes (KDIGO) clinical practice guidelines. All three classification systems are based on separate criteria for serum creatinine (S_{cr}) and urine output.
2. AKI is a common complication in hospitalized patients and is associated with high morbidity and mortality, especially in critically ill.
3. AKI is categorized based on three distinct types of injury: (a) prerenal—decreased renal blood flow, (b) intrinsic—structural damage within the kidney, and (c) postrenal—an obstruction is present within the urine collection system.
4. Conventional formulas used to determine estimated glomerular filtration rate (eGFR) and creatinine clearance should not be used to estimate renal function in patients with AKI. This may be especially true for medication dosing adjustments.
5. Prevention is of utmost importance since there are very few therapeutic options available for the treatment of established AKI.
6. Supportive management remains the primary approach to prevent or reduce the complications associated with AKI. Supportive therapies include renal replacement therapy (RRT), nutritional support, avoidance of nephrotoxins, and blood pressure and fluid management.
7. For those patients with prolonged or severe AKI, RRT is the cornerstone of support along with an aggressive approach to fluid, electrolyte, and waste management.
8. Drug dosing for AKI patients receiving continuous renal replacement therapy (CRRT) or sustained low-efficiency dialysis (SLED) is poorly characterized. Dosing regimens should be individualized and therapeutic drug monitoring utilized whenever possible.
9. Diuretic resistance is a common phenomenon in the patient with AKI and can be addressed with sodium restriction, combination diuretic therapy, or a continuous infusion of a loop diuretic.

INTRODUCTION

Acute kidney injury (AKI) is a clinical syndrome generally defined by an abrupt reduction in kidney function as evidenced by changes in laboratory values, serum creatinine (S_{cr}), blood urea nitrogen (BUN), and urine output. The consequences of AKI can be serious, especially in hospitalized patients, among whom complications and mortality are particularly high. Early recognition along with supportive therapy is the focus of management for those with established AKI, as there is no therapy that directly reverses the injury. Individuals at risk, such as those with history of chronic kidney disease (CKD), need to have their hemodynamic status carefully monitored and their exposure to nephrotoxins minimized. A thorough patient workup is often necessary and includes past medical and surgical history, medication use, physical examination, and multiple laboratory tests. Management goals include maintenance of blood pressure, fluid, and electrolyte homeostasis, all of which may be dramatically altered. Additional therapies designed to eliminate or minimize the insult that precipitated AKI include discontinuation of the offending drug (i.e., the nephrotoxin), aggressive hydration, maintenance of renal perfusion, and renal replacement therapy (RRT).

In this chapter, the definition, classification, epidemiology, and common etiologies of AKI are presented. Methods to recognize and assess the extent of kidney function loss are also discussed. Finally, preventive strategies for patients at risk and management approaches for those with established AKI are reviewed.

DEFINITION AND CLASSIFICATION OF ACUTE KIDNEY INJURY

1 Over the past 10 years, several efforts by a broad consensus of experts have been made to standardize the definition and classification of AKI. In 2004, the Acute Dialysis Quality Initiative (ADQI) group published a consensus-derived definition and classification system called the Risk, Injury, Failure, Loss of Kidney Function, and End-Stage Kidney Disease (RIFLE) classification.[1] In 2007, a modified version of RIFLE was developed by the Acute Kidney Injury Network (AKIN) and these criteria are presented in Table 28-1[2] (see Table 28-1 for an overview of all classification systems). Both classification systems are now widely accepted and have been validated to predict outcomes in thousands of patients

TABLE 28-1 RIFLE, AKIN, and KDIGO Classification Schemes for Acute Kidney Injury[a]

RIFLE Category	S_{cr} and GFR[b] Criteria	Urine Output Criteria
Risk	S_{cr} increase to 1.5-fold or GFR decrease >25% from baseline	<0.5 mL/kg/h for ≥6 hours
Injury	S_{cr} increase to twofold or GFR decrease >50% from baseline	<0.5 mL/kg/h for ≥12 hours
Failure	S_{cr} increase to threefold or GFR decrease >75% from baseline, or S_{cr} ≥4 mg/dL (≥354 μmol/L) with an acute increase of at least 0.5 mg/dL (44 μmol/L)	Anuria for ≥12 hours
Loss	Complete loss of function (RRT) for >4 weeks	
ESKD	RRT >3 months	
AKIN Criteria	**S_{cr} Criteria**	**Urine Output Criteria**
Stage 1	S_{cr} increase ≥0.3 mg/dL (≥27 μmol/L) or 1.5- to 2-fold from baseline	<0.5 mL/kg/h for ≥6 hours
Stage 2	S_{cr} increase >2- to 3-fold from baseline	<0.5 mL/kg/h for ≥12 hours
Stage 3	S_{cr} increase >3-fold from baseline, or S_{cr} ≥4 mg/dL (≥354 μmol/L) with an acute increase of at least 0.5 mg/dL (≥44 μmol/L), or need for RRT	<0.3 mL/kg/h for ≥24 hours or anuria for ≥12 hours
KDIGO Criteria	**S_{cr} Criteria**	**Urine Output Criteria**
Stage 1	S_{cr} increase ≥0.3 mg/dL (≥27 μmol/L) or 1.5–1.9 times from baseline	<0.5 mL/kg/h for 6–12 hours
Stage 2	S_{cr} increase 2–2.9 times from baseline	<0.5 mL/kg/h for ≥12 hours
Stage 3	S_{cr} increase three times from baseline, or S_{cr} ≥4 mg/dL (≥354 μmol/L), or need for RRT, or eGFR[c] <35 mL/min/1.73 m² (<0.34 mL/s/m²) in patients <18 years	Anuria for ≥12 hours

AKIN, Acute Kidney Injury Network; ESKD, end-stage kidney disease; eGFR, estimated glomerular filtration rate; h, hours; KDIGO, Kidney Disease: Improving Global Outcomes; RIFLE, Risk, Injury, Failure, Loss of Kidney Function, and End-Stage Kidney Disease; RRT, renal replacement therapy; S_{cr}, serum creatinine.

[a]For all staging systems, the criterion that leads to worst possible diagnosis should be used.
[b]GFR calculated using the Modification of Diet in Renal Disease (MDRD) equation.
[c]GFR calculated using the Schwartz formula.

worldwide.[3,4] While generally similar, there are a few noteworthy differences: RIFLE defines AKI as an abrupt (1 to 7 days) but sustained (>24 hours) decrease in renal function from baseline while AKIN designates a 48-hour period for the decrease to occur. Also, AKIN removed RIFLE's last two classification components (Loss of Kidney Function and End-Stage Kidney Disease [ESKD]) from the staging system and instead places all patients receiving RRT automatically into AKIN stage 3. Finally, AKIN removed all estimated glomerular filtration rate (eGFR) criteria from its staging system and lowered the absolute increase in S_{cr} from 0.5 mg/dL (44 μmol/L) designated for RIFLE-Risk class to 0.3 mg/dL (27 μmol/L) for AKIN stage 1.[1,2]

Even though the initial aim of RIFLE and the AKIN modification was to provide a standardized definition of AKI, they resulted in two distinct definitions that were not consistently applied across studies and thus have provided somewhat different epidemiologic findings. In order to provide a single definition of AKI for practice, research, and public health, a second modification of RIFLE and AKIN criteria was recently published by the Kidney Disease: Improving Global Outcomes (KDIGO) Clinical Practice Guidelines working group in 2012.[5]

KDIGO defines AKI as being present if any of the following three criteria are met: 1. Increase in S_{cr} by at least 0.3 mg/dL (27 μmol/L) within 48 hours, 2. Increase in S_{cr} by at least 1.5 times baseline within the prior 7 days, or 3. Decrease in urine volume to less than 0.5 mL/kg/h for 6 hours.

KDIGO staging of AKI is similar to the RIFLE and AKIN criteria with the notable addition of inclusion of pediatric patients (<18 years) to KDIGO Stage 3 for those with an estimated GFR of less than 35 mL/min/1.73 m² (0.34 mL/s/m²) as determined by the Schwartz formula.[5] Due to the very recent publication of KDIGO guidelines, it still remains to be seen if it will supersede RIFLE and AKIN criteria for the diagnosis and classification of AKI in the future.

Since all three staging systems depend on S_{cr} and urine output as the main diagnostic criteria, they are associated with the same inherent weaknesses. An increase in S_{cr} is usually evident about 1 or 2 days after development of AKI. This lag time in S_{cr} rise may significantly delay diagnosis of AKI and adversely affect patient outcomes. Urine output reduction emerges earlier in AKI but is a very nonspecific marker because it may not always be present. In fact, patients with AKI can be anuric (urine output <50 mL/day), oliguric (urine output <500 mL/day), or nonoliguric (urine output >500 mL/day). Urine output will also vary with volume status, diuretic administration, and presence of obstruction.[6] Further, since all criteria are based on detecting a decrease in S_{cr} from its baseline, a patient's renal function prior to the development of AKI needs to be known. If the baseline measure of S_{cr} is not available and the patient has no history of renal dysfunction, the ADQI, a workgroup composed of experts in nephrology and critical care, has suggested estimating the baseline S_{cr} value by using the four variable Modification of Diet in Renal Disease (MDRD) equation with an assumed normal GFR of 75 mL/min/1.73 m² (0.72 mL/s/m²).[1] However, this method needs to be interpreted with caution as it has been found to overestimate the incidence of AKI by as much as 40%.[7,8]

EPIDEMIOLOGY

The epidemiology of AKI varies widely depending on the patient population, geographical location, and the criteria used to evaluate the patient. AKI is generally considered to be an uncommon condition in the community-dwelling population, with an annual incidence of 520 per 100,000 person-years for nondialysis requiring AKI and 30 per 100,000 person-years for dialysis-requiring injury[9] (Table 28-2). AKI is more common in hospitalized individuals, with a reported incidence ranging from 2% to 20%.[10,11] Intensive care unit (ICU) patients have the highest risk of developing AKI, with 20% to 60% of critically ill patients being affected.[3,4]

2 Increased mortality and morbidity are two well-recognized complications of AKI. In particular, severity, duration, and frequency of AKI appear to be important predictors of poor patient outcomes. Any degree of AKI is associated with an increased risk of death, and the odds increase with the severity of the insult.[11,12] For survivors of AKI, the development of some degree of CKD and need for RRT are other important considerations.[13] In addition, AKI is associated with increased length of hospital stay, ventilator days, and need for posthospitalization care.[10,13]

TABLE 28-2 Incidence and Outcomes of AKI

	Community-Acquired AKI	Hospital-Acquired AKI	ICU-Acquired AKI
Incidence	Low (<1%)	Moderate (2–20%)	High (20–60%)
Cause	Usually single	Single or multiple	Multifactorial
Overall mortality rate	N/A	15–40%	30–90%
Common risk factors	Chronic comorbid conditions, elderly, male gender, sepsis, dehydration, infection, drugs (ACEIs, ARBs, diuretics)	Volume depletion, hypotension, sepsis, low cardiac output, nephrotoxic drugs, radiocontrast dyes	Septic shock, major surgery, multiorgan failure, hypotension, low cardiac output, nephrotoxic drugs

ACEIs, angiotensin-converting enzyme inhibitors; AKI, acute kidney injury; ARBs, angiotensin receptor blockers; ICU, intensive care unit; N/A, not available.

ETIOLOGY

❸ The etiology of AKI can be divided into broad categories based on the anatomic location of the injury associated with the precipitating factor(s). The management of patients presenting with this disorder is largely predicated on identification of the specific etiology responsible for the patient's AKI (Fig. 28-1). Traditionally, the causes of AKI have been categorized as (a) prerenal, which results from decreased renal perfusion in the setting of undamaged parenchymal tissue, (b) intrinsic, the result of structural damage to the kidney, most commonly the tubule from an ischemic or toxic insult, and (c) postrenal, caused by obstruction of urine flow downstream from the kidney (Fig. 28-2).

Community-acquired AKI most commonly occurs secondary to renal hypoperfusion from volume depletion (dehydration, vomiting, and diarrhea), sepsis, or medications (angiotensin-converting enzyme inhibitors [ACEIs], angiotensin receptor blockers [ARBs], and diuretics).[9,14,15] The most common cause of hospital- and

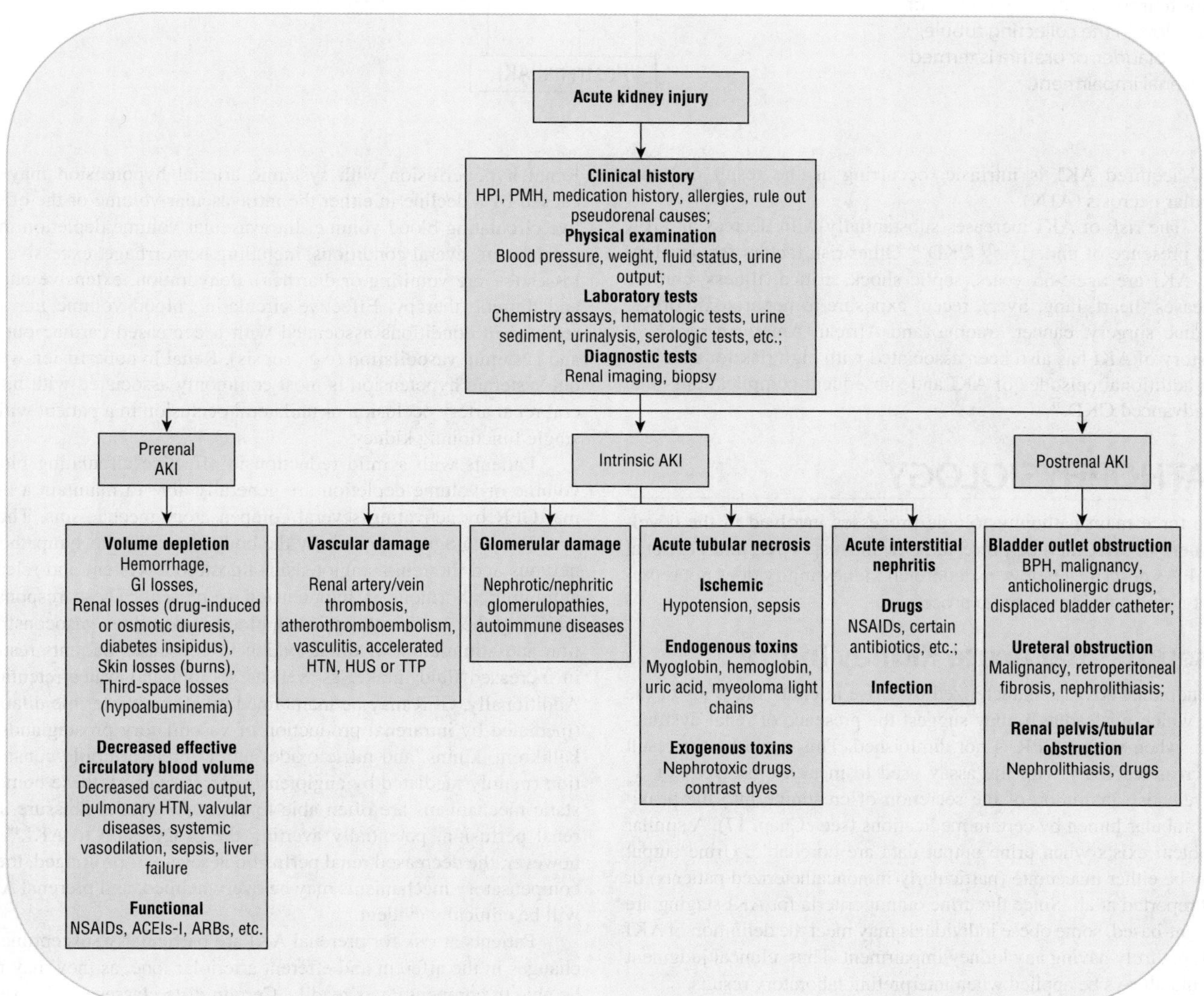

FIGURE 28-1 Classification of acute kidney injury (AKI) based on etiology. (ACEIs, angiotensin-converting enzyme inhibitors; ARBs, angiotensin receptor blockers; BPH, benign prostatic hyperplasia; HPI, history of present illness; HTN, hypertension; HUS, hemolytic uremic syndrome; NSAIDs, nonsteroidal antiinflammatory drugs; PMH, past medical history; TTP, thrombotic thrombocytopenic purpura.)

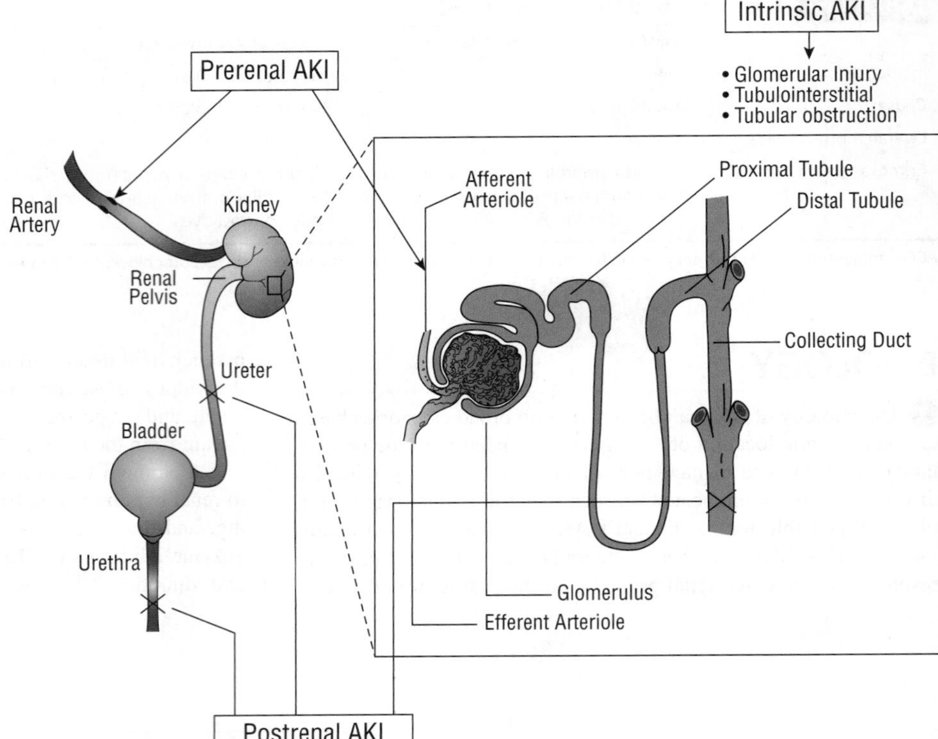

FIGURE 28-2 Physiologic classification of AKI. Blood flows through the afferent arteriole, to the glomerulus, and exits through the efferent arteriole. A decrease in blood flow and renal perfusion can lead to a prerenal reduction in renal function. Under conditions in which renal blood flow is diminished, the kidney maintains glomerular ultrafiltration by vasodilating the afferent arterioles and vasoconstricting the efferent arterioles. Medications that may interfere with these processes may result in an abrupt decline in glomerular filtration. Damage to the glomerular or tubular regions leads to intrinsic AKI. Obstruction of urine flow in the collecting tubule, ureter, bladder, or urethra is termed postrenal impairment.

ICU-acquired AKI is intrinsic, occurring as the result of acute tubular necrosis (ATN).

The risk of AKI increases substantially with decreasing GFR and presence of underlying CKD.[16] Other risk factors for developing AKI are age >65 years, septic shock, critical illness, chronic diseases (heart, lung, liver), recent exposure to nephrotoxic drugs, cardiac surgery, cancer, trauma, and African American race.[5,15,17] History of AKI has also been associated with high risk for developing additional episodes of AKI and subsequent complications such as advanced CKD.[18]

PATHOPHYSIOLOGY

The three main pathophysiologic processes involved in the development of AKI include prerenal AKI, intrinsic AKI, and postrenal AKI. As described below, pseudorenal kidney injury does not represent a true pathophysiologic process.

Pseudorenal Acute Kidney Injury

Pseudorenal AKI is characterized by a rise in either the BUN or the S_{cr}, which misleadingly may suggest the presence of renal dysfunction, when in fact GFR is not diminished. This could be the result of cross-reactivity with the assay used to measure the BUN or S_{cr} or selective inhibition of the secretion of creatinine into the proximal tubular lumen by certain medications (see eChap. 17). A similar problem exists when urine output data are unreliable. Urine output may be either inaccurate (particularly in noncatheterized patients) or not reported at all. Since the urine output criteria for AKI staging are weight-based, some obese individuals may meet the definition of AKI without truly having any kidney impairment. Thus, clinical judgment should always be applied when interpreting laboratory results.

Prerenal Acute Kidney Injury

Prerenal AKI or prerenal azotemia results from hypoperfusion of the renal parenchyma, with or without systemic arterial hypotension. Renal hypoperfusion with systemic arterial hypotension may be caused by a decline in either the intravascular volume or the effective circulating blood volume. Intravascular volume depletion may result from several conditions, including hemorrhage, excessive GI losses (severe vomiting or diarrhea), dehydration, extensive burns, and diuretic therapy. Effective circulating blood volume may be reduced in conditions associated with a decreased cardiac output and systemic vasodilation (e.g., sepsis). Renal hypoperfusion without systemic hypotension is most commonly associated with bilateral renal artery occlusion or unilateral occlusion in a patient with a single functioning kidney.

Patients with a mild reduction in effective circulating blood volume or volume depletion are generally able to maintain a normal GFR by activating several compensatory mechanisms. Those initial physiologic responses by the body stimulate the sympathetic nervous and the renin–angiotensin–aldosterone system and release antidiuretic hormone if hypotension is present. These responses work together to directly maintain blood pressure via vasoconstriction and stimulation of thirst, which in conscious patients results in increased fluid intake, as well as sodium and water retention. Additionally, GFR may be maintained by afferent arteriole dilation (mediated by intrarenal production of vasodilatory prostaglandins, kallikrein, kinins, and nitric oxide) and efferent arteriole constriction (mainly mediated by angiotensin II). In concert, these homeostatic mechanisms are often able to maintain arterial pressure and renal perfusion, potentially averting the progression to AKI.[19] If, however, the decreased renal perfusion is severe or prolonged, these compensatory mechanisms may be overwhelmed, and prerenal AKI will be clinically evident.

Patients at risk for prerenal AKI are particularly susceptible to changes in the afferent and efferent arteriolar tone, as they may not be able to compensate as readily. Certain drug classes can interfere with these renal adaptive responses that are normally responsible for maintaining adequate renal perfusion. The resulting reduction in the glomerular hydrostatic pressure precipitates an abrupt decline in GFR and is sometimes referred to as functional AKI. A common cause of this syndrome is a decrease in efferent arteriolar resistance as the result of initiation of an ACE inhibitor or ARB (see Chap. 31). For example, individuals with heart failure are often given an ACE inhibitor or ARB to help improve left ventricular function, but if the dose is titrated too rapidly, they may experience a decline in GFR. If the increase in the S_{cr} is less than 30% from baseline, the medication can generally be continued. Another classic example is initiation of ACE inhibitors or ARBs in patients with renovascular disease. It is estimated that ACE inhibitor–induced renal failure occurs in 6% to 23% of patients with bilateral renal artery stenosis and in 38% of patients with unilateral stenosis who have a single kidney.[20] As a result, administration of ACE inhibitor or ARB therapy in the presence of those conditions is contraindicated. Nonsteroidal anti-inflammatory drugs (NSAIDs) may also initiate AKI in susceptible individuals. NSAIDs inhibit renal prostaglandin production and afferent arteriolar vasodilation, which some patients rely on to maintain renal perfusion and GFR. Patients at risk for NSAID-induced AKI include those with CKD, volume depletion, and decreased effective circulating blood volume.[21]

If the causes of renal hypoperfusion are promptly corrected, prerenal AKI can be reversed and renal function returned to baseline in a matter of days. Prolonged prerenal azotemia, in contrast, can cause direct (and potentially irreversible) injury to the renal parenchyma and lead to development of ischemic ATN.[22]

Intrinsic Acute Kidney Injury

Intrinsic AKI results from direct damage to the kidney and is categorized on the basis of the injured structures within the kidney: the renal vasculature, glomeruli, tubules, and interstitium.

Renal Vasculature Damage

Occlusion of the larger renal vessels resulting in AKI is not common but can occur if large atheroemboli or thromboemboli occlude the bilateral renal arteries or one vessel of the patient with a single kidney. Atheroemboli most commonly develop during vascular procedures that cause atheroma dislodgement, such as angioplasty and aortic manipulations. Thromboemboli may arise from dislodgement of a mural thrombus in the left ventricle of a patient with severe heart failure or from the atria of a patient with atrial fibrillation. Renal artery thrombosis may occur in a similar fashion to coronary thrombosis, in which a thrombus forms in conjunction with an atherosclerotic plaque.

Although smaller vessels can also be obstructed by atheroemboli or thromboemboli, the damage is limited to the vessels involved, and the development of significant AKI is unlikely. However, these small vessels are susceptible to inflammatory processes that lead to microvascular damage and vessel dysfunction when the renal capillaries are affected. Neutrophils invade the vessel wall, causing damage that can include thrombus formation, tissue infarction, and collagen deposition within the vessel structure. Diffuse renal vasculitis can be mild or severe, with severe forms promoting concomitant ischemic ATN. The S_{cr} is usually elevated when the lesions are diffuse. Accelerated hypertension that is not treated may also compromise renal microvascular blood flow, causing diffuse renal capillary damage.

Glomerular Damage

Only 5% of the cases of intrinsic AKI are of glomerular origin. The glomerulus is one of two capillary beds in the kidney. It serves to filter fluid and solute into the tubules while retaining proteins and other large blood components in the intravascular space. Because the glomerulus is a capillary system, similar damage observed in the renal vasculature can additionally occur by the same mechanisms. The pathophysiology and specific therapeutic approaches to glomerulonephritis are described in detail in Chapter 32.

Tubular Damage

Approximately 85% of all cases of intrinsic AKI are caused by ATN, of which 50% are a result of renal ischemia, often arising from an extended prerenal state. The remaining 35% are the result of exposure to direct tubule toxins, which can be endogenous (myoglobin, hemoglobin, or uric acid) or exogenous (contrast agents, aminoglycosides, etc.). The tubules located within the medulla of the kidney are particularly at risk for ischemic injury, as this portion of the kidney is metabolically active and thus has high oxygen requirements, yet, as compared with the cortex, receives relatively low oxygen delivery. Thus, ischemic conditions caused by severe hypotension or exposure to vasoconstrictive drugs preferentially affect the tubules more than any other portion of the kidney.

The clinical evolution of ATN is characterized by three distinct phases: initiation, maintenance, and recovery. The hallmarks of the initiation phase are ischemic injury and GFR reduction, both of which occur as a result of the interplay between several different pathophysiologic processes. Ischemic injury causes tubular epithelial cell necrosis or apoptosis and is followed by an extension phase with continued hypoxia and an inflammatory response involving the nearby interstitium. The loss of epithelial cells between the filtrate and the interstitium leaves the basement membrane denuded and unable to appropriately regulate fluid and electrolyte transfer across the tubular lumen. As a result, the glomerular filtrate starts leaking back into the interstitium and is reabsorbed into the systemic circulation. Additionally, urine flow is obstructed by accumulation of sloughed epithelial cells, cellular debris, and formation of casts. The onset of ATN can occur over hours to days, depending on the factors responsible for the damage. Regardless of the etiology, tubular injury, back leakage, and obstruction lead to decreased urine-concentrating ability, decreased urine output, and, ultimately, reduced GFR. Continued kidney hypoxia or toxin exposure after the original insult kills more cells and propagates the inflammatory response. It also can extend the injury and delay the recovery process. With prolonged ischemia, the tubular epithelial cells in the corticomedullary junction are damaged and die.[22] When the toxin or ischemia is removed, a maintenance phase ensues and may last anywhere from a few weeks to several months. The maintenance phase is eventually followed by a recovery phase, during which new tubule cells are regenerated. The recovery phase is associated with a notable diuresis, which requires prompt attention to maintain fluid balance, or a secondary prerenal injury may occur. However, if the ischemia or injury is extremely severe or prolonged, cortical necrosis may occur, limiting tubule cell regrowth in the affected areas.[20]

Interstitial Damage

If the renal interstitium becomes severely inflamed and edematous, it can lead to development of acute interstitial nephritis (AIN). AIN may be caused by drugs (see Chap. 31), infections, and, rarely, autoimmune idiopathic diseases. Whatever the inciting event, acute interstitial injury is characterized by lesions composed of monocytes, eosinophils, macrophages, B cells, or T cells, clearly identifying an immunologic response as the injurious process affecting the interstitium. If AIN is caused by a drug hypersensitivity reaction, most patients will regain normal renal function within several weeks if the offending drug is promptly discontinued. If symptoms of AIN remain unrecognized, and the exposure to the causative agent continues, persistent renal dysfunction associated with interstitial fibrosis and tubular atrophy may develop.[23]

Postrenal Acute Kidney Injury

Postrenal AKI accounts for less than 5% of all cases of AKI and may develop as the result of obstruction at any level within the urinary collection system[22] (see Fig. 28-1). However, if the obstructing process is above the bladder, it must involve both kidneys (one kidney in a patient with a single functioning kidney) to cause clinically significant AKI, as one functioning kidney can generally maintain a near-normal GFR. Bladder outlet obstruction, the most common cause of obstructive uropathy, is often the result of a prostatic process (hypertrophy, cancer, or infection), producing a physical impingement on the urethra and thereby preventing the passage of urine. It may also be the result of an improperly placed urinary catheter. Blockage may also occur at the ureter level secondary to nephrolithiasis, blood clots, sloughed renal papillae, or physical compression by an abdominal process. Crystal deposition within the tubules from oxalate and some medications severe enough to cause AKI is uncommon, but it is possible in patients with severe volume contraction and in those receiving large doses of a drug with relatively low urine solubility (see Chap. 31). In these cases, patients have insufficient urine volume to prevent crystal precipitation in the urine. Extremely elevated uric acid concentrations from chemotherapy-induced tumor lysis syndrome can cause obstruction and direct tubular injury as well.[24] Wherever the location of the obstruction, urine will accumulate in the renal structures above the obstruction and cause increased pressure upstream. The ureters, renal pelvis, and calyces all expand, and the net result is a decline in GFR. If renal vasoconstriction ensues, a further decrement in GFR will be observed.

CLINICAL PRESENTATION

The initiating signs or symptoms prompting the clinical suspicion of AKI is highly variable and largely dependent on the underlying etiology. It may be a change in urinary habits (e.g., decreased urine output or urine discoloration), sudden weight gain, or severe abdominal or flank pain. Early recognition and cause identification are critical, as they directly affect the outcome of AKI. One of the first steps in the diagnostic process is to determine if the renal complication is acute, chronic, or the result of an acute change in a patient with known CKD (also called acute-on-chronic renal failure). Patients should also be promptly evaluated for any changes in their fluid and electrolyte status. Patients presenting with AKI in the outpatient environment may have very nonspecific or seemingly unrelated symptoms so that the time of onset of the injury can be difficult to determine. On the other hand, AKI in hospitalized patients is often detected much earlier in its course due to frequent laboratory studies and daily patient assessment.

Patient Assessment

The assessment of a patient with AKI starts with a thorough review of his or her medical records, with a particular focus on chronic conditions, medication history, laboratory studies, procedures, and surgeries. An exhaustive review of prescription and nonprescription medicines, herbal products, and recreational drugs may help determine if AKI was potentially precipitated by drug ingestion.

During the initial patient evaluation, presumptive signs and symptoms of AKI need to be differentiated from a potential new diagnosis of CKD. A past medical history for renal disease–related chronic conditions (e.g., poorly controlled hypertension and diabetes mellitus), previous laboratory data documenting the presence of proteinuria or an elevated S_{cr}, and the finding of bilateral small kidneys on renal ultrasonography suggest the presence of CKD rather than AKI. However, it is important to note that patients with CKD may develop episodes of AKI as well. In that case, an abrupt rise in the patient's baseline S_{cr} is one of the most useful indicators of the presence of an acute insult to the kidneys.

An acute change in urinary habits is another common and noticeable symptom associated with AKI. The presence of cola-colored urine is indicative of blood in the urine, a finding commonly associated with acute glomerulonephritis. In hospitalized patients, changes in urine output may be helpful in characterizing the cause of the patient's AKI. Acute anuria is typically caused by either complete urinary obstruction or a catastrophic event (e.g., shock or acute cortical necrosis). Oliguria, which often develops over several days, suggests prerenal azotemia, whereas nonoliguric renal failure usually results from acute intrinsic renal failure or incomplete urinary obstruction.

Depending on the underlying cause of AKI, patients may present with a variety of symptoms affecting virtually any organ system of the body. Constitutional symptoms such as nausea, vomiting, fatigue, malaise, and weight gain are common but nonspecific. The onset of flank pain is suggestive of a urinary stone; however, if bilateral, it may suggest swelling of the kidneys secondary to acute glomerulonephritis or AIN. Complaints of severe headaches may suggest the presence of severe hypertension and vascular damage. The presence of fever, rash, and arthralgias may be indicative of drug-induced AIN or lupus nephritis.

A thorough physical examination is an important step in evaluating individuals with AKI, as clues regarding the etiology can be evident from the patient's head (eye examination) to toe (evidence of dependent edema) assessment. Observations will either support or refute the cause as prerenal, intrinsic, or postrenal. Evaluation of the patient's volume and hemodynamic status is critical as well, as it will guide management. For example, patients with prerenal AKI can present with either volume depletion or fluid overload. Volume depletion may be evidenced by the presence of postural hypotension, decreased jugular venous pressure (JVP), and dry mucous membranes. Fluid overload, on the other hand, is often reflected by elevated JVP, pitting edema, ascites, and pulmonary crackles.

Conventional Markers of Kidney Function

4 The commonly available laboratory tests used to evaluate the patient with renal insufficiency are described in eChapter 17. Over the past 3 decades, S_{cr} has been the most widely used laboratory test for estimating creatinine clearance (CL_{cr}) and GFR. However, there are several limitations associated with its use. S_{cr} varies widely with a patient's age, gender, muscle mass, diet, and hydration status. For example, patients with reduced creatinine production, such as those with low muscle mass, may have very low S_{cr} values (<0.6 mg/dL [<53 μmol/L]); thus, the presence of a gradual S_{cr} rise to normal values (0.8 to 1.2 mg/dL [71 to 106 μmol/L]) may actually suggest the presence of AKI. However, in the presence of improved nutrition and a large muscle mass, a S_{cr} of 1.2 mg/dL (106 μmol/L) may be a true representation of a person's current renal status. Instead of using fixed numbers to determine renal function, changes in the value from a patient's baseline need to be considered. S_{cr} is normally inversely proportional to GFR. However, rapid changes in GFR (as they occur in AKI) disrupt this equilibrium and make S_{cr} a very insensitive marker. In fact, changes in S_{cr} will lag behind the GFR's decline by 1 to 2 days due to slow accumulation, increased tubular secretion, and increased extrarenal clearance.[25] This can lead to a significant overestimation of the patient's GFR in the early stages of AKI and consequently a potential delay in the diagnosis of the syndrome.

An example of this phenomenon is illustrated by an acute renal artery thrombus that results in abrupt cessation of GFR in one kidney as a consequence of the complete obstruction of blood flow to that kidney (Fig. 28-3). Although 5 minutes following the event GFR is decreased 50% (assuming the other kidney is functioning and unaffected), the S_{cr} remains unchanged. Assuming a standard daily creatinine production of ~20 mg/kg of lean body weight, one can expect ~1.4 g of creatinine production in a 24-hour period in

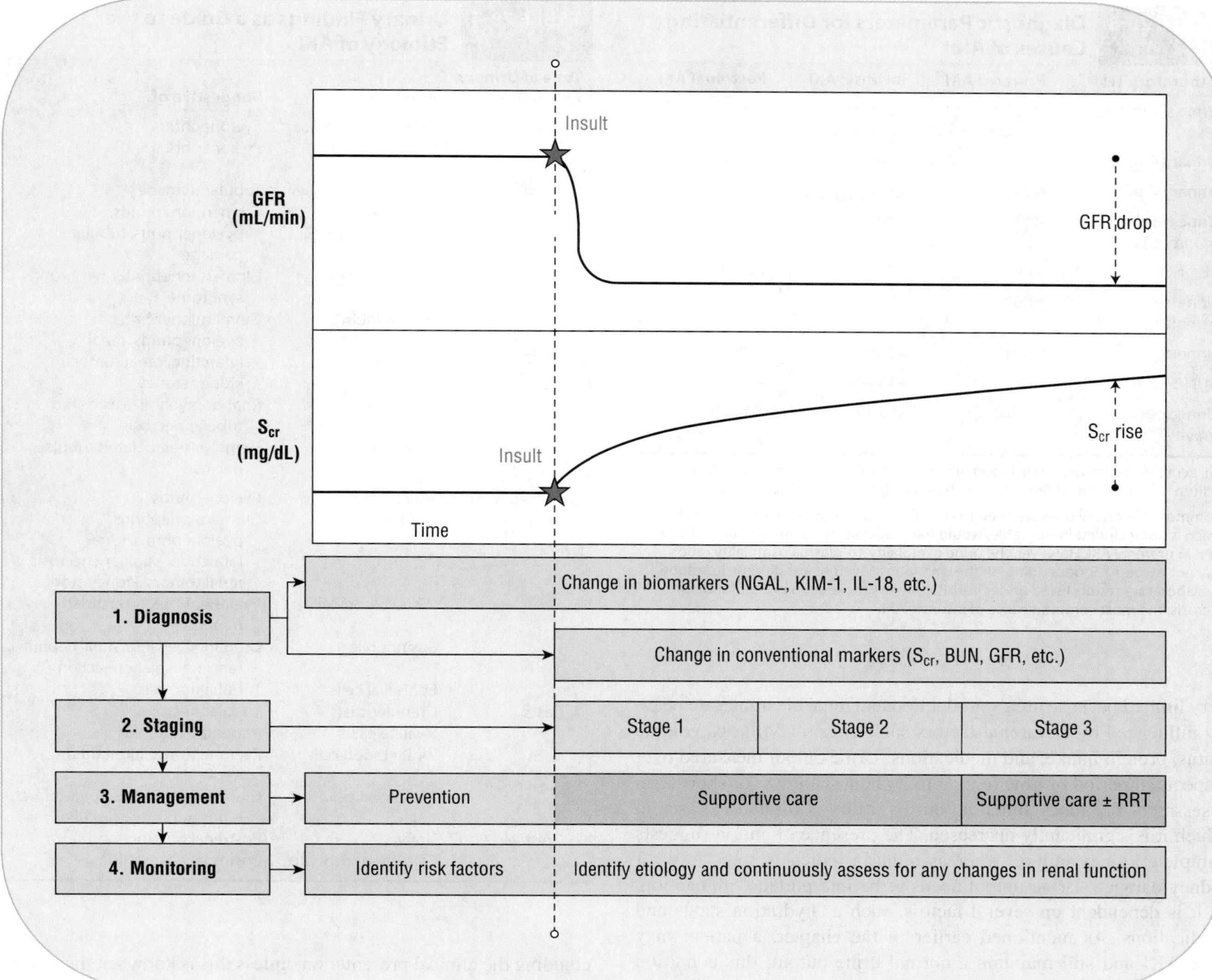

FIGURE 28-3 Glomerular filtration rate (GFR; mL/min) and serum creatinine (S_{cr}; mg/dL) versus time following the insult that leads to acute kidney injury (AKI). Prior to the renal insult, a patient's GFR and S_{cr} are at stable levels. After the renal insult has occurred, GFR readily declines while S_{cr} does not increase immediately, as it is dependent on creatinine production and attainment of steady-state serum concentrations. Novel biomarkers can detect AKI within a few hours after the injury has occurred while conventional biomarkers may take 1 to 2 days to detect a noticeable change. AKI can only be staged once S_{cr} has increased to a significant level. Patients at risk may benefit from prevention strategies; however, once AKI is diagnosed, supportive care and potentially renal replacement therapy should be implemented. Patients with established AKI should undergo further testing to determine the most likely etiology of AKI and need to be continuously monitored for any changes in their renal function. (BUN, blood urea nitrogen; IL-18, interleukin-18; KIM-1, kidney injury molecule 1; NGAL, neutrophil gelatinase–associated lipocalin.)

a 70-kg individual. In pharmacokinetic terms, daily creatinine production is analogous to a continuous infusion, and GFR determines the elimination rate of creatinine. In a patient with normal renal function (GFR of 120 mL/min [2 mL/s]), the half-life of creatinine is 3.5 hours, with 95% of steady state achieved in ~14 hours. If GFR declines to 50%, 25%, or 10% of normal, the half-life of creatinine increases, resulting in prolongation of the time to reach 95% of steady state, specifically taking 1, 2, and 4 days, respectively.

Because S_{cr} steady-state values are assumed when one uses several GFR calculation methods, such as the Cockcroft-Gault, MDRD, and Chronic Kidney Disease Epidemiology Collaboration (CKD-EPI) equations, should not be used in AKI patients with unstable renal function. These equations will typically overestimate GFR when the AKI is worsening and underestimate it when the AKI is resolving. Instead, it may be useful to evaluate changes in S_{cr} values from the patient's baseline and also consider the S_{cr} sequence values to determine if renal function is potentially improving (S_{cr} values declining) or worsening (S_{cr} values rising). The most recent S_{cr} reflects the time-averaged kidney function over the preceding time period. Several mathematical approaches to estimate GFR in patients with unstable S_{cr} that incorporate the principles of creatinine accumulation and elimination have been proposed and are discussed in detail in eChapter 17. However, these methods have not been extensively validated in the setting of acute alterations in renal function, and their value for adjusting medication dosing is questionable. Additionally, these equations are complex and are not commonly used in the clinical setting.

Two other widely available markers of renal function are BUN and urine output. BUN is widely used to assess hemodialysis adequacy in chronic hemodialysis patients. However, its use in AKI is

TABLE 28-3 Diagnostic Parameters for Differentiating Causes of AKI[a]

Laboratory Test	Prerenal AKI	Intrinsic AKI	Postrenal AKI
Urine sediment	Hyaline casts, may be normal	Granular casts, cellular debris	Cellular debris
Urinary RBC	None	2–4+	Variable
Urinary WBC	None	2–4+	1+
Urine Na (mEq/L or mmol/L)	<20	>40	>40
FE_{Na} (%)	<1	>2	Variable
Urine/serum osmolality	>1.5	<1.3	<1.5
Urine/S_{cr}	>40:1	<20:1	<20:1
BUN/S_{cr} (urea/S_{cr}, SI)	>20 (>80)	~15 (~60)	~15 (~60)
Urine specific gravity	>1.018	<1.012	Variable

AKI, acute kidney injury; BUN, blood urea nitrogen; FE_{Na}, fractional excretion of sodium; S_{cr}, serum creatinine; RBC, red blood cell; WBC, white blood cell.

[a]Common laboratory tests are used to classify the cause of AKI. Functional AKI, which is not included in this table, would have laboratory values similar to those seen in prerenal AKI. However, the urine osmolality-to-plasma osmolality ratios may not exceed 1.5, depending on the circulating levels of antidiuretic hormone. The laboratory results listed under intrinsic AKI are those seen in acute tubular necrosis, the most common cause of intrinsic AKI.

very limited because urea's production and renal clearance are heavily influenced by extrarenal factors such as critical illness, volume status, protein intake, and medications. Urine output measured over a specified period of time (e.g., 4 to 24 hours) allows for short-term assessment of kidney function, but its utility is limited to cases in which it is significantly decreased. The presence of anuria suggests complete kidney failure, whereas oliguria indicates some level of kidney damage. Urine output needs to be interpreted with caution, as it is dependent on several factors, such as hydration status and medications. As mentioned earlier in the chapter, a patient may have AKI and still maintain a normal urine output; this condition is referred to as nonoliguric AKI. Another approach to estimating renal function is to directly measure CL_{cr} over a short period of time, for example, 4 to 12 hours.[26] Although potentially precise and fairly simple to do, its accuracy is questionable if the urine output is low or the urine collection is incomplete.

In addition to BUN and S_{cr}, selected blood tests, urinary chemistry, and urinary sediment are routinely used to differentiate the cause of AKI and guide patient management. For example, a complete blood cell count with differential can help rule out infectious causes of AKI. Serum electrolyte values may be abnormal because of the acute decline of the kidney's ability to regulate electrolyte excretion. Particular attention should be paid to serum potassium and phosphorus values, which can be markedly elevated and cause life-threatening complications. In individuals with normal renal function, the ratio between BUN and S_{cr} is usually less than 15:1 using conventional units (60:1 using SI units). In the presence of prerenal AKI, reabsorption of BUN exceeds that of creatinine; thus, one often sees a ratio greater than 20:1 (80:1 using SI units).

Given the limited usefulness of solely using S_{cr} or BUN concentrations to differentiate the etiology of AKI, urinary electrolytes and osmolality should be determined, and both a microscopic and chemical analysis of the urine should be performed (Table 28-3). The finding of a high urinary specific gravity, in the absence of glucosuria or mannitol administration, suggests an intact urinary concentrating mechanism and that the cause of the patient's AKI is likely prerenal azotemia. The presence of urinary protein is often difficult to interpret, especially in the setting of acute or chronic renal failure. A patient with CKD may have a baseline proteinuria, thus

TABLE 28-4 Urinary Findings as a Guide to the Etiology of AKI

Type of Urinary Evaluation	Presence of	Suggestive of
Urinalysis	Leukocyte esterases	Pyelonephritis
	Nitrites	Pyelonephritis
	Protein	
	Mild (<0.5 g/day)	Tubular damage
	Moderate (0.5–3 g/day)	Glomerulonephritis, pyelonephritis, tubular damage
	Large (>3 g/day)	Glomerulonephritis, nephrotic syndrome
	Hemoglobin	Glomerulonephritis, pyelonephritis, renal infarction, renal tumors, kidney stones
	Myoglobin	Rhabdomyolysis-associated tubular necrosis
	Urobilinogen	Hemolysis-associated tubular necrosis
Urine sediment		
Cells	Microorganisms	Pyelonephritis
	Red blood cells	Glomerulonephritis, pyelonephritis, renal infarction, papillary necrosis, renal tumors, kidney stones
	White blood cells	Pyelonephritis, interstitial nephritis
	Eosinophils	Drug-induced interstitial nephritis, renal transplant rejection
	Epithelial cells	Tubular necrosis
Casts	Granular casts	Tubular necrosis
	Hyaline casts	Prerenal azotemia
	White blood cell casts	Pyelonephritis, interstitial nephritis
	Red blood cell casts	Glomerulonephritis, renal infarct, lupus nephritis, vasculitis
Crystals	Urate	Postrenal obstruction
	Calcium phosphate	Postrenal obstruction

clouding the clinical presentation, unless this is known at the time of AKI assessment. Classically, proteinuria is a hallmark of glomerular damage. However, tubular damage can also result in proteinuria, as the tubules are responsible for reabsorbing small proteins that are normally filtered by all glomeruli. The presence of blood also results in a positive urine protein test, so this confounder must always be assessed when a positive urine protein is obtained. Hematuria suggests acute intrinsic AKI secondary to glomerular injury, infection, or a kidney stone. On microscopic examination, the key findings are cells, casts, and crystals, and the presence of one or more of these may suggest specific etiologies of the AKI (Table 28-4). The finding of urinary crystals may indicate nephrolithiasis and a postrenal obstruction. If red blood cells or red blood cell casts are present, one should consider the presence of a physical injury to the glomerulus, renal parenchyma, or vascular beds. The finding of white blood cells or white blood cell casts suggests interstitial inflammation (i.e., interstitial nephritis), which can be secondary to an allergic, granulomatous, or infectious process.

Simultaneous measurement of urine and serum electrolytes is also helpful in the setting of AKI (see Table 28-3). From these values, a fractional excretion of sodium (FE_{Na}) can be calculated. The equation for the calculation of the FE_{Na} is as follows:

$$FE_{Na} = \frac{\text{excreted Na}}{\text{filtered Na}} \times 100 = \frac{U_{vol} \times U_{Na}}{GFR \times S_{Na}} \times 100$$

where

$$GFR = \frac{U_{vol} \times U_{cr}}{S_{cr} \times t}$$

Thus:

$$FE_{Na} = \frac{U_{Na} \times S_{cr} \times 100}{U_{cr} \times S_{Na}}$$

where U_{vol} is urine volume; U_{cr} is urine creatinine concentration; U_{Na} is urine sodium; S_{cr} is serum creatinine concentration; S_{Na} is serum sodium concentration, which usually does not vary much; GFR is the glomerular filtration rate; and *t* is the time period over which the urine is collected.

The FE_{Na} is one of the better diagnostic parameters to differentiate the cause of AKI. A low urinary sodium concentration (<20 mEq/L [<20 mmol/L]) and low FE_{Na} (<1%) in a patient with oliguria suggest that there is stimulation of the sodium-retentive mechanisms in the kidney and that tubular function is intact. These findings are most characteristic of prerenal azotemia. Unfortunately, diuretic use in the preceding days limits the usefulness of the FE_{Na} calculation by increasing natriuresis, even in hypovolemic patients. The fractional excretion of urea (FE_{Urea}), which can be calculated like FE_{Na}, is sometimes used as an alternative means to assess tubular function. The inability to concentrate urine results in a high FE_{Na} (>2%), suggesting tubular damage as the primary cause of the intrinsic AKI. However, this is also not an absolute finding, as there are some intrinsic causes that can be associated with a low FE_{Na} (e.g., contrast nephropathy, myoglobinuria, and interstitial nephritis). Highly concentrated urine (>500 mOsm/kg [>500 mmol/kg]) suggests stimulation of antidiuretic hormone and intact tubular function. These findings are consistent with prerenal azotemia.

Novel Biomarkers of Kidney Function

Diagnostic delays associated with creatinine-based methods have stimulated the search for novel biomarkers that are able to detect renal injury before a clinically evident decline in GFR occurs. Biomarkers that can detect renal injury more sensitively than S_{cr} would enable clinicians to identify AKI earlier and, as a result, initiate preventative strategies and other interventions more rapidly.

An ideal biomarker would be highly sensitive and specific for AKI, noninvasive, and reliably and easily measurable using standardized clinical assays. In addition, it would differentiate between different AKI etiologies, be unaffected by other comorbidities and biologic variables, and allow for monitoring of response to AKI interventions. Over the past 10 years, several biomarkers have been investigated in their ability to detect and predict the clinical outcomes of AKI.[27] Since no single marker fulfills all the criteria to be deemed "ideal," combining multiple biomarkers into a panel may serve as a future clinical application for early detection, differential diagnosis, prognosis, response, and recovery of AKI. Of note, since the area of biomarker research is still relatively novel, these tests are not routinely available at most clinical practice sites. Over the past 2 years, several clinical studies evaluated the diagnostic and prognostic value of AKI biomarkers in heterogeneous patient populations and overall demonstrated promising results. However, the transition to clinical application will still require further validation, standardization, and development of implementation strategies for their use in all practice settings. Table 28-5 summarizes the advantages and disadvantages of the four most promising biomarkers.

One such biomarker, serum cystatin C (see eChap. 17), is an endogenous cysteine proteinase that is released into the plasma by all nucleated cells in the body at a relatively constant rate and is then freely filtered by the glomerulus. It does not undergo any significant secretion or reabsorption, but is instead completely metabolized by the proximal renal tubules and undetectable in urine in normal kidney tissue.[28] However, if tubular injury occurs, plasma cystatin C levels will rise and urinary levels will become detectable. Serum cystatin C has been extensively studied as a marker of estimated GFR in patients with stable renal function, and its measurements are readily available using standardized assays.[29] Its performance in early detection and clinical outcome prediction for AKI has yielded varied results. While it does seem to outperform S_{cr}, it has not generally outperformed other novel biomarkers.[28] One of its main limitations is that, similarly to S_{cr}, cystatin C is a marker of GFR and not a direct marker of tissue injury. Therefore, the rise in its concentrations may be delayed compared with other biomarkers and it lacks specificity in differentiating AKI from CKD.[27] Also, cystatin C levels may be altered by certain disease states (e.g., thyroid dysfunction and systemic inflammation) and possibly patient demographics (age, weight, gender, etc.).[30,31]

Another relatively novel biomarker is neutrophil gelatinase–associated lipocalin (NGAL), a transporter protein found on cell surfaces of neutrophils and various epithelial cells. It is freely filtered by the glomeruli and reabsorbed by the proximal tubules.[32] As a result, if proximal tubular injury occurs, urinary NGAL levels are expected to rise. Studies indicate that NGAL is a valuable biomarker of AKI development across a range of clinical settings, including both pediatrics and adults, patients with contrast-induced nephropathy (CIN), critically ill, and cardiac surgery patients.[33] NGAL measurements may be elevated as early as 1 to 2 hours after renal injury in select populations and correlate well with the severity of AKI.[34] Also, the recent development of two standardized clinical assays, a chemiluminescent microparticle assay for urine NGAL and a point-of-care kit

TABLE 28-5 Advantages and Disadvantages of Novel Clinical Biomarkers of AKI

Biomarker	Source	Description	Advantages	Disadvantages
Cystatin C	Plasma Urine	Endogenous cysteine proteinase filtered by the glomeruli and catabolized by proximal tubules	Well studied as a marker of stable GFR Commercial assay available	Levels altered in the presence of systemic inflammation, thyroid disease, patient demographics Nonspecific marker of GFR Delayed increase in concentrations postinsult (8–12 hours) compared with other biomarkers
IL-18	Urine	Proinflammatory cytokine expressed by proximal tubules after renal injury	Marker of ischemic AKI	Inconsistent performance across different patient populations Unknown impact of systemic inflammation on urinary levels
KIM-1	Urine	Glycoprotein expressed by proximal tubules after renal injury	Commercial urine test available Early marker of ischemic AKI	Not widely studied in different patient populations
NGAL	Plasma Urine	Epithelial protein filtered by the glomeruli and reabsorbed by the proximal tubules	Commercial test available Highly sensitive and specific in select populations	Decreased specificity in patients with CKD and other comorbidities

AKI, acute kidney injury; CKD, chronic kidney disease; GFR, glomerular filtration rate; IL-18, interleukin-18; KIM-1, kidney injury molecule-1; NGAL, neutrophil gelatinase–associated lipocalin.

for plasma NGAL, will help increase the availability of this measure to assess the risk of AKI.[27] Although NGAL appears to be a very sensitive, specific, and early biomarker of AKI, its levels may be influenced by the presence of CKD and other comorbidities.[35]

Interleukin-18 (IL-18) is a proinflammatory cytokine produced by the proximal tubular epithelial cells in response to renal injury. It seems to be specific for ischemic ATN and can distinguish it from CKD, prerenal azotemia, nephrotic syndrome, and urinary tract infections.[36] Urinary IL-18 levels begin increasing as early as 4 to 6 hours after an ischemic insult, peak at 12 hours, and remain elevated for up to 48 hours.[37] Urinary IL-18 has been studied in several clinical settings with varied results. Its ability for early detection of AKI has proven more robust in patients with discrete ischemia reperfusion injury such as kidney transplantation or pediatric cardiopulmonary bypass and less favorable in critically ill patients or adults with comorbidities.[27,38] This finding may, in part, be explained by the potential confounding impact of systemic inflammatory states on IL-18 levels, but the extent of this association still remains largely unknown.[27] Even though the performance of IL-18 on early AKI detection has been inconsistent, recent studies suggest that IL-18 may be more useful as a prognostic marker of poor renal outcomes, including mortality.

Kidney injury molecule 1 (KIM-1) is a membrane glycoprotein expressed by the proximal tubular epithelial cells and released into the urine in response to ischemic renal injury. One advantage of KIM-1 is that it is not expressed in healthy kidney tissue or detected in plasma.[39] While KIM-1 does have detectable levels in patients with other renal diseases such as CKD and CIN, these concentrations are significantly lower compared with ischemic AKI.[27,32] This finding suggests that KIM-1 may be useful in differentiating ischemic AKI from other types of renal injury. Studies indicate that KIM-1 is a promising biomarker for early detection as its levels are elevated as early as 2 hours after renal injury.[40] In addition, a rapid urine dipstick test for KIM-1 is now available that provides semiquantitative results in 15 minutes and may serve as an additional tool for rapid and early diagnosis of AKI.[41]

Diagnostic Considerations

When the source of renal injury is unclear after a history, physical examination, and assessment of laboratory values, imaging techniques such as abdominal radiography, including the kidneys, ureters, and bladder (KUB), computed tomography (CT), and ultrasonography may be helpful. These may reveal small, shrunken kidneys indicative of CKD. Postrenal obstruction can often be identified with a renal ultrasonogram and/or CT scan. Renal ultrasonography is also useful in detecting obstruction or hydronephrosis. Nephrolithiases as small as 5 nm or a narrowing of the ureteral tract can be detected by ultrasonography or more sensitive tests, such as KUB and CT.

In cases in which the cause of AKI is not evident, renal biopsies are useful in determining the cause in the majority of patients. Because of the associated risk of bleeding, a renal biopsy is rarely undertaken and should only be performed in those circumstances when a definitive diagnosis is needed to guide therapy, such as the precise etiology of glomerulonephritis (see Chap. 32).

PREVENTION OF AKI

5 The preventive strategy will depend on the type of renal insult. Clearly, complete avoidance of all potential causes of injury is the most effective preventive method; however, it may not always be possible to implement. Sometimes, the risk of renal injury is predictable, such as decreased perfusion secondary to coronary bypass surgery or secondary to the administration of a radiocontrast dye prior to a diagnostic procedure. In these situations, the potential insult to the kidneys cannot be avoided but may be preventable with aggressive hydration and removal of any additional insults. In the outpatient setting, all healthcare professionals should educate the patient on preventive measures for AKI. Patients should receive counseling regarding their optimal daily fluid intake (~2 L/day) to avoid dehydration, especially if they are to receive a potentially nephrotoxic medication. In the inpatient setting, adequate hydration, standardized hemodynamic support in the critically ill, and avoidance of nephrotoxic medications are commonly recommended strategies for the prevention of AKI. Table 28-6 summarizes the recommendations published by KDIGO clinical practice guidelines regarding recommended and not recommended therapies for the prevention of AKI.[5,24]

Desired Outcome

The goals of AKI prevention are to (a) screen and identify patients at risk, (b) monitor high-risk patients until the risk has subsided, and (c) implement prevention strategies when appropriate.

TABLE 28-6 KDIGO Recommendations for Prevention and Treatment of AKI

Drug	Indication	Recommended for Prevention	Recommended for Treatment	Comments
ANP	AKI	No (2C)	No (2B)	
Diuretics	AKI	No (1B)	No (2C)	Acceptable if managing concurrent fluid overload
Dopamine (1–3 mcg/kg/min)	AKI	No (1A)	No (1A)	
Fenoldopam	AKI CI-AKI	No (2C) No (1B)	No (2C)	
Isotonic saline IV	AKI CI-AKI	Yes (2B) Yes (1A)	Yes (2B)	For AKI: recommended in the absence of hemorrhagic shock
NAC	AKI CI-AKI	No (2D) Yes (2D)		For CI-AKI: give in combination with isotonic saline
RRT	AKI CI-AKI	 No (2C)	Yes (NG)	
Sodium bicarbonate IV	CI-AKI	Yes (1A)		
Theophylline	CI-AKI	No (2C)		
Vasopressors	AKI	Yes (1C)	Yes (1C)	Recommended in combination with fluids in vasomotor shock

AKI, acute kidney injury; ANP, atrial natriuretic peptide; CI-AKI, contrast-induced acute kidney injury; KDIGO, Kidney Disease: Improving Global Outcomes; NAC, *N*-acetylcysteine; RRT, renal replacement therapy.
Strength of recommendation levels: 1, recommended; 2, suggested; NG, not graded.
Quality of supporting evidence: A, high; B, moderate; C, low; D, very low.

Nonpharmacologic Therapy

Several nonpharmacologic therapies have been explored for the prevention of AKI, including hydration and RRT.

Hydration

Hydration is one of the primary interventions that has consistently shown benefit and is routinely used in the prevention of AKI. Fluids have largely been studied in association with hemodynamic instability secondary to intravascular volume depletion as well as contrast administration before a radiologic procedure.

Hemodynamic instability increases the risk of AKI as it can lead to decreased renal perfusion and subsequent renal injury. Both isotonic crystalloids and colloid-containing solutions have been studied as means to replace intravascular volume. Among colloids, synthetic products such as hyperoncotic hydroxyethyl starch have been associated with renal dysfunction and should generally be avoided in patients at risk for AKI.[42] Albumin appears to be safe for the kidneys; however, it is more costly and does not provide better patient outcomes compared with isotonic saline.[43] As a result, KDIGO guidelines recommend isotonic crystalloids over colloids for intravascular volume expansion in patients at risk for AKI.[5]

CIN is a common cause of ATN in the inpatient setting (see Chap. 31 for a detailed discussion of CIN) and is typically characterized by an increase in S_{cr} starting at 12 hours to up to 5 days after the radiologic procedure.[5] It is associated with increased mortality especially in individuals with CKD, diabetes, volume depletion, concurrent nephrotoxic drug therapy, or hemodynamic instability.[44] Hydration is thought to counterbalance some of the deleterious effects of radiocontrast dyes by diluting the contrast media, preventing renal vasoconstriction that contributes to hypoxia and ischemia, and minimizing tubular obstruction.[45] Sodium bicarbonate infusion has also been evaluated for the prevention of CIN. The hypothesized mechanism for protection is that sodium bicarbonate may reduce the formation of oxygen free radicals by alkalinizing renal tubular fluid.[46] There is currently no agreement on which hydration regimen is more effective as some studies indicate lower incidences of CIN with sodium bicarbonate while others show lower CIN rates with isotonic saline.[47,48] The KDIGO guidelines currently recommend using either sodium bicarbonate or isotonic saline in high-risk individuals receiving radiocontrast media.[5]

Since there is no consensus on the optimal rate and duration of fluid infusions, CIN hydration protocols may vary slightly across different institutions. A common sodium bicarbonate regimen is 154 mEq/L (154 mmol/L) infused at 3 mL/kg/h for 1 hour before the procedure and at 1 mL/kg/h for 6 hours after the procedure.[46,48] The rate and duration of normal saline infusion vary, but one frequently cited regimen is 1 mL/kg/h for 12 hours before and 12 hours after the procedure.[48] The rate of administration may need to be adjusted depending on the patient's cardiopulmonary and volume status.

Renal Replacement Therapy

Prophylactic administration of RRT has been explored as another potential approach to prevent CIN in high-risk patients. Radiocontrast media are eliminated by the kidneys, but their clearance is delayed in patients with renal dysfunction, thereby increasing their risk for nephrotoxicity. RRT use is based on its ability to enhance radiocontrast dye clearance and thus potentially prevent nephrotoxicity. So far, there seems to be no overall benefit of RRT in decreasing the incidence of CIN.[43,49] In fact, there seems to be a significantly higher risk of harm among studies using prophylactic hemodialysis versus other RRT modalities such as hemofiltration.[43,49] There also may be a difference in renal outcomes based on the timing of RRT relative to contrast administration as well as the patients' degree of renal impairment. RRT has demonstrated most promising clinical benefit when hemofiltration was initiated both before and after the procedure in patients with advanced CKD (stage 4 or higher).[48,50] Other, more practical issues associated with using prophylactic RRT are cost and the labor-intensive and invasive nature of the procedure itself. Overall, due to a relatively uncertain benefit, KDIGO guidelines do not currently recommend RRT for prevention of CIN.[5] However, further investigation is needed to elucidate the mechanisms and timing of different RRT modalities and clarify the effect of underlying CKD on renal outcomes.

Pharmacologic Therapy

Several pharmacologic therapies have been investigated for the prevention of AKI with variable results.

Loop Diuretics

Loop diuretics are frequently used for the management of fluid overload in patients at risk for AKI as well as those with established renal injury. Early experimental studies proposed that loop diuretics had the following theoretical advantages: decreased risk of tubular obstruction secondary to an increased urine flow and flushing out of debris; increased urine output that may be beneficial in itself, as nonoliguric AKI is associated with better outcomes than oliguric AKI; decreased risk of ischemic injury as the result of inhibition of the sodium/potassium chloride cotransporter and thus a reduction in oxygen demand; and enhanced renal blood flow due to increased availability of renal prostaglandins.[28] However, clinical studies have found that even though the loop diuretics increase urine output, they neither reduce the incidence of AKI nor improve patient outcomes, such as mortality, need for RRT, and renal recovery.[28,51] There is even some evidence of potential harm associated with their use, in particular, ototoxicity and possibly mortality in certain clinical settings.[51] Proposed explanations for such lack of benefit are twofold. Loop diuretics may not be reaching the proximal tubule, their site of action, due to tubular obstruction from debris, increased extrarenal clearance secondary to hypoalbuminemia, and increased urinary protein binding due to albuminuria. Also, loop diuretics may actually decrease renal blood flow by reducing effective circulating arterial volume, which, in turn, may stimulate the adrenergic and the renin–angiotensin systems.[28] Therefore, the KDIGO guidelines recommend limiting the use of loop diuretics to the management of fluid overload and avoiding their use for the sole purpose of prevention or treatment of AKI.[5]

Vasodilator Therapy

Vasodilators studied for the prevention and treatment of AKI include dopamine, fenoldopam, anaritide, and nesiritide.

Dopamine Dopamine is a nonselective dopamine receptor agonist that, in high doses, also stimulates the adrenergic receptors. Low doses of IV dopamine (1 to 3 mcg/kg/min) increase renal blood flow, induce natriuresis and diuresis, and might be expected to increase GFR. Theoretically, this could be considered beneficial, as an increase in renal perfusion and oxygenation might limit ischemic cell injury, inhibition of sodium transport might reduce oxygen demand, and an enhanced GFR might flush nephrotoxins and casts from the tubules. Despite these theoretical suggestions, controlled studies have found that low-dose dopamine did not prevent AKI, need for dialysis, or mortality compared with placebo.[52] Thus, current evidence and KDIGO guidelines do not support the use of low-dose dopamine for prevention or treatment of noncardiogenic AKI.[5]

Fenoldopam Fenoldopam mesylate is a selective dopamine A1 receptor agonist that increases renal blood flow, natriuresis, and diuresis without systemic α- or β-adrenergic stimulation. Fenoldopam has largely been studied in critically ill and/or cardiac surgery patients. Some studies have demonstrated decreased inpatient mortality and need for RRT while others have not found any benefit.[53]

Due to a lack of large multicenter trials as well as risk of hypotension, current KDIGO guidelines do not recommend the use of fenoldopam for the prevention and treatment of AKI.[5]

Natriuretic Peptides Natriuretic peptides, specifically atrial natriuretic peptide (ANP) and brain natriuretic peptide (BNP), mediate vasodilation, diuresis, and natriuresis. ANP, which is released from the atrium in response to a rise in atrial stretch, dilates the afferent renal arteriole and constricts the efferent renal arteriole resulting in an increase in renal perfusion and GFR. Clinical studies on human recombinant ANP (anaritide) have varied in their findings, depending on the patient population and the anaritide dose under study. There is some evidence that anaritide may be beneficial in reducing the need for RRT in cardiac surgery patients but not in other patient populations.[54] Also, anaritide at low doses (50 to 100 ng/kg/min) seems to be associated with improved outcomes while doses above 100 ng/kg/min increase the risk of hypotension and arrhythmias.[5,54] On the other hand, studies using BNP (nesiritide) have largely demonstrated no benefit on the long-term survival and renal outcomes in patients at risk for AKI.[55] Due to the need for further research on appropriate dosing and duration as well as risk of adverse effects, both ANP and BNP are currently not recommended for prevention or treatment of AKI by the KDIGO Work Group.[5]

Antioxidants

Ascorbic acid and *N*-acetylcysteine (NAC) are two antioxidants that have been studied for the prevention of AKI.

Ascorbic Acid Ascorbic acid has mainly been studied in the prevention of CIN, as its antioxidant properties are thought to alleviate oxidative stress caused by CIN-associated ischemia reperfusion injury.[56] While its excellent safety profile and low cost make it an attractive option, clinical studies have reported inconsistent results on its protective effect against CIN.[57–59] One randomized, double-blind, placebo-controlled trial demonstrated that ascorbic acid, 3 g orally before the procedure and 2 g orally twice daily for two doses after the procedure, significantly diminished the incidence of CIN in patients undergoing coronary angiography/intervention.[58] However, several subsequent studies were unable to reproduce the same results and have largely found no difference from placebo.[57,59] While the KDIGO Work Group does not specifically provide recommendations on ascorbic acid, majority of studies indicate that ascorbic acid is expected to have little, if any, therapeutic benefit for the prevention of CIN.

***N*-Acetylcysteine** NAC is another antioxidant that has been widely studied in the prevention of CIN. However, a therapeutic benefit is thought to be quite modest and has not been consistently demonstrated.[47,60] When compared with ascorbic acid, NAC seemed to be more beneficial in preventing CIN, particularly in diabetic patients with preexisting CKD.[61] The recommended dosing regimen for prevention of CIN is 600 to 1,200 mg orally every 12 hours for 2 to 3 days, with the first two doses administered prior to contrast exposure. This dosing regimen is generally well tolerated and expected to have little adverse effects. NAC has also been evaluated for the prevention of AKI in postoperative setting as well as in critically ill patients with hypotension, but studies have failed to demonstrate any protective effect on renal function.[5,62]

Insulin

Glycemic control in critically ill patients is of utmost importance, as stress hyperglycemia and insulin resistance are common during critical illness. The causes of insulin resistance are multifactorial but include impaired glucose homeostasis due to loss of the kidney's metabolic function, and decreased hepatic and peripheral glucose uptake secondary to uremia. Hyperglycemia has also been associated with an increased risk of renal injury, but the exact mechanisms by which glucose may contribute to renal toxicity are not fully elucidated.[63] Experimental studies indicate increased sensitivity to renal ischemia reperfusion injury, glucose overload in the kidney causing tissue damage, and increased inflammation.[64] Patients may also be at higher risk for hypoglycemia, as the kidneys are the primary metabolic site of insulin.

Contrary to earlier findings, recent studies conducted in critically ill patients now indicate that intensive insulin therapy to maintain blood glucose of 80 to 110 mg/dL (4.4 to 6.1 mmol/L) is associated with more adverse effects compared with conventional insulin therapy (180 to 200 mg/dL [10 to 11.1 mmol/L] blood glucose).[65,66] The Normoglycemia in Intensive Care Evaluation and Survival Using Glucose Algorithm Regulation (NICE-SUGAR) trial, a large multicenter randomized study conducted in medical and surgical ICU patients, revealed that intensive glucose control was associated with significantly greater 90-day mortality rates and higher risk of hypoglycemia compared with conventional insulin therapy (144 to 180 mg/dL [8 to 10 mmol/L]). Although the study did not report the incidence of ICU-acquired AKI, no significant difference in the need for RRT between the two groups was noted.[65] A subsequent meta-analysis of 26 published trials conducted in ICUs found that intensive insulin therapy increased the risk of hypoglycemia by sixfold and did not provide an overall mortality benefit.[67] As a way to balance potential benefit and harm, current KDIGO guidelines suggest using insulin therapy to target plasma glucose of 110 to 149 mg/dL (6.1 to 8.3 mmol/L).[5]

Adenosine Receptor Antagonists

Adenosine is generated at enhanced rates in response to increased tubular sodium chloride transport or hypoxia. It subsequently binds to glomerular adenosine A1 receptors to lower GFR by constricting the afferent arteriole. Theophylline is a nonselective adenosine receptor antagonist and has mainly been studied for the prevention of CIN. Two systematic reviews reported a nonsignificant trend toward reduced incidence of CIN.[68,69] It is important to note that theophylline may have significant adverse effects such as tachycardia and tremor as well as a high potential for drug interactions. Due to the risk of adverse effects as well as a relatively small benefit, KDIGO guidelines suggest against using theophylline for prevention of CIN.[5]

Erythropoietin

Erythropoietin is a primary regulator of red blood cell production and is widely used to treat anemia in patients with CKD and cancer. Experimental models have demonstrated the tissue-protective role of erythropoietin against ischemic renal injury.[70] However, a subsequent double-blind, placebo-controlled trial found no difference in the outcome of AKI among ICU patients.[71] As a result, the KDIGO Work Group recommends against the use of erythropoietin for prevention and treatment of AKI.[5]

TREATMENT OF AKI

Identification and management of AKI should be prompt. Prerenal sources of AKI should be managed with hemodynamic support and volume replacement.[72] Postrenal therapy focuses on removing the cause of the obstruction. It is important to approach the treatment of established AKI with an understanding of the patient's comorbidities and baseline renal function. Loss of kidney function combined with other clinical conditions, such as cardiac and liver failure, is associated with higher mortality than that associated with the development of AKI alone.[73] At times, the most efficacious remedy for AKI is management of the comorbid precipitating event. Appreciation of the baseline renal function is also important at the outset of AKI management, because the preexisting level of renal function indicates the highest degree of recovery that can be attained.

Desired Outcomes

The desired outcome in patients with AKI is to facilitate renal recovery and minimize injury. Renal recovery is facilitated by ensuring that hemodynamic parameters and blood chemistries are monitored daily and maintained within normal range. Fluid status should be monitored by following fluid ins and outs and patient weight as both excessive and insufficient fluid administration can be detrimental to patient recovery. Renal injury can be minimized by careful daily review of patient medications with the goal of avoiding nephrotoxic drugs and adjusting the dosing of renally eliminated medications. Patients receiving RRT need to have their medication administration and serum concentration measurement times adjusted appropriately with regards to the timing and duration of their RRT.

Presence of CKD indicates that the kidneys have less reserve, and there is a greater likelihood that full recovery may not occur.

6 Supportive care is the mainstay of AKI management regardless of etiology. RRT may be necessary to maintain fluid and electrolyte balance while removing accumulating waste products or toxins.[72] The slow process of renal recovery cannot begin until insults are eliminated. The recovery process for ATN typically occurs within 10 to 14 days after insult resolution. This may be prolonged if the kidney is exposed to repeated insults.

Desired Outcomes

Short-term goals of AKI management include minimizing the degree of insult to the kidney, reducing extrarenal complications, and expediting the patient's recovery of renal function. The ultimate goal is to have the patient's renal function restored to his or her pre-AKI baseline. Table 28-6 summarizes the recommendations published in the KDIGO clinical practice guidelines regarding recommended and not recommended therapies for the treatment of AKI.[5]

Nonpharmacologic Therapy

Initial modalities to reverse or minimize prerenal AKI include eliminating medications associated with kidney damage and improving cardiac output and renal blood flow. If dehydration is evident, then appropriate fluid replacement therapy should be initiated. Moderately volume-depleted patients can be given oral rehydration fluids; however, if IV fluid is required, isotonic saline is preferred, and large volumes may be necessary for adequate fluid resuscitation. In septic patients, IV fluid challenges are initiated with up to 1,000 mL of isotonic saline over 30 minutes if tolerated with an assessment of the volume status after each challenge.[74] The patient should be monitored for pulmonary edema, peripheral edema, adequate blood pressure (target mean arterial pressure ≥65 mm Hg), normoglycemia, and electrolyte balance. Urine output ≥0.5 mL/kg/h is generally targeted during the initial fluid resuscitation phase.[74]

In patients with anuria or oliguria, slower rehydration, such as 250 mL boluses or 100 mL/h infusions of isotonic saline or a balanced crystalloid solution, should be considered to reduce the risk for pulmonary edema, especially if heart failure or pulmonary insufficiency exists. Isotonic saline has been associated with hyperchloremic metabolic acidosis and acid–base imbalance if the dehydration is accompanied by a severe electrolyte imbalance amenable to large and relatively rapid infusions. For example, dehydration resulting from severe diarrhea is often accompanied by metabolic acidosis caused by bicarbonate losses. A reasonable IV rehydration fluid in this situation would be 5% dextrose with 0.45% sodium chloride plus 50 mEq (50 mmol) of sodium bicarbonate per liter, administered as boluses as described above, followed by a brisk continuous infusion (200 mL/h) until rehydration is complete, acidosis corrected, and diarrhea resolved. This fluid will remain mostly in the intravascular space, providing the necessary perfusion pressure to the kidneys, as well as a substantial amount of bicarbonate to correct the acidosis.

If the prerenal AKI is a result of blood loss or is complicated by symptomatic anemia, red blood cell transfusion to a hematocrit no higher than 30% (0.30) is the treatment of choice.[74] Although albumin is sometimes used as a resuscitative agent, its use should be limited to individuals with severe hypoalbuminemia (e.g., liver disease and nephritic syndrome) who are resistant to crystalloid therapy. These patients have severe hypoalbuminemia-associated third spacing that complicates fluid management, and albumin may be useful in this setting.[75]

The most common interventions that must be made when treating patients with intrinsic or postobstructive AKI involve fluid and electrolyte management. Fluid and electrolyte status will need to be assessed regularly and individualized. At times, drug infusions and nutrition solutions may need to be maximally concentrated. Maintenance IV infusions should be minimized unless the patient is euvolemic or is receiving RRT to maintain fluid balance. Supportive care goals include maintenance of adequate cardiac output and blood pressure to allow adequate tissue perfusion. However, a fine balance must be maintained in anuric and oliguric patients unless the patient is hypovolemic or is able to achieve fluid balance via RRT. If fluid intake is not minimized, edema may rapidly develop, especially in hypoalbuminemic patients. Excessive fluid administration can also impair the function of other organ systems and reduce outcomes.[76] In critically ill patients with vasomotor shock, vasopressors such as norepinephrine, vasopressin, or dopamine may be used in conjunction with fluids in order to maintain adequate hemodynamics and renal perfusion.[5]

Renal Replacement Therapy

7 RRT can be administered either intermittently or continuously. The optimal mode for hemodialysis is unclear and varies depending on the clinical presentation of the patient.[5] Some recent data suggest that more aggressive approaches using RRT in a more liberal fashion or use of a bioartificial membrane consisting of renal proximal tubule cells may improve survival in critically ill patients with AKI.[77] Early RRT should be considered when life-threatening changes in fluid, electrolyte, and acid–base balance are present.[5,78] The choice of continuous versus intermittent RRTs is a matter of considerable debate and usually depends on physician preference and the resources available at the hospital. The most common indications for initiation of RRT are summarized in Table 28-7.

TABLE 28-7 Common Indications for Renal Replacement Therapy

Indication for Renal Replacement Therapy	Clinical Setting
A: *a*cid–base abnormalities	Metabolic acidosis resulting from the accumulation of organic and inorganic acids
E: *e*lectrolyte imbalance	Hyperkalemia, hypermagnesemia
I: *i*ntoxications	Salicylates, lithium, methanol, ethylene glycol, theophylline, phenobarbital
O: fluid *o*verload	Postoperative fluid gain/overload
U: *u*remia	Accumulation of uremic toxins

Clinical Controversy...

Controversy exists as to what is the optimal RRT modality for patients with AKI. As a result, selection of a particular type of RRT is largely determined by physician preference and/or hospital resources.

Intermittent Hemodialysis Intermittent hemodialysis (IHD) is the most frequently used RRT. IHD machines are readily available in most acute care facilities, and healthcare workers are commonly familiar with their use. Hemodialysis treatments usually last 3 to 4 hours, with blood flow rates to the dialyzer typically ranging from 200 to 400 mL/min. Advantages of IHD include rapid removal of volume and solute and correction of most of the electrolyte abnormalities associated with AKI. IHD can be scheduled to allow multiple treatments per day per machine. The primary challenge is hypotension, typically caused by rapid removal of intravascular volume over a short period of time. Venous access for dialysis can be difficult in hypotensive patients and can limit the effectiveness of IHD, leading to ineffective solute clearance, lack of acidosis correction, continued volume overload, and delayed recovery because of further ischemic insults to the kidneys. If hemodialysis is carefully monitored and hypotension avoided, better patient outcomes can be achieved.[79] Patients with CKD stage 5 generally achieve adequate solute and volume control with three times weekly dialysis, but hypercatabolic, fluid-overloaded patients with AKI may require daily hemodialysis treatments. The use of daily versus three times weekly IHD in the setting of AKI has been associated with a reduction in dialysis-related hypotension and a shorter period of time to full recovery of kidney function.[80] Chapter 30 provides a detailed explanation of the principles and processes of IHD.

Continuous Renal Replacement Therapy Continuous renal replacement therapy (CRRT) is a viable approach to manage hemodynamically unstable patients with AKI. Several CRRT variants have been developed, including continuous venovenous hemofiltration (CVVH), continuous venovenous hemodialysis (CVVHD), and continuous venovenous hemodiafiltration (CVVHDF). They differ in the degree of solute and fluid clearance that can be clinically achieved as a result of the use of diffusion, convection, or a combination of both. A greater amount of solute removal and higher mean arterial pressures are observed during CCRT compared with IHD in critically ill patients with AKI.[81] In CVVH, solute and fluid clearance is primarily a result of convection, in which passive diffusion of fluids containing solutes is removed, while volume absent of the solutes is replaced (Fig. 28-4). CVVHD provides extensive solute removal primarily by diffusion, in which solute molecules at a higher concentration (plasma) pass through the dialysis membrane to an area of lower concentration (dialysate). Also, some fluid is removed as a function of the ultrafiltration coefficient of the dialyzer. CVVHD potentially has a lower risk of clotting than CVVH because of reduced hemoconcentration, as there is less fluid removal during the process. CVVHDF combines both convection or hemofiltration and hemodialysis, achieving even higher solute and fluid removal rates (Fig. 28-4). The ultrafiltration rate is an important determinant of the effectiveness of all three forms of CRRT. In direct comparisons of ultrafiltration rates of 25 to 40 mL/kg/h or higher, no difference in mortality has been observed, and there was a tendency toward prolonged need for renal replacement in those who received the higher ultrafiltration rate.[82,83] Therefore, current KDIGO guidelines recommend an ultrafiltration rate of no more than 20 to 25 mL/kg/h during CRRT.[5]

Because of the reduced blood flow rates relative to IHD, CRRT-related thrombosis is a significant concern; thus, some form of anticoagulation during RRT is generally necessary for almost all patients. Typical anticoagulation is achieved by the administration of parenteral agents such as regional citrate (preferred if increased risk for bleeding is present), unfractionated heparin, low-molecular-weight heparin in some cases, or a direct thrombin inhibitor when other therapies are contraindicated.[5,84] Replacement fluids can be infused either just before or after the dialyzer/hemofilter. Infusing fluids after the hemofilter can result in hemoconcentration within the filter, a factor associated with an increased risk of thrombosis of the dialyzer. Replacing fluids before the filter reduces thrombosis risk, but it also reduces solute clearance.

Disadvantages of CRRT may include limited availability of the special equipment necessary to provide these treatments or the need for intensive nursing care, and the need to individualize the IV replacement, dialysate fluids, and drug therapy adjustments. There is also very little known about drug-dosing requirements for patients who are receiving CRRT.[85] CRRT use is most commonly considered for those patients with higher acuity because of their intolerance of IHD-associated hypotension. Current KDIGO guidelines suggest using CRRT over IHD in hemodynamically unstable patients.[5]

Hybrid Dialysis Therapies (8) Another alternative to CRRT is the hybrid extended-duration IHD that is also utilized in critically ill patients with AKI. Hybrid IHD therapies have a variety of names, with the two most common being sustained low-efficiency dialysis (SLED)[79] and slow, extended, daily dialysis (see Fig. 28-4).[86] These therapies use lower blood (150 to 200 mL/min) and dialysate (300 to 400 mL/min) flow rates with extended treatment periods of 6 to 12 hours. For critically ill patients with AKI, SLED appears comparable to CRRT for hemodynamic control.[79] Anticoagulation is still required, but the amount necessary compared with CRRT is lower.[86] Although the use of hybrid hemodialysis therapies is increasing, our knowledge of their impact on drug removal remains limited.[87] Daily delivery of SLED presents challenges to clinicians prescribing drug and nutrition therapy, as most of the dosing guidelines are based on IHD given three times per week in CKD patients. Thus, application of these guidelines in patients with AKI may potentially yield suboptimal outcomes.

IHD Compared with CRRT In addition to patient-specific differences, there are marked differences between IHD and the three primary types of CRRT—CVVH, CVVHD, and CVVHDF—with regard to drug removal.[85,87,88]

During CVVH, drug removal primarily occurs via convection/ultrafiltration (the passive transport of drug molecules at the concentration at which they exist in plasma water into the ultrafiltrate). Convective removal is most efficient for smaller agents, typically less than 15,000 Da (15 kDa) in size, and those that are primarily unbound in the plasma. The clearance of a drug by either of these methods is thus a function of the membrane permeability for the drug, which is called the sieving coefficient (SC), and the rate of ultrafiltrate formation (UFR). Alteration in the pore size of the filter and surface charge relative to the molecule being removed may vary between different dialyzers. If diffusion of the drug is not dependent on the filter pore size, then the SC can be calculated as follows:

$$\mathrm{SC} = \frac{2 \times C_{\mathrm{UF}}}{C_{\mathrm{a}} + C_{\mathrm{v}}}$$

where C_a and C_v are the concentrations of the drug in the plasma going into and returning from the dialyzer/hemofilter, respectively, and C_{UF} is the concentration in the ultrafiltrate. The SC is often approximated by the fraction unbound (f_u) because this information may be more readily available. Thus, the clearance by CVVH can be calculated as

$$\mathrm{Cl}_{\mathrm{CVVH}} = \mathrm{UFR} \times \mathrm{SC}$$

or approximated as

$$\mathrm{Cl}_{\mathrm{CVVH}} = \mathrm{UFR} \times f_{\mathrm{u}}$$

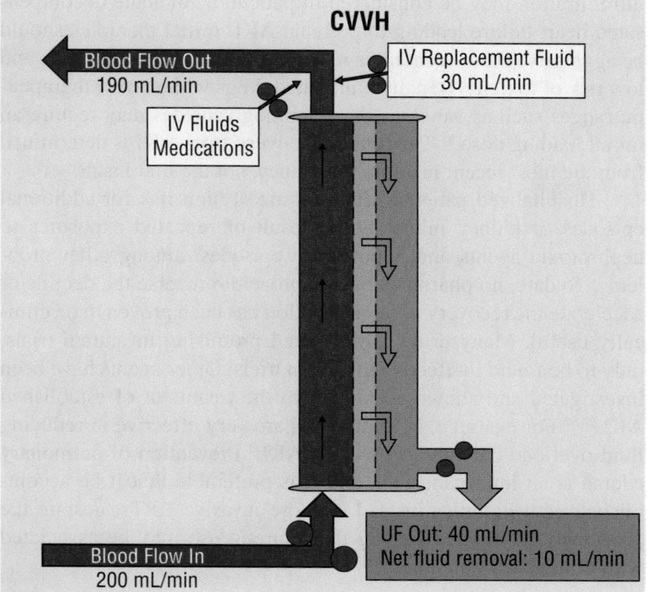

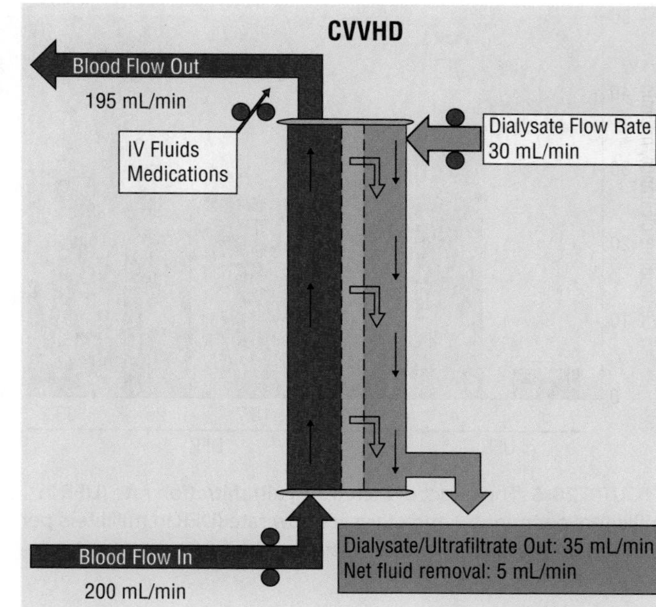

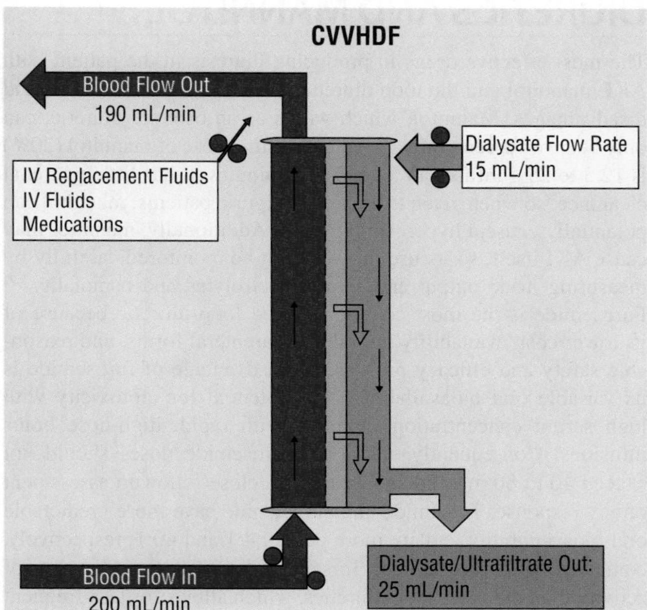

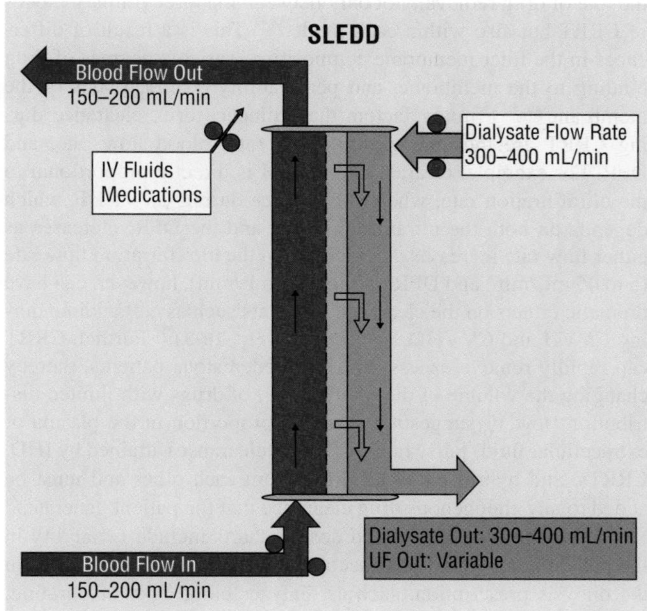

FIGURE 28-4 Several renal replacement therapies are commonly used in patients with AKI, including one of the three primary continuous renal replacement therapy (CRRT) variants: (a) continuous venovenous hemofiltration (CVVH), (b) continuous venovenous hemodialysis (CVVHD), (c) continuous venovenous hemodiafiltration (CVVHDF), and the hybrid intermittent hemodialysis therapy (d) sustained low-efficiency dialysis (SLED). The blood circuit in each diagram is represented in red, the hemofilter/dialyzer membrane is yellow, and the ultrafiltration/dialysate compartment is brown. Excess body water and accumulated endogenous waste products are removed solely by convection when CVVH is employed. With CVVHD, waste products are predominantly removed as the result of passive diffusion from the blood, where they are in high concentration to the dialysate. The degree of fluid removal that is accomplished by convection is usually minimal. CVVHDF uses convection to a degree similar to that employed during CVVH as well as diffusion, and thus is often associated with the highest clearance of drugs and waste products. Finally, SLED employs lower blood and dialysate flow rates than intermittent hemodialysis (IHD), but because of its extended duration, it is a gentler means of achieving adequate waste product and fluid removal.

In CVVHDF, clearance is a combination of both diffusion and convection. The Cl_{CVVHDF} can be mathematically approximated, providing the blood flow rate is greater than 100 mL/min and the dialysate flow rate (DFR) is between 8 and 33 mL/min, as

$$Cl_{CVVHDF} = (UFR \times f_u) + Cl_{diffusion}$$

where $Cl_{diffusion}$ is the clearance via diffusion from plasma water to the dialysate. In the clinical setting, it is not possible to separate these two components (UFR and DFR) of Cl_{CVVHDF}. In essence, the Cl_{CVVHDF} is calculated as the product of the combined ultrafiltrate and dialysate volume (V_{df}) and the concentration of the drug in this fluid (C_{df}) divided by the plasma concentration (C_p^{mid}) at the midpoint of the V_{df} collection period.

Individualization of therapy for a patient receiving CRRT is dependent on the patient's residual renal function and the clearance of the drug by the mode of CRRT. There are differences in

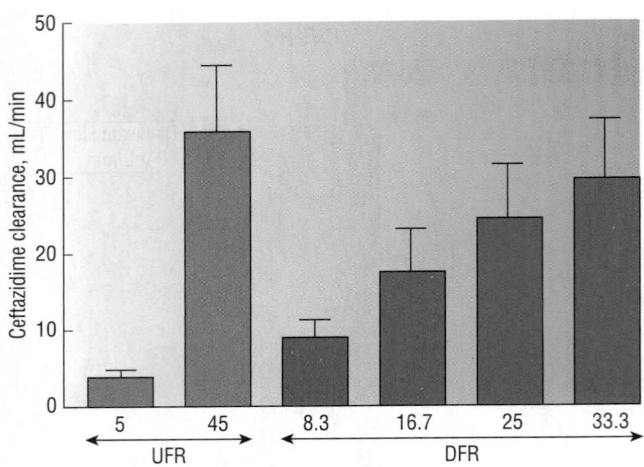

FIGURE 28-5 The effect of increasing ultrafiltration rate (UFR in milliliters per minute) and dialysate flow rate (DFR in milliliters per minute) on the clearance of ceftazidime. *(Adapted from reference 91.)*

the rate of drug removal, not only between the three primary modes of CRRT but also within each mode.[85,88] This is a result of differences in the filter membrane composition, variable degrees of drug binding to the membrane, and permeability characteristics of the membrane.[89–91] Primary factors that influence drug clearance during CRRT are thus the ultrafiltration rate, blood flow rate, and DFR. For example, clearance in CVVH is directly proportional to the ultrafiltration rate, whereas clearance during CVVHDF, which depends on both the ultrafiltration rate and the DFR, increases as either flow rate increases. An increase in the ultrafiltration flow rate (5 to 45 mL/min) and DFR (8.3 to 33.3 mL/min), however, can have dramatic effects on the clearance of agents such as ceftazidime during CVVH and CVVHD, respectively (Fig. 28-5).[91] Further, CRRT can rapidly remove excess fluid from edematous patients, thereby changing the volume of distribution (V_D) of drugs with limited distribution (low V_D suggesting a greater proportion in the plasma or extracellular fluid) fairly rapidly.[88] Drug clearances attained by IHD, CRRTs, and hybrid RRTs all differ from each other and must be added to any endogenous drug clearance that the patient generates.

Limitations of IHD-based dosing charts include variability in the patient's individual pharmacokinetic parameters, differences in the dialysis prescription, such as dialyzer blood flow or duration, and the use of new IHD dialyzers. The approach to hemodialysis may also change on a daily basis, especially in hemodynamically unstable individuals with AKI. This could include, for example, the type of dialyzer/filter used, the duration, the degree of hemofiltration compared with convection, and the blood flow rate. Individualization of a dosing regimen may require daily assessment of the clinical status of the patient and any planned or recently administered hemodialysis.

Overall, there are numerous potential pharmacokinetic and pharmacodynamic alterations to be aware of in the patient with AKI. Unfortunately, there is a dearth of data to quantify these changes, and even less evidence demonstrating that if one incorporates these considerations into patient care, the associated outcomes will be improved.

Pharmacologic Therapy

Once the kidney has been damaged by an acute insult, initial therapies should be directed to prevent further insults to the kidney, thereby minimizing extension of the injury.[5] Dosing considerations should include the drugs' volume of distribution and the volume status of the patient. If sepsis is present, antibiotic therapy regimens should be adjusted for decreased renal elimination. Diuretics or ultrafiltration may be considered in patients with acute decompensated heart failure leading to prerenal AKI. Initial therapies should be aggressive if the agent has a relatively wide therapeutic range and low risk of toxicity. Renally eliminated drugs with narrow therapeutic ranges such as vancomycin or aminoglycosides may require an initial loading dose.[88] The time to recovery from AKI is determined from the most recent insult to the kidney, not the first insult.

Hospitalized patients with AKI are at high risk for additional episodes of kidney injury as the result of repeated exposures to nephrotoxic agents and hypotensive episodes, among other problems. To date, no pharmacologic approach to reverse the decline or accelerate the recovery of renal function has been proven to be clinically useful. Many drugs have looked promising in animal trials, only to be found ineffective in human trials. Other agents have been investigated and shown no benefit in the treatment of established AKI.[28,51] For example, loop diuretics are very effective in reducing fluid overload but can also worsen AKI.[5] Prevention of pulmonary edema is an important goal, and it is preferable that it be accomplished with diuretics instead of more invasive RRTs, despite the previously mentioned finding that diuretic use may be associated with diminished outcomes.[5,28]

DIURETICS AND MANNITOL

The most effective drugs in producing diuresis in the patient with AKI, mannitol and the loop diuretics, have distinct advantages and disadvantages. Mannitol, which works as an osmotic diuretic, can only be given parenterally. A typical starting dose of mannitol (20%) is 12.5 to 25 g infused IV over 3 to 5 minutes. It has little nonrenal clearance, so when given to anuric or oliguric patients, mannitol can potentially cause a hyperosmolar state. Additionally, mannitol may cause AKI itself, so its use in AKI must be monitored carefully by measuring urine output and serum electrolytes and osmolality.[5,92] Furosemide is the most commonly used loop diuretic because of its lower cost, availability in oral and parenteral forms, and reasonable safety and efficacy profiles. A disadvantage of furosemide is its variable oral bioavailability and potential for ototoxicity with high serum concentrations attained with rapid, high-dose bolus infusions. Consequently, initial IV furosemide doses should not exceed 40 to 80 mg and should include close followup assessment of any response. Torsemide and bumetanide have more predictable oral bioavailability and are more potent, 4:1 and 40:1, respectively, compared with furosemide. Torsemide has a longer duration of activity than the other loop diuretics, which allows for less-frequent administration but may also make it more difficult to titrate the dose. Ethacrynic acid is typically reserved for patients who are allergic to sulfa compounds. Loop diuretics all work equally well provided that they are administered in equipotent doses. In a patient who is unresponsive to aggressive IV loop diuretic therapy, switching to another loop diuretic is unlikely to be beneficial.

Diuretic Resistance

9 The inability to respond to diuretics is common in AKI and is associated with poor patient outcomes.[28] An effective technique to overcome diuretic resistance is to administer loop diuretics via continuous infusion instead of intermittent boluses. Less natriuresis occurs when equal doses of loop diuretics are given as a bolus instead of as a continuous infusion. Furthermore, adverse reactions from loop diuretics (myalgia and hearing loss) occur less frequently in patients receiving continuous infusion compared with those receiving intermittent boluses, ostensibly because higher serum concentrations are avoided. An initial loading dose (equivalent to furosemide 40 to 80 mg) should be given prior to the initiation of a continuous infusion at 10 to 20 mg/h of furosemide or its equivalent. Patients with low CL_{cr} may have much lower rates of diuretic

TABLE 28-8 Common Causes of Diuretic Resistance in Patients with Acute Kidney Injury

Causes of Diuretic Resistance	Potential Therapeutic Solutions
Excessive sodium intake (sources may be dietary, IV fluids, and drugs)	Remove sodium from nutritional sources and medications
Inadequate diuretic dose or inappropriate regimen	Increase dose, use continuous infusion or combination therapy
Reduced oral bioavailability (usually furosemide)	Use parenteral therapy, switch to oral torsemide or bumetanide
Nephrotic syndrome (loop diuretic protein binding in tubule lumen)	Increase dose, switch diuretics, use combination therapy
Reduced renal blood flow	
Drugs (NSAIDs, ACEIs, vasodilators)	Discontinue these drugs if possible
Hypotension	Intravascular volume expansion and/or vasopressors
Intravascular depletion	Intravascular volume expansion
Increased sodium resorption	
Nephron adaptation to chronic diuretic therapy	Combination diuretic therapy, sodium restriction
NSAID use	Discontinue NSAID
Heart failure	Treat heart failure, increase diuretic dose, switch to better-absorbed loop diuretic
Cirrhosis	Paracentesis
Acute tubular necrosis	Increase diuretic dose, diuretic combination therapy

ACEIs, angiotensin-converting enzyme inhibitors; NSAIDs, nonsteroidal antiinflammatory drugs.

secretion into the tubular fluid; consequently, higher doses are generally used in patients with renal insufficiency.[28]

There are several reasons why certain patients develop diuretic resistance. Excessive sodium intake may override the ability of the diuretics to eliminate sodium. Patients with ATN have a reduced number of functioning nephrons on which the diuretic may exert its action. Other clinical states, such as glomerulonephritis, are associated with heavy proteinuria. Intraluminal loop diuretics cannot exert their effect in the loop of Henle because they are extensively bound to proteins present in the urine. Still other patients may have greatly reduced bioavailability of oral furosemide because of intestinal edema, often associated with high preload states, which further reduces oral furosemide absorption. Table 28-8 includes possible therapeutic options to counteract each form of diuretic resistance.

Combination therapy of loop diuretics plus a diuretic from a different pharmacologic class may be an alternative approach in the setting of AKI.[93,94] Loop diuretics increase the delivery of sodium chloride to the distal convoluted tubule and collecting duct. With time, these areas of the nephron compensate for the activity of the loop diuretic and increase sodium and chloride resorption. Diuretics that work at the distal convoluted tubule (chlorothiazide and metolazone) or the collecting duct (amiloride, triamterene, and spironolactone) may have a synergistic effect when administered with loop diuretics by blocking the compensatory increase in sodium and chloride resorption.[94] Of these combinations, oral metolazone is used most frequently because, unlike other thiazides, it produces effective diuresis at a GFR <20 mL/min (<0.33 mL/s). IV chlorothiazide (500 mg) has been used when oral metolazone is not feasible but is associated with notably higher cost. The combination of metolazone and a loop diuretic has been used successfully in the management of fluid overload in patients with heart failure, cirrhosis, and nephrotic syndrome.

Drug Dosing Considerations in AKI

Optimization of drug therapy for patients with AKI is often challenging. The multiple variables influencing responses to the drug regimen include the patient's residual drug clearance, fluid accumulation, and delivery of RRT. For renally eliminated drugs, particularly for agents with a narrow therapeutic range, serum drug concentration measurements and assessment of pharmacodynamic responses are likely to be necessary. If hepatic function is intact, choosing an agent eliminated primarily by the liver may be preferred. However, any renally eliminated active metabolites may accumulate to a point where they can elicit an undesired pharmacologic effect. Renal failure can also independently impair nonrenal drug elimination including metabolism.[95] Unfortunately, pharmacokinetic studies in patients with established AKI are fairly limited. Further, the use of dosing guidelines based on data derived from patients with stable CKD may not reflect the clearance and volume of distribution in critically ill AKI patients (see Chap. 33).[85] The inability to adequately dose drugs in critically ill patients with AKI requiring RRT may be one factor contributing to the lack of improving outcomes with newer RRT approaches.

Edema, which is common in AKI, can significantly increase the volume of distribution of many drugs, particularly water-soluble ones with relatively small volumes of distribution. Increased fluid distribution into the tissues (i.e., sepsis and anasarca in heart failure) can also contribute to a larger volume of distribution for many drugs and thereby reduce the proportion of drug in the plasma that is available to be removed by RRT. Because AKI frequently occurs in critically ill patients, multisystem organ failure is often an accompanying problem. In addition to volume overload, reductions in cardiac output or liver function can significantly alter the pharmacokinetic profile of many drugs, such as vancomycin, aminoglycosides, and low-molecular-weight heparins.[85,96,97]

If rapid onset of activity is desired, a loading dose may be necessary to promptly achieve desired serum concentrations because the expanded volume of distribution and the prolonged elimination half-life reextend the time (3.5 times the half-life) needed to reach steady-state concentrations. Maintenance dosing regimens should be reassessed frequently and be based on the patient's most current renal function. A dose that provides the desired serum concentration on one day may be inappropriate a few days later if the patient's fluid status, RRT prescription, or renal function has changed dramatically.

Drug therapy individualization for the AKI patient who is receiving any form of RRT is complicated by the fact that patients with AKI may have a higher residual nonrenal clearance than patients with CKD who have a similar CL_{cr}.[85] This has been reported with some drugs, such as ceftriaxone, imipenem, and vancomycin.[98–100] Alterations in the activity of some, but not all, cytochrome P450 enzymes have been demonstrated in patients with CKD.[95] The nonrenal clearance of imipenem in patients with AKI (91 mL/min [1.52 mL/s]) is between the values observed in stage 5 CKD patients (50 mL/min [0.84 mL/s]) and those with normal renal function (120 mL/min [2 mL/s]).[100] This may be the result of less accumulation of uremic waste products that may alter hepatic function. If a patient with AKI has higher than anticipated nonrenal clearance, this would result in lower than expected, possibly subtherapeutic, serum concentrations. For example, to maintain comparable serum concentrations, the imipenem dose requirement in patients with AKI would be 2,000 mg daily as compared with the recommended dosage for patients with ESRD of 1,000 mg daily.[100] As AKI persists, the nonrenal clearance values appear to approach those observed in patients with CKD.[99,100] Finally, the clearance of aminoglycosides has been reported to be higher and the elimination half-life shorter in those with severe AKI compared with ESRD patients requiring hemodialysis.[96] Another challenge is that much of the dosing-related data were acquired in patients with CKD, with initial pharmacokinetic assessments done after single-dose administration. The determination of pharmacokinetic parameters using a single-dose model may result in more rapid initial drug removal estimates secondary to distribution from the plasma to the tissue as well. Thus, application of dosing regimens derived from studies in patients with CKD and ESRD in addition to the use of more aggressive RRT approaches may result in underdosing of certain drugs and thereby contribute to less than optimal clinical outcomes.

Clinical **Controversy...**

There is a scarcity of data on how to appropriately dose medications in patients receiving CRRT or SLED. Some clinicians use dosing recommendations extrapolated from IHD data, while others believe that more aggressive dosing regimens are warranted.

Electrolyte Management

Hypernatremia and fluid retention are frequent complications of AKI. Total daily sodium intake should be monitored since excessive amounts may be a reason for diuretic therapy failure. Further, commonly administered IV antibiotics such as metronidazole, ampicillin, piperacillin, and fluconazole may contain significant amounts of sodium. As a result, the cumulative effect of a few sodium-containing medications and fluids can be significant.

In continuous and intermittent RRTs, there usually is less concern about hypernatremia developing because these therapies often incorporate isonatremic (135 to 140 mEq/L [135 to 140 mmol/L] of sodium) solutions as the dialysate or ultrafiltrate replacement solutions. Serum sodium concentrations should be monitored daily. Hyperkalemia, hyperphosphatemia, and, to a lesser extent, hypermagnesemia are electrolyte disorders that are frequently seen in patients with AKI. Higher ultrafiltration rates can potentially increase the risk for hyperphosphatemia. The shift in electrolytes is generally not a serious concern in those who are receiving RRT, but electrolytes should be monitored closely in all patients with AKI.

The most common electrolyte disorder encountered in AKI patients is hyperkalemia, as >90% of potassium is renally eliminated. Life-threatening cardiac arrhythmias may occur with serum potassium concentrations >6 mEq/L (>6 mmol/L), so frequent monitoring of potassium is essential. Some foods and medications such as oral phosphorous replacement powders (e.g., Neutra-Phos and Neutra-Phos-K) and alkalinizers (Polycitra) contain substantial amounts of potassium (see Chap. 36). Some medications may promote potassium retention by the kidneys and should also be avoided or closely monitored (see Chaps. 31 and 37).

Other electrolytes that require monitoring are phosphorus and magnesium. Both are eliminated by the kidneys and are not removed efficiently by dialysis. In the early stages of AKI, hyperphosphatemia may be more common than hypophosphatemia. Patients with significant tissue destruction (e.g., trauma, rhabdomyolysis, and tumor lysis syndrome) may have substantial amounts of phosphorus released from the destroyed tissue. Calcium-containing antacids should be avoided to prevent precipitation of calcium phosphate in the soft tissues. Typically, the dietary intake of phosphorus and magnesium needs to be restricted. However, patients receiving prolonged RRT can develop deficiency states, particularly pediatric patients as a result of reduced body stores. In contrast to the patient with CKD, AKI patients do not usually develop calcium imbalance secondary to the limited duration of the illness. One exception to this is seen in patients who are receiving CRRT with citrate as the anticoagulant. Citrate binds to serum calcium and is typically infused before the dialyzer/hemofilter. Calcium chloride or calcium gluconate is administered prior to returning the blood to the patient, while the citrate that reaches the systemic circulation is subsequently metabolized by the liver. The goals of citrate anticoagulation are to maintain the circuit ionized calcium between 0.8 and 1.6 mg/dL (0.2 and 0.4 mmol/L), and the patient's systemic ionized calcium between 4.4 and 5.2 mg/dL (1.1 to 1.3 mmol/L).[5] Since severe hypocalcemia can result in arrhythmias or even death, frequent monitoring of unbound serum calcium concentrations is essential.

Nutritional Considerations in AKI

Nutritional management of critically ill patients with AKI can be extremely complex, as it needs to account for metabolic derangements resulting from both renal dysfunction and underlying disease processes, as well as the effects of RRT on nutrient balance. Stress, inflammation, and injury lead to hypermetabolic and hypercatabolic states and may alter the nutritional requirements. In addition, severe malnutrition found in up to 42% of patients with AKI is a risk factor for increased hospital mortality and length of stay.[74] Thus, patient outcomes can be significantly improved if the nutritional status is optimized.

Loss of the normal physiologic and metabolic functions of the kidney and the hypercatabolic response to stress and injury will have a significant impact on the metabolism of nutrients. Derangements in glucose, lipid, and protein metabolism result in hyperglycemia and insulin resistance, hypertriglyceridemia, protein catabolism, and negative nitrogen balance. The latter, in particular, is problematic to manage, as increased amino acid turnover and skeletal muscle breakdown lead to muscle wasting and malnutrition and do not respond well to increasing exogenous protein supplementation. KDIGO guidelines currently recommend a caloric intake goal of 20 to 30 kcal/kg/day (84 to 126 kJ/kg/day) irrespective of the stage of renal impairment and preferentially through the enteral route.[5] In the setting of noncatabolic AKI without need for dialysis, 0.8 to 1 g/kg/day of protein is suggested and 1 to 1.5 g/kg/day if patient is receiving RRT.[5] CRRT is associated with an increased removal of small water-soluble molecules such as amino acids and certain nutrients. As a result, hypercatabolic patients receiving CRRT will typically have higher protein requirements up to a maximum of 1.7 g/kg/day.[5]

Another nutritional consideration for patients receiving CRRT is the heat loss as a consequence of the cooling of the patient's blood as it traverses the extracorporeal circuit.[101] Even though the blood cooling effect by CRRT is widely recognized in clinical practice, its prevention and effect on energy and nutritional requirements have not been well studied. The blood cooling effect is reported to occur more frequently with venovenous modalities, higher dialysate, and lower blood flow rates. Also, certain patient characteristics, such as female gender, low normal baseline temperature, and low body weight, have been identified as risk factors for hypothermia.[101,102] Overall, CRRT should be recognized as a potential source of heat loss. However, no recommendations are currently available for prevention or define the nutritional supplementation that may be necessary as the result of CRRT-induced blood cooling.

Personalized Pharmacotherapy

In the presence of AKI, several processes may exist that can alter drug response such as impaired elimination, RRT-related drug removal, or physiologic alterations in pharmacodynamic response. Guidance from clinical trials on how to appropriately adjust drug regimens is limited. Thus, continuous assessment is required when optimizing pharmacotherapeutic regimens. Changes in the patient's clinical presentation including renal replacement regimens may require clinicians to make frequent adjustments. Information from yesterday's medical record review may not reflect what is

TABLE 28-9 Key Monitoring Parameters for Patients with Established Acute Kidney Injury

Parameter	Frequency
Fluid ins/outs	Every shift
Patient weight	Daily
Hemodynamics (blood pressure, heart rate, mean arterial pressure, etc.)	Every shift
Blood chemistries	
Sodium, potassium, chloride, bicarbonate, calcium, phosphate, magnesium	Daily
Blood urea nitrogen/serum creatinine	Daily
Drugs and their dosing regimens	Daily
Nutritional regimen	Daily
Blood glucose	Daily (minimum)
Serum concentration data for drugs	After regimen changes and after renal replacement therapy has been instituted
Times of administered doses	Daily
Doses relative to administration of renal replacement therapy	Daily
Urinalysis	
Calculate measured creatinine clearance	Every time measured urine collection performed
Calculate fractional excretion of sodium	Every time measured urine collection performed
Plans for renal replacement	Daily

happening today or is being planned for tomorrow. Physiologic processes or metabolites that may have limited expression in normal renal function may elicit greater influence in AKI. Treating the patient may require more aggressive pharmacotherapy regimens initially that can be subsequently tapered back. Clinicians should keep the overall clinical status of the patient in mind when developing management plans. Key to optimal patient outcomes includes maximizing prevention, early identification of AKI, implementation of supportive therapies, and frequent assessments until the AKI has resolved.

EVALUATION OF THERAPEUTIC OUTCOMES

Vigilant monitoring of patients with AKI is essential, particularly in those who are critically ill. Table 28-9 summarizes the main monitoring parameters for patients with established AKI.

Once the laboratory-based tests (e.g., urinalysis and FE_{Na} calculations) have been conducted to diagnose the cause of AKI, they usually do not have to be repeated. In established AKI, daily measurements of urine output, fluid intake, and weight should be performed. Vital signs should be monitored at least daily, more often if the acuity of illness is high. Daily blood tests for electrolytes, BUN, and a complete blood cell count should be considered routine for hospitalized patients.

Therapeutic drug monitoring should be performed for drugs that have a narrow therapeutic window that can be measured by the hospital laboratory. If results from these serum drug concentrations cannot be obtained in a timely fashion (<24 hours), then their value is limited. When considering approaches to measuring serum concentrations, consensus is limited. Measuring a serum drug concentration prior to hemodialysis has the advantage of allowing time for the result to be reported and redosing done shortly after dialysis with minimal delay. This is especially important if the desired pharmacologic effects are lost during or after hemodialysis is complete because the serum concentrations have become subtherapeutic. Knowledge based on previous observations of how a particular agent is removed for a given dialysis approach and a prehemodialysis serum concentration can assist in estimating the amount of the drug removed and predict the need for any postdialysis doses. Serum concentrations drawn after hemodialysis may reflect plasma concentrations that are transiently depressed until the drug can reequilibrate from the tissues (plasma rebound effect). The advantage with an after-dialysis level is the greater accuracy in determining how much drug was cleared during hemodialysis, but this may delay reestablishing target effects. Greater therapeutic drug monitoring may be necessary in patients with AKI than what is done routinely for other patients because of the potential changes in hemodynamic status.

CLINICAL BOTTOM LINE

The unique characteristics of AKI compared with CKD can lead to notable differences in how renal function is measured and how treatment regimens are developed. Most management approaches involve both prevention and support strategies, so as to minimize the potential for additional harm to the kidney. Understanding the constantly changing status inherent to AKI and how to adjust management regimens is a key component to optimizing therapy.

ABBREVIATIONS

ACE	angiotensin-converting enzyme
ADQI	Acute Dialysis Quality Initiative
AIN	acute interstitial nephritis
AKI	acute kidney injury
AKIN	Acute Kidney Injury Network
ANP	atrial natriuretic peptide
ARB	angiotensin receptor blocker
ATN	acute tubular necrosis
BNP	brain natriuretic peptide
BUN	blood urea nitrogen
CIN	contrast-induced nephropathy
CKD	chronic kidney disease
CKD-EPI	Chronic Kidney Disease Epidemiology Collaboration
CL_{cr}	creatinine clearance
CRRT	continuous renal replacement therapy
CT	computed tomography
CVVH	continuous venovenous hemofiltration
CVVHD	continuous venovenous hemodialysis
CVVHDF	continuous venovenous hemodiafiltration
DFR	dialysate flow rate
eGFR	estimated glomerular filtration rate
ESKD	end-stage kidney disease
FE_{Na}	fractional excretion of sodium
FE_{Urea}	fractional excretion of urea
GFR	glomerular filtration rate
ICU	intensive care unit
IHD	intermittent hemodialysis
IL-18	interleukin-18
JVP	jugular venous pressure
KDIGO	Kidney Disease: Improving Global Outcomes
KIM-1	kidney injury molecule 1
KUB	kidneys, ureters, and bladder
MDRD	Modification of Diet in Renal Disease
NAC	*N*-acetylcysteine
NGAL	neutrophil gelatinase–associated lipocalin
NICE-SUGAR	Normoglycemia in Intensive Care Evaluation and Survival Using Glucose Algorithm Regulation
NSAID	nonsteroidal antiinflammatory drug

RIFLE	Risk, Injury, Failure, Loss of Kidney Function, and End-Stage Kidney Disease
RRT	renal replacement therapy
SC	sieving coefficient
S_{cr}	serum creatinine
SLED	sustained low-efficiency dialysis
UFR	ultrafiltrate formation

REFERENCES

1. Bellomo R, Ronco C, Kellum JA, et al. Acute renal failure—Definition, outcome measures, animal models, fluid therapy and information technology needs: The Second International Consensus Conference of the Acute Dialysis Quality Initiative (ADQI) Group. Crit Care 2004;8:R204–R212.
2. Mehta RL, Kellum JA, Shah SV, et al. Acute Kidney Injury Network: Report of an initiative to improve outcomes in acute kidney injury. Crit Care 2007;11:R31.
3. Bagshaw SM, George C, Dinu I, Bellomo R. A multi-centre evaluation of the RIFLE criteria for early acute kidney injury in critically ill patients. Nephrol Dial Transplant 2008;23:1203–1210.
4. Hoste EA, Clermont G, Kersten A, et al. RIFLE criteria for acute kidney injury are associated with hospital mortality in critically ill patients: A cohort analysis. Crit Care 2006;10:R73.
5. Kidney Disease: Improving Global Outcomes (KDIGO) Acute Kidney Injury Workgroup. KDIGO clinical practice guideline for acute kidney injury. Kidney Int Suppl 2012;2:1–138.
6. Ricci Z, Ronco C. Year in review 2007: Critical Care—Nephrology. Crit Care 2008;12:230.
7. Siew ED, Matheny ME, Ikizler TA, et al. Commonly used surrogates for baseline renal function affect the classification and prognosis of acute kidney injury. Kidney Int 2010;77:536–542.
8. Zavada J, Hoste E, Cartin-Ceba R, et al. A comparison of three methods to estimate baseline creatinine for RIFLE classification. Nephrol Dial Transplant 2010;25:3911–3918.
9. Hsu CY, McCulloch CE, Fan D, et al. Community-based incidence of acute renal failure. Kidney Int 2007;72:208–212.
10. Liangos O, Wald R, O'Bell JW, et al. Epidemiology and outcomes of acute renal failure in hospitalized patients: A national survey. Clin J Am Soc Nephrol 2006;1:43–51.
11. Uchino S, Bellomo R, Goldsmith D, et al. An assessment of the RIFLE criteria for acute renal failure in hospitalized patients. Crit Care Med 2006;34:1913–1917.
12. Liano F, Felipe C, Tenorio MT, et al. Long-term outcome of acute tubular necrosis: A contribution to its natural history. Kidney Int 2007;71:679–686.
13. Coca SG, Singanamala S, Parikh CR. Chronic kidney disease after acute kidney injury: A systematic review and meta-analysis. Kidney Int 2012;81:442–448.
14. Kaufman J, Dhakal M, Patel B, Hamburger R. Community-acquired acute renal failure. Am J Kidney Dis 1991;17:191–198.
15. Lameire N, Van Biesen W, Vanholder R. The changing epidemiology of acute renal failure. Nat Clin Pract Nephrol 2006;2:364–377.
16. Pannu N, James M, Hemmelgarn BR, et al. Modification of outcomes after acute kidney injury by the presence of CKD. Am J Kidney Dis 2011;58:206–213.
17. Pisoni R, Wille KM, Tolwani AJ. The epidemiology of severe acute kidney injury: From BEST to PICARD, in acute kidney injury: New concepts. Nephron Clin Pract 2008;109:c188–c191.
18. Thakar CV, Christianson A, Himmelfarb J, Leonard AC. Acute kidney injury episodes and chronic kidney disease risk in diabetes mellitus. Clin J Am Soc Nephrol 2011;6:2567–2572.
19. Badr KF, Ichikawa I. Prerenal failure: A deleterious shift from renal compensation to decompensation. N Engl J Med 1988;319:623–629.
20. Lameire N. The pathophysiology of acute renal failure. Crit Care Clin 2005;21:197–210.
21. Gambaro G, Perazella MA. Adverse renal effects of anti-inflammatory agents: Evaluation of selective and nonselective cyclooxygenase inhibitors. J Intern Med 2003;253:643–652.
22. Sharfuddin AA, Weisbord SD, Palevsky PM, Molitoris BA. Acute kidney injury. In: Brenner BM, ed. Brenner and Rector's The Kidney, 9th ed. Philadelphia: WB Saunders, 2011:1044–1100.
23. Kelly CJ, Neilson EG. Tubulointerstitial diseases. In: Brenner BM, ed. Brenner and Rector's The Kidney, 9th ed. Philadelphia: WB Saunders, 2011:1332–1355.
24. Frokiaer J, Zeidel ML. Urinary tract obstruction. In: Brenner BM, ed. Brenner and Rector's The Kidney, 9th ed. Philadelphia: WB Saunders, 2011:1382–1410.
25. Bagshaw SM, Bellomo R. Early diagnosis of acute kidney injury. Curr Opin Crit Care 2007;13:638–644.
26. Baumann TJ, Staddon JE, Horst HM, Bivins BA. Minimum urine collection periods for accurate determination of creatinine clearance in critically ill patients. Clin Pharm 1987;6:393–398.
27. Slocum JL, Heung M, Pennathur S. Marking renal injury: Can we move beyond serum creatinine? Transl Res 2012;159:277–289.
28. Herget-Rosenthal S, Marggraf G, Husing J, et al. Early detection of acute renal failure by serum cystatin C. Kidney Int 2004;66:1115–1122.
29. Inker LA, Okparavero A. Cystatin C as a marker of glomerular filtration rate: Prospects and limitations. Curr Opin Nephrol Hypertens 2011;20:631–639.
30. Knight EL, Verhave JC, Spiegelman D, et al. Factors influencing serum cystatin C levels other than renal function and the impact on renal function measurement. Kidney Int 2004;65:1416–1421.
31. Manetti L, Pardini E, Genovesi M, et al. Thyroid function differently affects serum cystatin C and creatinine concentrations. J Endocrinol Invest 2005;28:346–349.
32. Devarajan P. Neutrophil gelatinase-associated lipocalin: A promising biomarker for human acute kidney injury. Biomark Med 2010;4:265–280.
33. Haase M, Bellomo R, Devarajan P, et al. Accuracy of neutrophil gelatinase-associated lipocalin (NGAL) in diagnosis and prognosis in acute kidney injury: A systematic review and meta-analysis. Am J Kidney Dis 2009;54:1012–1024.
34. Bennett M, Dent CL, Ma Q, et al. Urine NGAL predicts severity of acute kidney injury after cardiac surgery: A prospective study. Clin J Am Soc Nephrol 2008;3:665–673.
35. Bagshaw SM, Bennett M, Haase M, et al. Plasma and urine neutrophil gelatinase-associated lipocalin in septic versus non-septic acute kidney injury in critical illness. Intensive Care Med 2010;36:452–461.
36. Parikh CR, Jani A, Melnikov VY, et al. Urinary interleukin-18 is a marker of human acute tubular necrosis. Am J Kidney Dis 2004;43:405–414.

37. Parikh CR, Mishra J, Thiessen-Philbrook H, et al. Urinary IL-18 is an early predictive biomarker of acute kidney injury after cardiac surgery. Kidney Int 2006;70:199–203.
38. Ho E, Fard A, Maisel A. Evolving use of biomarkers for kidney injury in acute care settings. Curr Opin Crit Care 2010;16:399–407.
39. van Timmeren MM, van den Heuvel MC, Bailly V, et al. Tubular kidney injury molecule-1 (KIM-1) in human renal disease. J Pathol 2007;212:209–217.
40. Liangos O, Tighiouart H, Perianayagam MC, et al. Comparative analysis of urinary biomarkers for early detection of acute kidney injury following cardiopulmonary bypass. Biomarkers 2009;14:423–431.
41. Vaidya VS, Ford GM, Waikar SS, et al. A rapid urine test for early detection of kidney injury. Kidney Int 2009;76: 108–114.
42. Wiedermann CJ, Dunzendorfer S, Gaioni LU, et al. Hyperoncotic colloids and acute kidney injury: A meta-analysis of randomized trials. Crit Care 2010;14:R191.
43. Perel P, Roberts I. Colloids versus crystalloids for fluid resuscitation in critically ill patients. Cochrane Database Syst Rev 2012;6:CD000567.
44. McCullough PA. Contrast-induced acute kidney injury. J Am Coll Cardiol 2008;28:1419–1428.
45. Weisbord SD, Palevsky PM. Prevention of contrast-induced nephropathy with volume expansion. Clin J Am Soc Nephrol 2008;3:273–280.
46. Caulfield JL, Singh SP, Wishnok JS, et al. Bicarbonate inhibits *N*-nitrosation in oxygenated nitric oxide solutions. J Biol Chem 1996;271:25859–25863.
47. Briguori C, Airoldi F, D'Andrea D, et al. Renal Insufficiency Following Contrast Media Administration Trial (REMEDIAL): A randomized comparison of 3 preventive strategies. Circulation 2007;115:1211–1217.
48. Klima T, Christ A, Marana I, et al. Sodium chloride vs. sodium bicarbonate for the prevention of contrast medium-induced nephropathy: A randomized controlled trial. Eur Heart J 2012;33:2071–2079.
49. Cruz DN, Goh CY, Marenzi G, et al. Renal replacement therapies for prevention of radiocontrast-induced nephropathy: A systematic review. Am J Med 2012;125:66–78.e3.
50. Marenzi G, Lauri G, Campodonico J, et al. Comparison of two hemofiltration protocols for prevention of contrast-induced nephropathy in high-risk patients. Am J Med 2006;119:155–162.
51. Ho KM, Sheridan DJ. Meta-analysis of frusemide to prevent or treat acute renal failure. BMJ 2006;333:420.
52. Friedrich JO, Adhikari N, Herridge MS, Beyene J. Meta-analysis: Low-dose dopamine increases urine output but does not prevent renal dysfunction or death. Ann Intern Med 2005;142:280–224.
53. Landoni G, Biondi-Zoccai GG, Tumlin JA, et al. Beneficial impact of fenoldopam in critically ill patients with or at risk for acute renal failure: A meta-analysis of randomized clinical trials. Am J Kidney Dis 2007;49: 56–68.
54. Nigwekar SU, Navaneethan SD, Parikh CR, Hix JK. Atrial natriuretic peptide for preventing and treating acute kidney injury. Cochrane Database Syst Rev 2009;(4):CD006028.
55. Lingegowda V, Van QC, Shimada M, et al. Long-term outcome of patients treated with prophylactic nesiritide for the prevention of acute kidney injury following cardiovascular surgery. Clin Cardiol 2010;33:217–221.
56. Cetin M, Devrim E, Serin Kilicoglu S, et al. Ionic high-osmolar contrast medium causes oxidant stress in kidney tissue: Partial protective role of ascorbic acid. Ren Fail 2008;30:567–572.
57. Boscheri A, Weinbrenner C, Botzek B, et al. Failure of ascorbic acid to prevent contrast-media induced nephropathy in patients with renal dysfunction. Clin Nephrol 2007;68:279–286.
58. Spargias K, Alexopoulos E, Kyrzopoulos S, et al. Ascorbic acid prevents contrast-mediated nephropathy in patients with renal dysfunction undergoing coronary angiography or intervention. Circulation 2004;110:2837–2842.
59. Zhou L, Chen H. Prevention of contrast-induced nephropathy with ascorbic acid. Intern Med 2012;28:531–535.
60. Amini M, Salarifar M, Amirbaigloo A, et al. *N*-Acetylcysteine does not prevent contrast-induced nephropathy after cardiac catheterization in patients with diabetes mellitus and chronic kidney disease: A randomized clinical trial. Trials 2009;10:45.
61. Jo SH, Koo BK, Park JS, et al. *N*-Acetylcysteine versus ascorbic acid for preventing contrast-induced nephropathy in patients with renal insufficiency undergoing coronary angiography NASPI study—A prospective randomized controlled trial. Am Heart J 2009;157:576–583.
62. Ho KM, Morgan DJ. Meta-analysis of *N*-acetylcysteine to prevent acute renal failure after major surgery. Am J Kidney Dis 2009;53:33–40.
63. Mehta RL. Glycemic control and critical illness: Is the kidney involved? J Am Soc Nephrol 2007;18:2623–2627.
64. Vanhorebeek I, Gunst J, Ellger B, et al. Hyperglycemic kidney damage in an animal model of prolonged critical illness. Kidney Int 2009;76(5):512–520.
65. Finfer S, Chittock DR, Su SY, et al. Intensive versus conventional glucose control in critically ill patients. N Engl J Med 2009;360:1283–1297.
66. Van den Berghe G, Wilmer A, Hermans G, et al. Intensive insulin therapy in the medical ICU. N Engl J Med 2006; 354:449–461.
67. Griesdale DE, de Souza RJ, van Dam RM, et al. Intensive insulin therapy and mortality among critically ill patients: A meta-analysis including NICE-SUGAR study data. CMAJ 2009;180:821–827.
68. Kelly AM, Dwamena B, Cronin P, et al. Meta-analysis: Effectiveness of drugs for preventing contrast-induced nephropathy. Ann Intern Med 2008;148:284–294.
69. Bagshaw SM, Ghali WA. Theophylline for prevention of contrast-induced nephropathy: A systematic review and meta-analysis. Arch Intern Med 2005;165:1087–1093.
70. Johnson DW, Pat B, Vesey DA, et al. Delayed administration of darbepoetin or erythropoietin protects against ischemic acute renal injury and failure. Kidney Int 2006;69:1806–1813.
71. Endre ZH, Walker RJ, Pickering JW, et al. Early intervention with erythropoietin does not affect the outcome of acute kidney injury (the EARLYARF trial). Kidney Int 2010;77: 1020–1030.
72. Joslin J, Ostermann M. Care of the critically ill emergency department patient with acute kidney injury. Emerg Med Int 2012;2012:760623.
73. Damman K, Navis G, Voors AA, et al. Worsening renal function and prognosis in heart failure: Systematic review and meta-analysis. J Card Fail 2007;13:599–608.
74. Dellinger RP, Levy MM, Carlet JM, et al. Surviving Sepsis Campaign: International guidelines for management of severe sepsis and septic shock: 2008. Crit Care Med 2008;36:296–327.
75. Vincent JL. Relevance of albumin in modern critical care medicine. Best Pract Res Clin Anaesthesiol 2009;23:183–191.

76. Bouchard J, Soroko SB, Chertow GM, et al. Fluid accumulation, survival and recovery of kidney function in critically ill patients with acute kidney injury. Kidney Int 2009;76:422–427.
77. Ding F, Humes HD. The bioartificial kidney and bioengineered membranes in acute kidney injury. Nephron Exp Nephrol 2008;109:e118–e122.
78. Hoste EA, Dhondt A. Clinical review: Use of renal replacement therapies in special groups of ICU patients. Crit Care 2012;16:201.
79. Fieghen HE, Friedrich JO, Burns KE, et al. The hemodynamic tolerability and feasibility of sustained low efficiency dialysis in the management of critically ill patients with acute kidney injury. BMC Nephrol 2010;11:32.
80. Schiffl H, Lang SM, Fischer R. Daily hemodialysis and the outcome of acute renal failure. N Engl J Med 2002;346:305–310.
81. Rabindranath K, Adams J, Macleod AM, Muirhead N. Intermittent versus continuous renal replacement therapy for acute renal failure in adults. Cochrane Database Syst Rev 2007;(3):CD003773.
82. Bellomo R, Cass A, Cole L, et al. Intensity of continuous renal-replacement therapy in critically ill patients. N Engl J Med 2009;361:1627–1638.
83. Casey ET, Gupta BP, Erwin PJ, et al. The dose of continuous renal replacement therapy for acute renal failure: A systematic review and meta-analysis. Ren Fail 2010;32:555–561.
84. Oudemans-van Straaten HM, Wester JP, de Pont AC, Schetz MR. Anticoagulation strategies in continuous renal replacement therapy: Can the choice be evidence based? Intensive Care Med 2006;32:188–202.
85. Heintz BH, Matzke GR, Dager WE. Antimicrobial dosing concepts and recommendations for critically ill adult patients receiving continuous renal replacement therapy or intermittent hemodialysis. Pharmacotherapy 2009;29:562–577.
86. Kumar VA, Craig M, Depner TA, Yeun JY. Extended daily dialysis: A new approach to renal replacement for acute renal failure in the intensive care unit. Am J Kidney Dis 2000;36:294–300.
87. Dager WE. Filtering out important considerations for developing drug-dosing regimens in extended daily dialysis. Crit Care Med 2006;34:240–241.
88. Churchwell MD, Mueller BA. Drug dosing during continuous renal replacement therapy. Semin Dial 2009;22:185–188.
89. Joy MS, Matzke GR, Frye RF, Palevsky PM. Determinants of vancomycin clearance by continuous venovenous hemofiltration and continuous venovenous hemodialysis. Am J Kidney Dis 1998;31:1019–1027.
90. Lau AH, Kronfol NO. Determinants of drug removal by continuous hemofiltration. Int J Artif Organs 1994;17:373–378.
91. Matzke GR, Frye RF, Joy MS, Palevsky PM. Determinants of ceftazidime clearance by continuous venovenous hemofiltration and continuous venovenous hemodialysis. Antimicrob Agents Chemother 2000;44:1639–1644.
92. Wade GN, Schneider JE, Friedman MI. Insulin-induced anestrus in Syrian hamsters. Am J Physiol 1991;260:R148–R152.
93. Karajala V, Mansour W, Kellum JA. Diuretics in acute kidney injury. Minerva Anestesiol 2009;75:251–257.
94. Jentzer JC, DeWald TA, Hernandez AF. Combination of loop diuretics with thiazide-type diuretics in heart failure. J Am Coll Cardiol 2010;56:1527–1534.
95. Vilay AM, Churchwell MD, Mueller BA. Clinical review: Drug metabolism and nonrenal clearance in acute kidney injury. Crit Care 2008;12:235.
96. Dager WE, King JH. Aminoglycosides in intermittent hemodialysis: Pharmacokinetics with individual dosing. Ann Pharmacother 2006;40:9–14.
97. Kane-Gill SL, Feng Y, Bobek MB, et al. Administration of enoxaparin by continuous infusion in a naturalistic setting: Analysis of renal function and safety. J Clin Pharm Ther 2005;30:207–213.
98. Heinemeyer G, Link J, Weber W, et al. Clearance of ceftriaxone in critical care patients with acute renal failure. Intensive Care Med 1990;16:448–453.
99. Macias WL, Mueller BA, Scarim SK. Vancomycin pharmacokinetics in acute renal failure: Preservation of nonrenal clearance. Clin Pharmacol Ther 1991;50:688–694.
100. Mueller BA, Scarim SK, Macias WL. Comparison of imipenem pharmacokinetics in patients with acute or chronic renal failure treated with continuous hemofiltration. Am J Kidney Dis 1993;21:172–179.
101. Yagi N, Leblanc M, Sakai K, et al. Cooling effect of continuous renal replacement therapy in critically ill patients. Am J Kidney Dis 1998;32:1023–1030.
102. Rickard CM, Couchman BA, Hughes M, McGrail MR. Preventing hypothermia during continuous veno-venous haemodiafiltration: A randomized controlled trial. J Adv Nurs 2004;47:393–400.

Chronic Kidney Disease

Joanna Q. Hudson and Lori D. Wazny

29

KEY CONCEPTS

1. Chronic kidney disease (CKD) is classified based on the cause of kidney disease, assessment of glomerular filtration rate, and extent of proteinuria.
2. Frequent complications of advanced CKD include altered sodium and water balance, hyperkalemia, metabolic acidosis, anemia, CKD-related mineral and bone disorder (CKD-MBD), and cardiovascular disease.
3. Reduction of kidney mass, development of glomerular hypertension, and intratubular proteinuria are key mechanisms responsible for the progression of CKD.
4. Anemia of CKD is primarily caused by a deficiency in the production of endogenous erythropoietin by the kidney with iron deficiency as a contributing factor.
5. CKD-MBD includes abnormalities in parathyroid hormone (PTH), calcium, phosphorus, the calcium–phosphorus product, vitamin D, bone turnover, and soft-tissue calcifications and contributes to extravascular calcifications.
6. Guidelines by the National Kidney Foundation Kidney Disease/Dialysis Outcomes Quality Initiative (NKF-KDOQI) and Kidney Disease: Improving Global Outcomes (KDIGO) provide information to assist healthcare providers in clinical decisions and the design of appropriate therapy to manage CKD progression and the associated complications.
7. Patient education plays a critical role in the appropriate management of patients with CKD and related complications. A multidisciplinary team structure is a rational approach to provide this education and effectively design and implement the extensive nonpharmacologic and pharmacologic interventions required.
8. Angiotensin-converting enzyme inhibitors (ACEIs) and angiotensin receptor blockers (ARBs) are key pharmacologic treatments of CKD because of their effects on renal hemodynamics and reduction of blood pressure, which help to limit kidney disease progression.
9. Management of anemia includes administration of erythropoietic-stimulating agents (ESAs) (epoetin alfa, darbepoetin alfa) and regular iron supplementation (oral or IV administration) to maintain hemoglobin and prevent the need for blood transfusions. There is evidence indicating a higher risk of cardiovascular events when hemoglobin is targeted to greater than 11 g/dL (110 g/L; 6.83 mmol/L).
10. Management of CKD-MBD includes dietary phosphorus restriction, phosphate-binding agents, vitamin D supplementation, and calcimimetic therapy.

Chronic kidney disease (CKD) is defined as abnormalities in kidney structure or function, present for 3 months or longer, with implications for health.[1] Structural abnormalities include albuminuria of more than 30 mg/day, presence of hematuria or red cell casts in urine sediment, electrolyte and other abnormalities due to tubular disorders, abnormalities detected by histology, structural abnormalities detected by imaging, or history of kidney transplantation. An abnormality in kidney function is usually indicated by a decrease in glomerular filtration rate (GFR).

(1) CKD is classified by cause of kidney disease, GFR category, and albuminuria level based on new recommendations from the Kidney Disease: Improving Global Outcomes (KDIGO) guidelines for evaluation and management of CKD.[1] This is referred to as CGA staging (*c*ause, *G*FR, *a*lbuminuria). Tables 29-1 and 29-2 outline the GFR and albuminuria categories. Table 29-1 also shows the corresponding staging terminology by the Kidney Disease Outcomes Quality Initiative (KDOQI).[2] For the purpose of this chapter, the KDOQI terminology for staging will be used since currently most studies and recommendations refer to the KDOQI staging system. When the GFR remains below 15 mL/min/1.73 m^2 (0.14 mL/s/m^2) renal replacement therapy, either dialysis (see Chap. 30) or transplantation (see Chap. 70), is indicated. The patient with stage 5 CKD requiring chronic dialysis or renal transplantation is said to have end-stage renal disease (ESRD). In this chapter, ESRD refers specifically to patients who are receiving chronic dialysis and transplantation and is covered in Chapters 30 and 70.

The prognosis of CKD can vary and is dependent on the following factors: (a) cause of kidney disease; (b) GFR at time of diagnosis; (c) degree of albuminuria; and (d) presence of other comorbid conditions. Patients with any of the following should be referred to a nephrologist for evaluation and collaborative management: GFR less than 30 mL/min/1.73 m^2 (0.29 mL/s/m^2), persistent and significant albuminuria, progression of CKD (e.g., drop in GFR category), presence of urinary red cell casts not readily explained, CKD and hypertension refractory to treatment (e.g., ≥4 antihypertensive agents), persistent abnormalities of serum potassium, recurrent or extensive nephrolithiasis, or hereditary kidney disease.[1]

(2) Often complications of CKD are unrecognized or are inappropriately managed, and for many patients this contributes to significant morbidity, premature mortality, or a poor prognosis by the time they reach ESRD. Frequent complications of advanced CKD include altered sodium and water balance, hyperkalemia, metabolic acidosis, anemia, CKD-related mineral and bone disorder (CKD-MBD), and cardiovascular disease (CVD). This chapter covers the pathophysiology and treatment of anemia and CKD-MBD with other complications briefly discussed at the end of the chapter. The reader is referred to Chapters 34, 36, and 37 for a

TABLE 29-1 GFR Categories[1,2]

KDIGO Category	GFR (mL/min/ 1.73 m² [mL/s/m²])	Terms	Corresponding KDOQI Category
G1	>90 (>0.87)	Normal or high	Stage 1 CKD
G2	60–89 (0.58–0.86)	Mildly decreased	Stage 2 CKD
G3a	45–59 (0.43–0.57)	Mildly to moderately decreased	Stage 3 CKD
G3b	30–44 (0.29–0.42)	Moderately to severely decreased	Stage 3 CKD
G4	15–29 (0.14–0.28)	Severely decreased	Stage 4 CKD
G5	<15 (<0.14)	Kidney failure	Stage 5 CKD (ESRD if requiring dialysis)

GFR, glomerular filtration rate; ESRD, end-stage renal disease.

TABLE 29-3 Other Complications of Chronic Kidney Disease

Organ System or Complication	Clinical Manifestations
Amyloidosis	Accumulation of β_2-microglobulin Carpal tunnel syndrome
Blood and immune disorders	Bleeding diathesis Impaired cell-mediated immunity Lymphopenia Platelet dysfunction
Endocrine	Hypoglycemic episodes (result of ↓ degradation of insulin by the kidney)
GI	Nausea, vomiting, anorexia (from uremia) Delayed gastric emptying Gastroesophageal reflux GI bleeding
Protein–energy wasting	Malnutrition
Neurologic	Peripheral neuropathies Restless leg syndrome Uremic encephalopathy

more detailed discussion of sodium and water balance, hyperkalemia, and metabolic acidosis. Table 29-3 lists other complications of advanced CKD not covered in detail in this chapter.

EPIDEMIOLOGY

Drawing from National Health and Nutrition Examination Survey (NHANES) data, the prevalence of CKD (not including the ESRD population) in the United States is estimated to affect over 25 million people, 13% of the U.S. population.[3] CKD is more likely in individuals over 60 years of age and in those with diabetes, hypertension, and CVD. In the National Kidney Foundation's Kidney Early Evaluation Program (KEEP), over 32,000 of the 124,041 participants (25%) had CKD.[4] The 2012 report of the United States Renal Data System (USRDS) indicates that in 2010, the latest year for which data are available, approximately 114,083 new cases of ESRD were reported (incidence) and the number of individuals with ESRD (prevalence) as of the end of 2010 was just over 593,086, including 413,725 patients on dialysis and 179,361 with a functioning kidney after transplantation.[3] Incidence rates of ESRD are higher in African Americans (3.4 times greater) and Native Americans (0.5 times greater) compared with whites and 1.5 times greater in Hispanics than in non-Hispanics.[3] In patients 75 years of age and older, the incidence and prevalence rates have increased since the year 2000 by 12% and 44%, respectively. Total Medicare costs for ESRD in 2010 were approximately $32.9 billion, an 8% increase from the previous year, which accounted for approximately 6% of the total Medicare budget.[3]

TABLE 29-2 Quantification of Proteinuria by Different Methods

	Albuminuria Category		
Urine Test	A1: Normal to Mildly Increased	A2: Moderately Increased	A3: Severely Increased[a]
Other terminology	Normoalbuminuria	Microalbuminuira	Macroalbuminuria
AER (mg/24 h)	<30	30–300	>300
PER (mg/24 h)	<150	150–500	>500
ACR			
mg/g	<30	30–300	>300
mg/mmol	<3	3–30	>30
PCR			
mg/g	<150	150–500	>500
mg/mmol	<15	15–50	>50
Protein reagent strip	Negative to trace	Trace to +	+ or greater

AER, albumin excretion rate (24-hour urine collection); PER, protein excretion rate (24-hour urine collection); ACR, albumin-to-creatinine ratio (spot urine sample), micrograms of albumin per gram of creatinine (SI units: milligrams of albumin per millimole of creatinine); PCR, protein-to-creatinine ratio (spot urine sample), milligrams of protein per gram of creatinine (SI units: milligrams of protein per millimole of creatinine).

[a]Includes nephrotic syndrome (defined as urine albumin excretion >2,200 mg/day or urine protein excretion >3,000 mg/day).

Reprinted by permission from Macmillan Publishers Ltd: Kidney Disease: Improving Global Outcomes (KDIGO) CKD Work Group. KDIGO 2012 Clinical Practice Guideline for the Evaluation and Management of Chronic Kidney Disease. Kidney Int Suppl 2013;3:1–150.

Mortality in the CKD population is 59% higher than in non-CKD patients when adjusted for age, gender, race, comorbidity, and prior hospitalizations.[3] The mortality rate in the ESRD population increases substantially with age and is much greater than age-matched individuals in the general population for every age group. In fact, ESRD patients have a mortality rate 6 to 8 times higher than age-matched individuals without kidney disease.[3] Associated predictors of mortality and hospitalization in hemodialysis patients include decreased serum albumin, elevated phosphorus, low hemoglobin (Hb) level, catheter use for dialysis access, and the presence of comorbidities, such as diabetes and CVD.[3,5] The association of mortality with these factors highlights the need to address complications as soon as they are detected, ideally prior to development of ESRD.

The prevalence of secondary complications at specific stages of CKD is difficult to ascertain because of limited data and use of various definitions. Data from the KEEP study targeting a higher-risk population reported that anemia (defined as a Hb of <13.5 g/dL [<135 g/L; <8.38 mmol/L] in men and <12 g/dL [<120 g/L; <7.45 mmol/L] in women) was present in over 20% of individuals with CKD with a much higher prevalence (approximately 60%) in those with stage 4 or 5 CKD.[4] Forty-five percent of CKD KEEP participants with an available parathyroid hormone (PTH) level had an elevated value. Other evaluations have reported elevated PTH (>65 pg/mL, [>65 ng/L; >7 pmol/L]) in 56% of individuals with an estimated GFR (eGFR) less than 60 mL/min/1.73 m².[6]

Although the number of patients with ESRD is substantial, it is projected that by the year 2020 the prevalence will significantly increase, with the majority of cases attributable to diabetes. CKD is one of the public health priorities for the nation and is one of the disease prevention and health promotion focus areas in Healthy People 2020.[7] The CKD goals are as follows: (a) reduce the proportion of the U.S. population with CKD, (b) increase the proportion of persons with CKD who know they have impaired kidney function, (c) increase the proportion of persons with diabetes and CKD who receive recommended medical evaluation, (d) increase the proportion of persons with diabetes and CKD who receive recommended medical treatment with angiotensin-converting enzyme inhibitors (ACEIs) or angiotensin II receptor blockers, (e) improve cardiovascular care in persons with CKD, (f) reduce the death rate among people with CKD, (g) reduce the rate of new cases of ESRD, (h) reduce kidney failure due to diabetes, (i) increase the proportion of CKD patients receiving care from a nephrologist at least 12 months before the start of renal replacement therapy, and (j) reduce deaths in persons with ESRD.

ETIOLOGY OF CKD

Susceptibility Factors

CKD susceptibility factors include advanced age, low income or education, and racial/ethnic minority status, as well as reduced kidney mass, low birth weight, family history of CKD, inflammation, and dyslipidemia.[8–11] Although most of these susceptibility factors are not amenable to pharmacologic or lifestyle interventions, they are useful for identifying individuals at high risk of CKD.

Initiation Factors

Initiation factors are conditions that directly result in kidney damage and are modifiable by pharmacologic therapy. Diabetes mellitus continues to be the leading cause of CKD and ultimately of ESRD in the United States and Canada, accounting for 45% of new ESRD cases in 2010.[3] Hypertension is the second leading cause of ESRD and it accounts for approximately 29% of new cases of ESRD.[3] Glomerulonephritis, which includes a wide variety of lesions caused by immunologic, vascular, and other idiopathic diseases (see Chap. 32), is the third leading cause of ESRD. Other diseases and conditions causing CKD are polycystic kidney disease, Wegener's granulomatosis, vascular diseases, and human immunodeficiency virus (HIV) nephropathy.

Progression Factors

Progression risk factors are those associated with further decline in kidney function. Persistence of the underlying initiation factors (e.g., diabetes mellitus, hypertension, glomerulonephritis) themselves may serve as the most important predictor of progressive CKD. Other factors associated with progression include those that may be consequent to the underlying kidney disease (e.g., hypertension, proteinuria) or independent of underlying kidney disease (e.g., smoking, obesity).

Diabetes Mellitus

Without treatment, nearly 80% of patients with type 1 diabetes and microalbuminuria will develop overt nephropathy and nearly 50% of those with type 1 diabetes, nephropathy, and hypertension will develop stage 5 CKD within 10 years.[12,13] In contrast, only 20% to 40% of those with type 2 diabetes for more than 15 years will demonstrate progressive disease.[12] A recent evaluation of participants in the Diabetes Control and Complications Trial (DCCT) and the Epidemiology of Diabetes Interventions and Complications (EDIC) studies suggests the historical estimates of diabetes with CKD may be inflated, since only 17% to 25% of the type 1 diabetic participants developed diabetes with CKD after 30 years.[14] It is not clear whether the lower incidence represents an improvement in overall care or simply is a by-product of enrollment in these studies. Progression of diabetes with CKD likely has multiple determinants including both hypertensive and glycemic control and therefore occurs at a variable rate.

Hypertension

Hypertension is both a cause of CKD and a result of CKD. Early treatment of hypertension and achievement of target blood pressure has been demonstrated to slow the rate of progression of CKD. The KDIGO guidelines for the management of blood pressure in CKD recommend the goal is to control blood pressure at all stages of CKD regardless of the underlying cause.[15]

Proteinuria

The importance of proteinuria in the progression of CKD has been well documented.[16] Proteinuria is also a strong risk factor for cardiovascular mortality and morbidity.[17] In diabetes with CKD, an albumin excretion rate higher than 30 mg per 24 hours strongly predicted the development of progression of CKD.[18] In the Modification of Diet in Renal Disease (MDRD) study, the baseline level of proteinuria also predicted progression of CKD in nondiabetic kidney disease.[19] The joint role of blood pressure and proteinuria on the progression of CKD was investigated in a meta-analysis that compared the efficacy of antihypertensive regimens for patients with predominantly nondiabetic kidney disease.[20] Patients with higher systolic blood pressures and proteinuria greater than 1 g/day had a significantly greater risk for progression of CKD.

Smoking

Smoking is associated with an acute reduction in GFR and an increase in urinary albumin excretion, heart rate, and blood pressure, likely secondary to nicotine exposure.[21] Data also suggest that smoking may promote initiation and progression of CKD in patients with type 1 and type 2 diabetes.[22,23] The "cigarette pack years" was an independent predictive factor for CKD progression among diabetic subjects.[24] In addition, smoking has been associated with the diagnosis of CKD in those with hypertension, especially among black patients, and with the development of stage 5 CKD.[21,25] Smoking has also been identified as a risk factor for CKD progression in patients with IgA nephropathy, polycystic kidney disease, and systemic lupus erythematosus.[22,26]

Obesity

Population data from Kaiser Permanente revealed an increased risk of stage 5 CKD in overweight and obese subjects.[27] The risk of stage 5 CKD was directly related to the magnitude of obesity and remained even after adjustment for diabetes and hypertension. Another study showed that a BMI $\geq$25 kg/m^2 at age 20 years is associated with a threefold increase in risk of CKD compared with a BMI lower than 25 kg/m^2. Obesity (BMI $\geq$30 kg/m^2) among men and morbid obesity (BMI $\geq$35 kg/m^2) among women were associated with threefold to fourfold increases in risk.[28] This finding has been supported by results of a meta-analysis where the presence of kidney disease was associated with higher BMI and obesity led to more progressive loss of kidney function.[29] Observational studies have also shown obesity to be an independent risk factor for onset of CKD.[30] The available data suggest the need to include weight reduction as part of the treatment of progressive kidney disease.

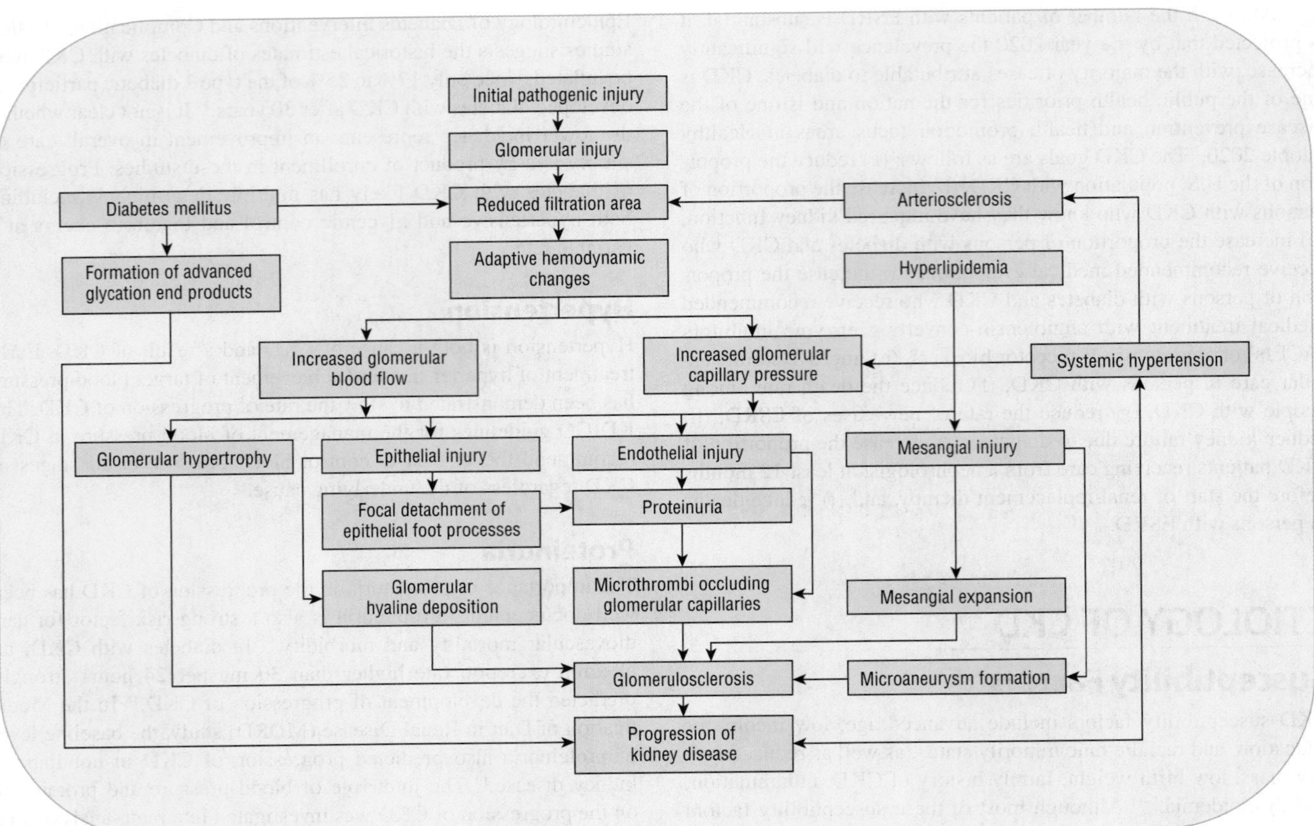

FIGURE 29-1 Proposed mechanisms for progression of kidney disease.

PATHOPHYSIOLOGY

Chronic Kidney Disease

3 Progression of CKD to ESRD occurs over years to decades in the majority of people, with the precise mechanism of kidney damage dependent on the etiology of the disease. As evidenced by the variety of initiation and progression factors, kidney damage can result from an array of heterogeneous causes. Diabetes with CKD is characterized by glomerular mesangial expansion. In hypertensive nephrosclerosis, the kidney's arterioles have arteriolar hyalinosis while with polycystic kidney disease renal cysts develop. While the initial structural damage depends on the primary disease affecting the kidney, the majority of progressive nephropathies share a final common pathway to irreversible renal parenchymal damage and ESRD (Fig. 29-1).[31] The key elements of this pathway are (a) loss of nephron mass, (b) glomerular capillary hypertension, and (c) proteinuria.

Exposure to any of the initiation risk factors can result in loss of nephron mass. The remaining nephrons hypertrophy to compensate for the loss of nephron mass and kidney function.[31] Initially, this compensatory hypertrophy may be adaptive; however, over time it can lead to the development of intraglomerular hypertension, possibly mediated by angiotensin II.[32] Angiotensin II is a potent vasoconstrictor of both afferent and efferent arterioles, but it preferentially affects the efferent arterioles, leading to increased pressure within the glomerular capillaries and consequent increased filtration fraction. The development of intraglomerular hypertension usually correlates with the development of systemic arterial hypertension. High intraglomerular capillary pressure impairs the size-selective function of the glomerular permeability barrier, resulting in increased urinary excretion of albumin and proteinuria.[32] Angiotensin II may also mediate CKD progression through nonhemodynamic effects.

Proteinuria alone may promote progressive loss of nephrons as a result of direct cellular damage.[31] Filtered proteins such as albumin, transferrin, complement factors, immunoglobulins, cytokines, and angiotensin II are toxic to kidney tubular cells. Numerous studies have demonstrated that the presence of these proteins in the renal tubule leads to increased production of inflammatory and vasoactive cytokines such as endothelin and monocyte chemoattractant protein-1 (MCP-1).[33] Proteinuria is also associated with the activation of complement components on the apical membrane of proximal tubules. Accumulating evidence now suggests that intratubular complement activation may be the key mechanism of damage in the progressive proteinuric nephropathies.[33] These events ultimately lead to scarring of the interstitium, progressive loss of structural nephron units, and a reduction in GFR.

Anemia of Chronic Kidney Disease

4 The primary cause of anemia in CKD patients is a decrease in production of erythropoietin, the glycoprotein hormone necessary for erythropoiesis (red blood cell production), by interstitial fibroblasts in the renal cortex of the kidney where approximately 90% of production occurs. In individuals with normal kidney function, plasma concentrations of erythropoietin increase exponentially in response to hypoxia; however, this response is lost as kidney disease progresses to stage 3 CKD and beyond. The result is a normochromic (normal colored red cell), normocytic (normal size red cell) anemia.[34]

Iron deficiency is common in individuals with stage 5 CKD due to decreased GI absorption of iron, inflammation, frequent blood testing, blood loss from hemodialysis, and increased iron demands from erythropoietic-stimulating agent (ESA) therapy,

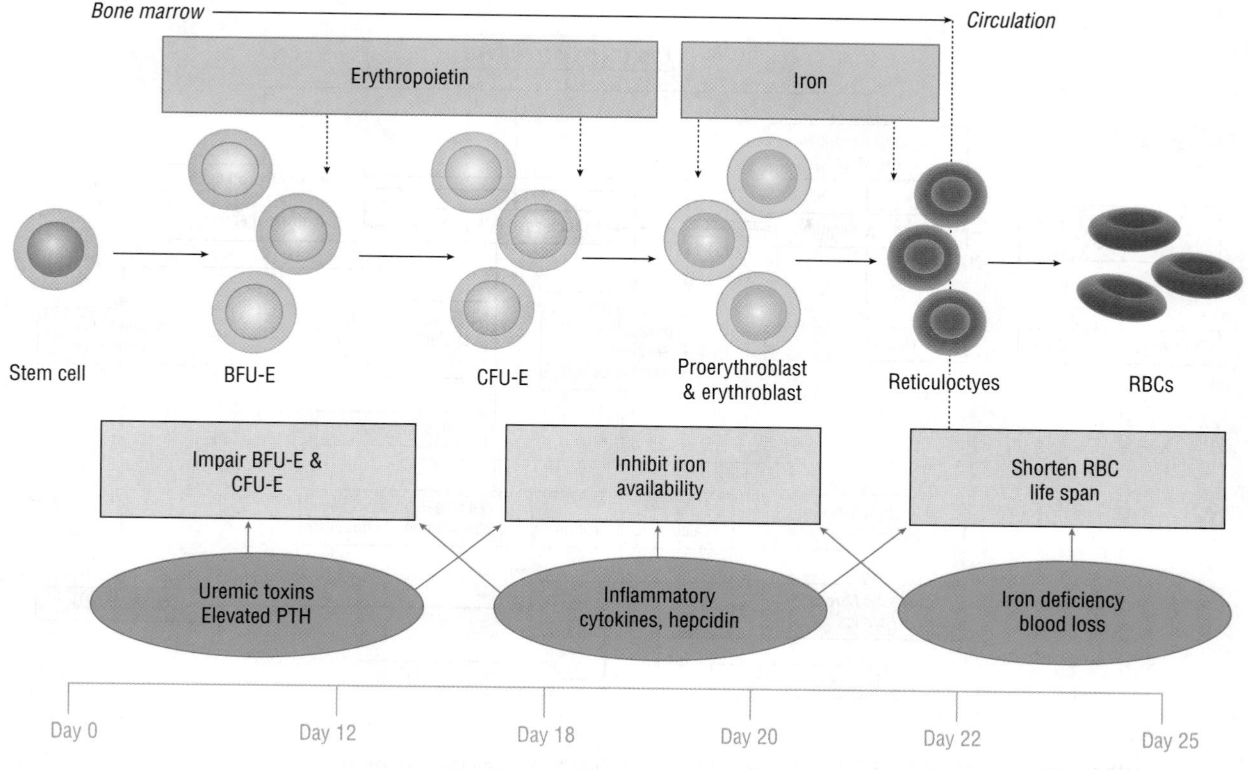

FIGURE 29-2 The process of red blood cell production (erythropoiesis) in the bone marrow requires erythropoietin and iron. This process is impaired due to factors that occur in advanced CKD such as accumulation of uremic toxins and inflammation (shown in rectangles and ovals). (BFU-E, burst-forming unit erythroid; CFU-E, colony-forming unit erythroid; RBC, red blood cells.) *(Reprinted from reference 35. Copyright © 2009, with permission from Elsevier.)*

making it the leading cause of resistance to ESAs.[35] Frequent iron supplementation is necessary to prevent and correct iron deficiency in both the ESRD and CKD populations. Hepcidin is a hormone produced by the liver that is responsible for regulation of iron. This hormone directly inhibits the protein ferroportin that transports iron out of storage cells. When iron stores are high, hepcidin production is increased to block the transfer of iron from enterocytes to the plasma. Conversely, hepcidin production is decreased when iron stores are low. Hepcidin production is also induced by inflammation or infection. As a result, the increase in hepcidin in inflammatory conditions may lead to a sequestering of iron and ineffective red blood cell production (e.g., iron-restricted erythropoiesis). The fact that hepcidin plays such a role in iron regulation has prompted the development of hepcidin antagonists to potentially alter iron transport. At this time there is no agent that is commercially available.[36]

Additional factors contributing to the development of anemia of CKD are the decreased red cell life span (from the normal of 120 days to approximately 60 days in individuals with stage 5 CKD) and vitamin B_{12} and folate deficiencies. A schematic of the process of red blood cell production is shown in Figure 29-2 that includes factors that impair this process in individuals with CKD.[35]

Anemia in the CKD population has been associated with decreased quality of life, increased hospitalizations, and CVD.[37] ESAs have been shown to reduce these morbidities; however, there is now increasing evidence that treatment of anemia to achieve Hb targets above 11 g/dL (110 g/L; 6.83 mmol/L) may lead to increased risk of cardiovascular events and death.[38–41] Thus, treatment approaches have shifted to less aggressive use of ESAs and more conservative Hb goals in the CKD population.[42]

CKD-Related Mineral and Bone Disorder

5 Disorders of mineral and bone metabolism are common in the CKD population and include abnormalities in PTH, calcium, phosphorus, the calcium–phosphorus product (Ca × P product), vitamin D, and bone turnover, as well as soft-tissue calcifications. Historically these abnormalities have been described as characteristics of secondary hyperparathyroidism (sHPT) and renal osteodystrophy (ROD). The more recently adopted term CKD-MBD encompasses the abnormalities in mineral and bone metabolism as well as associated calcifications.[43]

The pathophysiology of CKD-MBD is complex (Fig. 29-3). Calcium and phosphorus homeostasis is mediated through the effects of PTH, the precursor form of vitamin D known as 25-hydroxyvitamin D (25OHD), active vitamin D or 1,25-dihydroxyvitamin D (calcitriol), and fibroblast growth factor-23 (FGF-23) on bone, the GI tract, kidney, and the parathyroid gland. As kidney function declines, there is a decrease in phosphorus elimination, which results in hyperphosphatemia and a reciprocal decrease in serum calcium concentration. Hypocalcemia is the primary stimulus for secretion of PTH by the parathyroid glands. PTH secretion is suppressed by the interaction of ionized calcium with the calcium-sensing receptor on the chief cells of the parathyroid gland. Hyperphosphatemia also increases PTH synthesis and release through its direct effects on the parathyroid gland and production of prepro-PTH messenger RNA.[44] In an attempt to normalize ionized calcium, PTH decreases phosphorus reabsorption and increases calcium reabsorption by the proximal tubules of the kidney (at least until the GFR falls to less than approximately 30 mL/min/1.73 m^2 [0.29 mL/s/m^2]) and also increases calcium mobilization from bone. FGF-23 production

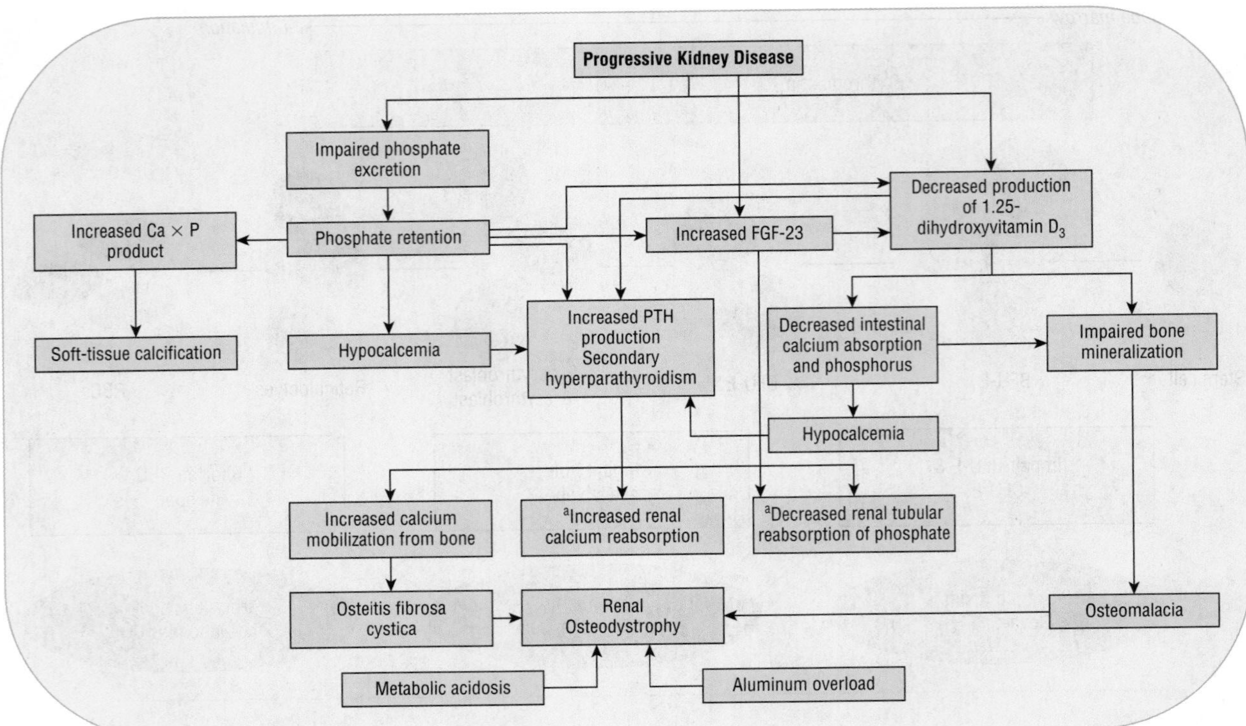

FIGURE 29-3 Pathophysiology of CKD-MBD. ([a]These adaptations are lost as kidney disease progresses.)

in bone also increases and this growth factor promotes phosphate excretion by the kidney. The result is a resetting of the calcium and phosphorus homeostasis set point, at least in the early stages of CKD; however, this occurs at the expense of an elevated PTH ("the trade-off hypothesis"). With advanced kidney disease, the kidney fails to respond to PTH or to FGF-23. The increase in PTH is most notable when GFR is less than 60 mL/min/1.73 m^2 (0.58 mL/s/m^2) (stage 3 CKD) and worsens as kidney function further declines.[44]

The most active form of vitamin D (1,25-dihydroxyvitamin D_3 or calcitriol) promotes increased intestinal absorption of calcium and phosphorus, which helps to normalize ionized calcium. Calcitriol also works directly on the parathyroid gland to suppress PTH production. The enzyme 1-α-hydroxylase is responsible for the final hydroxylation and conversion of the vitamin D precursor, 25OHD, to the active form in the kidney. As kidney disease progresses, the process is impaired due to decreased delivery of 25OHD to the kidney as GFR declines and loss of 1-α-hydroxylase activity. The resultant vitamin D deficiency leads to reduced intestinal calcium and phosphorus absorption and worsening hyperparathyroidism. Increases in FGF-23, which facilitate excretion of phosphorus, also promote calcitriol deficiency.[45] Calcitriol deficiency is observed at all levels of GFR, but is more prevalent in individuals with stage 4 or 5 CKD.[46] Deficiency in 25OHD (levels of <30 ng/mL [<75 nmol/L]) is also common in individuals with CKD due to decreased dermal synthesis of vitamin D, decreased exposure to sunlight, and reduced dietary intake of vitamin D and is a contributing factor to development of hyperparathyroidism.[46]

The abnormalities of CKD-MBD lead to bone abnormalities and other associated consequences. The continuous high rate of production of PTH by the parathyroid glands promotes parathyroid hyperplasia. Nodular tissue demonstrates more rapid growth potential and appears to be associated with fewer vitamin D and calcium-sensing receptors, resulting in resistance to the effects of calcium and vitamin D therapy.[44] Bone abnormalities are found almost universally in ESRD patients and in the majority of those with stage 3 to 5 CKD.[43] The bone abnormalities include osteitis fibrosa cystica (high bone turnover disease), osteomalacia (low bone turnover disease), and adynamic bone disease. Osteitis fibrosa cystica is most common and is characterized by areas of peritrabecular fibrosis. Bone marrow fibrosis and decreased erythropoiesis are also consequences of severe osteitis fibrosa cystica. Osteomalacia was historically noted in hemodialysis patients with aluminum toxicity, a finding less common today due to the decreased use of aluminum-containing phosphate binders and changes in the processing of dialysate solutions to decrease aluminum content. Adynamic lesions are characterized by low amounts of fibrosis or osteoid tissue and low bone formation rates. Multiple risk factors for the development of this bone disease have been identified: high concentrations of dialysate calcium along with high doses of calcium-containing phosphate binders, aggressive management with vitamin D therapy, diabetes, and aluminum toxicity.[43] Symptoms of CKD-MBD are often not evident until after significant skeletal damage has developed; consequently, prevention is the key to minimize the consequences of long-term complications. When symptoms such as bone pain and skeletal fractures occur, the disease is not easily amenable to treatment.

The morbidity and mortality of CKD patients is increased in individuals with PTH levels >495 pg/mL (>495 ng/L; >53 pmol/L).[47] Elevations of serum phosphorus, even within the upper limits of the normal range, have been associated with increased risk of cardiovascular events and/or mortality (all-cause or cardiovascular mortality) in patients with stage 3 to 5 CKD.[48] The incidence of calciphylaxis (also known as calcific uremic arteriolopathy [CUA]), which refers to rapid calcification of subcutaneous (SubQ) tissue, in patients with advanced kidney disease has increased over the last decade and has been associated with CKD-MBD and an elevated Ca × P product, although a direct cause and effect relationship has not been established.[49] Intake of calcium from calcium-based binders may also contribute to coronary artery calcification (CAC).[43] These data underscore the need to consider all the consequences of elevated PTH, calcium, and phosphorus, not just their effects on bone.

CLINICAL PRESENTATION Stage 4 or 5 Chronic Kidney Disease

Symptoms

- Uremic symptoms (fatigue, weakness, shortness of breath, mental confusion, nausea and vomiting, bleeding, and loss of appetite), as well as itching, cold intolerance, weight gain (from accumulation of fluid), and peripheral neuropathies are common in patients with stage 5 disease.

Signs

- Edema, changes in urine output (volume and consistency), "foaming" of urine (indicative of proteinuria), and abdominal distension.

Laboratory Tests

- *Decreased*: eGFR, bicarbonate (metabolic acidosis), Hb/hematocrit (Hct; anemia), iron indices (iron deficiency), vitamin D levels, albumin (malnutrition), glucose (may result from decreased degradation of insulin with impaired kidney function or poor oral intake), and calcium (in early stages of CKD).
- *Increased*: serum creatinine, cystatin C, blood urea nitrogen, potassium, phosphorus, PTH, FGF-23, ACR, PCR, blood pressure (hypertension is a common cause and result of CKD), glucose (uncontrolled diabetes is a cause of CKD), low-density lipoprotein and triglycerides, and calcium (in ESRD).
- *Other*: may be hemoccult-positive if GI bleeding occurs secondary to uremia.

Other Diagnostic Tests

- Urine sediment abnormalities (hematuria, red blood cell and white blood cell casts, renal tubular epithelial cells)
- Pathologic abnormalities indicating glomerular, vascular, tubulointerstitial disease, or cystic and congenital diseases
- Structural abnormalities such as polycystic kidneys, renal masses, renal artery stenosis, cortical scarring due to infarcts and pyelonephritis, or small kidneys (common in more severe CKD) detected by imaging studies (e.g. ultrasound, computed tomography, magnetic resonance imaging, angiography)

CLINICAL PRESENTATION

Chronic Kidney Disease

CKD is often asymptomatic, which is a reason many patients are not diagnosed with the disease until they reach stage 5 CKD and are at or near the point of requiring renal replacement therapy. This problem has prompted automated reporting by clinical labs of the eGFR as determined by the MDRD equation or Chronic Kidney Disease Epidemiology Collaboration equation (CKD-EPI equation) for the purpose of identifying individuals with CKD earlier (see eChap. 17). Clinicians must understand how to interpret the eGFR and values for urine albumin excretion to appropriately stage individuals with CKD (Tables 29-1 and 29-2). eChapter 17 provides a detailed discussion of the methods available for detection of urinary albumin and protein.

The albumin-to-creatinine ratio (ACR) is recommended as the preferred measurement for testing of urinary protein because it is relatively standardized and albumin is the most important protein lost in the urine in the majority of patients with CKD.[1] Some data suggest, however, that ACR is a poor predictor of 24-hour total protein loss compared with the protein-to-creatinine ratio (PCR) and it is not a better predictor of renal outcomes and mortality in patients with CKD.[1] Hence, there may be clinical reasons for a specialist to use PCR instead of ACR to quantify and monitor significant levels of proteinuria (e.g., patients with monoclonal gammopathies). For measurement of both ACR and PCR, an early morning urine sample is preferred since it correlates the best with 24-hour protein excretion and has relatively low intraindividual variability. A random urine sample is acceptable if an early morning urine sample is not available. Conditions that may transiently increase the ACR include menstrual blood, urinary tract infection, exercise, and those conditions that increase vascular permeability (e.g., sepsis).

Twenty-four-hour urine collection for protein remains the standard reference, but this urine collection process is prone to errors, particularly in the outpatient setting or in hospitalized patients who do not have a urinary catheter. Inaccuracies, such as missed collection of a urine sample during the 24-hour period, may contribute to underestimation of true proteinuria.

The subjective and objective findings of CKD that may be present in an individual are dependent on the severity of disease and are more likely to be observed in stage 4 or 5 CKD. Damage to the kidney has detrimental consequences for many other organ systems, particularly once patients develop ESRD. Anemia, CKD-MBD, malnutrition, and fluid and electrolyte abnormalities become more common as kidney function deteriorates. Secondary complications may even be recognized prior to making the diagnosis of CKD and presence of such complications warrants further workup.

Because patients are often asymptomatic, CKD should be suspected in individuals with conditions such as diabetes, hypertension, genitourinary abnormalities, and autoimmune diseases. In addition, individuals of older age and those with a family history of kidney disease should be considered for CKD screening. Recommended screening studies include serum creatinine and assessment of GFR, urinalysis, and/or imaging studies of the kidneys. Abnormal elevations of serum creatinine, reflecting decreases in GFR, or presence of urinary or imaging study abnormalities are indications for a full evaluation of CKD. The rate of GFR loss can vary in CKD because of differences in the underlying disease process and the extent of kidney damage, treatment responsiveness, and compliance with therapies.

DIAGNOSTIC CONSIDERATIONS FOR SECONDARY COMPLICATIONS

As two of the most common complications of CKD, anemia and CKD-MBD should be diagnosed early in the course of CKD.

Anemia of Chronic Kidney Disease

Signs and symptoms of anemia of CKD include fatigue, shortness of breath, cold intolerance, chest pain, tingling in the extremities, tachycardia, headaches, and general malaise. Despite associations of development of LVH with worsening anemia, there are no prospective studies demonstrating that early and aggressive treatment improves cardiovascular end points or reduces LVH in the CKD population. Improvements in quality of life have been observed with increases in Hb, but such improvements must be weighed against reported risks associated with using ESAs to achieve near-normal Hb levels in the CKD population.[50]

Since individuals with anemia of CKD may be asymptomatic, laboratory evaluation is commonly the initial approach to diagnosing anemia of CKD. According to the KDOQI guidelines for anemia management, the Hb should be measured in all individuals with CKD regardless of stage.[51] KDIGO recommends measuring Hb concentrations annually in stage 3 CKD patients, biannually in stage 4 to 5 CKD patients, and at least every 3 months in dialysis patients.[42] The diagnosis of anemia is made and further workup of anemia is required when the Hb is less than 13 g/dL (130 g/L; 8.07 mmol/L) for adult males and less than 12 g/dL (120 g/L; 7.45 mmol/L) for adult females using the KDIGO definition.[42] Iron deficiency is the primary cause of resistance to treatment of anemia with ESAs; therefore, assessment of the iron status is necessary. The iron indices transferrin saturation (TSat) and serum ferritin provide information on iron immediately available for use in the bone marrow for red blood cell production (TSat) and storage iron (serum ferritin). The TSat is calculated as follows: (serum iron/TIBC) × 100, where TIBC is the total iron-binding capacity. If the TSat and serum ferritin values are below the desired threshold (see Treatment section later in this chapter), iron supplementation is warranted.

Additional workup should be done to evaluate other causes of anemia such as blood loss, deficiencies in vitamin B_{12} or folate, or other disease states that contribute to anemia, including human immunodeficiency virus infection and malignancies. Red blood cell indices (mean corpuscular volume, mean corpuscular Hb concentration), white blood cell count, differential and platelet count, and absolute reticulocyte count should also be assessed. A stool guaiac test should be performed to rule out GI bleeding. Measurement of serum erythropoietin concentrations is not generally useful since levels may fall into what is considered a "normal" range, but are insufficient relative to the degree of decline in Hb.

CKD-Related Mineral and Bone Disorder

Patients with CKD-MBD are generally asymptomatic until bone manifestations such as prolonged high bone turnover develop or the patient experiences calcifications. Biochemical or imaging abnormalities typically precede clinical manifestations. The biochemical abnormalities of CKD-MBD that should be evaluated in patients with stage 3 CKD include serum phosphorus, calcium, Ca × P product, and PTH. The recommended frequencies of monitoring calcium, phosphorus, and PTH by CKD stage based on the KDOQI and KDIGO guidelines are shown in Table 29-4.[43,52] The KDIGO guidelines also recommend monitoring bone-specific alkaline phosphatase annually in stage 4 and 5 CKD patients. The frequency of monitoring these parameters may increase once a diagnosis of CKD-MDB is made, and further information is needed to assess the patient's response to treatment and to guide decisions about changes in therapy.

In addition to monitoring for biochemical abnormalities that define CKD-MBD, evaluation of bone architecture is also necessary in some cases. The gold standard test for diagnosing bone manifestations of CKD-MBD is a bone biopsy for histologic analysis; however, this is an invasive test that is not easily performed. KDOQI and KDIGO guidelines recommend bone biopsy only in patients in whom the etiology of symptoms is not clear or in individuals with more unique biochemical abnormalities.[43,52] This includes patients experiencing unexplained fractures, persistent hypercalcemia, and possible aluminum toxicity. If aluminum concentrations are elevated (60 to 200 mcg/L [2.2 to 7.4 μmol/L]), a deferoxamine test should be done. KDIGO also suggests a bone biopsy be considered in CKD patients prior to beginning treatment with bisphosphonates since adynamic bone disease is a contraindication to the use of these agents. Bone biopsy findings are described on the basis of turnover rate, mineralization, and volume. Bone mineral density testing is not generally recommended in patients with advanced CKD since this test has not been shown to predict fracture risk and does not indicate the type of ROD.[43]

Abnormalities in mineral metabolism are highly associated with vascular and soft-tissue calcifications, known risk factors for mortality; therefore, diagnostic testing for calcifications should be considered in the evaluation for CKD-MBD. Electron-beam computed tomography (EBCT) is a noninvasive and sensitive method available for detecting cardiovascular calcifications and has been used clinically and in studies in the CKD population. Other methods advocated include lateral abdominal radiographs to detect vascular calcification and echocardiogram to detect valvular calcification. KDIGO suggests these tests are reasonable alternatives to EBCT based on the sensitivity to detect calcifications and lower cost.[43]

TREATMENT

General Approach to Patient Care

Individuals with CKD should be evaluated frequently to assess the rate of progression of CKD, to diagnose secondary complications and comorbid conditions, and to receive treatment for these complications prior to development of ESRD. Historically, the common complications of anemia and CKD-MBD have not been diagnosed or appropriately managed in the earlier stages of CKD. Late referral to a nephrologist may in part account for this poor management; however, even in ideal clinical environments such as nephrology clinics, these secondary complications may not be recognized in the early stages of CKD.

6 Management of CKD should be based on the most current consensus guidelines and the best clinical practices such as those developed by the National Kidney Foundation Kidney Disease/Dialysis Outcomes Quality Initiative (NKF-KDOQI), KDIGO, and other relevant professional associations.[1,2] The KDOQI and KDIGO

TABLE 29-4 Recommended Frequency of Monitoring Calcium, Phosphorus, PTH, and 25OHD by Stage of CKD (KDOQI and KDIGO Guidelines)[43,52]

	Calcium and Phosphorus		PTH		25-Hydroxyvitamin D	
CKD Stage	**KDOQI**	**KDIGO**	**KDOQI**	**KDIGO**	**KDOQI**	**KDIGO**
3	Annually	Every 6–12 months	Annually	Baseline, and then based on level and CKD progression	If PTH above target	Baseline level; correct deficiencies as in general population
4	Every 3 months	Every 3–6 months	Every 3 months	Every 6–12 months		
5	Monthly	Every 1–3 months	Every 3 months	Every 3–6 months	Not measured	

KDIGO, Kidney Disease: Improving Global Outcomes; KDOQI, Kidney Disease Outcomes Quality Initiative; PTH, parathyroid hormone.

guidelines and recommendations were developed based on evidence, when available, and the recommendations of an expert group of individuals. With this in mind, these recommendations should not replace clinical judgment, but should provide a basis on which treatment decisions can be made in the context of both evidence and opinion. The secondary complications of CKD that are addressed in the currently available KDOQI guidelines include anemia of CKD, bone metabolism and disease, CVD in dialysis patients, dyslipidemias, hypertension, and nutrition. KDIGO clinical practice guidelines pertinent to CKD address evaluation and management of CKD, blood pressure MBD, anemia, lipid management, hepatitis C in CKD, and glomerulonephritis.

7 Appropriate management of CKD ideally involves a multidisciplinary approach to address the nonpharmacologic and pharmacologic interventions, dietary education, and social/financial concerns. The typical team in outpatient dialysis facilities includes physicians (nephrologists), nurses, dietitians, and social workers as mandated by the U.S. government. In some clinical settings pharmacists are also active members of the care team. ESRD patients are prescribed an average of 10 to 12 medications, which increases the potential for drug-related problems (DRPs).[3,53] Pharmacists involved with the CKD population have identified DRPs (e.g., inappropriate dose or indication for a medication, adverse drug reactions) that commonly occur in the CKD population and have demonstrated that clinical pharmacy services reduce such problems and improve patient's quality of life.[53] Patients with CKD who have access to an interdisciplinary team as opposed to a nephrologist alone have been shown to have increased Hb values, were more likely to receive ACEI, iron supplementation, and bicarbonate therapies, had a slower decline in eGFR (1.2 mL/min/1.73 m^2 vs. 2.5 mL/min/1.73 m^2), and had decreased mortality.[54–56] Interdisciplinary teams in these published studies consisted of nephrologists, nephrology nurses, dietitians, social workers, pharmacists, and diabetes educators.

Pharmacists must be prepared to provide Medication Therapy Management (MTM) for individuals with CKD since this population receives medications and care in the community settings. Drug-dosing guidelines based on the degree of kidney function should be followed, and a complete medication history of prescription and nonprescription medications, as well as herbals and nutritional supplements, should be obtained and routinely updated. Recommendations on drug dosing in patients with CKD are also available from a KDIGO conference that addressed this topic.[57] Appropriate measures should also be taken for hospitalized patients to decrease the risk of nephrotoxicity from radiocontrast agents and antibiotics such as aminoglycosides, as well as from nonsteroidal antiinflammatory drugs and ACEIs (see Chap. 31).

A summary of nonpharmacologic and pharmacologic recommendations that apply to all individuals with CKD is listed in Table 29-5.

Desired Outcome

The overall goal of therapy in individuals with CKD is to delay or prevent progression of the disease, thereby minimizing the development or severity of associated complications and ultimately limiting the progression to ESRD when hemodialysis, peritoneal dialysis, or kidney transplantation is required. Once a patient is diagnosed with CKD, implementation of therapy to address the primary cause (e.g., diabetes, hypertension, or glomerulonephritis) is a priority. Patients who reach stage 4 CKD almost inevitably experience progression to ESRD, and thus at some time in the near future will require dialysis or transplantation to sustain life. It is during stage 4 CKD that planning for renal replacement therapy (hemodialysis or peritoneal dialysis) should begin, including patient education about dialysis modalities and options for transplantation (see Chaps. 30 and 70). With ESRD the primary goal is to sustain a good quality of life and prevent adverse outcomes by aggressively managing complications of CKD.

TABLE 29-5 Recommendations for Individuals with CKD[1,15]

Nonpharmacologic
Exercise 30 minutes five times per week
Weight loss if BMI >25 kg/m^2
Smoking cessation
Alcohol: two standard drinks per day for men and one standard drink per day for women[a]
If hypertension: low-sodium diet (<2 g/day, <90 mmol/day)
Pharmacologic
Adjust medication doses for kidney function
Seek pharmacist or medical advice before using over-the-counter medicines or nutritional protein supplements
Herbal medicines are not recommended
Temporarily discontinue potentially nephrotoxic/renally excreted drugs if eGFR <60 mL/min/1.73 m^2 in patients who are acutely unwell or hypovolemic (e.g., metformin, RAAS blockers, diuretics, NSAIDs/COX II inhibitors, lithium, digoxin)
Vaccines: • Influenza yearly • Pneumococcal vaccine if eGFR <30 mL/min/1.73 m^2, nephrotic syndrome, diabetes, or receiving immunosuppression. Single booster dose at year 5 • Hepatitis B vaccine if eGFR <30 mL/min/1.73 m^2 and risk of progression of CKD
ASA for secondary prevention only
Avoid oral phosphate-containing bowel preparations in people with a GFR <60 mL/min/1.73 m^2 (<0.58 mL/s/m^2) or in those known to be at risk of phosphate nephropathy

See Abbreviations in text for definitions.

[a]Standard drink: 30 mL spirits, 100 mL wine, 285 mL full-strength beer, and 425 mL light beer.

Desired Outcomes

The overall goal of therapy in individuals with CKD is to delay or prevent progression of the disease, thereby minimizing the development or severity of associated complications and ultimately limiting the progression to ESRD when hemodialysis, peritoneal dialysis, or kidney transplantation is required.

The desired outcomes of anemia management are to increase oxygen-carrying capacity, improve the patient's quality of life, and decrease the need for blood transfusions.

The overall goal for management of CKD-MBD is to "normalize" the biochemical parameters and prevent the detrimental consequences, including bone manifestations, cardiovascular and extravascular calcifications, and the associated morbidity and mortality.

Nonpharmacologic Therapy

Diet Meta-analyses to determine the effect of protein restriction on the progression of CKD suggest only a relatively small benefit from dietary protein restriction.[58–60] Protein restriction to 0.8 g/kg/day is recommended only in patients with an eGFR less than 30 mL/min/1.73 m^2 with appropriate monitoring by a dietitian to avoid malnutrition. High sodium intake can increase blood pressure and proteinuria, blunt the response to renin–angiotensin system blockade, and induce glomerular hyperfiltration; therefore, decreasing salt intake to less than 2 g or 90 mEq (mmol) per day of sodium (corresponding to 5 g sodium chloride) is recommended, particularly in patients with hypertension or proteinuria.[1]

Smoking Cessation and Exercise Smoking cessation is encouraged to slow progression of CKD and to reduce the risk of CVD.[1] Clinicians should educate patients regarding the risks and institute appropriate therapeutic options, both nonpharmacologic and

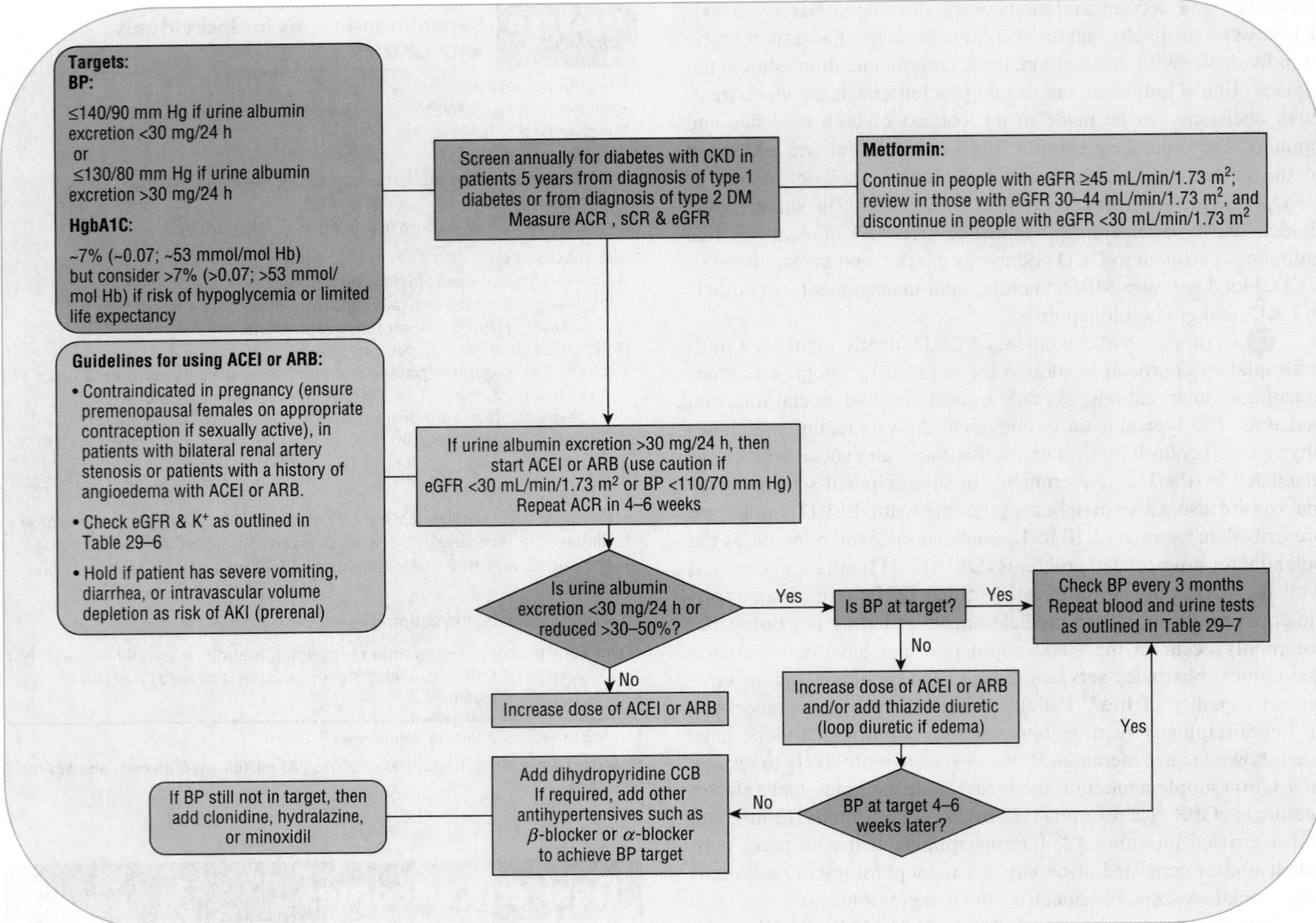

FIGURE 29-4 Diabetes with CKD algorithm. Strategy for screening and treatment of diabetes with CKD based on urine albumin excretion, target blood pressure, and eGFR. *(Data from National Kidney Foundation. KDOQI clinical practice guidelines and clinical practice recommendations for diabetes and chronic kidney disease. Am J Kidney Dis 2007;49(Suppl 2):S1–S180; reference 1.)*

pharmacologic, for smoking cessation. These options are discussed in further detail in Chapter 49. People with CKD are encouraged to exercise at least 30 minutes five times per week and achieve a healthy body weight to maintain a BMI of 20 to 25 kg/m^2.[1]

Pharmacologic Therapy

Diabetes with CKD Figure 29-4 provides an algorithm for the management of diabetes in patients with CKD. ACEI and/or an angiotensin receptor blocker (ARB) should be used as first-line therapy if the urine albumin excretion or equivalent test (Table 29-2) is >30 mg/24 h. The dose is usually increased until albuminuria is reduced by 30% to 50% or side effects such as a significant drop in eGFR or elevation in serum potassium occur (Table 29-6).

8 Evidence from clinical trials has confirmed the beneficial effects of ACEIs on kidney function for patients with diabetes, and both ACEIs and ARBs remain the mainstay of therapy.[61,62] These studies showed benefits of ACEI in individuals with both type 1 and type 2 diabetes with varying degrees of kidney damage. A meta-analysis that pooled several of the small and large randomized controlled studies showed beneficial effects of ACEI therapy on diabetes with CKD.[63] Progression to proteinuria was reduced by 65% for patients with diabetes mellitus and microalbuminuria, and progression of CKD (doubling of serum creatinine) was reduced by 40% for both diabetics and nondiabetics with macroalbuminuria.

ARBs have also been shown to slow the progression of diabetes in patients with CKD.[64–66] Currently, both ACEIs and ARBs reduce the rate of progression in type 2 diabetes, whereas only ACEIs have been adequately evaluated for patients with type 1 diabetes. However, in practice these agents are used interchangeably. Chapter 3 includes a thorough discussion of dose, dose titration, monitoring, and adverse effects of ACEI and ARB. Alternative drug treatments to reduce proteinuria are discussed below.

Figure 29-4 provides the current glycosylated hemoglobin (HgbA$_1$C) target in this patient population. However, it should be noted that HgbA$_1$C measurements are based on an assumed red blood cell life span of 90 days. In CKD, the red blood cell life span is decreased, so HgbA$_1$C values may be falsely low.[1] The HgbA$_1$C should be interpreted along with the patient's home blood glucose readings before making a determination of diabetic control. It is also important to note that patients with stage 3 and 4 CKD are at higher risk of developing hypoglycemia because the kidney metabolizes insulin. When GFR decreases, the degradation of endogenous or injected insulin is decreased and patients may require reduced doses of oral or injectable hypoglycemics. As a result, patients with eGFR <30 mL/min/1.73 m^2 should be educated on how to recognize and treat hypoglycemic episodes. Dose adjustments or avoidance of renally eliminated hypoglycemics is necessary. A thorough review of dosing, monitoring, and goals of therapies to treat diabetes mellitus is provided in Chapter 57.

TABLE 29-6 ACEI and ARB Drug Monitoring in CKD

Drug	Adverse Drug Reaction	Monitoring Parameter	Comments
ACEI or ARB	↓ GFR	sCr to calculate eGFR If eGFR ≥60 mL/min/1.73 m², repeat in 4–12 weeks If eGFR 30–59 mL/min/1.73 m², repeat in 2–4 weeks If eGFR <30 mL/min/1.73 m², repeat in ≤2 weeks	Dose adjustments: eGFR ↓ 0–15%, no dose change eGFR ↓ 15–30%, no dose change but repeat eGFR in 10–14 days eGFR ↓ 30–50%, reduce dose and repeat eGFR every 5–7 days until GFR within 30% of baseline eGFR ↓ >50%, discontinue ACEI or ARB and repeat eGFR every 5–7 days until GFR is within 15% of baseline value
	↑ serum K⁺	Serum K⁺ at same intervals as eGFR above	If K⁺ >5 mEq/L (mmol/L), advise dietary K⁺ restriction If K⁺ >6 mEq/L (mmol/L), prescribe loop diuretic if tolerated ± K⁺ resin binder

eGFR recommendations from KDIGO guidelines on management of blood pressure in CKD.[15]

Hypertension Figure 29-5 provides an algorithm for the recommended blood pressure goals based on the degree of albuminuria present and the choice of antihypertensive agent for CKD patients without diabetes mellitus. Previous guidelines suggested a target blood pressure of less than 130/80 mm Hg for all patients with CKD. A meta-analysis of 2,272 subjects with nondiabetic kidney disease concluded that no benefits in renal or cardiovascular outcomes or mortality were achieved in patients treated to a goal blood pressure of 125 to 130/75 to 80 mm Hg as compared with 140/90 mm Hg.[67] Subjects with proteinuria greater than 300 mg/day did benefit from the lower blood pressure target. The ongoing Systolic Blood Pressure Intervention Trial (SPRINT) may provide the evidence needed to determine whether an even lower blood pressure goal of 120 mm Hg systolic pressure is desirable in patients with nephrotic range proteinuria.[68] The KDIGO guidelines recommend a target blood pressure of ≤140/90 mm Hg if urine albumin excretion or equivalent (Table 29-2) is <30 mg/24 h.[15]

In patients with a urine albumin excretion >30 mg/24 h or equivalent (Table 29-2), the target blood pressure is ≤130/80 mm Hg and first-line therapy with an ACEI or ARB is recommended.[15] If this fails to achieve the target blood pressure, then thiazide diuretics may offer additional reduction of proteinuria in combination with an ARB.[69,70] It has been widely quoted that thiazide diuretics are not effective for blood pressure control when creatinine clearance is less than 30 mL/min (0.5 mL/s), but there is limited evidence to support this statement.[71] While salt and water excretion may initially account for their antihypertensive effect, long-term lowering of blood pressure appears to involve vasodilation that is not affected by reduced kidney function. While there is some controversy, a switch to a loop

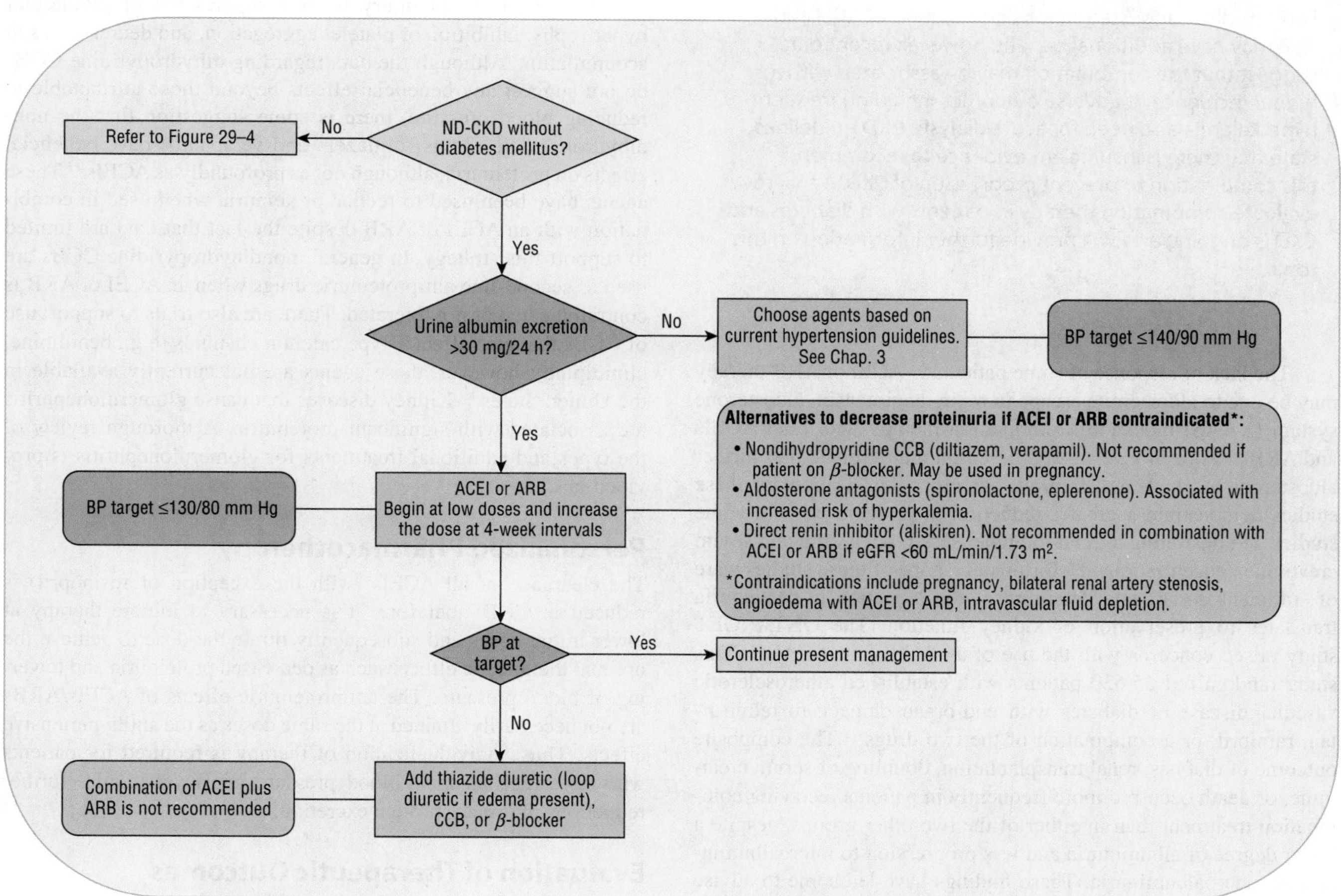

FIGURE 29-5 Treatment of hypertension in chronic kidney disease patients, nondialysis ND-CKD without diabetes mellitus. Strategy for treatment of hypertension based on urine albumin excretion and target blood pressure. *(Data from reference 1.)*

diuretic should be considered in patients with stage 4 or 5 CKD with inadequate blood pressure control while receiving a regimen that included a thiazide diuretic. The choice of additional antihypertensive agents should be based on concomitant disease states and other compelling indications as discussed in Chapter 3. At this time, there is insufficient evidence to recommend the combination of an ACEI plus an ARB to prevent progression of CKD.[1] Patients and clinicians should be aware that targeting a blood pressure of less than 130/80 mm Hg will often require three or more drugs.

Proteinuria The antiproteinuric effect of ACEIs and ARBs is a class effect and not specific to any one agent.[63,72] For patients with hypertension, the primary goal is to achieve the target blood pressure while a secondary goal is to control proteinuria. For normotensive patients, the ACEI/ARB dose should be titrated to reduce the degree of proteinuria. Patients with hypertension and proteinuria may experience adverse effects associated with blood pressure lowering, and drug doses should be titrated to achieve the maximum reduction of proteinuria without reducing blood pressure to a level associated with adverse events including further decline in kidney function. Specific dosing recommendations for ACEIs and ARBs have not been established; consequently, the lowest recommended dose should be initiated for the management of hypertension. In addition, one needs to consider the presence of other concomitant diseases and past history of treatment, as well as any adverse effects demonstrated with particular agents. If patients exhibit adverse effects such as cough with an ACEI, a switch to an ARB may be appropriate.

Clinical **Controversy...**

Early studies suggested that a combination of ACEI and ARB may have additional benefit; however, recent data suggest that the combination may be associated with a higher incidence of adverse outcomes including frequent hyperkalemia and need for acute dialysis. CKD guidelines state that there is insufficient evidence to recommend this combination to prevent progression of CKD. A trial to evaluate combination therapy in patients with diabetes and CKD is ongoing and will provide further information on this topic.

The lack of response of some patients to ACEI or ARB therapy may be due to aldosterone escape in renin–angiotensin–aldosterone system (RAAS) blockade. Combination therapy with both ACEIs and ARBs has been investigated based on the rationale that further aldosterone blockade may improve outcomes.[73–75] In summary, these studies demonstrate a greater reduction in proteinuria, with some studies demonstrating a trend to higher serum potassium and serum creatinine concentrations. Unfortunately, none of these studies were of sufficient duration to determine if the reduction in proteinuria translates to preservation of kidney function. The ONTARGET study raised concerns with the use of an ACEI plus an ARB. This study randomized 25,620 patients with established atherosclerotic vascular disease or diabetes with end-organ damage to telmisartan, ramipril, or a combination of the two drugs.[76] The composite outcome of dialysis, renal transplantation, doubling of serum creatinine, or death occurred more frequently in patients receiving combination treatment than in either of the two other groups, despite a lower degree of albuminuria and less progression to microalbuminuria or macroalbuminuria. These findings have led some to advise against the combination of these two agents; however, critics of the study have argued that these findings cannot be extrapolated to individuals with proteinuric kidney disease as only 4% of patients in the study had overt proteinuria.[77] Combination therapy with an ACEI and an ARB likely does have a role for patients with diabetes and CKD with macroalbuminuria and is being evaluated more closely in an ongoing randomized double-blind multicenter clinical trial of Veterans Administration patients (VA NEPHRON D).[78]

The concept of aldosterone escape has led to the search for other methods to suppress the RAAS in an effort to improve renal outcomes. A Cochrane systematic review examined the addition of an aldosterone antagonist (e.g., spironolactone, eplerenone) to an ACEI, ARB, or ACEI plus ARB mainly in patients with diabetes and CKD.[79] Significant decreases in proteinuria were observed; however, there was also a significant increase in the risk of hyperkalemia (relative risk [RR] 3.06, 95% CI 1.26 to 7.41). At this time, long-term effects on renal outcomes, mortality, and safety are unknown.

Aliskiren, a direct renin inhibitor, has been shown to reduce proteinuria when used in combination with an ARB or a diuretic.[80,81] While short-term benefits have been demonstrated, there are concerns regarding the use of aliskiren in combination with an ACEI or ARB. The ALTITUDE trial compared placebo or aliskiren 300 mg/day added to an ACEI or ARB in patients with diabetes who had either an increased urine albumin or an eGFR of 30 to 60 mL/min/1.73 m^2 and established CVD.[82] This trial was stopped early due to safety concerns that included an increase in hyperkalemia and hypotension in the aliskiren combination group with no benefit in the primary composite cardiovascular and renal outcomes. The FDA subsequently issued a warning that aliskiren in combination with an ACEI or ARB is contraindicated in patients with diabetes and that the use of aliskiren with an ACEI or ARB in patients with an eGFR <60 mL/min/1.73 m^2 should be avoided.[83]

Some CCBs decrease glomerular injury without negatively changing renal hemodynamics.[84] The postulated mechanisms for this decrease in renal injury include suppression of glomerular hypertrophy, inhibition of platelet aggregation, and decrease in salt accumulation. Although the data regarding dihydropyridine CCBs do not suggest any beneficial effects beyond those attributable to reducing blood pressure, there is some suggestion that the nondihydropyridine agents (diltiazem and verapamil) have beneficial effects on proteinuria, although not as profoundly as ACEIs.[85] These agents have been used to reduce proteinuria when used in combination with an ACEI or ARB despite the fact that data are limited to support this strategy. In general, nondihydropyridine CCBs are used as second-line antiproteinuric drugs when an ACEI or ARB is contraindicated or not tolerated. There are also trials to support use of CCBs that also affect T-type calcium channels (e.g., benidipine, clinidipine); however, these agents are not currently available in the United States.[86] Kidney diseases that cause glomerulonephritis are associated with significant proteinuria. A thorough review of the types and additional treatments for glomerulonephritis is provided in Chapter 32.

Personalized Pharmacotherapy

The clearance of all ACEIs (with the exception of fosinopril) is reduced in CKD; therefore, it is necessary to initiate therapy at lower initial doses and subsequently titrate the dose to achieve the optimal therapeutic effects such as decreased proteinuria and lowering of blood pressure. The antiproteinuric effects of ACEIs/ARBs are not necessarily attained at the same doses as the antihypertensive effects. Thus, individualization of therapy is required for patients who have reached their blood pressure goals yet require further reductions in urinary protein excretion.

Evaluation of Therapeutic Outcomes

A monitoring plan for ACEI and ARB therapy in the CKD population is outlined in Table 29-6 with some recommendations based on the KDOQI guidelines on hypertension in CKD.[87] Frequency of lab

TABLE 29-7 Recommended Outcome Measure Monitoring Intervals for Patients with CKD[1]

KDIGO GFR Stage	eGFR (mL/min/1.73 m²)	Albuminuria Stage		
		A1: 10–29 mg/g (1–2.9 mg/mmol)	A2: 30–299 mg/g (3–30 mg/mmol)	A3: >300 mg/g (>30 mg/mmol)
G1	≥90	12 months	12 months	6 months
G2	60–89	12 months	12 months	6 months
G3a	45–59	12 months	6 months	4 months
G3b	30–44	6 months	4 months	4 months
G4	15–29	4 months	4 months	2–3 months
G5	<15	1–3 months	1–3 months	1–3 months

Blood tests: CBC, Na, K, Cl, bicarbonate, urea, creatinine, and eGFR. If DKD, add $HgbA_1C$. Fasting lipid profile at least yearly. At stage G3b or later: also add albumin, calcium, phosphorus, parathyroid hormone, serum iron, TIBC, and ferritin.

Urine tests: ACR (or PCR if indicated), standard urinalysis, and urine culture and sensitivity only if symptoms suggestive of urinary tract infection.

and urine testing based on stage of CKD and degree of albuminuria as defined by KDIGO is shown in Table 29-7. The monitoring necessary for patients with hypertension and diabetes is the same in the CKD population as it is in the non-CKD population, and readers should refer to the appropriate chapters in this textbook for further information.

Anemia of Chronic Kidney Disease

Desired Outcome

The desired outcomes of anemia management are to increase oxygen-carrying capacity, decrease signs and symptoms of anemia, improve the patient's quality of life, and decrease the need for blood transfusions. Achievement of these goals requires a combination of an ESA and iron supplementation to promote and maintain erythropoiesis. Hb is the preferred monitoring parameter for red blood cell production because, unlike Hct, its concentration is not affected by blood storage conditions and instrumentation used for analysis. Table 29-8 lists the Hb and iron indices for nondialysis and dialysis-dependent CKD patients as suggested by KDOQI and KDIGO guidelines.

Target Hemoglobin and Use of ESAs

Initiation of ESA therapy should be considered in all CKD patients when Hb is between 9 and 10 g/dL (90 and 100 g/L; 5.59 and 6.21 mmol/L) and in nondialysis patients when the following additional criteria are met: (a) the rate of Hb decline indicates the likelihood of requiring a RBC transfusion and (b) reducing the risk of alloimmunization and/or other RBC-transfusion-related risks is a goal. According to the labeling for the available ESAs, the ESA dose should be decreased or interrupted when Hb is above 10 g/dL (100 g/L; 6.21 mmol/L) in CKD patients not receiving dialysis or above 11 g/dL (110 g/L; 6.83 mmol/L) in patients receiving dialysis. This is in contrast to the KDOQI and more recent KDIGO recommendations. On November 1, 2011, Centers for Medicare and Medicaid Services (CMS) removed the requirement that dialysis providers maintain Hb levels above 10 g/dL (100 g/L; 6.21 mmol/L) because no lower level of Hb was proven safe for patients treated with an ESA.[88] This change took effect in payment year 2013.

The target range for Hb in the CKD population is a topic of much debate. Observational studies and USRDS data have shown decreased hospitalizations, lower mortality, and improved quality of life with Hb levels above 11 g/dL (110 g/L; 6.83 mmol/L).[89,90] While these data support a higher Hb, targeting Hb levels above 13 g/dL (130 g/L; 8.07 mmol/L) with ESA therapy has resulted in increased risk of mortality and cardiovascular events compared with patients maintained in the 11 to 12 g/dL (110 to 120 g/L; 6.83 to 7.45 mmol/L) range. These conclusions were based on clinical trials (CHOIR and CREATE trials) that included individuals with early stage CKD and from previous data reported in the hemodialysis population (Normal Hematocrit Cardiac Trial [NHCT]).[38–41]

TABLE 29-8 Suggested Hb and Iron Indices in Adults with Anemia of Chronic Kidney Disease: KDOQI and KDIGO Guidelines[42,103]

Parameter	KDOQI		KDIGO	
	ND-CKD and PD-CKD	HD-CKD	ND-CKD[a]	HD and PD-CKD[a]
Hb	Hb 11–12 g/dL (110–120 g/L; 6.83–7.45 mmol/L) Do not use ESAs to exceed Hb of 13 g/dL (130 g/L; 8.07 mmol/L)	Hb 11–12 g/dL (110–120 g/L; 6.83–7.45 mmol/L) Do not use ESAs to exceed Hb of 13 g/dL (130 g/L; 8.07 mmol/L)	If Hb ≥10 g/dL (≥100 g/L; ≥6.21 mmol/L), do not initiate an ESA If Hb <10 g/dL (<100 g/L; <6.21 mmol/L), consider rate of fall of Hb, prior response to iron, risk of needing a transfusion, risk of ESA therapy, and presence of anemia symptoms before initiating an ESA Do not use ESAs to maintain Hb above 11.5 g/dL (115 g/L; 7.14 mmol/L)	Use ESAs to avoid drop in Hb to <9 g/dL (<90 g/L; <5.59 mmol/L) by starting ESA when Hb is between 9 and 10 g/dL (90 and 100 g/L; 5.59 and 6.21 mmol/L) Do not use ESAs to maintain Hb above 11.5 g/dL (115 g/L; 7.14 mmol/L)
TSat[b] (goal during ESA therapy)	>20% (>0.20)	>20% (>0.20)	>30% (>0.30)	>30% (>0.30)
Serum ferritin[b] (goal during ESA therapy)	>100 ng/mL (>100 mcg/L; >225 pmol/L)	>200 ng/mL (>200 mcg/L; >450 pmol/L)	>500 ng/mL (>500 mcg/L; >1,100 pmol/L)	>500 ng/mL (>500 mcg/L; >1,100 pmol/L)

ND-CKD, nondialysis CKD patients; PD-CKD, peritoneal dialysis patients; HD-CKD, hemodialysis patients; CKD, chronic kidney disease; Hb, hemoglobin; TSat, transferrin saturation.

[a]The KDIGO expert panel considered the quality of the evidence to be *low* or *very* low.

[b]If TSat and serum ferritin are below suggested levels, consider iron supplementation if goal is to increase Hb and/or decrease ESA dose. *Note*: Serum ferritin is an acute-phase reactant—use clinical judgment when above 500 ng/mL (500 mcg/L; 1,100 pmol/L).

TABLE 29-9 Trials Evaluating ESAs and Target Hb/Hct

Study	Study Population and End Points	ESA	Target Hb or Hct	Results	Comments
Normal Hematocrit Cardiac Trial (NHCT)[39,40]	1,265 ESRD patients with CHF or ischemic heart disease on hemodialysis *Primary end points*: Length of time to death or first MI	Epoetin alfa	Low Hct 32% (0.32) ($n = 631$) "Normal" Hct 42% (0.42) ($n = 634$)	Study was stopped before completion when the group randomized to a higher Hct target showed a trend toward higher mortality and nonfatal MI (relative risk [RR] 1.28, 95% CI 0.92–1.78)	Higher Hct target in the hemodialysis population with cardiovascular disease was not supported
Correction of Hb and Outcomes in Renal Insufficiency (CHOIR)[38]	1,432 stage 3–4 CKD patients *Primary end points*: Composite of death, MI, hospitalization for congestive heart failure, and stroke	Epoetin alfa	Low Hb 11.3 g/dL (113 g/L; 7.01 mmol/L) ($n = 717$) High Hb 13.5 g/dL (135 g/L; 8.38 mmol/L) ($n = 715$)	Study stopped before completion because of a higher risk of the composite of death, stroke, MI, and hospitalization for CHF in the group randomized to higher Hb target (hazard ratio 1.34; 95% CI 1.03–1.74)	Mean Hb for high Hb group was 12.6 g/dL (126 g/L; 7.82 mmol/L); mean Hb for low Hb group was 11.3 g/dL (113 g/L; 7.01 mmol/L) Those who reached the target Hb in the higher Hb group received larger doses of epoetin alfa (10,694 units) compared with those who achieved the target Hb in the lower Hb group (6,057 units)
Cardiovascular Risk Reduction by Early Anemia Treatment with Epoetin Beta (CREATE)[41]	603 CKD patients (primarily stage 4) *Primary end point*: Composite cardiovascular events	Epoetin beta	Partial anemia correction group: Hb 10.5–11.5 g/dL (105–115 g/L; 6.52–7.14 mmol/L) ($n = 302$) Complete anemia correction group: Hb 13–15 g/dL (130–150 g/L; 8.07–9.31 mmol/L) ($n = 301$)	No significant difference in the risk of a first cardiovascular event between the complete correction and partial correction groups (hazard ratio 0.78; 95% CI 0.53–1.14; $P = 0.20$)	More frequent dialysis initiation (42% vs. 37%, $P = 0.03$) and hypertension (30% vs. 20%, $P = 0.005$) in the group randomized to a higher Hb target
Trial to Reduce Cardiovascular Events with Aranesp Therapy (TREAT)[93]	4,038 stage 3–4 CKD patients with type 2 DM *Primary end points*: Time to the composite outcome of death or a cardiovascular event and the time to the composite outcome of death or ESRD	Darbepoetin alfa or placebo	13 g/dL (130 g/L; 8.07 mmol/L) for darbepoetin group ($n = 2,012$) Placebo group received darbepoetin as rescue therapy if Hb <9 g/dL (<90 g/L; <5.59 mmol/L) ($n = 2,026$)	No evidence of benefit with darbepoetin alfa and a trend toward harm: death or a cardiovascular event (hazard ratio for darbepoetin vs. placebo 1.05; 95% CI 0.94–1.17; $P = 0.41$). Death or ESRD (hazard ratio 1.06; 95% CI 0.95–1.19; $P = 0.29$). Fatal or nonfatal stroke (hazard ratio 1.92; 95% CI 1.38–2.68; $P < 0.001$).	Median Hb achieved was 12.5 g/dL (125 g/L; 7.76 mmol/L) in darbepoetin group and 10.6 g/dL (106 g/L; 6.58 mmol/L) in placebo group Patients with a history of cancer in the higher Hb group also had a higher risk of death

CHF, congestive heart failure; DM, diabetes mellitus; ESA, erythropoietic-stimulating agent; ESRD, end-stage renal disease.

A summary of these key trials is shown in Table 29-9. An increased risk of all-cause mortality with ESA treatment was also reported in a meta-analysis of nine randomized controlled trials that included over 5,100 CKD patients treated to Hb targets in the range of 12 to 16 g/dL (120 to 160 g/L; 7.45 to 9.93 mmol/L).[91] There was also a higher risk of dialysis access thrombosis and uncontrolled blood pressure in the higher Hb group. Subsequent analysis of the CHOIR trial has also shown an association between targeting a higher Hb and increased rate of progression of CKD.[92]

Results from the Trial to Reduce Cardiovascular Events with Aranesp Therapy (TREAT) (Table 29-9) also failed to support a higher Hb.[93] Despite the association between anemia and reduction in hospitalization and cardiovascular events that prompted many to expect positive outcomes from this study, individuals treated to the higher Hb target did not have a reduction in the primary end points. In addition, there was also an almost twofold increase in the risk of stroke (5% in the treatment group vs. 2.6% in the placebo group), a finding that was not associated with baseline characteristics of the patients or other potential risk factors.[94] Those patients with a history of cancer in the higher Hb group also had a higher risk of death, a finding that requires additional investigation.

Clinical **Controversy...**

The higher risk of mortality and cardiovascular events in CKD patients treated to achieve a higher Hb with an ESA has led to an update in targets for Hb. There are discrepancies, however, in the FDA-approved labeling for ESAs and the KDIGO and KDOQI guidelines in terms of when to initiate therapy and the target Hb. There are also practitioners who advocate that for patients without specific cardiovascular risk factors (e.g., atherosclerosis), a Hb of 11 to 12 g/dL (120 to 130 g/L) or greater achieved with low-dose ESA is reasonable. Healthcare providers must weigh the risks and benefits of ESA use in individual patients and consider the reimbursement structure for ESAs and iron in the practice environment when making decisions about anemia management.

The association of poor outcomes with the dose of ESA used in the aforementioned studies has raised concern. Subsequent analysis of the CHOIR study showed that high-dose ESA use was associated with greater risk of death.[95] Those individuals able to achieve the target Hb in the CHOIR study did not have worse outcomes. Further analysis of the NHCT data also showed a reduction in mortality by 60% for those individuals who responded to epoetin therapy compared with nonresponders.[96] Such findings have led to discussion of whether hyporesponsiveness to ESAs due to other conditions such as inflammation may explain the higher event rates in this group of individuals. The overall negative cardiovascular outcomes observed with higher Hb targets in the randomized trials have prompted much discussion about the potential causes, including not only ESA dose and Hb target but also the rate of rise in Hb and the variability in Hb over time (e.g., degree of fluctuation in Hb).[97]

Since the CHOIR and CREATE trials in 2006 and evaluation of subsequent reports calling into question the safety of ESAs, there have been several FDA advisories and changes made to ESA product labeling for more conservative use of ESAs. The most recent was in June 2011 when the FDA notified healthcare professionals of modified recommendations.[98] ESA manufacturers revised the precautions, black box warning, and dosing sections of ESA product labeling. The labeling for all ESAs warns that dosing ESAs to target Hb levels greater than 11 g/dL (110 g/L; 6.83 mmol/L) for CKD patients increases the risk for death, serious cardiovascular reactions, and stroke.[99–102] Practitioners are advised to consider ESAs in patients with CKD only when the Hb is below 10 g/dL (100 g/L; 6.21 mmol/L) and to individualize therapy to use the lowest ESA dose necessary to decrease the need for red blood cell transfusions.

Of note, recommendations in the revised product labeling differ from the target of 11 to 12 g/dL (110 to 120 g/L; 6.83 to 7.45 mmol/L) recommended in the KDOQI guidelines for management of anemia of CKD and from the previous labeling that recommended a target of 10 to 12 g/dL (100 to 120 g/L; 6.21 to 7.45 mmol/L) in ESA-treated patients with CKD.[103] KDIGO anemia guidelines from 2012 are shown in Table 29-8. It is important to consider that in making the recommendations regarding Hb targets listed in Table 29-8, the KDIGO expert panel considered the quality of the evidence to be *low* or *very* low. Clinicians should always take into account trends in Hb when adjusting ESA doses. Before making treatment decisions, prescribers must weigh the risks of ESA use and higher Hb values against the benefit of fewer blood transfusions and ensure that patients understand these risks and benefits.

Iron Status

Iron supplementation is required by most CKD patients receiving an ESA because of the increased iron demand that results from stimulation of red blood cell production. As CKD worsens, a progressive decline in Hb despite ESA therapy may be observed. Iron indices that should be monitored include the TSat, an indicator of iron immediately available for delivery to the bone marrow, and serum ferritin, an indirect measure of storage iron. The content of hemoglobin in reticulocytes (CHr) is also recommended as a parameter to assess iron status in hemodialysis patients, although it is not commonly used in clinical practice. Transferrin is the carrier protein for iron and, as a protein, may be affected by nutritional status. Serum ferritin is an acute-phase reactant, meaning it may be elevated under certain inflammatory conditions and give a false indication of storage iron. Previous versions of the KDOQI anemia guidelines recommended an upper level for TSat of 50% (0.50) and serum ferritin of 800 ng/mL (800 mcg/L; 1,800 pmol/L) to reduce the risk of iron overload. No upper level for these iron indices has been established in the current recommendations; however, the guidelines state that there is insufficient evidence to recommend routine administration of IV iron if the patient's serum ferritin level is greater than 500 ng/mL (500 mcg/L; 1,100 pmol/L).[51] KDIGO guidelines do not suggest stringent iron indices, but do recommend that iron supplementation be administered if TSat is ≤30% (≤0.30) and serum ferritin is ≤500 ng/mL (≤500 mcg/L; ≤1,100 pmol/L) if the goal is to increase the Hb or decrease the ESA dose (Table 29-8).[42] Since ferritin is an acute-phase reactant, the decision of whether to give IV iron in conditions of elevated ferritin must be based on objective parameters such as TSat and Hb in addition to the clinical condition of the patient (e.g., infection, inflammation).

Iron supplementation is required for *absolute iron deficiency*, when whole-body iron stores are low, but may also be required in individuals with *functional iron deficiency*. In the latter condition the individual with anemia may have a low TSat, but a serum ferritin at or above goal. In this situation iron stores fail to release iron rapidly enough to satisfy the demands for erythropoiesis. It has been shown that anemic hemodialysis patients with a TSat less than 25% (0.25) and serum ferritin between 200 and 1,200 ng/mL (200 and 1,200 mcg/L; 450 and 2,700 pmol/L) had an improved response to ESAs when they also received a 1 g course of IV iron.[104]

Nonpharmacologic Therapy

Nonpharmacologic therapy for anemia of CKD includes maintaining adequate dietary intake of iron as well as folate and B_{12}. Patients on hemodialysis or peritoneal dialysis should be routinely supplemented with water-soluble vitamins (vitamins B, C, and folic acid) as these vitamins are often depleted with dialysis therapy. A relatively small amount of dietary iron, approximately 1 to 2 mg (or approximately 10%), is absorbed each day, primarily in the duodenum. Although there is some debate as to whether GI absorption of iron is significantly altered in patients with severe CKD, it is clear that oral intake from dietary sources alone is insufficient to meet the increased iron requirements from initiation of ESA therapy.

Pharmacologic Therapy

9 Pharmacologic therapy for anemia of CKD is based on a foundation of ESA therapy to correct erythropoietin deficiency and iron supplementation to correct and prevent iron deficiency caused by ongoing blood loss and increased iron demands associated with the initiation of erythropoietic therapy. Iron supplementation is first-line therapy for anemia of CKD if iron deficiency is diagnosed, and for some patients the target Hb may be achieved without concomitant ESA therapy. For most individuals with advanced CKD, however, combined therapy with iron and an ESA is required.

Iron Supplementation Iron supplements provide the elemental iron required for production of Hb and its subsequent incorporation in red blood cells, the net result of which is an increase in the transportation of oxygen to tissues.

Therapeutic Options Options for iron supplementation include oral and IV therapy. Oral iron preparations include ferrous salts (ferrous sulfate, ferrous fumarate, and ferrous gluconate), polysaccharide iron complex, and a heme iron polypeptide formulation. Numerous nonprescription products are available and differ in their content of elemental iron. Approximately 10% of orally administered iron is absorbed in the duodenum and upper jejunum. Absorption of iron is decreased by food and achlorhydria. The heme form of oral iron binds to a different receptor in the GI tract than nonheme iron, is absorbed to a greater extent, and may be better tolerated.[105] Some oral iron formulations also include ascorbic acid to enhance iron absorption. Serum iron concentrations and the area under the curve are not useful to assess efficacy due to the complex regulation of iron uptake by erythrocytes and incorporation as iron stores following administration.[106]

TABLE 29-10 IV Iron Preparations[107–111]

Iron Compounds	Brand Names	Half-Life (Hours)	FDA-Approved Indications	FDA-Approved Dosing	Dose Ranges (mg)[a]
Iron dextran	INFeD[b] Dexferrum[b]	40–60	Patients with iron deficiency in whom oral iron is unsatisfactory	100 mg over 2 minutes (25-mg test dose required)	25–1,000[a]
Sodium ferric gluconate	Ferrlecit[c] Nulecit[c]	1	Adult and pediatric HD patients aged 6 years and older receiving ESA therapy	Adult: 125 mg over 10 minutes or 125 mg in 100 mL of 0.9% NaCl over 60 minutes Pediatric: 1.5 mg/kg in 25 mL of 0.9% NaCl over 60 minutes; maximum dose 125 mg per dose	62.5–1,000[a]
Iron sucrose	Venofer[d]	6	Adult and pediatric HD patients aged 2 years and older	Adult: 100 mg over 2–5 minutes or 100 mg in maximum of 100 mL of 0.9% NaCl over 15 minutes per consecutive HD session Pediatric: 0.5 mg/kg not to exceed 100 mg per dose over 5 minutes or diluted in 25 mL of 0.9% NaCl administered over 5–60 minutes	25–1,000[a]
			Adult and pediatric nondialysis CKD patients aged 2 years and older	Adult: 200 mg over 2–5 minutes on five different occasions within 14-day period Pediatric: see HD dosing above	
			Adult and pediatric PD patients aged 2 years and older	Adult: two infusions, 14 days apart, of 300 mg in a maximum of 250 mL of 0.9% NaCl over 1.5 hours, followed by one infusion, 14 days later, of 400 mg in a maximum of 250 mL of 0.9% NaCl over 2.5 hours Pediatric: see HD dosing above	
Ferumoxytol	Feraheme[e]	15	Adult patients with iron-deficiency anemia associated with chronic kidney disease	510 mg (17 mL) as a single dose, followed by a second 510 mg dose 3–8 days after the initial dose (rate of 1 mL or 30 mg/s)	510 mg

CKD, chronic kidney disease; ESA, erythropoietin-stimulating agent; HD, hemodialysis; PD, peritoneal dialysis.
[a]Small doses (e.g., 25–150 mg/wk) generally used for maintenance regimens. Larger doses (e.g., 1 g) should be administered in divided doses.
[b]Supplied in 1-mL (Dexferrum) and 2-mL (Dexferrum and InFeD) single-dose vials containing 50 mg of elemental iron/mL.
[c]Available in 5-mL glass ampules or vials containing 62.5 mg elemental iron.
[d]Supplied in 2.5-, 5-, and 10-mL single-dose vials containing 20 mg/mL.
[e]Supplied as a 17-mL single-use vial containing 510 mg elemental iron (30 mg/mL).

IV iron preparations are colloids that consist of an iron-containing core that is surrounded by a carbohydrate shell to stabilize the iron complex. Available agents differ in the size of the core and the composition of the surrounding carbohydrate. These differences affect the rate of dissociation of iron from the complex to phagocytes within the reticuloendothelial system where iron is either stored or released to the extracellular carrier protein transferrin, which transports iron to the bone marrow for red blood cell production.

Five IV iron products are currently available in the United States (see Table 29-10): two composed of iron dextran (INFeD®, molecular weight [MW] 96 kDa; and Dexferrum®, MW 265 kDa), sodium ferric gluconate (Ferrlecit® and Nulecit®, MW 350 kDa), iron sucrose (Venofer®, MW 43 kDa), and ferumoxytol (Feraheme®, MW 750 kDa).[107–112]

Either oral or IV administration of iron is recommended in stage 3 to 4 CKD patients and those receiving peritoneal dialysis. Oral iron supplementation is more convenient for those patients who do not have regular IV access; however, at some point they are likely to require IV iron supplementation to meet iron needs and correct absolute iron deficiency, especially if they are receiving an ESA. In HD patients with ESRD, GI absorption of iron is often inadequate to meet the increase in iron demand from ESA therapy and chronic blood loss. KDOQI guidelines recommend IV iron as the preferred route of administration in the HD population.[51] Parenteral iron improves the responsiveness to ESA therapy and thus lower doses can be used to maintain the target Hb in hemodialysis patients.

Iron administration in patients with functional iron deficiency is questionable. A trial of IV iron therapy may be warranted if the Hb is less than desired.[104]

Adverse Effects Adverse effects of oral iron are primarily GI in nature and include constipation, nausea, and abdominal cramping. These adverse effects are more likely as the dose is escalated and may be present in more than 50% of patients receiving 200 mg of elemental iron per day. These unfavorable effects often discourage patients from taking these medications on a chronic basis. Some of these GI side effects can be minimized if oral iron products are taken with food; however, food may decrease absorption of oral iron.

Adverse effects of IV iron include allergic reactions, hypotension, dizziness, dyspnea, headaches, lower back pain, arthralgia, syncope, and arthritis. Some of these reactions, in particular hypotension, can be minimized by decreasing the dose or rate of infusion of iron. The most concerning potential consequence of IV iron administration is anaphylaxis. Anaphylactic reactions to iron dextran have been reported in up to 1.8% of patients, with serious reactions including respiratory complications and cardiovascular collapse occurring in approximately 0.6% to 0.7% of patients.[42] Such reactions are believed to be partly a response to antibody formation to the dextran component. Adverse reactions have been reported more frequently in those receiving Dexferrum compared with INFeD.[42]

Sodium ferric gluconate, iron sucrose, and ferumoxytol have a better safety record than either of the iron dextran products, based on their history of use in Europe over the last 4 decades (sodium ferric gluconate and iron sucrose) and data in the United States since these products were approved. A comparison of adverse event rates reported to the FDA for IV iron products revealed that ferumoxytol had higher rates of adverse events than sodium ferric gluconate or iron sucrose.[113] Serious adverse events including anaphylactic-type reactions and cardiac arrest prompted a change in the product labeling postmarketing.[110] As a superparamagnetic oxide, ferumoxytol may affect the diagnostic ability of magnetic resonance imaging studies; therefore, these imaging studies should be done prior to administration of ferumoxytol when possible. These effects may persist for up to 3 months following administration of ferumoxytol. Ferumoxytol will not interfere with x-ray, computed tomography, positron emission tomography, single photon emission computed tomography, ultrasonography, or nuclear medicine imaging.[110]

Administration of IV iron also introduces a risk of iron overload. Deposition of excess iron may affect several organ systems, leading to hepatic, pancreatic, and cardiac dysfunction. Bone marrow biopsy provides the most definitive diagnosis of iron overload, but because it is an extremely invasive procedure, it is not widely employed in most clinical settings. Maintaining serum ferritin and TSat values that demonstrate efficacy in preventing iron deficiency, yet are safe, is the most reasonable approach to minimize the risk of iron toxicity. The challenge is in defining these upper limits, particularly for serum ferritin, which may be elevated in inflammatory conditions and not reflective of true iron stores in such situations. If symptomatic overload does occur, deferoxamine (Desferal), deferiprone (Ferriprox), or phlebotomy may be necessary.

Dosing and Administration If oral therapy is initiated, the recommended dose is 200 mg of elemental iron per day. With numerous oral agents to choose from, the best option is one that provides adequate elemental iron with the fewest number of dosage units required per day. KDIGO guidelines suggest a 1- to 3-month trial of oral therapy in the nondialysis CKD population.[42] For the hemodialysis population, administration of 1 g of IV iron is recommended to initially replete patients with an absolute iron deficiency. Typical repletion dosing regimens for IV iron are 100 mg as iron sucrose or iron dextran over 10 dialysis sessions, or 125 mg of sodium ferric gluconate over 8 dialysis sessions (see Table 29-10). Ferumoxytol is administered as 510 mg at a rate not to exceed 30 mg/s (1 mL/s) with a second dose given within 3 to 8 days, a higher dose and administration rate compared with other available IV iron formulations.[110] Without ongoing iron supplementation, many patients quickly become iron deficient. To prevent iron deficiency, maintenance doses of IV iron are administered in hemodialysis patients (e.g., iron sucrose or iron dextran 25 to 100 mg/wk; sodium ferric gluconate 62.5 to 125 mg/wk) based on evidence of improved Hb and lower ESA doses with these regimens.[42,51]

Administration of a 25 mg test dose is required for all iron dextran products. This test dose should be administered over at least 30 seconds for InFeD and 5 minutes for Dexferrum.[107,108] It is recommended that a period of ≥1 hour lapse before administering the remainder of the dose. Patients receiving any of the non-dextran IV iron agents should be closely observed for signs of hypersensitivity during and for at least 30 minutes after administration.[109–111] KDIGO guidelines advocate monitoring for 60 minutes following an infusion of any available IV iron product, with a stronger emphasis on this recommendation for iron dextran products.[42]

The safety and efficacy of high-dose IV iron regimens have been evaluated. Iron dextran has been safely administered to dialysis patients in total-dose infusions ranging from 400 mg to 2 g and to patients with stage 3 or 4 CKD at doses of up to 500 mg.[114,115] Sodium ferric gluconate has been safely administered at doses of 250 mg infused over 1 hour (4.2 mg/min).[116] Iron sucrose at doses of up to 500 mg administered over 3 hours on consecutive days has been successful in maintaining iron stores without causing serious adverse events.[117] Higher-dose regimens for iron sucrose have been approved in patients with early stage CKD and peritoneal dialysis patients (see Table 29-10), populations in whom administration of higher doses is more convenient as these patients are seen less frequently by healthcare providers than the hemodialysis population.[111] As a general practice, if IV iron doses higher than those currently approved are used in practice, they should be administered over at least 2 to 4 hours depending on the dose due to the risk of hypersensitivity reactions, hypotension, dizziness, and nausea.

Although there are conflicting reports, most clinicians believe that exposure to iron may contribute to the risk of bacterial infection because iron is used by microorganisms for metabolic functions. The association of IV iron with oxidative stress, acceleration of atherosclerosis, and other cardiovascular conditions has also been suggested.[118] These potential long-term risks of IV iron therapy are not clearly defined, and there are no data confirming unequivocally that aggressive use of IV iron in CKD patients treated with ESA therapy increases patient morbidity or mortality. KDIGO guidelines suggest that IV iron be avoided in patients with active systemic infections.[42]

Erythropoietic-Stimulating Agent Therapy

Since FDA approval of epoetin alfa in 1989, ESA therapy has become an integral part of the care for patients with CKD. ESAs available in the United States include epoetin alfa (distributed as Epogen and Procrit), and darbepoetin alfa (Aranesp).[99–101] Peginesatide, a synthetic, pegylated peptide that has no amino acid sequence homology to erythropoietin, was available in March 2012 and approved for use in dialysis patients, but was withdrawn from the market in early 2013 due to reports of serious adverse events.[102]

Pharmacology and Mechanism of Action Epoetin alfa is a glycoprotein manufactured by recombinant DNA technology that has the same amino acid sequence as endogenous erythropoietin. Darbepoetin alfa has two additional *N*-linked carbohydrate chains that decrease the affinity for the erythropoietin receptor, but yield a longer duration of activity compared with erythropoietin. All ESAs have the same biologic activity as endogenous erythropoietin in that they bind to and activate the erythropoietin receptor to stimulate erythropoiesis.

Pharmacokinetics and Pharmacodynamics All available ESAs may be administered by either the IV or the SubQ route. Although bioavailability is less with SubQ than with IV administration, the prolonged absorption phase leads to an extended half-life (see Table 29-11). The prolonged half-life with SubQ administration leads to a more sustained physiologic stimulation of erythroid precursors. Trials have shown that the same target Hb can be achieved and maintained at SubQ epoetin doses 15% to 30% lower than IV doses.[51,119] The prolonged half-life of darbepoetin offers the advantage of less-frequent dosing, starting at once a week or once every other week. This is of particular benefit in stage 4 and 5 CKD patients who are not yet receiving dialysis and those receiving peritoneal dialysis since these patients are not in a clinical setting as frequently as hemodialysis patients and do not have regular IV access.

The pharmacodynamics of ESAs is important to consider when evaluating response to therapy. With initiation of ESA therapy or a change in dose, the Hb may begin to rise as the result of demargination of reticulocytes; however, it takes approximately 10 days before erythrocyte progenitor cells mature and are released into the circulation. The Hb continues to increase until the life span of the cells stimulated by ESA therapy is reached (mean 2 months; range 1 to 4 months in patients with ESRD). At this point a new

TABLE 29-11 Erythropoietic-Stimulating Agents[99–101]

Drug Name	Brand Name(s)	Starting Dose in Adults	Route of Administration[a]	Half-Life (Hours)
Epoetin alfa	Epogen, Procrit	50–100 units/kg once weekly or every 2 weeks (ND-CKD) 50-100 units/kg one to three times per week (HD or PD-CKD)	IV or subcutaneous	8.5 (IV) 24 (subcutaneous)
Darbepoetin alfa	Aranesp	0.45 mcg/kg once every 4 weeks (ND-CKD) 0.45 mcg/kg once per week or 0.75 mcg/kg every 2 weeks (HD or PD-CKD)	IV or subcutaneous	25 (IV) 48 (subcutaneous)

[a]The IV route is recommended in the hemodialysis population.

steady state is achieved (i.e., the rate at which red blood cells are being produced equals the rate at which they are leaving the circulation). For this reason it is important to evaluate the Hb response over several weeks.

Efficacy Patients will generally respond to ESA therapy in a dose-related fashion. The most common causes of resistance are iron deficiency, acute illness, catheter insertion, hypoalbuminemia, elevated C-reactive protein, chronic bleeding, aluminum toxicity, malnutrition, hyperparathyroidism, cancer and chemotherapy, HIV, inflammation, and infection.[51] Deficiencies in folate and vitamin B_{12} should also be considered as potential causes of resistance to ESA therapy, as both are essential for optimal erythropoiesis.

Adverse Effects Hypertension is the most common adverse event reported with ESAs and may be associated with the rate of rise in Hb.[51] Protocols established in some clinical settings recommend withholding ESA therapy if blood pressure is above a defined threshold. KDOQI guidelines for anemia do not recommend withholding ESA therapy for elevated blood pressure, but instead advocate more judicious use of antihypertensive agents and dialysis to control blood pressure; however, according to FDA-approved product labeling, ESAs should not be used in those with uncontrolled blood pressure.[99–101] Seizures have occurred in patients treated with epoetin, particularly within the first 90 days of starting therapy. Vascular access thrombosis may also be more frequent during ESA therapy.[42] The potential for these adverse effects calls for close monitoring of the rate of rise in Hb, changes in blood pressure, and neurologic symptoms following initiation of therapy or a change in ESA dose.

Antibody-associated pure red cell aplasia (PRCA) was reported in the late 1990s and early in 2000, but there have been very few cases since that time. An evaluation for PRCA should be considered for patients receiving ESA therapy for more than 8 weeks who develop either a rapid decrease in Hb level (rate of 0.5 to 1 g/dL/wk [5 to 10 g/L/wk; 0.31 to 0.62 mmol/L/wk]) or require one to two blood transfusions per week, and have an absolute reticulocyte count of less than 10,000/μL (10×10^9/L) with a normal platelet and white blood cell count.[42] Discontinuation of ESA therapy is recommended in antibody-mediated PRCA because antibodies are cross-reactive and continued exposure may lead to anaphylactic reactions. Immunosuppressive therapy has been effective in up to 50% of patients with PRCA.[120] No cases of PRCA were reported with peginesatide in initial clinical trials and there is evidence that peginesatide stimulates erythropoiesis in conditions of PRCA or hyporesponsiveness due to antierythropoietin antibodies.[121]

Drug–Drug Interactions No significant drug interactions have been reported with the available ESAs.

Dosing and Administration Recommended starting doses of ESA are listed in Table 29-11. Less frequent dosing of epoetin alfa (e.g., every 1 to 2 weeks) is effective and may be preferred for stage 3 and 4 CKD patients since these patients are seen in the outpatient clinical setting on a relatively infrequent basis.[122] Subcutaneous dosing is also more convenient in this population and in peritoneal dialysis patients who do not have regular IV access. Conversion tables for patients who are to be switched from epoetin alfa (units per week) to darbepoetin alfa (micrograms per week) are available in the labeling information for darbepoetin.[101]

When starting an ESA, Hb levels should be monitored at least weekly until stable and then at least monthly. Dose adjustments should be made based on Hb response with consideration of data on risks associated with higher Hb levels and rate of rise in Hb. An acceptable rate of increase in Hb is 1 to 2 g/dL (10 to 20 g/L; 0.62 to 1.24 mmol/L) per month. As a general rule, ESA doses should not be increased more frequently than every 4 weeks, although decreases in dose may occur more frequently in response to a rapid rate of rise in Hb. Based on labeling for ESAs, the dose should be reduced by at least 25% if the Hb increases by more than 1 g/dL (10 g/L; 0.62 mmol/L) in a 2-week period. The dose should be reduced or temporarily discontinued if the Hb level approaches or exceeds 11 g/dL (110 g/L; 6.83 mmol/L) in dialysis patients (all ESAs) or 10 g/dL (100 g/L; 6.21 mmol/L) in patients with CKD not requiring dialysis. KDIGO recommendations advocate a decrease in dose as opposed to withholding the ESA when a decrease in Hb concentration is desired.[42] A 25% increase in dose may be considered if the Hb has not increased by 1 g/dL (10 g/L; 0.62 mmol/L) after 4 weeks of ESA treatment and if no causes of resistance to the ESA have been identified. For patients who do not respond adequately over a 12-week escalation period, an increase in ESA dose is unlikely to improve response and may increase risks. Initial hyporesponsiveness to ESAs should be considered when there is no increase in Hb from baseline after the first month of appropriate weight-based dosing. Acquired ESA hyporesponsiveness may be suspected when patients previously on a stable ESA dose require two increases in ESA doses up to 50% beyond the stable dose.[42] In these situations repeat escalations in ESA dose beyond double the initial weight-based dose should be avoided. The lowest dose of ESA should be used to maintain a Hb level sufficient to reduce the need for RBC transfusions.[99–101] Figure 29-6 provides an approach to management of anemia using ESAs and iron therapy in patients with CKD.

Transfusions and Adjunct Therapies Red blood cell transfusions carry many risks and therefore should only be used in select situations, such as acute management of symptomatic anemia, following significant acute blood loss, and prior to surgical procedures that carry a high risk of blood loss, with the goal of preventing inadequate tissue oxygenation or cardiac failure. L-Carnitine supplementation and vitamin C were previously suggested as adjunctive treatments of anemia associated with kidney disease, but are not recommended because of the lack of evidence supporting improved anemia management with these therapies.[42]

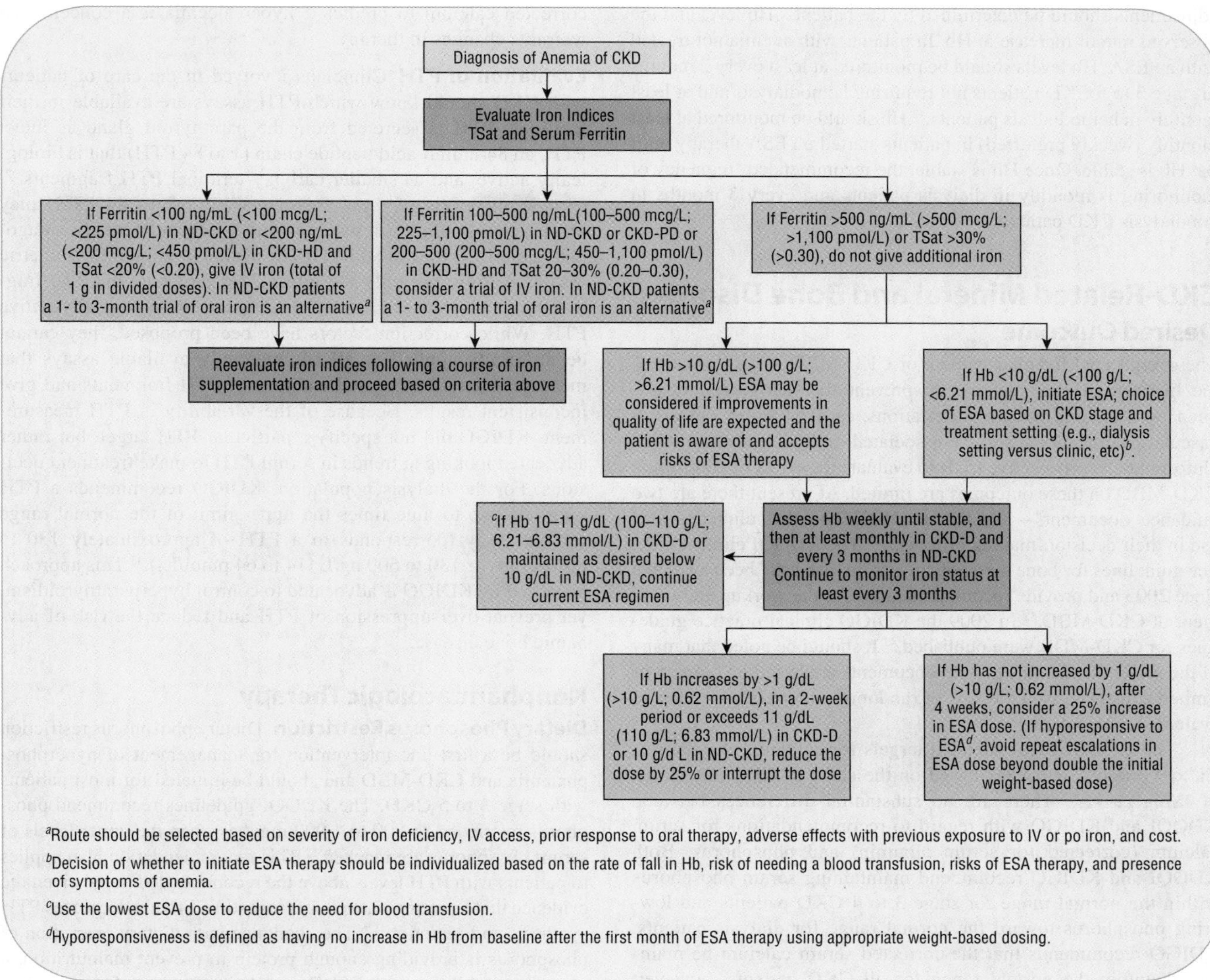

Diagnosis of Anemia of CKD
Evaluate Iron Indices TSat and Serum Ferritin
If Ferritin <100 ng/mL (<100 mcg/L; <225 pmol/L) in ND-CKD or <200 ng/mL (<200 mcg/L; <450 pmol/L) in CKD-HD and TSat <20% (<0.20), give IV iron (total of 1 g in divided doses). In ND-CKD patients a 1- to 3-month trial of oral iron is an alternative[a]
If Ferritin 100–500 ng/mL(100–500 mcg/L; 225–1,100 pmol/L) in ND-CKD or CKD-PD or 200–500 (200–500 mcg/L; 450–1,100 pmol/L) in CKD-HD and TSat 20–30% (0.20–0.30), consider a trial of IV iron. In ND-CKD patients a 1- to 3-month trial of oral iron is an alternative[a]
If Ferritin >500 ng/mL (>500 mcg/L; >1,100 pmol/L) or TSat >30% (>0.30), do not give additional iron
Reevaluate iron indices following a course of iron supplementation and proceed based on criteria above
If Hb >10 g/dL (>100 g/L; >6.21 mmol/L) ESA may be considered if improvements in quality of life are expected and the patient is aware of and accepts risks of ESA therapy
If Hb <10 g/dL (<100 g/L; <6.21 mmol/L), initiate ESA; choice of ESA based on CKD stage and treatment setting (e.g., dialysis setting versus clinic, etc)[b].
[c]If Hb 10–11 g/dL (100–110 g/L; 6.21–6.83 mmol/L) in CKD-D or maintained as desired below 10 g/dL in ND-CKD, continue current ESA regimen
Assess Hb weekly until stable, and then at least monthly in CKD-D and every 3 months in ND-CKD Continue to monitor iron status at least every 3 months
If Hb increases by >1 g/dL (>10 g/L; 0.62 mmol/L), in a 2-week period or exceeds 11 g/dL (110 g/L; 6.83 mmol/L) in CKD-D or 10 g/d L in ND-CKD, reduce the dose by 25% or interrupt the dose
If Hb has not increased by 1 g/dL (>10 g/L; 0.62 mmol/L), after 4 weeks, consider a 25% increase in ESA dose. (If hyporesponsive to ESA[d], avoid repeat escalations in ESA dose beyond double the initial weight-based dose)
[a]Route should be selected based on severity of iron deficiency, IV access, prior response to oral therapy, adverse effects with previous exposure to IV or po iron, and cost.
[b]Decision of whether to initiate ESA therapy should be individualized based on the rate of fall in Hb, risk of needing a blood transfusion, risks of ESA therapy, and presence of symptoms of anemia.
[c]Use the lowest ESA dose to reduce the need for blood transfusion.
[d]Hyporesponsiveness is defined as having no increase in Hb from baseline after the first month of ESA therapy using appropriate weight-based dosing.

FIGURE 29-6 Algorithm for management of anemia using iron and ESA therapy.[42]

Personalized Pharmacotherapy

Despite the fact that anemia is common in the CKD population and treatment guidelines are available, management cannot be standardized for all patients. The labeling changes for ESAs do not recommend a specific Hb target for all patients, but rather an individualized approach that considers risks of using ESAs, the rate of increase in Hb, the likelihood of requiring a blood transfusion, and other clinical conditions. For example, a lower ESA dose may be rational for a patient with a history of CVD, thromboembolism, or uncontrolled high blood pressure. The decision to withhold ESA therapy should be considered in patients with a history of malignancy (particularly active malignancy when cure is expected) or stroke. Conservative use of ESAs and lower Hb goals may also be desired in a patient with a high likelihood of a transplant where exposure to blood transfusions increases the risk of developing antibodies to multiple human leukocyte antigens and decreases their success in finding an appropriate donor match. While risks of targeting a Hb above 11 g/dL (110 g/L; 6.83 mmol/L) have been demonstrated, the precise Hb range to target and when to start therapy may also depend more on other factors including the patient-perceived quality of life. Improvements in patient-reported fatigue, energy level, sense of vitality, and physical functioning with anemia treatment have been demonstrated.[123] Patients should be informed of the risks of ESA therapy, but also the potential benefits from the patient perspective. This is one rationale for having ESAs under the REMS program.

The concerns for patient safety, the need for more stringent control of Hb levels, and cost of ESA therapy have also led to development of anemia management clinics. Pharmacist-managed clinics have shown Hb values within the target range and lower ESA usage compared with physician-based care and may be an ideal environment for an individualized approach to manage anemia of CKD.[124]

Evaluation of Therapeutic Outcomes

Iron status should be assessed at least every 3 months in patients receiving a stable ESA regimen or for those hemodialysis patients not treated with an ESA to detect iron deficiency as a cause for anemia.[42,51] Iron status should be monitored more frequently (e.g., every month) when initiating or increasing the ESA dose, following a course of IV iron, or when other factors put the patient at risk for iron loss (e.g., bleeding). For all ESAs, the initial dose and subsequent adjustments should be determined by the patient's Hb level and the observed rate of increase in Hb. In patients with anemia not treated with an ESA, Hb levels should be monitored at least every 3 months in stage 3 to 5 CKD patients not requiring hemodialysis and at least monthly in hemodialysis patients.[42] Hb should be monitored at least monthly (weekly preferred) in patients started on ESA therapy until the Hb is stable. Once Hb is stable, the recommended frequency of monitoring is monthly in dialysis patients and every 3 months in nondialysis CKD patients (see Fig. 29-6).

CKD-Related Mineral and Bone Disorder

Desired Outcome

The overall goal for management of CKD-MBD is to "normalize" the biochemical parameters and prevent the detrimental consequences, including bone manifestations, cardiovascular and extravascular calcifications, and the associated morbidity and mortality. Unfortunately, prospective trials to evaluate the effect of controlling CKD-MBD on these outcomes are limited. At present there are two guidance documents—KDOQI and KDIGO—that clinicians can use in their decision-making process.[43,52] The KDOQI clinical practice guidelines for bone metabolism and disease have been available since 2003 and provide recommendations for the workup and treatment of CKD-MBD.[52] In 2009 the KDIGO clinical practice guidelines for CKD-MDB were published.[43] It should be noted that many of the recommendations in both documents are based on opinion or limited evidence given the lack of randomized controlled studies to evaluate treatment outcomes.

The KDOQI-recommended targets for calcium, phosphorus, Ca × P product, and PTH based on the stage of CKD are shown in Table 29-12.[52] There are no substantial differences between KDOQI and KDIGO with regard to recommendations for serum calcium (corrected for serum albumin) and phosphorus. Both KDOQI and KDIGO recommend maintaining serum phosphorus within the normal range for stage 3 to 4 CKD patients and lowering phosphorus toward the normal range for dialysis patients. KDIGO recommends that the corrected serum calcium be maintained within the normal range for all CKD patients; however, KDOQI recommends a more conservative range in stage 5 CKD patients based on an increased risk of soft-tissue and vascular calcifications. The most appropriate strategy is to evaluate trends in corrected calcium to predict if hypercalcemia is a concern that warrants changes in therapy.

Evaluation of PTH Clinicians involved in the care of patients with CKD should know which PTH assays are available in their facilities. PTH is secreted from the parathyroid gland as intact PTH, an 84-amino-acid peptide chain (1 to 84 PTH) that is biologically active, and as smaller carboxy-terminal PTH fragments.[125] Circulating levels of these fragments (e.g., 7 to 84 PTH) may increase substantially in patients with CKD and actively antagonize the effects to 1 to 84 PTH. The available immunoradiometric assays measure not only the intact PTH molecule but also fragments, which may lead to overestimation of biologically active PTH. While correction factors have been proposed, they cannot be uniformly applied to all commercially available assays that measure different types and amounts of PTH fragments and give inconsistent results. Because of the variability in PTH measurement, KDIGO did not specify a particular PTH target, but rather advocated looking at trends in serum PTH to make treatment decisions. For the dialysis population, KDIGO recommends a PTH range of two to nine times the upper limit of the normal range for the assay (corresponds to a PTH of approximately 130 to 600 pg/mL or 130 to 600 ng/L [14 to 64 pmol/L]).[43] This approach proposed by KDIGO is advocated to control hyperparathyroidism, yet prevent oversuppression of PTH and reduce the risk of adynamic bone disease.

TABLE 29-12 Guidelines for Calcium, Phosphorus, Calcium–Phosphorus Product, and Parathyroid Hormone[43,52]

	Chronic Kidney Disease[a]		
Parameter	**Stage 3**	**Stage 4**	**Stage 5**
Corrected calcium	"Normal range"	"Normal range"	8.4–9.5 mg/dL[b] (2.10–2.38 mmol/L)
Phosphorus	2.7–4.6 mg/dL[c]	2.7–4.6 mg/dL[c]	3.5–5.5 mg/dL[d]
Ca × P product	<55 mg^2/dL^2[e]	<55 mg^2/dL^2[e]	<55 mg^2/dL^2[e]
Intact parathyroid hormone	35–70 pg/mL[f]	70–110 pg/mL[g]	150–300 pg/mL[h]

[a]Differences with Kidney Disease: Improving Global Outcomes (KDIGO) described in text (see Desired Outcome under CKD-Related Mineral and Bone Disorder in text).
[b]Recommend normal range for laboratory used, but keep target at lower end of range.
[c]SI units: 0.87–1.49 mmol/L.
[d]SI units: 1.13–1.78 mmol/L.
[e]SI units: 4.4 $mmol^2/L^2$.
[f]SI units: in ng/L or 3.7–7.5 pmol/L.
[g]SI units: in ng/L or 7.5–11.8 pmol/L.
[h]SI units: in ng/L or 16–32 pmol/L.

Nonpharmacologic Therapy

Dietary Phosphorus Restriction Dietary phosphorus restriction should be a first-line intervention for management of hyperphosphatemia and CKD-MBD and should be initiated for most patients with stage 3 to 5 CKD. The KDOQI guidelines recommend phosphorus restriction to 800 to 1,000 mg/day when the upper levels of serum phosphorus are reached.[52] This recommendation also applies to patients with PTH levels above the recommended range given the evidence that lowering phosphorus ingestion directly decreases PTH synthesis and secretion.[126] The challenge with dietary restriction of phosphorus is providing enough protein to prevent malnutrition, a common problem in the ESRD population because foods high in phosphorus are generally high in protein. Examples of foods or beverages that contain high amounts of phosphorus include meats, dairy products, dried beans, nuts, colas, peanut butter, and beer. Nutritional goals must be evaluated on an individual basis, preferably by a dietitian specializing in the care of CKD patients. Dialysis patients require a higher protein intake (1.2 to 1.3 g/kg/day), making restriction of phosphorus even more challenging.

One of the most common obstacles to dietary phosphorus restriction is patient nonadherence because of the poor palatability of the allowed foods. Regular counseling by a dietitian is necessary to design a realistic diet that works with the patient's lifestyle.

Dialysis Hemodialysis and peritoneal dialysis lower serum phosphorus and calcium, the extent of which is dependent on concentration of each in the dialysate and the duration of dialysis. The dialysate calcium concentration in hemodialysis or peritoneal dialysis should be between 2.5 and 3 mEq/L (1.25 and 1.5 mmol/L).[43,52] Removal of phosphorus does occur with peritoneal dialysis and hemodialysis (approximately 2 to 3 g/wk, dependent on the dialysis prescription); however, dialysis alone does not usually control hyperphosphatemia. Patients on daily hemodialysis or nocturnal hemodialysis who typically have longer and/or more frequent dialysis sessions may have better phosphorus control and require fewer phosphate-binding agents due to increased phosphorus removal.[127]

Parathyroidectomy Parathyroidectomy is a therapeutic option for patients with severe CKD-MBD who do not respond to pharmacologic therapy. Surgery is recommended for those patients with persistently elevated PTH (PTH >800 pg/mL [>800 ng/L; >86 pmol/L]) associated with hypercalcemia and/or hyperphosphatemia who are refractory to medical therapy.[52] Surgical approaches include either subtotal parathyroidectomy or total parathyroidectomy with autotransplantation of parathyroid tissue to an accessible site, such as the forearm. Postoperative hypocalcemia, hypophosphatemia, and hypomagnesemia may occur because of a marked increase in bone production in relation to bone absorption ("hungry bone syndrome"). Following surgery frequent monitoring of calcium and phosphorus is necessary. Treatment with supplemental calcium and vitamin D may be required for weeks or months.

Pharmacologic Therapy

Phosphate-Binding Agents Patients with CKD, especially those with ESRD, typically require phosphate-binding agents in addition to dietary interventions to control serum phosphorus.

Pharmacology and Mechanism of Action Drugs that bind dietary phosphorous in the GI tract form insoluble phosphate compounds that are excreted in feces, thus reducing dietary phosphorus absorption. A variety of phosphate-binding agents are available, including elemental calcium-, lanthanum-, aluminum-, and magnesium-containing compounds, and the nonelemental agent sevelamer carbonate (Table 29-13). Patients must be instructed to take these agents with meals to maximize the binding of phosphorus in the GI tract.

Efficacy Oral calcium compounds are well established as first-line agents for control of both serum phosphorus and calcium concentrations, at least in the early stages of CKD when hypocalcemia is more common. Calcium carbonate and calcium acetate are the primary preparations used; calcium citrate is also available but is used less frequently since the citrate component increases aluminum absorption, although this problem is much less likely today as exposure to sources of aluminum has been reduced in CKD patients. Calcium carbonate is marketed in a variety of dosage forms and is relatively inexpensive. Unfortunately, many calcium carbonate products are considered food supplements and thus do not meet United States Pharmacopeia (USP) disintegration and dissolution requirements. In general, nationally advertised brands do meet these requirements, but it is difficult to determine whether private labels or house brands conform to these standards. Variability in gastric pH may also affect disintegration or dissolution, and thus phosphate-binding efficacy. Calcium carbonate is more soluble in an acidic medium and therefore should be administered prior to meals when stomach acidity is highest. In addition, acid-suppressing agents such as ranitidine and proton pump inhibitors may reduce the phosphate-binding activity of calcium carbonate by increasing gastric pH. Calcium acetate binds approximately twice as much phosphorus as calcium carbonate at comparable doses of elemental calcium.[52] Increased binding potency limits GI calcium absorption; however, calcium acetate is more soluble and therefore better absorbed than calcium carbonate in an alkaline pH, which may explain the similar incidence of hypercalcemia with these agents. For patients with hypocalcemia, calcium carbonate or calcium acetate may also be given as a calcium supplement taken between meals to promote calcium absorption.

Although calcium-containing phosphate-binding agents continue to be used as first-line therapy, their chronic use may increase the risk for vascular and tissue calcification. KDOQI guidelines recommend that the total dose of elemental calcium provided by calcium-containing binders should not exceed 1,500 mg/day and the total daily intake of elemental calcium from all sources should not exceed 2,000 mg.[52] KDIGO guidelines are less specific and suggest restricting the dose of calcium-containing binders only if hypercalcemia is present or if arterial calcification or adynamic bone disease is evident.[43] Both of these recommendations regarding calcium intake are based primarily on opinion.

TABLE 29-13 Phosphate-Binding Agents for Treatment of Hyperphosphatemia in CKD Patients

Drug	Brand Name	Compound Content	Starting Doses	Dose Titration[a]	Comments
Calcium carbonate[b]	Tums, Os-Cal, Caltrate	40% elemental calcium	0.5–1 g (elemental calcium) three times a day with meals	Increase or decrease by 500 mg per meal (200 mg elemental calcium)	First-line agent; dissolution characteristics and phosphate binding may vary from product to product Approximately 39 mg phosphorus bound per 1 g calcium carbonate
Calcium acetate (25% elemental calcium)	PhosLo	25% elemental calcium (169 mg elemental calcium per 667 mg capsule)	0.5–1 g (elemental calcium) three times a day with meals	Increase or decrease by 667 mg per meal (169 mg elemental calcium)	First-line agent; comparable efficacy to calcium carbonate with lower dose of elemental calcium Approximately 45 mg phosphorus bound per 1 g calcium acetate
	Phoslyra	667 mg calcium acetate per 5 mL			
Sevelamer carbonate	Renvela	800 mg tablet 0.8 and 2.4 g powder for oral suspension	800–1,600 mg three times a day with meals (once-daily dosing also effective)	Increase or decrease by 800 mg per meal	First-line agent; also lowers low-density lipoprotein cholesterol Consider in patients at risk for extraskeletal calcification Associated with a lower risk of acidosis and GI adverse events than Renagel (sevelamer hydrochloride) that is no longer available
Lanthanum carbonate	Fosrenol	500, 750, and 1,000 mg chewable tablets	1,500 mg daily in divided doses with meals	Increase or decrease by 750 mg/day	First-line agent; potential for accumulation of lanthanum due to GI absorption (long-term consequences unknown)
Aluminum hydroxide[b]	AlternaGel	Content varies (range 100–600 mg/unit)	300–600 mg three times a day with meals	Not for long-term use requiring titration	Not a first-line agent; risk of aluminum toxicity; do not use concurrently with citrate-containing products Reserve for short-term use (4 weeks) in patients with hyperphosphatemia not responding to other binders

[a]Based on phosphorus levels, titrate every 2–3 weeks until phosphorus goal reached.
[b]Multiple preparations available that are not listed.

Sevelamer is a nonabsorbable, nonelemental hydrogel phosphate-binding agent that effectively lowers phosphorus and has also been shown to significantly lower LDL and increase HDL cholesterol.[43] Once-daily dosing of sevelamer carbonate powder has also been shown to significantly decrease phosphorus levels, although this regimen was not as effective as three times daily dosing.[128] Whether sevelamer lowers the risk of calcification compared with calcium-containing binders is an issue of some debate.[43,129,130] KDOQI guidelines suggest using a non–calcium-containing binder in dialysis patients with severe vascular or soft-tissue calcifications, although these are opinion-based recommendations.[52] KDIGO recommends that binder choice be made considering the stage of CKD and the risk of calcifications.[43]

Clinical **Controversy. . .**

Hyperphosphatemia and vascular calcifications are associated with higher mortality. There is evidence that calcium-containing phosphate binders promote progression of vascular calcification; however, not all studies support this finding and recent evidence suggests this effect may occur with non–calcium-containing binders as well. The effect of binder choice on mortality is also controversial. There is evidence of a survival benefit with sevelamer in hemodialysis patients, but this is not a uniform finding. Currently, KDIGO guidelines recommend that calcium-based phosphate binders be restricted in patients with hypercalcemia, vascular calcifications, and/or adynamic bone disease; however, more evidence is needed to help guide selection of phosphate binders.

Lanthanum carbonate is a phosphate binder approved for patients with ESRD and has demonstrated efficacy in controlling phosphorus and maintaining PTH in the target range with less risk of hypercalcemia than calcium-containing binders.[43] The initial daily dose of 1,500 mg (administered in divided doses with meals) is often titrated to a range of 1,500 to 3,000 mg to maintain target phosphorus. The poor GI absorption, which limits systemic effects, and high binding capacity with phosphorus make this an attractive phosphate-binding agent, particularly when calcium-containing binders are not recommended due to hypercalcemia. Lanthanum is available as a chewable tablet, which may be appealing for some patients. Lanthanum carbonate (2,250 to 3,000 mg/day) was as effective in lowering serum phosphorus as sevelamer hydrochloride (4,800 to 6,400 mg/day) in hemodialysis patients.[131]

Aluminum salts were widely used in the 1980s as phosphate-binding agents because of their high binding potency. They should no longer be used as first-line agents, but rather reserved for acute treatment of severe hyperphosphatemia or used at low doses in combination with either calcium-containing binding agents or sevelamer in cases of hyperphosphatemia that is not responding to therapy with a single agent. According to KDOQI guidelines, the duration of aluminum therapy should be limited to 4 weeks if these agents are used at all.[52]

Magnesium-containing antacids are also effective phosphate binders and may decrease the amount of calcium-containing binders necessary for control of phosphorus; however, their use is limited by the frequent occurrence of GI side effects (i.e., diarrhea) and the potential for magnesium accumulation.

Clinical trials of niacin and niacin derivatives have been conducted to evaluate their potential use as phosphate-binding agents. While significant reductions in serum phosphorus have been observed with these agents in patients with stage 2 to 3 CKD and in hemodialysis patients, flushing reactions will likely limit their use in clinical practice.[132]

Adverse Effects Adverse effects of all available phosphate binders are generally limited to GI side effects, including constipation, diarrhea, nausea, vomiting, and abdominal pain. The risk of hypercalcemia may necessitate restriction of calcium-containing binder use and/or a reduction in dietary intake. Aluminum binders have been associated with CNS toxicity and the worsening of anemia, whereas magnesium binder use may lead to hypermagnesemia and hyperkalemia; therefore, aluminum and magnesium are not recommended for regular use in patients with kidney disease.

Drug–Drug and Drug–Food Interactions Calcium-containing phosphate-binding agents interfere with the absorption of several oral medications that are commonly prescribed for CKD patients, including iron, zinc, and quinolone antibiotics. No drug interaction studies have been performed with sevelamer carbonate; however, studies with sevelamer hydrochloride have not shown interactions with digoxin, warfarin, metoprolol, enalapril, or iron. Coadministration with ciprofloxacin did, however, result in a 50% decrease in bioavailability of the antibiotic. This information is included in the labeling for sevelamer carbonate.[133] Potential interactions between sevelamer and cyclosporine (decreased bioavailability of cyclosporine) and altered phosphorus binding in the presence of agents that increase gastric pH (e.g., omeprazole) have been reported.[134,135] Coadministration of lanthanum with tetracyclines, fluoroquinolones, levothyroxine, or drugs known to bind with cationic antacids may result in decreased bioavailability of these agents. The bioavailability of warfarin, digoxin, and metoprolol was not affected by coadministration of lanthanum.[136] In general, it is rational to separate the administration time of oral medications for which a reduction in bioavailability has a clinically significant effect (e.g., quinolones) from phosphate binders by at least 1 hour before or 3 hours after administration of the phosphate binder. This is a key patient-counseling recommendation as patients are often switched from one phosphate binder to another, and it is easier for them to remember this general concept regarding phosphate binders and other medications. Many phosphate binders are marketed as antacids or calcium supplements, and often CKD patients do not know why they have been prescribed these agents. Regular patient counseling is essential to improve adherence and minimize the potential for drug interactions.

Dosing and Administration Initial dosing regimens for phosphate-binding agents and suggested dose titration schemes are shown in Table 29-13. Doses should be titrated to achieve the recommended serum phosphorus concentrations based on the patient's stage of CKD. The daily dose of elemental calcium should be limited in individuals with elevated calcium levels.

Vitamin D Therapy There are several vitamin D compounds available in the United States (see Table 29-14). Ergocalciferol (D_2) and cholecalciferol (D_3) must be converted to the active form in the kidney while vitamin D analogs do not require this conversion step.

Pharmacology and Mechanism of Action Calcitriol (1,25-dihydroxyvitamin D_3) suppresses PTH secretion by stimulating absorption of serum calcium by intestinal cells and through direct activity on the parathyroid gland to decrease PTH synthesis. As a result, the serum calcium concentration is raised and the parathyroid glands decrease the rate of formation and secretion of PTH. The set point for calcium (i.e., the calcium concentration at which PTH secretion is decreased by 50%), which is generally raised in CKD-MBD, is lowered when active vitamin D therapy is initiated. This indicates that a lower ionized calcium concentration is effective at suppressing secretion of PTH. All of these actions are mediated by the interaction of vitamin D with vitamin D receptors, which are located in many organs, including the parathyroid gland, GI tract, and kidney. Calcitriol also upregulates vitamin D receptors, which

TABLE 29-14 Vitamin D Agents

Generic Name	Brand Name	Form of Vitamin D	Dosage Forms	Initial Dose	Dosage Range	Frequency of Administration
Nutritional Vitamin D						
Ergocalciferol[a]	Generic	D_2	po	Varies based on 25OHD levels	400–50,000 international units	Daily (doses of 400–2,000 international units)
Cholecalciferol[a]	Generic	D_3	po			Weekly or monthly for higher doses (50,000 international units)
Active Vitamin D						
Calcitriol	Calcijex Rocaltrol	D_3	IV po	1–2 mcg 0.25 mcg	0.5–5 mcg 0.25–5 mcg	Three times per week Daily or three times per week
Vitamin D Analogs[146,147]						
Paricalcitol	Zemplar	D_2	po	CKD nondialysis: 1 mcg daily or 2 mcg three times per week if PTH ≤500 pg/mL (≤500 ng/L; ≤54 pmol/L); 2 mcg daily or 4 mcg three time per week if PTH >500 pg/mL (>500 ng/L; >54 pmol/L) Stage 5 CKD: mcg dose based on ratio of PTH/80 and administered three times per week	1–4 mcg	Daily or three times per week
			IV	Stage 5 CKD: 0.04–1 mcg three times per week	2.5–15 mcg	Three times per week
Doxercalciferol	Hectorol	D_2	po	CKD nondialysis: 1 mcg daily Stage 5 CKD: 10 mcg three times per week	5–20 mcg	Daily or three times per week
			IV	Stage 5 CKD: 4 mcg three times per week	2–8 mcg	Three times per week

[a]Multiple preparations are available that are not listed.

ultimately may reduce parathyroid hyperplasia. Unfortunately, the enhanced GI absorption of calcium and phosphorus with calcitriol therapy frequently leads to hypercalcemia and hyperphosphatemia and an increase in the Ca × P product, which is associated with soft-tissue and vascular calcifications.[52]

The unique interactions of vitamin D with the vitamin D receptors have led to the development of vitamin D analogs that vary in their affinity for the vitamin D receptors. Paricalcitol and doxercalciferol retain activity with vitamin D receptors on the parathyroid gland to effectively lower PTH, but have less risk of hypercalcemia and hyperphosphatemia. Paricalcitol differs from calcitriol by the absence of the exocyclic carbon 19 and the fact that it is a vitamin D_2 derivative (19-nor-1,25-dihydroxyvitamin D_2). Doxercalciferol is a prohormone that is activated by CYP27 in the liver to form the major active D_2 metabolite 1,25-dihydroxyvitamin D_2. These analogs are available in IV and oral forms.

D_2 and D_3 bind with vitamin D–binding protein in the circulation and are delivered to the liver where they are converted to 25OHD, by the 25-hydroxylase enzyme. The 25OHD form is converted to the biologically active form 1,25-dihydroxyvitamin D (either D_2 or D_3 depending on the parent compound) by the 1-α-hydroxylase enzyme. This conversion occurs primarily in the kidney, but this enzyme is also present in extrarenal tissues. It is not clear whether active vitamin D produced in extrarenal tissue exerts its effects only locally or contributes to the overall endocrine functions of active vitamin D. It is 25OHD (the precursor form of active vitamin D) that is measured clinically to diagnose vitamin D deficiency. Supplementation with nutritional vitamin D is recommended for patients with low vitamin D levels (defined as a 25OHD less than 30 ng/mL [75 nmol/L]). This recommendation primarily applies to patients with stage 3 and 4 CKD who may have greater ability to convert 25OHD to the active form by hydroxylation in the kidney.

Pharmacokinetics Oral absorption of calcitriol occurs rapidly; therefore, both oral and IV therapies are reasonable options for treatment of CKD-MBD. The half-life of active calcitriol ranges from 15 to 38 hours in patients with ESRD.[137] The half-life of paricalcitol when administered IV or orally is approximately 14 to 20 hours.[138] The mean half-life of doxercalciferol after oral administration is approximately 32 to 37 hours with a range of up to 96 hours. These agents are extensively bound to plasma proteins and not removed by dialysis.

Efficacy Calcitriol, paricalcitol, and doxercalciferol are all effective in lowering PTH in patients with CKD; however, the trade-off is the undesired effect of raising calcium and phosphorus concentrations due to increased intestinal absorption. Although these effects are less likely with the newer analogs (paricalcitol and doxercalciferol), elevated calcium concentrations have been observed with these agents as well. Although comparisons between vitamin D analogs are relatively limited, the incidence of hyperphosphatemia with paricalcitol was lower than with doxercalciferol when administered at high doses to hemodialysis patients.[139] A more rapid suppression of PTH was also observed in paricalcitol-treated patients compared with those who received calcitriol.[140] The more clinically significant finding from this study was the decrease in incidence of hypercalcemia and elevated Ca × P product in the paricalcitol-treated patients.

Nontraditional effects of vitamin D, including a potential survival benefit, have also been reported in both CKD and ESRD patients.[48,141] It must be noted that these are observational studies and that prospective, randomized controlled trials are required to better understand survival benefits associated with vitamin D therapy. When the effect of paricalcitol on left ventricular mass was evaluated in patients with CKD and mild to moderate left ventricular hypertrophy, there was no improvement in left ventricular mass after 48 weeks of therapy.[142] Antiproteinuric effects of paricalcitol have also been reported in patients with stage 4 and 5 CKD.[143] A significant reduction in the urinary ACR was observed in CKD patients with type 2 diabetes receiving 2 mg of oral paricalcitol daily compared with placebo. These findings are of interest when considering other potential effects of vitamin D beyond suppression of PTH.

A review and meta-analysis of available studies in CKD patients (including dialysis) found that nutritional vitamin D supplementation with D_2 and D_3 led to improvement in 25OHD levels and decreased PTH without significant hypercalcemia or hyperphosphatemia.[144] There were few randomized studies included in this analysis and no study evaluated objective measures of bone disease or mortality. In ESRD patients nutritional vitamin D resulted in increased levels of 1,25-dihydroxyvitamin D, which suggests a potential role of extrarenal pathways of vitamin D activation.[145]

Adverse Effects Although all agents are effective in suppressing PTH levels, they may cause hypercalcemia and hyperphosphatemia, an effect that is most likely with calcitriol. Monitoring of PTH, calcium, and phosphorus is necessary to evaluate these effects and make changes in drug therapy.

Drug–Drug and Drug–Food Interactions Cholestyramine may reduce the absorption of orally administered calcitriol and doxercalciferol. In vitro data suggest that paricalcitol is metabolized by the hepatic enzyme CYP3A4 and has the potential to interact with other agents that are metabolized by this enzyme. When ketoconazole, a CYP3A4 inhibitor, was given concomitantly, paricalcitol serum concentrations doubled.[146] Caution is also advised when CYP3A4 inhibitors are given to those receiving doxercalciferol since hydroxylation of this precursor agent may be inhibited. There is also a warning in the product labeling to avoid concomitant use of magnesium-containing antacids and doxercalciferol to prevent development of hypermagnesemia.[147]

Dosing and Administration Because deficiency in the vitamin D precursor, 25OHD, is common in patients with CKD, measuring 25OHD levels in patients with stage 3 or 4 CKD who have PTH values above the upper recommended ranges is reasonable (see Table 29-12). If the 25OHD level is less than 30 ng/mL (75 nmol/L), nutritional vitamin D (e.g., D_2 or D_3) is recommended. The dose and duration of treatment are dependent on the severity of the deficiency. To prevent vitamin D insufficiency, doses of 600 to 800 units/day of D_2 are recommended. Calcitriol, doxercalciferol, or paricalcitol should be administered when PTH remains elevated despite the achievement of adequate 25OHD levels. Based on evidence of extrarenal pathways of conversion of vitamin D to the active form, there may be some basis for supplementation of nutritional vitamin D in the ESRD population, although most of these patients require an active vitamin D sterol (calcitriol, doxercalciferol, or paricalcitol).

Administration of calcitriol by either the oral or the IV route may be based on daily dosing (usually 0.25 to 1 mcg/day) or pulse dosing (0.5 to 2 mcg two to three times per week). Logistically, IV dosing is more practical in hemodialysis patients, whereas oral therapy is more practical for nondialysis CKD and peritoneal dialysis patients. Recommended doses of doxercalciferol and paricalcitol are shown in Table 29-14. Prior to starting therapy, the serum calcium and phosphorus should be within the normal range to minimize the risk of hypercalcemia and an elevated Ca × P product. This does not mean that vitamin D therapy should be withheld or discontinued in all patients with a Ca × P product greater than 55 mg^2/dL^2 (4.4 $mmol^2/L^2$) unless they are well above this threshold. Rather, use of agents with a lower risk of hypercalcemia and hyperphosphatemia and more prudent use of phosphate binders to lower calcium and phosphorus may be necessary in such patients. Dose adjustments of vitamin D should be made every 2 to 4 weeks based on PTH concentrations and trends in calcium and phosphorus.

Calcimimetics

Pharmacology and Mechanism of Action Cinacalcet hydrochloride (Sensipar) is a calcimimetic agent approved for treatment of sHPT in patients with CKD on dialysis. This compound acts by increasing the sensitivity of the calcium-sensing receptor located on the surface of the chief cells of the parathyroid gland to extracellular calcium, subsequently reducing PTH secretion. Cinacalcet does not increase intestinal calcium and phosphorus absorption. In fact, the reduction in PTH with cinacalcet is associated with a decrease in serum calcium.[43]

Pharmacokinetics The maximum plasma concentration of cinacalcet is achieved in approximately 2 to 6 hours following oral administration. The half-life is approximately 30 to 40 hours. Cinacalcet has a large volume of distribution (approximately 1,000 L) and is 93% to 97% bound to plasma proteins, both characteristics indicating that removal by dialysis is negligible. It is metabolized by the liver, specifically by the cytochrome P450 isoenzymes CYP3A4, CYP2D6, and CYP1A2.[148]

Efficacy In clinical trials conducted predominantly in dialysis patients, cinacalcet significantly decreased PTH and the Ca × P product, regardless of the severity of sHPT.[43] Studies in CKD patients not on dialysis showed effective lowering of PTH, but a high incidence of hypocalcemia and hyperphosphatemia; thus, this agent is not approved in the nondialysis CKD population. Cinacalcet may be used as a single agent to control hyperparathyroidism in ESRD patients; however, combined therapy with vitamin D is an effective approach to achieve target PTH, calcium, and phosphorus as demonstrated in clinical trials.[43] The effect of cinacalcet on vascular calcification has also been evaluated. The ADVANCE Study assessed the effect of cinacalcet plus low-dose active vitamin D versus flexible dosing of active vitamin D on progression of CAC in hemodialysis patients.[149] This study showed that the increase in CAC scores was less in cinacalcet-treated patients, although changes were not significant for all scores evaluated. A decrease in all-cause and cardiovascular mortality was also suggested by results of an observational study in hemodialysis patients prescribed cinacalcet in addition to vitamin D compared with those on vitamin D alone.[150] While these findings were promising, they were not supported by the EVOLVE trial (the Evaluation of Cinacalcet Therapy to Lower Cardiovascular Events), a prospective study designed to evaluate whether treatment with cinacalcet reduced the risk of all-cause mortality and cardiovascular events in HD patients.[151] Although patients in the cinacalcet group had fewer events, the results were not statistically significant.

Adverse Effects The most frequently reported adverse events with cinacalcet were nausea and vomiting. Cinacalcet lowers serum calcium and may cause hypocalcemia; therefore, this agent should not be started if the serum calcium is less than the lower limit of normal, approximately 8.4 mg/dL (2.10 mmol/L). Serum calcium should be measured within 1 week after initiation or following a dose adjustment of cinacalcet. Once the maintenance dose is established, serum calcium should be measured approximately monthly. Potential manifestations of hypocalcemia include paresthesia, myalgia, cramping, tetany, and convulsions.

Drug–Drug and Drug–Food Interactions Because cinacalcet is partially metabolized by cytochrome P450 CYP3A4, there is potential for drug interactions with agents that inhibit this pathway. Coadministration of cinacalcet and ketoconazole, a strong inhibitor of CYP3A4, resulted in an increase in the area under the curve and maximum concentration of 2.3 and 2.2 times, respectively. Cinacalcet is also a potent inhibitor of the enzyme CYP2D6. As a result, dose adjustments of concomitant medications that are predominantly metabolized by this enzyme and have a narrow therapeutic index, such as flecainide, thioridazine, vinblastine, and most tricyclic antidepressants (e.g., amitriptyline), may be necessary.[148] Concurrent administration of cinacalcet with amitriptyline increased amitriptyline and nortriptyline (active metabolite) exposure by approximately 20% in CYP2D6-extensive metabolizers.[148]

Several agents commonly used in the CKD population have been evaluated for interactions with cinacalcet. Coadministration of calcium carbonate, sevelamer, and pantoprazole did not affect the pharmacokinetics of cinacalcet. Coadministration of cinacalcet with warfarin also did not affect the pharmacokinetics of warfarin.[148]

Food has been shown to increase absorption of cinacalcet by up to 81% compared with fasting; therefore, this medication should be taken with meals to achieve the maximal effect.

Dosing and Administration The recommended starting dose of cinacalcet is 30 mg once daily. Calcium and phosphorus should be measured within 1 week and PTH should be measured within 1 to 4 weeks after starting cinacalcet or adjusting the dose. The dose should be titrated every 2 to 4 weeks to a maximum dose of 180 mg once daily to achieve the desired PTH levels and to maintain near-normal serum calcium concentrations. Patients with hepatic disease may require lower doses, as studies have shown a decrease in metabolism of cinacalcet in this patient population. Cinacalcet is available as a film-coated tablet containing 30, 60, or 90 mg.

Personalized Pharmacotherapy

(10) Management of PTH, phosphorus, and calcium is important in preventing CKD-MBD and cardiovascular and extravascular calcifications. Patients with CKD-MBD usually require a combination of dietary intervention, phosphate-binding medications, vitamin D, and calcimimetic therapy (for ESRD patients) to achieve these goals. KDOQI clinical practice guidelines for bone metabolism and disease suggest specific target ranges for calcium, phosphorus, Ca × P product, and PTH defined based on opinion and evidence when available. Given the lack of randomized controlled trials to support specific target levels for calcium, phosphorus, and PTH, the KDIGO recommendations for target levels and treatment approaches are much more general. Despite the fact that protocols for management of CKD-MBD exist that follow KDOQI or KDIGO, individualization of therapy is necessary and the evidence supporting specific targets is not robust.

When individualizing therapy for a patient, clinicians will also have to take into account the recent changes in the bundling system of payment for outpatient dialysis centers. The financial reimbursement a dialysis unit receives per dialysis session includes IV vitamin D therapy and in 2016 will also include the oral vitamin D agents, cinacalcet, and phosphate binders. There are concerns in the nephrology community about the effect the new system would have on treatment for CKD-MBD. Dialysis providers may advocate changing patients from more expensive, noncalcemic phosphate binders (e.g., sevelamer carbonate and lanthanum carbonate) to less expensive calcium-containing binders. Calcitriol, which is more likely to cause hypercalcemia and hyperphosphatemia, may be used more in the ESRD population since both the IV and oral forms are less expensive than paricalcitol and doxercalciferol. It is also anticipated that the use of cinacalcet may be reduced because of the cost of this oral calcimimetic. These changes in prescribing to reduce cost burden on dialysis facilities could potentially increase the incidence of hypercalcemia, calcifications, and morbidity in the ESRD population.

OTHER COMPLICATIONS OF CKD

Cardiovascular Disease

Patients with CKD are at increased risk of CVD independent of the etiology of their kidney disease.[152] As a predominant comorbidity, cardiovascular disorders and their sequelae are the leading cause of death in the ESRD population.[3] Higher mortality and risk of cardiovascular events has also been observed in individuals with stage 3 to 5 CKD.[3] In addition to traditional cardiac risk factors such as hypertension and hyperlipidemia, diabetes, tobacco use, and physical inactivity, patients with kidney disease have other unique risk factors. Among these are hyperhomocysteinemia, elevated levels of C-reactive protein, increased oxidant stress, and hemodynamic overload.[153]

Screening for the presence of cardiovascular risk factors is a high priority in this population. Individuals with stage 4 CKD should be assessed for cardiovascular risk factors. Modifiable cardiovascular risk factors such as hypertension, diabetes mellitus, hyperlipidemia, and smoking should be aggressively managed.[152] The KDOQI CVD guidelines recommend that all patients starting dialysis be assessed for cardiomyopathy, coronary artery, valvular heart, cerebrovascular, and peripheral vascular disease. They should also be screened for traditional (e.g., hypertension) and nontraditional cardiovascular risk factors.[153] Recommendations for management of coronary artery disease, acute coronary syndromes, valvular heart disease, cardiomyopathy, dysrhythmias, cerebrovascular disease, and peripheral vascular disease are also included in the KDOQI guidelines as are differences in management of these disorders in dialysis patients compared with the general population. Guidelines for management of cardiovascular risk factors are also included.

Hyperlipidemia

CKD with or without nephrotic syndrome is frequently accompanied by abnormalities in lipoprotein metabolism. It is well established that dyslipidemias cause atherosclerotic CVD, and there are many compelling reasons to treat these disorders. A clear association between hypercholesterolemia, hypertriglyceridemia, and other lipoprotein changes in patients with CKD and CVD has not been demonstrated in large prospective studies because individuals with kidney disease are usually excluded from these trials. A low or declining serum cholesterol in patients with ESRD is associated with higher mortality, a paradoxical effect.[153] These findings beg the question of whether aggressive lipid lowering is warranted in this population.

Although the concentrations of LDL are not uniformly increased in patients with kidney disease, these patients appear to produce small, dense LDL particles that are more susceptible to oxidation and more atherogenic than larger LDL subfractions. Other lipoprotein abnormalities include changes in apoprotein content of lipoprotein molecules, low HDL, increased triglycerides, and increased very-low-density and intermediate-density lipoproteins.[154] For patients with CKD and a urinary protein excretion greater than 3 g/day, the major lipid abnormalities are elevation of plasma total and LDL cholesterol, with or without low HDL cholesterol (<35 mg/dL [<0.91 mmol/L]), and elevated triglycerides. Treatment of proteinuria resolves the hyperlipidemia in most patients with nephrotic syndrome.

Management of dyslipidemia in patients with CKD has been guided by recommendations from the National Cholesterol Education Program and the KDOQI guidelines for dyslipidemia.[154,155] Based on evidence of risk reduction and the benefits of lipid-lowering therapy in the general population, the consensus was that CKD patients should be treated aggressively to an LDL cholesterol goal below 100 mg/dL (2.59 mmol/L).[154,155] However, the KDIGO guidelines for lipid management in CKD published in 2013 do not support this goal since clinical trials have not proven the strategy of targeting a specific LDL level to be beneficial.[156] KDIGO recommends that a lipid profile be done for all adults with CKD to include LDL, HDL, and triglycerides.[154,156] Follow up lipid levels are not recommended unless the information may alter management (e.g., assessing adherence to therapy or assessing cardiovascular risk in a patient <50 years of age and not currently on a statin). Patients should also be evaluated for other conditions that are known to cause dyslipidemias (e.g., liver disease).

KDIGO acknowledges that reduction in the risk of adverse cardiovascular events in patients with CKD has only been demonstrated with regimens that include a statin or statin plus ezetimibe combination and recommendations focus on these agents for individuals at risk of cardiovascular events.

Statins in CKD

Statins have been shown to decrease mortality and cardiovascular events in patients with early stage CKD; however, data are not as compelling in the ESRD population.[157] Although observational studies in hemodialysis patients receiving statins indicated a significant benefit, findings from prospective studies have not been encouraging.[158,159] Results from a 4-year study evaluating the effect of atorvastatin therapy on cardiac mortality in more than 1,200 hemodialysis patients with type 2 diabetes showed no significant benefit in the composite end point compared with the placebo group.[158] In fact, there was a significantly greater RR of fatal stroke in the atorvastatin-treated patients. These findings do not support initiation of statin therapy in ESRD patients, especially those with type 2 diabetes. The AURORA trial assessed the impact of rosuvastatin 10 mg daily or placebo on the primary end points of death from cardiovascular causes, nonfatal MI, or nonfatal stroke.[159] Despite a 43% reduction in cholesterol in the rosuvastatin group, there was no difference in the primary end points. The recently published Study of Heart and Renal Protection (SHARP) trial evaluated the effects of combined simvastatin (20 mg) and ezetimibe (10 mg) compared with placebo on time to first major vascular event (nonfatal MI or cardiac death, any stroke, or revascularization) in patients with no history of MI or coronary revascularization and included patients with CKD (6,247) and ESRD (3,023).[160] In patients receiving combined therapy during the 4.9-year followup period, there was a 17% reduction in the RR of major vascular events compared with the placebo group. A 32% reduction in LDL (from 103 to 70 mg/dL [2.66 to 1.81 mmol/L]) was achieved in a population assessed as two-third compliant with therapy. While overall these results are positive, the study was not powered to evaluate whether the observed effect was significant in the ESRD patients as a separate group.

Based on the available evidence, the KDIGO guidelines for lipid management in CKD recommend treatment with a statin in adults aged 50 and older with stage 1 to 5 CKD (not on dialysis). The statin/ezetimibe combination may also be an option in patients in this age group in stage 3 to 5 CKD (not on dialysis). KDIGO only recommends statins in adults aged 18 to 49 years with stage 1 to 5 CKD (not on dialysis) who have one or more of the following: known coronary disease, diabetes mellitus, prior ischemic stroke, and an estimated 10-year incidence of coronary death or nonfatal myocardial infarction >10%. It is not recommended that statins or statin/ezetimibe be initiated in patients with stage 5 CKD on dialysis; however, therapy with these agents may be continued if patients were receiving these medications at the time of dialysis initiation.[156] Due to the risk of adverse events with statins and absence of safety data in patients with stage 3 to 5 CKD, KDIGO recommends using statins at doses shown to be beneficial in randomized studies conducted in this population (e.g., atorvastatin 20 mg, fluvastatin 80 mg, rosuvastatin 10 mg, simvastatin 20 mg).[156]

Nutritional Status

Protein–energy malnutrition is very common among patients with advanced CKD (stages 4 and 5).[161] Causes of malnutrition in these patients include inadequate food intake secondary to anorexia, altered taste sensation, and the unpalatability of prescribed diets. Other factors in the ESRD population, such as the effect of the dialysis procedure on removal of nutrients, hypercatabolism induced by other inflammatory conditions, and blood loss, are also contributory. Protein restriction as an intervention to potentially delay progression of kidney disease in patients with stage 4 CKD may also lead to protein malnutrition by the time a patient reaches ESRD; therefore, the risks versus the benefits of this intervention must be considered on an individual basis as hypoalbuminemia and malnutrition have a strong association with mortality in chronic dialysis patients.

Patients with ESRD have increased nutritional needs relative to the general population, based on the effect of the disease state and the dialysis procedures on nutritional status. The recommended dietary protein intake in chronic hemodialysis patients is 1.2 g/kg body weight per day.[161] The recommended intake for chronic peritoneal dialysis patients is at least 1.2 to 1.3 g/kg body weight per day, based on the increased protein loss that occurs with this dialysis modality. The recommended total daily energy intake in both hemodialysis and peritoneal dialysis patients is 35 kcal/kg (147 kJ/kg) body weight per day. For peritoneal dialysis patients, this includes intake from both diet and the glucose absorbed from peritoneal dialysate. For patients older than 60 years of age, this criterion differs, because increasing age is generally associated with reduced physical activity and lean body mass. Daily energy intake for these patients is 30 to 35 kcal/kg (126 to 147 kJ/kg) body weight per day. Nutritional support should be considered for those patients who cannot achieve these goals with oral intake alone. Another option for nutritional supplementation in patients on hemodialysis includes interdialytic parenteral nutrition.

Vitamin requirements for ESRD patients receiving dialysis differ from those of a healthy person because of dietary modifications, kidney dysfunction, and dialysis therapy. The plasma concentrations of vitamins A and E are elevated in ESRD, whereas those of the water-soluble vitamins (B_1, B_2, B_6, B_{12}, niacin, pantothenic acid, folic acid, biotin, and vitamin C) tend to be low in large part because many are dialyzable. The goal for vitamin supplementation should be to prevent subclinical and frank deficiency. Special vitamin supplements have been formulated for the dialysis population, which primarily include vitamins B and C and folic acid.

BOTTOM LINE

The number of patients with and at risk for CKD is increasing, with a substantial rise in the population with stage 5 CKD expected in the next decade. Although efforts to delay progression of CKD including prudent use of ACEIs and ARBs are paramount, measures to diagnose and manage the associated secondary complications and comorbid conditions early in the course of the disease are also essential. Common complications of stage 4 and 5 CKD include anemia and CKD-MBD. Cardiovascular complications are also prevalent in the population with CKD, and are the leading cause of mortality in patients with ESRD. Patient education plays a critical role in the appropriate management of CKD and related complications.

A multidisciplinary team structure is a rational approach to providing this education and effectively designing and implementing the required extensive nonpharmacologic and pharmacologic interventions. Pharmacists are among the healthcare providers who contribute substantially to this team as shown by their activities in MTM, improving patient adherence with drug therapy, and providing more cost-effective medication use in dialysis facilities. There are many opportunities for pharmacists to become involved in both the outpatient dialysis or ambulatory care settings and the inpatient environment to improve the management of patients with CKD and the associated complications.

ABBREVIATIONS

ACEI	angiotensin-converting enzyme inhibitor
ACR	albumin-to-creatinine ratio
AIDS	acquired immunodeficiency syndrome
ARB	angiotensin receptor blocker
Ca × P product	calcium–phosphorus product; serum calcium (corrected for albumin) multiplied by serum phosphorus
CAC	coronary artery calcification
CHr	content of hemoglobin in reticulocytes
CKD	chronic kidney disease
CKD-EPI equation	Chronic Kidney Disease Epidemiology Collaboration equation
MTM	Medication Therapy Management
CMS	Centers for Medicare and Medicaid Services
CUA	calcific uremic arteriolopathy
CVD	cardiovascular disease
D2	ergocalciferol
D3	cholecalciferol
DCCT	Diabetes Control and Complications Trial
DRP	drug-related problem
EBCT	electron-beam computed tomography
EDIC	Epidemiology of Diabetes Interventions and Complications
eGFR	estimated glomerular filtration rate
ESA	erythropoietic-stimulating agent
ESRD	end-stage renal disease
EVOLVE	Evaluation of Cinacalcet Therapy to Lower Cardiovascular Events
FGF-23	fibroblast growth factor-23
GFR	glomerular filtration rate
Hb	hemoglobin
Hct	hematocrit
$HgbA_1C$	glycosylated hemoglobin
KDIGO	Kidney Disease: Improving Global Outcomes
KDOQI	Kidney Disease Outcomes Quality Initiative
KEEP	Kidney Early Evaluation
MBD	mineral and bone disorder
MCP-1	monocyte chemoattractant protein-1
MDRD	Modification of Diet in Renal Disease
MW	molecular weight
NHANES	National Health and Nutrition Examination Survey
NHCT	Normal Hematocrit Cardiac Trial
NKF	National Kidney Foundation
25OHD	25-hydroxyvitamin D
PCR	protein-to-creatinine ratio
PRCA	pure red cell aplasia
PTH	parathyroid hormone
RAAS	renin–angiotensin–aldosterone system
ROD	renal osteodystrophy
RR	relative risk
SHARP	Study of Heart and Renal Protection
sHPT	secondary hyperparathyroidism
SPRINT	Systolic Blood Pressure Intervention Trial
TIBC	total iron-binding capacity
TREAT	Trial to Reduce Cardiovascular Events with Aranesp Therapy
TSat	transferrin saturation
USP	United States Pharmacopeia
USRDS	United States Renal Data System

REFERENCES

1. Kidney Disease: Improving Global Outcomes (KDIGO) CKD Work Group. KDIGO 2012 Clinical Practice Guideline for the Evaluation and Management of Chronic Kidney Disease. Kidney Int Suppl 2013;3:1–150.
2. National Kidney Foundation. K/DOQI clinical practice guidelines for chronic kidney disease: Evaluation, classification, and stratification. Am J Kidney Dis 2002;39:S1–S266.
3. U.S. Renal Data System, USRDS 2012 Annual Data Report: Atlas of Chronic Kidney Disease and End-Stage Renal Disease in the United States. Bethesda, MD: National Institutes of Health, National Institute of Diabetes and Digestive and Kidney Diseases, 2012.
4. Whaley-Connell AT, Vassalotti JA, Collins AJ, Chen SC, McCullough PA. National Kidney Foundation's Kidney Early Evaluation Program (KEEP) annual data report 2011. Am J Kidney Dis 2012;59:S1–S4.
5. Lacson E Jr, Wang W, Hakim RM, et al. Associates of mortality and hospitalization in hemodialysis: Potentially actionable laboratory variables and vascular access. Am J Kidney Dis 2009;53:79–90.
6. Levin A, Bakris GL, Molitch M, et al. Prevalence of abnormal serum vitamin D, PTH, calcium, and phosphorus in patients with chronic kidney disease: Results of the study to evaluate early kidney disease. Kidney Int 2007; 71:31–38.
7. US Department of Health and Human Services. Healthy People 2020 Objectives for Chronic Kidney Disease. 2012, *http://www.healthypeople.gov/2020/topicsobjectives2020/overview.aspx?topicid=6*.
8. Shoham DA, Vupputuri S, Kaufman JS, et al. Kidney disease and the cumulative burden of life course socioeconomic conditions: The Atherosclerosis Risk in Communities (ARIC) study. Soc Sci Med 2008;67:1311–1320.
9. Norris K, Nissenson AR. Race, gender, and socioeconomic disparities in CKD in the United States. J Am Soc Nephrol 2008;19:1261–1270.
10. Vikse BE, Irgens LM, Leivestad T, et al. Low birth weight increases risk for end-stage renal disease. J Am Soc Nephrol 2008;19:151–157.
11. McClellan WM, Satko SG, Gladstone E, et al. Individuals with a family history of ESRD are a high-risk population for CKD: Implications for targeted surveillance and intervention activities. Am J Kidney Dis 2009;53:S100–S106.
12. Dronavalli S, Duka I, Bakris GL. The pathogenesis of diabetic nephropathy. Nat Clin Pract Endocrinol Metab 2008;4:444–452.
13. Raile K, Galler A, Hofer S, et al. Diabetic nephropathy in 27,805 children, adolescents, and adults with type 1 diabetes: Effect of diabetes duration, A1C, hypertension, dyslipidemia, diabetes onset, and sex. Diabetes Care 2007;30:2523–2528.
14. Nathan DM, Zinman B, Cleary PA, et al. Modern-day clinical course of type 1 diabetes mellitus after 30 years' duration: The Diabetes Control and Complications Trial/Epidemiology of Diabetes Interventions and Complications and Pittsburgh epidemiology of diabetes complications experience (1983-2005). Arch Intern Med 2009;169: 1307–1316.
15. KDIGO Blood Pressure Work Group. KDIGO clinical practice guideline for the management of blood pressure in chronic kidney disease. Kidney Int Suppl 2012;2:337–414.
16. Bakris GL. Slowing nephropathy progression: Focus on proteinuria reduction. Clin J Am Soc Nephrol 2008;3 (Suppl 1):S3–S10.

17. Nathan DM, Cleary PA, Backlund JY, et al. Intensive diabetes treatment and cardiovascular disease in patients with type 1 diabetes. N Engl J Med 2005;353:2643–2653.
18. Keane WF. Proteinuria: Its clinical importance and role in progressive renal disease. Am J Kidney Dis 2000;35: S97–S105.
19. Klahr S, Levey AS, Beck GJ, et al. The effects of dietary protein restriction and blood-pressure control on the progression of chronic renal disease. Modification of Diet in Renal Disease Study Group. N Engl J Med 1994;330: 877–884.
20. Jafar TH, Stark PC, Schmid CH, et al. Progression of chronic kidney disease: The role of blood pressure control, proteinuria, and angiotensin-converting enzyme inhibition: A patient-level meta-analysis. Ann Intern Med 2003;139: 244–252.
21. Hogan SL, Vupputuri S, Guo X, et al. Association of cigarette smoking with albuminuria in the United States: The third National Health and Nutrition Examination Survey. Ren Fail 2007;29:133–142.
22. Orth SR. Effects of smoking on systemic and intrarenal hemodynamics: Influence on renal function. J Am Soc Nephrol 2004;15(Suppl 1):S58–S63.
23. Ejerblad E, Fored CM, Lindblad P, et al. Association between smoking and chronic renal failure in a nationwide population-based case–control study. J Am Soc Nephrol 2004;15:2178–2185.
24. Sawicki PT, Didjurgeit U, Muhlhauser I, et al. Smoking is associated with progression of diabetic nephropathy. Diabetes Care 1994;17:126–131.
25. Bakris G, Rahman M, Lea J, et al. Associations between cardiovascular risk factors and glomerular filtration rate at baseline in the African American Study of Kidney Disease (AASK) trial. J Am Soc Nephrol 1998;10:A0717.
26. Ward MM, Studenski S. Clinical prognostic factors in lupus nephritis. The importance of hypertension and smoking. Arch Intern Med 1992;152:2082–2088.
27. Hsu CY, McCulloch CE, Iribarren C, et al. Body mass index and risk for end-stage renal disease. Ann Intern Med 2006;144:21–28.
28. Ejerblad E, Fored CM, Lindblad P, et al. Obesity and risk for chronic renal failure. J Am Soc Nephrol 2006;17:1695–1702.
29. Wang Y, Chen X, Song Y, et al. Association between obesity and kidney disease: A systematic review and meta-analysis. Kidney Int 2008;73:19–33.
30. Eknoyan G. Obesity and chronic kidney disease. Nefrologia 2011;31(4):397–403.
31. Remuzzi G, Benigni A, Remuzzi A. Mechanisms of progression and regression of renal lesions of chronic nephropathies and diabetes. J Clin Invest 2006;116:288–296.
32. Lopez-Novoa JM, Martinez-Salgado C, Rodriguez-Pena AB, Lopez-Hernandez FJ. Common pathophysiological mechanisms of chronic kidney disease: Therapeutic perspectives. Pharmacol Ther 2010;128:61–81.
33. Abbate M, Zoja C, Remuzzi G. How does proteinuria cause progressive renal damage? J Am Soc Nephrol 2006;17: 2974–2984.
34. Jelkmann W. Regulation of erythropoietin production. J Physiol 2011;589:1251–1258.
35. Kalantar-Zadeh K, Streja E, Miller JE, Nissenson AR. Intravenous iron versus erythropoiesis-stimulating agents: Friends or foes in treating chronic kidney disease anemia? Adv Chronic Kidney Dis 2009;16:143–151.
36. Coyne DW. Hepcidin: Clinical utility as a diagnostic tool and therapeutic target. Kidney Int 2011;80: 240–244.
37. van Nooten FE, Green J, Brown R, et al. Burden of illness for patients with non-dialysis chronic kidney disease and anemia in the United States: Review of the literature. J Med Econ 2010;13:241–256.
38. Singh AK, Szczech L, Tang KL, et al. Correction of anemia with epoetin alfa in chronic kidney disease. N Engl J Med 2006;355:2085–2098.
39. Besarab A, Bolton WK, Browne JK, et al. The effects of normal as compared with low hematocrit values in patients with cardiac disease who are receiving hemodialysis and epoetin. N Engl J Med 1998;339:584–590.
40. Besarab A, Goodkin DA, Nissenson AR. The normal hematocrit study—Follow-up. N Engl J Med 2008;358: 433–434.
41. Drueke TB, Locatelli F, Clyne N, et al. Normalization of hemoglobin level in patients with chronic kidney disease and anemia. N Engl J Med 2006;355:2071–2084.
42. Kidney Disease: Improving Global Outcomes (KDIGO) Anemia Work Group. KDIGO clinical practice guideline for anemia in chronic kidney disease. Kidney Int Suppl 2012;2:279–335.
43. Kidney Disease: Improving Global Outcomes (KDIGO) CKD-MBD Work Group. KDIGO clinical practice guideline for the diagnosis, evaluation, prevention, and treatment of chronic kidney disease-mineral and bone disorder (CKD-MBD). Kidney Int Suppl 2009:S1–S130.
44. Cunningham J, Locatelli F, Rodriguez M. Secondary hyperparathyroidism: Pathogenesis, disease progression, and therapeutic options. Clin J Am Soc Nephrol 2011;6:913–921.
45. Quarles LD. Role of FGF23 in vitamin D and phosphate metabolism: Implications in chronic kidney disease. Exp Cell Res 2012;318:1040–1048.
46. Martin KJ, Gonzalez EA. Vitamin D supplementation in CKD. Clin Nephrol 2011;75:286–293.
47. Ganesh SK, Stack AG, Levin NW, et al. Association of elevated serum PO(4), Ca × PO(4) product, and parathyroid hormone with cardiac mortality risk in chronic hemodialysis patients. J Am Soc Nephrol 2001;12:2131–2138.
48. Block GA. Therapeutic interventions for chronic kidney disease-mineral and bone disorders: Focus on mortality. Curr Opin Nephrol Hypertens 2011;20:376–381.
49. Rogers NM, Coates PT. Calcific uraemic arteriolopathy: An update. Curr Opin Nephrol Hypertens 2008;17:629–634.
50. Foley RN, Curtis BM, Parfrey PS. Erythropoietin therapy, hemoglobin targets, and quality of life in healthy hemodialysis patients: A randomized trial. Clin J Am Soc Nephrol 2009;4:726–733.
51. KDOQI, National Kidney Foundation. Clinical practice guidelines and clinical practice recommendations for anemia in chronic kidney disease in adults. Am J Kidney Dis 2006;47:S16–S85.
52. Eknoyan G, Levin A, Levin NW. Bone metabolism and disease in chronic kidney disease. Am J Kidney Dis 2003;42:1–201.
53. Mason NA. Polypharmacy and medication-related complications in the chronic kidney disease patient. Curr Opin Nephrol Hypertens 2011;20:492–497.
54. Bayliss EA, Bhardwaja B, Ross C, et al. Multidisciplinary team care may slow the rate of decline in renal function. Clin J Am Soc Nephrol 2011;6:704–710.
55. Mendelssohn DC. Coping with the CKD epidemic: The promise of multidisciplinary team-based care. Nephrol Dial Transplant 2005;20:10–12.
56. Goldstein M, Yassa T, Dacouris N, McFarlane P. Multidisciplinary predialysis care and morbidity and mortality of patients on dialysis. Am J Kidney Dis 2004; 44:706–714.

57. Matzke GR, Aronoff GR, Atkinson AJ Jr, et al. Drug dosing consideration in patients with acute and chronic kidney disease—A clinical update from Kidney Disease: Improving Global Outcomes (KDIGO). Kidney Int 2011;80:1122–1137.
58. Fouque D, Laville M. Low protein diets for chronic kidney disease in non diabetic adults. Cochrane Database Syst Rev 2009;(3):CD001892.
59. Robertson L, Waugh N, Robertson A. Protein restriction for diabetic renal disease. Cochrane Database Syst Rev 2007;(4):CD002181.
60. Pan Y, Guo LL, Jin HM. Low-protein diet for diabetic nephropathy: A meta-analysis of randomized controlled trials. Am J Clin Nutr 2008;88:660–666.
61. Tylicki L, Lizakowski S, Rutkowski B. Renin–angiotensin–aldosterone system blockade for nephroprotection: Current evidence and future directions. J Nephrol 2012;25:900–910.
62. Effects of ramipril on cardiovascular and microvascular outcomes in people with diabetes mellitus: Results of the HOPE study and MICRO-HOPE substudy. Heart Outcomes Prevention Evaluation Study Investigators. Lancet 2000;355:253–259.
63. Kshirsagar AV, Joy MS, Hogan SL, et al. Effect of ACE inhibitors in diabetic and nondiabetic chronic renal disease: A systematic overview of randomized placebo-controlled trials. Am J Kidney Dis 2000;35:695–707.
64. Lewis EJ, Hunsicker LG, Clarke WR, et al. Renoprotective effect of the angiotensin-receptor antagonist irbesartan in patients with nephropathy due to type 2 diabetes. N Engl J Med 2001;345:851–860.
65. Parving HH, Lehnert H, Brochner-Mortensen J, et al. The effect of irbesartan on the development of diabetic nephropathy in patients with type 2 diabetes. N Engl J Med 2001;345:870–878.
66. Brenner BM, Cooper ME, de Zeeuw D, et al. Effects of losartan on renal and cardiovascular outcomes in patients with type 2 diabetes and nephropathy. N Engl J Med 2001; 345:861–869.
67. Upadhyay A, Earley A, Haynes SM, Uhlig K. Systematic review: Blood pressure target in chronic kidney disease and proteinuria as an effect modifier. Ann Intern Med 2011;154:541–548.
68. Systolic Blood Pressure Intervention Trial (SPRINT). 2009, *www.sprinttrial.org*.
69. Dussol B, Moussi-Frances J, Morange S, et al. A randomized trial of furosemide vs hydrochlorothiazide in patients with chronic renal failure and hypertension. Nephrol Dial Transplant 2005;20:349–353.
70. Turner JM, Bauer C, Abramowitz MK, et al. Treatment of chronic kidney disease. Kidney Int 2012;81:351–362.
71. Chan CY, Peterson EJ, Ng TM. Thiazide diuretics as chronic antihypertensive therapy in patients with severe renal disease—Is there a role in the absence of diuresis? Ann Pharmacother 2012;46:1554–1558.
72. Bakris G, Burgess E, Weir M, et al. Telmisartan is more effective than losartan in reducing proteinuria in patients with diabetic nephropathy. Kidney Int 2008;74: 364–369.
73. Jennings DL, Kalus JS, Coleman CI, et al. Combination therapy with an ACE inhibitor and an angiotensin receptor blocker for diabetic nephropathy: A meta-analysis. Diabet Med 2007;24:486–493.
74. Kunz R, Friedrich C, Wolbers M, Mann JF. Meta-analysis: Effect of monotherapy and combination therapy with inhibitors of the renin angiotensin system on proteinuria in renal disease. Ann Intern Med 2008;148:30–48.
75. MacKinnon M, Shurraw S, Akbari A, et al. Combination therapy with an angiotensin receptor blocker and an ACE inhibitor in proteinuric renal disease: A systematic review of the efficacy and safety data. Am J Kidney Dis 2006;48:8–20.
76. Mann JF, Schmieder RE, McQueen M, et al. Renal outcomes with telmisartan, ramipril, or both, in people at high vascular risk (the ONTARGET study): A multicentre, randomised, double-blind, controlled trial. Lancet 2008;372:547–553.
77. Ruggenenti P, Remuzzi G. Proteinuria: Is the ONTARGET renal substudy actually off target? Nat Rev Nephrol 2009;5:436–437.
78. Fried LF, Duckworth W, Zhang JH, et al. Design of combination angiotensin receptor blocker and angiotensin-converting enzyme inhibitor for treatment of diabetic nephropathy (VA NEPHRON-D). Clin J Am Soc Nephrol 2009;4:361–368.
79. Navaneethan SD, Nigwekar SU, Sehgal AR, Strippoli GF. Aldosterone antagonists for preventing the progression of chronic kidney disease. Cochrane Database Syst Rev 2009;(3):CD007004.
80. Parving HH, Persson F, Lewis JB, et al. Aliskiren combined with losartan in type 2 diabetes and nephropathy. N Engl J Med 2008;358:2433–2446.
81. Persson F, Rossing P, Reinhard H, et al. Renal effects of aliskiren compared with and in combination with irbesartan in patients with type 2 diabetes, hypertension, and albuminuria. Diabetes Care 2009;32:1873–1879.
82. Parving HH, Brenner BM, McMurray JJ, et al. Cardiorenal end points in a trial of aliskiren for type 2 diabetes. N Engl J Med 2012;367:2204–2213.
83. U.S. FDA. FDA Drug Safety Communication: New Warning and Contraindication for Blood Pressure Medicines Containing Aliskiren (Tekturna). Silver Spring, MD: U.S. FDA, 2012. http://www.fda.gov/drugs/drugsafety/ucm300889.htm
84. Dworkin LD, Benstein JA, Parker M, et al. Calcium antagonists and converting enzyme inhibitors reduce renal injury by different mechanisms. Kidney Int 1993;43: 808–814.
85. Hart P, Bakris GL. Calcium antagonists: Do they equally protect against kidney injury? Kidney Int 2008;73:795–796.
86. Abe M, Okada K, Maruyama N, et al. Comparison between the antiproteinuric effects of the calcium channel blockers benidipine and cilnidipine in combination with angiotensin receptor blockers in hypertensive patients with chronic kidney disease. Expert Opin Investig Drugs 2010;19: 1027–1037.
87. Abosaif NY, Arije A, Atray NK, et al. K/DOQI clinical practice guidelines on hypertension and antihypertensive agents in chronic kidney disease. Am J Kidney Dis 2004;43:S1–S290.
88. Centers for Medicare & Medicaid Servives (CMS), HHS. Medicare program; end-stage renal disease prospective payment system and quality incentive program; ambulance fee schedule; durable medical equipment; and competitive acquisition of certain durable medical equipment, prosthetics, orthotics and supplies. Final rule. Fed Regist 2011;76:70228–70316.
89. Finkelstein FO, Story K, Firanek C, et al. Health-related quality of life and hemoglobin levels in chronic kidney disease patients. Clin J Am Soc Nephrol 2009;4: 33–38.
90. U.S. Renal Data System, USRDS 2007 Annual Data Report: Atlas of End-Stage Renal Disease in the United States. Bethesda, MD: National Institutes of Health, National Institute of Diabetes and Digestive and Kidney Diseases, 2007.

91. Phrommintikul A, Haas SJ, Elsik M, Krum H. Mortality and target haemoglobin concentrations in anaemic patients with chronic kidney disease treated with erythropoietin: A meta-analysis. Lancet 2007;369:381–388.
92. Inrig JK, Barnhart HX, Reddan D, et al. Effect of hemoglobin target on progression of kidney disease: A secondary analysis of the CHOIR (Correction of Hemoglobin and Outcomes in Renal Insufficiency) Trial. Am J Kidney Dis 2012;60:390–401.
93. Pfeffer MA, Burdmann EA, Chen CY, et al. A trial of darbepoetin alfa in type 2 diabetes and chronic kidney disease. N Engl J Med 2009;361:2019–2032.
94. Skali H, Parving HH, Parfrey PS, et al. Stroke in patients with type 2 diabetes mellitus, chronic kidney disease, and anemia treated with darbepoetin alfa: The trial to reduce cardiovascular events with Aranesp therapy (TREAT) experience. Circulation 2011;124:2903–2908.
95. Szczech LA, Barnhart HX, Inrig JK, et al. Secondary analysis of the CHOIR trial epoetin-alpha dose and achieved hemoglobin outcomes. Kidney Int 2008;74:791–798.
96. Kilpatrick RD, Critchlow CW, Fishbane S, et al. Greater epoetin alfa responsiveness is associated with improved survival in hemodialysis patients. Clin J Am Soc Nephrol 2008;3:1077–1083.
97. Unger EF, Thompson AM, Blank MJ, Temple R. Erythropoiesis-stimulating agents—Time for a reevaluation. N Engl J Med 2010;362:189–192.
98. U.S. FDA. FDA Drug Safety Communication: Modified Dosing Recommendations to Improve the Safe Use of Erythropoiesis-Stimulating Agents (ESAs) in Chronic Kidney Disease. Silver Spring, MD: U.S. FDA, 2011, *http://www.fda.gov/Drugs/DrugSafety/ucm259639.htm.*
99. Epogen [package insert]. Thousand Oaks, CA: Amgen, 2011.
100. Procrit [package insert]. Raritan, NJ: Ortho Biotech, 2011.
101. Aranesp [package insert]. Thousand Oaks, CA: Amgen, 2011.
102. Omontys [package insert]. Palo Alto, CA: Affymax Inc, 2012.
103. KDOQI. KDOQI clinical practice guideline and clinical practice recommendations for anemia in chronic kidney disease: 2007 update of hemoglobin target. Am J Kidney Dis 2007;50:471–530.
104. Coyne DW, Kapoian T, Suki W, et al. Ferric gluconate is highly efficacious in anemic hemodialysis patients with high serum ferritin and low transferrin saturation: Results of the Dialysis Patients' Response to IV Iron with Elevated Ferritin (DRIVE) Study. J Am Soc Nephrol 2007;18:975–984.
105. Nissenson AR, Berns JS, Sakiewicz P, et al. Clinical evaluation of heme iron polypeptide: Sustaining a response to rHuEPO in hemodialysis patients. Am J Kidney Dis 2003;42: 325–330.
106. Geisser P, Burckhardt S. The pharmacokinetics and pharmacodynamics of iron preparations. Pharmaceutics 2011;3:12–33.
107. Dexferrum [package insert]. Shirley, NY: American Regent Laboratories Inc, 2008.
108. InFeD [package insert]. Florham Park, NJ: Watson Pharma, 2009.
109. Ferrlecit [package insert]. Bridgewater, NJ: Sanofi-Aventis, 2011.
110. Feraheme [package insert]. Lexington, MA: AMAG Pharmaceuticals Inc, 2012.
111. Venofer [package insert]. Shirley, NY: American Regent Laboratories Inc, 2012.
112. Danielson BG. Structure, chemistry, and pharmacokinetics of intravenous iron agents. J Am Soc Nephrol 2004;15 (Suppl 2):S93–S98.
113. Bailie GR. Comparison of rates of reported adverse events associated with i.v. iron products in the United States. Am J Health Syst Pharm 2012;69:310–320.
114. Auerbach M, Winchester J, Wahab A, et al. A randomized trial of three iron dextran infusion methods for anemia in EPO-treated dialysis patients. Am J Kidney Dis 1998;31: 81–86.
115. Dahdah K, Patrie JT, Bolton WK. Intravenous iron dextran treatment in predialysis patients with chronic renal failure. Am J Kidney Dis 2000;36:775–782.
116. Folkert VW, Michael B, Agarwal R, et al. Chronic use of sodium ferric gluconate complex in hemodialysis patients: Safety of higher-dose (> or =250 mg) administration. Am J Kidney Dis 2003;41:651–657.
117. Blaustein DA, Schwenk MH, Chattopadhyay J, et al. The safety and efficacy of an accelerated iron sucrose dosing regimen in patients with chronic kidney disease. Kidney Int Suppl 2003:S72–S77.
118. Hayat A. Safety issues with intravenous iron products in the management of anemia in chronic kidney disease. Clin Med Res 2008;6:93–102.
119. Besarab A. Optimizing anaemia management with subcutaneous administration of epoetin. Nephrol Dial Transplant 2005;20(Suppl 6):vi10–vi15.
120. Pollock C, Johnson DW, Horl WH, et al. Pure red cell aplasia induced by erythropoiesis-stimulating agents. Clin J Am Soc Nephrol 2008;3:193–199.
121. Macdougall IC, Rossert J, Casadevall N, et al. A peptide-based erythropoietin-receptor agonist for pure red-cell aplasia. N Engl J Med 2009;361:1848–1855.
122. Pergola PE, Gartenberg G, Fu M, et al. A randomized controlled study comparing once-weekly to every-2-week and every-4-week dosing of epoetin alfa in CKD patients with anemia. Clin J Am Soc Nephrol 2010;5:598–606.
123. Kliger AS, Fishbane S, Finkelstein FO. Erythropoietic stimulating agents and quality of a patient's life: Individualizing anemia treatment. Clin J Am Soc Nephrol 2012;7:354–357.
124. Aspinall SL, Cunningham FE, Zhao X, et al. Impact of pharmacist-managed erythropoiesis-stimulating agents clinics for patients with non-dialysis-dependent CKD. Am J Kidney Dis 2012;60:371–379.
125. Souberbielle JC, Roth H, Fouque DP. Parathyroid hormone measurement in CKD. Kidney Int 2010;77:93–100.
126. Martin KJ, Gonzalez EA. Prevention and control of phosphate retention/hyperphosphatemia in CKD-MBD: What is normal, when to start, and how to treat? Clin J Am Soc Nephrol 2011;6:440–446.
127. Walsh M, Manns BJ, Klarenbach S, et al. The effects of nocturnal compared with conventional hemodialysis on mineral metabolism: A randomized-controlled trial. Hemodial Int 2010;14:174–181.
128. Fishbane S, Delmez J, Suki WN, et al. A randomized, parallel, open-label study to compare once-daily sevelamer carbonate powder dosing with thrice-daily sevelamer hydrochloride tablet dosing in CKD patients on hemodialysis. Am J Kidney Dis 2010;55:307–315.
129. Kakuta T, Tanaka R, Hyodo T, et al. Effect of sevelamer and calcium-based phosphate binders on coronary artery calcification and accumulation of circulating advanced glycation end products in hemodialysis patients. Am J Kidney Dis 2011;57:422–431.
130. Qunibi W, Moustafa M, Muenz LR, et al. A 1-year randomized trial of calcium acetate versus sevelamer on progression of coronary artery calcification in hemodialysis patients with comparable lipid control: The Calcium Acetate

Renagel Evaluation-2 (CARE-2) study. Am J Kidney Dis 2008;51:952–965.
131. Sprague SM, Ross EA, Nath SD, et al. Lanthanum carbonate vs. sevelamer hydrochloride for the reduction of serum phosphorus in hemodialysis patients: A crossover study. Clin Nephrol 2009;72:252–258.
132. Aramwit P, Srisawadwong R, Supasyndh O. Effectiveness and safety of extended-release nicotinic acid for reducing serum phosphorus in hemodialysis patients. J Nephrol 2012;25:354–362.
133. Renvela [package insert]. Cambridge, MA: Genzyme Corporation, 2011.
134. Guillen-Anaya MA, Jadoul M. Drug interaction between sevelamer and cyclosporin. Nephrol Dial Transplant 2004;19:515.
135. Capitanini A, Lupi A, Osteri F, et al. Gastric pH, sevelamer hydrochloride and omeprazole. Clin Nephrol 2005;64: 320–322.
136. Fosrenol [package insert]. Wayne, PA: Shire U.S. Inc, 2011.
137. Bailie GR, Johnson CA. Comparative review of the pharmacokinetics of vitamin D analogues. Semin Dial 2002;15:352–357.
138. Zemplar Capsules [package insert]. Abbott Park, IL: Abbott Laboratories Inc, 2011.
139. Joist HE, Ahya SN, Giles K, et al. Differential effects of very high doses of doxercalciferol and paricalcitol on serum phosphorus in hemodialysis patients. Clin Nephrol 2006;65:335–341.
140. Sprague SM, Llach F, Amdahl M, et al. Paricalcitol versus calcitriol in the treatment of secondary hyperparathyroidism. Kidney Int 2003;63:1483–1490.
141. Melamed ML, Thadhani RI. Vitamin D therapy in chronic kidney disease and end stage renal disease. Clin J Am Soc Nephrol 2012;7:358–365.
142. Thadhani R, Appelbaum E, Pritchett Y, et al. Vitamin D therapy and cardiac structure and function in patients with chronic kidney disease: The PRIMO randomized controlled trial. JAMA 2012;307:674–684.
143. de Zeeuw D, Agarwal R, Amdahl M, et al. Selective vitamin D receptor activation with paricalcitol for reduction of albuminuria in patients with type 2 diabetes (VITAL study): A randomised controlled trial. Lancet 2010;376: 1543–1551.
144. Kandula P, Dobre M, Schold JD, et al. Vitamin D supplementation in chronic kidney disease: A systematic review and meta-analysis of observational studies and randomized controlled trials. Clin J Am Soc Nephrol 2011;6:50–62.
145. Jean G, Terrat JC, Vanel T, et al. Evidence for persistent vitamin D 1-alpha-hydroxylation in hemodialysis patients: Evolution of serum 1,25-dihydroxycholecalciferol after 6 months of 25-hydroxycholecalciferol treatment. Nephron Clin Pract 2008;110:c58–c65.
146. Zemplar Injection [package insert]. Abbott Park, IL: Abbott Laboratories Inc, 2011.
147. Hectorol Injection [package insert]. Cambridge, MA: Genzyme Corporation, 2010.
148. Sensipar (Cinacalcet HCl) Tablets [package insert]. Thousand Oaks, CA: Amgen Inc, 2011.
149. Raggi P, Chertow GM, Torres PU, et al. The ADVANCE study: A randomized study to evaluate the effects of cinacalcet plus low-dose vitamin D on vascular calcification in patients on hemodialysis. Nephrol Dial Transplant 2011;26:1327–1339.
150. Block GA, Zaun D, Smits G, et al. Cinacalcet hydrochloride treatment significantly improves all-cause and cardiovascular survival in a large cohort of hemodialysis patients. Kidney Int 2010;78:578–589.
151. EVOLVE Trial Investigators, Chertow GM, Block GA, et al. Effect of cinacalcet on cardiovascular disease in patients undergoing dialysis. N Engl J Med 2012;367:2482–2494.
152. Weir MR. Recognizing the link between chronic kidney disease and cardiovascular disease. Am J Manag Care 2011;17(Suppl 15):S396–S402.
153. K/DOQI Workgroup. K/DOQI clinical practice guidelines for cardiovascular disease in dialysis patients. Am J Kidney Dis 2005;45:16–153.
154. National Kidney Foundation. K/DOQI clinical practice guidelines for managing dyslipidemias in patients with chronic kidney disease. Am J Kidney Dis 2003;41:S1–S91.
155. Expert Panel on Detection, Evaluation, and Treatment of High Blood Cholesterol in Adults. Executive summary of the third report of the National Cholesterol Education Program (NCEP) Expert Panel on Detection, Evaluation, and Treatment of High Blood Cholesterol in Adults (Adult Treatment Panel III). JAMA 2001;285:2486–2497.
156. Kidney Disease: Improving Global Outcomes, Lipid Management Work Group. KDIGO clinical practice guideline for lipid management in CKD. In press.
157. Palmer SC, Craig JC, Navaneethan SD, et al. Benefits and harms of statin therapy for persons with chronic kidney disease: A systematic review and meta-analysis. Ann Intern Med 2012;157:263–275.
158. Wanner C, Krane V, Marz W, et al. Atorvastatin in patients with type 2 diabetes mellitus undergoing hemodialysis. N Engl J Med 2005;353:238–248.
159. Fellstrom BC, Jardine AG, Schmieder RE, et al. Rosuvastatin and cardiovascular events in patients undergoing hemodialysis. N Engl J Med 2009;360:1395–1407.
160. Baigent C, Landray MJ, Reith C, et al. The effects of lowering LDL cholesterol with simvastatin plus ezetimibe in patients with chronic kidney disease (Study of Heart and Renal Protection): A randomised placebo-controlled trial. Lancet 2011;377:2181–2192.
161. Clinical practice guidelines for nutrition in chronic renal failure. K/DOQI, National Kidney Foundation. Am J Kidney Dis 2000;35:S1–S140.

30

Hemodialysis and Peritoneal Dialysis

Kevin M. Sowinski, Mariann D. Churchwell, and Brian S. Decker

KEY CONCEPTS

1. Hemodialysis (HD) involves the perfusion of blood and dialysate on opposite sides of a semipermeable membrane. Solutes are removed from the blood by diffusion and convection. Excess plasma water is removed by ultrafiltration.
2. Native arteriovenous (AV) fistulas are the preferred access for HD because of fewer complications and a longer survival rate. Venous catheters are plagued by complications such as infection and thrombosis and often deliver low blood flow rates.
3. Adequacy of HD can be assessed by the *Kt/V* and urea reduction ratio (URR). The National Kidney Foundation's Kidney Disease Outcomes Quality Initiative minimum goal *Kt/V* is greater than 1.2 per treatment and the URR is greater than 65%.
4. During HD, patients commonly experience hypotension and cramps. Other more serious complications include infection and thrombosis of the vascular access.
5. Peritoneal dialysis (PD) involves the instillation of dialysate into the peritoneal cavity via a permanent peritoneal catheter. The peritoneal membrane lines the highly vascularized abdominal viscera and acts as the semipermeable membrane. Solutes are removed from the blood across the peritoneum via diffusion and ultrafiltration. Excess plasma water is removed via ultrafiltration created by osmotic pressure generated by various dextrose or icodextrin concentrations.
6. Patients on PD are required to instill and drain, manually or via automated systems, several liters of fresh dialysate each day. The more exchanges completed each day results in greater solute removal.
7. Peritonitis is a common complication of PD. Initial empiric therapy for peritonitis should include intraperitoneal (IP) antibiotics that are effective against both gram-positive and gram-negative organisms.
8. Nasal carriage of *Staphylococcus aureus* is associated with an increased risk of catheter-related infections and peritonitis. Prophylaxis with intranasal mupirocin (twice a day for 5 days every month) or mupirocin (daily) at the exit site can effectively reduce *S. aureus* infections.

INTRODUCTION

The three primary treatment options for patients with end-stage renal disease (ESRD) are hemodialysis (HD), peritoneal dialysis (PD), and kidney transplantation. The United States Renal Data System (USRDS) is the national system that "collects, analyzes, and distributes" data relating to patients with ESRD or Stage 5 chronic kidney disease (CKD) in the United States.[1] According to the 2011 USRDS, at the end of 2009, there are more than 550,000 patients in the United States with ESRD. Of these, 370,274 and 27,522 patients were being treated with HD and PD, respectively, and 172,553 had a functioning kidney transplant. In 2009, 116,395 new patients started therapy for ESRD (dialysis or transplantation) and more than 91,000 patients died. The vast majority of new dialysis patients are treated with HD. The number of patients treated with PD has steadily decreased since 2000.[1] Although the number of patients who have received a kidney transplant has risen, transplantation has not kept pace with the growing prevalence of ESRD in the United States.[1]

Since 1972, the treatment of ESRD (both dialysis and kidney transplantation) has been paid for by Medicare. The total cost of ESRD in 2009 was 42.5 billion dollars, this includes Medicare costs (29 billion), Medicare patient obligation costs (4.2 billion), and non-Medicare costs (9.3 billion). Total Medicare spending for ESRD in 2009 rose by 3.1%. The Medicare spending does not include Part D expenditures, which were 1.55 billion in 2008. ESRD consumes a vastly disproportionate amount of resources; approximately 1% of the patients in the Medicare program have ESRD, yet 6% of the budget is consumed by the ESRD program. Although total spending for ESRD treatment continues to climb, per-patient spending (after adjusting for inflation) was fairly flat recently.[1]

There are some positive signs as it relates to public health and ESRD. Although the total number of dialysis patients is increasing in the United States, the number of new dialysis patients per total population has stabilized or slightly decreased from the highest value observed in 1997. The prevalence of ESRD continues to climb, reflective of reduced mortality and enhanced patient care. The primary diagnosis for new patients with ESRD is diabetes.[1] Chapter 29 provides a thorough discussion on the epidemiology of CKD.

This chapter serves as a primer on the principles and practice of dialysis and the complications associated with the delivery of dialysis treatments. The chapter focuses on HD and PD as the modalities most commonly employed for the management of ESRD (see Chap. 28 for a discussion of the role of renal replacement therapies in the management of acute kidney injury). The pertinent factors that should be considered before the initiation of dialysis are described. The morbidity and mortality associated with HD and PD are compared, as these considerations may influence the dialysis method chosen by patients and clinicians. Because dialysis by either method is not a generic procedure, the variants of HD and PD are detailed. The multiple types of vascular and peritoneal access used to provide HD and PD, including various catheters and surgical techniques, are illustrated. The concept of dialysis adequacy for each modality is briefly reviewed. Finally, the clinical presentation of the common complications of both dialytic therapies is presented, along

TABLE 30-1 Patient-Related Videos Relative to Dialysis Procedures and Therapies

Source	Website (accessed 30 October 2012)
Baxter	http://www.youtube.com/renalinfo
Davita Inc.	http://www.davita.com/videos/
NxStage Medical, Inc.	https://www.nxstage.com/homehemodialysis/patientvideos
Fresenius Medical Care	http://www.ultracare-dialysis.com/Footer/LinksResources/VideoLibrary.aspx
National Kidney Foundation	http://www.youtube.com/watch?v=NHS0oyHR4vI&feature=plcp
NBC News	http://video.msnbc.msn.com/nightly-news/40856952#40856952

with pertinent nonpharmacologic and pharmacologic therapeutic approaches. Patient-related videos that describe living with CKD, dialysis, and associated dialysis therapies are shown in Table 30-1. This information is included to provide the reader with a patient perspective into the disease and its associated therapies.

MORBIDITY AND MORTALITY IN DIALYSIS PATIENTS

Morbidity in patients receiving dialysis can be assessed in a number of different ways including tabulation of the number of hospitalizations per patient-year, the number of days hospitalized per patient per year, or the incidence of certain complications. The number of all-cause hospital admissions in dialysis patients per patient-year (1.9 hospitalizations per patient-year) have changed little since 1993. However, the rate of hospitalizations fell in 2006, to a rate approximately 4% less than that in 1993. Trends in hospitalization demonstrate an increase in hospitalization as a consequence of infection and cardiovascular disease and a decrease in hospitalizations as a consequence of vascular access problems. Patients with a functioning kidney transplant have a lower rate of hospitalization and shorter length of stay. Hospitalizations are more frequent for whites than for blacks, and the frequency and duration increase with age in both dialysis modality groups.[1]

The life expectancy of U.S. dialysis patients is markedly lower than that of healthy subjects of the same age and sex. In those older than 65 years, the risk of dying is twofold higher in dialysis patients compared with those with diabetes, cancer, heart failure, and cardiovascular disease.[1] Approximately 50% of deaths in dialysis patients are cardiovascular related. In fact, those with CKD are more likely to die from cardiovascular disease before they reach ESRD. Infections, usually related to the dialysis access, are the second most common cause of death in dialysis patients. Although mortality is high in this patient population, improvement has been made and the overall patient mortality rate has fallen among dialysis patients since 1988. The changes in mortality rates are more impressive when the duration of a patient's time receiving dialysis is considered. In patients receiving dialysis for fewer than 2 years, mortality rates decreased 25% since 1988. However, in those treated for 5 years or more, mortality rates increased 10%. These changes suggest that death is occurring later in the course of dialysis therapy. Regardless, in the United States, nearly two thirds of all dialysis patients die within 5 years of initiation of dialysis treatment, a life expectancy worse than patients with heart failure or numerous cancers.[2]

In addition to the morbidity and mortality discussed above a dialysis patient's quality of life is generally poor. Quality-of-life assessments including the impact of dialysis treatment on these patients have been an area of considerable research.[3–6] Additionally, in an effort to understand how these patients manage the constraints and difficulties of their life situations health care providers and researchers have provided commentaries and papers.[7–11] For example, restrictions caused by thrice weekly HD and/or associated treatments have been shown to impact many areas of a patient's life. These include but are not limited to, physical endurance, sex life, employment, social life, and dietary restrictions. Patients often complain of fatigue and fear of the unknown related to their disease and its progression. Although, the authors of this chapter may be able to describe the disruption to a patient's life induced by this chronic disease only a kidney disease patient can adequately describe the three trips per week to the outpatient HD unit for a 3- to 4-hour HD session. The PD patient or the home HD patient may have some freedom from these restrictions, but this freedom comes with its own constraints (see the videos listed in Table 30-1).

INDICATIONS FOR DIALYSIS

The National Kidney Foundation's Kidney Disease Outcome Quality Initiative (NKF-K/DOQI) recommends that planning for dialysis begin when patients reach CKD stage 4 (estimated glomerular filtration rate [eGFR] or creatinine clearance [CL_{cr}] below 30 mL/min per 1.73 m^2 [0.29 mL/s/m^2]).[12] Beginning the preparation process at this point allows adequate time for proper education of the patient and family and for the creation of a suitable vascular or peritoneal access. For patients choosing HD, a permanent arteriovenous (AV) access (preferably a fistula) should be surgically created when Cl_{cr} or eGFR falls below 25 mL/min (0.42 mL/s), serum creatinine is greater than 4 mg/dL (354 μmol/L), or 1 year prior to the anticipated need for dialysis.[13]

The primary criterion for initiation of dialysis is the patient's clinical status: the presence of persistent anorexia, nausea, and vomiting, especially if accompanied by weight loss, fatigue, declining serum albumin concentrations, uncontrolled hypertension or congestive heart failure, and neurologic deficits or pruritus. Some nephrologists use critical lab values of serum creatinine or blood urea nitrogen as indicators of when to initiate dialysis. The 2006 update of the NKF-K/DOQI guidelines suggest that risks and benefits of dialysis should be evaluated when eGFR or CL_{cr} is <15 mL/min per 1.73 m^2 (<0.14 mL/s/m^2).[12,14] The advantages and disadvantages of HD and PD are depicted in Tables 30-2 and 30-3, respectively. These factors, along with the patients' concomitant diseases, personal preferences, and support environments, are the principal determinants of the dialysis mode they will receive.[2]

TABLE 30-2 Advantages and Disadvantages of Hemodialysis

Advantages

1. Higher solute clearance allows intermittent treatment
2. Parameters of adequacy of dialysis are better defined and therefore underdialysis can be detected early
3. Technique failure rate is low
4. Even though intermittent heparinization is required, hemostasis parameters are better corrected with HD than PD
5. In-center HD enables closer monitoring of the patient

Disadvantages

1. Requires multiple visits each week to the HD center, which translates into loss of patient independence
2. Disequilibrium, dialysis-induced hypotension, and muscle cramps are common. May require months before the patient adjusts to HD
3. Infections in HD patients may be related to the choice of membranes, the complement-activating membranes being more deleterious
4. Vascular access is frequently associated with infection and thrombosis
5. Decline of RRF is more rapid compared to PD

TABLE 30-3 Advantages and Disadvantages of Peritoneal Dialysis

Advantages
1. Hemodynamic stability due to slow ultrafiltration rate
2. Higher clearance of larger solutes, which may explain good clinical status in spite of lower urea clearance
3. Better preservation of RRF
4. Convenient IP route for administration of drugs such as antibiotics and insulin
5. Suitable for elderly and very young patients who may not tolerate HD well
6. Freedom from the "machine" gives the patient a sense of independence (for continuous ambulatory PD)
7. Less blood loss and iron deficiency, resulting in easier management of anemia or reduced requirements for erythropoietin and parenteral iron
8. No systemic heparinization required
9. Subcutaneous versus IV erythropoietin or darbepoetin may reduce overall doses and be more physiologic

Disadvantages
1. Protein and amino acid losses through peritoneum and reduced appetite from continuous glucose load and sense of abdominal fullness predispose patients to malnutrition
2. Risk of peritonitis
3. Catheter malfunction, exit site, and tunnel infection
4. Inadequate ultrafiltration and solute clearance in patients with a large body size, unless large volumes and frequent exchanges are employed
5. Patient burnout and high rate of technique failure
6. Risk of obesity with excessive glucose absorption
7. Mechanical problems such as hernias, dialysate leaks, hemorrhoids, or back pain are more common than HD
8. Extensive abdominal surgery may preclude PD
9. No convenient access for IV iron administration

Clinical **Controversy...**

There is debate over which dialysis treatment modality, HD or PD, is most desirable in terms of morbidity and mortality. Outcome studies have provided conflicting results. Although less than 10% of U.S. patients are treated with PD, nephrologists suggest many more ESRD patients could be treated with PD.

While the intent of this chapter is not to exhaustively compare and contrast HD and PD and the relative benefits of each, there is considerable debate in the literature regarding the mortality differences between HD and PD. A recent trial examining mortality in dialysis patients in the Netherlands found no difference between patients receiving either modality in the first 2 years. However after that mortality rates were higher in patients on PD.[14] Most observational trials suggest that PD is associated with a survival advantage early in therapy, which wanes with increased treatment time. Well-designed studies are extremely difficult to conduct in this population and thus the question of superiority of one modality over the other is controversial. Differences in outcomes may be related to a wide array of confounding factors, such as the dose of dialysis, baseline patient health status, physician bias in modality selection, patient compliance with dialysis and medication therapy, or other unknown factors. For example, healthier patients tend to be directed toward PD and factors such as age, duration of dialysis, and comorbidities play an important role in the complex relationship between patient outcomes and mortality.[15,16] Without clear distinction between modalities in terms of many important outcomes, the selection of the optimal therapy for a given patient is challenging. The NKF-K/DOQI guidelines recommend that the timing of dialysis initiation is a compromise between maximizing patient QOL by extending the dialysis-free period while avoiding complications that will decrease the length and quality of dialysis-assisted life.[12]

HEMODIALYSIS

Although HD was first successfully used in 1940, the procedure was not used widely until the Korean War in 1952. Permanent dialysis access was developed in the 1960s,[17] which allowed routine use of HD in patients with ESRD. Subsequent decades brought advances in dialysis technology, including the introduction of more efficient and biocompatible dialyzer membranes and safer techniques. HD is now the most common type of renal replacement therapy for patients with ESRD.

Principles of Hemodialysis

1 HD, simply stated, consists of the perfusion of blood and a physiologic solution on opposite sides of a semipermeable membrane.[18] Multiple substances, such as water, urea, creatinine, uremic toxins, and drugs, move from the blood into the dialysate, by either passive diffusion or convection as the result of ultrafiltration. Diffusion is the movement of substances down a concentration gradient; usually for endogenous waste products from the blood to dialysate; the rate of diffusion depends on the difference between the concentration of the solute in blood and dialysate, solute characteristics, that is size, water solubility, and charge, the dialyzer membrane composition, and blood and dialysate flow rates. Diffusive transport is rapid for small solutes, but slows with increasing molecular size. Other important diffusive solute transport factors include the membrane thickness, porosity, and the steric hindrance between the membrane pores and solute. Ultrafiltration is the movement of water across the dialyzer membrane as a consequence of hydrostatic or osmotic pressure and is the primary means for removal of excess fluid. Convection occurs when dissolved solutes are "dragged" across a membrane with fluid transport (if the pores in the dialyzer are large enough to allow them to pass). Convection can be maximized by increasing the hydrostatic pressure gradient across the dialysis membrane, or by changing to a dialyzer that is more permeable to water transport. These two processes of diffusion and convection can be controlled independently, and thus a patient's HD prescription can be individualized to attain the desired degree of solute and fluid removal.[18]

Hemodialysis Access

2 Obtaining and maintaining access to the circulation has been a challenge for long-term use and success of HD.[18] The AV fistula, AV graft, or venous catheter through which blood is obtained for dialysis is referred to as the dialysis access. Permanent access to the circulation may be accomplished by several techniques, including the creation of an AV fistula, an AV graft, or by the use of venous catheters (Fig. 30-1).[19] The native AV fistula is created by the anastomosis of a vein and artery (i.e., the radial artery to the cephalic vein or the brachial artery to the cephalic vein). The native AV fistula has many advantages over other access methods. Fistulas have the longest survival of all blood-access devices and are associated with the lowest rate of complications such as infection and thrombosis. In addition, patients with fistulas have increased survival and lower hospitalization rates compared to other HD patients. Finally, the use of AV fistulas is the most cost-effective in terms of placement and long-term maintenance. Ideally, the most distal site (the wrist) is used to construct the fistula. This fistula is the easiest to create, and in the case of access failure, more proximal sites on the arm are preserved. Unfortunately, fistulas require 1 to 2 months or more to mature before they can be routinely utilized for dialysis. In addition, creation of an AV fistula may be difficult in elderly patients and in patients with peripheral vascular disease (which is particularly common in patients with diabetes).

Synthetic AV grafts, usually made of polytetrafluoroethylene, are another option for permanent AV access. In general, grafts

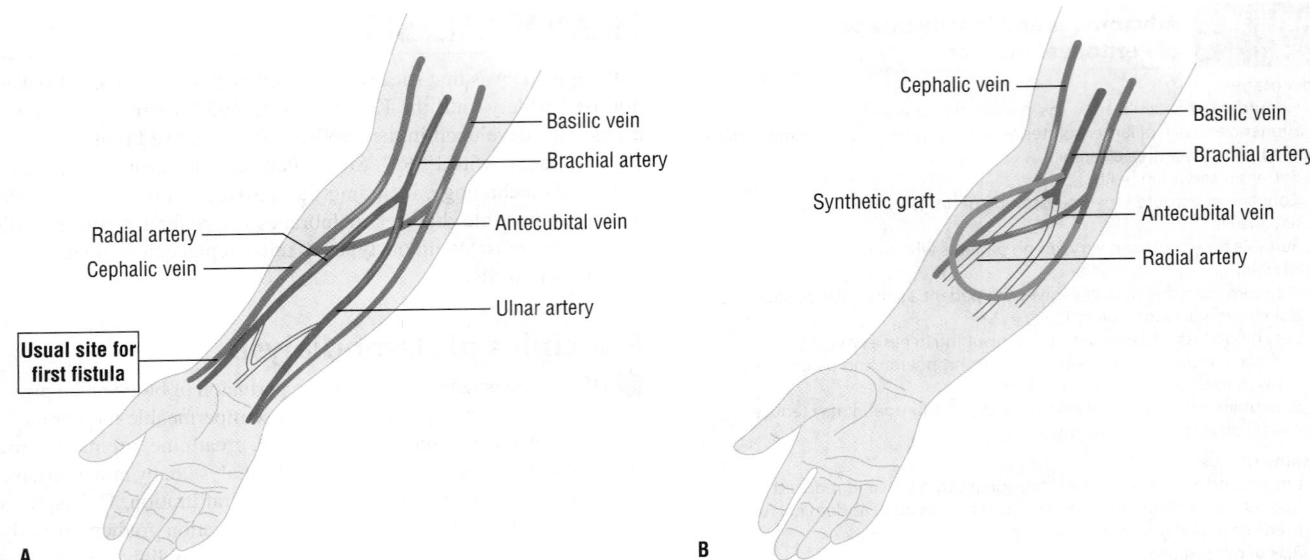

FIGURE 30-1 The predominant types of vascular access for chronic dialysis patients are (*A*) the AV fistula and (*B*) the synthetic AV forearm graft. The first primary AV fistula is usually created by the surgical anastomosis of the cephalic vein with the radial artery. The flow of blood from the higher-pressure arterial system results in hypertrophy of the vein. The most common AV graft (depicted in green) is between the brachial artery and the basilic or cephalic vein. The flow of blood may be diminished in the radial and ulnar arteries since it preferentially flows into the low pressure graft.

require only 2 to 3 weeks to endothelialize before they can be routinely used. The primary disadvantages of this type of access when compared to an AV fistula are shorter survival of the graft, and higher rates of infection and thrombosis. The least-desirable HD access is via central venous catheters (CVCs), which, unfortunately, are commonly used in chronic HD patients. Venous catheters can be placed in the femoral, subclavian, or internal jugular vein. The main advantage of catheters is that they can be used immediately. Catheters are often used in small children, diabetic patients with severe vascular disease, the morbidly obese, and patients who have no viable sites for permanent AV access. Late referrals to a nephrology specialist and delayed placement of a more appropriate long-term access contribute to the overuse of venous catheters in chronic HD patients. The major problem with all venous catheters is that they have a short life span and are more prone to infection and thrombosis than either AV grafts or fistulas. Furthermore, some catheters are not able to provide adequate blood flow rates, which can limit the dose of dialysis delivered.[19–23] Regardless, tunneled dialysis catheters are used frequently for a variety of reasons including ease of insertion, pain-free dialysis, and immediate use. They are however associated with increased morbidity, mortality, and increased cost.[24]

The ESRD Clinical Performance Measures (CPM) Project examined quality of dialysis care markers, including anemia management, serum albumin, vascular access (for HD), and adequacy of dialysis. The report evaluated a sample population of adult in-center patients, 8,915 HD patients and 1,469 PD patients.[25] At the end of 2005, 54% and 44% of incident and prevalent patients, respectively, were using AV fistulas for HD. The CPM Project's goal is that 50% and 40% of incident and prevalent HD patients, respectively, should be using an AV fistula. Unfortunately, 21% of HD patients were using chronic catheters in 2005. This percent of patients using catheters is much higher than the CPM Project's goal of <10%. The extensive use of catheters may be a result of the large population of patients who are not candidates for AV access, or that they are being used until permanent AV access can be accomplished. As noted earlier, timely referral to a nephrologist and vascular surgeon is necessary for the placement of the most appropriate access.

Hemodialysis Procedures

The HD system consists of an external vascular circuit through which the patient's blood is transferred in sterile polyethylene tubing to the dialyzer via a mechanical pump (Fig. 30-2).[26] The patient's anticoagulated blood then passes through the dialyzer on one side of the semipermeable membrane and is returned to the patient. The dialysate solution, which consists of purified water and electrolytes, is pumped through the dialyzer countercurrent to the flow of blood on the opposite side of the semipermeable membrane. In most cases, systemic anticoagulation (with heparin) is used to prevent clotting of the HD circuit. The process of dialysis results in the removal of metabolic waste products and water and replenishment of body buffers.[18] There are three broad categories of dialysis membranes: low flux, high efficiency, and high flux. Low-flux dialyzers, mostly made of cuprophane or cellulose acetate, have small pores that limit clearance to relatively small molecules (size ≤500 daltons) such as urea and creatinine. High-efficiency membranes have large surface areas and thus have a greater ability to remove water, urea, and other small molecules. High-flux membranes have larger pores that are capable of removing high-molecular-weight substances, such as β_2-microglobulin, and vancomycin in addition to other larger molecular weight drugs.[26,27] The primary reason to use high-efficiency and/or high-flux membranes is that clearance of both low- and high-molecular-weight substances is much greater than with the conventional membranes, allowing for shorter treatment times. To maximize the capacity or fully utilize the filter's high flux membrane, high-efficiency and high-flux dialysis require blood flow rates greater than 400 mL/min, dialysate flow rates greater than 500 mL/min, and the use of strict controls on the rate of fluid removal. Typically these dialyzers are composed of polysulfone, polymethylmethacrylate, polyamide, cellulose triacetate, and polyacrylonitrile.[26]

HD is usually prescribed three times weekly for 3 to 5 hours. The average duration of dialysis treatment session in the United States in 2005 was just over 3.5 hours.[25] Larger patients generally require longer treatment times for adequate solute removal. This is a substantial time commitment for any patient undergoing HD and

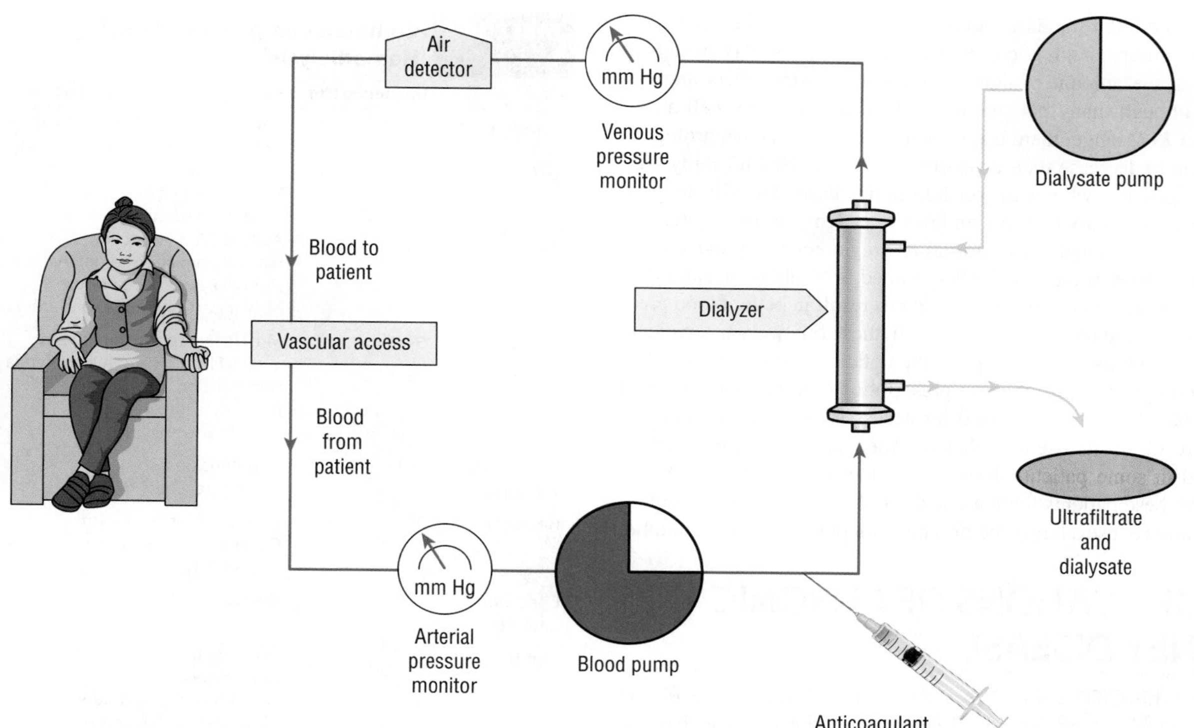

FIGURE 30-2 In HD, the patient's blood is pumped to the dialyzer at a rate of 300 to 600 mL/min. An anticoagulant (usually heparin) is administered to prevent clotting in the dialyzer. The dialysate is pumped at a rate of 500 to 1,000 mL/min through the dialyzer countercurrent to the flow of blood. The rate of fluid removal from the patient is controlled by adjusting the pressure in the dialysate compartment.

results in substantial loss of control over their life. Other types of HD have been explored in an effort to balance dialysis adequacy with patient outcomes and quality of life. Short daily HD, extended dialysis, and quotidian HD are all terms used to describe variants of HD in which dialysis is administered daily for shorter periods of time (2 to 2.5 hours) or as long, slow nocturnal treatments of up to 6 to 8 hours. The theoretical rationale for these treatments is to enhance the efficiency of HD and to reduce HD-induced hemodynamic instability. There is some evidence that these dialysis techniques result in improved clinical outcomes and that it may be a more cost-effective dialysis procedure.[28,29] Both of these therapeutic options are usually delivered in the home. The delivery of traditional HD in the home setting is more commonly used in some countries such as New Zealand and Canada. Despite the perceived advantages, the use of home HD is uncommon in the United States, with less than 1% of dialysis patients receiving HD care at home.[1] Prospective clinical trials are needed in this area to elucidate the role of these types of dialysis therapy.

Measures of Hemodialysis Adequacy

The optimal dose of HD for each individual patient varies and is that the amount of therapy above which there is no cost-effective increment in the patient's quality-adjusted life expectancy. The two primary goals of the dialysis prescription are to achieve a desired dry weight and the adequate removal of endogenous waste products such as urea. Dry weight is the target postdialysis weight at which the patient is normotensive and free of edema. Measurement of urea removal, while imperfect, is the typical way in which dialysis adequacy is quantified. Referred to as the "delivered dose" of dialysis, urea removal is utilized as the surrogate for removal of other toxins.

The delivered or desired dose of dialysis in terms of solute removal can be expressed as the URR or the *Kt*/*V* (pronounced "K-T-over-V"). The URR is a simple concept and is easily calculated as:

$$\text{URR} = \frac{\text{Predialysis BUN} - \text{Postdialysis BUN}}{\text{Predialysis BUN}} \times 100$$

The URR is frequently used to measure the delivered dialysis dose, however, it does not account for the contribution of convective removal of urea. The *Kt*/*V* is a unitless index based on the dialyzer clearance of urea (*K*) in L/h multiplied by the duration of dialysis (*t*) in hours, divided by the urea distribution volume of the patient (*V*) in liters.[30] *Kt*/*V* is thus the fraction of the patient's total body water that is cleared of urea during a dialysis session. Urea kinetic modeling, using computer software, is the optimal means to calculate the *Kt*/*V*.[31] An in-depth discussion of the pros and cons of various methods of calculating and interpreting *Kt*/*V* is beyond the scope of this chapter. The reader is referred to other sources for more in-depth information.[30,31]

3 The NKF-K/DOQI recommends that the minimally adequate delivered dose of dialysis is a *Kt*/*V* of 1.2 (equivalent to an average URR of 65%).[12] To achieve this goal, the recommended target prescribed *Kt*/*V* is 1.4 (equivalent to an average URR of 70%).[12] Lower levels of dialysis treatment are thought to be associated with increased morbidity and mortality.[18] Many nephrologists believe that even greater doses of dialysis would have positive outcomes in dialysis patients, and so the average dose of dialysis has been increasing in the United States. In 2004, the mean delivered *Kt*/*V* as reported by the CPM was 1.55.[25] The Hemodialysis (HEMO) Study was designed to determine the effects of high-dose dialysis and the use of high-flux HD membranes on morbidity and mortality.[32] The results of this prospective, randomized trial that assigned patients to either standard (*Kt*/*V* = 1.25) or high-dose (*Kt*/*V* = 1.65) dialysis with high-flux or low-flux membranes revealed that the risk of death was

similar in both the standard and high-dose therapy and the low- and high-flux groups. Thus there does not appear to be any benefit in increasing the amount of dialysis above the current recommendations. Although many patients in the United States are well above the target *Kt/V* range, there is no reason to believe that nephrologists will begin to decrease their dose of dialysis. The HEMO study only enrolled patients who were on traditional thrice-weekly dialysis, thus the applicability of these findings to patients on more intensive regimens, such as daily or nocturnal HD regimens that provide long, frequent dialysis, remains to be determined,[28,29,33] although early data indicate that these intensive HD regimens result in better blood pressure, anemia, and phosphate control.[28] In those relatively few patients who are below the adequacy goal, the deficiency may be related to patient compliance with dialysis prescription (ending dialysis early) or low blood flow rates caused by access stenosis or thrombosis, or as a result of the use of catheters. Adequate dialysis may not be achieved in some patients despite compliance and sufficient blood flow. For these patients there are really only two options to increase urea clearance: use a larger membrane or increase the treatment time.

COMPLICATIONS OF CHRONIC KIDNEY DISEASE

Patients with CKD defined as a glomerular filtration rate (GFR) <60 mL/min/1.73 m^2 (<0.58 mL/s/m^2) are more likely to have at least one additional comorbid disease such as diabetes, hypertension, cardiovascular disease (CVD), BMI ≥30 kg/m^2. CKD patients are also more likely to be older (age ≥60). The most recent NHANES III data (2005 to 2010) report the prevalence of these comorbid diseases in CKD patients as diabetes 19.3%, hypertension 14.8%, CVD 24.3%, and BMI ≥30 kg/m^2 11.7% with older age at 18.4%. When compared with the NHANES III 1988 to 1994 report the 2005 to 2010 report found that the largest increase in CKD patients was among those patients with CVD (25.4% to 40.8%) although the prevalence of CKD patients only increased from 12.3% to 14%.[34]

The pharmacotherapy management of CKD and any of these comorbid diseases requires multiple medications in addition to dietary restrictions and exercise. As CKD advances to ESRD the pill burden can substantially increase. The daily pill burden for ESRD patients is one of the highest for any chronic disease state. ESRD patients took a mean of 11 ± 4 medications (nine oral and two parenteral) which based on the oral medications resulted in a total pill burden of 19 pills (interquartile range 12) per day. This higher pill burden was associated with a lower quality of life and was not associated with better control of serum phosphorus, a major disease-related problem in ESRD patients.[35]

Patients receiving renal replacement therapy need to be compliant with not only diet and drugs but also dialysis whether this treatment is daily or three times a week. Compliance is essential to manage these diseases but can seem overwhelming for the patient. Therefore, a good working relationship with healthcare providers including their pharmacist can provide the information and support patients require to actively managing these diseases.

COMPLICATIONS OF HEMODIALYSIS

❹ Complications associated with HD therapy are significant and can limit therapy efficacy. These complications that occur during the actual therapy (intradialytic), as well as those associated with vascular access are discussed in this chapter.[36–38]

Intradialytic Complications

The most common complications that occur during the HD procedure include hypotension, cramps, nausea and vomiting, headache, chest pain, back pain, and fever or chills.[37,38] Table 30-4 lists these complications and their etiology and predisposing factors.

TABLE 30-4 Common Complications During Hemodialysis[38]

	Incidence (%)	Etiology/Predisposing Factors
Hypotension	20–30	Hypovolemia and excessive ultrafiltration Antihypertensive medications prior to dialysis Target dry weight too low Diastolic dysfunction Autonomic dysfunction Low calcium and sodium in dialysate High dialysate temperature Meal ingestion prior to or during dialysis
Cramps	5–20	Muscle hypoperfusion due to ultrafiltration and hypovolemia Hypotension Electrolyte imbalance Acid–base imbalance
Nausea and vomiting	5–15	Hypotension Dialyzer reaction
Headache	5	Disequilibrium syndrome Caffeine withdrawal due to dialysis removal
Chest and back pain	2–5	Unknown
Pruritus	5	Inadequate dialysis Skin dryness Secondary hyperparathyroidism Abnormal skin concentrations of electrolytes Histamine release Mast cell proliferation
Fever and chills	<1	Endotoxin release; infection of dialysis catheter

A decrease in blood pressure is often noted during HD, but a symptomatic decline in blood pressure that requires nursing or medical intervention can lead to a decrease in the effectiveness of this treatment.[37] Intradialytic hypotension (IDH) is primarily related to the rate and amount of fluid removed during[32] typical treatments, although other causes, as listed in Table 30-4, may also play a role.[39] Other symptoms such as nausea and cramping are often present during acute hypotensive episodes. The replacement of acetate with bicarbonate as the dialysate buffer, the use of volumetric ultrafiltration controllers, as well as individualized dialysate sodium concentrations and modeling have helped reduce the incidence of hypotension.[40–42]

Skeletal muscle cramps complicate 5% to 20% of HD treatments. Although the pathogenesis of cramps is multifactorial, plasma volume contraction and decreased muscle perfusion caused by excessive ultrafiltration are frequently the initiating events.[37,38] Another complication pruritus, which may appear to increase in severity during the HD treatment, is actually a complication of CKD and the management of this condition is discussed in Chapter 29.

Vascular Access Complications

The maintenance of vascular access patency is critical for HD patients since this access is essential for treatment. Aneurysm and stenosis have been reported with AV fistulas and grafts and resolution of this is primarily by surgical means. Thrombosis and infection are the most common vascular access complications with the highest occurrence found in patients with a cuff catheter compared with those with an AV graft or AV fistula.[38,43,44]

Vascular access dysfunction is usually identified by a decrease in blood flow through the access (blood flow <300 mL/min) over a period of days to weeks. Ultrasound, venography, or computed tomography scans can be used for a definitive diagnosis.[22,45,46] Catheter thrombosis can form either inside (intrinsic) or outside (extrinsic) the catheter. The occlusion can form within the lumen at the tip or develop a fibrin sleeve around the catheter where this fibrin sleeve can serve as a nidus for infection and ultimately require catheter removal.[47,48]

Infection is the second leading cause of mortality in HD patients.[49] The risk of sepsis-related death is 100 times greater in dialysis patients than the general population and those with an indwelling catheter have the highest risk.[50] Common skin flora such as *S. aureus* and coagulase-negative staphylococcus are frequently the source of infection, but gram-negative bacterial and fungal causes must not be overlooked. Catheter-related infections develop at the insertion site, hub, or both. The infection source for long-term catheters such as a tunneled catheter is usually the hub where bacteria can enter the blood leading to a bloodstream infection.[51,52] Overall HD access with a catheter is associated with higher rates of bacteremia, osteomyelitis, septic arthritis, endocarditis, and death as well as increased treatment costs compared with an AV fistula or AV graft.[43]

TABLE 30-5 Management of Hypotension

Acute treatment	Place patient in the Trendelenburg position Decrease ultrafiltration rate Give 100–200 mL bolus of normal saline IV Give 10–20 mL of hypertonic saline (23.4%) IV over 3–5 minutes 12.5 g mannitol
Prevention	
Nonpharmacologic	Accurately set "dry weight" Use steady constant ultrafiltration rate Keep dialysate sodium greater than serum sodium Lower dialysate temperatures Bicarbonate dialysate Avoid food before or during HD
Pharmacologic	Midodrine 2.5–10 mg orally 30 minutes before HD (start at 2.5 mg and titrate) Other options (limited evidence): Levocarnitine 20 mg/kg IV after HD Sertraline 50–100 mg daily Fludrocortisone 0.1 mg before HD DDAVP 1–2 intranasal sprays (150 mcg per spray)

MANAGEMENT OF HEMODIALYSIS COMPLICATIONS

Hypotension

Acute management of IDH includes placing the patient in the Trendelenburg position, decreasing the ultrafiltration rate, lowering the dialysate temperature, modifying dialysate electrolyte concentrations, and/or administering normal or hypertonic saline.[36–41] IDH may not occur during each HD session and patient intravariability could necessitate further HD customization. Hypertensive medications administered the day prior to HD therapy may contribute to IDH; therefore, a careful review of all medications including antihypertensive therapies is warranted. Patients with IDH should be counseled to take their blood pressure medications after HD.

IDH is generally related to an insufficient cardiac response to reduced circulating blood volume; therefore, most treatments are directed toward restoring or maintaining adequate blood vessel perfusion in these patients. For example decreasing the dialysate temperature to 36.5°C (97.7°F) may help reduce core body temperature, which can decrease vasodilation.[53,54] If nonpharmacologic interventions are not adequate to prevent or reduce the incidence of symptomatic IDH then pharmacologic interventions should be considered (Table 30-5). Several pharmacologic options are discussed in this section.

Midodrine, an α_1-adrenergic agonist prodrug (active metabolite desglymidodrine), with peripheral vasoconstrictive properties has been effective with managing IDH. Midodrine administered prior to HD in doses ranging from 2.5 to 10 mg resulted in postdialysis blood pressure elevations and improvement of symptoms. An average increase of systolic and diastolic blood pressures was 12.4 and 7.3 mm Hg above the values in control patients, respectively.[55] An 8-month long study found that midodrine 10 mg given 30 minutes prior to dialysis resulted in correction of hypotension without any adverse events.[56] Oral midodrine (5 mg) given twice daily can increase blood pressure in HD patients with chronic hypotension on nondialysis days.[57] It is important to note that the effects of midodrine are probably best in patients with hypotension related to autonomic dysfunction as opposed to other causes of hypotension. The main adverse effect related to midodrine is urinary retention, but patients with peripheral vascular disease should be monitored for digital or lower limb ischemia.[58]

Other potential therapeutic agents for IDH include levocarnitine, sertraline, and intranasal desmopressin acetate (DDAVP). The IV administration of levocarnitine (20 mg/kg at the end of each dialysis session) reduced hypotensive episodes from 17 to 7 (P <0.02) in a study of 38 patients.[59,60] The high cost and limited data on levocarnitine, however, preclude a strong recommendation for its use. Sertraline has demonstrated efficacy in some,[61,62] but not all studies.[63] A study of 17 IDH patients compared DDAVP to placebo (saline nasal spray).[64] Overall, the use of DDAVP increased post-HD blood pressure and decreased the incidence of IDH. In addition, fludrocortisone has been suggested as a potential agent for symptomatic hypotension.[65] These medications have limited clinical evidence and should be used with caution in patients with IDH.

Muscle Cramps

Nonpharmacologic interventions related to dialytic therapy may help alleviate muscle cramps. These measures include adjusting the ultrafiltration rate to avoiding hypotension, volume contraction, or hypoosmolality. Other methods to reduce muscle cramps are compression devices, moist heat, massage, exercise, stretching or muscle flexing and should be considered first to minimize adverse consequences (Table 30-6).[37,66]

Both vitamin E and quinine significantly reduce the incidence of muscle cramps.[67–69] Quinine is usually well tolerated, but rarely may cause temporary sight and hearing disturbances, thrombocytopenia, or GI distress. Furthermore, quinine tends to increase plasma digoxin concentrations and may enhance the effect of warfarin. This constellation of adverse events prompted the withdrawal of quinine from the over-the-counter market in 1995 and prescription quinine can no longer be marketed for leg cramps.

TABLE 30-6 Management of Cramps

Acute treatment	Give 100–200 mL bolus of IV normal saline Give 10–20 mL of IV hypertonic saline (23.4%) over 3–5 minutes Give 50 mL of 50% IV glucose (nondiabetic patients)
Prevention	
Nonpharmacologic	Accurately set "dry weight" Keep dialysate sodium greater than serum sodium Stretching exercises, massage, flexing, or compression devices
Pharmacologic	Vitamin E 400 international units at bedtime Quinine 324 mg daily (second-line therapy)

A randomized, double-blind, placebo-controlled trial demonstrated that both vitamin E (400 mg) and vitamin C (250 mg) reduce the frequency of cramps in dialysis patients.[70] The combination of these two drugs had an additive effect. Although these data further strengthen the case for vitamin E, it is unclear what role oral vitamin C would play since many patients are on a renal multiple vitamin containing vitamin C (the current study restricted all vitamin products for 1 month prior to the study). Furthermore, there is some concern that oxalate, a metabolite of vitamin C, may accumulate in dialysis patients and result in systemic oxalosis.

Exogenous administration of creatine might have some beneficial effects on muscle cramps in dialysis patients.[71] Ten patients with intradialytic muscle cramps were randomized to either creatine (12 mg before dialysis) or placebo. The frequency of muscle cramps decreased 60% in the creatine group, while there were no differences in the placebo group. Although serum creatinine concentrations rose in the treatment group, no side effects were noted.[71] Certainly more research in this area is needed before creatine supplementation can be recommended for the prevention and treatment of muscle cramps during HD.

The relationship of elevated calcium, phosphorus, and intact parathyroid hormone in relation to muscle pain, cramps, pruritus, and dry skin (xerosis) were evaluated in 1,469 HD and PD patients.[72] At baseline approximately 67% of patients suffered from at least one of these symptoms. After 4 years of follow-up, those patients with diminished or no symptoms had lower serum phosphorus concentrations.[72] This study suggests that adequate dialysis along with dietary controls can help reduce muscle pain, cramps, itching, and dry skin in dialysis patients.

Shakuyaku-kanzo-to, a combination of peony and licorice root from traditional Japanese and Chinese medicine, was studied in 23 HD patients for acute treatment of muscle cramps. The ultrafiltration rate was reduced to zero and shakuyaku-kanzo-to (2.5 gram granule) was administered when a patient complained of cramping during HD. These interventions resulted in a muscle cramp resolution rate of 88.5% that occurred between 5 and 10 minutes.[73] It is difficult to determine if muscle cramp cessation was due to stopping HD fluid removal, shakuyaku-kanzo-to, or the combination of both treatments. Previous studies have examined the use[45] of shakuyaku-kanzo-to for the frequency and severity of muscle cramps but the results were inconsistent and a few patients had an increase in symptoms.[74]

Pharmacologic interventions to diminish muscle cramps are limited and currently vitamin E has the strongest evidence-based clinical trials and its safety profile. Quinine sulfate is available as Qualaquin 324 mg capsule (URL Pharma, Philadelphia, PA) but is FDA approved only for malaria. The FDA has warned against the off-label use of quinine for muscle cramps because of potential serious side effects related to its use. The dosage for HD-related muscle cramps is one capsule (324 mg) either at bedtime or 1 to 2 hours prior to HD.

Vascular Access Thrombosis

Prevention of vascular access thrombus formation is a key component to maintain this lifeline for HD patients. Multiple oral and IV anticoagulant and antiplatelet agents and IV thrombolytic agents have been studied for vascular access patency. Several of these therapeutic options are discussed in this section.

Clinical **Controversy. . .**

The use of oral anticoagulant or antiplatelet agents to maintain vascular access patency is controversial since the risk may be greater than the benefit. Studies have reported conflicting results and serious adverse reactions in HD patients that may increase morbidity and mortality.

The use of oral antiplatelet agents to prevent vascular access thrombosis has been controversial since efficacy is not well-established and there is an increased risk of bleeding.[45,46,75] Extended-release dipyridamole with aspirin was studied in 649 patients with a newly placed arteriovenous graft (AVG). Patients received either treatment or placebo and were followed for 1 month after the loss of graft patency. At 1 year, unassisted patency was 28% in the treatment group compared to 23% in the placebo group. Adverse events were slightly higher in the treatment group (55% vs. 53%), but bleeding rates were similar between groups (12%).[76] Daily aspirin use has also been evaluated in the maintenance of AV fistula in HD patients.[77] This observational cohort study reported that consistent aspirin use was associated with a lower rate of AV fistula failure and no increase in new GI bleeding compared to patients not receiving aspirin. Consistent aspirin use was studied in this trial, but not aspirin dose. The use of warfarin to maintain vascular access patency for dialysis patients has become controversial with some trials suggesting an increase in morbidity and mortality with the use of warfarin.[78–81] Warfarin dosing regimens and adjusted international normalized ratio (INR) targets have also been examined in HD patients.[80] Much of the recent literature has suggested that warfarin should be used with caution in HD patients. These patients generally require a lower dose and are at a much higher risk of a major hemorrhagic event.[78,79,81]

The effect of fish oil supplementation for AVG patency was reported in HD patients (n = 201).[82] Patients were randomized to receive either a combination of eicosapentaenoic acid (EPA) 400 mg and docosahexaenoic acid (DHA) 200 mg or placebo for 12 months after AVG placement. The loss of native AVG patency was lower in the fish oil (48%) versus placebo (62%) groups, but the proportion of graft malfunction was not significantly different (P = 0.06). Fish oil may have some benefit for patients with an AVG since time to thrombus was longer and thrombus rates were about half that of placebo.[82]

Patients whose HD access is a venous catheter may benefit from a solution instilled in the catheter lumen between HD sessions. This is referred to as a catheter locking solution and has been used to maintain catheter patency.[45,83] Many HD centers use unfractionated heparin (UFH) as a catheter locking solution, but alternatives to UFH are being reported. The Citrate 4% versus heparin and the reduction of thrombosis study (CHARTS) was a prospective, randomized study examining sodium citrate 4% (n = 32) versus UFH (n = 29) and the reduction of catheter thrombosis in HD patients.[84] Catheter dysfunction occurred more often in the UFH (44.8%) versus the citrate (40.6%) groups (P = 0.799). Systemic bleeding events were significantly greater with UFH (n = 21) compared with citrate (n = 7; P = 0.035). Overall a catheter locking solution of sodium citrate 4% was as effective as UFH but may offer a better safety profile at a reduced cost.[84]

CVC patency was compared in HD patients (n = 225) randomized to receive either a catheter lock solution of regimen that alternated UFH and recombinant tissue plasminogen activator (rt-PA) or UFH alone.[85] Patients in the rt-PA group had rt-PA 1 mg instilled per catheter lumen (2 mg total) once a week and UFH 5,000 units/mL per lumen on the remaining treatment days. The heparin-only group received the same heparin lock solution dose after each HD session. Catheter malfunction occurred more often in the heparin-only (43.8%) versus rt-PA (20%) group (P = 0.02). A catheter lock solution regimen including rt-PA is considerably more expensive than an UFH-only regimen. The study investigators concluded that the increased drug cost is offset by decreasing catheter malfunction rates and possibly avoiding hospitalization for these patients.[85]

The therapeutic alternatives for venous catheter thrombosis are listed in Table 30-7. If a catheter-related thrombus is suspected, a forced saline flush should be used to clear the catheter, followed by installation of a thrombolytic. A number of studies have been published using alteplase[86–88] and reteplase[89,90] for thrombosed HD catheters. The initial

TABLE 30-7 Management of Hemodialysis Catheter Thrombosis

Nonpharmacologic therapy
Forced saline flush
Referral to vascular surgeon
Pharmacologic therapy
Alteplase: Instill 2 mg/2 mL per catheter lumen port; attempt to aspirate after 30 minutes; may repeat dose if catheter function is not restored in 120 minutes; longer durations of instillation have been used
Reteplase: Instill 0.4 units/0.4 mL in each lumen, attempt to aspirate after 20–30 minutes, may repeat if necessary

reperfusion rates for both alteplase and reteplase were approximately 90%. A systematic review of thrombolytics in HD catheters to restore function compared the efficacy, safety, and cost of alteplase, reteplase, and teneteplase.[91] The authors found the most evidence with alteplase, which is the only agent of the three agents, FDA approved, for venous catheter clearance. The venous catheter clearance rates were reteplase (88 ± 4%), alteplase (81 ± 37%), and tenecteplase (41 ± 5%). The cost analysis favored the use of reteplase: however to attain these savings reteplase must be batch prepared. It also can be stored frozen to extend its shelf-life.[91]

Alteplase is available commercially as a 2 mg/2 mL vial and can be administered as a short dwell for 30 to 60 minutes, as a long dwell or left in the catheter between treatments. A study evaluating patency rates between alteplase short-term (1 hour) and long-term (52 hours) dwells found no difference in patency rates between the short or long dwells.[92] Alteplase has also been given as a short infusion. Infusion doses reported in the literature include 2 mg per hour over 4 hours[93,94] for blocked catheter and 1 mg per hour over 4 hours for a sluggish blood flow.[93] Infusions may theoretically be more efficacious than the dwell technique because the thrombus is only exposed to the thrombolytic at the very tip of the catheter. Another consideration is dwell versus push techniques for thrombolytic therapy. A prospective, randomized study compared the efficacy of an alteplase dwell protocol (30 to 120 minutes) to a push protocol (30 minutes) for restoring occluded HD catheter function ($n = 82$).[95] Adequate blood flow was restored more often in the push protocol (32/39 catheters) compared with the dwell protocol (28/43 catheters). This study showed that a push protocol with alteplase was as effective and safe for managing HD catheter dysfunction and might be more practical than a dwell technique.[95]

Infection

HD patients who develop a fever during treatment should immediately be evaluated for infection; blood cultures should be collected prior to the administration of any prophylactic antibiotics. In cases when an AV fistula infection is suspected empiric broad-spectrum antibiotic therapy must be initiated usually with vancomycin plus an aminoglycoside. Antibiotic treatment should continue for a total of 6 weeks and therapy should be tailored to culture sensitivities. Unfortunately, a suspected infection in an AVG may require more than antibiotic therapy alone and a surgical procedure to remove the infected graft material may be needed. A suspected infection in a temporary catheter may warrant catheter removal and if possible obtain a culture of the catheter tip.[96–98] Since catheter-related infections are more common than infections with an AV fistula or AVG, preventative care approaches very important for HD patients. Treatment with systemic antibiotic plus an antimicrobial catheter lock solution may be needed. Preventative care includes minimizing the use and duration of catheters, proper disinfection and sterile technique, and the use of an antimicrobial ointment at the exit site (mupirocin 2%, povidone-iodine). Dialysis unit protocols that employ universal precautions, such as limit manipulation of the catheter, skin preparation with an antiseptic wash (tincture of iodine, chlorhexidine, etc.), and the use of face masks by the patient and caregiver, can significantly reduce the incidence of catheter-related bacteremia.[96,97,99] Topical application of 2% mupirocin ointment to a tunneled HD catheter exit site after each HD session was shown in one study to increase infection-free days from 55 (control group) to 108 (treatment group).[100] However, there are concerns that the use of mupirocin prophylaxis may lead to the development of resistant *S. aureus*. A 6-year study that prospectively monitored HD patient CVC infection rates used a once-a-week application of a topical polysporin triple ointment (bacitracin/gramicidin/polymyxin B) to CVC exit sites as part of standard CVC care did not report an increase in *S. aureus* resistance.[101] An alternative to mupirocin may be the use of topical medical grade *Leptospermum* honey (Medihoney™ Pty Ltd Derma Sciences, Inc., Princeton, NJ) to catheter exit sites. In a preliminary study medical-grade *Leptospermum* honey was found to be as effective as mupirocin in reducing catheter infections.[102]

The Infectious Disease Society of America (IDSA) has published comprehensive guidelines (2009 and 2011) regarding catheter care and the diagnosis and management of catheter-related infections.[97,99] The 2006 Kidney Dialysis Outcomes Quality Initiative (KDOQI) guidelines also provide an outline for patient care.[45] However, there are differences in what IDSA has proposed and what is practical in the outpatient chronic HD setting for HD patients with an indwelling catheter. In an effort to protect potential HD access sites peripheral blood draws are often avoided in HD patients. Blood cultures are generally obtained from the blood tubing connecting the catheter to the HD machine. A full-course of antimicrobial treatment is warranted if these blood cultures are found to be positive.[97,99] Empiric therapy with coverage for both gram-positive and gram-negative bacteria should be initiated after the blood cultures are obtained. The incidence of methicillin-resistant *Staphylococcus aureus* (MRSA) bacteremia is high enough to warrant initial treatment with vancomycin for gram-positive coverage and either an aminoglycoside or third-generation cephalosporin for gram-negative coverage.[97,99] Therapy should be adjusted once blood cultures identify an organism. For example if the isolated organism is methicillin-sensitive *S. aureus*, therapy may be changed to IV cefazolin (20 mg/kg, rounded to the nearest 500 mg) after each dialysis session.[103,104] Antibiotic selection should be based on bacterial coverage and optimizing the pharmacokinetics of administering a dose after a HD treatment session without requiring additional dosages between HD sessions. Examples of antimicrobial agents that meet these objectives are vancomycin, cefazolin, ceftazidime, daptomycin, and aminoglycosides.[97,103–106]

The IDSA guidelines recommend that the infected catheter should be removed if *S. aureus*, *Pseudomonas* species, or *Candida* species are identified as the infectious cause. Although removal of the catheter is warranted since up to 75% of patients have a recurrence of bacteremia after completing a course of antibiotics, this is not always possible in HD patients. Options such as replacing the catheter over a guidewire or using a catheter lock solution in conjunction with IV antibiotics have been used as an alternative.[97,99] Recent studies have suggested that between 62% and 70% of catheters can be salvaged using this technique (as defined by absence of fever without loss of catheter).[97,99] The IDSA guidelines recommend the use of catheter lock solutions as adjunctive therapy after each dialysis session for 10 to 14 days in patients that their catheter was not removed and bacteremia symptoms resolved in 2 to 3 days. The IDSA recommendations for antibiotic therapy are listed in Table 30-8.

As opposed to treatment, catheter locking has also been studied to prevent infection and thrombosis in HD catheters.[107] A meta-analysis of randomized control trials of catheter-related

TABLE 30-8 Management of Hemodialysis Access Infection

I. Primary AV fistula
  A. Treat as subacute bacterial endocarditis for 6 weeks
  B. Initial antibiotic choice should always cover gram-positive organisms (e.g., vancomycin 20 mg/kg IV with serum concentration monitoring or cefazolin 20 mg/kg IV three times per week or after each dialysis session)
  C. Gram-negative coverage is indicated for patients with diabetes, human immunodeficiency virus infection, prosthetic valves, or those receiving immunosuppressive agents, gentamicin 2 mg/kg IV with serum concentration monitoring

II. Synthetic AV grafts
  A. Local infection—empiric antibiotic coverage for gram-positive, gram-negative, and *Enterococcus* (e.g., gentamicin plus vancomycin then individualized after culture results available). Continue for 2 to 4 weeks.
  B. Extensive infection—antibiotics as above plus total resection
  C. If accesses is less than 1 month old, antibiotics as above plus remove the graft

III. Tunneled cuffed catheters (internal jugular, subclavian)
  A. Infection localized to catheter exit site.
    1. No drainage—topical antibiotics (e.g., mupirocin ointment)
    2. Drainage present—gram-positive antibiotic coverage (e.g., cefazolin 20 mg/kg IV three times per week)
  B. Bacteremia with or without systemic signs or symptoms
    1. Gram-positive antibiotic coverage as in III.A.2
    2. If symptomatic at 36 hours, remove the catheter
    3. If stable and asymptomatic, change catheter and provide culture-specific antibiotic coverage for a minimum of 3 weeks

bacteremia and antimicrobial lock solutions identified eight studies with 829 patients and more than 90,100 catheter days. Overall analysis found the use of an antimicrobial lock solution reduced the risk of a catheter-related infection (relative risk [RR] 0.32; 95% confidence interval [CI] 0.10 to 0.42).[108] A recent study not included in this meta-analysis compared lock solutions of UFH 1,000 units/mL to a combination of gentamicin 320 mcg/mL with 4% sodium citrate. The rate of blood stream infections was significantly lower ($P = 0.003$) and time to first bacteremia was significantly longer ($P = 0.005$) with combination solution of gentamicin and citrate compared with UFH.[109]

The data examining the use of catheter lock solutions for treatment and prevention of catheter-related infections are growing, but there is still a concern regarding antibiotic resistance with the wide use of antibiotics in catheter locks. Currently, NKF-K/DOQI does not recommend routine locking of catheters with antibiotics.

PERITONEAL DIALYSIS

Although the concept of peritoneal lavage has been described as far back as the 1700s, it wasn't until the 1920s that PD was first employed as an acute treatment for uremia. It was used infrequently during subsequent years until the concept of PD as a chronic therapy for ESRD was proposed in the 1960s. By the mid-1970s, PD was used relatively commonly and over the ensuing years the number of patients receiving PD increased slowly until the early 1980s. At that time, several innovations in PD delivery systems were introduced, such as improved catheters and dialysate bags. These innovations led to improved outcomes, decreased morbidity, and a corresponding increase in the use of PD as a viable alternative to HD for the treatment of ESRD. However, even with these proposed advantages, there has been a declining use of PD in the world over the past decade.[2] Some patients—such as those with more hemodynamic instability (e.g., hypotension) or significant residual kidney function, and perhaps patients who desire to maintain a significant degree of self-care may be better suited to PD rather than to HD. There is some debate over important outcomes for patients on PD. Table 30-3 describes some advantages and disadvantages of PD.

Principles of Peritoneal Dialysis

5 The three basic components of HD—namely, a blood-filled compartment separated from a dialysate-filled compartment by a semipermeable membrane—are also present in PD.[110] In PD, the dialysate-filled compartment is the peritoneal cavity, into which dialysate is instilled via a peritoneal catheter that traverses the abdominal wall. The contiguous peritoneal membrane surrounds the peritoneal cavity. The cavity, which normally contains about 100 mL of lipid-rich lubricating fluid, can expand to a capacity of several liters. The peritoneal membrane that lines the cavity functions as the semipermeable membrane, across which diffusion and ultrafiltration occur. The membrane is classically described as a monocellular layer of peritoneal mesothelial cells. However, the dialyzing membrane is also comprised of the basement membrane and underlying connective and interstitial tissue. The peritoneal membrane has a total area that approximates body surface area (approximately 1 to 2 m^2). Blood vessels supplying and draining the abdominal viscera, musculature, and mesentery constitute the blood-filled compartment.

Unlike HD, the crucial components of PD cannot be manipulated to maximize solute and fluid removal. Because the blood is not in intimate contact with the dialysis membrane as it is in HD, metabolic waste products must travel a considerable distance to the dialysate-filled compartment. In addition, unlike HD, there is no easy method to regulate blood flow to the surface of the peritoneal membrane, nor is there a countercurrent flow of blood and dialysate to increase diffusion and ultrafiltration via changes in hydrostatic pressure. Similarly there is no easy means available to manipulate the peritoneal membrane. Most of the control in dialysis dosing during PD involves alterations in dialysate volume, dwell time, and the number of exchanges per day. For these reasons, PD is a much-less-efficient process per unit time as compared with HD, and must, therefore, be a virtually continuous procedure to achieve acceptable goals for clearance of metabolic waste products.

Peritoneal Dialysis Access

Access to the peritoneal cavity is via the placement of an indwelling catheter. Many types are available and Figure 30-3 shows an example.[110] Most catheters are manufactured from silastic, which is soft, flexible, and biocompatible. A typical adult catheter is 40 to 45 cm long, 20 to 22 cm of which are inside the peritoneal cavity. Placement of the catheter is such that the distal end lies low in a pelvic gutter. The center section of the catheter has one or two cuffs made of a porous material. This section is tunneled inside the anterior abdominal wall so that the cuffs provide mechanical support and stability to the catheter, a mechanical barrier to skin organisms, and prevent their migration along the catheter into the peritoneal cavity. The cuffs are placed at different sites surrounding the abdominal rectus muscle. The remainder of the central section of the catheter is tunneled subcutaneously before exiting the abdominal surface, usually a few centimeters below and to one side of the umbilicus.

The placement of the catheter exit site is one of the factors related to the development or prevention of exit-site infections and peritonitis. The external section of most peritoneal catheters ends with a Luer-Lok connector, which can be connected to a variety of administration sets. These catheters can be used immediately if necessary, provided that small initial volumes are instilled; however, a maturation period of 2 to 6 weeks is preferred.

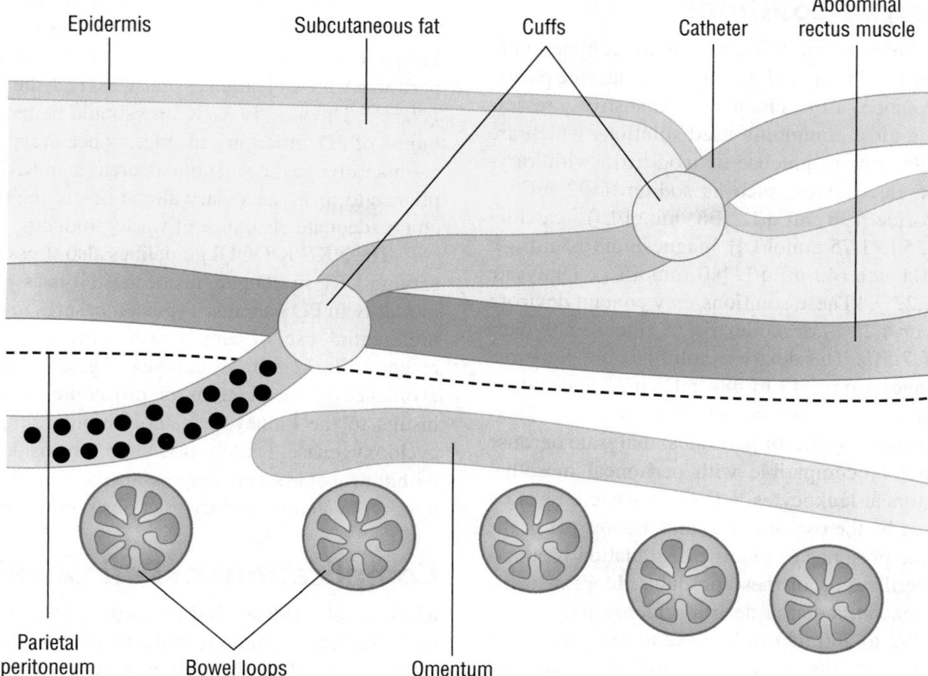

FIGURE 30-3 Diagram of the PD catheter placement through the abdominal wall into the peritoneal cavity.

Peritoneal Dialysis Procedures

6 In the United States, several variants of PD are clinically utilized. All variants of PD require the placement of a dialysis solution to dwell in the peritoneal cavity for some period, removing the spent dialysate, and then repeating the process. The prescribed dose of PD may be altered by changing the number of exchanges per day, by altering the volume of each exchange, or by altering the strength of dextrose in the dialysate for some or all exchanges. Increasing any one of these variables increases the effective osmotic gradient across the peritoneum, leading to increased ultrafiltration and diffusion (solute removal). If the dwell time is extended, equilibrium may be reached, after which time there will be no further water or solute removal. In fact, after a critical period, reverse water movement may occur.[110,111]

In a basic continuous ambulatory peritoneal dialysis (CAPD) system, the patient or caregiver is manually responsible for performing the prescribed number of dialysate exchanges. The patient is connected to a bag of prewarmed peritoneal dialysate via the PD catheter, by a length of tubing called a transfer set. The most common transfer set used is the Y transfer set. This consists of a Y-shaped piece of tubing that is attached at its stem to the patient's catheter, leaving the remaining two limbs of the Y attached to dialysate bags, one filled with fresh dialysate and the other empty. The spent dialysate from the previous dwell is drained into the empty bag, and the peritoneum is subsequently refilled from the bag containing fresh dialysate. The Y set is then disconnected and the bag containing the spent fluid and the empty bag that had contained fresh dialysate are detached and discarded. Typically a patient instills 2 to 3 L of dialysate three times during the day with each exchange lasting 4 to 6 hours, and then a single dialysate exchange overnight lasting 8 to 12 hours. At the end of the prescribed dwell period, a new Y set is attached and the process is repeated. The process of outflow, aseptic manipulation of the administration set and catheter, and inflow requires a total time of approximately 30 minutes.[111]

CAPD involves performing the dialysate exchanges manually, whereas automated systems, collectively termed automated peritoneal dialysis (APD), perform the exchanges with a device referred to as a cycler. APD systems are designed for patients who are unable or unwilling to perform the necessary aseptic manipulations, and for those who require more dialysis. APD provides an automated cycler that performs the exchanges. The device is set up in the evening, and the patient attaches the peritoneal catheter to it at bedtime. The machine performs several short-dwell exchanges (usually 1 to 2 hours) during the night. This permits a long cycle-free daytime dwell of up to 12 to 14 hours. Typical APD regimens involve total 24-hour exchanges of approximately 12 L, which include one or more daytime dwells.[112] This type of regimen is sometimes referred to as APD with a "wet" day. The APD variant, nightly intermittent PD, has a similar theme, except that the peritoneal cavity tends to be dialysate free during the day. This type of regimen is frequently referred to as APD with a "dry" day. A number of variants exist and depend largely on equipment availability, patient and prescriber preference, and whether the patient retains any residual renal function (RRF), which influences the quantity of dialysis prescribed.[111]

The APD systems include continuous cycling PD, tidal PD, and nightly intermittent PD.[111] The prototypic form of APD is usually a hybrid between CAPD and continuous cycling PD, in which some of the daily exchanges (usually the overnight exchanges) are completed using an automated device. Recent advances in PD procedures involve using continuous flow peritoneal dialysate.[113,114] This technique maintains a fixed IP volume and rapid, continuous movement of dialysate into and out of the peritoneal cavity. To accomplish this, two PD catheters (an inlet and outlet catheter) and a means of generating a large volume of sterile dialysate are required. Dialysate is generated via conventional HD equipment or sorbent technology. In continuous flow peritoneal dialysate, clearance of small solutes is three to eight times greater than with APD, and approximates that with daily HD.[113] Potential applications of continuous flow peritoneal dialysate include daily home dialysis, treatment of acute renal failure in the intensive care unit, and ultrafiltration of ascites.[113]

Peritoneal Dialysis Solutions

All forms of PD use dialysate solutions, which are commercially available in volumes of 1 to 3 L in flexible polyvinyl chloride plastic bags. It is beyond the scope of this chapter to exhaustively review all the options, but the most commonly used solutions which are commercially available contain glucose or icodextrin with varying concentrations of electrolytes, such as sodium (132 mEq/L [132 mmol/L]), chloride (96 mEq/L [96 mmol/L]), calcium (2.5 to 3.5 mEq/L [1.25 to 1.75 mmol/L]), magnesium (0.5 mEq/L [0.25 mmol/L]), and lactate (40 mEq/L [40 mmol/L]). Dialysate pH is maintained at 5.2.[66,110] These solutions may contain dextrose (1.5%, 2.5%, 3.86%, or 4.25%) or icodextrin (a glucose polymer) at a concentration of 7.5%. The dextrose solutions are hyperosmolar (osmolarity ranges from 345 to 484 mOsm/L) and induce ultrafiltration (removal of free water) by crystalline osmosis. Dextrose is not the ideal osmotic agent for peritoneal dialysate because these solutions are not biocompatible with peritoneal mesothelial cells or with peritoneal leukocytes.[83] The cytotoxic effects on these cells are mediated by the osmolar load and the low pH of the solutions, as well as the presence of glucose degradation products formed during heat sterilization of these products. Icodextrin PD solution contains icodextrin, a starch-derived glucose polymer. It has an osmolality of 282 to 286 mOsm/kg (282 to 286 mmol/kg), which is isoosmolar with serum. Icodextrin produces prolonged ultrafiltration by a mechanism resembling colloid osmosis resulting in ultrafiltration volumes similar to those with 4.25% dextrose. Icodextrin may have fewer of the metabolic effects associated with dextrose, such as hyperglycemia and weight gain. It is indicated for use during the long (8 to 16 hours) dwell of a single daily exchange in CAPD and APD patients.[115] Outside of North America, lower glucose degradation product dialysate solutions are also available with similar solute concentrations, but with a pH of 7.3.[110] These newer, biocompatible dialysate solutions are claimed to be less harmful to the peritoneal membrane and preserve RRF to a greater extent than currently available standard solutions.[116,117] Preservation of RRF in PD and HD patients is important as it has been shown to decrease mortality.[118] Moreover, preservation of RRF in PD patients has been shown to increase the time to the first episode of peritonitis.[119] However, the putative benefits of the biocompatible dialysate solutions have not been completely borne out. In a study that compared biocompatible to standard dialysate solutions, researchers found that the biocompatible solutions did not slow the rate of decline in GFR as compared to standard solutions, but they did delay the onset of anuria and reduced the incidence of peritonitis better.[120]

Measures of Peritoneal Dialysis Adequacy

The adequacy of PD is determined by clinical assessment, solute clearance determination, and fluid removal. As in HD, the clearance of urea, a product of protein catabolism, can be quantified by calculating *Kt*/*V*. The calculations determine a daily *Kt*/*V*, which is converted to a weekly value that is relevant for PD patients.[121]

PD adequacy is a major issue, which has received considerable attention during the last 10 years. The most recent NKF-K/DOQI guidelines recommend that patients on PD have at least a total *Kt*/*V* of 1.7 per week.[122,123] It is important to note that RRF may provide a significant component of the total *Kt*/*V*. Patients may commence PD with a residual CL_{cr} of approximately 9 to 12 mL/min, which contributes a renal *Kt*/*V* of 0.2 to 0.4. Over a period of 1 to 2 years, RRF tends to progressively deteriorate. Because total *Kt*/*V* is the sum of PD *Kt*/*V* and renal *Kt*/*V*, the total *Kt*/*V* will progressively diminish unless PD *Kt*/*V* is increased (by increasing the prescribed dose of PD) to compensate for the reduced renal *Kt*/*V*.

For patients producing <100 mL urine per day, the weekly *Kt*/*V* dose of 1.7 must be provided entirely by peritoneal clearance. For patients producing >100 mL urine per day, combined renal and peritoneal urea clearances must exceed the weekly *Kt*/*V* dose of 1.7.[122,123] The weekly *Kt*/*V* dose should be measured within the first month of PD initiation and at least once every 4 months thereafter. It is imperative to detect subtle decreases in RRF along with noncompliance to make necessary alterations to the prescribed PD dose to attain adequate clearance of waste products.

The NKF-K/DOQI guidelines also stress the importance of preserving RRF in PD patients because it is associated with decreased mortality in PD patients. Typical measures to maintain RRF include preferential use of angiotensin-converting enzyme inhibitors or receptor blockers in all patients, regardless of blood pressure, and avoidance of medications or procedures that are associated with insults to the kidney (e.g., nonsteroidal anti-inflammatory drugs, cyclooxygenase-2 inhibitors, aminoglycosides, radiocontrast dyes, withdrawal of immunosuppressant therapies from a transplanted kidney, hypovolemia, urinary tract obstruction, and hypercalcemia).[122]

Complications of Peritoneal Dialysis

Mechanical, medical, and infectious problems complicate PD therapy. Mechanical complications include kinking of the catheter and inflow and outflow obstruction; excessive catheter motion at the exit site, leading to induration and possible infection and aggravation of tissues; pain from impingement of the catheter tip on the viscera; or inflow pain resulting from a jet effect of too rapid dialysate inflow.

Table 30-9 lists the numerous medical complications of PD. An average PD patient absorbs up to 60% of the dextrose in each exchange. This continuous supply of calories leads to increased adipose tissue deposition, decreased appetite, malnutrition, and altered requirements for insulin in diabetic patients. Fibrin formation in dialysate is common and can lead to obstruction of catheter outflow. Infectious complications of PD are a major cause of morbidity and mortality and are the leading cause of technique failure and transfer from PD to HD. The two predominant infectious complications are peritonitis and catheter-related infections, which include both exit-site and tunnel infections.

Peritonitis

7 The incidence of peritonitis is influenced by connector technology, by the composition of patient populations, and by the use of APD versus CAPD. The incidence of peritonitis reported by most dialysis centers in the United States is about one episode every

TABLE 30-9 Medical Complications of Peritoneal Dialysis

Cause	Complication	Treatment
Glucose load	Exacerbation of diabetes mellitus	IP insulin
Fluid overload	Exacerbation of congestive heart failure Edema Pulmonary congestion	Increase ultrafiltration Diuretics, if the patient has RRF
Electrolyte abnormalities	Hypercalcemia/hypocalcemia	Alter dialysate calcium content
PD additives	Chemical peritonitis	Discontinue PD additives
Malnutrition	Albumin loss Loss of amino acids Muscle wasting Increased adipose tissue	Dietary changes Parenteral nutrition Discontinue PD
Unknown	Fibrin formation in dialysate	IP heparin

IP, intraperitoneal; PD, peritoneal dialysis.

CLINICAL PRESENTATION Peritoneal Dialysis-Related Peritonitis

General

- Patients generally present with abdominal pain and cloudy effluent

Symptoms

- The patient may complain of abdominal tenderness, abdominal pain, fever, nausea and vomiting, and chills

Signs

- Cloudy dialysate effluent may be observed
- Temperature may or may not be elevated

Laboratory Tests

- Dialysate white blood cell count >100/mm^3 (>10^8/L), of which at least 50% are polymorphonuclear neutrophils
- Gram stain of a centrifuged dialysate specimen

Other Diagnostic Tests

- Culture and sensitivity of dialysate should be obtained

24 patient-months, although it may be as low as one episode every 60 patient-months.[123] Within 1 year of starting CAPD, 40% to 60% of patients develop their first episode of peritonitis (although the incidence is significantly lower in APD patients).

Clinical Presentation Peritonitis is a major cause of catheter loss in PD patients. A statistically significant correlation between infectious complications and death rates has been reported. Of patients who had more than 1 peritonitis episode per year, 0.5 to 1 episode per year, or less than 0.5 episode per year, 50% died after 3, 4, and 5 years of therapy, respectively. It is important to note that these relationships are not necessarily cause and effect, as many of these patients succumb to cardiovascular events.[124]

Peritonitis has several imprecise definitions, but guidelines suggest that an elevated dialysate white blood cell count of greater than 100 per microliter (or 10^8/L) with at least 50% polymorphonuclear neutrophils indicates the presence of inflammation, of which peritonitis is the most likely cause. The patient who presents with abdominal pain and a cloudy effluent is usually given a provisional diagnosis of peritonitis. Inherent in this definition is a number of false-positive and false-negative diagnoses, because a small percentage of patients with culture-proven peritonitis will have clear dialysate, and some patients, such as menstruating females, may have cloudy PD effluent without clinical infection. Sterile culture peritonitis remains problematic; it is defined as an episode in which there is clinical suspicion of peritonitis, but for which the culture of the dialysate reveals no organism. There are several postulates for the high incidence (up to 20% of episodes) of culture-negative peritonitis. Many peritonitis-producing organisms are slime producers and may adhere to the peritoneal membrane or to the catheter surface and be protected from exogenous antibiotics. Sufficient numbers of these bacteria may proliferate to cause peritoneal membrane inflammation and clinical peritonitis, but an inadequate number may seed into the peritoneal cavity to be recovered by conventional microbiologic techniques. In addition, free-floating planktonic bacteria may be rapidly phagocytosed by peritoneal white blood cells, thereby rendering them unavailable for culture.[125]

Contemporary methods have increased the recovery rate of organisms and decreased the culture-negative rate. Centrifugation is currently recommended as the optimum culture method. Centrifugation of a large volume of dialysate (50 mL), resuspension of the sediment in 3 to 5 mL of sterile saline, and subsequent inoculation in culture media produce a culture-negative rate less than 5%. If centrifuge equipment is not available, blood culture bottles can be directly injected with 5 to 10 mL of dialysate effluent. However, this method results in a culture-negative rate of up to 20%.[126]

The majority of infections are caused by gram-positive bacteria, of which *Staphylococcus epidermidis* is the predominant organism. There is no single predominant gram-negative organism. Together, gram-positive and gram-negative organisms account for 80% to 90% of all episodes of peritonitis, and constitute the spectrum against which initial empiric therapy is directed.[127]

Catheter-Related Infections

PD patients experience an exit-site infection approximately once every 24 to 48 months. Patients with previous infections tend to have a higher subsequent incidence. The majority of exit-site infections are caused by *S. aureus*. In contrast to peritonitis, *S. epidermidis* accounts for less than 20% of exit-site infections. Although gram-negative organisms, such as *Pseudomonas*, are less common, they can result in significant morbidity. The diagnostic characteristics of these infections are somewhat vague but generally include the presence of purulent drainage, with or without erythema at the catheter exit site. The risk of exit-site infections is increased several-fold in patients who are nasal carriers of *S. aureus*.[128]

Management of Infectious Complications

Peritonitis

The International Society of Peritoneal Dialysis (ISPD) updated the PD-related infections recommendations in 2010, which provide guidelines for treatments such as peritonitis, tunneled, and exit-site infections. These PD-related infections are associated with dialysis modality treatment failures and substantial morbidity and mortality; therefore, appropriate pharmacotherapy treatment is essential (Fig. 30-4).[126] The ISDP guidelines specifically address the importance of dialysis center-specific antibiotic selection, the effect of RRF on antibiotic pharmacokinetics, and updated recommendations regarding the use of aminoglycosides and vancomycin in PD patients. In 2011, ISPD published a position statement on reducing the risks of PD-related infections.[129] The ISPD position statement includes updates to the prevention of exit-site infections and routine care for PD patients.

IP administration of antibiotics remains the preferred delivery route over IV therapy. Antimicrobial dosing recommendations provided in the ISPD guidelines distinguish between dosing for intermittent (one exchange per day) and continuous therapy (all exchanges). In addition, dosing recommendations are modified on the basis of the patient's PD modality (CAPD or APD) and whether the patient has RRF (urine output) >100 mL/day.[126,129]

Following a single IP antibiotic dose the drug concentrations achieved in dialysate and serum differ between intermittent and continuous methods. Intermittent therapy IP therapy necessitates that sufficient drug concentration transfers from the

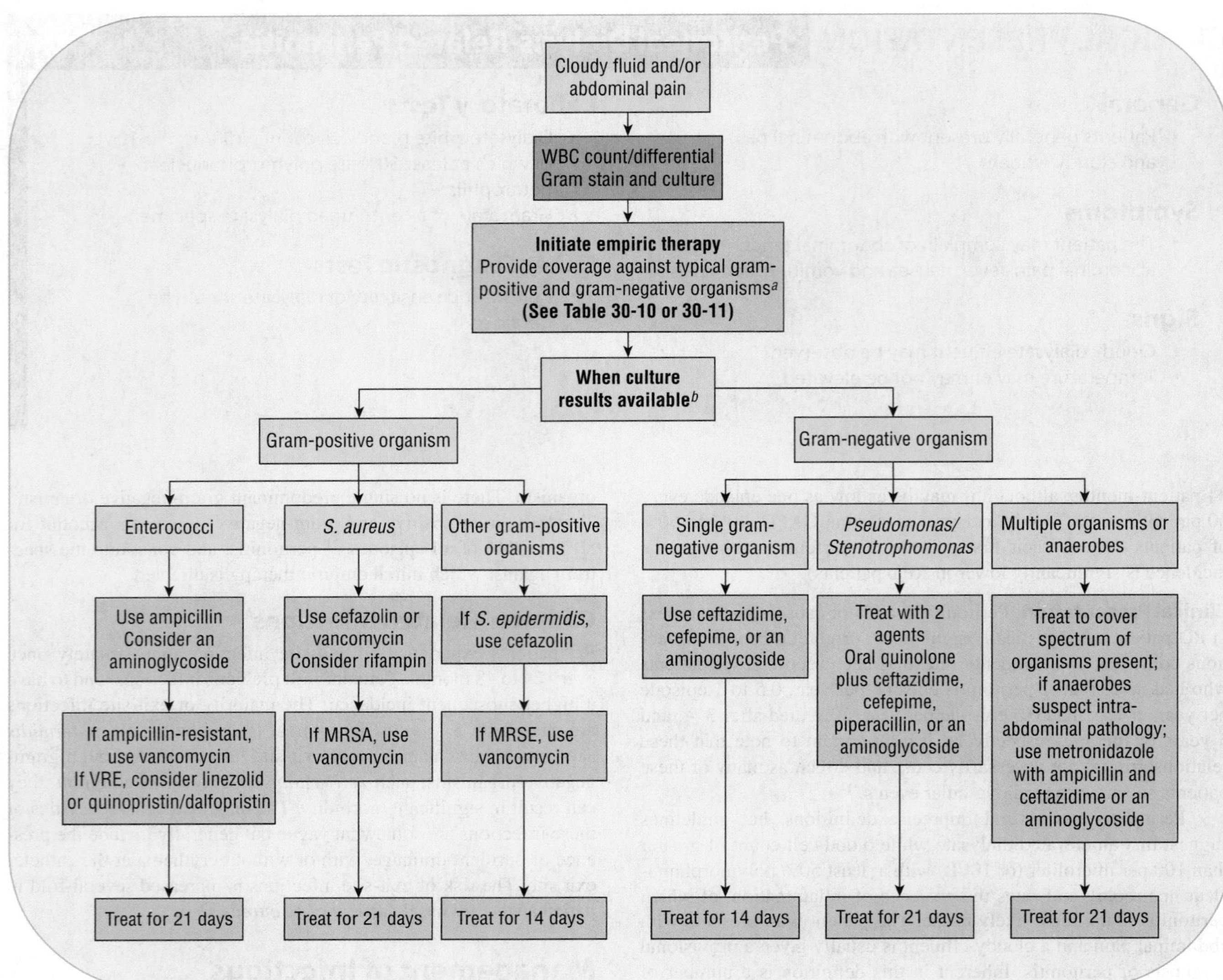

FIGURE 30-4 Pharmacotherapy recommendations for the treatment of bacterial peritonitis in PD patients. [a]Choice of empiric treatment should be made based on the dialysis center's and the patient's history of infecting organisms and their sensitivities. [b]Final choice of therapy should always be guided by culture and sensitivity results. (MRSA, methicillin-resistant *Staphylococcus aureus*; MRSE, methicillin-resistant *Staphylococcus epidermidis*; *S. aureus*, *Staphylococcus aureus*; *S. epidermidis*, *Staphylococcus epidermidis*; VRE, vancomycin-resistant enterococci; WBC, white blood cell.)

peritoneal cavity to systemic circulation thus allowing drug to diffuse back into the peritoneum during drug-free dialysate dwell time(s). Therefore, once daily dosing requires drug(s) be added to the exchange with the longest dwell time to ensure maximum bioavailability.

Continuous dosing recommendations may indicate the need for a loading dose with the very first IP dose with a maintenance dose for each subsequent exchange. Vancomycin, aminoglycoside, and cephalosporin agents generally can use either drug dosing method. It is recommended that a continuous dosing method be used for penicillins and fluoroquinolones. No matter which CAPD drug dosing method is used the goal is to deliver and maintain adequate peritoneum drug concentrations. Intermittent or continuous dosing is effective for CAPD patients but IP dosing for APD patients may require a different dosing schedule. The rapid overnight dialysate exchanges with APD will increase solute clearance over a short time period. This appears to be particularly important for first generation cephalosporin agents. The ISPD guidelines recommend continuous dosing of a first-generation cephalosporin because of concerns over inadequate IP drug concentration during the shorter APD dialysate dwells. Another consideration would be to switch a patient to a CAPD regimen until treatment for peritonitis is completed. With regard to RRF, in patients with daily urine output greater than 100 mL, the dose should be empirically increased by 25% for drugs that are renally eliminated. The ISPD dosing recommendations for IP antibiotics in CAPD and APD patients are shown in Tables 30-10 and 30-11, respectively.[126]

The compatibility and stability of antibiotics added to peritoneal dialysate is another important consideration. In dextrose solutions, most antibiotic additives appear to be stable (usually defined as retaining at least 90% of initial activity) for about 1 week if refrigerated, or 1 to 2 days if left at room temperature. Recent data suggest that cefazolin, ceftazidime, cefepime, vancomycin, gentamicin, tobramycin, netilmicin, and heparin are stable in icodextrin.[130–132] A concern with some compatibility and stability studies is that an assay of total drug concentration may include parent drug-degradation products in addition to active drug; therefore, the solution may not retain sufficient pharmacologic activity.

TABLE 30-10 Intraperitoneal Antibiotic Dosing Recommendations for Continuous Ambulatory Peritoneal Dialysis Patients[126]

Drug	Intermittent (Per Exchange, Once Daily)	Continuous (mg/L, All Exchanges)
Aminoglycosides		
Amikacin[a]	2 mg/kg	LD 25, MD 12
Gentamicin[a]	0.6 mg/kg	LD 8, MD 4
Netilmicin[a]	0.6 mg/kg	LD 8, MD 4
Tobramycin[a]	0.6 mg/kg	LD 8, MD 4
Cephalosporins		
Cefazolin[a]	15 mg/kg	LD 500, MD 125
Cefepime[a]	1,000 mg	LD 500, MD 125
Cephalothin[a]	15 mg/kg	LD 500, MD 125
Cephradine[a]	15 mg/kg	LD 500, MD 125
Ceftazidime[a]	1,000–1,500 mg	LD 500, MD 125
Ceftizoxime[a]	1,000 mg	LD 250, MD 125
Penicillins		
Azlocillin[a]	ND	LD 500, MD 250
Ampicillin[a]	ND	MD 125
Oxacillin[a]	ND	MD 125
Nafcillin[a]	ND	MD 125
Amoxicillin[a]	ND	LD 250–500, MD 50
Penicillin G[a]	ND	LD 50,000 units, MD 25,000 units
Quinolones		
Ciprofloxacin[a]	ND	LD 50, MD 25
Others		
Vancomycin[a]	15–30 mg/kg Q5-7d	LD 1,000, MD 25
Daptomycin	ND	LD 1,000, MD 250
Aztreonam[a]	ND	LD 100, MD 20
Teicoplanin	15 mg/kg	LD 400, MD 20
Linezolid		Oral 200–300 mg daily
Antifungals		
Amphotericin B	NA	MD 1.5
Fluconazole	200 mg IP every 24–48 hours	
Combinations		
Ampicillin/sulbactam[a]	2 g q 12 hours	LD 1,000, MD 100
Imipenem/cilastatin[a]	1 g twice daily	LD 500, MD 200
Quinupristin/dalfopristin[b]	25 mg/L in alternate bags	

LD, loading dose in mg; MD, maintenance dose in mg; NA, not applicable; ND, no data.

[a]Dosing of these drugs in patients with RRF (defined as more than 100 mL/day urine output) dose should be empirically increased by 25%.

[b]Given in conjunction with 500 mg IV twice daily.

The systemic toxicities of IP regimens remain unclear, but are likely similar to those associated with IV and oral antibiotic administration. Intermittent (once-daily) IP dosing of drugs, such as aminoglycosides, may reduce the risk of systemic toxicity (ototoxicity and nephrotoxicity).[126] Due to controversial/conflicting clinical trial data,[133,134] the current ISPD guidelines state that there is no convincing evidence that short courses of aminoglycosides lead to loss of RRF. Also, that prolonged or repeated courses are probably inadvisable if an alternative approach is available.[127] This latter controversial recommendation was based on the opinion of the committee and restated in a recent NKF-K/DOQI document. Since the preservation of RRF is very important for PD patients, routine use of aminoglycosides should be avoided in patients with significant RRF (producing >100 mL urine per day) if other antibiotic choices are available.[126]

TABLE 30-11 Intermittent Intraperitoneal Antibiotic Dosing Recommendations for Automated Peritoneal Dialysis Patients[126]

Drug	Intraperitoneal Dose
Vancomycin	LD: 30 mg/kg IP in longest dwell, repeat dosing 15 mg/kg IP in longest dwell every 3–5 days, following levels (aim to keep serum trough levels above 15 mcg/mL [mg/L; 10.4 μmol/L])
Tobramycin	LD: 1.5 mg/kg IP in longest dwell, then 0.5 mg/kg IP each day in longest day dwell
Fluconazole	200 mg IP in one exchange per day every 24–48 hours
Cefepime	1 g IP in longest dwell
Cefazolin	20 mg/kg IP every day, in longest dwell

IP, Intraperitoneal; LD, loading dose in mg; MD, maintenance dose in mg.

Clinical Controversy...

The ISPD guidelines for peritonitis treatment state that patients with significant RRF should not receive aminoglycosides if other antibiotic choices are available. Aminoglycosides were found to increase the rate of decline in RRF in one study. However, another study refuted this claim.

Initial empiric therapy for peritonitis, regardless of whether a Gram stain was performed or organisms were identified, should include agents effective against both gram-positive and gram-negative organisms. Antibiotic selection should be based on a dialysis center's antibiogram or resistance patterns, a history of the patient's infections, and the organism's antibiotic sensitivity profile. In many cases, a first-generation cephalosporin such as cefazolin in combination with a second drug that provides broader gram-negative coverage, such as ceftazidime, cefepime, or an aminoglycoside, will prove suitable. Patients with documented allergy to cephalosporin antibiotics can be treated with vancomycin and an aminoglycoside. High rates of methicillin resistance have been reported by many dialysis centers and vancomycin should be used as first-line therapy against gram-positive organisms for patients treated at these centers. Monotherapy with agents providing both gram-positive and gram-negative coverage is an alternative option. Both imipenem–cilastatin and cefepime are effective in treating CAPD-related peritonitis.[135]

After culture and sensitivity results are obtained, antibiotic therapy should be adjusted appropriately (see Fig. 30-4). Tables 30-10 and 30-11 list doses for antibiotics. Treatment should be continued for 14 to 21 days. If the patient does not show a sign of clinical improvement within 72 hours after antibiotic treatment is initiated, the culture should be repeated and the patient reevaluated. If the peritoneal dialysate white blood cell count remains high after 4 days of appropriate antibiotic therapy, clinicians should consider removing the peritoneal catheter, starting IV antibiotics and initiating HD for dialytic maintenance therapy.

Fungal peritonitis is associated with a poor prognosis and high morbidity and mortality. One problem with prospective assessment of antifungal regimens is the infrequency with which these infections occur. This makes it difficult to design and implement comparative studies. Most literature about antifungal treatment is therefore retrospective or limited to reports of local experience.[136] As a result, the ISPD recommendations for treatment of fungal peritonitis are somewhat vague and treatment should be based on culture and sensitivity results. However, one area that has been clarified is the question as to whether the PD catheter should be removed. The ISPD recommendations are to remove the catheter immediately after identifying fungi. If the Gram stain indicates the presence of yeast, treatment may be initiated with amphotericin B and oral flucytosine. Once culture and sensitivity results are available, fluconazole, caspofungin, or voriconazole may replace amphotericin B. Treatment with these agents should be continued orally for an additional 10 days after

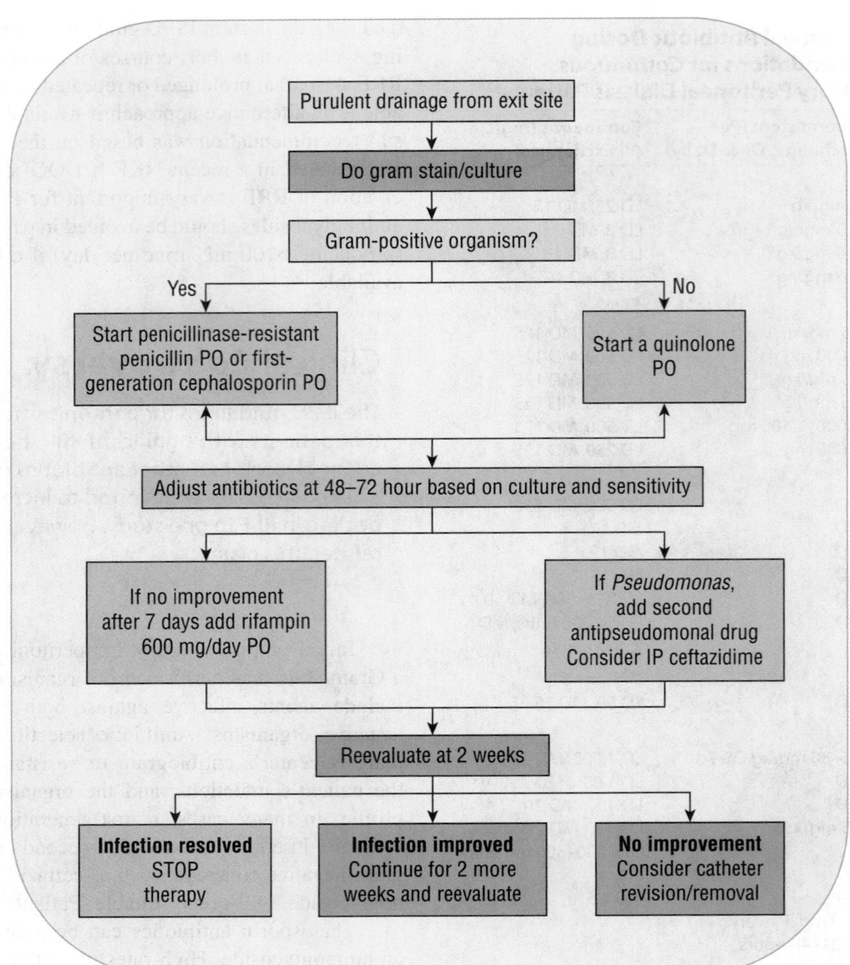

FIGURE 30-5 Management strategy of exit-site infections for PD patients. IP, intraperitoneal; PO, orally. *(From reference 128.)*

catheter removal. It remains unclear whether there is any benefit from fungal prophylaxis.[137] Recommendations are also provided for the treatment of mycobacterial, or tuberculous, peritonitis. Although this infection is a rare complication, it can be difficult to diagnose, and treatment requires multiple drugs.

Catheter-Site Infections

Topical antibiotics and disinfectants appear to be effective agents for the prevention of exit-site infections.[138–141] Gram-positive organisms should be treated with oral penicillinase-resistant penicillin or a first-generation cephalosporin such as cephalexin (Fig. 30-5). Rifampin may be added if necessary, in slowly resolving or particularly severe *S. aureus* infections. Vancomycin should be avoided in routine or empiric treatment of gram-positive catheter-related infections, but will be necessary for MRSA. Gram-negative organisms should be treated with oral quinolones. The effectiveness of oral quinolones may be diminished owing to the chelation drug interactions with divalent and trivalent metal ions, which are commonly taken by dialysis patients. Administration of quinolones should occur at least 2 hours prior to these drugs. In cases where *Pseudomonas aeruginosa* is the pathogen, a second antipseudomonal drug should be added. IP ceftazidime may be considered. In all cases antibiotics should be continued until the exit site appears normal; 2 to 3 weeks of therapy may be necessary. A patient with a catheter-related infection that progresses to peritonitis will usually require catheter removal.[126,129]

Prevention of Peritonitis and Catheter Exit-Site Infections

8 Attempts to prevent peritonitis and catheter-related infections have included refinement of connector system technology (Luer-Lok connectors), enhanced patient training techniques, and the use of prophylactic antibiotic regimens and vaccines.[142] Several studies have examined the impact of antibacterial agents as prophylaxis against both peritonitis and tunnel-related infections. Intermittent rifampin, 300 mg orally twice a day for 5 days, repeated every 3 months, appears to decrease the number of catheter-related infections, but not the incidence of peritonitis. The efficacy of other antibiotic prophylaxis for peritonitis and catheter-related infections is limited. Long-term, extended-duration prophylaxis with penicillins or cephalosporins is not effective.[126,129]

Nasal carriage of *S. aureus* is associated with an increased risk of catheter-related infections and peritonitis.[126,129] In addition, diabetic patients and those on immunosuppressive therapy are at increased risk for *S. aureus* catheter infections. Prophylaxis with intranasal mupirocin (twice daily for 5 to 7 days every month), mupirocin (daily) at the exit site, or oral rifampin can effectively reduce *S. aureus* exit-site infections. Because of the minimal toxicity of mupirocin and the risk of rifampin resistance, mupirocin regimens are preferred.[126,129] However, it is important to note that *S. aureus* isolates with a high degree of resistance to mupirocin have been isolated from PD patients using prophylactic mupirocin at the peritoneal catheter exit site.[143] However, a recent study did not observe resistance patterns with the use of mupirocin. Patients in this study applied mupirocin to the exit-site either once or thrice weekly. After three years exit-site infections and peritonitis rates were significantly lower in the thrice weekly application group.[144] In addition, gentamicin cream applied daily to the exit site has been found to effectively reduce both *S. aureus* and *P. aeruginosa* exit-site infection,[126,129] but a recent study comparing mupirocin 2% and gentamicin 0.1% creams for exit-site prophylaxis noted a decrease in gentamicin susceptibility patterns for *Enterobacteriaceace* (12%) and *Pseudomonas* (14%).[145]

A double-blinded, randomized controlled trial compared the use of the topical ointments mupirocin to polysporin triple (P^3; bacitracin, gramicidin, and polymyxin B) in PD patients (n = 201) for the prevention of PD-related infections. Patients applied the ointment to the exit site with each dressing change and were followed for up to 18 months. No significant difference was found between groups for time to first PD-related infections (P = 0.41) for either agent, but a significant increase in fungal infections was observed in the P^3 versus mupirocin group (7 vs. 0; P = 0.01). The authors concluded that the use of P^3 for PD-related infection prophylaxis was not superior to mupirocin and may increase the risk of fungal infections.[146]

PERSONALIZED THERAPY

Because of the limitation of available kidneys for transplantation, dialysis (HD and PD) remains the most widely available and commonly used ESRD treatments. Despite continual advances in dialysis and transplantation, kidney disease is associated with significant morbidity and mortality. Given the lack of a true cure for CKD, emphasis recently has been placed on the prevention and early detection of kidney disease. Goals set by the NKF-K/DOQI, the Healthy People 2010 initiative, and the Centers for Medicare and Medicaid Services' CPM Project provide guidance and direction for all healthcare practitioners. In fact, there have been some significant gains in recent years in terms of incidence rate of ESRD, optimal access placement, and mortality and morbidity.[45,147] For patients with ESRD, a focus on quality of life and rehabilitation may be a valuable and viable goal toward which the nephrology community should direct its research resources. Although prevention of ESRD is the primary goal for clinicians and adequate access to renal transplantation is secondary, dialysis will likely be a part of the treatment paradigm for ESRD for many years to come.

ACKNOWLEDGMENTS

The authors wish to acknowledge the contributions of Rowland Ewell, Pharm. D., Edward F. Foote, Pharm. D., and Harold J. Manley, Pharm. D., to the previous editions of this chapter.

ABBREVIATIONS

APD	automated peritoneal dialysis
AV	arteriovenous
CAPD	continuous ambulatory peritoneal dialysis
CL_{cr}	creatinine clearance
CPM	clinical performance measures
ESRD	end-stage renal disease
GFR	glomerular filtration rate
HD	hemodialysis
IP	intraperitoneal
ISPD	The International Society of Peritoneal Dialysis
NKF-K/DOQI	National Kidney Foundation's Kidney Disease/ Dialysis Outcome Quality Initiative
PD	peritoneal dialysis
RRF	residual kidney function
URR	urea reduction ratio

REFERENCES

1. USRDS 2011 Annual Data Report: Atlas of End-Stage Renal Diseases in the United States. Bethesda, MD: National Institutes of Health, National Institutes of Diabetes and Digestive and Kidney Diseases, 2011.
2. Khawar O, Kalantar-Zadeh K, Lo WK, Johnson D, Mehrotra R. Is the declining use of long-term peritoneal dialysis justified by outcome data? Clin J Am Soc Nephrol 2007;2:1317–1328.
3. Abdel-Kader K, Myaskovsky L, Karpov I, et al. Individual quality of life in chronic kidney disease: Influence of age and dialysis modality. Clin J Am Soc Nephrol 2009;4:711–718.
4. Abdel-Kader K, Unruh ML, Weisbord SD. Symptom burden, depression, and quality of life in chronic and end-stage kidney disease. Clin J Am Soc Nephrol 2009;4:1057–1064.
5. Kimmel PL, Patel SS. Quality of life in patients with chronic kidney disease: Focus on end-stage renal disease treated with hemodialysis. Semin Nephrol 2006;26:68–79.
6. Perlman RL, Finkelstein FO, Liu L, et al. Quality of life in chronic kidney disease (CKD): A cross-sectional analysis in the Renal Research Institute—CKD study. Am J Kidney Dis 2005;45:658–666.
7. Curtin RB, Johnson HK, Schatell D. The peritoneal dialysis experience: Insights from long-term patients. Nephrol Nurs J 2004;31:615–624.
8. Gregory DM, Way CY, Hutchinson TA, Barrett BJ, Parfrey PS. Patients' perceptions of their experiences with ESRD and hemodialysis treatment. Qual Health Res 1998;8:764–783.
9. Hagren B, Pettersen IM, Severinsson E, Lutzen K, Clyne N. Maintenance haemodialysis: Patients' experiences of their life situation. J Clin Nurs 2005;14:294–300.
10. Krespi R, Bone M, Ahmad R, Worthington B, Salmon P. Haemodialysis patients' beliefs about renal failure and its treatment. Patient Educ Couns 2004;53:189–196.
11. Tong A, Sainsbury P, Chadban S, et al. Patients' experiences and perspectives of living with CKD. Am J Kidney Dis 2009;53:689–700.
12. Hemodialysis Adequacy 2006 Work Group: Clinical practice guidelines for hemodialysis adequacy, update 2006. Am J Kidney Dis 2006;48:S2–S90.
13. Himmelfarb J, Chuang P, Schulman G. Hemodialysis. In: Brenner BM, Rector FC, eds. Brenner & Rector's the Kidney, Vol. 2, 8th ed. Philadelphia: Saunders/Elsevier; 2008:xxii, 2241, lxix.
14. Termorshuizen F, Korevaar JC, Dekker FW, Van Manen JG, Boeschoten EW, Krediet RT. Hemodialysis and peritoneal dialysis: Comparison of adjusted mortality rates according to the duration of dialysis: Analysis of the Netherlands Cooperative Study on the Adequacy of Dialysis 2. J Am Soc Nephrol 2003;14:2851–2860.
15. Miskulin DC, Meyer KB, Athienites NV, et al. Comorbidity and other factors associated with modality selection in incident dialysis patients: The CHOICE Study. Choices for Healthy Outcomes in Caring for End-Stage Renal Disease. Am J Kidney Dis 2002;39:324–336.
16. Vonesh EF, Snyder JJ, Foley RN, Collins AJ. The differential impact of risk factors on mortality in hemodialysis and peritoneal dialysis. Kidney Int 2004;66:2389–2401.
17. Himmelfarb J, Ikizler TA. Hemodialysis. N Engl J Med 2010;363:1833–1845.

18. Pastan S, Bailey J. Dialysis therapy. N Engl J Med 1998;338:1428–1437.
19. Hayashi R, Huang E, Nissenson AR. Vascular access for hemodialysis. Nat Clin Pract Nephrol 2006;2:504–513.
20. Allon M, Work J. Venous catheter access for hemodialysis. In: Daugirdas JT, Blake PG, Ing TS, eds. Handbook of Dialysis, 4th ed. Philadelphia: Lippincott Williams & Wilkins; 2007:87–104.
21. Kumor V, Depner TA, Besarab A, Ananthakrishnan S. Arteriovenous access for hemodialysis. In: Daugirdas JT, Blake PG, Ing TS, eds. Handbook of Dialysis, 4th ed. Philadelphia: Lippincott Williams & Wilkins; 2007: 105–126.
22. Saad TF, Vesely TM. Venous access for patients with chronic kidney disease. J Vasc Interv Radiol 2004;15:1041–1045.
23. Vanholder R. Vascular access. Int J Artif Organs 2002;25:347–353.
24. Chan MR, Yevzlin AS. Tunneled dialysis catheters: Recent trends and future directions. Adv Chronic Kidney Dis 2009;16:386–395.
25. 2006 Annual Report, End Stage Renal Disease Clinical Performance Measures Project. Department of Health and Human Services CMMS, Office of Clinical Standards and Quality, Baltimore, Maryland, January 2007. http://www.cms.gov/Medicare/End-Stage-Renal-Disease/CPMProject/downloads/ESRD2006AnnualReport.pdf. Accessed on April 1 2013.
26. Ahmad S, Misra M, Hoenich N, Daugirdas JT. Hemodialysis apparatus. In: Daugirdas JT, Blake PG, Ing TS, eds. Handbook of Dialysis, 4th ed. Philadelphia: Lippincott Williams & Wilkins, 2007:59–78.
27. Schulman G. Clinical application of high-efficiency hemodialysis. In: Nissenson AR, Fine RN, eds. Handbook of Dialysis Therapy, 4th ed. Philadelphia: Saunders/Elsevier, 2008.
28. Pierratos A. Daily (quotidian) hemodialysis. In: Nissenson AR, Fine RN, eds. Handbook of Dialysis Therapy, 4th ed. Philadelphia: Saunders/Elsevier, 2008.
29. Pierratos A, McFarlane P, Chan CT. Quotidian dialysis—update 2005. Curr Opin Nephrol Hypertens 2005;14:119–124.
30. Daugirdas JT, Van Stone JC. Physiologic principles and urea kinetic modeling. In: Daugirdas JT, Blake PG, Ing TS, eds. Handbook of Dialysis, 4th ed. Philadelphia: Lippincott Williams & Wilkins, 2007:25–58.
31. Daugirdas JT, C.M. K. Chronic hemodialysis prescription: A urea kinetic approach. In: Daugirdas JT, Blake PG, Ing TS, eds. Handbook of Dialysis, 4th ed. Philadelphia: Lippincott Williams & Wilkins, 2007:121–147.
32. Eknoyan G, Beck GJ, Cheung AK, et al. Effect of dialysis dose and membrane flux in maintenance hemodialysis. N Engl J Med 2002;347:2010–2019.
33. Kooistra MP. Frequent prolonged home haemodialysis: Three old concepts, one modern solution. Nephrol Dial Transplant 2003;18:16–9.
34. Centers for Disease Control and Prevention (CDC). National Center for Health Statistics (NCHS). National Health and Nutrition Examination Survey Data. Hyattsville, MD: U.S. Department of Health and Human Services, Centers for Disease Control and Prevention, 2010 http://wwwn.cdc.gov/nchs/nhanes/search/nhanes09_10.aspx.
35. Chiu YW, Teitelbaum I, Misra M, de Leon EM, Adzize T, Mehrotra R. Pill burden, adherence, hyperphosphatemia, and quality of life in maintenance dialysis patients. Clin J Am Soc Nephrol 2009;4:1089–1096.
36. Davenport A. Intradialytic complications during hemodialysis. Hemodial Int 2006;10:162–167.
37. Sarkar S, Kait Watcharachai C, Levin NW. Complications During Hemodialysis, 4th ed. New York: McGraw-Hill, 2005.
38. Sherman R, Daugirdas J, Ing T. Complications During Hemodialysis, 4th ed. Philadelphia: Lipincott Williams & Wilkins, 2007.
39. Leypoldt JK, Cheung AK, Delmez JA, et al. Relationship between volume status and blood pressure during chronic hemodialysis. Kidney Int 2002;61:266–275.
40. Zhou YL, Liu HL, Duan XF, Yao Y, Sun Y, Liu Q. Impact of sodium and ultrafiltration profiling on haemodialysis-related hypotension. Nephrol Dial Transplant 2006;21:3231–3237.
41. Gabutti L, Bianchi G, Soldini D, Marone C, Burnier M. Haemodynamic consequences of changing bicarbonate and calcium concentrations in haemodialysis fluids. Nephrol Dial Transplant 2009;24:973–981.
42. Sherman RA. Intradialytic hypotension: An overview of recent, unresolved and overlooked issues. Semin Dial 2002;15:141–143.
43. Lok CE. Fistula first initiative: Advantages and pitfalls. Clin J Am Soc Nephrol 2007;2:1043–1053.
44. Wasse H. Catheter-related mortality among ESRD patients. Semin Dial 2008;21:547–549.
45. Besarab A, Work J. NKF-K/DOQI Clinical Practice Guidelines for Vascular Access: 2006. Am J Kidney Dis. 2006;48(S1):S176–S247.
46. Allon M, Work J. Venous Catheter Access for Hemodialysis, 4th ed. Philadelphia: Lipincott Williams & Wilkins, 2007.
47. Piraino B. *Staphylococcus aureus* infections in dialysis patients: Focus on prevention. ASAIO J 2000;46:S13–S17.
48. Leehey DJ, Cannon JP, Lentino JR. Infections, 4th ed. Philadelphia: Lippincott Williams & Wilkins, 2007.
49. U.S. Renal Data System Annual Data Report: Atlas of chronic kidney disease and end-stage renal disease in the United States. Bethesda, MD: National Institutes of Health, National Institute of Diabetes and Digestive and Kidney Diseases, 2008.
50. Sarnak MJ, Jaber BL. Mortality caused by sepsis in patients with end-stage renal disease compared with the general population. Kidney Int 2000;58:1758–1764.
51. Maki DG, Stolz SM, Wheeler S, Mermel LA. Prevention of central venous catheter-related bloodstream infection by use of an antiseptic-impregnated catheter. A randomized, controlled trial. Ann Intern Med 1997;127:257–266.
52. Raad I, Umphrey J, Khan A, Truett LJ, Bodey GP. The duration of placement as a predictor of peripheral and pulmonary arterial catheter infections. J Hosp Infect 1993;23:17–26.
53. Chesterton LJ, Selby NM, Burton JO, McIntyre CW. Cool dialysate reduces asymptomatic intradialytic hypotension and increases baroreflex variability. Hemodial Int 2009;13:189–196.
54. Selby NM, McIntyre CW. A systematic review of the clinical effects of reducing dialysate fluid temperature. Nephrol Dial Transplant 2006;21:1883–1898.
55. Prakash S, Garg AX, Heidenheim AP, House AA. Midodrine appears to be safe and effective for dialysis-induced hypotension: A systematic review. Nephrol Dial Transplant 2004;19:2553–2558.
56. Cruz DN. Midodrine: A selective alpha-adrenergic agonist for orthostatic hypotension and dialysis hypotension. Expert Opin Pharmacother 2000;1:835–840.
57. Lin YF, Wang JY, Denq JC, Lin SH. Midodrine improves chronic hypotension in hemodialysis patients. Am J Med Sci 2003;325:256–261.
58. Rubinstein S, Haimov M, Ross MJ. Midodrine-induced vascular ischemia in a hemodialysis patient: A case report and literature review. Ren Fail 2008;30:808–812.

59. Ahmad S, Robertson HT, Golper TA, et al. Multicenter trial of L-carnitine in maintenance hemodialysis patients. II. Clinical and biochemical effects. Kidney Int 1990;38: 912–918.
60. Golper TA, Wolfson M, Ahmad S, et al. Multicenter trial of L-carnitine in maintenance hemodialysis patients. I. Carnitine concentrations and lipid effects. Kidney Int 1990;38:904–911.
61. Yalcin AU, Kudaiberdieva G, Sahin G, et al. Effect of sertraline hydrochloride on cardiac autonomic dysfunction in patients with hemodialysis-induced hypotension. Nephron Physiol 2003;93:P21–P28.
62. Yalcin AU, Sahin G, Erol M, Bal C. Sertraline hydrochloride treatment for patients with hemodialysis hypotension. Blood Purif 2002;20:150–153.
63. Brewster UC, Ciampi MA, Abu-Alfa AK, Perazella MA. Addition of sertraline to other therapies to reduce dialysis-associated hypotension. Nephrology (Carlton) 2003;8:296–301.
64. Beladi-Mousavi SS, Beladi-Mousavi M, Hayati F, Talebzadeh M. Effect of intranasal DDAVP in prevention of hypotension during hemodialysis. Nefrologia 2012;32:89–93.
65. Perazella MA. Pharmacologic options available to treat symptomatic intradialytic hypotension. Am J Kidney Dis 2001;38:S26–S36.
66. Crawford-Bonadio TL, Diaz-Buxo JA. Comparison of peritoneal dialysis solutions. Nephrol Nurs J 2004;31: 499–507, 520; quiz 508–509.
67. El-Hennawy AS, Zaib S. A selected controlled trial of supplementary vitamin E for treatment of muscle cramps in hemodialysis patients. Am J Ther 2010;17:455–459.
68. Kobrin SM, Berns JS. Quinine—A tonic too bitter for hemodialysis-associated muscle cramps? Semin Dial 2007;20:396–401.
69. Roca AO, Jarjoura D, Blend D, et al. Dialysis leg cramps. Efficacy of quinine versus vitamin E. ASAIO J 1992;38: M481–M485.
70. Khajehdehi P, Mojerlou M, Behzadi S, Rais-Jalali GA. A randomized, double-blind, placebo-controlled trial of supplementary vitamins E, C and their combination for treatment of haemodialysis cramps. Nephrol Dial Transplant 2001;16:1448–1451.
71. Chang CT, Wu CH, Yang CW, Huang JY, Wu MS. Creatine monohydrate treatment alleviates muscle cramps associated with haemodialysis. Nephrol Dial Transplant 2002;17: 1978–1981.
72. Noordzij M, Boeschoten EW, Bos WJ, et al. Disturbed mineral metabolism is associated with muscle and skin complaints in a prospective cohort of dialysis patients. Nephrol Dial Transplant 2007;22:2944–2949.
73. Hyodo T, Taira T, Takemura T, et al. Immediate effect of Shakuyaku-kanzo-to on muscle cramp in hemodialysis patients. Nephron Clin Pract 2006;104:c28–c32.
74. Hyodo T, Taira T, Kumakura M, et al. The immediate effect of Shakuyaku-kanzo-to, traditional Japanese herbal medicine, for muscular cramps during maintenance hemodialysis. Nephron 2002;90:240.
75. Tordoir J, Canaud B, Haage P, et al. EBPG on vascular access. Nephrol Dial Transplant 2007;22(Suppl 2):ii88–117.
76. Dixon BS, Beck GJ, Vazquez MA, et al. Effect of dipyridamole plus aspirin on hemodialysis graft patency. N Engl J Med 2009;360:2191–2201.
77. Hasegawa T, Elder SJ, Bragg-Gresham JL, et al. Consistent aspirin use associated with improved arteriovenous fistula survival among incident hemodialysis patients in the dialysis outcomes and practice patterns study. Clin J Am Soc Nephrol 2008;3(5):1373–1378.
78. Chan KE, Lazarus JM, Thadhani R, Hakim RM. Anticoagulant and antiplatelet usage associates with mortality among hemodialysis patients. J Am Soc Nephrol 2009;20:872–881.
79. Chan KE, Lazarus JM, Thadhani R, Hakim RM. Warfarin use associates with increased risk for stroke in hemodialysis patients with atrial fibrillation. J Am Soc Nephrol 2009;20:2223–2233.
80. Sood MM, Rigatto C, Bueti J, et al. Thrice weekly warfarin administration in haemodialysis patients. Nephrol Dial Transplant 2009;24:3162–3167.
81. Limdi NA, Beasley TM, Baird MF, et al. Kidney function influences warfarin responsiveness and hemorrhagic complications. J Am Soc Nephrol 2009;20:912–921.
82. Lok CE, Moist L, Hemmelgarn BR, et al. Effect of fish oil supplementation on graft patency and cardiovascular events among patients with new synthetic arteriovenous hemodialysis grafts: A randomized controlled trial. JAMA 2012;307:1809–1816.
83. Krediet RT, van Westrhenen R, Zweers MM, Struijk DG. Clinical advantages of new peritoneal dialysis solutions. Nephrol Dial Transplant 2002;17(Suppl 3):16–18.
84. Macrae JM, Dojcinovic I, Djurdjev O, et al. Citrate 4% versus heparin and the reduction of thrombosis study (CHARTS). Clin J Am Soc Nephrol 2008;3:369–374.
85. Hemmelgarn BR, Moist LM, Lok CE, et al. Prevention of dialysis catheter malfunction with recombinant tissue plasminogen activator. N Engl J Med 2011;364:303–312.
86. Daeihagh P, Jordan J, Chen J, Rocco M. Efficacy of tissue plasminogen activator administration on patency of hemodialysis access catheters. Am J Kidney Dis 2000;36: 75–79.
87. Little MA, Walshe JJ. A longitudinal study of the repeated use of alteplase as therapy for tunneled hemodialysis catheter dysfunction. Am J Kidney Dis 2002;39:86–91.
88. Savader SJ, Ehrman KO, Porter DJ, Haikal LC, Oteham AC. Treatment of hemodialysis catheter-associated fibrin sheaths by rt-PA infusion: Critical analysis of 124 procedures. J Vasc Interv Radiol 2001;12:711–715.
89. Castner D. The efficacy of reteplase in the treatment of thrombosed hemodialysis venous catheters. Nephrol Nurs J 2001;28:403–404, 407–410.
90. Hilleman DE, Dunlay RW, Packard KA. Reteplase for dysfunctional hemodialysis catheter clearance. Pharmacotherapy 2003;23:137–141.
91. Hilleman D, Campbell J. Efficacy, safety, and cost of thrombolytic agents for the management of dysfunctional hemodialysis catheters: A systematic review. Pharmacotherapy 2011;31:1031–1040.
92. Macrae JM, Loh G, Djurdjev O, et al. Short and long alteplase dwells in dysfunctional hemodialysis catheters. Hemodial Int 2005;9:189–195.
93. Davies J, Casey J, Li C, Crowe AV, McClelland P. Restoration of flow following haemodialysis catheter thrombus. Analysis of rt-PA infusion in tunnelled dialysis catheters. J Clin Pharm Ther 2004;29:517–520.
94. Davies J, Casey J, Li C, Crowe AV, McClelland P. Analysis of rt-PA infusion in tunnelled dialysis catheters. EDTNA ERCA J 2005;31:75–78.
95. Vercaigne LM, Zacharias J, Bernstein KN. Alteplase for blood flow restoration in hemodialysis catheters: a multicenter, randomized, prospective study comparing "dwell" versus "push" administration. Clin Nephrol. 2012;78(4):287–296.

96. Allon M. Treatment guidelines for dialysis catheter-related bacteremia: An update. Am J Kidney Dis 2009;54:13–17.
97. Mermel LA, Allon M, Bouza E, et al. Clinical practice guidelines for the diagnosis and management of intravascular catheter-related infection: 2009 Update by the Infectious Diseases Society of America. Clin Infect Dis 2009;49:1–45.
98. O'Grady NP, Alexander M, Burns LA, et al. Guidelines for the prevention of intravascular catheter-related infections. Am J Infect Control 2011;39:S1–S34.
99. O'Grady NP, Alexander M, Burns LA, et al. Guidelines for the prevention of intravascular catheter-related infections. Clin Infect Dis 2011;52:e162–193.
100. Johnson DW, MacGinley R, Kay TD, et al. A randomized controlled trial of topical exit site mupirocin application in patients with tunnelled, cuffed haemodialysis catheters. Nephrol Dial Transplant 2002;17:1802–1807.
101. Battistella M, Bhola C, Lok CE. Long-term follow-up of the Hemodialysis Infection Prevention with Polysporin Ointment (HIPPO) Study: A quality improvement report. Am J Kidney Dis 2011;57:432–441.
102. Johnson DW, van Eps C, Mudge DW, et al. Randomized, controlled trial of topical exit-site application of honey (Medihoney) versus mupirocin for the prevention of catheter-associated infections in hemodialysis patients. J Am Soc Nephrol 2005;16:1456–1462.
103. Allon M. Dialysis catheter-related bacteremia: Treatment and prophylaxis. Am J Kidney Dis 2004;44:779–791.
104. Fitzgibbons LN, Puls DL, Mackay K, Forrest GN. Management of gram-positive coccal bacteremia and hemodialysis. Am J Kidney Dis 2011;57:624–640.
105. Zvonar R, Natarajan S, Edwards C, Roth V. Assessment of vancomycin use in chronic haemodialysis patients: Room for improvement. Nephrol Dial Transplant 2008;23:3690–3695.
106. Salama NN, Segal JH, Churchwell MD, et al. Intradialytic administration of daptomycin in end stage renal disease patients on hemodialysis. Clin J Am Soc Nephrol 2009;4:1190–1194.
107. Poole CV, Carlton D, Bimbo L, Allon M. Treatment of catheter-related bacteraemia with an antibiotic lock protocol: Effect of bacterial pathogen. Nephrol Dial Transplant 2004;19:1237–1244.
108. Labriola L, Crott R, Jadoul M. Preventing haemodialysis catheter-related bacteraemia with an antimicrobial lock solution: A meta-analysis of prospective randomized trials. Nephrol Dial Transplant 2008;23:1666–1672.
109. Moran J, Sun S, Khababa I, Pedan A, Doss S, Schiller B. A randomized trial comparing gentamicin/citrate and heparin locks for central venous catheters in maintenance hemodialysis patients. Am J Kidney Dis 2012;59:102–107.
110. Sharma A, Blake PG. Peritoneal dialysis. In: Brenner BM, Rector FC, eds. Brenner & Rector's the Kidney, Vol. 2, 8th ed. Philadelphia: Saunders/Elsevier, 2008:xxii, 2241, lxix.
111. Brophy DF, Mueller BA. Automated peritoneal dialysis: New implications for pharmacists. Ann Pharmacother 1997;31:756–764.
112. Clinical practice recommendations for peritoneal dialysis adequacy. Am J Kidney Dis 2006;48:S130–S158.
113. Diaz-Buxo JA. Continuous-flow peritoneal dialysis: Update. Adv Perit Dial 2004;20:18–22.
114. Amerling R, Winchester JF, Ronco C. Continuous flow peritoneal dialysis: Update 2012. Contrib Nephrol 2012;178:205–215.
115. Frampton JE, Plosker GL. Icodextrin: A review of its use in peritoneal dialysis. Drugs 2003;63:2079–2105.
116. Thomas J, Teitelbaum I. Preservation of residual renal function in dialysis patients. Adv Perit Dial 2011;27:112–117.
117. Garcia-Lopez E, Lindholm B, Davies S. An update on peritoneal dialysis solutions. Nat Rev Nephrol 2012;8:224–233.
118. Canada-USA (CANUSA) Peritoneal Dialysis Study Group: Adequacy of dialysis and nutrition in continuous peritoneal dialysis: Association with clinical outcomes. J Am Soci Nephrol 1996;7:198–207.
119. Han SH, Lee SC, Ahn SV, et al. Reduced residual renal function is a risk of peritonitis in continuous ambulatory peritoneal dialysis patients. Nephrol Dial Transplant 2007;22:2653–2658.
120. Johnson DW, Brown FG, Clarke M, et al. Effects of biocompatible versus standard fluid on peritoneal dialysis outcomes. J Am Soc Nephrol 2012;23:1097–1107.
121. Smit W. Estimates of peritoneal membrane function—New insights. Nephrol Dial Transplant 2006;21(Suppl 2):ii16–19.
122. Peritoneal Dialysis Adequacy Work Group: Clinical practice guidelines for peritoneal dialysis adequacy. Am J Kid Dis 2006;48:S98–S129.
123. Troidle L, Finkelstein F. Treatment and outcome of CPD-associated peritonitis. Ann Clin Microbiol Antimicrob 2006;5:6.
124. Troidle L, Gorban-Brennan N, Finkelstein FO. Outcome of patients on chronic peritoneal dialysis undergoing peritoneal catheter removal because of peritonitis. Adv Perit Dial 2005;21:98–101.
125. Piraino B, Bernardini J, Bender FH. An analysis of methods to prevent peritoneal dialysis catheter infections. Perit Dial Int 2008;28:437–443.
126. Li PK, Szeto CC, Piraino B, et al. Peritoneal dialysis-related infections recommendations: 2010 update. Perit Dial Int 2010;30:393–423.
127. Piraino B, Bailie GR, Bernardini J, et al. Peritoneal dialysis-related infections recommendations: 2005 update. Perit Dial Int 2005;25:107–131.
128. Herwaldt LA, Boyken LD, Coffman S, Hochstetler L, Flanigan MJ. Sources of *Staphylococcus aureus* for patients on continuous ambulatory peritoneal dialysis. Perit Dial Int 2003;23:237–241.
129. Piraino B, Bernardini J, Brown E, et al. ISPD position statement on reducing the risks of peritoneal dialysis-related infections. Perit Dial Int 2011;31:614–630.
130. Elwell RJ, Volino LR, Frye RF. Stability of cefepime in icodextrin peritoneal dialysis solution. Ann Pharmacother 2004;38:2041–2044.
131. Robinson RF, Morosco RS, Smith CV, Mahan JD. Stability of cefazolin sodium in four heparinized and non-heparinized dialysate solutions at 38°C. Perit Dial Int 2006;26:593–597.
132. Voges M, Divino-Filho JC, Faict D, Somers F, Vermeulen P. Compatibility of insulin over 24 hours in standard and bicarbonate-based peritoneal dialysis solutions contained in bags made of different materials. Perit Dial Int 2006;26:498–502.
133. Baker RJ, Senior H, Clemenger M, Brown EA. Empirical aminoglycosides for peritonitis do not affect residual renal function. Am J Kidney Dis 2003;41:670–675.
134. Shemin D, Maaz D, St Pierre D, Kahn SI, Chazan JA. Effect of aminoglycoside use on residual renal function in peritoneal dialysis patients. Am J Kidney Dis 1999;34:14–20.
135. Wiggins KJ, Johnson DW, Craig JC, Strippoli GFM. Treatment of peritoneal dialysis-associated peritonitis: A systematic review of randomized controlled trials. Am J Kidney Dis 2007;50:967–988.
136. Felgueiras J, del Peso G, Bajo A, et al. Risk of technique failure and death in fungal peritonitis is determined mainly by duration on peritoneal dialysis: Single-center experience of 24 years. Adv Perit Dial 2006;22:77–81.

137. Williams PF, Moncrieff N, Marriott J. No benefit in using nystatin prophylaxis against fungal peritonitis in peritoneal dialysis patients. Perit Dial Int 2000;20:352–353.
138. Bernardini J, Bender F, Florio T, et al. Randomized, double-blind trial of antibiotic exit site cream for prevention of exit site infection in peritoneal dialysis patients. J Am Soc Nephrol 2005;16:539–545.
139. Mahajan S, Tiwari SC, Kalra V, et al. Effect of local mupirocin application on exit-site infection and peritonitis in an Indian peritoneal dialysis population. Perit Dial Int 2005;25:473–477.
140. Mahaldar A, Weisz M, Kathuria P. Comparison of gentamicin and mupirocin in the prevention of exit-site infection and peritonitis in peritoneal dialysis. Adv Perit Dial 2009;25:56–59.
141. Uttley L, Vardhan A, Mahajan S, Smart B, Hutchison A, Gokal R. Decrease in infections with the introduction of mupirocin cream at the peritoneal dialysis catheter exit site. J Nephrol 2004;17:242–245.
142. Bender FH, Bernardini J, Piraino B. Prevention of infectious complications in peritoneal dialysis: Best demonstrated practices. Kid Int Suppl 2006:S44–S54.
143. Berns JS. Infection with antimicrobial-resistant microorganisms in dialysis patients. Semin Dial 2003;16: 30–37.
144. Cavdar C, Saglam F, Sifil A, et al. Effect of once-a-week vs. thrice-a-week application of mupirocin on methicillin and mupirocin resistance in peritoneal dialysis patients: Three years of experience. Ren Fail 2008;30: 417–422.
145. Pierce DA, Williamson JC, Mauck VS, Russell GB, Palavecino E, Burkart JM. The effect on peritoneal dialysis pathogens of changing topical antibiotic prophylaxis. Perit Dial Int 2012;32(5):525–530.
146. McQuillan RF, Chiu E, Nessim S, et al. A randomized controlled trial comparing mupirocin and polysporin triple ointments in peritoneal dialysis patients: The MP3 Study. Clin J Am Soc Nephrol 2012;7:297–303.
147. Mujais S, Story K. Peritoneal dialysis in the US: Evaluation of outcomes in contemporary cohorts. Kid Int Suppl 2006:S21–S26.

31

Drug-Induced Kidney Disease

Thomas D. Nolin

KEY CONCEPTS

1. The initial diagnosis of drug-induced kidney disease (DIKD) typically involves detection of elevated serum creatinine and blood urea nitrogen, for which there is a temporal relationship between the toxicity and use of a potentially nephrotoxic drug.
2. DIKD is best prevented by avoiding the use of potentially nephrotoxic agents for patients at increased risk for toxicity. However, when exposure to these drugs cannot be avoided, recognition of risk factors and specific techniques, such as hydration, may be used to reduce potential nephrotoxicity.
3. Acute tubular necrosis is the most common presentation of DIKD in hospitalized patients. The primary agents implicated are aminoglycosides, radiocontrast media, cisplatin, amphotericin B, and osmotically active agents.
4. Angiotensin-converting enzyme inhibitors and nonsteroidal antiinflammatory drugs are associated with hemodynamically mediated kidney injury, the pathogenesis of which is a decrease in glomerular capillary hydrostatic pressure.
5. Acute allergic interstitial nephritis is observed in up to 27% of kidney biopsies performed for hospitalized patients with unexplained acute kidney injury. Clinical manifestations of AIN typically present approximately 14 days after initiation of therapy and include fever, maculopapular rash, eosinophilia, arthralgia, often with pyuria, hematuria, proteinuria, and oliguria.

INTRODUCTION

Numerous diagnostic and therapeutic agents have been associated with the development of drug-induced kidney disease (DIKD) or nephrotoxicity. It is a relatively common complication with variable presentations depending on the drug and clinical setting, inpatient or outpatient. Manifestations of DIKD include acid–base abnormalities, electrolyte imbalances, urine sediment abnormalities, proteinuria, pyuria, and/or hematuria. However, the most common manifestation of DIKD is a decline in the glomerular filtration rate (GFR), which results in a rise in serum creatinine (S_{cr}) and blood urea nitrogen (BUN) and several other indicators of acute and chronic kidney injury (see eChap. 18 and Chap. 28).[1] Initial diagnosis of DIKD is often delayed as it typically is based on the detection of elevated S_{cr} and BUN, for which there is a temporal relationship between the kidney injury and exposure to the potentially nephrotoxic drug. This is consistent with classic qualitative definitions of acute renal failure, which have relied on either an abrupt increase in S_{cr} or an abrupt decline in urine output (see eChap. 18 and Chap. 28). Historically, the clinical use of numerous definitions of acute renal failure and nephrotoxicity based on quantitative changes in the S_{cr} concentration and other clinical end points made it extraordinarily difficult to ascertain their true incidence.[2] During the last decade however, standard terminology (e.g., acute kidney injury, AKI) and diagnostic criteria based on a combination of physiologic measurements (e.g., S_{cr} and urine output) have been adopted and are now routinely used in clinical practice and research.[3,4] This will likely lead to new epidemiologic data about DIKD that are more accurate.

Nephrotoxicity is often reversible if one discontinues the use of the offending agent, but in some cases there may still be an AKI and progression to stage 5 chronic kidney disease (CKD), which includes end-stage renal disease (ESRD). Currently, many different mechanisms are responsible for the pathogenesis of DIKD, and the introduction of new drugs with novel mechanisms of action provides the potential for the identification of new presentations of AKI and CKD. This chapter reviews the epidemiology, pathophysiology, risk factors, and basic principles of prevention of DIKD. Detailed discussions of these issues plus management strategies are presented for the most commonly used agents that have been associated with a moderate to high likelihood of DIKD.

EPIDEMIOLOGY

The incidence and characteristics of outpatient or community-acquired DIKD are not well understood since mild toxicity is often unrecognized in this setting. However, the acquisition of data regarding the pharmacoepidemiology of these effects has become more important as care increasingly shifts to the outpatient setting. The incidence of community-based AKI that required dialysis was recently reported to be 29.5 per 100,000 person years and 522.4 per 100,000 person years for patients not requiring dialysis.[5] Although the incidence of drug-induced AKI was not specifically reported, earlier studies have implicated community-acquired DIKD in up to 20% of hospital admissions due to AKI.[6] Conversely, AKI has been reported in up to 7% of hospitalized patients,[7] and as many as 20% to 30% of critically ill patients may experience AKI during their hospitalization.[8,9] Drug-induced causes have been implicated in up to 60% of all cases of in-hospital AKI and as such are a recognized source of significant morbidity and mortality. Although the incidence of in-hospital antibiotic-induced AKI alone has been reported to be as high as 36%, it appears to be declining, while cases of in-hospital AKI due to nonselective nonsteroidal antiinflammatory drugs (NSAIDs), angiotensin-converting enzyme inhibitors (ACEIs), chemotherapeutic agents, and antiviral drugs are increasing.[1]

CLINICAL PRESENTATION Drug-Induced Kidney Disease

General

- The most common manifestation is a decline in GFR leading to a rise in S_{cr} and BUN
- Alterations in renal tubular function without loss of glomerular filtration may be evident

Symptoms

- Patients may complain of malaise, anorexia, vomiting, shortness of breath, or edema, particularly in the outpatient setting

Signs

- Decreased urine output may be an early sign of toxicity, particularly with radiographic contrast media, NSAIDs, and ACEIs, with progression to volume overload and hypertension
- Proximal tubular injury: Metabolic acidosis with bicarbonaturia; glycosuria in the absence of hyperglycemia; and reductions in serum phosphate, uric acid, potassium, and magnesium due to increased urinary losses
- Distal tubular injury: Polyuria from failure to maximally concentrate urine, metabolic acidosis from impaired urinary acidification, and hyperkalemia from impaired potassium excretion

Laboratory Tests

- An abrupt (within 48 hours) reduction in kidney function defined as an absolute increase in S_{cr} of ≥0.3 mg/dL (27 μmol/L), a percentage increase in S_{cr} of ≥50% (1.5-fold from baseline), or a reduction in urine output (documented oliguria of less than 0.5 mL/kg per hour for more than 6 hours),[13] when correlated temporally with the initiation of drug therapy may indicate drug-induced AKI

Other Diagnostic Tests

- Urinary excretion of *N*-acetyl-β-D-glucosaminidase, γ-glutamyl transpeptidase, glutathione *S*-transferase, and interleukin (IL)-18 are markers of proximal tubular injury and have been used for the early detection of AKI in critically ill patients
- Kidney injury molecule-1 (KIM-1) is expressed in the proximal tubule and is upregulated for patients with ischemic acute tubular necrosis, appearing in the urine within 12 hours after the ischemic insult
- Neutrophil gelatinase-associated lipocalin (NGAL) protein may be detected in the urine within 3 hours of ischemic injury

❶ Because the most common manifestation of DIKD is a decline in GFR leading to a rise in S_{cr} and BUN, the onset of toxicity in hospitalized, acutely ill patients is most often recognized by routine laboratory monitoring. Decreased urine output may also be an early sign of toxicity, particularly with radiographic contrast media, NSAIDs, and ACEIs. In the outpatient setting, nephrotoxicity is often recognized by the development of symptoms such as malaise, anorexia, vomiting, volume overload (shortness of breath or edema), and hypertension. S_{cr} or BUN concentrations and urine collection for creatinine clearance may subsequently be measured to quantify the degree of decline in GFR. Marked intrasubject between-day variability of S_{cr} values have been noted (±20% for values within the normal range; see eChap. 18). Furthermore, they may be altered as the result of dietary changes and initiation of drug therapy, which may interfere with the assay procedure. Thus changes in S_{cr} or urine output consistent with the diagnostic criteria for AKI (see Chap. 28),[10] when correlated temporally with the initiation of drug therapy, are a common threshold for the identification of DIKD.

Nephrotoxicity may also be evidenced by primary alterations in renal tubular function without a corresponding loss of glomerular filtration. In this setting, urinary enzymes and low-molecular-weight proteins may be used as earlier and more specific biomarkers of nephrotoxicity compared with S_{cr} and BUN, which are relatively insensitive markers of kidney injury.[11,12] S_{cr} and BUN are used as surrogates of kidney function, not injury per se, and typically significant kidney injury must have occurred days before a rise in either is evident. Urinary excretion of kidney injury molecule-1 (KIM-1), *N*-acetyl-β-glucosaminidase, γ-glutamyl transpeptidase, glutathione *S*-transferase, neutrophil gelatinase-associated lipocalin (NGAL), and interleukin-18 are markers of proximal tubular injury and have been used for the early detection of acute kidney damage in several patient populations.[11–14] For example, the transmembrane protein KIM-1 is upregulated for patients with ischemic acute tubular necrosis (ATN), appearing in the urine within 12 hours after the ischemic insult.[14] Urinary *N*-acetylglucosamine (NAG) concentrations are a highly sensitive indicator of AKI and have been shown to detect AKI in critically ill patients up to 4 days prior to a rise in S_{cr} was observed.[14] Similarly, urinary NGAL is an early marker of AKI, preceding a rise in S_{cr} by up to 3 days. In the future, urinary biomarkers such as KIM-1, NAG, and NGAL may facilitate the earlier detection of kidney injury and diagnosis of nephrotoxicity and minimize the long-term consequences of this common drug-induced disorder.[11,12,14]

PRINCIPLES FOR PREVENTION OF DRUG-INDUCED NEPHROPATHY

❷ The primary principle for prevention of DIKD is to avoid the use of nephrotoxic agents for patients at increased risk for toxicity. Therefore, an awareness of potentially nephrotoxic drugs and knowledge of risk factors that increase renal vulnerability is essential.[15] Exposure to these drugs often cannot be avoided, so several interventions have been proposed to reduce the potential for the development of nephrotoxicity, for example, adjustment of medication dosage regimens based on accurate estimates of kidney function, and careful and adequate hydration to establish high urine flow rates.[16] Other preventative strategies are still theoretical and/or investigational and relate directly to the specific nephrotoxic mechanisms of a given drug.

The several specific drug-induced renal structural–functional alterations that are responsible for the vast majority of cases of

TABLE 31-1 Drug-Induced Kidney Structural–Functional Alterations

Tubular epithelial cell damage	
Acute tubular necrosis	• Pentamidine
• Aminoglycoside antibiotics	• Foscarnet
• Radiographic contrast media	• Zoledronate
• Cisplatin, carboplatin	Osmotic nephrosis
• Amphotericin B	• Mannitol
• Cyclosporine, tacrolimus	• Dextran
• Adefovir, cidofovir, tenofovir	• IV immunoglobulin
Hemodynamically mediated kidney injury	
• Angiotensin-converting enzyme inhibitors	• Nonsteroidal antiinflammatory drugs (NSAIDs)
• Angiotensin II receptor blockers	• Cyclosporine, tacrolimus
	• OKT3
Obstructive nephropathy	
Intratubular obstruction	Nephrolithiasis
• Acyclovir	• Sulfonamides
• Sulfonamides	• Triamterene
• Indinavir	• Indinavir
• Foscarnet	Nephrocalcinosis
• Methotrexate	• Oral sodium phosphate solution
Glomerular disease	
• Gold	• NSAIDs, cyclooxygenase-2 inhibitors
• Lithium	• Pamidronate
Tubulointerstitial disease	
Acute allergic interstitial nephritis	Chronic interstitial nephritis
• Penicillins	• Cyclosporine
• Ciprofloxacin	• Lithium
• NSAIDs, cyclooxygenase-2 inhibitors	• Aristolochic acid
	Papillary necrosis
• Proton pump inhibitors	• NSAIDs, combined phenacetin, aspirin, and caffeine analgesics
• Loop diuretics	
Renal vasculitis, thrombosis, and cholesterol emboli	
Vasculitis and thrombosis	• Methamphetamines
• Hydralazine	• Cyclosporine, tacrolimus
• Propylthiouracil	• Adalimumab
• Allopurinol	• Bevacizumab
• Penicillamine	Cholesterol emboli
• Gemcitabine	• Warfarin
• Mitomycin C	• Thrombolytic agents

DIKD are listed in Table 31-1. This chapter discusses the pathophysiologic mechanisms responsible for the development of DIKD with these agents in detail, along with clinical presentation, prevention strategies, therapeutic management approaches, and relevant monitoring plans.

TUBULAR EPITHELIAL CELL DAMAGE

3 Drugs that lead to renal tubular epithelial cell damage typically do so via direct cellular toxicity or ischemia. Damage is most often localized in the proximal and distal tubular epithelia and is termed acute tubular necrosis when cellular degeneration and sloughing from proximal and distal tubular basement membranes are observed.[17] This classically manifests as cellular debris-filled, muddy-brown, granular casts in the urinary sediment.[17,18] Specific indicators of proximal tubular injury include metabolic acidosis with bicarbonaturia; glycosuria in the absence of hyperglycemia; and reductions in serum phosphate, uric acid, potassium, and magnesium as a result of increased urinary losses. Indicators of distal tubular injury include polyuria from failure to maximally concentrate urine (i.e., nephrogenic diabetes insipidus), metabolic acidosis from impaired urinary acidification, and hyperkalemia from impaired potassium excretion.

Acute Tubular Necrosis

ATN is the most common presentation of DIKD in the inpatient setting. The primary agents associated with this type of injury are aminoglycosides, radiocontrast media, cisplatin, amphotericin B, foscarnet, and osmotically active agents such as immunoglobulins, dextrans, and mannitol.[9,19]

Aminoglycoside Nephrotoxicity

Incidence Aminoglycoside antibiotic-associated nephrotoxicity has been reported to occur in between 10% and 25% of patients receiving a therapeutic course.[9,20,21] Critically ill patients appear to have a higher risk for nephrotoxicity with reported rates as high as 58%.[20] The large variance is in part a result of the use of different definitions of toxicity, variability between agents in the class, and the risk factors present in the study population.

Clinical Presentation Clinical evidence of aminoglycoside-associated nephrotoxicity is typically seen within 5 to 10 days after initiation of therapy and manifests as a gradual progressive rise in S_{cr} and BUN and decrease in creatinine clearance.[9] Patients usually present with nonoliguria, that is, they maintain urine volumes greater than 500 mL/day and sometimes have microscopic hematuria and proteinuria.[9,19] Although renal magnesium wasting can occur (i.e., daily excretion of more than 10 to 30 mg), the risk of symptomatic hypomagnesemia is generally low. Full recovery of kidney function is common if aminoglycoside therapy is discontinued immediately upon discovering signs of toxicity.[11] However, severe AKI may develop occasionally, and for these individuals renal replacement therapy may be required (see Chap. 28). The diagnosis of aminoglycoside-associated nephrotoxicity is often difficult, particularly in critically ill patients with multiple comorbidities and is confounded by other factors that are independently associated with the development of AKI.[20] For instance, concurrent dehydration, sepsis, hypotension, ischemia, and use of other nephrotoxic drugs frequently contribute to AKI in patients who are receiving aminoglycosides.[17]

Pathogenesis Aminoglycoside-associated ATN is primarily due to accumulation of high drug concentrations within proximal tubular epithelial cells, and subsequent generation of reactive oxygen species that produce mitochondrial injury, which leads to cellular apoptosis and necrosis.[10,19] This results in cell sloughing from proximal tubular basement membranes into the tubular lumen, which can result in tubular obstruction and back leakage of the glomerular filtrate across the damaged tubular epithelium. Toxicity is related to cationic charge of the drugs in this class, which facilitates their binding to negatively charged renal tubular epithelial membrane phospholipids in the proximal tubules, followed by intracellular transport and concentration in lysosomes. The number of cationic groups on the drug molecule appears to correlate with the degree of nephrotoxicity, which is consistent with the observation of higher rates of toxicity with neomycin versus gentamicin, followed by tobramycin, then amikacin.[9,15]

Risk Factors Multiple risk factors for aminoglycoside-associated nephrotoxicity have been identified: the aggressiveness of aminoglycoside dosing, synergistic toxicity as the result of combination drug therapy, and preexisting clinical conditions of the patient (Table 31-2).[9,15,20]

Prevention Aminoglycoside-associated ATN may be prevented by careful and cautious selection of patients and the use of alternative antibiotics whenever possible and as soon as microbial sensitivities are known. Commonly used alternatives include fluoroquinolones (e.g., ciprofloxacin or levofloxacin) and third- or fourth-generation cephalosporins (e.g., ceftazidime or cefepime). When aminoglycosides are necessary, gentamicin, tobramycin,

TABLE 31-2 Potential Risk Factors for Aminoglycoside Nephrotoxicity

(A) Related to aminoglycoside dosing:
Large total cumulative dose
Prolonged therapy
Trough concentration exceeding 2 mg/L[a]
Recent previous aminoglycoside therapy
(B) Related to synergistic nephrotoxicity. Aminoglycosides in combination with
Cyclosporine
Amphotericin B
Vancomycin
Diuretics
Iodinated radiographic contrast agents
Cisplatin
NSAIDs
(C) Related to predisposing conditions in the patient
Preexisting kidney disease
Diabetes
Increased age
Poor nutrition
Shock
Gram-negative bacteremia
Liver disease
Hypoalbuminemia
Obstructive jaundice
Dehydration
Hypotension
Potassium or magnesium deficiencies

[a]The equivalent concentration in SI molar units are 4.3 μmol/L for tobramycin, 4.2 μmol/L for gentamicin.

and amikacin are most commonly used, but therapy should be selected to optimize antimicrobial efficacy.[22] Furthermore, it is imperative to avoid volume depletion, limit the total aminoglycoside dose administered, and avoid concomitant therapy with other nephrotoxic drugs. Future therapeutic alternatives may include new aminoglycoside congeners that retain the desired bactericidal activity and yet are devoid of nephrotoxicity, and may also include concurrent use of antioxidant compounds such as vitamin E and *N*-acetylcysteine.[23,24]

Prospective, individualized pharmacokinetic monitoring has been used for more than three decades, and its use has been associated with a decrease in the incidence of aminoglycoside-associated nephrotoxicity.[25] These studies, however, were often small and statistically underpowered. High-dose intermittent dosing of aminoglycosides, termed once daily dosing, used in combination with other antibiotics, has been intensively investigated as a practical cost-effective method to maintain antimicrobial efficacy while reducing the risk of AKI.[24,26,27] The reduction in incidence may be the result of limited proximal tubular aminoglycoside uptake during the transient, high-peak serum concentrations, and because of the presence of low aminoglycoside concentrations for a greater proportion of the dosing interval, which facilitates excretion of the aminoglycoside.[22] Although greater clinical efficacy and reduced nephrotoxicity may be realized with once daily compared with standard dosing, seriously ill, immunocompromised, and elderly patients, as well as those with preexisting kidney disease, are not ideal candidates for this approach.[24]

Management Aminoglycoside use should be discontinued or the dosage regimen revised if AKI is evident (i.e., there is an S_{cr} increase of 0.5 mg/dL [44 μmol/L] or more that is not attributable to another cause). Other nephrotoxic drugs should be discontinued if possible, and the patient should be maintained adequately hydrated and hemodynamically stable.[26] Short-term renal replacement therapy may be necessary, but ESRD has rarely been reported to be solely the result of aminoglycoside toxicity.[28]

Radiographic Contrast Media Nephrotoxicity

Incidence The incidence of radiographic contrast media-induced nephrotoxicity (CIN) has declined over the past decade from approximately 15% to 7% of all patients receiving iodinated contrast; yet it remains the third leading cause of hospital-acquired AKI, accounting for up to 11% of cases.[29] The incidence varies depending on the population studied and presence of risk factors; rising from <2% for patients with normal kidney function up to 50% for patients with CKD or diabetes mellitus.[30] As the number of risk factors associated with CIN increases, there is a proportional increase in the incidence of nephrotoxicity and in hospital and postdischarge mortality rates.[29,31] A 5.5-fold increased risk of death has been reported for patients who develop CIN compared with those who do not, with the highest mortality rates observed for patients who developed AKI and required renal replacement therapy.[19,21] In-hospital and 2-year mortality rates of 36% and 81%, respectively, have been reported for patients who developed CIN and those that required dialysis. An in-hospital mortality rate of only 7% was observed in those with CIN not requiring dialysis.[29]

Clinical Presentation CIN is usually transient in nature, presenting most commonly as nonoliguria with kidney injury apparent within the first 24 to 48 hours after the administration of contrast. The S_{cr} concentration usually peaks between 3 and 4 days after exposure, with recovery after 7 to 10 days.[32,33] However, irreversible oliguric (urine volume <500 mL/day) AKI requiring dialysis has been reported in high-risk patients.[31] Urinalysis typically reveals tubular enzymuria with hyaline and granular casts but may also be completely void of casts. The urine sodium concentration and fractional excretion of sodium are frequently low, with the latter typically <1% (<0.01).

Pathogenesis The primary mechanisms by which contrast media induces nephrotoxicity are renal ischemia and direct cellular toxicity.[29] Renal ischemia likely results from systemic hypotension and simultaneous acute vasoconstriction caused by disruption of normal prostaglandin synthesis and the release of adenosine, endothelin, and other renal vasoconstrictors. Subsequently, a 50% sustained reduction in renal blood flow that lasts for several hours immediately following contrast administration may be evident.[29] This reduced renal blood flow leads to increased concentrations of contrast in the renal tubules and exacerbates the direct cytotoxicity. The extent of cellular toxicity is directly related to the duration of tubular cell exposure to contrast. Thus, preservation of high urinary flow rates with adequate hydration before, during, and after contrast administration is vital to keep renal blood flow as high as reasonably possible to minimize tubular cell exposure to the contrast agent.[29] In humans, plasma osmolality is normally between 275 and 290 mOsm/kg (275 and 290 mmol/kg). Since low- and high-osmolar contrast agents are hyperosmolar to plasma (i.e., 600 to 800 mOsm/kg [600 to 800 mmol/kg] and ~2,000 mOsm/kg [~2,000 mmol/kg], respectively), their use may result in osmotic diuresis, dehydration, renal ischemia, and increased blood viscosity caused by red blood cell aggregation. Oxidative stress has also been implicated in the development of ATN after contrast administration,[34] which may explain the possible benefit of the antioxidant *N*-acetylcysteine.[35]

Risk Factors Decreased renal blood flow exacerbates the ischemic and direct cytotoxic effects of contrast media on the renal tubules. Therefore, preexisting kidney disease, particularly in those with estimated GFR <60 mL/min/1.73 m^2, is the most important risk factor present in up to 60% of patients who develop CIN.[29] Other patient-specific risk factors include conditions associated with decreased renal blood flow (i.e., congestive heart failure, dehydration/volume depletion, and hypotension), and patients with atherosclerosis and reduced effective circulating arterial blood volume appear to also have an elevated risk.[33] Diabetes is also a significant risk factor, likely due to coexisting kidney disease (diabetic nephropathy). The presence of multiple myeloma has traditionally been considered a relative contraindication for contrast use, but the risk appears to be associated with concomitant dehydration, kidney disease, or hypercalcemia rather than the diagnosis itself. Larger volumes or doses of contrast and the use of low- as well as high-osmolar contrast agents are also independent predictors of CIN. Intraarterial administration of contrast confers greater risk than IV administration.[29] Lastly, concurrent use of nephrotoxins and drugs that alter renal hemodynamics such as NSAIDs and ACEIs also increases risk. Risk factors are additive, and there is a proportional increase in the incidence of CIN and associated mortality as the number of risk factors increases.[29,31]

Prevention CIN can be anticipated in the majority of patients who are at risk; so the use of preventative procedures is justified for virtually all patients. Table 31-3 lists the recommended interventions for prevention of contrast nephrotoxicity. All patients scheduled to receive contrast media should be assessed for risk factors, and the risk-to-benefit ratio should be considered.[29,33,36,37] High-risk patients can be identified by evaluating medical history and indication for the contrast study, along with their most recent S_{cr} concentrations. Nephrotoxicity is best prevented in high-risk patients by using alternative imaging procedures (e.g., ultrasound, noncontrast magnetic resonance imaging, and nuclear medicine scans).[36] However, if contrast media must be used, the smallest adequate volume should be administered. If the ratio of the volume of contrast to be infused relative to the patient's creatinine clearance is ≥3.7 (≥222 if creatinine clearance is expressed in units of milliliters per second), the likelihood of nephrotoxicity is markedly increased.[38] Therefore, in general, the volume of contrast administered should not be greater than twice the baseline estimated creatinine clearance.[29]

Low-osmolar (600 to 800 mOsm/kg; 600 to 800 mmol/kg) nonionic (iohexol and iopamidol) and ionic (ioxaglate) contrast agents may be used to minimize the incidence of nephrotoxicity. Standard hyperosmolar contrast media (e.g., low- and high-osmolar agent) are not reabsorbed in the kidney and cause osmotic diuresis, which contributes to the renal toxicity observed with these agents. Low-osmolar contrast agents have less than half the osmolality of high-osmolar (~2,000 mOsm/kg; ~2,000 mmol/kg) agents and are associated with less toxicity, especially when used for patients with preexisting kidney disease.[39] However, use of low-osmolar agents does not preclude the development of nephrotoxicity. Even low-osmolar agents are hyperosmolar relative to plasma, which is likely the reason they are associated with greater nephrotoxicity than the iso-osmolar nonionic contrast agent iodixanol. Iodixanol has been shown to have the lowest risk for CIN for patients with CKD and diabetes.[29,39]

Clinical **Controversy...**

Some clinicians believe that low- or iso-osmolar contrast media should be used for virtually all patients at risk for toxicity. Others believe that the cost-to-benefit ratio of using low-osmolar contrast agents to prevent nephrotoxicity is questionable except for patients at high risk.

Volume expansion and correction of dehydration prior to contrast administration is a mainstay of preventive therapy.[36,40] Parenteral hydration with isotonic saline before and after contrast administration reduces the incidence of toxicity, particularly in high-risk patients, and is currently the most widely accepted preventative intervention.[40] Volume expansion may exert its beneficial effects through dilution of contrast media, prevention of renal vasoconstriction leading to ischemia, preservation of high urine flow rates, decreased tubular cell exposure to contrast, and avoidance of tubular obstruction. Hydration with isotonic sodium bicarbonate has been shown to provide more protection than saline, perhaps by reducing the formation of pH-dependent oxygen free radicals,[41] but recent studies reported contradictory findings.[36,42] Larger, adequately powered studies are needed to confirm these findings and to demonstrate conclusively that bicarbonate-based hydration is superior to saline. The use of oral hydration regimens has also been proposed but requires further study to clarify its role and is not currently recommended in lieu of parenteral hydration.[40]

N-acetylcysteine is a thiol-containing antioxidant that may effectively reduce the risk of developing CIN for patients with preexisting kidney disease. Despite the publication of dozens of

TABLE 31-3 Recommended Interventions for Prevention of Contrast Nephrotoxicity[29,35,40,41,43]

Intervention	Recommendation	Recommendation Grade[a]
Contrast	• Minimize contrast volume/dose • Use nonjodinated contrast studies • Use low- or iso-osmolar contrast agents	A-1 A-2 A-2
Medications	• Avoid concurrent use of potentially nephrotoxic drugs, for example, NSAIDs, aminoglycosides	A-2
Isotonic sodium chloride (0.9%)	• Initiate infusion 3–12 hours prior to contrast exposure and continue 6–24 hours postexposure • Infuse at 1–1.5 mL/kg/h adjusting postexposure as needed to maintain a urine flow rate of ≥150 mL/h • Alternatively, in urgent cases, initiate infusion at 3 mL/kg/h, beginning 1 hour prior to contrast exposure, then continue at 1 mL/kg/h for 6 hours postexposure	A-1
Isotonic sodium bicarbonate (154 mEq/L [154 mmol/L])	• Initiate and maintain infusion as per isotonic sodium chloride above • Alternatively, initiate infusion at 3 mL/kg/h, beginning 1 hour prior to contrast exposure, then continue at 1 mL/kg/h for 6 hours postexposure	B-2
N-acetylcysteine	• Administer 600–1,200 mg by mouth (PO) every 12 hours, 4 doses beginning prior to contrast exposure (i.e., 1 dose prior to exposure and 3 doses postexposure)	B-1

[a]*Strength of recommendations*: A, B, and C are good, moderate, and poor evidence to support recommendation, respectively. *Quality of evidence*: 1, evidence from more than 1 properly randomized, controlled trial; 2, evidence from more than 1 well-designed clinical trial with randomization, from cohort or case-controlled analytic studies or multiple time series, or dramatic results from uncontrolled experiments; 3, evidence from opinions of respected authorities, based on clinical experience, descriptive studies, or reports of expert communities.

clinical trials and meta-analyses, a therapeutic benefit of NAC has not been consistently demonstrated, and its therapeutic role remains controversial.[43] Nevertheless, its use should be considered, along with hydration, for all patients who are at high risk of toxicity.[35,37,43] The recommended *N*-acetylcysteine dosing regimen for prevention of CIN is to give four doses of 600 mg to 1,200 mg orally every 12 hours, with the first dose administered prior to contrast exposure (see Table 31-3).[29,35,41] Finally, other nephrotoxic drugs should be discontinued if possible, and subsequent contrast studies appropriately timed to minimize cumulative toxicity.

Clinical **Controversy. . .**

Some clinicians believe that insufficient evidence exists to justify use of *N*-acetylcysteine for the prevention of contrast-induced nephrotoxicity, while others feel that its safety profile, ease of use, low cost, and potential for benefit are adequate justification for use for all patients.

Renal replacement therapy, including intermittent hemodialysis and continuous modalities, for example, continuous venovenous hemofiltration (CVVH), effectively removes iodinated contrast, and was considered by some to be a therapeutic option for the prevention of CIN.[44] However, because of the logistical issues (e.g., technical difficulty), high cost of renal replacement therapy, and lack of consistent clinical efficacy data, currently this approach is not recommended.[44,45]

Management Currently there is no specific therapy available for managing established CIN. Care is supportive as described in Chapter 28. Kidney function (e.g., S_{cr} and urine output), electrolytes (e.g., sodium and potassium), and volume status should be closely monitored.

Cisplatin Nephrotoxicity

Incidence Cisplatin is one of the most important and widely used antineoplastic drugs for the treatment of solid tumors, often demonstrating exceptional efficacy (i.e., cure rates over 90% in testicular cancers).[46,47] Unfortunately, the primary dose-limiting toxicity of platin-containing compounds is nephrotoxicity. Cisplatin nephrotoxicity occurs in 20% to 30% of patients and is a significant cause of morbidity.[46,48] Carboplatin, a second-generation platinum analog, is associated with a lower incidence of nephrotoxicity than cisplatin and thus is the preferred agent in high-risk patients.[49]

Clinical Presentation Cisplatin administration results in impaired tubular reabsorption and decreased urinary concentration ability, leading to increased excretion of salt and water (i.e., polyuria) within 24 hours of treatment. Polyuria persists, and a decrease in GFR evidenced by a rise in S_{cr} concentration may be seen within 72 to 96 hours after cisplatin administration.[47,48] S_{cr} peaks approximately 10 to 14 days after initiation of therapy, with recovery by 21 days. As many as 25% of patients may have reversible elevations in S_{cr} and BUN for 2 weeks after cisplatin treatment. However, kidney damage is dose related and cumulative with subsequent cycles of therapy, so the S_{cr} concentration may continue to rise, and irreversible kidney injury may result.[48,49] Hypomagnesemia is a hallmark finding of cisplatin nephrotoxicity, due to impaired magnesium reabsorption and thus increased urinary losses.[47] Hypomagnesemia is often accompanied by hypocalcemia and hypokalemia and may be severe, leading to seizures, neuromuscular irritability, or personality changes. Urinalysis typically reveals leukocytes, renal tubular epithelial cells, and granular casts.[48]

Pathogenesis The pathogenesis of cisplatin nephrotoxicity is multifactorial in nature and likely begins with cellular uptake and accumulation of the drug in proximal tubular epithelial cells to concentrations that may reach five times the serum concentration.[46,48] Tubular cell exposure to cisplatin then activates a series of cell signaling pathways, including the mitogen-activated protein kinase (MAPK) pathway, p53, caspase, and the generation of reactive oxygen species, that collectively promote tubular cell injury and death via necrosis and/or apoptosis.[49] Simultaneous production of proinflammatory cytokines such as tumor necrosis factor-α (TNF-α) within tubular cells activates an inflammatory response, which may worsen the renal insult.[46] Although tubular damage is evident in both the proximal and distal segments, the majority occurs in the proximal tubules and is followed by a progressive loss of glomerular filtration capacity and impaired distal tubular function. Renal biopsies generally reveal necrosis of proximal and distal tubules and collecting ducts, with no obvious morphological changes to the glomeruli.[48]

Risk Factors Risk factors include increased age, dehydration, renal irradiation, concurrent use of nephrotoxic drugs, large cumulative doses, and alcohol abuse.[47,48]

Prevention The best renoprotective strategy is a combination of interventions, including prospective dose reduction and decreased frequency of administration, which usually requires using the platin compounds in combination with other chemotherapeutic agents, avoiding concurrent use of other nephrotoxic drugs, and ensuring patients are euvolemic or somewhat hypervolemic prior to initiating treatment.[46,50] Vigorous hydration with isotonic saline should be used for all patients with a goal of maintaining at least 100 to 150 mL/h of urine output during and after cisplatin treatment. Hydration should be initiated 12 to 24 hours prior to and continued for 2 to 3 days after cisplatin administration at rates of 100 to 250 mL/h, as tolerated, to maintain a urine flow of 3 to 4 L/day.[47]

Amifostine, an organic thiophosphate that is converted to an active metabolite, chelates cisplatin in normal cells and reduces the nephrotoxicity, neurotoxicity, ototoxicity, and myelosuppression associated with cisplatin and carboplatin therapy. It is also thought to serve as a thiol donor, thereby reducing intracellular reactive oxygen species and corresponding oxidative stress that plays a critical role in the development of cellular injury.[23,46] Pretreatment with amifostine should be considered for patients who are at high risk for kidney injury, particularly patients who are elderly, volume depleted, have CKD, or are receiving other nephrotoxic drugs concurrently. The current recommended dose of amifostine is 910 mg/m^2 administered IV over 15 minutes, beginning 30 minutes prior to cisplatin administration.[51] Common toxicities include acute hypotension, nausea, and fatigue.

Other renoprotective strategies include the use of hypertonic saline (e.g., administration of each dose in 250 mL of 3% saline) to reduce tubular cisplatin uptake. Classic antioxidants such as ascorbic acid, thiol-based antioxidants such as α-lipoic acid and *N*-acetylcysteine, which reduce oxidative damage by acting as a sulfhydryl donor, and the disulfiram metabolite diethyldithiocarbamate to reduce cytochrome P450 2E1-mediated generation of hydroxyl radicals have also been evaluated.[52] Finally, reduced renal exposure can be achieved with the use of localized intraperitoneal administration in conjunction with systemic administration of sodium thiosulfate for those with peritoneal tumors.[47]

Management AKI caused by cisplatin therapy is usually partially reversible with time and supportive care, including dialysis. Kidney function indices should be closely followed, with S_{cr} and BUN concentrations checked daily. Serum magnesium, potassium, and calcium concentrations should be monitored daily and corrected as needed.[48,49] Hypocalcemia and hypokalemia may be difficult to reverse until hypomagnesemia is corrected. Progressive kidney disease caused by cumulative nephrotoxicity may be irreversible and in some cases may lead to ESRD and require chronic dialysis support.

Amphotericin B Nephrotoxicity

Incidence Variable rates of amphotericin B nephrotoxicity have been reported that correspond in large part to the cumulative dose administered. Nephrotoxicity may be seen in nearly 30% of patients receiving median cumulative doses as low as 240 mg and reaches an incidence of >80% when cumulative doses approach 5 g.[53,54] Although numerous studies demonstrate lower rates of nephrotoxicity with liposomal formulations compared with conventional amphotericin B, it is difficult to compare rates of toxicity between products and studies because of the variability in the study populations, doses administered, and inconsistent definitions of nephrotoxicity and methods of assessment.[55,56]

Clinical Presentation Dose-dependent nephrotoxicity is often evident after administration of cumulative doses of 2 to 3 g as nonoliguria, renal tubular potassium, sodium, and magnesium wasting, impaired urinary concentrating ability, and distal renal tubular acidosis.[9] Although the cumulative dose is a significant risk factor, the time to onset of kidney injury varies considerably, ranging from a few days to weeks.[53] Tubular dysfunction usually manifests 1 to 2 weeks after treatment is begun, and potassium and magnesium replacement may be necessary. This is typically followed by a decrease in GFR and a rise in S_{cr} and BUN concentrations. Consequently, kidney function indices should be closely followed, with S_{cr} and BUN concentrations checked daily, and serum magnesium, potassium, and calcium concentrations monitored every other day and corrected as needed.

Pathogenesis Amphotericin B nephrotoxicity occurs predominantly via two mechanisms. The first is direct tubular epithelial cell toxicity resulting from interaction of amphotericin B with ergosterol in the cell membrane, leading to increased tubular cell membrane permeability, lipid peroxidation, and eventual necrosis of proximal tubular cells.[53] Tubular injury appears to be exacerbated by ischemic injury, which is a result of a reduction in renal blood flow and GFR due to afferent arteriolar vasoconstriction.[9,53]

Risk Factors Risk factors that impact the likelihood of developing amphotericin B nephrotoxicity include preexisting kidney disease, large individual and cumulative doses, short infusion times, volume depletion, hypokalemia, increased age, and concomitant administration of diuretics and other nephrotoxins (cyclosporine in particular).[9,53]

Prevention Permanent decrements in GFR are best prevented by incorporating a low threshold (i.e., if S_{cr} reaches 2 mg/dL [177 μmol/L] on 2 consecutive days) for stopping amphotericin B or switching to a liposomal formulation. Several lipid formulations of amphotericin B (e.g., amphotericin B lipid complex, liposomal amphotericin B) are available and should be used in most high-risk patients as they reduce nephrotoxicity by enhancing drug delivery to sites of infection and reducing interaction with tubular epithelial cell membranes.[53,56] Nephrotoxicity can also be minimized by limiting the cumulative dose, increasing the infusion time, ensuring the patient is well hydrated, and avoiding concomitant administration of other nephrotoxins.[9] Administration of 1 L IV 0.9% sodium chloride daily during the course of therapy appears to reduce toxicity and a single infusion of saline 10 to 15 mL/kg prior to administration of each dose of amphotericin B are generally recommended.[53] A number of other antifungal agents such as itraconazole, voriconazole, and caspofungin are viable alternatives and are now routinely used in lieu of amphotericin B for patients at high risk of developing nephrotoxicity.[9]

Clinical **Controversy...**

Although liposomal formulations of amphotericin B are dramatically more expensive than conventional amphotericin B (i.e., $300 to $1,000 per day vs. $5 per day),[66] many clinicians recommend using liposomal formulations for all patients with CKD and those at risk for developing nephrotoxicity. Others maintain that the safety and efficacy of liposomal formulations are not yet established enough to warrant their use for all patients.

Management Amphotericin B nephrotoxicity is best treated by discontinuation of therapy and substitution of alternative antifungal therapy, if possible. Renal tubular dysfunction and glomerular filtration will improve gradually to some degree in most patients, but damage may be irreversible. Kidney function indices should be closely followed, with S_{cr} and BUN concentrations checked daily, and serum magnesium, potassium, and calcium concentrations should be monitored daily and corrected as needed.[9]

Osmotic Nephrosis

It is now known that several drugs, including mannitol, low-molecular-weight dextran, hydroxyethyl starch, and radiographic contrast media, or drug vehicles, such as sucrose, maltose, and propylene glycol, are associated with osmotic nephrosis, which may rarely lead to ATN and AKI.[9,57,58] Since osmotic nephrosis does not necessarily negatively affect proximal tubular function, its presence may often go undetected in patients without overt signs of ATN. This likely contributes to the extremely low incidence of osmotic nephrosis reported for causative agents.[57] IV immunoglobulin solutions containing hyperosmolar sucrose may cause osmotic nephrosis and AKI in 1% to 10% of cases, which is usually reversible shortly after discontinuing therapy.[57] Maltose-based IV immunoglobulin solutions have also been implicated in the development of osmotic nephrosis.[59] Although IV immunoglobulin-induced nephropathy is the modern prototype for osmotic nephrosis, it is understood that the vehicle (i.e., sucrose or maltose) is the culprit and not the immunoglobulins themselves.

Clinical Presentation and Pathogenesis

The clinical presentation of osmotic nephrosis is often subtle. While tubular proteinuria or vacuolated tubular cells may be observed on urinalysis for patients with AKI, the definitive diagnosis of osmotic nephrosis is only made via a kidney biopsy.[57] IV immunoglobulin-induced AKI typically presents as oliguria after 2 to 4 days of treatment and may persist for up to 2 weeks.[9] Kidney injury occurs via uptake of the offending agent through pinocytosis into proximal tubular epithelial cells, subsequent formation of vacuoles, and accumulation of lysosomes, which collectively results in an oncotic gradient and thus cellular swelling, tubular luminal occlusion, and compromised cellular integrity.[57] Renal replacement therapy may be necessary for up to 40% of patients developing osmotic nephrosis-associated AKI.[57] However, it is usually reversible, with nearly all patients recovering normal kidney function following withdrawal of the offending drug.[9]

Risk Factors

Risk factors for osmotic nephrosis include excessive doses of offending agents, preexisting kidney disease, ischemia, older age (>65 years), and concomitant use of other nephrotoxins. Nephrotoxicity may be prevented by limiting the dose, reducing the rate of infusion, and avoiding dehydration and concomitant nephrotoxins.[57]

HEMODYNAMICALLY MEDIATED KIDNEY INJURY

4 Hemodynamically mediated kidney injury generally refers to any cause of AKI resulting from an acute decrease in intraglomerular pressure, including "prerenal" states leading to reduced effective renal blood flow (e.g., hypovolemia, congestive heart failure) and medications that affect the renin–angiotensin system.[9,18] The kidneys receive approximately 25% of resting cardiac output, which renders them particularly susceptible to alterations in renal blood flow and enhances their exposure to circulating drugs.[15] Within each nephron, blood flow and pressure are regulated by glomerular afferent and efferent arterioles to maintain intraglomerular capillary hydrostatic pressure, glomerular filtration, and urine output. Afferent and efferent arteriolar vasoconstrictions are primarily mediated by angiotensin II, whereas afferent vasodilation is primarily mediated by prostaglandins (Fig. 31-1).[60] This specialized blood flow is precisely regulated by interrelations between arachidonic acid metabolites, natriuretic factors, nitric oxide, the sympathetic nervous system, the renin–angiotensin system, and the macula densa response to distal tubular solute delivery.[60,61] Drug-induced causes of hemodynamic kidney injury typically stem from constriction of glomerular afferent arterioles and/or dilation of glomerular efferent arterioles. ACEIs, angiotensin II receptor blockers (ARBs), and NSAIDs are the agents that have been most commonly implicated.[9]

Angiotensin-Converting Enzyme Inhibitors and Angiotensin II Receptor Blockers

These agents are extensively utilized for the management of hypertension and prevention of the progression of CKD even though they have been associated with the development of AKI.

Incidence

Patients with renal artery stenosis, volume depletion, and congestive heart failure and those with preexisting kidney disease, including diabetic nephropathy, are most likely to experience a significant decline in kidney function when therapy with one of these agents is initiated.[62] For example, between 20% and 25% of hospitalized patients with congestive heart failure develop AKI within weeks after treatment with ACEIs is initiated.[63,64] The incidence of ACEI-induced AKI may be as high as 23% for patients with bilateral renal artery stenosis and up to 38% for patients with unilateral renal artery stenosis.[8] Moreover, ACEIs and ARBs are among the most commonly implicated medications in emergency hospitalizations, contributing to nearly 3% of emergency room visits for adverse drug events.[65]

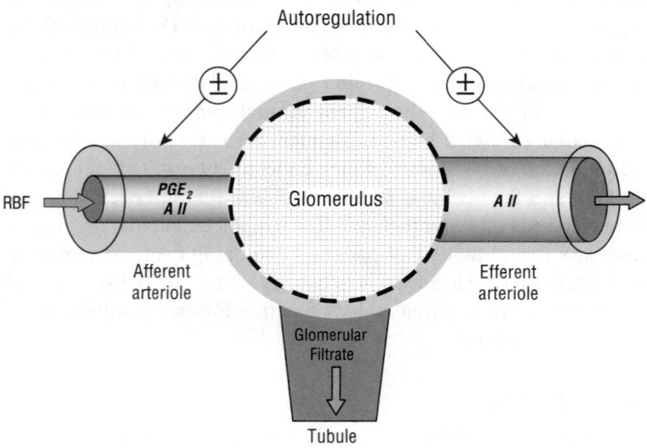

FIGURE 31-1 Normal glomerular autoregulation serves to maintain intraglomerular capillary hydrostatic pressure, glomerular filtration rate (GFR), and, ultimately, urine output. (A II, angiotensin II; PGE_2, prostaglandin E_2; RBF, renal blood flow.)

Clinical Presentation

Therapy with ACEIs and ARBs will acutely reduce GFR; so a moderate rise in S_{cr} after initiation of therapy should be anticipated.[62] Importantly, a distinction must be made between a potentially detrimental reduction in GFR and a normal, predictable rise in S_{cr}. An increase in S_{cr} of up to 30% is commonly observed within 3 to 5 days of initiating therapy and is an indication that the drug has begun to exert its desired pharmacologic effect.[9,62] The increase in S_{cr} typically stabilizes within 1 to 2 weeks and is usually reversible upon stopping the drug. Furthermore, an association exists between acute increases in S_{cr} of ≤30% from baseline that stabilize within the first 2 months of initiating therapy and preservation of kidney function. The S_{cr} threshold for discontinuation of ACEI or ARB therapy is unclear.[62] However, an increase in S_{cr} of more than 30% above baseline in the course of 1 to 2 weeks may necessitate discontinuation of the offending drug.

Pathogenesis

ACEI- or ARB-mediated kidney injury is primarily the result of disruption of normal autoregulation of intraglomerular capillary hydrostatic pressure.[9] Normally, the kidney attempts to maintain GFR by dilating the afferent arteriole and constricting the efferent arteriole in response to a decrease in renal blood flow. During states of reduced blood flow, the juxtaglomerular apparatus increases renin secretion. Plasma renin converts angiotensinogen to angiotensin I, and ultimately angiotensin II by angiotensin-converting enzyme. Angiotensin II constricts the afferent and efferent arterioles, but has a greater effect on the efferent arterioles, resulting in a net increase in intraglomerular pressure.[62] Additionally, renal prostaglandins, prostaglandin E_2 in particular, are released and induce a net dilation of the afferent arteriole, thereby improving blood flow into the glomerulus. Together these processes maintain GFR and urine output (Fig. 31-2).[18,60,61]

When ACEI therapy (e.g., enalapril or ramipril) is initiated, the synthesis of angiotensin II is decreased, thereby preferentially dilating the efferent arteriole. This reduces outflow resistance from the glomerulus and decreases hydrostatic pressure in the glomerular capillaries, which alters Starling forces across the glomerular capillaries to decrease intraglomerular pressure and GFR. This in turn often leads to nephrotoxicity, particularly in the setting of reduced renal blood flow or effective arterial blood volume (Fig. 31-3), that is, prerenal settings (e.g., congestive heart failure) in which glomerular afferent arteriolar blood flow is reduced and the efferent arteriole is vasoconstricted to maintain sufficient glomerular capillary hydrostatic pressure for ultrafiltration.[63,64]

Risk Factors

Patients at greatest risk are those dependent on angiotensin II and renal efferent arteriolar constriction to maintain blood pressure and GFR.[62] These include patients with bilateral renal artery stenosis or stenosis in a single kidney (i.e., renal transplant); patients with decreased effective arterial blood volume (i.e., prerenal states), especially those with decompensated congestive heart failure, volume depletion from excess diuresis or GI fluid loss, hepatic cirrhosis with ascites, and nephrotic syndrome; patients with preexisting kidney disease; and patients receiving concurrent nephrotoxic drugs, particularly other drugs that affect intraglomerular autoregulation such as NSAIDs.[9,62,66]

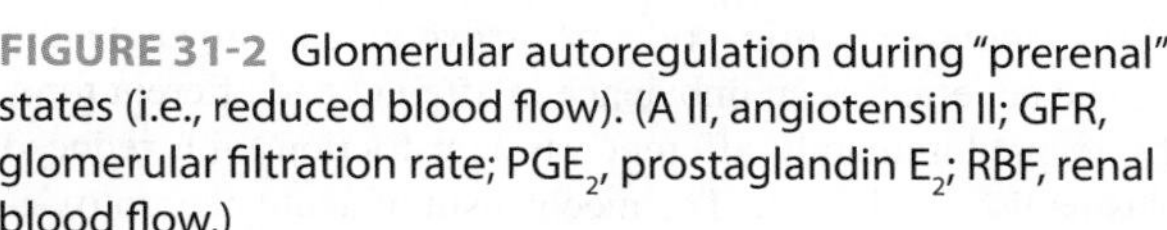

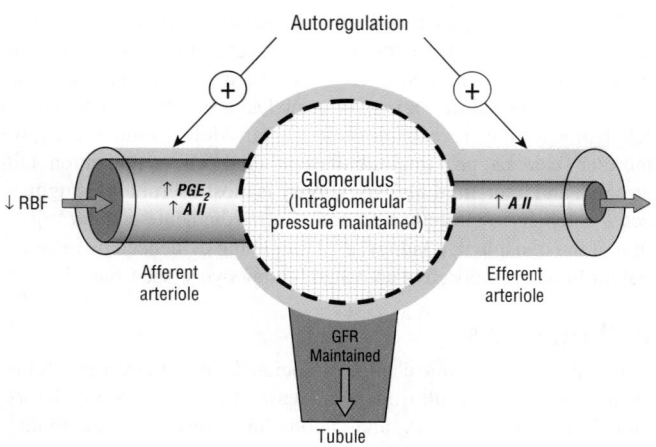

FIGURE 31-2 Glomerular autoregulation during "prerenal" states (i.e., reduced blood flow). (A II, angiotensin II; GFR, glomerular filtration rate; PGE_2, prostaglandin E_2; RBF, renal blood flow.)

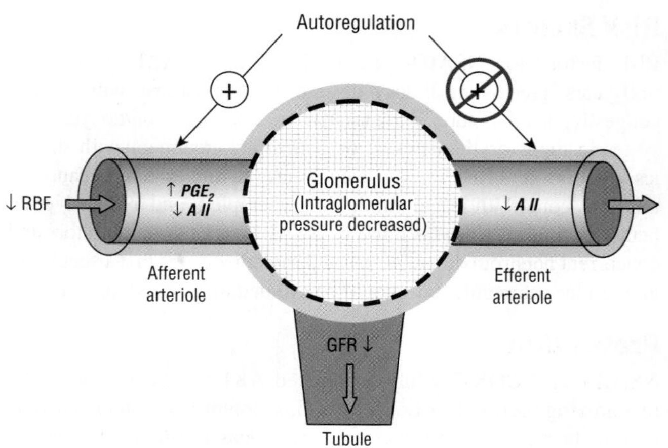

FIGURE 31-3 Pathogenesis of angiotensin-converting enzyme inhibitor (ACEI) nephropathy. (A II, angiotensin II; GFR, glomerular filtration rate; PGE_2, prostaglandin E_2; RBF, renal blood flow.)

Prevention

Hemodynamically mediated AKI caused by ACEIs or ARBs is frequently preventable by recognizing the presence of preexisting kidney disease or decreased effective renal blood flow as a result of volume depletion, heart failure, or liver disease. A common strategy for at-risk patients is to initiate therapy with very low doses of a short-acting ACEI (e.g., captopril 6.25 mg to 12.5 mg), then gradually titrate the dose upward and convert to a longer-acting agent after patient tolerance has been demonstrated. Outpatients may be started on low doses of long-acting ACEIs (e.g., enalapril 2.5 mg) with gradual dose titration every 2 to 4 weeks until the maximum dose or desired response is achieved. Kidney function indices and serum potassium concentrations must be monitored carefully, daily for hospitalized patients and every 2 to 3 days for outpatients. Monitoring may need to be more frequent during outpatient initiation of ACEI or ARB therapy for patients with preexisting kidney disease, congestive heart failure, or suspected renovascular disease. Use of concurrent hypotensive agents and other drugs that affect renal hemodynamics (e.g., NSAIDs, diuretics) should be discouraged and dehydration avoided.

Management

Acute decreases in kidney function and the development of hyperkalemia usually resolve over several days after ACEI or ARB therapy is discontinued. Occasionally patients will require management of severe hyperkalemia, as described in detail in Chapter 36.

ACEI or ARB therapy may frequently be reinitiated, particularly for patients with congestive heart failure, after intravascular volume depletion has been corrected or diuretic doses reduced. Slight reductions in kidney function (maintenance of a S_{cr} concentration of 2 to 3 mg/dL [177 to 265 μmol/L]) may be an acceptable trade-off for hemodynamic improvement in certain patients with severe congestive heart failure or renovascular disease not amenable to revascularization.

Nonsteroidal Antiinflammatory Drugs and Selective Cyclooxygenase-2 Inhibitors

The overall safety of NSAIDs is evidenced by the nonprescription availability in the United States of several drugs in the class (e.g., ibuprofen, naproxen, ketoprofen). Although potential adverse renal effects from nonprescription NSAIDs had been a concern, conventional nonselective NSAIDs and selective cyclooxygenase-2 (COX-2) inhibitors are unlikely to acutely affect kidney function in the absence of renal ischemia or excess renal vasoconstrictor activity.[9,67,68] Nevertheless, given their general safety and widespread availability, NSAIDs are among the most commonly used drugs. More than 30 million people take NSAIDs daily worldwide.[69]

Incidence

Although the incidence of NSAID-induced AKI is unclear, historical reports suggest that 500,000 to 2.5 million people develop some degree of NSAID nephrotoxicity in the United States annually.[70]

Clinical Presentation

NSAID- and COX-2-induced AKI can occur within days of initiating therapy, particularly with a short-acting agent such as ibuprofen, or within days of some other precipitating event (e.g., intravascular volume depletion). Patients typically present with complaints of diminished urine output, weight gain, and/or edema. Urine sodium concentrations (<20 mEq/L [<20 mmol/L]) and fractional excretion of sodium (<1% [0.01]) are usually low, and BUN, S_{cr}, potassium, and blood pressure are typically elevated.[17,69] The urine sediment is usually bland and unchanged from baseline but may show occasional granular casts.

Pathogenesis

The pathogenesis of NSAID- and COX-2-induced AKI lies in the disruption of normal intraglomerular autoregulation.[9,67,69] Specifically, NSAIDs inhibit cyclooxygenase (COX)-catalyzed synthesis of vasodilatory prostaglandins, including prostaglandins I_2 (prostacyclin) and E_2, from arachidonic acid.[67] These prostaglandins are synthesized in the renal cortex and medulla by vascular endothelial and glomerular mesangial cells, and their effects are primarily local and result in net afferent arteriolar vasodilation. Vasodilatory prostaglandins have limited activity in states of normal renal blood flow, but in states of decreased renal blood flow, their synthesis is increased and they serve a vital autoregulatory role in the protection against renal ischemia and hypoxia by antagonizing renal arteriolar vasoconstriction due to angiotensin II, norepinephrine, endothelin, and vasopressin.[67] Thus, administration of NSAIDs in the setting of reduced renal blood flow will blunt the usual compensatory increase in prostaglandin activity, altering the normal autoregulatory balance in favor of renal vasoconstrictors, thereby promoting renal ischemia and a reduction in glomerular filtration.[69]

Risk Factors

Risk factors for NSAID- and COX-2-induced AKI include age >60 years, preexisting kidney disease, hepatic disease with ascites, congestive heart failure, intravascular volume depletion/dehydration, systemic lupus erythematosus, or concurrent treatment with diuretics, ACEIs, or ARBs.[9,66] The elderly are at higher risk because of multiple comorbidities, multiple-drug therapies, and reduced renal hemodynamics.[68] Combined use of NSAIDs or COX-2 inhibitors and concurrent nephrotoxic drugs, particularly other drugs that affect intraglomerular autoregulation, should be avoided in high-risk patients.[9]

Prevention

NSAID- and COX-2 inhibitor-induced AKI can be prevented by recognizing high-risk patients, avoiding potent compounds such as indomethacin and using analgesics with less prostaglandin inhibition, such as acetaminophen, nonacetylated salicylates, aspirin, and possibly nabumetone.[9] Nonnarcotic analgesics (e.g., tramadol) may also be useful but do not provide antiinflammatory activity. When NSAID therapy is essential for high-risk patients, the minimal effective dose should be used for the shortest duration possible, and NSAIDs with short half-lives should be considered (e.g., sulindac) along with optimal management of predisposing medical problems and frequent kidney function monitoring.[9] Moreover, use of concurrent hypotensive agents and other drugs that affect renal hemodynamics (e.g., ACEIs, ARBs, diuretics) should be discouraged in high-risk patients and dehydration avoided.

Traditional, nonselective NSAIDs inhibit COX-1 and COX-2, whereas the selective drugs meloxicam, celecoxib, and valdecoxib preferentially inhibit COX-2. COX-2 inhibitors were anticipated to be beneficial in high-risk patients. However, recent data indicate that they affect kidney function similarly to nonselective NSAIDs, and thus caution is warranted with their use, particularly in high-risk patients.[9,68]

Management

NSAID-induced AKI is treated by discontinuation of therapy and supportive care. Kidney injury is rarely severe, and recovery is usually rapid. Occasionally, the hemodynamic insult is sufficiently severe to cause ATN, which can prolong injury.

Cyclosporine and Tacrolimus

The calcineurin inhibitors cyclosporine and tacrolimus have dramatically enhanced the success of solid-organ transplantation. As many as 94% of kidney transplant patients are prescribed a calcineurin inhibitor-based immunosuppressive regimen.[71] Nephrotoxicity, however, remains a major dose-limiting adverse effect of both drugs. Although delayed chronic interstitial nephritis has also been reported, acute hemodynamically mediated kidney injury is an important mechanism of calcineurin inhibitor-induced nephrotoxicity.

Incidence

Historically, reversible AKI occurred frequently in transplant recipients during the first 6 months of cyclosporine therapy. The 5-year risk of CKD after transplantation of a nonrenal organ ranges from 7% to 21%, depending on the type of organ transplanted, and the occurrence of CKD in these patients is associated with more than a fourfold increase in the risk of death.[72]

Clinical Presentation

The clinical presentation of acute nephrotoxicity associated with calcineurin inhibitors (i.e., hemodynamically mediated AKI) is quite different from the presentation of chronic nephrotoxicity (see Chronic Interstitial Nephritis below). AKI may occur within days of initiating therapy, manifesting as a rise in S_{cr} concentration and a corresponding decline in creatinine clearance.[9] Hypertension, hyperkalemia, sodium retention, oliguria, renal tubular acidosis, and hypomagnesemia are frequently observed in the absence of urine sediment abnormalities or morphologic lesions.[71] On the other hand, renal biopsy may reveal thickening of arterioles, mild focal glomerular sclerosis, proximal tubular epithelial cell vacuolization and atrophy, and interstitial fibrosis. Biopsy is most useful to distinguish acute calcineurin inhibitor nephrotoxicity from acute cellular rejection of the transplanted kidney, the latter being evidenced by interstitial infiltrates composed of activated lymphocytes (see Chap. 70).[73,74]

Pathogenesis

The acute hemodynamic changes associated with calcineurin inhibitor nephrotoxicity result from an increase in potent vasoconstrictors including thromboxane A_2 and endothelin, activation of the renin–angiotensin and sympathetic nervous systems, as well as a reduction in the vasodilators nitric oxide, prostacyclin, and prostaglandin E_2.[71,73,74] The net effect is an imbalance in afferent and efferent tone, resulting in predominantly afferent vasoconstriction with reduced renal plasma flow and GFR.[9] The mechanism of acute nephrotoxicity is generally thought to be dose related, since kidney function improves rapidly following dose reduction.[9]

Risk Factors

Risk factors include age over 65, higher dose, concomitant therapy with nephrotoxic drugs (particularly NSAIDs), and interacting drugs that inhibit calcineurin inhibitor metabolism and transport and thus increase systemic exposure, older kidney allograft age, salt depletion, diuretic use, and polymorphic expression of P-glycoprotein.[71,73] The incidence of AKI with potential progression to chronic nephropathy has decreased since the introduction of lower-dose-therapy regimens. Unfortunately, there has been no apparent reduction in the incidence of the slow, dose-dependent decline in glomerular filtration.[74]

Prevention

Because acute hemodynamically mediated kidney injury secondary to cyclosporine and tacrolimus appears to be concentration related, pharmacokinetic and pharmacodynamic monitoring is an important means of preventing toxicity.[71] However, the persistent presence of therapeutic or low cyclosporine concentrations does not totally preclude the development of nephrotoxicity. Calcium channel blockers may antagonize the vasoconstrictor effect of cyclosporine by dilating glomerular afferent arterioles and preventing acute decreases in renal blood flow and glomerular filtration.[71] Lastly, decreased doses of cyclosporine or tacrolimus, primarily when used in combination with other nonnephrotoxic immunosuppressants, may minimize the risk of toxicity, but this may increase the risk of chronic rejection.[74]

Management

AKI usually improves with dose reduction and treatment of contributing illness or the discontinuation of interacting drugs. CKD is usually irreversible, but progressive toxicity may be limited by discontinuation of cyclosporine (or tacrolimus) therapy or dose reduction, with the continuation of other immunosuppressants.[71,74] S_{cr} and BUN should be closely monitored (daily if possible), as should cyclosporine or tacrolimus concentrations, to ensure that serum concentrations are within the narrow therapeutic range.

INTRATUBULAR OBSTRUCTION

The precipitation of drug crystals in distal tubular lumens can lead to intratubular obstruction, interstitial nephritis, and occasionally superimposed ATN. Nephrolithiasis, the formation of stones within the kidney, results from abnormal crystal precipitation in the renal collecting system, potentially causing urinary tract obstruction with kidney injury. Numerous medications have been associated with development of crystal nephropathy.

Incidence

The incidence is unclear for most of the implicated agents.

Pathogenesis

Drugs may induce intratubular obstruction and AKI by direct (precipitation of the drug itself) and indirect means (i.e., promoting release and precipitation of tissue-degradation products or cellular casts). For example, antineoplastic drugs may cause acute renal tubular obstruction indirectly by inducing tumor lysis syndrome, hyperuricemia, and intratubular precipitation of uric acid crystals.[75] The diagnosis is supported by a urine uric acid-to-creatinine ratio greater than 1. Uric acid precipitation can be prevented by vigorous hydration with normal saline, beginning at least 48 hours prior to chemotherapy, to maintain urine output 100 mL/h in adults. Administration of allopurinol 100 mg/m^2 thrice daily (maximum of 800 mg/day) started 2 to 3 days prior to chemotherapy, and urinary alkalinization to pH 7 may also be of value.[76]

Drug-induced rhabdomyolysis is another form of indirect toxicity, which can lead to intratubular precipitation of myoglobin and, if severe, AKI.[77] The most common cause of drug-induced rhabdomyolysis is direct myotoxicity from 3-hydroxy-3-methylglutaryl-coenzyme A (HMG-CoA) reductase inhibitors or statins, including lovastatin and simvastatin. The risk of rhabdomyolysis is increased when these drugs are administered concurrently with gemfibrozil, niacin, or inhibitors of the CYP3A4 metabolic pathway (e.g., erythromycin and itraconazole).[78]

A newly recognized complication of warfarin therapy has been called warfarin-related nephropathy (WRN), which is characterized by glomerular hemorrhage with subsequent intratubular obstruction by red blood cell casts.[79] Patients with underlying CKD appear to be at greatest risk. The incidence of WRN may be as high as 33% in CKD versus 16.5% in non-CKD patients.[80] Other risk factors included age, diabetes mellitus, hypertension, and cardiovascular disease. WRN is also associated with an increased mortality rate. In a recent study, the 1-year mortality rate was 31.1% in patients with presumed WRN versus 18.9% in control subjects, an increased risk of 65%.[80]

Intratubular precipitation of drugs or their metabolites can also directly cause AKI. Precipitation of drug crystals is due primarily to supersaturation of a low urine volume with the offending drug or relative insolubility of the drug in either alkaline or acidic urine.[81,82] Volume depletion is an important risk factor for the development of AKI. Urine pH decreases to approximately 4.5 during maximal stimulation of renal tubular hydrogen ion secretion. Certain solutes can precipitate and obstruct the tubular lumen at this acid pH, particularly when urine is concentrated, such as for patients with volume depletion. For example, several antiviral drugs have been associated with intratubular precipitation and AKI.[81–84] Acyclovir is relatively insoluble at physiologic urine pH and is associated with intratubular precipitation in dehydrated oliguric patients.[81,82] Foscarnet complexation with ionized calcium may result in precipitation of calcium-foscarnet salt crystals in renal glomeruli, causing primarily a crystalline glomerulonephritis. The salt crystals may then secondarily precipitate in the renal tubules causing tubular necrosis. The protease inhibitor indinavir has been associated with crystalluria, crystal nephropathy, dysuria, urinary frequency, back and flank pain, or nephrolithiasis in approximately 8% of treated patients.[82,85] Intratubular indinavir crystal precipitation can be prevented in nearly 75% of treated patients if one assures that the patient consumes at least 2 to 3 L of fluid per day.[82] Sulfadiazine, when used at high doses, and methotrexate may also precipitate in acidic urine and can cause oligoanuric kidney injury.[81,82] Massive administration of ascorbic acid can also result in obstruction of renal tubules with calcium oxalate crystals, leading to "oxalate nephropathy".[81] Triamterene and the quinolone antibiotic ciprofloxacin may also precipitate in renal tubules and cause kidney injury.[82]

Kidney injury caused by intratubular precipitation of most tissue-degradation products or drugs and their metabolites can be largely prevented and possibly treated by administering the drug after vigorously prehydrating the patient, maintaining a high urine volume, and urinary alkalinization.[82]

NEPHROCALCINOSIS

Nephrocalcinosis is a clinical pathologic condition characterized by extensive tubulointerstitial precipitation and deposition of calcium phosphate crystals leading to marked tubular calcification.[81,86,87] It is most commonly seen in clinical conditions associated with hypercalcemia and hypercalciuria, such as hyperparathyroidism, malignancy, and less frequently increased intake of calcium or vitamin D. However, nephrocalcinosis can also result from hyperphosphatemia and hyperphosphaturia in the absence of hypercalcemia, as is known to occur for patients who have received oral sodium phosphate solution (OSPS) as a bowel preparation.[81,86,87]

Acute Phosphate Nephropathy

The term acute phosphate nephropathy was coined specifically to describe OSPS-induced nephrocalcinosis, as its pathogenesis is the result of increased phosphate intake rather than hypercalcemia.[87] During the last decade, several cases of nephrocalcinosis have been reported after use of OSPS for bowel preparation prior to GI procedures, and strong associations have recently been demonstrated between exposure to OSPS and a decline in kidney function, particularly in the elderly and those with preexisting kidney disease.[81,87–89]

Incidence The incidence of acute phosphate nephropathy is between 1 in 1,000 and 1 in 5,000 exposures, translating to roughly 1,400 to 7,000 new cases annually.[90]

Clinical Presentation Patients usually present with AKI several days to months after exposure to OSPS. Low-grade proteinuria (<1 g/day), normocalcemia, and bland urinary sediment are usually observed. Extensive deposition of calcium phosphate in the distal tubules and collecting ducts without glomerular or vascular injury is the hallmark of acute phosphate nephropathy.[81]

Risk Factors Risk factors include advanced age, preexisting kidney disease, female sex, hypertension, diabetes, bowel conditions associated with prolonged intestinal transit, high sodium phosphate dosage, volume depletion, and medications that affect renal perfusion or function (e.g., diuretics, lithium, NSAIDs, ACEIs, or ARBs).[87]

NEPHROLITHIASIS

Nephrolithiasis (formation of renal calculi or kidney stones) does not present as classic nephrotoxicity since GFR is usually not decreased. Drug-induced nephrolithiasis can be the result of abnormal crystal precipitation in the renal collecting system, potentially causing pain, hematuria, infection, or, occasionally, urinary tract obstruction with kidney injury. The overall prevalence of drug-induced nephrolithiasis is estimated to be 1%.[91]

Kidney stone formation, possibly also accompanied by intratubular precipitation of crystalline material, has been a rare complication of drug therapy. Until the acquired immune deficiency syndrome (AIDS) era, triamterene had been the drug most frequently associated with kidney stone formation, with a prevalence of 0.4%.[91] Sulfadiazine is a poorly soluble sulfonamide that has caused symptomatic acetylsulfadiazine crystalluria with stone formation and flank or back pain, hematuria, or kidney injury in up to 29% of patients treated with the drug.[81,82] A high urine volume and urinary alkalinization to pH >7.15 may be protective. Numerous other drugs have been implicated in the development of nephrolithiasis, including the antiviral drugs nelfinavir and foscarnet, the antibacterial agents ciprofloxacin, amoxicillin, and nitrofurantoin, and various products containing ephedrine, norephedrine, pseudoephedrine, and melamine.[92,93]

GLOMERULAR DISEASE

Proteinuria, particularly nephrotic range proteinuria (defined as urine protein excretion greater than 3.5 g/day per 1.73 m^2) with or without a decline in the GFR is a hallmark sign of glomerular injury (see Chap. 32).[94] Several different glomerular lesions may occur, including minimal change disease, focal segmental glomerulosclerosis (FSGS), and membranous nephropathy, mostly by immune mechanisms rather than direct cellular toxicity. Although drug-induced glomerular disease is uncommon, a variety of agents have been implicated.[95]

Minimal Change Glomerular Disease

Drug-induced minimal change glomerular disease is frequently accompanied by interstitial nephritis and is most common during NSAID therapy.[94] Lithium, quinolone antibiotics, and interferon-α have also been implicated.[19,95] Patients present abruptly with nephrotic range proteinuria, hypoalbuminemia, and hyperlipidemia and rarely with hematuria and hypertension.[19,94] The pathogenesis is unknown, but nephrotic range proteinuria as a consequence of NSAID therapy is frequently associated with a T-lymphocytic interstitial infiltrate, suggesting disordered cell-mediated immunity. Proteinuria usually resolves rapidly after discontinuation of the offending drug, and a 3- to 4-week course of corticosteroids may help resolve the lesion. More than 90% of adults achieve complete remission over the course of several months.[94]

Focal Segmental Glomerulosclerosis

FSGS is characterized by patchy areas (i.e., only some glomeruli are partially affected by the disease) of glomerular sclerosis with interstitial inflammation and fibrosis (see Chap. 32). FSGS is becoming the most common cause of nephrotic syndrome in African Americans and whites in the United States.[94] It represents a pattern of glomerular injury, not a disease per se, and is the final common pathway by which normal glomerular components are replaced by fibrous scar tissue. FSGS has been described in the setting of chronic heroin abuse (known as *heroin nephropathy*).[96] The pathogenesis is unknown but may include direct toxicity by heroin or adulterants and injury from bacterial or viral infections accompanying IV drug use. The bisphosphonates pamidronate and zoledronate, commonly used to treat osteoporosis, malignancy-associated hypercalcemia, and Paget's disease, are associated with the development of a particularly aggressive variant of FSGS called *collapsing glomerulopathy*.[97] It presents with massive proteinuria (>8 g/day), and it is typically characterized by rising S_{cr} at diagnosis and rapid progression to ESRD.[94] Patients receiving IV formulations, high doses, or prolonged therapy are at highest risk.[97]

Membranous Nephropathy

Membranous nephropathy is characterized by subepithelial immune complex formation along glomerular capillary loops and, although rarely seen, has classically been associated with gold therapy, penicillamine, captopril, and NSAID use.[19,95] Patients present with nephrotic range proteinuria and microscopic hematuria, with hypertension and elevated S_{cr} apparent for patients with more advanced disease.[94] The pathogenesis may involve damage to proximal tubule epithelium with antigen release, antibody formation, and glomerular immune complex deposition. Proteinuria usually resolves slowly after discontinuing the offending drug. Patients who remain nephrotic after 6 months should be treated with a 6- to 12-month course of immunosuppressive therapy, which typically consists of prednisone and cyclophosphamide.[94]

TUBULOINTERSTITIAL NEPHRITIS

Tubulointerstitial nephritis refers to diseases in which the predominant changes occur in the renal interstitium rather than the tubules. The presentation may be acute and reversible with interstitial edema, rapid loss of kidney function, and systemic symptoms or chronic and irreversible, associated with interstitial fibrosis and minimal to no systemic symptoms.[19,98]

Acute Allergic Interstitial Nephritis

Incidence

5 The incidence of drug-induced acute allergic interstitial nephritis (AIN) is unclear and likely varies with clinical setting. For example, the incidence has been estimated to be 0.7 cases per 100,000 young outpatient men but from 10% to 27% of kidney biopsies performed in hospitalized patients with unexplained AKI demonstrate AIN.[98,99] Multiple drugs have been implicated in the development of AIN (Table 31-4). It usually manifests 2 weeks after exposure to a drug but may occur sooner if the patient was previously sensitized.[98]

Clinical Presentation

Although methicillin-induced AIN is the prototype for AIN, it is now recognized that AIN is associated with all β-lactam antibiotics (including cephalosporins) and numerous other antimicrobials. Clinical signs present approximately 14 days after initiation of therapy and include (with their approximate incidence) fever (27% to 80%), maculopapular rash (15% to 25%), eosinophilia (23% to 80%), arthralgia (45%), and oliguria (50%).[98] Systemic hypersensitivity findings of the classic triad of fever, rash, and arthralgia, often along with eosinophilia and eosinophiluria, strongly suggest the diagnosis of AIN. However, this constellation of findings is not consistently reliable as one or more are frequently absent; so caution is warranted in basing diagnosis on hypersensitivity findings alone.[98] Eosinophiluria, an important marker of drug-induced AIN, is frequently absent, possibly because of fragility of eosinophils in urine and inadequate laboratory methodology. Anemia, leukocytosis, and elevated immunoglobulin E levels may occur. Tubular dysfunction may be manifested by acidosis, hyperkalemia, salt wasting, and concentrating defects.[98]

NSAID-induced AIN has a different clinical presentation than that seen with most other drugs.[98] Patients are typically over 50 years of age (reflecting NSAID use for degenerative joint disease), the onset is delayed a mean of 6 months from initiation of therapy compared with 2 weeks with β-lactams, and fever, rash, and eosinophilia are typically not observed in patients with NSAID-induced AIN.[98] Concomitant nephrotic syndrome (proteinuria >3.5 g/day) occurs in more than 70% of patients. Prompt diagnosis of

TABLE 31-4 Drugs Associated with Allergic Interstitial Nephritis

Antimicrobials	
Acyclovir	Indinavir
Aminoglycosides	Rifampin
Amphotericin B	Sulfonamides
β-Lactams	Tetracyclines
Erythromycin	Trimethoprim–sulfamethoxazole
Ethambutol	Vancomycin
Diuretics	
Acetazolamide	Loop diuretics
Amiloride	Triamterene
Chlorthalidone	Thiazide diuretics
Neuropsychiatric	
Carbamazepine	Phenytoin
Lithium	Valproic acid
Phenobarbital	
Nonsteroidal antiinflammatory drugs	
Aspirin	Ketoprofen
Indomethacin	Phenylbutazone
Naproxen	Diclofenac
Ibuprofen	Zomepirac
Diflunisal	Cyclooxygenase-2 inhibitors
Piroxicam	
Miscellaneous	
Acetaminophen	Lansoprazole
Allopurinol	Methyldopa
Interferon-α	Omeprazole
Aspirin	*P*-aminosalicylic acid
Azathioprine	Phenylpropanolamine
Captopril	Propylthiouracil
Cimetidine	Radiographic contrast media
Clofibrate	Ranitidine
Cyclosporine	Sulfinpyrazone
Glyburide	Warfarin sodium
Gold	

AIN is important as discontinuation of the offending drug may prevent irreversible renal damage. Renal biopsy is the most definitive method for diagnosis.

Pathogenesis

The pathogenesis of the majority of cases of AIN is considered to be an allergic hypersensitivity response. This is supported by the fact that AIN is characterized as a diffuse or focal interstitial infiltrate of lymphocytes, eosinophils, and occasional polymorphonuclear neutrophils.[98] Granulomas and tubular epithelial cell necrosis are relatively common with drug-induced AIN. Occasionally a humoral antibody-mediated mechanism is implicated by the presence of circulating antibody to a drug hapten–tubular basement membrane complex, low serum complement levels, and deposition of immunoglobulin G and complement in the tubular basement membrane. More commonly, a cell-mediated immune mechanism is suggested by the absence of these findings and the presence of a predominantly T-lymphocyte.[98]

Risk Factors

No specific risk factors have been identified because these are idiosyncratic hypersensitivity reactions. Individuals with other drug allergies may have increased risk and warrant close monitoring.

Prevention

No specific preventive measures are known because of the idiosyncratic nature of these reactions. Patients must be monitored carefully to recognize the signs and symptoms because promptly discontinuing the offending drug often leads to full recovery.[98]

Management

Corticosteroid therapy is beneficial and should be initiated immediately or soon after diagnosis of AIN along with discontinuance of the offending drug to avoid the risk of incomplete recovery of kidney function. While various regimens have been used, high-dose oral prednisone 1 mg/kg/day for 8 to 14 weeks with a stepwise taper has been used successfully.[99,100] Typical kidney function indices (e.g., S_{cr}, BUN) and signs and symptoms of AIN should be monitored closely for improvement.

Chronic Interstitial Nephritis

Lithium, analgesics, calcineurin inhibitors, aristolochic acid, and only a few other drugs have been reported to cause chronic interstitial nephritis, which is usually a progressive and irreversible lesion.

Lithium

Incidence The prevalence of non-dialysis-dependent CKD stemming from chronic lithium nephrotoxicity in the general population of patients treated with lithium was recently estimated to be 1.2%.[101,102] The prevalence of lithium-induced ESRD among all ESRD patients is between 0.2% and 0.8%.[101] Several renal tubular lesions are associated with lithium therapy: an impaired ability to concentrate urine (nephrogenic diabetes insipidus) is seen in up to 87% of patients with biopsy proven nephrotoxicity, and incomplete distal renal tubular acidosis is observed in up to 50% of these patients.[103]

Clinical Presentation Lithium-induced nephrotoxicity is typically asymptomatic and develops insidiously during years of therapy. Blood pressure is normal and urinary sediment is bland, making detection difficult until the disease progresses significantly.[104] It is usually recognized by rising BUN or S_{cr} concentrations or the onset of hypertension. Polydipsia (excessive thirst) and polyuria (excessive urination) are observed in 40% and 20%, respectively, of patients with nephrogenic diabetes insipidus (see Chap. 34).[103] Although interstitial fibrosis may be observed as early as 5 years after beginning therapy, lithium-induced CKD usually occurs after 10 to 20 years of lithium treatment.[104]

Pathogenesis The precise mechanism of chronic lithium-induced nephrotoxicity is not well characterized. Impaired ability to concentrate urine is a result of a decrease in collecting duct response to antidiuretic hormone, which may be related to downregulation of aquaporin 2 water channel expression during lithium therapy.[104] Chronic tubulointerstitial nephritis attributed to lithium is evidenced most commonly by biopsy findings of interstitial fibrosis, tubular atrophy, and glomerular sclerosis. The pathogenesis may involve cumulative direct lithium toxicity since duration of therapy correlates with the decline in the GFR.[104]

Risk Factors It is now established that long-term lithium therapy is associated with nephrotoxicity in the absence of episodes of acute intoxication, and that the duration of therapy is the major determinant of chronic nephrotoxicity. Increased age may also be a risk factor, but daily dose is not.[102,104]

Prevention Prevention of acute and chronic toxicity includes maintaining lithium concentrations as low as therapeutically possible, avoiding dehydration, and monitoring kidney function. It is unknown whether progression to CKD can be prevented by stopping lithium use when mild kidney injury is first recognized. This poses a dilemma as lithium is highly effective for affective disorders and the risks and potential benefits of discontinuing such a beneficial drug need to be carefully considered.[104] However, if lithium therapy is continued, kidney function must be monitored and therapy discontinued if it continues to decline. Amiloride has been used for prevention and treatment of lithium-induced nephrogenic diabetes insipidus, since it blocks epithelial sodium transport of lithium into the cortical collecting duct in the distal nephron.[104,105]

Management Symptomatic polyuria and polydipsia can be reversed by discontinuation of lithium therapy or ameliorated with amiloride 5 to 10 mg daily during continued lithium therapy (see Chap. 34).[103,105] If polyuria does not resolve within 7 to 10 days of therapy, then the amiloride dose should be increased to 20 mg daily. Progressive chronic interstitial nephritis is treated by discontinuation of lithium therapy, adequate hydration, and avoidance of other nephrotoxic agents. Lithium serum concentrations, as well as kidney function indices, including urine output, BUN, and S_{cr}, should be monitored closely for resolution of signs and symptoms of toxicity.[104]

Cyclosporine and Tacrolimus

Delayed chronic tubulointerstitial nephritis, considered the Achilles' heel of calcineurin inhibitor-based immunosuppressive regimens, has been reported after several months of therapy and can result in irreversible kidney disease.[71] Toxicity is progressive and usually manifests as a slowly rising S_{cr} concentration and decreased creatinine clearance that may not reflect the severity of histopathologic changes. All three compartments of the kidney can be affected, evidenced by typical biopsy findings that include arteriolar hyalinosis, glomerular sclerosis, and a striped pattern of tubulointerstitial fibrosis.[71,74,103] The pathogenesis appears to involve sustained renal arteriolar endothelial cell injury and increased extracellular matrix synthesis, which ultimately result in chronic ischemia of the tubulointerstitial compartment because of increased release of endothelin-1, decreased production of nitric acid, and upregulation of transforming growth factor-β.[71] Unlike acute nephrotoxicity, chronic toxicity is not dose dependent.

Aristolochic Acid

Incidence Although the true incidence of aristolochic acid nephropathy is unknown, approximately 3% to 5% of patients who consume the natural product develop interstitial fibrosis with tubular atrophy.[106]

Clinical Presentation Patients with aristolochic acid nephropathy typically present with mild-to-moderate hypertension, mild proteinuria, glucosuria, and moderately elevated S_{cr} concentrations.[106] Anemia and shrunken kidneys are also common on initial presentation. The overwhelming majority of cases reported to date have been in women. The main pathologic lesions observed in the kidneys are interstitial fibrosis with atrophy and destruction of proximal tubules throughout the renal cortex; in general, the glomeruli are not affected. Perhaps the most remarkable feature of aristolochic acid nephropathy is the rate at which it progresses. In most individuals, ESRD requiring dialysis or transplantation develops within 6 to 24 months of exposure. An alarming high prevalence (approximately 40% to 45%) of urothelial transitional cell carcinoma has been observed in Belgian patients who underwent renal transplantation.[106]

Pathogenesis Although the precise mechanism of aristolochic acid nephropathy and urothelial carcinoma has yet to be characterized. The major components of aristolochic acid are metabolized to mutagenic compounds called *aristolactam I* and *aristolactam II*, respectively, which have been demonstrated to form aristolochic acid–DNA adducts in humans. Recent data indicate that these adducts cause direct DNA damage and may lead to proximal tubular atrophy and apoptosis.[106]

Prevention The primary means of preventing aristolochic acid nephropathy appears to be the limitation of exposure to compounds containing aristolochic acids. Several countries, including the United Kingdom, Canada, Australia, and Germany, have banned the use of *Aristolochia*-containing herbs.[106]

Papillary Necrosis

Papillary necrosis is a form of chronic tubulointerstitial nephritis characterized by necrosis of the renal papillae, the regions of the kidney where the collecting ducts enter the renal pelvis, which leads to progressive kidney disease.[107] Papillary necrosis is associated with diabetes, sickle cell disease, obstruction and infection of the urinary tract, and most commonly analgesic use.[108]

Analgesic Nephropathy

Incidence Prototypical analgesic nephropathy is characterized by chronic tubulointerstitial nephritis with papillary necrosis.[108] Chronic excessive consumption of combination analgesics, particularly those containing phenacetin, was believed to be the major cause and led to the removal of phenacetin and phenacetin mixtures from most world markets. However, contemporary analgesics, particularly aspirin, acetaminophen, and NSAIDs, alone or in combination, are also associated with the development of analgesic nephropathy, but there is insufficient causative evidence to definitively link these nonphenacetin-containing analgesics with nephropathy.[107] The incidence of analgesic nephropathy has declined significantly since removal of phenacetin from many countries, with the prevalence estimated to now be <5% in the United States adult ESRD population.[108]

Clinical Presentation Analgesic nephropathy is a progressive disease that evolves slowly over several years.[108] It is difficult to recognize in the early stages of the disease because patients are often asymptomatic, and it may be underdiagnosed as a cause of ESRD. It is seen more commonly in women than men. Early manifestations are generally nonspecific and may include headache and upper GI symptoms; later manifestations include impaired urinary concentrating ability, dysuria, sterile pyuria, microscopic hematuria, mild proteinuria (<1.5 g/day), and lower back pain. As disease progresses, hypertension, atherosclerotic cardiovascular disease, renal calculi, and bladder stones are common, and pyelonephritis is a classic finding in advanced analgesic nephropathy.[107] The most sensitive and specific diagnostic criteria include (a) a history of chronic daily habitual analgesic ingestion (daily use for at least 3 to 5 years); (b) IV pyelography, renal ultrasound, or renal computed tomography imaging, which reveals decreased renal mass and bumpy renal contours; (3) elevated S_{cr}, that is, up to 4 mg/dL (354 µmol/L); and (4) papillary calcifications.[107,108]

Pathogenesis Analgesic nephropathy originates in the papillary tip as a result of accumulated toxins, drugs and metabolites, decreased blood flow, and impaired cellular energy production. The metabolism of phenacetin to acetaminophen, which is then oxidized to toxic free radicals that are concentrated in the papilla, appears to be the initiating factor that causes toxicity by mechanisms analogous to acetaminophen hepatotoxicity via glutathione depletion.[103] Cortical interstitial nephritis develops secondary to papillary necrosis. Salicylates potentiate these effects by also depleting renal glutathione, and inhibiting prostaglandin-mediated vasodilation, thus further predisposing the renal medulla to ischemic injury.[103]

Risk Factors The epidemiology of analgesic use and analgesic nephropathy continues to evolve. The classic concept persists that risk for ESRD increases with cumulative consumption of combination analgesics, phenacetin, or acetaminophen and aspirin or NSAIDs. Caffeine contained in combination analgesics may increase risk, but the role is not clear.[107,108] Chronic use of therapeutic doses of NSAIDs alone, but not aspirin or salicylates alone, can cause analgesic nephropathy. High-dose acetaminophen use alone is associated with an increased risk for ESRD. However, these associations remain inconclusive as a consequence of study design flaws, as acetaminophen has been the preferentially prescribed analgesic for patients with CKD.[107,108]

Prevention Prevention has depended primarily on public health efforts to restrict the sale of phenacetin and combination analgesics. This has effectively reduced analgesic nephropathy in Australia and Europe.[107] However, risk continues with ongoing availability of nonprescription combination analgesics containing aspirin, acetaminophen, and caffeine in the United States and throughout the world.

Individuals requiring chronic analgesic therapy may reduce risk by limiting the total dose, avoiding combined use of two or more analgesics, and maintaining good hydration to prevent renal ischemia and decrease the papillary concentration of toxic substances. Acetaminophen remains the preferred nonopiate analgesic for patients with preexisting kidney disease.

Management Treatment of established nephrotoxicity requires cessation of analgesic consumption.[103] This can prevent progression and may improve kidney function. Kidney function indices, including urine output, BUN, and S_{cr}, should be monitored every several months. Patients should also be monitored for the development of transitional cell carcinoma of the renal pelvis, calyces, ureters, and bladder, which may present years after analgesic nephropathy is diagnosed.

RENAL VASCULITIS, THROMBOSIS, AND CHOLESTEROL EMBOLI

Renal Vasculitis

Drug-induced renal vascular disease commonly presents as vasculitis, thrombotic microangiopathy, or cholesterol emboli.[109] Vasculitis implies inflammation of the vessel wall, capillaries, or glomeruli and is typically classified according to vessel size (i.e., small, medium, or large vessel vasculitis).[19] Small vessel vasculitides usually affect multiple organ systems, including the kidneys and lungs, and are associated with nonspecific inflammatory symptoms such as fever, malaise, myalgias, arthralgias, and weight loss.[94] Numerous drugs are associated with the development of renal vasculitis, including hydralazine, propylthiouracil, allopurinol, phenytoin, sulfasalazine, penicillamine, and minocycline (Table 31-1).[109,110] Most drug-induced cases of vasculitis, including hydralazine, propylthiouracil, allopurinol, penicillamine, and the anti-TNF-α drug adalimumab have been implicated in the development of antineutrophil cytoplasmic antibody (ANCA)-positive vasculitis.[109–111] Patients present with hematuria, proteinuria, oliguria, and red cell casts, frequently along with fever, malaise, myalgias, and arthralgias.[109] Treatment typically consists of withdrawing the offending drug and administration of corticosteroids or other immunosuppressive therapy, and usually leads to resolution of symptoms within weeks to months.[110]

Thrombotic Microangiopathy

Thrombotic microangiopathy is characterized clinically by microangiopathic hemolytic anemia, fragmented red cells, and thrombocytopenia and pathologically by vascular endothelial proliferation, endothelial cell swelling, and intraluminal platelet thrombi in the small vessels, particularly affecting the renal and cerebral capillaries and arterioles.[19,112] The absence of inflammation in vessel walls distinguishes thrombotic microangiopathy from vasculitis. Numerous medications, including oral contraceptive agents, cyclosporine, tacrolimus, muromonab-CD3, many cancer chemotherapeutic agents including mitomycin C, cisplatin, and gemcitabine, interferon-α, ticlopidine, clopidogrel, quinine, and several biological agents such as bevacizumab and sunitinib are associated with the development of thrombotic microangiopathy.[93,111,112] Patients may present with fever, neurological dysfunction, elevated S_{cr} and BUN, and hypertension, along with microangiopathic hemolytic anemia and thrombocytopenia.[19] Kidney injury can be severe and irreversible, although corticosteroids, antiplatelet agents, plasma exchange, plasmapheresis, and high-dose IV immunoglobulin G have each induced clinical improvement.

Cholesterol Emboli

Anticoagulants (particularly warfarin) and thrombolytics (e.g., urokinase, streptokinase, tissue-plasminogen activator) are associated with cholesterol embolization of the kidney.[113] These drugs act to remove or prevent thrombus formation over ulcerative plaques or may induce hemorrhage within clots, thereby causing showers of cholesterol crystals that lodge in small diameter arteries of the kidney (renal arterioles and glomerular capillaries). Cholesterol crystal emboli induce an endothelial inflammatory response, which leads to complete obstruction, ischemia, and necrosis of affected vessels within weeks to months after initiation of therapy.[113] Purple discoloration of the toes and mottled skin over the legs are important clinical clues. Treatment is supportive in nature, since kidney injury is generally irreversible.

PHARMACOECONOMICS

The pharmacoeconomic implications of DIKD are enormous. An increase in S_{cr} of ≥0.5 mg/dL (44 μmol/L) is independently associated with a 6.5-fold increase in the odds of death, a 3.5-day increase in length of hospital stay, and nearly $7,500 in excess hospital costs even after adjusting for age, sex, and measures of comorbidity.[7] Amphotericin B-induced AKI leads to a mean increased length of hospital stay of 8.2 days and adjusted additional costs of $29,823 per patient,[114] and the mean additional in-hospital cost for each episode of contrast-induced AKI has been estimated to be $10,345 per case.[29] The major driver of the increased costs associated with contrast-induced AKI was the cost of the longer initial hospital stay. The increased availability of automated clinical decision support systems and computer-guided medication dosing for hospital inpatients may improve the safety of potentially harmful drugs and minimize the occurrence of nephrotoxicity in this setting, thereby potentially lowering the corresponding economic consequences.[114,115]

ABBREVIATIONS

ACEI	angiotensin-converting enzyme inhibitor
AIDS	acquired immune deficiency syndrome
AIN	allergic interstitial nephritis
AKI	acute kidney injury
ARB	angiotensin II receptor blocker
BUN	blood urea nitrogen
CIN	contrast media-induced nephrotoxicity
CKD	chronic kidney disease
COX	cyclooxygenase

ESRD	end-stage renal disease
FSGS	focal segmental glomerulosclerosis
GFR	glomerular filtration rate
KIM-1	kidney injury molecule-1
NGAL	neutrophil gelatinase-associated lipocalin
NSAID	nonsteroidal antiinflammatory drug
OSPS	oral sodium phosphate solution
S_{cr}	serum creatinine
WRN	warfarin-related nephropathy

REFERENCES

1. Himmelfarb J, Ikizler TA. Acute kidney injury: changing lexicography, definitions, and epidemiology. Kidney Int 2007;71:971–976.
2. Zappitelli M, Parikh CR, Akcan-Arikan A, et al. Ascertainment and epidemiology of acute kidney injury varies with definition interpretation. Clin J Am Soc Nephrol 2008;3:948–954.
3. Ricci Z, Cruz D, Ronco C. The RIFLE criteria and mortality in acute kidney injury: a systematic review. Kidney Int 2008;73:538–546.
4. Slater MB, Anand V, Uleryk EM, Parshuram CS. A systematic review of RIFLE criteria in children, and its application and association with measures of mortality and morbidity. Kidney Int 2012;81:791–798.
5. Hsu CY, McCulloch CE, Fan D, et al. Community-based incidence of acute renal failure. Kidney Int 2007;72: 208–212.
6. Elasy TA, Anderson RJ. Changing demography of acute renal failure. Semin Dial 1996;9:438–443.
7. Chertow GM, Burdick E, Honour M, et al. Acute kidney injury, mortality, length of stay, and costs in hospitalized patients. J Am Soc Nephrol 2005;16:3365–3370.
8. Lameire N, Van Biesen W, Vanholder R. Acute renal failure. Lancet 2005;365:417–430.
9. Pannu N, Nadim MK. An overview of drug-induced acute kidney injury. Crit Care Med 2008;36:S216–S223.
10. Mehta RL, Kellum JA, Shah SV, et al. Acute Kidney Injury Network: report of an initiative to improve outcomes in acute kidney injury. Crit Care 2007;11:R31.
11. Goodsaid FM, Blank M, Dieterle F, et al. Novel biomarkers of acute kidney toxicity. Clin Pharmacol Ther 2009;86: 490–496.
12. Fuchs TC, Hewitt P. Biomarkers for drug-induced renal damage and nephrotoxicity—an overview for applied toxicology. AAPS J 2011;13:615–631.
13. Coca SG, Parikh CR. Urinary biomarkers for acute kidney injury: perspectives on translation. Clin J Am Soc Nephrol 2008;3:481–490.
14. Vaidya VS, Ferguson MA, Bonventre JV. Biomarkers of acute kidney injury. Annu Rev Pharmacol Toxicol 2008;48:463–493.
15. Perazella MA. Renal vulnerability to drug toxicity. Clin J Am Soc Nephrol 2009;4:1275–1283.
16. Naughton CA. Drug-induced nephrotoxicity. Am Fam Physician 2008;78:743–750.
17. Khalil P, Murty P, Palevsky PM. The patient with acute kidney injury. Prim Care 2008;35:239–264.
18. Abuelo JG. Normotensive ischemic acute renal failure. N Engl J Med 2007;357:797–805.
19. John R, Herzenberg AM. Renal toxicity of therapeutic drugs. J Clin Pathol 2009;62:505–515.
20. Oliveira JF, Silva CA, Barbieri CD, et al. Prevalence and risk factors for aminoglycoside nephrotoxicity in intensive care units. Antimicrob Agents Chemother 2009;53: 2887–2891.
21. Martinez-Salgado C, Lopez-Hernandez FJ, Lopez-Novoa JM. Glomerular nephrotoxicity of aminoglycosides. Toxicol Appl Pharmacol 2007;223:86–98.
22. Drusano GL, Ambrose PG, Bhavnani SM, et al. Back to the future: using aminoglycosides again and how to dose them optimally. Clin Infect Dis 2007;45:753–760.
23. Koyner JL, Sher Ali R, Murray PT. Antioxidants. Do they have a place in the prevention or therapy of acute kidney injury? Nephron Exp Nephrol 2008;109:e109–e117.
24. Balakumar P, Rohilla A, Thangathirupathi A. Gentamicin-induced nephrotoxicity: do we have a promising therapeutic approach to blunt it? Pharmacol Res 2010;62:179–186.
25. Greenwood BC, Szumita PM, Lowry CM. Pharmacist-driven aminoglycoside quality improvement program. J Chemother 2009;21:42–45.
26. Pagkalis S, Mantadakis E, Mavros MN, et al. Pharmacological considerations for the proper clinical use of aminoglycosides. Drugs 2011;71:2277–2294.
27. Stabler SN, Ensom MH. Extended-interval aminoglycoside therapy for adult patients with febrile neutropenia: a systematic review. Can J Hosp Pharm 2011;64:182–191.
28. Tzovaras V, Tsimihodimos V, Kostara C, et al. Aminoglycoside-induced nephrotoxicity studied by proton magnetic resonance spectroscopy of urine. Nephrol Dial Transplant 2011;26:3219–3224.
29. McCullough PA. Contrast-induced acute kidney injury. J Am Coll Cardiol 2008;51:1419–1428.
30. Brar SS, Shen AY, Jorgensen MB, et al. Sodium bicarbonate vs sodium chloride for the prevention of contrast medium-induced nephropathy in patients undergoing coronary angiography: a randomized trial. JAMA 2008;300: 1038–1046.
31. Rudnick M, Feldman H. Contrast-induced nephropathy: what are the true clinical consequences? Clin J Am Soc Nephrol 2008;3:263–272.
32. Weisbord SD, Palevsky PM. Contrast-induced acute kidney injury: short- and long-term implications. Semin Nephrol 2011;31:300–309.
33. Solomon R. Contrast-induced acute kidney injury (CIAKI). Radiol Clin North Am 2009;47:783–788.
34. Pflueger A, Abramowitz D, Calvin AD. Role of oxidative stress in contrast-induced acute kidney injury in diabetes mellitus. Med Sci Monit 2009;15:RA125–136.
35. Fishbane S. *N*-acetylcysteine in the prevention of contrast-induced nephropathy. Clin J Am Soc Nephrol 2008;3: 281–287.
36. Ellis JH, Cohan RH. Prevention of contrast-induced nephropathy: an overview. Radiol Clin North Am 2009;47:801–811.
37. Kelly AM, Dwamena B, Cronin P, et al. Meta-analysis: effectiveness of drugs for preventing contrast-induced nephropathy. Ann Intern Med 2008;148:284–294.
38. Laskey WK, Jenkins C, Selzer F, et al. Volume-to-creatinine clearance ratio: a pharmacokinetically based risk factor for prediction of early creatinine increase after percutaneous coronary intervention. J Am Coll Cardiol 2007;50: 584–590.
39. Heinrich MC, Haberle L, Muller V, et al. Nephrotoxicity of iso-osmolar iodixanol compared with nonionic low-osmolar contrast media: meta-analysis of randomized controlled trials. Radiology 2009;250:68–86.
40. Weisbord SD, Palevsky PM. Prevention of contrast-induced nephropathy with volume expansion. Clin J Am Soc Nephrol 2008;3:273–280.

41. Briguori C, Airoldi F, D'Andrea D, et al. Renal Insufficiency Following Contrast Media Administration Trial (REMEDIAL): a randomized comparison of 3 preventive strategies. Circulation 2007;115:1211–1217.
42. From AM, Bartholmai BJ, Williams AW, et al. Sodium bicarbonate is associated with an increased incidence of contrast nephropathy: a retrospective cohort study of 7977 patients at mayo clinic. Clin J Am Soc Nephrol 2008;3: 10–18.
43. Weisbord SD, Palevsky PM. Strategies for the prevention of contrast-induced acute kidney injury. Curr Opin Nephrol Hypertens 2010;19:539–549.
44. Weisbord SD, Palevsky PM. Iodinated contrast media and the role of renal replacement therapy. Adv Chronic Kidney Dis 2011;18:199–206.
45. Cruz DN, Goh CY, Marenzi G, et al. Renal replacement therapies for prevention of radiocontrast-induced nephropathy: a systematic review. Am J Med 2012; 125:66–78.
46. Pabla N, Dong Z. Cisplatin nephrotoxicity: mechanisms and renoprotective strategies. Kidney Int 2008;73:994–1007.
47. Launay-Vacher V, Rey JB, Isnard-Bagnis C, et al. Prevention of cisplatin nephrotoxicity: state of the art and recommendations from the European Society of Clinical Pharmacy Special Interest Group on Cancer Care. Cancer Chemother Pharmacol 2008;61:903–909.
48. Yao X, Panichpisal K, Kurtzman N, Nugent K. Cisplatin nephrotoxicity: a review. Am J Med Sci 2007;334:115–124.
49. Perazella MA. Onco-nephrology: renal toxicities of chemotherapeutic agents. Clin J Am Soc Nephrol 2012;7:1713–1721.
50. Perazella MA, Moeckel GW. Nephrotoxicity from chemotherapeutic agents: clinical manifestations, pathobiology, and prevention/therapy. Semin Nephrol 2010;30:570–581.
51. Hensley ML, Hagerty KL, Kewalramani T, et al. American Society of Clinical Oncology 2008 clinical practice guideline update: use of chemotherapy and radiation therapy protectants. J Clin Oncol 2009;27:127–145.
52. dos Santos NA, Carvalho Rodrigues MA, Martins NM, dos Santos AC. Cisplatin-induced nephrotoxicity and targets of nephroprotection: an update. Arch Toxicol 2012;86: 1233–1250.
53. Goldman RD, Koren G. Amphotericin B nephrotoxicity in children. J Pediatr Hematol Oncol 2004;26:421–426.
54. Bates DW, Su L, Yu DT, et al. Mortality and costs of acute renal failure associated with amphotericin B therapy. Clin Infect Dis 2001;32:686–693.
55. Ullmann AJ. Nephrotoxicity in the setting of invasive fungal diseases. Mycoses 2008;51(Suppl 1):25–30.
56. Safdar A, Ma J, Saliba F, et al. Drug-induced nephrotoxicity caused by amphotericin B lipid complex and liposomal amphotericin B: a review and meta-analysis. Medicine (Baltimore) 2010;89:236–244.
57. Dickenmann M, Oettl T, Mihatsch MJ. Osmotic nephrosis: acute kidney injury with accumulation of proximal tubular lysosomes due to administration of exogenous solutes. Am J Kidney Dis 2008;51:491–503.
58. Welles CC, Tambra S, Lafayette RA. Hemoglobinuria and acute kidney injury requiring hemodialysis following intravenous immunoglobulin infusion. Am J Kidney Dis 2010;55:148–151.
59. Huter L, Simon TP, Weinmann L, et al. Hydroxyethylstarch impairs renal function and induces interstitial proliferation, macrophage infiltration and tubular damage in an isolated renal perfusion model. Crit Care 2009;13:R23.
60. Kobori H, Nangaku M, Navar LG, Nishiyama A. The intrarenal renin–angiotensin system: from physiology to the pathobiology of hypertension and kidney disease. Pharmacol Rev 2007;59:251–287.
61. Cupples WA, Braam B. Assessment of renal autoregulation. Am J Physiol Renal Physiol 2007;292:F1105–F1123.
62. Ryan MJ, Tuttle KR. Elevations in serum creatinine with RAAS blockade: why isn't it a sign of kidney injury? Curr Opin Nephrol Hypertens 2008;17:443–449.
63. Chittineni H, Miyawaki N, Gulipelli S, Fishbane S. Risk for acute renal failure in patients hospitalized for decompensated congestive heart failure. Am J Nephrol 2007;27:55–62.
64. Cruz CS, Cruz LS, Silva GR, Marcilio de Souza CA. Incidence and predictors of development of acute renal failure related to treatment of congestive heart failure with ACE inhibitors. Nephron Clin Pract 2007; 105:c77–83.
65. Budnitz DS, Lovegrove MC, Shehab N, Richards CL. Emergency hospitalizations for adverse drug events in older Americans. N Engl J Med 2011;365:2002–2012.
66. Lapi F, Azoulay L, Yin H, et al. Concurrent use of diuretics, angiotensin converting enzyme inhibitors, and angiotensin receptor blockers with non-steroidal anti-inflammatory drugs and risk of acute kidney injury: nested case–control study. BMJ 2013;346:e8525.
67. House AA, Silva Oliveira S, Ronco C. Anti-inflammatory drugs and the kidney. Int J Artif Organs 2007;30: 1042–1046.
68. Winkelmayer WC, Waikar SS, Mogun H, Solomon DH. Nonselective and cyclooxygenase-2-selective NSAIDs and acute kidney injury. Am J Med 2008;121:1092–1098.
69. Cheng HF, Harris RC. Renal effects of non-steroidal anti-inflammatory drugs and selective cyclooxygenase-2 inhibitors. Curr Pharm Des 2005;11:1795–1804.
70. Whelton A. Nephrotoxicity of nonsteroidal anti-inflammatory drugs: physiologic foundations and clinical implications. Am J Med 1999;106:13S–24S.
71. Naesens M, Kuypers DR, Sarwal M. Calcineurin inhibitor nephrotoxicity. Clin J Am Soc Nephrol 2009;4:481–508.
72. Ojo AO, Held PJ, Port FK, et al. Chronic renal failure after transplantation of a nonrenal organ. N Engl J Med 2003;349:931–940.
73. Pallet N, Djamali A, Legendre C. Challenges in diagnosing acute calcineurin-inhibitor induced nephrotoxicity: from toxicogenomics to emerging biomarkers. Pharmacol Res 2011;64:25–30.
74. Liptak P, Ivanyi B. Primer: histopathology of calcineurin-inhibitor toxicity in renal allografts. Nat Clin Pract Nephrol 2006;2:398–404.
75. Lameire N, Van Biesen W, Vanholder R. Acute renal problems in the critically ill cancer patient. Curr Opin Crit Care 2008;14:635–646.
76. Tosi P, Barosi G, Lazzaro C, et al. Consensus conference on the management of tumor lysis syndrome. Haematologica 2008;93:1877–1885.
77. Bagley WH, Yang H, Shah KH. Rhabdomyolysis. Intern Emerg Med 2007;2:210–218.
78. Molden E, Skovlund E, Braathen P. Risk management of simvastatin or atorvastatin interactions with CYP3A4 inhibitors. Drug Saf 2008;31:587–596.
79. Brodsky SV, Satoskar A, Chen J, et al. Acute kidney injury during warfarin therapy associated with obstructive tubular red blood cell casts: a report of 9 cases. Am J Kidney Dis 2009;54:1121–1126.
80. Brodsky SV, Nadasdy T, Rovin BH, et al. Warfarin-related nephropathy occurs in patients with and without chronic

kidney disease and is associated with an increased mortality rate. Kidney Int 2011;80:181–189.
81. Herlitz LC, D'Agati VD, Markowitz GS. Crystalline nephropathies. Arch Pathol Lab Med 2012;136:713–720.
82. Yarlagadda SG, Perazella MA. Drug-induced crystal nephropathy: an update. Expert Opin Drug Saf 2008;7:147–158.
83. Kalyesubula R, Perazella MA. Nephrotoxicity of HAART. AIDS Res Treat 2011;2011:562790.
84. Jao J, Wyatt CM. Antiretroviral medications: adverse effects on the kidney. Adv Chronic Kidney Dis 2010;17:72–82.
85. Izzedine H, Harris M, Perazella MA. The nephrotoxic effects of HAART. Nat Rev Nephrol 2009;5:563–573.
86. Heher EC, Thier SO, Rennke H, Humphreys BD. Adverse renal and metabolic effects associated with oral sodium phosphate bowel preparation. Clin J Am Soc Nephrol 2008;3:1494–1503.
87. Markowitz GS, Perazella MA. Acute phosphate nephropathy. Kidney Int 2009;76:1027–1034.
88. Russmann S, Lamerato L, Motsko SP, et al. Risk of further decline in renal function after the use of oral sodium phosphate or polyethylene glycol in patients with a preexisting glomerular filtration rate below 60 ml/min. Am J Gastroenterol 2008;103:2707–2716.
89. Khurana A, McLean L, Atkinson S, Foulks CJ. The effect of oral sodium phosphate drug products on renal function in adults undergoing bowel endoscopy. Arch Intern Med 2008;168:593–597.
90. Markowitz GS, Radhakrishnan J, D'Agati VD. Towards the incidence of acute phosphate nephropathy. J Am Soc Nephrol 2007;18:3020–3022.
91. Daudon M, Jungers P. Drug-induced renal calculi: epidemiology, prevention and management. Drugs 2004;64:245–275.
92. Hau AK, Kwan TH, Li PK. Melamine toxicity and the kidney. J Am Soc Nephrol 2009;20:245–250.
93. Harbord N. Novel nephrotoxins. Adv Chronic Kidney Dis 2011;18:214–218.
94. Beck LH Jr, Salant DJ. Glomerular and tubulointerstitial diseases. Prim Care 2008;35:265–296.
95. Izzedine H, Launay-Vacher V, Bourry E, et al. Drug-induced glomerulopathies. Expert Opin Drug Saf 2006;5:95–106.
96. Jaffe JA, Kimmel PL. Chronic nephropathies of cocaine and heroin abuse: a critical review. Clin J Am Soc Nephrol 2006;1:655–667.
97. Perazella MA, Markowitz GS. Bisphosphonate nephrotoxicity. Kidney Int 2008;74:1385–1393.
98. Perazella MA, Markowitz GS. Drug-induced acute interstitial nephritis. Nat Rev Nephrol 2010;6:461–470.
99. Gonzalez E, Gutierrez E, Galeano C, et al. Early steroid treatment improves the recovery of renal function in patients with drug-induced acute interstitial nephritis. Kidney Int 2008;73:940–946.
100. Ricketson J, Kimel G, Spence J, Weir R. Acute allergic interstitial nephritis after use of pantoprazole. CMAJ 2009;180:535–538.
101. Bendz H, Schon S, Attman PO, Aurell M. Renal failure occurs in chronic lithium treatment but is uncommon. Kidney Int 2010;77:219–224.
102. Rej S, Herrmann N, Shulman K. The effects of lithium on renal function in older adults—a systematic review. J Geriatr Psychiatry Neurol 2012;25:51–61.
103. Braden GL, O'Shea MH, Mulhern JG. Tubulointerstitial diseases. Am J Kidney Dis 2005;46:560–572.
104. Grunfeld JP, Rossier BC. Lithium nephrotoxicity revisited. Nat Rev Nephrol 2009;5:270–276.
105. Bedford JJ, Weggery S, Ellis G, et al. Lithium-induced nephrogenic diabetes insipidus: renal effects of amiloride. Clin J Am Soc Nephrol 2008;3:1324–1331.
106. Debelle FD, Vanherweghem JL, Nortier JL. Aristolochic acid nephropathy: a worldwide problem. Kidney Int 2008;74:158–169.
107. Vadivel N, Trikudanathan S, Singh AK. Analgesic nephropathy. Kidney Int 2007;72:517–520.
108. De Broe ME, Elseviers MM. Over-the-counter analgesic use. J Am Soc Nephrol 2009;20:2098–2103.
109. Radic M, Martinovic Kaliterna D, Radic J. Drug-induced vasculitis: a clinical and pathological review. Neth J Med 2012;70:12–17.
110. Wiik A. Drug-induced vasculitis. Curr Opin Rheumatol 2008;20:35–39.
111. Perez-Alvarez R, Perez-de-Lis M, Ramos-Casals M. Biologics-induced autoimmune diseases. Curr Opin Rheumatol 2013;25:56–64.
112. Dlott JS, Danielson CF, Blue-Hnidy DE, McCarthy LJ. Drug-induced thrombotic thrombocytopenic purpura/hemolytic uremic syndrome: a concise review. Ther Apher Dial 2004;8:102–111.
113. Scolari F, Ravani P. Atheroembolic renal disease. Lancet 2010;375:1650–1660.
114. Hug BL, Witkowski DJ, Sox CM, et al. Occurrence of adverse, often preventable, events in community hospitals involving nephrotoxic drugs or those excreted by the kidney. Kidney Int 2009;76:1192–1198.
115. McCoy AB, Waitman LR, Gadd CS, et al. A computerized provider order entry intervention for medication safety during acute kidney injury: a quality improvement report. Am J Kidney Dis 2010;56:832–841.

Glomerulonephritis

Alan H. Lau

32

KEY CONCEPTS

1. Glomerulonephritis is a collection of glomerular diseases mediated by different immunologic pathogenic mechanisms, resulting in varied clinical presentation and therapeutic outcomes.
2. The signs and symptoms associated with glomerulonephritis can be nephritic in nature, characterized by inflammatory injury, or nephrotic in nature, characterized by proteinuria.
3. In the absence of specific and effective therapy for many types of glomerulonephritis, supportive treatments for edema, hypertension, hyperlipidemia, and intravascular thrombosis play important roles in reducing the complications associated with the disease.
4. To maximize therapeutic benefits and minimize drug-induced complications, patients have to be monitored closely to assess their therapeutic responses as well as the development of any treatment-induced toxicities.
5. Among all the types of glomerulonephritis, minimal-change nephropathy is most responsive to treatment. Steroids can induce good responses in most patients during initial treatment as well as relapse.
6. Because of the lack of consistently effective treatment for primary focal segmental glomerular sclerosis, angiotensin-converting enzyme inhibitors or angiotensin receptor blockers are commonly used for patients with mild disease to control symptoms. Steroids and immunosuppressive agents are reserved for patients with severe disease.
7. The optimal treatment for lupus nephritis depends on the underlying lesion and disease activity, as well as the severity and duration of the clinical presentation.
8. The treatment of poststreptococcal glomerulonephritis is mainly supportive and symptomatic. Antibiotic therapy does not prevent subsequent diseases but may reduce the severity.

The precise pathogenetic mechanisms of many glomerular diseases remain unknown, and the available therapeutic regimens are still far from optimal. This chapter provides an overview of the primary causes of glomerulonephritis with a focus on their etiology, the pathophysiologic mechanisms responsible for glomerular injury, and the clinical presentation of the eight predominant types of glomerulonephritis. Treatment options and monitoring approaches for each of these types of glomerulonephritis are also discussed. Diabetes mellitus is an important secondary cause of glomerular injury, and a thorough discussion of the pathophysiology and management of this condition can be found in Chapter 57.

NORMAL GLOMERULAR ANATOMY AND FUNCTION

The glomerulus, which is enclosed within the Bowman's capsule, consists of two important components: the filtration barrier and the mesangium (Fig. 32-1). The capillary wall, which serves as a filtration barrier, consists of three well-defined layers: fenestrated endothelium, glomerular basement membrane (GBM), and epithelial cell layer. The epithelial cells, also known as podocytes, have specialized foot processes embedded in the outer layer of the GBM. It is across this barrier that fluid flows and ultimately becomes the ultrafiltrate. Under normal conditions, the GBM functions as a compact hydrated gel of matrix proteins with a pore-like structure. The mesangium, which consists of mesangial cells embedded in an extracellular matrix, provides support for the glomerular capillaries and also modulates blood flow through the capillaries.

The unique capillary bed of the glomerulus allows small non-protein plasma constituents up to the size of inulin, which has a molecular weight of 5.2 kDa, to pass freely while excluding macromolecules equal to or larger than albumin, which has a molecular weight of 69 kDa. The ease of passage of solutes through the glomerular membrane is impacted by both the size and charge of the solute. Fixed, negatively charged sites are found within the glomeruli in all three layers of the capillary wall: the endothelium, the epithelium, and the GBM. The movement of negatively charged molecules is thus restricted more than that of neutral or positively charged molecules. Different glomerular diseases affect this size- and charge-selective barrier to different extents; consequently, glomerulopathies present with varied clinical features and solute-excretion patterns.

Some of the glomerular cells, such as the epithelial cells, have phagocytic function that can remove macromolecules trapped within the filtration barrier. They are also capable of synthesizing the GBM. In contrast, the mesangial cells regulate glomerular hemodynamics in response to angiotensin II and by producing prostaglandins. These cells also synthesize and respond to various cytokines and thus play a key role in immune-mediated glomerular diseases. Resident phagocytes in the mesangium are responsible for moving macromolecules trapped in the basement membrane into the urinary space. They are also involved in the development of both immune and nonimmune glomerular injury.

EPIDEMIOLOGY AND ETIOLOGY

In the United States in 2010, glomerulonephritis was the third most common cause of end-stage renal disease (ESRD), accounting for approximately 15% of all the living ESRD patients. About

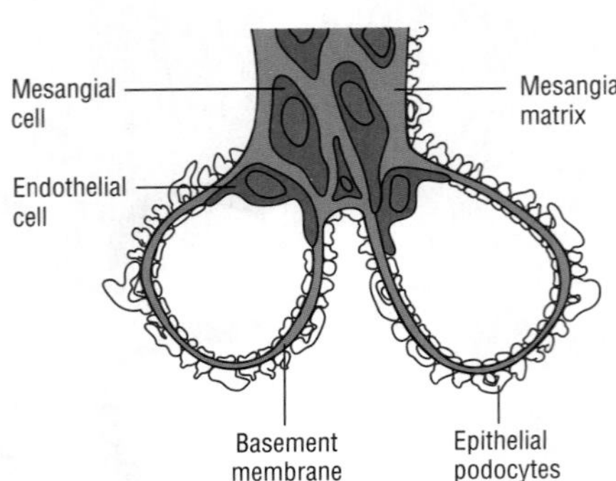

FIGURE 32-1 Microanatomy of the glomerulus.

7,300 patients (6.4% of all patients) develop stage 5 chronic kidney disease, which is also called ESRD, because of glomerulonephritis each year.[1]

Humoral and cellular immunologic mechanisms participate in the pathogenesis of most glomerulonephritis. Abnormalities in coagulation and metabolism, as well as hereditary and vascular diseases, also contribute to glomerular damage. The histopathologic manifestations vary substantially among the different types of glomerulonephritis. An overview of the primary pathogenetic mechanisms is presented in this section, and specific abnormalities for each of the primary types of glomerulonephritis are presented in subsequent sections.

PATHOPHYSIOLOGY

1 The glomerular lesion may be diffuse (involving all glomeruli), focal (involving some but not all glomeruli), or segmental, also known as local (involving part of the individual glomerulus). The pathologic manifestations may also be described as proliferative (overgrowth of epithelium, endothelium, or mesangium), membranous (thickening of GBM), and/or sclerotic.

The glomerular capillary wall is particularly susceptible to immune-mediated injury. Antigens and antibodies tend to localize in the glomerulus, probably because of its high blood flow and capillary hydrostatic pressure. Parenchymal damage can be induced as a result of humoral- and cell-mediated immune reactions. Antibodies and sensitized T lymphocytes are the primary mediators of glomerular injury.[2,3]

Production of antibodies to endogenous or exogenous antigens that are recognized as foreign by the host is the first step in humoral immunologic damage to the glomerulus. Endogenous antigens may be intrinsic glomerular antigens, such as Heymann antigen on the epithelial cell or Goodpasture antigen on the GBM, or previously sequestered antigens, such as DNA or thyroglobulin. Exogenous antigens are most often viral, bacterial, parasitic, or fungal in origin. Antineutrophil cytoplasmic autoantibodies (ANCAs) (i.e., autoantibodies that react to the cytoplasmic components of neutrophils and monocytes) are found in patients with idiopathic crescentic glomerulonephritis and also in the accompanying vasculitis.

Complexes of antigens and antibodies may be formed in the circulation and then passively entrapped in the glomerular capillary or mesangium. Alternately, experimental antibodies may combine with endogenous glomerular antigens or exogenous antigens entrapped in the glomerulus to form complexes locally, or in situ.[3] The type and extent of glomerular damage depend on the location of the immune complex formation and the rate at which it is removed. Impaired removal facilitates the growth of the complex and thus increases the likelihood of glomerular damage.

Subsequent to antigen–antibody formation, a series of biologic events is triggered that ultimately leads to glomerular injury. Noninflammatory lesions can result from the binding of noncomplement-fixing antibody to the glomerular epithelial cell (mechanism 1) or from the activation of the complement system to form the C5b-9 membrane attack complex (mechanism 2).[3] Both mechanisms can damage the glomerular epithelial cell and result in capillary wall injury and proteinuria. Inflammatory lesions are induced by glomerular infiltration of circulating inflammatory cells such as neutrophils, monocytes/macrophages, and platelets (mechanism 3) or by proliferation of resident glomerular mesangial cells (mechanism 4), resulting in GBM damage.[3] The migration of neutrophils and monocytes to the glomerular tufts is promoted by chemoattractants such as complement fragments (C3a and C5a), platelet-activating factor, interleukin-8, and monocyte chemotactic protein-1.[4] Various cytokines, chemokines, and growth factors are then released to participate in the inflammatory process.[2]

T cells sensitized to glomerular antigen, macrophages, and resident mesangial cells are important participants in cell-mediated injury. Sensitized T cells can cause glomerular hypercellularity in the absence of antibody deposition.[2–4] Cytotoxic T cells may bind with the target cells and destroy them. Alternatively, a delayed-type hypersensitivity reaction may be initiated by activated T cells through the release of lymphokines to attract, activate, and transform monocytes into macrophages.[3] These humoral and cellular mediators, in conjunction with a host of toxic molecular entities including reactive oxygen species, proteinases, eicosanoids, and procoagulants, which are secreted by neutrophils, macrophages, platelets, and resident glomerular cells, can alter the permeability, blood flow, and function of the glomeruli. Vascular constriction and occlusion follow and result in the eventual destruction of the glomeruli.

Acute forms of glomerular injury frequently lead to chronic and persistent renal dysfunction, even though the original immune factors that induced the initial glomerular injury have resolved. Experimental and clinical investigations suggest that a variety of factors may participate in the progression of renal injury. These factors include systemic and glomerular hypertension, high dietary protein intake, proteinuria, glomerular hypertrophy, hyperlipidemia, activation of the coagulation system, abnormalities of calcium and phosphorus balance, and tubulointerstitial injury. The degree of proteinuria not only is an index of the severity of glomerular disease but also has been associated with an increased rate of progression of renal injury. Heavy proteinuria is an indicator of poor prognosis in various glomerular diseases.

Proteinuria is also accompanied by an increased flux of macromolecules across the mesangium. The mesangial overload may then lead to structural damage. The passage of serum components, such as complement, across the GBM may have a pathophysiologic effect on the glomerular epithelial cells and alter the integrity of the glomerular filtration barrier. The damaging effects of macromolecules other than albumin, such as immunoglobulins, lipoproteins, transferrin, and complement, remain to be characterized.

CLINICAL PRESENTATION

2 Although patients with glomerular disease may present with an array of signs and symptoms, they are often categorized into one of two broad classifications: nephritic syndrome or nephrotic syndrome (Table 32-1). The unique clinical presentation characteristics of the predominant glomerulopathies are described in the individual disease sections, presented later in the chapter.

Nephritic syndrome reflects glomerular inflammation and frequently results in hematuria. White cells and cellular and

CLINICAL PRESENTATION Nephritic and Nephrotic Syndromes

General

- The patients are generally not in acute distress

Symptoms

- The patients may not experience any major symptoms

Nephritic Signs

- Hematuria
- Hypertension and edema as renal function declines

Nephrotic Signs

- Edema
- Weight gain
- Fatigue

Laboratory Tests

- Proteinuria up to 3 g/day
- Pus, cellular and granular casts in urine is common
- Hypoproteinemia
- Hypercoagulable state for some patients
- Proteinuria, >3.5 g/day/1.73 m^2
- Hyperlipidemia
- Lipiduria

granular casts are commonly found in the urine. In contrast, nephrotic syndrome reflects noninflammatory injury to the glomerular structures and results in few cells or cellular casts in the urine. Initially, there may be limited or no reduction in renal excretory function.

Hematuria occurs when red blood cells leak through the openings of the GBM. The presence of red cell casts is highly indicative of glomerulonephritis or vasculitis. The presence of dysmorphic red blood cells in the urine is suggestive of glomerular disease. The red blood cells are damaged as they pass through the openings in the GBM or the cells may sustain osmotic injury as they travel through the different osmotic environments within the lumen of the kidney tubules.

The presence of proteinuria indicates a defect of the size- and/or charge-selective barriers within the GBM. Normal urinary protein excretion is between 40 and 80 mg/day, with a maximum of 150 mg. Fewer than 20 mg of the excreted proteins are albumin. Most of the albumin that enters the glomerular filtrate is either reabsorbed or catabolized by the tubular epithelium. The dipsticks that are commonly used to identify proteinuria detect only albumin; they become positive when protein excretion is more than 300 to 500 mg/day. They are therefore unable to detect the early stages of renal injury secondary to diabetes mellitus or hypertension, which often result in microalbuminuria with urinary albumin excretion ranges between 30 and 300 mg/day. Chemstrip Micral-Test II (Roche Diagnostics, Indianapolis, IN), a simple immunoassay on a dipstick, permits specific and semiquantitative determination of urinary albumin concentrations at five levels: 0, 10, 20, 50, and 100 mg/L. Another qualitative test, Micro-Bumintest (Bayer Diabetes Care, Mishawaka, IN), registers a positive reading when the urine albumin concentration is greater than 40 mg/L.

Hypertension is common for patients with glomerular diseases, as a result of renal salt retention causing plasma volume expansion. In contrast, increased activity of vasoconstrictors such as angiotensin II is often the cause for patients with chronic glomerular diseases. Scarring of the glomerulus resulting in regional ischemia is thought to be responsible for the hypertension. Activation of the sympathetic nervous system and the release of vasoconstrictor substances may also contribute.

TABLE 32-1 Tendencies of Glomerular Diseases to Manifest Nephrotic and Nephritic Features

	Nephrotic Features	Nephritic Features
Minimal-change nephropathy	++++	–
Membranous nephropathy	++++	+
Diabetic glomerulosclerosis	++++	+
Amyloidosis	++++	+
Focal segmental glomerulosclerosis	+++	++
Mesangioproliferative glomerulonephritis	++	++
Membranoproliferative glomerulonephritis	++	+++
Proliferative glomerulonephritis	++	+++
Acute poststreptococcal glomerulonephritis	+	++++
Crescentic glomerulonephritis[a]	+	++++

[a]Can be immune complex-mediated, antiglomerular basement membrane antibody-mediated, or associated with antineutrophil cytoplasmic autoantibodies.

Nephritic Syndrome

Glomerular bleeding resulting in hematuria is typical in nephritic syndrome. Dysmorphic red cells, especially acanthocytes, are a sensitive and specific marker of glomerular bleeding. The presence of pus and cellular and granular casts in the urine is common. The extent of proteinuria is variable. Patients with severe nephritic glomerular injury have renal function impairment because of the reduced glomerular surface area available for filtration, as a result of constriction of the capillary lumen by proliferating mesangial cells or inflammatory cells.

Nephrotic Syndrome

Nephrotic syndrome is characterized by proteinuria greater than 3.5 g/day per 1.73 m^2, hypoproteinemia, edema, and hyperlipidemia. A hypercoagulable state may also be present in some patients. The syndrome may be the result of primary diseases of the glomerulus, or be associated with systemic diseases such as diabetes mellitus, lupus, amyloidosis, and preeclampsia. Hypoproteinemia, especially hypoalbuminemia, results from increased urinary loss of albumin and an increased rate of catabolism of filtered albumin by proximal tubular cells. The compensatory increase in hepatic synthesis of albumin is insufficient to replenish the protein loss, probably because of malnutrition.

Edema formation in patients with nephrotic syndrome was traditionally thought to be driven by the reduced plasma oncotic pressure secondary to hypoalbuminemia. If the oncotic pressure is low, the movement of fluid from the vascular space to the interstitial compartment results in a reduction of the plasma volume, which can trigger compensatory renal sodium and water retention through the activation of the renin–angiotensin–aldosterone axis, vasopressin, and the sympathetic nervous system (the "underfill" mechanism). However, experimental data reveal that the plasma volume is actually normal or elevated. Hypoalbuminemia may not cause edema until the serum albumin concentration is less than 2 g/dL (20 g/L). In addition, the transcapillary oncotic pressure gradient is not as high as previously thought because increased lymphatic flow reduces the interstitial oncotic pressure by removing protein and fluid from the interstitium, thereby reducing the transcapillary oncotic pressure gradient.[5] Instead, fluid retention is likely mediated by a primary increase in sodium reabsorption at the distal nephron, which is probably caused by tubular resistance to the action of atrial natriuretic peptide (the "overflow" mechanism).[6] It is likely that both mechanisms may contribute to nephrotic edema in different patients.[6]

Albuminuria greater than 3 g daily is associated with a significant increase in serum cholesterol concentrations for patients with primary glomerular disease.[7] Hyperlipidemia in nephrotic syndrome is characterized by elevated serum total cholesterol and triglyceride concentrations, with increased very-low-density lipoprotein (VLDL) and low-density lipoprotein (LDL) cholesterol concentrations. Lipoprotein (a) levels may also be increased. The reduced plasma oncotic pressure as a result of hypoalbuminemia may stimulate hepatic synthesis of lipids and lipoproteins. The increased VLDL production and increased liver cholesterol synthesis, along with a decrease in LDL receptor activity, can then lead to an increase in LDL cholesterol concentrations. In addition, reduced serum albumin or the loss of a liporegulatory substance may result in reduced VLDL clearance.[8] Nephrotic patients with hyperlipidemia, especially those with concomitant hypertension, are presumed to have an increased risk for atherosclerotic vascular disease. Hyperlipidemia also promotes the progression of glomerular injury, as evidenced by glomerulosclerosis, mesangial expansion, and hyalinosis.[8,9]

Many patients with nephrotic syndrome have a hypercoagulable state caused by defects of several control proteins in the coagulation cascade. The concentration of the coagulation inhibitor antithrombin III is reduced because of increased loss in the urine. A reduced amount of the coagulation inhibitors proteins C and S, along with increased concentrations of factors V and VIII, increased fibrinogen concentrations, and abnormal platelet function, may also contribute to the hypercoagulable state. The net result of these alterations in coagulation is an increased risk for arterial and venous thrombosis, especially in the deep veins and renal veins. As many as 25% of patients with membranous nephropathy may have renal vein thrombosis.

TABLE 32-2 Evaluation of Patients Suspected of Having Glomerular Disease

Medical history

To identify symptoms of medical conditions that may cause glomerular disease

- Diabetes mellitus
- Amyloidosis
- Systemic lupus erythematosus
- Other familial conditions associated with renal disease

To identify symptoms suggestive of nephrotic syndrome

- Reduced appetite
- Fatigue
- Weight gain
- Edema

Medication, environmental, and occupational histories

To identify possible exposure to potentially nephrotoxic drugs, toxins, or chemicals

Physical examination

To identify signs and symptoms associated with systemic diseases

- Hypertension
- Rash
- Arthritis
- Retinopathy
- Neuropathy
- Lymphadenopathy
- Hepatomegaly
- Malignancy

Laboratory evaluation

Urinalysis

- To determine nephrotic nature of glomerular disease
  - Proteinuria, >3.5 g/day/1.73 m^2
  - Lipiduria
- To determine nephritic nature of glomerular disease
  - Hematuria
  - Pyuria
  - Cellular, granular casts

Glomerular filtration rate

- To determine extent of glomerular damage

Other tests

- To identify type and etiology of glomerular disease
  - Serum complement concentration
  - Antinuclear and anti-DNA antibodies
  - Antistreptolysin antibodies
  - Circulating antiglomerular basement membrane antibodies
  - Cryoglobulins

Percutaneous renal biopsy

- To provide definitive diagnosis of glomerular disease

DIAGNOSTIC CONSIDERATIONS

Patients with suspected glomerular disease should have an extensive medical history obtained to identify potential systemic causes (Table 32-2). Medication, environmental, and occupational histories may also help identify possible exposure to potentially nephrotoxic agents. A carefully conducted physical examination and laboratory evaluation may reveal the presence of systemic diseases that may contribute to the development of glomerular disease (Fig. 32-2). In addition, the patient's age, gender, and ethnic background may be helpful in pinpointing the specific type of glomerular disease. Many of the conditions are more prevalent in certain age groups, although they may occur at any age. For example, proliferative glomerulonephritis is more common in those younger than 40 years of age, whereas the incidence of membranous glomerulonephritis is dramatically higher in those older than 50 years of age.

Laboratory evaluation such as urinalysis can help differentiate the nephrotic or nephritic nature of the disease. The glomerular filtration rate (GFR) may be used to determine the extent of glomerular damage. In the early stages of the disease, the GFR may remain normal. Initial injury to the glomerulus primarily lowers the permeability coefficient (K_f) of the GBM by reducing the surface area available for filtration and/or the unit permeability of the membrane. The reduced permeability is compensated by an elevation in the glomerular capillary hydrostatic pressure through afferent arteriolar dilation and efferent arteriolar constriction. Extensive glomerular damage may therefore be present before a substantial reduction of total GFR is evident.

Although the cause of glomerular disease may be established from clinical and laboratory evaluation, sometimes percutaneous renal biopsy may be needed to provide a definitive diagnosis.

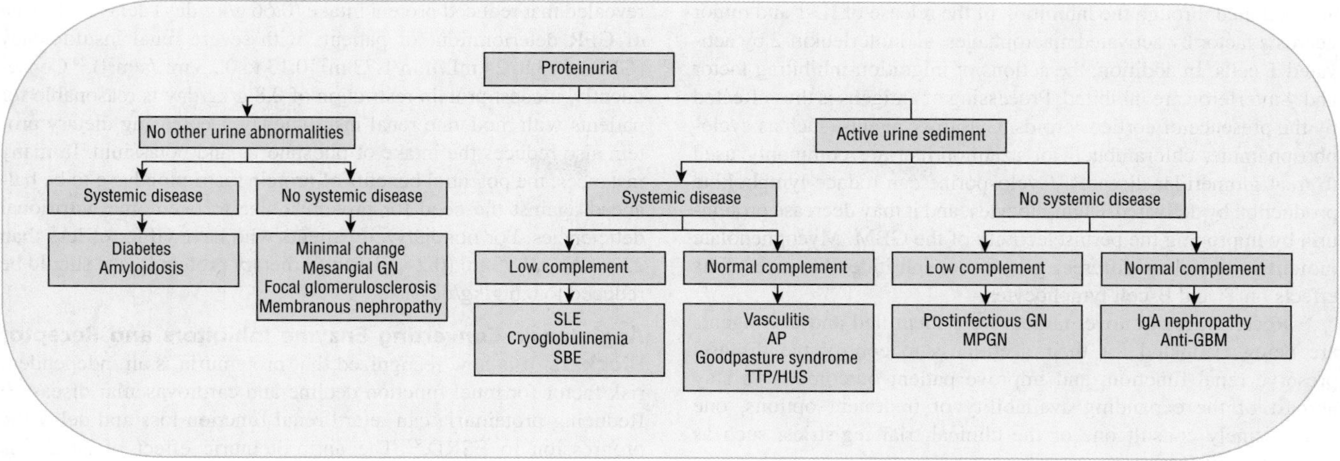

FIGURE 32-2 Clinical presentations of glomerulonephritis. (AP, anaphylactoid purpura; GBM, glomerular basement membrane; GN, glomerulonephritis; HUS, hemolytic uremic syndrome; IgA, immunoglobulin A; MPGN, membranoproliferative glomerulonephritis; SBE, subacute bacterial endocarditis; SLE, systemic lupus erythematosus; TTP, thrombotic thrombocytopenic purpura.)

TREATMENT

General Approach to Treatment

The course and prognosis of the different glomerular diseases are extremely variable and depend on the underlying etiology. In glomerular diseases with a secondary cause, such as poststreptococcal glomerulonephritis (PSGN), after the initiating factor is removed, the prognosis of the renal disease is often good. In contrast, the rates of renal function deterioration among the primary glomerulonephritides vary markedly. The majority of patients with minimal-change disease, IgA nephropathy, and membranous nephropathy have a fairly good prognosis. However, those with focal segmental glomerulosclerosis (FSGS) who are resistant to therapy, as well as those with rapidly progressive glomerulonephritis (RPGN) who are untreated, are likely to experience rapid loss of renal function. In some instances, half of the renal function may be lost within a 3-month period. Certain glomerulonephritides, such as minimal-change nephropathy, are very responsive to treatment while patients with membranous proliferative glomerulonephritis are rarely responsive to existing therapies.

Because of the variable courses exhibited by the different glomerulonephritides, specific treatment approaches have been developed for each disease. When natural history of the glomerulonephritis is well delineated, it is more likely that potential regimens can be designed and evaluated from both therapeutic and economic perspectives. The potential therapeutic benefits of treatment regimens should always be weighed against the risks to which the patients are being exposed. It is therefore imperative to identify patients who are most likely to benefit from treatment, especially those who have other risk factors that may contribute to the deterioration of their renal function. In those instances in which satisfactory regimens are not available to treat the primary disease, appropriate supportive measures should be employed. Optimization of systemic and glomerular blood pressure, reducing proteinuria, and possibly controlling hyperlipidemia may all improve the long-term outcome as well as the quality of life of these patients.

KDIGO (Kidney Disease: Improving Global Outcomes) is a global nonprofit foundation dedicated to improving the care and outcomes of kidney disease patients worldwide through promoting coordination, collaboration, and integration of initiatives to develop and implement clinical practice guidelines for many kidney diseases through its work groups of experts.[10] The quality of evidence and strength of recommendations were graded. Many of these clinical practice guidelines are referenced in the ensuing sections on the treatment of individual primary glomerular diseases.

Nonpharmacologic Therapy

3 For patients with nephrotic syndrome, dietary measures involve restriction of sodium intake to 50 to 100 mEq/day (50 to 100 mmol/day),[11] protein intake of 0.8 to 1 g/day,[11,12] and a low-lipid diet of less than 200 mg cholesterol. Total fat should account for less than 30% of daily total calories.[11] Sodium restriction is important not only in the control of edema, but also in the control of hypertension and proteinuria. Similarly, protein restriction not only helps to reduce proteinuria but also has a potential role in retarding the progression of renal disease. Patients should also stop smoking because a dose-dependent increase in risk for developing ESRD was observed in men with primary inflammatory (immunoglobulin A glomerulonephritis) or noninflammatory (polycystic kidney disease) renal diseases.[13]

Because many immune factors are implicated in the pathogenesis of glomerulonephritis, plasmapheresis may be used to remove these mediators. During the procedure, whole blood is removed from the body and centrifugation is used to separate the cellular elements from the plasma. The cells are then infused back to the patient after resuspension in saline or plasma substitute. The plasma proteins, presumably including the pathogenic immune factors, are thereby removed from the patient.

Pharmacologic Therapy

Immunosuppressive Agents

Immunosuppressive agents, alone or in combination, are commonly used to alter the immune processes that are responsible for the glomerulonephritides. Corticosteroids, in addition to their immunosuppressive effect, also possess antiinflammatory activities. They reduce the production and/or release of many substances that mediate the inflammatory process, such as prostaglandins, leukotrienes, platelet-activating factors, tumor necrosis factors, and interleukin-1 (IL-1). Movement of leukocytes and macrophages to the site of inflammation is also inhibited. The immunosuppressive effects of corticosteroids are mediated through the inhibition of the release of IL-1 and tumor necrosis factor by activated macrophages, and interleukin-2 by activated T cells. In addition, the actions of migration-inhibiting factor and γ-interferon are inhibited. Processing of antigens is thus affected by the presence of corticosteroids. Cytotoxic agents, such as cyclophosphamide, chlorambucil, or azathioprine, are commonly used to treat glomerular diseases. Cyclosporine can reduce lymphokine production by activated T lymphocytes, and it may decrease proteinuria by improving the permselectivity of the GBM. Mycophenolate mofetil is useful in different glomerulonephritides because of its effects on T- and B-cell lymphocytes.

Recently, many novel targets were identified and new agents are being evaluated for their usefulness to control the disease, preserve renal function, and improve patient outcome.[14] To stay abreast of the expanding availability of treatment options, one can routinely consult one of the clinical trial registries, such as *www.clinicaltrials.gov*.

Diuretics

Management of nephrotic edema involves salt restriction, bed rest, and use of support stockings and diuretics. However, severe salt restriction is difficult to achieve and prolonged bed rest can predispose nephrotic patients to thromboembolism. Hence the use of a loop diuretic such as furosemide is frequently required. Although the delivery of diuretic to the kidney tubules is normal, the presence of large amounts of protein in the urine promotes drug binding, and thereby reduces the availability of the diuretic to the luminal receptor sites. In addition, reduced sodium delivery to the distal tubule secondary to decreased glomerular perfusion may also alter diuretic effectiveness. Large doses of the loop diuretic, such as 160 to 480 mg of furosemide, may be needed for patients with moderate edema (see Chap. 34). In some instances, a thiazide diuretic or metolazone may be added to enhance natriuresis.[11,15] Alternatively, continuous IV infusion of a loop diuretic, such as furosemide 160 to 480 mg/day, may be employed.[16] For patients with morbid edema, albumin infusion may be used to expand plasma volume and increase diuretic delivery to the renal tubules, thus enhancing diuretic effect. However, it may precipitate congestive heart failure and may also reduce therapeutic response to steroid in minimal-change nephropathy. For patients with significant edema, the goal of treatment should be a daily loss of 1 to 2 lb (0.45 to 0.9 kg) of fluid until the patient's desired weight has been obtained.

Antihypertensive Agents

Optimal control of hypertension for patients with glomerular disease is important in reducing both the progression of renal disease and the risk for cardiovascular disease[12] (see Chaps. 3 and 29). The target blood pressure for patients with chronic kidney disease defined by GFR <60 mL/min (<1 mL/s) or albuminuria >300 mg/day is less than 130/80 mm Hg.[17] Angiotensin-converting enzyme inhibitors (ACEIs) and angiotensin II receptor blockers (ARBs) delay the loss of renal function for patients with diabetic and nondiabetic (primarily glomerulonephritis) renal diseases.[18] Nondihydropyridine calcium channel blockers (e.g., diltiazem, verapamil) reduce proteinuria and preserve renal function and could be used as an additional agent. In contrast, the dihydropyridine calcium channel blockers (e.g., nifedipine, amlodipine, or nisoldipine) are effective in lowering blood pressure, but without the benefit of proteinuria reduction.[19]

Antiproteinuria Agents

Dietary protein restriction reduces proteinuria and may retard renal function deterioration. Secondary analysis of the Modification of Diet in Renal Disease Study for patients with moderate renal insufficiency (GFR of 25 to 55 mL/min/1.73 m^2 [0.24 to 0.53 mL/s/m^2]) revealed that reduced protein intake (0.66 g/kg/day) delayed the rate of GFR deterioration for patients with severe renal insufficiency (GFR of 13 to 24 mL/min/1.73 m^2 [0.13 to 0.23 mL/s/m^2]).[20] Consequently, modest protein restriction of 0.8 g/kg/day is reasonable for patients with moderate renal insufficiency. Decreasing dietary protein also reduces the intake of phosphorus and potassium. In many instances, the potential benefits of protein restriction have to be balanced against the need for protein intake to overcome nutritional deficiencies. For nondialyzed patients who have GFRs of less than 25 mL/min/1.73 m^2 (0.24 mL/s/m^2), dietary protein intake should be reduced to 0.6 g/kg/day.[13]

Angiotensin-Converting Enzyme Inhibitors and Receptor Blockers It is now recognized that proteinuria is an independent risk factor for renal function decline and cardiovascular disease.[21] Reducing proteinuria can retard renal function loss and delay the progression to ESRD.[22] The antiproteinuric effect of ACEIs is associated with a fall in filtration fraction, suggesting a reduction in intraglomerular pressure. Recent studies show that ACEIs and ARBs may also have direct effects on podocytes, resulting in reduction of proteinuria and glomerular scarring.[23] In addition, angiotensin-converting enzyme (ACE) inhibition may also reduce the effect of angiotensin II on renal cell proliferation, thereby reducing sclerosis. These beneficial effects on proteinuria are beyond what can be attributed by the drug's antihypertensive effects (see Chaps. 3 and 29).[24,25]

Clinical **Controversy. . .**

Differences in the mechanism of action accountable for proteinuria reduction and renal protective effects of ACEs and ARBs have been espoused by some clinicians and thus combination therapy has been recommended. Others believe that at comparable doses their effects are similar and thus there is no benefit of combination therapy.

The combined use of an ACEI and an ARB reduces the rate of renal function decline more than either treatment alone.[18] A meta-analysis of 21 randomized, controlled studies revealed that combination therapy enhanced the reduction of proteinuria in both diabetic and nondiabetic patients.[26] Combination therapy maximizes blockade of the renin–angiotensin system by counteracting the effects of angiotensin II produced by non-ACE pathways. In addition, with the blockade of the angiotensin II type 1 receptor, the angiotensin II produced by the non-ACE pathways may still act on the angiotensin II type 2 receptors, further facilitating vasodilation.[27] An angiotensin II receptor antagonist should therefore be added to the regimen for those patients who do not attain full and persistent remission of proteinuria with an ACEI alone. A thorough review of the combined use of ACEs and ARBs for diabetic nephropathy and proteinuria reduction is found in Chapter 29.

Nonsteroidal Antiinflammatory Agents Nonsteroidal antiinflammatory drugs (NSAIDs) probably reduce proteinuria through prostaglandin E_2 inhibition, resulting in a reduction of intraglomerular pressure, a decrease in GFR, and restoration of the barrier size selectivity of the GBM.[12] Indomethacin and meclofenamate are the two most evaluated NSAIDs. Their antiproteinuric effect is comparable to that attained with ACEIs, and combined treatment with an ACEI results in additional proteinuria reduction.[28] However, adherence to a low-sodium diet or concurrent use of a diuretic is needed to maximize the antiproteinuric effect. Because of their potential for nephrotoxicity, especially for patients with poor renal function, long-term use of an NSAID for renoprotection is not preferred.[24]

Adrenocorticotropin A synthetic adrenocorticotropin (ACTH) analog has been used in Europe for proteinuria reduction associated with nephrotic syndrome. It was reported to have effects similar to alternating months of steroids and cyclophosphamide.[29] Instead of the synthetic analog, a natural, purified ACTH gel is available in the United States and is approved by the FDA for inducing a remission of proteinuria in the nephrotic syndrome without uremia of the idiopathic type or that due to lupus erythematosus. Favorable response was reported in an observation series of 21 patients in the United States.[30] However, the authors cautioned the interpretation of the results since the data were not derived from a controlled, randomized study. The patients had different glomerular diseases and the long-term effect was not reported.

Statins

An abnormal lipoprotein profile increases the risk of atherosclerosis and coronary heart disease for patients with nephrotic syndrome. It is therefore important to treat patients with persistent nephrotic syndrome and sustained dyslipidemia, especially those with high VLDL and LDL cholesterol levels in the presence of a normal or low high-density lipoprotein cholesterol level (see Chaps. 11 and 29). Therapy is especially needed for those with concurrent atherosclerotic cardiovascular disease, or with additional risk factors for atherosclerosis, such as smoking and hypertension.[8]

A low-fat diet is usually not sufficient to correct hyperlipoproteinemia.[12] β-Hydroxy-β-methylglutaryl-coenzyme A (HMG-CoA) reductase inhibitors, also known as "statins" such as lovastatin, pravastatin, simvastatin, and fluvastatin, are considered the treatment of choice.[12] They reduce total plasma cholesterol concentration, LDL cholesterol, and total plasma triglyceride concentrations.[8] Aside from the lipid-lowering effects, statins may confer renoprotection through different mechanisms, including reduction of cell proliferation and mesangial matrix accumulation and antiinflammatory and immunomodulatory effects.[31] Recent clinical studies show that they can reduce proteinuria and delay renal function loss.[32,33] The combined use of an ACEI with a statin may offer additional benefits in controlling nephrotic hyperlipidemia.[20]

Anticoagulants

Renal vein thrombosis, pulmonary emboli, or other thromboembolic events are serious and common complications of nephrotic syndrome, and are frequently seen in those with membranous nephropathy. Although patients who have documented thromboembolic episodes should be anticoagulated with warfarin until remission of nephrotic syndrome, the use of prophylactic anticoagulation is controversial. A decision analysis study suggested that prophylactic anticoagulation is beneficial for patients with membranous nephropathy.[34] Prophylactic anticoagulation is not recommended for all patients; rather, a "selective" approach or individualized assessment should be conducted to identify those at high risk (i.e., those with severe nephrotic syndrome and a serum albumin concentration <2 to 2.5 g/dL [<20 to 25 g/L]).[34] Also at risk are those who require prolonged bed rest, those receiving high-dose IV steroid therapy, and individuals who are dehydrated as well as postsurgical patients.[12]

Evaluation of Therapeutic Outcomes

The management of patients with glomerulonephritis involves specific pharmacologic therapy for the glomerular disease and supportive measures to prevent and/or treat the pathophysiologic sequelae, namely, hypertension, edema, and progression of renal disease. Although the course of the disease, as well as the specific treatment regimens, varies among the different glomerulonephritis, the monitoring parameters for efficacy assessment are similar. For patients with nephrotic syndrome, supportive therapy should also address the management of extrarenal complications of heavy proteinuria, namely, hypoalbuminemia, hyperlipidemia, and thromboembolism. Because patients with significant proteinuria tend to have more rapid decline of renal function, reduction of proteinuria thus becomes critical in delaying the rate of progression toward ESRD.

TABLE 32-3 Monitoring Parameters to Assess Response to Glomerulonephritis Treatment

Renal function
Serum creatinine concentration
24-h urine collection for creatinine clearance determination
24-h urine collection for urinary protein excretion
Urine protein-to-creatinine ratio
Clinical signs and symptoms
Nephrotic syndrome
Proteinuria
Serum lipid concentrations
Edema
Nephritic presentations
Hematuria
Urinalysis
Complete blood count
Blood pressure
General well-being: appetite, energy level
Kidney biopsy to assess disease progression and response to therapy
Assessment of drug therapy adverse reactions and toxicities

The frequency of monitoring is dependent on the specific glomerulopathy and severity of the disease.

4 Patients should be monitored closely for therapeutic response as well as the development of treatment-related toxicities. Although the rate of renal function deterioration is an important indicator of the long-term success of treatment, resolution of nephrotic and nephritic signs and symptoms associated with the glomerulopathies is an important short-term therapeutic target (see Table 32-3).

Serum creatinine concentration as well as creatinine clearance should be evaluated prior to and during treatment; 24-hour urine outflow should be collected to determine the extent of proteinuria. Alternatively, the daily urine protein excretion may be estimated from the urinary total protein-to-creatinine concentration ratio. After establishing the correlation between the 24-hour urinary protein excretion and the protein-to-creatinine ratio, single, random urine specimens may be used in place of a 24-hour urine collection. Blood pressure should be monitored periodically to assess the need for and the adequacy of antihypertensive therapy. The pressures should also be evaluated in conjunction with clinical signs and symptoms of edema and fluid overload to gauge the need for volume control as well as diuretic use. For patients with nephrotic syndrome, serum lipid concentrations should be monitored. If the patient has hematuria, urinalysis and a complete blood count should be obtained. The clinician should also be aware of the patient's appetite and energy level, because these are indicators of the patient's overall state of well-being. At times, renal biopsy is needed to assess response to treatment and disease progression, to determine future treatment strategy, and to confirm the initial diagnosis.

Patients receiving cytotoxic drug treatment should be evaluated for drug-related toxicities every week during the initial treatment period. After 1 month of treatment, the frequency of monitoring may be reduced. When the patient is on long-term steroid treatment, monthly visits are often required for assessment of both efficacy and toxicities. If a favorable response is obtained after a course of treatment, the patient may be evaluated every 3 to 4 months. The patient's renal function, proteinuria, urinalysis, blood pressure, lipid profile, and the overall state of health should be assessed during these regular follow-up visits.

Minimal-Change Nephropathy

Epidemiology and Etiology

Minimal-change nephropathy (also termed nil disease or minimal-change disease) is commonly found in children, accounting for about 85% to 90% of all cases of nephrotic syndrome in children between 1 and 4 years of age. The percentage drops gradually to less than 50% after age 10 years and accounts for less than 20% of all cases of idiopathic nephrotic syndrome in adults. Secondary causes of minimal-change nephropathy include drug administration (e.g., NSAIDs, lithium, interferons), lupus, and various T-cell–related disorders, such as Hodgkin's disease and leukemias.

Pathophysiology

Minimal-change disease is characterized by the absence of definitive pathologic changes observed under light and immunofluorescence microscopy. The characteristic lesion in patients with minimal-change disease, as visualized under electron microscopy, is the spreading and fusion of the foot processes of epithelial cells over an unchanged GBM. Lipoid nephrosis is another term that has been used to describe this type of glomerular disease because lipids, as well as renal tubular cells, are found in the urine. The pathogenesis of minimal-change disease is unknown. Altered cell-mediated immunologic response, specifically T-cell dysfunction or changes in the T-cell subpopulations, may be responsible. The activated lymphocytes are thought to secrete lymphokines that reduce the production of anions in the GBM. The permeability of the GBM to plasma albumin is increased through a reduction of electrostatic repulsion. The loss of anionic charges also results in fusion of the epithelial cell foot processes. Other vascular permeability factors, such as hemopexin, interleukin-4, and vascular endothelial growth factor, also have been suggested to be responsible.

Clinical Presentation

Most patients present initially with edema, frequently acute in onset, following a nonspecific upper respiratory tract infection, allergic reaction, or vaccinations, which might have activated the T lymphocytes. Nephrotic syndrome with massive proteinuria (substantially more than 40 mg/m^2/h for children and >3 to 3.5 g/day for adults), edema, hypoalbuminemia, and hyperlipidemia is common. The patient's weight may increase dramatically because of sodium and fluid retention. Nephritic features, such as gross hematuria, are uncommon. Hypertension and decreased renal function are uncommon in children but are more common in older adults.[35] For some patients, volume depletion may result in mild-to-moderate azotemia.

TREATMENT

Pharmacologic Therapy

Steroids

5 Minimal-change disease is most responsive to initial treatment with corticosteroids. In children, steroid therapy is expected to reduce proteinuria in approximately 90% of the patients, with >95% 10-year renal survival. Because of the excellent response to initial therapy with steroids and the prevalence of this glomerular disease in children, reduction of proteinuria secondary to steroid treatment is considered diagnostic for minimal-change disease without the need for biopsy. Prednisone is commonly administered at 60 mg/m^2 per day initially for 4 to 6 weeks. The dose is then reduced to 40 mg/m^2 per day every other day for another 4 to 6 weeks, with or without tapering afterward (Fig. 32-3).[36] Proteinuria will disappear in 50% of patients after 1 week and in 90% of patients after 4 weeks of treatment. Different

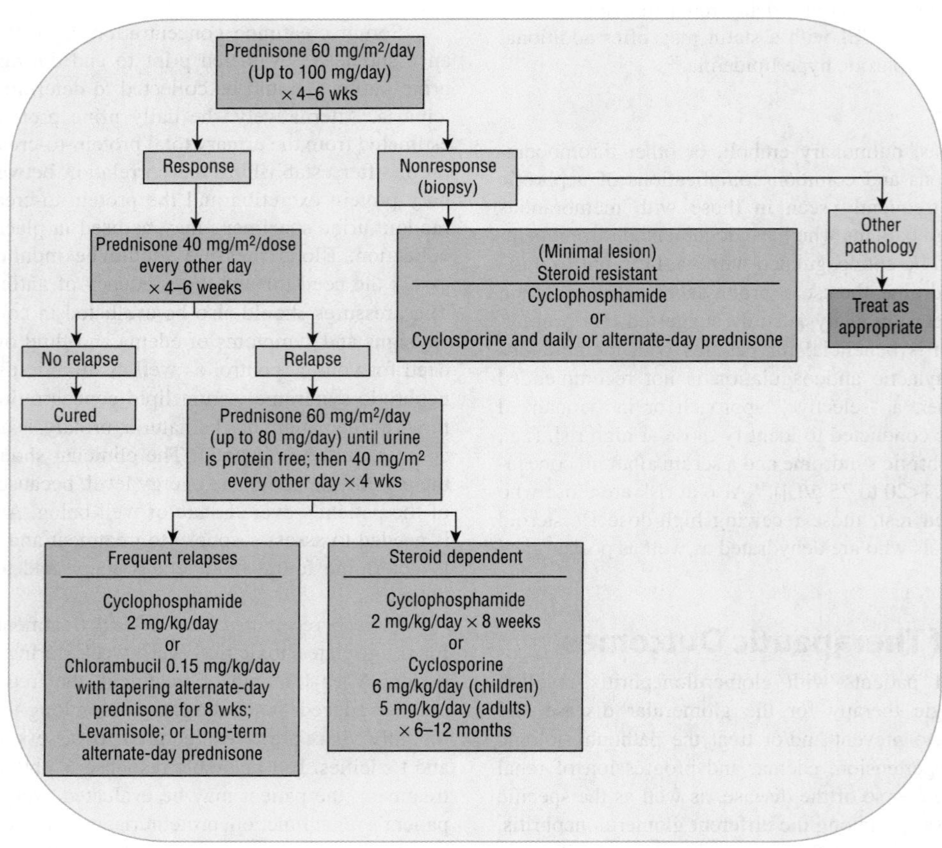

FIGURE 32-3 Treatment algorithm for minimal-change nephropathy. *(Reprinted by permission from Macmillan Publishers Ltd: from reference 36.)*

versions of the steroid regimen are available as there is no consensus on the optimal dose and duration. Studies are being conducted to identify the best strategy to induce remission, reduce disease recurrence, and minimize adverse effects of the therapy. Commonly, the initial episode is treated with an extended course (months) of therapy, followed by shorter treatment (weeks) for relapses.[37]

For adults, prednisone 1 mg/kg per day is given initially for 4 weeks with a reduction to 0.75 mg/kg every other day for the next 4 weeks. Proteinuria will disappear in 50% to 60% of patients after 8 weeks of treatment, and complete remission will be attained in 80% of patients after 28 weeks of therapy.[35]

Relapse As many as 85% of the patients who respond to initial steroid therapy (steroid sensitive) will experience a relapse of proteinuria, mostly within 6 to 12 months after disease onset. The risk of relapse is affected by the duration of initial steroid therapy.[12,36] Children who were asymptomatic with proteinuria diagnosed during routine urine screening tend to have less frequent relapses and a more favorable clinical course. In those who relapse, 50% to 65% may have steroid-responsive relapse episodes over the subsequent 3- to 5-year period. The dose and duration of steroid treatment for the relapse do not influence the subsequent rate of relapse.[12,36] Commonly, 60 mg/m^2 per day of prednisone is given until the urine is free of protein for 3 days, to be followed by 4 weeks of alternate-day prednisone at 40 mg/m^2 per dose.[36]

Frequent Relapse Approximately 10% to 20% of children that are responsive to steroid will experience three or four relapses. Half of them will then relapse frequently and become steroid dependent, requiring continuous low-dose alternate-day prednisone to maintain an extended relapse-free period.[36] A small number of patients eventually develop resistance to steroids, and a biopsy done at that time often reveals another pathology such as FSGS. It is controversial whether minimal-change disease progresses into FSGS or whether the glomerulosclerosis that was present at the time of initial diagnosis was inadvertently diagnosed as minimal-change nephropathy because of tissue-sampling error during the renal biopsy.

Cytotoxic Agents

Cytotoxic agents are often considered for patients who are steroid resistant, as well as for those who require large doses of steroids to sustain remission (steroid dependent). These agents are also beneficial for pediatric patients who experience growth inhibition secondary to chronic use of steroids.[12] Cytotoxic agents are effective in inducing remission and the duration of remission tends to be longer than that induced by steroids. In those patients who relapse after cytotoxic therapy, they may respond to steroids better than before.

Cyclophosphamide at 2 mg/kg per day for 10 to 12 weeks given alone or with prednisone (50 to 75 mg/m^2) is very effective in inducing remission and restoring steroid responsiveness for patients who were previously steroid dependent and then became steroid resistant. Alternatively, chlorambucil at 0.1 to 0.2 mg/kg per day may be used. This agent, however, is associated with more adverse effects than cyclophosphamide. Azathioprine has also been used; however, treatment for 6 to 12 months is often needed before any favorable response is apparent.

The immunosuppressive effect of cytotoxic agents, with or without the concurrent use of steroids, can result in serious infections, which are the primary cause of death for patients with minimal-change nephropathy. Other toxicities associated with cyclophosphamide include gonadal fibrosis, which results in sterility, hemorrhagic cystitis, alopecia, and a potential to develop malignancy in those on long-term treatment.

Calcineurin Inhibitors

Cyclosporine decreases lymphokine production by activated T lymphocytes and thereby reduces proteinuria by reversing the lymphokine-induced alterations in the anionic charge and permeability of the GBM to albumin. For patients with steroid-sensitive or steroid-dependent disease, cyclosporine induces remission in 80% to 85% of patients. However, the disease-free period is not often sustained, and relapse, which is usually not as responsive to cyclosporine retreatment, may occur as soon as the drug is tapered or discontinued. The steroid-sparing effect of cyclosporine is also useful for steroid-dependent patients, especially those who have experienced significant adverse effects.

Dosage The usual starting dose of cyclosporine for remission induction is 5 mg/kg per day for adults and 100 to 150 mg/m^2 per day for children. Similar dosages are used to maintain remission long term. The optimal cyclosporine blood concentrations, as well as the need to monitor them, are controversial. No correlation has been found between the severity of the cyclosporine-induced tubulointerstitial lesions and the mean dose or trough drug concentration. However, monitoring of the area under the serum concentration–time curve has been suggested and target exposures have been proposed.[38] Testing the in vitro sensitivity of peripheral blood lymphocytes to cyclosporine in the presence of a T-cell mitogen may offer a novel method to predict response and individualize therapy.[39]

Adverse Events Adverse events such as rise in serum creatinine, hypertrichosis, and gingival hyperplasia are quite common. Long-term therapy may result in persistent hypertension and progressive renal failure. Cyclosporine should not therefore be given for more than 4 months in the absence of any beneficial effect. Consequently, it is indicated for patients (a) who relapse frequently or are steroid dependent, after failing to respond to a course of cyclophosphamide; (b) for whom cyclophosphamide is contraindicated or when gonadal toxicity is a concern; (c) who are steroid dependent when a "steroid holiday" is needed for catch-up growth and puberty; or (d) who have steroid-resistant disease.[36]

Levamisole

Levamisole, an immunostimulant, can promote the maturation of young T cells and restore the function of T cells and phagocytes when the immune system is depressed. It may also inhibit the production of an immunosuppressive lymphokine. Levamisole was found to have a steroid-sparing effect and was capable of maintaining remission in children who had frequent relapse steroid-dependent nephrotic syndrome.[40] In addition, it is as effective as cyclophosphamide in reducing relapse rate and steroid dosages.[41] The adverse effect of levamisole are mild neutropenia, which is generally reversible, and GI upsets. At present the drug is no longer available in the United States; however, it is recommended by the KDIGO guidelines as a steroid-sparing agent.[10]

Mycophenolate Mofetil

Mycophenolate mofetil is an immunosuppressant that can suppress T- and B-cell lymphocyte proliferation, B-lymphocyte antibody production, and expression of adhesion molecules. It is reported to have steroid-sparing effects and is useful in frequently relapsing, steroid-dependent and steroid-resistant patients, as well as in those who fail cytotoxic therapy.[42]

Rituximab

Rituximab has been observed to induce long-term remission with repeated doses,[43] possibly through a direct effect on the podocyte actin cytoskeleton. However, its use is not recommended by the KDIGO clinical practice guidelines due to the lack of randomized trials and risk for serious adverse effects.[10]

Prognosis

The long-term prognosis of most patients with minimal-change disease is good. The majority of pediatric patients will not experience any relapse of the disease 10 years after the initial onset, and most will be free of the proteinuria after puberty. In adults, an 85% to 90% survival rate is seen 10 years after disease onset. Although this condition may spontaneously remit in up to 70% of untreated adults, life-threatening complications may be associated with untreated nephrotic syndrome. Significant deterioration in renal function is uncommon in both adult and pediatric patients and is observed only in those who are steroid resistant or steroid dependent. Because of the overall favorable outcome of the disease and the relatively uncommon progression into chronic renal failure, aggressive use of cytotoxic agents is not indicated even for most patients with frequent relapses. Toxicities associated with aggressive therapy do not justify the need to induce remission in those patients who fail to respond to steroids and the nonaggressive use of cytotoxic agents. Symptomatic therapy with diuretics to control edema, in conjunction with a low-salt diet and albumin infusion as needed for acute development of anasarca, is often a more rewarding therapeutic approach. NSAIDs and ACEIs may also be used to reduce the proteinuria.

Focal Segmental Glomerulosclerosis

Etiology and Epidemiology

FSGS is a clinicopathologic condition that can be idiopathic (primary) or secondary to a variety of causes. FSGS accounts for less than 20% of the cases of idiopathic nephrotic syndrome in children and approximately 40% in adults[44]; however, it may account for 36% to 80% of the cases in African Americans. The incidence of FSGS has been rapidly increasing, so that it now is the most common glomerular disease that ultimately leads to ESRD. Conditions such as sickle cell disease, cyanotic congenital heart disease, and morbid obesity can induce hemodynamic stress on an initially normal nephron population and result in FSGS. Severe glomerular injury can also be seen in patients with nephropathy associated with heroin abuse, human immunodeficiency virus (HIV) infection, and genetic mutations involving the podocin and WT1 genes. A recent case series identified the association of FSGS and proteinuria in bodybuilders after long-term anabolic steroid abuse.[45] In addition, heroin, pamidronate, and interferon have been associated with FSGS.[44] The primary and secondary sclerotic lesions may be morphologically similar, but they represent diseases with different courses and responses to therapy.

Pathophysiology

Sclerotic lesions are characteristically found in some of the glomeruli (focal) and usually involve only a portion of the glomeruli (segmental).[44] Similar to minimal-change disease, fusion of foot processes is commonly seen in those glomeruli that are not sclerotic. It is thought that both minimal-change disease and FSGS share similar pathogenetic mechanisms, with FSGS resulting in severe injury to the glomerular epithelial cells. During the early stage of FSGS, only a small number of glomeruli may have the segmental sclerotic lesion, and the disease may be confined to the juxtamedullary region. If an inadequate number of glomeruli are sampled during renal biopsy, the diagnosis of FSGS may be missed, or the patient may be thought to have minimal-change disease. Resistance to steroid therapy may thus be one of the first clues that the patient, indeed, has FSGS rather than minimal-change disease. Alternatively, a patient may have the steroid-sensitive minimal-change disease initially, which subsequently progresses to steroid-resistant FSGS.

Clinical Presentation

Almost all the patients present with proteinuria, and many of them have all the features of nephrotic syndrome. The proteinuria is nonselective, containing albumin and other higher-molecular-weight proteins, and is usually less severe when compared to patients who have minimal-change disease. Hypertension, microscopic hematuria, and renal dysfunction may be seen in up to half of the patients. Reduced renal function becomes more prevalent as the disease progresses.

The presenting clinical features in nephrotic adults with minimal-change nephropathy can be indistinguishable from that of FSGS, and renal biopsy is therefore critical in the diagnosis of adults with nephrotic syndrome. African Americans have a fourfold higher risk of developing FSGS than white or Asian patients. They tend to develop the disease earlier and present with nephrotic range proteinuria more often. They are less responsive to steroids and are more likely to experience a rapid decline in renal function, resulting in ESRD.

TREATMENT

Pharmacologic Therapy

The treatment of FSGS is controversial because of the lack of data from randomized, prospective, controlled trials.

Steroids

A course of prednisone (1 to 2 mg/kg/day) with tapering after 3 to 6 months of treatment is first used for nephrotic patients.[44] Urinary protein excretion and serum albumin concentration should be monitored to assess efficacy. The median time to induce complete remission is 3 to 4 months, although 5 to 9 months may be needed in some patients. In general, 30% to 50% of all patients are expected to be resistant to steroids, after at least 4 months of therapy. Patients with diffuse mesangial IgM deposition may be prone for steroid resistance.[46]

If the patient develops a relapse after an adequate response to the initial treatment, a second course of steroids is generally sufficient. However, if relapse occurs frequently, cytotoxic agents or cyclosporine would be indicated. For patients who are not nephrotic, their relatively favorable prognosis does not support using steroids or other immunosuppressive agents. However, close follow-up and good blood pressure control with ACEIs are necessary to minimize disease progression.[44]

Most of the studies conducted thus far include mostly white patients. In a retrospective review of 72 patients that included 65 African American patients, steroid use was not associated with renal survival or the induction of proteinuria remission.[47] The initial creatinine level, blood pressure, and severity of renal lesions are significant factors for renal survival. About one third of the patients who received steroids developed complications such as diabetes and significant weight gain.

Cytotoxic Agents

When used with steroids during initial therapy, cytotoxic agents were not found to offer any additional beneficial effect.[44,48] Randomized clinical trials are not available to support their use as first-line therapy.[10]

Calcineurin and Rapamycin Inhibitors

In steroid-resistant patients, cyclosporine therapy has produced a complete or partial remission in 70% of patients, with a relapse rate of 47%.[49] Tacrolimus may also be used with similar effects.[50] Therapy continued for 12 months before slow tapering is more likely to maintain remission. In patients with diabetes, psychiatric disorder, or severe osteoporosis, calcineurin inhibitor may be a first-line therapy due to the concern for steroid side effects.[44] The effect of sirolimus on proteinuria has been found to be conflicting; however, it may cause a rapid decline in GFR, and hence its use for FSGS is not recommended.[51]

Mycophenolate Mofetil

Mycophenolate mofetil has been reported to have favorable effects for patients who were steroid resistant. After inducing remission with high-dose IV methylprednisolone and oral cyclosporine, a combination of cyclosporine and mycophenolate, followed by mycophenolate alone, can sustain long-term remission, preserve renal function, and improve blood pressure control.[52] However, due to the varied experiences from different investigators, further studies are needed to define the role of this agent among the various treatment options.

ACEIs and ARBs

6 Because of the lack of a consistently effective regimen for primary FSGS, many patients with mild disease are treated conservatively. ACEIs and ARBs are effective in reducing proteinuria and stabilizing renal function in many patients with primary or secondary FSGS. Control of blood pressure and hyperlipidemia are important as well.[44] For patients who have nephrotic range proteinuria, an elevated serum creatinine concentration, and interstitial scarring on biopsy, corticosteroids with or without immunosuppressive agents are often used.

Prognosis

ESRD develops within 10 years in 10% or less of the 30% to 50% of adults and children who had attained complete remission.[49] For those patients who are resistant to therapy, the rate of renal function deterioration to ESRD may be rapid, within 1 year, or slow, over as long as 10 to 20 years; approximately 50% develop ESRD within 10 years. Those patients with severe proteinuria (>10 to 15 g/day), high serum creatinine concentration at diagnosis, initial steroid resistance, or interstitial fibrosis on renal biopsy are likely to have a more rapid decline in renal function. African American patients may also have a higher risk. Kidney transplantation is often indicated for those patients who develop ESRD; however, FSGS has recurred in 40% of the renal allografts soon after transplantation.[44] Children, nonblack race, and those with severe disease or rapid progression to ESRD prior to transplantation are more likely to experience a recurrence. The proteinuria may reappear within hours after transplantation, and graft failure may occur in one third to one half of the patients. The median time to recurrence was reported to be 14 days in one study. Although cyclosporine is ineffective in preventing the recurrence of nephrotic syndrome after transplantation, a high dose of the agent (up to 35 mg/kg/day) induces a remission of the recurrent disease. ACEIs and plasmapheresis are also used to prolong graft survival. The effectiveness of these therapies and the rapid recurrence of the disease in the transplanted kidney substantiate the possibility that a circulating humoral mediator is responsible for the nephropathy. Plasmapheresis to remove the mediator was found to be effective in inducing a remission.[44]

Membranous Nephropathy

Etiology and Epidemiology

Membranous nephropathy is the most common disorder responsible for idiopathic nephrotic syndrome in adults, accounting for about 20% to 25% of cases. It is also a frequent cause of renal failure secondary to glomerulonephritis. The hallmark histologic features of membranous nephropathy are glomerular capillary wall thickening with subepithelial deposits under light and electron microscopy. Autoimmunity is responsible for 70% to 80% of the cases. Autoantibodies toward phospholipase A2 receptor (PLA2R) and neutral endopeptidase (NEP) have been discovered recently.[53] The presence of bovine serum albumin (BSA) and anti-BSA antibodies in certain patients suggests that food antigens may be involved in the pathogenesis. Further anti-PLA2R antibodies appear to predict disease activity and response to therapy.[53]

About 25% of adults and 80% of children have secondary causes.[54] In the United States, the most common etiologies are autoimmune diseases (e.g., lupus), infection (e.g., hepatitis B and C), syphilis, neoplasm (e.g., carcinoma of the lung, breast, GI tract, or kidney), and medications (e.g., gold, penicillamine, or captopril). Malaria and schistosomiasis are common causes in other parts of the world. De novo membranous nephropathy can also occur in the allografts of renal transplant patients. Because the responses to therapy as well as the prognosis for idiopathic and secondary membranous nephropathy are different, it is important to identify any potential underlying causes for the nephropathy prior to treatment. Although this glomerular disease can occur at any age, the peak incidence is between ages 30 and 50 years and is especially likely in patients older than age 50 years who present with nephrotic syndrome.[54]

Pathophysiology

Examination of kidney tissue under light microscopy reveals normal mesangium and normocellularity. The glomerular capillary wall may be thickened in well-developed lesions. In the advanced stage, the epithelial side of the capillary wall is markedly thickened, and intramembranous deposits are found. Progressive changes in capillary lumen patency parallel those in the GBM, resulting in glomerulosclerosis with capillary collapse and tubular atrophy in end-stage membranous nephropathy. Immunofluorescence microscopy shows strong capillary wall staining of IgG and C3 on the epithelial side of the basement membrane. Antibody-mediated immune injury appears to be the main pathogenetic mechanism. The immune complex can be formed in situ or deposited from circulating immune complexes.

Clinical Presentation

Most patients with membranous nephropathy present with heavy proteinuria (exceeding 3.5 g/day). Those patients excreting large amounts of IgG and α_1-microglobulin, indicating more significant tubulointerstitial damage, have a lower remission rate, and are more likely to progress toward renal failure.[54]

The signs and symptoms are usually insidious in onset and may consist of anorexia, malaise, edema, anasarca, or ascites, and pericardial and pleural effusions may also be present. As a result of a hypercoagulable state, pulmonary embolism may develop but rarely results in death. The incidence of renal vein thrombosis varies from 5% to 62%, and membranous nephropathy should be suspected when there is a sudden onset of hematuria, loin pain, pulmonary embolus, fluctuating or worsening proteinuria or GFR, renal tubular acidosis, or an increase in leg edema. Hypertension is found in approximately 30% of patients and is more common with renal insufficiency or in advanced disease.

In addition to heavy proteinuria, urinalysis often reveals lipiduria and oval fat bodies. Microhematuria is seen in fewer than 25% of patients, and gross hematuria and red cell casts are rare. In idiopathic membranous nephropathy, the serum complement concentrations are normal. Low levels of complement should alert one to search for secondary causes, such as lupus, hepatitis B infection, or an alternative diagnosis. Similarly, antinuclear antibodies, anti-DNA antibodies, rheumatoid factor, hepatitis B serologies, and serum cryoglobulins are generally negative in idiopathic membranous nephropathy. Occult malignancy has been found in as many as 10% of elderly patients with membranous nephropathy.

TREATMENT

The treatment of idiopathic membranous nephropathy is controversial and ranges from supportive therapy to immunosuppression. Conservative management of patients with mild disease includes edema control with salt restriction and diuretics[5] and reduction of

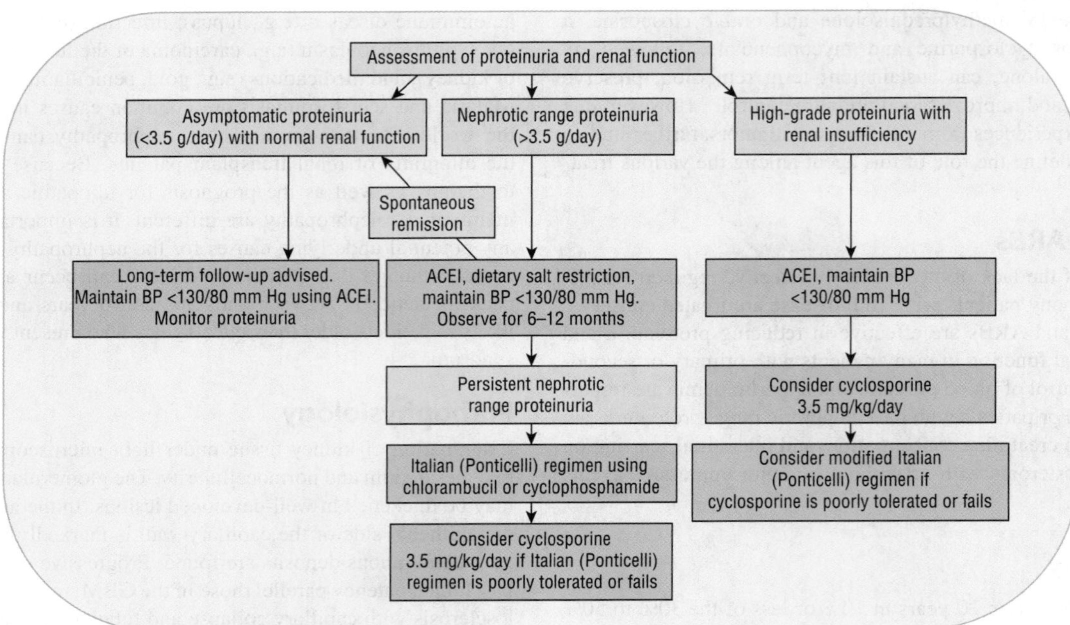

FIGURE 32-4 Treatment algorithm for idiopathic membranous nephropathy. *(Adapted from reference 55.)*

proteinuria with protein restriction and ACEIs (Fig. 32-4).[10,55] Management of hypertension and hyperlipidemia is required for most patients, whereas prophylactic anticoagulation, despite having benefits shown to outweigh the risks, is usually given only for patients with renal vein thrombosis or documented pulmonary embolus.[34,55]

Pharmacologic Therapy

Steroids

Remission of proteinuria, whether spontaneously or treatment related, may confer a good prognosis. Corticosteroids alone were ineffective in improving proteinuria remission rate in all controlled trials and in preventing progression.[56] The result of a meta-analysis also confirmed the lack of efficacy of steroids when used alone.[57]

Cytotoxic Agents

Cytotoxic agents, when used in conjunction with corticosteroids, are effective in increasing the remission rate of proteinuria and preserving renal function.[10] Ponticelli and colleagues devised such a regimen by combining IV methylprednisolone (1 g) for 3 days followed by oral methylprednisolone (0.4 mg/kg) for the subsequent 27 days of months 1, 3, and 5. Oral chlorambucil (0.2 mg/kg) is to be given daily in months 2, 4, and 6.[58] The 10-year renal survival was increased to 92% when compared with 60% in the control group. They later substituted cyclophosphamide (2.5 mg/kg/day) for chlorambucil, which resulted in similar rates of proteinuria remission and relapse, but with fewer serious side effects in those who received cyclophosphamide.[59]

Results from a recent meta-analysis of randomized, controlled trials affirmed that cytotoxic agents, but not steroids, are effective in reducing nephrotic-range proteinuria, with cyclophosphamide having fewer adverse effects than chlorambucil.[56]

Calcineurin Inhibitors

Cyclosporine is effective in reducing proteinuria and rate of renal function decline as well as inducing remission of nephrotic syndrome. Such effects were observed in patients with preserved, declining, or impaired renal function as well as those who are resistant to other immunosuppressants.[56] Results from a retrospective study indicate that using cyclosporine in combination with steroids was more effective in inducing remission than cytotoxic agents with steroids in inducing remission; however, there was more relapse associated with the cyclosporine regimen.[56] The concurrent use of small doses of prednisone tend to favor remission and reduce risk of relapse.[57] However, long-term use of calcineurin inhibitors may increase blood pressure and result in nephrotoxicity, especially in patients with preexisting renal function impairment.[10]

Tacrolimus has been studied by several investigators in small, noncontrolled trials and was found to have efficacy similar to cyclosporine.[10,56]

Alternative Therapeutic Options

Because spontaneous remission is common and only approximately 25% of patients with new-onset idiopathic membranous nephropathy ultimately develop ESRD in 20 to 30 years, it is prudent not to aggressively treat all patients at the onset of the disease. Patients who have a low risk for renal disease progression can be managed with observation and symptomatic therapy. Normalizing the blood pressure and reducing proteinuria with ACEIs and/or ARBs are important as both hypertension and proteinuria are independent risk factors for the progression of renal failure.[54] Patients with low risk for renal disease progression include children 2 to 16 years of age, adult males with proteinuria less than 2 g/day, or adult females with proteinuria less than 5 g/day and normal renal function.

In contrast, patients who have a high risk of developing renal failure, including those with proteinuria greater than 10 g/day with or without impaired renal function, and patients with symptomatic nephrotic syndrome with a plasma albumin of less than 2 g/dL (20 g/L) should be aggressively treated to induce remission. An alkylating agent such as cyclophosphamide or chlorambucil, combined with steroids, should be given to induce remission. Recently, rituximab was shown to be effective in several small studies; however, randomized, controlled trials are not available to elucidate its longer-term effects.[56,60] Treatment decisions should be made in light of the FDA black box warning fort potentially fatal mucocutaneous reactions as well as the risk for severe infection. The effect of eculizumab was evaluated in one trial and was not found to be beneficial.[61]

Favorable results have been reported for mycophenolate mofetil by some investigators with conflicting efficacy by others.[56]

However, it might be a reasonable alternative for patients experiencing significant adverse effects from steroids, alkylating agents, or calcineurin inhibitors. Tetracosactide, a synthetic analog of adrenocorticotropic hormone, has also been shown in small studies to offer results superior to the cytotoxic–steroid combination regimen.[10,29]

The cytotoxic–steroid combination regimen may be effective in inducing remission in the 30% to 40% of the medium-risk patients who relapse within 2 years after treatment discontinuation. Alternately, cyclosporine may be used with similar effectiveness.[54] The cyclophosphamide–steroid combination should also be used for relapse in high-risk patients.

Prognosis

The natural course of idiopathic membranous nephropathy is variable. Up to 30% of the patients experience spontaneous remission, commonly within 2 years of disease onset. Half of the remaining patients have persistent proteinuria with long-term preservation of renal function, while the other half has gradual loss of renal function.[54] Heavy proteinuria (>10 g/day), male gender, elevated serum creatinine concentration at the time of presentation; poorly controlled hypertension, advanced age at onset of disease, non-Asian race, certain human leukocyte antigen phenotypes, and tubulointerstitial fibrosis on initial renal biopsy are associated with progressive renal disease.[54] A predictive algorithm, incorporating the level of proteinuria, initial creatinine clearance, as well as the slope of renal function decline over 6 months, has been developed to determine the risk for disease progression.[54]

In general, patients with idiopathic membranous nephropathy have a relatively benign course with mean 10-year survival of approximately 70%. Those who present with persistent nonnephrotic proteinuria seldom develop renal insufficiency and have a normal life expectancy. Fewer than 10% of patients develop a remitting and relapsing course.[54] The prognosis for secondary membranous nephropathy depends on the underlying cause. Remission occurs when the infection resolves or when the causative medication is withdrawn. For patients with a transplanted kidney, both de novo and recurrent membranous nephropathy may occur. Patients with primary membranous nephropathy are more at risk. Recurrence is typically associated with nephrotic syndrome and a high risk of allograft failure from disease and/or rejection.

Membranoproliferative Glomerulonephritis

Etiology and Epidemiology

Membranoproliferative glomerulonephritis (MPGN) is one of the least-common renal morphologic entities that occur in older children and adults. Although it accounts for 7% to 10% of all case of biopsy-confirmed glomerulonephritis, MPGN is the third or fourth leading cause of ESRD among the primary glomerular diseases.[62] For some unclear reason, the incidence of MPGN has been decreasing over the past few decades in the United States and Europe. However, in Africa and Asia, idiopathic MPGN is still common, perhaps secondary to exposure to unrecognized infectious and parasitic agents.

Pathophysiology

MPGN is a "pattern of injury," rather than a specific disease, caused by many disorders.[10] The several types of MPGN are classified according to the pathologic features. Type I MPGN, also known as mesangiocapillary glomerulonephritis, is characterized by diffuse thickening of glomerular capillary walls and mesangial hypercellularity. Immune complexes are presumed to have a major role in the pathogenesis of type I MPGN, which is the most common type of primary, idiopathic MPGN.

Type II MPGN is also known as dense-deposit disease (DDD) because of the presence of dense deposits of C3 within the GBM, which gives rise to a ribbon-like appearance. Other variants of the disease include type III MPGN, which is seen rarely and consists of subendothelial and subepithelial deposits with lamination and disruption of the lamina densa of the GBM.

Clinical Presentation

Nephrotic syndrome is the most common presenting condition although some patients may also have a nephritic component (hematuria), hypertension, and progressive renal impairment. Hypocomplementemia is commonly seen.

TREATMENT

Pharmacological Treatment

Steroids and Cytotoxic Agents

Results from small uncontrolled studies suggest that certain patients may benefit from various immunosuppressive regimens. However, the lack of randomized, controlled studies makes it difficult to make strong treatment recommendations.[62] For patients with idiopathic MPGN, nephrotic syndrome, and progressive decline of kidney function, the KDIGO guidelines recommend using oral cyclophosphamide or mycophenolate plus low-dose alternate-day or daily steroids for initial therapy trial of no longer than 6 months.[10]

In those with normal kidney function, no active urinary sediment, and nonnephrotic range proteinuria, one may use ACEIs to control blood pressure and reduce proteinuria in light of the favorable long-term outcomes.[62] Patients with secondary MPGN should receive therapy directed against the primary etiology. Figure 32-5 presents an algorithm for a general approach for treatment and follow-up of MPGN.

Antiplatelet Agents

Although several studies have shown dipyridamole and aspirin to reduce proteinuria, reduction of GFR decline was not generally observed.[63] Consequently, the efficacy of antiplatelet therapy for idiopathic MPGN remains in doubt.[10] Similarly, the ability of heparin and warfarin, in combination with steroids and cytotoxic agents, to reduce renal function decline was not confirmed to be sustained.

Alternative Therapeutic Agents

Since steroids are not known to be effective for type II disease other yet-to-be-proven strategies such as rituximab, eculizumab, sulodexide, and plasma infusion or exchange may be considered.[64] It is difficult to conduct large-scale controlled trials for MPGN because of the low incidence of the disease. Based on the available studies, many of the drugs evaluated do not have any consistent, beneficial effect on renal function and proteinuria. Renal transplantation is an alternative; however, the recurrence rate is close to 100% for type II MPGN and is approximately 20% to 30% for type I MPGN. Half of the allografts ultimately fail.

Prognosis

Type I MPGN is a slowly progressive disease that accounts for 80% of all MPGN, but only 5% to 15% of all cases of nephrotic syndrome seen in pediatric and adult patients. It occurs most frequently for patients between 5 and 30 years of age, and because remissions are rare, many patients eventually develop ESRD. The renal survival is 60% to 65% at 10 years, and the presence of nephrotic syndrome, interstitial disease, and hypertension are poor prognostic indicators.[64] Type II MPGN is a more aggressive disease that constitutes approximately 15% of all patients with MPGN. Only 20%

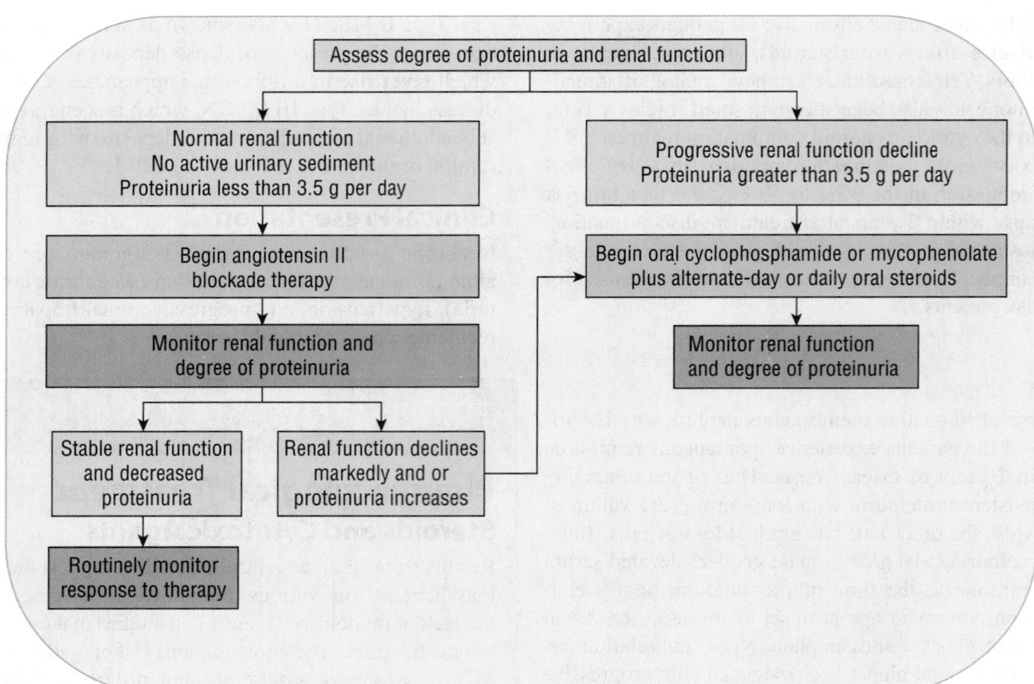

FIGURE 32-5 Treatment algorithm for membranoproliferative glomerulonephritis.

of patients remain stable for more than a few years, and the median time before the development of ESRD is 7 years.

Immunoglobulin A Nephropathy

Etiology and Epidemiology

IgA nephropathy, also known as *Berger's disease*, was first described by Jean Berger in France in 1968. It now is the most common primary glomerulonephritis in the world and accounts for 10% of patients with ESRD in many countries. The prevalence among patients with glomerulonephritis or patients who had kidney biopsy varies from 30% to 35% or as high as 45% in Asia to 30% to 40% in Europe. In the United States, the overall prevalence is approximately 10% to 15% but is as high as 35% among Native Americans living in New Mexico.[65] These differences in prevalence may reflect variations in genetic predisposition, as well as the criteria used for urinary screening and kidney biopsy. The high biopsy rate tends to correlate with high frequency of the disease.

IgA nephropathy is the most common primary glomerulapathy in young adult Caucasians[10] and is two to six times more common in males than in females. It is uncommon in blacks, both in the United States and in Africa.[65] IgA nephropathy was once thought to be a benign disease presenting with asymptomatic hematuria; however, its ability to present with any clinical syndrome associated with glomerular disease is now recognized. Some patients will develop ESRD over variable periods of time.

Pathophysiology

Primary IgA nephropathy is an immune-complex–mediated disease in which IgA deposits and other pathologic lesions are found in kidney tissues. In contrast, Henoch–Schönlein purpura, a systemic disease that is believed to be closely linked to IgA nephropathy, shares similar immunohistologic findings in the kidneys. Both typically have vasculitis affecting the joints, skin, and GI tract, which may result from the same pathologic process of IgA nephropathy. The diagnosis of IgA nephropathy is established by the presence of mesangial IgA deposits upon immunofluorescence examination of the kidney biopsy. The IgA immune complex, composed of IgA antibody bound with an environmental antigen, such as a virus, bacteria, or food substances, is presumed deposited from the systemic circulation. Alternately, the complex may be formed in situ, with the IgA antibody bound with an endogenous antigen in the mesangium. In the mesangium, IgA can bind with receptors on the mesangial cells to induce proliferation and cytokine production. In addition, IgA can activate complement through the alternate pathway to induce glomerular damage. The extent of the injury depends on the characteristics of the IgA that favor mesangial deposition, the susceptibility of the mesangium toward deposition, the ability of the patient to mount an inflammatory response to the deposits, and the response of the kidney to the injury in a way that favors progressive renal damage. The key abnormalities and their implications on treatment was reviewed recently by Boyd et al.[66]

The Oxford histologic classification system has been developed to provide a uniform approach to biopsy evaluation and disease classification.[66,67] Further studies are needed to elucidate its ability to predict renal function loss and response to treatment.

Clinical Presentation

IgA nephropathy commonly presents in the second and third decades of life, but it can occur at any age. Many patients have microscopic hematuria and proteinuria for years, persistently or intermittently, during the early stages of the disease. About half of the patients present with gross hematuria concurrent with an infection, commonly in the upper respiratory tract.[65] The hematuria may occur 1 to 2 days after the onset of infection symptoms, which is different from the 10- to 14-day delay seen after the pharyngitis in PSGN. Proteinuria is common, and nephrotic range often indicates advanced disease. Hypertension and edema are infrequent but are common in PSGN.

Renal dysfunction is uncommon at the initial presentation; however, approximately 10% to 20% of the patients develop ESRD within 10 years, and 30% develop it after 20 years. The extent of proteinuria is one of the strongest predictors of poor long-term outcomes.[68] Uncontrolled hypertension, GFR reduction at disease presentation, and obesity are additional risk factors for developing renal failure.[10,68]

TREATMENT

General Approach to Treatment

Normotensive patients with normal renal function, isolated microhematuria, and minor proteinuria should be observed closely without specific treatment (Fig. 32-6).[68] Patients with minimal proteinuria of 0.5 to 1 g/day should receive optimized supportive therapy, using ACEI or ARB to attain BP of <103/80 mm Hg and urinary protein excretion of <500 mg/day.[25] Combined ACEI and ARB seems to be more effective than monotherapy. For patients with persistent proteinuria ≥1 g/day, steroid therapy for 6 months should be used after 3 to 6 months of optimized supportive care. Fish oil may be used if desired. Immunosuppression should not be used for patients with GFR <30 to 50 mL/min because of the lack of trials to demonstrate beneficial effects.[68] Comprehensive support must be continued in these patients in an attempt to stabilize the renal function.

Nonpharmacologic Therapy

Low-Gluten Diet and Tonsillectomy

Restriction of dietary gluten is effective for patients with celiac disease but not for patients with no identifiable nephritogenic antigens. Removal of the tonsils, which produce IgA_1 and may contribute to IgA nephropathy, may reduce proteinuria and hematuria, as shown in several small, nonrandomized trials in Japan.[66] However, such benefits were not seen in studies in Caucasians. Results from recent meta-analysis does not reveal efficacy when used alone.[69] The KDIGO guidelines therefore do not suggest using tonsillectomy for IgA nephropathy.[10] However, it may be helpful for patients who developed recurrent macroscopic hematuria as provoked by bacterial tonsillitis.

Pharmacological Therapy

Steroids

Corticosteroids with or without immunosuppressive agents have been used to treat IgA nephropathy for many years. A recent meta-analysis showed that steroid therapy is associated with reduction in proteinuria, risk for progression to ESRD, as well as the rate of renal function deterioration.[70] However, optimal antiproteinuric and antihypertensive therapy were not given in some of the studies.[10] Low-dose, short-term (<3 months) steroid therapy is not expected to yield favorable results. In contrast, larger doses of steroids (IV methylprednisolone 1 g/day for 3 days at months 1, 3, and 5 and oral prednisone 0.5 mg/kg every other day for 6 months) were able to reduce proteinuria and renal function deterioration.[71] However, the risk for toxicity with such high doses of steroid might be considered high by some, yet the side effects were reported as minor.[71] The KDIGO guidelines therefore suggest a 6-month course of steroid for patients with persistent proteinuria ≥1 g/day, despite 3 to 6 months of optimized supportive care and GFR of >50 mL/min per 1.73 m^2.[10]

Cytotoxic Agents and Mycophenolate Mofetil

Several studies have evaluated the efficacy of azathioprine and cyclophosphamide. In some of the studies, cyclophosphamide was used in conjunction with dipyridamole, heparin, and warfarin. It is difficult to assess which of these agents contributed to the limited favorable effects observed. In addition, in many of these studies, blood pressure control and ACE inhibition were not always optimal. At present, there is no clear evidence to support the use of these cytotoxic agents for IgA nephropathy.[68] The KDIGO guidelines do not therefore suggest using these agents.[10]

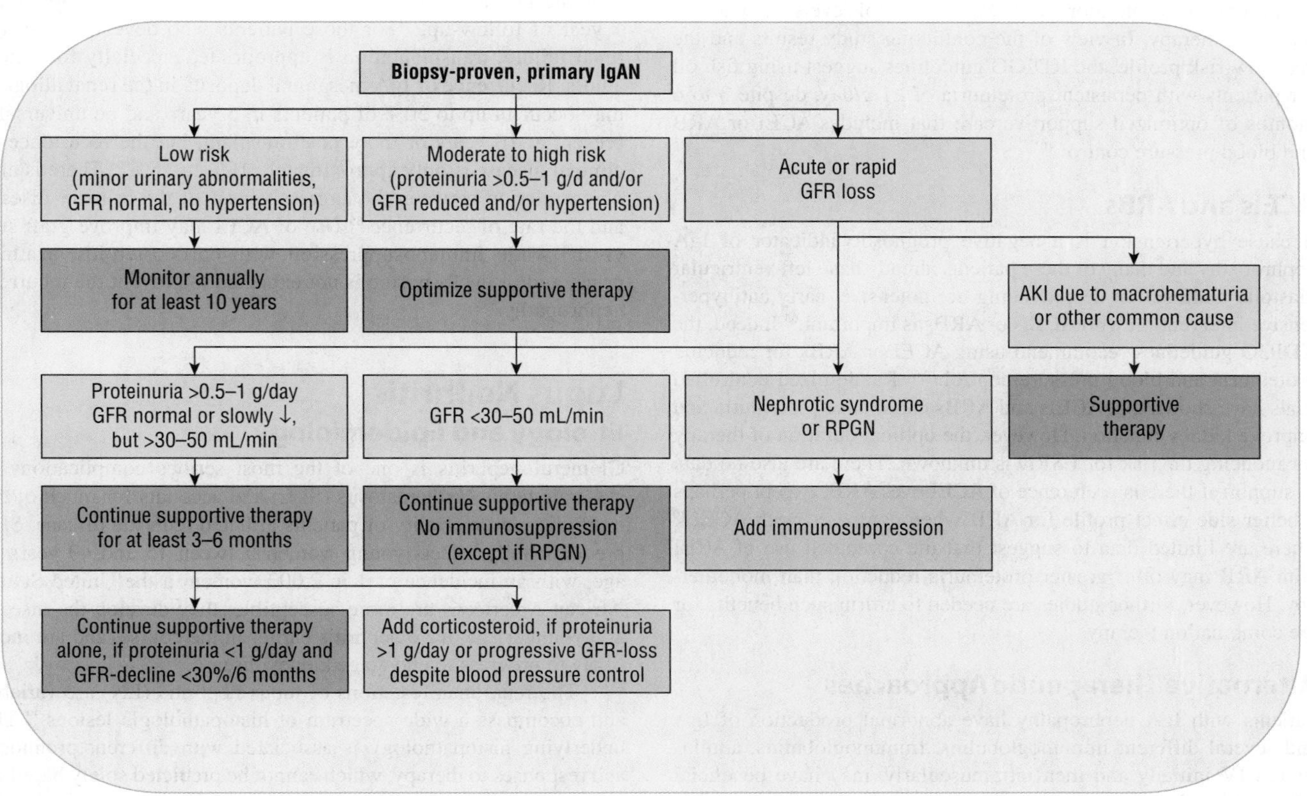

FIGURE 32-6 Treatment algorithm for biopsy-proven IgA nephropathy. *(Adapted from reference 68.)*

Clinical Controversy...

Fish oil has been recommended by some while others have advocated the first-line use of mycophenolate mofetil for the management of patients with IgA nephropathy.

Mycophenolate mofetil have been evaluated for treating IgA nephropathy on the premise that it may reduce IgA synthesis and mesangial uptake and/or suppress the effects of proinflammatory or profibrogenic mediators.[72] Favorable results were observed in two studies in China; however, no such beneficial effects were seen in studies in Belgium and in the United States.[10,69] These heterogeneous results and the potential for adverse effects preclude recommendation to use mycophenolate for IgA nephropathy.[10]

Fish Oil

The third approach is to reduce glomerular inflammation and glomerulosclerosis induced by IgA deposits. Antiinflammatory agents, antiplatelet drugs, and anticoagulants have been tried without success to decrease the production or action of mediators responsible for IgA immune-complex–induced glomerular damage. However, the *n*-3 fatty acids in fish oil reduce the production or action of prostaglandins and leukotrienes, thus limiting the renal damage caused by inflammation, platelet aggregation, and vasoconstriction.[25] In a controlled trial on patients with heavy proteinuria and mildly impaired renal function, daily use of fish oil delayed the progression of renal failure with modest reduction in proteinuria.[73] A meta-analysis of five controlled studies indicated that a minor, but not statistically significant, beneficial effect on renal function may be observed.[74] Results from several recent studies failed to confirm the beneficial effects reported earlier, and further studies are needed to confirm the role as well as the optimal dose. In many of the studies, 4 to 12 g/day were given for two or more years. Some of the fish oil preparations are rich in cholesterol; thus, it is appropriate to monitor the LDL cholesterol levels for patients receiving therapy. In view of the conflicting study results and the very low-risk profile, the KDIGO guidelines suggest using fish oil for patients with persistent proteinuria of ≥1 g/day, despite 3 to 6 months of optimized supportive care that includes ACEI or ARB and blood pressure control.[10]

ACEIs and ARBs

Because hypertension is a negative prognostic indicator of IgA nephropathy and many of these patients already have left ventricular diastolic malfunction despite being normotensive, early antihypertensive intervention with ACEIs or ARBs is important.[65] Indeed, the KDIGO guidelines recommend using ACEI or ARBs for reducing proteinuria and blood pressure control.[10,68] Randomized controlled trials have shown that ACEIs and ARBs can reduce proteinuria and improve kidney function. However, the optimal duration of therapy for reducing the risk for ESRD is unknown. There are also no data to support if there is preference of ACEI over ARB, except perhaps a better side effect profile for ARB when compared with ACEI.[10] There are limited data to suggest that the combined use of ACEI with ARB may offer greater proteinuria reduction than monotherapy. However, further studies are needed to affirm such benefits for the combination therapy.

Alternative Therapeutic Approaches

Patients with IgA nephropathy have abnormal production of IgA and several different immunoglobulins. Immunoglobulins, administered IV initially and then intramuscularly, may have beneficial effects through immunomodulation, increased catabolism of autoantibodies, and blockade of receptors.[75] While favorable results were reported in one trial, large randomized controlled trials are needed to substantiate its efficacy.

Urokinase, danazol, dapsone, sodium cromoglycate, and plasma exchange have also been evaluated, but none is consistently effective nor shown to affect renal function. Cyclosporine, tacrolimus, sirolimus, and mizoribine have been evaluated in a limited number of studies; available results do not support its use for IgA nephropathy.

Antiplatelet agents are commonly used in Japan and rarely outside of Asia for IgA nephropathy.[76] A recent meta-analysis of seven trials (four in Japan and three in Hong Kong) revealed that these agents reduced proteinuria and stabilized renal function.[74] In view of the different agents and concurrent immunosuppressive regimens used among the trials, it would not be possible to derive a recommendation and the KDIGO guidelines do not recommend using these agents.[10]

Prognosis

The majority of the patients with IgA nephropathy have a clinically inconspicuous course and some may experience spontaneous remission. However, others may have an increase in proteinuria and decline in renal function. It is therefore important to follow the patients over a long period of time since progressive disease may appear in 30% of the patients.[68] Spontaneous remission is seen in only 10% to 25% of children and 5% to 7.5% of adults. Unfortunately, no therapy is known to be consistently effective for the treatment of IgA nephropathy. Because of the slow progression of the disease to ESRD, it is very difficult to conduct trials to evaluate the long-term effectiveness of specific treatments. Since the pathophysiological mechanisms of this disease are not well defined, it has been difficult to design and evaluate results of clinical trials.[66]

Urinary protein excretion and the mean arterial blood pressure at follow-up correlate well with the progression of disease. The risk of developing ESRD is proportional to the amount of proteinuria, under the influence of ACEI and ARB therapy, after 1 year of follow-up.[77] For those patients who develop end-stage renal failure, transplantation is appropriate, especially for young adults. Recurrence of IgA mesangial deposits in the renal allograft may occur in up to 50% of patients in 5 years and be universally present at 10 years or more posttransplant, but the recurrence of clinical disease is only approximately 10% to 15%.[65] There is also no correlation between the aggressiveness of the primary disease and the rate of recurrence.[65] Use of ACEI may improve graft survival[78] while immunosuppression with corticosteroids, azathioprine, and/or cyclosporine is not expected to prevent the recurrent nephropathy.[68]

Lupus Nephritis

Etiology and Epidemiology

Glomerulonephritis is one of the most serious complications of systemic lupus erythematosus (SLE) and accounts for much of the morbidity and mortality of patients afflicted with the disease. SLE predominantly affects young women between 15 and 40 years of age, with an incidence of 1 in 2,000 women in the United States. African Americans are more susceptible; they develop the disease at a younger age, have nephritis earlier in the course, and are more likely to progress to end-stage kidney disease.

The renal manifestations of lupus nephritis (LN) are variable and encompass a wide spectrum of histopathologic lesions.[79] The underlying histopathology is associated with different prognoses and responses to therapy, which cannot be predicted solely based on clinical manifestations. Thus, a renal biopsy is required to assess the severity of the disease and to predict the short-term and long-term outcomes associated with therapy. Drugs, such as hydralazine and procainamide, are known to precipitate a lupus syndrome; however, they are unlikely to cause disease that affects the kidney.

Pathophysiology

Immune complex deposits, whether formed in the circulation or in situ, can be found in various regions of the glomerulus, as well as the peritubular interstitium and vasculature outside the glomerulus. Based on light, immunofluorescence, and electron microscopy findings, LN can be categorized into six ISN/RPS (International Society of Nephrology/Renal Pathology Society) classifications: I, minimal-mesangial LN; II, mesangial-proliferative LN; III, focal LN; IV, diffuse LN; V, membranous LN; and VI, advanced sclerosing LN.[80]

The hallmark feature in the pathogenesis of SLE is B-cell hyperactivity and the dysregulated production of autoantibodies against multiple antigens in the body, including DNA and various ribonucleoproteins.[79,81] The size and location of the immune complexes in the glomerulus correlate with the nature and severity of renal injury. Deposition of small numbers of stable immune complexes of intermediate size in the mesangium tends to produce less severe inflammation in the glomerulus. The sequestration of the immune complexes in the mesangium prevents them from activating inflammatory mediators. Hence, the lesion is noninflammatory in nature. In contrast, large numbers of intermediate-sized or large immune complexes result in infiltration of inflammatory cells and release of necrotizing enzymes. In addition, the kidney may also sustain damage through mechanisms related to thrombotic microangiopathy.

Clinical Presentation

Females have a higher risk for developing lupus, especially in the adult years. Nephritis is commonly seen within the first 4 years of diagnosis of SLE but may also be the first manifestation of the disease. The clinical presentation ranges from minimal hematuria and proteinuria to severe, rapidly progressive diffuse glomerulonephritis. Proteinuria is very common, and nephrotic syndrome is seen in most patients with membranous lesions. Microscopic hematuria is almost always present, whereas macroscopic hematuria, which commonly indicates severe renal involvement, is rare. Active urinary sediments (red cell casts, dysmorphic red cells, and hematuria) are suggestive of the diffuse proliferative lesion.[79] Hypertension is present in 25% to 45% of patients and is associated with a worse prognosis. Poor prognosis and higher risk for renal involvement were observed among African American, Hispanic, and Asian patients, compared with white and Puerto Rican–Hispanic patients.[10,82] Other conditions found to be associated with poor prognosis include elevated serum creatinine concentration, heavy proteinuria, anemia (hematocrit <26% [<0.26]), and disease onset during childhood or in those >60 years of age. Most patients have hypocomplementemia and increased antibody titers for anti-double-stranded DNA, particularly those with focal or diffuse proliferative lesions. Serum creatinine concentration at the time of diagnosis is most predictive of short-term outcome.

TREATMENT

General Approach to Treatment

7 The choice of therapy depends on the underlying lesion and the activity, as well as the chronicity indices. Acute life-threatening disease involving multiple organs requires induction treatment that can suppress the disease promptly. In contrast, long-term management of chronic indolent disease requires therapy with more acceptable side-effect profiles. Corticosteroids are the cornerstone of therapy. However, for severe LN, primarily the diffuse proliferative type, alkylating agents may be needed to reduce or prevent the progression to ESRD. Newer alternatives with fewer side effects are now available.

Optimal blood pressure control is important. ACEIs or ARBs are commonly used to reduce proteinuria and blood pressure. It may also slow disease progression through reduction of inflammation and glomerular injury.[83] Patients with normal renal function and nonnephrotic range proteinuria (class I LN and II LN) typically do not require therapy, except for the management of extrarenal lupus manifestations.[10,83] The prognosis of these patients is generally good, and renal biopsy can be delayed. However, close follow-up of renal function and urinalysis is required.

Acute Induction Treatment

Steroids and Cytotoxic Agents

Patients with nephrotic range proteinuria, deteriorating renal function, and/or active urinary sediments require a renal biopsy to define the underlying lesion and determine the activity and chronicity of disease. Patients with class III LN and class IV LN should be treated with steroids: oral prednisone of up to 1 mg/kg, followed by tapering over 6 to 12 months or pulse IV methylprednisolone followed by low-dose oral steroids.[10]

Cyclophosphamide is used concurrently because it is a powerful B-cell inhibitor and can suppress the resynthesis of autoantibodies to normal levels. Combined use of IV cyclophosphamide and methylprednisolone is more effective than either agent alone in inducing remission.[10,84] Alternately, cyclophosphamide may be given orally, but it results in more adverse effects because of higher cumulative exposure.[83] It is uncertain whether IV administration or oral therapy is more effective. Azathioprine has also been used instead; however, it was reported to result in higher relapse rate and renal function decline.[10] The risk for adverse events, such as infection, gonadal damage, amenorrhea, and cervical dysplasia, and malignancy is increased with the cytotoxic regimens.[81]

Mycophenolate Mofetil

Several trials have found that mycophenolate mofetil with concurrent steroid therapy is an effective agent for induction therapy.[85] It was as effective as cyclophosphamide in inducing remission but with fewer side effects. A recent meta-analysis of the literature corroborates to the fact that it is an excellent agent for the induction of remission and that continued use may reduce risk for death or development of ESRD.[82] Several recent trials that included African Americans, who are known to have a poorer prognosis, also show that mycophenolate mofetil was more efficacious than IV cyclophosphamide and resulted in fewer adverse effects.[83,86] Based on these data, mycophenolate mofetil is now considered an alternative to cyclophosphamide as initial therapy for patients with class III LN and class IV LN. However, cyclophosphamide may be preferred for severe class III/IV LN since the long-term outcome may be more favorable than mycophenolate[10] (Fig. 32-7).

Clinical Controversy...

Is mycophenolate mofetil preferred over cyclophosphamide for acute induction treatment of LN?

Chronic Maintenance Treatment

Steroids and Cytotoxic Agents

Oral steroid is commonly used as a component of maintenance treatment (≤10 mg/day prednisolone).[10,83] Alternate-day regimens

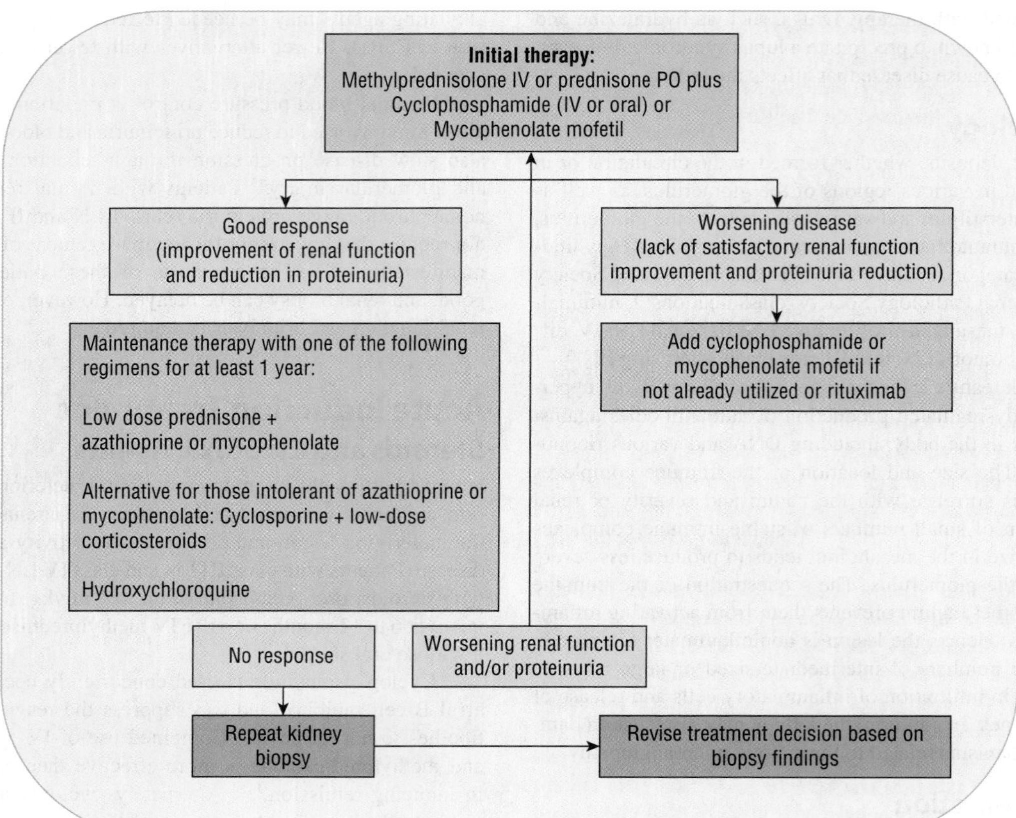

FIGURE 32-7 Treatment algorithm for class III (focal) and class IV (diffuse) lupus nephritis.

are often used in children to minimize growth retardation. Monthly pulse IV steroids in conjunction with cyclophosphamide resulted in more sustained remission, fewer relapses, and no significant increase in side effects.[87] Meta-analysis shows this combination to be more beneficial than steroid or cyclophosphamide alone. Cyclophosphamide, because of its bladder and gonadal toxicity, has been given as monthly and then bimonthly IV injection, instead of daily administration, for two or more years. However, toxicity is still a concern.

The efficacy of mycophenolate or azathioprine as maintenance therapy was evaluated against cyclophosphamide. Patients receiving mycophenolate or azathioprine were found to have better outcome and fewer side effects than cyclophosphamide. They are recommended by the KDIGO guidelines for maintenance therapy.[10] Depending on the study, mycophenolate was found to be either equivalent or better than azathioprine.[88,89] However, the drug should not be used during pregnancy since many lupus patients are women of child-bearing age.

Calcineurin Inhibitors

Cyclosporine may reduce proteinuria and lupus activity, stabilize renal function, and improve kidney morphology. It has been shown to have comparable efficacy and safety with azathioprine in preventing relapse for patients with diffuse proliferative LN.[90] It is recommended by the KDIGO guidelines for those intolerant of the side effects of azathioprine or mycophenolate.

Hydroxychloroquine

The antimalarial agent hydroxychloroquine can inhibit the toll-like receptors that contribute to autoimmunity. It was reported to be protective against the onset of LN, relapse of the disease, development of ESRD, venous thrombosis, and also a beneficial effect on lipid profiles.[10] Hydroxychloroquine is recommended by KDIGO guidelines for all patients of any class for patients receiving the drug should have annual eye examination for possible retinal toxicity, especially after 5 years of continuous use.

Alternative Therapeutic Agents

Many new agents have been developed to target the various pathways, costimulatory molecules, and immune mediators responsible for the pathologic autoantibody production.[82] Ocrelizumab is an anti-CD20 monoclonal antibody being evaluated as an adjunctive induction agent.[83] Abatacept, a selective T-cell co-stimulation modulator, is being studied as add-on induction therapy to cyclophosphamide or mycophenolate regimens. Belimumab, a monoclonal antibody that inhibits B-lymphocyte stimulating protein, appears to be efficacious for SLE treatment but not for LN.[91] Also being studied are acthar gel, an ACTH formulation[29] and laquinimod (TV-5600 or ABR-215062), a oral immunomodulator that is a quinoline-3-carboxamide derivative.[83]

Prognosis

The prognosis of patients with class II disease is generally good, and often no specific treatment is needed. For patients with class V disease, steroids alone commonly induce partial or complete remission. Immunosuppressive agents can be used for those who are not responsive to steroids. The survival of patients with classes III and IV disease has improved during the last two to three decades to approximately 74% to 80% at 10 years.[79] With the recent use of mycophenolate mofetil, better understanding of the optimal cytotoxic regimens, the use of lower steroid dosages, and better management of complications such as hypertension, infections, hyperlipidemia, and other metabolic complications of the disease, the long-term outcome has become more favorable. Lupus patients with end-stage kidney disease on dialysis fare as well as those with nonlupus-related renal disease. In those patients who received a renal transplant, the allograft outcome of patients with LN is favorable and comparable to those without lupus. Recurrence of lupus in the renal allograft can occur but is usually of minor clinical importance.

Rapidly Progressive Glomerulonephritis

Etiology and Epidemiology

RPGN describes a clinicopathologic syndrome of rapid loss of renal function—usually a greater than 50% decrement of the GFR within 3 months. The predominant histologic finding of RPGN is extensive crescent formation, usually in more than 50% of the glomeruli. Hence, it is also known as *crescentic* glomerulonephritis. RPGN accounts for 2% to 7% of all renal biopsy findings and is responsible for up to 5% of patients with end-stage kidney disease. The age ranges of susceptible patients vary with the type of RPGN. For example, types I and II RPGN are more common in younger patients, whereas type III is seen more frequently in older individuals.

RPGN is not a single disease entity. A variety of glomerulonephritides with or without systemic diseases may present as RPGN, including anti-GBM glomerulonephritis, Goodpasture's syndrome, LN, PSGN, MPGN, IgA nephropathy, polyarteritis nodosa, Wegener's granulomatosis, and idiopathic crescentic glomerulonephritis.

Primary RPGN is categorized according to the immunofluorescence microscopic findings, indicating different immunopathogenesis, therapeutic approaches, and clinical outcomes. Type I is characterized by the linear localization of immunoglobulins, mainly IgG, along the GBM, signifying anti-GBM antibody-induced injury. Type II is defined by the coarse granular deposition of immunoglobulins and complement within the capillary walls and mesangium, indicating immune-complex–mediated injury. Type III is characterized by scanty or complete lack of immune complex deposits; consequently, it is also known as *pauci-immune RPGN*. Circulating ANCAs are often detected in type III RPGN.

Pathophysiology

Different etiologic factors are implicated as the cause of RPGN: toxins, drugs, viral and bacterial infections, neoplasms, autoimmune mechanisms, and various immunogenetic factors.[92] Regardless of the etiology and type of RPGN, damage in the glomerular capillary wall by both humoral and cellular pathways of inflammation is common. Activation of the terminal C5b-9 (membrane-attacking complex) of the complement system produces severe capillary wall injury. Proteinases and reactive oxygen species released by neutrophils and macrophages may result in severe glomerular injury. Platelets and the coagulation system are activated and result in capillary thrombosis. The ruptured capillaries release fibrinogen and procoagulants that may come into contact with thrombogenic tissue debris and lead to fibrinoid changes. In anti-GBM glomerulonephritis, the direct attack of the anti-GBM antibody on the GBM is responsible for the capillary wall injury.[92] For patients with ANCA-associated disease, the interaction of ANCAs with neutrophils and monocytes, which have been primed by concurrent infections or inflammatory processes, can lead to activation of these leukocytes and release of toxic oxygen species and lytic enzymes, resulting in vascular injury.

The disruption of the capillary wall allows movement of macrophages and other plasma constituents into Bowman's space and stimulates the formation of crescents, which are composed mainly of parietal epithelial cells, as well as macrophages and fibroblasts. Crescent formation indicates the severity of the glomerular capillary disease but not its pathogenesis.

Clinical Presentation

Among the crescentic glomerulonephritides, the pauci-immune RPGN (type III) is the most frequent, accounting for more than 50% of cases, whereas the anti-GBM antibody-mediated RPGN (type I) is the least frequent, occurring in roughly 10% to 20% of patients. Of patients with type I RPGN, 60% to 70% may have concurrent pulmonary hemorrhage and Goodpasture's syndrome, which is caused by antibodies directed against the pulmonary alveolar basement membrane. Most patients with immune-complex–mediated RPGN (type II) have collagen vascular disease, systemic infections, or a severe form of primary glomerular disease. Approximately 70% of patients with type III RPGN also present with evidence of systemic vasculitis, such as Wegener's granulomatosis and polyarteritis nodosa. Some patients have only renal manifestations and are said to have idiopathic crescentic glomerulonephritis or renal vasculitis.

The clinical presentation is dominated by progressive renal insufficiency with complaints of tea-colored urine, malaise, anorexia, low-grade fever, and migratory polyarthropathy. Type I RPGN is more common in younger patients, whereas patients with ANCA-mediated disease tend to be older.[93] Urinalysis commonly shows nephritic sediments with hematuria, erythrocyte casts, and proteinuria. However, overt nephrotic syndrome is rare.

Serologic analysis is very useful in distinguishing the different types of RPGN. The detection of serum anti-GBM antibodies with the appropriate clinical presentation confirms the diagnosis of anti-GBM glomerulonephritis. More than 80% of patients with pauci-immune or idiopathic crescentic glomerulonephritis have circulating ANCAs. ANCAs are autoantibodies specific for the cytoplasmic constituents of neutrophil granules and monocyte lysosomes. Patients with ANCA-associated disease limited to renal involvement often have P-ANCA (perinuclear staining), whereas patients with Wegener's granulomatosis tend to have C-ANCA (cytoplasmic staining). Both the anti-GBM antibody and the ANCAs are absent in patients with type II RPGN. Measurements of circulating immune complexes are not useful for making a specific diagnosis, but detection of specific serum antibodies known to mediate immune-complex–associated nephritis is helpful, using anti-DNA antibody as a marker for LN and elevated antistreptolysin O (ASO) titers for PSGN.

TREATMENT

General Approach to Treatment

Early aggressive therapy has improved the renal prognosis of patients with crescentic glomerulonephritis. The rapid deterioration of renal function and the paucity of a large number of patients make randomized controlled studies very difficult to conduct. Based on the available data, immunosuppressive therapy alone appears to be ineffective for type I RPGN, while types II and III RPGN respond well to high-dose steroid therapy.[92,94] Because of the differences in response, the therapeutic approaches for each type of RPGN are presented separately below.

Specific Approaches to Treatment

Antiglomerular Basement Membrane Glomerulonephritis (Type I)

Steroids and cyclophosphamide, in conjunction with plasma exchange, are recommended by the KDIGO guidelines in all patients with anti-GBM glomerulonephritis except those who are dialysis-dependent, have 100% crescent in biopsy sample, and do not have pulmonary hemorrhage.[10] Plasma exchanges remove the pathogenic anti-GBM antibodies in circulation and are conducted for 2 weeks or until the antibodies disappear. Steroids (prednisolone 1 mg/kg/day, tapered over 6 months) and cyclophosphamide (2 to 3 mg/kg/day for 3 months) are then given to prevent new antibody production.[93,94] Patients with mild disease generally respond well to plasma exchange alone or immunosuppression (steroid and/or cytotoxic agents). For patients with severe disease (poor renal function and extensive crescent formation), most are expected to respond to the combination of plasma exchange and steroid/cytotoxic drug therapy. Pulse IV administration of corticosteroids (methylprednisolone 30 mg/kg/day for 3 days) has been used successfully to alleviate pulmonary hemorrhage, but the results are not as convincing for glomerulonephritis.[92,94] Because of the rapid decline in renal function, diagnosis should be established early so that therapy can proceed without delay. When the serum creatinine concentration is 6 mg/dL (530 μmol/L) or above or the patient is oliguric or requires dialysis, the response to therapy is usually poor, and the patient should be treated conservatively.[93,94] Poor response should also be expected when crescents are found in more than 85% of the glomeruli.

Immune-Complex–Mediated Glomerulonephritis (Type II)

Patients with postinfectious RPGN generally have a favorable prognosis even without treatment. Complete spontaneous recovery occurs in 50% of cases, whereas chronic renal failure develops in 32%.[92] Pulse doses of methylprednisolone (30 mg/kg/day, every other day × 3), followed by oral prednisone (1 mg/kg/day, tapered over several months) and then tapering, are beneficial in type II RPGN, with a response rate of 85% for patients with acute disease and 70% in those with more chronic disease.[92,94] Plasmapheresis does not appear to provide any additional benefit.[94]

Antineutrophil Cytoplasmic Autoantibody-Associated Glomerulonephritis (Type III)

Combined use of high-dose corticosteroids and cyclophosphamide induces remission in more than 90% of patients.[95] IV cyclophosphamide, possibly because of the lower cumulative dose administered, is associated with fewer infectious complications while being as effective as the oral route in inducing remission; however, the risk of relapse may be higher.[96] Because approximately 30% of the patients may relapse, cyclophosphamide also has been used for maintenance therapy. Rituximab and corticosteroids are recommended by the KIDGO guidelines as an alternative initial treatment in patients without severe disease or in whom cyclophosphamide is contraindicated.[10]

Maintenance therapy, using azathioprine or mycophenolate mofetil, is recommended for at least 18 months in patients who remain in remission, except those who are dialysis-dependent and have no extrarenal manifestation of disease.[10] Trimethoprim–sulfamethoxazole is suggested to be used as an adjunct in patients with upper respiratory disease. However, etanercept is not recommended.

Mycophenolate mofetil and methotrexate are also being used, and they have been shown in limited studies to be effective.[94,96] Plasmapheresis is indicated for those with advanced kidney failure or diffuse pulmonary hemorrhage. However, its benefits for patients with better kidney function and mild to moderate disease is not clear.[10,96]

Renal Transplantation

Anti-GBM nephritis may recur in up to 55% of patients who received a renal transplant. However, only 25% of these patients showed clinical disease activity, with rare allograft failure. Because the frequency of recurrence and its severity are related to the presence of circulating anti-GBM antibody, it is recommended that transplantation should not be performed until the anti-GBM antibody is undetectable for at least 6 to 12 months. The recurrence rate of ANCA-associated nephritis is 17%, with the average time to relapse from transplantation of 31 months.[97]

Prognosis

Regardless of the type of RPGN, poor response to therapy and an ominous renal survival are expected if the patient presents with oliguria, has a serum creatinine concentration greater than 6 or 7 mg/dL (530 or 619 μmol/L), is dialysis dependent, or has a renal biopsy showing advanced chronic parenchymal disease.[95] For those patients who had received kidney transplant, recurrence of the disease is common.

Poststreptococcal Glomerulonephritis

Etiology and Epidemiology

PSGN and glomerulonephritis caused by other infectious agents, such as bacteria, viruses, and parasites, were once common. Improved sanitation, personal hygiene, medical care, and public health measures helped to decrease the incidence of group A streptococcal infection both in the United States and in other developed countries, resulting in a decline of PSGN. In contrast, glomerulonephritis secondary to other infectious agents, such as hepatitis C and HIV, is seen with increasing frequency.

PSGN is now the most common form of glomerulonephritis in children but is less common than the other types of glomerulonephritis in adults. PSGN is seen mostly in children aged between 5 and 15 years and is uncommon in children younger than 2 years of age and in adults older than 50 years of age. It normally follows pharyngeal or skin infection caused by the nephritogenic strains of group A streptococci; however, other strains of streptococci, such as groups C and G, have also been reported to cause PSGN. Streptococcal pharyngitis is more common in winter and early spring, whereas skin infection is frequently found in the summer. The risk for developing acute glomerulonephritis secondary to the nephritogenic strains of bacteria is approximately 10% to 15% for infected patients. However, three to four times more patients may experience a subclinical form of the disease.

Pathophysiology

Streptococcal antigens may induce changes in the glomerular components rendering them immunogenic or autologous IgG may be altered to become antigenic. Alternately, the streptococcal antigens may induce antibodies that react with glomerular antigens. In situ immune complexes are then formed and result in a complement-mediated inflammatory response. The kinin and coagulation cascades are activated, and chemotactic factors are released to recruit neutrophils and monocytes, resulting in acute glomerular lesions.

Examination of the acute PSGN kidneys reveals hypercellular glomeruli with proliferation of mesangial and endothelial cells. Infiltration of neutrophils, monocytes, and eosinophils is apparent within the capillary lumen and also in the mesangial areas. Crescent formation may be seen for patients with severe disease, and if found in more than 30% of the glomeruli, RPGN may be present concurrently.[98] The prognosis is generally poor for these patients, and complete recovery is unlikely. Immunofluorescence examination reveals diffuse granular deposits of IgG and C3 along the GBM and also in the mesangium.

Clinical Presentation

The nephritis is preceded by a latent period following a streptococcal infection. The latent period is commonly 7 to 14 days for pharyngitis and 14 to 28 days for skin infection. An acute nephritic syndrome then develops, commonly with hematuria and edema. Gross hematuria is seen in 70% of patients, and microscopic hematuria can be found in all patients. Hypertension is usually mild to moderate and results from sodium and water retention. Many patients have signs and symptoms associated with volume overload, which include dyspnea, orthopnea, and cough. Urinalysis of patients with PSGN reveals hematuria, dysmorphic red blood cells, and red cell casts. Proteinuria is common but often not in the nephrotic range. Renal function is frequently mildly impaired.

Throat or skin culture may be positive for group A streptococci, despite the latent period following the initial infection. However, antibiotic therapy may render the culture result negative. Serologic measurements of antibodies to different streptococcal antigens can confirm recent exposure to the infection. Titers that can be measured include ASO, antistreptokinase, antihyaluronidase (AHase), antideoxyribonuclease B (ADNase B), and antinicotyladenine dinucleotidase (NADase).[99] For most patients with streptococcal pharyngitis, the ASO titers begin to rise about 10 to 14 days later, peak at 3 to 4 weeks, and persist for several months before decreasing. The rise in ASO titers can be reduced by antibiotic treatment and may not be seen for patients with streptococcal skin infection in whom the streptolysin may be bound to skin lipids. ADNase B and AHase titers should be used instead because they are specific and are positive in the majority of patients. The streptozyme test is a combined assay for ASO, ADNase B, NADase, and AHase. Antibodies to other antigens such as zymogen, streptococcal cationic proteinase exotoxin B (SPEB), and plasmin receptor (Plr) were evaluated recently.[100]

Serum complement levels are often decreased for patients with PSGN. If the C3 level is depressed for more than 6 to 8 weeks, MPGN, LN, or glomerulonephritis related to endocarditis or occult visceral abscess should be suspected. Renal biopsy is not normally indicated unless the patient has prolonged hematuria, proteinuria, or depressed C3 level. Renal biopsy is needed to detect other types of glomerulonephritis such as lupus, RPGN, or MPGN.

TREATMENT

General Approach to Treatment

8 The treatment of PSGN is mainly supportive and symptomatic. Early antibiotic therapy does not prevent subsequent PSGN, but it may reduce the severity of the disease. It can, however, prevent the spread of the streptococcal infection to other family members. Antibiotic prophylaxis is not recommended because infected patients will develop long-lasting, often lifelong immunity against the strain of streptococci. Exposure to another nephritogenic strain of streptococci is possible, but unlikely.

Supportive measures should be used to control fluid volume and blood pressure. Because the hypertension is of the low-renin type, ACEIs and β-blockers are not expected to be useful. If the patient has crescentic disease, use of pulse steroids and/or immunosuppressive agents can be considered; however, the efficacy and safety of these agents have not been established for this condition.

Prognosis

The acute manifestations of PSGN are normally self-limited, and for more than 95% of patients renal function has returned to baseline within 3 to 6 weeks. Diuresis usually begins 7 to 10 days after onset of the acute episode, whereas hypertension and azotemia resolve in 1 to 2 weeks. Gross hematuria lasts for 1 to 2 weeks, and proteinuria usually resolves within 6 months in more than 90% of children. However, microscopic hematuria may persist for up to 2 years. In general, children have more rapid recovery than adults. Prognosis is often better when PSGN occurs during an epidemic than in cases found sporadically. Most of the children will recover fully and be free from chronic complications of PSGN if they have no preexisting renal disorder, heavy proteinuria, or crescentic glomerular lesions or did not require hospitalization during the acute episode. In contrast, adult patients have a less favorable long-term outcome. As many as 50% of the patients may develop persistent proteinuria, hypertension, and renal insufficiency, with some resulting in end-stage renal failure.

CLINICAL BOTTOM LINE

A better understanding of the pathogenetic mechanisms leading to glomerular injury has led to marked improvements in the treatment of glomerulonephritis. However, the glomerulopathies are a heterogeneous group of immune disorders with different clinical courses, prognoses, and responses to current immunologic and nonimmunologic therapies. The clinician should understand the natural history and prognosis of each subgroup of glomerulonephritis, the efficacy of different immunomodulation regimens in inducing disease remission and preserving renal function, and the characteristics of at-risk patients who warrant aggressive therapy. Judicious use of immunosuppressive agents with careful monitoring of their adverse effects cannot be overemphasized. In addition, treatment of the disease complications and control of factors that lead to progression of renal disease are important in reducing the morbidity and mortality of patients with glomerulonephritis. The KDIGO guidelines for the first time offer clinicians many evidence-based recommendations that are useful for making individual patient treatment decisions.

ABBREVIATIONS

ACE	angiotensin-converting enzyme
ADNase B	antideoxyribonuclease B
AHase	antihyaluronidase
ANCA	antineutrophil cytoplasmic autoantibody
ARB	angiotensin II receptor blocker
ASO	antistreptolysin O
ESRD	end-stage renal disease
GBM	glomerular basement membrane
GFR	glomerular filtration rate
FSGS	focal segmental glomerulosclerosis
HIV	human immunodeficiency virus
HMG-CoA	β-hydroxy-β-methylglutaryl-coenzyme A
LDL	low-density lipoprotein (cholesterol)
MPGN	membranoproliferative glomerulonephritis
NADase	antinicotyladenine dinucleotidase
PSGN	poststreptococcal glomerulonephritis
RPGN	rapidly progressive glomerulonephritis
SLE	systemic lupus erythematosus
VLDL	very-low-density lipoprotein (cholesterol)

REFERENCES

1. U.S. Renal Data System 2012 Annual Data Report. Minneapolis, MN: USRDS Coordinating Center, 2012, http://www.usrds.org.
2. Schena FP, Gesualdo L, Grandaliano G, Montinaro V. Progression of renal damage in human glomerulonephritides: Is there sleight of hand in winning the game? Kidney Int 1997;52:1439–1457.
3. Couser WG. Mediation of immune glomerular injury. J Am Soc Nephrol 1990;1:13–29.
4. Remuzzi G, Zoja C, Perico N. Proinflammatory mediators of glomerular injury and mechanisms of activation of autoreactive T cells. Kidney Int Suppl 1994;44:S8–S16.
5. Humphreys MH. Mechanisms and management of nephrotic edema. Kidney Int 1994;45:266–281.
6. Schrier RW, Fassett RG. A critique of the overfill hypothesis of sodium and water retention in the nephrotic syndrome. Kidney Int 1998;53:1111–1117.

7. Warwick GL, Fox JG, Boulton-Jones JM. The relationship between urinary albumin excretion rate and serum cholesterol in primary glomerular disease. Clin Nephrol 1994;41:135–137.
8. Wheeler DC, Bernard DB. Lipid abnormalities in the nephrotic syndrome: Causes, consequences, and treatment. Am J Kidney Dis 1994;23:331–346.
9. Kaysen GA, De Sain-van der Verlden M. New insights into lipid metabolism in the nephrotic syndrome. Kidney Int Suppl 1999;71:S18–S21.
10. Cattran DC, Feehally J, et al. KDIGO clinical practice guidelines for glomerulonephritis. Kidney Int Suppl 2012;2: 139–274.
11. Ponticelli C, Passerini P. Treatment of the nephrotic syndrome associated with primary glomerulonephritis. Kidney Int 1994;46:595–604.
12. Klahr S, Levey A, Beck G, et al. The effects of dietary protein restriction and blood pressure control on the progression of chronic renal disease. N Engl J Med 1994;330:877–884.
13. Orth SR, Stockmann A, Conradt C, et al. Smoking as a risk factor for end-stage renal failure in men with primary renal disease. Kidney Int 1998;54:926–931.
14. Nachman PH, Martin J. Developments in the immunotherapy of glomerular disease. J Pharm Pract 2002;15:472–489.
15. Fliser D, Schroter M, Neubeck M. Coadministration of thiazides increases the efficacy of loop diuretics even in patients with advanced renal failure. Kidney Int 1994;46:482–488.
16. Rudy DW, Voelker JR, Greene PK, et al. Loop diuretics for chronic renal insufficiency: A continuous infusion is more efficacious than bolus therapy. Ann Intern Med 1991;115: 360–366.
17. Chobanian AV, Bakris GL, Black HR, et al. The seventh report of the joint national committee on prevention, detection, evaluation and treatment of high blood pressure: The JNC 7 report. JAMA 2003;289:2560–2572.
18. Ruggenenti P, Remuzzi G. Is therapy with combined ACE inhibitor and angiotensin receptor antagonist the new gold standard of treatment for nondiabetic, chronic proteinuric nephropathies? NephSAP 2003;2:235–237.
19. Gashti CN, Bakris GL. The role of calcium antagonists in chronic kidney disease. Curr Opin Nephrol Hypertens 2004;18:155–161.
20. Levey AS, Adler S, Caggiula AW, et al. Effects of dietary protein restriction on the progression of advanced renal disease in the Modification of Diet in Renal Disease Study. Am J Kidney Dis 1996;27:652–663.
21. Toto R. Proteinuria reduction: Mandatory consideration or option when selecting an antihypertensive agent? Curr Hypertens Rep 2005;7:374–378.
22. The GISEN group (Gruppo Italiano di Studi Epidemiologici in Nefrologia). Randomized placebo-controlled trial effect of ramipril on decline in glomerular filtration rate and risk of terminal renal failure in proteinuric, non-diabetic nephropathy. Lancet 1997;349:1857–1863.
23. Jefferson JA, Shank SJ. Glomerular disease: The podocyte is ready for prime time and may already be center stage. NephSAP 2006;331–338.
24. Vogt L, Navis G, de Zeeuw D. Renoprotection: A matter of blood pressure reduction or agent-characteristics? J Am Soc Nephrol 2002;13(Suppl 3):S202–S207.
25. Alexopoulos E. Treatment of primary IgA nephropathy. Kidney Int 2004;65:341–355.
26. MacKinnon M, Shurraw S, Akbari A, Knoll GA, Jaffey J, Clark HD. Combination therapy with an angiotensin receptor blocker and an ACE inhibitor in proteinuric renal disease: A systematic review of the efficacy and safety data. Am J Kidney Dis 2006;48:8–20.
27. Taal MV, Brenner BM. Combination ACEI and ARB therapy: Additional benefit in renoprotection? Curr Opin Nephrol Hypertens 2002;11:377–381.
28. Perico N, Remuzzi A, Sangalli F, et al. The antiproteinuric antagonism in human IgA nephropathy is potentiated by indomethacin. J Am Soc Nephrol 1998;9:2308–2317.
29. Ponticelli C, Passerini P, Salvadori M, et al. A randomized pilot trial comparing methylprednisolone plus a cytotoxic agent versus synthetic adrenocorticotropic hormone in idiopathic membranous nephropathy. Am J Kidney Dis 2006;47:233–240.
30. Bomback AS, Tumlin JA, Baranski J, et al. Treatment of nephrotic syndrome with adrenocorticotropic hormone (ACTH) gel. Drug Des Devel Ther 2011;5:147–153.
31. Oda H, Keane WF. Recent advances in statins and the kidney. Kidney Int Suppl 1999;71:S2–S5.
32. Tonelli M, Moyé L, Sacks FM. Effect of pravastatin on loss of renal function in people with moderate chronic renal insufficiency and cardiovascular disease. J Am Soc Nephrol 2003;14:1605–1613.
33. Agarwal R. Effects of statins on renal function. Am J Cardiol 2006;97:748–755.
34. Glassock RJ. Prophylactic anticoagulation in nephrotic syndrome: A clinical conundrum. J Am Soc Nephrol 2007;18:2221–2225.
35. Nolasco F, Cameron JS, Heywood EF, et al. Adult-onset minimal-change nephrotic syndrome: A long-term follow-up. Kidney Int 1986;29:1215–1223.
36. Bargman JM. Management of minimal lesion glomerulonephritis: Evidence-based recommendations. Kidney Int Suppl 1999;70:S3–S16.
37. Tune BM, Mendoza SA. Treatment of the idiopathic nephrotic syndrome: Regimens and outcomes in children and adults. J Am Soc Nephrol 1997;8:824–832.
38. Rinaldi S, Sesto A, Barsotti P, Faraggiana T, Sera F, Rizzoni G. Cyclosporine therapy monitored with abbreviated area under curve in nephrotic syndrome. Pediatr Nephrol 2005;20:25–29.
39. Yoshida M, Yoshikawa N, Akashi M, et al. Lymphocyte drug sensitivity is useful for prediction of the antiproteinuric effect and relapse rate in cyclosporine treatment for frequent-relapse minimal change nephrotic syndrome. Kidney Blood Press Res 2005;28:226–229.
40. Fu LS, Shien CY, Chi CS. Levamisole in steroid-sensitive nephrotic syndrome children with frequent relapses and/or steroid dependency: Comparison of daily and every-other-day usage. Nephron Clin Pract 2004;97:c137–c141.
41. Alsaran K, Grisaru S, Stephens D, et al. Levamisole vs. cyclophosphamide for frequently-relapsing steroid-dependent nephrotic syndrome. Clin Nephrol 2001;56: 289–294.
42. Li Z, Duan C, He J, et al. Mycohenolate mofetil therapy for children with steroid-resistant nephrotic syndrome. Pediatr Nephrol 2010;25:883–888.
43. Kemper MJ, Gellermann J, Habbig S, et al. Long-term follow-up after rituximab for steroid-dependent idiopathic nephrotic syndrome. Nephrol Dial Transplant 2012;27: 1910–1915.
44. D'Agati VD, Kaskel FJ, Falk RJ. Focal segmental glomerulosclerosis. N Engl J Med 2011;365:2398–2411.
45. Herlitz LC, Markowitz GS, Farris AB, et al. Development of focal segmental glomerulosclerosis after anabolic steroid abuse. J Am Soc Nephrol 2010;21:163–172.

46. Mubarak M, Kazi JI, Shakeel S, et al. Clinicopathologic characteristics and steroid response of IgM nephropathy in children presenting with idiopathic nephritic syndrome. APMIS 2011;119:180–186.
47. Crook ED, Habeeb D, Gowdy O, et al. Effects of steroids in focal segmental glomerulosclerosis in a predominantly African-American population. Am J Med Sci 2005;330: 19–24.
48. Goumenos DS, Tsagalis G, El Nahas AM, et al. Immunosuppressive treatment of idiopathic focal segmental glomerulosclerosis: A five-year follow-up study. Nephron Clin Pract 2006;104:c75–c82.
49. Frassinetti Castelo Branco Camurça Fernandes P, Bezerra Da Silva G Jr, De Sousa Barros FA, et al. Treatment of steroid-resistant nephrotic syndrome with cyclosporine: Study of 17 cases and a literature review. J Nephrol 2005;18:711–720.
50. Roberti I, Vyas S. Long-term outcome of children with steroid-resistant nephrotic syndrome treated with tacrolimus. Pediatr Nephrol 2010;25:1117–1124.
51. Cho ME, Hurley JK, Kopp JB. Sirolimus therapy of focal segmental glomerulosclerosis is associated with nephrotoxicity. Am J Kidney Dis 2007;49:310–317.
52. Gellermann J, Ehrich JH, Querfeld U, et al. Sequential maintenance therapy with cyclosporin A and mycophenolate mofetil for sustained remission of childhood steroid-resistant nephrotic syndrome. Nephrol Dial Transplant 2012;27: 1970–1978.
53. Herrmann SMS, Sethi S, Fervenza FC. Membranous nephropathy: The start of a paradigm shift. Curr Opin Nephrol Hypertens 2012;21:203–210.
54. Cattran D. Management of membranous nephropathy: When and what for treatment. J Am Soc Nephrol 2005;16:1188–1194.
55. Geddes CC, Cattran DC. The treatment of idiopathic membranous nephropathy. Semin Nephrol 2000;20:299–308.
56. Waldman M, Austin III HA. Controversies in the treatment of idiopathic membranous nephropathy. Nat Rev Nephrol 2009;5:469–479.
57. Ponticelli C, Passerini P. Management of idiopathic membranous nephropathy. Expert Opin Pharmacother 2010;11:2163–2175.
58. Ponticelli C, Zucchelli P, Passerini P, et al. A 10-year follow-up of a randomized study with methylprednisolone and chlorambucil in membranous nephropathy. Kidney Int 1995;48:1600–1604.
59. Ponticelli C, Altieri P, Scolari F, et al. A randomized study comparing methylprednisolone plus chlorambucil versus methylprednisolone plus cyclophosphamide in idiopathic membranous nephropathy. J Am Soc Nephrol 1998;9: 444–450.
60. Jayne D. Role of Rituximab therapy in glomerulonephritis. J Am Soc Nephrol 2010;21:14–17.
61. Appel G, Nachman P, Hogan S, et al. Eculizumab (C5 complement inhibitor) in the treatment of idiopathic membranous nephropathy [abstract]. J Am Soc Nephrol 2002;13:668A.
62. Sethi S, Fervenza FC. Membranoproliferative glomerulonephritis—A new look at an old entity. New Engl J Med 2012; 366:1119–1131.
63. Levin A. Management of membranoproliferative glomerulonephritis: Evidence-based recommendations. Kidney Int Suppl 1999;70:S41–S46.
64. Smith RJ, Alexander J, Barlow PN, et al. New approaches to the treatment of dense deposit disease. J Am Soc Nephrol 2007;18:2447–2456.
65. Donadio JV, Grande JP. Immunoglobulin A nephropathy. N Engl J Med 2002;347:738–748.
66. Boyd JK, Cheung CK, Molyneux K, et al. An update on the pathogenesis and treatment of IgA nephropathy. Kidney Int 2012;81:831–843.
67. Barbour SJ, Reich HN. Risk stratification of patients with IgA nephropathy. Am J Kidney Dis 2012;59:865–873.
68. Floege J, Eitner F. Current therapy for IgA nephropathy. J Am Soc Nephrol 2011;22:1785–1794.
69. Wang Y, Chen J, Wang Y, et al. A meta-analysis of the clinical remission rate and long-term efficacy of tonsillectomy in patients with IgA nephropathy. Nephrol Dial Transplant 2011;26:1923–1931.
70. Samuels JA, Strippoli GF, Craig JC, et al. Immunosuppressive treatments for immunoglobulin A nephropathy: A meta-analysis of randomized controlled trials. Nephrology (Carlton) 2004;9:177–185.
71. Pozzi C, Andrulli S, Del Vecchio L, et al. Corticosteroids effectiveness in IgA nephropathy: Long-term results of a randomized, controlled trial. J Am Soc Nephrol 2004;15: 157–163.
72. Lai KN. Future directions in the treatment of IgA nephropathy. Nephron 2002;92:263–270.
73. Donadio JV Jr, Grande JP, Bergstralh EJ, et al. The long-term outcome of patients with IgA nephropathy treated with fish oil in a controlled trial. Mayo Nephrology Collaborative Group. J Am Soc Nephrol 1999;10:1772–1777.
74. Dillon JJ. Fish oil therapy for IgA nephropathy: Efficacy and interstudy variability. J Am Soc Nephrol 1997;8: 1739–1744.
75. Rasche FM, Keller E, Lepper PM, et al. High-dose intravenous immunoglobulin pulse therapy in patients with progressive immunoglobulin A nephropathy: A long-term follow-up. Clin Exp Immunol 2006;146:47–53.
76. Taji Y, Kuwahara T, Shikata S, et al. Meta-analysis of antiplatelet therapy for IgA nephropathy. Clin Exp Nephrol 2006;10:268–273.
77. Donadio JV, Bergstralh EJ, Grande JP, et al. Proteinuria patterns and their association with subsequent end-stage renal disease in IgA nephropathy. Nephrol Dial Transplant 2002;17:1197–1203.
78. Courtney AE, McNamee PT, Nelson WE, Maxwell AP. Does angiotensin blockade influence graft outcome in renal transplant recipients with IgA nephropathy? Nephrol Dial Transplant 2006;21:3550–3554.
79. Contreras G, Roth D, Pardo V, et al. Lupus nephritis: A clinical review for practicing nephrologists. Clin Nephrol 2002;57:95–107.
80. Weening JJ, D'Agati VD, Schwartz MM, et al. The classification of glomerulonephritis in systemic lupus erythematosus revisited. Kidney Int 2004;65:521–530.
81. Waldman M, Appel GB. Update on the treatment of lupus nephritis. Kidney Int 2006;70:1403–1412.
82. Tsokos G. Systemic lupus erythematous. New Engl J Med 2011;365:2110–2121.
83. Bomback AS, Appel GB. Updates on the treatment of lupus nephritis. J Am Soc Nephrol 2010;21:2028–2035.
84. Gourley MF, Austin HA, Scott D, et al. Methylprednisolone and cyclophosphamide, alone or in combination, in patients with lupus nephritis. A randomized, controlled trial. Ann Intern Med 1996;125:549–557.
85. Walsh M, James M, Jayne D, Tonelli M, Manns BJ, Hemmelgarn BR. Mycophenolate mofetil for induction therapy of lupus nephritis: A systematic review and meta-analysis. Clin J Am Soc Nephrol 2007;2:968–975.
86. Appel GB, Contreras G, Dooley MA, et al. Mycophenolate mofetil versus cyclophosphamide for induction treatment of lupus nephritis. J Am Soc Nephrol 2009;20:1103–1112.

87. Illei GG, Austin HA, Crane M, et al. Combination therapy with pulse cyclophosphamide plus pulse methylprednisolone improves long-term renal outcome without adding toxicity in patients with lupus nephritis. Ann Intern Med 2001;135: 248–257.
88. Houssiau FA, D'Cruz D, Sangle S. Azathioprine versus mycophenolate mofetil for long-term immunosuppression in lupus nephritis: Results from the MAINTAIN Nephritis Trial. Ann Rheum Dis 2010;69:2083–2089.
89. Dooley MA, Jayne D, Ginzler EM. Mycophenolate versus azathioprine as maintenance therapy for lupus nephritis. N Engl J Med 2011;365:1886–1895.
90. Griffiths B, Emery P, Ryan V. The BILAG multi-centre open randomized controlled trial comparing ciclosporin vs azathioprine in patients with severe SLE. Rheumatology (Oxford) 2010;49:723–732.
91. Boyce EG, Fusco BE. Belimumab: Review of use in systemic lupus erythematous. Clin Ther 2012;34(5): 1006–1022.
92. Couser WG. Rapidly progressive glomerulonephritis: Classification, pathogenetic mechanisms, and therapy. Am J Kidney Dis 1988;11:449–464.
93. Little MA, Pusey CD. Rapidly progressive glomerulonephritis: Current and evolving treatment strategies. J Nephrol 2004;17:10–19.
94. Bolton WK. Treatment of glomerular disease: ANCA-negative RPGN. Semin Nephrol 2000;20:244–255.
95. Jennette JC. Rapidly progressive crescentic glomerulonephritis. Kidney Int 2003;63:1164–1177.
96. de Groot K, Adu D, Savage CO. The value of pulse cyclophosphamide in ANCA-associated vasculitis: Meta-analysis and critical review. Nephrol Dial Transplant 2001;16:2018–2027.
97. Nachman PH, Segelmark M, Westman K, et al. Recurrent ANCA-associated small-vessel vasculitis after transplantation: A pooled analysis. Kidney Int 1999;56:1544–1550.
98. Couser WG, Johnson RJ. Postinfective glomerulonephritis. In: Neilson EG, Couser WG, eds. Immunologic Renal Diseases, 2nd ed. Philadelphia, PA: Lippincott-Raven, 2001:899–929.
99. Rodriguez-Iturbe B, Parra G. Glomerulonephritis associated with infection: Poststreptococcal glomerulonephritis. In: Massry SG, Glas-sock RJ, eds. Massry & Glassock's Textbook of Nephrology, 4th ed. Philadelphia, PA: Lippincott Williams & Wilkins, 2001:667–671.
100. Rodriguez-Iturbe B. Nephritis-associated streptococcal antigens: Where are we now? J Am Soc Nephrol 2004;15:1961–1962.

Drug Therapy Individualization for Patients with Chronic Kidney Disease

33

Rima A. Mohammad and Gary R. Matzke

KEY CONCEPTS

1. Chronic kidney disease (CKD) results in minimal alterations in the absorption or bioavailability of most drugs.
2. The volume of distribution (V_D) of many drugs is increased in the presence of acute and chronic kidney disease as a consequence of volume expansion and/or reduced protein binding.
3. In addition to the expected decrement in renal clearance, nonrenal clearance (i.e., GI and hepatic drug metabolism) of several drugs is also reduced in patients with CKD.
4. Individualization of a drug dosage regimen for a patient with reduced kidney function is based on the pharmacodynamic/pharmacokinetic characteristics of the drug and the patient's degree of residual renal function.
5. The drug dosing guidelines for patients with CKD in many drug information resources are highly variable and many are not optimal for clinical use.
6. The effect of hemodialysis or peritoneal dialysis on drug elimination is dependent on the characteristics of the drug and the dialysis prescription.
7. Hemodialysis clearance data can be used to guide the initial drug dosage regimen recommendation for hemodialysis patients; however, prospective monitoring of serum concentrations is often warranted especially for those with a narrow therapeutic index.

Chronic kidney disease (CKD) is a common condition characterized by the presence of kidney damage, a urine albumin-to-creatinine ratio greater than 30 mg/g (3.4 mg/mmol) or a glomerular filtration rate (GFR) of less than 60 mL/min (1 mL/s) for greater than 3 months. It is estimated that 10% of adults, greater than 20 million people, in the United States have CKD.[1] Between 2000 and 2008, the incidence of CKD has more than doubled in adults 65 years old and older.[1] The combination of CKD, age-related reductions in renal function, and the high utilization of medications in these patients increases their risk of adverse effects particularly if their drug regimen is not appropriately individualized.[2,3] Furthermore a marked reduction in kidney function in adults of any age, whether acute or chronic, has been noted to affect the pharmacokinetics of many medications.[4–12] Thus patients with CKD are often prescribed an extensive array of medications for CKD-related and other comorbid conditions (see Chap. 29). These factors necessitate that clinicians individualize drug therapy to maximize therapeutic outcomes and to minimize therapeutic misadventures.

Drug excretion is markedly effected by CKD. Medications which are predominantly renally eliminated unchanged (f_e) may accumulate in patients with CKD, which can complicate existing conditions and increase the risk of adverse effects. If 30% or more of a drug is renally eliminated unchanged, it will have a high likelihood, >70%, of requiring dosage regimen adjustment in patients with CKD. The pharmacokinetics of drugs with an f_e less than 30% also may be affected and a recent study indicated that 20% to 37.5% of such drugs approved in the United States from 1998 to 2010 had a dosage adjustment for patients in the product labeling.[13] If there is no official recommendation in the product labeling a dosage regimen adjustment may be calculated on the basis of the drug's f_e and the ratio of the patient's residual renal function relative to an age and gender normal value for estimated creatinine clearance (CL_{cr}) or GFR.[14] However, for medications that are extensively metabolized or for which dramatic changes in protein binding and/or distribution volume (V_D) have been noted, a more complex adjustment strategy may need to be employed.[4,15] Furthermore, physiologic and biochemical changes associated with CKD may also independently impact drug dosing and serum drug concentrations.[4]

Clinicians thus will often need to proactively design individualized therapeutic regimens to optimize achievement of the desired outcomes while minimizing adverse events, if they use basic pharmacokinetic principles combined with the drug's disposition characteristic and the patient's clinical status. In this chapter, the influence of CKD on drug pharmacokinetic properties is characterized and the most commonly used medications that are affected are discussed. In addition, a general guide for individualizing drug therapy in patients with CKD is presented along with dosage recommendations for the most commonly used drugs in this patient population. Finally, the impact of chronic renal replacement therapy (i.e., peritoneal dialysis and hemodialysis) on drug disposition is discussed and dosage recommendations for selected drugs are presented. Drug dosage regimen adjustment strategies for patients with acute kidney injury (AKI) including those who are receiving continuous renal replacement therapy are presented in Chapter 28.

EFFECT OF CHRONIC KIDNEY DISEASE ON DRUG DISPOSITION

Prior to the 1990s, there were no regulatory guidelines regarding when and how pharmacokinetic/pharmacodynamic studies of drugs in patients with renal insufficiency should be conducted as part of the new drug application process.[16,17] Thus much of the pharmacokinetic/pharmacodynamic data in patients with renal insufficiency published during the 1970s through much of the 1990s were derived from postmarketing studies. Unfortunately, the utility of these studies were often limited by small sample sizes, which led to inconsistent and sometimes conflicting results. Furthermore it was rare that detailed information was incorporated into the official (i.e., FDA) prescribing information. The FDA published the first guidance for industry on renal impairment studies in 1998 and since then, the frequency and quality of renal impairment studies as part of drug development has increased.[13,18,19] A proposed revision to the 1998 guidance on renal impairment studies was recently circulated for comment which recommended: (a) conducting studies in nonrenally as well as renally eliminated drugs, (b) conducting studies in patients receiving hemodialysis, (c) conducting studies to evaluate pharmacokinetics of therapeutic proteins in patients with renal insufficiency, (d) categorizing renal function based on estimated GFR (using the modification of diet in renal disease [MDRD] equation) or CL_{cr} (using the Cockcroft–Gault [C–G] equation), and (e) modifications to how the results of renal impairment studies are presented in the official drug label.[20–22] Although this revision has not been "officially" implemented by the FDA, it appears to be impacting how the industry considers the design of renal pharmacokinetic/pharmacodynamic studies.

Drug Absorption

1 There is little quantitative information regarding the influence of CKD on drug absorption and bioavailability. Many studies evaluating bioavailability of oral medications in CKD patients were not designed to provide an assessment of the drug's absolute bioavailability (e.g., they did not include a comparison of the area under the concentration–time curve (AUC) after oral and IV administration of the drug). Rather, the principal outcomes that were documented were alterations in the peak concentration (C_{max}), time at which the peak concentration was attained (t_{max}), or in the fractional amount of drug recovered in the urine in a finite time period. Unfortunately, this limited information has been extrapolated by some into a general conclusion that drug absorption is slowed and/or that the extent of absorption is reduced in patients with CKD.[23,24]

Both CKD and comorbid conditions associated with CKD (e.g., diabetes mellitus and cardiovascular disease) may contribute to changes in drug absorption. Some patients present with changes in GI transit time and gastric pH (e.g., gastroparesis associated with diabetes mellitus), edema of the GI tract, persistent vomiting and diarrhea, and phosphate binder administration have all been proposed as a rationale for alterations in the bioavailability of drugs in CKD patients.[2,8] For example, patients with uremic-induced vomiting, now only occasionally observed in patients with severe renal insufficiency, may decrease a medication's time in the GI tract and thereby limit absorption of that drug. Edema of the GI tract, secondary to cirrhosis or congestive heart failure, can decrease the bioavailability of some medications such as oral furosemide.[2,25] A reduction in gastric acidity associated with the concomitant administration of antacids and phosphate binders has been associated with a reduction in bioavailability of several medications including several antibiotics and digoxin.[26–29]

However, there are only a few drugs (e.g., some β-blockers, dextropropoxyphene, dihydrocodeine, felodipine, sertraline, and cyclosporine) with documented increases in bioavailability in patients with CKD as a result of a reduction in metabolism during the drug's first pass through the GI tract and liver.[4,30–35] Although the bioavailability of several of these compounds is increased in the presence of CKD, clinical consequences (development of excessive or unexpected adverse effects) have only been demonstrated with dextropropoxyphene and dihydrocodeine.[31,32] For some agents, those metabolized by cytochrome P450 (CYP) 3A4, the bioavailability may be dramatically increased when the medications are taken along with grapefruit juice: felodipine by 184% and cyclosporine by 20%.[33,34]

Drug Distribution

The V_D of many drugs is increased in patients with moderate to severe CKD as well as those with preexisting CKD who develop AKI (Table 33-1) and lead to a reduction in serum drug concentrations.[4,8–10,36] This increase in V_D may be the result of pathophysiologic alterations in body composition, fluid overload secondary to excessive IV fluid administration, decreased protein binding, or increased tissue binding. Decreased tissue binding of drugs in patients with CKD may result in a reduction in V_D, which has been reported for only a few medications (e.g., digoxin and pindolol).[9,10]

TABLE 33-1 Volume of Distribution of Selected Drugs in Patients with End-Stage Renal Disease

Drug	Normal (L/kg)	ESRD (L/kg)	Change From Normal (%)
Increased			
Amikacin	0.20	0.29	45
Cefazolin	0.13	0.17	31
Cefoxitin	0.16	0.26	63
Ceftriaxone	0.28	0.48	71
Cefuroxime	0.20	0.26	30
Doripenem	0.25	0.47	88
Dicloxacillin	0.08	0.18	125
Erythromycin	0.57	1.09	91
Furosemide	0.11	0.18	64
Gentamicin	0.20	0.32	60
Isoniazid	0.6	0.8	33
Minoxidil	2.6	4.9	88
Phenytoin	0.64	1.4	119
Trimethoprim	1.36	1.83	35
Vancomycin	0.64	0.85	33
Decreased			
Chloramphenicol	0.87	0.60	−31
Digoxin	7.3	4	−45
Ethambutol	3.7	1.6	−57

Data from references 8–10, 59, and 73.

Variability in fluid status is a common issue in patients with CKD, especially those that are critically ill. Many of these critically ill patients receive large volumes of IV fluids for various clinical conditions (e.g., resuscitation from shock), and develop edema, pleural effusions, or ascites as a result thereof. These therapeutic interventions, in addition to renal insufficiency that can result in reduced water excretion, can result in an increase in V_D and alterations in drug serum concentrations, especially with hydrophilic drugs.[3] For example the V_D of aminoglycosides has been noted to be increased by 1.34- to 1.66-fold in postsurgical patients with septic shock.[37] Interstitial fluid concentration of piperacillin was also reported to be three- to fourfold lower in patients undergoing heart surgery and in patients with sepsis.[37] These marked reductions in drug concentration may be due to increased capillary permeability following fluid accumulation in the interstitial space.[37]

Effect of Altered Protein Binding

2 The unbound fraction of many acidic drugs increases in CKD patients as the result of a decrease in protein binding and this is associated with an increase in the apparent V_D.[8] A new equilibrium is ultimately established as a result of increased drug elimination/distribution, such that the unbound concentrations remain comparable to those observed in patients with normal renal function despite the fact that total concentrations are reduced. Thus, the net effect is an alteration in the relationship between total drug concentration and pharmacodynamic effect. For example, protein binding of phenytoin (90% protein-bound, primarily to albumin) is significantly reduced

and this change alters the relationship between total phenytoin concentration and desired and toxic effects.[8,38] The resulting increase in unbound fraction, from values of 10% in those with normal renal function to approximately 20% or more in those with stage 5 CKD, results in increased hepatic clearance and decreased total concentrations. Thus, in patients with CKD, the therapeutic range based on total phenytoin concentration is shifted downward from normal values of 10 to 20 mg/L (10 to 20 mcg/mL; 40 to 79 mmol/L) to values as low as 4 to 8 mg/L (4 to 8 mcg/mL; 16 to 32 mmol/L). Since the unbound concentration therapeutic range is the same for all patients, 1 to 2 mg/L (1 to 2 mcg/mL; 4 to 8 mmol/L), such a measurement provides the best target for individualizing phenytoin therapy in patients with CKD.

The decrease in plasma protein binding of acidic drugs (e.g., phenytoin) has been attributed to qualitative changes in the binding sites, accumulation of endogenous inhibitors of binding, and/or decreased concentrations of albumin. The first two of these mechanisms appear to account for most of the observed changes in binding. In addition, the high concentrations of metabolites of some compounds that accumulate in patients with end-stage renal disease (ESRD) may compete for protein binding sites with the parent compound.[39]

The principal binding protein for several basic drugs is α_1-acid glycoprotein, an acute-phase reactant protein whose plasma concentrations are increased in CKD patients.[4,8] As a result of this increase, the unbound fraction of some basic drugs (e.g., bepridil, disopyramide) may be significantly decreased and the V_D increased in CKD patients, especially renal transplant and hemodialysis patients.[4,8]

Effect of Altered Tissue Binding

Altered tissue binding may also result in a reduction of the apparent V_D of a drug. For example, the V_D of digoxin has been reported to be reduced by 30% to 50% from the normal values in patients with stage 5 CKD, as well as in hemodialysis patients.[40] This reduction in V_D may be a result of decreased tissue binding, the presence of acidosis, or digoxin-like immunoreactive substances.[9,41] In this case, the absolute amount of digoxin bound to the receptor is reduced and the resultant serum digoxin concentration is higher than anticipated. Thus, in patients with renal insufficiency, particularly in those with stage 5 CKD, a "normal" total drug concentration may be associated with either an adverse reaction secondary to elevated unbound drug concentrations, or a subtherapeutic response because of an altered plasma-to-tissue drug concentration ratio. The monitoring of unbound drug concentrations in CKD patients is thus warranted for those drugs that have a narrow therapeutic range, are highly protein bound (free fraction of <20%), and for which marked variability in the free fraction has been reported (e.g., phenytoin and disopyramide).

Effect of V_D Calculation Method

Finally, the method used to calculate the volume of distribution may be influenced by renal insufficiency. The three most commonly used volume of distribution terms are: volume of the central compartment (V_c), volume of the terminal phase (V_β and V_{area}), and volume of distribution at steady state (V_{ss}). The V_c for many drugs approximates extracellular fluid volume and thus may be increased or decreased by acute changes. Oliguric acute renal failure is often accompanied by fluid overload and a resultant increased V_c for many drugs. The V_{area} or V_β represents the proportionality constant between plasma concentrations in the terminal elimination phase and the amount of drug remaining in the body. V_β is affected by both distribution characteristics, as well as by the terminal elimination rate constant. V_β and V_{ss} will often be similar in magnitude, with V_β being slightly larger. Because V_{ss} has the advantage of being independent of drug elimination, it is the most appropriate volume term to use when one desires to compare drug distribution volumes between patients with renal insufficiency and those with normal renal function.[42]

Drug Metabolism

Accumulation of Metabolites

There are only a few drugs that are eliminated completely unchanged via the kidneys and thus most drugs are metabolized to some extent. Patients with severe renal insufficiency who are receiving chronic drug therapy may experience accumulation of metabolite(s) as well as the parent compound. Metabolites of several drugs have been reported to have significant pharmacologic and/or toxicologic activity.[43] However, the pharmacokinetics and pharmacodynamics of metabolites are not often fully elucidated. In a sense, the patient with severe CKD is being exposed to a new pharmacologic entity since the sum of the serum concentrations of the metabolite and the parent compound are markedly different than those reported in patients with normal renal function.

The metabolite may have pharmacologic activity similar to that of the parent drug and thus contribute significantly to clinical response; that is true, for example, of oxypurinol. Alternatively, the metabolite may have qualitatively dissimilar pharmacologic action; for example, normeperidine has CNS stimulatory activity that reportedly produces seizures, whereas meperidine has CNS depressant actions.[44,45] Because of the multiplicity of potential interactions of compounds that are primarily metabolized, the practical consequences of metabolite accumulation are difficult to predict and are most often identified in those patients at risk by trial and error.

Alterations of CYP 450 Enzyme Activity

3 A decrease in the renal clearance of drugs in patients with CKD is well appreciated. However, there is now good preclinical and emerging clinical evidence which suggests that CKD may lead to alterations in nonrenal clearance of many medications as the result of alterations in the activities of uptake and efflux transporters as well as CYP enzymes in the liver and other organs[8–12,46] (Table 33-2). The effect(s) of renal insufficiency on nonrenal drug clearance appear to depend on whether the reduction in renal function is acute or chronic in nature. For example, higher residual

TABLE 33-2 Impact of ESRD on Nonrenal Clearance of Selected Drugs

Decrease		
Acyclovir	Imipenem	Procainamide
Aztreonam	Isoniazid	Quinapril
Bupropion	Ketorolac	Raloxifene
Captopril	Losartan	Repaglinide
Carvedilol	Lovastatin	Rosuvastatin
Cefotaxime	Metoclopramide	Simvastatin
Ceftriaxone	Minoxidil	Valsartan
Cimetidine	Morphine	Vancomycin
Ciprofloxacin	Nicardipine	Verapamil
Doripenem	Nimodipine	Warfarin
Erythromycin	Nortriptyline	
Increase		
Bumetanide	Nifedipine	
Fosinopril		
No Change		
Acetaminophen	Lidocaine	Theophylline
Clonidine	Metoprolol	
Insulin	Pentobarbital	

Data from references 8–10.

TABLE 33-3 Major Pathways of Nonrenal Drug Clearance

CL_{NR} Pathway	Selected Substrates
Oxidative Enzymes	
CYP	
1A2	Polycyclic aromatic hydrocarbons, caffeine, imipramine, theophylline
2A6	Coumarin
2B6	Nicotine, bupropion
2C8	Retinoids, paclitaxel, repaglinide
2C9	Celecoxib, diclofenac, flurbiprofen, indomethacin, ibuprofen, losartan, phenytoin, tolbutamide, *S*-warfarin
2C19	Diazepam, *S*-mephenytoin, omeprazole
2D6	Codeine, debrisoquine, desipramine, dextromethorphan, fluoxetine, paroxetine, duloxetine, nortriptyline, haloperidol, metoprolol, propranolol
2E1	Ethanol, acetaminophen, chlorzoxazone, nitrosamines
3A4/5	Alprazolam, midazolam, cyclosporine, tacrolimus, nifedipine, felodipine, diltiazem, verapamil, fluconazole, ketoconazole, itraconazole, erythromycin, lovastatin, simvastatin, cisapride, terfenadine
Conjugative Enzymes	
UGT	Acetaminophen, morphine, lorazepam, oxazepam, naproxen, ketoprofen, irinotecan, bilirubin
NAT	Dapsone, hydralazine, isoniazid, procainamide
Transporters	
OATP	
1A2	Bile salts, statins, fexofenadine, methotrexate, digoxin, levofloxacin
1B1	Bile salts, statins, fexofenadine, repaglinide, valsartan, olmesartan, irinotecan, bosentan
1B3	Bile salts, statins, fexofenadine, telmisartan, valsartan, olmesartan, digoxin
2B1	Statins, fexofenadine, glyburide
P-gp	Digoxin, fexofenadine, loperamide, irinotecan, doxorubicin, vinblastine, paclitaxel, erythromycin
MRP	
2	Methotrexate, etoposide, mitoxantrone, valsartan, olmesartan
3	Methotrexate, fexofenadine

nonrenal clearance for vancomycin, meropenem, and imipenem has been documented in patients with AKI compared to patients with CKD, who have comparable CL_{cr}.[47] In humans with renal insufficiency, the activities of CYPs appear to be relatively unaffected. It was reported that CYP3A4 activity was reduced,[7,9–12] but recent data indicate that organic anion-transporting polypeptide (OATP) uptake activity is reduced and thus the perceived changes in CYP3A4 activity were likely due to altered transporter activity, not an alteration in CYP activity. The reduction of nonrenal clearance of several drugs that exhibit overlapping CYP and transporter substrate specificity in patients with stage 4 or stage 5 CKD supports this premise (Table 33-3). These studies must be interpreted with caution, however, because concurrent drug intake, age, smoking status, and alcohol intake were often not taken into consideration. Furthermore, pharmacogenetic variations in drug-metabolizing enzymes that may have been present in the individual before the onset of AKI or CKD must be considered, if known.[7,9–12] This differential effect on individual enzymes may help to explain some of the conflicting reports of whether drug metabolism is altered in the presence of CKD. Cytochrome P450 enzyme 3A activity as measured by the erythromycin breath test (EBT) is 28% lower in ESRD patients as compared with healthy controls.[48] Although baseline CYP3A activity was lower in these patients, the increase in CYP3A activity observed following enzyme induction with rifampin was similar.[48] Nolin and colleagues have recently shown that EBT results are reduced more in those ESRD patients with higher blood urea nitrogen concentrations and that hemodialysis is associated with an acute improvement in the patient's metabolic activity.[10] These data indicate that CKD has a detrimental effect on this important pathway of hepatic drug metabolism in humans.

Prediction of the effect of renal insufficiency on the metabolism of a particular drug is however difficult and there is currently no quantitative strategy to predict changes for one drug based on data from another even if they are in the same pharmacologic class. However, some qualitative insight can be gained if one knows what enzyme is involved in the metabolism of the drug of interest and how the enzyme(s) or transporter(s) is affected by the presence of CKD.

EFFECT OF CHRONIC KIDNEY DISEASE ON RENAL TRANSPORTERS

Renal clearance (CL_R) of a drug is the composite of GFR, tubular secretion, and reabsorption ($CL_R = [GFR \times f_u] + [CL_{secretion} - CL_{reabsorption}]$), where f_u is the fraction of the drug unbound to plasma proteins. Drug elimination by filtration occurs by diffusion; while tubular secretion and reabsorption are bidirectional processes that involve carrier-mediated renal transport systems.[49] Renal transport systems have been broadly classified on the basis of substrate selectivity into the anionic and cationic renal transport systems, which are responsible for the transport of a number of organic acidic and basic drugs, respectively (see eChap. 18 and Table 33-3).[8] Several drugs are actively secreted by one or more of these transporter families, which include organic cationic (e.g., famotidine, trimethoprim, and dopamine), organic anionic (e.g., ampicillin, cefazolin, and furosemide), nucleoside (e.g., zidovudine), and P-glycoprotein transporters (e.g., digoxin, vinca alkaloids, and steroids).[50,51] Alterations in filtration, secretion, or reabsorption, secondary to CKD may have a dramatic effect on drug disposition: for drugs that are primarily filtered, a reduction in GFR will result in a proportional decrease in renal drug clearance.

ESTIMATION OF RENAL FUNCTION

In the absence of data delineating the contribution of tubular function to renal clearance, the clinical measurement or estimation of CL_{cr} or GFR remains the guiding factor for drug dosage regimen design.[4,6,12] The importance of an alteration in renal function on drug elimination depends on two factors: the fraction of drug normally eliminated by the kidney unchanged and the degree of renal insufficiency. Quantitation of the patient's renal function can be accomplished by measurement of CL_{cr} or GFR or estimation of CL_{cr} or GFR based on the stable serum creatinine concentration (see eChap. 18). Because of the time delay involved and problems in obtaining complete urine collections, measured CL_{cr} or GFR values are infrequently used for initial drug dosage regimen design. Therefore the calculation of initial drug dosage regimens relies on the estimation of CL_{cr} or GFR in adults and children from such routinely available clinical data as age, gender, height, weight, and serum creatinine or serum cystatin C. The best method to use for adults remains controversial with many supporters of the C–G equation and others who support the use of the MDRD or chronic kidney disease epidemiology collaboration equation (CKD-EPI) approach[52–54] (see eChap. 18).

Recently, there is considerable debate regarding the use of C–G or MDRD equation to guide drug dosing adjustment in patients with CKD. Recommendations as to when to adjust drug dosage regimens for currently approved medications are largely (greater than 95%) based on relationships between drug clearance and CL_{cr} calculated by the C–G equation.[55] Several studies have shown that when compared to drug dosing based on C–G, the use of MDRD equation resulted in conflicting drug dosing recommendations in 40% of patients.[56–58] A recent systematic comparison between C–G and MDRD equations showed that the classification of renal function with each equation was generally similar.[59] However, using the MDRD equation resulted in conflicting drug dosing recommendations (higher or lower dosing categories) in 12% of patients and resulted in higher dosing recommendations in patients with a combination of advanced age (age > 80 years), low weight (<55 kg), and modest elevations of serum creatinine (>0.7 and ≤1.5 mg/dL [>62 and ≤133 μmol/L]).[59]

The introduction of the 2009 CKD-EPI creatinine equation complicates things further.[60] Reports showed that the CKD-EPI creatinine equation was more accurate in those with higher mean measured GFRs (estimated to be >60 mL/min per 1.73 m^2); however, the MDRD equation was more accurate in those with GFRs less than 60 mL/min per 1.73 m^2.[52] In 2012, there were two variations of the CKD-EPI equation (CKD-EPI cystatin C equation and CKD-EPI creatinine–cystatin C equation) reported, which utilize cystatin C with or without serum creatinine to estimate GFR. One study showed that the CKD-EPI creatinine-cystatin C equation performed better and resulted in more accurate estimates of GFR compared to equations that used creatinine or cystatin C alone (CKD-EPI cystatin C or CKD-EPI creatinine equations).[54] Although, recent data show improved accuracy of estimating GFR, especially with the CKD-EPI creatinine-cystatin C equation, there is extremely little data regarding the use of these equations to guide drug dosing in CKD patients. As such, drug dosing recommendations should continue to be based on CL_{cr} estimated by C–G for the present.[55]

DRUG DOSAGE REGIMEN DESIGN FOR PATIENTS WITH CHRONIC KIDNEY DISEASE

4 The initial or "loading" dose for should be the same for patients with impaired renal function as those with normal renal function unless the volume of distribution is known to be altered in the presence of renal insufficiency or a concomitant disease (Table 33-1). Maintenance dosage regimen guidelines for CKD patients in FDA or European Medicines Agency (EMA) approved product labeling should be the foundation for ongoing therapy. If such information is not available or if there is marked variance between these two agencies' recommendations the approach depicted in Table 33-4 for designing a dosage regimen for a patient with CKD can be utilized. In either case the design of the optimal dosage regimen is dependent on the availability of an accurate characterization of the relationship between the pharmacokinetic parameters of the drug and renal function and an accurate assessment of the patient's renal function.

Most dosage-adjustment guidelines have proposed the use of a fixed dose or interval for patients with broad ranges of renal function that are different from those that are the foundation of the CKD staging scheme (see Chap. 29).[3,8,15,36,61–63] Indeed, normal renal function has often been ascribed to anyone who has a CL_{cr} >80 to 90 mL/min (>1.34 to 1.50 mL/s), even though the population normal CL_{cr} values range from 115 to 125 mL/min per 1.73 m^2 (>1.11 to 1.20 mL/s/m^2). The recent dosage adjustment guidelines and references often use different ranges to represent mild, moderate, and severe renal insufficiency.[55] The predominant ranges for mild, moderate, and severe renal insufficiency can be defined as a CL_{cr} of 60 to 89 mL/min (1 to 1.49 mL/s), CL_{cr} of 30 to 59 mL/min (0.5 to 0.99 mL/s), and CL_{cr} of 10 to 30 mL/min (0.17 to 0.5 mL/s), respectively. ESRD is usually defined as a CL_{cr} of less than 10 mL/min (0.17 mL/s). Each of these categories encompasses a broad range in renal function, and thus the calculated drug regimen may not be optimal for all patients whose renal function lies within the given category of renal function.

TABLE 33-4 Stepwise Approach to Adjust Drug Dosage Regimens for Patients with Renal Insufficiency

Step 1	Obtain history and relevant demographic/clinical information	Record demographic information, obtain past medical history including history of renal disease, and record current laboratory information (e.g., serum creatinine)
Step 2	Estimate creatinine clearance	Use the Cockcroft–Gault equation to estimate creatinine clearance, or calculate creatinine clearance from timed urine collection
Step 3	Review current medications	Identify drugs for which individualization of the treatment regimen will be necessary
Step 4	Calculate individualized treatment regimen	Determine treatment goals (see the text); calculate dosage regimen based on pharmacokinetic characteristics of the drug and the patient's renal function (see Table 33-6)
Step 5	Monitor	Monitor parameters of drug response and toxicity; monitor drug levels if available/applicable
Step 6	Revise regimen	Adjust regimen based on drug response or change in patient status (including renal function) as warranted

5 Secondary references, such as the American Hospital Formulary Service Drug Information Service,[61] Goodman and Gilman's the Pharmacological Basis of Therapeutics,[36] the British National Formulary,[62] and Drug Prescribing in Renal Failure,[63] are excellent sources of information about a drug's pharmacokinetic characteristics in subjects with normal and impaired renal function. Marked variation in recommendations along with the paucity of details of the methods used to generate the dosing advice have resulted in some cautioning against their routine clinical use.[64] In addition, none of these sources consistently provide the explicit relationships of the kinetic parameters of interest (total body clearance [CL], elimination rate constant [k], and V_D) with a continuous index of renal function, such as CL_{cr}. To find this information, one may need to identify the original research study that assessed the drug's disposition or a comprehensive review article on the class of drugs of interest. This is a time-consuming process that may be difficult to carry out for each drug and patient combination in real time. Ideally, one should be able to identify a relationship between CL and k with an estimated GFR or CL_{cr}, such as those depicted in Table 33-5. This information, along with the patient's estimated CL_{cr} or GFR, is the foundation upon which one can formulate a therapeutic regimen to attain the desired therapeutic outcome.

If specific literature recommendations and/or the relationship of kinetic parameters to estimated GFR or CL_{cr} are not available, then one can estimate the CL or k of the patient with the method of Rowland and Tozer,[14] provided the fraction of the drug that is eliminated renally unchanged (f_e) in subjects with normal renal function is known.[65] This approach assumes that the change in CL and k are proportional to CL_{cr}, that the renal disease does not alter the drug's metabolism, that the metabolites, if formed, are inactive and nontoxic, that the drug obeys first-order (linear) kinetic principles, and that it is adequately described by a one-compartment model. If these

TABLE 33-5 Relationship Between Creatinine Clearance and Total Body Clearance and Terminal Elimination Rate Constant of Selected Drugs

Drug	Elimination Rate Constant	Total Body Clearance[a]
Acyclovir		$CL = 3.37 (CL_{cr}) + 0.41$
Amikacin	$k = (0.0024 \times CL_{cr}) + 0.01$	$CL = 0.6 (CL_{cr}) + 9.6$
Aztreonam		$CL = 0.8 (CL_{cr}) + 26.6$
Cefazolin	$k = (0.0028 \times CL_{cr}) + 0.022$	$CL = 0.34 (CL_{cr}) + 6.6$
Ceftazidime	$k = (0.004 \times CL_{cr}) + 0.004$	$CL = 1.15 (CL_{cr}) + 10.6$
Ciprofloxacin		$CL = 2.83 (CL_{cr}) + 363$
Digoxin		$CL = 0.88 (CL_{cr}) + 23$
Ganciclovir		$CL = 1.24 (CL_{cr}) + 8.57$
Gentamicin	$k = (0.0029 \times CL_{cr}) + 0.015$	$CL = 0.983 (CL_{cr})$
Imipenem		$CL = 1.42 (CL_{cr}) + 54$
Lithium		$CL = 0.20 (CL_{cr})$
Ofloxacin		$CL = 1.04 (CL_{cr}) + 38.7$
Piperacillin	$k = (0.0049 \times CL_{cr}) + 0.21$	$CL = 1.36 (CL_{cr}) + 1.50$
Tobramycin	$k = (0.0029 \times CL_{cr}) + 0.01$	$CL = 0.801 (CL_{cr})$
Vancomycin	$k = (0.00083 \times CL_{cr}) + 0.0044$	$CL = 0.69 (CL_{cr}) + 3.7$

CL, total body clearance; CL_{cr}, creatinine clearance.

[a]Clearance in mL/min can be converted to mL/s through multiplication by 0.0167.

assumptions are true, then the kinetic parameter/dosage-adjustment factor (Q) can be calculated as:

$$Q = 1 - [f_e(1 - KF)]$$

where KF is the ratio of the patient's CL_{cr} or GFR to the assumed normal value of 120 mL/min (equivalent to 2 mL/s). Thus for a drug that is 85% eliminated renally unchanged in a patient who has a CL_{cr} of 10 mL/min (0.17 mL/s), the Q factor would be:

$$\begin{aligned} Q &= 1 - \{0.85[1 - (10/120)]\} \\ &= 1 - [0.85(0.92)] \\ &= 1 - 0.78 \\ &= 0.22 \end{aligned}$$

The best method for dosage regimen adjustment must then be selected. Specifically, one must determine whether the desired goal is the maintenance of a similar peak, trough, or average steady-state drug concentration or if there is a clearly defined pharmacodynamics endpoint such as the time above the minimum inhibitory concentration (MIC) or the ratio of the AUC relative to the MIC. If there is a significant relationship between peak concentration and clinical response[66] (e.g., aminoglycosides) or toxicity[67] (e.g., phenobarbital and phenytoin), then attainment of the specific target values is critical. If, however, no specific target values for peak or trough concentrations have been reported (e.g., antihypertensive agents and benzodiazepines), then a regimen goal of attaining the same average steady-state concentration is likely to be appropriate.

Although several methods have been proposed to attain the desired average steady-state concentration profile, the principal choices are to decrease the dose or prolong the dosing interval. If the size of the dose is reduced while the dosing interval remains unchanged, the desired average steady-state concentration will be similar; however, the peak will be lower and the trough higher (Fig. 33-1). Alternatively, if the dosing interval is increased and the dose size remains unchanged, the peak and trough concentrations in the patient with reduced renal function will be similar to those in the patient with normal renal function. This dosage adjustment method is often recommended because it is likely to yield cost savings as a result of a reduction in nursing and pharmacy time, as well as a reduction in the supplies associated with frequent drug administration. Finally, the dose and dosing interval may both need to be changed to allow the administration of a clinically feasible dose (500 mg vs. a calculated value of 487 mg) or a practical dosing interval, for example, 12 hours instead of 17 hours.

If the relationship between the pharmacokinetic parameters of the drug and renal function are known, the first step in the process is to estimate the drug disposition parameters in the patient with renal insufficiency. The dosage-adjustment factor (Q) can then be calculated as the ratio of the estimated k or CL of the patient relative to subjects with normal renal function defined as a CL_{cr} = 120 mL/min (2 mL/s) by Rowland and Tozer.[14] The dosage adjustment factor is then used to determine the dose or dosing interval alterations

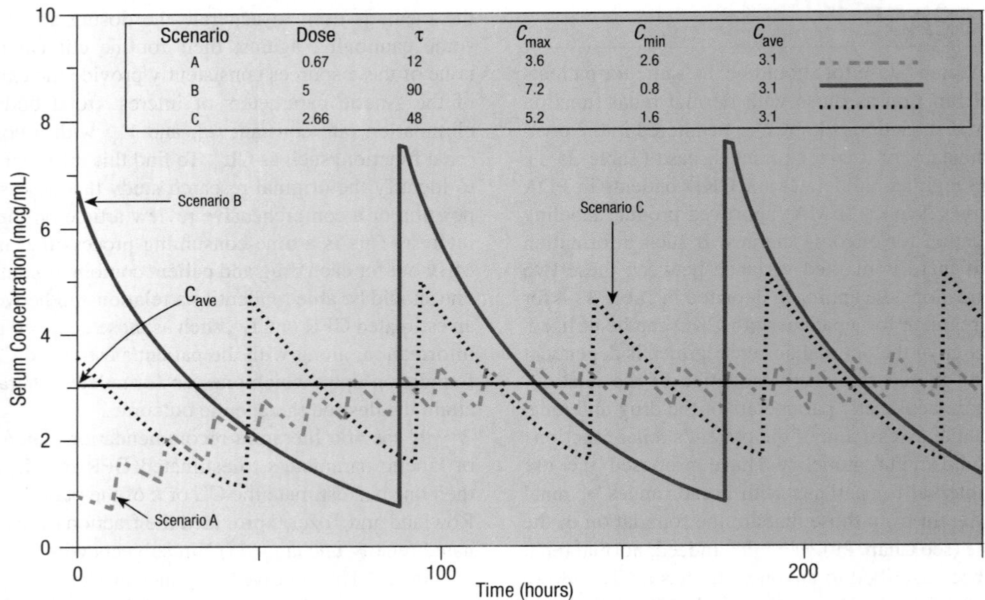

FIGURE 33-1 Although the average steady-state concentrations (C_{ave}) are identical regardless of which dosage-adjustment strategy one decides to implement, the concentration–time profile will be markedly different if one changes the dose and maintains the dosing interval (τ) constant (*Scenario A*), versus changing the dosing interval and maintaining the dose constant (*Scenario B*) or changing both (*Scenario C*).

TABLE 33-6 Stepwise Approach to Calculating a Dosage Regimen Based on Drug's Pharmacokinetic Characteristics and Patient's Renal Function

	Steps	Calculation Examples with Cefazolin
Step 1	Calculate total body clearance of drug in a subject with normal renal function (CL_{norm}); CL_{cr} = 120 mL/min	$CL_{norm} = [0.34 (CL_{cr})] + 6.6$ $CL_{norm} = [0.34(120)] + 6.6$ $CL_{norm} = 47.4$ mL/min per 1.8 m^2
Step 2	Calculate total body clearance of drug in a subject with renal insufficiency (CL_{fail})	In patient with $CL_{cr} = 15$ mL/min $CL_{fail} = [0.34(CL_{cr})] + 6.6$ $CL_{fail} = [0.34(15)] + 6.6$ $CL_{fail} = 11.7$ mL/min per 1.8 m^2
Step 3	Calculate the quotient (Q) for a subject with renal insufficiency	$Q = CL_{fail}/CL_{norm}$ $Q = 11.7/47.4$ $Q = 0.25$
Step 4	Calculate the maintenance dose (D_f) or adjusted dosing interval (τ_f) in a subject with renal insufficiency; D_n = normal dose; τ_n = normal dosing interval	$D_n = 1{,}000$ mg; $\tau_n = 8$ h $D_f = D_n \times Q$ $D_f = 1{,}000 \text{ mg} \times 0.25$ $D_f = 250$ mg $\tau_f = \tau_n/Q$ $\tau_f = 8/0.25$ $\tau_f = 32$ h
Step 5	Choose dosing adjustment: 1. Maintain D_n and use τ_f 2. Maintain τ_n and use D_f	Dosing adjustments: 1. 1,000 mg every 32 h 2. 250 mg every 8 h
Step 6	Calculate D_f based on practical dosing interval (τ_p), which is selected	$D_n = 1{,}000$ mg; $\tau_f = 32$ h; $\tau = 12$ h (selected to limit missed doses) $D_f = (D_n \times Q \times \tau_p)/\tau_n$ $D_f = (1{,}000 \text{ mg} \times 0.25 \times 12)/32$ $D_f = 375$ mg
Step 7	Recommend dosing regimen (dependent on product availability and limited risk of missed doses)	375 mg every 12 h

CL_{cr}, creatinine clearance.

Creatinine clearance in mL/min can be converted to mL/s through multiplication by 0.0167. Clearance in mL/min per 1.73 m^2 can be converted to mL/s/m^2 through multiplication by 0.00963.

necessary for the patient. Table 33-6 provides an example application of the stepwise approach of calculating a dosage regimen based on pharmacokinetic characteristics of the drug and the patient's renal function.

The relationship between drug clearance and CL_{cr} (expressed in conventional units of mL/min) has been reported for several drugs (Table 33-5). How one can apply the relationship between a patient's renal function and pharmacokinetic characteristics of cefazolin, a commonly used antibiotic for the treatment of infections in CKD and dialysis patients to develop and individualized dosage recommendation are illustrated in Table 33-6 and briefly highlighted here. The first step is to calculate the CL of cefazolin for a subject with normal renal function (CL_{norm}) and CL for the patient with renal insufficiency (CL_{fail}) to obtain the ratio of the predicted clearance values (Q) which can be used to calculate the new dosing regimen.

It is also important to consider other characteristics of cefazolin, such as MICs and concentrations associated with toxicities and adverse events, before modifying a dosage regimen. For cefazolin, the rate of cell kill is optimized by maintaining the concentration of drug above the MIC of the organism for at least 40% of the dosing interval. In general, this means that lower doses given more frequently would be expected to achieve target attainment to a greater degree than high doses given less often. The intermittent dose method may also achieve high concentrations of cefazolin which could result in dose-dependent toxicities such as seizures.[68] Therefore, in the example shown in Table 33-6, the maintenance dose (D_f) for a patient with renal insufficiency and the adjusted dosing interval (τ_f) are calculated from the relationships between the Q value and the normal dose (D_n) and normal dosing interval (τ_n).

If the V_D of a drug is significantly altered in CKD patients or in whom one desires to attain a specific maximum or minimum concentration, the estimation of a dosage regimen becomes more complex. If the relationship between V_D and CL_{cr} has been characterized, then V_D may be estimated. If one assumes that a one-compartment linear model can describe the drug, the predicted V_D may then be used with the predicted k of the drug to yield an adjusted-dosing interval and IV dose.

For orally administered drugs, the τ_f can be calculated and the dose can be approximated as:

$$\tau_f = \{(-1/k_f)[\ln(C_{min}/C_{max})]\} + t_{peak}$$

$$\text{Dose}_{po} = [FC^t{}_p V_D(k_a - k)]/[k_a(e^{-kt}/1 - e^{-k\tau})(e^{-k_a t}/1 - e^{-k_a \tau})]$$

where F equals bioavailability, C^t_p equals the desired plasma concentration at time t, and k_a is the absorption rate constant. This approach allows for the individualization of an oral dosage regimen for attainment of specific peak and trough serum concentrations. If the drug is absorbed extremely rapidly, one can approximate the τ_f and the dose using equations originally proposed for IV dosing as:

$$\tau_f = (-1/k_f)[\ln(C_{min}/C_{max})]$$

$$\text{Dose}_{po} = V_D \times (C_{max} - C_{min})$$

These principles have been used by many investigators to derive dosage recommendations for commonly used drugs for patients with CKD (Tables 33-7 and 33-8).[61,63,68–75]

DRUG DOSAGE REGIMEN DESIGN FOR PATIENTS RECEIVING RENAL REPLACEMENT THERAPY

Continuous renal replacement therapies are used for the management of fluid overload and the removal of uremic toxins in patients with AKI and other conditions.[69] Several forms of continuous renal replacement therapy in clinical use today are extensively described in Chapter 28 and several dosage regimen individualization approaches are presented and critiqued. Which of these therapies will be optimal for a given patient is dependent on several factors, including bleeding risk, degree of hypercatabolism, acid–base balance, and experience of the healthcare provider team. The rationale for and approaches for delivery of renal replacement therapy on an intermittent and occasionally continuous basis for those with ESRD are described in Chapter 30.

Peritoneal Dialysis

Peritoneal dialysis, like other dialysis modalities, has the potential to affect drug disposition; however, drug therapy individualization is often less complicated in these patients as a result of the limited drug clearances achieved with the variants of this procedure (see Chap. 30). In general, hemodialysis is more effective in removing drugs than peritoneal dialysis such that if a drug is not removed by hemodialysis, it is unlikely to be significantly removed by peritoneal dialysis. Many of the factors that are important in determining drug dialyzability for other treatment modalities pertain to peritoneal dialysis as well.[76,77] Factors that influence drug dialyzability by peritoneal dialysis include drug-specific characteristics such as molecular weight, solubility, degree of ionization, protein binding, and V_D. The intrinsic properties of the peritoneal membrane that affect drug removal include blood flow and peritoneal membrane surface area, which is

TABLE 33-7 Drug Dosing Guidelines for Nonantibiotics Commonly Used by CKD Patients

		Glomerular Filtration Rate (mL/min)[a]			
Drug	**Usual Dose**	**30–50**	**10–30**	**<10**	**IHD Dosing**
Amlodipine	5–10 mg daily	100%	100%	100%	100%
Atenolol	50–100 mg daily	100%	50 mg q24 h,	25 mg q24 h	25–50 mg three times weekly
Atorvastatin	10 mg daily	100%	100%	100%	100%
Bumetanide	0.5–2 mg q 8–12 h	100%	100%	100%	100%
Digoxin	Indication: dependent; LD: 1–1.5 mg MD: 0.125–0.5 mg q 24 h	LD: 100%, MD: 25–50% q 24 h	LD: 100%, MD: 25–75% q 24 h	LD: 50%, MD: 10–25% q 48 h	LD: 50%, MD: 10–25% q 48 h
Diltiazem	30 mg q 6–8 h (oral regular)	100%	100%	100%	100%
Esomeprazole	20–40 mg daily	100%	100%	100%	100%
Exenatide (immediate release)	5–10 mcg q 12 h	100%[b]	Avoid	Avoid	Avoid
Famotidine	20–40 mg daily	50% daily	50% daily	25–50% daily	25–50% daily or 20–40 mg q 48–72 h
Furosemide	Individualize	100%	100%	100%	100%
Gabapentin	300–600 mg q 8 h	200–700 mg q 12 h	200–700 mg q 24	100–300 mg q 24	LD: 300 mg, MD: 100–300 mg q 24 Post-HD:100–300 mg
Glipizide	5–10 mg daily	50%	50%	50%	50%
Glyburide	2.5–5 mg daily	Avoid	Avoid	Avoid	Avoid
Hydralazine (oral)	25–50 mg q 6 h	q 8 h	q 8 h	q 8–12 h	q 8–12 h
Hydrochlorothiazide	25–50 mg daily	100%	Avoid[c]	Avoid[c]	Avoid[c]
Insulin	Variable	75%	75%	50%	50%
Lansoprazole	15–60 mg daily	100%	100%	100%	100%
Lisinopril	10 mg daily	50–75%	50%	25%	25%
Metformin	0.5–1 g q 12 h	25–50%	25%	Avoid	Avoid
Metoprolol	25–200 mg q 12 h	100%	100%	100%	100%
Olmesartan	20–40 mg daily	100%	100%	100%	100%
Pantoprazole (oral)	40 mg q 12 h	100%	100%	100%	100%
Pravastatin	10–40 mg daily	100%	10 mg q 24 h	10 mg q 24	10 mg q 24
Pregabalin	300 mg/day	50%	25%	10–25%	10–25% Post-HD:50–75 mg
Ranitidine	150–300 mg daily (oral)	150 mg q 24 h	150 mg q 24 h	75 mg q 24 h	75 mg q 24 h
Rosuvastatin	5–40 mg daily	100%	5–10 mg daily[d]	5–10 mg daily[d]	5–10 mg daily[d]
Simvastatin	10–40 mg daily	100%	100%	5 mg q 24 h	5 mg q 24
Sitagliptin	100 mg daily	50%	25%	25%	25%
Spironolactone	50–100 mg/daily	Usual dose, q 12–24 h	Usual dose, q 12–24 h	Avoid	Avoid

IHD, intermittent hemodialysis; LD, loading dose; MD, maintenance dosing.

[a]The range following glomerular filtration rate (GFR) indicates the use of the dose that corresponds to that range of GFR in patients not on dialysis. GFR in mL/min can be converted to mL/s through multiplication by 0.0167.

[b]Caution should be used when initiating or escalating dose.

[c]Should not be used with Cl_{cr} <30 mL/min (<0.5 mL/s), but are effective with loop diuretics.

[d]Initial dose should be 5 mg daily and titrate as needed to a maximum dose of 10 mg daily.

Data from references 46, 48, 54, 74, and 75.

approximately equal to the body surface area. There is an inverse relationship between peritoneal drug clearance and molecular weight, protein binding, and V_D. In addition, drug compounds that are ionized at physiologic pH will diffuse across the membrane more slowly than unionized compounds. Detailed reviews of the disposition of several drugs in chronic peritoneal dialysis patients are reported elsewhere.[76,78] Antiinfective agents are the most commonly studied drugs because of their primary role in the treatment of peritonitis.[76,79] The treatment priorities for peritoneal dialysis peritonitis and the recommended drug regimens are presented in detail in Chapter 30 (see Tables 30-10 and 30-11).

Peritoneal dialysis, in current practice, is often prescribed to attain a urea clearance of approximately 10 mL/min (0.17 mL/s), so it is unlikely to significantly impact the CL of any drug by more than 10 mL/min (0.17 mL/s).[6] In addition, since most medications have a larger molecular size than urea, their resultant CL will likely be even lower: probably between 5 and 7.5 mL/min (0.08 to 0.13 mL/s). Therefore, drug dosing recommendations for the management of conditions other than peritonitis, reported for patients with estimated CL_{cr} or GFR of 10 to 15 mL/min (0.17 to 0.25 mL/s), are likely suitable for patients receiving peritoneal dialysis.[63]

Hemodialysis

Although many new hemodialyzers have been introduced in the last 20 years and more than 100 different ones were available in the United States in 2013, the effect of hemodialysis on drug disposition is rarely reevaluated after it is initially reported. Thus, most of the

TABLE 33-8 Antibiotic Drug Dosing Recommendations

Drug	Regimen for Normal Renal Function	Glomerular Filtration Rate (mL/min)[a]			
		30–50	10–30	<10	IHD Dosing
Amoxicillin	0.5–1.0 g q8	q 8–12 h	q 12 h	q 24 h	0.25–0.5 g q 24 h
Amoxicillin/clavulanate	500/125 mg q 8 h	q 8–12 h	q 12 h[b]	q 12 h[b]	q 12–24 h[b]
Ampicillin	1–2 g q 6 h	q 6–12	q 6–12	q 12–24	1 g q 12 h
Ampicillin/sulbactam	1.5–3 g q 6–8 h	q 8 h	q 12 h	q 12–24 h	q 12–24 h
Azithromycin	250–500 mg q 24 h	100%	100%	100%	100%
Cefazolin	1–2 g q 8 h	q 8–12 h	0.5–1 g q 12 h	0.5–1 g q 24 h	15–20 mg/kg q 48–72
Cefepime	2 g q 8–12 h	q 12–24 h	1–2 g q 24 h	0.5–1 g q 24 h	1–2 g q 48–72 h
Ceftriaxone	1 g q 24 h	100%	100%	100%	100%
Cephalexin	250–1,000 mg q 6 h	500 mg q 8–12 h	500 mg q 8–12 h	250–500 mg q 12–24 h	250 mg q 12–24 h
Ciprofloxacin	400 mg q 8–12 h (IV) 500–750 mg q 12 h (oral)	q 8–12 h 50–75%	q 24 h 50–75%	q 24 h 50%	200–400 q 24 50%
Doripenem	500 mg q 8 h	250 mg q 8 h	250 mg q 12 h	250 mg q 12 h	250 mg q 24 h[c]
Ertapenem	1g q 24 h	100%	50%	50%	50%
Fluconazole	200–800 mg q 24 h	50–75%	50%	50%	200–400 mg q 48–72 h
Imipenem	0.5 g q 6 h	0.5 g q 8 h	0.5 g q 12 h	0.25 g q 12 h	0.25–0.5 g q 12 h
Levofloxacin	500–750 mg q 24 h	50% q 24 h	50% q 24–48 h	25–50% q 48 h	25–50% q 48–72 h
Meropenem	1 g q 8 h	1 g q 12 h	0.5–1 g q 12 h	0.5 g q 24 h	1 g q 48–72 h
Moxifloxacin	400 mg q 24 h	100%	100%	100%	100%
Penicillin G	1–4 million U q 4–6 h	75%	75%	25–50%	LD: usual dose MD: 25–50% q 4–6 h or 50–100% q 8–12 h
Piperacillin/tazobactam[d]	3.375–4.5 g q 6 h	2.25–3.375 g q 6 h	2.25–3.375 g q 8–12 h	2.25 g q 8–12	125 g q 8–12 h
Tobramycin[e]	5–7 mg/kg q 24 h	5–7 mg/kg q 36–48 h	IND	IND	1.5–2 mg/kg q 48–72 h and then IND
Trimethoprim/ sulfamethoxazole[f]	2.5–5 mg/kg q 6–12 h	q 6–12 h	q 12–24 h	q 24 h	2.5–10 mg/kg/day or 5–20 mg/kg three times weekly
Vancomycin[e,g]	15–20 mg/kg q 8–12 h	q 24 h	IND	IND	LD: 15–25 mg/kg MD: 5–10 mg/kg (after IHD)

IND, individualize based on concentration monitoring; IHD, intermittent hemodialysis; LD, loading dose; MD, maintenance dosing; MU, million units; NC, no change.

[a]The range following glomerular filtration rate (GFR) indicates the use of the dose that corresponds to that range of GFR in patients not on dialysis. GFR in mL/min can be converted to mL/s through multiplication by 0.0167.

[b]Extended release and 875 mg tablets are not recommended.

[c]For infection caused by *Pseudomonas aeruginosa*, should be dosed 500 mg IV q 12 h on day 1, then 500 mg IV q 24 h.

[d]First dosage modification should be made at a GFR of ≤40 mL/min (≤0.67 mL/s). Second dosage modification should be made at a GFR of <20 mL/min (<0.33 mL/s).

[e]Dosing in critically ill patients should be individualized based on pharmacokinetic monitoring.

[f]Dosed based on trimethoprim component.

[g]A vancomycin loading dose of 25–30 mg/kg (based on actual body weight) should be considered for all patients. In patients with a GFR ≤ 30 mL/min (≤0.5 mL/s), subsequent doses of 15 to 20 mg/kg should be given when the serum concentration falls below 10 mg/L or 20 mg/L (6.9 or 14 μmol/L) (depending on the site of infection and MIC of organism)

Data from references 53, 64, and 75–78.

literature, especially for older medications, probably represents an underestimation of the impact of hemodialysis on its disposition.[80,81]

6 The impact of hemodialysis on a patient's drug therapy is dependent on several factors, including the characteristics of the drug, the dialysis conditions, and the clinical situation for which dialysis is performed. Drug-related factors that affect dialyzability include the molecular weight or size, degree of protein binding, and V_D.[4] The vast majority of dialysis filters in use in the United States up until the mid-1990s were composed of cellulose, cellulose acetate, or regenerated cellulose (cuprophane), and they were generally impermeable to drugs with a molecular weight greater than 1,000 Da.[82] Drugs that are small but highly protein bound also are not well dialyzed because both of the principal binding proteins, α_1-acid glycoprotein and albumin, have a very high molecular weight. Finally, those drugs that are widely distributed, V_D greater than 2 L/kg, are poorly removed by hemodialysis.

The hemodialysis procedure, be it acute for the management of AKI, intermittent three times a week or daily for an extended period or some combination thereof for the management of ESRD can dramatically affect the dialysis clearance of a medication.[81] The primary factors that vary between patients are the composition of the dialysis filter, the filter surface area, the blood, dialysate and ultrafiltration flow rates, and whether or not the dialysis unit reuses the dialysis filter. Dialysis membranes in the 21st century are predominantly composed of semisynthetic or synthetic materials (e.g., polysulfone, polymethylmethacrylate, or polyacrylonitrile). High-flux dialysis membranes have larger pore sizes and more closely mimic the filtration characteristics of the human kidney. This allows the passage of most solutes, including drugs (e.g., vancomycin) that have a molecular weight of 20,000 Da or less.[80,82] An increase in removal has also been reported with several other drugs that have lower molecular weights (Table 33-9).[80]

TABLE 33-9 Drug Disposition during Dialysis Depends on Dialyzer Characteristics

	Hemodialysis Clearance (mL/min)[a]		Half-Life during Dialysis (h)	
Drug	**Conventional**	**High Flux**	**Conventional**	**High Flux**
Cefazolin	15.1	30–38	NR	NR
Ceftazidime	60	155[b]	3.3	1.2[b]
Cefuroxime	NR	103[c]	3.8	1.6[c]
Foscarnet	183	253[c]	NR	NR
Gentamicin	58.2	116[c]	3	4.3[c]
Netilmicin	46	87–109	5–5.2	2.9–3.4
Ranitidine	43.1	67.2[c]	5.1	2.9[c]
Vancomycin	9–21	40–150[c]	35–38	4.5–11.8[c]

NR, not reported.
[a]Clearance in mL/min can be converted to mL/s through multiplication by 0.0167.
[b]Polyamide filter.
[c]Polysulfone filter.
Adapted from reference 59.

Overall, the impact of hemodialysis on drug therapy is highly variable and thus one cannot assume that a certain percentage of a drug is removed with each dialysis session; neither should a "yes" answer regarding the dialyzability of drugs be considered sufficient information to make therapeutic decisions, since this provides no quantification of the impact of hemodialysis. Characteristics of the dialysis procedure that was utilized in the drug study, such as membrane composition and surface area and blood and dialysis flow rates, are thus critical data that should be known before one uses the hemodialysis clearance data to prospectively design a drug dosing regimen for a hemodialysis patient.

The quantitative impact of hemodialysis on drug disposition can be calculated in several ways.[4] The most commonly utilized means for assessing the effect of hemodialysis is to calculate the dialyzer clearance (CL_D) of the drug. The CL_D can be calculated by several approaches. The CL_D^b from blood can be calculated as $CL_D^b = Q_b [(A_b - V_b)/A_b]$, where Q_b is the blood flow through the dialyzer, A_b is the concentration of drug in blood going into the dialyzer, and V_b is the blood concentration of the drug leaving the dialyzer. This equation, also known as the "*A–V* difference method," is valid only if the drug concentrations are measured in whole blood and if the drug rapidly and completely distributes into red blood cells. Because drug concentrations are generally determined in plasma, the previous equation is usually modified to $CL_D^p = Q_p [(A_p - V_p)/A_p]$, where p represents plasma and Q_p is the plasma flow, which equals Q_b (1 – hematocrit). This clearance calculation most accurately reflects dialysis drug clearance as most drugs do not significantly penetrate red blood cells or bind to formed blood elements. However, for drugs that readily partition into and out of erythrocytes, this equation could likely underestimate hemodialysis clearance. Furthermore, one must keep in mind that venous plasma concentrations may be artificially high and CL_D^p will be low if plasma water is removed from the blood at a faster rate than the drug. This tends to occur when extensive ultrafiltration is performed simultaneously with diffusion during dialysis.[6]

The recovery clearance approach remains the benchmark for the determination of dialyzer clearance and it can be calculated as:[4]

$$CL_D^r = R/AUC_{0-t}$$

where, R is the total amount of drug recovered unchanged in the dialysate and AUC_{0-t} is the area under the predialyzer plasma concentration–time curve during the period of time that the dialysate was collected. To determine the AUC_{0-t}, at least two and preferably three to four plasma concentrations should be obtained during dialysis.

The hemodialysis clearance values reported in the literature may vary significantly depending on which of these methods were used to calculate CL_D. The principal reason for this is that for most medications we do not know the degree and rapidity with which the drug crosses the red blood cell membrane. Because the CL_D^r method incorporates no assumption of the degree of red blood cell permeability, it can be reliably used as the benchmark value. The primary limitation of this calculation is that the concentrations of the drug in the dialysate may be below the sensitivity limits of the assay.

The following principles may be used to generate a drug dosage regimen recommendation for hemodialysis patients by using a value of CL_D that is reported in the literature.[4,80] Because clearance terms are additive, the total clearance during dialysis can be calculated as the sum of the patient's residual renal and nonrenal clearance during the interdialytic period (CL_{RES}) and dialyzer clearance (CL_D):

$$CL_T = CL_{RES} + CL_D$$

The half-life during the period between dialysis treatments and during dialysis can then be calculated from the following relationships using an estimate of the drug's V_D, which can be obtained from the literature:[65]

$$t_{1/2,\text{off HD}} = 0.693(V_D/CL_{RES})$$
$$t_{1/2,\text{on HD}} = 0.693(V_D/CL_{RES} + CL_D)$$

Once the key pharmacokinetic parameters have been estimated/calculated, they may be used to simulate the plasma concentration–time profile of the drug for the individual patient and then one can ascertain how much drug to administer and when. This approach to drug therapy individualization can be accomplished in a stepwise fashion assuming first-order elimination of the drug and a one-compartment model.

For example, a 54-year-old critically ill female with ESRD was transferred to a medical intensive care unit from the general medical unit, where she was febrile with a temperature of 39°C (102.2°F). Her weight was 64 kg (141 lb) and her height was 65 inches (165 cm). She had a residual CL_{cr} of 3 mL/min (0.05 mL/s), and was receiving high-flux dialysis (F80 polysulfone dialyzer) for 4 hours on Mondays, Wednesdays, and Fridays. She was started on vancomycin for a methicillin-resistant *Staphylococcus aureus* (MRSA) catheter-associated bacteremia and her first dose of 1,000 mg was administered at the end of her hemodialysis treatment at the referring hospital. The first step is to estimate this patient's pharmacokinetic parameters of vancomycin on the basis of published population data.[83] The V_D in this patient can be estimated to be 54.4 L (0.85 L/kg × 64 kg), and her residual total body clearance (CL_{RES}) estimated from the relationship between CL and CL_{cr} [$CL_{RES} = (0.69 \times CL_{cr}) + 3.7$] is 7.15 mL/min (0.12 mL/s) or 0.43 L/h. The k can be approximated as:

$$\begin{aligned} k &= CL_{RES}/V_D \\ &= 0.43\ \text{L/h}/54.4\ \text{L} \\ &= 0.0079\ \text{h}^{-1} \end{aligned}$$

The hemodialysis clearance of vancomycin (CL_D) is dependent on the dialyzer and a value of 120 mL/min (2 mL/s; 7.2 L/h) is a reasonable estimate for this dialyzer.[84]

One now can predict what the plasma concentrations of vancomycin will be over the next 24 to 48 hours, assuming the infusion time for the drug (t') was 1 hour. The concentration at the end of the 1-hour infusion (C_{max}) would be:

$$\begin{aligned} C_{max} &= \frac{(\text{Dose}/t')(1 - e^{-kt'})}{CL_{RES}} \\ &= \frac{(1{,}000\ \text{mg/h})(1 - e^{-(0.0079)1})}{0.43\ \text{L/h}} \\ &= (2{,}325.58\ \text{mg/L})(0.0078) \\ &= 18.1\ \text{mg/L} \end{aligned}$$

The plasma concentration prior to the next dialysis session (C_{bD}), which is 44 hours away, and the concentration 4 hours later after dialysis (C_{aD}) can be calculated as:

$$\begin{aligned} C_{bD} &= C_{max} \times e^{-(CL_{RES}/V_D) \times t} \\ &= 18.1 \times e^{-0.0079 \times 44} \\ &= 12.8 \text{ mg/L} \\ C_{aD} &= C_{bD} \times e^{-[(CL_{RES} + CL_D)/V_D] \times t} \\ &= 12.8 \times e^{-[(0.43 + 7.2)/54.4] \times 4} \\ &= 12.8 \times e^{-0.14 \times 4} \\ &= 7.3 \text{ mg/L} \end{aligned}$$

On the basis of these data, the second dose which should be administered after the second dialysis session should be increased as one generally desires to maintain vancomycin trough concentrations between 15 and 20 mg/L (10 to 14 μmol/L) for a MRSA catheter-associated bacteremia.[70,85] The patient received a vancomycin dose of 1,500 mg 4 hours after the end of the second dialysis session. The increase in serum concentration at the end of this 1-hour infusion (C_{change}) would be:

$$\begin{aligned} C_{change} &= \frac{(\text{Dose}/t')(1 - e^{-kt'})}{CL_{RES}} \\ &= \frac{(1{,}500 \text{ mg/h})(1 - e^{-(0.0079)1})}{0.43 \text{ L/h}} \\ &= (3{,}488.4 \text{ mg/L})(0.0078) \\ &= 27.2 \text{ mg/L} \end{aligned}$$

Thus the C_{max} would be approximately 34 mg/L (24 μmol/L), the sum of the residual concentration from the first dose of approximately 7 mg/L (5 μmol/L) and the C_{change}. The plasma concentration prior to the third dialysis session (C_{bD}), which is 40 hours away, and the concentration 4 hours later after the third dialysis (C_{aD}) can be estimated as:

$$\begin{aligned} C_{bD} &= C_{max} \times e^{-(CL_{RES}/V_D) \times t} \\ &= 34 \text{ mg/L} \times e^{-0.0079 \times 40} \\ &= 24.8 \text{ mg/L} \\ C_{aD} &= C_{bD} \times e^{-[(CL_{RES} + CL_D)/V_D] \times t} \\ &= 24.8 \times e^{-[(0.43 + 7.2)/54.4] \times 4} \\ &= 24.8 \times e^{-0.14 \times 4} \\ &= 14.2 \text{ mg/L} \end{aligned}$$

This higher dose would be considered by many to have achieved too high of concentrations since the lowest value during the majority of the dosing interval exceeded 24.8 mg/L (17.1 μmol/L). Thus the serum concentration data from the several blood samples, which were collected to characterize this patient's residual vancomycin clearance, V_D, and the clearance of vancomycin during dialysis should be analyzed to generate a new dose estimate for administration after the second dialysis session. Blood samples were collected at the following times after the first dose of 1,000 mg so that the patient's pharmacokinetic parameters for vancomycin could be determined:

Day 1: 8 pm (4 hours after dose)	25 mg/L or mcg/mL (17 μmol/L)
Day 2: 9 am (39 hours after dose; just before dialysis)	18 mg/L or mcg/mL (12 μmol/L)
Day 3: 1 pm (immediately after dialysis)	10 mg/L or mcg/mL (6.9 μmol/L)

The elimination rate during the interdialytic period (k_{ID}) and during dialysis (k_{DD}), and the V_D can be calculated as:

$$\begin{aligned} k_{ID} &= (\ln C_1/C_2)/\Delta t \\ &= (\ln 25/18)/35 \\ &= 0.0094 \text{ h}^{-1} \end{aligned}$$

$$\begin{aligned} V_D &= \frac{\text{Dose}}{C_{max} - C_{min}} \\ &= \frac{1{,}000 \text{ mg}}{25 \text{ mg/L} - 0 \text{ mg/L}} \\ &= 40 \text{ L} \end{aligned}$$

$$\begin{aligned} k_{DD} &= (\ln C_2/C_3)/\Delta t \\ &= (\ln 18/10)/4 \\ &= 0.1496 \text{ h}^{-1} \end{aligned}$$

where Δt is the time in hours between the two measured concentrations and C_{min} the vancomycin concentration in plasma prior to the administration of the first dose is zero. The patient's residual clearance (CL_{RES}) and dialyzer clearance (CL_D) of vancomycin can then be calculated as:

$$\begin{aligned} CL_{RES} &= V_D \times k_{ID} \\ &= 40 \text{ L} \times 0.0094 \\ &= 0.376 \text{ L/h or } 6.26 \text{ mL/min } (0.10 \text{ mL/s}) \\ CL_D &= CL_T - CL_{RES} \\ &= (k_{DD} \times V_D) - 6.26 \text{ mL/min} \\ &= (5.88 \text{ L/h or } 97.9 \text{ mL/min}) - 6.26 \text{ mL/min} \\ &= 91.64 \text{ mL/min } (1.53 \text{ mL/s}) \end{aligned}$$

Analysis of the measured serum concentrations obtained after the first dose yielded pharmacokinetic parameters that were significantly less than those projected based on population data: the patient's residual clearance was 12.5% lower and the volume of distribution was 26.5% lower. Thus the serum peak concentration was 6.9 mg/L (4.8 μmol/L) higher than desired and the concentration prior to the second dialysis session was almost 30% higher than desired. These measured values in clinical practice could now be utilized to plan the dosage to be administered after the third dialysis session.

For medications with a narrow therapeutic index (e.g., vancomycin and gentamicin), therapeutic drug monitoring (e.g., plasma concentration measurements and dialyzer clearance estimation) should be utilized to guide drug dosing.[6] The ultimate reason for measuring the plasma concentrations of aminoglycosides, vancomycin, and several other antibacterial agents is to individualize the patient's dosage regimen to achieve a bacteriologic cure while preserving residual renal function. Thus there remains one important step in our evaluation: the calculation of the dose this patient should receive after the second dialysis session. The two factors that enter into this decision are the desired peak and trough concentrations. Vancomycin dosing is primarily based on attaining desired trough concentrations, usually between 15 and 20 mg/L (10 to 14 μmol/L). Peak concentrations are rarely used and not recommended to derive dosing recommendations and adjustments; however, for this patient example, a desired peak concentration [20 to 40 mg/L (14 to 28 μmol/L)] could be utilized to calculate a dose.[70] In addition to considering desired vancomycin concentrations, it is important to consider the timing of vancomycin sample collections relative to the time of dialysis. If vancomycin levels are obtained after hemodialysis, it is recommended to wait at least 3 hours to check a level because vancomycin concentrations have been noted to reach the maximum rebounded concentration within 3 hours after the end of hemodialysis.[86]

Assuming the desired peak concentration was 30 mg/L (21 μmol/L) and trough concentration was 15 mg/L (10 micromol/L), the postdialysis dose this patient would need can then be calculated using the simplified approach below, because the $t_{1/2}$ is extremely prolonged relative to the infusion time, and thus minimal drug is eliminated during the infusion period:

$$\begin{aligned}\text{Dose} &= V_D \times (C_{max} - C_{min}) \\ &= 40\ \text{L} \times (30 - 15) \\ &= 600\ \text{mg}\end{aligned}$$

7 It is common practice in most hemodialysis units to administer drugs after the patient has received dialysis on the premise that it is desirable to minimize the loss of drug that would result from the additional clearance during hemodialysis. Certainly, administration of antihypertensive agents and vasoactive drugs should be avoided in the hours prior to a hemodialysis session to minimize the likelihood of hypotension. However, emerging pharmacokinetic and pharmacodynamic considerations suggest that this may not be the optimal approach for several other agents, such as aminoglycosides[87–89] and vancomycin.[90–92] Two evaluations of predialysis and one of intradialytic dosing of aminoglycosides indicate that similar peak concentrations, a prime indicator of efficacy, can be obtained in these scenarios relative to those observed with postdialysis dosing.[87,88] The AUC during the dosing interval and the subsequent predialysis concentrations were noted to be significantly reduced and thus the risk of ototoxicity and further renal injury may be minimized. The best dosing schedule, a dose roughly twice that traditionally employed for postdialysis administration, in the 26 patients evaluated by Teigen et al., resulted in the achievement of the desired peak and AUC in approximately 90% of patients.[88] The administration of traditional doses of tobramycin (1.5 mg/kg) or vancomycin (1,000 mg) during dialysis has been associated with markedly lower areas under the concentration–time curve than those observed when the same dose was administered postdialysis; consequently, higher dosage regimens are usually necessary to compensate for the additional loss of drug during the dialysis procedure. It is highly recommended that aminoglycoside and vancomycin concentrations in hemodialysis patients should be measured after the first dose and dialysis session and so that the dosage regimen can be individualized accordingly using Bayesian methodology whenever possible.

CLINICAL BOTTOM LINE

Subtherapeutic or supratherapeutic responses to drugs in patients with renal insufficiency are often misinterpreted and not recognized. The adverse outcomes associated with inappropriate drug dosing have not been quantified but do warrant future investigations. The utilization of FDA or EMA drug dosage recommendations in official prescribing information should be used for the initiation of therapy in most clinical situations. Critically ill individuals especially those with renal insufficiency likely have marked pharmacokinetic variability and may require the use of sound pharmacokinetic principles in concert with reliable population pharmacokinetic estimates to project the optimal approach to drug dosage regimen design. Individualization of all drugs with a narrow therapeutic index for AKI and CKD patients should be undertaken whenever clinical therapeutic monitoring tools are available. The key action step is to use the knowledge we have to improve patient outcomes. The recent study of van Dijk et al. is an unfortunate reminder of how far we still have to go to optimize the therapy of patients with renal insufficiency.[93] They observed that although dosage adjustments based on renal function were warranted in 24% of the prescriptions of the patients with CL_{cr} less than 51 mL/min (0.85 mL/s), such adjustments were only performed in 59% of cases.

ABBREVIATIONS

A_b	concentration of drug in blood going into the dialyzer (arterial side)
AKI	acute kidney injury
A_p	concentration of drug in plasma going into the dialyzer (arterial side)
$AUC_{0\text{-}t}$	the area under the predialyzer plasma concentration–time curve during hemodialysis
C_{aD}	plasma concentration after dialysis
C_{bD}	plasma concentration prior to the next dialysis session
C–G	Cockcroft–Gault
CKD	chronic kidney disease
CKD-EPI	chronic kidney disease epidemiology collaboration equation
CL	total body clearance
CL_D^b	dialyzer clearance from blood
CL_{cr}	creatinine clearance
CL_D	dialyzer clearance
CL_{fail}	clearance of a drug in patients with impaired renal function
CL_{norm}	clearance of a drug in patients with normal renal function
CL_D^p	dialyzer clearance from plasma
CL_R	net renal excretion
CL_D^r	recovery clearance of dialyzer
$CL_{reabsorption}$	tubular reabsorption
CL_{RES}	residual drug clearance in a dialysis patient
$CL_{secretion}$	tubular secretion
CL_T	total clearance during dialysis
C_{max}	peak drug concentration
C_{min}	trough drug concentration
C_{ss}	average steady-state plasma concentration
CYP	cytochrome P450
D_f	maintenance dose for a patient with renal insufficiency
D_n	dose for a patient with normal renal function
EBT	erythromycin breath test
ESRD	end-stage renal disease
f_e	fraction of drug eliminated unchanged in the urine
f_u	fraction of drug unbound to plasma proteins
GFR	glomerular filtration rate
k	elimination rate constant
k_{DD}	elimination rate constant during dialysis
KF	ratio of the patient's CL_{cr} to the assumed normal value of 120 mL/min (2 mL/s)
k_{ID}	elimination rate constant between dialysis sessions (interdialytic)
MDRD	modification of diet in renal disease equation
MIC	minimum inhibitory concentration
MRSA	methicillin-resistant *Staphylococcus aureus*
Q	kinetic parameter/dosage-adjustment factor
Q_b	blood flow through the dialyzer
Q_p	plasma flow through the dialyzer = Q_b (1 – hematocrit)
R	the total amount of drug recovered unchanged in the dialysate
t'	infusion time of drug
Δt	time in hours between two measured concentrations
$t_{1/2}$	half-life
$t_{1/2,\text{on HD}}$	half-life during dialysis
$t_{1/2,\text{off HD}}$	half-life off dialysis
τ_f	dosing interval in a patient with renal failure
τ_p	practical dosing interval for a patient with renal failure
τ_n	dosing interval in a patient with normal renal function
t_{max}	time-to-peak drug concentration
V_{area}	volume of distribution area

V_b blood concentration of drug leaving the dialyzer
V_β volume of terminal phase (serum protein)
V_c volume of the central compartment
V_D volume of distribution
V_{ss} volume of distribution at steady state

REFERENCES

1. National Kidney and Urologic Diseases Information Clearinghouse (NKUDIC). Kidney Disease Statistics for the United States. U.S. Department of Health and Human Services, New Release, November 2012, *http://kidney.niddk.nih.gov/kudiseases/pubs/kustats/*
2. Olyaei AJ, Steffl JL. A quantitative approach to drug dosing in chronic kidney disease. Blood Purif 2011;31:138–145.
3. Olyaei AJ, Bennett WM. Drug dosing in the elderly patients with chronic kidney disease. Clin Geriatr Med 2009;25:459–527.
4. Matzke GR, Comstock TJ. Influence of renal disease and dialysis on pharmacokinetics. In: Evans WE, Schentag JJ, Burton ME, eds. Applied Pharmacokinetics: Principles of Therapeutic Drug Monitoring, 4th ed. Baltimore, MD: Lippincott Williams & Wilkins, 2005:187–212.
5. Ritschel WA, Denson DD. Influence of disease on bioavailability. In: Ritschel WA, ed. Pharmacokinetics: Regulatory, Industrial, Academic Perspectives. New York, NY: Marcel Dekker, 1995.
6. Matzke GR, Aronoff GR, Atkinson AJ Jr, et al. Drug dosing consideration in patients with acute and chronic kidney disease—A clinical update from Kidney Disease: Improving Global Outcomes (KDIGO). Kidney Int 2011;80:1122–1137.
7. Naud J, Nolin TD, Leblond FA, Pichette V. Current understanding of drug disposition in kidney disease. J Clin Pharmacol 2012;52:10S–22S.
8. Verbeeck RK, Musuamba FT. Pharmacokinetics and dosage adjustment in patients with renal dysfunction. Eur J Clin Pharmacol 2009;65:757–773.
9. Dreisbach AW. The influence of chronic renal failure on drug metabolism and transport. Clin Pharmacol Ther 2009;86: 553–556.
10. Nolin TD. Altered nonrenal drug clearance in ESRD. Curr Opin Nephrol Hypertens 2008;17:555–559.
11. Momper JD, Venkataramanan R, Nolin TD. Nonrenal drug clearance in CKD: Searching for the path less traveled. Adv Chronic Kidney Dis 2010;17:384–391.
12. Nolin TD, Unruh ML. Clinical relevance of impaired nonrenal drug clearance in ESRD. Semin Dial 2010;23: 482–485.
13. Matzke GR, Marks SA, Dowling TC, Murphy JE, Burckart GJ. Influence of Kidney Disease on Drug Pharmacokinetics: An assessment of industry studies submitted to FDA for New Molecular Entities 1999–2010. Presented at 45th Annual Meeting of The American Society of Nephrology, November 3, 2012, San Diego, CA.
14. Rowland M, Tozer TN. Clinical Pharmacokinetics: Concepts and Applications, 3rd ed. Philadelphia, PA: Lea & Febiger, 1995:156–183.
15. Matzke GR, Dowling TD. Dosing concepts in renal dysfunction. In: Murphy JE, ed. Clinical Pharmacokinetics Pocket Reference, 5th ed. Bethesda, MD: American Society of Health-System Pharmacists, 2011:427–443.
16. Ibrahim S, Honig P, Huang SM, et al. Clinical pharmacology studies in patients with renal impairment: Past experience and regulatory perspectives. J Clin Pharmacol 2000;40(1):31–38.
17. Huang SM, Temple R, Xiao S, et al. When to conduct a renal impairment study during drug development: US Food and Drug Administration perspective. Clin Pharmacol Ther 2009:86:475–479.
18. Anonymous. Characterization of the relationship between the pharmacokinetics and pharmacodynamics of a drug and renal function. U.S. Department of Health and Human Services, FDA Guidance, May 1998, *http://www.fda.gov/cber/guidelines.htm.*
19. Zhang Y, Zhang L, Abraham S, et al. Assessment of the impact of renal impairment on systematic exposure of new molecular entities: Evaluation of recent new drug applications. Clin Pharmacol Ther 2009;85:305–311.
20. Anonymous. Pharmacokinetics in patients with impaired renal function—Study design, data analysis, and impact on dosing and labeling. U.S. Department of Health and Human Services, Draft FDA Guidance, March 2010, *http://www.fda.gov/cber/guidelines.htm.*
21. Zhang L, Xu N, Xiao S, et al. Regulatory perspective on designing pharmacokinetic studies and optimizing labeling recommendations for patients with chronic kidney disease. J Clin Pharmacol 2012;52:79S–90S.
22. Tortorici MA, Cutler D, Zhang L, Pfister M. Design, conduct, analysis, and interpretation of clinical studies in patients with impaired kidney function. J Clin Pharmacol 2012;52:109S–118S.
23. Cusack BJ. Pharmacokinetics in older persons. Am J Geriatr Pharmacother 2004;2(4):274–302.
24. Ritschel WA, Denson DD. Influence of disease on bioavailability. In: Ritschel WA, ed. Pharmacokinetics: Regulatory, Industrial, Academic Perspectives. New York, NY: Marcel Dekker, 1995.
25. Bellomo R, Prowle JR, Echeverri JE. Diuretic therapy in fluid-overloaded and heart failure patients. Contrib Nephrol 2010;164:153–163.
26. Hurwitz A. Antacid therapy and drug kinetics. Clin Pharmacokinet 1977;2:269–280.
27. Maton PN, Burton ME. Antacids revisited: A review of their clinical pharmacology and recommended therapeutic use. Drugs 1999;57:855–870.
28. Craig RM, Murphy P, Gibson TP, et al. Kinetic analysis of d-xylose absorption in normal subjects and in patients with chronic renal failure. J Lab Clin Med 1983;101:496–506.
29. Craig RM, Carlson S, Ehrenpreis ED. d-xylose kinetics and hydrogen breath tests in functionally anephric patients using the 15-gram dose. J Clin Gastroenterol 2000;31:55–59.
30. Matzke GR, Frye RF. Drug administration in patients with renal insufficiency: Minimizing renal and extrarenal toxicity. Drug Saf 1997;16:205–231.
31. Gibson TP, Giacomini KM, Briggs WA, et al. Propoxyphene and norpropoxyphene plasma concentrations in the anephric patient. Clin Pharmacol Ther 1980;27:665–670.
32. Barnes JN, Williams AJ, Tomson MJ, et al. Dihydrocodeine in renal failure: Further evidence for an important role of the kidney in the handling of opioid drugs. BMJ 1985;290: 740–742.
33. Bailey DG, Arnold JM, Munoz C, Spence JD. Grapefruit juice—Felodipine interaction; mechanism, predictability, and effect of naringin. Clin Pharmacol Ther 1993;53(6):637–642.
34. Min Dl, Ku YM, Perry PJ, et al. Effect of grapefruit juice on cyclosporine pharmacokinetics in renal transplant patients. Transplantation 1996;62:123–125.
35. Ueda N, Yoshimura R, Umene-Nakano W, et al. Grapefruit juice alters plasma sertraline levels after single ingestion of sertraline in healthy volunteers. World J Biol Psychiatry 2009;10:832–835.

36. Thummel KE, Shen DD, Isoherranen N. Appendix II. Design and optimization of dosage regimens: Pharmacokinetic data. In: Brunton LL, Chabner BA, Knollmann BC, eds. Goodman & Gilman's The Pharmacological Basis of Therapeutics, 12th ed. New York, NY: McGraw-Hill, 2011, *http://www.accessmedicine.com/content.aspx?aID=16683174*.
37. Alvarez-Lerma F, Grau S. Management of antimicrobial use in the intensive care unit. Drugs 2012;72:447–470.
38. Winter ME. Phenytoin and fosphenytoin. In: Murphy JE, ed. Clinical Pharmacokinetics Pocket Reference, 5th ed. Bethesda, MD: American Society of Health-System Pharmacists, 2011:247–259.
39. Meijers BKI, Bemmers B, Verbeke B, et al. A review of albumin binding in CKD. Am J Kidney Dis 2008;51:839–850.
40. Job ML. Digoxin. In: Murphy JE, ed. Clinical Pharmacokinetics Pocket Reference, 5th ed. Bethesda, MD: American Society of Health-System Pharmacists, 2011:139–147.
41. Malini PL, Strocchi E, Feliciangeli G, et al. Digitalis receptors and digoxin sensitivity in renal failure. Clin Exp Pharmacol Physiol 1985;12:115–120.
42. Koup J. Disease states and drug pharmacokinetics. J Clin Pharmacol 1989;29:674–679.
43. Yuan R, Venitz J. Effect of chronic renal failure on the disposition of highly hepatically metabolized drugs. Int J Clin Pharmacol Ther 2000;38:245–253.
44. Szeto HH, Inturrisi CE, Houde R, et al. Accumulation of normeperidine, an active metabolite of meperidine, in patients with renal failure of cancer. Ann Intern Med 1977;86:738–741.
45. Murphy EJ. Acute pain management for the patient with concurrent renal or hepatic disease. Anaesth Intensive Care 2005;33:311–322.
46. Nolin DT, Frye RF, Le P, et al. ESRD impairs nonrenal clearance of fexofenadine but not midazolam. J Am Soc Nephrol 2009;20:2269–2276.
47. Vilay AM, Churchwell MD, Mueller BA. Drug metabolism and clearance in acute kidney injury. Crit Care 2008;12:235.
48. Dowling TC, Briglia AE, Fink JC, et al. Characterization of hepatic cytochrome P4503 A activity in patients with end-stage renal disease. Clin Pharmacol Ther 2003;73:427–434.
49. Lee W, Kim RB. Transporters and renal drug elimination. Annu Rev Pharmacol Toxicol 2004;44:137–166.
50. Sun H, Frassetto L, Benet LZ. Effects of renal failure on drug transport and metabolism. Pharmacol Ther 2006;109:1–11.
51. Masereeuw R, Russel FGM. Therapeutic implications of renal anionic drug transporters. Pharmacol Ther 2010;126:200–216.
52. Earley A, Miskulin D, Lamb EJ, et al. Estimating equations for glomerular filtration rate in the era of creatinine standardization. Ann Intern Med 2012;156:785–795.
53. Steffl JL, Bennett W, Olyaei AJ. The old and new methods of assessing kidney function. J Clin Pharmacol 2012;52:63S–71S.
54. Inker LA, Schmid CH, Tighiouart H, et al. Estimating glomerular filtration rate from serum creatinine and cystatin C. N Engl J Med 2012;367:20–29.
55. Dowling TC, Matzke GR, Murphy JE, Burckart GJ. Evaluation of renal drug dosing: Prescribing information and clinical pharmacist approaches. Pharmacotherapy 2010;30:776–786.
56. Wargo KA, Eiland EH, Hamm W, et al. Comparison of the modification of diet in renal disease and Cockcroft–Gault equations for antimicrobial dosing adjustments. Ann Pharmacother 2006;40:1248–1253.
57. Golik MV, Lawrence KR. Comparison of dosing recommendations for antimicrobial drugs based on two methods for assessing kidney function: Cockcroft–Gault and modification of diet in renal disease. Pharmacotherapy 2008;28:1125–1132.
58. Hermsen ED, Maiefski M, Florescu MC, et al. Comparison of the modification of diet in renal disease and Cockcroft–Gault equations for dosing antimicrobials. Pharmacotherapy 2009;29:649–655.
59. Park EJ, Wu K, Mi Z, Dong T, et al. A systematic comparison of Cockcroft–Gault and modification of diet in renal disease equations for classification of kidney dysfunction and dosage adjustment. Ann Pharmacother 2012;46:1174–1187.
60. Levey AS, Stevens LA, Schmid CH, et al. CKD-EPI (Chronic Kidney Disease Epidemiology Collaboration). A new equation to estimate glomerular filtration rate. Ann Intern Med 2009;150:604–612.
61. McEvoy GK, Snow EK, Miller J, et al. American Hospital Formulary Service, Drug Information. Bethesda, MD: American Society of Health-System Pharmacists, 2012.
62. Joint Formulary Committee. British National Formulary, 64th ed. London: British Medical Association and Royal Pharmaceutical Society of Great Britain, 2004. *http://www.bnf.org/bnf/*.
63. Aronoff GR, Bennett WM, Berns JS, et al. Drug Prescribing in Renal Failure: Dosing Guidelines for Adults and Children, 5th ed. Philadelphia, PA: American College of Physicians-American Society of Internal Medicine, 2007.
64. Vidal L, Shavit M, Fraser A, et al. Systematic comparison of four sources of drug information regarding adjustment of dose for renal function. BMJ 2005;331:263–266.
65. Matzke GR, Clermont G. Clinical pharmacology and therapeutics. In: Murray PT, Brady HR, Hall JB, eds. Intensive Care in Nephrology. Boca Raton, FL: Taylor & Francis, 2006:245–265.
66. Craig WA. Pharmacokinetic/pharmacodynamic parameters: Rationale for antibacterial dosing of mice and men. Clin Infect Dis 1998;26:1–12.
67. Murphy JE. Clinical Pharmacokinetics Pocket Reference, 5th ed. Bethesda, MD: American Society of Health-System Pharmacists, 2011.
68. Drusano GL. Pharmacokinetic optimisation of β-lactams for the treatment of ventilator-associated pneumonia. Eur Respir Rev 2007;16:45–49.
69. Heintz BH, Matzke GR, Dager WE. Antimicrobial dosing concepts and recommendations for critically ill adult patients receiving continuous renal replacement therapy or intermittent hemodialysis. Pharmacotherapy 2009;29:562–577.
70. Rybak MJ, Lomaestro BM, Rotschafer JC, Moellering RC Jr, et al. Therapeutic monitoring of vancomycin in adults summary of consensus recommendations from the American Society of Health-System Pharmacists, the Infectious Diseases Society of America, and the Society of Infectious Diseases Pharmacists. Pharmacotherapy 2009;29:1275–1279.
71. Munar MY, Singh H. Drug dosing adjustments in patients with chronic kidney disease. Am Fam Physician 2007;75:1487–1496.
72. Micromedex® Healthcare Series. Thomson Reuters (Healthcare) Inc., 2012, *http://www.thomsonhc.com*.
73. Mandell GL, Bennett JE, Dolin R, eds. Mandell, Douglas, and Bennett's Principles and Practice of Infectious Disease,

7th ed. Philadelphia, PA: Churchill Livingstone Elsevier, 2010.

74. Shah A, Lettieri J, Blum R, et al. Pharmacokinetics of intravenous ciprofloxacin in normal and renally impaired subjects. J Antimicrob Chemother 1996;38:103–116.
75. Gilbert B, Robbins P, Livornese LL Jr. Use of antibacterial agents in renal failure. Infect Dis Clin North Am 2009;23:899–924.
76. Manley HJ, Bailie GR. Treatment of peritonitis in APD: Pharmacokinetic principles. Semin Dial 2002;15:418–421.
77. Veltri MA, Neu AM, Fivush BA, et al. Drug dosing during intermittent hemodialysis and continuous renal replacement therapy: Special considerations in pediatric patients. Pediatr Drugs 2004;6:45–65.
78. Taylor CA, Abdel-Rahman E, Zimmerman SW, Johnson CA. Clinical pharmacokinetics during continuous ambulatory peritoneal dialysis. Clin Pharmacokinet 1996;31:293–308.
79. Li PKT, Szeto CC, Piraino B, et al. Peritoneal dialysis-related infections recommendations: 2010 update. Perit Dial Int 2010;30:393–423.
80. Matzke GR. Status of hemodialysis of drugs in 2002. J Pharm Pract 2002;15:405–418.
81. Secker BS, Mueller BA, Sowinski KM. Drug dosing considerations in alternative hemodialysis. Adv Chronic Kidney Dis 2007;14:e17–e26.
82. Cheung AK. Hemodialysis and hemofiltration. In: Greenberg A, Cheung AK, Coffman TM, Falk RJ, Jennette JC, eds. Primer on Kidney Disease, 5th ed. Philadelphia, PA: WB Saunders, 2008.
83. Matzke GR, Buby J. Vancomycin. In: Murphy JE, ed. Clinical Pharmacokinetics Pocket Reference, 5th ed. Bethesda, MD: American Society of Hospital Pharmacists, 2011.
84. Launay-Vacher V, Izzedine H, Mercadal L, Deray G. Clinical review: Use of vancomycin in haemodialysis patients. Crit Care 2002;6:313–316.
85. Liu C, Bayer A, Cosgrove SE, et al. Clinical practice guidelines by the infectious diseases society of America for the treatment of methicillin-resistant *Staphylococcus aureus* infections in adults and children: Executive summary. Clin Infect Dis 2011;52(3):285–292.
86. Welage LS, Mason NA, Hoffman EJ, et al. Influence of cellulose triacetate hemodialyzers on vancomycin pharmacokinetics. J Am Soc Nephrol 1995;6:1284–1290.
87. Matsuo H, Hayashi J, Ono K, et al. Administration of aminoglycosides to hemodialysis patients immediately before dialysis: A new dosing modality. Antimicrob Agents Chemother 1997;41:2597–2601.
88. Teigen MMB, Duffull S, Dang L, Johnson DW. Dosing of gentamicin in patients with end-stage renal disease receiving hemodialysis. J Clin Pharmacol 2006;46:1259–1267.
89. Mohamed OHK, Wahba IM, Watnick S, et al. Administration of tobramycin in the beginning of the hemodialysis session: A novel intradialytic dosing regimen. Clin J Am Soc Nephrol 2007;2:694–699.
90. Scott MK, Macias WL, Kraus MA, et al. Effects of dialysis membrane on intradialytic vancomycin administration. Pharmacotherapy 1997;17(2):256–262.
91. Ariano RE, Fine A, Sitar DS, et al. Adequacy of a vancomycin dosing regimen in patients receiving high-flux hemodialysis. Am J Kidney Dis 2005:46;681–687.
92. Crawford BS, Largen RF, Walton T, Doran JJ. Once-weekly vancomycin for patients receiving high-flux hemodialysis. Am J Health-Syst Phar 2008;65:1248–1253.
93. van Dijk EA, Drabbe NRG, Kruijtbosch M, De Smet PAGM. Drug dosage adjustments according to renal function at hospital discharge. Ann Pharmacother 2006;40:1254–1260.

Disorders of Sodium and Water Homeostasis

34

Katherine Hammond Chessman and Gary R. Matzke

KEY CONCEPTS

1. Blood volume and plasma osmolality are tightly regulated in the human body because they are essential for normal cellular function. Water balance determines the serum sodium concentration, and sodium balance determines the water status.
2. Hypovolemic hypotonic hyponatremia is relatively common in patients taking thiazide diuretics; however, thiazide-induced hyponatremia is usually mild and relatively asymptomatic.
3. Euvolemic (isovolemic) hyponatremia is most often caused by the syndrome of inappropriate secretion of antidiuretic hormone (SIADH). Common causes of SIADH include some cancers, central nervous system (CNS) and pulmonary disorders, and certain drugs.
4. Symptoms of hypo- or hypernatremia are usually neurologic and range from weakness, lethargy, restlessness, irritability, and confusion to twitching, seizures, coma, and death. Symptom severity depends on both the magnitude of the change in the serum sodium concentration and the rate at which it changes.
5. Treatment goals in patients with either hypo- or hypernatremia should include cautious correction of the serum sodium concentration and, when appropriate, restoration of a normal extracellular fluid (ECF) volume. Too rapid correction of the serum sodium can result in cerebral edema, seizures, neurologic damage, osmotic demyelination syndrome, and possibly death. To minimize the risk of these complications, the serum sodium concentration should be corrected at a rate not to exceed 6 to 12 mEq/L (6 to 12 mol/L) in 24 hours, depending on the rate of change in the serum sodium concentration.
6. Asymptomatic or mildly symptomatic hyponatremia should be managed conservatively with treatment directed at the underlying cause. IV infusion of 0.9% NaCl solution is most often used to correct the serum sodium concentration in patients with moderate to severe symptoms from hypovolemic hypotonic hyponatremia. A 3% NaCl infusion can be cautiously used in patients with moderate to severe symptoms and euvolemic or hypervolemic hypotonic hyponatremia (along with a loop diuretic).
7. Hypernatremia is always hypertonic and most commonly occurs when increased water or hypotonic fluid losses are not offset by increased water intake or administration.
8. Hypovolemic hypernatremia is relatively common in patients taking loop diuretics. After symptoms of hypovolemia are corrected with 0.9% NaCl solution, free water should be replaced.
9. Patients with central diabetes insipidus (DI) can be treated with desmopressin acetate, with a goal to decrease urine volume to less than 2 L per day while maintaining the serum sodium concentration between 137 and 142 mEq/L (137 and 142 mmol/L). Patients with nephrogenic DI should be treated by correcting the underlying cause, when possible, and sodium restriction in conjunction with a thiazide diuretic to decrease the ECF volume by approximately 1 to 1.5 L.
10. Edema develops as a primary defect in renal sodium handling or as a response to a decreased effective circulating volume. It is usually first detected in the feet or pretibial areas of ambulatory patients. Pulmonary edema, evidenced by auscultatory crackles, can be life threatening.
11. Diuretics are the primary pharmacologic means for minimizing edema and improving organ function. Diuretic resistance often can be overcome by using an increased dose or by using a combination of a loop diuretic and a thiazide or thiazide-like diuretic.

1 Both blood volume and plasma osmolality are tightly regulated in the human body because they are essential for normal cellular function. Blood volume is a determinant of effective tissue perfusion which is required to deliver oxygen and nutrients to and remove metabolic waste products from tissues. Plasma osmolality, the primary determinant of which is sodium concentration, is an important determinant of intracellular fluid (ICF) volume. Maintenance of normal ICF volume is particularly critical in the brain, which is 80% water, and where alterations, especially rapid changes, can result in significant dysfunction and potentially death.

Simply put, water balance determines the serum sodium concentration, and sodium balance determines the volume status. Thus, the homeostatic mechanisms for controlling blood volume are focused on controlling sodium balance, and, in contrast, the homeostatic mechanisms for controlling plasma osmolality are focused on controlling water balance. Disorders of sodium and water homeostasis are common, caused by a variety of diseases, conditions, and drugs, and potentially serious. This chapter reviews the etiology, classification, clinical presentation, and therapy for disorders of sodium and water homeostasis.

SODIUM AND WATER HOMEOSTASIS

Hypo- and hypernatremia are syndromes of altered plasma tonicity and cell volume that reflect a change in the ratio of total exchangeable body sodium to total body water (TBW). TBW is distributed primarily into two compartments: the intracellular compartment (ICF; 60% of TBW) and the extracellular compartment

TABLE 34-1 Composition of Common IV Solutions

Solution	Dextrose	[Na^+] (mEq/L or mmol/L)	[Cl^-] (mEq/L or mmol/L)	Tonicity	Distribution % ECF	Distribution % ICF	Free water/L
D_5W	5 g/dL (50 g/L)	0	0	Hypotonic	40	60	1,000 mL
0.45% sodium chloride[a]	0	77	77	Hypotonic	73	37	500 mL
Ringer's lactate	0	130	105	Isotonic	97	3	0 mL
0.9% sodium chloride[b]	0	154	154	Isotonic	100	0	0 mL
3% sodium chloride[c]	0	513	513	Hypertonic	100	0	−2,331 mL

Cl^-, chloride; D_5W, 5% dextrose in water; ECF, extracellular fluid; ICF, intracellular fluid; Na^+, sodium.

[a]Also referred to as "half normal saline."

[b]Also referred to as "normal saline."

[c]This solution will result in osmotic removal of water from the intracellular space.

or extracellular fluid (ECF; 40% of TBW). Sodium and its accompanying anions (chloride and bicarbonate) comprise more than 90% of the total osmolality of the ECF; whereas ICF osmolality is primarily determined by the concentration of potassium and its accompanying anions (mostly organic and inorganic phosphates). The intra- and extracellular sodium and potassium concentrations are maintained by the sodium–potassium–adenosine triphosphatase (Na^+-K^+-ATPase) pump. Most cell membranes are freely permeable to water, and thus the osmolalities of the ICF and the ECF are equal.

Effective osmoles are solutes that cannot freely cross cell membranes, such as sodium and potassium. The ECF concentration of effective osmoles determines its tonicity, which directly affects the distribution of water between the extra- and intracellular compartments. Addition of an isotonic solution (e.g., 0.9% sodium chloride [NaCl] solution) to the ECF will result in no change in intracellular volume because there will be no change in the effective ECF osmolality. However, addition of a hypertonic solution (e.g., 3% NaCl) to the ECF will result in a decrease in ICF (cell) volume, and addition of a hypotonic solution (e.g., 0.45% NaCl) to the ECF will result in an increase in cell volume. Table 34-1 summarizes the composition of commonly used IV solutions and their respective distribution into the ICF and ECF compartments following IV administration.

Edelman's equation defines serum sodium as a function of the total exchangeable sodium and potassium in the body and the TBW: $Na_S = Na_{total\ body} + K_{total\ body}/TBW$, where Na_S is the serum sodium concentration; $Na_{total\ body}$ is the total body sodium content; $K_{total\ body}$ is the total body potassium content; and TBW is the total body water in liters.[1] The serum sodium concentration is tightly regulated and thus usually varies by no more than 2% to 3%. Regulation of the serum sodium concentration occurs indirectly via mechanisms that control its determinants: plasma osmolality and blood volume. The kidney regulates water excretion through a hypothalamic feedback mechanism, such that the serum osmolality remains relatively constant (275 to 290 mOsm/kg [275 to 290 mmol/kg]) despite day-to-day variations in water intake. Plasma osmolality is primarily determined by the sodium concentration, but serum glucose and blood urea nitrogen (BUN) may contribute significantly at times. Serum osmolality can be estimated as:

$$Osm_S = (2 \times Na_S) + (Glucose_S/18) + (BUN/2.8)$$

where Osm_S is the serum osmolality in mOsm/kg; Na_S is the serum sodium concentration in mEq/L; $Glucose_S$ is the serum glucose concentration in mg/dL; and BUN is the blood urea nitrogen concentration in mg/dL. Alternatively, when using SI units the equation becomes:

$$Osm_S = (2 \times Na_S) + (Glucose_S) + (BUN)$$

where Osm_S is the serum osmolality in mmol/kg; Na_S is the serum sodium concentration in mmol/L; $Glucose_S$ is the glucose concentration in mmol/L; and BUN is the blood urea nitrogen concentration in mmol/L.

Arginine vasopressin (AVP), commonly known as antidiuretic hormone (ADH), is synthesized in the hypothalamus and released from the posterior pituitary as a result of both osmotic and nonosmotic regulators. When the plasma osmolality increases by 1% to 2% or more AVP is released and binds to the vasopressin 2 (V2) receptors on the basolateral surface of renal tubular epithelial cells, resulting in the insertion of water channels (aquaporin 2) into the apical tubular lumen surface of the cell.[2] Water can then pass through the cell into the peritubular capillary space where it is reabsorbed into the systemic circulation. As serum osmolality increases, even as little as 1%, AVP is released and thirst is stimulated. The combined effects of increased water intake and decreased water excretion (kidney's response to AVP) result in a decrease in the serum osmolality and inhibition of further AVP secretion, once the normal plasma osmolality is restored.

Nonosmotic AVP release occurs when osmoreceptors in the brain detect a 6% to 10% reduction in the effective circulating blood volume or arterial blood pressure. The effective circulating volume is that part of the ECF responsible for organ perfusion. A decrease in the effective circulating volume (more accurately, the pressure associated with that volume) activates arterial baroreceptors in the carotid sinus and glomerular afferent arterioles, resulting in stimulation of the renin–angiotensin system and increased angiotensin II synthesis. Angiotensin II stimulates both nonosmotic AVP release and thirst. This volume stimulus can override osmotic inhibition of AVP release. Conservation of water then restores the effective circulating volume and blood pressure at the expense of producing a decreased serum osmolality and hyponatremia.[2] Although hyponatremia and hypernatremia can be associated with conditions of high, low, or normal ECF sodium and volume, both conditions most commonly result from abnormalities of water homeostasis.

HYPONATREMIA

Epidemiology and Etiology

Hyponatremia, usually defined as a serum sodium concentration less than 135 mEq/L (135 mmol/L), is the most common electrolyte abnormality encountered in clinical practice in both adults and children.[1,3–6] Although the prevalence is not well established and varies with the patient population studied, it has been estimated to be as high as 28% in patients admitted to an acute care hospital.[7] Mild hyponatremia (serum sodium concentration less than 136 mEq/L [136 mmol/L]) was observed in 42.6%, while 6.2% of patients had values less than 126 mEq/L (126 mmol/L), and 1.2% had values less than 116 mEq/L (116 mmol/L). The incidence has

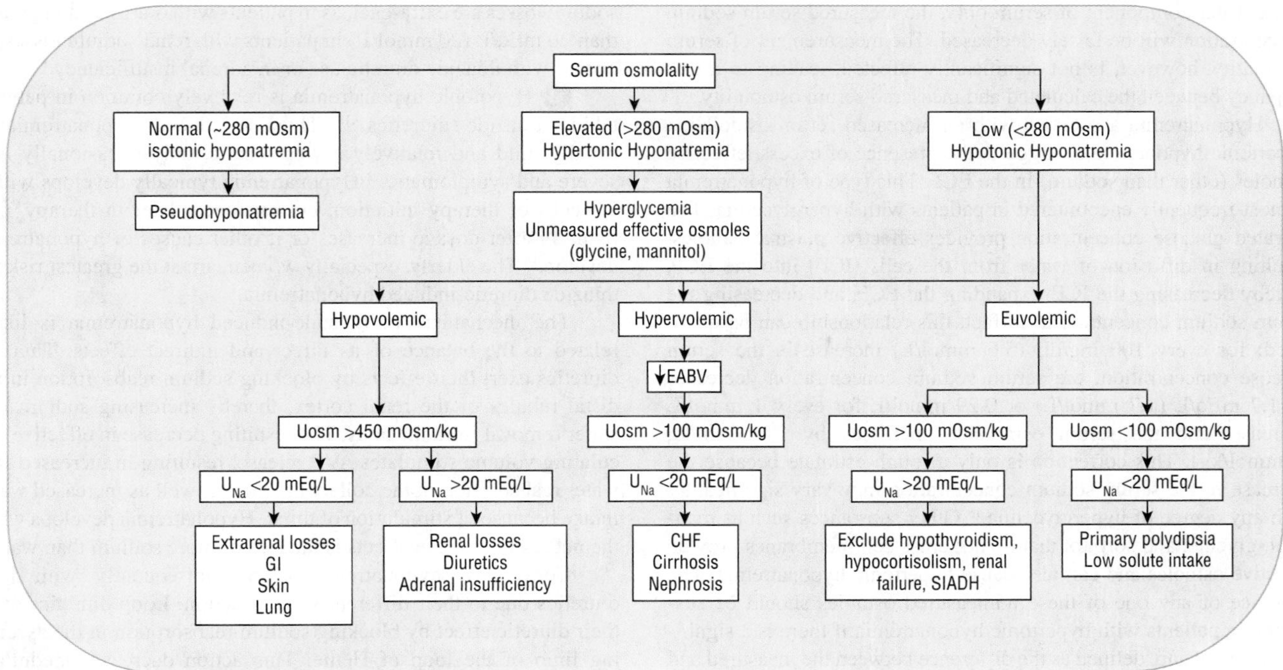

FIGURE 34-1 Diagnostic algorithm for the evaluation of hyponatremia. (CHF, congestive heart failure; SIADH, syndrome of inappropriate secretion of antidiuretic hormone; UNa, urine sodium concentration [values in mEq/L are numerically equivalent to mmol/L]; Uosm, urine osmolality [values in mOsm/kg are numerically equivalent to mmol/kg].)

been reported to be as high as 21% in patients seen in ambulatory hospital clinics, and 7% in community clinics.[7] Drug-induced hyponatremia especially that associated with thiazide diuretics,[8,9] and psychotropic medications,[10,11] is common. Advancing age (older than 30 years) is also a risk factor for hyponatremia, independent of sex.[7]

Residents in nursing homes have a twofold higher incidence of hyponatremia than that observed in age-matched, community-dwelling individuals.[3] More than 75% of these hyponatremic episodes were precipitated by increased intake of hypotonic oral or IV fluids. Similarly, ingestion of excessive fluid volumes has been identified as a key risk factor in the development of hyponatremia in marathon runners. Although women had a threefold higher rate of hyponatremia, smaller body size and longer racing time, not sex, appear to be the principal factors accounting for the increased incidence.[11]

Recognition of the high prevalence of hyponatremia is essential because this condition is associated with significant morbidity and mortality.[2,12–15] Transient or permanent brain dysfunction can result from either the acute effects of hypoosmolality or too rapid correction of hypoosmolality in patients with hyponatremia. Hyponatremia is predominantly the result of an excess of extracellular water relative to sodium because of impaired water excretion. The kidney normally has the capacity to excrete large volumes of dilute urine after ingestion of a water load. Nonosmotic AVP release, however, can lead to water retention and a drop in the serum sodium concentration, despite a decrease in both serum and intracellular osmolality. The causes of nonosmotic AVP release include hypovolemia, decreased effective circulating volume as seen in patients with chronic heart failure (HF), nephrosis, and cirrhosis. The syndrome of inappropriate secretion of antidiuretic hormone (SIADH), a common cause of hyponatremia, is associated with some oncologic diseases, especially small cell lung cancer, and CNS damage (e.g., head trauma, meningitis). The pathophysiology, clinical features, and management of hyponatremia are detailed below.

Pathophysiology

Hyponatremia can be associated with normal, increased, or decreased plasma osmolality, depending on its cause. Figure 34-1 provides an algorithm for diagnosing patients with hyponatremia. Hyponatremia in patients with normal serum osmolality can be caused by hyperlipidemia or hyperproteinemia. This form of hyponatremia, termed pseudohyponatremia, is an artifact of a specific laboratory method (flame photometry) used to measure serum sodium concentration. This laboratory method is used rarely today, replaced by the use of ion-specific electrodes to measure the serum sodium concentration. If flame photometry is used, the serum volume will be overestimated because the elevated lipids or proteins account for a greater proportion of the total sample volume (Fig. 34-2). Because sodium is distributed

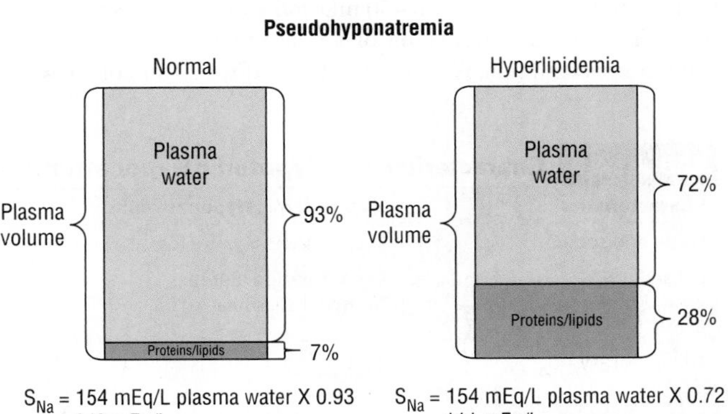

FIGURE 34-2 Elevated lipids or proteins result in a larger discrepancy between the volume of the sample and plasma water, leading to a falsely low measurement of the serum sodium concentration when using the method of flame photometry. (S_{Na}, serum sodium concentration [values in mEq/L are numerically equivalent to mmol/L].)

in the water component of serum only, the measured serum sodium concentration will be falsely decreased. The measurement of serum osmolality, however, is not significantly affected, leading to a discrepancy between the calculated and measured serum osmolality.

Hyponatremia associated with an increased serum osmolality, hypertonic hyponatremia, suggests the presence of excess, effective osmoles (other than sodium) in the ECF. This type of hyponatremia is most frequently encountered in patients with hyperglycemia. The elevated glucose concentration provides effective plasma osmoles, resulting in diffusion of water from the cells (ICF) into the ECF, thereby decreasing the ICF, expanding the ECF, and decreasing the serum sodium concentration. In fact, this relationship can be quantified: for every 100 mg/dL (5.6 mmol/L) increase in the serum glucose concentration, the serum sodium concentration decreases by 1.7 mEq/L (1.7 mmol/L) or 0.29 mmol/L for every 1 mmol/L decrease, and the serum osmolality increases by 2 mOsm/kg (2 mmol/kg). This correction is only a rough estimate because the decrease in the serum sodium concentration may vary significantly with any degree of hyperglycemia.[15] Other substances such as mannitol, glycine, and sorbitol that do not cross cell membranes provide effective osmoles and can also cause hypertonic hyponatremia. The presence of any one of these unmeasured osmoles should be suspected in patients with hypertonic hyponatremia if there is a significant osmolal gap, defined as the difference between the measured and calculated plasma osmolality.

Hyponatremia associated with decreased plasma osmolality, hypotonic hyponatremia, is the most common form of hyponatremia and has many potential causes (see Table 34-2). Clinical assessment of ECF volume is an important step in the diagnostic evaluation of a patient with hypotonic hyponatremia. Categorization of these patients into one of three groups (decreased, increased, or clinically normal ECF volume) is essential in identifying the pathophysiologic mechanisms responsible for the hyponatremia and developing an appropriate treatment plan.

Hypovolemic Hypotonic Hyponatremia

Most patients with ECF volume contraction lose fluids that are hypotonic relative to plasma and thus can become transiently hypernatremic. This includes patients with fluid losses caused by diarrhea, excessive sweating, and diuretics. This transient hypernatremic hyperosmolality results in osmotic AVP release and stimulation of thirst. If sodium and water losses continue, the resultant hypovolemia results in more AVP release. Patients who then drink water (a hypotonic fluid) or who are given hypotonic IV fluids retain water, and hyponatremia develops. These patients typically have a urine osmolality greater than 450 mOsm/kg (450 mmol/kg), reflecting AVP action and formation of a concentrated urine. The urine sodium concentration is less than 20 mEq/L (20 mmol/L) when sodium losses are extrarenal, as in patients with diarrhea, and greater than 20 mEq/L (20 mmol/L) in patients with renal sodium losses, as occurs with thiazide diuretic use or in adrenal insufficiency.[17]

2 Hypotonic hyponatremia is relatively common in patients taking thiazide diuretics.[9,18] Thiazide-induced hyponatremia is usually mild and relatively asymptomatic; only occasionally is it severe and symptomatic.[18] Hyponatremia typically develops within 2 weeks of therapy initiation, but can occur later in therapy, particularly after dosage increases or if other causes of hyponatremia develop.[18] The elderly, especially women, are at the greatest risk for thiazide diuretic-induced hyponatremia.

The mechanism of thiazide-induced hyponatremia is likely related to the balance of its direct and indirect effects. Thiazide diuretics exert their effects by blocking sodium reabsorption in the distal tubules of the renal cortex, thereby increasing sodium and water removal from the body. The resulting decrease in effective circulating volume stimulates AVP release, resulting in increased free water reabsorption in the collecting duct, as well as increased water intake because of stimulation of thirst. Hyponatremia develops when the net result of these effects is the loss of more sodium than water.

Conversely, hyponatremia occurs infrequently with loop diuretics due to their different sites of action. Loop diuretics exert their diuretic effect by blocking sodium reabsorption in the ascending limb of the loop of Henle. This action decreases medullary osmolality. Thus, when the loop diuretics decrease effective circulating volume and stimulate AVP release, less water reabsorption occurs in the collecting ducts than would occur if the osmolality of the renal medulla were normal. Thiazide diuretics do not alter medullary osmolality because their site of action is in the renal cortex not the medulla. In addition, most loop diuretics have a shorter half-life than the thiazides, and patients can usually replete the urinary sodium and water losses prior to taking the next dose, thereby minimizing AVP stimulation.

Euvolemic Hypotonic Hyponatremia

3 Euvolemic (isovolemic) hypotonic hyponatremia is associated with a normal or slightly decreased ECF sodium content and increased TBW and ECF volume. The increase in ECF volume is usually not sufficient to cause peripheral or pulmonary edema or other signs of volume overload, and thus patients appear clinically euvolemic. Euvolemic hyponatremia is most often caused by SIADH.

In SIADH, water intake exceeds the kidney's capacity to excrete water, either because of increased AVP release via nonosmotic and/or nonphysiologic processes or enhanced sensitivity of the kidney to AVP. In patients with SIADH, the urine osmolality is generally greater than 100 mOsm/kg (100 mmol/kg), and the urine sodium concentration is usually greater than 20 mEq/L (20 mmol/L) due to the ECF volume expansion (Table 34-2).

TABLE 34-2 Characteristics of Hypotonic Hyponatremic States

Characteristics	Hypovolemic Hyponatremia	Euvolemic (Isovolemic) Hyponatremia	Hypervolemic Hyponatremia
Water and sodium	Sodium loss >> water loss	Water gain only	Water gain > sodium gain, heart failure
Causes	Renal: thiazide diuretics Nonrenal: diarrhea	Syndrome of inappropriate antidiuretic hormone (SIADH)	Heart failure Liver cirrhosis Kidney failure
Effect on TBW	↓↓	↑	↑↑
Effect on TBNa	↓	↔	↑↑
Laboratory findings in addition to hyponatremia	Renal: UOsm high, UNa high Nonrenal: UOsm high, UNa low	Renal: UOsm low, UNa variable Nonrenal: UOsm high, UNa variable	UOsm high, UNa high
Clinical presentation	Orthostasis, hypotension, tachycardia, dry mucous membranes, CNS changes	Depends on severity of hyponatremia: seizures, lethargy	Peripheral and pulmonary edema, variable blood pressure
Treatment	0.9% NaCl until vital signs stable; then maintenance fluid replacement (D5/0.45% NaCl)	Water restriction; demeclocycline; loop diuretics; vaptan	Sodium restriction; water restriction; loop diuretics; vaptan

TABLE 34-3 Potential Causes of SIADH

Drug-induced		Non-drug Induced
Increased ADH release		
Nicotine	Haloperidol	Malignancy (lung, pancreatic, duodenal)
Clofibrate	Thioridazine	CNS (trauma, tumor, meningitis, hemorrhage, stroke)
Barbiturates	Opioids	Pulmonary (pneumonia, ARDS, TB)
Thiothixene	Bromocriptine	Postoperative state
Tricyclic antidepressants	Monoamine oxidase inhibitors	Nausea
Vinca alkaloids	Cisplatin	Anxiety
Carboplatin		
Increased sensitivity to ADH		
Acetaminophen	Oxytocin	
ADH analogs (desmopressin)	NSAIDs	
	Chlorpropamide	
Carbamazepine	Tolbutamide	
Lamotrigine		
Mixed or uncertain mechanism		
Omeprazole	Cyclophosphamide	
Ectasy	Angiotensin-converting enzyme (ACE) inhibitors	
Moxifloxacin	Selective serotonin receptor inhibitors (SSRIs)	

TABLE 34-4 Clinical Presentation of Hyponatremia

General
- Patients are usually asymptomatic.
- Symptoms are primarily neurologic.
- Presence and severity of symptoms depend on the magnitude and rapidity of onset of hyponatremia.
- Other symptoms may be present depending on the etiology of the hyponatremia (e.g., dry mucous membranes, tachycardia, and hypotension with hypovolemia).

Symptoms
- Mild: nausea and malaise
- Moderate: headache, lethargy, restlessness, and disorientation
- Severe: seizures, coma, respiratory arrest, brainstem herniation, and death

Laboratory tests
- Serum sodium concentration less than 135 mEq/L (135 mmol/L)
- Plasma osmolality and urine sodium concentration can be helpful.
- Other tests: serum glucose and lipids and kidney and thyroid function tests

The most common causes of SIADH include tumors such as small cell lung or pancreatic cancer, CNS disorders (e.g., head trauma, stroke, meningitis, pituitary surgery), and pulmonary disease (e.g., tuberculosis, pneumonia, acute respiratory distress syndrome). Patients with kidney and adrenal insufficiency or hypothyroidism can also present with euvolemic hyponatremia, and the evaluation of patients with suspected SIADH should always include consideration of these disorders as the etiology. A variety of drugs can cause SIADH by enhancing AVP release, the effect of AVP on the kidney, or by other unknown mechanisms[10,14,15,20] (Table 34-3). The differential diagnosis of euvolemic hypotonic hyponatremia also includes primary or psychogenic polydipsia. Patients with this disorder drink more water (usually more than 20 L/day) than the kidneys can excrete as solute-free water. However, unlike in SIADH, AVP secretion is suppressed, resulting in a urine osmolality that is less than 100 mOsm/kg (100 mmol/kg). The urine sodium is typically low (less than 15 mEq/L [15 mmol/L]) as a result of dilution.[11] Hyponatremia can develop even with more modest water intakes in patients who are ingesting very low-solute diets.

Hypervolemic Hypotonic Hyponatremia

Hyponatremia associated with ECF volume expansion occurs in conditions in which the kidney's sodium and water excretion are impaired. Patients with cirrhosis, HF, or nephrotic syndrome have an expanded ECF volume and edema, but a decreased effective arterial blood volume (EABV). This decreased volume results in renal sodium retention, and eventually ECF volume expansion and edema. At the same time, there is nonosmotic stimulation of AVP release and water retention in excess of sodium retention, which perpetuates the hyponatremic state.

Clinical **Controversy. . .**

Some clinicians advocate using combinations of diuretics in cases of diuretic-resistant edema associated with nephrotic syndrome, while others prefer to use larger-than-average doses of single agents to overcome enhanced protein binding in the tubular lumen associated with proteinuria.

Clinical Presentation

4 The clinical presentation of patients with hyponatremia is summarized in Table 34-4. Patients with chronic (defined as lasting longer than 48 hours), mild hyponatremia (serum sodium concentration 125 to 134 mEq/L [125 to 134 mmol/L]) are usually asymptomatic, with hyponatremia being discovered incidentally when serum electrolytes are measured for other purposes.[21] However, mild symptoms of hyponatremia are frequently unnoticed by both clinicians and patients.[22] Chronic, mild hyponatremia is associated with impairment of attention, posture, and gait, all of which contribute to a substantially increased fall risk. Even "asymptomatic" patients, when formally tested, have impaired attention and gait to a degree that is comparable to symptoms seen with a blood alcohol level of 0.06% (13 mmol/L).[23,24]

Patients with moderate (serum sodium concentration 115 to 124 mEq/L [115 to 124 mmol/L]), severe (serum sodium concentration 110 to 114 mEq/L [110 to 114 mmol/L]), or rapidly developing hypotonic hyponatremia often present with a range of neurologic symptoms resulting from hypoosmolality-induced brain cell swelling. Classic neurologic symptoms include nausea, malaise, headache, lethargy, restlessness, and disorientation. In severe cases, seizures, coma, respiratory arrest, brainstem herniation, and death can occur.

The presence of these symptoms and their severity depend on both the magnitude of the hyponatremia and the rate at which the hyponatremia develops. The magnitude of the hyponatremia is important because serum osmolality decreases in direct proportion to the serum sodium concentration, and water movement into brain cells increases as serum osmolality decreases. The rate of change of the serum osmolality is an important factor because brain cells are able to adjust their intracellular osmolality to minimize cellular volume changes in response to volume changes, but time is required for this adaptation to occur.[25] When a decline in plasma osmolality causes water movement into brain cells, inorganic Cl^- and K^+, and organic osmolytes, such as taurine, glutamate, and myoinositol, move out of the cells to decrease intracellular osmolality and minimize intracellular water shifts.[26] Organic osmolytes, such as myoinositol, a osmotically active substances contribute substantially to controlling intracellular osmolality in the brain without directly altering cellular function.[25,26] The various components of this adaptive mechanism occur over different time frames, with sodium and potassium efflux occurring within minutes to several hours and organic osmolyte efflux occurring within hours to several days.[25,26] Maximal compensation for decreased plasma osmolality typically requires up to 48 hours. Thus, acute changes in plasma osmolality are more likely to be associated with symptoms. Concurrent respiratory failure and hypoxemia increase the risk of adverse neurologic outcomes because hypoxemia diminishes the brain's capacity to actively transport solute out of cells, leading to a higher incidence of cerebral edema.[25,26] Children and women have poorer clinical outcomes than adults and males, respectively. For example, post-menopausal women have a 25-fold higher risk of death or permanent neurological damage with acute hypervolemic hypotonic hyponatremia than men.[27] Hyponatremia is a severe risk factor for morbidity and mortality in patients with HF and cirrhosis.[2]

In addition to neurologic symptoms, patients with hypovolemic hyponatremia can present with signs and symptoms of hypovolemia, including dry mucous membranes, decreased skin turgor, tachycardia, decreased jugular venous pressure, hypotension, and orthostatic hypotension. These findings often are helpful in identifying the type of hyponatremia present.

5 The brain's adaptation to a chronic change in the plasma osmolality leads to development of neurologic symptoms if hyponatremia (hypoosmolality) is corrected too rapidly. The combination of the adaptive decrease in intracellular osmolality and rapid increase in serum osmolality results in excessive movement of water out of the brain cells and ICF volume depletion. Too rapid correction of the serum sodium concentration can lead to an acute decrease in brain cell volume, which contributes to the pathogenesis of *osmotic demyelination syndrome* (ODS),[2,28] also known as central pontine myelinolysis, because the demyelinated lesions, which appear on magnetic resonance imaging, most often occur in the central pons; however, it can extend to extrapontine structures.[1] Patients with this complication might develop hyperreflexia, para- or quadriparesis, parkinsonism, pseudobulbar palsy, *locked-in syndrome* (a condition in which a patient is aware and awake but cannot move or communicate verbally due to complete paralysis of nearly all voluntary muscles in the body except for the eyes), or death approximately 1 to 7 days after treatment.[1,12,29] Patients with a significant degree of cerebral adaptation (e.g., chronic serum sodium concentration less than 110 mEq/L [110 mmol/L]) to hypotonic hyponatremia are at highest risk of developing this syndrome because these patients have lower intracellular osmolalities at the initiation of therapy, resulting in a greater decrease in intracellular volume in brain cells when the plasma osmolality is raised too rapidly.[28] Other conditions that increase the risk of ODS include alcoholism, liver failure, orthotopic liver transplantation, potassium depletion, and malnutrition. Thus, if duration of hyponatremia is unknown; then it is generally safer to treat as if it is chronic when developing an initial treatment plan.[1]

TREATMENT

6 The following principles serve as general guidelines for the treatment of patients with hyponatremia:[1,18,21,30] (a) It is important for both short- and long-term management to treat the underlying cause of hyponatremia. (b) Appropriate treatment of hypotonic hyponatremia requires balancing the risks of hyponatremia versus the risk of ODS. In general, patients who acutely developed moderate to severe hyponatremia and/or patients who have severe symptoms are at greatest risk and potentially benefit most from more rapid correction of hyponatremia. (c) Correction of hypovolemic hypotonic hyponatremia is usually best accomplished with 0.9% NaCl solution, as these patients have both sodium and water deficits. (d) Active correction of euvolemic and hypervolemic hypotonic hyponatremia in patients who do not require rapid correction is usually best accomplished by water restriction. Demeclocycline, AVP vasopression 2 receptor antagonists (*vaptans*), or 0.9% NaCl solution plus a loop diuretic (furosemide, bumetanide) can be used if the initial response to water restriction is not adequate. (e) In patients with severe symptoms, 3% NaCl solution (possibly combined with a loop diuretic) should initially be used to more rapidly correct the hyponatremia. A loop diuretic such as furosemide can be administered concurrently with 3% NaCl to enhance the serum sodium correction by increasing free water excretion. (f) Long-term management will be required for patients in whom the underlying cause of hyponatremia cannot be corrected. Depending on the cause, water restriction, increasing sodium intake, and/or the use of an AVP antagonist (vaptan) can be used. Application of these principles to the treatment of patients with various forms of hypotonic hyponatremia is discussed in the following sections.

Desired Outcome

Regardless of the type or cause of hyponatremia, the goals of treatment for all patients are to resolve the underlying cause of the sodium and ECF volume imbalance, if possible, and to safely correct the sodium and water derangements. The treatment plan for patients with hyponatremia depends on the underlying cause of the hyponatremia and the severity of the patient's symptoms. Patients with an acute onset of hyponatremia or severe symptoms require more aggressive therapy to correct the hypotonicity. The initial goal for these patients is to increase plasma tonicity just enough to control severe symptoms; this typically requires only a small increase (5%) in serum sodium concentration. Once severe symptoms have abated, then continued correction of the serum sodium concentration should be achieved at a controlled rate. Patients who are asymptomatic or who have only mild to moderate symptoms do not require rapid correction of the serum sodium concentration. Treatment is dictated by the underlying etiology. In all cases the goal is to avoid an increase in the serum sodium concentration of more than 12 mEq/L (12 mmol/L) in 24 hours or 0.5 mEq/L (0.5 mmol/L) per hour.[1,2,21,30] However, because of the usual uncertainty regarding duration of hyponatremia, correction of no more than 6 to 8 mEq/L (6 to 8 mmol/L) or 0.33 mEq/L/h (0.33 mmol/L/h) is prudent to avoid ODS.[1]

ACUTE OR SEVERELY SYMPTOMATIC HYPOTONIC HYPONATREMIA

A patient who has or is at high risk of experiencing severe symptoms caused by hyponatremia should receive either 3% NaCl (513 mEq/L [513 mmol/L]) or 0.9% NaCl (154 mEq/L [154 mmol/L]) solution until severe symptoms resolve.[1,3,18,22,32] Resolution of severe symptoms frequently requires only a small (~5%) increase in serum sodium concentration; although, some clinicians suggest that the initial safe target should be a serum sodium concentration of approximately 120 mEq/L (120 mmol/L).[3,33] The relative concentrations of urine sodium and potassium (osmotically effective urine cations) must be compared with those of the infusate in planning a treatment regimen for patients with hypotonic hyponatremia. For the serum sodium concentration to increase after infusion of a sodium chloride solution, the sodium concentration of the infusate must exceed the sum of the urinary sodium and potassium concentrations to produce an effective net free-water excretion.

Patients with SIADH often have urinary concentrations of osmotically effective cations that exceed the sodium concentration of 0.9% NaCl. In this case, use of isotonic sodium chloride can actually worsen hyponatremia.[31] These patients should be preferentially treated with 3% NaCl solution. The relatively high urinary sodium concentration in patients with SIADH is due to ECF expansion, which minimizes sodium reabsorption along the nephron. When the urine osmolality exceeds 300 mOsm/kg (300 mmol/kg), it is generally advisable to administer an IV loop diuretic, not only to increase solute-free water excretion but also to prevent volume overload, which can result from infusion of hypertonic sodium chloride. IV furosemide, 20–40 mg every 6 hours, or bumetanide, 0.5 to 1 mg/dose every 2 to 3 hours for two doses, is generally sufficient to prevent volume overload and to decrease the urinary concentration of osmotically active cations to less than 150 mEq/L (150 mmol/L). If intermittent loop diuretic doses are not sufficient to manage edema, then continuous infusions have been used. Furosemide, 20 to 40 mg, given IV, followed by a 10 to 40 mg/h infusion, or bumetanide 1 mg given IV followed by a 0.5 to 2 mg/h infusion have been used.

Patients with hypovolemic hypotonic hyponatremia can be treated with 0.9% NaCl solution. In contrast to patients with SIADH, patients with this condition avidly reabsorb sodium throughout the nephron because the effective circulating blood volume is decreased. Thus, the urine sodium concentration is often less than 20 mEq/L (20 mmol/L), substantially less than the sodium content of 0.9% NaCl solution. While the use of 3% NaCl solution will correct hyponatremia in these patients, it will not correct the hypovolemia; thus, its use should be reserved for patients with severe symptoms requiring very rapid correction of the serum sodium concentration.

Acute hypervolemic hypotonic hyponatremia is particularly problematic to manage because the sodium and volume needed to minimize the risk of cerebral edema or seizures can worsen already compromised liver, heart, or kidney function. These patients generally should be treated with 3% NaCl and initiation of fluid (water) restriction. Loop diuretic therapy will also likely be required to facilitate urinary free water excretion.

Determination of a Sodium Chloride Infusion Regimen

Several methods for determining the correct sodium chloride solution infusion regimen for a patient with hyponatremia have been proposed.[1,2,18,29,32,33] These empiric approaches provide only an initial estimate of the correct infusion regimen. More complex equations have been derived, but improved outcomes using these equations have not been demonstrated.[18,29]

One common approach to acute treatment of hyponatremia is to estimate the change in serum sodium concentration resulting from the infusion of 1 L of 3% or 0.9% NaCl solution. An example of this approach is shown in Box 34-1. Another method involves calculating the sodium deficit, then replacing one-third of the deficit in the first 6 hours with the remaining two thirds being replaced over the following 24 to 48 hours. Sodium deficit can be calculated using the following equation:

$$\text{Na deficit (mEq)} = [(\text{Na}_D - \text{Na}_S) \times \text{TBW}]$$

where Na_D is the goal serum sodium (usually 125 to 130 mEq/L [125 to 130 mmol/L] to avoid too rapid correction); Na_S is the patient's

BOX 34-1 Assessment and Treatment of Euvolemic Hyponatremia

Calculating the change in serum sodium concentration after an IV fluid bolus:

$$\Delta \text{Na}_S = [\text{Na}_{IV} - \text{Na}_S]/(\text{TBW} + \text{Vol}_{IV})$$

where ΔNa_S is the change in serum sodium concentration; Na_{IV} is the sodium concentration of infusate (e.g., 154 mEq/L [154 mmol/L] for 0.9% NaCl; 513 mEq/L [513 mmol/L] for 3% NaCl); Na_S is the initial serum sodium concentration; TBW is the total body water (in liters); and Vol_{IV} is the volume of infused fluid in liters

TBW can be estimated as follows:

Children and men younger than 70 years: 0.6 L/kg × wt (kg)
Men older than 70 years and women younger than 70 years: 0.5 L/kg × wt (kg)
Women older than 70 years: 0.45 L/kg × wt (kg)
Dehydrated, older patients: 0.4 L/kg × wt (kg)
where wt is the current body weight

Clinical Example

A 66-year-old woman (weight, 60 kg [132 lb]; height, 170 cm [5 ft 7 in]) presents with nausea, vertigo, and disorientation which developed over several days. Ten days ago, she began taking carbamazepine for trigeminal neuralgia. Her serum sodium concentration on admission to the emergency room was 108 mEq/L (108 mmol/L). She receives the diagnosis of SIADH.

Plan of Care

1. Discontinue carbamazepine (the likely etiology of her SIADH)
2. Admit to hospital for correction of hyponatremia
3. Increase serum sodium concentration to no higher than 120 mEq/L (120 mmol/L) during the first 24 hours. Limit increase to 6 to 12 mEq/L (6 to 12 mmol/L) during first 24 hours
4. Due to degree of hyponatremia and presence of symptoms, give 3% NaCl solution. Calculate change in serum sodium after 1 L bolus as follows:
   ΔNa_S = (513 mEq/L – 108 mEq/L)/[(0.5 L/kg × 60 kg) + 1 L] = 13.1 mEq/L or 1.31 mEq/100 mL
   [Note: In SI units, the calculation is the same using mmol/L rather than mEq/L.]

Infusion of 1 L of 3% NaCl solution will result in a 13.1 mEq/L (13.1 mmol/L) rise in the serum sodium concentration. A 12 mEq/L (12 mmol/L) increase is desired; thus, the appropriate infusion volume is 916 mL [(12 mEq/L/13.1 mEq/L) × 1,000 mL] or [(12 mmol/L/13.1 mmol/L) × 1,000 mL]. (Note: The approach to this calculation would be similar if 0.9% NaCl was used, except that for each 1 L infusion, the expected increase in serum sodium concentration would be only 1.5 mEq/L (1.5 mmol/L), and an infusion volume of approximately 8 L would be required to achieve the targeted serum sodium concentration.)

5. Moderate to severe symptoms: serum sodium concentration should be increased by ~1.5 mEq/L/h (1.5 mmol/L/h) over the first 2 to 4 hours of treatment for a total of 3 to 6 mEq/L [3 to 6 mmol/L] or until the symptoms have resolved. An initial infusion rate of 114 mL/h for the first 2 to 4 hours is needed.
6. Check serum sodium concentration every 2 to 3 hours
7. Once symptoms subside, continue infusion rate at ~23 to 31 mL/h for the next 20 to 22 hours, to slowly correct hyponatremia. Monitor serum sodium concentration every 4 hours or more often if serum sodium is rapidly changing

current serum sodium concentration; and, TBW is the patient's current total body water calculated as shown in Box 34-1. The appropriate infusion volume for a given patient can then be estimated using the desired proportion of the estimated change that would result from a 1-L infusion or the amount of fluid needed to provide the calculated sodium deficit. The final step is to calculate an appropriate infusion rate for the calculated volume that will control the rate of increase of the serum sodium concentration to 6 to 12 mEq/L (6 to 12 mmol/L) in 24 hours (Box 34-1). Using desmopressin in combination with 3% NaCl solution to minimize the risk of treating hyponatremia has been suggested but is generally not recommended.[1]

Clinical **Controversy...**

Clinicians often disagree whether or not to administer 3% NaCl to patients with symptomatic hypotonicity. Advantages of 3% NaCl include more rapid correction of serum sodium concentration with smaller infusion volumes. The disadvantage of 3% NaCl is a higher risk of too rapid correction of serum sodium concentration causing ODS. The clinician must carefully consider the cause and the rapidity of development of the patient's hyponatremia as well as the relative risk of slower correction of the hyponatremia versus the development of ODS.

Evaluation of Therapeutic Outcomes

Patients with severely symptomatic hypotonic hyponatremia should be admitted to the intensive care unit (ICU) or other setting where frequent monitoring of neurologic and volume status is feasible. Examination of the heart, lungs, and neurologic status should be performed frequently during the initial 12 hours of therapy. The serum sodium concentration should be measured every 2 to 4 hours, and the urine osmolality, sodium, and potassium should be measured every 4 to 6 hours over the first day of therapy so that the infusion rate can be adjusted to avoid increasing the serum sodium too rapidly.[1]

NONEMERGENT HYPOVOLEMIC HYPOTONIC HYPONATREMIA

Most patients with hypovolemic hypotonic hyponatremia are either asymptomatic or have only mild-to-moderate symptoms so they do not require rapid correction of their hyponatremia. Many of these patients are at higher risk of developing ODS if serum sodium correction occurs too rapidly because they have chronic hyponatremia that has been maximally compensated for by the brain's osmotic adaptation. Treatment of these patients should include correction of the underlying condition, if possible, and administration of 0.9% NaCl solution to correct hypovolemia. This solution effectively replaces the sodium and water deficits that exist in these patients, and its use carries a lower risk of an excessive rate of correction than using a 3% NaCl solution.

The ECF deficit can be estimated based on sex, change in body weight, and age. One method to estimate the ECF deficit and an example of its use is shown in Box 34-2. If the patient's previous weight is not known, the ECF deficit can be roughly estimated based on clinical signs and symptoms. The presence of hyponatremia suggests an ECF deficit of 5% or more, whereas the presence of orthostatic hypotension suggests an ECF deficit of at least 10% to 15%. A 0.9% NaCl solution or Lactated Ringers soluton, isotonic fluids, would be optimal to correct the patient's volume deficit because 100% of it will remain in the ECF space (Table 34-1). The overriding initial treatment goal is to restore effective circulating volume; thus, it might be necessary to infuse 0.9% NaCl at 200 to 400 mL/h until symptoms of hypovolemia improve. The infusion rate can then be decreased to 100 to 150 mL/h so that the serum sodium concentration increases by no more than 6 to 12 mEq/L (6 to 12 mmol/L) or 0.5 to 1 mEq/L/h over the initial 24 hours. Infusion of 0.9% NaCl at a rate greater than 250 mL/h should be used cautiously in patients with left ventricular dysfunction or kidney insufficiency.

It is important to recognize that the rate of increase in the serum sodium concentration can substantially increase once hypovolemia has been corrected if infusion rates are not adjusted appropriately.[1] When the ECF volume is restored, AVP secretion will cease, and a rapid water diuresis can ensue, which can

BOX 34-2 Assessment and Treatment of Hypotonic Hypovolemic Hyponatremia

$$\text{ECF deficit (mL)} = \text{ECF}_{normal} - \text{ECF}_{current}$$

OR

$$\text{ECF deficit (mL)} = (0.33 \times \text{TBW}_{normal}) - (0.33 \times \text{TBW}_{current})$$

Clinical Example

A 56-year-old woman (height, 173 cm [5 ft 8 in]; weight, 62 kg [137 lb]) was started on hydrochlorothiazide 25 mg once daily 10 days ago for hypertension. She presents with complaints of mild nausea and dizziness when she stands up. Her current weight is 55.5 kg (122 lb). Physical examination reveals dry mucous membranes and orthostatic hypotension. Her serum sodium concentration is 125 mEq/L (125 mmol/L).

Her ECF deficit can be estimated as follows:

$$\text{ECF deficit} = [0.33 \times 62 \text{ kg} \times 0.5 \text{ L/kg}] - [0.33 \times 55.5 \text{ kg} \times 0.5 \text{ L/kg}]$$

$$\text{ECF deficit} = [62 \text{ kg} \times 0.5 \text{ L/kg} \times 0.33] - [55.3 \text{ kg} \times 0.5 \text{ L/kg} \times 0.33]$$

$$\text{ECF deficit} = 10.2 \text{ L} - 9.1 \text{ L} = 1.1 \text{ L}$$

The expected increase in the serum sodium concentration following the infusion of 1 L of 0.9% NaCl can be estimated as (see Box 34-1):

$$\Delta Na_S \text{ with 1 L of infusate} = [154 \text{ mEq/L} - 125 \text{ mEq/L}]/[(0.5 \text{ L/kg} \times 55.3 \text{ kg}) + 1 \text{ L}] = 1.0 \text{ mEq/L (mmol/L)}$$

The patient's serum sodium concentration will be 126 mEq/L (mmol/L) [(125 mEq/L (mmol/L) + 1 mEq/L (mmol/L)] following the infusion of 1 L 0.9% NaCl.

Treatment goals: restore effective circulating volume and correct serum sodium concentration

Treatment plan:

1. Infuse 0.9% NaCl at 200 to 400 mL/h until symptoms of hypovolemia improve; then decrease infusion to 100 to 150 mL/h so that the serum sodium concentration increases by no more than 6 to 12 mEq/L (6 to 12 mmol/L) or 0.5 to 1 mEq/L/h (0.5 to 1 mmol/L/h) over the initial 24 hours.
2. Hold thiazide diuretic until volume status is restored.
3. Consider restarting diuretic at lower dose, e.g., 12.5 mg once daily.

potentially result in an increase in the serum sodium concentration at a rate greater than desired. Estimation of the patient's ECF deficit at the initiation of therapy can be helpful. If the serum sodium concentration is observed to be increasing at a rate greater than 0.5 mEq/L/h (0.5 mmol/L/h), the infusate can be changed to 0.45% NaCl, and the infusion rate set to one that slows the rate of increase in the serum sodium concentration. Caution should be exercised if 0.45% NaCl is infused alone as this solution is hypoosmolar (osmolality is 154 mOsm/L) and may result in hemolysis. Most often, Dextrose 5%/0.45% NaCl is infused to provide an isoosmolar solution. Potassium depletion or repletion can also affect hyponatremia and its correction. One mEq of retained potassium equals 1 mEq retained sodium; thus, if concomitant hypokalemia is corrected at the same time as the hyponatremia, too rapid correction of hyponatremia can occur.[1]

Evaluation of Therapeutic Outcomes

Patients presenting with evidence of volume depletion should be reexamined frequently during the initial few hours of therapy. The serum sodium concentration should be measured every 2 to 4 hours to allow timely adjustment of the rate and composition of IV fluids to avoid too rapid increase in the serum sodium concentration. IV 0.9% NaCl solution should be administered judiciously in patients with a history of HF or kidney insufficiency, with frequent cardiopulmonary assessments so that the infusion rate can be appropriately decreased at the earliest sign of pulmonary congestion.

NONEMERGENT EUVOLEMIC HYPOTONIC HYPONATREMIA

The fact that an individual's neurological performance is restored to normal with correction of their hyponatremia provides a rationale for therapeutic management of all patients to maintain their serum sodium concentration at or above 130 mEq/L (130 mmol/L). Long-term management is thus required for patients in whom the underlying cause of hyponatremia is not readily correctable.

The treatment of SIADH always involves restricting water and correcting the underlying cause, if possible (Table 34-2). Drugs that could be contributing should be identified and discontinued. The goal of treatment is to induce negative water balance by restricting water intake to less than 1,000 to 1,200 mL/day, such that water losses from insensible sources (skin and lung) and from obligate urine and stool losses exceed intake. Daily insensible water losses via skin and lungs are approximately 900 mL/day; whereas approximately 200 mL and a minimum of 500 mL/day is lost in stool and in urine output, respectively. Because approximately 850 mL of water per day is ingested in food, and an additional 350 mL are generated from oxidative processes, this degree of water restriction should result in a negative water balance of several hundred milliliters per day. Other therapy goals include keeping the serum sodium concentration between 125 and 130 mEq/L (125 and 130 mmol/L) to prevent symptoms of hypotonicity and avoiding iatrogenic hypo- or hypervolemia.

Patients with chronic SIADH who are unable to restrict water sufficiently to maintain the serum sodium at least between 120 and 125 mEq/L (120 and 125 mmol/L) can be treated by increasing solute intake with sodium chloride and/or administration of a loop diuretic. Sodium chloride tablets increase the obligatory daily solute excretion, which augments the kidney's capacity for water excretion. The goal is to increase the daily solute intake and excretion to approximately 900 mOsm (900 mmol) per day. Because an average diet contains approximately 600 mOsm (600 mmol), 9 g of sodium chloride would be required to increase the osmolar excretion to 900 mOsm/day (900 mmol/day) (each 1 g sodium chloride tablet contains 17 mmol of sodium and 17 mmol of chloride). Because extracellular volume expansion is an expected adverse effect, a loop diuretic should be administered concurrently to avoid pulmonary and peripheral edema. Loop diuretics also enhance water excretion by limiting the formation of the medullary concentration gradient.

Demeclocycline is another treatment option for SIADH in patients whose sodium is not adequately controlled by water restriction alone or to replace water restriction. Demeclocycline causes nephrogenic diabetes insipidus by inhibiting tubular AVP activity, resulting in increased water excretion. The usual demeclocycline dosage is 300 mg given orally two to four times daily. Because of its delayed onset of action (3 to 6 days), this agent has no role in the acute management of severe hyponatremia, and dosage adjustments should be made no more frequently than every 3 to 4 days.[34] Demeclocycline should not be used in patients with liver disease or compromised fluid intake, who are at high risk for demeclocycline-induced renal tubular toxicity and acute kidney failure,[34,35] in children younger than 8 years of age because it can interfere with tooth and bone development, and in pregnant women.

The usual therapeutic options of water restriction, loop diuretic therapy, and increased sodium intake have recently been augmented with the introduction of the vaptans. These agents can be used to treat SIADH, as well as other causes of euvolemic and hypervolemic hypotonic hyponatremia.[34,36–40] Vaptans should not be used for emergency treatment of hyponatremia or in patients with hypovolemia.

Blockade of AVP binding can occur at one or more of its three distinct AVP receptors: V1, predominantly found in the liver, CNS, and cardiomyocytes; V2, located in the distal nephron; and V3, localized in the anterior pituitary and pancreas. Selective V2 receptor antagonism prevents aquaporin-2 water channel transport to the apical surface, thereby decreasing AVP-dependent water reabsorption in the collecting duct. The inhibition of AVP activity leads to excretion of large volumes of water, decreased urine osmolality, and an increase in the serum sodium concentration.[2] These positive outcomes are achieved without significantly increasing electrolyte excretion; thus, these agents also have been called "aquaretics." While several new compounds are currently under investigation, only two vaptans are currently marketed in the United States.

Conivaptan (Vaprisol®, Astellas Pharma US, Inc., North Brook, IL), a mixed vasopressin V1- and V2-receptor antagonist, is FDA-labeled for use in the treatment of acute euvolemic hyponatremia in hospitalized patients. Its utility in the treatment of chronic hyponatremia is limited because it is available only for IV administration and is not labeled for use in patients with HF.

Tolvaptan (Samsca®, Otsuka Pharmaceutical Co, Ltd, Tokyo, Japan) is an oral, nonpeptide selective AVP V2-receptor blocker with a greater affinity for the V2 receptor than endogenous AVP. It is FDA-labeled for use in the treatment of clinically significant (serum sodium concentration less than 125 mEq/L [125 mmol/L]) euvolemic or hypervolemic hyponatremia or less marked symptomatic hyponatremia that is unresponsive to other therapeutic interventions in patients with HF, cirrhosis, and SIADH. It appears to be safe and effective when given alone at promoting aquaresis and raising serum sodium concentration in both short- and intermediate-term studies (SALT-1 and SALT-2), respectively.[40] In addition, when used alone, it is superior to furosemide or water restriction, and when given in combination with furosemide, synergistic effects have been noted.[41] Tolvaptan is primarily metabolized to inactive metabolites by CYP3A4 enzymes and less than 1% is eliminated unchanged in the urine; thus clinicians should avoid its use in those receiving potent inhibitors of CYP3A4 (e.g., ketaconazole, clarithromycin, itraconazole, ritonivir). Concomitant therapy with P-glycoprotein inhibitors and grapefruit juice has also been noted to result in increased serum tolvaptan concentrations. For example, digoxin steady-state concentrations increased 20%, peak concentrations increased ~30%, and renal clearance decreased 59% when given concomitantly with tolvaptan (60 mg/day).[42] Conversely, the optimal benefits of tolvaptan therapy may not be realized and its dosage may need to be increased in patients who are receiving potent CYP3A4 inducers (e.g., phenytoin, phenobarbital, St. John's Wort). Dose linearity has been observed within the therapeutic range, and based on its terminal half-life (5 to 12 hours after 7 days or more of therapy), minimal accumulation occurs.[43,44] The usual starting tolvaptan dosage is 15 mg given orally once daily. Tolvaptan has an oral bioavailabilty of about 56%. For patients who can not take tolvaptan tablets orally, the tablets can be crushed, suspended in water and administered via a nasogastric tube, but a 25% mean decrease in the tolvaptan area under the concentration-time curve has been demonstrated in healthy adults with this administration method.[45] If, after 24 hours, a greater increase in serum sodium concentration is needed, the dosage may be increased to 30 mg once daily and after another 24 hours, to a maximum of 60 mg once daily. Tolvaptan therapy is contraindicated in those needing rapid correction of their serum sodium concentration, those unable to sense or respond appropriately to thirst, patients with hypovolemic hyponatremia, patients taking strong CYP3A4 inhibitors, and patients who are anuric. Among clinical trial participants who had a serum sodium concentration less than 125 mEq/L (125 mmol/L) at the start of tolvaptan therapy, the most common adverse events were thirst, dry mouth, weakness, constipation, hyperglycemia, and urinary frequency; although, these adverse events have rarely necessitated therapy discontinuation. Reversible elevations in hepatic transaminases have also been reported. However, irreversible liver damage with the potential to cause death or require a liver transplant was reported in three patients in a large clinical trial evaluating the use of tolvaptan in patients with autosomal dominant polycystic kidney disease.[46] As a result of this finding, the FDA issued a warning that tolvaptan should not be used for more than 30 days, should not be used by anyone with cirrhosis, and if any sign of liver disease occurs, it should be stopped. The FDA-approved labeling includes a boxed warning stating that tolvaptan therapy should begin or resume only in a hospital where the patient's serum sodium concentration can be closely monitored. To reduce the ODS risk, the initial FDA-approved labeling required that each patient should receive a medication guide with each prescription as part of a Risk Evaluation and Mitigation Strategy (REMS). This information is now included in the package insert given to all patients, and the medication guide is not required.

The vaptans have dramatic effects on water excretion, and the marketing of tolvaptan represented the first significant breakthrough in the therapy of hyponatremia and disorders of fluid homeostasis since the introduction of loop diuretics. However, the role of vaptans in the clinical management of patients with SIADH, HF, and cirrhosis is still unclear, especially given their cost. It is important to recognize that AVP receptor antagonists are contraindicated in patients with hypovolemia as their use would worsen the hypovolemia.

Evaluation of Therapeutic Outcomes

The serum sodium concentration should be measured every 24 to 48 hours after water restriction is initiated until it stabilizes at a concentration at or above 125 mEq/L (125 mmol/L). A continued decline in the serum sodium concentration would indicate either nonadherence to the prescribed water restriction or the need for a stricter restriction. Once the serum sodium concentration is stable at 125 mEq/L (125 mmol/L) or higher, the patient should be evaluated every 2 to 4 weeks to assess neurologic status and to obtain serum and urine sodium, potassium, and osmolality. Volume status (e.g., blood pressure, mucous membranes, skin turgor, and heart and lung examination) should also be assessed, particularly in patients who are being treated with sodium chloride tablets and/or loop diuretics.

NONEMERGENT HYPERVOLEMIC HYPOTONIC HYPONATREMIA

The initial treatment goals for patients with asymptomatic or minimally symptomatic hypotonic hyponatremia and an expanded ECF volume include achieving a negative water balance while minimizing rapid changes in cell volume until the serum sodium concentration is at or above 125 mEq/L (125 mmol/L). This involves correction of the underlying cause, when possible, as well as water restriction to an intake of less than 1,000 to 1,200 mL/day. Dietary sodium intake should be restricted to 1,000 to 2,000 mg/day, depending on the degree of ECF volume expansion and edema.

Patients with hypervolemic hypotonic hyponatremia caused by HF should be treated with measures that can potentially improve cardiac contractility and improve the effective circulating volume, thereby limiting nonosmotic AVP release. Therapeutic options include digitalis or afterload reduction with angiotensin-converting enzyme inhibitors (ACEIs) or angiotensin II receptor blockers (ARBs). Of these, only ACEIs have been shown in clinical trials to be of benefit in partially correcting hyponatremia in patients with HF;[48] however, correction of sodium with ACEIs has not been shown to lead to better outcomes.[49] No specific ACEI offers any particular advantage for this indication, and the dosage should be titrated to keep the systolic blood pressure between 110 and 130 mm Hg. Dose-limiting adverse effects of ACEIs include hyperkalemia (serum potassium concentration greater than 5.5 mEq/L [5.5 mmol/L]), as well as a decline in kidney function. The benefits and risks of continuing ACEI use must be weighed carefully in each case, but a decrease in glomerular filtration rate (GFR) of less than 30% that stabilizes within 2 months of beginning ACEI therapy generally does not require ACEI dosage reduction or discontinuation.[46]

Other potentially treatable causes of asymptomatic hyponatremia associated with an expanded ECF volume include nephrotic syndrome and cirrhosis. ACEIs can be used to decrease proteinuria in patients with nephrotic syndrome, leading to partial correction of hypoalbuminemia and to a decrease in nonosmotic AVP release. Patients with advanced cirrhosis can benefit from placement of a transjugular intrahepatic portosystemic shunt, which can increase the effective circulating volume and thus reduce nonosmotic AVP release. This procedure can potentially exacerbate or precipitate hepatic encephalopathy and should be avoided in patients with a history of encephalopathy.

Vaptans have also been used for the treatment of hypervolemic hypotonic hyponatremia in patients with HF or cirrhosis.[36,38,50,51] The effectiveness of tolvaptan use in the short-term management of patients with HF with hypervolemic hyponatremia has been evidenced by decreased body weight, increased urine output, decreased pulmonary capillary wedge pressure, and decreases in urine osmolality.[52–57] Long-standing beneficial effects, reduction in hospitalization or death, or progression of HF have not been observed in several pivotal trials.[54,56,58] Prolonged tolvaptan use leads to an increased endogenous AVP concentration and this overstimulation of V1A receptors could lead to increased afterload and progression of HF.[59] However, no worsening of left ventricular dilatation has been observed after 52 weeks of tolvaptan therapy (30 mg daily).[58]

Evaluation of Therapeutic Outcomes

Patients being treated for hypervolemic hypotonic hyponatremia should initially be evaluated on a daily basis for lung congestion,

TABLE 34-5 Characteristics of Hypernatremic States

Characteristics	Hypovolemic Hypernatremia	Euvolemic (Isovolemic) Hypernatremia	Hypervolemic Hypernatremia
Water and sodium	Water loss >> sodium loss	Water loss only	Sodium gain > water gain
Causes	Renal: osmotic diuresis, diuretic use, postoperative diuresis, high-output acute tubular necrosis	Congenital or acquired DI Nephrogenic DI Primary polydipsia	Sodium overload (e.g., 3% NaCl, sodium bicarbonate, salt tablets, concentrated tube feedings, hypertonic dialysate, sodium-containing medications)
Effect on TBW	↓↓	↓	↑
Effect on TBNa	↓	↔	↑↑
Laboratory findings in addition to hypernatremia	Renal: UOsm high, UNa high Nonrenal: UOsm high, UNa low	Renal: UOsm low, UNa variable Nonrenal: UOsm high, UNa variable	UOsm high, UNa high
Clinical presentation	Orthostasis, hypotension, tachycardia, dry mucous membranes	Depends on severity of hypernatremia; seizures, lethargy	Peripheral and pulmonary edema, variable blood pressure
Treatment	0.9% NaCl until vital signs stable, then free water replacement	Free water replacement, vasopressin	Free water replacement with loop diuretic; may require hemodialysis to remove volume

ascites, peripheral edema, and signs or symptoms of hyponatremia. The serum sodium concentration should be measured daily until it stabilizes at or above 125 mEq/L (125 mmol/L) following initiation of water restriction. Patients should then be assessed 1 week following discharge, and then every 2 to 4 weeks to assess compliance with the water restriction and other treatment measures, volume status, and hyponatremia-related symptoms.

HYPERNATREMIA

Epidemiology and Etiology

7 Hypernatremia, defined as a serum sodium concentration greater than 145 mEq/L [145 mmol/L], is always associated with hypertonicity and cellular dehydration, resulting from a deficit of water relative to ECF sodium content. A hypertonic state is a potent stimulus for AVP secretion and activation of the thirst mechanism. Therefore, hypernatremia is most commonly observed in patients with an impaired thirst response or in those without access to water. Young infants and children, comatose patients, the elderly, and disabled patients with an impaired sensorium or functional status are therefore at highest risk for this disorder.[60] The incidence of hypernatremia in general medical–surgical hospitalized patients and patients in ICUs has been estimated to be at least 1% and 4% to 8%, respectively.[61–63] In 92% of 130 ICU cases, hypernatremia was iatrogenic: the result of too little free water and too much hypertonic solution along with increased renal water loss.[64]

Outcome in patients with hypernatremia generally depends on the severity of the decrease and the rapidity with which it developed. In children, mortality from acute hypernatremia developing in less than 72 hours ranges from 10% to 70%. In contrast, chronic hypernatremia, defined as that which develops over 3 or more days, has a mortality rate of only 10%.[65] In adults, an acute increase in serum sodium concentration to greater than 160 mEq/L (160 mmol/L) is associated with a 75% mortality rate.[33] In contrast to children, adults in whom hypernatremia developed at a slower rate still have a high mortality rate of approximately 60%. Hypernatremia in adults is often associated with a serious underlying illness, which likely contributes to the higher mortality rate.

Pathophysiology

Hypernatremia most often results from water loss by either renal or extrarenal mechanisms. Less commonly, hypernatremia can result from administration of hypertonic fluids or excess sodium ingestion. Patients develop hypovolemic, hypervolemic, or isovolemic hypernatremia depending on the relative magnitude of sodium and water loss or gain caused by the underlying condition (Table 34-5).

Water loss commonly occurs as a result of insensible losses (evaporative water loss through the skin and lungs) in patients deprived of water. Hospitalized patients who are febrile or receiving mechanical ventilation are often treated with IV fluids containing insufficient free water to replace insensible losses. Hypernatremia can be observed in patients with hypotonic GI losses (diarrhea or vomiting) or in patients who have been exposed to high temperatures who suffer large water losses from both sweat and insensible losses.

A water diuresis can also be caused by diabetes insipidus (DI), which can be classified as either central DI (decreased AVP secretion) or nephrogenic DI (decreased kidney response to AVP). Patients with untreated DI excrete large volumes (3 to 20 L/day) of dilute urine, resulting in hypernatremia. Possible causes of DI are listed in Table 34-6.

Administration of hypertonic sodium chloride can result in hypernatremia and an expanded ECF volume. This type of hypernatremia is typically iatrogenic and can follow excess sodium bicarbonate administration, use of hypertonic sodium chloride enemas, or intrauterine injection of hypertonic sodium chloride. Isotonic

TABLE 34-6 Causes of Diabetes Insipidus

Central	Nephrogenic
Familial[a] Unreplaced insensible losses • Skin • Lung Hypodipsia Neurogenic • Neurosurgery • Tuberculosis • Head trauma • CNS malignancy/cyst • Hypoxic encephalopathy • Ethanol ingestion (transient) • Sarcoidosis • Sheehan syndrome[b]	Familial • Inherited aquaporin-2 defect • Inherited vasopressin V2-receptor defect Hypercalcemia (chronic) Hypokalemia Kidney disease Drug-induced • Cidofovir • Lithium toxicity • Amphotericin B • Demeclocycline • Foscarnet • Ifosfamide • Vasopressin V2-receptor antagonists • Methoxyflurane

AVP, arginine vasopressin; DI, diabetes insipidus.

[a]60 mutations in the AVP gene cause neurohypophyseal DI from U.S. National Library of Medicine. Genetics Home Reference. AVP. *http://ghr.nlm.nih.gov/gene/AVP*.
[b]Postpartum hypopituitarism caused by severe bleeding during childbirth.

TABLE 34-7 Clinical Presentation of Hypernatremia

General
- Increase in serum sodium concentration and osmolality causes acute water movement from the ICF to the ECF.
- Decreased volume in the brain can cause cerebral vein rupture, leading to focal intracerebral and subarachnoid hemorrhages and possible irreversible neurologic damage.

Symptoms
- Mild: lethargy, weakness, confusion, restlessness, and irritability
- Moderate: twitching
- Severe: seizures, coma, and death; usually requires an acute elevation in the plasma sodium concentration to 160 mEq/L (160 mmol/L) or higher
- Serum sodium concentration greater than 180 mEq/L (>180 mmol/L) is associated with a high mortality rate.
- Other symptoms depend on etiology of hypernatremia: postural hypotension, tachycardia, dry mucous membranes, diminished skin turgor, reduced or increased urine output
- Signs and symptoms may be difficult to detect because many patients with this condition have neurologic disease.

Laboratory tests
- Serum sodium concentration greater than 145 mEq/L (145 mmol/L)
- Urine osmolality may be helpful in diagnosing the cause.

sodium chloride solutions can lead to sodium accumulation if dilute urine is excreted.[66] Patients with hyperaldosteronism rarely spontaneously present with an expanded ECF and mild hypernatremia. A common cause of hypernatremia in the ICU is sodium intake from IV and enteral fluids and medications.[67] Sodium balance should be carefully monitored in critically ill patients to avoid iatrogenic hypernatremia.

Clinical Presentation

Hypernatremia results in movement of water from the ICF to the ECF. Patients with central DI often present with sudden onset of polyuria, whereas patients with nephrogenic DI develop polyuria more gradually. Symptoms seen in patients with hypernatremia (Table 34-7) are primarily caused by a decrease in neuronal (brain) cell volume and can include weakness, lethargy, restlessness, irritability, and confusion. Symptoms of more severe or rapidly developing hypernatremia include twitching, seizures, coma, and death. As discussed in the hyponatremia section, neurons can adapt to ECF tonicity changes by adjusting ICF osmolality by decreasing or increasing the concentration of inorganic (potassium, chloride) and organic osmolytes (glutamate, taurine, and myoinositol).[26] ECF hypertonicity results in generation of intracellular organic osmolytes within 24 hours of onset leading to an increase in ICF tonicity that then draws water into the neurons, limiting the decrease in cell volume. Patients with chronic hypernatremia are therefore less likely to present with symptoms compared to patients with acute onset hypernatremia.

Hypernatremia is often associated with serious underlying illness, and signs and symptoms related to the illness are often present. Patients with a history of severe diarrhea or vomiting can present with ECF volume depletion. Elderly patients deprived of water after sustaining a stroke or hip fracture often present with mental status changes and other signs of ECF volume depletion. Clinically detectable ECF volume depletion, however, might not be evident until the serum sodium concentration exceeds 160 mEq/L (160 mmol/L) because these patients primarily have water loss, two thirds of which is derived from the ICF. The urine is concentrated, osmolality often exceeds 450 mOsm/kg (450 mmol/kg), as a result of both osmotic and nonosmotic AVP release. The first step in evaluating patients with hypernatremia is the clinical assessment of the ECF and urine volume and the serum and urine osmolality (Fig. 34-3).

Patients with a contracted ECF volume and a low urine output include those who have sustained insensible water losses that exceed intake, as well as those with extrarenal losses of hypotonic fluids. On physical examination, the patient will have postural hypotension, diminished skin turgor, and delayed capillary refill. The daily urine output is typically less than 1 L.

A multicenter, case–control study examined the clinical presentation of hypernatremia in 150 elderly patients in geriatric care facilities.[68] Low blood pressure, tachycardia, dry oral mucosa,

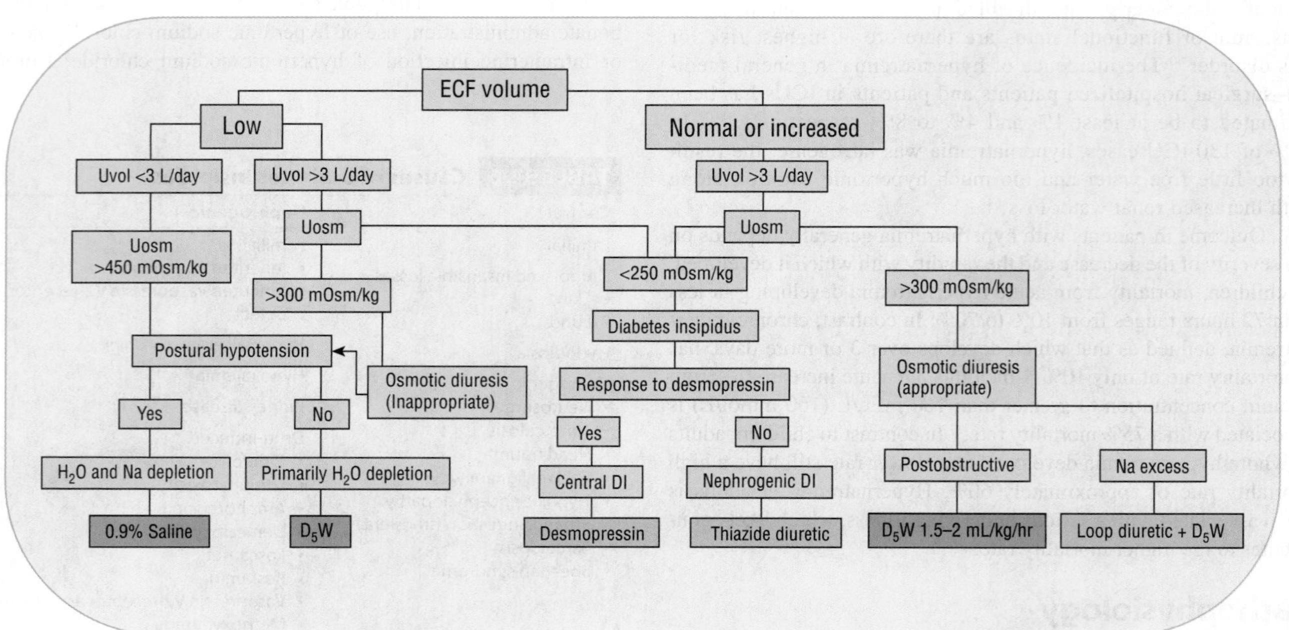

FIGURE 34-3 Diagnostic and treatment algorithm for hypernatremia. (D_5W, 5% dextrose in water; ECF, extracellular fluid; H_2O, water; Na, sodium; Uosm, urine osmolality [values in mOsm/kg are numerically equivalent to mmol/kg]; Uvol, daily urine volume.) See the text for guidelines regarding calculations of infusion rates for IV solutions.

decreased skin turgor, and recent changes in consciousness were all more common in patients with hypernatremia than in controls. In this mixed patient population, the presence of signs of dehydration was variable, with orthostatic hypotension and decreased subclavicular and forearm skin turgor present in at least 60% of patients. Abnormal subclavicular and thigh skin turgor, dry oral mucosa, and recent change in consciousness were significantly and independently associated with hypernatremia.

Osmotic Diuresis

In the presence of an ongoing osmotic diuresis, patients will have a urine volume greater than 3 L/day. Excessive urinary excretion of glucose, sodium, urea, or an exogenously administered solute (e.g., mannitol) is identified either by history or by direct measurement of serum and urinary concentrations of the suspected solute. Patients with postobstructive diuresis, such as those with bladder outlet obstruction caused by prostatic hypertrophy, are usually volume expanded as a result of retained excess solute because of a decline in the GFR. The osmotic diuresis that follows alleviation of the obstruction is appropriate in that it promotes excretion of the excess retained solute.

Patients with severe hyperglycemia, conversely, present with signs of volume depletion, and the diuresis is inappropriate as it further exacerbates the degree of ECF volume contraction associated with hyperglycemia. The estimated serum sodium concentration can be calculated by adding 1.7 mEq/L (1.7 mmol/L) for every 100 mg/dL (5.6 mmol/L) increase in the serum glucose concentration before estimating the water deficit.[3]

Diabetes Insipidus

Patients with DI tend to maintain a normal ECF volume as long as they are conscious and have free access to water. Patients typically have only a slight elevation in the serum sodium concentration (usually141 to 145 mEq/L [141 to 145 mmol/L]), and a daily urine volume greater than 3 L.

A water deprivation test is sometimes recommended to aid in the differential diagnosis.[33,66] This diagnostic test consists of depriving a patient of water for 8 to 12 hours. Urine osmolality, urine volume, and body weight are then measured before and after subcutaneous administration of 5 mcg of desmopressin acetate. Patients with central DI will show a prompt increase in urine osmolality to approximately 600 mOsm/kg (600 mmol/kg) and a decrease in urine volume after desmopressin administration. In those with nephrogenic DI, the urine osmolality will not increase above 300 mOsm/kg (300 mmol/kg).

The value of performing a water deprivation test in patients with polyuria and hypernatremia has recently been questioned.[69] Because hypernatremia provides a maximal stimulus for AVP secretion, discriminating between nephrogenic and central DI can be based on the plasma AVP concentration and urinary response to desmopressin without the need for water deprivation. The water deprivation test is likely to be of diagnostic value only in patients with polyuria and a normal serum sodium concentration.

Sodium Overload

Patients who have ingested large amounts of sodium (more than four tablespoons table salt [1,400 mEq or 1,400 mmol sodium]) or who have received more than 5 L of hypertonic fluids are volume expanded; although this may not always be clinically evident as edema. This volume expansion results in an osmotic diuresis, polyuria, and a urine osmolality greater than 300 mOsm/kg (300 mmol/kg). The excess sodium will be excreted in the urine in patients with normal perfusion and kidney function. With organ dysfunction, volume expansion will occur.

Clinical Controversy. . .

The relative merits of the various drug treatment options, including NSAIDs and amiloride, for nephrogenic DI have not been well studied. Choice of agents is therefore subject to clinician preference. It is unclear if there is a significant difference among these agents in the risk of clinically important decreases in GFR when they are used to produce mild ECF volume decreases.

TREATMENT

Desired Outcome

Treatment goals for patients with hypernatremia include correcting the serum sodium concentration to 145 mEq/L (145 mmol/L) at a rate that restores and maintains brain cell volume as close to normal as possible and normalizing the ECF volume, if indicated. Adequate treatment should result in the resolution of symptoms associated with hypovolemia. Careful titration of fluids and medications should minimize the adverse effects from too rapid correction of the serum sodium concentration. Rapid correction can result in movement of excessive water into the brain cells, resulting in cerebral edema, seizures, neurologic damage, and potentially death. Restriction of dietary sodium intake and water replacement can be necessary to prevent recurrence of hypernatremia.

Physical examination with attention to volume status and measurement of serum and urine sodium concentrations and osmolalities should be completed every 2 to 3 months during chronic therapy. A 24-hour urine collection to measure urine volume and sodium excretion will help guide therapy with diuretics and determine adherence to sodium restriction.

Pharmacologic Therapy

Hypovolemic Hypernatremia

8 Patients with hypovolemic hypernatremia should be treated initially with 0.9% NaCl until hemodynamic stability is restored. An initial infusion rate of 200 to 300 mL/h will likely be appropriate for most adults; children generally receive 10 to 20 mL/kg/h. Once intravascular volume is restored, 0.45% NaCl or 5% dextrose in water (D_5W) can then be infused to correct the water deficit. The ECF volume deficit can be estimated as:

$$\text{ECF (water) deficit} = \text{TBW}_{\text{current}} \times [1 - (140/\text{Na}_{\text{S1}})]$$

where $\text{TBW}_{\text{current}}$ is the current total body water; Na_{S1} is the initial serum sodium concentration (in mEq/L [mmol/L]); and 140 is the normal or goal serum sodium concentration in mEq/L (mmol/L). Although this formula provides an adequate estimate of the water deficit caused by pure water loss, it underestimates the deficit in patients with hypotonic fluid loss. The formula is not useful when sodium and potassium must be prescribed in addition to water.[1]

The appropriate rate of correction depends on the rapidity with which the hypernatremia developed. Hypernatremia that has developed over a period of only a few hours can be initially corrected at a rate of approximately 1 mEq/L (1 mmol/L) per hour, whereas a rate of 0.5 mEq/L (0.5 mmol/L) per hour or less should be used when hypernatremia has developed more slowly.[1,21] The rate of correction should generally be limited to no more than 10 to 12 mEq/L (10 to 12 mmol/L) per day.[1,30]

The serum sodium concentration and fluid status should be monitored every 2 to 3 hours during the first 24 hours of treatment in patients with symptomatic hypernatremia to permit appropriate adjustment of the rate of infusion of hypotonic fluids. After symptoms resolve and the serum sodium concentration is less than 148 mEq/L (148 mmol/L), serum sodium determinations every 6 to 12 hours and fluid status assessment every 8 to 24 hours are generally sufficient to monitor therapy.

Treatment of hyperglycemia-induced osmotic diuresis consists of correcting the hyperglycemia with insulin, as well as administering 0.9% NaCl until signs of ECF volume depletion resolve. Once hemodynamic stability is restored, the free water deficit should be corrected as described above.

Hypernatremia in patients undergoing a postobstructive diuresis should be treated with infusion of hypotonic fluids (e.g., 0.45% NaCl) at a maintenance rate of approximately 1.5 mL/kg per hour. Because this solution is hypotonic, care should be taken to avoid infusing it alone to prevent hemolysis. Administering fluids to replace urine output on a 1:1 volume basis tends to perpetuate the diuresis and should be avoided. Some clinicians use a 0.5:1 volume replacement to avoid this complication.

Central Diabetes Insipidus

9 Patients with central DI should generally receive AVP replacement therapy with desmopressin, an AVP analog.[1,21] Because of variable absorption of orally administered desmopressin, central DI is best treated with the intranasal formulation, 1-desamino-8-D-arginine vasopressin (DDAVP); however, oral tablets are available and are useful in some patients. The initial intranasal dose should be 10 mcg once daily, titrating up to 10 mcg twice daily based on serum sodium concentration. Each insufflation of intranasal DDAVP (100 mcg/mL) delivers 10 mcg of desmopressin acetate. Additionally, several medications with antidiuretic properties have been used successfully in the management of central and nephrogenic DI (Table 34-8). They can be used as adjunctive therapy with DDAVP or as an alternative to DDAVP.

The desmopressin dose should be adjusted to achieve adequate urinary concentration during sleep to prevent nocturia, a daily urine volume of approximately 1.5 to 2 L, and a serum sodium concentration between 137 and 142 mEq/L (137 and 142 mmol/L). The serum sodium concentration should be measured every 3 to 4 days during the initial dose titration period, and then every 2 to 4 months. Desmopressin administration results in nonsuppressible AVP activity and presents a risk of water intoxication with excess water retention. Patients using desmopressin should therefore be monitored for signs and symptoms of both hyponatremia and hypervolemia. It has been suggested that patients who experience water intoxication can minimize the risk of a second episode by delaying one desmopressin dose each week until polyuria and thirst develop, thus demonstrating the continued need for desmopressin therapy.[21]

TABLE 34-8 Drugs Used to Manage Central and Nephrogenic Diabetes Insipidus

Drug	Indication	Dose
Desmopressin acetate	Central and nephrogenic	5–20 mcg intranasally every 12–24 h
Chlorpropamide	Central	125–250 mg orally daily
Carbamazepine	Central	100–300 mg orally twice a day
Clofibrate	Central	500 mg orally four times a day
Hydrochlorothiazide	Central and nephrogenic	25 mg orally q 12–24 h
Amiloride	Lithium-related nephrogenic	5–10 mg orally daily
Indomethacin	Central and nephrogenic	50 mg orally q 8–12 h

Nephrogenic Diabetes Insipidus

In patients with nephrogenic DI, concomitant hypercalcemia and hypokalemia, if present, should be corrected, and any medications that potentially contribute to the pathogenesis should be discontinued, if possible.[70,71] One key goal in treating nephrogenic DI is to induce a mild ECF deficit (1 to 1.5 L) with a thiazide diuretic and dietary sodium restriction (85 mEq [85 mmol] Na^+ or 2,000 mg NaCl per day), which often can decrease urine volume by as much as 50% (Table 34-8). This ECF deficit will increase proximal tubule water reabsorption, decrease the volume of filtrate delivered to the distal nephron, and decrease urine volume. Indomethacin at a dosage of 50 mg given orally three times daily potentiates AVP activity and thus can be used as adjunctive therapy.

Sodium Overload

Treatment of sodium overload consists of administration of loop diuretics to facilitate excretion of the excess sodium and IV D_5W. The volume of infusate needed to correct the water deficit and hypernatremia at an appropriate rate can be estimated as described previously. Furosemide, 20 to 40 mg given IV every 6 hours, should also be administered.

The serum sodium concentration should initially be measured at least every 2 to 4 hours, and the diuretic continued until signs of ECF volume overload (pulmonary congestion and edema) resolve. The serum sodium concentration can be determined every 6 to 12 hours once the concentration is less than 148 mEq/L (148 mmol/L) and symptoms of hypertonicity have resolved.

EDEMA

10 The development of edematous states is usually due to heart, kidney, or liver failure, or a combination of these conditions; although, it can develop secondary to a rapid decrease in serum albumin concentration along with excess fluid intake in the setting of burns or trauma.[72,73] The body closely monitors blood volume to help ensure adequate tissue perfusion. A decline in the effective circulating volume (actually the blood pressure resulting from that volume) results in decreased kidney sodium and water excretion. Under these conditions, the kidneys retain all the water and sodium ingested until the effective circulating volume is restored to near normal. An increase in dietary sodium is accompanied by an increase in water intake caused by the initial increase in serum osmolality and stimulation of thirst. The resultant increase in ECF volume augments kidney perfusion, effecting a transient increase in GFR which leads to enhanced sodium filtration and excretion. These homeostatic mechanisms are crucial for maintaining sodium balance, as retention of just a few milliequivalents (mmoles) of sodium per day can eventually lead to an expanded ECF volume and edema formation.

Pathophysiology

Edema can be defined as a clinically detectable increase in interstitial fluid volume. In adults, edema formation generally requires an interstitial volume increase of at least 2.5 to 3 L. Edema develops when excess sodium is retained either as a primary defect in renal sodium excretion or as a response to a decrease in the effective circulating volume despite a normal or expanded ECF volume. An increase in the capillary hydrostatic pressure because of ECF volume expansion or an increase in central venous pressure can lead to edema formation. Edema may also occur when there is an alteration in Starling forces within the capillary.[72] The Starling equation denotes the relationship between factors affecting the movement of fluid between the capillary and interstitium and is discussed in detail in Chapter 13.

Edema may develop rapidly in those with an acute decompensation in myocardial contractility which leads to an elevation in pulmonary venous pressure that is transmitted back to the pulmonary capillaries and ultimately results in acute pulmonary edema. Edema may also develop insidiously as in the case of renal sodium and water retention due to diminished effective circulating volume which leads to a rise in the ECF volume and edema formation in both peripheral and pulmonary interstitial tissues.

Edema is the classical presentation in patients with nephrotic syndrome. There are two theories posited to explain edema in nephrotic syndrome: the *underfill* and the *overfill* hypothesis.[72] The underfill hypothesis states that decreased oncotic pressure from hypoalbuminemia (most pronounced with a serum albumin concentration less than 2 g/dL [20 g/L]) leads to excess filtration of fluid from the intravascular space to the interstitial space (*third spacing*) causing hypovolemia, kidney hypoperfusion, activation of the renin–angiotensin–aldosterone system, and secondary renal sodium retention. The overfill hypothesis is simply that primary renal sodium retention leads to edema.

Patients with cirrhosis initially develop ascites as a result of splanchnic vasodilation resulting in an increase in the pressure in the portal circulation (i.e., portal hypertension). The combination of portal hypertension and splanchnic vasodilation increases capillary pressure and permeability and facilitates the accumulation of ascites (fluid in the abdominal cavity; third spacing). Ascites can cause a decrease in effective circulating ECF volume and activation of the sympathetic nervous system and the renin–angiotensin–aldosterone system, leading to secondary hyperaldosteronism. The subsequent renal sodium retention leads to worsened ascites and edema.[72]

Clinical Presentation

Edema is usually first detected in the feet or pretibial area of ambulatory patients and in the presacral area of bed-bound individuals. Edema is described as "pitting" when a depression created by exerting pressure for several seconds over a bony prominence such as the tibia does not rapidly refill. The severity of the edema should be rated on a semi-quantitative scale of 1+ to 4+ depending on the depth of the pit: 1+ = 2 mm; 2+ = 4 mm; 3+ = 6 mm; and 4+ = 8 mm.

The extent of the edema should also be quantified according to the areas involved. Pretibial edema, for example, should be quantified according to how far it extends up the lower leg (e.g., one-third up the lower leg). Pulmonary edema, an increase in lung interstitial and alveolar water, is often evidenced by crackles (rales) upon auscultation. Rales should be quantified according to how far the crackles extend from the dependent portion of the lung(s). So, for example, edema limited to the ankles and feet would indicate less severe edema than edema that extends halfway up the lower legs, and crackles limited to the base of both lungs in an upright person would indicate less severe pulmonary edema than crackles throughout both lung fields.

TREATMENT

General Approach to Treatment

The goals of therapy for hypervolemic hypernatremia are to minimize edema and to improve organ function, as well as to relieve accompanying symptoms (e.g., dyspnea, abdominal distention). Importantly, the presence of edema does not always dictate the need for pharmacologic (diuretic) therapy. Severe pulmonary edema requires immediate pharmacologic treatment because it is life-threatening. Other forms of edema may be treated gradually, with a comprehensive approach that includes not only diuretics but also sodium and water restriction and treatment of the underlying disease. Sodium intake should generally be restricted to 1,000 to 2,000 mg/day. A slow, more judicious approach in non-life–threatening situations will help to minimize complications of diuretic therapy and excessive diuresis, including impaired perfusion, azotemia, and impaired cardiac output due to a fall in the left ventricular end-diastolic filling pressure.

Pharmacologic Therapy

11 Diuretics are the primary pharmacologic therapy for edema management when treatment of the underlying disease and sodium and water restriction are insufficient to reduce the expanded ECF volume and relieve edema. Diuretics can be categorized according to the site in the nephron where sodium reabsorption is inhibited. Loop diuretics (furosemide, bumetanide, torsemide and ethacrynic acid) inhibit the sodium–potassium–chloride (Na^+–K^+–$2Cl^-$) carrier in the loop of Henle, while thiazide diuretics (hydrochlorothiazide, chlorthalidone, and metolazone) inhibit the Na^+–Cl^- carrier in the distal tubule. Potassium-sparing diuretics inhibit the sodium channel in the cortical collecting duct either directly (triamterene and amiloride) or by interfering with aldosterone activity (spironolactone and eplerenone). A diuretic's efficacy depends on: (a) the amount of filtered sodium normally reabsorbed at its site of action; (b) the amount of sodium reabsorbed distal to its site of action; (c) adequate delivery of the drug to its site of action; and (d) the amount of sodium reaching its site of action in a given patient.

All diuretics act by inhibiting sodium reabsorption in the renal tubules; thus increase fractional excretion of sodium (FeNa). Loop diuretics are the most potent diuretics, as evidenced by the fact that they increase peak FeNa from normal of 1% (0.01) or less to 20% to 25% (0.20 to 0.25). Thiazide- and potassium-sparing diuretics are less potent and increase peak FeNa only to 3% to 5% (0.03 to 0.05) and 1% to 2% (0.01 to 0.02), respectively.[19] Although a large portion of the filtered sodium is reabsorbed in the proximal nephron, the efficacy of proximal-acting diuretics (e.g., acetazolamide) is limited by reabsorption of excess fluid and sodium in the loop of Henle. Furthermore, sodium reabsorption by the distal tubule can compensate for reduced reabsorption in the loop of Henle when sodium intake is high.

The effectiveness of thiazide and loop diuretics is dependent on drug concentration in the tubular lumen. These diuretics are delivered to the tubular lumen via active transport by the proximal tubular cells. Osmotic diuretics are freely filtered into the tubular lumen in the proximal tubule; whereas, spironolactone gains access to mineralocorticoid receptors in the cortical collecting duct through diffusion from the systemic circulation.

A threshold concentration of loop or thiazide diuretic must be delivered to the respective site of action to achieve a natriuresis.[19] Once this concentration is achieved, a further diuretic dose increase will not elicit an increase in diuretic response. Thus, a "ceiling dose" for these diuretics is recognized. Administration of 40 mg of IV furosemide to a normal subject will result in excretion of 200 to 250 mEq (200 to 250 mmol) of sodium in 3 to 4 L of urine over a 3- to 4-hour period.[19]

Loop diuretics except torsemide have a rapid action but short half-life requiring administration every 2 to 3 hours while thiazide diuretics have a longer half-life allowing for less frequent (once daily) dosing. Table 34-9 lists the maximal effective doses and dosing intervals for loop diuretics in patients with cirrhosis, HF, nephrotic syndrome, and those with reduced kidney function.

Patients with kidney insufficiency often require larger diuretic doses to achieve adequate drug concentrations at the site of action. The natriuretic response is decreased in patients with kidney insufficiency because the filtered sodium load falls proportionately as GFR declines. This decrease in the GFR can be partially overcome by administering diuretics more frequently or by

TABLE 34-9 Maximal Effective Dose[a] and Dosing Interval for Edema Management with Loop Diuretics

Diuretic	Dosing Interval	Normal	Cirrhosis	CHF	Nephrotic Syndrome	GFR (10–50 mL/min [0.17–0.84 mL/s])	GFR (<10 mL/min [<0.17 mL/s])
Furosemide							
IV	6–8 h	10–40 mg	40 mg	40–80 mg	120 mg	80 mg	200 mg
Oral	6–8 h	20–80 mg	80 mg	80–160 mg	240 mg	160 mg	320–400 mg
Bumetanide							
IV/Oral	6–8 h	1 mg	1 mg	2–3 mg	3 mg	2–3 mg	8–10 mg
Torsemide							
IV/Oral	24 h	15–20 mg	10–20 mg	20–50 mg	50 mg	20–50 mg	50–100 mg

CHF, congestive heart failure; GFR, glomerular filtration rate.

[a]Although these doses are considered maximal doses, higher doses may be required due to insufficient quantities in the renal tubular fluid.[73]

using a continuous infusion, a method commonly used in critically ill patients. The latter will limit the effect of postdiuretic sodium retention in the distal nephron. Table 34-10 lists initial continuous infusion rates for patients based on their creatinine clearance. Patients with diuretic-resistant edema can be treated with both a loop and a thiazide-type diuretic.

Loop diuretic resistance can be caused by pronounced sodium reabsorption in the distal sites of the nephron when sodium absorption in the loop of Henle is blocked. If sodium intake is not restricted, this distal sodium reabsorption can compensate entirely for the loop-diuretic induced sodium loss. Another mechanism of diuretic resistance is impaired diuretic delivery to the site of action. Patients with HF and a normal GFR may have impaired oral furosemide absorption. An adequate diuresis is most readily sustained by increasing the frequency of diuretic administration, but a higher dose may also be effective (Fig. 34-4). Absorption of orally administered loop diuretics can be compromised by GI edema, gastroparesis, and delayed gastric emptying, findings often seen in critically ill patients. Inadequate drug concentrations at the site of action can also be caused by decreased perfusion as might be seen in patients with decompensated HF or those with decreased kidney perfusion. Due to extensive binding to serum albumin (more than 95%), very little of these agents reach the tubule lumen by filtration, and they are almost exclusively transported into the proximal tubule lumen by active secretion via the organic acid secretory pathway.[19] Human studies, however, have demonstrated that when albumin binding is inhibited by concurrent sulfasoxazole administration, diuretic resistance persists, suggesting a decrease in intrinsic tubular sensitivity to loop diuretics.[75] This impaired natriuretic response can be overcome by using higher diuretic doses to increase the delivery of free drug to the secretory site in the nephron.[76] Decreased intrinsic diuretic activity with repeated dosing may also play a role in the development of diuretic resistance. Whether this is mediated by the first two mechanisms or as a mechanism to prevent hypovolemia is not well understood. Combinations of loop diuretics with distally acting diuretics are generally necessary to promote a natriuresis that exceeds distal tubular sodium reabsorption for those with nephrotic syndrome (Fig. 34-5).

TABLE 34-10 Continuous Infusion Rates for Loop Diuretics

Drug	Initial Infusion Rate based on Creatinine Clearance		
	<25 mL/min (0.42 mL/s)	25–75 mL/min (0.42–1.25 mL/s)	>75 mL/min (>1.25 mL/s)
Bumetanide	1–2 mg/h	0.5–1 mg/h	0.5 mg/h
Furosemide	20–40 mg/h	10–20 mg/h	10 mg/h
Torsemide	10–20 mg/h	5–10 mg/h	5 mg/h

Secondary hyperaldosteronism from activation of the renin–angiotensin–aldosterone system plays a major role in the pathogenesis of edema in patients with cirrhosis. Therefore, these patients should initially be treated with an aldosterone antagonist (e.g., spironolactone) in the absence of impaired GFR and hyperkalemia (Fig. 34-6). Thiazides can then be added for patients with a creatinine clearance greater than 50 mL/min (0.84 mL/s). For those whose edema remains diuretic resistant, a loop diuretic can be used instead of the thiazide. Patients with impaired GFR (creatinine clearance less than 40 mL/min [0.67 mL/s]) can require a loop diuretic, with addition of a thiazide in those who do not achieve adequate diuresis.[73,75]

Complications of loop and thiazide diuretic therapy include hypokalemia, excess ECF volume loss, calcium imbalance, hyponatremia, hypomagnesemia, metabolic alkalosis, and hyperuricemia. Patients with refractory edema treated with high-dose synergistic combinations are at high risk for developing hypokalemia.[8] Thiazides can also cause hypercalcemia, particularly in patients with mild subclinical hyperparathyroidism. Loop diuretics cause hypercalciuria and can lead to bone disorders when used chronically. Chronic therapy with potassium-sparing diuretics (i.e., triamterene, amiloride, and spironolactone) can cause a mild metabolic acidosis and hyperkalemia. Patients with moderate to severe kidney dysfunction or those receiving nonsteroidal antiinflammatory drugs (NSAIDs), ACEIs, or angiotensin receptor blockers are at highest risk for hyperkalemia. In addition, spironolactone can cause reversible gynecomastia in about 10% of men receiving it,

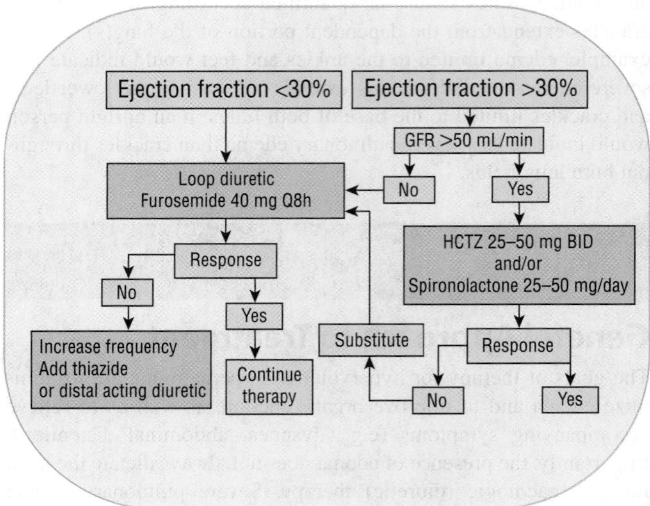

FIGURE 34-4 Therapeutic algorithm for diuretic use in patients with heart failure. (GFR, glomerular filtration rate [50 mL/min is equivalent to 0.84 mL/s]; HCTZ, hydrochlorothiazide.)

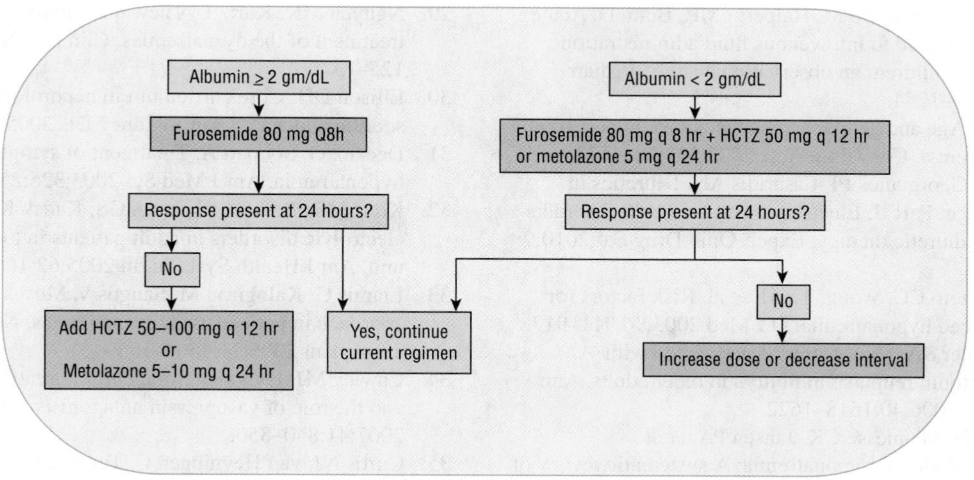

FIGURE 34-5 Therapeutic algorithm for diuretic therapy in patients with nephrotic syndrome. Albumin concentration of 2 g/dL is equivalent to 20 g/L. (HCTZ, hydrochlorothiazide.)

and in about 50% of men receiving 150 mg/day or more. This side effect, however, has not been associated with eplerenone, another aldosterone antagonist.[77]

EVALUATION OF THERAPEUTIC OUTCOMES

Patients should be monitored by careful history and intermittent physical examinations to detect signs and symptoms of edema as well as adverse effects of treatment. Physical examination should include measurement of blood pressure and pulse in either supine or seated positions and after standing for 2 to 3 minutes. ECF volume can be estimated based on the height of the jugular venous pressure, extent of edema, auscultation of the heart and lungs, and skin turgor. Follow-up monitoring (10 to 14 days after therapy initiation) should include determinations of serum sodium, potassium, chloride, bicarbonate, magnesium, calcium, BUN, serum creatinine, and uric acid. A new steady state will have developed over that time period and further fluctuations in ECF volume and electrolyte balance generally do not occur in the absence of a change in clinical status, diuretic dosage, or dietary intake. Repeated blood tests are not necessary at every visit unless there is a change in the patient's clinical status.

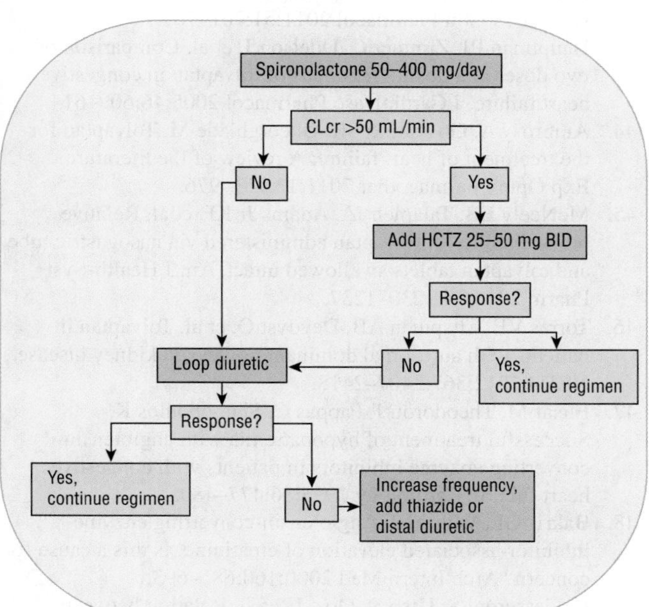

FIGURE 34-6 Therapeutic algorithm for diuretic use in patients with cirrhosis. (CLcr, creatinine clearance [50 mL/min is equivalent to 0.84 mL/s]; HCTZ, hydrochlorothiazide.)

ABBREVIATIONS

ACEI	angiotensin-converting enzyme inhibitor
AVP	arginine vasopressin, also known as vasopressin, antidiuretic hormone, or ADH
ATPase	adenosine triphosphatase
BUN	blood urea nitrogen
D_5W	5% dextrose in water
DDAVP	1-desamino-8-D-arginine vasopressin
DI	diabetes insipidus
ECF	extracellular fluid
FeNa	fractional excretion of sodium
GFR	glomerular filtration rate
HF	heart failure
ICU	intensive care unit
NSAID	nonsteroidal antiinflammatory drug
ODS	osmotic demyelination syndrome
SIADH	syndrome of inappropriate secretion of antidiuretic hormone
TBW	total body water
Vaptan	vasopression 2 receptor antagonist

REFERENCES

1. Androgué HJ, Madias NE. The challenge of hyponatremia. J Am Soc Nephrol 2012;23:1140–1148.
2. Schrier RW. The science behind hyponatremia and its clinical manifestations. Pharmacotherapy 2011;31(5 Pt 2):9S–17S.
3. Upadhyay A, Jaber BL, Madias NE. Incidence and prevalence of hyponatremia. Am J Med 2006;119(7A):S30–S35.
4. Upadhyay A, Jaber BL, Madias NE. Epidemiology of hyponatremia. Semin Nephrol 2009;29(3):227–238.
5. Patterson JH. The impact of hyponatremia. Pharmacother 2011;31 (5 Pt 2):5S–8S.

6. Hoorn EJ, Geary D, Robb M, Halperin ML, Bohn D. Acute hyponatremia related to intravenous fluid administration in hospitalized children: an observational study. Pediatr 2004;113:1279–1284.
7. Hawkins RC. Age and gender as risk factors for hyponatremia and hypernatremia. Clin Chim Acta 2003;337:169–172.
8. Sarafidis PA, Georgianos PI, Lasaridis AN. Diuretics in clinical practice. Part II: Electrolyte and acid-base disorders complicating diuretic therapy. Expert Opin Drug Saf 2010;9: 259–273.
9. Chow KM, Szeto CC, Wong, TY-H, et al. Risk factors for thiazide-induced hyponatremia. Q J Med 2003;96:911–917.
10. Jacob S, Spinler SA. Hyponatremia associated with selective serotonin reuptake inhibitors in older adults. Ann Pharmacother 2006;40:1618–1622.
11. Meulendijks D, Mannesse CK, Jansen PA, et al. Antipsychotic-induced hyponatremia: A systematic review of the published evidence. Drug Saf 2010;33:101–114.
12. Almond CSD, Shin AY, Fortescue EB, et al. Hyponatremia among runners in the Boston Marathon. N Engl J Med 2005;352:1550–1556.
13. Koczmara C, Wade AW, Skippen P, et al. Hospital-acquired acute hyponatremia and reports of pediatric deaths. Dynamics 2010;21:21–26.
14. Asadollahi K, Beeching N, Gill G. Hyponatremia as a risk factor for hospital mortality. Q J Med 2006;99:877–880.
15. Kacprowicz RF, Lloyd JD. Electrolyte complications of malignancy. Emerg Med Clin North Am 2009;27:257–269.
16. Nzerue CM, Baffoe-Bonnie H, You W, et al. Predictors of outcome in hospitalized patients with severe hyponatremia. J Natl Med Assoc 2003;95:335–343.
17. Kurtz I, Nguyen MK. Evolving concepts in the quantitative analysis of the determinants of the plasma water sodium concentration and the pathophysiology and treatment of dysnatremias. Kidney Int 2005;68:1982–1993.
18. Reynolds RM, Seckl JR. Hyponatremia for the clinical endocrinologist. Clin Endocrinol 2005;63:366–374.
19. Sarafidis PA, Georgianos PI, Lasaridis AN. Diuretics in clinical practice. Part I: Mechanisms of action, pharmacological effects and clinical indications of diuretic compounds. Expert Opin Drug Saf 2010;9:243–257.
20. Liamis G, Milionis H, Elisaf M. A review of drug-induced hyponatremia. Am J Kidney Dis 2008;52:144–153.
21. Reynolds RM, Padfield PL, Seckl JR. Disorders of sodium balance. BMJ 2006;332:702–705.
22. Decaux G. Is asymptomatic hyponatremia really asymptomatic? Am J Med 2006;119(7A):S79–S82.
23. Kinsella S, Moran S, Sullivan MO, et al. Hyponatremia independent of osteoporosis is associated with fracture occurrence. Clin J Am Soc Nephrol 2010;5:275–280.
24. Ayus JC, Morits ML. Bone disease as a new complication of hyponatremia: Moving beyond brain injury. Clin J Am Soc Nephrol 2010;5:167–168.
25. Sterns RH, Silver SM. Brain volume regulation in response to hypoosmolality and its correction. Am J Med 2006;119(7A):S12–S16.
26. Fisher SK, Heacock AM, Keep RF, Foster DJ. Receptor regulation of osmolyte homeostasis in neural cells. J Physiol 2010;18:3355–3364.
27. Ayus JC, Arrief AI. Chronic hyponatremic encephalopathy in post-menopausal women—Association of therapies with morbidity and mortality. JAMA 1999;281:2299–2304.
28. Murase TM, Sugimura Y, Takefuji S, et al. Mechanisms and therapy of osmotic demyelination. Am J Med 2006;119(7A): S69–S73.
29. Nguyen MK, Kurtz I. A new quantitative approach to the treatment of the dysnatremias. Clin Exp Nephrol 2003;7: 125–137.
30. Ellison DH. Core curriculum in nephrology: Disorders of sodium and water. Am J Kidney Dis 2005;46:356–361.
31. Decaux G, Soupart A. Treatment of symptomatic hyponatremia. Am J Med Sci 2003;326:25–30.
32. Kraft MD, Btaiche IF, Sacks GS, Kudsk KA. Treatment of electrolyte disorders in adult patients in the intensive care unit. Am J Health Syst Pharm 2005;62:1663–1682.
33. Liamis G, Kalogirou M, Saugos V, Moses E. Therapeutic approach in patients with dysnatremias. Nephrol Dial Transplant 2006;21:1564–1569.
34. Cawley MJ. Hyponatremia: current treatment strategies and the role of vasopressin antagonists. Ann Pharmacother 2007;41:840–850.
35. Curtis NJ, van Heyningen C, Turner JJ. Irreversible nephrotoxicity from demeclocycline in the treatment of hyponatremia. Age Ageing 2002;31:151–152.
36. Greenberg A, Verbalis JG. Vasopressin receptor antagonists. Kidney Int 2006;69:2124–2130.
37. Palm CP, Pistrosch F, Herbrig K, Gross P. Vasopressin antagonists as aquaretic agents for the treatment of hyponatremia. Am J Med 2006;119(7A):S87–S92.
38. Schrier RW, Gross P, Gheorghiade M, et al. Tolvaptan, a selective oral vasopressin V2-receptor antagonist, for hyponatremia. N Engl J Med 2006;355:2099–2112.
39. Oghlakian G, Klapholz M. Vaospressin and vasopressin receptor antagonists in heart failure. Cardiol Rev 2009; 17:10–15.
40. Costello-Boerrigter LC, Boerrigter G, Burnett JC. Pharmacology of vasopressin antagonists. Heart Fail Rev 2009;14:75–82.
41. Shoaf SE, Graumer SL, Briemont P, et al. Pharmacokinetic and pharmacodynamic interaction between tolvaptan, an onopeptide AV antagonist and furosemide or hydrochlorthiazide. J Cardiovasc Pharmacol 2007;50:213–222.
42. Shoaf SE, Ohzone Y, Ninomiya S, et al. In vitro P-glycoprotein interactions and steady-state pharmacokinetic interactions between tolvaptan and digoxin in healthy subjects. J Clin Pharmacol 2011:51:761–769.
43. Hauptman PJ, Zimmer C, Udelson J, et al. Comparison of two doses and dosing regimens of tolvaptan in congestive heart failure. J Cardiolvasc Pharmacol 2005;46:609–614.
44. Ambrosy A, Goldsmith SR, Gheorghiade M. Tolvaptan for the treatment of heart failure: A review of the literature. Exp Opin Pharmacother 2011;12:961–976.
45. McNeely EB, Talameh JA, Adams Jr KF, et al. Relative bioavailability of tolvaptan administered via nasogastric tube and tolvaptan tablets swallowed intact. Am J Health-Syst Pharm 2013;70:1230–1237.
46. Torres VE, Chapman AB, Devuyst O, et al. Tolvaptan in patients with autosomal dominant polycystic kidney disease. NEJM 2012;367:2407–2418.
47. Elisaf M, Theodorou J, Pappas C, Siamopoulos K. Successful treatment of hyponatremia with angiotensin-converting enzyme inhibitors in patients with congestive heart failure. Cardiology 1995;86:477–480.
48. Bakris GL, Weir MR. Angiotensin-converting enzyme inhibitor-associated elevation of creatinine: Is this a cause for concern? Arch Intern Med 2000;160:685–693.
49. Baldasseroni S, Urso R, Orso F, et al. Relation between serum sodium levels and prognosis in outpatients with chronic heart failure: neutral effect of treatment with beta-blockers and angiotensin-converting enzyme inhibitors: data

from the Italian network on congestive heart failure (IN-CHF database). J Cardiovasc Med 2011;12:723–731.

50. Gerbes AL, Gulberg V, Gines P, et al. Therapy of hyponatremia in cirrhosis with a vasopressin receptor antagonist: A randomized double-blind multicenter trial. Gastroenterology 2003;124:933–939.
51. Berl T, Quittnet-Pelletier F, Verbalis JG, et al. Oral tolvaptan is safe and effective in chronic hyponatremia. J Am Soc Nephrol 2010;21:705–712.
52. Dixon MB, Lien YH. Tolvaptan and its potential in the treatment of hyponatremia. Therapeut Clin Risk Management 2008;4:1149–1155.
53. Gheorghaide M, Niazi I, Quyang J, et al. Vasopressin V2-receptor blockage with tolvaptan in patients with chronic heart failure: Results from a double-blind randomized trial. Circulation 2003;107:2690–2696.
54. Gheorghaide M, Gattis WA, O'Connor CM, et al. Effects of tolvaptan, a vasopressin antagonist, in patients hospitalized with worsening heart failure: A randomized controlled trial. JAMA 2004;291:1963–1971.
55. Gheorghiade M, Konstam MA, Burnett JC Jr, et al. Short-term clinical effects of tolvaptan, an oral vasopressin antagonist, in patients hospitalized for heart failure: The EVEREST Clinical Status Trials. JAMA 2007;297:1332–1343.
56. Konstam MA, Gheorghiade M, Burnett JC Jr, et al. Effects of oral tolvaptan in patients hospitalized for worsening heart failure: The EVEREST Outcome Trial. JAMA 2007;297: 1319–1331.
57. Udelson JE, Orlandi C, Quyang J, et al. Acute hemodynamic effects of tolvaptan, a vasopressin V2 receptor blocker, in patients with symptomatic heart failure and systolic dysfunction: an international, multicenter, randomized, placebo-controlled trial. J Am Coll Cardiol 2008;52:1540–1545.
58. Udelson JE, McGrew FA, Flores E, et al. Multicenter, randomized, double-blind, placebo-controlled study on the effect of oral tolvaptan on left ventricular dilation and function in patients with heart failure and systolic dysfunction. J Am Coll Cardiol 2005;49:2151–2159.
59. Costello-Boerrigter LC, Smith WB, Boerrigter G, et al. Vasopressin-2-receptor antagonism augments water excretion without changes in renal hemodynamics or sodium and potassium excretion in human heart failure. Am J Physiol Renal Physiol 2005;290:F273–F278.
60. Al-Absi A, Gosmanova EO, Wall BM. A clinical approach to the treatment of chronic hypernatremia. Am J Kidney Dis 2012;60:1032–1038.
61. Waite MD, Fuhrman SA, Badawi O, Zuckerman IH, Franey CS. Intensive care unit-acquired hypernatremia is an independent predictor of increased mortality and length of stay. J Crit Care 2013;. *http://dx.doi.org/10.1016/j.jcrc.2012.11.013*.
62. Palevsky PM, Bhagrath R, Greenberg A. Hypernatremia in hospitalized patients. Ann Intern Med 1996;124:197–203.
63. Aiyagari V, Deibert E, Diringer MN. Hypernatremia in the neurologic intensive care: How high is too high? J Crit Care 2006;21:163–172.
64. Hoom EJ, Betjes MG, Weigel J, Zietse R. Hypernatremia in critically ill patients: Too little water and too much salt. Nephrol Dial Transplant 2008;23:1562–1568.
65. Moritz ML, Ayus JC. The changing pattern of hypernatremia in hospitalized children. Pediatrics 1999;104:435–439.
66. Lindner G, Funk GC. Hypernatremia in critically ill patients. J Crit Care 2012. *http://dx.doi.org/10.1016/j.jcrc.2012.05.001*.
67. Buckley MS, Leblanc JM, Cawley MJ. Electrolyte disturbances associated with commonly prescribed medications in the intensive care unit. Crit Care Med 2010;38:S253–S264.
68. Chassagne P, Druesne L, Capet C, Menard JF, Bercoff E. Clinical presentation of hypernatremia in elderly patients: A case control study. J Am Geriatr Soc 2006;54:1225–1230.
69. Moritz ML. A water deprivation test is not indicated in the evaluation of hypernatremia [letter]. Am J Kidney Dis 2005;46:1150–1151.
70. Sands JM, Bichet DG. Nephrogenic diabetes insipidus. Ann Intern Med 2006;144:186–194.
71. Garofeanu CG, Weir M, Rosas-Arellano P, et al. Causes of reversible nephrogenic diabetes insipidus: A systematic review. Am J Kidney Dis 2005;45:626–637.
72. Siddall EC, Radhakrishnan J. The pathophysiology of edema formation in the nephrotic syndrome. Kidney Int 2012;82:635–642.
73. Somberg JC, Molnar J. Therapeutic approaches to the treatment of edema and ascites: The use of diuretics. Am J Ther 2009:16:98–101.
74. Asare K. Management of loop diuretic resistance in the intensive care unit. Am J Health-Syst Pharm 2009;66: 1635–1640.
75. Agarwal R, Gorski JC, Sundblad K, Brater DC. Urinary protein binding does not affect response to furosemide in patients with nephrotic syndrome. J Am Soc Nephrol 2000;11:1100–1105.
76. Ellison DH. Edema and the clinical use of diuretics. In: Greenberg A, ed. Primer on Kidney Diseases, 5th ed. Philadelphia, PA: WB Saunders, 2009:135–147.
77. Nappi JM, Sieg A. Aldosterone receptor antagonists in patients with chronic heart failure. Vasc Heal Risk Manag 2011;7:353–363.

Disorders of Calcium and Phosphorus Homeostasis

35

Amy Barton Pai

KEY CONCEPTS

1 Severe acute hypercalcemia can result in cardiac arrhythmias, whereas chronic hypercalcemia can lead to calcium deposition in soft tissues including blood vessels and the kidney.

2 The correction of hypercalcemia can include multiple pharmacotherapeutic modalities such as hydration, diuretics, bisphosphonates, and steroids, depending on the etiology and acuity of the hypercalcemia.

3 Hypocalcemia is typically associated with an insidious onset; however, some drugs such as cinacalcet are associated with rapid decreases in serum calcium.

4 Acute treatment of hypocalcemia requires calcium supplementation whereas chronic management may require other therapies such as vitamin D to maintain serum calcium values.

5 Hyperphosphatemia occurs most frequently in patients with chronic kidney disease (CKD).

6 Treatment of nonemergent hyperphosphatemia includes the use of phosphate binders to decrease absorption of phosphorus from the GI tract.

7 Hypophosphatemia is a relatively common complication among critically ill patients.

8 Treatment of acute hypophosphatemia usually requires IV supplementation of phosphorous salts.

INTRODUCTION

Disorders of calcium and phosphorus are common complications of multiple acute and chronic diseases. These disorders are frequently seen in the acute care setting; however, they are also often present in ambulatory patients, usually in a less severe state. The consequences of electrolyte disorders can range from asymptomatic to life-threatening, requiring hospitalization and emergent treatment. The maintenance of fluid and electrolyte homeostasis requires adequate functioning and modulation by multiple hormones on tissues of multiple organ systems.

There are many common drug therapies that can disturb the normal homeostatic mechanisms that maintain calcium and phosphorous balance. In addition, with some drug therapies, toxicity is enhanced when underlying electrolyte disorders are present. Drug-induced disorders typically respond well to discontinuation of the offending agent(s); however, additional therapies are sometimes required to correct the disorder. This chapter reviews the etiology, classification, clinical presentation, and therapy for the most common disorders of calcium and phosphorus homeostasis.

DISORDERS OF CALCIUM HOMEOSTASIS

The maintenance of physiologic calcium concentrations in the intracellular and extracellular spaces is vital for the preservation and function of cell membranes; propagation of neuromuscular activity; regulation of endocrine and exocrine secretory functions; blood coagulation cascade; platelet adhesion process; bone metabolism; muscle cell excitation/contraction coupling; and mediation of the electrophysiologic slow-channel response in cardiac and smooth-muscle tissue.

The disorders of calcium homeostasis are related to the calcium content of the extracellular fluid (ECF), which is tightly regulated and comprises less than 0.5% of the total body stores of calcium. Skeletal bone contains more than 99% of total body stores of calcium.[1] ECF calcium is moderately bound to plasma proteins (46%), primarily albumin.[2] Ionized or free calcium is the physiologically active form and is the fraction that is homeostatically regulated.[3] Extracellular calcium, however, is most commonly measured as the total serum calcium level, which includes both bound and unbound calcium.[2] The normal total calcium serum concentration range is 8.5 to 10.5 mg/dL (2.13 to 2.63 mmol/L).[3]

Proper assessment of total serum calcium concentrations includes measurement of the patient's serum albumin concentration. Hypoalbuminemia, which can be associated with many chronic disease states, is probably the most common cause of "laboratory hypocalcemia." Patients remain asymptomatic because the unbound or ionized fraction of serum calcium remains normal (normal range, 4.4 to 5.4 mg/dL [1.10 to 1.35 mmol/L]). A corrected total serum calcium (S_{ca}) concentration can be calculated based on the measured total serum calcium and the difference between a patient's measured albumin concentration and the normative value of 4 g/dL (40 g/L) by the following equations:

$$\text{Corrected } S_{ca} \text{ (mg/dL)} = \text{Measured } S_{ca} \text{ (mg/dL)} + (0.8 \times [4 \text{ g/dL} - \text{measured albumin (g/dL)}])$$

or

$$\text{Corrected } S_{ca} \text{ (mmol/L)} = \text{Measured } S_{ca} \text{ (mmol/L)} + (0.02 \times [40 \text{ g/L} - \text{measured albumin (g/L)}])$$

The concentration of ionized calcium is closely regulated by the interactions of parathyroid hormone (PTH), phosphorus, vitamin D, and calcitonin (Fig. 35-1). PTH increases serum calcium concentrations by stimulating calcium release from bone, increasing renal tubular reabsorption, and enhancing absorption in the GI tract secondary to increased renal production of 1,25-dihydroxy vitamin D_3. Vitamin D directly increases serum calcium, as well

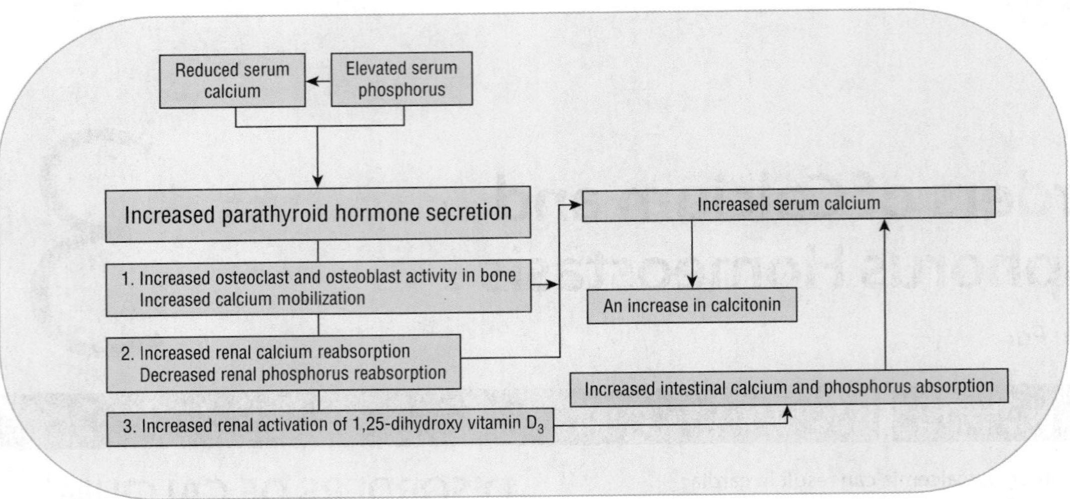

FIGURE 35-1 Homeostatic mechanisms to maintain serum calcium concentrations.

as phosphorus concentrations, by increasing GI absorption. Indirectly, it can also lead to calcium release from bone and reduced renal excretion. Calcitonin inhibits osteoclastic bone resorption. Its plasma concentrations are increased when ionized calcium concentrations are high as the body attempts to return the calcium level to the normal range. Disruption of these homeostatic mechanisms results in the clinical manifestations of hypercalcemia or hypocalcemia.

Alteration of the concentration of albumin or its binding of calcium can be expected to change the unbound fraction of total serum calcium. The most significant cause of changes in calcium binding to albumin is a change in ECF pH. In the presence of acute metabolic alkalosis the fraction of calcium bound to albumin is increased, thus reducing the plasma concentration of ionized calcium. This can result in symptomatic hypocalcemia; that is, paresthesia, muscle cramping and spasms, memory loss, and seizures.[1] Conversely, metabolic acidosis decreases calcium binding to albumin and results in increased ionized calcium. Hypoalbuminemic states are probably the most common cause of "laboratory hypocalcemia." When the albumin level is decreased, the ionized calcium concentration can be normal, although total serum calcium concentration is low. Each 1 g/dL (10 g/L) drop in the serum albumin concentration below 4 g/dL (40 g/L) will result in a decrease of total serum calcium concentration by 0.8 mg/dL (0.20 mmol/L).[1,2] This approach of calculating an albumin-adjusted calcium concentration has been found to overestimate the degree of hypercalcemia and usually fails to identify hypocalcemia in critically ill patients; therefore, ionized calcium values should be used to assess calcium status in these patients.[4,5]

HYPERCALCEMIA

There are multiple and diverse causes of hypercalcemia (total serum calcium >10.5 mg/dL [>2.62 mmol/L]) (Table 35-1). The most common causes of hypercalcemia are cancer and primary hyperparathyroidism.

Epidemiology and Etiology

The reported incidence of primary hyperparathyroidism in the United States ranges from 10 to 30 cases per 100,000 people.[6] Hypercalcemia of cancer occurs in approximately 20% to 40% of cancer patients at some time during the course of their disease.[7] Cancer-associated hypercalcemia is predominantly encountered in hospitalized patients, whereas primary hyperparathyroidism accounts for the vast majority of cases in the outpatient setting.[8,9]

Pathophysiology

Hypercalcemia is the result of one or a combination of three primary mechanisms: increased bone resorption, increased GI absorption, or increased tubular reabsorption by the kidneys (see Fig. 35-1).

Many tumors secrete PTH-related protein (PTHrP), which binds to the PTH receptors in bone and renal tissues, leading to increased bone resorption and renal tubular reabsorption.[11] Tumors can also secrete substances such as vitamin D, transforming growth factor, interleukins, prostaglandins, interferon, tumor

TABLE 35-1 Etiologies of Hypercalcemia

Neoplasms	**Medications**
Bone metastasis	Thiazides
Breast	Lithium
Multiple myeloma	Vitamin D
Lymphoma	Vitamin A
Leukemia	Calcium
Humoral induced	Aluminum/magnesium antacids
Ovary	Theophylline
Kidney	Tamoxifen
Pheochromocytoma	Ganciclovir
Multiple endocrine neoplasia	**Granulomatous disease**
Lung	Sarcoidosis
Head and neck	Tuberculosis
Esophagus	Cryptococcus
Cervix	Berylliosis
Lymphoproliferative disease	Histoplasmosis
Hyperparathyroidism	Coccidioidomycosis
Primary	Leprosy
Tertiary	**Endocrine disease**
Miscellaneous	Adrenal insufficiency
Immobilization	Hyperthyroidism
Paget's disease	Acromegaly
Familial hypocalciuric hypercalcemia	
Adolescence	
Rhabdomyolysis	

necrosis factor, and granulocyte-macrophage colony-stimulating factor, which are associated with the development of hypercalcemia.[7] Hypercalcemia of malignancy is a common complication of squamous cell carcinomas of the lung, head, and neck, hematologic malignancies such as multiple myeloma and T-cell lymphomas, and carcinomas of ovary, kidney, bladder, and breast. The most frequent types of malignancy associated with hypercalcemia are carcinomas of the lung and breast.[7] Breast and squamous cell lung carcinomas secrete PTHrP which binds to the type I PTH receptor (PTHR1) and enhances bone resorption.[10,11] In contrast, up to 40% of patients with multiple myeloma develop hypercalcemia principally as the result of osteoclast-mediated bone destruction.[7]

Primary hyperparathyroidism is the most common cause of chronic hypercalcemia in the general population. Benign parathyroid adenomas account for 80% to 85% of these cases of hyperparathyroidism, parathyroid hyperplasia accounts for 15%, and parathyroid carcinoma is the cause in less than 1% of cases.[9]

Other causes of chronic hypercalcemia include medications, endocrine and granulomatous disorders, physical immobilization, high bone-turnover states (adolescence and Paget's disease), and rhabdomyolysis. Increased GI absorption can be the result of excessive ingestion of vitamin D analogs, calcium supplements, and lithium. Lithium and vitamin A therapy can increase bone resorption, whereas increased renal tubular reabsorption of calcium can occur with thiazide and lithium therapy. The exact mechanism of lithium-induced hypercalcemia is not known but may include competitive inhibition of calcium influx into cells, increasing the threshold sensitivity of the calcium-sensing receptor (CaSr) and subsequent inhibition of PTH gene transcription.[8] Addison's disease, acromegaly, and thyrotoxicosis are endocrine disorders that can lead to hypercalcemia because of increased renal tubular reabsorption and increased bone resorption. Finally, the granulomatous disorders (sarcoidosis, tuberculosis, histoplasmosis, and leprosy) are associated with hypercalcemia caused by an increase in GI and renal tubular absorption secondary to granuloma production of 1,25-dihydroxy vitamin D_2.[12] Milk-alkali syndrome is the term applied to those situations where an individual develops hypercalcemia following the ingestion of calcium and absorbable alkali (e.g., calcium carbonate) and is an important cause of hypercalcemia in patients who are not on dialysis.[13,14]

Clinical Presentation

Patients with mild-to-moderate hypercalcemia, that is, total serum calcium concentrations above the upper threshold of normal but less than 13 mg/dL (<3.25 mmol/L) or ionized calcium concentrations less than 6 mg/dL (<1.50 mmol/L) can often be asymptomatic. This is typically the case for the vast majority of patients who have drug-induced hypercalcemia or primary hyperparathyroidism.[8,15,16] In fact, one study noted normocalcemia in approximately 20% of patients with a diagnosis of primary hyperparathyroidism, suggesting target tissue resistance to PTH.[16]

1 The presenting signs and symptoms of severe hypercalcemia that occur if the total serum calcium concentration is >13 mg/dL (>3.25 mmol/L) may differ depending on the acuity of onset.[2] Hypercalcemia of malignancy usually develops quickly and is accompanied by a classic symptom complex of anorexia, nausea and vomiting, constipation, polyuria, polydipsia, and nocturia.[15] Polyuria and nocturia secondary to a urinary-concentrating defect constitute some of the most frequent renal effects of hypercalcemia.[15] Hypercalcemic crisis is characterized by an acute elevation of total serum calcium to a value >15 mg/dL (>3.75 mmol/L), acute renal insufficiency, and obtundation (inability to arouse).[15] If untreated, hypercalcemic crisis can progress to oliguric renal failure, coma, and life-threatening ventricular arrhythmias.[15] The primary complications associated with chronic hypercalcemia (hyperparathyroidism) include metastatic calcification, hypercalciuria, and chronic renal insufficiency secondary to interstitial nephrocalcinosis.[15]

Calcium and/or calcium–phosphorus complex deposition in blood vessels and multiple organs is a complication of chronic hypercalcemia and/or concomitant hyperphosphatemia and hyperparathyroidism. Calcium deposits in atherosclerotic lesions contribute to cardiac disease.[17] Intracardiac and arterial calcifications have been found in patients with Paget's disease who have normal renal function. It is hypothesized that similar calcification processes occur in both bone and vascular tissue, leading to cardiovascular diseases including heart failure, systolic hypertension, and ischemic heart disease.[18]

The electrocardiographic changes associated with hypercalcemia include shortening of the QT interval and coving of the ST-T wave.[15] Very high serum calcium concentrations can cause T-wave widening, indicating a repolarization defect that may be associated

CLINICAL PRESENTATION Hypercalcemia

General

- The signs and symptoms of hypercalcemia depend on the severity and on the rapidity of onset

Symptoms

- Symptoms include fatigue, weakness, anorexia, depression, anxiety, cognitive dysfunction, vague abdominal pain, and constipation. Renal symptoms can include polyuria, polydipsia, and nocturia. Rarely, severe hypercalcemia leads to acute pancreatitis

Signs

- Renal: Nephrolithiasis; renal tubular dysfunction, particularly decreased concentrating ability; and acute and chronic renal insufficiency
- Cardiovascular: Hypercalcemia also directly shortens the myocardial action potential, which is reflected in a shortened QT interval and coving of the ST–T wave. Spontaneous ventricular tachyarrhythmias and elevations in blood pressure have also been reported. Chronic hypercalcemia can lead to cardiac calcification
- Musculoskeletal: Rheumatologic complaints related to hyperparathyroidism include gout, pseudogout, and chondrocalcinosis

Laboratory Tests

- Serum calcium concentrations of >10.5 mg/dL (>2.63 mmol/L) are considered to represent hypercalcemia. Patients with values up to 13 mg/dL (3.25 mmol/L) are generally considered to have mild or moderate hypercalcemia, whereas those with values greater than this indicate the presence of severe hypercalcemia with spontaneous ventricular tachyarrhythmias.[15] Hypertension and arrhythmias have occurred in the setting of hypercalcemia. The effects of digoxin on cardiac conduction including lowering of the excitation threshold, shortening of the effective refractory period, and increased atrioventricular refractoriness can be potentiated by hypercalcemia.[19]

Nephrolithiasis (kidney stones) and nephrocalcinosis (calcium deposits in the kidney) are the primary renal complications arising from long-standing hypercalcemia, as the result of primary hyperparathyroidism. Stone formation is dependent on a favorable milieu within the kidney or urinary tract, such as oversaturation of the urine and/or reduced concentrations of endogenous inhibitors of crystal formation (e.g., citrate or pyrophosphate). It is estimated that hyperparathyroidism accounts for 2% to 8% of all patients with calcium stones.[20,21] Of note, in those patients with low glomerular filtration rates (GFRs), the 24-hour urinary calcium will actually diminish secondary to decreased production of 1,25-dihydroxy vitamin D_2. However, the fractional excretion of calcium might increase.[21] Sarcoidosis is the other hypercalcemic condition frequently associated with calcium stones.[20] Other causes of nephrolithiasis with calcium-containing stones include hypocitraturia, renal tubular acidosis, hyperoxaluria, and hyperuricosuria.[22,23] Stone formers who have primary hyperparathyroidism are more likely to be female, older than 50 years of age, and have a family history of multiple endocrine disorders.[20] High dietary sodium intake can also raise urinary calcium concentrations, perhaps due to a reduction in calcium reabsorption in the kidney, thus predisposing patients to calcium stones. Although chronic renal failure can be the ultimate result of persistent stones, it is the primary cause of renal disease in <2% of the end-stage renal disease population.

TREATMENT

Desired Outcome

The indications for the treatment of acute hypercalcemia are dependent on the severity of hypercalcemia, acuity of its development, and presence or absence of symptoms requiring emergent treatment (e.g., necrotizing pancreatitis). The therapeutic intervention plan should be crafted to reverse signs and symptoms, restore normocalcemia, and correct or manage the underlying cause of hypercalcemia.

General Approach to Treatment

Chronic hypercalcemia is usually caused by an underlying medical condition or prescribed pharmacotherapies that can be resolved by successful treatment of the condition or withdrawal of the offending agent. Acute hypercalcemic episodes induced by malignancies may be mitigated by chemotherapy and/or radiation treatment. Effective surgical or drug treatment of primary hyperparathyroidism should reduce serum calcium concentrations as well as reduce the development of long-term complications such as vascular complications, chronic kidney disease (CKD), and kidney stones.

Nonpharmacologic Therapy

Hypercalcemic crisis and acute symptomatic severe hypercalcemia should be considered medical emergencies and treated immediately (Fig. 35-2).

These patients may require immediate-acting interventions to promptly reduce the serum calcium concentration if they are experiencing ECG changes, neurologic manifestations, or pancreatitis. Pharmacologic therapy consisting of volume expansion and enhancement of urinary calcium excretion with loop diuretics is usually the initial management strategy. Hemodialysis against a zero- or low-calcium dialysate solution should be considered for patients with severely impaired renal function (CKD stage 4 or 5) who cannot tolerate large fluid loads and in whom diuretics have limited efficacy.[22]

Effective treatment of moderate to severe hypercalcemia in the absence of life-threatening symptoms begins with attention to the underlying disorder and correction of associated fluid and electrolyte abnormalities. Patients with primary hyperparathyroidism may require surgery, particularly if they have systemic manifestations.

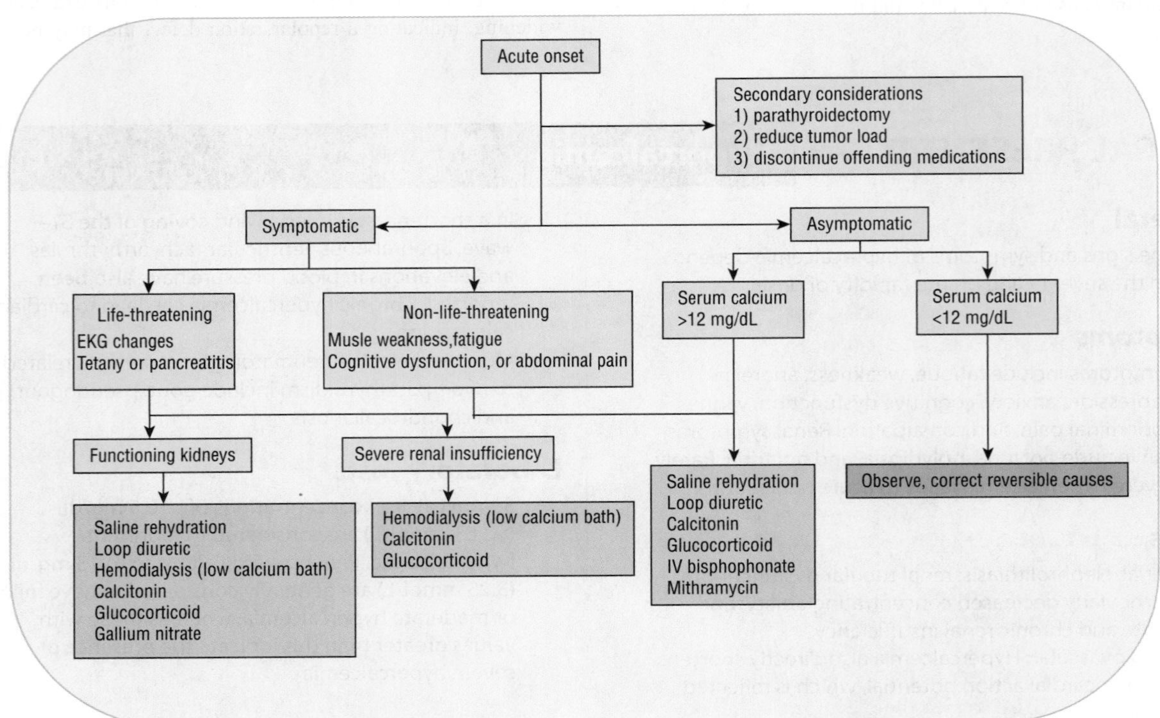

FIGURE 35-2 Pharmacotherapeutic options for the acutely hypercalcemic patient. Serum calcium of 12 mg/dL is equivalent to 3 mmol/L.

TABLE 35-2 Drug Dosing Table for Hypercalcemia

Drug/Brand Name	Starting Dosage	Time Frame to Initial Response	Special Population Considerations
0.9% saline ± electrolytes/NA	200–300 mL/h	24–48 hours	CI in renal insufficiency; congestive heart failure
Loop diuretics Furosemide/Lasix® Bumetandide/Bumex® Torsemide/Demadex®	40–80 mg IV q 1–4 h	N/A	CI in patients with allergy to sulfas (use ethacrynic acid)
Calcitonin/Miacalcin®	4 units/kg q 12 h SC/IM 10–12 units/h IV	1–2 hours	CI in patients with allergy to calcitonin
Pamidronate/Aredia®	30–90 mg IV over 2–24 hours	2 days	CI in renal insufficiency
Etidronate/Didronel®	7.5 mg/kg/day IV over 2 hours	2 days	CI in renal insufficiency
Zoledronate/Zometa®	4–8 mg IV over 15 minutes	1–2 days	CI in renal insufficiency
Ibandronate/Boniva®	2–6 mg IV bolus	2 days	CI in renal insufficiency
Gallium nitrate/Ganite®	200 mg/m²/day	?	CI in severe renal insufficiency
Mithramycin/Mithracin®	25 mcg/kg IV over 4–6 hours	12 hours	CI in decreased liver function; renal insufficiency; thrombocytopenia
Glucocorticoids	40–60 mg oral prednisone equivalents daily	3–5 days	CI in patients with serious infections; hypersensitivity

SC, subcutaneous; CI, contraindicated.

Clinical **Controversy...**

For patients with primary hyperparathyroidism, emerging data suggest that treatment with cinacalcet may be appropriate as a first-line intervention over parathyroidectomy.

Patients with malignancy often require surgical or chemotherapeutic reduction of tumor load to control the exogenous supply of cytokines and hormones (e.g., PTHrP) that cause hypercalcemia. In contrast, patients with drug-induced hypercalcemia generally respond to discontinuation of the offending agent.[23]

Pharmacologic Therapy

❷ For those patients with normal to moderately impaired renal function (CKD stages 3 and 4), the cornerstone of initial treatment of severe hypercalcemia or hypercalcemic crisis is volume expansion with normal saline to increase natriuresis and ultimately urinary calcium excretion (see Table 35-2). Patients with symptomatic hypercalcemia are often extracellular volume depleted secondary to vomiting and polyuria; thus rehydration with saline-containing fluids is necessary to interrupt the stimulus for sodium and calcium reabsorption in the renal tubule.[24] Rehydration can be accomplished by the infusion of normal saline at rates of 200 to 300 mL/h, until the patient is fluid resuscitated and serum calcium approaches the upper limit of the normal range. The precise rate depends on concomitant conditions (primarily cardiovascular and renal) and magnitude of hypercalcemia. The saline infusion rate can be decreased to a rate that approximates the patient's intake of oral or IV fluids. (see Chap. 34 for a thorough discussion of how to calculate water deficit.) Adequacy of hydration is assessed by measuring fluid intake and output or by central venous pressure monitoring.[9] Loop diuretics such as furosemide (40 to 80 mg IV every 1 to 4 hours) or ethacrynic acid (for patients with sulfa allergies) can also be instituted to increase urinary calcium excretion and to minimize the development of volume overload from the administration of saline[9] (Fig. 35-2 and Table 35-2). Loop diuretics such as furosemide block calcium (and sodium) reabsorption in the thick ascending limb of the loop of Henle and augment the calciuric effect of saline alone. The importance of rehydration prior to loop diuretic use is critical because if dehydration persists or becomes worse, the serum calcium can actually increase because of enhanced proximal tubule calcium reabsorption.[2] Potassium chloride, 10 to 20 mEq/L (10 to 20 mmol/L), should be added to the saline solution after rehydration is accomplished to maintain normokalemia in the presence of diuretic therapy. Serum magnesium levels should also be monitored, and magnesium replacement instituted if magnesium levels fall below 1.8 mg/dL (0.74 mmol/L) (Table 35-3). Rehydration with saline and administration of furosemide can result in a decrease of 2 to 3 mg/dL (0.50 to 0.75 mmol/L) in total serum calcium within 24 to 48 hours.[9]

Alternative Drug Treatments

Calcitonin

In those patients in whom saline hydration therapy is contraindicated (e.g., those with severe chronic heart failure [CHF] or moderate-to-severe renal dysfunction), short-term therapy with calcitonin is a viable alternative agent to initiate reduction of serum calcium levels within 24 to 48 hours. Calcitonin has a rapid onset of action (within 1 to 2 hours); however, the degree and extent of serum calcium level reduction are often unpredictable.[2]

Subcutaneous administration of salmon calcitonin, 50 to 100 international units daily or three times weekly, has been used to manage mild hypercalcemia in patients with Paget's disease.[25]

TABLE 35-3 Hypercalcemia Drug Monitoring Table

Drug	Adverse Effects
0.9% saline ± electrolytes	Electrolyte abnormalities; fluid overload
Loop diuretics	Electrolyte abnormalities
Calcitonin	Facial flushing, nausea/vomiting, allergic reaction
Pamidronate	Fever
Etidronate	Fever
Zoledronate	Fever, fatigue, skeletal pain
Ibandronate	Fever, musculoskeletal pain
Gallium nitrate	Nephrotoxicity; hypophosphatemia; nausea/vomiting/diarrhea; metallic taste
Mithramycin	Nausea/vomiting; stomatitis; thrombocytopenia; nephrotoxicity; hepatotoxicity
Glucocorticoids	Diabetes; osteoporosis; infection

TABLE 35-4 Treatment of Nephrolithiasis Associated with Chronic Hypercalcemia and Hypercalciuria

Intervention	Indications	Comments
Extracorporeal Shock Wave Lithotripsy		
Uses sound waves to break up stones, which then can pass spontaneously	Obstruction of the urinary tract, especially with stones >5 mm	Consider adjunctive use of potassium citrate to inhibit aggregation of residual fragments
Prevention of Stone Formation		
Alkalinizing agents	Treatment for nonemergent active stones. Can also be used for prevention	Potassium citrate preferred over sodium citrate as it decreases urinary calcium, inhibits calcium oxalate precipitation, and increases urinary citrate more
Potassium citrate PO 20 mEq twice daily		
Sodium citrate PO 20–30 mEq twice daily		
Decrease Urinary Calcium Excretion		
Thiazide diuretics	Prevention	Drug of choice in patients with low bone density
Hydrochlorothiazide (Hydrodiuril®) PO 50 mg every day		
Indapamide (Lozol®) PO 25 mg every day		
Chlorthalidone (Hygroton®) PO 25 mg every day		
Binding Intestinal Calcium		
Cellulose sodium phosphate (Calcibind)	Prevention for those with absorptive hypercalciuria	Alternative to thiazides if intolerant or ineffective, monitor bone density
Calcium binding ion-exchange resin that decreases GI absorption of calcium: PO 5 g twice daily with oxalate restriction		
Inhibition of Crystal Formation		
Phyllanthus niruri plant extract	Prevention, after shock wave lithotripsy	Commercial preparations with *P. niruri* as the sole ingredient can be difficult to obtain
Inhibits calcium oxalate stone formation by incorporating glycosaminoglycans into the calculi: PO 2 g daily		
Low-Calcium Diet		
Less than 400 mg/day	Prevention	Monitor bone density prior to and periodically during treatment, limit oxalate restriction, can increase hyperoxaluria, data suggest that high calcium intake may actually be more beneficial

The intranasal formulation of calcitonin has been used in doses of 200 to 400 international units daily; unfortunately, this has resulted in only mild decreases in serum calcium. The lack of significant efficacy of the synthetic intranasal formulation is the result of the lower potency and shorter duration of action as compared to salmon calcitonin. Patients who develop nephrolithiasis from hypercalciuria are most often treated with sodium citrate to prevent stone formation, thiazide diuretics to decrease urinary calcium excretion, or shock wave lithotripsy (Table 35-4).

Pharmacology Calcitonin decreases serum calcium concentrations, primarily by inhibiting bone resorption. It can also reduce renal tubular reabsorption of calcium, thus promoting calciuresis.[26] Recently, the calcitonin receptor has been shown to play an important role in calcium homeostasis, particularly in states of calcium stress (e.g., vitamin D toxicity).[26] Calcitonin from salmon sources is most commonly administered subcutaneously or intramuscularly (for larger volumes) in a starting dose of 4 units/kg every 12 hours.

Adverse Effects The side effects from IV administered calcitonin (facial flushing, nausea, and vomiting) limit patient acceptability. Allergic reactions, although rare, do occur; therefore, a test dose (intradermal injection of 0.1 mL of a 10 units/mL solution) is recommended prior to starting therapy. If marked erythema and/or wheal formation does not occur within 15 minutes after administration, therapy can begin. Salmon calcitonin therapy is associated with tachyphylaxis caused by antibody formation to foreign proteins or molecules resembling the calcitonin polypeptide.[26] Tachyphylaxis has been primarily documented in patients receiving therapy for more than 4 months and thus might not be clinically significant in the acute care setting. The addition of corticosteroid therapy or conversion to human calcitonin increases effectiveness.[2]

Bisphosphonates

Bisphosphonates block bone resorption very efficiently, render the hydroxyapatite crystal of bone mineral resistant to hydrolysis by phosphatases, and also inhibit osteoclast precursors from attaching to the mineralized matrix, thus blocking their transformation into mature functioning osteoclasts.[15,27] The antiresorptive properties of this class of agents can provide long-term control of serum calcium and are the first-line therapy for cancer-associated hypercalcemia.

Pharmacology and Dosing Pamidronate is very effective in controlling hypercalcemia associated with malignancy and slightly more effective than etidronate.[7] The usual dose of pamidronate is 30 to 90 mg as an IV infusion given over 2 to 24 hours. Pamidronate also has the advantage of single-day therapy.[9] Etidronate, when administered in doses of 7.5 mg/kg per day by slow IV infusion over at least 2 hours for 3 days, is effective in the therapy of hypercalcemia of malignancy.[9] Zoledronate and ibandronate are newer, high-potency bisphosphonates with demonstrated effectiveness in the treatment of hypercalcemia of malignancy. Complete response has been reported in 88.4% to 86.7% of zoledronate- versus 69.7% of pamidronate-treated patients.[28,29] Zoledronate IV doses of 4 to 8 mg given over 5 minutes have resulted in normalization of serum calcium concentrations.[29] IV infusions of 0.02 or 0.04 mg/kg diluted in 5% dextrose (given over 20 to 50 minutes) have also been effective.[30] A similar hypocalcemic response has been noted with ibandronate in comparison with pamidronate (76.5% vs. 75.8%); however, the time period to a relapse of hypercalcemia was longer with ibandronate (14 vs. 4 days), suggesting a therapeutic advantage for ibandronate.[31] In contrast to other bisphosphonates, ibandronate can be administered by bolus injection. Single doses of 4 to 6 mg when administered every 3 to 4 weeks have been effective in managing hypercalcemia of malignancy.[32] The onset of serum calcium concentration decline is slower with bisphosphonate therapy (concentrations begin to decline in 2 days and reach a nadir in 7 days); thus calcitonin therapy can be necessary if rapid serum level reduction is required.[9,32] Duration of normocalcemia varies, but usually does not exceed 2 to 3 weeks. It appears to be dependent on the severity and treatment response of the underlying malignancy.[2] The duration of response has been suggested to be longer with zoledronate (4 to 5 weeks), although the data are sparse.[30]

Adverse Effects Fever is a common side effect of IV bisphosphonate therapy. Although oral bisphosphonates are useful for the treatment of bone turnover in Paget's disease, there are insufficient data to suggest their use for the initial treatment of hypercalcemia. The use of oral bisphosphonates for maintenance therapy in patients predisposed to hypercalcemia (malignancy) has been successful in some cases.[33] The safety of continuous bisphosphonate therapy in patients with moderate-to-severe renal insufficiency is currently unknown. Renal function monitoring (serum creatinine) is advised with the use of bisphosphonates, as cases of acute tubular necrosis have been reported.[34,35] Although there are no published guidelines for frequency of serum creatinine monitoring, it is advisable to evaluate serum creatinine within a week after the infusion and just prior to the next scheduled dose.

Denosumab

Denosumab is a monoclonal antibody that inhibits the receptor activator of nuclear factor kappa-light-chain-enhancer of activated B cells (NF-κB) ligand (RANKL), a principal mediator of osteoclast survival. Denosumab is FDA approved for the treatment of osteoporosis.

Denosumab has been investigated in patients with malignancies and bone metastases (without hypocalcemia) who were either bisphosphonate naïve or who had previous exposure to bisphosphonates. Patients were randomized to receive an IV bisphosphonate every 4 weeks (91% received zoledronic acid) or a fixed dose of denosumab every 4 weeks (30, 120, and 180 mg) or every 12 weeks (60 and 180 mg) to investigate the effect on the primary outcome measure of urinary-*N*-telopeptide, a marker for bone turnover. Patients who were bisphosphonate naïve had similar decline in markers of bone turnover. In patients with previous exposure to bisphosphonates, treatment with denosumab produced significantly greater reductions in bone turnover compared with an IV bisphosphonate.[36] A recent clinical trial in breast cancer patients that were randomized to subcutaneous denosumab 120 mg or IV zolendronic acid 4 mg and placebo every 4 weeks showed that denosumab therapy prolonged time to first skeletal-related event or hypercalcemia by 18%.[37] These data indicate utility of denosumab in hypercalcemia of malignancy, particularly in patients who do not have an optimal response to bisphosphonates.[38] Denosumab has also been reported to successfully treat hypercalcemia after successful stem cell transplantation and restitution of osteoclast function in patients with osteopetrosis, a heritable disorder associated with defective osteoclast function.[39]

Gallium Nitrate

Gallium nitrate is indicated for the treatment of symptomatic hypercalcemia of malignancy not responsive to hydration therapy.[40] However, because of its adverse side-effect profile, it is generally reserved for those who fail to respond to less toxic agents. Gallium nitrate inhibits bone resorption, and may be superior to calcitonin in inducing normocalcemia. The initial dose is usually a continuous IV infusion of 200 mg/m^2 per day for five consecutive days. Gallium nitrate can be more effective in achieving normocalcemia in patients with epidermoid (squamous) cancers.[41] Because gallium nitrate is nephrotoxic, the initial dose should be conservative and the patient's renal function should be closely monitored.

Mithramycin

Mithramycin (plicamycin) is a potent cytotoxic antibiotic that inhibits osteoclast-mediated bone resorption and thereby reduces hypercalcemia. Mithramycin can be administered via IV infusion (25 mcg/kg) over 4 to 6 hours in saline or 5% dextrose solutions. This therapy can be repeated daily for 3 to 4 days or on alternating days for three to eight doses.[9,42] Serum calcium levels begin to fall within 12 hours of a mithramycin dose, with the peak effect generally occurring over 48 to 96 hours.[2,9] Common dose-related adverse effects of mithramycin include nausea, vomiting, stomatitis, thrombocytopenia, inhibition of platelet function, and renal and hepatotoxicity.

Corticosteroids

Prednisone or an equivalent agent is usually effective in the treatment of hypercalcemia resulting from multiple myeloma, leukemia, lymphoma, sarcoidosis, and hypervitaminoses A and D.[2,27,42] These agents are effective because they reduce GI calcium absorption.[42] Corticosteroids may also prevent tachyphylaxis to salmon calcitonin.[26] Daily doses of 40 to 60 mg of prednisone or the equivalent are effective at reducing serum calcium within 3 to 5 days followed by a reduction in urinary calcium excretion within 7 to 10 days. The disadvantages of corticosteroid therapy are its relatively slow onset of action and the potential for diabetes mellitus, osteoporosis, and increased susceptibility to infection.[43]

Cinacalcet

The calcimimetic agent cinacalcet HCl is approved for management of parathyroid carcinoma.[44,45] It binds to the CaSr, and increases the sensitivity for receptor activation by extracellular calcium. This results in reduced PTH and serum calcium concentrations.[44,45] Cinacalcet HCl administered at a starting dose of 30 mg orally twice daily has been used for the treatment of hypercalcemia secondary to parathyroid carcinoma. The dosage is titrated every 2 to 4 weeks in 30-mg increments until the desired serum calcium level is achieved. The maximum approved dosage is 90 mg three to four times daily. Patients should have serum calcium measured within 1 week after starting or increasing the dose of this agent.[46]

HYPOCALCEMIA

3 Hypocalcemia occurs infrequently in the outpatient setting and is most common in elderly, malnourished patients and those who have received sodium phosphate as a bowel preparation agent.

Incidence

The incidence of hypocalcemia in intensive care unit patients ranges from 70% to 90% based on total serum calcium values less than 8.5 mg/dL (<2.13 mmol/L) to 15% to 50% based on the observation of ionized calcium concentrations less than 4.4 mg/dL

(<1.10 mmol/L).[3] Emergent treatment of hypocalcemia is rarely warranted unless life-threatening symptoms are present (e.g., frank tetany or seizures).

Pathophysiology

Hypocalcemia is the result of alterations in the effect of PTH and vitamin D on the bone, gut, and kidney (see Fig. 35-1). The primary causes of hypocalcemia are postoperative hypoparathyroidism and vitamin D deficiency. Other causes include magnesium deficiency, thyroid surgery, medications, hypoalbuminemia, blood transfusions, peripheral blood progenitor cell harvesting, tumor lysis syndrome, and mutations in the CaSr.[47–52] PTH concentrations are elevated in conditions of hypocalcemia, with the exception of hypoparathyroidism and hypomagnesemia.[53]

Vitamin D Deficiency

Vitamin D and its metabolites play an important role in the maintenance of extracellular calcium concentrations and in normal skeletal structure and mineralization. Vitamin D is necessary for the optimal absorption of calcium and phosphorus. On a worldwide basis, the most common cause of chronic hypocalcemia is nutritional vitamin D deficiency. In malnourished populations, manifestations include rickets and osteomalacia. Nutritional vitamin D deficiency is uncommon in Western societies because of the fortification of milk with ergocalciferol. The most common cause of vitamin D deficiency in Western societies is GI disease.[15] Gastric surgery, chronic pancreatitis, small-bowel disease, intestinal resection, and bypass surgery are associated with decreased concentrations of vitamin D and its metabolites.[15] Vitamin D replacement therapy might need to be administered by the IV route if poor oral bioavailability is noted. Decreased production of 1,25-dihydroxyvitamin D_3 can occur as a result of a hereditary defect resulting in vitamin D-dependent rickets.[53] Recently, polymorphisms of the vitamin D receptor have been identified, and these genetic variations can contribute to increased risk of rickets associated with vitamin D and calcium deficient diets, especially in certain African and East Asian populations.[54] It also can occur secondary to CKD if there is insufficient production of the 1-α-hydroxylase enzyme for the production of the most active metabolite, 1,25-dihydroxy vitamin D_3. Treatment of hypocalcemia associated with CKD is reviewed in Chapter 29.

Hypomagnesemia

Hypomagnesemia of any cause can be associated with severe symptomatic hypocalcemia that is unresponsive to calcium replacement therapy (see Chap. 36). Reduced serum magnesium concentrations can impair PTH secretion and induce resistance of target organs to the actions of PTH.[15] Normalization of serum calcium concentrations in these patients is thus dependent on appropriate replacement of magnesium.

Hungry Bone Syndrome

An acute, symptomatic rapid fall in total serum calcium concentration (to values <7 mg/dL [<1.75 mmol/L]) is common in patients who have recently had a parathyroidectomy or thyroidectomy. Hypocalcemia in these postsurgical patients is generally transient in nature.[53] The "hungry bone syndrome" is a condition of profound hypocalcemia whereby the bone avidly incorporates calcium and phosphorus from the blood in an attempt to recalcify bone.[55] Serum calcium concentrations should be monitored every 6 hours during the 24 to 48 hours following such surgeries, and pharmacologic doses of calcium can be necessary to prevent or minimize the drop in serum calcium. Additionally, mild-to-moderate hypocalcemia can be a long-term consequence of parathyroidectomy in hemodialysis patients.[53]

Drug-Induced Hypocalcemia

Drug-induced hypocalcemia has been reported in patients receiving furosemide, calcitonin, bisphosphonates, gallium nitrate, mithramycin, cinacalcet, fluoride, ketoconazole, and pentamidine.[46,56]

Clinical **Controversy. . .**

Some data have shown that animal source vitamin D_3 (cholecalciferol) is more efficacious at raising serum 25(OH) D concentrations compared with plant source vitamin D_2 (ergocalciferol).

Oral phosphorus therapy, commonly used to treat patients with malabsorption syndromes caused by GI diseases, can also result in hypocalcemia. The anticonvulsants phenobarbital and phenytoin cause hypocalcemia by increasing catabolism of vitamin D and thereby impairing calcium release from bone and reducing intestinal calcium absorption.[47] Drugs that cause hypomagnesemia (aminoglycosides, amphotericin B, cyclosporine, diuretics, foscarnet, and cisplatin) are also associated with an increased risk of hypocalcemia. Chelating agents in blood (citrate) and in radiographic contrast media (ethylenediaminetetraacetate) can also cause transient hypocalcemia.[47,48,57] Concentrated citrate is increasingly being used in hemodialysis catheter locks and to anticoagulate the dialysis circuit during continuous renal replacement therapy. Symptomatic hypocalcemia (ionized calcium <2.4 mg/dL [<0.60 mmol/L]) has been reported in patients exposed to citrate solutions, which appears to be related to the concentration of the citrate solution.[58] Injection of citrate solutions greater than the volume of the dead space of the catheter lumen or accidental injection of citrate catheter lock solutions that are not intended for systemic administration have been associated with serious cardiovascular problems such as hypotension or cardiac arrest.[59]

Hypoparathyroidism

Hypoparathyroidism can be caused by autoimmune disease, congenital defects, or iatrogenically by inadvertent removal during thyroidectomy or from damage with radiation therapy. Chronic hypothyroidism produces an insidious development of hypocalcemia and thus most patients remain asympotomatic. The chronic hypocalcemia may ultimately present as visual impairment secondary to cataracts.[60]

Clinical Presentation

The clinical manifestations of hypocalcemia are quite variable. The more acute the drop in ionized calcium concentration, the more likely the patient will develop symptoms.[51] Increases in plasma pH enhance the binding of calcium to albumin and thus alkalosis can result in rapid decreases in ionized calcium. Concomitant hypomagnesemia, hypokalemia, hyponatremia, and additive side effects from prescribed medications also increase the likelihood of symptomatic presentation.

Hypocalcemia can manifest as neuromuscular, CNS, dermatologic, and cardiac sequelae.[15] Acute hypocalcemia is more likely to manifest as neuromuscular (paresthesia, muscle cramps, tetany, and laryngeal spasm) and cardiovascular symptoms, whereas chronic hypocalcemia often presents as CNS (e.g., depression, anxiety, memory loss, confusion, hallucinations, and tonic–clonic seizures) and dermatologic symptoms (hair loss, grooved and brittle nails, and eczema).[47] The hallmark sign of acute hypocalcemia is tetany caused by enhanced peripheral neuromuscular irritability.[15] Tetany manifests as paresthesia around the mouth and in the extremities,

CLINICAL PRESENTATION Hypocalcemia

General

- Acute hypocalcemia may result in rapid decreases in serum ionized calcium. Parathyroidectomy and thyroidectomy are also associated with a rapid reduction in serum calcium. In chronic hypocalcemia vitamin D deficiency should be considered

Symptoms

- The symptoms of hypocalcemia include tetany, paresthesia, muscle cramps, and laryngeal spasms. Chronic hypocalcemia is usually associated with depression, anxiety, memory loss, and confusion

Signs

- Neurologic: The hallmark of acute hypocalcemia is tetany, which is characterized by neuromuscular irritability including seizure potential. Extrapyramidal disorders, mainly parkinsonism but also dystonia, hemiballismus, choreoathetosis, and oculogyric crises occur in 5% to 10% of patients with idiopathic hypoparathyroidism. Chvostek's and/or Trousseau's signs can be elicited during physical examination
- Dermatologic: The skin can be dry, puffy, and coarse. Other dermatologic manifestations can include hyperpigmentation, dermatitis, eczema, and psoriasis. Hair and skin signs including coarse, brittle, and sparse hair with patchy alopecia and brittle nails can also appear
- Ophthalmologic: Cataract development has been reported to occur with hypocalcemia
- Dental manifestations: These are usually associated with the presence of chronic hypocalcemia in early development. Signs include dental hypoplasia, failure of tooth eruption, defective enamel and root formation, and abraded carious teeth
- Cardiovascular: Hypotension, decreased myocardial performance, and CHF have been reported. A prolonged QT interval, arrhythmias, and bradycardia can also occur but are more common with acute or very severe hypocalcemia
- GI: Steatorrhea can be associated with chronic hypocalcemia
- Musculoskeletal: Myopathy has been reported
- Endocrine: Hypocalcemia alone can impair insulin release. In addition, idiopathic hypoparathyroidism can be associated with polyglandular autoimmune syndromes

Laboratory Tests

- Serum calcium levels of less than 8.5 mg/dL (<2.13 mmol/L) are considered to represent hypocalcemia if ionized calcium values are also less than 4.4 mg/dL (<1.1 mmol/L)

muscle spasms and cramps, carpopedal (hands and feet) spasms, and rarely as laryngospasm and bronchospasm.[15] Chvostek's and/or Trousseau's signs can be elicited during physical examination.[47] Chvostek's sign is elicited by tapping the facial nerve anterior to the ear and eliciting twitching of facial muscles. Trousseau's sign is elicited by inflating a blood pressure cuff above systolic blood pressure for 3 minutes and observing whether a carpal spasm is induced.

The cardiovascular manifestations of hypocalcemia result in electrocardiographic changes characterized by a prolonged QT interval and symptoms of decreased myocardial contractility often associated with congestive heart failure (CHF).[47] Both acute and chronic hypocalcemia can result in a reversible syndrome characterized by acute myocardial failure or refractory CHF. Other cardiovascular manifestations include arrhythmias, bradycardia, and hypotension that are unresponsive to fluid and pressor administration.[47]

TREATMENT

Desired Outcome

❹ The goals of therapy for patients with normal renal function are the resolution of signs and symptoms of hypocalcemia, restoration of normocalcemia, management of associated electrolyte abnormalities, and treatment of the underlying cause of hypocalcemia. The goals for patients with CKD are different and are discussed in detail in Chapter 29. Asymptomatic hypocalcemia associated with hypoalbuminemia requires no treatment because ionized (physiologically active) plasma calcium concentrations are normal. Treatment of hypocalcemia is dependent on identification of the pathogenesis of the underlying disorder, acuteness of onset, and presence and severity of symptoms. Acute symptomatic hypocalcemia requires parenteral administration of soluble calcium salts (Fig. 35-3).

Pharmacologic Therapy

Acute Treatment

The initial therapeutic intervention for patients with acute symptomatic hypocalcemia is to administer 100 to 300 mg of elemental calcium IV over 5 to 10 minutes.[61] This can be accomplished by the administration of 1 g of calcium chloride (27% elemental calcium) or 2 to 3 g of calcium gluconate (9% elemental calcium). Calcium gluconate is generally preferred over calcium chloride for peripheral venous administration because calcium gluconate is less irritating to veins. The use of calcium gluconate provides a less predictable and slightly smaller increase in plasma ionic calcium compared with calcium chloride. Calcium should not be infused at a rate greater than 60 mg of elemental calcium per minute because severe cardiac dysfunction, including ventricular fibrillation, can result.[61] IV calcium administration should be used with caution in patients receiving digitalis glycosides because of the possibility of bradycardia or atrioventricular (A–V) block.[3] The bolus dose of calcium is only effective for 1 to 2 hours and should be followed by a continuous infusion of elemental calcium at a rate of 0.5 to 2 mg/kg per hour.[3] The calcium concentrations should be monitored every 4 to 6 hours during the IV infusions. The ionized calcium concentration usually normalizes within 4 hours, and the maintenance infusion rate of elemental calcium can then be decreased to 0.3 to 0.5 mg/kg per hour to maintain the desired calcium concentration.[1] Calcium should not

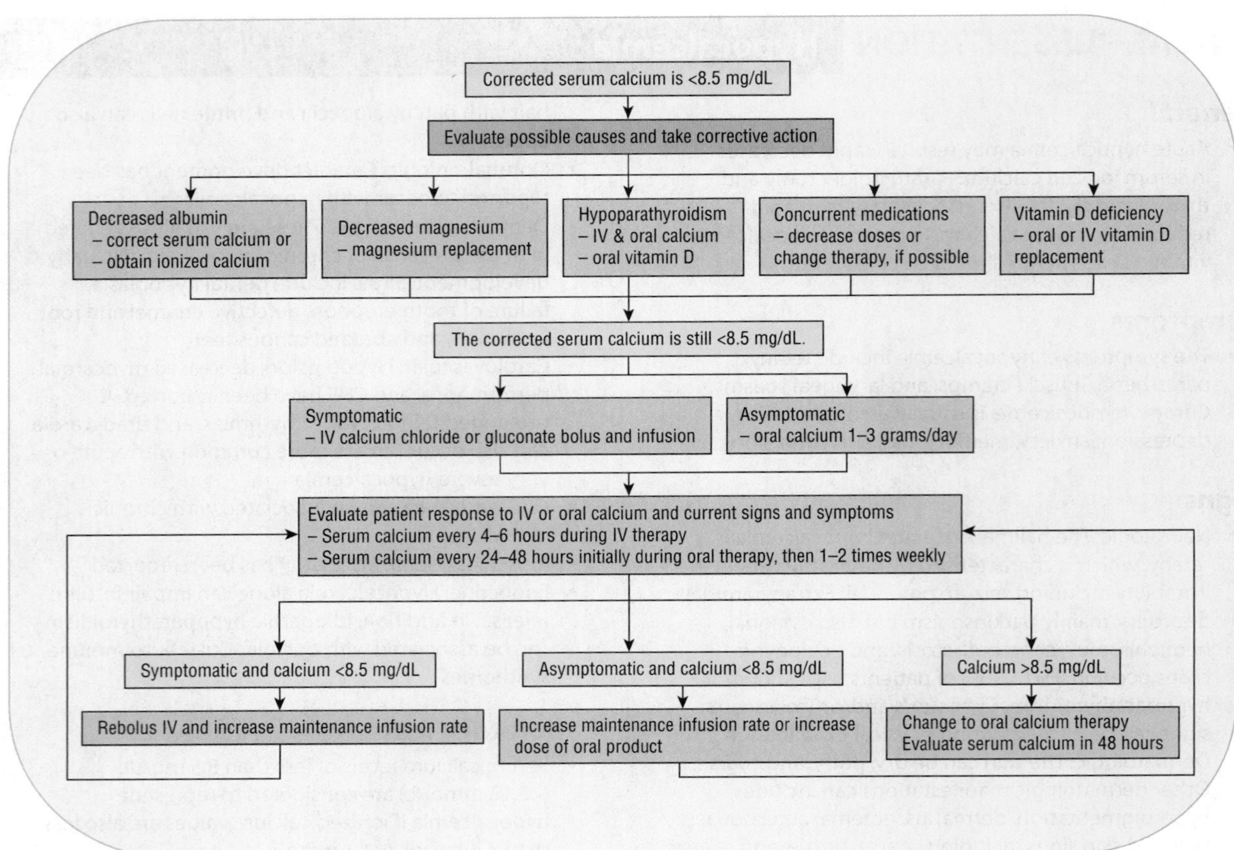

FIGURE 35-3 Hypocalcemia diagnostic and treatment algorithm. Serum calcium of 8.5 mg/dL is equivalent to 2.13 mmol/L.

be added to bicarbonate- or phosphate-containing solutions because of the possibility of precipitation.

Chronic Treatment

Once acute hypocalcemia is corrected by parenteral administration, further treatment modalities should be individualized according to the cause of hypocalcemia. If hypomagnesemia is present, magnesium supplementation is indicated (see Chap. 36). Hypocalcemia secondary to hungry bone syndrome following parathyroidectomy has been attenuated by pretreatment with bisphosphonates.[62] Asymptomatic and chronic hypocalcemia associated with hypoparathyroidism and vitamin D-deficient states can be managed by oral calcium and vitamin D supplementation (see Chap. 29). Therapy is begun with 1 to 3 g/day of elemental calcium.[1] Average maintenance doses range from 2 to 8 g of elemental calcium per day in divided doses. If serum calcium does not normalize, a vitamin D preparation may need to be added.

Personalized Pharmacotherapy

Treatment of hypocalcemia associated with vitamin D-deficient states should be individualized. In patients with malabsorption, vitamin D requirements vary markedly, and large doses can be required. In contrast, vitamin D deficiency associated with anticonvulsant medication can be corrected with smaller doses of vitamin D. Oral doses of 1,25-dihydroxy vitamin D_3 usually range from 0.5 to 3 mcg daily. The usual initial oral dose of ergocalciferol is 50,000 international units daily.[61] Vitamin D doses are usually adjusted approximately every 4 weeks. Vitamin D deficiency is highly prevalent especially in areas of low sun exposure and limited dietary sources of vitamin D.[63] New data suggest that current dietary recommendations are not sufficient to maintain 25-hydroxy vitamin D_3 concentrations at or above 32 mcg/L (80 nmol/L).[63] The treatment of vitamin D deficiency associated with CKD generally requires the administration of 1,25-dihydroxy vitamin D_3 or another synthetic vitamin D_2 analog such as paricalcitol or doxercalciferol. Patients who have reduced 25-hydroxylase activity (e.g., hepatic disease) can also require treatment with calcitriol (1,25-dihydroxy vitamin D_3). The newer vitamin D_2 analogs (paricalcitol and doxercalciferol) were developed to preferentially suppress PTH secretion with less effect on serum calcium concentration and thus their efficacy for the management of hypocalcemia may be minimal. In selected cases, increasing calcium ingestion can be required if vitamin D replacement alone is ineffective in returning calcium concentrations to normal.

Clinical **Controversy. . .**

Several single nucleotide polymorphisms have been identified in the CaSr gene. The effect of these polymorphisms on the pharmacodynamic profile and the risk of hypocalcemia associated with cinacalcet and other calcimimetics remains to be elucidated.

Adverse Effects

Adverse effects of oral calcium and vitamin D supplementation include hypercalcemia and hypercalciuria, especially in the hypoparathyroid patient, in whom the renal calcium-sparing effect of PTH is absent. Hypercalciuria can increase the risk of calcium stone formation and nephrolithiasis in susceptible patients. One maneuver to help prevent calcium stones is to maintain the urine calcium excretion below 300 mg per day. Intermittently monitoring 24-hour urine collections for total calcium excretion can help to minimize the occurrence of hypercalciuria. The addition of thiazide diuretics for patients at risk for stone formation can result in an increase in tubular calcium reabsorption and reduction of vitamin D requirements.[61]

DISORDERS OF PHOSPHORUS HOMEOSTASIS

Inorganic phosphorus in the form of phosphate is an essential element in phospholipid cell membranes, nucleic acids, and phosphoproteins, which are required for mitochondrial function.[64] Phosphorus regulates the intermediary metabolism of carbohydrates, fats, and proteins. Phosphorus also regulates enzymatic reactions including glycolysis, ammoniagenesis, and the 1-hydroxylation of 25-hydroxyvitamin D_3.[64] In addition, phosphorus is required for the generation of 2,3-diphosphoglycerate (2,3-DPG) in red blood cells, which is required for normal oxygen–hemoglobin dissociation and delivery of oxygen to the tissues.[65] Phosphorus is the source of the high-energy bonds of adenosine triphosphate (ATP), thus fueling a wide variety of physiologic processes, including muscle contractility, electrolyte transport, neurologic function, and other important biochemical reactions.[64] Considering its diverse biologic importance, it is not difficult to appreciate the clinical implications of disorders of phosphorus homeostasis.

Phosphate, the major intracellular anion, is present in living organisms mainly as organic phosphate esters such as 2,3-DPG, adenosine, guanosine triphosphate, and fructose 1,6-diphosphate.[64] Only a small fraction of intracellular phosphorus exists as inorganic phosphate; however, this fraction is critical because it is the source from which ATP is resynthesized.[64] The majority of inorganic phosphate is located in the extracellular space where it is the prime determinant of intracellular phosphate; thus, small increments in the organic phosphate levels can profoundly alter both the extracellular and intracellular phosphate levels. Metabolic disturbances (acidosis, alkalosis, and ketoacidosis), hydrogen ion shifts, and hormones (PTH, calcitonin, cortisol, and vitamin D) all can cause transcellular shifts in phosphorus concentrations. Because of these phenomena, the serum phosphorus level does not accurately reflect total body stores.[65]

The typical Western diet provides a daily intake of 800 to 1,600 mg of phosphorus. Approximately 60% to 80% of this is absorbed in the GI tract by passive and active transport (vitamin D mediated). PTH, 1,25-dihydroxy vitamin D_3, and low-phosphate diets mediate increased absorption. Decreased absorption occurs under conditions of increased dietary intake of phosphorus and magnesium, glucocorticoid therapy, and hypothyroidism. The normal serum phosphorus concentration in adults is 2.5 to 4.5 mg/dL (0.81 to 1.45 mmol/L) and for children younger than 12 years old it is 4 to 5.6 mg/dL (1.29 to 1.81 mmol/L). Influx via the GI tract and bone and tubular reabsorption by the kidney are the most important regulators of steady-state serum phosphorus concentrations. Renal excretion of phosphorus is a two-step process: glomerular filtration and proximal tubular reabsorption by passive transport coupled to sodium. Under normal conditions, 85% to 90% of filtered phosphate is reabsorbed, the majority in the early proximal tubule. Renal tubular reabsorption of phosphate is inhibited by PTH and 1,25-dihydroxy vitamin D_3.[64] There are increasing data in the literature that indicate fibroblast growth factor 23 (FGF23) is a key regulator of phosphate homeostasis.[66,67] FGF23 acts principally to decrease tubular reabsorption of phosphate and inhibit 1-α-hydroxylase, thereby reducing the concentration of active vitamin D. FGF23-mediated receptor activation requires klotho, a transmembrane protein. The tissue specificity for FGF23 effects appears to be defined by klotho–FGF23 coexpression. Conversely, phosphate reabsorption in the renal tubule is increased by growth hormone, insulin, and insulin-like growth factor 1.[64] Internal phosphorus balance (transcellular phosphate distribution) is also of importance in the maintenance of normal serum phosphate. The serum phosphate level can vary by as much as 2 mg/dL (0.65 mmol/L) throughout the day, primarily as the result of changes in carbohydrate intake, insulin secretion, and diurnal variation.[64]

Hyperphosphatemia

Hyperphosphatemia typically results from either renal failure or endogenous intracellular phosphate release. Hyperphosphatemia occurs frequently in patients with acute renal failure and is a nearly universal finding in those with advanced stages of CKD (e.g., stages 4 and 5). Tumor lysis syndrome is a complication of chemotherapy associated with massive lysis of cells and release of intracellular contents. The incidence of tumor lysis syndrome has been reported to be as high as 40% in patients treated for non-Hodgkin's lymphoma.[64] Other causes of hyperphosphatemia include hemolysis and rhabdomyolysis.

Pathophysiology

5 The most common cause of hyperphosphatemia is a failure of renal tubular reabsorption to maintain serum phosphate when GFR is markedly inpaired (e.g., GFR <25 mL/min/1.73 m^2 [<0.24 mL/s/m^2]).[64] Retention of phosphate decreases vitamin D synthesis and induces hypocalcemia, which leads to an increase in PTH, a finding that can be seen in those with stage 2 to 3 CKD. This physiologic response inhibits further tubular reabsorption of phosphorus as the kidney attempts to correct hyperphosphatemia and normalize serum calcium concentrations. Patients with excessive exogenous phosphate administration or who experience massive tissue breakdown or cell lysis in the setting of acute renal failure can rapidly develop moderate-to-severe hyperphosphatemia (serum phosphate >6.5 mg/dL [>2.10 mmol/L]).[64] Severe hyperphosphatemia (serum phosphate >7 mg/dL [>2.26 mmol/L]) is commonly encountered in patients with CKD, especially those with GFRs less than 15 mL/min per 1.73 m^2 (0.14 mL/s/m^2) (see Chap. 29).

Hyperphosphatemia caused by an increase in renal tubular reabsorption associated with hypoparathyroidism and associated decreases in PTH is usually less severe than that observed in patients with severe renal failure or excessive exogenous or endogenous introduction of phosphate into the ECF. Acromegaly (mediated by growth hormone) and thyrotoxicosis (mediated by catecholamines) can also cause hyperphosphatemia by increasing tubular phosphate reabsorption.

Exogenous Phosphate Loads Iatrogenic causes of hyperphosphatemia have been widely reported, and clinicians should be aware of the phosphorus content of IV, oral, and rectally administered products. Large doses of phosphate administered IV to treat hypercalcemia can ultimately result in severe life-threatening hyperphosphatemia. Although less-well recognized, oral and rectal administration of phosphate-containing solutions such as sodium phosphate (Fleet Phospho-Soda) can also result in severe and life-threatening hyperphosphatemia, especially in patients with moderate and severe renal insufficiency.[68,69] The risk of mortality is dependent on the amount of phosphorus absorbed from the administered product; however, fatalities have occurred at lower phosphate concentrations.[68] Acute phosphate nephropathy and renal failure have also been reported with the use of oral sodium phosphate bowel preparations. Recently the FDA issued a safety warning regarding the use of these products in patients at risk (the elderly, those with CKD) or on medications known to effect renal hemodynamics (e.g., diuretics, nonsteroidal antiinflammatory drugs [NSAIDs], or renin–angiotensin–aldosterone system inhibitors).[70] IV or oral vitamin D therapy can increase absorption of phosphorus in the GI tract by up to 50%. Acute phosphorus poisoning as a result of ingestion of laundry detergents is a rare and often unrecognized cause of elevated phosphate concentrations.

Rapid Tissue Catabolism Any disorder that results in necrosis of skeletal muscle (i.e., rhabdomyolysis) can generate the release of large amounts of intracellular phosphate into the systemic circulation. This condition is frequently associated with acute kidney injury (see Chap. 28) and thus severe hyperphosphatemia can develop because of increased endogenous phosphate release coupled with the impaired proximal tubule reabsorption such that phosphaturic hormones (e.g., PTH, FGF23) become ineffective. Bowel infarction, malignant hyperthermia, and severe hemolysis are also conditions that can increase endogenous release of phosphate.

Moderate hyperphosphatemia is also commonly observed in patients undergoing treatment for acute leukemia and lymphomas.[50] Chemotherapeutic treatment of acute lymphoblastic leukemia can result in the release of large amounts of phosphate into the systemic circulation secondary to lysis of lymphoblasts. Initiation of chemotherapy for Burkitt's lymphoma results in tumor lysis syndrome, a rapid lysis of malignant cells that results in hyperphosphatemia, hyperuricemia, hyperkalemia, and hypocalcemia.[50]

Acid–Base Disorders Lactic acidosis and diabetic ketoacidosis can trigger the transcellular shift of endogenous intracellular phosphate into the extracellular space and thereby dramatically increases serum phosphorous concentrations. In one study, hyperphosphatemia was present in more than 90% of patients with diabetic ketoacidosis prior to the initiation of treatment.[74] After the institution of treatment, serum phosphate levels should be checked hourly as they can decrease rapidly, and patients can ultimately develop hypophosphatemia.

Clinical Presentation

The severe acute onset of hyperphosphatemia can result in calcium and phosphate complexation and lead to the precipitation of calcium phosphate into soft tissues, intrarenal calcification, nephrolithiasis, or obstructive uropathy. Other symptoms associated with moderate-to-severe hyperphosphatemia include nausea, vomiting, diarrhea, lethargy, and seizures. The major effects of long-term hyperphosphatemia are related to the development of hypocalcemia (caused by phosphate inhibition of renal 1-α-hydroxylase) and its related consequences, as well as vascular and organ damage resulting from the deposition of calcium-phosphate crystals. Extravascular calcification can result in band keratopathy, "red eye," pruritus, and periarticular calcification, especially in CKD patients. In addition, soft-tissue calcifications in the conjunctiva, skin, heart, cornea, lung, gastric mucosa, and kidney have been observed, primarily in CKD patients with chronic disordered mineral metabolism.[65] Hyperphosphatemia associated with CKD can result in renal osteodystrophy because of overproduction of PTH. This condition is discussed in detail in Chapter 29.

TREATMENT

Desired Outcome

Management of patients with acutely elevated serum phosphate should be directed at avoiding GI and neurologic symptoms and preventing deposition in the urinary tract to avoid the development of acute renal failure. The treatment of hyperphosphatemia is focused on returning serum phosphate concentrations to the normal or near normal (for those with CKD) range, with the hope that one can minimize the long-term cardiovascular consequences of calcium-phosphate crystal deposition in the vasculature. Calcium-phosphate crystals are likely to form in vivo when the product of the serum calcium and phosphate concentrations exceeds 50 to 60 mg^2/dL^2 (4 to 4.8 mmol^2/L^2). Serum phosphate concentrations greater than 6.5 mg/dL (2.10 mmol/L) have been independently associated with increased morbidity and mortality in patients on maintenance hemodialysis.[71] The Kidney Disease Improving Global Outcomes (KDIGO) clinical practice guidelines suggest that for patients with CKD stages 3 to 5, serum phosphorus should be maintained in the normal range. In dialysis-dependent patients with stage 5 CKD, KDIGO suggests lowering elevated phosphorus levels toward the normal range.[72]

Pharmacologic Therapy

Severe symptomatic hyperphosphatemia manifesting as hypocalcemia and tetany should be treated by the IV administration of calcium salts. Although this can seem counterintuitive in a patient with a phosphate of 16 mg/dL (5.17 mmol/L) and a calcium of 7 mg/dL (1.75 mmol/L) (the calcium–phosphorus product is 112 mg^2/dL^2 [9 mmol^2/L^2]), correction of severe hypocalcemia is of primary importance because of the critical nature of this disorder. If calcium concentrations are not critically low, the initial management strategy should include limitation of all exogenous sources of phosphate and efforts to block further absorption should be initiated. Dialysis can be initiated if the patient remains symptomatic despite these interventions.

Drug Treatments of First Choice

6 In general, the most effective way to treat nonemergent hyperphosphatemia is to decrease phosphate absorption from the GI tract by the use of phosphate-binding agents.[64] Antacids containing divalent and trivalent cations (calcium, lanthanum, magnesium, and aluminum), or sevelamer are the agents most frequently used in the prevention and treatment of hyperphosphatemia (see Table 29-13).[73] Long-term treatment with aluminum hydroxide and aluminum carbonate should be discouraged because the use of these agents has been associated with anemia, CNS disorders, and bone disease.[73]

CLINICAL PRESENTATION Hyperphosphatemia

General

- Serum phosphate concentration is primarily determined by the ability of the kidneys to reabsorb phosphate; therefore, hyperphosphatemia is uncommon in patients with normal kidney function

Symptoms

- Acute symptoms include GI disturbances, lethargy, obstruction of the urinary tract, and rarely seizures. Symptoms associated with chronic hyperphosphatemia are associated with deposition of calcium-phosphate crystals and include "red eye" and pruritus

Signs

- The elevated calcium-phosphate product results in precipitation in arteries, joints, soft tissues, and the viscera. This can result in tissue necrosis, termed calciphylaxis or calcemic uremic arteriopathy

Laboratory Tests

- Serum phosphate levels >4.5 mg/dL (>1.45 mmol/L) represent hyperphosphatemia

Short-term therapy with these agents is effective and safe. Aluminum and calcium are available in oral suspension formulations, which can aid administration in acutely ill patients with G-tubes. The most frequent adverse effect from phosphate-binding agents (especially calcium) is constipation. Calcium salts are the preferred phosphate-binding agents except when there is concomitant hypercalcemia. Therapy with the polymer agent (sevelamer) or lanthanum carbonate might avoid the detrimental effects associated with aluminum, magnesium, or calcium therapy.

Hypophosphatemia

Mild-to-moderate hypophosphatemia is usually asymptomatic and associated with serum phosphate concentrations of 1 to 2 mg/dL (0.32 to 0.65 mmol/L), whereas severe hypophosphatemia that is frequently symptomatic is correlated with serum phosphorus concentrations of less than 1 mg/dL (0.32 mmol/L).[65] Hypophosphatemia has been observed in approximately 1% to 3% of the laboratory screening panels of patients who have been admitted to a hospital.[65] The incidence in hospitalized critically ill patients is 18% to 28%.[64] Unlike its severe form, mild or moderate hypophosphatemia seldom causes recognizable signs and symptoms.[73]

Pathophysiology

7 Hypophosphatemia can be the result of decreased GI absorption, reduced tubular reabsorption, or extracellular to intracellular redistribution.[64] Although mild-to-moderate hypophosphatemia is common and can occur in inpatients and outpatients, severe hypophosphatemia is predominantly encountered in the acute care setting and can be associated with life-threatening symptoms, including seizures, coma, and rhabdomyolysis (Table 35-5).

Decreased GI Absorption Phosphate-binding substances such as sucralfate, calcium carbonate, sevelamer, lanthanum carbonate, and aluminum- or magnesium-containing antacids have the potential to bind large amounts of phosphorus in the gut, thereby preventing absorption. If phosphate-binding agents are ingested on a chronic basis in conjunction with a dietary phosphorus deficiency, hypophosphatemia can result.[74] Patients who are receiving long-term phosphate-binding agents, those with peptic ulcer disease or CKD, and those who may be predisposed to moderate hypophosphatemia (alcoholics) are at highest risk for the development of severe hypophosphatemia. Hyperparathyroidism can cause hypophosphatemia as a result of decreased GI absorption of dietary phosphorus.

Decreased Tubular Reabsorption Reduced tubular reabsorption of phosphate can occur in hyperparathyroid (primary and secondary) patients with normal renal function and those with vitamin D deficiency or elevated FGF23 concentrations. Elevated PTH levels lead to an increase in serum calcium concentrations and decreased serum phosphate concentrations. Serum phosphorus is decreased as the result of a reduction in renal tubular reabsorption.[75] Recovery from extensive third degree burns is associated with development of an anabolic state as stress levels decrease and nutritional therapies take effect as well as a marked diuretic phase associated with an impressive renal loss of phosphate.[75] Because phosphate is rapidly incorporated into the new cells, this can contribute to the severity of the hypophosphatemia. Drugs that cause increased renal elimination of phosphate include diuretics (acetazolamide and osmotic diuretics), glucocorticoids, and sodium bicarbonate.[74]

Cellular Shifts Rapid refeeding of malnourished patients with high-carbohydrate, high-calorie diets with inadequate amounts of supplemental phosphate can result in severe symptomatic hypophosphatemia. This phenomenon is especially prevalent in patients with other underlying risk factors for the development of hypophosphatemia, such as alcoholism.[75] The etiology of severe hypophosphatemia associated with hyperalimentation and nutritional recovery can be separated into two phases: acute, rapid hypophosphatemia secondary to intracellular shifts of phosphate resulting from glucose-induced insulin secretion; and the gradual decrease in serum phosphate concentration over 5 to 10 days secondary to tissue repair in the presence of phosphate deprivation.[76] The development of severe hypophosphatemia secondary to hyperalimentation can be prevented by the administration of 12 to 15 mmol of phosphate per liter of hyperalimentation solution or 15 mmol per 1,000 calories (4.2 kJ) of dextrose.[76] Transcellular shifts in phosphate also occur after parathyroidectomy, causing severe hypocalcemia and hypophosphatemia because of hungry bone syndrome (deposition of phosphate and calcium in the bone).

Severe and prolonged respiratory alkalosis (a result of hyperventilation, pain, anxiety, and sepsis) can cause hypophosphatemia.[65] Respiratory alkalosis is thought to contribute significantly to the hypophosphatemia observed during alcohol withdrawal.[68] Although patients with diabetic ketoacidosis may present with hyperphosphatemia, the institution of therapy to correct it can cause serum phosphate concentrations to decrease rapidly as phosphate shifts back into the intracellular compartment. In addition, the acidosis associated with the diabetic ketoacidotic state can cause a decomposition of organic compounds inside the cell and a release

TABLE 35-5 Conditions Associated with the Development of Hypophosphatemia

Decreased GI absorption
Phosphate-binding drugs
Sucralfate
Calcium carbonate
Aluminum/magnesium antacids
Sevelamer
Lanthanum carbonate
Decreased dietary phosphorus intake
Glucocorticoids
Vitamin D deficiency/resistance
Hypoparathyroidism
Chronic diarrhea
Steatorrhea
Reduced tubular reabsorption
Hyperparathyroidism (primary and secondary)
Elevated FGF23
Recovery from burns
Rickets
Malignant neoplasms
Fanconi's syndrome
Acute volume expansion
Metabolic acidosis
Renal transplantation
Vitamin D deficiency and/or resistance
Diuretics
Acetazolamide
Osmotic agents
Glucocorticoids
Sodium bicarbonate
Internal redistribution
Refeeding syndrome
Parenteral nutrition
Parathyroidectomy (hungry bone syndrome)
Alcoholism
Respiratory alkalosis
Diabetic ketoacidosis (correction)
Dextrose solutions
Insulin
Catecholamines
Anabolic steroids
Glucagon
Calcitonin
Erythropoietin

of inorganic phosphate into the plasma and subsequently into the urine.[64] The combination of intracellular phosphate breakdown and the shift of phosphate into cells on initiation of treatment can lead to severe hypophosphatemia. Drugs associated with transcellular shifts in phosphate include dextrose solutions, glucagon, insulin, catecholamines, calcitonin, erythropoietic agents, and anabolic steroids.

Chronic ethanol abusers are prone to a variety of serum electrolyte disorders including hypocalcemia, hypomagnesemia, hypokalemia, and hypophosphatemia. The etiology of hypophosphatemia in the alcoholic patient is multifactorial. Malnutrition, poor dietary intake, diarrhea, vomiting, and the use of phosphate-binding antacids can all contribute to the hypophosphatemia of alcoholism.[64] In addition, serum phosphate concentrations may decrease after hospitalization in the alcoholic patient with the institution of dextrose-containing IV fluids as a result of an intracellular shift of phosphate.[64,76] Hyperventilation associated with the alcohol withdrawal syndrome can also contribute to the development of hypophosphatemia.[76] Alcoholic patients are particularly susceptible to the complications of hypophosphatemia such as rhabdomyolysis, which is often seen during withdrawal or refeeding.[76] Thus, serum phosphate concentrations should be routinely monitored in alcoholic patients.

Clinical Presentation

The clinical manifestations of severe hypophosphatemia are diverse and many organ systems can be affected. It is likely that two primary biochemical abnormalities are responsible for most of the clinical manifestations of severe hypophosphatemia.[64] First, intracellular energy stores may be decreased secondary to depletion of intracellular ATP. This can result in disruptions in cellular function. Second, reduced red blood cell 2,3-DPG concentrations are associated with a shift to the left of the oxyhemoglobin saturation curve. This shift is associated with a decrease in the release of oxygen to peripheral tissues (increased oxygen affinity for hemoglobin) and may result in tissue hypoxia.[65] These metabolic disorders can be seen in a wide variety of organ systems.

Neurologic (CNS) manifestations of severe hypophosphatemia result in a metabolic encephalopathy syndrome. This progressive syndrome of irritability, apprehension, weakness, numbness, paresthesia, dysarthria, confusion, obtundation, seizures, and coma has been described in patients with severe hypophosphatemia.[75,76] Neuropsychiatric disturbances include apathy, delirium, hallucinations, and paranoia. Peripheral neuropathy and symptoms resembling Guillain–Barré syndrome have also been reported.[76]

Severe hypophosphatemia can result in significant dysfunction of skeletal muscle ranging from myalgia, bone pain, and weakness, with chronic hypophosphatemia, to potentially fatal rhabdomyolysis with severe acute hypophosphatemia.[75] Laboratory evaluations can help to distinguish between chronic and acute on chronic hypophosphatemia. Elevated alkaline phosphatase, normal creatine phosphokinase, and normal to low phosphate and calcium are present in cases of chronic hypophosphatemia. In contrast, hyperkalemia, hyperuricemia, elevated blood urea nitrogen and creatinine, hypercalcemia, and myoglobinuria are often present in cases in which rhabdomyolysis complicates the acute or chronic hypophosphatemia.[75] Hypophosphatemia can result in acute respiratory failure secondary to respiratory muscle weakness and diaphragmatic contractile dysfunction. Thus, frequent assessment of serum phosphate concentration is indicated in patients at risk for respiratory failure. Likewise, adequate treatment of hypophosphatemia in respiratory failure can aid in successful weaning from the ventilator.[65] Dysphagia and ileus have also been attributed to hypophosphatemia.[65]

Myocardial dysfunction has been reported to be impaired in the setting of hypophosphatemia and has resulted in congestive cardiomyopathy. This has been reported in alcoholics, and postoperative and intensive care patients. Depletion of cardiac ATP stores has been hypothesized as the cause of this syndrome.[72] Arrhythmias have also been reported in patients with hypophosphatemia. Because hypophosphatemia is a potentially reversible cause of heart failure, it should be considered in patients who experience an acute deterioration in ventricular function.

CLINICAL PRESENTATION Hypophosphatemia

General

- Major conditions associated with symptomatic hypophosphatemia are chronic alcoholism, IV hyperalimentation without adequate phosphate supplementation, and the chronic ingestion of antacids. Severe hypophosphatemia can also be seen during treatment of diabetic ketoacidosis and with prolonged hyperventilation

Symptoms

- Except for the effects on mineral metabolism, the symptoms of hypophosphatemia are caused by two consequences (reduction of red cell 2,3-DPG and reduction of intracellular ATP levels), and can impact virtually all organ systems. The symptoms are predominantly neurological and can include irritability, apprehension, weakness, numbness, paresthesia, and confusion. Severe acute development of hypophosphatemia can result in seizures or coma

Signs

- The initial response of bone to hypophosphatemia contributes to hypercalcemia and hypercalciuria. Prolonged hypophosphatemia can also result in rickets and osteomalacia
- Neurologic: Severe hypophosphatemia can lead to a metabolic encephalopathy
- Cardiopulmonary: Impaired myocardial contractility, respiratory failure secondary to ATP depletion, CHF, new onset or worsening of an existing condition
- Musculoskeletal: Proximal myopathy, dysphagia, and ileus have been reported. Acute hypophosphatemia superimposed on preexisting severe phosphate depletion can lead to rhabdomyolysis
- Hematologic: Alterations in the hematopoietic system can also occur, resulting in hemolysis, reduction in phagocytotic and granulocyte chemotactic ability, as well as defective clot retraction and thrombocytopenia

Laboratory Tests

- Serum phosphate levels <2.4 mg/dL (<0.78 mmol/L) are indicative of hypophosphatemia; however, symptomatic hypophosphatemia typically is not evident until serum phosphate <1 mg/dL (<0.32 mmol/L)

Hematologic manifestations of hypophosphatemia include decreased levels of 2,3-DPG, decreased red blood cell ATP, and membrane rigidity.[64] When red blood cell ATP decreases to below 15% of normal, cells become spherocytic and rigid, and are trapped and destroyed in the spleen.[65] Therefore, hemolysis can be a manifestation of severe hypophosphatemia. Reduction in ATP content of white blood cells can result in mobility, chemotaxis, phagocytosis, and bactericidal dysfunction.[76] These changes can contribute to an increased risk of infection in hypophosphatemic patients.

Finally, prolonged hypophosphatemia may result in osteopenia and osteomalacia because of enhanced osteoclastic resorption of bone and limited crystallization constituents (phosphate), respectively. Glucose intolerance from hypophosphatemia caused by tissue insensitivity to insulin has also been described.

TREATMENT

Desired Outcome

The goals of therapy are the reversal of signs and symptoms of hypophosphatemia, normalization of serum phosphate concentrations, and management of underlying conditions. Awareness of the clinical situations in which hypophosphatemia is anticipated (alcoholism, diabetic ketoacidosis, and parenteral nutrition) is of vital importance in preventing iatrogenic hypophosphatemia. The routine addition of phosphate (12 to 15 mmol/L) to IV hyperalimentation solutions is of utmost importance for the prevention of severe hypophosphatemia in hospitalized patients.

Pharmacologic Therapy

Severe Hypophosphatemia

8 Severe (<1 mg/dL [<0.32 mmol/L]) or symptomatic hypophosphatemia should be treated with parenteral phosphate replacement. Oral phosphate supplementation is usually reserved for patients who are asymptomatic or who exhibit mild-to-moderate hypophosphatemia. Estimation of total body phosphate deficit is difficult because phosphate is an intracellular electrolyte. Dosage and infusion recommendations, as well as response to parenteral phosphate replacement, are highly variable.[77] The infusion of 15 mmol of phosphate in 250 mL of 5% dextrose or 0.9% sodium chloride over 3 hours is a safe and effective treatment for severe hypophosphatemia.[77] Mean increases in serum phosphate of 0.5 to 0.8 mg/dL (0.16 to 0.26 mmol/L) have been reported. Doses of 15 to 30 mmol of phosphate can be given over 1 to 3 hours in patients without hypercalcemia (serum calcium >10.5 mg/dL [>2.63 mmol/L]).[78] Other authors recommend a wider dosage range of 0.08 to 0.64 mmol/kg body weight (5 to 45 mmol in a 70-kg [154 lb] patient) given over 4 to 12 hours.[79] IV phosphate therapy produces the desired increase in serum phosphate at 24 hours in 20% to 80% of patients. Response is dependent on the degree of phosphate depletion and replacement dose administered.[65] Furthermore, the initial success is often followed in 48 to 72 hours by recurrent hypophosphatemia, necessitating close monitoring of serum phosphate and repeated administration of phosphate products as warranted.

Adverse Effects of Parenteral Phosphate Parenteral phosphate supplementation is associated with risks of hyperphosphatemia, metastatic soft tissue deposition of calcium-phosphate product, hypomagnesemia, hypocalcemia, and hyperkalemia or hypernatremia (caused by IV phosphate salt). Inappropriate administration of large doses of parenteral phosphate over relatively short time periods has resulted in symptomatic hypocalcemia and soft-tissue calcification.[64] The rate of infusion and choice of initial dosage should therefore be based on severity of hypophosphatemia, presence of symptoms, and coexistent medical conditions. Patients should be closely monitored with frequent (every 6 hours) serum phosphate determinations for 48 to 72 hours after starting IV therapy. It can be necessary to continue administration of IV phosphate for several days in some patients, although other patients may be able to tolerate an oral maintenance regimen. Monitoring should also include assessment of serum potassium, calcium, and magnesium concentrations. Hypomagnesemia secondary to intracellular shifts occurs frequently (27% to 80%) in severely hypophosphatemic patients.[77] Therapy with parenteral phosphate should be undertaken with great caution and at reduced dosage for patients with hypercalcemia or renal dysfunction.[76]

TABLE 35-6 Phosphorus Replacement Therapy

Product (Salt)	Phosphate Content	Initial Dosing Based on Serum K
Oral Therapy (Potassium Phosphate + Sodium Phosphate)		
Neutra-Phos® (7 mEq/packet each of Na and K)	250 mg (8 mmol)/packet	One packet three times daily[a]
Neutra-Phos-K® (14.25 mEq/packet of K)	250 mg (8 mmol)/packet	Serum K >5.5 mEq/L (>5.5 mmol/L); not recommended
K-Phos Neutral® (13 mEq/tablet Na and 1.1 mEq/tablet K)	250 mg (8 mmol)/tablet	Serum K >5.5 mEq/L (>5.5 mmol/L) one tablet three times daily
Uro-KP-Neutral® (10.9 mEq/tablet Na and 1.27 mEq/tablet K)	250 mg (8 mmol)/tablet	Serum K >5.5 mEq/L (>5.5 mmol/L) one tablet three times daily
Fleets Phospho-soda® (sodium phosphate solution)	4 mmol/mL	Serum K >5.5 mEq/L (>5.5 mmol/L) 2 mL three times daily
IV Therapy		
Sodium PO_4 (4 mEq/mL Na)	3 mmol/mL	Serum K >3.5 mEq/L (>3.5 mmol/L) 15–30 mmol IVPB
Potassium PO_4 (4.4 mEq/mL K)	3 mmol/mL	Serum K <3.5 mEq/L (<3.5 mmol/L) 15–30 mmol IVPB

IVPB, IV piggyback; K, potassium; Na, sodium; PO_4, phosphate.

[a]Monitor serum K closely + IV piggy back.

Mild-to-Moderate Hypophosphatemia

Mild-to-moderate or asymptomatic hypophosphatemia can be treated by the administration of oral phosphate salts in doses of 1.5 to 2 g (50 to 60 mmol) daily in divided doses (see Table 35-6). Phosphate concentrations should be monitored daily, with the goal of correcting the reduced phosphate concentration in approximately 7 to 10 days. The primary dose-limiting adverse effect associated with oral phosphate replacement is the development of osmotic diarrhea. Patients with mild-to-moderate hypophosphatemia and moderate-to-severe renal insufficiency should receive reduced daily oral doses (i.e., 1 g or approximately 30 mmol of phosphate) with careful monitoring of serum phosphate concentration because they are predisposed to phosphate retention. In addition to phosphate supplementation for hypophosphatemia, dipyridamole can decrease renal phosphate leaking and increase serum phosphate. Doses of 75 mg four times daily have resulted in increases in serum 1,25-dihydroxy vitamin D_3 and decreases in serum calcium and urolithiasis events.[80]

CLINICAL BOTTOM LINE

Clinicians play an integral part in the management of fluid and electrolyte abnormalities. Initial treatment strategy should be based on acuity of onset and severity of symptoms. Because the etiologies of calcium and phosphate disorders are diverse, it is important to integrate the known or anticipated pathophysiologic disease course into the treatment strategy. The patient's medication history should be comprehensively assessed to determine whether the electrolyte abnormality may be drug induced. After resolution or treatment of the calcium or phosphate disorder, the medication regimen should be evaluated periodically. This proactive interventional approach will facilitate the management of mild disorders in the community and can reduce the need for hospitalization.

ABBREVIATIONS

ATP	adenosine triphosphate
CHF	congestive heart failure
CKD	chronic kidney disease
FGF23	fibroblast growth factor 23
2,3-DPG	2,3-diphosphoglycerate
NSAID	nonsteroidal antiinflammatory drug
PTH	parathyroid hormone
PTHrP	PTH-related protein
S_{ca}	serum calcium

REFERENCES

1. Copper MS, Gittoes NJL. Diagnosis and management of hypocalcemia. BMJ 2008;336:1298–1302.
2. Nussbaum SR. Pathophysiology and management of severe hypercalcemia. Endocrinol Metab Clin North Am 1993;22:343–362.
3. Dickerson RN. Treatment of moderate to severe acute hypocalcemia in critically ill trauma patients. J Parenter Enteral Nutr 2007;21:228–233.
4. Slomp J, van der Voort PH, Gerritsen RT, et al. Albumin-adjusted calcium is not suitable for diagnosis of hyper- and hypocalcemia in the critically ill. Crit Care Med 2003;31: 1389–1393.
5. Byrnes MC, Huynh K, Helmer SD, et al. A comparison of corrected serum calcium levels to ionized calcium levels among critically ill surgical patients. Am J Surg 2005;189: 310–314.
6. Marcocci C, Cetani F. Clinical practice. Primary hyperparathyroidism. N Engl J Med. 2011;365(25): 2389–2397.
7. Lumachi F, Brunello A, Roma A, et al. Medical treatment of malignancy-associated hypercalcemia. Curr Med Chem 2008;15:415–421.
8. Rifai MA, Moles JK, Harrington DP. Lithium-induced hypercalcemia and parathyroid dysfunction. Psychosomatics 2001;42:359–361.
9. Fraser WD. Hyperparathyroidism. Lancet 2009;374: 145–158.
10. McMahan J. A case of resistant hypercalcemia of malignancy with a proposed treatment algorithm. Ann Pharmacother 2009;43:1532–1538.
11. McCauley LK, Martin TJ. Twenty-five years of PTHrP progress: From cancer hormone to multifunctional cytokine. J Bone Miner Res 2012;27(6):1231–1239.
12. French S, Subauste J, Geraci S. Calcium abnormalities in hospitalized patients. South Med J 2012;105(4):231–237.
13. Picolis MK, Lavis VR, Orlander PR. Milk-alkali is a major cause of hypercalcemia. Clin Endocrinol (Oxf) 2005;63: 566–576.
14. Beall DP, Henslee HB, Webb HR, et al. Milk-alkali syndrome: A historical review and description of the modern version of the syndrome. Am J Med Sci 2006;331: 233–242.
15. Moe SM. Disorders involving calcium, phosphorus and magnesium. Prim Care 2008;35:215–237, v–vi.
16. Shlapack MA, Rizvi AA. Normocalcemic primary hyperparathyroidism: Characteristics and clinical significance of an emerging entity. Am J Med Sci 2012;343(2):163–166.
17. Karwowski W, Naumnik B, Szczepański M, Myśliwiec M. The mechanism of vascular calcification—A systematic review. Med Sci Monit 2012;18(1):RA1–RA11.
18. Towler DA, Demer LL. Thematic series on the pathobiology of vascular calcification: An introduction. Circ Res 2011;108(11):1378–1380.
19. Vella A, Gerber TC, Hayes DL, et al. Digoxin, hypercalcemia and cardiac conduction. Postgrad Med 1999;75:554–556.
20. Rejnmark L, Vestergaard P, Mosekilde L. Nephrolithiasis and renal calcifications in primary hyperparathyroidism. J Clin Endocrinol Metab 2011;96(8):2377–2385.
21. Yamashita H, Noguchi S, Uchino S, et al. Influence of renal function on clinicopathological features of primary hyperparathyroidism. Eur J Endocrinol 2003;148: 597–602.
22. Ralston SH, Coleman R, Fraser WD, et al. Medical management of hypercalcemia. Calcif Tissue Int 2004;74: 1–11.
23. Lumachi F, Brunello A, Roma A, Basso U. Cancer-induced hypercalcemia. Anticancer Res 2009;29:1551–1555.
24. Davey RA, Turner AG, McManus JF, et al. Calcitonin plays a physiological role to protect against hypercalcemia in mice. J Bone Miner Res 2008;23:1182–1193.
25. Inzerillo AM, Zaidi M, Huang CL. Calcitonin: Physiological actions and clinical applications. J Pediatr Endocrinol Metab 2004;17:931–940.
26. Grauer A, Ziegler R, Raue F. Clinical significance of antibodies against calcitonin. Exp Clin Endocrinol Diabetes 1995;103:345–351.
27. Stewart AF. Hypercalcemia associated with cancer. N Engl J Med 2005;352:373–379.
28. Wellington K, Goa KL. Zoledronic acid: A review of its use in the management of bone metastases and hypercalcemia of malignancy. Drugs 2003;63:417–437.
29. Major P, Lortholary A, Hon J, et al. Zoledronic acid is superior to pamidronate in the treatment of hypercalcemia of malignancy: A pooled analysis of two randomized, controlled clinical trials. J Clin Oncol 2001;19:558–567.
30. Body JJ, Lortholary A, Romieu G, et al. A dose-finding study of zoledronate in hypercalcemic cancer patients. J Bone Miner Res 1999;14:1557–1561.
31. Pecherstorfer M, Steinhauer EU, Rizzoli R, et al. Efficacy and safety of ibandronate in the treatment of hypercalcemia of malignancy: A randomized multicenter comparison to pamidronate. Support Care Cancer 2003;11:539–547.
32. Guay DR. Ibandronate, an experimental intravenous bisphosphonate for osteoporosis, bone metastases and hypercalcemia of malignancy. Pharmacotherapy 2006;26: 655–673.
33. Costa L, Lipton A, Coleman RE. Role of bisphosphonates for the management of skeletal complications and bone pain from skeletal metastases. Support Cancer Ther 2006;3: 143–153.
34. Banerjee D, Asif A, Striker L, et al. Short-term, high-dose pamidronate-induced acute tubular necrosis: The postulated mechanisms of bisphosphonate nephrotoxicity. Am J Kidney Dis 2003;41:E18.

35. Markowitz GS, Fine PL, Stack JI, et al. Toxic acute tubular necrosis following treatment with zoledronate (Zometa). Kidney Int 2003;64:281–289.
36. Body JJ, Lipton A, Gralow J, et al. Effects of denosumab in patients with bone metastases, with and without previous bisphosphonate exposure. J Bone Miner Res 2010;25: 440–446.
37. Martin M, Bell R, Bourgeois H, et al. Bone-related complications and quality of life in advanced breast cancer: Results from a randomized phase III trial of denosumab versus zoledronic acid. Clin Cancer Res 2012;18(17): 4841–4849.
38. Boikos SA, Hammers HJ. Denosumab for the treatment of bisphosphonate-refractory hypercalcemia. J Clin Oncol 2012;30(29):e299. doi: 10.1200/JCO.2012.41.7923.
39. Shroff R, Beringer O, Rao K, Hofbauer LC, Schulz A. Denosumab for post-transplantation hypercalcemia in osteopetrosis. N Engl J Med 2012;367(18):1766–1767.
40. Leyland-Jones B. Treatment of cancer-related hypercalcemia: The role of gallium nitrate. Semin Oncol 2003;30(2 Suppl 5):13–19.
41. Cvitkovic F, Armand JP, Tubiana-Hulin M, et al. Randomized, double-blind, phase II trial of gallium nitrate compared with pamidronate for acute control of cancer-related hypercalcemia. Cancer J 2006;12:47–52.
42. Ziegler R. Hypercalcemic crisis. J Am Soc Nephrol 2001;12(Suppl 17):S3–S9.
43. Silverman SL, Lane NE. Glucocorticoid-induced osteoporosis. Curr Osteoporos Rep 2009;7:23–26.
44. Silverberg SJ, Rubin MR, Faiman C, et al. Cinacalcet hydrochloride reduces the serum calcium concentration in inoperable parathyroid carcinoma. J Clin Endocrinol Metab 2007;92:3803–3808.
45. Messa P, Alfieri C, Brezzi B. Clinical utilization of cinacalcet in hypercalcemic conditions. Expert Opin Drug Metab Toxicol 2011;7(4):517–528.
46. Sensipar® (cinacalcet HCl) [package insert]. Thousand Oaks, CA: Amgen, Inc., 2004–2011.
47. Khan A, Fong J. Hypocalcemia: Updates in diagnosis and management for primary care. Can Fam Physician 2012;58(2):158–162.
48. Jawan B, de Villa V, Luk HN, et al. Ionized calcium changes during living-donor liver transplantation in patients with and without administration of blood-bank products. Transpl Int 2003;16:510–514.
49. Kishimoto M, Ohto H, Shikama Y, et al. Treatment for the decline of ionized calcium levels during peripheral blood progenitor cell harvesting. Transfusion 2002;42: 1340–1347.
50. Firwana BM, Hasan R, Hasan N, et al. Tumor lysis syndrome: A systematic review of case series and case reports. Postgrad Med 2012;124(2):92–101.
51. Alvarez-Hernandez D, Santamaria I, Rodriguez-Garcia M, et al. A novel mutation in the calcium-sensing receptor responsible for autosomal dominant hypocalcemia in a family with two uncommon parathyroid hormone polymorphisms. J Mol Endocrinol 2003;31: 255–262.
52. Hu J, Mora S, Colussi G, et al. Autosomal dominant hypocalcemia caused by a novel mutation in the loop 2 region of the human calcium receptor extracellular domain. J Bone Miner Res 2002;17:1461–1469.
53. Peacock M. Calcium metabolism in health and disease. Clin J Am Soc Nephrol 2010;5:S23–S30.
54. Kitanaka S, Isojima T, Takaki M, et al. Association of vitamin D-related gene polymorphisms with manifestation of vitamin D deficiency in children. Endocr J 2012;59(11):1007–1014.
55. Tachibana S, Sato S, Yokoi T, et al. Severe hypocalcemia complicated by postsurgical hypoparathyroidism and hungry bone syndrome in a patient with primary hyperparathyroidism, Graves' disease, and acromegaly. Intern Med 2012;51(14):1869–1873.
56. Maalouf NM, Heller HJ, Odvina CV, et al. Bisphosphonate-induced hypocalcemia: Report of 3 cases and review of the literature. Endocr Pract 2006;12:48–53.a
57. Choyke PL, Knopp MV. Pseudohypocalcemia with MR imaging contrast agents: A cautionary tale. Radiology 2003;227:639–646.
58. Uhl L, Maillet S, King S, Kruskall MS. Unexpected citrate toxicity and severe hypocalcemia during apheresis. Transfusion 1997;37:1063–1065.
59. Polaschegg HD, Sodemann K. Risks related to catheter locking solutions containing concentrated citrate. Nephrol Dial Transplant 2003;18:2688–2689.
60. Maeda SS, Fortes EM, Oliveira UM, et al. Hypoparathyroidism and pseudohypoparathyroidism. Arq Bras Endocrinol Metabol 2006;50(4):664–673.
61. Dickerson RN. Treatment of hypocalcemia in critical illness—Part 2. Nutrition 2007;23:436–437.
62. Lee I, Sheu WH, Tu ST, et al. Bisphosphonate pretreatment attenuates hungry bone syndrome postoperatively in subjects with primary hyperparathyroidism. J Bone Miner Metab 2006;24:255–258.
63. Hollis BW. Circulating 25-hydroxy vitamin D levels indicative of vitamin D sufficiency: Implications for establishing a new effective dietary intake recommendation for vitamin D. J Nutr 2005;135:317–322.
64. DeMeglio LA, White KE, Econs MJ. Disorders of phosphate metabolism. Endrocrinol Metab Clin North Am 2000;29:591–609.
65. Uribarri J. Phosphorus homeostasis in normal health and in chronic kidney disease patients with special emphasis on dietary phosphorus. Semin Dial 2007;20: 295–301.
66. Liu S, Quarles LD. How fibroblast growth factor 23 works. J Am Soc Nephrol 2007;18:1637–1647.
67. Prie D, Torres PU, Friedlander G. Latest findings in phosphate homeostasis. Kidney Int 2009;75: 882–889.
68. Adamcewicz M, Bearelly D, Porat G, Friedenberg FK. Mechanism of action and toxicities of purgatives used for colonoscopy preparation. Expert Opin Drug Metab Toxicol 2011;7(1):89–101.
69. Aydogan T, Kanbay M, Uz B, et al. Fatal hyperphosphatemia secondary to a phosphosoda bowel preparation in a geriatric patient with normal renal function. J Clin Gastroenterol 2006;40:177.
70. FDA requires new safety measures for oral sodium phosphate products to reduce risk of acute kidney injury risk associated with both prescription and over-the-counter (OTC) products. *http://www.fda.gov/NewsEvents/Newsroom/PressAnnouncements/2008/ucm116988.htm*
71. Block GA, Klassen PS, Lazarus JM, et al. Mineral metabolism, mortality and morbidity in maintenance hemodialysis. 2004;15:2208–2218.
72. KDIGO Clinical Practice Guidelines for the Diagnosis, Evaluation, Prevention, and Treatment of Chronic Kidney Disease-Mineral and Bone Disorder (CKD-MBD). Chapter 4.1: Treatment of CKD-MBD targeted at lowering high serum phosphorus and maintaining serum calcium. Kidney Int 2009;76(Suppl 113):S50–S99.

73. Hutchison AJ, Smith CP, Brenchley PE. Pharmacology, efficacy and safety of oral phosphate binders. Nat Rev Nephrol 2011;7(10):578–589.
74. Liamis G, Milionis HJ, Elisaf M. Medication-induced hypophosphatemia: A review. QJM 2010;103(7):449–459.
75. Subramanian R, Khardori R. Severe hypophosphatemia. Pathophysiologic implications, clinical presentation, and treatment. Medicine (Baltimore) 2000;79:1–78.
76. Amanzadeh J, Reilly RF. Hypophosphatemia: An evidence-based approach to its clinical consequences and management. Nat Clin Pract Nephrol 2006;2:136–148.
77. Perreault MM, Ostrop NJ, Tierney MG. Efficacy and safety of intravenous phosphate replacement in critically ill patients. Ann Pharmacother 1997;31:683–688.
78. Charron T, Bernard F, Skrobik Y, et al. Intravenous phosphate in the intensive care unit: More aggressive repletion regimens for moderate and severe hypophosphatemia. Intensive Care Med 2003;29: 1273–1278.
79. Clark CL, Sacks GS, Dickerson RN, et al. Treatment of hypophosphatemia in patients receiving specialized nutrition support using a graduated dosing scheme: Results from a prospective clinical trial. Crit Care Med 1995;23: 1504–1511.
80. Prie D, Blanchet FB, Essig M, et al. Dipyridamole decreases renal phosphate leak and augments serum phosphorus in patients with low renal phosphate threshold. J Am Soc Nephrol 1998;9:1264–1269.

Disorders of Potassium and Magnesium Homeostasis

36

Donald F. Brophy

KEY CONCEPTS

1. Potassium regulates many biochemical processes in the body and is a key cation for electrical action potentials across cellular membranes.
2. In patients with concomitant hypokalemia and hypomagnesemia, it is imperative to correct the hypomagnesemia before the hypokalemia.
3. Potassium chloride is the preferred potassium supplement for the most common causes of hypokalemia.
4. Hyperkalemia is a common occurrence in patients with acute or chronic kidney disease.
5. Hypomagnesemia is commonly caused by excessive GI or renal magnesium wasting.
6. Hypermagnesemia is predominantly observed in patients with acute or chronic kidney disease.

Potassium and magnesium are electrolytes that are responsible for numerous metabolic activities. Disorders of these electrolytes are frequently seen in both the acute care and community ambulatory care settings. Therefore, clinicians need a firm understanding of the etiology, pathophysiology, symptoms, pharmacotherapy, and monitoring of these disorders. This chapter describes the homeostatic mechanisms that are responsible for the maintenance of normal potassium and magnesium serum concentrations. The clinical disorders responsible for the development of hyperkalemia, hypermagnesemia, hypokalemia, and hypomagnesemia are also reviewed.

POTASSIUM

Potassium is the most abundant cation in the body, with estimated total-body stores of 3,000 to 4,000 mEq (3,000 to 4,000 mmol).[1] Ninety-eight percent of this amount is contained within the intracellular compartment, and the remaining 2% is distributed within the extracellular compartment. The sodium-potassium adenosine triphosphatase (Na^+-K^+-ATPase) pump located in the cell membrane is responsible for the compartmentalization of potassium. This pump is an active transport system that maintains increased intracellular stores of potassium by transporting sodium out of the cell and potassium into the cell at a ratio of 3:2. Consequently, the pump maintains a higher concentration of potassium inside the cell.

The normal serum concentration range for potassium is 3.5 to 5 mEq/L (3.5 to 5 mmol/L), whereas the intracellular potassium concentration is usually approximately 150 mEq/L (150 mmol/L).[2] Approximately 75% of the intracellular potassium is located in skeletal muscle; the remaining 25% is located in the liver and red blood cells. Extracellular potassium is distributed throughout the serum and interstitial space. Potassium is dynamic in that it is constantly moving between the intracellular and extracellular compartments according to the body's needs. Thus, the serum potassium concentration alone does not accurately reflect the total-body potassium content.

1 Potassium has many physiologic functions within cells, including protein and glycogen synthesis and cellular metabolism and growth. It is also a determinant of the electrical action potential across the cell membrane.[1] The ratio of the intracellular-to-extracellular potassium concentration is the major determinant of the resting membrane potential across the cell membrane. Thus, the resting membrane potential is greatly affected by variations in extracellular potassium concentration. Serum potassium concentrations outside the normal range can have disastrous effects on neuromuscular activity, in particular cardiac conduction. Hypo- and hyperkalemia are both associated with potentially fatal cardiac arrhythmias, along with other neuromuscular disturbances. Finally, potassium is integral to maintaining healthy blood pressure balance, prevention of stroke, and potentially other cardiovascular diseases.[3] Both the National High Blood Pressure Education Program and the Institute of Medicine recommend potassium supplementation as strategies for preventing and treating hypertension.[4–6]

Control of Potassium Homeostasis

Potassium homeostasis, the maintenance of serum potassium within the normal range, is affected by dietary intake, GI and urinary excretion, hormones, acid–base balance, body fluid tonicity, and a highly integrated feedback mechanism.[7,8] The recommended daily allowance for dietary potassium intake in the United States is approximately 50 mEq/day (50 mmol/day); however, the Seventh Report of the Joint National Committee on Prevention, Detection, Evaluation, and Treatment of High Blood Pressure guidelines recommends a daily intake of 100 mEq (100 mmol) for prevention of hypertension and other cardiovascular complications.[9] Potassium is found in abundance in fruits, vegetables, and meats. The typical American ingests approximately 50 to 150 mEq (50 to 150 mmol) of potassium daily. Nearly all of this is absorbed, with only 10 to 20 mEq/day (10 to 20 mmol/day) eliminated in feces. The amount eliminated in the feces increases, however, in patients with diarrhea and in those with chronic kidney disease (CKD).[8]

The kidney is the primary route of potassium elimination. Potassium is freely filtered, but almost all of it is reabsorbed passively in the proximal tubule and the thick ascending limb of the loop of Henle.[10] Therefore, urinary potassium excretion is primarily determined by potassium secretion from the luminal cells of the distal tubule and collecting duct. Although the amount of potassium filtered by the glomerulus approaches 700 mEq (700 mmol) per day, only approximately 10% to 20% is actually excreted in the urine.[10] However, this amount can vary based on dietary intake, serum potassium concentration, and aldosterone activity. For example, more potassium is renally excreted in conditions that result in high aldosterone activity (e.g., dehydration) when the body is attempting to conserve sodium or when there is an increase in dietary potassium intake.

Hormones such as insulin, catecholamines, and aldosterone dramatically affect potassium homeostasis. Insulin is the most important hormonal mediator of potassium balance because it stimulates the cellular Na^+-K^+-ATPase pump to increase transport of potassium into liver, muscle, and adipose tissue.[7] There is a complex negative feedback loop in which insulin secretion tightly regulates serum potassium concentrations: an increase of only a few tenths of a milliequivalent (mmol) of potassium stimulates pancreatic insulin secretion in an attempt to prevent hyperkalemia from developing.[1] If hyperkalemia does occur, glucagon is released from the liver to protect against insulin-induced hypoglycemia. Conversely, hypokalemia inhibits insulin secretion, a finding that explains why some patients receiving diuretics develop hyperglycemia.

An elevation in circulating catecholamines such as epinephrine usually results in the intracellular movement of potassium by two mechanisms.[10] They stimulate the β-receptor, which directly activates the Na^+-K^+-ATPase pump. Second, they stimulate glycogenolysis, which raises blood glucose concentrations, thereby increasing insulin secretion. This dual mechanism is often used therapeutically in patients with hyperkalemia to normalize serum potassium concentrations.

Aldosterone, a mineralocorticoid that is secreted from the adrenal glands in response to high serum potassium concentrations, promotes urinary potassium excretion. Aldosterone works in the distal tubule and collecting duct to promote the reabsorption of sodium and water in exchange for potassium. Aldosterone may also have extrarenal activity by stimulating cellular Na^+-K^+-ATPase pump activity.[10]

Changes in acid–base status significantly affect the serum potassium concentration. For example, the infusion of metabolic inorganic acids, such as hydrochloric acid, results in an increase in serum potassium. The body compensates for excessive hydrogen ions by moving them from the serum into the cell in exchange for intracellular potassium, to maintain electroneutrality. The processes by which this occurs are highly complex, and involve cellular H^+-K^+-ATPase pumps and both Na^+-HCO_3^- and K^+-HCO_3^- cotransporters.[11] The efflux of potassium into the serum can result in hyperkalemia. A commonly quoted approximation of the pH effect is that for every 0.1 unit decrease in pH, there is a corresponding increase in serum potassium of 0.6 to 0.8 mEq/L (0.6 to 0.8 mmol/L) (with a wide range of 0.2 to 1.7).[6] This is often referred to as *false hyperkalemia* because there is not a true excess of total-body potassium. Metabolic acidosis associated with lactic acidosis and ketoacidosis does not result in hyperkalemia, because both cations and anions enter the cell, thus maintaining electroneutrality.[1] Respiratory acidosis also does not significantly affect the serum potassium concentration.

Conversely, metabolic alkalosis has been associated with hypokalemia. As a result of a net loss of hydrogen ion from the serum, intracellular hydrogen ions enter the serum to increase the acidity of the blood. To maintain electroneutrality, extracellular potassium ions are shifted intracellularly. This creates a relative deficiency of potassium in the serum. Serum potassium decreases approximately 0.6 mEq/L (0.6 mmol/L) for each 0.1 unit increase in blood pH. This is frequently termed *false hypokalemia* because there is not a true deficiency in total-body potassium.

Finally, hyperosmolality can result in enhanced movement of potassium from the cell into the extracellular fluid. This occurs most likely because of the associated cell shrinkage and water loss, which increases the intracellular-to-extracellular potassium gradient.[4] This is seen most commonly in conditions such as diabetic ketoacidosis. Conversely, hypoosmolality does not seem to affect potassium distribution.

HYPOKALEMIA

Epidemiology

Hypokalemia (defined as a serum potassium concentration <3.5 mEq/L [<3.5 mmol/L]) is a commonly encountered electrolyte abnormality in clinical practice. Hypokalemia can be categorized as mild (serum potassium 3.1 to 3.5 mEq/L [3.1 to 3.5 mmol/L]), moderate (serum potassium 2.5 to 3 mEq/L [2.5 to 3 mmol/L]), or severe (<2.5 mEq/L [<2.5 mmol/L]).[12] When hypokalemia is detected, a diagnostic workup that evaluates the patient's comorbid disease states and concomitant medications should be initiated. Hypokalemia is virtually nonexistent in healthy adults. This is due in part to the relatively high potassium content in the typical Western diet as well as the body's effective potassium-sparing mechanisms, which tightly regulate the serum potassium concentration. However it has been estimated that as many as 50% of patients who receive thiazide or loop diuretics have serum potassium concentrations less than 3.5 mEq/L (3.5 mmol/L).[13]

While hypokalemia may be thought of as merely a laboratory abnormality, there are serious potential consequences associated with persistent hypokalemia. Recent data suggest that hypokalemia increases mortality in patients with chronic heart failure and in those with CKD, a population typically thought to be more sensitive to the effects of hyperkalemia.[14] In fact, even mild hypokalemia in patients with CKD appears to confer a greater risk of dying compared with those with mild to moderate hyperkalemia.[15]

Etiology and Pathophysiology

Hypokalemia results when there is a total-body potassium deficit, or when serum potassium is shifted into the intracellular compartment. Total-body deficits occur in the setting of poor dietary intake of potassium, or when there are excessive renal and GI losses of potassium. Maintaining a consistent dietary intake of potassium is important because the body has no effective method for storing potassium. At steady state, potassium excretion matches potassium intake; approximately 90% of ingested potassium is renally excreted, whereas 10% is excreted in feces.[10] This underscores the importance of eating a well-balanced diet. Elderly patients with chronic diseases and those undergoing surgery are at increased risk for developing hypokalemia because of insufficient intake or losses resulting from surgery.

Many drugs can cause hypokalemia by a variety of mechanisms including intracellular potassium shifting and increased renal or stool losses (Table 36-1). The most common cause of drug-induced hypokalemia is loop and thiazide diuretic administration as these agents inhibit renal sodium reabsorption, which results in increased sodium delivery to the distal tubule. Consequently, hypokalemia develops because the distal tubule selectively reabsorbs sodium, and excretes potassium down its concentration gradient. Second, because diuretics result in volume contraction, aldosterone is secreted that further promotes the renal excretion of potassium. If concomitant potassium supplements are not provided to patients receiving loop and thiazide diuretics, mild to moderate hypokalemia is inevitable.

The second most common etiology of hypokalemia is excessive loss of potassium-rich GI fluid as a result of diarrhea and/or vomiting. The typical potassium loss in feces is approximately 10 mEq (10 mmol) per day.[8] In diarrheal states, this amount increases proportionally with the volume of stool output. Vomiting also accounts for substantial potassium losses, which have been

TABLE 36-1 Mechanism of Drug-Induced Hypokalemia

Transcellular Shift	Enhanced Renal Excretion	Enhanced Fecal Elimination
β_2-Receptor agonists	**Diuretics**	**Laxatives**
Epinephrine	Acetazolamide	Sodium polystyrene sulfonate
Albuterol	Thiazides	Phenolphthalein
Terbutaline	Indapamide	Sorbitol
Fomoterol	Metolazone	
Salmeterol	Furosemide	
Isoproterenol	Torsemide	
Ephedrine	Bumetanide	
Pseudoephedrine	Ethacrynic acid	
Tocolytic agents	**High-dose penicillins**	
Ritodrine	Nafcillin	
Nylidrin	Ampicillin	
Theophylline	Penicillin	
Caffeine	**Mineralocorticoids**	
Insulin overdose	**Miscellaneous**	
	Aminoglycosides	
	Amphotericin B	
	Cisplatin	

estimated to be as high as 30 to 50 mEq (30 to 50 mmol) per liter of vomitus.[13] Metabolic alkalosis can also occur in cases of severe diarrhea and vomiting as a result of loss of these bicarbonate-rich fluids. This causes an intracellular shifting of potassium, which lowers the serum concentration of potassium even further. Prolonged diarrhea and vomiting can significantly affect children and elderly patients because their kidneys are unable to effectively maintain adequate fluid status.

❷ Hypomagnesemia, which is present in more than 50% of cases of clinically significant hypokalemia, contributes to the development of hypokalemia because it reduces the intracellular potassium concentration and promotes renal potassium wasting.[16] While the precise mechanism of the accelerated renal loss is unknown, many believe that the intracellular potassium concentration may decrease because hypomagnesemia impairs the function of the Na^+-K^+-ATPase pump thereby promoting K^+ wasting. Alternatively, the combination of increased sodium delivery to the distal tubule, elevated aldosterone concentrations, and hypomagnesemia may cause the renal outer medullary potassium channels to excrete potassium.[16] What is clear is that hypokalemia and hypomagnesemia often coexist as a result of drugs (diuretic administration) or disease states (diarrhea). When concomitant hypokalemia and hypomagnesemia occur, the magnesium deficiency should be corrected first, otherwise full repletion of the potassium deficit is difficult.

TREATMENT

Desired Outcome

The goals of hypokalemia management are to prevent and/or treat serious life-threatening complications, normalize the serum potassium concentration, identify and correct the underlying cause of hypokalemia, and finally prevent overcorrection of the serum potassium concentration.

General Approach to Therapy

The general approach to therapy depends on the degree and rapidity with which hypokalemia developed and the presence of symptoms. Serum potassium concentrations between 3.5 and 4 mEq/L (3.5 and 4 mmol/L) are a sign of early potassium depletion. No pharmacologic therapy is recommended at this point; however, these patients should be encouraged to increase their dietary intake of potassium-rich foods. When the serum potassium concentration is between 3 and 3.5 mEq/L (3 and 3.5 mmol/L), the patient's concomitant conditions and therapies will largely determine whether pharmacologic therapy should be initiated. Oral potassium supplementation should be initiated in patients with underlying cardiac conditions that predispose them to cardiac arrhythmias. This includes patients receiving concomitant digoxin therapy. Patients with serum potassium concentrations below 3 mEq/L (3 mmol/L) should always be treated to achieve values between 4 and 4.5 mEq/L (4 and 4.5 mmol/L). In asymptomatic patients, oral therapy is the preferred route of administration. IV potassium can be necessary in symptomatic patients with severe depletion, or in patients who are intolerant to oral supplementation. In patients with concomitant moderate to severe hypomagnesemia, the magnesium deficit should be corrected before potassium supplementation.[10,12]

CLINICAL PRESENTATION Hypokalemia

General

- The signs and symptoms of hypokalemia are usually nonspecific and highly variable between patients

Symptoms

- Symptoms are highly dependent on the degree of hypokalemia and its rapidity of onset
- Mild hypokalemia is often asymptomatic
- Moderate hypokalemia is associated with cramping, weakness, malaise, and myalgias

Signs

- Cardiovascular: In severe hypokalemia, ECG changes often include ST-segment depression or flattening, T-wave inversion, and U-wave elevation. Clinical arrhythmias include heart block, atrial flutter, paroxysmal atrial tachycardia, ventricular fibrillation, and digitalis-induced arrhythmias
- Musculoskeletal: Cramping and impaired muscle contraction

Laboratory Tests

- Serum potassium concentration below 3.5 mEq/L (3.5 mmol/L) is diagnostic. Hypomagnesemia (serum magnesium concentration below 1.7 mg/dL [1.4 mEq/L; 0.70 mmol/L]) can also be present

TABLE 36-2 Foods that are High in Potassium

High content (>250 mg/100 g)	Highest content (>1,000 mg/100 g)
Vegetables	Dried figs
Spinach	Molasses
Tomatoes	**Very high content (>500 mg/100 g)**
Broccoli	Dried fruits (dates, prunes)
Squash	Nuts
Beets	Avocados
Cauliflower	Bran cereals
Carrots	Lima beans
Potatoes	
Fruits	
Bananas	
Cantaloupe	
Kiwi	
Oranges	
Mangos	
Meats	
Ground beef	
Steak	
Pork	
Lamb	
Veal	

TABLE 36-3 General Consensus Guidelines for Potassium Replacement

Guideline	Comment
Potassium replacement therapy should accompany dietary consumption of potassium-rich foods	Potassium-rich foods often cannot completely replace potassium associated with chloride losses (vomiting, diuretics, or nasogastric suction) because it is almost entirely coupled to phosphate. Furthermore, increasing dietary intake of these foods can lead to unwanted weight gain
Potassium replacement is recommended for sodium-sensitive and hypertensive patients	A high-sodium diet often results in excessive urinary potassium excretion
Potassium replacement is recommended in patients who are subject to vomiting, diarrhea, or diuretic/laxative abuse	These conditions promote excessive renal and GI potassium loss
Potassium supplementation is best administered orally in divided doses over several days to achieve full repletion	
Laboratory measurement of serum potassium is convenient, but not always accurate	Clinicians should be aware of the factors that result in transcellular potassium shifts. Monitoring 24-hour urinary potassium excretion can be necessary in high-risk patients
Patient adherence to potassium replacement can be increased with compliance-enhancing regimens	Microencapsulated products have no bitter smell or aftertaste and have much better GI tolerance. Regimens should be made as simple as possible to follow
A potassium dosage of 20 mEq/day (20 mmol/day) is usually sufficient to prevent hypokalemia from occurring. Doses of 40–100 mEq (40–100 mmol) are usually sufficient to treat hypokalemia	

Nonpharmacologic Therapy

The best and most abundant source of potassium supplementation comes from dietary sources, in particular, fresh fruits and vegetables, fruit juices, and meats. Table 36-2 lists foods that are excellent sources of potassium. Salt substitutes that contain potassium chloride are another effective, inexpensive source of potassium. Increased dietary intake of foods with high potassium content, however, is not recommended long term because it can add unwanted calories to the patient's diet. Moreover, dietary potassium is almost entirely coupled with phosphate, rather than chloride, so it is not as effective in correcting potassium loss associated with hypochloremic conditions such as vomiting, nasogastric suctioning, and diuretic therapy.

Pharmacologic Therapy

Formal guidelines for potassium supplementation were last published by the National Council on Potassium in Clinical Practice in 2000 (Table 36-3).[17] These guidelines provided a comprehensive framework for potassium administration as a prophylactic and therapeutic replacement in many distinct patient populations. When deciding how to design the optimal regimen, one must consider: (a) the patient's normal baseline potassium concentration; (b) underlying medical conditions that can affect potassium balance; (c) concomitant medications that can affect potassium balance; (d) the patient's dietary and salt intake; and (e) the patient's ability to comply with the therapeutic regimen.[17]

A general rule for potassium replacement is that for every 1 mEq/L (1 mmol/L) decrease of potassium below 3.5 mEq/L (3.5 mmol/L), there is a corresponding total-body potassium deficit of 100 to 400 mEq (100 to 400 mmol). Because of the wide variance in projected deficits, each patient's therapy must be individualized and adjustments made on the basis of the patient's signs, symptoms, and frequent measurements of serum potassium. In patients receiving chronic loop or thiazide diuretic therapy, 40 to 100 mEq (40 to 100 mmol) of oral potassium supplementation can correct mild to moderate potassium deficits. Doses up to 120 mEq (120 mmol) can be required in more severe deficiencies. When providing oral potassium supplementation, the total daily dose should be divided into three to four doses to minimize the development of GI side effects. Patients receiving diuretics can become chronically hypokalemic and can benefit from combination potassium-sparing diuretic therapy.

3 Whenever possible, potassium supplementation should be administered by mouth. Three salts are available for oral potassium supplementation: chloride, phosphate, and bicarbonate. Potassium phosphate should be used when patients are both hypokalemic and hypophosphatemic; potassium bicarbonate is most commonly used when potassium depletion occurs in the setting of metabolic acidosis. Potassium chloride, however, is the primary salt form used because it is the most effective treatment for the most common causes of potassium depletion (i.e., diuretic-induced and diarrhea-induced) as these conditions are associated with potassium and chloride losses.

Potassium chloride can be administered in either tablet or liquid formulations (Table 36-4). The liquid forms are generally less expensive; however, patient compliance can be low because of their strong, unpleasant taste. Two sustained-release solid dosage forms are currently available in the United States: a wax-matrix formulation, and a microencapsulated formulation. The microencapsulated tablet is generally preferred because it disintegrates better in the stomach and is associated with less GI irritation. IV potassium use should be limited to: (a) severe cases of hypokalemia (serum

TABLE 36-4 Differentiation of Available Potassium Supplements

Supplement	Comment
Controlled-release microencapsulated tablet	Disintegrates better in GI tract; fewer GI erosions as compared to wax-matrix tablets
Encapsulated controlled-release microencapsulated particles	Fewer erosions as compared to wax-matrix tablets
Potassium chloride elixir	Inexpensive, poor taste, poor compliance, immediate effect
Potassium chloride effervescent tablets for solution	More expensive than elixir, convenient
Wax-matrix extended-release tablets	Easier to swallow; more GI erosions as compared to other therapies

concentration <2.5 mEq/L [<2.5 mmol/L]); (b) patients exhibiting signs and symptoms of hypokalemia such as electrocardiogram (ECG) changes or muscle spasms; or (c) patients unable to tolerate oral therapy. IV supplementation is more dangerous than oral therapy because it is more likely to result in hyperkalemia, phlebitis, and pain at the site of infusion.

The vehicle in which IV potassium is administered is important. Whenever possible, potassium should be prepared in saline-containing solutions (e.g., 0.9% or 0.45% sodium chloride [NaCl]). Dextrose-containing solutions stimulate insulin secretion, which can cause intracellular shifting of potassium, worsening the patient's hypokalemia, and should be avoided whenever possible. Generally, 10 to 20 mEq (10 to 20 mmol) of potassium is diluted in 100 mL 0.9% NaCl for IV administration. These concentrations are safe when administered through a peripheral vein over 1 hour. When infusion rates exceed 10 mEq/h (10 mmol/h) ECG monitoring should be performed to detect cardiac changes. The serum potassium concentration should be evaluated following the infusion of each 30 to 40 mEq (30 to 40 mmol) to direct further potassium replacement requirements. Multiple doses of potassium can be repeated as needed until the serum potassium concentration normalizes. To allow adequate time for the potassium to equilibrate between the intra- and extracellular spaces, the clinician should wait at least 30 minutes from the end of each infusion before obtaining a serum concentration. Care should be taken to avoid sampling from the same line in which the potassium was infused, as this can result in a spuriously high potassium concentration.

In cases of severe potassium depletion, patients can require as much as 300 to 400 mEq/day (300 to 400 mmol/day). In this instance, it is common practice to dilute 40 to 60 mEq (40 to 60 mmol) in 1,000 mL 0.45% NaCl and infuse at a rate not exceeding 40 mEq/h (40 mmol/h). This should be performed in an intensive care unit under continuous ECG monitoring. Because of the high potassium concentration, and the risk for burning pain and peripheral venous sclerosis, the infusion should be through a central venous catheter into a large vein (e.g., superior vena cava) but care must be taken not to place the tip of the catheter into the right atrium.[18] Directly delivering high potassium concentrations into the heart can result in cardiac arrhythmias. Given the volume required to infuse this dose of potassium, this infusion strategy might be impractical in certain clinical situations (e.g., patients requiring fluid restriction). A reasonable approach is to split the potassium dose between the oral and IV routes. For example, if a symptomatic patient requires 120 mEq (120 mmol) of potassium, the clinician can give 60 mEq (60 mmol) as the immediate-release potassium liquid, and the other 60 mEq (60 mmol) can be given through the IV route (20 mEq/100 mL/h [20 mmol/100 mL/h] in three doses). When giving large potassium doses, serum monitoring should be performed following the administration of half the dose to guide the clinician as to the need for additional potassium. This can also help avoid the development of hyperkalemia.

In the rare circumstances when cardiac arrest from hypokalemia is imminent, IV bolus dosing of potassium 10 mEq (10 mmol) over 5 minutes can be initiated and repeated once, if necessary.[18]

Alternative Therapies

Potassium-sparing diuretics are an alternative to chronic exogenous potassium supplementation, especially when patients are concomitantly receiving drugs that are known to deplete potassium (e.g., diuretics or amphotericin B). Spironolactone inhibits the effect of aldosterone in the distal convoluted tubule, thereby decreasing potassium elimination in the urine. Spironolactone is especially effective as a potassium-sparing agent in patients with primary or secondary hyperaldosteronism. Amiloride and triamterene act by an aldosterone-independent mechanism; however, the precise mechanism of their potassium sparing is unknown.

Spironolactone is available as 25-, 50-, and 100-mg tablets. The usual starting dose is 25 to 50 mg daily, and can be titrated to a maximum dose of 400 mg/day. The potassium-retaining effects generally take approximately 48 hours to occur. Important side effects include hyperkalemia, gynecomastia, breast tenderness, and impotence in men. Triamterene is available as 50- and 100-mg capsules. The usual starting dose is 50 mg twice daily, which can be titrated to 100 mg twice daily. Triamterene 50 mg is available as a combination product with hydrochlorothiazide 25 mg and is commonly used for the treatment of hypertension. Common side effects include hyperkalemia, sodium depletion, and metabolic acidosis. Amiloride is available as a 5-mg tablet. The usual starting dose is 5 mg daily; however, 10 mg can be given in those with severe hypokalemia. This is also available as a combination product with hydrochlorothiazide 50 mg. The most common side effects are hyperkalemia and metabolic acidosis.

Concomitant use of potassium supplementation with potassium-sparing diuretics is not necessary. There is a significant risk of hyperkalemia during combination therapy, especially in patients with underlying renal insufficiency or diabetes mellitus.

Evaluation of Therapeutic Outcomes

Serum potassium concentrations should be monitored regularly while the patient is receiving potassium supplementation. For patients receiving prophylactic potassium supplementation during diuretic therapy, the serum potassium and magnesium concentrations, as well as renal function should be monitored every 1 to 2 months in stable patients. In hospitalized patients receiving oral therapy for mild hypokalemia, the potassium concentration should be monitored every 2 to 3 days. Generally, the potassium concentration begins to increase within 72 hours. If it does not increase by at least 1 mEq/L (1 mmol/L) within 96 hours, the clinician should suspect concomitant magnesium depletion. Patients receiving IV potassium supplementation require close ECG monitoring if the infusion rate is greater than 20 mEq/h (20 mmol/h): doses greater than this should be administered only in the presence of continuous ECG monitoring. Additionally, the patient should have potassium concentrations obtained halfway through, and 30 minutes following completion of the total potassium dose to guide further potassium dosing. Finally, the patient should be assessed for adverse effects such as pain at the infusion site or phlebitis.

Clinical Bottom Line

Hypokalemia is a frequent medical condition caused by both biological processes as well as drug therapy. While mild hypokalemia is frequently asymptomatic, severe hypokalemia can cause fatal cardiac dysrhythmias, particularly in patients receiving concomitant medications such as digoxin. Patients receiving drugs that cause potassium wasting, e.g., thiazide or loop diuretics, should be closely followed for the development of hypokalemia and appropriate potassium supplementation should be started when necessary. Generally oral potassium is sufficient for mild hypokalemia; IV potassium is reserved for severe deficiency, and its use should be monitored closely.

HYPERKALEMIA

Hyperkalemia, defined as a serum potassium concentration greater than 5 mEq/L (5 mmol/L), can be further classified according to its severity: mild hyperkalemia (5.1 to 5.9 mEq/L [5.1 to 5.9 mmol/L]), moderate hyperkalemia (6 to 7 mEq/L [6 to 7 mmol/L]), and severe hyperkalemia (above 7 mEq/L [7 mmol/L]).[17]

Epidemiology

❹ Hyperkalemia is much less common than hypokalemia. In fact, if all patients with acute and chronic kidney disease were excluded, the true prevalence of hyperkalemia would be insignificant. The incidence of hyperkalemia in hospitalized patients is highly variable, and reports have ranged from 1.4% to 10%.[17] Most cases of hyperkalemia are the result of overcorrection of hypokalemia with IV potassium supplements. Severe hyperkalemia occurs more commonly in elderly patients with renal insufficiency who receive chronic oral potassium supplementation.

Etiology and Pathophysiology

Hyperkalemia develops when potassium intake exceeds excretion (true hyperkalemia) (i.e., elevated total-body stores), or when the transcellular distribution of potassium is disturbed (i.e., normal total-body stores). The four primary causes of hyperkalemia—(a) increased potassium intake, (b) decreased potassium excretion, (c) tubular unresponsiveness to aldosterone, and (d) redistribution of potassium into the extracellular space—are discussed below.

Hyperkalemia Associated with Increased Potassium Intake

Hyperkalemia in this setting is almost always associated with renal insufficiency. Patients with stage 4 or 5 CKD and dialysis patients who are noncompliant with dietary potassium restrictions often present with life-threatening hyperkalemia. Many of these patients do not realize that fresh fruits and vegetables contain large amounts of potassium. Anecdotally, in many dialysis centers the incidence of hyperkalemia peaks during the summer months, when fresh garden produce is available. Another common dietary source associated with the development of hyperkalemia is potassium chloride salt substitutes. Many dialysis patients are instructed to use salt substitutes to avoid excessive sodium intake in an attempt to control volume overload. These patients unwittingly become hyperkalemic because these products contain approximately 10 to 15 mEq (10 to 15 mmol) potassium per gram, or 200 mEq (200 mmol) per tablespoon. Finally, many over-the-counter herbal and alternative medicine products may contain significant concentrations of potassium. It is essential for patients with CKD to receive education regarding dietary sources of potassium as well as information on the potassium content of herbal products because the ingestion of these can lead to hyperkalemia.

Hyperkalemia Associated with Decreased Renal Potassium Excretion

Normally functioning kidneys excrete 80% of the daily potassium intake. Therefore, when the kidney is unable to excrete potassium appropriately, as in acute kidney injury (AKI) and stage 4 to 5 CKD, potassium is retained and often results in hyperkalemia. Finally, many drugs can inhibit the kidney's ability to excrete potassium by inhibiting aldosterone and thus contribute to an increase in serum potassium concentrations.

Severe hyperkalemia is more common in AKI than in CKD because patients are often hypercatabolic and can have underlying disorders, such as rhabdomyolysis or tumor lysis syndrome, which result in release of potassium from injured or lysed cells.[19] Severe hyperkalemia is rare in stable CKD patients, perhaps because of enhanced GI and renal potassium excretion.[20] Data suggest that hyperkalemia directly stimulates renal K^+ excretion through an effect that is independent of, and additive to, that of aldosterone.[20] Although the overall incidence of hyperkalemia is higher in patients with CKD when compared with patients without CKD, due to these adaptive mechanisms and their decreased susceptibility to cardiac effects of chronic hyperkalemia, it has been associated with a lower mortality rate.[21] Renal excretion of potassium is also inhibited by various endocrinologic disorders, including adrenal insufficiency, Addison's disease, and selective hypoaldosteronism. All of these disorders involve a decreased production of aldosterone, which results in the retention of potassium.

Several drugs have profound effects on the kidney's ability to regulate potassium. Five drug classes in particular have specific effects on the kidney: angiotensin-converting enzyme inhibitors (ACEIs), angiotensin-II receptor blockers (ARBs), direct renin inhibitors, potassium-sparing diuretics, and prostaglandin inhibitors such as nonsteroidal antiinflammatory drugs (NSAIDs). Although hyperkalemia with these drugs is typically dose dependent, the rates of hyperkalemia have been reported to range from 5% to 10% in most clinical trials. Other commonly used drugs that can cause hyperkalemia are digoxin, cyclosporine, tacrolimus, trimethoprim–sulfamethoxazole, heparin, and pentamidine.

Tubular Unresponsiveness to Aldosterone

Certain medical conditions, such as sickle cell anemia, systemic lupus erythematosus, and amyloidosis, can produce a defect in tubular potassium secretion, possibly as the result of an alteration in the aldosterone-binding site.

Redistribution of Potassium into the Extracellular Space

The efflux of potassium from within the cell into the extracellular fluid, which is associated with no change in total-body potassium stores, is to be expected in the presence of metabolic acidosis, diabetes mellitus, chronic renal failure, or lactic acidosis. *β*-Blockers can also result in a transcellular potassium shift.

The serum potassium concentration can also be falsely elevated in some conditions, and not reflect the actual in vivo potassium concentration, that is, pseudohyperkalemia. Pseudohyperkalemia occurs most commonly in the setting of extravascular hemolysis of red blood cells. When a blood specimen is not processed promptly and cellular destruction occurs, intracellular potassium is released into the serum. It can also occur in conditions of thrombocytosis or leukocytosis. If severe hyperkalemia is found in a patient who is asymptomatic with an otherwise normal laboratory report, the hyperkalemia is most likely pseudohyperkalemia, and a repeat blood sample should be evaluated. Truly elevated

CLINICAL PRESENTATION Hyperkalemia

General

- Related to the effects of excessive potassium on neuromuscular, cardiac, and smooth muscle cell function

Symptoms

- Frequently asymptomatic
- The patient might complain of heart palpitations or skipped heartbeats

Signs

- ECG changes (see Fig. 36-1 for description)

Laboratory Tests

- Serum potassium concentration above 5.5 mEq/L (5.5 mmol/L)

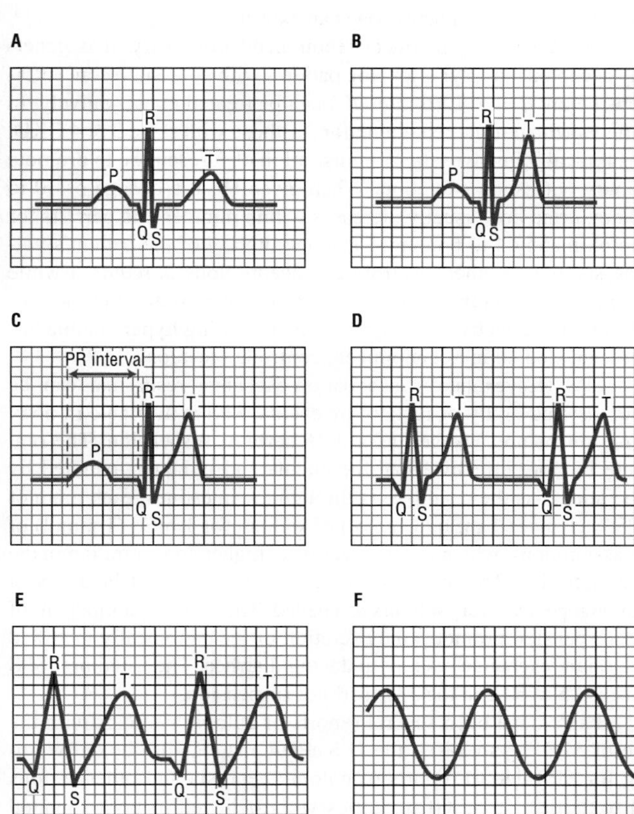

FIGURE 36-1 The earliest electrocardiographic manifestation of hyperkalemia is an increase in the rate of ventricular repolarization, which results in a peaking of the T wave at serum potassium concentrations of ~5.5 to 6 mEq/L (~5.5 to 6 mmol/L) (*B*), relative to the normal ECG presentation (*A*). Further increases in the serum potassium concentration above 6 mEq/L (6 mmol/L) result in conduction delays through the His-Purkinje system, the atrial myocardium, and the ventricular myocardium. The ECG manifestations of these conduction delays and the sequence in which they occur are a widening of the PR interval (*C*), delay through the His-Purkinje system, a loss of the P wave (*D*), delay through the atrial myocardium, a widening of the QRS complex (*E*), and delay through the ventricular myocardium. Finally, there is a merging of the QRS complex with the T wave (*F*), which results in a sine-wave appearance.

potassium concentrations are normally associated with other laboratory abnormalities, such as low carbon dioxide (acidosis) or elevated blood urea nitrogen and creatinine concentrations (indicating renal insufficiency).

TREATMENT

Desired Outcome

The goals of therapy for the treatment of hyperkalemia are to antagonize adverse cardiac effects, reverse signs and symptoms that are present, and return the serum and total-body stores of potassium to normal. The design of the treatment approach is determined by the severity of hyperkalemia, the rapidity of its development, and the patient's clinical condition. Although ECG changes are directly proportional to the plasma potassium concentration and its rate of increase, they may not be present in all patients. In contrast, ventricular fibrillation may be the first cardiac manifestation of hyperkalemia in some patients.[22] Asymptomatic patients with mild hyperkalemia usually require no specific therapy other than dietary education to control intake, and monitoring of serum potassium daily if an inpatient or weekly if an outpatient to assure resolution. Severe hyperkalemia (above 7 mEq/L [7 mmol/L]) or moderate hyperkalemia (6 to 6.9 mEq/L [6 to 6.9 mmol/L]), when associated with clinical symptoms or ECG changes, requires immediate treatment. Initial treatment of severe and moderate symptomatic hyperkalemia is focused on antagonism of the cardiac membrane actions of hyperkalemia (e.g., with calcium). Secondarily, one should attempt to decrease extracellular potassium concentration by promoting its intracellular movement (e.g., with glucose, insulin, β_2-receptor agonists, or sodium bicarbonate) or enhance its removal from the body by hemodialysis, the oral administration of cation-exchange resins, and/or the use of loop diuretics. In any case, the underlying cause of hyperkalemia should be identified and reversed, and exogenous potassium must be withheld.

General Approach to Treatment

A general treatment approach for patients with hyperkalemia is outlined in Figure 36-2. In patients who have acute ECG changes, IV calcium should be administered to prevent or treat any cardiac manifestations of hyperkalemia. At the same time, the serum potassium concentration should be rapidly decreased to below 5 mEq/L (5 mmol/L) within minutes by administering drugs that cause an intracellular shift, followed by those that increase the elimination of potassium from the body.[22] If the patient is asymptomatic, rapid correction may not be necessary, and will likely depend on the clinical context associated with the rise in serum potassium concentration. If one anticipates the need to reduce total-body potassium stores, an ion exchange resin (e.g., sodium polystyrene sulfonate [SPS]) that results in removal of potassium from the body over several hours to days may be initiated shortly after the emergent care has been instituted. SPS use is contraindicated in patients with bowel dysfunction.

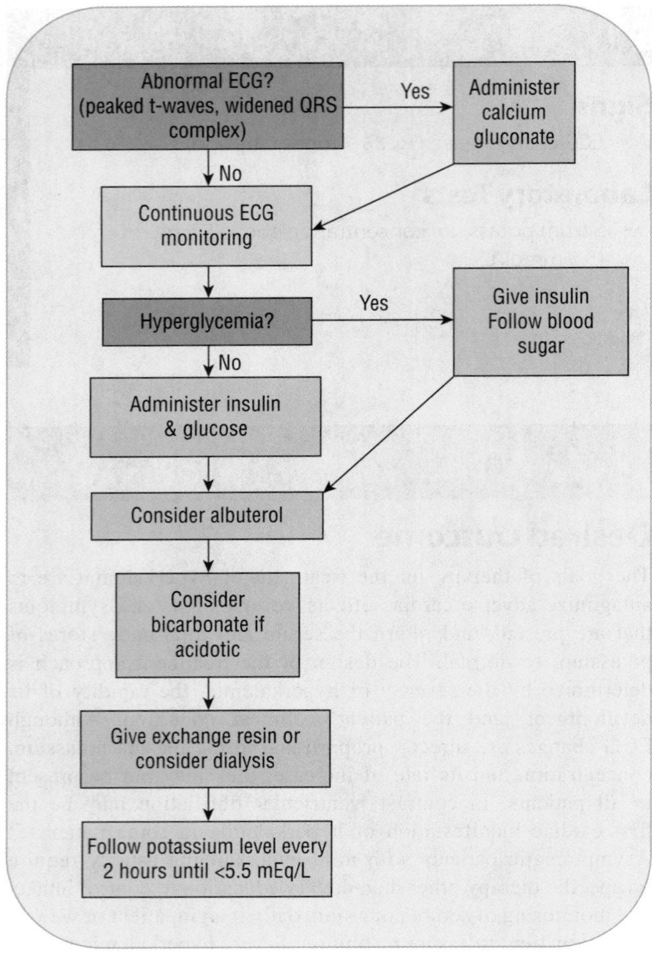

FIGURE 36-2 Treatment approach for hyperkalemia. (Serum potassium of 5.5 mEq/L is equivalent to 5.5 mmol/L.)

Nonpharmacologic Therapy

A recent study suggested that hemodialysis patients who ingested foods supplemented with glycyrrhetinic acid, the active ingredient in licorice, were better able to maintain plasma potassium concentrations within the normal range compared with hemodialysis patients given placebo.[23,24] Glycyrrhetinic acid inhibits the enzyme 11β-hydroxy-steroid dehydrogenase II, thereby increasing cortisol availability in the colon. The net result is enhanced potassium elimination in the feces. Other nonpharmacologic therapies, specifically available for dialysis-dependent patients with end-stage renal disease (ESRD), are the institution of intermittent dialysis or hemofiltration therapy.

Pharmacologic Therapy

Various drug therapies have been used to lower the serum potassium concentration. The optimal regimen for a given patient is dependent on the rapidity and degree of lowering that is necessary. Table 36-5 provides an overview of the available therapies, and their respective onset and duration of action one can expect.

While specific treatment recommendations vary, it is generally accepted that asymptomatic patients with potassium concentrations below 6 mEq/L (6 mmol/L) can be treated conservatively. In patients with normal renal function, or those with stage 3 or 4 CKD, this typically involves the administration of furosemide to promote urinary potassium excretion. When given IV at a dosage of 40 to 80 mg, urine flow usually increases within minutes and persists for approximately 4 to 6 hours. Close monitoring of the patient's volume status and other electrolyte concentrations is required while the patient is receiving furosemide or other loop diuretic therapy. Of note, the effectiveness of diuretics in treating hyperkalemia has not been studied in a randomized, controlled fashion.

SPS (Kayexalate®) is a cation-exchange resin that can be administered orally or rectally by enema. SPS is available in powder form or prepackaged as a 33% sorbitol suspension. The oral route is more effective than the enema and is better tolerated by the patient. As the resin passes through the intestines, each gram of SPS exchanges 1 mEq (1 mmol) of sodium for 1 mEq (1 mmol) of potassium ions, which are in a relatively higher concentration in the large intestine. The onset of action of SPS is within 1 hour, and it can be repeated every 4 hours as needed. The sorbitol component of the suspension promotes the excretion of the cationically modified potassium exchange resin by inducing diarrhea. The usual oral SPS dose is 15 to 60 g in the 33% sorbitol suspension.

There have been several reports of colonic necrosis with the use of SPS.[25,26] In 2009, the U.S. FDA mandated a boxed warning for SPS due to reports of colonic necrosis and other serious GI toxicities.[27] The GI toxicities were believed to be associated

TABLE 36-5 Therapeutic Alternatives for the Management of Hyperkalemia

Medication	Dose	Route of Administration	Onset/Duration of Action	Acuity	Mechanism of Action	Expected Result
Calcium	1 g	IV over 5–10 minutes	1–2 min/10–30 min	Acute	Raises cardiac threshold potential	Reverses electrocardiographic effects
Furosemide	20–40 mg	IV	5–15 min/4–6 h	Acute	Inhibits renal Na^+ reabsorption	Increased urinary K^+ loss
Regular insulin	5–10 units	IV or SC	30 min/2–6 h	Acute	Stimulates intracellular K^+ uptake	Intracellular K^+ redistribution
Dextrose 10%	1,000 mL (100 g)	IV over 1–2 hours	30 min/2–6 h	Acute	Stimulates insulin release	Intracellular K^+ redistribution
Dextrose 50%	50 mL (25 g)	IV over 5 minutes	30 min/2–6 h	Acute	Stimulates insulin release	Intracellular K^+ redistribution
Sodium bicarbonate	50–100 mEq (50–100 mmol)	IV over 2–5 minutes	30 min/2–6 h	Acute	Raises serum pH	Intracellular K^+ redistribution
Albuterol	10–20 mg	Nebulized over 10 minutes	30 min/1–2 h	Acute	Stimulates intracellular K^+ uptake	Intracellular K^+ redistribution
Hemodialysis	4 hours	N/A	Immediate/variable	Acute	Removal from serum	Increased K^+ elimination
Sodium polystyrene sulfonate	15–60 g	Oral or rectal	1 h/variable	Nonacute	Resin exchanges Na^+ for K^+	Increased K^+ elimination

with the 70% sorbitol; however, there are also reports of GI toxicity with the 33% sorbitol solution. A common finding in these reports was that toxicity occurred most commonly in patients who recently underwent GI surgery or had a current or previous history of bowel dysfunction. This FDA warning was updated in 2011. A recent commentary provided some needed perspective on the role of SPS in treating hyperkalemia.[28] While the authors echoed the FDA warning, they found little risk to using the SPS 33% sorbitol suspension or SPS powder mixed in water for oral administration. They also noted that necrosis was most commonly found when SPS was administered as a retention enema in patients who had recent GI surgery, or bowel dysfunction. These authors recommended that the retention enema route of administration be abandoned given the risk of side effects and the fact that the enema route appears to be less effective compared with oral administration.

In symptomatic patients, or in those with severe hyperkalemia, emergency care is indicated. Initial therapy in this setting is the administration of IV calcium chloride or gluconate 1 g to protect the heart from life-threatening arrhythmias.[22] Calcium antagonizes the cardiac membrane effect of hyperkalemia by reducing the electrical threshold potential for cardiac myocytes and reverses ECG changes within minutes. IV calcium should not be given to patients receiving digoxin as it can lead to digoxin toxicity. Its duration of action is 30 to 60 minutes, and it can be repeated as needed based on ECG findings. IV calcium can be given as either the chloride or gluconate salt; each is available as a 10% solution by weight. Calcium chloride provides approximately three times more calcium than equal volumes of the gluconate salt; however, it can cause tissue necrosis if extravasation occurs. For this reason, calcium gluconate is more commonly administered, with the standard dose being 10-mL IV bolus over 5 to 10 minutes.

Rapid correction of hyperkalemia may necessitate the administration of drugs that result in an intracellular shift of potassium, such as insulin and dextrose, sodium bicarbonate, and a β_2-adrenergic receptor agonist (e.g., albuterol or terbutaline). The treatment of choice depends on the underlying medical disorders accompanying hyperkalemia. For example, in patients with concomitant metabolic acidosis, a sodium bicarbonate bolus or infusion of 50 to 100 mEq (50 to 100 mmol) is the preferred therapy (see Chap. 37 for additional information). Sodium bicarbonate helps us to correct the metabolic acidosis by raising the extracellular pH, in addition to causing a rapid intracellular potassium shift. It should be noted that sodium bicarbonate is much less effective when hyperkalemia is not related to metabolic acidosis.[1] Sodium bicarbonate is also less effective in patients with ESRD, in whom a decrease in serum potassium may not be seen for as long as 4 hours. Sodium bicarbonate can also lead to sodium and volume overload in patients with stage 4 or 5 CKD. Administration of a fast-acting (e.g., Insulin Lispro) or regular insulin (5 to 10 units IV and dextrose (10% or 50%) is an effective method of reducing potassium. Insulin increases the activity of the Na^+-K^+-ATPase pump, thereby intracellularly shifting potassium. Glucose should be given with insulin unless the serum glucose is above 250 mg/dL (13.9 mmol/L) because hypoglycemia can develop as a result of the effects of the insulin therapy. An IV bolus of 10 units of regular insulin and 25 g of dextrose usually lowers the serum potassium concentration by 0.6 mEq/L (0.6 mmol/L) in dialysis-dependent patients.[22] β_2-Adrenergic agonists have a dual mechanism for lowering serum potassium. First, they stimulate the Na^+-K^+-ATPase pump to promote intracellular potassium uptake. Second, they stimulate pancreatic β-receptors to increase insulin secretion. Albuterol can be administered via IV (0.5 mg given over 15 minutes) or via nebulizer (10 to 20 mg nebulized over 10 minutes); however, it should be noted that injectable albuterol is not available in the United States. In ESRD patients, decreases in plasma potassium concentration of 0.6 mEq/L (0.6 mmol/L) and 1 mEq/L (1 mmol/L) can be anticipated after inhalation of 10 and 20 mg of albuterol, respectively. Of note, the doses of inhaled albuterol used for hyperkalemia are at least four times higher than those typically used for bronchospasm. There are important limitations with albuterol therapy, most notably variable bioavailability via the inhaled route (leading to potential over- or under-dosing and unpredictability of response) and second, cardiac side effects such as tachycardia, which are undesirable in patients who already have an abnormal ECG. Furthermore, as many as 40% of patients may be resistant to the hypokalemic effects of albuterol and patients already receiving a nonselective β_2-receptor antagonist may not respond. Therefore, albuterol should not be used alone for the urgent treatment of hyperkalemia in CKD patients.[22] The use of subcutaneous terbutaline has also been shown to be effective in a small group of dialysis patients with hyperkalemia.[29]

A Cochrane Review evaluated the emergency treatment of hyperkalemia.[30] Many of the reviewed studies were small, and not all intervention groups had sufficient data for meta-analysis to be performed. However, given these limitations, inhaled and nebulized β-agonists, and IV insulin-and-glucose were all deemed effective. The combination of nebulized β-agonists with IV insulin and glucose appeared to be more effective than either agent alone. The meta-analysis results were equivocal for IV bicarbonate, and notably, SPS was not effective by 4 hours.

A major problem with drawing conclusions from this meta-analysis is the heterogeneity of the study population. Most of the data were from nonrandomized, noncontrolled observational studies and case reports. Doses of the drugs were not standardized and follow-up was often lacking. Therefore, the clinician should exercise caution when extrapolating these findings to his or her clinical practice. This underscores the need for clinicians to be able to interpret the limitations of the published literature. Nonetheless, the Cochrane database review corroborates the approach detailed in Figure 36-2.

Clinical **Controversy...**

SPS is commonly prescribed to both inpatients and outpatients for the management of hyperkalemia. Recent data, however, question its clinical effectiveness. Also, emerging data suggest its use may be associated with GI necrosis, especially in patients who recently underwent GI surgery or have current bowel injury.

Evaluation of Therapeutic Outcomes

The evaluation of therapeutic outcomes differs based on the severity of hyperkalemia. For example, mild or moderate asymptomatic hyperkalemia is observed much more frequently compared with symptomatic, severe hyperkalemia. Many drugs such as ACEIs, ARBs, direct renin inhibitors, and spironolactone result in asymptomatic hyperkalemia. In patients with normal renal function, once these drugs are initiated and the dose titrated, clinicians should check the potassium concentration at least monthly. For those patients with renal dysfunction, monitoring should be more frequent, such as biweekly until the dose is stabilized. In the case where the patient has been on a stable dose for a long period of time and hyperkalemia develops, the clinician should attempt to downward titrate the dose or switch to another medication without hyperkalemia as a side effect (e.g., calcium channel blocker).

In patients who have acute symptomatic hyperkalemia (e.g., ECG changes), frequent potassium concentration and ECG monitoring is warranted. The patient should receive continuous ECG telemetry monitoring until the serum potassium concentration decreases below 5 mEq/L (5 mmol/L), and the ECG abnormalities resolve. Similarly, while the patient is receiving emergent therapy, serial serum potassium concentrations should be obtained hourly until the potassium concentration decreases below 5 mEq/L (5 mmol/L). For patients who receive insulin and dextrose therapy for hyperkalemia, blood glucose monitoring should be performed hourly or more frequently if patients demonstrate signs and symptoms of hypoglycemia. For patients who receive large doses of sodium bicarbonate therapy for hyperkalemia, an arterial blood gas or serum chemistry profile should be obtained to assess their acid–base status. Furthermore, the patient should be evaluated for signs of fluid overload secondary to the high sodium load. Patients receiving albuterol or terbutaline therapy should be questioned regularly regarding the development of palpitations and tachycardia. The patient's medication records should be reviewed to assure the patient is not receiving drug therapy that increases the serum potassium concentration. Furthermore, the patient should be questioned regarding the occurrence of diarrheal stool output.

Clinical Bottom Line

Hyperkalemia commonly occurs in patients with reduced kidney function or other metabolic disturbances. It can rapidly evolve into a medical emergency; therefore, prompt identification and appropriate pharmacotherapy is needed. In patients with mild hyperkalemia, potassium binding resins or loop diuretics may be useful, and should be used as first-line therapy. In severe hyperkalemia with ECG changes, IV calcium should be given to protect against cardiac dysrhythmias. Additionally rapid-acting therapies such as IV insulin and dextrose are indicated to move potassium intracellularly.

DISORDERS OF MAGNESIUM HOMEOSTASIS

Magnesium plays a central role in cellular function and is an important cofactor in more than 300 biochemical reactions in the body, especially those systems that are dependent on adenosine triphosphate. Mitochondrial function, protein synthesis, cell membrane function, parathyroid hormone (PTH) secretion, and glucose metabolism are just a few important functions affected by magnesium.[31] It is the fourth most abundant extracellular cation and the second most abundant intracellular cation, after potassium. Disorders of magnesium homeostasis are commonly encountered in clinical situations and most frequently are manifested as alterations in cardiovascular and neuromuscular function. Life-threatening conditions such as paralysis and cardiac arrhythmias can occur, making the proper recognition and treatment of these problems of paramount importance. Altered magnesium balance also plays a key role in chronic disease states such as diabetes mellitus, CKD, osteoporosis, development of kidney stones, as well as heart and vascular disease.[32]

Magnesium is principally distributed in bone (67%) and muscle (20%). Because of its predominantly intracellular distribution, measurement of magnesium in the extracellular compartment may not accurately reflect the total-body magnesium content. The majority of magnesium in the extracellular fluid is in the ionized form as only 20% is bound to serum proteins. The normal range for serum magnesium is 1.4 to 1.8 mEq/L [1.7 to 2.3 mg/dL or 0.70 to 0.95 mmol/L].

The recommended daily dietary magnesium intake for adults is approximately 420 mg/day and 320 mg/day for men and women, respectively. The maintenance of magnesium homeostasis depends on the balance between intake and output. Thirty percent to 40% of ingested magnesium is absorbed in the small bowel. The absorption of magnesium decreases as the dietary intake increases. Reductions in absorption have also been noted in the elderly and those with CKD. A small amount is present in intestinal secretions and reabsorbed in the sigmoid colon. The kidneys play a major role in maintaining magnesium balance. Approximately 95% of the filtered magnesium is reabsorbed, thus in most patients less than 5% is excreted in the urine.[32] Renal magnesium handling is unique in that approximately 20% of the filtered magnesium is reabsorbed in the proximal tubule; the majority of reabsorption occurs in the thick ascending limb of the loop of Henle. This explains why loop diuretics often cause profound urinary magnesium wasting. Unlike most other important electrolytes, there is no hormonal regulation of the distribution of magnesium between bone and circulating or intracellular magnesium pools. Because of this, both hypomagnesemia and hypermagnesemia commonly occur.

HYPOMAGNESEMIA

Epidemiology

Hypomagnesemia is a common problem in both ambulatory and hospitalized patients. Although the exact prevalence is difficult to estimate, it has been reported that up to 65% of intensive care unit patients are magnesium deficient. Although serum magnesium concentrations are not a reliable index of total-body magnesium content, they remain the primary diagnostic tool to evaluate body stores.

Etiology and Pathophysiology

5 Hypomagnesemia is usually associated with disorders of the intestinal tract or kidney.[33] Drugs or conditions that interfere with intestinal absorption or increase renal excretion of magnesium can result in hypomagnesemia (Table 36-6). Decreased intestinal absorption as a result of small bowel disease is the most common cause of hypomagnesemia worldwide. These disorders include regional enteritis; radiation enteritis; ulcerative colitis; acute and chronic diarrhea; pancreatic insufficiency and other malabsorptive syndromes; small-bowel bypass surgery; and chronic laxative abuse. Hypomagnesemia is commonly associated with alcoholism. The etiology is often multifactorial, including reduced intake, pancreatic insufficiency, chronic vomiting and diarrhea, and urinary magnesium wasting. In addition, patients who are hospitalized for acute alcohol withdrawal often receive IV glucose and can experience even greater reductions in their serum magnesium concentration.

Primary renal magnesium wasting can be caused by a defect in renal tubular magnesium reabsorption, or inhibition of sodium reabsorption in those segments in which magnesium transport follows passively. The former condition is associated with hypercalciuria, nephrolithiasis, and progressive renal disease, while the latter is associated with Gitelman's and Bartter's syndromes.[33] Much more common than these is renal magnesium wasting secondary to thiazide and loop diuretics. Other commonly used drugs that can cause renal magnesium wasting include aminoglycosides, amphotericin B, cyclosporine, digoxin, tacrolimus, cisplatin, pentamidine, and foscarnet.

TREATMENT

Desired Outcome

The treatment goals in the management of hypomagnesemia are (a) resolution of the signs and symptoms, (b) restoration of normal magnesium concentrations, (c) correction of concomitant electrolyte

TABLE 36-6 Causes of Hypomagnesemia

GI
Reduced intake
Protein-calorie malnutrition
Prolonged parenteral fluid administration without magnesium
Alcoholism
Reduced absorption
Primary hypomagnesemia
Malabsorption syndromes (e.g., tropical sprue, celiac disease, radiation enteritis, or intestinal lymphectasia)
Short-bowel syndrome (e.g., small-bowel resection or ileal bypass)
Pancreatic insufficiency
Increased loss
Excessive vomiting
Prolonged nasogastric suction
Excessive laxative use
Intestinal and biliary fistulas
Prolonged diarrhea (ulcerative colitis, Crohn's disease, or cancer of the colon)
Renal
Primary tubular disorders
Primary renal magnesium wasting
Bartter's syndrome
Renal tubular acidosis
Diuretic phase of acute tubular necrosis
Postobstructive dieresis
Postrenal transplant dieresis
Glomerulonephritis
Pyelonephritis
Drug-induced renal losses
Aminoglycosides
Amphotericin B
Cyclosporine
Tacrolimus
Diuretics
Digitalis
Cisplatin
Pentamidine
Forscarnet
Hormone-induced renal losses
Primary hyperparathyroidism
Hyperthyroidism
Aldosteronism
"Hungry bone syndrome" after parathyroidectomy
Internal redistribution
Diabetic ketoacidosis
Glucose, amino acid, or insulin administration
Massive blood transfusion (citrate)
Pancreatitis with lipidemia (magnesium soap)
Other
Excessive sweating and lactation
Hypercalcemia and hypercalciuria
Phosphate depletion
Chronic alcoholism
Extracellular fluid volume expansion

abnormalities, and (d) identification and correction of the underlying cause of magnesium depletion.

General Approach to Treatment

Nearly all of the data regarding magnesium replacement therapy have been derived from relatively old data in acutely ill, hospitalized patients. Magnesium supplementation can be given by the oral, intramuscular (IM), or IV route. The severity of the magnesium depletion and the presence of severe signs and symptoms should dictate the route of administration. Because IM administration is painful, it should be reserved for those patients with severe hypomagnesemia and limited venous access. IV bolus administration is associated with flushing, sweating, and a sensation of warmth; thus bolus administration should be avoided if possible. Additionally, because calcium forms a complex with the sulfate moiety, which is then excreted, large amounts of IV magnesium sulfate should be administered with caution to hypocalcemic patients, as it can further exacerbate calcium deficiency.[32] There have been no clinical trials assessing the optimal regimen for magnesium replacement; however, it is widely accepted that 8 to 12 g of magnesium sulfate be administered in the first 24 hours followed by 4 to 6 g per day for 3 to 5 days to adequately replete body stores.[34] Even if severe magnesium depletion is present, approximately 50% of the administered dose is excreted in the urine. Consequently, magnesium replacement should be performed over 3 to 5 days, and continued supplementation should be provided for patients unable to eat and for those patients with continued magnesium wasting. Table 36-7 lists the commonly used magnesium oral supplements and their respective elemental magnesium content.

Nonpharmacologic Therapy

There are currently no nonpharmacologic options for the management of hypomagnesaemia.

Pharmacologic Therapy

It is currently controversial whether all asymptomatic patients require magnesium supplementation. However, should treatment be warranted, those patients with serum magnesium concentrations greater than 1 mEq/L (1.2 mg/dL [0.5 mmol/L]) can be treated with oral supplements. Oral supplementation is preferred because magnesium uptake is a slow process that may require prolonged administration. Several magnesium products are available, including magnesium-containing antacids or laxatives, comprised of a variety of magnesium salts in tablet or capsule formulations. Many of the oral products contain very little magnesium, which necessitates three or four doses per day. As expected, diarrhea is the most

CLINICAL PRESENTATION Hypomagnesemia

General

- The dominant organ systems affected by hypomagnesemia are the neuromuscular and cardiovascular systems

Symptoms

- Neuromuscular symptoms such as tetany, twitching, and generalized convulsions are common
- Cardiac symptoms include heart palpitations

Signs

- Neuromuscular: Presence of Chvostek's sign, Trousseau's sign, tremor, and tetany
- Cardiovascular: Cardiac arrhythmias (ventricular fibrillation, torsade de pointes, or digoxin-induced arrhythmias), sudden cardiac death, and hypertension can be present. ECG abnormalities include widened QRS complex and peaked T waves with mild hypomagnesemia; and prolonged PR interval, progressive widening of QRS complex, and flattened T waves with moderate to severe hypomagnesemia

Laboratory Tests

- Serum magnesium concentration less than 1.4 mEq/L (1.7 mg/dL [0.70 mmol/L]). Serum potassium and calcium concentrations can also be low

TABLE 36-7 Common Magnesium Products and Their Elemental Magnesium Content

Product	Elemental Magnesium Content
Magnesium oxide	242 mg in a 400-mg tablet
Magnesium hydroxide	167 mg in a 400-mg tablet or 5-mL oral suspension
Magnesium chloride	143 mg tablet
Magnesium citrate	48 mg in the 290 mg/5 mL oral solution
Magnesium gluconate	27 mg in a 500-mg tablet
Magnesium lactate	84 mg in an 84 mg-tablet

common dose-limiting side effect of oral therapy, which can greatly reduce patient compliance. Therefore, sustained release magnesium products are preferred as they not only improve patient compliance, but also reduce the occurrence of GI side effects.

In cases of severe magnesium depletion (serum concentrations <1 mEq/L [<1.2 mg/dL; <0.5 mmol/L]), or if signs and symptoms are present regardless of the serum concentration, IV magnesium should be administered. A dose of 4 to 6 grams should be administered over 12 to 24 hours and repeated as necessary in order to maintain magnesium concentrations above 1 mEq/L (1.2 mEq [0.5 mmol/L]). Doses of 2 to 4 grams infused over 1 hour are frequently used clinically; however, these result in transient benefit because of the extensive renal excretion. Therapy should be continued until the signs and symptoms have completely resolved. In patients with renal insufficiency, the dose should be reduced by 25% to 50%.

Evaluation of Therapeutic Outcomes

In patients with acute, asymptomatic mild to moderate hypomagnesemia receiving therapy, serum magnesium concentrations should be obtained at least daily during their hospitalization. Patients receiving oral magnesium therapy should be questioned regarding GI tolerance and the occurrence of diarrhea. Patients being treated for symptomatic severe hypomagnesemia should have their serum magnesium concentration monitored hourly until the serum concentration reaches 1.5 mEq/L (1.8 mg/dL [0.75 mmol/L]) and the symptoms resolve. At that point, the serum magnesium concentration can be monitored every 6 to 12 hours for the next 24 hours while receiving magnesium supplementation. Once the magnesium concentration is stable in the normal range, a concentration can be obtained daily. It should be reiterated that it typically takes 3 to 5 days to fully replete total-body magnesium stores. Patients receiving oral magnesium-containing antacids or supplements should be asked regularly about the occurrence of diarrhea.

Clinical Bottom Line

Hypomagnesemia is generally associated with kidney or GI tract disorders. In cases of mild, chronic magnesium loss, oral magnesium preparations can be used; however, the dose-limiting side effect is diarrhea. For more severe cases of hypomagnesemia, IV magnesium sulfate can be safely administered. Repeated doses may be needed as IV magnesium is rapidly eliminated in urine. In such cases, close monitoring of serum magnesium concentrations is needed.

HYPERMAGNESEMIA

Epidemiology

6 Hypermagnesemia (serum magnesium >2 mEq/L [>2.4 mg/dL; >1 mmol/L]) is a rare occurrence that is generally seen in patients with stage 4 or 5 CKD when magnesium intake exceeds the excretory capacity of the kidneys. Elderly patients are prone to hypermagnesemia because of their reduced glomerular filtration rate (GFR) and because of their tendency to consume magnesium-containing antacids and vitamins.

Etiology and Pathophysiology

Because absolute magnesium excretion decreases as GFR declines, serum magnesium concentrations tend to increase in patients with moderate to severe CKD. Indeed, magnesium concentrations steadily increase as the GFR decreases below 30 mL/min/1.73 m^2 (0.29 mL/s/m^2). As long as the patient maintains a normal diet, the serum magnesium concentration typically stabilizes at approximately 2.5 mEq/L (3 mg/dL [1.25 mmol/L]). If patients with stage 4 or 5 CKD are taking concomitant magnesium-containing antacids, the serum concentration can approach 6 mEq/L (7.3 mg/dL [3 mmol/L]), a value associated with signs and symptoms of toxicity. Critically ill patients with multiorgan system failure receiving enteral or parenteral nutrition are also prone to develop hypermagnesemia. Finally, the parenteral treatment of eclampsia with magnesium sulfate can lead to hypermagnesemia. Table 36-8 lists other causes of hypermagnesemia.

Clinical Presentation

The signs and symptoms of hypermagnesemia reflect magnesium's action on the neuromuscular and cardiovascular systems.[34,35] The main symptoms include lethargy, confusion, dysrhythmias, and muscle weakness. Symptoms are rare when the serum concentration is below 4 mEq/L (4.9 mg/dL [2 mmol/L]) (Fig. 36-3).

TREATMENT

Desired Outcome

The goals of therapy are to (a) reverse the neuromuscular and cardiovascular manifestations of hypermagnesemia, (b) decrease the magnesium concentration toward normal values, and (c) identify and treat the underlying cause of hypermagnesemia.

Nonpharmacologic Therapy

There are currently no nonpharmacologic options for the management of hypermagnesemia.

Pharmacologic Therapy

There are three primary means of treating hypermagnesemia: (a) reduce magnesium intake, (b) enhance elimination of magnesium, and (c) antagonize the physiologic effects of magnesium. The

TABLE 36-8 Causes of Hypermagnesemia

Decreased renal excretion
Acute renal failure
CKD with exogenous intake

Excessive intake
Treatment of toxemia of pregnancy
Ureteral irrigants (hemiacidrin)
Cathartics

Other
Lithium therapy
Hypothyroidism
Milk-alkali syndrome
Addison's disease
Viral hepatitis
Acute diabetic ketoacidosis

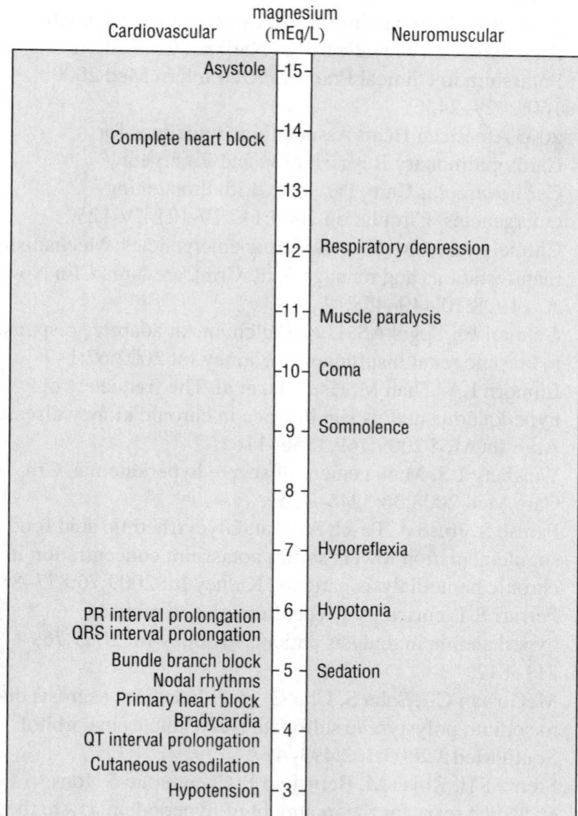

FIGURE 36-3 Clinical findings associated with hypermagnesemia. (Serum magnesium levels in mmol/L can be determined by multiplying the serum magnesium value expressed in mEq/L by 0.5.)

optimal treatment regimen for the management of hypermagnesemia depends on the severity of the patient's signs and symptoms and the degree of serum concentration elevation. IV elemental calcium doses of 100 to 200 mg directly antagonize the neuromuscular and cardiovascular effects of hypermagnesemia. Oral calcium is not effective because of its relatively poor bioavailability and slow onset of action. The clinical effect of calcium is immediate, but the effect is transient; hence, repeated IV doses of 100 to 200 mg of elemental calcium (e.g., 2 g of calcium gluconate) might need to be administered hourly until the signs or symptoms abate and the magnesium concentration is normalized. Supportive care with cardiac pacing, vasopressors, and mechanical ventilation can be necessary in life-threatening situations. In patients with normal renal function, or those with stage 1, 2, or 3 CKD, forced diuresis with 0.45% NaCl and loop diuretics can promote magnesium elimination. An initial IV bolus of furosemide 40 mg or a similar equivalent can be used. Subsequent dosing can be determined based on the patient's clinical response. Patients with CKD can require long-term loop diuretic therapy to maintain adequate fluid and electrolyte balance. In dialysis patients, their hemodialysis prescription should be changed to employ magnesium-free dialysate.

Evaluation of Therapeutic Outcomes

Patients who are receiving IV calcium salts for the treatment of severe, symptomatic hypermagnesemia should have their serum magnesium concentration evaluated hourly until symptoms abate and the magnesium concentration decreases below 4 mg/dL (3.3 mEq/L [1.64 mmol/L]). Furthermore, the patient should be continuously monitored to detect ECG changes. In CKD patients who can produce urine, forced diuresis with saline and furosemide should reduce the serum magnesium concentration within 6 to 12 hours. Close monitoring of the urine output and physical examination for signs of volume overload are important. Emergency hemodialysis will usually correct the hypermagnesemia within 4 hours and is a reasonable option for those who are currently receiving hemodialysis. To prevent further episodes of hypermagnesemia, the patient should receive dietary education regarding foods and beverages that contain large quantities of magnesium (Table 36-9).

TABLE 36-9 Magnesium Content of Selected Foods

Food	Elemental Magnesium Content (mg)
Halibut, cooked, 3 oz (85 g)	90
Almonds, dry roasted, 1 oz (28 g)	80
Cashews, dry roasted, 1 oz (28 g)	75
Spinach, one-half cup (120 mL)	75
Shredded wheat cereal, two biscuits	55
Instant oatmeal, 1 cup (240 mL)	55
Baked potato with skin (medium)	50
Peanuts, dry roasted, 1 oz (28 g)	50
Yogurt, plain, skim milk, 8 oz (227 g)	45
Brown rice, long-grained, one-half cup (120 mL)	40
Banana (medium)	30

Clinical Bottom Line

Hypermagnesemia is generally associated with advanced CKD. Severe cases of hypermagnesium can result in neurologic symptoms or cardiac dysrhythmias. Should these symptoms occur, IV calcium can counteract these effects. Forced diuresis with saline and loop diuretics is useful in lowering magnesium in patients with mild to moderate renal dysfunction; hemodialysis should be reserved for ESRD patients.

PERSONALIZED PHARMACOTHERAPY

As discussed throughout the chapter, there are numerous patient considerations that must be taken into account when designing appropriate pharmacotherapy for potassium and magnesium disorders. At this time, there are no genetic, genomic, or pharmacokinetic factors that are used to personalize pharmacotherapy for the treatment of these electrolyte disorders.

ABBREVIATIONS

ACEI	angiotensin-converting enzyme inhibitor
AKI	acute kidney injury
ARB	angiotensin-II receptor blocker
CKD	chronic kidney disease
ECG	electrocardiogram
ESRD	end-stage renal disease
NSAID	nonsteroidal antiinflammatory drug
PTH	parathyroid hormone
SPS	sodium polystyrene sulfonate

REFERENCES

1. Palmer BF, Dubose TD. Disorders of potassium metabolism. In: Schrier RW, ed. Renal and Electrolyte Disorders, 7th ed. Philadelphia, PA: Lippincott Williams & Wilkins, 2010: 137–165.
2. Schaefer TJ, Wolford RW. Disorders of potassium. Emerg Med Clin North Am 2005;23:723–747.
3. D'Elia L, Barba G, Cappuccio FP, Strazzullo P. Potassium intake, stroke, and cardiovascular disease: A meta-analysis of prospective studies. J Am Coll Cardiol 2011;57:1210–1219.
4. Whelton PK, He J, Appel LJ, et al. Primary prevention of hypertension: Clinical and public health advisory from the National High Blood Pressure Education Program. JAMA 2002;288:1882–1888.
5. Food and Nutrition Board, Institute of Medicine. Panel on Dietary Reference Intakes for Electrolytes and Water. Dietary Reference Intakes for Water, Potassium, Sodium, Chloride, and Sulfate. Washington, DC: National Academies Press, 2005.
6. Adrogue HJ, Madias NE. Sodium and potassium in the pathogenesis of hypertension. N Engl J Med 2007;356: 1966–1978.
7. Greenlee M, Wingo CS, McDonough AA, Youn JH, Kone BC. Narrative review: Evolving concepts in potassium homeostasis and hypokalemia. Ann Intern Med 2009;150:619–625.
8. Sterns RH, Emmett M. Fluid, electrolyte and acid–base disturbances: Hypokalemia. In: Sterns RH, Emmett M, eds. NephSAP® Nephrology Self-Assessment Program. Washington, DC: American Society of Nephrology, 2011:117–125.
9. Chobanian AV, Bakris GL, Black HR, et al. The Seventh Report of the Joint National Committee on prevention, detection, evaluation, and treatment of high blood pressure: The JNC 7 report. JAMA 2003;289:2560–2572.
10. Malnic G, Muto S, Giebisch G. Regulation of potassium excretion. In: Alpern RJ, Hebert SC, eds. Seldin and Giebisch's the Kidney, 4th ed. Amsterdam: Elsevier, 2008:1301–1347.
11. Aronson PS, Giebisch G. Effects of pH on potassium: new explanations for old observations. J Am Soc Nephrol 2011;22:1981–1989.
12. Gennari FJ. Disorders of potassium homeostasis: Hypokalemia and hyperkalemia. Crit Care Clin 2002;18:273–288.
13. Gennari FJ. Hypokalemia. N Engl J Med 1998;339: 451–458.
14. Bowling CB, Pitt B, Ahmed MI, et al. Hypokalemia and outcomes in patients with chronic heart failure and chronic kidney disease. Circ Heart Fail 2010;3:253–260.
15. Korgaonkar S, Tilea A, Gillespie BW, et al. Serum potassium and outcomes in CKD: Insights from the RRI CKD cohort study. J Am Soc Nephrol 2010;5:762–69.
16. Huang CL, Kuo E. Mechanism of hypokalemia in magnesium deficiency. J Am Soc Nephrol 2007;18: 2649–2652.
17. Cohn JN, Kowey PR, Whelton PK, Prisant LM. New guidelines for potassium replacement in clinical practice: A contemporary review by the National Council on Potassium in Clinical Practice. Arch Intern Med 2000; 160:2429–2436.
18. 2005 American Heart Association Guidelines for Cardiopulmonary Resuscitation and Emergency Cardiovascular Care. Part 10.1. Life threatening emergencies. Circulation 2005;112:IV-121–IV-125.
19. Chmielewski CM. Hyperkalemic emergencies: Mechanisms, manifestations and management. Crit Care Nurs Clin North Am 1998;10:449–458.
20. Gennari FJ, Segal AS. Hyperkalemia: An adaptive response in chronic renal insufficiency. Kidney Int 2002;62:1–9.
21. Einhorn LA, Zhan M, Hsu VD, et al. The frequency of hyperkalemia and its significance in chronic kidney disease. Arch Int Med 2009;169:1156–1162.
22. Weisberg LS. Management of severe hyperkalemia. Crit Care Med 2008;36:3246–3251.
23. Farese S, Jruse A, Pasch A, et al. Glycyrrhetinic acid food supplementation lowers serum potassium concentration in chronic hemodialysis patients. Kidney Int 2009;76;877–884.
24. Ferrari P. Licorice: A sweet alternative to prevent hyperkalemia in dialysis patients? Kidney Int 2009;76; 811–812.
25. McGowan CE, Saha S, Chu G, et al. Intestinal necrosis due to sodium polystyrene sulfonate (Kayexalate) in sorbitol. South Med J 2009;102:493–497.
26. Sterns RH, Rojas M, Bernstein P, Chennupati S. Ion-exchange resin for the treatment of hyperkalemia: Are they safe and effective? J Am Soc Nephrol 2010;21:733–735.
27. Kayexalate (Sodium Polystyrene Sulfonate) Powder Boxed Warning. 2012, http://www.fda.gov/Safety/MedWatch/SafetyInformation/ucm186845.htm.
28. Watson M, Abbott KC, Yuan CM. Damned if you do, damned if you don't: Potassium binding resins in hyperkalemia. Clin J Am Soc Nephrol 2010;5:1723–1726.
29. Sowinski KM, Cronin D, Mueller BA, Kraus MA. Subcutaneous terbuatline use in CKD to reduce potassium concentrations. Am J Kidney Dis 2005;45:1040–1045.
30. Mahoney BA, Smith WAD, Lo DS, et al. Emergency interventions for hyperkalemia. Cochrane Database Syst Rev 2005;18:CD003235.
31. Spiegel DM. Normal and abnormal magnesium metabolism. In: Schrier RW, ed. Renal and Electrolyte Disorders, 7th ed. Philadelphia, PA: Lippincott Williams & Wilkins, 2010; 229–250.
32. Musso CG. Magnesium metabolism in health and disease. Int Urol Nephrol 2009;41:357–362.
33. Martin KJ, Gonzalez EA, Slatopolsky E. Clinical consequences and management of hypomagnesemia. J Am Soc Nephrol 2009;20:2291–2295.
34. Topf JM, Murray PT. Hypomagnesemia and hypermagnesemia. Rev Endocr Metab Disord 2003;4: 195–206.
35. Moe SM. Disorders involving calcium, phosphorus and magnesium. Primary Care 2008;35:215–237.

37

Acid–Base Disorders

John W. Devlin and Gary R. Matzke

KEY CONCEPTS

1 The kidney plays a central role in the regulation of acid–base homeostasis through the excretion or reabsorption of filtered bicarbonate (HCO_3^-), the excretion of metabolic fixed acids, and generation of new HCO_3^-.

2 Arterial blood gases (ABGs), along with serum electrolytes, physical findings, medical and medication history, and the clinical condition of the patient, are the primary tools to determine the cause of an acid–base disorder and to design and monitor a course of therapy.

3 Metabolic acidosis and metabolic alkalosis are generated by a primary change in the serum bicarbonate concentration. In metabolic acidosis, bicarbonate is lost or a nonvolatile acid is gained, whereas metabolic alkalosis is characterized by a gain in bicarbonate or a loss of nonvolatile acid.

4 Renal tubular acidosis (RTA) refers to a group of disorders characterized by impaired tubular renal acid handling despite normal or near-normal glomerular filtration rates. These patients often present with hyperchloremic metabolic acidosis.

5 Respiratory compensation for a primary metabolic acidosis begins rapidly (within 15 to 30 minutes) but does not reach a steady state for 12 to 24 hours after the onset of metabolic acidosis.

6 Primary therapy of most acid–base disorders must include treatment or elimination of the underlying cause, not just correction of the pH and electrolyte disturbances.

7 Potassium supplementation is always necessary for patients with chronic metabolic acidosis, as the bicarbonaturia resulting from alkali therapy increases the renal potassium wasting.

8 Effective treatment of the underlying cause of some organic acidoses (e.g., ketoacidosis) can result in the regeneration of bicarbonate within hours, thus mitigating the need for alkali therapy.

9 Loss of gastric acid from vomiting or nasogastric suctioning is often responsible for the development of a metabolic alkalosis, characterized by hypochloremia and hyperbicarbonatemia.

10 Aggressive diuretic therapy can produce a metabolic alkalosis, and the accompanying hypokalemia can be serious.

11 The patient's response to volume replacement can be predicted by the urine chloride concentration and permits the differential diagnosis of metabolic alkalosis.

12 Management of these disorders usually consists of treatment of the underlying cause of mineralocorticoid excess. In patients in whom the mineralocorticoid excess cannot be corrected, chronic pharmacologic therapy can be required.

13 In most cases of acute metabolic acidosis, such as following cardiopulmonary arrest, sodium bicarbonate therapy is not indicated and can be detrimental. Blood gas analysis should guide therapy.

INTRODUCTION

Acid–base disorders are common and often serious disturbances that can result in significant morbidity and mortality. This chapter reviews the mechanisms responsible for the maintenance of acid–base balance and the laboratory analyses that aid clinicians in their assessment of acid–base disorders. The pathophysiology of the four primary acid–base disturbances is presented, evidence-based therapeutic options are reviewed, and management guidelines to optimize the outcome of patients with one of these disorders are presented. Given that medications are a frequent cause of acid–base abnormalities and that acid–base abnormalities are often preventable, clinicians must anticipate drug-related problems to avoid or minimize the clinical consequences of acid–base disorders, and when necessary, design appropriate treatment regimens.

ACID–BASE CHEMISTRY

An acid (in this equation, hydrochloric acid) is a substance that can *donate* protons (hydrogen ion [H^+]):

$$\text{(acid) } HCl \rightarrow H^+ + \text{chloride ion } (Cl^-)$$

A base (in this equation, ammonia [NH_3]) is a substance that can *accept* protons (hydrogen ion [H^+]):

$$\text{Ammonia } (NH_3) + H^+ \rightarrow NH^+_4 \text{ (base)}$$

The acid–base pairs commonly encountered in clinical practice are listed in Table 37-1.

The acidity of body fluids is quantified in terms of the hydrogen ion concentration. By convention, the degree of acidity is expressed

TABLE 37-1 Acid–Base Pairs

Carbonic acid/bicarbonate	H_2CO_3/HCO_3^-
Monobasic/dibasic phosphate	H_2PO_4/HPO_4^-
Ammonium/ammonia	NH_4^+/NH_3
Lactic acid/lactate	$H_6C_3O_3/H_5C_3O_3^-$

as pH, or the negative logarithm (base 10) of the hydrogen ion concentration. Thus, hydrogen ion concentration and pH are inversely related. Normally, the pH of blood is maintained at 7.40 ($[H^+]$ of 4×10^{-8} M) with a range of 7.35 to 7.45. A pH of less than 6.7 ($[H^+]$ of 2×10^{-7} M), representing a fivefold increase in hydrogen ion concentration, or greater than 7.7 ($[H^+]$ of 2×10^{-8} M), representing a 50% decrease in hydrogen ion concentration, is considered incompatible with life.

The hydrogen ion concentration in blood may not be indicative of that in other body compartments. For example, the pH within cells, within the cerebrospinal fluid, or on the surface of bone can all be altered without causing an alteration in blood pH.[1] Recognizing this caveat, the acid–base status of the body is usually analyzed based on measurement of blood pH. Alterations in blood pH serve as the basis for the diagnosis of acid–base disorders.

Because the dissociation of acid–base pairs is an equilibrium reaction, the relationship between hydrogen ion concentration or pH and the relative concentrations of the acid and base can be described mathematically in terms of the dissociation constant for the acid–base buffer pair. When expressed as a logarithmic relationship, where p*K* is the negative logarithm of the dissociation constant *K*, this is known as the Henderson–Hasselbalch equation:

$$pH = pK + \log([base]/[acid])$$

BUFFERS

The ability of a weak acid and its corresponding anion (base) to resist change in the pH of a solution on the addition of a strong acid or base is referred to as *buffering*. An acid–base pair is most efficient in functioning as a buffer at a pH close to its p*K*. The principal extracellular buffer is the carbonic acid/bicarbonate (H_2CO_3/HCO_3^-) system. Other physiologic buffers include plasma proteins, hemoglobin, and phosphates. Because the isohydric principle requires that all buffer systems remain in chemical equilibrium, the complex buffering of biologic fluids can be analyzed based on a single buffer pair.

The carbonic acid/bicarbonate buffer system plays a unique role in acid–base homeostasis. In addition to being the most abundant extracellular buffer, the components of this buffer pair are under dynamic regulation by the body. In the presence of carbonic anhydrase, carbonic acid, $[H_2CO_3]$, is in equilibrium with carbon dioxide (CO_2) gas. Changes in ventilation that alter the partial pressure of CO_2 (P_{CO_2}) in the blood regulate the carbonic acid level in the blood. The bicarbonate concentration is independently regulated by the kidney. Because the p*K* for the carbonic acid/bicarbonate system is 6.1, the relationship between pH, carbonic acid, and bicarbonate concentrations can be described by the Henderson–Hasselbalch equation. The concentration of carbonic acid is directly proportional to the amount of CO_2 dissolved in blood, which is equal to the product of P_{CO_2} and its solubility in physiologic fluids ($P_{CO_2} \times 0.03$ for P_{CO_2} expressed in mm Hg or $P_{CO_2} \times 0.226$ for P_{CO_2} expressed in kPa). This term can, therefore, be substituted into the equation below in place of $[H_2CO_3]$.

$$pH = 6.1 + ([HCO_3^-]/[H_2CO_3])$$
$$pH = 6.1 + \log([HCO_3^-]/(P_{CO_2} \times 0.03)) \text{ for } P_{CO_2} \text{ in mm Hg}$$

or

$$pH = 6.1 + \log([HCO_3^-]/(P_{CO_2} \times 0.226)) \text{ for } P_{CO_2} \text{ in kPa}$$

Thus, hydrogen ion concentration and pH are determined not by the absolute amounts of bicarbonate and P_{CO_2}, but by their ratio.[1] Under normal physiologic conditions, the kidneys maintain the serum bicarbonate at approximately 24 mEq/L (24 mmol/L), whereas the lungs maintain the P_{CO_2} at approximately 40 mm Hg (5.3 kPa). The normal physiologic pH is thus 7.4:

$$pH = 6.1 + \log[24/(0.03 \times 40)] \text{ (or } pH = 6.1 + \log[24/(0.226 \times 5.3)])$$
$$pH = 6.1 + 1.3 = 7.4$$

If, in response to an acid load, the serum bicarbonate concentration were to decrease to 12 mEq/L (12 mmol/L), the predicted pH would be:

$$[HCO_3^-] = 12 \text{ mEq/L (12 mmol/L)}$$
$$P_{CO_2} = 40 \text{ mm Hg (5.3 kPa)}$$
$$pH = 6.1 + \log[12/0.03 \times 40] \text{ or}$$
$$pH = 6.1 + \log[12/(0.226 \times 5.3)]$$
$$pH = 6.1 + 1.0 = 7.1$$

However, the normal respiratory response to an acid load is hyperventilation. As a result, if the P_{CO_2} decreased to approximately 26 mm Hg (3.5 kPa), the change in pH would be less:

$$[HCO_3^-] = 12 \text{ mEq/L (12 mmol/L)}$$
$$P_{CO_2} = 26 \text{ mm Hg (3.5 kPa)}$$
$$pH = 6.1 + \log[12/0.03 \times 26]$$
$$\text{(or } pH = 6.1 + \log[12/(0.226 \times 3.5)])$$
$$pH = 6.1 + 1.19 = 7.29$$

Thus, the physiologic regulation of both P_{CO_2} and $[HCO_3^-]$ permits the carbonic acid/bicarbonate system to provide more effective buffering of the extracellular fluids (ECFs) than could be achieved on the basis of chemical buffering alone.

REGULATION OF ACID–BASE HOMEOSTASIS

Cellular metabolism results in the production of large quantities of hydrogen that need to be excreted to maintain acid–base balance. In addition, small amounts of acid and alkali are also presented to the body through the diet. The bulk of acid production is in the form of CO_2, with the average adult producing approximately 15,000 mmol of CO_2 each day from the catabolism of carbohydrate, protein, and fat.[2] When respiratory function is normal, the amount of CO_2 produced metabolically is equal to the amount lost by respiration, and the blood CO_2 concentration remains constant.

Digestion of dietary substances and tissue metabolism also result in the production of nonvolatile acids. These acids are derived primarily from the sulfur-containing amino acids cysteine and methionine, as well as from ingested sulfur. In addition, phosphates are generated from the metabolism of proteins and phospholipids. Neutral substances such as glucose can also be incompletely metabolized to intermediates, such as lactic and pyruvic acid, and fatty acids can be incompletely metabolized to acetoacetic acid and β-hydroxybutyric acid. These dietary and metabolic fixed acids are excreted, primarily by the kidney, to maintain acid–base homeostasis. On average, daily fixed acid excretion is approximately 0.8 mEq/kg per day (0.8 mmol/kg per day).[3]

Three mechanisms, each of which varies in its onset, collectively maintain acid–base balance: extracellular buffering, ventilatory regulation of carbon dioxide elimination, and renal regulation of hydrogen ion and bicarbonate excretion. Extracellular buffering occurs rapidly and is the body's first defense against a sudden increase in hydrogen ion concentration. Hyperventilation will then result in a decrease in P_{CO_2}, returning blood pH toward normal. Finally, the kidney will excrete the excess hydrogen ion, with the resultant return of acid–base balance to normal over a period of day(s).

Extracellular Buffering

The body's buffering system can be divided into three components: bicarbonate/carbonic acid, proteins, and phosphates. The bicarbonate buffer is the most important of the body's buffers, because (a) there is more bicarbonate present in the ECF than any other buffer component; (b) the supply of carbon dioxide is unlimited; and (c) the acidity of ECF can be regulated by controlling either the bicarbonate concentration or the Pco_2.

Carbonic acid represents the respiratory component of the buffer pair because its concentration is directly proportional to the Pco_2, which is determined by ventilation. Bicarbonate represents the metabolic component because the kidney may alter its concentration by reabsorption, generating new bicarbonate, or altering elimination.[4] The bicarbonate buffer system easily adapts to changes in acid–base status by alterations in ventilatory elimination of acid (Pco_2) and/or renal elimination of base (HCO_3^-).

The phosphate buffer system consists of serum inorganic phosphate (3.5 to 5 mg/dL [1.13 to 1.62 mmol/L]), intracellular organic phosphate, and calcium phosphate in bone. Extracellular phosphate is present only in low concentrations, so its usefulness as a buffer is limited; however, as an intracellular buffer, phosphate is more useful. Calcium phosphate in bone is relatively inaccessible as a buffer, but prolonged metabolic acidosis will result in the release of phosphate from bone.

Intracellular and extracellular proteins also act as buffering systems. The charged side chains of amino acids provide the buffering action. Because the concentration of protein is much greater intracellularly than extracellularly, protein is much more important as an intracellular buffer.

Respiratory Regulation

The second mechanism for maintenance of acid–base homeostasis is control of ventilation. Both the rate and depth of ventilation can be varied to allow for excretion of CO_2 generated by diet and tissue metabolism. Medullary chemoreceptors in the brainstem sense changes in Pco_2 and in pH and modulate the control of breathing. Increasing minute ventilation (the total amount of air exhaled over a 1-minute period), by increasing respiratory rate and/or tidal volume (the amount of air exhaled in one breath), will increase CO_2 excretion and decrease the blood Pco_2. Conversely, decreasing minute ventilation decreases CO_2 excretion and increases blood Pco_2. This system rapidly adjusts within minutes to changes in acid–base balance.[2]

Renal Regulation

1 Because bicarbonate is a small ion, it is freely filtered at the glomerulus. The bicarbonate load delivered to the nephron is approximately 4,500 mEq/day (4,500 mmol/day). To maintain acid–base balance, this entire filtered load must be reabsorbed. Bicarbonate reabsorption occurs primarily in the proximal tubule (Fig. 37-1). In the tubular lumen, filtered bicarbonate combines with hydrogen ion secreted by the apical sodium ion (Na^+)–H^+-exchanger to form carbonic acid. The carbonic acid is rapidly broken down to CO_2 and water by carbonic anhydrase located on the luminal surface of the brush border membrane. The CO_2 then diffuses into the proximal tubular cell, where it reforms carbonic acid in the presence of intracellular carbonic anhydrase. The carbonic acid dissociates to form hydrogen ions that can again be secreted into the tubular lumen, and bicarbonate that exits the cell across the basolateral membrane and enters the peritubular capillary.

Excretion of metabolic fixed acids and generation of new HCO_3^- is achieved through renal ammoniagenesis and distal tubular hydrogen ion secretion. Ammoniagenesis plays a critical role in acid–base homeostasis, with ammonium (NH_4^+) excretion comprising approximately 50% of renal net acid excretion. Ammonium is generated from the deamination of glutamine in the proximal tubule. For each ammonium ion excreted in the urine, one bicarbonate ion is regenerated and returned to the circulation.[5]

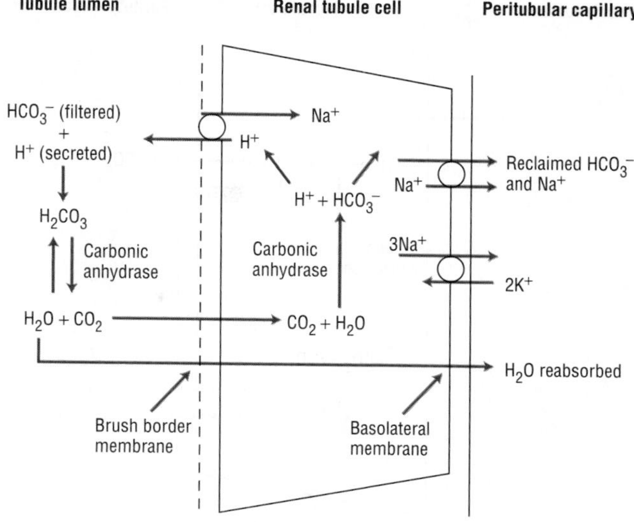

FIGURE 37-1 Proximal tubular bicarbonate reabsorption. In the tubular lumen, filtered bicarbonate (HCO_3^-) combines with hydrogen ion (H^+) secreted by an apical sodium ion (Na^+)–H^+ exchanger to form carbonic acid (H_2CO_3). The carbonic acid is rapidly broken down to carbon dioxide (CO_2) and water by carbonic anhydrase located on the luminal surface of the brush border membrane. The CO_2 then diffuses into the proximal tubular cell, where it reforms carbonic acid in the presence of intracellular carbonic anhydrase. The carbonic acid dissociates the former hydrogen ion that can again be secreted into the tubular lumen, and bicarbonate that exits the cell across the basolateral membrane and enters the peritubular capillary.

Distal tubular hydrogen ion secretion accounts for the remaining 50% of net acid excretion (Fig. 37-2). In the distal tubular cell, CO_2 combines with water in the presence of intracellular carbonic anhydrase to form carbonic acid, which dissociates to H^+ and HCO_3^-. The H^+ is actively transported into the tubular lumen by a H^+–adenosine triphosphatase (ATPase). The bicarbonate exits the cell across the basolateral membrane and enters the circulation.[5]

ACID–BASE DISTURBANCES

2 Alterations in blood pH are designated by the suffix "-emia"; *acidemia* is an arterial blood pH <7.35 and *alkalemia* is an arterial blood pH >7.45. The pathophysiologic processes that result in alterations in blood pH are designated by the suffix "-osis." These disturbances are classified as either metabolic or respiratory in origin. In metabolic acid–base disorders, the primary disturbance is in the plasma bicarbonate concentration. Metabolic acidosis is characterized by a decrease in the plasma bicarbonate concentration whereas in metabolic alkalosis the plasma bicarbonate concentration is increased. Respiratory acid–base disorders are caused by alterations in alveolar ventilation that produce corresponding changes in the partial pressure of carbon dioxide from arterial blood ($Paco_2$). In respiratory acidosis, the $Paco_2$ is elevated; in respiratory alkalosis, it is decreased. Each disturbance has a compensatory (secondary) response that attempts to correct the HCO_3^--to-$Paco_2$ ratio toward normal and mitigate the change in pH (Table 37-2). Although the time course of the respiratory compensatory responses to metabolic disturbances is rapid, the metabolic compensation for respiratory disturbances is slow. As a result, respiratory disturbances are characterized as acute (minutes

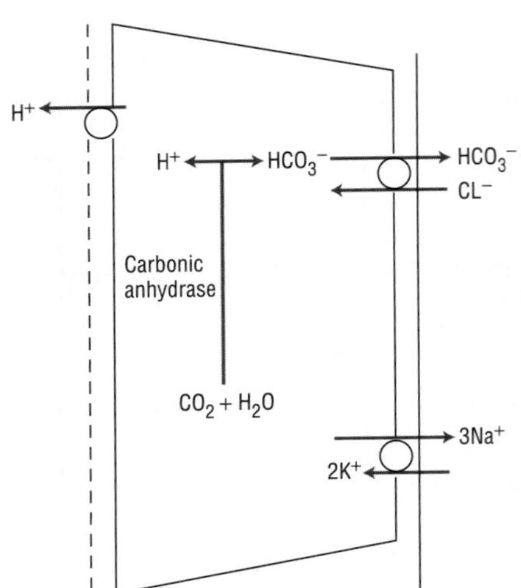

FIGURE 37-2 Collecting duct acid excretion. Hydrogen ion (H^+) and bicarbonate (HCO_3^-) are generated intracellularly from carbon dioxide (CO_2) and water, in the presence of intracellular carbonic anhydrase. The hydrogen ion is actively secreted into the tubular lumen by H^+–ATPase located in the apical (luminal) membrane. Bicarbonate exits the cell across the basolateral membrane and enters the peritubular capillary. (Cl^-, chloride ion; Na^+, sodium ion.)

to hours in duration), indicating that there has not been sufficient time for metabolic compensation, or chronic (days), indicating that sufficient time for metabolic compensation has elapsed.

CLINICAL ASSESSMENT OF ACID–BASE STATUS

3 Blood gases are measured to determine the patient's oxygenation and acid–base status. Under normal circumstances, there is no clinically significant difference in pH between arterial and mixed venous blood. Arterial samples are designated with the letter "a" (e.g., partial pressure of oxygen from arterial blood [Pao_2] and $Paco_2$), whereas mixed venous samples are labeled with the letter "v" or not labeled (e.g., partial pressure of oxygen from venous blood [Pvo_2] and partial pressure of carbon dioxide from venous blood [$Pvco_2$]). The normal values for arterial and venous blood gases are shown in Table 37-3. Arterial blood reflects how well the blood is being oxygenated by the lungs (an accurate measurement of Pao_2), whereas venous blood reflects how much oxygen tissues are using. Arterial blood rather than venous blood should be used whenever possible because venous blood obtained from an extremity can provide misleading information. If metabolism in the extremity is altered by hypoperfusion, exercise, infection, or some other cause, the difference in the amount of dissolved oxygen between arterial and venous blood can be dramatic. The venous pH and Pco_2 during cardiopulmonary resuscitation might be significantly lower and higher, respectively, than the arterial pH and arterial Pco_2. This indicates a severe tissue acidosis from CO_2 accumulation caused by hypoperfusion.

TABLE 37-2 Interpretation of Simple Acid–Base Disorders

Acid–Base Disorder	pH	Primary Disturbances	Compensation
Acidosis			
Respiratory	Decrease	Increase $Paco_2$	Increase HCO_3^-
Metabolic	Decrease	Decrease HCO_3^-	Decrease $Paco_2$
Alkalosis			
Respiratory	Increase	Decrease $Paco_2$	Decrease HCO_3^-
Metabolic	Increase	Increase HCO_3^-	Increase $Paco_2$

HCO_3^-, bicarbonate; $Paco_2$, partial pressure of carbon dioxide from arterial blood.

TABLE 37-3 Normal Blood Gas Values

	Arterial Blood	Mixed Venous Blood
pH	7.40 (7.35–7.45)	7.38 (7.33–7.43)
Po_2	80–100 mm Hg (10.6–13.3 kPa)	35–40 mm Hg (4.7–5.3 kPa)
Sao_2	95% (0.95)	70–75% (0.70–0.75)
Pco_2	35–45 mm Hg (4.7–6.0 kPa)	45–51 mm Hg (6.0–6.8 kPa)
HCO_3^-	22–26 mEq/L (22–26 mmol/L)	24–28 mEq/L (24–28 mmol/L)

HCO_3^-, bicarbonate; Pco_2, partial pressure of carbon dioxide; Po_2, partial pressure of oxygen; Sao_2, saturation of arterial oxygen.

Analysis of Arterial Blood Gas Data

ABGs provide an assessment of the patient's acid–base status.[6] Low pH values (<7.35) indicate an acidemia, whereas high pH values (>7.45) indicate an alkalemia (Fig. 37-3). In a metabolic acidosis, the pH is decreased in association with a decreased serum bicarbonate concentration and a compensatory decrease in $Paco_2$. In a respiratory acidosis, the pH is decreased; the $Paco_2$, however, is elevated. The serum bicarbonate concentration is variable, depending on whether it is an acute disturbance (minimal increase in serum bicarbonate) or a chronic respiratory acidosis (substantial increase in serum bicarbonate). In a metabolic alkalosis, the pH is elevated in association with an increased bicarbonate concentration and a compensatory increase in $Paco_2$. In a respiratory alkalosis, the pH is also elevated; the $Paco_2$, however, is decreased. As with respiratory acidosis, the metabolic compensation is variable: a minimal decrease in serum bicarbonate is often noted in acute respiratory alkalosis while a larger decrease in [HCO_3^-] is common with chronic respiratory alkalosis. Although each measurement has a normal range (see Table 37-3), it is often easiest to consider the midpoint of each range as the normal value. This would correlate to a pH of 7.4, $Paco_2$ of 40 mm Hg (5.3 kPa), and HCO_3^- of 24 mEq/L (24 mmol/L). Steps in acid–base interpretation are described in Table 37-4.

When ABGs differ significantly from those expected on the basis of the patient's clinical condition and previous laboratory determinations, additional venous blood samples should be drawn to assess plasma electrolyte concentrations. The bicarbonate calculated from the patient's $Paco_2$ and pH of the blood gas should be compared with the measured total CO_2 content (the amount of CO_2 gas extractable from plasma, consisting of HCO_3^-, H_2CO_3, and Pco_2). Ordinarily, the blood gas bicarbonate value is approximately 1 to 2 mEq/L (1 to 2 mmol/L) less than total CO_2 content.[3] If these values do not correspond, the results should be interpreted with caution because the difference can reflect an error in the blood collection or storage of the sample, or in the calibration of the blood gas analyzer.

METABOLIC ACID–BASE DISORDERS

Metabolic Acidosis

Metabolic acidosis is characterized by a decrease in pH as the result of a primary decrease in serum bicarbonate concentration.

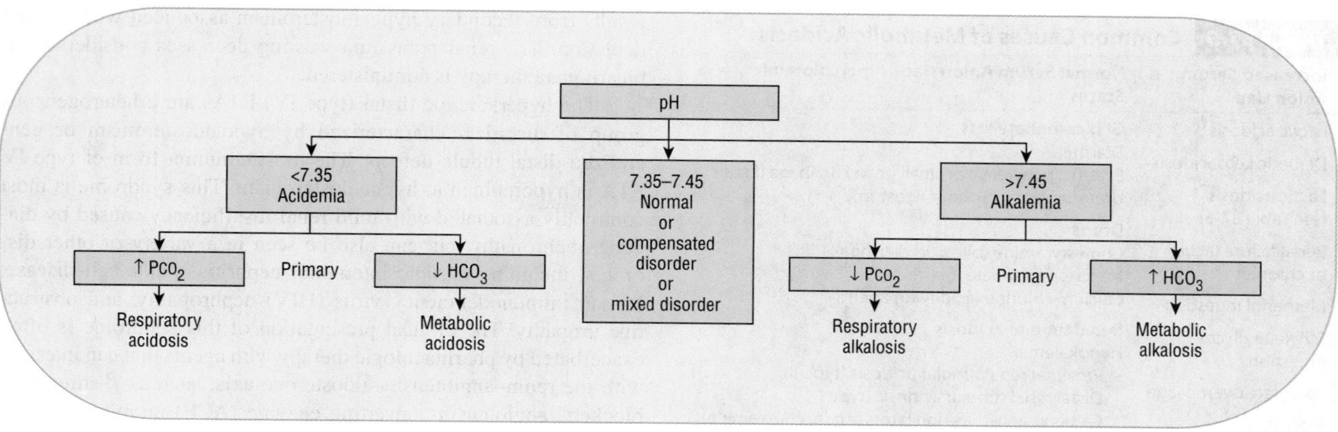

FIGURE 37-3 Analysis of arterial blood gases. (HCO_3^-, bicarbonate; Pco_2, partial pressure of carbon dioxide.)

Pathophysiology

Metabolic acidosis can result from the buffering (consumption of HCO_3^-) of an exogenous acid, an organic acid accumulating because of a metabolic disturbance (e.g., lactic acid or ketoacids), or the progressive accumulation of endogenous acids secondary to impaired renal function (e.g., phosphates and sulfates).[7] The serum HCO_3^- can also be decreased as the result of a loss of bicarbonate-rich body fluids (e.g., diarrhea, biliary drainage, or pancreatic fistula) or occur secondary to the rapid administration of non-alkali–containing IV fluids (dilutional acidosis).[8]

The serum anion gap (SAG), as defined below, can be used to infer whether an organic or mineral acidosis is present.

$$SAG = [Na^+] - [Cl^-] - [HCO_3^-]$$

To maintain electroneutrality, the total concentration of cations in the serum must equal the total concentration of anions.

$$[Na^+] + [UCs] = ([Cl^-] + [HCO_3^-]) + [UAs]$$

The cation concentration is equal to the sodium concentration plus that of "unmeasured" cations (UCs), predominantly magnesium, calcium, and potassium. The anion concentration is equal to the concentrations of chloride, bicarbonate, and "unmeasured" anions (UAs), including proteins, sulfates, phosphates, and organic anions. Therefore, as the result of the combination of the two equations above, the SAG can be expressed as:

$$SAG = [UAs] - [UCs]$$

The normal SAG is approximately 9 mEq/L (9 mmol/L), with a range of 3 to 11 mEq/L (3 to 11 mmol/L). This value is lower than the value of 12 mEq/L (12 mmol/L) cited in the literature in the past because of changes in the instrumentation for measurement of serum electrolytes.[7] Increases in the anion gap (AG) to values in excess of 17 to 20 mEq/L (17 to 20 mmol/L) are indicative of the accumulation of unmeasured anions in ECF.

These unmeasured anions are generated as the result of the consumption of HCO_3^- by endogenous organic acids such as lactic acid, acetoacetic acid, or β-hydroxybutyric acid or from the ingestion of toxins such as methanol or ethylene glycol. The degree of elevation in the SAG is dependent on the clearance of the anion, as well as the multiple factors that influence HCO_3^- concentrations. Thus, the SAG is a relative rather than an absolute indication of the cause of metabolic acidosis. The SAG can also be elevated in the metabolic acidosis because of renal failure, as the result of the accumulation of various organic anions, phosphates, and sulfates.

In hyperchloremic metabolic acidosis, bicarbonate losses from the ECF are replaced by chloride, and the SAG remains normal. This decrease in bicarbonate may be due to GI tract losses, dilution of bicarbonate in the ECF as the result of the addition of sodium chloride solutions or chloride-containing acids. Common causes of metabolic acidosis with an increased or a normal SAG are listed in Table 37-5.

Hyperchloremic Metabolic Acidosis

Hyperchloremic metabolic acidosis can result from increased GI bicarbonate loss, renal bicarbonate wasting, impaired renal acid excretion, or exogenous acid gain. GI disorders such as diarrhea, biliary, or pancreatic drainage through either a surgical drain or fistula can result in the loss of large volumes of bicarbonate-containing fluids. Severe diarrhea, the most common cause of hyperchloremic metabolic acidosis, can lead to a daily loss of 5 to 10 L of fluid containing 100 to 140 mEq/L (100 to 140 mmol/L) of sodium, 20 to 40 mEq/L (20 to 40 mmol/L) of potassium, 80 to 100 mEq/L (80 to 100 mmol/L) of chloride, and 30 to 50 mEq/L (30 to 50 mmol/L) of bicarbonate.[4] Patients who have undergone ureteral diversion into the sigmoid colon or isolated ileal loop can also develop a hyperchloremic metabolic acidosis. This is the result of a net loss of bicarbonate given that chloride is reabsorbed and bicarbonate is secreted by GI epithelial cells in the presence of the urine that is retained in the colon or bowel loop.

Hyperchloremic metabolic acidosis caused by renal bicarbonate wasting is the defining disturbance in proximal RTA and is a complication of therapy with carbonic anhydrase inhibitors, particularly when they are administered for more than 24 to 48 hours. During the treatment of diabetic ketoacidosis, renal loss of β-hydroxybutyrate and acetoacetate, which would otherwise be metabolized to yield bicarbonate, can contribute to the development of hyperchloremic metabolic acidosis. Impaired renal acid

TABLE 37-4 Steps in Acid–Base Diagnosis

1. Obtain ABGs and electrolytes simultaneously
2. Compare [HCO_3^-] on ABG and electrolytes to verify accuracy
3. Calculate SAG
4. Is acidemia (pH <7.35) or alkalemia (pH >7.45) present?
5. Is the primary abnormality respiratory (alteration in $Paco_2$) or metabolic (alteration in HCO_3)?
6. Estimate compensatory response (Table 37-7)
7. Compare change in [Cl^-] with change in [Na^+]

[Cl^-], chloride ion; [HCO_3^-], bicarbonate; [Na^+], sodium ion; $Paco_2$, partial pressure of carbon dioxide from arterial blood; SAG, serum anion gap.

TABLE 37-5 Common Causes of Metabolic Acidosis

Increased Serum Anion Gap	Normal Serum Anion Gap/Hyperchloremic States
Lactic acidosis	**GI bicarbonate loss**
Diabetic ketoacidosis	Diarrhea
	External pancreatic or small bowel drainage (fistula)
Lactic acidosis (see Table 37-6)	Ureterosigmoidostomy, ileostomy
	Drugs
Renal failure (acute or chronic)	Cholestyramine (bile acid diarrhea)
	Magnesium sulfate (diarrhea)
Methanol ingestion	Calcium chloride (acidifying agent)
Ethylene glycol ingestion	**Renal tubular acidosis**
	Hypokalemia
	Proximal renal tubular acidosis (type II)
Salicylate overdosage	Distal renal tubular acidosis (type I)
Starvation	Carbonic anhydrase inhibitors (e.g., acetazolamide)
	Hyperkalemia
	Generalized distal nephron dysfunction (type IV)
	Mineralocorticoid deficiency or resistance
	Tubulointerstitial disease
	Drug-induced hyperkalemia
	Potassium-sparing diuretics (amiloride, spironolactone, triamterene)
	Trimethoprim
	Pentamidine
	Heparin
	ACE inhibitors and receptor blockers
	NSAIDs
	Cyclosporin A
	Other
	Acid ingestion (ammonium chloride, hydrochloric acid, hyperalimentation)
	Expansion acidosis (rapid saline administration)

excretion that occurs as a result of distal tubular dysfunction in patients with distal RTAs can also occur in patients with moderate to severe renal insufficiency from other causes. The metabolic acidosis of renal insufficiency is initially hyperchloremic but can progress to an anion-gap acidosis as the renal insufficiency worsens and sulfates, phosphates, and other anions accumulate. Hyperchloremic metabolic acidosis can also result from the exogenous administration of acid (hydrochloric acid, ammonium chloride) or the unbuffered administration of acid salts from the amino acids in total parenteral nutrition fluids.

Renal Tubular Acidosis

(4) Renal tubular disorders can involve the proximal tubule, with a resultant failure to reabsorb filtered bicarbonate, or affect acid excretion in the distal tubule. The distal RTAs are the most common, and are all characterized by impaired net acid excretion. The distal RTAs are subdivided into those that are associated with hypokalemia (type I) and those associated with hyperkalemia (type IV). Patients with classic distal (type I) RTA have impaired hydrogen ion secretion and are unable to excrete the daily acid load necessary to maintain acid–base balance.[4] These patients are unable to maximally acidify their urine (i.e., attain urine pH <5.5), even in the face of an acid challenge. Type I RTA may be the result of a primary tubular defect or develop secondary to a wide variety of disorders including hypercalcemia, multiple myeloma, systemic lupus erythematosus, Sjögren's syndrome, sickle-cell disease, and renal transplant rejection, or following the administration of amphotericin B or ingestion of toluene. The primary form of this disorder usually occurs in children and can result in severe acidosis, slowed growth, nephrocalcinosis, and kidney stones.[7,9] In adults, clinical complications include osteomalacia, nephrocalcinosis, and recurrent kidney stones. The hypokalemia associated with classic distal (type I) RTA results from secondary hypoaldosteronism associated with volume depletion. The renal potassium wasting decreases considerably if bicarbonate therapy is administered.

The hyperkalemic distal (type IV) RTAs are a heterogeneous group of disorders characterized by hypoaldosteronism or generalized distal tubule defects. The most common form of type IV RTA is hyporeninemic hypoaldosteronism. This syndrome is most commonly associated with mild renal insufficiency caused by diabetic nephropathy, but can also be seen in a variety of other disorders, including chronic interstitial nephritis, sickle-cell disease, human immunodeficiency virus (HIV) nephropathy, and obstructive uropathy. The clinical presentation of this syndrome is often exacerbated by pharmacologic therapy with agents that can interfere with the renin–angiotensin–aldosterone axis, such as β-adrenergic blockers, angiotensin-converting enzyme (ACE) inhibitors, angiotensin receptor blockers, and nonsteroidal antiinflammatory drugs (NSAIDs). Heparin can induce the syndrome by inhibiting adrenal aldosterone biosynthesis. Patients with this form of RTA are able to maximally acidify their urine (urine pH <5.5).[9] The primary defect in acid excretion is impaired ammoniagenesis caused by mild renal insufficiency. Hyperaldosteronism predisposes to the development of hyperkalemia, which results in further impairment of ammoniagenesis. Treatment to control the hyperkalemia is usually sufficient to reverse the metabolic acidosis, and mineralocorticoid replacement is frequently unnecessary.

Hyperkalemic distal (type IV) RTA resulting from generalized distal tubule defects is less common than hyporeninemic hypoaldosteronism but is more common than classic distal (type I) RTA. Patients with this defect have impaired tubular potassium secretion in addition to impaired urinary acidification (urine pH >5.5, despite acidemia or acid loading). Urinary obstruction is the most frequent cause of this disorder, which can also be associated with sickle-cell nephropathy, systemic lupus erythematosus, HIV nephropathy, analgesic abuse nephropathy, amyloidosis, renal transplant rejection, and chronic cyclosporine nephrotoxicity.

Proximal (type II) RTA is characterized by defects in proximal tubular reabsorption of bicarbonate. Normally, more than 85% of filtered bicarbonate is reabsorbed in the proximal tubule. Defects in proximal tubular bicarbonate reabsorption result in increased delivery of bicarbonate to the distal nephron, which has a limited capacity for bicarbonate reabsorption. As a result, at a normal serum bicarbonate concentration, the filtered bicarbonate load is incompletely reabsorbed, and is lost in the urine. As the serum bicarbonate concentration decreases, the filtered load of bicarbonate is proportionately decreased. A new equilibrium is established in which the kidney is able to reabsorb the filtered bicarbonate load, albeit at a reduced serum bicarbonate concentration. Thus, patients with proximal RTA present with a chronic, nonprogressive hyperchloremic metabolic acidosis. These patients are able to acidify their urine in response to an acid load, but develop bicarbonaturia at a reduced serum bicarbonate concentration following bicarbonate loading. The impaired bicarbonate reabsorption results in salt wasting and secondary hyperaldosteronism. Hypokalemia, which can be severe, usually develops as a result of the hyperaldosteronism and bicarbonaturia.[4,7] Unlike patients with classic distal (type I) RTA, the hyperkalemia if present in proximal RTA is exacerbated by alkali replacement. Proximal RTA can develop as an isolated defect, or it can be associated with generalized proximal tubular dysfunction (Fanconi's syndrome), with impaired proximal tubular glucose, phosphate, and amino acid reabsorption. Proximal RTA usually presents as an acquired disorder, secondary to a variety of diseases (amyloidosis, multiple myeloma, or nephrotic syndrome) or exposure to toxins (lead, cadmium, mercury, or outdated tetracyclines). Pharmacologic therapy with carbonic anhydrase inhibitors produces an iatrogenic form of proximal RTA.

Elevated Anion Gap Metabolic Acidosis

Metabolic acidosis with an increased SAG commonly results from increased endogenous organic acid production.[7] In lactic acidosis, lactic acid accumulates as a by-product of anaerobic metabolism. Accumulation of the ketoacids β-hydroxybutyric acid and acetoacetic acid defines the ketoacidosis of uncontrolled diabetes mellitus, alcohol intoxication, and starvation (see Table 37-5). In advanced renal failure, accumulation of phosphate, sulfate, and organic anions is responsible for the increased SAG, which is usually less than 24 mEq/L (24 mmol/L).[7] The severe metabolic acidosis seen in myoglobinuric acute renal failure caused by rhabdomyolysis may be caused by the metabolism of large amounts of sulfur-containing amino acids released from myoglobin.

The presence of mild elevations in the SAG cannot be automatically attributed to the presence of a high SAG metabolic acidosis. Elevations in the SAG are commonly seen in hospitalized patients, especially those who are critically ill.[7,10] A variety of factors can contribute to this nonspecific elevation in the SAG, including the presence of alkalemia, which increases the anionic charge of albumin and other plasma proteins. The usefulness of the SAG as a marker of acid–base status is dependent on proper interpretation of a patient's clinical status.[5,11] Despite these limitations, when the SAG exceeds 20 to 25 mEq/L (20 to 25 mmol/L) a significant organic acidosis is likely to be present.

High anion gap metabolic acidosis can develop in many clinical settings, including uncontrolled diabetes mellitus (see Chap. 57), alcohol intoxication (see Chaps. 24 and 49), and starvation (see Chap. 47). Toxic ingestions of methanol and ethylene glycol are also associated with high anion gap metabolic acidosis and can be differentiated from other causes of SAG because of the presence of an elevated osmolar gap. The mechanisms responsible for the development of acidosis in these settings are diverse.[7,12]

Lactic Acidosis Lactic acidosis is one of the most common causes of high SAG metabolic acidosis and can impact approximately 1% of hospitalized patients. Lactic acid is the end product of anaerobic metabolism of glucose (glycolysis).[7] In normal individuals, lactic acid derived from pyruvate enters the circulation in small amounts and is promptly removed by the liver. In the liver, and to a lesser extent in the kidney, lactic acid is reoxidized to pyruvic acid, which is then metabolized to CO_2 and H_2O. The normal plasma lactate concentration in healthy subjects is approximately 1 mEq/L (1 mmol/L).[3,7,12] The diagnosis of lactic acidosis should be considered in all patients with metabolic acidosis associated with an increased SAG. Lactic acidosis is considered to be present when lactate concentrations exceed 4 to 5 mEq/L (4 to 5 mmol/L) in an acidemic patient.

Classically, lactic acidosis has been differentiated into disorders associated with tissue hypoxia (type A lactic acidosis) and disorders associated with deranged oxidative metabolism (type B lactic acidosis), although the distinction between them is blurred (Table 37-6).[7,11,12] The etiologies of lactic acidosis can also be categorized on the basis of changes in lactate production and/or utilization.[7,12] Metabolic disturbances can result in increased tissue pyruvate production or impaired utilization, with proportional increases in lactate concentrations. Increased lactate production is more commonly associated with alterations in tissue redox state, resulting in preferential conversion of pyruvate to lactate. During anaerobic metabolism, reduced nicotinamide adenine dinucleotide accumulates, driving the conversion of pyruvate to lactate and increasing the lactate-to-pyruvate ratio. States of enhanced metabolic activity (e.g., grand mal seizures, strenuous exercise, or hyperthermia), decreased tissue oxygen delivery (e.g., severe anemia, hypoxia, circulatory shock, or carbon monoxide poisoning), or impaired oxygen utilization (e.g., cyanide toxicity) all are associated with lactic acidosis. Impaired hepatic clearance of lactate, as seen in hypoperfusion states, liver failure, and alcohol intoxication, can also result in lactic acidosis.

TABLE 37-6 Causes of Lactic Acidosis

Primary decrease in tissue oxygenation
Shock
Severe anemia
Congestive heart failure
Asphyxia
Carbon monoxide poisoning
Deranged oxidative metabolism
Medications
Catecholamines
Linezolid
Metformin
Nalidixic acid
NRTIs (didanosine, stavudine, zidovudine)
Overdose (iron, isoniazid, salicylates, theophylline)
Propofol infusion syndrome
Propylene glycol toxicity (IV lorazepam, IV pentobarbital)
Sodium nitroprusside (secondary to cyanide toxicity)
Streptozocin
Diabetes mellitus
Malignancy
Seizures
Methanol, ethanol, or ethylene glycol
Disorders associated with inborn errors of metabolism

Cardiovascular and septic shock, with resultant tissue hypoperfusion, are the most common causes of lactic acidosis. Poor tissue perfusion and hypoxia influence enzymatic pyruvate and lactate metabolism to stimulate anaerobic glycolysis and to decrease lactate utilization. This leads to hyperlactatemia and lactic acidosis. The mortality rate of this type of lactic acidosis can be as high as 80% and correlates with the degree of hyperlactatemia.

Lactic acidosis associated with liver disease, toxins, and congenital enzyme deficiency can be caused by deranged oxidative metabolism or impaired lactate clearance.[4,7,12] The exact role of diabetes mellitus in the induction of lactic acidosis is not clear. It may involve a decrease in pyruvate dehydrogenase activity, the enzyme responsible for pyruvate metabolism. Lactic acidosis in neoplastic disease is uncommon and reported mostly in patients with myeloproliferative disorders. Leukocytes and neoplastic cells in general have high rates of glycolysis. In the case of a large tumor or tightly packed bone marrow, oxygenation can be decreased, favoring the accumulation of lactate. Lactic acidosis has been reported in patients with massive liver tumors, and it has been postulated that the liver uptake of lactate is decreased in these patients. Lactic acidosis associated with seizures is usually transient and occurs because of excessive muscle activity.[13]

A number of medications can cause lactic acidosis.[13–23] Two of the most common medications associated with the development of lactic acidosis are nucleoside-analog reverse transcriptase inhibitors (NRTIs) (3.9 cases per 1,000 person-years) and metformin (0.03 cases per 1,000 person-years).[15–17] The proposed mechanism of NRTI-induced lactic acidosis is the inhibition of the enzyme DNA polymerase gamma that is responsible for mitochondrial DNA synthesis.[15] Disruption of this enzyme can inhibit the transport of lactate into the mitochondria, leading to an accumulation in the cytoplasm. Stavudine is the NRTI most frequently associated with lactic acidosis; however, the combination of stavudine and didanosine confers the highest risk.

The primary suspected mechanism for metformin-induced lactic acidosis is inhibition of liver gluconeogenesis as the result of its inhibitory effects on pyruvate carboxylase which is necessary for the conversion of pyruvate to glucose.[16,17] Other possible pathways for metformin-associated lactic acidosis include a decrease in both hepatic intracellular pH and cardiac output and an increase in lactate production in the gut and increased renal loss of bicarbonate.[13] Risk factors for metformin-induced lactic acidosis include renal insufficiency, liver disease, dehydration, advanced age, alcohol consumption, and supratherapeutic dosing. Metformin should be discontinued during periods of tissue hypoxia (e.g., myocardial infarction, sepsis), for 3 days after contrast media has been administered or 2 days before general anesthesia administration. In the latter two cases, metformin should only be reinstituted when the patient's renal function is stable.

Propylene glycol is commonly used as a solubilizing agent in IV drug preparations (e.g., lorazepam, pentobarbital) and is predominantly metabolized to lactic acid via the hepatic enzyme alcohol dehydrogenase. The administration of large doses of propylene glycol, particularly to patients with renal or liver insufficiency, can lead to a lactic acidosis with an osmolar gap and thus serial measurement of the osmolar gap can be used to detect propylene glycol accumulation.[18,19]

Reports of the association between propofol and lactic acidosis were initially described in children.[20] This association is now recognized in adults and has come to be known as the propofol-related infusion syndrome. In addition to lactic acidosis, cardiac failure, rhabdomyolysis, and renal failure have been observed primarily because of uncoupling of oxidative phosphorylation and impaired oxidation of free fatty acids. This syndrome is most frequently seen in patients receiving propofol at high doses (>5 mg/kg/h) for more than 2 days.

Clinical Presentation

Chronic metabolic acidosis is usually not associated with severe acidemia and is relatively asymptomatic. The major manifestations are in the bones, where chronic acidemia causes bone demineralization with the development of rickets in children and osteomalacia and osteopenia in adults.[26] In infants and children, chronic metabolic acidosis is associated with growth failure and short stature and can be associated with nonspecific symptoms including anorexia, nausea, weight loss, and muscle weakness.

Severe metabolic acidosis is usually associated with acute processes. The manifestations of severe acidemia (pH <7.20) involve the cardiovascular, respiratory, and CNS. Hyperventilation is often the first sign of metabolic acidosis. At a pH of 7.2, pulmonary ventilation increases approximately fourfold, and an eightfold increase has been noted at a pH of 7.[24,25] Respiratory compensation can occur as Kussmaul respirations—the deep, rapid respirations seen commonly in patients with diabetic ketoacidosis. In extremely severe acidosis (pH <6.8), CNS function is disrupted to such a degree that the respiratory center is depressed.

CNS depression correlates more closely with spinal fluid pH than with blood pH. For this reason, neurologic symptoms tend to occur more frequently and to a greater degree in patients with respiratory acidosis because the CO_2 accumulated in the respiratory form readily crosses the blood–brain barrier to cause acidosis in the CNS.[1] Because of the slow penetration of administered bicarbonate into the CNS, the CNS pH fails to normalize as rapidly as blood pH. Therefore patients continue to hyperventilate because of sustained CNS acidity, and severe respiratory alkalosis can occur. Sustained lowering of the $Paco_2$ within 12 to 36 hours is to be anticipated during the correction of any metabolic acidosis.[1]

Systemic acidosis can cause peripheral arteriolar dilatation, characterized by flushing, a rapid heart rate, and wide pulse pressure. Initially, cardiac output can be increased, but as acidosis becomes more severe, myocardial contractility becomes impaired, and cardiac output decreases. The effects of vagal stimulation are also enhanced at pH levels lower than 7.1, probably as a consequence of inhibition of acetylcholinesterase. This increases the danger of vagally mediated bradycardia and heart block during acidosis.

GI symptoms of metabolic acidosis include loss of appetite, nausea, and vomiting. Severe acidosis (pH <7.1) interferes with carbohydrate metabolism and insulin utilization, and results in hyperglycemia. Metabolic acidosis alters potassium homeostasis and contributes to the development of hyperkalemia. The magnitude of the effect on serum potassium depends on the type of acidosis: Acidosis caused by mineral acids (e.g., hydrochloric acid) is associated with a greater change in potassium levels than acidosis caused by organic acids (e.g., lactic acidosis), in which the increase in potassium attributable to the acidosis per se is minimal.

Compensation

5 The patient's primary means to compensate for metabolic acidosis is to increase carbon dioxide excretion by increasing the respiratory rate. This results in a decrease in $Paco_2$. This ventilatory compensation results from stimulation of the respiratory center by changes in cerebral bicarbonate concentration and pH.[1] For

CLINICAL PRESENTATION Metabolic Acidosis

General

- The patient is usually relatively asymptomatic if the acidosis is acute and mild. In those with severe acidemia (pH <7.15–7.20), the cardiovascular, respiratory and central nervous systems can be affected

Symptoms

- The patient may complain of loss of appetite, nausea, and vomiting

Signs

- Cardiac: Flushing, a rapid heart rate, wide pulse pressure, and an increase in cardiac output can be seen initially. This can be followed by a reduction in cardiac output, blood pressure, and liver and kidney blood flow
- Cerebral: Obtundation or coma
- Metabolic: Insulin resistance; increased protein degradation; increased metabolic demands
- GI: Nausea, vomiting, loss of appetite
- Respiratory: Dyspnea, hyperventilation with deep, rapid respirations is seen in those with severe acidosis
- Chronic acidemia causes bone demineralization with the development of rickets in children and osteomalacia and osteopenia in adults

Laboratory Tests

- Serum CO_2 is low. Hyperglycemia and hyperkalemia are common. Patients with a pH of <7.2 are deemed to have a severe acidosis

TABLE 37-7 Guidelines for Initial Interpretation of Acid–Base Disorders

Acidosis	
Metabolic	Pa_{CO_2} (in mm Hg) should decrease by 1.3 times the fall in plasma [HCO_3^-] (in mEq/L or mmol/L)
Acute respiratory	The plasma [HCO_3^-] should increase by 0.1 times the increase in Pa_{CO_2} ± 3 (in mm Hg)
Chronic respiratory	The plasma [HCO_3^-] should increase by 0.35 times the increase in Pa_{CO_2} ± 4 (in mm Hg)
Alkalosis	
Metabolic	Pa_{CO_2} (in mm Hg) should increase by 0.4–0.6 times the rise in plasma [HCO_3^-] (in mEq/L or mmol/L)
Acute respiratory	The plasma [HCO_3^-] should decrease by 0.2 times the decrease in Pa_{CO_2} (in mm Hg), but usually not to less than 18 mEq/L (mmol/L)
Chronic respiratory	The plasma [HCO_3^-] should fall by 0.35 times the decrease in Pa_{CO_2} (in mm Hg), but usually not to less than 14 mEq/L (mmol/L)

HCO_3^-, bicarbonate; Pa_{CO_2}, partial pressure of carbon dioxide from arterial blood.
Adapted from reference 4.

every 1-mEq/L (1 mmol/L) decrease in bicarbonate concentration below the average of 24, the Pa_{CO_2} decreases by approximately 1 to 1.5 mm Hg (0.13 to 0.20 kPa) from the normal value of 40 (5.3 kPa) (Table 37-7).

The anticipated Pa_{CO_2} associated with a given bicarbonate concentration for patients with uncomplicated metabolic acidosis can be calculated as[25]:

$$Pa_{CO_2} = (1.5 \times [HCO_3^-]) + 8] \pm 2 \text{ for } Pa_{CO_2} \text{ in mm Hg}$$
$$(Pa_{CO_2} = (0.2 \times [HCO_3^-]) + 1.1] \pm 0.3 \text{ for } Pa_{CO_2} \text{ in kPa})$$

For example, 95% of patients with a plasma bicarbonate of 16 mEq/L (16 mmol/L) should have an arterial P_{CO_2} of 30 to 34 mm Hg (4.0 to 4.5 kPa). An observed arterial P_{CO_2} within this range is consistent with physiologic respiratory compensation for a metabolic acidosis and suggests that there is no respiratory disturbance. In contrast, if the P_{CO_2} is less than 30 mm Hg (4.0 kPa), a superimposed respiratory alkalosis can be present, whereas if the P_{CO_2} is greater than 34 mm Hg (4.5 kPa), a superimposed respiratory acidosis is likely present.

TREATMENT

Chronic Metabolic Acidosis

6 Asymptomatic patients with mild to moderate degrees of acidemia (plasma bicarbonate of 12 to 20 mEq/L ([12 to 20 mmol/L]; pH 7.2–7.4) do not require emergent therapy. They can usually be managed with gradual correction of the acidemia, over a period of days to weeks, using oral sodium bicarbonate or other alkali preparations (Table 37-8). In all forms of chronic metabolic acidosis, primary therapy should be directed at treating the underlying disease state. GI pathology should be treated to reduce ongoing bicarbonate losses, and factors that exacerbate RTA should be treated. If acidemia persists, alkali therapy should be instituted with the goal of normalization of blood pH. The loading dose (LD) of alkali to initially correct the acidemia can be calculated as follows:

$$\text{LD (mEq or mmol/L)} = (V_D\ HCO_3^- \times \text{body weight [BW]}) \times (\text{desired } [HCO_3^-] - \text{current } [HCO_3^-])$$

where V_D is the volume of distribution of bicarbonate.[7]

For a 60-kg patient with a serum bicarbonate of 15 mEq/L (15 mmol/L), the LD is calculated thus:

$$\begin{aligned}\text{LD (mEq)} &= (0.5 \text{ L/kg} \times 60 \text{ kg}) \times (24 \text{ mEq/L} - 15 \text{ mEq/L}) \\ &= 30 \text{ L} \times 9 \text{ mEq/L} \\ &= 270 \text{ mEq/L (270 mmol/L)}\end{aligned}$$

The calculated LD of alkali should be administered over several days to avoid volume overload from the accompanying sodium load. For this scenario, a regimen of 60 to 70 mEq (60 to 70 mmol) three times a day for 3 to 5 days should result in an increase in HCO_3^- levels toward normal. In addition to the calculated LD, supplemental alkali must also be provided to replace ongoing losses, which can be approximated to be 2 mEq/kg (2 mmol/kg) per day or 40 mEq (40 mmol) three times a day. In patients with associated volume depletion, bicarbonate replacement can be provided simultaneous with volume resuscitation by substituting bicarbonate for chloride in IV crystalloid solutions.

TABLE 37-8 Therapeutic Alternatives for Oral Alkali Replacement

Generic Name	Trade Name(s)	Milliequivalents of Alkali	Dosage Form(s)	Comment
Shohl's solution (sodium citrate/citric acid)	Bicitra (Willen)	1 mEq Na/mL; equivalent to 1 mEq bicarbonate	Solution (500 mg Na citrate, 334 mg citric acid/5 mL)	Citrate preparations increase absorption of aluminum
Sodium bicarbonate	Various (e.g., Sodamint)	3.9 mEq bicarbonate/tablet (325 mg)	325 mg tablet	Bicarbonate preparations can cause bloating because of CO_2 production
		7.8 mEq bicarbonate/tablet (650 mg)	650 mg tablet	
	Baking soda (various)	60 mEq bicarbonate/tsp (5 g/tsp)	Powder	
Potassium citrate	Urocit-K (Mission)	5 mEq citrate/tablet	5 mEq tablet	See above
Potassium bicarbonate/ potassium citrate	K-Lyte (Bristol)	25 mEq bicarbonate/tablet	25 mEq tablet (effervescent)	
	K-Lyte DS (Bristol)	50 mEq bicarbonate/tablet (double strength)	50 mEq tablet (effervescent)	See above
Potassium citrate/ citric acid	Polycitra-K (Willen)	2 mEq K/mL; equivalent to 2 mEq bicarbonate	Solution (1,100 mg K citrate, 334 mg citric acid/5 mL)	See above
		30 mEq bicarbonate/unit dose packet	Crystals for reconstitution (3,300 mg K citrate, 1,002 mg citric acid/unit dose packet)	
Sodium citrate/ potassium citrate/ citric acid	Polycitra (Willen) Polycitra-LC (Willen)	1 mEq K, 1 mEq Na/mL; equivalent to 2 mEq bicarbonate	Syrup (Polycitra) solution (Polycitra-LC) (Both contain 550 mg K citrate, 500 mg Na citrate, 334 mg citric acid/5 mL)	See above

In patients with chronic metabolic acidosis because of GI bicarbonate losses, maintenance therapy should provide sufficient alkali to replace ongoing bicarbonate losses. The magnitude of this replacement is variable and can be substantial (>10 mEq/kg [>10 mmol/kg] per day). In addition, associated losses of other electrolytes, such as potassium and magnesium, may need to be replaced (see Chap. 36).

Proximal (type II) RTA is a bicarbonate-wasting disorder that requires the administration of large maintenance doses of alkali (10 to 15 mEq/kg [10 to 15 mmol/kg] per day). As alkali replacement raises the serum bicarbonate concentration toward normal, the proximal tubule's capacity to reabsorb bicarbonate is overwhelmed, and renal bicarbonate wasting increases. In children, aggressive therapy of proximal RTA is necessary to avoid growth retardation and osteopenia. Because this is generally a mild, nonprogressive acidosis in adults, the benefit of alkali therapy is frequently outweighed by the risks of increased potassium wasting. In patients with classic distal (type I) RTA, maintenance therapy usually requires only enough alkali to buffer the amount of acid generated from dietary intake and metabolism. This usually approximates 1 to 3 mEq/kg per day (1 to 3 mmol/kg per day).

7 After initial potassium deficits are replaced, ongoing potassium supplementation may not be required, as renal potassium losses decrease following initiation of appropriate alkali therapy. The use of potassium alkali salts can, however, be desirable in patients with associated nephrolithiasis, because sodium salts can increase urinary calcium excretion.

The metabolic acidosis associated with hyperkalemic distal (type IV) RTA with hyporeninemic-hypoaldosteronemia that is often seen in patients with diabetes mellitus can be corrected by the treatment of hyperkalemia alone (see Chap. 36). The use of supplemental alkali (1 to 2 mEq/kg [1 to 2 mmol/kg] per day) to increase sodium intake and stimulate distal tubular potassium secretion can be beneficial. A minority of patients require the administration of pharmacologic amounts of fludrocortisone.[7] Type IV RTA resulting from a generalized distal tubular disorder often responds to low doses of alkali (1.5 to 2.0 mEq/kg [1.5 to 2.0 mmol/kg] per day).[27] Corrections of the acidosis along with modest dietary potassium restriction (to 1 mEq/kg [1 mmol/kg] per day) will often result in the maintenance of serum potassium levels of 5 mEq/L (5 mmol/L) or less.

Acute Severe Metabolic Acidosis

8 The management of patients with life-threatening acute metabolic acidosis (plasma bicarbonate of 8 mEq/L [8 mmol/L] and pH <7.20) is dependent on the underlying cause and the patient's cardiovascular status. In some cases, patients will require emergent hemodialysis therapy (see Chap. 30). Patients with hyperchloremic acidosis (e.g., diarrhea-induced) are unable to regenerate bicarbonate, and the generation of new bicarbonate by the kidneys can require several days before one can observe a meaningful change in their status.[11] Thus IV alkali therapy is often required for these patients.

Although conventional wisdom recommends the use of alkali replacement in patients with severe acidemia because of the deleterious effects of acidemia on circulatory function,[6,7,10,11] studies have not demonstrated that its administration improves patient outcomes.[28–31] Alkali therapies may either improve or worsen clinically relevant endpoints such as [H+], $Paco_2$, lactate concentrations, and cardiac output. The specific patient populations most likely to benefit or be harmed from alkalinizing therapy are presented in Table 37-9.

There are several therapeutic alternatives available for the acute correction of severe metabolic acidosis. Sodium acetate, sodium citrate, and sodium lactate are unreliable sources of alkali because their alkalinizing effect is dependent on their oxidative conversion to bicarbonate. This process is often impaired in critically ill patients, especially those with liver disease or circulatory failure. Although sodium bicarbonate is the most widely used IV alkalotic agent,[7] several studies suggest that it is frequently ineffective and can actually be deleterious, especially in patients with lactic acidosis.[28–31] Two of the three remaining alternatives (Carbicarb and dichloroacetate [DCA]) are investigational and not available in most clinical settings. Tromethamine, or THAM, is a carbon dioxide-consuming, commercially available solution that buffers respiratory as well as metabolic acids.

TABLE 37-9 Patient Populations Likely to Benefit or Suffer from Alkalinizing Therapy

Patients with Potential for Benefit	Patients with Potential for Harm
Distal (type 1) renal tubular acidosis	Hypernatremia
Severe hypochloremic metabolic acidosis secondary to diarrhea or surgical diversion	Hypervolemia Acute renal failure Congestive heart failure
Specific poisonings and intoxications (e.g., salicylate overdose with metabolic acidosis)	Pulmonary disease resulting in decreased ventilation Acute lung injury where lung-protective ventilation strategy is used Diabetic ketoacidosis

Clinical **Controversy...**

The role of alkali therapy in patients with severe lactic acidosis is controversial. Treatment should be directed at the underlying causes as serial bicarbonate administration is often not effective and in some settings can be deleterious.

Sodium Bicarbonate

While sodium bicarbonate administration provides fluid and electrolyte replacement and increases arterial pH, neither animal nor clinical studies demonstrate an improvement in cardiac function, organ perfusion, or intracellular pH.[28–31] In addition, sodium bicarbonate administration can actually have paradoxical adverse effects on intracellular pH. When bicarbonate is given by IV infusion, the carbon dioxide generated diffuses more readily than bicarbonate across cell membranes and into cerebrospinal fluid. Therefore, the intracellular pH can actually be decreased by administration of bicarbonate.[4]

Excessive sodium bicarbonate administration can result in (a) a shift of the oxyhemoglobin saturation curve to the left, thereby impairing oxygen release from hemoglobin to tissues; (b) sodium and water overload, with subsequent pulmonary congestion and hypernatremia; (c) paradoxical tissue acidosis as a result of the production of CO_2 that freely diffuses into myocardial and cerebral cells[32]; and (d) decreased ionized calcium with a resultant decrease in myocardial contractility. If there is an endogenous source of bicarbonate, such as can occur in the case of ketoacidosis or lactic acidosis, a bicarbonate "overshoot" can develop because the ketoacids (acetoacetic acid and β-hydroxybutyric acid) or lactic acid are converted in the liver to bicarbonate once the underlying cause of acidosis is corrected.[10,11,33] Alkalosis can also result if too much sodium bicarbonate is administered too quickly.

If IV sodium bicarbonate is used, one must be mindful that the goals are to increase, not normalize, pH (to approximately 7.20) and plasma bicarbonate (to 8 to 10 mEq/L [8 to 10 mmol/L]). There is no calculative method that will assure attainment of these goals with a given dose of sodium bicarbonate because of the multiplicity of competing processes that can affect acid–base status (e.g., vomiting, potential increases in endogenous acid production, and renal failure) and the marked variability in the volume of distribution of bicarbonate (50% of body weight in patients with mild acidosis to approximately 100% in those with severe acidosis).[10,32–33] Kraut and Madias[7] recommend that the dose of sodium bicarbonate be calculated using a distribution volume of 50% of body weight for all patients to avoid overtreatment. The total dose calculated as described previously in the RTA section should be administered as an infusion over one-half to several hours. Follow-up monitoring of ABGs, beginning no sooner than 30 minutes after the end of the infusion, should be used to guide further therapeutic decisions.

Clinical **Controversy...**

Although it has been recommended that sodium bicarbonate be administered to raise the arterial pH to approximately 7.20, in an effort to prevent complications such as ventricular tachyarrhythmia, there are no controlled clinical trials demonstrating that sodium bicarbonate administration is significantly better than general supportive care in reducing morbidity and mortality in these patients.[30,31,34]

Bicarbonate therapy is generally not necessary for patients with cardiac arrest, even if the initial arrest was unmonitored. The American Heart Association's Advanced Cardiac Life Support (ACLS) provider manual states that sodium bicarbonate is not useful or effective during resuscitation in hypoxic patients with lactic acidosis.[34] Additionally, sodium bicarbonate is considered to be not useful or effective in those who are undergoing prolonged resuscitation with effective ventilation.[34] Furthermore, if sodium bicarbonate is used, it should be used only after defibrillation, cardiac compression, support of ventilation including intubation, and drug therapies such as epinephrine and antiarrhythmic agents have been employed.[34] The initial dose of sodium bicarbonate in this situation is (1 mEq/kg [1 mmol/kg]) administered by rapid, direct IV injection.[35] Subsequent doses of sodium bicarbonate should be based on measurements of arterial blood pH and $Paco_2$ given the propensity for it to cause alkalemia.[36]

Tromethamine

THAM, available as a 0.3 N solution, is a highly alkaline, sodium-free organic amine that acts as a proton acceptor to prevent or correct acidosis.[7,28] THAM combines with hydrogen ions from carbonic acid to form bicarbonate and a cationic buffer. THAM also acts as an osmotic diuretic to increase urine flow, urine pH, and the excretion of fixed acids, CO_2, and electrolytes. At pH 7.4, 30% of THAM is not ionized and therefore can penetrate into cells and neutralize acidic anions of the intracellular fluid. Intracellular pH increases have been noted within 1 hour after the infusion of THAM. There is, however, no clinical or physiologic evidence that this action is beneficial, or that THAM is more efficacious than sodium bicarbonate.[28,37]

When THAM is used, it must be administered slowly, with careful monitoring to avoid alkalosis. The usual empiric dosage range for THAM is 1 to 5 mmol/kg administered IV over 1 hour, but doses up to 1.25 mmol/kg can be given over 5 to 15 minutes in acute situations. The dose of THAM can be individualized using the following equation[35]:

$$\text{Dose of THAM (in mL)} = 1.1 \times \text{BW (in kg)} \times \text{base deficit}$$

where base deficit = normal $[HCO_3^-]$ – current $[HCO_3^-]$.

The need for additional THAM is determined by serial measurements of the serum bicarbonate concentration and calculation of the base deficit. Large doses can cause respiratory depression as a result of an increase in blood pH and a decrease in $Paco_2$ concentration.[35] THAM solution is highly alkaline and can cause severe inflammation, vascular spasm, or tissue damage (necrosis, sloughing, pain, chemical phlebitis, or thrombosis) if infiltration occurs. Hyperkalemia, hypoglycemia, hypocalcemia, and impaired coagulation have also been reported.[28,35] This agent should only be used with extreme caution in patients with severe liver or kidney failure.

Carbicarb

Carbicarb is an equimolar mixture of sodium carbonate (Na_2CO_3) and sodium bicarbonate ($NaHCO_3$).[38,39] Given that the carbonate ion is a stronger base than bicarbonate, Carbicarb preferentially buffers hydrogen ions resulting in the formation of bicarbonate rather than CO_2. Thus Carbicarb limits, but does not eliminate, the generation of CO_2. Unlike bicarbonate, which can produce a paradoxical intracellular acidosis and thereby impair cardiac function, Carbicarb appears to correct intracellular acidosis if present.[40,41] Despite these effects, there are no consistent data on the effects of Carbicarb on hemodynamic endpoints and this agent is not available for use in humans.[28]

Dichloroacetate

DCA, another investigational agent, facilitates aerobic lactate metabolism by stimulating the activity of lactate dehydrogenase, thus reversing hyperlactatemia and elevating blood pH.[42,43] DCA, when compared to conventional management in controlled studies, however, has not been shown to improve hemodynamic parameters or clinical outcomes.[42–44] DCA can cause mild drowsiness and peripheral neuropathy that can be ameliorated or prevented with thiamine supplementation.[45] The future role of DCA in the management of metabolic acidosis, particularly lactic acidosis, remains to be clarified.[28]

Metabolic Alkalosis

Pathophysiology

Metabolic alkalosis is a simple acid–base disorder that presents as alkalemia (increased arterial pH) with an increase in plasma bicarbonate. It is an extremely common entity in hospitalized patients with acid–base disturbances. Under normal circumstances, the kidney is readily able to excrete an alkali load. Thus evaluation of patients with metabolic alkalosis must consider two separate issues: (a) the initial process that generates the metabolic alkalosis; and (b) alterations in renal function that maintain the alkalemic state.[46,47]

9 The generation of metabolic alkalosis can also result from excessive losses of hydrogen ions from the kidneys or stomach or from a gain secondary to the ingestion or administration of bicarbonate-rich fluids. Gastric juice, rich in chloride and hydrogen ions, is secreted at a rate of less than 50 mL/h in the basal state, but can increase up to fivefold with stimulation.[8] In the gastric parietal cells, the hydrogen ion and bicarbonate are generated from CO_2 and water.[46] The hydrogen ion is secreted into gastric fluid, and the bicarbonate is retained in the ECF. Normally, an amount of bicarbonate equal to the bicarbonate generated in the stomach is eliminated in the alkaline pancreatic and small-bowel secretions, maintaining hydrogen ion balance. With vomiting and nasogastric suctioning, the hydrogen ion is lost externally and metabolic alkalosis results. Diarrhea, as seen with secretory villous adenomas and other secretory diarrheas, often results in excessive GI losses of chloride-rich, bicarbonate-poor fluid, and thus leads to the generation of metabolic alkalosis.

10 Diuretic agents acting on the thick ascending limb of the loop of Henle (e.g., furosemide, bumetanide, and torsemide) and distal convoluted tubule (e.g., thiazides) have most commonly been associated with the generation of metabolic alkalosis.[47,48] These agents promote the excretion of sodium and potassium almost exclusively in association with chloride, without a proportionate increase in bicarbonate excretion. Collecting duct hydrogen ion secretion is stimulated directly by the increased luminal flow rate and sodium delivery, and indirectly by intravascular volume contraction, which

results in secondary hyperaldosteronism. Renal ammoniagenesis can also be stimulated by concomitant hypokalemia, further augmenting net acid excretion.

Increased renal acid excretion can also be the result of excess mineralocorticoid activity. Elevated mineralocorticoid levels directly stimulate collecting duct hydrogen ion secretion and indirectly increase ammoniagenesis by causing hypokalemia.[46] Increased mineralocorticoid activity can result from Cushing's syndrome, primary hyperaldosteronism, or hyperaldosteronism secondary to increased renin activity (e.g., malignant hypertension). In Bartter's and Gitelman's syndromes, defects in sodium transport in the loop of Henle (Bartter) or distal convoluted tubule (Gitelman) lead to hypokalemia, secondary hyperaldosteronism, and metabolic alkalosis.[46] In Liddle's syndrome, enhanced sodium reabsorption by the cortical collecting duct epithelial sodium channel results in a syndrome of pseudohyperaldosteronism.[46] Administration of high doses of penicillins (e.g., ticarcillin) can produce metabolic alkalosis because they act as nonreabsorbable anions. High concentrations of poorly reabsorbable anions in the distal renal tubule increase luminal flow rate and luminal electronegativity, which enhances the secretion of potassium and hydrogen ions and results in hypokalemia and metabolic alkalosis.

Metabolic alkalosis can also be generated by the gain of exogenous alkali. This can be seen as a result of bicarbonate administration or from the infusion of organic anions that are metabolized to bicarbonate, such as acetate, lactate, and citrate. The milk-alkali syndrome was historically a common cause of metabolic alkalosis in patients with peptic ulcer disease secondary to the ingestion of large quantities of milk products and antacids. With the advent of alternative therapies for dyspeptic syndromes that are far more effective than milk, this syndrome is now rarely seen.

Metabolic alkalosis is predominantly maintained because of an abnormality in renal function. Normally, the kidneys are capable of excreting all of the excess bicarbonate presented to them, even during periods of increased bicarbonate loads.[4] As the serum bicarbonate concentration increases, the filtered bicarbonate load exceeds the maximal rate for bicarbonate reabsorption, and the excess bicarbonate is excreted in the urine. Under normal circumstances, the excess bicarbonate is rapidly excreted, and metabolic alkalosis does not occur or is corrected in a matter of hours.[46]

11 Several mechanisms can impair renal bicarbonate excretion and contribute to the maintenance phase of metabolic alkalosis.[46] In general, these mechanisms can be divided into volume-mediated processes (sodium chloride-responsive) and volume-independent processes (sodium chloride-resistant) that are predominantly associated with excess mineralocorticoid activity and hypokalemia (Table 37-10). Intravascular volume depletion maintains metabolic alkalosis through a number of mechanisms. Decreases in the glomerular filtration rate reduce the filtered load of bicarbonate at any given serum concentration, thereby decreasing the kidney's ability to excrete a bicarbonate load. Although this can play a role in patients with chronic kidney disease, it is also an important factor in patients in whom intravascular volume contraction accompanies metabolic alkalosis. Decreased effective arterial blood volume also enhances proximal and distal tubular sodium reabsorption. Sodium reabsorption must be coupled with reabsorption of an anion, such as chloride or bicarbonate, or exchange with a cation, such as potassium or hydrogen, to maintain charge neutrality. In the proximal tubule, increased sodium reabsorption stimulates bicarbonate reabsorption. In the distal nephron, enhanced sodium reabsorption, particularly in the setting of hypokalemia, stimulates hydrogen ion secretion.

Mineralocorticoid excess also plays a significant role in the maintenance of metabolic alkalosis. In patients with volume-responsive metabolic alkalosis, intravascular volume depletion stimulates aldosterone secretion. As discussed earlier, excess mineralocorticoid activity can also underlie the generation of metabolic alkalosis. In either situation, the increased mineralocorticoid effect stimulates collecting duct hydrogen ion secretion. Metabolic alkalosis can also be maintained by persistent hypokalemia, enhancing proximal tubular bicarbonate reabsorption, stimulating ammoniagenesis, and increasing distal tubular hydrogen ion secretion.[46]

TABLE 37-10 Causes of Metabolic Alkalosis Differentiated on the Basis of Their Responsiveness to Sodium Chloride

Sodium chloride-responsive (urinary chloride concentration <10 mEq/L [<10 mmol/L])
GI disorders
Vomiting
Gastric drainage
Villous adenoma of the colon
Chloride diarrhea
Diuretic therapy
Correction of chronic hypercapnia
Cystic fibrosis
Excessive bicarbonate therapy of an organic acidosis
Mild/moderate potassium deficiency
Sodium chloride-resistant (urinary chloride concentration >20 mEq/L [>20 mmol/L])
Excess mineralocorticoid activity
Hyperaldosteronism
Cushing's syndrome
Bartter's syndrome
Gitelman's syndrome
Excessive black licorice intake
Profound potassium depletion
Magnesium deficiency
Liddle's syndrome
Estrogen therapy
Unclassified
Alkali administration
Milk-alkali syndrome
Massive blood or plasma protein fraction transfusion
Nonparathyroid hypercalcemia
Carbohydrate refeeding after starvation
Large doses of penicillin

Clinical Presentation

There are no unique signs or symptoms associated with mild to moderate metabolic alkalosis, but patients may complain of symptoms related to the underlying cause of the disorder (e.g., muscle weakness with hypokalemia or postural dizziness with volume depletion). They may have a history of vomiting, gastric drainage, or diuretic use, all of which contribute to the development of metabolic alkalosis. Severe alkalemia (blood pH >7.60) has been associated with cardiac arrhythmias, particularly in patients with heart disease, hyperventilation, and hypoxemia.[46] Neuromuscular irritability can be present, with signs of tetany or hyperactive reflexes, possibly caused by the decreased ionized calcium concentration that occurs secondary to the increase in pH. This decrease in ionized calcium may be caused by a conformational change in the albumin molecules to which the calcium is bound, resulting in increased binding, or by decreased competition from hydrogen ions for binding sites on the albumin molecule. Mental confusion, muscle cramping, and paresthesia can also occur. Lastly, patients will be more difficult to liberate from mechanical ventilation.

Compensation

The respiratory response to metabolic alkalosis is hypoventilation, which results in an increased $Paco_2$. Respiratory compensation is initiated within hours when the central and peripheral chemoreceptors sense an increase in pH. The $Paco_2$ increases 6 to 7 mm Hg (0.8 to 0.9 kPa) for each 10 mEq/L (10 mmol/L) increase in

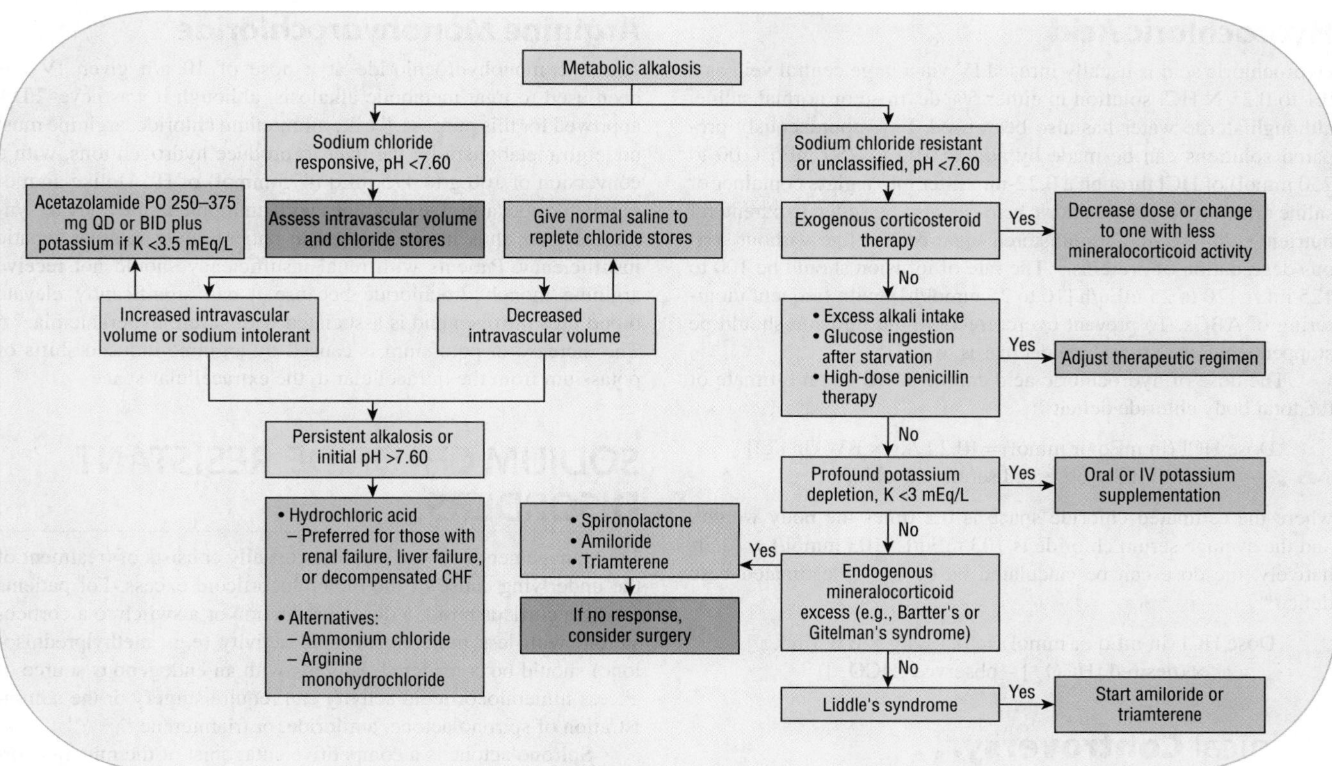

FIGURE 37-4 Treatment algorithm for patients with primary metabolic alkalosis. (BID, twice daily; CHF, chronic heart failure; K, potassium [serum potassium in mEq/L is numerically equivalent to mmol/L]; PO, orally; QD, every day.)

bicarbonate, up to a $PaCO_2$ of approximately 50 to 60 mm Hg (6.7 to 8.0 kPa) (see Table 37-7) before hypoxia sensors react to prevent further hypoventilation. If the $PaCO_2$ is normal or less than normal, one should consider the presence of a superimposed respiratory alkalosis, which can be secondary to fever, gram-negative sepsis, or pain.

TREATMENT

Because the body tolerates alkalemia far less well than acidemia, treatment of metabolic alkalosis is nearly always required and should be aimed at correcting the factor(s) responsible for the maintenance of the alkalosis.[46] For example, vomiting should be treated with antiemetics, gastric losses of hydrogen ions during nasogastric suction can be modulated by giving histamine blockers such as ranitidine or proton pump inhibitors such as omeprazole, and reducing or discontinuing diuretic therapy.[46,49] Metabolic alkalosis will persist until the renal mechanism responsible for maintaining the disorder is corrected, despite the fact that the original cause of the elevated plasma bicarbonate may have resolved. For example, hypovolemia should be treated with sodium chloride (i.e., diuretic abuse or nasogastric suction) to allow excretion of bicarbonate by the kidney. However, patients with severely compromised cardiovascular function may not be able to tolerate this therapeutic approach. In situations such as this and/or the presence of life-threatening alkalosis, some have advocated reduction in pH by control of ventilation.[4] Although controlled hypoventilation, sometimes using inspired CO_2 with supplemental oxygen to prevent hypoxia can be lifesaving,[4] this approach is not universally accepted.[33] Therapy for metabolic alkalosis can be conceptualized on the basis of the sodium chloride responsiveness of the disorders as shown in Figure 37-4.

SODIUM CHLORIDE-RESPONSIVE DISORDERS

Sodium chloride-responsive disorders usually result from volume depletion and chloride loss, which can accompany severe vomiting, prolonged nasogastric suction, and diuretic therapy. Initially, therapy is directed at expanding intravascular volume and replenishing chloride stores. Sodium and potassium chloride-containing solutions should be administered to patients who can tolerate the volume load.[46] Patients with metabolic alkalosis who are volume overloaded or intolerant to volume administration because of congestive heart failure can benefit from the carbonic anhydrase inhibitor acetazolamide. This agent inhibits the action of carbonic anhydrase, thereby inhibiting renal bicarbonate reabsorption. Unfortunately, it also increases the renal losses of potassium and phosphate. Administration of acetazolamide (250 to 375 mg once or twice daily) can promote a sufficient bicarbonate diuresis and return the pH toward normal.[50] However, because the clinical effectiveness of the drug declines as the HCO_3^- concentration decreases, only rarely will this approach fully correct the alkalosis.[46]

Acidifying agents including hydrochloric acid, ammonium chloride, and arginine monohydrochloride can be used to treat severe (pH >7.6) symptomatic metabolic alkalosis.[51] In general, this management is reserved for patients who are unresponsive to conventional fluid and electrolyte management or who are unable to tolerate the requisite volume load because of decompensated congestive heart failure or advanced renal failure.[46] Alternatively, hemodialysis using a low-bicarbonate dialysate can be used for the rapid correction of metabolic alkalosis.

Hydrochloric Acid

Hydrochloric acid is usually infused IV via a large central vein as a 0.1 to 0.25 N HCl solution in either 5% dextrose or normal saline, although sterile water has also been used. Extemporaneously prepared solutions can be made by adding 100 to 250 mEq (100 to 250 mmol) of HCl through a 0.22-mm filter into a glass container of saline or dextrose. Hydrochloric acid can also be added to parenteral nutrient solutions and administered via a central line without serious degradation of proteins.[52] The rate of infusion should be 100 to 125 mL/h (10 to 25 mEq/h [10 to 25 mmol/h]), with frequent monitoring of ABGs. To prevent overcorrection, the infusion should be stopped when the arterial pH decreases to 7.50.[46]

The dose of hydrochloric acid can be based on an estimate of the total body chloride deficit[35]:

$$\text{Dose HCl (in mEq or mmol)} = [0.2 \text{ L/kg} \times \text{BW (in kg)}] \times [103 - \text{observed serum chloride}]$$

where the estimated chloride space is 0.2 times the body weight, and the average serum chloride is 103 mEq/L (103 mmol/L). Alternatively, the dose can be calculated based on the estimated base deficit[46]:

$$\text{Dose HCl (in mEq or mmol)} = [0.5 \text{ L/kg} \times \text{BW (in kg)}] \times (\text{desired } [HCO_3^-] - \text{observed } [HCO_3^-])$$

Clinical **Controversy...**

At present, there are no comparative data that address the relative accuracy of these two formulas for determining the dose of hydrochloric acid.

The dose of hydrochloric acid is usually infused IV over 12 to 24 hours.[35] A severe transient respiratory acidosis can occur if the hydrochloric acid is infused too quickly because of a slower reduction of the elevated bicarbonate concentration in the cerebrospinal fluid than in the ECF. Improvement is usually seen within 24 hours of initiating therapy. ABGs and serum electrolytes should be drawn every 4 to 8 hours to evaluate and adjust therapy.

Ammonium Chloride

Ammonium chloride has a limited role in the treatment of metabolic alkalosis. The liver converts ammonium chloride (NH_4Cl) to urea and free hydrochloric acid[35]:

$$2NH_4Cl + 2HCO_3^- \rightarrow CO(NH_2)_2 + CO_2 + 3H_2O + 2Cl^-$$

The dose of ammonium chloride can be calculated on the basis of the chloride deficit using the same method as for HCl and assuming that 20 g ammonium chloride will provide 374 mEq (374 mmol) of H^+. However, only one half of the calculated dose of ammonium chloride should be administered so as to avoid ammonia toxicity. Ammonium chloride is available as a 26.75% solution containing 100 mEq (100 mmol) of H^+ in 20 mL, which should be further diluted prior to administration. A dilute solution can be prepared by adding 20 mL of ammonium chloride to 500 mL of normal saline and infusing the solution at a rate of no more than 1 mEq/min (1 mmol/min). Improvement in metabolic status is usually seen within 24 hours. CNS toxicity, marked by confusion, irritability, seizures, and coma, has been associated with more rapid rates of administration. Ammonium chloride must be administered cautiously to patients with renal or hepatic impairment. In patients with hepatic dysfunction, impaired conversion of ammonia to urea can result in increased ammonia levels and worsened encephalopathy. In patients with renal failure, the increased urea synthesis can exacerbate uremic symptoms.[35]

Arginine Monohydrochloride

Arginine monohydrochloride at a dose of 10 g/h given IV has been used to treat metabolic alkalosis, although it was never FDA approved for this purpose.[35] Like ammonium chloride, arginine must undergo metabolism by the liver to produce hydrogen ions, with a conversion of 100 g to 475 mEq (475 mmol) of H^+. Unlike ammonium chloride, arginine combines with ammonia in the body to synthesize urea; thus it can be used in patients with relative hepatic insufficiency. Patients with renal insufficiency should not receive arginine monohydrochloride because it can significantly elevate blood urea nitrogen and is associated with severe hyperkalemia.[35,46] The increase in potassium is caused by arginine-induced shifts of potassium from the intracellular to the extracellular space.

SODIUM CHLORIDE-RESISTANT DISORDERS

12 Management of these disorders usually consists of treatment of the underlying cause of the mineralocorticoid excess. For patients taking a corticosteroid, a dosage reduction or a switch to a corticosteroid with less mineralocorticoid activity (e.g., methylprednisolone) should be considered. Patients with an endogenous source of excess mineralocorticoid activity can require surgery or the administration of spironolactone, amiloride, or triamterene.[46,48,53,54]

Spironolactone is a competitive antagonist of the mineralocorticoid receptor. Amiloride and triamterene are potassium-sparing diuretics that inhibit the epithelial sodium channel in the distal convoluted tubule and collecting duct. All three agents inhibit aldosterone-stimulated sodium reabsorption in the collecting duct. In addition, spironolactone directly inhibits aldosterone stimulation of the hydrogen ion secretory pump. Thus, most patients with mineralocorticoid excess, including Bartter's and Gitelman's syndromes, respond to therapy with these agents.[46,53–56] Liddle's syndrome, which is a form of pseudohypoaldosteronism caused by overactivity of the epithelial sodium channel, is not responsive to spironolactone but can be treated with either amiloride or triamterene. Although experience is limited, some patients with Bartter's and Gitelman's syndromes may respond to NSAIDs or ACE inhibitors.[53–56] Finally, aggressive potassium repletion can correct the alkalosis in those who have not responded to the approaches outlined above.

RESPIRATORY ACID–BASE DISORDERS

As with the metabolic acid–base disturbances, there are two cardinal respiratory acid–base disturbances: respiratory acidosis and respiratory alkalosis. These disorders are generated by a primary alteration in carbon dioxide excretion, which changes the concentration of carbon dioxide, and therefore the carbonic acid concentration in body fluids. A primary reduction in $Paco_2$ causes an increase in pH (respiratory alkalosis), and a primary increase in $Paco_2$ causes a decrease in pH (respiratory acidosis). Unlike the metabolic disturbances, for which respiratory compensation is rapid, metabolic compensation for the respiratory disturbances is slow. Hence, these disturbances can be further divided into acute disorders, with a duration of minutes to hours, and where metabolic compensation has yet to occur, and chronic disorders that have been present long enough for metabolic compensation to be complete.

Respiratory Alkalosis

Respiratory alkalosis is characterized by a primary decrease in $Paco_2$ that leads to an elevation in pH. The $Paco_2$ decreases when

TABLE 37-11 Causes of Respiratory Alkalosis

Central stimulation of respiration
Anxiety
Pain
Fever
Brain tumors, vascular accidents
Head trauma
Pregnancy
Progesterone
Catecholamines, theophylline, nicotine
Salicylates
Hypoxemia or tissue hypoxemia
High altitude
Decreased $Paco_2$
Pneumonia
Pulmonary edema
Severe anemia
Peripheral stimulation of respiration
Pulmonary emboli
Asthma

$Paco_2$, partial pressure of carbon dioxide from arterial blood.

the excretion of CO_2 by the lungs exceeds the metabolic production of CO_2. It is the most frequently encountered acid–base disorder, occurring physiologically in normal pregnancy and in persons living at high altitudes.[56,57] Respiratory alkalosis also occurs frequently among hospitalized patients (Table 37-11).

Pathophysiology

A decrease in $Paco_2$ occurs when ventilatory excretion exceeds metabolic production. Because endogenous production of CO_2 is relatively constant, negative CO_2 balance is primarily caused by an increase in ventilatory excretion of CO_2 (hyperventilation). The metabolic production of CO_2, however, can be increased during periods of stress or with excess carbohydrate administration (e.g., parenteral nutrition). Hyperventilation can develop from an increase in neurochemical stimulation via either central or peripheral mechanisms, or be the result of voluntary or mechanical (iatrogenic) hyperventilation.

A decrease in $Paco_2$ can occur in patients with cardiogenic, hypovolemic, or septic shock because oxygen delivery to the carotid and aortic chemoreceptors is reduced. This relative deficit in Pao_2 stimulates an increase in ventilation. The hyperventilation in sepsis is also mediated via a central mechanism. Hyperventilation-induced respiratory alkalosis with an elevation in cardiac index and hypotension without peripheral vasoconstriction can therefore be an early sign of sepsis.

Clinical Presentation

Although most patients are asymptomatic, respiratory alkalosis can cause adverse neuromuscular, cardiovascular, and GI effects.[56] During periods of decreased $Paco_2$, there is a decrease in cerebral blood flow, which can be responsible for symptoms of lightheadedness, confusion, decreased intellectual functioning, syncope, and seizures. Nausea and vomiting can occur, probably as a result of cerebral hypoxia. In severe respiratory alkalosis, cardiac arrhythmias can occur because of sensitization of the myocardium to the arrhythmogenic effects of circulating catecholamines.[2] Acute respiratory alkalosis has no effect on blood pressure or cardiac output in awake individuals. Anesthetized patients, however, can experience a decrease in both cardiac output and blood pressure, possibly owing to the lack of a tachycardic response.[56]

The concentration of serum electrolytes can also be altered secondary to the development of respiratory alkalosis. The serum chloride concentration is usually slightly increased, and serum potassium concentration can be slightly decreased. Clinically significant hypokalemia can be a consequence of extreme respiratory alkalosis, although the effect is usually very small or negligible.[2,56] Serum phosphorus concentration can decrease by as much as 1.5 to 2.0 mg/dL (0.48 to 0.65 mmol/L) because of the shift of inorganic phosphate into cells. Reductions in the blood ionized calcium concentration can be partially responsible for symptoms such as muscle cramps and tetany. Approximately 50% of calcium is bound to albumin, and an increase in pH results in an increase in binding.[56]

Compensation

The initial response of the body to acute respiratory alkalosis is chemical buffering: hydrogen ions are released from the body's buffers—intracellular proteins, phosphates, and hemoglobin—and titrate down the serum bicarbonate concentration. This process occurs within minutes. Acutely, the bicarbonate concentration can be decreased by a maximum of 3 mEq/L (3 mmol/L) for each 10-mm Hg (1.3 kPa) decrease in $Paco_2$[24] (see Table 37-7). When only physicochemical buffering has occurred, the disturbance is referred to as acute respiratory alkalosis.

Metabolic compensation occurs when respiratory alkalosis persists for more than 6 to 12 hours. In response to the alkalemia, proximal tubular bicarbonate reabsorption is inhibited, and the serum bicarbonate concentration decreases. Renal compensation is usually complete within 1 to 2 days. The renal bicarbonaturia, as well as decreased NH_4^+ and titratable acid excretion, are direct effects of the reduced $Paco_2$ and pH on renal reabsorption of chloride and bicarbonate.[2] The acuity of the respiratory alkalosis can be assessed on the basis of the degree of renal compensation (see Table 37-7). In fully compensated respiratory alkalosis, the bicarbonate concentration

CLINICAL PRESENTATION Respiratory Alkalosis

General

- The patient is usually asymptomatic if the condition is chronic and mild

Symptoms

- The patient may complain of light-headedness, confusion, muscle cramps and tetany, and decreased intellectual functioning
- Nausea and vomiting can occur, probably as a result of cerebral hypoxia

Signs

- In severe respiratory alkalosis pH >7.60
- Syncope and seizures
- Cardiac arrhythmias
- Hyperventilation

Laboratory Tests

- Serum chloride concentration is usually slightly increased. Serum ionized calcium, potassium, and phosphorus concentration can be decreased decreases by 4 mEq/L (4 mmol/L) below 24 for each 10-mm Hg (1.3 kPa) drop in $Paco_2$. For example, a sustained decrease in $Paco_2$ of 20 mm Hg (2.7 kPa) will lower serum bicarbonate from 24 to 14 mEq/L (24 to 14 mmol/L) with a resultant pH of 7.46. Bicarbonate concentrations differing from those anticipated using the preceding guidelines suggest a mixed acid–base disorder.

TREATMENT

Because most patients with respiratory alkalosis, especially chronic cases, have few or no symptoms and pH alterations are usually mild (pH not exceeding 7.50), treatment is often not required.[56,57] The first consideration in the treatment of acute respiratory alkalosis with pH >7.50 is the identification and correction of the underlying cause. Relief of pain, correction of hypovolemia with IV fluids, treatment of fever or infection, treatment of salicylate overdose, and other direct measures can prove effective. A rebreathing device, such as a paper bag, can be useful in controlling hyperventilation in patients with the anxiety/hyperventilation syndrome.[57] Oxygen therapy should be initiated in patients with severe hypoxemia. Patients with life-threatening alkalosis (pH >7.60), particularly if it is a mixed respiratory and metabolic condition, tend to have complications, such as arrhythmias or seizures, which can require mechanical ventilation with sedation and/or paralysis to control hyperventilation.

Respiratory alkalosis in patients receiving mechanical ventilation is usually iatrogenic. It can often be corrected by decreasing either the set respiratory rate or tidal volume, although other measures can also be employed. The use of a capnograph and spirometer in the breathing circuit enables a more precise adjustment of the ventilator settings. Another method of treating respiratory alkalosis is to increase the amount of dead space in the ventilator circuit by placing a known length of tubing between the artificial airway and the "Y" piece of the ventilator. This results in "rebreathing" of expired gas, and therefore an increase in the inspired carbon dioxide concentration, which should increase the carbon dioxide tension of the patient, correcting the respiratory alkalosis. In patients breathing more rapidly than the ventilator settings, sedation with or without paralysis can be employed.

Respiratory Acidosis

Pathophysiology

Respiratory acidosis occurs when the lungs fail to excrete carbon dioxide resulting in a lower pH. This can be the result of conditions that centrally inhibit the respiratory center, diseases that interfere with pulmonary perfusion or neuromuscular function, and intrinsic airway or parenchymal pulmonary disease (Table 37-12). Acute respiratory acidosis with hypoxemia, hypercarbia, and acidosis is life-threatening. Those disorders that produce an increase in $Paco_2$ and hypoxemia to a degree compatible with life (e.g., chronic obstructive pulmonary disease), with or without oxygen therapy, can result in chronic respiratory acidosis (Table 37-13). These patients can function normally without noticeable neurologic defects with $Paco_2$ concentrations in the range of 90 to 100 mm Hg (12 to 13.3 kPa) (normal, 40 mm Hg [5.3 kPa]), provided that adequate oxygenation is maintained.[56]

TABLE 37-12 Causes of Acute Respiratory Acidosis

Central
Drugs (anesthetics, opioids, sedatives)
Stroke
Head injury
Infection
Status epilepticus
Perfusion abnormalities
Massive pulmonary embolism
Cardiac arrest
Airway and pulmonary abnormalities
Airway obstruction: Foreign body, laryngeal edema
Aspiration of vomitus
Asthma
Chronic pulmonary obstructive disease (COPD)
Severe pulmonary edema
Severe pneumonia
Adult respiratory distress syndrome (ARDS)
Smoke inhalation
Pneumothorax
Neuromuscular abnormalities
Brainstem or cervical cord injury
Guillan–Barré syndrome
Myasthenia gravis
Mechanical ventilator
Ventilator malfunction
Inadequate frequency or tidal volume settings
Large dead space
Total parenteral nutrition (increased CO_2 production)

Clinical Presentation

Respiratory acidosis can produce neurologic symptoms, including altered mental status, abnormal behavior, seizures, stupor, and coma. Hypercapnia can mimic stroke or CNS tumors by producing headache, papilledema, focal paresis, and abnormal reflexes. These CNS symptoms are attributable to the vasodilator effects of CO_2 in the brain that result in an increase in cerebral blood flow.[2]

CLINICAL PRESENTATION Respiratory Acidosis

General

- The patient is usually symptomatic

Symptoms

- The patient may complain of confusion or difficulty thinking and headache

Signs

- In severe respiratory acidosis:
- Cardiac: Increased cardiac output if moderate that decreases if severe. Refractory hypotension can be present in some patients
- CNS: Abnormal behavior, seizures, stupor, and coma. Papilledema, focal paresis, and abnormal reflexes can also be present

Laboratory Tests

- Serum potassium concentration can be modestly increased. Hypercapnia can be moderate ($Paco_2$ of 50 to 55 mm Hg [6.7–7.3 kPa]) to severe ($Paco_2$ of >80 mm Hg [>10.6 kPa]). Hypoxia (Pao_2 is <70 mm Hg [<9.3 kPa]) is often present

TABLE 37-13 Causes of Chronic Respiratory Acidosis
Neuromuscular abnormalities
Brainstem infarct
Obesity-hypoventilation (Pickwickian) syndrome
Tumors
Poliomyelitis
Multiple sclerosis
Diaphragmatic paralysis
Pulmonary abnormalities
Chronic obstructive pulmonary disease
Kyphoscoliosis
Interstitial pulmonary disease
Overzealous parenteral feeding

The CNS response to hypercapnia is extremely variable between patients and is most influenced by the acuity of presentation. Given that chronic hypercapnia blunts the usual respiratory stimulus of an elevated $Paco_2$, hypoxemia rather than hypercapnia provides the primary ventilatory stimulus in patients with severe chronic respiratory acidosis.[56]

The degree to which cardiac contractility and heart rate are altered depends on the severity of the acidosis and the rapidity with which it develops. Modest acute hypercapnia ($Paco_2$ of 50 to 55 mm Hg [6.7 to 7.3 kPa]) stimulates a stress-like response, with elevated catecholamines and corticosteroid hormone levels, and can result in increased cardiac output and pulmonary artery pressure.[56] As the severity increases, cardiac output declines and vascular resistance decreases leading to refractory hypotension in some patients.[2]

In respiratory acidosis, the serum potassium concentration increases modestly secondary to cellular shifts. The increases are less than those seen with inorganic metabolic acidosis and are difficult to predict for individual patients.

Compensation

The body responds to acute respiratory acidosis with chemical buffering. The increase in $Paco_2$ results in increased carbonic acid levels. The carbonic acid dissociates, releasing hydrogen ions, which are buffered by nonbicarbonate buffers (i.e., proteins, phosphate, and hemoglobin) and bicarbonate. Thus, on the basis of physicochemical factors, increases in $Paco_2$ raise the serum bicarbonate concentration. In general, in acute respiratory acidosis, the bicarbonate concentration increases by 1 mEq/L (1 mmol/L) above 24 for each 10-mm Hg (1.3 kPa) increase in $Paco_2$ above 40 (5.3 kPa) (see Table 37-7).

Metabolic compensation occurs when respiratory acidosis is prolonged beyond 12 to 24 hours. In response to hypercapnia and acidemia, proximal tubular bicarbonate reabsorption, ammoniagenesis, and distal tubular hydrogen secretion are enhanced, resulting in an increase in the serum bicarbonate concentration that raises the pH toward normal. Renal compensation for chronic hypercapnia generally results in the plasma bicarbonate concentration increasing by 4 mEq/L (4 mmol/L) above 24 for each 10-mm Hg (1.3 kPa) increase in $Paco_2$ above 40 (5.3 kPa) (see Table 37-7). The new steady state in acid–base values is generally achieved within 5 days of the onset of hypercapnia in dogs; the time interval necessary for compensation in humans has not been established.

TREATMENT

The treatment of respiratory acidosis is dependent on the chronicity of the patient's condition. Respiratory decompensation in patients with chronic elevations in $Paco_2$ is frequently seen in those with acute infections and those recently started on narcotic analgesics or oxygen therapy.[56] Aggressive treatment of these conditions can offer considerable benefit and should be initiated. Furthermore, tranquilizers and sedatives should be avoided and supplemental oxygen, if used, should be minimized.

Acute Respiratory Acidosis

13 When carbon dioxide excretion is severely impaired ($Paco_2$ >80 mm Hg [>10.6 kPa]) and/or life-threatening, hypoxia is present (Pao_2 <40 mm Hg [<5.3 kPa]); the immediate therapeutic goal is to provide adequate oxygenation. Under these circumstances, hypoxia, not acidemia, is the principal threat to life. A patent airway needs to be established, which can necessitate intubation. Excessive secretions must be cleared from the airway and oxygen administered to restore adequate oxygenation. Mechanical ventilation is usually required.

The underlying cause of the acidosis should be treated aggressively (e.g., bronchodilators for treatment of severe bronchospasm; narcotic or benzodiazepine antagonists to reverse the deleterious effects of these agents on the respiratory center). Bicarbonate administration is rarely necessary in the treatment of respiratory acidosis. Furthermore, rapid correction of acidosis with bicarbonate can eliminate the patient's respiratory drive or precipitate metabolic alkalosis. Cautious use of alkali (bicarbonate or THAM) can restore the responsiveness of bronchial muscles to β-adrenergic agonists and thus can be beneficial for those patients with severe bronchospasm.[56] ABGs should be monitored closely to ensure that the respiratory acidosis is resolving without creating a metabolic alkalosis as the result of compensatory elevation in HCO_3^- and decrease in $Paco_2$. ABGs should be obtained every 2 to 4 hours during the acute phase and less frequently (every 12 to 24 hours) as the acidosis improves.

Acute Respiratory Acidosis in a Compensated Chronic Respiratory Acidotic Patient

Patients with a history of chronic respiratory acidosis (e.g., those with chronic obstructive pulmonary disease) can experience an acute worsening of their respiratory acidosis. This can result in severe life-threatening hypoxemia. As with acute respiratory acidosis, the goals of therapy are maintenance of a patent airway and adequate oxygenation. Individuals with chronic respiratory acidosis are routinely able to tolerate a low Pao_2 and an elevated $Paco_2$ because of compensation (increased number of red blood cells, hemoglobin content, and 2,3-diphosphoglycerate). The drive to breathe in these patients is dependent on hypoxemia rather than hypercarbia. Administration of oxygen to a patient with chronic respiratory acidosis can eliminate this drive to breathe and result in the syndrome of carbon dioxide narcosis. In this case, if the Pao_2 is 50 mm Hg (6.7 kPa), no oxygen treatment is necessary. If the Pao_2 is <50 mm Hg (<6.7 kPa), oxygen therapy should be initiated carefully using a controlled flow of oxygen.[2]

ABGs should be checked periodically to ensure adequate oxygenation. If the $Paco_2$ increases during oxygen therapy, it can be a sign of impending carbon dioxide narcosis and oxygen therapy may need to be discontinued. The underlying cause of the acute exacerbation should be aggressively managed. Pulmonary infections should be treated with the appropriate antibiotics and bronchodilators administered as necessary. Excess secretions should be cleared from the airway to allow proper gas exchange. This can involve increasing oral fluid intake to decrease the viscosity of secretions, deep breathing, and postural drainage, suction, or bronchoscopy.

MIXED ACID–BASE DISORDERS

Diagnosis

The diagnosis of a mixed disorder depends on an understanding of the appropriate quantitative response of the compensatory mechanisms for each of the simple acid–base disturbances. To diagnose mixed disorders, one must know how each of the four simple disorders alters pH, $Paco_2$, and $[HCO_3^-]$ (see Table 37-7). If a given set of blood gases does not decrease within the range of expected responses for a simple acid–base disturbance, a mixed disorder should be suspected. In addition to laboratory information, a thorough history and physical examination of the patient will often lead to the diagnosis, even before the laboratory data are available. Examples of common mixed disturbances follow.

Mixed Respiratory Acidosis and Metabolic Acidosis

In mixed respiratory and metabolic acidosis, there is a failure of compensation. The respiratory disorder prevents the compensatory decrease in $Paco_2$ expected in the defense against metabolic acidosis. The metabolic disorder prevents the buffering and renal mechanisms from raising the bicarbonate concentration as expected in the defense against respiratory acidosis. In the absence of these compensatory mechanisms, the pH decreases markedly.

Mixed respiratory and metabolic acidosis may develop in patients with cardiorespiratory arrest, in those with chronic lung disease who are in shock, and in metabolic acidosis patients who develop respiratory failure. When treating this mixed disorder, clinicians need to respond to both the respiratory and metabolic acidosis. Improved oxygen delivery must be initiated to improve hypercarbia and hypoxia. Mechanical ventilation may be needed to reduce $Paco_2$. During the initial stage of therapy, appropriate amounts of alkali should be given to reverse the metabolic acidosis (see Treatment, Metabolic Acidosis above).

Mixed Respiratory Alkalosis and Metabolic Alkalosis

The combination of respiratory and metabolic alkalosis is the most common mixed acid–base disorder. This mixed disorder occurs frequently in critically ill surgical patients with respiratory alkalosis caused by mechanical ventilation, hypoxia, sepsis, hypotension, neurologic damage, pain, or drugs, and with metabolic alkalosis caused by vomiting or nasogastric suctioning and massive blood transfusions. It can also occur in patients with hepatic cirrhosis who hyperventilate, receive diuretics, or vomit, as well as in patients with chronic respiratory acidosis and an elevated plasma bicarbonate concentration who are placed on mechanical ventilation and undergo a rapid decrease in $Paco_2$.

The renal excretion of bicarbonate that usually occurs as compensation for the respiratory alkalosis is prevented by the complicating metabolic alkalosis. Likewise, the retention of $Paco_2$ expected to compensate for metabolic alkalosis is prevented by the primary respiratory alkalosis. The failure of compensation that occurs with mixed respiratory and metabolic alkalosis can result in a severe alkalemia.

Administration of sodium chloride and potassium chloride solutions will help correct the metabolic component of this disorder and adjustment of the ventilator and/or treatment of an underlying disorder that is causing hyperventilation can correct or ameliorate the respiratory component of this mixed disorder.

Mixed Metabolic Acidosis and Respiratory Alkalosis

This mixed disorder is often seen in patients with advanced liver disease, salicylate intoxication, and pulmonary-renal syndromes. The respiratory alkalosis will decrease the $Paco_2$ beyond the appropriate range for the respiratory compensation usually seen with metabolic acidosis. The plasma bicarbonate concentration also decreases below the level expected in compensation for a simple respiratory alkalosis. In a sense, the defense of pH for either disorder alone is enhanced; thus the pH can be normal or close to normal, with a low $Paco_2$ and a low $[HCO_3^-]$. Treatment of this disorder should be directed at the underlying cause. Because of the enhanced compensation, the pH is usually closer to normal than in either of the two simple disorders.

Mixed Metabolic Alkalosis and Respiratory Acidosis

This mixed disorder often occurs in patients with chronic obstructive pulmonary disease and chronic respiratory acidosis who are treated with salt restriction, diuretics, and possibly glucocorticoids. When diuretics are initiated, the plasma bicarbonate may increase because of increased renal bicarbonate generation and reabsorption, providing mechanisms for both generating and maintaining metabolic alkalosis. The elevated pH diminishes respiratory drive and may therefore worsen the respiratory acidosis.

Although the pH may not deviate significantly from normal, treatment may need to be initiated to maintain Pao_2 and $Paco_2$ at acceptable levels. Because it is often difficult to correctly identify this mixed disorder, it is helpful to observe the patient's response to discontinuation of diuretics and administration of sodium and potassium chloride.[2] If the patient has a simple metabolic alkalosis, the $Paco_2$ will normalize, but it will only minimally affect the $Paco_2$ if it is a mixed disorder. Treatment should be aimed at decreasing the plasma bicarbonate with sodium and potassium chloride therapy, thereby allowing the renal excretion of retained bicarbonate from the diuretic-induced metabolic alkalosis. This therapy should be used cautiously to avoid exacerbating any underlying congestive heart failure.

CLINICAL BOTTOM LINE

Because acid–base disorders are such a common and widespread problem, pharmacists can play a key role in identifying, preventing, and properly treating acid–base abnormalities. Acid–base disorders do not occur only in the intensive care unit setting. Patients in ambulatory and extended care settings have many chronic conditions and drug therapies that commonly affect acid–base balance. Thus pharmacists in all practice settings should use their knowledge to identify patients at high risk for developing drug-related problems that affect acid–base balance and to undertake appropriate prevention and treatment measures to improve the quality of life of the patients they care for.

ABBREVIATIONS

BW	body weight
DCA	dichloroacetate
ECF	extracellular fluid
H^+	hydrogen ion
HCO_3^-	bicarbonate
H_2CO_3	carbonic acid
HIV	human immunodeficiency virus
NH_4^+	ammonium
$Paco_2$	partial pressure of carbon dioxide from arterial blood
Pao_2	partial pressure of oxygen from arterial blood
pH	the negative logarithm (base 10) of the hydrogen ion concentration
pK	the negative logarithm of the dissociation constant
$Pvco_2$	partial pressure of carbon dioxide from venous blood
Pvo_2	partial pressure of oxygen from venous blood
RTA	renal tubular acidosis
SAG	serum anion gap
THAM	tromethamine (Tris[hydroxymethyl]-aminomethane)
UCs	unmeasured cations
UAs	unmeasured anions

REFERENCES

1. Stewart PA. Goals, definitions and basic principles. In: Kellum JA, Ebers Paul WG, eds. Stewart's Textbook of Acid–Base, 2nd ed. Amsterdam: Elsevier, 2007:36–62.
2. Constable P. Clinical acid–base chemistry. In: Ronco C, ed. Critical Care Nephrology, 2nd ed. Philadelphia, PA: Elsevier, 2009:581–614.
3. Eckardt KU. Disorders of acid–base balance. In: Bremmer BM, ed. Bremmer and Rector's The Kidney, 9th ed. New York: Saunders, 2012:619–679.
4. Kamel S, Razeen-Davids M, Lin SH, et al. Interpretation of electrolytes and acid–base parameters in blood and urine. In: Bremmer BM, ed. Bremmer and Rector's The Kidney, 9th ed. New York: Saunders, 2012:906–928.
5. Morgan TJ. Unmeasured ions and the strong ion gap. In: Kellum JA, Ebers PWG, eds. Stewart's Textbook of Acid–Base, 2nd ed. Amsterdam: Elsevier, 2007:324–335.
6. Boniatti MM, Cardozo PR, Castilho RK, et al. Acid–base disorders evaluation in critically ill patients: We can improve our diagnostic ability. Intensive Care Med 2009;35(8): 1377–1382.
7. Kraut JA, Madias NE. Metabolic acidosis: Pathophysiology, diagnosis and management. Nat Rev Nephrol 2010;6: 274–285.
8. Ayers P, Dixon C. Simple acid–base tutorial. J Parentr Enteral Nutr 2012;36:18–23.
9. Reddy P. Clinical approach to renal tubular acidosis in adult patients. Int J Clin Pract 2011;65:350–360.
10. Dzierba AL, Abraham P. A practical approach to understanding acid–base abnormalities in critical illness. J Pharm Pract 2011;24:17–26.
11. Morris CG, Low J. Metabolic acidosis in the critically ill: Part 1. Classification and pathophysiology. Anaesthesia 2008;63(3):294–301.
12. Adrogue A, Gennari FJ, Galla JH, et al. Assessing acid–base disorders. Kidney Int 2009;76:1239–1247.
13. Liamis G, Milionis HJ, Elisaf M. Pharmacologically-induced metabolic acidosis: A review. Drug Saf 2010;33:371–391.
14. Levine M, Brooks DE, Truitt CA, et al. Toxicology in the ICU: Part 1: General overview and approach to treatment. Chest 2011;140:795–806.
15. Diamini J, Ledwaba L, Mokwena N, et al. Lactic acidosis and symptomatic hyperlactataemia in a randomized trial of first-line therapy in HIV-infected adults in South Africa. Antivir Ther 2011;16:605–609.
16. Salpeter SR, Greyber E, Pasternak GA, et al. Risk of fatal and nonfatal lactic acidosis with metformin use in type 2 diabetes mellitus. Cochrane Database Syst Rev 2010;20:CD002967.
17. Lalau JD. Lactic acidosis induced by metformin: Incidence, management and prevention. Drug Saf 2010;33:727–740.
18. Horinek EL, Kiser TH, Fish DN, et al. Propylene glycol accumulation in critically ill patients receiving intravenous lorazepam infusions. Ann Pharmacother 2009;43:1964–1971.
19. Pillai U, Hothi JC, Bhat ZY. Severe propylene glycol toxicity secondary to use of anti-epileptics. Am J Ther 2012 Oct 19 (epub ahead of press).
20. Deidrich DA, Brown DR. Analytic reviews: Propofol infusion syndrome in the ICU. J Intensive Care Med 2011;26:59–72.
21. Zietse R, Zoutendijk R, Hoorn EJ. Fluid, electrolyte and acid–base disorders associated with antibiotic therapy. Nat Rev Nephrol 2009;5(4):193–202.
22. Kato K, Sugiura S, Yano K, et al. The latent risk of acidosis in commercially available total parenteral nutrition (TPN) products: A randomized clinical trial in postoperative patients. J Clin Biochem Nutr 2009;45(1):68–73.
23. Mirza NS, Alfirevic A, Jorgensen A, et al. Metabolic acidosis with topiramate and zonisamide: An assessment of its severity and predictors. Pharmacogenet Genomics 2011;21:297–302.
24. Adrogues HJ. Mixed acid–base disturbances. J Nephrol 2006;19(Suppl 9):S97–S103.
25. Albert MS, Dell RB, Winters RW. Quantitative displacement of acid–base equilibrium in metabolic acidosis. Ann Intern Med 1964;66:312–322.
26. Chauhan V, Kelepouris E, Chauban N, et al. Current concepts and management strategies in chronic kidney disease—Mineral and bone disorders. South Med J 2012;1045:479–485.
27. Chadra V, Alon US. Hereditary renal tubular disorders. Semin Nephrol 2009;29(4):399–411.
28. Thomas KW, Schmidt GA. Alkanizing therapy in the management of acid–base disorder. In: Ronco C, ed. Critical Care Nephrology, 2nd ed. Philadelphia, PA: Elsevier, 2009: 685–713.
29. Rachoin JS, Weisberg LS, McFadden CB. Treatment of lactic acidosis: Appropriate confusion. J Hosp Med 2010;5:E1–E7.
30. Cooper DJ, Walley KR, Wiggs BR, Russell JA. Bicarbonate does not improve hemodynamics in critically ill patients who have lactic acidosis: A prospective controlled clinical study. Ann Intern Med 1990;112:492–498.
31. Boyd JH, Walley KR. Is there a role for sodium bicarbonate in treating lactic acidosis from shock? Curr Opion Crit Care 2008;14:379–383.
32. Adrogue HJ, Rashad MN, Gorin AB, et al. Assessing acid–base status in circulatory failure: Differences between arterial and central venous blood. N Engl J Med 1989;320: 1312–1316.
33. Kellum JA. Disorders of acid–base balance. Crit Care Med 2007;35(11):2630–2636.
34. Neumar RW, Otto CW, Link MS, et al. Part 8: Adult advanced cardiovascular life support: 2010 American Heart Association Guidelines for Cardiopulmonary Resuscitation and Emergency Cardiovascular Care. Circulation 2010;122:S729–S767.
35. McEvoy GK, Litvak K, Welsh OH, et al. American Hospital Formulary Service, Drug Information. Bethesda, MD: American Society of Health-System Pharmacists, 2012.
36. Geraci MJ, Klipa D, Heckman MG, et al. Prevalence of sodium bicarbonate-induced alkalemia in cardiopulmonary arrest patients. Ann Pharmacother 2009;43:1245–1250.
37. Hoste EA, Colpaert K, Vanholder RC, et al. Sodium bicarbonate versus THAM in ICU patients with mild metabolic acidosis. J Nephrol 2005;18(3):303–307.
38. Leung JM, Landow L, Franks M, et al. Safety and efficacy of intravenous Carbicarb in patients undergoing surgery: Comparison with sodium bicarbonate in the treatment of mild metabolic acidosis. Crit Care Med 1994;22: 1540–1549.
39. Shapiro JI. Functional and metabolic responses of the isolated heart during acidosis: Effects of sodium bicarbonate and Carbicarb. Am J Physiol 1990;258:H1835–H1839.
40. Shapiro JI. Pathogenesis of cardiac dysfunction during metabolic acidosis: Therapeutic implications. Kidney Int 1997;51:47–51.
41. Bersin RM, Arieff AI. Improved hemodynamic function during hypoxia with Carbicarb, a new agent for the management of acidosis. Circulation 1988;77:227–233.
42. Stacpoole PW, Wright EC, Baumgartner TG, et al. A controlled clinical trial of dichloroacetate for treatment of lactic acidosis. N Engl J Med 1992;327:1564–1569.

43. Stacpoole PW, Nagaraja NV, Hutson AD. Efficacy of dichloroacetate as a lactate-lowering drug. J Clin Pharmacol 2003;43:683–691.
44. Vary TC, Siegel JH, Zechnich A, et al. Pharmacologic reversal of abnormal glucose regulation, BCAA utilization, and muscle catabolism in sepsis by dichloroacetate. J Trauma 1988;28:1301–1311.
45. Shangraw RE, Lohan-Mannion D, Hayes A, et al. Dichloroacetate stabilizes the intraoperative acid–base balance during liver transplantation. Liver Transpl 2008; 14(7):989–998.
46. Khanna A, Kurtzman NA. Metabolic alkalosis. J Nephrol 2006;19 (Suppl 9):S86–S96.
47. Gennari FJ. Pathophysiology of metabolic alkalosis: A new classification based on the centrality of stimulated collecting duct ion transport. Am J Kidney Dis 2011;58:626–636.
48. Mikhalidis G, Mikhailidis DP, Elisaf M. Acid–base and electrolyte abnormalities observed in patients receiving cardiovascular drugs. J Cardiovasc Pharmacol Ther 2003; 8:267–279.
49. Barton CH, Vaziri ND, Ness RL, et al. Cimetidine in the management of metabolic alkalosis induced by nasogastric drainage. Arch Surg 1979;1:70–74.
50. Mazur JE, Devlin JW, Peters MJ, et al. Single versus multiple doses of acetazolamide for metabolic alkalosis in critically ill medical patients: A randomized, double-blind trial. Crit Care Med 1999;27(7):1257–1261.
51. Rowlands BJ, Tindall SF, Elliot DJ. The use of dilute hydrochloric acid and cimetidine to reverse severe metabolic alkalosis. Postgrad Med J 1978;54:118–123.
52. Mirtallo JM, Rogers KR, Johnson JA, et al. Stability of amino acids and the availability of acid in total parenteral nutrition solutions containing hydrochloric acid. Am J Hosp Pharm 1981;38:1729–1731.
53. Graziani G, Fedeli C, Moroni L, Cosmai L, Badalamenti S, Ponticelli C. Gitelman syndrome: Pathophysiological and clinical aspects. QJM 2010;103:741–748.
54. Hene RJ, Koomans HA, Dorhout Mees EJ, et al. Correction of hypokalemia in Bartter's syndrome by enalapril. Am J Kidney Dis 1987;9:200–205.
55. Vinci JM, Gill JR Jr, Bowden RE, et al. The Kallikrein-Kinin system in Bartter's syndrome and its response to prostaglandin synthetase inhibition. J Clin Invest 1987;61: 1671–1682.
56. Effros RM, Swenson ER. Acid–base balance. In: Mason RJ, Broaddus CV, Martin TR, et al. Murray & Nadel's Textbook of Respiratory Medicine, 5th ed. Philadelphia, PA: Saunders/ Elsevier, 2010.
57. Foster GT, Vaziri ND, Sassoon CS. Respiratory alkalosis. Respir Care 2001;46:384–391.

38 Alzheimer's Disease

Patricia W. Slattum, Emily P. Peron, and Angela Massey Hill

KEY CONCEPTS

1. Alzheimer's disease (AD) is the most common form of dementing illness, and the prevalence of AD increases with each decade of life.
2. The etiology of AD is unknown, and current pharmacotherapy neither cures nor arrests the pathophysiology.
3. Neuritic plaques and neurofibrillary tangles are the pathologic hallmarks of AD; however, the definitive cause of this disease is yet to be determined.
4. AD affects multiple areas of cognition and is characterized by a gradual onset with a slow, progressive decline.
5. A thorough physical examination (including neurologic examination), as well as laboratory and imaging studies, is required to rule out other disorders and diagnose AD before considering drug therapy.
6. Pharmacotherapy for AD focuses on impacting three domains: cognition, behavioral and psychiatric symptoms, and functional ability.
7. Nondrug therapy and social support for the patient and family are the primary treatment interventions for AD.
8. Cholinesterase inhibitors and memantine are used to treat cognitive symptoms of AD; other medications have been suggested to be beneficial because of their potential preventive or cognitive effects.
9. Appropriate management of vascular disease risk factors may reduce the risk for developing AD and may prevent the worsening of dementia in patients with AD.
10. A thorough behavioral assessment and plan with careful examination of environmental factors should be conducted before initiating drug therapy for behavioral symptoms.

"I now begin the journey that will lead me into the sunset of my life."
Ronald Reagan

Alzheimer's disease (AD), first characterized by Alois Alzheimer in 1907, is a gradually progressive dementia affecting cognition, behavior, and functional status. The exact pathophysiologic mechanisms underlying AD are not entirely known, and no cure exists.[1] Although drugs may reduce AD symptoms for a time, the disease is eventually fatal.

AD profoundly affects the family as well as the patient. The need for supervision and assistance increases until the late stages of the disease, when AD patients become totally dependent on a caregiver for all of their basic needs. These are the all-too-common experiences of the millions of people in the United States who care for someone with AD. To address the growing AD crisis facing the United States, the first national strategic plan, the National Alzheimer's Plan, was released in 2012 with the goals of coordinating efforts across the federal government to prevent and treat AD, increase public awareness, and improve the quality of care and support for patients and their caregivers.[2]

EPIDEMIOLOGY

1 AD is the most common cause of dementia, accounting for 50% to 60% of cases of late-life cognitive dysfunction. Its prevalence among dementia patients increases to 80% if AD lesions in conjunction with other pathologic brain lesions are considered.[3–5] Table 38-1 lists the most common types of dementia. Dementia can result from multiple etiologies. This chapter focuses exclusively on dementia of the Alzheimer's type. However, the reader is encouraged to use the nonpharmacologic approaches and management of behavioral problems outlined in this chapter as a general treatment approach for other types of dementia that may share similar features with AD.

Approximately 5.4 million Americans have AD.[4,5] By the year 2050, one in five people will be older than age 65 years, and the number of AD patients is projected to be 13.2 million (Fig. 38-1). Most cases present in persons older than age 65 years, but approximately 4% of cases occur in persons younger than age 65 years. Onset can be as early as age 30 years, resulting in the arbitrary age classifications of younger-onset (age less than 65 years) and late-onset (age 65 years and older).[4]

Increasing age is the greatest risk factor for AD, but AD is not a normal part of aging. The prevalence of AD increases exponentially with age, affecting approximately 4% of people <65 years, 6% of individuals age 65 to 74 years, 44% of those age 75 to 84 years, and 46% of persons age 85 years and older.[4] Factors determining age of onset and rate of progression remain largely undefined.

Survival following AD diagnosis is typically 4 to 8 years, but may be as long as 20 years. It is the fifth leading cause of death for those age 65 years and older in the United States. AD may not cause death directly. The most common cause of death in patients with AD is pneumonia, possibly resulting from swallowing difficulties and

TABLE 38-1 Common Types of Dementia in Late Life

Alzheimer's disease
Vascular dementia
Lewy body dementia
Mixed dementia
Other (Parkinson's disease, Frontotemporal dementia, Huntington's disease, Creutzfeldt–Jakob disease)
Potentially reversible causes of dementia (e.g., normal-pressure hydrocephalus, thyroid dysfunction, vitamin B_{12} deficiency, depression, Wernicke–Korsakoff syndrome)

Data from Rubin[128] and the Alzheimer's Association.[4]

immobility in the terminal stage of the disease.[4] Those diagnosed with AD spend, on average, more years in the most severe stage of the disease than any other stage, and much of this time is spent in a nursing home.[4]

Etiology and Genetics

2 The exact etiology of AD is unknown; however, several genetic and environmental factors have been explored as potential causes of AD. Dominantly inherited forms of AD account for less than 1% of cases.[6,7] More than half of young-onset, dominantly inherited cases of AD can be attributed to alterations on chromosomes 1, 14, or 21. The majority and most aggressive young-onset cases are attributed to mutations of a gene located on chromosome 14, which produces a protein called presenilin 1.[8] A structurally similar protein, presenilin 2, is produced by a gene on chromosome 1. Both presenilin 1 and presenilin 2 encode for membrane proteins that may be involved in amyloid precursor protein (APP) processing. Scientists have identified more than 160 mutations in presenilin genes, and these mutations appear to result in reduced activity of γ-secretase, an enzyme important in β-amyloid peptide (Aβ) formation.[8] APP is encoded on chromosome 21. Only a small number of young-onset familial AD cases have been associated with mutations in the *APP* gene, resulting in overproduction of Aβ or an increase in the proportion of Aβ ending at residue 42.[8]

Genetic susceptibility to late-onset AD is primarily linked to the apolipoprotein E (*APOE*) genotype.[6–9] Thus far, the contribution

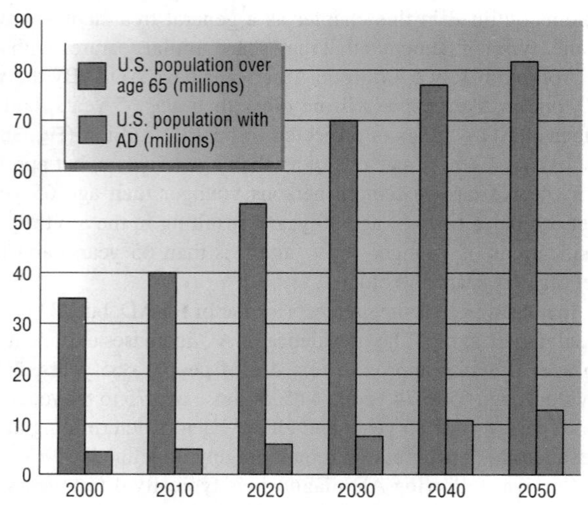

FIGURE 38-1 Our aging population. The percentage of U.S. population older than age 65 years and the percentage with AD projected from years 2000 to 2050. *(Estimates based on data from references 1 and 134.)*

of other candidate genes appears to be minor, although AD may be a heterogeneous disease resulting from complex interactions among multiple susceptibility genes and environmental factors. There are three major subtypes or alleles of *APOE* (e.g., **2*, **3*, and **4*). Inheritance of the *APOE*4* allele is believed to account for much of the genetic risk in late-onset AD. The mechanism through which *APOE*4* confers an increased risk is unknown, although *APOE*4* is associated with factors that may contribute to AD pathology, such as abnormalities in mitochondria, cytoskeletal dysfunction, and low glucose usage.[5] The risk for AD is two- to threefold higher in individuals with one *APOE*4* allele and 12-fold higher in individuals with two *APOE*4* alleles compared to those with no *APOE*4* alleles.[9] Moreover, onset of symptoms occurs at a relatively younger age as compared with patients having zero or only one copy of *APOE*4* in their genotype.[9] The strength of association is not the same across all races however.[1,4] The *APOE*4* allele is not diagnostic or even essential for disease presence.

Genetic factors have been linked to both younger- and late-onset AD. Genetic explanatory factors continue to be investigated.[6–8] Epigenetic modifications, particularly DNA methylation, have been reported in AD, and this is an emerging area of research that may help explain the pathologic complexity of AD and aging as a risk factor for the development of AD.[10]

Environmental and Other Factors

A number of environmental factors are associated with an increased risk of AD, including age, decreased reserve capacity of the brain (reduced brain size, low educational level, and reduced mental and physical activity in late life), head injury, Down's syndrome, depression, mild cognitive impairment (MCI), and risk factors for vascular disease (hypercholesterolemia, hypertension, atherosclerosis, coronary heart disease, smoking, elevated homocysteine, obesity, metabolic syndrome, and diabetes).[4,5,11] Whether these vascular risk factors are true causal risk factors for AD contributing to AD pathology, or whether they result in cerebrovascular pathology that, in turn, contributes to the symptoms of AD, remains to be established.

The incidence of AD rises with increasing age and AD may develop in individuals over the course of decades,[4] suggesting that AD is a disease most people are in the process of developing throughout adulthood. The debate about whether dementia is a distinct disease or part of aging remains unresolved. An in-depth discussion of the aging—AD controversy is not possible in this chapter; it is reviewed elsewhere.[12–14]

PATHOPHYSIOLOGY

3 The signature lesions in AD are amyloid plaques and neurofibrillary tangles (NFTs) located in the cortical areas and medial temporal lobe structures of the brain.[3] Along with these lesions, degeneration of neurons and synapses, as well as cortical atrophy occurs. Plaques and NFTs may also be present in other diseases, even in normal aging, but at least in younger demographics there tends to be a higher burden of plaques and NFTs in AD-affected subjects than there is in age-matched controls. Several mechanisms have been proposed to explain changes in the brain that result in symptoms of AD, including misfolding of proteins (Aβ aggregation and deposition leading to the formation of plaques and hyperphosphorylation of tau protein leading to NFT development); synaptic failure and depletion of neurotrophin and neurotransmitters; and mitochondrial dysfunction (oxidative stress, impaired insulin signaling in the brain, vascular injury, inflammatory processes, loss of calcium regulation, and defects in cholesterol metabolism).[3]

Amyloid Cascade Hypothesis

Amyloid plaques are extracellular lesions found in the brain and cerebral vasculature. Plaques largely consist of Aβ. Aβ peptides consisting of 36 to 43 amino acids are produced via processing of a larger protein, APP. Aβ_{42} is less common than other Aβ peptides, but is prone to aggregation and plaque formation.[3] The amyloid cascade hypothesis states that there is an imbalance between the production and clearance of Aβ peptides resulting in aggregation that causes accumulation of Aβ ultimately leading to AD.[3] Studies on younger-onset AD and Down's syndrome led to the formulation of the amyloid cascade hypothesis. Recent versions of the amyloid cascade hypothesis assume Aβ that is not sequestered in plaques actually drives the disease.[3] Even so, the amyloid cascade hypothesis seems most applicable in cases of younger-onset, autosomal dominant AD. It is not clear whether it is reasonable to etiologically extrapolate to the late-onset form (which afflicts the vast majority of those affected). Whether individuals with late-onset AD also carry genetic variations that promote a primary Aβ amyloidosis remains to be shown. If this turns out not to be the case, the possibility that amyloidosis in late-onset AD is secondary to a more upstream event will require consideration. Before this conceptual conundrum is laid to rest, however, the amyloid cascade hypothesis will likely undergo a therapy-based practical test. If treatments that efficiently reduce Aβ production or remove brain Aβ fail to arrest disease progression, it would argue amyloidosis is not the primary pathology in most of those with AD.

Neurofibrillary Tangles

As Aβ was being identified in plaques, other researchers showed that NFTs are commonly found in the cells of the hippocampus and cerebral cortex in persons with AD and are composed of abnormally hyperphosphorylated tau protein. Tau protein provides structural support to microtubules, the cell's transportation and skeletal support system.[3] When tau filaments undergo abnormal phosphorylation at a specific site, they cannot bind effectively to microtubules, and the microtubules collapse. Without an intact system of microtubules, the cell cannot function properly and eventually dies. The density of the NFTs correlates with the severity of the dementia.[3] NFTs are found in other dementing illnesses besides AD, and may represent a common method by which various inciting factors culminate in cell death.[3]

Inflammatory Mediators

Inflammatory or immunologic paradigms are often viewed as a corollary of the amyloid cascade hypothesis. Certainly, brain amyloid deposition associates with local inflammatory and immunologic alterations. This led some to propose that inflammation is relevant to AD neurodegeneration.[3] Inflammatory/immunologic hypotheses argue that although Aβ may have direct neurotoxicity, at least some of its toxicity might actually be an indirect consequence of an Aβ protofibril-induced microglia activation and astrocyte recruitment. This inflammatory response may represent an attempt to clear amyloid deposition. However, it is also associated with release of cytokines, nitric oxide, and other radical species, and complement factors that can both injure neurons and promote ongoing inflammation.[3] Indeed, levels of multiple cytokines and chemokines are elevated in AD brains, and certain proinflammatory gene polymorphisms are reported to be associated with AD.[3]

Consistent with these molecular observations are epidemiologic data suggesting that exposure to nonsteroidal antiinflammatory drugs (NSAIDs) may reduce AD risk.[15,16] However, multiple prospective short duration trials of NSAIDs in AD prevention and of NSAIDs as AD treatment have been disappointing.[3,17]

The Cholinergic Hypothesis

Multiple neuronal pathways are destroyed in AD. Neuronal damage can be seen in conjunction with plaque structures.[3] Widespread cell dysfunction or degeneration results in a variety of neurotransmitter deficits, with cholinergic abnormalities being the most prominent.[3] Loss of cholinergic activity correlates with AD severity. In the late stage of AD, the number of cholinergic neurons is reduced, and there is loss of nicotinic receptors in the hippocampus and cortex. Presynaptic nicotinic receptors control the release of acetylcholine, as well as other neurotransmitters important for memory and mood, including glutamate, serotonin, and norepinephrine.[3]

The discovery of vast cholinergic cell loss led to the development of a cholinergic hypothesis of the pathophysiology of AD. The cholinergic hypothesis targeted cholinergic cell loss as the source of memory and cognitive impairment in AD. Consequently, it was presumed that increasing cholinergic function would improve symptoms of memory loss. This approach is flawed because cholinergic cell loss appears to be a secondary consequence of Alzheimer's pathology, not the disease-producing event, and cholinergic neurons are only one of many neuronal pathways destroyed in AD. Simple addition of acetylcholine cannot compensate for the loss of neurons, receptors, and other neurotransmitters lost during the course of the illness. Thus the goal is to minimize or improve symptoms through augmentation of neurotransmission at remaining synapses.

Other Neurotransmitter Abnormalities

Although the cholinergic system has received particular attention in AD pharmaceutical research, deficits also exist in other neuronal pathways. For example, serotonergic neurons of the raphe nuclei and noradrenergic cells of the locus ceruleus are lost, while monoamine oxidase type B activity is increased. Monoamine oxidase type B is found predominantly in the brain and in platelets, and is responsible for metabolizing dopamine. In addition, abnormalities appear in glutamate pathways of the cortex and limbic structures, where a loss of neurons leads to a focus on excitotoxicity models as possible contributing factors to AD pathology.

Glutamate is the major excitatory neurotransmitter in the cortex and hippocampus. Many neuronal pathways essential to learning and memory use glutamate as a neurotransmitter, including the pyramidal neurons (a layer of neurons with long axons carrying information out of the cortex), hippocampus, and entorhinal cortex. Glutamate and other excitatory amino acid neurotransmitters have been implicated as potential neurotoxins in AD.[18] Dysregulated glutamate activity is thought to be one of the primary mediators of neuronal injury after stroke or acute brain injury. Although intimately involved in cell injury, the role of excitatory amino acids in AD is as yet unclear; however, blockade of *N*-methyl-D-aspartate (NMDA) receptors decreases activity of glutamate in the synapse and may hypothetically lessen the degree of cellular injury in AD.

Brain Vascular Disease and High Cholesterol

There is growing evidence of a causal association between cardiovascular disease and its risk factors and the incidence of AD. Cardiovascular risk factors that are also risk factors for dementia include hypertension, elevated low-density lipoprotein cholesterol, low high-density lipoprotein cholesterol, and diabetes.[19] Brain vascular disease may augment the cognitive impairment observed for a given amount of AD pathology in the brain. Dysfunctional blood vessels may impair nutrient delivery to neurons and reduce clearance of Aβ from the brain.[3] Vascular disease may accelerate amyloid deposition and increase amyloid toxicity to neurons.[3] Midlife diastolic hypertension is adversely associated with AD, while late-life hypertension may show an inverse association with AD.[20] Diabetes may increase the risk of dementia through factors related to "metabolic syndrome" (dyslipidemia and hypertension), effects of potentially toxic glucose metabolites on the brain and vasculature, and through insulin itself.[19] Disturbances in insulin-signaling pathways, both in the periphery and the brain, have been linked to AD. Insulin may also regulate the metabolism of Aβ and tau protein.[3]

Research has found multiple links between cholesterol and AD. APOE is synthesized in the liver, central nervous system, and cerebrospinal fluid (CSF) and is responsible for transporting cholesterol in the blood through the brain. It is carried by low-density lipoprotein into neurons and binds to NFTs. APOE*4 is associated with increasing deposition of Aβ and is thought to act as an accelerating modulator in vascular dementia. Elevated cholesterol levels in brain neurons may alter membrane functioning and result in the cascade leading to plaque formation and AD.

Other Mechanisms

Other hypotheses proposed to explain AD pathogenesis include oxidative stress, mitochondrial dysfunction, and loss of estrogen. Each of these mechanisms may contribute to AD pathogenesis, but the extent of the contribution is uncertain. There is a growing body of evidence of a role for oxidative stress and the accumulation of free radicals in the brain of AD patients.[3] Some epidemiologic studies suggest vitamin E, and possibly the combination of vitamin E and vitamin C, may reduce AD risk while others do not.[3] Mitochondrial dysfunction may result in disruption of energy metabolism in the neuron.[3,21,22] The role of estrogen in cognitive aging and dementia continues to be an active area of investigation. Despite convincing evidence that estrogens affect the brain in ways that would be expected to improve cognitive aging and reduce the risk of AD, the results of clinical studies have been largely disappointing.[21] A single common mechanism for producing AD does not exist. Regardless of the source, however, the features remain the same: degeneration of neurons in higher brain areas; accumulation of NFTs and amyloid plaques; profound destruction of cholinergic pathways; and an insidious dementia, slowly progressive until death.

CLINICAL PRESENTATION OF ALZHEIMER'S DISEASE

4 The onset of AD is almost imperceptible, without abrupt changes in cognition or function. Deficits occur progressively over time, affecting multiple areas of cognition.[4,22] For treatment and assessment purposes, it is helpful to divide AD symptoms into two basic categories: cognitive symptoms and noncognitive (behavioral) symptoms. Cognitive symptoms are present throughout the illness, whereas behavioral symptoms are less predictable. Table 38-2 summarizes the stages of AD.

Diagnosis

A family member often first brings memory complaints to the attention of a primary care clinician. Up to 50% of patients who meet criteria for dementia are not given a diagnosis in the primary care setting, leading some to believe that an appropriate screening tool may be helpful in aiding diagnosis and leading to earlier treatment.[23,24] Despite the phenomenon of underdiagnosis, the United States Preventative Services Task Force concluded that there are insufficient data to recommend for or against cognitive screening for AD, because it could not be determined if the benefits outweigh the risks.[23] Screening is being promoted as part of the Medicare Annual Wellness Visit by the Alzheimer's Association (AA).[25]

Until recently the only way to confirm a clinical diagnosis of AD was through direct examination of brain tissue at autopsy or biopsy. Several criteria have been used in clinical practice and research for the detection and diagnosis of dementia, including the *Diagnostic and Statistical Manual of Mental Disorders*, Fifth Edition (DSM-5) criteria,[26] the Agency for Healthcare Research and Quality (AHRQ) Guidelines,[27] the American Academy of Neurology Guidelines,[28] the National Institute of Neurological Disorders and Stroke (NINDS) criteria,[29] and the National Institute of Neurological and Communicative Disorders and Stroke (NINCDS), and the Alzheimer's Disease and Related Disorders Association (ADRDA) Criteria.[30] In 2011, revisions to the NINCDS and ADRDA Criteria

CLINICAL PRESENTATION Alzheimer's Disease

General

- The patient may have vague memory complaints initially, or the patient's significant other may report that the patient is "forgetful." Cognitive decline is gradual over the course of illness. Behavioral disturbances may be present in moderate stages. Loss of daily function is common in advanced stages

Symptoms

Cognitive

- Memory loss (poor recall and losing items)
- Aphasia (circumlocution and anomia)
- Apraxia
- Agnosia
- Disorientation (impaired perception of time and unable to recognize familiar people)
- Impaired executive function

Noncognitive

- Depression, psychotic symptoms (hallucinations and delusions)
- Behavioral disturbances (physical and verbal aggression, motor hyperactivity, uncooperativeness, wandering, repetitive mannerisms and activities, and combativeness)

Functional

- Inability to care for self (dressing, bathing, toileting, and eating)

Laboratory Tests

- Rule out vitamin B_{12} and folate deficiency
- Rule out hypothyroidism with thyroid function tests
- Blood cell counts, serum electrolytes, and liver function tests

Other Diagnostic Tests

- CT or MRI scans may aid diagnosis

TABLE 38-2 Stages of Alzheimer's Disease

Mild (MMSE score 26–18)	Patient has difficulty remembering recent events. Ability to manage finances, prepare food, and carry out other household activities declines. May get lost while driving. Begins to withdraw from difficult tasks and to give up hobbies. May deny memory problems
Moderate (MMSE score 17–10)	Patient requires assistance with activities of daily living. Frequently disoriented with regard to time (date, year, and season). Recall for recent events is severely impaired. May forget some details of past life and names of family and friends. Functioning may fluctuate from day to day. Patient generally denies problems. May become suspicious or tearful. Loses ability to drive safely. Agitation, paranoia, and delusions are common
Severe (MMSE score 9–0)	Patient loses ability to speak, walk, and feed self. Incontinent of urine and feces. Requires care 24 hours a day, 7 days a week

MMSE, Mini-Mental Status Examination.

Data from Feldman and Woodward,[129] Alzheimer's Association,[4] and Reisberg et al.[130]

for the clinical diagnosis of AD were recommended by the National Institute on Aging (NIA) and the AA[25,31] DSM-5 provides criteria for diagnosis of minor and major neurocognitive disorders, with specific criteria for neurocognitive disorders due to AD.[32] The new NIA-AA criteria view AD as a spectrum beginning with a preclinical phase progressing to increasingly severe clinical stages of AD. Three workgroups formulated diagnostic criteria for the dementia phase,[33] the symptomatic, predementia phase (MCI),[34] and the asymptomatic, preclinical phase of AD.[35] At this time, AD is still primarily a clinical diagnosis, but this is expected to change in coming years as brain imaging, CSF, and other AD biomarkers are validated and available for routine clinical use. The patient's examination should suggest that cognitive decline from a previously higher baseline has occurred. The history should corroborate this, and further indicate that cognitive decline has reached the point where changes in social or occupational functioning are present. It is possible to administer a sophisticated exam that defines cognitive domain strengths and weaknesses and enables a neuroanatomic localization of the observed deficits. When approached in this way, the exam can indicate a pattern of cognitive decline that is consistent with AD, and assist with rendering a diagnosis that is as much a diagnosis of inclusion as it is of exclusion.

Objectively defining social or occupational dysfunction can prove tricky in the older patient who may be retired, and who may also lead a socially restricted lifestyle for reasons of frailty. For such patients, the minimal requirement is to establish a change in activities of daily living. Early on, this usually involves a change in instrumental activities of daily living (handling finances, organizing medications) rather than basic activities of daily living (hygiene, dressing). Some AD subspecialists use a detailed, standardized, semistructured interview of a nonpatient informant as the most critical piece of the diagnostic evaluation.[36]

5 For patients who meet criteria for dementia (whether the underlying cause is ultimately felt to be AD or not), current recommendations from the American Academy of Neurology include a neuroimaging study (computed tomography or magnetic resonance imaging), as well as a serologic evaluation that includes blood cell counts, serum electrolytes, liver function tests, a test of thyroid function, and a vitamin B_{12} level.[28] When circumstances suggest AD is not the leading entity on the differential diagnosis, other neurologic tests such as CSF analysis or electroencephalogram can occasionally be justified. Neuropsychological testing is also optional, but can prove quite useful for the diagnosis of AD by helping to establish a neuroanatomical localization for the patient's cognitive deficits.

Almost any medication can contribute to cognitive impairment in vulnerable individuals, but certain classes of medication are more commonly implicated. Benzodiazepines and other sedative hypnotics, anticholinergics, opioid analgesics, antipsychotics, and anticonvulsants have been associated with cognitive impairment.[37,38] NSAIDs, histamine H_2-receptor antagonists, digoxin, amiodarone, antihypertensives, and corticosteroids have been implicated in cases of delirium.[37] Because medications are a reversible cause of cognitive symptoms, medication review and management are essential.

Efforts to define the role of other AD diagnostic tests are ongoing. Positron emission tomography scanning may reveal a pattern of hypometabolism typical of AD, but by itself the diagnostic accuracy of positron emission tomography scanning still lags behind that of the clinical examination and history.[39] *APOE* genotyping by itself is also insufficient to make or break a diagnosis of AD, but demonstrating an *APOE*4* allele in a suspected patient increases the specificity of the diagnosis and can help predict which patients with MCI are most likely to progress to a diagnosis of AD over the next several years.[40] Unless the patient developed dementia prior to age 60 years and also had a parent that developed AD before age 60 years, presenilin 1, presenilin 2, or *APP* genotyping is usually not indicated.

Mild Cognitive Impairment

It has long been recognized that aging individuals experience changes in cognitive function. MCI constitutes a syndromic designation that categorizes patients with cognitive complaints insufficient to warrant a diagnosis of dementia. The NIA-AA diagnostic criteria specifically address the diagnosis of MCI.[34] Persons diagnosed with MCI carry a 10% to 15% chance per year of progressing to an AD diagnosis.[41] What clinicians are likely seeing in most people with MCI is the initial manifestation of a progressive degenerative dementia that will eventually meet AD diagnostic criteria.[34,41] However, it is important to note that not everyone meeting MCI criteria will have AD. As the MCI designation is increasingly applied, MCI criteria continue to evolve.[34,41]

TREATMENT

Desired Outcomes

6 The primary goal of treatment in AD is to symptomatically treat cognitive difficulties and preserve patient function as long as possible. Secondary goals include treating the psychiatric and behavioral sequelae. Current AD treatments have not been shown to prolong life, cure AD, or halt or reverse the pathophysiologic processes of the disorder.[36]

General Treatment Approach

Clinical trials have consistently demonstrated modest benefits of early and continuous treatment with cholinesterase inhibitors.[42] Memantine added in moderate to severe disease may also provide benefit. Following this approach allows for maximal maintenance of cognition and activities of daily living. A symptomatic approach is used to treat behavioral symptoms as they arise.

Provision of education to the patient and family at the time of diagnosis, including discussion of the course of illness, realistic expectations of treatment, and the importance of legal and financial planning, are essential to appropriate treatment.

Nonpharmacologic Therapy

7 AD has a profound effect on both the patient and family, so appropriate treatment is needed. Nonmedication interventions are the current primary interventions for management of AD, and

TABLE 38-3 Basic Principles of Care for the Alzheimer's Patient

- Consider vision, hearing, or other sensory impairments
- Find optimal level of autonomy and adjust expectations for patient performance over time
- Avoid confrontation. Remain calm, firm, and supportive if the patient becomes upset
- Maintain a consistent, structured environment with stimulation level appropriate to the individual patient
- Provide frequent reminders, explanations, and orientation cues. Employ guiding, demonstration, and reinforcement
- Reduce choices, keep requests and demands of the patient simple, and avoid complex tasks that lead to frustration
- Bring sudden declines in function and the emergence of new symptoms to professional attention

Data from Alzheimer's Association,[4] Rubin,[128] and Lyketsos et al.[84]

medications should be used in the context of multimodal interventions. Behavioral and psychiatric symptoms are among the most challenging and distressing symptoms of the disease and may be the determining factor in a family's decision to seek institutional care. Symptoms such as sleep disturbances, wandering, urinary incontinence, agitation, and aggression in patients with dementia are best managed using behavioral interventions rather than medications whenever possible.[42–44]

Upon initial diagnosis, the patient and caregiver should be educated on the course of illness, prognosis, available treatments, legal decisions, and quality-of-life issues. Caregiving strategies, including stress-management techniques and support group options, should also be discussed. Caregiver education and support programs have been shown to improve caregiver skill, knowledge, confidence, and quality of life, and, in some cases, delay time to nursing home placement.[45,46] Table 38-3 lists basic principles of care for the AD patient. The general approach to nonmedication strategies for behavioral symptoms is to identify the symptom, identify causative factors, and adapt the caregiving environment to remedy the situation.[4] Environmental triggers may include noise, glare, an insecure space, and too much background distraction, including television. Personal discomfort may also trigger behaviors, so it is important to monitor for pain, hunger, thirst, constipation, full bladder, fatigue, infections, skin irritation, comfortable temperature, fears, and frustrations.[4] Medical comorbidity is a major source of functional and cognitive impairment in patients with AD, so general health maintenance is warranted.[4] Interventions should redirect the patient's attention rather than be confrontational and should specifically address known triggers. Creating a calm environment and removing stressors and triggers is key. Other nonpharmacological approaches include exercise, light therapy, music therapy, reminiscence therapy, aroma therapy, relaxation techniques, validation therapy, massage and touch therapy, and multisensory stimulation.[47] Caregivers should be referred to support services, such as the AA, for assistance in developing nonpharmacologic strategies for managing difficult behaviors.

The caregiver must be prepared to face the changes in life that will occur, and acceptance of this does not come easily. Denial on the part of the patient and rationalization on the part of the family are common. The clinician should encourage the family to address legal and financial matters and designate a durable power of attorney for execution of financial and medical decisions once the patient is incompetent. The caregiver will need to address issues such as respite services to provide time for rest, relaxation, and conduct of personal business. Eventually, the caregiver will need to face critical and difficult questions with respect to institutionalization. Local resources, such as the AA, can provide detailed information regarding support services. Table 38-4 lists this and other referral sources for caregivers.

TABLE 38-4 Resources for Caregivers of Persons with Alzheimer's Disease

The following organizations provide educational literature and information on diagnosis, treatment, social support, and ongoing research in Alzheimer's disease:

U.S. Administration on Aging, National Family Caregiver Support Program
http://www.aoa.gov

National Institute on Aging Alzheimer's Disease Education & Referral Center (ADEAR)
http://www.nia.nih.gov/alzheimers

The Alzheimer's Association
http://www.alz.org

The Alzheimer's Research Forum
http://www.alzforum.org

AARP
http://www.aarp.org

National Family Caregivers Association
http://www.thefamilycaregiver.org

ElderCare Online
http://www.ec-online.net

Education, communication, and planning are key nonpharmacologic components of caring for a patient with AD. Preparation in the early stages of illness may lessen some of the caregiver stress as the illness progresses.

Pharmacologic Therapy

Pharmacotherapy for Cognitive Symptoms

8 Table 38-5 presents a treatment algorithm for managing cognitive symptoms in AD. Cholinesterase inhibitors and NMDA-receptor antagonists are indicated for treatment of AD. The latest treatment guidelines recommend the use of cholinesterase inhibitors for AD, with no preference for a specific agent.[48–50] Donepezil, rivastigmine, and galantamine are indicated in mild to moderate AD, while donepezil is also indicated in severe disease. Memantine is indicated for moderate to severe AD; current evidence does not support its use in earlier stages of the disease.[51] Additional benefit may be achieved when memantine is added to cholinesterase inhibitor therapy in moderate to severe AD.[52] There is no evidence supporting combination therapy of more than one cholinesterase inhibitor. No head-to-head trials comparing memantine monotherapy to cholinesterase inhibitor therapy have been conducted to date.

Disagreement exists about how best to determine effectiveness of treatments for AD. Selection of qualitative versus quantitative assessment may bias a clinician's impression of response. Subtle changes are often detected only by psychometric testing. Because no standard has been suggested to define the effectiveness

TABLE 38-5 Treatment Options for Cognitive Symptoms in Alzheimer's Disease

- In mild to moderate disease, consider therapy with a cholinesterase inhibitor:
  - Donepezil or
  - Rivastigmine or
  - Galantamine
- Titrate to recommended maintenance dose as tolerated
- In moderate to severe disease, consider adding antiglutamatergic therapy:
  - Memantine
- Titrate to recommended maintenance dose as tolerated
- Alternatively, consider memantine or cholinesterase inhibitor therapy alone
- Behavioral symptoms may require additional pharmacologic approaches

Data from Ballard et al.[1] and Lyketsos et al.[84]

of medications for AD, great variation exists between clinicians, and the duration of treatment ranges from months to years. Realistic expectations for treatment success may include slowed decline in behavioral, functional, and cognitive abilities and delayed long-term care placement.[53]

Unfortunately, clinical trials have failed to provide answers to key questions in treating AD patients. Information from clinical trials is insufficient to know if a cholinesterase inhibitor dose–response relationship exists, or if additional cognitive improvement may be gained by increasing to the maximum tolerated dose, rather than continuing with the usual recommended daily dosage. Guidance in extrapolating data related to changes in cognition is needed, so that a reasonable duration of clinical treatment with cholinesterase inhibitors and NMDA-antagonists can be determined. One concern is that those who respond to treatment may lose the benefits of that treatment once the medication is stopped.[54,55] Moreover, gaps in treatment have been linked with worse outcomes in open-label trials;[56,57] however, in a more recent large observational study there was no increased risk of institutionalization or death associated with gaps in cholinesterase inhibitor therapy.[58] Regardless, dosing regimens should be simplified and patient/caregiver preferences considered in an effort to improve adherence and persistence.

In natural disease progression studies, scores on the Alzheimer's Disease Assessment Scale—Cognition (ADAS-cog) have been shown to worsen (increase) by an average of less than or equal to five points over 1 year in mild dementia and 7 to 11 points annually in moderate dementia. Based on these findings, the general consensus is that a four-point change in the ADAS-cog represents a clinically significant change.[42] Therefore, if a pharmacotherapeutic agent decreases the ADAS-cog score by four points, one could think of this as having delayed progression of disease symptoms by 6 months. The usefulness of the ADAS-cog in clinical practice is limited because of the time required for administration; it is much more practical to assess changes in disease severity using the Mini-Mental Status Examination (MMSE). An untreated patient has an average decline of two to four points in MMSE score per year. Successful treatment would reflect a decline of less than two points a year. It is reasonable to change to a different cholinesterase inhibitor if the decline in MMSE score is greater than two to four points after 1 year with the initial agent.[59]

8 Cholinesterase Inhibitors In the early 1980s, researchers began to examine means to enhance cholinergic activity in patients with AD by inhibiting the hydrolysis of acetylcholine through reversible inhibition of cholinesterase. Tacrine was the first such drug to be examined in a systematic fashion. However, tacrine was fraught with significant side effects, including hepatotoxicity, which severely limited its usefulness. Tacrine is no longer available in the US market, having been replaced by safer, more tolerable cholinesterase inhibitors. The newer cholinesterase inhibitors donepezil, rivastigmine, and galantamine show similar symptomatic improvement in cognitive, global, and functional outcomes in patients with mild to moderate AD, and duration of benefit varies from 3 to 12 months.[60–62]

The mechanism of action differs slightly between drugs in this class.[59] Donepezil specifically and reversibly inhibits acetylcholinesterase. Rivastigmine inhibits both butyrylcholinesterase and acetylcholinesterase. Galantamine is a selective, competitive, reversible acetylcholinesterase inhibitor and also enhances the action of acetylcholine on nicotinic receptors. The clinical relevance of these differences is unknown.

Choice of cholinesterase inhibitor therapy for an individual patient is based on ease of use, patient preference, cost, and safety issues, such as potential for drug interactions.[48,49] Pharmacokinetic properties should also be considered, as rivastigmine and galantamine have short half-lives (1.5 and 7 hours, respectively) as compared to donepezil (70 hours). As such, if rivastigmine or galantamine treatment is interrupted for several days or longer, the patient should be restarted at the lowest dose and titrated to the current dose. This is true for all formulations of these drugs, including the Exelon® patch.[63–66] Dosing strategies for cholinesterase inhibitors and memantine are summarized in Table 38-6.

TABLE 38-6 Dosing of Drugs Used for Cognitive Symptoms

Drug	Brand Name	Initial Dose	Usual Range	Special Population Dose	Other
Cholinesterase Inhibitors					
Donepezil	Aricept®, Aricept® ODT®	5 mg daily in the evening	5–10 mg daily in mild to moderate AD 10-23 mg daily in moderate to severe AD		Available as: tablet, orally disintegrating tablet (ODT) Can be taken with or without food Weight loss associated with 23 mg daily dose
Rivastigmine	Exelon®, Exelon® Patch	1.5 mg twice daily (capsule, oral solution) 4.6 mg/day (transdermal patch)	3–6 mg twice a day (capsule, oral solution) 9.5–13.3 mg/day (transdermal patch)	Moderate to severe renal impairment, mild to moderate hepatic impairment, or low body weight (<50 kg [110 lb]): consider maximum daily dose of 4.6 mg every 24 hours (transdermal patch)	Available as: capsule, oral solution, transdermal patch Take with meals Also indicated for dementia associated with Parkinson's disease Application of multiple transdermal patches at same time associated with hospitalization and death
Galantamine	Razadyne®, Razdyne® ER	4 mg twice daily (tablet, oral solution) 8 mg daily in the morning (extended-release capsule)	8–12 mg twice a day (tablet, oral solution) 16–24 mg (extended-release capsule)	Moderate renal or hepatic impairment: maximum daily dose of 16 mg Severe renal or hepatic impairment: not recommended	Available as: tablet, oral solution, extended-release capsule Take with meals
***N*-Methyl-d-Aspartate (NMDA) Receptor Antagonist**					
Memantine	Namenda®, Namenda® XR	5 mg daily 7 mg daily (extended-release capsule)	10 mg twice daily 28 mg daily (extended-release capsule)	Severe renal impairment: target maintenance dose of 5 mg twice daily (tablet, oral solution) or 14 mg daily (extended-release capsule)	Available as: tablet, oral solution, extended-release capsule Can be taken with or without food

ODT, orally disintegrating tablet.

Data from References 63–66, 72, and 73.

TABLE 38-7 Monitoring Drug Therapy for Cognitive Symptoms

Drug	Adverse Drug Reaction	Monitoring Parameter	Comments
Cholinesterase inhibitors	Dizziness, syncope, bradycardia, atrial arrhythmias, myocardial infarction, angina, seizures, sinoatrial and atrioventricular block	Report of dizziness or falls, pulse, blood pressure, and postural blood pressure change	Dizziness is usually mild, transient, and not related to cardiovascular problems Routine pulse checks at baseline, monthly during titration, and every 6 months thereafter
Cholinesterase inhibitors	Nausea, vomiting, diarrhea, anorexia, and weight loss	Weight and GI complaints	Take with food to decrease GI upset Usually transient, dose-related GI adverse effects seen with drug initiation, dosage titration, or drug switch Debilitated patients or those weighing <55 kg (121 lb) may be more likely to experience GI adverse effects and significant weight loss, particularly when rivastigmine is prescribed or when titrating to donepezil 23 mg GI adverse effects less prominent with transdermal versus oral rivastigmine
Cholinesterase inhibitors	Peptic ulcer disease, GI bleeding	Signs or symptoms of active or occult GI bleeding	Of particular concern for patients at increased risk of developing ulcers, such as those with a history of ulcer disease or concurrently taking NSAIDs
Cholinesterase inhibitors	Insomnia, vivid/abnormal dreams, nightmares	Complaints of sleep disturbances, daytime drowsiness	Donepezil can be taken in the morning to decrease risk of sleep disturbances
Memantine	Headache, confusion, dizziness, hallucinations	Report of dizziness or falls, hallucinations	Confusion may be observed during dose titration and is usually transient Memantine may mitigate GI adverse effects associated with cholinesterase inhibitor therapy
Memantine	Constipation	GI complaints	

NSAIDs, nonsteroidal antiinflammatory drugs.

Data from Alzheimer's Association,[4] Rowland et al.,[131] Farlow and Cummings,[70] Qaseem et al.,[48] Sadowsky and Galvin,[42] and references 63–66, 72, and 73.

Adverse drug reactions and corresponding monitoring parameters are described in Table 38-7. Cholinesterase inhibitors have similar adverse event profiles, and this class of drugs is generally well-tolerated. The most frequent adverse events associated with these agents are mild to moderate GI symptoms (e.g., nausea, vomiting, and diarrhea).[52] Gradual dose titration over several months can improve tolerability.[50] Alternatives to the immediate-release tablet/capsule dosage form are available for patients who have complex dosing regimens, tolerability issues, or difficulty swallowing, though cost may be prohibitive until they are generically available. Patients and caregivers should be cautioned against abrupt discontinuation of cholinesterase inhibitor therapy, as this can lead to worsening cognition and behavior in some patients.[67,68] Concurrent use of anticholinergic medications with cholinesterase inhibitors should also be avoided.[69] Depending on individual patient response, tolerability, and preference, switching to an alternate dosage form of cholinesterase inhibitor agent may be necessary during the course of AD treatment. Manufacturer recommendations for switching between dosage forms of the same drug are specified in the prescribing information, but the optimal procedure for switching between agents remains uncertain. Length of the washout period when switching from one cholinesterase to another may vary based on drug pharmacokinetics; however, 1 week is generally sufficient.[70]

8 Antiglutamatergic Therapy Memantine is the only NMDA-antagonist currently available. At concentrations achieved at least under in vitro conditions, memantine blocks glutamatergic neurotransmission by antagonizing NMDA receptors. Glutamate is an excitatory neurotransmitter in the brain implicated in long-term potentiation, a neuronal mechanism important for learning and memory.[71] Blocking NMDA receptors can mitigate excitotoxic neurotoxicity and provide neuroprotection. There is currently no clinical evidence to indicate memantine confers neuroprotection in AD.[42,51,71]

Memantine is currently indicated for use in moderate to severe AD. Its use has been studied in patients with moderate and severe AD as monotherapy and in combination with donepezil with favorable results on cognition and function.[51] Studies of memantine alone and in combination with cholinesterase inhibitors in mild AD performed to date have provided insufficient evidence to support an indication for mild AD.[42]

In its tablet or oral solution form, memantine should be initiated at 5 mg once a day and titrated weekly in 5 mg intervals to the target maintenance dose of 10 mg twice daily. The extended-release capsule form of memantine is to be initiated at 7 mg daily and titrated up to a maximum of 28 mg daily. Dose titration is achieved in 7 mg intervals with at least 1 week between dose adjustments. Dosing of 5 mg twice daily (tablet, oral solution) or 14 mg daily (extended-release capsule) is recommended in patients with severe renal impairment (creatinine clearance of 5 to 29 mL/min [0.08 to 0.49 mL/s]).

Overall, memantine has been well-tolerated in clinical trials. The most common adverse events include headache, constipation, confusion, and dizziness.[72,73] Memantine has 100% bioavailability regardless of administration with or without food. Protein binding is relatively low (45%). Memantine is not metabolized by the liver and does not inhibit cytochrome P450 activity. It is primarily excreted unchanged in the urine, and the half-life of memantine ranges from 60 to 80 hours.[72,73]

Role of Combination Therapy Combination therapy with memantine added to cholinesterase inhibitor therapy is generally prescribed for patients with moderate to severe AD. The rationale for this add-on therapy is that the drug classes have different mechanisms of action. In an observational study, memantine plus a cholinesterase inhibitor was compared to cholinesterase inhibitor monotherapy and to no treatment with either. Combination therapy slowed cognitive and functional decline to a statistically significant degree compared to the other groups; this was a 4-year sustained effect that appeared to increase over time.[74] A randomized controlled trial (RCT) randomized patients with moderate to severe AD already receiving stable donepezil treatment to either memantine or placebo. At the end of this 6-month trial, patients randomized to memantine (combination therapy) had significantly better outcomes in measures of cognition, function, behavior, and global status than those randomized to placebo (donepezil monotherapy). The group randomized to receive memantine also had a lower rate of discontinuation due to adverse events versus placebo.[75] Based on data from this study and others, memantine may have a role in mitigating GI adverse events associated with cholinesterase inhibitors.[42,75]

Effect of Current Treatments on Neurodegenerative Processes AD is a progressive disorder. Affected individuals typically experience some degree of cognitive decline and histologic change years (if not decades) before a diagnosis is made. Therefore, the ideal treatment will be one that not only reverses symptoms by enhancing cognitive function (a symptomatic treatment), but also arrests the neurodegeneration-relevant molecular processes that underlie cognitive decline (a disease-modifying treatment).

Clinical trials for AD prompt consideration of whether positive outcomes suggest either a symptomatic or disease-modifying effect. Any rapid performance improvement on cognitive ability, activities of daily living, or behavioral end points is indicative of a symptomatic effect. All cholinesterase inhibitor agents and memantine demonstrate this pattern. On the other hand, arrest of decline or a sustained reduction in the slope of decline would argue the presence of a disease-modifying effect. It has not been possible to unequivocally demonstrate this in trials of the currently approved treatments. Long-duration, double-blind, placebo-controlled trials to evaluate whether cholinesterase inhibitors, with or without memantine, have disease-modifying effects are difficult to perform, because doing so would require continuing a placebo arm over an extended period, well beyond demonstration of symptomatic benefit. Also, subject attrition over an extended study would complicate both intent-to-treat and observed cases analyses.

With the currently approved AD drug treatments, pivotal placebo-controlled trials were followed by open-label extension studies. Published studies have lasted as long as 5 years, and as part of these studies, decline in the treatment group was compared with "projected" placebo groups based on the placebo groups followed during the 6-month randomized phase of the efficacy study, as well as natural history cohorts from the precholinesterase inhibitor therapy era. Although analyses of this sort conclude that, for up to at least 5 years, persons receiving treatment exceed their projected nontreatment cognitive performance, no convincing evidence of a disease-modifying effect emerges.[76–80]

Clinical **Controversy...**

In light of the irreversible nature of AD, the question of whether to intervene at the time of AD diagnosis or earlier (when patients are asymptomatic or exhibit symptoms of MCI) remains controversial. Some studies suggest cognitive benefits in patients with MCI treated with cholinesterase inhibitors. However, cholinesterase inhibitors have not been shown to prevent conversion from normal cognition or MCI to AD. Despite inconclusive evidence for early intervention, cholinesterase inhibitors are commonly prescribed off-label prior to formal diagnosis of AD.[81–83]

Management of Brain Vascular Health

9 Guidelines for the care of patients with AD support the management of vascular brain disease and its associated risk factors as part of the treatment of AD.[84] There is a growing body of evidence that brain vascular disease may play a role in the progression of dementia. For a given level of Alzheimer's pathology, vascular disease in the brain may add to the degree of cognitive impairment.[84] Management of brain vascular disease includes monitoring blood pressure, glucose, cholesterol, and homocysteine and initiation of appropriate interventions.[84] Guidelines recommend low-dose aspirin therapy in patients with AD with significant brain vascular disease.[84] Elevated homocysteine levels correlate with decreased performance on cognitive tests, but there remains insufficient evidence of a benefit of B vitamin supplementation (B_6, B_{12}, and folic acid) on cognitive function in patients with AD.[1] The Alzheimer's Association's Maintain Your Brain campaign recommends staying physically, mentally, and socially active; adopting a low-fat, low-cholesterol diet rich in dark vegetables and fruit; and managing body weight, blood pressure, cholesterol, and blood sugar to reduce the risk of heart disease, stroke, and diabetes.[4] Appropriate management of vascular disease risk factors may reduce the risk for developing AD,[85] although currently insufficient evidence exists to draw definitive conclusions on the association between risk factor modification and risk of AD.[11]

Other Potential Treatment Approaches

Estrogen Estrogen replacement has been studied extensively for the treatment and prevention for AD. Most, but not all, retrospective epidemiologic studies show a lower incidence of AD in women who took estrogen replacement therapy postmenopausally. Prospective clinical trials have not supported the use of estrogen as a treatment for cognitive decline and longer trials tend to suggest harm. Overall, the evidence does not support the use of estrogen to treat or prevent dementia.[49,86]

Antiinflammatory Agents Retrospective epidemiologic studies suggest a protective effect against AD in patients who have taken NSAIDs. The benefits of antiinflammatory agents have been less compelling in prospective clinical studies. NSAIDs have had no cognitive benefit in AD patients or else benefits so minimal the risk of harm exceeds the potential benefit.[17] Because there is a lack of compelling data and also a significant incidence of adverse effects, particularly gastritis and the possibility of GI bleeds, NSAIDs and prednisone are not recommended for general use in the treatment or prevention of AD.[17]

Lipid-Lowering Agents An AD protective effect has been postulated for lipid-lowering agents, particularly the 3-hydroxy-3-methylglutaryl-coenzyme A-reductase inhibitors. Longitudinal epidemiologic studies suggest an association between elevated midlife total cholesterol levels and AD.[19] Increased risk of dementia does not appear to be associated with hypercholesterolemia in late life however.[19] Other studies note that the incidence of AD is lower in patients who have taken either a statin or another lipid-lowering agent, but not in patients who were taking other cardiovascular medications.[19] It is important to note that not all epidemiologic studies suggest an association between cholesterol and AD.[19]

RCTs of statin therapy given in late life to patients at risk for vascular disease indicate that statins do not prevent AD.[87] Several RCTs of statins for the treatment of mild to moderate AD have been completed or are ongoing. Thus far, these trials have not demonstrated a significant benefit of statin therapy, but results of ongoing trials should help to clarify the role of statins in the treatment of AD.[88] Interestingly, cognitive impairment has been recognized as a rare adverse event associated with statin therapy. The extent of cognitive impairment may depend on the lipid solubility of the drug, regulating the amount of drug that is able to cross the blood–brain barrier. As simvastatin and lovastatin have the highest lipophilicity, they may be the most likely candidates to cause memory impairment.[89] More research is needed to understand the complex relationship between cholesterol, statin therapy, and cognitive functioning. For now these agents should be reserved for patients who have other indications for their use.[84]

Dietary Supplements

Dietary supplements are widely used for the prevention and treatment of AD and available evidence has been recently reviewed.[90–93] A detailed discussion of the many nutraceuticals, herbal products, and medical foods that have been promoted for the prevention and treatment of AD is beyond the scope of this chapter. The more commonly used dietary supplements are described here.

Vitamin E Based on pathophysiologic theories involving oxidative stress and the accumulation of free radicals in AD, significant interest has evolved regarding the use of antioxidants in the treatment of AD. Vitamin E was frequently recommended as adjunctive treatment for AD patients based on data from a clinical trial evaluating the time to critical end points (e.g., death, institutionalization, loss of ability to perform activities of daily living, or severe dementia) in patients treated with vitamin E, selegiline, the combination, or placebo.[94] Although vitamin E and selegiline were superior to placebo, this study has been criticized because of differences in baseline cognitive severity, calling the validity of the results into question. Side effects observed with vitamin E administration include impaired hemostasis, fatigue, nausea, diarrhea, abdominal pain, and falls.[94] A meta-analysis found that high-dose vitamin E increases mortality in supplemented subjects.[95] In addition, vitamin E had no benefit in patients with MCI in the progression to AD.[83] In light of these findings, vitamin E supplementation is no longer recommended for the treatment of AD. Vitamin E remains under investigation for the prevention of AD.

Ginkgo biloba *G. biloba* for the prevention and treatment of AD has been extensively studied. Proposed mechanisms for Ginkgo's use in AD include its potential to increase blood flow, decrease blood viscosity, antagonize platelet-activating factor receptors, increase anoxia tolerance, inhibit monoamine oxidase, and serve as an antioxidant. Active ingredients in *G. biloba* include flavonoids, the Ginkgo flavone glycosides and bioflavonoids. Most studies reporting benefit in patients with AD have studied a standardized extract, EGb 761, in doses of 120 mg per day for at least 4 to 6 weeks. The clinical significance of the modest benefits detected is unclear and direct comparisons to cholinesterase inhibitors or memantine are lacking. Those advocating the use of Ginkgo for AD suggest doses of 120 to 240 mg of the standard leaf extract twice per day be used, and note 12 weeks of consistent dosing may be needed to observe an effect.[96] However, a large trial of *G. biloba* in which the 120 mg twice a day dose was studied did not reduce either the overall incidence rate of dementia or AD incidence in elderly individuals with normal cognition or MCI.[97] Another recent large trial found that the long-term use of *G. biloba* extract did not reduce the risk of progression to AD among older adults suffering from memory complaints compared with placebo.[98] Side effects reported from EGb 761 studies were typically mild, including nausea, vomiting, diarrhea, headaches, dizziness, palpitations, restlessness, and weakness. Because EGb also has a potent antiplatelet effect, it should be avoided by individuals taking anticoagulant or antiplatelet therapies, and should be used cautiously in patients taking NSAIDs.[96,99] Current practice guidelines do not recommend Ginkgo for the prevention or treatment of AD.[84]

Huperzine A It is an alkaloid isolated from the Chinese club moss, *Huperzia serrata.* It reversibly inhibits acetylcholinesterase and is administered orally in doses of 50 to 200 mcg two to four times daily. Clinical studies suggest huperzine A may have efficacy in the symptomatic treatment of AD, but more studies are needed to determine its place in therapy. In a medium-sized, randomized, double-blind, placebo-controlled, multicenter study in patients with mild to moderate AD performed in China, treatment with huperzine A at doses of 400 mcg/day for 12 weeks resulted in improvement in cognition by an average of 4.6 points assessed by ADAS-cog ($P = 0.000$), 2.7 points on the MMSE, and 1.5 points on the Alzheimer's Disease Assessment Scale—noncognition ($P = 0.008$).[100] Replication of these study results are still pending. The current consensus is that huperzine A has not been adequately studied for use in AD, its consistency in commercially available products remains a concern, and potential side effects could be significant, especially in those taking cholinesterase inhibitors.[96,101]

Polyphenols Several epidemiological studies have demonstrated that moderate ingestion of wine, but not distilled spirits, is associated with a lower incidence of AD.[91] One of the components of red wine, resveratrol, has been the focus of research related to dementia. Resveratrol, a phenolic compound with antioxidant properties, is found commonly in foods such as grapes, peanuts, chocolate, blueberries, and red wine. Resveratrol's proposed benefits in AD are to prevent reactive oxygen species-induced Aβ production and apoptosis-mediated neurodegeneration.[91] Resveratrol 500 mg daily for 13 weeks followed by 1,000 mg daily for 39 weeks is currently under evaluation for the treatment of mild to moderate AD in a randomized, double-blind, placebo-controlled study.[102]

The polyphenol curcumin (turmeric) is a spice used in Indian curry that has antioxidant and antiinflammatory properties and has been proposed as one explanation for the lower incidence of AD in India compared to the United States.[89] Curcumin may prevent or treat AD by decreasing amyloid plaque formation, clearing existing plaques, and chelating metal ions.[89] Early studies with curcumin in AD did not provide evidence supporting its benefit in AD, but this may have been due to the poor oral availability of curcumin, insufficient dosing, and short duration of the trials. Synthetic formulations of curcumin as well as pharmaceutical modifications of the naturally occurring curcumin are being developed to improve the bioavailability of curcumin.[91] Studies are ongoing to evaluate the efficacy, safety, and dosing of curcumin for the treatment of AD.

Medical Foods Several medical foods have been studied for the treatment of AD. Medical foods constitute a unique category that consists of ingestible entities specifically intended for the treatment of diseases that have "specific nutritional requirements" and in which the medical food may manipulate disease-relevant pathophysiology. Although medical foods regulatory approval standards are not as rigorous as those required for approvals of new medications, medical foods are obtained only by prescription. AC1202 (Axona®) is a mixture of medium-chain fatty acids, consisting primarily of the C8 fatty acid, caprylic acid. AC1202 is converted by the liver to a ketone body, β-hydroxybutyrate, which is released into the blood stream. β-Hydroxybutyrate crosses the blood–brain barrier and can be used as an oxidative phosphorylation substrate by neuronal mitochondria. Support for AC1202 efficacy in the treatment of AD comes mostly from a phase IIb trial in which subjects randomized to 40 mg per day of AC1202 for 45 days performed relatively better on the ADAS-cog than did subjects randomized to a placebo.[103] A subanalysis of these data revealed that this benefit was entirely driven by subjects who did not have an *APOE*4* allele. For *APOE*4* carriers, ADAS-cog performance between subjects receiving AC1202 and placebo were comparable at all time points studied. GI-related side effects were common, but in general side effects were felt to be mild. Coconut oil is a source of caprylic acid, but does not contain sufficient quantities to meet the needs of a person with AD.[90] Coconut oil continues to be used by some patients as a less expensive alternative to AC1202 however.

Souvenaid® with Fortasyn Connect™ is a medical food with clinical trial data supporting it use in AD but is not yet commercially available. This product is administered once daily and contains omega-3 fatty acids, phospholipids, choline, uridine monophosphate, vitamin E, vitamin C, selenium, vitamin B_{12}, vitamin B_6, and folic acid. The nutrients in this product are at levels above what could be obtained from a normal diet. It is believed that these ingredients provide precursors that increase phosphatides that, along with synaptic proteins, comprise synaptic membranes.[90] In a randomized, double-blind, multicenter trial in treatment-naïve patients with mild to moderate AD receiving Souvenaid® with Fortasyn Connect™, improvement was seen after 12 weeks in one of two primary outcome measures of cognitive function.[90] GI events were the most commonly reported adverse events. A second 24-week, randomized, controlled, double-blind, parallel-group, multicountry trial in treatment naïve patients with mild AD confirmed these findings.[104]

Clinical **Controversy...**

The use of medical foods in patients with AD remains controversial. Limited laboratory and clinical data are available on these products. Also, there is no postapproval safety monitoring required for products that are classified as medical foods. At this time there are no studies comparing the efficacy and safety of these products with other established cognitive-enhancing treatment options. Controversy exists between those who advocate for availability of dietary supplements to consumers and those who advocate for the exclusive application of evidence-based medicine. The major concern is the marketing of potentially ineffective products to those suffering from memory loss or dementia. Despite the lack of a clear evidence base, patient interest in these products continues. This may in part be driven by the limitations of currently available therapies for AD.

Tramiprosate Tramiprosate (homotaurine), or Alzhemed®, showed promise as a treatment for AD in early development. In animal studies, homotaurine demonstrated the ability to interfere with amyloid plaque formation and subsequent degeneration of neuronal cells. Phase III trials were disappointing, and the FDA declined to approve marketing of homotaurine as a prescription drug. Homotaurine is naturally occurring in seaweed, and is now available as the dietary supplement, Vivimind® for age-associated memory impairment.[105]

Omega-3 Fatty Acids Arguments that omega-3 fatty acids found in fish oil, such as docosahexaenoic acid and eicosapentaenoic acid, could benefit AD subjects have existed for some years. A large prospective, placebo-controlled trial of docosahexaenoic acid in AD subjects was recently reported. For the most part, results were disappointing, and although it could not be ruled out that population subsets did benefit, the primary study end points were negative.[106] There is insufficient evidence at this time to recommend docosahexaenoic acid for the treatment of AD.

Drugs and Treatment Strategies in Development

New drug development is focused on disease modifying and prevention strategies and falls broadly into several categories: treatments designed to reduce levels of brain Aβ or manipulate its configuration, treatments targeting tau protein, antiinflammatory approaches, and therapies to address insulin resistance in the brain.

Reducing Aβ Formation To reduce brain amyloid levels, approaches to both reducing Aβ production and enhancing its removal have been and still are undergoing evaluation. Aβ is produced through enzymatic processing of APP by two enzyme complexes, the β- and γ-secretases. β-Secretase inhibitors have entered phase II and III human trials. Agents that specifically inhibit γ-secretase could prove problematic from a side-effect perspective, as γ-secretase is also critical for processing Notch3, a protein of developmental importance and perhaps brain maintenance. Certain NSAIDs (ibuprofen and flurbiprofen) influence γ-secretase, but do not inhibit it outright. In general, these NSAIDs alter where γ-secretase cuts the APP protein. An enantiomer of flurbiprofen, tarenflurbil, completed a large phase III efficacy trial in which no evidence of efficacy was seen.[107] Stimulation of α-secretase blocks the formation of Aβ and generates neuroprotective peptide that is another strategy to reduce Aβ. Therapies aimed at activating α-secretase are currently under investigation.[107]

Increasing Aβ Clearance Immunotherapy approaches have been studied as a way to enhance Aβ removal. The most extensive investigation involved AN1792, a Aβ-based vaccine. A phase II trial in humans was prematurely halted after a substantial percentage of those mounting a robust immune response to the vaccine experienced encephalitis, a potentially life-threatening brain inflammation. The most comprehensive, long-term clinicopathologic study of subjects receiving AN1792 later concluded that vaccinated subjects show a predictable rate of cognitive decline and that despite reducing brain plaque burdens, AN1792 vaccination is unlikely to meaningfully benefit those with the common form of late-onset, sporadic AD.[108] Despite these failures, second-generation active immunization vaccines are undergoing Phase II trials that, hopefully, will not trigger encephalitis. Clinical development of two of the most promising Aβ monoclonal antibodies, bapineuzumab and solanezumab, was discontinued after disappointing results in Phase III clinical trials.[109] The usefulness of treating AD subjects with IV immunoglobulin preparations, which naturally contain antibodies to Aβ, is under evaluation.[107]

Preventing Aβ Aggregation Proponents of the amyloid cascade hypothesis claim the species of Aβ that is most likely to prove relevant to AD neurodegeneration are Aβ oligomers formed through limited aggregation of Aβ monomers. Tramiprosate was designed to prevent Aβ oligomer formation and tested clinically in a large phase III trial. No evidence of efficacy was seen.[107] Other agents targeted at this mechanism remain under clinical investigation. Metals such as zinc, copper, and iron play a role in Aβ aggregation. Metal chelators are also being developed for potential treatment of AD.[107]

Targeting Tau Targeting tau has been challenging, and thus far there are few therapeutic options in clinical trials. One approach is inhibition of kinase-mediated phosphorylation since tau hyperphosphorylation leads to tau dysfunction and aggregation. Agents under investigation include lithium and valproate.[107] Protein phosphates are also being targeted to reduce hyperphosphorylation. Metformin and selenium are currently under investigation for this purpose. Tau aggregation inhibitors are also under study, including methylene blue.[107]

Reducing Oxidative Stress and Inflammation in the Brain Inflammation, oxidative stress, and mitochondrial dysfunction in chronic neurodegenerative disorders contribute to the neuronal dysfunction and loss that occurs in these conditions. Production of Aβ and hyperphosphorylated tau may simply be downstream cell responses to the cycle of inflammation and oxidative stress that eventually overwhelms the neuron's ability to compensate. Targeting the upstream oxidative stress and inflammation is an active area of investigation. Nutriceuticals and vitamins, as well as antiinflammatory medications (etanercept, prednisone, ibuprofen, indomethacin, naproxen, celecoxib, rofecoxib, atorvastatin, simvastatin, rosuvastatin, pravastatin, rosiglitazone, and the mitochondrial stabilizer latrepirdine) have shown promising results in preclinical studies and early clinical investigations, but subsequent clinical trials have often been conflicting or negative.[107] One possible explanation is that the benefit from these agents may be in primary prevention before damage is severe enough that symptoms of cognitive decline are evident.[107]

Targeting Insulin Resistance in the Brain Low levels of insulin and insulin resistance in the brain are associated with cognitive impairment and AD. Individuals with type 2 diabetes have a twofold higher risk of developing AD.[110] One of the actions of insulin in the brain is to modulate the levels of Aβ, leading researchers to explore this area for potential treatment opportunities. One promising approach is a new class of diabetes medications, glucagon-like peptide-1 receptor agonists. Liraglutide has been shown to reduce amyloid production and protect neurons from resulting damage in animal models.[110] Early clinical studies with intranasal insulin showed improvement in memory and daily functioning in patients with MCI and mild or moderate AD.[111] A large multicenter trial of this treatment strategy is scheduled to begin in 2013.[110]

Suggestions of efficacy in phase II trials in no way ensures efficacy will be seen in phase III trials. This caveat seems especially pertinent in AD drug development, as phase II trials of flurbiprofen, tramiprosate, rosiglitazone, latrepirdine, bapineuzumab, and solanezumab all reported some evidence of efficacy that did not bear out in phase III studies. Obviously, successful development of new AD treatments depends on elucidating AD's true underlying pathophysiology. One reason for the failure of so many AD therapeutics may be that current strategies do not target the pathways that ultimately result in AD. Another reason may be that medications are being initiated when the disease has already progressed too far to be reversed.[110] New approaches include studying amyloid-blocking agents in patients with genetic predisposition to young-onset AD before symptoms are present and studying patients with biomarkers of disease risk or presymptomatic signs of disease to determine the potential value of new treatments.[109]

Pharmacotherapy of Noncognitive Symptoms

Most patients with AD manifest noncognitive symptoms at some point in the illness.[112] These symptoms can be roughly divided into three categories: psychotic symptoms, inappropriate or disruptive behavior, and depression. Effective management of these problems is important because behavioral symptoms are distressing to both the patient and the caregiver, necessitate increased caregiver supervision and patience, and are a leading reason for nursing home placement.

(10) Strategies for treatment of psychotic or behavioral symptoms should include environmental interventions first, then pharmacologic interventions only when necessary. Behaviors such as agitation, aggression, delusions, hallucinations, repetitive vocalizations, and wandering may be caused by medications, medical illness (e.g., pain, constipation, dehydration, and infection), environmental precipitants, poor caregiving, physical/verbal abuse, and unmet physical or psychological needs. These possible underlying causes should be explored and corrected when possible before initiating drug therapies.[25] The need for medications may exist when neuropsychiatric symptoms are of sufficient severity to cause significant distress to the patient or caregiver, interfere with function or cause disability, impede delivery of necessary care, or pose a danger to self or others.[49,84,112] The balance between risks of the medication and expected benefits must be acceptable to the patient or surrogate decision maker. Medications should be used cautiously, with adequate monitoring for efficacy and adverse events.

Despite the high prevalence of noncognitive symptoms in AD, relatively little research has been conducted in these patients. Data from clinical trials of antidepressants, cholinesterase inhibitors, and antipsychotics are emerging, but more research is needed. To date, no drug has been approved by the U.S. FDA for the treatment of behavioral disturbances in patients with dementia. Because of limited clinical data, treatment is primarily empiric, with side-effect profiles used as a guide in selecting the appropriate treatment. Psychotropic medications with anticholinergic effects should be avoided because they may actually worsen cognition and interfere with cholinesterase inhibitor therapy.

TABLE 38-8 Medications Used for Noncognitive Symptoms of Dementia

Drugs	Starting Dose (mg)	Maintenance Dose in Dementia (mg/day)	Target Symptoms
Antipsychotics			Psychosis: hallucinations, delusions, suspiciousness Disruptive behaviors: agitation, aggression
Aripiprazole	10–15	30 (maximum)	
Olanzapine	2.5	5–10	
Quetiapine	25	100–400	
Risperidone	0.25	0.5–2	
Antidepressants			Depression: poor appetite, insomnia, hopelessness, anhedonia, withdrawal, suicidal thoughts, agitation, anxiety
Citalopram	10	10–20	
Escitalopram	5	10 (maximum)	
Fluoxetine	10	10–20	
Paroxetine	10	10–40	
Sertraline	12.5	150 (maximum)	
Mirtazapine	15	15–30	
Trazodone	25	75–150	
Anticonvulsants			Agitation or aggression
Carbamazepine	100	300–600	
Valproic acid	125	500–1,500	

Data from Sadowsky and Galvin,[42] Benoit et al.,[132] and Geriatrics at Your Fingertips.[133]

General guidelines governing therapy can be summarized as follows: use reduced doses, monitor closely, titrate dosage slowly, and document carefully. Treatment should be considered as temporary.[113] Caregivers often have erroneous expectations regarding the effects of psychotropic medications, and the anticipated benefits and risks of therapy should be clearly explained. Disruptive behaviors and delusions wax and wane with disease progression. Attempts to slowly taper and discontinue medication should be undertaken regularly in minimally symptomatic patients, because some patients improve on medication withdrawal.[84] Table 38-8 outlines suggested doses of medications.

Cholinesterase Inhibitors and Memantine

Clinical trials with cholinesterase inhibitors have consistently reported modest benefit in managing neuropsychiatric symptoms, although these are generally not the primary outcomes studied in the trials.[114–117] Any benefits in symptoms such as agitation may accrue gradually over time, since cholinesterase inhibitors may not significantly reduce agitation when administered to patients experiencing acute agitation.[118] Memantine shows modest behavioral benefits as well, either alone or in combination with cholinesterase inhibitors, and may also spare the use of antipsychotics to treat agitation.[114,115,117] These treatments can provide modest short-term improvement and possibly slow the development and progression of behavioral symptoms. Cholinesterase inhibitors also have a small beneficial effect on caregiver burden and active time use among caregivers of persons with AD.[119] These benefits should be considered along with cognitive benefits in treatment decisions. Long-term effects on behavior have not been demonstrated to date, and further research is needed.

Antipsychotics

Antipsychotics are widely used in the management of neuropsychiatric symptoms in AD. There is modestly convincing evidence that most of the atypical antipsychotics provide some benefit for particular neuropsychiatric symptoms, but these data have been insufficient to gain FDA approval as an indication for the management of behavioral symptoms in AD. Based on a meta-analysis, only 17% to 18% of dementia patients show a treatment response to atypical antipsychotics.[120] In a double-blind, placebo-controlled trial of 421 outpatients with AD and psychosis, aggression, or agitation randomized to receive olanzapine, quetiapine, risperidone, or placebo for up to 36 weeks, there were no significant differences among the treatments in time to discontinuation of treatment or improvement in the Clinical Global Impression of Change scale. The investigators concluded that adverse effects offset advantages in the efficacy of atypical antipsychotic drugs for treatment of psychosis, aggression, or agitation in patients with AD.[120] A recent systematic review and meta-analysis found small but statistically significant benefits in global behavioral symptom scores in elderly patients with dementia for aripiprazole, olanzapine, and risperidone.[121] Adverse events are common with atypical and typical antipsychotics in patients with AD. These adverse events associated with atypical antipsychotics include somnolence, extrapyramidal symptoms, abnormal gait, worsening cognition, cerebrovascular events, and increased risk of death.[122] These findings resulted in a FDA-mandated "black box warning" concerning the use of atypical antipsychotics in the treatment of AD. Typical antipsychotics may also be associated with a small increased risk of death, as well as more severe extrapyramidal effects and hypotension. Chapter 50 includes a more detailed discussion of antipsychotic adverse events. Overall, there is a modest expectation of treatment benefit and potential for significant harm associated with antipsychotic use in patients with AD. Individual risk and benefit must be considered when initiating therapy. Prescribing of antipsychotics in AD should be restricted to patients with severe symptoms that have not responded to other measures and treatment should rarely be continued beyond 12 weeks.[123] Diligent monitoring during treatment is essential along with frequent reassessment of continued need.

Antidepressants

Depressive symptoms are common in patients with AD. Apathy is seen in 48% to 92% of individuals with dementia, and clinically significant depression occurs in approximately 32% with mild dementia, 23% with moderate disease, and 18% in the severe stage of the dementia.[117] Some trials have studied the efficacy of antidepressants in treating depression in patients with AD, but the results are conflicting.[124] Small sample size, short duration of treatment, and differing measures of therapy outcomes limit comparison across studies and may account in part for conflicting study results.[117] Improvement in patients receiving placebo is also common. In practice, treatment with selective serotonin reuptake inhibitors (SSRIs) is initiated most commonly in patients with AD, based on side-effect profile and evidence of efficacy,[49,125] however a recent study comparing sertraline, mirtazapine, and placebo found no benefit for these agents in treating depression in patients with dementia.[126] Among the SSRIs, the best evidence exists for sertraline and citalopram.[115] Serotonergic function may also play a role in some of the other behavioral symptoms of AD, and some studies support the use of SSRIs in the management of these behaviors, even in the absence of depression.[115] Tricyclic antidepressants have efficacy similar to the SSRIs, but should generally be avoided because of their anticholinergic activity.[49] There is little evidence for the use of trazodone to manage behavioral or depressive symptoms, but it is commonly recommended to treat insomnia in patients with AD.[49]

Chapter 51 has a more complete discussion of treatment of depression.

Miscellaneous Therapies

Because antipsychotic and antidepressant therapy has shown only modest efficacy and poses a risk of undesirable side effects, medications traditionally used to treat disruptive behaviors and aggression in other psychiatric and neurologic disorders have been suggested as potential alternatives. These alternatives include benzodiazepines and antiepileptics.[117,123]

Benzodiazepines have been used to treat anxiety, agitation, and aggression, but the benefit is generally modest.[49] There are no RCTs that have investigated the use of benzodiazepines for the management of behavioral disturbances in AD. Because benzodiazepines impair cognition, worsen breathing disorders, and may increase the risk of falls in AD patients, their routine use is not advised, except on an "as needed basis" for infrequent episodes of agitation.[49,117] "Mood stabilizer" anticonvulsants such as carbamazepine, valproic acid, or gabapentin may be appropriate alternatives, but evidence is conflicting.[115,117] Clearly, more rigorous placebo-controlled studies are needed to determine the relative efficacy and place in therapy for these medication alternatives.

Noncognitive symptoms are often the most difficult aspect of AD for the caregiver. When nonpharmacologic approaches fail, selected antipsychotics and antidepressants have been useful for effective management of behavioral, psychotic, and depressive symptoms, thereby easing caregiver burden and allowing the patient to spend additional time at home. Alternative treatments are available when initial choices are not successful. Adverse events remain an important concern in this population.

Clinical **Controversy. . .**

The appropriate use of medications in the management of behavioral disturbances in patients with dementia continues to be controversial. Nonpharmacologic approaches are considered first-line therapy, but evidence for individual nonpharmacologic strategies is often lacking, and there are many barriers to implementing these approaches consistently. Nonpharmacologic strategies require caregiver education and training, sufficient staffing resources in facilities or caregiver time at home, and availability of necessary supplies or equipment. Overcoming these barriers is challenging, but an important step in minimizing the use of medications for managing behavioral disturbances in AD.

PERSONALIZED THERAPY

At this time there are no specific recommendations regarding the choice of agent or dosing regimen for current cognitive enhancing therapies based on genotype or other biomarkers. There is a great deal of attention among AD researchers to identify biomarkers for AD, and recommendations are likely to evolve over time as we better understand the underlying pathophysiology of AD and the predictors of patient response. Recommendations for patients with renal or hepatic dysfunction or low body weight are detailed in Table 38-6. It is important to consider that most patients with AD are older adults and therefore may be taking multiple medications for other acute and chronic health conditions. The potential for adverse events due to drug interactions increases as the number of medications increases.

EVALUATION OF THERAPEUTIC OUTCOMES

An evaluation of therapeutic outcomes in the patient with AD begins with a thorough assessment at baseline and a clear definition of therapeutic goals. Cognitive status, physical status, functional performance, mood, and behavior all need to be evaluated before initiation of drug therapy. The clinician should interview both the patient and the caregiver to assess response to drug therapy. In evaluating response to cognitive agents, the clinician should ask questions about the patient's ability to perform daily functional tasks and about mood and behavior, as well as questions about memory and orientation. Objective assessments such as MMSE for cognition assessment, the Physical Self-Maintenance Scale for assessment of activities of daily living, and the Neuropsychiatric Inventory Questionnaire for assessment of behavioral disturbances can be used to quantify changes in symptoms and function.[127]

Because target symptoms of psychiatric disorders may respond differently in dementia patients, a detailed list of symptoms to be treated should be documented in the pharmacotherapy plan to aid in monitoring. These could include, for example, "striking at spouse because patient believes spouse is an impostor," "verbal threats and refusal to allow clothes to be changed," and so on, as opposed to documenting vague symptoms such as "aggression" or "delusions." To make an accurate assessment of depression, multiple symptoms (e.g., sleep, appetite, and activity and interest levels) need to be assessed in addition to the patient's stated mood.

The patient should be observed carefully for potential side effects of drug therapy. The specific side effects to be monitored and the method and frequency of monitoring should be documented. Patients should be monitored for therapeutic effect 8 weeks after initiation of therapy and least every 6 months thereafter.[127] However, patients need to be treated for an adequate duration to see a therapeutic effect from a given intervention. Because the effects of cognition-enhancing medications are not great, a treatment period of several months to a year may be necessary before it can be determined whether therapy is beneficial. Cognitive effects of the drug are often noticed only as a plateauing during treatment or as deterioration following drug discontinuation. In general, cognitive agents should be continued if the patient is demonstrating no change in clinical status. However, if there is doubt, the medication can be slowly tapered and discontinued, and the patient monitored off the drug for 4 to 6 weeks to determine the need for continued therapy.

ABBREVIATIONS

AA	Alzheimer's Association
Aβ	β-Amyloid peptide
AD	Alzheimer's disease
ADAS-cog	Alzheimer's Disease Assessment Scale—Cognition
ADRDA	Alzheimer's Disease and Related Disorders Association
AHRQ	Agency for Healthcare Research and Quality
APOE	apolipoprotein E
APP	amyloid precursor protein
CSF	cerebrospinal fluid
DSM-5	Diagnostic and Statistical Manual of Mental Disorders, Fifth Edition
FDA	Food and Drug Administration
MCI	mild cognitive impairment
MMSE	Mini-Mental Status Examination
NFT	neurofibrillary tangle
NIA	National Institute on Aging
NINCDS	National Institute of Neurological and Communicative Disorders and Stroke
NINDS	National Institute of Neurological Disorders and Stroke
NMDA	*N*-methyl-D-aspartate
NSAID	nonsteroidal antiinflammatory drug
RCT	randomized controlled trial
SSRI	selective serotonin reuptake inhibitor

REFERENCES

1. Ballard C, Gauthier S, Corbett C, et al. Alzheimer's disease. Lancet 2011;377:1019–1031.
2. Alzheimer's Association. 2013, *http://napa.alz.org/*.
3. Querfurth HW, LaFerla FM. Alzheimer's disease. N Engl J Med 2010;362:329–344.
4. Alzheimer's Association. 2012 Alzheimer's Disease Facts and Figures. Alzheimers Dement 2012;8:131–168.
5. Reitz C, Brayne C, Mayeux R. Epidemiology of Alzheimer disease. Nat Rev Neurol 2011;7:137–152.
6. Bertram L, Tanzi RE. Genome-wide association studies in Alzheimer's disease. Hum Mol Genet 2009;18: R137–R145.
7. Betram L, Tanzi RE. The genetics of Alzheimer's disease. Prog Mol Biol Transl Sci 2012;107:79–100.
8. Williamson J, Goldman J, Marder KS. Genetic aspects of Alzheimer's disease. Neurologist 2009;15:80–86.
9. Kim J, Basak J, Holtzman DM. The role of apolipoprotein E in Alzheimer's disease. Neuron 2009;63: 287–303.
10. Mastroeni D, Grover A, Delvaux E, et al. Epigenetics mechanisms in Alzheimer's disease. Neurobiol Aging 2011;32:1161–1180.
11. Daviglus ML, Plassman BL, Pirzada A, et al. Risk factors and preventive interventions for Alzheimer Disease. Arch Neurol 2011;68:1185–1190.
12. Swerdlow RH. Is aging part of Alzheimer's disease, or is Alzheimer's disease part of aging? Neurobiol Aging 2007;28:1465–1480.
13. Kern A, Behl C. The unsolved relationship of brain aging and late-onset Alzheimer disease. Biochim Biophys Acta 2009;1790:1124–1132.
14. Duncan GW. The aging brain and neurodegenerative diseases. Clin Geriatr Med 2011;27:629–644.
15. McGreer PL, McGreer EG. NSAIDs and Alzheimer disease: Epidemiological, animal model and clinical studies. Neurobiol Aging 2007;28:639–647.
16. Vlad SC, Miller DR, Kowall NW, et al. Protective effects of NSAIDs on the development of Alzheimer disease. Neurology 2008;70:1672–1677.
17. Jaturapatporn D, Isaac MGEKN, McCleery J, et al. Aspirin, steroidal and non-steroidal anti-inflammatory drugs for the treatment of Alzheimer's disease. Cochrane Database Syst Rev 2012;2:CD006378.
18. Parsons CG, Stöffler A, Danysz W. Memantine: A NMDA receptor antagonist that improves memory by restoration of homeostasis in the glutamatergic system—to little activation is bad, too much is even worse. Neuropharmacology 2007;53:699–723.
19. Dickstein DL, Walsh J, Brautigam H, et al. Role of vascular risk factors and vascular dysfunction in Alzheimer's disease. Mt Sinai J Med 2010;77:82–102.
20. Power MC, Weuve J, Gagne JJ, et al. The association between blood pressure and incident Alzheimer disease. Epidemiology 2011;22:646–659.
21. Henderson VW. Action of estrogens in the aging brain: Dementia and cognitive aging. Biochim Biophys Acta 2010;1800:1077–1083.
22. Galvin JE, Sadowsky CH. Practical guidelines for the recognition and diagnosis of dementia. J Am Board Fam Med 2012;25:367–382.
23. Boustani M, Peterson B, Hanson L, et al. Screening for dementia in primary care: A summary of the evidence for the U.S. Preventive Services Task Force. Ann Intern Med 2003;138:927–937.

24. Milne A, Cluverwell A, Guss R, et al. Screening for dementia in primary care: A review of the use, efficacy and quality of measures. Int Psychogeriatr 2008;20;911–926.
25. Alzheimer's Association. Alzheimer's Disease and Dementia | Alzheimer's Association. *http://www.alz.org/*. Accessed February 8, 2013.
26. American Psychiatric Association. Diagnostic and Statistical Manual of Mental Disorders, 5th ed. Washington, DC: American Psychiatric Association, 2013.
27. Costa PT Jr, Williams TF, Somerfield M, et al. Early Identification of Alzheimer's Disease and Related Dementias. Clinical Practice Guidelines, Quick Reference Guide for Clinicians, No. 19. Rockville, MD: U.S. Department of Health and Human Services, Public Health Service, Agency for Health Care Policy and Research, 1996.
28. Knopman DS, DeKosky ST, Cummings JL, et al. Practice parameter: Diagnosis of dementia (an evidence-based review): Report of the Quality Standards Subcommittee of the American Academy of Neurology. Neurology 2001;56:1143–1153.
29. Roman GC, Tatemichi TK, Erkinjuntti T, et al. Vascular dementia: Diagnostic criteria for research studies. Report of the NINDS-AIREN International Workshop. Neurology 1993;43:250–260.
30. McKhann G, Drachman D, Folstein M, et al. Mental and clinical diagnosis of Alzheimer's disease: Report of the NINCDS-ADRDA Work Group under the auspices of the Department of Health and Human Services Task Force on Alzheimer's disease. Neurology 1984;34:939–944.
31. Jack CR, Albert M, Knopman DS, et al. Introduction to revised criteria for the diagnosis of Alzheimer's disease: National Institute on Aging and the Alzheimer Association workgroups. Alzheimers Dement 2011;7:257–262.
32. Reiman EM, McKhann GM, Albert MS, et al. Alzheimer's disease: Implications of the updated diagnostic and research criteria. J Clin Psychiatry 2011;72:1190–1196.
33. McKhann GM, Knopman DS, Chertkow H, et al. The diagnosis of dementia due to Alzheimer's disease: Recommendations from the National Institute on Aging–Alzheimer's Association Workgroups on Diagnostic Guidelines for Alzheimer's disease. Alzheimers Dement 2011;7:263–269.
34. Albert MS, DeKosky ST, Dickson D, et al. The diagnosis of mild cognitive impairment due to Alzheimer's disease: Recommendations from the National Institute on Aging–Alzheimer's Association Workgroups on Diagnostic Guidelines for Alzheimer's disease. Alzheimers Dement 2011;7:270–279.
35. Sperling RA, Aisen PS, Beckett LA, et al. Toward defining the preclinical stages of Alzheimer's disease: Recommendations from the National Institute on Aging–Alzheimer's Association Workgroups on Diagnostic Guidelines for Alzheimer's disease. Alzheimers Dement 2011;7:280–292.
36. Fillenbaum GG, Peterson B, Morris JC. Estimating the validity of the Clinical Dementia Rating Scale: The CERAD experience. Consortium to Establish a Registry for Alzheimer's Disease. Aging 1996;8:379–385.
37. Moore AR, O'Keeffe ST. Drug-induced cognitive impairment in the elderly. Drugs Aging 1999;15:15–28.
38. Boustani M, Campbell N, Munger S. Impact of anticholinergics on the aging brain: a review and practical application. Aging Health 2008;4:311–320.
39. Bloudek LM, Spackman DE, Blankenburg M, Sullivan SD. Review and meta-analysis of biomarkers and diagnostic imaging in Alzheimer's disease. J Alzheimers Dis 2011;26:627–645.
40. Schipper HM. Apolipoprotein E: Implications for AD neurobiology, epidemiology and risk assessment. Neurobiol Aging 2009;32:778–790.
41. Geda YE. Mild cognitive impairment in older adults. Curr Psychiatry Rep 2012;14:320–327.
42. Sadowsky CH, Galvin JE. Guidelines for the management of cognitive and behavioral problems in dementia. J Am Board Fam Med 2012;25:350–366.
43. Gitlin LN, Kales HC, Lyketsos CG. Nonpharmacologic management of behavioral symptoms in dementia. JAMA 2012;308:2020–2029.
44. Ballard C, Khan Z, Clack H, et al. Nonpharmacological treatment of Alzheimer's disease. Can J Psychiatry 2011;56:589–595.
45. Elliott AF, Burgio LD, DeCoster J. Enhancing caregiver health: Findings from the resources for enhancing Alzheimer's caregiver health II intervention. J Am Geriatr Soc. 2010;58:30–37.
46. Mittelman MS, Haley WE, Clay OJ, Roth DL. Improving caregiver well-being delays nursing home placement of patients with Alzheimer's disease. Neurology 2006;67: 1592–1599.
47. Olazaran J, Reisberg B, Clara L, et al. Nonpharmacological therapies in Alzheimer's disease: A systematic review of efficacy. Dement Geriatr Cogn Disord 2010;30:161–178.
48. Qaseem A, Snow V, Cross JT Jr, et al. Current pharmacologic treatment of dementia: A clinical practice guideline from the American College of Physicians and the American Academy of Family Physicians. Ann Intern Med 2008;148:370–378.
49. APA Work Group on Alzheimer's Disease and other Dementias; Rabins PV, Blacker D, Rovner BW, et al. American Psychiatric Association practice guideline for the treatment of patients with Alzheimer's disease and other dementias, second edition. Am J Psychiatry 2007;164:5–56.
50. Birks J. Cholinesterase inhibitors for Alzheimer's disease. Cochrane Database Syst Rev 2006;1:CD005593.
51. McShane R, Areosa Sastre A, Minakaran N. Memantine for dementia. Cochrane Database Syst Rev 2009:CD003154.
52. Farrimond LE, Roberts E, McShane R. Memantine and cholinesterase inhibitor combination therapy for Alzheimer's disease: A systematic review. BMJ Open 2012;2: e000917.
53. Farlow MR, Miller ML, Pejovic V. Treatment options in Alzheimer's disease: Maximizing benefit, managing expectations. Dement Geriatr Cogn Disord 2008;25(5): 408–422.
54. Holmes C, Wilkinson D, Dean C, et al. The efficacy of donepezil in the treatment of neuropsychiatric symptoms in Alzheimer disease. Neurology 2004;63(2):214.
55. Rainer M, Muche HA, Kruger-Rainer C, et al. Cognitive relapse after discontinuation of drug therapy in Alzheimer's disease: Cholinesterase inhibitors versus nootropics. J Neural Transm 2001;108(11):1327.
56. Greenberg SM, Tennis MK, Brown LB, et al. Donepezil therapy in clinical practice: A randomized crossover study. Arch Neurol 2000;57(1):94–99.
57. Rogers SL, Farlow MR, Doody RS, et al. A 24-week, double-blind, placebo-controlled trial of donepezil in patients with Alzheimer's disease: Donepezil Study Group. Neurology 1998;50(1):136–145.
58. Pariente A, Fourrier-Reglat A, Bazin, et al. Effect of treatment gaps in elderly patients with dementia treated with cholinesterase inhibitors. Neurology 2012;78: 957–963.
59. Massoud F, Desmarais JE, Gautheir S. Switching cholinesterase inhibitors in older adults with dementia. In Psychogeriatr 2011;23:372–378.

60. Birks J, Grimley Evans J, Iakovidou V, et al. Rivastigmine for Alzheimer's disease. Cochrane Database Syst Rev 2009;2:CD001191.
61. Birks J, Harvey R J. Donepezil for dementia due to Alzheimer's disease. Cochrane Database Syst Rev 2009:CD001190.
62. Loy C, Schneider L. Galantamine for Alzheimer's disease and mild cognitive impairment. Cochrane Database Syst Rev 2006:CD001747.
63. Aricept (donepezil hydrochloride) [package insert]. Woodcliff Lake, NJ: Eisai Inc., 2012.
64. Exelon (rivastigmine tartrate) [package insert]. East Hanover, NJ: Novartis Pharmaceuticals, 2006.
65. Exelon Patch (rivastigmine transdermal system) [package insert]. East Hanover, NJ: Novartis Pharmaceuticals, 2012.
66. Razadyne (galantamine hydrobromide) [package insert]. Titusville, NJ: Ortho-McNeil-Janssen Pharmaceuticals, 2011.
67. Singh S, Dudley C. Discontinuation syndrome following donepezil cessation. Int J Geriatr Psychiatry 2003;18: 282–284.
68. Lee J, Monette J, Sourial N, et al. The use of a cholinesterase inhibitor review committee in long-term care. J Am Med Dir Assoc 2007;8:243–247.
69. Sink KM, Thomas J, Xu H, et al. Dual use of bladder anticholinergics and cholinesterase inhibitors: Long-term functional and cognitive outcomes. J Am Geriatr Soc 2008;56:847–853.
70. Farlow MR, Cummings JL. Effective pharmacologic management of Alzheimer's disease. Am J Med 2007;120:388–397.
71. Herrmann N, Li A, Lanctot K. Memantine in dementia: A review of the current evidence. Expert Opin Pharmacother 2011;12:787–800.
72. Namenda (memantine hydrochloride) [package insert]. St. Louis, MO: Forest Laboratories, 2011.
73. Namenda extended-release capsules (memantine hydrochloride) [package insert]. St. Louis, MO: Forest Laboratories, 2010.
74. Atri A, Shaughnessy LW, Locascio JJ, Growdon JH. Long-term course and effectiveness of combination therapy in Alzheimer disease. Alzheimer Dis Assoc Disord 2008;22:209–221.
75. Tariot PN, Farlow MR, Grossberg GT, et al. Memantine treatment in patients with moderate to severe Alzheimer disease already receiving donepezil: A randomized controlled trial. JAMA 2004;291:317–324.
76. Rogers SL, Doody RS, Pratt RD, Ieni JR. Long-term efficacy and safety of donepezil in the treatment of Alzheimer's disease: Final analysis of a US multicentre open-label study. Eur Neuropsychopharmacol 2000;10(3):195–203.
77. Raskind MA, Peskind ER, Truyen L, et al. The cognitive benefits of galantamine are sustained for at least 36 months: A long-term extension trial. Arch Neurol 2004;61:252–256.
78. Farlow MR, Lilly ML; ENA713 B352 Study Group. Rivastigmine: An open-label, observational study of safety and effectiveness in treating patients with Alzheimer's disease for up to 5 years. BMC Geriatr 2005;5:3.
79. Reisberg B, Doody R, Stoffler A, et al. A 24-week open-label extension study of memantine in moderate to severe Alzheimer's disease. Arch Neurol 2006;63:49–54.
80. Doody RS, Geldmacher DS, Gordon B, et al. Open-label, multicenter, phase 3 extension study of the safety and efficacy of donepezil in patients with Alzheimer disease. Arch Neurol 2001;58:427–433.
81. Roberts JS, Karlawish JH, Uhlmann WR, et al. Mild cognitive impairment in clinical care: A survey of American Academy of Neurology members. Neurology 2010;75: 425–431.
82. Peters O, Lorenz D, Fesche A, et al. A combination of galantamine and memantine modifies cognitive function in subjects with amnestic MCI. J Nutr Health Aging 2012;16:544–548.
83. Petersen RC, Thomas RG, Grunchman M, et al. Vitamin E and donepezil for the treatment of mild cognitive impairment. N Eng J Med 2005;352:2379–2388.
84. Lyketsos CG, Colenda CC, Beck C, et al. Position statement of the American Association for Geriatric Psychiatry regarding principles of care for patients with dementia resulting from Alzheimer's disease. Am J Geriatr Psychiatry 2006;14:561–573.
85. Middleton LE, Yaffe K. Promising strategies for the prevention of dementia. Arch Neurol 2009;66:1210–1215.
86. Barrett-Conner E, Laughlin GA. Endogenous and exogenous estrogen, cognitive function and dementia in postmenopausal women: Evidence from epidemiologic studies and clinical trials. Semin Reprod Med 2009;27: 275–282.
87. McGuinness B, Bullock CD, Passmore P. Statins for the prevention of dementia [review]. Cochrane Database Syst Rev 2009;2:CD003160.
88. McGuiness B, O'Hare J, Craig D, et al. Statins for the treatment of dementia. Cochrane Database Syst Rev 2010;8:CD007514.
89. Rojas-Fernandez CH, Cameron JC. Is statin-associated cognitive impairment clinically relevant? A narrative review and clinical recommendations. Ann Pharmacother 2012;46:549–557.
90. Wollen KA. Alzheimer's disease: The pros and cons of pharmaceutical, nutraceutical, botanical, and stimulatory therapies, with a discussion of treatment strategies from the perspective of patients and practitioners. Altern Med Rev 2010;15:223–244.
91. Shah RC. Medical foods for Alzheimer's disease. Drugs Aging 2011;28:421–428.
92. Howes M-JR, Perry E. The role of phytochemicals in the treatment and prevention of dementia. Drugs Aging 2011;28:439–468.
93. Kim HG, Oh MS. Herbal medicines for the prevention and treatment of Alzheimer's disease. Curr Pharm Des 2012;18:57–75.
94. Isaac MGEKN, Quinn R, Tabet N. Vitamin E for Alzheimer's disease and mild cognitive impairment. Cochrane Database Syst Rev 2008;3:CD002854.
95. Miller ER 3rd, Pastor-Barriuso R, Riemersma RA, et al. Meta-analysis: High-dosage vitamin E supplementation may increase all-cause mortality. Ann Intern Med 2005;142: 37–46.
96. Kelley BJ, Knopman DS. Alternative medicine and Alzheimer disease. Neurologist 2008;14:299–306.
97. DeKosky ST, Williamson JD, Fitzpatrick AL, et al. *Ginkgo biloba* for prevention of dementia. A randomized controlled trial. JAMA 2008;300:2253–2262.
98. Vellas B, Coley N, Ousset P, et al. Long-term use of standardized *Ginkgo biloba* extract for the prevention of Alzheimer's disease (GuidAge): A randomized placebo-controlled trial. Lancet Neurol 2012;11:851–859.
99. Weinmann S, Roll S, Schwarzbach C, et al. Effects of *Ginkgo biloba* in dementia: Systematic review and meta-analysis. BMC Geriatr 2012;10:14.

100. Zhang Z, Wang X, Chen Q, et al. Clinical efficacy and safety of huperzine Alpha in treatment of mild to moderate Alzheimer disease, a placebo-controlled, double-blind, randomized trial. Zhonghua Yi Xue Za Zhi 2002;82:941–944.
101. Li J. Wu HM, Zhou GJ, et al. Huperzine A for Alzheimer's disease. Cochrane Database Syst Rev 2008;2:CD005592.
102. Resveratrol for Alzheimer's Disease. 2012, *http://clinicaltrials.gov/ct2/show/NCT01504854*.
103. Henderson ST, Vogel JL, Barr LJ, et al. Study of the ketogenic agent AC-1202 in mild to moderate Alzheimer's disease: a randomized, double-blind, placebo-controlled, multicenter trial [abstract]. Nutr Metab 2009;6:31.
104. Scheltens P, Twisk JWR, Blesa R, et al. Efficacy of Souvenaid in mild Alzheimer's disease: Results from a randomized, controlled trial. J Alzheimers Dis 2012;31:225–236.
105. Herrmann N, Chau SA, Kircankski I, et al. Current and emerging drug treatment options for Alzheimer's disease. Drugs 2011;71:2031–2065.
106. Quinn JF, Raman R, Thomas RG, et al. Docosahexaenoic acid supplementation and cognitive decline in Alzheimer's disease: A randomized trial. JAMA 2010;304:1903–1911.
107. Haas C. Strategies, development, and pitfalls of therapeutic options for Alzheimer's disease. J Alzheimers Dis 2012;28:241–281.
108. Holmes C, Boche D, Wilkinson D, et al. Long-term effects of Abeta42 immunisation in Alzheimer's disease: Follow-up of a randomized, placebo-controlled phase I trial. Lancet 2008;372:216–223.
109. Callaway E. Alzheimer's drugs take a new tack. Nature 2012;489:13–14.
110. Friedrich MJ. New research on Alzheimer treatment ventures beyond plaques and tangles. JAMA 2012;308: 2553–2555.
111. Craft S, Baker LD, Montine TJ, et al. Intranasal insulin therapy for Alzheimer disease and amnestic mild cognitive impairment: A pilot clinical trial. Arch Neurol 2012;69:29–38.
112. Azermai M, Petrovic M, Elseviers MM, et al. Systematic appraisal of dementia guidelines for the management of behavioural and psychological symptoms. Ageing Res Rev 2012;11:78–86.
113. Alves L, Correia ASA, Miguel R, et al. Alzheimer's disease: A clinical practice-oriented review. Front Neur 2012;3:63. doi: 10.3389/fneur.2012.00063.
114. Cummings JL, Mackell J, Kaufer D. Behavioral effects of current Alzheimer's disease treatments: A descriptive review. Alzheimer Dement 2008;4:49–60.
115. Passmore MJ, Gardner DM, Polak Y, et al. Alternatives to atypical antipsychotics for the management of dementia-related agitation. Drugs Aging 2008;25:381–398.
116. Rodda J, Morgan S, Walker Z. Are cholinesterase inhibitors effective in the management of the behavioral and psychological symptoms of dementia in Alzheimer's disease? A systematic review of randomized, placebo-controlled trials of donepezil, rivastigmine and galantamine. Int Psychogeriatr 2009;21:813–824.
117. Desai AK, Schwartz L, Grossberg GT. Behavioral disturbance in dementia. Curr Psychiatry Rep 2012;14: 298–309.
118. Howard RJ, Juszczak E, Ballard CG, et al. Donepezil for the treatment of agitation in Alzheimer's disease. N Engl J Med 2007;357:1382–1392.
119. Lingler JH, Martire LM, Schulz R. Caregiver-specific outcomes in antidementia clinical drug trials: A systematic review and meta-analysis. J Am Geriatr Soc 2005;53: 983–990.
120. Schneider LS, Tariot PN, Dagerman KS, et al. Effectiveness of atypical antipsychotic drugs in patients with Alzheimer's disease. N Engl J Med 2006;355:1525–1538.
121. Maher AR, Maglione M, Bagley S, et al. Efficacy and comparative effectiveness of atypical antipsychotic medications for off-label uses in adults. JAMA 2011;306:1359–1369.
122. Schneider LS, Dagerman K, Insel PS. Efficacy and adverse effects of atypical antipsychotics for dementia: Meta-analysis of randomized, placebo-controlled trials. Am J Geriatr Psychiatry 2006;14:191–210.
123. Ballard C, Corbett A. Management of neuropsychiatric symptoms in people with dementia. CNS Drugs 2010;24:729–739.
124. Seitz DP, Adunuri N, Gill SS, et al. Antidepressants for agitation and psychosis in dementia. Cochrane Database Syst Rev2011;2: CD008191. doi: 10.1002/14651858. CD008191.pub2.
125. Henry G, Williamson D, Tampi RR. Efficacy and tolerability of antidepressants in the treatment of behavioral and psychological symptoms of dementia, a literature review of evidence. Am J Alzheimers Dis Other Demen 2011;26: 169–183.
126. Banerjee S, Hellier J, Dewey M, et al. Sertraline or mirtazapine for depression in dementia (HTA-SADD): A randomized, multicentre, double-blind, placebo-controlled trial. Lancet 2011;378:403–411.
127. Raetz J. Monitoring therapy for patients with Alzheimer's disease. Am Fam Phys 2007;75:1703–1704.
128. Rubin CD. The primary care of Alzheimer's disease. Am J Med Sci 2006;332:314–333.
129. Feldman HH, Woodward M. The staging and assessment of moderate to severe Alzheimer disease. Neurology 2005;65:S10–S17.
130. Reisberg B, Jamil IA, Khan S, et al. Staging Dementia. In: Abou-Saleh MT, Katona C, Kumar A (eds.) Principles and Practice of Geriatric Psychiatry, 3rd ed. Hoboken, NJ: Wiley-Blackwell 2011:162–169.
131. Rowland JP, Rigby J, Harper AC, Rowland R. Cardiovascular monitoring with acetylcholinesterase inhibitors: A clinical protocol. Adv Psychiatr Treat 2007;13:178–184.
132. Benoit M, Arbus C, Blanchard F, et al. Professional consensus on the treatment of agitation, aggressive behaviour, oppositional behaviour and psychotic disturbances in dementia. J Nutr Health Aging 2006;10:410–415.
133. American Geriatrics Society. Geriatrics at Your Fingertips. 2012, *http://www.geriatricsatyourfingertips.org/*.
134. U.S. Census Bureau, Population Division. U.S. Interim Projections by Age, Sex, Race, and Hispanic Origin: 2000–2050; Table 2a, Projected Population of United States, by Age and Sex: 2000–2050. *http://www.census.gov/population/www/projections/usinterimproj/*.

39

Multiple Sclerosis

Jacquelyn L. Bainbridge, Augusto Miravalle, and John R. Corboy

KEY CONCEPTS

1. The etiology of multiple sclerosis (MS) is unknown, but it appears to be autoimmune in nature. Currently there is no cure.
2. MS is characterized by CNS demyelination and axonal damage.
3. MS is classified by the nature of progression over time into several categories, which have different clinical presentations and responses to therapy.
4. Although studies do not support the general use of any of the FDA-approved disease-modifying therapies (DMTs) in patients with progressive forms of the illness, information derived from multiple studies suggests younger patients with progressive illness and those with either superimposed acute relapses or enhancing lesions on magnetic resonance imaging (MRI) scans may benefit from some of the presently used DMTs.
5. Diagnosis of MS requires evidence of dissemination of lesions over time and in multiple parts of the CNS and/or optic nerve, and is made primarily on the basis of clinical symptoms and examination. Diagnostic criteria also allow for the use of MRI, spinal fluid evaluation, optical coherence tomography, and evoked potentials to aid in the diagnosis.
6. Exacerbations or relapses of MS can be disabling. When this is the case exacerbations and relapses are treated with high-dose glucocorticoids, such as methylprednisolone IV, with onset of clinical response typically within 3 to 5 days.
7. Treatment of relapsing-remitting multiple sclerosis (RRMS) with the DMTs interferon-β (IFN-β) (Avonex, Betaseron, Rebif, Extavia), glatiramer acetate (Copaxone), natalizumab (Tysabri), mitoxantrone (Novantrone), fingolimod (Gilenya), teriflunomide (Aubagio), and dimethyl fumarate (Tecfidera) can reduce annual relapse rate, lessen severity of relapses, slow progression of changes on MRI scans, slow progression of disability, and slow cognitive decline. In addition, they have been shown to reduce the likelihood of developing a second attack after a first clinically isolated syndrome (CIS) consistent with MS.
8. In most cases, treatment with DMTs should begin promptly after the diagnosis of relapsing-remitting MS, or after a CIS if the brain MRI is suggestive of high risk of further attacks. Natalizumab and other choices that have been associated with problematic adverse events should be reserved for those patients who have failed one or more standard therapies and those with poor prognostic signs.
9. The definition of treatment inadequacy for RRMS remains unclear, and therapy changes after "treatment failure" should be individualized.
10. Patients suffering with MS frequently have symptoms such as spasticity, bladder dysfunction, fatigue, neuropathic pain, cognitive dysfunction, and depression that can require treatment. Patients must be counseled that therapies such as IFN-β and glatiramer acetate will not relieve these symptoms. Depression is common in MS and can pose the risk of suicide.

Multiple sclerosis (MS) is an inflammatory disease of the CNS that affects approximately 1 in 200 women and fewer men in the United States.[1] The term "multiple sclerosis" refers to two characteristics of the disease: numerous affected areas of the brain and spinal cord (CNS) producing multiple neurologic symptoms that accrue over time, and the characteristic plaques or sclerosed areas that are the hallmark of the disease.

1 Although MS was first described almost 140 years ago, the cause remains a mystery, and a cure is still unavailable. Nevertheless, many advances have been made in treating and managing the disease complications and improving the quality-of-life of affected individuals.

EPIDEMIOLOGY

Epidemiologic aspects of MS have been reviewed in many publications.[1–5] MS affects approximately 400,000 people in the United States and 2.5 million people worldwide.[6] MS is usually diagnosed between the ages of 15 and 45 years; peak incidence occurs in the fourth decade. Approximately 10,000 new cases are diagnosed per year in the United States. Women are afflicted more than men by a ratio of 2:1. Men usually develop the first signs of MS at a later age than women, and are more likely to develop a progressive form of the disease. The most important factors in determination of risk for developing the disease are geography, age, environmental influences, and genetics. In general, disease prevalence is higher the greater the distance from the equator; within the United States the prevalence of MS is higher in states above the 37th parallel. Recent studies, however, suggest a waning latitude gradient as demonstrated by a substantial increase in MS incidence in Mediterranean regions. Rising incidence of MS in females appears to be associated with urbanization. As an example, recent reports suggest that MS incidence markedly rose on Crete among female subjects residing in urban settings or relocating at a young age from rural areas; this suggests that an environmental factor yet to be identified might play a role in changing disease susceptibility.[7]

MS occurs more frequently in whites of Scandinavian ancestry than in other ethnic groups. In addition, an inverse relationship between MS risk and 25-hydroxyvitamin D levels has been proposed.[1,8]

Etiology

It is thought that genetically susceptible individuals ≤15 years of age who have lived in a high-risk area for at least 2 years and were exposed to a crucial environmental agent are at risk for developing MS. Interestingly, an individual who migrates from a low- to high-risk area prior to the age of 15 years acquires the same chance of developing MS as those who live in a high-risk area all their lives.[2] If the move is made from a high- to a low-risk area, the individual retains the high risk if the move is made after the age of 15 years, but acquires the lower risk if the move is made prior to this age.[2] Smoking cigarettes has been associated with both an increased risk of developing MS and with more severe progression of disability.[5,9]

Viral or bacterial infections may be an important environmental cause of MS. Although no clear association has been identified, certain infections might participate in the pathogenesis of MS by initiating or activating autoreactive immune cells in genetically susceptible individuals, leading to subsequent demyelination. Evidence to support a viral etiology includes increased immunoglobulin G (IgG) synthesis in the CNS, increased antibody titers to certain viruses, and epidemiologic studies that indicate a childhood exposure factor, suggesting that "viral" infections may precipitate exacerbations. In addition, viruses have been shown to cause diseases with prolonged incubation periods, myelin destruction, and a relapsing-remitting course in both humans and experimental animal models.[1,10]

Although numerous viruses have a proposed association with MS, the greatest evidence supports Epstein–Barr virus (EBV). Links of EBV infection to MS pathology are yet largely hypothetical. Autoreactive T-cells could be activated by EBV through molecular mimicry, whereby sequence similarities between EBV and self-peptides are sufficient to result in the cross-activation of autoreactive T- or B-cells. Other potential mechanisms of demyelination include enhanced breakdown and presentation of self-antigens, expression of viral superantigens, or bystander activation.[11] Antibody titers to Epstein–Barr nuclear antigen (EBNA) complex are higher in MS patients versus controls, especially if blood is collected ≥5 years before onset. These titers increase over time in MS patients (controls are unchanged), and a fourfold increase in EBNA titers over time results in a threefold increased risk of developing MS (almost an 18-fold increase in those with first samples before age 20).[12] Interestingly, one paper notes individuals positive for *HLA DRB1*1501* have a 24-fold increased risk of developing MS when they also have antibodies to certain epitopes within EBNA-1 compared with others.[13] This is consistent with a genetic-environmental interaction. In addition, anti-EBNA titers have been associated with relapsing-remitting multiple sclerosis (RRMS), conversion of clinically isolated syndrome (CIS) to clinically definite multiple sclerosis (CDMS, confirmed diagnosis of MS), and with magnetic resonance imaging (MRI) measures such as gadolinium-enhancing lesions, change in T_2 lesion volume ($r = 0.27$; $P = 0.044$), and Expanded Disability Status Scale (EDSS) score ($r = 0.3$; $P = 0.035$). Zivadinov et al. also found anti-EBNA and anti-vascular cell adhesion (VCA) titers associated with gray matter atrophy in MS.[14] While Serafini et al. have claimed to identify evidence of abortive infection in a significant number of MS patients,[15] others have not been able to replicate these findings.[16] The majority of data would lead to a conclusion that exposure to EBV is somehow associated with developing MS, but does not support the concept of an active or aborting EBV infection directly causing MS.

The familial recurrence rate of MS is approximately 5%, with siblings being the most commonly reported relationship,[4] and a concordance rate among monozygotic twins of approximately 25%. This is consistent with the idea that an environmental agent is important in the etiology of MS, but also suggests a role for one or more genes. Genes that lie within the major histocompatibility complex (MHC), which is located on the sixth chromosome in humans, have been linked to MS.[1,4] Recent data show a significant association of risk with mutations in the interleukin-2α (IL-2α) and interleukin-7α (IL-7α) receptor genes.[17–19] African Americans are significantly less likely to be diagnosed with MS compared with whites, although there is emerging evidence that they are more likely to have a severe disease course[20] and respond less well to interferon (IFN) therapy.[21] A locus on chromosome 1 may be associated with increased susceptibility in African Americans.[22]

PATHOPHYSIOLOGY

2 The basic physiologic derangement in MS is stripping of the myelin sheath surrounding CNS axons. This activity is associated with an inflammatory, perivenular infiltrate consisting of T and B lymphocytes, macrophages, antibodies, and complement.[10] Demyelination renders axons susceptible to damage, which becomes irreversible when they are severed. Irreversible axonal damage correlates with disability and can be visualized as hypointense lesions, or "black holes," on T_1-weighted MRI.[23,24]

It is well accepted that MS lesions are heterogeneous, which may be due in part to differences in the stage of evolution of the lesions over time, differences in underlying immunopathogenesis, or a combination. Briefly stated, acute lesions show demyelination and axonal destruction with lymphocytic activity consistent with an inflammatory state. In contrast, more chronic lesions display less inflammatory lymphocytes with active remyelination.[10] Although traditional descriptions have focused on white matter as the sole location of MS lesions, more recent studies have clearly identified cortical and subcortical gray matter lesions both pathologically[25] and radiographically.[26] In addition, a subset of patients with progressive MS are noted to have abnormalities consistent with B-cell follicles in the meninges.[27]

Just as the full dimensions of the neuropathology are uncertain, so is the pathogenesis of the MS lesion. Substantial evidence suggests it is an autoimmune process directed against myelin and oligodendrocytes, the cells that make myelin[10] (Fig. 39-1). A new concept of T-cell entry into the CNS suggests that the initial lymphocyte invasion in MS may proceed through the ventricles, toward the choroid plexus along a CCL 20 gradient that attracts activated Th17 cells.[28] The actual mediator of myelin and axonal destruction has not been established, but may reflect a combination of macrophages, antibodies, destructive cytokines, and reactive oxygen intermediates. The exact trigger for activation of T-cells in the periphery remains unclear, but the T-cells in MS patients recognize myelin basic protein (MBP), proteolipid protein, myelin oligodendrocyte glycoprotein, and myelin-associated glycoprotein. T-helper subtypes can be either pathogenic or protective in MS. Furthermore, theory holds that certain T-cell subsets are not terminally differentiated, but instead engender a level of plasticity that allows for their conversion from pathogenic to protective and vice versa under certain conditions (Fig. 39-2).[29] In patients with stable or mild disease, increased numbers of cells are found that express messenger RNA (mRNA) for transforming growth factor-β (TGF-β) and interleukin-10 (IL-10) compared with patients with severe disease. Conversely, a reduction in the number of T-regulatory (Treg) cells, which exhibit suppressor activity, is associated with

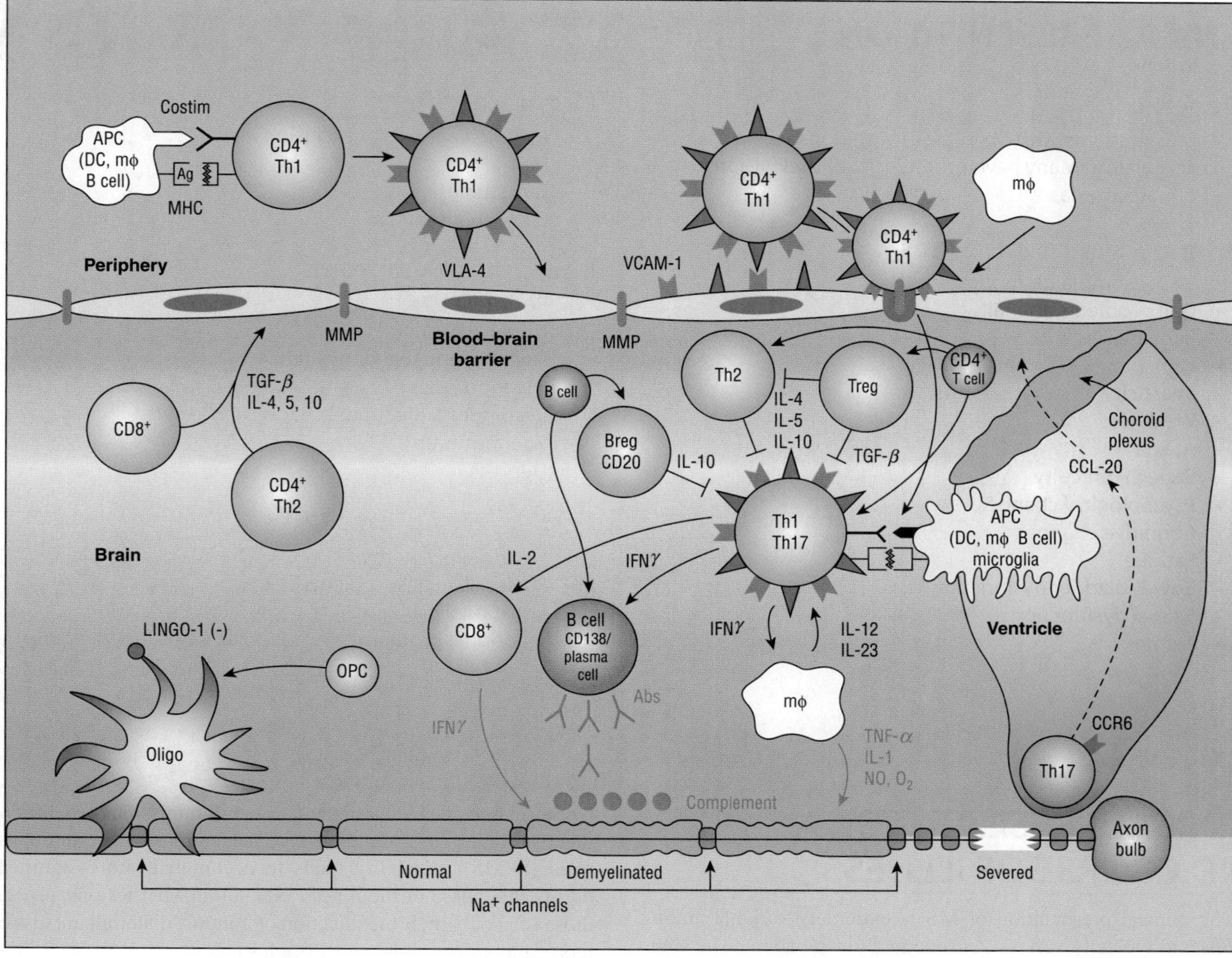

FIGURE 39-1 Autoimmune theory of the pathogenesis of multiple sclerosis (MS). In MS, the immunogenic cells tend to be more myelin-reactive, and these T-cells produce cytokines mimicking a Th1-mediated proinflammatory reaction. T-helper cells (CD4+) appear to be key initiators of myelin destruction in MS. These autoreactive CD4+ cells, especially of the T-helper cell type 1 (Th1) subtype, are activated in the periphery, perhaps following a viral infection. The activation of T- and B-cells requires two signals. The first signal is the interaction between MHC and APC (macrophage, dendritic cell, B-cell). The second signal consists of the binding between B7 on the APC and CD28 on the T-cell for T-cell activation. Similarly, CD40 expressed on APCs and CD40L expressed on T-cells interact to signal the proliferation of B-cells within the blood–brain barrier following the entry to T-cells. The T-cells in the periphery express adhesion molecules on their surfaces that allow them to attach and roll along the endothelial cells that constitute the blood–brain barrier. The activated T-cells also produce MMP that help to create openings in the blood–brain barrier, allowing entry of the activated T-cells past the blood–brain barrier and into the CNS. Once inside the CNS, the T-cells produce proinflammatory cytokines, especially interleukins (ILs) 1, 2, 12, 17, and 23, tumor necrosis factor-α (TNF-α), and interferon-γ (INF-γ), which further create openings in the blood–brain barrier, allowing entry of B-cells, complement, macrophages, and antibodies. The T-cells also interact within the CNS with the resident microglia, astrocytes, and macrophages, further enhancing production of proinflammatory cytokines and other potential mediators of CNS damage, including reactive oxygen intermediates and nitric oxide. The role of modulating, or downregulating, cytokines such as IL-4, IL-5, IL-10, and transforming growth factor-β (TGF-β) also has been described. These cytokines are the products of CD4+, CD8+, and Th1-cells.[10] New pathogenic mechanisms involve, but are not limited to, receptor-ligand mediated T-cell entry via choroid plexus (CCR6-CCL20 axis),[28] coupling of key receptor-ligands for inhibition of myelination/demyelination (LINGO-1/NOGO66/p75 or TROY complex, Jagged-Notch signaling).(Ag, antigens; APC, antigen presenting cell; DC, dendrite cell; IgG, immunoglobulin G; MΦ, macrophage; Na+, sodium ion; MMP, matrix metalloproteinases; MHC, major histocompatibility complex; OPC, oligodendrocyte precursor cell; VLA, very late antigen; VCAM, vascular cell adhesion molecule.)

active MS and can be found in patients with progressive disease. It should be noted, however, that Treg ratios do not always correlate with disease activity. Of note, experimental evidence associates high 25-hydroxyvitamin D levels with improved Treg function, favoring the Th2 phenotype in the Th1/Th2 balance.[30] Finally, the significance of one of the immunological hallmarks of MS, the intrathecal synthesis of multiple clones of immunoglobulins, remains unclear. The antigen(s) against which these immunoglobulins are directed remain unknown, but do not appear to include common CNS myelin antigens.[31] The complex interplay of a variety of cells, antibodies, and cytokines remains to be elucidated.

CLINICAL PRESENTATION Multiple Sclerosis

General

- Most patients with MS present with nonspecific complaints. Many have problems with their vision or paresthesias

Primary Symptoms/Signs

- Visual complaints/optic neuritis
- Gait problems and falls
- Paresthesias
- Pain
- Spasticity
- Weakness
- Ataxia
- Speech difficulty
- Psychological changes
- Cognitive changes
- Fatigue
- Bowel/bladder dysfunction
- Sexual dysfunction
- Tremor

Laboratory Tests

- MS is a diagnosis of exclusion
- MRI
- CSF studies
- Evoked potentials

Secondary Symptoms

- Recurrent UTIs
- Urinary calculi
- Decubiti and osteomyelitis
- Osteoporosis
- Respiratory infections
- Poor nutrition
- Depression

Tertiary Symptoms

- Financial problems
- Personal/social problems
- Vocational problems
- Emotional problems

CLINICAL PRESENTATION AND COURSE OF ILLNESS

❸ The clinical presentation of MS is extremely variable among patients and typically varies over time in a given patient. The signs and symptoms of MS can be divided into three categories. Primary symptoms are a direct consequence of conduction disturbances produced by demyelination and axonal damage, and reflect the area of the CNS that is damaged. Secondary symptoms are complications resulting from primary symptoms. For example, urinary retention, a primary symptom, can lead to frequent urinary tract infections (UTIs), a secondary symptom. Tertiary symptoms relate to the effect of the disease on the patient's everyday life.[32]

The clinical course of CDMS is classified into four categories.[33] At the onset of symptoms, about 85% of patients have exacerbations—new symptoms lasting at least 24 hours and separated from other new symptoms by at least 30 days—followed by remissions (complete or incomplete). Exacerbations are frequently referred to as relapses or attacks. This course is called RRMS; the first clinical presentation is typically CIS. During the RRMS phase, there is a correlation between new brain MRI lesions and clinical attacks, but typically there are many more new MRI lesions than new clinical symptoms. In RRMS patients, attack frequency tends to decrease over time and becomes independent of the development of progressive disabilities.[34] Neurologic recovery following an exacerbation is often quite good early in the disease course, but following repeated relapses, recovery tends to be less complete. In addition, there is a new concept of a radiologically isolated syndrome (RIS), referring to individuals who have clinical scenarios not typical of MS, yet obtain MRI scans for other reasons (e.g., headache) and have radiological signs suggestive of MS. Some percentage of these patients convert to RRMS over time,[35] although when to start treatment remains unclear and varies by practice.

Up to 10% to 20% of RRMS patients have a benign course, characterized by few relapses, often sensory, with minimal disability accruing over time. Most RRMS patients eventually enter a progressive phase in which attacks and remissions are difficult to identify. This is referred to as secondary-progressive multiple sclerosis (SPMS). Disability tends to accumulate more significantly during this phase of the illness. New brain MRI lesions, especially those seen only after the injection of contrast material, are less common, and brain atrophy and T1 holes increase.[36]

❹ Approximately 15% of patients never have attacks and remissions but have progressive disease from the outset, known as primary-progressive multiple sclerosis (PPMS). These patients will have symptoms, especially spastic paraparesis that may worsen rapidly or relatively slowly over time, and accrue progressively more disability. Patients with PPMS are diagnosed at a later age, with the number of males roughly equal to that of females. In general, PPMS patients tend to have a worse prognosis than those who present initially with RRMS, although more recent data suggest progression is variable.[37] Many clinical trials have suggested that a significant portion of patients with PPMS do not receive benefit from studied therapies. However, a recent article using rituximab suggests a subgroup of PPMS patients who are <51 years of age and have at least one gadolinium-enhancing lesion may benefit from this therapy.[38] Finally, a small percentage of patients may have a mixture of both progression and relapses, referred to as progressive-relapsing multiple sclerosis (PRMS). These patients are generally treated as relapsing patients.

Progression of the illness throughout the lifetime can be measured in many ways. The most widely used clinical rating scale is the EDSS, which uses a numerical value ranging from 0 (no disability) to 10 (death) to evaluate neurologic functions.[39] The limitations of this scale are the relative insensitivity to clinical changes not involving impairment of ambulation, such as changes in cognition, fatigue, and affect. Other tools, such as the multiple sclerosis functional composite (MSFC), are being evaluated for increased sensitivity and utility in describing changes in MS-related disability over time.[40] Increasingly, MRI is being used as an index of both disease activity and progression.[10] Specifically, the appearance of new lesions or changes in lesion number, size, and volume are being used as outcome measures in research studies. Optical coherence

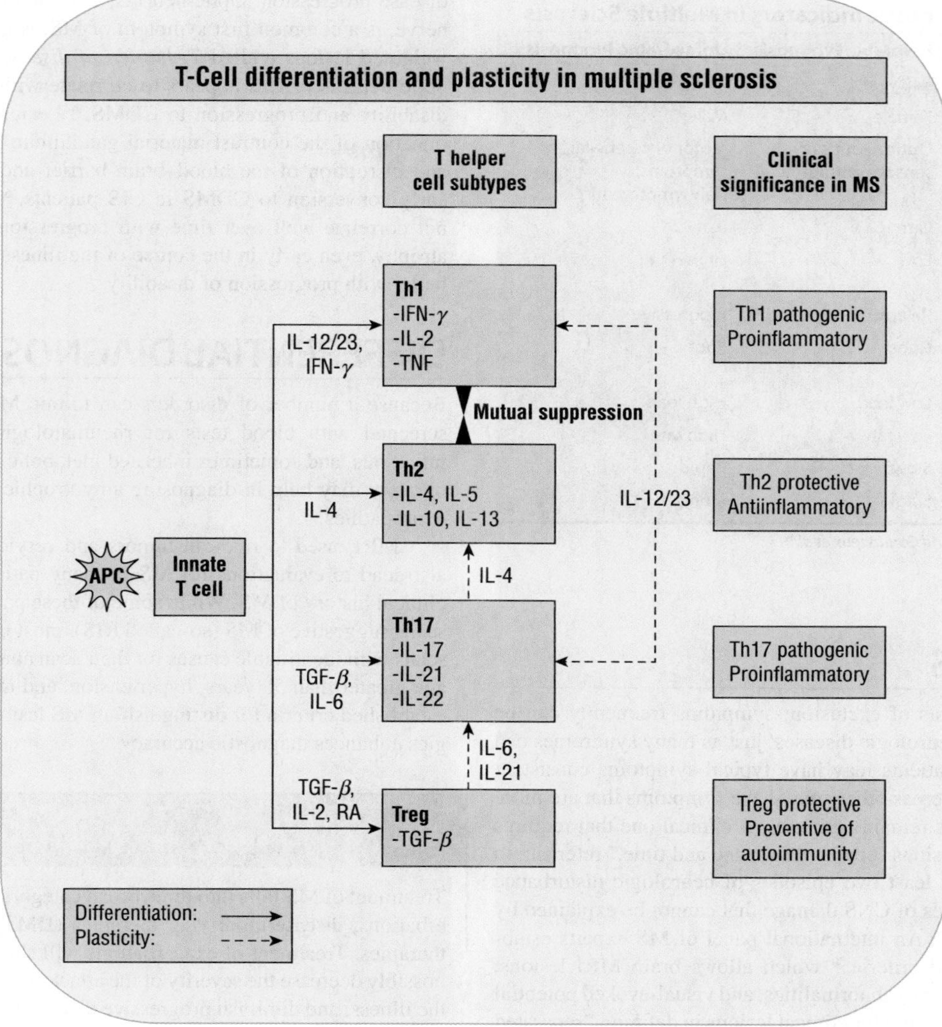

FIGURE 39-2 Upon interaction with an antigen-laden APC and specific cytokines, the innate T-cells undergo differentiation into a few lineages (subtypes). Four subtypes significant for MS pathophysiology are illustrated here (Th1, Th2, Th17, and Treg). Th1 and Th17 are proinflammatory, Th2 is anti-inflammatory, and Treg is regulatory. Th1 and Th2 are mutually suppressive and are relatively stable differentiated subtypes. In contrast, Th17 and Treg subtypes are recently found to exhibit "plasticity." In other words, they can undergo phenotypic conversion to another T-cell subtype (Th1 or Th2) in the presence of specific cytokine conditions. This plasticity of Th17 and Treg is the immunologic basis for development of therapeutic agents to favor the production of suitable Th subtypes for combating microbial invasion and also concurrently achieving neurocellular recovery after an infection.[29] (APC, antigen presenting cell.)

tomography measures the retinal neural fiber layer thickness, and may also be a measurable sign of pathological progression over time.[41]

The unpredictable nature of MS makes it impossible to anticipate when an exacerbation will occur. However, certain factors, including infections, heat (including fever), sleep deprivation, stress, malnutrition, anemia, concurrent organ dysfunction, exertion, and childbirth, may aggravate symptoms or lead to an attack. Interestingly, many patients experience a significant reduction in relapses during the third trimester of pregnancy, followed by a relative increase postpartum.[42] Between 60% and 80% of individuals diagnosed with the MS have been reported to be sensitive to environmental heat.

Clinically, increased body temperature might result in worsening of previous neurological deficits, including fatigue and decreased muscular endurance. Blurred vision, known as Uthoff's phenomenon, is caused by increased body temperature due to physical exercise or physical restraint. Body temperature influences nerve impulses, which are blocked or slowed down in a damaged nerve. After normalization of the temperature, signs and symptoms improve or disappear.

MS usually does not directly diminish life expectancy. The development of secondary complications such as pneumonia or septicemia (secondary to aspiration in those with swallowing difficulties, decubitus ulcers, or UTIs) or rapid progression of primary lesions affecting respiratory function can lead to a shorter than expected life span. Most of the decrease in life span is seen in patients with rapidly progressive disease. Suicide rates as high as seven times that seen in the general population have been reported.[43] Clinical and demographic factors used to predict prognosis of MS are listed in Table 39-1.[5,44] Several MRI features also have been shown to correlate with progression of disease (see below).[45–47]

TABLE 39-1 Prognostic Indicators in Multiple Sclerosis

Indicator	Favorable Prognosis	Unfavorable Prognosis
Age at onset	<40 years	>40 years
Gender	Female	Male
Initial symptoms	Optic neuritis or sensory symptoms	Motor or cerebellar symptoms; polysymptomatic
Disability	Late	Early
Attack frequency in early disease	Low	High
Course of disease	Relapsing/remitting	Progressive
Recovery after first event	Good	Poor
T_2 lesions	Low load	High load
T_1 black hole lesions	Low rate	High rate
Growth of lesions	Slow	Rapid
Locations of lesions	Single	Multiple

Data From Fisniku et al.[48] and Confavreux et al.[49]

DIAGNOSIS

5 MS is a diagnosis of exclusion; symptoms frequently can be attributed to other neurologic diseases, just as many syndromes can mimic MS. Some patients may have typical symptoms consistent with classic CIS, whereas others may have symptoms that are more vague. The diagnosis remains primarily a clinical one that requires demonstration of "lesions separated in space and time," referring to the occurrence of at least two episodes of neurologic disturbance reflecting distinct sites of CNS damage that cannot be explained by another mechanism.[50] An international panel of MS experts established the McDonald criteria,[50] which allows brain MRI lesions, cerebrospinal fluid (CSF) abnormalities, and visual-evoked potential (VEP) studies to substitute for clinical lesions in defining "separated in space and time." A reevaluation of the McDonald criteria has simplified the use of these laboratory studies.[45] In the new scheme, diagnostic categories are MS, possible MS (for those individuals at high risk of developing MS), and not MS; these new criteria allow for earlier diagnosis.[45] Newer, simpler MRI criteria defining dissemination in time and space may be somewhat more sensitive and equally specific.[51–53] A consensus panel of the American Association of Neurology endorses the utility of MRI for diagnostic purpose,[47] and the U.S. FDA has approved several of the immunotherapies to be used after a single attack (CIS) of demyelination in the context of an appropriately abnormal brain MRI. A proposed set of criteria now being considered will allow for earlier diagnosis in patients with CIS to establish "dissemination in time and space" with a single MRI. Therefore, patients will need to have lesions in different areas of their CNS with at least one enhancing lesion that correlates with clinical symptomatology. By fulfilling these criteria, a patient can be diagnosed with CDMS.

Laboratory Studies

To date, there are no tests specific for MS. Evidence provided by MRI of the brain and spine,[46,47] CSF evaluation (presence of increased oligoclonal bands and increased IgG), evoked potentials,[45,50] and optic coherence tomography,[54] used in conjunction with the physical examination and history, aids in establishing the diagnosis of MS. MRI, the most valuable diagnostic tool, produces images of the brain and spine that reflect damage that is characteristic of MS plaques in multiple areas of the CNS. MRI is the preferred technique for establishing a diagnosis, prognosis, and for following disease progression. Optic neuritis, a lesion or lesions on the optic nerve, is a common first symptom of MS. A greater number of T_2-weighted lesions (called *T_2 burden of disease*) on MRI following optic neuritis or CIS appears to correlate with the development of disability and progression to CDMS.[46] Lesions that enhance after injection of the contrast material gadolinium indicate new lesions and disruption of the blood–brain barrier and are associated with early conversion to CDMS in CIS patients.[46,55] However, they do not correlate well over time with progression of disability. Brain atrophy, even early in the course of the illness, probably correlates better with progression of disability.[47]

DIFFERENTIAL DIAGNOSIS

Because a number of disorders can mimic MS, most patients are screened with blood tests for rheumatologic, collagen-vascular, infectious, and sometimes inherited metabolic diseases. Electromyography may help in diagnosing amyotrophic lateral sclerosis and neuropathies.

MRI, used to rule out tumors and cervical spondylosis, may also lead to evaluations for MS in many patients with little or no clinical history of MS. While some of these patients may have MRI scans suggestive of MS (so-called RIS), most have nonspecific MRI scans with identifiable causes for their scan abnormalities, including age greater than 50 years, hypertension, and migraine.[56] The use of established criteria for distinguishing MS lesions from other etiologies enhances diagnostic accuracy.

TREATMENT

Treatment of MS falls into three broad categories: treatment of exacerbations, disease-modifying therapies (DMTs), and symptomatic therapies. Treatment of exacerbations will shorten the duration and possibly decrease the severity of the attack. DMTs alter the course of the illness, and diminish progressive disability over time. Symptomatic management of the disease is of utmost importance to maintain the patient's quality-of-life. Although different treatment modalities have been studied in the last 30 years, many older trials had flawed designs. As there are no universally accepted treatment algorithms, treatments vary among clinicians and centers. Perhaps more importantly, treatment decisions are frequently based on the wishes and goals of individual patients rather than evidence-based algorithms. One potential algorithm for the immunotherapy of CDMS is shown in Figure 39-3.

Desired Outcomes

The main goals of treatment are to improve patients overall quality-of-life and minimize long-term disability. Treatment goals are attained by altering MS exacerbations or relapses, decreasing the number of white matter lesions and black holes on MRI, averting brain atrophy, and ultimately halting disease progression. This can be achieved by early recognition of the disease (CIS) and immediate utilization of FDA-approved drugs.

General Approach to Treatment

The severity of symptoms at initial presentation will determine whether an induction or escalation algorithm will be assigned to an individual patient. When FDA-approved drugs do not alter the naturally progressive disease, investigational agents or non–FDA-approved medications, such as rituximab, may be used. As a general rule, MS affects patients in their most productive years of life. Practitioners must work with their patients to set realistic expectations over their lifetime and develop a long-term treatment and

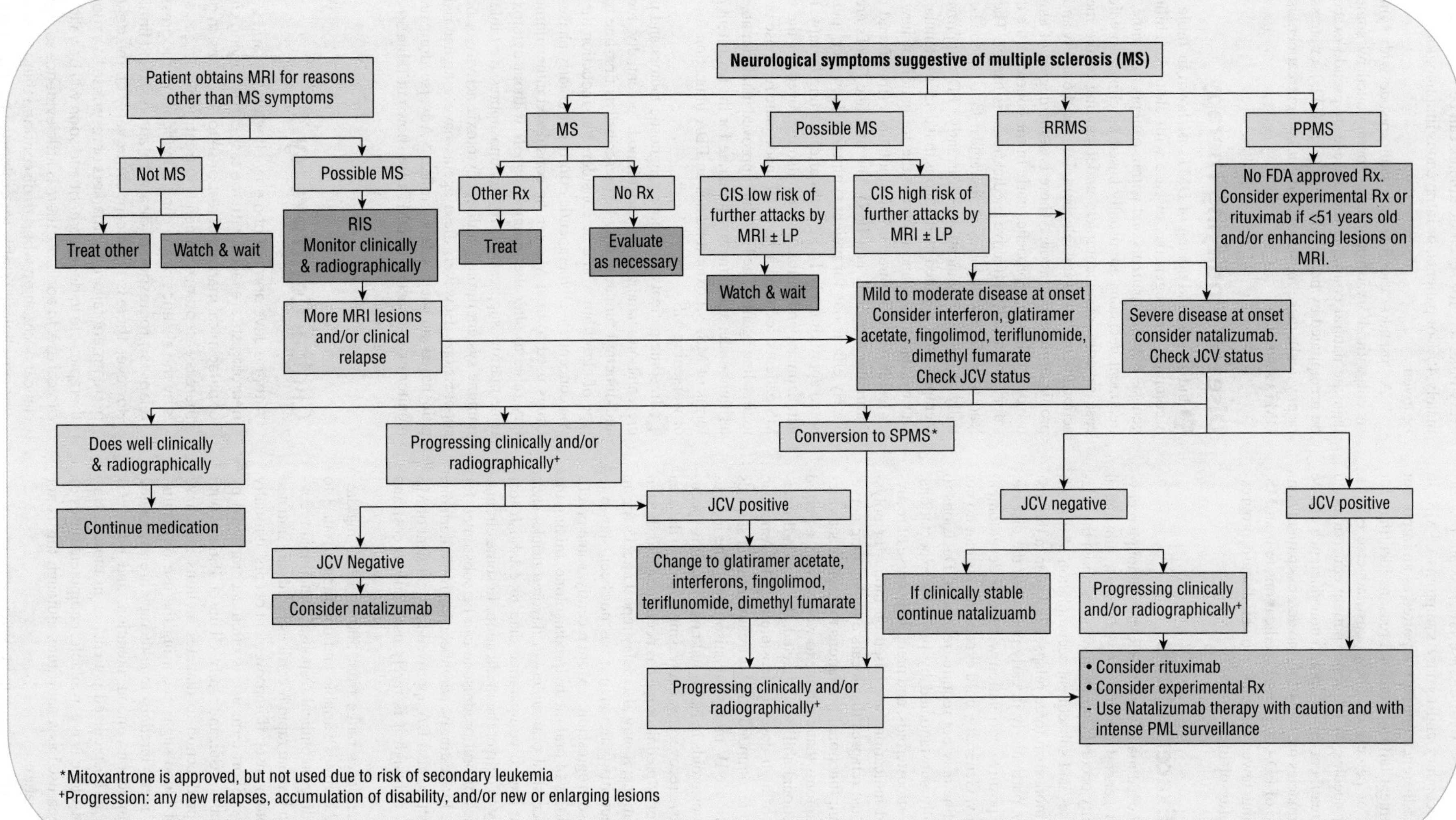

FIGURE 39-3 Algorithm for management of clinically definite multiple sclerosis. (ABC-R, interferon β_{1a} [Avonex], interferon β_{1b} [Betaseron, Extavia], glatiramer acetate [Copaxone], and interferon β_{1a} [Rebif]; IVIG, intravenous immunoglobulin.)

management plan. Patients may require external support and assistance to accept their diagnosis. With disease progression, patients are likely to acquire secondary and tertiary symptoms of MS. In clinical trials, high nonadherence rates are reported as an important issue for potential treatment failure. Potential reasons identified for nonadherence are lack of perceived benefit, cost, adverse effects, depression, and fear of needles. With proper patient education and therapy management, treatment failure due to nonadherence can be avoided. Specialty pharmacies may be useful to address patient concerns. With the advance of FDA-approved medications to treat MS, patients are experiencing fewer relapses, slower disease progression, and improved quality-of-life.

Treatment of Exacerbations

6 Exacerbations are the hallmark of early RRMS. Although recovery after relapses is in general complete, over time a substantial accumulation of disability occurs. Controversy exists about the relationship between relapses and subsequent accumulation of disability. Frequent relapses (more than three relapses per year in the first 2 years after diagnosis), particularly in early phases of the disease, have shown consistent positive correlation with later development of neurological disability. Generally, mild exacerbations that do not produce functional decline may not require treatment. Decisions to treat relapses are usually substantiated by patient's expectations, prior experience with corticosteroids, and predicted course of recovery. Generally accepted indications are based on mono- or polysymptomatic presentations; relapses that localize to the optic nerve, spinal cord, or brainstem; functional limitations that affect activities of daily living; and symptoms that continue to worsen over a period of 2 weeks. When functional ability is affected, the standard intervention is IV injection of high-dose corticosteroids. The American Academy of Neurology recommends that if treatment with steroids is warranted, it is best to use IV methylprednisolone.[57] The mechanism of action for corticosteroids in MS is unknown, but it is speculated that steroids improve recovery by decreasing edema in the area of demyelination. IV methylprednisolone has been shown to shorten the duration of exacerbations; it may also delay repeat attacks for up to 2 years after optic neuritis,[57] although it has not been shown to definitively affect disease progression.[58] More recently, some practitioners are using high doses of oral methylprednisolone, mixing the lyophilized powder or crushed oral tablets in flavored drinks such as smoothies, but there are no comparative data to establish that this is an equivalent way to deliver the medication. In some circumstances, equipotent doses of oral prednisone can be substituted for IV methylprednisolone. Interestingly, adrenocorticotropic hormone (ACTH) is the only agent that is FDA approved for treatment of MS exacerbation treatment, although it is rarely used due to cost and availability.

Methylprednisolone doses range from 500 to 1,000 mg/day, given IV. Duration of therapy is variable and can range from 3 to (rarely) 10 days, depending on clinical response. Functional recovery after an exacerbation is more rapid if corticosteroids are initiated within 2 weeks of symptom onset. If improvement occurs, it usually begins after 3 to 5 days. Short-term use is often accompanied by sleep disturbance, a metallic taste, and rarely, GI upset. Patients with diabetes mellitus or a predilection to diabetes mellitus may have significant elevations of blood sugar, requiring the use of insulin. Longer durations of IV methylprednisolone therapy are associated with acne and fungal infections, mood alteration, and rarely, GI hemorrhage (especially in hospitalized patients or in those taking aspirin). If methylprednisolone is not available, equipotent doses of dexamethasone have been used as a substitute, although this is not well supported in the literature.

A small number of patients have more severe attacks, manifested by hemiplegia, paraplegia, or quadriplegia. If these patients fail to improve with aggressive steroid therapy, plasma exchange every other day for seven treatments can be beneficial for approximately 40% of patients, or intravenous immunoglobulin (IVIG) can be given.

A "pseudo-exacerbation" is an episode with symptoms consistent with an exacerbation, but precipitated by something other than the natural course of the disease. A pseudo-exacerbation can be precipitated by heat, infections (e.g., UTIs), or stress (emotional or physical); these must be ruled out before treatment is initiated or DMTs altered.

Disease-Modifying Therapy

7 Indications and dosing of DMTs is shown in Table 39-2. MS is a complex, heterogeneous disease with clear variability in pathogenesis between patients and within patients over time. As a result, treatment decisions are usually based on clinical predictors of disease severity, our incomplete understanding of the mechanism of action of currently available therapies, and the safety and tolerability profile of the medications. There is some degree of agreement that use of escalation approaches early in the course of the disease, with safer yet partially effective medications, is useful. These concepts lead to various categories of therapies: first-, second-, and potentially third-line medications. Currently, FDA-approved first-line therapies (self-injected medications that decrease annualized relapse rate by about 30% and decrease the formation of new white matter lesion) include three IFN formulations (four brand names), and glatiramer acetate (a non-IFN). The first-line DMTs are not immediately efficacious for patient symptoms. However, their efficacy is noted approximately 1 to 2 years after starting therapy. Fingolimod, natalizumab, and mitoxantrone, also approved for the treatment of MS patients, are used in cases of inadequate response or intolerance to first-line agents. The FDA has approved natalizumab, fingolimod, teriflunomide, and dimethyl fumarate for the treatment of relapsing forms of MS. Mitoxantrone has an FDA indication for progressive or worsening MS.

8 In some patients with poor prognostic factors and poor clinical presentation, natalizumab, fingolimod, potentially teriflunomide, and dimethyl fumarate may be prescribed as first-line therapy. This type of algorithm would be considered an induction therapy, where you concentrate all therapeutic efforts in the early phases of disease. Drugs used to treat MS can be considered either immunomodulatory (able to alter the immune signals without cytotoxic effect or bone marrow suppression) or immunosuppressive (able to alter the immune system through a direct cytotoxic activity or bone marrow suppression). However, these agents have a higher risk-to-benefit ratio based on their safety profile.[59] Adverse drug reactions and monitoring parameters of DMTs are shown in Table 39-3.

Clinical **Controversy. . .**

With the development of highly effective therapies, neurologists are faced with the task of identifying clinical or paraclinical markers of response to therapies. In general there is acceptance on defining treatment success, and that is by the absence of any clinical evidence of progression (e.g., relapses, progression of disability, and new MRI findings). However, there is significant controversy on the definition of treatment failure. Biomarkers of response to various therapies are in development and soon will be validated for clinical use. In addition, there is little evidence to support the clinical decision on when to discontinue therapies in patients who are clinically stable for prolonged periods of time.

TABLE 39-2 Disease Modifying Therapy

Drug	Brand Name	Indication	Initial Dose	Usual Dose	Comment
Interferon-β_{1a}	Avonex	Relapsing forms of MS	30 mcg (6 million international units) IM once weekly	30 mcg IM once weekly	Avonex is considered as a low potency interferon
Interferon-β_{1a}	Rebif	Relapsing forms of MS	22 mcg SQ three times a week	22 or 44 mcg SQ three times a week	Rebif is considered as a high potency interferon
Interferon-β_{1b}	Betaseron, Extavia	Relapsing forms of MS	250 mcg (8 million international units) SQ every other day	250 mcg SQ every other day	Betaseron/Extavia is considered as a high potency interferon Pregnancy category C Cost per year[a]: $36,010 (Avonex), $38,475 (Betaseron/Extavia), $38,761 (Rebif)
Glatiramer acetate	Copaxone	CIS, RRMS	20 mg SQ once daily	20 mg SQ once daily	Pregnancy category B Cost per year[a]: $40,187
Mitoxantrone	Novantrone	SPMS, PRMS, and worsening RRMS	12 mg/m^2 IV every 3 months	12 mg/m^2 IV every 3 months	Life time dose should not exceed 140 mg/m^2 Pregnancy category D
Natalizumab	Tysabri	Relapsing forms of MS	300 mg IV every 4 weeks	300 mg IV every 4 weeks	REMS Pregnancy category C Cost per year[a]: $42,312
Fingolimod	Gilenya	Relapsing forms of MS	0.5 mg orally once daily	0.5 mg orally once daily	REMS Pregnancy category C Cost per year[a]: $48,000
Teriflunomide	Aubagio	Relapsing forms of MS	7 mg orally once daily	7 or 14 mg orally once daily	Pregnancy category X Cost per year[a]: $48,000 Cholestyramine and charcoal accelerate teriflunomide elimination
Dimethyl fumarate	Tecfidera	Relapsing forms of MS	120 mg delayed release twice daily × 7 days	240 mg delayed release twice daily	Pregnancy category C Cost per year: $54,000

CIS, clinically isolated syndrome; IM, intramuscular; PRMS: primary relapsing multiple sclerosis; REMS, Risk Evaluation and Mitigation Strategy; RRMS, relapsing remitting multiple sclerosis; SPMS, secondary progressive multiple sclerosis; SQ, subcutaneous.

Cost[a]: Cost does not include nursing, pharmacy, and technical fees.

TABLE 39-3 Adverse Drug Reactions and Monitoring Parameters

Drug	Adverse Drug Reaction	Monitoring Parameter	Comments
Interferon-β_{1a}	Depression, leukopenia, flu-like symptoms, injection site reactions	Electrolytes, CBC, LFTs, thyroid function, LVEF, depression LFTs at baseline, 1 month, and every 3 months for a year, and every 6 months thereafter	Avoid use in untreated severe depression
Interferon-β_{1b}	Depression, injection site reactions, flu-like symptoms	Electrolytes, CBC, LFTs, thyroid function, depression	Avoid use in untreated severe depression More frequent injection site reactions reported
Glatiramer acetate	Injection site reactions, infection, hypersensitivity, chest tightness, flushing, urticaria	MRI, tissue necrosis, post injection reaction	Chest tightness, flushing, urticaria can occur at any dose
Mitoxantrone	Bone marrow suppression, neutropenia, cardiotoxicity, AML, nausea, vomiting, diarrhea	CBC, ECG, LVEF	Secondary leukemia Life time maximum dose due to cardiac toxicity
Natalizumab	PML, depression, fatigue, respiratory infection, arthralgia	JCV antibody, infection, MRI, LFTs	Risk of PML Risk of IRIS when discontinued due to PML
Fingolimod	Lymphocytopenia, macular retinal edema, AV block, infection	CBC, ECG, varicella zoster antibody, blood pressure, ophthalmic examination, LFTs	Requires first dose observation Contraindicated in patients receiving Class I and III antiarrhythmic drugs and those with recent cardiac disease,[a] second and third degree AV block Ketoconazole increases fingolimod serum concentration (3A4 inhibition) Vaccine efficacy may be decreased
Teriflunomide	Steven–Johnson syndrome, liver failure, neutropenia, respiratory infection, activation of TB, alopecia, neuropathy	CBC, LFTs, blood pressure, pregnancy, TB test	Contraindicated in severe hepatic impairment Possibility of TB reactivation Active metabolite of leflunomide
Dimethyl fumarate	Flushing, rash, pruritus, GI discomfort, lymphocytopenia, increased LFTs, albuminuria	CBC, LFTs	Taking with food decreases incidence of flushing

AML, acute myeloid leukemia; CBC, complete blood count; ECG, electrocardiogram; LVEF, left ventricular ejection fraction; PML, progressive multifocal leukoencephalopathy; LFT, liver function test.

[a]Cardiac disease including myocardiac infarction, unstable angina, stroke, transient ischemic attack, and heart failure NYHA Class III/IV.

TABLE 39-4 Evidenced-Based Recommendations for Disease Modifying Treatment of Multiple Sclerosis

Recommendations	Recommendation Grades[a]
Interferon-β	
• Interferon-β has been shown to reduce attack rates in patients with MS or those with CIS who are at high risk of developing MS	A-I
• It is appropriate to consider IFN-β for any patient with clinically definite MS or who already has RRMS or SPMS and is still experiencing relapses	A-I
• The effectiveness of IFN-β in patients with SPMS but without relapses is uncertain	U-I
• Route of administration of IFN-β products is probably not clinically important with regards to efficacy; however, the side effect profile does differ	B-II
• Rate of production of neutralizing antibodies is probably less with IFN-β_{1a} than with IFN-β_{1b}	B-I
• Presence of neutralizing antibodies may be associated with a reduction in the clinical effectiveness of IFN-β treatment	C-I
Glatiramer acetate	
• Glatiramer acetate has been shown to reduce the attack rate in patients with RRMS	A-I
• Treatment with glatiramer acetate may slow sustained disability progression in RRMS	C-I
Mitoxantrone	
• Mitoxantrone probably reduces the attack rate in patients with relapsing forms of MS	B-II, III
• Mitoxantrone may have a beneficial effect on disease progression in MS	C-II, III
Natalizumab	
• Natalizumab decreases clinical relapse rate, Gd-enhancing lesions, and new T_2 lesions	A-I
• Natalizumab in RRMS positively changes measures of disease severity such as EDSS progression rate and changes lesions on MRI in RRMS	A-I

CIS, Clinically isolated syndrome; RCT, randomized controlled trial; RRMS, relapsing-remitting multiple sclerosis; SPMS, secondary-progressive multiple sclerosis.

[a]Strength of recommendations: A: established. B: probable. C: possible. U: inadequate data to support recommendation.

Quality of evidence: Class I, evidence from one or more prospective, randomized, controlled clinical trial; Class II, evidence from cohort or RCT not meeting criteria for class I; Class III, evidence from other controlled trials; Class IV, evidence from uncontrolled studies, case reports, case series, or expert opinion.

Reprinted with permission from Goodin et al.[60] and data from Goodin et al. Assessment: the use of natalizumab (Tysabri) for the treatment of multiple sclerosis (an evidence-based review): report of the Therapeutics and Technology Assessment Subcommittee of the American Academy of Neurology. Neurology 2008;71:766–773.

Interferon-β_{1b} and Interferon-β_{1a}

IFN-β_{1b} (Betaseron and Extavia) was the first agent proven to favorably alter the natural course of the illness.[60] In Table 39-4, DMTs are listed with evidence-based recommendations from the American Academy of Neurology.[60] Although the exact mechanism of action is unknown, IFN-β_{1b}'s effect in MS may be caused by its immunomodulating properties, including the ability to augment suppressor cell function and reduce IFN-γ secretion by activated lymphocytes, its macrophage-activating effect, and its ability to downregulate the expression of IFN-γ–induced class II MHC gene products on antigen-presenting glial cells. IFN suppresses T-cell proliferation and may decrease blood–brain barrier permeability by decreasing matrix metalloproteinases.[60] IFN-β also increases the production of regulatory CD56 (bright) natural killer cells and Treg cells.[61] In general, all IFNs exert these actions in the periphery and at the blood–brain barrier level.

IFN-β_{1b} is a nonglycosylated synthetic analog of recombinant IFN-β that is produced in *Escherichia coli*. IFN-β_{1b} is administered subcutaneously every other day at a dose of 250 mcg (8 million international units). Clinical trials have demonstrated that at these doses, IFN-β_{1b} significantly reduces annual relapse rate and MRI burden of disease compared with placebo. No significant differences were noted between the IFN- and placebo-treated groups with respect to clinical disability.[60] Betaseron is packaged in partially premixed syringes with a new formulation that does not require refrigeration and can be used with an autoinjector. In 2009, an additional IFN product was introduced with the trade name Extavia; Extavia is the same medicinal product as Betaseron.

IFN-β_{1a} (Avonex and Rebif) is a natural-sequence glycosylated IFN produced in Chinese hamster ovary cells. Avonex is administered as a 30-mcg dose (6 million international units) intramuscularly once weekly. The prefilled syringes (33 mcg/0.5 mL, four per package) should be refrigerated, but can be kept at room temperature for 30 days. Rebif is made in a very similar fashion to Avonex but given as either 22 or 44 mcg (0.5 mL) subcutaneously three times weekly. It is supplied in a 0.5-mL prefilled syringe with an autoinjector. Rebif should also be kept refrigerated, but is stable at room temperature for 30 days. A new formulation may have lower immunogenicity and a slightly better side-effect profile.[62]

When given 30 mcg intramuscularly once weekly for 2 years, patients receiving IFN-β_{1a} (Avonex) demonstrated, compared with placebo, statistically significant reductions (approximately one-third) in annual relapse rate as well as disease progression, defined as a confirmed decrease of one point on the EDSS.[63] When disease progression was assessed by MRI studies, patients receiving active drug had significantly fewer new enhancing lesions compared with placebo-treated patients. Similar results were seen with higher dose (44 mcg), more frequent administration (three times weekly), and subcutaneous injection of IFN-β_{1a} (Rebif).[60] Other studies reveal significant effects on slowing brain atrophy[64] and the progression of cognitive decline[63] in patients treated with Avonex. Taken together, these observations show that IFN-β possesses significant disease-modifying activity.

Side effects are similar with all the IFNs. Baseline complete blood counts, platelet determinations, and liver function tests should be documented before starting therapy, at 1 month, then every 3 months for 1 year, and every 6 months thereafter. Small percentages of patients develop depressed cell counts and liver enzyme elevations that are usually transient and respond to discontinuation of therapy. Rarely patients have developed true liver failure requiring liver transplant, and package inserts for IFN-β products have been altered to reflect this risk. The most common adverse effects include injection-site redness, swelling, menstrual irregularities, flu-like symptoms (e.g., fever, chills, and myalgias), and rarely necrosis. These symptoms can be mild or severe and are seen in most patients. The flu-like side effects typically occur for up to 24 hours after injection and typically abate within 1 to 3 months after starting the injections, but they persist in some patients. Injection-site reactions are probably worse with IFN-β_{1b}, can occur at any time, and can be lessened by using appropriate injection technique, including site rotation (thighs and buttocks), topical lidocaine, application of ice before and after the injection, or use of an autoinjector (usually free from drug manufacturer). Injecting the medications at body temperature (place under armpits to warm) will decrease injection-site pain. By taking the injection at night prior to bed time the patient may sleep through most of the flu-like symptoms; nonsteroidal anti-inflammatory agents or acetaminophen taken before and at regular intervals for 24 hours after administration may alleviate the flu-like symptoms. Initiation of one-quarter or one-half the standard dose, with increase to full dosage over 1 to 2 months, also may be beneficial in reducing flu-like side effects.[65] Some authors suggest that because of the transient immune activation that can occur following the introduction of IFN-β, a short burst of oral prednisone can alleviate some adverse effects.[65]

Less commonly reported and transient side effects include shortness of breath, tachycardia, thyroid dysfunction, and neutralizing antibodies. Although depression is a common finding in MS patients, all the IFNs, especially IFN-β_{1b}, can produce depressive symptoms. Clinicians must monitor patients carefully for signs of depression and treat accordingly. Patients who develop depression should be monitored closely for suicide risk. Most patients will not feel better or have improvement in symptoms when taking IFNs, and many will experience side effects; thus, adherence can become a major issue. Finally, safety data on IFN-β in pregnancy and lactation are lacking. Abortifacient activity in primates has been noted, and until adequate safety data are available, women should be counseled as to appropriate contraception while using these products. In general, pregnancy tends to protect patients from MS exacerbation.

Although the adverse-effect profile of IFN-β_{1a} resembles that of IFN-β_{1b}, intramuscular IFN-β_{1a} (Avonex) may hold several advantages, including fewer local injection-site reactions and once-weekly administration versus subcutaneous injection every other day (or 3 days per week) with Rebif.

Glatiramer Acetate (Copaxone)

Glatiramer acetate (Copaxone, formerly known as copolymer-1) is a synthetic polypeptide consisting of L-alanine, L-glutamic acid, L-lysine, and L-tyrosine. Although the precise mechanism of action of this compound is unknown, glatiramer acetate appears to mimic the antigenic properties of MBP.[66] This agent also may act by directly binding to MHC class II receptors and inhibiting binding of MBP peptides to T-cell receptor complexes.[66] Glatiramer acetate has demonstrated that it induces Th2 (anti-inflammatory) lymphocytes in experimental allergic encephalomyelitis.[66] This is thought to contribute to "bystander" suppression at the site of the MS lesion and thereby reduction of inflammation, demyelination, and axonal damage.[60] Glatiramer acetate may also suppress T-cell activation; recent studies suggest that it may be associated with a neuroprotective effect by inducing brain-derived neurotrophic factor.[67]

Given as a daily 20-mg subcutaneous dose, glatiramer acetate appears to have a relatively mild adverse effect profile. Mild pain and pruritus at the injection site are the most frequent patient complaints. Approximately 10% of patients experience a one-time transient reaction consisting of chest tightness, flushing, and dyspnea beginning several minutes after injection and lasting usually no longer than 20 minutes. The postinjection reaction can occur with any dose, and is not limited to the first injection. If patients have no history or evidence of coronary artery disease, they may be assured these reactions are almost always self-limited and benign. Several adverse effects associated with the IFNs, including flu-like symptoms and depression, do not appear to be provoked by glatiramer acetate. Multicenter trials with glatiramer acetate have demonstrated significant reductions in mean annual relapse rate (approximately 29%), comparable with the IFNs.[60] An extension trial, completed after the original, pivotal 2-year study, suggests that glatiramer acetate may slow the progression of disability in patients with RRMS.[60] Glatiramer acetate also delays development of T_1 holes on brain MRIs;[68] long-term uncontrolled data show that it remains safe and effective for individuals who continue to take it over 10 years.[69] Glatiramer acetate is available as 20 mg/mL prefilled syringes, and needs to be stored in the refrigerator but can be kept at room temperature for up to 1 week.

Natalizumab (Tysabri)

Natalizumab is a partially humanized monoclonal antibody directed at the cell surface adhesion molecule $\alpha_4\beta$-integrin (also known as very-late antigen 1, VLA-1). Natalizumab works by attaching to VLA-1 and blocking its interaction with its ligand on CNS endothelium vascular cell adhesion molecule (VCAM-1). Thus, activated lymphocytes are denied entry past the blood–brain barrier. In a phase II study, compared with placebo, natalizumab significantly reduced the number of new gadolinium-enhancing lesions by more than 90%, and diminished relapses as well.[70] In a 2-year phase III trial (A Randomized, Placebo-Controlled Trial of Natalizumab for Relapsing Multiple Sclerosis [AFFIRM]), compared with placebo, annual relapse rate was reduced by more than 60%, gadolinium-enhancing lesions were lessened by more than 90%, and progression of disability was significantly delayed.[71] In a separate 2-year, phase III trial (The Safety and Efficacy of Natalizumab in Combination with Interferon Beta-1a in Patients with Relapsing Remitting Multiple Sclerosis [SENTINEL]) in patients already taking IFN-β_{1a} (Avonex), those who had natalizumab added had a relapse rate reduction of more than 50% and gadolinium-enhancing lesion reduction of 84% compared with patients who continued with IFN-β_{1a} alone.[72] In these trials, natalizumab was injected IV every 4 weeks and was relatively well tolerated, although approximately 1% of patients developed infusion reactions, and 6% developed neutralizing antibodies that diminished the efficacy of the drug.

On November 23, 2004, the FDA approved natalizumab for use in relapsing MS in patients with inadequate response or intolerance to other MS therapies with the stipulation that the studies would continue. In February 2005, Biogen and Elan voluntarily removed natalizumab from the market after receiving reports of two patients (one patient from the SENTINEL trial, and one patient in a Crohn's disease study), who died after developing progressive multifocal leukoencephalopathy (PML), a rare brain infection most commonly seen in patients with human immunodeficiency virus.[73–75] One other patient who developed PML in the SENTINEL trial survived.[73–75] Further safety analysis did not identify other cases, so on March 9, 2006, an FDA advisory panel reviewing the data suggested reapproval of natalizumab for use in relapsing patients with a mandatory Risk Evaluation and Mitigation Strategy (REMS) program called TOUCH. On June 5, 2006, the FDA reapproved use of natalizumab in the United States with a black-box warning about PML. As of September 2012, 271 cases of PML have been identified, all in patients using the medication for 8 months or longer. The estimated risk for developing PML is low. Three factors appear to impact the overall risk of developing PML while receiving natalizumab therapy: duration of treatment (24 months or longer), history of John Cunningham virus (JCV) infection, and prior use of immunosuppressive therapies (mycophenolate mofetil, alemtuzumab, efalizumab, and rituximab).[76,77] A two-step enzyme-linked immunosorbent assay (ELISA, STRATIFY TEST) is available for qualitative detection of serum antibodies to the JCV, offering a false-negative rate of 2.5%.[76,77]

Plasma exchange (PLEX) has been utilized to help clear the drug more rapidly from the blood of patients who develop PML.[78] An acute syndrome, referred to as immune reconstitution inflammatory syndrome, has been associated with acute neurological deterioration after PLEX, requiring the use of steroids.[79]

Natalizumab is indicated for relapsing forms of MS to delay the accumulation of physical disability and decrease the number of relapses in patients who have a documented inadequate response or intolerance to traditional MS therapies. Patients receiving natalizumab must be enrolled in the TOUCH program. The overall predicted seroconversion rate for JCV is 2% to 3% per year. For that reason, the current recommendation is to screen patients at baseline and every 6 months with a JCV test while receiving natalizumab therapy.[80]

Fingolimod (Gilenya)

Approved September 21, 2010, fingolimod is the first oral DMT for MS. It has a unique mechanism of action as a sphingosine 1-phosphate receptor agonist. Fingolimod exhibits its immunosuppressant properties by sequestering circulating lymphocytes into secondary lymphoid organs and reduces the infiltration of T lymphocytes and macrophages into the CNS. It may have neuroprotective effects. In clinical trials it decreased annualized relapse rates by approximately

52% compared to IFN-β_{1a}. After 7 years of continuous fingolimod therapy, approximately 92% of patients were free of gadolinium-enhancing lesions, although these data used the 1.25 mg dose. The recommended dose approved by the FDA is 0.5 mg once daily.

Major side effects include pronounced first dose bradycardia and, rarely, bradyarrhythmia or atrioventricular block, infections, macular edema, a decrease in forced expiratory volume over 1 second in patients with previously compromised lung function, elevation of liver enzymes, and a sustained increase of approximately 1 to 2 mm Hg in systolic and diastolic blood pressure. Rare cases of lymphoma have also been identified. The reversal of lymphopenia can take 2 to 4 weeks after discontinuation of the drug. The cumulative number of deaths in patients receiving fingolimod, either during clinical trials or postmarketing use, is 31 patients as of February 2012. Extensive evaluation of patient deaths of apparently cardiovascular or unknown origin concluded that for each of the deaths, any contribution of fingolimod treatment was unclear, and the rate of death among MS patients treated with fingolimod was not higher than the rate of death for MS patients not receiving the drug. Nevertheless, the FDA announced a series of label updates. It is recommended that all patients starting fingolimod treatment be monitored for signs of bradycardia for at least 6 hours after the first dose. The FDA also recommends hourly pulse and blood pressure monitoring for all patients starting treatment, with electrocardiogram monitoring prior to dosing and at the end of the observation period; monitoring should continue until all symptoms resolve. The period should extend past 6 hours in patients at higher risk, in some cases overnight. Additionally, the package insert requires a new 6-hour observation period in patients who have discontinued and wish to restart therapy. The recommendation varies depending on the time of discontinuation and days of therapy missed. To reduce risks related to bradycardia or atrioventricular block, extended monitoring is now recommended in patients with certain preexisting conditions such as QT prolongation. This is also a concern in patients receiving concomitant drugs that slow the heart rate or atrioventricular conduction, drugs that cause QT interval prolongation, and those who have a known risk for torsades. The following class Ia and class III antiarrhythmic agents are contraindicated with concurrent use of fingolimod: quinidine, procainamide, disopyramide, amiodarone, bretylium, sotalol, ibutilide, azimilide, dofetilide, and dronedarone.[81]

Additional monitoring recommendations include baseline complete blood counts, liver function tests, ophthalmologic examinations, and electrocardiogram in patients with known heart problems. To date, one important drug interaction has been reported with concomitant use of ketoconazole and fingolimod. Ketoconazole has been shown to increase the area under the curve by 70%. If a live vaccine is to be administered to a patient (Zostavax, Flumist, YF-VAX, etc.), consider doing so prior to starting fingolimod or wait until 2 months after discontinuation. The degree to which fingolimod's oral delivery may alter the likelihood of a patient using, or continuing to use, a self-injectable medication remains to be seen.

Teriflunomide (Aubagio)

Teriflunomide (Aubagio) is an immunomodulatory agent, which was FDA approved on September 12, 2012 for the treatment of relapsing forms of MS. The medication works by inhibiting dihydroorotate dehydrogenase to prevent the proliferation of peripheral lymphocytes (T and B cells). The reduction of activated lymphocytes in the CNS reduces the inflammation and demyelination, which occurs in patients with MS. Teriflunomide is the active metabolite of leflunomide, an agent approved for the treatment of rheumatoid arthritis; however, teriflunomide is dosed as 7 or 14 mg orally once daily. This medication is available for distribution by specialty pharmacies.

O'Connor et al. studied 1,088 patients with CDMS. The patients were randomized to receive 7 or 14 mg of teriflunomide or placebo. Patients receiving 7 and 14 mg daily of teriflunomide had a statistically significant reduction in annualized relapse rate compared with placebo (relative risk reductions: 31.2% and 31.5%; $P = 0.0002$ and 0.0005, respectively). The risk of disability progression was statistically significantly reduced for those receiving 14 mg of teriflunomide daily (hazard ratio reduction: 29.8%; $P = 0.0279$).[82]

In a 36-week randomized, double-blinded, placebo-controlled study in MS subjects with relapse, 179 patients were randomized to 7 or 14 mg of teriflunomide or placebo. The primary outcome was the average number of unique active lesions per MRI scan during treatment. A statistically significant reduction in the primary endpoint was reported for both 7 and 14 mg of teriflunomide compared with placebo (0.98 and 1.06; $P = 0.0052$ and 0.0234, respectively).[83]

Key pharmacokinetic parameters of teriflunomide are displayed in Table 39-5. Although teriflunomide is not metabolized by CYP 450 enzymes, it inhibits CYP2C8 and induces CYP1A2. This medication is also a substrate for the breast cancer resistant protein (BCRP). Thus, inhibitors of BCRP (cyclosporine) may increase serum concentrations of teriflunomide. Additionally, teriflunomide inhibits OATP1B1 and OAT3. However, the significance of these drug interactions is unknown at this time. Studies found that concomitant use of warfarin and teriflunomide resulted in a 25% decrease in international normalized ratio (INR), rendering the need for close monitoring. When teriflunomide is coadministered with estradiol and levonorgestrel, the mean maximum serum concentration and area under the curve are increased.

TABLE 39-5 Pharmacokinetic Parameters of Teriflunomide

Time to maximum serum concentrations	1–4 hours
Protein binding	>99%
Metabolism	Hydrolysis, oxidation, *N*-acetylation, and sulfate conjunction
Half-life of elimination	18 and 19 days for 7 and 14 mg, respectively. Time to steady state is about 3 months

The most common adverse effects seen with teriflunomide are increases in liver function tests, alopecia, nausea, diarrhea, influenza, headache, and paresthesias.

Teriflunomide carries a black-box warning because of the risk of hepatotoxicity and teratogenicity (based on animal data). Monitoring for teriflunomide includes liver function tests (within 6 months prior to initiating teriflunomide and monthly for the first 6 months). Animal studies have found that oral teriflunomide resulted in fetal malformations and embryolethality in female rats as well as reduced sperm count in male rats. Based on these data, teriflunomide is not recommended in pregnancy. Females taking this medication should be placed on birth control. Patients who become pregnant during therapy or within 2 years after discontinuation of therapy should enroll in the Aubagio Pregnancy Registry and consider a cholestyramine washout. Additionally, men taking this medication with partners who wish to become pregnant may consider a cholestyramine washout to reduce serum drug levels as this drug may remain in the blood for up to 2 years after discontinuation. Teriflunomide may activate tuberculosis so a negative skin test or treatment of the disease must be documented prior to starting therapy. Overall, teriflunomide's efficacy is about that of the IFN products and glatiramer acetate.

Dimethyl Fumarate (Tecfidera)

Dimethyl fumarate has an unknown mechanism of action; however, it is an in vitro nicotinic acid receptor agonist and an in vivo activator of the nuclear factor (erythroid-derived 2)-like 2 (Nrf2) pathway that is involved in cellular response to oxidative stress. It is approved by the FDA for relapsing forms of MS. Dimethyl fumarate is metabolized by esterases in the GI tract, blood, and tissues. There are no known drug interactions. It is classified in pregnancy category C. Dimethyl fumarate is dosed initially at 120 mg (delayed release) orally twice daily. After 7 days, the dose should be increased to 240 mg (delayed release) orally twice daily. Laboratory monitoring includes a complete blood count prior to starting therapy and within 6 months of initiating treatment and annually. Side effects include lymphocytopenia (2% to 6%), increased liver function tests, and flushing (40%), which should improve over 1 month and is decreased by taking it with food. Rash, abdominal pain, diarrhea, nausea, and vomiting have also been reported. GI side effects decrease over 1 month.

In the "Efficacy and Safety Study of Oral Dimethyl Fumarate (BG-12) with Active Reference in Relapsing Remitting Multiple Sclerosis (CONFIRM)" dimethyl fumarate decreased the annualized relapse rate by 44% and 51% with twice daily or three times daily dosing, respectively. In "The Determination of the Efficacy and Safety of Oral BG-12 in Relapsing-Remitting MS" the annualized relapse rate decreased by 47% and 52% with 240 mg twice daily or three times daily dosing, respectively.

Mitoxantrone (Novantrone)

Mitoxantrone (Novantrone), a member of the anthracenedione family, is approved by the FDA for reducing neurologic disability and the frequency of clinical relapses in patients with SPMS (chronic), PRMS, or worsening RRMS.[84] The MRI outcomes, however, were not as robust as those typically seen in the trials of relapsing patients alone.[85] Mitoxantrone is administered as a brief (5- to 15-minute) IV infusion dosed at 12 mg/m^2 every 3 months. An evaluation of left ventricular ejection fraction and electrocardiogram are required prior to administration of each dose, and if signs or symptoms of congestive heart failure develop. The maximum allowable lifetime cumulative dose of mitoxantrone is 140 mg/m^2. Other potential side effects noted are nausea, alopecia, menstrual disorder, amenorrhea, upper respiratory tract infection, UTIs, and leukemia. The role that mitoxantrone will ultimately play in the treatment of MS remains unclear because potential cardiac toxicity limits its long-term use. More recent estimates also suggest the risk of leukemia may be as high as 1 in 145 patients, which has significantly decreased interest in its use for MS patients.[86] In addition, although patients with SPMS were included in the mitoxantrone in multiple sclerosis (MIMS—effect of mitoxantrone on MRI in progressive MS) trial, resulting in FDA approval for use in SPMS, there was no substudy documenting slowing of progression specifically in this subgroup of patients.[84,85] Thus, support for use of mitoxantrone in this context is less strong.[86]

Remaining Questions for Disease-Modifying Therapy

9 Despite encouraging results from well-conducted clinical trials, several relevant issues remain. The most important question in the use of the DMTs is when to begin therapy. The Medical Advisory Board of the National Multiple Sclerosis Society has adopted recommendations regarding the use of the current MS DMTs (Table 39-6).[87]

Decisions about the use of any medication rest on determination of the severity of the illness, the efficacy of the medication, and the side effects and costs related to the therapy. Clearly, these drugs slow the course of the illness but do not suppress it completely, and in some individuals, there is no apparent benefit. There is now, however, overwhelming evidence that the vast majority of untreated patients will have progressive disease over time. Pathologic data clearly show that even in acute lesions there is significant axonal damage that is essentially irreversible. MRI data show that 80% to 90% of all new enhancing lesions are asymptomatic, suggesting that a "quiet" clinical course does not necessarily mean there is not ongoing disease activity that ultimately will be reflected in cognitive problems and progressive spastic paraparesis.

TABLE 39-6 Disease Management Consensus Statement

- Initiation of therapy with an IFN-β medication (Avonex, Betaseron, Rebif, and Extavia) or glatiramer acetate is advised as soon as possible following a definite diagnosis of MS with active, relapsing disease, and can also be considered for selected patients with a first attack who are at high risk of MS
- Natalizumab is FDA approved for patients who have had an inadequate response to, or are not able to tolerate other MS therapies
- Mitoxantrone can be considered for patients with relapsing worsening disease or patients with secondary-progressive MS who are worsening, whether or not relapses are occurring
- Patients' access to medication should not be limited by the frequency of relapses, age, or level of disability
- Treatment is not to be stopped during evaluation for continuing treatment
- Therapy is to be continued indefinitely, unless there is clear lack of benefit, intolerable side effects, new data that reveal other reasons for cessation, or better therapy becomes available
- Interferon-β medications, glatiramer acetate, mitoxantrone, and natalizumab are all FDA approved for patients with MS and should be included in formularies and covered by third-party payers so that physicians and patients can determine the most appropriate agent on an individual basis
- Movement from one immunomodulating drug to another should be permitted for medical reasons
- None of these agents are approved for use in women trying to become pregnant, who are pregnant, or nursing mothers

Data from Miller et al.[87] with permission.

Furthermore, it is now known that very early therapy is effective. In patients with CIS and two or more T_2 lesions on brain MRI (i.e., at high risk for developing CDMS), placebo-controlled studies with all three of the IFN agents and glatiramer acetate have shown significant delay in a second attack and positive outcomes on a variety of MRI measures (BENEFIT, Betaseron in Newly Emerging Multiple Sclerosis for Initial Treatment; CHAMPS, Controlled High Risk Subjects Avonex Multiple Sclerosis Prevention Study; and ETOMS, Early Treatment of Multiple Sclerosis).[60,88] Thus, very early therapy is potentially warranted, and IFN-β_{1b}, IFN-β_{1a} (Avonex), and glatiramer acetate are approved by the FDA for use after CIS in those patients with abnormal MRIs consistent with demyelination, suggestive of high risk of further demyelinating events. The National Multiple Sclerosis Society recommends that patients with relapsing disease should be placed on Avonex, Betaseron (or Extavia), Copaxone, or Rebif (ABC-R) therapy immediately after the diagnosis.[87]

A second major issue is which drug to use in which patient. There has not been a single, randomized study comparing all four ABC-R drugs with one another in a similar patient population at the same time.[89] The pivotal placebo-controlled trials produced results that were more similar than different when comparing across trials, including a nearly identical one-third reduction in relapse rate for all four drugs over 2 years. A small number of studies have suggested higher dose, more frequent administration of IFN may be more efficacious than lower dose, less frequent administration,[90,91] but these differences appear modest. Other studies argue against this,[92,93] and recent studies note no significant difference in outcomes between standard and double dose IFN-β_{1b} and glatiramer acetate,[94] and no difference between IFN-β_{1a} (Rebif) and glatiramer acetate.[95]

A concern with all three IFN products that further muddies our understanding of the clinical differences between the IFN products is the development of neutralizing antibodies. In clinical trials, 30% to 40% of patients receiving IFN-β_{1b} developed antibodies directed against the drug.[97] In these patients, the exacerbation rate was similar to that in placebo-treated patients. In patients on IFN-β_{1b}, neutralizing antibodies can occur as early as 3 to 6 months and as late as 18 months. This product tends to be the most antigenic.[96] With IFN-β_{1a}, neutralizing antibodies were found in 22% of early trials of Avonex, but later studies reported that only 2% to 5% of treated patients developed antibodies; this decrease was caused by a formulation change of the drug making it the least antigenic.[93,96] Percentages of antibody formation for Rebif (approximately 12%) are intermediate, therefore moderately antigenic, and this can occur in the first 9 to 15 months of treatment, which is the same time frame for antibody production with Avonex.[60,96,97] The long-term clinical significance of these findings, however, is still not completely clear, although three recent studies have further confirmed the effect of neutralizing antibodies on relapses, MRI lesions, and progression of disability.[97–100] Whether these antibodies are truly cross-reactive between products is unknown, as is the duration during which antibodies can be detected. There are no general consensus guidelines regarding when to test for neutralizing antibodies, which assay to use, or what titer cutoff to apply to patients in clinical settings.[101] An important question is whether production of antibodies might be diminished with treatments such as corticosteroids. Another concern of practitioners is the relationship between active ingredients and varying excipients or particulate matter of IFN therapies and the production of neutralizing antibodies. Neutralizing antibodies are seen in approximately 6% of patients treated with natalizumab, and the antibodies seem to diminish efficacy.[72]

8 We now have experience for more than a decade with MS patients taking DMTs, yet continuing to have more relapses, more lesions on MRI, more disability, and ongoing slippage into SPMS.[102] There is no accepted definition of treatment inadequacy, although the Canadian Multiple Sclerosis Research Council has suggested a relatively simple approach that incorporates the elements of relapse rate, new MRI lesions, and change on the EDSS.[103] If a patient develops significant and persistent IFN antibodies, movement to a non-IFN (glatiramer acetate, natalizumab, fingolimod, teriflunomide, dimethyl fumarate, mitoxantrone, or possibly rituximab[104]) is reasonable. When failing low-dose IFN, options include changing to a higher dose, more frequent administration of IFN, or changing to a non-IFN. A second option is addition of an immunosuppressant agent, such as monthly methylprednisolone,[105] azathioprine, methotrexate, or mycophenolate. As noted above, the addition of natalizumab to IFN-β_{1a} was effective, but produced rare cases of PML, and thus, this combination should not be used. The addition of a statin agent may worsen MS[106] although these results are not definitive.

Symptomatic Management

10 Many of the symptoms of MS do not require pharmacologic management or do not respond to it. This section addresses the primary symptoms in which pharmacologic management may be of benefit (Table 39-7).[32,103,107–110,112] See the preceding section on the treatment of exacerbations for a discussion of optic neuritis.

Clinical **Controversy...**

In MS, there is no clear role for combination DMTs. Because of potential additive immunosuppression, all DMTs are currently used as monotherapy. There may be theoretical potential therapeutic benefit in adding an immunomodulator and an immunosuppressive agent, but the risk can be far greater (e.g., natalizumab plus interferon showed increased risk of PML). A recent clinical trial utilizing interferon and glatiramer acetate (CombiRX) demonstrated that there is minimal benefit of using the two in combination. However, other potential DMT combinations are yet to be studied.

TABLE 39-7 Treatment of Selected Primary MS Symptoms

Spasticity	Bladder Symptoms	Sensory Symptoms	Fatigue
Baclofen	Propantheline	Carbamazepine	Amantadine
Dantrolene	Oxybutynin	Phenytoin	Antidepressants
Diazepam	Dicyclomine	Amitriptyline or other TCAs	Modafinil
Tizanidine	DDAVP	Gabapentin	Methylphenidate
Tiagabine	Self-catheterization	Lamotrigine	Dextro-amphetamine
Gabapentin	Imipramine or amitriptyline	Pregabalin	Armodafinil
Pregabalin	Prazosin		
Botulinum toxin type A	Botulinum toxin type A		
Dalfampridine	Solifenacin		
	Darifenacin		
	Trospium		
	Hyoscyamine		

DDAVP, desmopressin acetate; TCA, tricyclic antidepressant.

Data from Schapiro,[32] Freedman et al.,[103] Mitchell,[107] Goodman et al.,[108] Stenager et al.,[110] and National MS Society.[122]

Gait Difficulties and Spasticity

Problems with gait can be caused by spasticity, weakness, ataxia, defective proprioception, or a combination of these factors. Spasticity often presents late in disease and is amenable to pharmacologic intervention, whereas physical therapy may be required in treating gait disturbances caused by other factors. Spasticity is encountered commonly and tends to affect the legs more markedly than the arms. Spasticity can result in falls; however, in the later stages of the disease, the increased muscle tone of a spastic limb often lends pseudo strength to patients with underlying weakness. Therefore, when using muscle relaxants, one must be careful not to decrease the tone to an extent that ambulation is actually hindered.[32,107] Baclofen (Lioresal), a γ-aminobutyric acid (GABA) analog, is the preferred agent and usually is started in dosages of 10 mg three times daily and titrated upward to achieve the desired response. Most patients achieve a satisfactory response with dosages between 40 and 80 mg/day; however, dosages higher than the recommended daily maximum of 80 mg are required by some patients.[32,107] A wearing-off is common, due to the relatively short duration of action. A longer-acting version of Lioresal is under study. Continuous intrathecal administration of baclofen may be an option for patients unable to tolerate or unresponsive to oral therapy. Baclofen should not be discontinued abruptly to avoid the possibility of seizures.[107] Small doses of diazepam (Valium) (e.g., 0.5 to 1 mg) often are added to baclofen in patients in whom optimal response has not been achieved.

Another effective agent with a different mechanism of action is tizanidine (Zanaflex). This short-acting, α-adrenergic agonist acts in the CNS to reduce spasticity by increasing presynaptic inhibition of motor neurons. It appears to have efficacy comparable with that of baclofen.[107] Dosage must be titrated slowly over 2 to 4 weeks, starting with 4 mg at bedtime, with adjustments based on clinical response. Effective tolerated dosages have ranged from 2 to 36 mg/day. Sedation, dizziness, and dry mouth are the most commonly reported adverse effects, but hypotension also can occur, as well as a rare but severe hepatotoxicity. Tizanidine can be added in small dosages to baclofen, sometimes creating better results and making possible smaller doses of each drug.

In patients who are unable to tolerate baclofen or tizanidine, diazepam (Valium; 2 to 10 mg/day), clonazepam (Klonopin; 1 to 3 mg/day), or dantrolene sodium (Dantrium; 100 to 400 mg/day) may be considered as alternatives, but they generally are less effective than either baclofen or tizanidine. Mild spasticity also may respond to moderately high doses of gabapentin (Neurontin; 1,800 to 3,600 mg/day). Tiagabine (Gabitril 8 to 56 mg/day) may be useful in some patients with spasticity, but side effects can prohibit its use. Pregabalin (Lyrica; 75 to 300 mg/day) has similar features and mechanism of actions as gabapentin, although pregabalin is approximately three times more potent and does not saturate the L-transporter system in the GI tract, so it may prove useful in the treatment of spasticity in MS patients.

Botulinum toxin type A (Botox; dose depending on the muscles injected) has been shown to be effective in improving spasticity.[32] The amount of toxin required to exert an effect on spasticity is often too excessive to use safely in the larger muscles; therefore, its use is best limited to smaller areas of focal muscle spasm.

An alternative approach to gait disruption employs K^+ channel blockers such as 4-aminopyridine (4-AP). However, at the FDA-approved dose, the blockade of K+ channels is negligible. Regardless, dalfampridine can potentiate synaptic transmission and increase muscle twitch tension. Recent studies have shown that 4-AP may modestly improve walking speed.[108,109] In early 2010, the FDA approved the use of a long-acting proprietary version of 4-AP, dalfampridine (Ampyra; 20 mg/day), for use in the United States. Dalfampridine is approved as a treatment to improve walking in patients with MS. It has been shown to increase walking speed by approximately 25% in responders.[108,109] In other countries, dalfampridine is referred to as fampridine.[109] A REMS program is in place to manage risks associated with dalfampridine use.

Safety concerns with the use of dalfampridine include the risk of seizures, particularly when patients exceed the maximum dose of 10 mg twice daily. The medication is contraindicated in patients with a history of seizures. It is important that patients are educated on not taking compounded 4-AP with dalfampridine, which is an extended release product. Additionally, the drug should not be chewed, crushed, or cut. If the patient misses a dose, they should take it immediately upon recognition and never double up on the dose, due to the risk of seizures. Commonly reported side effects of dalfampridine include UTIs, insomnia, dizziness, headaches, and balance disorders.

Tremor

Cerebellar symptoms such as tremor can be troubling and difficult to control. Medications that can be helpful include propranolol, primidone, and isoniazid.

Bowel and Bladder Symptoms

Patients commonly complain of incontinence, urgency, frequency, and nocturia, which are indications of a hyperreflexic bladder (i.e., inability to store urine). A number of anticholinergic agents, including oxybutynin chloride (Ditropan; 10 to 20 mg/day), tolterodine (Detrol; 2 to 4 mg/day), propantheline bromide (Pro-Banthine; 45 to 90 mg/day), hyoscyamine (Levsin; 0.75 to 1.5 mg/day), and dicyclomine hydrochloride (Bentyl; 30 to 80 mg/day) are used to treat this problem if symptoms are mild. Ditropan is available in an extended-release formulation (5 and 10 mg). In addition, tricyclic antidepressants, such as imipramine (Tofranil) and amitriptyline (Elavil), have been used for their anticholinergic properties to treat this condition. With all anticholinergic agents, great care must be used to avoid falls, decreased cognition, and constipation, which is worsened by the patient's natural instinct to limit fluid intake. Antimuscarinic agents such as trospium chloride (Sanctura; 40 mg/day), solifenacin succinate (Vesicare; 5 to 10 mg/day), darifenacin hydrobromide (Enablex; 7.5 to 15 mg/day), and fesoterodine (Toviaz; 4 to 8 mg/day) are also used to treat incontinence. In June 2012, the FDA approved mirabegron (Myrbetriq), a β_3 adrenergic agonist for the treatment of overactive bladder. As an alternative, the synthetic antidiuretic hormone preparation desmopressin acetate (DDAVP; 0.2 to 0.6 mg/day) has been reported to be effective in the treatment of urgency and incontinence. Use of DDAVP is best limited to bedtime to improve sleep and prevent significant problems with hyponatremia and seizures if overused. Patients with significant sphincter detrusor dyssynergia may benefit from the oral use of α-adrenergic blockers such as prazosin (Minipress; 10 to 40 mg/day), tamsulosin (Flomax), or intramuscular use of botulinum toxin type A (Botox; dose depends on the muscles injected) to relax the internal sphincter.

Intermittent self-catheterization and the crede maneuver with or without a concomitant anticholinergic agent is recommended in patients with large postvoid residual volumes (>100 mL) or when the urinary problem is hyporeflexic in nature (failure to empty). Cholinergic agents (bethanechol) may be useful in patients with a hyporeflexive bladder. Patients with large postvoid residual volumes are at risk for developing UTIs and often are prescribed urinary acidifiers such as vitamin C or antiseptics such as methenamine mandelate to prevent infections. Antibiotics used for UTI prophylaxis include sulfamethoxazole/trimethoprim, cephalexin, cinoxacin, and nitrofurantoin.

Constipation is the most common bowel complaint. Many medications (e.g., narcotics, anticholinergics) in common use may worsen this problem, as may voluntary water restriction in those patients with urinary urgency and incontinence. Increases in dietary fiber and hydration may alleviate this problem, but in some instances laxatives or enemas may be necessary.

Major Depression

Major depression is common in patients with MS, and the risk of suicide may be increased markedly compared with healthy subjects.[110] Patients should be monitored closely for the development of major depressive symptomatology and treated accordingly (see Chap. 51). IFN products and natalizumab should be used cautiously in patients with significant depression.

Sensory Symptoms

Numbness and paresthesia are frequent sensory complaints but usually do not require treatment. Some MS patients may develop acute or chronic pain syndromes[107] such as trigeminal neuralgia and painful dysesthesias, for which treatment is necessary. Carbamazepine (Tegretol; 400 to 1,200 mg/day) is the preferred agent for the treatment of trigeminal neuralgia. Other agents also commonly used for neuropathic pain include amitriptyline and related tricyclic antidepressants, gabapentin, pregabalin, and duloxetine.

Sexual Dysfunction

Sexual dysfunction in both men and women are common in MS, and counseling should be offered to both partners. Sildenafil citrate (Viagra), tadalafil (Cialis), and vardenafil (Levitra) are very effective for men with MS who have erectile dysfunction. Other options for men include alprostadil injection (Caverject) or intraurethral suppositories (MUSE). Viagra is currently being studied in females with MS and sexual dysfunction. In patients needing antidepressant therapy for whom sexual dysfunction is a concern, bupropion is preferable to selective serotonin reuptake inhibitors as it has a much lower incidence of sexual side effects.

Fatigue

Fatigue, one of the most common complaints in MS patients, can be severely disabling, but treatment is often overlooked. Typically present in the mid to late afternoon, it can increase with heat exposure, exertion, intercurrent infection, spasticity, weakness, and depression. Amantadine hydrochloride (100 mg twice daily) is used often and may offer significant relief.[32,103] Methylphenidate (Ritalin) and related products, and dextroamphetamine (Dexedrine) are used commonly for fatigue in MS. Modafinil (Provigil), at 200 mg daily, up to 400 mg daily may be helpful for MS-related fatigue. The *R*-enantiomer of modafinil is armodafinil (Nuvigil) dosed at 150 or 250 mg daily, which reaches peak concentrations more quickly with potentially fewer side effects than modafinil. In patients suffering from both depression and fatigue, a more activating antidepressant such as fluoxetine may be employed.

Cognition

Cognitive dysfunction is common in MS, affecting up to 50% or more of patients. It generally manifests itself as word-finding difficulties and problems with concentration and short-term memory. Cognitive dysfunction can be treated with stimulants or cholinesterase inhibitors.

Pseudobulbar Palsy

Pseudobulbar palsy is a condition, which is caused by progressive degeneration of the corticobulbar tract in patients with MS. Patients with this condition have dysarthria, dysphonia, and dysphagia. Additionally, sudden, uncontrollable, emotional outbursts such as crying or laughing occur inappropriately. Dextromethorphan/quinidine 20 mg/10 mg is used for the treatment of this pseudobulbar affect. The recommended dosing for this combination medication is one capsule daily for 1 week, followed by one capsule twice daily. Although the mechanism of action is unknown, the rationale for utilization of this combination drugs is that dextromethorphan is rapidly metabolized by CYP2D6, and quinidine inhibits the CYP2D6 enzyme to increase the serum concentration of dextromethorphan.

Complementary and Alternative Therapies for MS

A large percentage of patients with MS use complementary and alternative medicine (CAM) instead of, or in addition to, disease-modifying and symptomatic therapies. Common CAM therapies include diet and dietary supplements, such as vitamins, minerals, and herbs. Antioxidant supplements vitamin A, C, E, α-lipoic acid, coenzyme Q10, grape seed, pine bark extracts, mangosteen, and acai have suggestive evidence of benefiting MS patients. However, for patients with MS, there is a theoretical risk associated with taking antioxidant supplements owing to their ability to stimulate the immune system (T-cells and macrophages). Stimulating the immune system in patients with MS could be counterproductive, possibly worsening or exacerbating their disease, and may counteract the effects of immunomodulators. Other immune-stimulating supplements that should be used with caution are garlic, ginseng (Asian and Siberian), Echinacea, cat's claw, astragalus, alfalfa, and stinging nettle. A few agents that may pose a problem in MS, but may have benefit when taken in moderation, are zinc, melatonin (for insomnia), and dehydroepiandrosterone.[111]

In general, insufficient data support the effectiveness and safety of CAM therapies for MS. However, for patients with MS who are willing to try new approaches with limited evidence, CAM may be a consideration in some cases. Healthcare providers can be a source of objective information regarding the use of CAM for MS and can assist their patients in making the best decision.[111]

Vaccine Recommendations

A yearly flu shot is recommended for all patients with MS, including patients on any of the DMTs. The intranasal influenza vaccine, FluMist, which is a live, attenuated vaccine, is not recommended for patients with MS, however. As DMTs suppress the immune system, a patient taking one of these medications is at increased risk for developing an infection of the strain of virus given in the vaccine. Live virus vaccines are also more likely to cause an increase in MS disease activity than inactivated virus vaccines. Finally, it is unknown whether there are any direct interactions between DMTs and the intranasal influenza vaccine.[112] This information can likely be extrapolated to other vaccines, so if a patient is in need of a vaccination of any kind, "killed" virus vaccines are recommended.

Patients opting to take fingolimod who are varicella zoster virus antibody negative should consider receiving the varicella zoster virus immunization (even though it is a live attenuated vaccine) at least 2 months prior to beginning fingolimod. This should allow time to mount an antibody response prior to immunosuppression with fingolimod.

PERSONALIZED PHARMACOTHERAPY

The initial presentation of MS differs between individuals. When a patient is newly diagnosed modifiable risk factors may be considered prior to selecting therapy. Some of these modifiable risk factors include vitamin D deficiency, excess body weight, and smoking. Vitamin D deficiency has been associated with the risk of developing MS, and higher vitamin D levels may reduce MRI brain activity and thus reduce relapse rates.[8] Excess body weight is also associated with a higher risk of developing MS.[113] Smoking is associated with the development of MS, disability, MRI abnormalities, and conversion to CDMS (51% to 75% in 3 years).[9,114]

Treatments available for MS need to be individualized based on the initial symptomatology, MRI presentation, and the risk associated with the chosen therapy. Essentially when patients present, they can be given a modestly effective therapy with a low side effect profile (e.g., IFNs and glatiramer acetate) or a more aggressive therapy with a higher risk profile (natalizumab, fingolimod, or dimethyl fumarate). The weighing of the risks and benefits is ultimately dependent on a patient's presentation or progression of disease.

The importance of adherence cannot be underestimated in patients taking first-line DMTs. Nonadherence has been reported anywhere between 17% and 50%. The reason many patients stop taking their first-line DMTs is multifactorial, and includes perceived lack of efficacy, side effects, fear of needles, and depression. Patients who remain adherent to their first-line DMTs generally remain employed full-time in the work force compared with those who are nonadherent. It is crucial that we emphasize and establish realistic expectations for our patients on first-line DMTs. Overall, untreated MS patients generally relapse about every 6 months, whereas treated patients relapse about every 2 to 5 years. Adherence is the key to successful treatment of MS.

EVALUATION OF THERAPEUTIC OUTCOMES

Response to treatment of acute exacerbations of MS is commonly seen within days. With respect to DMTs, it is important for the clinician to recognize that over the short term (days to weeks), little or no apparent benefit may be noted by either patient or clinician. Evaluation of therapeutic outcomes, such as decreased MS exacerbations and hospitalizations or perhaps slowed disease progression and disability (as measured using scales such as EDSS), must be conducted over a period of months to years. Patients should be provided with realistic goals and expectations of these treatment options and encouraged to participate in the evaluation of therapeutic response. Initially, it may be important to reevaluate patients at relatively short time intervals to monitor for adverse effects.

Safety monitoring of patients on IFN includes regular laboratory monitoring, patient observation, and questioning for adverse effects or changing disability, and regular neurologic examinations. Specific laboratory monitoring for individuals on IFN therapy should include a complete blood count, platelet count, and liver function tests. These should be completed at baseline, every 3 months for 1 year, and every 6 months thereafter. Glatiramer acetate requires no laboratory monitoring. Teriflunomide requires a transaminase, bilirubin, complete blood count, tuberculin skin test, and blood pressure prior to initiating therapy and alanine aminotransferase monthly for 6 months after starting. Teriflunomide is associated with renal failure and increased potassium; therefore, patients should be monitored as needed. Dimethyl fumarate requires a complete blood count prior to starting therapy and within 6 months of treatment initiation and annually and liver function tests. Natalizumab and fingolimod have REMS programs to monitor safety. In addition to counseling patients regarding the adverse effects associated with these drugs, clinicians should actively encourage patients to comply with their prescribed regimens.

ABBREVIATIONS

4-AP	4-aminopyridine
ABC-R	Avonex, Betaseron, Copaxone, and Rebif
BCRP	breast cancer resistant protein
CAM	complementary and alternative medicine
CDMS	clinically definite multiple sclerosis
CIS	clinically isolated syndrome
CSF	cerebrospinal fluid
DDAVP	desmopressin
DMT	disease-modifying therapy
EBNA	Epstein–Barr nuclear antigen
EBV	Epstein–Barr virus
EDSS	expanded disability status scale
GABA	γ-aminobutyric acid
HLA	human leukocyte antigen
IFN	interferon
IL-2	interleukin-2
IL-10	interleukin-10
JCV	John Cunningham virus
MHC	major histocompatibility complex
MBP	myelin basic protein
MRI	magnetic resonance imaging
MS	multiple sclerosis
MSFC	multiple sclerosis functional composite
PML	progressive multifocal leukoencephalopathy
PPMS	primary-progressive multiple sclerosis
PRMS	Progressive-relapsing multiple sclerosis
REMS	Risk Evaluation and Mitigation Strategy
RIS	radiologically isolated syndrome
RRMS	relapsing-remitting multiple sclerosis
SPMS	secondary-progressive multiple sclerosis
TGF-β	transforming growth factor-β
Treg	T-regulatory cells
UTI	urinary tract infection
VCAM	vascular cell adhesion molecule
VEP	visual-evoked potential
VLA-1	very-late antigen 1

ACKNOWLEDGMENTS

The authors acknowledge Caleb Y. Oh, PharmD, Anne E. Eudy, PharmD, Karrine D. Roberts, PharmD candidate, Lisa Hong, PharmD candidate, and Joan Kaufman, illustrator, for their contributions to this chapter.

REFERENCES

1. Ascherio A, Munger K. Epidemiology of multiple sclerosis: From risk factors to prevention. Semin Neurol 2008;28: 17–28.
2. Goodin DS. The causal cascade to multiple sclerosis: A model for MS pathogenesis. PLoS One 2009;4:e4565.
3. Oksenberg JR, Baranzini SE, Sawcer S, Hauser SL. The genetics of multiple sclerosis: SNPs to pathways to pathogenesis. Nat Rev Genet 2008;9:516–526.
4. Ebers GC. Environmental factors and multiple sclerosis. Lancet Neurol 2008;7:268–277.
5. Healy BC, Ali EN, Guttmann CRG, et al. Smoking and disease progression in multiple sclerosis. Arch Neurol 2009;66:858–864.
6. National MS Society. Fact sheet multiple sclerosis; 2011. *http://www.nationalmssociety.org/chapters/mnm/mediacenter/factsheetmultiplesclerosis/index.aspx.*
7. Kotzamani D, Panou T, Mastorodemos V, et al. Rising incidence of multiple sclerosis in females associated with urbanization. Neurology 2012;78(22):1728–1735.
8. Munger KL, Levin LI, Hollis BW. Serum 25-hydroxyvitamin D levels and risk of multiple sclerosis. JAMA 2006;296: 2832–2838.
9. Zivadinov R, Weinstock-Guttman B, Hashmi K, et al. Smoking is associated with increased lesion volumes and brain atrophy in multiple sclerosis. Neurology 2009;73(7): 504–510.
10. Frohman EM, Racke MK, Raine CS. Multiple sclerosis—The plaque and its pathogenesis. N Engl J Med 2006;354: 942–955.
11. Owens GP, Bennett JL. Trigger, pathogen, or bystander: The complex nexus linking Epstein–Barr virus and multiple sclerosis. Mult Scler 2012;18(9):1204–1248.
12. Levin LI, Munger KL, Rubertone MV, et al. Temporal relationship between elevation of Epstein–Barr virus antibody titers and initial onset of neurological symptoms in multiple sclerosis. JAMA 2005;293:2496–2500.
13. Sundstrom P, Nystrom M, Ruuth K, et al. Antibodies to specific EBNA-1 domains and HLA DRB1*1501 interact as risk factors for multiple sclerosis. J Neuroimmunol 2009;215(1-2):102–107.
14. Zivadinov R, Zorzon M, Weinstock-Guttman B, et al. Epstein–Barr virus is associated with grey matter atrophy in multiple sclerosis. J Neurol Neurosurg Psychiatry 2009;80(6):620–625.
15. Serafini B, Rosicarelli B, Franciotta D, et al. Dysregulated Epstein–Barr virus infection in the multiple sclerosis brain. J Exp Med 2007;204:2899–2912.
16. Willis SN, Stadelmann C, Rodig SJ, et al. Epstein–Barr virus infection is not a characteristic feature of multiple sclerosis brain. Brain 2009;132:3318–3328.
17. Hafler DA, Compston A, Sawcer S, et al. Risk alleles for multiple sclerosis identified by a genomewide study. N Engl J Med 2007;357:851–862.
18. D'Netto MJ, Ward H, Morrison KM, et al. Risk alleles for multiple sclerosis in multiplex families. Neurology 2009;72:1984–1988.
19. Maier LM, Lowe CE, Cooper J, et al. IL2RA genetic heterogeneity in multiple sclerosis and type 1 diabetes susceptibility and soluble interleukin-2 receptor production. PLoS Genet 2009;5:e1000322.
20. Cree BA, Khan O, Bourdette D, et al. Clinical characteristics of African Americans versus Caucasian Americans with multiple sclerosis. Neurology 2004;63: 2039–2045.

21. Cree BA, Al-Sabbagh A, Bennett R, et al. Response to interferon beta-1a treatment in African American multiple sclerosis patients. Arch Neurol 2005;62:1681–1683.
22. Reich D, Patterson N, DeJager PL, et al. A whole-genome admixture scan finds a candidate locus for multiple sclerosis susceptibility. Nat Genet 2005;37:1113–1118.
23. Trapp BD, Peterson J, Ransohoff RM, et al. Axonal transection in the lesions of multiple sclerosis. N Engl J Med 1998;338:278–285.
24. Truyen L, van Wuesberghe JHTM, Barkof F, et al. Accumulation of hypointense lesions ("black holes") on T_1 spin echo MRI correlates with disease progression in multiple sclerosis. Neurology 1996;47:1469–1476.
25. Pirko I, Lucchinetti CF, Sriram S, Bakshi R. Gray matter involvement in multiple sclerosis. Neurology 2007;68: 634–642.
26. Zivadinov R, Minagar A. Evidence for gray matter pathology in multiple sclerosis: A neuroimaging approach. J Neurol Sci 2009;282:1–4.
27. Magliozzi R, Howell O, Vora A, et al. Meningeal B-cell follicles in secondary progressive multiple sclerosis associate with early onset of disease and severe cortical pathology. Brain 2007;130:1089–1104.
28. Reboldi A, Coisne C, Baumjohann D, et al. C-C chemokine receptor 6-regulated entry of T_H-17 cells into the CNS through the choroid plexus is required for the initiation of EAE. Nat Immunol 2009;10:514–523.
29. Zhou L, Chong MMW, Littman DR. Plasticity of CD4+ T-cell lineage differentiation. Immunity 2009;30:646–655.
30. Smolders J, Thewissen M, Peelen E, et al. Vitamin D status is positively correlated with regulatory T cell function in patients with multiple sclerosis. PLoS One 2009;4:e6635.
31. Owens GP, Bennett JL, Lassmann H, et al. Antibodies produced by clonally expanded plasma cells in multiple sclerosis cerebrospinal fluid. Ann Neurol 2009;65:639–649.
32. Schapiro RT. Managing symptoms of multiple sclerosis. Neurol Clin 2005;23:177–187.
33. Weinshenker BG. Natural history of multiple sclerosis. Ann Neurol 1994;36:S6–S11.
34. Confavreux C, Vukusic S. Natural history of multiple sclerosis: A unifying concept. Brain 2006;129(3):606–616.
35. Lebrun C, Bensa C, Debouverie M, et al. Association between clinical conversion to multiple sclerosis in radiologically isolated syndrome and magnetic resonance imaging, cerebrospinal fluid, and visual evoked potential: Follow-up of 70 patients. Arch Neurol 2009;66;841–846.
36. Zivadinov R, Zorzon M. Is gadolinium enhancement predictive of the development of brain atrophy in multiple sclerosis? A review of the literature. J Neuroimaging 2002;12:302–309.
37. Tremlett H, Paty D, Devonshire V. The natural history of primary progressive MS in British Columbia, Canada. Neurology 2005;65:1919–1923.
38. Hawker K, O'Connor P, Freedman MS, et al. Rituximab in patients with primary progressive multiple sclerosis: Results of a randomized double-blind placebo-controlled multicenter trial. Ann Neurol 2009;66:460–471.
39. Kurtzke JF. Rating neurologic impairment in multiple sclerosis: An expanded disability status scale (EDSS). Neurology 1983;33:1444–1452.
40. Rudick RA, Cutter G, Reingold S. The multiple sclerosis functional composite: A new clinical outcome measure for multiple sclerosis trials. Mult Scler 2002;8:359–365.
41. Gordon-Lipkin E, Chodkowski B, Reich DS, et al. Retinal nerve fiber layer is associated with brain atrophy in multiple sclerosis. Neurology 2007;69:1603–1609.
42. Lee M, O'Brien P. Pregnancy and multiple sclerosis. J Neurol Neurosurg Psychiatry 2008;79:1308–1311.
43. Sadovnick AD, Eisen K, Ebers GC, Paty DW. Cause of death in patients attending multiple sclerosis clinics. Neurology 1991;41:1193–1196.
44. Swanson JW. Multiple sclerosis: Update in diagnosis and review of prognostic factors. Mayo Clin Proc 1989;64: 577–586.
45. Polman CH, Reingold SC, Edan G, et al. Diagnostic criteria for multiple sclerosis: 2005 revisions to the "McDonald Criteria." Ann Neurol 2005;58:840–846.
46. Frohman EM, Goodin DS, Calabresi PA, et al. The utility of MRI in suspected MS. Report of the Therapeutics and Technology Assessment Subcommittee of the American Academy of Neurology. Neurology 2003;61:1332–1338.
47. Fisher E, Rudick R, Simon J, et al. Eight-year follow-up study of brain atrophy in patients with MS. Neurology 2002;59:1412–1420.
48. Fisniku LK, Brex PA, Altmann DR, et al. Disability and T2 MRI lesions: A 20-year follow-up of patients with relapse onset of multiple sclerosis. Brain 2008;131(Pt3):808–817.
49. Confavreux C, Vukusic S. Accumulation of irreversible disability in multiple sclerosis from epidemiology to treatment. Clin Neurol Neurosurg 2006;108(3):327–332.
50. McDonald W, Compston A, Edan G, et al. Recommended diagnostic criteria for multiple sclerosis: Guidelines from the international panel on diagnosis of multiple sclerosis. Ann Neurol 2001;50:121–127.
51. Dalton C, Brex P, Miszkiel K, et al. New T_2 lesions enable an earlier diagnosis of multiple sclerosis in clinically isolated syndromes. Ann Neurol 2003;53:673–676.
52. Swanton JK, Rovira A, Tintore M, et al. MRI criteria for multiple sclerosis in patients presenting with clinically isolated syndromes: A multicentre retrospective study. Lancet Neurol 2007;6:677–686.
53. Lo CP, Kao HW, Chen SY, et al. Prediction of conversion from clinically isolated syndrome to clinically definite multiple sclerosis according to baseline MRI findings: A comparison of revised McDonald criteria and Swanton modified criteria. J Neurol Neurosurg Psychiatry 2009;80:1107–2209.
54. Galetta KM, Calabresi PA, Frohman EM, Balcer LJ. Optical coherence tomograph (OCT): Imaging the visual pathway as a model for neurodegeneration. Neurotherapeutics 2011;8(1):117–132.
55. Berger T, Rubner P, Schautzer F, et al. Antimyelin antibodies as a predictor of clinically definite multiple sclerosis after a first demyelinating event. N Engl J Med 2003;349:139–145.
56. Carmosino MJ, Brousseau KM, Arciniegas DB, et al. Initial evaluations for multiple sclerosis in a university multiple sclerosis center: Outcomes and role of magnetic resonance imaging in referral. Arch Neurol 2005;62: 585–590.
57. Kaufman DI, Trobe JD, Eggenberger ER, Whitaker JN. Practice parameter: The role of corticosteroids in the management of acute monosymptomatic optic neuritis. Report of the Quality Standards Subcommittee of the American Academy of Neurology. Neurology 2000;54: 2039–2044.
58. Zivadinov R, Rudick RA, De Masi R, et al. Effects of IV methylprednisolone on brain atrophy in relapsing-remitting MS. Neurology 2001;57:1239–1247.
59. Kinkel PR, Miravalle A. Current guidelines and standard treatments of RR-MS. 2011. Addressing Unmet Medical Needs in Relapsing-Remitting Multiple Sclerosis. *http://www.futuremedicine.com*. doi:10.2217/ebo.11.111:6–25.

60. Goodin DS, Frohman EM, Garmany GP, et al. Disease-modifying therapies in multiple sclerosis: Report of the Therapeutics and Technology Assessment Subcommittee of the American Academy of Neurology and the Multiple Sclerosis Council for Clinical Practice Guidelines. Neurology 2002;58:169–178.
61. Vandebark AA, Huan J, Agotsch M, et al. Interferon-beta-1a increases CD56(bright) natural killer cells and CD4+CD25+ Foxp3 expression in subjects with multiple sclerosis. J Neuroimmunol 2009;215:125–128.
62. Giovannoni G, Barbarash O, Casset-Semanaz F, et al. Safety and immunogenicity of a new formulation of interferon beta-1a (Rebif New Formulation) in a Phase IIIb study in patients with relapsing multiple sclerosis: 96-week results. Mult Scler 2009;15:219–228.
63. Fischer JS, Priore RL, Jacobs LD, et al. Neuropsychological effects of interferon-β-la in relapsing multiple sclerosis. Ann Neurol 2000;48:885–892.
64. Simon JH, Jacobs L, Campion M, et al. A longitudinal study of brain atrophy in relapsing MS. Neurology 1999;58: 139–145.
65. Frohman E, Phillips T, Kokel K, et al. Disease-modifying therapy in multiple sclerosis: Strategies for optimizing management. Neurology 2002;8:227–236.
66. Racke MK, Lovett-Racke AE, Karandikar NJ. The mechanism of action of glatiramer acetate treatment in multiple sclerosis. Neurology 2010;74(Suppl 1): S25–S30.
67. Azoulay D, Vachapova V, Shihman B, et al. Lower brain-derived neurotrophic factor in serum of relapsing remitting MS. Reversal by glatiramer acetate. J Neuroimmunol 2005;167:215–218.
68. Fillippi M, Rovaris M, Rocca MA, et al. Glatiramer acetate reduces the proportion of new MS lesions evolving into "black holes." Neurology 2001;57:731–733.
69. Ford CC, Johnson KP, Lisak RP, et al. A prospective open-label study of glatiramer acetate: Over a decade of continuous use in multiple sclerosis patients. Mult Scler 2006;12:309–320.
70. Miller DH, Khan OA, Sheremata WA, et al. A controlled trial of natalizumab for relapsing multiple sclerosis. N Engl J Med 2003;348:15–23.
71. Polman CH, O'Conor PW, Havrdova E, et al. A randomized, placebo-controlled trial of natalizumab for relapsing multiple sclerosis (AFFIRM). N Engl J Med 2006;354: 899–910.
72. Rudick RA, Stuart WH, Calabresi PA, et al. Natalizumab plus interferon beta-1a for relapsing multiple sclerosis (SENTINEL). N Engl J Med 2006;354:911–923.
73. Kleinschmidt-DeMasters BK, Tyler KL. Progressive multifocal leukoencephalopathy complicating treatment with natalizumab and interferon beta-1a for multiple-sclerosis. N Engl J Med 2005:353;369–374.
74. Langer-Gould A, Atlas SW, Green AJ, et al. Progressive multifocal leukoencephalopathy in a patient treated with natalizumab. N Engl J Med 2005;353:375–381.
75. Van Assche G, Van Ranst M, Sclot R, et al. Progressive multifocal leukoencephalopathy after natalizumab therapy for Crohn's disease. N Engl J Med 2005;353:362–368.
76. Gorelik L, Lerner M, Bixler S, et al. Anti-JC virus antibodies: Implications for PML risk stratification. Ann Neurol 2010;68:295–303.
77. Bozic C, Richman S, Plavina T, et al. Anti-John Cunningham virus antibody prevalence in multiple sclerosis patients: Baseline results of STRATIFY-1. Ann Neurol 2011;70(5):742–750.
78. Khatri BO, Man S, Giovannoni G, et al. Effect of plasma exchange in accelerating natalizumab clearance and restoring leukocyte function. Neurology 2009;72:402–409.
79. Lindå H, von Heijne A, Major EO, et al. Progressive multifocal leukoencephalopathy after natalizumab monotherapy. N Engl J Med 2009;361:1081–1087.
80. Sadiq SA, Puccio LM, Brydon EW. JCV detection in multiple sclerosis patients treated with natalizumab. J Neurol 2010;257:954–958.
81. U.S. Food and Drug Administration. FDA Drug Safety Communication: Revised recommendations for cardiovascular monitoring and use of multiple sclerosis drug Gilenya fingolimod. FDA 2011, *http://www.fda.gov/Drugs/DrugSafety/ucm303192.htm*.
82. O'Connor P, Wolinsky JS, Confavreux C, et al. Randomized trial of oral teriflunomide for relapsing multiple sclerosis. N Engl J Med 2011;365(14):1293–1303.
83. O'Connor PW, Li D, Freedman MS, et al. A Phase II study of the safety and efficacy of teriflunomide in multiple sclerosis with relapses. Neurology 2006;66(6): 894–900.
84. Hartung HP, Gonsette R, Konig N, et al. Mitoxantrone in progressive multiple sclerosis, a placebo-controlled, double-blind, randomized, multicentre trial. Lancet 2002;360: 2018–2025.
85. Krapf H, Morrissey SP, Zenker O, et al. Effect of mitoxantrone on MRI in progressive MS. Results of the MIMS trial. Neurology 2005;65:690–695.
86. Martinelli V, Bellantonio P, Bergamaschi R, et al. Incidence of acute leukaemia in multiple sclerosis patients treated with mitoxandrone: A multicentre retrospective Italian study. Neurology 2009;73:330–333.
87. Miller A, Lisak R, Bohen B, et al. National Multiple Sclerosis Society (NMSS). Disease Management Consensus Statement: Expert Opinion Paper. New York: National MS Society, 2007:1–8. *http://www.nationalmssociety.org/docs/HOM/Exp_Consensus.pdf*.
88. Freedman MS, Kappos L, Polman CH, et al. Betaseron in newly emerging multiple sclerosis for initial treatment (BENEFIT): Clinical outcomes. Neurology 2006; (Suppl 2):A61.
89. Vartanian T. An examination of the results of the EVIDENCE, INCOMIN, and phase III studies of interferon beta products in the treatment of multiple sclerosis. Clin Ther 2003;1:105–118.
90. Durelli L, Verdun E, Bergui M, et al. Every-other-day interferon-β-1b versus once-weekly interferon-β-1a for multiple sclerosis: Results of a 2-year prospective randomized multicentre study (INCOMIN). Lancet 2002;359:1453–1460.
91. Panitch H, Goodin D, Francis G, et al. Randomized, comparative study of interferon-β-1a treatment regimens in MS. The EVIDENCE Trial. Neurology 2002;59: 1496–1506.
92. Koch-Henriksen N, Sorensen PS, Christensen T, et al. A randomized study of two interferon-beta treatments in relapsing-remitting multiple sclerosis. Neurology 2006;66:1056–1060.
93. Clanet M, Radue E, Kappos L, et al. A randomized, double-blind, dose-comparison study of weekly interferon-β-1a in relapsing MS. Neurology 2002;59:1507–1517.
94. O'Connor P, Filippi M, Arnason B, et al. 250 mcg or 500 mcg interferon beta-1b versus 20 mg glatiramer acetate in relapsing-remitting multiple sclerosis: A prospective, randomised, multicentre study. Lancet Neurol 2009;8: 889–897.

95. Mikol DD, Barkhof F, Chang P, et al. Comparison of subcutaneous interferon beta-1a with glatiramer acetate in patients with relapsing multiple sclerosis (the Rebif vs. Glatiramer Acetate in Relapsing MS Disease [REGARD] study): A multicentre, randomised, parallel, open-label trial. Lancet Neurol 2008;7:903–914.
96. Namaka M, Pollitt-Smith M, Gupta A, et al. The clinical importance of neutralizing antibodies in relapsing-remitting multiple sclerosis. Curr Med Res Opin 2006;22:223–239.
97. Bertolotto A. Neutralizing antibodies to interferon beta: Implications for the management of multiple sclerosis. Curr Opin Neurol 2004;17:241–246.
98. Francis GS, Rice GP, Alsop JC, et al. Interferon beta 1a in MS. results following development of neutralizing antibodies in PRISMS. Neurology 2005;65:48–55.
99. Kappos L, Clanet M, Sandberg-Wollheim M, et al. Neutralizing antibodies and efficacy of interferon beta-1a: A 4-year controlled study. Neurology 2005;65:40–47.
100. Giovannoni G, Goodman A. Neutralizing anti-IFN-beta antibodies: How much more evidence do we need to use them in practice? Neurology 2005;65:6–8.
101. Goodin DS, Frohman EM, Hurwitz B, et al. Neutralizing antibodies to interferon beta: Assessment of their clinical and radiographic impact: An evidence report. Neurology 2007;67:977–984.
102. Kappos L, Polman C, Pozzilli C, et al. Final analysis of the European multicenter trial on IFNβ-1b in secondary-progressive MS. Neurology 2001;57:1969–1975.
103. Freedman MS, Patry DG, Grand'Maison F, et al. Treatment optimization in multiple sclerosis. Can J Neurol Sci 2004;31:157–168.
104. Hauser SL, Waubant E, Arnold DL, et al. B-cell depletion with rituximab in relapsing-remitting multiple sclerosis. N Engl J Med 2008;358:676–688.
105. Sorensen PS, Mellgren SI, Svenningsson A, et al. NORdic trial of oral methylprednisolone as add-on therapy to interferon beta-1a for treatment of relapsing-remitting multiple sclerosis (NORMIMS study): A randomised, placebo-controlled trial. Lancet Neurol 2009;8: 519–529.
106. Birnbaum G, Cree B, Altafullah I, et al. Combining beta interferon and atorvastatin may increase disease activity in multiple sclerosis. Neurology 2008;71:1390–1395.
107. Mitchell G. Update on multiple sclerosis therapy. Med Clin North Am 1993;77:231–249.
108. Goodman AD, Brown TR, Krupp LB, et al. Sustained-release oral fampridine in multiple sclerosis: A randomised, double-blind, controlled trial. Lancet 2009;373: 732–738.
109. Egeberg M, Oh CY, Bainbridge JL. Clinical overview of dalfampridine: The agent with a novel mechanism of action to help with gait disturbances. Clinical Therapeutics 2012;34:2185–2194.
110. Stenager EN, Stenager E, Koch Henriksen N, et al. Suicide and multiple sclerosis: An epidemiological investigation. J Neurol Neurosurg Psychiatry 1992;55:542–545.
111. Bowling AC. Complementary and Alternative Medicine in Multiple Sclerosis, 2nd ed. New York, NY: Demos, 2007.
112. National MS Society. News Detail. 2009, *http://nationalmssociety.org/news/news-detail/index.aspx?nid=2115.*
113. Munger KL, Chitnis T, Ascherio A. Body size and risk of MS in two cohorts of US women. Neurology 2009;73(19): 1543–1550.
114. Hedstrom AK, Baarnhielm M, Olsson T, Alfredsson L. Tobacco smoking, not Swedish snuff use, increases the risk of multiple sclerosis. Neurology 2009;73(9): 696–701.

40

Epilepsy

Susan J. Rogers and Jose E. Cavazos

KEY CONCEPTS

1. Patient-specific treatment goals should be identified as early as possible.
2. Accurate diagnosis and classification of seizure/syndrome type is critical to selection of appropriate pharmacotherapy.
3. Patient characteristics such as age, comorbid conditions, ability to comply with the prescribed regimen, and presence or absence of insurance coverage can also influence the choice of antiepileptic drugs (AEDs).
4. Pharmacotherapy of epilepsy is highly individualized and requires titration of the dose to optimize AED therapy (maximal seizure control with minimal or no side effects). Approximately 50% to 70% of patients can be maintained on one AED.
5. If the therapeutic goal is not achieved with monotherapy, a second drug can be added or a switch to an alternative single AED can be made. If a second AED is added it should have a different mechanism of action from the first, although there is no clear evidence in humans to support this.
6. Some patients eventually can discontinue AED therapy. Several factors predict successful withdrawal of AEDs.
7. Surgery is the treatment of choice in selected patients with refractory focal epilepsy.
8. The appropriate use of AEDs requires a thorough understanding of their clinical pharmacology, including mechanism of action, pharmacokinetics, adverse reactions, and drug interactions, as well as available dosage forms.

Epilepsy is a disorder that is best viewed as a symptom of disturbed electrical activity in the brain, which may have many etiologies. It is a collection of many different types of seizures that vary widely in severity, appearance, cause, consequence, and management. Seizures that are prolonged or repetitive can be life-threatening. Epilepsy is defined by the occurrence of at least two unprovoked seizures separated by 24 hours.[1] The effect epilepsy has on patients' lives can be significant and extremely frustrating. It is also important to recognize that seizures can be just one (albeit the most obvious) symptom of an epileptic disorder. Not uncommonly, patients have other comorbid disorders, including depression, anxiety, and potentially neuroendocrine disturbances. Patients with epilepsy also may display neurodevelopmental delay, memory problems, and/or cognitive impairment. Although, by convention, the focus of drug treatment is on the abolition of seizures, clinicians must also try to address these common comorbidities.

EPIDEMIOLOGY

Each year, 120 per 100,000 people in the United States come to medical attention because of a newly recognized seizure.[1] At least 8% of the general population will have at least one seizure in a lifetime. However, it is common to have a seizure and not have epilepsy. The rate of recurrence of a first unprovoked seizure within 5 years ranges between 23% and 80%. Children with an idiopathic first seizure and a normal electroencephalogram (EEG) have a particularly favorable prognosis. Some seizures occur as single events resulting from withdrawal of CNS depressants (e.g., alcohol, barbiturates, and other drugs) or during acute neurologic illnesses or systemic toxic conditions (e.g., uremia or eclampsia). Some patients will have seizures only associated with fever. These febrile seizures do not constitute epilepsy.[1]

The age-adjusted incidence of epilepsy is 44 per 100,000 person-years. Each year, approximately 125,000 new epilepsy cases occur in the United States; only 30% are in people younger than 18 years of age at the time of diagnosis. There is a bimodal distribution in the occurrence of the first seizure, with one peak occurring in newborn and young children and the second peak occurring in patients older than 65 years of age. The relatively high frequency of epilepsy in the elderly is now being recognized.

ETIOLOGY

Seizures occur because a group of cortical neurons discharge abnormally in synchrony. Anything that disrupts the normal homeostasis or stability of neurons can trigger hyperexcitability and seizures. Thousands of medical conditions can cause epilepsy, from genetic mutations to traumatic brain injury. A genetic predisposition to seizures has been observed in many forms of primary generalized epilepsy. Patients with mental retardation, cerebral palsy, head injury, or strokes are at an increased risk for seizures and epilepsy. The more profound the degree of mental retardation as measured by the intelligence quotient (IQ), the greater is the incidence of epilepsy. In the elderly, the onset of seizures is typically associated with focal neuronal injury induced by strokes, neurodegenerative disorders (e.g., Alzheimer's disease), and other conditions. In some cases, if an etiology of seizures can be identified and corrected, the patient may not require chronic antiepileptic drug (AED) treatment. Patients can also present with unprovoked seizures that do not have an identifiable cause, and thus by definition have idiopathic or cryptogenic epilepsy. *Idiopathic etiology* is the term used for suspected genetic cause, whereas *cryptogenic etiology* is used if no obvious cause is found for focal-onset seizures.

Many factors have been shown to precipitate seizures in susceptible individuals. Hyperventilation can precipitate absence seizures. Excessive sleep, sleep deprivation, sensory stimuli, emotional stress, and hormonal changes occurring around the time of menses, puberty, or pregnancy have been associated with the onset of or an increased frequency of seizures. A careful drug history should be obtained from patients presenting with seizures because theophylline, alcohol, high-dose phenothiazines, antidepressants (especially maprotiline or bupropion), and street drug use have been associated with provoking seizures. Perinatal injuries and small gestational weight at birth are also risk factors for the development of partial-onset seizures. Immunizations have not been associated with an increased risk of epilepsy.

PATHOPHYSIOLOGY

Seizures result from excessive excitation, or in the case of absence seizures, from disordered inhibition of a large population of cortical neurons.[2] This is reflected on EEG as a sharp wave or *spike*. Initially, a small number of neurons fire abnormally. Normal membrane conductances and inhibitory synaptic currents break down, and excess excitability spreads, either locally to produce a focal seizure or more widely to produce a generalized seizure. This onset propagates by physiologic pathways to involve adjacent or remote areas. The clinical manifestations depend on the site of the focus, the degree of irritability of the surrounding area of the brain, and the intensity of the impulse.[2]

There are multiple mechanisms that might contribute to synchronous hyperexcitability, including: (a) alterations in the distribution, number, type, and biophysical properties of ion channels in the neuronal membranes; (b) biochemical modifications of receptors; (c) modulation of second messaging systems and gene expression; (d) changes in extracellular ion concentrations; (e) alterations in neurotransmitter uptake and metabolism in glial cells; and (f) modifications in the ratio and function of inhibitory circuits. In addition, local neurotransmitter imbalances could be a potential mechanism for focal epileptogenesis. Transitory imbalances between the main neurotransmitters, glutamate (excitatory) and γ-aminobutyric acid (GABA) (inhibitory), and neuromodulators (e.g., acetylcholine, norepinephrine, and serotonin) might play a role in precipitating seizures in susceptible patients.[2]

Control of abnormal neuronal activity with AEDs is accomplished by elevating the threshold of neurons to electrical or chemical stimuli or by limiting the propagation of the seizure discharge from its origin. Raising the threshold most likely involves stabilization of neuronal membranes, whereas limiting the propagation involves depression of synaptic transmission and reduction of nerve conduction.[2]

Prolonged seizures and continued exposure to glutamate can result in neuronal injury in vulnerable neuronal populations resulting in functional deficits, primarily in memory, and in permanent changes of wiring of the neuronal circuitry. Sprouting and reorganization of neuronal projections might lead to a chronic susceptibility to seizures, neuronal destruction, and brain damage. However, limited degree of neurogenesis in the hippocampal pathways has been induced by epileptic seizures. The role of these newly born neurons is not well understood.

CLINICAL PRESENTATION

The International League Against Epilepsy has proposed two major schemes for the classification of seizures and epilepsies: the International Classification of Epileptic Seizures and the International Classification of the Epilepsies and Epilepsy Syndromes.[3,4] The International Classification of Epileptic Seizures (Table 40-1) combines the clinical description with certain electrophysiologic

CLINICAL PRESENTATION Epilepsy

General

In most cases, the healthcare provider will not be in a position to witness a seizure. Many patients (particularly those with CP or GTC seizures) are amnestic to the actual seizure event. Obtaining an adequate history and description of the ictal event (including time course) from a witness is critically important. With treatment the typical clinical presentation of the seizure may change

Symptoms

Symptoms of a specific seizure will depend on seizure type. Although seizures can vary between patients, they tend to be stereotyped within an individual

- CP seizures can include somatosensory or focal motor features
- CP seizures are associated with altered consciousness
- Absence seizures can be almost nondetectable with only very brief (seconds) periods of altered consciousness
- GTC seizures are major convulsive episodes and are always associated with a loss of consciousness

Signs

Interictally (between seizure episodes), there are typically no objective or pathognomonic signs

Laboratory Tests

There are currently no diagnostic laboratory tests for epilepsy. In some cases, particularly following GTC (or perhaps CP) seizures, serum prolactin levels can be transiently elevated. Laboratory tests can be done to rule out treatable causes of seizures (e.g., hypoglycemia, altered electrolyte concentrations, infections, etc.) that do not represent epilepsy

Other Diagnostic Tests

- EEG is very useful in the diagnosis of various seizure disorders
- An epileptiform EEG is found in only approximately 50% of the patients who have epilepsy
- A prolactin serum level obtained within 10 to 20 minutes of a tonic–clonic seizure can be useful in differentiating seizure activity from pseudoseizure activity but not from syncope[5]
- Although magnetic resonance imaging (MRI) is very useful (especially imaging of the temporal lobes), a computed tomography (CT) scan typically is not helpful except in the initial evaluation for a brain tumor or cerebral bleeding

TABLE 40-1 International Classification of Epileptic Seizures

I. Partial seizures (seizures begin locally)
   A. Simple (without impairment of consciousness)
      1. With motor symptoms
      2. With special sensory or somatosensory symptoms
      3. With psychic symptoms
   B. Complex (with impairment of consciousness)
      1. Simple partial onset followed by impairment of consciousness—with or without automatisms
      2. Impaired consciousness at onset—with or without automatisms
   C. Secondarily generalized (partial onset evolving to generalized tonic–clonic seizures)
II. Generalized seizures (bilaterally symmetrical and without local onset)
   A. Absence
   B. Myoclonic
   C. Clonic
   D. Tonic
   E. Tonic–clonic
   F. Atonic
   G. Infantile spasms
III. Unclassified seizures
IV. Status epilepticus

Data from Commission on the Classification and Terminology of the International League Against Epilepsy.[3,4]

findings to classify epileptic seizures. Seizures are divided into two main pathophysiologic groups—partial seizures and generalized seizures—by EEG recordings and clinical symptomatology.

Partial (focal) seizures begin in one hemisphere of the brain and—unless they become secondarily generalized—result in an asymmetric motor manifestation. Partial seizures manifest as alterations in motor functions, sensory or somatosensory symptoms, or automatisms. Partial seizures with no loss of consciousness are classified as *simple partial* (SP). In some cases, patients will describe somatosensory symptoms as a "warning" prior to the development of a generalized tonic–clonic (GTC) seizure. These warnings are, in fact, SP seizures and frequently are termed auras.

Partial seizures with an alteration of consciousness are described as *complex partial* (CP). With CP seizures, the patient can have automatisms, periods of memory loss, or aberrations of behavior. Some patients with CP epilepsy have been mistakenly diagnosed as having psychotic episodes. CP seizures also can progress to GTC seizures. Patients with CP seizures typically are amnestic to these events. A partial seizure that becomes generalized is referred to as a *secondarily generalized seizure*.

Generalized seizures have clinical manifestations that indicate involvement of both hemispheres. Motor manifestations are bilateral, and there is a loss of consciousness. Generalized seizures can be further subdivided by EEG and clinical manifestations. Generalized absence seizures are manifested by a sudden onset, interruption of ongoing activities, a blank stare, and possibly a brief upward rotation of the eyes. They generally occur in young children through adolescence. It is important to differentiate absence seizures from CP seizures.

With GTC seizures there is a sudden sharp tonic contraction of muscles followed by a period of rigidity and clonic movements. During the seizure, the patient may cry or moan, lose sphincter control, bite the tongue, or develop cyanosis. After the seizure, the patient may have altered consciousness, drowsiness, or confusion for a variable period of time (postictal period) and frequently goes into a deep sleep. Tonic and clonic seizures can also occur separately.

Brief shock-like muscular contractions of the face, trunk, and extremities are known as *myoclonic jerks*. They can be isolated events or rapidly repetitive. A sudden loss of muscle tone is known as an *atonic seizure*, which may present as a head drop, the dropping of a limb, or a slumping to the ground. These patients often wear protective head ware to prevent trauma.

The International Classification of Epilepsies and Epilepsy Syndromes adds components such as age of onset, intellectual development, findings on neurologic examination, and results of neuroimaging studies to define epilepsy syndromes more fully. Syndromes can include one or many different seizure types (e.g., Lennox–Gastaut syndrome). The syndromic approach includes seizure type(s) and possible etiologic classifications (e.g., idiopathic, symptomatic, or unknown). *Idiopathic* describes syndromes that are presumably genetic but also those in which no underlying etiology is documented or suspected. A family history of seizures is commonly present, and neurologic function is essentially normal except for the occurrence of seizures. *Symptomatic* cases involve evidence of brain damage or a known underlying cause. A *cryptogenic* syndrome is assumed to be symptomatic of an underlying condition that cannot be documented. Unknown or undetermined is used when no cause can be identified. This syndromic classification requires more information and is more important for prognostic determinations and response to treatment than for a classification based simply on seizure type.

TREATMENT

Desired Outcomes

1 The ideal goal of treatment for epilepsy is complete elimination of seizures and no side effects with an optimal quality of life (QOL). Data from a large systematic review found that optimal QOL in epilepsy patients is defined by decreasing their seizure frequency and severity as well as addressing comorbid conditions, especially anxiety and depression.[6] A large multicenter study found that in pharmacoresistant epilepsy patients, the adverse effects of their AEDs and depressive comorbidity were far more important in determining QOL than reducing the frequency of their seizures when seizure freedom cannot be obtained.[7] In addition, other factors that can impact QOL in epilepsy patients include issues about driving, economic security, forming relationships, safety, social isolation, and social stigma.

The American Academy of Neurology (AAN) has developed eight quality performance measures for the clinician that define a high quality of care of these patients.[8] In a recent survey of practicing neurologists, poor performance was found on three of these eight—counseling patients about AED side effects, discussion about depression, and their knowledge about referral of the intractable epilepsy patient for surgery.[9] Lastly in helping to address QOL in epilepsy patients, an international consensus group has recently developed evidenced-based and practice-based statements to provide guidance on the management of neuropsychiatric conditions associated with epilepsy including depression.[10]

Clinical **Controversy. . .**

A significant amount of accumulating data suggests that treatment-resistant epilepsy may be intertwined with the presence of anxiety and/or depression in many epilepsy patients. In some patients the presence of bilateral hippocampal atrophy, diffuse cortical atrophy, or both in those persons with a history of depressive disorder at time of onset of epilepsy may provide a possible explanation for a very poor treatment response to AEDs. In addition, the issue of increased suicide rate seen in patients on AEDs may be influenced by the presence of these conditions. Until more valid data are collected in this area, it is the responsibility of the clinician treating the patient to make sure these conditions are carefully taken into account when selecting the appropriate AED therapy.

General Approach to Treatment

2 The general approach to treatment involves assessment of seizure type and frequency, identification of treatment goals, development of a care plan, and a plan for followup evaluation. During the assessment phase, it is critical to establish an accurate diagnosis of the seizure type and classification in order to select the appropriate initial AEDs. Patient-specific treatment goals must be identified, and these can change over time. Despite appropriate AED treatment, approximately 30% to 35% of patients are refractory to treatment. In this setting, seizure freedom may not be obtained, and more obtainable goals should be established (e.g., decrease in the number of seizures and minimized drug adverse effects).

3 Patient characteristics such as age, medical condition, ability to comply with a prescribed regimen, and insurance coverage also should be explored because these can influence AED choices or help to explain nonadherence to the regimen, a lack of response, or unexpected adverse effects.

Once the assessment is complete, for patients with new-onset seizures, the choice is whether to use drug therapy and, if so, which one. For a patient with long-standing epilepsy, adequacy of the current medication regimen must be evaluated. An AED should not be considered ineffective unless the patient has experienced unacceptable adverse effects with continued seizures.

4 If a decision is made to start AED therapy, monotherapy is preferred, and approximately 50% to 70% of all patients with epilepsy can be maintained on one drug.[11] However, many of these patients are not seizure free. The percentage of patients who are seizure free on one drug varies by seizure type. After 12 months of treatment, the percentage who are seizure free is highest for those who have only GTC seizures (48% to 55%), lowest for those who have only CP seizures (23% to 26%), and intermediate for those with mixed seizure types (25% to 32%).[11] Combining AEDs with different mechanisms of action to achieve freedom from seizures may be advantageous, although this approach is as yet unproven. Approximately 65% of patients can be expected to be maintained on one AED and be considered well controlled, although not necessarily seizure free.

5 Of the 35% of patients with unsatisfactory control, 10% will be well controlled with a two-drug treatment. Of the remaining 25%, 20% will continue to have unsatisfactory control despite multiple drug treatment. There may be a genetic predisposition to epilepsy that is refractory to drug therapy. Some of these patients may become candidates for surgery or vagal nerve stimulator.

Once the care plan is established, an AED is selected. Patient education and assurance of patient understanding of the plan are essential. Detailed directions regarding titration, what to do in the event of a treatment-emergent side effect, and what to do if a seizure occurs must be provided to patients. Documentation of the assessment, care plan, and educational process is essential. Providing the patient with a seizure and side-effect diary will assist in the followup and evaluation phase. At the followup stage of treatment (which can be done in the hospital, clinic, pharmacy, or by phone), the treatment goals must be reviewed. If the goal has been achieved, new goals should be identified. For example, if the GTC seizures are now controlled, the goal may be to control partial seizures. If a patient fails to respond to the first AEDs, trials with other AEDs should be attempted as appropriate. Completion of the evaluation often requires a reassessment of the patient and development of a new care plan taking into account patient compliance, efficacy, and safety of the initial treatment.

Medication noncompliance can be the single most common reason for treatment failure. It is estimated that up to 60% of patients with epilepsy are noncompliant.[12] The rate of noncompliance is increased by the complexity of the drug regimen and by doses taken three and four times a day. Frequent uncontrolled seizures can also predispose a patient to noncompliance secondary to confusion over whether the drug was taken. Noncompliance is not influenced by age, sex, psychomotor development, or seizure type.[12]

TABLE 40-2 Recurrence Risk for Patients Experiencing One Unprovoked Seizure

Type of Patient	First-Year Risk (%)	Fifth-Year Risk (%)
Adults with single unproved seizure		34
No CNS insult	10	29
Influence of family history		
Sibling with seizure	29	46
No sibling with seizures	7	27
EEG patterns		
GSW on EEG	15	58
Normal EEG	9	26
Occurrence of previous seizure	10	39
Caused by an illness or childhood febrile seizure		
Remote symptomatic	26	48
With Todd's paresis	41	75
Status epilepticus at onset	37	56
Prior acute seizure	60	80
Idiopathic	10	29

EEG, electroencephalogram; GSW, generalized spikes and waves.
Data from Leppik[13] and Gross-Tsur et al.[15]

Difference of opinion exists on the most appropriate time to initiate AED therapy. Treatment decisions vary depending on individual patient clinical characteristics and circumstances. Some clinicians start AED treatment after the first seizure, whereas others do not initiate treatment until a second, unprovoked seizure has occurred. Still others initiate prophylactic treatment following a CNS insult thought likely to cause epilepsy eventually (e.g., stroke or head trauma). Drug treatment may not be indicated when seizures have minimal impact on patients' lives or when there has been only a single seizure. If a patient presents after a single isolated seizure, one of three treatment decisions can be made: treat, possibly treat, or do not treat. These decisions are based on the probability of the patient having a second seizure (Table 40-2). For patients with no risk factors, the probability of a second seizure is less than 10% in the first year and approximately 24% by the end of 2 years. If risk factors are present, the recurrence rate can be as high as 80% after 5 years.[13] The decision on whether to start AED therapy often depends on patient-specific factors such as epilepsy syndrome, seizure etiology, presence of a neuroanatomic defect, and the EEG, as well as, the patient's lifestyle and preferences. Patients who have had two or more seizures generally should be started on AEDs.

When to Stop Antiepileptic Drugs

The AEDs used to control seizures may not need to be given for a lifetime. Polypharmacy can be reduced, and some patients can discontinue AEDs altogether. The drug considered less appropriate for the seizure type (or the agent deemed most responsible for adverse effects) should be discontinued first. In some cases, decreasing the number of AEDs can decrease side effects and increase cognitive abilities. This improvement in cognition may be small, especially if the patient is on a drug that primarily affects psychomotor speed with less effect on higher-order cognitive functioning.

6 Factors favoring successful withdrawal of AEDs include a seizure-free period of 2 to 4 years, complete seizure control within 1 year of onset, an onset of seizures after age 2 but before age 35,

and a normal neurologic examination and EEG. Factors associated with a poor prognosis in discontinuing AEDs, despite a seizure-free interval, include a history of a high frequency of seizures, repeated episodes of status epilepticus (SE), a combination of seizure types, and development of abnormal mental functioning. A 2-year seizure-free period is suggested for absence and rolandic epilepsy, whereas a 4-year seizure-free period is suggested for SP, CP, and absence seizures associated with tonic–clonic seizures. AED withdrawal generally is not suggested for patients with juvenile myoclonic epilepsy (JME), absence with clonic–tonic–clonic seizures, or clonic–tonic–clonic seizures. The AAN has issued guidelines for discontinuing AEDs in seizure-free patients.[14] After assessing the risks and benefits to both the patient and society, AED withdrawal can be considered in a patient meeting the following profile: seizure free for 2 to 5 years, a history of a single type of partial seizure or primary GTC seizures, a normal neurologic exam and normal IQ, and an EEG that has normalized with treatment. When these factors are present, the relapse rate is expected to be less than 32% for children and 39% for adults.

AED withdrawal should be done gradually, especially in patients with profound developmental disabilities. Some patients will have a recurrence of seizures as the AEDs are withdrawn. Sudden withdrawal is associated with the precipitation of SE. Withdrawal seizures are of particular concern for agents such as benzodiazepines and barbiturates. Seizure relapse has been reported to be more common if these AEDs are withdrawn over 1 to 3 months compared to over 6 months.

The risk of seizure relapse has been estimated at 10% to 70%. A meta-analysis determined that the relapse rate was 25% after 1 year and 29% after 2 years. Recurrence of seizures tends to occur early with at least one-half of the recurrences within 6 months of AED withdrawal and 60% to 90% within 1 year. Patients who relapse will generally become seizure free and in remission after AEDs are restarted although not necessarily immediately. The underlying epilepsy syndrome appears to determine prognosis for long-term remission.[15]

Clinical **Controversy...**

It is not entirely clear which patients with epilepsy will require lifelong treatment. Although many clinicians feel that AED therapy is lifelong, others would argue that certain patients with idiopathic epilepsy and a normal neurologic examination and EEG are candidates for AED withdrawal following a prolonged period of seizure freedom (e.g., greater than 2 to 3 years). A large amount of the data supporting discontinuing AEDs has been obtained from children. Some adults will be reticent to discontinue AED therapy even if the clinician is in favor of it because of the fear of having a seizure and the consequences (e.g., loss of driver's license) that it would entail. The patient should agree and must be a willing participant in the plan to reduce or withdraw AED therapy.

Nonpharmacologic Therapy

Nonpharmacologic therapy for epilepsy includes diet, surgery, and vagus nerve stimulation (VNS). A vagal nerve stimulator is an implanted medical device that is Food and Drug Administration (FDA) approved for use as adjunctive therapy in reducing the frequency of seizures in adults and adolescents older than 12 years of age with partial-onset seizures that are refractory to AEDs. It is also used off-label in the treatment of refractory primary generalized epilepsy. The mechanisms of antiseizure actions of VNS are unknown. Human clinical studies have shown that VNS changes the cerebrospinal fluid (CSF) concentration of inhibitory and stimulatory neurotransmitters and activates specific areas of the brain that generate or regulate cortical seizure activity through increased blood flow. There is experimental evidence to suggest that the anticonvulsant effect of VNS is mediated by the locus coeruleus.[16]

The VNS device is relatively safe. It may also have a positive effect on mood and behavior, often independent of seizure reduction. The most common side effect associated with stimulation is hoarseness, voice alteration, increased cough, pharyngitis, dyspnea, dyspepsia, and nausea. Serious adverse effects reported include infection, nerve paralysis, hypoesthesia, facial paresis, left vocal cord paralysis, left facial paralysis, left recurrent laryngeal nerve injury, urinary retention, and low-grade fever. In the VNS studies, the percentage of patients who achieved a 50% or greater reduction in their seizure frequency (responders) ranged from 23% to 50%.

7 Surgery is the treatment of choice in selected patients with refractory focal epilepsy, especially those patients with seizures originating from the temporal lobe.[17] The Early Randomized Surgery for Epilepsy trial resulted in freedom from seizures in 78% of newly refractory temporal lobe epilepsy patients, and none were seizure free in the group on standard drug therapy. Surgery reduces the risk of epilepsy-associated death, and it may also improve depression and anxiety in refractory epilepsy patients.[18,19] A systematic review/meta-analysis of published evidence of temporal lobe patients with pharmacoresistant epilepsy concluded that the combination of surgery with medical treatment is four times as likely as medical treatment alone to achieve freedom from seizures.[20] A National Institutes of Health Consensus Conference identified three absolute requirements for surgery. They are (a) an absolute diagnosis of epilepsy, (b) failure on an adequate trial of drug therapy, and (c) definition of the electroclinical syndrome. A focus in the temporal lobe has the best chance for a positive outcome; however, extratemporal foci can be excised successfully in more than 75% of patients. The procedure is not without risk. Learning and memory can be impaired postoperatively, and general intellectual abilities are also affected in a small number of patients. Surgery may be particularly useful in children with intractable epilepsy. Patients may need to continue AED therapy for a period of time following successful epilepsy surgery, but dosage reduction may be achieveable.[21]

The ketogenic diet, devised in the 1920s, is high in fat and low in carbohydrates and protein, and it leads to acidosis and ketosis. Protein and calorie intake are set at levels that will meet requirements for growth. Most of the calories are provided in the form of heavy cream and butter. No sugar is allowed. Vitamins and minerals are supplemented. Medium-chain triglycerides can be substituted for the dietary fats. Fluids are also controlled. It requires strict control and parent compliance. Although some centers find the diet useful for refractory patients, others have found that it is poorly tolerated by patients. Long-term effects include kidney stones, increased bone fractures, and adverse effects on growth.[22] An international consensus statement has been published, which offers recommendations employing various forms of the ketogenic diet which may be more tolerable, including the use of the modified Atkins diet and the Low Glycemic Index Treatment.[23] Subsequent data support the use of these variations in the ketogenic diet, as well as the medium chain triglyceride ketogenic diet in select patients.[24]

Pharmacologic Therapy

Optimal management of epilepsy requires that AED treatment be individualized. Different patient groups (e.g., children, women of child-bearing potential, and the elderly) may be better suited to receive one AED than another by virtue not only of seizure type

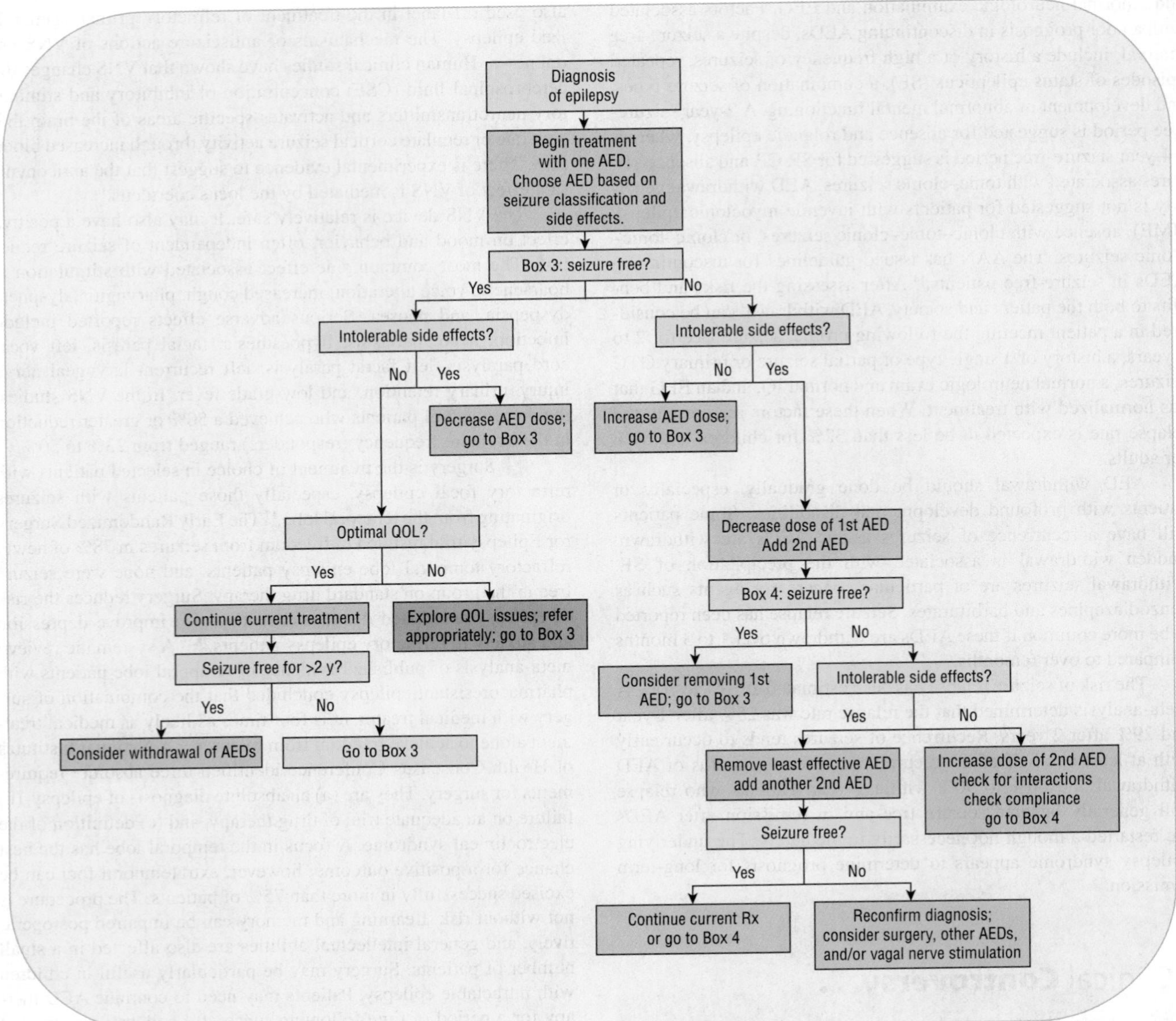

FIGURE 40-1 Algorithm for the treatment of epilepsy. (AED, antiepileptic drug; QOL, quality of life.)

but also of susceptibility or relative risk for certain adverse effects. These issues are highlighted further below.

8 Selection and optimization of AED therapy require not only an understanding of drug mechanism(s) of action and spectrum of clinical activity, but also an appreciation of pharmacokinetic variability and patterns of drug-related adverse effects. An AED must be effective for the specific seizure type being treated. The drug treatments of first choice depend on the type of epilepsy, drug-specific adverse effects, and patient preferences. Ultimately, AED effectiveness is the result of the interaction of each of these factors. A suggested algorithm for a general approach to the treatment of epilepsy is shown in Figure 40-1.

Table 40-3 provides evidenced-based treatment recommendations by three professional/regulatory bodies.[25–28] In addition, recommendations from a U.S. panel of experts, which included more recent drug treatment data compared to the AAN–American Epilepsy Society (AES) recommendations are included.[29]

The mechanism of action of most AEDs can be categorized as (a) affecting ion channel kinetics, (b) augmenting inhibitory neurotransmission, or (c) modulating excitatory neurotransmission. Augmentation in inhibitory neurotransmission includes increasing CNS concentrations of GABA, whereas efforts to decrease excitatory neurotransmission are primarily focused on decreasing (or antagonizing) glutamate and aspartate neurotransmission. AEDs that are effective against GTC and partial seizures probably reduce sustained repetitive firing of action potentials by delaying recovery of sodium channels from activation. Drugs that reduce corticothalamic T-type calcium currents are effective against generalized absence seizures. Myoclonic seizures respond to drugs that enhance $GABA_A$-receptor inhibition. In addition to mechanism of action, awareness of pharmacokinetic properties (Table 40-4), adverse effects (Table 40-5), and AED metabolic pathway as well as inducer or inhibitory effects on liver (Table 40-6) can aid in the optimization of AED therapy. Pharmacokinetic interactions are a common complicating factor in AED selection. Interactions can occur in any of the pharmacokinetic processes: absorption, distribution, metabolism, or elimination. Caution should be used when AEDs are added to or withdrawn from a drug regimen.

TABLE 40-3 Drugs of Choice for Specific Seizure Disorders

Seizure Type	First-Line Drugs	Alternative Drugs[a]	Comments
Partial seizures (newly diagnosed)			
U.S. guidelines[25,26]	*Adults and adolescents:* Carbamazepine Gabapentin Oxcarbazepine Phenobarbital Phenytoin Topiramate Valproic acid		*FDA approved:* Carbamazepine Lacosamide Phenobarbital Phenytoin Topiramate Valproic acid
U.K. guidelines[27]	Carbamazepine Lamotrigine	Levetiracetam Oxcarbazepine Valproic acid	
ILAE guidelines[28]	*Adults:* Carbamazepine Phenytoin Valproic acid *Children:* Oxcarbazepine *Elderly:* Gabapentin Lamotrigine	*Adults:* Gabapentin Lamotrigine Oxcarbazepine Phenobarbital Topiramate *Children:* Phenobarbital Phenytoin Topiramate Valproic acid *Elderly:* Carbamazepine	
U.S. Expert Panel 2005[29]	Carbamazepine Lamotrigine Oxcarbazepine	Levetiracetam	
Partial seizures (refractory monotherapy)			
U.S. guidelines[25,26]	Lamotrigine Oxcarbazepine Topiramate		*FDA approved:* Carbamazepine Lamotrigine Oxcarbazepine Phenobarbital Phenytoin Topiramate Valproic acid
U.K. guidelines[27]	Lamotrigine Oxcarbazepine Topiramate		
Partial seizures (refractory adjunct)			
U.S. guidelines[25,26]	*Adults:* Gabapentin Lamotrigine Levetiracetam Oxcarbazepine Tiagabine Topiramate Zonisamide *Children:* Gabapentin Lamotrigine Oxcarbazepine Topiramate		*FDA approved:* Carbamazepine Gabapentin Lamotrigine Levetiracetam Oxcarbazepine Phenobarbital Phenytoin Pregabalin Tiagabine Valproic acid Vigabatrin Zonisamide
U.K. guidelines[27]	Carbamazepine Clobazam Gabapentin Lamotrigine Levetiracetam Oxcarbazepine Valproic acid Topiramate	Lacosamide Phenobarbital Phenytoin Pregabalin Tiagabine Vigabatrin Zonisamide	
Generalized seizures absence (newly diagnosed)			
U.S. guidelines[25,26]	Lamotrigine		*FDA approved:* Ethosuximide Valproic acid
U.K. guidelines[27]	Ethosuximide Lamotrigine Valproic Acid	Clobazam Clonazepam Levetiracetam Topiramate Zonisamide	
ILAE guidelines[28]	None	Ethosuximide Lamotrigine Valproic acid	
U.S. Expert Panel 2005[29]	Ethosuximide Valproic acid	Lamotrigine	
Primary generalized (tonic–clonic)			
U.S. guidelines[25,26]	Topiramate		*FDA approved:* Lamotrigine Levetiracetam Topiramate
U.K. guidelines[27]	In following order: Valproic acid Lamotrigine Carbamazepine Oxcarbazepine	Clobazam Levetiracetam Topiramate	
ILAE guidelines[28]	None	*Adults:* Carbamazepine Lamotrigine Oxcarbazepine Phenobarbital Phenytoin Topiramate Valproic acid Children: Carbamazepine Phenobarbital Phenytoin Topiramate Valproic acid	
U.S. Expert Panel 2005[29]	Valproic acid	Lamotrigine Topiramate	
Juvenile myoclonic epilepsy			*FDA approved:* Levetiracetam (myoclonic seizures)
U.K guidelines[27]	Ethosuximide Lamotrigine Valproic acid	Clobazam Clonazepam Levetiracetam Topiramate Zonisamide	
ILAE[28]	None	Clonazepam Lamotrigine Levetiracetam Topiramate Valproic acid Zonisamide	
U.S. Expert Panel 2005[29]	Valproic acid	Levetiracetam Topiramate Zonisamide	

ILAE, International League Against Epilepsy.

[a]Includes possibly effective drugs.

Data from French et al.,[25,26] National Institute for Clinical Excellence,[27] Glauser et al.,[28] and Karceski et al.[29]

TABLE 40-4 Antiepileptic Drug Pharmacokinetic Data

AED	$t_{1/2}$ (Hours)	Time to Steady State (Days)	Unchanged (%)	V_D (L/kg)	Clinically Important Metabolite	Protein Binding (%)
Carbamazepine	12 M; 5–14 Co	21–28 for completion of autoinduction	<1	1–2	10,11-epoxide	40–90
Clobazam	36–42	7–14	3	1.4	*N*-desmethyl clobazam	80–90
Ethosuximide	A 60; C 30	6–12	10–20	0.67	No	0
Ezogabine	7–11	3–4	36%	2–3	*n*-Acetylmetabolite	80
Felbamate	16–22	5–7	50	0.73–0.82	No	~25
Gabapentin[a]	5–40[b]	1–2	100	0.65–1.04	No	0
Lacosamide	13	3	40	0.6	No	<15
Lamotrigine	25.4 M	3–15	0	1.28	No	40–50
Levetiracetam	7–10	2		0.7	No	<10
Oxcarbazepine	3–13	2		0.7	10-Hydroxy-carbazepine	40
Phenobarbital	A 46–136; C 37–73	14–21	20–40	0.6	No	50
Phenytoin	A 10–34; C 5–14	7–28	<5	0.6–8.0	No	90
Pregabalin	A 6–7[b]	1–2	90	0.5	No	0
Primidone	A 3.3–19; C 4.5–11	1–4	40	0.43–1.1	PB	80
Rufinamide	6–10	2	4	0.8-1.2	No	26–35
Tiagabine	5–13		Negligible		No	95
Topiramate	18–21	4–5	50–70	0.55–0.8 (male); 0.23–0.4 (female)	No	15
Valproic acid	A 8–20; C 7–14	1–3	<5	0.1–0.5	May contribute to toxicity	90–95 binding saturates
Vigabatrin	5–8	N/A	<2	0.8	No	0
Zonisamide	24–60	5–15		0.8–1.6	No	40–60

A, adult; AED, antiepileptic drug; C, child; Co, combination therapy; M, monotherapy; N/A, not applicable since effect depends on inhibiting enzyme; PB, phenobarbital; V_D, volume of distribution.

[a]The bioavailability of gabapentin is dose-dependent.

[b]Half-life depends on renal function.

Data from Faught,[30] Leppik,[31] Patsalos et al.,[32] Onfi [package insert],[33] and Potiga [package insert].[34]

Adverse effects of AEDs can be divided into acute and chronic (see Table 40-5). Acute effects can be dose/serum concentration-related or idiosyncratic. Concentration-dependent effects are common and troublesome but not usually life-threatening. Neurotoxic adverse effects are encountered commonly and can include sedation, dizziness, blurred or double vision, difficulty with concentration, and ataxia. In many cases, these effects can be alleviated by decreasing the dose or avoided in some cases by titrating the dose upward very slowly. Most idiosyncratic reactions are mild, but they can be more serious if the hypersensitivity involves one or more organ systems. Other idiosyncratic side effects including hepatitis or blood dyscrasias are serious but rare.

Acute organ failure, when it occurs, generally occurs within the first 6 months of AED therapy. Unfortunately, laboratory screening evaluations of blood and urine typically are not helpful in predicting or detecting the early stage of severe reactions and generally are not recommended in asymptomatic patients. An exception to this is in the screening of patients of Southeast Asian heritage for HLA-B*1502 antigen who are to receive carbamazepine and possibly phenytoin, lamotrigine, and oxcarbazepine. There is a strong association between the presence of this antigen and Stevens–Johnson syndrome as well as toxic epidermal necrolysis.[38] In addition the HLA genotype HLA-A*3101 has been found to be associated with multiple carbamazepine-induced cutaneous reactions in Chinese, Japanese, and European populations.[38] In any patient, laboratory assessment, including white blood cell (WBC) counts and liver function tests, may be reasonable if the patient reports an unexplained illness (e.g., lethargy, vomiting, fever, or rash).[7] It is important to note that patients dosed and maintained within "therapeutic ranges" are also capable of experiencing toxicities to AEDs.[32] Another potential long-term adverse effect of AED treatment is osteomalacia and osteoporosis.[39,40] The bone disorders associated with AED use are a heterogeneous group of disorders, ranging from asymptomatic high-turnover disease, with findings of normal bone mineral density, to markedly decreased bone mineral density sufficient to warrant the diagnosis of osteoporosis. While the etiology of these osteopathies is uncertain, it has been hypothesized that certain drugs, including phenytoin, phenobarbital, carbamazepine, oxcarbazepine, felbamate, and valproic acid, may interfere with vitamin D metabolism; at least for the CYP3A4 inducers this activity may be explained by recent findings of an inducible CYP3A4-dependent vitamin D pathway.[41] Whether the other AEDs cause these effects is unknown, however, current evidence suggests that lamotrigine does not. Common laboratory findings in these patients include elevated bone-specific alkaline phosphatase concentration, intact parathyroid hormone, and decreased serum calcium and 25-OH vitamin D concentrations. Patients receiving these drugs should receive supplemental vitamin D and calcium, as well as bone mineral density testing if other risk factors for osteoporosis are present.

Comparative data now exist between some of the older AEDs, carbamazepine, phenytoin, and valproic acid and the newer agents, levetiracetam, lamotrigine, and topiramate (low dose) that suggest the older agents increase circulatory vascular risk markers, which may contribute to acceleration of atherosclerosis and that this effect is treatment duration dependent.[42,43]

The comparative effects of AEDs on cognition have been difficult to evaluate because of differences or inconsistencies in study design, seizure types studied, control for serum drug concentrations,

TABLE 40-5 Antiepileptic Drug Side Effects and Monitoring

Drug	Adverse Drug Reaction Acute Side Effects: Concentration Dependent	Adverse Drug Reaction Acute Side Effects: Idiosyncratic	Chronic Side Effects
Carbamazepine	Diplopia Dizziness Drowsiness Nausea Unsteadiness Lethargy	Blood dyscrasias Rash (HLA antigen testing may be relevant to avoid Stevens–Johnson or toxic epidermal necrolysis)	Hyponatremia Metabolic bone disease (monitor vit D and serum calcium)
Clobazam	Somnolence Sedation Pyrexia Ataxia	Drooling Aggression Irritability Constipation	
Ethosuximide	Ataxia Drowsiness GI distress (avoid by multiple daily dosing) Unsteadiness Hiccoughs	Blood dyscrasias Rash	Behavior changes Headache
Ezogabine	Dizziness Somnolence Fatigue Confusion Vertigo Tremors Blurred vision	Urinary retention QT prolongation (get baseline EKG and during treatment) Euphoria	Not established
Felbamate	Anorexia Nausea Vomiting Insomnia Headache	Aplastic anemia (follow CBC) Acute hepatic failure (follow liver enzymes)	Not established
Gabapentin	Dizziness Fatigue Somnolence Ataxia	Pedal edema	Weight gain
Lacosamide	Dizziness Vertigo Headache Nausea Vomiting PR interval increase (get baseline EKG and during treatment)	Liver enzyme elevation	Not established
Lamotrigine	Diplopia Dizziness Unsteadiness Headache	Rash (slower titration of dose may decrease chance of occurrence)	Not established
Levetiracetam	Sedation Behavioral disturbance	Psychosis (rare but more common in elderly or persons with mental illness)	Not established
Oxcarbazepine	Sedation Dizziness Ataxia Nausea	Rash	Hyponatremia
Phenobarbital	Ataxia Hyperactivity Headache Unsteadiness Sedation Nausea	Blood dyscrasias Rash	Behavior changes Connective tissue disorders Intellectual blunting Metabolic bone disease Mood change Sedation
Phenytoin	Ataxia Nystagmus Behavior changes Dizziness Headache Incoordination Sedation Lethargy Cognitive impairment Fatigue Visual blurring	Blood dyscrasias Rash (HLA antigen testing may be relevant to avoid Stevens–Johnson or toxic epidermal necrolysis) Immunologic reaction	Behavior changes Cerebellar syndrome (occurs high serum levels) Connective tissue changes Skin thickening Folate deficiency Gingival hyperplasia Hirsutism Coarsening of facial features Acne Cognitive impairment Metabolic bone disease (monitor vit D and serum calcium) Sedation

(*continued*)

TABLE 40-5 Antiepileptic Drug Side Effects and Monitoring (*Continued*)

Drug	Adverse Drug Reaction Acute Side Effects: Concentration Dependent	Adverse Drug Reaction Acute Side Effects: Idiosyncratic	Chronic Side Effects
Pregabalin	Dizziness Somnolence Incoordination Dry mouth Blurred vision	Pedal edema Creatine kinase elevation Decrease platelets	Weight gain
Primidone	Behavior changes Headache Nausea Sedation Unsteadiness	Blood dyscrasias Rash	Behavior change Connective tissue disorders Cognitive impairment Sedation
Rufinamide	Dizziness Nausea Vomiting Somnolence	Multiorgan hypersensitivity Status epilepticus Leukopenia QT shortening	Not established
Tiagabine	Dizziness Fatigue Difficulties concentrating Nervousness Tremor Blurred vision Depression Weakness	Spike-wave stupor	Not established
Topiramate	Difficulties concentrating Psychomotor slowing Speech or language problems Somnolence, fatigue Dizziness Headache	Metabolic acidosis Acute angle glaucoma Oligohydrosis	Kidney stones Weight loss
Valproic acid	GI upset Sedation Unsteadiness Tremor Thrombocytopenia	Acute hepatic failure Acute pancreatitis Alopecia	Polycystic ovary-like syndrome (increase incidence in females <20 years or overweight) Weight gain Hyperammonemia Menstrual cycle irregularities
Vigabatrin	Permanent vision loss Fatigue Somnolence Weight gain Tremor Blurred vision	Abnormal MRI brain signal changes (infants with infantile spasms) Peripheral neuropathy Anemia	Permanent vision loss (greater frequency, adults vs. children vs. infants)
Zonisamide	Sedation Dizziness Cognitive impairment Nausea	Rash (is a sulfa drug) Metabolic acidosis Oligohydrosis	Kidney stones Weight loss

Data from French et al.,[25,26] Leppik,[31] Halford and Lapointe,[35] Cada et al.,[36] Sabril [package insert],[37] Onfi [package insert],[33] and Potiga [package insert].[34]

and the neuropsychologic tests used. In general, there are not large differences between the older drugs, although the barbiturates, phenobarbital and primidone, appear to cause more cognitive impairment than other commonly used AEDs.[44,45] Phenytoin, particularly when serum concentrations are above the commonly accepted therapeutic range, may have a greater effect on motor function and speed. Among the older AEDs, valproic acid may cause less impairment of cognition. Improvement in cognition has been reported in patients switched from phenytoin or phenobarbital to valproic acid. However, these improvements are subtle if patients are in the same relative area of the therapeutic range. Patients changed from polytherapy to monotherapy also may demonstrate improvement in cognition. Some of the newer agents are believed to cause fewer neurobehavioral or cognitive effects. Among the newer AEDs, gabapentin and lamotrigine have been shown in several studies to cause fewer cognitive impairments compared with older agents, such as carbamazepine.[46–48] Conversely, topiramate may cause substantial cognitive impairment, particularly when used at high doses or during rapid dose escalation.[48] In addition, these patients may not be fully aware of their deficits.[49,50] AED treatment itself may sometimes worsen seizures due to improper AED selection for a specific seizure type or syndrome or can represent a paradoxical toxic effect of the drug.[51]

Because most adult patients have localization-related (partial-onset) seizures, the most widely used AEDs traditionally have been carbamazepine, phenobarbital, phenytoin, and valproic acid. For CP seizures, these AEDs have similar efficacy.[52,53] Of these, carbamazepine and phenytoin are the most commonly prescribed AEDs for partial seizures in the United States. This preference is largely based on data derived from two landmark trials conducted through the Veterans Administration (VA) Epilepsy Cooperative Study Group. In the first of these trials, patients with new-onset partial or generalized epilepsy were randomized to receive either carbamazepine, phenobarbital, phenytoin, or primidone.[52] After 3 years, patients who received either carbamazepine or phenytoin were equally likely, and patients on phenobarbital or primidone were least likely to have remained on their originally assigned treatment. Thus, carbamazepine and phenytoin were considered the drugs of first choice in patients with new-onset partial or generalized

TABLE 40-6 Antiepileptic Drugs Elimination Pathways and Major Effects on Hepatic Enzymes

Antiepileptic Drugs	Major Hepatic Enzymes	Renal Elimination (%)	Induced	Inhibited
Carbamazepine	CYP3A4; CYP1A2; CYP2C8	<1	CYP1A2; CYP2C; CYP3A; GT	None
Clobazam	CYP3A4; CYP2C19; CYP2B6	0	CYP3A4 (weak)	CYP2D6
Ethosuximide	CYP3A4	12–20	None	None
Ezogabine	GT; acetylation	85	None	None
Felbamate	CYP3A4; CYP2E1; other	50	CYP3A4	CYP2C19; β-oxidation
Gabapentin	None	Almost completely	None	None
Lacosamide	CYP2C19	70	None	None
Lamotrigine	GT	10	GT	None
Levetiracetam	None (undergoes nonhepatic hydrolysis)	66	None	None
Oxcarbazepine (MHD is active oxcarbazepine metabolite)	Cytosolic system	1 (27 as MHD)	CYP3A4; CYP3A5; GT	CYP2C19
Phenobarbital	CYP2C9; other	25	CYP3A; CYP2C; GT	None
Phenytoin	CYP2C9; CYP2C19	5	CYP3A; CYP2C; GT	
Pregabalin	None	100	None	None
Rufinamide	Hydrolysis	2	CYP3A4 (weak)	CYP2E1 (weak)
Tiagabine	CYP3A4	2	None	None
Topiramate	Not known	70	CYP3A (dose dependent)	CYP2C19
Valproate	GT; β-oxidation	2	None	CYP2C9; GT epoxide hydrolase
Vigabatrin	None	Almost completely	CYP2C9	None
Zonisamide	CYP3A4	35	None	None

CYP, cytochrome P450 isoenzyme system; GT, glucuronyltransferase.

Data from Faught,[30] Leppik,[31] Patsalos et al.,[32] Halford and Lapointe,[35] Cada et al.,[36] Sabril [package insert],[37] Onfi [package insert],[33] and Potiga [package insert].[34]

seizures. Carbamazepine was associated with fewer side effects. A followup study using almost identical methods compared carbamazepine and valproic acid.[53] Carbamazepine- and valproic acid-treated groups had equal retention rates for tonic–clonic seizures. Carbamazepine was superior to valproic acid for efficacy in the treatment of partial seizures. Valproic acid caused slightly more adverse effects.

Based primarily on these trials, carbamazepine has been recognized as the AED of first choice for partial seizures. Several of the newer generation AEDs are now proving to be reasonable alternatives. The newer AEDs were first approved as adjunctive therapy for patients with refractory partial seizures. Monotherapy trials with several of these newer agents including lamotrigine, gabapentin, topiramate, oxcarbazepine, and levetiracetam have now been completed.[54–56] Comparisons between lamotrigine and older agents, including carbamazepine and phenytoin as initial monotherapy for partial seizures have been conducted in Europe, and the results suggest comparable effectiveness and perhaps better tolerability for lamotrigine, particularly in elderly patients. In a large, unblinded, randomized, controlled trial in hospital-based outpatient clinics in the United Kingdom, lamotrigine was found to be clinically better than carbamazepine for time to treatment failure outcomes in newly diagnosed patients with partial seizures; lamotrigine was determined to be a cost-effective alternative to carbamazepine. Other drugs studied in this trial were gabapentin, oxcarbazepine, and topiramate.[57] Results from a VA cooperative trial designed to compare gabapentin, lamotrigine, and carbamazepine in newly diagnosed elderly patients with partial seizures found that lamotrigine efficacy is comparable with that of both gabapentin and carbamazepine, and is better tolerated than carbamazepine but equal to gabapentin in this population.[58] Clinical data suggest that in newly diagnosed patients, oxcarbazepine is as effective as phenytoin, valproic acid, and immediate-release carbamazepine, with perhaps fewer adverse effects. Close examination of the conversion to monotherapy trials suggests that oxcarbazepine demonstrates efficacy even in patients who previously had an inadequate response to carbamazepine, in spite of their structural similarity. Lastly, levetiracetam in a 1-year study was found to have equal efficacy and tolerability when studied against controlled-release carbamazepine.[59]

In addition, several monotherapy trials using an active control or pseudoplacebo design also have been conducted. Although these study designs provide evidence of efficacy for the newer drugs, because the comparison is between active drug and placebo in patients who continue to have seizures in spite of current treatment with standard AEDs, it is difficult to compare the efficacy of the newer drugs directly with the older AEDs. Generally speaking, the newer AEDs appear to have comparable efficacy to the older agents and are perhaps better tolerated. A recent systematic review and meta-analysis attempted to compare the efficacy and tolerability of the newer AEDs in treatment of refractory partial epilepsy as add on therapy with another AED or placebo; although the results provided indirect evidence, the authors found topiramate and probably levetiracetam more efficacious in controlling seizure frequency and gabapentin less efficacious compared to all other new AEDs. In addition, tolerability was poorer with oxcarbazepine and topiramate whereas gabapentin and levetiracetam were better tolerated with the most common side effects comparable between the new AEDs.[60]

To date, among the newer generation agents, lamotrigine, oxcarbazepine, and topiramate have received FDA approval for use as monotherapy in patients with partial seizures. Phenobarbital and primidone are also useful in partial seizures, but sedation and cognitive adverse effects limit their utility. Felbamate, which has monotherapy approval, is effective but has been associated with some significant side effects. Interpretation of monotherapy trials with the newer AEDs can be daunting owing to the unique study designs and specific patient populations employed. Withholding an effective AED (i.e., giving placebo) in patients with epilepsy is generally considered unethical. Primarily generalized seizures such as absence seizures may respond differently pharmacologically than other seizure types. Phenytoin, phenobarbital, and carbamazepine, although effective in GTC and partial seizures, are ineffective for absence seizures, and in some cases, can precipitate an increase in seizure frequency. Absence seizures are best treated with ethosuximide, valproic acid, and perhaps lamotrigine. For levetiracetam, topiramate, and zonisamide, additional data are needed to confirm efficacy. Oxcarbazepine, gabapentin, and tiagabine do not appear to be effective in treating absence seizures, and can worsen this condition in some patients. If the patient has a combination of absence and other generalized or partial seizures, valproic acid or lamotrigine is the preferred first choice because they are effective for absence and other seizure types. If valproic acid is ineffective in treating a mixed seizure disorder that includes absence, ethosuximide could be used in combination with another AED.

The traditional treatment of tonic–clonic seizures is phenytoin; however, carbamazepine and valproic acid are increasingly used because these AEDs have a lower incidence of side effects with equal efficacy. Valproic acid generally is considered the drug of first choice for atonic seizures and for JME. Lamotrigine and perhaps topiramate and zonisamide can be alternative agents for these seizure types. Levetiracetam is FDA approved as adjunctive treatment of myoclonic seizures in patients with JME.

Results of a large, unblinded, randomized, controlled trial conducted in patients with new-onset generalized and unclassified epilepsy outpatients in the United Kingdom has helped to define the role of the newer generation drugs. These researchers found that for idiopathic generalized epilepsy, valproic acid was significantly better tolerated than topiramate and more efficacious than lamotrigine.[61] A post hoc analysis of this trial delineated clinical factors significant in influencing treatment failure and in achieving a 12 month remission.[62]

Serum concentrations of the older AEDs should be viewed as a tool with which to optimize therapy for an individual patient, not as a therapeutic end point in itself. The serum concentration is a target that should be correlated with clinical response. The desired outcome is the cessation of seizures without side effects. Seizure control can occur before the "minimum" of the published therapeutic range is achieved, and side effects can appear before the "maximum" of the range is achieved. Some patients may need and tolerate concentrations beyond the maximum. The therapeutic range for AEDs can be different for different seizure types. Serum concentrations may need to be higher to control CP seizures than to control tonic–clonic seizures. Clinicians should define a therapeutic range for an individual patient above which there are side effects and below which the patient experiences seizures. Then serum levels can be useful to document lack of efficacy, loss of efficacy, noncompliance, and to determine how much room there is to increase a dose based on expected toxicity. Depending on the AED, serum levels can also be useful in patients with significant renal and/or hepatic disease, patients taking multiple drugs, and women who are pregnant or taking oral contraceptives (OCs). Therapeutic concentration ranges have not been clearly defined for some of the second-generation AEDs.

Therapeutic Considerations in the Elderly and Young

Use of AEDs in the elderly and young can pose special challenges.[32] Avoidance of AEDs that interact with other medications that the elderly are often taking is of upmost importance. Many of the AEDs are inducers or inhibitors of the cytochrome P450 (CYP450) system, which can adversely affect the drug level of concomitantly administered drugs. Hypoalbuminemia is common in the elderly, and can make monitoring and adjustment of serum drug levels of highly albumin-bound AEDs, such as phenytoin, valproic acid, and tiagabine, problematic. The elderly also experience body mass changes, such as an increase in fat to lean body mass or decrease in body water, which can affect the volume of distribution of some drugs, and therefore possibly the elimination half-life. In addition, declining renal and/or hepatic function can occur in the elderly, which can require a lower dose of the AED. Lastly, the pharmacodynamic response to AEDs can change with aging such that elderly patients may be more sensitive to various neurocognitive adverse effects. Also, elderly patients' seizures may be controlled at relatively lower total serum concentrations.

For neonates and infants, an increase in the total body water to fat ratio and a decrease in serum albumin and α-acid glycoprotein can result in volume of distribution changes that can affect the elimination half-life of the AEDs. In addition, newborns up to the age of 2 to 3 years display decreased efficiency in renal elimination, with newborns being the most affected. Hepatic activity is also reduced in this population. However, by age 2 to 3 years, hepatic activity is more robust than that seen in adults. Therefore, children require higher doses of many of the AEDs than adults, whereas neonates and infants require lower doses. Lastly, rapidly changing and sometimes inconsistent metabolism in the patient groups above make therapeutic drug monitoring especially important even though the definition of therapeutic blood level is less certain in these patients than in adults.

Therapeutic Considerations in Women (and Men)

Many hormones influence brain electrical excitability, and estrogen and progesterone may interact in complex ways to alter neuronal excitability and protein synthesis. Estrogen has a slight proconvulsant effect, whereas progesterone exerts a mild anticonvulsant effect. Estrogen has a mild inhibitory effect on GABA receptors, potentiates excitatory glutaminergic activity, and can promote the development of kindling. Progesterone has the opposite effect and appears to potentiate GABA receptor activity and reduce neuronal discharge rates. AEDs, especially hepatic metabolizing enzyme inducers, increase the metabolism of these hormones and induce the production of sex hormone-binding globulin. This may lead to decreases in the unbound fraction of the hormone. Enzyme-inducing AEDs, including topiramate and oxcarbazepine at higher doses, can cause treatment failures in women taking OCs owing to induction of the metabolism of ethinyl estradiol and progestin. This may also be an issue with rufinamide, lamotrigine, clobazam, and felbamate, all which have a small effect in decreasing the bioavailability of OCs. A supplemental form of birth control, in addition to OCs, is advised if breakthrough bleeding occurs. However medroxyprogesterone depot injection, copper intrauterine devices, and hormone-releasing intrauterine systems are not affected by AEDs. There are no data available on the efficacy of the transdermal contraceptive patch or the emergency contraceptive pill in patients taking these AEDs, but it has been suggested that women use twice the normal dose of the postcoital pill.[63] Valproic acid, benzodiazepines, except clobazam, and most of the newer AEDs, such as gabapentin, levetiracetam, tiagabine, zonisamide, vigabatrin, and lacosamide, are not enzyme inducers and have not been implicated in reducing contraceptive effectiveness. Of note, OCs lower lamotrigine's serum level significantly and lower valproic acid's level about 20%.[32]

In some women, vulnerability to seizures is highest just before and during the menstrual flow (catamenial seizures) and at the time of ovulation. The increased susceptibility to seizures during those catamenial periods is associated with a slight increase of estrogen relative to progesterone. The risk of catamenial epilepsy is estimated at 12.5%, but it may be as high as 50% in women with epilepsy. This pattern of seizure exacerbation can also be related to progesterone withdrawal and changes in the estrogen-to-progesterone ratio. Conventional AEDs should be used as primary agents but intermittent supplementation with higher dose of AED or benzodiazepines should be considered. Acetazolamide also has been used during catamenial periods but with variable and limited success. Hormonal therapy with progestational agents, particularly cyclic natural progesterone therapy, may be effective.

Reproductive endocrine disorders are common in women with epilepsy and include menstrual irregularity, infertility, sexual dysfunction, and in some patients polycystic ovary syndrome (PCOS).[64] Potential mechanisms for these disturbances include disruption of the hypothalamic–pituitary–adrenal (HPA) axis via seizure discharges in limbic structures and/or AEDs.[64] AEDs, particularly the enzyme-inducing agents (e.g., carbamazepine, phenytoin, and phenobarbital), also may affect HPA function by altering the metabolism of the neuroactive sex hormones, including testosterone. Valproic acid is associated with increasing changes in sex hormone concentrations that causes hyperandrogenism and polycystic changes regardless if the patient has epilepsy, especially in women who have gained weight or those who start valproic acid at age less than 20 years.[64]

During pregnancy there may be increased maternal seizures, pregnancy complications, and adverse fetal outcome.[65] Approximately 25% to 30% of pregnant women have increased seizures, whereas seizures decrease in a similar number. However, the risk of seizures is significantly less if the patient has been seizure free 12 months prior to the pregnancy.[66] Increased seizure frequency may result from either a direct effect on seizure threshold or a reduction in AED concentration. An increase in clearance has been reported for phenytoin, carbamazepine, phenobarbital, ethosuximide, lamotrigine, oxcarbazepine, levetiracetam, topiramate, and clorazepate during pregnancy. Protein binding may also be reduced. The altered disposition of AEDs can begin as early as the first 10 weeks of pregnancy, and may require up to 4 weeks postpartum to normalize (longer for carbamazepine and phenobarbital than for phenytoin).

Women with epilepsy have a higher incidence of adverse pregnancy outcomes. Although the risk of congenital malformations is 4% to 6% (twice as high as in nonepileptic women), more than 90% of pregnancies in epileptic mothers have satisfactory outcomes. Older data, much of which included AED polytherapy, indicated that barbiturates and phenytoin may cause congenital heart malformations, orofacial clefts, and other malformations. From these data the risk of neural tube defect with valproic acid and carbamazepine was estimated to be 0.5% to 1%, respectively, and appeared to be related to drug exposure during gestational days 0 to 28. Other adverse pregnancy outcomes associated with maternal seizures, but not necessarily caused by AEDs, are growth, psychomotor, and mental retardation. Women with epilepsy are also more likely to have miscarriages, and 10% to 20% of infants are born with low birth weight. Updated practice parameters are available to aid in the counseling and management of pregnant women with epilepsy.[67–69]

Although data exist which question the effectiveness of folic acid supplementation, it is currently believed that some teratogenic effects may be prevented by adequate folate intake; therefore, prenatal vitamins with folic acid (0.4 to 5 mg/day) should be given to any woman of child-bearing potential who is taking AEDs.[65] Also, that higher folate doses should be used in women with a history of a previous pregnancy with a neural tube defect or taking valproic acid. Higher AED doses and serum concentrations, polytherapy, and a family history of birth defects appear to increase the teratogenic risk of AEDs. Deciding on the most effective single-drug treatment prior to conception is vitally important. Current data strongly suggest that an increased risk of adverse outcomes in women with epilepsy is due to teratogenic effects of AEDs and not epilepsy since studies show that epileptic women who do not take AEDs have the same risk of birth defects as infants born to control, seizure free women.[70] The most concerning effects are found with the use of valproic acid in the pregnant patient. Data gathered from pregnancy registries and long-term studies suggest that valproic acid exposure is associated with a 1% to 2% risk of neural tube defects, a 10- to 20-fold increase over the general population, and an increased risk of neurodevelopmental deficits, reduced verbal abilities, and poorer attentional tasks; it appears that these effects are dose-dependent with major congenital malformation risk significantly increasing at 600 mg/day and largest risk observed at doses that exceed 1,000 mg/day. However, individual susceptibility is genetically determined, and teratogenicity can occur at much lower doses in some persons. Data are still limited on the newer agents, although topiramate may have a negative effect on birth weight and cause an increase risk in oral cleft and hypospadias in the fetus.[70] Some AEDs can cause neonatal hemorrhagic disorder, which can be prevented by administrating 10 mg/day vitamin K orally to the mother during the last month of pregnancy and/or administering parenteral vitamin K to the newborn at delivery.[69]

Most AEDs pass into the breast milk, and concentrations are measureable in breastfeeding infants. In general, the degree of protein binding of a given AED allows for prediction of its concentration in breast milk. AEDs with less protein binding accumulate more in breast milk. Treatment with AEDs is not necessarily a reason to discourage breastfeeding. In fact, an argument could be made that since AEDs should rarely be discontinued abruptly, breastfeeding is a reasonable way to allow for a downward titration of a medication that the baby was exposed to for the past 9 months. Infants born to women taking any AED (particularly barbiturates or benzodiazepines) should be closely observed for signs of excess sedation, irritability, or poor feeding.[65] An ongoing multicenter observational study of breastfeeding women taking AED monotherapy has failed to show significant cognitive effects in children exposed in utero to various AEDs—carbamazepine, lamotrigine, phenytoin, or valproic acid, although there was some negative effect on cognition noted for phenytoin.[71]

The perimenopausal period can be associated with worsening of seizures. At menopause, seizures often improve in frequency, particularly in women with a catamenial seizure pattern. According to current data, conjugated equine estrogens plus 2.5 mg of medroxyprogesterone acetate may increase the frequency of epileptic seizures. It is suggested that a combination of single estrogenic compound such as 17-β-estradiol along with a natural progesterone should be considered in women who need hormone replacement therapy for disruptive menopausal symptoms.[72] Data suggest that men with epilepsy have reduced fertility, and that carbamazepine, oxcarbazepine, and valproic acid are associated with sperm abnormalities in these men while levetiracetam appears to slightly increase serum testosterone.[73] In addition, valproic acid seems to cause testicular atrophy resulting in reduced testosterone volume.[74]

Clinical Considerations with Specific Drugs

Tables 40-4 through 40-7 list specific data (including pharmacokinetics, adverse effects, metabolism, and dosing) for each of the commonly used AEDs. Below we summarize the pharmacology, advantages and disadvantages, and perspectives on the place in therapy of some specific AED.

Carbamazepine

Pharmacology and Mechanism of Action Carbamazepine is believed to act primarily by enhancing fast inactivation of voltage-gated sodium channels. In addition, interaction with voltage-gated calcium and potassium channels might also contribute to its activity.[75]

Pharmacokinetics The absorption of carbamazepine from immediate-release tablets is slow and erratic because of its low water solubility. There is also large variability in the peak-to-trough concentrations of up to 40%. There is no first-pass metabolism. Food, especially fat, may enhance the bioavailability of carbamazepine. Carbamazepine suspension is absorbed faster than the tablets.[76] Controlled-release (Tegretol-XR) and sustained-release (Carbatrol) preparations are also available, and they are bioequivalent in twice-daily (every 12 hours) dosing to immediate-release carbamazepine

TABLE 40-7 Antiepileptic Drugs Dosing and Target Serum Concentration Ranges

Drug	Brand Name	Initial or Starting Dose	Usual Range or Maximum Dose	Comments Target Serum Concentration Range
Barbiturates				
Phenobarbital	Various	1–3 mg/kg/day (10–20 mg/kg LD)	180–300 mg	10–40 mcg/mL (43–172 μmol/L)
Primidone	Mysoline	100–125 mg/day	750–2,000 mg	5–10 mcg/mL (23-46 μmol/L)
Benzodiazepines				
Clobazam	Onfi	≤30 kg 5 mg/day; >30 kg 10 mg/day	≤30 kg up to 20 mg; >30 kg up to 40 mg	0.03–0.3 ng/mL (0.1–1.0 nmol/L)
Clonazepam	Klonopin	1.5 mg/day	20 mg	20–70 ng/mL (0.06–0.22 μmol/L)
Diazepam	Valium	PO: 4–40 mg IV: 5–10 mg	PO: 4–40 mg IV: 5–30 mg	100–1,000 ng/mL (0.4–3.5 μmol/L)
Lorazepam	Ativan	PO: 2–6 mg IV: 0.05 mg/kg IM: 0.05 mg/kg	PO: 10 mg IV: 0.05 mg/kg	10–30 ng/mL (31–93 nmol/L)
Hydantoin				
Phenytoin	Dilantin	PO: 3–5 mg/kg (200–400 mg) (15–20 mg/kg LD)	PO: 500–600 mg	Total: 10–20 mcg/mL (40–79 μmol/L) Unbound: 0.5–3 mcg/mL (2–12 μmol/L)
Succinimide				
Ethosuximide	Zarontin	500 mg/day	500–2,000 mg	40–100 mcg/mL (282–708 μmol/L)
Other				
Carbamazepine	Tegretol	400 mg/day	400–2,400 mg	4–12 mcg/mL (17–51 μmol/L)
Ezogabine	Potiga	300 mg/day	1,200 mg	Not defined
Felbamate	Felbatol	1,200 mg/day	3,600 mg	30–60 mcg/mL (126–252 μmol/L)
Gabapentin	Neurontin	300–900 mg/day	4,800 mg	2–20 mcg/mL (12–117 μmol/L)
Lacosamide	Vimpat	100 mg/day	400 mg	Not defined
Lamotrigine	Lamictal	25 mg every other day if on VPA; 25–50 mg/day if not on VPA	100–150 mg if on VPA; 300–500 mg if not on VPA	4–20 mcg/mL (16–78 μmol/L)
Levetiracetam	Keppra Keppra XR	500–1,000 mg/day	3,000–4,000 mg	12–46 mcg/mL (70–270 μmol/L)
Oxcarbazepine	Trileptal	300–600 mg/day	2,400–3,000 mg	3–35 mcg/mL (MHD) (12–139 μmol/L)
Pregabalin	Lyrica	150 mg/day	600 mg	Not defined
Rufinamide	Banzel	400–800 mg/day	3,200 mg	Not defined
Tiagabine	Gabitril	4–8 mg/day	80 mg	0.02–0.2 mcg/mL (0.05–0.5 μmol/L)
Topiramate	Topamax	25–50 mg/day	200–1,000 mg	5–20 mcg/mL (15–59 μmol/L)
Valproic acid	Depakene Depakene SR Depakote Depakote ER Depacon	15 mg/kg (500–1,000 mg)	60 mg/kg (3,000–5,000 mg)	50–100 mcg/mL (347–693 μmol/L)
Vigabatrin	Sabril	1,000 mg/day	3,000 mg	0.8–36 mcg/mL (6–279 μmol/L)
Zonisamide	Zonegran	100–200 mg/day	600 mg	10–40 mcg/mL (47–188 μmol/L)

IM, intramuscular; LD, loading does; MHD, 10-monohydroxy-derivative; PO, orally; VPA, valproic acid.

Data from Patsalos et al.,[32] Halford and Lapointe,[35] Cada et al.,[36] Sabril [package insert],[37] Onfi [package insert],[33] and Potiga [package insert].[34]

dosed four times daily (every 6 hours). Compared with immediate-release carbamazepine, both these formulations have lower peaks and higher troughs, which may decrease side effects and improve seizure control. Carbatrol can improve QOL measurements compared to the immediate-release product.[77] Patients should be told to take Tegretol-XR with food and that the casing will be excreted in the feces. It cannot be broken or crushed. Tegretol-XR and Carbatrol appear to be bioequivalent; however, there is less variability in the absorption of Carbatrol.[76]

Carbamazepine is a neutral and highly lipophilic drug that is highly protein bound to α_1-acid glycoprotein and albumin. The major metabolite of carbamazepine is carbamazepine-10,11-epoxide, which has anticonvulsant activity in animals and humans. The formation of the 10,11-epoxide is influenced by concurrent use of other enzyme-inducing or enzyme-inhibiting drugs; thus the 10,11-epoxide concentration may change with the administration of other drugs (e.g., valproate and felbamate) with no change in parent carbamazepine concentration.

Carbamazepine induces its own metabolism (autoinduction), thereby decreasing its half-life after chronic therapy. The presence of enzyme-inducing drugs reduces the half-life even more. The enzyme-induction effect begins within 3 to 5 days of starting therapy and takes 21 to 28 days to complete. Therefore, it is possible to achieve initial concentrations that are within the therapeutic range but have concentrations fall despite continued therapy and good compliance. Some patients who respond well to initial therapy may be labeled refractory or noncompliant if the autoinduction phenomenon is not considered. The autoinduction reverses rapidly if carbamazepine is discontinued. Carbamazepine also displays diurnal variation in its serum level with evening levels lower than morning levels. It appears that carbamazepine is cleared significantly faster in females than males and in Caucasians compared to African Americans, and therefore variable dosing may be needed.[77]

Adverse Effects Carbamazepine side effects can parallel the rise and decline of serum concentrations daily. Neurosensory side effects are the most common (35% to 50% of patients). These side effects are more common during initiation of therapy and can dissipate with continued treatment. Carbamazepine can also cause nausea, which can be caused by a local effect of the drug on the GI tract, in which case food may help, or it can be caused by an effect on the brainstem, which may ultimately require discontinuation of the drug. Dosage manipulation, including the use of the controlled- or sustained-release preparations, should be tried before the patient is considered to be intolerant of carbamazepine. Carbamazepine can cause hyponatremia, the incidence of which increases with age, however, its occurrence is lower than that seen with oxcarbazepine. Periodic determinations of serum sodium concentration are recommended, especially in the elderly.[76]

Leukopenia is the most common hematologic side effect, with an incidence as high as 10%. It usually is transient, even when the drug is continued, and can be caused by a redistribution of WBCs rather than a decrease in their production.[76] In about 2% of patients, leukopenia is persistent, but even patients with WBC counts of 3,000/mm^3 (3×10^9/L) or less do not seem to have an increased incidence of infection. A clinical guide is to continue carbamazepine therapy unless the WBC count drops to less than 2,500/mm^3 (2.5×10^9/L) and the absolute neutrophil count drops to less than 1,000/mm3 (1×10^9/L).

Drug Interactions Because of concentration-dependent efficacy and side effects, drug interactions with carbamazepine often are very significant. Drugs that inhibit CYP3A4 potentially may increase carbamazepine serum concentrations. Carbamazepine can induce the metabolism of other drugs.

Dosing and Administration The variable contributions of the 10,11-epoxide metabolite and free-carbamazepine concentrations have restricted a precise definition of the therapeutic range. Loading doses of carbamazepine are indicated only for critically ill patients. During dosage titration, it must be remembered that carbamazepine clearance increases with time. Doses may be started at one-fourth to one-third the anticipated maintenance dose and increased every 2 to 3 weeks. Because of the auto- and heteroinduction of carbamazepine metabolism, it is necessary to administer the drug two to four times per day. Carbamazepine tablets should not be stored in places where they would be exposed to high heat or high humidity.[76]

Advantages Carbamazepine has been well studied. Oral solid and liquid dosage forms are available. The oral solid dosage form is available as an immediate-release tablet, as a sustained-release capsule, and a controlled-release tablet. The sustained- and controlled-release dosage forms allow for twice-daily dosing to reduce the peak-to-trough fluctuations. Compared with other first-generation AEDs, carbamazepine causes minimal cognitive impairment.

Disadvantages Carbamazepine has an active metabolite that can contribute to efficacy and toxicity. Other drugs can alter the concentration of this metabolite without changing the concentration of the parent carbamazepine. It induces its own metabolism, which complicates dosage titration. It also induces the metabolism of other medications, and other drugs may interact with it and/or its active metabolite. There is no parenteral formulation. There are clinically meaningful CNS side effects including sedation and nausea. One prospective study, however, found fewer side effects with the sustained-release formulation compared to the immediate-release formulation.[78] When ingested during the first trimester of pregnancy, carbamazepine has been associated with a slight risk of spina bifida. Chronic carbamazepine use has also been associated with decreases in bone mineral density and 25-hydroxy (OH) vitamin D. The generic formulations of immediate-release tablets have been associated with breakthrough seizures when brands have been switched.

Place in Therapy Carbamazepine is considered a first-line therapy for patients with newly diagnosed partial seizures and for patients with primary generalized convulsive seizures who are not in an emergent situation.

Clobazam

Pharmacology and Mechanism of Action Clobazam is a 1,5-chlorinated benzodiazepine derivative. The drug potentiates GABA's effect at the GABA receptor, increasing chloride current by increasing channel opening; the α subunit of GABA-A is especially important in the drug's activity.

Pharmacokinetics Clobazam is 80% to 90% protein bound. The drug is metabolized in the liver to *N*-desmethylclobazam primarily, which is an active metabolite; the metabolite achieves plasma concentrations three to five times higher than clobazam, but it has 1/5 the activity. Clobazam and *N*-desmethylclobazam have elimination half-lifes of 36 to 42 hours and 71 to 82 hours, respectively.

Adverse Effects CNS effects are the most common side effects with clobazam. With abrupt discontinuation, a withdrawal syndrome can be seen which consists of convulsions, psychosis, hallucinations, behavioral disorder, tremor, and anxiety; milder symptoms can present as dysphoria, anxiety, and insomnia.

Drug Interactions Clobazam inhibits CYP2D6; therefore, drugs metabolized by this enzyme may require dosage reduction. It is a weak inducer of CYP3A4 and may lower the serum levels of some OC's, which are metabolized by this enzyme.

Dosing and Administration Dosing is weight based, so patients who are less than or equal to 30 kg are started at 5 mg/day and increased slowly to 20 mg/day, while those weighing more than 30 kg are started at 10 mg/day and increased slowly to 40 mg/day; doses greater than 5 mg should be given in two divided doses. Dosing in geriatric patients is initiated as in patients weighing less than or equal to 30 kg, but increased up to 40 mg depending on the weight of the patient. Poor metabolizers of CYP2C19 are dosed like geriatric patients.

Advantages Clobazam is a potent chlorinated benzodiazepine that is more efficacious than clonopin in the treatment of Lennox–Gastaut. As with other benzodiazepines, tolerance can develop to its effectiveness in treatment of epilepsy, however 30% of patients do not develop tolerance, so the drug can often be used for years.

Disadvantages It is a class IV controlled substance. Patients must be carefully weaned off the drug to avoid a significant withdrawal symptoms. The drug is much less effective than clonazepam in treatment of myoclonic jerks and absence seizures. There is no liquid or parenteral formulation available.

Place in Therapy Adjunctive treatment of seizures associated with Lennox–Gastaut syndrome.

Ethosuximide

Pharmacology and Mechanism of Action Ethosuximide is believed to exert its primary action through inhibition of T-type calcium channels.[75]

Pharmacokinetics Metabolism occurs in the liver by hydroxylation, and the metabolites are believed to be inactive. There is some evidence of nonlinear pharmacokinetics at higher concentrations.

Adverse Effects The most frequently reported side effects are nausea and vomiting (up to 40% of patients), which may be minimized by administration of smaller and more frequent doses.[79]

Drug Interactions Because ethosuximide is not protein bound, displacement interactions do not occur. Valproic acid may inhibit the metabolism of ethosuximide, but only if the metabolism of ethosuximide is near saturation.

Dosing and Administration A loading dose is not required. Titration over 1to 2 weeks to maintenance doses of 20 mg/kg per day usually results in therapeutic concentrations. Data suggest that patients can be managed successfully on once-a-day therapy; however, GI distress appears to be dose related, and the total daily dose is usually divided into two equal doses.[79]

Advantages This drug is very effective in the treatment of absence seizures. It is generally well tolerated and has few pharmacokinetic interactions.

Disadvantages Ethosuximide has a very narrow spectrum of activity.

Place in Therapy Ethosuximide is still a first-line treatment for absence seizures.

Ezogabine

Pharmacology and Mechanism of Action The primary mechanism of action of ezogabine is as a selective positive allosteric modulator (opener) of KCNQ2-5 channels, which stabilizes the resting membrane potential and reduces brain excitability.[80]

Pharmacokinetics Ezogabine's oral bioavailability is 60%; high fat food does not affect the extent of its absorption but increases its maximal blood drug concentration (C_{max}) 38% and delays its time to maximal blood drug concentration (T_{max}) by 0.75 hour. Ezogabine has a 30% lower trough serum level in the evening than in the morning. The drug undergoes glucuronidation and acetylation with the major metabolite, *n*-acetyl metabolite (NAMR) being less active than the parent drug in animal models. Elderly subjects show a 40% to 50% higher area under the drug concentration time curve (AUC) and a 30% higher half-life compared to younger subjects, and therefore dosage reduction is recommended.

Adverse Effects CNS effects are the most common side effects seen with ezogabine. More concerning is urinary retention, which occurs usually within the first 6 months, but onset can be later; special caution is advised if the drug is used in persons with benign prostatic hypertrophy, those already on anticholinergics, or those persons unable to communicate clinical symptoms. In addition, the drug can cause QT prolongation, with increased occurrence within 3 hours of administration. Caution is advised in those already taking drugs that can increase the QT interval and persons with congestive heart failure, ventricular hypertrophy, hypokalemia, or hypomagnesemia.

Drug Interactions Ezogabine can increase lamotrigine clearance by 22% and decrease AUC by 18% while NAMR may inhibit renal clearance of digoxin. Ezogabine serum levels may be reduced 35% by phenytoin and 31% by carbamazepine. Lastly, alcohol may increase systemic exposure, C_{max} and AUC, of ezogabine, resulting in an increase in adverse drug effects.

Dosing and Administration The drug must be titrated up slowly to avoid CNS effects and given three times a day. If the drug is discontinued, it should be titrated down over at least 3 weeks.

Advantages Ezogabine works by an entirely different mechanism, and therefore may be valuable when added to another AED as adjunctive therapy.

Disadvantages It is a class V controlled substance. The drug may interfere with both urine and serum bilirubin clinical lab assays causing falsely elevated readings. Its tendency to cause urinary retention and QT prolongation in some patients requires special vigilance when prescribing the drug. There are no liquid or parenteral formulations available, and the drug must be taken three times per day.

Place in Therapy Given the drug's novel mechanism of action, it should be used adjunctively in select patients who fail to respond optimally to other AEDs for treatment of partial seizures.

Felbamate

Pharmacology and Mechanism of Action At therapeutic doses, felbamate appears to act by blocking *N*-methyl-D-aspartate (NMDA) synaptic responses and by modulating $GABA_A$ receptors. At higher doses it may modulate sodium channels and inhibit high-voltage activated calcium channels.[75]

Pharmacokinetics Felbamate is rapidly and well absorbed. The absorption is unaffected by food or antacids. Approximately 40% to 50% of a dose of felbamate is metabolized by hydroxylation and conjugation pathways in the liver, and the remainder is excreted unchanged in the urine. It displays linear pharmacokinetics.[80]

Adverse Effects The most frequently reported side effects prior to marketing were anorexia, weight loss, insomnia, nausea, and headache (sometimes severe). Anorexia and weight loss may be especially problematic in children and in patients with diminished caloric intake. After marketing, felbamate was found to be associated with aplastic anemia and acute liver failure. The onset was between 68 and 354 days of therapy. The approximate rate of occurrence of aplastic anemia is 1 in 3,000 and of hepatitis is 1 in 10,000. Data suggest a possible increased risk for aplastic anemia in patients, especially women, with a history of cytopenia, AED allergy or significant toxicity, viral infection, and/or immunologic problems.[25,26,81]

Drug Interactions Felbamate can induce or inhibit the metabolism of the older AEDs. Interactions between warfarin and felbamate have also been reported.[80]

Dosing and Administration The starting dose of felbamate is increased at 2-week intervals.

Advantages Felbamate has a broad spectrum of activity and a unique mechanism of action. It is approved for treating atonic seizures in patients with the Lennox–Gastaut syndrome and is also effective in treating patients with partial seizures.

Disadvantages The use of felbamate is limited by the association with aplastic anemia and hepatotoxicity, as well as multiple drug interactions.

Place in Therapy It should be reserved for patients not responding to other AEDs.

Gabapentin

Pharmacology and Mechanism of Action Gabapentin was designed to be a GABA agonist but does not react at the GABA receptor, alter GABA uptake, or interfere with GABA transaminase. Gabapentin appears to bind to an amino acid carrier protein and to act at a unique receptor. It inhibits high-voltage activated calcium channels.[75] It elevates human brain GABA levels, possibly via alterations in GABA synthesis or reversal of the neuronal GABA transporter, resulting in nonvesicular release of GABA.[82]

Pharmacokinetics Gabapentin is a substrate of the L-amino acid carrier protein in the gut (system L) and in the CNS.[83] This carrier protein transports the drug across the gut membrane by an active process. The binding of gabapentin to this system is saturable, and gabapentin therefore displays dose-dependent bioavailability that appears to vary considerably between individuals.[84] Food, including protein-rich meals, does not appear to interfere with gabapentin oral absorption.[85,86] Concentrations in human CSF are 5% to 35% of plasma levels, and tissue concentrations are approximately 80% of plasma levels.

Because gabapentin is eliminated exclusively by the kidneys, dosage adjustments are necessary in patients with significantly impaired renal function.

Adverse Effects CNS effects, as well as weight gain, are the most common side effects seen with gabapentin. Aggressive behavior has been reported in children.[87] A withdrawal reaction characterized by anxiety, insomnia, nausea, sweating, and increased pain has also been reported with abrupt discontinuation in patients taking it for pain.

Drug Interactions Gabapentin does not induce or inhibit liver enzymes; therefore, drug interactions are not likely to occur. There is a 10% reduction in the clearance of gabapentin in patients taking cimetidine and a 20% reduction in the bioavailability if aluminum antacids are taken simultaneously with gabapentin. These interactions are unlikely to be clinically significant.

Dosing and Administration Typical starting doses of gabapentin are 300 mg at bedtime on the first day, increasing to 900 mg/day over 3 days. Faster titration rates (e.g., starting at 300 to 900 mg three times daily) have been well tolerated.[87] Data suggest gabapentin should be given at least four times a day when the total daily dose is 3,600 mg or greater.[88] It does not appear to be absorbed rectally. Patients with end-stage renal disease maintained on hemodialysis should receive an initial 300- to 400-mg dose with 200 to 300 mg gabapentin given after every 4 hours of hemodialysis.

Advantages Gabapentin has multiple mechanisms of action and is mechanistically different from first-generation AEDs. It is not metabolized and is excreted unchanged by the kidney. It has a broad therapeutic index with minimal CNS adverse effects and few drug interactions. Doses can be escalated rapidly. It is available in liquid dosage form.

Disadvantages Gabapentin is absorbed by an active process that saturates at higher doses. This may require more frequent daily dosing for patients who need doses greater than 3,600 mg/day. Doses exceeding the 3,600 mg/day maximum listed in the package insert may be required in some patients to achieve seizure remission. There is no parenteral formulation.

Place in Therapy Gabapentin is a second-line agent for patients with partial seizures who have failed initial treatment. In addition, although monotherapy has no proven efficacy in previously diagnosed refractory patients, it may have a role in patients with less severe seizure disorders, such as new-onset partial epilepsy, particularly in the elderly. Gabapentin also has been shown to be useful for chronic pain and other nonepileptic conditions.

Lacosamide

Pharmacology and Mechanism of Action Lacosamide is a functionalized amino acid with unknown mechanism of action, but two mechanisms are suggested.[35] It selectively enhances slow inactivation of voltage-gated sodium channels, resulting in stabilization of hyper-excitable neuronal membranes and inhibition of repetitive neuronal firings. In addition, it binds to collapsin response mediator protein (CRMP-2), a phosphoprotein mainly expressed in the CNS, and it is involved in neuronal differentiation and control of axonal outgrowth. The role of CRMP-2 binding in seizure control is unknown.

Pharmacokinetics Lacosamide is rapidly and almost completely absorbed after oral administration, and food does not affect its bioavailability. There is a linear relationship between daily doses and serum concentrations up to 800 mg/day. No dosage adjustment is necessary in children or the elderly. Moderate hepatic and renal impairment have both been shown to increase systemic drug exposure up to approximately 40%.[35]

Adverse Effects CNS and GI effects are the most common side effects seen with lacosamide, and they are dose related. The drug can also cause a small increase in median PR interval (5 to 9 milliseconds) on the electrocardiogram (ECG).

Drug Interactions The blood level of lacosamide is decreased by approximately 15% to 20% by enzyme-inducing AEDs.[33] It is a substrate of CYP2C19; however, there are no known drug interactions between lacosamide and drugs metabolized by CYP2C19. The drug does not appear to affect the serum concentration of OCs containing ethinyl estradiol and levonorgestrel.[35]

Dosing and Administration The starting dose is 100 mg/day in two divided doses, with dose increase by 100 mg/day every week until a daily dose of 200 to 400 mg has been reached. Studies have shown that a dose of 600 mg daily may be efficacious for some patients, but at the expense of more CNS side effects.

Advantages There is an IV form of lacosamide available for short-term replacement that appears to be safe, well tolerated, and easy to administer as well as a liquid dosage form. It does not affect the serum level of other AEDs, and its serum level is minimally affected by enzyme-inducing AEDs. It has novel mechanism(s) of action.

Disadvantages Lacosamide is a class V controlled substance.

Place in Therapy It is a potent second-line agent that should be considered in those patients who have failed first-line AEDs.

Lamotrigine

Pharmacology and Mechanism of Action Lamotrigine inhibits voltage-dependent sodium channels; it also inhibits high voltage-activated calcium channels and attenuates release of glutamate and to a lesser extent, GABA and dopamine.[75]

Pharmacokinetics Lamotrigine is completely and rapidly absorbed, with a bioavailability of 98%. Food does not significantly affect absorption. It is also absorbed following rectal administration, but the bioavailability is approximately 50% of that of oral dosage forms. Lamotrigine clearance is higher in children and lower in the elderly compared with young adults. There are only modest differences in the pharmacokinetics of lamotrigine in the elderly versus younger subjects. Hepatic disease, depending on severity, can influence lamotrigine pharmacokinetics. Approximately 17% of a lamotrigine dose can be removed by hemodialysis, with the half-life being reduced to approximately 13 hours. For patients on dialysis, the half-life is much more prolonged between dialyses. The half-life is prolonged in patients with renal failure.

Adverse Effects CNS effects, including headache, are the most frequently reported side effects seen with lamotrigine. Adverse effects are more common when lamotrigine is given in combination with other AEDs (e.g., diplopia when given concomitantly with carbamazepine or tremor with valproic acid) compared with monotherapy, and they can be pharmacodynamic in nature. Lamotrigine can cause rash, which usually appears in the first 3 to 4 weeks of therapy. Patients who have developed a rash with another AED are more likely to develop a rash with lamotrigine.[89] The rash typically is generalized, erythematous, and morbilliform. However, a Stevens–Johnson reaction also has been reported. Some rashes, especially those which develop early, can necessitate the withdrawal of lamotrigine.[90] Risk factors for the emergence of more serious rashes appear to be concomitant use of valproic acid and situations where high initial doses or rapid dosage escalation is used. Data from several European monotherapy trials suggest that when dosed appropriately, the incidence of rash from lamotrigine is similar to that of older agents such as carbamazepine and phenytoin. The incidence is higher in children than in adults.

Drug Interactions Lamotrigine does not inhibit liver enzymes and has a low potential for pharmacokinetic interactions with other drugs. It has been found to decrease the bioavailability of the progesterone component (levonorgestrel) of a combination OC by 19%. The clinical relevance of this interaction has not been determined.[91]

Concomitant treatment with OCs can lead to a reduction in the serum concentrations of lamotrigine because of an induction of lamotrigine glucuronidation by ethinyl estradiol.[92] In addition, lamotrigine serum levels can significantly increase during the week off OC treatment in some patients.[93]

Valproic acid substantially inhibits the metabolism of lamotrigine, with maximal inhibition occurring at valproic acid doses and serum concentrations of 500 mg/day and 40 to 50 mcg/mL (280 to 350 μmol/L), respectively.[94] A pharmacodynamic interaction can occur with concurrent carbamazepine therapy, causing an increase in CNS side effects.

Dosing and Administration In patients who are taking enzyme-inducing drugs, lamotrigine can be started more rapidly than in patients receiving valproic acid. The maintenance doses are also different. Managing dosing is critical owing to the relationship between rash, concomitant valproic acid treatment, and the dose escalation rate. Removal of inducers from a lamotrigine regimen may necessitate decreases in lamotrigine dose, whereas removal of valproic acid can necessitate an increase in the lamotrigine dose. Dispersible and oral disintegrating tablets are available for patients who cannot swallow an oral solid tablet.

Advantages Lamotrigine is potentially a broad-spectrum AED, having efficacy in partial seizures and several types of generalized seizures. Pediatric dosage forms are available as a chewable dispersible tablet and an oral disintegrating tablet. It is also available as an extended release product for once daily dosing. It neither induces nor inhibits the metabolism of other AEDs. Lamotrigine has linear pharmacokinetics and is not highly protein bound. It is generally well tolerated in both children and elderly patients and does not cause weight gain.

Disadvantages Lamotrigine is associated with rash, especially in patients who start at a high dose, have rapid dose escalation, and/or are taking concurrent valproic acid. Therefore, the initial doses must be low (especially if the patient is on valproic acid) and escalated slowly to maximize safety. There is no parenteral dosage form.

Place in Therapy Lamotrigine is useful as both adjunctive treatment in patients with partial seizures and as monotherapy. Lamotrigine monotherapy appears to have comparable effectiveness with more traditional AEDs such as carbamazepine and phenytoin. In addition, it may be a useful alternative for primary generalized seizure types such as absence and as adjunctive therapy for primary GTC seizures, the latter of which is an approved indication.

Levetiracetam

Pharmacology and Mechanism of Action The mechanism of action of levetiracetam has yet to be delineated; however, the drug is not active in the classic models used to test AEDs. The drug binds in the brain to the synaptic vesicle protein SV2A, which is believed to be important in its activity.[95] Limited animal data suggest that levetiracetam may have *antiepileptogenic effects*, meaning that it may prevent the development of epilepsy under certain circumstances, however confirmation of this research is needed.[96]

Pharmacokinetics Absorption of levetiracetam is rapid and complete following oral administration, and it is not significantly affected by food or enteral nutrition formulas.[97] Renal elimination of unchanged parent drug accounts for the majority of clearance (66%), with the remainder being metabolized via nonhepatic enzymatic hydrolysis to inactive metabolites. This pathway involves neither the CYP450 or UGT isozyme systems. Because it is eliminated renally, clinicians should anticipate age-related reductions in clearance in elderly patients. Conversely, levetiracetam clearance appears to be approximately 40% higher in children than in adults. In addition, patients with severe liver cirrhosis should initially receive one-half the recommended starting dose because of a 57% decrease in clearance.[98] Levetiracetam is excreted into breast milk in potentially clinically important amounts.[99] Data are sparse regarding serum concentration–effect relationships.

Adverse Effects CNS effects are the most common side effects seen with levetiracetam, and they are usually mild. In children and young adults, agitation, irritability, or somnolence/lethargy are the most frequently reported CNS side effects.[100] The mechanism underlying these effects is unknown.

Drug Interactions Levetiracetam neither inhibits nor induces the CYP450, UGT, or epoxide hydrolase enzyme systems, and in vitro data predict a low potential for pharmacokinetic interactions. It does not appear to significantly interact with other AEDs, warfarin, digoxin, or OCs.

Dosing and Administration Levetiracetam is available orally and parenterally. The IV product has not been tested for intramuscular (IM) use, and therefore, should not be administered IM. Typically the initial dose is given twice daily, with dosage increments every 2 weeks. To minimize CNS side effects, dosing may be initiated at one-half the suggested initial dose, given once a day. The IV formulation should be given at the same frequency and dose as the oral product. Although not FDA approved, the oral dose of levetiracetam has been titrated up rapidly to 3,000 mg in 3 days in some intractable seizure patients with improvement seen after day 2.[101]

Advantages Levetiracetam is felt to have a novel, although unknown, mechanism of action. It has linear pharmacokinetics and is not metabolized by the CYP450 system. No significant drug interactions, including with OCs, have been reported. Initial doses may be effective. The drug appears to be well tolerated, with transient sedation being the most troublesome adverse effect.

Disadvantages Dose adjustments are needed for patients with decreased renal function, and slower dose escalation may be needed to avoid CNS adverse effects. Behavioral problems can limit therapy in some patients.

Place in Therapy Levetiracetam is indicated for patients with partial seizures who have failed initial therapy. Its role as monotherapy for partial seizures remains to be clarified. It is approved for adjunctive treatment of myoclonic seizures in patients with JME and as adjunctive treatment of primarily generalized seizures in patients with idiopathic generalized epilepsy.

Oxcarbazepine

Pharmacology and Mechanism of Action Oxcarbazepine, which is structurally related to carbamazepine, is a prodrug that is rapidly converted to the active 10-monohydroxy derivative (MHD). The mechanism of action of oxcarbazepine is similar to that of carbamazepine. Oxcarbazepine and MHD block voltage-sensitive sodium channels, modulate the voltage-activated calcium currents, and increase potassium conductance. Oxcarbazepine can display differing affinities for both sodium channels and Ca^{2+} channels compared with older drugs such as carbamazepine.[102] Whereas carbamazepine may modulate L-type Ca^{2+} channels, oxcarbazepine appears to modulate N- and P-type Ca^{2+} channels.[103] Whether these differences lead to differing patterns of clinical effectiveness is uncertain. It has no significant interactions with neurotransmitters or modulation of receptor sites.

Pharmacokinetics Oxcarbazepine is absorbed completely, and MHD is inactivated by glucuronide conjugation and eliminated by the kidneys. Oxcarbazepine and its active metabolite do not undergo autoinduction. The relationship between dose and serum concentration is linear. Children 2 to 6 years of age need larger doses (per kg) to achieve the same serum concentration, suggesting a more rapid clearance. C_{max} and bioavailability of MHD in elderly volunteers were higher than in younger volunteers, and the elimination rate was slower, possibly reflecting decreased renal elimination. Patients with significant renal impairment may require a dosage reduction.

Adverse Effects CNS effects are the most frequent side effects seen with oxcarbazepine. In comparative trials, oxcarbazepine generally caused fewer side effects than phenytoin, valproic acid, or carbamazepine. Dizziness may be more common in elderly patients than in young adults. CNS adverse effects appear to be far more common at doses greater than 1,200 mg/day. Hyponatremia, defined as a plasma sodium concentration of less than 125 mmol/L, has been reported in up to 25% of patients taking oxcarbazepine and occurs more often in elderly patients. Clinicians should be particularly watchful in patients receiving concomitant sodium-depleting drugs such as diuretics. Hyponatremia appears to occur less frequently in children. Clinicians should consider monitoring serum sodium levels following the initiation of oxcarbazepine, and they should instruct patients regarding the symptoms of hyponatremia. Approximately 25% to 30% of patients who develop a rash with carbamazepine will experience a similar reaction with oxcarbazepine.[25,26,81] The tolerability of oxcarbazepine has not been compared with that of extended-release formulations of carbamazepine that have lower peaks and potentially fewer side effects than immediate-release carbamazepine formulations.

Drug Interactions Oxcarbazepine decreases the bioavailability of ethinyl estradiol and levonorgestrel.[104] Women concurrently taking OCs should be counseled about the potential for contraceptive failure. Unlike carbamazepine, there are no interactions between cimetidine, erythromycin, or warfarin and oxcarbazepine. The administration of oxcarbazepine in doses greater than 1,200 mg with phenytoin has resulted in a 40% increase in the concentration of phenytoin, consistent with inhibition of CYP 2C19. Oxcarbazepine treatment may modestly reduce lamotrigine serum concentrations, suggesting induction of UGT isozymes.[105]

The replacement of carbamazepine with oxcarbazepine may result in a drug interaction because an enzyme-inducing drug is being removed.

Dosing and Administration Doses and titration schedules differ regarding whether the drug is used for mono- or adjunctive therapy in adults versus children. Although not FDA approved, doses up to 60 mg/kg/day have been used in infants and children younger than 4 years of age to successfully control partial-onset seizures.[106] In patients being converted from carbamazepine, the typical maintenance dose of oxcarbazepine is 1.5 times the carbamazepine dose or less, if patients are on large doses of carbamazepine, due to autoinduction of carbamazepine but not oxcarbazepine.

Advantages The efficacy of oxcarbazepine is comparable with that of carbamazepine, phenytoin, and valproic acid. It may be better tolerated than phenytoin as monotherapy and therefore, less likely to be discontinued.[107] There is broad international experience with this drug.

Disadvantages About 30% of patients who have experienced a rash with carbamazepine have a cross-reaction with oxcarbazepine. There are more reports of hyponatremia with oxcarbazepine, especially in patients at risk. Replacing carbamazepine with oxcarbazepine can result in interactions owing to the removal of an enzyme inducer. Enzyme-inducing drugs can increase the clearance of MHD.

Place in Therapy Oxcarbazepine is indicated for use as monotherapy or adjunctive therapy in the treatment of partial seizures in adults and children as young as 4 years of age. It is also a potential first-line drug for patients with primary generalized convulsive seizures. Oxcarbazepine may also be effective in patients not demonstrating a response to carbamazepine.

Phenytoin

Pharmacology and Mechanism of Action The primary mechanism of action of phenytoin is believed to be its ability to inhibit voltage-dependent sodium channels.[75]

Pharmacokinetics The pharmacokinetics of phenytoin are complex. For a more in-depth understanding, the reader is referred to a more extensive review.[108] The oral absorption of phenytoin is almost complete. Dissolution is the rate-limiting step, and absorption may be saturable at higher doses, such as those used for oral loading. Absorption following IM administration of phenytoin is erratic and delayed, and IM injections are painful; however, IM absorption following fosphenytoin is rapid and well tolerated.

Phenytoin enters the brain rapidly and is redistributed to other body tissues, including breast milk and the placenta. Phenytoin competes for albumin sites with other highly protein-bound drugs. It is essential to know the patient's serum albumin level in interpreting the serum concentrations of phenytoin.[109] Patients with significant renal dysfunction will have altered phenytoin protein binding. Obesity increases the volume of distribution.

Phenytoin is metabolized in the liver by parahydroxylation. The major isoforms responsible for the metabolism of phenytoin are CYP2C9 and CYP2C19; the former displays polymorphism, which may affect the response to phenytoin.[75] Phenytoin displays Michaelis–Menten pharmacokinetics, and the metabolism of phenytoin saturates at doses used clinically. The clinical importance of this is that a small change in dose can result in a disproportionally large increase in serum concentrations, potentially leading to toxicity. In some patients the metabolism of phenytoin can saturate even at low serum concentrations within the therapeutic range. The long-held belief that the metabolism of phenytoin decreases with age in adults has been challenged.[110]

Adverse Effects CNS effects are the most frequent side effects seen with phenytoin. Most of these effects usually are transient and can be minimized by slow dosage titration. At very high concentrations of greater than 50 mcg/mL (200 μmol/L), phenytoin can exacerbate seizures.

It is unclear whether the chronic side effects of phenytoin are concentration or duration dependent. One of the more common chronic side effects is gingival hyperplasia. Good oral hygiene can minimize gingival hyperplasia and should be encouraged. Other chronic effects include vitamin D deficiency, osteomalacia, carbohydrate intolerance, immunologic disturbances, hypothyroidism, and peripheral neuropathy. Phenytoin is associated with rare hypersensitivity or idiosyncratic reactions resulting in rashes, Stevens–Johnson syndrome, pseudolymphoma, bone marrow suppression, lupus-like reactions, and hepatitis.[111]

Drug Interactions Phenytoin is associated with numerous drug interactions involving altered absorption, metabolism, and protein binding that can enhance or reduce its effects. It is an inducer of both CYP450 and UGT isozymes. The absorption of phenytoin can be increased or decreased with the administration of food depending on the composition of the meal. The bioavailability of phenytoin suspension can be decreased in patients receiving continuous enteral nutrient tube feedings. However, a single-dose study of simultaneous administration of enteral feeding found no difference in phenytoin bioavailability, suggesting that the mechanism was something other than physical contact.[108]

Phenytoin decreases folic acid absorption. Replacement of folic acid can reduce phenytoin concentration and result in loss of efficacy.[108]

Dosing and Administration Four oral dosage forms are available, and changing dosage forms can lead to changes in phenytoin serum concentrations. Whether or not a dosage form uses the parent drug or salt form should be considered when changing from one dosage form to another. One hundred milligrams of phenytoin acid is equal to 92 mg of phenytoin sodium. Phenytoin capsules are designated as immediate-release or extended-release. Only the extended-release capsules should be used in once-daily dosing. Particle size rather than formulation may determine the rate of absorption.

If oral administration is not feasible, IV administration of phenytoin is preferred, as IM administration can cause tissue necrosis. Fosphenytoin is a prodrug for phenytoin and is available as a parenteral dosage form. Fosphenytoin is ordered in phenytoin equivalents (PE), the actual dose of phenytoin acid desired. It is very water-soluble and is converted rapidly to phenytoin systemically. Fosphenytoin can be given rapidly IV and IM with reliable absorption and minimal pain. It is significantly better tolerated than phenytoin.

Because of saturable absorption, an oral loading dose, such as 20 mg/kg, should be divided into four equal doses and given at 6-hour intervals. Subsequent dosage adjustments should be done cautiously owing to its nonlinear elimination. One author has suggested that if the serum concentration is less than 7 mcg/mL (28 μmol/L), the daily dose should be increased by 100 mg; if the serum concentration is between 7 and 12 mcg/mL (28 and 48 μmol/L), the daily dose can be increased by 50 mg; and if the serum concentration is greater than 12 mcg/mL (48 μmol/L), the daily dose can be increased by 30 mg or less. These increases are reported to result in less than 10% of patients achieving a phenytoin serum concentration greater than 25 mcg/mL (99 μmol/L).[112]

Advantages After more than 66 years, phenytoin's risk-to-benefit ratio is well established. It is available in oral solid, oral liquid, extended-release oral solid, and parenteral (phenytoin and fosphenytoin) dosage forms, allowing flexibility in dosing and use in emergent situations. In some patients, the extended-release dosage form can be given once a day with good seizure control.

Disadvantages Phenytoin displays Michaelis–Menten pharmacokinetics, meaning that the metabolism saturates at doses given clinically thus complicating dose titration. Also, phenytoin is an inducer of CYP450 isozymes, is metabolized by CYP450 enzymes, and is highly protein bound. Therefore, many drug interactions are associated with coadministration of this agent. It also has multiple significant adverse effects.

Place in Therapy Phenytoin has long been a first-line AED for primary generalized convulsive and partial seizures. However, its place in therapy is being reevaluated as more experience is gained with newer AEDs.

Pregabalin

Pharmacology and Mechanism of Action It is proposed that pregabalin's binding to the subunit of the voltage-gated calcium channel may be responsible in large part for the drug's activity. This binding results in a decrease in the release of several excitatory neurotransmitters, including glutamate, noradrenaline, substance P, and calcitonin gene-related peptide.[113]

Pharmacokinetics Pregabalin is a substrate of the L-amino acid carrier protein in the CNS. It does not display dose-dependent bioavailability. Food decreases the rate of absorption but not the bioavailability of the drug.[114]

Pregabalin is eliminated primarily by renal excretion as an unchanged drug, and therefore dosage adjustment is required in patients with significantly impaired renal function. In anuric patients, 50% of the dose is removed by 4 hours of hemodialysis.

Adverse Effects CNS effects, as well as weight gain, are the most frequently reported side effects seen with pregabalin. It is unknown if pregabalin causes aggressive behavior in children. A withdrawal reaction characterized by anxiety, nervousness, and irritability has been noted in patients being treated for generalized anxiety upon abrupt discontinuation of the drug.[115]

Drug Interactions Because pregabalin is predominantly excreted unchanged in the urine and undergoes negligible metabolism, drug interactions are unlikely.

Dosing and Administration Starting doses of pregabalin are divided into twice or thrice daily intervals. The manufacturer recommends that patients with end-stage renal disease maintained on hemodialysis receive a 25 to 75 mg daily dose with 25 to 75 mg given after every 4 hours of hemodialysis.

Advantages Pregabalin is somewhat more potent than gabapentin without the dose-limited GI absorption properties. It has minimal CNS side effects and no drug interactions.

Disadvantages It is a class V controlled substance. Like gabapentin it can cause weight gain and peripheral edema, especially as the dose is increased. There is no parenteral formulation available.

Place in Therapy Pregabalin is a second-line agent for patients with partial seizures who have failed initial treatment. It is also useful for chronic neuropathic pain and generalized anxiety disorder.[115]

Rufinamide

Pharmacology and Mechanism of Action Rufinamide suppresses neuronal hyperexcitability through prolongation of the inactivation phase of voltage-gated sodium channels.[116]

Pharmacokinetics Oral absorption is relatively slow with a T_{max} of 4 to 6 hours. At low doses (600 mg), the drug is relatively well absorbed (85%) when taken with food; however, the percentage of drug absorbed decreases with higher doses. Twice-daily dosing is recommended due to the slow absorption properties and the drug's short half-life (6 to 10 hours).[36] It is extensively metabolized with no active metabolites, with primary biotransformation by carboxylesterases. Although clinical data indicate that children and adults have similar pharmacokinetics, population pharmacokinetic modeling suggests that in the absence of interacting comedication the drug may have a higher clearance in children.[116]

Adverse Effects CNS effects are the most common side effects seen with rufinamide. These effects are dose-dependent. Rufinamide may increase the incidence of convulsions in some patients, and may precipitate SE. Multiorgan hypersensitivity has occurred within 4 weeks of starting treatment in patients younger than 12 years of age.

Drug Interactions Rufinamide is a weak inhibitor of CYP2E1 and a weak inducer of CYP3A4; the later effect may be responsible for modestly lower levels of carbamazepine and triazolam when given concomitantly with rufinamide. It may decrease the AUC of combination OCs containing ethinyl estradiol and norethindrone; however, it is not known if this is due to induction of CYP3A4 or uridine diphosphate glucuronosyl transferase (UDP-GT), or both. Rufinamide is responsible for a modest increase in the clearance of lamotrigine, phenobarbital, and phenytoin, and the effect is greater in children than adults. Carbamazepine, phenytoin, primidone, and phenobarbital significantly increase the clearance of rufinamide; however, it is believed this interaction is not entirely due to

CYP450 enzyme induction. Valproic acid significantly decreases the clearance of rufinamide and elevates serum levels of rufinamide by 70%.

Dosing and Administration The initial dose of rufinamide is 400 to 800 mg/day given in divided doses with an increase in dose every other day until a maximum dose of 45 mg/kg/day or 3,200 mg/day (whichever is less) is obtained.

Advantages The drug is effective for seizures associated with Lennox–Gastaut syndrome without causing cognitive and psychiatric adverse effects. The dose can be rapidly escalated.

Disadvantages Drug interactions are common with rufinamide, and patients with Lennox–Gastaut are usually on multiple medications. It displays decreased absorption at higher doses and when taken on an empty stomach. The drug has caused convulsions and SE in some patients.

Place in Therapy As an adjunctive agent in controlling seizures in Lennox–Gastaut syndrome after patients have failed valproic acid, topiramate, and lamotrigine.

Tiagabine

Pharmacology and Mechanism of Action Tiagabine is a potent specific inhibitor of GABA uptake into neuronal elements, thus, enhancing the action of GABA by decreasing its removal from the synaptic space.[117]

Pharmacokinetics Tiagabine is absorbed quickly and nearly completely after oral administration. There is a linear relationship between dose and serum concentrations. Children eliminate tiagabine slightly faster than adults. Hepatic impairment causes higher and more prolonged plasma concentrations of total and unbound drug. Renal dysfunction does not change its pharmacokinetics.[117] Tiagabine displays diurnal variation in its serum level, with evening levels lower than morning levels.

Adverse Effects CNS and GI effects are the most frequent side effects seen with tiagabine. Adverse events usually are mild to moderate and transient, and most occur during dose titration.[118] CNS side effects can be diminished by taking tiagabine with food, thus slowing the absorption rate. It has increased the incidence of nonconvulsive SE in patients with chronic refractory partial epilepsy.[119] In addition, there are reports of SE or new-onset seizures occurring in patients without a history of epilepsy.

Drug Interactions Food decreases the rate but not the extent of absorption. Tiagabine is displaced from protein by naproxen, salicylates, and valproate. However, tiagabine does not displace phenytoin, valproic acid, amitriptyline, tolbutamide, or warfarin.[117]

Dosing and Administration A clear dose–response has been demonstrated, and the minimal effective adult dose level is 30 mg/day. The initial dose is increased weekly.

Advantages Tiagabine has a known mechanism of action. It is the first drug marketed in the United States that acts only on GABA reuptake. It has linear pharmacokinetics and is not reported to interact with other drugs.

Disadvantages Initially high and rapid dosage escalation is associated with increased CNS side effects. Therefore, the drug must be started at a low dose and titrated gradually to response. Lower doses may be needed in patients with liver disease. Tiagabine is metabolized by CYP3A4 enzymes, and other drugs may alter its clearance. There is no parenteral formulation.

Place in Therapy Tiagabine is second-line therapy for patients with partial seizures who have failed initial therapy. It does not appear to have a role in primary generalized seizure types.

Topiramate

Pharmacology and Mechanism of Action Topiramate has multiple modes of action involving voltage-dependent sodium channels, GABA-receptor subunits, high-voltage calcium channels, and kainate/α-amino-3-hydroxy-5-methylisoxazole-4-propionic acid (AMPA) subunits.[75] It also inhibits carbonic anhydrase, which likely is not a major mechanism of action.[75]

Pharmacokinetics Although generally considered to have linear absorption and elimination pharmacokinetics, a greater than proportional increase in both C_{max} and AUC has been observed and probably is explained by saturable binding to erythrocytes.[120] Approximately 50% of the dose is excreted renally unchanged; however, its metabolism is increased by approximately 50% when given with enzyme-inducing AEDs. Renal tubular reabsorption may be involved prominently in the renal handling of topiramate.

Adverse Effects CNS effects are the most frequent side effects reported with topiramate, including "thinking abnormally," which rarely has included psychosis. Most of these occurred during rapid titration and at higher doses.[121] Word-finding difficulties can be a problem with topiramate and can occur in a significant number of patients, especially patients with left posterior temporal lobe epilepsy or SP seizures.[122] Concomitant therapy with topiramate, valproic acid, or phenobarbital can cause cognitive dysfunction. Nephrolithiasis has occurred in 1.5% of patients receiving topiramate, which is two to four times the incidence in the general population. Patients should be encouraged to maintain adequate fluid intake in order to minimize this problem. Topiramate can cause metabolic acidosis at doses as low as 50 mg/day. Risk factors for this condition include renal disease, severe respiratory disorders, SE, diarrhea, surgery, and the ketogenic diet. Metabolic acidosis in part may explain the anorexia and weight loss seen with this drug.[82]

Drug Interactions Oral clearance of digoxin is slightly increased when topiramate is added. Topiramate coadministration can cause increased phenytoin serum concentrations in some patients. The variable response can be explained by the intersubject variability in the proportion of phenytoin clearance attributed to CYP2C19 metabolism and whether the patient is a homozygous or heterozygous carrier of the mutant allele responsible for the CYP2C9 and/or CYP2C19 "poor metabolizer" phenotype. Topiramate can modestly increase the oral clearance of valproic acid and increase formation of the 4-ene-valproic acid metabolite. However, the clinical significance of this interaction is unclear. Topiramate increases the clearance of ethinyl estradiol in a dose-dependent manner. Topiramate doses of less than 200 mg/day are unlikely to alter OC pharmacokinetics.[123]

Dosing and Administration Topiramate should be titrated slowly to avoid adverse events with dosage increments every 1 to 2 weeks. For patients on other AEDs, doses greater than 600 mg/day do not appear to lead to improved efficacy and can cause increased adverse effects; however, higher doses may prove beneficial to individual patients who tolerate them.[124]

Advantages Topiramate has multiple mechanisms of action and is a broad-spectrum AED. Elimination is primarily renal, but hepatic metabolism occurs, especially if given concomitantly with enzyme inducers. It has linear pharmacokinetics and few drug interactions.

Disadvantages With rapid dosage escalation, topiramate can compromise cognitive functioning, including impaired word finding and impaired short-term memory. Therefore, initial doses should be low, and titration must be slow. Renal stones and weight loss have been associated with topiramate use. The dose should be decreased in patients with renal impairment. There is no parenteral formulation.

Place in Therapy Topiramate is a first-line AED for partial seizures as an adjunct and/or monotherapy. It is also approved for the treatment of tonic–clonic seizures in primary generalized epilepsy.

Valproic Acid/Divalproex Sodium

Pharmacology and Mechanism of Action Alterations of the synthesis and degradation of GABA do not fully explain the antiseizure activity of valproic acid. Valproic acid may potentiate postsynaptic GABA responses, may have a direct membrane-stabilizing effect, and may affect potassium channels.[125]

Pharmacokinetics Valproic acid appears to be absorbed completely from available oral dosage forms when administered on an empty stomach.[125] However, the rate of absorption differs among preparations. Peak concentrations occur in 0.5 to 1 hour with the syrup, 1 to 3 hours with the capsule, and 2 to 6 hours with the enteric-coated tablet.[125] The extended-release formulation (Depakote-ER) is FDA approved for patients with migraine headache and epilepsy. The bioavailability of this formulation is approximately 15% less than that of enteric-coated divalproex sodium (Depakote).

Valproic acid is extensively bound to albumin, and this binding is saturable. Accordingly, the valproic acid free fraction will increase as the total serum concentration increases. Because of this saturable binding, measurement of unbound serum concentrations may be a better monitoring parameter than the total valproic acid serum concentration, especially at higher concentrations or in patients with hypoalbuminemia.

The primary route of valproic acid metabolism is β-oxidation, although up to 40% of a dose may be excreted as the glucuronide. At least 10 metabolites of valproic acid have been identified. Some of these may have weak anticonvulsant activity, and at least one metabolite may be responsible for the hepatotoxicity reported. One of the lesser oxidative metabolites, 4-ene-VPA, causes hepatotoxicity in rats. The formation of this metabolite is increased when valproic acid is given with enzyme-inducing drugs.[125] Valproic acid displays diurnal elimination with lower evening serum levels occurring than morning levels. It crosses into the placenta, and concentrations may be up to five times higher in cord serum blood than in the mother due to higher binding in the fetal compartment.[126]

Adverse Effects The most frequently reported side effects are GI (up to 20%), including nausea, vomiting, anorexia, as well as weight gain. Pancreatitis is rare. GI complaints may be minimized, but not totally alleviated, with the enteric-coated formulation or by giving the drug with food. Alopecia and hair changes are temporary, and hair growth returns even with continued dosing. Weight gain can be significant for many patients and is associated with an increase in fasting insulin and leptin serum levels.[127] The increase in serum insulin is believed to be caused by the inhibition of metabolism of insulin by the liver.[128] This has led to the development of insulin resistance in obese male and female subjects.[125] Valproic acid causes minimal cognitive impairment.[125]

The most serious side effect reported with valproic acid is hepatotoxicity. Hyperammonemia is common (50%) but does not necessarily imply liver damage. Most liver failure deaths have occurred in patients who were younger than 2 years of age, had mental retardation, and received multiple AEDs. Hepatotoxicity occurred early in the course of therapy. Patients who complain of nausea, vomiting, lethargy, anorexia, and edema in the first 6 to 12 months of therapy should have liver function evaluated. Multiple AEDs can alter the metabolism of valproic acid, leading to increased formation of the potentially liver-toxic 4-ene-VPA. Valproic acid has been shown to alter carnitine metabolism, and it has been postulated that a deficiency of carnitine alters fatty acid oxidation that could lead to both liver toxicity and hyperammonemia.[129] However, valproic acid hepatotoxicity has occurred in a patient taking supplemental carnitine, and a prospective study demonstrated no effect on well-being when carnitine was added. Although carnitine can ameliorate hyperammonemia in part, it is expensive, and there are only limited data to support routine supplemental use in patients taking valproic acid.[130]

Thrombocytopenia and alterations in platelet aggregation occur in the patients receiving valproic acid, and these phenomena are related to serum concentration. These blood coagulopathies may occur more frequently in children than in adults.[131]

Drug Interactions Because it is highly protein bound, other highly protein-bound drugs (e.g., free fatty acids and aspirin) can displace valproic acid.

Valproic acid can inhibit specific CYP450 isozymes, epoxide hydrolase, and UGT isozymes. The addition of valproic acid to phenobarbital results in a 30% to 50% decrease in phenobarbital clearance and significant toxicity if the dose of phenobarbital is not reduced. Data also suggest that combination OCs may increase the clearance of valproic acid and lower serum levels by 20%.[32] In addition, carbapenems, especially meropenem, can lower valproic acid levels.[132]

Dosing and Administration Valproic acid in some patients may have a half-life long enough for once-daily dosing with enteric-coated divalproex, but more frequent dosing is the norm. Based on half-life data, twice-daily dosing is feasible with any valproic acid dosage form; however, children and patients taking enzyme inducers can require dosing three to four times daily. The serum concentration–dose relationship is curvilinear (e.g., the concentration–dose ratio decreases with increasing dose) probably because of increasing free concentrations and a resulting increase in clearance.

Valproic acid is available as a soft gelatin capsule, an enteric-coated tablet, a syrup, a "sprinkle capsule," an extended-release formulation designed for once-daily dosing, and an IV formulation for replacement of oral therapy or in situations where rapid loading is necessary.[125] This parenteral formulation must not be given IM because it can cause tissue necrosis. The sprinkle capsule, designed to be opened and mixed with food, has a slower rate of absorption, which results in fewer fluctuations in the peak-to-trough ratio. The syrup is absorbed more rapidly than any solid dosage form. The enteric-coated divalproex tablet is not sustained release. It must be metabolized in the gut to valproic acid. The enteric coating reduces GI distress. The enteric coating causes delayed absorption, although once the enteric coating dissolves, sodium divalproex has absorption, metabolism, and elimination rates similar to those of the gelatin capsule. If a patient is switched from Depakote to Depakote-ER, the dose should be increased by 14% to 20%. Depakote-ER may be given once daily.

Advantages Valproic acid is available in multiple dosage formulations. The IV formulation is especially well tolerated. It has a wide therapeutic index and is considered a broad-spectrum AED. It is also used in other neurologic or psychiatric disorders (e.g., migraine headache, bipolar disorder).

Disadvantages Some patients report significant weight gain with valproic acid, which may limit compliance. It has other side effects, such as alopecia, tremor, pancreatitis, PCOS, and thrombocytopenia. It has been associated with hepatic necrosis in young children. As an enzyme inhibitor, it is involved in multiple drug–drug interactions.

Place in Therapy Valproic acid is first-line therapy for primary generalized seizures, including myoclonic, atonic, and absence seizures. It can be used as both monotherapy and adjunctive therapy for partial seizures, and it can be very useful in patients with mixed seizure disorders.

Vigabatrin

Pharmacology and Mechanism of Action Vigabatrin is an amino acid that is a structural analog of GABA. It is a racemic mixture consisting of two enantiomers with only the *S*(+)-enantiomer active. Vigabatrin is a selective, irreversible inhibitor of GABA-transaminase, the enzyme that degrades GABA, thereby increasing GABA levels in the CNS.[133]

Pharmacokinetics Vigabatrin undergoes virtually no metabolism and is excreted unchanged in the urine. It is rapidly absorbed from the GI tract, and food has no effect on its absorption. Serum vigabatrin levels are linearly related to dosage, but therapeutic levels are not related to duration of effect; duration of effect is directly related to regeneration of the enzyme which metabolizes GABA. Since vigabatrin undergoes virtually no metabolism and is excreted renally, dosage adjustment is necessary in renally impaired patients. Children have a higher vigabatrin clearance than adults and therefore require higher mg/kg doses.[32]

Adverse Effects Vigabatrin may aggravate seizures, particularly absence and myoclonic seizures in patients with generalized epilepsies. Patients with history of depression, psychosis, or behavioral disturbances may be at greater risk to develop psychiatric effects.[133] Vigabatrin causes progressive, irreversible, bilateral concentric visual field constriction in a high percentage of patients. It may also reduce visual acuity in a dose-related and life exposure-related manner. Vigabatrin is associated with weight gain and edema, peripheral neuropathy, somnolence, and fatigue. In up to 11% of patients (up to age 3 years) treated with high doses of the drug for infantile spasms, magnetic resonance imaging (MRI) findings have been strongly suggestive of intramyelinic edema in select brain areas. These findings appear to be reversible, and their significance is unclear.[134]

Drug Interactions Vigabatrin induces CYP2C and therefore decreases phenytoin plasma levels by approximately 20%. One study noted at least a 10% increase in serum carbamazepine levels in the majority of patients started on adjunctive therapy with vigabatrin, which has not been supported in clinical trials.

Dosing and Administration Vigabatrin's initial dose in adults for refractory CP seizures is 1,000 mg/day given in two divided doses with an increase by 500 mg/day weekly until 3,000 mg/day is reached. Initial dose in infants and children for infantile spasms is 50 mg/kg/day given in two divided doses with an increase by 25 to 50 mg/kg/day every 3 days to a maximum dose of 150 mg/kg/day.

Advantages Vigabatrin has been widely studied and used in numerous countries throughout the world.

Disadvantages Adverse effects are sizeable and significant. It is available only through a restricted distribution program (SHARE program), which requires providers and patients to register. Vision should be checked at baseline and every 3 months for up to 3 to 6 months after drug discontinuation.

Place in Therapy Vigabatrin is a first-line agent for infantile spasms, particularly those with tuberous sclerosis as the etiology. It is a third-line adjunctive agent for refractory partial epilepsy.

Zonisamide

Pharmacology and Mechanism of Action Zonisamide, a sulfonamide, is believed to exert its antiepileptic effect by inhibition of slow sodium channels, by blockade of T-type Ca^{2+} channels, and possibly by inhibition of glutamate release. It also has a weak carbonic anhydrase inhibitory effect.[135]

Pharmacokinetics Zonisamide is well absorbed and reaches a maximum concentration in 2 to 5 hours. It is metabolized by CYP3A4 and to a much lesser extent by CYP2C19 and CYP3A5. Approximately 30% is excreted unchanged in the urine. Zonisamide is distributed to most tissues, but the drug is concentrated in the red blood cells. It crosses the placenta. The concentration in breast milk is similar to that in the plasma.[135]

Adverse Effects CNS effects, including word-finding problems and irritability, as well as GI effects are the most common side effects seen with zonisamide. Adverse effects may be more common during rapid dose escalation. Because it is structurally related to sulfonamides, hypersensitivity reactions can occur (0.02% of patients), and zonisamide should be used with caution (if at all) in patients with a confirmed allergy to sulfonamide compounds. A 2.6% incidence of symptomatic kidney stones has been reported in patients treated in the United States.[136] Because of reports of modest, reversible declines in renal function in some patients, monitoring of renal function may be advisable for certain patients. Oligohidrosis has been reported. In addition, modest weight loss has been reported with this agent.[25,26,81]

Drug Interactions Zonisamide does not inhibit or induce the CYP450 system.

Dosing and Administration Zonisamide is given once or twice daily, however, once-daily dosing causes greater fluctuations in serum concentrations and perhaps more side effects. The dose should be increased every 2 weeks to response. Zonisamide is stable for 48 hours when mixed with water, apple juice, or pudding.

Advantages Zonisamide has multiple mechanisms of action and may be a broad-spectrum AED. There is broad international experience with this drug. It has a very long half-life, which is suitable for once- or twice-daily dosing. Patients may experience modest weight loss.

Disadvantages The dose of zonisamide should be titrated slowly to patient response. Renal stones and oligohidrosis have been reported. In addition, cognitive impairment can occur, especially if the dosage is escalated rapidly. It should be avoided in patients allergic to "sulfa drugs."

Place in Therapy Zonisamide is approved for the adjunctive treatment of partial seizures. Zonisamide is potentially effective in a variety of partial and primary generalized seizure types.

Clinical **Controversy. . .**

The place in therapy of the newer drugs is still being determined. The cost of the newer AEDs generally is much higher than that of the older drugs. Given that, in general, the efficacy of the newer drugs is comparable with that of the older agents, many clinicians (and patients) have been slow to adopt this newer generation of drugs, however this is changing as more generic new AEDs become available. It is important to recognize that overall effectiveness encompasses both efficacy and tolerability assessments. Generally speaking, the newer generation of AEDs possess fewer adverse effects and seems to be better tolerated than older, far less expensive agents such as the barbiturates. Some may also have less costly long-term adverse effects such as effects on bone metabolism or the fetus, and they may cause fewer drug interactions, which require higher doses of drugs to avoid treatment failures. These differences may well justify the shrinking difference in cost. Whether to switch to newer generation AEDs needs to be determined on an individual patient basis.

PERSONALIZED PHARMACOTHERAPY

The most important aspect in the use of AEDs in persons with epilepsy is to tailor the choice of drug to the patient's seizure type(s), concomitant medical problem(s) including concurrent medications, the patient's economic status, and age. Evaluation of the patient's renal and hepatic function is key to employing the best AED(s) in the treatment. The use of a generic AED may work well in one patient, but not in another. Assessment of QOL in the individual patient ultimately may be more meaningful than measuring blood levels of the AEDs. It is clear that the cheapest drug in epilepsy (e.g., phenobarbital) is not the best because of the number of side effects. Because epilepsy treatment continues to be highly individualized, the drug or combination of drugs that controls seizures with the least number of side effects will be the drug of choice for that patient, no matter how expensive the drug acquisition cost.

Since many patients with epilepsy require minimal variation in blood concentrations to prevent seizures and avoid side effects, generic prescribing for epilepsy remains controversial. Issues related to generic use have been clearly delineated in the literature.[137,138] What has yet to be determined is whether bioequivalence translates into therapeutic equivalence in the use of generic AEDs and whether there is a subset of patients where this is not true.

Just as important is treating the epileptic pregnant patient, since this requires special knowledge of which AEDs' pharmacokinetic profiles are affected by pregnancy, so dosage adjustment can be instituted to avoid breakthrough seizures.

In recent years much progress has been made in delineating patients who are at greater risk to develop severe adverse hypersensitivity reactions such as Stevens–Johnson syndrome and toxic epidermal necrolysis through HLA allele testing (see Pharmacologic Therapy section). Ongoing work is also being done to identify patients who may be at risk to develop multiorgan hypersensitivity syndrome using lymphocyte testing, although a test is not yet commercially available.

To date, there are very few epileptic syndromes that can be identified by genetic testing; however, research is still ongoing in this area. The genetic risk of epilepsy is quite complex, that is, multiple genetic and environmental factors seem to contribute to epilepsy risk. In addition, reliable genetic markers for drug efficacy have not been identified, since the occurrence of AED resistance is probably multifactorial.

EVALUATION OF THERAPEUTIC OUTCOMES

A therapeutic range should be established for each patient to define concentrations that result in minimal side effects and optimal seizure control. This therapeutic plasma concentration range should be used to identify the appropriate patient-specific dose. Patients should be monitored long term for seizure control, comorbid conditions, social adjustment (including QOL assessments), drug interactions, compliance, and adverse effects. Periodic screening for comorbid neuropsychiatric disorders such as depression and anxiety is also important. Clinical response is more important than the serum drug concentrations.

Outcomes can be assessed by regular clinical monitoring, drug utilization review, and QOL assessments. Clinical monitoring involves identifying the number and type of seizures. Patients should record the severity and the frequency of seizures in a seizure diary. There should be a decrease in the number and/or severity of seizures. Patients and family should be questioned regularly to determine whether they are truly seizure free.

ABBREVIATIONS

AAN	American Academy of Neurology
AED	antiepileptic drug
AES	American Epilepsy Society
AMPA	α-amino-3-hydroxy-5-methylisoxazole-4-propionic acid
AUC	area under the drug concentration time curve
CP	complex partial
C_{max}	maximal blood drug concentration
CSF	cerebrospinal fluid
CT	computed tomography
ECG	electrocardiogram
EEG	electroencephalogram
GABA	γ-aminobutyric acid
GTC	generalized tonic–clonic
HPA	hypothalamic–pituitary–adrenal
IM	intramuscular
ILAE	International League Against Epilepsy
IQ	intelligence quotient
JME	juvenile myoclonic epilepsy
MHD	monohydroxy derivative
MRI	magnetic resonance imaging
NMDA	*N*-methyl-D-aspartate
OC	oral contraceptive
PCOS	polycystic ovary syndrome
QOL	quality of life
SE	status epilepticus
SP	simple partial
T_{max}	time to maximal blood drug concentration
VNS	vagus nerve stimulation
WBC	white blood cell

REFERENCES

1. Sander JW. The epidemiology of epilepsy revisited. Curr Opin Neurol 2003;16:165–170.
2. Najm IM, Moddel G, Janigro D. Mechanisms of epileptogenesis and experimental models of seizures. In: Wyllie E, ed. The Treatment of Epilepsy, 4th ed. Philadelphia, PA: Lippincott Williams & Wilkins, 2006:91–102.
3. Commission on Classification and Terminology of the International League Against Epilepsy. Proposal for revised clinical and electroencephalographic classification of epileptic seizures. Epilepsia 1981;22:489–501.
4. Commission on Classification and Terminology of the International League Against Epilepsy. Proposal for revised classification of epilepsies and epileptic syndromes. Epilepsia 1989;30:389–399.
5. Chen DK, So YT, Fisher RS. Use of serum prolactin in diagnosing epileptic seizures. Report of the therapeutic and technology assessment subcommittee of the American Academy of Neurology. Neurology 2005;65:668–675.
6. Taylor RS, Sander JW, Taylor RJ, et al. Predictors of health-related quality of life and costs in adults with epilepsy: A systematic review. Epilepsia 2011;52:2168–2180.
7. Luoni C, Bisulli F, Canevini MP, et al. Determinants of health-related quality of life in pharmacoresistant epilepsy: Results from a large multicenter study of consecutively enrolled patients using validated quantitative assessments. Epilepsia 2011;52:2181–2191.
8. Fountain NB, Van Ness PC, Swain-Eng R, et al. Quality improvement in neurology: AAN epilepsy quality measures: Report of the Quality Measurement and Reporting Subcommittee of the American Academy of Neurology. Neurology 2011;76:94–99.

9. Wasade VS, Spanaki M, Iyengar R, et al. AAN Epilepsy Quality Measures in clinical practice: A survey of neurologists. Epilepsy Behav 2012;24:468–473.
10. Kerr MP, Mensah S, Besag F, et al. International consensus clinical practice statements for the treatment of neuropsychiatric conditions associated with epilepsy. Epilepsia 2011;52:2133–2138.
11. Mattson RH. Antiepileptic drug monotherapy in adults: Selection and use in new-onset epilepsy. In: Levy RH, Mattson RH, Meldrum BS, eds. Antiepileptic Drugs, 5th ed. Philadelphia, PA: Lippincott Williams & Wilkins, 2002: 72–95.
12. Garnett WR. Antiepileptic drug treatment: Outcomes and adherence. Pharmacotherapy 2000;20:191S–199S.
13. Leppik IE. Contemporary Diagnosis and Management of the Patient with Epilepsy, 6th ed. Newton, PA: Handbooks in Health Care, 2006:66–76.
14. Quality Standards Subcommittee of the American Academy of Neurology. Practice parameter: A guideline for discontinuing antiepileptic drugs in seizure free patients [summary statement]. Neurology 1996;47:600–602.
15. Gross-Tsur V, O'Dell C, Shinnar S. Initiation and discontinuation of antiepileptic drugs. In: Wyllie E, ed. The Treatment of Epilepsy, 4th ed. Philadelphia, PA: Lippincott Williams & Wilkins, 2006:681–694.
16. Krahl SE, Clark KB, Smith DC, et al. Locus coeruleus lesions suppress the seizure-attenuating effects of vagus nerve stimulation. Epilepsia 1998;39:709–714.
17. Engel J, McDermott MP, Wiebe S, et al. Early surgical therapy for drug-resistant temporal lobe epilepsy. JAMA 2012;307:922–930.
18. Sperling MR, Harris A, Nei M, et al. Mortality after epilepsy surgery. Epilepsia 2005;46(Suppl 11):49–53.
19. Devinsky O, Barr WB, Vickrey BG, et al. Changes in depression and anxiety after resective surgery for epilepsy. Neurology 2005;65:1744–1749.
20. Schmidt D, Stavem K. Long-term seizure outcome of surgery versus no surgery for drug-resistant partial epilepsy: A review of controlled studies. Epilepsia 2009;50:1301–1309.
21. Berg AT, Vickrey GB, Langfitt JT, et al. Reduction of AEDs in postsurgical patients who attain remission. Epilepsia 2006;47;64–71.
22. Groesbeck DK, Bluml RM, Kossoff EH. Long-term use of the ketogenic diet: Outcomes of 28 children with over 6 years diet duration. Neurology 2006;66(Suppl 2):A41.
23. Dossoff EH, Zupec-Kania BA, Amark PE, et al. Optimal clinical management of children receiving the ketogenic diet: Recommendations of the International Ketogenic Diet Study Group. Epilepsia 2009;50:304–317.
24. Miranda MJ, Turner Z, Magrath G. Alternative diets to the classical ketogenic diet—Can we be more liberal? Epilepsy Res 2012;100:278–285.
25. French JA, Kanner AM, Bautista J, et al. Efficacy and tolerability of the new antiepileptic drugs: I. Treatment of new onset epilepsy. Neurology 2004;62:1252–1260.
26. French JA, Kanner AM, Bautista J, et al. Efficacy and tolerability of the new antiepileptic drugs: II. Treatment of refractory epilepsy. Neurology 2004;62:1261–1273.
27. Nunes VD, Sawyer L, Neilson J, et al. Diagnosis and management of the epilepsies in adults and children: Summary of updated NICE guidance. BMJ 2012;344:e281.
28. Glauser T, Ben-Menachem E, Bourgeois B, et al. ILAE treatment guidelines: Evidenced-based analysis of antiepileptic drug efficacy and effectiveness as initial monotherapy for epileptic seizures and syndromes. Epilepsia 2006;47:1094–1120.
29. Karceski S, Morrell MJ, Carpenter D. Treatment of epilepsy in adults: Expert opinion. Epilepsy Behav 2005;7: S1–S64.
30. Faught E. Pharmacokinetic considerations in prescribing antiepileptic drugs. Epilepsia 2001;42(Suppl 4):19–23.
31. Leppik IE. Contemporary Diagnosis and Management of the Patient with Epilepsy, 6th ed. Newton, PA: Handbooks in Health Care, 2006:92–149.
32. Patsalos PN, Berry DJ, Bourgeois BFD, et al. Antiepileptic drugs-best practice guidelines for therapeutic drug monitoring: A position paper by the subcommission on therapeutic drug monitoring, ILAE Commission on Therapeutic Strategies. Epilepsia 2008;49:1239–1276.
33. Onfi [package insert]. Deerfield, IL: Lundbeck Inc., October 2011.
34. Potiga [package insert]. Research Triangle Park, NC: GlaxoSmithKline and Valeant Pharmaceuticals North America, June 2011.
35. Halford JJ, Lapointe M. Clinical perspectives on lacosamide. Epilepsy Curr 2009;9:1–9.
36. Cada DJ, Levien TL, Baker DE. Rufinamide. Hosp Pharm 2009;44:412–422.
37. Sabril [package insert]. Deerfield, IL: Lundbeck Inc., August 2009.
38. Perucca P, Gilliam FG. Adverse effects of antiepileptic drugs. Lancet 2012;11:792–802.
39. Pack AM, Morrell MJ, McMahon DJ, et al. Bone health in young women with epilepsy after one year of antiepileptic drug monotherapy. Neurology 2008;70:1586–1593.
40. Lado F, Spiegel R, Masur JH, et al. Value of routine screening for bone demineralization in an urban population of patients with epilepsy. Epilepsy Res 2008;78: 155–160.
41. Wang Z, Lin YS, Zheng XE, et al. An inducible cytochrome P4503A4-dependent vit D catabolic pathway. Mol Pharmacol 2012;81:498–509.
42. Chuang Y-C, Chuang H-Y, Lin T-K, et al. Effects of long-term antiepileptic drug monotherapy on vascular risk factors and atherosclerosis. Epilepsia 2012;53;120–128.
43. Mintzer S, Skidmore CT, Rankin SJ, et al. Conversion from enzyme-inducing antiepileptic drugs to topiramate: Effects on lipids and C-reactive protein. Epilepsy Res 2012;98: 88–93.
44. Meador KJ, Gilliam FG, Kanner AM, Pellock JM. Cognitive and behavioral effects of antiepileptic drugs. Epilepsy Behav 2001;2:S1–S17.
45. Vermeulen J, Aldenkamp AP. Cognitive side-effects of chronic anti-epileptic drug treatment: A review of 25 years of research. Epilepsy Res 1995;22:65–95.
46. Meador KJ, Loring DW, Ray PG, et al. Differential cognitive effects of carbamazepine and gabapentin. Epilepsia 1999;40:1279–1285.
47. Meador KJ, Loring DW, Ray PG. Differential cognitive effects of carbamazepine and lamotrigine [abstract]. Neurology 2000;54:A84.
48. Martin R, Kuzniecky R, Ho S, et al. Cognitive effects of topiramate, gabapentin and lamotrigine in healthy young adults. Neurology 1999;52:321–327.
49. Fritz N, Glogau S, Hoffman J, et al. Efficacy and cognitive side effects to tiagabine and topiramate in patients with epilepsy. Epilepsy Behav 2005;6:373–381.
50. Salinsky MC, Storzbach D, Spencer DC, et al. Effects of topiramate and gabapentin on cognitive abilities in healthy volunteers. Neurology 2005;64:792–798.
51. Sazgar M, Bourgeois B. Aggravation of epilepsy by antiepileptic drugs. Pediatr Neurol 2005;33:227–234.

52. Mattson RH, Cramer JA, Collins JF, et al. Comparison of carbamazepine, phenobarbital, phenytoin, and primidone in partial and secondarily generalized tonic–clonic seizures. N Engl J Med 1985;313:145–151.
53. Mattson RH, Cramer JA, Collins JF, et al. A comparison of valproate with carbamazepine for the treatment of complex partial seizures and secondarily generalized tonic–clonic seizures in adults. N Engl J Med 1992;327:765–771.
54. Beydoun A, Kutluay E. Conversion to monotherapy: Clinical trials in patients with refractory partial seizures. Neurology 2003;60(Suppl 4):S13–S25.
55. French JA, Kanner AM, Bautista J, et al. Efficacy and tolerability of the new antiepileptic drugs: I. Treatment of new-onset epilepsy. Epilepsia 2004:45;401–409.
56. French JA, Kanner AM, Bautista J, et al. Efficacy and tolerability of the new antiepileptic drugs: II. Treatment of refractory epilepsy. Epilepsia 2004:45;410–423.
57. Marson AG, Al-Kharusi AM, Alwaidh M, et al. The SANAD study of effectiveness of carbamazepine, gabapentin, lamotrigine, oxcarbazepine, or topiramate for treatment of partial epilepsy: An unblinded randomized controlled trial. Lancet 2007;369(9566):1000–1015.
58. Rowan AJ, Ramsay ER, Collins JF, et al. New onset geriatric epilepsy: A randomized study of gabapentin, lamotrigine, and carbamazepine. Neurology 2005;64:1868–1873.
59. Brodie MJ, Perucca E, Ryvlin P, et al. Comparison of levetiracetam and controlled-release carbamazepine in newly diagnosed epilepsy. Epilepsy 2007;68:402–408.
60. Costa J, Fareleira F, Ascencão R, et al. Clinical comparability of the new antiepileptic drugs in refractory partial epilepsy: A systematic review and meta-analysis. Epilepsia 2011;52:1280–1291.
61. Marson AG, Al-Karusi AM, Alwaidh M, et al. The SANAD study of effectiveness of valproate, lamotrigine, or topiramate for generalized and unclassifiable epilepsy: An unblinded randomized controlled trial. Lancet 2007;369(9566):1016–1026.
62. Bonnett L, Smith CT, Smith D, et al. Prognostic factors for time to treatment failure and time to 12 months of remission for patients with focal epilepsy: Post-hoc, subgroup analyses of data from the SANAD trial. Lancet Neurol 2012;11:331–340.
63. Crawford PM. Managing epilepsy in women of childbearing age. Drug Saf 2009;32:293–307.
64. Verrotti A, D'Egidio C, Mohn A, et al. Antiepileptic drug, sex hormones, and PCOS. Epilepsia 2011;52:199–211.
65. Yerby MS, Kaplan P, Tran T. Risks and management of pregnancy in women with epilepsy. Cleve Clin J Med 2004;71:S25–S37.
66. Vajda FJ, Hitchcock A, Graham J, et al. Seizure control in antiepileptic drug-treated pregnancy. Epilepsia 2008;49: 172–176.
67. Harden CL, Hopp J, Ting TY, et al. Management issues for women with epilepsy—Focus on pregnancy (an evidence-based review): 1. Obstetrical complications and change in seizure frequency. Epilepsia 2009;50:1229–1236.
68. Harden CL, Meador KJ, Pennell PB, et al. Management issues for women with epilepsy—Focus on pregnancy (an evidence-based review): II. Teratogenesis and perinatal outcomes. Epilepsia 2009;50:1237–1246.
69. Harden CL, Pennell PB, Koppel BS, et al. Management issues for women with epilepsy-Focus on pregnancy (an evidence-based review): III. Vitamin K, folic acid, blood levels, and breast-feeding. Epilepsia 2009;50:1247–1255.
70. Wlodarczyk BJ, Palacios AM, George TM, Finnell RH. Antiepileptic drugs and pregnancy outcomes. Am J Med Gene Part A 2012;158A:2071–2090.
71. Meador KJ, Baker GA, Browning N, et al. Effects of breastfeeding in children of women taking antiepileptic drugs. Neurology 2010;75:1954–1960.
72. Erel T, Guralp O. Epilepsy and menopause. Arch Gynecol Obstet 2011;284:749–755.
73. Harden CL, Nikolov BG, Kandula P, et al. Effect of levetiracetam on testosterone levels in male patients. Epilepsia 2010;51:2348–2351.
74. Isojaervi JIJ, Loefgren E, Juntunen KST, et al. Effect of epilepsy and antiepileptic drugs on male reproductive health. Neurology 2004;62:247–253.
75. Ferraro TN, Buono RJ. The relationship between the pharmacology of antiepileptic drugs and human gene variation: An overview. Epilepsy Behav 2005;7:18–36.
76. Garnett WR, Bainbridge JL, Johnson SL. Carbamazepine. In: Murphy J, ed. Clinical Pharmacokinetics, 4th ed. Bethesda, MD: American Society of Health-Systems Pharmacists, 2008:121–138.
77. Marino SE, Birbaum AK, Leppik IE, et al. Steady-state carbamazepine pharmacokinetics following oral and stable-labeled intravenous administration in epilepsy patients: effects of race and sex. Clin Pharmacol Ther 2012;91:483–488.
78. Ficker DM, Privitera M, Krauss G, et al. Improved tolerability and efficacy in epilepsy patients with extended-release carbamazepine. Neurology 2005;65:593–595.
79. Garnett WR, Bainbridge JL, Johnson SL. Ethosuximide. In: Murphy J, ed. Clinical Pharmacokinetics. Bethesda, MD: American Society of Health-Systems Pharmacists, 2008:153–159.
80. Gunthorpe MJ, Large CH, Sankar R. The mechanism of action of retigabine (ezogabine), a first-in-class K+ channel opener for the treatment of epilepsy. Epilepsia 2012;53: 412–424.
81. Pellock JM, Perhach JL, Sofia RD. Felbamate. In: Levy RH, Mattson RH, Meldrum BS, et al., eds. Antiepileptic Drugs, 5th ed. Philadelphia, PA: Lippincott Williams & Wilkins, 2002:301–318.
82. LaRoche SM, Helmers SL. The new antiepileptic drugs: Scientific review. JAMA 2004;291:605–614.
83. Taylor CP, Gee NS, Su TZ, et al. A summary of mechanistic hypothesis of gabapentin pharmacology. Epilepsy Res 1998;29:233–249.
84. Luer MS, Hamani C, Dujovny M, et al. Saturable transport of gabapentin at the blood–brain barrier. Neurol Res 1999;21:559–562.
85. Gidal BE, Radulovic LL, Kruger S, et al. Inter- and intrasubject variability in gabapentin (GBP) absorption and absolute bioavailability. Epilepsy Res 2000;40:123–127.
86. Gidal BE, Maly MM, Kowalski J, et al. Gabapentin absorption: Effect of mixing with foods of varying macronutrient content. Ann Pharmacother 1998;32:405–408.
87. Lee DO, Steingard RJ, Cesena M, et al. Behavioral side effects of gabapentin in children. Epilepsia 1996;37:87–90.
88. McLean MJ, Gidal BE. Gabapentin in the treatment of epilepsy: A dosing review. Clin Ther 2003;25:1382–1406.
89. Gidal BE, DeCerce J, Bockbrader HR, et al. Gabapentin bioavailability: Effect of dose and frequency of administration in adult patients with epilepsy. Epilepsy Res 1998;31:91–99.
90. Hirsch LJ, Weintraub DB, Buchsbaum R, et al. Predictors of lamotrigine-associated rash. Epilepsia 2006;47:318–322.
91. Messenheimer JA. Rash in adult and pediatric patients treated with lamotrigine. Can J Neurol Sci 1998;25:S14–S18.
92. Sidhu J, Bulsara S, Job S, Philipson R. A bi-directional pharmacokinetic interaction study of lamotrigine and the combined oral contraceptive pill in healthy subjects [abstract]. Epilepsia 2004;45(Suppl 7):330.

93. Christensen J, Petrenaite V, Atterman J, et al. Oral contraceptives induce lamotrigine metabolism: Evidence from a double-blind, placebo-controlled trial. Epilepsia 2007;48:484–489.
94. Gilman JT. Lamotrigine: An antiepileptic agent for the treatment of partial seizures. Ann Pharmacother 1995;29:144–151.
95. Lynch BA, Lambeng N, Nocka K, et al. The synaptic vesicle protein SV2A in the binding site for the antiepileptic drug levetiracetam. Proc Natl Acad Sci USA 2004;101: 9861–9866.
96. Loscher W, Honack D, Rundfeldt C. Antiepileptogenic effects of the novel anticonvulsant levetiracetam (ucb LO59) in the kindling model of temporal lobe epilepsy. J Pharmacol Exp Ther 1998;284:474–479.
97. Fay MA, Sheth RD, Gidal BE. Oral absorption kinetics of levetiracetam: The effect of mixing with food or enteral nutrition. Clin Ther 2005:27:594–598.
98. Brockmoeller J, Thomsen T, Wittstock M, et al. Pharmacokinetics of levetiracetam in patients with moderate to severe liver cirrhosis (Child-Pugh classes A, B and C): Characterization by dynamic liver function tests. Clin Pharmacol Ther 2005;77:529–541.
99. Harden CL, Pennell PB, Koppel BS, et al. Practice parameter update: Management issues for women with epilepsy—Focus on pregnancy (an evidence-based review): vitamin K, folic acid, blood levels, and breastfeeding. Neurology 2009;73:142–149.
100. Coppola G, Mangano S, Tortorella G, et al. Levetiracetam during 1-year follow-up in children, adolescents, and young adults with refractory epilepsy. Epilepsy Res 2004;59: 35–42.
101. Stefan H, Wang-Tilz Y, Pauli E, et al. Onset of action of levetiracetam: A RCT trial using therapeutic intensive seizure analysis (TISA). Epilepsia 2006;47:516–522.
102. Ambrosio AF, Soares-Da-Silva P, Carvalho CM, Carvalho AP. Mechanisms of action of carbamazepine and its derivatives, oxcarbazepine, BIA 2-093 and BIA 2-024. Neurochem Res 2002;27:121–130.
103. Ambrosio AF, Silva AP, Malva JO, et al. Carbamazepine inhibits L-type Ca^{2+} channels in cultured rat hippocampal neurons stimulated with glutamate receptor agonists. Neuropharmacology 1999;38:1349–1359.
104. Kalis MM, Huff NA. Oxcarbazepine, an antiepileptic agent. Clin Ther 2001;23:680–700.
105. May TW, Ramback B, Jurgens U. Influence of oxcarbazepine and methsuximide on lamotrigine concentrations in epileptic patients with and without valproic acid comedication: Results of a retrospective study. Ther Drug Monit 1999;21:175–181.
106. Pina-Garza JE, Espinoza R, Nordli D, et al. Oxcarbazepine adjunctive therapy in infants and young children with partial seizures. Neurology 2005;65:1370–1375.
107. Muller M, Marson AG, Williamson PR. Oxcarbazepine versus phenytoin monotherapy for epilepsy. Cochrane Database Syst Rev 2006;2:CD003615.
108. Tozer TN, Winter ME. Phenytoin. In: Evans WE, Schentag JJ, Jusko WJ, eds. Applied Pharmacokinetics, 3rd ed. Spokane, WA: Applied Therapeutics, 1992:1–44 [chapter 25].
109. Anderson GD, Pak C, Doane KW, et al. Revised Winter-Tozer equation for normalized phenytoin concentrations in trauma and elderly patients with hypoalbuminemia. Ann Pharmacother 1997;31:279–284.
110. Ahn JE, Cloyd JC, Brundage RC, et al. Phenytoin half-life and clearance during maintenance therapy in adults and elderly patients with epilepsy. Neurology 2008;71:38–43.
111. Bruni J. Phenytoin and other hydantoins: Adverse effects. In: Levy RH, Mattson RH, Meldrum BS, et al., eds. Antiepileptic Drugs, 5th ed. Philadelphia, PA: Lippincott Williams & Wilkins, 2002:605–610.
112. Privitera MD. Clinical rules for phenytoin dosing. Ann Pharmacother 1993;27:1169–1173.
113. Ben-Menachem E. Pregabalin pharmacology and its relevance to clinical practice. Epilepsia 2004;45(Suppl 6):13–18.
114. Bialer M, Johannessen SI, Kupferberg HJ, et al. Progress report on new antiepileptic drugs: A summary of the seventh EILAT conference (EILAT VII). Epilepsy Res 2004;61:1–48.
115. Shneker BF, McAuley JW. Pregablin: A new neuromodulator with broad therapeutic indications. Ann Pharmacother 2005;39:2029–2037.
116. Perucca E, Cloyd J, Critchley D, et al. Rufinamide: Clinical pharmacokinetics and concentration–response relationships in patients with epilepsy. Epilepsia 2008;49:1123–1120.
117. Schachter SC. Tiagabine: Current status and potential clinical applications. Expert Opin Investig Drugs 1996;5: 1377–1387.
118. Leppik IE. Tiagabine: The safety landscape. Epilepsia 1995;36:S10–S13.
119. Koepp MJ, Edwards M, Collins J, et al. Status epilepticus and tiagabine therapy revisited. Epilepsia 2005;46:1625–1632.
120. Gidal BE, Lensmeyer GL. Therapeutic drug monitoring of topiramate: Evaluation of the saturable distribution between erythrocytes and plasma in whole blood using an optimized HPLC method. Ther Drug Monit 1999;21:567–576.
121. Shorvon SD. Safety of topiramate: Adverse events and relationship to dosing. Epilepsia 1996;37(Suppl 2):S18–S22.
122. Mula M, Trimble M, Thompson P, et al. Topiramate and word-finding difficulties in patients with epilepsy. Neurology 2003;60:1104–1107.
123. Gidal BE. Topiramate: Drug interactions. In: Levy RH, Mattson RH, Meldrum BS, et al., eds. Antiepileptic Drugs, 5th ed. Philadelphia, PA: Lippincott Williams & Wilkins, 2002:735–739.
124. Privitera M, Fincham R, Penry J, et al. Topiramate placebo-controlled dose-ranging trial in refractory partial epilepsy using 600-, 800-, and 1,000-mg daily dosages. Neurology 1996;46:1678–1683.
125. Davis R, Peters DH, McTavish D. Valproic acid: A reappraisal of its pharmacological properties and clinical efficacy in epilepsy. Drugs 1994;47:332–372.
126. Ornoy A. Valproic acid in pregnancy: How much are we endangering the embryo and fetus? Reprod Toxicol 2009;28:1–10.
127. Greco R, Latini G, Chiarelli F, et al. Leptin, ghrelin, and adiponectin in antiepileptic patients treated with valproic acid. Neurology 2005;65;1808–1809.
128. Pylvanen V, Pakarinen A, Knip M, Isojaervi J. Characterization of insulin secretion in valproate-treated patients with epilepsy. Epilepsia 2006;47:1460–1464.
129. Genton P, Gelissse P. Valproic acid: Adverse effects. In: Levy RH, Mattson RH, Meldrum BS, et al. Antiepileptic Drugs, 5th ed. Philadelphia, PA: Lippincott Williams & Wilkins, 2002:837–851.
130. Gidal BE, Inglese CM, Meyer JM, et al. Diet and valproate mediated transient hyperammonemia: Effect of L-carnitine supplementation in children with epilepsy. Pediatr Neurol 1997;16:301–305.
131. Gerstner T, Teich M, Bell N, et al. Valproate-associated coagulopathies are frequent and variable in children. Epilepsia 2006;47:1136–1143.
132. Comparison of carbapenem antibiotics. Pharmacist's Lett/Prescriber's Lett 2007;23(12):231205.

133. Ben-Menachem E, Dulac O, Chiron C. Vigabatrin. In: Engel J, Pedley TA, eds. Epilepsy: A Comprehensive Textbook, 2nd ed. Philadelphia, PA: Lippincott Williams & Wilkins, 2008:1683–1693.
134. Shorvon SD. Drug treatment of epilepsy in the century of the ILAE: The second 50 years, 1959–2009. Epilepsia 2009;50(Suppl 3):93–130.
135. Welty TE. Zonisamide. In: Wyllie E, ed. The Treatment of Epilepsy, 4th ed. Philadelphia, PA: Lippincott Williams & Wilkins, 2006:891–899.
136. Lee BI. Zonisamide: Adverse effects. In: Levy RH, Mattson RH, Meldrum BS, et al., eds. Antiepileptic Drugs. Philadelphia, PA: Lippincott Williams & Wilkins, 2002; 892–898.
137. Gidal BE, Tomson T. Debate: Substitution of generic drugs in epilepsy: Is there cause for concern? Epilepsia 2008;49(Suppl 9):56–62.
138. Privitera MD. Generic antiepileptic drugs: Current controversies and future directions. Epilepsy Curr 2008;8:113–117.

41

Status Epilepticus

Stephanie J. Phelps and James W. Wheless

KEY CONCEPTS

1. Status epilepticus (SE) is a neurologic emergency that is associated with significant morbidity and mortality.
2. Generalized convulsive status epilepticus (GCSE) is defined as any recurrent or continuous seizure activity lasting longer than 30 minutes in which the patient does not regain baseline mental status. Any seizure that does not stop within 5 minutes should be treated as impending SE.
3. There are two types of SE, GCSE and nonconvulsive status epilepticus (NCSE). GCSE is the most common type.
4. Most GCSE develops in patients with no history of epilepsy; however, a patient with preexisting epilepsy may experience GCSE as a result of acute anticonvulsant withdrawal, metabolic disorder, concurrent illness, or progression of neurologic disease.
5. Although the pathophysiology of GCSE is unknown, experimental models have shown that there is a dramatic decrease in γ-aminobutyric acid–mediated inhibitory synaptic transmission and that glutamatergic excitatory synaptic transmission sustains the seizures.
6. General treatment includes patient stabilization, adequate oxygenation, preservation of cardiorespiratory function, management of systemic complications, and aggressive assessment of underlying causes.
7. The main purpose of treatment is to prevent or decrease morbidity and mortality of prolonged seizures. Pharmacologic treatment needs to be rapid and aimed at terminating both electrical and clinical seizures. The probability of poorer outcomes increases with increased length of electrographic seizure activity.
8. Lorazepam is the preferred benzodiazepine in treatment of GCSE because of its efficacy and long duration of action in the CNS. Midazolam is the preferred benzodiazepine for intramuscular (IM) administration.
9. Currently, the hydantoins (phenytoin and fosphenytoin) are the long-acting anticonvulsants used most frequently. Either phenytoin or fosphenytoin should be given concurrently with benzodiazepines.
10. The maximum rate of infusion for phenytoin and fosphenytoin in adults is 50 mg/min and 150 mg PE/min, respectively.
11. If GCSE is not controlled by two first-line agents (benzodiazepine plus hydantoin or phenobarbital), the GCSE is considered to be refractory. In these cases, anesthetic doses of midazolam, pentobarbital, or propofol may be used.

INTRODUCTION

❶ Status epilepticus (SE) is a common neurologic emergency that is associated with brain damage and death. ❷ The traditional definition defines SE as (a) any seizure lasting longer than 30 minutes whether or not consciousness is impaired or (b) recurrent seizures without an intervening period of consciousness between seizures.[1] Clinically, this definition has limited use, as the average seizure is less than 2 minutes; and only 40% of seizures lasting 10 to 29 minutes cease without treatment.[2,3] Pharmacoresistance[4] and mortality[3] significantly increase with prolonged seizure duration. ❷ Therefore, aggressive treatment of seizures lasting 5 minutes or more is strongly recommended. ❸ SE can present in several forms (Table 41-1), including generalized convulsive status epilepticus (GCSE) and nonconvulsive status epilepticus (NCSE).[1]

NCSE occurs in 25% of those with SE and is characterized by a fluctuating or continuous "epileptic twilight" state that produces altered consciousness and/or behavior (e.g., lethargy, decreased mental function). An electroencephalogram (EEG) is the most important diagnostic and management tool.[5] In most instances, a benzodiazepine and/or valproate remain drugs of choice.[5] Although IV hydantoin, levetiracetam, or phenobarbital can be tried in nonresponders, general anesthesia is usually not appropriate.[5]

This chapter will focus on GCSE, which is the most common and severe form of SE. It is characterized by repeated primary or secondary generalized seizures that involve both hemispheres of the brain and are associated with a persistent postictal state.[4]

EPIDEMIOLOGY

The worldwide and United States incidence ranges between 1.2 to 5 million and 100,000 to 152,000 cases each year, respectively.[4] GCSE has no predilection for gender or socioeconomic status but does occur more frequently in nonwhites across all ages.[6] Most GCSE occurs in individuals with no history of epilepsy; however, approximately 5% of adults and 10% to 25% of children with epilepsy will develop GCSE.[7] The incidence of GCSE is highest in those younger than 1 year of age and in those older than 60 years of age.

ETIOLOGY

Precipitating events for GCSE vary and generally reflect different populations and referral patterns. ❹ Most episodes in individuals with epilepsy occur because of acute anticonvulsant withdrawal, a metabolic disorder or concurrent illness, or progression of a preexisting neurologic disease. Common etiologies and mortality

TABLE 41-1 International Classification of Status Epilepticus

Convulsive		Nonconvulsive	
International	**Traditional Terminology**	**International**	**Traditional Terminology**
Generalized SE • Tonic–clonic[a,b] • Tonic[c] • Clonic[c] • Myoclonic[b] • Erratic[d]	Grand mal, epilepticus convulsivus	Absence[c]	Petit mal, spike-and-wave stupor, spike and-slow-wave or 3/s spike-and-wave, epileptic fugue, epilepsia minora continua, epileptic twilight, minor SE
Secondary generalized SE[a,b] • Tonic • Partial seizures with secondary generalization		Partial SE[a,b] Simple partial Somatomotor Dysphasic Other types Complex partial	Focal motor, focal sensory, epilepsia partialis continua, adversive SE Elementary Temporal lobe, psychomotor, epileptic fugue state, prolonged epileptic stupor, prolonged epileptic confusional state, continuous epileptic twilight state

SE, status epilepticus.

[a]Most common in older children.
[b]Most common in adolescents and adults.
[c]Most common in infants and young children.
[d]Most common in neonates.

rates are shown in Table 41-2.[6,8] Precipitating events are divided into those with and without neurologic structural lesions or those with a precipitating injury or insult. Cases with structural lesions or those with a specific neurologic insult are associated with a poor prognosis.

TABLE 41-2 Etiology and Mortality for Pediatric and Adult Cases of Status Epilepticus

Etiology	Mortality Number of Cases (%) $n = 200$ Cases of Pediatric SE	Mortality Number of Cases (%) $n = 512$ Cases of Adult SE
Type I (no Structural Lesion)		
Infection	55 (5)	6 (35)
CNS infection	11 (0)	2 (20)
Metabolic	20 (5)	12 (36)
Low AED levels	16 (0)	24 (7)
Alcohol	0 (0)	13 (8)
Idiopathic	6 (0)	13 (18)
Type II (Structural Lesion)		
Anoxia/hypoxia	27 (13)	14 (65)
CNS tumor	3 (50)	5 (22)
CVA	5 (0)	26 (27)
Drug overdose	5 (0)	3 (23)
Hemorrhage	5 (11)	4 (35)
Trauma	13 (0)	3 (23)
Remote causes[a]	33 (5)	7 (13)

AED, antiepileptic drug; CVA, cerebrovascular accident; SE, status epilepticus.

Percentages do not add up to 100% because some patients had multiple etiologies.
[a]More than half of remote causes were congenital malformations and CVA in pediatric and adult patients, respectively.

Data from references 6 and 8.

There are major differences in etiologies for pediatric and adult patients (see Table 41-2). During their first few weeks of life, infants who are born to addicted mothers can develop drug withdrawal seizures. Other neonates can develop GCSE because of pyridoxine deficiency, which should resolve within hours following IV pyridoxine (100 mg). Acute encephalopathy and metabolic disorders are the major causes of GCSE in those younger than 1 year of age. In young children, the cause is often a nonspecific illness such as fever and/or a viral illness. The most frequent precipitating events in adults are cerebrovascular disease, rapid anticonvulsant withdrawal, and low anticonvulsant serum concentrations. Cerebrovascular disease is the leading cause in those who have their first seizures after age 60. Prescription, over-the-counter, and recreational drugs should be considered in anyone with new-onset GCSE.

MORBIDITY AND MORTALITY

GCSE is harmful to the brain. While most contend that the GCSE is responsible for the damage, it is unknown if the morbidity results from the underlying etiology or the GCSE. Regardless of the inducing stimulus, neuronal damage in animal models is evident following 30 to 60 minutes of GCSE, and most progress to develop epilepsy following a prolonged seizure. Interestingly, inhibiting the seizure-induced neuronal damage does not prevent the development of epilepsy, suggesting that the seizures themselves may be harmful. It is hard to establish a relationship between GCSE and long-term outcomes because it is difficult to weigh the effects of seizure type, etiology, duration, concurrent physiologic events, and therapy or lack thereof. It has been shown that patients with a history of prolonged febrile seizures who later developed epilepsy share similar histopathologic changes (i.e., hippocampal sclerosis) to those found in animal models of GCSE.[9,10] In these cases, the period between the initial GCSE and the first epileptic seizure may be months to decades, suggesting a possible link between GCSE and the development of epilepsy. Importantly, studies of GCSE show that the currently available anticonvulsants do not reproducibly prevent the development of epilepsy following prolonged seizures.[9,11]

Patients who develop epilepsy following prolonged GCSE are less likely to experience remission of their seizures and may have decreased cognitive and memory function, mental retardation, or neurologic deficits when compared to those who develop epilepsy and subsequently have GCSE.[4] Most studies have found that younger children, the elderly, and those with preexisting epilepsy have a higher propensity for sequelae. Unless accompanied by an underlying neurologic abnormality, febrile status epilepticus is less likely to be associated with sequelae.

Estimated mortality in the United States following GCSE ranges between 22,000 and 42,000 individuals per year,[8] with rates up to 16% in children,[12] 20% in adults,[4] and 38% in the elderly.[6] When compared with other populations, neonates have a higher mortality and more neurologic sequelae.

Table 41-2 summarizes the etiology and corresponding mortality rates for GCSE.[6,8] Interestingly, the mortality associated with many etiologies is significantly greater in adults than in children. Unresponsive patients may die from GCSE, but more frequently they die from the acute illness that precipitated the GCSE. For example, patients with serious CNS structural changes (e.g., hemorrhage, stroke) have a poor prognosis, compared to those with no structural lesion.

Outcome is affected by the time between onset of GCSE and the initiation of treatment and the duration of the seizure. Mortality significantly increases with increased seizure duration (e.g., 2.6% for seizures 10 to 29 minutes, 19% for seizures lasting >30 minutes, and 32% for seizures lasting greater than 60 minutes).[2,8] Mortality has decreased over the past decade and probably reflects a recognition of the need to initiate sequenced therapy using large doses as soon as possible.

PATHOGENESIS

Seizures occur when the excitatory neurotransmission overcomes inhibitory impulses in one or more brain regions. Most seizures are brief (less than 5 minutes), largely because the brain's inhibitory mechanisms restore the balance of normal neurotransmission.[4] Although it is unknown why the mechanisms that control normal brain homeostasis fail, when seizures occur in close succession or the magnitude of the proconvulsant stimulus is severe, compensatory mechanisms can be overwhelmed.

5 While the exact cellular mechanisms are unknown, it appears that seizure initiation is caused by an imbalance between excitatory (e.g., glutamate, calcium, sodium, substance P, and neurokinin B) and inhibitory neurotransmission (e.g., γ-aminobutyric acid [GABA], adenosine, potassium, neuropeptide Y, opioid peptides, and galanin).[13]

Most of what is known has focused on gated ion channels.[13] GCSE is largely caused by glutamate acting on postsynaptic *N*-methyl-D-aspartate (NMDA) and α-amino-3-hydroxy-5-methylisoxazole-4-propionate (AMPA)/kainate receptors. During GCSE, glutamate activation of the NMDA and AMPA receptors causes opening of the gated calcium and sodium channels, which lead to neuronal depolarization. Sustained depolarization may maintain GCSE and eventually cause neuronal death through calcium-, free radical-, and kinase-mediated events.[9] Although drugs acting as NMDA and AMPA receptor antagonists seem attractive, it is likely that glutamate is not the sole mechanism for GCSE and that other mechanisms become increasingly important as the duration of seizures increases.

Little is known about second messenger systems (e.g., metabotropic glutamate receptors) and the development of GCSE. $GABA_A$ postsynaptic receptors control chloride channels to produce hyperpolarization (inhibition) of the postsynaptic cell membrane. These receptors have binding sites for GABA and select anticonvulsants (e.g., phenobarbital and benzodiazepines) and enhance $GABA_A$-mediated chloride inhibitory currents. It was previously thought that a decrease in presynaptic GABA led to prolonged seizures; however, it is currently held that GABA concentrations increase during the early phases of GCSE and continue to be elevated during late GCSE. Prolonged seizures lead to decreased inhibitory $GABA_A$-receptor density because of postsynaptic receptor endocytosis. Additionally, modification of $GABA_A$ receptors during SE may decrease response to both endogenous GABA and GABA agonists.[10] Clinically, the relative potencies of benzodiazepines and phenobarbital can be reduced up to 10-fold if seizures persist for more than 30 minutes.[10] A similar phenomenon occurs with sodium channel antagonists (phenytoin); however, the magnitude of resistance is less.

PATHOPHYSIOLOGY

As GCSE persists, there are systemic alterations, progression of motor phenomena, and development of specific EEG findings.[14] Two distinct and predictable phases have been identified. Phase I occurs during the first 30 minutes of seizure activity, and phase II immediately follows. Although these systemic complications affect the prognosis of GCSE, a prolonged seizure can destroy neurons independent of these events.[9] In fact, the systemic effects of induced seizures in animals can be blocked, but the damage to the neocortex, cerebellum, and hippocampus persists.

During phase I, each seizure markedly increases plasma epinephrine, norepinephrine, and steroid concentrations, which can cause hypertension, tachycardia, and cardiac arrhythmias.[15] Within minutes, arterial systolic pressures can rise to above 200 mm Hg, and heart rate can increase by 83 beats per minute. Mean arterial pressure does not fall below 60 mm Hg; hence, cerebral perfusion pressure is not compromised. In animals, cerebral blood flow is also increased, thereby protecting neurons from hypoxic injury.

In the presence of a hypoxic myocardium, seizure-induced increases in sympathetic and parasympathetic stimulation of the heart can result in ventricular arrhythmias. Autonomic neuron stimulation can cause a release of insulin and glucagon. Concurrently, circulating catecholamines cause an elevation of hepatic cyclic adenosine monophosphate, producing glycogenolysis. Although the patient can be hyperglycemic initially, serum glucose begins to fall.

Seizure-induced muscular contractions and hypoxia cause lactic acid release, which can produce severe acidosis that maybe accompanied by hypotension and shock. Muscle contractions can be so severe that rhabdomyolysis with secondary hyperkalemia and acute tubular necrosis can occur. The airway can be obstructed, causing the patient to become cyanotic or hypoxic. Additionally, an increase in salivation and tracheal and pulmonary secretions can cause aspiration pneumonia. Although transient pleocytosis can develop, it should not be attributed to SE until infectious causes have been eliminated. Between seizures, the EEG slows, and blood pressure normalizes. Although metabolic demands are increased, the brain is able to adequately compensate.

When seizures exceed 30 minutes (phase II), the EEG ictal discharge and clonic motor activity become continuous, and the patient begins to decompensate. Despite elevated levels of catecholamines, the patient can become hypotensive. During this time, autoregulation of cerebral blood flow becomes dependent on mean arterial pressure and begins to fail. There continues to be an excessive consumption of oxygen and glucose; however, compensatory mechanisms are no longer able to meet demands.

During Phase II, the serum glucose concentration may be normal or decreased. Profound hypoglycemia, secondary to hyperinsulinemia, can occur in those with hepatic dysfunction or reduced glycogen stores. Hyperthermia and respiratory deterioration with hypoxia and ventilatory failure can develop. Metabolic and biochemical complications, including respiratory and metabolic acidosis, hyperkalemia, hyponatremia, and azotemia, may develop. There is increased sweating and salivation.

CLINICAL PRESENTATION AND DIAGNOSIS

Accurate diagnosis requires observation, physical examination, laboratory assessment, EEG, and neurologic imaging. The nature and duration of the seizure should be obtained, but a diagnosis of GCSE should not be made until a clinician has observed a seizure. Most patients have an altered consciousness that ranges from obtunded to marked lethargy and somnolence with pronounced eyes-open unresponsiveness and waxy rigidity. Motor features can include muscle contractions, extensor or flexor posturing, and spasms. Over time, the clinical manifestations become less apparent. This has important ramifications in that seizures appear to have terminated without treatment or when an ineffective therapy is given.

In addition to an assessment of language and cognitive abilities, the physical and neurological examinations should assess motor, sensory, and reflex abnormalities, pupillary response, asymmetry, and posturing. The patient should also be examined for secondary injuries (e.g., tongue lacerations, shoulder dislocations, and head and facial trauma).

Laboratory tests are essential to the diagnosis of various etiologies. Hypoglycemia, hyponatremia, hypernatremia, hypomagnesemia, hypocalcemia, and renal failure all can cause seizures. A urine

CLINICAL PRESENTATION GCSE

Symptoms

- Impaired consciousness (e.g., lethargy to coma)
- Disorientation once GCSE is controlled
- Pain associated with injuries (e.g., tongue lacerations, shoulder dislocations, back pain, myalgias, headache, head trauma)

Early Signs

- Generalized convulsions
- Acute injuries or CNS insults that cause extensor or flexor posturing
- Hypothermia or fever suggestive of intercurrent illnesses (e.g., sepsis or meningitis)
- Incontinence
- Normal blood pressure or hypotension and respiratory compromise

Late Signs

- Clinical seizures may or may not be apparent
- Pulmonary edema with respiratory failure
- Cardiac failure (dysrhythmias, arrest, cardiogenic shock)
- Hypotension or hypertension
- Disseminated intravascular coagulation, multisystem organ failure
- Rhabdomyolysis
- Hyperpyrexia

Initial Laboratory Tests

- Complete blood count (CBC) with differential
- Serum chemistry profile (e.g., electrolytes, calcium, magnesium, glucose, serum creatinine, alanine aminotransferase [ALT], aspartate aminotransferase [AST])
- Urine drug/alcohol screen
- Blood cultures
- Arterial blood gas to assess for metabolic and respiratory acidosis, oxygenation
- Serum drug concentration if previous anticonvulsant suspected or known

Other Diagnostic Tests

- Spinal tap if CNS infection suspected
- EEG should be obtained on presentation and once clinical seizures are controlled
- CT with and without contrast
- MRI
- Radiograph if indicated to diagnose fractures

drug screen can help eliminate illicit drug use or drug overdose. Serum drug concentration(s) should be obtained in those on chronic anticonvulsants, as low concentrations can reflect partial adherence or rapid drug withdrawal. A baseline serum concentration is necessary to determine whether a loading dose of a specific anticonvulsant is required. Assessment of other laboratory parameters (e.g., hematology and chemistries to include albumin, renal function, and hepatic function) that affect anticonvulsant dosing also can be useful. An EEG is a valuable diagnostic tool, particularly in those with prolonged GCSE in whom clinically apparent seizures are not always evident, but therapy should not be delayed while awaiting testing or results.

Once seizures have stopped, it is important to determine if the patient is febrile or has a systemic or CNS infection. Many physiologic consequences of GCSE (e.g., leukocytosis, pleocytosis, and hyperthermia) produce symptoms that can be confused with other conditions. If a CNS infection is suspected, a spinal tap should be performed, and empiric antibiotics should be started. If vascular, neoplastic, or infectious etiologies are suspected, computed tomography (CT) or magnetic resonance imaging (MRI) should be obtained once the seizures are controlled.

TREATMENT

Various treatments are available for the management of GCSE. These range from abortion of impending SE with rescue medications to the use of pharmacologic and nonpharmacologic therapies for GCSE and refractory/resistant SE.

Desired Outcomes

Short-term desired outcomes include (a) immediate termination of all clinical and electrical seizure activity, (b) no clinically significant adverse effects, and (c) lack of recurrent seizure activity. The long-term outcomes involve minimizing or avoiding pharmacoresistant epilepsy and/or the development of neurologic sequelae that significantly impact quality of life.

Nonpharmacologic Therapy

The time of seizure onset should be noted. Vital signs should be assessed, an adequate and protected airway should be established, ventilation should be maintained, and oxygen should be administered. Frequent arterial blood gas determinations should assess for metabolic acidosis, which should be treated with sodium bicarbonate if the pH is less than 7.2. Assisted ventilation should be used to correct respiratory acidosis. Hyperthermia, if present, should be aggressively treated (e.g., rectal acetaminophen, cooling blanket).

Because electrical seizures may persist in the absence of overt clinical motor manifestations, an EEG should be performed in anyone who continues to have altered consciousness after clinical control of their seizures. Although hypoglycemia rarely causes GCSE, adults and children with a blood glucose less than 60 mg/dL (less than 3.3 mmol/L) should receive 50 mL of a 50% dextrose solution, and 1 mL/kg of a 25% dextrose solution, respectively.[4,7] Because Wernicke's encephalopathy can develop in alcoholics, adults should receive IV thiamine (100 mg) prior to glucose.[4] Serum glucose concentration should be determined to assess the need for further supplementation.

Pharmacologic Therapy

When a seizure does not stop within 5 minutes, or when doubt exists regarding the diagnosis, patients should be treated as if they have GCSE (Fig. 41-1). 6 7 There are four immediate goals: (a) patient stabilization, including adequate oxygenation, preservation

TABLE 41-4 Adverse Drug Reactions and Monitoring of Patients Receiving Drugs for GCSE

Drug	Adverse Drug Reaction	Monitoring Parameters	Comments
Diazepam	Hypotension and cardiac arrhythmias	Vital signs and electrocardiogram (ECG) during administration	Propylene glycol causes hypotension and cardiac arrhythmias when administered too rapidly; hypotension may occur with large doses
Fosphenytoin	Hypotension and cardiac arrhythmias; paresthesia, pruritus	Vital signs and ECG during administration	Hypotension is less than that noted with phenytoin, as this product does not contain propylene glycol; pruritus generally involves the face and groin areas, is dose and rate related, and subsides 5–10 minutes after infusion
Lidocaine	Fasciculations, visual disturbances, tinnitus, seizures		Occur at serum concentrations between 6 and 8 mg/L (25.6–34.1 μmol/L); seizures >8 mg/L (34.1 μmol/L)
Lorazepam	Apnea, hypotension, bradycardia, cardiac arrest, respiratory depression, metabolic acidosis, and renal toxicity	Vital signs and ECG during administration; HCO_3 and serum creatinine; cumulative dose of propylene glycol	Accumulation of propylene glycol during prolong continuous infusions may cause acidosis
Pentobarbital	Hypotension	Vital signs and ECG during administration	Rate of infusion should be slower or dopamine should be added if hypotension occurs
Phenytoin	Hypotension and cardiac arrhythmia; nystagmus	Vital signs and ECG during administration	Propylene glycol causes hypotension and cardiac arrhythmias when administered too rapidly. Large loading doses are generally not given to elderly individuals with preexisting cardiac disease or in critically ill patients with marginal blood pressure. The infusion rate should be slowed if the QT interval widens or if hypotension or arrhythmias develop; horizontal nystagmus suggests serum concentration above the reference range and toxicity; if a serum phenytoin concentration validates this, the dose should be decreased
Phenobarbital	Hypotension, respiratory, and CNS depression	Vital signs and mental status; EEG if used in anesthesia doses	Contains propylene glycol; if hypotension occurs, slow the rate of administration or begin dopamine; apnea and hypopnea can be more profound in patients treated initially with benzodiazepines
Propofol	Progressive metabolic acidosis, hemodynamic instability, and bradyarrhythmias	Vital signs, ECG, osmolar gap; EEG if used in anesthesia doses	Referred to as propofol infusion related syndrome, which can be fatal
Topiramate	Metabolic acidosis	Acid base status (serum bicarbonate)	Extremely rare

CNS, central nervous system; ECG, electrocardiogram; EEG, electroencephalogram.

Clinical **Controversy...**

The choice of long-acting anticonvulsant to give following the initial benzodiazepine is controversial. According to the Working Group on Status Epilepticus, phenytoin should be used in seizures that recur after treatment with a benzodiazepine.[15] Although this has been the practice for decades; no studies have documented the superiority of a hydantoin over other anticonvulsants. Thus, it is questionable if a hydantoin should be administered alone, in larger doses, or at all when seizures recur following benzodiazepine administration. This issue is further complicated by the frequent shortage of some of these medications, and emerging data suggesting that valproate may be as effective.

Phenytoin

9 A hydantoin is the second-line agent in GCSE that is unresponsive to the benzodiazepines or in seizures that recur after successful treatment with a benzodiazepine.[4] Although it is effective in terminating seizures in 40% to 91% of patients,[15] it can be inferior to lorazepam, phenobarbital, or diazepam plus phenytoin at stopping GCSE within 20 minutes of their infusion.[18,19]

Phenytoin has a long half-life (20 to 36 hours) and causes less respiratory depression and sedation than the benzodiazepines or phenobarbital[15]; however, it cannot be delivered rapidly enough to be considered a first-line single agent. Injectable phenytoin should be diluted to less than or equal to 5 mg/mL in normal saline. Microcrystals will precipitate if it is mixed in a glucose-containing solution. The vehicle (40% propylene glycol) can cause administration-related hypotension and cardiac arrhythmias (Table 41-4).[15] 10 For this reason, the maximum rate of infusion is limited (Table 41-3).[4]

Suggested IV loading doses are provided in Table 41-3.[15] A reduction in the loading dose is recommended for elderly patients,[15] and a larger loading dose is required in obese individuals.[20] If the patient has been on phenytoin prior to admission and the serum concentration is known, this should be considered in determining a loading dose. Although some advocate the administration of an additional 5 mg/kg in those with unresponsive GCSE, there is no evidence that this will be beneficial. This practice can cause concentrations to exceed the reference range and produce toxicity. Because phenytoin has poor lipid solubility and enters the brain slowly, it can take up to 60 minutes before the pharmacodynamic effect is apparent. This delay is important when considering administration of a second loading dose. Therapeutic serum concentrations, 10 to 20 mg/L (40 to 79 μmol/L), generally do not persist more than 24 hours; hence, maintenance doses (see Table 41-3) should be started within 12 to 24 hours of the loading dose.

Phenytoin has an alkaline pH, which may cause pain and burning during infusion; phlebitis can occur with chronic infusion, and tissue necrosis is likely on infiltration. IM administration is not recommended because absorption is delayed and erratic, and phenytoin can crystallize in tissue. Although oral loading doses have been used in patients not actively seizing, it may take 4 to 12 hours before adequate serum concentrations are obtained; thus, this practice is not recommended.

Fosphenytoin

Fosphenytoin, a water-soluble phosphate ester, has no known pharmacologic activity.[21] It is converted rapidly (7 to 15 minutes) and completely (100%) to phenytoin by blood and tissue phosphatases after IV and IM dosing.[21] The conversion delay was a concern initially; however, this time is offset by high protein binding, saturable binding at high concentrations, and the rapid rate of infusion.[21] It does not contain propylene glycol and is compatible with most common IV fluids.

Fosphenytoin should be dosed using phenytoin equivalents (PE), thereby obviating the need for interconversion between phenytoin and fosphenytoin. The loading dose and rates of administration of fosphenytoin can be found in Table 41-3. Because of delays in achieving adequate phenytoin serum concentrations, a loading dose should not be given IM unless IV access is impossible.

Fosphenytoin serum concentrations have no value. Serum phenytoin concentrations should be used for therapeutic drug monitoring, and the desired serum concentration range is the same as that for phenytoin. Fosphenytoin cross reacts with some phenytoin immunoassays causing an overestimation of phenytoin concentration; hence, blood should not be obtained for at least 2 hours after IV and 4 hours after IM administration.[21]

Clinical **Controversy...**

The debate continues as to which hydantoin is preferred in GCSE. Although phenytoin has been used for decades, it is associated with a variety of problems related to its formulation. Conversely, fosphenytoin is associated with less infusion pain and IV-site complications and fewer hemodynamic effects than phenytoin. Although most practitioners believe that fosphenytoin is clearly a "better" formulation, many struggle with the advantages of fosphenytoin, given its cost.

Phenobarbital

Phenobarbital has biphasic distribution into body organs.[22] During phase I, the drug distributes into highly vascular organs, but does not distribute into the brain. With the exception of fat, phenobarbital distributes throughout the body during phase II[22]; hence, lean body mass should be used in calculating doses in obese patients.[22] Although the highest brain concentrations occur 12 to 60 minutes after an IV dose,[22] seizures are controlled within minutes of the loading dose.[19] Despite two studies that found phenobarbital to be as effective as phenytoin, lorazepam, or diazepam plus phenytoin in patients with GCSE,[18] the Working Group on Status Epilepticus recommends that phenobarbital be given after a benzodiazepine plus phenytoin has failed.[15]

The loading and maintenance dose are given in Table 41-3. When necessary, larger loading doses (30 mg/kg) have been used in neonates without adverse effects. If the initial loading dose does not stop the seizures within 20 to 30 minutes, an additional 10 to 20 mg/kg can be given. If seizures continue, a third 10 mg/kg load can be given.[23] Phenobarbital exhibits first-order linear pharmacokinetics, and there is no maximum dose beyond which further doses are likely to be ineffective.[23] Once GCSE is controlled, the maintenance dose should be started within 12 to 24 hours.

Although injectable phenobarbital contains propylene glycol, it can be given more rapidly than phenytoin (see Table 41-3). It can be given IM, but its rate of absorption is too slow to be effective. Adverse drug reactions and monitoring can be found in Table 41-4.[4,15]

Clinical **Controversy...**

There are three different opinions regarding the use of phenobarbital in GCSE. Because barbiturates cause CNS and respiratory depression, as well as hypotension, most contend that phenobarbital should be the third-line agent when a benzodiazepine plus phenytoin has failed. Others suggest that the barbiturates are as safe and effective as other anticonvulsants and should be the drug of choice following a benzodiazepine. Still others support continuous-infusion midazolam as the third-line anticonvulsant before the barbiturates. Currently, most practitioners agree that phenobarbital is the long-acting anticonvulsant of choice in patients with hypersensitivity to the hydantoins or in those with cardiac conduction abnormalities.

Refractory GCSE

⓫ When adequate doses of a benzodiazepine, hydantoin, or barbiturate have failed, the condition is termed *refractory*. Approximately 10% to 15% of patients will develop refractory GCSE, and approximately 30% whose seizures are "clinically" controlled will have persistent electrical manifestations after administration of these anticonvulsants. When a patient develops refractory GCSE, an intense search should be performed for an acute or progressive cause.

While the goal is to stop electrical epileptiform activity, there is no consensus regarding the anticonvulsant of choice, sequencing of therapy, or treatment of refractory GCSE. Most recommend the administration of anesthetic doses of midazolam, pentobarbital, or propofol, while other approaches include the continuous infusion of a benzodiazepine, valproate, lacosamide, levetiracetam, topiramate, or lidocaine. Doses for these agents can be found in Table 41-5. A meta-analysis compared midazolam, propofol, and pentobarbital in refractory GCSE.[24] Overall response rates were significantly greater in those treated with pentobarbital (92%) compared to midazolam (80%) and propofol (73%). Seizure recurrence was more commonly observed with midazolam (51%) versus propofol (15%) and pentobarbital (12%). Although pentobarbital had a greater response rate, clinically significant hypotension was more common. Mortality rates were similar for the three drugs.

Benzodiazepines

Some advocate that anesthetic doses of midazolam should be the first-line agent in refractory GCSE. Table 41-5 shows the loading and maintenance doses of midazolam.[24] Most patients respond to these doses within an hour. Successful discontinuation is enhanced by maintaining the patient's phenytoin and phenobarbital serum concentration(s) above 20 mg/L (79 μmol/L) and 40 mg/L (172 μmol/L), respectively. Because of midazolam's short half-life, patients can return to consciousness more rapidly than those receiving larger doses of more sedating anticonvulsants (e.g., phenytoin, phenobarbital). Generally, continuous-infusion midazolam has been well tolerated, with few cases of hypotension and respiratory depression. Hypotension and poikilothermia can occur and can require supportive therapies.

Large-dose continuous-infusion lorazepam also has been used successfully,[25] but can be associated with adverse drug reactions due to propylene glycol.[26]

Pentobarbital

If there is an inadequate response to large doses of midazolam, anesthetizing the patient to suppress the cerebral ictal discharge is recommended.[15,27] Although it is likely that the patient is already being mechanically ventilated, intubation and respiratory support

TABLE 41-5 Dosing of Medications Used to Treat Refractory GCSE

Drug (Brand Name)	Initial Dose (Maximum Dose)	Maintenance Dose	Comments
Lacosamide (Vimpat)			
Adult	200–400 mg	200 mg bid	Administer IV over 15 minutes
Pediatric	2.5–3 mg/kg	6–8 mg/kg/day, given twice a day	
Levetiracetam (Keppra plus generics)			
Adult	2,000–3,000 mg	1,000 mg thrice a day	Administer IV over 5–15 minutes
Pediatric	40–60 mg/kg	40–60 mg/kg/day	
Lidocaine (generics)			
Adult	50–100 mg	1.5–3.5 mg/kg/h	Administer IV in ≤2 minutes
Pediatric	1 mg/kg (maximum 3–5 mg/kg in the first hour)	1.2–3 mg/kg/h	
Midazolam (Versed plus generic)			
Adult	200 mcg/kg[a]	50–500 mcg/kg/h[b]	Initial dose may be given IM; administer IV over 0.5–1 mg/min; continuous-infusion rate should be increased every 15 minutes in those who do not respond and should be guided by EEG response; development of tachyphylaxis can require frequent increases in dose; decrease dose by 1 mcg/kg/min every 2 hours once GCSE is controlled
Pediatric	150 mcg/kg[a]	60–120 mcg/kg/h[b]	
Pentobarbital (generics)			
Adult	10–20 mg/kg	1–5 mg/kg/h[b]	Over 1–2 hours, rate of infusion should be slowed or dopamine should be added if hypotension occurs; gradually titrated dose upward until there is evidence of burst suppression on EEG (i.e., isoelectric EEG) or prohibitive adverse effects occur. Twelve hours after a burst suppression is obtained, the rate should be titrated downward every 2–4 hours
Pediatric	15–20 mg/kg	1–5 mg/kg/h[b]	
Propofol (Diprivan plus generic)			
Adult	2 mg/kg	5–10 mg/kg/h[b]	Over 10 seconds in adults and 20–30 seconds in pediatric patients
Pediatric	3 mg/kg	2–18 mg/kg/h[c]	
Topiramate (Topamax plus generic)			
Adult	300–500 mg	400–1,600 mg/day	Given orally in divided dose every 12 hours. Doses as large as 25 mg/kg/day for 2–5 days have been used in children
Pediatric	5–10 mg/kg	5–10 mg/kg/day	
Valproate (Depacon plus generic)			
Adult	15–30 mg/kg	1–4 mg/kg/h[b]	Administer at 3 mg/kg/min; and follow by a continuous or intermittent infusion; larger doses may be required in those on hepatic enzyme inducers
Pediatric	20–25 mg/kg	1–4 mg/kg/h[b]	

EEG, electroencephalogram; GCSE, generalized convulsive status epilepticus; IM, intramuscular; IV, intravenous.
[a]Doses can be repeated twice at 10 to 15 minute intervals until the maximum dosage is given.
[b]Titrate dose as needed.
[c]Generally recommended not to exceed a dose of 4 mg/kg/h and a duration of 48 hours.

are mandatory during barbiturate coma, along with continuous EEG monitoring (Table 41-4). A short-acting barbiturate (usually either pentobarbital or thiopental) generally is preferred because it allows a more rapid reversal of coma.

Several sources note that the initial loading dose of pentobarbital is 5 mg/kg.[15] However, this dose is inadequate to achieve the serum concentrations (40 mg/L; 172 μmoL/L) necessary to induce an isoelectric EEG (Table 41-5).[27] Although the duration of barbiturate coma in most studies has been 2 to 3 days, it has been used safely for 53 days in an 18-year-old patient.[28] To avoid complications (e.g., pneumonia, pulmonary edema), the pentobarbital should be discontinued as soon as possible. It is important to have other anticonvulsants at therapeutic amounts before pentobarbital is withdrawn so that the risk of seizure recurrence is minimized. Because pentobarbital is a potent hepatic enzyme inducer, doses of most concurrent anticonvulsants will need to be larger than usual maintenance doses. The patient will need to be monitored for side effects as deinduction occurs and anticonvulsant concentrations increase. This can take up to a month after pentobarbital's discontinuation.

Propofol

Propofol is extremely lipid soluble, has a large volume of distribution, and has a very rapid onset of action. Its extremely short half-life promotes rapid awakening on drug discontinuation. Propofol's efficacy is comparable to midazolam for refractory GCSE.[27,29] Adverse drug reactions and doses can be found in Tables 41-4 and 41-5,[30] respectively. Finally, a normal adult dose can provide over 1,000 calories (4,186 J) per day as lipid at a cost to the patient that may exceed $800 per day.

Valproate

The IV dosage form approved by the FDA is not labeled for GCSE. A number of loading and continuous-infusion doses (see Table 41-5) have been used in both adult and pediatric patients.[24,31,32] A recent study showed that IV valproate and continuous infusion diazepam were comparable in GCSE. Although the manufacturer originally recommended IV valproate be given no faster than 20 mg/min, much faster rates have been studied (40 mg/min; 2 to 10 mg/kg/min) and are used for administration of the loading dose.[24,31] One study suggested the need to consider the effects of enzyme-inducing anticonvulsants when dosing and recommended that the continuous-infusion rate be determined by the presence of concurrent anticonvulsants (no inducers present, 1 mg/kg/h; one or more inducers [e.g., phenytoin, phenobarbital], 2 mg/kg/h; and inducers and pentobarbital coma, 4 mg/kg/h).[33] In general, IV valproate has been well tolerated, with no cases of respiratory depression. Hemodynamic instability is extremely rare, but patients' vital signs should be monitored closely during the loading dose.

Other Agents

Topiramate has been given orally in adults and in children with GCSE (Table 41-5), but may be associated with adverse drug reaction (Table 41-4).[13,26,34–37] Crushing the tablets and dissolving them in small amounts of water are necessary, as no liquid formulation is available. Response tends to be delayed hours to days. Once seizures are controlled, doses should be tapered to a tolerable maintenance dose.

Oral levetiracetam has been given in case series for GCSE.[38] However, IV levetiracetam should be used (Table 41-5), but doses larger than 3,000 mg/day do not add additional efficacy.[13,26,39–42] Levetiracetam is not hepatically metabolized and is minimally protein bound, which makes drug–drug interactions unlikely. There have been two case reports of lacosamide used in refractory GCSE and NCSE.[42–44] Like levetiracetam, its lack of effect on the metabolism on other medications makes it attractive for use. Neither levetiracetam nor lacosamide has been associated with toxicities (respiratory depression, hypotension) noted with the older anticonvulsants.

Lidocaine has been used in refractory GCSE, but is not recommended unless other agents have failed.[45] It is administered IV (Table 41-5) and has a rapid onset of action. Although the reference serum concentration range for the antiarrhythmic effects of lidocaine is 2 to 6 mg/L (8.5 to 25.6 μmol/L), the reference range for GCSE has not been established. Serum lidocaine concentrations should be monitored to avoid drug accumulation and toxicity (Table 41-4).

Halothane, isoflurane, ketamine, and other inhaled anesthetics can produce EEG suppression; however, these gases are difficult to deliver outside the operating room and require an anesthesiologist. No proven advantages have been shown over traditional anticonvulsants (e.g., barbiturate coma or continuous-infusion benzodiazepine), and these gases can increase intracranial pressure. If used, dosing is titrated to obtain EEG burst suppression. Finally, it is also prudent to validate that the patient does not have a low serum-magnesium concentration, because magnesium deficiency can lower the seizure threshold.

Personalized Pharmacotherapy

If the patient has been on phenytoin, phenobarbital, or valproate prior to admission, a stat serum concentration should be obtained and the results considered in determining a loading dose or redosing. A serum concentration should be obtained in any patient who is unresponsive to therapy or who exhibits concentration-associated adverse drug reactions. Pharmacogenetics produces differences in metabolic pathways and rate of drug metabolism, which can influence efficacy or toxicity. Obviously, a patient who is a poor metabolizer would theoretically have changes in drug metabolism based on expression of specific isoenzymes. For example, many Orientals have decreased CYP 2C19 activity; therefore, they may respond to lower doses of diazepam. If one were concerned about benzodiazepine-associated adverse effects in this population, lorazepam would be preferred.

Although a patient may have an alteration in gene expression that could be important in development of refractory SE or in response to various anticonvulsants, there is no information to support that this is important in GCSE. While HLA-B*1502 has been associated with severe skin reactions in patients receiving phenytoin, this is applicable to chronic and not acute, single dose therapy. Some studies have noted an association between P-glycoprotein and refractory epilepsy; however, no reports have suggested that this finding is important in GCSE. There is currently no evidence to support a change in protocol based on underlying genetics.

EVALUATION OF THERAPEUTIC OUTCOMES

Initial success is defined as termination of all clinical and electrical seizure activity, but ultimate success is measured by the patient's subsequent quality of life. The morbidity and mortality associated with GCSE are affected by the underlying etiology; however, morbidity and mortality can be minimized by the rapid implementation of a rational therapeutic plan. An EEG is an extremely important tool that not only allows practitioners to determine when abnormal electrical activity has been aborted, but also can assist in determining which anticonvulsant was effective. Because many of the anticonvulsants affect the cardiorespiratory system, it is imperative that vital signs (e.g., heart rate, respiratory rate, and blood pressure) be monitored during drug loading and infusion. Finally, it is imperative that the infusion site be assessed for any evidence of infiltration before and during administration of phenytoin. Information regarding the patient's past medical and drug history and imaging studies (e.g., MRI) also can help to determine if there is a defined etiology for the original episode of GCSE. This information then can be used to guide future medication therapy, as well as help in determining if the patient is at risk for a poor outcome.

ABBREVIATIONS

AMPA	α-amino-3-hydroxy-5-methyl-isoxazole-4-propionate
CT	computed tomography
EEG	electroencephalogram, electroencephalography
GABA	γ-aminobutyric acid
GCSE	generalized convulsive status epilepticus
MRI	magnetic resonance imaging
NCSE	nonconvulsive status epilepticus
NMDA	*N*-methyl-D-aspartate
PE	phenytoin equivalents
SE	status epilepticus

REFERENCES

1. Commission on Classification of Terminology, International League Against Epilepsy. Proposal for revised clinical and electroencephalographic classification of epileptic seizures. Epilepsia 1981;22:489–501.
2. DeLorenzo RJ, Garnett LK, Towne AR, et al. Comparison of status epilepticus with prolonged seizure episodes lasting from 10 to 29 minutes. Epilepsia 1999;40:164–169.
3. Jenssen S, Gracely EJ, Sperling MR. How long do most seizures last? A systematic comparison of seizures recorded in the epilepsy monitoring unit. Epilepsia 2006;47: 1499–1503.
4. Lowenstein DH, Alldredge BK. Status epilepticus. N Engl J Med 1998;338:970–976.
5. Maganti R, Gerber P, Drees C, Chung S. Nonconvulsive status epilepticus. Epilepsy Behav 2008;12:572–586.
6. DeLorenzo RJ, Pellock JM, Towne AR, Boggs J. Epidemiology of status epilepticus. J Clin Neurophysiol 1995;12:316–325.
7. Shorvon S. The management of status epilepticus. J Neurol Neurosurg Psychiatry 2001;70(Suppl 2):II22–II27.
8. DeLorenzo RJ, Towne AR, Pellock JM, Ko D. Status epilepticus in children, adults, and the elderly. Epilepsia 1992;33:S15–S25.
9. Pitkanen A. Efficacy of current antiepileptics to prevent neurodegeneration in epilepsy models. Epilepsy Res 2002;50:141–160.
10. Wasterlain CG, Mazarati AM, Naylor D, et al. Short-term plasticity of hippocampal neuropeptides and neuronal circuitry in experimental status epilepticus. Epilepsia 2002;45(Suppl 5):20–29.
11. Temkin NR. Antiepileptogenesis and seizure prevention trials with anti-epileptic drugs: Meta-analysis of controlled trials. Epilepsia 2001;42:515–524.
12. Singh RK, Gaillard WD. Status epilepticus in children. Curr Neurol Neurosci Rep 2009;9:137–144.
13. Wasterlain CG, Chen JWY. Mechanistic and pharmacologic aspects of status epielpticus and its treatment with new antiepileptic drugs. Epilepsia 2008;49:63–73.

14. Lothman E. The biochemical basis and pathophysiology of status epilepticus. Neurology 1990;40:13–23.
15. Working Group on Status Epilepticus. Treatment of convulsive status epilepticus: Recommendations of the Epilepsy Foundation of America's Working Group on Status Epilepticus. JAMA 1993;270:854–859.
16. Appleton R, Macleod S, Martland T. Drug management for acute tonic–clonic convulsions including convulsive status epilepticus in children. Cochrane Database Syst Rev 2008;16:CD001905.
17. Shlbergleit R, Durkalski V, Lowenstein D, et al. Intramuscular versus intravenous therapy for prehospital status epilepticus. N Engl J Med 2012;366:591–600.
18. Shaner DM, McCurdy SA, Herring MO, Gabor AJ. Treatment of status epilepticus: A prospective comparison of diazepam and phenytoin versus phenobarbital and optional phenytoin. Neurology 1988;38:202–207.
19. Treiman DM, Meyers PD, Walton NY, et al. A comparison of four treatments for generalized convulsive status epilepticus. Veterans Affairs Status Epilepticus Cooperative Study Group. N Engl J Med 1998;339:792–798.
20. Abernethy DR, Greenblatt DJ. Phenytoin disposition in obesity: Determination of loading dose. Arch Neurol 1985;42:468–471.
21. Fischer JH, Patel TV, Fischer PA. Fosphenytoin: Clinical pharmacokinetics and comparative advantages in the acute treatment of seizures. Clin Pharmacokinet 2003;42:33–58.
22. Dodson WE, Rust RS. Phenobarbital: Absorption, distribution, and excretion. In: Levy R, Mattson R, Meldrum B, eds. Antiepileptic Drugs, 4th ed. New York: Raven Press, 1995: 379–387.
23. Crawford TO, Mitchell WG, Fishman LS, Snodgrass SR. Very-high-dose phenobarbital for refractory status epilepticus in children. Neurology 1988;38:1035–1040.
24. Abend NS, Diugos DJ. Treatment of refractory status epilepticus: Literature review and a proposed protocol. Pediatr Neurol 2008;38:377–390.
25. Labar DR, Ali A, Root J. High-dose IV lorazepam for the treatment of refractory status epilepticus. Neurology 1994;44:1400–1403.
26. Yaucher NE, Fish JT, Smith HW, Wells JA. Propylene glycol-associated renal toxicity from lorazepam infusion. Pharmacotherapy 2003;23:1094–1099.
27. Claassen J, Hirsch LJ, Emerson RG, Mayer SA. Treatment of refractory status epilepticus with pentobarbital, propofol, or midazolam: A systematic review. Epilepsia 2002;43: 146–153.
28. Mirski MA, Williams MA, Hanlet DF. Prolonged pentobarbital and phenobarbital coma for refractory generalized status epilepticus. Crit Care Med 1995;23:400–404.
29. Brown LA, Levin GM. Role of propofol in refractory status epilepticus. Ann Pharmacother 1998;32:1053–1059.
30. Timpe EM, Eichner SF, Phelps SJ. Propofol-related infusion syndrome in critically ill pediatric patients: Coincidence, association, or causation? J Pediatr Pharmacol Ther 2006;11:17–42.
31. Chen WB, Gao R, Su Y, et al. Valproate versus diazepam for generalized status epilepticus: A pilot study. Eur J Neurol 2011;18:1391–1396.
32. Wheless JW, Trieman DM. The role of the newer antiepileptic drugs in the treatment of generalized convulsive status epilepticus. Epilepsia 2008;49(Suppl 9):74–78.
33. Hovinga CA, Chicella MF, Rose DF, et al. Use of IV valproate in three pediatric patients with nonconvulsive or convulsive status epilepticus. Ann Pharmacother 1999;33: 579–584.
34. Kahriman M, Minecan D, Kutluay E, et al. Efficacy of topiramate in children with refractory status epilepticus. Epilepsia 2003;44:1353–1356.
35. Towne AR, Garnett LK, Waterhouse EJ, et al. The use of topiramate in refractory status epilepticus. Neurology 2003;60:332–334.
36. Blumkin L, Lerman-Sagie T, Houri T, et al. Pediatric refractory partial status epilepticus responsive to topiramate. J Child Neurol 2005;20:239–241.
37. Conway JM, Birnbaum AK, Kriel RL, Cloyd JC. Relative bioavailability of topiramate administered rectally. Epilepsy Res 2003;54:91–96.
38. Rossetti AO, Bromfield EB. Determinants of success in the use of oral levetiracetam in status epilepticus. Epilepsy Behav 2006;8:651–654.
39. Möddel G, Bunten S, Dobis C, et al. Intravenous levetiracetam: A new treatment alternative for refractory status epilepticus. J Neurol Neurosurg Psychiatry 2009;80: 689–692.
40. Gallentine WB, Hunnicutt AS, Husain AM. Levetiracetam in children with refractory status epilepticus. Epilepsy Behav 2009;14:215–218.
41. Kirmani BF, Crisp ED, Kayani S, Rajab H. Role of intravenous levetiracetam in acute seizure management of children. Pediatr Neurol 2009;41:37–39.
42. Trinka E. What is the evidence to use new intravenous AEDs in status epilepticus? Epilepsia 2011;52(Suppl 8): 35–38.
43. Tilz C, Resch R, Hofer T, Eggers C. Successful treatment for refractory convulsive status epilepticus by parenteral lacosamide. Epilepsia 2010;51:316–317.
44. Kellinghaus C, Berning S, Besselmann M. Intravenous lacosamide as successful treatment for nonconvulsive status epilepticus after failure of first line therapy. Epilepsy Behav 2009;14:429–431.
45. Aggarwal P, Wali JP. Lidocaine in refractory status epilepticus: A forgotten drug in the emergency department. Am J Emerg Med 1993;2:243–244.

Acute Management of the Brain Injury Patient

42

Bradley A. Boucher and G. Christopher Wood

KEY CONCEPTS

1. Cerebral ischemia is the key pathophysiologic event triggering secondary neuronal injury following severe traumatic brain injury (TBI). Intracellular accumulation of calcium is postulated to be a central pathophysiologic process in amplifying and perpetuating secondary neuronal injury via inhibition of cellular respiration and enzyme activation.
2. *Guidelines for the Management of Severe Brain Injury*, published by the Brain Trauma Foundation (BTF)/American Association of Neurological Surgeons (AANS), serve as the foundation on which clinical decisions in managing adult neurotrauma patients are based; comparable guidelines for infants, children, and adolescents have also been published.
3. Correcting and preventing early hypotension (systolic blood pressure less than 90 mm Hg) and hypoxemia (Pao_2 less than 60 mm Hg [8.0 kPa]) are primary goals during the initial resuscitative and intensive care of severe TBI patients.
4. Nonpharmacologic treatment in the management of intracranial hypertension includes raising the head of the bed 30°, short-term mild hyperventilation ($Paco_2$ 30 to 35 mm Hg [4.0 to 4.7 kPa]), ventricular drainage if a ventriculostomy is present, and decompressive surgery.
5. The principal monitoring parameter for severe TBI patients within the intensive care environment is intracranial pressure (ICP). Cerebral perfusion pressure (CPP) is also a critical monitoring parameter and should be maintained between 50 and 70 mm Hg (6.7 and 9.3 kPa) (greater than 40 mm Hg [5.3 kPa] in pediatric patients) through the use of fluids, vasopressors, and/or ICP normalization therapy.
6. Nonspecific pharmacologic treatment in the management of intracranial hypertension should include analgesics, sedatives, antipyretics, and paralytics under selected circumstances.
7. Specific pharmacologic treatment in the management of intracranial hypertension includes mannitol, hypertonic saline, furosemide, and high-dose pentobarbital. Neither routine use of corticosteroids nor aggressive hyperventilation (i.e., $Paco_2$ less than 25 mm Hg [3.3 kPa]) should be used in the management of intracranial hypertension.
8. Use of phenytoin for the prophylaxis of posttraumatic seizures usually should be discontinued after 7 days if no seizures are observed.
9. Numerous investigational strategies (e.g., calcium antagonists, glutamate antagonists, antioxidants, free-radical scavengers, and progesterone) targeted at interrupting the pathophysiologic cascade of events occurring following severe TBI have been employed, but no proven therapeutic benefits have been identified.

Traumatic brain injury (TBI) is currently the leading cause of death and disability among children and young adults in the industrialized world.[1] A focus on TBI prevention, and improved acute care and rehabilitation must remain national priorities. This chapter summarizes TBI epidemiology and pathophysiology, and highlights the major guidelines and systematic reviews of the literature pertaining to the management of severe TBI patients.

EPIDEMIOLOGY

It is estimated that approximately 1.7 million persons sustain a TBI each year in the United States.[2] Among these individuals, 275,000 require hospital admission and 52,000 die annually.[2] Importantly, over 3.1 million Americans currently live with disabilities as a result of their TBI, highlighting the enormous physical and emotional toll of this health care problem.[3] The economic effects of acute neurotrauma are also enormous, with estimates of spending on TBI patients requiring hospitalization of $60 billion in the United States in 2000.[4] Economic costs to society from lost productivity are also massive, especially considering the young age of many TBI patients.[5] Falls are the leading cause of TBI (35.2%) while motor vehicle accidents result in the greatest number of TBI-related hospitalizations and deaths overall.[2] Death rates from TBI are highest in patients 75 years of age or older.[2]

PRIMARY AND SECONDARY BRAIN INJURY PATHOPHYSIOLOGY

The neurologic sequelae of brain trauma can occur instantaneously as a consequence of the primary injury or can result from secondary injuries that follow within minutes, hours, or days.[1] Primary injury involves the external transfer of kinetic energy to various structural components of the brain (e.g., neurons, nerve synapses, glial cells, axons, and cerebral blood vessels). The biomechanical forces responsible for primary brain injury can be classified broadly as contact (e.g., blunt-object blow, penetrating-missile injuries) and acceleration/deceleration (e.g., instantaneous brain movements following motor vehicle accidents).[1] Contact forces commonly result in skull fractures, brain contusions, and/or hemorrhages. Primary injuries are categorized further as focal (e.g., contusions, hematomas) or diffuse.[5] The latter usually are associated with shearing or stretch forces, which primarily affect axons within the brain (i.e., diffuse axonal injury).[6] The type of primary injury (i.e., focal vs. diffuse) is a major factor as to which of the secondary injury mechanisms discussed below will predominate following a TBI; however, many patients, especially those involved in high-speed accidents, sustain both types of injury.[7]

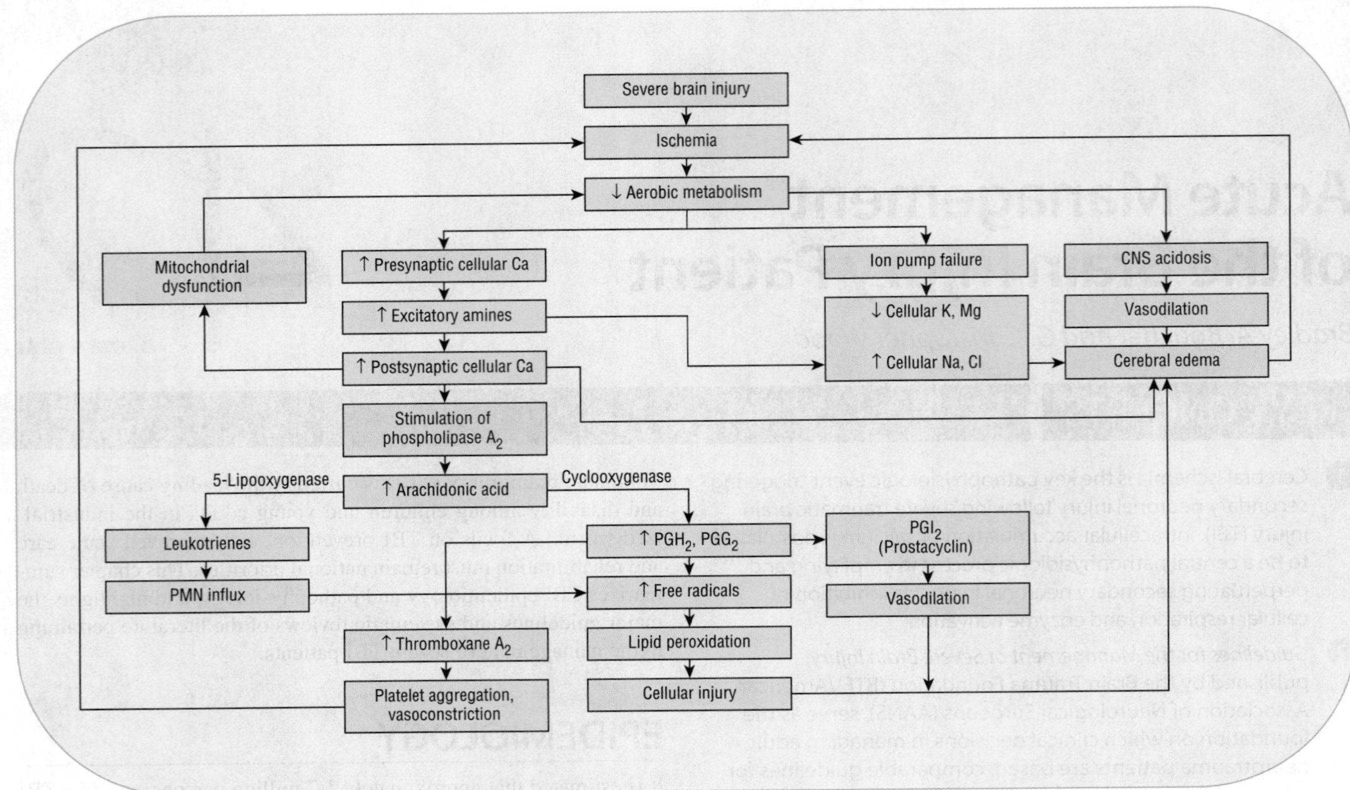

FIGURE 42-1 Schematic illustration of the cascade of biochemical events proposed to occur following severe neurotrauma (secondary brain injury). (Ca, calcium; CNS, central nervous system; K, potassium; Mg, magnesium; Na, sodium; Cl, chloride; PMN, polymorphonucleocyte; PG, prostaglandin.)

❶ A complex sequence of pathophysiologic events precipitated by primary brain injury may seriously disrupt the normal CNS balance between oxygen supply and demand.[7] Hypotension during the early posttraumatic period is a major contributor to this imbalance and a primary determinant of outcome.[1,6] The end result of this imbalance may be cerebral ischemia, the key pathophysiologic event triggering secondary injury.[7,8] Figure 42-1 is a simplified schematic of the processes that constitute secondary brain injury and their various interrelationships. The brain is particularly susceptible to ischemia because of its normally high resting energy requirement and its limited capacity to store oxygen, glucose, and adenosine triphosphate (ATP).[8] Vasospasm also can occur in approximately one-fourth to one-third of TBI patients.[6] These phenomena can result in imbalances in cerebral oxygen delivery (CDo_2) and consumption ($CMRo_2$), processes that are closely autoregulated under normal circumstances. Factors that can diminish cerebral oxygen supply following brain injury include cerebral edema, expanding mass lesions (e.g., epidural, subdural, and intracerebral hematomas), cerebral vasospasm, and loss of vasoregulatory control. Vasogenic cerebral edema can develop as a consequence of cerebral capillary endothelial damage and disruption of the blood–brain barrier.[7,8] Cytotoxic cerebral edema is a consequence of loss of cell wall integrity that accompanies ischemia or hypoxia.[8] With cytotoxic and vasogenic edema comes expansion of the intracellular and extracellular fluid spaces, respectively. Elevated intracranial pressure (ICP) is the most detrimental consequence of cerebral edema formation and occurs as the brain tissue volume increases within the nondistensible skull. A significant increase in ICP may further compromise cerebral blood flow (CBF) and extend cytotoxic edema. Hence an increase in ICP can be self-perpetuating unless this cycle is reversed. Hypoxemia can further exacerbate local decreases in cerebral oxygen supply following acute respiratory failure and systemic hypotension. Metabolic demand also can increase following neurotrauma secondary to seizures, agitation, and temperature elevation.[8] Brain tissue affected by focal ischemia can have a dense core surrounded by a marginally viable region.[8] If adequate CBF is restored, the affected tissue may recover; however, sustained ischemia can result in further loss of cellular integrity and eventual cell death.

The two distinctive end points along the spectrum of secondary neuronal injury are: (a) cellular necrosis characterized by membrane cell lysis, edema, and inflammation, and (b) apoptosis that leads to cell shrinkage and cell membrane dissolution.[7,8] Apoptosis, which is also known as programmed cell death, requires a cascade of intracellular events for completion of cell death.[7] The loss of ionic homeostasis is postulated to be a key event in fostering secondary brain injury following cerebral ischemia. Cellular influx of sodium, chloride, magnesium, and water with a corresponding efflux of potassium secondary to cytotoxic edema and Na^+-K^+-ATPase pump dysfunction.[7,8] An influx of calcium into the presynaptic terminal ends of damaged neurons is mediated by N-type voltage-sensitive calcium channels. This influx is postulated to stimulate excessive release of the excitatory amines glutamate and aspartate from the affected neurons. These amines then accumulate in the neuronal synaptic cleft in the presence of cellular energy failure.[8] The result is ongoing stimulation of postsynaptic cells, which can result in an extension of neurotoxicity and cell death. Influx of calcium and additional sodium is stimulated by activation of ionophore receptors including the *N*-methyl-D-aspartate (NMDA) receptor.[7,8] Calcium influx and its intracellular accumulation initiate a number of events that amplify and perpetuate secondary neuronal injury. High intracellular concentrations of calcium result in mitochondrial dysfunction, which further inhibits cellular respiration, a process already affected by ischemic and/or hypoxic insults.[7] A second major deleterious effect of calcium

CLINICAL PRESENTATION Acute Brain Injury

General

- Level of consciousness on admission ranges from awake and alert to completely unresponsive (i.e., GCS 15 to 3, respectively)

Symptoms

- Posttraumatic amnesia (e.g., greater than 1 hour), increasing dizziness, a moderate-to-severe headache, nausea/vomiting, limb weakness, or paresthesia may indicate more severe injury

Signs

- CSF otorrhea or rhinorrhea and seizures may indicate more severe injury
- A rapid deterioration in mental status strongly suggests the presence of an expanding lesion within the skull
- Severe TBI may be accompanied by significant alterations or instability in vital signs, including abnormal breathing patterns (e.g., apnea, Cheyne–Stokes respiration, tachypnea), hypertension, or bradycardia

Laboratory Tests

- ABGs indicating hypoxia (i.e., decreased Pao_2) or hypercapnia (i.e., increased $Paco_2$) may indicate compromised ventilation
- A positive blood ethanol concentration and/or positive urine drug screen indicates that drug intoxication may be affecting the patient's mental status in addition to the TBI
- Electrolyte disturbances can cause alterations in mental status, and their effects may interfere with assessment of neurological status relative to brain lesion

Other Diagnostic Tests

- CT of the head is an important diagnostic tool for detecting the presence of mass lesions

GCS, Glasgow Coma Scale; CSF, cerebrospinal fluid; TBI, traumatic brain injury; ABG, arterial blood gas; Pao_2, partial pressure of arterial blood oxygen; $PaCO_2$, partial pressure of arterial blood carbon dioxide; CT, computed tomography

is to stimulate activation of autodestructive enzymes, including phospholipases, endonucleases, and proteases, such as the caspase family of enzymes.[7,8] The effect of phospholipase A_2 stimulation includes formation of several arachidonic acid metabolites derived from membrane lipids: thromboxane A_2, prostaglandins, and leukotrienes.[7,8] The subsequent effects of these metabolites are lipid peroxidation and the formation of reactive oxygen species.[1,7,8] Data suggest that this event occurs very early after injury (e.g., before hospitalization), which may limit the effectiveness of exogenously administered antioxidants.

Cell-mediated injury involving inflammatory mediators (e.g., proinflammatory cytokines) and nitric oxide activation is yet another possible mechanism involved in secondary neuronal injury.[7] Among the cell lines implicated are polymorphonuclear neutrophils, platelets, endothelial cells, and macrophages. Noteworthy is that limited data suggest that activation of some inflammatory mediators may actually be beneficial such that the relative balance of the mediators versus absolute concentrations may be the most significant pathophysiologic factor following TBI. Stimulation of platelet aggregation, vasodilation, and vasoconstriction also may occur.

CLINICAL PRESENTATION

The Glasgow Coma Scale (GCS) is the most widely used system to grade the arousal and functional capacity of the cerebral cortex.[6] The GCS defines the level of consciousness according to eye opening, motor response, and verbal response (Table 42-1). A GCS score of 15 corresponds to a normal neurologic examination. A GCS score of 3 to 8, 9 to 12, and 13 to 15 is consistent with severe, moderate, and mild or minor brain injury, respectively.[6] The possibility of ethanol or drug intoxication, hypotension, hypoxia, postictal state, or hypothermia altering the neurologic examination always should be considered. Because opiates, sedatives, and neuromuscular blockers affect the neurologic examination, they should not be administered until the initial examination is complete if at all possible. Simple, rapidly attainable clinical variables that are predictive of survival include patient age, presence of hypotension, increased ICP, elevated GCS score (especially the motor score), pupillary reactivity, and findings on a computed tomographic (CT) scan of the head that include the presence and size of a hematoma, subarachnoid hemorrhage, midline shift, and compression of the ventricular cisterns.[9]

GENERAL TRAUMATIC BRAIN INJURY TREATMENT PRINCIPLES

2 In July 1995, the Brain Trauma Foundation (BTF) published an extensive document entitled *Guidelines for the Management of Severe Brain Injury* as a joint initiative with the Guidelines Committee of

TABLE 42-1 Glasgow Coma Scale

Response	Score
Eyes	
Open spontaneously	4
To verbal command	3
To pain	2
No response	1
Best Motor Response	
To verbal command	
Obeys	6
To painful stimulus (pressure to nailbeds)	
Localizes pain	5
Flexion, withdrawal	4
Flexion, abnormal (decorticate rigidity)	3
Extension (decerebrate rigidity)	2
No response	1
Best Verbal Response	
(Arouse patient with painful stimulus if necessary)	
Oriented and converses	5
Disoriented and converses	4
Inappropriate words	3
Incomprehensible sounds	2
No response	1
Total	3–15

the American Association of Neurological Surgeons (AANS) and the Joint Section on Neurotrauma and Critical Care of the AANS and the Congress of Neurological Surgeons, with subsequent revision in 2000.[10] A third revision was released in 2007.[11] This landmark publication constitutes the most widely accepted series of evidence-based standards, guidelines, and options for the care of severe TBI patients. Recommendations are reported as Level I (standards), Level II (guidelines), or Level III (options) based on the corresponding classes of evidence. As important are the data documenting that compliance with the BTF/AANS guidelines can result in improved outcomes relative to mortality rate, functional outcome scores, length of hospitalization, and cost.[12] Since then, guidelines addressing prehospital TBI management,[13] surgical management,[14] and management of penetrating brain injury have been published. Furthermore, TBI management guidelines for infants, children, and adolescents have been developed.[15] The recommendations emanating from these published guidelines on TBI management and various published systematic reviews will be highlighted throughout the remaining portion of this chapter. Until further clinical studies become available, recommendations from the published guidelines should serve as the foundation on which all clinical decisions in managing severe TBI are based. Nonetheless, it should be noted that the majority of the guidelines are based on Class II evidence (primarily prospective clinical trials) and Class III evidence (primarily retrospective clinical trials). Few Class I evidence studies (i.e., prospective, randomized, controlled trials) are available for treatment of TBI. The pharmacologic management of TBI is summarized in Table 42-2. Recommendations provided in this chapter pertain to adults and children unless specifically noted to the contrary.

Desired Outcomes

The overall goal in TBI management is not only reduction in morbidity and mortality, but also optimization of long-term functional outcome for these patients. This requires careful attention to the following short-term therapeutic goals: (a) establishment of an adequate airway and maintenance of ventilation and circulation during the initial period of resuscitation and evaluation, (b) maintenance of balance between CDo_2 and $CMRo_2$, (c) prevention or attenuation of secondary neuronal injury, and (d) prevention and/or treatment of associated medical complications.

Initial Resuscitation

The first priority in the unconscious patient is the establishment of an airway, which ensures adequate oxygenation and prevents aspiration.[6] **3** Thereafter, restoration of circulating blood volume and maintenance of systolic arterial pressure (SBP) greater than 90 mm Hg are of utmost importance.[1,11] In pediatric patients, the SBP goal should be greater than 70 mm Hg + (2 × age in years).[15] Correcting and preventing early hypotension (SBP less than 90 mm Hg) and hypoxia (Pao_2 less than 60 mm Hg [8.0 kPa]) are essential because these two factors are among the most powerful predictors of outcome.[9,11] Isotonic saline (0.9% normal saline) and lactated Ringer's solution have been traditionally used as initial resuscitation fluids of choice in TBI patients.[10] However, some clinicians believe that hypertonic saline (e.g., 3% or 7.5% saline) is beneficial in the resuscitation of TBI patients. Clinical studies have yielded equivocal results relative to superiority over isotonic solutions.[1,16] Regardless, no clear consensus exists as to the optimal initial resuscitation fluid. While albumin therapy may be considered as an alternative to crystalloid fluid resuscitation, a retrospective analysis of 460 TBI patients revealed an increase in mortality (33.2%) compared with those patients receiving 0.9% normal saline.[17] Vasopressors and inotropic agents may be needed to maintain an adequate mean arterial pressure (MAP) if hypotension persists after adequate restoration of intravascular volume. Figure 42-2 is an algorithm summarizing treatment priorities in the initial management of acute TBI.

TABLE 42-2 Pharmacologic Management of Traumatic Brain Injury

Hyperosmolar therapy
Mannitol is effective for control of raised intracranial pressure at doses of 0.25–1 g/kg body weight (Level II)
Hypertonic saline is effective in small studies, but no guideline recommendation is given
Infection prophylaxis
Periprocedural antibiotics for intubation should be administered to reduce the incidence of pneumonia (based largely on a single study) (Level II)
Routine prophylactic antibiotic use for ventricular catheter placement is not recommended to reduce infection (Level III)
Deep venous thrombosis prophylaxis
Low molecular weight heparin (LMWH) or low dose unfractionated heparin should be used in combination with mechanical prophylaxis. However, there is an increased risk of expansion of intracranial hemorrhage (Level III)
Anesthetics, analgesics, and sedatives
Prophylactic administration of barbiturates to reduce burst suppression electroencephalogram is not recommended (Level II)
High-dose barbiturate administration is recommended to control elevated ICP refractory to maximum standard medical and surgical treatment. Hemodynamic stability is essential before and after barbiturate therapy (Level II)
Propofol is recommended for the control of ICP, but not for improvement in mortality or 6-month outcomes. High-dose propofol can produce significant morbidity (Level II)
Antiseizure prophylaxis
Prophylactic use of phenytoin or valproate is not recommended for preventing late posttraumatic seizures (PTS) (greater than 7 days) (Level II)
Anticonvulsants are indicated to decrease the incidence of early PTS (within 7 days of injury) (Level II)
Corticosteroids
The use of steroids is not recommended for improving outcome or reducing intracranial pressure. In patients with moderate or severe TBI, high-dose methylprednisolone is associated with increased mortality and is contraindicated. (Level II)

ICP, intracranial pressure; LMWH, low molecular weight heparin; PTS, posttraumatic seizures; TBI, traumatic brain injury.

Level I: Recommendation based on a high level of clinical certainty from Class I evidence (e.g., good quality randomized controlled trial [RCT]).
Level II: Recommendation based on a moderate level of clinical certainty from Class II evidence (e.g., moderate quality RCT; good quality cohort; good quality case–control).
Level III: Clinical certainty has not been established based on Class III evidence (e.g., poor quality RCT; moderate or poor quality cohort; moderate or poor quality case–control; case series, databases, or registries).

Data from Reference 11.

Postresuscitative Care

Following successful resuscitation, priorities shift toward diagnostic evaluation of intracranial and extracranial injuries and emergent surgical intervention as needed. In many patients, evacuation of intracranial hematomas (i.e., epidural, subdural, and intracerebral hematomas) is essential to control ICP and improve outcome. Elevation of depressed skull fractures and debridement of penetrating wound tracts are other important emergent surgical procedures in TBI patients. **4** Decompressive craniectomies (i.e., removal of variable amount of skull bone) with or without temporal or frontal lobectomy may be considered in patients with increases in ICP refractory to more conservative measures.[1] The beneficial effects of routine decompressive surgery in adult TBI patients to date are controversial.[18] However, a recent pivotal randomized trial, while demonstrating acute effectiveness in ICP control using decompressive craniectomy, also found worse long-term outcomes compared with controls. This latter study calls into question the routine use of decompressive craniectomy in patients with refractory ICP.[19] Continuous ICP monitoring (e.g., intraventricular catheter, intraparenchymal fiberoptic catheter) is indicated in salvageable patients with

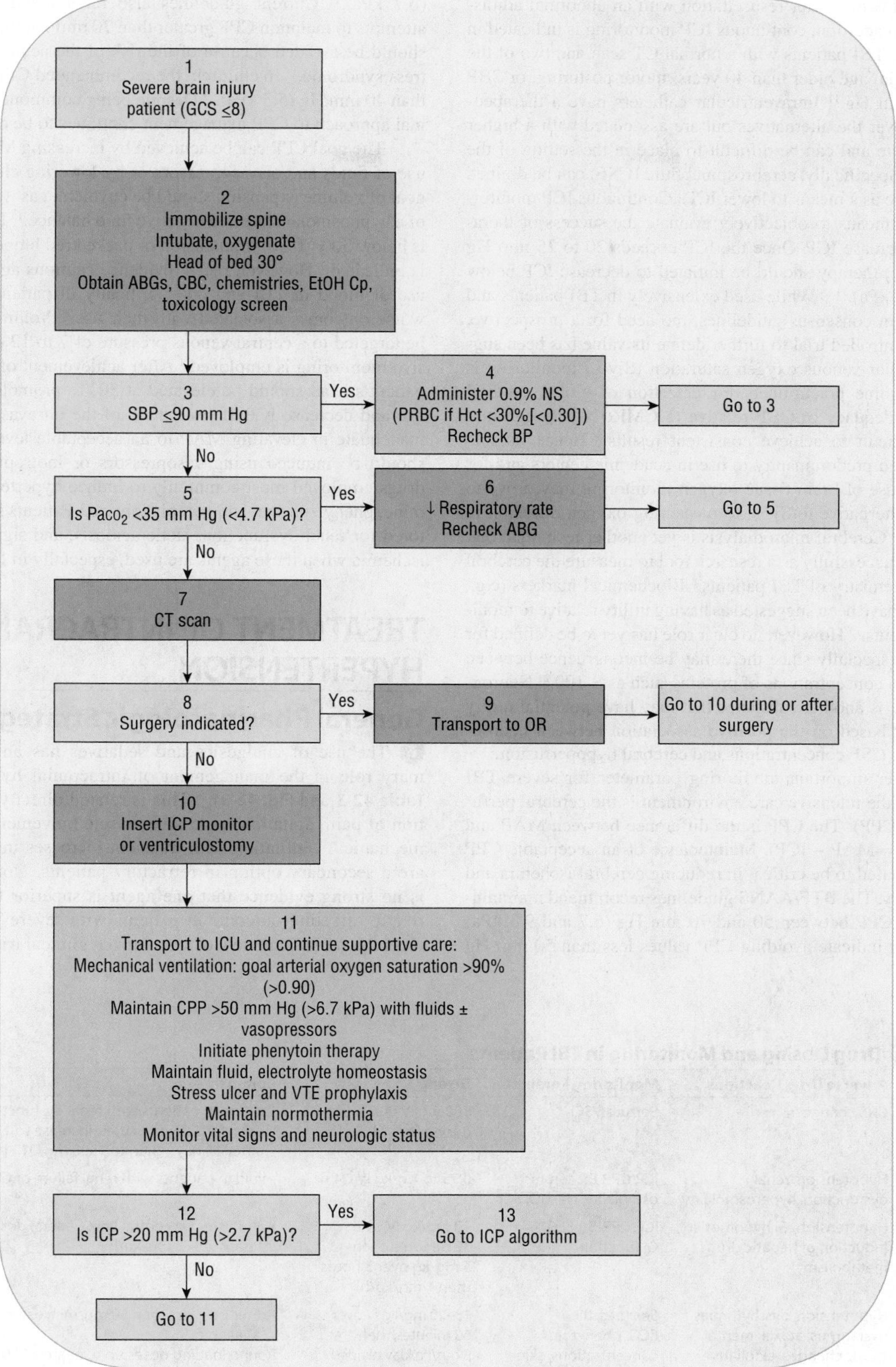

FIGURE 42-2 Algorithm for the acute management of the TBI patient. (GCS, Glasgow coma scale; BP, blood pressure; ABG, arterial blood gas; CBC, complete blood count; EtOH Cp, ethanol plasma concentration; SBP, systolic blood pressure; NS, normal saline; PRBC, packed red blood cells; Hct, hematocrit; $Paco_2$, partial pressure of arterial blood carbon dioxide; ICP, intracranial pressure; CT, computed tomography; OR, operating room; ICU, intensive care unit; CPP, cerebral perfusion pressure; CSF, cerebral spinal fluid.) *(Adapted with permission from Wood CG, Boucher BA. Management of Acute Traumatic Brain Injury. In: Richardson M, Chant C, Chessman KH, et al., eds. Pharmacotherapy Self-Assessment Program, 7th ed. Neurology and Psychiatry. Lenexa, KS: American College of Clinical Pharmacy, 2012:143, Figure 1-1.)*

a GCS score of 3 to 8 after resuscitation with an abnormal admission CT scan. In addition, continuous ICP monitoring is indicated in high-risk severe TBI patients with a normal CT scan and two of the following criteria: age older than 40 years, motor posturing, or SBP less than 90 mm Hg.[11] Intraventricular catheters have a therapeutic advantage over the alternatives but are associated with a higher complication rate and can be difficult to place in the setting of the swollen brain. Specifically, cerebrospinal fluid (CSF) can be drained using this device as a means to lower ICP.[1] Continuous ICP monitoring is the only means to objectively evaluate the success of therapies used to decrease ICP. Once the ICP exceeds 20 to 25 mm Hg (2.7 to 3.3 kPa), therapy should be initiated to decrease ICP below 20 mm Hg (2.7 kPa).[11,15] While used extensively in TBI patients and advocated within consensus guidelines, the need for a prospective, randomized, controlled trial to further define its value has been suggested.[20,21] Jugular venous oxygen saturation ($Sjvo_2$) monitoring is advocated by some practitioners for detection of global cerebral hypoxia (i.e., adequacy of CBF relative to $CMRo_2$), although it is technically difficult to achieve consistent results.[8] Hence its role remains confined predominantly to use in academic centers and for research.[8] The use of brain tissue oxygen monitoring may prove to be a superior alternative to $Sjvo_2$ to measuring oxygen diffusion in TBI patients.[8,22] Cerebral microdialysis is yet another technique that has been used successfully as a research tool to measure the cerebral extracellular chemistry of TBI patients.[8] Biochemical markers (e.g., S-100 protein) have been suggested as having utility relative to monitoring TBI patients.[23] However, no clear role has yet to be defined for such markers, especially since there may be incongruence between serum and brain concentrations of proteins such as S-100.[24] Neuron-specific enolase is another substance that may have potential utility as a biomarker based on the positive association between neuron-specific enolase CSF concentrations and cerebral hypoperfusion.[25]

5 Another important monitoring parameter for severe TBI patients within the intensive care environment is the cerebral perfusion pressure (CPP). The CPP is the difference between MAP and ICP (i.e., CPP = MAP − ICP). Maintenance of an acceptable CPP has been postulated to be critical in reducing cerebral ischemia and secondary injury. The BTF/AANS guidelines recommend maintaining a range of CPP between 50 and 70 mm Hg (6.7 and 9.3 kPa) and specifically indicate avoiding CPP values less than 50 mm Hg (6.7 kPa).[11] Current guidelines also recommend that aggressive attempts to maintain CPP greater than 70 mm Hg (9.3 kPa) in adults should be avoided because of the risk of the acute respiratory distress syndrome.[11] In children, the recommended CPP goal is greater than 40 mm Hg (5.3 kPa).[15] Despite being commonly used, the optimal approach to CPP management continues to be debated.[26]

The goal CPP can be achieved by increasing MAP through the use of fluids and/or vasopressors or by lowering elevated ICP. The goal of volume expansion should be euvolemia as well as avoidance of a hypoosmolar state and negative fluid balance.[15] If the hematocrit is below 30% (0.30), transfusion of packed red blood cells (PRBCs) is indicated.[1] However, recent evidence cautions against the liberal use of blood in TBI and other critically ill patients secondary to worse outcomes associated with their use.[27] Volume status should be targeted to a central venous pressure of 7 to 12 cm H_2O if invasive monitoring is employed.[1] After achievement of euvolemia, the patient's head should be elevated at 30° to promote venous drainage and decrease ICP. If restoration of the intravascular volume is inadequate in elevating MAP to an acceptable level, hypertension should be induced using vasopressors or inotropic support. The drugs employed most commonly to induce hypertension are dopamine, phenylephrine, and norepinephrine.[1] Patients should be monitored for renal dysfunction, lactic acidosis, and signs of peripheral ischemia when these agents are used, especially in large doses.

TREATMENT OF INTRACRANIAL HYPERTENSION

General Pharmacologic Strategies

6 The use of analgesics and sedatives has an important primary role in the management of intracranial hypertension (see Table 42-3 and Fig. 42-3).[28] This is related directly to the association of pain, agitation, excessive muscle movement, and resisting mechanical ventilation with transient increases in ICP. Paralytics are a secondary option in refractory patients. Nonetheless, there is no strong evidence that one agent is superior to another relative to affecting outcome in patients with severe TBI based on a recent systematic review of randomized clinical trials.[29] Effects on

TABLE 42-3 Drug Dosing and Monitoring in TBI Patients

Drug	Adverse Drug Reactions	Monitoring Parameter	Dosing	Comments
Levetiracetam (Keppra)	CNS changes	Seizures, SCr	500 mg IV Q12 h (dose during first 14 days)	Caution in patients with renal dysfunction If used for active seizures: increase to 1,000 mg Q12 h after 14 days, then to 1500 mg Q12 h after 28 days
Mannitol (Generic)	Hypotension, renal dysfunction, hyperosmolality	ICP, CPP, BP, serum osmolality, Na, UO, SCr	0.25 to 1 g/kg IV Q4 h	Avoid in patients with renal failure or CHF
Pentobarbital (Nembutal)	Hypotension, GI hypomotility, induction of hepatic drug metabolism	ICP, CPP, BP, EEG, GI function	10 mg/kg IV over 30 minutes, then 5 mg/kg over 3 hours, then 1 mg/kg/h	Administer via central line. General dose range for infusion is 1–3 mg/kg/h
Phenytoin (Dilantin)	Hypotension, dysrhythmias, nystagmus, ataxia, mental status changes, exfoliative dermatitis	Seizures, BP, ECG, phenytoin concentrations, skin	15–20 mg/kg IV over 60 minutes, then 5 mg/kg/day divided Q8 h or Q12 h	Administer less than 50 mg/min; use central line if available Round loading doses up to nearest 250 mg, round maintenance doses up to nearest 25 mg Trauma patients often require higher doses (i.e., >6 mg/kg/day) to achieve therapeutic concentrations
Propofol (Diprivan)	Hypotension, hyperkalemia, metabolic, acidosis, rhabdomyolysis, renal failure, hepatomegaly, lipemia	ICP, CPP, BP, SCr, K, arterial pH, triglycerides, lactate	General range: 0.5–3 mg/kg/h titrated to desired effect	Avoid doses greater than 5 mg/kg/hr or prolonged infusions; not approved for use in children

SCr, serum creatinine; ICP, intracranial pressure; CPP, cerebral perfusion pressure; BP, blood pressure; Na, sodium; UO, urine output; CHF, congestive heart failure; EEG, electroencephalogram; ECG, electrocardiogram; K, potassium.

The reader is referred to other appropriate chapters regarding other drugs not listed in this table.

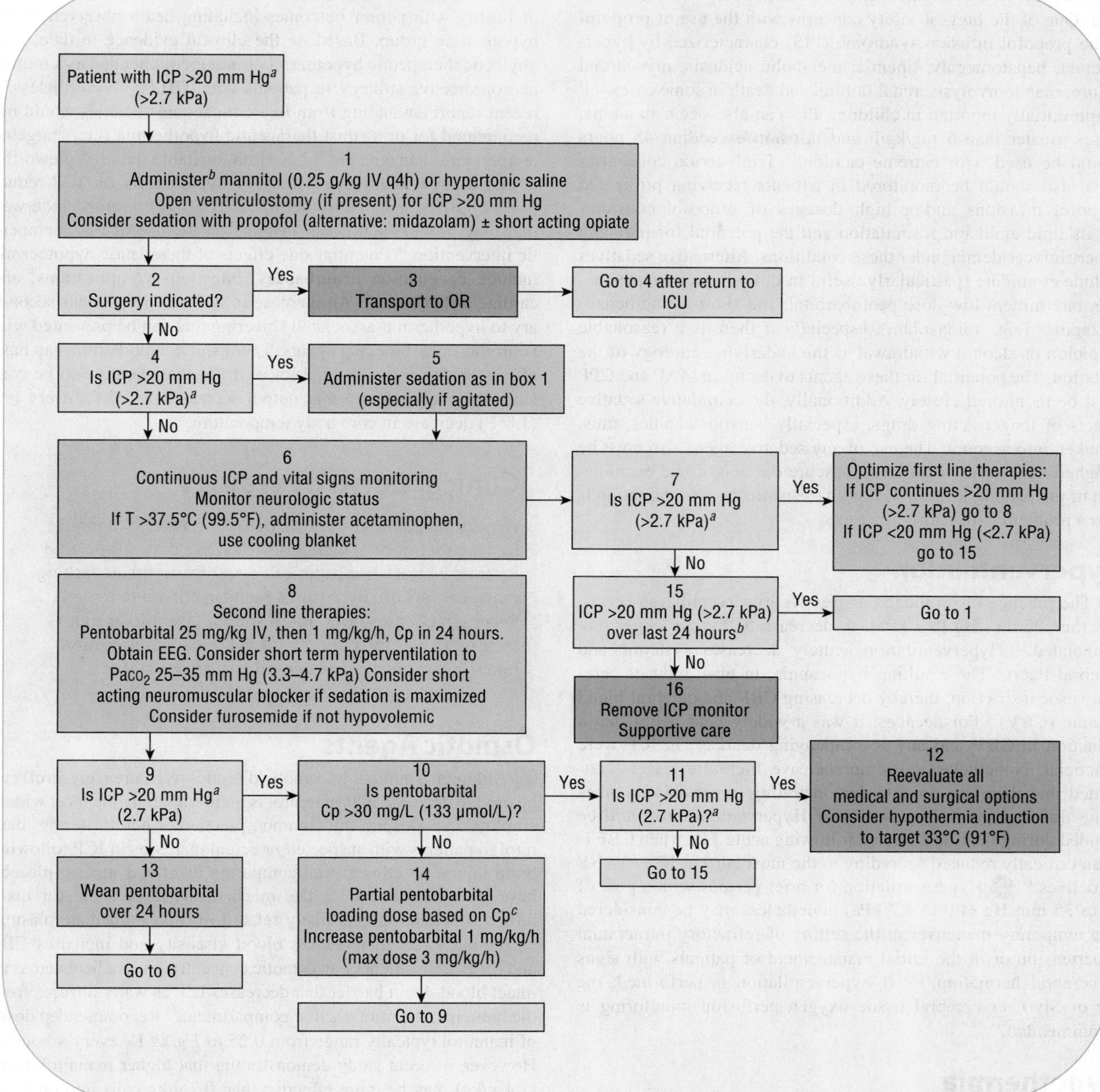

FIGURE 42-3 Algorithm for the management of increased ICP. [a]Treatment thresholds: ICP 20 to 29 mm Hg (2.7 to 3.9 kPa) for >15 minutes; ICP 30 to 39 mm Hg (4.0 to 5.2 kPa) for >2 minutes; ICP ≥ 40 mm Hg (≥5.3 kPa) for >1 minute. Note: Transient increases may occur following respiratory procedures (e.g., suctioning, chest physiotherapy, bronchoscopy, and intubation). [b]Hold if serum osmolality >320 mOsm/kg (320 mmol/kg). [c]Partial pentobarbital loading dose (mg) = (30 mg/L − measured Cp) (1 L/kg × wt(kg)) (pentobarbital concentration in μmol/L must first be divided by 4.439 to convert to mg/L). (Cp, plasma concentration; CT, computed tomography; OR, operating room; ICP, intracranial pressure; ICU, intensive care unit; T, temperature; CSF, cerebral spinal fluid; EEG, electroencephalogram; RR, respiratory rate; $Paco_2$, partial pressure of arterial blood carbon dioxide.) *(Adapted with permission from Wood CG, Boucher BA. Management of Acute Traumatic Brain Injury. In: Richardson M, Chant C, Chessman KH, et al., eds. Pharmacotherapy Self-Assessment Program, 7th ed. Neurology and Psychiatry. Lenexa, KS: American College of Clinical Pharmacy, 2012:144, Figure 1-2.)*

ICP, CPP, and MAP are variable.[29] Morphine sulfate is the most commonly used analgesic and sedative in this setting.[11,30] Noteworthy is that bolus doses of opiates may increase ICP by increasing CBF.[30] However, while continuous infusions of fentanyl and sufentanil are gaining in popularity, their use also may be associated with mild elevations in ICP.[11,30] Propofol has become the sedative of choice in TBI patients among many clinicians because of its ease of titration, rapidly reversible effects on discontinuation, and possible neuroprotective effects.[11] Although it is used for sedation in infants and children who are mechanically ventilated in the intensive care unit (ICU) setting, the FDA requires that the manufacturer labeling contains specific information that propofol is not approved for sedation of pediatric patients admitted to an ICU. One of the biggest safety concerns with the use of propofol is the propofol infusion syndrome (PIS) characterized by hyperkalemia, hepatomegaly, lipemia, metabolic acidosis, myocardial failure, rhabdomyolysis, renal failure, and death in some cases.[11,31] While initially reported in children, PIS can also occur in adults. Doses greater than 5 mg/kg/h and infusion exceeding 48 hours should be used with extreme caution.[11] Triglyceride concentrations also should be monitored in patients receiving prolonged propofol infusions and/or high dosages of propofol considering its lipid emulsion formulation and the potential for inducing hypertriglyceridemia under these conditions. Alternative sedatives include etomidate (particularly useful in rapid-induction anesthesia), intermittent low-dose pentobarbital, and short-acting benzodiazepines (e.g., midazolam), especially if there is a reasonable suspicion of alcohol withdrawal as the underlying etiology of the agitation. The potential for these agents to decrease MAP and CPP must be monitored closely. Additionally, the cumulative sedative effects of longer-acting drugs, especially benzodiazepines, must be taken into account. The use of any sedative agent also must be weighed against its potential to obscure the neurologic examination of the patient. Interference with the neurologic examination is also a problem with paralytic agents.

Hyperventilation

4 The practice of prolonged aggressive hyperventilation ($Pa{CO_2}$ less than 25 mm Hg [3.3 kPa]) to decrease ICP is no longer recommended.[11] Hyperventilation acutely decreases systemic and cerebral $Pa{CO_2}$. The resulting hypocapnia, in turn, induces cerebral vasoconstriction, thereby decreasing CBF and cerebral blood volume (CBV).[8] For decades, it was a widely held belief that a reduction in CBV and any accompanying decrease in ICP were beneficial. Nonetheless, a comprehensive literature review concluded that there are no data demonstrating improved outcomes using this therapeutic intervention.[32] Hyperventilation should be avoided during the first 24 hours following acute TBI when CBF is often critically reduced according to the most current BTF/AANS guidelines.[11] 7 Hyperventilation for brief periods with a goal of 30 to 35 mm Hg (4.0 to 4.7 kPa) nonetheless may be considered as a temporary maneuver in the setting of refractory intracranial hypertension or in the initial management of patients with signs of cerebral herniation.[11,15] If hyperventilation is performed, the use of $Sj{VO_2}$ or cerebral tissue oxygen perfusion monitoring is recommended.[11]

Hypothermia

Therapeutic hypothermia has been an attractive strategy for attempting to minimize secondary brain injury after TBI for decades. The mechanism underlying a protective effect of hypothermia is likely multifactorial, although a reduction in $CM{RO_2}$ is offered most frequently as the basis of any therapeutic benefits. Early TBI studies suggested promise for therapeutic hypothermia. In addition, some other patient populations with brain ischemia (e.g., cardiac arrest patients) have improved outcomes with hypothermia. Unfortunately, data from recent clinical trials of prophylactic therapeutic hypothermia in TBI patients have not shown improved outcomes. The first of two large randomized clinical trials of therapeutic hypothermia in 392 patients with nonpenetrating TBI using a targeted temperature of 33°C (91°F) revealed no improvement in outcome compared with the normothermic group.[11] In addition, more hypotension was observed in the therapeutic hypothermia group. The second major multicenter study focused on early cooling (i.e., less than or equal to 2.5 hours) to 35°C (95°F), then 48 hours at 33°C (91°F) followed by gradual rewarming.[33] The control group was treated under normothermia conditions. This study was discontinued after enrollment of 108 patients because of futility with poorer outcomes including death observed in the hypothermic group. Based on the clinical evidence to date, prophylactic therapeutic hypothermia is not recommended as a routine neuroprotective strategy in patients with TBI.[34–36] Nevertheless, a recent report emanating from five critical care societies would not recommend for or against therapeutic hypothermia (i.e., "targeted temperature management") based on available data.[37] Noteworthy is that a large, multicenter study of hypothermia for ICP reduction in TBI patients (Eurotherm3235Trial) is currently underway that may provide additional insights on the use of this therapeutic intervention.[38] Potential side effects of therapeutic hypothermia include coagulation disturbances, infectious complications, and cardiac arrhythmias.[35] An increase in ICP also may occur secondary to hypothermia-associated shivering that can be prevented with neuromuscular blocking agents. Therapeutic hypothermia can have effects on the pharmacokinetics of drugs that should also be considered. Specifically, cardiac output decreases by 7% for every 1°C (1.8°F) decrease in core body temperature.[39]

Clinical **Controversy. . .**

Hypertonic saline is an attractive alternative to mannitol for the treatment of increased ICP. While data supporting its effectiveness and superiority over mannitol are lacking, many centers use hypertonic saline in TBI management. Selection of an osmotic agent should take into account factors such as the patient's intravascular volume, renal function, serum electrolytes, and acid/base status.

Osmotic Agents

7 Although a number of osmotic diuretics (e.g., urea, glycerol) can be used to decrease ICP, mannitol is unquestionably the most widely employed.[1,11] Despite the common practice of administering mannitol to patients with suspected or actual increases in ICP following brain injury, no clinical trial comparing its effects against placebo have been performed.[30,40] The mechanisms responsible for mannitol's beneficial effects likely relate to (a) an immediate plasma-expanding effect that reduces blood viscosity and increases CBF and (b) establishment of an osmotic concentration gradient across an intact blood–brain barrier that decreases ICP as water diffuses from the brain into the intravascular compartment.[11] Recommended doses of mannitol typically range from 0.25 to 1 g/kg IV every 4 hours.[11] However, a recent study demonstrating that higher mannitol doses (1.4 g/kg) may be more effective than 0.7 g/kg calls into question this dosing recommendation.[41] Increased ICP is reduced within minutes following mannitol administration, and the duration of action ranges from 90 minutes to 6 hours depending on the dose and the clinical conditions that are present.[11] In order to maximize benefit and minimize adverse events, it was previously recommended that mannitol be administered as a bolus and not as a continuous infusion in this setting.[1,10] However, more recent analyses conclude that there is no demonstrable benefit using one administration approach over the other.[11]

Several adverse effects are associated with mannitol. In addition to hypotension resulting from its diuretic effect, a reversible acute renal dysfunction may occur in patients with previously normal renal function after long-term, large-dose administration, especially if the serum osmolality and serum sodium exceed 320 mOsm/kg (320 mmol/kg) and 160 meq/L (160 mmol/L), respectively.[1] Hence monitoring and maintaining the serum osmolality and sodium, and replacing urinary fluid losses are important to minimize this adverse event. Mannitol should be avoided in patients with renal failure.[15] Acute exacerbation of underlying congestive heart failure and pulmonary edema also may occur following rapid intravascular volume expansion. Furosemide is recommended as an alternative diuretic for lowering ICP in these latter patient groups.

While hypertonic saline solutions have been advocated by some as a resuscitative fluid following TBI as previously mentioned, solutions ranging from concentrations of 3% to 23.4% have also been used to acutely lower increased ICP.[16] Not only do hypertonic saline solutions create an osmotic gradient in favor of reducing cerebral edema, but evidence suggests that they may also have beneficial vasoregulatory, immunologic, and neurochemical effects as well. Plasma expansion may also lead to an increase in CBF. It is noteworthy, however, that the 2007 BTF guidelines do not recommend hypertonic saline due to a lack of supporting evidence.[42] Nonetheless, a crossover study of 20% mannitol versus 7.5% hypertonic saline and 6% dextan-70 in nine TBI patients with ICP greater than 20 mm Hg (greater than 2.7 kPa) demonstrated a significantly greater decrease in ICP and a longer duration of effect following the hypertonic saline infusions.[43] A recent meta-analysis also suggested that hypertonic saline may be modestly more effective than mannitol.[44] In contrast, two recent studies of equimolar doses of mannitol versus 7.45% and 15% hypertonic saline, respectively, revealed similar effects between the regimens in TBI patients.[45,46] If used, serum sodium concentrations should not be allowed to increase by more than 12 mEq/L (12 mmol/L) in a 24-hour period (0.5 mEq/L [0.5 mmol/L] per hour) to avoid neurologic adverse events. Furthermore, hypertonic saline should not be used if the serum sodium concentration exceeds 155 to 160 mEq/L (155 to 160 mmol/L).

Barbiturates

7 High-dose barbiturate therapy (i.e., *barbiturate coma*) has been used for decades in the management of increased ICP despite a lack of evidence documenting beneficial effects on patient morbidity and mortality.[47] Nonetheless, based largely on beneficial outcomes observed in a randomized clinical trial published in 1988, BTF/AANS and pediatric guidelines recommend that high-dose barbiturate therapy be considered in hemodynamically stable severe TBI patients refractory to maximal medical ICP-lowering therapy and decompressive surgery.[11,15] A recent study indicated survival at a discharge of 40% and good functional outcomes in 68% of survivors at 1 year in this TBI patient subset receiving high-dose barbiturate therapy.[48] Prophylactic use of barbiturates is not advocated in light of insufficient evidence supporting this practice and the potential for adverse events (e.g., hypotension).[11,15,47] Several mechanisms responsible for the cerebral protective effects of barbiturates have been proposed. These include (a) lowering the regional $CMRo_2$ with a coupled reduction in CBF to these areas, (b) inhibition of lipid peroxidation, and (c) alteration of cerebral vascular tone.[1,28] Prior to inducing a barbiturate coma, the severe TBI patient must be mechanically ventilated with continuous monitoring of arterial blood pressure, electrocardiogram (ECG), and ICP. Pentobarbital is the most commonly used barbiturate for this indication, although thiopental also has been used. Pentobarbital should be administered as an IV loading infusion totaling 25 mg/kg (i.e., 10 mg/kg over 30 minutes and then 5 mg/kg per hour for 3 hours), followed by a maintenance infusion of 1 to 2 mg/kg per hour.[1,11] If the systolic blood pressure falls during the loading or maintenance infusions, the rate should be slowed temporarily and blood pressure support initiated. The goal of a barbiturate coma is to maintain ICP and CPP at the previously discussed target thresholds in addition to achieving a pentobarbital steady-state concentration of between 30 and 40 mg/L (133 and 178 μmol/L) (despite poor correlation between serum concentrations and outcome) and EEG burst suppression.[11] Initiation of barbiturate therapy withdrawal can occur when ICP has been controlled satisfactorily for 24 to 48 hours. Barbiturates should be tapered over 24 to 72 hours to prevent ICP spikes.

Side effects associated with high-dose barbiturate therapy involve primarily the cardiovascular system. Hypotension caused by peripheral vasodilation may occur, necessitating decreasing the barbiturate dose or the administration of fluids and vasopressors to maintain blood pressure. A systematic review of the literature suggested that one of every four patients receiving barbiturate therapy will develop hypotension.[47] GI effects of barbiturates include decreased GI muscular tone and decreased amplitude of contraction. On emergence from coma, there may be a period of GI hypermotility. Care should be taken to avoid extravasation of pentobarbital and thiopental solutions because severe tissue damage may occur. Barbiturates should be administered by continuous infusion through a central line dedicated for this purpose. The potential for barbiturates to induce the hepatic drug metabolism of concurrent medications should be also considered. Lastly, the potential for prolonged interference with the neurologic examination of TBI patients must be considered prior to the initiation of high-dose barbiturate therapy.

Corticosteroids

7 Although corticosteroids are effective in preventing or reducing cerebral edema in patients with nontraumatic conditions producing vasogenic edema, studies in TBI patients have not demonstrated the ability of corticosteroids to lower ICP or improve outcome.[11,49] Specifically, use of corticosteroids following TBI has been associated with increased mortality and complications, including GI bleeding, glucose intolerance, electrolyte abnormalities, and infection. The largest investigation to date was known as the corticosteroid randomization after significant head injury (CRASH) study.[50] In this study, 10,008 patients with a GCS score less than or equal to 14 were randomized to receive a 48-hour continuous infusion of methylprednisolone or placebo. Results of this study indicated a higher risk of death within 2 weeks of enrollment (relative risk 1.18) in those patients receiving corticosteroids compared with patients receiving placebo ($P < 0.001$).[50] Based on this and several other major randomized trials, the BTF/AANS adult and pediatric guidelines recommend that high-dose corticosteroids not be used in patients with moderate to severe TBI.[11,15]

Clinical **Controversy...**

The role of levetiracetam in the treatment of TBI patients is uncertain. It continues to gain in popularity for the prevention of seizures despite the lack of data supporting its use for this indication.

TREATMENT AND PROPHYLAXIS OF COMPLICATIONS

Posttraumatic Seizures

It is generally agreed that patients who have experienced one or more seizures following a moderate-to-severe TBI should receive anticonvulsant therapy to avoid increases in $CMRo_2$ that occur with the onset of subsequent seizures and to prevent the development of (sometimes subclinical) status epilepticus with associated increase in mortality. Initial therapy in these persons should consist of incremental IV doses of diazepam (5 to 40 mg adults, 0.1 to 0.5 mg/kg infants and children) or lorazepam (2 to 8 mg adults, 0.03 to 0.1 mg/kg infants and children) to terminate any active seizure activity followed by IV phenytoin to prevent seizure recurrence. Phenytoin dosing regimens for adults and pediatric patients include an IV loading dose of 15 to 20 and 10 to 15 mg/kg, respectively, followed by a maintenance dose of 5 mg/kg per day. Alternatively, fosphenytoin, a water-soluble phosphate ester of phenytoin, can be administered IV or intramuscularly using the same doses, specified as phenytoin equivalents (PE). The merits of preventive anticonvulsant therapy in patients who have not had a seizure postinjury historically have been more controversial. Risk factors for early posttraumatic seizures (less than 7 days after injury) include a GCS score of less than 10, a cortical contusion, a depressed skull fracture, a subdural hematoma, an epidural hematoma, an intracerebral hematoma, a penetrating head wound, or a seizure within the first 24 hours of injury.[11] In a landmark randomized, placebo-controlled study, the incidence of early posttraumatic seizures in patients receiving placebo was 14.2% compared with 3.6% in patients receiving phenytoin (P <0.05) without a significant increase in drug-related side effects.[51] 8 A systematic review of the literature corroborated these findings, estimating an improved pooled relative risk for early seizure prevention of 0.34 (95% confidence interval [CI]: 0.21 to 0.54) in patients receiving anticonvulsants.[52] Thus, it is recommended that phenytoin (or alternatively carbamazepine) should be used to prevent seizures in TBI patients at high risk for the first 7 days after injury.[11,15,51] Valproate therapy is not recommended based on a trend for higher mortality in a study comparing valproate-treated patients with those receiving phenytoin short-term therapy.[51] Levetiracetam is a potentially attractive option[53]; however, the drug should be used cautiously because is not approved as monotherapy for seizures, and effectiveness in patients with TBI has not been studied in a large randomized clinical trial. Furthermore, the cost-effectiveness of levetiracetam versus phenytoin favors phenytoin.[54,55] A high-quality, randomized, clinical trial demonstrating superiority is needed before levetiracetam displaces phenytoin as the drug of choice following TBI. Nonetheless, if used in TBI patients, the potential for increased levetiracetam systemic clearance should be considered in dosing this agent.[56] The benefits of prophylactic anticonvulsants beyond 7 days have not been demonstrated, and thus their use for this indication is not recommended.[11] Unfortunately, despite reducing the incidence of early seizures following brain injury, no beneficial effects have been documented for anticonvulsants on patient mortality or long-term disability.[11,51] This is particularly disconcerting considering that the long-term risk of epilepsy after TBI has been documented up to 10 years or longer based on the results of a recent population-based cohort study.[57]

Clinical **Controversy. . .**

Prevention of deep venous thrombosis is of major importance in TBI patients. However, controversy remains relative to how early to initiate systemic anticoagulants in TBI patients with CT evidence of intracranial hemorrhage. Currently, the best available data suggest that pharmacologic prophylaxis can be started after a follow-up CT scan shows no worsening of the intracranial hemorrhage in patients who have stable ICP control and who did not have a severe hemorrhage on admission.

Supportive Care

While normalizing ICP and maintaining an adequate CPP are the highest priorities in preventing secondary injury following severe TBI, attention also must be given to preventing and/or treating systemic and extracranial complications.[11] One such complication is systemic hypertension. While several antihypertensives can be used, nicardipine is commonly used in TBI patients because of its effectiveness and lack of adverse effects on brain tissue oxygenation.[58] Fluid and electrolyte management is another important area of focus in the critically ill TBI patient.[16] Common electrolyte disturbances in TBI patients that should be monitored and treated aggressively include hyponatremia, hypomagnesemia, hypokalemia, and hypophosphatemia. Aggressive nutritional support of the TBI patient is another important therapeutic consideration. Evidence suggests that early feeding of TBI patients (i.e., by 7 days) may be associated with a trend toward better outcomes in terms of survival and disability.[11,59] Early enteral nutrition, in particular, within 48 hours is associated with better survival and better outcome at one month postinjury based on a recent retrospective study of severe TBI patients compared with matched controls who did not receive early enteral nutrition.[60] Hyperglycemia (glucose greater than or equal to 160 mg/dL [8.9 mmol/L]) is also common in patients with TBI and is associated with worse outcomes.[61] Nevertheless, intensive insulin therapy versus conventional glucose control should not be used since it is associated with adverse effects on brain glucose metabolism[62] and poor outcomes.[63] Infectious complications commonly encountered in severe TBI patients include nosocomial pneumonia, sepsis, urinary tract infections, and meningitis.[1] Treatment of these potentially devastating infections should be aggressive, with careful attention being paid to antibiotic blood–brain barrier penetration for intracranial infections. Hyperthermia also should be avoided in TBI patients because patients with elevated temperatures have poorer outcomes than normothermic patients.[1,64] Hence aggressive maintenance of a core temperature of less than 37.5°C (99.5°F) using acetaminophen, nonsteroidal antiinflammatory drugs (NSAIDs), and cooling blankets is indicated for patients following severe TBI. Other important therapeutic interventions include acute gastritis prophylaxis, and prevention of decubiti and contractures. Prevention of thromboembolic events is also extremely important supportive care in TBI patients since the incidence of a deep venous thrombosis is higher in TBI patients compared with patients without brain injury.[1,65] This can be accomplished with the use of graduated compression stockings or intermittent pneumatic compression devices initially. Thereafter, the decision to start systemic therapy (e.g., low-molecular weight heparin) depends on multiple factors. Generally, patients who had relatively minor bleeding on the initial CT scan and good ICP control can have pharmacological prophylaxis started immediately or shortly (1 to 3 days) after a follow-up CT scan shows no worsening of bleeding. Prophylaxis is continued until they are ambulatory.[11,66,67] However, systemic anticoagulation must be used with caution in patients with more severe intracerebral hemorrhage, or in patients who may need to undergo craniotomy early in their course. Monitoring for a coagulopathy is important in any severe TBI patient, since the incidence is high (greater than 30%), and coagulopathy is associated with a significantly longer ICU length of stay and an almost 10-fold increase in mortality based on data from a recent study.[68] Reversal of coagulopathy with recombinant factor VIIa in critically ill trauma patients with TBI is gaining in popularity among some practitioners despite lacking an approved indication or large clinical trials demonstrating its safety and efficacy in TBI patients.[69,70] Tranexamic acid is a more inexpensive hemostatic alternative to recombinant factor VIIa. However, more data are needed to determine the role of this agent in TBI patients before it is used routinely.[71]

Clinical Pathways/Guideline Implementation

Use of clinical pathways and formal TBI management guidelines have been demonstrated to improve TBI patient outcomes and reduce institutional resource utilization.[72,73] A cost–benefit analysis revealed that adoption of the BTF guidelines resulted in an increase of more than 3,600 adult severe TBI patients surviving at least 1 day from the more than 23,000 patients with severe TBI admitted annually to U.S. hospitals. Furthermore, patients having a good outcome based on their Glasgow Outcome Scale (GOS) increased from 35% to 66% with an overall estimated annual cost savings exceeding $4 billion.[74] Few practitioners would dispute the overall importance of integrating current evidence-based management guidelines into clinical practice as a means to optimize care and improve the functional outcome of TBI patients.

Investigational Therapy

9 The steady decrease in morbidity and mortality following severe neurotrauma over the last 30 years can be attributed largely to expeditious and aggressive management of events resulting in secondary injury (i.e., ischemia, hypoxia, increased ICP) using conventional treatment strategies. Numerous neuroprotective agents targeting specific pathophysiologic processes that are theorized to occur following severe TBI have been investigated over the last decade in an attempt to further enhance the prospects for a meaningful recovery. Prominent among these strategies have been attempts to modulate calcium influx through the administration of calcium antagonists[75,76] and glutamate antagonists including magnesium,[75,77–80] and the use of antioxidants/free radical scavengers.[75] Inhibitors of inflammatory mediators also are under consideration as neuroprotective agents.[81,82] Unfortunately, none of these agents to date has demonstrated a significant reduction in morbidity or mortality following severe TBI in phase III clinical trials. Noteworthy is that a Phase II pilot study demonstrated a decrease in mortality in 100 TBI patients randomized to receive a three-day infusion of progesterone compared with placebo.[83] A follow-up independently conducted, double-blinded clinical trial of progesterone in 159 TBI patients also improved outcome at 6 months postinjury.[84] Two Phase III trials of this promising pharmacologic strategy are currently underway[85] consistent with clinical data revealing a pooled relative risk for mortality for progesterone in TBI patients of 0.61 (95% CI 0.40 to 0.93).[86] Another recent prospective clinical trial comparing the erythropoiesis-stimulating agent (ESA), darbepoetin alfa, in severe TBI patients also demonstrated significantly improved survival in those receiving the darbepoetin compared with matched patients not receiving an ESA.[87] In light of such positive clinical trial results, the search is likely to continue for neuroprotective agents that eventually may improve the long-term outcome in severe TBI patients.[88] Other agents that have may have beneficial effects in TBI based on limited clinical or epidemiologic data include 3-hydroxy-3-methylglutaryl (HMG) coenzyme A reductase inhibitors[85,89] and β-blockers.[90,91] However, neither drug class has been studied in a published prospective, randomized, clinical trial in TBI patients. Miscellaneous agents being considered as viable neuroprotective agents based on experimental TBI studies including calpain inhibitors, inhibitors of caspases (enzymes involved in apoptosis), and the immunosuppressant, cyclosporine.[85]

Other Treatment Strategies

The concept of administering commercially available CNS-active agents for nonapproved indications in TBI patients should presently be considered investigative therapy. One example is the use of CNS stimulants in the management and rehabilitation of TBI patients. A comprehensive review of the use of methylphenidate relative to improving cognition following TBI was recently conducted. It was the opinion of the author that the literature does provide a degree of support for improvements in memory, attention, concentration, and mental processing in this patient subset, although results and study designs were highly variable for those investigations included in the analysis.[92] Another example is the use of Parkinson's disease medications (e.g., amantadine, bromocriptine, carbidopa/levodopa) in severe TBI patients in an attempt to enhance dopamine release and inhibit reuptake within the injured region of the brain. The results of a multicenter, prospective, double-blind, randomized, placebo controlled trial of amantadine, which was conducted in nonpenetrating TBI patients, were recently published.[93] Patients were enrolled 4 to 16 weeks after their TBI. The amantadine-treated patients had a significantly faster recovery and favorable rehabilitation outcomes compared with placebo. Unfortunately, the two groups became indistinguishable relative to neurologic improvement following taper of amantadine. Regardless, this agent holds excellent promise in TBI patients during the postinjury rehabilitation period. Cholinergic agents such as donepezil have also undergone limited investigation in TBI patients.[94,95] Antidepressants represent yet another class of agents that has been studied in TBI patients.[94] While intuitively appealing, use of psychostimulants to improve cognitive outcomes in TBI patients should be done cautiously with perhaps the lone exception of amantadine until large, well-controlled studies demonstrating beneficial effects are available. Additionally, the timing of administration of these drugs is controversial; the potential for cardiovascular side effects in the face of uncertain benefit would suggest that these drugs should be reserved for the postacute phase of treatment (i.e., weeks to months postinjury).

EVALUATION OF THERAPEUTIC OUTCOMES

The process for evaluation of therapeutic outcomes is summarized in Table 42-4. Patients with severe TBI require ICU monitoring initially with the goals of maintaining or reestablishing neurologic and systemic homeostasis as well as readily detecting any neurologic deterioration. This requires frequent evaluation of the patient's

TABLE 42-4 Evaluation of Therapeutic Outcomes

General	GCS: Record hourly initially, decrease frequency as neurologic status stabilizes Vital signs (BP, HR, RR, temperature): Record hourly initially, decrease frequency as neurologic status stabilizes Urine output: Record hourly initially, decrease frequency as neurologic status stabilizes Arterial oxygen saturation: Continuously while in ICU
Risk of increased ICP	ICP: Record hourly, decrease frequency as ICP stabilizes less than 20 mm Hg (2.7 kPa) (usually not until 48–72 hours postinjury at a minimum) CPP: Record hourly, decrease frequency as CPP stabilizes in the desired range[a]
Laboratory tests	Ethanol concentration and urine drug screen: On admission ABGs: Daily at a minimum while intubated, repeated as needed based on pulmonary instability requiring ventilator setting changes CBC: Daily while in ICU Serum electrolytes (Na, K, Cl): Daily while in ICU. Serum sodium and osmolality may be monitored as frequently as every 6 hours if osmotherapy (mannitol, furosemide, hypertonic saline) is being utilized Minerals (Mg, Ca, P): Daily initially until concentrations stable
Radiologic procedures	CT scan: Postresuscitation initially with repeat scan(s) as needed based on degree of neurologic instability (e.g., decrease in GCS) or initial CT appearance

GCS, Glasgow Coma Scale; BP, blood pressure; HR, heart rate; RR, respiratory rate; CSF, cerebrospinal fluid; TBI, traumatic brain injury; ICP, intracranial pressure; CPP, cerebral perfusion pressure; ABG, arterial blood gas; CBC, complete blood count; Na, sodium; K, potassium; Cl, chloride; Mg, magnesium; Ca, calcium; P, phosphorus; CT, computed tomography.

[a]Continuous monitoring mandated initially if technologically feasible.

neurologic status (e.g., GCS) and measurement of vital signs, urine output, and arterial oxygen saturation (as well as ICP in patients with an ICP monitor in place). Furthermore, careful attention must be paid to the potential for development of a variety of electrolyte, mineral, and acid–base disturbances; coagulopathies; and infections by obtaining various laboratory tests on a daily basis initially. The intensity of monitoring will be a function of the relative degree of neurologic and hemodynamic stability of the patient in the hours and days following the neurologic insult. Lastly, radiologic tests (e.g., CT scans) are essential not only for the initial diagnostic evaluation of TBI patients but also as means to evaluate the etiology for any subsequent neurologic deterioration.

PERSONALIZED PHARMACOTHERAPY

There are several opportunities for personalized pharmacotherapy in severe TBI patients. The most common general pharmacokinetic challenge is that TBI patients have a larger volume of distribution and more rapid hepatic clearance of drugs than most other patient populations.[96] These pharmacokinetic changes often make the optimizing of phenytoin and, less commonly, pentobarbital concentrations very difficult. As such, recommendations for phenytoin and pentobarbital dosing are weight based, and in the case of phenytoin, usually higher than the 300 mg/day dose is commonly seen in ambulatory patients. Pharmacodynamically, there can be wide interpatient variability in the efficacy of pharmacologic and nonpharmacologic interventions for ICP control. For some patients, there is a high degree of trial and error to find the best combination of interventions that are effective and not contraindicated by other factors. Lastly, the decision to start pharmacologic deep venous thrombosis prophylaxis may also be highly personalized depending on CT findings, neurologic progress, ICP control, and the possible need for surgery.

ABBREVIATIONS

AANS	American Association of Neurological Surgeons
ATP	adenosine triphosphate
BTF	Brain Trauma Foundation
CBF	cerebral blood flow
CBV	cerebral blood volume
CDo_2	cerebral oxygen delivery
$CMRo_2$	cerebral oxygen consumption
CPP	cerebral perfusion pressure
CSF	cerebrospinal fluid
CT	computed tomography
ECG	electrocardiogram
ESA	erythropoiesis-stimulating agent
GCS	Glasgow Coma Scale
GOS	Glasgow Outcome Scale
HMG	3-hydroxy-3-methylglutaryl
ICP	intracranial pressure
ICU	intensive care unit
MAP	mean arterial pressure
NMDA	*N*-methyl-D-aspartate
NSAID	nonsteroidal antiinflammatory drug
PIS	propofol infusion syndrome
PRBCs	packed red blood cells
SBP	systolic blood pressure
$Sjvo_2$	jugular venous oxygen saturation
TBI	traumatic brain injury

ACKNOWLEDGMENTS

The authors would like to acknowledge Shelly D. Timmons, MD, PhD, FACS, for her contributions to previous editions of this chapter.

REFERENCES

1. Cohen SM, Marion DW. Traumatic brain injury. In: Fink MP, Abraham E, Vincent JL, Kochanek PM, eds. Textbook of Critical Care, 5th ed. Philadelphia: Elsevier/Saunders; 2005:377–389.
2. Faul M, Xu L, Wald MM, Coronado V. Traumatic Brain Injury in the United States: Emergency Department Visits, Hospitalizations and Deaths 2002–2006. National Center for Injury Prevention and Control: Centers for Disease Control and Prevention, 2010:1–74.
3. Zaloshnja E, Miller T, Langlois JA, Selassie AW. Prevalence of long-term disability from traumatic brain injury in the civilian population of the United States, 2005. J Head Trauma Rehabil 2008;23(6):394–400.
4. Finkelstein E, Corso P, Miller T. The Incidence and Economic Burden of Injuries in the United States. New York: Oxford University Press, 2006.
5. Ling GS, Marshall SA. Management of traumatic brain injury in the intensive care unit. Neurol Clin 2008;26(2):409–426.
6. Chang CWJ. Neurologic injury: Prevention and initial care. In: Gabrielli A, Layon AJ, Yu M, eds. Civetta, Taylor, & Kirby's Critical Care, 4th ed. Philadelphia: Wolters Kluwer/Lippincott Williams & Wilkins, 2007:1245–1260.
7. Clark RSB, Jenkins L, Lai YC, et al. Biochemical, cellular, and molecular mechanisms of neuronal death and secondary brain injury in critical care. In: Fink MP, Abraham E, Vincent JL, Kochanek PM, eds. Textbook of Critical Care, 5th ed. Philadelphia: Elsevier/Saunders, 2005:263–273.
8. Manno EM, Rabinstein AA. Central nervous system. In: Gabrielli A, Layon AJ, Yu M, eds. Civetta, Taylor, & Kirby's Critical Care. Philadelphia: Wolters Kluwer/Lippincott Williams & Willkins, 2007:649–665.
9. Tasaki O, Shiozaki T, Hamasaki T, et al. Prognostic indicators and outcome prediction model for severe traumatic brain injury. J Trauma 2009;66(2):304–308.
10. Bullock R, Chesnut RM, Clifton GL, et al. Brain Trauma Foundation, Inc., American Association of Neurological Surgeons. Part 1: Guidelines for the Management of Severe Head Injury. New York: Brain Trauma Foundation, Inc., 2000.
11. Bratton SL, Chestnut RM, Ghajar J, et al. Guidelines for the managment of severe head injury. The Brain Trauma Foundation. The American Association of Neurological Surgeons. The Joint Section on Neurotrauma and Critical Care. J Neurotrauma 2007;24(Suppl 1):S1–S106.
12. Fakhry SM, Trask AL, Waller MA, Watts DD. Management of brain-injured patients by an evidence-based medicine protocol improves outcomes and decreases hospital charges. J Trauma 2004;56(3):492–499.
13. Gabriel EJ, Ghajar J, Jagoda A, et al. Guidelines for prehospital management of traumatic brain injury. J Neurotrauma 2002;19(1):111–174.
14. Bullock MR, Chesnut R, Ghajar J, et al. Guidelines for the surgical management of traumatic brain injury. Neurosurgery 2006;58(3):S2 1–62.
15. Adelson PD, Bratton SL, Carney NA, et al. Guidelines for the acute medical management of severe traumatic brain injury in infants, children, and adolescents. Crit Care Med 2003;31(6):S417–S491.

16. Rhoney DH, Parker D, Jr. Considerations in fluids and electrolytes after traumatic brain injury. Nutr Clin Pract 2006;21(5):462–478.
17. Myburgh J, Cooper DJ, Finfer S, et al. Saline or albumin for fluid resuscitation in patients with traumatic brain injury. N Engl J Med 2007;357(9):874–884.
18. Sahuquillo J, Arikan F. Decompressive craniectomy for the treatment of refractory high intracranial pressure in traumatic brain injury. Cochrane Database Syst Rev 2006(1):CD003983.
19. Cooper DJ, Rosenfeld JV, Murray L, et al. Decompressive craniectomy in diffuse traumatic brain injury. N Engl J Med 2011;364(16):1493–1502.
20. Shafi S, Diaz-Arrastia R, Madden C, Gentilello L. Intracranial pressure monitoring in brain-injured patients is associated with worsening of survival. J Trauma 2008;64(2): 335–340.
21. Smith M. Monitoring intracranial pressure in traumatic brain injury. Anesth Analg 2008;106(1):240–248.
22. Rosenthal G, Hemphill JC, 3rd, Sorani M, et al. Brain tissue oxygen tension is more indicative of oxygen diffusion than oxygen delivery and metabolism in patients with traumatic brain injury. Crit Care Med 2008;36(6):1917–1924.
23. Korfias S, Stranjalis G, Boviatsis E, et al. Serum S-100B protein monitoring in patients with severe traumatic brain injury. Intensive Care Med 2007;33(2):255–260.
24. Kleindienst A, Ross Bullock M. A critical analysis of the role of the neurotrophic protein S100B in acute brain injury. J Neurotrauma 2006;23(8):1185–1200.
25. Stein DM, Kufera JA, Lindell A, et al. Association of CSF biomarkers and secondary insults following severe traumatic brain injury. Neurocrit Care 2011;14(2):200–207.
26. White H, Venkatesh B. Cerebral perfusion pressure in neurotrauma: A review. Anesth Analg 2008;107(3):979–988.
27. Salim A, Hadjizacharia P, DuBose J, et al. Role of anemia in traumatic brain injury. J Am Coll Surg 2008;207(3):398–406.
28. Maas AIR, Stocchetti N. Intensive care after neurosurgery. In: Fink MP, Abraham E, Vincent JL, Kochanek PM, eds. Textbook of Critical Care, 5th ed. Philadelphia: Elsevier/Saunders, 2005.
29. Roberts DJ, Hall RI, Kramer AH, et al. Sedation for critically ill adults with severe traumatic brain injury: A systematic review of randomized controlled trials. Crit Care Med 2011;39(12):2743–2751.
30. Meyer MJ, Megyesi J, Meythaler J, et al. Acute management of acquired brain injury part II: An evidence-based review of pharmacological interventions. Brain Inj 2010;24(5): 706–721.
31. Otterspoor LC, Kalkman CJ, Cremer OL. Update on the propofol infusion syndrome in ICU management of patients with head injury. Curr Opin Anaesthesiol 2008;21(5): 544–551.
32. Meyer MJ, Megyesi J, Meythaler J, et al. Acute management of acquired brain injury part I: An evidence-based review of non-pharmacological interventions. Brain Inj 2010;24(5):694–705.
33. Clifton GL, Valadka A, Zygun D, et al. Very early hypothermia induction in patients with severe brain injury (the National Acute Brain Injury Study: Hypothermia II): A randomised trial. Lancet Neurol 2011;10(2):131–139.
34. Bratton SL, Chestnut RM, Ghajar J, et al. Guidelines for the management of severe traumatic brain injury. III. Prophylactic hypothermia. J Neurotrauma 2007;24(Suppl 1): S21–S25.
35. Peterson K, Carson S, Carney N. Hypothermia treatment for traumatic brain injury: A systematic review and meta-analysis. J Neurotrauma 2008;25(1):62–71.
36. Sydenham E, Roberts I, Alderson P. Hypothermia for traumatic head injury. Cochrane Database Syst Rev 2009(2):CD001048.
37. Nunnally ME, Jaeschke R, Bellingan GJ, et al. Targeted temperature management in critical care: A report and recommendations from five professional societies. Crit Care Med 2011;39(5):1113–1125.
38. Andrews PJ, Sinclair HL, Battison CG, et al. European society of intensive care medicine study of therapeutic hypothermia (32–35°C) for intracranial pressure reduction after traumatic brain injury (the Eurotherm3235Trial). Trials 2011;12:8.
39. Varon J. Therapeutic hypothermia: Implications for acute care practitioners. Postgrad Med 2010;122(1):19–27.
40. Wakai A, Roberts I, Schierhout G. Mannitol for acute traumatic brain injury. Cochrane Database Syst Rev 2005(4):CD001049.
41. Sorani MD, Morabito D, Rosenthal G, et al. Characterizing the dose–response relationship between mannitol and intracranial pressure in traumatic brain injury patients using a high-frequency physiological data collection system. J Neurotrauma 2008;25(4):291–298.
42. Bratton SL, Chestnut RM, Ghajar J, et al. Guidelines for the management of severe traumatic brain injury. II. Hyperosmolar therapy. J Neurotrauma 2007;24 (Suppl 1): S14–S20.
43. Battison C, Andrews PJ, Graham C, Petty T. Randomized, controlled trial on the effect of a 20% mannitol solution and a 7.5% saline/6% dextran solution on increased intracranial pressure after brain injury. Crit Care Med 2005;33(1): 196–202; discussion 257–258.
44. Kamel H, Navi BB, Nakagawa K, et al. Hypertonic saline versus mannitol for the treatment of elevated intracranial pressure: A meta-analysis of randomized clinical trials. Crit Care Med 2011;39(3):554–559.
45. Francony G, Fauvage B, Falcon D, et al. Equimolar doses of mannitol and hypertonic saline in the treatment of increased intracranial pressure. Crit Care Med 2008;36(3): 795–800.
46. Sakellaridis N, Pavlou E, Karatzas S, et al. Comparison of mannitol and hypertonic saline in the treatment of severe brain injuries. J Neurosurg 2011;114(2):545–548.
47. Roberts I. Barbiturates for acute traumatic brain injury. Cochrane Database Syst Rev 2012;12:CD00033.
48. Marshall GT, James RF, Landman MP, et al. Pentobarbital coma for refractory intra-cranial hypertension after severe traumatic brain injury: Mortality predictions and one-year outcomes in 55 patients. J Trauma 2010;69(2):275–283.
49. Alderson P, Roberts I. Corticosteroids for acute traumatic brain injury. Cochrane Database Syst Rev 2005;1:CD000196.
50. Roberts I, Yates D, Sandercock P, et al. Effect of intravenous corticosteroids on death within 14 days in 10008 adults with clinically significant head injury (MRC CRASH trial): Randomised placebo-controlled trial. Lancet 2004;364(9442):1321–1328.
51. Temkin NR. Preventing and treating posttraumatic seizures: The human experience. Epilepsia 2009; 50(Suppl 2):10–13.
52. Schierhout G, Roberts I. Anti-epileptic drugs for preventing seizures following acute traumatic brain injury. Cochrane Database Syst Rev 2012;6:CD000173.
53. Szaflarski JP, Sangha KS, Lindsell CJ, Shutter LA. Prospective, randomized, single-blinded comparative trial of intravenous levetiracetam versus phenytoin for seizure prophylaxis. Neurocrit Care 2010;12(2):165–172.

54. Cotton BA, Kao LS, Kozar R, Holcomb JB. Cost-utility analysis of levetiracetam and phenytoin for posttraumatic seizure prophylaxis. J Trauma 2011;71(2):375–379.
55. Pieracci FM, Moore EE, Beauchamp K, et al. A cost-minimization analysis of phenytoin versus levetiracetam for early seizure pharmacoprophylaxis after traumatic brain injury. J Trauma Acute Care Surg 2012;72(1): 276–281.
56. Spencer DD, Jacobi J, Juenke JM, et al. Steady-state pharmacokinetics of intravenous levetiracetam in neurocritical care patients. Pharmacotherapy 2011;31(10): 934–941.
57. Christensen J, Pedersen MG, Pedersen CB, et al. Long-term risk of epilepsy after traumatic brain injury in children and young adults: A population-based cohort study. Lancet 2009;373(9669):1105–1110.
58. Narotam PK, Puri V, Roberts JM, et al. Management of hypertensive emergencies in acute brain disease: Evaluation of the treatment effects of intravenous nicardipine on cerebral oxygenation. J Neurosurg 2008;109(6):1065–1074.
59. Cook AM, Peppard A, Magnuson B. Nutrition considerations in traumatic brain injury. Nutr Clin Pract 2008;23(6): 608–620.
60. Chiang YH, Chao DP, Chu SF, et al. Early enteral nutrition and clinical outcomes of severe traumatic brain injury patients in acute stage: A multi-center cohort study. J Neurotrauma 2012;29(1):75–80.
61. Liu-DeRyke X, Collingridge DS, Orme J, et al. Clinical impact of early hyperglycemia during acute phase of traumatic brain injury. Neurocrit Care 2009;11(2): 151–157.
62. Vespa P, McArthur DL, Stein N, et al. Tight glycemic control increases metabolic distress in traumatic brain injury: A randomized controlled within-subjects trial. Crit Care Med 2012;40(6):1923–1929.
63. Graffagnino C, Gurram AR, Kolls B, Olson DM. Intensive insulin therapy in the neurocritical care setting is associated with poor clinical outcomes. Neurocrit Care 2010;13(3): 307–312.
64. Badjatia N. Hyperthermia and fever control in brain injury. Crit Care Med (Review) 2009;37(7 Suppl):S250–S257.
65. Reiff DA, Haricharan RN, Bullington NM, et al. Traumatic brain injury is associated with the development of deep vein thrombosis independent of pharmacological prophylaxis. J Trauma 2009;66(5):1436–1440.
66. Koehler DM, Shipman J, Davidson MA, Guillamondegui O. Is early venous thromboembolism prophylaxis safe in trauma patients with intracranial hemorrhage. J Trauma 2011;70(2):324–329.
67. Scudday T, Brasel K, Webb T, et al. Safety and efficacy of prophylactic anticoagulation in patients with traumatic brain injury. J Am Coll Surg 2011;213(1):148–153.
68. Talving P, Benfield R, Hadjizacharia P, et al. Coagulopathy in severe traumatic brain injury: A prospective study. J Trauma 2009;66(1):55–61; discussion 61–62.
69. DeLoughery EP, Lenfesty B, DeLoughery TG. A retrospective case control study of recombinant factor VIIa in patients with intracranial haemorrhage caused by trauma. Br J Haematol 2011;152(5):667–669.
70. Perel P, Roberts I, Shakur H, et al. Haemostatic drugs for traumatic brain injury. Cochrane Database Syst Rev 2010;(1):CD007877.
71. Roberts I, Shakur H, Ker K, Coats T. Antifibrinolytic drugs for acute traumatic injury. Cochrane Database Syst Rev 2011;(1):CD004896.
72. Marion DW. Evidenced-based guidelines for traumatic brain injuries. Prog Neurol Surg 2006;19:171–196.
73. Hesdorffer DC, Ghajar J. Marked improvement in adherence to traumatic brain injury guidelines in United States trauma centers. J Trauma 2007;63(4):841–847.
74. Faul M, Wald MM, Rutland-Brown W, et al. Using a cost–benefit analysis to estimate outcomes of a clinical treatment guideline: Testing the Brain Trauma Foundation guidelines for the treatment of severe traumatic brain injury. J Trauma 2007;63(6):1271–1278.
75. Farin A, Marshall LF. Why have therapeutic trials in head injury been unable to demonstrate benefits? In: Valadka AB, Andrews BT, eds. Neurotrauma Evidence-Based Answers to Common Questions. New York: Thieme, 2005:124–131.
76. Vergouwen MD, Vermeulen M, Roos YB. Effect of nimodipine on outcome in patients with traumatic subarachnoid haemorrhage: A systematic review. Lancet Neurol 2006;5(12):1029–1032.
77. Arango MF, Mejia-Mantilla JH. Magnesium for acute traumatic brain injury. Cochrane Database Syst Rev 2006;(4):CD005400.
78. Kalia LV, Kalia SK, Salter MW. NMDA receptors in clinical neurology: Excitatory times ahead. Lancet Neurol 2008;7(8):742–755.
79. Schouten JW. Neuroprotection in traumatic brain injury: A complex struggle against the biology of nature. Curr Opin Crit Care 2007;13(2):134–142.
80. Temkin NR, Anderson GD, Winn HR, et al. Magnesium sulfate for neuroprotection after traumatic brain injury: A randomised controlled trial. Lancet Neurol 2007;6(1):29–38.
81. Doppenberg EM, Choi SC, Bullock R. Clinical trials in traumatic brain injury: Lessons for the future. J Neurosurg Anesthesiol 2004;16(1):87–94.
82. Shakur H, Andrews P, Asser T, et al. The BRAIN TRIAL: A randomised, placebo controlled trial of a Bradykinin B2 receptor antagonist (Anatibant) in patients with traumatic brain injury. Trials 2009;10:109.
83. Wright DW, Kellermann AL, Hertzberg VS, et al. ProTECT: A randomized clinical trial of progesterone for acute traumatic brain injury. Ann Emerg Med 2007;49(4):391–402.
84. Xiao G, Wei J, Yan W, et al. Improved outcomes from the administration of progesterone for patients with acute severe traumatic brain injury: A randomized controlled trial. Crit Care 2008;12(2):R61.
85. Loane DJ, Faden AI. Neuroprotection for traumatic brain injury: Translational challenges and emerging therapeutic strategies. Trends Pharmacol Sci 2010;31(12):596–604.
86. Junpeng M, Huang S, Qin S. Progesterone for acute traumatic brain injury. Cochrane Database Syst Rev 2011;(1):CD008409.
87. Talving P, Lustenberger T, Inaba K, et al. Erythropoiesis-stimulating agent administration and survival after severe traumatic brain injury: A prospective study. Arch Surg 2012;147(3):251–255.
88. Stoica B, Byrnes K, Faden AI. Multifunctional drug treatment in neurotrauma. Neurotherapeutics 2009;6(1): 14–27.
89. Wible EF, Laskowitz DT. Statins in traumatic brain injury. Neurotherapeutics 2010;7(1):62–73.
90. Cotton BA, Snodgrass KB, Fleming SB, et al. Beta-blocker exposure is associated with improved survival after severe traumatic brain injury. J Trauma 2007;62(1):26–33.
91. Schroeppel TJ, Fischer PE, Zarzaur BL, et al. Beta-adrenergic blockade and traumatic brain injury: Protective? J Trauma 2010;69(4):776–782.

92. Siddall OM. Use of methylphenidate in traumatic brain injury. Ann Pharmacother 2005;39(7–8):1309–1313.
93. Giacino JT, Whyte J, Bagiella E, et al. Placebo-controlled trial of amantadine for severe traumatic brain injury. N Engl J Med 2012;366(9):819–826.
94. Tenovuo O. Pharmacological enhancement of cognitive and behavioral deficits after traumatic brain injury. Curr Opin Neurol 2006;19(6):528–533.
95. Meyer MJ, Megyesi J, Meythaler J, et al. Acute management of acquired brain injury. Part III: An evidence-based review of interventions used to promote arousal from coma. Brain Inj 2010;24(5):722–729.
96. Boucher BA, Wood GC, Swanson JM. Pharmacokinetic changes in critical illness. Crit Care Clin 2006;22(2):255–271.

43

Parkinson's Disease

Jack J. Chen and David M. Swope

KEY CONCEPTS

1. Thoughtful consideration of selection of initial therapy, management of drug dosing, and use of adjunctive therapies throughout the course of idiopathic Parkinson's disease (PD) is necessary to optimize long-term therapeutic outcomes and minimize adverse effects.
2. The optimal time to start drug therapy in PD varies, but in general, treatment should be initiated when the disease begins to interfere with activities of daily living, employment, or quality of life.
3. Surgery is reserved for patients who require additional symptomatic relief or control of motor complications despite receiving medically optimized therapy.
4. Anticholinergic medication is useful for mild tremor-predominant PD but should be used with caution in the elderly and in those with preexisting cognitive difficulties.
5. As monotherapy, amantadine and monoamine oxidase type B (MAO-B) inhibitors provide benefits in early PD, but the symptomatic effect is less than that of dopamine agonists and carbidopa/levodopa (L-dopa).
6. Carbidopa/L-dopa is the most effective medication for symptomatic treatment, and eventually all patients with PD will require it.
7. Most carbidopa/L-dopa–treated patients will develop motor complications (e.g., fluctuations and dyskinesias).
8. MAO-B inhibitors and catechol-*O*-methyl-transferase inhibitors attenuate motor fluctuations in carbidopa/L-dopa–treated patients.
9. Dopamine agonists are effective and, compared to L-dopa, associated with less risk of developing motor complications but more risk to cause psychiatric symptoms, such as hallucinations and impulse control disorders.

The presence of tremor at rest, rigidity, bradykinesia, and postural instability (instability of balance) are considered the hallmark motor features of idiopathic Parkinson's disease (PD). These clinical features of PD were adeptly described in 1817 by James Parkinson.[1]

EPIDEMIOLOGY

Up to 1 million individuals in the United States have PD. The approximate annual incidence of PD (i.e., number of persons diagnosed with PD per year) is age-dependent and ranges from 10 per 100,000 persons in the sixth decade of life (i.e., 50 to 59 years of age) to 120 per 100,000 persons in the ninth decade of life (i.e., 80 to 89 years of age).[2] Likewise, the prevalence of PD also increases with age, affecting 1% of people older than age 65 years and 2.5% of those older than age 80 years. The usual age at time of diagnosis ranges between 55 and 65 years. A higher incidence is reported among males, with a male-to-female ratio of up to 2:1.

ETIOLOGY

The true etiology of PD is unknown, but is likely the result of interactions between aging, genetic constitution, and environmental factors. In PD, a key histopathologic feature is degeneration of dopaminergic neurons in the substantia nigra that project to the striatum (i.e., the nigrostriatal pathway).[3] Additionally, neuronal vulnerability in PD extends beyond the nigrostriatal pathway and includes specific neurons in autonomic ganglia, basal ganglia, spinal cord, and neocortex.[4] In humans and primates, administration of the compound 1-methyl-4-phenyl-1,2,3,6-tetrahydropyridine (MPTP) results in a form of parkinsonism. The MPTP compound is converted by monoamine oxidase (MAO)-B to 1-methyl-4-phenylpyridinium ion (MPP^+), a potent neurotoxin. MPP^+ is toxic to neurons by inhibiting mitochondrial complex 1 of the electron transport chain, which results in the generation of excessive reactive oxygen species and cell death.[5] Several synthetic pesticides have a molecular structure similar to that of MPTP. Although PD is sporadic, extensive epidemiologic research associates environmental factors, such as chronic exposure to pesticides, with an elevated risk for lifetime development of PD.[6–8] Interestingly, epidemiologic studies have consistently associated an inverse correlation between cigarette smoking and caffeine consumption for development of PD.[9,10]

Intrinsically, the substantia nigra pars compacta (SNc) is a region characterized by high levels of oxidative stress because free radicals are generated from dopamine degradation (mediated by MAO; Figure 43-1). Several antioxidative molecules (e.g., glutathione) are present in the SNc to limit damage produced by free-radical reactions, but in PD, such protection might be overwhelmed or impaired. Thus, cellular damage from oxidant stress has long been discussed as an etiopathologic component of PD.[11] The SNc is also rich in iron and copper, essential cofactors in the biosynthesis and metabolism of dopamine. The oxidation–reduction cycle of iron can also generate free radicals and toxic metabolites (Fig. 43-1). In addition, apoptosis (programmed cell death), excitotoxicity, inflammation, mitochondrial dysfunction, nitric oxide toxicity, proteosomal dysfunction, and autophagic cellular mechanisms are also implicated etiopathologic mechanisms in PD.

Genetic susceptibility also plays a role. Although rare, several forms of familial parkinsonism have been linked to specific genetic mutations.[12,13] For example, autosomal dominant forms of parkinsonism are associated with mutations of the α-synuclein: *PARK1/PARK4* and *leucine-rich repeat kinase 2* (*LRRK:PARK8*) gene loci. Autosomal recessive forms are associated with mutations of *parkin:PARK2*

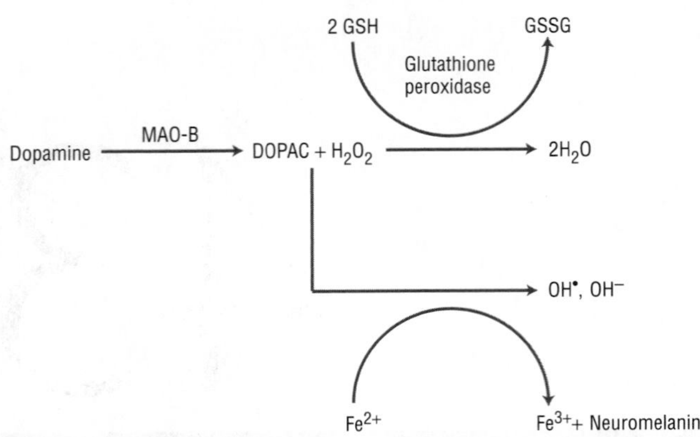

FIGURE 43-1 Dopamine metabolism results in hydrogen peroxide (H_2O_2) formation. If the glutathione system is deficient or excess hydrogen peroxide is present, hydrogen peroxide accepts an electron from ferrous iron (Fe^{2+}), forming ferric iron (Fe^{3+}), and the hydroxyl free radical ($OH^{\cdot}$). The hydroxyl free radical can cause lipid peroxidation, thereby damaging neuronal cell membranes. (DOPAC, 3,4-dihydroxyphenylacetic acid; GSH, glutathione; GSSG, glutathione disulfide; H_2O, water; OH^-, the hydroxide ion; MAO-B, monoamine oxidase B.)

and *PTEN-induced putative kinase 1 (PINK1:PARK6)* gene loci. Although less well defined, ongoing studies indicate that genetic polymorphisms also modify an individual's risk for idiopathic PD.

PATHOPHYSIOLOGY

In the SNc, the two hallmark histopathologic features of PD are depigmentation of dopamine-producing neurons (i.e., loss of SNc neurons) and presence of Lewy bodies (neuronal cytoplasmic filamentous aggregates composed of the presynaptic protein α-synuclein) in the remaining SNc neurons. Lewy bodies appear in degenerating neurons in association with adjacent gliosis and the distribution of pathology is proposed to occur in stages.[4] In the premotor stage of PD, Lewy bodies are initially found in the medulla oblongata, locus coeruleus, raphe nuclei, and olfactory bulb. This may correlate with observations that anxiety, depression, and impaired olfaction are detectable in premotor stages of PD. As PD progresses, Lewy pathology ascends to the midbrain (particularly the SNc) and accounts for development of motor features. In advanced stages, Lewy pathology spreads to the cortex, and this may correlate with cognitive and additional behavior changes. The observation that Lewy pathology can spread into adjacent healthy neurons has given rise to the postulate that prion-like propagation of α-synuclein aggregates may be occurring.

Pathologic findings reveal a correlation between the extent of nigrostriatal dopamine loss and the severity of certain PD motor features (e.g., bradykinesia). The threshold for onset of clinically detectable PD appears to be the loss of 70% to 80% of SNc neurons.[14] Functional neuroimaging studies suggest compensatory responses, such as upregulation of dopamine synthesis and downregulation of synaptic dopamine reuptake, occur as adaptive mechanisms beginning in the premotor stage of PD. These adaptive responses may help to explain why the motor features are not clinically detectable until profound depletion (70% to 80%) of SNc neurons has occurred.

Dopaminergic projections from the SNc to the striatum (putamen and caudate) synapse on two major populations of dopamine receptor-mediated efferent neurons (referred to as the direct and indirect pathways), which, in turn, mediate motor activity via a complex neuronal circuit involving the extrapyramidal system (Fig. 43-2). In PD, the degeneration of the SNc neurons results in reduced activity within these two efferent pathways. The direct pathway involves activation of striatal dopamine$_1$ (D_1) dopamine receptors (which are coupled to adenylate cyclase) and stimulates the inhibitory γ-aminobutyric acid (GABA)/substance P efferents to the globus pallidus interna (GPi) and substantia nigra pars reticulata. The GPi and substantia nigra pars reticulata efferents are inhibitory to the thalamus.[15] In PD, the reduced activation of D_1 receptors results in greater inhibition of the thalamus. The indirect pathway involves activation of striatal dopamine$_2$ (D_2) dopamine receptors (which are coupled to a guanosine triphosphate-binding protein that opens potassium channels to hyperpolarize neurons, thereby reducing the excitability of the neuron).[15] Activation of striatal D_2 receptors inhibits GABA/enkephalin efferents (medium spiny neurons) to the globus pallidus externa. The globus pallidus externa projects GABA neurons to the subthalamic nucleus. Here, excitatory glutamatergic neurons project to the GPi. GPi output is inhibitory on the glutamatergic thalamic projections. In PD, the reduced activation of D_2 receptors translates into greater inhibition of the thalamus. In PD,

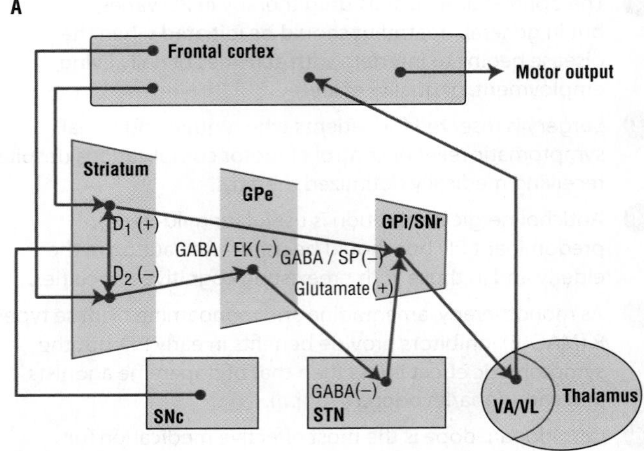

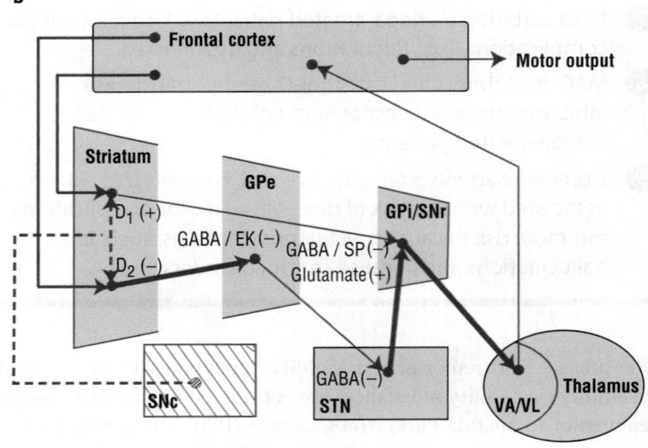

FIGURE 43-2 *A.* The normal balance of the basal ganglia–thalamocortical circuit. *B.* With nigrostriatal degeneration (*dashed line*), there is loss of inhibition of the GPi by the direct pathway and activation of the GPi via the indirect pathway, resulting in decreased activation of the cortex. See the text for details. (GPe, globus pallidus externa; GPi, globus pallidus interna; SNc, substantia nigra pars compacta; SNr, substantia nigra pars reticulata; STN, subthalamic nucleus; VA, ventroanterior nuclei of the thalamus; VL, ventrolateral nuclei of the thalamus.)

CLINICAL PRESENTATION Idiopathic Parkinson's Disease

General Features

- The patient exhibits bradykinesia and at least one of the following: resting tremor, rigidity, or postural instability. Asymmetry of motor features is supportive

Motor Symptoms

- The patient experiences decreased manual dexterity, difficulty arising from a seated position, diminished arm swing during ambulation, dysarthria (slurred speech), dysphagia (difficulty with swallowing), festinating gait (tendency to pass from a walking to a running pace), flexed posture (axial, upper/lower extremities), "freezing" at initiation of movement, hypomimia (reduced facial animation), hypophonia (reduced voice volume), and micrographia (diminution of handwritten letters/symbols; Fig. 43-3)

Autonomic and Sensory Symptoms

- The patient experiences bladder and anal sphincter disturbances, constipation, diaphoresis, fatigue, olfactory disturbance, orthostatic blood pressure changes, pain, paresthesia, paroxysmal vascular flushing, seborrhea, sexual dysfunction, and sialorrhea (drooling)

Mental Status Changes

- The patient experiences anxiety, apathy, bradyphrenia (slowness of thought processes), confusional state, dementia, depression, hallucinosis/psychosis (typically drug induced), and sleep disorders (excessive daytime sleepiness, insomnia, obstructive sleep apnea, and rapid eye movement sleep behavior disorder)

Sleep Disturbances

- The patient experiences excessive daytime sleepiness, insomnia, obstructive sleep apnea, and rapid eye movement sleep behavior disorder

Laboratory Tests

- No laboratory tests are available to diagnose PD

Other Diagnostic Tests

- Genetic testing is not routinely helpful
- Neuroimaging may be useful for excluding other diagnoses
- Medication history should be obtained to rule out drug-induced parkinsonism

restoring activity at the D_2 receptor appears to be of more importance than the D_1 receptor for mediating clinical improvements. Overall, loss of the presynaptic nigrostriatal dopamine neurons in PD results in inhibition of thalamic activity and reduced activation of the motor cortex. Dopaminergic therapies help to restore motor activity.

In addition to dopamine, the synaptic organization of the basal ganglia also involves a variety of other neurotransmitters and neuromodulators, including acetylcholine, adenosine, enkephalins, GABA, glutamate, serotonin, and substance P. The potential role for drug modulation of these other neurotransmitters and receptor types is an active area of research and novel drug discovery for PD.[16]

Atypical parkinsonian disorders such as multiple system atrophy and progressive supranuclear palsy are characterized by damage to postsynaptic striatal neurons and dopamine receptors. Therefore, dopaminergic therapies provide less robust efficacy in atypical parkinsonism.

CLINICAL PRESENTATION

Although PD is unmistakable in its advanced form, recognizing PD during the early stages can be challenging. The clinical diagnosis of PD is based on the presence of bradykinesia and at least one of three other features: muscular rigidity, resting tremor, and postural instability (Table 43-1).[17] Asymmetry of motor features is a supportive finding. It is important to note that tremor is not always present at the time of diagnosis, and postural instability typically occurs in later stages of PD. Overall, a diagnosis of PD can be made with a high level of confidence in a patient who has bradykinesia (along with rest tremor and/or rigidity), prominent asymmetry, and a good response to dopaminergic therapy. For the diagnosis of PD, other conditions must be reasonably excluded (Table 43-1). Medication-induced parkinsonism can mimic PD, so it is important to establish if such medications have been used (especially drugs that block D_2 receptors, such as antipsychotics, metoclopramide, or phenothiazine antiemetics).[18] Neurologic conditions that can be mistaken for PD include atypical parkinsonisms (e.g., corticobasal ganglionic degeneration, forms of multiple system atrophy, progressive supranuclear palsy) and essential tremor. Because the management and prognosis of PD differs from these other conditions, an accurate diagnosis is important. When the diagnosis is in doubt, referral to a movement disorders specialist is recommended.

PD develops insidiously and progressively worsens. Over many years, symptoms can worsen to the point of severe disability, necessitating placement in a skilled nursing facility (especially with the development of dementia or frequent falling). However, the majority of patients remain community dwelling.

Tremor of an upper extremity occurring at rest (and occasionally an action or postural tremor) is often the sole presenting complaint; however, only two thirds of patients with PD have tremor on diagnosis, and some never develop this sign. Tremor in PD is present most commonly in the hands, sometimes with a characteristic pill-rolling motion. Less commonly, tremor may involve the jaw or legs. Like other motor features of PD, resting tremor often begins unilaterally and becomes bilateral with disease progression. Stressful or emotional (either negative or positive) situations often increase the tremor amplitude and severity. Usually, volitional movement abolishes resting tremor, and tremor is absent during sleep. Although resting tremor is visibly noticeable in PD and may cause social embarrassment for the patient, it often is the least physically disabling of the motor features.

Rigidity is the increased muscular resistance to passive range of motion and commonly affects the upper and lower extremities. If tremor is present in the affected extremity, the rigidity is associated with a cogwheel or ratchet-like quality upon examination. Facial

TABLE 43-1 Diagnostic Criteria for Parkinson's Disease and Differential Diagnosis

Parkinson's disease

Step 1: Presence of bradykinesia and at least one of the following: resting tremor, rigidity, or postural instability

Step 2: Exclude other types of parkinsonism or tremor disorders (see Differential diagnosis)

Step 3: Presence of at least three supportive positive criteria:

- Asymmetry of motor signs/symptoms
- Unilateral onset
- Progressive disorder
- Resting tremor
- Excellent response to carbidopa/L-dopa
- L-dopa response for five years or longer
- Presence of L-dopa dyskinesias

Differential diagnosis

Essential tremor

Pharmacotoxicity (drug induced)
- Antiemetics (e.g., metoclopramide, prochlorperazine)
- Antipsychotics (e.g., phenothiazines, haloperidol, olanzapine, risperidone)
- Other drugs (α-methyldopa, cinnarizine, flunarizine, tetrabenazine)

Environmental toxicity (e.g., manganese, organophosphates)

Infections (e.g., human immunodeficiency virus, subacute sclerosing panencephalitis)

Metabolic disorder (e.g., hypothyroidism, parathyroid abnormalities)

Neoplasms, strokes, traumatic lesions involving the nigrostriatal pathways

Normal-pressure hydrocephalus

Parkinsonism with other neuronal system degenerations
- Corticobasal ganglionic degeneration
- Dementia with Lewy bodies
- Multiple-system atrophies
- Progressive supranuclear palsy
- Familial (hereditary) parkinsonism
  - Autosomal dominant
    - α-Synuclein gene mutation (PARK1 and PARK4)
    - Levodopa responsive dystonia
    - Leucine-rich repeat kinase 2 (LRRK2) mutation
    - Rapid-onset dystonia parkinsonism (DYT12)
    - Spinocerebellar ataxias (SCA2, SCA3)
  - Autosomal recessive
    - Wilson's disease
    - Young-onset parkinsonism (DJ-1, parkin, PINK1)
  - X-linked recessive
    - Fragile X tremor/ataxia syndrome (FXTAS)
    - Lubag (DYT3 or Filipino dystonia parkinsonism)

muscles also are affected, resulting in hypomimia (masking of facial expressions) that may be erroneously interpreted as apathy, depression, or unfriendliness.

Bradykinesia refers to slowness of movement. Movement in PD is often slow throughout an intended action, and difficulty with the initiation of movement also occurs. A progressive slowing and decline in dexterity may impair tasks such as hand clapping, finger tapping, and handwriting (Fig. 43-3). Intermittent immobility (*freezing*) is another common characteristic. Freezing is especially likely to occur in situations such as when walking through a narrow doorway or initiating a turn. Patients also may experience a slow shuffling gait with difficulty halting their steps while in motion (festinating gait).

Postural instability, most common in advanced stages of PD, is one of the most disabling problems of PD because it increases the fall risk and is least amenable to pharmacotherapy. Testing for impaired postural responses by means of the pull test (in which a patient is unable to recover balance after sudden backward displacement at the shoulders) can help to identify the risk for falling. Many patients with impaired postural responses also have tendencies for propulsive gait (festination) and freezing, which also increases the risk of falling.

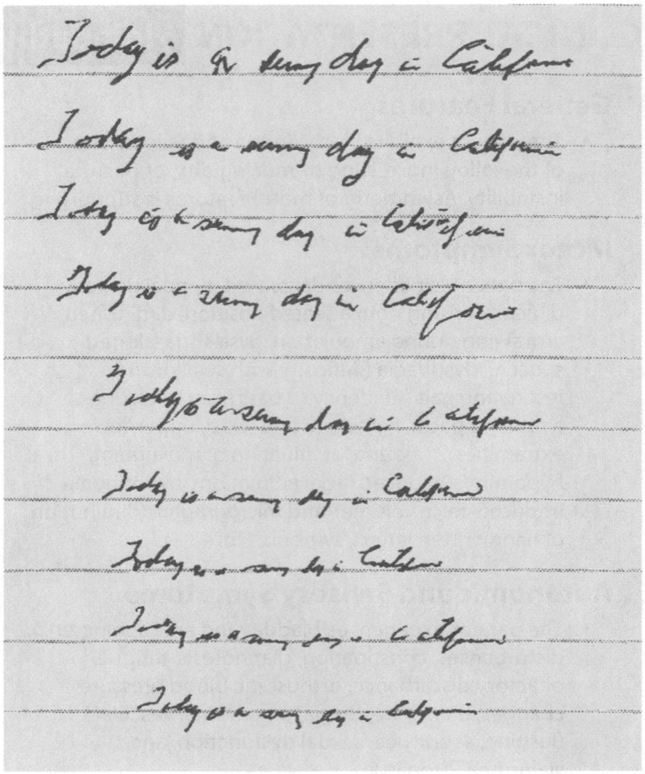

FIGURE 43-3 Example of micrographia in a patient with PD. As the sentence, "Today is a sunny day in California" is repeatedly handwritten, progressive diminution of letter size occurs (micrographia). The height of each lined row is approximately 5/16 inches (8 mm). *(Courtesy of Jack J. Chen, PharmD, and David M. Swope, MD.)*

Although PD is known predominantly as a movement disorder, neuropsychiatric abnormalities also develop. Cognitive deterioration is not inevitable in PD; however, some patients deteriorate in a manner indistinguishable from Alzheimer's disease and other dementing conditions.[19] PD patients are also at increased risk for anxiety and depression.[20] Although the disabilities of PD may provoke depression in some instances, the underlying biochemical changes in the brain associated with PD pathophysiology also predisposes for endogenous depression.

TREATMENT

Desired Outcomes

The goal in the management of PD is to improve motor and nonmotor symptoms so that patients are able to maintain the best possible quality of life.[21] Specific objectives to consider when selecting an intervention include preservation of the ability to perform activities of daily living; improvement of mobility; minimization of adverse effects, treatment complications, putative disease modification; and improvement of nonmotor features such as cognitive impairment, depression, fatigue, and sleep disorders. To accomplish some of these objectives, consultation with

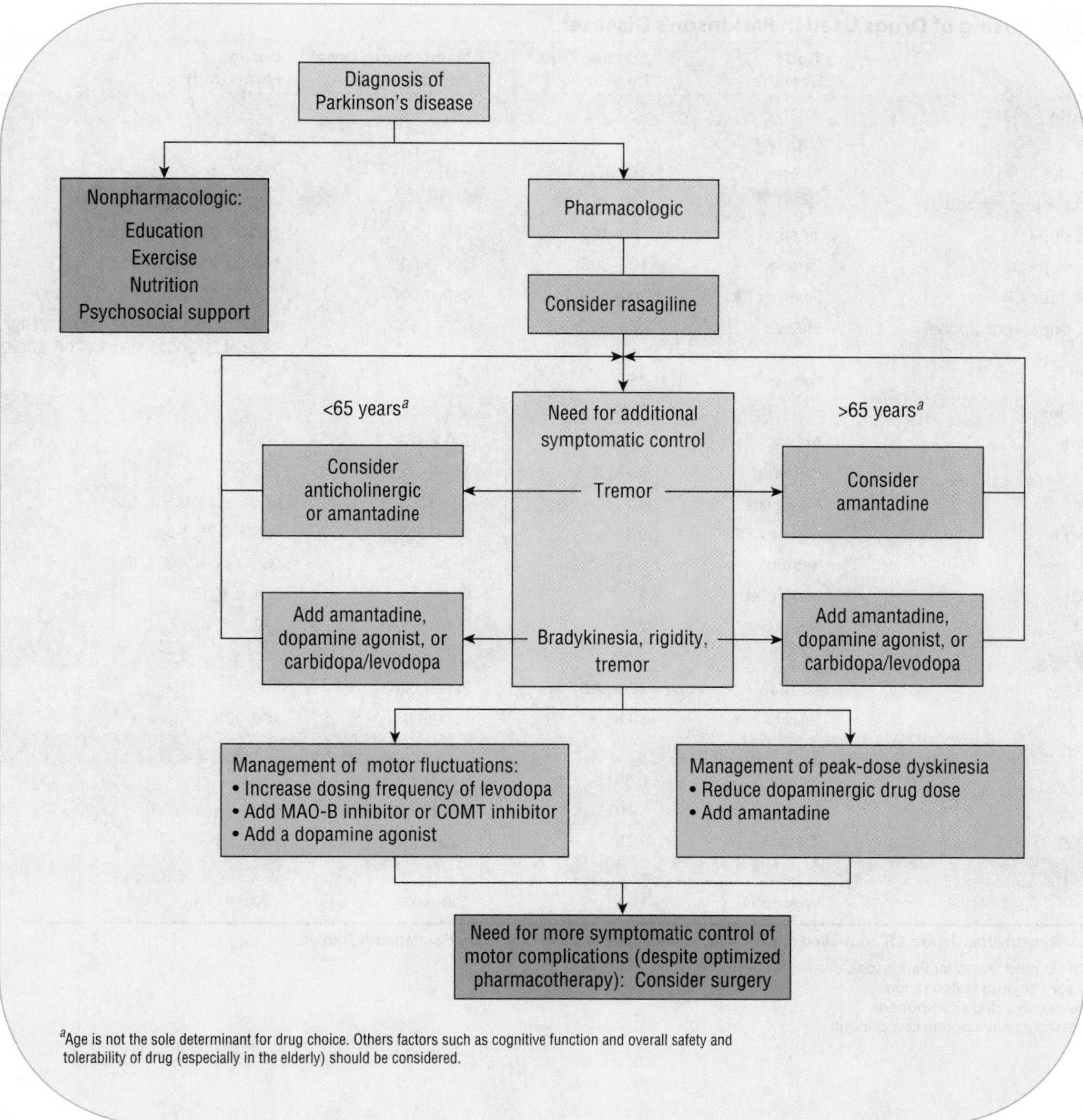

FIGURE 43-4 General approach to the management of early to advanced Parkinson's disease.

a specialist is helpful (e.g., movement disorders, physical therapy, psychiatry, and sleep medicine).

General Approach to Treatment

❶ ❷ Once a correct diagnosis of PD is made, nonpharmacologic and pharmacologic interventions must be considered. Thoughtful consideration of selection of initial therapy, management of drug dosing, and use of adjunctive therapies throughout the course of PD is necessary to optimize long-term therapeutic outcomes and minimize adverse effects. The optimal time to start drug therapy in PD varies, but in general, treatment should be initiated when the disease begins to interfere with activities of daily living, employment, or quality of life. Figure 43-4 illustrates a general treatment approach for early and advanced PD, Table 43-2 summarizes antiparkinsonian medications and mechanisms of action, and Table 43-3 summarizes monitoring parameters for potential adverse effects. Treatment guidelines and monographs are updated frequently to keep up with new information and changes in treatment paradigms.[22–26]

Clinical **Controversy . . .**

The question of when to initiate L-dopa therapy is a matter of debate. Generally, initial therapy with a non–L-dopa agent is often recommended for patients younger than 65 years of age. Proponents for initiating non-L-dopa agents first and then adding L-dopa at a later point, cite evidence suggesting that long-term L-dopa therapy is associated with an increased risk of motor complications that can be disabling and challenging to manage. Additionally, drugs such as rasagiline and dopamine agonists provide sufficient symptom control for mild to moderate PD. The counterargument is that L-dopa is inexpensive, more effective, and the development of motor complications is an acceptable trade-off. Age alone should not be the major deciding factor, and ultimately, individualized considerations of a patient's disability should guide all interventions for PD.

TABLE 43-2 Dosing of Drugs Used in Parkinson's Disease[a]

Generic Name	Trade Name	Starting Dose[b] (mg/day)	Maintenance Dose[b] (mg/day)	Dosage Forms (mg)
Anticholinergic Drugs				
Benztropine	Cogentin	0.5–1	1–6	0.5, 1, 2
Trihexyphenidyl	Artane	1–2	6–15	2, 5, 2/5 mL
Carbidopa/Levodopa Products				
Carbidopa/L-dopa	Sinemet	100–300[c]	300–1,000[c]	10/100, 25/100, 25/250
Carbidopa/L-dopa ODT	Parcopa	100–300[c]	300–1,000[c]	10/100, 25/100, 25/250
Carbidopa/L-dopa CR	Sinemet CR	200–400[c]	400–1,000[c]	25/100, 50/200
Carbidopa/L-dopa/entacapone	Stalevo	200–600[d]	600–1,600[d]	12.5/50/200, 18.75/75/200, 25/100/200, 31.25/125/200, 37.5/150/200, 50/200/200
Carbidopa	Lodosyn	25	25–75	25
Dopamine Agonists				
Apomorphine	Apokyn	1–3	3–12	30/3 mL
Bromocriptine	Parlodel	2.5–5	15–40	2.5, 5
Pramipexole	Mirapex	0.125	1.5–4.5	0.125, 0.25, 0.5, 1, 1.5
Pramipexole ER	Mirapex ER	0.375	1.5–4.5	0.375, 0.75, 1.5, 3, 4.5
Ropinirole	Requip	0.75	9–24	0.25, 0.5; 1, 2, 3, 4, 5
Ropinirole XL	Requip XL	2	8–24	2, 4, 6, 8, 12
Rotigotine	Neupro	2	2–8	1, 2, 3, 4, 6, 8
COMT Inhibitors				
Entacapone	Comtan	200–600	200–1,600	200
Tolcapone	Tasmar	300	300–600	100, 200
MAO-B Inhibitors				
Rasagiline	Azilect	0.5–1	0.5–1	0.5, 1
Selegiline	Eldepryl	5–10	5–10	5
Selegiline ODT	Zelapar	1.25	1.25–2.5	1.25, 2.5
Miscellaneous				
Amantadine	Symmetrel	100	200–300	100, 50/5 mL

COMT, catechol-*O*-methyltransferase; CR, controlled release; MAO, monoamine oxidase; ODT, orally disintegrating tablet.

[a]Marketed in the United States for Parkinson's disease.
[b]Dosages may vary beyond stated range.
[c]Dosages expressed as L-dopa component.
[d]Dosages expressed as entacapone component.

Nonpharmacologic Therapy

Surgical Therapy

3 Currently, surgery should be considered as an adjunct to pharmacotherapy when patients are experiencing frequent motor fluctuations or disabling dyskinesia or tremor despite an optimized medical regimen. There are several patient-selection criteria for surgery, including a diagnosis of levodopa (L-dopa)–responsive PD. Anatomic targets include the thalamus, GPi, and the subthalamic nucleus. Bilateral, chronic, high-frequency electrical stimulation of a target site, also known as deep-brain stimulation (DBS), is the preferred surgical modality.[27]

In DBS surgery, a battery-powered neurostimulator (pacemaker-like device) is implanted subcutaneously below the clavicle and provides constant electrical stimulation, via electrode wires, to the targeted brain structure. Thalamic DBS is very effective for suppressing tremor (specifically arm tremor), but it does not significantly improve the other parkinsonian features (bradykinesia, rigidity, motor fluctuations, or dyskinesias). Although debatable, subthalamic nucleus DBS is favored over GPi DBS because it is considered more effective. Subthalamic nucleus DBS is associated with improvements in tremor, rigidity, bradykinesia, motor fluctuations, and dyskinesia, as well as lowering of antiparkinsonian medications. However, problems with gait and postural instability may not improve significantly with DBS (or pharmacotherapy).

DBS procedures require routine adjustment of the electrical stimulation parameters (e.g., voltage, frequency, and pulse width) to achieve optimal control while minimizing side effects. The electrical stimulation parameters (or "electrical dosage") are adjusted via a programmable handheld device to meet each patient's needs and are performed by physicians as well as other trained individuals, including nurse practitioners and clinical pharmacists.

In recent years, cell-based restorative procedures have appeared promising (implantation of dopamine-producing cells such as human fetal mesencephalon tissue or retinal pigmented epithelial cells into the striatum) but have yielded disappointing clinical results.[28] Gene-based therapies are currently under investigation and remain highly experimental.[29]

Pharmacologic Therapy

Anticholinergic Medications

4 Because dopamine provides negative feedback to acetylcholine neurons in the striatum, the degeneration of nigrostriatal dopamine neurons also results in a relative increase of striatal cholinergic interneuron activity. This increased cholinergic activity (caused by

TABLE 43-3 Monitoring of Potential Adverse Reactions to Drug Therapy for Parkinson's Disease

Generic Name	Adverse Drug Reaction	Monitoring Parameter	Comments
Amantadine	Confusion	Mental status; renal function	Reduce dosage; adjust dose for renal impairment
	Livedo reticularis	Lower extremity examination; ankle edema	Reversible upon drug discontinuation
Benztropine	Anticholinergic effects, confusion, sedation	Dry mouth, mental status, constipation, urinary retention	Reduce dosage; avoid in elderly; history of constipation, memory impairment, urinary retention
Trihexyphenidyl	See benztropine	See benztropine	See benztropine
Carbidopa/L-dopa	Drowsiness	Daytime drowsiness	Reduce dose
	Dyskinesias	Abnormal involuntary movements	Reduce dose; add amantadine
	Nausea	Nausea	Take with food
COMT Inhibitors			
Entacapone	Augmentation of L-dopa side effects; also diarrhea	See carbidopa/L-dopa; also bowel movements	Reduce dose of L-dopa; antidiarrheal agents
Tolcapone	See entacapone; also liver toxicity	See carbidopa/L-dopa; also ALT/AST	See carbidopa/L-dopa; also at start of therapy and for every dose increase, ALT and AST levels at baseline and every 2–4 weeks for the first 6 months of therapy; afterward monitor based on clinical judgment.
Dopamine agonists			
Apomorphine	Drowsiness	Mental status	Reduce dose
	Nausea	Nausea	Premedicate with trimethobenzamide
	Orthostatic hypotension	Blood pressure, dizziness upon standing	Reduce dose
Bromocriptine	Confusion	Mental status	Reduce dose
	Drowsiness	Mental status	Reduce dose
	Hallucinations/delusions	Mental status	Reduce dose
	Nausea	Nausea	Titrate dose upward slowly; take with food
	Orthostatic hypotension	Blood pressure, dizziness upon standing	Reduce dose
	Pulmonary fibrosis	Chest radiograph	Chest radiograph at baseline and once yearly
Pramipexole	Confusion	Mental status	Reduce dose
	Drowsiness	Mental status	Reduce dose
	Hallucinations/delusions	Mental status	Reduce dose
	Impulsivity	Behavior	Reduce dose
	Nausea	Nausea	Titrate dose upward slowly; take with food
	Orthostatic hypotension	Blood pressure, dizziness upon standing	Reduce dose
Ropinirole	See pramipexole	See pramipexole	See pramipexole
Rotigotine	See pramipexole; also skin irritation at site of patch application	See pramipexole; also skin examination	See pramipexole; rotate patch application site
MAO-B inhibitors			
Rasagiline	Nausea	Nausea	Take with food
Selegiline	Confusion	Mental status	Reduce dose
	Insomnia	Mental status	Administer dose earlier in day
	Hallucinations	Mental status	Reduce dose
	Orthostatic hypotension	Blood pressure, dizziness upon standing	Reduce dose

ALT, alanine aminotransferase; AST, aspartate aminotransferase; COMT, catechol-*O*-methyltransferase; MAO, monoamine oxidase.

dopamine depletion) is believed to contribute to the tremor of PD. The anticholinergic drugs (e.g., benztropine and trihexyphenidyl) are considered effective against tremor, but no more so than dopaminergic agents.[22] Sometimes dystonic symptoms associated with PD are also improved by anticholinergic agents. Use of anticholinergic agents is limited due to the development of intolerable side effects, necessitating dosage reduction or drug discontinuation. Common adverse effects include blurred vision, confusion, constipation, dry mouth, memory difficulty, sedation, and urinary retention (Table 43-3). Younger patients are better able to tolerate anticholinergic side effects, whereas patients with preexisting cognitive deficits and advanced age are less tolerant. Anticholinergic drugs can be used alone or in conjunction with L-dopa and other antiparkinson agents.

Amantadine

5 Amantadine provides modest symptomatic benefit for tremor, as well as rigidity and bradykinesia. The precise mechanism of action of amantadine is unknown, but enhancement of dopamine release from presynaptic terminals and inhibition of glutamatergic *N*-methyl-D-aspartate (NMDA) receptors are implicated. Amantadine is typically administered 300 mg/day in divided doses. Amantadine is also useful for suppressing L-dopa–induced dyskinesia.[25] The antidyskinetic properties of amantadine are presumed to be mediated by antiglutamate activity which, in the setting of dyskinesias, appears to dominate over dopaminergic activity. Amantadine is eliminated renally, and a reduced dose should be administered when renal dysfunction is present (100 mg/day with creatinine clearances of 30 to 50 mL/min [0.50 to 0.84 mL/s], 100 mg every other day for creatinine clearances of 15 to 29 mL/min [0.25 to 0.49 mL/s], and 200 mg every 7 days for creatinine clearances of less than 15 mL/min [0.25 mL/s], and patients on hemodialysis).

Common side effects of amantadine include confusion, dizziness, dry mouth, and hallucinations. The elderly are particularly prone to develop confusion. Not uncommonly, amantadine may

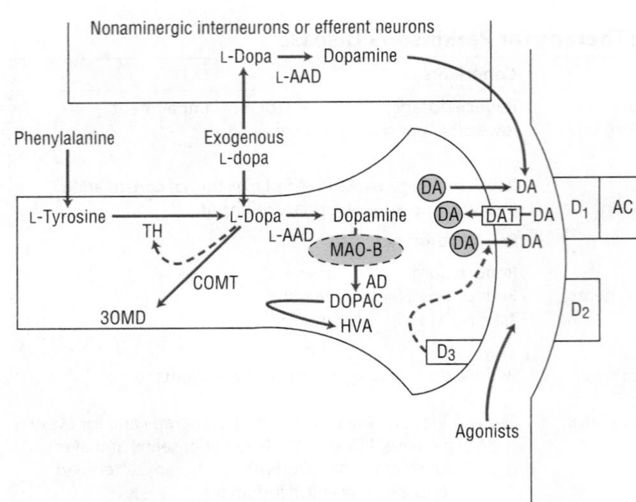

FIGURE 43-5 Dopamine metabolism in presynaptic dopamine neuron. (3OMD, 3-*O*-methyldopa; AC, adenylate cyclase; AD, aldehyde dehydrogenase; COMT, catechol-*O*-methyl transferase; D_1–D_3, dopamine receptors; DA, dopamine; DAT, dopamine transporter; DOPAC, 3,4-dihydroxyphenylacetic acid; HVA, homovanillic acid; L-AAD, L-aromatic amino acid decarboxylase; MAO-B, monoamine oxidase B; TH, tyrosine hydroxylase.)

cause livedo reticularis, a reversible condition characterized by diffuse mottling of the skin affecting the upper or lower extremities and often accompanied by lower-extremity edema (Table 43-3).

Carbidopa/L-Dopa

6 L-Dopa is the immediate precursor of dopamine and, in combination with a peripherally acting L-amino acid decarboxylase inhibitor (carbidopa or benserazide), remains the most effective drug for the symptomatic treatment of PD.[22] L-Dopa crosses the blood–brain barrier, whereas dopamine, carbidopa, and benserazide do not. The combination of L-dopa with carbidopa or benserazide reduces the unwanted peripheral conversion of L-dopa to dopamine. As a result, increased amounts of L-dopa are transported into the brain, and peripheral adverse effects of dopamine, such as nausea, are reduced. In the SNc, L-dopa is converted, via decarboxylation, to dopamine by the enzyme L-amino acid decarboxylase (Fig. 43-5). The converted dopamine is stored in the presynaptic SNc neurons until stimulated to be released into the synaptic cleft whereupon it binds to the D_1 and D_2 postsynaptic receptors. Dopamine activity is terminated primarily by reuptake back into the presynaptic neuron by means of a dopamine transporter. The enzymes MAO and catechol-*O*-methyltransferase (COMT) also inactivate dopamine.

6 Regardless of what the initial therapeutic agent is, ultimately all patients with PD will require L-dopa at some point. An initial maintenance L-dopa regimen of 300 mg/day (in divided doses and in combination with carbidopa or benserazide) often is adequate. With regard to carbidopa, about 75 mg/day is required to sufficiently inhibit the peripheral activity of L-amino acid decarboxylase, but some patients require more. Therefore, the usual initial maintenance carbidopa/L-dopa regimen is 25/100 mg three times daily. As the motor features of PD become progressively more severe, use of higher dosages is required. There is no maximum allowable total daily L-dopa dose; however, the usual maximal dose needed by patients, even those with severe PD, is 800 to 1,000 mg/day. Slow buildup of dose (e.g., increments of 100 mg L-dopa per week) can help to minimize treatment emergent side effects, such as drowsiness, nausea, postural hypotension, vivid dreaming, and vomiting (Table 43-3).

For patients with difficulty swallowing tablets, an orally disintegrating tablet preparation of carbidopa/L-dopa is available. Although this formulation rapidly dissolves on contact with saliva, the carbidopa/L-dopa does not undergo transmucosal absorption and must reach the proximal duodenum for absorption.

Pharmacokinetics There is marked intra- and intersubject variability in the time to peak plasma concentrations after oral L-dopa, and this may in part be attributed to differences in gastric emptying. L-Dopa is absorbed primarily in the proximal duodenum by a saturable large neutral amino acid transport system. Competition for this transporter by dietary or supplemental large neutral amino acids (e.g., leucine, phenylalanine) can interfere with L-dopa bioavailability.

L-Dopa is not bound to plasma proteins. Active transport across the blood–brain barrier occurs by the large neutral amino acid transporter system. Because large amounts of dietary large neutral amino acids may compete for transport across the blood–brain barrier and interfere with the clinical response to L-dopa, separation of L-dopa administration from high protein meals or amino acid dietary supplements have been recommended. However, in patients with early PD, this interaction is generally not significant. In advanced PD, special diets involving protein restriction or redistribution may improve L-dopa responsiveness and are sometimes implemented. A metabolite of L-dopa, 3-*O*-methyldopa, also competes for transport, but it is not clear how this affects L-dopa clinical response.

When peripheral decarboxylation of L-dopa is inhibited by carbidopa or benserazide, 3-*O*-methylation (via COMT) becomes the predominant catabolic pathway. The elimination half-life of L-dopa is about 1 hour, and this is extended to about 1.5 hours with the addition of carbidopa or benserazide. With the addition of a COMT inhibitor such as entacapone to carbidopa/L-dopa, the elimination half-life is extended to about 2 to 2.5 hours.

7 **Motor Complications of L-Dopa** Long-term L-dopa therapy is associated with a variety of motor complications, of which end-of-dose "wearing off" (motor fluctuations) and L-dopa peak-dose dyskinesias are the two most commonly encountered.[30] These motor complications can be disabling and challenging to manage. The approximate risk of developing either motor fluctuations or dyskinesia is 10% per year of L-dopa therapy.[31,32] However, motor complications can occur as early as 5 to 6 months after starting L-dopa therapy, especially if excessive doses are used initially.[33] Table 43-4 lists the motor complications associated with long-term treatment with L-dopa and suggested initial management strategies. Initiating

TABLE 43-4 Common Motor Complications and Possible Initial Treatments

Effect	Possible Treatments
End-of-dose "wearing off" (motor fluctuation)	Increase frequency of carbidopa/L-dopa doses; add either COMT inhibitor or MAO-B inhibitor or dopamine agonist
"Delayed on" or "no on" response	Give carbidopa/L-dopa on empty stomach; use carbidopa/L-dopa ODT; avoid carbidopa/L-dopa CR; use apomorphine subcutaneous
Start hesitation ("freezing")	Increase carbidopa/L-dopa dose; add a dopamine agonist or MAO-B inhibitor; utilize physical therapy along with assistive walking devices or sensory cues (e.g., rhythmic commands, stepping over objects)
Peak-dose dyskinesia	Provide smaller doses of carbidopa/L-dopa; add amantadine

COMT, catechol-*O*-methyltransferase; CR, controlled release; MAO, monoamine oxidase; ODT, orally disintegrating tablet.

therapy with the controlled-release (CR) form of carbidopa/L-dopa does not reduce the development of motor complications compared with standard-release carbidopa/L-dopa.[23]

7 ***End-of-Dose Wearing Off*** The terms "off" and "on" refer to periods of poor movement (i.e., return of tremor, rigidity, or slowness) and good movement, respectively. End-of-dose wearing off prior to a dose of medication is a common type of response fluctuation. This phenomenon is related to the increasing loss of neuronal storage capability for dopamine as well as the short half-life of L-dopa. Initially, exogenous L-dopa is taken up by the remaining SNc neurons, converted to dopamine, and stored in synaptic vesicles. With progressive loss of SNc neurons, storage capacity, and synthesis of endogenously derived dopamine, patients become more dependent on exogenous L-dopa. Hence the peripheral pharmacokinetic properties of L-dopa increasingly become the determinant of central dopamine synthesis. With advancing PD, the duration of action of a single carbidopa/L-dopa dose progressively shortens, and in some cases may produce benefits for as little as 1 hour. As a result, carbidopa/L-dopa needs to be given more frequently so as to minimize daytime off episodes and to maximize on time. In addition to administering L-dopa doses more frequently, other options are available (see Table 43-4). In particular, the addition of the COMT inhibitor entacapone or the MAO-B inhibitor rasagiline extends the action of L-dopa, and either should be considered.[23] A CR L-dopa product is available, but is not considered very effective for management of motor fluctuations.[23] Currently, a reformulated extended-release carbidopa/L-dopa capsule (i.e., IPX066) is investigational and expected to be available in the near future.

A dopamine agonist (e.g., pramipexole, ropinirole, and rotigotine) also can be added to a carbidopa/L-dopa regimen in an attempt to minimize the occurrence of wearing off. For acute off episodes, a subcutaneously administered short-acting dopamine agonist, apomorphine, is available and possesses a rapid onset of effect (within 20 minutes). It is administered as needed.[34] Alternatively, chronic subcutaneous apomorphine infusion (not available in the United States) provides stable and continuous systemic and central drug concentrations and improves motor fluctuations and dyskinesias. Long-term therapy is limited by injection site skin reactions.[35] In addition, a carbidopa/L-dopa intestinal (jejunal) gel (not yet available in the United States) has been demonstrated to be an effective and safe therapy for patients with persistent, on/off fluctuations.[36] Although not commonly performed, sipping small amounts of carbidopa/L-dopa solution very frequently throughout the day is also a method for managing on/off fluctuations. A solution that is stable for 72 hours at room temperature can be prepared by adding 10 crushed tablets of carbidopa/L-dopa 10/100 (or 25/100) mg and 2 g crystalline ascorbic acid to 1 L of water.[37]

Often, off episodes occur during the night, and patients will awaken in an off state (as a consequence of an overnight decline of drug levels). Bedtime administration of a dopamine agonist or a drug formulation that provides sustained drug levels overnight (e.g., carbidopa/L-dopa CR, ropinirole XL, pramipexole ER, rotigotine transdermal patch) can help reduce nocturnal off episodes and improve functioning upon awakening.

Nonadherence to medications also contributes to the frequency of off episodes. Therefore, engaging and supporting patients and caregivers in overcoming barriers to medication adherence is important.

"Delayed-On" and "No-On" Response "Delayed-on" or "no-on" (a delayed or absent onset of drug effect, respectively) responses to individual doses of carbidopa/L-dopa can be a result of delayed gastric emptying or decreased absorption in the duodenum. Chewing a tablet or crushing it and then drinking a full glass of water, or using the orally disintegrating tablet formulation on an empty stomach, can help mitigate effects of delayed gastric emptying. Additionally, subcutaneously administered apomorphine may be used as rescue therapy from delayed-on or no-on periods. A drug-free period ("drug holiday") has been investigated in an attempt to modify postsynaptic dopamine receptors and thus decrease unpredictable off states. Although not commonly performed because of discomfort (to the patient) and medical risks, when drug holidays are performed, it should be under close medical supervision.

Freezing "Freezing," or a sudden, episodic inhibition of lower-extremity motor function, may occur and will interfere with ambulation and increase the risk of falls. Patients may report that their "feet suddenly feel stuck to the floor" during ambulation or that they have difficulty initiating steps (start hesitation) or turns (turn hesitation). Freezing often is exacerbated by anxiety or when perceived obstacles (e.g., doorways, turnstiles) are encountered. Although changes to the antiparkinson drug regimen may be attempted, improvements are unlikely. Physical therapy along with assistive walking devices and sensory cues are helpful.

Dyskinesias Another complication of L-dopa therapy is "on" period dyskinesias (involuntary choreiform movements involving usually the neck, trunk, and lower/upper extremities). If patients report "shakiness," it is important to clarify if they are referring to tremor or dyskinesias. Dyskinesias usually are associated with peak striatal dopamine levels (peak-dose dyskinesia) and, simplistically, can be thought of as too much movement secondary to extension of the pharmacologic effect resulting in excessive striatal dopamine receptor stimulation. Less commonly, dyskinesias also can develop during the rise and fall of L-dopa effects (the dyskinesia–improvement–dyskinesia or diphasic pattern of response). In the case of peak-dose dyskinesias, use of lower individual doses of L-dopa is beneficial. With the lowering of the L-dopa dose, dyskinesias improve but at the cost of returning parkinsonian features, thereby necessitating an increase in dosage frequency or addition of another agent to counteract the effects of using a lower L-dopa dose. Glutamate overactivity may also be involved, as suggested by the antidyskinesia effect of amantadine (NMDA receptor antagonist) and positive results of investigational studies of antiglutamate ligands in animal models.[38] For severe dyskinesias (despite pharmacologically optimized therapy), surgery should be considered.

"Off-Period" Dystonia In PD, dystonias (sustained muscle contractions) can occur and more commonly affect a distal lower extremity (e.g., clenching of toes or involuntary turning of a foot). Dystonias often occur in the early morning hours (as a result of waning drug levels) and improve with the first L-dopa dose of the day. Remedies for early morning dystonia include bedtime administration of a long acting dopamine agonist, sustained-release carbidopa/L-dopa, baclofen, or focal injections of botulinum toxin type A or B (for persistent focal dystonia).

Monoamine Oxidase B Inhibitors

5 Two selective MAO-B inhibitors, rasagiline and selegiline, are available in the United States for management of PD. The selective inhibition of MAO-B in the brain interferes with the degradation of dopamine and results in prolonged dopaminergic activity. Both drugs contain a propargylamine moiety, which is essential for conferring irreversible inhibition of MAO-B. At therapeutic doses, these agents preferentially and irreversibly inhibit MAO-B over MAO-A.

A common concern with use of these agents is the potential for interactions with drugs that possess serotonergic activity. Concomitant use of MAO-B inhibitors with meperidine and other selected opioid analgesics is contraindicated because of a small risk of serotonin syndrome. However, concomitant use of other agents that enhance serotonin levels (e.g., antidepressants) is not contraindicated, and these drugs can be used concomitantly when clinically warranted.[39]

5 8 Selegiline, also known as L-deprenyl, is marketed for extending L-dopa effects and is typically administered 5 mg twice daily. Selegiline is also available as an orally disintegrating tablet formulation administered 1.25 to 2.5 mg once daily. A transdermal formulation of selegiline is also available but is not indicated for PD. As monotherapy in early PD, conventional selegiline provides modest improvements in motor function.[22] In more advanced PD, the adjunctive use of conventional selegiline can provide up to 1 hour of extended on time for patients with wearing off, although the data are inconsistent.[23] This inconsistent effect of conventional selegiline may be explained, in part, by poor and erratic bioavailability of the parent drug.

As an amphetamine pharmacophore, selegiline undergoes first-pass hepatic metabolism (predominantly via cytochrome P450 [CYP450] 2B6 and 2C19) to end products of L-methamphetamine and L-amphetamine. Adverse effects of selegiline are minimal but can include insomnia (especially if administered at bedtime), hallucinations, and jitteriness (Table 43-3). Selegiline also increases the peak effects of L-dopa and can worsen preexisting dyskinesias or psychiatric symptoms such as delusions. With the selegiline orally disintegrating tablet formulation, first-pass hepatic metabolism is bypassed as a consequence of transmucosal absorption of the drug. Hence, bioavailability characteristics of the parent drug are improved and formation of amphetamine metabolites is reduced. Thus, the selegiline orally disintegrating tablet formulation may provide an improved response relative to conventional selegiline.

5 8 Rasagiline is a second-generation, irreversible, selective MAO-B inhibitor administered at 0.5 or 1 mg once daily.[40] Rasagiline is effective as monotherapy in early PD and also as add-on therapy for managing motor fluctuations in advanced PD. In a large, placebo-controlled, 18-month, delayed-start clinical trial, patients initiated on rasagiline monotherapy early in PD had less functional decline than did patients whose treatment was delayed for 9 months.[41] This suggests that earlier initiation with rasagiline (even before the onset of functional impairment) may be associated with better long-term outcomes. For the management of patients with motor fluctuations, the efficacy of rasagiline appears similar to that of entacapone, offering approximately 1 hour of extra on time during the day.[42] Consequently, when an adjunctive agent is required for managing motor fluctuations, rasagiline is considered a first-line agent (as is entacapone).[23] Overall, rasagiline is well tolerated with minimal GI or neuropsychiatric side effects. Rasagiline is metabolized by hepatic CYP1A2 to aminoindan, which is inactive and devoid of amphetamine-like properties.[40]

MAO-B inhibitors with a propargylamine molecular scaffolding have been investigated for neuroprotective properties (clinically referred to as disease modification). These agents inhibit the oxidative deamination of dopamine, which generates hydrogen peroxide and, ultimately, oxyradicals capable of damaging nigrostriatal neurons (see Fig. 43-1). Because MAO-B inhibition diverts dopamine catabolism to an alternate route that does not generate peroxide, MAO-B inhibitor therapy may spare neurons from oxidative stress. Additionally, MAO-B inhibitors have demonstrated antiapoptotic properties in laboratory experiments, further suggesting the possibility of disease modification. Clinical studies to demonstrate disease modification with selegiline have yielded inconclusive results, perhaps contributed in part by selegiline amphetamine metabolites as well as inadequate study methodology. Results with rasagiline 1 mg/day from a clinical study utilizing methodology (i.e., delayed start) intended to demonstrate disease modification were positive, but the issue of disease-modifying properties of rasagiline is surrounded by controversy.[41]

Clinical **Controversy . . .**

Great interest and debate surround the putative disease-modifying effects of the MAO-B inhibitors. A large clinical study demonstrated that earlier initiation of rasagiline is associated with better outcomes as compared to delaying therapy, and this was attributed to a disease-modifying effect (as opposed to a symptomatic effect). Whether this is a class effect of MAO-B inhibitors is not known. However, selegiline is metabolized to amphetamine derivatives, which have been demonstrated to neutralize neuroprotective effects in various preclinical studies. In a clinical study of the dopamine agonist pramipexole in patients with early PD, no benefit of earlier initiation over delayed initiation was observed.

COMT Inhibitors

8 Two COMT inhibitors, entacapone and tolcapone, have been developed to extend the effects of L-dopa and are indicated for managing wearing off.[23] Both reduce the peripheral conversion of L-dopa to dopamine, thus enhancing central L-dopa bioavailability. Consequently, in the absence of L-dopa, they have no effect on PD symptoms. For patients with wearing off, these agents can decrease off-time significantly by increasing the L-dopa area under the curve by approximately 35%.[43] COMT inhibition is considered more effective than CR carbidopa/L-dopa in providing consistent extension of L-dopa effect.[23] A triple-combination product of carbidopa/L-dopa/entacapone offers convenience for some patients (i.e., fewer tablets to administer).

Tolcapone inhibits both peripheral and central COMT. Its use is limited by reports of fatal hepatotoxicity, such that strict monitoring of hepatic function, especially during the first 6 months of therapy, is required (Table 43-3).[39] Because of the hepatotoxicity risk, tolcapone is reserved for patients with fluctuations that are not responding to other therapies.

Entacapone has a shorter half-life than tolcapone, and 200 mg needs to be given with each dose of carbidopa/L-dopa up to a maximum of eight times per day. In clinical trials, both tolcapone and entacapone increased total daily on time by about 1 to 2 hours.[44,45] Dopaminergic adverse effects may occur and generally are manageable by reduction of the carbidopa/L-dopa dosage. With both agents, brownish-orange urinary discoloration may occur. Also, delayed onset of diarrhea (weeks to months later) can occur in up to 5% of patients. Unlike tolcapone, entacapone is not associated with hepatotoxicity, and if an adjunctive agent is needed for managing motor fluctuations, entacapone is considered one of the first choices.[23]

Dopamine Agonists

Dopamine agonists fall into two pharmacologic subtypes: ergot-derived agonists (bromocriptine) and the nonergot agonists (pramipexole, ropinirole, and rotigotine). The nonergot dopamine agonists are safer than the ergot-derived agonists[46] and are useful as monotherapy in mild-moderate PD, and also as adjuncts to L-dopa therapy in patients with motor fluctuations.[22,23] The dopamine agonists reduce the frequency of off periods and may allow reductions in L-dopa dosage.

9 Investigations comparing initial monotherapy with either L-dopa or a dopamine agonist in patients with PD have revealed a significantly reduced risk of developing motor complications associated with dopamine agonists.[47,48] Younger patients are more likely to develop motor complications; consequently, dopamine agonists are preferred over L-dopa. Older patients are more likely to experience

TABLE 43-5 Stepwise Approach to Management of Drug-Induced Hallucinosis and Psychosis in Parkinson's Disease

1. General measures such as evaluating for electrolyte disturbance (especially hypercalcemia or hyponatremia), hypoxemia, or infection (especially encephalitis, sepsis, or urinary tract infection)
2. Simplify the antiparkinsonian regimen as much as possible by discontinuing or reducing the dosage of medications with the highest risk-to-benefit ratio first[a]
   (a) Discontinue anticholinergics, including other nonparkinsonian medications with anticholinergic activity such as antihistamines or tricyclic antidepressants
   (b) Taper and discontinue amantadine
   (c) Discontinue monoamine oxidase-B inhibitor
   (d) Taper and discontinue dopamine agonist
   (e) Consider reduction of L-dopa (especially evening doses) and discontinuation of catechol-*O*-methyltransferase inhibitors
3. Consider atypical antipsychotic medication if disruptive hallucinosis or psychosis persists
   (a) Quetiapine 12.5–25 mg at bedtime; gradually increase by 25 mg each week if necessary, until hallucinosis or psychosis improved or
   (b) Clozapine 12.5–50 mg at bedtime; gradually increase by 25 mg each week if necessary until hallucinosis or psychosis improved (requires frequent monitoring for leukopenia)

[a]If dosage reduction or medication discontinuation is either infeasible or undesirable, go to step 3.

intolerable side effects (e.g., confusion, hallucinations, and orthostatic hypotension) from the dopamine agonists; consequently, carbidopa/L-dopa is preferred, particularly if cognitive problems or dementia is present.

Common adverse effects of dopamine agonists include nausea, confusion, hallucinations, light-headedness, lower-extremity edema, postural hypotension, sedation, and vivid dreaming (Table 43-3). Less common but serious adverse effects include impulsive behaviors (e.g., pathologic gambling or shopping, hypersexuality), psychosis, and sleep attacks (sudden, unexpected episodes of sleep). Hallucinations and delusion can be managed using a stepwise approach (Table 43-5) that often involves the use of an atypical antipsychotic medication, such as clozapine or quetiapine.[20] The addition of a dopamine agonist to L-dopa therapy also can increase the frequency and severity of L-dopa–induced dyskinesias, especially in patients with preexisting dyskinesias.

Initiation of a dopaminergic agonist is best performed by slow titration to minimize side effects. Pramipexole is initiated at a dose of 0.125 mg three times a day and increased every 5 to 7 days, as tolerated, to a maximum of 1.5 mg three times a day. An extended-release pramipexole formulation is also available. Immediate-release ropinirole is initiated at 0.25 mg three times a day and increased by 0.25 mg three times a day on a weekly basis to a maximum of 24 mg/day. An extended-release ropinirole formulation also is available.

Pramipexole is renally excreted with an 8- to 12-hour half-life. The initial dosage must be adjusted in renal insufficiency (0.125 mg twice daily for creatinine clearances of 35 to 59 mL/min [0.58 to 0.99 mL/s], 0.125 mg once daily for creatinine clearances of 15 to 34 mL/min [0.25 to 0.57 mL/s]). Ropinirole has a 6-hour half-life and is metabolized by CYP1A2. Potent inhibitors (e.g., fluoroquinolone antibiotics) and inducers (e.g., cigarette smoking) of this enzyme likely will lead to alterations in ropinirole clearance. Rotigotine transdermal patch is initiated at 2 mg once daily and increased weekly by 2 mg increments to achieve desired therapeutic effect. The rotigotine transdermal patch provides continuous release of drug over a 24-hour period.[49] Patch application sites should be rotated to minimize skin irritation and rash. Rotigotine disposition is not affected by hepatic or renal impairment and CYP-mediated drug interactions are not significant.

Apomorphine is an injectable nonergot dopamine agonist. It is an aporphine alkaloid originally derived from morphine but lacks narcotic properties.[34] Because of extensive hepatic first-pass metabolism, apomorphine is not suitable for oral administration and is administered subcutaneously. Apomorphine should not be injected IV. For patients with advanced PD who are experiencing intermittent off episodes despite optimized therapy, administration of subcutaneous apomorphine effectively triggers an "on" response within 20 minutes.[34] The effective dose ranges from 2 to 6 mg per injection, with most patients requiring approximately 0.06 mg/kg. Sites of injection (abdomen, upper arm, and upper thigh) should be rotated to avoid development of subcutaneous nodules. The metabolic pathway of apomorphine remains unknown. Apomorphine elimination half-life is approximately 40 minutes, and the duration of benefit can be up to 100 minutes. Nausea and vomiting are common side effects, and prior to the initiation of apomorphine, patients should be premedicated with the antiemetic trimethobenzamide.

PERSONALIZED PHARMACOTHERAPY

Currently, there are no pharmacogenomic parameters utilized to guide PD pharmacotherapy. Personalized therapy should take into account patient-specific factors including age, level of functional impairment, disability, desired therapeutic outcomes, comorbidities, employment status, drug tolerability, presence of motor complications, fall risk, cognitive impairment, need for skilled assistance, health-related economics, and patient preferences. The definition of functional impairment is highly patient specific. The lowest dose of anti-PD medication that provides satisfactory symptomatic results should be used and, for patients already on carbidopa/L-dopa, optimization of the L-dopa regimen should be attempted before adding adjunctive agents. As side effects and the severity, level of disability, and related comorbidities increase, therapy adjustments are expected and desired therapeutic endpoints should be reassessed.

For mild functional impairment, initial monotherapy may be initiated with an MAO-B inhibitor, such as rasagiline, with the addition of other therapeutic agents as PD motor symptoms progressively worsen. Therapy with rasagiline in early stage PD provides sufficient symptomatic benefit and is well tolerated. Dopamine agonist monotherapy is more potent than rasagiline or amantadine and provides greater symptomatic benefit for patients with greater than mild to moderate impairment. However, dopamine agonists are less well tolerated in older patients. For patients who are older, cognitively impaired, intolerant of dopamine agonists, or experiencing moderate or severe functional impairment, L-dopa (e.g., carbidopa/levodopa) is preferred. Ultimately, all patients will require the use of L-dopa (either as monotherapy or in combination with other agents). With the development of motor fluctuations, patients should administer L-dopa more frequently. Alternatively, addition of a COMT inhibitor, MAO-B inhibitor, or dopamine agonist to the L-dopa regimen should be considered. For management of L-dopa induced peak-dose dyskinesias, a reduction in L-dopa dose should be attempted. Alternatively, addition of amantadine should be considered. Surgery is considered only in patients who need more symptomatic control or who are experiencing severe motor complications despite pharmacologically optimized therapy.

The treatment plan evolves as the disease progresses and must include consideration of short-term symptomatic relief as well as long-term effects. Patient education should be communicated with realistic optimism. For example, it should be explained that although there is no cure for PD, modern medicine has many medications that can provide relief of symptoms. Nonpharmacologic interventions

TABLE 43-6 Monitoring Parkinson's Disease Therapy

1. Monitor medication administration times. Educate the patient that immediate-release carbidopa/L-dopa is absorbed best on an empty stomach but is commonly taken with food to minimize nausea. Avoid administration of conventional selegiline in the late afternoon or evening to minimize insomnia
2. Monitor to ensure that the patient and/or caregivers understand the prescribed medication regimen. For example, they should understand that catechol-*O*-methyltransferase inhibitors work by enhancing the effect of L-dopa and that the patient should not discontinue medication without notifying the clinician
3. Monitor and inquire specifically about dose-by-dose effects of medication, including response to doses of medication and the presence of dyskinesias, wearing-off effects, dizziness, nausea, or visual hallucinations. Offer suggestions to help alleviate these, or encourage the patient to discuss them with the clinician
4. Monitor and inquire about concerns that caregivers may have about the patient, such as presence of abnormal behaviors, dyskinesias, falls, hallucinations, memory problems, mood changes, and sleep disorders
5. Monitor for nonadherence and, if present, inquire for possible reasons (e.g., dosing convenience, financial issues, and adverse effects) and offer suggestions
6. Monitor for presence of drugs that can exacerbate idiopathic Parkinson's disease motor features (e.g., D_2 receptor blockers), and evaluate whether the presence of an anticholinergic agent is causing cognitive impairment

such as exercise should be encouraged, and problematic nonmotor features of PD should always be addressed.

EVALUATION OF THERAPEUTIC OUTCOMES

1 Pharmaceutical care related to PD improves patient outcomes.[50] Table 43-6 lists the monitoring parameters for PD therapy. Patient and caregiver satisfaction is an important component of evaluating therapeutic outcomes. Toward this end, establishing appropriate treatment expectations is important, patients and caregivers should be educated that PD is a neurodegenerative disease that progresses with time, and that some features will respond less well to pharmacotherapy (e.g., freezing, gait, and postural instability). Patients and caregivers can participate in treatment by recording medication administration times as well as the duration of on and off times that can be reviewed at each visit. Periodic review of all medications that the patient is taking should be performed to identify use of medications (e.g., D_2-receptor blockers) that can exacerbate PD motor features. If the patient reports memory problems, the medication profile should be screened for medications with anticholinergic properties and, if present, eliminated when possible. Assessment of the patient's general level of functioning, including activities of daily living and mobility, is important to determine when medication adjustments or physical therapy interventions are needed. Screening for anxiety or depressive disorders will help to determine if antidepressant or antianxiety therapy is needed. If falling is a problem, it is important to investigate whether falls are secondary to insufficient motor control or drug side effects, such as dizziness and orthostatic hypotension. The former may necessitate an increase in dose of antiparkinson agents, and the latter a reduction in drug dosage. Physical therapy is also helpful for strengthening ambulation and balance skills to minimize falls. The patient should be questioned about any difficulties with their antiparkinson medications, including presence of adverse effects. Recommendations always should be made in view of the patient's perception of the severity of symptoms and effect on quality of life.

ABBREVIATIONS

COMT	catechol-*O*-methyltransferase
CR	controlled release
D_1	dopamine receptor subtype 1
D_2	dopamine receptor subtype 2
DBS	deep-brain stimulation
GABA	γ-aminobutyric acid
GPi	globus pallidus interna
PD	idiopathic Parkinson's disease
L-dopa	levodopa
MAO	monoamine oxidase
MPP^+	1-methyl-4-phenylpyridinium
MPTP	1-methyl-4-phenyl-1,2,3,6-tetrahydropyridine
NMDA	*N*-methyl-D-aspartate
SNc	substantia nigra pars compacta

REFERENCES

1. Parkinson J. An essay on the shaking palsy. London: Sherwood, Neely, and Jones, 1817:1–66.
2. Kasten M, Chade A, Tanner CM. Epidemiology of Parkinson's disease. Handb Clin Neurol 2007;83:129–151.
3. Sulzer D. Multiple hit hypotheses for dopamine neuron loss in Parkinson's disease. Trends Neurosci 2007;30:244–250.
4. Halliday G, McCann H, Shepherd C. Evaluation of the Braak hypothesis: How far can it explain the pathogenesis of Parkinson's disease? Expert Rev Neurother 2012;12:673–686.
5. Gerlach M, Riederer P, Przuntek H, et al. MPTP mechanisms of neurotoxicity and their implications for Parkinson's disease. Eur J Pharmacol 1991;208:273–286.
6. Migliore L, Coppedè F. Genetics, environmental factors and the emerging role of epigenetics in neurodegenerative diseases. Mutat Res 2009;667:82–97.
7. Dick FD, De Palma G, Ahmadi A, et al.; Geoparkinson study group. Environmental risk factors for Parkinson's disease and parkinsonism: The Geoparkinson study. Occup Environ Med 2007;64:666–672.
8. Hancock DB, Martin ER, Mayhew GM, et al. Pesticide exposure and risk of Parkinson's disease: A family-based case–control study. BMC Neurol 2008;8:6.
9. Costa J, Lunet N, Santos C, et al. Caffeine exposure and the risk of Parkinson's disease: A systematic review and meta-analysis of observational studies. J Alzheimers Dis 2010;20(Suppl 1):S221–S238.
10. Chen H, Huang X, Guo X, et al. Smoking duration, intensity, and risk of Parkinson disease. Neurology 2010;74:878–884.
11. Muñoz P, Huenchuguala S, Paris I, Segura-Aguilar J. Dopamine oxidation and autophagy. Parkinsons Dis 2012;2012:920953. doi:10.1155/2012/920953.
12. Lesage S, Brice A. Role of Mendelian genes in "sporadic" Parkinson's disease. Parkinsonism Relat Disord 2012;18(Suppl 1):S66–S70.
13. Coppedè F. Genetics and epigenetics of Parkinson's disease. Scientific World J 2012;2012:489830.
14. Bernheimer H, Birkmayer W, Hornykiewicz O, et al. Brain dopamine and the syndromes of Parkinson's and Huntington: Clinical, morphological, and neurochemical correlations. J Neurol Sci 1973;20:415–455.
15. Smith Y, Bevan MD, Shink E, Bolam JP. Microcircuitry of the direct and indirect pathways of the basal ganglia. Neuroscience 1998;86:353–387.
16. Poewe W, Mahlknecht P, Jankovic J. Emerging therapies for Parkinson's disease. Curr Opin Neurol 2012;25:448–459.

17. Hughes AJ, Ben-Shlomo Y, Daniel SE, Lees AJ. What features improve the accuracy of clinical diagnosis in Parkinson's disease: A clinicopathologic study. Neurology 1992;42:1142–1146.
18. López-Sendón JL, Mena MA, de Yébenes JG. Drug-induced parkinsonism in the elderly: Incidence, management and prevention. Drugs Aging 2012;29:105–118.
19. Emre M. Dementia associated with Parkinson's disease. Lancet Neurol 2003;2:229–237.
20. Chen JJ. Anxiety, depression, and psychosis in Parkinson's disease: Unmet needs and treatment challenges. Neurol Clin 2004;22(Suppl 3):S63–S90.
21. Chen JJ, Swope DM. Pharmacotherapy for Parkinson's disease. Pharmacotherapy 2007;27(12 Pt 2):161S–173S.
22. Olanow CW, Stern MB, Sethi K. The scientific and clinical basis for the treatment of Parkinson's disease (2009). Neurology 2009;72(21 Suppl 4):S1–S136.
23. Pahwa R, Factor SA, Lyons KE, et al. Quality Standards Subcommittee of the American Academy of Neurology. Practice parameter: Treatment of Parkinson's disease with motor fluctuations and dyskinesia (an evidence-based review): Report of the Quality Standards Subcommittee of the American Academy of Neurology. Neurology 2006;66:983–995.
24. Miyasaki JM, Shannon K, Voon V, et al. Quality Standards Subcommittee of the American Academy of Neurology. Practice Parameter: Evaluation and treatment of depression, psychosis, and dementia in Parkinson's disease (an evidence-based review): Report of the Quality Standards Subcommittee of the American Academy of Neurology. Neurology 2006;66:996–1002.
25. Fox SH, Katzenschlager R, Lim SY, et al. The Movement Disorder Society Evidence-Based Medicine Review Update: Treatments for the motor symptoms of Parkinson's disease. Mov Disord 2011;26(Suppl 3):S2–S41.
26. Seppi K, Weintraub D, Coelho M, et al. The Movement Disorder Society Evidence-Based Medicine Review Update: Treatments for the non-motor symptoms of Parkinson's disease. Mov Disord 2011;26(Suppl 3):S42–S80.
27. Kluger BM, Klepitskaya O, Okun MS. Surgical treatment of movement disorders. Neurol Clin 2009;27:633–677.
28. Ma Y, Peng S, Dhawan V, Eidelberg D. Dopamine cell transplantation in Parkinson's disease: Challenge and perspective. Br Med Bull 2011;100:173–189.
29. Feng LR, Maguire-Zeiss KA. Gene therapy in Parkinson's disease: Rationale and current status. CNS Drugs 2010;24:177–192.
30. Khan TS. Off spells and dyskinesias: Pharmacologic management of motor complications. Cleve Clin J Med 2012;79(Suppl 2):S8–S13.
31. Stocchi F. Prevention and treatment of motor complications. Parkinsonism Relat Disord 2003;9(Suppl 2):S73–S81.
32. Pahwa R, Lyons KE. Options in the treatment of motor fluctuations and dyskinesias in Parkinson's disease: A brief review. Neurol Clin 2004;22(Suppl 3):S35–S52.
33. Parkinson Study Group. Levodopa and the progression of Parkinson's disease. N Engl J Med 2004;351:2498–2508.
34. Chen JJ, Obering C. Apomorphine in the management of motor fluctuations associated with Parkinson's disease. Clin Ther 2005;27;1710–1724.
35. Antonini A, Tolosa E. Apomorphine and levodopa infusion therapies for advanced Parkinson's disease: Selection criteria and patient management. Expert Rev Neurother 2009;9:859–867.
36. Devos D, French DUODOPA Study Group. Patient profile, indications, efficacy and safety of duodenal levodopa infusion in advanced Parkinson's disease. Mov Disord 2009;24:993–1000.
37. Pappert EJ, Buhrfiend C, Lipton JW, et al. Levodopa stability in solution: Time course, environmental effects, and practical recommendations for clinical use. Mov Disord 1996;11:24–26.
38. Johnson KA, Conn PJ, Niswender CM. Glutamate receptors as therapeutic targets for Parkinson's disease. CNS Neurol Disord Drug Targets 2009;8:475–491.
39. Chen JJ. Pharmacologic safety concerns in Parkinson's disease: Facts and insights. Int J Neurosci 2011;121(Suppl 2):45–52.
40. Chen JJ, Swope DM, Dashtipour K. Comprehensive review of rasagiline, a second-generation monoamine oxidase inhibitor, for the treatment of Parkinson's disease. Clin Ther 2007;29:1825–1849.
41. Olanow CW, Rascol O, Hauser R; ADAGIO Study Investigators. A double-blind, delayed-start trial of rasagiline in Parkinson's disease. N Engl J Med 2009;361: 1268–1278.
42. Rascol O, Brooks DJ, Melamed E, et al. Rasagiline as an adjunct to levodopa in patients with Parkinson's disease and motor fluctuations (LARGO, Lasting effect in Adjunct therapy with Rasagiline Given Once daily, study): A randomised, double-blind, parallel-group trial. Lancet 2005;365:947–954.
43. Ruottinen HM, Rinne UK. COMT inhibition in the treatment of Parkinson's disease. J Neurol 1998;245(Suppl 3):25–34.
44. Holm KJ, Spencer CM. Entacapone: A review of its use in Parkinson's disease. Drugs 1999;58:159–177.
45. Keating GM, Lyseng-Williamson KA. Tolcapone. A review of its use in the management of Parkinson's disease. CNS Drugs 2005;19:165–184.
46. Zanettini R, Antonini A, Gatto G, et al. Valvular heart disease and the use of dopamine agonists for Parkinson's disease. N Engl J Med 2007;356:39–46.
47. Rascol O, Brooks DJ, Korczyn AD, et al. A five-year study of the incidence of dyskinesia in patients with early Parkinson's disease who were treated with ropinirole or levodopa. 056 Study Group. N Engl J Med 2000;342: 1484–1491.
48. Parkinson Study Group. Pramipexole vs levodopa as initial treatment for Parkinson's disease: A 4-year randomized controlled trial. Arch Neurol 2004;61:1044–1053.
49. Chen JJ, Swope DM, Dashtipour K, Lyons KE. Transdermal rotigotine: A clinically innovative dopamine receptor agonist for the management of Parkinson's disease. Pharmacotherapy 2009;29:1452–1467.
50. Schröder S, Martus P, Odin P, Schaefer M. Impact of community pharmaceutical care on patient health and quality of drug treatment in Parkinson's disease. Int J Clin Pharm 2012;34:746–756.

Pain Management

Terry J. Baumann, Chris M. Herndon, and Jennifer M. Strickland

44

KEY CONCEPTS

1. It is important, whenever possible, to ask patients if they have pain, to identify the source of pain, and to assess the characteristics of the pain.
2. Doses must be individualized for each patient and administered for an adequate duration of time. Around-the-clock regimens should be considered for acute and chronic pain. As-needed regimens should be used for breakthrough pain or when acute pain displays wide variability and/or has subsided greatly.
3. For chronic pain that has a neuropathic component, anticonvulsants, topical analgesics, tricyclic antidepressants, serotonin–norepinephrine reuptake inhibitors, and opioids should be considered based on evidence-based recommendations when available.
4. Oral analgesics are preferred over other dosage forms whenever feasible, but it is important to adjust the route of administration to the needs of the patient.
5. Equianalgesic doses are useful as a guide when converting from one agent to another, but further dose titration usually is required to achieve treatment goals.
6. Patients taking analgesics should be monitored for response and side effects, particularly sedation and constipation associated with the opioids.
7. Care should be taken to identify and avoid potential drug–drug interactions with analgesics when possible, as increased adverse effects may occur (e.g., opioids and benzodiazepines).
8. Whenever possible, a multidisciplinary approach and nonpharmacologic strategies should be used.
9. Etiology of pain may not always be identifiable.

If we know that pain and suffering can be alleviated, and do nothing about it, then we ourselves, become the tormentors.
Primo Levi[1]

Humans have always known and sought relief from pain.[2] Today, pain's impact on society still is great, and indeed pain complaints remain a primary reason patients seek medical advice.[3]

Regrettably, many healthcare providers do not receive adequate training in this area, and new information is not widely disseminated and/or understood. Clearly, pain management is enhanced when a multidisciplinary approach is applied. Thus, understanding the pathophysiology of pain therapy and maintaining a working knowledge of pain regimens are important factors in addressing pain control.

DEFINITION

The accepted current definition of pain is: "an unpleasant sensory and emotional experience associated with actual or potential tissue damage or described in terms of such damage."[4] Pain often is so subjective, however, that many clinicians define pain as whatever the patient says it is. The best care is achieved when the patient comes first.

EPIDEMIOLOGY

Data presented in the recently released Institute of Medicine report, "Relieving Pain in America" suggests that greater than 100 million persons in the United States live with chronic pain.[5] Given that greater than 50% of persons with low back pain in the previous 3 months reported interference with basic and complex activity, it is not surprising that the estimated economic burden of just chronic pain alone exceeds 500 billion dollars (US) annually.[5] In 1 year, an estimated 25 million Americans will experience acute pain due to injury or surgery, and one third of Americans will experience severe chronic pain at some point in their lives.[3] Unfortunately, despite much public attention, considerable focused education, and a number of consensus guidelines, pain often remains inadequately or inappropriately treated.[3,5–10]

PHYSIOLOGY AND PATHOPHYSIOLOGY

The pathophysiology of pain involves a complex array of neural networks in the brain that are acted on by afferent stimuli to produce the experience we know as pain. It can be physiologic and protective (nociceptive) or pathophysiologic and harmful (e.g., neuropathic).[11]

Nociceptive Pain

Nociceptive pain, which can be considered protective and physiologic,[11] typically is classified as either somatic (arising from skin, bone, joint, muscle, or connective tissue) or visceral (arising from internal organs such as the large intestine or pancreas).[11] Whereas somatic pain often presents as throbbing and well localized, visceral pain can manifest as pain feeling as if it is coming from other structures (referred) or as a more localized phenomenon.[11] We can think of nociception in terms of transduction, transmission, perception, and modulation.[11]

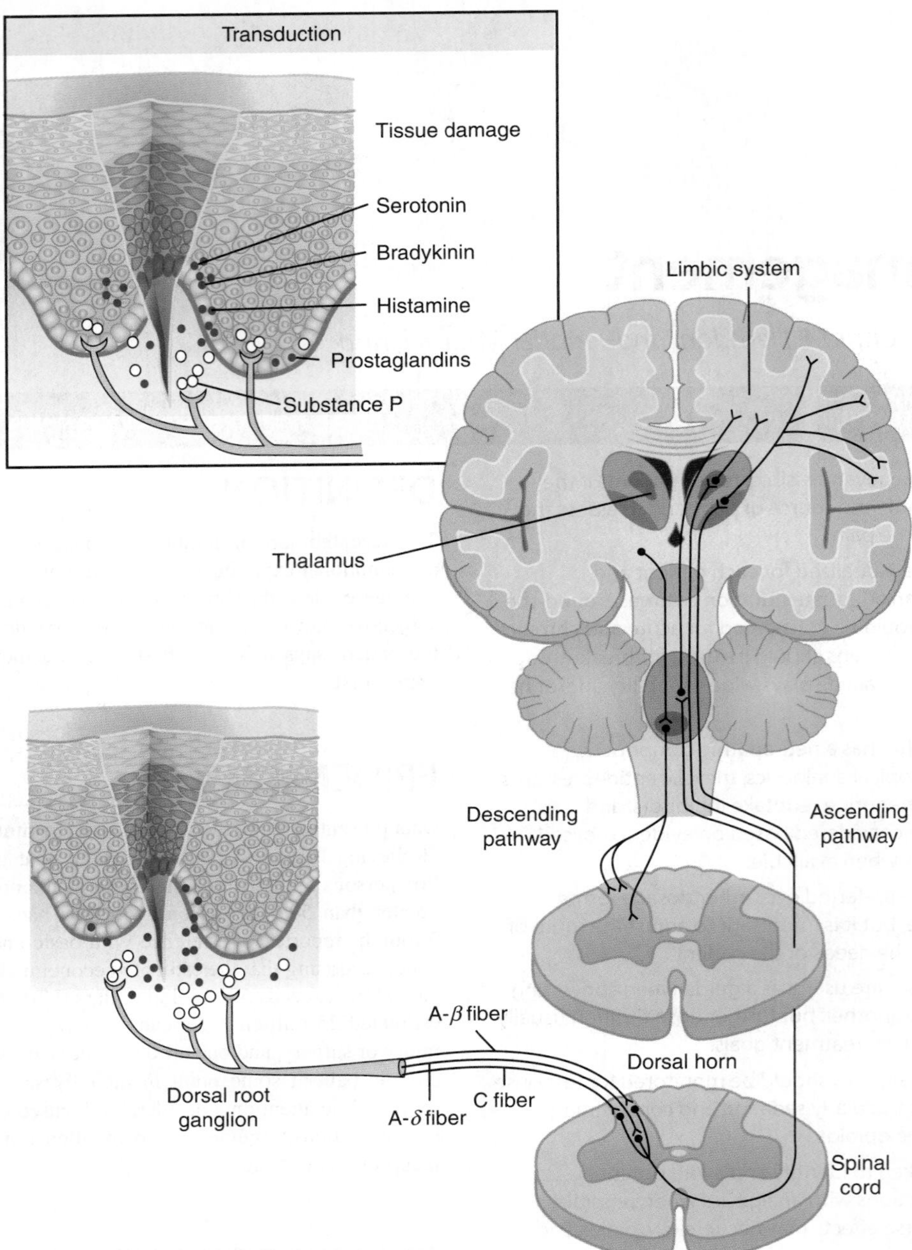

FIGURE 44-1 Schematic representation of nociceptive pain. *(Used with permission from, Pasero C, Portenoy R. Neurophysiology of pain and analgesia and the pathophysiology of neuropathic pain. In: McCaffery M, Pasero C, eds. Pain Assessment and Pharmacologic Management. St. Louis: Mosby, 2011:4–5, Figure 1-2.)*

Transduction

The first step leading to the sensation of pain is stimulation of free nerve endings known as *nociceptors*. These receptors are found in both somatic and visceral structures. They distinguish between noxious and innocuous stimuli, and they are activated and sensitized by mechanical, thermal, and chemical impulses.[11] The underlying mechanism of these noxious stimuli (which in and of themselves may sensitize/stimulate the receptor) may be the release/activation of bradykinins, nerve growth factor, prostaglandins, histamine, interleukins, tumor necrosis factor α, serotonin, and substance P (among others) that sensitize and/or activate the nociceptors.[11,12] Receptor activation (which also involves voltage-gated sodium channels) leads to action potentials that are transmitted along afferent nerve fibers to the spinal cord[11,12] (Fig. 44-1).

Transmission

Nociceptive transmission takes place in A-δ and C-afferent nerve fibers.[11] Stimulation of large-diameter, sparsely myelinated A-δ fibers evokes sharp, well-localized pain, whereas stimulation of unmyelinated, small-diameter C fibers produces aching, poorly localized pain.[11]

These afferent, nociceptive pain fibers synapse in various layers (laminae) of the spinal cord's dorsal horn, releasing a variety of neurotransmitters, including glutamate, substance P, and aspartate.[13] The complex array of events that influence pain can be explained in part by the interactions between neuroreceptors and neurotransmitters that take place in this synapse. For example, by stimulating sensory myelinated fibers that intraconnect in the dorsal horn with pain fibers, nonnoxious stimuli can have an inhibitory effect on pain transmission. These pain-initiated processes reach the brain through a complex array of ascending spinal cord pathways, which include the spinothalamic tract.[13] Information other than pain is also carried along these pathways. Thus, pain is influenced by many factors supplemental to nociception and precludes simple schematic representation. It is postulated that the thalamus acts as a relay station, as these pathways ascend and pass the impulses to central structures where pain can be processed further.[14]

Perception

At this point in transmission, pain is thought to become a conscious experience that takes place in higher cortical structures. The physiology surrounding perception is complex and not well understood, but we know cognitive and behavioral functions can modify pain. Thus relaxation, distraction, meditation, and guided mental imagery may strongly influence pain perception[11] and decrease pain. In contrast, a change in our neurobiochemical makeup that results in states such as depression or anxiety may worsen pain.

Modulation

The body modulates pain through a number of complex processes. One, known as the *endogenous opiate system*, consists of neurotransmitters (e.g., enkephalins, dynorphins, and β-endorphins) and receptors (e.g., μ, δ, and κ) that are found throughout the central and peripheral nervous system (CNS and PNS).[11,15] Like exogenous opioids, endogenous peptides bind to opioid receptor sites and modulate the transmission of pain impulses.[11] Other receptor types also can influence this system. Blockade of *N*-methyl-D-aspartate (NMDA) receptors, found in the dorsal horn, may increase the μ-receptors' responsiveness to opiates.[15]

The CNS also contains a highly organized descending system for the control of pain transmission. This system, which at least partially originates in the periaqueductal gray region of the midbrain, can inhibit synaptic pain transmission at the dorsal horn via modulation of the raphe nuclei in the brainstem.[11,16] Important neurotransmitters here include endogenous opioids, serotonin, norepinephrine, and γ-aminobutyric acid (GABA).[11,16]

Pathophysiologic Pain

Pathophysiologic pain is distinctly different from nociceptive pain in that it becomes disengaged from noxious stimuli or healing[11] and often is described in terms of chronic pain. This type of pain is a result of damage or abnormal functioning of the PNS and/or CNS.[11] A number of pain syndromes (e.g., postherpetic neuralgia, diabetic neuropathy, fibromyalgia, irritable bowel syndrome, sympathetic induced pain, chronic headaches, and some noncardiac chest pain) fall into this category. These pain syndromes are often under-recognized and difficult to treat. In addition, the pain reported often is not commensurate with physical exam findings or imaging results.

The mechanism responsible for pain of this nature may be the nervous system's endogenous dynamic nature. Nerve damage or certain disease states evoke both peripheral (e.g., alteration in nociceptive nerve fibers sensitivity, alterations in sodium channels, collateral sprouting of nerve fibers) and central (e.g., hyperexcitability of central neurons or central sensitization, NMDA receptor activation, central disinhibition) mechanisms leading to these changes.[11,17] Pain circuits rewire themselves both anatomically and biochemically.[18] This produces a mismatch between pain stimulation and inhibition and a potential progressive increase in the discharge of dorsal horn neurons.[18]

Clinically, patients present with episodic or continuous pain transmission (often described as burning, tingling, shock like, or shooting) exaggerated painful response to normally noxious stimuli (hyperalgesia), and/or painful response to normally nonnoxious stimuli (allodynia).[3,18] This change over time may help to explain why this type of pain often manifests long after the actual nerve-related injury or when no actual injury is identified.

TABLE 44-1 Characteristics of Acute and Chronic Pain

Characteristic	Acute Pain	Chronic Pain
Relief of pain	Highly desirable	Highly desirable
Dependence and tolerance to medication	Unusual	Common
Psychological component	Usually not present	Often a major problem
Organic cause	Common	May not be present
Environmental/family Issues	Small	Significant
Insomnia	Unusual	Common component
Treatment goal	Pain reduction	Functionality
Depression	Uncommon	Common

Data from Stimmel[2] and Approaches to Pain Managment.[73]

CLASSIFICATION OF PAIN

It is helpful in understanding pain to subdivide the presenting symptoms into acute pain, chronic pain, and cancer pain.

Acute Pain

Acute pain can be a useful physiologic process, warning individuals of disease states and potentially harmful situations. Unfortunately, severe, unremitting, undertreated acute pain, when it outlives its biologic usefulness, can produce many deleterious effects. Aside from unnecessary suffering, untreated and undertreated acute pain has also been shown to increase one's risk for the development of chronic pain syndromes.[19] Acute pain is usually nociceptive in nature with common causes, including surgery, acute illness, trauma, labor, and medical procedures.[3]

Chronic Pain

Under normal conditions, acute pain subsides quickly as the healing process decreases the pain-producing stimuli; however, in some instances, pain persists for months to years, leading to a chronic pathophysiologic pain state with features quite different from those of acute pain (Table 44-1).[3] Chronic pain can be classified as either being associated with cancer (cancer pain) or from noncancer etiologies (chronic noncancer pain). It often is a result of changes to nerve function and transmission thus making treatment difficult.[20]

Cancer Pain

Pain associated with potentially life-threatening conditions is often called malignant pain or in the case of cancer, cancer pain.[3] This type of pain includes both chronic and acute (e.g., breakthrough pain) components and often has multiple etiologies. It is pain caused by the disease itself (e.g., tumor invasion, organ obstruction), treatment (e.g., chemotherapy, radiation, and surgical incisions), or diagnostic procedures (e.g., biopsy).[3]

CLINICAL PRESENTATION

A patient-oriented approach is essential, and evaluation methods should not differ from those used in other medical conditions.[21] ❶ Therefore, a comprehensive history and physical examination are imperative to evaluate underlying diseases and possible other

CLINICAL PRESENTATION Pain

Acute Pain

General

- Obvious distress (e.g., trauma), infants may present with changes in feeding habits, increased fussiness. Those with dementia may exhibit changes in eating habits, increased agitation, calling out. Attention also must be given to mental/emotional factors that alter the pain threshold. Anxiety, depression, fatigue, anger, and fear in particular, are noted to lower this threshold, whereas rest, mood elevation, sympathy, diversion, and understanding raise the pain threshold

Symptoms

- Can be described as sharp, dull, shock like, tingling, shooting, radiating, fluctuating in intensity, and varying in location (these occur in a timely relationship with an obvious noxious stimuli)

Signs

- Hypertension, tachycardia, diaphoresis, mydriasis, and pallor, but these signs are *not diagnostic*
- In some cases there are no obvious physical signs
- Comorbid conditions usually not present
- Outcome of treatment generally predictable

Laboratory Tests

- Pain is always subjective
- There are no specific laboratory tests for pain
- Pain is best diagnosed based on patient description and history

Chronic Pain

General

- Can appear to have no noticeable suffering. Attention also must be given to mental/emotional factors that alter the pain threshold. Anxiety, depression, fatigue, anger, and fear in particular, are noted to lower this threshold; whereas rest, mood elevation, sympathy, diversion, and understanding raise the pain threshold

Symptoms

- Can be described as sharp, dull, shock-like, tingling, shooting, radiating, fluctuating in intensity, and varying in location (these often occur *without* a temporal relationship with an obvious noxious stimuli)
- Over time, the pain stimulus may cause symptoms that completely change (e.g., sharp to dull, obvious to vague).

Signs

- Hypertension, tachycardia, diaphoresis, mydriasis, and pallor are seldom present
- In most cases there are *no* obvious signs
- Comorbid conditions often present (e.g., insomnia, depression, and anxiety)
- Outcome of treatment often unpredictable

Laboratory Tests

- Pain is always subjective
- Pain is best diagnosed based on patient description and history
- There are *no* specific laboratory tests for pain; however, history and/or diagnostic proof of past trauma (e.g., computed tomography) may be helpful in diagnosing etiology. General labs that may be considered include vitamin D, thyroid stimulating hormone (generalized or widespread pain), and B12 (neuropathic pain)

Data from Twycross,[22] American Pain Society,[29] Huang et al.,[64] Hagen et al.,[65] Matoushek et al.,[66] Okumus et al.,[67] and Porche.[72]

contributing factors.[2] This includes asking if the patient has pain and identifying the source of pain when possible, however, the absence of a discreet etiology should not preclude pain treatment.[2] A baseline characterization of pain can be obtained by assessing the attributes outlined in Table 44-2.[22]

TREATMENT

Desired pain management outcomes include both nonpharmacologic and pharmacologic strategies.

Desired Outcomes

The primary goal of pain treatment depends on the type of pain present and should be tailored to individual patients and circumstances. **2** **3** For example, in acute pain, rapid pain relief or reduction in pain intensity is usually the desired target. In comparison, the goal in chronic noncancer pain is to improve or maintain the patient's level of day-to-day functioning, decrease the rate of physical deterioration, decrease pain perception, improve the patient's sense of well-being, improve family and social relationships, and decrease dependency on drug therapy.[2] And finally in cancer pain or other forms of malignant pain, the goal is to provide patients with adequate

TABLE 44-2 Pain Attributes

Onset and duration	When did pain begin and how long has it been since the pain began?
Palliative factors	What makes the pain better?
Provocative factors	What makes the pain worse?
Quality	Describe the pain
Location	Where is the pain?
Severity/intensity	How does this pain compare with other pain you have experienced?
Temporal factors	Does the intensity of the pain change with time?

Data from Twycross[22] and Berry et al.[3]

pain relief that allows them to tolerate diagnostic and therapeutic manipulation and permit the patient to function at a level that will allow freedom of movement and choice.[23]

Nonpharmacologic Therapy

Various nonpharmacologic therapies have been found to be beneficial in the management of acute and chronic pain, including physical manipulation, application of heat or cold, massage, biofeedback, cognitive behavioral therapy, relaxation, acupuncture, and exercise.[24–26] Spinal cord stimulators have also been found to be somewhat beneficial in some chronic pain conditions.[27]

Some commonly used nonpharmacologic therapies, including TENS (transcutaneous electrical nerve stimulation) and lumbar supports in back pain, have limited evidence or have been shown to be ineffective in the management of chronic pain.[26]

Simple interventions (e.g., education or introductory information about expected discomfort or pain after certain procedures) reduce patient distress and greatly reduce postprocedure suffering.[28] Some psychological techniques, including cognitive-behavioral therapy, relaxation training, imagery, and hypnosis, have proven effective in numerous types of pain, including postprocedure pain, low back pain, and cancer-related pain.[23,25,26,28] Nonpharmacologic therapies should be considered when possible.

Pharmacologic Treatment

Pharmacologic treatment is often considered the cornerstone of pain management.

Nonopioid Agents

Analgesia should be initiated with the most effective analgesic agent having the fewest side effects. Acetaminophen and nonsteroidal antiinflammatory drugs (NSAIDs) often are preferred first-line therapies, in the treatment of mild-to-moderate pain (Table 44-3). The exact mechanism of acetaminophen is not completely understood. NSAIDs inhibit formation of varying prostaglandins produced in response to noxious stimuli, thereby decreasing the pain impulses received by the CNS.[29] Acetaminophen is indicated as a first-line therapy in some pain-related disease states, such as osteoarthritis.

TABLE 44-3 Adult FDA-Approved Nonopioid Analgesics

Class and Generic Name	Brand Name	Initial Dose (mg)	Usual Dose Range in mg and (Maximal Dose in mg/day)	Special Population	Other
Salicylates					
Acetylsalicylic acid[a]—aspirin	Various	325–1,000	325–1,000 every 4–6 hours (4,000)		
Choline and magnesium trisalicylate	Various	500–1,500	500–1,500 every 8–12 hours (4,500)	750 every 8 hours (elderly)	
Diflunisal	Various	500–1,000	250–500 every 8–12 hours (1,500)		
Acetaminophen					
	Oral—Tylenol, various	325–1,000	325–1,000 every 4–6 hours (4,000[b])		
	Parenteral—Ofirmev	1,000	1,000 every 6 hours (4,000[b])	If <50 kg, 15 mg/kg every 6 hours, 750 mg maximum single dose	
Anthranilic Acids					
Meclofenamate	Various	50–100	50–100 every 4–6 hours (400)		
Mefenamic acid	Ponstel	500	250 every 6 hours (1,000[c])		Maximum 7 days
Indolacetic Acid					
Etodolac (immediate release)	Various	200–400	200–400 every 6–8 hours (1,000)		
Phenylacetic Acids					
Diclofenac potassium	Cataflam, various	25–50, in some patients, initial 100	Capsule-25 four times daily Tablet 50 three times a day (150[d])		
Diclofenac epolamine (patch)	Flector (patch)	One patch	Patch to be applied twice daily to painful area		Intact skin only
Diclofenac sodium (gel, solution)	Voltaren, Pennsaid			Gel and solution dosing joint specific for osteoarthritis and actinic keratoses	
Propionic Acids					
Ibuprofen[a]	Motrin, Advil, various	200–400	200–400 every 4–6 hours (1,200[e]) (2,400[f])		
	Caldolor (parenteral)	400–800	(3,200[f]) Injectable, 400–800 every 6 hours (3,200[f])		Infused over 30 minutes
Fenoprofen	Nalfon, various	200	200 every 4–6 hours (3,200)		
Ketoprofen	Various	25	25–50 every 6–8 hours (300)		
Naproxen	Naprosyn, various	250–500	250–500 every 12 hours (1,000)	For Osteoarthritis	
Naproxen sodium[a]	Aleve, Anaprox, various	275–550	550 every 12 hours or 275 every 6–8 hours (1,100[g])	For acute pain	

(continued)

TABLE 44-3 Adult FDA-Approved Nonopioid Analgesics (*Continued*)

Class and Generic Name	Brand Name	Initial Dose (mg)	Usual Dose Range in mg and (Maximal Dose in mg/day)	Special Population	Other
Pyrrolacetic Acids					
Ketorolac—parenteral	Various (parenteral)	30[h]–60 (single IM dose only) 15[h]–30 (single IV dose only)	15[h]–30 IV every 6 hours (60[h]–120)		Maximum 5 days
Ketorolac—oral	Various	10[h]–20	10 every 4–6 hours (40)		Maximum 5 days, which includes parenteral doses. Indicated for continuation with parenteral only
Ketorolac—nasal spray	Various	One spray in one[h] or each nostril	One spray, that is, 15.75 mg in each nostril every 6–8 hours (63[h]–126)	Elderly and weight <50 kg One spray (15.75 mg) in one nostril every 6–8 hours	Maximum 5 days
Cox-2 Selective					
Celecoxib	Celebrex	Initial 400 12 hours later followed by another 200 on first day	200 twice daily (400)		Note some recommend maintenance doses of 200 mg/day due to cardiac concerns

FDA, Food and Drug Administration; IM, intramuscular.

[a]Available both as an over-the-counter preparation and as a prescription drug.
[b]Some experts believe 4,000 mg may be too high. OTC max dose 3,000 mg daily.
[c]Up to 1,250 mg on the first day.
[d]Up to 200 mg on the first day.
[e]Over-the-counter dose.
[f]Some individuals may respond better to 3,200 mg as opposed to 2,400 mg, although well-controlled trials show no better response; consider risk versus benefits when using 3,200 mg/day, parenteral maximum daily dose = 3,200 mg.
[g]Initial daily dose may go to 1,375 mg.
[h]Dose for elderly and those under 50 kg (110 lbs).

Data from American Pain Society,[29] Facts and Comparisons,[44] Lexicomp Online,[68] and Watkins et al.[70]

NSAIDs may be particularly useful in the management of cancer-related bone pain and for short-term relief in the management of chronic low back pain.[23,30]

Studies comparing the efficacy of individual NSAIDs have failed to identify greater efficacy of any NSAID compared to any other. Therefore, the choice of a particular agent often depends on availability, cost, pharmacokinetics, pharmacologic characteristics, and the side-effect profile. Because of the large interpatient variability in response to individual NSAIDs, it is considered rational therapy to switch to another member of this class if there is inadequate response after a sufficient therapeutic trial of any single agent.[29] The duration of a sufficient trial has not been well defined; however, typically, a NSAID should be continued for a minimum of 1 month prior to evaluating the need to switch agents. Chronic use of NSAIDs, including selective inhibitors of cyclooxygenase 2 (COX-2 inhibitors), may be limited by adverse effects, including GI, renal, and cardiac effects. Topical NSAIDs may offer similar efficacy as oral NSAIDs in some patients with improved safety and tolerability.[31] Patient selection is critical to ensure optimal benefit from NSAID therapy while minimizing potential adverse effects.

Opioid Agents

Opioids are often the next logical step in the management of acute pain and cancer-related chronic pain. They also may be an effective treatment option in the management of chronic noncancer pain; however, this continues to be somewhat controversial. Many times a trial of opioids is warranted, but such a trial should not be done without a complete assessment of the pain complaint, including an assessment of the patient's functionality and risk factors for opioid misuse and abuse.[32]

The classification of these agents, their equianalgesic doses, relative histamine-releasing characteristics, pharmacokinetics, and dosing guidelines are outlined in Tables 44-4 and 44-5. Opioid choice should be based on patient acceptance; analgesic effectiveness; and pharmacokinetic, pharmacodynamic, and side-effect profiles (Tables 44-4 and 44-6).

The pharmacologic activity of opioids depends on their affinity for and action at central and peripheral opiate receptors.[33] Therapeutic activities and side effects range from those exhibited by the opiate agonists (e.g., morphine) to those seen with the opiate antagonists (e.g., naloxone). Partial agonists and antagonists (e.g., nalbuphine) compete with agonists for opiate receptor sites and, depending on the inherent agonist and antagonist properties, exhibit mixed agonist–antagonist activity.[33] This may result in analgesia with fewer undesirable side effects. Efficacy and side effects also may further differ among agents because of receptor subtype variability.[34] This μ-receptor subtype variability may explain why some patients respond differently to certain opioids, specifically μ-receptor agonists.[34]

The effects of the opioid analgesics are relatively selective, and at normal therapeutic concentrations, do not affect other sensory modalities.[33] While sensations of touch and proprioception are preserved; undesirable side effects may increase as the dose is escalated (Table 44-6).[33] Patients in severe pain may receive high doses of opioids with no unwanted side effects, but as the pain subsides, even very low doses may not be tolerated.[35] Frequently, when opioids are administered, pain is not eliminated, but its unpleasantness is decreased.[33] Patients report that although their pain is still present, it no longer bothers them.

Opioids share related pharmacologic attributes and exert a profound effect on the CNS and GI tract.[33] Mood changes, sedation, nausea, vomiting, decreased GI motility, constipation, respiratory

TABLE 44-4 Opioid Analgesics, Central Analgesics, Opioid Antagonist

Class and Generic Name (Brand Name)	Chemical Source	Relative Histamine Release	Route	Equianalgesic Dose in Adults (mg)	Approximate Onset (minutes)/Half-Life (hours)
Phenanthrenes (Morphine-Like Agonists)					
Morphine (various)	Naturally occurring	+++	IM PO	10 30	10–20[a]/2–4
Hydromorphone (Dilaudid, Exalgo, various)	Semisynthetic	+	IM PO	1.5 7.5	10–20[a]/2–3
Oxymorphone (Opana, various)	Semisynthetic	+	IM PO	1 10	10–20[a]/2
Levorphanol (various)	Semisynthetic	+	PO	Variable	30–60/12–15
Codeine (various)	Naturally occurring	+++	IM PO	15–30[b] 15–30[b]	 10–30/3
Hydrocodone (available as combination)	Semisynthetic	N/A	PO	30	30–60/4
Oxycodone (OxyContin, Oxecta, Roxicodone, various)	Semisynthetic	+	PO	20	30–60[a]/2–3
Phenylpiperidines (Meperidine-Like Agonists)					
Meperidine (Demerol, various)	Synthetic	+++	IM PO	100 300[c]	10–20/2–6
Fentanyl (Sublimaze, Duragesic, Lazanda, Abstral, Fentora, Subsys, Actiq, Onsolis, various)	Synthetic	+	IM Transdermal Buccal, transmucosal, sublingual, nasal inhaled	0.1 Variable[d] Variable[e]	7–15[a]/3–4
Diphenylheptanes					
Methadone (Dolophine, various)	Synthetic	+	IM/IV PO IM PO	Variable[f] (acute) Variable[f] (acute) Variable[f] (chronic) Variable[f] (chronic)	 30–60/8–59
Agonist–Antagonist or Partial Agonists					
Pentazocine (Talwin)	Synthetic	N/A	IM PO	Not recommended 50[b]	 15–30/2–3
Butorphanol (various)	Synthetic	N/A	IM Intranasal	2[b] 1[b] (one spray)	10–20/3–4
Nalbuphine (various)	Synthetic	N/A	IM	10[b]	<15/5
Buprenorphine (Buprenex, Butrans, Subutex, various)	Synthetic	N/A	IM Transdermal Sublingual	0.3 Variable 0.4	10–20/2–6
Antagonist					
Naloxone (Narcan, various)	Synthetic	N/A	IV	0.4–2[g]	1–2 (IV)/2–5 (IM) onset slightly longer than IV and if no response within 5 minutes repeat dose/0.05–1.5
Central Analgesics					
Tramadol (Ultram, Rybix, Ryzolt, ConZip, various)	Synthetic	N/A	PO	120	<60[a]/5–7
Tapentadol (Nucynta)	Synthetic	N/A	PO	N/A	Within 60[a]/4

IM, intramuscular; N/A, not available; PO, oral.

[a]Onset of action may differ for long-acting formulations.
[b]Starting dose only (equianalgesia not shown).
[c]Not recommended.
[d]Equivalent PO morphine dose = variable.
[e]For breakthrough pain only. Equianalgesic dose conversion should be avoided for Transmucosal Immediate Release Fentanyl (TIRF) products.
[f]The equianalgesic dose of methadone when compared with other opioids will decrease progressively the higher the previous opioid dose. Caution should be exercised when initiating in opioid naïve patients.
[g]Starting doses to be used in cases of opioid overdose.

Data from American Pain Society,[29] McPherson,[36] American Hospital Formulary Service,[43] Facts and Comparisons,[44] Tapentadol,[48] Lexicomp Online,[68] Li,[69] and Pasero et al.[77]

TABLE 44-5 Dosing Guidelines

Drug(s)	Initial Dose and Usual Range (Use lowest effective dose, titrate up or down based on patient response, opioid-tolerant patients may need dose modification)	Comments
NSAIDs/ acetaminophen/ aspirin	LOWEST effective dose should be used for the SHORTEST period of time with judicious evaluation of risk factors (see Table 44-3).	• Used in mild-to-moderate pain • May use in conjunction with opioid agents to decrease doses of each • Regular alcohol use with acetaminophen use may result in liver toxicity • Care must be exercised to avoid overdose when combination products containing these agents are used • With NSAIDs underlying renal impairment, hypovolemia, and CHF may predispose to nephrotoxicity
Morphine	PO 5–30 mg every 4 hours[a] IM 5–10 mg every 4 hours[a]	• Drug of choice in severe pain • May use immediate-release product with controlled release product to control breakthrough pain in cancer pain
	IV 2–5 mg every 3–4 hours[a]	• Typical patient-controlled analgesia IV dose is 1 mg with a 10-minute lockout interval
	SR 15–30 mg every 12 hours (may need to be every 8 hours in some patients)	• Every 24-hour products available (Avinza should not exceed doses of 1,600 mg/day)
	Rectal 10–20 mg every 4 hours[a]	• morphine liposomal (DepoDur) at 10, 15 mg/mL is available for epidural administration
Hydromorphone	PO 2–4 mg every 4–6 hours[a]	• Use in severe pain • More potent than morphine; otherwise, no advantages • Typical patient-controlled analgesia IV dose is 0.2 mg with a 10-minute lockout interval
	IM 0.8–1 mg every 4–6 hours[a]	• Every 24-hour product (Exalgo) available but only through a REMS program
	IV 0.2–0.6 mg every 2–3 hours[a] Rectal 3 mg every 6–8 hours[a]	
Oxymorphone	IM/SQ 1–1.5 mg every 4–6 hours[a] IV 0.5 mg initial dose	• Use in severe pain • May use immediate-release product with controlled release product to control breakthrough pain in cancer pain
	PO immediate-release 5–10 mg every 4–6 hours[a] PO extended-release 5–10 mg every 12 hours	• Extended-release reformulated to deter misuse
Levorphanol	PO 2 mg every 6–8 hours	• Use in severe pain • Extended half-life useful in cancer patients • In chronic pain, wait 3 days between dosage adjustments
Codeine	PO 15–30 mg every 4–6 hours[a] Maximum 360 mg day IM 15–30 mg every 4 hours[a]	• Use in mild to moderate pain • Weak analgesic; use with NSAIDs, aspirin, or acetaminophen, analgesic prodrug • Should not be used in children
Hydrocodone	PO 5–10 mg every 4–6 hours[a]	• Use in moderate/severe pain • Most effective when used with NSAIDs, aspirin, or acetaminophen • Only available as combination product with other ingredients for pain
Oxycodone	PO 5–15 mg every 4–6 hours[a] Controlled release 10 mg every 12 hours	• Use in moderate/severe pain • Most effective when used with NSAIDs, aspirin, or acetaminophen • May use immediate-release product with controlled release product to control breakthrough pain in cancer pain • CR reformulated to deter misuse
Meperidine	IM 50–100 mg every 3–4 hours[a] IV 5–10 mg every 5 minutes as needed[a]	• Use in severe pain • Oral not recommended • Do not use in renal failure • May precipitate tremors, myoclonus, and seizures • Use with monoamine oxidase inhibitors can induce hyperpyrexia and/or seizures or opioid overdose symptoms

(continued)

TABLE 44-5 Dosing Guidelines (*Continued*)

Drug(s)	Initial Dose and Usual Range (Use lowest effective dose, titrate up or down based on patient response, opioid-tolerant patients may need dose modification)	Comments
Fentanyl	IV 25–50 mcg/h IM 50–100 mcg every 1–2 hours[a] Transdermal 25 mcg/h every 72 hours Transmucosal (Actiq lollipop) 200 mcg. Must wait 4 hours prior to redosing. However, at any time during therapy may repeat previous dose × 1, 30 minutes after start of previous dose for that episode of breakthrough pain. Transmucosal (Onsolis buccal film) 200 mcg. Must wait 2 hours prior to redosing. Transmucosal (Fentora Buccal Tablet) 100 mcg. Must wait 4 hours prior to redosing. However, at any time during therapy may repeat previous dose × 1, 30 minutes after dose for that episode of breakthrough pain. Intranasal (Lazanda Spray) 100 mcg (one spray) in one nostril. Wait 2 hours prior to redosing. Sublingual (Subsys Spray) 100 mcg (one spray). Must wait 4 hours prior to redosing. However, at any time during therapy may repeat previous dose × 1, 30 minutes after dose for that episode of breakthrough pain. Sublingual (Abstral Tablet,) 100 mcg. Must wait 2 hours prior to redosing. However, at any time during therapy may repeat previous dose × 1, 30 minutes after dose for that episode of breakthrough pain.	• Used in severe pain • Do not use transdermal in acute pain • With transmucosal, intranasal, sublingual dosing, always start with lowest dose despite daily opioid intake. Product-specific titration and maximum dose recommendations exist • Transmucosal, intranasal, sublingual for breakthrough cancer pain in patients already receiving or tolerant to opioids • Transmucosal, intranasal, sublingual fentanyl dosage forms are only available through a REMS program.
Methadone	PO 2.5–10 mg every 8–12 hours IM 2.5–10 mg every 8–12 hours	• Effective in severe chronic pain • Sedation can be major problem • Some chronic pain patients can be dosed every 12 hours • Equianalgesic dose of methadone when compared with other opioids will decrease progressively the higher the previous opioid dose. • Avoid dose titrations more frequently than every 2 weeks
Pentazocine	IM, IV 30 mg every 3–4 hours[b] (maximum 360 mg day) PO 50–100 mg every 3–4 hours[b] (maximum 600 mg daily, for those 50 mg tablet containing 0.5 mg of naloxone) PO 25 mg every 4 hours[b] (maximum 150 mg daily, for those 25 mg tablet containing 650 mg of acetaminophen)	• Third-line agent for moderate-to-severe pain • May precipitate withdrawal in opiate-dependent patients • Parenteral doses not recommended
Butorphanol	IM 1–4 mg every 3–4 hours[b] IV 0.5–2 mg every 3–4 hours[b] Intranasal 1 mg (one spray) every 3–4 hours[b] If inadequate relief after initial spray, may repeat in other nostril × 1 in 60–90 minutes. Maximum two sprays (one per nostril) every 3–4 hours[b]	• Second-line agent for moderate-to-severe pain • May precipitate withdrawal in opiate-dependent patients
Nalbuphine	IM, IV 10 mg every 3–6 hours[b] (maximum 20 mg dose, 160 mg daily)	• Second-line agent for moderate-to-severe pain • May precipitate withdrawal in opiate-dependent patients
Buprenorphine	IM 0.3 mg every 6 hours[b] May repeat × 1, 30–60 minutes after initial dose IM 0.6 mg single dose may be given Slow IV 0.3 mg every 6 hours[b] May repeat × 1, 30–60 minutes after initial dose Transdermal delivery systems (5, 10, 20 mcg/h) available for every 7 day administration	• Second-line agent for moderate-to-severe pain • May precipitate withdrawal in opiate-dependent patients • Detailed manufacturer dosing conversion recommendations exist • Naloxone may not be effective in reversing respiratory depression • Infuse IV dose over at least 2 minutes
Naloxone	IV 0.4–2 mg may repeat × 1, 30–60 minutes after initial dose	• When reversing opiate side effects in patients needing analgesia, dilute and titrate (0.1–0.2 mg every 2–3 minutes) so as not to reverse analgesia • Duration of action of some opioids may outlast duration of naloxone; in these cases we may need to repeat doses
Tramadol	PO 50–100 mg every 4–6 hours[a] If rapid onset not required, start 25 mg/day and titrate over several days Extended-release PO 100 mg every 24 hours	• Maximum dose for nonextended-release, 400 mg/24 h, if more than 75 years old 300 mg/24 h, if creatinine clearance less than 30 mL/min 200 mg/24 h; maximum for extended-release, 300 mg/24 h • Decrease dose in patient with renal impairment and in the elderly
Tapentadol	PO 50–100 mg every 4–6 hours[a] Extended-release PO 50 mg every 12 hours	• First day of therapy may administer second dose after the first as soon as 1 hour after the first dose • Maximum dose first day 700 mg, maximum dose thereafter 600 mg (maximum dose for CR 500 mg) • REMS required

CHF, congestive heart failure; CR, Controlled Release; HCL, hydrochloride; IM, intramuscular; NSAID, nonsteroidal antiinflammatory drug; PO, oral; REMS, risk evaluation and mitigation strategies; SQ, subcutaneous; SR, sustained release.

[a]May start with an around-the-clock regimen and switch to as needed if/when the painful signal subsides or is episodic.
[b]Limited analgesic effect.

Data from American Pain Society,[29] Yaksh,[33] Facts and Comparisons,[44] and Lexicomp Online.[68]

TABLE 44-6 Analgesic Drug Monitoring

Drug (class)	Adverse Reaction	Monitoring Parameter	Comments
Opioids	Respiratory depression	Respiratory rate OR end-tidal capnography	Capnography considered more sensitive; however, equipment may be expensive to incorporate. Higher risk—Obstructive sleep apnea, chronic obstructive pulmonary disease
	Constipation	Bowel movement frequency and consistency	Constipation may be assessed using Bristol Scale
	Sedation	Sedation scale	Will decrease over time
	Nausea, vomiting	Nausea, vomiting	Will decrease over time
	Tolerance	Regular efficacy Monitoring	With chronic use, may lead to need for larger doses
	Dependence	Regular efficacy Monitoring	Will develop with chronic use
	Addiction/abuse	Regular efficacy Monitoring	Seldom problem with acute pain. In chronic pain use specified time trials with opioids, targeted functional end points, screening tools, and frequent monitoring
	Histamine release	Monitor for Uticaria, pruritus, bronchospasm	Incidence varies among agents
	Increase in sphincter tone	Monitor for biliary spasm, urinary retention	Incidence varies among agents
	Hypogonadism	Monitor fatigue, depression, sexual dysfunction, amenorrhea (women)	Problem with chronic use
NSAIDs	Upper GI bleeding	Complete blood count, stool guaiac (if symptoms such as black tarry stools, warrant)	One of leading causes of hospitalizations due to drug-related adverse effects in the United States
	Acute renal failure	Serum creatinine	
Acetaminophen	Hepatotoxicity	Serum transaminases (ALT/AST)	Elevated transaminases may occur even at doses less than 4000 mg daily
		Liver synthesis tests (PT/INR, albumin)	
		Acetaminophen serum concentration	

NSAIDs, nonsteroidal antiinflammatory drugs; ALT/AST, alanine transaminase/aspartate transaminase; PT/INR, prothrombin time/International normalized ratio.

Yaksh and Wallace,[33] Anonymous,[68] Watkins et al.,[70] and Herndon et al.[71]

depression, dependence, and tolerance are evident in varying degrees with all agents.[3,33] Tolerance to side effects (except to constipation) often develops over time.[3] Some differences exist between the opioids in regards to incidence of side effects, which may assist in selection of the most appropriate agent. (4) The route of administration depends on individual patient needs, with the oral route being preferred. However, the onset of analgesic effects for oral medications is approximately 45 minutes, and the peak effect usually occurs 1 to 2 hours after administration.[29] This delay must be a consideration when immediate relief is needed in the management of acute pain. Therefore, in some scenarios, such as acute severe pain (e.g., pain crisis) or when the patient is unable to take oral medications, alternative routes of therapy (e.g., IV) may be preferred. The relative potency, defined by the equianalgesic dose, of opioids differs greatly (Table 44-4). (5) Equianalgesic dose tables are often based on single-dose studies without regard for patient variability and should be used only as a guide.[36]

True opioid allergies are rare, but Table 44-4 also can be used when treating a patient who is allergic to opiates. Most reactions to opioids, such as itching or rash, are due to the associated histamine release from cutaneous mast cells, not a true allergic or immunoglobulin-E (IgE) or T-cell response.[37] Although caution is always advised, a decrease in potential cross-sensitivity is thought to exist when moving from one opioid structural class to another.[37] The classes are phenanthrenes (morphine-like agonists), phenylpiperidines (meperidine-like agonists), and diphenylheptanes (methadone-like agonists). When considering cross-sensitivity, the mixed agonist–antagonist and partial agonists class acts much like the morphine-like agonists.[37]

(2) (6) In the initial stages of acute pain, analgesics should be given around the clock. This should commence after administering a typical starting dose and titrating up or down, depending on the patient's degree of pain and demonstrated side effects (e.g., sedation).[29] As-needed schedules often produce wide swings in analgesic plasma concentrations that create wide swings in pain and sedation. This may initiate a vicious cycle where increasing amounts of pain medications are needed for relief. (2) As the painful state subsides and the need for medication decreases, as-needed schedules may be appropriate. As-needed schedules also may be useful in patients who present with pain that is intermittent or sporadic in nature (Fig. 44-2). When opioids are used in the management of persistent chronic pain, around-the-clock administration schedules should be utilized. As-needed or prn opioids should be used in conjunction with around-the-clock regimens and when patients experience breakthrough pain. Breakthrough pain is a brief, transitory, exacerbation of moderate to severe pain typically occurring in patients with underlying persistent pain that may otherwise be controlled.[36]

Continuous IV methods of opioid infusion are effective for some postoperative pain, but the probability of unwanted side effects is high, and this technique should be reserved for opioid-tolerant patients.[29] An alternative method is patient-controlled analgesia (PCA). With this technique, patients can self-administer a preset dose of an IV opioid via a pump electronically interfaced with a timing device. Compared with traditional as-needed opioid dosing, PCA yields better pain control, improved patient satisfaction, and relatively few differences in side effects.[38,39]

Administration of opioids directly into the CNS (e.g., epidural and intrathecal/subarachnoid routes) has shown considerable promise in the control of acute, chronic noncancer, and cancer pain (Table 44-7);[33,40] and is common in both large and small institutions throughout the United States. Because of reports of respiratory depression, pruritus, nausea, vomiting, urinary retention, and hypotension,[40] these methods of analgesia require careful monitoring and are best used by experienced practitioners. Respiratory depression

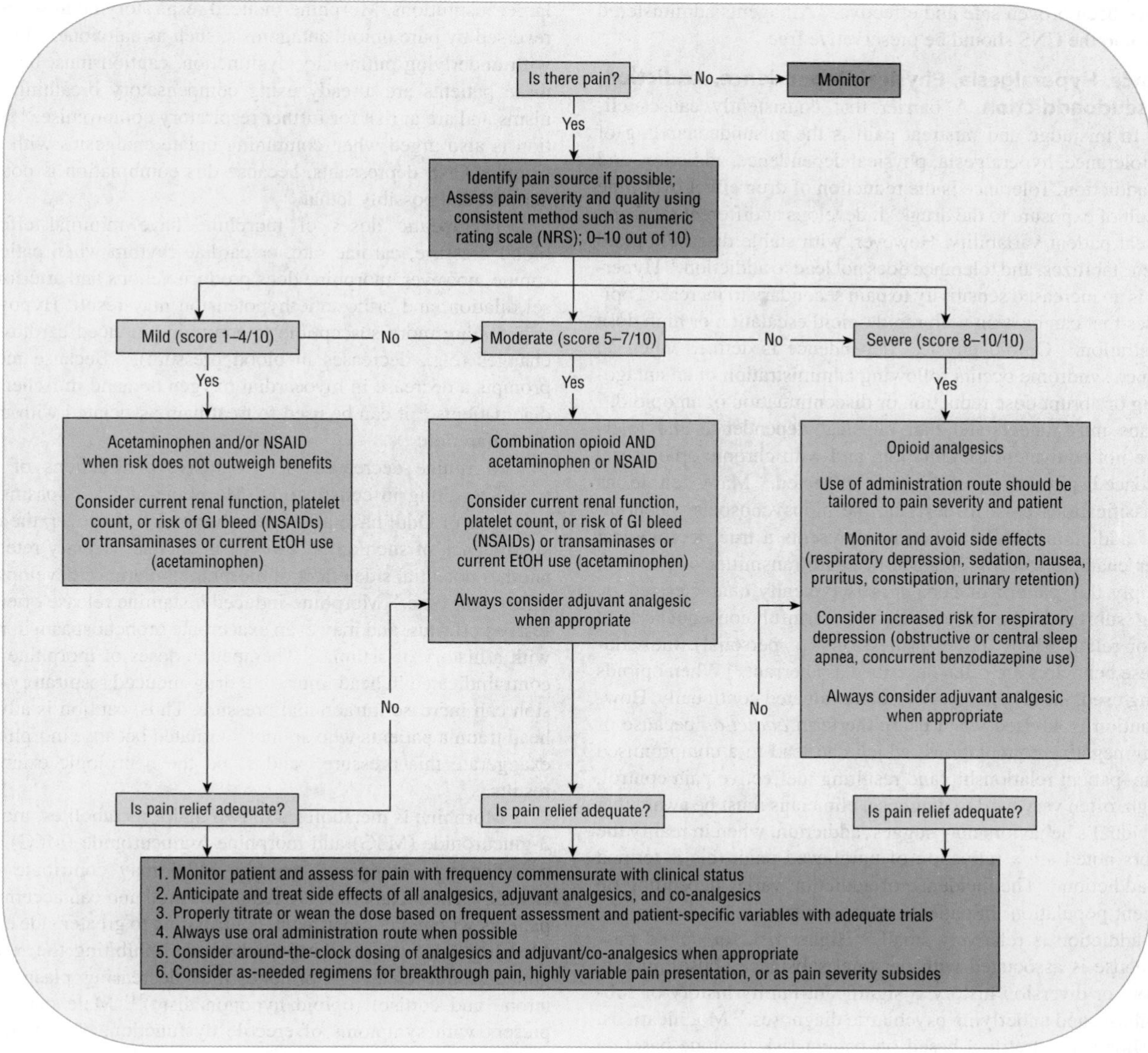

FIGURE 44-2 Algorithm for acute pain. *(Data modified from Omnicare, Inc., Acute Pain Pathway.)*

is of concern and can occur within minutes with intrathecal fentanyl or manifest as late as 19 hours after a single dose of intrathecal morphine.[40] Guidelines mandate respiratory monitoring for at least 24 hours after a single dose of intrathecal or epidural morphine with standing orders for naloxone (opioid antagonist) for full or partial reversal.[41] Analgesia and side effects are evident at lower doses when opioids are administered intrathecally instead of epidurally. This form of analgesia is often administered as a continuous-infusion and/or on a patient-controlled basis. When given simultaneously with intrathecal or epidural local anesthetics such as bupivacaine,

TABLE 44-7 Intraspinal Opioids

Agent	Single Dose (mg)	Onset of Pain Relief (minutes)	Duration of Pain Relief—Single Dose (hours)	Continual Infusion Dose (mg/h)
Epidural Route				
Morphine	1–6	30	6–24	0.1–1
Hydromorphone	0.8–2	5–15	4–16	0.1–0.3
Fentanyl	0.025–0.1	5	2–8	0.025–0.1
Sufentanil	0.01–0.06	5	2–4	0.01–0.05
Subarachnoid Route (Intrathecal)				
Morphine	0.1–0.3	15	8–34	N/A
Fentanyl	0.005–0.025	5	3–6	N/A

Note: Doses above should not be interpreted as equianalgesic doses for conversion to or from the specific opioid or route of administration.

Data from American Pain Society[29] and Yaksh and Wallace.[33]

they have been proven safe and effective.[40] All agents administered directly into the CNS should be preservative free.

Tolerance, Hyperalgesia, Physical Dependence, Addiction, and Pseudoaddiction A barrier that consistently causes clinicians to misjudge and mistreat pain is the misunderstanding of opioid tolerance, hyperalgesia, physical dependence, addiction, and pseudoaddiction. Tolerance is the reduction of drug effect over time as a result of exposure to the drug.[35] It develops at different rates and with great patient variability. However, with stable disease, opioid use often stabilizes, and tolerance does not lead to addiction.[35] Hyperalgesia is an increased sensitivity to pain secondary to increased opioid doses that can be seen with rapid opioid escalation or high dose administration.[35] Opioid physical dependence is defined when an abstinence syndrome occurs following administration of an antagonist drug or abrupt dose reduction or discontinuation of an opioid.[35] Clinicians must understand that physical dependence and tolerance are not equivalent to addiction; and with chronic opioid use, dependence is physiologic and is to be expected.[29] Many definitions and classifications exist to describe the biopsychosocial phenomenon of addiction. While addiction represents a true neurological disorder characterized by changes in neurotransmitter expression, put simply this pattern of behaviors is typically characterized by ongoing substance use *despite* known harmful consequences to health or relationships (either professional or personal). Individually, these behaviors are often described as aberrant.[35] When opioids are being used, these behaviors must be evaluated continually. However, caution is advised when using the term *addiction* because of its many negative connotations, which can lead to a compromised clinician–patient relationship and resulting ineffective pain control. Although, often very hard to diagnose, clinicians must be aware that an individual's behaviors may suggest addiction, when in reality the behaviors noted are a reflection of unrelieved pain, this is termed pseudoaddiction.[35] The incidence of addiction varies depending on the patient population. In patients with no history of addiction, the risk of addiction is relatively small.[35] Higher risk for opioid misuse or abuse is associated with personal substance abuse, misuse, addiction, or diversion history, a significant family history of substance abuse, and underlying psychiatric diagnoses.[32] Modifications, which should be stratified based on patient risk, include baseline and random drug screens, patient–provider treatment agreements, pill counts, a smaller prescription supply, and regular assessment of aberrant behaviors.[32] Combining these approaches with regular and ongoing assessments of pain and functionality may result in improved outcomes.[32]

Morphine and Congeners Despite the availability of several newer agents, morphine remains the prototype opiate analgesic. As new opioid and nonopioid compounds are developed, their efficacy and side-effect profiles are typically compared against morphine as the standard. Many clinicians consider morphine the first-line agent when treating moderate-to-severe pain.

Side effects can be numerous, particularly when morphine is first initiated or when doses are significantly increased. Morphine causes nausea and vomiting through direct stimulation of the chemoreceptor trigger zone, decreased peristalsis, and probably through a vestibular mechanism.[33] Opioid-induced nausea subsides over time.[3] Although euphoria and dysphoria have been reported, morphine's unpleasant effects are more prominent when administered to patients not experiencing pain.[33] As doses of morphine are increased, the respiratory center becomes less responsive to carbon dioxide, causing progressive respiratory depression.[33] This effect is less pronounced in patients being treated for severe or chronic pain.[3] Respiratory depression often manifests as a decrease in respiratory rate (although minute volume and tidal exchange also are affected) and is further compounded because the cough reflex is also depressed.[33] More recently, end-tidal capnography has become commonplace in larger institutions. Morphine-induced respiratory depression can be reversed by pure opioid antagonists, such as naloxone.[33] In patients with underlying pulmonary dysfunction, caution must be used, as these patients are already using compensatory breathing mechanisms and are at risk for further respiratory compromise.[33] **7** Caution is also urged when combining opiate analgesics with alcohol or other CNS depressants, because this combination is potentially harmful and possibly lethal.[33]

Therapeutic doses of morphine have minimal effects on blood pressure, cardiac rate, or cardiac rhythm when patients are supine; however, morphine does produce venous and arteriolar vessel dilation, and orthostatic hypotension may result. Hypovolemic patients are more susceptible to morphine-induced cardiovascular changes (e.g., decreases in blood pressure).[33] Because morphine prompts a decrease in myocardial oxygen demand in ischemic cardiac patients,[33] it can be used to treat pain associated with myocardial infarction.

Morphine decreases the propulsive contractions of the GI tract[33] resulting in constipation. Morphine-induced spasms of the sphincter of Oddi have also been observed.[33] However, the clinical significance of such an occurrence is unclear. Urinary retention is another potential side effect of morphine; tolerance develops to this effect over time.[33] Morphine-induced histamine release often manifests as pruritus, and may even exacerbate bronchospasm in patients with a history of asthma.[33] Therapeutic doses of morphine are not contraindicated in head injury, but drug-induced respiratory depression can increase intracranial pressure. Thus, caution is advised in head trauma patients who are not ventilated because morphine may exaggerate this pressure[33] and cloud the neurologic examination results.

Morphine is metabolized to two major metabolites, morphine-3-glucuronide (M3G) and morphine-6-glucuronide (M6G).[33] M6G contributes to analgesia, whereas M3G may contribute to side effects.[33] The metabolites are renally cleared and can accumulate in patients with renal impairment, contributing to greater side effects.[33] Morphine also affects the hypothalamus inhibiting the release of gonadotropin-releasing hormone, thus decreasing plasma testosterone and cortisol (opioid hypogonadism).[33] Male patients may present with symptoms of erectile dysfunction, decreased libido, and decreased analgesic efficacy of the opioid. Women may experience alopecia, amenorrhea, depressed mood, and decreased analgesic efficacy. Recommendations for clinical replacement of these hormones in patients using chronic opioid therapy are not well defined.[42] While the clinical meaning has not clearly been elucidated, morphine and other opioids, depending on the situation being used, may either enhance or inhibit the immune system.[33]

Hydromorphone is more potent than morphine, but its overall pharmacologic profile parallels that of morphine. Some clinicians believe hydromorphone is associated with fewer side effects, especially pruritus, compared with other opioids. However, the research is limited and does not conclusively demonstrate this difference. Oxymorphone can be administered orally and by injection. Although extended-release and immediate-release oral products are available, making oxymorphone useful in chronic and acute pain, it offers no pharmacologic advantage over morphine. Levorphanol has an extended half-life, but its overall therapeutic effects are similar to the other agents in this class.

Codeine is a commonly used opiate in the treatment of mild-to-moderate pain. It often is combined with other analgesic products (e.g., acetaminophen). Unfortunately, it has the same propensity to produce side effects as morphine. Hydrocodone is another commonly prescribed opiate and is available for pain only in combination products with other analgesic agents (e.g., acetaminophen, ibuprofen). Its pharmacologic properties are similar to those of morphine. Oxycodone is a useful oral analgesic for moderate-to-severe pain. This is especially true when the product is used in combination with nonopioids. Although oxycodone shares basic morphine characteristics, the availability of an immediate-release and controlled-release oral dosage form also makes it very useful in chronic pain as well as acute pain.

Meperidine and Congeners (Phenylpiperidines) The prototype phenylpiperidine, meperidine, has a pharmacologic profile comparable with that of morphine; however, it is not as potent and has a shorter analgesic duration. Meperidine offers no analgesic advantage over morphine, has greater toxicity (CNS hyperirritability caused by its renally eliminated metabolite normeperidine),[43] and should be limited in use. In particular, avoid long-term usage and use in patients at greatest risk for toxicity (e.g., elderly patients and those with renal dysfunction).

Fentanyl is a synthetic opioid structurally related to meperidine that is used often in anesthesiology as an adjunct to general anesthesia.[43] This agent is more potent and faster acting than meperidine (Table 44-4). It can be administered parenterally, transmucosally, sublingually, intranasally, and transdermally.

Methadone and Congeners Methadone has gained considerable popularity because of its oral efficacy, extended duration of action, and low cost. Although methadone is effective in acute pain,[44] it has gained particular prominence in treating cancer pain[32] and has increasingly been used in the management of chronic noncancer pain.[32] This despite the fact that, it has an unpredictable half-life, it can cause excessive sedation, and it is difficult to titrate. Properties unique to methadone, compared with other opioids, include the D-isomer's ability to antagonize NMDA receptors, agonist effects at κ- and δ-opioid receptors, and blockade of serotonin and norepinephrine reuptake.[36,45] These properties may prove useful in the treatment of neuropathic and chronic pain. However, few trials have thoroughly evaluated methadone's risks versus benefits.[32] Epidemiologic studies suggest a growing number of methadone-related deaths, and cardiac arrhythmias have been associated with methadone, particularly at higher doses or when used concurrently with other agents that prolong QTc intervals.[32] Recommendations exist for specific echocardiogram monitoring for methadone; however, concerns exist regarding their applicability.[46] The equianalgesic dose of methadone may decrease with higher doses of the previous opioid,[36] complicating conversions from other opioids to methadone.

Opioid Agonist–Antagonist Derivatives Analgesic agents that stimulate the analgesic portion of opioid receptors while blocking or having no effect on the toxicity portion would be considered ideal. The agonist–antagonist derivatives were developed with this in mind. This analgesic class produces analgesia and has the potential for less respiratory depression than opioid agonists.[33] These agents are considered to have a lower abuse potential than morphine, but psychotomimetic responses (e.g., hallucinations and dysphoria, as seen with pentazocine), limited analgesic effect, and a propensity to initiate withdrawal in opioid-dependent populations[29,33,44] have diminished their widespread clinical use.

Opioid Antagonists The opioid antagonist naloxone binds competitively to opioid receptors but does not produce an analgesic or opioid side-effect response. Therefore, it is used most often to reverse the toxic effects of agonist- and agonist–antagonist-derived opioids. Other opioid antagonists exist, including naltrexone and methylnaltrexone. Naltrexone's use is primarily limited to addiction medicine, while methylnaltrexone is used for opioid-induced constipation.[44]

Central Analgesics

Tramadol and tapentadol are the only centrally acting analgesics currently available in the United States. Tramadol binds to μ-opiate receptors and inhibits norepinephrine and serotonin reuptake. Tapentadol also binds the μ-opiate receptor, but inhibits largely norepinephrine reuptake. Tramadol is indicated for the relief of moderate to moderately severe pain, while tapentadol is indicated for moderate-to-severe acute pain and diabetic peripheral neuropathy.[44]

Both tramadol and tapentadol have side-effect profiles similar to that of the previously mentioned opioid analgesics (e.g., dizziness, nausea, somnolence, and constipation).[47,48] Tapentadol is a schedule II controlled substance, while tramadol is not scheduled federally, although it is a schedule IV in some states.[47] Tapentadol has not been systematically evaluated in patients with seizures, and it should be used with caution in seizure patients.[44] Seizure risk may be elevated in patients taking tramadol.[44] Tramadol may have a place in treating patients with chronic pain, especially neuropathic pain,[49] while tapentadol may be useful in the management of acute pain and when using the controlled release format in chronic pain[44] (e.g., diabetes-related nerve pain).[50]

Adjuvant Analgesics

Adjuvant analgesics represent a diverse group of pharmacologic agents with individual characteristics that make them useful in the management of pain but that typically are not classified as analgesics. Examples of adjuvant analgesics include antidepressants and anticonvulsants. 3 Chronic pain that has a neuropathic component (e.g., diabetic neuropathy) often requires adjuvant analgesic therapy (Table 44-8). Anticonvulsants (e.g., gabapentin, pregabalin, which may decrease neuronal excitability), tricyclic antidepressants, serotonin and norepinephrine reuptake inhibitor antidepressants (e.g., nortriptyline, duloxetine—which block the reuptake of serotonin and norepinephrine, thus enhancing pain inhibition), and topically applied local anesthetics (which decrease nerve stimulation) all have demonstrated efficacy in managing various chronic pain conditions.[49]

In the management of cancer pain, radiopharmaceuticals (e.g., strontium-89 or samarium), corticosteroids, and bisphosphonates

TABLE 44-8 Pharmacologic Management of Chronic Noncancer Pain

Type of Pain	Nonopioids	Opioids	Other Medications	Comments
Chronic low back pain	Acetaminophen NSAIDs (long-term use evidence weak)	Short-term use for mild-to-moderate flare-ups Not first line	Tramadol, TCAs, AEDs	Acetaminophen, NSAIDs first; tramadol or opioids in selected patients; AEDs or TCAs may be considered if neuropathic symptoms (evidence weak)
Fibromyalgia	Acetaminophen	Not recommended	Tramadol, AEDs (pregabalin), SNRIs (duloxetine, milnacipran)	Acetaminophen considered first (evidence weak); tramadol (evidence weak) AEDs, SNRIs (stronger evidence)
Neuropathic pain	Acetaminophen NSAIDs are rarely effective	Considered second-line therapy, are tried after AEDs, SNRIs, and/or TCAs	TCAs, AEDs, SNRIs, central analgesics, topical (e.g., 5% lidocaine patch, capsaicin)	TCAs, SNRIs, AEDs, 5% lidocaine patch considered first line; central analgesics, and opioids considered second-line agents; capsaicins considered third line

AED, antiepileptic drug; NSAIDs, nonsteroidal antiinflammatory drugs; SNRI, serotonin–norepinephrine reuptake inhibitor; TCA, tricyclic antidepressant.

Data from Dworkin and O'Connor,[49] Schwartz et al.,[50] Carville et al.,[73] Traynor et al.,[74] Chou et al.,[75] and Chou.[76]

TABLE 44-9 Injectable Local Anesthetics[a]

Agent (Brand Name)	Onset (minutes)	Duration (hours)
Esters		
Procaine (Novocain)	2–5	0.25–1
Chloroprocaine (Nesacaine, various)	6–12	0.5
Tetracaine (Pontocaine, various)	≤15	2–3
Amides		
Articaine[b] (Septicaine)	1–6	1
Mepivacaine (Polocaine, various)	3–5	0.75–1.5
Bupivacaine (Marcaine, various)	5	2–4
Bupivacaine liposomal (Exparel—local infiltration only)	Variable	24 local 96 systemic
Lidocaine (Xylocaine, various)	<2	0.5–1
Prilocaine (Citanest, various)	<2	≥1
Ropivacaine[c] (Naropin)	10–30	0.5–6

[a]Unless otherwise indicated, values are for infiltrative anesthesia.
[b]Product contains epinephrine.
[c]Epidural administration.
Data from Anonymous.[44,68]

are useful adjuvant analgesics in treating bone pain.[51] Although antihistamines and amphetamines have been used as adjuvant pain medications,[23] they have demonstrated only limited success.

Multimodal Therapy

Multimodal therapy is the concomitant use of different therapeutic interventions with the intent of obtaining additive therapeutic effects. Multimodal analgesia, one type of multimodal therapy, includes combining medications from different classes (e.g., combination therapy with opioids and nonopioids or adjuvant analgesics).[11] This often results in analgesia superior to that produced by either agent alone.[11] Multimodal analgesia may also permit the use of lower doses and provide a more favorable side-effect profile.[11] Multimodal therapy is useful for the management of both acute and chronic pain.

Regional Analgesia

Regional analgesia with properly administered local anesthetics can provide relief of both acute and chronic pain (Table 44-9).[3,40] These agents can be positioned by injection (e.g., in joints, in the epidural or intrathecal space, along nerve roots, or in a nerve plexus) or topically. Lidocaine in the form of a patch has proven effective in treating focal neuropathic pain.[49] Regional application of local anesthetics relieve pain by blocking nerve impulses.[44] High plasma concentrations can cause CNS excitation and depression, including dizziness, tinnitus, drowsiness, disorientation, muscle twitching, seizures, and respiratory arrest.[43] Cardiovascular effects include myocardial depression, hypotension, decreased cardiac output, heart block, bradycardia, arrhythmias, and cardiac arrest.[44] Disadvantages of such methods include the need for skillful technical application, need for frequent administration, and highly specialized followup procedures.

Special Considerations in Acute Pain

❶ ❷ ❹ ❻ ❽ The World Health Organization (WHO) recommends a three-step ladder approach using the simplest dosage schedules and medications with the least amount of potential harm based on pain intensity ratings from mild, to moderate, to severe.[23] An acute pain algorithm outlining how to use these principles is given in Figure 44-2. The importance of reassessment and titration during this process cannot be overemphasized.[28,52] Empiric or preemptive analgesia to prevent pain when anticipated should be considered particularly prior to procedures.[39]

Special Considerations in Cancer Pain

Managing the pain of cancer encompasses both acute and chronic management techniques. ❽ Thus, pharmacologic treatment and psychological therapies are best combined with surgical methods, anesthetic procedures, and supportive care measures in a multidisciplinary approach to pain relief. Assessment of the factors given in Table 44-2 also applies to cancer patients. Special attention must be given to continual reassessment of the painful state, adverse effects with medications, and aberrant behaviors. ❷ Individualization of therapy is always required.[23,29,53] Supportive care, in and outside the hospital, using programs such as hospice is one of the cancer patient's greatest allies, not only in coping with pain but also in accepting the disease. The positive effect this has on the patient cannot be overstated. Pharmacologic management is the mainstay of therapy, and a typical progression of analgesic use in oncology patients is outlined in Figure 44-3.

Special Considerations in Chronic Noncancer Pain

❽ Chronic noncancer pain is complex and therapeutic management should be multidisciplinary. Evaluation objectives include establishing an accurate diagnosis, identifying iatrogenic factors, obtaining a comprehensive psychiatric and psychosocial assessment, paying special attention to family and social problems, obtaining a description of factors that alleviate or exacerbate pain, and establishing effective goals of therapy.[2] ❾ In many cases the exact etiology of pain may not always be identifiable. ❽ In all cases of chronic noncancer pain, an integrated systematic approach (such as that often provided by specialty pain providers), with a strong emphasis on patient–clinician relationships, is essential. Patients and clinicians must realize that maximally effective treatment may take months or even years. The pharmacologic approach to common types of chronic noncancer pain is outlined in Table 44-8. Although opioids continue to be commonly utilized in the management of chronic noncancer pain and are often effective for individual patients, limited data have been published supporting long-term use of opioids. Thus, there is some debate regarding the benefit of chronic opioid therapy for chronic pain. However, when opioids are used, appropriate patient selection is critical to ensure optimal efficacy and minimal risks or negative outcomes. Steps should be taken to identify and manage risks prior to therapy and may include screening for risk of opioid misuse/abuse, utilizing treatment agreements that outline patient and provider expectations and responsibilities, and distinctly outlining the treatment plan with patients.[32] "Universal precautions" for pain management have been suggested as a method to standardize the assessment and ongoing management of chronic pain with opioids and incorporate many of these principles.[54]

Clinical **Controversy...**

Some clinicians believe that daily opioid doses in chronic noncancer patients should be limited because the risk of potential abuse and adverse effects may out-weigh the benefits. In fact, some guidelines have even incorporated recommendations to limit doses to less than 120 mg of morphine or its daily equivalent. Other clinicians believe by careful screening of patients for risks of abuse, frequent monitoring, identifying targeted pain symptoms, utilizing pain treatment "agreements," and distinctly outlining the treatment plans with patients, opioids can be titrated to effect, based on symptoms with no defined maximum dose.

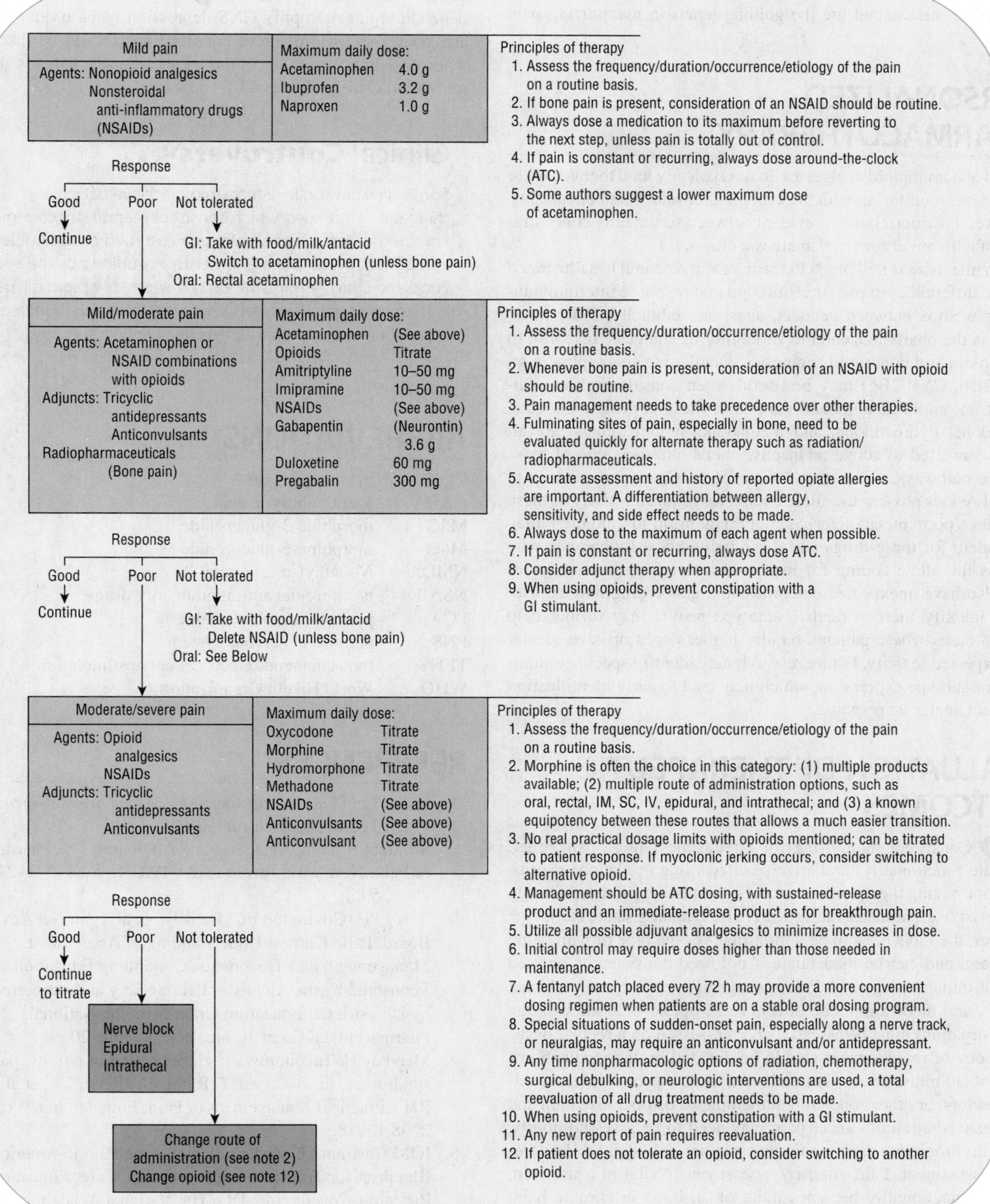

FIGURE 44-3 Algorithm for pain management in oncology patients. *(Data modified from the Kaiser Permanente Algorithm for Pain Management in Patients with Advanced Malignant Disease).*

Special Populations

The elderly and the young are at a higher risk for under-treatment because of inability to communicate or rate their pain. It is in these cases that parent or caregiver input becomes paramount to identify changes in behavior which might suggest pain (e.g., fussy, inconsolable, changes in eating patterns, crying out, or agitation). When patients cannot verbalize their pain (e.g., coma), monitoring behaviors (e.g., agitation) and physiologic signs and symptoms (e.g., heart rate) is appropriate.

3 8 In addition, those living with chronic, debilitating, and life-threatening illnesses need specialized pain control and care that is palliative in nature.[55] Although care must be taken in these populations to ensure that proper individualized treatment plans follow

accepted guidelines,[55–58] the key concepts in pain management as outlined in this chapter are the guiding tenets in maximizing pain control.

PERSONALIZED PHARMACOTHERAPY

Opioid and nonopioid analgesics do not typically lend themselves to serum level monitoring with the exception of select anticonvulsants. However, little correlation is evident between serum drug concentrations of anticonvulsants and analgesic efficacy.

While there is still much to learn, recent research has illustrated genetic differences in pain transmission and response interindividually as well as between genders, ages, and ethnicity. More interesting is the pharmacogenomic variability of analgesic response to both opioid and nonopioid analgesics. Qualitative genotyping (e.g., CYP 2D6, CYP 2B6) may be useful when considering the addition of an opioid metabolized via one of these enzymes. Codeine, oxycodone, hydrocodone, and methadone, among others, are all either converted to active or inactive metabolites via one of these enzyme pathways. Given that 1% to 3% of Caucasians and up to 30% of Asians possess the allele coding for reduced activity of these enzymes (poor metabolizer), genotyping prior to initiation may be prudent for these drugs and these individuals. Individuals who possess the allele coding for increased activity of these enzymes may also have unexpected outcomes, and genotyping may be useful to identify these patients. Genotype results may further help explain cases where patients require higher doses or have greater than expected toxicity. Future research may identify specific opioid-receptor subtype expression, which may lead to early identification of opioid analgesic response.[59]

EVALUATION OF THERAPEUTIC OUTCOMES

❷ ❻ Consistent monitoring for effectiveness (e.g., pain relief, adequate functionality) and adverse effects (e.g., sedation) is critical in optimizing therapeutic outcomes. Numerous validated scoring tools exist (e.g., numeric rating scale, visual analog scale, etc.);[3,60–62] however, the tools need to be appropriate for the type of pain being evaluated, and can be inadequate if not used consistently, or used without clinical judgment. Pain management efficacy, any change in pain, and medication side effects (e.g., opioid-induced sedation or constipation) must be assessed and reassessed on a regular basis. Frequency of reassessment should be dictated by the medication's route of administration, duration of action, various pharmacokinetic factors, or other concomitant therapies. Postoperative pain and acute exacerbation of cancer pain may need to be assessed hourly, whereas chronic noncancer pain may require only daily or less frequent assessment. Pain intensity assessment is vital in acute pain, whereas functionality becomes more of an issue in chronic pain. Quality of life must be assessed on a regular basis in all patients. Many advocate using the four "A"s (analgesia, activity, aberrant drug behavior, and adverse effects) as key assessment measures for any patient with chronic pain.[63]

It is important to note that often objective signs are lacking for pain evaluation. Acute pain may result in increased sympathetic tone (e.g., hypertension, tachycardia, and tachypnea); however, this response is usually diminished as acute pain progresses to chronic pain. The clinician must rely on the patient's description of their pain.[29]

❻ All opioids can cause constipation. The best management of constipation is prevention. Patients should be counseled on the proper intake of fluids and fiber. A stimulating laxative should be added with chronic opioid use. ❼ CNS depressants (e.g., alcohol, benzodiazepines) amplify CNS depression when used with opioid analgesics, and use of these combinations should be discouraged when possible. When the combinations are used, patients should be monitored closely (Tables 44-5 and 44-6).

Clinical **Controversy. . .**

Some clinicians believe that opioid risk evaluation and mitigation strategies, which consist of mandatory care-giver enrollment, prescriber training, patient medication guides, and patient prescriber agreements, as outlined by the Federal Food and Drug Administration will decrease opioid misuse and lead to better patient care. Others feel this leads to increased costs and becomes a barrier to effective pain therapy.

ABBREVIATIONS

COX-2	cyclooxygenase-2
GABA	γ-aminobutyric acid
M3G	morphine-3-glucuronide
M6G	morphine-6-glucuronide
NMDA	*N*-methyl-D-aspartate
NSAIDs	nonsteroidal antiinflammatory drugs
PCA	patient-controlled analgesia
PNS	peripheral nervous system
TENS	transcutaneous electrical nerve stimulation
WHO	World Health Organization

REFERENCES

1. Primo Levi Quote. *http://www.medscape.org/viewarticle/461612*. Last accessed July 2012.
2. Stimmel B. Pain, Analgesia and Addiction: The Pharmacology of Pain. New York: Raven Press, 1983:1, 2, 63, 241–245, 259, 266.
3. Berry PH, Covington EC, Dahl JL, et al. Editorial Advisory Board. Pain: Current Understanding of Assessment, Management, and Treatments. Continuing Education Sponsored by the American Pain Society and supported by Unrestricted Education Grant from the National Pharmaceutical Council, Inc. Release June 2006.
4. Merskey H. Taxonomy and classification of chronic pain syndromes. In: Benzon HT, Rathmell JP, Wu CL, et al., eds. Raj's Practical Management of Pain. Philadelphia, PA: Mosby, 2008:13–18.
5. IOM (Institute of Medicine). Relieving Pain in America: A Blueprint for Transforming Prevention, Care, Education, and Research. Washington, DC: The National Academic Press, 2011.
6. Health, United States, 2006 with Chartbook on Trends in the Health of Americans, Special Feature: Pain: 68–91. *http://www.cdc.gov/nchs/data/hus/hus06.pdf*. Last accessed May 2013.
7. Hahn KL. A decade of pain wasting away. Practical Pain Manag 2008;8:40–44.
8. Mandala M, Moro C, Labianca R, et al. Optimizing use of opiates in the management of cancer pain. Ther Clin Risk Manag 2006;2(4):447–453.
9. Decker SA, Culp KR, Cacchione PZ. Evaluation of musculoskeletal pain management practices in rural nursing

homes compared with evidence-based criteria. Pain Manag Nurs 2009;10(2):58–64.
10. Manchikanti L, Helm S, Fellows B, et al. Opioid epidemic in the United States. Pain Physician 2012;15(Suppl 3): ES9–ES38.
11. Pasero C, Portenoy R. Neurophysiology of pain and analgesia and the pathophysiology of neuropathic pain. In: McCaffery M, Pasero C, eds. Pain Assessment and Pharmacologic Management. St. Louis: Mosby, 2011:1–12.
12. Gold MS, Gebhart GF. Peripheral pain mechanisms and nociceptor sensitization. In: Fishman SM, Ballantyne JC, Rathmell JP, eds. Bonica's Pain Management. Baltimore, MD, Philadelphia, PA: Wolters Kluwer Health/Lippincott Williams & Wilkins, 2010:24–34.
13. High KN. Pain pathways: Peripheral, spinal, ascending, and descending pathways. In: Benzon HT, Rathmell JP, Wu CL, et al., eds. Raj's Practical Management of Pain. Philadelphia, PA: Mosby, 2008:119–134.
14. Lorenz J, Hauck M. Supraspinal mechanisms of pain and nociception. In: Fishman SM, Ballantyne JC, Rathmell JP, eds. Bonica's Pain Management. Baltimore, MD, Philadelphia, PA: Wolters Kluwer Health/Lippincott Williams & Wilkins, 2010:61–73.
15. Cortazzo MH, Fishman SM. Major opioids and chronic opioid therapy. In: Benzon HT, Rathmell JP, Wu CL, et al., eds. Raj's Practical Management of Pain. Philadelphia, PA: Mosby, 2008:597–611.
16. Randich A, Ness T. Modulation of spinal nociceptive processing. In: Fishman SM, Ballantyne JC, Rathmell JP, eds. Bonica's Pain Management. Baltimore, MD, Philadelphia, PA: Wolters Kluwer Health/Lippincott Williams & Wilkins, 2010:48–60.
17. Woolf CJ. Central sensitization: Implications for the diagnosis and treatment of pain. Pain 2011;152 (Suppl 3):S2–S15.
18. Apkarian A. Pain and brain changes. In: Benzon HT, Rathmell JP, Wu CL, et al., eds. Raj's Practical Management of Pain. Philadelphia, PA: Mosby, 2008:151–173.
19. Hanley MA, Jensen MP, Smith DG, et al. Preamputation pain and acute pain predict chronic pain after lower extremity amputation. J Pain 2007;8:102–109.
20. Latremoliere A, Woolf CJ. Central sensitization: A generator or pain hypersensitivity by central neural plasticity. J Pain 2009;10:895–926.
21. Breivik H, Borchgrevink PC, Allen SM, et al. Assessment of pain. Br J Anaesth 2008;101(1):17–24.
22. Twycross RG. Pain and analgesics. Curr Med Res Opin 1978;5:497–505.
23. Clinical Practice Guideline No. 9. Management of Cancer Pain. Publication No. 94-0592. Rockville, MD: Department of Health, Public Health Service, Agency for Health Care Policy and Research [now called Agency for Healthcare Research and Quality], 1994.
24. Grobios M, Benny B, Chan KT. Yaksh TL. Physical medicine techniques in pain management. In: Benzon HT, Rathmell JP, Wu CL, et al., eds. Raj's Practical Management of Pain. Philadelphia, PA: Mosby, 2008:135–149.
25. Turk D, Swanson K. Psychological interventions. In: Benzon HT, Rathmell JP, Wu CL, et al., eds. Raj's Practical Management of Pain. Philadelphia, PA: Mosby, 2008:739–755.
26. Chou R, Huffman LH. Nonpharmacologic therapies for acute and chronic low back pain: A review of the evidence for an American Pain Society/American College of Physicians Clinical Practice Guideline. Ann Intern Med 2007;147:492–504.
27. Simpson EL, Duenas A, Holmes, et al. Spinal cord stimulation for chronic pain of neuropathic or ischaemic origin: Systematic review and economic evaluation. Health Technol Assess 2009;13(1):1–154.
28. Clinical Practice Guideline. Acute Pain Management: Operative or Medical Procedures and Trauma. Publication No. 92-0032. Rockville, MD: Department of Health and Human Services, Public Health Service, Agency for Health Care Policy and Research [now called Agency for Healthcare Research and Quality], 1992.
29. American Pain Society. Principles of Analgesic Use in the Treatment of Acute Pain and Cancer Pain, 6th ed. Glenview, IL: American Pain Society, 2008.
30. Roelofs PD, Deyo RA, Koes BW, et al. Nonsteroidal anti-inflammatory drugs for low back pain: An updated Cochrane review. Spine 2008;33(16):1766–1774.
31. Roth SH, Fuller P. Diclofenac topical solution compared with oral diclofenac: A pooled safety analysis. J Pain Res 2011;4:159–167.
32. Chou R, Fanciullo GJ, Fine PG, et al. Clinical guidelines for the use of chronic opioid therapy in chronic noncancer pain. J Pain 2009;10:113–130.
33. Yaksh TL, Wallace MS. Opioids, analgesia, and pain management. In: Brunton LL, Chabner BA, Knollman BC, eds. The Pharmacological Basis of Therapeutics, 12th ed. New York: McGraw-Hill, 2011:481–525.
34. Pasternak G. Molecular insights into [mu] opioid pharmacology: From the clinic to the bench. Clin J Pain 2010:26;S3–S9.
35. Pasero C, Quinn TE, Portenoy RD, et al. Physiology and pharmacology of opioid analgesics. In: McCaffery M, Pasero C, eds. Pain Assessment and Pharmacologic Management. St. Louis: Mosby, 2011:283–300.
36. McPherson ML. Demystifying Opioid Conversion Calculations. A Guide For Effective Dosing. Bethesda, MD: American Society of Health-System Pharmacists, 2010.
37. Analgesic options for patients with allergic-type opioid reactions. Pharmacist's Lett/Prescriber's Lett 2006;22:220201.
38. Momeni M, Crucitti M, DeKock M. Patient controlled analgesia in the management of postoperative pain. Drugs 2006;66:2321–2337.
39. Pasero C, Quinn TE, Portenoy RD, et al. Key concepts in analgesic therapy. In: McCaffery M, Pasero C, eds. Pain Assessment and Pharmacologic Management. St. Louis: Mosby, 2011:301–322.
40. Melton S, Spencer S. Regional anesthesia techniques for acute pain management. In: Fishman SM, Ballantyne JC, Rathmell JP, eds. Bonica's Pain Management. Baltimore, MD, Philadelphia, PA: Wolters Kluwer Health/Lippincott Williams & Wilkins, 2010:723–754.
41. Horlocker TT, Burton AW, Connis RT, et al. Practice guidelines for the prevention, detection and management of respiratory depression associated with neuraxial opioid administration. Anesthesiology 2009;110:218–230.
42. Smith HS, Elliot JA. Opioid-induced androgen deficiency (OPIAD). Pain Physician 2012;15:ES145–E156.
43. American Hospital Formulary Service. In: McVoy GK, ed. Drug Information. Bethesda, MD: American Society of Health-System Pharmacists, 2009.
44. Facts and Comparisons On Line eAnswers. Wolters Kluwer Health. *http://online.factsandcomparisons.com/index.aspx.* Last accessed May 2013.
45. Pasero C, Quinn TE, Portenoy RD, et al. Guidelines for opioid drug selection. In: McCaffery M, Pasero C, eds. Pain Assessment and Pharmacologic Management. St. Louis: Mosby, 2011:323–367.

46. Krantz MJ, Martin J, Stimmel B, et al. QTc interval screening in methadone treatment. Ann Intern Med 2009; 150:387–395.
47. Tramadol [package insert]. Raritan, NJ: Ortho-McNeil, 2007.
48. Tapentadol [package insert]. Raritan NJ: PriCara, Division of Ortho-McNeil-Janssen Pharmaceuticals, Inc., 2009.
49. Dworkin RH, O'Connor AB, Audette J, et al. Recommendation for the pharmacologic management of neuropathic pain: An overview and literature update. May Clinic Proc 2010;85:S3–S14.
50. Schwartz S, Etropolski M, Shapir DY, et al. Safety and efficacy of tapentadol ER in patients with painful diabetic peripheral neuropathy: Results of a randomized-withdrawal, placebo-controlled trial. Curr Med Res Opin 2011;27(1):151–162.
51. Mitra R, Jones S. Adjuvant analgesics in cancer pain: A review. Am J Hosp Palliative Care 2012;29(1):70–79.
52. Practice Guidelines for Acute Pain Management in the Perioperative Setting. An updated report by the American Society of Anesthesiologists task force on acute pain management. Anesthesiology 2012;116:248–273.
53. National Comprehensive Cancer Network. Clinical Practice Guideline in Adult Cancer Pain, Version I, 2012.
54. Gourlay DL, Heit HA, Almahrezi A. Universal precautions in pain medicine: A rational approach to the treatment of chronic pain. Pain Med 2005;6(2):107–112.
55. Clinical Practice Guidelines for Quality Palliative Care, 2nd ed. National Consensus Project for Quality Palliative Care, 2009. *www.nationalconcensusproject.org*. Last accessed October 2012.
56. Clinical Practice Guideline, American Geriatrics Society Panel on Persistent Pain in Older Persons. The management of persistent pain in older persons. J Am Geriatr Soc 2009;57: 1331–1346.
57. American Academy of Pediatrics and American Pain Society. The assessment and management of acute pain in infants, children and adolescents. Pediatrics 2001;108:793–797.
58. Lago P, Garetti E, Merazzi D, et al. Guidelines for procedural pain in the newborn. Acta Paediatr 2009;98:932–939.
59. Muralidharan A, Smith MT. Pain, analgesia and genetics. J Pharm Pharmacol 2011;63:1387–1400.
60. National Institute of Health Pain Consortium. Pain Intensity Scales (last reviewed 1/17/2007). *http://painconsortium.nih.gov/pain_scales/index.html*. Last Accessed October 2012.
61. Calmels P, Mick G, Perrouin-Verbe B, et al. Neuropathic pain in spinal cord injury: Identification, classification, evaluation. Ann Phys Rehabil Med 2009;52:83–102.
62. Anderson KO. Assessment tools for the evaluation of pain in the oncology patient. Curr Pain Headache Rep 2007;11: 259–264.
63. Passik SD, Kirsh KL. Protecting your practice: Appropriate documentation for pain management. In: McCarbert BH, Passik SD, eds. Expert Guide to Pain Management. Philadelphia, PA: ACP Press, 2005:299–310.
64. Huang W, Shah S, Long Q, et al. Improvement of pain, sleep, and quality of life in chronic pain patients with vitamin D supplementation. Clin J Pain 2013;29(4):341–347.
65. Hagen K, Bjoro T, Zwart J, et al. Do high TSH values protect against chronic musculoskeletal complaints? The Nord-Trondelag Health Study (HUNT). Pain 2005;113:416–421.
66. Matoushek TA, Kearney TC, Lindsay TJ, et al. Loss of antinociceptive effectiveness of morphine and oxycodone following titration of levothyroxine: Case reports and a brief review of published literature. J Opioid Manag 2012;3: 193–198.
67. Okumus M, Ceceli E, Tuncay F, et al. The relationship between serum trace elements, vitamin B12, folic acid and clinical parameters in patients with myofascial pain syndrome. Back Musculoskelet Rehabil 2010;23(4):187–191.
68. Lexicomp Online. Wolters Kluwer Health. *https://online.lexi.com/lco/action/home;jsessionid=f0470bd1a69f3d8efec2b4892c36*. Last accessed May 2013.
69. Li F. Pharmacologically induced histamine release: Sorting out hypersensitivity reactions to opioids. Drug Therapy Topics 2006;35:1, 14–16.
70. Watkins PB, Kaplowitz N, Slattery TJ, et al. Aminotransferase elevations in healthy adults receiving 4 grams of acetaminophen daily: A randomized controlled trial. JAMA 2006;296:87–93.
71. Herndon CM, Hutchison RW, Berdine HJ, et al. Management of chronic nonmalignant pain with nonsteroidal anti-inflammatory drugs. Pharmacotherapy 2008;28:788–805.
72. Porche RA, ed. Approaches to pain management, an essential guide for clinical leaders. Oakbrook Terrace, IL: Joint Commission Resources, 2010:3–4.
73. Carville SF, Arendt-Nielsen SA, Biddal H, et al. EULAR evidence based recommendations for the management of fibromyalgia syndrome. Ann Rheu Dis 2008;67:536–541.
74. Traynor LM, Thiessen CN, Traynor AP. Pharmacotherapy of fibromyalgia. Am J Health-Sys Pharm 2011;68:1307–1319.
75. Chou R, Qaseem A, Snow V, et al. Diagnosis and treatment of low back pain: A Joint Clinical Practice Guideline from the American College of Physicians and American Pain Society. Ann Intern Med 2007;147:478–491.
76. Chou R. Pharmacologic management of low back pain. Drugs 2010;70:387–402.
77. Pasero C, Quinn TE, Portenoy RD, et al. Initiating Opioid Therapy. In: McCaffery M, Pasero C, eds. Pain Assessment and Pharmacologic Management. St. Louis: Mosby, 2011:442–461.

45

Headache Disorders

Deborah S. Minor and Marion R. Wofford

KEY CONCEPTS

1. Acute migraine therapies should provide consistent, rapid relief and enable the patient to resume normal activities at home, school, or work.
2. A stratified care approach, in which the selection of initial treatment is based on headache-related disability and symptom severity, is the preferred treatment strategy for the migraineur.
3. Strict adherence to maximum daily and weekly doses of antimigraine medications is essential.
4. Preventive therapy should be considered in the setting of recurring migraines that produce significant disability; frequent attacks requiring symptomatic medication more than twice per week; symptomatic therapies that are ineffective or contraindicated, or produce serious side effects; and uncommon migraine variants that cause profound disruption and/or risk of neurologic injury.
5. The selection of an agent for headache prophylaxis should be based on individual patient response, tolerability, convenience of the drug formulation, and coexisting conditions.
6. Each prophylactic medication should be given an adequate therapeutic trial (usually 6 months) to judge its maximal efficacy.
7. A general wellness program and avoidance of headache triggers should be included in the management plan.
8. After an effective abortive agent and dose have been identified, subsequent treatments should begin with that same regimen.

Headache is one of the most common complaints encountered by healthcare practitioners and among the top three principal reasons given by adults 18 years of age and over for visiting U.S. emergency departments.[1] It can be symptomatic of a distinct pathologic process or can occur without an underlying cause. In 2004, the International Headache Society (IHS) updated its classification system and diagnostic criteria for headache disorders, cranial neuralgias, and facial pain[2] (Table 45-1). Designed to facilitate headache diagnosis in clinical practice and research, the IHS classification provides more precise definitions and standardized nomenclature for both the primary (tension-type, migraine, and cluster headache) and secondary (symptomatic of organic disease) headache disorders. This chapter focuses on the management of the primary headache disorders.

Most recurrent headaches are the result of a benign chronic primary headache disorder.[3] Less often, headaches are symptomatic of a serious underlying medical condition, such as infection, cerebral hemorrhage, or brain mass lesion. The peak prevalence of tension-type and migraine headache, the most common of the primary headache disorders, occurs during the most productive years of life (18 to 59 years of age).[3,4] Despite the prevalence of these disorders and their associated disability, studies indicate that most headache sufferers do not seek appropriate medical care for their headaches.[4,5] An improved understanding of the diagnosis and pathophysiologic mechanisms of the primary headache disorders, particularly migraine, has led to the development of medications capable of providing rapid relief from moderate to severe attacks. However, a thorough evaluation of the headache history is essential to establish an accurate headache diagnosis and identify patients who can benefit from these specific therapeutic options.

MIGRAINE HEADACHE

Epidemiology

Results of the American Migraine Prevalence and Prevention Study indicate that 17.1% of women and 5.6% of men in the United States experience one or more migraine headaches per year. The prevalence of migraine varies considerably by age and gender, but the epidemiologic profile has remained stable over the past 15 years. After age 12, females are two to three times more likely than males to suffer from migraine. Gender differences in migraine prevalence have been linked to menstruation, but these differences persist beyond menopause. Prevalence is highest in both men and women between the ages of 30 and 49 years.[4] In the American Migraine Prevalence and Prevention Study, 93% of those with migraine reported some headache-related disability, and 54% were severely disabled or needed bedrest during an attack.[4] A number of neurologic and psychiatric disorders as well as cardiovascular diseases, including stroke, epilepsy, major depression, sleep apnea, obesity, and anxiety disorder, show increased comorbidity with migraine.[5–7] Whether this relationship is causal or representative of a common pathophysiologic mechanism is unknown. The economic burden of migraine is substantial; however, the indirect costs from work-related disability far exceed the direct costs associated with treatment.[7,8]

Etiology and Pathophysiology

The etiologic and pathophysiologic mechanisms of migraine are not completely understood. According to earlier theories, the migraine aura was caused by intracerebral arterial vasoconstriction followed by reactive extracranial vasodilation and associated headache. Studies of regional blood flow in the brain do not support this hypothesis, and previous vascular and neural theories of migraine development have merged into a combined theory of neurovascular mechanisms. Most clinicians now believe that the pathogenesis of migraine may be related to complex dysfunctions in neuronal and broad sensory processing.[2,5,9]

TABLE 45-1 International Headache Society Classification System: Focus on Migraine Headache

Migraine
Migraine without aura
Migraine with aura
Typical aura with migraine headache (aura lasting less than 1 hour)
Typical aura with nonmigraine headache
Typical aura without headache
Familial hemiplegic migraine
Sporadic hemiplegic migraine
Basilar-type migraine
Childhood periodic syndromes that are commonly precursors of migraine
Cyclic vomiting (self-limiting episodic condition)
Abdominal migraine (episodic midline abdominal pain attacks lasting 1–72 hours)
Benign paroxysmal vertigo of childhood (brief episodic vertigo)
Retinal migraine (repeated attacks of monocular visual disturbance)
Complications of migraine
Chronic migraine (occurring on 15 or more days/mo for more than 3 months)
Status migrainous (debilitating attack lasting for more than 72 hours)
Persistent aura without infarction (symptoms persisting for more than 1 week)
Migrainous infarction (aura symptoms associated with an ischemic brain lesion)
Migraine-triggered seizure
Probable migraine
Probable migraine without aura
Probable migraine with aura
Probable chronic migraine
Tension-type headache
Cluster headache and other trigeminal autonomic cephalalgias
Other primary headaches
Headache attributed to head and/or neck trauma
Headache attributed to cranial or cervical vascular disorder
Headache attributed to nonvascular intracranial disorder
Headache attributed to a substance or its withdrawal
Headache attributed to infection
Headache attributed to disorder of homeostasis
Headache or facial pain attributed to disorder of cranium, neck, eyes, ears, nose, sinuses, teeth, mouth, or other facial or cranial structures
Headache attributed to psychiatric disorder
Cranial neuralgias and central causes of facial pain
Other headache, cranial neuralgia, central or primary facial pain

Adapted with permission from reference 2.

The pain and symptoms of migraine may be understood as a combination of altered perceptions resulting from neural suppression and activation of subcortical structures and trigeminal systems. Migraine pain is believed to result from activity within the trigeminovascular system, a network of visceral afferent fibers that arises from the trigeminal ganglia and projects peripherally to innervate the pain-sensitive intracranial extracerebral blood vessels, dura mater, and large venous sinuses[10] (Fig. 45-1). These fibers also project centrally, terminating in the trigeminal nucleus caudalis in the brain stem and upper cervical spinal cord, and thus provide a pathway for nociceptive transmission from meningeal blood vessels into higher centers of the CNS. Activation of trigeminal sensory nerves triggers the release of vasoactive neuropeptides, including calcitonin gene–related peptide (CGRP), neurokinin A, and substance P, from perivascular axons. The released neuropeptides interact with dural blood vessels to promote vasodilation and dural plasma extravasation, resulting in neurogenic inflammation. Orthodromic conduction along trigeminovascular fibers transmits pain impulses to the trigeminal nucleus caudalis, where information is relayed further to higher cortical pain centers. Continued afferent input can result in sensitization of these central sensory neurons, producing a hyperalgesic state that responds to previously innocuous stimuli and maintains the headache.[5,9–11]

Aura occurs in a subgroup of migraineurs and also with the other primary headache disorders. The neurologic changes of the aura parallel those that occur during cortical spreading depression, a neuronal event characterized by a wave of depressed electrical activity that advances across the brain cortex at a rate consistent with the spread of aura symptoms.[5,9] Cortical spreading depression can cause inflammation and activation of the trigeminal nucleus caudalis. It is not clear whether this cortical spreading depression and the aura are the substrate of pain or actually trigger the presentation of migraine.[5,11]

Genetic factors seem to play an important role in susceptibility to migraine attacks. Studies in monozygotic twins suggest approximately 50% heritability of migraine with a multifactorial polygenic basis.[12] Although it is possible for any individual to experience a migraine attack, it is recurrence in the migraineur that is abnormal. Attack occurrence and frequency are governed by CNS sensitivity to migraine-specific triggers or environmental factors. Migraineurs appear to have a lowered threshold of response to specific environmental circumstances as a result of genetic factors that govern the balance of CNS excitation and inhibition at various levels.[12] Thus, trigger factors can be viewed as modulators of the genetic set point that predisposes to migraine headache. The hyperresponsiveness of the migrainous brain may be the result of an inherited abnormality in calcium and/or sodium channels and sodium/potassium pumps that regulate cortical excitability through the release of serotonin (5-hydroxytryptamine [5-HT]) and other neurotransmitters. Increased levels of excitatory amino acids such as glutamate and alterations in levels of extracellular potassium also can affect the migraine threshold and initiate and propagate the phenomenon of cortical spreading depression.[5,12,13]

5-HT has long been implicated as an important mediator of migraine headache. Specific populations of 5-HT receptor subfamilies appear to be involved in the pathophysiology and treatment of migraine headache. Acute antimigraine drugs such as the ergot alkaloids and triptan derivatives are agonists of vascular and neuronal 5-HT_1 receptor subtypes, resulting in vasoconstriction of meningeal blood vessels and inhibition of vasoactive neuropeptide release and pain signal transmission.[5,14] Drugs used for migraine prophylaxis also modulate neurotransmitter systems.[9] These actions and benefits in migraine management are consistent with the current understanding of migraine pathophysiology and neurovascular disorders.

Clinical Presentation

The migraine attack has been divided into several phases. *Premonitory symptoms* are experienced by 12% to 79% of migraineurs in the hours or days before the onset of headache.[2,5,15] The previously popular terms *prodrome* and *warning symptoms* should be avoided because these are often used mistakenly to include aura.[2] Premonitory symptoms vary widely among migraineurs but usually are consistent within an individual. Neurologic symptoms (e.g., allodynia, phonophobia, photophobia, hyperosmia, and difficulty concentrating) are common, but psychological (e.g., anxiety, depression, euphoria, irritability, drowsiness, fatigue, hyperactivity, and restlessness), autonomic (e.g., polyuria, diarrhea, and constipation), and constitutional (e.g., stiff neck, yawning, thirst, food cravings, and anorexia) symptoms also are reported.[2,5,15]

The migraine *aura*, a complex of positive and negative focal neurologic symptoms that precedes or accompanies an attack, is experienced by approximately 25% of migraineurs on some occasions.[2,15] The aura typically evolves over 5 to 20 minutes and lasts less than 60 minutes. Headache usually occurs within 60 minutes of the end of the aura. Occasionally, aura symptoms begin at the onset of headache or during the attack. The aura is most often visual and frequently affects half the visual field.[2] Visual auras vary in their complexity and can include both positive (scintillations, photopsia, teichopsia, or fortification spectrum) and negative (scotoma,

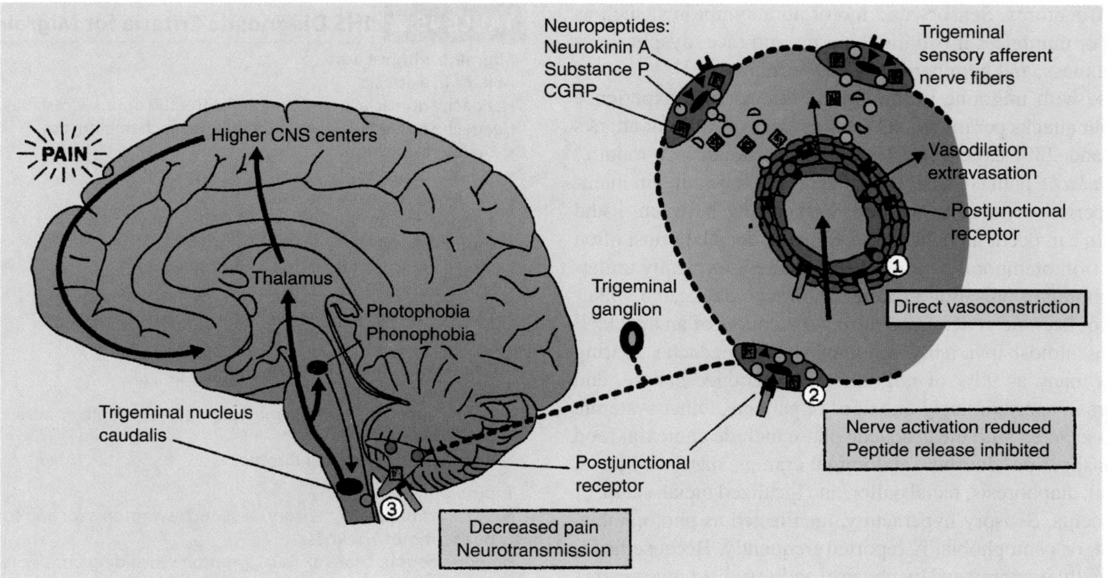

FIGURE 45-1 The pathophysiology of migraine headache. Vasodilation of intracranial extracerebral blood vessels (possibly the result of an imbalance in the brain stem) results in the activation of the perivascular trigeminal nerves that release vasoactive neuropeptides to promote neurogenic inflammation. Central pain transmission may activate other brain stem nuclei, resulting in associated symptoms (nausea, vomiting, photophobia, phonophobia). The antimigraine effects of the 5-HT1B/ID receptor agonists are highlighted at areas 1, 2, and 3. (CGRP, calcitonin gene–related peptide.) *(Reprinted from reference 10, Copyright © 1998, with permission from Elsevier.).*

CLINICAL PRESENTATION Migraine Headache

General

- Migraine is a common, recurrent, severe headache that interferes with normal functioning. It is a primary headache disorder divided into two major subtypes, migraine without aura and migraine with aura.

Symptoms

- Migraine is characterized by recurring episodes of throbbing head pain, frequently unilateral, that when untreated can last from 4 to 72 hours. Migraine headaches can be severe and associated with nausea, vomiting, and sensitivity to light, sound, and/or movement. Not all symptoms are present at every attack.
- In the headache evaluation, diagnostic alarms should be identified. These include: acute onset of the "first" or "worst" headache ever, accelerating pattern of headache following subacute onset, onset of headache after age 50 years, headache associated with systemic illness (e.g., fever, nausea, vomiting, stiff neck, and rash), headache with focal neurologic symptoms or papilledema, and new-onset headache in a patient with cancer or human immunodeficiency virus (HIV) infection.

Signs

- A stable pattern, absence of daily headache, positive family history for migraine, normal neurologic examination, presence of food triggers, menstrual association, long-standing history, improvement with sleep, and subacute evolution are all signs of migraine headache. Aura can signal the migraine headache but is not required for diagnosis.

Laboratory Tests

- In selected circumstances and secondary headache presentation, serum chemistries, urine toxicology profiles, thyroid function tests, Lyme's disease studies, and other blood tests such as a complete blood count, antinuclear antibody titer, erythrocyte sedimentation rate, and antiphospholipid antibody titer can be considered.

Diagnostic Tests

- Perform a general medical and neurologic physical examination. Check for abnormalities: vital signs (fever, hypertension), funduscopy (papilledema, hemorrhage, and exudates), palpation and auscultation of the head and neck (sinus tenderness, hardened or tender temporal arteries, trigger points, temporomandibular joint tenderness, bruits, nuchal rigidity, and cervical spine tenderness), and neurologic examination (identify abnormalities or deficits in mental status, cranial nerves, deep tendon reflexes, motor strength, coordination, gait, and cerebellar function). Consider neuroimaging studies in patients with abnormal neurologic examination findings of unknown etiology and in those with additional risk factors warranting imaging.

hemianopsia) features. Sensory and motor aura symptoms, such as paresthesias or numbness involving the arms and face, dysphasia or aphasia, weakness, and hemiparesis, also are reported.[2,15]

Of those with migraine in the United States, 14% experience more than four attacks per month, 63% experience one to four attacks per month, and 23% experience less than one attack per month.[4] Migraine *headache* pain is usually gradual in onset, peaking in intensity over a period of minutes to hours and lasting between 4 and 72 hours. Pain can occur anywhere in the face or head but most often involves the frontotemporal region. The headache is typically unilateral and throbbing or pulsating in nature; however, pain can be bilateral at onset or become generalized during the course of an attack.[2,15] GI symptoms almost invariably accompany the headache. During an attack, as many as 90% of migraineurs experience nausea, and emesis occurs in approximately one third of patients. Other systemic symptoms associated with the headache phase include anorexia, food cravings, constipation, diarrhea, abdominal cramps, nasal stuffiness, blurred vision, diaphoresis, facial pallor, and localized facial, scalp, or periorbital edema. Sensory hyperacuity, manifested as photophobia, phonophobia, or osmophobia, is reported frequently. Because headache pain usually is aggravated by physical activity, most migraineurs seek a dark, quiet room for rest and relief. Impaired concentration, depression, irritability, fatigue, or anxiety often accompanies the headache. Once headache pain wanes, patients may experience a *resolution phase* characterized by feeling tired, exhausted, irritable, or listless. Impaired concentration may continue, as well as scalp tenderness or mood changes. Some patients experience depression and malaise, whereas others can feel unusually refreshed or euphoric.[2,15] The reader is referred to the IHS classification and recent reviews for descriptions of the classic migraine variants and other migraine subtypes[2,15] (Table 45-1).

Although headaches have many potential causes, most are considered to be primary headache disorders. A comprehensive headache history is the most important element in establishing the clinical diagnosis of migraine.[5,16] A thorough headache history always should be obtained, and information collected should include age at onset, attack frequency and timing, duration of attacks, precipitating or aggravating factors, ameliorating factors, description of neurologic symptoms, characteristics of the headache pain (quality, intensity, location, and radiation), associated signs and symptoms, treatment history, family and social history, and the impact of headaches on daily life.

Secondary headache can be identified or excluded based on the headache history, as well as the results of general medical and neurologic examinations. Diagnostic and laboratory testing also can be warranted in the setting of suspicious headache features or an abnormal examination. The routine use of neuroimaging (computed tomography or magnetic resonance imaging) generally is not indicated in patients with migraine and a normal neurologic examination, but should be considered in patients with an unexplained abnormal neurologic examination or an atypical headache history.[2,3,15] Because migraine headaches usually begin by the second or third decade of life, headaches beginning after age 50 years suggest an organic etiology such as a mass lesion, cerebrovascular disease, or temporal arteritis. Table 45-2 lists the IHS diagnostic criteria for migraine with and without aura.[2]

TABLE 45-2 IHS Diagnostic Criteria for Migraine

Migraine without aura
At least five attacks
Headache attack lasts 4–72 hours (untreated or unsuccessfully treated)
Headache has at least two of the following characteristics:
- Unilateral location
- Pulsating quality
- Moderate or severe intensity
- Aggravation by or avoidance of routine physical activity (i.e., walking or climbing stairs)

During headache at least one of the following:
- Nausea, vomiting, or both
- Photophobia and phonophobia
- Not attributed to another disorder

Migraine with aura (classic migraine)
At least two attacks
Migraine aura fulfills criteria for typical aura, hemiplegic aura, or basilar-type aura
Not attributed to another disorder

Typical aura
Fully reversible visual, sensory, or speech symptoms (or any combination) but no motor weakness
Homonymous or bilateral visual symptoms including positive features (e.g., flickering lights, spot, lines) or negative features (e.g., loss of vision) or unilateral sensory symptoms including positive features (e.g., visual loss, pins and needles) or negative features (i.e., numbness), or any combination
At least one of the following:
- At least one symptom that develops gradually over a minimum of 5 minutes or different symptoms that occur in succession or both
- Each symptom lasts for at least 5 minutes and for no longer than 60 minutes
- Headache that meets criteria for migraine without aura begins during the aura or follows aura within 60 minutes

IHS, International Headache Society.
Adapted with permission from reference 2.

TREATMENT
Migraines

Desired Outcome

Clinicians who care for migraineurs must appreciate the impact of this painful and debilitating disorder on the life of the patient, the patient's family, and the patient's employer. Treatment strategies must address both immediate and long-term goals. (1) Acute migraine therapies should provide consistent, rapid relief and enable the patient to resume normal activities at home, school, or work. Recurrence of symptoms and treatment-related adverse effects should be minimal. Ideally, patients should be able to manage their own headaches effectively without a medical visit. In addition, migraineurs should take an active role in the creation of a long-term formal management plan. An individualized approach to treatment can result in a reduction in attack frequency and severity, thus minimizing headache-related disability and emotional distress and improving the patient's quality of life. Goals of long-term and acute treatment of migraine are listed in Table 45-3.[14,16]

TABLE 45-3 Goals of Therapy in Migraine Management

Goals of long-term migraine treatment
Reduce migraine frequency, severity, and disability
Reduce reliance on poorly tolerated, ineffective, or unwanted acute pharmacotherapies
Improve quality of life
Prevent headache
Avoid escalation of headache medication use
Educate and enable patients to manage their disease
Reduce headache-related distress and psychological symptoms

Goals for acute migraine treatment
Treat migraine attacks rapidly and consistently without recurrence
Restore the patient's ability to function
Minimize the use of backup and rescue medications[a]
Optimize self-care for overall management
Be cost-effective in overall management
Cause minimal or no adverse effects

[a]Rescue medications are defined as medications used at home when other treatments fail that permit the patient to get relief without a visit to the physician's office or emergency department.
Data from references 14, 16, and 17.

General Approach to Treatment

Nonpharmacologic and pharmacologic interventions are available for the management of migraine headache; however, drug therapy remains the mainstay of treatment for most patients. Pharmacotherapeutic management of migraine can be acute (i.e., symptomatic or abortive) or preventive (i.e., prophylactic). When choosing acute or preventive therapies, the clinician should consider the patient's response to specific medications and their tolerability, as well as coexisting illnesses that can limit treatment choices. Abortive or acute therapies can be migraine-specific (e.g., ergots and triptans) or nonspecific (e.g., analgesics, antiemetics, nonsteroidal antiinflammatory drugs [NSAIDs], and corticosteroids) and are most effective at relieving pain and associated symptoms when administered at the onset of migraine[14,16,17] (Table 45-4). 2 A stratified care approach in which the selection of initial treatment is based on headache-related disability and symptom severity is the preferred treatment strategy for the migraineur.[14,16]

TABLE 45-4 Drug Dosing Table—Acute Migraine Therapies[a]

Drug	Dose	Usual Range/Comments
Analgesics		
Acetaminophen (Tylenol)	1,000 mg at onset; repeat every 4–6 hours as needed	Maximum daily dose is 4 g
Acetaminophen 250 mg/aspirin 250 mg/caffeine 65 mg (Excedrin Migraine)	2 tablets at onset and every 6 hours	Available as nonprescription medication as Excedrin Migraine
Nonsteroidal Antiinflammatory Drugs		
Aspirin	500–1,000 mg every 4–6 hours	Maximum daily dose is 4 g
Ibuprofen (Motrin)	200–800 mg every 6 hours	Avoid doses >2.4 g/day
Naproxen sodium (Aleve, Anaprox)	550–825 mg at onset; can repeat 220 mg in 3–4 hours	Avoid doses >1.375 g/day
Diclofenac (Cataflam, Voltaren)	50–100 mg at onset; can repeat 50 mg in 8 hours	Avoid doses >150 mg/day
Ergotamine Tartrate		
Oral tablet (1 mg) with caffeine 100 mg (Cafergot)	2 mg at onset; then 1–2 mg every 30 minutes as needed	Maximum dose is 6 mg/day or 10 mg/wk; consider pretreatment with an antiemetic
Sublingual tablet (2 mg) (Ergomar)		
Rectal suppository (2 mg) with caffeine 100 mg (Cafergot, Migergot)	Insert 0.5 to 1 suppository at onset; repeat after 1 hour as needed	Maximum dose is 4 mg/day or 10 mg/wk; consider pretreatment with an antiemetic
Dihydroergotamine		
Injection 1 mg/mL (D.H.E. 45)	0.25–1 mg at onset IM, IV, or subcutaneous; repeat every hour as needed	Maximum dose is 3 mg/day or 6 mg/wk
Nasal spray 4 mg/mL (Migranal)	One spray (0.5 mg) in each nostril at onset; repeat sequence 15 minutes later (total dose is 2 mg or four sprays)	Maximum dose is 3 mg/day; prime sprayer four times before using; do not tilt head back or inhale through nose while spraying; discard open ampules after 8 hours
Serotonin Agonists (Triptans)		
Sumatriptan (Imitrex)		
Injection	6 mg subcutaneous at onset; can repeat after 1 hour if needed	Maximum daily dose is 12 mg
Oral tablets	25, 50, 85, or 100 mg at onset; can repeat after 2 hours if needed	Optimal dose is 50–100 mg; maximum daily dose is 200 mg; combination product with naproxen, 85/500 mg
Nasal spray	5, 10, or 20 mg at onset; can repeat after 2 hours if needed	Optimal dose is 20 mg; maximum daily dose is 40 mg; single-dose device delivering 5 or 20 mg; administer one spray in one nostril
Zolmitriptan (Zomig, Zomig-ZMT)		
Oral tablets	2.5 or 5 mg at onset as regular or orally disintegrating tablet; can repeat after 2 hours if needed	Optimal dose is 2.5 mg; maximum dose is 10 mg/day
		Do not divide ODT dosage form
Nasal spray	5 mg (one spray) at onset; can repeat after 2 hours if needed	Maximum daily dose is 10 mg/day
Naratriptan (Amerge)	1 or 2.5 mg at onset; can repeat after 4 hours if needed	Optimal dose is 2.5 mg; maximum daily dose is 5 mg
Rizatriptan (Maxalt, Maxalt-MLT)	5 or 10 mg at onset as regular or orally disintegrating tablet; can repeat after 2 hours if needed	Optimal dose is 10 mg; maximum daily dose is 30 mg; onset of effect is similar with standard and orally disintegrating tablets; use 5-mg dose (15 mg/day maximum) in patients receiving propranolol
Almotriptan (Axert)	6.25 or 12.5 mg at onset; can repeat after 2 hours if needed	Optimal dose is 12.5 mg; maximum daily dose is 25 mg
Frovatriptan (Frova)	2.5 or 5 mg at onset; can repeat in 2 hours if needed	Optimal dose 2.5–5 mg; maximum daily dose is 7.5 mg (three tablets)
Eletriptan (Relpax)	20 or 40 mg at onset; can repeat after 2 hours if needed	Maximum single dose is 40 mg; maximum daily dose is 80 mg
Miscellaneous		
Metoclopramide (Reglan)	10 mg IV at onset	Useful for acute relief in the office or emergency department setting
Prochlorperazine (Compazine)	10 mg IV or IM at onset	Useful for acute relief in the office or emergency department setting

ODT, orally disintegrating tablet.

[a]Limit use of symptomatic medications to fewer than 10 days/mo when possible to avoid medication-misuse headache.

Data from references 14, 18, and 28.

Because attack severity varies in individuals, patients may be advised to use nonspecific agents for mild to moderate headache not causing disability while reserving migraine-specific medications for more severe attacks. The absorption and efficacy of orally administered drugs can be compromised by gastric stasis or nausea and vomiting that accompany migraine. Pretreatment with antiemetic agents or the use of nonoral treatment (e.g., suppositories, nasal sprays, or injections) is advisable when nausea and vomiting are severe.[14,18]

The frequent or excessive use of acute migraine medications can result in a pattern of increasing headache frequency and drug consumption known as *medication-overuse headache* (or *rebound headache*).[2,5,19] The syndrome appears to evolve as a self-sustaining headache–medication cycle in which the headache returns as the medication wears off, leading to the consumption of more drug for relief. The headache history often reflects the gradual onset of an atypical daily or near-daily headache with superimposed episodic migraine attacks. Medication overuse is one of the most common causes of chronic daily headache.[19] Agents most commonly implicated in this syndrome include simple and combination analgesics and opiates. Triptans are also implicated but only in men with a high frequency of headaches.[2,5,19] Discontinuation of the offending agent leads to a gradual decrease in headache frequency and severity and a return of the original headache characteristics. Although detoxification usually can be accomplished on an outpatient basis, hospitalization can be necessary for the control of refractory rebound headache and other withdrawal symptoms (e.g., nausea, vomiting, asthenia, restlessness, and agitation). **3** Regulation of nociceptive systems and renewed responsiveness to therapy usually occur within 2 months following medication withdrawal.[2] Most experts recommend limiting use of acute migraine therapies to *fewer than 10 days per month* to avoid the development of medication-misuse headache.[20]

Preventive migraine therapies are administered on a daily basis to reduce the frequency, severity, and duration of attacks and improve responsiveness to symptomatic migraine therapies[8,21,22] (Table 45-5).

TABLE 45-5 Drug Dosing Table—Prophylactic Migraine Therapies

Drug	Initial Dose	Usual Range	Comments
β-Adrenergic Antagonists			
Atenolol[a] (Tenormin)	50 mg/day	50–200 mg/day	
Metoprolol[b] (Toprol, Toprol XL)	100 mg/day in divided doses	100–200 mg/day in divided doses	Dose short-acting four times a day and long-acting two times a day; available as extended release
Nadolol[a] (Corgard)	40–80 mg/day	80–240 mg/day	
Propranolol[b] (Inderal, Inderal LA)	40 mg/day in divided doses	40–160 mg/day in divided doses	Dose short-acting two to three times a day and long-acting one to two times a day; available as extended release
Timolol[b] (Blocadren)	20 mg/day in divided doses	20–60 mg/day in divided doses	
Antidepressants			
Amitriptyline[a] (Elavil)	10 mg at bedtime	20–50 mg at bedtime	
Venlafaxine[a] (Effexor, Effexor XR)	37.5 mg/day	75–150 mg/day	Available as extended release; increase dose after 1 week
Anticonvulsants			
Topiramate[b] (Topamax)	25 mg/day	50–200 mg/day in divided doses	As effective as amitriptyline, propranolol, or valproate; increase by 25 mg/wk
Valproic acid/divalproex sodium[b] (Depakene, Depakote, Depakote ER)	250–500 mg/day in divided doses, or daily for extended release	500–1,500 mg/day in divided doses, or daily for extended release	Monitor levels if compliance is an issue
Nonsteroidal Antiinflammatory Drugs			
Ibuprofen[a] (Motrin)	400–1,200 mg/day in divided doses	Same as initial dose	Use intermittently, such as for menstrual migraine prevention; daily or prolonged use may lead to medication-overuse headache and is limited by potential toxicity
Ketoprofen[a] (Orudis)	150 mg/day in divided doses	Same as initial dose	
Naproxen sodium[a] (Aleve, Anaprox)	550–1,100 mg/day in divided doses	Same as initial dose	
Serotonin Agonists (Triptans)			
Frovatriptan[b] (Frova)	2.5 or 5 mg/day in divided doses	Same as initial dose	Taken in the perimenstrual period to prevent menstrual migraine
Naratriptan[a] (Amerge)	2 mg/day in divided doses	Same as initial dose	
Zolmitriptan[a] (Zomig)	5–7.5 mg/day in divided doses	Same as initial dose	
Miscellaneous			
Histamine[a] (Histatrol)	1–10 ng two times per week	Same as initial dose	May cause transient itching and burning at injection site
Magnesium[a]	400 mg/day	800 mg/day in divided doses	May be more helpful in migraine with aura and menstrual migraine
MIG-99[a] (feverfew)	10–100 mg/day in divided doses	Same as initial dose	Withdrawal may be associated with increased headaches
Petasites[b]	100–150 mg/day in divided doses	150 mg/day in divided doses	Use only commercial preparations; plant is carcinogenic
Riboflavin[a]	400 mg/day in divided doses	400 mg/day in divided doses	Benefit only after 3 months

[a]Level B—probably effective (one Class I or two Class II studies).
[b]Level A—established efficacy (≥2 Class I studies).

Per American Academy of Neurology therapeutic classification of evidence, and references 21 and 31.
Data from references 8, 21–23, and 31.

4 Preventive therapy should be considered in the setting of recurring migraines that produce significant disability despite acute therapy; frequent attacks occurring more than twice per week with the risk of developing medication-overuse headache; symptomatic therapies that are ineffective or contraindicated, or produce serious side effects; uncommon migraine variants that cause profound disruption and/or risk of permanent neurologic injury (e.g., hemiplegic migraine, basilar migraine, and migraine with prolonged aura); and patient preference to limit the number of attacks.[8,23] Preventive therapy also may be administered preemptively or intermittently when headaches recur in a predictable pattern (e.g., exercise-induced migraine or menstrual migraine).[7] The evidence to support the various agents used for migraine prophylaxis has recently been reviewed. Only propranolol, timolol, divalproex sodium, and topiramate are currently approved by the FDA for the indication, although other agents have established or probable efficacy. **5** Guidelines identify which agents might be effective, but there is insufficient evidence as to how to choose one therapy over another. Thus, the selection of an agent typically is based on its side effect profile and the patient's coexisting/comorbid conditions.[16,21] **6** A therapeutic trial of 2 to 3 months is necessary to achieve clinical benefit, but some reduction in attack frequency can be evident by the first month of therapy. Maximal benefits are typically observed by 6 months of treatment.[7,8,21] Drug therapy should be initiated with low doses and gradually increased until a therapeutic effect is achieved or side effects become intolerable. Drug doses for migraine prophylaxis are often lower than those necessary for other indications.[7,8] Overuse of acute headache medications will interfere with the effects of preventive treatment.[16,19] Prophylactic treatment usually is continued for at least 6 to 12 months after the frequency and severity of headaches have diminished. After that time, based on discussions with the patient, gradual tapering or discontinuation may be reasonable.[8,21] Many migraineurs experience fewer and less severe attacks for lengthy periods following discontinuation of prophylactic medications or taper to a lower dose. Figures 45-2 and 45-3 identify treatment and management algorithms for migraine headache.

Nonpharmacologic Therapy

Nonpharmacologic therapy of acute migraine headache is limited but can include application of ice to the head and periods of rest or sleep, usually in a dark, quiet environment. Preventive management of migraine should begin with the identification and avoidance of factors that consistently provoke migraine attacks in susceptible individuals[2,3,16,24] (Table 45-6). Changes in estrogen levels associated with menarche, menstruation, pregnancy, menopause, oral contraceptive use, and other hormone therapies can trigger, intensify, or alleviate migraine.[7] A headache diary that records the frequency, severity, and duration of attacks can facilitate identification of migraine triggers. **7** Patients also can benefit from adherence to a wellness program that includes regular sleep, exercise, and eating habits, smoking cessation, and limited caffeine intake. Behavioral interventions, such as relaxation therapy, biofeedback (often

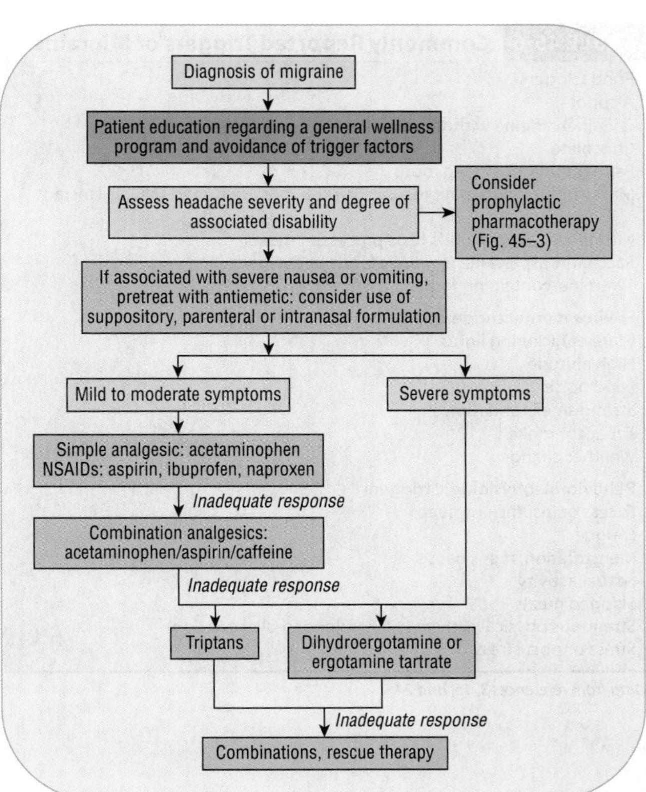

FIGURE 45-2 Treatment algorithm for migraine headaches.

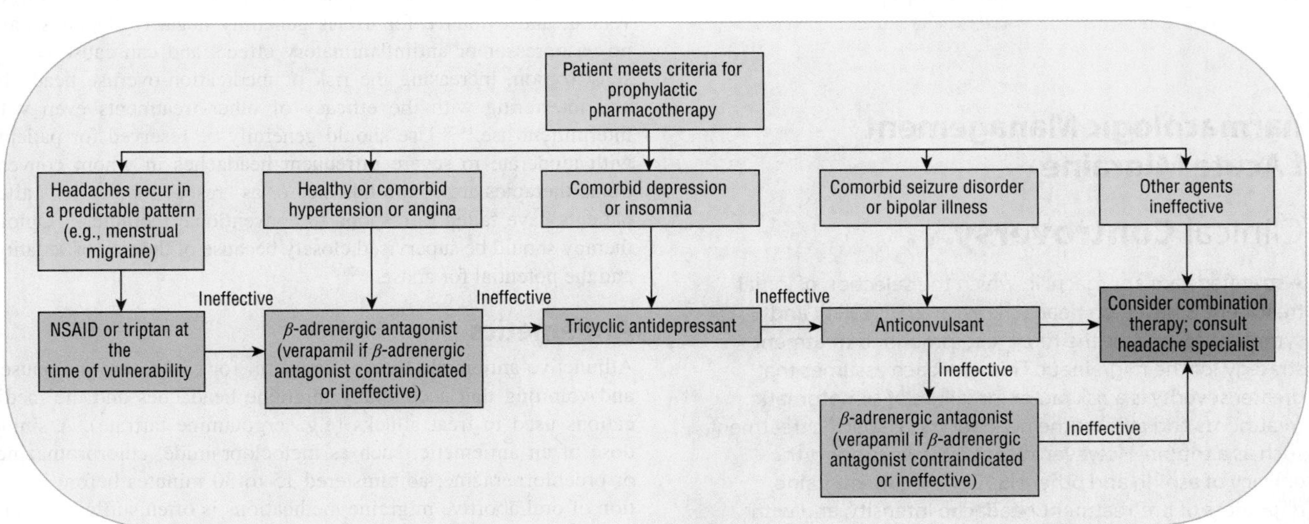

FIGURE 45-3 Treatment algorithm for prophylactic management of migraine headaches. (NSAID, nonsteroidal antiinflammatory drug.)

TABLE 45-6 Commonly Reported Triggers of Migraine

Food triggers
Alcohol
Caffeine/caffeine withdrawal
Chocolate
Fermented and pickled foods
Monosodium glutamate (e.g., in Chinese food, seasoned salt, and instant foods)
Nitrate-containing foods (e.g., processed meats)
Saccharin/aspartame (e.g., diet foods or diet sodas)
Tyramine-containing foods
Environmental triggers
Glare or flickering lights
High altitude
Loud noises
Strong smells and fumes
Tobacco smoke
Weather changes
Behavioral–physiologic triggers
Excess or insufficient sleep
Fatigue
Menstruation, menopause
Sexual activity
Skipped meals
Strenuous physical activity (e.g., prolonged overexertion)
Stress or post stress

Data from references 3, 16, and 24.

used in combination with relaxation therapy), and cognitive therapy, are preventive treatment options for patients who prefer nondrug therapy or when symptomatic therapies are poorly tolerated, contraindicated, or ineffective.[16]

Clinical **Controversy. . .**

Most migraineurs have triggers for the acute attack, at least occasionally, and are generally advised to avoid these as part of management to reduce the frequency of attacks. However, the complexity and usefulness of trigger avoidance is poorly understood by many patients and clinicians. Triggers may change over time in the life of the migraineur and be modified by preventive medication. Trigger avoidance can also impose severe lifestyle restrictions and more stress. Avoidance may ultimately not allow for desensitization from the trigger and the subsequent development of relative immunity.[24]

Pharmacologic Management of Acute Migraine

Clinical **Controversy. . .**

A stratified care approach, in which the selection of initial treatment is based on headache-related disability and symptom severity, is the most recommended treatment strategy for the migraineur. This approach assumes that greater severity is a risk factor for failure of symptomatic treatments and reflects the need for more specific treatment, such as a triptan. However, recent reviews support the efficacy of aspirin and other NSAIDs in acute migraine, regardless of pretreatment headache intensity, and with efficacy comparable to oral triptans.[25,26]

Analgesics and NSAIDs

Simple analgesics and NSAIDs are effective medications for the management of many migraine attacks (Table 45-4). They offer a reasonable first-line choice for treatment of mild to moderate migraine attacks or severe attacks that have been responsive in the past to similar NSAIDs or nonopiate analgesics. Of the NSAIDs, aspirin, diclofenac, ibuprofen, ketorolac, naproxen sodium, tolfenamic acid, and the combination of acetaminophen plus aspirin and caffeine have demonstrated the most consistent evidence of efficacy.[14,18] Evidence for other NSAIDs is either limited or inconsistent. Although some patients may observe benefits, acetaminophen alone is not generally recommended for migraine because the scientific support is not optimal.[17] Comparisons with other pharmacotherapeutic classes are limited; however, studies support the comparable efficacy of NSAIDs and triptans in acute migraine. Baseline headache intensity does not predict the success or failure of aspirin or other NSAIDs.[25,26] There are no studies comparing the relative efficacy of different NSAIDs.[18]

NSAIDs appear to prevent neurogenically mediated inflammation in the trigeminovascular system through the inhibition of prostaglandin synthesis. Metoclopramide can speed the absorption of analgesics and alleviate migraine-related nausea and vomiting.[14] Suppository analgesic preparations are an option when nausea and vomiting are severe.[18] Acute NSAID therapy is associated with GI (e.g., dyspepsia, nausea, vomiting, and diarrhea) and CNS (e.g., somnolence, dizziness) side effects. NSAIDs should be avoided or used cautiously in patients with previous ulcer disease, renal disease, or hypersensitivity to aspirin.[17,18]

The nonprescription combination of acetaminophen, aspirin, and caffeine was approved for the treatment of migraine in the United States because of its proven efficacy in relieving migraine pain and associated symptoms.[14,17] Aspirin and acetaminophen are also available in prescription combination products containing a short-acting barbiturate (butalbital) or narcotic (codeine). No randomized, placebo-controlled studies support the efficacy of butalbital-containing products in the treatment of migraine. The use of butalbital-containing analgesics or narcotics should be limited because of concerns about overuse, medication-overuse headache, and withdrawal.[17,18,20] Although frequent consumption of aspirin or acetaminophen alone can result in medication-overuse headache, combination analgesics appear to pose a greater risk.[18,20]

Opiate Analgesics

The use of narcotic analgesic drugs (e.g., meperidine, butorphanol, oxycodone, and hydromorphone) in migraine treatment is controversial, and evidence for use is generally negative. Opiates have no vasopressor or antiinflammatory effects and can cause central sensitization, increasing the risk of medication-overuse headache and interfering with the efficacy of other treatments even with intermittent use.[14,20] Use should generally be reserved for patients with moderate to severe infrequent headaches in whom conventional therapies are contraindicated or as "rescue medication" after patients have failed to respond to conventional therapies.[17] Opioid therapy should be supervised closely because of the risk of sedation and the potential for abuse.[14,20]

Antiemetics

Adjunctive antiemetic therapy is useful for combating the nausea and vomiting that accompany migraine headaches and the medications used to treat attacks (e.g., ergotamine tartrate). A single dose of an antiemetic, such as metoclopramide, chlorpromazine, or prochlorperazine, administered 15 to 30 minutes before ingestion of oral abortive migraine medications is often sufficient. Suppository preparations are available when nausea and vomiting are particularly prominent. Metoclopramide is also useful to reverse gastroparesis and improve absorption from the GI tract during severe attacks.[14,17]

In addition to antiemetic effects, dopamine antagonist drugs also have been used successfully as monotherapy for the treatment of intractable headache (Table 45-4). Prochlorperazine administered by the IV and intramuscular routes and IV metoclopramide provided more effective pain relief than placebo. Chlorpromazine and droperidol also have provided relief of migraine headache when administered parenterally at doses of 12.5 to 37.5 and 2.5 to 5 mg, respectively. The precise mechanism of action for these agents is unknown. The dopamine antagonists offer an alternative to the narcotic analgesics for the treatment of refractory migraine. Drowsiness and dizziness were reported occasionally, and extrapyramidal side effects were reported infrequently in migraine trials. Droperidol has a risk for QT prolongation.[17,18,20]

Miscellaneous Nonspecific Medications

Corticosteroids can be considered as rescue therapy for status migrainous (a severe, continuous migraine that can last up to 1 week).[17] IV or intramuscular dexamethasone at a dose of 10 to 25 mg has also been used as an adjunct to abortive therapy.[27]

Limited studies suggest a role for intranasal lidocaine in the treatment of acute migraine headache. Intranasal lidocaine, one to four drops of a 4% solution, provides rapid pain relief within 15 minutes of administration, but headache recurrence is common. Adverse effects generally are limited to local irritation, an unpleasant taste, and numbness of the throat.[17]

IV valproate 500 to 1,000 mg and magnesium sulfate 1,000 mg are nonsedating options for use in acute migraine treatment.[20] Future studies might establish a more defined role for these agents in migraine management.

Ergot Alkaloids and Derivatives

Ergotamine tartrate and dihydroergotamine are useful and can be considered for the treatment of moderate to severe migraine attacks (Table 45-4). These drugs are nonselective 5-HT_1 receptor agonists that constrict intracranial blood vessels and inhibit the development of neurogenic inflammation in the trigeminovascular system.[14] Central inhibition of the trigeminovascular pathway is also reported as well as agonist activity at dopaminergic receptors. Venous and arterial constriction occur with therapeutic doses, but ergotamine tartrate exerts more potent arterial effects than dihydroergotamine.[14,18,20]

Ergotamine tartrate is available for oral, sublingual, and rectal administration. Oral and rectal preparations contain caffeine to enhance absorption and potentiate analgesia. Ergotamine use is limited because of issues of efficacy and side effects. Dosage requirements should be titrated strictly to establish an effective but subnauseating dose for future attacks. Despite clinical use since 1926, evidence supporting the efficacy of ergotamine in migraine is inconsistent.[18]

Dihydroergotamine is available for intranasal and parenteral administration by the intramuscular, subcutaneous, and IV routes.[20] Parenteral dihydroergotamine was viewed previously as inpatient or emergency department treatment for moderate to severe migraine or intractable headache, but patients can be trained to self-administer dihydroergotamine intramuscularly or subcutaneously. Mixing with 1% or 2% lidocaine can reduce burning at the injection site. Clinical opinion suggests its use is relatively safe and effective when compared with other migraine therapies.[14,17]

Nausea and vomiting (resulting from stimulation of the chemoreceptor trigger zone) are among the most common adverse effects of the ergotamine derivatives. Pretreatment with an antiemetic agent should be considered with ergotamine and IV dihydroergotamine therapy. Other common side effects include abdominal pain, weakness, fatigue, paresthesias, muscle pain, diarrhea, and chest tightness. Rarely, symptoms of severe peripheral ischemia (ergotism), including cold, numb, painful extremities, continuous paresthesias, diminished peripheral pulses, and claudication, can result from the vasoconstrictor effects of the ergot alkaloids. Gangrenous extremities, myocardial infarction, hepatic necrosis, and bowel and brain ischemia have also been reported. Dihydroergotamine is rarely associated with such side effects. Triptans and ergot derivatives should not be used within 24 hours of each other.[14,18] Ergotamine derivatives are contraindicated in patients with renal or hepatic failure; coronary, cerebral, or peripheral vascular disease; uncontrolled hypertension; and sepsis; and in women who are pregnant or nursing. Dihydroergotamine does not appear to cause rebound headache, but dosage restrictions for ergotamine tartrate should be observed strictly to prevent this complication.[18,20]

Serotonin Receptor Agonists (Triptans)

Introduction of the 5-HT receptor agonists, or triptans, represented a significant advance in migraine pharmacotherapy. The first member of this class, sumatriptan, and the second-generation agents zolmitriptan, naratriptan, rizatriptan, almotriptan, frovatriptan, and eletriptan are selective agonists of the 5-HT_{1B} and 5-HT_{1D} receptors. Relief of migraine headache is the result of three key actions: normalization of dilated intracranial arteries through enhanced vasoconstriction, inhibition of vasoactive peptide release from perivascular trigeminal neurons, and inhibition of transmission through second-order neurons ascending to the thalamus.[14,28] These agents also display varying affinity for 5-HT_{1A}, 5-HT_{1E}, and 5-HT_{1F} receptors. The triptans are appropriate first-line therapy for patients with mild to severe migraine and are used for rescue therapy when nonspecific medications are ineffective.[28]

Sumatriptan, the most extensively studied acute therapy, is available for subcutaneous, oral, and intranasal administration. Subcutaneous sumatriptan is consistently superior to placebo in alleviating migraine headache and associated symptoms, with relief reported in 70% of patients at 2 hours in a meta-analysis of placebo-controlled studies.[28] In addition to enhanced efficacy, subcutaneous sumatriptan has a more rapid onset of action when compared with the oral formulation. The subcutaneous injection is packaged as an autoinjector device for self-administration by patients. Intranasal sumatriptan provides a faster onset of effect than the oral formulation and produces similar rates of response in placebo-controlled studies.[18,28]

Selection of a triptan is based on characteristics of the headache, convenience of dosing, and the patient's preference. At all marketed doses, the oral triptans are effective and well tolerated. The triptans differ in their pharmacokinetic and pharmacodynamic profiles (Table 45-7). In general, triptans can be divided into those with a faster onset and higher efficacy and those with a slower onset and lower efficacy. A recent meta-analysis summarizes the efficacy and tolerability of the oral triptans across published and unpublished studies. Using 100 mg of sumatriptan as the reference dose and based on 2-hour response rates, at doses recommended by the manufacturer, most of the triptans evaluated had similar therapeutic gains; frovatriptan and naratriptan were the exceptions with lower efficacy. Compared with other triptans, frovatriptan and naratriptan have the longest half-lives, the slowest onset of action, and less headache recurrence. This may make them more suitable for patients who have migraine attacks of a slow onset and longer duration. Faster-acting triptans are more efficacious when a rapid onset is necessary. Subcutaneous, intranasal, or orally dissolving tablets may be useful in patients with prominent early nausea or vomiting or those who have difficulty in swallowing tablets. Despite the fact that oral absorption can be delayed during migraine attacks, most patients prefer oral formulations.[14,20,25,28]

Clinical response to the triptans can vary considerably among individual patients. Individual responses cannot be predicted, and

TABLE 45-7 Pharmacokinetic Characteristics of Triptans

Drug	Half-Life (Hours)	Time to Maximal Concentration (t_{max})	Bioavailability (%)	Elimination
Almotriptan	3–4	1.4–3.8 hours	80	MAO-A, CYP3A4, CYP2D6
Eletriptan	4–5	1–2 hours	50	CYP3A4
Frovatriptan	25	2–4 hours	24–30	Mostly unchanged, CYP1A2
Naratriptan	5–6	2–3 hours	63–74	Largely unchanged, CYP450 (various isoenzymes)
Rizatriptan	2–3		45	MAO-A
Oral tablets		1–1.2 hours		
Disintegrating		1.6–2.5 hours		
Sumatriptan	2			MAO-A
SC injection		12–15 minutes	97	
Oral tablets		2.5 hours	14	
Nasal spray		1–2.5 hours	17	
Zolmitriptan	3		40–48	CYP1A2, MAO-A
Oral		2 hours		
Disintegrating		3.3 hours		
Nasal		4 hours		

CYP, cytochrome P450; MAO-A, monoamine oxidase type A.

Data from references 14, 20, and 28.

if one triptan fails, a patient can be switched successfully to another triptan.[14] ❽ After an effective agent and dose have been identified, subsequent treatments should begin with that same regimen. Combination therapy may also improve response rates and diminish migraine recurrence. A proprietary formulation of sumatriptan 85 mg plus naproxen 500 mg in a single tablet was more effective in clinical trials for headache relief and sustained pain-free response than either agent as monotherapy.[14,18]

Side effects to the triptans are common but usually mild to moderate in nature and of short duration. Adverse effects are consistent among the class and include paresthesias, fatigue, dizziness, flushing, warm sensations, and somnolence. Local side effects are reported with the subcutaneous (minor injection site reactions) and intranasal (taste perversion, nasal discomfort) routes. Up to 25% of patients receiving a triptan consistently report "triptan sensations," including tightness, pressure, heaviness, or pain in the chest, neck, or throat. The mechanism of these symptoms is unknown, but a cardiac source of pain seems unlikely in most patients.[28] However, all triptans are partial agonists of human 5-HT coronary artery receptors in vitro, resulting in a small but significant vasoconstrictor response. Adverse cardiac events are rare with only isolated cases of myocardial infarction and coronary vasospasm with ischemia reported. The triptans are contraindicated in patients with a history of ischemic heart disease (e.g., angina pectoris, Prinzmetal's angina, or previous myocardial infarction), uncontrolled hypertension, and cerebrovascular disease. Patients at risk for unrecognized coronary artery disease should use triptans with caution. Postmenopausal women, men older than 40 years of age, and patients with uncontrolled risk factors should receive a cardiovascular assessment prior to triptan use and have initial doses administered under medical supervision. Triptans are also contraindicated in patients with hemiplegic and basilar migraine and should not be used routinely in pregnancy.[18,28] The triptans should not be given within 24 hours of the ergotamine derivatives. Administration of sumatriptan, rizatriptan, and zolmitriptan within 2 weeks of therapy with monoamine oxidase inhibitors (MAOIs) is not recommended. Eletriptan should not be administered with cytochrome P450 3A4 inhibitors such as macrolide antibiotics, antifungals, and some antiviral therapies. Concomitant therapy with the selective serotonin reuptake inhibitors (SSRIs) or serotonin–norepinephrine reuptake inhibitors (SNRIs) (e.g., duloxetine, venlafaxine, and mirtazapine) can potentially cause 5-HT syndrome. Regulatory agencies caution against concurrent administration, although it appears the likelihood of CNS adverse events is extremely low. The potential risk of these combinations should be carefully considered and discussed with the patient.[14,18,29] Frequent use of the triptans has been associated with the development of medication-misuse headache.[17,28]

Prophylactic Pharmacologic Therapy

Clinical **Controversy. . .**

To determine maximal clinical benefits, a therapeutic trial of 6 months is recommended when initiating treatment for episodic migraine prevention. Despite this recommendation, most migraine prevention studies have relatively brief treatment durations of only 12 to 16 weeks. Long-term scientifically sound assessments and evaluations of migraine preventive treatments are needed to further define their role in clinical care.[21]

β-Adrenergic Antagonists

β-Adrenergic antagonists are among the most widely used drugs for migraine prophylaxis. Metoprolol, propranolol, and timolol have established efficacy in controlled clinical trials, reducing the frequency of attacks by 50% in greater than 50% of patients.[8,21] Atenolol and nadolol are also probably effective, while nebivolol and pindolol are possibly effective (Table 45-5).[21] Because the relative efficacy of the individual agents has not been established, selection of a β-blocker can be based on β-selectivity, convenience of the formulation, and tolerability. β-Blockers with intrinsic sympathomimetic activity are typically ineffective for migraine prophylaxis.[18] Although their precise mechanism of antimigraine action is unknown, β-blockers may raise the migraine threshold by modulating adrenergic or serotonergic neurotransmission in cortical or subcortical pathways. Although not first-line treatment for hypertension or anxiety, β-blockers may be useful along with other therapy in patients with comorbid hypertension or angina.[7] Side effects can include drowsiness, fatigue, sleep disturbances, vivid dreams, memory disturbance, depression, impotence, bradycardia, and hypotension. β-Blockers should be used with caution in patients with congestive heart failure, peripheral vascular disease, atrioventricular conduction disturbances, asthma, depression, and diabetes.[7,8,21]

Antidepressants

The beneficial effects of antidepressants in migraine are independent of their antidepressant activity and may be related to downregulation of central 5-HT_2 receptors, increased levels of synaptic norepinephrine, and enhanced endogenous opioid receptor actions.[30] The tricyclic antidepressant (TCA) amitriptyline and SNRI venlafaxine have demonstrated efficacy in placebo-controlled and comparative studies and are classified as probably effective for migraine prophylaxis (Table 45-5).[8,21] Use of other antidepressants is based primarily on clinical and anecdotal experience. There are insufficient or conflicting data to support or refute the efficacy of other antidepressants, such as protriptyline, fluoxetine, or fluvoxamine, for migraine prophylaxis.[21]

Anticholinergic side effects are common with TCAs and limit use of these agents in patients with benign prostatic hyperplasia and glaucoma. Evening doses are preferred because of associated sedation. Increased appetite and weight gain can occur. Orthostatic hypotension and cardiac toxicity (slowed atrioventricular conduction) also are reported occasionally.[8,21] The most common side effects reported with venlafaxine are nausea, vomiting, and drowsiness. Again, the potential risk of 5-HT syndrome should be considered in patients using SSRIs or SNRIs along with a triptan.[21,29]

MAOIs, such as phenelzine, have been used in the management of refractory headache, but their complex adverse effect profile limits their use to experienced prescribers. Strict adherence to a tyramine-free diet is necessary to avoid potentially life-threatening hypertensive crisis.[8,16] The reader is referred to Chapter 51 for dietary and concurrent medication restrictions for patients taking MAOIs.

Anticonvulsants

Anticonvulsant medications have emerged as important therapeutic options for migraine prophylaxis with valproate, divalproex, and topiramate all having established efficacy.[21] The beneficial effects of these agents are likely caused by multiple mechanisms of action, including enhancement of γ-aminobutyric acid (GABA)–mediated inhibition, modulation of the excitatory neurotransmitter glutamate, and inhibition of sodium and calcium ion channel activity.[30] Anticonvulsants are particularly useful in migraineurs with comorbid seizures, anxiety disorder, or bipolar illness.[8,21] The efficacy of sodium valproate and divalproex sodium (a 1:1 molar combination of valproate sodium and valproic acid) has been demonstrated in multiple placebo-controlled studies. In most trials for headache prophylaxis, there were no significant differences in treatment-emergent side effects between these agents and placebo. Nausea and vomiting, the most common early side effects, are self-limited and appear to be less common with divalproex sodium and gradual titration of doses. Alopecia, tremor, asthenia, somnolence, and weight gain are also complaints.[8,21,23] The extended-release formulation of divalproex sodium is administered once daily and is better tolerated than the enteric-coated formulation.[22] Hepatotoxicity is the most serious side effect of valproate therapy, but the risk appears to be low in migraineurs (e.g., patients older than 10 years of age who are receiving monotherapy and have no underlying metabolic or neurologic disorder). Baseline liver function tests should be obtained, but routine followup studies are not necessary in asymptomatic adults on monotherapy. Regular followup is necessary, however, for dosage adjustments and monitoring of effects.[8,21] Valproate is contraindicated in pregnant women (owing to potential teratogenicity) and patients with a history of pancreatitis or chronic liver disease.[21,22]

Topiramate is the most extensively studied medication to date for migraine prophylaxis. Efficacy and improvements in health-related quality of life including daily work, home, and social activities have been demonstrated in several placebo-controlled studies.[8,16] To minimize adverse effects, topiramate should be initiated at a low dose and slowly titrated upward. The benefits of topiramate are observed as early as 2 weeks after initiation of therapy, with significant reductions in migraine frequency within the first month. Approximately 50% of patients treated to target doses are responders (50% or greater reduction in mean headache frequency). Treatment-emergent adverse events associated with topiramate include paresthesia, fatigue, anorexia, diarrhea, weight loss, hypesthesia, difficulty with memory, language problems, taste perversion, and nausea. Paresthesia is the most common adverse event, occurring in about half of patients at target doses. Weight loss, occurring in 9% to 12% of patients, is a unique adverse effect, as weight gain is a common reason to discontinue other preventive medications. Topiramate should be used with caution or avoided in patients with a history of kidney stones or cognitive impairment.[8,21,23]

Preliminary studies suggest a role for other anticonvulsants for migraine prevention. Carbamazepine is possibly effective, and a recent study evaluated gabapentin, but data are insufficient to determine efficacy. Lamotrigine is classified as possibly or probably ineffective.[8,21]

NSAIDs

NSAIDs are modestly effective for reducing the frequency, severity, and duration of migraine attacks, but potential GI and renal toxicity limit the daily or prolonged use of these agents.[22] Consequently, NSAIDs have been used intermittently to prevent headaches that recur in a predictable pattern, such as menstrual migraine. Administration of NSAIDs in the perimenstrual period can be beneficial in women with true menstrual migraine. NSAIDs should be initiated 1 to 2 days prior to the expected onset of headache and continued during the period of vulnerability.[7,23] If long-term NSAID therapy is initiated, monitoring of renal function and occult blood loss is necessary. For migraine prevention, the evidence for efficacy is strongest for naproxen and weakest for aspirin.[21,23]

Triptans

Triptans are also useful for the prevention of menstrual migraine. Frovatriptan has established efficacy, while naratriptan and zolmitriptan are probably effective. The triptan is usually started 1 or 2 days before the expected onset of headache and continued during the period of vulnerability.[21,23] A separate indication for pure menstrual migraine is currently being deliberated by regulatory authorities.[21]

Miscellaneous Prophylactic Agents

At least two placebo-controlled studies show that petasites, an extract from the butterbur plant *Petasites hybridus*, is an effective preventive treatment for migraine.[8,23,31] A double-blind, placebo-controlled study demonstrated the probable efficacy of riboflavin (vitamin B_2) 400 mg daily in migraine prophylaxis. Riboflavin was well tolerated and associated with 50% or greater improvement in attack frequency in 54% of patients. However, the benefits of therapy became significant only after 3 months.[8,23,31] The relatively stable extract of feverfew (*Tanacetum parthenium*), MIG-99, is the most studied herbal preparation for migraine prevention. MIG-99 is classified as probably effective, reducing migraine frequency by 1.9 attacks per month.[8,23,31] Clinical trials evaluating various formulations of magnesium for migraine prevention have yielded mixed results, though overall probable efficacy.[23,31] CNS levels of magnesium are known to be significantly low during migraine attacks. Magnesium supplementation may be particularly effective for prevention of menstrual migraine and in migraine patients with aura.[8,23] Subcutaneous histamine has been compared with placebo, sodium valproate, and topiramate, with favorable results indicating probable efficacy in improving headache frequency, duration, and intensity. Transient burning and itching at the injection site were the only reported side effects with histamine administration.[31]

Other agents are possibly effective and may be considered for migraine prevention.[21,31] The angiotensin-converting enzyme inhibitor lisinopril and the angiotensin II receptor blocker candesartan provided effective migraine prophylaxis in recent double-blind, placebo-controlled, crossover studies of these agents.[21,23] Although use is limited by side effects, clonidine and guanfacine have also demonstrated possible efficacy.[21] Coenzyme Q10 was effective for migraine prevention and well tolerated in a small, randomized, double-blind, controlled study.[8,23,31] In one study, cyproheptadine (4 mg/day) was as effective as propranolol (80 mg/day) in reducing migraine frequency, duration, and severity, while the combination was more effective in attack frequency reduction.[21,31]

The calcium channel blockers, primarily verapamil, have been widely used for preventive treatment, although evidence supporting their use is inadequate or conflicting.[8,21,23] Extensive clinical experience and the ease of use of verapamil suggest a possible role in migraine prevention. Side effects of verapamil can include constipation, hypotension, bradycardia, atrioventricular block, and exacerbation of congestive heart failure.[8,21]

Localized injections of botulinum toxin type A have been used for various conditions and pain syndromes, including migraine headache. However, no consistent, statistically significant benefits have been found with migraine. The American Academy of Neurology concludes that botulinum toxin is probably ineffective.[23,32] Further study is needed to confirm the clinical utility and comparative efficacy for many of these miscellaneous agents in the prevention of migraine.

Personalized Pharmacotherapy

Although migraine is widely recognized as a disease that exacts an enormous toll on the sufferer, healthcare providers often do not recognize the degree and scope of functional impairment imposed by migraine on the individual.[16] In 2004, only half of those surveyed with clear symptoms of migraine were diagnosed by a physician. Although most episodic migraine sufferers take medications for their headaches, 21% use opioids or compounds containing barbiturates, and only 24% use a triptan. Just 13% use medications specifically to prevent migraine, although 26% meet criteria to be offered prophylaxis, and an additional 13% should be considered for treatment.[5] Because many migraineurs who receive inadequate care experience substantial levels of pain and disability, improvement in migraine diagnosis, care, and treatment potentially could result in lower direct and indirect costs of the disease.

Effective communication and education of headache patients regarding required behavior changes and appropriate use of acute and prophylactic pharmacotherapy is essential. Healthcare professionals should inquire about and address coexisting conditions that may contribute to headache presentation or successful acute and preventive management. Decisions for treatment should be individualized, with consideration for frequency and severity of headache episodes, level of disability, trigger factors, coexisting conditions, tolerability of the available agents, and the patient's lifestyle and preferences.[16,21]

Medications with the highest level of efficacy should be used for treatment. Migraine management should be individualized on the basis of the patient's clinical presentation and medical history. Therapy should usually be initiated with the lowest effective dose and then titrated upward until clinical benefits are achieved, in the absence of adverse events. Medications that increase headache frequency or severity should be avoided. Many patients try nonpharmacologic or nonprescription treatments for headache management either before or concurrently with other drug therapy. Patients may not know how to take these products optimally and often need instructions and dosing limits.

Analgesics and NSAIDs can be considered the drugs of choice if effective for infrequent mild to moderately severe attacks. The triptans or dihydroergotamine can be used if initial therapies prove ineffective or as first-line therapy in moderate to severe migraine headache. Abortive therapy should be instituted early in the course of the attack to optimize efficacy and minimize migraine-related pain and disability. Preventive therapy should be considered in the setting of recurring migraines that produce significant disability; frequent attacks requiring symptomatic medication more than twice per week; symptomatic therapies that are ineffective or contraindicated, or produce serious side effects; and uncommon migraine variants that cause risk of neurologic injury. Efficacy of a prescribed prophylactic regimen should be reassessed periodically. Therapeutic interventions require an adequate trial to achieve clinical benefit and often as long as 6 months for assessment of maximal benefit. A prolonged headache-free interval could allow for gradual dosage reduction and discontinuation of therapy.

A formal management plan and maintaining a headache diary are necessary for the patient and provider to evaluate therapy, headache impact, and medication consumption. Oversights can lead to decreased efficacy of medications resulting in repeat dosing and polypharmacy, decreased compliance, increased emergency visits, increased "doctor shopping," and, perhaps, increased use of expensive diagnostic procedures and inpatient services. Patients with stratified care targeted to their needs have higher headache response rates, shorter disability times, less health service utilization, and less loss of productivity.[18,23,31,32]

TENSION-TYPE HEADACHE

Epidemiology

Tension-type headache is the most common type of primary headache, with an estimated 1-year prevalence ranging from 31% to 86%.[3,33] Prevalence peaks in the fourth decade and is higher among women. The incidence decreases with age.[33] Although an estimated 60% of tension-type headache sufferers experience some degree of functional impairment during their attacks, less than 15% of sufferers seek medical attention, likely because most have infrequent attacks. Infrequent episodic tension-type headache (defined as fewer than one episode per month) is experienced by 64% of sufferers, while 22% have frequent episodic tension-type headache (episodes on 1 to 14 days/mo). The prevalence of chronic tension-type headache (15 or more days/mo, perhaps without recognizable episodes) is estimated at 0.9% to 2.2%. Risk factors associated with a poor outcome in tension-type headache include coexisting migraine, sleep problems, not being married, and the presence of chronic tension-type headache.[33,34]

Pathophysiology

Although tension-type headache is the most common type of headache, it is the least studied of the primary headache disorders, and there is limited understanding of key pathophysiologic concepts.[2,33] Some evidence supports that migraine and tension-type headaches represent a continuum of headache severity with similarities in mechanisms and pathophysiology. However, more recently, tension-type headache has been recognized as a distinct disorder.[2] The mechanism of pain in chronic tension-type headache is thought to originate from myofascial factors and peripheral sensitization of nociceptors. Central mechanisms also are involved, with heightened sensitivity of pain pathways in the CNS.[33] Mental stress, nonphysiologic motor stress, a local myofascial release of irritants, or a combination of these may be the initiating stimulus. Following activation of supraspinal pain perception structures, a self-limiting headache results in most individuals owing to central modulation of the incoming peripheral stimuli. Chronic tension-type headache can evolve from episodic tension-type headache in predisposed individuals due to a change in central circuits and nociceptive processing along the brain stem reflex pathway and subsequent sensitization of the CNS.[33,34] It is likely that other pathophysiologic mechanisms also contribute to the development of tension-type headache.

Clinical Presentation

Premonitory symptoms and aura are absent with tension-type headache. The pain usually is mild to moderate in intensity and often is described as a dull, nonpulsatile tightness or pressure.[2,33] Bilateral pain is most common, but the location can vary (frontal and temporal pain are most common; occipital and parietal regions also may be affected).[2] The pain is classically described as having a "hatband" pattern. Associated symptoms generally are absent, but mild photophobia or phonophobia may be reported. The disability associated with tension-type headache typically is minor in comparison with migraine headache, and routine physical activity does not affect headache severity.[2,33] Palpation of the pericranial or cervical muscles can reveal tender spots or localized nodules in some patients.[2] Tension-type headache is classified as either episodic (infrequent or frequent) or chronic based on the frequency and duration of the attacks.[2]

TREATMENT
Tension-Type Headaches

General Approach to Treatment

The vast majority of episodic tension-type headache sufferers self-medicate with nonprescription medications and do not consult a healthcare professional. Although pharmacologic and nonpharmacologic treatments are available, simple analgesics and NSAIDs are the mainstay of acute therapy. Most agents used for tension-type headache have not been studied in controlled clinical trials.[35]

Nonpharmacologic Therapy

Psychophysiologic therapy and physical therapy have been used in the management of tension-type headache. Behavioral treatments can consist of cognitive-behavioral therapy (i.e., stress management), relaxation training, and biofeedback. These therapies (alone, in combination, or with pharmacotherapy) can result in a 33% to 64% reduction in headache activity. Relaxation training combined with biofeedback is more effective than other behavioral therapy options.[36] Evidence supporting physical therapeutic options, such as heat or cold packs, ultrasound, electrical nerve stimulation, stretching, exercise, massage, acupuncture, manipulations, ergonomic instruction, and trigger point injections or occipital nerve blocks, is somewhat inconsistent. However, individual patients may benefit from selected modalities in reducing the frequency of tension-type headache or during an acute episode.[35,36]

Pharmacologic Therapy

Simple analgesics (alone or in combination with caffeine) and NSAIDs are effective for the acute treatment of most mild to moderate tension-type headaches. Acetaminophen, aspirin, diclofenac, ibuprofen, naproxen, ketoprofen, and ketorolac have demonstrated efficacy in placebo-controlled and comparative studies.[35] Failure of nonprescription agents can warrant therapy with prescription drugs. High-dose NSAIDs and the combination of aspirin or acetaminophen with butalbital or, rarely, codeine are effective options. Use of butalbital and codeine combinations should be avoided when possible owing to the high potential for overuse and dependency. Acute medications should be taken for episodic tension-type headache no more than 3 days (butalbital-containing), 9 days (combination analgesics), or 15 days (NSAIDs) per month to prevent the development of chronic tension-type headache.[35] There is no evidence to support the efficacy of muscle relaxants in the management of episodic tension-type headache.[35] Preventive treatment is appropriate for most patients with chronic tension-type headache and should be considered in those with frequent episodic tension-type headache if frequency (more than 2 per week), duration (greater than 3 to 4 hours), or severity results in medication overuse or substantial disability.[36] The principles of preventive treatment for tension-type headache are similar to those for migraine headache. TCAs are prescribed most often for prophylaxis, but other drugs also can be selected after consideration of comorbid medical conditions and respective side effect profiles. SSRIs are not effective in patients with tension-type headache who do not have depression. Limited studies support the use of the SNRIs mirtazapine and venlafaxine in patients with chronic tension-type headache and without depression.[34,36] Topiramate and gabapentin may have benefits in chronic tension-type headache; however, confirmation is needed from randomized clinical trials. Injection of botulinum toxin into pericranial muscles has demonstrated inconsistent efficacy in the prophylaxis of tension-type headache and because of this, it is not recommended for use.[32,36]

CLUSTER HEADACHE

Epidemiology

Cluster headache, the most severe of the primary headache disorders, is characterized by attacks of excruciating, unilateral head pain that occur in series lasting for weeks or months (i.e., cluster periods) separated by remission periods usually lasting months or years.[2,37] Cluster headaches can be episodic or chronic.[2] Cluster headache is relatively uncommon among the primary headache disorders, but the exact prevalence is uncertain. Estimates from pooled population studies show a lifetime prevalence of 124 per 100,000 or 0.12%.[38] The male-to-female ratio for cluster headache is approximately 3:1 with age of onset typically in the third decade for men and at a slightly younger age for women. Greater than 65% of patients with cluster headache are tobacco smokers or have a history of smoking. Tobacco cessation does not, however, seem to improve the course of cluster headaches. Recent genetic epidemiologic surveys support a predisposition for cluster headache can exist in certain families.[37,38]

Pathophysiology

The etiologic and pathophysiologic mechanisms of cluster headache are not completely understood. Neuroimaging studies performed during acute attacks have demonstrated activation of the ipsilateral hypothalamic gray area, implicating the hypothalamus as a modulator of cluster headaches. The hypothalamus secondarily activates trigeminal-autonomic reflexes, leading to the ipsilateral pain and cranial autonomic features characteristic of cluster headache.[37,39] The cyclic nature of attacks implicates a pathogenesis of hypothalamic dysfunction with resulting alterations in circadian rhythms.[39] There is some evidence that cluster headache may result from inflammation of the nerves traversing the cavernous sinus resulting in injury to sympathetic fibers of the internal carotid artery.[39]

Clinical Presentation

One hallmark of cluster headaches is the circadian rhythm of painful attacks. Episodic cluster headaches are the most common cluster headache subtype in both men and women, occurring in 80% of patients.[38] In episodic cluster headaches, attacks occur daily for

2 weeks to several months, followed by long pain-free intervals.[37,39] Periods of remission average 2 years in length but have been reported to be from 2 months to 20 years in duration. Approximately 10% of patients have chronic symptoms with attacks recurring for over 1 year without remission or with remission periods of less than 1 month.[37,39]

Cluster headache attacks occur commonly at night and more commonly in the spring and fall. Attacks occur suddenly, with pain peaking quickly after onset and generally lasting 15 to 180 minutes.[37] The pain is excruciating, penetrating, and of a boring intensity in orbital, supraorbital, and temporal unilateral locations.[37,39] The headache is accompanied by cranial autonomic symptoms such as conjunctival injection, lacrimation, nasal stuffiness, rhinorrhea, eyelid edema, facial sweating, and miosis/ptosis, which resolve with resolution of the headache. Most sufferers of cluster headaches also describe restlessness or agitation. Whereas migraine patients retreat to a quiet, dark room, cluster headache patients generally sit and rock or pace about the room clutching their head.[37] Auras are not present with cluster headaches. During the cluster period, attacks occur from once every other day to eight times per day.[37,39] Specific diagnostic criteria for cluster headaches are provided within the IHS classification system.[2]

TREATMENT
Cluster Headaches

As in migraine, therapy for cluster headaches involves both abortive and prophylactic therapy. Abortive therapy is directed at managing the acute attack. Prophylactic therapies are started early in the cluster period in an attempt to induce remission. Patients with chronic cluster headache can require prophylactic medications indefinitely.

Abortive Therapy
Oxygen

The standard acute treatment of cluster headache is inhalation of 100% oxygen by nonbreather facial mask at a rate of at least 12 L/min for 15 to 30 minutes.[40,42] Repeat administration can be necessary because of recurrence, as oxygen appears to merely delay, rather than abort, the attack in some patients.[40] No side effects have been reported with the use of oxygen, but caution should be used for those who smoke or have chronic obstructive pulmonary disease.

Triptans

The quick onset of subcutaneous and intranasal triptans makes them safe and effective abortive agents for cluster headaches. Subcutaneous sumatriptan (6 mg) is the most effective agent. Nasal sprays are less effective but may be better tolerated in some patients. Adverse events reported in cluster headache patients are similar to those seen in migraineurs. Orally administered triptans have limited use in cluster attacks because of their relatively slow onset of action; oral zolmitriptan (10 mg), however, was beneficial in patients with episodic cluster headache, with 60% experiencing mild or no pain at 30 minutes.[40–42]

Ergotamine Derivatives

All forms of ergotamine have been used in cluster headaches, although no controlled clinical trials support their use.[41,42] In clinical use, IV dihydroergotamine results in the quickest response, and repeated administration for 3 to 7 days can break the cycle of frequent attacks.[40] Ergotamine tartrate also has provided effective relief of cluster headache attacks when administered sublingually or rectally, but the pharmacokinetics of these preparations frequently limit their clinical utility.[41] Dosing guidelines are similar to those for migraine headache therapy.

Prophylactic Therapy
Verapamil

The preferred first-line treatment for prevention of cluster headaches is verapamil, a calcium channel blocker with antianginal and antiarrhythmic properties.[40,42] The beneficial effects of verapamil often appear after 1 week of therapy. A typical suggested dosage range is from 360 to 720 mg/day. Rarely, patients with refractory cluster headaches are treated with doses as high as 1,200 mg/day. In such patients, an electrocardiogram should be obtained as the dose is increased, due to concerns for bradycardia or heart block.[40,42]

Lithium

Lithium carbonate is effective for episodic and chronic cluster headache attacks and can be used as an alternative to or in combination with verapamil.[42] A positive response is seen in up to 78% of patients with chronic cluster headache, and in up to 63% of patients with episodic cluster headache.[40] The usual dose is 600 to 1,200 mg/day, with a suggested starting dose of 300 mg twice daily.[42] Optimal plasma lithium levels for prevention of cluster headache have not been established, but levels should be monitored and maintained between 0.6 and 1.2 mEq/L (0.6 and 1.2 mmol/L).[40]

Initial side effects are mild and include tremor, lethargy, nausea, diarrhea, and abdominal discomfort. Thyroid and renal function must be monitored during lithium therapy. Lithium should be administered with caution to patients with significant renal or cardiovascular disease, dehydration, pregnancy, or concomitant diuretic or NSAID use.[42]

Corticosteroids

Although there are few clinical trials evaluating the use of corticosteroids in cluster headache management, they have been used effectively for inducing remission.[40] Therapy is initiated with 40 to 60 mg/day prednisone and tapered over approximately 3 weeks. Relief appears within 1 to 2 days of initiating therapy. To avoid steroid-induced complications, long-term use is not recommended. Headaches can recur when therapy is tapered or discontinued.

Miscellaneous Agents

Other therapies that have been used in the acute management of cluster headache include intranasal lidocaine, hyperbaric oxygen, and subcutaneous octreotide. Limited studies or case reports also support the use of divalproex sodium, topiramate, gabapentin, intranasal civamide, intranasal capsaicin, tizanidine, baclofen, melatonin, transdermal clonidine, leuprolide, and intramuscular botulinum toxin for cluster prophylaxis.[41]

Neurosurgical interventions to relieve chronic cluster headaches in patients refractory to pharmacologic therapy should be considered for some with debilitating headaches.[37,42] Neurostimulation has gained attention in the last several years.[43] Deep brain stimulation of the posterior hypothalamus and occipital nerve stimulation studies have shown positive results in small clinical trials.[43]

EVALUATION OF THERAPEUTIC OUTCOMES

Patients should be monitored for frequency, intensity, and duration of headaches, as well as any change in the headache pattern. To this end, patients should be encouraged to keep a headache diary to document the frequency, severity, and duration of attacks, as well as response to medication and potential trigger factors. Careful monitoring is essential to initiate the most appropriate pharmacotherapy, document therapeutic successes and failures, identify medication contraindications, and prevent or minimize adverse events. Patients using acute therapies should be monitored for frequency of use of prescription and nonprescription medications to identify potential medication-misuse headache. Patient counseling is necessary to allow for proper medication use (e.g., self-injection with sumatriptan), to encourage early use of medications in the headache cycle, and to enhance patient compliance. Strict adherence to dosing guidelines should be stressed to minimize potential toxicity. Patterns of abortive medication use can be documented to establish the need for prophylactic therapy. Prophylactic therapies also should be monitored closely for adverse reactions, abortive therapy needs, adequate dosing, and compliance. Consultation with other healthcare practitioners should be encouraged when changes in headache patterns or medication use occur.

ABBREVIATIONS

CGRP	calcitonin gene–related peptide
GABA	γ-aminobutyric acid
5-HT	serotonin, 5-hydroxytryptamine
HIV	human immunodeficiency virus
IHS	International Headache Society
MAOIs	monoamine oxidase inhibitors
NSAIDs	nonsteroidal antiinflammatory drugs
SNRI	serotonin–norepinephrine reuptake inhibitor
SSRI	selective serotonin reuptake inhibitor
TCA	tricyclic antidepressant

REFERENCES

1. National Center for Health Statistics. Health, United States, 2008 with Chartbook. Hyattsville, MD: National Center for Health Statistics, 2009:62–63.
2. Headache Classification Committee of the International Headache Society. The international classification of headache disorders, 2nd ed. Cephalalgia 2004;24(Suppl 1): 1–151.
3. Bajwa ZH, Wootton RJ. Evaluation of headache in adults. UpToDate 2012;6:1–13, *www.uptodate.com*.
4. Lipton RB, Bigal ME, Diamond M, et al. Migraine prevalence, disease burden, and the need for preventive therapy. Neurology 2007;68:343–349.
5. Bigal ME, Ferrari M, Silberstein SD, et al. Migraine in the triptan era: Lessons from epidemiology, pathophysiology, and clinical science. Headache 2009;49:S21–S33.
6. Bigal ME, Kurth T, Hu H, et al. Migraine and cardiovascular disease. Neurology 2009;72:1864–1871.
7. Silberstein SD, Dodick D, Freitag F, et al. Pharmacological approaches to managing migraine and associated comorbidities—Clinical considerations for monotherapy versus polytherapy. Headache 2007;47:585–599.
8. Bigal ME, Lipton RB. The preventive treatment of migraine. Neurologist 2006;12(4):204–213.
9. Sprenger T, Goadsby PJ. Migraine pathogenesis and state of pharmacological treatment options. BMC Med 2009; 7(71):1–5.
10. Ferrari MD. Migraine. Lancet 1998;351:1043–1051.
11. Akerman S, Holland PR, Goadsby PJ. Diencephalic and brainstem mechanisms in migraine. Nature 2011;12: 570–584.
12. Gardner KL. Genetics of migraine: An update. Headache 2006;46(Suppl 1):S19–S24.
13. Wessman M, Terwindt GM, Kaunisto MA, et al. Migraine: A complex genetic disorder. Lancet Neurol 2007;6:521–532.
14. Da Silva AN, Tepper SJ. Acute treatment of migraines. CNS Drugs 2012;10:823–839.
15. Cutrer FM, Bajwa ZH, Sabahat A. Pathophysiology, clinical manifestations, and diagnosis of migraine in adults. UpToDate 2012;12:1–23, *www.uptodate.com*.
16. Buse DC, Rupnow FT, Lipton RB. Assessing and managing all aspects of migraine: Migraine attacks, migraine-related functional impairment, common comorbidities, and quality of life. Mayo Clin Proc 2009;84(5):422–435.
17. Matchar DB, Young WB, Rosenberg JA, et al. Evidence-Based Guidelines for Migraine Headache in the Primary Care Setting: Pharmacological Management of Acute Attacks. The U.S. Headache Consortium. 2000, *www.aan.com/professionals/practice/guidelines*.
18. Bajwa ZH, Sabahat A. Acute treatment of migraine in adults. UpToDate 2012;15:1–23, *www.uptodate.com*.
19. Bigal ME, Lipton RB. Modifiable risk factors for migraine progression. Headache 2006;46:1334–1343.
20. Tepper SJ, Spears RC. Acute treatment of migraine. Neurol Clin 2009;27:417–427.
21. Silberstein SD, Holland S, Freitag F, et al. Evidence-based guideline update: Pharmacological treatment for episodic migraine prevention in adults: Report of the Quality Standards Subcommittee of the American Academy of Neurology and the American Headache Society. Neurology 2012;78: 1337–1345.
22. Evans RW, Bigal ME, Grosberg B, Lipton RB. Target doses and titration schedules for migraine preventive medications. Headache 2006;46:160–164.
23. Bajwa ZH, Sabahat A. Preventive treatment of migraine in adults. UpToDate 2012;14:1–13, *www.uptodate.com*.
24. Kelman L. The triggers or precipitants of the acute migraine attack. Cephalalgia 2007;27(5):394–402.
25. Magis D, Schoenen J. Treatment of migraine: Update on new therapies. Curr Opin Neurol 2011;24:203–210.
26. Lampl C, Voelker M, Steiner TJ. Aspirin is first-line treatment for migraine and episodic tension-type headache regardless of headache intensity. Headache 2012;52:48–56.
27. Colman I, Friedman BW, Brown MD, et al. Parenteral dexamethasone for acute severe migraine headache: Meta-analysis of randomised controlled trials for preventing recurrence. BMJ 2008;336(7657):1359–1361.
28. Loder E. Triptan therapy in migraine. N Engl J Med 2010; 363:63–70.
29. Center for Drug Evaluation and Research. FDA Public Health Advisory: Combined Use of 5-Hydroxytryptamine Receptor Agonists (Triptans), Selective Serotonin Reuptake Inhibitors (SSRIs) or Selective Serotonin/Norepinephrine Reuptake Inhibitors (SNRIs) May Result in Life-Threatening Serotonin Syndrome. 2011, *www.fda.gov/cder/drug/advisory*.
30. Matthew NT. Dynamic optimization of chronic migraine treatment. Neurology 2009;72(Suppl 1):S14–S20.
31. Holland S, Silberstein SD, Freitag F, et al. Evidence-based guideline update: NSAIDs and other complementary treatments for episodic migraine prevention in adults: Report of the Quality Standards Subcommittee of the American Academy of Neurology and the American Headache Society. Neurology 2012;78:1346–1353.
32. Naumann M, So Y, Argoff CE, et al. Assessment: Botulinum neurotoxin in the treatment of autonomic disorders and pain (an evidence-based review): Report of the Therapeutics and Technology Assessment Subcommittee of the American Academy of Neurology. Neurology 2008;70: 1707–1714.

33. Taylor FR. Tension-type headache in adults: Pathophysiology, clinical features, and diagnosis. UpToDate 2012;3:1–16, *www.uptodate.com*.
34. Bendtsen L, Jensen R. Tension-type headache: The most common, but also the most neglected, headache disorder. Curr Opin Neurol 2006;19(3): 305–309.
35. Taylor FR. Tension-type headache in adults: Acute treatment. UpToDate 2012;14:1–12, *www.uptodate.com*.
36. Taylor FR. Tension-type headache in adults: Preventive treatment. UpToDate 2012;5:1–12, *www.uptodate.com*.
37. Nesbitt AD, Goadsy PJ. Cluster headache. BMJ 2012;344:e2407.
38. Broner SW, Cohen JM. Epidemiology of cluster headache. Curr Pain Headache Rep 2009;13:141–146.
39. May A. Cluster headache: Epidemiology, clinical features, and diagnosis. UpToDate 2012;4:1–12, *www.uptodate.com*.
40. May A. Cluster headache: Acute and preventive treatment. UpToDate 2012;12:1–15, *www.uptodate.com*.
41. Tyagi A, Matharu M. Evidence base for the medical treatments used in cluster headache. Curr Pain Headache Rep 2009;13:168–178.
42. Tfelt-Hansen PC, Jensen RH. Management of cluster headache. CNS Drugs 2012;26(7):571–580.
43. Wolter T, Kaube H. Neurostimulation for chronic cluster headache. Ther Adv Neurol Disord 2012;5(3):175–180.

Attention Deficit/ Hyperactivity Disorder

46

Julie A. Dopheide and Stephen R. Pliszka

KEY CONCEPTS

1. Untreated or ineffectively treated childhood attention deficit/hyperactivity disorder (ADHD) can lead to poor school performance, poor socialization, and increased risk for traffic accidents, psychiatric comorbidities, unemployment, and incarceration during adolescence and adulthood.
2. ADHD is 80% genetic in origin, and it is associated with decreased brain volume, a delay in cortical thickening, and dysregulation of the "default mode network," a brain system that regulates attention, prioritization of information, memory, and impulse control.
3. Symptoms of inattention or hyperactivity and impulsivity or all three must be present during childhood and cause functional impairment in two different settings for 6 months to meet diagnostic criteria for ADHD.
4. Pretreatment assessment of overall physical and mental health, psychiatric comorbidities, and goals of treatment must be set prior to initiating pharmacotherapy.
5. Preschoolers, school-age children, adolescents, and adults with ADHD all can benefit from nonpharmacologic interventions that include a healthy diet, education on ADHD, and potentially effective cognitive and behavioral treatments.
6. The psychostimulants, methylphenidate or amphetamine salts, are the most effective pharmacologic treatment options for all ages with a rapid therapeutic effect, typically within 1 or 2 hours of an effective dose.
7. α_2-Adrenergic agonists such as extended-release preparations of guanfacine and clonidine are less effective than stimulants in monotherapy and are used as adjuncts to improve symptom control, particularly oppositional behaviors and insomnia.
8. When ADHD coexists with bipolar disorder, it is necessary to first stabilize the mood with lithium, an anticonvulsant, or an atypical antipsychotic before adding an ADHD-specific medication such as a psychostimulant.
9. When ADHD coexists with other psychiatric conditions, such as anxiety disorders, major depression, or Tourette's disorder, it is optimal to treat the most functionally impairing disorder first (whether it is ADHD or the co-occurring condition) and then treat the second disorder.
10. Atomoxetine is a good option to manage ADHD symptoms in adolescents and adults with substance abuse disorders. It has a delayed onset of effect (2 to 4 weeks), but it has no abuse potential.

INTRODUCTION

Once considered primarily a childhood disorder, attention deficit/hyperactivity disorder (ADHD) is now known to persist into adolescence for 75% and into adulthood for approximately 50% of individuals.[1,2] The American Academy of Pediatrics (AAP) considers ADHD a chronic condition that requires ongoing management.[1] Functionally impairing inattention, impulsivity, and hyperactivity in the ADHD brain have been correlated with neuroanatomical and functional brain changes.[3,4] It is unusual for an individual to display signs of the disorder in all settings or even in the same setting at all times; however, there is a persistent pattern of symptoms that persists for 6 months or more.[3,5] Co-occurring anxiety, mood disorders, learning disabilities, medical conditions, and substance abuse must be considered in assessment and treatment. Behavioral interventions and medications are effective for all ages, but there are special considerations for treatment plan development and monitoring in each age group.[1–3]

The psychiatric assessment of a child requires obtaining information from the child, parents, caregivers, and teachers.[1] Treating children with psychotropic drugs requires a very different approach than treating adults. Children undergo neurologic, physiologic, and psychosocial changes throughout development. Age-related pharmacodynamic and pharmacokinetic differences can alter drug disposition and response. Psychotropic drug treatment of children is intended to control symptoms or behaviors that impair learning and development.[1,3] Children may not be able to articulate symptom response or adverse effects of a medication. (1) Adolescents and adults with ADHD may not have been diagnosed and treated during childhood, putting them at greater risk for the psychosocial consequences of ADHD including unemployment, unstable relationships, substance abuse, and incarceration.[1–3,6,7]

EPIDEMIOLOGY

In 2010, 5 million children in the United States aged 3 to 17 years had ADHD (8%). Boys (11%) were about twice as likely as girls (6%) to have ADHD. Non-Hispanic white and black children were more likely to have ADHD compared with children of Hispanic or Asian descent.[8] Worldwide rates of ADHD in children range from 4% to 12%.[3] Several epidemiologic studies, including surveys conducted by the National Institutes of Health (NIH), have documented rates of adult ADHD between 3% and 5% with comparable rates in men and women.[2,3]

Prescriptions for ADHD medication increased in all age groups from 1998 to 2005, particularly in adolescents and young adults.[3,9] A National Poison Control Center study estimated that between 1998 and 2005, prescriptions for teenagers and preteenagers increased 133% for amphetamine products, 52% for methylphenidate products, and 80% for both.[9] The FDA used prescription records from 59,000 retail pharmacies to analyze prescribing rates in 2010 compared with those in 2002 in children aged 0 to 17 years for several therapeutic areas including antibiotics, proton-pump inhibitors, antidepressants, and ADHD medications. Overall pediatric prescribing decreased 7% over the 8 years studied, but prescriptions for ADHD medications increased by 46%. Methylphenidate was the most commonly prescribed drug in the ADHD category, but usage remained constant from 2002 to 2010, whereas usage of amphetamine products dropped by 15%.[10] Usage of dexmethylphenidate, lisdexamfetamine, and guanfacine increased from 2004 to 2010, while usage of atomoxetine in youth decreased.[10]

ETIOLOGY AND PATHOPHYSIOLOGY

❷ Both genetic and nongenetic factors are implicated in the pathogenesis. First-degree relatives of an individual with ADHD have a fourfold to eightfold increased chance of developing ADHD compared with the general population; mean heritability (the proportion of variance due to genetics) is around 80%.[11] Candidate gene studies have implicated the dopamine transporter and receptor genes as well as the SNAP25 and COMT genes, but they have been found to account for only a small portion of the variance in ADHD symptoms. Genome-wide association studies (GWAS) have suggested that 40 to 80 different genes might be involved in ADHD, each conveying a small degree of risk.[12]

GWAS studies have previously focused on *common variants*, assuming a small number of genetic alterations, common in the population, accounted for most of the genetic risk in ADHD; this is clearly not the case.[13] Recently genetic studies have focused on multiple rare variants, that is, hundreds or even thousands of genetic variants might be involved in ADHD, such that each patient has a unique genetic pattern. Patients might have copies or deletions in the genome that cover multiple genes called copy number variants (CNV). These CNV studies have implicated a number of systems in ADHD: cholinergic receptors, cholesterol metabolism, and genes for CNS development,[14] an area of chromosome 15q13,[15] as well as glutamate metabotropic receptors.[16] Thus, the pathophysiology of ADHD may go well beyond the catecholamine systems that have been the focus of most studies to date.

Environmental factors may be involved in the etiology of ADHD, as well. Children with fetal alcohol syndrome, lead poisoning, and meningitis have a higher incidence of ADHD symptomatology.[3,17] ADHD is associated with a variety of environmental risks, including obstetric adversity, maternal smoking, and adverse parent–child relationships.[3,17]

❷ Although there are no definitive pathophysiologic markers for ADHD, imaging studies show subjects with ADHD have decreased total brain volume relative to controls in multiple brain regions (right prefrontal cortex, caudate nucleus, anterior cingulate gyrus, and cerebellum). Global thinning of the cortex has been observed in children with ADHD, and comparative studies show there is a delay in cortical thickening in ADHD brains relative to age-matched controls.[3] There is evidence showing that adults with ADHD whose symptoms remitted over time have increased cortical thickening and greater brain volume in key regions controlling attention and behavior than those with residual ADHD symptoms across adulthood.[18]

Functional magnetic resonance imaging (MRI) studies during inhibitory control tasks in patients with ADHD show reduced activity in prefrontal and anterior cingulate cortex, deficits which may be reversed with stimulant treatment.[19,20] Adults and children with ADHD show decreased activation of the ventral striatum when anticipating reward.[21,22] ❷ Alterations in the "default mode" attention network have been found in adults with ADHD.[3] The default mode network consists of the medial prefrontal cortex, medial parietal lobe or precuneus, as well as the posterior cingulate. These areas are active during the "resting state" when attention is not engaged; this system is actively suppressed during active attention. A lack of connectivity between the prefrontal cortex and precuneus (located in the midline of the parietal lobe) is associated with failure of suppression of the default mode network, causing lapses in attention and inhibitory control.[23] Recently, methylphenidate has been shown to decrease aberrant default mode network activation in children with ADHD.[24]

CLINICAL PRESENTATION

The AAP guideline for the diagnosis, evaluation, and treatment of ADHD in children and adolescents recommends an evaluation for any child 4 to 18 years of age who presents with academic or behavioral problems and symptoms of inattention, hyperactivity, or impulsivity.[1] ❸ At least six symptoms of inattention or hyperactivity and impulsivity causing impairment in more than one major setting for 6 months and an onset of symptoms before age 7 are currently required by the *Diagnostic and Statistical Manual of Mental Disorders, Fourth Edition, Text Revision* (DSM-IV-TR) for a diagnosis of ADHD.[5] Validated rating scales, such as the Connors Rating Scales—revised (CRS-revised), are recommended for objective symptom ratings from parents and teachers in different age groups.[1,3,7] The age criteria will likely be raised to 12 years old in the fifth edition of the DSM (DSM-5), given that cases of ADHD without prominent hyperactivity may be missed in childhood.[25] The DSM-5 may lower the number of symptoms required to make a diagnosis in adolescents and adults, given that epidemiologic studies have shown that adolescents and adults have fewer numbers of symptoms than children, but the symptoms are just as impairing.[2,7,26] These proposed changes in the DSM-5 are controversial, as some are concerned that they may result in a dramatic increase in diagnosis of ADHD and an increase in the prescribing of ADHD medications.[27] To make a diagnosis of ADHD, the clinician should rule out alternative causes of symptoms (learning disability, situational stressor) and assess for other conditions that may coexist with ADHD including oppositional defiant and conduct disorders, tics, and sleep and mood disorders.

Clinical **Controversy. . .**

The DSM-5 will likely lower the number of symptoms required to make a diagnosis in adolescents and adults, given that epidemiologic studies have shown that adolescents and adults have fewer numbers of symptoms than children, but the symptoms are just as impairing. These proposed changes in the DSM-5 are controversial to some who are concerned that they may result in a dramatic increase in the diagnosis of ADHD and an increase in the prescribing of ADHD medications.[7,26,27]

CLINICAL PRESENTATION ADHD

General

- Onset of symptoms must be before 7 years of age.

Symptoms

- Six or more of the symptoms must be present for 6 months; significant impairment must be seen in two or more settings (e.g., home and school); symptoms must be documented by parent, teacher, and clinician.
- *Inattention:*
  - Often fails to give close attention to details or makes careless mistakes in schoolwork or other activities
  - Often has difficulty sustaining attention
  - Often has difficulty organizing tasks and activities
  - Avoids tasks that require sustained mental effort
  - Often does not seem to listen when spoken to directly
  - Often does not follow through on instructions and fails to finish schoolwork, chores, or duties in the workplace
  - Is easily distracted by extraneous stimuli
  - Is often forgetful in daily activities
  - Loses things necessary for activities
- *Hyperactivity and impulsivity:*
  - Often fidgets with hands or feet or squirms in seat
  - Often leaves seat when remaining seated is expected
  - Often runs about or climbs excessively at inappropriate times
  - Often has difficulty playing quietly
  - Often interrupts or intrudes on others

Data from American Psychiatric Association. Disorders usually first evident in infancy, childhood or adolescence. In: Diagnostic and Statistical Manual of Mental Disorders, Fourth Edition, Text Revision. Washington, DC: American Psychiatric Association, 2000:39–134.

Preschoolers (3 to 5 Years)

The DSM-IV-TR diagnostic criteria for ADHD can be applied to preschool-age children, although it may be difficult to document symptoms in multiple settings with different caregivers if the child does not attend preschool.[28,29] Enrollment in a qualified preschool and a parent training program is often recommended. Both can help parents develop reasonable expectations for their child's development and foster the development of management skills for problem behaviors. Although methylphenidate has been found safe and effective for ADHD in 4- and 5-year-olds, behavioral interventions are recommended first. Medications can be considered when the child has moderate to severe symptoms unresponsive to behavioral interventions. The clinician needs to weigh the risks of starting medication at an early age against the harm of delaying diagnosis and treatment.[1]

School Age (6 to 11 Years)

Most cases of ADHD are first realized during ages 6 to 9 years, with the child having difficulty academically and/or socially in school and at home. Most children have combined inattentive and hyperactive or impulsive symptoms that cause functional impairment. This period is crucial to the child's success in school, socialization, and the development of his or her sense of self; therefore, accurate diagnosis and treatment is critical. Comorbid oppositional defiant disorder (ODD), conduct disorder, and aggression are indicators that the child is at greater risk for delinquency and substance abuse in adolescence.[30,31] This is the most well-studied age group, with strong data showing benefits of recognition and treatment with behavioral interventions and medications.[1]

Adolescents (12 to 18 Years)

Hyperactivity decreases in adolescents, and inattention and impulsivity are the more prominent functionally impairing symptoms. There may be fewer numbers of symptoms of ADHD in adolescence, but the symptoms present cause significant functional impairment.[26] Higher rates of delinquency, drug and alcohol use, and psychiatric comorbidity have been documented in adolescents with ADHD compared with in those without ADHD.[1,6,7,26] Assessment for substance abuse and risk of diversion must be considered before starting stimulant medications. Speeding and increased motor vehicle accidents occur at higher rates in teens with ADHD compared within those without the disorder.[1,6]

Adults

The presence of multiple comorbid conditions, particularly conduct or mood disorder, can increase the likelihood of ADHD chronicity into adulthood. DSM-IV-TR criteria for ADHD in childhood also apply to adults. Inattentive symptoms are the most common and functionally impairing in adults, but hyperactive and impulsive symptoms are experienced by many and are associated with higher rates of bipolar disorder and psychosis.[2] Cognitive deficits (e.g., executive functioning, working memory, task prioritization, lower IQ) have been documented in adults with ADHD in addition to a greater risk for unstable relationships, unemployment, psychiatric hospitalization, and incarceration compared with those without ADHD.[2,7,32] An ADHD screening tool is available to facilitate assessment in adults not diagnosed during childhood (*http://www.addcoach4u.com/documents/adultadhdscreenertest1.pdf*).[33]

TREATMENT

ADHD-specific cognitive and behavioral interventions are increasingly recognized as necessary components of an overall treatment plan aimed at symptom relief and optimal functioning. Several studies show combining medications with behavioral interventions produces the greatest symptom relief and the best outcomes.

Desired Outcomes

4 Specific goals of treatment or desired outcomes must be identified (e.g., able to sit in chair for 20 minutes; completes homework assignments, or no longer blurts out comments in class without being called upon). For adults, the desired outcome may be to read an entire newspaper before starting another project, improving safety while driving, or successfully completing tasks on time at work.[2,17,32]

TABLE 46-1 Behavioral Interventions for ADHD

Age	Description of Intervention	Typical Outcomes
Preschool and school age	Parent and family education on ADHD Training on behavioral modification Classroom management instruction for teachers	Improved parental understanding and satisfaction Improved compliance with parental commands Improved teacher satisfaction
Adolescent	Break up homework assignments into manageable segments. Structured schedule; organizer	Completion of assignments improves; improved self-esteem and sense of self
Adolescent and adult	ADHD-specific cognitive behavioral therapy Metacognitive therapy	Improved productivity and vocational success Improved relationships

From references 1, 3, 17, 34, and 35.

Nonpharmacologic Therapy

Educational, Cognitive, and Behavioral Interventions

5 Education on ADHD as a biologic disorder with brain-derived causes is essential for destigmatizing ADHD and improving treatment acceptance. Parent training and behavioral interventions such as positive rewards for good behavior and structured limit setting are recommended as first-line interventions before medication trials in preschoolers (3- to 5-year-olds) with ADHD. Behavioral interventions for ADHD are described in Table 46-1. It is crucial to get parents, teachers, and clinicians involved to coordinate care and provide consistent behavioral management for the child at home and at school. School-age children (6 to 11) also benefit from these behavioral interventions in addition to strategies, such as breaking up homework assignments into shorter, manageable segments. Although it varies by state, children and adolescents with ADHD may qualify for an individualized educational program (IEP) that allows for more time to take an exam, preferred seating, and modified work assignments.[1,28] It is noteworthy that most studies comparing behavioral intervention with stimulant therapy in youth found a much stronger effect on ADHD core symptoms from stimulants.[1,3,4] Combined behavioral and stimulant therapy resulted in greater improvements on academic and conduct measures in some studies with greater parent and teacher satisfaction ratings. Combining behavioral interventions with stimulants may allow for lower doses of stimulant that can reduce the risk of adverse effects.[1]

5 Recommended behavioral interventions for adolescents and adults include keeping an external organizer (e.g., smart phone, notebook with "to-do" lists) and breaking up activities into short, manageable tasks. Recognizing triggers for distraction and making a point of thinking before acting are useful interventions and are recommended during cognitive behavioral therapy (CBT) sessions designed to manage adult ADHD.[34,35] Establishing a regular schedule that includes exercise and relaxation can be beneficial as well. Controlled studies have shown that ADHD-specific CBT was more effective than psychoeducation and relaxation in adults with ADHD whose symptoms were only partially responsive to medication.[34] Similarly, adults with ADHD that partially responded to medications benefited more from a group-administered metacognition program (2 h/wk over 12 weeks) compared with supportive therapy sessions administered for the same amount of time.[35] The metacognitive therapy was designed to develop organizational skills and executive function self-management skills. Yoga, meditation, and some dietary supplements have been recommended for ADHD as well, but they should not take the place of more established effective treatments, such as medications and cognitive interventions.

Dietary Interventions

Extensive research has evaluated dietary interventions for ADHD, primarily in children with some adolescent data. When iron and zinc are supplemented in youth with known deficiencies, the therapeutic benefit of stimulant therapy can be enhanced, frequently allowing lower effective doses.[36,37] Omega-3 supplements can benefit some individuals with few side effects, but results are not consistently better than placebo. Additive-free and oligoantigenic elimination diets (e.g., omitting red/orange food dye in lunch meat and hot dogs; avoiding allergenic foods such as dairy and wheat) have been found useful only in small numbers of children who do not respond to other interventions. Although scientific evidence is lacking, there is a universal belief among families that the avoidance of sugar and artificial sweeteners improves ADHD symptoms. The attention paid to sugar avoidance and healthy diet is the more likely reason for improved behavior. An overall healthy diet with the proper balance of protein, fresh produce, and fiber is recommended.[37]

Pharmacologic Therapy

Figure 46-1 provides an algorithm for drug selection in the treatment of ADHD.

Stimulants

Stimulants are considered first-line therapy in most cases of ADHD; however, comorbid conditions impact the drug selection process. Pharmacotherapy should be considered whenever a thorough diagnostic assessment results in a diagnosis of ADHD. Several studies demonstrate the superiority of stimulants over behavioral interventions in alleviating core symptoms of ADHD.[3,38,39] Several studies show improvement in academic performance in medicated children with ADHD versus those unmedicated. A NIH study of 594 fifth graders with ADHD showed those medicated (greater than 90% took stimulants) had 2.9 points higher math scores and 5.4 points higher reading scores compared with unmedicated children.[39] Another study involving 363 ten- to 18-year-olds with ADHD showed medication improved but did not normalize cognition.[40]

6 Stimulants (e.g., methylphenidate, dexmethylphenidate, mixed amphetamine salts, and dextroamphetamine) are the most effective drug treatment options, with an effect size of 0.9 compared with nonstimulant drug treatment options whose effect sizes range from 0.5 to 0.7 signifying lower efficacy.[1,3,41] Methylphenidate and amphetamines block dopamine and norepinephrine reuptake; amphetamines also increase catecholamine release.[42] Both drugs inhibit monoamine oxidase (MAO), amphetamines more potently than methylphenidate.[42] Because different stimulants work through slightly different mechanisms, the lack of response to one chemical class of stimulant (e.g., methylphenidate or dexmethylphenidate) does not preclude response to another class (e.g., dextroamphetamine including lisdexamfetamine or mixed amphetamine salts).[3,4]

Stimulant dosing should be titrated for maximum individual efficacy and minimum side effects (see Table 46-2).[3,4,43–45]

With immediate-release stimulants, most patients require a two or three times daily dosing schedule because of the short half-lives

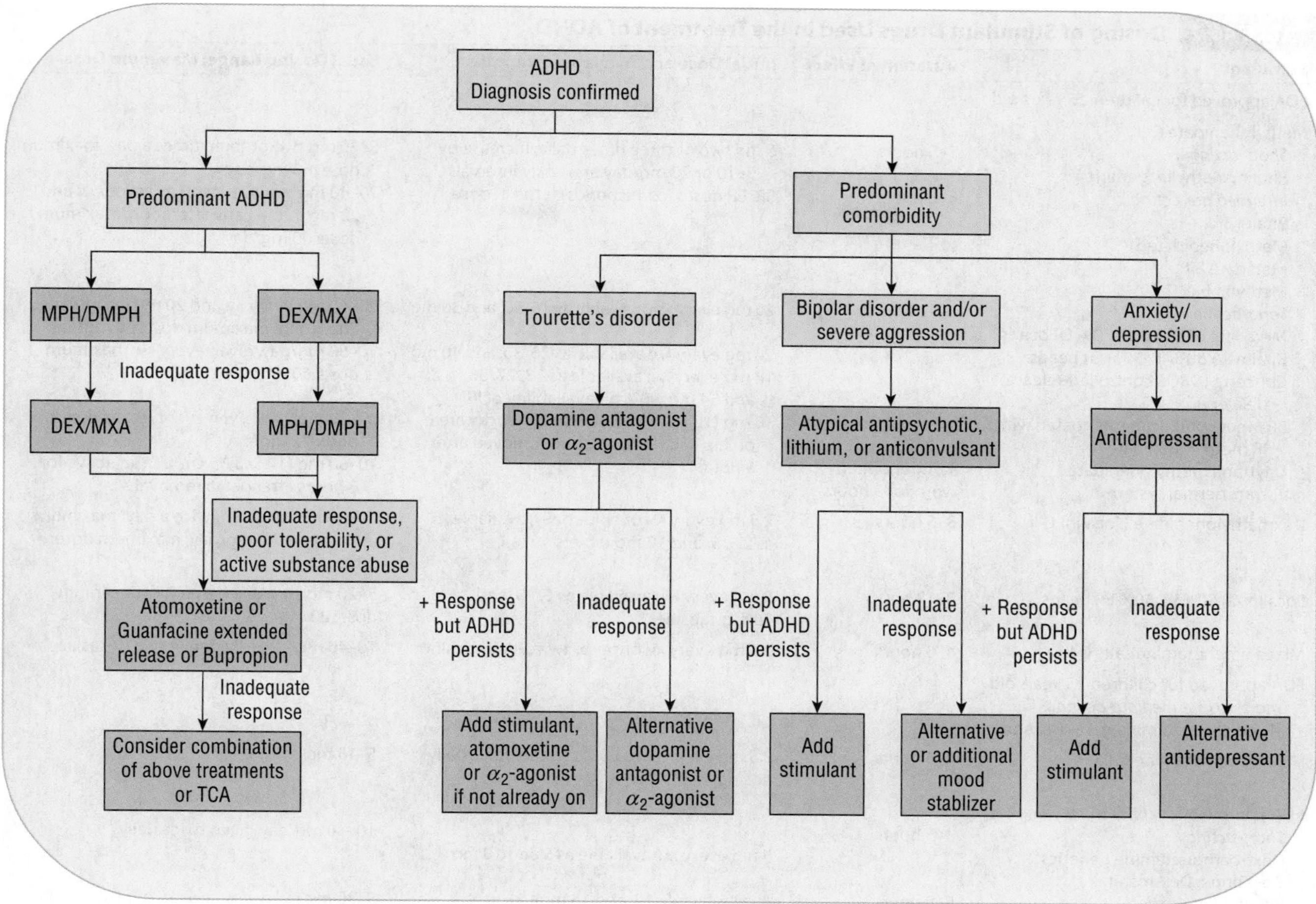

FIGURE 46-1 Algorithm for drug selection in the management of attention deficit/hyperactivity disorder (ADHD). Treat predominant disorder first, reassess, and consider alternative or adjunct medications for optimal symptom control. (DEX, dextroamphetamine; DMPH, dexmethylphenidate; MPH, methylphenidate; MXA, mixed amphetamine salts; TCA, tricyclic antidepressant.)
(Data from references 3, 17, 45, 61, 63, 64, and 68.)

of these drugs (2 to 4 hours for methylphenidate and dexmethylphenidate and ~4 to 6 hours for dextroamphetamine or mixed amphetamine salts).[3,4,17,45] Drug response is maximal during the absorption phase, is evident in 15 to 30 minutes, and lasts 2 to 6 hours.[3,4,17,45]

Drug delivery systems of once-daily products (amphetamine aspartate, amphetamine sulfate, dextroamphetamine sulfate, and dextroamphetamine saccharate [Adderall XR]; methylphenidate [Concerta]; methylphenidate [Daytrana]; dexmethylphenidate [Focalin XR]; methylphenidate [Metadate CD]; and methylphenidate long-acting [Ritalin LA]) provide 8 to 12 hours of symptom control.[3,4,17,41,45,46] Concerta uses an oral osmotic (OROS) controlled-release delivery system, whereas other oral preparations use combinations of immediate-release and extended-release beads.[3,4,45] Concerta is a nondeformable tablet, and it should not be given to children with GI narrowing because of the risk of obstruction. Methylphenidate transdermal system provides 12 hours of symptom control when worn for 9 hours.[41,45,46] Older wax-matrix sustained-release (SR) products (e.g., Ritalin SR) are less effective and infrequently used.[3,4,17] Once-daily stimulant formulations are the preferred treatment for ADHD in most individuals due to convenience and better medication adherence.[3,4,17,47] Immediate-release formulations have the advantage of lower cost, less insomnia, and potentially fewer growth effects versus extended-release products.[3,48] Adolescents and adults with ADHD are also responsive to stimulants.[2,3,45,49] Methylphenidate is effective in adolescents and adults in doses up to 1.5 mg/kg daily.[2,3,17] Lisdexamfetamine is a prodrug conjugated to an amino acid that requires cleavage during metabolism to the active dextroamphetamine. It has a longer time to onset of effect but may provide a smoother blood level compared with extended-release formulations. It is intended to pose less abuse potential.[41]

Administration of stimulant medications with food can delay the absorption and subsequently delay the onset of therapeutic effect by 30 minutes to 1 hour for immediate-release preparations, and 1 to 2 hours for extended-release preparations.[43] Total bioavailability of stimulant can be decreased by 10% to 30% with coadministration of food, more so for beaded formulations of extended-release stimulant compared with OROS methylphenidate or lisdexamfetamine.[43]

Adverse Effects The most common adverse effects of stimulants and their management strategies are listed in Table 46-3. Uncommon to rare but potentially serious adverse effects are discussed in the following sections.

Psychiatric The FDA has added warnings to the labeling of all stimulants and atomoxetine. Hundreds of postmarketing reports of three broad categories of psychiatric adverse events have been associated with stimulants: psychosis or mania, aggression or violent behavior, and severe anxiety or panic attacks. All of these reactions require dose reduction or cessation of stimulant therapy and supportive treatment.[3,50] An analysis of placebo-controlled trials in children showed a rate of stimulant-induced psychosis of 1.49 per 100 person years with no psychosis occurring in the placebo group. Hallucinations involving visual or tactile sensations of insects,

TABLE 46-2 Dosing of Stimulant Drugs Used in the Treatment of ADHD

Stimulant	Duration of Effect	Initial Dose and Available Strengths	Usual Dosing Range; Maximum Dose
FDA approved for children ≥6 years old			
Methylphenidate C-II[a]			
Short-acting IR	3–5 hours	5 mg two or three times daily; increase by 5–10 or 20 mg/day at weekly intervals	5–20 mg two or three times a day; maximum dose: 60 mg/day
Ritalin, methylin, generics			
Intermediate-acting	3–8 hours	SR, ER doses; corresponds to the IR dose	20–40 mg every AM or 40 mg every AM and 20 mg in the early afternoon; maximum dose: 60 mg/day
Ritalin SR			
Methylphenidate SR			
Metadate ER			
Methylin ER			
Long-acting	8–12 hours	20 mg every AM; available as 10, 20, and 30 mg	20–40 mg every AM and 20 mg in the early afternoon; maximum dose: 60 mg/day
Metadate CD 30% IR, 70% ER beads			
Ritalin LA 50% IR, 50% ER beads		20 mg every AM; available as 20, 30, and 40 mg	20–60 mg/day, given every AM; maximum dose: 60 mg/day
Concerta (OROS controlled-release delivery)		18 mg every AM; available as 18, 27, 36, and 54 mg; 90% bioavailability of IR	
ER inner compartments coated with IR methylphenidate		10 mg (12.5 cm²) applied to clean, dry area on hip each morning and removed after 9 hours	27–72 mg/day, given every AM; maximum dose: 72 mg/day
Daytrana methylphenidate transdermal system	12 hours when worn for 9 hours		10–30 mg (12.5–37.5 cm²). Drug active for 3 hours after patch removal
Dexmethylphenidate (Focalin) C-II	3–5 hours	2.5 mg every AM or twice daily; available as 2.5, 5, and 10 mg tablets	5–10 mg/day given twice a day; maximum initial dose: 7.5 mg/day; maximum dose: 20 mg/day
Focalin XR 50% IR, 50% ER beads	8–12 hours	5 mg every AM; available as 5, 10, and 20 mg capsules	5–20 mg/day, given every AM maximum dose: 20 mg/day
Mixed amphetamine salts C-II	4–6 hours	2.5 mg every AM once- or twice-daily dosing	10–40 mg/day (divided in two doses)
FDA approved for children ≥3 years old			
Short- to intermediate-acting			
Mixed amphetamine generics, Adderall			
Dextroamphetamine C-II	4–6 hours	2.5 mg every AM to two or three times daily dosing	5–15 mg twice daily
FDA approved for children ≥6 years old			
Short-acting	3–5 hours		10–40 mg/day given twice daily
Dextroamphetamine generics		5 mg every AM; available as 5 and 10 mg	
Dexedrine, Dextrostat			
Intermediate-acting	5–8 hours	Available as 5, 10, and 15 mg	5–30 mg every day or 5–15 mg twice daily; maximum: 40 mg/day
Dexedrine Spansule	8–12 hours		
Long-acting	8–12 hours		Start at low end; titrate weekly to response; give in AM
Lisdexamfetamine (prodrug converted to dextroamphetamine)		Available as 20, 30, 40, 50, 60, and 70 mg capsules	Longer onset compared with other dextroamphetamine products
FDA approved for children >6 years old			
Adderall XR 50% IR beads, 50% ER beads		Available as 5, 10, 20, and 30 mg capsules	5–30 mg once daily in the morning; maximum: 30 mg/day

ER, extended release; IR, immediate release; OROS, osmotically released oral delivery system; SR, sustained release; XR, extended release.

[a]The Drug Enforcement Administration label C-II, schedule II refers to significant abuse potential.

Data from references 1, 3, 17, and 45.

TABLE 46-3 Stimulant Adverse Effects and Their Management

Adverse Effect	Recommendation/Management Strategy
Common	
Reduced appetite, weight loss	Give high-calorie meal when stimulant effects are low (at breakfast or at bedtime), or consider cyproheptadine at bedtime
Stomachache	Administer stimulant on a full stomach; lower dose if possible
Insomnia	Give dose earlier in the day; lower the last dose of the day or give it earlier; consider a sedating medication at bedtime (guanfacine, clonidine, melatonin, or cyproheptadine)
Headache	Divide dose, give with food, or give an analgesic (e.g., acetaminophen or ibuprofen)
Rebound symptoms	Consider longer-acting stimulant trial, atomoxetine, or antidepressant
Irritability/jitteriness	Assess for comorbid condition (e.g., bipolar disorder); reduce dosage; consider mood stabilizer or atypical antipsychotic
Uncommon to Rare	
Dysphoria	Reduce dosage; reassess diagnosis; consider alternative therapy
Zombie-like state	Reduce dosage or change stimulant medication
Tics or abnormal movements	Reduce dosage; consider alternative medication
Hypertension, pulse fluctuations	Reduce dosage; change medication
Hallucinations	Discontinue stimulant; reassess diagnosis; mood stabilizer and/or antipsychotic may be needed

Data from references 1, 3, and 17.

snakes, or worms were typical in children. Stimulants should not be given to manage attention in individuals with primary psychotic illnesses such as schizophrenia or schizoaffective disorder due to the high risk of worsening psychosis.[50,51]

Cardiac A boxed warning for cardiovascular risks including sudden unexplained death has been added to ADHD stimulant drug labeling.[52,53] Clinical trial data show that children who take stimulants for ADHD can have an increased heart rate by ~5 beats/min and/or increased blood pressure by 2 to 7 mm Hg.[54] A 10-year review showed a 20% increased risk for emergency department visits for cardiac symptoms in those taking either methylphenidate or amphetamine.[54] Of note, these individuals were more likely to have a coexisting anxiety disorder.

In order to assess the risk of adverse cardiac outcomes, two studies of large healthcare databases compared rates of sudden cardiac death, heart attack, and stroke in those taking stimulants compared with in those not taking stimulants. The first study of 1.2 million 2- to 24-year-olds (mean age at baseline 11.1 years) taking stimulants for an average of 2.1 years showed that 3.1 per 100,000 experienced a serious cardiac event. This was no greater than rates in the general population. The second study included 150,000 users of stimulants aged 25 to 64 years old matched to 2 nonusers of stimulants (443,000). Duration of stimulant use was tracked by electronic prescription records and calculated in "person years" with an average of 107,000 person years in the stimulant user group. This study in adults found no greater risk of sudden death, heart attack, or stroke in stimulant users versus nonstimulant users. The relatively short duration of use and overall good health of those studied may have biased the results. These studies add to earlier findings showing no increased risk of serious cardiac events with stimulant use, and, therefore, no restriction in stimulant use has been recommended.[52,53]

Stimulant products generally should be used with caution in pediatrics or adults with known structural cardiac abnormalities. The American Heart Association recommends careful screening of all children and adolescents prior to initiating pharmacologic therapy for ADHD, including a medical and family history and physical examination.[55] The physician should consider a baseline electrocardiogram (ECG) if history suggests cardiovascular disease, but a routine ECG is not necessary.[4] The FDA did not find the risk of sudden unexplained death to be greater in those taking stimulants than in the general population; therefore, no restriction in stimulant use has been recommended.[4,45,49]

Growth Two reviews that analyzed approximately 32 studies indicated that stimulant treatment of ADHD can affect growth, but the effects are minimal or insignificant for most children. A study of 579 children showed a decrease of ~1 cm/y (~0.5 in) in height over 1 to 3 years of continuous treatment with methylphenidate and a weight deficit of 3 kg (6.6 lb) in the first year of treatment and 1.2 kg (2.6 lb) in the second year of treatment.[3] Amphetamine products may be associated with more growth effects than methylphenidate according to separate studies.[3] Proposed mechanisms of stimulant effects on growth include alterations in growth hormone or growth factor, decreased thyroxine secretion, and suppression of appetite leading to reduced caloric intake.[3,48] Two case–control studies, with approximately 140 boys and 110 girls, assessed growth effects after taking stimulant medication over a 10-year period and found no significant effect on growth in boys or girls taking stimulants compared with matched controls not taking stimulant. The average duration of stimulant use was 7.5 years.[56]

In most cases, children should be given a drug-free trial every year.[3,17,45] Time off stimulant appears to lessen stimulant growth suppressant effects, but evidence is lacking to firmly determine the impact of drug holidays on growth.[3,49] Consideration must be given to the risks of negative effects on learning, socialization, and self-image while off stimulant therapy when determining the frequency and duration of the drug-free trial. Annual drug holidays provide time to reassess the need for continued treatment.[3,49] Drug dosage often varies from year to year, largely because of age-related pharmacokinetic changes. As a child develops, hepatic metabolism slows, and volume of distribution increases.[43]

Nonstimulants

Extended-release guanfacine, extended-release clonidine, and atomoxetine are less effective alternatives to the stimulants for treatment of ADHD in children and adolescents. Atomoxetine is also approved in adults. Their potential benefits relative to stimulants include no abuse potential, less potential for growth effects, and less sleep disturbance.[3] See Table 46-4 for dosing.

Atomoxetine Atomoxetine is a selective norepinephrine reuptake inhibitor that should be taken in divided doses in the morning or late afternoon by children for improved tolerability. Adults can take it once daily, usually in the morning.[2,3] Placebo-controlled, short-term trials (6 to 12 weeks) have shown that atomoxetine is effective in reducing ADHD symptoms in children, teens, and adults, and long-term studies show ongoing benefit and safety for children and adolescent responders out to 4 years.[57] A controlled trial comparing atomoxetine, OROS methylphenidate, and placebo over 6 weeks in 6- to 16-year-old patients showed that both drugs were significantly better than placebo at improving ADHD symptoms, but OROS methylphenidate was superior to atomoxetine.[3,49] There was evidence for a preferential response to atomoxetine in some individuals.[49]

Atomoxetine has a significantly slower onset of therapeutic effect than stimulants (2 to 4 weeks vs. 1 to 2 hours with an effective stimulant dose), and full benefit may not be seen for 6 to 8 weeks.[3,49] Atomoxetine is sometimes combined with a stimulant in partially responsive patients based on limited data from open trials and case series describing fewer late-day rebound effects and better sleep when atomoxetine is given in the evening; however, adverse effects are additive.[3,49]

Atomoxetine Adverse Effects Possible adverse effects of atomoxetine, and their management, are similar to those of stimulants, including upset stomach, and psychiatric and cardiac adverse effects (see Table 46-4). Atomoxetine has less growth suppression risk compared with stimulants, but it has a greater risk of fatigue, sedation, and dizziness compared with stimulants or bupropion. Unlike stimulants, atomoxetine labeling includes a bolded warning of potential for severe liver injury following reports in two patients. Continuation studies have not shown evidence for liver toxicity with long-term use; however, a case of idiosyncratic liver toxicity requiring liver transplantation in a 10-year-old boy was reported.[57,58] Also, it is the only FDA-approved ADHD medication with a labeled warning for new-onset suicidality, 0.4% in atomoxetine-treated patients versus 0% in patients receiving placebo.[3] Sexual side effects, primarily decreased libido, have been reported in adults taking atomoxetine.[49]

α_2-Adrenergic Agonists Guanfacine and clonidine are central α_2-adrenergic agonists, acting both presynaptically to inhibit norepinephrine release and postsynaptically to increase blood flow in the prefrontal cortex. Increased blood flow in the prefrontal cortex has been shown to enhance working memory and executive functioning. Both interact with a multitude of neurotransmitter systems, including catecholamine, indolamine, and α_2-receptors on parasympathetic neurons, opioids, imidazole, and amino acid systems.[42]

Guanfacine has a longer elimination half-life and duration of action (18 hours) compared with clonidine (12 hours), and its greater selectivity for the α_{2a}-receptor, compared with clonidine, imparts less sedation and dizziness.[59] (7) Clonidine and guanfacine are not as effective as stimulants for monotherapy treatment. In addition to being approved as monotherapy, extended-release clonidine and guanfacine are FDA approved as adjuncts to stimulants and

TABLE 46-4 Dosing and Adverse Effect Monitoring of Nonstimulant Drugs for ADHD

Drug	Dosing Range and Titration Schedule	Adverse Effect Monitoring
Atomoxetine (Strattera)	≤70 kg (≤154 lb): start at 0.3–0.5 mg/kg every AM or twice daily, maximum: 1.4 mg/kg/day; ≥70 kg (≥154 lb): start at 40 mg every AM or divided twice daily, maximum: 100 mg/day	Nausea, anorexia, ↑ blood pressure, ↑ pulse, insomnia, fatigue, sedation, severe liver injury, suicidality
Bupropion (Wellbutrin SR, XL)	50–300 mg/day; 3 mg/kg/day by end of week 1; can increase to 6 mg/kg/day or maximum of 300 mg/day as tolerated	Nausea, insomnia, rash, tics; dose-related risk of seizures
Tricyclic antidepressants: imipramine, desipramine, or nortriptyline	50–150 mg/day; start at 0.5–1 mg/kg/day; increase as tolerated to 2–3 mg/kg/day; maximum: 300 mg/day of desipramine (adults only) or 150 mg/day nortriptyline	Sedation, dizziness, constipation, heart block (check ECG), weight gain, overdose toxicity, rapid heartbeat
Antipsychotics (for comorbid aggression or mood disorders only)		
Aripiprazole[a] (Abilify)	2–5 mg daily; can titrate weekly as tolerated to response (usual range: 5–20 mg/day)	Nausea, restlessness, insomnia extrapyramidal symptoms, dizziness, sedation
Haloperidol[a] (Haldol)	0.5–1 mg twice daily; can titrate every 3–4 days as tolerated to response (usual range: 0.5–5 mg/day)	Extrapyramidal symptoms, dizziness, ↑ serum prolactin, sedation
Olanzapine[a] (Zyprexa)	2.5–5 mg every day; can titrate every 3–4 days as tolerated to response (usual range: 7.5–15 mg/day)	Sedation, severe weight gain, restlessness, extrapyramidal symptoms Diabetes, marked hyperlipidemia (never a first-line treatment)
Quetiapine[a] (Seroquel)	25–50 mg twice daily; can titrate every 3–4 days as tolerated to response (usual range: 200–600 mg/day)	Sedation, dizziness, weight gain, diabetes, hyperlipidemia
Risperidone[a] (Risperdal)	0.25–0.5 mg twice daily; can titrate every 3–4 days as tolerated to response (1–4 mg/day)	Extrapyramidal symptoms, dizziness, ↑ serum prolactin, hepatotoxicity, weight gain Diabetes, hyperlipidemia
Ziprasidone[a] (Geodon)	10–20 mg twice daily; can titrate every 3–4 days as tolerated to response (usual range: 40–160 mg/day)	Nausea, restlessness, insomnia extrapyramidal symptoms, sedation, QTc prolongation
Other		
Clonidine (Catapres) or clonidine extended release XR (Kapvay)	0.05 mg two or four times daily; can increase as tolerated to 0.1–0.4 mg/day. For XR, give 0.1 mg at bedtime; may increase by 0.1 mg weekly; maximum: 0.4 mg/day given twice a day if dose >0.2 mg/day	Sedation, dizziness, heart block (check ECG), constipation, headache, upper abdominal pain
Guanfacine (Tenex) or guanfacine extended release XR (Intuniv)	0.5 once or twice daily; can increase as tolerated to 1–4 mg/day. For XR, give 1 mg in the AM; titrate weekly to response	Same as above with potentially lower risk of sedation. Effective dose higher in heavier children

ADHD, attention deficit/hyperactivity disorder; ECG, electrocardiogram; SR, sustained release; XL, extended-length.

[a]Short-term use (1–4 months) only for severe aggression associated with ADHD.

Data from references 3, 17, 63, and 64.

have been shown to further decrease ADHD symptoms in children and adolescents only partially responsive to stimulants. Both are prescribed frequently as adjuncts to reduce disruptive behavior, control aggression, or improve sleep in youth.[3,49,59] Neither have been studied sufficiently for ADHD in adults.

Guanfacine XR can be given once daily during monotherapy while clonidine XR should be given twice daily for optimal symptom coverage. Both are considered acceptable second-line agents for children and adolescents unresponsive to or unable to tolerate stomach upset or insomnia with stimulant medications. Extended-release guanfacine and clonidine are more sedating than stimulants or atomoxetine; therefore, sleepiness during the school day requires careful monitoring.[59]

α_2-Adrenergic Agonist Adverse Effects The most common side effects of clonidine and guanfacine are dose-dependent sedation, hypotension, and constipation.[3,45,59] Sedation usually subsides after 2 to 3 weeks of therapy.[3,17,59] Of concern are reports of bradycardia, syncope, rebound hypertension, heart block, and sudden death with immediate-release clonidine.[3,49,59] Four children have died on the combination of methylphenidate and immediate-release clonidine; however, complicating factors make it impossible to link the drug combination directly with the cause of death.[59] Extended-release guanfacine and clonidine appear to pose a lower risk of cardiac adverse effects according to available safety data.[59,60]

Bupropion and Tricyclic Antidepressants Bupropion, a monocyclic antidepressant, is a weak dopamine and norepinephrine reuptake inhibitor with no significant direct effect on serotonin or MAO. Its active metabolites augment noradrenergic and dopaminergic function. Investigations with bupropion in children demonstrated efficacy greater than placebo in two controlled trials and efficacy comparable with methylphenidate (n = 15 children) in another controlled trial.[3,17] Bupropion has been found beneficial for adolescents with depression and ADHD. For adults with ADHD, the number needed to treat (NNT) is between 4 and 5 compared with "2" with stimulant therapy.[46] Bupropion causes less appetite suppression and weight loss compared with stimulants but has a greater risk of seizures.[3,46,49]

Bupropion and Tricyclic Antidepressant Adverse Effects Bupropion's adverse effects include nausea, which can resolve over time or with slower dosage titration, and rash, which can require discontinuation of therapy if severe (see Table 46-4). Bupropion should not be used in children with a seizure or eating disorder because of unacceptable risk of seizures in these patients. It can cause or exacerbate tics.[3,49]

Possible CNS adverse effects of tricyclic antidepressants (TCAs) include dizziness, aggressiveness, excitement, nightmares, insomnia, forgetfulness, and irritability. Similar to other antidepressants, TCAs carry a warning of the risk of new-onset suicidality in pediatric patients and young adults up to the age of 24 years.[61] TCAs should be taken throughout the week and not just on school days. TCA-withdrawal effects are severe in children and include nausea, vomiting, and diarrhea.[61] Signs of CNS toxicity are confusion, impaired concentration, hallucinations, and delusions.

TCAs are last-line agents because they are the most dangerous in overdose and pose the greatest risk for cardiovascular side effects.[17,49] Imipramine and desipramine are the most systematically studied TCAs in the treatment of ADHD, although nortriptyline is also effective.[17] The onset of TCA clinical response occurs within the first 2 to 4 weeks.[17]

Lithium and Anticonvulsants Lithium and anticonvulsants are used increasingly to control aggression and explosive behavior in patients with a diagnosis of ADHD. Some patients actually can have childhood-onset bipolar disorder or combined ADHD–bipolar disorder.[3,62] (8) Lithium, valproate, and carbamazepine are effective for explosive behavior, aggression, and impulsivity, but they are not beneficial treatments for a child with the inattentive subtype of ADHD. Dosing starts in low divided doses with titration over 1 to 2 weeks to therapeutic response.[62,63]

Antipsychotics Conventional antipsychotics such as chlorpromazine and haloperidol can improve symptoms of hyperactivity and impulsivity but can have negative effects on learning and cognitive functioning and can cause extrapyramidal side effects (e.g., dystonia and tardive dyskinesia) that limit their usefulness.[3,64] Second-generation antipsychotics such as risperidone, olanzapine, quetiapine, ziprasidone, and aripiprazole have been used to control severe aggression in refractory cases of ADHD, particularly if conduct disorder or bipolar disorder coexists. They pose a lower risk of extrapyramidal side effects compared with conventional agents, but they can cause metabolic side effects such as hyperlipidemia, hyperglycemia, and weight gain.[63,64] Ziprasidone has the lowest risk of metabolic side effects among these second-generation antipsychotics.

Comorbidity

(9) Individuals with ADHD often present with comorbidities (Fig. 46-1). If multiple drugs are started simultaneously, it is impossible to determine the impact of each drug. The predominance and urgency of symptoms guide the drug selection process. For example, if a child presents as severely anxious or depressed with associated attentional problems, then an antidepressant should be initiated first with monitoring to determine if attentional symptoms improve.[3,45] When a child presents with severe ADHD and associated anxiety or depression, a stimulant should be initiated to treat the more severe ADHD. If ADHD symptoms improve significantly, but anxiety or depression persists, then an antidepressant can be added.[3,45] Studies show that stimulants do not routinely make anxiety disorders worse, but they might not improve symptoms either.[3,4,49] In a child with epilepsy, methylphenidate is safe and effective; however, the child should be stabilized and seizure-free on an anticonvulsant prior to initiation of the stimulant.[65]

ADHD and Substance Abuse

Genetics, age (16 to 25 years old), psychosocial factors, and comorbidities all influence one's risk for drug and alcohol abuse.[66] ADHD itself is a known risk factor for the development of a substance use disorder, and the most commonly abused substances are alcohol and marijuana. A 3-year outcome study of children diagnosed with ADHD showed that they were at least twice as likely to engage in substance abuse (alcohol, cigarettes, marijuana) compared with youth from their same school system without ADHD. The rate of abusing alcohol, cigarettes, and/or marijuana was 17.4% in those diagnosed with ADHD compared with 7.4% in those without ADHD. Children receiving stimulant medication did not have higher rates of abuse compared with those not receiving a stimulant.[67]

Parents frequently express concern that treating their child with a stimulant, particularly early treatment, may increase the risk of substance abuse. Followup studies show that stimulant therapy for ADHD neither increases nor decreases the risk of subsequent drug or alcohol abuse. One study showed that later onset of stimulant initiation (age 8 to 12) was associated with more substance use compared with those starting treatment earlier. In this study, the subgroup with early treatment (before the age of 8) did not differ from comparison subjects in lifetime rates of nonalcohol substance use (27% vs. 29%, respectively). It is possible that early stimulant treatment of ADHD has a protective effect toward the emergence of conduct disorder, which usually precedes antisocial personality disorder and increases the risk for delinquency and drug abuse.

Having conduct disorder along with ADHD further increases an individual's risk of substance abuse. In a prospective study of 11-year-old twins with ADHD and conduct disorder (760 female and 752 male twins) from the Minnesota Twin Family study, having conduct disorder and the hyperactive/impulsive subtype of ADHD predicted substance abuse (nicotine, cannabis, alcohol) at age 14, whereas the inattentive subtype of ADHD had a much lower risk of substance abuse. Youth with aggression combined with hyperactive and inattentive symptoms had greater rates of substance abuse compared with healthy youth or those with only inattentive symptoms. Alcohol and drug use was significantly greater in those with both aggression and inattentive symptoms. Treatment plans targeting aggression and conduct disorder are needed to lower the risk of substance abuse.

(10) Atomoxetine, α_2-agonist, or bupropion is a preferred agent for individuals with ADHD and active substance abuse disorders. If an individual is in recovery, a stimulant can be utilized with close supervision.

Clinical **Controversy. . .**

The use of stimulants to treat ADHD in individuals with a substance use disorder or history of drug or alcohol abuse is controversial. A diagnosis of ADHD confers at least a twofold greater risk of adolescent and adult substance abuse. The risk is greater if conduct disorder, antisocial personality, or bipolar disorder coexists. There is the risk that the individual with ADHD may abuse the stimulant, particularly if he or she is prone to substance abuse. Vigilance among prescribers and careful risk versus benefit assessment is necessary.[3,67]

ADHD and ODD/Conduct Disorder

ODD associated with ADHD in children is responsive to stimulant medication treatment, and once treated, ODD may be less likely to develop into the more severe conduct disorder. A study in aggressive 6- to 13-year-olds with ADHD found that systematic weekly methylphenidate titration to an average dose of 52 mg/day along with behavioral therapy resulted in optimal symptom control without the need for antiaggressive medications such as risperidone or quetiapine. This prevents exposure to the risk of atypical antipsychotic side effects such as weight gain, diabetes, hyperprolactinemia, and extrapyramidal side effects. Studies in adolescents taking OROS methylphenidate found most of them needed between 54 and 72 mg/day for optimal therapeutic benefit.[44] Studies in adolescents and adults with ADHD show that doses of stimulant above the recommended daily maximum are frequently needed for optimal symptom control prompting the American Academy of Child and Adolescent Psychiatry to publish an "off-label maximum dosage of 100 mg/day for methylphenidate and 60 mg/day for dextroamphetamine and mixed amphetamine salts." These dosage ranges appear in the academy's practice parameter on the treatment of ADHD.[2,17]

Tourette's and ADHD

Pharmacotherapy with stimulants increases dopaminergic and noradrenergic activity, which has the potential to aggravate or precipitate tics, although short- and long-term studies in 71 children showed no worsening of tics with methylphenidate dosed up to 0.5 mg/kg/day.[3] Studies examining the comparative effects of methylphenidate and dextroamphetamine on tics in children found the majority experienced improvement in ADHD symptoms with acceptable effects on tics. Methylphenidate was better tolerated than dextroamphetamine.[3,4]

A double-blind, placebo-controlled trial compared methylphenidate or clonidine monotherapy with combination methylphenidate and clonidine in patients with ADHD and Tourette's disorder. Combination therapy demonstrated the greatest benefit in reducing symptoms of ADHD and tics ($P < 0.0001$).[3] Clonidine appeared most helpful for impulsivity and hyperactivity, whereas methylphenidate was most helpful for inattention. All treatments were well tolerated, but sedation was common (28%) in those receiving clonidine.[3] Patients and caregivers should be aware of the risks of using stimulants in children with Tourette's disorder (see ADHD and Substance Abuse above); careful monitoring is essential.[3]

A controlled trial of atomoxetine versus placebo in 117 children with ADHD and Tourette's disorder over 18 weeks showed treatment with atomoxetine 0.5 to 1.5 mg/kg/day improved symptoms of both, with overall good tolerability. Treatment-emergent nausea, decreased appetite, decreased body weight, and increased heart rate occurred significantly more often in those receiving atomoxetine compared with in those receiving placebo.[3]

Clonidine or guanfacine alone is a less effective alternative to stimulants in the treatment of children with Tourette's disorder and ADHD. Guanfacine was administered to 34 children (mean age 10.4 years), with ADHD and tic disorder during an 8-week placebo-controlled trial at a dose of 1.5 to 3 mg/day. Tic severity decreased by 31% in the guanfacine group compared with 0% in the placebo group.[3] There was a mean improvement of 37% on the teacher-rated ADHD scale compared with 8% improvement with placebo. Clonidine and guanfacine's cardiovascular effects warrant careful clinical monitoring.[3,68]

Methylphenidate, clonidine, guanfacine, and atomoxetine appear to reduce ADHD symptoms in children with tics. Although stimulants have not been shown to worsen tics in most people with tic disorders, they may nonetheless exacerbate tics in individual cases. In these instances, treatment with α-agonists or atomoxetine may be an alternative.[68]

Personalized Pharmacotherapy

Factors that should be taken into account to personalize pharmacotherapy for ADHD include age, co-occurring conditions including substance abuse, effectiveness of treatment, side effect sensitivities, and patient or family preference. An individual's ability to metabolize a drug and the drug's pharmacokinetic profile and drug interaction potential should also be considered. To date, genomic studies have not provided information to guide therapy.

Pharmacokinetic and Drug Interactions

Methylphenidate is de-esterified prior to elimination and is less likely to have metabolic drug interactions compared with mixed amphetamine salts. Gender has been shown to influence the absorption of methylphenidate, with males having increased bioavailability compared with females.[43] Variability in dosage requirements for amphetamine salts, atomoxetine, bupropion, and TCAs can be due to interpatient variability in plasma concentration achieved at a given dose. All are metabolized via cytochrome P450 (CYP) 2D6, and bioavailability and half-life can be four to eight times greater in those taking a CYP2D6 inhibitor (e.g., bupropion, fluoxetine, or paroxetine) or in poor metabolizers. For example, atomoxetine's half-life is 5 hours in extensive metabolizers and 19 hours in poor metabolizers.[3] Bupropion is metabolized faster in prepubertal children, making twice-daily dosing optimal for efficacy (even for bupropion SR).[3] Twice-daily dosing of atomoxetine is optimal in children and adolescents to improve tolerability.[3] Once-daily dosing of bupropion or atomoxetine is possible for most adults. If tolerance develops after months of therapy, a dosage adjustment can be necessary to compensate for age-related changes in distribution and metabolism.

EVALUATION OF THERAPEUTIC OUTCOMES

Careful documentation of baseline symptoms and complaints over a 1-month predrug period is essential to the evaluation of therapeutic and adverse outcomes. Investigation regarding family history of psychiatric disorders and cardiac disease is essential to determine risk for related adverse drug reactions and to implement appropriate monitoring.[3,45,49] Baseline symptoms can be measured using videotapes, clinician rating scales (e.g., ADHD Rating Scale IV, Vanderbilt ADHD Diagnostic Scale), or both. In addition, height, weight, and eating, and sleeping patterns should be recorded at baseline and every 3 months.[3,45,49]

After the initiation and titration of any drug treatment, it is necessary that parents, teachers, and clinicians assess the overall functioning of the child or adult using standardized rating scales to determine if significant therapeutic benefit justifies continuing medication.[3,45,49] There is a lack of standardized assessment tools for adults; however, the adult ADHD screening tool can be useful.[33] Therapeutic effects of the stimulants include decreased motor activity and impulsivity and increased attention span.[3,45,49] This suggests that stimulants are indicated for ADHD symptoms and not for primary learning disorders. The benefits of drug therapy must outweigh the potential for adverse effects to justify continued treatment.[3,45,49]

Atomoxetine and bupropion also require monitoring to detect changes in appetite, weight, and sleep patterns, as well as pulse and blood pressure. An adequate trial of atomoxetine or bupropion consists of 6 weeks at maximum tolerated doses unless response occurs at a lower dose.[3,45,49]

When guanfacine or clonidine is given, careful clinical monitoring for fatigue, dizziness, and autonomic changes (e.g., blood pressure and pulse) is recommended.[3,45,59] The American Heart Association has stated that electrocardiographic monitoring is not required for clonidine treatment in children, although many clinicians continue to assess for ECG changes.[55] When discontinuing treatment, clonidine and guanfacine should be withdrawn slowly (0.05 mg clonidine/0.5 mg guanfacine reductions every 3 to 7 days) to prevent rebound hypertension or behavioral dyscontrol.[59,60] A therapeutic trial requires 1 to 2 months to assess therapeutic response, although increased sleep usually occurs immediately.

The effects of TCAs on the ECG should be monitored carefully. Of more concern are reports of sudden death in children taking desipramine or imipramine.[3,49,61] Children and adolescents given TCAs should have pretreatment and followup ECGs to assess the effects of TCA therapy on cardiac rate and rhythm.[61]

ABBREVIATIONS

AAP	American Academy of Pediatrics
ADHD	attention deficit/hyperactivity disorder
CBT	cognitive behavioral therapy
CNV	copy number variants
CRS-revised	Connor's Rating Scales—revised
CYP	cytochrome P450
DSM-5	*Diagnostic and Statistical Manual of Mental Disorders* (fifth edition)
DSM-IV-TR	*Diagnostic and Statistical Manual of Mental Disorders, Fourth Edition, Text Revision*
ECG	electrocardiogram
GWAS	genome-wide association studies
IEP	individualized educational program
MAO	monoamine oxidase
MRI	magnetic resonance imaging
NIH	National Institutes of Health
NNT	number needed to treat
ODD	oppositional defiant disorder
OROS	osmotically released oral delivery system
SR	sustained-release
TCA	tricyclic antidepressant

REFERENCES

1. American Academy of Pediatrics, Subcommittee on Attention-Deficit/Hyperactivity Disorder, Steering Committee on Quality Improvement and Management. ADHD: Clinical practice guideline for the diagnosis, evaluation, and treatment of attention-deficit/hyperactivity disorder in children and adolescents. Pediatrics 2011;128:1007–1022.
2. Wilens TE, Morrison NR, Prince J. An update on the pharmacotherapy of attention deficit/hyperactivity disorder in adults. Expert Rev Neurother 2011;11(10): 1443–1465.
3. Dopheide JA, Pliszka SR. Attention deficit hyperactivity disorder: An update. Pharmacotherapy 2009;29(6): 656–679.
4. Pliszka SR. Psychostimulants. In: Rosenberg DR, West GS, eds. Pharmacotherapy of Child and Adolescent Psychiatric Disorders. Sussex, UK: Wiley-Blackwell, 2012:65–104.
5. American Psychiatric Association. Diagnostic and Statistical Manual of Mental Disorders, Fourth Edition, Text Revision. Washington, DC: American Psychiatric Association, 2000:39–134.
6. Bussing R, Mason DM, Bell L, et al. Adolescent outcomes of childhood ADHD in a diverse community sample. J Am Acad Child Adolesc Psychiatry 2010;49(6): 595–605.
7. Biederman J, Petty CR, Monuteaux MC, et al. Adult psychiatric outcomes of girls with ADHD: 11 year follow-up in a longitudinal case–control study. Am J Psychiatry 2010;167:409–417.
8. Bloom B, Cohen RA, Freeman G. Summary health statistics for U.S. children: National Health Interview Survey, 2010. National Center for Health Statistics. Vital Health Stat 2011;10:250.
9. Setlik J, Bond GR, Ho M. Adolescent prescription ADHD medication abuse is rising along with prescriptions for these medications. Pediatrics 2009;124(3):875–879.
10. Chai G, Governale L, McMahon AW, et al. Trends of outpatient prescribing in US children, 2002-2010. Pediatrics 2012;130(1):23–31.
11. Thapar A, Cooper M, Jefferies R, et al. What causes attention deficit hyperactivity disorder? Arch Dis Child 2012;97: 260–265.
12. Poelmans G, Pauls DL, Buitelaar JK, et al. Integrated genome-wide association study findings: Identification of a neurodevelopmental network for attention deficit hyperactivity disorder. Am J Psychiatry 2011;168: 365–377.
13. Ross RG. Advances in the genetics of ADHD. Am J Psychiatry 2012;169:115–117.
14. Stergiakouli E, Hamshere M, Holmans P, et al. Investigating the contribution of common genetic variants to the risk and pathogenesis of ADHD. Am J Psychiatry 2012;169: 186–194.
15. Williams NM, Franke B, Mick E, et al. Genome-wide analysis of copy number variants in attention deficit hyperactivity disorder: The role of rare variants and duplications at 15q13.3. Am J Psychiatry 2012;169: 195–204.
16. Elia J, Glessner JT, Wang K, et al. Genome-wide copy number variation study associates metabotropic glutamate receptor gene networks with attention deficit hyperactivity disorder. Nat Genet 2012;44:78–84.
17. Pliszka SR, Bernet W, Bukstein O, et al., for the American Academy of Child and Adolescent Psychiatry Work Group on Quality Issues. Practice parameter for the assessment and treatment of children and adolescents with attention deficit/ hyperactivity disorder. J Am Acad Child Adolesc Psychiatry 2007;46:894–921.
18. Proal E, Riesse PT, Klein RT, et al. Brain gray matter deficits at 33-year follow-up in adults with ADHD established in childhood. Arch Gen Psychiatry 2011;68(11):1122–1134.
19. Cubillo A, Halari R, Smith A, et al. A review of fronto-striatal and fronto-cortical brain abnormalities in children and adults with attention deficit hyperactivity disorder (ADHD) and new evidence for dysfunction in adults with ADHD during motivation and attention. Cortex 2012;48:194–215.
20. Rubia K, Halari R, Cubillo A, et al. Methylphenidate normalises activation and functional connectivity deficits in attention and motivation networks in medication-naive children with ADHD during a rewarded continuous performance task. Neuropharmacology 2009;57:640–652.
21. Plichta MM, Vasic N, Wolf RC, et al. Neural hyporesponsiveness and hyperresponsiveness during immediate and delayed reward processing in adult attention-deficit/hyperactivity disorder. Biol Psychiatry 2009;65:7–14.
22. Scheres A, Milham MP, Knutson B, et al. Ventral striatal hyporesponsiveness during reward anticipation in attention-deficit/hyperactivity disorder. Biol Psychiatry 2007;61(5):720–724.
23. Andrews-Hanna JR, Riedler JS, Huang C, et al. Evidence for the default network's role in spontaneous cognition. J Neurophysiol 2010;104:322–335.
24. Liddle EB, Hollis C, Batty MJ, et al. Task-related default mode network modulation and inhibitory control in ADHD: Effects of motivation and methylphenidate. J Child Psychol Psychiatry 2011;52:761–771.
25. American Psychiatric Association. DSM-5 Development. 2012, *http://www.dsm5.org/ProposedRevision/Pages/proposedrevision.aspx?rid=383*.
26. Molina BSG, Hinshaw SP, Swanson JM, et al. The MTA at 8-years: Prospective follow-up of children treated for combined-type ADHD in a multisite study. J Am Acad Child Adolesc Psychiatry 2009;48(5):484–500.
27. Bastra L, Allen F. DSM-5 further inflates ADHD. J Nerv Ment Dis 2012;200(6):486–488.

28. Kaplan A, Adesman A. Clinical diagnosis and management of ADHD in preschool children. Curr Opin Pediatr 2011;23:684–692.
29. Tandon M, Si X, Luby J. Preschool onset ADHD: Course and predictors of stability over 24 months. J Child Adolesc Psychopharmacol 2011;21(4):321–330.
30. Jester JM, Nigg JT, Buu A, et al. Trajectories of childhood aggression and inattention/hyperactivity: Differential effects on substance abuse in adolescents. J Am Acad Child Adolesc Psychiatry 2008;47:1158–1165.
31. Mannuzza S, Klein RG, Truong NL, et al. Age of methylphenidate treatment initiation in children with ADHD and later substance abuse: Prospective follow-up into adulthood. Am J Psychiatry 2008;165:604–609.
32. Hirvikovski T, Waaler E, Alfredsson J, et al. Reduced ADHD symptoms in adults with ADHD after structured skills training group: Results from a randomized controlled trial. Behav Res Ther 2011;49:175–185.
33. New York University Medical School, Harvard Medical School, World Health Organization. Adult ADHD Screening Test for Symptoms of ADHD. 2012, *http://www.help4adhd.org/documents/adultadhdselfreportscale-asrs-v1-1.pdf*.
34. Safren SA, Sprich S, Mimiaga MJ, et al. Cognitive behavioral therapy vs. relaxation with educational support for medication-treated adults with ADHD and persistent symptoms. JAMA 2010;304(8):875–880.
35. Solanto MV, Marks DJ, Wasserstein J, et al. Efficacy of meta-cognitive therapy for ADHD. Am J Psychiatry 2010;167:958–968.
36. Turner CA, Xie D, Zimmerman BM, Carlarge CA. Iron status in toddlerhood predicts sensitivity to psychostimulants in children. J Atten Disord 2012;16(4) 295–303.
37. Millichap JG, Yee MM. The diet factor in attention deficit hyperactivity disorder. Pediatrics 2012;129:330–337.
38. Semrud-Clikeman M, Pliszka S, Liotti M. Executive functioning in children with ADHD: Combined type with and without a stimulant medication history. Neuropsychology 2008;22:329–340.
39. Scheffler RM, Brown TT, Fulton BD, et al. Positive association between attention-deficit/hyperactivity disorder medication use and academic achievement during elementary school. Pediatrics 2009;123:1273–1279.
40. Gualitieri CT, Johnson L. Medications do not necessarily normalize cognition in ADHD patients. J Atten Disord 2008;11:459–469.
41. Brams M, Moon E, Pucci M, et al. Duration of effect of long-acting stimulant preparations throughout the day. Curr Med Res Opin 2010;26(8):1809–1825.
42. Wilens TE. Mechanism of agents used for ADHD. J Clin Psychiatry 2006;67(Suppl 8):32–37.
43. Ermer JC, Adeyi BA, Pucci ML. Pharmacokinetic variability of long-acting stimulants in the treatment of children and adults with attention-deficit hyperactivity disorder. CNS Drugs 2010;24:1009–1025.
44. Blader JC, Pliszka SR, Jensen PS, et al. Stimulant-responsive and stimulant-refractory aggressive behavior among children with ADHD. Pediatrics 2010;126:e796–e806.
45. AAP Algorithm Pediatrics. Implementing the key action statements: An algorithm and explanation for process of care for evaluation, diagnosis, treatment, and monitoring ADHD in children and adolescents. Pediatrics 2011;(Suppl):S11–S21. *http://pediatrics.aappublications.org/content/suppl/2011/10/11/peds.2011*. Acessed (8-1-12).
46. Faraone SV, Glatt SJ. A comparison of the efficacy of medications for adult ADHD using meta-analyses of effect sizes. J Clin Psychiatry 2010;71(6):754–763.
47. Palli SR, Kamble PS, Chen H, Aparasu RR. Persistence of stimulants in children and adolescents with attention-deficit/hyperactivity disorder. J Child Adolesc Psychopharmacol 2012;22(2):139–148.
48. Correll CU, Carlson HE. Endocrine and metabolic adverse effects of psychotropic medications in children and adolescents. J Am Acad Child Adolesc Psychiatry 2006;45(7):771–791.
49. Kaplan G, Newcorn JH. Pharmacotherapy for child and adolescent attention-deficit hyperactivity disorder. Pediatr Clin North Am 2011;58:99–120.
50. Mosholder AD, Gelperin K, Hammad TA, et al. Hallucinations and other psychotic symptoms associated with the use of ADHD drugs in children. Pediatrics 2009;123(2):611–616.
51. Kraemer M, Uekerman J, Wiltfang J, et al. Methylphenidate-induced psychosis in adult ADHD: Report of 3 new cases and review of the literature. Clin Neuropharmacol 2010;33(4):204–206.
52. Cooper WO, Habel LA, Sox CM, et al. ADHD drugs and serious cardiovascular events in children and young adults. N Engl J Med 2011;365:1896–1904.
53. Habel LA, Cooper WO, Sox CM, et al. ADHD medications and risk of serious cardiovascular events in young and middle-aged adults. JAMA 2011;306(24):2673–2683.
54. Winterstein AG, Gerhard T, Shuster J, et al. Cardiac safety of methylphenidate versus amphetamine salts in the treatment of ADHD. Pediatrics 2009;124:e75–e80.
55. Vetter VL, Elia J, Erickson C, et al. Cardiovascular monitoring of children and adolescents with heart disease receiving stimulant drugs: A scientific statement from the American Heart Association Council on Cardiovascular Disease in the Young, Congenital Cardiac Defects Committee, and the Council on Cardiovascular Nursing. Circulation 2008;117:2407–2423.
56. Biederman J, Spencer TJ, Monuteaux MC, Faraone SV. A naturalistic 10-year prospective study of height and weight in children with ADHD grown up: Sex and treatment effects. Pediatrics 2010;157:635–640.
57. Donnelly C, Bangs M, Trzepacz P, et al. Safety and tolerability of atomoxetine over 3 to 4 years in children and adolescents with ADHD. J Am Acad Child Adolesc Psychiatry 2009;48(2):176–185.
58. Erdogen A, Ozcay F, Piskin E. Idiosyncratic liver failure probably associated with atomoxetine. J Child Adolesc Psychopharmacol 2011;21(2):295–297.
59. Croxtall JD. Clonidine extended release in attention-deficit hyperactivity disorder. Pediatr Drugs 2001;13(5):3209–3336.
60. Sallee F, McGough J, Wigal T, et al. Longterm safety of guanfacine extended release in children and adolescents with attention-deficit hyperactivity disorder. J Child Adolesc Psychopharmacol 2009;19:215–226.
61. Dopheide JA. Recognizing and treating depression in children and adolescents. Am J Health Syst Pharm 2006;63:233–243.
62. Geller B, Tillman R, Bolhofner K, et al. Pharmacologic and non-drug treatment of child bipolar 1 disorder during prospective 8-year follow-up. Bipolar Disord 2010;12:164–171.
63. Kowatch RA, Strawn JR, Sorter MT. Clinical trials support new algorithm for treating pediatric bipolar mania. Curr Psychiatry 2009;8(11):19–33.
64. Seida JC, Schouten JR, Boylan K, et al. Antipsychotics for children and young adults: A comparative effectiveness review. Pediatrics 2012;129:e771–e784.

65. Tan M, Appleton R. ADHD, methylphenidate, and epilepsy. Arch Dis Child 2005;90:57–59.
66. Substance Abuse and Mental Health Services Administration. Results from the 2010 National Survey on Drug Use and Health: Summary of National Findings. NSDUH Series H-41, HHS Publication No. (SMA) 11-4658. Rockville, MD: Substance Abuse and Mental Health Services Administration, 2011.
67. Wilens TE, Morrison NR. The intersection of ADHD and substance abuse. Curr Opin Psychiatry 2011;24: 280–285.
68. Pringsheim T, Steeves T. Pharmacological treatment for attention deficit hyperactivity disorder (ADHD) in children with comorbid tic disorders. Cochrane Database Syst Rev 2011;(4):CD007990. doi:10.1002/14651858. CD007990.pub2.

47

Eating Disorders

Steven C. Stoner and Valerie L. Ruehter

KEY CONCEPTS

1. The identification and acceptance of eating disorders as a psychiatric illness is increasingly common. They remain difficult to treat as effectiveness trials are limited, and patients are inherently resistant to accepting treatment.
2. Eating disorder not otherwise specified is currently the most commonly diagnosed form of eating disorder; however, proposed changes to the diagnostic criteria in the fifth edition of the *Diagnostic and Statistical Manual of Mental Disorders* would separate binge eating disorder as a stand-alone diagnosis.
3. Despite strong genetic associations for the development of eating disorders as established in monozygotic and dizygotic twin studies, a clear association with a specific genetic link mutation has not been identified.
4. Shifting between eating disorder diagnostic categories is possible, especially when symptom remission is not achieved with treatment.
5. Psychiatric comorbidities are common with all forms of eating disorders, and the differential diagnosis should generally include evaluation for depression, schizophrenia, generalized anxiety, and obsessive–compulsive and personality disorders.
6. During the process of caloric restoration, calories must be gradually introduced to prevent the potentially fatal complication known as refeeding syndrome.
7. Mortality resulting from suicide in eating disorders is not uncommon, and clinicians must monitor closely for suicidality and educate appropriately as they would during the treatment of patients with major depressive disorder with antidepressant therapy.
8. The current preferred treatment approach for anorexia nervosa includes a minimum of 6 months of psychotherapy, preferably cognitive behavioral therapy.
9. Data supporting the use of medication in anorexia nervosa are largely inconclusive. Primary limitations are small sample sizes and a bias in clinical trials because more highly motivated patients participate in studies.

Eating disorders are widely accepted as serious mental illnesses. The spectrum of eating disorders encompasses several complex diseases, sharing the pathologic feature of overevaluation of body shape and weight. Eating disorders arise from the interaction between environmental, societal, developmental, psychosocial, genetic, and biologic factors. It is estimated that 5 to 10 million women and 1 million men in the United States alone have an eating disorder. The urbanization of society, social pressure, and obsession with perfection and being thin have led to an increasing prevalence of eating disorders, with the peak onset being between 16 and 20 years of age.[1–4] Anorexia nervosa (AN), bulimia nervosa (BN), and eating disorders not otherwise specified (EDNOS) are the primary disorders that have been identified.[5]

(1) Despite an improved understanding of these cognitively and emotionally disabling and potentially fatal disorders, management remains difficult. Pharmacologic intervention is a small part of a comprehensive plan that emphasizes cognitive behavioral therapy (CBT) and psychotherapy.

EPIDEMIOLOGY

Anorexia Nervosa

AN occurs predominantly in girls and young women (90%) and usually presents in late adolescence (median onset 17 years of age), with new cases rarely diagnosed after age 40. The estimated prevalence of the disorder in the general population is 0.9% of females and 0.3% of males.[6] Longitudinal management of AN is difficult, as patients are often resistant to weight restoration plans. Rates of relapse requiring hospitalization within 1 year exceed 30%, and crude mortality rates are estimated at 4%.[7,8]

The promotion of the virtues of being thin is also a potentially negative environmental factor. Many websites, for example, inappropriately promote healthy lifestyle aspects of anorexia and being thin as a means of being in control, successful, and coping with life's pressures.[9]

Bulimia Nervosa

BN also occurs predominantly in girls and young women (90%) and usually presents in adolescence or early adult life.[6] Between 1% and 4.6% of adolescent and young adult females meet the diagnostic criteria for BN, with lifetime prevalence estimates of 1.5% of females and 0.5% of men.[3,5,6,10,11]

Eating Disorder Not Otherwise Specified

EDNOS is also described in the American Psychiatric Association's *Diagnostic and Statistical Manual of Mental Disorders, Fourth Edition, Text Revision* (*DSM-IV-TR*).[3,5] Originally designed to capture eating disorder cases that did not meet diagnostic criteria of AN or BN, it has instead developed into a diagnosis of indifference. (2) The overall prevalence of EDNOS is estimated at 3.5% among women and 2% in men, the highest prevalence of the eating disorders.[6] An estimated 50% of patients with an eating disorder admitted to tertiary care settings are believed to have this condition.[12] These individuals present with symptoms characteristic of eating disorders but do not meet specific diagnostic criteria. Two examples of EDNOS are night eating syndrome (NES) and binge eating disorder (BED).

NES is common in obesity clinic populations, often accompanied by depressive symptoms. The syndrome is defined by early morning anorexia, hyperphagia in the evening, nighttime insomnia, and subsequent early morning awakening.[5,13] NES affects an estimated 1.5% of the general population and 8.9% to 27% of patients in obesity clinics.[14–16] Patients with NES are reported to benefit from antidepressant therapy, most notably sertraline 50 to 200 mg daily.[13]

The diagnostic criteria for BED describe recurrent episodes of binge eating without compensatory behaviors (e.g., purging, excessive exercise, or fasting). BED typically presents later in life (older than 40 years of age), and approximately one fourth of BED patients are male.[12,17] CBT and interpersonal psychotherapy are the preferred treatments, although antidepressant therapy has also demonstrated limited benefits.[17]

ETIOLOGY AND PATHOPHYSIOLOGY

While the exact etiology of eating disorders is not known, it is most likely a combination of genetic, biologic, developmental, and environmental factors. The biologic basis for eating disorders is difficult to delineate because it is unclear if the biologic changes are caused by or are a result of the aberrant eating behavior.

Abnormalities of the hypothalamic–pituitary–gonadal, hypothalamic–pituitary–adrenal, and hypothalamic–pituitary–thyroid axes are described as potential causes of AN. Amenorrhea is found in the majority of females with anorexia, providing support for the association with gonadotropin.[11]

Serotonin, norepinephrine, and dopamine have been studied extensively with well-described roles in controlling eating behaviors, with more emphasis placed on the role of serotonin. Complicating the study of these abnormalities is that their dysfunction is thought to be secondary to weight loss. There is evidence suggesting serotonin and dopamine function remain abnormal after weight restoration.[18,19] Another molecular genetic target of study is brain-derived neurotrophic factor (BDNF), which is also being studied in disease states such as depression.[20]

3 There are strong genetic influences in AN and likely associations in both BN and BED. In addition, there is a high degree of premorbid anxiety and obsessive tendencies, which are also symptoms of disorders with suspected genetic associations. Twin studies have shown concordance of ~55% and 35% in monozygotic twins and 5% and 30% in dizygotic twins for AN and BN, respectively.

One of the most common areas of research has centered on the roles of serotonin, dopamine, and norepinephrine. Serotonin is the most commonly studied neurotransmitter in patients with eating disorders, but its study is complicated by the fact that it is affected by other factors including sex hormones. In addition, reduced dietary intake of food leads to reduced levels of tryptophan, which is required for the development of serotonin.[18–20] Serotonin activity is abnormally high in patients recovered from AN. In addition, serotonin 2A receptors are reduced after recovery, while dopamine receptors are increased.[18–20]

Genetic-based linkage studies have examined multiple single nucleotide peptides to identify predictors for developing AN, which may subsequently help identify appropriate pharmacologic treatments. Studies to date have identified possible associations with chromosomes #1, #2, #3, #4, and #13; however, there are no consistent findings to date, and studies are limited by low sample size.[18,21,22] Genetic mutation studies have focused on polymorphisms of the serotonin 2A receptor.[17] One acquired hereditary abnormality being studied is the presence of low-function alleles associated with the serotonin transporter (*5-HTTLPR*) and serotonin 2A receptor gene (*–1438G/A*), with findings suggesting an association with poor treatment response.[23] Recent work has also associated estrogen receptor I gene (ESRI) with the restrictive form of AN.[24]

Emphasis is also placed on environmental factors such as social stress and psychological and developmental issues related to dysfunctional family relationships triggering abnormal eating behavior.[3,11,12,25] Athletes are at risk for eating disorders, especially female gymnasts, ballet dancers, figure skaters, distance runners, swimmers, male wrestlers, and body builders.[26]

DIAGNOSTIC CRITERIA AND CLINICAL PRESENTATION

AN and BN occur together in ~30% to 64% of patients with eating disorders, and they may not be distinct diagnostic entities, but rather a continuum of symptoms. Thus, careful medical and psychiatric assessment at baseline is essential.[27–30] **4** Patients who initially present with either AN or BN may alternate from one to the other, especially in cases where remission is not achieved. Figure 47-1 demonstrates similar and unique features of both disorders.

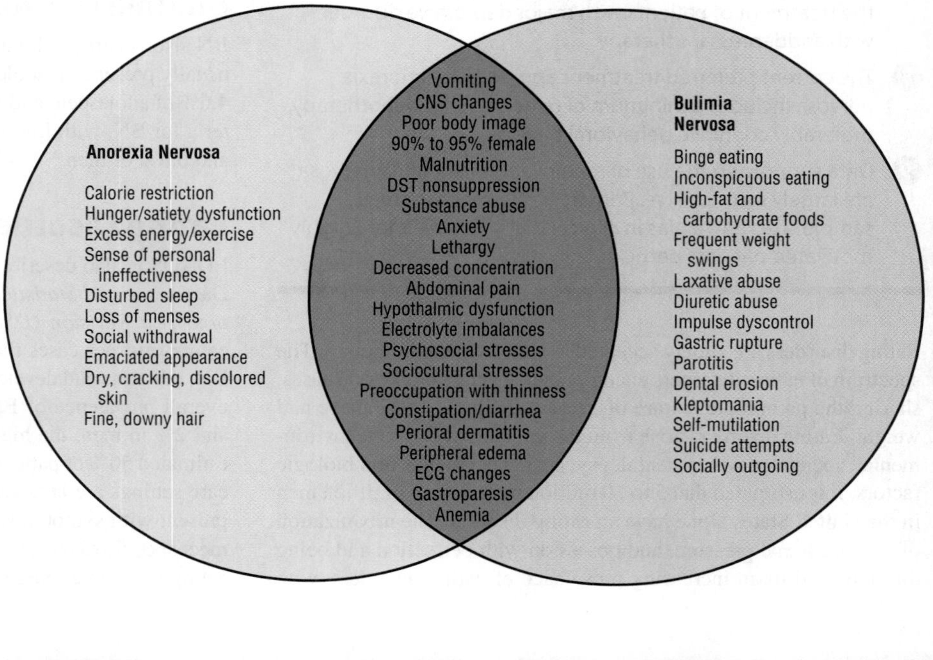

FIGURE 47-1 Signs and symptoms of anorexia nervosa and bulimia nervosa. (DST, dexamethasone suppression test; ECG, electrocardiogram.)

The use of purging methods is not limited to BN. Self-induced vomiting is the most common form of purging behavior.[31] Laxative abuse is another form of purging common in both AN and BN, used by an estimated 3% to 70% of patients.[31–33] Although ineffective as a weight-loss strategy, laxative abuse is often used in combination with other behaviors, including exercise, diuretics, enemas, and saunas. Within the diagnostic framework of AN, laxative abuse is most common in those identified with the purging subtype.[31] Psychiatric symptoms of depression, anxiety, and borderline personality disorder are also reported in those who abuse laxatives.[31–33]

Depression, schizophrenia, obsessive–compulsive disorder (OCD), and conversion disorders should be included in the differential diagnosis of AN and BN, as eating abnormalities can be a component of these illnesses. The salient differences are the overriding drive for thinness, disturbed body image, increased energy directed at losing weight, and binge eating episodes that are relatively specific for eating disorders. Most patients with eating disorders experience relief of psychiatric symptoms on refeeding.[12]

Anorexia Nervosa

The presentation of AN includes a recent period of weight loss as well as associated behaviors to promote this such as vomiting, limiting food intake, and excessive exercise. Current diagnostic criteria for AN include the refusal to maintain a minimal normal body weight, failure to make expected weight gains, intense fear and obsession about weight gain or being "fat," distorted body image, and amenorrhea for at least three consecutive cycles.[5] Patients typically lack an appreciation for the degree of weight loss experienced or are preoccupied with the idea that a part of their body is too large, despite evidence to the contrary. The *DSM-IV-TR* further classifies AN as restricting type (restricting food intake with no binge eating or purging behavior) or binge eating/purging type, in which patients regularly participate in bingeing or purging.[5] The anorexic patient has difficulty sensing when he or she is full (satiety) and commonly complains of feeling bloated after eating. Patients also describe not feeling in control of various aspects of their life, particularly caloric intake. Comorbid psychiatric conditions, such as major depression, are frequent but should initially be considered secondary to starvation and not a true mood disorder.

The fifth edition of the *Diagnostic and Statistical Manual of Mental Disorders* (*DSM-V*) is scheduled for release in 2013. A *DSM-V* work group is recommending a number of changes to the diagnosis of AN.[34] These include the following: elimination of descriptive examples for body weight maintenance, adding behavior as a symptom for failing to gain weight, removal of amenorrhea as a diagnostic component, and limiting the subclassifications of AN to symptoms exhibited in the prior 3 months.[22,34,35]

5 Psychiatric comorbidity is common, as up to 75% of patients have a primary mood disorder, and there is also an association with personality disorders and anxiety disorders, such as social phobia and OCD.[36] The lifetime prevalence of OCD in patients with AN is reported to be as high as 40%; the lifetime prevalence in the general population is 2.5%.[36–38] The impact that psychiatric comorbidity has on treatment outcomes of AN is unknown, but it is important to understand that deprivation of food may contribute to both mood and cognitive fluctuations.

Bulimia Nervosa

The core feature of BN is recurrent episodes of binge eating (an excessive intake of calorie-laden food over a short period of time). Persons with BN are overly sensitive about their weight and have a distorted body image. Most have normal weight, although they might fluctuate between being underweight and overweight. Patients lack control over their eating and participate in recurrent compensatory behavior to prevent weight gain. These behaviors may include self-induced vomiting; misuse of laxatives, diuretics, enemas, or other medications; strict dieting or fasting; or excessive exercise. To meet *DSM-IV-TR* criteria, the binges and compensatory behaviors must occur on average at least twice weekly for 3 months.[5] BN can further be differentiated by purging type (regularly engages in self-induced vomiting or the misuse of laxatives, diuretics, or enemas) or nonpurging type (uses other inappropriate compensatory behaviors, such as fasting or excessive exercise, but does not engage in purging activities).[5]

The *DSM-V* work group has proposed standardization of the frequency of symptoms for BN and BED, reducing the requirement of binges and compensatory behavior to one time per week for 3 consecutive months.[34] Subclassifications of BN would be eliminated in the new edition, with BN including what was formerly recognized as the purging form. The nonpurging form would now fall under the category of BED. By broadening the criteria, the size of the population in the EDNOS category should be reduced.

CLINICAL PRESENTATION Anorexia Nervosa

General

- Patients refuse to maintain body weight and have distorted perceptions about their body.

Symptoms

- Patients have obsessions and fears about eating and gaining weight.
- They complain about feeling full even when they have eaten very little food.
- Denial of symptoms and low self-esteem are the norm. Patients often feel ineffective and have a lack of self-control.

Signs

- Weakness, lethargy, cachexia, amenorrhea, vomiting, restricted food intake, inappropriate exercise, delayed sexual development, edema, delayed gastric emptying, constipation, bradycardia, hypotension, osteoporosis, dry cracking skin, lanugo, callus on dorsum of hand, perioral dermatitis, and erosion of dental enamel

Laboratory Abnormalities

- Hypokalemia, hypokalemic alkalosis, hypomagnesemia, leukopenia, QT interval prolongation, ST segment depression, U waves, hypercholesterolemia, and anemia

Other Diagnostic Tests

- Nonspecific electroencephalogram (EEG) changes

CLINICAL PRESENTATION Bulimia Nervosa

General

- Patients binge eat and stop when they have abdominal pain or self-induced vomiting or are interrupted by another person.
- They have a pattern of severe dieting followed by binge eating episodes.
- They are concerned about their body image but do not have the drive to thinness, which is characteristic of AN.

Symptoms

- Patients do not eat regular meals and do not feel satiety at the end of a meal.
- They may use laxatives for weight control.
- They have guilt, depression, and self-disparagement after binges.
- Social isolation can result from frequent bingeing.
- Chaotic and troubled personal relationships and substance abuse are common.

Signs

- Bingeing, vomiting, salivary gland inflammation, erosion of dental enamel, callus on dorsum of hand, perioral dermatitis, dental caries, parotid gland enlargement, abdominal pain, upper end of normal body weight or slightly overweight, frequent weight fluctuations, and diminished masticatory ability

Laboratory Abnormalities

- Hypokalemia, hypochloremic metabolic acidosis, and elevated serum amylase

Other Diagnostic Tests

- None

Patients typically binge and vomit at least once daily. Caloric intake varies, but patients can consume between 5,000 and 20,000 cal (20,929 and 83,716 J) during a single binge. Patients tend to consume foods that are easy to ingest, do not require much chewing or preparation, and are high in carbohydrates or fat. Binge eating is typically secretive and precipitated by a stressful event, followed by postbinge remorse. Binges often last less than 2 hours but can extend to more than 8 hours. To compensate for the excessive caloric intake, many patients fast for prolonged periods, exercise compulsively, purge, or abuse laxatives.

Psychiatric comorbidity includes depression (up to 80%), poor impulse control, and substance abuse. Approximately 30% to 37% of bulimic patients have a personal history of substance abuse.[39] Kleptomania and borderline and avoidant personality disorders are also frequently observed.[36,40] Patients also commonly steal laxatives and comfort items, such as candies and clothes.[11]

Binge Eating Disorder

Patients with BED present with recurrent episodes of bingeing without the compensatory behaviors associated with AN or BN. It is estimated that 5% to 10% of patients seeking treatment for obesity have BED. Comorbid psychotic disorders are common and reported in greater than 70% of BED patients.[41] Major depressive disorder and low self-esteem are common, although the self-deprecating focus on body image is less severe than in AN or BN.[15,38] Diagnostic criteria require that episodes of bingeing occur at least twice weekly over a period of 6 months.[5]

Proposed changes in the *DSM-V* are to separate out BED from the EDNOS category and change the diagnostic criteria for bingeing frequency to only once weekly.[22,34] In addition, what was formerly recognized as nonpurging BN would now be classified as BED.

MEDICAL COMPLICATIONS OF EATING DISORDERS

The potential medical complications of eating disorders involve multiple organ systems. The type of medical complication encountered is dependent on the type and frequency of the eating disorder behavior. Cardiac complications may occur and can include wasted cardiac muscle, orthostatic hypotension, decreased cardiac output, arrhythmia, and QTc interval prolongation.[42] 6 During caloric restoration, there is a potential risk for developing refeeding syndrome, which can progress to fatal cardiovascular collapse. This risk is reduced by the gradual versus rapid reintroduction of calories.

Metabolic (metabolic acidosis, metabolic alkalosis) and electrolyte disturbances (e.g., hypokalemia, hypomagnesemia, and hypocalcemia) and dehydration are often seen. Elevations in bicarbonate levels during periods of hypokalemia can be an indication that the patient is inducing vomiting or using dietary weight-loss medications. Non–anion-gap acidosis has also been reported with the abuse of laxative agents. Additionally, both acute and chronic renal failures have been reported.

GI, oropharyngeal, and dental complications are frequent, as are general complaints of lethargy and fatigue. Evidence of Russell's sign may be present signified by skin lesions on the fingers used to induce vomiting.

Hormonal changes related to the hypothalamic–pituitary–gonadal axis resulting from starvation are seen. These abnormalities include effects on estradiol, the gonadotropins (e.g., luteinizing hormone, follicle-stimulating hormone, and gonadotropin-releasing hormone), thyroid function, adrenal function, and growth hormone.[11,42] Specific to female athletes is the female athlete triad, defined by the development of irregular menses, osteoporosis, and disordered eating.[42,43] An athlete may experience only one or two components of the triad, or all three conditions.[44] Osteopenia, osteoporosis, and infertility are potential long-term complications of suppressed estrogen. The restoration of weight, specifically in AN, reverses the bone loss, although estrogen supplementation does not appear to be effective.[45] In all cases, the preferred method to address these issues is the normalization of nutrition. The impact on female fertility is not well studied, although the ability to carry a pregnancy to term or to give birth to a child of average birth weight appears reduced.

Chronic starvation can contribute to brain atrophy. Decreases in white matter and cerebrospinal fluid volumes return to normal after a healthy weight is achieved, but gray matter loss can persist.[12,46,47] A thorough physical and laboratory evaluation, as described in Table 47-1, is essential to determine the severity of medical complications.[5,25,48]

TABLE 47-1 Physical and Laboratory Assessment of Eating Disorders

Evaluation	Target Symptoms
Pulse	Bradycardia
Blood pressure	Hypotension, orthostasis
Height/weight	Underweight for size and age/body mass index
Respiratory rate	Rapid if heart failure occurs during refeeding
Temperature	Hypothermia, cold intolerance
Electrocardiogram	ST depression, flat T waves, U waves, increased QT interval, atrioventricular block
GI	Hypoactive bowel sounds, gastritis, abdominal distention
Skin	Dryness, scaling, lanugo, hair loss, calluses on fingers and hands
Menses	Amenorrhea
Complete blood count	Leukopenia, anemias, thrombocytopenia
Electrolytes	Hypokalemia, hypomagnesemia, hypophosphatemia, or hyperphosphatemia
pH	Metabolic alkalosis (acidosis if laxative abuse)
Amylase	Elevated; pancreatitis rare
Liver	Hypoalbuminemia, γ-glutamyl transferase if alcohol abuse
Thyroid	Low to low normal, but not true disease
Cortisol	Elevated with lack of suppression on dexamethasone suppression test
Bone density	Osteoporosis

From references 5, 12, 25, and 56.

TREATMENT

Desired Outcomes

The goals for patients with eating disorders are to reduce distorted body image; restore and maintain healthy body weight; establish normal eating patterns; improve psychological, psychosocial, and physical problems; resolve contributory family problems; enhance compliance; and prevent relapse.[12] Specific to BED is the additional goal of weight loss.

Prognosis

Anorexia Nervosa

The long-term prognosis of patients with AN is not clear, as studies focus only on patients receiving treatment. The course of the disorder most commonly consists of a single episode with subsequent return to normal weight, although patients can still experience issues with disturbed body image, disordered eating, and other psychiatric problems.[12] Some patients experience an unremitting course leading to death, whereas others suffer episodically. Remission rates appear to be a function of time in treatment as the lowest rates of remission are reported in shorter-duration followup trials, while remission rates near 80% have been reported in longer-term followup studies at 8 and 16 years.[30] Despite this, it is estimated that up to 20% remain chronically ill despite weight normalization, return of menses, and improved eating behaviors.[49] The prognosis is more favorable with longer followup care and younger age of onset, whereas a poorer prognosis is associated with chronic illness, lower initial weight, poor family relationships, obsessive–compulsive personality symptoms, and the presence of bulimia or purging behavior.[17,49–51] ⑦ Crude mortality rates appear to be lower than historically projected at a current estimated rate of 2.8% to 4%, although when associated death occurs, it is most often the result of cardiac arrest or suicide.[5,30,49]

Bulimia Nervosa

The prognosis of BN, although not well studied, appears to be better than that of AN. Patients with milder presenting symptoms who are treated as outpatients tend to do better, whereas those with electrolyte imbalances, esophagitis, dental caries, and salivary gland enlargement have a more complicated course.[11] The presence of psychiatric comorbidity and greater general psychiatric symptom severity have been determined to be poor prognostic indicators. Longer rates of followup tend to have higher rates of remission, reaching 70% or higher with 5 to 20 years of followup. However, it is important to note that even in cases in which patients respond, they continue to exhibit symptoms that wax and wane, sometimes meeting full criteria for diagnosis of BN or less severe symptoms of EDNOS. Total absence of symptoms is an uncommon outcome, and residual symptoms predispose the patient to relapse.[30] The actual definition of recovery varies, as once-a-month binge–purge episodes are considered by some to be recovery if their episodes were previously more frequent, whereas other clinicians consider a patient recovered only when there is complete absence of these behaviors.[51]

Binge Eating Disorder

Of all of the eating disorders, BED has the least amount of long-term followup data associated with it. Studies to date suggest higher remission rates (25% to 80%) in 1- and 4-year followup studies compared with findings in AN and BN longitudinal studies. These numbers are irrespective of treatment selected and treatment during the followup time frame studied. Estimated crude mortality rates range from 0% to 3% with a cumulative mortality rate reported at 0.5%.[30]

General Approach to Treatment

Treatment plans are individualized based on the severity of specific core features of the eating disorder and comorbid medical and psychiatric conditions. Psychiatrists, physician assistants, nurses, nutrition specialists, psychologists, and pharmacists play a role in the care of these complex patients. The absence of an adequate support system of family and friends can contribute to failed treatment. A critical first step is to determine the severity of illness, as that drives both the intensity and the setting for delivery of care. Hospitalization is generally reserved for the most severely ill patients. Some criteria for hospitalization are outlined in Table 47-2.[17,25,26] Medications are rarely indicated as a sole treatment for eating disorders, and many patients refuse medication, although they remain part of the comprehensive treatment strategy.[52–54] Comparative, double-blind, placebo-controlled trials are sparse, and most are limited by small sample sizes, ambivalent patient attitudes toward treatment, medical complications, and high dropout rates.[55]

Clinical **Controversy. . .**

Many clinicians believe that extrapolation of study results to AN patients in the clinic is tenuous at best. Most patients in the clinic have a low desire to improve their overall health and well-being, based on an abnormal perception of their body image. Study results have a natural bias, as they include those patients willing to try and get better.

TABLE 47-2 Criteria for Hospitalization of Patients with Eating Disorders

- Significant weight loss of 20% or more of normal weight, particularly if weight loss has been recent and rapid, severe starvation symptoms are present, or the patient has been ill for more than 2 years
- Reduced oral intake of food (sudden and persistent)
- Medical complications (e.g., edema) and metabolic abnormalities (e.g., hypoproteinemia) from bingeing, purging, and starvation (e.g., heart rate <40 beats/min, blood pressure <90/60 mm Hg, glucose <60 mg/dL [<3.33 mmol/L], potassium <3 mEq/L [<3 mmol/L], or inability to maintain core temperature)
- Co-occurring psychiatric symptoms, notably suicidal ideation, psychotic depression, or substance abuse and dependence
- Nonresponsive to outpatient treatment (after 3–4 months) and poor motivation to recover
- Demoralization or nonfunctional family
- Denial of severity of abnormal eating behaviors
- Continuous supervision required to prevent purging (vomiting or laxative abuse)

From references 5, 12, 17, 25, 26, and 56.

Anorexia Nervosa

Nonpharmacologic Treatments

8 Evidence supports that nonpharmacologic treatments have the greatest likelihood of eliciting a response in AN patients.[12,52] This includes CBT, dialectical behavioral therapy, behavioral management, interpersonal psychotherapy, nutritional counseling, and family therapy.[12,25,35,56] Current guidelines suggest at least 6 months of psychotherapy is preferred.[56] CBT helps the patient overcome distorted thinking, including self-worth as measured by body image, feelings of being fat despite evidence to the contrary, and denial. CBT also teaches patients how to use strategies besides eating to cope.

Interpersonal psychotherapy focuses on interpersonal relationships and functioning, whereas CBT provides positive reinforcement for weight gain.[37] A combined approach of interpersonal psychotherapy and CBT is also a reasonable treatment approach.[35] The benefit of treatment based on an addiction model (12-step program) is not supported by the literature.[12,17] Many psychiatric symptoms in an acutely ill patient, such as depression and anxiety, diminish or disappear with weight restoration. Initial treatment is directed toward restoring a healthy weight (greater than 90% of normal weight for age-matched controls) and treating food phobias.[57] After achieving medical stability and appropriate weight, therapy can be redirected toward addressing ongoing interpersonal problems, weight maintenance, cognitive restructuring, and skill development for relapse prevention.[58] Oral refeeding, initially with liquid formulas if necessary, is the most common approach to weight restoration.

In severe cases when a patient refuses to eat, nasogastric refeeding is preferred over IV bolus dosing.[12] Total parenteral nutrition is reserved only for the management of severely malnourished patients and if other refeeding methods fail. The decision to administer total parenteral nutrition must be made carefully, because of the potentially devastating psychological effect on patients who do not wish to gain weight.

Current clinical evidence suggests a controlled weight gain of 0.9 to 1.4 kg (2 to 3 lb) per week in inpatient settings and 0.2 to 0.5 kg (0.5 to 1 lb) per week in outpatient settings.[5,54,57] Recommendations vary; however, it is considered acceptable for patients to begin refeeding at 1,000 to 1,600 cal/day (4186 to 6697 J/day) (30 to 40 cal/kg/day [126 to 167 J/kg]) with slow titration upwards until they begin to demonstrate sustained weight gain.[12,56,59] This can require the intake of an additional 3,500 to 7,000 cal (14,650 to 29,301 J) per week.[56] Slow refeeding is important to minimize the risk of psychological and medical consequences, including refeeding syndrome, which can result in death.

Pharmacologic Therapy

Antidepressants Although many studies examined the role of antidepressants in the treatment of AN, they often have small sample sizes and large confidence intervals.[60] Antidepressants currently have no role in the acute treatment of AN, unless there is another clinical indication present.[12,17,52]

9 Data suggest that medication is ineffective if a patient weighs less than 85% of his or her expected weight. Thus, antidepressants should be initiated only if depression, anxiety, obsessions, or compulsions persist after the target weight is achieved.[17,57,61] The duration of treatment when antidepressants are used in this manner is unclear, but one study showed benefit in treated patients for 1 year, and current guidelines suggest 9 to 12 months of therapy.[3,12,56] Antidepressants, along with psychotherapy, have been used to help maintain weight and prevent relapse, but data supporting this are limited.[62] Most clinicians prefer the selective serotonin reuptake inhibitor (SSRI) antidepressants because they are better tolerated and have greater cardiovascular safety than tricyclic antidepressants (TCAs) and monoamine oxidase inhibitors (MAOIs).[12,63] Because these patients are sensitive to anticholinergic and cardiovascular effects, if TCAs or MAOIs are used, low starting doses and slow titration toward an effective dose are appropriate. The risk of cardiotoxicity in a malnourished population must not be underestimated, and a baseline electrocardiogram (ECG) should be obtained before initiation of these agents.

Fluoxetine continues to be the most widely studied SSRI in AN. Most clinicians initiate at low doses, for example, 20 mg/day, and increase to a maximum of 60 mg/day based on response and tolerability.[59,60,62] Some controversy exists regarding when antidepressant therapy should be initiated. During the starvation phases of anorexia, the majority of clinical trials suggest that antidepressants are ineffective, and there is debate as to their effectiveness once weight restoration has occurred. Evidence from a 52-week, randomized, placebo-controlled clinical trial of 93 patients with the treatment arm receiving doses from 20 to 80 mg/day after weight restoration showed no difference between fluoxetine and placebo for time to relapse.[64]

Antipsychotics First- and second-generation antipsychotics have been utilized as a treatment for AN, specifically targeting anxiety, and obsessive and paranoid thoughts related to weight gain. First-generation antipsychotics contributed to body mass index (BMI) gains, but provided little benefit overall at reducing other core symptoms, and the associated adverse events were considered to outweigh the benefits. Second-generation antipsychotics have provided an additional alternative for treating AN, with reports of improvement in weight gain and reductions in symptoms such as depression, anxiety, and obsessive–compulsiveness. Most of the data are from case reports or small trials in both adolescents and adults using risperidone 0.5 to 2.5 mg daily, olanzapine 2.5 to 15 mg daily, and quetiapine 50 to 800 mg daily.[65–68] Notably, olanzapine in combination with day hospital treatment was found to be more effective than day hospital treatment alone in achieving greater weight gain and reducing obsessive symptoms.[68] While some benefits have been reported, not all positive findings have been replicated, and caution is urged in patients as there is likely an increased susceptibility to some of the physiologic effects of antipsychotic medications. Optimal treatment duration is unknown, as most of the larger studies are less than or equal to 3 months in duration.

Miscellaneous Agents Metoclopramide can be helpful in reducing bloating, early satiety, and abdominal pain commonly found in AN, but it does not affect weight gain.[12] Low-dose, short-acting benzodiazepines (0.25 mg alprazolam or 0.5 mg lorazepam) given before meals are useful when severe anxiety limits eating.[12] Estrogen replacement has been used, but restoring menses through refeeding is a preferred approach to minimize bone density loss. Supplementation with zinc is also being studied to assist with weight restoration.[35]

Clinical **Controversy. . .**

Many clinicians believe that both diagnosis and research would be advanced by eliminating the subcategories and standardizing the number of bingeing episodes required for the diagnosis of BN. Likely this would decrease the number of individuals who currently fall into the category of EDNOS.

Bulimia Nervosa

Nonpharmacologic Therapy

Outpatient-based treatment is most often recommended except in extreme cases (see Table 47-2). The nondrug strategies used in BN are similar to those used with AN, and they are equally critical to success. CBT has the strongest evidence supporting its benefit in managing BN.[56] Current treatment guidelines suggest that CBT should consist of 16 to 20 sessions over a 4- to 5-month period.[56] Interpersonal psychotherapy also plays a role and has a moderate degree of evidence to support its use, but it is considered less effective than CBT.[12,17] Nutritional counseling, planned meals, and self-monitoring can help interrupt the binge–purge cycle. Family therapy in bulimic patients is less critical than with AN, as these patients tend to be older. A recent study suggested that CBT-guided self-care was a more effective treatment approach in adolescents than family therapy. Programs using motivational teaching and self-help guides based on CBT have shown promise.[25,69–71] When such programs have been combined with medication, for example, fluoxetine, enhanced response has been reported.[72,73] Data support the use of 12-step programs, but they should not be used as monotherapy.[12,17] Adjunctive interventions, such as acupuncture and yoga, targeting symptoms of anxiety and depression need further study.[74,75]

Pharmacologic Therapy

Antidepressants Antidepressants are used in the acute and maintenance phases of BN adjunctively with nonpharmacologic approaches. A wide array of antidepressants, including TCAs, MAOIs, trazodone, serotonin–norepinephrine reuptake inhibitors (SNRIs), bupropion, and SSRIs, have been studied. Additionally, several reviews analyzing this body of literature have been published, although there continues to be limited placebo-controlled, randomized, double-blind clinical studies.[17,52,76] Antidepressants are reported to reduce depression, anxiety, obsessions, and impulsive behaviors, such as binge eating and purging, and improve eating habits, although their impact on body dissatisfaction remains unclear. The presence of comorbid mood disorders is not necessary for an antidepressant response.

The benefit appears to be more robust in the acute phase of the illness, as relapse despite continued antidepressant use is common in patients who are in or near remission.[17,25,54] Antidepressant response usually occurs in 6 to 8 weeks, and reduction in frequency of binge–purge behavior has been as high as 73% and as low as zero.[52] Abstinence rates (elimination of bingeing and purging behaviors) with short-term use range from zero to 68%. More data are needed to determine the long-term benefits of antidepressants for preventing relapse of bulimia symptoms. One trial evaluating the impact of fluoxetine versus placebo in the maintenance phase showed a better outcome in patients receiving fluoxetine 60 mg/day, although high dropout rates in both groups blurred the overall benefit.[77]

SSRIs are the preferred agents because of their tolerability and because they have been studied in the largest number of patients. Fluoxetine remains the only medication with FDA approval for BN. Efficacy of other SSRI agents is still lacking, but an alternative SSRI may be considered in clinical practice for patients who do not respond to fluoxetine.[76] Tolerability is the primary criterion for selecting an antidepressant in the treatment of BN because of patients' heightened sensitivity to adverse effects and the lack of a clear difference in efficacy between the classes. Even though there is a suggestion that MAOIs produce the most robust effect, the risk of using these medications in impulsive patients limits their use.[54] SNRIs have shown promising results; however, the data supporting their use are limited to case reports. Bupropion, a norepinephrine–dopamine reuptake inhibitor, is contraindicated in bulimic patients because of the increased risk of seizures.

Before initiating pharmacologic therapy, a careful baseline physical examination, ECG, and laboratory workup are essential. Underlying ECG changes secondary to hypokalemia or bradycardia and atrioventricular block from starvation can be present. There is potential for fatal outcomes secondary to cardiac arrest or suicide. All antidepressants can cause seizures; thus, a careful risk–benefit assessment is warranted if the patient has predisposing factors such as a personal or family history of seizures, cerebrovascular disease, or alcohol or sedative–hypnotic withdrawal.

Doses in the treatment of BN are similar to those in patients treated for depression, although at the higher end of the range. Readers are referred to Chapter 51 for antidepressant dosing ranges. For fluoxetine, the higher end of the dosing range, 60 mg/day, can be necessary for response.[78] With all agents, most clinicians initially target the bottom to the middle of the dosing range and increase the dose if there is an inadequate response. Slow titration is needed to allow time to develop tolerance to adverse effects. If TCAs are used, serum concentration monitoring is recommended to ensure that absorption is not compromised by purging.

The time for antidepressant onset of effect in BN is unclear. In the absence of data, the definition of a therapeutic trial from the depression literature (4 to 8 weeks at a therapeutic dose) should be used. A 2010 report by Sysko et al. identified that response (defined as greater than 60% reduction in binge eating or vomiting frequency) by week 3 is a positive predictor of eventual treatment response.[79] Because the majority of subjects will not experience a complete remission, and there are few data on predictors of response or whether switching to another class will improve response, a clear and specific target should be stated initially.[18]

Optimal duration of treatment after response is poorly defined, although most clinicians treat for 9 months to 1 year and then reevaluate. The evidence is mixed as to whether any early benefit is sustained; hence, the decision to continue treatment should be made based on both initial response and the maintenance of that benefit. If the symptoms return within a few months after antidepressant discontinuation, then the treatment might need to be reinitiated.

Figure 47-2 describes criteria for medication use in BN, but it must be noted that no evidence-based consensus for treatment has been endorsed, even with the recent guidelines, meta-analyses, and reviews of the literature.[3,12,17,52,54,56,63]

Miscellaneous Agents Because of the lack of evidence demonstrating their benefit, lithium and traditional anticonvulsants are reserved for bulimic patients with a comorbid bipolar affective disorder.[12,80] Randomized, placebo-controlled trials with topiramate have demonstrated reduced binge/purge frequency

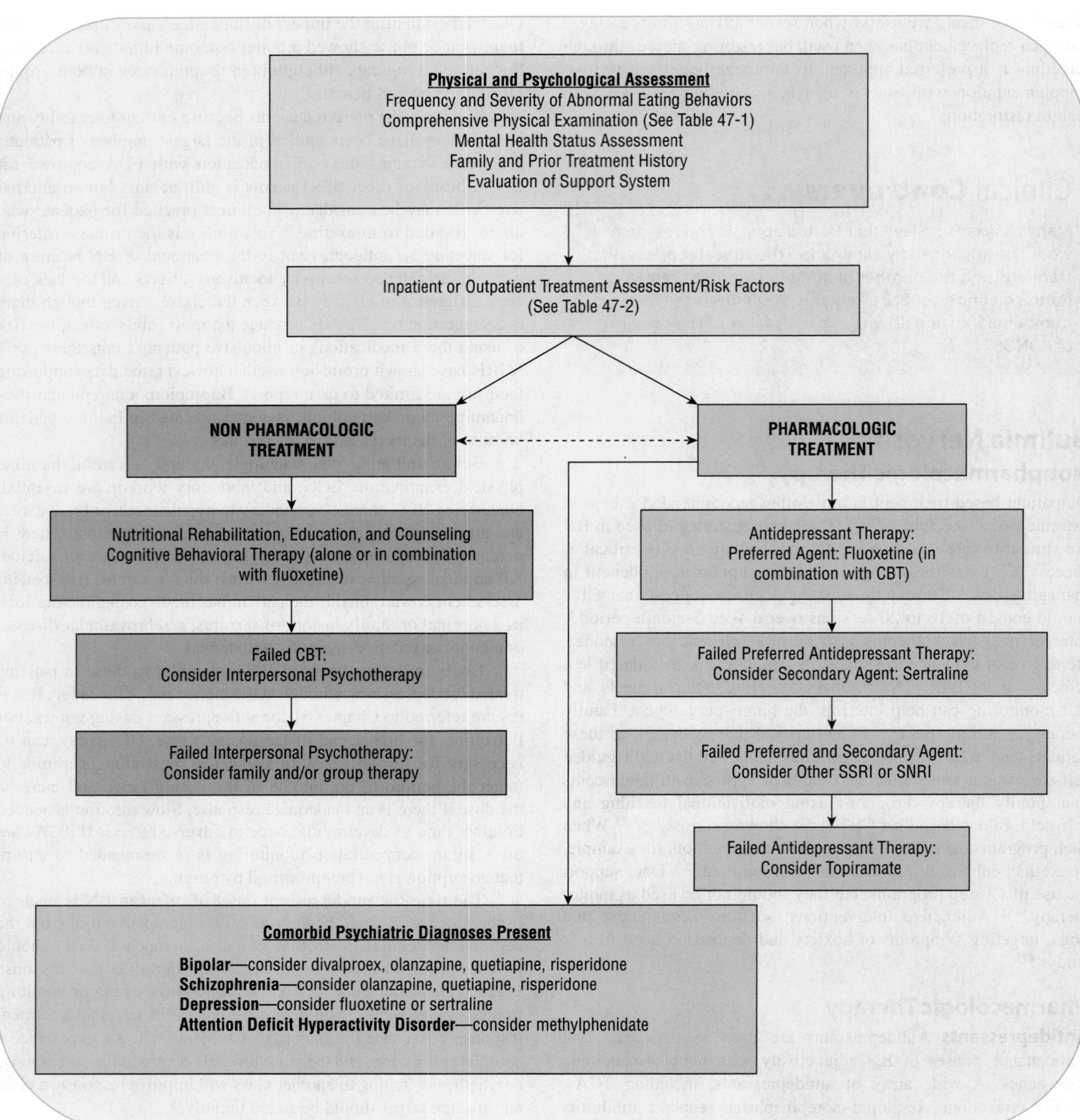

FIGURE 47-2 Bulimia nervosa treatment algorithm. (CBT, cognitive behavioral therapy; SNRI, serotonin–norepinephrine reuptake inhibitor; SSRI, selective serotonin reuptake inhibitor.)

and weight loss versus placebo, although side effects including cognitive impairment and paresthesia may hinder medication adherence.[81,82] Low-dose benzodiazepines before meals can help reduce anxiety associated with refeeding, although long-term use is not warranted because of the risk of abuse and dependence. One double-blind trial with ondansetron has shown benefit, but there are insufficient data to recommend a specific role for this agent.[83] Data are conflicting on the opiate antagonist naltrexone with only modest improvement seen at high doses, but naltrexone is not recommended due to risk of elevated hepatic transaminases.[65] Antipsychotics and appetite suppressants do not play a role in managing core symptoms of BN.[17]

Nonpharmacologic versus Pharmacologic Approaches

The combination of pharmacologic and nonpharmacologic measures appears to produce the best chance for a positive outcome for patients with BN.[56] Antidepressants, specifically SSRIs, are the drug class of choice in bulimic patients, whereas other medications are reserved for patients with comorbid psychiatric conditions. Only in unusual circumstances should patients be treated with antidepressants alone. Evidence suggests the greatest benefit is during the acute phase of treatment, whereas data are mixed regarding their role in the prevention of relapse.

Binge Eating Disorder

As in AN and BN, CBT and interpersonal psychotherapy seem to be the most effective interventions.[17] Antidepressants and anticonvulsants are the pharmacologic agents with the greatest promise in BED, but data are limited, trials are short in duration (20 weeks or less), and whether there is sustained benefit is unclear.[84] Although reports are mixed, antidepressants have demonstrated efficacy as monotherapy at reducing binge eating, decreasing BMI, and improving depressed mood during the acute phases of the illness compared with placebo, but they can also be used in combination with CBT to augment response.[17,65,85–87] The results from two different meta-analyses suggest that antidepressants have higher remission rates when compared with placebo.[76] The majority of the data are with SSRIs given at antidepressant doses.[83] Additionally, atomoxetine has been studied in the dose range of 40 to 120 mg daily and was associated with reduced binge eating and BMI.[88] Topiramate 25 to 300 mg daily has produced benefit at reducing binge frequency, body weight, and BMI, with remission rates higher when combined with CBT.[89,90] Zonisamide (100 to 600 mg/day) alone and in combination with CBT over the course of 16-week and 1-year studies has also demonstrated efficacy at reducing binge eating and weight loss; however, in both instances there have been high dropout rates due to intolerability.[76]

Orlistat 120 mg given three times daily, along with a calorie-restricted diet, has produced weight reduction in obese patients with BED.[91]

In summary, the question of where BED fits on the diagnostic spectrum continues to be explored. Current literature suggests that two different types of pharmacologic agents (SSRIs and topiramate) hold promise in the short term, but long-term data are lacking. As with other eating disorders, nonpharmacologic treatments are the key to a successful outcome.

Personalized Pharmacotherapy

Results from genetic variation studies are largely inconclusive at the present time. While serotonin has been the most widely studied neurotransmitter among the eating disorders, there is not an overwhelmingly consistent response to the serotonin-enhancing medications. Often response is simply a reduction in behaviors such as bingeing and purging, but not a complete amelioration of symptoms. To date, there is no widely accepted pharmacogenomic or pharmacokinetic predictors of medication response to AN, BN, BED, or any EDNOS.

EVALUATION OF THERAPEUTIC OUTCOMES

Anorexia Nervosa

A combination of subjective and objective measures is used to assess response in patients with AN. A reduction in the frequency and severity of abnormal eating habits, normalized exercise patterns and laboratory tests, and a sustained weight close to age-matched normals are key indicators of response. A diary recording exercise frequency, menses, food intake, patterns of eating, and associated feelings while eating is a useful tool to track progress, especially in the outpatient setting. Weekly weigh-ins on the same scale, preferably at a clinician's office, help monitor progress early in treatment and reduce the focus on weight and anxiety caused by the variability found among different scales. Followup laboratory tests and ECGs are not part of routine monitoring unless the patient is restricting food intake, is purging, or continues to lose weight despite treatment. Inpatients require daily assessment of weight and caloric intake, vital signs, and urine output because of the severity of their illness. They also can need monitoring of bathroom privileges early in their care. A healthy weight gain of no more than 0.2 to 0.5 kg (0.4 to 1.1 lb) per week toward a goal of 90% to 95% of normal weight or a BMI greater than 18.5 kg/m^2 is a critical sign of treatment success. A patient's use of coping skills and contingencies for dealing with stress, other than manipulating food consumption, also should be assessed. Antidepressants can assist in alleviation of persistent depression, anxiety, and obsessions, after weight restoration. Improvement in mood is expected to occur within 8 weeks. Patients receiving TCAs should be evaluated for dry mouth, constipation, hypotension, and sedation. Patients receiving SSRIs should be monitored for agitation, drug-induced anorexia, nausea, weight loss, and insomnia. The decision to use long-term medication must be based on specific and sustained improvement in the target symptoms, balanced against adverse effects.

Bulimia Nervosa

An individualized treatment and monitoring plan begins with a thorough assessment describing the baseline frequency and severity of treatment-responsive target symptoms and other associated findings. The assessment must be comprehensive, as a patient can hide his or her illness by shifting from one type of behavior to another (e.g., exercise to purging).

A comprehensive assessment includes a description of psychiatric symptoms, physical findings, frequency and severity of binge–purge episodes, laxative and ipecac use, exercise patterns, and laboratory and ECG abnormalities. Interpersonal and relationship problems should also be evaluated. Some findings indicating a more chronic course of illness, such as salivary gland inflammation and erosion of dental enamel, can take months to reverse or might never normalize. Hence, these are not sensitive indicators of early treatment response. Data describing a patient's baseline level of functioning and previous response to treatment should be used to set goals in the current treatment plan.

Antidepressant response usually occurs within 4 to 8 weeks after the onset of treatment. If response does not occur, binge–purge behavior should be considered as a factor potentially contributing to the malabsorption of medication. If this behavior is not present, then every attempt should be made to maximize the dose. Serum concentration monitoring, when appropriate as with TCAs, should be done periodically (every 3 to 6 months if a patient is responding and tolerating the medication, or more frequently if clinically indicated). Evaluation of previously described adverse effects also should be part of the monitoring plan. If the patient responds, he or she should be followed for 6 to 12 months, and then reassessed for the need for ongoing medication. If the patient relapses on medication discontinuation, then the medication should be restarted.

Ambulatory eating disorder patients present a particular challenge to clinicians. Impulsivity associated with BN can increase the risk for suicide. Prescriptions should be limited to small supplies. In addition, pharmacists should be alert to persons who make large or frequent purchases of laxatives or ipecac syrup, as this is an indicator of possible bulimic behaviors.

ABBREVIATIONS

AN	anorexia nervosa
BDNF	brain-derived neurotrophic factor
BED	binge eating disorder
BMI	body mass index
BN	bulimia nervosa
CBT	cognitive behavioral therapy
DSM-IV-TR	*Diagnostic and Statistical Manual of Mental Disorders, Fourth Edition, Text Revision*

DSM-V	*Diagnostic and Statistical Manual of Mental Disorders* (fifth edition)
ECG	electrocardiogram
EDNOS	eating disorder not otherwise specified
EEG	electroencephalogram
ESRI	estrogen receptor I gene
MAOI	monoamine oxidase inhibitor
NES	night eating syndrome
OCD	obsessive–compulsive disorder
SNRI	serotonin–norepinephrine reuptake inhibitor
SSRI	selective serotonin reuptake inhibitor
TCA	tricyclic antidepressant

ACKNOWLEDGMENTS

The authors acknowledge the contributions of Patricia A. Marken, PharmD, and Roger W. Sommi, PharmD, authors of Chapter 66 in the seventh edition of *Pharmacotherapy: A Pathophysiologic Approach.*

REFERENCES

1. Bulik CM, Tozzi FC, Anderson C, et al. The relationship between eating disorders and components of perfectionism. Am J Psychiatry 2003;160:366–368.
2. McKnight Investigators. Risk factors for the onset of eating disorders in adolescent girls: Results of the McKnight longitudinal risk factor study. Am J Psychiatry 2003;160:248–254.
3. Favaro A, Ferrara S, Santonastaso P. The spectrum of eating disorders in young women: A prevalence study in a general population sample. Psychosom Med 2003;65:701–708.
4. Striegel-Moore RH, Dohm FA, Kraemer HC, et al. Eating disorders in white and black women. Am J Psychiatry 2003;160:1326–1331.
5. American Psychiatric Association. Diagnostic and Statistical Manual of Mental Disorders, Fourth Edition, Text Revision. Washington, DC: American Psychiatric Press, 2000:583–596.
6. Hudson JI, Hiripi E, Pope HG Jr, Kessler RC. The prevalence and correlates of eating disorders in the national comorbidity survey replication. Biol Psychiatry 2007;61:348–358.
7. Pike KM. Long-term course of anorexia nervosa: Response, relapse, remission, and recovery. Clin Psychol Rev 1998;18: 447–475.
8. Crow SJ, Peterson CV, Swanson SA, et al. Increased mortality in bulimia nervosa and other eating disorders. Am J Psychiatry 2009;166:1342–1346.
9. Norris ML, Boydell KM, Pinhas L, Katzman DK. Ana and the Internet: A review of pro-anorexia websites. Int J Eat Disord 2006;39:443–447.
10. Hoek H, van Hoeken D. Review of the prevalence and incidence of eating disorders. Int J Eat Disord 2003;34: 383–386.
11. Sadock BJ, Sadock VA, eds. Kaplan and Sadock's Synopsis of Psychiatry: Behavioral Sciences/Clinical Psychiatry, 9th ed. Philadelphia: Lippincott Williams & Wilkins, 2003:739–750.
12. American Psychiatric Association. Treatment of patients with eating disorders, third edition. Am J Psychiatry 2006; 163(7 Suppl):4–54.
13. O'Reardon JP, Allison KC, Martino NS, et al. A randomized, placebo-controlled trial of sertraline in the treatment of night eating syndrome. Am J Psychiatry 2006;163:893–898.
14. Gluck ME, Geliebter A, Satov T. Night eating syndrome is associated with depression, low self-esteem, reduced daytime hunger, and less weight loss in obese outpatients. Obes Res 2001;9:264–267.
15. Rand CS, MacGreggor AMC, Stunkard AJ. The night eating syndrome in the general population and among postoperative obesity surgery patients. Int J Eat Disord 1997;22:65–69.
16. Stunkard AJ, Berkowitz R, Wadden T, et al. Binge eating disorder and the night eating syndrome. Int J Obes Relat Metab Disord 1996;20:1–6.
17. Fairburn CG, Harrison PJ. Eating disorders. Lancet 2003; 361:407–416.
18. Kaye WH. Neurobiology of anorexia and bulimia nervosa. Physiol Behav 2008;94:121–135.
19. Frank GK, Bailer UF, Henry SE, et al. Increased dopamine D2/D3 receptor binding after recovery from anorexia nervosa measured by positron emission tomography and [11c]raclopride. Biol Psychiatry 2005;58:908–912.
20. Ribases M, Gratacos M, Fernandez-Aranda F, et al. Association of BDNF with anorexia, bulimia, age of onset of weight loss in six European populations. Hum Mol Genet 2004;13(12):1205–1212.
21. Pinheiro AP, Bulik CM, Thornton LM, et al. Association study of 182 candidate genes in anorexia nervosa. Am J Med Genet B Neuropsychiatr Genet 2010;153B:1070–1080.
22. Grave RD. Eating disorders: Progress and challenges. Eur J Intern Med 2011;22:153–160.
23. Steiger H, Joober R, Gauvin L, et al. Serotonin-system polymorphisms (5-HTTLPR and −1438G/A) and responses of patients with bulimic syndromes to multimodal treatments. J Clin Psychiatry 2008;69:1565–1571.
24. Versini A, Ramoz N, Le Strat Y, et al. Estrogen receptor I gene is associated with restrictive anorexia nervosa. Neuropsychopharmacology 2010;35:1818–1825.
25. Halmi K. Eating disorders. In: Sadock BJ, Sadock VA, eds. Comprehensive Textbook of Psychiatry, 7th ed. Philadelphia: Lippincott Williams & Wilkins, 2000:1663–1676.
26. Powers PS. Initial assessment and early treatment options for anorexia nervosa and bulimia nervosa. Psychiatr Clin North Am 1996;19:639–655.
27. Casper RC, Hedeker D, McClough JF. Personality dimensions in eating disorders and their relevance for subtyping. J Am Acad Child Adolesc Psychiatry 1992;31: 830–840.
28. Eckert ED, Halmi KA, Marchi P, et al. Ten-year follow-up of anorexia nervosa: Clinical course and outcome. Psychol Med 1995;25:143–156.
29. Garner DM, Garfinkel PE, O'shaughnessy M. Validity of the distinction between bulimia with and without anorexia nervosa. Am J Psychiatry 1985;142:581–587.
30. Keel PK, Brown TA. Update on course and outcome in eating disorders. Int J Eat Disord 2010;43:195–204.
31. Tozzi F, Thornton LM, Mitchell J, et al. Features associated with laxative abuse in individuals with eating disorders. Psychosom Med 2006;68:470–477.
32. Garner DM, Garner MV, Rosen LW. Anorexia nervosa "restrictors" who purge: Implications for subtyping anorexia nervosa. Int J Eat Disord 1993;13:171–185.
33. Shroff H, Reba L, Thornton LM, et al. Features associated with excessive exercise in women with eating disorders. Int J Eat Disord 2006;39:454–461.
34. American Psychiatric Association, DSM-V Study Work Group. *www.dsm5.org*.
35. Yager J, Devlin MJ, Halmi KA, et al. Guideline Watch (August 2012): Practice Guideline for the Treatment of Patients with Eating Disorders, 3rd ed. http://psychiatryonline.org/pdfaccess.ashx?ResourceID=5391825&PDF. Accessed April 3, 2013.

36. Jordan J, Joyce PR, Carter FA, et al. Specific and nonspecific comorbidity in anorexia nervosa. Int J Eat Disord 2008;41:47–56.
37. Halmi KA. Eating disorders: Anorexia nervosa, bulimia nervosa, and obesity. In: Hales RE, Yudofsky SC, eds. Essentials of Clinical Psychiatry, 3rd ed. Washington, DC: American Psychiatric Press, 1999:667–685.
38. Braun DL, Sunday SR, Halmi KA. Psychiatric comorbidity in patients with eating disorders. Psychol Med 1994;24: 859–867.
39. Herzog DB, Keller MB, Sacks NR, et al. Psychiatric comorbidity in treatment seeking anorexics and bulimics. J Am Acad Child Adolesc Psychiatry 1992;31:810–818.
40. O'Brien KM, Vincent NK. Psychiatric comorbidity in anorexia and bulimia nervosa: Nature, prevalence, and causal relationships. Clin Psychol Rev 2003;23:53–74.
41. Grilo CM, White MA, Masheb RM. DSM-IV psychiatric disorder comorbidity and its correlates in binge eating disorder. Int J Eat Disord 2009;42(3):228–234.
42. Rome ES, Ammerman, S. Medical complications of eating disorders: An update. J Adolesc Health 2003;33:418–426.
43. Birch K. Female athlete triad. Br Med J 2005;330(7485): 244–246.
44. Mendelsohn FA, Warren MP. Anorexia, bulimia, and the female athlete triad: Evaluation and management. Endocrinol Metab Clin North Am 2010;39:155–167.
45. Mehler PS, MacKenzie TD. Treatment outcomes of osteopenia and osteoporosis in anorexia nervosa: A systematic review of the literature. Int J Eat Disord 2009;42(3):195–201.
46. Kingston K, Szmukler G, Andrews D, et al. Neuropsychological and structural brain changes in anorexia nervosa before and after refeeding. Psychol Med 1996;26:15–28.
47. Lambe EK, Katzman DK, Mikulis DJ, et al. Cerebral gray matter volume deficits after weight recovery from anorexia nervosa. Arch Gen Psychiatry 1997;54:537–542.
48. Carney CP, Anderson AE. Eating disorders: Guide to medical evaluation and complications. Psychiatr Clin North Am 1996;19:657–679.
49. Steinhausen HC. The outcome of anorexia nervosa in the 20th century. Am J Psychiatry 2002;159(8):1284–1293.
50. Fichter MM, Quadflieg N. Six year course of bulimia nervosa. Int J Eat Disord 1997;22:361–384.
51. Herzog DB, Nussbaum KM, Marmor AK. Comorbidity and outcome in eating disorders. Psychiatr Clin North Am 1996;19:843–859.
52. Mitchell JE, de Zwaan M, Roerig JL. Drug therapy for patients with eating disorders. Curr Drug Targets CNS Neurol Disord 2003;2:17–29.
53. Bacaltchuk J, Hay P. Antidepressants versus placebo for people with bulimia nervosa. Cochrane Database Syst Rev 2003;(4):CD003391 [updated November 2005].
54. Nakash-Eisikovits O, Dierberger A, Westen D. A multidimensional meta-analysis of pharmacotherapy for bulimia nervosa: Summarizing the range of outcomes in controlled clinical trials. Harv Rev Psychiatry 2002;10: 190–211.
55. Halmi KA, Agras WS, Crow S, et al. Predictors of treatment acceptance and completion in anorexia nervosa: Implications for future study designs. Arch Gen Psychiatry 2005;62: 776–781.
56. National Collaborating Centre for Mental Health. Eating Disorders: Core Interventions in the Treatment and Management of Anorexia Nervosa, Bulimia Nervosa and Related Eating Disorders. London: British Psychological Society and Royal College of Psychiatrists, 2004:1–36.
57. Zerbe KJ. Multimodal treatment of severe eating disorders. Essent Psychopharmacol 2000;3:1–17.
58. Kleifield EI, Wagner S, Halmi KA. Cognitive-behavioral treatment of anorexia nervosa. Psychiatr Clin North Am 1996;19:715–737.
59. Yager J, Anderson AE. Anorexia nervosa. N Engl J Med 2005;353(14):1481–1488.
60. Bulik CM, Berkman ND, Brownley KA, et al. Anorexia nervosa treatment: A systematic review of randomized controlled trials. Int J Eat Disord 2007;40:310–320.
61. Bergh C, Eriksson M, Lindberg G, Sodersten P. Selective serotonin reuptake inhibitors in anorexia. Lancet 1996; 348:1459–1460.
62. Kaye WH, Nagata T, Weltzin TE, et al. Double-blind placebo-controlled administration of fluoxetine in restricting- and restricting-purging-type anorexia nervosa. Biol Psychiatry 2001;4:644–652.
63. Jimerson DC, Wolfe BE, Brotman AW, Metzger ED. Medication in the treatment of eating disorders. Psychiatr Clin North Am 1996;19:739–754.
64. Walsh BT, Kaplan AS, Attia E, et al. Fluoxetine after weight restoration in anorexia nervosa: A randomized controlled trial. JAMA 2006;295(22):2605–2612.
65. Flament MF, Bissada H, Spettigue W. Evidence-based pharmacotherapy of eating disorders. Int J Neuropsychopharmacol 2012;15:189–207.
66. Dunican KC, DelDotto D. The role of olanzapine in the treatment of anorexia nervosa. Ann Pharmacother 2007;41: 111–115.
67. Mehler-Wex C, Romanos M, Kirchheiner J, Schulze UME. Atypical antipsychotics in severe anorexia nervosa in children and adolescents—Review and case reports. Eur Eat Disord Rev 2008;16:100–108.
68. Bissada H, Tasca GA, Barber AM, Bradwejn J. Olanzapine in the treatment of low body weight and obsessive thinking in women with anorexia nervosa: A randomized, double-blind, placebo-controlled trial. Am J Psychiatry 2008;165:1281–1288.
69. Schmidt U, Lee S, Beecham J, et al. A randomized controlled trial of family therapy and cognitive behavior therapy guided self-care for adolescents with bulimia nervosa and related disorders. Am J Psychiatry 2007;164:591–598.
70. Mitchell JE, Agras S, Crow S, et al. Stepped care and cognitive-behavioural therapy for bulimia nervosa: Randomized trial. Br J Psychiatry 2011;198:391–397.
71. Wilson GT, Zandberg LJ. Cognitive-behavioral guided self-help for eating disorders: Effectiveness and scalability. Clin Psychol Rev 2012;32:343–357.
72. Mitchell JE, Fletcher L, Hanson K, et al. The relative efficacy of fluoxetine and manual-based self-help in the treatment of outpatients with bulimia nervosa. J Clin Psychiatry 2001;21:298–304.
73. Walsh BT, Fairburn CG, Mickley D, et al. Treatment of bulimia nervosa in a primary care setting. Am J Psychiatry 2004;161:556–561.
74. Fogarty S, Harris D, Zaslawski C, et al. Acupuncture as an adjunct therapy in the treatment of eating disorders: A randomized cross-over pilot study. Complement Ther Med. 2010;18:233–240.
75. Carei TR, Fyfe-Johnson AL, Breuner CC, Brown MA. Randomized controlled clinical trial of yoga in the treatment of eating disorders. J Adolesc Health 2010;46: 346–351.
76. Hay PJ, Claudino AM. Clinical psychopharmacology of eating disorders: A research update. Int J Neuropsychopharmacol 2012;15:209–222.

77. Romano SJ, Halmi KA, Sarkar NP, et al. A placebo-controlled study of fluoxetine in continued treatment of bulimia nervosa after successful fluoxetine treatment. Am J Psychiatry 2002;159:96–102.
78. Fluoxetine Bulimia Nervosa Collaborative Study Group. Fluoxetine in the treatment of bulimia nervosa: A multicenter, placebo-controlled, double-blind trial. Arch Gen Psychiatry 1992;49:139–147.
79. Sysko R, Sha N, Wang Y, et al. Early response to antidepressant treatment in bulimia nervosa. Psychol Med 2010;40:999–1005.
80. McElroy SL, Kotwal R, Hudson JI, et al. Zonisamide in the treatment of binge eating disorder: An open-label, prospective trial. J Clin Psychiatry 2004;65(1):50–56.
81. Hoopes SP, Reimherr FW, Hedges DW, et al. Treatment of bulimia nervosa with topiramate in a randomized, double-blind, placebo-controlled trail, part 1: Improvement in binge and purge measures. J Clin Psychiatry 2003;64(11):1335–1341.
82. Nickel C, Tritt K, Muehlbacher M, et al. Topiramate treatment in bulimia nervosa patients: A randomized, double-blind, placebo-controlled trial. Int J Eat Disord 2005;38(4):295–300.
83. Faris PL, Kim SW, Meller WH, et al. Effect of decreasing afferent vagal activity with ondansetron on the symptoms of bulimia nervosa: A randomized double-blind trial. Lancet 2000;355:792–797.
84. Carter WP, Hudson JI, Lalonde JK, et al. Pharmacologic treatment of binge eating disorder. Int J Eat Disord 2003;34:S74–S88.
85. Devlin MJ, Goldfein JA, Petkova E, et al. Cognitive behavioral therapy and fluoxetine as adjuncts to group behavioral therapy for binge eating disorder. Obes Res 2005;13(6):1077–1088.
86. Kaplan AS. Academy for Eating Disorders international conference on eating disorders. Expert Opin Investig Drugs 2003;12:1441–1443.
87. McElroy SL, Casuto LS, Nelson EB, et al. Placebo-controlled trial of sertraline in the treatment of binge eating disorder. Am J Psychiatry 2000;157:1004–1006.
88. McElroy SL, Guerdjikova A, Kotwal R, Welge JA, et al. Atomoxetine in the treatment of binge-eating disorder: A randomized controlled trial. J Clin Psychiatry 2007;68:390–398.
89. McElroy SL, Hudson JI, Capece JA, et al. Topiramate for the treatment of binge-eating disorder associated with obesity: A placebo-controlled study. Biol Psychiatry 2007;61:1039–1048.
90. Claudino AM, de Oliveira IR, Appolinario JUC, et al. Double-blind, randomized, placebo-controlled trial of topiramate plus cognitive-behavior therapy in binge-eating disorder. J Clin Psychiatry 2007;8:1324–1332.
91. Golay A, Laurent-Jaccard A, Habicht F, et al. Effect of orlistat in obese patients with binge eating disorder. Obes Res 2005;13(10):1701–1708.

Substance-Related Disorders I: Overview and Depressants, Stimulants, and Hallucinogens

48

Paul L. Doering and Robin Moorman Li

KEY CONCEPTS

1. Problems related to abuse of chemical substances can occur acutely (e.g., respiratory arrest from using heroin) or after some length of time (e.g., dependence or withdrawal from continued use of an opiate). The treatment approach is distinctly different depending on the type of problem.
2. Certain drugs of abuse are marketed via the Internet and other unregulated outlets using names that would not immediately identify the substances as a dangerous drug. Health professionals must stay abreast of the latest marketing ruse to conceal the true nature of the substance.
3. Synthetic chemists are constantly developing new drugs of abuse with pharmacology that mimics that of established controlled substances. Often, the dangers of these substances are greater than that of the parent compound.
4. For a few drugs, there is a specific antidote that can be used in cases of overdoses. For others, treatment is symptomatic and supportive. Early recognition and treatment of acute drug intoxications can make a huge difference in the ultimate outcome for the patient.
5. Withdrawal from certain classes of drugs (e.g., benzodiazepines or barbiturates) can be life-threatening, and steps must be taken to ensure that withdrawal is gradual and that it takes place in closely supervised settings.
6. While there is much research focusing on drugs to treat the underlying addictive processes, to date the successes have been few. Whereas methadone, levo-α-acetylmethadol (LAAM), and now buprenorphine are used for narcotic maintenance, the logical approach at present should center on prevention.
7. While the goal of therapy for substance dependence is to wean patients from a drug or drug category altogether, this is often difficult to do. For some, the treatment strategy is to manage the chemical dependency to allow the patient to lead as normal a life as is possible. This may require the substitution of one drug for the primary drug of dependency.
8. Pharmacotherapy of substance-related disorders is most often adjunctive to other modes of therapy such as counseling and intense psychotherapy.

The book of *Ecclesiastes* wisely reminds us that "[W]hat has been will be again, what has been done will be done again; there is nothing new under the sun."[1] It is doubtful that the author of these sage words was referring to the repeating cycle of substance abuse, but when it comes to this subject there rarely *is* anything new under the sun, and this metaphor aptly applies.

Psychoactive drug use dates back to prehistoric times and the Neolithic era (8500 to 4000 BC) where the earliest human use of psychoactive substances consisted almost exclusively of plants and fruits whose mood-altering qualities were accidentally discovered but subsequently deliberately grown.[2]

Ancient civilizations (4000 BC to AD 400) such as the Sumerians, Egyptians, Indians, Chinese, and South Americans used opium, alcohol, cannabis, peyote, psychedelic mushrooms, and coca leaves. The Middle Ages (400 to 1400) saw the use of psychoactive plants such as belladonna and psilocybin mushroom, used by witches and shamans for healing and spiritual purposes, and distilled alcohol and coffee, tea, and opium spread along the trade routes.[2]

Almost 5,000 years ago at the Temple of Imhotep, a center for treating mental illness, opium was used in an attempt to cure the mentally ill by inducing vision, performing rituals, and praying to the gods.[2] Hippocrates, the father of medicine, recommended opium as a painkiller and as a treatment of female hysteria.[2] Evidence of the inhalation of cannabis smoke can be found in the 3rd millennium BC, as indicated by charred cannabis seeds found in a ritual fire at an ancient burial site in present-day Romania.[3] In 2003, a leather basket filled with cannabis leaf fragments and seeds was found next to a 2,500- to 2,800-year-old mummified shaman in the northwestern Xinjiang Uygur Autonomous Region of China.[4] Thousands of years later, nearly every one of these drugs is still used today in one form or another for their mind-altering effects.

For any textbook to remain relevant, it must give emphasis to *current* information in any given content area. This means that space previously budgeted to one subject must give way to more recent trends. For example, if this chapter was written in the late 1960s, great attention would be given to the use and abuse of lysergic acid diethylamide (LSD) or methamphetamine.[5,6] If it was written in the late 1970s, the epidemic abuse of hydromorphone (Dilaudid) would be featured.[7]

In the mid- to late 1970s great attention would be given to the abuse of methaqualone (Quaalude).[8] Somewhere along the way, the abuse of pentazocine would take center stage.[9] Amphetamine abuse has come, gone, and come back again.[10] γ-Hydroxybutyric acid (GHB) made a sudden and dramatic appearance on the scene, but its use has lessened in the past years.[11] The current epidemic of prescription drug abuse has skyrocketed its way into prominence. Hallucinogens such as dimethyltryptamine (DMT) and phenylethylamine derivatives are making a strong comeback.

By no means does this suggest that these above-mentioned drugs have disappeared, but instead many have taken a back seat to other, more commonly encountered drugs. For this reason, this rewrite of the present chapter and the one to follow will leave out some of the information from previous editions. The interested reader should consult prior editions of this textbook for information about these substances.

The lack of a common vocabulary in substance abuse treatment and prevention leads to several problems. Wide arrays of terms are in common use, many without precise meaning. This lack of universal agreement on language hampers effective communication among professionals and leads to difficulties in formulating public policy and administering third-party reimbursement programs.

In 2003, the Liaison Committee on Pain and Addiction, a collaborative effort of the American Academy of Pain Medicine, the American Pain Society, and the American Society of Addiction Medicine, developed definitions related to the use of medications for the treatment of pain consistent with current understanding of relevant neurobiology, pharmacology, and appropriate clinical practice. The definitions have been approved by each of the three collaborating organizations. The following definitions resulted from this consensus development committee[12]:

1. *Addiction* is a primary, chronic, neurobiologic disease, with genetic, psychosocial, and environmental factors influencing its development and manifestations. It is characterized by behaviors that include one or more of the following five C's: *c*hronicity, impaired *c*ontrol over drug use, *c*ompulsive use, *c*ontinued use despite harm, and *c*raving.
2. *Drug abuse* is a maladaptive pattern of substance use characterized by repeated adverse consequences related to the repeated use of the substance. Examples include failure to fulfill important obligations at work, school, or home; repeated use creating physical danger, such as driving under the influence; legal problems; and social or interpersonal problems such as arguments and fights.
3. *Physical dependence* is a state of adaptation that is manifested by a drug class–specific withdrawal syndrome that can be produced by abrupt cessation, rapid dose reduction, decreasing blood level of the drug, and/or administration of an antagonist.
4. *Tolerance* is a state of adaptation in which exposure to a drug induces changes that result in a diminution of one or more of the drug's effects over time.

EPIDEMIOLOGY

National Survey on Drug Use and Health

The National Survey on Drug Use and Health (NSDUH)[13] is the primary source of statistical information on the use of illegal drugs by the U.S. population. Conducted by the federal government since 1971, the survey collects data from a representative sample of the population at their place of residence.

In 2011, it was estimated 22.5 million Americans aged 12 or older were current illicit drug users, which was defined by using an illicit drug during the month prior to the survey interview. This survey also found that marijuana continues to be the most commonly used illicit drug and has increased from 17.4 million past month users in 2010 to 18.1 million past month users in 2011. About 6.1 million Americans (2.4% of the population) admitted they abused prescription drugs in the past month in 2011, which is slightly lower than the 2010 data (7 million Americans), but still a monumental problem in our country.[13]

Monitoring the Future Study

Every year the Institute for Social Research at the University of Michigan conducts its Monitoring the Future Study (MTFS), supported under a series of research grants from the National Institute on Drug Abuse.[14]

A main purpose of this research is to study changes in the beliefs, attitudes, and behavior of young people in the United States, which requires frequent reassessment to identify the rapidly changing patterns.[14]

The 2012 samples included 45,449 students located in 395 secondary schools.[14] After 4 straight years of increasing use among teens, annual marijuana use showed no further increase in any of the three grades surveyed in 2012. The 2012 annual prevalence rates (i.e., percent using in the prior 12 months) were 11%, 28%, and 36% for 8th, 10th, and 12th graders, respectively.

Daily use of marijuana, which had also been rising in all three grades in recent years, remained essentially flat between 2011 and 2012 at relatively high levels. The recent increases have been substantial—up by one quarter to one-third compared with their low points reached between 2006 and 2008 for the three grades. Today 1 in every 15 high school seniors (6.5%) is a daily or near-daily marijuana user. Researchers postulate that the increase of smoking marijuana is partly attributable to the national debate over medical use of cannabis, which may make the drugs seem safer to teenagers.[14]

Synthetic marijuana (see below) that contains designer chemicals included in the cannabinoid family (common names are K2, Spice, and Blaze) has been of increasing concern because of both its adverse effects and its high rates of use, first documented by this study in 2011. The annual prevalence rate held level among 12th graders in 2012—the second year of measurement—at 11.3%. Synthetic marijuana use was measured for the first time this year in 8th and 10th grades, and their annual prevalence rates were 4.4% and 8.8%, respectively. Aside from alcohol and tobacco, this is the second most widely used drug among 10th and 12th graders after marijuana, and the third most widely used among 8th graders after marijuana and inhalants.[14]

Illicit or street drug use has declined over the past decade (when marijuana use is not factored in). Unfortunately, the gradual decline has leveled off since 2010, and use has remained steady rather than declining when comparing 2011 data with 2008 data. The abuse of prescription drugs including sedatives, tranquilizers, and narcotic drugs other than heroin (most of which are analgesics) also continues to be a problem within this population group even though use has remained steady at 15.2% since 2008. Even though the use of these agents is not currently increasing in this specific population, they continue to be an important part of the nation's drug abuse problem.[14]

Substance Abuse Emergencies: The DAWN Program

Since the early 1970s, the Drug Abuse Warning Network (DAWN),[15] an ongoing national survey of hospital emergency departments (EDs), has collected information on patients seeking hospital ED treatment related to their use of an illegal drug or the nonmedical use of a legal drug. These data allow healthcare professionals to be better prepared to react to medical emergencies arising from illegal drug use and to target prevention and education programs to specific drug-using groups or populations.[15]

DAWN defines a *drug-related episode* as an ED visit that was induced by or related to the use of an illegal drug(s) or the nonmedical use of a legal drug for patients aged 6 to 97 years. In 2010, hospitals in the United States delivered a total of 136.1 million ED visits,[16] and DAWN estimates that 2,201,050 ED visits were associated with drug misuse or abuse. This is a 94% increase since 2004—2.5 million visits in 2004 in comparison to 4.9 million visits in 2010.[15] Of those ED visits, some key findings include the following:

1. 23.8% involved illicit drugs only
2. 27.4% involved pharmaceuticals only
3. 3.8% involved alcohol only in patients under the age of 21
4. 11.5% involved alcohol with other drugs

ECONOMIC IMPACT OF SUBSTANCE ABUSE

Substance abuse and addiction have an enormous impact on the economy. Over the years, the National Center on Addiction and Substance Abuse (CASA) at Columbia University has conducted studies aimed at quantifying the costs to local, state, and federal governments and agencies. The most recent figures[17] are based on 2005 spending because that was the most recent year for which data were available over the course of the latest study.

Substance abuse and addiction cost federal, state, and local governments at least $467.7 billion in 2005 alone. The CASA report found that of $373.9 billion in federal and state spending, 95.6% ($357.4 billion) went to "shovel up the consequences and human wreckage of substance abuse and addiction"[17]; only 1.9% went to prevention and treatment, 0.4% to research, 1.4% to taxation and regulation, and 0.7% to interdiction.

ACUTE VERSUS CHRONIC PROBLEMS

1 Misuse of chemical substances causes problems of two types: those that occur acutely and those that arise after continued use of a drug. Acute problems are usually predictable, given the pharmacology of the drug. Chronic abuse of chemical substances can cause a wide array of physical, psychological, and psychiatric morbidities. The substance-induced disorders discussed here mainly include intoxication and withdrawal.

1 The essential feature of substance dependence is the continued use of the substance despite adverse substance-related problems. The criteria for substance dependence are the same for each of the drugs or drug classes, varying only to fit the unique pharmacologic properties of each drug. Patients who take prescribed drugs for appropriate medical indications and in correct doses may still show tolerance, physical dependence, and withdrawal symptoms if the drug is stopped abruptly rather than being tapered. Tolerance and physical dependence are inevitable consequences of chronic treatment with opioids and certain other drugs, but by themselves, tolerance and physical dependence do not imply "addiction." To meet *Diagnostic and Statistical Manual of Mental Disorders, Fourth Edition, Text Revision* (*DSM-IV-TR*) criteria[18] for the diagnosis of substance dependence, at least three of the following must be present at any time in a 12-month period:

1. Tolerance.
2. Withdrawal, indicated by the appearance of the characteristic withdrawal syndrome or the use of the same or related drug to relieve or avoid withdrawal symptoms.
3. Substance is taken in larger amounts or over a longer period of time than was intended.
4. Patient has a persistent desire or unsuccessful efforts to cut down or control substance use.
5. Considerable time is spent in activities necessary to obtain the substance, use the substance, or recover from its effects.
6. Social, occupational, or recreational activities are given up or reduced because of substance use.
7. Substance use is continued despite knowledge of having a persistent or recurrent physical or psychological problem caused or exacerbated by the substance.

The characteristic feature of *substance abuse* is a maladaptive pattern of substance use indicated by repeated adverse consequences related to the repeated use of the substance.[18] Examples include failure to fulfill important obligations at work, school, or home; repeated use in situations in which it is physically dangerous, such as driving under the influence; legal problems; and social or interpersonal problems such as arguments and fights.[18] *Intoxication* refers to the development of a substance-specific syndrome after recent ingestion and presence in the body of a substance, and it is associated with maladaptive behavior during the waking state caused by the effect of the substance on the CNS. Examples include belligerence, mood lability, impaired judgment, and impaired social or occupational functioning. Evidence for recent intake of the substance can be obtained from the history, physical examination, or laboratory examination. The most common changes involve disturbances in perception, wakefulness, attention, thinking, judgment, motor behavior, and interpersonal behavior.

As with most illnesses, the course and prognosis of the disorders of substance use and dependence are variable. Getting patients who are drug dependent to stop using drugs is very difficult, and many patients return to drug use even after treatment. It has been reported that as many as 75% of treated, substance-dependent patients will relapse at least once. Many patients, however, are able to obtain recovery with treatment and continued care in 12-step programs such as Alcoholics Anonymous or Narcotics Anonymous (NA). Substance dependence or addiction can be viewed as a chronic illness that can be controlled successfully with treatment but cannot be cured and is associated with a high relapse rate. Without treatment, the course can progress to life-threatening severity, resulting from the effects of the drug, drug contaminants, or medical complications of use.[18] Recently, the definitions used in the *DSM-IV-TR* criteria have been criticized.[19] Although an in-depth discussion of the mechanism of drug addiction is beyond the scope of this chapter, the interested reader is directed to a review article that presents the current understanding of the biology of drug addiction.[20]

CNS DEPRESSANTS

Opiates and Opioids

Deaths from prescription opioids have reached epidemic levels in the past decade. The number of overdose deaths is now greater than those of deaths from heroin and cocaine combined. In 2010, about 12 million Americans (age 12 or older) reported nonmedical use of narcotic analgesics in the past year. Nearly one third of people aged 12 and over who used drugs for the first time in 2009 began by using a prescription drug nonmedically.[21] The Centers for Disease Control and Prevention (CDC) recently noted that, between 1997 and 2007, drug company distribution of prescription opioid analgesics increased 627%. The quantity of prescription painkillers sold to pharmacies, hospitals, and doctors' offices was four times larger in 2010 than in 1999. According to the CDC, current distribution levels would allow "for every American to take 5 mg of Vicodin every 4 hours for 3 weeks."[22] Stated alternatively, enough prescription opioids were prescribed in 2010 to medicate every American adult around-the-clock for a month.[21] Distribution by drug companies rose from 96 mg/person in 1997 to 698 mg/person in 2007. Although most of these drugs were prescribed for a medical purpose, many ended up in the hands of people who misused or abused them. Medical users in the last month numbered 9 million, while nonmedical users totaled 5.3 million.[22]

Nearly 15,000 people die every year of overdoses involving opioid analgesics. This is more than three times the people killed by these drugs in 1999. Nearly half a million ED visits in 2009 were due to people misusing or abusing prescription painkillers. For every overdose death there are 3 abuse treatment admissions, 35 ED visits for misuse or abuse, 161 people with abuse/dependence, and 461 nonmedical users. Nonmedical use of opioid analgesics costs health insurers up to $72.5 billion annually in direct healthcare costs.[22]

In the year 2000, retail pharmacies dispensed 174 million prescriptions for opioids, and by 2009, 257 million prescriptions were dispensed, which is an increase of 48%.[23]

Many states report problems with "pill mills," where doctors prescribe large quantities of opioids to people without medical justification. Some people also obtain prescriptions from multiple prescribers by "doctor shopping."

Clinical **Controversy. . .**

There is considerable debate about the appropriate use of prescribed opiates and how this might contribute to the overuse or abuse of these same drugs for nonmedicinal purposes. Not all decisions that physicians and other prescribers make are going to be correct. Likewise, pharmacists are going to occasionally make the wrong decision by either declining to fill a prescription that is proper and appropriate or filling one that is bogus. In the final analysis, mistakes in judgment are going to be made in both directions. Given this fact, in which direction should the health professional err? Should health practitioners give the patient the benefit of the doubt, writing or filling the prescription, even if their decision ultimately turns out to be wrong? Or should the mandate be in the other direction: refuse to prescribe pain medicines or refuse to fill the prescriptions, even when, in truth, the prescription is appropriate and valid? Most healthcare professionals assume that complaints of pain are real and prescribe accordingly.

Some states have a bigger problem with diversion and abuse of opioid analgesics than others. Prescription painkiller sales per person were more than three times higher in Florida, which has the highest rate, in comparison to Illinois, which has the lowest rate. From 2003 to 2009, a total of 16,550 drug overdose deaths were recorded by Florida medical examiners. The annual number of deaths increased 61%, from 1,804 to 2,905, and the death rate increased 47.5%, from 10.6 to 15.7 per 100,000 population. In 2009, approximately eight drug overdose deaths occurred each day. During 2003 to 2009, 85.9% of drug overdose deaths were unintentional, 11.1% were suicides, 2.6% were of undetermined intent, and 0.4% were homicides or pending. Prescription medications were implicated in 76.1% of all drug overdose deaths.[24] Further, opiate overdoses, once almost always due to heroin use, are now increasingly due to abuse of prescription painkillers.[25]

Nearly every state has authorized prescription drug monitoring programs (PDMPs), and most are operational at this time. PDMPs are electronic systems for the monitoring of controlled substances and drugs of concern dispensed in the state or dispensed to an address in the state. They aim to detect and prevent the diversion and abuse of prescription drugs at the retail level, where no other automated information collection system exists, and to allow for the collection and analysis of prescription data more efficiently than states without such a program can accomplish.

The NSDUH indicated that illicit drug use is 16.2% among pregnant teens and 7.4% among pregnant women aged 18 to 25 years.[13] Accordingly, in 2009, there were more than 13,000 babies born with neonatal abstinence syndrome (NAS) after being exposed to opioids in utero, a threefold increase since 2000.[26] Between 2000 and 2009, the incidence of NAS among newborns increased from 1.20 (95% CI, 1.04 to 1.37) to 3.39 (95% CI, 3.12 to 3.67) per 1,000 hospital births per year. Antepartum maternal opiate use also increased from 1.19 to 5.63 (per 1,000 hospital births per year). In 2009, newborns with NAS were more likely than all other hospital births to have low birth weight (19.1% vs. 7%), and respiratory complications (30.9% vs. 8.9%), and to be covered by Medicaid (78.1% vs. 45.5%). Mean hospital charges for discharges with NAS increased from $39,400 in 2000 to $53,400 in 2009. By 2009, 77.6% of charges for NAS were billed to state Medicaid programs.

Methadone

More than 30% of prescription opioid deaths involve methadone, even though only 2% of painkiller prescriptions are for this drug.[27]

Studies using medical examiner data suggested that more than three quarters of methadone overdoses involved persons who were not enrolled in programs treating opioid addiction with methadone and that most persons who overdosed were using it without a prescription.[27] Recent analyses have shown that methadone was involved in one in three opioid-related deaths in 2008.[28] Analysis of ED data[29,30] indicates that the estimated number of ED visits resulting from nonmedical use of methadone alone or in combination with other drugs in 2009 (n = 63,031) was significantly greater than the estimated number in 2004 (n = 36,806).

Six times as many people died of methadone overdoses in 2009 than a decade before.[31] More than 4 million methadone prescriptions were written for pain in 2009, despite US FDA warnings about the risks associated with methadone.

Methadone has pharmacologic properties unique among opioids, and as a result, a lack of knowledge about methadone among practitioners and patients has been identified as a factor contributing to the increased number of deaths observed in recent years.[32] Methadone's elimination half-life (8 to 59 hours) is longer than its duration of analgesic action (4 to 8 hours). In an FDA advisory issued in November 2006,[33] healthcare professionals were reminded that methadone's peak respiratory depressant effects typically occur later, and persist longer than its peak analgesic effects. The advisory notes that during treatment initiation, methadone's full analgesic effect is usually not attained until 3 to 5 days of dosing.

Deaths have been reported during conversion from chronic, high-dose treatment with other opioid agonists to methadone. It is critical to understand the pharmacokinetics of methadone when converting patients from other opioids to methadone. Particular vigilance is necessary during treatment initiation, during conversion from one opioid to another, and during dose adjustments. Also, there are pharmacokinetic and pharmacodynamic drug interactions between methadone and many other drugs. Thus, drugs administered concomitantly with methadone should be evaluated for interaction potential.[33]

Benzodiazepines and Other Sedative–Hypnotics

ED visits involving benzodiazepines clearly outnumber those involving any of the other types of psychotherapeutic agents. DAWN estimates that 408,021 ED visits associated with nonmedical use of pharmaceuticals involved benzodiazepines in 2010.[15] This is a dramatic increase from 2004 in which there were 170,471 ED visits attributed to benzodiazepines.

Because all benzodiazepines have abuse and dependence liability, patients cannot be switched from one benzodiazepine to another in hopes of decreasing a pattern of drug abuse or dependence behavior. Zolpidem, a nonbenzodiazepine, nonbarbiturate sedative, has been suggested to have little liability for physical dependence, but tolerance and withdrawal have been reported in association with its use as well.[15] Recent reports in the lay press have linked use of

CLINICAL PRESENTATION Benzodiazepine Intoxication and Withdrawal

General

- The intoxicated patient may be in acute distress in overdoses or when benzodiazepines are combined with alcohol.
- Patients in withdrawal may also be in acute distress and should be treated with a benzodiazepine taper to prevent seizures.

Symptoms

- The patient may experience memory impairment, drowsiness, visual disturbances, confusion, and GI disturbances. Patients may appear intoxicated, with slurred speech, poor coordination, swaying, and bloodshot eyes, with or without the odor of alcohol.

Signs

- Hypotension or nystagmus may be observed, and urinary retention may occur.

Laboratory Tests

- Qualitative testing to confirm presence of benzodiazepines is useful for diagnostic purposes, but quantitative plasma concentrations are usually not clinically useful.

zolpidem to sleep walking, erratic driving, binge eating, and other similarly bizarre activities.

Benzodiazepines generally do not cause life-threatening respiratory depression (unless taken with other sedatives), as do the barbiturate-like drugs.[16] Long-term use of even therapeutic doses of benzodiazepines can cause physical dependence and withdrawal symptoms after abrupt discontinuation.[16] Occurrence of hallucinations or seizures would indicate severe physical withdrawal.

Gradual tapering of dosage is also associated with less withdrawal and rebound anxiety than abrupt discontinuation. Dependence on sedative–hypnotics and benzodiazepines is summarized in Table 48-1. For additional information on benzodiazepine withdrawal, refer to Chapter 53.

Carisoprodol

Carisoprodol is a prescription drug marketed since 1959 and used in primary care settings for the treatment of musculoskeletal conditions associated with muscle spasms and back pain. Its effectiveness for this use has been questioned.[35] It is marketed in the United States as Soma as well as many generic versions. It is both structurally and pharmacologically related to meprobamate, a Schedule IV substance. In fact, a substantial percentage of the drug is metabolized to meprobamate,[35] a drug with barbiturate-like properties.

In legitimate medical practice, carisoprodol is used as an adjunct to rest, physical therapy, and other measures for relief of acute, painful musculoskeletal conditions.[35] Adverse effects are mostly related to the CNS: drowsiness, dizziness, vertigo, ataxia, tremor, agitation, irritability, headache, depressive reactions, syncope, and insomnia. Carisoprodol may also adversely affect cardiovascular (tachycardia, postural hypotension, and facial flushing), GI (nausea, vomiting, hiccup, and epigastric distress), and hematologic systems. Carisoprodol overdose has resulted in stupor, coma, shock, respiratory depression, and death.[35]

Recognizing that prolonged abuse of carisoprodol at high dosage can lead to tolerance, dependence, and withdrawal symptoms in humans,[36] U.S. Drug Enforcement Administration (DEA) issued a final rule to classify carisoprodol as a Schedule IV Controlled Substance effective January 11, 2012.[36]

The number of carisoprodol-related ED visits involving misuse or abuse by patients aged 50 or older tripled between 2004 and 2009 (from 2,070 to 7,115 visits). The majority of ED visits involving carisoprodol also involved other pharmaceuticals (77%); the most common combinations involved narcotic pain relievers (55%) and benzodiazepines (47%).[15]

TABLE 48-1 Pharmacologic Treatment of Substance Intoxication

Drug Class	Nonpharmacologic Therapy	Pharmacologic Therapy	Level of Evidence[a,b]
Benzodiazepines	Support vital functions	Flumazenil 0.2 mg/min IV initially; repeat up to 3 mg maximum	A1
Alcohol, barbiturates, and sedative–hypnotics (nonbenzodiazepines)	Support vital functions	None	B3
Opiates	Support vital functions	Naloxone 0.4–2 mg IV every 3 minutes	A1
Cocaine and other CNS stimulants	Monitor cardiac function	Lorazepam 2–4 mg IM every 30 minutes to 6 hours as needed for agitation	B2
		Haloperidol 2–5 mg (or other antipsychotic agent) every 30 minutes to 6 hours as needed for psychotic behavior	B3
Hallucinogens, marijuana, and inhalants	Reassurance; "talk-down therapy"; support vital functions	Lorazepam and/or haloperidol as above	B3
Phencyclidine	Minimize sensory input	Lorazepam and/or haloperidol as above	B3

[a]Strength of recommendations, evidence to support recommendation: A, good; B, moderate; C, poor.
[b]Quality of evidence: 1, evidence from more than one properly randomized controlled trial; 2, evidence from more than one well-designed clinical trial with randomization, from cohort or case–control analytic studies or multiple time series, or dramatic results from uncontrolled experiments; 3, evidence from opinions of respected authorities, based on clinical experience, descriptive studies, or reports of expert communities.

Data from references 34 and 83.

Dextromethorphan

Dextromethorphan abuse is one of the most common (and most dangerous) examples of nonprescription drug abuse.[37] Intoxication from consuming large doses of cough syrup is known on the street as "robodosing" or "robotripping." Handsful of cough and cold remedies are sometimes called "skittles" because they look similar to the popular fruit candy. Dextromethorphan creates a depressant and sometimes profound hallucinogenic effect when taken in large doses. Since it is a nonprescription drug, it is easily procured by adolescents. Those who use the cough syrup to get high are sometimes called "syrup heads."

High doses induce effects that include hyperexcitability, lethargy, ataxia, slurred speech, diaphoresis, hypertension, nystagmus, and mydriasis. When taken at much higher doses, it acts as a dissociative anesthetic, similar to phencyclidine (PCP, "angel dust") and ketamine ("Special K"). These are the effects sought by those who use the drug to get high. At these high doses, dextromethorphan also is a CNS depressant.[37]

The recommended treatment for acute overdoses of dextromethorphan is naloxone. Although reports of its efficacy are mixed, it may be helpful in reversing the CNS depressant and neurologic effects.[38]

CNS STIMULANTS

Cocaine

Cocaine is perhaps the most behaviorally reinforcing of all drugs of abuse. Clinicians estimate that approximately 10% of people who begin to use the drug recreationally will go on to serious, heavy use. Once having tried cocaine, an individual cannot predict or control the extent to which he or she will continue to use the drug.

The most characteristic pharmacologic effect of cocaine is stimulation of the CNS. In the CNS, cocaine appears to mediate its effects primarily by blocking reuptake of catecholamine neurotransmitters such as norepinephrine and dopamine.

Cocaine is absorbed rapidly from virtually all sites of application. For many years, cocaine has been administered as the hydrochloride salt form, usually by inhalation, but also by injection. In the last 18 to 20 years, as the purity of cocaine hydrochloride obtained on the street declined, many users converted the cocaine hydrochloride to cocaine base, also known as "crack" or "rock." Smoking the drug leads to almost instant absorption and intense euphoria. Peak plasma concentrations of more than 900 ng/mL (mcg/L; 3 μmol/L) have been achieved following inhalation of cocaine base vapors, compared with concentrations of only 150 to 200 ng/mL (mcg/L; 0.49 to 0.66 μmol/L) achieved after inhalation of similar amounts of pure cocaine hydrochloride powder.[39] The high from snorting can last 15 to 30 minutes, whereas that from smoking can last 5 to 10 minutes. Increased use can reduce the period of stimulation. An appreciable tolerance to the high can develop, and many addicts report that they seek but fail to achieve as much pleasure as they did from their first exposure. Scientific evidence suggests that the powerful neuropsychological reinforcing property of cocaine is responsible for an individual's continued use despite harmful physical and social consequences.

Research has helped clarify certain patterns of cocaine use, such as combining cocaine and alcohol. Such drug use would seem counterintuitive because cocaine is a CNS stimulant, and alcohol a CNS depressant. In the presence of alcohol, cocaine is metabolized to cocaethylene, a longer-acting but potent psychoactive compound compared with the parent drug.[40] The risk of death from cocaethylene is greater than from cocaine.[41] The cocaine–alcohol combination is one of the most commonly identified among individuals who come to hospital EDs with acute substance abuse problems.

Cocaine is metabolized and eliminated rapidly. The elimination half-life of cocaine is approximately 1 hour, and the duration of effect is very short.[39] The short duration of effect provides a powerful incentive for repeated use of the drug. Many users experience intense drug use cycling, sometimes lasting days, characterized by rapidly repeating doses of cocaine until their supply is exhausted. Laboratory monkeys, given a choice between food and cocaine around-the-clock for 8 days, consistently choose cocaine.

Complications of cocaine use frequently involve cardiovascular events.[42,43] Cocaine is a psychotomimetic drug, sometimes even at nontoxic doses. A kindling phenomenon has been described with cocaine in which neuronal function becomes altered with each dose of the drug. The psychosis is qualitatively very similar to a paranoid schizophrenic psychosis.[44] Although there is some controversy as to whether cocaine is associated with physical withdrawal on abrupt discontinuation, most clinicians feel that there is a characteristic syndrome of withdrawal effects, although they are not life-threatening.

Amphetamine, Methamphetamine, and Other Stimulants

The physiologic and psychological effects of amphetamines and other stimulants are qualitatively similar to those of cocaine—they diminish fatigue, increase alertness, and suppress appetite. Pharmacologically, amphetamines increase the activity of catecholamine neurotransmitters (e.g., norepinephrine and dopamine) by increasing release and by inhibiting the degradative enzyme monoamine oxidase.[36]

Methamphetamine is used orally, intranasally, rectally, by IV injection, and by smoking. Immediately after inhalation or IV injection, the methamphetamine user experiences an intense sensation, called a "rush" or "flash," that lasts only a few minutes and is described as extremely pleasurable.

Because methamphetamine elevates mood, people who experiment with it tend to use it with increasing frequency and in increasing doses, although this was not their original intent. The timing and intensity of the "rush" that accompanies the use of methamphetamine, which is a result of the release of high levels of dopamine in the brain, depend in part on the method of administration. Specifically, the effect is almost instantaneous when smoked or injected, whereas it takes approximately 5 minutes after snorting or 20 minutes after oral ingestion. Prolonged use of methamphetamine can result in a tolerance for the drug and increased use at higher dosage levels, creating dependence. Such continual use of the drug with little or no sleep may lead to an extremely irritable and paranoid state. Discontinuing use of methamphetamine often results in a state of depression, as well as fatigue, anergia, and some types of cognitive impairment that can last from 2 days to several months.

Negative consequences of methamphetamine abuse range from anxiety and insomnia to convulsions, paranoia, and brain damage. Methamphetamine-induced caries, or "meth mouth," is a characteristic pattern of dental decay commonly observed in patients who smoke methamphetamine.[45]

In addition to the many direct effects on methamphetamine users are the indirect impacts on individuals and society. Flammable ingredients that include acetone, red phosphorous, ethyl alcohol, and lithium metal are used in methamphetamine cookers, often with disastrous results. Fires and explosions often ensue, resulting in severe burns and uncovering laboratories to local law enforcement. Children of methamphetamine abusers are at high risk of neglect and abuse, and pregnant women's use of methamphetamine can cause growth retardation, premature birth, and developmental disorders in neonates. Treatment for methamphetamine dependence is very difficult, and has a low success rate.[46] The expanding global market is fed by an increase in clandestine manufacture

CLINICAL PRESENTATION Amphetamine Intoxication and Withdrawal

General

- Amphetamine intoxication is an acute condition that may result in death. Pharmacotherapy may be indicated for symptomatic control of seizures.
- Patients may experience withdrawal symptoms for several days, but are usually not in acute distress. Treatment is supportive in nature. Pharmacotherapy is not effective to treat the symptoms of amphetamine withdrawal.

Symptoms

- Depression, altered mental status, drug craving, dyssomnia, and fatigue are all symptoms of withdrawal.
- Amphetamine intoxication may present as increased wakefulness, increased physical activity, decreased appetite, increased respiration, hyperthermia, and euphoria. Other CNS effects include irritability, insomnia, confusion, tremors, convulsions, anxiety, paranoia, chest pain, and aggressiveness. Hyperthermia and convulsions can result in death.

Signs

- Patients with amphetamine intoxication may present with tachycardia, hypertension, or stroke.

Laboratory Tests

- A qualitative drug of abuse urine screening is used for diagnostic purposes. Confirmatory blood tests with gas chromatography and mass spectrophotometry may be used for verification.

of methamphetamine. Not only are there more laboratories in more countries, but their size and sophistication are also increasing. The number of reported domestic methamphetamine laboratory seizures in 2010 (6,768) represents a 12% increase over the total number of methamphetamine laboratories seized in 2009 (6,032).[46] An increasing number of methamphetamine laboratories seized in the United States are small-scale operations capable of producing less than 2 oz (about 60 g) of the drug per production cycle. At least 81% of the laboratories seized every year since 2006 were small-scale. Most of the remaining laboratories seized were also relatively small, with capacities between 2 and 8 oz (about 60 and 230 g) per production cycle.[46]

Methamphetamine is manufactured using the ephedrine or pseudoephedrine reduction method. In this process, ephedrine or pseudoephedrine is extracted from nonprescription cold and allergy tablets. Pharmacists should be wary of persons wishing to purchase large quantities of products containing nonprescription sympathomimetic products. As a precaution, federal legislation now mandates that pseudoephedrine-containing products be kept behind a counter, and suitable identification must be shown before they can be purchased.

Ecstasy and Other Methamphetamine Analogs

Several dozen analogs of amphetamine and methamphetamine are mildly hallucinogenic. Two methamphetamine analogs of most concern are 3,4-methylenedioxyamphetamine (MDA) and especially 3,4-methylenedioxymethamphetamine (MDMA or Ecstasy). The annual prevalence of Ecstasy declined significantly in 2012 in all three grades. Over the past dozen years, the use of Ecstasy has changed quite a bit, with rates being high in the early 2000s and decreasing through the mid-2000s. The 2012 annual prevalence rates are 1.1%, 3%, and 3.8% in grades 8, 10, and 12—less than half the peak rates observed in 2001.[14]

The effects of MDMA usually last approximately 4 to 6 hours. Users of the drug say that it produces profoundly positive feelings, empathy for others, elimination of anxiety, and extreme relaxation. MDMA is also said to suppress the need to eat, drink, or sleep, enabling users to endure 2- to 3-day parties. Consequently, MDMA use sometimes results in severe dehydration or exhaustion. MDMA generally reduces inhibitions and creates a sense of euphoria, but it also can evoke anxiety and paranoia. Heavier doses generate depression, irrationality, and psychosis. Users claim they experience feelings of closeness with others and a desire to touch them.

MDMA use can result in a variety of acute psychiatric disturbances, including panic, anxiety, depression, and paranoid thinking. Physical symptoms include muscle tension, nausea, blurred vision, faintness, chills, and sweating. MDMA also increases the heart rate and blood pressure. Other effects include hyperthermia, dehydration, vomiting, tremors, loss of control over body movements, insomnia, convulsions, rapid eye movements (REMs), and teeth and jaw clenching.

MDMA is perceived to be a harmless drug by many of its users, based in part on the fact that the risk of death is low compared with that with other drugs such as heroin and cocaine. However, mounting evidence points to neurotoxic effects of MDMA, involving a complex and incompletely understood mechanism. MDMA has been shown to destroy serotonin-producing neurons in animals, but further research is needed to understand the mechanism behind this loss of serotonin following MDMA exposure.

Researchers have found that heavy MDMA users have memory problems that persist for at least 2 weeks after they have stopped using the drug.[47,48] McCann et al.[49,50] conducted several studies to determine the effects of MDMA use on cognitive performance. MDMA users and controls were found to perform similarly on several cognitive tasks. However, MDMA subjects had significant performance deficits on a sustained-attention task requiring arithmetic calculations, a task requiring complex attention and incidental learning, a task requiring short-term memory, and a task of semantic recognition and verbal reasoning. The authors believe that their data provide further evidence that MDMA is neurotoxic to brain serotonin neurons in humans, and the behavioral data suggest that brain serotonin injury is associated with subtle but significant cognitive deficits.

Manufacturers of illicit drugs sometimes substitute other, potentially more dangerous substances for the one the buyer is expecting. Other suppliers produce products adulterated with chemical by-products of the incomplete processing of active ingredients. One such chemical, *para*-methoxyamphetamine, is a drastically more potent hyperthermic agent than MDMA, and deaths have been attributed to this agent.[51]

Synthetic Cathinones (aka Bath Salts)

2 Bath salts are a family of structurally related sympathomimetic, synthetic, designer drugs, known collectively as cathinones. Despite being marketed as "bath salts" or "plant food" and labeled "not for human consumption," people use these substances for their amphetamine or cocaine-like effects. The name "bath salts" appears to have been selected to disguise the true nature of these substances. They are available in small quantities (milligram or 0.5 g packages) and are not the same as legitimate commercial bath products that are used for taking a soothing bath. Since the time of their appearance in the recreational drug market, there have been numerous confirmed cases of abuse, dependence, severe intoxication, and deaths related to the consumption of synthetic cathinones.

Catha edulis (khat) is an evergreen slow-growing shrub or tree native to Ethiopia and cultivated in East Africa and the South West Arabian Peninsula that in recent years has been grown widespread in Europe as well.[52] In areas where it is grown people use the fresh vegetable material (leaves, stems, flower buds) of this plant for its stimulant effects. The fresh khat leaves contain 62 alkaloids, and 2 of these, cathine and cathinone, have been demonstrated to have amphetamine-like effects. Like amphetamines, cathine and cathinone are CNS stimulants, but their potency is less. Several studies have shown that the chronic use of this plant may produce various harmful effects, such as increased incidence of acute coronary vasospasm and myocardial infarction, esophagitis, gastritis, oral keratotic lesions, and liver toxicity.

Most of the synthetic cathinones, first appearing as recreational drugs in the mid-2000s, are a ring-substituted cathinone closely related to the phenethylamine family. The synthetic cathinones are the β-keto analogs of natural cathinone and differ from amphetamines by the presence of a ketone oxygen group at the β-position.

3 The pharmacology of these substances has not been extensively studied, but available information shows that these molecules may also inhibit monoamine oxidase.[53] Within the class of synthetic cathinones there are considerable differences in pharmacology. The synthetic cathinones pyrovalerone and MDPV are highly potent and selective catecholamine transporter inhibitors but not substrate releasers. Mephedrone, methylone, ethylone, butylone, and naphyrone act as nonselective monoamine uptake inhibitors, similar to cocaine and, with the exception of naphyrone, also release serotonin, similar to MDMA. Cathinone and methcathinone are selective catecholamine uptake inhibitors and releasers, similar to their non–β-keto analogs amphetamine and methamphetamine.

Case reports have revealed a variety of adverse effects associated with the use of bath salts, including tachycardia, hypertension, diabetic ketoacidosis, delusions, paranoid psychosis, hyperthermia, dizziness, agitation, headaches, hyponatremia, acute liver failure, and suicide. Fatal intoxication has been associated with members of this class of drugs.[54,55]

On July 9, 2012, President Barack Obama signed a law that classifies synthetic cathinones and classes of related chemicals as Schedule I Controlled Substances.[56]

HALLUCINOGENS

LSD

The drugs commonly classified as hallucinogens are LSD, psilocybin, DMT, mescaline, and other related compounds. LSD is one of the most potent mood-changing chemicals. It is manufactured from lysergic acid, which is found in ergot, a fungus that grows on rye and other grains.

Pharmacologically, LSD and related drugs stimulate both presynaptic (5-hydroxytryptamine [5-HT_{1A} and 5-HT_{1B}]) and postsynaptic (5-HT_2) serotonin receptors in the brain, which functionally can cause either agonist or antagonist effects on serotonin activity. Precisely how the hallucinogens exert their effects remains unclear. LSD is an extraordinarily potent compound, producing observable CNS effects at doses as low as 25 mcg. For an in-depth review of LSD the reader is directed to a review by Passie et al.[57]

Designer Drugs

2 The past few years has witnessed the (re)-emergence of a number of very potent substances from three categories of drugs: the phenethylamines, the piperazines, and the tryptamines.[58] These drugs are marketed largely through Internet sales, and are abused by people of all ages. They are illegally manufactured or synthesized in clandestine laboratories; many designer drugs are offered as a "research chemical," "not for human consumption."

Phenethylamines are ingested for their stimulant and hallucinogenic effects on the CNS. One group of the phenethylamine category that has received attention in recent years contains 2,5-dimethoxy or 2C derivatives, such as 4-bromo-2,5-dimethoxyphenethylamine (2C-B) or 2,5-dimethoxy-4-iodophenethylamine (2C-I).

Due to their stimulant and hallucinogenic effects, piperazines have entered the club or party scene. Piperazines of concern include *N*-benzylpiperazine (BZP), 1-(3-trifluoromethylphenyl)-piperazine (TFMPP), and 1-(3-chlorophenyl)-piperazine (*meta*-chlorophenylpiperazine [mCPP]). While mCPP is found in the illicit market, it is also a metabolite and starting material for the synthesis of several prescription drugs (e.g., trazodone, nefazadone).

Many of these emerging drugs have been added to DEA's drugs and chemicals of concern list, and 2 drugs—BZP and TFMPP—appeared on the list of top 25 drugs reported to National Forensic Laboratory Information System (NFLIS) in 2008 (BZP only), 2009, and 2010.[78] For example, *N,N*-DMT occurs naturally. South American snuffs and brews such as ayahuasca, prepared from a jungle vine (*Banisteriopsis caapi*), have been used in ancient medicinal and ritualistic practices that continue today. Like piperazines, tryptamines are hallucinogenic substances that are taken orally, or more rarely by smoking, snorting, or injection. Commonly abused tryptamines include DMT and 5-methoxy-*N,N*-diisopropyltryptamine (5-MeO-DIPT). Several of the drugs presented in this NFLIS Special Report have been named and federally scheduled under the Controlled Substances Act.

MARIJUANA

Marijuana continues to be the most commonly used illicit drug among U.S. residents aged 12 and older.[13] In 2011, an estimated 29.7 million residents reported using marijuana in the past year, a statistically significant increase from 25.9 million in 2008. According to the most recent MTFS,[14] annual marijuana prevalence peaked among 12th graders in 1979 at 51%, following a rise that began during the 1960s. Then use declined fairly steadily for 13 years, bottoming at 22% in 1992—a decline of more than half. The 1990s, however, saw a resurgence of use. After a considerable increase (one that actually began among 8th graders a year earlier than among 10th and 12th graders), annual prevalence rates peaked in 1996 at 8th grade and in 1997 at 10th and 12th grades. After these peak years, use declined among all three grades through 2006, 2007, or 2008; since then there has been an upturn in use in all three grades, indicating another possible resurgence in use, although in 2011 there was some decline in use among 8th graders. In 2010 there was a significant increase in daily use in all three grades, followed by a nonsignificant increase in 2011 reaching 1.3%, 3.6%, and 6.6% in grades 8, 10, and 12, respectively. The rate for 12th graders is the highest rate since 1981, when it was 7%.

Most users smoke marijuana in hand-rolled cigarettes (joints), while some use pipes or water pipes (bongs). Marijuana cigars

CLINICAL PRESENTATION Marijuana Intoxication

General Symptoms

- Patients intoxicated with marijuana may experience euphoria, sensory intensification, increased appetite, apathy, hallucinations, and dry mouth. Occasionally, marijuana use produces anxiety, fear, distrust, or panic.

Signs

- Tachycardia and conjunctival congestion may be observed in patients intoxicated with marijuana.

Laboratory Tests

- Although the duration of effect of marijuana may be only several hours, THC is detectable on toxicologic screening for up to 4 to 5 weeks, especially in chronic users.

called blunts have also become popular.[14] To make blunts, users slice open cigars and replace the tobacco with marijuana.

Marijuana's effects begin immediately after the drug enters the brain and last from 1 to 3 hours. If marijuana is consumed in food or drink, the short-term effects begin more slowly, usually within 30 minutes to 1 hour, and last longer, for as long as 4 hours. Smoking marijuana delivers several times more of its major active ingredient, delta-9-tetrahydrocannabinol (THC), into the blood than does eating or drinking the drug.

Marijuana Potency

The principal psychoactive component of marijuana is THC. Hashish, the dried resin of the top of the plant, is much more potent than the plant itself. Increasingly sophisticated growing techniques have resulted in plants of greater potency. In 1976, an analysis of DEA seizures found an average THC content of 0.5% to 1%. In 2011, that figure was nearing 12%, with some samples containing THC levels above 20% and 30%.[59]

Harmful Effects of Marijuana

Marijuana has been used widely and is believed by many to be a relatively harmless, nonaddictive intoxicant. Chronic low doses of marijuana usually are not associated with significant physical withdrawal on abrupt discontinuation, but many chronic users exhibit compulsive drug-seeking and drug-use behaviors characteristic of addiction or dependence.

In point of fact, scientific research has found that 1 in 10 marijuana users will become addicted to the drug. And if one begins in adolescence, that number rises to one in six.[60] Acutely, marijuana has many of the effects of alcohol—sedation, a decrease in reactivity and ability to perform complex tasks, and disinhibition. Endocrine effects including amenorrhea, decreased testosterone production, and inhibition of spermatogenesis have been demonstrated. Marijuana is associated with an amotivational syndrome characterized by a behavioral pattern of apathy, dullness, impaired judgment, decreased concentration and memory, loss of interest in personal hygiene, and a general reduction of goal-directed behavior.[61]

Science confirms[62] that the adolescent brain, particularly the part of the brain that regulates the planning of complex cognitive behavior, personality expression, decision making, and social behavior, is not fully developed until the early to mid-20s. Developing brains are especially susceptible to all of the negative effects of marijuana and other drug use.[62]

One of the most well-designed studies[63] on marijuana and intelligence, released in 2012, found that marijuana use reduces IQ by as much as eight points by age 38 among people who started using marijuana regularly before age 18 but then stopped. The purpose of the study was to test the association between persistent cannabis use and neuropsychological decline and determine whether decline is concentrated among adolescent-onset cannabis users. Participants were members of the Dunedin Study, a prospective study of a birth cohort of 1,037 individuals followed from birth (1972/1973) to age 38 years. Cannabis use was ascertained in interviews at ages 18, 21, 26, 32, and 38 years. Neuropsychological testing was conducted at age 13 years, before initiation of cannabis use, and again at age 38 years, after a pattern of persistent cannabis use had developed. Persistent cannabis use was associated with neuropsychological decline broadly across domains of functioning, even after controlling for years of education. Informants also reported noticing more cognitive problems for persistent cannabis users. Impairment was concentrated among adolescent-onset cannabis users, with more persistent use associated with greater decline. Further, cessation of cannabis use did not fully restore neuropsychological functioning among adolescent-onset cannabis users. Findings are suggestive of a neurotoxic effect of cannabis on the adolescent brain and highlight the importance of prevention and policy efforts targeting adolescents.[63]

Marijuana and Driving

Along with the increased prevalence of marijuana smoking, rates of driving under the influence of cannabis have also risen in recent year. Studies show that approximately 6% to 11% of fatal accident victims test positive for THC. In many of these cases alcohol is detected as well.[64] A recent systematic review and meta-analysis[65] was conducted to determine whether the acute consumption of cannabis by drivers increases the risk of motor vehicle collisions. The report included nine studies. The authors conclude that acute cannabis consumption is associated with an increased risk of a motor vehicle crash, especially for fatal collisions. An earlier meta-analysis[66] showed that estimated odds ratios relating marijuana use to crash risk reported in included studies ranged from 0.85 to 7.16.

A double-blind, placebo-controlled, randomized, three-way crossover study[67] was conducted to assess the effects of orally administered, normal therapeutic doses of dronabinol (10 and 20 mg) on driving performance in a standardized on-the-road driving test performed in normal traffic. About 25% of heavy users displayed driving impairments comparable to or worse than a blood alcohol concentration of 0.5 mg/mL (0.05 g%; 11 mmol/L).

Medical Marijuana

Since 1996, 18 states and the District of Columbia in the United States have enacted legislation to decriminalize marijuana for medical use.[68] Some believe that the widespread use of medical marijuana is a thinly veiled strategy for the future legalization for recreational as well as medicinal use. Vague state laws governing medical marijuana have allowed recreational users of the drug to take advantage of marijuana dispensaries. Obtaining a license to use marijuana is not difficult. For example, on the boardwalk of Venice Beach, California, pitchmen dressed in marijuana green clothing approach passersby with offers of a $35, 10-minute evaluation for a medical marijuana recommendation for everything from cancer to appetite loss.[69]

Clinical **Controversy. . .**

The mere mention of the words "medical marijuana" is bound to evoke strong emotions among laypersons and healthcare professionals alike. While the federal government continues to enforce laws that make possession and use of marijuana illegal, regardless of the intended purpose, at last count 18 of the U.S. states have legalized medical marijuana, and 2 have legalized recreational use of the drug. While the safety and efficacy of marijuana to treat certain identifiable medical conditions has been confirmed, many other uses are supported by anecdote or limited clinical experience. However, the debate involves much more than whether cannabis works or not to treat illness. Instead, there are political, social, economic, and religious considerations that cloud the controversy over whether marijuana should be legalized for medical purposes. This debate will continue for years to come.

Designing and conducting adequate research studies of the beneficial effects of marijuana present some methodologic challenges.[70,71] Smoked marijuana varies by dose, due to individual differences in absorption and metabolism in the liver, as well as puff frequency, depth of inhalation, and retention of inhaled smoke. Two comprehensive and dispassionate reviews[72,73] of medical marijuana have been published, and the reader is encouraged to consult these for further information.

In the November 2012 election, both Colorado and Washington states passed laws allowing recreational use of marijuana, allowing adults to possess and grow marijuana with state regulation and taxation. The legalization measure in Oregon was defeated. Arkansas voters rejected the use of medicinal marijuana, but voters in Massachusetts joined 17 other states and the District of Columbia in supporting "medical" marijuana. Montana retained their "medical" marijuana law with more restrictions. Under federal law, any marijuana use is still illegal. Time will tell how this dilemma will be handled.

Synthetic Cannabinoids

3 Over the past several years, recreational use of synthetic cannabinoid compounds has been increasing in the United States. Known colloquially as "K2," "Spice," "Aroma," "Mr. Smiley," "Zohai," "Eclipse," "Black Mamba," "Red X Dawn," "Blaze," and "Dream," these products were not listed as controlled substances until recently. As a result, they were available at gas stations and convenience stores, and on the Internet.

Following identification of THC in 1964 and the CB1 and CB2 cannabinoid receptors in the 1980s, there was a pharmaceutical effort to synthesize cannabinoid receptor agonists for potential therapeutic indications such as nausea and pain. The largest structural group of synthetic cannabinoid receptor agonists are the JWH compounds named after John W. Huffman, an organic chemist at Clemson University, who synthesized many of these compounds.[74] The vast majority of these efforts never reached commercial fruition. However, independent chemists now use this publicly available research to produce synthetic cannabinoids.

3 Currently there are over 100 compounds referred to as "synthetic marijuana."[75] The finished salable products consist of psychoactively inert dry plant material sprayed with these synthetic cannabinoid receptor agonists.[76,77]

NFLIS reported a dramatic increase in spice-related events, jumping from 15 in 2009 to 2,977 in 2010. Similarly, in 2011 there were a total of 6,959 calls to poison centers about exposures to synthetic marijuana, and from January 1, 2012 to October 31, 2012 alone, there were 4,710 calls.[79]

Symptoms of synthetic cannabinoid toxicity are similar to the euphoric and psychoactive effects of marijuana with additional sympathomimetic symptoms, including severe agitation and anxiety, extreme tachycardia, hypertension, nausea and vomiting, muscle spasms, seizures, tremors, diaphoresis, and restlessness. Intense hallucinations and psychotic episodes and suicidal and other harmful thoughts and/or actions have also been reported.[80]

Gunderson et al. have published a systematic review of the effects of synthetic cannabinoids and their psychosocial implications.[81]

INHALANTS

Inhalants are a diverse group of substances that include volatile solvents, gases, and nitrites that are sniffed, snorted, huffed, or bagged to produce intoxicating effects similar to those of alcohol. These substances are found in common household products such as glues, lighter fluid, cleaning fluids, paint products, nail polish remover, gasoline, rubber glue, waxes, and varnishes. Chemicals found in these products include toluene, benzene, methanol, methylene chloride, acetone, methyl ethyl ketone, methyl butyl ketone, trichloroethylene, and trichloroethane. The gas used as a propellant in canned whipped cream and in small metallic containers called "whippets" (used to make whipped cream) is nitrous oxide or "laughing gas."

Space limitation prevents an in-depth discussion of inhalants, and the interested reader is referred to past editions of this text.

TREATMENT

Acute Drug Intoxications

Treatment of drug intoxication, summarized in Table 48-1, is primarily supportive. Vital functions are maintained while waiting for the drug to be eliminated. Whenever possible, drug therapy should be avoided because psychotropic drug therapy has the potential for worsening a toxic reaction to another psychoactive agent; however, when patients are agitated, combative, assaultive, hallucinating, or delusional, drug therapy may be required. Toxicology screens are useful in the evaluation and treatment process, but knowledge of the metabolism of the suspected drug and its excretion patterns is important for proper interpretation of test results.

4 Flumazenil can be used to reverse toxic effects of benzodiazepines. Naloxone can be used to reverse the effects of opiates. The usual dosage for naloxone in acute opiate toxicity is 0.4 to 2 mg IV, given approximately every 3 minutes as necessary. In some instances a naloxone infusion could be administered since the half-life of the opiate is likely to be longer than that of naloxone (see Table 48-2). Although naloxone is effective in reversing opiate overdose, it also can precipitate physical withdrawal in physically dependent patients. An excellent comprehensive review of the management of opioid analgesic overdose was recently published.[83]

CLINICAL PRESENTATION Opioid Intoxication and Withdrawal

General

- Onset of the acute phase of withdrawal ranges from a few hours after stopping heroin to 3 to 5 days after stopping methadone. The duration of withdrawal ranges from 3 to 14 days.
- Opioid withdrawal is not fatal unless there is a concurrent medical problem of major concern.
- The presence of delirium should raise the question of concurrent withdrawal from another drug, such as alcohol, or another cause of delirium possibly secondary to drug use.

Symptoms

- During withdrawal, patients can experience piloerection, insomnia, muscle aches, and yawning. While intoxicated, patients can experience euphoria, dysphoria, apathy, sedation, or attention impairment.

Signs

- Fever, lacrimation, diaphoresis, or diarrhea may be observed during withdrawal. Motor retardation, slurred speech, and miosis may be observed during intoxication.

Laboratory Tests

- Treatment is based more on clinical presentation because plasma opioid levels may not be clinically useful.

Other Diagnostic Tests

- Arterial blood gases, pulse oximetry, and pulmonary function tests are useful to assess respiratory depression.

Intoxication with stimulants, including cocaine, is treated pharmacologically only if the patient is overtly psychotic and agitated.[42,84] Injectable benzodiazepines, usually lorazepam 2 to 4 mg intramuscularly every 30 minutes to 6 hours as necessary, can be used for agitation. Antipsychotic drugs can be used on a short-term basis, primarily in patients with psychotic symptoms, and usually at relatively low doses, such as haloperidol 2 to 5 mg intramuscularly every 30 minutes to 6 hours as necessary, followed by 5 to 15 mg orally per day in single or divided doses if the patient is still psychotic after initial treatment.[42]

An evidence-based guideline gives precise recommendations for treating the cardiovascular complications of cocaine abuse and provides insight into the epidemiology, pathophysiology, treatment, and prognosis of the cardiac effects of cocaine.[43] Seizures generally are treated supportively. IV lorazepam or diazepam can be used if seizures progress to status epilepticus.[42]

Hallucinogen intoxication is treated in a manner similar to stimulant intoxication. Drug therapy often can be avoided because patients can respond to careful reassurance, or so-called talk-down therapy. When necessary, short-term antianxiety and/or antipsychotic drug therapy can be used, as described previously.

TABLE 48-2 How to Use a Naloxone Infusion

1. If a naloxone bolus (start with 0.04 mg IV and titrate) is successful, administer two thirds of the effective bolus dose per hour by IV infusion; frequently reassess the patient's respiratory status
2. If respiratory depression is not reversed after the bolus dose:
   Intubate the patient, as clinically indicated
   Administer up to 10 mg of naloxone as an IV bolus. If the patient does not respond, do not initiate an infusion
3. If the patient develops withdrawal after the bolus dose:
   Allow the effects of the bolus to abate
   If respiratory depression recurs, administer half of this new bolus dose and begin an IV infusion at two thirds of the initial bolus dose per hour. Frequently reassess the patient's respiratory status
4. If the patient develops withdrawal signs or symptoms during the infusion:
   Stop the infusion until the withdrawal symptoms abate
   Restart the infusion at half the initial rate; frequently reassess the patient's respiratory status
   Exclude withdrawal from other xenobiotics
5. If the patient develops respiratory depression during the infusion:
   Readminister half of the initial bolus and repeat until reversal occurs
   Increase the infusion by half of the initial rate; frequently reassess the patient's respiratory status
   Exclude continued absorption, readministration of opioid, and other etiologies as the cause of the respiratory depression

Data from reference 82, with permission.

Withdrawal

5 Treatment of drug withdrawal is the primary indication for drug therapy in substance-related disorders. Goals of drug therapy include prevention of progression of withdrawal to life-threatening severity and enabling the patient to be sufficiently comfortable and functional to participate in a behavioral treatment program and supportive drug therapy. The clinician should remember that withdrawal is usually part of a substance dependence disorder. In drug therapy for withdrawal, it is important to avoid reinforcing the patient's drug-seeking and drug-use behavior to the extent possible. Patients must be educated to deal with the stress of withdrawal without seeking drugs. Treatment of drug withdrawal is summarized in Table 48-3.

CNS Depressant Withdrawal

Benzodiazepines

5 Treatment of benzodiazepine withdrawal is very similar to the treatment of alcohol withdrawal. The major difference in management is the length of treatment.[85] The onset of withdrawal symptoms in patients physically dependent on the long-acting benzodiazepines can be delayed up to 7 days after discontinuation of the drug. A common approach in detoxification of such patients is to initiate treatment at usual dosages (chlordiazepoxide orally 50 mg three times a day; lorazepam orally 2 mg three times a day) and to maintain the initial dosage for 5 days, with gradual tapering over an additional 5 days. Detoxification in patients physically dependent on shorter-acting benzodiazepines is similar to treatment of alcohol withdrawal.[85]

Among the benzodiazepines, alprazolam has been suggested to be more difficult to taper and discontinue than the other benzodiazepines.[85] A longer, more gradual taper of the benzodiazepine used for detoxification can be needed. With all benzodiazepines,

CLINICAL PRESENTATION Cocaine Intoxication and Withdrawal

General

- In overdoses, cocaine is a CNS and cardiac stimulant. Cocaine-related deaths are often a result of cardiac arrest or seizures followed by respiratory arrest.

Symptoms

- Symptoms of intoxication include motor agitation, elation, euphoria, grandiosity, loquacity, hypervigilance, sweating or chills, nausea, and vomiting.
- Symptoms of withdrawal include fatigue, sleep disturbances, nightmares, depression, and changes in appetite.
- High doses of cocaine and/or prolonged use can trigger paranoia.

Signs

- Tachycardia, mydriasis, and either elevated or lowered blood pressure may be observed with overdose. Cardiac abnormalities (e.g., arrhythmias) and respiratory depression may be observed with overdose. Bradyarrhythmias, myocardial infarction, and tremors may be observed in acute withdrawal. Prolonged cocaine snorting can result in ulceration of the mucous membranes of the nose and can damage the nasal septum enough to cause it to collapse.

Laboratory Tests

- Qualitative drugs of abuse urine screening tests are useful, followed by confirmatory testing if necessary. Levels of the primary metabolite, benzoylecgonine, may help diagnose acute cocaine toxicity.

Other Diagnostic Tests

- Abnormal electroencephalograms may be observed with patients in acute withdrawal.

TABLE 48-3 Treatment of Withdrawal from Some Common Drugs of Abuse

Drug or Drug Class	Pharmacologic Therapy	Level of Evidence[a,b]
Benzodiazepines		
Short- to intermediate-acting	Lorazepam 2 mg three to four times a day; taper over 5–7 days	A1
Long-acting	Lorazepam 2 mg three to four times a day; taper over additional 5–7 days	A1
Barbiturates	Pentobarbital tolerance test; initial detoxification at upper limit of tolerance test; decrease dosage by 100 mg every 2–3 days	B3
Opiates	Methadone 20–80 mg orally daily; taper by 5–10 mg daily or buprenorphine 4–32 mg orally daily, or clonidine 2 mcg/kg three times a day × 7 days; taper over additional 3 days	A1 (methadone and buprenorphine) B1 (clonidine)
Mixed-substance withdrawal		
Drugs are cross-tolerant	Detoxify according to treatment for longer-acting drug used	B3
Drugs are not cross-tolerant	Detoxify from one drug while maintaining second drug (cross-tolerant drugs), and then detoxify from second drug	B3
CNS stimulants	Supportive treatment only; pharmacotherapy often not used; bromocriptine 2.5 mg three times a day or higher may be used for severe craving associated with cocaine withdrawal	B2

[a]Strength of recommendations, evidence to support recommendation: A, good; B, moderate; C, poor.
[b]Quality of evidence: 1, evidence from more than one properly randomized controlled trial; 2, evidence from more than one well-designed clinical trial with randomization, from cohort or case–control analytic studies or multiple time series, or dramatic results from uncontrolled experiments; 3, evidence from opinions of respected authorities, based on clinical experience, descriptive studies, or reports of expert communities.
Data from references 34, 83, and 86.

protracted minor abstinence symptoms—such as anxiety, insomnia, irritability, sensitivity to light and sound, and muscle spasms—can remain for several weeks in patients with a history of long exposure, even after the acute phase of benzodiazepine withdrawal is complete.

Opiates

Opiate withdrawal syndrome is similar to a severe case of influenza. It is not life-threatening unless there is a concurrent life-threatening medical condition. Observable signs of withdrawal should be noted before initiation of drug therapy. Characteristic signs and symptoms of opiate withdrawal include pupillary dilation, lacrimation, rhinorrhea, piloerection ("gooseflesh"), yawning, sneezing, anorexia, nausea, vomiting, and diarrhea. Seizures do not occur. Onset and duration of withdrawal symptoms and the time of peak occurrence depend on the half-life of the drug involved. Typically heroin withdrawal reaches a peak within 36 to 72 hours of discontinuation and can last for 7 to 10 days. For methadone, symptoms peak at 72 hours but can last for 2 weeks or more.[87]

In the past, drug therapy for opioid withdrawal had typically been methadone, a synthetic opiate. Methadone is administered in decreasing doses over a period not exceeding 30 days (short-term detoxification) or 180 days (long-term detoxification). With methadone there were limited provisions for take-at-home dosing because of concern about the diversion of these drugs to illicit use.[88]

Use of Buprenorphine in Opiate Withdrawal and Maintenance

5 In 2002, buprenorphine was approved for opioid withdrawal. Prior to the passage of the federal Drug Addiction Treatment Act (DATA) of 2000,[89] office-based management of opioid dependence was illegal because existing federal laws prohibited physicians from prescribing narcotics for the sole purpose of maintaining a patient in a narcotic-addicted state.

The first of two formulations approved, Subutex, contains only buprenorphine and is intended for use at the beginning of treatment. The other, Suboxone, contains both buprenorphine and the opiate antagonist naloxone, and is intended to be used in maintenance treatment of opiate addiction. When buprenorphine with naloxone is administered sublingually, the naloxone component produces no clinically significant effect; however, after parenteral administration, naloxone-induced opioid antagonism occurs resulting in symptoms of withdrawal.[90,91]

To qualify, physicians must be board certified in addiction medicine/psychiatry or hold other special credentials, and physicians are required to obtain 8 hours of authorized training before they can prescribe medications for office-based treatment of opioid dependence.[90] DATA 2000, as amended in December 2006, specifies that an individual physician may have a maximum of 30 patients on opioid therapy at any one time for the first year. One year after the date on which a physician submitted the initial notification, the physician may submit a second notification of the need and intent to treat up to 100 patients.[90,91]

Medically supervised withdrawal with buprenorphine consists of an induction phase and a dose-reduction phase. Best practice guidelines collectively called Treatment Improvement Protocols (TIPs) are periodically issued for treatment of substance use disorders. TIP 40 (the guideline for the use of buprenorphine in the treatment of opioid addiction)[92] provides consensus- and evidence-based guidance on the use of buprenorphine.

The statement recommends that patients dependent on short-acting opioids (e.g., hydromorphone, oxycodone, heroin) be inducted directly onto buprenorphine/naloxone tablets. The use of buprenorphine (as either buprenorphine monotherapy or buprenorphine/naloxone combination treatment) to taper off long-acting opioids should be considered only for those patients who have evidence of sustained medical and psychosocial stability, and should be undertaken in conjunction and in coordination with patients' overall opioid treatment programs.

6 While there is much research focusing on drugs to treat the underlying addictive processes, to date the successes have been few. Whereas methadone, levo-α-acetylmethadol (LAAM), and now buprenorphine are used for narcotic maintenance, the logical approach at present should center on prevention. 7 Maintenance treatment with buprenorphine for opioid addiction consists of three phases: (a) induction, (b) stabilization, and (c) maintenance.[92] Induction is the first stage of buprenorphine treatment and involves helping patients begin the process of switching from the opioid of abuse to buprenorphine. The goal of the induction phase is to find the minimum dose of buprenorphine at which the patient discontinues or markedly diminishes use of other opioids and experiences no withdrawal symptoms, minimal or no side effects, and no craving for the drug of abuse. The consensus panel recommends that the buprenorphine/naloxone combination be used for induction treatment (and for stabilization and maintenance) for most patients. The consensus panel further recommends that initial induction doses be administered as observed treatment; further doses may be thereafter provided via prescription. To minimize the chances of precipitating withdrawal, patients who are transferring from long-acting opioids (e.g., methadone, sustained-release morphine, sustained-release oxycodone) to buprenorphine should be inducted using buprenorphine monotherapy, but switched to buprenorphine/naloxone soon thereafter. Induction protocols are shown in Figure 48-1.

The stabilization phase begins when a patient is experiencing no withdrawal symptoms, is experiencing minimal or no side effects, and no longer has uncontrollable cravings for opioid agonists. Dosage adjustments may be necessary during early stabilization, and frequent contact with the patient increases the likelihood of compliance. The longest period that a patient is on buprenorphine is the maintenance phase. This period may be indefinite. During the maintenance phase, attention must be focused on the psychosocial and family issues that have been identified during the course of treatment as contributing to a patient's addiction.[92]

Some other issues related to opioid abuse that need to be addressed during maintenance treatment include, but are not limited to, the following[92]:

1. Psychiatric comorbidity
2. Somatic consequences of drug use
3. Family and support issues
4. Structuring of time in prosocial activities
5. Employment and financial issues
6. Legal consequences of drug use
7. Other drug and alcohol abuse

A recent systematic review[93] evaluating the withdrawal component of buprenorphine treatment, including 22 studies involving 1,736 participants, was published. The major comparisons for buprenorphine were with methadone (5 studies) and clonidine or lofexidine (12 studies). Five studies compared different rates of buprenorphine dose reduction.

The authors concluded that severity of withdrawal is similar for withdrawal managed with buprenorphine and withdrawal managed with methadone, but withdrawal symptoms may resolve more quickly with buprenorphine. It appears that completion of withdrawal treatment may be more likely with buprenorphine relative to methadone (RR 1.18; 95% CI, 0.93 to 1.49; $P = 0.18$), but more studies are required to confirm this.[93]

5 A rapid detoxification technique has been developed that is designed to shorten detoxification by precipitating withdrawal through the administration of opioid antagonists such as naloxone or naltrexone.[93] This approach is thought to have the advantage of getting patients through detoxification rapidly, minimizing the risk of relapse, and initiating treatment more quickly with naltrexone maintenance combined with suitable psychosocial interventions. Ultrarapid detoxification represents a variant of this technique in which patients undergo opioid antagonist–precipitated withdrawal while under general anesthesia or heavy sedation. In the United States, there has been a rapid proliferation of programs offering ultrarapid detoxification, with some programs charging up to $15,000 per treatment. Rapid detoxification remains unproven and controversial.

Antagonist-induced withdrawal is more intense but less prolonged than withdrawal managed with reducing doses of methadone, and doses of naltrexone sufficient for blockade of opioid effects can be established significantly more quickly with antagonist-induced withdrawal than withdrawal managed with clonidine and symptomatic medications. The level of sedation does not affect the intensity and duration of withdrawal, although the duration of anesthesia may influence withdrawal severity. There is a significantly greater risk of adverse events with heavy, compared with light, sedation (RR 3.21, 95% CI, 1.13 to 9.12, $P = 0.03$) and probably with this antagonist-induced withdrawal compared with other forms of detoxification.[93]

The potential risks and high cost of using opioid-blocking drugs during heavy sedation or anesthesia to bring on withdrawal outweigh the benefits.[93]

DESIRED OUTCOMES

Substance Dependence

8 The treatment of drug dependence is primarily behavioral. The patient generally is taught that complete abstinence is the only realistic alternative to a life of uncontrollable drug use and despair that ultimately will end in death, and that there is no intermediate, controllable level of drinking or use of another drug. There may be an extremely few individuals who can return to controllable levels of drinking alcohol, but it is impossible to predict who these individuals are. The prospect of life without alcohol or other drugs

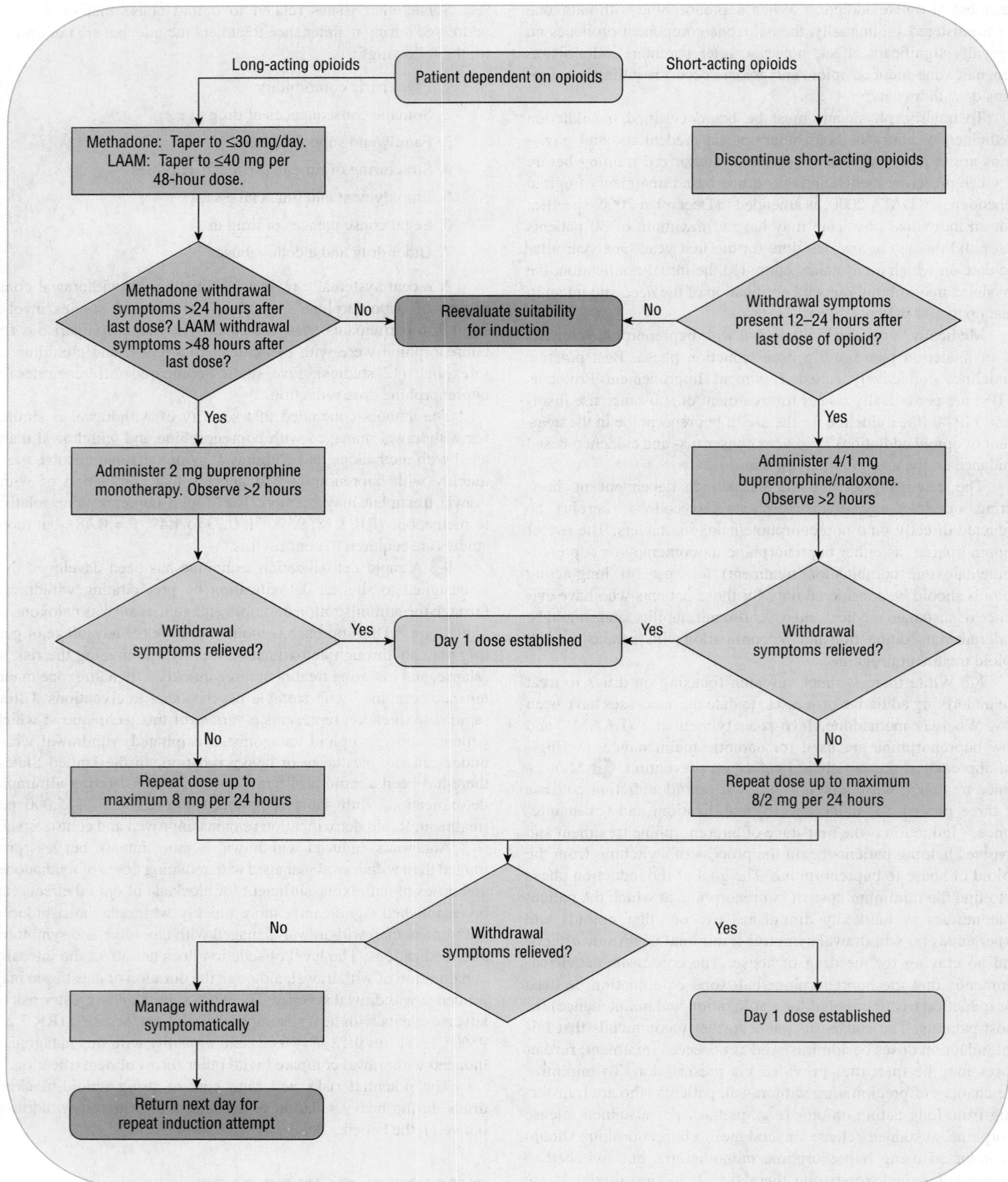

FIGURE 48-1 Determining the induction dose for days 1–2 of buprenorphine therapy.

is incomprehensible to many patients. Entry into treatment often is facilitated by some type of leverage that the drug-dependent person associates with negative consequences, such as potential loss of job, divorce, legal problems, or deteriorating physical health. Early treatment is directed at penetrating the denial of a problem that is always present. The patient must be educated as to the disease of addiction, the effects of drugs, and the permanence of the condition.

As evidenced by the approval of the two buprenorphine products, there has been a trend toward outpatient treatment for drug dependence, caused in part by cost-containment efforts. Inpatient treatment programs can cost as much as $20,000 for a 4-week stay. When withdrawal symptoms are mild to moderate and there are no other medical indications for hospitalization, outpatient treatment can be an attractive alternative to inpatient treatment. One critical criterion for outpatient treatment is the patient's compliance with complete abstinence from the dependence-producing drug during the treatment experience.

Families must be involved in treatment. The course of the patient's illness often has a devastating effect on other family members. Severely depleted self-esteem, denial of the family member's addiction, feelings of responsibility for the family member's drug use, and other behaviors that parallel the addiction process are often present.

8 Because at present there are no drugs to effectively treat the underlying addictive processes of drug dependence, treatment must be a lifelong process. Aftercare, or what is now being called *continued care*, should include regular and frequent treatment in some form. Most drug-dependence treatment programs embrace a treatment approach based on the 12 steps to recovery. Among chemically dependent healthcare professionals, treatment that incorporates both 12-step and peer-led self-help groups can be most effective.

PERSONALIZED PHARMACOTHERAPY

The notion of using pharmacogenetic testing to individualize the treatment of substance abuse disorders is relatively new, but studies of several genes have yielded significant findings.[94] Several gene variants have been shown to influence individual response to pharmacotherapy for drug addiction, notably in the μ-opioid receptor gene OPRM1 A118G (rs561720), polymorphisms of CYP2A6, and ANKK1 Taq1A. It remains to be seen how this genetic information will be incorporated into clinical practice. Prospective studies evaluating the use of genetic testing in a clinical setting and the effect on treatment outcome are warranted to further evaluate the benefits and risks of this approach.[94]

ABBREVIATIONS

BZP	*N*-benzylpiperazine
CASA	Center on Addiction and Substance Abuse
CDC	Centers for Disease Control and Prevention
DATA	Drug Addiction Treatment Act
DAWN	Drug Abuse Warning Network
DEA	U.S. Drug Enforcement Administration
DMT	dimethyltryptamine
DSM-IV-TR	*Diagnostic and Statistical Manual of Mental Disorders, Fourth Edition, Text Revision*
ED	emergency department
GHB	γ-hydroxybutyric acid
5-HT	5-hydroxytryptamine
LAAM	levo-α-acetylmethadol
LSD	lysergic acid diethylamide
5-MeO-DIPT	5-methoxy-*N*,*N*-diisopropyltryptamine
mCPP	*meta*-chlorophenylpiperazine
MDA	3,4-methylenedioxyamphetamine
MDMA	3,4-methylenedioxymethamphetamine
MTFS	Monitoring the Future Study
NA	Narcotics Anonymous
NAS	neonatal abstinence syndrome
NFLIS	National Forensic Laboratory Information System
NSDUH	National Survey on Drug Use and Health
PCP	phencyclidine
PDMP	prescription drug monitoring program
REM	rapid eye movement
TFMPP	1-(3-trifluoromethylphenyl)-piperazine
THC	delta-9-tetrahydrocannabinol
TIPs	Treatment Improvement Protocols

REFERENCES

1. Ecclesiastes 1:9 New International Version. *http://www.biblegateway.com/passage/?search=Ecclesiastes%201:9&version=NIV*.
2. Inaba DS, Cohen WE. Uppers, Downers, All Arounders: Physical and Mental Effects of Psychoactive Drugs, 7th ed. Medford, OR: CNS Productions Inc, 2011:1.1.
3. Rudgley R. The Lost Civilizations of the Stone Age. New York: Free Press, 2000:138.
4. Jiang HE, Xiao Li X, Zhaod YX, et al. A new insight into *Cannabis sativa* (Cannabaceae) utilization from 2500-year-old Yanghai Tombs, Xinjiang, China. J Ethnopharmacol 2006;108:414–422.
5. Frosch WA, Robbins ES, Stern M. Untoward reactions to lysergic acid diethylamide (LSD) resulting in hospitalization. N Engl J Med 1965;273(23):1235–1239.
6. James IP. A methylamphetamine epidemic? Lancet 1968;1(7548):916.
7. Lindberg DK. A word of warning: Marked increase in hydromorphone (Dilaudid) addiction. J Fla Med Assoc 1978;65:822.
8. Bridge TP, Ellinwood EH Jr. Quaalude alley: A one-way street. Am J Psychiatry 1973;130:217–219.
9. Finkelstein IS. Pentazocine abuse. JAMA 1973;224:249.
10. Derlet RW, Rice P, Horowitz BZ, Lord RV. Amphetamine toxicity: Experience with 127 cases. J Emerg Med 1989;7(2):157–161.
11. Bechtel LK, Holstege CP. Criminal poisoning: Drug-facilitated sexual assault. Emerg Med Clin North Am 2007;25:499–525.
12. Savage SR, Joranson DE, Covington EC, et al. Definitions related to the medical use of opioids: Evolution towards universal agreement. J Pain Symptom Manage 2003;26:655–667.
13. Substance Abuse and Mental Health Services Administration. Results from the 2011 National Survey on Drug Use and Health: National Findings. Series H-44, HHS Publication No. (SMA) 12-4713. Rockville, MD: Substance Abuse and Mental Health Services Administration, 2012.
14. Johnston LD, O'Malley PM, Bachman JG, Schulenberg JE. Monitoring the Future National Results on Adolescent Drug Use: Overview of Key Findings, 2012. Ann Arbor, MI: Institute for Social Research, the University of Michigan, 2013.
15. Substance Abuse and Mental Health Services Administration, Center for Behavioral Health Statistics and Quality. The DAWN Report: Highlights of the 2010 Drug Abuse Warning Network (DAWN) Findings on Drug-Related Emergency Department Visits. Rockville, MD: Substance Abuse and Mental Health Services Administration, July 2, 2012.
16. National Center for Health Statistics. National Hospital Ambulatory Medical Care Survey: 2009 Emergency Department Summary Tables. *http://www.cdc.gov/nchs/data/ahcd/nhamcs_emergency/2009_ed_web_tables.pdf and http://www.cdc.gov/nchs/fastats/ervisits.htm*.
17. National Center on Addiction and Substance Abuse at Columbia University. "You've Got Drugs!" V: Prescription Drug Pushers on the Internet. A CASA White Paper. New York, NY: National Center on Addiction and Substance Abuse at Columbia University, July 2008.
18. American Psychiatric Association. Diagnostic and Statistical Manual of Mental Disorders, Fourth Edition, Text Revision. Washington, DC: American Psychiatric Association, 2000:212–214.

19. Heit HA, Gourlay DL. DSM-V and the definitions: Time to get it right. Pain Med 2009;10:784–786.
20. Koob GF, Volkow ND. Neurocircuitry of addiction. Neuropsychopharmacology 2010;35:217–238 [Erratum. Neuropsychopharmacology 2010;35:1051].
21. Centers for Disease Control and Prevention. Prescription Painkiller Overdoses in the US. *http://www.cdc.gov/VitalSigns/pdf/2011-11-vitalsigns.pdf.*
22. Centers for Disease Control and Prevention. Public Health Grand Rounds. February 17, 2011, *http://www.cdc.gov/about/grand-rounds/archives/2011/pdfs/PHGRRx17feb2011.pdf.*
23. Based on Data from SDI, Vector One: National. Years 2000-2009. Extracted June 2010, *http://www.fda.gov/downloads/AdvisoryCommittees/CommitteesMeetingMaterials/Drugs/AnestheticAndLifeSupport DrugsAdvisoryCommittee/UCM217510.pdf.*
24. Centers for Disease Control and Prevention. Drug overdose deaths—Florida, 2003-2009. MMWR Morb Mortal Wkly Rep 2011;60(26):869–872.
25. Unintentional Drug Poisoning in the United States, National Center for Injury Prevention and Control, Centers for Disease Control and Prevention. July 2010, *http://www.cdc.gov/homeandrecreationalsafety/pdf/poison-issue-brief.pdf.*
26. Patrick SW, Schumacher RE, Benneyworth BD, et al. Neonatal abstinence syndrome and associated health care expenditures: United States, 2000-2009. JAMA 2012;307:1934–1940 [Epub April 30, 2012].
27. Substance Abuse and Mental Health Services Administration. Data Summary: Methadone Mortality, A 2010 Reassessment. Rockville, MD: US Department of Health and Human Services, Substance Abuse and Mental Health Services Administration, 2010, *http://www.dpt.samhsa.gov/pdf/methadone_mortality_data_2010.pdf.*
28. Warner M, Chen L, Makuc D, et al. Drug Poisoning Deaths in the United States, 1980–2008. NCHS Data Brief, No. 81. Hyattsville, MD: National Center for Health Statistics, 2011, *http://www.cdc.gov/nchs/data/databriefs/db81.htm.*
29. Substance Abuse and Mental Health Services Administration, Center for Behavioral Statistics and Quality. The DAWN Report: Methadone-Related Emergency Department Visits Involving Nonmedical Use. Rockville, MD: Substance Abuse and Mental Health Services Administration, 2012, *http://www.samhsa.gov/data/2k12/web_dawn_022/methadone_er_nonmedical.pdf.*
30. Warner M, Chen LH, Makuc DM, et al. Drug poisoning deaths in the United States, 1980-2008. NCHS Data Brief. 2011;81:1–8.
31. Vital signs: Risk for overdose from methadone used for pain relief—United States, 1999-2010. MMWR Morb Mortal Wkly Rep 2012;61:493–497.
32. Methadone-Associated Overdose Deaths; Factors Contributing to Increased Deaths and Efforts to Prevent Them. United States Government Accounting Office Report to Congressional Requesters. GAO-09-341. March 26, 2009, *http://www.gao.gov/new.items/d09341.pdf.*
33. U.S. Food and Drug Administration. Information for Healthcare Professionals: Methadone. Issued November 27, 2006, *http://www.fda.gov/Drugs/DrugSafety/PostmarketDrugSafetyInformationforPatientsandProviders/ucm142841.htm.*
34. Ruiz P, Strain EC. Lowinson and Ruiz's Substance Abuse: A Comprehensive Textbook, 5th ed. Riverwoods, IL: Lippincott Williams & Wilkins, 2011:1074.
35. Fass JA. Carisoprodol legal status and patterns of abuse. Ann Pharmacotherapy 2010;44:1962–1967 [Epub November 9, 2010].
36. Department of Justice, Drug Enforcement Administration. 21 CFR Part 1308. Schedules of Controlled Substances: Placement of Carisoprodol into Schedule IV 21. *http://www.deadiversion.usdoj.gov/fed_regs/rules/2011/fr1212_10.htm.*
37. Reissig CJ, Carter LP, Johnson MW, et al. High doses of dextromethorphan, an NMDA antagonist, produce effects similar to classic hallucinogens. Psychopharmacology (Berl) 2012;223(1):1–15 [Epub April 13, 2012].
38. Chyka PA, Erdman AR, Manoguerra AS, et al. American Association of Poison Control Centers. Dextromethorphan poisoning: An evidence-based consensus guideline for out-of-hospital management. Clin Toxicol (Phila) 2007;45: 662–677.
39. Carrera MR, Meijler MM, Janda KD. Cocaine pharmacology and current pharmacotherapies for its abuse. Bioorg Med Chem 2004;12:5019–5030.
40. Laizure SC, Parker RB. Pharmacodynamic evaluation of the cardiovascular effects after the coadministration of cocaine and ethanol. Drug Metab Dispos 2009;37:310–314.
41. Farooq MU, Bhatt A, Patel M. Neurotoxic and cardiotoxic effects of cocaine and ethanol. J Med Toxicol 2009;5: 134–138.
42. Phillips K, Luk A, Soor GS, et al. Cocaine cardiotoxicity: A review of the pathophysiology, pathology, and treatment options. Am J Cardiovasc Drugs 2009;9:177–196.
43. McCord J, Jneid H, Hollander JE, et al. American Heart Association Acute Cardiac Care Committee of the Council on Clinical Cardiology. Management of cocaine-associated chest pain and myocardial infarction: A scientific statement from the American Heart Association Acute Cardiac Care Committee of the Council on Clinical Cardiology. Circulation 2008;117:1897–1907 [Epub March 17, 2008].
44. Mahoney JJ III, Kalechstein AD, De La Garza R II, et al. Presence and persistence of psychotic symptoms in cocaine-versus methamphetamine-dependent participants. Am J Addict 2008;17:83–98.
45. Hamamoto DT, Rhodus NL. Methamphetamine abuse and dentistry. Oral Dis 2009;15:27–37.
46. U.S. Department of Justice National Drug Threat Assessment. 2011, *http://www.justice.gov/archive/ndic/pubs44/44849/44849p.pdf.*
47. Skelton MR, Williams MT, Vorhees CV. Developmental effects of 3,4-methylenedioxymethamphetamine: A review. Behav Pharmacol 2008;19:91–111.
48. Indlekofer F, Piechatzek M, Daamen M. Reduced memory and attention performance in a population-based sample of young adults with a moderate lifetime use of cannabis, ecstasy and alcohol. J Psychopharmacol 2009;23(5): 495–509.
49. McCann UD, Kuwabara H, Kumar A, et al. Persistent cognitive and dopamine transporter deficits in abstinent methamphetamine users. Synapse 2008;62: 91–100.
50. McCann UD, Szabo Z, Vranesic M, et al. Positron emission tomographic studies of brain dopamine and serotonin transporters in abstinent (+/–)3,4-methylenedioxymethamphetamine ("ecstasy") users: Relationship to cognitive performance. Psychopharmacology (Berl) 2008;200:439–450.
51. Lamberth PG, Ding GK, Nurmi LA. Fatal paramethoxy-amphetamine (PMA) poisoning in the Australian Capital Territory. Med J Aust 2008;188:426.
52. Coppola M, Mondola R. Synthetic cathinones: Chemistry, pharmacology and toxicology of a new class of designer drugs of abuse marketed as "bath salts" or "plant food". Toxicol Lett 2012;211:144–149 [Epub March 21, 2012].

53. Simmler LD, Buser TA, Donzelli M, et al. Pharmacological characterization of designer cathinones in vitro. Br J Pharmacol 2013;168(2):458–470. doi:10.1111/j.1476-5381.2012.02145.x [Epub ahead of print].
54. Loeffler G, Hurst D, Penn A, Yung K. Spice, bath salts, and the U.S. military: The emergence of synthetic cannabinoid receptor agonists and cathinones in the U.S. Armed Forces. Mil Med 2012;177(9):1041–1048.
55. Prosser JM, Nelson LS. The toxicology of bath salts: A review of synthetic cathinones. J Med Toxicol 2012;8(1):33–42.
56. One Hundred Twelfth Congress of the United States of America. Synthetic Drug Abuse Prevention Act of 2012. Senate Bill 3187, the Food and Drug Administration Section 1152. Addition of Synthetic Drugs to Schedule I of the Controlled Substances Act. January 3, 2012.
57. Passie T, Halpern JH, Stichtenoth DO, Emrich HM, Hintzen A. The pharmacology of lysergic acid diethylamide: A review. CNS Neurosci Ther 2008;14(4):295–314.
58. National Forensic Laboratory Information System Special Report: Emerging 2C-Phenethylamines, Piperazines, and Tryptamines in NFLIS, 2006-2011. Springfield, VA: U.S. Drug Enforcement Administration, Office of Diversion Control. 2012, *http://www.deadiversion.usdoj.gov/nflis/spec_rpt_emerging_2012.pdf*.
59. High potency marijuana concerns authorities. Star News Online May 21, 2012, *http://www.starnewsonline.com/article/20120521/ARTICLES/120529958?template=printart*.
60. Wagner FA, Anthony JC. From first drug use to drug dependence; developmental periods of risk for dependence upon cannabis, cocaine, and alcohol. Neuropsychopharmacology 2002;26:479–488.
61. Cherek DR, Lane SD, Dougherty DM. Possible amotivational effects following marijuana smoking under laboratory conditions. Exp Clin Psychopharmacol 2002;10:26–38.
62. Mills KL, Lalonde F, Clasen L, Giedd JN, Blakemore SJ. Developmental changes in the structure of the social brain in late childhood and adolescence. Soc Cogn Affect Neurosci 2012 [Epub ahead of print].
63. Meier MH, Caspi A, Ambler A, et al. Persistent cannabis users show neuropsychological decline from childhood to midlife. Proc Natl Acad Sci U S A 2012;109(40): E2657–E2664. doi:10.1073/pnas.1206820109 [Epub August 27, 2012].
64. Sewell RA, Poling J, Sofuoglu M. The effect of cannabis compared with alcohol on driving. Am J Addict 2009;18:185–193.
65. Asbridge M, Hayden JA, Cartwright JL. Acute cannabis consumption and motor vehicle collision risk: Systematic review of observational studies and meta-analysis. BMJ 2012;344:e536. doi:10.1136/bmj.e536.
66. Li MC, Brady JE, DiMaggio CJ, et al. Marijuana use and motor vehicle crashes. Epidemiol Rev 2012;34(1):65–72 [Epub October 4, 2011].
67. Bosker WM, Kuypers KP, Theunissen EL, et al. Medicinal Δ(9)-tetrahydrocannabinol (dronabinol) impairs on-the-road driving performance of occasional and heavy cannabis users but is not detected in Standard Field Sobriety Tests. Addiction 2012;107(10):1837–1844. doi:10.1111/j.1360-0443.2012.03928.x [Epub July 12, 2012].
68. ProCon.org. Medical Marijuana. January 9, 2011, *http://medicalmarijuana.procon.org/view.resource.php?resourceID=000881*.
69. Onishi N. Marijuana only for the sick? A farce, some Angelenos say. New York Times October 7, 2012, *http://www.nytimes.com/2012/10/08/us/california-fight-to-ensure-marijuana-goes-only-to-sick.html?_r=0*.
70. Cerdá M, Wall M, Keyes KM, et al. Medical marijuana laws in 50 states: Investigating the relationship between state legalization of medical marijuana and marijuana use, abuse and dependence. Drug Alcohol Depend 2012;120(1–3): 22–27 [Epub November 17, 2011].
71. Gorelick DA, Heishman SJ. Methods for clinical research involving cannabis administration. In: Onaivi ES, ed. Methods in Molecular Medicine: Marijuana and Cannabinoid Research: Methods and Protocols. New Jersey: Humana Press, 2006.
72. Medical marijuana: Answers to your burning questions. Pharmacist's Letter/Prescriber's Letter 2010;26:260906.
73. Seamon MJ, Fass JA, Maniscalco-Feichtl M, Abu-Shraie NA. Medical marijuana and the developing role of the pharmacist. Am J Health Syst Pharm 2007;64:1037–1044.
74. Federation of American Scientists. Synthetic Drugs: Overview and Issues for Congress. *http://www.fas.org/sgp/crs/misc/R42066.pdf*.
75. European Monitoring Centre for Drugs and Drug Addiction. Action on New Drugs Briefing Paper: Understanding the 'Spice' Phenomenon. 2009, *http://www.emcdda.europa.eu/drugsituation/new-drugs*.
76. Wells DL, Ott CA. The "new" marijuana. Ann Pharmacother 2011;45(3):414–417.
77. Hudson S, Ramsey J, King L, et al. Use of high-resolution accurate mass spectrometry to detect reported and previously unreported cannabinomimetics in "herbal high" products. J Anal Toxicol 2010;34(5):252–260.
78. U.S. Drug Enforcement Administration, Office of Diversion Control. National Forensic Laboratory Information System Special Report: Synthetic Cannabinoids and Synthetic Cathinones Reported in NFLIS, 2009-2010. Springfield, VA: U.S. Drug Enforcement Administration, 2011.
79. American Association of Poison Control Centers. Synthetic Marijuana. *http://www.aapcc.org/alerts/synthetic-marijuana*.
80. Cohen J, Morrison S, Greenberg J, Saidinejad M. Clinical presentation of intoxication due to synthetic cannabinoids. Pediatrics 2012;129:e1064-e1067. doi:10.1542/peds.2011-1797 [Epub March 19, 2012].
81. Gunderson EW, Haughey HM, Ait-Daoud N, et al. "Spice" and "K2" herbal highs: A case series and systematic review of the clinical effects and biopsychosocial implications of synthetic cannabinoid use in humans. Am J Addict 2012;21:320–326. doi:10.1111/j.1521-0391.2012.00240.x [Epub April 23, 2012].
82. Nelson LS, Olsen D. Opioids. In: Nelson LS, Olsen D, eds. Goldfrank's Toxicologic Emergencies, 9th ed. New York: McGraw-Hill, 2011, *http://www.accesspharmacy.com/content.aspx?aID=6511222* [chapter 38].
83. Boyer EW. Management of opioid analgesic overdose. N Engl J Med 2012;367:146–155.
84. Mathias S, Lubman DI, Hides L. Substance-induced psychosis: A diagnostic conundrum. J Clin Psychiatry 2008;69:358–367.
85. Lader M, Tylee A, Donoghue J. Withdrawing benzodiazepines in primary care. CNS Drugs 2009;23: 19–34. doi:10.2165/0023210-200923010-00002.
86. Shoptaw SJ, Kao U, Heinzerling K, Ling W. Treatment for amphetamine withdrawal. Cochrane Database Syst Rev 2009;(2):CD003021.
87. Soyka M, Kranzler HR, van den Brink W, et al. The World Federation of Societies of Biological Psychiatry (WFSBP) guidelines for the biological treatment of substance use and related disorders. Part 2: Opioid dependence. WFSBP Task

Force on Treatment, Guidelines for Substance Use Disorders. World J Biol Psychiatry 2011;12:160–187.

88. Amato L, Minozzi S, Davoli M, Vecchi S. Psychosocial and pharmacological treatments versus pharmacological treatments for opioid detoxification. Cochrane Database Syst Rev 2011;(9):CD005031.
89. Drug Addiction Treatment Act of 2000 (DATA), Title XXXV of the Children's Health Act of 2000 (Public Law No. 106-310, 116 Stat 1222). *http://buprenorphine.samhsa.gov/fulllaw.html*.
90. CSAT Buprenorphine Information Center. The Center for Substance Abuse Treatment (CSAT), Substance Abuse and Mental Health Services Administration (SAMHSA). *http://buprenorphine.samhsa.gov/*.
91. Orman JS, Keating GM. Buprenorphine/naloxone: A review of its use in the treatment of opioid dependence. Drugs 2009;69:577–607.
92. TIP 40 Center for Substance Abuse Treatment. Clinical Guidelines for the Use of Buprenorphine in the Treatment of Opioid Addiction. Treatment Improvement Protocol (TIP) Series 40. DHHS Publication No. (SMA) 04-3939. Rockville, MD: Substance Abuse and Mental Health Services Administration, 2004, *http://www.ncbi.nlm.nih.gov/bookshelf/br.fcgi?book=hssamhsatip&part=A72248*.
93. Gowing L, Ali R, White JM. Opioid antagonists under heavy sedation or anesthesia for opioid withdrawal. Cochrane Database Syst Rev 2010;(1):CD002022. doi:10.1002/14651858.CD002022.pub3.
94. Sturgess JE, George TP, Kennedy JL, et al. Pharmacogenetics of alcohol, nicotine and drug addiction treatments. Addict Biol 2011;16(3):357–376. doi:10.1111/j.1369-1600.2010.00287.x [Epub March 1, 2011].

Substance-Related Disorders II: Alcohol, Nicotine, and Caffeine

49

Paul L. Doering and Robin Moorman Li

KEY CONCEPTS

1. Tobacco is the number one preventable cause of death in the United States.
2. Nearly 17 million Americans report current heavy alcohol use or alcohol abuse.
3. Pharmacogenomic studies have identified genotypic and functional phenotypic variants that either serve to protect patients or predispose them toward alcohol dependence.
4. Alcohol is a CNS depressant that shares many pharmacologic properties with the nonbenzodiazepine sedative–hypnotics.
5. The metabolism of alcohol is considered to follow zero-order pharmacokinetics, and this has important implications for the time course in which alcohol can exert its effects.
6. Benzodiazepines are the treatment of choice for alcohol withdrawal.
7. Disulfiram, naltrexone, and acamprosate are FDA-approved drug therapies for the treatment of alcohol dependence. The clinical utility of these agents to improve sustained abstinence remains controversial. Relapse is common.
8. More than three quarters of smokers are nicotine dependent. Tobacco dependence is a chronic condition that requires repeated interventions.
9. Use of nicotine replacement therapy along with behavioral counseling doubles cessation rates.
10. Bupropion and varenicline are efficacious alone and in combination with nicotine replacement therapy for smoking cessation.

(1) Alcohol, nicotine, and caffeine are considered by most to be socially acceptable drugs, yet they impose an enormous social and economic cost on our society. Approximately 443,000 deaths each year are attributable to tobacco use, making tobacco the number one preventable cause of death and disease in this country.[1,2] The three leading causes of death attributable to smoking include lung cancer, chronic obstructive pulmonary disease, and ischemic heart disease.[3]

(2) In 2011, heavy drinking was reported by 6.2% of the population aged 12 or older, or 15.9 million people,[4] a decrease from the previous year's data in which 16.9 million people were heavy drinkers. Approximately one quarter (22.6%) of persons aged 12 or older participated in binge drinking at least once in the 30 days prior to the National Survey on Drug Use and Health (NSDUH) in 2011.[4]

The World Health Organization estimates that there are approximately 2 billion people worldwide who consume alcoholic beverages, and 76.3 million with diagnosable alcohol-use disorders.[5] Long-term alcohol abuse often leads to chronic disease. A causal relationship between alcohol abuse and at least 60 types of chronic disease or injury has been established (e.g., esophageal cancer, liver cancer, and cirrhosis of the liver, epileptic seizures, homicide, and motor vehicle accidents) worldwide.[5] Nationally, according to the Drug Abuse Warning Network 2010 survey,[6] 687,574 emergency department visits involved either alcohol in combination with other drugs (for patients of all ages) or alcohol only for patients aged 20 or younger.

(2) Worldwide, alcohol abuse leads to 1.8 million deaths annually.[5] Nationally, according to the Alcohol-Attributable Deaths Report, 80,374 U.S. citizens with medium and high average daily alcohol consumption die each year because of alcohol-related causes, including traffic collisions and cirrhosis of the liver.[7] Direct and indirect health and social costs of alcoholism to the nation are estimated to be $223.5 billion annually,[8] and governments pay more than 60% of their healthcare costs.

Caffeine is currently the most widely used psychoactive substance in the world. In the United States, 80% to 90% of adults regularly consume behaviorally active doses of caffeine.

ALCOHOL

Epidemiology of Alcohol Use

Approximately half of Americans aged 12 or older reported being current drinkers of alcohol according to the NSDUH 2011 (51.8%). This translates to an estimated 133.4 million people, which is similar to the 2010 estimate of 131.3 million people (51.8%).[4] In 2011 heavy drinking was reported by 6.2% of the population aged 12 or older, meaning that they drank five or more drinks on the same occasion on at least 5 different days in the past month.[4]

The Disease Model of Addiction as Applied to Alcoholism

The disease concept of addiction, using alcoholism as a model, states that addiction is a disease, and that individuals who suffer from the disease do not choose to contract the disease any more than someone who suffers from heart disease or diabetes mellitus chooses to contract that illness. A *disease* is defined as "any deviation from or interruption of the normal structure or function of any part, organ, or system (or combination thereof) of the body that is manifested by a characteristic set of symptoms and signs and whose etiology, pathology, and prognosis may be known or unknown."[9] Diagnostic criteria for alcoholism do not specify frequency of drinking or amount of alcohol consumed. The key determinant is whether drinking is compulsive, out of control, and consequential when one drinks.[10]

(3) It has long been recognized that alcoholism is heritable, as 50% to 60% of first-degree relatives of alcoholics become alcohol

TABLE 49-1 Genotypic, Phenotypic, and Environmental Factors that Increase Alcohol-Dependence Risk

Susceptibility Genes	Phenotype	Environment
Regions on chromosomes 1 and 4 that code for the following receptors:	Personality traits that include:	Religious background
$GABA_A$	Novelty seeking	Urban residence (vs. rural)
Serotonin 1b	Impulsivity	History of sexual abuse
DRD4	Aggression	Being single
Tryptophan hydroxylase	Depression	Having deceased parents
Neuropeptide Y	Maximum number of alcoholic drinks consumed per day	
Gene that codes for:		
ALDH2		
5HTTLPR		

ALDH2, aldehyde dehydrogenase 2; DRD4, type 4 dopamine receptor gene; GABA, γ-aminobutyric acid; 5HTTLPR, 5 hydroxytryptamine transporter.

Data from references 12–15.

dependent themselves.[11] Research has identified several traits (or phenotypes) that attenuate one's risk of alcohol dependence. Initially based on data from preclinical studies, pharmacogenomic studies have identified genotypic and functional phenotypic variants that either serve to protect patients or predispose them toward alcohol dependence.[12] Large-scale pharmacoepidemiologic studies have further elucidated the environmental risk factors that are associated with either protective effects or predisposition toward alcoholism.[13] The known susceptibility genes, phenotypic characteristics, and environmental risk factors are summarized in Table 49-1.[11–15]

Pharmacology and Pharmacokinetics of Alcohol

Alcohol as a Drug

4 Alcohol is a CNS depressant that affects the CNS in a dose-dependent fashion, producing sedation that progresses to sleep, unconsciousness, coma, surgical anesthesia, and finally fatal respiratory depression and cardiovascular collapse. Alcohol affects endogenous opiates and several neurotransmitter systems in the brain, including γ-aminobutyric acid (GABA), glutamine, and dopamine. Alcohol is available in a variety of concentrations in various alcoholic beverages. There is approximately 14 g of alcohol in a 12-oz (355 mL) can of beer (approximately 5%), 4 oz (118 mL) of nonfortified wine (approximately 10% to 14%), or one shot (1.5 oz [44 mL]) of 80-proof whiskey (40%). Full consumption of this amount will cause an increase in blood alcohol level of approximately 20 to 25 mg/dL (4.3 to 5.4 mmol/L) in a healthy 70-kg (154 lb) male, although this varies with the time frame over which the alcohol is consumed, the type of alcoholic beverage, whether food is consumed along with it, and many patient variables. The lethal dose of alcohol in humans is variable, but deaths generally occur when blood alcohol levels are greater than 400 to 500 mg/dL (87 to 109 mmol/L).[16]

Pharmacokinetics

Absorption of alcohol begins in the stomach within 5 to 10 minutes of oral ingestion. The onset of clinical effects follows fairly rapidly. Peak serum concentrations of alcohol usually are achieved 30 to 90 minutes after finishing the last drink, although it is variable depending on the type of alcoholic beverage consumed, what and when the person last ate, and other factors.[17]

More than 90% of alcohol in the plasma is metabolized in the liver by three enzyme systems that operate within the hepatocyte. The remainder is excreted by the lungs and in urine and sweat. Alcohol is metabolized to acetaldehyde by alcohol dehydrogenase in the cell. In turn, acetaldehyde is metabolized to carbon dioxide and water by the enzyme aldehyde dehydrogenase. A second pathway for oxidation of alcohol uses catalase, an enzyme located in the peroxisomes and microsomes. The third enzyme system, the microsomal alcohol oxidase system, has a role in the oxidation of alcohol to acetaldehyde. These last two mechanisms are of lesser importance than the alcohol dehydrogenase–aldehyde dehydrogenase system.[17]

5 The metabolism of alcohol generally is said to follow zero-order pharmacokinetics.[17] This can, in fact, be an oversimplification because at very high or very low concentrations of alcohol the metabolism can follow first-order pharmacokinetics.[18] On average, the blood alcohol concentration (BAC) is lowered from 15 to 22.2 mg/dL (3.3 to 4.8 mmol/L) per hour in the nontolerant individual, assuming that the individual is in the postabsorptive state (Table 49-2). Alcohol has a volume of distribution of 0.6 to 0.8 L/kg, representing the total body water.[17]

Clinical Indicators of Chronic Alcohol Abuse

The CAGE questionnaire is a tool for detecting individuals more likely to be abusing alcohol and therefore at greater risk for alcohol withdrawal. CAGE is a mnemonic for four questions: (a) Do you ever feel the need to *c*ut down on your alcohol use? (b) Have you ever been *a*nnoyed by others telling you that you drink too much? (c) Have you ever felt *g*uilty about your drinking or something you did while drinking? (d) Do you ever have an "*e*ye opener"? A positive response to two or more of these four questions suggests an

TABLE 49-2 Specific Effects of Alcohol Related to BAC

BAC (%)[a] (mmol/L)	Effect
0.02–0.03 (4–8)	No loss of coordination, slight euphoria, and loss of shyness
0.04–0.06 (9–14)	Feeling of well-being, relaxation, lower inhibitions, sensation of warmth. Euphoria. Some minor impairment of reasoning and memory, lowering of caution
0.07–0.09 (15–21)	Slight impairment of balance, speech, vision, reaction time, and hearing. Euphoria. Judgment and self-control are reduced, and caution, reason, and memory are impaired. It is illegal to operate a motor vehicle in some states at this level
0.10–0.125 (22–27)	Significant impairment of motor coordination and loss of good judgment. Speech can be slurred; balance, vision, reaction time, and hearing impaired. Euphoria. It is illegal to operate a motor vehicle at this level of intoxication
0.13–0.15 (28–34)	Gross motor impairment and lack of physical control. Blurred vision and major loss of balance. Euphoria is reduced, and dysphoria is beginning to appear
0.16–0.20 (35–43)	Dysphoria (anxiety, restlessness) predominates; nausea can appear. The drinker has the appearance of a "sloppy drunk"
0.25 (54)	Needs assistance in walking; total mental confusion. Dysphoria with nausea and some vomiting
0.30 (65)	Loss of consciousness
≥0.40 (>87)	Onset of coma, possible death caused by respiratory arrest

BAC, blood alcohol concentration.

[a]Grams of ethyl alcohol per 100 mL of whole blood.

increased likelihood of alcohol abuse with an average sensitivity of 0.71 (71%) and an average specificity of 0.90 (90%).[19]

Acute Effects of Alcohol

At lower serum concentrations, euphoria and disinhibition may be noted. Slurred speech, altered perception of the environment, impaired judgment, ataxia, incoordination, nystagmus, and hyperreflexia may occur. As plasma levels increase, combative and destructive behavior may occur. With higher levels still, somnolence and respiratory depression may ensue. The typical effects of various BACs are shown in Table 49-2, although effects vary from individual to individual.

Alcohol Poisoning

Acute alcohol poisoning usually occurs with rapid consumption of large quantities of alcoholic beverages. With sustained drinking of moderate amounts of alcohol, the user passes out before a toxic dose of alcohol can be ingested, and/or the person vomits to rid the stomach of its toxic reservoir. With rapid drinking, the person may fall asleep or pass out without vomiting, allowing continued alcohol absorption from the GI tract until fatal BACs are achieved.

Laboratory Studies

In the emergency room, a BAC should be ordered in any patient in whom alcohol ingestion is suspected, regardless of the presenting complaint. For clinical purposes, most laboratories report BAC in units of mg/dL or mmol/L. In legal cases, results are reported in percentage (grams of ethyl alcohol per 100 mL of whole blood). If the diagnosis is unclear, if the intoxication seems atypical, or when there is suspicion of multiple drug ingestions, a complete toxicologic screen to rule out the presence of other substances may be useful.

TREATMENT
Alcohol-Related Disorders

Desired Outcomes

Goals for alcohol-dependent persons trying to decrease or discontinue alcohol intake include: (a) the prevention and treatment of withdrawal symptoms (including seizures and delirium tremens) and medical or psychiatric complications, (b) long-term abstinence after detoxification, and (c) entry into ongoing medical and alcohol-dependence treatment.

Alcohol Withdrawal

Pharmacologic Therapy

6 Symptom-triggered treatment with a benzodiazepine is the current standard of care in alcohol detoxification to manage and minimize symptoms and avoid progression to the more severe stages of withdrawal. A meta-analysis was performed to provide evidence-based recommendations on the pharmacologic management of alcohol withdrawal.[20] A similar study was done to develop treatment strategies for alcohol withdrawal delirium.[21] Trials comparing different benzodiazepines demonstrated that all appear similarly efficacious in reducing signs and symptoms of withdrawal.[20,21]

Clinical Controversy. . .

Some clinicians believe that chlordiazepoxide is the "drug of choice" for alcohol withdrawal because some of the earliest literature reported successful use of this drug. Symptom-triggered treatment with a benzodiazepine is the current standard of care in alcohol detoxification to manage and minimize symptoms and avoid progression to the more severe stages of withdrawal. However, substantial evidence exists that no specific drug in this class is better than the others. Despite this, many practitioners still believe that chlordiazepoxide is superior to other benzodiazepines.

A Cochrane review[22] of the effectiveness and safety of benzodiazepines in the treatment of alcohol withdrawal symptoms was published in 2010. According to this report "the available data show that benzodiazepines are effective against alcohol withdrawal seizures when compared to placebo, but data on safety outcomes are sparse and fragmented. There is a need for larger, well-designed studies in this field."

CLINICAL PRESENTATION Alcohol Intoxication and Withdrawal

General

- Acute alcohol detoxification and withdrawal after chronic alcohol abuse is a serious condition that can require hospitalization and adjunctive pharmacotherapy. If the BAC gets high enough, death is possible.

Symptoms

- The intoxicated patient can present with slurred speech and ataxia. The patient can be sedated or unconscious. As BACs decrease rapidly, nausea, vomiting, and hallucinations can ensue. Delirium and seizures are the most severe symptoms.

Signs

- The intoxicated patient can present with nystagmus.
- In withdrawal, the patient can present with tachycardia, diaphoresis, or hyperthermia.

Laboratory Tests

- In the emergency department, a BAC should be ordered when alcohol ingestion is suspected. Most laboratories report BAC in units of milligrams per deciliter. A whole blood alcohol level of 150 mg/dL (33 mmol/L) reported in the hospital corresponds to 0.15% BAC obtained by law enforcement.
- A complete toxicologic screen to rule out the presence of other substances can be useful.

Other Diagnostic Tests

- Differentiate acute alcohol intoxication from other medical illnesses (e.g., head trauma).
- Use computed tomography (CT) on any patient with focal neurologic findings, failure to improve, new-onset seizures, or mental status out of proportion to degree of intoxication.

Treatment Regimens

Symptom-Triggered Therapy With symptom-triggered therapy, medication is given only when the patient has symptoms. This approach results in treatment that is shorter, potentially avoiding oversedation and allowing the clinician to focus on specific therapy for alcohol dependence.[20,21] A typical regimen would include lorazepam 2 mg administered every hour as needed when a structured assessment scale—for example, the Clinical Institute Withdrawal Assessment–Alcohol, Revised (CIWA-AR)—indicates that symptoms are moderate to severe (Table 49-3).[23]

Fixed-Schedule Therapy Over the years, benzodiazepines given regularly at a fixed dosing interval have been used for alcohol withdrawal. The major problem with this approach is underdosing of the benzodiazepine because of cross-tolerance (see Table 49-3). Current guidelines take exception with this rigid approach, urging clinicians to allow for some degree of individualization within fixed-schedule therapy.[20,21]

Treatment of Alcohol Withdrawal Seizures Alcohol withdrawal seizures do not require treatment with an anticonvulsant drug

TABLE 49-3 Dosing and Monitoring of Pharmacologic Agents Used in the Treatment of Alcohol Withdrawal

Drug	Dose Per Day (Unless Otherwise Stated)	Indication	Monitoring	Duration of Dosing	Level of Evidence for Efficacy[a]
Multivitamin	1 tablet	Malnutrition	Diet	At least until eating a balanced diet at caloric goal	B3
Thiamine	50–100 mg	Deficiency	CBC, WBC, nystagmus	Empiric × 5 days. More if evidence of deficiency	B2
Crystalloid fluids (typically D5–0.45 NS with 20 mEq of KCl per liter)	50–100 mL/h	Dehydration	Weight, electrolytes, urine output, nystagmus if dextrose	Until intake and outputs stabilize and oral intake is adequate	A3
Clonidine oral (Catapres)	0.05–0.3 mg Consider dose reduction in the elderly	Autonomic tone rebound and hyperactivity	Shaking, tremor, sweating, blood pressure	3 days or less	B2
Clonidine transdermal (Catapres-TTS)	TTS-1 to TTS-3 Consider dose reduction in the elderly	Autonomic tone rebound and hyperactivity	Shaking, tremor, sweating, blood pressure	1 week or less. One patch only	B3
Labetalol	20 mg IV every 2 hours as needed; dosage reduction (e.g., by about 50% for oral dosage) is advised in patients with hepatic impairment	Hypertensive urgencies and above	Blood pressure target	Individual doses as needed	B3
Antipsychotics, haloperidol (Haldol)	2.5 to 5 mg every 4 hours	Agitation unresponsive to benzodiazepines, hallucinations (tactile, visual, auditory, or otherwise), or delusions	Subjective response plus rating scale (CIWA-AR or equivalent)	Individual doses as needed	B1
Antipsychotics, atypical		Agitation unresponsive to benzodiazepines, hallucinations, or delusions in patients intolerant of conventional antipsychotics	Subjective response plus rating scale (CIWA-AR or equivalent)	Individual doses as needed in addition to scheduled antipsychotic	C3
Quetiapine (Seroquel)	25–200 mg; dosage adjustment is necessary in hepatic impairment				
Aripiprazole (Abilify)	5–15 mg				
Benzodiazepines		Tremor, anxiety, diaphoresis, tachypnea, dysphoria, seizures	Subjective response plus rating scale (CIWA-AR or equivalent)	Individual doses as needed. Underdosing is more common than overdosing	A2
Lorazepam (Ativan)	0.5–2 mg				
Chlordiazepoxide (Librium)	5–25 mg				
Clonazepam (Klonopin)	0.5–2 mg				
Diazepam (Valium)	2.5–10 mg				
Alcohol oral		Prevent withdrawal	Subjective signs of withdrawal	Wide variation	C3
Alcohol IV		Prevent withdrawal	Subjective signs of withdrawal	Wide variation	C3

CBC, complete blood count; CIWA-AR, Clinical Institute Withdrawal Assessment for Alcohol, Revised; D5, dextrose 5%; KCl, potassium chloride; NS, normal saline; WBC, white blood cell count.

[a]Strength of recommendations, evidence to support recommendation: A, good; B, moderate; C, poor.

Quality of evidence: 1, evidence from more than one properly randomized controlled trial; 2, evidence from more than one well-designed clinical trial with randomization, from cohort or case–control analytic studies or multiple time series, or dramatic results from uncontrolled experiments; 3, evidence from opinions of respected authorities, based on clinical experience, descriptive studies, or reports of expert communities.

Data from references 20 and 21.

unless they progress to status epilepticus because seizures usually end before diazepam or another drug can be administered.[21] Phenytoin, which is not cross-tolerant to alcohol, does not prevent or treat withdrawal seizures, and without an IV loading dose, therapeutic blood levels of phenytoin are not reached until acute withdrawal is complete. Patients experiencing seizures should be treated supportively. An increase in the dosage and slowing of the tapering schedule of the benzodiazepine used in detoxification or a single injection of a benzodiazepine can be necessary to prevent further seizure activity. Patients with a history of withdrawal seizures can be predicted to experience an especially severe withdrawal syndrome. In such patients, a higher initial dosage of a benzodiazepine and a slower tapering period of 7 to 10 days are advisable.

Treatment of Nutritional Deficits and Electrolyte Abnormalities Fluid status should be carefully assessed, and fluid, electrolyte, and vitamin abnormalities should be corrected. Hydration can be necessary in patients with vomiting, diarrhea, increased body temperature, or severe agitation. Alcoholics often have electrolyte imbalances because of inadequate nutrition and fluid volume related to antidiuretic hormone inhibition. Hypokalemia can be corrected with oral potassium supplementation as long as renal function is adequate. Thiamine (vitamin B_1) is often depleted in alcoholics, and supplementation is standard because it can prevent the development of the Wernicke-Korsakoff syndrome (e.g., mental confusion, eye movement disorders, and ataxia [poor motor coordination]). An initial dose of 100 mg IV or IM is commonly used. In practice, thiamine is usually given 100 mg once daily orally, IV, or intramuscularly for 3 to 5 days (see Table 49-3).

Alcohol hypoglycemia usually occurs in the absence of overt liver disease, and it is more likely if the patient is fasting or exercising or is sensitive to alcohol; it is less likely if the patient is obese. The alcohol directly interferes with hepatic gluconeogenesis but not glycogenolysis. The energy required for metabolism of alcohol is diverted away from the energy needed to take up lactate and pyruvate—substrates for gluconeogenesis. So, patients who drink alcohol can become hypoglycemic once glycogen stores are depleted. Neurologic symptoms of hypoglycemia can be confused with alcohol intoxication, and in the inpatient setting, blood glucose should be monitored regularly.

Treatment Settings Alcohol withdrawal treatment can take place in hospitals, inpatient detoxification units, or outpatient settings. Only patients with mild to moderate symptoms should be considered for outpatient treatment, and it is a good idea to have a responsible, sober person available to help the patient monitor symptoms and administer medications. Patients with a strong craving for alcohol, those concurrently using other drugs, and those with a history of seizures or delirium tremens are not good candidates for outpatient treatment. Pharmacologic agents used in the treatment of alcohol withdrawal are summarized in Table 49-3.

Pharmacologic Management of Alcohol Dependence

7 In the United States, disulfiram, naltrexone, once-monthly injectable extended-release naltrexone, and acamprosate are the only four drugs that are FDA-approved for the treatment of alcohol dependence. Disulfiram acts as a deterrent to the resumption of drinking, and naltrexone is a competitive opioid antagonist that has been shown to reduce cravings for alcohol. Acamprosate is a GABAergic agonist that modulates alcohol cravings (Table 49-4). Other drugs, including nalmefene, bupropion, various serotonergic agents (including selective serotonin reuptake inhibitors and vascular serotonin-3 [5-HT_3] receptor antagonists), topiramate, and lithium, also have been used either abroad or in the United States off-label for alcohol dependence.

Disulfiram

Disulfiram deters a patient from drinking by producing an aversive reaction if the patient drinks. In the absence of alcohol, disulfiram has minimal effects. Disulfiram inhibits aldehyde dehydrogenase in the biochemical pathway for alcohol metabolism, allowing acetaldehyde to accumulate. The resulting increase in acetaldehyde causes severe facial flushing, throbbing headache, nausea and vomiting, chest pain, palpitations, tachycardia, weakness, dizziness, blurred vision, confusion, and hypotension. Severe reactions including myocardial infarction, congestive heart failure, cardiac arrhythmia, respiratory depression, convulsions, and death can occur, particularly in vulnerable individuals.[24]

TABLE 49-4 Dosing and Monitoring of Pharmacologic Agents Used in the Treatment of Alcohol Dependence

Drug	Dosage Range Per Day	Indication	Monitoring	Duration of Dosing	Level of Evidence for Efficacy[a]
Disulfiram (Antabuse)	250–500 mg; used with extreme caution in patients with hepatic cirrhosis or insufficiency	Deterrence	Facial flushing, liver enzymes	Indefinite	B2
Acamprosate (Campral)	999–1,998 mg and higher (333 mg tablets) Dosage adjustment necessary in renal impairment	Craving	Patient-reported craving, renal function	Indefinite	A1
Naltrexone (ReVia)	50–100 mg; dosage adjustment may be needed in renal and liver impairment	Craving	Patient-reported craving	Indefinite	A1
Mood stabilizers (e.g., lamotrigine [Lamictal], topiramate [Topamax], carbamazepine [Tegretol], valproic acid [Depakote])	Seizure disorder doses	Craving	Patient-reported craving, plasma drug levels	Indefinite	B2
Antidepressants (e.g., clomipramine [Anafranil], bupropion [Wellbutrin], doxepin [Sinequan], fluoxetine [Prozac])	Depression doses	Craving, depression, anxiety	Patient-reported craving	Indefinite	B2

[a]Strength of recommendations: A, B, and C, good, moderate, and poor evidence to support recommendation, respectively.

Quality of evidence: 1, evidence from more than one properly randomized controlled trial; 2, evidence from more than one well-designed clinical trial with randomization, from cohort or case–control analytic studies or multiple time series, or dramatic results from uncontrolled experiments; 3, evidence from opinions of respected authorities, based on clinical experience, descriptive studies, or reports of expert communities.

Data from references 24 and 26.

Naltrexone

Naltrexone, an opiate antagonist available in the United States since 1984 for the treatment of opioid dependence, blocks the effects of exogenous opioids. In 1994, the FDA approved its use in the treatment of alcohol dependence. Naltrexone is thought to attenuate the reinforcing effects of alcohol, and those who consume alcohol while taking naltrexone report feeling less intoxicated and having less craving for alcohol.[25] Evidence suggests that genetics plays a role in the clinical response to naltrexone. Carriers of the Asp40 polymorphism in the μ-opioid receptor gene show increased response to naltrexone with lower rates of relapse to heavy drinking.

Naltrexone should not be given to patients currently dependent on opiates because it can precipitate a severe withdrawal syndrome. Naltrexone is associated with dose-related hepatotoxicity, but this generally occurs at doses higher than those recommended for treatment of alcohol dependence. Nevertheless, it is considered contraindicated in patients with hepatitis or liver failure, and liver function tests should be monitored monthly for the first 3 months and every 3 months thereafter.

Nausea is the most common side effect of naltrexone, occurring in approximately 10% of patients. Other side effects are headache, dizziness, nervousness, fatigue, insomnia, vomiting, anxiety, and somnolence. If dosed daily, naltrexone 50 mg is sufficient to effectively block μ-opioid receptors.

In April 2006, the FDA approved Vivitrol, a once-monthly intramuscular naltrexone formulation. The usual effective dose is 380 mg IM each month.[26,27] Extended-release formulations reduce the likelihood of forgetting or choosing not to take medication, assuring that once the patient receives an injection, he or she will be "adherent" for the next month.[26]

Criticism has been leveled at the extended-release dosage form, suggesting that naltrexone's benefit may be limited to less severe alcohol dependence, and exclusively to reduction in heavy drinking rather than abstinence. Pettinati et al.[27] report the results of a study in alcohol-dependent patients who had higher baseline severity, as measured by: (a) the Alcohol Dependence Scale (ADS) or (b) having been medically detoxified in the week before randomization. Higher severity alcohol-dependent patients, when receiving 380 mg ($n = 50$) of the extended-release compound compared with placebo ($n = 47$), had significantly fewer heavy-drinking days during the study (hazard ratio = 0.583; $P = 0.0049$) and showed an average reduction of 37.3% in heavy-drinking days compared with 27.4% for placebo-treated patients ($P = 0.039$). The authors contend that their data support the efficacy of extended-release naltrexone 380 mg in relatively higher severity alcohol dependence for both reduction in heavy drinking and maintenance of abstinence.

Acamprosate

Acamprosate is a glutamate modulator at the *N*-methyl-D-aspartate (NMDA) receptor that reduces alcohol craving. Acamprosate, approved in the United States in 2004, had been available in Europe for many years. Patients treated with acamprosate are more successful in maintaining abstinence from alcohol versus placebo. Acamprosate is well tolerated, with GI adverse effects most common.

A Cochrane review of 24 randomized controlled trials (RCTs) with 6,915 participants[28] found that, compared with placebo, acamprosate significantly reduced the risk of any drinking (RR 0.86 [95% CI 0.81 to 0.91]; NNT 9.09 [95% CI 6.66 to 14.28]) and significantly increased the cumulative abstinence duration (mean difference 10.94 [95% CI 5.08 to 16.81]), while secondary outcomes did not reach statistical significance. Diarrhea was the only side effect that was more frequently reported with acamprosate than placebo (risk difference 0.11 [95% 0.09 to 0.13]; NNTB 9.09 [95% CI 7.69 to 11.11]). See Table 49-4 for dosing information for this and the other options used in treating alcohol dependence.

NICOTINE

Clinical guidelines for tobacco use and dependence were released in 2000 and updated in 2008.[29] Telephone quitlines are available in every state, and more patient are now referred to smoking cessations counseling services. There also is a growing number of Internet and mobile phone text messaging programs that have been developed to reach the teenage and young adult population to promote smoking cessation.[30,31] The number of adults who smoke has decreased from 42.4% in 1965 to 19.3% in 2010, and now there are more former smokers than current smokers.

Despite this encouraging news, cigarette smoking continues to be the leading cause of preventable morbidity and mortality in the United States. Data from the 2010 National Health Interview Survey (NHIS)[32] found that the overall percent of current smokers from the years 2005 to 2010 in adults ≥18 years old decreased from 20.9 to 19.3. It was determined this represents 3 million fewer smokers in 2010 compared with those in 2005, but this decline has not been uniform across all subsets of the population. The Healthy People 2020 target is currently set for the prevalence of smoking to be less than or equal to 12%, and based on the current rate of decline, this target will not be met. Healthy People 2020 also calls for greater utilization of tobacco use counseling within ambulatory settings to improve smoking cessation rates.[33]

Epidemiology of Tobacco Use

The NSDUH reported in 2011 that an estimated 26.5% (68.2 million) of the U.S. population 12 years of age and older used a tobacco product at least once in the month prior to being interviewed. In addition, 56.8 million Americans were current cigarette smokers, 12.9 million smoked cigars, 8.2 million used smokeless tobacco, and 2.1 million smoked pipes.[4] Comparing age groups, adults between the ages of 18 and 25 years have the highest rate of cigarette use (39.5%), but it is encouraging to see the rates continue to decrease each year since 2002 when 40.8% of young adults were using cigarettes. Within youth aged 12 to 17, use of cigarettes also continued to decline from 15.2% in 2002 to 10% in 2011.[4]

Data trends from the 2011 NSDUH continue to show smoking prevalence varies based on the level of education. The highest percentage of adults who admitted to smoking were adults who had not completed high school (33.7%). The lowest rate of smoking was seen in adults who graduated from college (11.7%). Results from the NSDUH also showed cigarette smoking was higher in unemployed adults (40.7%) in comparison to adults who were employed full time (23.3%).[4]

Economic Impact of Smoking

The direct healthcare expenditures associated with smoking total approximately $298 billion a year, which includes factors such as lost productivity, premature death, and direct medical expenditures.[34] Medicaid patients' smoking rates are substantially higher in comparison to the general population. Smoking-attributable medical expenditures are estimated at 11% of Medicaid program expenditures.[35]

HEALTH RISKS OF SMOKING

Cigarette smoking substantially increases the risk of (a) cardiovascular diseases such as stroke, sudden death, and heart attack; (b) nonmalignant respiratory diseases including emphysema, asthma, chronic bronchitis, and chronic obstructive pulmonary disease; (c) lung cancer; and (d) other cancers.[33]

Exposure to environmental tobacco smoke (*passive exposure*) has been cited as the cause of 3,400 lung cancer deaths and 46,000 heart disease–related deaths in the United States every year.[36] Children who are exposed to environmental smoke have a higher risk of respiratory infection, asthma, and middle ear infections than those who are not exposed. Sudden infant death syndrome occurs more often in infants whose mothers smoked during pregnancy than in offspring of nonsmoking mothers.[36] The harmful effects of smoking on reproduction and pregnancy include reduced fertility and fetal growth, as well as increased risk of ectopic pregnancy and spontaneous abortion.[36]

PHARMACOLOGY OF NICOTINE

Nicotine is a ganglionic cholinergic agonist with pharmacologic effects that are highly dependent on dose. These effects include central and peripheral nervous system stimulation and depression, respiratory stimulation, skeletal muscle relaxation, catecholamine release by the adrenal medulla, peripheral vasoconstriction, and increased blood pressure, heart rate, cardiac output, and oxygen consumption. Cigarette smoking or low doses of nicotine produce an increased alertness and increased cognitive functioning by stimulating the cerebral cortex. At higher doses, nicotine stimulates the "reward" center in the limbic system of the brain.[37]

When nicotine is ingested, a feeling of pleasure and relaxation can occur. Repetitive exposure to nicotine leads to neuroadaptation, which builds tolerance to the initial effects. An accumulation of nicotine in the body leads to a more substantial withdrawal reaction if cessation is attempted.[38] Common symptoms experienced during withdrawal can include anxiety, difficulties concentrating, irritability, and strong cravings for tobacco. Onset of these withdrawal symptoms usually occurs within 24 hours and can last for days, weeks, or longer.[38] This powerful force of nicotine addiction is one reason smokers who attempt to achieve smoking cessation have a high rate of relapse, and only 3% remain abstinent 6 months following the quit date.[39]

TREATMENT

Desired Outcomes

Ideally, we would hope that more and more people stop smoking altogether and that young people never take up the habit. This is unlikely to happen. The Healthy People 2020 target setting the prevalence of smoking to be less than or equal to 12% discussed above is a realistic and achievable goal.

Nicotine Dependence

Agency for Healthcare Research and Quality Clinical Practice Guideline: Treating Tobacco Use and Dependence

The Agency for Healthcare Research and Quality (AHRQ) periodically convenes expert panels to develop clinical guidelines for healthcare practitioners. Because of the widespread prevalence of smoking-related illnesses, its related morbidity and mortality, and the economic burden imposed, the agency convened a panel of experts in 1994 to develop guidelines on the treatment of tobacco addiction. The resultant guideline for smoking cessation was updated in 2008,[29] and no further updates have been released at the time of this writing.

The revised guideline suggests strategies for providing appropriate treatments for every patient. Because effective treatments for tobacco dependence now exist, every patient should receive at least minimal treatment every time he or she visits a clinician (Figs. 49-1 and 49-2).

The guideline identified a number of key findings that clinicians should use:

1. (8) Tobacco dependence is a chronic condition that often requires repeated intervention. However, effective treatments exist that can produce long-term or permanent abstinence.
2. Because effective tobacco-dependence treatments are available, every patient who uses tobacco should be offered at least one of these treatments.
3. It is essential that clinicians and healthcare delivery systems (including administrators, insurers, and purchasers) institutionalize the consistent identification, documentation, and treatment of every tobacco user who is seen in a healthcare setting.
4. Brief tobacco-dependence treatment is effective, and every patient who uses tobacco should be offered at least brief treatment.
5. There is a strong dose–response relationship between the intensity of tobacco-dependence counseling and its effectiveness. Treatments involving person-to-person contact (via individual, group, or proactive telephone counseling) are consistently effective, and their effectiveness increases with treatment intensity (e.g., minutes of contact).
6. Three types of counseling and behavioral therapies were found to be especially effective and should be used with all patients who are attempting tobacco cessation:
   - Provision of practical counseling (problem-solving/skills training)
   - Provision of social support as part of treatment (intra-treatment social support)
   - Help in securing social support outside treatment (extra-treatment social support)

Numerous effective pharmacotherapy options for smoking cessation now exist (Table 49-5). Seven first-line pharmacotherapy options reliably increase long-term smoking abstinence rates: sustained-release (SR) bupropion, nicotine gum, nicotine inhaler,

CLINICAL PRESENTATION Nicotine Withdrawal

General

- The patient may experience anxiety but may not be in acute distress. Symptoms can wax and wane over time.

Symptoms

- The patient may complain of cravings, difficulty concentrating, frustration, irritability, and impatience. Hostility, insomnia, and restlessness can also occur.

Signs

- Increased skin temperature can be present.

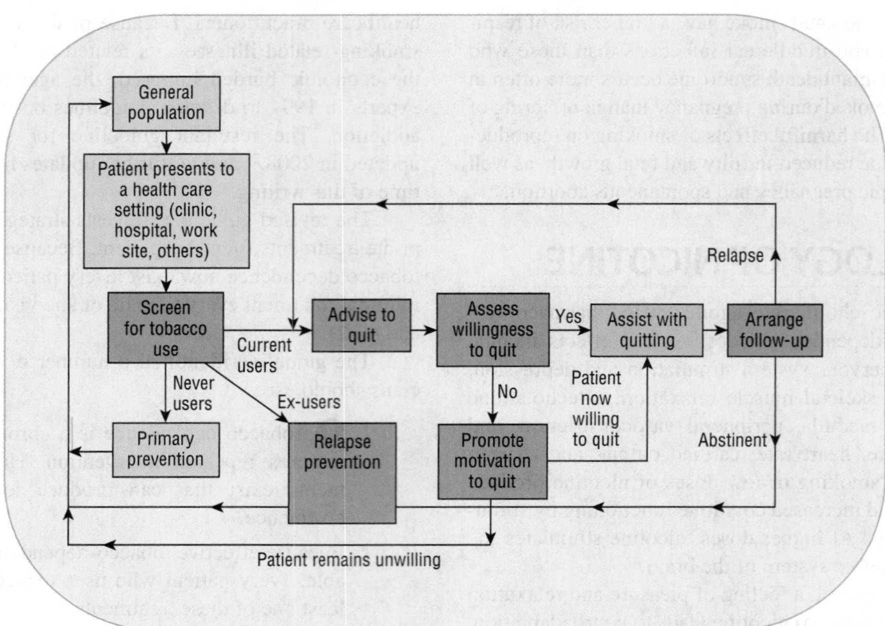

FIGURE 49-1 Model for treatment of tobacco use and dependence.

nicotine lozenge, nicotine nasal spray, nicotine patch, and varenicline. Combinations of these should be considered if a single agent has failed.

Two second-line pharmacotherapy options are considered efficacious and can be considered by clinicians if first-line options are not effective: clonidine and nortriptyline.

Tobacco-dependence treatments are both clinically effective and cost-effective relative to other medical and disease prevention interventions. As such, insurers and purchasers should ensure all insurance plans include as a reimbursed benefit the counseling and pharmacotherapeutic treatments that are identified as effective in this guideline, as well as clinician reimbursement for providing tobacco-dependence treatment just as they are reimbursed for treating other chronic conditions.

Other Factors Important to the Success of a Smoking-Cessation Strategy

The AHRQ expert panel emphasized the importance of the type and intensity of the contact with the counselor to the success of the intervention. When interventions last for more than 10 minutes, the increase in cessation rates is much better than when interventions do not involve contact with a professional. Group and individual counseling is more effective than no intervention in increasing abstinence rates. Self-help materials (e.g., handouts, pamphlets, and brochures) without any direct physical contact are not effective.[40] Interventions are more successful when they include social support and training in general problem-solving skills, stress management, and relapse prevention. The number of treatment sessions offered is also important. Providing at least four or more sessions, longer than 10 minutes in length, and if possible providing treatments from multiple types of clinicians have proven higher success rates compared with less intensive interventions.[29] Although comprehensive behavioral interventions have been shown to be more effective in helping people quit smoking and remain abstinent, less intensive treatments are beneficial as well. Even minimal contacts lasting less than 3 minutes and simple advice to quit are more successful in increasing cessation rates than intervention involving no contact.[29] A recent study also showed physicians offering assistance to all

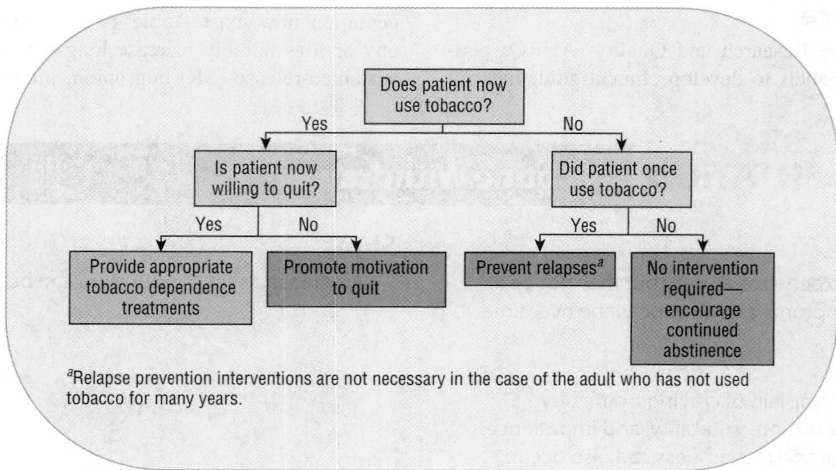

FIGURE 49-2 Algorithm for treating tobacco use.

TABLE 49-5 Dosing and Monitoring of Pharmacologic Agents Used for Smoking Cessation

Drug	Place in Therapy	Dosage Range	Duration	Comments/Monitoring Parameters	LOEE[a]
Bupropion SR[b,c] (Zyban)	First-line	Titrate up to 150 mg orally twice daily. May require reduced initial dose in elderly	3–6 months	Patients receiving both bupropion and a nicotine patch should be monitored for hypertension	A1
Clonidine[c,d] (Catapres)	Second-line	Titrate to response; 0.2–0.75 mg/day. Consider dose reduction in the elderly	6–12 months	Monitor baseline electrolyte and lipid profiles, renal function, uric acid, complete blood count, and blood pressure	B2
Nicotine polacrilex (gum)[b] (Nicorette)	First-line	Initial dose depends on smoking history: 2–4 mg every 1–8 hours	12 weeks (taper down over time)	Heart rate and blood pressure should be monitored periodically during nicotine replacement therapy	A1
Nicotine inhaler[b] (Nicotrol)	First-line	24–64 mg/day (total daily dose)	3–6 months (taper down over time)	Heart rate and blood pressure should be monitored periodically during nicotine replacement therapy	A1
Nicotine nasal spray[b] (Nicotrol NS)	First-line	8–40 mg/day (total daily dose)	14 weeks (taper down over time)	Heart rate and blood pressure should be monitored periodically during nicotine replacement therapy	A1
Nicotine patch[b] (NicoDerm, Nicotrol)	First-line	Initial dose depends on smoking history: 7–21 mg topically once daily	6 weeks (taper down over time)	Heart rate and blood pressure should be monitored periodically during nicotine replacement therapy	A1
Nortriptyline[c,d] (Aventyl)	Second-line	Titrate up to 75–100 mg orally daily	6–12 months	Dry mouth, blurred vision, and constipation are dose-dependent adverse effects	B2
Varenicline[c] (Chantix)	First-line	Titrate up to 1 mg orally twice daily. If CrCl <30 mL/min, 0.5 mg once per day	3–6 months	Monitor renal function, especially in elderly patients. Nausea, headache, insomnia are dose-dependent adverse effects	A1

LOEE, level of evidence for efficacy.

[a]Strength of recommendations, evidence to support recommendation: A, good; B, moderate; C, poor.
Quality of evidence: 1, evidence from more than one properly randomized controlled trial; 2, evidence from more than one well-designed clinical trial with randomization, from cohort or case–control analytic studies or multiple time series, or dramatic results from uncontrolled experiments; 3, evidence from opinions of respected authorities, based on clinical experience, descriptive studies, or reports of expert communities.
[b]Nicotine replacement therapies can be combined with each other and/or bupropion to increase long-term abstinence rates.
[c]Do not abruptly discontinue. Taper up initially, and taper off once therapy is complete.
[d]Clonidine and nortriptyline are not FDA-approved for smoking cessation.

Data from reference 29.

smoking patients to achieve smoking cessation is much more effective than only offering assistance to patients who are interested in smoking cessation.[41]

Motivational interviewing is a form of counseling to help patients identify barriers for making a behavior change. A meta-analysis[42] of 14 studies published between 1997 and 2008, including over 10,000 smokers who underwent motivational interviewing as part of the smoking cessation program, found that motivational interviewing with standard care or brief cessation advice did improve quit rates modestly. Subgroup analysis found that motivational interviewing was most effective when completed in longer sessions by primary care physicians and counselors.

Counseling alone can be effective, but counseling efficacy is further augmented by the addition of pharmacotherapy. In a meta-analysis that included 111 trials with more than 43,000 participants using one or more of the five forms of nicotine replacement therapy (NRT) including nicotine gum, nasal spray, patches, lozenges, or inhaler, it was found that the use of NRT significantly increased the rate of cessation compared with placebo.[43]

Pharmacologic Therapy for Smoking Cessation

All patients attempting to quit should be encouraged to use effective pharmacotherapy agents for smoking cessation except in the presence of special circumstances. As with other chronic diseases, the most effective treatment of tobacco dependence encompasses multiple modalities. Pharmacotherapy is a vital element of a multicomponent smoking cessation program that should always include nonpharmacologic components. The role of pharmacotherapy in smoking cessation is summarized in Table 49-5.

Nicotine Replacement Therapy

9 In 2009, a systematic review[43] was performed to determine the effectiveness of the different forms of NRT (e.g., chewing gum, transdermal patches, nasal spray, inhalers, and tablets) in achieving abstinence or a sustained reduction in the amount smoked. The review showed that all of the commercially available forms of NRT were effective for smoking cessation. Use of NRT doubled the odds of quitting.

A head-to-head placebo-controlled trial[44] comparing 5 smoking cessation pharmacotherapies was done in 1,504 smokers who had smoked at least 10 cigarettes per day for 6 months. Patients were randomized to receive SR bupropion, nicotine patch, nicotine lozenge, nicotine patch plus nicotine lozenge, bupropion plus nicotine lozenge, or placebo. At 6 months it was found the quit rates were 40.1% for the nicotine patch plus nicotine lozenge, 34.4% for the nicotine patch, 33.5% for the nicotine lozenge, 33.2% for bupropion plus nicotine lozenge, 31.8% for bupropion alone, and 22.2% for placebo.

Nicotine Gum Clinicians should offer 4-mg rather than 2-mg nicotine gum to highly dependent smokers.[29] The 2-mg gum is recommended for patients smoking fewer than 25 cigarettes per day, whereas the 4-mg gum is recommended for patients smoking 25 or more cigarettes per day. Generally, the gum should be used for up to 12 weeks, no more than 24 pieces chewed per day.

Gum should be chewed slowly until a peppery or minty taste emerges and then "parked" between cheek and gums to facilitate nicotine absorption through the oral mucosa. Acidic beverages (e.g., coffee, juices, or soft drinks) interfere with the buccal absorption of nicotine, so eating and drinking anything except water should be avoided for 15 minutes before and during chewing. Instructions to chew the gum on a fixed schedule (at least one piece every 1 to 2 hours) for at least 1 to 3 months can be more beneficial than ad libitum use.[29]

Nicotine Patch The nicotine patch is available both as a nonprescription medication and as a prescription drug, and it approximately doubles long-term abstinence rates over those produced by placebo interventions.[43] Treatment of 8 weeks or less has been shown to be as efficacious as longer treatment periods. The 16- and 24-hour patches are of comparable efficacy. Clinicians should consider starting treatment on a lower patch dose in patients smoking 10 or fewer cigarettes per day.[29]

A patch should be applied as soon as the patient wakes on the quit day and at the start of each day thereafter. The patient should place a new patch on a relatively hairless location, typically between the neck and waist. There are no restrictions on activity while using the patch. Patients who experience sleep disruption should remove the 24-hour patch prior to bedtime or use the 16-hour patch.

Nicotine Nasal Spray Nicotine nasal spray more than doubles long-term abstinence rates when compared with a placebo spray. It is available exclusively as a prescription medication. A dose of nicotine nasal spray consists of one 0.5-mg delivery to each nostril (1 mg total). Initial dosing should be one to two doses per hour, increasing as needed for symptom relief. The minimum recommended treatment is 8 doses per day, with a maximum limit of 40 doses per day (5 doses per hour). Recommended duration of therapy is 3 to 6 months. Patients should not sniff, swallow, or inhale through the nose while administering doses because this increases irritating effects.[29]

Nicotine Lozenge The nicotine lozenge is available as a 2-mg and a 4-mg dose. The 2-mg lozenge is recommended for patients who normally smoke their first cigarette later than 30 minutes after awakening, and the 4-mg lozenge is recommended for smokers who smoke within 30 minutes of waking. The duration of treatment is 12 weeks. It is recommended no more than 20 lozenges should be used in 1 day.[29] The most common side effect of the lozenge is nausea. As with the nicotine gum, acidic beverages (e.g., coffee, juices, or soft drinks) interfere with the buccal absorption of nicotine, so eating and drinking anything except water should be avoided for 15 minutes before and during use of the lozenge.[29]

Instructing Patients in the Use of NRT Compliance with NRT improves when the patient is presented a clear rationale for its use and a realistic expectation about the response. It should be explained to the patient that nicotine is responsible for addiction and that discontinuation of the nicotine causes craving for cigarettes, tension, irritability, sadness, problems with sleep, and difficulty concentrating. The patient should be told that using the patch results in less desire to smoke and provides an opportunity for a new nonsmoker to practice all the new nonsmoking skills without being burdened by craving. The patient should understand that with smoking, there are naturally peaks and valleys in the amount of nicotine in the bloodstream. With the patch there is a steady gradual rise in the blood nicotine concentration that levels off and remains constant for much of the day and then gradually decreases while the person is asleep.[29]

Side Effects Nicotine replacement products have relatively few side effects. Nausea and light-headedness are possible symptoms of nicotine overdose that warrant a reduction of the nicotine dose.

The most frequent side effect with the nicotine patch is skin irritation related to the adhesive or the medium containing nicotine and not to the nicotine itself. Approximately 50% of patients report skin irritation during the course of treatment with the patch. The patch site can be rotated to diminish this problem. Switching to a different brand of patch can alleviate the problem because different products use different adhesives or media. The gum can be used instead of the patch when the skin irritation is severe. Less than 5% of patients were forced to discontinue therapy because of skin reactions.[29]

Duration Those who commit to quitting smoking using NRT should be told that treatment for up to 3 months is common.[45] However, some patients will experience severe withdrawal even beyond this time period; thus, long-term use of NRT might be indicated. Long-term use of NRT has not been linked to any safety concerns and is supported by the 2008 updated U.S. Public Health Service Guidelines.[29]

Non-Nicotine Options

Bupropion ⑩ Bupropion inhibits neuronal reuptake and potentiates the effects of norepinephrine and dopamine. Although its precise mechanism in smoking cessation is not well understood, dopamine has been associated with the rewarding effects of addictive substances. The AHRQ panel concluded that SR bupropion is an efficacious smoking cessation treatment that patients should be encouraged to use.[29]

Contraindications for bupropion use include current or past seizure disorders, a history of monoamine oxidase inhibitor use over the last 14 days, and a history of anorexia nervosa or bulimia. Along with multiple other precautions listed in the product labeling, current alcohol use, use of medications that lower seizure threshold (e.g., antidepressants, antipsychotics), and depression are possible concerns when using this medication.[28] In 2009, the FDA required manufacturers of Zyban (bupropion) and generic manufacturers to add new boxed warnings and to develop a medication guide highlighting the risk of serious neuropsychiatric symptoms in patients using this product. Possible symptoms include depressed mood, agitation, anxiety, hostility, changes in behavior, suicidal thoughts and behavior, and attempted suicide.[29]

A double-blind, placebo-controlled, randomized multicenter trial was conducted in which healthy smokers received either SR bupropion 150 mg twice daily or a placebo daily for 7 weeks and were subsequently seen for counseling and followup for a total of 52 weeks. The primary end points were biochemically confirmed continuous abstinence at weeks 7 and 52. The authors specifically conducted this trial in the primary care setting to verify the general applicability of the results to the intended end users. Results of this study showed bupropion was efficacious, with an absolute 25% of participants continuously abstinent at 1 year; it doubled the odds of continuous abstinence from week 4 to 7 and from week 4 to 52 compared with placebo.[46]

A meta-analysis[47] involving 49 trials utilizing bupropion for smoking cessation showed that bupropion significantly increased the incidence of long-term cessation when used as a sole agent in 36 separate trials. Other trials that used bupropion as an add-on agent with NRT did not show additional benefit in improving cessation rates.[47]

⑩ For smoking cessation, the manufacturer recommends a dosage of 150 mg once daily for 3 days and then twice daily for 7 to 12 weeks or longer, with or without NRT. Patients are instructed to stop smoking during the second week of treatment and are encouraged to use counseling and support services along with the medication. For maintenance therapy, consider SR bupropion 150 mg twice daily for up to 6 months.[29]

Varenicline (Chantix) Varenicline acts at sites in the nicotine-affected brain in two ways: by providing nicotine effects to ease withdrawal symptoms and by blocking the effects of nicotine from cigarettes if they resume smoking. Specifically, varenicline is a partial agonist that binds selectively to α_4-β_2-nicotinic acetylcholine receptors with a greater affinity than nicotine. When bound to the receptor, the drug blocks nicotine from binding and also evokes a response but to a lesser degree than nicotine. The stimulation of the receptor results in release of dopamine and thus provides a type of "reward" that can decrease craving and withdrawal symptoms.[48]

The recommended dosage for varenicline is 0.5 mg daily for 3 days, increase to 0.5 mg twice daily for 3 days, and then increase to 1 mg twice daily for a standard 12-week treatment. If abstinence has not been achieved after the 12-week treatment, then a second 12-week treatment may be prescribed.[48]

Varenicline is listed as a first-line agent in the 2008 clinical guidelines on treating tobacco use and dependence. Eleven trials comparing varenicline with placebo, three of which also had a comparison with bupropion, were reviewed in a meta-analysis.[49] Varenicline resulted in a twofold to threefold increased likelihood of long-term smoking cessation compared with nonpharmacologic treatment. Most studies were only 12 weeks, so efficacy beyond this time period needs further study.

Since 2006, when varenicline was approved by the FDA, alarming numbers of adverse effects, including suicidal thoughts, erratic behavior, and aggressive behavior, have been reported. The large number of reports led to the release of a Public Health Advisory by the FDA in February 2008.[50] The advisory stressed the importance of screening for any type of psychiatric illness or any behavior changes after starting varenicline. A boxed warning along with an update of the medication guide from the manufacturer was required by the FDA.[51]

The FDA sponsored two epidemiologic studies that evaluated the neuropsychiatric adverse events linked to the use of varenicline. These studies had multiple limitations, and although the studies did not show an increased risk of hospitalization secondary to neuropsychiatric events, it is important for both healthcare professionals and patients to be aware of the possible risks associated with the use of varenicline.[52]

Specific warnings stress patients should report any history of psychiatric illness and any changes in behavior or mood immediately to their prescribing practitioner.[50] There have also been concerns with the risk of cardiovascular events associated with the use of varenicline, and the FDA requested a systematic review of all randomized clinical trials to identify if there was an associated cardiovascular risk with the use of varenicline.[53]

Clinical **Controversy. . .**

Concerns have been voiced regarding cardiovascular adverse events related to varenicline use. The FDA reviewed a clinical trial that showed a small increase in cardiovascular events in varenicline-treated patients with cardiovascular disease compared with placebo-treated patients.[53] In light of the fact that cigarette smoking substantially increases the risk of cardiovascular diseases,[38] and varenicline has been shown to cause a twofold to threefold increase in the likelihood of long-term smoking cessation,[51] the benefits in most cases may outweigh the risks. It is important for healthcare providers to educate patients with cardiovascular disease of the risks and benefits of varenicline to allow them to make an informed decision.

Seven hundred patients who smoked and also suffered from cardiovascular disease were randomized to either varenicline or placebo and followed for 12 weeks of therapy and another 40 weeks following treatment. It was shown varenicline was more effective in helping patients to achieve smoking cessation and maintain abstinence for up to 1 year than placebo. It was found that varenicline may be associated with a small increase in risk of cardiovascular events, but the benefit of smoking cessation in this patient population is very important and must be considered when evaluating the risk-to-benefit ratio.[53]

Prochaska and Hilton[54] published a meta-analysis that included all 22 trials published up to May 2012. The study focused on events occurring during drug exposure. Rates of treatment emergent, cardiovascular serious adverse events were 0.63% (34/5,431) in the varenicline groups and 0.47% (18/3,801) in the placebo groups. The summary estimate for the risk difference, 0.27% (95% confidence interval −0.10 to 0.63; $P = 0.15$), based on all 22 trials, was neither clinically nor statistically significant.

Comparison of NRT and Non-Nicotine Options

A systematic review and multiple treatment meta-analysis was performed using a Baysean model to evaluate the effect of high-dose and standard-dose NRT, combination NRT, bupropion, and varenicline.[55] The primary outcome included smoking abstinence at 4, 12, 26, and 52 weeks following the set quit date. The standard- and high-dose NRT patch, bupropion, and varenicline were shown to be superior to placebo and controls on a consistent basis. Varenicline was shown to be statistically more effective in achieving smoking abstinence compared with the other agents except at 6 months when compared with high-dose NRT patches and combination therapy. It is difficult to identify which agent is more effective over another at this time, since other considerations such as cost and specific patient factors must also be taken into account.[55]

Second-Line Medications

Second-line medications are pharmacotherapies for which there is evidence of efficacy for treating tobacco dependence, but which have a more limited role than first-line medications because (a) the FDA has not approved them for treatment of tobacco dependence and (b) there are more concerns about potential side effects than with first-line medications.[29] Second-line treatments should be considered for use on a case-by-case basis after first-line treatments have been used or considered.

Clonidine Clonidine has been found to be efficacious as a smoking cessation treatment. It can be used off-label as a second-line agent to treat tobacco dependence. A meta-analysis[56] of six trials showed that clonidine increased smoking cessation rates by 11% (OR 1.89; CI 1.30 to 2.14). There was a high incidence of dose-dependent side effects, particularly dry mouth and sedation.[56] It should be noted that abrupt discontinuation of clonidine can result in symptoms such as nervousness, agitation, headache, and tremor, accompanied or followed by a rapid rise in blood pressure and elevated catecholamine levels.

Doses have varied significantly, from 0.15 to 0.75 mg/day orally and from 0.1 to 0.2 mg/day transdermally, without a clear dose–response relationship to cessation. Most commonly reported side effects include dry mouth, drowsiness, dizziness, sedation, and constipation. Clonidine will lower blood pressure in most patients; thus, blood pressure should be monitored.[29]

Nortriptyline Nortriptyline is also considered to be efficacious as a second-line agent for tobacco dependence. Therapy is initiated 10 to 28 days before the quit date to allow it to reach steady state at the target dose. Trials have initiated treatment at a dose of 25 mg/day, increasing gradually to a target dose of 75 to 100 mg/day. Duration of treatment used in smoking cessation trials has been approximately 12 weeks. Most commonly reported side effects include sedation, dry mouth, blurred vision, urinary retention, light-headedness, and tremor.[29]

Future Treatments Work continues on the development of vaccines to treat nicotine addiction. Vaccines are designed to produce antibodies that bind to nicotine and prevent it from entering the brain. As a result, the positive stimulus in the brain that is normally caused by nicotine is no longer present, thereby taking away the physical motivation for smoking.[57]

Currently there are four vaccines in development, but only NicVAX and NIC002 have any information published in the peer-reviewed literature. Based on the published Phase I/II trials and one unpublished Phase III trial, these vaccines were able to induce an immune response even when the patient was currently smoking, and tolerability was favorable. However, these studies have not been shown to improve abstinence rates over placebo. Further research is needed to determine if these vaccines will become an option for smoking cessation in the future.[57]

Personalized Pharmacotherapy Personalized pharmacotherapy might be a future option in improving the smoking cessation rates that continue to be low. Genome-wide association studies attempted to identify several genetic determinants of smoking behavior, and a phenotype may have been discovered that might identify patients who are at higher risk for developing nicotine dependence.[58] Examples of areas being studied include identifying genes directly related to nicotine reward and metabolism pathways,[39] identifying ways to anticipate response to various smoking cessation treatments based on cytochrome P450 systems, and nicotine metabolite ratios, all of which could lead to selecting the most effective smoking cessation treatment for each individual patient.[58]

CAFFEINE

Caffeine is the most widely consumed behaviorally active substance in the world, generating an increased sense of well-being, happiness, energy, alertness, and sociability.[59] Caffeinism is the term coined to describe the clinical syndrome produced by acute or chronic overuse of caffeine. The syndrome usually is characterized by CNS and peripheral manifestations, most notably anxiety, psychomotor alterations, sleep disturbances, mood changes, and psychophysiologic complaints. As many as one in five adults consume doses of caffeine generally considered large enough to cause clinical symptoms.[59]

Pharmacologically, the risk of developing meaningful clinical manifestations becomes high when intake exceeds 500 mg/day. This places 20% to 30% of North Americans at risk.[59] Caffeine has been proposed as a "model of drug abuse" despite the facts that its sale is largely unrestricted and that heavy consumption of caffeine-containing beverages is not considered to be drug abuse. The information below represents a broad overview of dependence, withdrawal, and tolerance. The reader interested in more information is urged to consult the exhaustive review by Juliano et al.[59]

Epidemiology of Caffeine Use and Abuse

Approximately 173 million consumers drink tea and 183 million consumers drink coffee.[60] The National Coffee Association reports that 40% of 18- to 24-year-olds are drinking coffee each day, while 54% of adults aged 25 to 39 reported drinking coffee daily.

The majority of caffeine users progress to a pattern of frequent or daily consumption. Participants in a study reported consuming a mean of 547.8 mg of caffeine per day. They reported daily consumption of soft drinks (74%), roasted or ground coffee (56%), cocoa/chocolate (36%), bag or leaf tea (34%), instant tea (10%), instant coffee (7%), and caffeine-containing medications (6%). Most participants (81%) reported having their first caffeinated product within 60 minutes of waking. The mean age of onset of regular caffeine consumption was 15.9 years. Results of a recent study showed that, according to their parents, children aged 5 to 7 years old consumed approximately 52 mg of caffeine per day, and children aged 8 to 12 years old consumed approximately 109 mg.[61]

Energy Drinks

A number of energy drinks containing caffeine, taurine, vitamins, and sugar have found their way onto the American market. Sold under brand names such as Red Bull, Monster Energy, Rockstar, and Full Throttle, these products are especially popular with adolescents and emerging adults. Over half of college students surveyed reported drinking at least one energy drink per month.[62] They are generally marketed to enhance alertness or provide a short-term energy boost. Common energy drinks contain approximately 80 mg caffeine per 8 oz (~250 mL) serving, but commercially available energy drinks are often sold in 16-oz (~500 mL) containers and can contain up to 505 mg of caffeine.[62]

Additionally, several manufacturers have marketed alcoholic beverages that have caffeine as an additional ingredient. Some have other ingredients such as guarana, taurine, and ginseng. The Center for Science in the Public Interest has chosen to call these beverages "alcospeed."[63] A novel website calling itself the "Energy Fiend—The Caffeine Fix"[64] lists 577 caffeinated beverages and their respective caffeine content. At least 130 contained more than the 0.02% caffeine limit for soft drinks imposed by the FDA.

Differential Diagnosis

Caffeine intoxication is the only official diagnosis associated with caffeinism in the *Diagnostic and Statistical Manual of Mental Disorders, Fourth Edition, Text Revision* (*DSM-IV-TR*).[10] Caffeine-induced anxiety can manifest as restlessness, nervousness, excitement, insomnia, diuresis, flushing, GI disturbance, muscle twitching, irritability, and jitteriness. If caffeine-induced insomnia requires specific treatment, caffeine-induced sleep disorder is an appropriate *DSM-IV-TR* diagnosis.[10]

Because excessive caffeine consumption is so widespread, a thorough history of caffeine use should be included in the routine assessment of all new patients in primary care medical settings. In this manner, the practitioner can use the information gathered to uncover high levels of caffeine intake and then use the information to pinpoint the cause of clinical signs and symptoms typical of caffeinism. Clinical manifestations of caffeinism almost always lessen in intensity or disappear completely within 1 to 2 weeks after removing the drug.

Pharmacology of Caffeine

Caffeine is rapidly and completely absorbed from the GI tract, reaching a peak blood level within 30 to 45 minutes of oral ingestion. It easily crosses the blood–brain barrier, and levels achieved in the brain are proportional to the dose administered.

The half-life of caffeine in humans is approximately 3.5 to 5 hours. Serious problems rarely result from overdoses of caffeine. In fact, the amount of caffeine needed to cause death in an average adult male is 5 to 10 g, the equivalent of 50 to 100 cups of regular brewed coffee. Thus, the risk of overdose from dietary sources of caffeine is virtually nonexistent.

Caffeine increases the heart rate and force of contraction. It also has a strong diuretic effect. The key factor promoting caffeine use and dosage increases can be the drug's reinforcing effect on pleasure and reward centers of the brain. Caffeine's pharmacologic actions appear comparable (although less potent) with those of other stimulants, such as amphetamines and cocaine.

Caffeine Dependence

Research has shown that abstinence from caffeine induces a distinct withdrawal syndrome. Evidence for this was presented by Strain et al.[65] In a structured psychiatric interview, subjects who self-identified as having problems with caffeine use were evaluated for features of a *DSM-IV-TR* diagnosis of drug dependence. Those judged as caffeine dependent manifested at least three of four criteria (i.e., tolerance, withdrawal, persistent desire, or an unsuccessful

CLINICAL PRESENTATION Excessive Caffeine Intake

General

- The patient may not be in acute distress.

Symptoms

- The patient may complain of nausea, vomiting, diarrhea, and psychomotor agitation, and can appear restless, nervous, and excited.

Signs

- The patient can present with facial flushing, diuresis, and muscle twitching.
- Tachycardia or cardiac arrhythmias can also occur.

Laboratory Tests

- Caffeine serum concentrations are rarely used clinically.

attempt to reduce consumption and persistent use despite adverse psychological or physical consequences). Of 99 people screened, 27 were evaluated by means of a structured psychiatric interview modified for the diagnosis of caffeine dependence; 16 of those subjects (59%) met the criteria. In a second phase of the study, 11 of the 16 caffeine-dependent individuals participated in a 2-day double-blind crossover study of caffeine deprivation. Nine showed evidence of caffeine withdrawal during the placebo phase.

Caffeine Withdrawal

The frequency of the caffeine withdrawal syndrome is not well known, but it may be common. Withdrawal can occur when individuals who previously consumed caffeine on a regular basis suddenly discontinue its intake.[66] The syndrome is characterized by the occurrence of headache, drowsiness, fatigue, and sometimes impaired psychomotor performance, difficulty concentrating, nausea, excessive yawning, and craving. These symptoms usually appear within 18 to 24 hours of discontinuation, corresponding to the time required for the drug to leave the body.

The caffeine withdrawal headache is somewhat unique, starting with a sense of fullness in the head and progressing to throbbing and diffuse pain that is made worse by movement. The maximum intensity of the pain occurs 3 to 6 hours after beginning.

When caffeine is reintroduced, relief of withdrawal symptoms tends to occur within 30 to 60 minutes. At present, this appears to be the most effective "treatment" for the caffeine withdrawal syndrome.

Effect on Sleep

Caffeine interferes with sleep in most nontolerant individuals.[59] Tolerant people are much less likely to self-report sleep abnormalities, or they may sense that the insomnia has disappeared altogether. To illustrate, 53% of those consuming less than 250 mg/day agreed that caffeine before bedtime would prevent sleep, compared with 43% of those consuming 250 to 749 mg/day, and only 22% of those taking 750 mg/day or more. Even though the higher-level consumers denied that caffeine interferes with their sleep, studies done in the sleep laboratory confirm that caffeine consumers do have greater sleep latency, more frequent awakenings, and altered sleep architecture, and that these effects are dose related.

Caffeine During Pregnancy

Over the years there has been much discussion on whether or not caffeine intake during pregnancy is harmful to the developing fetus. Results of research have been mixed, but, in general, caffeine has not been shown to be a potent and consistent teratogen. Kuczkowski[67] published an evidence-based review highlighting the implications of caffeine intake in pregnancy and offering recommendations for practitioners providing peripartum care to expectant mothers who consume caffeine. The author concluded that, for the healthy pregnant adult, moderate daily caffeine intake at a dose level up to 400 mg/day is not associated with adverse effects such as general toxicity, cardiovascular effects, effects on bone status and calcium balance, changes in adult behavior, increased incidence of cancer, or effects on fertility. The study did not identify any significant positive associations between maternal caffeine consumption and cardiovascular malformations.

The March of Dimes advises women to limit their caffeine intake to less than 200 mg/day. This recommendation was prompted by the results of a population-based prospective cohort study published in March 2008[68] showing that pregnant women consuming 200 mg or more of caffeine a day had double the risk of miscarriage compared with those who had no caffeine. Criticism of this study was swift to follow, and its conclusions have been called into question.

A Cochrane systematic review[69] points out that authors of some observational studies have concluded that caffeine intake is harmful to the fetus. The review concludes that there is insufficient evidence from RCTs to support any reason to avoid caffeine during pregnancy. Unfortunately, this review is based on only one published controlled trial.

Caffeine and Headaches

A Norwegian study[70] investigated the association between caffeine consumption and headache in the general adult population. Results were based on cross-sectional data from 50,483 (55%) out of 92,566 invited participants aged greater than or equal to 20 years. A weak but significant association (OR 1.16; 95% CI 1.09 to 1.23) was found between high caffeine consumption and infrequent headaches. In contrast, headache for greater than 14 days/mo was less likely among individuals with high caffeine consumption compared with those with low caffeine consumption. The authors speculate that their results may indicate that high caffeine consumption changes chronic headache into infrequent headache due to the analgesic properties of caffeine. Alternatively, chronic headache sufferers tend to avoid intake of caffeine to not aggravate their headaches, whereas individuals with infrequent headache are less aware that high caffeine use can be a cause.

TREATMENT

Desired Outcomes

Many people drink coffee, tea, and other caffeinated beverages without problems. When adverse health effects do occur (e.g., insomnia, headaches, anxiety, palpitations), it may be necessary to cut down on the amount of caffeine ingested or to eliminate it altogether to achieve the goal of elimination of these symptoms.

Caffeinism

Caffeinism is treated by reducing or discontinuing the drug. It may be necessary to wean the patient off the drug gradually because going "cold turkey" can produce such serious symptoms that the drug must be restarted. Decaffeinated beverages can be substituted slowly for the caffeinated type. However, relapses are less likely to occur when the drug is discontinued all at once, probably because of the considerable self-discipline required to continue weaning the drug when one knows that an increase in dose will cause the symptoms to abate.

ABBREVIATIONS

ADS	Alcohol Dependence Scale
AHRQ	Agency for Healthcare Research and Quality
BAC	blood alcohol concentration
CIWA-AR	Clinical Institute Withdrawal Assessment for Alcohol, Revised
CT	computed tomography
DSM-IV-TR	*Diagnostic and Statistical Manual of Mental Disorders, Fourth Edition, Text Revision*
GABA	γ-aminobutyric acid
5-HT_3	serotonin-3
NHIS	National Health Interview Survey
NMDA	*N*-methyl-D-aspartate
NRT	nicotine replacement therapy
NSDUH	National Survey on Drug Use and Health
RCT	randomized controlled trial
SR	sustained release

REFERENCES

1. Centers for Disease Control and Prevention. State-specific smoking-attributable mortality and years of potential life lost—United States, 2000–2004. MMWR Morb Mortal Wkly Rep 2009;58:29–33.
2. Centers for Disease Control and Prevention. Health, United States, 2008. Hyattsville, MD: Centers for Disease Control and Prevention, National Center for Health Statistics, 2009.
3. Center for Disease Control and Prevention. The Health Consequences of Smoking: A Report from the Surgeon General. Atlanta, GA: U.S. Department of Health and Human Services, CDC, 2004.
4. Substance Abuse and Mental Health Services Administration. Results from the 2011 National Survey on Drug Use and Health: Summary of National Findings, NSDUH Series H-44 HHS Publication No. (SMA) 12-4713. Rockville, MD: Substance Abuse and Mental Health Services Administration, 2012.
5. World Health Organization, Department of Mental Health and Substance Abuse. Global Status Report on Alcohol and Health. Geneva: World Health Organization. *http://www.who.int/substance_abuse/publications/global_alcohol_report/msbgsruprofiles.pdf.*
6. Substance Abuse and Mental Health Services Administration, Center for Behavioral Health Statistics and Quality. The DAWN Report: Highlights of the 2010 Drug Abuse Warning Network (DAWN) Findings on Drug-Related Emergency Department Visits. Rockville, MD: Substance Abuse and Mental Health Services Administration, July 2, 2012.
7. Alcohol-Related Disease Impact (ARDI) Dataset. National Center for Chronic Disease Prevention and Health Promotion, Alcohol and Public Health, Centers for Disease Control and Prevention. *http://apps.nccd.cdc.gov/DACH_ARDI/Default/Default.aspx.*
8. Bouchery EE, Harwood HJ, Sacks JJ, et al. Economic costs of excessive alcohol consumption in the U.S., 2006. Am J Prev Med 2011;41:516–524.
9. Genung V. Understanding the neurobiology, assessment, and treatment of substances of abuse and dependence: A guide for the critical care nurse. Crit Care Nurs Clin North Am 2012;24:117–130.
10. American Psychiatric Association. Diagnostic and Statistical Manual of Mental Disorders, Fourth Edition, Text Revision. Washington, DC: American Psychiatric Association, 2000:212–214.
11. Enoch MA. The influence of gene–environment interactions on the development of alcoholism and drug dependence. Curr Psychiatry Rep 2012;14:150–158.
12. Bierut LJ. Genetic vulnerability and susceptibility to substance dependence. Neuron 2011;69:618–627.
13. Agrawal A, Verweij KJ, Gillespie NA, et al. The genetics of addiction—A translational perspective. Transl Psychiatry 2012;2:e140. doi:10.1038/tp.2012.54.
14. Luo X, Kranzler HR, Zuo L, et al. Diplotype trend regression analysis of the ADH gene cluster and the ALDH2 gene: Multiple significant associations with alcohol dependence. Am J Hum Genet 2006;78:973–987.
15. Krystal JH, Staley J, Mason G, et al. Gamma-aminobutyric acid type A receptors and alcoholism: Intoxication, dependence, vulnerability, and treatment. Arch Gen Psychiatry 2006;63:957–968.
16. Kugelberg FC, Jones AW. Interpreting results of ethanol analysis in postmortem specimens: A review of the literature. Forensic Sci Int 2007;165:10–29.
17. Zakhari S. Overview: How is alcohol metabolized by the body? Alcohol Res Health 2006;29:245–254.
18. Jones AW. Evidence-based survey of the elimination rates of ethanol from blood with applications in forensic casework. Forensic Sci Int 2010;200:1–20 [Epub March 20, 2010].
19. Dhalla S, Kopec JA. The CAGE questionnaire for alcohol misuse: A review of reliability and validity studies. Clin Invest Med 2007;30:33–41.
20. Mayo-Smith MF. Pharmacological management of alcohol withdrawal. A meta-analysis and evidence-based practice guideline. American Society of Addiction Medicine Working Group on Pharmacological Management of Alcohol Withdrawal. JAMA 1997;278:144–151.
21. Mayo-Smith MF, Beecher LH, Fischer TL, et al. Working Group on the Management of Alcohol Withdrawal Delirium, Practice Guidelines Committee, American Society of Addiction Medicine. Management of alcohol withdrawal delirium. An evidence-based practice guideline. Arch Intern Med 2004;164:1405–1412 [Erratum. Arch Intern Med 2004;164:2068].
22. Amato L, Minozzi S, Vecchi S, Davoli M. Benzodiazepines for alcohol withdrawal. Cochrane Database Syst Rev 2010;(3):CD005063.
23. McMicken D, Liss JL. Alcohol-related seizures. Emerg Med Clin North Am 2011;29:117–124.
24. Garbutt JC. The state of pharmacotherapy for the treatment of alcohol dependence. J Subst Abuse Treat 2009;36: S15–S23 [quiz S24–S25].
25. Unterwald EM. Naltrexone in the treatment of alcohol dependence in the treatment of alcohol dependence. J Addict Med 2008;2:121–127.
26. Garbutt JC, Kranzler HR, O'Malley SS, et al. Vivitrex Study Group. Efficacy and tolerability of long-acting injectable naltrexone for alcohol dependence: A randomized controlled

trial. JAMA 2005;293:1617–1625 [Erratum. JAMA 2005;293:1978; Erratum. JAMA 2005;293:2864].

27. Pettinati HM, Silverman BL, Battisti JJ, et al. Efficacy of extended-release naltrexone in patients with relatively higher severity of alcohol dependence. Alcohol Clin Exp Res 2011;35(10):1804–1811. doi:10.1111/j.1530-0277.2011.01524.x [Epub May 16, 2011].
28. Rösner S, Hackl-Herrwerth A, Leucht S, et al. Acamprosate for alcohol dependence. Cochrane Database Syst Rev 2010;(9):CD004332.
29. Fiore MC, Baily WC. Treating Tobacco Use and Dependence. Clinical Practice Guidelines. Rockville, MD: U.S. Department of Health and Human Services, Public Health Service, June 2000 [updated May 2008].
30. Pierce J, Cummins S. Quitlines and nicotine replacement for smoking cessation: Do we need to change policy? Annu Rev Public Health 2012;33:341–356.
31. Jamal A, Dube SR, Malarcher AM, Shaw L, Engstrom MC; Centers for Disease Control and Prevention. Tobacco use screening and counseling during physician office visits among adults—National Ambulatory Medical Care Survey and National Health Interview Survey, United States, 2005-2009. MMWR Morb Mortal Wkly Rep 2012;61(Suppl):38–45.
32. Centers for Disease Control and Prevention. Vital signs: Current cigarette smoking among adults aged ≤ 18 years—United States, 2005-2010. MMWR Morb Mortal Wkly Rep 2011;60(35):1207–1212.
33. Centers for Disease Control and Prevention. Quitting smoking among adults—United States, 2001–2010. MMWR Morb Mortal Wkly Rep 2011;60:1513–1519.
34. Runberger J, Hollenbeak C, Kline D. Potential Costs and Benefits of Smoking Cessation: An Overview of the Approach to State Specific Analysis. 2010, *http://www.lung.org/stop-smoking/tobacco-control-advocacy/reports-resources/cessation-economic-benefits/reports/US.pdf*.
35. Armour BS, Finkelstein EA. State-level Medicaid expenditures attributable to smoking. Prev Chronic Dis 2009;6:A84.
36. U.S. Department of Health and Human Services. The Health Consequences of Involuntary Exposure to Tobacco Smoke: A Report of the Surgeon General. Atlanta, GA: U.S. Department of Health and Human Services, Centers for Disease Control and Prevention, Coordinating Center for Health Promotion, National Center for Chronic Disease Prevention and Health Promotion, Office on Smoking and Health, 2006, *http://www.surgeongeneral.gov/library/secondhandsmoke/report/citation.pdf*.
37. Balfour DJ. Neuroplasticity within the mesoaccumbens dopamine system and its role in tobacco dependence. Curr Drug Targets CNS Neurol Disord 2002;1:413–421.
38. Benowitz NL. Clinical pharmacology of nicotine implications for understanding, preventing, and treating tobacco addiction. Clin Pharmacol Ther 2008;83:531–541.
39. Benowitz N. Pharmacology of nicotine: Addiction, smoking-induced disease, and therapeutics. Annu Rev Pharmacol Toxicol 2009;49:57–71.
40. Ranney L, Melvin C. Systematic review: Smoking cessation intervention strategies for adults and adults in special populations. Ann Intern Med 2006;145:845–856.
41. Aveyard P, Begh R, Parsons A, West R. Brief opportunistic smoking cessation interventions: A systematic review and meta analysis to compare advice to quit and offer of assistance. Addiction 2012;107:1066–1073.
42. Lai DT, Cahill K, Qin Y, Tang JL. Motivational interviewing for smoking cessation. Cochrane Database Syst Rev 2010;(1):CD006936.
43. Perera S, Bullen C. Nicotine replacement therapy for smoking cessation [review]. Cochrane Collaboration 2009;4:1–163.
44. Piper ME, Smith SS. A randomized placebo-controlled clinical trial of 5 smoking cessation pharmacotherapies. Arch Gen Psychiatry 2009;66:1253–1262.
45. McRobbie H, Thornley S. The importance of treating tobacco dependence. Rev Esp Cardiol 2008;6:620–628.
46. Fossati R, Apolone G. A double-blind placebo-controlled randomized trial of bupropion for smoking cessation in primary care. Arch Intern Med 2007;167:1791–1797.
47. Hughes JR, Stead LF. Antidepressants for smoking cessation. Cochrane Database Syst Rev 2011;(2):CD000031.
48. Williams J. Review of varenicline for tobacco dependence: Panacea or plight? Expert Opin Pharmacother 2011;12: 1799–1812.
49. Cahill K, Stead LF, Lancaster T. Nicotine receptor partial agonists for smoking cessation. Cochrane Database Syst Rev 2011;4:CD006103.
50. FDA Public Health Advisory. Important Information on Chantix (Varenicline). 2008, *http://www.fda.gov/Drugs/DrugSafety/PostmarketDrugSafetyInformationforPatientsandProviders/DrugSafetyInformationforHeathcareProfessionals/PublicHealthAdvisories/ucm051136.htm*.
51. FDA Public Health Advisory. FDA Requires New Boxed Warnings for the Smoking Cessation Drugs Chantix and Zyban. 2009, *http://www.fda.gov/Drugs/DrugSafety/PostmarketDrugSafetyInformationforPatientsandProviders/DrugSafetyInformationforHeathcareProfessionals/PublicHealthAdvisories/ucm169988.htm*.
52. FDA. FDA Drug Safety Communication: Safety Review Update of Chantix (Varenicline) and Risk of Neuropsychiatric Adverse Events. October 24, 2011, *http://www.fda.gov/Drugs/DrugSafety/ucm276737.htm*.
53. Food and Drug Administration. FDA Drug Safety Communication: Chantix (Varenicline) may Increase the Risk of Certain Cardiovascular Adverse Events in Patients with Cardiovascular Disease. July 2011, *http://www.fda.gov/Drugs/Drugsafety/ucm259161.htm*.
54. Prochaska JJ, Hilton JF. Risk of cardiovascular serious adverse events associated with varenicline use for tobacco cessation: Systematic review and meta-analysis. BMJ 2012;344:e2856. doi:10.1136/bmj.e2856.
55. Mills E, Wu P, Lockhart I, Thorlund K, Puhan M, Ebbert JO. Comparisons of high dose and combination nicotine replacement therapy, varenicline, and bupropion for smoking cessation: A systematic review and multiple treatment meta-analysis. Ann Med 2012;44:588–597.
56. Gourlay SG, Stead LF, Benowitz NL. Clonidine for smoking cessation. Cochrane Database Syst Rev 2004;(3):CD000058.
57. Raupach T, Hoogsteder PH, Onno van Schayck CP. Nicotine vaccines to assist with smoking cessation: Current status of research. Drugs 2012;72:e1–e16.
58. Ho MK, Tyndale RF. Overview of the pharmacogenomics of cigarette smoking. Pharmacogenomics J 2007;7:81–98.
59. Juliano LM, Evatt DP, Richards BD, Griffiths RR. Characterization of individuals seeking treatment for caffeine dependence. Psychol Addict Behav 2012;26:948–954. doi:10.1037/a0027246.
60. Packaged Facts Market Research Group. *http://www.packagedfacts.com/about/release.asp?id=2601*.
61. Warzak WJ, Evans S, Floress MT, et al. Caffeine consumption in young children. J Pediatr 2011;158:508–509.
62. Malinauskas BM, Aeby VG, Overton RF, et al. A survey of energy drink consumption patterns among college students. Nutr J 2007;6:35.

63. ALCOSPEED (Alcoholic Energy Drinks). Center for Science in the Public Interest. *http://www.cspinet.org/new/pdf/alcospeedfactsheet.pdf*.
64. The Energy Fiend. *http://www.energyfiend.com/the-caffeine-database*.
65. Strain EC, Mumford GK, Silverman K, Griffiths RR. Caffeine dependence syndrome. Evidence from case histories and experimental evaluations. JAMA 1994;272:1043–1048.
66. Juliano LM, Huntley ED, Harrell PT, Westerman AT. Development of the Caffeine Withdrawal Symptom Questionnaire: Caffeine withdrawal symptoms cluster into 7 factors. Drug Alcohol Depend 2012;124:229–234 [Epub February 15, 2012].
67. Kuczkowski KM. Caffeine in pregnancy. Arch Gynecol Obstet 2009;280:695–698.
68. Weng X, Odouli R, Li DK. Maternal caffeine consumption during pregnancy and the risk of miscarriage: A prospective cohort study. Am J Obstet Gynecol 2008;198:279.e1–279.e8.
69. Jahanfar S, Jaafar SH. Effects of restricted caffeine intake by mother on fetal, neonatal and pregnancy outcome. Cochrane Database Syst Rev 2009;2:CD006965. doi:10.1002/14651858.CD006965.pub2.
70. Hagen K, Thoresen K, Stovner LJ, Zwart JA. High dietary caffeine consumption is associated with a modest increase in headache prevalence: Results from the Head-HUNT Study. J Headache Pain 2009;10:153–159.

50

Schizophrenia

M. Lynn Crismon, Tami R. Argo, and Peter F. Buckley

KEY CONCEPTS

1. Although multiple neurotransmitter dysfunctions are involved in schizophrenia, the etiology is more likely mediated by multiple subcellular processes that are influenced by different genetic polymorphisms.
2. The clinical presentation of schizophrenia is characterized by positive symptoms, negative symptoms, and impairment in cognitive functioning.
3. Comprehensive care for individuals with schizophrenia must occur in the context of a multidisciplinary mental healthcare environment that offers comprehensive psychosocial services in addition to psychotropic medication management.
4. A thorough patient evaluation (e.g., history, mental status examination, physical examination, psychiatric diagnostic interview, and laboratory analysis) should occur to establish a diagnosis of schizophrenia and to identify potential co-occurring disorders, including substance abuse and general medical disorders.
5. Given that it is challenging to differentiate among antipsychotics based on efficacy, side effect profiles become important in choosing an antipsychotic for an individual patient.
6. Pharmacotherapy guidelines should emphasize monotherapies with antipsychotics of optimal efficacy-to-side effect ratios and progress to medications with greater side effect risks, and combination regimens should only be used in the most treatment-resistant patients.
7. Adequate time on a given medication at a therapeutic dose is the most important variable in predicting medication response.
8. Long-term maintenance antipsychotic treatment is necessary for the vast majority of patients with schizophrenia in order to prevent relapse.
9. Thorough patient and family psychoeducation should be implemented, and methods such as motivational interviewing that focus on patient-driven outcomes that allow patients to achieve life goals should be employed.
10. Pharmacotherapy decisions should be guided by systematic monitoring of patient symptoms, preferably with the use of brief symptom rating scales and systematic assessment of potential adverse effects.

Schizophrenia is one of the most complex and challenging of psychiatric disorders. It represents a heterogeneous syndrome of disorganized and bizarre thoughts, delusions, hallucinations, inappropriate affect, and impaired psychosocial functioning. From the time that Kraepelin first described dementia praecox in 1896 until publication of the *Diagnostic and Statistical Manual of Mental Disorders, Fourth Edition, Text Revision* (*DSM-IV-TR*) in 2000, the description of this illness has continuously evolved.[1] Scientific advances that increase our knowledge of CNS physiology, pathophysiology, and genetics will likely improve our understanding of schizophrenia in the future.

EPIDEMIOLOGY

According to the Epidemiologic Catchment Area Study, the lifetime prevalence of schizophrenia using strict diagnostic criteria ranges from 0.6% to 1.9%. If a broader definition is used, the lifetime rate rises to 2% to 3%.[2] The worldwide prevalence of schizophrenia is remarkably similar among most cultures. Schizophrenia most commonly has its onset in late adolescence or early adulthood and rarely occurs before adolescence or after the age of 40 years. Although the prevalence of schizophrenia is equal in males and females, the onset of illness tends to be earlier in males. Males most frequently have their first episode during their early 20s, whereas with females it is usually during their late 20s to early 30s.[1,3]

ETIOLOGY

Although the etiology of schizophrenia is unknown, research has demonstrated various abnormalities in brain structure and function.[4] However, these changes are not consistent among all individuals with schizophrenia. The cause of schizophrenia is likely multifactorial, that is, multiple pathophysiologic abnormalities can play a role in producing the similar but varying clinical phenotypes we refer to as schizophrenia.

A neurodevelopmental model has been evoked as one possible explanation for the etiology of schizophrenia.[4] This model proposes that schizophrenia has its origins in some as yet unknown in utero disturbance, possibly occurring during the second trimester of pregnancy. Evidence for this is provided by the abnormal neuronal migration demonstrated in studies of schizophrenic brains. This "schizophrenic lesion" can result in abnormalities in cell shape, position, symmetry, connectivity, and functionally to the development of abnormal brain circuits.[4] Changes are consistent with a cell migration abnormality during the second trimester of pregnancy, and some studies associate upper respiratory infections during the second trimester of pregnancy with a higher incidence of schizophrenia.[5] Other studies associate low birth weight (LBW; less than 2.5 kg [5.5 lb]), obstetric complications, or neonatal hypoxia with schizophrenia.[2] Maternal stress, perhaps related to the effects of circulating glucocorticoids in utero, may be a risk factor for schizophrenia. Maternal "stress" could derive from a variety of external and internal noxious events (malnutrition, infection, etc.).

The resulting secondary "synaptic disorganization" associated with such insults is thought not to produce overt clinical manifestations of psychosis until adolescence or early adulthood because this is the corresponding time period of neuronal maturation.

Although studies have shown decreased cortical thickness and increased ventricular size in the brains of many patients with schizophrenia, this occurs in the absence of widespread gliosis.[4] One hypothesis is that obstetric complications and hypoxia, in combination with a genetic predisposition, could activate a glutamatergic cascade that results in increased neuronal pruning. It is hypothesized that this genetic predisposition may be related to genes controlling *N*-methyl-D-aspartate (NMDA) receptor activity. As a part of the normal neurodevelopmental process, pruning of dendrites occurs. In normal individuals, approximately 35% of the peak number of dendrites at 2 years of age are pruned by midadolescence. Some studies have shown a higher percentage of pruning in individuals with schizophrenia. Furthermore, synaptic pruning predominantly involves glutamatergic dendrites. Hypoxia or other prenatal insult can result in a decreased number of basal neurons from which to start, and glutamatergic activation can exaggerate the pruning process.[4,5] There is also renewed interest in the immune system and schizophrenia. Studies have shown an increased susceptibility to immune/autoimmune disorders in schizophrenia, as well as abnormalities of autoantibodies and cytokine functioning.[6] The immune hypothesis of schizophrenia also emphasizes integration of mental and physical well-being.

Numerous studies have shown neuropsychological abnormalities and impairment in reaching normal motor milestones and abnormal movements in young children who later develop schizophrenia.[3] Abnormalities in brain function occur long before the onset of psychotic symptomatology and provide empirical evidence for schizophrenia being a neurodevelopmental disorder.[4] However, the progressive clinical deterioration in many patients suggests that this illness can also have a neurodegenerative component. This is consistent with recent brain imaging studies that show deteriorative brain changes in patients with frequent relapses.[2,4,7] These changes may be most pronounced among adolescents with early onset schizophrenia.[8] Schizophrenia may be an illness exhibiting neurodegenerative propensity based on a vulnerable neurodevelopmental predisposition.[2,9,10] Although a specific abnormality has not been discovered, evidence suggests a genetic basis for schizophrenia. Although the risk of developing schizophrenia is 0.6% to 1.9% in the U.S. population, the risk is approximately 10% if a first-degree relative has the illness and 3% if a second-degree relative has the illness.[2,11] If both parents have schizophrenia, the risk of producing an offspring with schizophrenia increases to approximately 40%. Twin studies in dizygotic twins report that the risk of the second twin developing schizophrenia if one twin has the illness is between 12% and 14%. However, in monozygotic twins the risk increases to 48%.[11] Numerous adoption studies indicate that the risk for schizophrenia lies with the biologic parents, and change in the environment during the child's developmental stages does not alter this. If schizophrenia occurs in siblings, the onset of illness tends to occur at the same age in each, thus lessening the possibility of an environmental precipitant.

Numerous approaches have been utilized to study the genetics of schizophrenia, including genome-wide association studies (GWAS), copy number variant (CNV) studies, and gene candidate studies.[12] Genetic etiologies in schizophrenia are likely heterogeneous, but present with similar clinical phenotypes, and involve epigenetic interactions.[12] GWAS have identified nearly 20 genetic loci that reach genome-wide significance ($P = 5 \times 10^{-8}$), but only some of these have been replicated in multiple studies.[13] GWAS indicate susceptible genes for schizophrenia on chromosome 6, and common genes underlying psychosis on ZNF804A, CACN1A2, NRGN, and PBRM1.[12] Risk for schizophrenia has been demonstrated in CNV studies for deletions on chromosomes 1, 15, and 22. Polymorphism in the *VAL/MET* alleles of the catecholamine-*O*-methyl transferase gene may explain some of the frontal lobe functional deficits in a subset of individuals with schizophrenia.[11] Other recent studies have shown abnormalities in several genes that code for neurodevelopment and for trophic factors.[11,14] For example, dysbindin is a neurodevelopmental protein gene that is found on chromosome 6, and it has been termed a NMDA-related schizophrenia susceptibility gene.[15] Alleles associated with decreased dysbindin RNA in the dorsolateral prefrontal cortex have been reported in patients with schizophrenia and their families.[15] Another recent GWAS of a large pedigree showed increased signal at chromosome 8p, close to the gene that encodes for neuregulin—another neurodevelopmental gene. Interest is burgeoning regarding how genetic vulnerability might interact with environmental stressors, such as cannabis abuse.[16]

PATHOPHYSIOLOGY

Advances in imaging technology and changes in research methodology have resulted in varying results from brain imagining studies over time, although most recent studies have found decreases in gray matter and increases in ventricular size. A recent meta-analysis of systematic reviews conducted since the year 2000 found consistent decreases in gray matter in multiple brain areas, including the frontal lobes, cingulate gyri, and medial temporal regions among others. A corresponding increase in ventricular size was also observed as well as decreased white matter in the corpus callosum.[17] Changes in hippocampal volume may correspond with impairment in neuropsychological testing.[2] Rather than a decrease in the number of neurons in affected brain areas, a decrease in axonal and dendritic communications between cells can result in a loss of connectivity that can be important with respect to neuronal adaptivity and CNS homeostasis.[2,4] These changes are likely consistent with the evidence for abnormal neuronal pruning.[4] Four dopaminergic pathways and five major dopamine (DA) receptor subtypes are of primary interest. Table 50-1 outlines the origin, innervation, and primary functional activity of each pathway, as well as the effects of DA antagonists.[18]

TABLE 50-1 Dopaminergic Tracts and Effects of Dopamine Antagonists

Dopamine Tract	Origin	Innervation	Function	Dopamine Antagonist Effect
Nigrostriatal	Substantia nigra (A9 area)	Dorsal striatum	Extrapyramidal system, movement	Movement disorders
Mesolimbic	Midbrain ventral tegmentum (A10 area)	Nucleus accumbens, hippocampus, and amygdala	Emotional functioning, motivational behavior	Relief of psychosis
Mesocortical	Midbrain ventral tegmentum (A10 area)	Frontal and prefrontal lobe cortex	Cognition, executive function	Relief of psychosis? Akathisia?
Tuberohypophyseal	Hypothalamus	Pituitary gland	Regulates prolactin release	Increased prolactin concentrations

Data from reference 18.

Evidence supports the presence of a DA-receptor defect in schizophrenia. Numerous positron emission tomography (PET) studies have shown regional brain abnormalities, including increased glucose metabolism in the caudate nucleus and decreased blood flow and glucose metabolism in the frontal lobe and left temporal lobe.[3] This can indicate dopaminergic hyperactivity in the head of the caudate nucleus and dopaminergic hypofunction in the frontotemporal regions. PET studies using dopamine-2 (D_2)-specific ligands suggest increased densities of D_2 receptors in the head of the caudate nucleus with decreased densities in the prefrontal cortex.[3,4] However, a recent meta-analysis showed an increase in presynaptic DA synthesis and release in the striatum with only a small increase in $D_{2/3}$ receptor availability.[19] PET studies assessing dopamine-1 (D_1) function suggest that subpopulations of schizophrenics may have decreased densities of D_1 receptors in the caudate nucleus and the prefrontal cortex. Hypofrontality can be associated with lack of volition and cognitive dysfunction, core features of schizophrenia. It is unknown whether these changes represent a primary event or secondary processes related to other pathophysiologic abnormalities in schizophrenia. Because of the heterogeneity in the clinical presentation of schizophrenia, it has been suggested that the DA hypothesis may be more applicable to "neuroleptic-responsive psychosis," with multiple different etiologies possibly being responsible for causing schizophrenia.[2] Attempts have been made to develop relationships between these abnormal findings and behavioral symptoms present in schizophrenic patients. The positive symptoms are possibly more closely associated with DA-receptor hyperactivity in the mesocaudate, whereas negative symptoms and cognitive impairment are most closely related to DA-receptor hypofunction in the prefrontal cortex. Presynaptic D_1 receptors in the prefrontal cortex are thought to be involved in modulating glutamatergic activity, and this can be important with regard to working memory in individuals with schizophrenia.[2]

The glutamatergic system is one of the most widespread excitatory neurotransmitter systems in the brain. Alterations in its function, either hypoactivity or hyperactivity, can result in toxic neuronal reactions.[3] Dopaminergic innervation from the ventral striatum decreases the limbic system's inhibitory activity (perhaps through γ-aminobutyric acid [GABA] interneurons); thus, dopaminergic stimulation increases arousal. The corticostriatal glutamate pathways have the opposite effect, inhibiting dopaminergic function from the ventral striatum, therefore allowing the limbic system to have increased inhibitory activity. Descending glutamatergic tracts interact with dopaminergic tracts directly as well as through GABA interneurons. Glutamatergic deficiency produces symptoms similar to those of dopaminergic hyperactivity and possibly those seen in schizophrenia. Clinical support for this comes from the fact that phencyclidine, a potent psychotomimetic, is a noncompetitive antagonist at the NMDA receptor, a major glutamate receptor. Similarly, abuse of ketamine, a veterinary anesthetic, can resemble schizophrenia. Ketamine, a competitive antagonist at glutamatergic NMDA receptors, has been shown to lead to reduction in D_1 neurotransmission through glutamatergic inhibition of DA release.[20] It is proposed that schizophrenia may involve some in utero assault that leads to a developmental defect in NMDA receptor function—so-called NMDA hypofunction. This defect is proposed to have latent clinical expression with the psychotic manifestations from NMDA hypofunction not being seen until late adolescence or early adulthood. MicroRNAs, small noncoding RNAs, are critical to neurodevelopment as well as to regulation of adult neuronal processes. NMDA-regulated microRNA miR-132 is significantly downregulated in individuals with schizophrenia as compared with controls. Several genes are regulated by miR-132, and this altered expression may be related to NMDA hypofunction and the abnormal synaptic pruning seen in the brains of individuals with schizophrenia.[21]

Serotoninergic receptors are present on dopaminergic axons, and stimulation of these receptors decreases DA release, at least in the striatum.[22] Although somewhat more diffuse, the distribution of serotonergic neurons is similar to that of dopaminergic neurons, thus allowing these two neurotransmitter systems to innervate the same areas. In fact, 5-hydroxytryptamine$_2$ (serotonin-2; 5-HT$_2$) receptors and D_4 receptors have been found to be colocalized in the cortex.[2,22] Patients with schizophrenia with abnormal brain scans have higher whole-blood serotonin (5-HT) concentrations, and these concentrations are correlated with increased ventricular size.[22]

❶ Schizophrenia is a complex disorder, and multiple etiologies likely exist. Based on current knowledge, it is naive to think that any currently proposed etiology can adequately explain the genesis of this complex disease. Molecular research involving genetically determined subtle changes in microRNA, G proteins, protein metabolism, and other subcellular processes can eventually identify the biologic disturbances associated with schizophrenia.[2,4,9,21]

CLINICAL PRESENTATION

Schizophrenia is the most common functional psychosis, and great variability occurs in clinical presentation. Despite numerous attempts to portray a stereotype in movies and on television, the stereotypic schizophrenic essentially does not exist. Moreover, schizophrenia is not a "split personality." It is a chronic disorder of thought and affect with the individual having a significant disturbance in interpersonal relationships and ability to function in society.

The first psychotic episode can be sudden in onset with few premorbid symptoms, or commonly can be preceded by withdrawn, suspicious, peculiar behavior (schizoid). During acute psychotic episodes, the patient loses touch with reality, and in a sense, the brain creates a false reality to replace it. Acute psychotic symptoms can include hallucinations (especially hearing voices), delusions (fixed false beliefs), and ideas of influence (beliefs that one's actions are controlled by external influences). Thought processes are disconnected (loose associations), the patient may not be able to carry on logical conversation (alogia), and can have simultaneous contradictory thoughts (ambivalence). The patient's affect can be flat (no emotional expression), or it can be inappropriate and labile. The patient is often withdrawn and inwardly directed (autism). Uncooperativeness, hostility, and verbal or physical aggression can be seen because of the patient's misperception of reality. Self-care skills are impaired, and the patient is frequently dirty and unkempt, and in general has poor hygiene. Sleep and appetite are often disturbed. When the acute psychotic episode remits, the patient typically has residual features. This is an important point in differentiating schizophrenia from other psychotic disorders. Although residual symptoms and their severity vary, patients can have difficulty with anxiety management, suspiciousness, and lack of volition, motivation, insight, and judgment. Therefore, they often have difficulty living independently in the community. Because of poor anxiety management and suspiciousness, they are frequently withdrawn socially, and have difficulty forming close relationships with others. In addition, impaired volition and motivation contribute to poor self-care skills and make it difficult for the patient with schizophrenia to maintain employment.

Patients with schizophrenia frequently experience a lack of historicity, or difficulty in learning from their experiences. They can repeatedly make the same mistakes in social conduct and situations requiring judgment. They have difficulty understanding the importance of treatment, including medications, in maintaining their ability to function in society. Therefore, they tend to discontinue medications and other treatments, and this increases the risk of relapse and rehospitalization. The co-occurrence of substance abuse (predominantly alcohol or polysubstance—alcohol, cannabis,

TABLE 50-2 *DSM-IV-TR* Diagnostic Criteria for Schizophrenia

A. Characteristic symptoms: Two or more of the following, each persisting for a significant portion of at least a 1-month period:
   1. Delusions
   2. Hallucinations
   3. Disorganized speech
   4. Grossly disorganized or catatonic behavior
   5. Negative symptoms

Note: Only one criterion A symptom is required if delusions are bizarre or if hallucinations consist of a voice keeping a running commentary on the person's behavior or two or more voices conversing with each other

B. Social/occupational dysfunction: For a significant portion of the time since onset of the disorder, one or more major areas of functioning such as work, interpersonal relations, or self-care are significantly below the level prior to onset
C. Duration: Continuous signs of the disorder for at least 6 months. This must include at least 1 month of symptoms fulfilling criterion A (unless successfully treated). This 6-month period may include prodromal or residual symptoms
D. Schizoaffective or mood disorder has been excluded
E. Disorder is not due to a medical disorder or substance use
F. If a history of a pervasive developmental disorder is present, there must be symptoms of hallucinations or delusions present for at least 1 month

DSM-IV-TR, Diagnostic and Statistical Manual of Mental Disorders, Fourth Edition, Text Revision.

Reprinted with permission from the Diagnostic and Statistical Manual of Mental Disorders. 4th ed. Text Revision (Copyright © 2000). American Psychiatric Association.

cocaine) in patients with schizophrenia is very common and is another frequent reason for relapse and hospitalization.[1,2] This effect can be caused by direct toxic effects of these drugs on the brain,[23] but is also caused by the medication nonadherence that is associated with substance abuse.

Although the course of schizophrenia is variable, the long-term prognosis for many patients is poor. It is marked by intermittent acute psychotic episodes and impaired psychosocial functioning between acute episodes, with most of the deterioration in psychosocial functioning occurring within 5 years after the first psychotic episode.[23] By late life, the patient can appear "burned out," that is, the patient ceases to have acute psychotic episodes, but residual symptoms persist. In a subpopulation of patients, probably 5% to 15%, psychotic symptoms are nearly continuous, and response to antipsychotics is poor.[23]

Schizophrenia is a chronic disorder, and the patient's history must be carefully assessed for dysfunction that has persisted for longer than 6 months. After their first episode, patients with schizophrenia rarely have a level of adaptive functioning as high as before the onset of the disorder. Table 50-2 summarizes the *DSM-IV-TR* criteria for schizophrenia.[1]

❷ The *DSM-IV-TR* classifies the symptoms of schizophrenia into two categories: positive and negative. Recently greater emphasis has been placed on a third symptom category, cognitive dysfunction (Table 50-3).[23] The areas of cognition found to be abnormal in schizophrenia include attention, working memory, and executive function. Positive symptoms have traditionally attracted the most attention and are the ones most improved by antipsychotics.

TABLE 50-3 Schizophrenia Symptom Clusters

Positive	Negative	Cognitive
Suspiciousness	Affective flattening	Impaired attention
Unusual thought content (delusions)	Alogia	Impaired working memory
Hallucinations	Anhedonia	Impaired executive function
Conceptual disorganization	Avolition	

Data from references 1, 24, and 131.

However, negative symptoms and impairment in cognition are more closely associated with poor psychosocial function. Along with these characteristic features of schizophrenia, many patients also have comorbid psychiatric and general medical disorders.[23] These include depression, anxiety disorders, substance abuse, and general medical disorders such as respiratory disorders, cardiovascular disorders, and metabolic disturbances. These comorbidities substantially complicate the clinical presentation and course of schizophrenia.

It has been suggested that symptom complexes can correlate with prognosis, cognitive functioning, structural abnormalities in the brain, and response to antipsychotic drugs. Negative symptoms and cognitive impairment can be more closely associated with prefrontal lobe dysfunction and positive symptoms with temporolimbic abnormalities. Many patients demonstrate both positive and negative symptoms. Patients with negative symptoms frequently have more antecedent cognitive dysfunction, poor premorbid adjustment, low level of educational achievement, and a poorer overall prognosis.[23]

TREATMENT

Desired Outcome

Pharmacotherapy is the mainstay of treatment in schizophrenia, and it is impossible in most patients to implement effective psychosocial rehabilitation programs in the absence of antipsychotic treatment.[23] ❸ A pharmacotherapeutic treatment plan should be developed that delineates drug-related aspects of therapy. Most deterioration in psychosocial functioning occurs during the first 5 years after the initial psychotic episode, and treatment should be particularly assertive during this period.[23] The individualized treatment plan created for each patient should have explicit end points defined, including realistic goals for the target symptoms most likely to respond, and the relative time course for response.[23,24] Other desired outcomes include avoiding unwanted side effects, integrating the patient back into the community, increasing adaptive functioning to the extent possible, and preventing relapse.

Nonpharmacologic Therapy

Psychosocial rehabilitation programs oriented toward improving patients' adaptive functioning are the mainstay of nondrug treatment for schizophrenia. These programs can include case management, psychoeducation, targeted cognitive therapy, basic living skills, social skills training, basic education, work programs, supported housing, and financial support. In particular, programs aimed at employment and housing have been the more effective interventions and are considered "best practices." Programs that involve families in the care and life of the patient have been shown to decrease rehospitalization and improve functioning in the community. For particularly low-functioning patients, assertive intervention programs, referred to as *active community treatment* (ACT), are effective in improving patients' functional outcomes. ACT teams are available on a 24-hour basis and work in the patient's home and place of employment to provide comprehensive treatment, including medication, crisis intervention, daily living skills, and supported employment and housing.[23,24] Medication treatment cannot be successful without proper attention to these other aspects of care. People with schizophrenia need comprehensive care, with coordination of services across psychiatric, addiction, medical, social, and rehabilitative services. The level of coordination in the United States is often insufficient, and patients become at risk to "fall through the cracks." National policy documents have called for greater coordination of care.[25] Additionally, emphasis is growing on the role that the patient plays in a recovery-based system of

TABLE 50-4 Psychotherapeutic Approaches to the Treatment of Schizophrenia

Individual	Group	Cognitive Behavioral
Supportive/counseling Personal therapy Social skills therapies Vocational sheltered employment rehabilitation therapies	Interactive/social	Cognitive behavioral therapy Compliance therapy

care, where the person's lifetime aspirations and goals become the center of care, rather than symptom reduction being the primary focus. This recovery-based approach recognizes the strengths and resilience of people with schizophrenia.[26] It also acknowledges how people with schizophrenia can also be a support to others who are coping with the illness.[27] It is important to frame clinical decision making in the context of a mutual process involving patient and clinician—rather than a unilateral "here's a prescription ... please take these tablets" approach. It is increasingly recognized that cognitive behavioral therapy can help some patients. A list of psychotherapeutic approaches to the treatment of schizophrenia is given in Table 50-4.

Pharmacologic Therapy

4 The importance of initial accurate diagnostic assessment cannot be overemphasized. A thorough mental status examination (MSE), psychiatric diagnostic interview, physical and neurologic examination, complete family and social history, and laboratory workup must be performed to confirm the diagnosis and exclude general medical or substance-induced causes of psychosis. Laboratory tests, biologic markers, and commonly available brain imaging techniques do not assist in the diagnosis of schizophrenia or selection of medication. A pretreatment patient workup not only is important in excluding other pathology but also serves as a baseline for monitoring potential medication-related side effects, and should include vital signs, complete blood count, electrolytes, hepatic function, renal function, electrocardiogram (ECG), fasting serum glucose, serum lipids, thyroid function, and urine drug screen.

Both first-generation antipsychotics (FGAs) and second-generation antipsychotics (SGAs) (with the exception of clozapine) are first-line agents in the treatment of schizophrenia.[24,28] No absolute criterion distinguishes atypical (second-generation) from typical (traditional or FGA) antipsychotics, and no universally accepted definition exists for an atypical antipsychotic.[22] Therefore, *second-generation antipsychotic* is a more appropriate term. Common to all definitions is the ability of the drug to produce antipsychotic response with few or no acutely occurring extrapyramidal side effects (EPS). Other attributes that have been ascribed to SGAs include enhanced efficacy (particularly for negative symptoms and cognition), absence or near absence of propensity to cause tardive dyskinesia, and lack of effect on serum prolactin.[22] To date, the only approved SGA that fulfills all of these criteria is clozapine.[22] Although early studies suggested that SGAs might have a superior effect on negative symptoms and cognition, this has not been confirmed in more recent studies.[2,24] The major factor in distinguishing among antipsychotics is adverse effects.[29] The major advantage of SGAs is their lower risk of neurologic side effects, particularly effects on movement. However, this is offset by increased risk of metabolic side effects with some SGAs, including weight gain, hyperlipidemias, and diabetes mellitus. 5 Side effect profiles differ among antipsychotics, and this information in combination with individual patient characteristics should be used in deciding which drug to use in an individual patient.

Results from the Clinical Antipsychotic Trials of Intervention Effectiveness (CATIE) study indicate that olanzapine, compared with quetiapine, risperidone, ziprasidone, and the FGA perphenazine, has modest, but not statistically significant, superiority in maintenance therapy when treatment persistence is the primary clinical outcome.[29] However, increased metabolic adverse effects occurred with olanzapine.

No known differences exist in efficacy between low- and high-potency FGAs. Previous patient or family history of response to an antipsychotic is helpful in the selection of an agent. Table 50-5 lists antipsychotics and their usual dosage ranges.

Published Guidelines and an Algorithm Example

6 Figure 50-1 outlines a suggested pharmacotherapeutic algorithm for schizophrenia. This algorithm is based on the compilation of three evidence-based guidelines, the 2009 update of the practice guideline from the American Psychiatric Association (APA),[30] the 2009 update of the Patient Outcomes Research Team (PORT) guidelines,[28] and the 2012 update of the guidelines from the World Federation of Biological Psychiatry.[31]

Stage 1A of the treatment algorithm applies to those patients experiencing their first acute episode of schizophrenia. All available antipsychotics except clozapine are recommended for monotherapy treatment in stage 1A. The clinician needs to evaluate the relative risk of EPS with FGAs versus the risk of metabolic side effects with different SGAs in making a decision for drug selection. The World Federation favors SGAs because of the reduced risk of EPS.[31] The 2009 PORT recommendations advise against the use of olanzapine in first episode because of weight gain and metabolic side effects.[28,31] Compared with SGAs, haloperidol produced more pseudoparkinsonism and a higher 1-year discontinuation rate in the European First Episode Schizophrenia Trial (EUFEST).[30,31] If an FGA is used, it is better to use a moderate-potency antipsychotic such as loxapine or perphenazine. Among the more established SGAs, aripiprazole and ziprasidone produce the least weight gain. Because of the sensitivity to antipsychotic-induced EPS in first-episode patients, antipsychotic dosing should be initiated at the lower end of the dose range.[31]

Clinical **Controversy...**

With no clear difference in efficacy among first-line antipsychotics, adverse effect profiles become the primary variable in choosing an antipsychotic. While the World Federation of Psychiatry Guidelines favor the SGAs as first-line antipsychotics, the PORT guidelines offer no preference, but do not recommend olanzapine in first psychotic break patients.

Stage 1B addresses those patients who have been previously treated with an antipsychotic, are currently off medications, and are experiencing a recurrent acute psychotic episode. Any antipsychotic monotherapy except clozapine is recommended. However, an antipsychotic that previously produced nonresponse or intolerance should not be used.[31]

Stage 2 addresses pharmacotherapy in a patient who had inadequate clinical improvement with the antipsychotic used in stage 1A or 1B. Stage 2 recommends an alternate antipsychotic monotherapy with the exception of clozapine.[28,31] Because of safety concerns and the need for white blood cell (WBC) monitoring, it is recommended that patients be tried on two different monotherapy antipsychotic trials before proceeding to a trial of

TABLE 50-5 Available Antipsychotics and Dosage Ranges

Generic Name	Trade Name	Starting Dose (mg/day)	Usual Dosage Range (mg/day)	Comments
First-Generation Antipsychotics				
Chlorpromazine	Thorazine	50–150	300–1,000	Most weight gain among FGAs
Fluphenazine	Prolixin	5	5–20	
Haloperidol	Haldol	2–5	2–20	Higher dropout rate in first episode
Loxapine	Loxitane	20	50–150	
Loxapine inhaled	Adasuve	10	10	Maximum 10 mg per 24 hours Approved REMS program only
Perphenazine	Trilafon	4–24	16–64	
Thioridazine	Mellaril	50–150	100–800	Significant QTc prolongation
Thiothixene	Navane	4–10	4–50	
Trifluoperazine	Stelazine	2–5	5–40	
Second-Generation Antipsychotics				
Aripiprazole	Abilify	5–15	15–30	
Asenapine	Saphris	5	10–20	Sublingual only
Clozapine	Clozaril	25	100–800	Check plasma level before exceeding 600 mg
Iloperidone	Fanapt	1–2	6–24	Care with dosing in CYP2D6 slow metabolizers
Lurasidone	Latuda	20–40	40–120	
Olanzapine	Zyprexa	5–10	10–20	Avoid in first episode because of weight gain
Paliperidone	Invega	3–6	3–12	Bioavailability increased when administered with food
Quetiapine	Seroquel	50	300–800	
Risperidone	Risperdal	1–2	2–8	
Ziprasidone	Geodon	40	80–160	Take with food

Note: In first-episode patients, starting dose and target dose should generally be 50% of the usual dose range. See Long-Acting Injectable Antipsychotics in text for dosing for these agents.

Data from reference 31.

clozapine (stage 3).[28,31] However, clozapine has superior efficacy in decreasing suicidal behavior, and it should be considered at stage 2 for the suicidal patient.[28] Clozapine can also be considered at stage 2 in patients with a history of violence or comorbid substance abuse.[28]

If partial or poor adherence contributes to inadequate clinical improvement, then long-acting injectable antipsychotics should be considered.[24,28,31] In addition to individuals who are identified as partially adherent, some patients may elect long-acting injections instead of taking daily oral medication.

In stage 3, treatment failure on two different antipsychotics from different classes meets the definition of treatment resistance, and the recommended treatment is clozapine.[28,30,31]

In stage 4, only minimal evidence exists for any treatment options for those patients who do not have adequate symptom improvement with clozapine. Additional treatment options that are tried, again with minimal evidence, include electroconvulsive therapy augmentation, mood stabilizer augmentation, and another antipsychotic combined with clozapine.[28,31] The use of antipsychotic combinations is controversial, as limited evidence supports increased efficacy for combination antipsychotic treatment.[28,31]

Predictors of Response

Obtaining a thorough medication history is important, and previous antipsychotic treatment should help guide the selection of drug therapy, in that either a good prior response favors the use of the same agent or a negative prior response suggests the selection of a dissimilar drug. Nonprescription and illicit drug use can influence psychiatric presentation and thus diagnosis or antipsychotic response. Amphetamines and other CNS stimulants, cocaine, corticosteroids, digitalis glycosides, indomethacin, marijuana, pentazocine, phencyclidine, and other drugs can induce psychosis in susceptible individuals or exacerbate psychosis in patients with preexisting psychiatric illness.[32] Patients with schizophrenia who continue to abuse alcohol or drugs usually have a poor response to medications and a poor prognosis. Alcohol, caffeine, and nicotine use potentially results in drug interactions.

Individual differences in patient response have been either proposed or identified, which can be clinically useful predictors of response.[23,24] Acute onset and short duration of illness, presence of acute stressors or precipitating factors, later age of onset, family history of affective illness, and good premorbid adjustment as reflected in stable interpersonal relationships or employment are all predictors of good response.[23,24]

Although controversial, affective symptoms can correlate with an overall good response. Negative symptoms and neuropsychological deficits related to cognition and neurologic soft signs can correlate with poor antipsychotic response.[23,24] A patient's subjective response within the first 48 hours after being administered an FGA can be associated with drug responsiveness.[33] An initial dysphoric response, demonstrated by stating a dislike of the medication, or feeling worse or zombie-like, combined with anxiety or akathisia-like symptoms, is associated with poor drug response, adverse effects, and nonadherence.

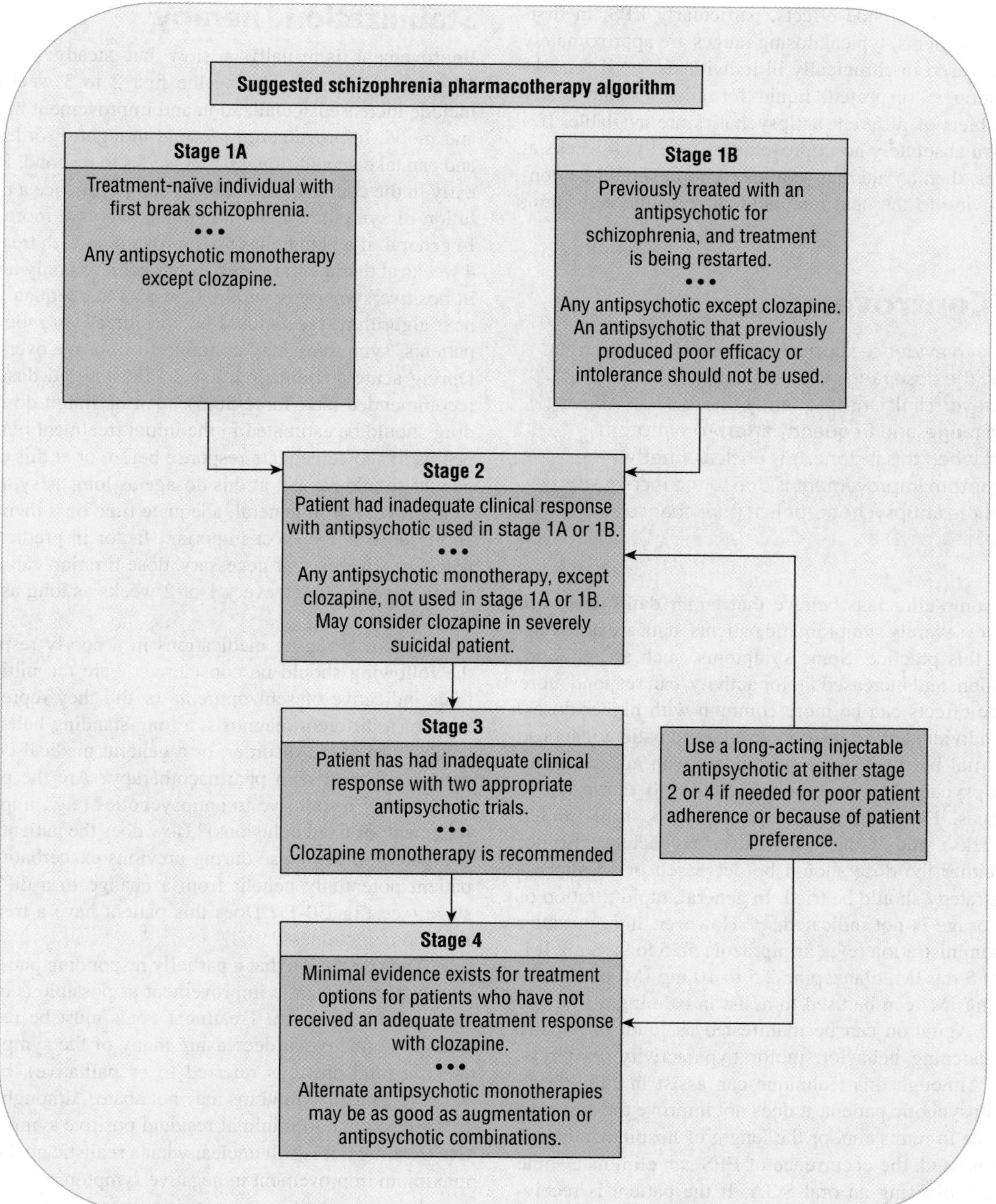

FIGURE 50-1 Suggested pharmacotherapy algorithm for treatment of schizophrenia. Schizophrenia should be treated in the context of an interprofessional model that addresses the psychosocial needs of the patient, necessary psychiatric pharmacotherapy, psychiatric comorbidities, treatment adherence, and any medical problems the patient may have. See the text for a description of the algorithm stages. *(Data from references 28, 30, and 31.)*

The importance of developing a therapeutic alliance between the patient and the clinician cannot be underestimated. Patients who form positive therapeutic alliances are more likely to be adherent with all aspects of therapy, experience a better outcome at 2 years, and require smaller antipsychotic doses.

A certain minority of patients fail to benefit from antipsychotic therapy, and their psychosocial functioning can actually worsen. Unfortunately, no accepted method is available to identify these people before treatment.[23,24] Recent evidence suggests that pharmacogenetics can play a role in predicting treatment response, both with respect to symptom improvement and with liability to develop side effects.[34,35] However, insufficient information is available to recommend routine clinical testing.

Initial Treatment in an Acute Psychotic Episode

The goals during the first 7 days of treatment should be decreased agitation, hostility, combativeness, anxiety, tension, and aggression, and normalization of sleep and eating patterns. The usual recommendation is to initiate therapy and to titrate dose over the first few days to an average effective dose, unless the patient's physiologic status or history indicates that this dose can result in unacceptable adverse effects. Because of its strong α_1-antagonism and resulting risk of hypotension, iloperidone and clozapine should be titrated more slowly than other antipsychotics. Table 50-5 lists the usual dosage range, and an average dose is typically midrange. Because of increased sensitivity to side effects, particularly EPS, in first-episode psychotic patients, typical dosing ranges are approximately 50% of the doses used in chronically ill individuals.[28,31] If "cheeking" of medication is suspected, liquid formulations and orally disintegrating tablets of different antipsychotics are available. If a patient has shown absolutely no improvement after 2 to 4 weeks at therapeutic doses, then an alternative antipsychotic should be considered (i.e., moving to the next treatment stage in the algorithm; see Fig. 50-1).[22,23]

Clinical **Controversy. . .**

Minimal research evidence supports the use of antipsychotic doses beyond the dose range in the FDA-approved product labeling. However, clinicians frequently titrate doses above the approved range, and frequently attest to symptom improvement when this is done. It is unclear whether the observed symptom improvement is due to the increased dose, time on the antipsychotic, or just pure chance.

Although some clinicians believe that larger daily doses are necessary in more severely symptomatic patients, data are not available to support this practice. Some symptoms, such as agitation, tension, aggression, and increased motor activity, can respond more quickly, but side effects can be more common with higher doses. However, interindividual differences in dosage and patient response do occur. In partial but inadequate responders who are tolerating the chosen antipsychotic, it may be reasonable to titrate above usual dose ranges. However, this tactic should be time-limited (i.e., 2 to 4 weeks), and if the patient does not achieve further improvement, either the dose should be decreased or an alternative treatment strategy should be tried. In general, rapid titration of antipsychotic dosage is not indicated.[23,28] However, intramuscular antipsychotic administration (e.g., aripiprazole 5.25 to 9.75 mg IM, haloperidol 2 to 5 mg IM, olanzapine 2.5 to 10 mg IM, or ziprasidone 10 to 20 mg IM) can be used to assist in calming a severely agitated patient. Agitation can be manifested as loud, physically or verbally threatening behavior, motor hyperactivity, or physical aggression. Although this technique can assist in calming an acutely agitated psychotic patient, it does not improve the extent of remission, or time to remission, or the length of hospitalization. If haloperidol IM is used, the occurrence of EPS can eliminate some of the advantages of using an oral SGA. If the patient is receiving an antipsychotic within the usual therapeutic range, the use of lorazepam 2 mg IM as needed in combination with the maintenance antipsychotic is a rational alternative to an injectable antipsychotic. Hypotension, respiratory depression, CNS depression, and death are possible when injectable lorazepam is used in combination with either olanzapine or clozapine; thus, this parenteral combination is not recommended.[30,31]

The initial Risk Evaluation and Mitigation Strategy (REMS) for inhaled loxapine powder was approved by the FDA with an indication of treatment of acute agitation associated with schizophrenia or bipolar disorder. Because of the risk of bronchospasm, pulmonary distress, and pulmonary arrest, the medication can only be administered in a healthcare facility and through the FDA-approved REMS. Before administration, patients must be screened for a history of asthma, chronic obstructive pulmonary disease, or other lung disease associated with bronchospasm, and use is limited to one 10 mg inhaled dose per 24-hour period.[36] It is not known whether inhaled loxapine offers any therapeutic advantages in acute agitation compared with currently available IM or oral products. Similarly, the safety of this product when used in routine clinical practice is unclear.

Stabilization Therapy

Improvement is usually a slow but steady process over 6 to 12 weeks or longer. During the first 2 to 3 weeks, goals should include increased socialization and improvement in self-care habits and mood. Improvement in formal thought disorder should follow and can take an additional 6 to 8 weeks to respond. Patients who are early in the course of their illness can experience a more rapid resolution of symptoms than individuals who are more chronically ill. In general, if a patient has no improvement with treatment after 2 to 4 weeks at therapeutic doses, or has achieved only a partial decrease in positive symptoms within 12 weeks at adequate doses, then the next algorithm stage should be considered. In more chronically ill patients, symptoms may continue to improve over 3 to 6 months. During acute stabilization, usual FDA-labeled doses of SGAs are recommended (see Table 50-5).[24] An optimum dose of the chosen drug should be estimated in the initial treatment plan. If the patient begins to show adequate response before or at this dosage, then the patient should remain at this dosage as long as symptoms continue to improve. **7** In general, adequate time on a therapeutic antipsychotic dose is the most important factor in predicting medication response. However, if necessary, dose titration can continue within the therapeutic range every 1 or 2 weeks as long as the patient has no side effects.

Before changing medications in a poorly responding patient, the following should be considered: Were the initial target symptoms indicative of schizophrenia or did they represent manifestations of a different diagnosis, a long-standing behavioral problem, a substance abuse disorder, or a general medical condition? Is the patient adherent with pharmacotherapy? Are the persistent symptoms poorly responsive to antipsychotics (e.g., impaired insight or judgment, or fixed delusions)? How does the patient's current status compare with response during previous exacerbations? Would this patient potentially benefit from a change to a different treatment stage (see Fig. 50-1)? Does this patient have a treatment-resistant schizophrenic illness?

The conclusion that a partially responding patient has achieved as much symptomatic improvement as possible is one that must be made with great care. Treatment goals must be realistic. Medications are effective at decreasing many of the symptoms of schizophrenia (and are thus referred to as palliative), but they are not curative, and all symptoms may not abate. Although one should aim to achieve none to minimal residual positive symptoms with effective treatment, it is still unclear what a realistic goal is with regard to maximum improvement in negative symptoms.

It is important to screen patients for co-occurring mental disorders, and their presence can become more apparent during the stabilization or maintenance phases of schizophrenia treatment. Examples include substance abuse disorders, depression, obsessive-compulsive disorder, and panic disorder. As co-occurring disorders will limit symptom and functional improvement and increase the risk of relapse, it is critical that treatment for the co-occurring disorder be implemented in combination with evidence-based treatment for schizophrenia.

Maintenance Treatment

Maintenance drug therapy prevents relapse, as shown in numerous double-blind studies. The average relapse rate after 1 year is 18% to 32% with active drug (including some nonadherent patients) versus 60% to 80% for placebo.[24,37] Avoiding relapses is thus a major goal of treatment.[38]

After treatment of the first psychotic episode in a patient with schizophrenia, medication should be continued for at least 12 months after remission.[24,29,31] **8** Many schizophrenia experts recommend that patients with robust medication response be treated for at least 5 years. In chronically ill individuals, continuous or lifetime pharmacotherapy is necessary in the majority of patients to prevent relapse. This should be approached with the lowest effective dose of the antipsychotic that is likely to be tolerated by the patient.[24,29,31]

Antipsychotics should be tapered slowly before discontinuation. Abrupt discontinuation of antipsychotics, especially clozapine, can result in withdrawal symptoms, felt to be a manifestation of rebound cholinergic outflow. Insomnia, nightmares, headaches, GI symptoms (e.g., abdominal cramps, stomach pain, nausea, vomiting, and diarrhea), restlessness, increased salivation, and sweating are reported. Although available evidence does not indicate a best way to switch from one antipsychotic to another, it is often recommended to taper and discontinue the first antipsychotic over at least 1 to 2 weeks while the second antipsychotic is initiated and the dose titrated.[24,31] Tapering needs to occur more slowly with clozapine.[24]

Long-Acting Injectable Antipsychotics

Long-acting antipsychotics are recommended for patients who are unreliable in taking oral medication on a daily basis, and thus are not usually used as first-line therapy. Before a long-acting antipsychotic is initiated, it should be determined whether the patient's medication nonadherence is because of side effects. If so, an alternative medication with a more favorable side effect profile should be considered before a long-acting injectable antipsychotic. The patient's motivation for treatment is a major factor influencing outcome. Conversion from oral therapy to a long-acting injectable is most successful in patients who have been stabilized on oral therapy. The ideal patient for a long-acting injectable is the individual who does not like the daily reminder of oral medication or is unreliable in taking medications.

Paliperidone palmitate is a long-acting injectable that has the advantage of once-monthly injections and easy conversion from oral to IM treatment.[39] Olanzapine pamoate monohydrate is a long-acting injectable that is administered every 2 or 4 weeks. It is associated with a postinjection sedation/delirium syndrome occurring in approximately 2% of patients.[40] The risk of occurrence does not appear related to dose or duration of treatment. One hypothesis is that its occurrence may be associated with accidental entry of the drug into the bloodstream.[40] The product labeling contains an FDA black box warning regarding this syndrome. Olanzapine pamoate is subject to a REMS, and the FDA labeling restricts the availability of long-acting olanzapine to a restricted distribution program. The injection must be administered in a registered healthcare facility, and the patient must be observed by a health professional for at least 3 hours after administration.[41] A long-acting formulation of aripiprazole is under FDA review at the time of publication, and a once-weekly oral formulation is in development.

Conversion from an oral antipsychotic to a long-acting medication should start with stabilization on an oral dosage form of the same agent, for a short trial (3 to 7 days), to determine whether the patient tolerates the medication without significant side effects. With long-acting risperidone, measurable serum concentrations are not seen until approximately 3 weeks after single-dose administration. Thus, it is important that the oral antipsychotic be administered for at least 3 weeks after beginning the injections. Dose adjustments are recommended to be made no more often than once every 4 weeks.[42] The recommended starting dose with risperidone long-acting injection is 25 mg, and clinical experience suggests that titration to doses greater than or equal to 37.5 mg per injection may be necessary for maintenance treatment. Long-acting risperidone has demonstrated efficacy, with an optimum dose range between 25 and 50 mg given IM every 2 weeks. Doses above 50 mg every 2 weeks are not recommended, as research indicates no greater efficacy but more EPS.[42]

Paliperidone palmitate can be injected into either the deltoid or the gluteal muscle, and treatment is initiated with 234 mg on day 1 and 156 mg a week later. No overlap with oral drug is necessary. Monthly IM doses are then titrated according to response within a range of 39 to 234 mg.[39] Olanzapine pamoate monohydrate is recommended for deep gluteal injection, and the initial injectable dose varies from 210 to 405 mg depending on the oral olanzapine daily maintenance dose and the frequency of injectable administration. The official product information should be consulted regarding preparation and administration information.[40,41]

For fluphenazine decanoate, the simplest dosing conversion method recommends 1.2 times the oral fluphenazine daily dose for stabilized patients, rounding up to the nearest 12.5-mg interval, administered in weekly doses for the first 4 to 6 weeks; or 1.6 times the oral daily dose for more acutely ill patients.[43] Subsequently, fluphenazine decanoate can be administered once every 2 to 3 weeks. Oral fluphenazine can be overlapped for 1 week. For haloperidol decanoate, a factor of 10 to 15 times the oral haloperidol daily dose is commonly recommended, rounding up to the nearest 50-mg interval, administered in a once-monthly dose with an oral haloperidol overlap for the first month. A more assertive conversion method recommends 20 times the oral daily dose, but dividing the injection into consecutive doses of 100 to 200 mg every 3 to 7 days until the entire amount is given.[44] With this method, oral medication overlap is unnecessary. The haloperidol decanoate dose is decreased by 25% at both second and third months.

Methods to Enhance Patient Adherence

It is often challenging for individuals with chronic illnesses to maintain appropriate medication adherence, and partial compliance is a reality in the treatment of all chronic illnesses.[31] Individuals with serious mental disorders have somewhat higher nonadherence rates than those with general medical disorders, with the following explanations provided: denial of illness, lack of insight, grandiosity or paranoia, no perceived need for medication, perceived lack of input into choice of medication or dosage, side effects, misperceived "allergies," or the number of medications prescribed or doses received daily. It is estimated that half of patients with schizophrenia or schizoaffective disorder take their medication less than 70% of the time.[31] Clinicians should expect partial medication compliance to be the norm. This should be approached in a nonjudgmental manner, with the clinician actively engaging the patient in care and using motivational interviewing techniques as mechanisms to enhance therapeutic alliance and patient adherence.

Numerous different methods have been used in an attempt to improve treatment adherence of patients with schizophrenia. Interventions that provide continuous focus on adherence and that are of long duration have shown benefit. These should incorporate problem solving techniques and be accompanied by technical learning aids. Pharmacy-based interventions and ones using nurse case managers have shown promise in improving adherence.[45] It has been suggested that programs need to include a focus on patient-driven outcomes, and not just medication adherence. For example, interventions should include efforts to allow patients to achieve life goals and function. This requires that programs be tailored to the needs of individual patients.[45] Psychoeducation strategies should include motivational interview techniques in individual counseling as well as group activities. 9

Some studies suggest that compliance therapy, targeted cognitive behavioral therapy focusing on medication adherence, can improve patient adherence, but the success seen in early studies has not been consistently replicated.[45]

Groups facilitated by trained individuals who have the illness are alleged to be more effective in enhancing awareness and acceptance of schizophrenia and necessary treatment than groups led only by professionals. Active involvement of family members further increases the likelihood of patient adherence with treatment. In addition to programs provided by community mental health centers, support groups operated by consumer groups such as the

National Alliance on Mental Illness (NAMI) are available in most urban areas. In the hospital, self-medication administration can reinforce the patient's perception of his or her active role in his or her own treatment. When patients miss outpatient appointments, active outreach interventions must be implemented to enhance patient engagement in treatment.[24,45]

Management of Treatment-Resistant Schizophrenia

In general, "treatment resistant" describes a patient who has had inadequate symptom response from multiple antipsychotic trials.[24] Traditionally, treatment resistance has been defined as lack of improvement in positive symptoms, but it can be defined by poor improvement in negative symptoms, or even by medication intolerance. Between 10% and 30% of patients receive minimal symptomatic improvement after multiple FGA monotherapy trials.[24] An additional 30% to 60% of patients have partial but inadequate improvement in symptoms or unacceptable side effects associated with antipsychotic use.[24,31] In those patients failing two or more pharmacotherapy trials, a treatment-refractory evaluation should be performed to reexamine diagnosis, substance abuse, medication adherence, and psychosocial stressors. Targeted cognitive behavioral therapy or other psychosocial augmentation strategies should be considered.[31]

Clozapine

Only clozapine has shown superiority over other antipsychotics in randomized clinical trials for the management of treatment-resistant schizophrenia. Most other SGAs have either not been studied in treatment-refractory patients or been evaluated in small open trials. In a seminal study, clozapine was effective in approximately 30% of patients with treatment-resistant schizophrenia, compared with only 4% treated with a combination of chlorpromazine and benztropine.[46] The criteria for treatment resistance require two treatment failures, and include both FGAs and SGAs. Other treatment candidates for clozapine include those patients who cannot tolerate neurologic side effects of even conservative doses of other antipsychotics.

Clinical **Controversy...**

Although clozapine is the only treatment that has evidence of proven benefit in patients with treatment-resistant schizophrenia, and its use in treatment-resistant schizophrenia is recommended in all treatment guidelines, it is underutilized by clinicians in practice. Although the reasons for its underutilization are not totally understood, factors may include clinician fear of clozapine's potential adverse effects, the WBC monitoring required by the FDA, and mental health treatment systems that do not support use of the drug.

Symptomatic improvement with clozapine in the treatment-resistant patient often occurs slowly, and as many as 60% of patients may improve if clozapine is used for up to 6 months. This, in combination with clozapine's adverse effect profile, provides sufficient information to conclude that clozapine is not a panacea for schizophrenia. Polydipsia and hyponatremia (psychogenic water drinking) is a frequent problem among treatment-resistant patients, and clozapine reportedly decreases water drinking and increases serum sodium in such patients.[47]

Because of the risk of orthostatic hypotension, clozapine is usually titrated more slowly than other antipsychotics, particularly on an outpatient basis. If a 12.5-mg test dose does not produce hypotension, then clozapine 25 mg at bedtime is recommended, increased to 25 mg twice a day after 3 days, and then increased in 25 to 50 mg/day increments every 3 days until a dose of at least 300 mg/day is reached. Because high doses are associated with significantly increased side effects, including seizures, a clozapine serum concentration is recommended before exceeding 600 mg/day. If the clozapine serum concentration is less than 350 ng/mL (350 mcg/L; 1.07 μmol/L), then the dose should be increased as side effects allow to achieve this serum concentration.[31]

Augmentation and Combination Strategies

Little empirical evidence exists to guide treatment decisions for patients who do not respond to clozapine.[28,31] Augmentation therapy involves the addition of a nonantipsychotic drug to an antipsychotic drug in a poorly or partially responsive patient, whereas combination treatment involves using two antipsychotics simultaneously.

Mood stabilizers are frequently used as an augmentation strategy. Lithium does not enhance antipsychotic effect but may improve labile affect and agitated behavior in selected patients.[48] Valproic acid and carbamazepine have also been used. A large placebo-controlled trial supports faster symptom improvement, but no difference in maintenance treatment, when divalproex was used in combination with either olanzapine or risperidone.[49] Enzyme induction with carbamazepine can cause a decrease in antipsychotic serum concentrations and potentially worsen psychotic symptoms in some patients.[24,31] The 2009 PORT recommendations do not endorse the use of mood stabilizer augmentation in treatment-resistant patients.[28]

Only limited data are available to support antidepressant augmentation of antipsychotics.[31] Consistently positive results have been reported when using selective serotonin reuptake inhibitors (SSRIs) to treat obsessive-compulsive symptoms that worsen or arise during clozapine treatment.

Combining an FGA with an SGA and combining different SGAs have been suggested as intervention strategies for treatment-resistant patients. Pharmacodynamically, there is limited rationale for explaining how combinations of antipsychotics would produce enhanced efficacy, and increased side effects, particularly increased EPS, metabolic effects, and hyperprolactinemia, are possible results.[50] Clinically, no evidence exists to prove that antipsychotic combinations are superior to monotherapy, and the 2009 PORT recommendations do not support their use.[28] However, a recent meta-analysis did find a modest benefit for the use of polypharmacy in schizophrenia.[51] This remains a highly contentious area and one where clinicians' practice is not aligned with available evidence. In general, a series of antipsychotic monotherapies, including clozapine, are preferred over antipsychotic combinations.[28] However, when clozapine fails to produce desired outcomes, a time-limited combination trial is sometimes considered.[31] Such antipsychotic combination treatment trials should be time-limited (e.g., maximum 12 weeks) and the patient carefully evaluated with rating scales for changes in symptomatology. If no apparent improvement is observed, then one of the medications should be tapered and discontinued. However, if the patient has a partial response (greater than or equal to 20% improvement in positive symptoms) after 12 weeks with combination treatment, medications should be titrated to doses at the upper end of the therapeutic range, and treatment should continue for an additional 12 weeks before a change in treatment is considered.

Clinical **Controversy...**

Although insufficient evidence exists to support the use of antipsychotic combination treatment and guidelines such as PORT do not recommend this practice, antipsychotic polypharmacy is common. It is well known that clinicians frequently do not follow evidence-based treatment guidelines.

Patients with Schizophrenia who are Violent

Most patients with schizophrenia do not exhibit violent behavior—perhaps this is even surprising given the severity and stress of hearing voices, being paranoid, etc. That said, there are nevertheless patients who do become violent, and then, as a group, patients with schizophrenia are more likely to be violent than the general population. Risk factors for violence include those associated with violence in the general population (e.g., childhood trauma and exposure to violence, alcohol and substance abuse, psychopathy, access to firearms) and (to some lesser extent) psychotic symptoms.[52] Patients are at risk to become violent when they relapse and so keeping patients with schizophrenia clinically stable is a major consideration. Some states even have outpatient commitment laws where patients at risk of violence are "forced" to get ongoing care, and if they default, they are sent back to the hospital. Patients who are really dangerous are invariably contained either in the legal system itself or legally as "forensic" patients where they are held by court order in a psychiatric facility.

Antipsychotic Mechanism of Action

The exact mechanism of action of antipsychotics is unknown. It has been suggested that antipsychotics be classified into three different categories: (a) typical or traditional (high D_2 antagonism and low 5-HT_{2A} antagonism); (b) atypical (moderate to high D_2 antagonism and high 5-HT_{2A} antagonism); and (c) atypical clozapine-like (low D_2 antagonism and high 5-HT_{2A} antagonism).[53,54] With the exception of aripiprazole, all current SGAs have a greater affinity for 5-HT_{2A} receptors than D_2 receptors.

Studies of antipsychotic receptor binding in humans have used PET scans to examine neurotransmitter receptor binding at steady state, 12 hours postdose in small numbers of individuals. At least 60% to 65% D_2 receptor occupation is necessary to decrease positive psychotic symptoms, whereas blockade of approximately 77% or more of D_2 receptors is associated with EPS.[53,55] FGAs are DA receptor antagonists with high affinity for D_2 receptors. During chronic treatment with these agents, between 70% and 90% of D_2 receptors in the striatum are usually occupied. In contrast, during clozapine treatment only 38% to 47% of D_2 receptors are occupied, even with high doses. Newer SGAs have variable D_2 binding. With low-dose risperidone (2 to 5 mg/day), D_2 binding ranges from 60% to 79%, but with doses greater than 6 mg daily, binding commonly exceeds the 77% threshold associated with the development of EPS. Risperidone 2 mg/day produces 5-HT_{2A} binding greater than 70%, and with 4 mg/day it is nearly 100%.[53,56] Olanzapine 10 to 20 mg/day produces D_2 binding ranging from 71% to 80%, whereas at 30 to 40 mg/day, it ranges from 83% to 88%. At 5 mg/day, 5-HT_{2A} receptors are near saturation of binding.[53] Ziprasidone has the highest 5-HT_{2A}-to-D_2 affinity ratio of any of the currently available antipsychotics. It is also a potent 5-HT_{1A} agonist.[57]

Quetiapine has the lowest D_2 binding. At doses of 300 to 600 mg/day, 12-hour postdose D_2 binding ranges from 0% to 27%. Even at quetiapine 800 mg/day, only 30% of D_2 receptors are occupied. At these same daily doses, 45% to 90% of 5-HT_{2A} receptors are occupied. However, when quetiapine D_2 binding is examined 2 to 3 hours postdose, 58% and 64% of receptors were occupied with 400 and 450 mg, respectively. Transient blockade of DA receptors may be adequate to produce antipsychotic effect, but long-term D_2 blockade is required for production of EPS and sustained hyperprolactinemia. Low D_2 binding, and thus atypicality, can be directly associated with how rapidly the antipsychotic disassociates from the D_2 receptor.[53,56] The availability of aripiprazole, a partial agonist at D_2 receptors, represents a further elaboration of the DA hypothesis of antipsychotic action.[54,58] It is proposed that aripiprazole works as a functional partial agonist. Aripiprazole is a rather weak 5-HT_{2A} antagonist but a potent 5-HT_{1A} agonist.[54,58]

Iloperidone has high affinity for D_2, D_3, and 5-HT_{2A} receptors, and moderate affinity for D_4, 5-HT_6, 5-HT_7, and α_1-receptors.[59] Asenapine has high affinity for 5-HT_{2A} and D_2 receptors as well as for α_1- and histamine-1 receptors. D_2 occupancy of approximately 80% is predicted to occur with a sublingual dose of 5 to 10 mg twice daily.[60] It is clear that the SGAs differ in their mechanisms of action and most likely in the manner in which they produce an atypical clinical profile.

The primary therapeutic effects of FGAs are thought to occur in the limbic system, including the ventral striatum, whereas EPS are thought to be related to DA blockade in the dorsal striatum. 5-HT_{2A} antagonism in combination with modest D_2 blockade leads to release of DA in the prefrontal cortex, and this is one explanation for the decrease in negative symptoms and improvement in cognition reported with atypical antipsychotics.

Antipsychotics vary in their effects on other neurotransmitter receptor systems.[53,54,56] Although the significance of these different mechanisms on efficacy is unclear, they do potentially explain differences in side effect profiles. These differences in pharmacodynamic profiles point out that the SGAs are not all alike, and patients obtaining an inadequate clinical response (either efficacy or side effects) with one antipsychotic may have a superior response on an alternate drug. Thus, serial SGA monotherapy trials should be tried in patients receiving a suboptimal clinical response (see Fig. 50-1).

Pharmacokinetics

As a class, antipsychotics are highly lipophilic and highly bound to membranes and plasma proteins. They distribute readily into most tissues with a high blood supply and can accumulate in tissues; therefore, they have large volumes of distribution.[61] Most antipsychotics are largely metabolized, primarily through the cytochrome P450 (CYP) pathways in the liver, except for ziprasidone, which is largely metabolized by aldehyde oxidase. Fluphenazine, perphenazine, and risperidone are metabolized through CYP2D6, and thus are susceptible to polymorphic metabolism.[62] This is also one of the major pathways for the metabolism of aripiprazole and iloperidone.[59] Thirty percent to 35% of Africans and Asians are slow to intermediate metabolizers. Approximately 0% to 5% of African Americans, 1% of Asians, and 5% to 10% of whites are poor metabolizers.[62,63] In addition, some people of Swedish descent and up to 30% of those from Northern Africa may be ultrarapid metabolizers.[63] Polymorphism in CYP1A2 can potentially result in a decrease in the metabolic rate of clozapine, and increased clozapine metabolic rate in smokers has been linked to a specific genotype.[62] The possibility of genetic polymorphism should be considered when dosing and monitoring the clinical effects of antipsychotics. Table 50-6 outlines the prominent metabolic pathways of selected antipsychotics.

Asenapine is unique in that it has less than 2% bioavailability after oral administration, but has a bioavailability of approximately 35% sublingually—the FDA-approved route of administration. Eating and drinking within 10 minutes after sublingual administration will reduce bioavailability.[60]

Most antipsychotics have fairly long elimination half-lives, generally 24 hours or more, with the exception of quetiapine and ziprasidone, which have short half-lives.[58,61] Among the SGAs, only clozapine has an established therapeutic serum concentration, with efficacy being associated with a clozapine plasma concentration greater than 350 ng/mL (350 mcg/L; 1.07 μmol/L).[61] Whether a potential maximum therapeutic clozapine serum concentration exists is unknown. Clozapine serum concentration should be obtained before exceeding 600 mg daily, in patients who develop unusual or severe adverse side effects, in patients who are taking concomitant

TABLE 50-6 Pharmacokinetic Parameters of Selected Antipsychotics

Drug	Bioavailability (%)	Half-Life	Major Metabolic Pathways	Active Metabolites
Selected First-Generation Antipsychotics (FGAs)				
Chlorpromazine	10–30	8–35 hours	FMO3, CYP3A4	7-Hydroxy, others
Fluphenazine	20–50	14–24 hours	CYP2D6	?
Fluphenazine decanoate		14.2 ± 2.2[a] days	CYP2D6	
Haloperidol	40–70	12–36 hours	CYP1A2, CYP2D6, CYP3A4	Reduced haloperidol
Haloperidol decanoate		21 days	CYP1A2, CYP2D6, CYP3A4	Reduced haloperidol
Perphenazine	20–25	8.1–12.3 hours	CYP2D6	7-OH-perphenazine
Second-Generation Antipsychotics (SGAs)				
Aripiprazole	87	48–68 hours	CYP2D6, CYP3A4	Dehydroaripiprazole
Asenapine	<2 orally 35 SL Nonlinear	13–39 hours	UGT1A4, CYP1A2	None known
Clozapine	12–81	11–105 hours	CYP1A2, CYP3A4, CYP2C19	Desmethylclozapine
Iloperidone	96	18–33 hours	CYP2D6, CYP3A4	P88
Lurasidone	10–20	18 hours	CYP3A4	ID-14233 and ID-14326
Olanzapine	80	20–70 hours	CYP1A2, CYP3A4, FMO3	*N*-Glucuronide; 2-OH-methyl; 4-*N*-oxide
Paliperidone ER	28	23 hours	Renal unchanged (59%) CYP3A4 and multiple pathways	None known
Paliperidone palmitate		25–49 days	Renal unchanged (59%) CYP3A4 and multiple pathways	None known
Quetiapine	9 ± 4	6.88 hours	CYP3A4	7-OH-quetiapine
Risperidone	68	3–24 hours	CYP2D6	9-OH-risperidone
Risperidone Consta		3–6 days	CYP2D6	9-OH-risperidone
Ziprasidone	59	4–10 hours	Aldehyde oxidase, CYP3A4	None

[a]Based on multiple-dose data. Single-dose data indicate a β-half-life of 6–10 days.

Data from references 39, 42–44, 58–63, 127, and 128.

medications that can cause drug interactions, in patients who have age or pathophysiologic changes suggesting a change in pharmacokinetics, or for assessment of patient adherence.[37,61]

Adverse Effects

Table 50-7 presents the relative incidence of common categories of antipsychotic side effects. Side effects are discussed below with respect to organ system affected. A general approach to monitoring and assessing side effects requires prospective monitoring by clinicians, preferably using a thorough review of systems approach. Patient-oriented self-rated side effect scales can be helpful, as many patients with schizophrenia do not readily complain of side effects.

With the variety of antipsychotics currently available, using an alternative antipsychotic should be considered in patients who complain of poorly tolerated side effects. Because medication side effects are one of the primary predictors of patient nonadherence, the clinician should take advantage of the treatment options currently available in an attempt to improve patient outcomes. As we learn more about relative side effect risks (e.g., weight gain, glucose intolerance, QTc prolongation, acute EPS, and tardive dyskinesia), it will be necessary to regularly reconsider which antipsychotics should be considered first-line treatment alternatives.

Endocrine System

DA blockade in the tuberoinfundibular tract results in increased prolactin levels as DA is the major prolactin-inhibiting factor. Hyperprolactinemia may occur in up to 87% of patients treated with FGAs, risperidone, or paliperidone. The major side effects associated with hyperprolactinemia are gynecomastia, galactorrhea, menstrual irregularities, decreased libido, and sexual dysfunction. Although not conclusive, chronic hyperprolactinemia has been associated with decreased bone mineral density. Tolerance does not appear to develop to antipsychotic-induced hyperprolactinemia. Newer antipsychotics including asenapine, iloperidone, and lurasidone have not been shown to induce clinically meaningful changes in prolactin levels.[59,60,64] Switching to an SGA that has minimal sustained effect on prolactin is a reasonable treatment option.[65]

Weight gain is frequently reported in both adults and children receiving antipsychotics.[65,66] Although the exact mechanism is uncertain, weight gain has been associated with antihistaminic effects, antimuscarinic effects, and blockade of 5-HT_{2C} receptors including 5-HT_{2C} receptor polymorphism. However, dietary factors and activity levels can play a significant role in this population, as does renourishment after a period of poor self-care. In particular, significant weight gain, as defined by greater than or equal to 7% of the baseline body weight, after 1 year of treatment has been seen in as many as 80% of patients treated with olanzapine, 58% treated with risperidone, 50% treated with quetiapine, and 21% treated with iloperidone.[65,67] The risk of weight gain may be greater in patients with their first psychotic episode. Ziprasidone and aripiprazole, as well as newer agents asenapine and lurasidone, are associated with minimal weight gain.[60,64]

The risk of cardiovascular-related mortality is higher in individuals with schizophrenia,[65,68] and this is further aggravated by drug-related weight gain and the high prevalence of smoking. Additionally, obesity is a risk factor for diabetes mellitus.[65] Weight gain during treatment is concerning for patients and a major reason for poor medication adherence.[69]

TABLE 50-7 Relative Side Effect Incidence of Commonly Used Antipsychotics[a,b]

	Sedation	EPS	Anticholinergic	Orthostasis	Weight Gain	Prolactin
Aripiprazole	+	+	+	+	+	+
Asenapine	+	++	±	++	+	+
Chlorpromazine	++++	+++	+++	++++	++	+++
Clozapine	++++	+	++++	++++	++++	+
Fluphenazine	+	++++	+	+	+	++++
Haloperidol	+	++++	+	+	+	++++
Iloperidone	+	±	++	+++	++	+
Lurasidone	+	+	+	+	±	±
Olanzapine	++	++	++	++	++++	+
Paliperidone	+	++	+	++	++	++++
Perphenazine	++	++++	++	+	+	++++
Quetiapine	++	+	+	++	++	+
Risperidone	+	++	+	++	++	++++
Thioridazine	++++	+++	++++	++++	+	+++
Thiothixene	+	++++	+	+	+	++++
Ziprasidone	++	++	+	+	+	+

EPS, extrapyramidal side effects. Relative side effect risk: ±, negligible; +, low; ++, moderate; +++, moderately high; ++++, high.

[a]Side effects shown are relative risk based on doses within the recommended therapeutic range.

[b]Individual patient risk varies depending on patient-specific factors.

Several different genetic variations have been correlated with predisposition for antipsychotic-associated weight gain. Recent meta-analysis of all genetic studies looking at the −759 C/T promoter region polymorphism of the 5-HT_{2C} receptor gene confirmed an association of 5-HT_{2C} in antipsychotic-induced weight gain.[70] Polymorphisms in leptin and leptin receptor genes have also been linked with clozapine- and olanzapine-associated weight gain.[71,72] Alfa-2a-adrenergic receptor gene, G protein β_3 subunit gene, and brain-derived neurotrophic factor (BDNF) gene have been genetic targets; however, results are inconsistent as to whether a relationship exists with these polymorphisms and antipsychotic-associated weight gain.[73–76]

Several approaches have been recommended to address weight gain. Stroup et al. have shown that switching the antipsychotic to another agent with less weight gain liability is one choice.[77] Another choice is to add one of the weight-reducing agents.[78–80] Dietary restriction, exercise, and behavior modification programs are reported to be successful in small short-term studies.[81] An American Diabetes Association consensus task force recommends consideration of a change in antipsychotic if a patient gains more than 5% of baseline body weight after starting the drug.[82]

Clinical **Controversy...**

Although weight gain with antipsychotics is a major challenge in psychiatry, no clear consensus currently exists regarding how to address weight gain in these patients.

Patients with schizophrenia have a higher prevalence of type 2 diabetes than the nonschizophrenic population. Beyond this, antipsychotics may adversely affect glucose levels in diabetic patients. The extent to which these effects are related to drug-induced weight increase is unclear.[66,81] Data collected from the FDA MedWatch Drug Surveillance System for clozapine, olanzapine, quetiapine, and risperidone indicate that nearly 60% of the new-onset diabetes reported occurred within the first 6 months of treatment initiation.[65] Clozapine and olanzapine have the highest risk of new-onset diabetes followed by risperidone and then quetiapine. Although likely less than with the other SGAs, inadequate data are available to accurately estimate the risk with ziprasidone and aripiprazole.[65] The 2009 PORT recommendations do not recommend olanzapine as a first-line antipsychotic option.[28] In March 2004, the FDA issued a safety alert requiring revisions in the labeling of all SGAs that describes the increased risk of diabetes mellitus in patients taking atypical antipsychotics.[83] Designing care models and standards for managing diabetes in patients with schizophrenia is important in addressing this major health problem.

Cardiovascular System

Orthostatic Hypotension Orthostatic hypotension is thought to be caused by α-adrenergic blockade, and may occur in up to 75% of treated patients.[84] Clozapine, iloperidone, quetiapine, and risperidone appear to have the greatest risk and should have their doses titrated over several days to decrease the risk of symptomatic hypotension.[85] Antipsychotic combination treatment may result in a greater risk of orthostasis.[84] Orthostatic hypotension can occur in any patient, but diabetic patients with preexisting cardiovascular disease and the elderly seem particularly predisposed. Other risk factors may include dehydration and presence of alcoholic neuropathy.[85] Patients should be advised to slowly move to the standing position to allow for adaptation. Tolerance to this effect may occur within 2 to 3 months. If not, lower doses or a change to an antipsychotic with less α-blockade can be attempted. Fluid resuscitation or increasing salt intake may also help minimize orthostatic blood pressure changes.[85]

Electrocardiographic Changes Among the antipsychotics, thioridazine, clozapine, iloperidone, and ziprasidone are most likely to cause ECG changes. ECG changes include increased heart rate (through sinus tachycardia from anticholinergic effects, or reflex tachycardia from α-adrenergic blockade), flattened T waves, ST segment depression, and prolongation of QT and PR intervals. The most clinically important of these potential changes is prolongation of the QTc, which has been associated with ventricular arrhythmias, including torsade de pointes syndrome. This is thought to occur as a result of blockade of the cardiac delayed potassium rectifier channel.[86] Thioridazine has been shown to prolong the QTc on average approximately 20 milliseconds longer than haloperidol, risperidone, olanzapine, or quetiapine.[84,86] Thioridazine's effect on QTc prolongation is dose related, and has led to a black box warning in the FDA-approved product labeling. In the same study, ziprasidone prolonged the QTc by approximately 10 milliseconds or about one half of the effect of thioridazine.[84] Widespread clinical use suggests that ziprasidone's effects on the ECG are not commonly associated with clinical sequelae, unless the patient has baseline risk factors.[84] Iloperidone has a dose-related effect on QTc, with an average prolongation of about 9 milliseconds at a dose of 20 to 24 mg/day.[59] Iloperidone is subject to polymorphic metabolism and there may be an increased risk of QTc prolongation in CYP2D6 slow metabolizers.[87] High IV doses of haloperidol elevate the risk of prolonged QTc, which also carries a black box warning in the FDA-approved product labeling.[88] Although the precise point at which QTc prolongation becomes clinically dangerous is unclear, it has been recommended to discontinue a medication associated with QTc prolongation if the interval consistently exceeds 500 milliseconds.

Greater caution regarding antipsychotic choice and use is necessary in the elderly, in patients with preexisting cardiac or cerebrovascular disease (including bradycardia and second- or third-degree AV block), and in patients taking diuretics or medications that may prolong the QTc.[84,88] Being female confers a longer QTc, and twice the risk of medication-induced torsade de pointes.[88] In patients older than 50 years of age, a pretreatment ECG is recommended, as are baseline serum potassium and magnesium levels. These factors should be considered in antipsychotic selection.

Sudden Cardiac Death A large retrospective analysis found that the risk of sudden cardiac death (SCD) with use of FGAs and SGAs was twice that of nonusers,[84,89] with risk increasing with escalated dose. It has been estimated that 15 cases of SCD occur per 10,000 years of antipsychotic exposure.[86] Further meta-analysis has conferred a lack of evidence for differential effects on cardiovascular mortality favoring one class of antipsychotics over the other.[84,89] Further prospectively designed studies are needed to confirm a dose-dependent increase in cardiovascular sudden death with antipsychotic use, and to determine whether certain antipsychotics are associated with a greater risk than others.

Lipid Changes

Treatment with at least some SGAs and phenothiazines appears associated with elevations in serum triglycerides and cholesterol. Oxidation of apolipoprotein B lipoproteins and elevations in sterol regulatory element binding protein-controlled gene expression are among the purported mechanisms by which these lipid changes occur during antipsychotic treatment.[90,91] Among the SGAs, less risk for change in serum lipid or cholesterol levels can occur with risperidone, ziprasidone, aripiprazole, asenapine, iloperidone, and lurasidone.[60,64,65,67,68] In the CATIE trial, olanzapine was associated with greater and significant adverse effects on metabolic parameters, including lipids, blood glucose, and body weight versus the other study treatments, but these differences in tolerability did not affect discontinuation rates.[29]

The occurrence of weight gain, diabetes, and lipid abnormalities during antipsychotic therapy is consistent with the development of metabolic syndrome (i.e., syndrome X). Cohorts of patients with schizophrenia have shown elevated prevalence of metabolic syndrome as compared with general population cohorts. Prevalence rates of metabolic syndrome in U.S. populations treated with antipsychotics range from 28% to 60%, with 40.9% reported in the prospectively designed CATIE trial.[92]

Metabolic syndrome consists of raised triglycerides (greater than or equal to 150 mg/dL [1.70 mmol/L]), low HDL cholesterol (less than or equal to 40 mg/dL [1.03 mmol/L] for males, less than or equal to 50 mg/dL [1.29 mmol/L] for females), elevated fasting glucose (greater than or equal to 100 mg/dL [5.6 mmol/L]), blood pressure elevation (greater than or equal to 130/85 mm Hg), and weight gain (abdominal circumference greater than 102 cm [40 in] for males, greater than 88 cm [35 in] in females).[65,68] These abnormalities dictate an important role for general health screening and monitoring in patients with schizophrenia, and prompt intervention when such abnormalities occur. The propensity of individual antipsychotics to produce metabolic disturbances should be considered in the context of individual patient risk factors at the time of drug selection.

Anticholinergic Effects

Patients receiving antipsychotics or antipsychotics in combination with anticholinergics can experience anticholinergic side effects (e.g., dry mouth, constipation, tachycardia, blurred vision, inhibition or impairment of ejaculation, urinary retention, or impaired memory). This is particularly so with low-potency FGAs, and the elderly are especially sensitive to these effects. Of the SGAs, clozapine and olanzapine have moderately high rates of causing anticholinergic effects. Constipation, caused by slowed peristaltic movement and decreased intestinal fluid content, should be closely monitored and treated, especially in the elderly. Paralytic ileus and necrotizing enterocolitis can also occur.

CNS

Extrapyramidal System

Dystonia Dystonia is a state of abnormal tonicity, sometimes described simplistically as a severe "muscle spasm."[93,94] More accurately, dystonias are prolonged tonic contractions, with a rapid onset, usually within 24 to 96 hours of dosage initiation or dosage increase. They can be life-threatening, as in the case of pharyngeal–laryngeal dystonias, and can contribute to patient nonadherence. Types of dystonic reactions include trismus, glossospasm, tongue protrusion, pharyngeal–laryngeal dystonia, blepharospasm, oculogyric crisis, torticollis, and retrocollis. Dystonic reactions occur primarily with FGAs. Risk factors include younger patients (especially males), the use of high-potency agents, and high dosage. The overall incidence from the 1960s to the mid-1970s ranged from 2.3% to 10%, but as higher-potency traditional antipsychotics became more widely used, the rate increased to as high as 64%.

Intramuscular or IV anticholinergics (Table 50-8) or benzodiazepines are the treatments of choice for dystonia. Benztropine 2 mg or diphenhydramine 50 mg can be given intramuscularly or IV. Diazepam 5 to 10 mg by slow IV push or lorazepam 1 to 2 mg intramuscularly is a treatment alternative. Relief is typically seen within 15 to 20 minutes of an intramuscular injection and within 5 minutes of IV administration. The antipsychotic can be continued, with concomitant short-term use of oral anticholinergic agents. In general, prophylactic anticholinergic medications are not recommended routinely with all FGAs. However, prophylaxis is reasonable when using high-potency FGAs (e.g., haloperidol or fluphenazine) in young men, and in patients with a history of dystonia.[94] Dystonias can also be minimized by the use of lower initial FGA doses. Anticholinergics are good choices for prophylaxis, whereas amantadine has not been proven effective for this purpose. The risk of dystonia is greatly reduced with SGAs.

Akathisia Akathisia is defined as the inability to sit still and as being functionally motor restless. The most accurate diagnosis is made by combining subjective complaints with objective symptoms (pacing, shifting, shuffling, or tapping feet). Subjectively, patients may describe a feeling of inner restlessness or disquiet or a

TABLE 50-8 Agents Used to Treat Extrapyramidal Side Effects

Generic Name	Equivalent Dose (mg)	Daily Dosage Range (mg)
Antimuscarinics		
Benztropine[a]	1	1–8[b]
Biperiden[a]	2	2–8
Trihexyphenidyl	2	2–15
Antihistaminic		
Diphenhydramine[a]	50	50–400
Dopamine Agonist		
Amantadine	NA	100–400
Benzodiazepines		
Lorazepam[a]	NA	1–8
Diazepam	NA	2–20
Clonazepam	NA	2–8
β-Blockers		
Propranolol	NA	20–160

NA, not applicable

[a]Injectable dosage form can be given intramuscularly for relief of acute dystonia.
[b]In treatment-refractory cases, dosage can be titrated to 12 mg/day with careful monitoring; nonlinear pharmacokinetics have been reported.

compulsion to move or remain in constant motion. Akathisia occurs in 20% to 40% of patients treated with high-potency FGAs.[93,94] It is frequently accompanied by dysphoria.

Akathisia responds poorly to anticholinergics.[93,94] Traditionally, reduction in antipsychotic dosage has been considered the best intervention; however, this might not be a realistic goal in an acutely psychotic patient. A logical alternative is to switch to an antipsychotic with a lower risk of akathisia, or an antipsychotic previously used in the patient without adverse effect. Akathisia can occasionally occur with SGAs, particularly aripiprazole and risperidone. Quetiapine and clozapine appear to have the lowest risk of producing akathisia.[93,94]

Benzodiazepines have been used for treatment of akathisia, but the high prevalence of co-occurring substance abuse in schizophrenia discourages their prescribing.[94] The β-blockers (e.g., propranolol in doses up to 160 mg daily, nadolol in doses up to 80 mg daily, and metoprolol in β_2-selective doses of 100 mg daily or less) are reported as effective.[94]

Pseudoparkinsonism Pseudoparkinsonism, produced by D_2 blockade in the nigrostriatum, resembles idiopathic Parkinson's disease. A patient with pseudoparkinsonism can present with any of four cardinal symptoms: (a) akinesia, bradykinesia, or decreased motor activity including difficulty initiating movement, as well as extreme slowness, mask-like facial expression, micrographia, slowed speech, and decreased arm swing; (b) tremor, known as pill-rolling type, that is predominant at rest and decreases with movement, usually involving the fingers and hands, although tremors can also be seen in the arms, legs, neck, head, and chin; (c) cogwheel rigidity, seen as the patient's limbs yielding in jerky, ratchet-like fashion when passively moved by the examiner; and (d) postural abnormalities and instability manifested as stooped posture, difficulty in maintaining stability when changing body position, and a gait that ranges from slow and shuffling to festinating. Fatigue and weakness can be noted, as well as oral abnormalities including dysphagia, dysarthria, and abnormal palmomental and glabellar reflexes. The overall incidence of pseudoparkinsonism from FGAs ranges from 15.4% to 36%, depending on the drug and dose. Akinesia alone can be seen in 59% of patients on high-potency FGAs. Other risk factors include increasing age and possibly female gender. The onset of symptoms is typically 1 to 2 weeks after initiation of antipsychotic therapy or a dose increase.

The efficacy of anticholinergic medications in treating symptoms of pseudoparkinsonism is well established.[93,94] Interestingly, recent meta-analyses and trial data, such as a secondary analysis of data from the CUtLASS-1 and CATIE studies, are not reporting marked differences in rates of EPS between FGAs and SGAs when FGA treatments are accompanied by appropriate use of anticholinergic medications.[95]

Benztropine's long half-life allows once- to twice-daily dosing. Typical dosing is 1 to 2 mg twice a day up to a usual maximum dosage of 8 mg daily. Trihexyphenidyl (2 to 5 mg three times a day), diphenhydramine (25 to 50 mg three times a day), and biperiden (2 mg three times a day) usually require thrice-daily administration. Diphenhydramine produces more sedation than the other agents. All of the anticholinergics have been abused for their euphoriant effects.[96] Symptoms typically begin to resolve within 3 to 4 days after initiation of treatment, but a minimum of at least 2 weeks of treatment is normally required for full response. Amantadine is generally as efficacious for pseudoparkinsonism as anticholinergics, with significantly less effect on memory function.[94] The need for prophylactic use of these agents against pseudoparkinsonism is less convincing than with dystonias, and is unnecessary when using SGAs.[94] The long-term treatment of pseudoparkinsonism with antiparkinsonism medication is somewhat controversial, and an attempt should be made to taper and discontinue these agents 6 weeks to 3 months after symptom resolution. If symptoms reappear, then switching to an SGA should be considered. The risk of pseudoparkinsonism with SGAs is low. When risperidone is used in doses greater than 6 mg/day, the risk of pseudoparkinsonism symptoms approaches that with FGAs. Quetiapine, aripiprazole, and clozapine are reasonable alternatives in a patient experiencing EPS with other SGAs.[58,93,94]

Tardive Dyskinesia Tardive dyskinesia is a syndrome characterized by abnormal involuntary movements occurring late in onset in relation to initiation of antipsychotic therapy. It is sometimes irreversible and continues to be a controversial issue.

The classic description of tardive dyskinesia is the buccal–lingual–masticatory (BLM) syndrome, or orofacial movements. The onset of BLM movements is usually insidious. Typically, they are the first detectable signs of tardive dyskinesia and begin with mild forward, backward, or lateral movements of the tongue. If the disorder progresses, more obvious or frank BLM movements appear, including tongue thrusting, rolling, or fly-catching movements, and chewing or lateral jaw movements. Tardive dyskinesia symptoms can interfere with the patient's ability to chew, speak, or swallow. Further complications include oral ulcerations, inability to wear dentures, and inflammation and loosening of mandibular joints. Eating difficulties and malnutrition can be severe complications. Weight loss can be seen in patients with esophageal or respiratory manifestations. Facial movements include frequent blinking, brow arching, grimacing, upward deviation of the eyes, and lip smacking. Involvement of the extremities sometimes occurs, with the appearance of restless choreiform and distal athetosis of limbs including twisting, spreading, flexion and extension of fingers, toe tapping, and toe dorsiflexion. Unusual posture, hyperextension, pelvic thrusting, axial hyperkinesia ballismus, exaggerated lordosis, rocking, and swaying are occasionally observed. Among the differential diagnoses are withdrawal dyskinesias occurring after short-term use of antipsychotics, spontaneous orofacial dyskinesias in the elderly, orofacial dyskinesias in the edentulous, stereotypic movements in schizophrenics, Huntington's disease, and congenital torsion dystonia. Orofacial movements are more common in older patients, whereas the truncal axial movements are classically reported in young adults. Movements can worsen with stress, decrease with sedation, and disappear during sleep. Concentration on motor tasks or attempts to suppress the movements can actually increase them.

Early signs of tardive dyskinesia can be reversible but if allowed to persist, they can become irreversible, even with drug discontinuation. When the antipsychotic dose is decreased or tapered and discontinued, worsening of abnormal movements can occur, followed by possible slow improvement after months or years if the patient remains on lower doses or discontinues treatment. No standardized diagnostic criteria for tardive dyskinesia are available. Abnormal involuntary movements can be detected early through physical assessment and the use of rating scales. Available rating scales include the Abnormal Involuntary Movement Scale (AIMS) and the Dyskinesia Identification System: Condensed User Scale (DISCUS).[97] Neither scale is diagnostic in itself.

Risk factors include increasing age, the occurrence of acute EPS, poor antipsychotic drug response, diagnosis of organic mental disorder, diabetes mellitus, mood disorders, and possibly female gender.[93] Duration of antipsychotic therapy, daily dosage, and possibly total cumulative dosage are probably the most significant risk factors. Polymorphisms of the DA D_3 receptor, 5-HT_{2C} receptor, and the superoxide dismutase-2 genes have all been implicated in varying the risk of TD with antipsychotic use.[98] Overall morbidity and mortality are greater in tardive dyskinesia patients.

With FGAs, the reported prevalence of tardive dyskinesia ranges from 0.5% to 62%.[93] In a first episode of schizophrenia, the incidence is estimated at about 5% per year, with the overall prevalence ranging from 20% to 25% with long-term treatment. Among the elderly, the overall risk of tardive dyskinesia is higher.[93,94] Tardive dyskinesia is not always permanent, with remission of symptoms observed in 25% of patients after 5 years of continued treatment.[31,93,94]

The risk of tardive dyskinesia with SGAs may be significantly lower.[93] A systematic review of 12 studies with SGAs lasting 1 year or more found an overall risk of tardive dyskinesia to be approximately 2.98% per year in nonelderly adults as compared with 7.7% for FGAs.[99] Although lower than the FGAs, the PORT guidelines report no difference in the risk of tardive dyskinesia among SGAs.[28,31]

Prevention of tardive dyskinesia is important, as treatment of the movements once they occur is difficult. One of the more compelling arguments for the first-line use of SGAs is their lower risk of tardive dyskinesia.[31,100] Regular neurologic examinations (AIMS or other scales) should be performed at baseline and at least quarterly to assess for possible early signs of tardive dyskinesia. At the first signs of tardive dyskinesia, the need for continuing antipsychotic treatment should be reassessed. In such situations, if the patient is taking an FGA and continuing treatment is indicated, the medication should be switched to an SGA.

Numerous drugs have been used in an attempt to treat tardive dyskinesia. In two controlled trials lasting 22 to 52 weeks, clozapine decreased abnormal involuntary movements.[28,31,96] Switching antipsychotic therapy to clozapine is a favored first-line pharmacotherapeutic strategy in patients with moderate to severe dyskinesias.[31,96]

Sedation and Cognition Chlorpromazine, thioridazine, clozapine, olanzapine, and quetiapine are the most sedating antipsychotics. Administration of most or all of the daily dosage at bedtime can decrease daytime sedation and in some patients eliminate the need for hypnotic agents. Sedation occurs early in treatment and can decrease over time. Oversedation can play a large role in cognitive, perceptual, and motor dysfunction. However, positive effects of medication on cognition are seen with chronic administration, evidenced by improvements in tasks involving visual motor skills, attention to task, and working memory. Compared with FGAs, several studies have shown cognitive benefits of SGAs. However, results from the CATIE trial showed no differences in cognitive improvement between SGAs and the FGA perphenazine.[101] Comparative effects of different SGAs on cognition are as yet unclear, but available studies suggest that different SGAs can have effects on varying cognitive domains.[31]

As discussed in Long-Acting Injectable Antipsychotics above, olanzapine pamoate monohydrate injectable is associated with a postinjection sedation/delirium syndrome.[40,41]

Seizures An increased risk of drug-induced seizures occurs in all patients treated with antipsychotics. However, this risk is greater if the following predisposing factors are present: preexisting seizure disorder, history of drug-induced seizure, abnormal electroencephalogram (EEG), and preexisting CNS pathology or head trauma. Seizures are more closely associated with the use of higher doses, rapid dosage increases, and on initiation of treatment. When an isolated seizure occurs, a dosage decrease is first recommended; routine prophylactic use of anticonvulsant therapy is not recommended. Although spontaneously occurring seizures have been reported with most antipsychotics, the highest potential risk for an antipsychotic-related seizure is with clozapine or chlorpromazine. If a change in antipsychotic therapy is required because of a drug-induced seizure, risperidone, thioridazine, haloperidol, pimozide, trifluoperazine, and fluphenazine are associated with the lowest potential.[94]

Thermoregulation Poikilothermia, the body temperature adjusting to the ambient temperature, can be a serious side effect of antipsychotic therapy in temperature extremes.[102] Hyperpyrexia can be a danger in hot weather or during exercise. Inhibition of sweating, a result of anticholinergic properties impairing the peripheral mechanisms of heat dissipation, can contribute to this problem, which in its severest form can lead to heat stroke. Hypothermia is a risk in cold temperatures, particularly in the elderly. All patients receiving antipsychotics should be educated about these potential problems. Thermoregulatory problems are reportedly more common with the use of low-potency FGAs and can occur with the more anticholinergic SGAs.

Neuroleptic Malignant Syndrome Neuroleptic malignant syndrome (NMS) occurs in 0.5% to 1% of patients receiving FGAs. NMS can occur more frequently in patients receiving high-potency FGAs, injectable or depot FGAs, and in patients who are dehydrated, with physical exhaustion, or organic mental disorders. Although less common, NMS has been reported with SGAs, including clozapine. The onset of symptoms varies from early in treatment to months later. It develops rapidly, over the course of 24 to 72 hours. NMS can occur after antipsychotic discontinuation, especially when depot agents are used. Possible mechanisms of NMS include disruption of the central thermoregulatory process or excess production of heat secondary to skeletal muscle contractions. The differential diagnosis includes heat stroke, lethal catatonia, anesthetic-associated malignant hyperthermia, anticholinergic toxicity, and monoamine oxidase inhibitor drug interactions. Cardinal signs and symptoms of NMS are body temperature exceeding 38°C (100.4°F), altered level of consciousness, autonomic dysfunction (tachycardia, labile blood pressure, diaphoresis, tachypnea, or urinary or fecal incontinence), and rigidity. Laboratory evaluation, although nonspecific, frequently shows leukocytosis with or without a left shift, increases in creatine kinase (CK), aspartate aminotransferase, alanine aminotransferase, lactate dehydrogenase, and myoglobinuria.[94]

Treatment should begin with antipsychotic discontinuation and supportive care. In many cases that alone is effective. The role of adjunctive agents is unclear, yet they are often used. The DA agonist bromocriptine reduces rigidity, fever, or CK in up to 94% of patients, whereas the use of amantadine has been successful in up to 63% of patients. Dantrolene has been used as a skeletal muscle relaxant, with positive effects on temperature, heart rate, respiratory rate, and CK in up to 81% of patients.[94] Wide recognition and rapid antipsychotic discontinuation has drastically reduced mortality from 20% 25 years ago to 4% in the mid-1990s.

Many patients with schizophrenia, despite having had NMS, will require future antipsychotic pharmacotherapy. A review of antipsychotic rechallenges suggests that the risk of rechallenge is acceptable in most patients, provided that the patient is observed for an extended period of time (2 weeks or more is suggested) without antipsychotics, that there is careful monitoring and slow dose titration, and that the patient is maintained on the lowest possible dose.[94] A different antipsychotic, an SGA or a low-potency FGA, should be used for rechallenge following an episode of NMS.

Psychiatric Side Effects Antipsychotic-induced akathisia, akinesia, and dysphoria can have unfortunate sequelae, resulting in what has been termed "behavioral toxicity."[33] Akinesia, characterized by "diminished spontaneity," results in symptoms of apathy and withdrawal, often mistaken for the negative symptoms of schizophrenia; these patients can actually appear depressed. Delirium and psychosis are reported with larger doses of FGAs or combinations of anticholinergics with FGAs. Chronic confusion and disorientation can occur in the elderly as a result of antipsychotic treatment.[103] Unfortunately, the link is not always made with antipsychotic therapy, and the patient is misdiagnosed with delirium from a different etiology. This clinical presentation, called a *pseudodementia*, may be reversible on discontinuation of the antipsychotic.

Ophthalmologic Effects Anticholinergic effects of antipsychotics or concomitant antiparkinson medications can exacerbate narrow-angle (angle-closure) glaucoma. Antipsychotics with low anticholinergic effects should be used in such individuals, and they should be appropriately monitored.[104]

Opaque deposits in the cornea and lens occur with chronic phenothiazine treatment, most frequently with chlorpromazine. Although visual acuity is not usually affected, periodic slit-lamp ophthalmologic examinations are frequently recommended in patients receiving long-term treatment with phenothiazines, as fully formed cataracts are a possibility.[104]

Because of cataract development and lenticular changes in animals, baseline and periodic eye examinations are recommended in the product labeling for quetiapine.[105] However, clinical use of quetiapine since marketing has not shown a significant risk of cataracts.[105] Retinitis pigmentosa can result from use of thioridazine doses greater than 800 mg daily. It is caused by melanin deposits and can result in permanent visual impairment or blindness.

Genitourinary System

Urinary hesitancy and retention, secondary to anticholinergic effects, are reported with low-potency FGAs and with clozapine. Men with benign prostatic hypertrophy are especially prone to this effect.[106]

Urinary incontinence is thought to be caused by α-blockade, and among the SGAs, it appears to be particularly problematic with clozapine. The incidence has been reported to be as high as 44%, and it can be persistent in 25% of patients.[107]

Although inadequately studied, multiple mechanisms are likely responsible for sexual dysfunction, including dopaminergic blockade, hyperprolactinemia, histaminergic blockade (sedation), anticholinergic effects, and α-adrenergic blockade. Unmedicated individuals with schizophrenia report decreased libido. Most but not all studies show a relationship between hyperprolactinemia and sexual dysfunction, including decreased libido, erectile dysfunction, difficulty achieving orgasm, and ejaculatory abnormalities. Risperidone produces at least as much sexual dysfunction as FGAs; other SGAs, with weak effects on prolactin, produce less sexual dysfunction. Patients experiencing sexual dysfunction with FGAs or risperidone should be switched to an SGA with less effect on prolactin.[108]

Priapism, a sustained and painful erection which is unprovoked and persists for longer than an hour, is increasingly reported with antipsychotic medication use. This is believed to occur as a result of α_1-adrenergic receptor blockade, leading to intracavernosal blood stasis.[109] This can evolve into a urologic emergency, due to the ischemic nature of the priapism. Patients on antipsychotics with other risk factors, including sickle-cell disease and history of prolonged erections,[109] and perhaps those patients taking other medications with α_1-blocking properties should be counseled regarding this rare but important adverse reaction. If left untreated, priapism may lead to permanent impotence.

Hematologic System

Transient leukopenia can occur during initial treatment with antipsychotics; however, it typically does not progress to be clinically significant.[110] The three antipsychotics with highest relative risk of neutropenic are in rank order clozapine, chlorpromazine, and olanzapine.[111] If the WBC count is less than 3,000/mm^3 (3×10^9/L), or if the absolute neutrophil count (ANC) is less than 1,000/mm^3 (1×10^9/L), the antipsychotic should be discontinued, and the WBC monitored closely until it returns to normal. Agranulocytosis reportedly occurs in 0.01% of patients receiving FGAs, and more frequently with chlorpromazine and thioridazine. The onset is usually within the first 8 weeks of therapy. Agranulocytosis can initially manifest as a local infection, with sore throat, leukoplakia, erythema, and ulcerations of the pharynx. These symptoms in any patient receiving antipsychotics should signal the immediate need for a WBC count. If either the WBC count or ANC falls below these parameters, the drug should be discontinued immediately and the patient monitored closely for the development of secondary infections. Isolated rare cases of thrombocytopenia and eosinophilia have also been reported.

Agranulocytosis with clozapine significantly limits the usefulness of this agent. The risk of developing neutropenia or agranulocytosis with clozapine is approximately 3% and 0.8%, respectively.[111] Increasing age and female gender are associated with greater risk. The time period for greatest risk is between months 1 and 6 of treatment, and weekly WBC monitoring for the first 6 months of therapy is mandated in the FDA-approved product labeling. After the first 6 months, the labeling allows the frequency of WBC monitoring to be decreased to every 2 weeks for months 7 to 12, after which it can be decreased to monthly if all WBCs are normal. If the total WBC count drops to less than 2,000/mm^3 (2×10^9/L), or the ANC is less than 1,000/mm^3 (1×10^9/L), clozapine should be discontinued and the patient monitored closely. Granulocyte colony-stimulating factor filgrastim has been used to hasten recovery. In cases of moderate neutropenia (granulocytes 2,000 to 3,000/mm^3 [2×10^9/L to 3×10^9/L], or ANC 1,000 to 1,500/mm^3 [1×10^9/L to 1.5×10^9/L]), which occurs in up to 2% of patients, clozapine should be discontinued with daily monitoring of complete blood counts until values return to normal.

Dermatologic System

Allergic reactions are rare and usually occur within 8 weeks of initiating therapy, manifesting as maculopapular, erythematous, pruritic rashes that are evident on the face, neck, trunk, or extremities. Contact dermatitis, including the oral mucosa, can occur in patients or medical personnel. For patients, mixing the antipsychotic concentrate in a sufficient quantity of a nonacidic liquid and swallowing it quickly decreases problems in susceptible patients. Care should be taken in the handling and preparation of liquid FGAs.

Phenothiazine can absorb ultraviolet light, resulting in the formation of free radicals, which can have damaging effects on the skin. All antipsychotics can cause photosensitivity. Erythema and severe sunburns can occur. Exposure to sunlight should be limited, and patients should be educated about the use of a maximally blocking sunscreen, hats, protective clothing, and sunglasses.[112]

Blue-gray or purplish skin coloration in areas exposed to sunlight occurs in patients receiving higher doses of low-potency phenothiazines during long-term administration, especially with chlorpromazine. It commonly occurs with concurrent corneal or lens pigmentation.

Miscellaneous Adverse Effects

A sometimes troubling side effect with clozapine is sialorrhea, which can occur in up to 54% of patients. The mechanism of clozapine-induced drooling is unclear. Although both anticholinergics and α-agonists have been used to treat clozapine-related sialorrhea, research evidence is insufficient to make specific recommendations.[113]

Toxicity with Overdose

Acute overdose with antipsychotics rarely results in serious symptomatology. Mild intoxication manifests as sedation, hypotension, and miosis, whereas with severe intoxication, agitation and delirium can typically progress to motor retardation, seizures, cardiac arrhythmias, respiratory arrest, and coma. Dystonias and pseudoparkinsonism symptoms also occur. Supportive measures, gastric lavage, and activated charcoal are recommended. Induction of emesis can be difficult because of effects on the chemoreceptor trigger zone, and dialysis is ineffective because of the degree of drug–protein binding. Phenytoin or sodium bicarbonate is useful in the treatment of quinidine-like cardiac conduction effects on the QRS or QTc. Physostigmine is not generally recommended to reverse anticholinergic toxicity because of deleterious effects on arrhythmias and seizure threshold.[112]

Use in Pregnancy and Lactation

Minimal data exist regarding the effects of pregnancy on schizophrenia. However, disorganized thought processes, impaired cognition, and negative symptoms can have a detrimental effect on the functioning and self-care of the mother, and therefore adversely affect the fetus.[114] Currently available data assessing the risk of teratogenesis with antipsychotic agents are insufficient. Epidemiologic studies show a slightly increased risk of birth defects with low-potency FGAs. Haloperidol is the best studied of all antipsychotics, and no relationship between its use and teratogenicity has been found. One study indicates a greater than twofold elevated risk of preterm birth in women with schizophrenia taking FGAs as compared with unaffected mothers not taking antipsychotics.[114]

SGAs have increasing information regarding safety in pregnancy; however, very few large studies and very few prospective studies have been performed to evaluate possible teratogenicity of SGAs. Two prospectively designed nonrandomized, observational studies have reported no increased risk of teratogenic birth defects with SGA exposure.[115,116] One large registry data study performed in Sweden found a significantly increased risk of cardiovascular defects with FGA or SGA exposure[117]; however, when stratifying by antipsychotic class, it was found that all defects were found in those exposed to FGAs, while no cardiovascular defects were reported with SGAs.[118] Definitive data are still lacking.

Studies have shown differing results in regard to infant outcomes in fetuses exposed to SGAs. Women with schizophrenia taking SGAs showed no significant risk of LBW, preterm birth, or infant considered small or large for gestational age (LGA) when compared with infants born to unaffected and unexposed mothers.[114] One prospectively designed study found a higher rate of LBW infants in mothers taking SGAs (10%) than in the reference group (2%),[115] while another prospective study reported higher rates of LGA infant births in women taking SGAs compared with those in the FGA and reference groups.[119]

Other potential interests in studying early and late exposure to antipsychotics include postnatal and gestational complications. Weight gain associated with olanzapine and clozapine and the potential risk of gestational diabetes should be considered in drug selection.[120] A recent retrospective cohort study reported nearly twofold odds of gestatational diabetes in women who used antipsychotics during pregnancy.[120]

Risk of neonatal EPS is increased with in utero exposure to FGAs, with effects in the infant lasting for 3 to 12 months after birth.[121] In February 2011, the FDA issued a safety announcement informing healthcare professionals that the pregnancy section of drug labels had been updated for the entire class of antipsychotics, highlighting the potential risk for EPS and withdrawal symptoms in newborns whose mothers were treated with antipsychotics during their third trimester.[121] Symptoms of neonatal withdrawal reported to the FDA included agitation, hypertonia, hypotonia, tremor, somnolence, respiratory distress, and feeding disorder.

The risk of antipsychotic use must be weighed against the benefits of pharmacotherapy in pregnant women experiencing disorganized thoughts, delusions about change in body image or pregnancy, or who are unable to provide adequate prenatal care.[114,121]

Antipsychotics appear in breast milk with milk-to-plasma ratios of 0.5:1. However, 1 week after delivery, clozapine milk concentrations were found to be as much as 279% of serum concentrations. Its use during breast-feeding is not recommended.[122] Overall, little is known about breast-feeding and the potential effects of antipsychotics on the neonate. Although not contraindicated, the lowest dosage should be used in the mother, and the infant carefully monitored.

Drug Interactions

Most drug interactions occur because of pharmacodynamic or pharmacokinetic interactions. Common examples of pharmacodynamic interactions resulting in enhanced effect include the excess sedation that can occur when antipsychotics are used concomitantly with other medications that have sedative side effects. Additive antimuscarinic effects of antipsychotics used with other medications with antimuscarinic effects can result in urinary retention, constipation, blurred vision, or other anticholinergic side effects.[33,123] Both combined sedative and anticholinergic effects from multiple medications can result in impaired cognition, particularly in the elderly and other patients predisposed to such problems.[123] Patients are more likely to experience symptomatic orthostatic hypotension when an antipsychotic is used with other medications that cause orthostasis. Although metoclopramide is prescribed for treating esophageal reflux, it is a DA antagonist, and patients are more likely to experience akathisia and other EPS if it is used concomitantly with antipsychotics.[124] Although some SSRIs can interact with antipsychotics through enzyme inhibition, they can also interact through pharmacodynamic mechanisms. 5-HT_2 receptors are present on the presynaptic dopaminergic neuron, and their activation leads to decreased DA release from the presynaptic terminal. Increased availability of 5-HT through SSRI effect can activate these receptors, decrease DA release, and add to the dopaminolytic effects of antipsychotics.[124] In the absence of enzyme inhibition, SSRIs can still precipitate akathisia or EPS when added to a patient stabilized on an antipsychotic. A potentially more dangerous interaction can occur when medications that slow myocardial conduction and thus prolong the QTc are used in combination with antipsychotics that significantly prolong the QTc.[124] Medications that prolong the QTc should be monitored carefully in patients taking concomitant diuretics.[124] These effects can all increase the risk of clinically significant adverse effects.

Asenapine inhibits CYP2D6, and is the only SGA that has been shown to significantly affect the pharmacokinetics of other medications.[60] Table 50-6 lists the known major pathways involved in the metabolism of SGAs. Risperidone is metabolized primarily by

CYP2D6 to its active metabolite, 9-OH-risperidone (paliperidone), which is thought to have a similar pharmacodynamic profile.[124] Although paliperidone is primarily eliminated renally unchanged, potent inducers of CYP3A4 can cause a potential need for dosage adjustment.[63,125] CYP1A2 is the primary isoenzyme for metabolism of asenapine with CYP3A4 also being a significant pathway.[63]

Based on current information, inhibitors of CYP1A2 have the greatest potential for causing interactions with clozapine and olanzapine.[126] Examples include cimetidine, fluvoxamine, and fluoroquinolone antibiotics (e.g., ciprofloxacin) to varying degrees. To date, however, no serious inhibition interactions have been reported with olanzapine, which may be a result of olanzapine's wide therapeutic index. Carbamazepine has been reported to increase olanzapine elimination by as much as 50%.[126] Cigarette smoking is a potent inducer of CYP1A2, and one would expect lower mean olanzapine serum concentrations in smokers compared with those in nonsmokers.

Because of the risk of seizures with higher clozapine tissue concentrations, interactions that inhibit clozapine's metabolism are potentially significant. In particular, fluvoxamine increases clozapine serum concentrations by an average of twofold to threefold and up to fivefold.[126,127] Fluoxetine and erythromycin can increase clozapine serum concentrations to a lesser degree.[126,127] Mean clozapine serum concentrations are reported to be 32% lower in smokers compared with those in nonsmokers.[126] If a patient taking clozapine stops smoking, the resulting increase in clozapine serum concentration could be associated with seizures.[63] Carbamazepine can induce clozapine metabolism and lead to lower serum concentrations.[110]

A study with the potent CYP3A4 inhibitor ketoconazole showed minimal effects on ziprasidone single-dose pharmacokinetics, with only a 33% mean increase in the ziprasidone area under the time-versus-concentration curve.[124] These results are consistent with data suggesting that aldehyde oxidase is the major metabolic pathway for ziprasidone, with only 30% to 35% being metabolized by CYP3A4.[128]

Modest elevations of aripiprazole serum concentration occur in the presence of ketoconazole or quinidine, which inhibit CYP3A4 and 2D6, respectively. Carbamazepine has been reported to decrease aripiprazole serum concentrations.[58,127]

Since iloperidone is metabolized through CYP2D6 and 3A4, its clearance can be impaired by inhibitors of these pathways. Since iloperidone prolongs the QTc interval, these types of interactions have the potential to be clinically significant. For example, it is recommended that the iloperidone dose be decreased by 50% when used with CYP2D6 inhibitors such as fluoxetine or paroxetine.[59]

Table 50-9 summarizes potential antipsychotic drug interactions.

Personalized Pharmacotherapy

Pharmacotherapy must be individualized for each person with schizophrenia. With the possible exception of iloperidone, no laboratory tests are generally available that will predict a patient's response to treatment. Past response to treatment, potential adverse effects, patient personal preference, and medication price are the primary variables that should be used in selecting an antipsychotic for a patient being treated at stages 1 or 2 of the treatment algorithm. In the CATIE study, the number one reason for drug discontinuation was the patient not wanting to take that medication any more, and the second most common reason was adverse effects.[29] These two factors should be carefully considered in antipsychotic selection. Medication dosage must also be individualized within the usual dose ranges. Careful consideration must also be given to concomitant medications that may interact with the antipsychotic and necessitate a change in dosage.

Preliminary data suggest a relationship between different genetic markers and clinical improvement as well as QTc prolongation in patients treated with iloperidone. Another study showed some of these markers to be associated with response to risperidone.[34,87] It is too early to conclude whether these or other genetic markers will have a clinically useful role to play in the treatment of persons with schizophrenia.

Given that no antipsychotic has proven superiority with regard to efficacy in the treatment of schizophrenia (with the exception of clozapine in treatment resistance), cost should be a factor in antipsychotic selection. Olanzapine, quetiapine, risperidone, and all FGAs have generic equivalents available, and this should be a factor in selecting an antipsychotic at stage 1 of the treatment algorithm.

EVALUATION OF THERAPEUTIC OUTCOMES

Assessment of response has traditionally been done subjectively or empirically (a relative sense of how the clinician feels the patient is doing). A formal MSE is used to structure the patient interview and focus on items related to appearance, mood, sensorium, intellectual functioning, and thought processes. However, the MSE is neither specific nor quantitative for the measurement of drug response. **10** Clinicians should be trained to use simple, standardized psychiatric rating scales to assist in objectively rating patient drug responses.[130] The Brief Psychiatric Rating Scale (BPRS) and the Positive and Negative Symptom Scale (PANSS) were developed for use in clinical trials as research tools to quantify symptom improvement seen with antipsychotic treatment.[130] Objectively, the use of a numeric indicator (e.g., 20%, 30%, or 40% reduction in BPRS score) has been used to quantify overall symptom reduction and classify patients according to different degrees of response. However, these types of rating scales are too long and unwieldy to be routinely used within the time constraints of most clinical practices. Symptom scales used in clinical practice must be sufficiently brief to be used during an ordinary clinic visit (e.g., 15 to 30 minutes) while measuring both positive and negative symptoms, and being sufficiently representative of overall symptomatology. The four-item Positive Symptom Rating Scale (PSRS) and the Brief Negative Symptom Assessment are brief scales that meet such criteria (Table 50-10).[131] A brief rating scale of positive symptoms, such as the PSRS, should be used at baseline before starting pharmacotherapy, and at each time response to pharmacotherapy is assessed.

Clinical **Controversy...**

Psychiatry is one of the few specialties in medicine in which measurement is not a routine component of patient care. Although biologic measures do not currently exist in psychiatry, symptoms associated with a patient's illness can be measured and quantified. Although increasing evidence attests to the benefits of quantifying symptom severity, the use of symptom rating scales remains uncommon in clinical practice.

Similarly, the pharmacotherapeutic plan should include specific monitoring parameters for side effects (see Table 50-11). The plan should include how the potential side effect will be evaluated, and the frequency of assessment. Given the risk of weight gain, diabetes, and lipid abnormalities associated with many of the SGAs, a consensus task force led by the American Diabetes Association recommends the following baseline parameters before beginning antipsychotics: family history, weight, height, body mass index,

TABLE 50-9 Common Potential Drug Interactions with Antipsychotic Medications

Mechanism of Interaction	Examples of Interacting Drugs or Other Substances			Clinical Effect
Pharmacodynamic Drug Interactions with Antipsychotics				
Muscarinic receptor blockade	*Anticholinergics* Benztropine Diphenhydramine Trihexyphenidyl			↑ anticholinergic SE Blurred vision Constipation Impaired Cognition Urinary retention
Additive or synergistic sedation	*Sedatives* Benzodiazepines Concomitant AP Diphenhydramine Melatonin and melatonin agonists Mirtazapine Trazodone TCAs Zaleplon Zolpidem *Anticholinergics* Benztropine Diphenhydramine Trihexyphenidyl Mirtazapine			↑ sedation Lethargy Impaired cognition Impaired psychomotor activity ↑ risk of accidents
DA antagonist use for different indication	Metoclopramide			↑ EPS
Cardiovascular interactions				
Additive effects on QTc	*TCA antidepressants* Amitriptyline Clomipramine Imipramine	Procainamide Quinidine		↑ *risk of ECG changes and dysrhythmias*
Electrolyte changes	Diuretics			↑ *risk of ECG changes and dysrhythmias*
Stimulation of presynaptic 5-HT receptors on DA neuron	SSRIs			↑ *EPS*
Sympatholytics: α-blockade-↓ NE release	Clonidine Methyldopa Prazosin			↑ hypotension
↑ DA receptor binding	*Antipsychotics*			↑ SEs, particularly EPS
Pharmacokinetic Drug Interactions with Antipsychotics				
Substrate Antipsychotic and Mechanism of Action		***Inhibitor or Inducer***		***Clinical Effect***
Aripiprazole and iloperidone				
Inhibition of AP metabolism (CYP2D6, CYP3A4)	*Antidepressants* Bupropion Clomipramine Doxepin Duloxetine Fluoxetine Fluvoxamine Paroxetine Sertraline *HIV protease inhibitors* Indinavir Nelfinavir Ritonavir	*Anti-infectives* Ciprofloxacin Clarithromycin Erythromycin Fluconazole Ketoconazole Itraconazole *Antipsychotics* Asenapine Chlorpromazine Haloperidol Perphenazine Thioridazine	*Miscellaneous* Ciprofloxacin Chlorpheniramine Cimetidine Cocaine Diltiazem Diphenhydramine Cimetidine Grapefruit juice Haloperidol Hydroxyzine Methadone Quinidine Ticlopidine Verapamil	↑ AP effect ↑ SE
Induction of AP metabolism	*Antiepileptics* Carbamazepine Oxcarbazepine Phenobarbital Phenytoin	*Anti-infectives* Rifampin *Miscellaneous* Glucocorticoids Modafinil	*Herbals* St. John's wort	↓ AP effect
Asenapine				
Eating food or drinking liquids within 10 minutes of asenapine sublingual administration will decrease bioavailability				
Inhibition of AP metabolism (CYP1A2)	*Antidepressants* Fluvoxamine	*Anti-infectives* Ciprofloxacin Fluroquinolones	*Miscellaneous* Amidarone Cimetidine	↑ AP effect ↑ SE
Induction of AP metabolism	*Anti-infectives* Nafcillin	*Miscellaneous* Broccoli Brussels sprouts Chargrilled meat Smoking tobacco	*Miscellaneous* Insulin Modafinil Omeprazole	↓ AP effect

(*continued*)

TABLE 50-9 Common Potential Drug Interactions with Antipsychotic Medications (*Continued*)

Mechanism of Interaction	Examples of Interacting Drugs or Other Substances			Clinical Effect
Pharmacokinetic Drug Interactions with Antipsychotics				
Substrate Antipsychotic and Mechanism of Action		***Inhibitor or Inducer***		***Clinical Effect***
Clozapine Inhibition of AP metabolism (CYP3A4, CYP1A2, CYP2C19)	*Antidepressants* Fluoxetine Fluvoxamine *HIV protease inhibitors* Indinavir Nelfinavir Ritonavir *Anticonvulsants* Felbamate Oxcarbazepine	*Anti-infectives* Ciprofloxacin Clarithromycin Erythromycin Fluconazole Ketoconazole Itraconazole Nafcillin	*Miscellaneous* Amidarone Diltiazem Cimetidine Grapefruit juice Haloperidol Modafinil Omeprazole Ticlopidine Topiramate Verapamil Cimetidine	↑ AP effect ↑ SE
Induction of AP metabolism	*Antiepileptics* Carbamazepine Phenobarbital Phenytoin	*Anti-infectives* Rifampin *Miscellaneous* Glucocorticoids Insulin Modafinil Omeprazole	*Herbals* St. John's wort	↓ AP effect
Haloperidol Inhibition of AP metabolism (CYP2D6, OP3A4, CYP1A2)	*Antidepressants* Bupropion Doxepin Duloxetine Fluoxetine Fluvoxamine Paroxetine Sertraline *HIV protease inhibitors* Indinavir Nelfinavir Ritonavir Sequinavir	*Anti-infectives* Ciprofloxacin Clarithromycin Erythromycin Fluoconazole Fluoroquinolones Ketoconazole Itraconazole *Antipsychotics* Chlorpromazine Perphenazine	*Miscellaneous* Amiodarone Chlorpheniramine Cimetidine Diltiazem Diphenhydramine Quinidine Diphenhydramine Cimetidine Grapefruit juice Hydroxyzine Methadone Quinidine Verapamil	↑ AP effect ↑ SE
Induction of AP metabolism	*Anticonvulsants* Carbamazepine Oxcarbazepine Phenobarbital Phenytoin	*Anti-infectives* Nafcillin Rifampin *Miscellaneous* Broccoli Brussels sprouts Chargrilled meat Glucocorticoids Insulin Modafinil Omeprazole Modafinil	*Herbals* St. John's wort Tobacco smoking	↓ AP effect
Iloperidone (see Aripiprazole above)				
Olanzapine Inhibition of AP metabolism (CYP3A4 and CYP1A2)	*Antidepressants* Fluoxetine (norfluoxetine) Fluvoxamine *HIV protease inhibitors* Indinavir Nelfinavir Ritonavir	*Anti-infectives* Ciprofloxacin Clarithromycin Erythromycin Fluoconazole Fluoroquinolones Ketoconazole Itraconazole	*Miscellaneous* Amiodarone Cimetidine Diltiazem Cimetidine Grapefruit juice Verapamil	↑ AP effect ↑ SE
Induction of AP metabolism	*Antiepileptics* Carbamazepine Oxcarbazepine Phenobarbital Phenytoin *HIV protease inhibitors* Efavirenz Nevirapine	*Anti-infectives* Nafcillin Rifampin Miscellaneous Broccoli Brussels sprouts Chargrilled meat Glucocorticoids Insulin Modafinil Omeprazole	*Herbals* St. John's wort Smoking tobacco	↓ AP effect
Paliperidone The bioavailability of paliperidone is significantly increased when it is taken with food. Although this could increase paliperidone effect, including adverse effects, the clinical significance is undetermined. Only potent CYP3A4 (e.g., carbamazepine, rifampin, St. John's wort) inducers appear to increase paliperidone metabolism and affect dose requirements				

(*continued*)

TABLE 50-9 Common Potential Drug Interactions with Antipsychotic Medications (*Continued*)

Mechanism of Interaction	Examples of Interacting Drugs or Other Substances			Clinical Effect
Pharmacokinetic Drug Interactions with Antipsychotics				
Substrate Antipsychotic and Mechanism of Action		***Inhibitor or Inducer***		***Clinical Effect***
Lurasidone and quetiapine	*Antidepressants*	*Anti-infectives*	*Miscellaneous*	↑ AP effect
Inhibition of AP metabolism (CYP3A4)	Fluoxetine (norfluoxetine) Fluvoxamine Nefazodone *HIV protease inhibitors* Indinavir Nelfinavir Ritonavir Sequinavir	Ciprofloxacin Clarithromycin Erythromycin Fluoconazole Ketoconazole Itraconazole	Amiodarone Cimetidine Diltiazem Grapefruit juice Verapamil	↑ SE
Induction of AP metabolism	*Antiepileptics* Carbamazepine Oxcarbazepine Phenobarbital Phenytoin *HIV protease inhibitors* Efavirenz Nevirapine	*Anti-infectives* Rifampin *Miscellaneous* Glucocorticoids Modafinil	*Herbals* St. John's wort	↓ AP effect
Perphenazine and risperidone				
Note: Because risperidone's metabolite formed through CYP2D6 metabolism is active (paliperidone), the clinical significance of metabolic drug interactions with risperidone is undetermined				
Inhibition of AP metabolism (CYP2D6)	*Antidepressants* Bupropion Clomipramine Doxepin Duloxetine Fluoxetine Paroxetine Sertraline *Antipsychotics* Chlorpromazine Haloperidol (reduced haloperidol) Perphenazine	*Miscellaneous* Amiodarone Cimetidine Chlorpheniramine Cocaine Diphenhydramine Cimetidine Haloperidol Hydroxyzine Methadone Quinidine		↑ AP effect ↑ SE
Induction of AP metabolism (via CYP3A34, a minor pathway for risperidone)	Dexamethasone Rifampin			↓ AP effect
Ziprasidone				
The bioavailability of ziprasidone is increased twofold when it is taken with food. Consistent administration with food is recommended				

AP, antipsychotic; DA, dopamine; EPS, extrapyramidal symptoms; 5-HT, serotonin; SE, side effect; SSRI, serotonin selective reuptake inhibitor; TCAs, tricyclic antidepressants.

Data from references 59, 60, 63, 123, 125–129.

TABLE 50-10 Brief Clinical Assessments for Monitoring Antipsychotic Response in Schizophrenia

4-Item Positive Symptom Rating Scale (PSRS)								
Use each item's anchor points to rate the patient								
1. Suspiciousness	NA[a]	1	2	3	4	5	6	7
2. Unusual thought content	NA	1	2	3	4	5	6	7
3. Hallucinations	NA	1	2	3	4	5	6	7
4. Conceptual disorganization	NA	1	2	3	4	5	6	7
Each item is scored from 1 (not present) to 7 (extremely severe)							SCORE: ______	
Brief Negative Symptom Assessment (BNSA)								
Use each item's anchor points to rate the patient								
1. Prolonged time to respond	1	2	3	4	5	6		
2. Emotion: Unchanging facial expression, blank, expressionless face	1	2	3	4	5	6		
3. Reduced social drive	1	2	3	4	5	6		
4. Poor grooming and hygiene	1	2	3	4	5	6		
Each item is scored from 1 (normal) to 6 (severe)					SCORE: ______			

[a]NA, not able to be assessed.

Data from reference 131.

TABLE 50-11 Antipsychotic Adverse Effects and Monitoring Parameters

Adverse Reaction	Monitoring Parameter	Frequency	Comments
Adverse Effect Monitoring Parameters for all Antipsychotic Medications			
Akathisia	Ask about restless or anxiety. Observe patient for restlessness. Barnes Akathisia Scale can also be used	Every visit	
Anticholinergic side effects	Ask patient about constipation, blurry vision, urinary retention, or unusual dry mouth	Every visit	
Glucose intolerance	FBS or HbA1c	At baseline, after 3 months, and if normal, then annually	
Hyperlipidemia	Lipid profile	At baseline, after 3 months, and if normal, then annually	
Orthostatic hypotension	Ask patient about dizziness on standing. If present, check BP and HR in sitting and standing positions	Every visit	The degree of orthostatic change in BP to produce symptoms varies. In general, a BP change of 20 mm Hg or more is significant
Hyperprolactinemia	In women, ask about expression of milk from the breast and menstrual irregularities. In men, ask about breast enlargement or expression of milk from nipples. If symptoms present, check serum prolactin level	Every visit	In the absence of symptoms, there is no need to monitor serum prolactin
Sedation	Ask patient about unusual sedation or sleepiness	Every visit	
Sexual dysfunction	Ask patient about decreased sexual desire, difficulty being aroused, or problems with orgasm	Every visit	Patients with schizophrenia have more sexual dysfunction than the normal population. Compare symptoms with medication-free state
Tardive dyskinesia	Standardized rating scale such as the AIMS or the DISCUS	At baseline, and then every 3 months for FGAs and every 6 months for SGAs	
Weight gain	Measure body weight, BMI, and waist circumference	At baseline, monthly for the first 3 months, and then quarterly	Waist circumference is the single best predictor of cardiac morbidity
Adverse Effect Monitoring Parameters for Specific Antipsychotics			
Agranulocytosis	White blood cell (WBC) and absolute neutrophil counts (ANC)	At baseline, weekly for 6 months, then every 2 weeks for 6 months, and then monthly	Clozapine only
Sialorrhea or excess drooling	Ask patient about problems with excess drooling, waking in the morning with a wet ring on his or her pillow. Visual observation of the patient for drooling	Every visit	Clozapine only
Bronchospasm, respiratory distress, respiratory depression, respiratory arrest	Before administration, patients must be screened for a history of asthma, chronic obstructive pulmonary disease, or other lung disease associated with bronchospasm. Monitor patient every 15 minutes for a minimum of 1 hour after drug administration for signs and symptoms of bronchospasm (i.e., vital signs and chest auscultation). Only one 10 mg dose can be given every 24 hours	Every dose administration	Inhaled Loxitane only. Can only be administered in approved healthcare facilities registered in REMS program
Postinjection sedation/delirium syndrome	Observation of the patient for at least 3 hours after drug administration. Monitor for possible sedation, altered level of consciousness, coma, delirium, confusion, disorientation, agitation, anxiety, or other cognitive impairment	Every dose administration	Long-acting olanzapine pamoate monohydrate only. Can only be administered in approved healthcare facilities registered in REMS program

waist circumference, blood pressure, fasting plasma glucose, and fasting lipid profile.[82] They also recommend followup monitoring of these parameters after beginning or changing SGAs. Weight should be monitored monthly for the first 3 months, and quarterly thereafter. The other parameters should be assessed at the end of 3 months and then annually. Self-assessments can be a useful adjunct in treating the patient. Although the patient with schizophrenia may not always be accurate in evaluating symptom severity, the use of patient self-assessments increases patient engagement in care, enhances therapeutic alliance, and gives the clinician an opportunity to identify misconceptions the patient may have regarding symptoms associated with the illness, medication side effects, and the like.[130,132] Traditionally, clinicians have often accepted partial symptom response in schizophrenia as success, and have not been aggressive in attempting to achieve greater symptomatic remission. The advent of multiple different SGAs with varying side effect profiles should encourage clinicians to be more assertive in attempting to achieve symptom remission. This is consistent with an increasing focus on remission as a goal of treatment and evolving recovery movements with an emphasis on consumerism in the care of the severely mentally ill.[25] A recent study showing how the Internet can be used to aid relapse prevention efforts gives us a glimpse of how consumerism may enhance and influence the care for schizophrenia in the future.[133]

ABBREVIATIONS

ACT	active community treatment
AIMS	Abnormal Involuntary Movement Scale
ANC	absolute neutrophil count
APA	American Psychiatric Association
BDNF	brain-derived neurotrophic factor
BLM	buccal–lingual–masticatory
BPRS	Brief Psychiatric Rating Scale
CATIE	Clinical Antipsychotic Trials of Intervention Effectiveness
CK	creatine kinase
CNV	copy number variant
CYP	cytochrome P450
D_1	dopamine-1
D_2	dopamine-2
DA	dopamine
DISCUS	Dyskinesia Identification System: Condensed User Scale
DSM-IV-TR	*Diagnostic and Statistical Manual of Mental Disorders, Fourth Edition, Text Revision*
ECG	electrocardiogram
EEG	electroencephalogram
EPS	extrapyramidal side effect
EUFEST	European First Episode Schizophrenia Trial
FGA	first-generation antipsychotic
GABA	γ-aminobutyric acid
GWAS	genome-wide association studies
5-HT	serotonin
LBW	low birth weight
LGA	large for gestational age
MSE	mental status examination
NAMI	National Alliance on Mental Illness
NMDA	*N*-methyl-D-aspartate
NMS	neuroleptic malignant syndrome
PANSS	Positive and Negative Symptom Scale
PET	positron emission tomography
PORT	Patient Outcomes Research Team
PSRS	Positive Symptom Rating Scale
REMS	Risk Evaluation and Mitigation Strategy
SCD	sudden cardiac death
serotonin-2, 5-HT_2	5-hydroxytryptamine$_2$
SGA	second-generation antipsychotic
SSRI	selective serotonin reuptake inhibitor
WBC	white blood cell

REFERENCES

1. American Psychiatric Association. Schizophrenia and other psychotic disorders. In: Diagnostic and Statistical Manual of Mental Disorders, Fourth Edition, Text Revision. Washington, DC: American Psychiatric Association, 2000:297–319.
2. Os JV, Kapur S. Schizophrenia. Lancet 2009;374:635–645.
3. Jones P, Buckley P. Schizophrenia. London: Mosby, 2006.
4. Weinberger D. Schizophrenia as a neurodevelopmental disorder. In: Weinberger DR, Hirsch SR, eds. Schizophrenia. Oxford, UK: Blackwell Science, 2003:326–348.
5. Miller BJ, Culpepper N, Rapaport MH, Buckley P. Prenatal inflammation and neurodevelopment in schizophrenia: A review of human studies. Prog Neuropsychopharmacol Biol Psychiatry 2013;42:92–100 [Epub ahead of print].
6. Benros ME, Nielsen PR, Nordentoft M, et al. Autoimmune diseases and severe infections as risk factors for schizophrenia: A 30-year population-based register study. Am J Psychiatry 2011;168:1303–1310.
7. Ho BC, Andreasen NC, Nopoulos P, et al. Progressive structural brain abnormalities and their relationships to clinical outcome: A longitudinal magnetic resonance imaging study early in schizophrenia. Arch Gen Psychiatry 2003;60:585–594.
8. Arango C, Rapado-Castro M, Reig S, et al. Progressive brain changes in children and adolescents with first-episode psychosis. Arch Gen Psychiatry 2012;69(1):16–26.
9. Van OS J. From schizophrenia metafacts to non-schizophrenia facts. Schizophr Res 2011;127(1–3): 16–17.
10. Keshavan MS, Nasrallah HA, Tandon R. Schizophrenia, "just the facts" 6. Moving ahead with the schizophrenia concept: From the elephant to the mouse. Schizophr Res 2011;127(1–3):3–13.
11. McDonald C, Murphy KC. The new genetics of schizophrenia. Psychiatr Clin North Am 2003;26:41–63.
12. Lee KW, Woon PS, Teo YY, Sim K. Genome wide studies (GWAS) and copy number variation (CNV) studies of the major psychoses: What have we learnt? Neurosci Biobehav Rev 2012;36:556–571.
13. Bergen SE, Petryshen TL. Genome-wide association studies of schizophrenia: Does bigger lead to better. Curr Opin Psychiatry 2012;25:76–82.
14. The International Schizophrenia Consortium, Stone JL, O'Donovan MC, et al. Rare chromosomal deletions and duplications increase risk of schizophrenia. Nature 2008;455:237–241.
15. Kantrowitz J, Javitt DC. Glutamatergic transmission in schizophrenia: From basic research to clinical practice. Curr Opin Psychiatry 2012;25:96–102.
16. Zammit S, Owen MJ, Evans J, et al. Cannabis, COMT and psychotic experiences. Br J Psychiatry 2011;199:380–385.
17. Shepherd AM, Laurens KR, Matheson SL, et al. Systematic meta-review and quality assessment of the structural brain alterations in schizophrenia. Neurosci Biobehav Rev 2012;36:1342–1356.
18. Vauquelin G, Bostoen S, Vanderheyden P, Seeman P. Clozapine, atypical antipsychotics and the benefits of fast-off D_2 dopamine receptor antagonism. Naunyn Schmiedebergs Arch Pharmacol 2012;385:337–372.
19. Howes OD, Kambeitz J, Kim E, et al. The nature of dopamine dysfunction in schizophrenia and what this means for treatment. Arch Gen Psychiatry 2012;69:776–786.
20. Narendran R, Frankle WG, Keefe R, et al. Altered prefrontal dopaminergic function in chronic recreational ketamine users. Am J Psychiatry 2005;162:2352–2359.
21. Miller BH, Zeier Z, Lanz TA, et al. MicroRNA-132 dysregulation in schizophrenia has implications for both neurodevelopment and adult brain function. PNAS 2012;109:3125–3130.
22. Meltzer HY, Massey BW. The role of serotonin receptors in the action of atypical antipsychotic drugs. Curr Opin Pharmacol 2011;11(1):59–67.
23. Castle DJ, Buckley PF. Schizophrenia. Oxford, UK: Oxford University Press, 2008.
24. Lehman AF, Lieberman JA, Dixon LB, et al.; American Psychiatric Association; Steering Committee on Practice Guidelines. Practice guideline for the treatment of patients with schizophrenia, second edition. Am J Psychiatry 2004;161(Suppl 2):1–56.
25. Committee on Crossing the Quality Chasm: Adaptation to Mental Health and Addictive Disorders. Improving the Quality of Health Care for Mental and Substance-Use Conditions: Quality Chasm Series. Rockville, MD: Institute of Medicine, National Academies Press, 2005.

26. Substance Abuse and Mental Health Services Administration. National Consensus Statement on Mental Health Recovery. Rockville, MD: U.S. Department of Health and Human Services, 2006.
27. Davidson L, Chinman M, Sells D, et al. Peer support among adults with mental illness: A report from the field. Schizophr Bull 2006;32:443–450.
28. Buchanan RW, Kreyenbuhl J, Kelly DL, et al. The 2009 schizophrenia PORT psychopharmacological treatment recommendations and summary statements. Schizophr Bull 2010;36:71–93.
29. Lieberman JA, Stroup S. The NIMH-CATIE schizophrenia study: What did we learn? Am J Psychiatry 2011;168: 770–775.
30. Dixon LB, Perkins B, Calmas C. Guideline watch (September 2009): Practice guideline for the treatment of patients with schizophrenia. Psychiatry Online. *http://psychiatryonline.org/content.aspx?bookid=28§ionid=1682213*.
31. Hasan A, Falkai P, Wobrock T, et al. World Federation of Societies of Biological Psychiatry (WFSBP) guidelines for the biological treatment of schizophrenia, part 1: Update 2012 on the acute treatment of schizophrenia and the management of treatment resistance. World J Biol Psychiatry 2012;13:318–378.
32. Buckley PF, Miller BJ, Lehrer DS, Castle DJ. Psychiatric comorbidities and schizophrenia. Schizophr Bull 2009;35(2):383–402.
33. Van Putten T, Marder SR. Behavioral toxicity of antipsychotic drugs. J Clin Psychiatry 1987;48(Suppl 9):13–19.
34. Fijal BA, Stauffer VL, Kinon BJ, et al. Analysis of gene variants previously associated with iloperidone response in patients with schizophrenia who are treated with risperidone. J Clin Psychiatry 2012;73:367–371.
35. Miller D, Ellingrod V, Holman TL, et al. Clozapine-induced weight gain associated with 5HT2C receptor −759C/T polymorphism. Am J Med Genet B Neuropsychiatr Genet 2005;133:97–100.
36. Initial REMS Approval. NDA 022549, ADASUVE (Loxapine) Inhalation Powder. Approved Risk and Mitigation Strategies (REMS). U.S. Food and Drug Administration. *http://www.fda.gov/downloads/AdvisoryCommittees/CommitteesMeetingMaterials/Drugs/PsychopharmacologicDrugsAdvisoryCommittee/UCM282900.pdf*.
37. Leucht S, Barnes TR, Kissling W, et al. Relapse prevention in schizophrenia with new-generation antipsychotics: A systematic review and exploratory meta-analysis of randomized, controlled trials. Am J Psychiatry 2003;160:1209–1222.
38. Schennach R, Naber D, Rüther E, et al. Predictors of relapse in the year after hospital discharge among patients with schizophrenia. Psychiatr Serv 2012;63:87–90.
39. Citrome L. Paliperidone palmitate—A review of the efficacy, safety and cost of a new second-generation depot antipsychotic medication. Int J Clin Pract 2010;64:216–239.
40. Frampton JE. Olanzapine long-acting injection: A review of its use in the treatment of schizophrenia. Drugs 2010;70:2289–2213.
41. Prescribing information. Zyprexa Relprevv. Indianapolis, IN: Lilly USA, July 5, 2011.
42. Harrison TS, Goa KL. Long-acting risperidone: A review of its use in schizophrenia. CNS Drugs 2004;18:113–132.
43. Ereshefsky L, Saklad SR, Jann MW, et al. Future of depot neuroleptic therapy: Pharmacokinetics and pharmacodynamic approaches. J Clin Psychiatry 1984;45(5 pt 2):50–59.
44. Ereshefsky L, Toney G, Saklad SR, Seidel DR. A loading dose strategy for converting from oral to depot haloperidol. Hosp Community Psychiatry 1993;44:1155–1161.
45. Barkhof E, Meijer CJ, de Sonneville LMJ, et al. Interventions to improve adherence to antipsychotic medications in patients with schizophrenia—A review of the past decade. Eur Psychiatry 2012;27:9–18.
46. Kane J, Honigfeld G, Singer J, et al. Clozapine for the treatment-resistant schizophrenic: A double-blind comparison with chlorpromazine. Arch Gen Psychiatry 1988;45:789–796.
47. Spears NM, Leadbetter RA, Shutty MS. Clozapine treatment in polydipsia and intermittent hyponatremia. J Clin Psychiatry 1996;57:123–128.
48. Leucht S, Kissling W, McGrath J. Lithium for schizophrenia revisited: A systematic review and meta-analysis of randomized controlled trials. J Clin Psychiatry 2004;65: 177–186.
49. Casey DE, Daniel DG, Wassef AA, et al. Effect of divalproex combined with olanzapine or risperidone in patients with an acute exacerbation of schizophrenia. Neuropsychopharmacology 2003;28:182–192.
50. Kapur S, Roy P, Daskalakis J, Remington G. Increased dopamine D_2 receptor occupancy and elevated prolactin level associated with addition of haloperidol to clozapine. Am J Psychiatry 2001;158:311–314.
51. Correll CU, Rummel-Kluge C, Corves C, et al. Antipsychotic combinations vs. monotherapy in schizophrenia: A meta-analysis of randomized controlled trials. Schizophr Bull 2009;35(2):443–457.
52. Buckley P, Citrome L, Nichita C, Vitacco M. Psychopharmacology of aggression in schizophrenia. Schizophr Bull 2011;37:930–936.
53. Kapur S, Mamo D. Half a century of antipsychotics and still a central role for dopamine D_2 receptors. Prog Neuropsychopharmacol Biol Psychiatry 2003;27:1081–1090.
54. Meltzer L, Li Z, Kaneda Y, Ichikawa J. Serotonin receptors: Their key role in drugs to treat schizophrenia. Prog Neuropsychopharmacol Biol Psychiatry 2003;27:1159–1172.
55. Nyberg S, Eriksson B, Oxenstierna G, et al. Suggested minimal effective dose of risperidone based on PET measured D_2 and 5-HT_{2A} receptor occupancy in schizophrenic patients. Am J Psychiatry 1999;156:869–875.
56. Kapur S, Zipursky RB, Remington G. Clinical and theoretical implications of 5-HT_2 and D_2 receptor occupancy of clozapine, risperidone, and olanzapine in schizophrenia. Am J Psychiatry 1999;156:286–293.
57. Stahl SM, Shayegan DK. The psychopharmacology of ziprasidone: Receptor-binding properties and real-world psychiatric practice. J Clin Psychiatry 2003;64(Suppl 19):6–12.
58. DeLeon A, Patel NC, Crismon ML. Aripiprazole: A comprehensive review of its pharmacology, clinical efficacy, and tolerability. Clin Ther 2004;26:649–666.
59. Citrome L. Iloperidone for schizophrenia: A review of the efficacy and safety profile for this newly commercialized second-generation antipsychotic. Int J Clin Pract 2009;63:1237–1248.
60. Citrome L. Asenapine for schizophrenia and bipolar disorder: A review of the efficacy and safety profile for this newly approved sublingually absorbed second-generation antipsychotic. Int J Clin Pract 2009;63:1762–1784.
61. Mauri MC, Volonteri LS, Colasanti A, et al. Clinical pharmacokinetics of atypical antipsychotics: A critical review of the relationship between plasma concentrations and clinical response. Clin Pharmacokinet 2007;46:359–388.

62. Zhou SF, Liu JP, Chowbay B. Polymorphism of human cytochrome P450 enzymes and its clinical impact. Drug Metab Rev 2009;41:89–295.
63. Preskorn SH. Clinically important differences in the pharmacokinetics of the ten newer atypical antipsychotics: Part 2. Metabolism and elimination. J Psychiatr Practice 2012;18:361–368.
64. Citrome L. Lurasidone for schizophrenia: A review of the efficacy and safety profile for this newly approved second-generation antipsychotic. Int J Clin Pract 2011;65: 189–210.
65. Monteleone P, Martiadis V, Maj M. Management of schizophrenia with obesity, metabolic and endocrinological disorders. Psychiatr Clin North Am 2009;32:775–794.
66. Correll CU, Manu P, Olshanskiy V, et al. Cardiometabolic risk of second-generation antipsychotic medications during first-time use in children and adolescents. JAMA 2009;302:1765–1773.
67. Crabtree BL, Montgomery J. Iloperidone for the management of adults with schizophrenia. Clin Ther 2011;33:330–345.
68. Ganguli R, Strassing M. Prevention of metabolic syndrome in serious mental illness. Psychiatr Clin North Am 2011;34(1):109–125.
69. Velligan DI, Weiden PJ, Sajatovic M, et al. The expert consensus guideline series: Adherence problems in patients with serious and persistent mental illness. J Clin Psychiatry 2009;70:1–48.
70. De Luca V, Mueller DJ, de Bartolomeis A, et al. Association of the HTR2C gene and antipsychotic induced weight gain: A meta-analysis. Int J Neuropsychopharmacol 2007;10(5):697–704.
71. Ellingrod VL, Bishop JR, Moline J, et al. Leptin and leptin receptor gene polymorphisms and increases in body mass index (BMI) from olanzapine treatment in persons with schizophrenia. Psychopharmacol Bull 2007;40(1):57–62.
72. Reynolds GP. The pharmacogenetics of symptom response to antipsychotic drugs. Psychiatry Investig 2012;9(1): 1–7.
73. Wang YC, Bai YM, Chen JY, et al. Polymorphism of the adrenergic receptor alpha 2a –1291C>G genetic variation and clozapine-induced weight gain. J Neural Transm 2005;112(11):1463–1468.
74. Bishop JR, Ellingrod VL, Moline J, Miller D. Pilot study of the G-protein beta3 subunit gene (C825T) polymorphism and clinical response to olanzapine or olanzapine-related weight gain in persons with schizophrenia. Med Sci Monit 2006;12(2):BR47–BR50.
75. Zhang XY, Zhou DF, Wu GY, et al. BDNF levels and genotype are associated with antipsychotic-induced weight gain in patients with chronic schizophrenia. Neuropsychopharmacology 2008;33(9):2200–2205.
76. Kuo PH, Kao CF, Chen PY, et al. Polymorphisms of INSIG2, MC4R, and LEP are associated with obesity- and metabolic-related traits in schizophrenic patients. J Clin Psychopharmacol 2011;31:705–711.
77. Stroup TS, McEvoy JP, King KD, et al. Schizophrenia trials network. A randomized trial comparing the effectiveness of switching from olanzapine, quetiapine, or risperidone to aripiprazole to reduce metabolic risk: Comparison of antipsychotics for metabolic problems (CAMP). Am J Psychiatry 2011;168:947–956.
78. McElroy SL, Winstanley E, Mori N, et al. A randomized, placebo-controlled study of zonisamide to prevent olanzapine-associated weight gain. J Clin Psychopharmacol 2012;32:165–172.
79. Hoffmann VP, Case M, Jacobson JG. Assessment of treatment algorithms including amantadine, metformin, and zonisamide for the prevention of weight gain with olanzapine: A randomized controlled open-label study. J Clin Psychiatry 2012;73(2):216–223.
80. Wu RR, Jin H, Gao K, et al. Metformin for treatment of antipsychotic-induced amenorrhea and weight gain in women with first-episode schizophrenia: A double-blind, randomized, placebo-controlled study. Am J Psychiatry 2012;169:813–821.
81. Pramyothin P, Khaodhiar L. Metabolic syndrome with the atypical antipsychotics. Curr Opin Endocrinol Diabetes Obes 2010;17:460–466.
82. American Diabetes Association. Consensus development conference on antipsychotic drugs and obesity and diabetes. Diabetes Care 2004;27:596–601.
83. 2004 Safety Alerts for Human Medical Products. MedWatch. U.S. Food and Drug Administration, U.S. Department of Health and Human Services, 2004, *http://www.fda.gov/Safety/MedWatch/SafetyInformation/SafetyAlertsforHumanMedicalProducts/ucm152982.htm.*
84. Mackin P. Cardiac side effects of psychiatric drugs. Hum Psychopharmacol 2008;23:3–14.
85. Gugger J. Antipsychotic pharmacotherapy and orthostatic hypotension: Identification and management. CNS Drugs 2011;25:659–671.
86. Nielsen J, Graff C, Kanters J, et al. Assessing QT interval prolongation and its associated risks with antipsychotics. CNS Drugs 2011;25:473–490.
87. Dopheide JA. Iloperidone: Does it have a meaningful place in therapy? Am J Health Syst Pharm 2011;68:297.
88. Wenzel-Seifert K, Wittmann M, Haen E. QTc prolongation by psychotropic drugs and the risk of torsade de pointes. Dtsch Arztebl Int 2011;108:687–693.
89. Weinmann S, Read J, Aderhold V. Influence of antipsychotics on mortality in schizophrenia: Systematic review. Schizophr Res 2009;113(1):1–11.
90. Ferno J, Skrede S, Vik-Mo AO, et al. Lipogenic effects of psychotropic drugs: Focus on the SREBP system. Front Biosci 2011;16:49–60.
91. Sarandol A, Kirli S, Akkaya C, et al. Coronary artery disease risk factors in patients with schizophrenia: Effects of short term antipsychotic treatment. J Psychopharmacol 2007;21(8):857–863.
92. McEvoy JP, Meyer JM, Goff DC, et al. Prevalence of the metabolic syndrome in patients with schizophrenia: Baseline results from the Clinical Antipsychotic Trials of Intervention Effectiveness (CATIE) schizophrenia trial and comparison with national estimates from NHANES III. Schizophr Res 2005;80(1):19–32.
93. Pierre JM. Extrapyramidal symptoms with atypical antipsychotics. Drug Saf 2005;28:191–208.
94. Haddad PM, Dursun SM. Neurological complications of psychiatric drugs: Clinical features and management. Hum Psychopharmacol 2008;23:15–26.
95. Peluso M, Lewis S, Barnes T, et al. Extrapyramidal motor side-effects of first and second-generation antipsychotic drugs. Br J Psychiatry 2012;200:387–392.
96. Caplan JP, Epstein LA, Quinn DK, et al. Neuropsychiatric effects of prescription drug abuse. Neuropsychol Rev 2007;17:363–380.
97. Sprague RL, Kalachnik JE. Reliability, validity, and a total score cutoff for the Dyskinesia Identification System Condensed User Scale (DISCUS) with mentally ill and mentally retarded populations. Psychopharmacol Bull 1991;27:51–58.

98. Reynolds GP. The impact of pharmacogenetics on the development and use of antipsychotic drugs. Drug Discov Today 2007;12(21–22):953–959.
99. Correll CU, Schenk EM. Tardive dyskinesia and new antipsychotics. Curr Opin Psychiatry 2008;21:151–156.
100. Tarsy D, Lungu C, Baldessarini R. Epidemiology of tardive dyskinesia before and during the era of modern antipsychotic drugs. Handb Clin Neurol 2011;100:601–616.
101. Keefe RS, Bilder RM, Davis SM, et al. Neurocognitive effects of antipsychotic medications in patients with chronic schizophrenia in the CATIE trial. Arch Gen Psychiatry 2007;64:633–647.
102. Martin-Latry K, Goumy MP, Latry P, et al. Psychotropic drug use and the risk of heat-related hospitalization. Eur Psychiatry 2007;22:335–338.
103. Jackson N, Doherty J, Coulter S. Neuropsychiatric complications of commonly used palliative care drugs. Postgrad Med J 2008;84:121–126.
104. Li J, Tripathi RC, Tripathi BJ. Drug-induced ocular disorders. Drug Saf 2008;31:127–141.
105. Fraunfelder FW. Twice-yearly exams unnecessary for patients taking quetiapine. Am J Ophthalmol 2004;138: 870–871.
106. Verhamme KM, Sturkenboom MC, Stricker BH, Bosch R. Drug-induced urinary retention: Incidence, management, and prevention. Drug Saf 2008;31:373–388.
107. Tsakiri P, Oelke M, Michel MC. Drug-induced urinary incontinence. Drugs Aging 2008;25:541–549.
108. Rettenbacher MA, Hofer A, Ebenbichler C, et al. Prolactin levels and sexual adverse effects in patients with schizophrenia during antipsychotic treatment. J Clin Psychopharmacol 2010;30:711–715.
109. Andersohn F, Schmedt N, Weinmann S, et al. Priapism associated with antipsychotics: Role of alpha1 adrenoceptor affinity. J Clin Psychopharmacol 2010;30:68–71.
110. Hall RL, Smith AG, Ewards JG. Haematological safety of antipsychotic drugs. Expert Opin Drug Saf 2003;2:395–399.
111. Flanagan RJ, Dunk L. Haematological toxicity of drugs used in psychiatry. Hum Psychopharmacol 2008;23:27–41.
112. Perry PJ, Alexander B, Liskow B. Psychotropic Drug Handbook, 8th ed. Washington, DC: American Psychiatric Press, 2007:1–139.
113. Syed R, Au K, Cahill C, et al. Pharmacological interventions for clozapine-induced hypersalivation. Cochrane Database Syst Rev 2008;(3):CD005579.
114. Lin HC, Chen IJ, Chen YH, et al. Maternal schizophrenia and pregnancy outcome: Does the use of antipsychotics make a difference? Schizophr Res 2010;116(1):55–60.
115. McKenna K, Koren G, Tetelbaum M, et al. Pregnancy outcome of women using atypical antipsychotic drugs: A prospective comparative study. J Clin Psychiatry 2005;66(4):444–449.
116. Coppola D, Russo LJ, Kwarta RF Jr, et al. Evaluating the postmarketing experience of risperidone use during pregnancy: Pregnancy and neonatal outcomes. Drug Saf 2007;30(3):247–264.
117. Reis M, Källén B. Maternal use of antipsychotics in early pregnancy and delivery outcome. J Clin Psychopharmacol 2008;28(3):279–288.
118. Einarson A, Boskovic R. Use and safety of antipsychotic drugs during pregnancy. J Psychiatr Pract 2009;15(3):183–192.
119. Newham JJ, Thomas SH, MacRitchie K, et al. Birth weight of infants after maternal exposure to typical and atypical antipsychotics: Prospective comparison study. Br J Psychiatry 2008;192(5):333–337.
120. Bodén R, Lundgren M, Brandt L, et al. Antipsychotics during pregnancy: Relation to fetal and maternal metabolic effects. Arch Gen Psychiatry 2012;69:715–721.
121. Antipsychotics and Pregnancy, Safety Announcement. U.S. Food and Drug Administration, 2011, *http://www.fda.gov/Drugs/DrugSafety/ucm243903.htm.*
122. Ernst CL, Goldberg JF. The reproductive safety profile of mood stabilizers, atypical antipsychotics, and broad-spectrum psychotropics. J Clin Psychiatry 2002;63 (Suppl 4):42–55.
123. Ereshefsky L. Drug–drug interactions with the use of psychotropic medications. CNS Spectr 2009;14(Suppl 8):1–8.
124. Miller AL, Dassori A, Ereshefsky L, Crismon ML. Recent issues and developments in antipsychotic use. In: Dunner DL, Rosenbaum JF, eds. Psychiatric Clinics of North America Annual Review of Drug Therapy 2001. Philadelphia, PA: WB Saunders, 2001;8:209–235.
125. Prescribing information. Invega Sustenna (paliperidone palmitate). Titusville, NJ: Janssen Pharmaceuticals, August 2012.
126. DeVane CL, Markowitz JS. Antipsychotics. In: Levy RH, Thummel KE, Trager WF, et al., eds. Metabolic Drug Interactions. Philadelphia, PA: Lippincott Williams & Wilkins, 2000:245–258.
127. Spina E, de Leon J. Metabolic drug interactions with newer antipsychotics: A comparative review. Basic Clin Pharmacol Toxicol 2007;100:4–22.
128. Urichuk L, Prior TI, Dursun S, Baker G. Metabolism of atypical antipsychotics: Involvement of cytochrome P450 enzymes and relevance for drug–drug interactions. Curr Drug Metab 2008;9:410–418.
129. Flockhart DA. Drug Interactions: Cytochrome P450 Drug Interaction Table. *http://medicine.iupui.edu/clinpharm/ddis/table.asp.*
130. Miller AL, Chiles JA, Chiles JK, et al. The TMAP schizophrenia algorithms. J Clin Psychiatry 1999;60:649–657.
131. Argo TR, Crismon ML, Miller AL, et al. Schizophrenia Treatment Algorithms, Texas Medication Algorithm Project Procedural Manual. Austin, TX: Texas Department of State Health Services, 2008:62 pp.
132. Toprac MG, Rush AJ, Conner TM, et al. The Texas Medication Algorithm Project patient and family education program: A consumer-guided initiative. J Clin Psychiatry 2000;61:477–486.
133. Spaniel F, Vohlidka P, Hrdlicka J, et al. ITAREPS: Information technology aided relapse prevention programme in schizophrenia. Schizophr Res 2008;98(1–3):312–317.

51

Major Depressive Disorder

Christian J. Teter, Judith C. Kando, and Barbara G. Wells

KEY CONCEPTS

1. Extensive treatment guidelines are available to assist in the treatment of major depressive disorder, including medication management. Clinicians treating individuals with major depressive disorder should be familiar with these guidelines.
2. When evaluating a patient for the presence of depression, it is essential to rule out medical causes of depression and drug-induced depression.
3. The goal of pharmacologic treatment of depression is the resolution of current symptoms (i.e., remission) and the prevention of further episodes of depression (i.e., relapse or recurrence).
4. When counseling patients with depression who are receiving antidepressant medications, the patient should be informed that adverse effects might occur immediately, while resolution of symptoms may take 2 to 4 weeks or longer. Adherence to the treatment plan is essential to a successful outcome, and tools to help increase medication adherence should be discussed with each patient.
5. Antidepressants are generally considered equally efficacious in groups of patients with major depressive disorder. Therefore, other factors, such as age, side effect profile, and past history of response, are used to guide the selection of antidepressants.
6. When determining if a patient has been nonresponsive to a particular pharmacotherapeutic intervention, it must be determined whether the patient has received an adequate dose for an adequate duration and whether the patient has been medication adherent.
7. Pharmacogenetic tests (e.g., the FDA-approved AmpliChip to evaluate CYP2D6 and CYP2C19 polymorphisms) are now commercially available. However, there are no standard or well-accepted recommendations for the use of pharmacogenetic testing as it relates to antidepressant treatment of major depressive disorder.
8. When evaluating response to an antidepressant, in addition to target signs and symptoms, the clinician must consider quality-of-life issues, such as role, social, and occupational functioning. In addition, the tolerability of the agent should be assessed because the occurrence of side effects may lead to medication nonadherence, especially given the chronicity of the disease and need for long-term medication management.

A diagnosis of major depressive disorder (MDD) is given when an individual experiences one or more major depressive episodes without a history of manic, mixed, or hypomanic episodes. A major depressive episode is defined by the criteria listed in the *Diagnostic and Statistical Manual of Mental Disorders, Fourth Edition, Text Revision* (*DSM-IV-TR*).[1] Depression is associated with significant functional disability, morbidity, and mortality. Newer generations of antidepressants, such as the selective serotonin reuptake inhibitors (SSRIs), are effective and better tolerated than older agents, such as the tricyclic antidepressants (TCAs) and the monoamine oxidase inhibitors (MAOIs). In addition, substantial efforts have been undertaken to improve the ability of clinicians to recognize and appropriately treat the signs and symptoms of depression. This chapter focuses exclusively on the diagnosis and treatment of MDD.

1 In the absence of well-accepted evidence-based medicine for the medication management of MDD, the reader is referred to the *Practice Guideline for the Treatment of Patients with Major Depressive Disorder*, which is available at *www.psych.org*. This extensive document (now available in its third iteration) is a practical guide to the management of depression based on the best available data as well as clinical consensus.[2]

EPIDEMIOLOGY

The true prevalence of depressive disorders in the United States is unknown. The National Comorbidity Survey Replication found that 16.2% of the population studied had a history of MDD in their lifetime, and more than 6.6% had an episode within the past 12 months.[3] Women have a higher risk of depression than men from early adolescence until their mid-50s, with a lifetime rate that is 1.7 to 2.7 times greater.[4] Although depression can occur at any age, adults 18 to 29 years of age experience the highest rates of major depression during any given year.[3] The estimated lifetime prevalence of major depression in individuals aged 65 to 80 recently was reported to be 20.4% in women and 9.6% in men.[5] Depressive disorders are common during adolescence, with comorbid substance abuse, suicide attempts, and deaths occurring frequently in these young patients.[6,7] Depressive disorders and suicide tend to occur within families. For example, approximately 8% to 18% of patients with major depression have at least one first-degree relative (father, mother, brother, or sister) with a history of depression, compared with 5.6% of the first-degree relatives of those without depression.[8] Furthermore, first-degree relatives of patients with depression are 1.5 to 3 times more likely to develop depression than normal controls.[1,8,9] A recent meta-analysis found that the heritability of liability for major depression was 37%, whereas the remaining 63% of the variance in liability was due to individual-specific environment.[10] Therefore, MDD is relatively common, occurs more frequently in

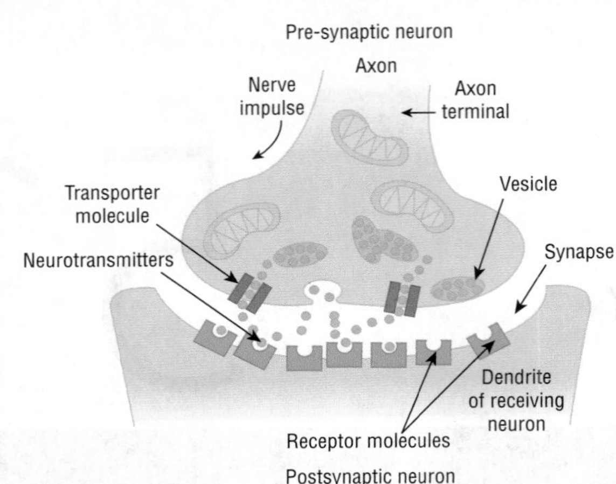

FIGURE 51-1 Monoamine neurotransmitter (NT) regulation at the neuronal level. NTs carry messages between cells. Each NT generally binds to a specific receptor, and this coupling initiates a cascade of events. NTs are reabsorbed back into nerve cells by reuptake pumps (i.e., transporter molecules) at which point they may be recycled for later use or broken down by enzymes. For their primary mechanism of action, most antidepressants are thought to inhibit the transporter molecules and allow more NT to remain in the synapse. *(Data from U.S. Department of Health and Human Services, National Institutes of Health, National Institute on Drug Abuse, Office of Science Policy and Communications, Science Policy Branch; figure reproduced from the Mind Over Matter educational series.)*

women than in men, and prevalence is influenced by both genetic and environmental factors.

ETIOLOGY

The etiology of depressive disorders is too complex to be totally explained by a single social, developmental, or biologic theory. Several factors appear to work together to cause or precipitate depressive disorders. The symptoms reported by patients with MDD consistently reflect changes in brain monoamine neurotransmitters (NTs), specifically norepinephrine (NE), serotonin (5-HT), and dopamine (DA).[11–13] See Figure 51-1 for a visual explanation of how these monoamine NTs are regulated at the level of the neuron and within the synapse.

PATHOPHYSIOLOGY

Several years before the introduction of antidepressants, the cause of depression was linked to decreased brain levels of the NTs NE, 5-HT, and DA, although the actual cause remains unknown. This biogenic amine hypothesis evolved as a result of several observations made in the early 1950s. It was noted that the antihypertensive drug reserpine depleted neuronal storage granules of NE, 5-HT, and DA and produced clinically significant depression in 15% or more of patients.[14]

Although the reuptake blockade of monoamines (e.g., NE, DA, and 5-HT) occurs immediately on administration of an antidepressant, the clinical antidepressant effects (i.e., measurable improvement) are generally delayed by weeks.[11,15] This delay may be the result of a cascade of events from receptor occupancy to gene transcription.[16] This delay in onset of action has caused researchers to focus on the adaptive changes induced by antidepressants.[12] Accordingly, theories that focus on adaptive (or chronic) changes in amine receptor systems have emerged. In the mid-1970s, it was recognized that chronic, but not acute, administration of antidepressants to animals caused desensitization of NE-stimulated cyclic adenosine monophosphate synthesis. In fact, for most antidepressants, downregulation of β-adrenergic receptors accompanies this desensitization.[17] Studies of many antidepressants have demonstrated that either desensitization or downregulation of NE receptors corresponds to a clinically relevant time course for antidepressant effects.[11] Other studies have revealed desensitization of presynaptic 5-HT_{1A} autoreceptors following chronic administration of antidepressants.[18] Thus, a theory based on changes in receptor sensitivity provides a cogent explanation of the delayed onset of therapeutic response of antidepressant drugs.[11] The dysregulation hypothesis incorporates the diversity of antidepressant activity with the adaptive changes occurring in receptor sensitization over several weeks. In this theory, emphasis is placed on a failure of homeostatic regulation of NT systems rather than on absolute increases or decreases in their activities. According to this hypothesis, effective antidepressant agents restore efficient regulation to the dysregulated NT system.[19]

It is apparent that no single NT theory of depression is adequate. The 5-HT/NE link hypothesis maintains that both the serotonergic and noradrenergic systems are involved in an antidepressant response.[17] This hypothesis is also consistent with the rationale of the postsynaptic alteration theory of depression, which emphasizes the importance of β-adrenergic receptor downregulation for achieving an antidepressant effect.[17] Furthermore, both serotonergic and noradrenergic medications downregulate β-adrenergic receptors, and there is a link between 5-HT and NE.[17] This implies that medications that are effective in the treatment of depression act at both of these NT systems.

Traditional explanations of the biologic basis of depressive disorders have focused largely on NE and 5-HT; however, most of the evidence that coalesced into the biogenic amine hypothesis of depression does not clearly distinguish between NE and DA. There is an abundance of evidence suggesting that DA transmission is decreased in depression and that agents that increase dopaminergic transmission have been found to be effective antidepressants.[20] Specifically, studies suggest that increased DA transmission in the mesolimbic pathway accounts for at least part of the mechanism of action of antidepressant medications.[20] The mechanisms by which antidepressant drugs alter DA transmission remain unclear, but may be mediated indirectly by primary actions at NE or 5-HT terminals. The complexity of the interaction between 5-HT, NE, and possibly DA is gaining greater appreciation, but a more in-depth understanding of the precise mechanism is needed.

More recent insight into the possible mechanisms underlying depressive disorders comes from studies on brain-derived neurotrophic factor (BDNF). BDNF is a growth factor protein that regulates the differentiation and survival of neurons. A growing body of evidence suggests this process might be disrupted in depressive disorders. More specifically, chronic stress and an associated increase in glucocorticoids such as cortisol may cause a disruption of BDNF expression in the hippocampus. This process may be prevented, or possibly even reversed, by antidepressant medications.[21] This is a relatively recent theory, which has not been firmly established. However, if proven valid, it demonstrates that antidepressants may help prevent deleterious effects of chronic stress and depressive symptoms.

Biologic Markers

Investigators continue to search for biologic or pharmacodynamic (PD) markers to assist in the diagnosis and treatment of depressed patients. Although no biologic marker has been discovered, several biologic abnormalities are present in many depressed patients.

Approximately 45% to 60% of patients with major depression have a neuroendocrine abnormality, including hypersecretion of cortisol or a lack of cortisol suppression after dexamethasone administration (i.e., a positive dexamethasone suppression test). In fact, it has been suggested that the inability of the brain to suppress the hypothalamic–pituitary–adrenal (HPA) axis and the associated stress response could lead to the pathophysiology and symptoms of depression.[22] According to this theory, there is a disruption somewhere in the normal negative feedback system that controls cortisol levels (see Fig. 59-3 for a visual display of this negative feedback system). There are many potential negative consequences of excess circulating cortisol, including disruption in BDNF expression as discussed above.

Unfortunately, the high rate of false-positive and false-negative results associated with neuroendocrine abnormalities in depressed patients limits the usefulness of testing for these markers, and has led to their relative lack of use in clinical practice. However, they still provide a clue as to the potential pathophysiology of depressive disorders, which may lead us to more effective treatment options.

CLINICAL PRESENTATION

2 When a patient presents with depressive symptoms, it is necessary to investigate the possibility of a contributing medical or drug-induced etiology. All depressed patients should have a complete physical examination, mental status examination, and basic laboratory workup, including a complete blood count with differential, thyroid function tests, and electrolyte determinations, to identify any potential medical problems. A listing of all possible medical conditions associated with depression is beyond the scope of this chapter. The *DSM-IV-TR* describes a diagnostic category for both "Mood Disorder due to a General Medical Condition" and "Substance-Induced Mood Disorder,"[1] which are common causative factors for depressive symptoms. For example, up to 40% of patients with certain neurologic disorders (e.g., stroke, Alzheimer's disease) develop depressive symptoms at some point during the course of their illness.[1] Furthermore, individuals experiencing withdrawal from substances of abuse (e.g., cocaine) commonly present with depressive symptoms.[23]

Table 51-1 lists medications commonly associated with causing or exacerbating depressive symptoms.[2,24,25] A complete medication review should be performed because several medications (in addition to those listed in Table 51-1) may contribute to depressive symptoms. Once a medical condition or concomitant medication has been ruled out as the cause of the depressive symptoms, the patient should be evaluated for MDD. According to the *DSM-IV-TR*, a single major depressive episode is characterized by five or more of the symptoms described in Table 51-2. At least one of the symptoms is depressed mood (often an irritable mood in children or adolescents) or loss of interest or pleasure in nearly all activities.[1] These symptoms must have been present nearly every day for at least 2 weeks and must represent a change from the patient's previous level of functioning. The 5th edition of the *Diagnostic and Statistical Manual omits* the bereavement exclusion that appears as item D in Table 51-2. Some feel that this omission opens the door to misdiagnosis of normal grief as major depressive disorder. The diagnostic code for major depressive disorder is determined by whether this is a single or recurrent depressive episode, current severity, presence of psychotic features, and remission status. The diagnosis can be followed by specifiers that apply to the current episode. The possible specifiers include anxious distress, mixed features (i.e., presence of some manic/hypomanic features), melancholic features, atypical features, mood-congruent psychotic features, catatonia, peripartum onset, and seasonal pattern. The clinician must consider presenting symptoms, their duration, and the patient's current level of social, occupational, or other important areas of functioning. Significant stressors or life events may trigger depression in some individuals but not others, and there may be an important precipitant at the beginning of the disorder.[1] A patient diagnosed with MDD may

TABLE 51-1 Selected Medications Associated with Drug-Induced Depressive Symptoms

Acne treatment
Isotretinoin

Anticonvulsants
Levetiracetam
Topiramate
Vigabatrin

Antimigraine agents
Triptans

Cardiovascular medications
β-Blocker
Clonidine
Methyldopa
Reserpine

Hormonal therapy
Gonadotropin-releasing hormone
Oral contraceptives
Steroids (e.g., prednisone)
Tamoxifen

Immunologic agents
Interferons

Smoking cessation drugs
Varenicline

Data from references 2, 24, and 25.

TABLE 51-2 *DSM-IV-TR* Criteria for Major Depressive Episode

A. Five (or more) of the following symptoms have been present during the same 2-week period and represent a change from previous functioning; at least one of the symptoms is either (1) depressed mood or (2) loss of interest or pleasure
   Note: Do not include symptoms that are clearly due to a general medical condition or mood-incongruent delusions or hallucinations
   1. Depressed mood most of the day nearly every day
   2. Markedly diminished interest or pleasure in all, or almost all, activities most of the day nearly every day
   3. Significant weight loss when not dieting or weight gain (e.g., a change of more than 5% of body weight in a month), or decrease or increase in appetite nearly every day
   4. Insomnia or hypersomnia nearly every day
   5. Psychomotor agitation or retardation nearly every day (observable by others, not merely subjective feelings of restlessness or being slowed down)
   6. Fatigue or loss of energy nearly every day
   7. Feelings of worthlessness or excessive or inappropriate guilt nearly every day
   8. Diminished ability to think or concentrate, or indecisiveness, nearly every day
   9. Recurrent thoughts of death (not just fear of dying), recurrent suicidal ideation without a specific plan, or a suicide attempt or a specific plan for committing suicide

B. The symptoms cause clinically significant distress or impairment in social, occupational, or other important areas of functioning

C. The symptoms are not due to the direct physiologic effects of a substance (e.g., a drug of abuse, a medication) or a general medical condition (e.g., hypothyroidism)

D. The symptoms are not better accounted for by bereavement i.e., after the loss of a loved one, the symptoms persist for longer than 2 months or are characterized by marked functional impairment, morbid preoccupation with worthlessness, suicidal ideation, psychotic symptoms, or psychomotor retardation

Reprinted with permission from the Diagnostic and Statistical Manual of Mental Disorders. 4th ed. Text Revision (Copyright © 2000). American Psychiatric Association.

have one or more recurrent episodes of major depression during his or her lifetime.

Depression Rating Scales

Instruments to assess the severity of depressive symptoms can be used for both clinical and research purposes. For example, the Montgomery-Åsberg Depression Rating Scale (MADRS) is a clinician-administered scale that is commonly used in drug trials given its sensitivity to change.[26] Other depression rating scales are self-administered. For example, the Beck Depression Inventory (BDI) takes only 5 to 10 minutes to complete by the respondent.[27] For a more detailed explanation for both of these instruments, as well as other rating scales and evaluation approaches, please refer to eChapter 19.

Emotional Symptoms

A major depressive episode is characterized by a persistent, diminished ability to experience pleasure. A loss of interest and pleasure in usual activities, hobbies, or work is common. Patients appear sad or depressed, and they are often pessimistic and believe that nothing will help them feel better. The presence of feelings of worthlessness or inappropriate guilt may identify patients at risk for suicide.[28] Anxiety symptoms are present in almost 90% of depressed outpatients. Patients often have guilt feelings that are unrealistic, and these may reach delusional proportions. Patients may feel that they deserve punishment and may view their present illness as a punishment. A patient suffering from major depression with psychotic features may hear voices (auditory hallucinations) saying that he or she is a bad person and that he or she should commit suicide. Depression with psychotic features may require hospitalization, especially if the patient becomes a danger to self or others.

Physical Symptoms

Physical symptoms often motivate patients, especially the elderly, to seek medical attention. Chronic fatigue is a common complaint, with a decreased ability to perform normal daily tasks. Fatigue often appears worse in the morning and does not improve with rest. Complaints of pain, especially headache, often accompany fatigue.

Sleep disturbances generally present as frequent early morning awakening with difficulty returning to sleep. This may coexist with difficulty falling asleep and frequent nighttime awakening. Less frequently, depressed patients complain of increased sleep (hypersomnia), although they experience daytime exhaustion or fatigue.

Appetite disturbances, including complaints of decreased appetite, often result in substantial weight loss, especially in the elderly.[29] Some patients lose 2 lb (0.9 kg) or more per week without dieting. Other patients, especially in the ambulatory setting, may overeat and gain weight, although they actually may not enjoy eating. Some patients exhibit GI complaints, others cardiovascular complaints, especially palpitations. Patients frequently present with a loss of sexual interest or libido.[30]

Intellectual or Cognitive Symptoms

Intellectual or cognitive symptoms include a decreased ability to concentrate, slowed thinking, and a poor memory for recent events. Patients may appear confused and indecisive. Depression should be considered when cognitive symptoms are present in the elderly.[29]

Psychomotor Disturbances

Patients may appear noticeably slowed or retarded in physical movements, thought processes, and speech (psychomotor retardation). Conversely, depression may be accompanied by psychomotor agitation, manifesting as purposeless, restless motion (e.g., pacing, wringing of hands, or outbursts of shouting).

SUICIDE RISK EVALUATION AND MANAGEMENT

The Centers for Disease Control and Prevention lists suicide as the 11th leading cause of death among Americans and the 2nd leading cause of death among 25- to 34-year-olds. In 2006, there were 91 suicides per day in the United States.[31] All patients diagnosed with MDD should be assessed for suicidal thoughts. Factors associated with an increased risk for suicide include psychiatric and substance use disorders, adolescence and younger age adults, physical illness, recent stressful life event, childhood trauma, hopelessness, and male gender.[32] Those with a higher level of risk have high degrees of suicidal intent and describe more specific plans, in particular, plans that are violent and irreversible.[32] It is important to remember that the risk of suicide in those recovering from major depression may increase as they develop the energy and capacity to act on a plan made earlier in a course of illness. Additionally, despite factors to help identify those at greatest risk, it remains very difficult to predict suicidality in any given individual. Therefore, when suicidal intent is suspected, it is important to ask, "Are you thinking about harming or killing yourself?" If the risk is significant, the patient must be referred immediately to an appropriate healthcare professional. Additionally, certain depression rating scales, such as the MADRS discussed above, include questions that target suicidality, which may help identify those patients at risk.

In September 2004, the FDA required manufacturers of antidepressants to add a boxed warning stating that antidepressants increase the risk of suicidal thinking and behavior in short-term studies in children and adolescents with depressive disorders. These risks have become a new source of concern among those treating their patients with antidepressants. In order to help deal with the confusion these risks have caused, experts have recommended the following[33]:

1. It is especially important to closely monitor patients for suicidal ideation and behavior at the beginning of treatment and among younger patients.
2. Discuss the possibility that adverse events may occur, including behavioral agitation or anger, and encourage patients to seek help should this occur.
3. Deal with the subject of suicide directly.

It is important to note that there is little evidence to suggest that withholding antidepressant treatment decreases the risk of eventual suicide and may actually increase the risk. Furthermore, it may be that longer-term medication is needed for any protective effects against suicidality.[33]

In May 2007, the FDA released additional requests to the makers of antidepressants that the black box warning regarding suicidality be expanded to include warnings about the increased risk of suicidality (thinking and behavior) in young adults 18 to 24 years of age, during the initial stages of treatment.

In contrast to some of the concerns discussed above, recent evidence suggests that fluoxetine and venlafaxine may be associated with a "protective" effect from suicidality among adults and older patients; however, among youth, the medications lacked this apparent protective effect. It should be noted that Gibbons et al. did not find that fluoxetine and venlafaxine increased the risk of suicidality among youth.[34] The complex relationships between antidepressant use and suicidality will continue to be explored with the hopes of more unequivocal recommendations.

TREATMENT

Desired Outcomes

The goals of treatment are to reduce the symptoms of acute depression, facilitate the patient's return to a level of functioning like that before the onset of illness, and prevent further episodes of depression. Whether or not to hospitalize the patient is often the first decision that is made in consideration of the patient's risk of suicide, physical state of health, social support system, and presence of a psychotic depression.

General Approach to Treatment

❸ There are three phases of treatment for patients with MDD: (a) the *acute* phase lasting approximately 6 to 12 weeks in which the goal is remission (i.e., absence of symptoms); (b) the *continuation* phase lasting 4 to 9 months after remission is achieved, in which the goal is to eliminate residual symptoms or prevent relapse (i.e., return of symptoms within 6 months of remission); and (c) the *maintenance* phase lasting at least 12 to 36 months in which the goal is to prevent recurrence (i.e., a separate episode of depression).[2,35] The risk of recurrence increases as the number of past episodes increases. The duration of antidepressant therapy depends on the risk of recurrence. Some investigators recommend lifelong maintenance therapy for persons at greatest risk for recurrence (persons younger than 40 years of age with two or more prior episodes and persons of any age with three or more prior episodes).[2]

❹ Educating the patient and their support system (e.g., family and friends) regarding the delay in antidepressant effects and the importance of adherence should occur before and during the entire course of treatment. The treatment of MDD generally includes nonpharmacologic and pharmacologic strategies, which are discussed in further detail below.

Nonpharmacologic Therapy

In addition to pharmacologic interventions, psychotherapy should be employed whenever the patient is able and willing to participate. Psychotherapy alone is not recommended for the acute treatment of patients with severe and/or psychotic MDD. However, if the depressive episode is mild to moderate in severity, psychotherapy may be the first-line therapy.[36] The effects of psychotherapy and antidepressant medications are considered to be additive. Combined treatment may be advantageous for patients with partial responses to either treatment alone and for those with a chronic course of illness. However, for uncomplicated, nonchronic MDD, combined treatment may provide no unique advantage.[36] Although not extensively evaluated, cognitive therapy, behavioral therapy, and interpersonal psychotherapy appear equally effective.[36] Maintenance psychotherapy as the sole treatment to prevent recurrence generally is not recommended. Often, medication alone may prevent a depressive recurrence during the maintenance phase.[36]

Electroconvulsive therapy (ECT) is a safe and effective treatment for certain severe mental illnesses, including MDD. Patients with depression are candidates for ECT when a rapid response is needed, risks of other treatments outweigh potential benefits, there is a history of poor response to antidepressants and a history of good response to ECT, and the patient expresses a preference for ECT.[37] Guidelines developed by the American Psychiatric Association (APA) include indications and contraindications for the appropriate use of ECT, procedures for obtaining informed consent, and issues in administering ECT.[37] A more recent nonpharmacologic approach is repetitive transcranial magnetic stimulation (rTMS), which has demonstrated efficacy in treating MDD and does not require anesthesia as does ECT.[38]

Pharmacologic Therapy

Antidepressants can be classified in several ways, including by chemical structure and the presumed mechanism of antidepressant activity. Although the link between the presumed mechanism of drug action and antidepressant response is tenuous, this classification has the advantage of being based on established pharmacology and clearly explains some of the common, but expected, adverse effects. The knowledgeable clinician can use these facts to tailor treatment to individual patient needs and thereby optimize treatment outcome. Currently available antidepressants, including dosing guidance, are provided in Table 51-3.[2,15,35,39–42]

❺ Studies have found that antidepressants are of *equivalent efficacy* in groups of patients when administered in comparable doses. Because one cannot predict which antidepressant will be the most effective in an individual patient, the initial choice is made empirically. Factors that often influence the choice of an antidepressant include the patient's history of response, history of familial antidepressant response, patient's concurrent medical illnesses and medications, presenting symptoms (e.g., fatigue as compared with psychomotor agitation), potential for drug–drug interactions, adverse events profile, patient preference, and drug cost. Although the pathophysiology of major depression remains elusive, the clinician can now select from multiple approved drug therapies with presumed different mechanisms of action[2] as highlighted in Table 51-4.[15,35,41–44] Failure to respond to one antidepressant class or one antidepressant drug within a class does not predict a failed response to another drug class or another drug within the same class. Approximately 65% to 70% of patients with varying types of depression improve with drug therapy, compared with 30% to 40% who improve with placebo.

Antidepressant Medication Classes

Selective Serotonin Reuptake Inhibitors

The efficacy of SSRIs is superior to placebo and comparable to other classes of antidepressants in treating patients with major depression.[2,35] SSRIs are generally chosen as *first-line antidepressants* due to their safety in overdose and improved tolerability. Furthermore, the decision as to which SSRI to use *within* the class is typically based on the nuances of each medication, such as differences in drug interaction profile and pharmacokinetic (PK) parameters (e.g., half-life), or due to cost considerations. These concepts will be discussed in greater detail later in this chapter.

Serotonin–Norepinephrine Reuptake Inhibitors (SNRIs)

Tricyclic Antidepressants Although TCAs are effective in treating all depressive subtypes, their use has diminished greatly due to the availability of equally effective therapies that are much safer in overdose and better tolerated. All TCAs potentiate the activity of NE and 5-HT by blocking their reuptake. However, the potency and selectivity of TCAs for the inhibition of reuptake of NE and 5-HT vary greatly among these agents (Table 51-4). Because TCAs affect other receptor systems including the cholinergic, neurologic, and cardiovascular systems, adverse events are reported frequently during TCA therapy.[15]

Newer-Generation SNRIs Venlafaxine inhibits 5-HT reuptake at low doses, and NE reuptake at higher doses; thus, it is referred to as an SNRI. Desvenlafaxine, the primary active metabolite of venlafaxine, is also an SNRI and has been approved to treat depressive disorders. Duloxetine is an SNRI with both 5-HT and NE reuptake inhibition across all doses. Some studies suggest that the

TABLE 51-3 Adult Dosing Guidance for Currently Available Antidepressant Medications

Drug	Brand Name	Initial Dose (mg/day)	Usual Dosage Range (mg/day)	Comments (e.g., Maximum Daily Dosage, Suggested Therapeutic Plasma Concentration)[a]
Selective Serotonin Reuptake Inhibitors (SSRIs)				
Citalopram	Celexa	20	20–40	Doses greater than 40 mg/day not recommended due to QT prolongation risk; maximum 20 mg/day for CYP2C19 poor metabolizers or coadministration with CYP2C19 inhibitors
Escitalopram	Lexapro	10	10–20	Maximum 20 mg/day; dose may be increased to maximum daily dose after at least 1 week if needed; 5 mg tablet available for unique circumstances
Fluoxetine	Prozac	20	20–60	Maximum 80 mg/day; dose may be increased in 20 mg increments; doses of 5 or 10 mg/day have been used as initial therapy; doses >20 mg/day may be given in a single daily dose or divided twice daily
Fluvoxamine	Luvox	50	50–300	Maximum 300 mg/day; daily doses >100 mg total dose should be divided twice daily, with the larger dose given at night
Paroxetine	Paxil	20	20–60	Maximum 50 mg/day (IR); titrate 10 mg/day increments weekly Maximum 62.5 mg/day (CR); titrate 12.5 mg/day increments weekly
Sertraline	Zoloft	50	50–200	Maximum 200 mg/day; titrate 25 mg/day increments weekly
Serotonin–Norepinephrine Reuptake Inhibitors (SNRIs)				
Newer-generation SNRIs				
Desvenlafaxine	Pristiq	50	50	Doses up to 400 mg/day have been studied; however, AEs are increased and no additional benefit has been shown at doses exceeding 50 mg/day
Duloxetine	Cymbalta	30	30–90	Maximum 120 mg/day (given once or twice daily); doses exceeding 60 mg/day not shown to provide increased efficacy for the treatment of MDD
Venlafaxine	Effexor	37.5–75	75–225	Maximum 375 mg/day (IR); maximum 225 mg/day (ER); may increase in increments up to 75 mg/day at a minimum of every 4 days. Dose reductions may be required if sustained hypertension occurs
Tricyclic antidepressants (TCAs)				
Amitriptyline	Elavil	25	100–300	Maximum 300 mg/day for MDD; may be given as a single daily dose at bedtime or in divided doses throughout the day Therapeutic serum level 100–250 ng/mL (370–925 nmol/L); parent drug plus metabolite (i.e., nortriptyline)
Desipramine	Norpramin	25	100–300	Maximum 300 mg/day Suggested therapeutic concentration range for combined imipramine + desipramine: 150–300 ng/mL (550–1,100 nmol/L)
Doxepin	Sinequan	25	100–300	Maximum 300 mg/day; may be given in a single daily dose at bedtime (if tolerated) or in divided doses throughout the day; a single dose should not exceed 150 mg
Imipramine	Tofranil	25	100–300	Maximum 300 mg/day; may be given in a single daily dose at bedtime (if tolerated) or in divided doses throughout the day Suggested therapeutic concentration range for combined imipramine + desipramine: 150–300 ng/mL (550–1,100 nmol/L)
Nortriptyline	Pamelor	25	50–150	Maximum 150 mg/day; total daily may be given as a single daily dose (if tolerated) or 25 mg doses given three to four times daily Therapeutic serum level 50–150 ng/mL (190–570 nmol/L)
Norepinephrine and Dopamine Reuptake Inhibitor (NDRI)				
Bupropion	Wellbutrin	150	150–300	Please see text for proper dosing, which can help decrease seizure risk Maximum 450 mg/day (IR, ER), 400 mg/day (SR); ER dosed once daily; SR dosed once or twice daily; IR may be dosed up to three times daily
Mixed Serotonergic Effects (Mixed 5-HT)				
Nefazodone	Serzone	100	300–600	Maximum 600 mg/day; daily doses should be divided twice daily
Trazodone	Desyrel; Oleptro	50	150–300	Maximum 600 mg/day; IR daily dose should be divided three times daily and may increase by 50 mg/day increments every 3–7 days; ER dose titration initiated at 150 mg at bedtime and can be increased 75 mg/day every 3 days
Vilazodone	Viibryd	10	40	Target dose = 40 mg/day unless coadministered with CYP3A4 inhibitor (dose not to exceed 20 mg/day); doses greater than 40 mg/day have not been assessed Dose titration: 10 mg/day for 7 days, 20 mg/day for 7 days, and then 40 mg/day
Serotonin and α_2-Adrenergic Antagonist				
Mirtazapine	Remeron	15	15–45	Maximum 45 mg/day; may increase dose no more frequently than every 1–2 weeks; dose adjustment may be required for renal impairment
Monoamine Oxidase Inhibitors (MAOIs)				
Phenelzine	Nardil	15	30–90	Early phase recommended dosing: 15 mg three times daily; dosing may be increased to 90 mg/day based on tolerance and response Maintenance phase: dose should be reduced over several weeks to a daily dose as low as 15 mg/day or 15 mg every other day
Selegiline (transdermal)	Emsam	6	6–12	Not to exceed 12 mg/24 hours; dose may be increased by 3 mg/day increments every 2 weeks; transdermal delivery system designed to deliver dose continuously over a 24-hour period
Tranylcypromine	Parnate	10	20–60	Maximum 60 mg/day; divided dosing; if no response after 2 weeks, increase by 10 mg increments at 1- to 3-week intervals Medication cross-taper: allow at least 1 medication-free week, an then initiate tranylcypromine at 50% of usual starting dose for at least 1 week

AE, adverse effects; CR, continuous release; ER, extended release; IR, immediate release; MDD, major depressive disorder; SR, sustained release.

[a]SI conversion for cases where reference ranges are for a mixture of parent drug and active metabolite is calculated based on a 1:1 ratio.

Data from references 2, 15, 35, 39–42.

TABLE 51-4 Relative Potencies of Norepinephrine and Serotonin Reuptake Blockade and Selected Side Effect Profile of Antidepressants

	Reuptake Antagonism		Anticholinergic Effects	Sedation	Orthostatic Hypotension	Seizures[a]	Conduction Abnormalities[a]
	Norepinephrine	Serotonin					
Selective Serotonin Reuptake Inhibitors (SSRIs)							
Citalopram	0	++++	0	+	0	++	++
Escitalopram	0	++++	0	0	0	0	0
Fluoxetine	0	+++	0	0	0	++	0
Fluvoxamine	0	++++	0	+	0	++	0
Paroxetine	0	++++	+	+	0	++	0
Sertraline	0	++++	0	0	0	++	0
Serotonin–Norepinephrine Reuptake Inhibitors (SNRIs)							
Duloxetine[b]	++++	++++	+	0	+	0	0
Venlafaxine[c] and desvenlafaxine	++++	++++	+	+	0	++	+
Tricyclic Antidepressants (TCAs)							
Amitriptyline	++	++++	++++	++++	+++	+++	+++
Desipramine	++++	+	++	++	++	++	++
Doxepin	++	++	+++	++++	++	+++	++
Imipramine	+++	+++	+++	+++	++++	+++	+++
Nortriptyline	+++	++	++	++	+	++	++
Mixed Serotonergic (Mixed 5-HT)							
Nefazodone	0	++	0	+++	+++	++	+
Trazodone	0	++	0	++++	+++	++	+
Vilazodone	0	++++	0	+	0	++	0
Norepinephrine and Dopamine Reuptake Inhibitor (NDRI)							
Bupropion[d]	+	0	+	0	0	++++	+
Serotonin and α_2-Receptor Antagonist							
Mirtazapine	0	0	+	++	++	0	+

++++, high; +++, moderate; ++, low; +, very low; 0, absent.

[a]These are uncommon side effects of antidepressant drugs, particularly when used at normal therapeutic doses; they may be dose-dependent, resulting in corresponding dose restrictions (e.g., citalopram 40 mg/day maximum due to QTc prolongation concerns).

[b]Duloxetine: balanced 5-HT and NE reuptake inhibition.

[c]Venlafaxine: primarily 5-HT at lower doses, NE at higher doses, and DA at very high doses.

[d]Bupropion: also blocks dopamine reuptake.

Data from references 15, 35, 41–44.

SNRIs may be associated with higher rates of response and remission than other antidepressants; however, most of these studies involved venlafaxine, and not all studies support this conclusion.[43] A recent report from the Agency for Healthcare Research and Quality (AHRQ) found that discontinuation rates secondary to lack of efficacy are 34% lower (odds ratio = 0.66, 95% CI = 0.47 to 0.93) for venlafaxine compared with those for SSRIs.[45]

Mixed Serotonergic Medications (Mixed 5-HT)

Trazodone and nefazodone have dual actions on serotonergic neurons, acting as both 5-HT_2 antagonists and 5-HT reuptake inhibitors. They may also enhance 5-HT_{1A}-mediated neurotransmission.[15] Trazodone blocks α_1-adrenergic and histaminergic receptors leading to increased side effects (e.g., dizziness and sedation) that limit its use as an antidepressant. Recently, a longer-acting extended-release preparation of trazodone was approved by the FDA. However, its place in the treatment of MDD is yet to be determined. Nefazodone's use as an antidepressant has declined as well after reports of hepatic toxicity began to emerge. The FDA-approved nefazodone labeling includes a black box warning describing rare cases of liver failure.[46] Trazodone and nefazodone are effective agents in treating major depression; however, both of them carry risks that limit their usefulness as antidepressants.

Recently, vilazodone became the first combination SSRI and 5-HT_{1A} receptor partial agonist to be approved for the treatment of MDD based on two 8-week, placebo-controlled MDD trials.[47] Vilazodone's place in therapy has yet to be determined.

Norepinephrine and Dopamine Reuptake Inhibitor (NDRI)

Bupropion has no appreciable effect on the reuptake of 5-HT, but it inhibits both the NE and DA reuptake pumps.[18,44] These pharmacologic properties make bupropion unique among all currently available antidepressants.

Serotonin and α_2-Adrenergic Receptor Antagonists

Mirtazapine enhances central noradrenergic and serotonergic activity through the antagonism of central presynaptic α_2-adrenergic autoreceptors and heteroreceptors.[48] Furthermore, it antagonizes 5-HT_2 and 5-HT_3 receptors as well as histamine receptors. The antagonism of 5-HT_2 and 5-HT_3 receptors has been linked to lower anxiety and GI side effects, respectively. Blockade of histamine receptors is associated with the sedative properties of mirtazapine.[18]

Monoamine Oxidase Inhibitors

MAOIs increase the concentrations of NE, 5-HT, and DA within the neuronal synapse through inhibition of the MAO enzyme. Similar to TCAs, chronic therapy causes changes in receptor sensitivity (i.e., downregulation of β-adrenergic, α-adrenergic, and serotonergic receptors).[49] The MAOIs phenelzine and tranylcypromine are nonselective inhibitors of MAO-A and MAO-B. A selegiline transdermal patch was approved by the FDA for treatment of MDD that allows inhibition of MAO-A and MAO-B in the brain, yet has reduced effects on MAO-A in the gut[39] (see tyramine interactions with MAOIs below).

Clinical **Controversy. . .**

Ketamine is a dissociative anesthetic that has received a great deal of attention in recent years for its apparent rapid efficacy at reducing depressive symptoms in patients with treatment-resistant depression.[50] Given that ketamine is not FDA-approved for depression, is available only IV, and is a known substance of abuse, use of this drug to treat depressive symptoms will require much more study. Currently, ketamine is an experimental pharmacotherapy for MDD.

Adverse Effects

Selective Serotonin Reuptake Inhibitors

The SSRIs have a low affinity for histaminic, α_1-adrenergic, and muscarinic receptors, and therefore they produce fewer anticholinergic and cardiovascular adverse effects than the TCAs, and are not usually associated with significant weight gain.[51–53] The most common adverse effects, which generally are mild and short-lived, are GI symptoms (e.g., nausea, vomiting, and diarrhea), sexual dysfunction in both males and females, headache, and insomnia.[52] A discontinuation or withdrawal syndrome may occur if SSRIs are abruptly discontinued. However, the longer the half-life of the drug and its active metabolite, the less likely a withdrawal syndrome will occur.[53,54] Although SSRIs are known to improve the anxiety symptoms associated with depression, a few patients experience an increase in anxiety symptoms or agitation early in treatment. Lastly, despite their excellent safety profile, there have been growing concerns with the SSRIs. For example, citalopram has been linked to a dose-dependent increase in QT interval that requires careful attention to maximum dosages.[55]

Serotonin–Norepinephrine Reuptake Inhibitors

The TCAs affect several NTs and produce a wide range of pharmacologic actions, including several unwanted, but expected, adverse effects. The most commonly occurring side effects are dose-related and are associated with blockade of cholinergic receptors (anticholinergic effects) and include dry mouth, constipation, blurred vision, urinary retention, dizziness, tachycardia, memory impairment, and, at higher doses, delirium.[49] Although some tolerance does develop to these adverse effects, they have the potential to impact patient adherence, particularly in the elderly and those receiving long-term maintenance therapy. Orthostatic hypotension is a common, dose-related, and potentially problematic adverse effect that has been attributed to the affinity of the TCAs for adrenergic receptors.[56] TCAs also cause cardiac conduction delays and may induce heart block in patients with a preexisting conduction disorder. TCA overdose can produce severe arrhythmias.[56] Furthermore, the FDA released a warning in December 2009 that the desipramine prescribing information will be changed to reflect an increased risk of death in patients receiving desipramine who have a *family history* of sudden cardiac death, cardiac dysrhythmias, and cardiac conduction disturbances. More on this reaction can be found at the FDA's MedWatch website. Therefore, caution should be exercised when prescribing these agents, especially in higher doses, to patients with clinically significant cardiac disease, and to patients with a family history of a cardiac event. Additional adverse effects that may lead to TCA nonadherence include weight gain and sexual dysfunction.[57]

The most commonly reported adverse effects with venlafaxine are similar to those of SSRIs and may be dose-related; they include nausea, sexual dysfunction, and activation.[2] However, recent evidence strongly suggests that venlafaxine is associated with a higher incidence of nausea and vomiting compared with the SSRIs.[45] Venlafaxine may also cause a dose-related increase in diastolic blood pressure, and baseline blood pressure is not a useful predictor of the occurrence of this phenomenon. Blood pressure should be monitored regularly during venlafaxine therapy, and dosage reduction or discontinuation may be necessary if sustained hypertension occurs.[58] Duloxetine was relatively well tolerated in short-term clinical trials; however, experience in long-term studies and in a larger population of patients will more clearly define its risks and benefits. The most commonly reported adverse events were nausea, dry mouth, constipation, decreased appetite, insomnia, and increased sweating.[43,59] According to the AHRQ report cited above, there were higher discontinuation rates secondary to side effects associated with both duloxetine and venlafaxine compared with the SSRI class of antidepressants.[45]

Mixed Serotonergic Medications

Trazodone and nefazodone have minimal anticholinergic effects and 5-HT agonist side effects, but they can cause orthostatic hypotension. Sedation, cognitive slowing, and dizziness are the most frequent dose-limiting side effects associated with trazodone.[49] Common adverse effects associated with nefazodone include lightheadedness, dizziness, orthostatic hypotension, somnolence, dry mouth, nausea, and asthenia (weakness). Due to the previously discussed potential for hepatic injury associated with nefazodone use, treatment should not be initiated in individuals with active liver disease or with elevated baseline serum transaminases.[46] A rare but potentially serious adverse effect of trazodone is priapism, which is reported to occur in approximately 1 in 6,000 male patients. Some cases have required surgical intervention (1 in 23,000), and permanent impotence may result.[60] There have been no reports of priapism associated with nefazodone use in men, but there is a published case report of nefazodone-induced clitoral priapism.[60]

Norepinephrine and Dopamine Reuptake Inhibitor

Adverse effects associated with bupropion include nausea, vomiting, tremor, insomnia, dry mouth, and skin reactions. The occurrence of seizures in patients taking bupropion appears to be strongly dose-related, and may be increased by predisposing factors such as history of prior seizure activity, severe alcohol withdrawal, head trauma, and CNS tumor. Additionally, bupropion use is contraindicated in patients with eating disorders such as bulimia and anorexia, as these patients are prone to electrolyte abnormalities and are therefore at higher risk for seizure activity. At daily doses of 450 mg (the FDA-approved maximum dose) or less, the incidence of seizures is 0.4%.[61] Due to its pharmacologic profile (i.e., proadrenergic), bupropion may cause activation or agitation in some patients.[18] Bupropion is associated with less sexual dysfunction compared with the SSRIs.[45]

Serotonin and α_2-Adrenergic Receptor Antagonists

The most common adverse effects of mirtazapine are somnolence, weight gain, dry mouth, and constipation. Interestingly, side effects such as weight gain may be less with larger mirtazapine doses due to different mechanisms of action at different doses,[53] such as increased noradrenergic transmission as the dose is increased. Weight gain associated with mirtazapine after 6 to 8 weeks is in the range of 0.8 to 3 kg.[45]

Monoamine Oxidase Inhibitors

The most common adverse effect of MAOIs is postural hypotension; this is more likely to occur with phenelzine than with tranylcypromine and may be minimized through divided dosage scheduling. Other common adverse effects include weight gain and sexual side effects (e.g., decreased libido, anorgasmia).[2] Phenelzine has mild to moderate sedating effects, while tranylcypromine may exert a stimulating effect, and therefore insomnia can occur. In addition, fever, myoclonic jerking, and brisk deep tendon reflexes may occur.[62] Hypertensive crisis, a potentially serious and life-threatening but rare adverse reaction, may occur when MAOIs are taken concurrently with certain foods, especially those high in tyramine, or some medications. Examples of potentially high tyramine foods and medications that should be avoided or used with caution are provided in Table 51-5.[41,63,64] Ten milligrams of tyramine can cause a marked pressor effect, and 25 mg can result in a serious hypertensive crisis.[65] These incidents may culminate in cerebrovascular accident and death. Symptoms of hypertensive crisis include occipital headache, stiff neck, nausea, vomiting, sweating, and sharply elevated blood pressure. Hypertensive crises can be treated with antihypertensive agents such as captopril.[66] Education of patients taking MAOIs regarding dietary and medication restrictions is extremely important. Notably, according to the FDA-approved prescribing information for the transdermal selegiline patch, patients receiving the 6-mg/24-hour dose are not required to modify their diet. However, patients receiving the 9- or 12-mg/24-hour dose are still required to follow the dietary restrictions similar to the other MAOIs.

Serotonin Syndrome (SS)

Any antidepressant that increases serotonergic neurotransmission can be associated with SS. The typical triad of symptoms seen in SS includes mental status changes, autonomic instability, and neuromuscular abnormalities. However, SS has been identified in cases without all three of these symptoms being present. Therefore, alternative approaches to the well-accepted SS triad have been suggested. For example, it has been proposed that the presence of any of the following symptom clusters is highly diagnostic of SS: (a) tremor + hyperreflexia, (b) spontaneous clonus, (c) muscle rigidity + temperature >38°C (100.4°F) + ocular clonus or inducible clonus, (d) ocular clonus + agitation or diaphoresis, and (e) inducible clonus + agitation or diaphoresis.[67]

TABLE 51-5 Dietary and Medication Restrictions for Patients Taking Monoamine Oxidase Inhibitors[a]

Foods	
Aged cheeses[b]	Liver (chicken or beef, more than 2 days old)
Sour cream[c]	Raisins
Yogurt[c]	Pods of broad beans (fava beans)
Cottage cheese[c]	Yeast extract and other yeast products
American cheese[c]	Soy sauce
Mild Swiss cheese[c]	Chocolate[e]
Wine[d] (especially Chianti and sherry)	Coffee[e]
Beer	Ripe avocado
Sardines	Sauerkraut
Canned, aged, or processed meats	Licorice
Monosodium glutamate	
Medications	
Amphetamines	Levodopa
Appetite suppressants	Local anesthetics containing sympathomimetic vasoconstrictors
Asthma inhalants	Meperidine
Buspirone	Methyldopa
Carbamazepine	Methylphenidate
Cocaine	Other antidepressants[f]
Cyclobenzaprine	Other MAOIs
Decongestants (topical and systemic)	Reserpine
Dextromethorphan	Rizatriptan
Dopamine	Stimulants
Ephedrine	Sumatriptan
Epinephrine	Sympathomimetics
Guanethidine	Tryptophan

[a]According to the FDA-approved prescribing information for the transdermal selegiline patch, patients receiving the 6-mg/24-hour dose are not required to modify their diet. However, patients receiving the 9- or 12-mg/24-hour dose are still required to follow the dietary restrictions similar to the other MAOIs.
[b]Clearly warrants absolute prohibition (e.g., English Stilton, blue, Camembert, cheddar).
[c]Up to 2 oz daily is acceptable.
[d]Three ounce white wine or a single cocktail is acceptable.
[e]Up to 2 oz daily is acceptable: larger amounts of decaffeinated coffee are acceptable.
[f]Tricyclic antidepressants may be used with caution by experienced clinicians in treatment-resistant populations.

Data from references 41, 63, and 64.

Pharmacokinetics and Pharmacodynamics

The PK of the antidepressants is summarized in Table 51-6.[41–43,68–70] The diversity of SSRIs is evident not only in their chemical structures but also in their PK profiles.[68,71] The unique PK attributes of each SSRI can be used to guide treatment. For example, the long half-life of fluoxetine and its active metabolite norfluoxetine may be beneficial in instances of partial nonadherence (e.g., missed doses). Conversely, caution must be taken to monitor for drug–drug interactions prior to combining another medication with fluoxetine. SSRIs are extensively distributed to the tissues, and all, with the possible exception of citalopram and sertraline, may have a nonlinear pattern of drug accumulation with long-term administration.[51,71] Therefore, the relationship between the dose and observed effect (e.g., side effect) may change over time for the nonlinear SSRIs, and this needs to be considered during treatment.

Bioavailability is low (30% to 70%) for most TCAs as a result of the first-pass hepatic effect, which shows great interindividual variation.[72] The TCAs have a large volume of distribution and concentrate in brain and cardiac tissue in laboratory animals. They are bound extensively and strongly to plasma albumin, erythrocytes, α_1-acid glycoprotein, and lipoprotein.[72] The major metabolic pathways are demethylation, aromatic and aliphatic hydroxylation, and glucuronide conjugation. Enterohepatic cycling has been described.[72,73] Metabolism of TCAs is linear within the usual dosage range. The elimination half-lives of the TCAs can vary greatly among individual patients.[72]

Venlafaxine is metabolized to an active metabolite, O-desmethylvenlafaxine, which contributes to the overall pharmacologic effect,[74] and has received FDA approval as an antidepressant. Venlafaxine has the lowest plasma protein binding of any antidepressant (27% to 30%), which reduces the likelihood of drug interactions via this mechanism. As might be expected, different formulations of venlafaxine with different PK profiles have led to different adverse effect profiles. For example, venlafaxine extended-release formulation, with its sustained plasma concentrations, has been associated with higher rates of sexual dysfunction among men (37%) compared with the immediate-release formulation (6%).[74]

TABLE 51-6 Pharmacokinetic Properties of Antidepressants

Generic Name	Elimination Half-Life[a]	Time of Peak Plasma Concentration (Hours)	Plasma Protein Binding (%)	Percentage Bioavailable	Clinically Important Metabolites
Selective Serotonin Reuptake Inhibitors (SSRIs)					
Citalopram	33 hours	2–4	80	≥80	None
Escitalopram	27–32 hours	5	56	80	None
Fluoxetine	4–6 days[b]	4–8	94	95	Norfluoxetine
Fluvoxamine	15–26 hours	2–8	77	53	None
Paroxetine	24–31 hours	5–7	95		None
Sertraline	27 hours	6–8	99	36[c]	None
Serotonin–Norepinephrine Reuptake Inhibitors (SNRIs)					
Desvenlafaxine	11 hours	7.5	30	80	None
Duloxetine	12 hours	6	90	50	None
Venlafaxine	5 hours	2	27–30	45	*O*-Desmethylvenlafaxine
TCAs					
Amitriptyline	9–46 hours	1–5	90–97	30–60	Nortriptyline
Desipramine	11–46 hours	3–6	73–92	33–51	2-Hydroxydesipramine
Doxepin	8–36 hours	1–4	68–82	13–45	Desmethyldoxepin
Imipramine	6–34 hours	1.5–3	63–96	22–77	Desipramine
Nortriptyline	16–88 hours	3–12	87–95	46–70	10-Hydroxynortriptyline
Mixed Serotonergic (Mixed 5-HT)					
Nefazodone	2–4 hours	1	99	20	*meta*-Chlorophenylpiperazine
Trazodone	6–11 hours	1–2	92	[d]	*meta*-Chlorophenylpiperazine
Vilazodone	25 hours	4–5	>95	72[e]	
Norepinephrine/Dopamine Reuptake Inhibitor (NDRI)					
Bupropion	10–21 hours	3	82–88	[d]	Hydroxybupropion Threohydrobupropion Erythrohydrobupropion
Serotonin and α_2-Adrenergic Antagonists					
Mirtazapine	20–40 hours	2	85	50	None

[a]Biologic half-life in slowest phase of elimination.
[b]Four to 6 days with chronic dosing; norfluoxetine, 4–16 days.
[c]Increases 30–40% when taken with food.
[d]No data available.
[e]Take with food to increase area under the curve concentrations.

Data from references 41–43, 68–70.

Bupropion is metabolized to multiple active metabolites (see Table 51-6). There are currently three formulations of bupropion (immediate release, sustained release, and extended release), which are considered bioequivalent.[75] The bupropion peak plasma concentrations are lower for the sustained-release formulation of bupropion, and it is believed this may contribute to a lower seizure risk with that formulation.[76]

Mirtazapine undergoes extensive biotransformation to several metabolites[77] and is primarily eliminated in the urine (renal elimination). However, these metabolites are present at such low plasma concentrations as to minimally contribute to the overall pharmacologic profile of mirtazapine.

Altered Pharmacokinetics

In patients with cirrhosis, the half-lives of fluoxetine and norfluoxetine increased to 7.6 and 12 days, respectively.[71] Patients with hepatic impairment had a twofold increase in plasma concentrations of paroxetine.[78] Similarly, in patients with mild stable cirrhosis, the half-life of sertraline was 2.5 times greater than in patients without liver disease.[79] Patients with renal impairment had a twofold to fourfold increase in paroxetine plasma concentrations compared with normal volunteers.[78] Plasma concentrations of SSRIs in the elderly are reported to be greater than in younger patients.[71]

Factors that influence TCA plasma concentrations include disease states, genetics, age, cigarette smoking, and concurrent drug administration. Hepatic disease may result in increased TCA plasma concentrations.[40] Renal failure does not alter nortriptyline metabolism, but the 10-hydroxy metabolite may accumulate, and protein binding may be diminished, with resulting enhanced sensitivity to the drug.[72] Clinicians should be alert to the possibility of higher-than-expected plasma concentrations of some TCAs in the elderly.

The clearance of venlafaxine, mirtazapine, and their metabolites may be reduced among patients with hepatic or renal disease,[69] and doses should be adjusted accordingly. Elderly patients may require a dose reduction with mirtazapine.[69]

Plasma Concentration and Clinical Response

Studies in acutely depressed patients have demonstrated a correlation between antidepressant effect and plasma concentrations for some TCAs. However, the patient's clinical response, not plasma concentration, dictates dosage adjustments. Some patients with plasma concentrations outside the suggested therapeutic plasma concentration range respond, whereas others are nonresponsive regardless of their plasma concentration. See Table 51-3 for a listing of suggested therapeutic plasma concentration ranges. There are four TCAs (amitriptyline, nortriptyline, desipramine, and imipramine) with evidence to support an association between plasma concentrations and clinical response. However, the best established therapeutic range is for nortriptyline (50 to 150 ng/mL [190 to 570 nmol/L]),[40] which appears to demonstrate a curvilinear plasma concentration–response relationship.

For the newer antidepressants, a correlation has not been established between plasma concentration and clinical response or adverse effects.

Plasma Concentration Monitoring

Because of interindividual variations in plasma concentrations achieved by a given dose, interpretation of plasma concentrations can be very difficult for the TCAs.[40] Although plasma level monitoring is not performed routinely, some indications include inadequate response, relapse, serious or persistent adverse effects, use of higher-than-standard doses, suspected toxicity, elderly patients, pregnant patients, cardiac disease, suspected nonadherence, suspected PK drug interactions, and change in the manufacturer of the product. If plasma concentration monitoring is used to detect nonadherence, a cutoff as low as 30 ng/mL (~110 nmol/L) for the TCAs has been suggested to avoid confusion with low bioavailability or unusually rapid metabolism. Plasma concentrations should be obtained at steady state, usually after a minimum of 1 week at constant dosage. Sampling should be performed during the drug elimination phase, usually in the morning, 12 hours after the last dose. Samples collected in this manner are comparable for patients on once-, twice-, or thrice-daily regimens.[72]

Drug Interactions

Drug–drug interactions fall into two broad categories: PK or PD drug interactions. In contrast to the SSRIs, which have potential for both PK and PD interactions, other newer-generation antidepressants such as venlafaxine, duloxetine, mirtazapine, and bupropion have drug interactions that are primarily PD. This may be partly explained by the relative lack of cytochrome P450 inhibition among these newer agents compared with that among SSRIs (see Table 51-7).[41,42,51,68–70]

Pharmacokinetic

Because the TCAs are metabolized in the liver through the cytochrome P450 system, they may interact with other drugs that modify hepatic enzyme activity or hepatic blood flow. TCAs are also extensively protein bound, which can cause drug interactions through displacement from protein-binding sites. Many commonly used medications can interact when given concurrently with TCAs. Due to their frequent coadministration, a common drug interaction occurs between the TCAs and certain SSRIs, such as paroxetine and fluoxetine. These drugs are known to inhibit cytochrome P450 (e.g., CYP2D6) with the resultant increase in TCA plasma concentrations. Drug–drug interactions may occur when an SSRI is coadministered with another drug metabolized through the cytochrome P450 system. Two of the isoenzymes of the cytochrome P450 system, 2D6 and 3A4, are responsible for the metabolism of more than 80% of currently marketed drugs.[70] The ability of an SSRI, or any antidepressant, to inhibit or induce the activity of these enzymes will be a significant contributory factor in determining its capability to cause a PK drug interaction when administered concomitantly. Table 51-7 shows the cytochrome P450 enzyme inhibitory potential of the second- and third-generation antidepressant agents. In patients receiving a stable dose of any medication known to interact with SSRIs, if an SSRI is to be initiated, the starting dose should be low and titrated carefully to evaluate the potential importance of the interaction. As nefazodone use has been severely limited due to its potential to induce liver toxicity, and trazodone is primarily used as a non–FDA-approved hypnotic at low doses, neither of these agents are likely to be involved in clinically significant drug interactions. However, it should be noted that nefazodone is a potent inhibitor of cytochrome P450 3A4.[70]

TABLE 51-7 Second- and Third-Generation Antidepressants and Cytochrome (CYP) P450 Enzyme Inhibitory Potential

	CYP Enzyme			
Drug	**1A2**	**2C**	**2D6**	**3A4**
Bupropion	0	0	+	0
Citalopram	0	0	+	NA
Duloxetine	0	0	+++	0
Escitalopram	0	0	+	0
Fluoxetine	0	++	++++	++
Fluvoxamine	++++	++	0	+++
Mirtazapine	0	0	0	0
Nefazodone	0	0	0	++++
Paroxetine	0	0	++++	0
Sertraline	0	++	+	+
(des)Venlafaxine	0	0	0/+	0

++++, high; +++, moderate; ++, low; +, very low; 0, absent.

Data from references 41, 42, 51, 68–70.

Pharmacodynamic

Certain PD drug interactions that may occur with SSRIs are concerning and require close monitoring. For example, the combination of an SSRI with another drug that augments serotonergic function (e.g., linezolid) can lead to SS, which is characterized by symptoms such as clonus, hyperthermia, and mental status changes,[67] although these symptoms are not unanimously agreed upon; therefore, a washout period of 2 to 5 weeks (depending on the half-life of the SSRI) may be necessary before the initiation of another serotonergic medication. Lastly, the TCAs, SNRIs, and SSRIs can also potentially be involved in SS as described within Adverse Effects above and in Table 51-8.[41,42,63,64]

Clinical **Controversy...**

Recent research, in both mice and humans, suggests the possibility that NSAIDs may lessen the efficacy of SSRIs. A recent editorial in the *American Journal of Psychiatry* provided a thoughtful discussion on the topic.[80] At this time evidence is insufficient to draw firm conclusions. However, given the volume of prescriptions for both NSAIDs and SSRIs, this is an area of pharmacotherapy that certainly deserves further research and thoughtful prescribing practices.

Lastly, refer to Monoamine Oxidase Inhibitors under Adverse Effects above and Table 51-5 to read more about the hypertensive crisis that may result following the coadministration of MAOIs and other medications that increase vasopressor response (e.g., amphetamines). Notably, MAOIs and TCAs may be coadministered safely in refractory patients with apparent increased efficacy compared with monotherapy; however, severe reactions (e.g., hypertensive crisis) and fatalities have occurred.[2,72] Therefore, this combination should be used sparingly by experienced clinicians and monitored extremely carefully.

TABLE 51-8 Selected Drug Interactions of Newer-Generation Antidepressants

Antidepressant	Interacting Drug/Drug Class	Effect
Selective Serotonin Reuptake Inhibitors		
Citalopram and escitalopram	MAOIs	Potential for hypertensive crisis, serotonin syndrome, delirium
	Linezolid (*MAOI effects*)	Serotonin syndrome
	Sibutramine	Serotonin syndrome
	Triptans	Serotonin syndrome
Fluoxetine	Alprazolam	Increased plasma concentrations and half-life of alprazolam; increased psychomotor impairment
	Antipsychotics (e.g., haloperidol and risperidone)	Increased antipsychotic concentrations; increased extrapyramidal side effects
	β-Adrenergic blockers	Increased metoprolol serum concentrations; increased bradycardia; possible heart block
	Carbamazepine	Increased plasma concentrations of carbamazepine; symptoms of carbamazepine toxicity
	Linezolid (*MAOI effects*)	Serotonin syndrome
	MAOIs	Potential for hypertensive crisis, serotonin syndrome, delirium
	Phenytoin	Increased plasma concentrations of phenytoin; symptoms of phenytoin toxicity
	TCAs	Markedly increased TCA plasma concentrations; symptoms of TCA toxicity
	Sibutramine	Serotonin syndrome
	Triptans	Serotonin syndrome
	Thioridazine	Thioridazine C_{max} increased; prolonged QTc interval
Fluvoxamine	Alosetron	Increased alosetron AUC (sixfold) and half-life (threefold)
	Alprazolam	Increased AUC of alprazolam by 96%, increased alprazolam half-life by 71%; increased psychomotor impairment
	β-Adrenergic blockers	Fivefold increase in propranolol serum concentration; bradycardia and hypotension
	Carbamazepine	Increased plasma concentrations of carbamazepine; symptoms of carbamazepine toxicity
	Clozapine	Increased clozapine serum concentrations; increased risk for seizures and orthostatic hypotension
	Diltiazem	Bradycardia
	MAOIs	Potential for hypertensive crisis, serotonin syndrome, delirium
	Methadone	Increased methadone plasma concentrations; symptoms of methadone toxicity
	Ramelteon	Increased AUC (190-fold) and C_{max} (70-fold)
	Sibutramine	Serotonin syndrome
	TCAs	Increased TCA plasma concentration; symptoms of TCA toxicity
	Theophylline and caffeine	Increased serum concentrations of theophylline or caffeine; symptoms of theophylline or caffeine toxicity
	Thioridazine	Thioridazine C_{max} increased; prolonged QTc interval
	Warfarin	Increased hypoprothrombinemic response to warfarin
Paroxetine	Antipsychotics (e.g., haloperidol, perphenazine)	Increased antipsychotic concentrations; increased CNS and extrapyramidal side effects
	β-Adrenergic blockers	Increased metoprolol serum concentrations; increased bradycardia; possible heart block
	Linezolid (*MAOI effects*)	Serotonin syndrome
	MAOIs	Potential for hypertensive crisis, serotonin syndrome, delirium
	TCAs	Markedly increased TCA plasma concentrations; symptoms of TCA toxicity
	Sibutramine	Serotonin syndrome
	Triptans	Serotonin syndrome
	Thioridazine	Thioridazine C_{max} increased; prolonged QTc interval
Sertraline	Linezolid (*MAOI effects*)	Serotonin syndrome
	MAOIs	Potential for hypertensive crisis, serotonin syndrome, delirium
	Sibutramine	Serotonin syndrome
	Triptans	Serotonin syndrome
Serotonin–Norepinephrine Reuptake Inhibitors		
Venlafaxine and desvenlafaxine	MAOIs	Potential for hypertensive crisis, serotonin syndrome, delirium
	Sibutramine	Serotonin syndrome
	Triptans	Serotonin syndrome
Duloxetine	MAOIs	Potential for hypertensive crisis, serotonin syndrome, delirium
	Sibutramine	Serotonin syndrome
	Thioridazine	Thioridazine C_{max} increased; prolonged QTc interval
	Triptans	Serotonin syndrome
Serotonin and α-2-Adrenergic Antagonist		
Mirtazapine	Carbamazepine	Mirtazapine concentration decreased (60%)
	MAOIs	Theoretically central serotonin syndrome could occur
Norepinephrine and Dopamine Reuptake Inhibitor		
Bupropion	MAOIs	Potential for hypertensive crisis
	Medications that lower seizure threshold	Increased incidence of seizures

AUC, area under the time concentration curve; C_{max}, maximum concentration; MAOI, monoamine oxidase inhibitor.

Data from references 41, 42, 63, and 64.

Adjunct to Pharmacotherapy

The APA Task Force on Complementary and Alternative Medicine (CAM) recently provided consensus-based recommendations on the use of CAM for the treatment of MDD.[81] While these recommendations are not the focus of this chapter, clinicians treating patients with MDD should be cognizant of them.

Omega-3 Fatty Acids

It appears from the literature reviewed by the task force that eicosapentaenoic acid (EPA) and docosahexaenoic acid (DHA) omega-3 fatty acids can be used as augmentation in the treatment of MDD. Furthermore, EPA alone or the combination of EPA/DHA is likely more effective than DHA alone.

St. John's Wort

There is a lack of consensus regarding St. John's wort for the treatment of MDD. Furthermore, St. John's wort induces hepatic metabolic enzymes and is associated with significant drug interactions. Therefore, the APA Task Force conservatively states that St. John's wort may be reasonable for some individuals with mild to moderate MDD.

S-Adenosyl-L-Methionine (SAMe)

The use of SAMe received a favorable review by the APA Task Force. However, the final consensus was that more rigorous studies need to confirm the efficacy of SAMe for treating MDD.

Folate

The three compounds in this category are (a) folic acid, (b) folinic acid, and (c) 5-methyltetrahydrofolate (5-MTHF). These folate compounds are involved in the synthesis of key NTs, such as 5-HT. The task force states that augmentation with these compounds is reasonable, but more work is needed to clarify which subgroup of patients may achieve the greatest response. For example, in one study, only women responded to folic acid augmentation of fluoxetine treatment.

Exercise

Physical activity has long been recommended for individuals with many ailments, and recent data suggest benefits in depressed patients. For example, positive preliminary findings led to the Treatment with Exercise Augmentation for Depression (TREAD) study, which is a study designed to confirm the promising initial findings. Recently published findings from this study showed that 16 kcal (67 kJ) per kilogram per week (KKW) exercise was associated with greater remission rates compared with 4 KKW, when both were used as augmentation to an SSRI.[82] The task force concluded that integrating exercise into the MDD treatment plan is medically appropriate and confers many well-accepted health benefits.

Special Populations

Elderly Patients

Depression in the elderly is a major public health problem. Many elderly depressed patients are inadequately treated, or depression is missed or mistaken for another disorder, such as dementia. In the elderly, depressed mood, the typical signature symptom of depression, may be less prominent than other depressive symptoms such as loss of appetite, cognitive impairment, sleeplessness, anergia, and loss of interest in and enjoyment of the normal pursuits of life.[83] Older adults may not recognize common symptoms associated with depression such as anhedonia (inability to experience pleasure), fatigue, and concentration difficulties. Somatic (physical) complaints are quite frequently the presenting symptoms in elderly depressed patients. Appropriate recognition and treatment of depression in the elderly is extremely important. In fact, individuals 65 years of age and older have a very high rate of suicidality.[83] Increased suicidal attempts in the depressed elderly may be due to access to firearms, diminished cognitive functioning, sleep disruptions, poor social interactions, and inattention among primary caregivers.[84]

Before initiating antidepressant treatment, a complete physical examination should be performed. In prescribing antidepressants, elderly patients may be either overtreated or undertreated. Overtreatment occurs when age-related PK and PD factors are overlooked. Undertreatment results from an overly conservative approach as a result of the patient's advanced age or concurrent medical problems. SSRIs are usually selected as first-choice antidepressants in the elderly, and this may enable the clinician to avoid some of the problematic adverse effects commonly associated with TCAs (e.g., sedative, anticholinergic, and cardiovascular side effects). Furthermore, there is evidence to suggest that the long-term use of antidepressants such as SSRIs in the elderly, administered with either psychotherapy or clinical management, may prevent a depressive relapse.[85] Bupropion and venlafaxine are often selected because of milder anticholinergic and less frequent cardiovascular side effects.[86] Mirtazapine has been shown to be an effective antidepressant in the elderly (at least 65 years of age) and better tolerated than the SSRI paroxetine. Furthermore, secondary measures of anxiety and sleep were improved following mirtazapine administration.[87]

Pediatric Patients

Accumulating evidence indicates that childhood depression occurs quite commonly. Symptoms of depression in the young may vary from accepted diagnostic criteria and include several nonspecific symptoms such as boredom, anxiety, failing adjustment, and sleep disturbance.[88]

Data collected under controlled conditions that support the efficacy of antidepressants in children and adolescents are sparse, and no antidepressant, except fluoxetine, is FDA-approved for the treatment of depression in patients younger than 18 years of age, although other antidepressants (e.g., sertraline) have been studied in this population.[89]

The use of antidepressants in children and adolescents was complicated when, in March 2004, the FDA issued a black box warning in the product labeling for antidepressant medications warning clinicians and patients of the increased risk for suicidal ideation and behavior when antidepressants are used in this population. However, several retrospective longitudinal reviews of the use of antidepressants in children found no significant increase in the risk of suicide attempts or deaths.[90–92] Furthermore, adolescents suffering from depression who remain untreated may successfully commit suicide.[93,94] Further study is needed to resolve this important clinical dilemma.

Several cases of sudden death have been reported in children and adolescents taking antidepressants, such as desipramine. A baseline electrocardiogram (ECG) is recommended before initiating treatment with a TCA in children and adolescents, and many clinicians recommend an additional ECG when steady-state plasma concentrations are achieved.[95]

The treatment of depression in children remains challenging, as depression can be difficult to diagnose and treat once identified. Antidepressants are used to treat depressed children and adolescents because no other definitive effective therapies are currently available. Also, demonstration of efficacy in this population, as well as in adults, is confounded by a high placebo response rate. However, the TCAs and several of the SSRIs remain viable treatment options when prescribed and monitored appropriately.

Pregnant and Lactating Patients

Approximately 14% of pregnant women develop a serious depression during pregnancy.[96] The data presented in several recent publications should be considered when making treatment decisions for pregnant women suffering from major depression.[96–98] The first evaluation looked at the risk of discontinuing antidepressant therapy in pregnant women suffering from depression and found a significant risk of relapse. In this study, women who discontinued antidepressant therapy were five times more likely to have a relapse during their pregnancy than were women who continued treatment.[98] Another study utilized population health data to determine whether exposure to SSRIs and depression in pregnant women differs from exposure to maternal depression alone. The authors found that prenatal exposure to SSRIs was associated with an increased risk of low birth weight and respiratory distress, and that this relationship remained after accounting for maternal illness severity.[96] A study by Chambers et al. reported a sixfold greater likelihood of the occurrence of persistent pulmonary hypertension of newborn infants exposed to an SSRI after the 20th week of gestation.[97] A recent editorial on the use of antidepressants in pregnancy lists four therapeutic principles to guide the clinician in treating women during pregnancy: (a) Pregnancy does not protect against the occurrence of depression, and the likelihood of relapse is very high in untreated women with recurrent illness. (b) Maternal depression adversely affects child development, and prenatal depression may adversely affect the offspring. (c) When attempting to balance benefit and risk, transient postnatal behavioral abnormalities in the offspring of treated mothers must not be assumed to portend long-term compromise. (d) SSRIs, the most commonly used and best-tolerated treatment for depression, carry a small but significant risk for a serious medical consequence.[99]

In September 2009, the APA and the American College of Obstetricians and Gynecologists released a report discussing the treatment of depression during pregnancy. One of the prominent conclusions of this report was that *both* antidepressant treatment and untreated depression have been associated with potential problems during pregnancy. However, studies to date have not been able to adequately control for all the necessary variables involved in birth outcomes (e.g., maternal depressive disorder) and more work needs to be done.[100]

In summary, the risks and benefits of drug therapy during pregnancy must always be weighed, and concerns about the risks of untreated depression during pregnancy should be considered. These include the possibility of low birth weight secondary to poor maternal weight gain, suicidality, potential for hospitalization, potential for marital discord, inability to engage in appropriate obstetric care, and difficulty caring for other children.[101] Several different approaches exist for dealing with pregnancy and antidepressant use. First, discontinuation of an antidepressant before conception is an option for women who are stable and appear likely to remain well while not taking antidepressant medication. Second, continuation of the antidepressant until conception may be reasonable. For those who have a history of depressive relapse after medication discontinuation, the antidepressant should be continued throughout pregnancy. Further evaluations of the newer antidepressant agents are needed to fully understand the risks associated with their use at various stages of the gestational period. Again, the risks of not treating depression in a pregnant woman should not be underestimated or minimized.

There is a great deal of uncertainty regarding long-term antidepressant exposure during breastfeeding due to the lack of data. However, both sertraline and paroxetine appear in relatively low concentrations in breast milk and in samples taken from infants.[102]

Relative Resistance and Treatment-Resistant Depression

The majority of "treatment-resistant" depressed patients are likely the result of inadequate therapy (relative resistance). This theory is supported by data from the National Institute of Mental Health (NIMH) Sequenced Treatment Alternatives to Relieve Depression (STAR*D) study, which is generally considered to be one of the premier antidepressant trials among patients with depressive disorders.[103] This study showed that one in three depressed patients who previously did not achieve remission using an antidepressant became symptom free with the help of an additional medication (e.g., bupropion SR) and one in four achieved remission after switching to a different antidepressant (e.g., venlafaxine XR).[103] Furthermore, patients can be switched to another medication within the same class. For example, patients in the STAR*D study not responding to an initial SSRI were shown to be as likely to respond to another SSRI as they were to a medication from a different class.[104]

Although several different definitions for treatment-resistant depression have been proposed, the most widely accepted is depression, which has not achieved remission even after two optimal antidepressant trails.[105] More than 40% of patients with MDD being treated with antidepressants meet these criteria.[105] Three pharmacologic approaches that have been used with success for treatment-resistant depression include the following:

1. The current antidepressant may be stopped and a trial with another agent initiated (i.e., switching). For example, the STAR*D trial compared switching to mirtazapine (up to 60 mg/day) versus nortriptyline (up to 200 mg/day) after two consecutive failed medication treatments.[106] In the mirtazapine group, 12.3% of patients met the remission criterion of a score of 7 or less on the Hamilton Rating Scale for Depression (HAM-D), while 19.8% of nortriptyline patients met this criterion at the end of 14 weeks.
2. The current antidepressant can be augmented by the addition of another agent such as lithium, or another antidepressant can be added (i.e., combination antidepressant treatment). For example, the STAR*D trial evaluated the addition of lithium or triiodothyronine (T_3) to current antidepressant treatment. After approximately 10 weeks, T_3 augmentation resulted in higher remission rates (24.7%) compared with lithium (15.9%). However, the differences between these two augmentation strategies were modest and not statistically significant.[105]
3. The use of atypical antipsychotic agents to augment the antidepressant response. Aripiprazole was the first atypical antipsychotic to receive FDA approval for adjunctive use in adults with MDD. Additionally, olanzapine *in combination* with fluoxetine (Symbyax) was approved for treatment-resistant depression. Please refer to the FDA website for additional information on FDA approvals.

The APA practice guideline for the treatment of patients with MDD offers guidance for managing patients who fail to respond. These guidelines advise that if patients fail to respond to medication after 6 to 8 weeks, a reappraisal of the treatment regimen should be considered.[2] Partial responders should consider changing the dose, augmenting the antidepressant, or adding psychotherapy or ECT. For those with no response, options include changing to a second antidepressant or the addition of psychotherapy or ECT. Comorbid medical or psychiatric conditions should be identified and treated because they may complicate treatment.

6 Before changing a patient's treatment, the clinician is advised to evaluate the adequacy of the medication dosage and adherence with the prescribed regimen. Issues to be addressed in assessing the patient who has not responded to treatment include the following:

1. Is the diagnosis correct?
2. Does the patient have a psychotic depression?
3. Has the patient received an adequate dose and adequate duration of treatment?
4. Do adverse effects preclude adequate dosing?

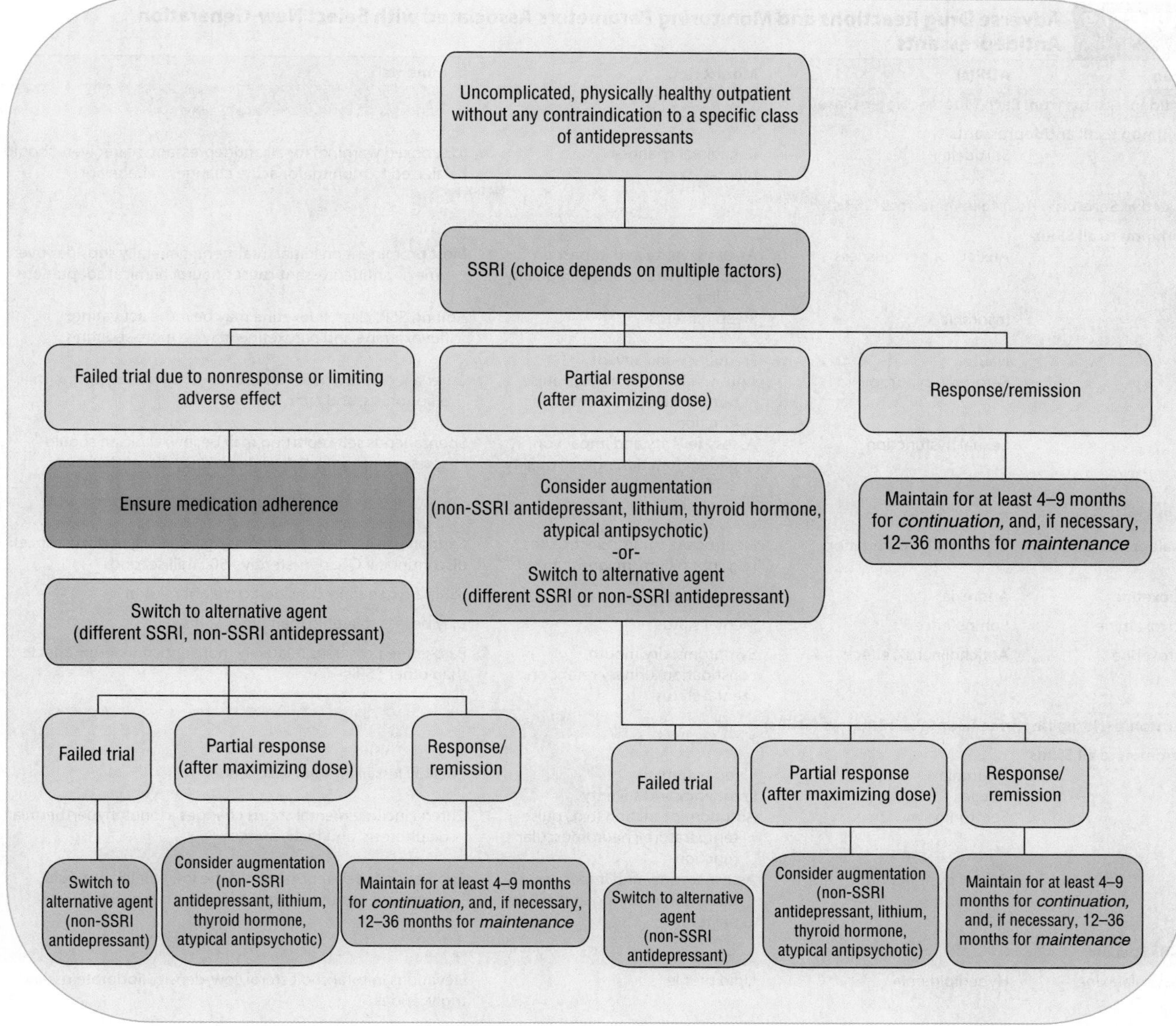

FIGURE 51-2 Algorithm for treatment of uncomplicated MDD. (SSRI, selective serotonin reuptake inhibitor.)

5. Has the patient adhered to the prescribed regimen?
6. Was a stepwise approach to treatment used?
7. Was treatment outcome adequately measured?
8. Is there a coexisting or preexisting medical or psychiatric disorder?
9. Are there other factors that interfere with treatment?

Clinical Application

A suggested algorithm for the management of uncomplicated MDD is shown in Figure 51-2. Recommended initial doses and dosage ranges are shown in Table 51-3. Antidepressant doses are generally titrated upwards depending on symptom response and adverse effects. Table 51-3 provides some medication-specific guidelines for dose titration. It is important to remember that 3 to 4 weeks is usually required before a mood-elevating response is seen. A 6-week trial at a maximum dosage is considered an adequate trial.[2] It is crucial to counsel the patient about the expected lag time before the onset of clinical response. Patients uneducated in this regard often fail to adhere to their prescribed regimens.

Some antidepressant dosing regimens are particularly important from a safety standpoint. For example, bupropion must be carefully dosed in order to reduce seizure risk. Bupropion is usually initiated at 75 mg twice daily, and this dose may be increased to 100 mg three times daily after a few days. Most patients will respond at 300 mg/day; however, an increase to 450 mg/day, given as 150 mg three times daily, may be considered in patients with no or partial response after several weeks of treatment at 300 mg/day. Additionally, both a 12-hour and a 24-hour sustained-release formulation are available, allowing for less frequent dosing.

Caution is urged when dosing antidepressants in special populations. For example, in elderly patients, as a general rule, dosing is initiated at one half the initial dose administered to younger adults, and the dose is increased at a slower rate.

Personalized Pharmacotherapy

7 Pharmacogenetic applications in psychiatry have been explored for some time. Pharmacogenetic tests (e.g., the FDA-approved AmpliChip to evaluate CYP2D6 and CYP2C19 polymorphisms) are now available. However, there are no standard or well-accepted

TABLE 51-9 Adverse Drug Reactions and Monitoring Parameters Associated with Select New-Generation Antidepressants

Drug	ADR(s)	Monitoring	Comments
Antidepressants from Each Pharmacologic Class			
Common to all antidepressants			
	Suicidality	Behavioral changes Mental status	(U.S. boxed warning) for all antidepressants; caregivers should be alerted to monitor for acute changes in behavior
Selective Serotonin Reuptake Inhibitors (SSRIs)			
Common to all SSRIs			
	Anxiety or nervousness	Assess severity and impact on patient functioning and quality of life	Most prominent on initial treatment; generally subsides over time as antidepressant causes neurochemical adaptations
	Insomnia	Sleep patterns	Among SSRI class: fluoxetine may be more activating; fluvoxamine and paroxetine may be more sedating
	Nausea	Frequency and severity	
	Serotonin syndrome	Autonomic function (e.g., pulse, temperature); neuromuscular function	Criteria include mental status change, clonus, hyperthermia, diaphoresis, and tachycardia
	Sexual dysfunction	Assess severity and impact on patient functioning and quality of life	Spontaneous self-reporting may be low; clinician should assess symptoms; reversible on drug discontinuation
SSRI-Specific			
Citalopram	QT interval prolongation	Electrocardiogram; electrolytes (e.g., potassium, magnesium)	Caution use in "at-risk" patients (e.g., electrolyte disturbance); discontinue if QTc persistently >500 milliseconds
Fluoxetine	Anorexia	Weight (over time)	SSRIs are generally considered weight neutral
Fluvoxamine	Somnolence	Mental status	May be less tolerable than other SSRIs
Paroxetine	Anticholinergic effects	Symptoms: dry mouth, constipation, urinary retention, mental status	Paroxetine possesses relatively more anticholinergic effects than other SSRIs
Serotonin–Norepinephrine Reuptake Inhibitors (SNRIs)			
Common to all SNRIs			
	Insomnia	Sleep patterns	Possibly less likely with duloxetine
	Nausea	Frequency and severity	
	Serotonin syndrome	Autonomic function (e.g., pulse temperature); neuromuscular function	Criteria include mental status changes, clonus, hyperthermia, diaphoresis, and tachycardia
	Sexual dysfunction	Assess severity and impact on patient functioning and quality of life	Spontaneous self-reporting may be low; clinician should assess symptoms; reversible on drug discontinuation
SNRI-Specific			
Desvenlafaxine	Hyperlipidemia	Lipid profile	Elevations in total cholesterol, low-density lipoproteins, and triglycerides
Duloxetine	Orthostatic *hypo*-tension	Blood pressure, pulse	Initial treatment or on dose increase
Venlafaxine	Dose-related *hyper*-tension	Blood pressure, pulse	May need to lower dose or discontinue
Mixed Serotonergic Effects (Mixed 5-HT)			
Nefazodone	Liver toxicity	Liver function tests	Nefazodone use is extremely limited in the United States due to concerns about liver toxicity
Trazodone	Orthostatic hypotension	Blood pressure, pulse	May be more severe as compared with other antidepressants; rate-limiting side effect
	Priapism	Patient report of sexual side effects, especially painful erection	Patient should seek medical attention for prolonged erection (i.e., >4 hours)
Vilazodone	Serotonin syndrome	Autonomic function (e.g., pulse temperature); neuromuscular function	Criteria include mental status changes, clonus, hyperthermia, diaphoresis, and tachycardia
Serotonin and α_2-Adrenergic Antagonist			
Mirtazapine	Weight gain	Body weight	Frequently occurring and significant (>7%) weight gain among adults
Norepinephrine and Dopamine Reuptake Inhibitor (NDRI)			
Bupropion	Seizure activity	Electroencephalogram	See text for proper dosing, which can help decrease seizure risk; caution use in patients with eating disorders or alcohol use disorders

Data from references 2, 41, 42, and 64.

guidelines for the use of pharmacogenetic testing as it relates to antidepressant treatment.[107] In contrast, PK parameters have long been one of the primary considerations when choosing among the antidepressants, particularly within a medication class.[2] For example, PK parameters help the clinician choose a particular SSRI (e.g., longer fluoxetine half-life for partial nonadherence).

EVALUATION OF THERAPEUTIC OUTCOMES

8 Several monitoring parameters, in addition to plasma concentrations, are useful in managing patients (Table 51-9).[2,41,42] Patients must be monitored for adverse effects, such as sedation and anticholinergic effects, and for remission of previously documented target symptoms. The presence of side effects does not necessarily indicate adequate dosage. In addition, changes in social and occupational functioning should be assessed. Patients receiving venlafaxine should have their blood pressure monitored at regular intervals. Patients older than 40 years of age should receive a pretreatment ECG before starting TCA therapy, and followup ECGs should be performed periodically. Patients should be monitored for the emergence of suicidal ideation after initiation of any antidepressant. Weight gain and sexual dysfunction, common events associated with most antidepressants, are associated with nonadherence and should be monitored and discussed with the patient.

In addition to the clinical interview, psychometric rating instruments (such as those highlighted earlier in this chapter and in eChap. 19) allow for rapid and reliable measurement of the nature and severity of depressive and associated symptoms. It is helpful to administer the rating scales prior to treatment, 6 to 8 weeks after initiation of therapy, and periodically thereafter. Interviewing a family member or friend (with the patient's permission) regarding symptoms and daily functioning also can assist in assessment of progress. Patients should be monitored at more frequent intervals early in treatment. Monitoring is then continued at regular intervals throughout the continuation and maintenance phases of treatment. Regular monitoring for reemergence of target symptoms should be continued for several months after antidepressant therapy is discontinued.

Finally, one useful set of criteria that can be used with a variety of psychometric scales was suggested by Mann.[35] Following these criteria, the following definitions are used: (a) *nonresponse* is less than 25% decrease in baseline symptoms, (b) *partial response* is a 26% to 49% decrease in baseline symptoms, and (c) *partial remission or response* is greater than a 50% decrease in baseline symptoms. Consistent with other recommendations, *remission* is a return to baseline functioning with no symptoms present.[2]

COLLABORATIVE PRACTICE

Significant evidence exists to show that depression is common and chronic, and causes significant morbidity and mortality. Pharmacists, in conjunction with other healthcare providers, can play a crucial role in the screening, recognition, and treatment of this disorder. In fact, the U.S. Preventive Services Task Force recommends screening adults for depression in clinical practices that have systems in place to ensure accurate diagnosis, effective treatment, and followup.[108] In addition, pharmacists and other healthcare clinicians play a crucial role in ensuring adherence to medication regimens through assessment of a patient's willingness and ability to take a medication, including an assessment of financial viability, and through patient education regarding dosing, side effects and drug interactions, and guidance regarding followup appointments with prescribing clinicians.[109]

ABBREVIATIONS

AHRQ	Agency for Healthcare Research and Quality
APA	American Psychiatric Association
BDI	Beck Depression Inventory
BDNF	brain-derived neurotrophic factor
CAM	complementary and alternative medicine
DA	dopamine
DHA	docosahexaenoic acid
DSM-IV-TR	*Diagnostic and Statistical Manual of Mental Disorders, Fourth Edition, Text Revision*
ECG	electrocardiogram
ECT	electroconvulsive therapy
EPA	eicosapentaenoic acid
5-HT	serotonin
HAM-D	Hamilton Rating Scale for Depression
HPA	hypothalamic–pituitary–adrenal
KKW	kilocalories per kilogram per week
5-MTHF	5-methyltetrahydrofolate
MADRS	Montgomery-Åsberg Depression Rating Scale
MAOI	monoamine oxidase inhibitor
MDD	major depressive disorder
NDRI	norepinephrine and dopamine reuptake inhibitor
NE	norepinephrine
NIMH	National Institute of Mental Health
NT	neurotransmitter
PD	pharmacodynamic
PK	pharmacokinetic
rTMS	repetitive transcranial magnetic stimulation
SAMe	*S*-adenosyl-L-methionine
SNRI	serotonin–norepinephrine reuptake inhibitor
SS	serotonin syndrome
SSRI	selective serotonin reuptake inhibitor
STAR*D	Sequenced Treatment Alternatives to Relieve Depression
T_3	triiodothyronine
TCA	tricyclic antidepressant
TREAD	Treatment with Exercise Augmentation for Depression

REFERENCES

1. American Psychiatric Association. Diagnostic and Statistical Manual of Mental Disorders, Fourth Edition, Text Revision. Arlington, VA: American Psychiatric Association. 2000.
2. American Psychiatric Association. Practice Guideline for the Treatment of Patients with Major Depressive Disorder, 3rd ed. Arlington, VA: American Psychiatric Association, 2010.
3. Kessler RC, Berglund P, Demler O, et al. The epidemiology of major depressive disorder: Results from the National Comorbidity Survey Replication (NCS-R). JAMA 2003; 289(23):3095–3105.
4. Burt VK, Stein K. Epidemiology of depression throughout the female life cycle. J Clin Psychiatry 2002;63(Suppl 7): 9–15.
5. Steffens DC, Skoog I, Norton MC, et al. Prevalence of depression and its treatment in an elderly population: The Cache County study. Arch Gen Psychiatry 2000;57(6): 601–607.
6. Kessler RC, Walters EE. Epidemiology of DSM-III-R major depression and minor depression among adolescents and young adults in the National Comorbidity Survey. Depress Anxiety 1998;7(1):3–14.

7. Larsson B, Ivarsson T. Clinical characteristics of adolescent psychiatric inpatients who have attempted suicide. Eur Child Adolesc Psychiatry 1998;7(4):201–208.
8. Weissman MM, Gershon ES, Kidd KK, et al. Psychiatric disorders in the relatives of probands with affective disorders. The Yale University—National Institute of Mental Health Collaborative Study. Arch Gen Psychiatry 1984;41(1):13–21.
9. Warner V, Weissman MM, Mufson L, Wickramaratne PJ. Grandparents, parents, and grandchildren at high risk for depression: A three-generation study. J Am Acad Child Adolesc Psychiatry 1999;38(3):289–296.
10. Sullivan PF, Neale MC, Kendler KS. Genetic epidemiology of major depression: Review and meta-analysis. Am J Psychiatry 2000;157(10):1552–1562.
11. Stahl SM. Blue genes and the mechanism of action of antidepressants. J Clin Psychiatry 2000;61(3): 164–165.
12. Delgado PL. Depression: The case for a monoamine deficiency. J Clin Psychiatry 2000;61(Suppl 6):7–11.
13. Hirschfield R. History and the evolution of the monoamine hypothesis of depression. J Clin Psychiatry 2000;61(Suppl 6): 4–6.
14. Delgado PL, Moreno FA, Potter R, et al. Norepinephrine and serotonin in antidepressant action: Evidence from neurotransmitter depletion studies. In: Briley M, Montgomery SA, eds. Antidepressant Therapy at the Dawn of the Third Millennium. London: Marin Dunitz, 1997: 141–163.
15. Baldessarini RJ. Drugs and the treatment of psychiatric disorders: Depression and anxiety disorders. In: Hardman JG, Limbrid LE, Goodman A, et al., eds. Goodman and Gilman's The Pharmacological Basis of Therapeutics, 10th ed. New York: McGraw-Hill, 2000:447–484.
16. Stahl SM. Blue genes and the monoamine hypothesis of depression. J Clin Psychiatry 2000;61(2):77–78.
17. Feighner JP. Mechanism of action of antidepressant medications. J Clin Psychiatry 1999;60(Suppl 4):4–11.
18. Stahl SM. Basic psychopharmacology of antidepressants, part 1: Antidepressants have seven distinct mechanisms of action. J Clin Psychiatry 1998;59(Suppl 4):5–14.
19. Siever LJ, Davis KL. Overview: Toward a dysregulation hypothesis of depression. Am J Psychiatry 1985;142(9): 1017–1031.
20. Ordway GA, Klimek V, Mann JJ. Neurocircuitry of mood disorders. In: Davis KL, Charney D, Coyle JT, Nemeroff C, eds. Neuropsychopharmacology: The Fifth Generation of Progress. Brentwood, TN: American College of Neuropsychopharmacology, 2002:1051–1064.
21. Berton O, Nestler EJ. New approaches to antidepressant drug discovery: Beyond monoamines. Nat Rev Neurosci 2006;7(2):137–151.
22. Thase M. Mood disorders. In: Sadock BJ, Sadock VA, eds. Neurobiology. Kaplan & Sadock's Comprehensive Textbook of Psychiatry. Philadelphia, PA: Lippincott Williams & Wilkins, 2004.
23. Sofuoglu M, Dudish-Poulsen S, Poling J, et al. The effect of individual cocaine withdrawal symptoms on outcomes in cocaine users. Addict Behav 2005;30(6): 1125–1134.
24. Patten SB, Barbui C. Drug-induced depression: A systematic review to inform clinical practice. Psychother Psychosom 2004;73(4):207–215.
25. Botts S, Ryan M. Depression. Drug-Induced Diseases: Prevention, Detection, and Management, 2nd ed. Bethesda, MD: American Society of Health-System Pharmacists, 2010.
26. Montgomery SA, Asberg M. A new depression scale designed to be sensitive to change. Br J Psychiatry 1979; 134:382–389.
27. Beck AT, Ward CH, Mock J, Erbaugh J. An inventory for measuring depression. Arch Gen Psychiatry 1961;4:561–571.
28. McGirr A, Renaud J, Seguin M, et al. An examination of DSM-IV depressive symptoms and risk for suicide completion in major depressive disorder: A psychological autopsy study. J Affect Disord 2007;97(1–3):203–209.
29. Lebowitz BD, Pearson JL, Schneider LS, et al. Diagnosis and treatment of depression in late life. Consensus statement update. JAMA 1997;278(14):1186–1190.
30. Trivedi MH. The link between depression and physical symptoms. Prim Care Companion J Clin Psychiatry 2004; 6(Suppl 1):12–16.
31. Centers for Disease Control and Prevention, National Center for Injury Prevention and Control. Suicide: Facts at a Glance. Summer 2009, *http://www.cdc.gov/violenceprevention/pdf/Suicide-DataSheet-a.pdf*.
32. Jacobs DG, Baldessarini RJ, Fawcett JA, et al. Practice guidelines for the assessment and treatment of patients with suicidal behaviors. Am J Psychiatry 2003;160(Suppl 11): 1–60.
33. Fawcett JA, Baldessarini RJ, Coryell WH. Defining and managing suicidal risk in patients taking psychotropic medications. J Clin Psychiatry 2009;70(6):782–789.
34. Gibbons RD, Brown CH, Hur K, et al. Suicidal thoughts and behavior with antidepressant treatment: Reanalysis of the randomized placebo-controlled studies of fluoxetine and venlafaxine. Arch Gen Psychiatry 2012;69(6):580–587.
35. Mann JJ. The medical management of depression. N Engl J Med 2005;353:1819–1834.
36. Blackbum IM, Moore RG. Controlled acute and follow-up trial of cognitive therapy and pharmacotherapy in outpatients with recurrent depression. Br J Psychiatry 1997;171: 328–334.
37. Klapheke MM. Electroconvulsive therapy consultation: An update. Convuls Ther 1997;13:227–241.
38. Gaynes BN, Lux L, Lloyd S, et al. Nonpharmacologic Interventions for Treatment-Resistant Depression in Adults. Comparative Effectiveness Review No. 33 (Prepared by RTI International–University of North Carolina (RTI-UNC) Evidence Based Practice Center under Contract No. 290-02-0016I). AHRQ Publication No. 11-EHC056-EF. Rockville, MD: Agency for Healthcare Research and Quality, September 2011, *www.effectivehealthcare.ahrq.gov/reports/final.cfm*.
39. Patkar AA, Pae C-U, Masand PS. Transdermal selegiline: The new generation of monoamine oxidase inhibitors. CNS Spectr 2006;11:363–375.
40. Watanabe MD, Winter ME. Tricyclic antidepressants: Amitriptyline, desipramine, imipramine, and nortriptyline. In: Winter ME, ed. Basic Clinical Pharmacokinetics, 4th ed. Baltimore, MD: Lippincott Williams & Wilkins, 2004: 423–437.
41. Medscape Reference. Copyright © 1994-2012 by WebMD LLC. *http://reference.medscape.com/psychiatry*.
42. Lexi-Comp Online [Internet]. Hudson, OH: Lexi-Comp Inc, 2011.
43. Stahl SM, Grady MM, Moret C, Briley M. SNRIs: Their pharmacology, clinical efficacy, and tolerability in comparison with other classes of antidepressants. CNS Spectr 2005;10:732–747.
44. Horst WD, Preskorn SH. Mechanism of action and clinical characteristics of three atypical antidepressants: Venlafaxine, nefazodone, bupropion. J Affect Disord 1998;51:237–254.

45. Gartlehner G, Hansen RA, Morgan LC, et al. Second-Generation Antidepressants in the Pharmacologic Treatment of Adult Depression: An Update of the 2007 Comparative Effectiveness Review (Prepared by the RTI International–University of North Carolina Evidence-Based Practice Center, Contract No. 290-2007-10056-I). AHRQ Publication No. 12-EHC012-EF. Rockville, MD: Agency for Healthcare Research and Quality, December 2011, *www.effectivehealthcare.ahrq.gov/reports/final.cfm*.
46. Ables AZ, Baughman OL III. Antidepressants: Update on new agents and indications. Am Fam Physician 2003;67:547–554.
47. Citrome L. Vilazodone for major depressive disorder: A systematic review of the efficacy and safety profile for this newly approved antidepressant—What is the number needed to treat, number needed to harm and likelihood to be helped or harmed? Int J Clin Pract 2012;66(4):356–368.
48. Gorman JM. Mirtazapine: Clinical overview. J Clin Psychiatry 1999;60(Suppl 17):9–13.
49. Bryant SG, Brown CS. Current concepts in clinical therapeutics: Major affective disorders, part 2. Clin Pharmacol 1986;5:385–395.
50. Mathew SJ, Shah A, Lapidus K, et al. Ketamine for treatment-resistant unipolar depression. CNS Drugs 2012; 26(3):189–204.
51. Preskorn SH. Clinically relevant pharmacology of selective serotonin reuptake inhibitors: An overview with emphasis on pharmacokinetics and effects on oxidative drug metabolism. Clin Pharmacokinet 1997;32(Suppl 1):1–21.
52. Goldstein BJ, Goodnick PJ. Selective serotonin reuptake inhibitors in the treatment of affective disorders: III. Tolerability, safety and pharmacoeconomics. J Psychopharmacol 1998;12(3 Suppl B):S55–S87.
53. Masand PS, Gupta S. Long-term side effects of newer-generation antidepressants: SSRIs, venlafaxine, nefazodone, bupropion, and mirtazapine. Ann Clin Psychiatry 2002;14: 175–182.
54. Westenberg HG, Sander C. Tolerability and safety of fluvoxamine and other antidepressants. Int J Clin Pract 2006;60(4):482–491.
55. FDA Drug Safety Communication: Revised Recommendations for Celexa (Citalopram Hydrobromide) Related to a Potential Risk of Abnormal Heart Rhythms with High Doses. *http://www.fda.gov/Drugs/DrugSafety/ucm297391.htm*.
56. Nemeroff CB. The burden of severe depression: A review of diagnostic challenges and treatment alternatives. J Psychiatr Res 2007;41:189–206.
57. Settle ED Jr. Antidepressant drugs: Disturbing and potentially dangerous adverse effects. J Clin Psychiatry 1998;59(Suppl 16):25–30.
58. Feighner JP. Cardiovascular safety in depressed patients: Focus on venlafaxine. J Clin Psychiatry 1995;56:574–579.
59. Bauer M, Moller HJ, Schneider E. Duloxetine: A new selective and dual-acting antidepressant. Expert Opin Pharmacother 2006;7(4):421–427.
60. Stimmel GL, Gutierrez MA. Counseling patients about sexual issues. Pharmacotherapy 2006;26(11):1608–1615.
61. Johnston JA, Lineberry CG, Ascher JA. A 102 center prospective study of seizures in association with bupropion. J Clin Psychiatry 1991;52:450–456.
62. Rabkin JG, Quitkin FM, McGrath P, et al. Adverse reactions to monoamine oxidase inhibitors: II. Treatment correlates and clinical management. J Clin Psychopharmacol 1985;5:2–9.
63. Anonymous. Lexi-Comp Online™ Interaction Analysis. Lexi-Comp Online, Lexi-Comp Inc. *http://online.lexi.com*.
64. Anonymous. Drug interactions. Thomson MICROMEDEX Healthcare Series. *https://www.thomsonhc.com*.
65. Neil JF, Licata SM, May SJ, Himmelhock JM. Dietary noncompliance during treatment with tranylcypromine. J Clin Psychiatry 1979;40:33–37.
66. Varon J, Marik PE. The diagnosis and management of hypertensive crises. Chest 2000;118:214–227.
67. Boyer EW, Shannon M. Current concepts: The serotonin syndrome. N Engl J Med 2005;352:1112–1120.
68. Hemeryck A, Belpaire FM. Selective serotonin reuptake inhibitors and cytochrome P-450 mediated drug–drug interactions: An update. Curr Drug Metab 2002;3: 13–37.
69. Kent JM. SNaRIs, NaSSAs, and NaRIs: New agents for the treatment of depression. Lancet 2000;355:911–918.
70. DeVane CL. Differential pharmacology of newer antidepressants. J Clin Psychiatry 1998;59(Suppl 20): 85–93.
71. DeVane CL. Metabolism and pharmacokinetics of the selective serotonin reuptake inhibitors. Cell Mol Neurobiol 1999;19:443–466.
72. Wells BG. Tricyclic antidepressants. In: Taylor WJ, Caviness MHD, eds. A Textbook for the Clinical Application of Therapeutic Drug Monitoring. Irving, TX: Abbott Laboratories, 1986:449–465.
73. Rudorfer MV, Potter WZ. Metabolism of tricyclic antidepressants. Cell Mol Neurobiol 1999;19:373–409.
74. Olver JS, Burrows GD, Norman TR. The treatment of depression with different formulations of venlafaxine: A comparative analysis. Hum Psychopharmacol 2004;19: 9–16.
75. Jefferson JW, Pradko JF, Muir KT. Bupropion for major depressive disorder: Pharmacokinetic and formulation considerations. Clin Ther 2005;27:1685–1695.
76. Dunner DL, Zisook S, Billow AA, et al. A prospective safety surveillance study for bupropion sustained-release in the treatment of depression. J Clin Psychiatry 1998;59:366–373.
77. Timmer CJ, Sitsen JM, Delbressine LP. Clinical pharmacokinetics of mirtazapine. Clin Pharmacokinet 2000;38:461–474.
78. Krastev Z, Terzivoanov D, Vlahov V, et al. The pharmacokinetics of paroxetine in patients with liver cirrhosis. Acta Psychiatry Scand 1989;350(Suppl):91–92.
79. Demolis JL, Angebaud P, Grange JD, et al. Influence of liver cirrhosis on sertraline pharmacokinetics. Br J Clin Pharmacol 1996;42:394–397.
80. Shelton RC. Does concomitant use of NSAIDs reduce the effectiveness of antidepressants? Am J Psychiatry 2012;169(10):1012–1015.
81. Freeman MP, Fava M, Lake J, et al. Complementary and alternative medicine in major depressive disorder: The American Psychiatric Association Task Force report. J Clin Psychiatry 2010;71(6):669–681.
82. Trivedi MH, Greer TL, Church TS, et al. Exercise as an augmentation treatment for nonremitted major depressive disorder: A randomized, parallel dose comparison. J Clin Psychiatry 2011;72(5):677–684.
83. Otong D. The art of prescribing. Antidepressants in late-life depression: Prescribing principles. Perspect Psychiatr Care 2006;42(2):149–153.
84. Turvey CL, Conwell Y, Jones MP, et al. Risk factors for late-life suicide. A prospective, community-based study. Am J Geriatr Psychiatry 2002;10:398–406.
85. Reynolds CF 3rd, Dew MA, Pollock BG, et al. Maintenance treatment of major depression in old age. N Engl J Med 2006;354(11):1130–1138.

86. Kohn R, Epstein-Lubrow G. Course and outcomes of depression in the elderly. Curr Psychiatr Rep 2006;8(1): 34–40.
87. Schatzberg AF, Kremer C, Rodrigues HE, Murphy GM Jr; Mirtazapine vs. Paroxetine Study Group. Double-blind, randomized comparison of mirtazapine and paroxetine in elderly depressed patients. Am J Geriatr Psychiatry 2002;10:541–550.
88. Cosgrave E, McGorry P, Allen N, Jackson H. Depression in young people: A growing challenge for primary care. Aust Fam Physician 2000;29:123–127.
89. Wagner KD, Ambrosini P, Rynn M, et al. Efficacy of sertraline in the treatment of children and adolescents with major depressive disorder. JAMA 2003;290:1033–1041.
90. Olfson M, Marcus SC, Shaffer D. Antidepressant drug therapy and suicide in severely depressed children and adults: A case–control study. Arch Gen Psychiatry 2006;63(8):865–872.
91. Valuck RJ, Libby AM, Sills MR, et al. Antidepressant treatment and risk of suicide attempt by adolescents with major depressive disorder: A propensity-adjusted retrospective cohort study. CNS Drugs 2004;18(15): 1119–1132.
92. Simon GE, Savarino J, Operskalski B, Wang PS. Suicide risk during antidepressant treatment. Am J Psychiatry 2006;163(1):41–47.
93. Hallfors DD, Waller MW, Ford CA, et al. Adolescent depression and suicide risk: Association with sex and drug behavior. Am J Prev Med 2004;27(3):224–231.
94. Haavisto A, Sourander A, Ellila H, et al. Suicidal ideation and suicide attempts among child and adolescent psychiatric inpatients in Finland. J Affect Disord 2003;76(1–3):211–221.
95. Leonard HL, Meyer HC, Swedo SE, et al. Electrocardiographic changes during desipramine and clomipramine treatment in children and adolescents. J Am Acad Child Adolesc Psychiatry 1995;34:1460–1468.
96. Oberlander TF, Warburton W, Misri S, et al. Neonatal outcomes after prenatal exposure to selective serotonin reuptake inhibitor antidepressants and maternal depression using population-based linked health data. Arch Gen Psychiatry 2006;63:898–906.
97. Chambers CD, Hernandex-Diaz S, Van Marter LJ, et al. Selective serotonin-reuptake inhibitors and risk of persistent pulmonary hypertension of the newborn. N Engl J Med 2006;354(6):579–587.
98. Cohen LS, Altshuler LL, Harlow BL, et al. Relapse of major depression during pregnancy in women who maintain or discontinue antidepressant treatment. JAMA 2006;295(5):499–507.
99. Rubinow, DR. Antidepressant treatment during pregnancy: Between Scylla and Charybdis. Am J Psychiatry 2006;163(6):954–955.
100. Yonkers KA, Wisner KL, Stewart DE, et al. The management of depression during pregnancy: A report from the American Psychiatric Association and the American College of Obstetricians and Gynecologists. Gen Hosp Psychiatry 2009;31:403–413.
101. Hendrick V, Altshuler L. Management of major depression during pregnancy. Am J Psychiatry 2002;159:1667–1673.
102. Freeman MP. Breastfeeding and antidepressants: Clinical dilemmas and expert perspectives. J Clin Psychiatry 2009;70:291–292.
103. Sequenced Treatment Alternatives to Relieve Depression (STAR*D). *http://www.edc.pitt.edu/stard.*
104. Rush AJ, Trivedi MH, Wisniewski SR, et al. Bupropion-SR, sertraline, or venlafaxine-XR after failure of SSRIs for depression. N Engl J Med 2006;354:1231–1242.
105. Nierenberg AA, Fava M, Trivedi MH, et al. A comparison of lithium and T3 augmentation following two failed medication treatments for depression: A STAR*D Report. Am J Psychiatry 2006;163:1519–1530.
106. Fava M, Rush AJ, Wisniewski SR, et al. A comparison of mirtazapine and nortriptyline following two consecutive failed medication treatments for depressed outpatients: A STAR*D report. Am J Psychiatry 2006;163(7):1161–1172.
107. Martin J, Lee KC. Pharmacogenomics of antidepressants for major depressive disorder. Ment Health Clin 2012;1(9):17. *http://cpnp.org/resource/mhc/2012/03/pharmacogenomics-antidepressants-major-depressive-disorder.*
108. U.S. Preventive Services Task Force. Screening for Depression. Rockville, MD: Agency for Healthcare Research and Quality, May 2002, *http://www.ahrq.gov/clinic/3rduspstf/depression/.*
109. Finely P, Rens HR, Pont JT, et al. Impact of a collaborative pharmacy practice model on the treatment of depression in primary care. Am J Health Syst Pharm 2002;59:1518–1526.

52

Bipolar Disorder

Shannon J. Drayton and Christine M. Pelic

KEY CONCEPTS

1. Bipolar disorder is a cyclic mental illness with recurrent mood episodes that occur over a person's lifetime. The symptoms, course, severity, and response to treatment differ among individuals.
2. Bipolar disorder is likely caused by genetic factors, environmental triggers, and the dysregulation of neurotransmitters, neurohormones, and second messenger systems in the brain.
3. Clinicians should be sure to obtain a detailed history, including potential substance use and medical illness, to avoid a delay in the diagnosis and treatment of bipolar disorder.
4. The goal of therapy for bipolar disorder should be to improve patient functioning by reducing mood episodes. This is accomplished by maximizing adherence to therapy and limiting adverse effects.
5. Patients and family members should be educated about bipolar disorder and treatments. Long-term monitoring and adherence to treatment are major factors in obtaining stabilization of the disorder.
6. Lithium and valproate are the mainstays of treatment for both acute mania and prophylaxis for recurrent manic and depressive episodes. Anticonvulsants (such as lamotrigine, carbamazepine, and oxcarbazepine) and second-generation antipsychotics (such as aripiprazole, olanzapine, risperidone, quetiapine, and ziprasidone) are alternative or adjunctive treatments for bipolar disorder. Anticonvulsants may be more effective than lithium in several mood subtypes (e.g., mixed states and rapid cycling). The use of lithium, valproate, or quetiapine for acute bipolar depression should be considered as a first-line treatment option.
7. Baseline and followup laboratory tests are required for some medications to monitor for adverse effects.
8. Some patients can be stabilized on one mood stabilizer, but others may require combination therapies or adjunctive agents during an acute mood episode. If possible, adjunctive agents should be tapered and discontinued when the acute mood episode remits and the patient is stabilized. Adjunctive agents may include benzodiazepines, additional mood stabilizers or antipsychotics, and/or antidepressants.

❶ Bipolar disorder is a common, chronic, and often severe cyclic mood disorder characterized by recurrent fluctuations in mood, energy, and behavior.[1–3] It differs from recurrent major depression (or unipolar depression) in that a manic, hypomanic, or mixed episode occurs during the course of the illness.[1] Bipolar disorder is a lifelong illness with a variable course and requires both nonpharmacologic and pharmacologic treatments for mood stabilization.[1,2]

EPIDEMIOLOGY

The overall prevalence of bipolar disorder was 4.5% in a U.S. comorbidity study: 1% meeting criteria for bipolar I, 1.1% for bipolar II, and 2.4% of patients with subthreshold recurrent mood cycling (i.e., cyclothymia, bipolar disorder not otherwise specified [NOS]).[4] Symptom onset for depression or (hypo)mania in bipolar disorder typically occurs in late adolescence or early adulthood, with greater than two thirds developing symptoms before 18 years of age.[5] Bipolar I disorder occurs equally in men and women, whereas bipolar II disorder is more common in women.[1,2] Depression and mixed presentations may occur more frequently in women.[6–8]

ETIOLOGY AND PATHOPHYSIOLOGY

❷ The exact etiology of bipolar disorder is unknown. Bipolar disorder is thought to be a complex disease that is influenced by developmental, genetic, neurobiologic, and psychological factors.[9] Many theories have been proposed regarding the pathophysiology of mood disorders. Family, twin, and adoption studies report an increased lifetime prevalence risk of having mood disorders among first-degree relatives of patients with bipolar disorder.[10,11] Genetic linkage studies suggest multiple gene loci can be involved in the heredity of mood disorders.[12–14] Neuroimaging studies have found neurochemical, anatomic, and functional abnormalities in bipolar patients.[15] Many researchers suspect that altered synaptic and circuit functioning accounts for mood and cognitive changes seen in bipolar disorder, rather than dysfunction of individual neurotransmitters.[16] Environmental or psychosocial stressors, immunologic factors, and sleep dysregulation all have been associated with bipolar disorder and can negatively influence the course of illness.[17–21]

CLINICAL PRESENTATION AND DIAGNOSIS

❶ The essential feature of bipolar spectrum disorders is a history of mania or hypomania that is not caused by any other medical condition, substance, or psychiatric disorder.[1,2] The *Diagnostic and Statistical Manual of Mental Disorders, Fourth Edition, Text Revision* (*DSM-IV-TR*) of the American Psychiatric Association (APA) details the present understanding of mood disorders.[1] Bipolar disorder is divided into four subtypes based on the identification of specific mood episodes: bipolar I, bipolar II, cyclothymic disorder, and bipolar disorder NOS. See Table 52-1 for a definition of mood disorders by type of episode. Bipolar I and II can further be specified to reflect the most recent mood state (i.e., hypomanic or major

TABLE 52-1 Mood Disorders Defined by Episodes

Disorder Subtype	Episode(s)[a]
Major depressive disorder, single episode	Major depressive episode
Major depressive disorder, recurrent	Two or more major depressive episodes
Bipolar disorder, type I[b]	Manic episode ± major depressive or mixed episode
Bipolar disorder, type II[c]	Major depressive episode + hypomanic episode
Dysthymic disorder	Chronic subsyndromal depressive episodes
Cyclothymic disorder[d]	Chronic fluctuations between subsyndromal depressive and hypomanic episodes (2 years for adults and 1 year for children and adolescents)
Bipolar disorder not otherwise specified	Mood states do not meet criteria for any specific bipolar disorder

[a]The length and severity of a mood episode and the interval between episodes vary from patient to patient. Manic episodes are usually briefer and end more abruptly than major depressive episodes. The average length of untreated manic episodes ranges from 4 to 13 months. Episodes can occur regularly (at the same time or season of the year) and often cluster at 12-month intervals. Women have more depressive episodes than manic episodes, whereas men have a more even distribution of episodes.
[b]For bipolar I disorder, 90% of individuals who experience a manic episode later have multiple recurrent major depressive, manic, hypomanic, or mixed episodes alternating with a normal mood state.
[c]Approximately 5–15% of patients with bipolar II disorder will develop a manic episode over a 5-year period. If a manic or mixed episode develops in a patient with bipolar II disorder, the diagnosis is changed to bipolar I disorder.
[d]Patients with cyclothymic disorder have a 15–50% risk of later developing a bipolar I or II disorder.

Data from references 1–3.

depressive episode). See Table 52-2 for the evaluation and diagnostic criteria of mood episodes. Bipolar disorder is a cyclic mood disorder, and patients may sequentially experience different types of episodes with or without a period of normal mood (euthymia) between. Persons with bipolar disorder can have mood fluctuations that continue for months, or after one episode they can sometimes go years without recurrence of any type of mood episode. Comorbid conditions associated with bipolar disorder include, but are not limited to, substance abuse, personality disorders, anxiety disorders, eating disorders, and a higher incidence of several medical conditions.[1–3,22–26]

DIAGNOSTIC DIFFICULTY

Episodes of mania or depression may be induced or caused by medical illness, medications, or substance intoxication or withdrawal (see Table 52-3 for causes of mania and Table 51-1 for causes of depression).[1,2] A complete medical, psychiatric, and medication history; physical examination; and laboratory testing are necessary to rule out any organic causes of mania or depression.[2] An accurate diagnosis is important because some psychiatric and neurologic disorders present with manic-like or depressive-like symptoms.[2,3] Bipolar disorder commonly co-occurs with substance use disorders and may be difficult to diagnose in the presence of cocaine use.[37] When making the diagnosis of new-onset bipolar disorder in a geriatric population, clinicians should be particularly aware of secondary causes of mania and depression that may impact treatment.[38]

TABLE 52-2 Evaluation and Diagnosis of Mood Episodes

Diagnosis Episode	Impairment of Functioning or Need for Hospitalization[a]	*DSM-IV-TR* Criteria[b]
Major depressive	Yes	>2-Week period of either depressed mood or loss of interest or pleasure in normal activities, associated with at least five of the following symptoms: • Depressed, sad mood (adults); can be irritable mood in children • Decreased interest and pleasure in normal activities • Decreased appetite, weight loss • Insomnia or hypersomnia • Psychomotor retardation or agitation • Decreased energy or fatigue • Feelings of guilt or worthlessness • Impaired concentration and decision making • Suicidal thoughts or attempts
Manic	Yes	>1-Week period of abnormal and persistent elevated mood (expansive or irritable), associated with at least three of the following symptoms (four if the mood is only irritable): • Inflated self-esteem (grandiosity) • Decreased need for sleep • Increased talking (pressure of speech) • Racing thoughts (flight of ideas) • Distractible (poor attention) • Increased activity (socially, at work, or sexually) or increased motor activity or agitation • Excessive involvement in activities that are pleasurable but have a high risk for serious consequences (buying sprees, sexual indiscretions, poor judgment in business ventures)
Hypomanic	No	At least 4 days of abnormal and persistent elevated mood (expansive or irritable), associated with at least three of the following symptoms (four if the mood is only irritable): • Inflated self-esteem (grandiosity) • Decreased need for sleep • Increased talking (pressure of speech) • Racing thoughts (flight of ideas) • Increased activity (socially, at work, or sexually) or increased motor activity or agitation • Excessive involvement in activities that are pleasurable but have a high risk for serious consequences (buying sprees, sexual indiscretions, poor judgment in business ventures)
Mixed	Yes	Criteria for both a major depressive episode and a manic episode (except for duration) occur nearly every day for at least a 1-week period
Rapid cycling	Yes	>4 major depressive or manic episodes (manic, mixed, or hypomanic) in 12 months

[a]Impairment in social or occupational functioning; need for hospitalization because of potential self-harm, harm to others, or psychotic symptoms.
[b]The disorder is not caused by a medical condition (e.g., hypothyroidism) or substance-induced disorder (e.g., antidepressant treatment, medications, electroconvulsive therapy).

Data from reference 1.

TABLE 52-3 Secondary Causes of Mania

Medical conditions that induce mania
- CNS disorders (brain tumor, strokes, head injuries, subdural hematoma, multiple sclerosis, systemic lupus erythematosus, temporal lobe seizures, Huntington's disease)
- Infections (encephalitis, neurosyphilis, sepsis, human immunodeficiency virus)
- Electrolyte or metabolic abnormalities (calcium or sodium fluctuations, hyperglycemia or hypoglycemia)
- Endocrine or hormonal dysregulation (Addison's disease, Cushing's disease, hyperthyroidism or hypothyroidism, menstrual-related or pregnancy-related or perimenopausal mood disorders)

Medications or drugs that induce mania
- Alcohol intoxication
- Drug withdrawal states (alcohol, α_2-adrenergic agonists, antidepressants, barbiturates, benzodiazepines, opiates)
- Antidepressants (MAOIs, TCAs, 5-HT and/or NE and/or DA reuptake inhibitors, 5-HT antagonists)
- DA-augmenting agents (CNS stimulants: amphetamines, cocaine, sympathomimetics; DA agonists, releasers, and reuptake inhibitors)
- Hallucinogens (LSD, PCP)
- Marijuana intoxication precipitates psychosis, paranoid thoughts, anxiety, and restlessness
- NE-augmenting agents (α_2-adrenergic antagonists, β-agonists, NE reuptake inhibitors)
- Steroids (anabolic, adrenocorticotropic hormone, corticosteroids)
- Thyroid preparations
- Xanthines (caffeine, theophylline)
- Nonprescription weight loss agents and decongestants (ephedra, pseudoephedrine)
- Herbal products (St. John's wort)

Somatic therapies that induce mania
- Bright light therapy
- Deep brain stimulation
- Sleep deprivation

DA, dopamine; 5-HT, serotonin; LSD, lysergic acid diethylamide; MAOI, monoamine oxidase inhibitor; NE, norepinephrine; PCP, phencyclidine; TCA, tricyclic antidepressant.

Data from references 1, 27–36.

Another disease state that has a similar presentation to bipolar disorder is schizoaffective disorder. This disease is a mix between schizophrenia and bipolar disorder. Patients with schizoaffective disorder have mood episodes, but the distinguishing factor from bipolar disorder is that these patients experience psychosis even between mood episodes during periods of euthymia. Clinicians must rely on family members or others who know the patient well to determine if the patient is psychotic between mood episodes. It can be difficult for clinicians to obtain a full psychiatric history on patients, thus making schizoaffective disorder widely diagnosed. Schizoaffective disorder is treated with mood stabilizers and antipsychotics as maintenance therapy.

COURSE OF ILLNESS

3 Bipolar disorder is frequently not recognized and treated for many years because of its fluctuating course and episodic mood states.[2,3] Patients may have delays in treatment ranging 8 to 13 years from onset of index mood episode until initiation of mood stabilizer.[39] This delay confers a risk of poor social functioning, increased hospitalizations, and a greater likelihood of lifetime suicide attempts.[40] Onset of illness in early childhood tends to be associated with increased mood episodes, rapid cycling, and comorbid psychiatric conditions as well as a stronger family history of mood disorders.[41] Gender differences may influence a patient's course of illness, tolerability of medication, and response to treatment. Women are more likely to have increased depressive symptoms, older age of onset, better compliance, complex management in pregnancy, and higher association with physical illness such as thyroid abnormalities than men are. In men there may be increased incidence of mania and substance use.[42]

The kindling theory is used to explain why bipolar disorder progresses over one's life and why preventative treatment is imperative. Episodes can become longer in duration and more frequent with aging.[2] Usually there is a period of normal functioning between episodes, but approximately 20% to 30% of patients with bipolar I disorder and 15% with bipolar II disorder have no period of euthymia because of mood lability, residual mood symptoms, or a direct switch to the opposite polarity.[1]

Rapid cycling (more than four mood episodes per year) is more common in females and occurs in approximately 10% to 20% of bipolar I and II disorder patients.[2,3,43,44] Frequent and severe episodes of depression appear to be the most common hallmark of rapid cycling. Use of alcohol, stimulants, antidepressants, sleep deprivation, hypothyroidism, and seasonal changes can play a role in rapid cycling.[3,44,45] Seasonal patterns of mania in the summer and depression during the winter have been observed. Rapid-cycling patients have a poorer long-term prognosis and often require combination therapies.[3]

Fluctuations in hormones and neurotransmitters during the luteal phase of the menstrual cycle, postpartum period, and perimenopause (starting ~10 years before menopause) can precipitate mood changes and increase cycling.[1,43,46] Women with bipolar I disorder are at greater risk for relapse into mania or depression during the postpartum period.[2] If a severe mood episode occurs postpartum, there is an increased risk for recurrences during subsequent postpartum periods.[2]

Alcohol and substance abuse is common among patients with bipolar disorder and can have a significant impact on the age of onset, course of the illness, and response to treatment.[3,22,23] Alcohol and drug abuse or dependence has been reported in 46% and 41% of bipolar patients, respectively.[2,22] Patients with substance use disorders are more likely to have an earlier onset of their illness, mixed states, higher rates of relapse, a poorer response to treatment, comorbid personality disorders, increased suicide risk, and more psychiatric hospitalizations.[3] Bipolar patients often self-medicate with substances such as alcohol or cocaine during episodes, resulting in further impairment of judgment, poor impulse control, treatment nonadherence, and a worsening of the clinical course.[2,3,47]

More than one half (55% to 65%) of bipolar I patients have some degree of functional disability after the onset of their illness, and approximately 10% to 20% of bipolar patients have severe impairment in their psychosocial and occupational functioning.[2,3,48] In a 1-year longitudinal study in 258 bipolar patients, two thirds had four or more mood episodes a year despite comprehensive pharmacologic treatment, and approximately 33.2% of the year was spent being depressed compared with 10.8% of the time in a manic phase.[48]

Compared with the general population, individuals with bipolar disorder have a 2.3 times higher mortality rate. Suicide attempts occur in up to 50% of patients with bipolar disorder, and approximately 10% to 19% of individuals with bipolar I disorder commit suicide.[1–3,49] Studies suggest patients with bipolar II disorder have more suicide attempts than bipolar I patients.[49]

The best predictor for level of functioning during a person's lifetime is adherence with medication treatment. Medication discontinuation occurs in up to 50% of patients secondary to intolerance of drug-induced side effects.[50] Failure to recognize the disorder, reluctance to acknowledge it, or poor adherence with treatment are reasons an estimated two thirds of patients with bipolar disorder do not receive appropriate treatment. Nonadherence with pharmacologic treatment and substance abuse are major factors in relapse and hospitalizations.[2,3]

TABLE 52-4 General Principles for the Management of Bipolar Disorder

Goals of treatment
- Eliminate mood episode with complete remission of symptoms (i.e., acute treatment)
- Prevent recurrences or relapses of mood episodes (i.e., continuation phase treatment)
- Return to complete psychosocial functioning
- Maximize adherence with therapy
- Minimize adverse effects
- Use medications with the best tolerability and fewest drug interactions
- Treat comorbid substance use and abuse
- Eliminate alcohol, marijuana, cocaine, amphetamines, and hallucinogens
- Minimize nicotine use and stop caffeine intake at least 8 hours prior to bedtime
- Avoidance of stressors or substances that precipitate an acute episode

Monitor for
- Mood episodes: document symptoms on a daily mood chart (document life stressors, type of episode, length of episode, and treatment outcome); monthly and yearly life charts are valuable for documenting patterns of mood cycles
- Medication adherence (missing doses of medications is a primary reason for nonresponse and recurrence of episodes)
- Adverse effects, especially sedation and weight gain (manage rapidly and vigorously to avoid noncompliance)
- Suicidal ideation or attempts (suicide completion rates with bipolar I disorder are 10–15%; suicide attempts are primarily associated with depressive episodes, mixed episodes with severe depression, or presence of psychosis)

Data from references 2, 22, and 51.

TREATMENT

Desired Outcome

4 The desired outcome in treating bipolar disorder is to effectively resolve acute manic, hypomanic, and depressive episodes, prevent further episodes, maintain good functioning, promote treatment adherence, and minimize side effects.[2,3] The general principles and goals for the management of bipolar disorder are found in Table 52-4.

General Approach to Treatment

5 Treatment of bipolar disorder must be individualized because the clinical presentation, severity, and frequency of episodes vary widely among patients. Treatment approaches should include both nonpharmacologic and pharmacologic strategies.[3] Patients and family members should be educated about bipolar disorder (e.g., symptoms, causes, and course) and treatment options. Long-term adherence to treatment is the most important factor in achieving stabilization of the disorder.

6 The treatment of bipolar disorder can vary depending on what type of episode the patient is experiencing. Once diagnosed with bipolar disorder, patients should remain on a mood stabilizer (e.g., lithium, valproate) for their lifetime. During acute episodes, medications can be added and then tapered once the patient is stabilized and euthymic. For example, when treating a patient for mania with psychotic features, the patient should be on a mood stabilizer and an antipsychotic. If the antipsychotic is the patient's maintenance therapy, the dose should be increased or perhaps the medication should be changed altogether if the patient goes into a manic episode. If treating a patient for a severe depressive episode, a clinician may need to maximize the dose of the mood stabilizer or add another medication (e.g., quetiapine).

Nonpharmacologic Therapy

The basics of nonpharmacologic approaches should address issues of adequate nutrition, sleep, exercise, and stress reduction.[3] Sleep deprivation, high stress, and deficiencies in dietary essential amino acids, fatty acids, vitamins, and minerals can exacerbate mood episodes and result in poorer outcomes.[3] Mood charting is an effective strategy in detecting early signs and symptoms of mania and depression. Another effective treatment is to combine medications with adjunctive psychoeducational programs, supportive counseling, insight-oriented psychotherapy (individual or group), couples or family therapy, cognitive behavioral therapy, and communication enhancement training.[2,3,22,52]

Pharmacologic Therapy

6 Pharmacotherapy is crucial for the acute and maintenance treatment of bipolar disorder and includes lithium, valproate, carbamazepine, lamotrigine, first-generation antipsychotics (FGAs) and second-generation antipsychotics (SGAs), and adjunctive agents such as antidepressants and benzodiazepines. General treatment guidelines for the acute treatment of mood episodes in patients with bipolar I disorder are found in Table 52-5.

Product information, dosing, and administration of agents used in the treatment of bipolar disorder are found in Table 52-6.

6 The term *mood stabilizer* is often used to describe the class of medications used in the treatment of bipolar disorder, but this may not be accurate as some medications are more effective for acute mania, some for the depressive episode, and others for the maintenance phase.[54] Lithium, valproate (or divalproex sodium), extended-release carbamazepine, aripiprazole, asenapine, olanzapine, quetiapine, risperidone, and ziprasidone are currently approved by the U.S. FDA for the treatment of acute mania in bipolar disorder; only lithium, divalproex sodium, aripiprazole, olanzapine, and lamotrigine are approved for the maintenance treatment of bipolar disorder. Quetiapine is the only monotherapy antipsychotic that is FDA-approved for bipolar depression. Lithium is the drug of choice for bipolar disorder with euphoric mania, whereas valproate has better efficacy for mixed states and irritable/dysphoric mania compared with lithium.[2]

Combination therapies (e.g., lithium plus valproate or carbamazepine; lithium or valproate plus a SGA) can provide better acute response and long-term prevention of relapse and recurrence than monotherapy in some bipolar patients, particularly those with mixed states or rapid cycling.[2,54] The majority of patients hospitalized for an acute episode will be on combination therapy.

Several guidelines and algorithms have been published regarding the treatment of bipolar disorder, and these are generally based on the best available data and clinical consensus of experts. The Canadian Network for Mood and Anxiety Treatments (CANMAT) and International Society for Bipolar Disorders (ISBD) published updated treatment guidelines in 2009.[53] In addition, an international task force of the World Federation of Societies of Biological Psychiatry (WFSBP) has published guidelines for the treatment of acute bipolar depression and mania.[55,56] The WFSBP mania and depression guidelines were updated in 2009 and 2010, respectively; maintenance (2003) guidelines have yet to be updated.

Based on the CANMAT and ISBD guidelines and available research, an example treatment algorithm and guidelines for acute mood episodes in adult patients with bipolar I disorder are listed in Table 52-5. Because newer anticonvulsants, SGAs, and combination therapies are under investigation for bipolar disorder, published guidelines, algorithms, and decision trees can quickly become out of date as new scientific knowledge evolves. Selection of treatments for acute mood episodes (e.g., manic or mixed, depressive, or rapid cycling) and for maintenance strategies to prevent relapses of mood episodes should be individualized. Treatment plans should be based

TABLE 52-5 Algorithm and Guidelines for the Acute Treatment of Mood Episodes in Patients with Bipolar I Disorder

Acute Manic or Mixed Episode		Acute Depressive Episode	
General Guidelines		**General Guidelines**	
Assess for secondary causes of mania or mixed states (e.g., alcohol or drug use) Discontinue antidepressants Taper off stimulants and caffeine if possible Treat substance abuse Encourage good nutrition (with regular protein and essential fatty acid intake), exercise, adequate sleep, stress reduction, and psychosocial therapy		Assess for secondary causes of depression (e.g., alcohol or drug use) Taper off antipsychotics, benzodiazepines, or sedative–hypnotic agents if possible Treat substance abuse Encourage good nutrition (with regular protein and essential fatty acid intake), exercise, adequate sleep, stress reduction, and psychosocial therapy	
Hypomania	**Mania**	**Mild to Moderate Depressive Episode**	**Severe Depressive Episode**
First, optimize current mood stabilizer or initiate mood-stabilizing medication: lithium,[a] valproate,[a] carbamazepine,[a] or SGAs Consider adding a benzodiazepine (lorazepam or clonazepam) for short-term adjunctive treatment of agitation or insomnia if needed Alternative medication treatment options: oxcarbazepine **Second**, if response is inadequate, consider a two-drug combination: • Lithium[a] **plus** an anticonvulsant or an SGA • Anticonvulsant **plus** an anticonvulsant or SGA	**First**, two- or three-drug combinations (lithium,[a] valproate,[a] or SGA) **plus** a benzodiazepine (lorazepam or clonazepam) and/or antipsychotic for short-term adjunctive treatment of agitation or insomnia; lorazepam is recommended for catatonia Do not combine antipsychotics Alternative medication treatment options: carbamazepine[a]; if patient does not respond or tolerate, consider oxcarbazepine **Second**, if response is inadequate, consider a three-drug combination: • Lithium[a] **plus** an anticonvulsant **plus** an antipsychotic • Anticonvulsant **plus** an anticonvulsant **plus** an antipsychotic **Third**, if response is inadequate, consider ECT for mania with psychosis or catatonia,[d] or add clozapine for treatment-refractory illness	**First**, initiate and/or optimize mood-stabilizing medication: lithium[a] or quetiapine Alternative anticonvulsants: lamotrigine,[b] valproate[a]; antipsychotics: fluoxetine/olanzapine combination	**First**, optimize current mood stabilizer or initiate mood-stabilizing medication: lithium[a] or quetiapine Alternative fluoxetine/olanzapine combination If psychosis is present, initiate an antipsychotic in combination with above Do not combine antipsychotics Alternative anticonvulsants: lamotrigine,[b] valproate[a] **Second**, if response is inadequate, consider carbamazepine[a] or adding antidepressant **Third**, if response is inadequate, consider a three-drug combination: • Lithium **plus** lamotrigine[b] **plus** an antidepressant • Lithium **plus** quetiapine **plus** antidepressant[c] **Fourth**, if response is inadequate, consider ECT for treatment-refractory illness and depression with psychosis or catatonia[d]

ECT, electroconvulsive therapy; SGA, second-generation antipsychotic.

[a]Use standard therapeutic serum concentration ranges if clinically indicated; if partial response or breakthrough episode, adjust dose to achieve higher serum concentrations without causing intolerable adverse effects; valproate is preferred over lithium for mixed episodes and rapid cycling; lithium and/or lamotrigine is preferred over valproate for bipolar depression.

[b]Lamotrigine is not approved for the acute treatment of depression, and the dose must be started low and slowly titrated up to decrease adverse effects if used for maintenance therapy of bipolar I disorder. Lamotrigine may be initiated during acute treatment with plans to transition to this medication for long-term maintenance. A drug interaction and a severe dermatologic rash can occur when lamotrigine is combined with valproate (i.e., lamotrigine doses must be halved from standard dosing titration).

[c]Controversy exists concerning the use of antidepressants, and they are often considered third line in treating acute bipolar depression, except in patients with no recent history of severe acute mania or potentially in bipolar II patients.

[d]ECT is used for severe mania or depression during pregnancy and for mixed episodes; prior to treatment, anticonvulsants, lithium, and benzodiazepines should be tapered off to maximize therapy and minimize adverse effects.

Data from references 2, 51, and 53.

on patient-specific characteristics, comorbid psychiatric and medical conditions, and avoidance of drug interactions and adverse effects.[2]

Specific Pharmacologic Therapies

Lithium Lithium was first used in 1949 as a treatment for mania and was approved in 1972 in the United States for the treatment of acute mania and for maintenance therapy. Despite numerous investigations into the biologic and clinical properties of lithium, there is no unified theory for its mechanism of action.[22,57–59] Chronic lithium administration may modulate gene expression and have neuroprotective effects. Lithium has unique pharmacokinetics because it is a monovalent cation. It is rapidly absorbed, is widely distributed with no protein binding, is not metabolized, and is excreted unchanged in the urine and in other body fluids.[60]

Efficacy Lithium was the first established mood stabilizer, and is still considered a first-line agent for acute mania, acute bipolar depression, and maintenance treatment of bipolar I and II disorders.[53] Early placebo-controlled studies with lithium reported up to a 78% response rate in aborting an acute manic or hypomanic episode, but more recent studies suggest a slower onset of action and a more moderate effectiveness when compared with other agents.[2,3,61] In placebo-controlled studies in bipolar depression, lithium has been found to have efficacy, but there can be a 6- to 8-week delay for its antidepressant effects.[2] Lithium is more effective for pure or elated (classic) mania, and can be less effective for mania with psychotic features, mixed episodes, rapid or continuous cycling, alcohol and drug abuse, and in organic-induced mood states.[2,3,62]

Long-term lithium therapy is more effective in patients with fewer prior episodes, with a history of euthymia or good functioning between episodes, and with a family history of bipolar illness with a positive response to lithium. Lithium produces a prophylactic response in up to two thirds of patients and reduces suicide risk by 8- to 10-fold.[2,61–63]

Clinical **Controversy...**

What is the role of lithium in a patient with suicidality? An observational study demonstrated a reduction in suicide risk in patients on continued lithium treatment. However, this study does not address how and when lithium should be initiated in patients who are currently suicidal. Lithium overdose can be fatal. Therefore, the role of lithium in preventing suicidal behavior during mood episodes is unclear.

TABLE 52-6 Products, Dosage and Administration, and Clinical Use of Agents Used in the Treatment of Bipolar Disorder

Drug	Initial Dosing	Usual Dosing; Special Population Dosing	Comments
"Brand name"			
Lithium salts: FDA-approved for bipolar disorder			
Lithium carbonate[a,b] "Eskalith" "Eskalith CR" "Lithobid" Lithium citrate[a,b] "Cibalith-S"	300 mg twice daily	900–2,400 mg/day in two to four divided doses, preferably with meals Renal impairment: lower doses required with frequent serum monitoring There is wide variation in the dosage needed to achieve therapeutic response and trough serum lithium concentration (i.e., 0.6–1.2 mEq/L [mmol/L] for maintenance therapy and 1–1.2 mEq/L [mmol/L] for acute mood episodes taken 8–12 hours after the last dose)	Use alone or in combination with other drugs (e.g., valproate, carbamazepine, antipsychotics) for the acute treatment of mania and for maintenance treatment
Anticonvulsants: FDA-approved for bipolar disorder			
Divalproex sodium[a] "Depakote" "Depakote ER" Valproic acid[a] "Stavzor"	250–500 mg twice daily A loading dose of divalproex (20–30 mg/kg/day) can be given	750–3,000 mg/day (20–60 mg/kg/day) given once daily or in divided doses Titrate to clinical response Dose adjustment needed with hepatic impairment	Use alone or in combination with other drugs (e.g., lithium, carbamazepine, antipsychotics) for the acute treatment of mania and for maintenance treatment Use caution when combining with lamotrigine because of potential drug interaction
Lamotrigine[b] "Lamictal"	25 mg daily	50–400 mg/day in divided doses. Dosage should be slowly increased (e.g., 25 mg/day for 2 weeks, then 50 mg/day for weeks 3 and 4, and then 50-mg/day increments at weekly intervals up to 200 mg/day) Dose adjustment needed with hepatic impairment	Use alone or in combination with other drugs (e.g., lithium, carbamazepine) for long-term maintenance treatment for bipolar I disorder
Carbamazepine "Equetro[a]"	200 mg twice daily	200–1,800 mg/day in two to four divided doses Titrate to clinical response Dose adjustment needed with hepatic impairment	Use alone or in combination with other medications (e.g., lithium, valproate, antipsychotics) for the acute and long-term maintenance treatment of mania or mixed episodes for bipolar I disorder. APA guidelines recommend reserving it for patients unable to tolerate or who have inadequate response to lithium or valproate Extended-release tablets should be swallowed whole and not be broken or chewed
Anticonvulsants: not FDA-approved for bipolar disorder			
Carbamazepine "Tegretol" "Epitol" "Tegretol-XR" "Carbatrol"	200 mg twice daily	200–1,800 mg/day in two to four divided doses Titrate to clinical response Dose adjustment needed with hepatic impairment	Carbatrol capsules can be opened and contents sprinkled over food
Valproic acid "Depakene" Valproate sodium "Depacon"	250–500 mg twice daily A loading dose of divalproex (20–30 mg/kg/day) can be given	750–3,000 mg/day (20–60 mg/kg/day) given once daily or in divided doses Titrate to clinical response Dose adjustment needed with hepatic impairment	Use caution when combining with lamotrigine because of potential drug interaction
Oxcarbazepine "Trileptal"	300 mg twice daily	300–1,200 mg/day in two divided doses Titrate based on clinical response Dose adjustment required with severe renal impairment	Use after patients have failed treatment with carbamazepine or have intolerable side effects May have fewer adverse effects and be better tolerated than carbamazepine
Atypical antipsychotics: FDA-approved for bipolar disorder			
Aripiprazole[a,b] "Abilify"	10–15 mg daily	10–30 mg/day once daily	May be used in combination with lithium, valproate, or carbamazepine for the acute treatment of mania or mixed states (primarily with psychotic features) for bipolar I disorder
Asenapine[a] "Saphris"	5–10 mg twice daily sublingually	5–10 mg twice daily sublingually	
Olanzapine[a,b] "Zyprexa," "Zyprexa Zydis"	2.5–5 mg twice daily	5–20 mg/day once daily or in divided doses	
Olanzapine and fluoxetine[c] "Symbyax"	6 mg olanzapine and 25 mg fluoxetine daily	6–12 mg olanzapine and 25–50 mg fluoxetine daily	
Quetiapine[a,b] "Seroquel"	50 mg twice daily	50–800 mg/day in divided doses or once daily when stabilized	
Risperidone[a] "Risperdal" "Risperdal M-Tab"	0.5–1 mg twice daily	0.5–6 mg/day once daily or in divided doses	
Ziprasidone[a] "Geodon"	40–60 mg twice daily	40–160 mg/day in divided doses. Administer with food	
Benzodiazepines	Dosage should be slowly adjusted up and down according to response and adverse effects		Use in combination with other medications (e.g., antipsychotics, lithium, valproate) for the acute treatment of mania or mixed episodes Use as a short-term adjunctive sedative–hypnotic agent

FDA-approved agents may be used as monotherapy in various phases of the illness as noted in table footnotes.[a,b,c]

[a]FDA-approved for acute mania.
[b]FDA-approved for maintenance.
[c]FDA-approved for acute bipolar depression.

Data from references 2, 3, 22, and 53.

Patients maintained on standard serum concentrations of lithium (0.8 to 1 mEq/L [mmol/L]) may have fewer relapses than patients maintained on lower serum concentrations (0.4 to 0.6 mEq/L [mmol/L]).[2,3] Abrupt discontinuation or noncompliance with lithium therapy can increase the risk of relapse.[2,3] Discontinuation-induced refractoriness has been reported in approximately one fifth of patients who previously were stabilized on lithium.[2,3]

Lithium augmentation of carbamazepine, lamotrigine, and valproate can improve treatment response in bipolar I disorder.[2,64] Concomitant use of lithium with valproate or carbamazepine appears to be well tolerated but can increase the risk of sedation, weight gain, GI complaints, and tremor.

Lithium is frequently combined with either FGAs or SGAs for treatment of euphoric acute mania with psychotic features. Case reports of neurotoxicity (e.g., delirium, cerebellar dysfunction, extrapyramidal symptoms, and severe tremors) have been published in elderly patients receiving lithium and FGAs.[60] Combining lithium with calcium channel blockers is not recommended because of reports of neurotoxicity and severe bradycardia with verapamil or diltiazem.[60] Acute neurotoxicity and delirium have been reported in patients receiving electroconvulsive therapy (ECT) with lithium (even at reduced dosages); therefore, lithium should be withdrawn and discontinued at least 2 days before ECT and should not be resumed until 2 to 3 days after the last treatment.

Adverse Effects Approximately 35% to 93% of patients treated with lithium will experience adverse effects. These are divided into those that occur early in therapy but are generally innocuous and transient, those that occur with long-term therapy and are usually not dose-related, and toxic effects that occur with high serum concentrations.[2,60]

Initial side effects are often dose-related and are worse at peak serum concentrations (1 to 2 hours postdose).[2] Standard approaches for minimizing adverse effects include lowering the dose, taking smaller doses with food, using extended-release products, and trying once-daily dosing at bedtime.[2] GI distress (e.g., nausea, vomiting, dyspepsia, and diarrhea) can be minimized by the standard approaches or by adding antacids or antidiarrheal agents.[2] Diarrhea can sometimes be managed by switching from tablet or capsule formulation to liquid formulation. Diarrhea produced by lithium is commonly an osmotic diarrhea, and therefore switching to a formulation that clears the gut quickly can ameliorate symptoms. Muscle weakness and lethargy develop in about 30% of patients, but these symptoms are usually transient. Polydipsia with polyuria and nocturia occurs in up to 70% of patients and can be managed by changing to once-daily bedtime dosing.

A fine hand tremor can be evident in up to 50% of patients. Stress, concomitant use of antidepressants or antipsychotics, caffeine, sympathomimetics, and impending toxicity can exacerbate the tremor. Strategies to reduce the tremor include standard approaches (e.g., switch to long-acting preparation, lower dose if possible) or adding a β-adrenergic antagonist (e.g., propranolol 20 to 120 mg/day).

Lithium reduces the kidney's ability to concentrate urine and can cause a nephrogenic diabetes insipidus characterized by low urine specific gravity and a low osmolality polyuria (urine volumes greater than 3 L/day).[2,60] Lithium-induced nephrogenic diabetes insipidus is treated with loop diuretics, thiazide diuretics, or triamterene. If a thiazide diuretic is used (e.g., hydrochlorothiazide 50 mg/day), lithium doses should be decreased by 50%, and potassium levels should be monitored.[2] Amiloride, a potassium-sparing diuretic, has weaker natriuretic effects than thiazides and appears to be relatively safe with minimal effect on lithium clearance. Potassium supplements have been suggested as another treatment for lithium-induced polyuria.[22] Fluid restriction is not recommended because dehydration increases the risk of lithium toxicity. If edema occurs, treatment approaches include lowering sodium intake or using a diuretic (e.g., spironolactone); close monitoring for lithium toxicity is necessary because these treatments often increase lithium concentrations.

Patients on long-term lithium therapy have a 10% to 20% risk of developing morphologic renal changes (e.g., glomerular sclerosis, tubular atrophy, and interstitial nephritis) that is associated with impairment of water resorption and increased serum creatinine concentrations.[2] Lithium rarely causes nephrotoxicity if patients are maintained on the lowest effective dose, if once-daily dosing is used, if adequate hydration is maintained, and if toxicity is avoided.[22] Lithium should be avoided in patients with preexisting renal disease unless there is frequent monitoring.

Lithium is concentrated in the thyroid gland, interferes with thyroid hormone synthesis, and can induce the formation of thyroid antibodies.[60] Up to 30% of patients on maintenance lithium therapy develop transiently elevated thyroid-stimulating hormone concentrations, and 5% to 35% of patients develop a goiter and/or hypothyroidism.[2] Lithium-induced hypothyroidism is not dose-related, is observed 10 times more frequently in women (particularly in those with rapid cycling), and usually occurs after 6 to 18 months of therapy.[2] Hypothyroidism does not require discontinuation of lithium, because exogenous thyroid hormone (i.e., levothyroxine) can be added to the regimen. When lithium is discontinued, the need for exogenous thyroid hormone should be reassessed, because hypothyroidism can be reversible.

Lithium can cause a variety of benign and reversible cardiac effects, particularly T-wave flattening or inversion (in up to 30% of patients), atrioventricular block, and bradycardia.[2,22,60] If a patient has significant preexisting cardiac disease, consultation with a cardiologist and an electrocardiogram is recommended at baseline and during lithium therapy.

Other late-appearing lithium side effects include benign reversible leukocytosis and a variety of dermatologic effects (e.g., acne and acneiform eruptions, exacerbation of psoriasis, pruritic dermatitis).[3] Weight gain is common (~20% of patients gain >10 kg [22 lb]) and can be related to fluid retention, the consumption of high-calorie beverages as a result of polydipsia, or a decreased metabolic rate because of hypothyroidism.[22,62] Severe neurologic disturbances such as coarse hand tremors, ataxia, slurred speech, myasthenia gravis, extrapyramidal syndrome, pseudotumor cerebri, and papilledema are occasionally observed.

Lithium is an extremely toxic drug if accidentally or intentionally taken in overdose. Lithium toxicity can occur with blood levels greater than 1.5 mEq/L (mmol/L), but elderly patients can have symptoms of toxicity at therapeutic levels.[2] Severe lithium intoxication occurs when concentrations are higher than 2 mEq/L (mmol/L), and there is a worsening in several key symptoms: *GI* (e.g., vomiting, diarrhea, or incontinence), *coordination* (e.g., severe fine to coarse hand tremor, unstable gait, slurred speech, and muscle twitching), and *cognition* (e.g., poor concentration, drowsiness, disorientation, apathy, and coma).[2] Several reports of seizures, cardiac dysrhythmia, permanent neurologic impairments with ataxia and deficits in memory, and kidney damage with reduced glomerular filtration rate have been reported after lithium intoxication.[2]

Situations that predispose patients to lithium toxicity include sodium restriction, dehydration, vomiting, diarrhea, age greater than 50, heart failure, cirrhosis, and drug interactions that decrease lithium clearance. Heavy exercise, sauna baths, hot weather, and fever can promote sodium loss. Patients should be cautioned to maintain adequate sodium and fluid intake (2.5 to 3 qt [~2.5 to 3 L] per day of fluids) and to avoid the excessive use of coffee, tea, cola, and other caffeine-containing beverages and alcohol.

If lithium toxicity is suspected, the person should go to an emergency room to be monitored, and lithium should be discontinued.[2] Gastric lavage and IV fluids may be needed, and the patient should be monitored for fluid balance, renal and electrolyte status, and neurologic changes. When lithium concentrations are above

3.5 to 4 mEq/L (mmol/L), intermittent hemodialysis (12 hours on and 12 hours off) can be started and continued until the lithium concentration is below 1 mEq/L (mmol/L) when taken 12 hours after the last dialysis.

Drug–Drug Interactions Thiazide diuretics, nonsteroidal anti-inflammatory drugs, cyclooxygenase-2 inhibitors, angiotensin-converting enzyme inhibitors, and salt-restricted diets can elevate lithium levels.[2] Neurotoxicity can occur when lithium is combined with carbamazepine, diltiazem, losartan, methyldopa, metronidazole, phenytoin, and verapamil.[2,60] Analgesics such as acetaminophen or aspirin and loop diuretics are less likely to interfere with lithium clearance. Caffeine and theophylline can enhance the renal elimination of lithium. Because lithium has no effect on hepatic metabolizing enzymes, it has fewer drug–drug interactions compared with carbamazepine, oxcarbazepine, and valproate.

Dosing and Administration Lithium dosing depends on the patient's age and weight, tolerance to adverse effects, and the acuity of the illness. Dosing is generally titrated up to achieve steady-state serum lithium concentrations of 0.6 to 1.2 mEq/L (mmol/L).[2] Lithium therapy is usually initiated with low to moderate doses (600 mg/day) for prophylaxis and higher doses (900 to 1,200 mg/day) for acute mania, using a two- to three-times daily dosing regimen.[2,60] Immediate-release lithium preparations should be given in two or three divided daily doses, whereas extended-release products can be given once or twice daily. In clinical practice many clinicians dose the immediate-release and extended-release preparations once daily. It can be best to initially begin a patient on divided dosing, but once stabilized many patients are able to switch to once-daily dosing without decompensating.

Lithium levels are considered to be at steady state at approximately day 5, and serum samples should be drawn 12 hours postdose. Once a desired serum concentration has been achieved, levels should be drawn in 2 weeks and then if stable every 3 to 6 months or as clinically indicated. Maintenance lithium serum concentrations are usually measured every 3 months, but can be adjusted to every 6 months for stabilized patients, and every 1 to 2 months for patients with frequent mood episodes.[2] Lithium clearance rates increase by 50% to 100% during pregnancy and return to normal postpartum; thus, lithium levels should be determined monthly during pregnancy and weekly the month before delivery. At delivery, rapid fluid changes can significantly increase lithium levels; thus, a reduction to prepregnancy lithium doses and adequate hydration are recommended.[2]

The recommended guidelines for baseline and routine laboratory testing for lithium are listed in Table 52-7. The dose should be adjusted based on the steady-state serum concentration drawn 12 hours (±30 minutes) after the last dose.[61] A therapeutic trial for outpatients should last a minimum of 4 to 6 weeks with lithium

TABLE 52-7 Guidelines for Baseline and Routine Laboratory Tests and Monitoring for Agents Used in Treatment of Bipolar Disorder

	Baseline: Physical Examination and General Chemistry[a]	Hematologic Tests[b]		Metabolic Tests[c]		Liver Function Tests[d]		Renal Function Tests[e]		Thyroid Function Tests[f]		Serum Electrolytes[g]		Dermatologic[h]	
	Baseline	Baseline	6–12 months	Baseline	6–12 months	Baseline	6–12 months	Baseline	6–12 months	Baseline	6–12 months	Baseline	6–12 months	Baseline	6–12 months
SGAs[i]	X			X	X										
Carbamazepine[j]	X	X	X			X	X	X				X	X	X	X
Lamotrigine[k]	X													X	X
Lithium[l]	X	X	X	X	X			X	X	X	X	X	X	X	X
Oxcarbazepine[m]	X											X	X		
Valproate[n]	X	X	X	X	X	X	X							X	X

[a]Screen for drug abuse and serum pregnancy.
[b]Complete blood cell count (CBC) with differential and platelets.
[c]Fasting glucose, serum lipids, and weight.
[d]Lactate dehydrogenase, aspartate aminotransferase, alanine aminotransferase, total bilirubin, and alkaline phosphatase.
[e]Serum creatinine, blood urea nitrogen, urinalysis, urine osmolality, and specific gravity.
[f]Triiodothyronine, total thyroxine, thyroxine uptake, and thyroid-stimulating hormone.
[g]Serum sodium.
[h]Rashes, hair thinning, and alopecia.
[i]Second-generation antipsychotics: Monitor for increased appetite with weight gain (primarily in patients with initial low or normal body mass index); monitor closely if rapid or significant weight gain occurs during early therapy; cases of hyperlipidemia and diabetes reported.
[j]Carbamazepine: Manufacturer recommends CBC and platelets (and possibly reticulocyte counts and serum iron) at baseline, and that subsequent monitoring be individualized by the clinician (e.g., CBC, platelet counts, and liver function tests every 2 weeks during the first 2 months of treatment, and then every 3 months if normal). Monitor more closely if patient exhibits hematologic or hepatic abnormalities or if the patient is receiving a myelotoxic drug; discontinue if platelets are <100,000/mm^3 (<100 × 10^9/L), if white blood cell (WBC) count is <3,000/mm^3 (<3 × 10^9/L), or if there is evidence of bone marrow suppression or liver dysfunction. Serum electrolyte levels should be monitored in the elderly or those at risk for hyponatremia. Carbamazepine interferes with some pregnancy tests.
[k]Lamotrigine: If renal or hepatic impairment, monitor closely and adjust dosage according to manufacturer's guidelines. Serious dermatologic reactions have occurred within 2–8 weeks of initiating treatment and are more likely to occur in patients receiving concomitant valproate, with rapid dosage escalation, or using doses exceeding the recommended titration schedule.
[l]Lithium: Obtain baseline electrocardiogram for patients older than 40 years or if preexisting cardiac disease (benign, reversible T-wave depression can occur). Renal function tests should be obtained every 2–3 months during the first 6 months, and then every 6–12 months; if impaired renal function, monitor 24-hour urine volume and creatinine every 3 months; if urine volume >3 L/day, monitor urinalysis, osmolality, and specific gravity every 3 months. Thyroid function tests should be obtained once or twice during the first 6 months, and then every 6–12 months; monitor for signs and symptoms of hypothyroidism; if supplemental thyroid therapy is required, monitor thyroid function tests and adjust thyroid dose every 1–2 months until thyroid function indices are within normal range, and then monitor every 3–6 months.
[m]Oxcarbazepine: Hyponatremia (serum sodium concentrations <125 mEq/L [mmol/L]) has been reported and occurs more frequently during the first 3 months of therapy; serum sodium concentrations should be monitored in patients receiving drugs that lower serum sodium concentrations (e.g., diuretics or drugs that cause inappropriate antidiuretic hormone secretion) or in patients with symptoms of hyponatremia (e.g., confusion, headache, lethargy, and malaise). Hypersensitivity reactions have occurred in approximately 25–30% of patients with a history of carbamazepine hypersensitivity and require immediate discontinuation.
[n]Valproate: Weight gain reported in patients with low or normal body mass index. Monitor platelets and liver function during first 3–6 months if evidence of increased bruising or bleeding. Monitor closely if patients exhibit hematologic or hepatic abnormalities or in patients receiving drugs that affect coagulation, such as aspirin or warfarin; discontinue if platelets are <100,000/mm^3/L (<100 × 10^9/L) or if prolonged bleeding time. Pancreatitis, hyperammonemic encephalopathy, polycystic ovary syndrome, increased testosterone, and menstrual irregularities have been reported; not recommended during first trimester of pregnancy due to risk of neural tube defects.

Data from references 2, 22, 60, 65–69.

serum concentrations of 0.6 to 1.2 mEq/L (mmol/L). Acutely manic patients can require serum concentrations of 1 to 1.2 mEq/L (mmol/L), and some need up to 1.5 mEq/L (mmol/L) to achieve a therapeutic response. Although serum concentrations less than 0.6 mEq/L (mmol/L) are associated with higher rates of relapse, some patients can do well at 0.4 to 0.7 mEq/L (mmol/L).[2] For bipolar prophylaxis in elderly patients, serum concentrations of 0.4 to 0.6 mEq/L (mmol/L) are recommended because of increased sensitivity to adverse effects.[2]

Anticonvulsants

Divalproex sodium (also known as sodium valproate) was marketed in 1995 for the acute treatment of mania in adults and is now the most prescribed mood stabilizer in the United States. It is FDA-approved only for the treatment of acute manic or mixed episodes; however, it is commonly used in clinical practice as maintenance monotherapy for bipolar disorder. Limited data support its use in acute bipolar depression. Carbamazepine is commonly used for both acute and maintenance therapy. The only formulation approved in the United States for bipolar disorder is extended-release carbamazepine, although other formulations can be used. Some data support the use of oxcarbazepine, a 10-keto analogue of carbamazepine, in the treatment of bipolar disorder; however, it is not approved for the treatment of bipolar disorder in the United States. Valproate, carbamazepine, and oxcarbazepine all have a wide range of neurologic, GI, electrolyte, and hematologic adverse effects that requires regular assessment and routine blood work.

Lamotrigine is FDA-approved for the maintenance treatment of bipolar I disorder. Lamotrigine add-on or monotherapy has been used for treatment-refractory bipolar depression.[64] This medication appears to be most effective in the prevention of relapse of depression and does not appear to have efficacy for treatment of acute depression, mania, mixed states, or rapid cycling in bipolar I.[70] Lamotrigine is associated with hypersensitivity reactions and rare life-threatening skin rashes and requires slow dosage titration.[2]

Valproate Sodium and Valproic Acid The exact mechanism of action of valproic acid is not known. It is a branched-chain fatty acid and was originally used as an organic solvent before it was discovered in the 1960s to have anticonvulsant properties. Valproate has antimigraine, mood-stabilizing, and antiaggressive effects.[65] In 1995, the enteric-coated formulation divalproex sodium (sodium valproate) was approved for the acute treatment of mania. Several controlled studies have shown valproate to be as effective as lithium and olanzapine in patients with pure mania, and it can be more effective than lithium in certain subtypes of bipolar disorder (e.g., rapid cycling, mixed states, bipolar disorder with comorbid substance abuse).[2,3,22,44,71] Placebo- and lithium-controlled and open studies report that valproate reduces or prevents recurrent manic, depressive, and mixed episodes.[2,3,22]

Giving lithium, carbamazepine, antipsychotics, or benzodiazepines with valproate can augment its antimanic effects. The addition of valproate to lithium can have synergistic effects in treatment-refractory rapid cycling and mixed states, and the combination has demonstrated efficacy in maintenance therapy for bipolar I disorder.[43] Combinations of valproate and carbamazepine can have synergistic effects, but the potential drug interactions make blood level monitoring of both agents essential.[22] Adding adjunctive SGAs to valproate can be effective for breakthrough mania or if there is incomplete or partial response to monotherapy. Clozapine, olanzapine, and quetiapine can increase the risk of sedation and weight gain when combined with valproate. The combination of valproate and lamotrigine can be effective, but there is an increased risk of rashes, ataxia, tremor, sedation, and fatigue.[65,72]

Adverse Effects The most frequent dose-related adverse effects with valproate are GI complaints (anorexia, nausea, indigestion, vomiting, mild diarrhea, and flatulence), fine hand tremors, and sedation.[2,22,65] The GI complaints are usually transient, but giving the medication with food, using lower initial doses with gradual increases in doses, or switching to divalproex sodium extended-release tablets can minimize them.[2,22] Reduction of the dose or the addition of a β-blocker can alleviate tremors, and giving the total daily dose at bedtime can minimize daytime sedation.[2,22]

Other adverse effects of valproate include ataxia, lethargy, alopecia, changes in the texture or color of hair, pruritus, prolonged bleeding because of inhibition of platelet aggregation, transient increases in liver enzymes, and hyperammonemia.[22,65] Increased appetite and weight gain occurs in approximately 50% of patients on long-term valproate therapy. Thrombocytopenia can occur at higher doses, and patients should be monitored for bleeding and bruising. Lowering the valproate dose can restore platelet counts to normal levels.[2] Fatal necrotizing hepatitis is a rare idiosyncratic, non–dose-related adverse effect that has occurred in children with epilepsy receiving multiple anticonvulsants.[22,65] A life-threatening hemorrhagic pancreatitis has been reported in both children and adults.[2,22,65] An in-depth discussion of adverse effects can be found in Chapter 40.

Drug–Drug Interactions A summary of drug–drug interactions for valproate can be found in Chapter 40.

Dosing and Administration For healthy inpatient adults with acute mania, the initial starting dosage of valproate is typically 20 mg/kg/day in divided doses over 12 hours. The daily dose is adjusted by 250 to 500 mg every 1 to 3 days based on clinical response and tolerability. Maximum recommended dosing is 60 mg/kg/day (see Table 52-6).[2,22,65] For outpatients who are hypomanic or euthymic, or for elderly patients, the initial starting dose is generally lower (5 to 10 mg/kg/day in divided doses) and gradually titrated to avoid adverse effects. Once an optimal dose has been achieved, the total daily dose can be given twice daily or at bedtime if tolerated.[2,22,65] Extended-release divalproex can be administered once daily, but bioavailability can be 15% lower than that of immediate-release products, thus requiring slightly higher doses.[2] In clinical practice, patients with bipolar disorder who are stable can be switched between formulations without having to change the dose. This is not the case for patients with seizure disorder.

Recommended baseline and routine laboratory tests for valproate are listed in Table 52-7. Although therapeutic serum concentrations of valproic acid have not been established in bipolar disorder, most clinicians use the anticonvulsant therapeutic serum range of 50 to 125 mcg/mL (347 to 866 μmol/L) taken 12 hours after the last dose.[2,22] In one study patients with valproate levels greater than 94.1 mcg/mL (652 μmol/L) had greater efficacy for bipolar mania.[73] Patients with cyclothymia or mild bipolar II disorder can have a therapeutic response to lower doses and blood levels, whereas some patients with a more severe form of bipolar disorder can require up to 150 mcg/mL (1,040 μmol/L). Serum valproic acid levels are most useful when assessing for compliance and toxicity.

Carbamazepine Carbamazepine, a dibenzazepine derivative, is structurally related to tricyclic antidepressants (TCAs).[22] The precise mechanism of action of carbamazepine in affective disorders remains to be elucidated.[63] Carbamazepine is not a first-line agent for bipolar disorder, and is generally reserved for lithium-refractory patients, rapid cyclers, or mixed states.[2,22] It has acute antimanic effects comparable to lithium and chlorpromazine, but its long-term effectiveness is unclear.[2,22] One comparison trial in hospitalized manic patients indicated that carbamazepine was less effective and needed more rescue adjunctive medications than valproate.[2] Other comparison studies with lithium have reported carbamazepine to be less effective than lithium for maintenance therapy.[2] In a double-blind, placebo-controlled, crossover study and in an open study, carbamazepine showed efficacy in the treatment of bipolar depression.[2,22] Studies with treatment-refractory patients have reported that carbamazepine has both acute and long-term prophylactic effects.[3,22] A gradual loss of efficacy over time (similar to lithium and valproate) has been reported in some patients.[3,22]

The combination of carbamazepine with lithium, valproate, and antipsychotics is often used for treatment-resistant patients experiencing a manic episode.[22] Carbamazepine plus olanzapine was not found to be more effective than carbamazepine alone in the treatment of acute mania or mixed episodes.[53] Carbamazepine increases the hepatic metabolism of antidepressants, anticonvulsants, and antipsychotics; thus, dosage increases can be necessary (see Drug–Drug Interactions below).[22,66] Calcium channel blockers (e.g., verapamil and diltiazem) increase carbamazepine blood levels; thus, combination therapy should be closely monitored.[66] The combination of carbamazepine with nimodipine for treatment-refractory bipolar illness can have potential benefit.[74]

Adverse Effects A summary of adverse effects for carbamazepine can be found in Chapter 40. Acute overdoses of carbamazepine are potentially lethal, and serum levels above 15 mcg/mL (63 μmol/L) are associated with ataxia, choreiform movements, diplopia, nystagmus, cardiac conduction changes, seizures, and coma.[2] Gastric lavage, hemoperfusion, and symptomatic treatment are recommended for the management of carbamazepine toxicity.

Drug–Drug Interactions Carbamazepine significantly induces the hepatic cytochrome P450 isoenzyme 3A4 and to a lesser degree 1A2, 2C9/10, and 2D6, which increases the metabolism of many medications.[2,3,66] Women taking oral contraceptives who receive carbamazepine require alternative contraceptive methods.[3]

Carbamazepine is metabolized to an active 10,11-epoxide metabolite; thus, medications that inhibit 3A4 isoenzymes can result in carbamazepine toxicity (e.g., cimetidine, diltiazem, erythromycin, fluoxetine, fluvoxamine, isoniazid, itraconazole, ketoconazole, nefazodone, propoxyphene, and verapamil).[2,3,22,66] When carbamazepine is combined with valproate, the carbamazepine dose should be reduced because valproate displaces carbamazepine from protein-binding sites, thus increasing free levels.[3,22] Combining clozapine and carbamazepine is not recommended because of the possibility of bone marrow suppression with both agents.[22]

Dosing and Administration During an acute manic episode in most hospitalized patients, carbamazepine can be started at 400 to 600 mg/day in divided doses with meals and increased by 200 mg/day every 2 to 4 days up to 10 to 15 mg/kg/day. In outpatients the initial dose of carbamazepine should be lower and titrated gradually in order to avoid adverse effects. In clinical practice many patients are able to tolerate once-daily dosing of carbamazepine once their mood episode has stabilized. The dose of carbamazepine should be gradually increased until response is achieved or there is evidence of toxicity. During the first month of therapy, serum concentrations of carbamazepine may be affected due to autoinduction of cytochrome P450 3A4 enzymes.[66]

Carbamazepine serum levels are usually obtained every 1 to 2 weeks during the first 2 months, and then every 3 to 6 months during maintenance therapy. Serum levels should be drawn 10 to 12 hours after the dose (trough levels) and at least 4 to 7 days after a dosage change. Although there is no correlation between carbamazepine serum concentration and degree of antimanic or antidepressant response, most clinicians attempt to maintain levels between 6 and 10 mcg/mL (25 and 42 μmol/L) (although some treatment-resistant patients can require serum concentrations of 12 to 14 mcg/mL [51 to 59 μmol/L]). Recommended baseline and routine laboratory tests for carbamazepine are listed in Table 52-7.

Oxcarbazepine Oxcarbazepine, a 10-keto analogue of carbamazepine, blocks voltage-sensitive sodium channels, modulates voltage-activated calcium currents, and increases potassium conductance.[67] Initial trials suggested oxcarbazepine has mood-stabilizing effects similar to those of carbamazepine, with the advantages of milder adverse effects, no autoinduction of liver enzymes, and potentially fewer drug interactions.[2] There are currently less data supporting the use of oxcarbazepine than carbamazepine in the treatment of bipolar disorder.

Adverse Effects Oxcarbazepine has dose-related adverse effects of dizziness, sedation, headache, ataxia, fatigue, vertigo, abnormal vision, diplopia, nausea, vomiting, and abdominal pain.[67] In one study, hyponatremia was reported to occur in patients taking oxcarbazepine and carbamazepine at rates of 29.9% and 13.5%, respectively.[75] Severe hyponatremia (sodium less than or equal to 128 mEq/L [mmol/L]) was reported by Dong et al. as 12.4% and 2.8% of patients for oxcarbazepine and carbamazepine, respectively.[75] An in-depth discussion of adverse effects can be found in Chapter 40.

Drug–Drug Interactions Oxcarbazepine, a cytochrome P450 2C19 enzyme inhibitor and a 3A3/4 enzyme inducer, has the potential for causing drug interactions.[67] It induces the metabolism of oral contraceptives; thus, alternative contraceptive measures are required.[3,76]

Dosing and Administration Initial dosing is usually 150 to 300 mg twice daily, and daily doses can be increased by 300 to 600 mg every 3 to 6 days up to 1,200 mg/day in divided doses (with or without food).[67]

Lamotrigine Lamotrigine blocks voltage-sensitive sodium channels, modulates or decreases glutamate and aspartate release, and has antikindling properties.[3,64,68,72,77]

Efficacy The effectiveness of lamotrigine for the maintenance treatment of bipolar I disorder in adult patients was established in two multicenter, double-blind, placebo-controlled studies.[2] Doses of 200 mg/day were more effective than lower doses, and there were no advantages to using 400 mg/day. Lamotrigine has both antidepressant and mood-stabilizing effects; it may have augmenting properties when combined with lithium or valproate, and has low rates of switching patients to mania.[72,78] Although lamotrigine is less effective for acute mania compared with standard mood stabilizers, it may be beneficial in the maintenance therapy of treatment-resistant bipolar I and II disorders, in rapid-cycling dysphoric mania, and in mixed states.[2,3,72] Lamotrigine seems to be most effective for the prevention of bipolar depression; therefore, clinically it is often used in the treatment of patients with bipolar II. There are case reports of possible lamotrigine-induced mania when added to lithium, carbamazepine, and valproate.[79] In each of the cases reported, the patients had depressive mood symptoms or rapid mood changes requiring additional therapy.[79]

Adverse Effects Common adverse effects include headache, nausea, dizziness, ataxia, diplopia, drowsiness, tremor, rash, and pruritus.[68,72] Approximately 10% of patients in premarketing clinical trials developed a maculopapular rash and required discontinuation of therapy.[68,72] Although most rashes are self-limiting and resolve with continued treatment, some cases progressed to life-threatening conditions such as Stevens-Johnson syndrome. The incidence of rash appears to be greatest with coadministration of valproate, with higher than recommended initial doses, and with rapid dose escalation.[68] Patients should be warned about the rash, and the need for discontinuing lamotrigine if the rash is diffuse, involves mucosal membranes, and is accompanied by a fever or sore throat. For an in-depth discussion of the adverse effects of lamotrigine, see Chapter 40.

Drug–Drug Interactions Valproate decreases the clearance of lamotrigine (i.e., more than doubles the half-life), and lamotrigine must be administered at a reduced dosage (approximately half the standard dose).[68] For an in-depth discussion of drug–drug interactions with lamotrigine, see Chapter 40.

Dosing and Administration For the maintenance treatment of bipolar disorder, the usual dosage range of lamotrigine is 50 to 300 mg/day. The target dose is generally 200 mg/day (100 mg/day in combination with valproate and 400 mg/day in combination with carbamazepine).[68,72] For patients not taking medications that affect lamotrigine's clearance, the dose is 25 mg/day for the first 2 weeks of therapy, 50 mg/day for weeks 3 and 4, 100 mg/day for week 5, and 200 mg/day for week 6 and beyond.[2,68,72] Patients who stop lamotrigine therapy for more than a few days should be restarted on the recommended dosage escalation titration schedule.

Antipsychotics

FGAs that block dopamine-2 (DA_2) receptors and SGAs that block both DA_2 and serotonin 2A ($5\text{-}HT_{2A}$) receptors are used to decrease dopamine (DA) activity in the treatment of mania and mixed states. FGAs and SGAs such as aripiprazole, asenapine, haloperidol, olanzapine, quetiapine, risperidone, and ziprasidone are effective as monotherapy or adjunctive therapy in the treatment of acute mania.[80] Controlled studies in acute mania with lithium or valproate plus an antipsychotic suggest greater efficacy with combination therapies compared with that with any of these agents alone.[2,80] FGAs (e.g., chlorpromazine and haloperidol) are effective in up to 70% of patients with acute mania, particularly those with psychosis and psychomotor agitation. SGAs have demonstrated similar efficacy for the treatment of acute mania associated with agitation, aggression, and psychosis.[2,80]

Treating acute bipolar depression is very challenging, and some antipsychotics may play a useful role. Four large randomized controlled trials support use of quetiapine as a monotherapy treatment option for bipolar depression.[53] Data also support use of combined fluoxetine/olanzapine in treating bipolar depression.

Long-term safety of antipsychotics as monotherapy or as an adjunctive therapy for bipolar maintenance treatment still needs to be evaluated.[2,53,80] Risks versus benefits must be weighed due to the long-term adverse effects (e.g., obesity, type 2 diabetes, hyperlipidemia, hyperprolactinemia, and tardive dyskinesia) antipsychotics may cause.[80,81] Aripiprazole, olanzapine, and risperidone long-acting injection are effective monotherapy options for maintenance treatment in bipolar disorder.[53] Some data reported in abstract form support quetiapine for maintenance treatment. First-generation depot antipsychotics (e.g., haloperidol decanoate, fluphenazine decanoate) can have a place in maintenance treatment of bipolar disorder in patients who are noncompliant or treatment-resistant.[2]

Clozapine monotherapy has acute and long-term mood-stabilizing effects in refractory bipolar disorder, including conditions with mixed mania and rapid cycling, but requires regular white blood cell monitoring for agranulocytosis.[2,22,80]

Clinical **Controversy...**

What is the role of SGAs in bipolar disorder?

The use of SGAs in bipolar disorder does not come without risk. Metabolic side effects should be considered when weighing risks and benefits of various acute and chronic treatment options. The optimal management of weight gain and its consequences on physical and mental health is important. Clinicians must make prescribing decisions in collaboration with patients concerning the treatment of bipolar disorder, weighing the risks of antipsychotics versus traditional mood stabilizers (e.g., lithium or valproate).

Adverse Effects A summary of adverse effects for antipsychotics can be found in Chapter 50.

Drug–Drug Interactions A summary of drug interactions with antipsychotics can be found in Chapter 50.

Dosing and Administration For acute mania, higher initial doses of antipsychotics can be required (e.g., olanzapine 20 mg/day in hospitalized patients). Once acute mania is controlled (usually within 7 to 28 days), the antipsychotic can be gradually tapered and discontinued, and the patient maintained on the mood stabilizer monotherapy.

Monitoring

7 Recommendations for baseline and routine laboratory testing for patients receiving carbamazepine, lamotrigine, lithium, oxcarbazepine, SGAs, and valproate are found in Table 52-7.

Alternative Medication Treatments

8 **Benzodiazepines** Weighing the risk-to-benefit ratio, high-potency benzodiazepines such as clonazepam and lorazepam are commonly used as an alternative to or in combination with antipsychotics when patients are experiencing acute mania, agitation, anxiety, panic, and insomnia, or cannot take mood stabilizers (e.g., during the first trimester of pregnancy).[2,3,82,83] Lorazepam is available for intramuscular injection and is useful in the acute management of agitation. Benzodiazepines cause minimal adverse effects compared with antipsychotics, and at higher doses, rapidly sedate agitated patients.[3] They can cause CNS depression, sedation, cognitive and motor impairment, dependence, and withdrawal reactions. When no longer required, benzodiazepines should be gradually tapered and discontinued to avoid withdrawal symptoms.

Antidepressants For many years antidepressants were recommended as adjunctive therapy for acute bipolar depression. Data from the Systematic Treatment Enhancement Program for Bipolar Disorder (STEP-BD) suggest that adjunctive antidepressants may be no better than placebo for acute bipolar depression when combined with mood stabilizers.[84] Controversy exists concerning the use of antidepressants, and many clinicians consider them third line in treating acute bipolar depression, except in patients with no history of severe and/or recent mania or potentially in bipolar II patients.[85] The concern of mood switching (i.e., rapidly switching from depression to mania or hypomania) with the use of antidepressants is valid, although not common. Data show that the rate of mood switch with selective serotonin reuptake inhibitors (SSRIs) is around 3.8%, similar to placebo, when combined with mood stabilizers. The rate of mood switch with dual-acting agents (e.g., TCAs or venlafaxine) is higher, and thus these agents should be used with caution.[85,86] It is very important that before initiating therapy with an antidepressant, the patient should be on a therapeutic dosage or blood level of a primary mood stabilizer.[2] Patients who have a history of mania after a depressive episode or who have frequent cycling should be treated cautiously with antidepressants.[2,3] In general, the antidepressant should be gradually withdrawn 2 to 6 months after remission, and the patient maintained on a mood-stabilizing agent.[87,88] For more information, see Chapter 51 for comparisons among antidepressants.

Calcium Channel Antagonists Calcium channel antagonists inactivate voltage-sensitive calcium channels, thus inhibiting neurotransmitter synthesis and release and neuronal signal transmission.[22,77] Verapamil, a nondihydropyridine, has demonstrated mood-stabilizing properties in some studies, but negative results were found in other trials.[2,3,22,89] Nimodipine, a dihydropyridine, can be more effective than verapamil for rapid-cycling bipolar disorder because of its anticonvulsant properties, high lipid solubility, and good penetration into the brain.[2,3,22,45,77,89] Calcium channel blockers are generally well tolerated, and the most common adverse effects are bradycardia and hypotension. These are seldom used in everyday clinical practice.

Newer Anticonvulsants Third-generation anticonvulsants have been investigated for treating bipolar disorder with the hope that a different mechanism of action would be beneficial for mood stabilization. Gabapentin, levetiracetam, tiagabine, topiramate, and zonisamide have negative or limited positive data supporting their use in bipolar disorder. Topiramate has been used as an add-on weight-reduction medication, but there are no randomized controlled trials supporting its use in bipolar disorder.[90]

Special Populations

The approach for treating bipolar disorder in special populations (e.g., comorbid medical or psychiatric disorders, pregnancy) can vary among clinicians. Patients with comorbid medical conditions or concomitant substance abuse, those older than 65 or younger than 18 years of age, and pregnant patients can require different treatment approaches. Women have a high risk of relapse postpartum; therefore, prophylaxis with mood stabilizers is recommended immediately postpartum to decrease the risk of relapse.[91]

Prophylactic medications such as lithium or valproate can prevent postpartum episodes in women with bipolar disorder.[2] Pharmacotherapy during pregnancy is complicated, and the risk-to-benefit ratio must be weighed. Infants whose mothers took lithium during the first trimester of pregnancy may have a lower incidence of cardiovascular defects (particularly Ebstein's anomaly) than was previously thought.[2,22] Current estimates of this malformation when given lithium during the first trimester are estimated between 1:1,000 and 1:2,000.[91] Lithium freely crosses the placenta and is found in equal concentrations in maternal and fetal blood.[60] When lithium is used during pregnancy, it should be tapered down to the lowest effective dose necessary to decrease the risk of relapse. Lithium can cause "floppy" infant syndrome (e.g., low Apgar scores, lethargy, hypotonia, bradycardia, cyanosis, shallow respiration, and poor sucking), hypothyroidism, and nontoxic goiters. Milk concentrations of lithium range from 30% to 50% of the mother's serum concentration, and serum concentrations in the nursing infant are 10% to 50% of the mother's; thus, breastfeeding is usually discouraged.[2,92] If using lithium during pregnancy, dose adjustments and close monitoring of serum levels will be needed due to changes in glomerular filtration rates and renal perfusion rates during pregnancy and immediately after delivery.[93]

Neural tube defects cause the most concern for clinicians treating pregnant patients during their first trimester. Data from the North American Antiepileptic Drug Pregnancy Registry show the risk of neural tube defects is about 1 in 1,500 for nonexposed babies.[94] Carbamazepine's risk of neural tube defects is estimated to be 0.5% to 1%.[77] Carbamazepine is excreted in breast milk (the milk-to-maternal plasma ratio of carbamazepine is ~0.4).[3] Craniofacial abnormalities, developmental delays, microcephaly, and other abnormalities are also of concern when using anticonvulsants. For pregnant patients treated with lamotrigine, major malformation rates are similar to those in the general population (2.9% vs. 2% to 3%, respectively), but data for lamotrigine are limited compared with those for some older anticonvulsants.[93] The International Lamotrigine Pregnancy Register reports 12 major congenital malformations from 414 first-trimester exposures.[93] Valproate is usually not recommended during the first trimester of pregnancy because the risk of neural tube birth defects is about 1 in 20 exposed babies.[94] Australian registry data in patients with epilepsy show dose-related teratogenicity with doses greater than 1,100 mg/day of valproate.[95] Administration of folate can reduce the risk of neural tube defects; therefore, the risks versus benefits of using valproate during pregnancy must be discussed with the patient.[22] Women of childbearing age on valproic acid and pregnant women should receive folic acid supplementation. Valproic acid is excreted into human breast milk in low concentrations (less than 1% to 10% of the mother's serum level), so is considered to be compatible with breastfeeding.[3] One case report of thrombocytopenia and anemia from valproate exposure has been reported in a nursing infant. If the mother receives valproate during breastfeeding, mother and infant should have identical laboratory monitoring.

Caution should be used when prescribing antipsychotics during pregnancy. There are far more data on the use of FGAs than those on the use of SGAs during pregnancy. Some data are available for haloperidol and low-dose chlorpromazine, and these data show no elevated rate of physical malformations during first-trimester exposure.[96] Higher doses of chlorpromazine used in treating psychiatric illness may be associated with neonatal withdrawal and extrapyramidal symptoms.[96] Data on other FGAs are limited. Data on the SGAs are more limited, but do not show an overall increased risk of fetal abnormalities.[96] Most of the data are for olanzapine, risperidone, and quetiapine.[96] There are limited reports with clozapine, aripiprazole, and ziprasidone.[96] There is still a paucity of human data with antipsychotics, and therefore risk-to-benefit ratio must be weighed.

There are few controlled studies in children and adolescents with bipolar disorder; thus, little is known about the long-term efficacy and safety of specific agents or for combination therapies in this population.[10,97] Lithium, valproic acid, and carbamazepine are all used in pediatric bipolar disorder. Data are limited, supporting their use with only six double-blind studies completed in the pediatric population.[98] Lithium is the only medication approved as a mood stabilizer for children older than 12 years of age.[99] Aripiprazole and risperidone are FDA-approved for bipolar mania in patients aged 13 to 17 years.[100] Quetiapine is approved as monotherapy or adjunct to lithium or divalproex in patients aged 10 to 17 years during a manic episode.[100] It did not show efficacy in a small pilot study of adolescent bipolar depression.[101] Olanzapine is approved for use in patients with manic or mixed episodes aged 13 to 17 years.[100] Ziprasidone has support of an FDA advisory panel for pediatric acute mania, but it does not yet have FDA approval.[102] Long-term data are still needed for all of these agents. Published guidelines for treatment of bipolar disorder in children and adolescents include the *Practice Parameters for the Assessment and Treatment of Children and Adolescents with Bipolar Disorder* by the American Academy of Child and Adolescent Psychiatry.[10]

Patients with bipolar illness are more likely to have medical comorbidities than the general population (64.3% vs. 48.3%).[103] As people age, medical comorbidities tend to increase, which complicates the management of bipolar disorder in elderly patients. Renal clearance decreases, and elimination half-life nearly doubles for lithium in elderly patients.[104] Half-life of valproate has been reported to increase with aging.[105] Patients with dementia can have increased sensitivity to the side effects of mood stabilizers and antipsychotics. No prospective, randomized, placebo-controlled trials have been published examining efficacy of lithium or valproate in elderly patients.[106]

Personalized Pharmacotherapy

New information is quickly evolving in the area of pharmacogenetics and pharmacogenomics that may help clinicians individualize treatment for patients with bipolar disorder. Genetic testing is available to determine if patients are poor or rapid metabolizers of cytochrome P450 2D6 and 2C19, thus helping predict potential response as well as adverse effects. The use of carbamazepine requires genetic testing for the human leukocyte antigen (HLA) allele, HLA-B 1502, in patients of Asian ancestry to help detect a higher risk of Stevens-Johnson syndrome and toxic epidermal necrolysis.

EVALUATION OF THERAPEUTIC OUTCOMES

The establishment and maintenance of a therapeutic alliance between the patient and clinician is essential in monitoring a patient's psychiatric status and safety; enhancing treatment adherence; promoting good nutrition, sleep, and exercise; identifying stressors; recognizing new mood episodes; and minimizing adverse reactions and drug interactions.[2] Patients who have a partial response or nonresponse to established bipolar therapies should be reassessed for an accurate diagnosis, concomitant medical or psychiatric conditions, and medications or substances that exacerbate mood symptoms. Nonadherence to medication treatment, delusional symptoms, alcohol or substance abuse, rapid cycling, or mixed states are often associated with poorer treatment outcomes.

ABBREVIATIONS

APA	American Psychiatric Association
CANMAT	Canadian Network for Mood and Anxiety Treatments
DA	dopamine
DA_2	dopamine-2
DSM-IV-TR	*Diagnostic and Statistical Manual of Mental Disorders, Fourth Edition, Text Revision*
ECT	electroconvulsive therapy
FGAs	first-generation antipsychotics
5-HT_{2A}	serotonin 2A
HLA	human leukocyte antigen
ISBD	International Society for Bipolar Disorders
NOS	not otherwise specified
SGAs	second-generation antipsychotics
SSRI	selective serotonin reuptake inhibitor
STEP-BD	Systematic Treatment Enhancement Program for Bipolar Disorder
TCA	tricyclic antidepressant
WFSBP	World Federation of Societies of Biological Psychiatry

REFERENCES

1. American Psychiatric Association. Diagnostic and Statistical Manual of Mental Disorders, Fourth Edition, Text Revision. Washington, DC: American Psychiatric Association, 2000:345–401.
2. American Psychiatric Association. Practice guideline for the treatment of patients with bipolar disorder (revision). Am J Psychiatry 2002;159:1–50.
3. Goldberg JF, Harrow M, eds. Bipolar Disorders: Clinical Course and Outcome. Washington, DC: American Psychiatric Press, 1999.
4. Merikangas KE, Akiskal HS, Angst J, et al. Lifetime and 12-month prevalence of bipolar spectrum disorder in the National Comorbidity Survey replication. Arch Gen Psychiatry 2007;64:543–552.
5. Perlis RH, Miyahara S, Marangell LB, et al. Long-term implications of early onset in bipolar disorder: Data from the first 1000 participants in the Systematic Treatment Enhancement Program for Bipolar Disorder (STEP-BD). Biol Psychiatry 2004;55(9):875–881.
6. Nivoli AM, Pacchiarotti I, Rosa AR, et al. Gender differences in a cohort study of 604 bipolar patients: The role of predominant polarity. J Affect Disord 2011;133(3):443–449.
7. Suppes T, Mintz J, McElroy SL, et al. Mixed hypomania in 908 patients with bipolar disorder evaluated prospectively in the Stanley Foundation Bipolar Treatment Network: A sex-specific phenomenon. Arch Gen Psychiatry 2005;62(10): 1089–1096.
8. Sherazi R, McKeon P, McDonough M, et al. What's new? The clinical epidemiology of bipolar I disorder. Harv Rev Psychiatry 2006;14(6):273–284.
9. Miklowitz DJ, Cicchetti D. Toward a life span developmental psychopathology perspective on bipolar disorder. Dev Psychopathol 2006;18(4):935–938.
10. McClellan J, Kowatch R, Findling RL; Work Group on Quality Issues. Practice parameters for the assessment and treatment of children and adolescents with bipolar disorder. J Am Acad Child Adolesc Psychiatry 2007;46:107–125.
11. Smoller JW, Finn CT. Family, twin, and adoption studies of bipolar disorder. Am J Med Genet C Semin Med Genet 2003;123:48–58.
12. Baum AE, Akula N, Cabanero M, et al. A genome wide association study implicates diacylglycerol kinase eta (DGKH) and several other genes in the etiology of bipolar disorder. Mol Psychiatry 2008;13:197–207.
13. Newberg AR, Catapano LA, Zarate CA, et al. Neurobiology of bipolar disorder. Expert Rev Neurother 2008;8:93–110.
14. Kato T. Molecular genetics of bipolar disorder and depression. Psychiatry Clin Neurosci 2007;61:3–19.
15. Hallahan B, Newell J, Soares JC. Structural magnetic resonance imaging in bipolar disorder: An international collaborative mega-analysis of individual adult patient data. Biol Psychiatry 2011;69:326–335.
16. Martinowich K, Schloesser RJ, Manji HK. Bipolar disorder: From genes to behavior pathway. J Clin Invest 2009;119: 726–736.
17. Beyer JL, Kuchibhatla M, Cassidy F, Krishnan KR. Stressful life events in older bipolar patients. Int J Geriatr Psychiatry 2008;23(12):1271–1275.
18. Miklowitz DJ, Johnson SL. Social and familial factors in the course of bipolar disorder: Basic processes and relevant interventions. Clin Psychol (New York) 2009;16(2):281–296.
19. Goldstein BI, Kemp DE, Soczynska JK, et al. Inflammation and the phenomenology, pathophysiology, comorbidity, and treatment of bipolar disorder: A systematic review of the literature. J Clin Psychiatry 2009;70:1078–1090.
20. Drexhage RC, Kniijff EM, Padmos RC, et al. The mononuclear phagocyte system and its cytokine inflammatory networks in schizophrenia and bipolar disorder. Expert Rev Neurother 2010;10:59–76.
21. Gruber J, Miklowitz DJ, Harvey AG, et al. Sleep matters: Sleep functioning and course of illness in bipolar disorder. J Affect Disord 2011;134:416–429.
22. Goodnick PJ, ed. Mania: Clinical and Research Perspectives. Washington, DC: American Psychiatric Press, 1998.
23. Ostacher MJ, Perlis RH, Nierenberg AA, et al. Impact of substance use disorders on recovery from episodes of depression in bipolar disorder patients: Prospective data from the Systematic Treatment Enhancement Program for Bipolar Disorder (STEP-BD). Am J Psychiatry 2010;167:289–297.
24. Coryell W, Solomon DA, Fiedorowicz JG, Endicott J, Schettler PJ, Judd LL. Anxiety and outcome in bipolar disorder. Am J Psychiatry 2009;166:1238–1243.
25. McElroy SL, Guerdjikova A, Lavanier S, O'Melia A. Bipolar disorder with co-occurring eating disorders: Prevalence and pharmacotherapeutic indications. FOCUS J Lifelong Learn Psychiatry 2011;9(4):435–448.
26. Weber NS, Fisher JA, Cowan DN, Niebuhr DW. Psychiatric and general medical conditions comorbid with bipolar disorder in the National Hospital Discharge Survey. Psychiatr Serv 2011;62(10):1152–1158.

27. Ceïde ME, Rosenberg PB. Brief manic episode after rituximab treatment of limbic encephalitis. J Neuropsychiatry Clin Neurosci 2011;23(4):E8.
28. Chopra A, Tye SJ, Lee KH, et al. Underlying neurobiology and clinical correlates of mania status after subthalamic nucleus deep brain stimulation in Parkinson's disease: A review of the literature. J Neuropsychiatry Clin Neurosci 2012;24(1):102–110.
29. Dias RS, Lafer B, Russo C, et al. Longitudinal follow-up of bipolar disorder in women with premenstrual exacerbation: Findings from STEP-BD. Am J Psychiatry 2011;168(4): 386–394.
30. Goldsmith M, Singh M, Chang K. Antidepressants and psychostimulants in pediatric populations: Is there an association with mania? Pediatr Drugs 2011;13(4): 225–243.
31. Habek M, Brina M, Brina VV, et al. Psychiatric manifestations of multiple sclerosis and acute disseminated encephalomelitis. Clin Neurol Neurosurg 2006;108(3): 290–294.
32. Navinés R, Castellví P, Solà R, Martín-Santos R. Peginterferon- and ribavirin-induced bipolar episode successfully treated with lamotrigine without discontinuation of antiviral therapy. Gen Hosp Psychiatry 2008;30(4):387–389.
33. Plante DT, Winkelman JW. Sleep disturbance in bipolar disorder: Therapeutic implications. Am J Psychiatry 2008;165(7):830–843.
34. Santos CO, Caeiro L, Ferro JM, Figueira ML. Mania and stroke: A systematic review. Cerebrovasc Dis 2011;32(1): 11–21.
35. Spiegel DS, Weller AL, Pennell K, et al. The successful treatment of mania due to acquired immunodeficiency syndrome using ziprasidone: A case series. J Neuropsychiatry Clin Neurosci 2010;22(1):111–114.
36. Valentí M, Pacchiarotti I, Bonnín CM, et al. Risk factors for antidepressant-related switch to mania. J Clin Psychiatry 2012;73(2):e271–e276.
37. Goldberg JF, Garno JL, Callahan AM, et al. Overdiagnosis of bipolar disorder among substance use disorder inpatients with mood instability. J Clin Psychiatry 2008;69:1751–1757.
38. Brooks JO, Hoblyn JC. Secondary mania in older adults. Am J Psychiatry 2005;162(11):2033–2038.
39. Drancourt N, Etain B, Lajnef M, et al. Duration of untreated bipolar disorder: Missed opportunities on the long road to optimal treatment. Acta Psychiatr Scand 2013;127:136–144. doi:10.1111/j.1600-0447.2012.01917.x [Epub ahead of print].
40. Goldberg JF, Ernst CL. Features associated with the delayed initiation of mood stabilizers at illness onset in bipolar disorder. J Clin Psychiatry 2002;63(11):985–991.
41. Leverich GS, Post RM, Keck PE Jr, et al. The poor prognosis of childhood onset bipolar disorder. J Pediatr 2007;150: 485–490.
42. Vega P, Barbeito S, Ruiz de Azúa S. Bipolar disorder differences between genders: Special considerations for women. Womens Health 2011;7(6):663–676.
43. Freeman MP, Wosnitzer Smith K, Freeman SA, et al. The impact of reproductive events on the course of bipolar disorder in women. J Clin Psychiatry 2002;63:284–287.
44. Calabrese JR, Shelton MD, Rapport DJ, et al. Current research on rapid cycling bipolar disorder and its treatment. J Affect Disord 2001;67:241–255.
45. Barrios C, Chaudhry TA, Goodnick PJ. Rapid cycling bipolar disorder. Expert Opin Pharmacother 2001;2: 1963–1973.
46. Rasgon N, Bauer M, Glenn T, et al. Menstrual cycle related mood changes in women with bipolar disorder. Bipolar Disord 2003;5:48–52.
47. Sherwood Brown E, Suppes T, Adinoff B, Rajan Thomas N. Drug abuse and bipolar disorder: Comorbidity or misdiagnosis? J Affect Disord 2001;65:105–115.
48. Post RM, Denicoff KD, Leverich GS, et al. Morbidity in 258 bipolar outpatients followed for 1 year with daily prospective ratings on the NIMH life chart method. J Clin Psychiatry 2003;64:680–690.
49. Abreu LN, Lafer B, Baca-Garcia E, Oquendo MA. Suicidal ideation and suicide attempts in bipolar disorder type I: An update for the clinician. Rev Bras Psiquiatr 2009;31(3):271–280.
50. Lingam R, Scott J. Treatment non-adherence in affective disorders. Acta Psychiatr Scand 2002;105:164–172.
51. Suppes T, Dennehy EB, Hirschfeld RM, et al. The Texas implementation of medication algorithms: Update to the algorithms for treatment of bipolar I disorder. J Clin Psychiatry 2005;66:870–886.
52. Miklowitz DJ, Otto MW, Frank E, et al. Psychosocial treatments for bipolar depression; a 1-year randomized trail from the Systematic Treatment Enhancement Program. Arch Gen Psychiatry 2007;64:419–427.
53. Yatham LN, Kennedy SH, Schaffer A, et al. Canadian Network for Mood and Anxiety Treatments (CANMAT) and International Society for Bipolar Disorders (ISBD) collaborative update of CANMAT guidelines for the management of patients with bipolar disorder: Update 2009. Bipolar Disord 2009;11:225–255.
54. Bauer MS, Mitchner L. What is a "mood stabilizer"? An evidence-based response. Am J Psychiatry 2004;161:3–18.
55. Grunze H, Vieta E, Goodwin G, et al. World Federation of Societies of Biological Psychiatry (WFSBP) guidelines for biological treatment of bipolar disorders: Update 2010 on the treatment of acute bipolar depression. World J Biol Psychiatry 2010;11:81–109.
56. Grunze H, Vieta E, Goodwin GM, et al. The World Federation of Societies of Biological Psychiatry (WFSBP) guidelines for the biological treatment of bipolar disorders: Update 2009 on the treatment of acute mania. World J Biol Psychiatry 2009;10:85–116.
57. Kelso JR. Arguments for the genetic basis of the bipolar spectrum. J Affect Disord 2003;73:183–197.
58. Manji HK, Moore GJ, Chen G. Bipolar disorder: Leads from the molecular and cellular mechanisms of action of mood stabilizers. Br J Psychiatry Suppl 2001;41:S107–S119.
59. Shaldubina A, Agam G, Belmaker RH. The mechanism of lithium action: State of the art, ten years later. Prog Neuropsychopharmacol Biol Psychiatry 2001;25:855–866.
60. McEvoy GK, Miller J, Snow EK, et al. Lithium Salts. AHFS Drug Information 2007. Bethesda, MD: American Society of Health-System Pharmacists, 2007:2566–2575.
61. Baldessarini RJ, Tondo L, Hennen J, Viguera AC. Is lithium still worth using? An update of selected recent research. Harv Rev Psychiatry 2002;10:59–75.
62. Goodwin FK. Rationale for long-term treatment of bipolar disorder and evidence for long-term lithium treatment. J Clin Psychiatry 2002;63(Suppl 10):5–12.
63. Baldessarini RJ, Tondo L, Hennen J. Lithium treatment and suicide risk in major affective disorders: Update and new findings. J Clin Psychiatry 2003;64(Suppl 5):44–52.
64. Calabrese JR, Huffman RF, White RL, et al. Lamotrigine in the acute treatment of bipolar depression: Results of five double-blind, placebo controlled clinical trials. Bipolar Disord 2008;10:323–333.

65. McEvoy GK, Miller J, Snow EK, et al. Valproate Sodium, Valproic Acid, Divalproex Sodium. AHFS Drug Information 2007. Bethesda, MD: American Society of Health-System Pharmacists, 2007:2255–2262.
66. McEvoy GK, Miller J, Snow EK, et al. Carbamazepine. AHFS Drug Information 2007. Bethesda, MD: American Society of Health-System Pharmacists, 2007:2220–2225.
67. McEvoy GK, Miller J, Snow EK, et al. Oxcarbazepine. AHFS Drug Information 2007. Bethesda, MD: American Society of Health-System Pharmacists, 2007:2244–2246.
68. McEvoy GK, Miller J, Snow EK, et al. Lamotrigine. AHFS Drug Information 2007. Bethesda, MD: American Society of Health-System Pharmacists, 2007:2233–2239.
69. American Diabetes Association, American Psychiatric Association, American Association of Clinical Endocrinologists, et al. Consensus development conference on antipsychotic drugs and obesity and diabetes. Diabetes Care 2004;27:596–601.
70. Amann B, Born C, Crespo JM, et al. Lamotrigine: When and where does it act in affective disorders? A systematic review. J Psychopharmacol 2010;25(10):1289–1294.
71. Macritchie K, Geddes JR, Scott J, et al. Valproate for acute mood episodes in bipolar disorder. Cochrane Database Syst Rev 2003;(1):CD004052.
72. Malhi GS, Adams D, Berk M. Medicating mood with maintenance in mind: Bipolar depression pharmacotherapy. Bipolar Disord 2009;11:55–76.
73. Allen MH, Hirschfeld RM, Wozniak PJ, et al. Linear relationship of valproate serum concentration to response and optimal serum levels for acute mania. Am J Psychiatry 2006;163:272–275.
74. Pazzaglia PJ, Post RM, Ketter TA, et al. Nimodipine monotherapy and carbamazepine augmentation in patients with refractory recurrent affective illness. J Clin Psychopharmacol 1998;18:404–413.
75. Dong X, Leppik IE, White J, Rarick J. Hyponatremia from oxcarbazepine and carbamazepine. Neurology 2005;65:1976–1978.
76. Perucca E. Clinically relevant drug interactions with antiepileptic drugs. Br J Clin Pharmacol 2005;61:246–255.
77. Manji HK, Bowden CL, Belmaker RH, eds. Bipolar Medications: Mechanisms of Action. Washington, DC: American Psychiatric Press, 2000.
78. Malhi GS, Mitchell PB, Salim S. Bipolar depression: Management options. CNS Drugs 2003;17:9–25.
79. Raskin S, Teitelbaum A, Zislin J, Durst R. Adjunctive lamotrigine as a possible mania inducer in bipolar patients. Am J Psychiatry 2006;163:159–160.
80. Tohen M, Vieta E. Antipsychotic agents in the treatment of bipolar mania. Bipolar Disord 2009;11:45–54.
81. Marder SR, Essock SM, Miller AL, et al. Physical health monitoring of patients with schizophrenia. Am J Psychiatry 2004;161:1334–1349.
82. McEvoy GK, Miller J, Snow EK, et al. Benzodiazepines. AHFS Drug Information 2007. Bethesda, MD: American Society of Health-System Pharmacists, 2007:2508–2518.
83. Alderfer BS, Allen MH. Treatment of agitation in bipolar disorder across the life cycle. J Clin Psychiatry 2003;64(Suppl 4):3–9.
84. Sachs GS, Nierenberg AA, Calabrese JR, et al. Effectiveness of adjunctive antidepressant treatment for bipolar disorder. N Engl J Med 2007;356:1711–1722.
85. Gigsman HJ, Geddes JR, Rendell JM, et al. Antidepressants for bipolar depression: A systematic review of randomized, controlled trials. Am J Psychiatry 2004;161:1537–1547.
86. Post RM, Altshuler LL, Leverich GS, et al. Mood switch in bipolar depression: Comparison of adjunctive venlafaxine, bupropion, and sertraline. Br J Psychiatry 2006;189:124–131.
87. Sachs GS, Koslow CL, Ghaemi SN. The treatment of bipolar depression. Bipolar Disord 2000;2:256–260.
88. Sachs GS, Printz DJ, Kahn DA, et al. The expert consensus guideline series: Medication treatment of bipolar disorder 2000. Postgrad Med 2000;Spec No:1–104.
89. Levy NA, Janicak PG. Calcium channel antagonists for the treatment of bipolar disorder. Bipolar Disord 2000;2: 108–119.
90. Aronne LJ, Segal KR. Weight gain in the treatment of mood disorders. J Clin Psychiatry 2003;64(Suppl 8):22–29.
91. Yonkers KA, Wisner KL, Stowe Z, et al. Management of bipolar disorder during pregnancy and the postpartum period. Am J Psychiatry 2004;161:608–620.
92. Ernst CL, Goldberg JF. The reproductive safety profile of mood stabilizers, atypical antipsychotics, and broad-spectrum psychotropics. J Clin Psychiatry 2002;63(Suppl 4):42–55.
93. Dodd S, Berk M. The safety of medications for the treatment of bipolar disorder during pregnancy and the puerperium. Curr Drug Saf 2006;1:25–33.
94. US Food and Drug Administration. Information for Healthcare Professionals: Risk of Neural Tube Birth Defects Following Prenatal Exposure to Valproate. December 3, 2009, *http://www.fda.gov/Drugs/DrugSafety/PostmarketDrugSafetyInformationforPatientsandProviders/DrugSafetyInformationforHeathcareProfessionals/ucm192649.htm.*
95. Vajda FJE, Hitchcock A, Graham J, et al. The Australian register of antiepileptic drugs in pregnancy: The first 1002 pregnancies. Aust N Z J Obstet Gynaecol 2007;47:468–474.
96. Einarson A, Boskovic R. Use and safety of antipsychotic drugs during pregnancy. J Psychiatr Pract 2009;15:183–192.
97. Chang KD, Ketter TA. Special issues in the treatment of pediatric bipolar disorder. Expert Opin Pharmacother 2001;2: 613–622.
98. Liu HY, Potter MP, Woodworth KY, et al. Pharmacologic treatments for pediatric bipolar disorder: A review and meta-analysis. J Am Acad Child Adolesc Psychiatry 2011;50(8): 749–762.
99. Madaan V, Chang KD. Pharmacotherapeutic strategies for pediatric bipolar disorder. Expert Opin Pharmacother 2007;8: 1801–1819.
100. Gentile S. Clinical usefulness of second-generation antipsychotics in treating children and adolescents diagnosed with bipolar or schizophrenic disorders. Pediatr Drugs 2011;13(5):291–302.
101. Zuddas A, Zanni R, Usala T. Second generation antipsychotics (SGAs) for non-psychotic disorders in children and adolescents: A review of the randomized controlled studies. Eur Neuropsychopharmacol 2011;21:600–620.
102. Kuehn BM. FDA panel OKs 3 antipsychotic drugs for pediatric use, cautions. JAMA 2009;302:833–834.
103. McIntyre RS, Konarski JZ, Soczynska JK, et al. Medical comorbidity in bipolar disorder: Implications for functional outcomes and health service utilization. Psychaitr Serv 2006;57(8):1140–1144.
104. Hardy BG, Shulman KI, Mackenzie SE. Pharmacokinetics of lithium therapy. J Clin Psychopharmacol 1987;4:201–205.
105. Bryson SM, Verma N, Scott PJW, et al. Pharmacokinetics of valproic acid in young and elderly subjects. Br J Clin Psychiatry 1983;16:104–105.
106. Young RC. Evidence-based pharmacological treatment of geriatric bipolar disorder. Psychiatr Clin North Am 2005;28:837–869.

Anxiety Disorders I: Generalized Anxiety, Panic, and Social Anxiety Disorders

53

Sarah T. Melton and Cynthia K. Kirkwood

KEY CONCEPTS

1. The long-term goal in treatment of generalized anxiety disorder is remission with minimal or no anxiety symptoms and no functional impairment.
2. Antidepressants are the agents of choice for the management of generalized anxiety disorder.
3. Antidepressants have a lag time of 2 to 4 weeks or longer before antianxiety effects occur in generalized anxiety disorder.
4. When monitoring the effectiveness of antidepressants in panic disorder, it is important to allow an adequate amount of time (8 to 12 weeks) to achieve full therapeutic response.
5. Clonazepam and alprazolam extended-release are alternatives to alprazolam immediate-release for patients with panic disorder having breakthrough panic symptoms at the end of a dosing interval.
6. The optimal duration of panic therapy is unknown; 12 to 24 months of pharmacotherapy is recommended before gradual drug discontinuation over 4 to 6 months is attempted.
7. Social anxiety disorder is a chronic long-term illness requiring extended therapy. After improvement, at least a 1-year medication maintenance period is recommended.
8. The selective serotonin reuptake inhibitors or venlafaxine are considered first-line pharmacotherapy for social anxiety disorder.
9. An adequate trial of antidepressants in generalized social anxiety disorder lasts at least 8 weeks, and maximal benefit may not be seen until 12 weeks.
10. The three principal domains in which improvement should be observed in generalized social anxiety disorder are symptoms, functionality, and well-being.

Anxiety is an emotional state commonly caused by the perception of real or perceived danger that threatens the security of an individual. It allows a person to prepare for or react to environmental changes. Everyone experiences a certain amount of nervousness and apprehension when faced with a stressful situation. This is an adaptive response and is transient in nature.

Anxiety can produce uncomfortable and potentially debilitating psychological (e.g., worry or feeling of threat) and physiologic arousal (e.g., tachycardia or shortness of breath) if it becomes excessive. Some individuals experience persistent, severe anxiety symptoms and possess irrational fears that significantly impair normal daily functioning. These persons often suffer from an anxiety disorder.[1]

Anxiety disorders are among the most frequent mental disorders encountered in clinical practice. Healthcare professionals often mistake anxiety disorders for physical illnesses, and only one quarter of patients receive appropriate treatment.[2] Failure to diagnose and manage anxiety disorders results in negative outcomes including overuse of healthcare resources, increased morbidity, and mortality.[3] Individuals with anxiety disorders develop cardiovascular, cerebrovascular, gastrointestinal, and respiratory disorders at a significantly higher rate than the general population.[4]

To treat anxiety appropriately, the clinician must make a reliable diagnosis. It is essential that the distinction between short-term symptoms of anxiety and anxiety disorders be understood. Common or situational anxiety is a normal response to a stressful circumstance. Although symptoms can be severe, they are temporary and usually last no more than 2 or 3 weeks. Although short-term, "as-needed" treatment with an anxiolytic agent such as a benzodiazepine is common and can provide some symptomatic relief, prolonged drug therapy is not recommended for situational anxiety.[5]

EPIDEMIOLOGY

Anxiety disorders, as a group, are the most commonly occurring psychiatric disorders. According to the National Comorbidity Survey Replication of the prevalence, severity, and comorbidity estimates of mental disorders in the United States, the most recent 1-year prevalence rate for anxiety disorders was 19.1% in persons aged 18 years and older. Specific phobias were the most common anxiety disorder, with a 12-month prevalence of 9.1%. The 1-year prevalence of generalized anxiety disorder (GAD) was 2.7%, that of panic disorder was 2.7%, and that of social anxiety disorder (SAD) was 7.1%.[6]

In general, anxiety disorders are a group of heterogeneous illnesses that develop before age 30 years and are more common in women, individuals with social issues, and those with a family history of anxiety and depression. Patients often develop another anxiety disorder, major depression, or substance abuse.[1–3] The clinical picture of mixed anxiety and depression is much more common than an isolated anxiety disorder.[7]

ETIOLOGY

The differential diagnosis of anxiety disorders includes medical and psychiatric illnesses and certain drugs.[7] Hypotheses on the etiology of anxiety disorders are based on interactions between a combination of factors including vulnerability (e.g., genetic predisposition and early childhood adversity) and stress (e.g., occupational and traumatic experience). The vulnerability may be associated with genetic factors and neurobiologic adaptations of the central nervous system (CNS).[8]

TABLE 53-1 Common Medical Illnesses Associated with Anxiety Symptoms

Cardiovascular Angina, arrhythmias, cardiomyopathy, congestive heart failure, hypertension, ischemic heart disease, myocardial infarction
Endocrine and metabolic Cushing's disease, diabetes, hyperparathyroidism, hyperthyroidism, hypothyroidism, hypoglycemia, hyponatremia, hyperkalemia, pheochromocytoma, vitamin B_{12} or folate deficiencies
Neurologic Migraine, seizures, stroke, neoplasms, poor pain control
Respiratory system Asthma, chronic obstructive pulmonary disease, pulmonary embolism, pneumonia
Others Anemias, cancer, systemic lupus erythematosus, vestibular dysfunction

Data from references 4, 9, and 10.

TABLE 53-2 Drugs Associated with Anxiety Symptoms

Anticonvulsants: carbamazepine, phenytoin
Antidepressants: selective serotonin reuptake inhibitors, bupropion, serotonin–norepinephrine reuptake inhibitors
Antihypertensives: clonidine, felodipine
Antibiotics: quinolones, isoniazid
Bronchodilators: albuterol, theophylline
Corticosteroids: prednisone
Dopamine agonists: amantadine, levodopa
Herbals: ma huang, ginseng, ephedra
Illicit substances: ecstasy, marijuana
Nonsteroidal antiinflammatory drugs: ibuprofen, indomethacin
Stimulants: amphetamines, methylphenidate, nicotine, caffeine, cocaine
Sympathomimetics: pseudoephedrine, phenylephrine
Thyroid hormones: levothyroxine
Toxicity: anticholinergics, antihistamines, digoxin

Data from references 1 and 10.

Medical Diseases Associated with Anxiety

Anxiety symptoms are an inherent part of the initial clinical presentation of several diseases, thus complicating the distinction between anxiety disorders and medical disorders.[4,7] Anxiety disorders are strongly and independently associated with chronic medical illness, low levels of physical health-related quality of life (QOL), and physical disability.[4] If anxiety symptoms are secondary to a medical illness, they usually will subside as the medical situation stabilizes. However, the knowledge that one has a physical illness can trigger anxious feelings and further complicate therapy. Persistent anxiety subsequent to a physical illness requires further assessment for an anxiety disorder. Common somatic symptoms of anxiety that frequently present in medical disorders include abdominal pain, palpitations, tachycardia, sweating, flushing, tremor, chest pain or tightness, and shortness of breath. Although less specific, symptoms of muscle tension, headache, and fatigue are also common manifestations of anxiety. Medical disorders most closely associated with anxiety are listed in Table 53-1.[4,9,10]

Psychiatric Diseases Associated with Anxiety

Anxiety can be a presenting feature of several major psychiatric illnesses. Anxiety symptoms are extremely common in patients with mood disorders, schizophrenia, dementia, and substance-use disorders. Most psychiatric patients will have two or more concurrent psychiatric disorders (comorbidity) within their lifetime.[6] It is important to diagnose and treat all comorbid psychiatric conditions in patients with anxiety disorders.

Drug-Induced Anxiety

Drugs are a common cause of anxiety symptoms (Table 53-2). Anxiety occurs during the use of CNS-stimulating drugs in a dose-dependent manner, but ingestion of minimal amounts can result in marked anxiety, including panic attacks, in some individuals. The onset of drug-induced anxiety is usually rapid after the initiation of therapy. A thorough medication history evaluating for a recent drug or dosage change is important to rule out a drug-induced etiology for the anxiety.

Anxiety occurs occasionally during the use of CNS depressants, especially in children and the elderly; however, anxiety complaints are more common as complications of drug withdrawal after the abrupt discontinuation of these agents.[7,10]

PATHOPHYSIOLOGY

Data from biochemical and neuroimaging studies indicate that the modulation of normal and pathologic anxiety states is associated with multiple regions of the brain and abnormal function in several neurotransmitter systems, including norepinephrine (NE), γ-aminobutyric acid (GABA), serotonin (5-HT), corticotropin-releasing factor (CRF), and cholecystokinin.[11] Current neuroanatomic models of fear (i.e., the response to danger) and anxiety (i.e., the feeling of fear that is disproportionate to the actual threat) include some key brain areas. The amygdala, a temporal lobe structure, plays a critical role in the assessment of fear stimuli and learned response to fear.[11,12] The locus ceruleus (LC), located in the brain stem, is the primary NE-containing site, with widespread projections to areas responsible for implementing fear responses (e.g., vagus, lateral and paraventricular hypothalamus). The hippocampus is integral in the consolidation of traumatic memory and contextual fear conditioning. The hypothalamus is the principal area for integrating neuroendocrine and autonomic responses to a threat.[11,12]

Neurochemical Theories

Noradrenergic Model

The basic premise of the noradrenergic theory is that the autonomic nervous system of anxious patients is hypersensitive and overreacts to various stimuli. Many anxious patients clearly display symptoms of peripheral autonomic hyperactivity. In response to threat or fearful situations, the LC serves as an alarm center, activating NE release and stimulating the sympathetic and parasympathetic nervous systems. Chronic central noradrenergic overactivity down-regulates α_2-adrenoreceptors in patients with GAD. This receptor is hypersensitive in some patients with panic disorder.[11] By administering drugs that have a relatively specific effect on the LC, researchers have further explored the NE theory of anxiety and panic disorder. Drugs with anxiogenic effects (e.g., yohimbine [an α_2-adrenergic receptor antagonist]) stimulate LC firing and increase noradrenergic activity. NE in turn increases glutamate release (an excitatory neurotransmitter).[11] This produces subjective feelings of anxiety and can precipitate a panic attack in those with panic disorder, but not in normal volunteers.[11] Drugs with anxiolytic or antipanic effects (e.g., benzodiazepines and antidepressants) inhibit LC firing, decrease noradrenergic activity, and block the effects of anxiogenic drugs.[11]

GABA Receptor Model

There are two superfamilies of GABA protein receptors: $GABA_A$ and $GABA_B$. Drugs that reduce anxiety and produce sedation target the $GABA_A$ receptor. The $GABA_B$ receptor is a G-protein–coupled receptor postulated to be involved in the presynaptic inhibition of GABA release.[11–13] $GABA_A$ receptors are ligand-gated ion channels composed of five protein subunits. Several classes of subunits (i.e., α_{1-6}, β_{1-3}, γ_{1-3}, δ, ε, θ, π, ρ_{1-3}) surround a central pore, and the receptor is connected to the cytoskeleton.[14] Benzodiazepine ligands enhance the inhibitory effects of GABA.[14] GABA, the major inhibitory neurotransmitter in the CNS, has a strong regulatory or inhibitory effect on the 5-HT, NE, and dopamine (DA) systems. When GABA binds to the $GABA_A$ receptor, neuronal excitability is reduced.

The specific role of the GABA receptors in anxiety disorders has not been established. The number of $GABA_A$ receptors can change with alterations in the environment (e.g., chronic stress), and the subunit expression can be altered by hormonal changes.[14] In patients with GAD, benzodiazepine binding in the left temporal lobe is reduced.[14] Abnormal sensitivity to antagonism of the benzodiazepine binding site and decreased binding was demonstrated in panic disorder.[11,14] This is consistent with the suggestion that panic disorder is secondary to a lack of central inhibition that results in uncontrolled elevations in anxiety during panic attacks.[13] Examination of whole brain and regional GABA in patients with SAD using proton magnetic resonance spectroscopy showed impairment of the GABA system.[15]

Serotonin Model

Although there are data suggesting that the 5-HT system is dysregulated in patients with anxiety disorders, definitive evidence that shows a clear abnormality in 5-HT function is lacking. 5-HT is primarily an inhibitory neurotransmitter that is used by neurons originating in the raphe nuclei of the brain stem and projecting diffusely throughout the brain (e.g., cortex, amygdala, hippocampus, and limbic system). Abnormalities in serotonergic functioning through release and uptake at the presynaptic autoreceptors ($5\text{-}HT_{1A/1D}$), the serotonin reuptake transporter (SERT) site, or effect of 5-HT at the postsynaptic receptors (e.g., $5\text{-}HT_{1A}$, $5\text{-}HT_{2A}$, and $5\text{-}HT_{2C}$) may play a role in anxiety disorders.[11,13] Preclinical models suggest that greater 5-HT function facilitates avoidance behavior; however, primate studies show that reducing 5-HT increases aggression.[11,13] It is postulated that greater 5-HT activity reduces NE activity in the LC, inhibits defense/escape response via the periaqueductal gray (PAG) region, and reduces hypothalamic release of CRF. The selective serotonin reuptake inhibitors (SSRIs) acutely increase 5-HT levels by blocking the SERT to increase the amount of 5-HT available postsynaptically, and are efficacious in blocking the manifestations of panic and anxiety.[11]

Low 5-HT activity may lead to a dysregulation of other neurotransmitters. NE and 5-HT systems are closely linked, and interactions between the two are reciprocal and vary. NE may act at presynaptic 5-HT terminals to decrease 5-HT release, and its activity at postsynaptic receptors can cause increased 5-HT release.

Buspirone is a selective $5\text{-}HT_{1A}$ partial agonist that is effective for GAD but not for panic disorder. Because the selective $5\text{-}HT_{1A}$ partial agonists reduce serotonergic activity, GAD symptoms may reflect excessive 5-HT transmission or overactivity of the stimulatory 5-HT pathways.[16] There is circumstantial evidence for the involvement of serotonergic and dopaminergic systems in the pathophysiology of generalized SAD.[17]

Neuroimaging Studies

Functional neuroimaging studies support the crucial role of the amygdala, anterior cingulate cortex (ACC), and insula in the pathophysiology of anxiety.[12] In GAD there is an abnormal increase in the brain's fear circuitry, as well as increased activity in the prefrontal cortex, which appears to have a compensatory role in reducing GAD symptoms.[18] Patients with panic have abnormalities of midbrain structures, including the PAG. Neuroimaging studies have shown activation of insula and upper brain stem (including the PAG), as well as deactivation of the ACC during experimental panic attacks.[19] Patients with SAD have greater activity than matched comparison subjects in the amygdala and insula, structures linked to negative emotional responses.[20,21] Both pharmacotherapy and psychotherapy decreased cerebral blood flow in the amygdala, hippocampus, and surrounding cortical areas in patients with SAD.[21]

CLINICAL PRESENTATION

The *Diagnostic and Statistical Manual of Mental Disorders, Fourth Edition, Text Revision* classifies anxiety disorders into several categories: GAD, panic disorder (with or without agoraphobia), agoraphobia, SAD, specific phobia, obsessive-compulsive disorder (OCD), posttraumatic stress disorder (PTSD), and acute stress disorder.[1] The characteristic features of these illnesses are anxiety and avoidance behavior. Anxiety symptoms must cause significant distress and impairment in social, occupational, or other areas of functioning, and should not be secondary to a drug or illicit substance or a general medical disorder, or occur solely as part of another psychiatric disorder.[1] OCD and PTSD are discussed in Chapter 54.

Generalized Anxiety Disorder

The diagnostic criteria for GAD require persistent symptoms for most days for at least 6 months.[1] The essential feature of GAD is unrealistic or excessive anxiety and worry about a number of events or activities.[1] The anxiety or apprehensive expectation is accompanied by at least three psychological or physiologic symptoms. Anxiety and worry are not confined to features of another psychiatric illness (e.g., having a panic attack, being embarrassed in public).[1]

The onset, course of illness, and comorbid conditions of GAD are important considerations. GAD has a gradual onset with an

CLINICAL PRESENTATION Generalized Anxiety Disorder

Psychological and Cognitive Symptoms

- Excessive anxiety
- Worries that are difficult to control
- Feeling keyed up or on edge
- Poor concentration or mind going blank

Physical Symptoms

- Restlessness
- Fatigue
- Muscle tension
- Sleep disturbance
- Irritability

Data from references 1 and 22.

CLINICAL PRESENTATION A Panic Attack

Psychological Symptoms
- Depersonalization
- Derealization
- Fear of losing control, going crazy, or dying

Physical Symptoms
- Abdominal distress
- Chest pain or discomfort
- Chills
- Dizziness or light-headedness
- Feeling of choking
- Hot flushes
- Palpitations
- Nausea
- Paresthesias
- Shortness of breath
- Sweating
- Tachycardia
- Trembling or shaking

Data from references 1, 22, and 23.

average age of 21 years; however, there is a bimodal distribution. Onset occurs earlier when GAD is the primary presentation and later when GAD is secondary. GAD can be exacerbated or precipitated in later life by severe psychological stressors. Most patients present between the ages of 35 and 45 years, with women twice as likely to have GAD as men. The course of the illness is chronic (i.e., episodes can last for a decade or longer); there is a high percentage of relapse and low rates of recovery. The likelihood of remission at 2 years is 25%.[1] Patients report substantial interference with their lives and have a high probability of seeking treatment.[9] Lifetime comorbidity with another psychiatric disorder occurs in 90% of patients with GAD, with depression being found in over 60%.[9]

Panic Disorder

Panic disorder begins as a series of unexpected (spontaneous) panic attacks involving an intense, terrifying fear similar to that caused by life-threatening danger. The unexpected panic attacks are followed by at least 1 month of persistent concern about having another panic attack, worry about the possible consequences of the panic attack, or a significant behavioral change related to the attacks.[1] During an attack, patients describe at least four physiologic and physical symptoms. Panic attacks usually last no more than 20 to 30 minutes, with the peak intensity of symptoms within the first 10 minutes. Often patients seek help at a physician's office or emergency department, only to have their symptoms resolve before or on arrival. Because panic symptoms mimic those present in several medical conditions, patients often are misdiagnosed, and multiple referrals are common.[1]

Secondary to the panic attacks, up to 70% of patients develop agoraphobia.[23,24] Agoraphobia is anxiety about being in places or situations in which escape might be difficult or where help might not be available in the event of a panic attack.[1] As a result, patients often avoid specific situations (e.g., being in a crowd or flying) in which they fear a panic attack might occur.[1]

Complications of panic disorder include depression (10% to 65% have major depressive disorder), alcohol abuse, and high use of health services and emergency rooms.[1] Patients with panic disorder have a high lifetime risk for suicide attempts compared with the general population.[23,24] The usual course is chronic but waxing and waning.

Social Anxiety Disorder

SAD is characterized by an intense, irrational, and persistent fear of being negatively evaluated or scrutinized in at least one social or performance situation. Exposure to the feared circumstance usually provokes an immediate situation-related panic attack. In generalized SAD, fear and avoidance extend to various social situations, whereas in the nongeneralized form of SAD, fear is confined to only one or two social situations. Blushing is the principal physical indicator and distinguishes SAD from other anxiety disorders. Adults with SAD usually recognize their fear is excessive and unreasonable; however, they are unable to overcome it without

CLINICAL PRESENTATION Social Anxiety Disorder

Fears of Being
- Scrutinized by others
- Embarrassed
- Humiliated

Some Feared Situations
- Eating or writing in front of others
- Interacting with authority figures
- Speaking in public
- Talking with strangers
- Use of public toilets

Physical Symptoms
- Blushing
- "Butterflies in the stomach"
- Diarrhea
- Sweating
- Tachycardia
- Trembling

Types
- Generalized: fear and avoidance extend to a wide range of social situations
- Nongeneralized: fear limited to one or two situations

Data from references 1, 25, and 26.

treatment. If necessary, the feared situation is avoided or endured with significant distress.[1] In individuals younger than 18 years of age, the duration of symptoms must be at least 6 months to meet the diagnostic criteria.[1]

The mean age of onset of SAD is during the mid-teens. Rates of SAD are slightly higher among women than among men and more frequent in younger cohorts. It is a chronic disorder with a mean duration of 20 years.[1] People with SAD can be reluctant to seek professional help despite the existence of beneficial treatments because consultation with a clinician is perceived as a feared social interaction.[25]

Differentiating SAD from other anxiety disorders can be difficult. Panic attacks occur in both SAD and panic disorder, but the distinction between the two is the rationale behind fear; fear of anxiety symptoms is characteristic of panic disorder, whereas fear of embarrassment from social interaction typifies SAD.[1,26] A majority of SAD patients eventually develop a concurrent mood, anxiety, or substance abuse disorder.[25,26]

Specific Phobia

Specific phobia is marked and persistent fear of a circumscribed object or situation (e.g., insects or heights). Apart from contact with the feared object or situation, the patient is usually free of symptoms. Most persons simply avoid the feared object and adjust to certain restrictions on their activities.[1]

TABLE 53-3 Drug Choices for Anxiety Disorders

Anxiety Disorder	First-Line Drugs	Second-Line Drugs	Alternatives
Generalized anxiety disorder	Duloxetine Escitalopram Paroxetine Sertraline Venlafaxine XR	Benzodiazepines Buspirone Imipramine Pregabalin	Hydroxyzine Quetiapine
Panic disorder	SSRIs Venlafaxine XR	Alprazolam Citalopram Clomipramine Clonazepam Imipramine	Phenelzine
Social anxiety disorder	Escitalopram Fluvoxamine CR Paroxetine Sertraline Venlafaxine XR	Clonazepam Citalopram	Gabapentin Phenelzine Pregabalin

CR, controlled-release; SSRI, selective serotonin reuptake inhibitor; XR, extended-release.

Data from references 3, 9, 22, 26–29.

TREATMENT

Generalized Anxiety Disorder

Desired Outcomes

The goals of therapy in the acute management of GAD are to reduce the severity and duration of the anxiety symptoms and to improve overall functioning. ❶ The long-term goal in GAD is remission with minimal or no anxiety symptoms, no functional impairment, and increased QOL.[9] Prevention of recurrence is another long-term consideration.

General Approach to Treatment

Once GAD is diagnosed, a patient-specific treatment plan, which usually consists of both psychotherapy and drug therapy, is developed. The plan depends on the severity and chronicity of symptoms, age, medication history, and comorbid medical and psychiatric conditions.[9] Factors such as anticipated adverse effects, history of prior response in the patient or family member, patient preference, and cost should be considered when treatment is initiated. Psychotherapy is the least invasive and safest treatment modality. Antianxiety medication is indicated for patients experiencing symptoms severe enough to produce functional disability. Table 53-3 lists drug choices for GAD, panic disorder, and SAD.

Nonpharmacologic Therapy

Nonpharmacologic treatment modalities in GAD include psychoeducation, short-term counseling, stress management, psychotherapy, meditation, or exercise. Psychoeducation includes information on the etiology and management of GAD. Anxious patients should be instructed to avoid caffeine, nonprescription stimulants, diet pills, and excessive use of alcohol. Most patients with GAD require psychological therapy, alone or in combination with antianxiety drugs, to overcome fears and to learn to manage their anxiety and worry.[5] Cognitive behavioral therapy (CBT) is the most effective psychological therapy in GAD patients. CBT for GAD includes self-monitoring of worry, cognitive restructuring, relaxation training, and rehearsal of coping skills.[5] Psychotherapy or medication alone has comparable efficacy in acute treatment.[22] The relapse rate with CBT is less than with other types of psychological modalities.[22] Controlled trials comparing the efficacy of combining drug and psychotherapy over long-term treatment are lacking.[22] Advantages of CBT over pharmacotherapy include patient preference and lack of troubling adverse effects. However, CBT is not widely available, requires specialized training, and entails weekly sessions for an extended time period (i.e., 12 to 20 weeks).[5]

Pharmacologic Therapy

The benzodiazepines are the most effective and commonly prescribed drugs for the rapid relief of acute anxiety symptoms (Table 53-4). All benzodiazepines are equally effective anxiolytics, and consideration of pharmacokinetic properties and the patient's clinical situation will assist in the selection of the most appropriate agent.[5,33]

Because of the lack of dependency and tolerable adverse effect profile, antidepressants have emerged as the treatment of choice for the management of chronic anxiety, especially in the presence of comorbid depressive symptoms. Buspirone is an additional anxiolytic option (Table 53-5) in patients without comorbid depression or other anxiety disorders (e.g., panic disorder and SAD). Because of the high risk of adverse effects and toxicity, barbiturates, antipsychotics, antipsychotic–antidepressant combinations, and antihistamines generally are not indicated in the treatment of GAD.[3] The benzodiazepines are more effective in treating the somatic and autonomic symptoms of GAD as opposed to the psychic symptoms (e.g., apprehension and worry), which are reduced by antidepressants.[3]

The most recent treatment guidelines from the World Federation of Societies of Biological Psychiatry and the National Institute for Health and Clinical Evidence are evidence-based.[3,28] A descriptive flowchart with recommendations based on levels of evidence from the International Psychopharmacology Algorithm Project for the psychosocial and pharmacologic management of GAD is shown in Figure 53-1.[40]

Alternative Drug Treatments

Hydroxyzine, pregabalin, and atypical antipsychotics are alternatives.[9,22,34] The antihistamine hydroxyzine was effective in studies

TABLE 53-4 Benzodiazepine Antianxiety Agents

Drug	Brand Name	Approved Dosage Range (mg/day)	Maximum Dosage for Geriatric Patients (mg/day)	Approximate Equivalent Dose (mg)	Comments
Alprazolam[a]	Niravam,[b] Xanax Xanax XR	0.75–4 1–10[c]	2	0.5	Associated with interdose rebound anxiety
Chlordiazepoxide[a]	Librium	25–400	40	10	
Clonazepam[a]	Klonopin Klonopin Wafer[b]	1–4[c]	3	0.25–0.5	
Clorazepate[a]	Tranxene	7.5–60	30	7.5	
Diazepam[a]	Valium	2–40	20	5	
Lorazepam[a]	Ativan	0.5–10	3	1	Preferred in elderly
Oxazepam[a]	Serax	30–120	60	30	Preferred in elderly

XR, extended-release.

[a]Available generically.
[b]Orally disintegrating formulation.
[c]Panic disorder dose.

Dosing and equivalence data from references 30–32.

conducted for as long as 12 weeks in patients with GAD. Hydroxyzine is commonly used in the primary care setting, but it is considered be to be a second-line agent because of adverse effects and lack of efficacy for comorbid disorders.[9] Pregabalin, which binds to the $\alpha_2\delta$ subunit of voltage-gated calcium channels to reduce nerve terminal calcium influx, acts on "hyperexcited" neurons. Pregabalin produced anxiolytic effects similar to lorazepam, alprazolam, and venlafaxine in acute efficacy trials.[33] Quetiapine extended-release 150 mg/day monotherapy was superior to placebo in three studies, and as effective as paroxetine 20 mg/day and escitalopram 10 mg/day but with an earlier onset of action.[34] In a 52-week treatment of GAD, quetiapine extended-release was superior to placebo in the prevention of anxiety relapse.[34] Quetiapine is not FDA-approved for GAD, and the long-term risks and benefits of atypical antipsychotics in the treatment of GAD are unclear.[34] Analysis of data from a pooled sample of trials found kava kava to be no more effective than placebo.[41] Because of reports of hepatotoxicity, kava kava is not recommended as an anxiolytic.[41] Although valerian, St. John's wort, and passionflower have been used to manage GAD, there is insufficient evidence of their effectiveness and safety.[42]

Clinical **Controversy. . .**

Pregabalin is classified as first-line treatment for GAD in evidence-based guidelines and is approved for treatment of anxiety in Europe. However, pregabalin is not approved for GAD in the United States, and experts with the IPAP pharmacologic algorithm do not support the first-line position of pregabalin because of lack of clinical experience and lack of data to establish efficacy for comorbid conditions.

TABLE 53-5 Nonbenzodiazepine Antianxiety Agents for Generalized Anxiety Disorder

Drug	Brand Name	Initial Dose	Usual Range (mg/day)[a]	Comments
Antidepressants				
Duloxetine	Cymbalta	30 or 60 mg/day	60–120	FDA-approved
Escitalopram	Lexapro	10 mg/day	10–20	FDA-approved, available generically
Imipramine	Tofranil	50 mg/day	75–200	Available generically
Paroxetine	Paxil Pexeva	20 mg/day	20–50	FDA-approved, available generically, avoid in pregnancy
Sertraline	Zoloft	50 mg/day	50–200	Available generically
Venlafaxine XR	Effexor XR	37.5 or 75 mg/day	75–225[b]	FDA-approved, available generically
Azapirone				
Buspirone	BuSpar	7.5 mg twice daily	15–60[b]	FDA-approved, available generically
Diphenylmethane				
Hydroxyzine	Vistaril	25 or 50 mg four times daily	200–400	FDA-approved, available generically, approved in children for anxiety and tension in divided daily doses of 50–100 mg
Anticonvulsant				
Pregabalin	Lyrica	50 mg three times daily	150–600	Dosage adjustment required in renal impairment
Atypical antipsychotic				
Quetiapine XR	Seroquel XR	50 mg at bedtime	150–300	

XR, extended-release.

[a]Elderly patients are usually treated with approximately one half of the dose listed.
[b]No dosage adjustment is required in elderly patients.

Data from references 3, 33–39.

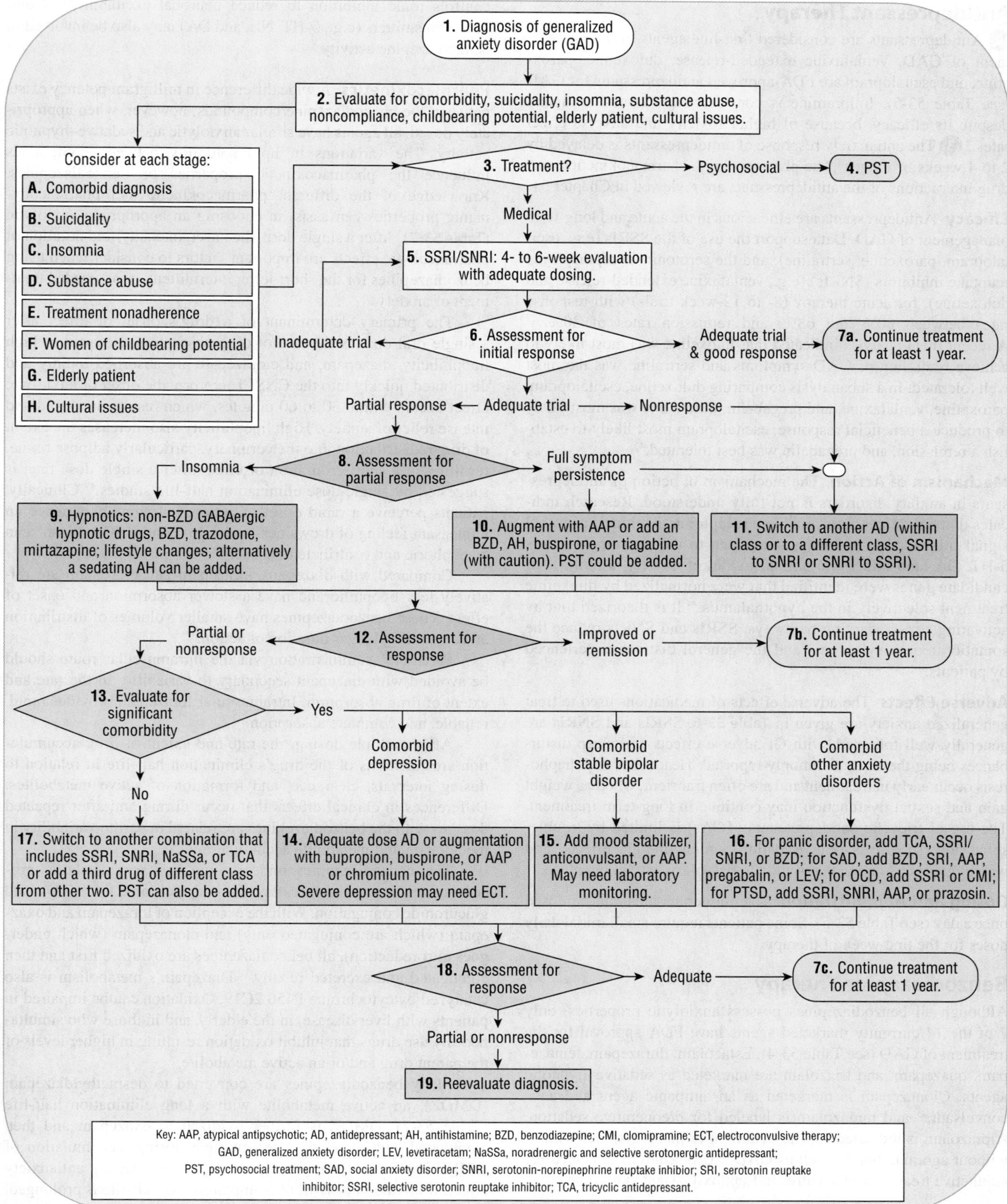

FIGURE 53-1 International Psychopharmacology Algorithm Project (IPAP) generalized anxiety disorder (GAD) algorithm flowchart. Yellow, first-line treatment (nodes 3–6); green, second-line treatment (nodes 8–12); blue, third-line treatment, no comorbidity (nodes 13–16); orange, third-line treatment, with comorbidity (nodes 14–16); light green, assessment and evaluation. Levels of evidence used in development of the flowchart were: 1, more than one placebo-controlled trial with sample sizes over 30; 2, one placebo-controlled trial (or active vs. active drug comparison) with sample size of 30 or greater; 3, one or small (n <30) placebo-controlled trial; 4, case reports or open-label trials; and 5, expert consensus without published evidence. *(Flowchart is used by permission of the International Psychopharmacology Algorithm Project, http://www.ipap.org.[40])*

Antidepressant Therapy

❷ Antidepressants are considered first-line agents in the management of GAD. Venlafaxine extended-release, duloxetine, paroxetine, and escitalopram are FDA-approved antidepressants for GAD (see Table 53-5). Imipramine is considered a second-line agent, despite its efficacy, because of higher toxicity and adverse effect rates.[3] ❸ The antianxiety response of antidepressants is delayed by 2 to 4 weeks or longer.[3] The pharmacology, pharmacokinetics, and drug interactions of the antidepressants are reviewed in Chapter 51.

Efficacy Antidepressants are efficacious in the acute and long-term management of GAD. Data support the use of the SSRIs (e.g., escitalopram, paroxetine, sertraline), and the serotonin–norepinephrine reuptake inhibitors (SNRIs) (e.g., venlafaxine extended-release and duloxetine), for acute therapy (8- to 12-week trials) with response rates between 60% and 68%, and remission rates of 30%.[3,22] A recent meta-analysis indicated that fluoxetine was most likely to achieve remission of GAD symptoms and sertraline was the most well tolerated. In a subanalysis comparing duloxetine, escitalopram, paroxetine, venlafaxine, and pregabalin, duloxetine was most likely to produce a beneficial response, escitalopram most likely to establish a remission, and pregabalin was best tolerated.[43]

Mechanism of Action The mechanism of action of antidepressants in anxiety disorders is not fully understood. Research indicates that antidepressants modulate receptor activation of neuronal signal transduction pathways connected to the neurotransmitters 5-HT, DA, and NE. In an animal model of anxiety, a number of candidate genes were identified that were normalized by fluoxetine treatment selectively in the hypothalamus.[44] It is theorized that by activating stress-adapting pathways, SSRIs and SNRIs reduce the somatic anxiety symptoms and the general distress experienced by patients.

Adverse Effects The adverse effects of medications used to treat generalized anxiety are given in Table 53-6. SSRIs and SNRIs are generally well tolerated, with GI adverse effects and sleep disturbances being the most commonly reported. Headaches and diaphoresis occur early in treatment and are often transient, whereas weight gain and sexual dysfunction may continue in long-term treatment. The use of tricyclic antidepressants (TCAs) is limited by troublesome adverse effects (e.g., sedation, anticholinergic effects, and weight gain) in some patients and the risk of toxicity in overdose.

Dosing and Administration The antidepressants can be dosed once a day (see Table 53-5). Some patients require small initial daily doses for the first week of therapy.

Benzodiazepine Therapy

Although all benzodiazepines possess anxiolytic properties, only 7 of the 14 currently marketed agents have FDA approval for the treatment of GAD (see Table 53-4). Estazolam, flurazepam, temazepam, quazepam, and triazolam are marketed as sedative–hypnotic agents. Clonazepam is marketed as an antipanic agent and anticonvulsant,[45] and midazolam is labeled for preoperative sedation. Alprazolam is indicated for the treatment of panic disorder with or without agoraphobia, as well as GAD.[46] Clobazam in indicated for adjunctive treatment of seizures in Lennox-Gastaut syndrome.[32]

Pharmacology and Mechanism of Action The GABA receptor model of anxiety theorizes that benzodiazepines ameliorate anxiety through potentiation of the inhibitory activity of GABA.[14] Benzodiazepines bind on the $GABA_A$ receptor at the α_1, α_2, α_3, and α_5 subunits in combination with a β subunit and the γ_2 subunit.[14] The anxiolytic effects of benzodiazepines are mediated at the α_2 site, while sedative effects result from binding at the α_1 subunit. The binding sites of benzodiazepines and GABA are at the receptor interfaces of α/β and α/γ_2, respectively. The GABA receptor controls tonic inhibition to reduce neuronal excitability.[14] Other neurotransmitters (e.g., 5-HT, NE, and DA) may also be involved in benzodiazepine activity.

Pharmacokinetics A wide difference in milligram potency exists between the benzodiazepine compounds; however, when appropriately dosed, all agents have similar anxiolytic and sedative–hypnotic activity. The variations in lipid solubility between compounds influence the pharmacokinetic properties of benzodiazepines. Knowledge of the different pharmacokinetic and pharmacodynamic properties can assist in choosing an appropriate anxiolytic (Table 53-7). After a single dose, the onset, intensity, and duration of pharmacologic effects are important factors to consider when using benzodiazepines for the short-term, intermittent, or as-needed treatment of anxiety.

The primary determinant of a drug's onset of effect after a single oral dose is the rate of drug absorption. Because of high lipophilicity, diazepam, and clorazepate are absorbed rapidly and distributed quickly into the CNS. Therefore, the onset of anxiolytic effect occurs within 30 to 60 minutes, which results in a rapid and intense relief of anxiety. High lipophilicity also increases the extent of drug redistribution into the periphery, particularly adipose tissue, resulting in a shorter duration of effect after a single dose than is suggested by single-dose elimination half-life studies.[47] Clinically, patients perceive a rapid onset of action, but some experience an unpleasant feeling of drowsiness or loss of control. This "rush" can be euphoric and contribute to abuse.

Compared with diazepam, lorazepam and oxazepam are relatively less lipophilic and have a slower absorption and onset of effect. These benzodiazepines have smaller volumes of distribution and a resulting longer duration of action.[47]

Parenteral administration via the intramuscular route should be avoided with diazepam secondary to variability in the rate and extent of drug absorption. Intramuscular lorazepam provides rapid, reliable, and complete absorption.

After multiple dosing, the rate and extent of drug accumulation are functions of the drug's elimination half-life in relation to dosing intervals, clearance, and formation of active metabolites. Differences in clinical effects that occur during and after repeated dosages with the benzodiazepines are related in part to variability in metabolism and metabolite accumulation.[47]

The benzodiazepines undergo two primary metabolic processes, hepatic oxidation (catalyzed by cytochrome P450 3A4) and glucuronide conjugation. With the exception of lorazepam and oxazepam (which are conjugated only) and clonazepam (which undergoes nitroreduction), all benzodiazepines are oxidized first and then conjugated and excreted renally.[47] Diazepam's metabolism is also catalyzed by cytochrome P450 2C19. Oxidation can be impaired in patients with liver disease, in the elderly, and in those who simultaneously use drugs that inhibit oxidation resulting in higher levels of the parent drug and/or an active metabolite.

Many benzodiazepines are converted to desmethyldiazepam (DMDZ), an active metabolite with a long elimination half-life (Table 53-7). DMDZ is further oxidized to oxazepam and then conjugated and excreted. After multiple dosing, accumulation of DMDZ is slow and extensive, providing a long-lasting antianxiety effect. If oxidation of DMDZ is impaired, the half-life is prolonged, and extensive drug accumulation can result with repeated dosing.

Clorazepate is a prodrug and possesses no anxiolytic effects until metabolized to DMDZ. Before absorption, clorazepate is metabolized rapidly in the stomach through a pH-dependent process under acidic conditions.

Benzodiazepines with shorter half-lives (e.g., alprazolam, lorazepam, and oxazepam) reach steady-state plasma concentrations rapidly, and drug accumulation after repeated dosing is minimal. Oxazepam and lorazepam have no active metabolites.

TABLE 53-6 Monitoring of Adverse Effects Associated with Medications Used in the Treatment of Anxiety Disorders

Medication Class/Drug	Adverse Drug Reaction	Monitoring Parameter	Comments
Selective Serotonin Reuptake Inhibitors			
	Jitteriness syndrome	Patient interview	
	Suicidality	Patient interview	Monitor weekly in first few weeks in patients with comorbid depression and patients under age 25
	Nausea, diarrhea	Patient interview	Typically transient
	Headache	Patient interview	Typically transient
	Weight gain	Body weight, BMI, waist circumference	Paroxetine may be more likely to cause weight gain
	Sexual dysfunction	Patient interview	Significant reason for nonadherence
	Hyponatremia	Basic metabolic panel	Monitor at baseline and periodically thereafter. More frequent monitoring required in high-risk groups, especially the elderly (>65 years)
	Thrombocytopenia	Complete blood count	Reported with citalopram
	Teratogenicity	Pregnancy test at baseline	Avoid paroxetine in pregnancy; Pregnancy Category D
	QT prolongation	ECG	Before starting citalopram, consider ECG and measurement of QT interval in patients with cardiac disease
	Discontinuation syndrome	Patient interview	Avoid abrupt discontinuation in all but fluoxetine
Serotonin–Norepinephrine Reuptake Inhibitors			
	Jitteriness syndrome	Patient interview	
	Suicidality	Patient interview	Monitor weekly in first few weeks in patients with comorbid depression and patients under age 25
	Nausea, diarrhea	Patient interview	Typically transient
	Headache	Patient interview	Typically transient
	Elevated blood pressure	Blood pressure	Monitor blood pressure on initiation and regularly during treatment
	Sexual dysfunction	Patient interview	Significant reason for nonadherence
	Discontinuation syndrome	Patient interview	Avoid abrupt discontinuation
Tricyclic Antidepressants			
	Jitteriness syndrome	Patient interview	
	Suicidality	Patient interview	Monitor weekly in first few weeks in patients with comorbid depression and patients under age 25
	Anticholinergic effects	Patient interview	Contraindicated with narrow-angle glaucoma, prostatic hypertrophy, and urinary retention
	Weight gain	Body weight, BMI, waist circumference	
	Sexual dysfunction	Patient interview	Significant reason for nonadherence
	Sedation	Patient interview	Administer dosage at bedtime when feasible
	Arrhythmia	ECG	At baseline and periodically in children and patients >40 years of age
	Orthostatic hypotension	Blood pressure with position changes	
	Cholinergic rebound	Patient interview	Avoid abrupt discontinuation; taper doses
Benzodiazepines			
	Drowsiness, fatigue	Patient interview	Avoid operating large machinery; tolerance to sedation develops after repeated dosing
	Anterograde amnesia and memory impairment	Patient interview	Risk of anterograde amnesia is worsened with concomitant intake of alcohol
	Dependence	Patient interview; Prescription Monitoring Program	Monitor for early refills or escalation of dosage
	Withdrawal symptoms	Physical examination; patient interview	Taper doses on discontinuation
	Respiratory depression	Respiratory rate	Avoid administering with other CNS depressants (i.e., opioids, alcohol)
	Psychomotor impairment	Physical examination	Increased risk of falls
	Paradoxical disinhibition	Physical examination; family report	Increase in anxiety, irritability, or agitation may be seen in the elderly or children
Other Drugs			
Buspirone	Nausea, abdominal pain	Patient interview	Typically transient
	Drowsiness, dizziness	Patient interview	Typically transient
Phenelzine	Jitteriness syndrome	Patient interview	
	Suicidality	Patient interview	Monitor weekly in first few weeks in patients with comorbid depression and patients under age 25
	Hypertensive crisis	Blood pressure	Tyramine-free diet and avoidance of drug interactions required
	Orthostatic hypotension	Blood pressure with position changes	
Pregabalin	Dizziness, somnolence	Patient interview	
	Peripheral edema	Physical examination	
	Thrombocytopenia	Complete blood count	
	Weight gain	Body weight	
Quetiapine	Sedation	Patient interview	
	Metabolic syndrome	Body weight, BMI, waist circumference, fasting lipids and glucose	Fasting labs at baseline and then periodically
	Akathisia	Patient interview	
	Tardive dyskinesia	Abnormal Involuntary Movement Scale	
	Orthostatic hypotension	Blood pressure with position changes	

ECG, electrocardiogram; BMI, body mass index.

TABLE 53-7 Pharmacokinetics of Benzodiazepine Antianxiety Agents

Drug	Time to Peak Plasma Level (Hours)	Elimination Half-Life, Parent (Hours)	Metabolic Pathway	Clinically Significant Metabolites	Protein Binding (%)
Alprazolam	1–2	12–15	Oxidation	—	80
Chlordiazepoxide	1–4	5–30	*N*-Dealkylation	Desmethylchlordiazepoxide	96
			Oxidation	Demoxepam	
				DMDZ[a]	
Clonazepam	1–4	30–40	Nitroreduction	—	85
Clorazepate	1–2	Prodrug	Oxidation	DMDZ	97
Diazepam	0.5–2	20–80	Oxidation	DMDZ	98
				Oxazepam	
Lorazepam	2–4	10–20	Conjugation	—	85
Oxazepam	2–4	5–20	Conjugation	—	97

[a]Desmethyldiazepam (DMDZ) half-life 50–100 hours.

Data from references 32 and 47.

Benzodiazepine protein binding is extensive, especially for the drugs with a long elimination half-life. After a single dose of a benzodiazepine with a long elimination half-life, the expected duration of clinical activity may not parallel the drug's pharmacokinetic half-life because of drug redistribution.[47] After multiple dosing, drugs with long elimination half-lives and active metabolites require 1 to 2 weeks to reach steady state.

Efficacy Clinical trials of benzodiazepines show that 65% to 75% of patients with GAD have a marked to moderate response, with most of the improvement occurring in the first 2 weeks of therapy.[28,29] Benzodiazepines are more effective on the somatic symptoms of anxiety and fail to obviate the cognitive or psychic symptoms (e.g., worry).

Adverse Effects The most common adverse events associated with benzodiazepine therapy involve CNS depression (Table 53-6). This is manifested clinically as drowsiness, sedation, psychomotor impairment, and ataxia.[48] A transient mild drowsiness is experienced commonly by patients during the first few days of treatment; however, tolerance often develops. Disorientation, depression, confusion, irritability, aggression, and excitement are reported.[48]

Impairment of memory and recall also can occur during benzodiazepine treatment. The memory loss induced by the benzodiazepines typically is limited to events occurring after drug ingestion (anterograde amnesia).[48] Anterograde amnesia is secondary to disordered consolidation processes that store information and is not impairment in the perception or retrieval of information.[2] Benzodiazepines with high affinity for binding to the benzodiazepine receptor (e.g., alprazolam) appear to possess a higher potential for amnesia.[48]

Abuse, Dependence, Withdrawal, and Tolerance Two serious complications of benzodiazepine therapy are the potential for abuse and development of physical dependence. Benzodiazepine abuse is rare in the general population of users; however, individuals with a history of multiple drug abuse (e.g., alcohol or sedatives) are at the greatest risk for becoming benzodiazepine abusers.[5,48]

Because of the chronicity of illness, persons with GAD and panic disorder are at high risk of developing benzodiazepine dependence. Benzodiazepine dependence is a physiologic phenomenon demonstrated by the appearance of a predictable abstinence syndrome (withdrawal symptoms) on abrupt discontinuation of therapy.[48] Withdrawal symptoms can result because of the sudden dissociation of a benzodiazepine from its receptor site. After abrupt discontinuation, an acute decrease in GABA neurotransmission results, producing a less inhibited CNS.

Benzodiazepine Discontinuation After benzodiazepine therapy is discontinued suddenly, several events can occur. Rebound anxiety represents an immediate but transient return of original symptoms having an increased intensity compared with baseline. Recurrence or relapse is the return of original symptoms with similar intensity as before treatment.

Withdrawal symptoms are the emergence of new symptoms and a worsening of preexisting symptoms after benzodiazepine discontinuation. Symptoms can persist for days to weeks and resolve gradually over months.

Common symptoms of benzodiazepine withdrawal include anxiety, insomnia, restlessness, muscle tension, and irritability. Less frequently occurring symptoms are nausea, malaise, coryza, blurred vision, diaphoresis, nightmares, depression, hyperreflexia, and ataxia. Tinnitus, confusion, paranoid delusions, hallucinations, and seizures occur rarely. Withdrawal seizures can occur with both therapeutic and high doses of benzodiazepines with a short elimination half-life, usually within 3 days of drug discontinuation. They can occur approximately 1 week after discontinuation of agents with a long elimination half-life. High benzodiazepine doses, a long duration of therapy, and concurrent ingestion of drugs that lower the seizure threshold are risk factors for withdrawal seizures.

The onset of withdrawal symptoms in patients ingesting benzodiazepines with short elimination half-lives occurs much earlier (within 24 to 48 hours) than in those taking benzodiazepines with long elimination half-lives (within 3 to 8 days). Other factors associated with an increased incidence and severity of benzodiazepine withdrawal include high doses and long-term benzodiazepine therapy.

A strategy to minimize the severity of benzodiazepine withdrawal is a 25% per week reduction in dosage until 50% of the dose is reached, and then dosage reduction by one eighth every 4 to 7 days.[49] If therapy exceeds 8 weeks, a slow dosage taper over 2 to 3 weeks is recommended; however, if the duration of treatment is 6 months, a taper over 4 to 8 weeks should ensue.[49] Long-term use of benzodiazepines (i.e., 1 year or longer) requires a 2- to 4-month slow taper.[49] Tapering will not eliminate the emergence of withdrawal symptoms entirely but will prevent severe withdrawal. Slow drug taper is extremely important for the drugs with a short elimination half-life, because some individuals have greater difficulty with discontinuation. Withdrawal symptoms with short half-life benzodiazepines were no more severe than with longer half-life agents; therefore, switching from a short- to long-acting benzodiazepine before gradual taper is not supported.[48,49] The addition of CBT facilitated benzodiazepine tapering in patients with GAD.[50] Adjunctive use of carbamazepine or pregabalin can help reduce withdrawal severity during the benzodiazepine taper.[49,51] Patients should avoid the intake of alcohol and stimulants during the withdrawal process. Although tolerance develops to the sedative, muscle relaxant, and anticonvulsant activities, the benzodiazepines do not appear to lose anxiolytic or antipanic efficacy. However, the anxiolytic efficacy of benzodiazepines in long-term clinical trials (greater than 6 to 8 months of chronic use) has not been documented.[5]

Drug Interactions Drug interactions with the benzodiazepines generally fall into two categories: pharmacodynamic and pharmacokinetic. Simultaneous use of alcohol and a benzodiazepine results in additive CNS depressant effects. In addition, concurrent use of a benzodiazepine and other drugs with CNS depressant properties (e.g., opioids, antipsychotics, and antihistamines) can potentiate the adverse sedative effects. When ingested alone in an overdose attempt, benzodiazepines are rarely life-threatening; however, the combination of benzodiazepines with alcohol or other CNS depressant agents is potentially fatal.

Concurrent use of medications that inhibit cytochrome P450 3A4 (e.g., ketoconazole, nefazodone, and ritonavir) can increase the blood levels of alprazolam and diazepam. Drugs that induce cytochrome P450 3A4 (e.g., carbamazepine, St. John's wort) can reduce benzodiazepine levels. Consult a drug interaction website (*http://www.factsandcomparisons.com/facts-comparisons-online.aspx*) for further information.

Dosing and Administration Benzodiazepine dosage requirements vary widely among patients and must be individualized. Therapy should be initiated using low doses (e.g., alprazolam 0.25 mg three times a day or equivalent doses of other benzodiazepines) and titrated upward to relieve anxiety symptoms and avoid adverse events. After an initial treatment response is achieved, agents with long elimination half-lives can be dosed at bedtime. Dosage adjustments should be made weekly. Three to 4 weeks of a daily dose at the maximum dose constitutes an adequate clinical trial (see Table 53-4).[5]

The duration of benzodiazepine therapy for the acute management of anxiety should be limited to 2 to 4 weeks. In general, benzodiazepines should be used with a regular dosing regimen and not on an as-needed basis.[9] Only in the treatment of short-term distress (e.g., air travel, dental phobia) as-needed use may be justified.[3,9] Individuals with persistent symptoms should be managed with antidepressants because of the risk of dependence with continued benzodiazepine therapy.

Patient education should include the anticipated length of drug therapy, potential side effects, and consequences of the ingestion of alcohol and other CNS depressants. Patients should understand that benzodiazepines provide symptomatic relief but do not solve underlying psychological problems. Patients should be instructed not to decrease or discontinue benzodiazepine usage without contacting their prescriber.

Buspirone Therapy

Buspirone is a nonbenzodiazepine anxiolytic that lacks anticonvulsant, muscle relaxant, hypnotic, motor impairment, and dependence properties. It is considered to be a second-line agent for GAD because of inconsistent reports of efficacy (particularly long term), delayed onset of effect (i.e., 2 weeks or longer), and lack of efficacy for other potential concurrent depressive and anxiety disorders.[52] Unlike benzodiazepines, buspirone is effective for the psychic symptoms of anxiety.[52]

Pharmacology and Mechanism of Action Buspirone's anxiolytic mechanism of action is unknown. It is thought to exert its anxiolytic effect through partial agonist activity at the 5-HT_{1A} presynaptic receptors, thus reducing the firing of 5-HT neurons.[47]

Pharmacokinetics After an oral dose, buspirone is absorbed rapidly and completely and undergoes extensive first-pass metabolism. The mean elimination half-life is 2.5 hours, and it must be dosed two to three times daily, which adversely affects adherence to the drug regimen.[47]

Adverse Effects Adverse events include dizziness, nausea, and headaches[47] (Table 53-6).

Drug Interactions Drugs that inhibit cytochrome P450 3A4 (e.g., verapamil, itraconazole, fluvoxamine) can increase buspirone levels. Rifampin caused a 10-fold reduction in buspirone levels. Buspirone reportedly elevates blood pressure in patients taking a monoamine oxidase inhibitor (MAOI).

Dosing and Administration The dose of buspirone can be titrated in increments of 5 mg/day every 2 to 3 days as needed.[47] The onset of improvement in psychic symptoms precedes the relief of somatic symptoms; maximum therapeutic benefit might not be evident for 4 to 6 weeks.

Buspirone is a treatment option for patients with GAD, particularly for patients with uncomplicated GAD, in patients who fail other anxiolytic therapies, or in patients with substance abuse. It is not useful in clinical situations requiring immediate anxiolysis or for situations requiring as-needed anxiolytic therapy.[47] Evidence suggests that buspirone may have less efficacy in patients who have previously used benzodiazepines.[29]

Special Populations

The management of anxiety in patients with substance abuse, pregnant women, children, elderly patients, and those patients with adherence problems requires special consideration in the choice of anxiolytic. Patients with GAD may misuse alcohol, cannabis, or other substances to manage anxiety. The symptoms of GAD are similar to those of withdrawal, and it is difficult to confirm the diagnosis of GAD until after abstinence is obtained. Benzodiazepine therapy should be avoided in this population.

There is evidence that maternal anxiety during pregnancy and the postpartum period potentially pose significant risk to the child. Clinical practice guidelines for anxiety disorders recommend use of fluoxetine, sertraline, or citalopram; however, jitteriness, myoclonus, and irritability in the neonate and premature infant have been reported.[53] Paroxetine (Pregnancy Category D) should be avoided in pregnant women because of risk of cardiovascular malformations.[35]

Cleft lip, cleft palate, and other teratogenic effects are associated with benzodiazepine use, but a causal relationship is inconclusive. Clinicians should avoid benzodiazepine use during the first trimester, use the lowest dosage for the shortest period of time, divide the total daily dosage into two or three doses to prevent high peak plasma levels, and use the agent as monotherapy.[9,53] Benzodiazepine risks during the third trimester include sedation, withdrawal symptoms, and "floppy baby syndrome" (e.g., hypotonia, low Apgar scores, hypothermia). Alprazolam should be avoided during pregnancy because of neonatal withdrawal. Should benzodiazepines be required during pregnancy, the preferred agents are diazepam and chlordiazepoxide.[54] The antidepressants are favored for GAD during pregnancy based on safety considerations. Diazepam and clonazepam should not be used in nursing mothers because infants can experience sedation, lethargy, and weight loss.[9]

There are few controlled clinical trials of drugs in children and adolescents with GAD. CBT alone or in conjunction with antidepressants can have long-term benefits.[9] Randomized controlled trials of fluvoxamine, fluoxetine, sertraline, and venlafaxine extended-release indicate short-term efficacy[3,55]; however, behavioral activation was reported with clonazepam.[3] No antidepressant is FDA-indicated for GAD in children or adolescents. Increased monitoring for behavioral activation with benzodiazepines and suicide-related adverse effects with antidepressants is necessary if these agents are prescribed.

Patients with hepatic disease are at risk for drug accumulation and subsequent complications. Duloxetine use should be avoided in patients with hepatic insufficiency.[36] Drug accumulation of benzodiazepines can result in the elderly secondary to a decreased capacity for oxidation and alterations in the volume of distribution. Therefore, intermediate- or short-acting benzodiazepines without active metabolites are preferred for chronic use. Elderly patients are also sensitive to the CNS adverse effects of benzodiazepines (regardless of half-life), and their use is associated with a high frequency of falls and hip fractures. Recent studies of buspirone, duloxetine, escitalopram, sertraline, venlafaxine, and pregabalin showed efficacy in elderly patients with GAD.[3,56–58]

Personalized Pharmacotherapy

The need for treatment is determined by patient-specific factors including severity and duration of symptoms, degree of disability, and the presence of coexisting disorders (i.e., mood or other anxiety disorders). The patient should be assessed for response to or intolerance of previous treatment approaches. The selection of a specific treatment modality should be based on concurrent medical conditions, contraindications, patient's preference of treatment, and the availability of potential treatment options. The clinician should consider FDA warnings (e.g., QTc prolongation for citalopram) and potential for adverse events with medical disease (e.g., anticholinergic effects and weight gain with paroxetine in patients with diabetes, obesity, or benign prostatic hyperplasia) when selecting an agent. Increased risk of suicidality should be considered in patients taking antidepressants who are less than 25 years of age. All patients should receive education that includes information about GAD, treatment choices, and resources for support in the community. The patient should be an integral part of decision making and should be informed about effectiveness, common adverse effects, duration of treatment, cost associated with treatment, and what to expect when treatment is discontinued.[29]

Evaluation of Therapeutic Outcomes

Initially, anxious patients should be monitored once every 2 weeks for a reduction in the frequency, duration, and severity of anxiety symptoms and improvement in functioning.[29] The clinician should assess the patient for response to treatment by asking about specific target symptoms of anxiety and emergence of adverse events. Ideally, the patient should have no or minimal anxiety or depressive symptoms and no functional impairment. Use of an objective measurement of remission of GAD (e.g., Hamilton Rating Scale for Anxiety score less than or equal to 7 and a Sheehan Disability Scale score less than or equal to 1 on each item) can assist in the evaluation of drug response.[9,29] The definition of treatment resistance is defined as a poor, partial, or lack of response with at least two antidepressants from different classes. Treatment strategies for patients who do not achieve an appropriate response with a first-line agent include increasing the dose of the SSRI/SNRI, changing to a different agent in the same class, changing to a different agent of a different class, or augmentation of therapy. At any point of nonresponse or loss of previous response, the clinician should assess for (a) symptoms (e.g., psychotic symptoms) that may suggest a need for additional medications or (b) reasons for treatment nonadherence (e.g., adverse effects, cost of medications, limited understanding of the illness or treatments).[9] Patients should also be assessed for concurrent substance abuse, concurrent illnesses, and suicidal thoughts. Once a patient has responded to pharmacotherapy, the regimen should be continued for at least 1 year.[9] Early discontinuation is associated with a greater risk of relapse.[9]

TREATMENT
Panic Disorder

Desired Outcomes

The goal of therapy in panic disorder is remission. Patients should be free of panic attacks, have no or minimal anticipatory anxiety and agoraphobic avoidance, and have no functional impairment.[27]

General Approach to Treatment

Therapeutic options include single or combined pharmacologic agents, concurrent psychotherapy, or psychotherapy followed by pharmacotherapy. Most patients without agoraphobic avoidance will improve with pharmacotherapy alone; however, if avoidance is present, CBT typically is initiated concurrently. With all effective drug therapies, resolution of agoraphobic avoidance tends to occur slowly. A meta-analysis comparing the use of SSRIs and venlafaxine in panic disorder showed response to be similar among treatments.[59] Adding psychosocial treatment to pharmacotherapy may improve long-term outcomes by reducing the likelihood of relapse when pharmacotherapy is stopped.[27]

Nonpharmacologic Therapy

Patients should be educated to avoid substances that can precipitate panic attacks, including caffeine, nicotine, alcohol, drugs of abuse, and nonprescription stimulants.[1,27] Epidemiologic data suggest that daily smoking increases risk for panic attacks and may be a causal or exacerbating factor in some individuals with panic disorder.[27] Preliminary evidence suggests that aerobic exercise (e.g., walking for 60 minutes or running for 20 to 30 minutes 4 days/wk) may benefit patients with panic disorder.[28] CBT is associated with short-term improvement in 80% to 90% of patients and 6-month improvement in 75% of patients. A course of CBT for panic disorder is 16 to 20 hours in length conducted over a period of 4 months.[28] Bibliotherapy (the use of self-help books), exercise, and Internet-based CBT are other options.[27]

Pharmacologic Therapy

Panic disorder is treated effectively with several drugs including the SSRIs, the SNRI venlafaxine, the TCA imipramine, and the benzodiazepines alprazolam and clonazepam[27,28] (Table 53-8). Alprazolam, clonazepam, fluoxetine, paroxetine, sertraline, and venlafaxine are approved for this indication. SSRIs are the first-line agents because of their tolerability and efficacy in acute and long-term studies[3,27]; however, the benzodiazepines are the most commonly used drugs for panic disorder.[27] In a meta-analysis of the pharmacotherapy of panic disorder, the following antidepressants were significantly superior to placebo with the following increasing order of effectiveness: citalopram, sertraline, paroxetine, fluoxetine, and venlafaxine for panic symptoms and paroxetine, fluoxetine, fluvoxamine, citalopram, venlafaxine, and mirtazapine for overall anxiety symptoms.[59] Imipramine is effective for panic disorder; however, it is considered to be a second-line agent because of the significant cardiovascular and anticholinergic effects associated with it. Five practice guidelines are published.[3,22,27–29] An algorithm for the pharmacologic therapy of panic disorder appears in Figure 53-2.

Benzodiazepines are considered second-line agents. Because of the risk of dependency, benzodiazepines should be used only after several trials of antidepressants have failed.[3,27] Because of potential emergence of depressive symptoms during treatment, benzodiazepines should not be used as monotherapy in a patient who is clinically depressed or has a history of depression. In

TABLE 53-8 Drugs Used in the Treatment of Panic Disorder

Class/Generic Name	Brand Name	Starting Dose	Antipanic Dosage Range (mg)	Comments
Selective Serotonin Reuptake Inhibitors				
Citalopram	Celexa	10 mg/day	20–40	Dosage used in clinical trials; maximum dose limited by QT prolongation; available generically
Escitalopram	Lexapro	5 mg/day	10–20	Dosage used in clinical trials; available generically
Fluoxetine	Prozac	5 mg/day	10–30	Available generically
Fluvoxamine	Luvox	25 mg/day	100–300	Available generically
Paroxetine	Paxil	10 mg/day	20–60	FDA-approved; available generically
	Pexeva			
	Paxil CR	12.5 mg/day	25–75	
Sertraline	Zoloft	25 mg/day	50–200	FDA-approved; available generically
Serotonin–Norepinephrine Reuptake Inhibitor				
Venlafaxine XR	Effexor XR	37.5 mg/day	75–225	FDA-approved; available generically
Benzodiazepines				
Alprazolam	Xanax	0.25 mg three times a day	4–10	FDA-approved; available generically
	Xanax XR	0.5–1 mg/day	1–10	
Clonazepam	Klonopin	0.25 mg once or twice per day	1–4	FDA-approved; available generically
Diazepam	Valium	2–5 mg three times a day	5–20	Dosage used in clinical trials; available generically
Lorazepam	Ativan	0.5–1 mg three times a day	2–8	Dosage used in clinical trials; available generically
Tricyclic Antidepressant				
Imipramine	Tofranil	10 mg/day	75–250	Dosage used in clinical trials; available generically
Monoamine Oxidase Inhibitor				
Phenelzine	Nardil	15 mg/day	45–90	Dosage used in clinical trials

Data from references 3, 23, and 27.

patients whose illness is complicated by a history of alcohol or drug abuse, benzodiazepine use should be avoided.[27] Controlled trials have established that the short-term (4- to 6-week) addition of alprazolam or clonazepam to antidepressants produces a more rapid therapeutic response, with discontinuation of the benzodiazepine by week 7 of therapy.[29]

Alternative Drug Treatments

Buspirone, trazodone, bupropion, antipsychotics, antihistamines, and β-blockers are ineffective in panic disorder.[3,22,27] The majority of studies assessing the efficacy of MAOIs in treating panic disorder were open-labeled, and lacked adequate sample sizes. MAOIs are reserved for the most refractory or difficult patients.[27]

Antidepressant Therapy

Tricyclic Antidepressants

Efficacy Imipramine is the most studied TCA, alleviating panic attacks in 75% of patients with panic disorder. Imipramine effectively blocks panic attacks within at least 4 weeks; however, maximal improvement (including antiphobic response) does not occur until 8 to 12 weeks.[27]

Adverse Effects The adverse effects of medications used to treat panic disorder are found in Table 53-6. Up to 40% of patients experience stimulant-like effects, including anxiety, insomnia, and jitteriness.[27] These adverse effects often affect patient adherence, prevent medication dosage increases, and interfere with the overall treatment outcome.

Other problems with TCA use in panic disorder are well documented and include anticholinergic effects, orthostatic hypotension, delayed onset of antipanic effects, and toxicity in overdose.[27] Approximately 25% of patients reportedly discontinue treatment because of side effects, especially weight gain.[27]

Dosing and Administration When using imipramine, treatment should be slowly increased by 10 mg every 2 to 4 days as tolerated (Table 53-8).

Selective Serotonin Reuptake Inhibitors

Efficacy Clinical studies indicate that all SSRIs are effective in panic disorder.[27] The percentage of patients who become panic-free ranges between 60% and 80%.[27] (4) The antipanic effect of SSRIs is delayed for at least 4 weeks, and some patients do not respond for 8 to 12 weeks.[27]

Adverse Effects Typical antidepressant doses of SSRIs can cause side effects of insomnia, jitteriness, restlessness, and agitation, and lead to drug discontinuation in patients with panic disorder. Other adverse effects associated with SSRI use in panic disorder are listed in Table 53-6.

Dosing and Administration Low initial doses of SSRIs are recommended (see Table 53-8) to avoid stimulatory side effects (e.g., insomnia or nervousness), and should be maintained for the first week of therapy. Doses at the upper end of the dosing range can be necessary to achieve response.[28]

Serotonin–Norepinephrine Reuptake Inhibitors

Efficacy Approximately 54% to 60% of patients were panic-free on venlafaxine extended-release 75 or 150 mg daily. The remission rates were 44% for both dosages in acute efficacy studies.[60]

Adverse Effects The most common adverse effects of venlafaxine extended-release in panic trials were nausea, dry mouth, constipation, anorexia, insomnia, somnolence, tremors, sweating, and sexual dysfunction.[27]

Dosing and Administration The dosage of venlafaxine extended-release is 37.5 mg/day for the first 3 to 7 days, and then increased

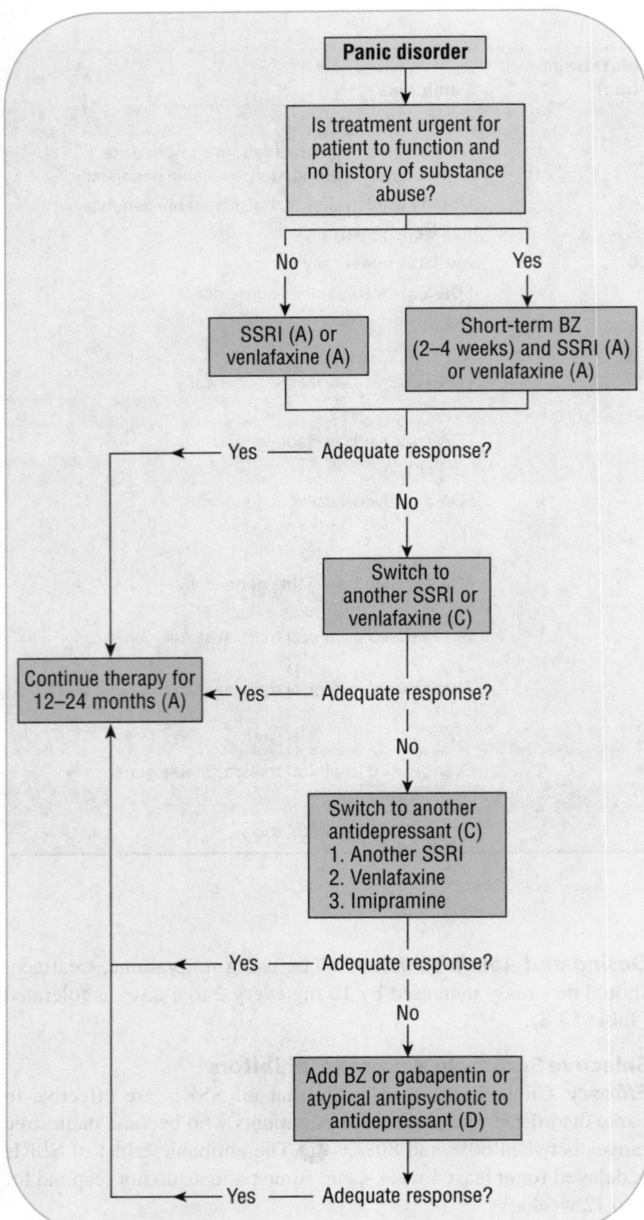

FIGURE 53-2 Algorithm for the pharmacotherapy of panic disorder. Strength of recommendations: A, directly based on category I evidence (i.e., meta-analysis of randomized controlled trials [RCT] or at least one RCT); B, directly based on category II evidence (i.e., at least one controlled study without randomization or one other type of quasi-experimental study); C, directly based on category III evidence (i.e., nonexperimental descriptive studies); D, directly based on category IV evidence (i.e., expert committee reports or opinions and/or clinical experience of respected authorities). (BZ, benzodiazepine; SSRI, selective serotonin reuptake inhibitor.) *(Data from references 27 and 28.)*

to a minimum of 75 mg/day (Table 53-8). Increasing the dose to 150 mg/day after initial nonresponse or partial response is recommended. A dose–response relationship was not evident in clinical trials.[38]

Benzodiazepines

Efficacy The high-potency benzodiazepines clonazepam and alprazolam are the preferred agents.[27,28] Diazepam and lorazepam are possibly effective in treating panic disorder when taken in sufficiently high doses.[27] Alprazolam provides rapid relief for patients in distress, but because of its short half-life, multiple daily dosing is required and often results in profound withdrawal symptoms with missed doses.[27] Therapeutic response to benzodiazepines occurs in 1 to 2 weeks. Relapse rates of 50% or higher are common despite slow drug tapering.[49]

Adverse Effects Patient acceptance of benzodiazepines usually is not a problem, and except for sedation, side effects are reported rarely (Table 53-6).

Dosing and Administration Doses of clonazepam can be increased by 0.25 or 0.5 mg every 3 days to 4 mg/day if needed.[45] Alprazolam can be slowly increased over several weeks to reach an ideal dose. **5** The duration of action of immediate-release alprazolam can be as little as 4 to 6 hours with resulting breakthrough symptoms; use of the extended-release alprazolam or clonazepam will avoid this problem. Most patients require 3 to 6 mg/day of alprazolam, and some need higher doses to obtain a full therapeutic (antipanic and antiphobic) response.

Clinical **Controversy. . .**

The role of long-term benzodiazepine use in the treatment of anxiety disorders is controversial. Most experts and regulatory guidelines recommend that use of benzodiazepines be limited to short-term in treatment of anxiety disorders because of the risk for tolerance, dose escalation, and dependence. Other experts argue that the benefits of long-term benzodiazepine use outweigh the potential adverse effects for most patients.

Treatment Resistance Common reasons for treatment failures are comorbid psychiatric disorders, rapid dosage increases with resulting intolerable side effects, and underdosage.[27] All standard treatments should be tried before using augmentation strategies. In patients with a partial response to one agent, a low dose of another antipanic agent (e.g., a TCA, benzodiazepine, or an SSRI) can be added.[27]

Phases of Therapy

Acute Phase The main goal of therapy in the acute phase is reduction of symptoms (e.g., resolution of panic attacks, reduction in anxiety and phobic fears, resumption of the patient's usual activities).[22,27] The duration of this phase is generally 1 to 3 months depending on the choice of drug. Therapy should be altered if there is no response after 6 to 8 weeks of an adequate dose.

The guiding principle for SSRIs and SNRIs in panic disorder is to start with low doses (approximately one fourth to one half of the starting doses for depression), use an adequate dose, and treat for about 12 weeks.[22,27] Adverse effects, often from too high an initial dose, can prevent achievement of an optimal dosage, compromise treatment response, and contribute to patient nonadherence.

The duration of the acute phase with benzodiazepines is approximately 1 month because response is rapid. A regular dosing schedule rather than an "as-needed" schedule is preferred for patients with panic disorder who are taking benzodiazepines, where the goal is to prevent panic attacks rather than reduce symptoms once an attack has already occurred.[27]

Maintenance Phase and Discontinuation **6** The optimal length of therapy is unknown; however, the total duration of therapy appears to be 12 to 24 months before drug discontinuation over 4 to 6 months is attempted.[27] The dose used in the acute phase is continued into the maintenance phase.[27] When drugs are discontinued too early, a high rate of relapse occurs; thus, longer periods of treatment are associated with a more sustained response. Reinstitution of drug usually results in renewed clinical response.[27] Pharmacotherapy, even at long duration, might not prevent relapse, and many patients require long-term therapy.

The most important determinant of adherence with maintenance therapy is the tolerability of adverse events.[27] Some adverse events that are experienced short term become unbearable during long-term management (e.g., sexual dysfunction and weight gain). TCAs, SSRIs (except fluoxetine), and venlafaxine can be associated with discontinuation symptoms.

The primary risk of long-term benzodiazepine use is the development of dependence and withdrawal reactions on discontinuation. Abuse of benzodiazepines usually is confined to patients with a personal or family history of substance or alcohol abuse.[5,48] The approach to benzodiazepine discontinuation involves a slow and gradual tapering of the dose because withdrawal symptoms and rebound anxiety may occur during discontinuation. Benzodiazepines should be tapered over 2 to 4 months at rates no higher than 10% of the dose per week.[27,49] Patients receiving benzodiazepines and antidepressants should be told not to decrease or discontinue therapy unless authorized by their clinician.[28]

Special Populations

Elderly patients with panic disorder have fewer, less intense symptoms and avoidant behavior than younger patients.[61] Youth often present with fear that they are dying or being smothered, and agoraphobia can be manifested as a fear of leaving home.[55] CBT is effective in both populations. If pharmacotherapy is used, antidepressants, especially the SSRIs, are preferred for management of panic disorder, and benzodiazepines are second-line agents because of potential problems with disinhibition in these two populations.

Personalized Pharmacotherapy

Research is evolving regarding pharmacogenetic properties related to benzodiazepine agents. While all benzodiazepines bind to the $GABA_A$ receptor, they have different physiochemical properties, most notably lipid solubility, which influence their pharmacokinetics, including rate of absorption and diffusion. Pharmacogenomic studies of benzodiazepines have focused on metabolizing enzymes. In particular, benzodiazepines are biotransformed by different cytochrome P450 isoforms and also by different UDP-glucuronosyltransferase subtypes. Evaluation of these factors in patients with genetic alterations in metabolism is an important part of personalized therapy. The most recent data available regarding research on the effects of pharmacogenetic properties of the benzodiazepines can be located online at The Pharmacogenomics Knowledgebase.[62]

Considerations that guide selection of the treatment modality for panic disorder include patient preference, past treatment history, the presence of co-occurring medical or other psychiatric conditions, cost, and treatment availability. Psychosocial treatment in the form of CBT is recommended for patients who prefer nonpharmacologic therapy and who are able to invest the effort and time to attend weekly sessions and between-session homework exercises. Pharmacotherapy with a first-line agent is recommended for patients who prefer medications or who do not have access to or resources to engage in CBT. Combination with psychotherapy and pharmacotherapy is appropriate for patients who have failed monotherapy with medication or CBT.

Providing education about the disorder may relieve some of the symptoms of panic by helping the patient to realize that the symptoms are neither life-threatening nor uncommon. Patients should be informed regarding the lag time before a therapeutic response will occur and any problematic side effects that might affect early adherence (i.e., jitteriness syndrome). Many patients are reluctant to take drugs for fear that their illness will worsen or that they will become addicted. Adverse events are often perceived as a worsening of the illness and can contribute to nonadherence or prevent necessary dosage increases. A strong therapeutic alliance between the clinician and the patient is important in supporting the patient through the aspects of the treatment that may provoke anxiety.

Evaluation of Therapeutic Outcomes

During the first few weeks of the acute phase of therapy, patients with panic disorder should be seen every 1 to 2 weeks when starting a new medication, and then every 2 to 4 weeks to adjust drug dosages based on improvement in panic symptoms and to monitor for adverse events.[27,28] After the dose is stabilized and symptoms have decreased, visits every 2 months should suffice.[28] The patient should be counseled to maintain a diary to record the date, time, frequency, duration, and intensity of panic episodes, level of anticipatory anxiety or agoraphobic avoidance, and the severity of distress and impairment related to the panic disorder. Treatment outcomes can be assessed objectively by use of the Panic Disorder Severity Scale. Remission is defined as equal to or less than 3 with no or mild agoraphobic avoidance, anxiety, disability, or depressive symptoms. Treatment response is indicated by a 40% or greater reduction in overall score.[29]

At scheduled visits, the clinician can inquire about the level of disability experienced by the patient and have the patient complete the Sheehan Disability Scale (with a goal of less than or equal to 1 point on each item). During drug discontinuation, the frequency of appointments should be increased to evaluate for emergence of potential withdrawal symptoms and monitor for relapse.

TREATMENT
Social Anxiety Disorder

Desired Outcomes

The goals of therapy in the acute phase of treatment are to reduce physiologic symptoms of anxiety (e.g., tachycardia, flushing, and sweating), social anxiety, and phobic avoidance. The duration of this phase is 4 to 12 weeks, depending on the drug therapy.

The goals of therapy in the continuation phase (3 to 6 months) are to extend the therapeutic benefits, especially the patient's ability to participate in social activities, and improve QOL. Although the primary goal of treatment is to reduce anxiety symptoms to manageable levels, even modest reductions in avoidance and discomfort can be highly valued by patients.[25]

7 At least a 1-year medication maintenance period is recommended to maintain improvement and decrease the rate of relapse.[2,26,29] Situations suggesting a possible need for long-term treatment include the presence of unresolved symptoms or comorbidity, an early onset of disease, and a prior history of relapse.[25] The long-term goal in the treatment of SAD is remission with the disappearance of the core symptoms of social anxiety, little or no anxiety, and no functional impairment or concurrent depressive symptoms.[25]

General Approach to Treatment

Patients with generalized SAD should be treated aggressively. Obstacles to effective treatment include patient avoidance of therapy secondary to fear and shame, treatment directed toward somatic symptoms or concurrent conditions, and financial barriers.[25,63] Patients with SAD often respond more slowly and less completely than patients with other anxiety disorders. Therefore, it is important to set reasonable expectations for response to therapy. Consideration of current symptoms, prior treatments, concurrent conditions, and history of substance abuse guide treatment selection.

CBT and pharmacotherapy are effective in the treatment of SAD.[3,25,63] Pharmacotherapy is often the most practical choice because CBT might not be available outside of large urban areas. Acute treatment outcomes for CBT and pharmacotherapy are equal.[3,29] Drug therapy is superior in reducing subjective general anxiety acutely, although CBT has a greater likelihood of maintaining response after termination.[29,63]

There are no data to predict which patients will respond best to pharmacotherapy, CBT, or a combination, or maintain gains after discontinuing pharmacotherapy. The only significant indication of treatment response in pharmacotherapy is duration of treatment.[25,26] Some patients elect lifelong therapy, and many are reluctant to attempt drug discontinuation because of fear of relapse.

Nonpharmacologic Therapy

Patients should be educated about SAD and support groups. Self-help group programs that focus on effective communication can benefit people with public speaking phobia.

CBT consists of exposure therapy, cognitive restructuring, relaxation training techniques, and social skills training.[3,25,26] Through CBT, patients learn to overcome anxiety in social situations and alter the beliefs and responses that maintain this anxiety. Therapy usually lasts several months and often is conducted in groups. In clinical trials, one-half to two-thirds of patients responded at 12 weeks.[25]

Clinical **Controversy...**

The question of which component of CBT is the most effective in the treatment of SAD is controversial. Recent evidence suggests that including a cognitive component is crucial. Individual therapy may be more effective than group therapy. Additional research is needed to determine the efficacy of CBT in the context of real-world experiences.

Pharmacologic Therapy

Antidepressant Therapy

8 The SSRIs and venlafaxine are beneficial for concurrent depression, and are safe when used in patients with substance abuse. Paroxetine, sertraline, venlafaxine extended-release, and fluvoxamine extended-release are approved for the treatment of generalized SAD, and are considered first-line agents because of efficacy and tolerability (Table 53-9). Controlled trials comparing different SSRIs, or SSRIs and an SNRI, demonstrated equivalent efficacy between agents.[25,63] TCAs are not effective in SAD.[25] Evidence-based guidelines for the treatment of SAD were published by the World Federation of Societies of Biological Psychiatry, the British Association for Psychopharmacology, the National Institute for Health and Clinical Excellent, and the Canadian Psychiatric Association.[3,22,29,64] An algorithm for the pharmacotherapy of generalized SAD appears in Figure 53-3.

Selective Serotonin Reuptake Inhibitors

Efficacy Large trials of escitalopram, fluvoxamine (immediate- and controlled-release), paroxetine, sertraline, and venlafaxine extended-release have shown efficacy and tolerability. Results of studies with fluoxetine have been inconsistent. The onset of effect was delayed 4 to 8 weeks, and maximum benefit was often not observed until 12 weeks or longer. Large relapse prevention trials with escitalopram, paroxetine, and sertraline demonstrated relapse rates of 4% to 14% with continued drug treatment, compared with 36% to 39% with placebo.[26]

Dosing and Administration SSRIs should be initiated at doses similar to those used for the treatment of depression and administered as a single daily dose (see Table 53-9). If the patient suffers from comorbid panic disorder, the SSRI dose should be started at one-fourth or one-half of the dose. The dose–response curve for SSRIs tends to be relatively flat, but individual patients can require

TABLE 53-9 Drugs Used in the Treatment of Generalized Social Anxiety Disorder

Drug	Brand Name	Initial Dose	Usual Range (mg/day)	Comments
Selective Serotonin Reuptake Inhibitors				
Citalopram	Celexa	20 mg/day	20–40	Dosage used in clinical trials; maximum dose of 40 mg limited by QT prolongation; available generically
Escitalopram	Lexapro	5 mg/day	10–20	Dosage used in clinical trials; available generically
Fluvoxamine CR	Luvox CR	100 mg	100–300	FDA-approved; available generically
Paroxetine	Paxil	10 mg/day	10–60	FDA-approved; available generically
Paroxetine CR	Paxil CR	12.5 mg/day	12.5–37.5	FDA-approved; available generically
Sertraline	Zoloft	25–50 mg/day	50–200	FDA-approved; available generically
Serotonin–Norepinephrine Reuptake Inhibitor				
Venlafaxine XR	Effexor XR	75 mg/day	75–225	FDA-approved; available generically
Benzodiazepine				
Clonazepam	Klonopin	0.25 mg/day	1–4	Dosage used in clinical trials; used as augmenting agent; available generically
Monoamine Oxidase Inhibitor				
Phenelzine	Nardil	15 mg at bedtime	60–90	Dosage used in clinical trials
Alternative Agents				
Buspirone	BuSpar	10 mg twice per day	45–60	Dosage used in clinical trials; used as augmenting agent; available generically
Gabapentin	Neurontin	100 mg three times a day	900–3,600	Dosage used in clinical trials; dosage adjustment required in renal impairment
Pregabalin	Lyrica	100 mg three times a day	600	Dosage used in clinical trials
Quetiapine	Seroquel	25 mg at bedtime	25–400	Dosage used in clinical trials

XR, extended-release; CR, controlled-release.

Data from references 3, 25, 26, and 64.

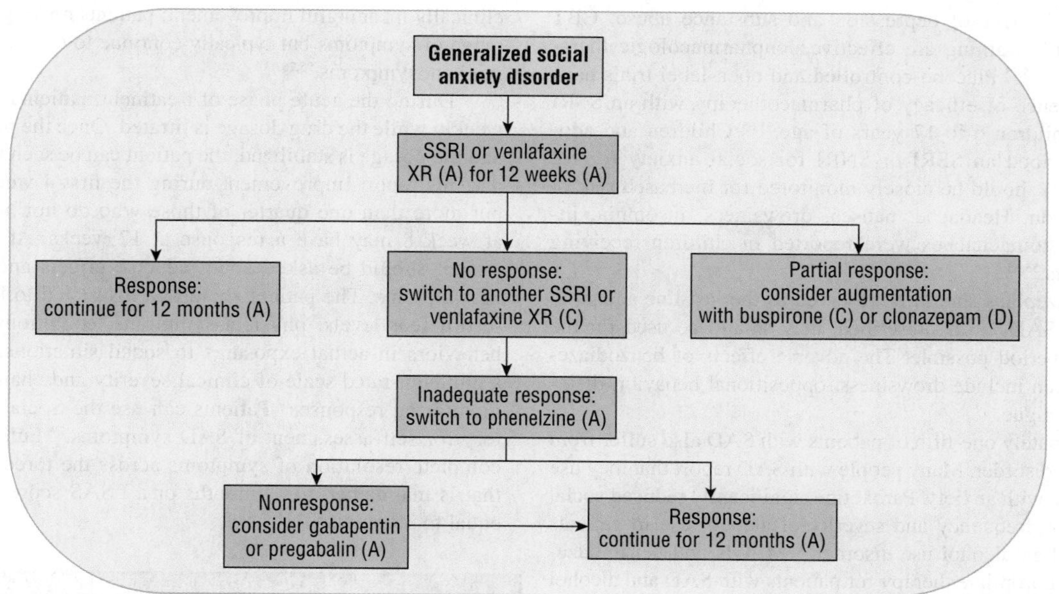

FIGURE 53-3 Algorithm for the pharmacotherapy of generalized social anxiety disorder. Strength of recommendations: A, directly based on category I evidence (i.e., meta-analysis of randomized controlled trials [RCT] or at least one RCT); B, directly based on category II evidence (i.e., at least one controlled study without randomization or one other type of quasi-experimental study); C, directly based on category III evidence (i.e., nonexperimental descriptive studies); D, directly based on category IV evidence (i.e., expert committee reports or opinions and/or clinical experience of respected authorities). (SSRI, selective serotonin reuptake inhibitor.) *(Data from references 3 and 26.)*

higher doses. Increase the dose as tolerated in patients who have not responded after 4 weeks of therapy.[26,63] When discontinuing an SSRI, the dosage should be tapered monthly (i.e., decreasing sertraline by 50 mg or paroxetine by 10 mg) to reduce the risk of relapse and discontinuation symptoms.

Venlafaxine

Efficacy The efficacy of venlafaxine extended-release was established in four double-blind, parallel-group, 12-week, multicenter, placebo-controlled, flexible-dose studies and one double-blind, parallel-group, 6-month, placebo-controlled, fixed/flexible-dose study.[38] Efficacy was assessed with the Liebowitz Social Anxiety Scale (LSAS). In these five trials, venlafaxine extended-release was significantly more effective than placebo on change from baseline to end point on the LSAS total score.[38]

Adverse Effects Adverse effects included anorexia, dry mouth, nausea, insomnia, and sexual dysfunction (Table 53-6).

Dosing and Administration Additional therapeutic benefits of venlafaxine extended-release above 75 mg/day were not shown.[38] Venlafaxine should be tapered slowly (i.e., decreasing by 37.5 mg/mo) to decrease the risk of relapse during discontinuation.

Alternative Agents

Benzodiazepines Benzodiazepines are commonly used in the treatment of patients who cannot tolerate or fail to respond to antidepressants. They are not considered first-line therapy for SAD because of concerns over the adverse effects, potential for dependence, the possibility of rebound anxiety, and ineffectiveness in the treatment of depression. Clonazepam is the most extensively studied benzodiazepine for the treatment of generalized SAD.[29]

If clonazepam is prescribed, the acute phase of therapy is about 1 month. Patients should be instructed not to decrease or discontinue clonazepam without consulting their clinician because of the risks of rebound anxiety and withdrawal symptoms. Patients on clonazepam for 6 months who were slowly tapered over 5 months maintained their treatment response.[26] Clonazepam should be gradually tapered at a rate not to exceed 0.25 mg every 2 weeks.

Anticonvulsants Gabapentin and pregabalin were effective in controlled trials, whereas levetiracetam was ineffective.[26]

β-Blockers β-Blockers decrease the perception of anxiety by blunting the peripheral autonomic symptoms of arousal (e.g., rapid heart rate, sweating, blushing, and tremor), and they are often used to decrease anxiety in performance-related situations. For patients with specific SAD, 10 to 80 mg of propranolol or 25 to 100 mg of atenolol can be taken 1 hour before a performance as needed.[25] A test dose should be taken at home before the presentation to assure that β-blockade is sufficient and there are no adverse events. Controlled trials with β-blockers do not support daily use in generalized SAD.[3,29]

Treatment Resistance 9 An adequate antidepressant trial usually consists of 8 to 12 weeks (at maximum dosages).[3,25,29] Subsequent options include a trial of a second SSRI or venlafaxine extended-release. Some patients experience clinical benefit during the first 4 weeks of therapy.[3,25,29] If nonresponsiveness continues, a trial of an alternative agent is warranted.

There are little data on the choice of treatments if antidepressants fail. Published studies offer preliminary support for the combination of an SSRI with a benzodiazepine, but not with pindolol.[26]

Atypical antipsychotics and MAOIs are options in treatment-resistant SAD. Quetiapine monotherapy showed a large effect size on the Social Phobia Inventory when compared with placebo.[63] Although phenelzine is effective in 77% of patients with SAD,[3,29] dietary restrictions, potential drug interactions, and adverse effects (e.g., weight gain and hypertensive crisis) have limited its use. If a patient is switched from another antidepressant to phenelzine, an appropriate washout period should be followed.

Special Populations

SAD can present in children of preschool to elementary school age. If the disorder is not treated, it can persist into adulthood and increase the risk of depression and substance abuse. CBT and social skills training are effective nonpharmacologic therapies in children.[55,65] Placebo-controlled and open-label trials have provided evidence of efficacy of pharmacotherapy with an SSRI or SNRI in children 6 to 17 years of age.[55,65] Children and adolescents prescribed an SSRI or SNRI for social anxiety (or for other purposes) should be closely monitored for increased risk of suicidal ideation. Headache, nausea, drowsiness, insomnia, jitteriness, and stomachaches were reported in children receiving antidepressants.[55,65]

Benzodiazepines should be reserved as the last-line agents in children with SAD.[55,65] If prescribed, they should be used for the shortest time period possible. The adverse effects of benzodiazepines in children include drowsiness, oppositional behavior, disinhibition, and fatigue.

Approximately one-fifth of patients with SAD also suffer from an alcohol use disorder. Many people with SAD report that they use alcohol to cope with anxiety. Paroxetine significantly reduced social anxiety and the frequency and severity of alcohol use in patients with SAD and an alcohol use disorder.[66] MAOIs and benzodiazepines are not appropriate therapy for patients with SAD and alcohol use disorder. SSRIs are the drugs of choice.

Personalized Pharmacotherapy

Despite the availability of effective treatments for social anxiety, most adults in the United States with social anxiety do not receive mental healthcare for their symptoms. Often the symptoms that patients desire to relieve interfere with the ability to seek treatment. Patients often feel embarrassed of what others might think or say about them. It is important to develop an alliance with the patient and offer reassurance throughout the treatment process.

Certain complications may influence the choice of first-line pharmacotherapy. Comorbid depression or suicidal ideation requires careful evaluation and close monitoring. Patients with comorbid substance abuse on presentation may require postponing pharmacotherapy until after detoxification and avoidance of use of benzodiazepines as part of treatment.

Patient-specific education about treatment is important. Patients should be instructed about the gradual onset of effect, when to expect full therapeutic benefit, and that long-term therapy is required. When drug therapy is discontinued, the dosage needs to be gradually decreased over several months, and the patient should be seen more frequently to monitor for signs and symptoms of relapse or withdrawal.

It is important to remember that although pharmacotherapy usually leads to improvement in social and occupational functioning, most patients do not achieve a full remission. Many patients require additional treatment, often in the form of CBT.

There is little evidence available to predict response to pharmacotherapy for social anxiety. Variation in a functional polymorphism known to influence 5-HT reuptake is associated with SSRI response in patients with generalized SAD. In a trial that evaluated whether variation in the 5-HT transporter gene promoter (5HTTLPR) influences the efficacy of SSRIs, a trend was seen for a linear association between 5HTTLPR genotype and likelihood of response to SSRI.[67] Reduction in social anxiety symptoms during SSRI treatment was significantly associated with 5HTTLPR genotype using either the diallelic or triallelic classification.[67]

Evaluation of Therapeutic Outcomes

10 The pharmacotherapy of SAD can be monitored in three principal domains: SAD symptoms (e.g., fears and physical symptoms), functionality, and well-being or overall improvement.[25,26,63] Response to pharmacotherapy in SAD is defined as a stable, clinically meaningful improvement; patients no longer have the full range of symptoms but typically continue to experience more than minimal symptoms.[25,26,63]

During the acute phase of treatment, patients should be seen weekly while the drug dosage is titrated. Once the patient responds and the dosage is stabilized, the patient can be seen monthly. Many patients report improvement during the first 4 weeks of therapy, but more than one quarter of those who do not have a response at week 8 may have a response at 12 weeks. At each visit, the patient should be asked about adverse effects and improvement in symptoms. The patient should be instructed to keep a diary to record fear levels, physical symptoms, cognitions, and anxious behaviors in actual exposures to social situations. The LSAS is a clinician-rated scale of clinical severity and change in SAD for monitoring response.[29] Patients can use the Social Phobia Inventory for self-assessment of SAD symptoms.[29] Full remission is a complete resolution of symptoms across the three SAD domains that is maintained for 3 months or a LSAS score of less than or equal to 30 points.[29]

TREATMENT
Specific Phobia

Specific phobia is considered unresponsive to drug therapy, although highly responsive to CBT. The use of benzodiazepines or paroxetine in patients who failed CBT is supported by limited data. Benzodiazepines can be detrimental in patients with specific phobias treated with CBT.[22]

CONCLUSIONS

Anxiety disorders are common in the population and occur concurrently with other psychiatric disorders. The proper management of anxiety disorders begins with the correct diagnosis; not all patients should receive antianxiety agents. Nonpharmacologic interventions often are effective alone or when combined with drug therapy.

There are several subtypes of anxiety disorders, and the diagnosis determines the type of drug and nonpharmacologic intervention selected. Although benzodiazepines remain the drugs of choice for situational anxiety, antidepressants have emerged as first-line therapy for GAD, panic disorder, and SAD. Benzodiazepines are reserved for use in situations requiring immediate anxiety relief during the first 2 to 4 weeks of therapy with a long-term agent such as an antidepressant. Antidepressants, including the SSRIs and SNRIs, and the benzodiazepines clonazepam and alprazolam are used extensively in patients with GAD, panic disorder, and SAD.

The long-term goal of therapy for GAD, panic disorder, and SAD is remission of core anxiety symptoms with no impairment in functionality, minimal anxiety, and no depressive symptoms. Augmentation with anticonvulsants and atypical antipsychotics show some promise in treatment-resistant cases.

ABBREVIATIONS

ACC	anterior cingulate cortex
CBT	cognitive behavioral therapy
CRF	corticotropin-releasing factor
DA	dopamine
DMDZ	desmethyldiazepam
GABA	γ-aminobutyric acid
GAD	generalized anxiety disorder
5-HT	serotonin

LC	locus ceruleus
LSAS	Liebowitz Social Anxiety Scale
MAOI	monoamine oxidase inhibitor
NE	norepinephrine
OCD	obsessive-compulsive disorder
PAG	periaqueductal gray
PTSD	posttraumatic stress disorder
QOL	quality of life
SAD	social anxiety disorder
SERT	serotonin reuptake transporter
SNRI	serotonin–norepinephrine reuptake inhibitor
SSRI	selective serotonin reuptake inhibitor
TCA	tricyclic antidepressant

REFERENCES

1. American Psychiatric Association. Diagnostic and Statistical Manual of Mental Disorders, Fourth Edition, Text Revision. Washington, DC: American Psychiatric Association, 2000: 429–484.
2. Craske MG, Roy-Byrne PP, Stein MB, et al. Treatment for anxiety disorders: Efficacy to effectiveness to implementation. Behav Res Ther 2009;47(11):931–937.
3. Bandelow B, Zohar J, Hollander E, et al. World Federation of Societies of Biological Psychiatry (WFSBP) guidelines for the pharmacological treatment of anxiety, obsessive-compulsive and post-traumatic stress disorders—First revision. World J Biol Psychiatry 2008;9(4):248–312.
4. Roy-Byrne PP, Davidson KW, Kessler RC, et al. Anxiety disorders and comorbid medical illness. Gen Hosp Psychiatry 2008;30:208–225.
5. Katzman MA. Current considerations in the treatment of generalized anxiety disorder. CNS Drugs 2009;23(2): 103–120.
6. National Comorbidity Survey Replication (NCS-R) Lifetime and 12-Month Prevalence Estimates. Data Updated July 9, 2007, *http://www.hcp.med.harvard.edu/ncs/index.php*.
7. Brandish EK, Baldwin DS. Anxiety disorders. Medicine 2012;40(11):599–606.
8. Smoller JW, Block SR, Young MM. Genetics of anxiety disorders: The complex road from DSM to DNA. Depress Anxiety 2009;26(11):965–975.
9. Davidson JR, Zhang W, Connor KM, et al. A psychopharmacological treatment algorithm for generalized anxiety disorder (GAD). J Psychopharm 2010;24(1):3–26.
10. Rogers MP, Wolfe DJ. Anxiety in the medical patient. Psychiatric Times 2007;24(3):1–4.
11. Martin EI, Ressler KJ, Binder E, et al. The neurobiology of anxiety disorders: Brain imaging, genetics, and psychoneuroendocrinology. Psychiatr Clin North Am 2009;32:549–575.
12. Damsa C, Losel M, Moussally J. Current status of brain imaging in anxiety disorders. Curr Opin Psychiatry 2009;22(1):96–110.
13. Matthew SJ, Price RB, Charney DS. Recent advances in the neurobiology of anxiety disorders: Implications for novel therapeutics. Am J Med Genet C Semin Med Genet 2008;148C(2):89–98.
14. Möhler H. GABA(A) receptor diversity and pharmacology. Cell Tissue Res 2006;326:505–516.
15. Pollack MH, Jensen JE, Simon NM, et al. High-field MRS study of GABA, glutamate and glutamine in social anxiety disorder: Response to treatment with levetiracetam. Prog Neuropsychopharmacol Biol Psychiatry 2008;32(3): 739–743.
16. Akimova E, Lanzenberger R, Kasper S. The serotonin-1A receptor in anxiety disorders. Biol Psychiatry 2009;66(7): 627–635.
17. van der Wee NJ, van Veen JF, Stevens H, et al. Increased serotonin and dopamine transporter binding in psychotropic medication-naive patients with generalized social anxiety disorder shown by 123I-beta-(4-iodophenyl)-tropane SPECT. J Nucl Med 2008;49(5):757–763.
18. Stein MB. Neurobiology of generalized anxiety disorder. J Clin Psychiatry 2009;70(Suppl 2):15–19.
19. Graeff FG, Del-Ben CM. Neurobiology of panic disorder: From animal models to brain neuroimaging. Neurosci Biobehav Rev 2008;32(7):1326–1335.
20. Etkin A, Wager TD. Functional neuroimaging of anxiety: A meta-analysis of emotional processing in PTSD, social anxiety disorder, and specific phobia. Am J Psychiatry 2007;164:1476–1488.
21. Freitas-Ferrari MC, Hallak JE, Trzesniak C, et al. Neuroimaging in social anxiety disorder: A systematic review of the literature. Prog Neuropsychopharmacol Biol Psychiatry 2010;34(4):565–580.
22. Baldwin DS, Anderson IM, Nutt DJ, et al. Evidence-based guidelines for the pharmacological treatment of anxiety disorders: Recommendations from the British Society for Psychopharmacology. J Psychopharmacol 2005;19: 567–596.
23. Katon WJ. Panic disorder. N Engl J Med 2006;354:2360–2367.
24. Perugi G, Frare F, Toni C. Diagnosis and treatment of agoraphobia with panic disorder. CNS Drugs 2007;21(9): 741–764.
25. Schneier FR. Social anxiety disorder. N Engl J Med 2006;355(10):1029–1036.
26. Stein MB, Stein DJ. Social anxiety disorder. Lancet 2008; 371:1115–1125.
27. American Psychiatric Association. Practice Guideline for the Treatment of Patients with Panic Disorder. Arlington, VA: American Psychiatric Association, 2009, *http://www.psychiatryonline.com/pracGuide/pracGuideTopic_9.aspx*.
28. National Institute for Clinical Excellence. Generalised Anxiety Disorder and Panic Disorder (with or without Agoraphobia) in Adults. Management in Primary, Secondary, and Community Care. NICE Clinical Guideline 113. January 2011, *http://guidance.nice.org.uk/CG113*.
29. Canadian Psychiatric Association. Clinical practice guidelines: Management of anxiety disorders. Can J Psychiatry 2006;51(8 Suppl 2):9S–91S.
30. Bostwick JR, Cusher MI, Yasugi S. Benzodiazepines: A versatile clinical tool. Clin Psychiatry 2012;11(4):55–64.
31. Benzodiazepine toolkit. Pharmacist's Letter/Prescriber's Letter 2011;27(4):270406.
32. Benzodiazepines. Facts and Comparisons® eAnswers (Online). Wolters Kluwer Health Inc, 2012, *http://www.factsandcomparisons.com/facts-comparisons-online.aspx*.
33. Lydiard RB, Rickels K, Herman B, et al. Comparative efficacy of pregabalin and benzodiazepines in treating the psychic and somatic symptoms of generalized anxiety disorder. Int J Neuropsychopharmacol 2010;13:229–241.
34. Gao K, Sheehan DV, Calabrese JR. Atypical antipsychotics in primary generalized anxiety disorder or comorbid with mood disorders. Expert Rev Neurother 2009;9(8):1147–1158.
35. Paxil [package insert]. Research Triangle Park, NC: GlaxoSmithKline, February 2012.
36. Cymbalta [package insert]. Indianapolis, IN: Eli Lily and Company, October 2012.
37. Lexapro [package insert]. St. Louis, MO: Forest Pharmaceuticals Inc, May 2011.

38. Effexor XR [package insert]. Philadelphia, PA: Wyeth Pharmaceuticals Inc, a subsidiary of Pfizer Inc, October 2012.
39. Vistaril [package insert]. New York: Pfizer Labs, February 2010.
40. The International Psychopharmacology Algorithm Project. IPAP—Generalized Anxiety Disorder Algorithm. *http://www.ipap.org/gad/index.php*.
41. Connor KM, Payne V, Davidson JRT. Kava in generalized anxiety disorder: Three placebo-controlled trials. Int Clin Psychopharmacol 2006;21:249–253.
42. Zoberti K, Pollard CA. Treating anxiety without SSRIs. J Fam Pract 2010;59(3):148–154.
43. Baldwin D, Woods R, Lawson R, Taylor D. Efficacy of drug treatments for generalized anxiety disorder: Systematic review and meta-analysis. BMJ 2011;342:d1199. doi:10.1136/bmj.d1199.
44. David DJ, Samuels BA, Rainer Q, et al. Neurogenesis-dependent and –independent effects of fluoxetine in an animal model of anxiety/depression. Neuron 2009;62(4): 479–493.
45. Klonopin [package insert]. San Francisco, CA: Genentech, August 2011.
46. Xanax XR [package insert]. New York, NY: Pharmacia and Upjohn Company Inc, August 2011.
47. Labbate LA, Fava M, Rosenbaum JF, Arana GW. Handbook of Psychiatric Therapy, 6th ed. Philadelphia, PA: Lippincott Williams & Wilkins, 2010:163–192.
48. Lader M. Benzodiazepines revisited—Will we ever learn? Addiction 2011;106:2086–2109.
49. Lader M, Tylee A, Donoghue J. Withdrawing benzodiazepines in primary care. CNS Drugs 2009;23(1): 19–34.
50. Gosselin P, Ladouceur R, Morin CM, et al. Benzodiazepine discontinuation among adults with GAD: A randomized trial of cognitive-behavioral therapy. J Consult Clin Psychol 2006;74:908–919.
51. Denis C, Fatseas M, Lavie E, et al. Pharmacological interventions for benzodiazepine mono-dependence in outpatient settings. Cochrane Database Syst Rev 2006;(3):CD005194.
52. Chessick C, Allen M, Thase M, et al. Azapirones for generalized anxiety disorder. Cochrane Database Syst Rev 2006;(3):CD006115.
53. Oyebode F, Rastogi A, Berrisford G, et al. Psychotropics in pregnancy: Safety and other considerations. Pharmacocol Ther 2012;135(1):71–77.
54. Bellantuono C, Tofani S, Di Sciascio G, Santone G. Benzodiazepine exposure in pregnancy and risk of major malformations: A critical overview. Gen Hosp Psychiatry 2013;35:3–8. doi:10.1016/j.genhosppsych.2012.09.003.
55. American Academy of Child and Adolescent Psychiatry. Practice parameter for the assessment and treatment of children and adolescents with anxiety disorders. J Am Acad Child Adolesc Psychiatry 2007;46(2):267–283.
56. Carter NJ, McCormack PL. Duloxetine: A review of its use in the treatment of generalized anxiety disorder. CNS Drugs 2009;23(6):523–541.
57. Mokhber N, Azarpazhooh MR, Khajehdaluee M, et al. Randomized, single-blind, trial of sertraline and buspirone for treatment of elderly patients with generalized anxiety disorder. Psychiatry Clin Neurosci 2010;64(2):128–133.
58. Montgomery S, Chatamra K, Pauer L, et al. Efficacy and safety of pregabalin in elderly people with generalised anxiety disorder. Br J Psychiatry 2008;193(5):389–394.
59. Andrisano C, Chiesa A, Serretti A. Newer antidepressants and panic disorder: A meta-analysis. Int Clin Psychopharmacol 2012;28:33–45.
60. Pollack MH, Lepola U, Koponen H, et al. A double-blind study of the efficacy of venlafaxine extended-release, paroxetine and placebo in the treatment of panic disorder. Depress Anxiety 2007;24:1–14.
61. Giacobbe P, Flint A. Panic disorder in the elderly. Aging Health 2007;3(2):245–255.
62. PharmGKB: The Pharmacogenomic Database. *http://www.pharmgkb.org/index.jsp*.
63. Jörstad-Stein EC, Heimberg RG. Social phobia: An update on treatment. Psychiatr Clin North Am 2009;32(3):641–663.
64. National Institute for Clinical Excellence. Social Anxiety Disorder: Recognition, Assessment and Treatment of Social Anxiety Disorder. NICE Clinical Guideline Draft. December 2012, *http://guidance.nice.org.uk/CG/Wave24/1#keydocs*.
65. Khan-Khalid S, Santibanez MP, McMicken C, Rynn MA. Social anxiety disorder in children and adolescents: Epidemiology, diagnosis, and treatment. Pediatr Drugs 2007;9(4):227–237.
66. Book SW, Thomas SE, Randall PK, Randall CL. Paroxetine reduces social anxiety in individuals with a co-occurring alcohol use disorder. J Anxiety Disord 2008;22(2):310–318.
67. Stein MB, Seedat S, Gelermter J. Serotonin transporter gene promotor polymorphism predicts SSRI response in generalized social anxiety disorder. Psychopharmacology 2006;187:68–72.

Anxiety Disorders II: Posttraumatic Stress Disorder and Obsessive-Compulsive Disorder

54

Cynthia K. Kirkwood, Sarah T. Melton, and Barbara G. Wells

KEY CONCEPTS

1. The short-term goal in posttraumatic stress disorder (PTSD) is reduction in core symptoms, while the long-term goal is remission.
2. Cognitive behavioral therapy and eye movement desensitization and reprocessing are the most effective nonpharmacologic methods to reduce symptoms of PTSD.
3. The selective serotonin reuptake inhibitors (SSRIs) and venlafaxine are considered first-line treatments for PTSD.
4. An adequate trial of SSRIs in PTSD requires appropriate dosing and duration of treatment.
5. Patients with PTSD who respond to pharmacotherapy should continue treatment for at least 12 months.
6. SSRIs are the drugs of choice for the treatment of obsessive-compulsive disorder (OCD).
7. Augmentation of SSRI treatment with low doses of antipsychotics may be helpful.
8. If an inadequate response to an SSRI for OCD occurs after 4 to 6 weeks at the maximum dose, switch to another SSRI.
9. Medication taper can be considered after 1 to 2 years of treatment in patients with OCD.

Traumatic world or local events (e.g., wars, terrorist attacks, natural disasters, kidnappings, interpersonal violence) can lead to development of posttraumatic stress disorder (PTSD). Initially diagnosed in veterans of war, PTSD is now acknowledged as a significant psychiatric illness in the civilian population and more recently among deployed service personnel of the Afghanistan and Iraq campaigns in whom the suicide rate has escalated.[1–3] PTSD continues to be poorly recognized and diagnosed in clinical practice.[4] Because of its co-occurrence with other anxiety disorders, depression, substance abuse, and traumatic brain injury, the overlapping symptoms can lead to diagnostic uncertainty. Advances in the science and treatment of PTSD can assist clinicians in all fields of healthcare to screen patients for a history of trauma and effectively manage PTSD if it is present.

Intrusive obsessive thoughts and compulsive ritualistic behaviors characterize obsessive-compulsive disorder (OCD). OCD can be severely debilitating and impair functioning in social, family, and work settings, with an overall decrease in quality of life (QOL). OCD is associated with an increased risk of suicide, with 15% of patients reporting a previous history of suicide attempt.[5] Increased understanding of symptom dimensions and treatment response can improve QOL in patients suffering from OCD.

EPIDEMIOLOGY

The estimated lifetime prevalence of PTSD is 6.8% in the U.S. population.[6] Lifetime prevalence of OCD has been estimated at 2.3% in the general population and 2% to 4% in the pediatric population.[7,8]

PTSD is associated with the incidence of trauma. It is estimated that approximately 60% of men and 50% of women are exposed to a life-threatening traumatic event.[6] Of these individuals 8.2% of men and 20% of women will develop PTSD. Previous exposure to a trauma and the intensity of response to the event increase the risk of PTSD. Men tend to be assaulted more frequently, but women have a higher rate of PTSD after assaults being more likely to experience rape and sexual abuse.[6] Genetic factors can increase vulnerability to PTSD if an individual is exposed to a traumatic event. Offspring of Holocaust survivors had a higher lifetime prevalence rate of PTSD compared with a control group.[6]

The epidemiology of OCD is influenced by age and gender. OCD typically begins early in life, with 20% of cases occurring in childhood, 29% in adolescence, and 49% of cases occurring by age 20.[1] Age of onset has a bimodal distribution with peaks around 10 and 21 years.[7] The onset of illness is earlier in men than in women.[8] Higher rates of other anxiety disorders are reported in first-degree relatives of patients with OCD.[9] Early age of onset has been associated with higher probabilities of comorbid impulse control, somatoform, eating, and tic disorders.[10] Heredity is stronger when there is an early age of onset or comorbidity with tic disorder.[11]

ETIOLOGY

The exact etiologies of PTSD and OCD are not known. It is likely that abnormalities in several areas of brain functioning interact to cause these chronic anxiety disorders. Genetics may play a role in expression of PTSD and OCD, but environmental factors likely are also involved. A genome-wide association study did not detect any single nucleotide polymorphisms (SNPs) associated with OCD but there was a significant enrichment of methylation quantitative trait loci (mQTLs) and frontal lobe expression of quantitative trait loci (eQTLs) in the highest ranked autosomal SNPs, suggesting that these signals may influence gene expression and perhaps the etiology of OCD.[11] Genetic etiologies of both PTSD and OCD are current research areas.

Controversy exists over the existence of a subtype of OCD characterized as a pediatric autoimmune neuropsychiatric disorder associated with streptococcal infections (PANDAS). A relationship between the sudden onset of OCD and chronic tic disorder with an age of onset between 3 years and puberty with possible exacerbations and remissions, and a temporal association with streptococcal infection associated with symptoms of OCD or neurologic abnormalities has been proposed.[12] Although most patients with OCD do not have a streptococcal etiology, an accurate medical history regarding onset of illness is imperative because specific treatment strategies are indicated.

PATHOPHYSIOLOGY

Research findings in the areas of neuroendocrinology, neurobiology, and neuroimaging have advanced a number of theories on the pathophysiology of anxiety disorders. Neuroendocrine changes in the hypothalamic–pituitary–adrenal (HPA) axis are implicated in the pathophysiology of PTSD.[13] As reviewed in Chapter 53, data from neurochemical and neuroimaging studies indicate that the modulation of normal and pathologic anxiety states is associated with multiple regions of the brain (e.g., amygdala, hippocampus, thalamus, and prefrontal cortex).[13,14] Abnormal function in several neurotransmitter systems, including norepinephrine (NE), γ-aminobutyric acid (GABA), glutamate, dopamine (DA), and serotonin (5-HT), may affect the manifestations of anxiety disorders.[13,15]

Neuroendocrine Theories

Neuroendocrine studies provide data that abnormalities occurring pretrauma, during trauma, and posttrauma contribute to PTSD. Normally the immediate reaction to stress occurs as an automatic response from the amygdala to the sympathetic and parasympathetic systems and the HPA axis.[13] The release of corticotropin-releasing factor (CRF) stimulates cortisol secretion from the adrenal gland. Both catecholamines and cortisol levels rise in tandem. Cortisol reduces the stress response by tempering the sympathetic reaction through negative feedback on the pituitary and hypothalamus.[13] These systems return to normal after a few hours.

Recent data implicate a role for the neuropeptides CRF and neuropeptide Y (NPY) in PTSD. Patients with PTSD have a hypersecretion of CRF but demonstrate subnormal levels of cortisol at the time of trauma and chronically.[13] Lower plasma cortisol concentrations were associated with greater severity of PTSD symptoms in nonmilitary patients.[15] Dysregulation of the HPA axis is postulated to be a risk factor for eventual development of PTSD.[13] Higher plasma concentrations of NPY were found in combat-exposed men who did not develop PTSD and could play a role in resiliency.[15]

Neurochemical Theories

Several neurotransmitters may be involved in the pathophysiology of PTSD. 5-HT, NE, and glutamate are associated with the processing of emotional and somatic contents of memories in the amygdala. The cortex and hippocampus are involved in storing the facts and related cues of memory.[15] The noradrenergic theory posits that the autonomic nervous system of anxious patients is hypersensitive and overreacts to stimuli. The alarm center, the locus ceruleus, releases NE to stimulate the sympathetic and parasympathetic nervous systems. Hyperactive noradrenergic signaling in patients with PTSD is a consistent research finding and includes increased 24-hour catecholamine excretion.[15] Glutamate signaling abnormalities may result in distortion of amygdala-dependent emotional processing under stress.[13,15] Dysregulation of the processing of sensory input and memories may contribute to the dissociative and hypervigilant symptoms in PTSD. Abnormalities of GABA inhibition may lead to increased awareness or response to stress, as seen in PTSD.[15]

Both 5-HT and DA are implicated in the pathogenesis of OCD. Selective and potent serotonergic reuptake inhibitors have consistently been shown effective for symptoms of the illness.[16–19] A recent meta-analysis concluded that higher doses of selective serotonin reuptake inhibitors (SSRIs) were associated with improved efficacy in the treatment of OCD.[19] A Cochrane systematic review of 17 studies found that SSRIs were more effective than placebo in treating symptoms of OCD, and that SSRIs were similar to each other in efficacy.[18] DA dysregulation may contribute to some forms of OCD. Neurologic symptoms (e.g., tics) are part of the clinical presentation in some patients with OCD. Tourette's disorder, a disorder of DA function, is often a concurrent disease.[1] Augmentation with antipsychotic drugs may improve symptoms in patients with OCD who are partially responsive to SSRIs.[20]

Neuroimaging Studies

Neuroimaging studies suggest that certain areas of the brain are altered by psychological trauma. In PTSD most functional neuroimaging studies have involved the amygdala, ventromedial prefrontal cortex (vmPFC), dorsal anterior cingulate cortex (dACC), and hippocampus. Findings of increased activation of the amygdala after trauma-related imagery, sounds, or smells indicate that this structure plays a role in the persistence of traumatic memory.[14] Decreased amygdala activation is correlated with resilience to PTSD and response to cognitive behavioral therapy (CBT).[14] Hypofunctioning of the vmPFC is theorized to prevent extinction in patients with PTSD and is inversely correlated with severity of symptoms.[14] Hyperresponsivity of the dACC and the insular cortex may correlate with impaired response to emotional stimuli or those that predict threat. The most consistent findings are decreased hippocampus volumes and *N*-acetylaspartate levels in patients with PTSD.[13,14] In twin studies, the unaffected twin of patients with PTSD also demonstrated smaller hippocampi compared with twins without PTSD. These findings suggest that lower hippocampal volumes in patients with PTSD are likely a precursor associated with vulnerability for subsequent development of PTSD.[13]

Neuroimaging studies suggest that dysfunction in the cortical–striatal–thalamic circuits is responsible for impulsive behavior and inability to regulate socially acceptable behaviors.[21] Drugs that decrease hyperactivity in the cortical–striatal–thalamic circuits decrease symptoms of OCD.[11,22] Glutamate may play a role in OCD symptomatology.[23]

CLINICAL PRESENTATION

The *Diagnostic and Statistical Manual of Mental Disorders, Fourth Edition, Text Revision* classifies anxiety disorders into several categories: generalized anxiety disorder, panic disorder (with or without agoraphobia), social anxiety disorder, specific phobia, OCD, PTSD, and acute stress disorder (ASD).[1] The characteristic features of these illnesses are anxiety and avoidance behavior. Generalized anxiety disorder, panic disorder, and social anxiety disorder are discussed in Chapter 53.

Posttraumatic Stress Disorder

Exposure to a traumatic event is required for a diagnosis of PTSD.[1] The person must have witnessed, experienced, or been confronted with a situation that involved definite or threatened death or serious injury, or possible harm to himself or herself or others. The patient's response to the trauma must include intense fear, helplessness, or horror.[1] Some examples of traumatic events include physical attacks by an intimate partner, traffic accidents, military combat, earthquakes, being held hostage, child sexual abuse, and witnessing a murder or injury of another.

The resulting PTSD symptoms include persistent reexperiencing of the traumatic event, avoidance of stimuli associated with the trauma, numbing of general responsiveness, and persistent symptoms of hyperarousal. Patients must have at least one reexperiencing symptom, at least three signs or symptoms of persistent avoidance

CLINICAL PRESENTATION Posttraumatic Stress Disorder

Reexperiencing Symptoms

- Recurrent, intrusive distressing memories of the trauma
- Recurrent, disturbing dreams of the event
- Feeling that the traumatic event is recurring (e.g., dissociative flashbacks)
- Physiologic reaction to reminders of the trauma

Avoidance Symptoms

- Avoidance of conversations about the trauma
- Avoidance of thoughts or feelings about the trauma
- Avoidance of activities that are reminders of the event
- Avoidance of people or places that arouse recollections of the trauma
- Inability to recall an important aspect of the trauma
- Anhedonia
- Estrangement from others
- Restricted affect
- Sense of a foreshortened future (e.g., does not expect to have a career, marriage)

Hyperarousal Symptoms

- Decreased concentration
- Easily startled
- Hypervigilance
- Insomnia
- Irritability or anger outbursts

Subtypes

- Acute: duration of symptoms is less than 3 months
- Chronic: symptoms last for longer than 3 months
- With delayed onset: onset of symptoms is at least 6 months posttrauma

Data from references 1 and 25.

of stimuli associated with the trauma, and at least two symptoms of increased arousal.[1] Symptoms from each category need to be present for longer than 1 month and cause significant distress or impairment in functioning. Most persons diagnosed with PTSD also meet criteria for another mental disorder.[1]

Anxiety and dissociative symptoms (e.g., absence of emotional responsiveness, derealization, inability to recall important features of the trauma) emerging within 1 month after exposure to a traumatic stressor are classified as ASD. Symptoms of ASD are experienced during or immediately after the trauma, last for at least 2 days, and resolve within 4 weeks.[1]

The age of onset and course of PTSD are variable. PTSD can occur at any age. The presentation is not predictable because symptoms are related to the duration and intensity of the trauma, the presence of other psychiatric disorders, and how the patient deals with the trauma. Symptoms emerge soon after a traumatic event and either dissipate or chronically persist in survivors.[24] About 95% of patients who recover do so within a year, and 40% have persistent symptoms 6 years later. PTSD co-occurs with mood, anxiety, and substance use disorders. The course of illness is fluctuating, worsening with life stressors.[24]

Obsessive-Compulsive Disorder

Patients with OCD exhibit a great variety of symptoms on presentation to clinicians. The diversity and oddity of symptoms that manifest can obscure accurate diagnosis and delay appropriate treatment of the disorder. Patients can be secretive about symptoms and purposefully refuse to report symptoms.[5] Patients can present in a seemingly incongruous manner to nonpsychiatrists for other complaints—dermatologists for eczema or chapped skin, pediatricians for parental concerns over a child's compulsive hand washing, neurologists for tics, or dentists for gum lesions from compulsive teeth brushing.

The diagnostic criteria for OCD require the presence of obsessions and/or compulsions (although most patients have both) that are severe enough to cause marked distress, to be time-consuming (occupy more than 1 hour/day), and to cause significant impairment in social or occupational functioning.[1] An obsession is a recurrent, persistent idea, thought, impulse, or image that is experienced as intrusive and inappropriate and produces marked anxiety. Common obsessions involve thoughts about contamination (e.g., concern with germs or dirt) and repeated doubts.[1]

CLINICAL PRESENTATION Obsessive-Compulsive Disorder

Obsessions

- Repetitive thoughts (e.g., feeling contaminated after touching an object, doubting whether the stove was turned off)
- Repetitive images (e.g., recurrent sexually explicit pictures)
- Repetitive impulses (e.g., need for symmetry or putting things in specific order, impulse to shout out obscenities in a church)

Compulsions

- Repetitive activities (e.g., hand washing, checking, ordering, need to ask, need to confess)
- Repetitive mental acts (e.g., counting, repeating words silently, praying)

Data from references 1 and 5.

Individuals must recognize that their obsessions or compulsions are excessive or unreasonable. Obsessions must be acknowledged as products of the individual's own mind, and attempts must be made to ignore or suppress them. The obsessions produce marked feelings of anxiety and are not simply excessive worry about a real-life situation.[1]

A compulsion is defined as a repetitive behavior or mental act generally performed in response to an obsession. Diagnostically, compulsive behavior is not pleasurable and is designed to prevent discomfort or the occurrence of a dreaded event that is often unknown. For example, many patients are obsessed with feelings of doubt (e.g., whether a door was left unlocked), causing them marked distress and leading to repetitive checking (or compulsive behaviors). These behaviors are usually performed according to certain rules or in a stereotyped fashion. Because patients recognize their compulsive behavior as silly or senseless, they become extremely adept at denying symptoms, disguising their rituals, and concealing their illness from friends and family.[1]

Patients with OCD often have concurrent depression, other anxiety disorders, and substance abuse. It is a chronic illness in most patients, with severity of symptoms varying in intensity over time. Many patients with OCD have significantly impaired QOL and ability to function.[5]

TREATMENT
Posttraumatic Stress Disorder

Desired Outcome

❶ The short-term goal of therapy in the management of PTSD is reduction in core symptoms (i.e., intrusive reexperiencing, avoidance, and hyperarousal). Patients should also have improvements in disability, concurrent psychiatric conditions, and QOL. The long-term goal in PTSD is remission.

General Approach to Treatment

In general, patients who seek treatment acutely after a trauma and are in intense distress should receive therapy based on their presenting symptoms (e.g., a nonbenzodiazepine hypnotic for difficulty sleeping). Short courses of exposure-based, trauma-focused cognitive behavioral therapy (TFCBT) can be helpful to prevent chronic PTSD in patients who present during the first 3 months of the event.[26] If symptoms (e.g., hyperarousal, avoidance, dissociation, sleep difficulties, or depressed mood) persist for 3 to 4 weeks and the patient experiences marked social, occupational, and/or interpersonal impairment, they can be treated with pharmacotherapy, psychotherapy, or both. Many patients with PTSD will improve substantially with pharmacotherapy but retain some symptoms. Treatment regimens usually combine psychoeducation, psychosocial support and/or treatment, and pharmacotherapy.[24,25]

Nonpharmacologic Therapy

Psychotherapy can be used when a patient suffers from mild symptoms, in patients who prefer not to use medications, or in conjunction with drugs in patients with severe symptoms to improve response. Patients who have experienced trauma should be educated that they can experience anxiety, depression, nightmares, and even flashbacks as a reaction to the event. Brief courses of prolonged exposure, a form of CBT, in close proximity to the traumatic event resulted in lower rates of PTSD 3 and 6 months later.[4,26] Single-session critical incident stress debriefing was not shown to be effective in preventing development of PTSD and actually can cause harm.[26,27]

❷ Psychotherapies for treating PTSD include stress management, TFCBT, eye movement desensitization and reprocessing (EMDR), and psychoeducation.[28] Short-term reductions in symptoms can be achieved with stress management, group therapy, hypnosis, or psychodynamic therapy.[27,28] The cognitive and behavioral approaches of TFCBT and EMDR are more effective than stress management or group therapy to reduce symptoms of PTSD.[28] Psychoeducation includes information about the disease state, treatment options, and avoidance of excessive use of alcohol and other substances of abuse. Novel nonpharmacologic approaches (e.g., interpersonal psychotherapy, narrative exposure therapy, imagery modification) and delivery methods (e.g., telemedicine, computer-delivered CBT) are under study.[29]

Pharmacologic Therapy

❸ Antidepressants are the major pharmacotherapeutic treatment for PTSD. In addition to their efficacy in PTSD, these agents are also effective for concurrent depression and anxiety disorders. SSRIs and venlafaxine are the first-line pharmacotherapy of PTSD.[27,30–32] The tricyclic antidepressants (TCAs) and monoamine oxidase inhibitors (MAOIs) can also be effective, but they have less favorable side effect profiles (Table 54-1). Both sertraline and paroxetine are approved for the acute treatment of PTSD,[33,34] and sertraline is approved for the long-term (i.e., 52 weeks) management of PTSD.[34] A number of drugs can be used as augmentation agents (e.g., antiadrenergic drugs and atypical antipsychotics).[31,32] Benzodiazepines are not effective for PTSD.[31,32] A number of treatment guidelines are published.[35] Table 54-2 provides a summary of key points from the treatment guidelines for PTSD. An algorithm for the treatment of PTSD appears in Figure 54-1.

Antidepressant Therapy

Selective Serotonin Reuptake Inhibitors SSRIs act pharmacologically to enhance serotonergic functioning. Large prospective studies documented the efficacy of sertraline and paroxetine in the acute management of PTSD. Approximately 60% of the patients show

TABLE 54-1 Dosing of Antidepressants in the Treatment of Posttraumatic Stress Disorder

Drug	Brand Name	Initial Dose	Usual Range (mg/day)	Comments
Selective Serotonin Reuptake Inhibitors				
Fluoxetine[a]	Prozac®	10 mg/day	10–40[b]	
Paroxetine[a]	Paxil®, Pexeva®	10–20 mg/day	20–40[b]	Maximum dose is 50 mg/day[c]
Sertraline[a]	Zoloft®	25 mg/day	50–100	Maximum dose is 200 mg/day[c]
Other Agents				
Amitriptyline[a]	Elavil®	25 or 50 mg/day	75–200[b]	
Imipramine[a]	Tofranil®	25 or 50 mg/day	75–200[b]	
Mirtazapine[a]	Remeron®	15 mg/night	30–60[b]	
Phenelzine[a]	Nardil®	15 or 30 mg every night	45–90[b]	
Venlafaxine extended-release[a]	Effexor XR®	37.5 mg/day	75–225[b]	

[a]Available generically.
[b]Dosage used in clinical trials but not FDA-approved.
[c]Dosage is FDA-approved.

Data from references 31, 33, and 34.

TABLE 54-2 Summary of Key Points in Treatment Guidelines for the Pharmacologic Treatment of Posttraumatic Stress Disorder

Recommendation	Level of Evidence	Comments
First-line Treatments		
SSRIs: fluoxetine, paroxetine, sertraline	I	At 4 weeks if there is partial response, continue for another 4 weeks. At 8 weeks, if no improvement, increase dose to maximum tolerated or switch to another first-line treatment
SNRIs: venlafaxine	I	
Second-line Treatments		
TCAs: amitriptyline, imipramine	II	The risk of adverse effects and potential for fatalities in a TCA overdose are higher than with SSRIs or SNRIs
Other: mirtazapine	II	
Augmentation with prazosin for sleep/nightmares	II[27]	Recommended in the VA guidelines[27]
Augmentation with risperidone	II[31]	The VA guidelines[27] recommend against using risperidone as an augmenting agent secondary to metabolic adverse effects. There is insufficient evidence to support use of other atypical antipsychotics
Third-Line treatments		
MAOIs: phenelzine	IV[31]	The VA guidelines[27] recommend phenelzine to be used cautiously (Level III)

Levels of evidence: I, strong recommendation, full evidence from controlled trials; II, recommended, limited positive evidence from controlled trials; III, may be recommended, evidence from uncontrolled trials or case reports/expert opinion; IV, evidence is insufficient to recommend, inconsistent findings.

Data from references 27 and 31.

improvement.[30] In general, SSRIs reduced the numbing symptoms of PTSD, whereas other drugs did not. Adverse reactions reported in patients with PTSD treated with SSRIs include GI symptoms, sexual dysfunction, insomnia, and agitation. Long-term use of SSRIs (durations of 9 to 12 months) was effective in preventing relapse.[30–32]

Other Antidepressants The serotonin–norepinephrine reuptake inhibitor (SNRI) venlafaxine has shown efficacy in PTSD. In a 12-week, placebo-controlled trial comparing venlafaxine extended-release and sertraline, venlafaxine was effective in reducing the avoidance/numbing and hyperarousal clusters of PTSD, whereas sertraline improved all PTSD symptom clusters.[36] The remission rates for venlafaxine extended-release were 30.2% after 12 weeks[36] and 50.1% after 6 months.[37]

Other antidepressants have been studied in controlled trials. Mirtazapine was effective on global ratings of symptoms in 64% of patients with PTSD in doses up to 45 mg/day and is considered a second-line agent.[27,31] Bupropion sustained-release was not effective in patients with chronic PTSD.[38]

The TCAs amitriptyline and imipramine are also considered second-line agents, and the MAOI phenelzine is considered a third-line antidepressant if therapeutic trials of SSRIs or venlafaxine have failed. TCAs are associated with a higher burden of adverse effects compared with SSRIs (e.g., daytime drowsiness, toxicity in overdose, and poor compliance).[27,31]

Alternative Drug Treatments

Atypical antipsychotics, α_1-adrenergic antagonists, antidepressants, mood stabilizers, and anticonvulsants can be used as augmenting agents for persistent symptoms, in cases of partial response to SSRI therapy after 4 to 6 weeks, or for comorbidities.[39] Risperidone reduced PTSD symptoms in combat veterans on antidepressants with and without psychosis.[40] Olanzapine added adjunctively to SSRIs decreased PTSD symptoms and significantly improved sleep compared with placebo. Patients gained an average of 13.2 lb

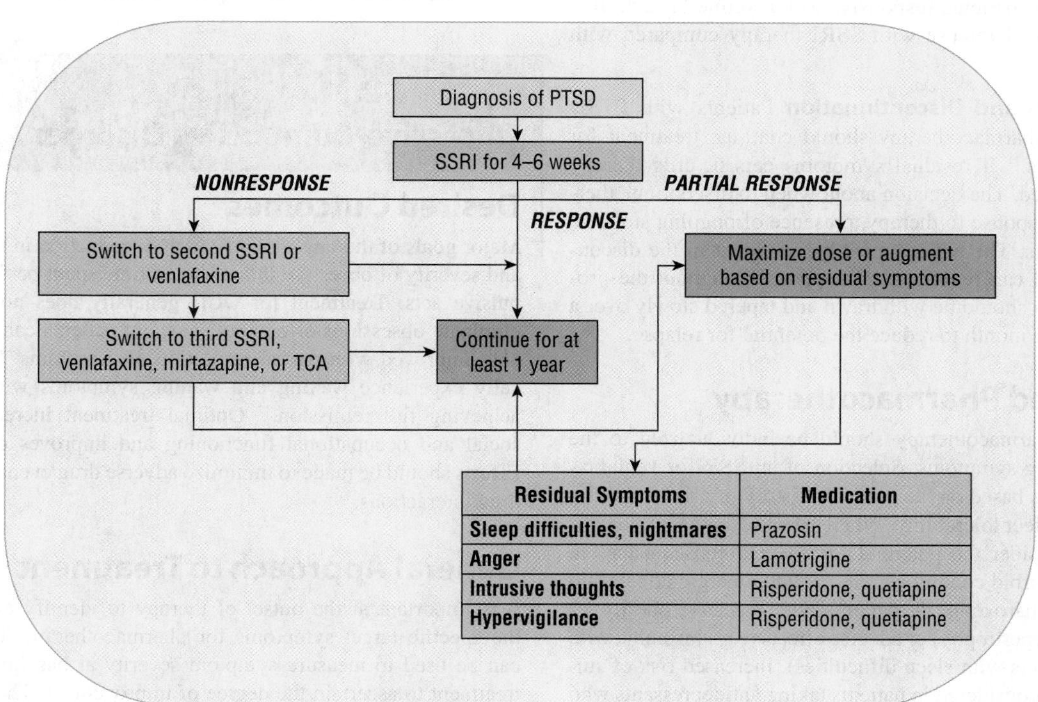

FIGURE 54-1 Algorithm for the pharmacotherapy of posttraumatic stress disorder (PTSD). *(Data from references 27 and 31.)*

(6 kg) over the course of the 8-week trial.[40] Quetiapine reduced core PTSD symptoms over an 8-week period when added to concurrent therapy.[41] Overall there is a modest positive effect of risperidone and quetiapine in double-blind trials with intrusive and hypervigilance symptoms showing the most improvement.[42]

Prazosin can be useful in some patients with PTSD. It decreased nightmares and sleep disturbances and improved the core PTSD symptoms in daily doses of 1 to 4 mg. Its presumed mechanism of action is reduction of noradrenergic transmission.[43,44] Other options for persistent sleep disturbances with less evidence include trazodone, mirtazapine, and atypical antipsychotics.[44]

Anticonvulsants can assist in reducing impulsive anger and can also be used in patients with comorbid bipolar disorder. Some data support efficacy of lamotrigine as an augmenting agent. Data with other anticonvulsants are inconsistent.[39] The use of an anticonvulsant is not recommended as monotherapy.[27]

Special Populations

Children who experience stress and trauma (e.g., sexual or physical abuse or loss of a parent) are predisposed to develop mood and anxiety disorders. SSRIs are the initial pharmacologic agents of choice in this patient population. Psychotherapy is also a treatment option (e.g., play therapy).[45]

Dosage and Administration

Acute Phase PTSD symptoms respond slowly to pharmacotherapy, and some patients never experience full resolution. SSRIs should be started 3 to 4 weeks after exposure to a trauma in patients with no improvement in their acute stress response. The initiation of an SSRI should be at a low dose with gradual titration upward toward antidepressant doses. ❹ Eight to 12 weeks is an appropriate duration of antidepressant therapy to determine response.[27,46]

Continuation Phase Many patients are undergoing psychotherapy during the continuation phase of therapy, and dosages can vary as patients deal with past traumatic experiences. During this phase symptoms continue to improve, and the maximal drug benefit (i.e., improvement of disability) accrues.[46] Six-month relapse prevention trials in patients responsive to fluoxetine or sertraline indicate low rates of relapse with SSRI therapy compared with placebo.[46]

❺ **Maintenance and Discontinuation** Patients with PTSD who respond to pharmacotherapy should continue treatment for at least 12 months.[31] If residual symptoms persist, drug therapy should be continued. The decision about when to discontinue therapy is based on response to therapy, presence of ongoing stresses, and adverse effects. The patient must be confident in the discontinuation plan and can require extra support throughout the process. Drug therapy should be withdrawn and tapered slowly over a period of at least 1 month to reduce the potential for relapse.

Personalized Pharmacotherapy

The choice of pharmacotherapy should be individualized to the patient's presenting symptoms. Selection of an SSRI or venlafaxine monotherapy is based on the patient's history of prior response, safety, and side effect tolerability. When selecting an agent, the clinician should consider the potential for adverse consequences in patients with comorbid conditions (e.g., anticholinergic effects and weight gain with paroxetine in patients with diabetes, obesity, or benign prostatic hypertrophy) or adverse effects (e.g., insomnia with fluoxetine in patients with sleep difficulties). Increased risk of suicidality should be considered in patients taking antidepressants who are less than 25 years of age. If symptoms of insomnia or nightmares continue, prazosin can be added to provide relief. Risperidone or quetiapine can be added for patients who fail to respond or have a partial response to antidepressant therapy.

Clinical **Controversy...**

It is unknown how long a patient with PTSD should be treated with an SSRI or venlafaxine to achieve a maximal response. The initial SSRI trial duration most clinicians use is 4 to 6 weeks, although sometimes up to 12 weeks is required.

Evaluation of Therapeutic Outcomes

During the acute phase of therapy, patients should be seen frequently. During months 3 to 6 of therapy, the patient can be seen monthly, and in months 6 to 12, visits can be extended to every 2 months. On each visit the patient should be asked about previously identified target symptoms of PTSD as well as other symptoms including insomnia, suicidal ideation, anger outbursts, irritability, psychosis, ongoing trauma, and disability. The Clinician-Administered PTSD Scale (CAPS) can be used by the clinician to assess symptom severity at visits.[27] A remission in patients with PTSD is defined as a 70% or greater reduction in symptoms. Patients who have a 50% response or greater reduction in symptoms are considered to have an adequate response, while those with a 25% to 50% reduction in symptoms are considered partial responders. Before deciding that a patient is not responsive to pharmacotherapy, the clinician should ensure that the medication trial has been adequate in both dose and duration.

Many patients with PTSD are sensitive to the adverse effects of drugs. They should be monitored carefully for adverse reactions that can delay the escalation of drug dosages or cause the patient distress. See Chapter 51 for details on monitoring antidepressants. Routine assessment of the metabolic profile is necessary if an atypical antipsychotic is used concurrently.[31] When pharmacotherapy is discontinued, patients should be seen more frequently and monitored carefully for signs of relapse or withdrawal.

TREATMENT
Obsessive-Compulsive Disorder

Desired Outcomes

Major goals of therapy for OCD include reduction in the frequency and severity of obsessive thoughts and time spent performing compulsive acts. Treatment for OCD generally does not completely eliminate obsessions or compulsions, but patients can feel remarkably improved with partial resolution of symptoms. Patients typically experience waxing and waning symptoms with only 20% achieving full remission.[47] Optimal treatment increases psychosocial and occupational functioning and improves overall QOL. Efforts should be made to minimize adverse drug events and prevent drug interactions.

General Approach to Treatment

It is important at the outset of therapy to identify and document the specific target symptoms for pharmacotherapy. Rating scales can be used to measure symptom severity at baseline and during treatment to ascertain the degree of improvement. The Yale-Brown Obsessive-Compulsive Scale (YBOCS) is the most widely used clinician-administered scale. A QOL scale can assist the clinician in identifying other areas to target for treatment (e.g., depression and reduced physical well-being).[48]

The FDA has approved five antidepressants for the management of OCD: clomipramine, fluoxetine, fluvoxamine, paroxetine, and sertraline. CBT and SSRIs are considered effective first-line treatment modalities.[49] Initial therapy may include CBT alone, SSRI monotherapy, or the combination of CBT and an SSRI, and is based on clinical judgment of symptom severity and patient preferences.[49] CBT alone can be used in cooperative patients who do not desire drug therapy, or those with mild anxiety or depressive symptoms. Patients unable to participate in CBT or with a prior history of medication therapy response should be treated with SSRI monotherapy. Combined CBT and SSRIs is recommended in patients with failure on an SSRI alone or in those with severe OCD. If a combination of CBT and an SSRI is unsuccessful, another SSRI should be tried before augmentation therapy. If there is no response or partial response to combined CBT and three adequate antidepressant trials (one of which is clomipramine), augmentation with another drug and more intensive CBT can be tried.[49] Augmentation with antipsychotics has proven efficacious in some patients with partial response.[20,49]

Table 54-3 provides a summary of key points from the treatment guidelines for OCD. Although some OCD symptoms can improve over the first 4 to 6 weeks of therapy, an adequate trial of any medication is considered to be 8 to 12 weeks.

Nonpharmacologic Therapy

A number of nonpharmacologic treatments are effective for OCD. CBT with behavioral techniques (i.e., exposure and response prevention [ERP]) is the most common initial nonpharmacologic treatment of choice. ERP is preferred for patients with mild symptoms, particularly children and adolescents, and in those without a psychiatric comorbidity or desire to avoid medications.[50] Clinicians can use motivational interviewing techniques to assist patients with treatment acceptance.[49]

Other options are deep brain stimulation (DBS) and ablative neurosurgery.[51] DBS is FDA-approved as a humanitarian device for severe, treatment-resistant OCD. It should not be used alone as first-line treatment but may be added to CBT or used in refractory patients. Surgery should be reserved for rare cases.[49,51]

Pharmacologic Therapy

Practice guidelines for the treatment of patients with OCD were published by the American Psychiatric Association.[49]

(6) SSRIs are considered to be the drugs of choice for patients with OCD.[49] While not FDA-approved, escitalopram has also shown efficacy in reduction of OCD symptoms.[52] Clomipramine, a TCA with strong 5-HT reuptake inhibition, has an active metabolite, desmethylclomipramine, which inhibits NE reuptake.[49,53] Meta-analytic findings of greater efficacy of clomipramine than SSRIs are not consistent with comparative trial data.[49]

Alternative Drug Treatments

Recent studies have examined novel augmentation approaches. Augmentation with the drugs that modulate the excitatory neurotransmitter glutamate (e.g., riluzole, memantine, and topiramate) have shown initial promising results.[47,50] Ondansetron, dextroamphetamine, and D-cycloserine as possible augmentation agents in refractory OCD patients have had mixed results. These alternative augmenting treatments are reserved for refractory patients.[47,49]

Special Populations

Children and Adolescents OCD affecting children and adolescents is prevalent. There are symptom and treatment similarities and differences between OCD developing earlier in life and that which develops later. Younger patients exhibit poorer insight regarding obsessions, have more obsessions involving fear of harm and separation, and possess more rituals involving family members.[7] CBT weekly or daily and including family members has also been effective.[50] ERP is preferred as the first-line treatment for children and adolescents with milder symptom severity and less comorbidity.[50] Effects of pediatric ERP have been reported to last up to 2 years.[50] CBT and SSRI treatment are considered first-line for pediatric patients.[54]

TABLE 54-3 Summary of Key Points in Treatment Guidelines for Obsessive-Compulsive Disorder

Recommendation	Level of Evidence	Comments
First-Line Treatments		
CBT alone	I	13–20 sessions
SSRI alone	I	8–12 weeks, at least 4–6 weeks at maximum tolerated dose
CBT + SSRI	I	13–20 CBT sessions and 8- to 12-week SSRI with 4–6 weeks at maximum tolerated dose If monotherapy with CBT or SSRI alone does not provide adequate response, combination therapy with CBT + SSRI should be tried before augmentation with another pharmacologic agent
Second-Line Treatments		
Switch to another SSRI or clomipramine	I	
Augmentation with antipsychotic	II	
Third-Line Treatments		
Switch to another antipsychotic augmenting agent	II	
Augmentation of SSRI with clomipramine	III	
Maintenance and Discontinuation Phase		
After 1–2 years, gradual taper over several months	I	
Periodic CBT booster sessions for 3–6 months	II	

Levels of evidence: I, recommended with substantial clinical confidence; II, recommended with moderate clinical confidence; III, may be recommended on the basis of individual circumstances.

Data from reference 49.

Clomipramine, fluvoxamine, sertraline, paroxetine, and fluoxetine are approved by the FDA for treatment of OCD in children and adolescents.[49] Childhood and adult OCD appear to respond similarly to drug therapy. SSRIs are effective (50% to 56% respond to the initial agent) and well tolerated in the treatment of OCD and are generally considered first-line agents.[49,54] In children, the most commonly described side effects of SSRI therapy include sedation, nausea, diarrhea, insomnia, anorexia, tremor, and hyperstimulation.[54] The starting dose of clomipramine in children is 25 mg daily in divided doses. The dose can be increased over the first 2 weeks up to 3 mg/kg or 100 mg, whichever is smaller. Over the next several weeks, the dose can be increased up to 3 mg/kg with a maximum of 200 mg daily.[53] The risk of suicidality in youth is discussed in Chapter 51.

Hepatic and Renal Disease Clomipramine and the SSRIs are extensively metabolized in the liver, and patients with significant liver disease should be prescribed these drugs cautiously and in lower doses than those used in healthy subjects. The pharmacokinetics of sertraline is not altered in patients with significant renal dysfunction, and dosage adjustment is not necessary in these patients.[34] Increased plasma concentrations of paroxetine occur in subjects with renal impairment.[33] The initial dose of paroxetine should be reduced in patients with severe renal impairment, and upward titration should occur more slowly.[33] No dosage adjustment is necessary for patients with renal impairment receiving clomipramine.[53]

Elderly Little information is available on treating OCD in the elderly. Case reports and anecdotal information suggest that the antiobsessional drugs are likely to be equally effective in the elderly and in younger adults.[55] Selection of medication for an elderly person with OCD, however, should be based on history of response and adverse side effect profile. Treatment should be initiated with low doses in elderly patients, and doses should be increased slowly, with vigilance for emergence of side effects.[49] Because of clomipramine's sedative and anticholinergic side effects, it is not usually chosen as first-line therapy for elderly OCD patients.[49] The use of SSRIs in elderly patients is discussed in Chapter 51.

Pregnancy Risk–benefit analysis should be made by practitioners when deciding to use pharmacotherapy options during pregnancy.[49] The use of SSRIs in pregnancy and lactation is discussed in Chapter 51.

Antidepressant Therapy

Serotonergic Antidepressants The only potent 5-HT reuptake inhibitors consistently demonstrating efficacy in controlled trials are the TCA clomipramine and the SSRIs fluoxetine, fluvoxamine, paroxetine, and sertraline.

Current evidence indicates that 5-HT is important for the antiobsessional effects of medication.[11,54] SSRIs and clomipramine inhibit 5-HT reuptake into the presynaptic neuron. Inhibiting reuptake of 5-HT makes more 5-HT available to postsynaptic receptors and reduces formation of the 5-HT metabolite 5-hydroxyindoleacetic acid. Although other antidepressants, such as imipramine and amitriptyline, inhibit 5-HT reuptake, they are less potent and selective than SSRIs. Prolonged exposure to increased amounts of 5-HT after chronic antidepressant treatment (2 to 3 weeks) leads to altered responsiveness of postsynaptic 5-HT receptors or presynaptic autoregulatory receptors that govern 5-HT release in specific brain regions. An improvement in obsessional symptoms may correlate with plasma concentrations of clomipramine but not desmethylclomipramine, the metabolite of clomipramine with less selectivity for 5-HT reuptake inhibition.

Most experts agree that SSRIs are better tolerated than clomipramine. SSRIs are less likely to cause cardiovascular, sedative, anticholinergic, and weight-gain side effects, and to reduce the seizure threshold. Clomipramine is less likely than SSRIs to cause insomnia, akathisia, nausea, and diarrhea. Antidepressant side effects can be more severe when larger doses are used and with faster dose escalation. Tolerance to antidepressant adverse effects often develops over 6 to 8 weeks of treatment, and tolerance is more likely to develop to nausea, diarrhea, sedation, diminished libido and/or orgasm, anxiety, restlessness, insomnia, and anticholinergic side effects than to akathisia.[55]

Pharmacokinetics Clomipramine is rapidly absorbed after oral administration. Maximum plasma concentrations occur within 2 to 6 hours. Clomipramine is highly protein-bound (97%) in the blood and has a half-life of 19 to 37 hours.[53] The drug is metabolized to desmethylclomipramine, which is pharmacologically active. The pharmacokinetics of SSRIs is discussed in Chapter 51.

Efficacy SSRIs are effective in the treatment of OCD. Well-designed trials comparing these medications with placebo, head-to-head comparative trials, and meta-analyses have established that fluoxetine, fluvoxamine, paroxetine, sertraline, citalopram, and escitalopram are equally effective and that clomipramine may be somewhat more effective.[16,52] Forty percent to 60% of patients with OCD respond to a serotonergic antidepressant, with remission occurring in 8% to 37% of patients. Most patients continue to have symptoms that limit their functioning.[56]

Other Antidepressants Venlafaxine, which acts as a 5-HT and NE reuptake inhibitor, may be effective for OCD.[50,55]

Augmentation with Antipsychotics 7 Augmentation of SSRI treatment with low doses of antipsychotics may be helpful. Typical antipsychotics are generally not recommended because of an increased risk for extrapyramidal symptoms.[47,55] One-third to one-half of treatment-refractory patients with OCD responded to antipsychotic augmentation.[20,47] Evidence supports augmentation with low-dose risperidone or aripiprazole in short-term efficacy trials.[20,57] The efficacy for olanzapine and quetiapine is inconclusive.[20,58] The long-term use of second-generation antipsychotic augmentation resulted in modest improvement and higher rates of adverse effects (i.e., sedation, weight gain, increased blood glucose).[59] The benefits and risks of using second-generation antipsychotic augmentation should be evaluated carefully.

Dosage and Administration Table 54-4 summarizes dosing guidelines for SSRIs and clomipramine. The dose to achieve response in OCD is often higher than doses used in other indications.[49,60] If there is inadequate response to an average dose, then it should be incrementally increased to the maximum dose within 5 to 9 weeks from the start of treatment. 8 If there is an inadequate response after 4 to 6 weeks at the maximum dose, then another SSRI should be tried.[49] Eight to 12 weeks is considered an adequate trial before changing to another agent. Experts recommend waiting for a 3-month trial of an antidepressant before augmenting with a second-generation antipsychotic.[20,60]

Although the appropriate maintenance dose of antidepressants is unknown, gradual dose reduction can occur in some patients without loss of efficacy.[47]

Personalized Pharmacotherapy

The choice of an SSRI for treatment is based on history of prior response, safety, and side effect tolerability of the patient. All SSRIs are considered to be equally efficacious, but a patient may respond better to one agent over another.[49] When selecting pharmacotherapy, the clinician should consider FDA warnings (e.g., QTc prolongation for citalopram), potential for adverse consequences in patients with comorbid conditions (e.g., anticholinergic effects and weight gain with paroxetine in patients with diabetes, obesity, or benign

TABLE 54-4 Dosing of Serotonin Reuptake Inhibitors in the Treatment of OCD

Drug	Brand Name	Initial Dose	Usual Range	Comments
Citalopram[a,b]	Celexa®	20 mg daily	20–40 mg daily	Maximum dose is 40 mg in adults daily to prevent QTc prolongation; maximum dose of 20 mg daily in elderly patients, CYP2C19 poor metabolizers, or use with concurrent moderate-to-strong CYP2C19 inhibitors (e.g., cimetidine, omeprazole)
Clomipramine[a]	Anafranil®	25 mg daily	100–250 mg daily	Plasma levels (clomipramine and desmethylclomipramine) should be less than 500 ng/mL (500 mcg/L; ~1.7 μmol/L) (12 hours postdose to prevent conduction delays and seizures)
Escitalopram[a,b]	Lexapro®	10 mg daily	10–20 mg daily	Doses up to 40 mg may be needed in some patients
Fluoxetine[a]	Prozac®	20 mg daily	40–60 mg daily	Doses of 80 mg or higher may be needed in some patients
Fluvoxamine[a]	Luvox CR®	50 mg daily	50–200 mg daily	For initial doses use generic immediate-release. Doses up to 300 mg daily have been used in some patients
Paroxetine[a]	Paxil®, Pexeva®	20 mg daily	40–60 mg daily	Higher doses may be needed in some patients
Sertraline[a]	Zoloft®	50 mg daily	50–200 mg daily	Higher doses may be needed in some patients

[a]Available generically.
[b]Not FDA-approved for treatment of obsessive-compulsive disorder. Optimal dosing guidelines are not well established.
Data from references 33, 34, 47, 49, and 53.

prostatic hypertrophy), or adverse effects (e.g., insomnia with fluoxetine in patients with sleep difficulties). Increased risk of suicidality should be considered in patients taking SSRIs who are less than 25 years of age. Drug interactions should be avoided—citalopram, escitalopram, and sertraline have the least potential for inhibition of CYP450 isoenzymes (see Chap. 51).

Risks to consider with clomipramine include lethality in overdose in patients with suicidal ideation, anticholinergic effects in patients with constipation, narrow-angle glaucoma, or urinary hesitancy, and potential for seizures in patients with epilepsy. Clomipramine use is associated with the risk of QTc prolongation when used alone and in combination with other agents that prolong the QTc interval.[53]

Clinical **Controversy. . .**

When a patient with OCD has a partial response to an SSRI, it is unclear whether a second-generation antipsychotic should be used preferentially to increasing the dose of the SSRI or to augmenting with another agent, such as clomipramine. Many practitioners will increase the SSRI dose if well tolerated before adding in a low dose of an antipsychotic because of the risk of adverse effects.

TABLE 54-5 Monitoring of Patients Being Treated for Obsessive-Compulsive Disorder

Drug	Adverse Drug Reaction	Monitoring Parameter	Comments
Clomipramine	Dry mouth, constipation, nausea, dyspepsia, anorexia, somnolence, tremors, dizziness, nervousness	Patient interview	Tolerance should occur in 2 weeks
	Seizures	Patient interview	
	Orthostatic hypotension, tachycardia, ECG changes	Vital signs, ECG	Obtain baseline ECG in patients over 40 years of age and those with cardiovascular disease
	Suicidality	Patient interview	Highest risk is in patients below 25 years of age
	Agranulocytosis, leukopenia	CBC with differential	Labs if patient complains of sore throat, fever
	Weight gain	Patient body weight	Assess at each visit

CBC, complete blood count; ECG, electrocardiogram.

Evaluation of Therapeutic Outcomes

Target symptoms of OCD should be monitored closely. The degree of response can indicate a need to modify dosage, change drug, or augment therapy. Rating scales can be used to monitor symptom response to therapy for OCD (e.g., YBOCS) and changes in QOL. The clinician should inquire about and address problematic adverse effects (including the emergence of suicidal ideation) reported by the patient and the amount of time the patient spends obsessing and performing compulsions. Changes in social and occupational functioning should be assessed.

Table 54-5 details the monitoring of clomipramine pharmacotherapy in patients with OCD. Monitoring of SSRIs can be found in Chapter 51 and antipsychotics in Chapter 50. After patients have responded to the acute phase of treatment, treatment gains are maintained with maintenance-phase strategies.

9 Monthly followup visits are recommended for at least 3 to 6 months, and a medication taper can be considered after 1 to 2 years of treatment. Medication should not be rapidly discontinued, and booster CBT sessions can reduce the risk of relapse when medication is withdrawn. The drug dosage can be decreased by 10% to 25% every 1 to 2 months with careful observation for symptom relapse.[49] Some patients require lifelong medication therapy.

ABBREVIATIONS

ASD acute stress disorder
CAPS Clinician-Administered Posttraumatic Stress Disorder Scale
CBT cognitive behavioral therapy
CRF corticotropin-releasing factor
dACC dorsal anterior cingulate cortex
DA dopamine

DBS	deep brain stimulation
eQTLs	expression of quantitative trait loci
EMDR	eye movement desensitization and reprocessing
ERP	exposure and response prevention
GABA	γ-aminobutyric acid
5-HT	serotonin
HPA	hypothalamic–pituitary–adrenal
mQTLs	methylation quantitative trait loci
MAOI	monoamine oxidase inhibitor
NE	norepinephrine
NPY	neuropeptide Y
OCD	obsessive-compulsive disorder
PANDAS	pediatric autoimmune neuropsychiatric disorder associated with streptococcal infection
PTSD	posttraumatic stress disorder
QOL	quality of life
SNP	single nucleotide polymorphism
SNRI	serotonin–norepinephrine reuptake inhibitor
SSRI	selective serotonin reuptake inhibitor
TCA	tricyclic antidepressant
TFCBT	trauma-focused cognitive behavioral therapy
vmPFC	ventromedial prefrontal cortex
YBOCS	Yale-Brown Obsessive-Compulsive Scale

REFERENCES

1. American Psychiatric Association. Diagnostic and Statistical Manual of Mental Disorders, Fourth Edition, Text Revision. Washington, DC: American Psychiatric Association, 2000:429–484.
2. Hoge CW, Auchterlonie JL, Milliken CS. Mental health problems, use of mental health services, and attrition from military services after returning from Iraq or Afghanistan. JAMA 2006;295:1023–1032.
3. Sher L, Braquehais M, Casas M. Posttraumatic stress disorder, depression, and suicide in veterans. Cleve Clin J Med 2012;79(2):92–97.
4. Wisco BE, Marx BP, Keane TM. Screening, diagnosis and treatment of post-traumatic stress disorder. Mil Med 2012;177(Suppl 8):7–13.
5. Fenske JN, Schwenk TL. Obsessive-compulsive disorder: Diagnosis and management. Am Fam Physician 2009;80(3):239–245.
6. Klein S, Alexander DA. Epidemiology and presentation of post-traumatic disorders. Psychiatry 2006;8:282–287.
7. Geller D. Obsessive-compulsive and spectrum disorders in children and adolescents. Psychiatr Clin North Am 2006;29:353–370.
8. Ruscio AM, Stein DA, Chiu WT, Kessler RC. The epidemiology of obsessive-compulsive disorder in the National Comorbidity Survey Replication. Mol Psychiatry 2010;15(1):53–63.
9. Grabe HJ, Ruhrmann S, Ettelt S, et al. Familiality of obsessive–compulsive disorder in nonclinical and clinical subjects. Am J Psychiatry 2006;163: 1986–1992.
10. de Mathis MA, do Rosario MC, Diniz JB, et al. Obsessive–compulsive disorder: Influence of age at onset on comorbidity patterns. Eur Psychiatry 2008;23: 187–194.
11. Nestadt G, Grados M, Samuels JF. Genetics of OCD. Psychiatr Clin North Am 2010;33(1):141–158.
12. Shulman ST. Pediatric autoimmune neuropsychiatric disorders associated with streptococci (PANDAS): Update. Curr Opin Pediatr 2009;21:127–130.
13. Sherin JE, Nemeroff CB. Posttraumatic stress disorder: The neurobiological impact of psychological trauma. Dialogues Clin Neurosci 2011;13:263–278.
14. Shin LM, Liberzon I. The neurobiology of fear, stress and anxiety disorders. Neuropsychopharmacology 2010;35: 169–191.
15. Martin EI, Ressler KJ, Binder E, Nemeroff CB. The neurobiology of anxiety disorders: Brain imaging, genetics and psychoneuroendocrinology. Psychiatr Clin North Am 2009;32:549–575.
16. Rabinowitz I, Baruch Y, Barak Y. High-dose escitalopram for the treatment of obsessive-compulsive disorder. Int Clin Psychopharmacol 2008;23:49–53.
17. Koran LM, Aboujaoude E, Ward H, et al. Pulse-loaded intravenous clomipramine in treatment-resistant obsessive-compulsive disorder. J Clin Psychopharmacol 2006;26(1):79–83.
18. Soomro GM, Altman D, Rajagopal S, Oakley-Browne M. Selective serotonin re-uptake inhibitors (SSRIs) versus placebo for obsessive compulsive disorder (OCD). Cochrane Database Syst Rev 2008;(1):CD001765.
19. Bloch MH, McGuire J, Landeros-Weisenberger A, et al. Meta-analysis of the dose–response relationship of SSRIs in obsessive-compulsive disorder. Mol Psychiatry 2010;15:850–855.
20. Bloch MH, Landeros-Weisenberger A, Kemendi B, et al. A systematic review: Antipsychotic augmentation with treatment refractory obsessive-compulsive disorder. Mol Psychiatry 2006;11:622–632.
21. Friedlander L, Desrocher M. Neuroimaging studies of obsessive-compulsive disorder in adults and children. Clin Psychol Rev 2006;26:32–49.
22. Maia TV, Cooney RE, Peterson BS. The neural bases of obsessive-compulsive disorder in children and adults. Dev Psychopathol 2008;20:1251–1283.
23. MacMaster FP. Translational neuroimaging research in pediatric obsessive-compulsive disorder. Dialogues Clin Neurosci 2010;12:165–174.
24. Shalev AY. Posttraumatic stress disorder and stress-related disorders. Psychiatr Clin North Am 2009;32: 687–704.
25. Canadian Psychiatric Association. Clinical practice guidelines: Management of anxiety disorders. Can J Psychiatry 2006;51(Suppl 2):9S–91S.
26. Bisson JI. Post-traumatic stress disorder. Occup Med 2007;57:399–403.
27. U.S. Department of Veterans Affairs. VA/DoD Clinical Practice Guideline: Management of Post-Traumatic Stress Disorder and Acute Stress Reaction: Guideline Summary, Version 2.0. Washington, DC, 2010, *http://www.healthquality.va.gov/ptsd/CPG_Summary_FINAL_MgmtofPTSDfinal11612.pdf*.
28. Bisson J, Andrew M. Psychological treatment of post-traumatic stress disorder (PTSD). Cochrane Database Syst Rev 2007;(3):CD003388. doi:10.1002/14651858.CD003388.pub3.
29. Bomyea J, Lang AJ. Emerging interventions for PTSD: Future directions for clinical care and research. Neuropharmacology 2012;62:607–616.
30. Stein DJ, Ipser JC, Seedat S. Pharmacotherapy for post traumatic stress disorder (PTSD). Cochrane Database Syst Rev 2006;(1):CD002795. doi:10.1002/14651858.CD002795.pub2.
31. Bandelow B, Sher L, Bunevicius R, et al. Guidelines for the pharmacological treatment of anxiety disorders, obsessive-compulsive disorder, and post-traumatic stress

disorder in primary care. Int J Psychiatry Clin Pract 2012;16:77–84.
32. Ipser JC, Stein DJ. Evidence-based pharmacotherapy of post-traumatic stress disorder. Int J Neuropsychopharmacol 2012;15(6):825–840.
33. Paxil [package insert]. Research Triangle Park, NC: GlaxoSmithKline, July 2011.
34. Zoloft [package insert]. New York, NY: Pfizer Inc, May 2012.
35. Bajor LA, Ticlea AN, Osser DN. The Psychopharmacology Algorithm Project at the Harvard South Shore Program: An update on posttraumatic stress disorder. Harv Rev Psychiatry 2011;19:240–258.
36. Davidson J, Rothbaum BO, Tucker P, et al. Venlafaxine extended release in posttraumatic stress disorder: A sertraline- and placebo-controlled study. J Clin Psychopharmacol 2006;26:259–267.
37. Davidson J, Baldwin D, Stein DJ, et al. Treatment of posttraumatic stress disorder with venlafaxine extended release: A 6-month randomized controlled trial. Arch Gen Psychiatry 2006;63:1158–1165.
38. Becker ME, Hertzberg MA, Moore SD, et al. A placebo-controlled trial of bupropion SR in the treatment of chronic posttraumatic stress disorder. J Clin Psychopharmacol 2007;27:193–197.
39. Berger W, Mendlowicz MV, Marques-Portella C, et al. Pharmacologic alternatives to antidepressants in posttraumatic stress disorder: A systematic review. Prog Neuropsychopharmacol Biol Psychiatry 2009;33:169–180.
40. Pae C, Lim H, Peindl K, et al. The atypical antipsychotics olanzapine and risperidone in the treatment of posttraumatic stress disorder: A meta-analysis of randomized, double-blind, placebo-controlled clinical trials. Int Clin Psychopharmacol 2008;23:1–8.
41. Ahern EP, Mussey M, Johnson C, et al. Quetiapine as an adjunctive treatment for post-traumatic stress disorder: An 8-week open-label study. Int Clin Psychopharmacol 2006;21:29–33.
42. Ahern EP, Juergens T, Cordes T, et al. A review of atypical antipsychotic medications for posttraumatic stress disorder. Int Clin Psychopharmacol 2011;26:193–200.
43. Aurora RN, Zak RS, Auerbach SH, et al. Best practice guide for the treatment of nightmare disorder in adults. J Clin Sleep Med 2010;6(4):389–401.
44. Nappi CM, Drummond SPA, Hall JMH. Treating nightmares and insomnia in posttraumatic stress disorder: A review of current evidence. Neuropharmacology 2012;62:576–585.
45. Ipser JC, Stein DJ, Hawkridge S, Hoppe L. Pharmacotherapy for anxiety disorders in children and adolescents. Cochrane Database Syst Rev 2009;(3):CD005170. doi:10.1002/14651858.CD005170.pub2.
46. Davidson JRT. Pharmacologic treatment of acute and chronic stress following trauma. J Clin Psychiatry 2006;67(Suppl 2): 34–39.
47. Stein DJ, Koen N, Fineberg N, et al. A 2012 evidence-based algorithm for the pharmacotherapy for obsessive-compulsive disorder. Curr Psychiatry Rep 2012;14:211–219.
48. Rush A, First M, Blacker D. Handbook of Psychiatric Measures, 2nd ed. Washington, DC: American Psychiatric Association, 2008, *http://www.R2library.com/marc_frame.aspx?*
49. American Psychiatric Association. Practice Guideline for the Treatment of Patients with Obsessive-Compulsive Disorder. Arlington, VA: American Psychiatric Association, 2007, *http://www.psych.org/psych_pract/treatg/pg/prac_guide.cfm*.
50. Walsh KH, McDougle CJ. Psychotherapy and medication management for obsessive-compulsive disorder. Neuropsychiatr Dis Treat 2011;7:485–494.
51. Greenberg BD, Rauch SL, Haber SN. Invasive circuitry-based neurotherapeutics: Stereotactic ablation and deep brain stimulation for OCD. Neuropsychopharmacology 2010;35:317–336.
52. Dougherty DD, Jameson M, Deckersbach T, et al. Open-label study of high (30 mg) and moderate (20 mg) dose escitalopram for the treatment of obsessive-compulsive disorder. Int Clin Psychopharmacol 2009;24:306–311.
53. Anafranil [package insert]. Hazelwood, MO: Mallinckrodt Inc, October 2012.
54. Kalra SK, Swedo SE. Children with obsessive-compulsive disorder: Are they just "little adults"? J Clin Invest 2009;119:737–746.
55. Denys D. Pharmacotherapy of obsessive-compulsive disorder and obsessive-compulsive spectrum disorders. Psychiatr Clin North Am 2006;29:553–584.
56. McGuire JF, Lewin AB, Horng B, et al. The nature, assessment, and treatment of obsessive-compulsive disorder. Postgrad Med 2012;124(1):152–165.
57. Muscatello MRA, Bruno A, Pandolfo G, et al. Effect of aripiprazole augmentation of selective serotonin reuptake inhibitors or clomipramine in treatment-resistant obsessive-compulsive disorder: A double-blind, placebo-controlled study. J Clin Psychopharmacol 2011;31: 174–179.
58. Diniz JB, Shavitt RG, Fossaluza V, et al. A double-blind, randomized, controlled trial of fluoxetine plus quetiapine or clomipramine versus fluoxetine plus placebo for obsessive-compulsive disorder. J Clin Psychopharmacol 2011;31: 763–768.
59. Matsunga H, Nagata T, Hayashida K, et al. A long-term trial of the effectiveness and safety of atypical antipsychotic agents in augmenting SSRI-refractory obsessive-compulsive disorder. J Clin Psychiatry 2009;70(6):863–868.
60. Bandelow B, Zohar J, Hollander E, et al. World Federation of Societies of Biological Psychiatry (WFSBP) guidelines for the pharmacological treatment of anxiety, obsessive-compulsive and post-traumatic stress disorders—First revision. World J Biol Psychiatry 2008;9(4):248–312.

55

Sleep Disorders

John M. Dopp and Bradley G. Phillips

KEY CONCEPTS

1. Common causes of insomnia include concomitant psychiatric disorders, significant psychosocial stressors, excessive alcohol use, caffeine intake, and nicotine use.
2. Good sleep hygiene, including relaxing before bedtime, exercising regularly, establishing a regular bedtime and wake-up time, and discontinuing alcohol, caffeine, and nicotine, alone and in combination with drug therapy, should be part of patient education and treatments for insomnia.
3. Long-acting benzodiazepines should be avoided in the elderly.
4. Benzodiazepine tolerance and dependence are avoided by using low-dose therapy for the shortest possible duration.
5. Obstructive sleep apnea may be an independent risk factor for the development of hypertension. When hypertension is present, it is often refractory to drug therapy until sleep-disordered breathing is alleviated.
6. Nasal continuous positive airway pressure is the first-line therapy for obstructive sleep apnea, and weight loss should be encouraged in all obese patients.
7. Pharmacologic management of narcolepsy is focused on two primary areas: treatment of excessive daytime sleepiness and rapid eye movement (REM) sleep abnormalities.
8. Short-acting benzodiazepine receptor agonists, ramelteon, or melatonin taken at appropriate target bedtimes for east or west travel reduce jet lag and shorten sleep latency.
9. Dopamine agonists are effective for restless legs syndrome and have replaced levodopa as first-line therapy.

Approximately 70 million Americans suffer with a sleep-related problem, and as many as 60% of those experience a chronic disorder.[1] In a study by the National Institute on Aging, of 9,000 patients aged 65 years and older, more than 80% report a sleep-related disturbance.[1]

INTRODUCTION TO SLEEP

Sleep Cycles

Sleep is divided into two phases: nonrapid eye movement (NREM) sleep and rapid eye movement (REM) sleep. Each night humans typically experience four to six cycles of NREM and REM sleep, with each cycle lasting between 70 and 120 minutes.[2] There are four stages of NREM sleep. Healthy sleep will typically progress through the four stages of NREM sleep prior to the first REM period. From wakefulness, sleep typically progresses quickly through stages 1 and 2. Stage 1 of NREM sleep is the stage between wakefulness and sleep, and individuals describe this experience as being awake, being drowsy, or being asleep. During stages 3 and 4 NREM, both metabolic activity and brain waves slow. This slow-wave sleep occurs most frequently early in the sleep period. Stages 3 and 4 sleep are called *delta sleep*, as the sleep is characterized by high-amplitude slow activity known as delta waves (0.5 to 3 Hz) with no eye movements and low tonic muscle activity.

REM sleep involves a dramatic physiologic change from NREM sleep, to a state in which the brain becomes electrically and metabolically activated.[2] REM occurs in bursts and is accompanied by a 62% to 173% increase in cerebral blood flow, generalized muscle atonia, bursts of bilateral REMs, poikilothermia, dreaming, and fluctuations in respiratory and cardiac rate.[2] REM cycles tend to lengthen in the later stages of the sleep cycle.[2]

Circadian Rhythm

At birth human infants spend up to 20 hours a day sleeping. At 3 to 6 months of age there is a differentiation between REM and NREM sleep. By age 3 years the ultradian sleep–wake rhythm changes to a circadian pattern. The suprachiasmatic nucleus of the brain serves as the biologic clock and paces the circadian rhythm. Although the length of a day is 24 hours, in environments devoid of light cues, the sleep–wake cycle lasts about 25 hours.[3] In midlife, there is a gradual decline in sleep efficiency and sleep time.[2] The elderly have lighter and more fragmented sleep, with intermittent arousals, shifts in the sleep stages, and a gradual reduction of slow-wave sleep.

Neurochemistry

The neurochemistry of sleep is complex, as sleep cannot be localized to either a specific area of the brain or a neurotransmitter. NREM sleep appears to be controlled by the basal forebrain, the lower brain stem to the thalamus, and hypothalamus.[3] Numerous neurotransmitters mediate NREM sleep, including γ-aminobutyric acid (GABA) and adenosine.[3] REM sleep appears to be turned on by cholinergic cells in the mesencephalic, medullary, and pontine gigantocellular regions. REM sleep appears to be turned off by the dorsal raphe nucleus, the locus coeruleus, and the nucleus parabrachialis lateralis, the latter two of which are primarily noradrenergic. The ascending reticular activating system and the posterior hypothalamus facilitate arousal and wakefulness.[4] Dopamine has an alerting effect; decreases in dopamine promote sleepiness.[5] Neurochemicals involved in wakefulness include norepinephrine and acetylcholine in the cortex and histamine and neuropeptides such as substance P and corticotropin-releasing factor in the hypothalamus.[5,6]

Polysomnography

Sleep is typically measured and observed in sleep laboratories using an electroencephalogram (EEG), electrooculograms of each eye, electrocardiogram, electromyogram, air thermistors, abdominal and thoracic strain belts, and oxygen saturation monitor. This study is named polysomnography (PSG) and is used to assess and record variables that characterize sleep and aid in diagnosis of sleep disorders. Variables obtained during PSG include sleep onset, arousals, sleep stages, eye movements, leg and jaw movements, arrhythmias, airflow during sleep, respiratory effort, and oxygen desaturations. Home sleep monitoring that measures variables such as electrocardiogram, oxygen saturation, airflow, and respiratory effort is also increasingly used to diagnose sleep apnea.

CLASSIFICATION OF SLEEP DISORDERS

The *Diagnostic and Statistical Manual of Mental Disorders, Fourth Edition, Text Revision* (*DSM-IV-TR*) classifies sleep disorders into four categories based on etiology and requires a symptom duration of at least 1 month before a sleep disorder can be diagnosed.[7,8] Primary sleep disorders are those disorders in which there is no other etiology (mental disorder, substance-related disorder, or medical condition) responsible for the disorder. They appear to be based on an endogenous abnormality of the sleep–wake cycle or circadian rhythm, and they are divided into dyssomnias (abnormality in the amount, quality, or timing of sleep) and parasomnias (abnormal behavioral or physiologic events associated with sleep, e.g., sleepwalking and REM behavior disorder). Dyssomnias include sleep disorders such as insomnia, narcolepsy, obstructive sleep apnea (OSA), and circadian rhythm disorders.

Insomnia

Insomnia is the most common complaint in general medical practice.[9] It causes distress, frequently because of a fear or a feeling of not being able to fall asleep at bedtime, and can impair work-related productivity because of daytime fatigue or drowsiness. Insomnia is subjectively characterized as a complaint of difficulty falling asleep, difficulty maintaining sleep, or experiencing nonrestorative sleep.[7,8] Insomnia lasting two or three nights is considered to be transient insomnia, whereas short-term insomnia usually resolves in less than 3 weeks. Insomnia, according to the *DSM-IV-TR*, is considered to be chronic when it lasts longer than 1 month.[8]

Epidemiology

Primary insomnia usually begins in early or middle adulthood and is rare in childhood or adolescence. Symptoms of insomnia occur in 33% to 50% of the adult population.[9] A 1-year prevalence study of insomnia in the United States reports that one third of the individuals surveyed complained of insomnia, and 17% reported that the symptoms were serious.[1] Conservative estimates of chronic insomnia range from 9% to 12% in adulthood and up to 20% in the elderly.[1,10] Although young adults are more likely to complain that they have difficulty falling asleep, middle-aged and elderly adults are more likely to complain that they have middle-of-the-night awakening or early morning awakening. Women complain of insomnia twice as frequently as men. Individuals who are elderly, unemployed, separated, or widowed, and those with a lower socioeconomic status report a significantly higher incidence of insomnia than the general population. Forty percent of individuals with insomnia also have a concurrent psychiatric disorder (anxiety, depression, or substance abuse).[11]

TABLE 55-1 Common Etiologies of Insomnia

Situational
Work or financial stress, major life events, interpersonal conflicts
Jet lag or shift work
Medical
Cardiovascular (angina, arrhythmias, heart failure)
Respiratory (asthma, sleep apnea)
Chronic pain
Endocrine disorders (diabetes, hyperthyroidism)
GI (gastroesophageal reflux disease, ulcers)
Neurologic (delirium, epilepsy, Parkinson's disease)
Pregnancy
Psychiatric
Mood disorders (depression, mania)
Anxiety disorders (e.g., generalized anxiety disorder, obsessive-compulsive disorder)
Substance abuse (alcohol or sedative–hypnotic withdrawal)
Pharmacologically induced
Anticonvulsants
Central adrenergic blockers
Diuretics
Selective serotonin reuptake inhibitors
Steroids
Stimulants

Approximately 10% to 20% of those with insomnia use nonprescription drugs or alcohol to self-treat.

Differential Diagnosis

Primary insomnia is considered to be an endogenous disorder caused by either a neurochemical or a structural disorder affecting the sleep–wake cycle. Individuals with primary insomnia can be light sleepers who are easily aroused by noise, temperature, or anxiety. Some studies suggest that primary insomnia is a "hyperarousal state," in that insomnia patients have increased metabolic rates compared with controls and thus take longer to fall asleep.[2] Comorbid or secondary insomnia is frequently a symptom or manifestation of another medical disorder. Evaluation of patients with a complaint of transient or short-term insomnia should focus on recent stressors, such as a separation, a death in the family, a job change, or college exams.

1 Chronic insomnia is frequently comorbid with psychiatric or medical conditions. A complete diagnostic examination should be completed in these individuals and should include routine laboratory tests, physical and mental status examinations, as well as ruling out any medication- or substance-related causes.[12] Special consideration should also be given to other sleep disorders that can have a similar presentation, including restless legs syndrome (RLS), periodic limb movements of sleep (PLMS), and sleep apnea. Common causes of insomnia are listed in Table 55-1.

TREATMENT

Desired Outcomes

The goals of treatment of insomnia are to correct the underlying sleep complaint, consolidate sleep, improve daytime functioning and sleepiness, and avoid adverse effects from selected therapies. Drug therapy should be used in the lowest possible dose, for the shortest possible time period.

Treatment Principles

Therapeutic management of insomnia is initially based on whether the individual has experienced a transient, short-term, or chronic sleep disturbance. Clinical history should assess the onset, duration,

TABLE 55-2 Nonpharmacologic Recommendations for Management of Insomnia

Stimulus control procedures

1. Establish regular times to wake up and to go to sleep (including weekends)
2. Sleep only as much as necessary to feel rested
3. Go to bed only when sleepy. Avoid long periods of wakefulness in bed. Use the bed only for sleep or intimacy; do not read or watch television in bed
4. Avoid trying to force sleep; if you do not fall asleep within 20–30 minutes, leave the bed and perform a relaxing activity (e.g., read, listen to music, or watch television) until drowsy. Repeat this as often as necessary
5. Avoid daytime naps
6. Schedule worry time during the day. Do not take your troubles to bed

Sleep hygiene recommendations

1. Exercise routinely (three to four times weekly) but not close to bedtime because this can increase wakefulness
2. Create a comfortable sleep environment by avoiding temperature extremes, loud noises, and illuminated clocks in the bedroom
3. Discontinue or reduce the use of alcohol, caffeine, and nicotine
4. Avoid drinking large quantities of liquids in the evening to prevent nighttime trips to the restroom
5. Do something relaxing and enjoyable before bedtime

and frequency of the symptoms; effect on daytime functioning; sleep hygiene habits; and history of previous symptoms or treatment.[13] Management of all patients with insomnia should include identifying the cause of the insomnia, patient education on sleep hygiene, and stress management. Any unnecessary pharmacotherapy should be eliminated.[10] Transient insomnia, which occurs as a result of an acute stressor, is expected to resolve quickly and should be treated with good sleep hygiene and careful use of sedative–hypnotics.[11] Short-term insomnia, associated with situational, personal, or medical stress, can be treated similarly.[13] Chronic insomnia requires careful assessment for possible underlying medical causes, nonpharmacologic approaches, and careful use of sedative–hypnotics.[12]

Nonpharmacologic Therapy

❷ In many cases insomnia can be treated without sedative–hypnotics. Education about normal sleep and habits for good sleep hygiene are important for all patients with insomnia. Nonpharmacologic interventions for insomnia frequently consist of short-term cognitive behavioral therapies, most commonly stimulus control therapy, sleep restriction, relaxation therapy, cognitive therapy, paradoxical intention, biofeedback, and education on good sleep hygiene (Table 55-2).[10,14] In patients aged 55 and older, research indicates that cognitive behavioral therapy may be more effective than pharmacologic therapy at improving certain measures of insomnia.[15,16]

Pharmacologic Therapy

Miscellaneous Agents

Antihistamines exhibit sedating properties and are included in many nonprescription sleep agents. They are effective in the treatment of mild insomnia and are generally safe.[13] Diphenhydramine and doxylamine are more sedating than pyrilamine. Patients quickly experience tolerance to sedative effects, and increasing the dose of antihistamines will not produce a linear increase in response. Antihistamines are considered to be less effective than benzodiazepines, and they have the disadvantages of anticholinergic side effects, which are especially troublesome in the elderly.[13,17]

Antidepressants are alternatives for patients with nonrestorative sleep who should not receive benzodiazepines, especially those who have depression, pain, or a risk of substance abuse. Using antidepressants for insomnia without depression is common but not well studied, and the doses used for treating insomnia are not effective antidepressant doses.[9,13,14] Sedating antidepressants such as amitriptyline, doxepin, and nortriptyline are effective for inducing sleep continuity, although daytime sedation and side effects can be significant.[9,13] Anticholinergic activity, adrenergic blockade, and cardiac conduction prolongation can be problematic, especially in the elderly and in overdose situations.[9] Low-dose doxepin (3 to 6 mg) was recently FDA-approved for the treatment of sleep maintenance insomnia. Mirtazapine is a sedating antidepressant that may help patients sleep, but it may also cause daytime sedation and weight gain.

Trazodone in doses of 25 to 100 mg at bedtime is sedating and can improve sleep continuity.[11] Trazodone is popular for the treatment of insomnia in patients prone to substance abuse, as dependence is not a problem with trazodone, and in patients with selective serotonin reuptake inhibitor and bupropion-induced insomnia.[11] Other side effects include carryover sedation and α-adrenergic blockade. Orthostasis can occur at any age, but it is more dangerous in the elderly. Priapism is a rare but serious side effect.[18]

Ramelteon is a melatonin receptor agonist approved for the treatment of sleep-onset insomnia. It is selective for the MT1 and MT2 melatonin receptors that are thought to regulate the circadian rhythm and sleep onset. The recommended dose is 8 mg taken at bedtime to induce sleep. Although generally well tolerated, the most common adverse events reported are headache, dizziness, and somnolence. Ramelteon is not a controlled substance and can be a viable option for patients with a history of substance abuse. It effectively treats sleep-onset difficulties in patients with chronic obstructive pulmonary disease and sleep apnea.[19,20]

Valerian is a herbal sleep remedy that has been studied for its sedative–hypnotic properties in patients with insomnia. The mechanism of action is not fully understood but may involve increasing concentrations of GABA. The recommended dose for insomnia ranges from 300 to 600 mg. An equivalent dose of dried herbal valerian root is 2 to 3 g soaked in one cup of hot water for 20 to 25 minutes.[21]

Benzodiazepine Receptor Agonists

The most commonly used treatments for insomnia have been the benzodiazepine receptor agonists (BZDRAs). BZDRAs are effective as sedative–hypnotics and are FDA-labeled for the treatment of insomnia (Table 55-3). The FDA requires BZDRA labeling to include a caution regarding anaphylaxis, facial angioedema, and complex sleep behaviors (e.g., sleep driving, phone calls, sleep eating, etc.). The BZDRAs consist of the newer nonbenzodiazepine $GABA_A$ agonists and the traditional benzodiazepines. All BZDRAs bind to $GABA_A$ receptors in the brain, resulting in agonist effects on GABAergic transmission and hyperpolarization of neuronal membranes. Traditional benzodiazepines have sedative, anxiolytic, muscle relaxant, and anticonvulsant properties; newer nonbenzodiazepine GABA agonists possess only sedative properties.

Benzodiazepine Hypnotics

Benzodiazepines relieve insomnia by reducing sleep latency and increasing total sleep time. They increase stage 2 sleep while decreasing delta sleep.[11] Benzodiazepine hypnotics should not be prescribed for individuals who are pregnant or who have untreated sleep apnea or a history of substance abuse. Patients should be instructed to avoid alcohol and other CNS depressants.

Adverse Effects Side effects are dose dependent and vary according to the pharmacokinetics of the individual benzodiazepine. High doses with long or intermediate elimination half-lives have a greater potential for producing daytime sedation, psychomotor incoordination, and cognitive deficits. Most traditional benzodiazepines maintain hypnotic efficacy for 1 month. However, tolerance can develop with time.

TABLE 55-3 Pharmacokinetics of Benzodiazepine Receptor Agonists

Generic Name (Brand Name)	t_{max}[a] (Hours)	Half-Life[b] (Hours)	Daily Dose Range (mg)	Metabolic Pathway	Clinically Significant Metabolites
Estazolam (ProSom)	2	12–15	1–2	Oxidation	—
Eszopiclone (Lunesta)	1–1.5	6	2–3	Oxidation Demethylation	—
Flurazepam (Dalmane)	1	8	15–30	Oxidation *N*-Dealkylation	Hydroxyethylflurazepam, flurazepam aldehyde *N*-Desalkylflurazepam[c]
Quazepam (Doral)	2	39	7.5–15	Oxidation, *N*-dealkylation	2-Oxo-quazepam, *N*-desalkylflurazepam[c]
Temazepam (Restoril)	1.5	10–15	15–30	Conjugation	—
Triazolam (Halcion)	1	2	0.125–0.25	Oxidation	—
Zaleplon (Sonata)	1	1	5–10	Oxidation	—
Zolpidem (Ambien; Intermezzo)	1.6	2–2.6	1.75–10[d]	Oxidation	—

[a]Time to peak plasma concentration.
[b]Half-life of parent drug.
[c]*N*-Desalkylflurazepam, mean half-life 47–100 hours.
[d]Oral and sublingual dosing 5–10 mg, sublingual tablets for middle-of-the night dosing 1.75–3.5 mg (1.75 for women, 3.5 mg for men).

Anterograde amnesia, an impairment of memory and recall of events occurring after the dose is taken, has been reported with most BZDRAs (it is more likely to occur with short-acting agents).[11] Rebound insomnia, characterized by increased wakefulness beyond baseline amounts that last for one to two nights after abrupt discontinuation, occurs with BZDRAs. The lowest effective dosage should be used to minimize rebound insomnia and avoid adverse effects on memory.

3 Benzodiazepine half-lives are prolonged in older patients, increasing the potential for drug accumulation and the incidence of CNS side effects, including prolonged sedation and cognitive and psychomotor impairment. BZDRAs with long elimination half-lives (e.g., flurazepam and quazepam) are generally not first-line agents in these patients. Benzodiazepine use is associated with increased risk of falls and hip fractures in the elderly, but since insomnia itself increases fall and fracture risk, it is unclear if benzodiazepines increase risk independent of sleep problems.[22]

Clinical **Controversy. . .**

Recent population studies suggest that use of sedative–hypnotics may be associated with increased mortality. Even though causality cannot be established based on the evidence to date, these studies raise important concerns. Although the evidence does not warrant discontinuation of hypnotics, it reemphasizes the importance of using sedative–hypnotics prudently at the lowest dose possible, for the shortest duration necessary.

Nonbenzodiazepine $GABA_A$ Agonists

Zolpidem, zaleplon, and eszopiclone are nonbenzodiazepine hypnotics that selectively bind to $GABA_A$ receptors and effectively induce sleepiness. Zolpidem has a duration of action of 6 to 8 hours.[23] It is comparable in efficacy to benzodiazepine hypnotics and is effective for reducing sleep latency and nocturnal awakenings and increasing total sleep time. It does not appear to have significant effects on next-day psychomotor performance. Sustained-release, sublingual, and reduced-strength (1.75 and 3.5 mg) formulations of zolpidem are available and are used to increase total sleep time, to reduce sleep latency, and for middle-of-the night rescue dosing, respectively.

Zolpidem is less disruptive of sleep stages than benzodiazepines. Adverse effects are dose related and can include drowsiness, amnesia, dizziness, headache, and GI complaints.[23] Sleep eating during zolpidem therapy can result in significant weight gain.[23] The recommended daily dose of zolpidem is 10 or 5 mg in elderly patients and those with hepatic impairment. Because food decreases its absorption, zolpidem should be taken on an empty stomach.[24]

Zaleplon has a rapid onset of action and a half-life of 1 hour, and it is metabolized to inactive metabolites.[25] It is effective for decreasing time to sleep onset but not for reducing nighttime awakening or for increasing total sleep time.[26] Because of its short half-life, zaleplon has no effect on next-day psychomotor performance and can be used as a sleep aid for middle-of-the-night awakenings.[27] The recommended dose is 10 mg in adults and 5 mg in the elderly.[25] The most common adverse effects with zaleplon are dizziness, headache, and somnolence. There are two drug interactions of note: zaleplon plasma levels are increased when combined with cimetidine and decreased with rifampin.[23]

Eszopiclone is effective at reducing time to sleep onset, wake time after sleep onset, and number of awakenings, and increasing total sleep time and sleep quality. Eszopiclone's duration of action is up to 6 hours,[28] so it can be a good option for treatment of sleep maintenance insomnia or early morning awakenings. The most common adverse effects with eszopiclone are somnolence, unpleasant taste, headache, and dry mouth.[28] Eszopiclone is labeled for long-term use and may be taken nightly for up to 6 months.[28,29]

Other Considerations

In general, the nonbenzodiazepine hypnotics seem to be associated with less withdrawal, tolerance, and rebound insomnia than the benzodiazepine hypnotics. None of the nonbenzodiazepine $GABA_A$ agonists have significant active metabolites.

Evaluation of Therapeutic Outcomes

An algorithm for the evaluation and treatment of dyssomnias is shown in Figure 55-1. Patients with short-term or chronic insomnia should be evaluated after 1 week of therapy to assess for drug efficacy, adverse effects, and adherence to nonpharmacologic recommendations.

Patients should be instructed to keep a sleep diary. The diary requires daily recording of bedtime, wake time, latency of sleep onset, number and duration of awakenings, medication ingestion, naps, and an index of sleep quality. For patients with chronic insomnia, possible medical, psychiatric, and pharmacologic causes

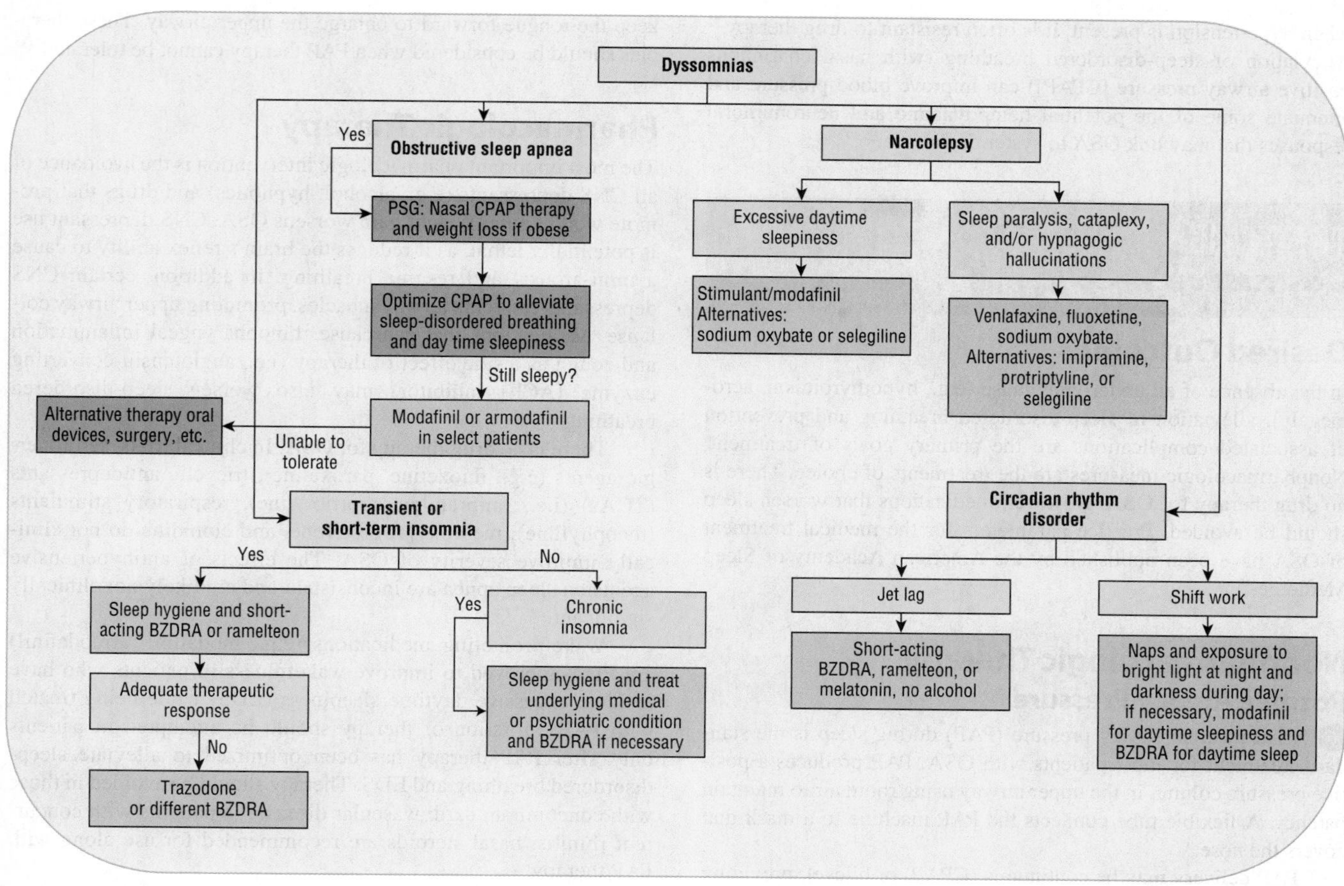

FIGURE 55-1 Algorithm for treatment of dyssomnias. (BZDRA, benzodiazepine receptor agonist; CPAP, continuous positive airway pressure.) *(Adapted with permission from reference 30.)*

should be identified and managed.[11] Patients with insomnia should receive education about possible medication side effects and their management.

4 Clinicians should educate patients about the concepts of tolerance, withdrawal, and rebound insomnia. Tolerance and dependence can be avoided by using hypnotics at the lowest possible dose, intermittently, and for the shortest duration possible. Patients should receive instruction about frequency of drug use and the expected duration of therapy, to help prevent development of dependence. Withdrawal symptoms can be diminished by tapering the dosage gradually.

SLEEP APNEA

Sleep apnea is a common disease, affecting 20 to 25 million Americans. It has a higher prevalence in men, particularly in African American and Hispanic populations.[31,32] Sleep apnea also occurs in children and adolescents. It is characterized by repetitive episodes of cessation of breathing during sleep followed by blood oxygen desaturation and brief arousal from sleep to restart breathing. As a result, individuals with sleep apnea experience fragmented sleep, poor sleep architecture, and periods of apnea and hypopnea. PSG is used to diagnose and quantify sleep apnea as central, obstructive, or mixed. Central sleep apnea (CSA) involves impairment of the respiratory drive, whereas OSA is caused by upper airway collapse and obstruction. Patients with mixed sleep apnea experience both CSA and OSA. Severity of sleep apnea is determined by the number of apnea (total cessation of airflow) and hypopnea (partial airway closure with blood oxygen desaturation) episodes documented by PSG, which is expressed as the respiratory disturbance index (RDI). Mild sleep apneics have an RDI of between 5 and 15 episodes/h, moderate 15 to 30 episodes/h, whereas individuals with severe OSA exhibit more than 30 episodes/h.

OSA is associated with motor vehicle accidents, depression, increased cancer risk, stroke, and cardiovascular disease.[33–36] Alleviation of sleep-disordered breathing may improve patient outcomes, particularly those related to cardiovascular disease.[36]

Obstructive Sleep Apnea

OSA is characterized by partial or complete closure of the upper airway, posterior from the nasal septum to the epiglottis, during inspiration. The reason for the loss of upper airway patency is not fully understood and is likely caused by several competing factors. Anatomical factors including neck obesity, narrow airway, and fixed upper airway lesions (e.g., polyps, enlarged tonsils) can narrow the upper airway. Intraluminal negative pressure generated during each inspiration also promotes collapse of the upper airway that competes with dilating forces, primarily the pharyngeal dilator muscle. Acromegaly, amyloidosis, and hypothyroidism as well as neurologic conditions that impair upper airway muscle tone may cause OSA. The hallmarks of OSA are witnessed apneas, gasping, or both. Other recognized signs, symptoms, and considerations of sleep apnea include obesity, snoring, daytime sleepiness, family history, and hypertension.

5 OSA is increasingly linked to cardiovascular and cerebrovascular morbidity and mortality, independent of other risk factors.[36] Individuals with OSA are at risk for developing hypertension, and

when hypertension is present, it is often resistant to drug therapy.[37] Alleviation of sleep-disordered breathing (with nasal continuous positive airway pressure [CPAP]) can improve blood pressure and attenuate some of the potential hemodynamic and neurohumoral responses that may link OSA to systemic disease.[38,39]

TREATMENT
Obstructive Sleep Apnea

Desired Outcomes

In the absence of an underlying cause (e.g., hypothyroidism, acromegaly), alleviation of sleep-disordered breathing and prevention of associated complications are the primary goals of treatment. Nonpharmacologic measures are the treatments of choice. There is no drug therapy for OSA. However, medications that worsen sleep should be avoided. Practice parameters for the medical treatment of OSA have been published by the American Academy of Sleep Medicine.[40]

Nonpharmacologic Therapy

Positive Airway Pressure

❻ Nasal positive airway pressure (PAP) during sleep is the standard treatment for most patients with OSA. PAP produces a positive pressure column in the upper airway using room air to maintain patency. A flexible tube connects the PAP machine to a mask that covers the nose.

PAP delivery may be continuous (CPAP) or bilevel, providing a reduced applied pressure during expiration. During PSG, the pressure setting is increased (up to 20 cm H_2O) until sleep-disordered breathing is eliminated. Barriers to PAP adherence, such as ill-fitted mask and nasal dryness, can be managed. PAP nonadherence for one night results in a complete reversal of the gains made in daytime alertness.[41] In the clinical setting, poor PAP adherence may impact blood pressure control and management in patients with OSA and hypertension.

Weight Reduction

Obesity can worsen sleep apnea, and weight management should be implemented for all overweight patients with OSA. OSA can predispose to weight gain, and in obese patients with mild OSA weight loss alone can be effective.[42] Individuals who are morbidly obese and have severe OSA can undergo gastric stapling for weight loss.

Surgery

Surgical therapy (uvulopalatopharyngoplasty) opens the upper airway by removing the tonsils, trimming and reorienting the posterior and anterior tonsillar pillars, and removing the uvula and posterior portion of the palate. This is not a first-line option because it is invasive. In very severe cases tracheostomy may be necessary. This procedure can be indicated for select individuals who are morbidly obese, have severe facial skeletal deformity, experience severe drops in oxygen saturation (e.g., less than 70%), or have significant cardiac arrhythmias associated with their OSA.

Other Therapies

For individuals who experience OSA only during certain sleep positions (e.g., when lying on their back), positional therapies can be effective alone but are usually used in conjunction with PAP therapy. Oral appliances can be used to advance the lower jawbone and to keep the tongue forward to enlarge the upper airway. These therapies should be considered when PAP therapy cannot be tolerated.[43]

Pharmacologic Therapy

The most important pharmacologic intervention is the avoidance of all CNS depressants (e.g., alcohol, hypnotics) and drugs that promote weight gain. Weight gain worsens OSA. CNS depressant use is potentially lethal, as it reduces the brain's reflex ability to cause a mini-arousal and resume breathing. In addition, certain CNS depressants can relax airway muscles, promoting upper airway collapse. Medications that can cause rhinopharyngeal inflammation and cough as a side effect of therapy (i.e., angiotensin-converting enzyme [ACE] inhibitor) may also worsen sleep-disordered breathing.

There is no drug therapy for OSA. In clinical trials, serotonergic agents (e.g., fluoxetine, paroxetine), tricyclic antidepressants (TCAs) (i.e., imipramine, protriptyline), respiratory stimulants (theophylline), medroxyprogesterone, and clonidine do not clinically improve severity of OSA. The effects of antihypertensive agents on sleep apnea are inconsistent and are likely not clinically significant.

Wake-promoting medications (e.g., modafinil, armodafinil) are FDA-approved to improve wakefulness in patients who have residual excessive daytime sleepiness (EDS) while being treated with PAP. Initiation of therapy should be attempted in patients only after PAP therapy has been optimized to alleviate sleep-disordered breathing and EDS. Therapy should be avoided in those with concomitant cardiovascular disease. In patients with concurrent rhinitis, nasal steroids are recommended for use along with PAP therapy.

Evaluation of Therapeutic Outcomes

Individuals with sleep apnea should be evaluated after 1 to 3 months of treatment for improvement in alertness and daytime symptoms (e.g., sleepiness, memory, and irritability) and weight reduction. Individuals experiencing symptoms (e.g., daytime sleepiness, snoring, loss of blood pressure control) despite PAP therapy should have PSG repeated. Symptoms can recur if patients gain weight, requiring a higher pressure setting. Conversely, PAP pressure settings can be decreased if weight loss is achieved. Patient adherence to PAP therapy can be monitored by assessing the built-in compliance meter that measures the hours used at effective pressure.

Central Sleep Apnea

CSA causes fragmented sleep and consequent daytime somnolence. However, unlike OSA, arousals from sleep are not required to initiate airflow. During PSG, there is an absence of airflow out of the mouth and nose with no activation of the inspiratory muscles. The prevalence of CSA is not well established and is less than OSA. CSA can be idiopathic but more commonly is caused by underlying autonomic nervous system lesions (e.g., cervical cordotomy), neurologic diseases (e.g., poliomyelitis, encephalitis, and myasthenia gravis), high altitudes, opioid abuse, and congestive heart failure. For these reasons, potential underlying causes for CSA should be evaluated and treated. For example, worsening CSA in heart failure patients can signal the need to optimize heart failure therapies. Practice parameters for the treatment of CSA have been published by the American Academy of Sleep Medicine.[44]

Drug therapy for CSA is limited and is individualized for each patient, based on underlying etiology. Acetazolamide, which induces a metabolic acidosis that stimulates respiratory drive, and theophylline, which improves severity of CSA, have been studied but have minimal effects on clinical variables.[45,46]

CLINICAL PRESENTATION Narcolepsy

Symptoms

- Patients may complain of EDS and disrupted nighttime sleep; often they have some accompanying REM sleep abnormality, sleep paralysis, cataplexy, and/or hallucinations.

Laboratory Tests

- Although not routinely tested, there is a high incidence of human leukocyte antigen (HLA) haplotypes DR2 and HLA-DQ6/DQB1 in narcolepsy.

Other Diagnostic Tests

- Narcolepsy is definitively diagnosed using the multiple sleep latency test (nap test). The patient takes four to five naps in a day, and narcolepsy is diagnosed if the patient falls asleep quickly (within less than 5 minutes) and goes into REM sleep in two of those nap periods.

NARCOLEPSY

Narcolepsy is a severely debilitating neurologic disease that affects between 0.03% and 0.06% of adult Americans.[47] Despite the debilitating nature of the disease, it can be undiagnosed or misdiagnosed for years. It is equal or somewhat higher in men compared with women, and it develops during adolescence. It is commonly recognized in the second decade of life and increases in severity through the third and fourth decades.[47] Individuals with narcolepsy complain of EDS, and in the sleep laboratory, individuals with narcolepsy exhibit impairment of both the onset and the offset of REM and NREM sleep and have arousals and disturbed sleep during the night.

Four characteristic symptoms differentiate narcolepsy from other sleep disorders and are known as the *narcolepsy tetrad*: EDS, cataplexy, hallucinations, and sleep paralysis. Cataplexy, a sudden bilateral loss of muscle tone of varying severity and duration without the loss of consciousness, occurs in 70% to 80% of people with narcolepsy.[47] Patients can suffer subtle changes, such as jaw or head slumping, or severe weakness, such as knee buckling or collapsing to the ground. Cataplexy is often precipitated by situations characterized by high emotion (e.g., laughter, anger, excitement). Cataleptic episodes can be brief, lasting seconds, or can last for several minutes. Sleep paralysis is an episodic loss of voluntary muscle tone that occurs when the individual is falling asleep or waking. Individuals are conscious but not able to move or speak. Hallucinations while falling asleep (i.e., hypnagogic) and on awakening (i.e., hypnopompic) are brief, dream-like experiences that intrude into wakefulness and are experienced by nearly 70% of narcoleptics. Unfortunately, these symptoms sometimes lead to an incorrect diagnosis of mental illness.[47] Cataplexy, sleep paralysis, and hypnagogic hallucinations can be caused by REM sleep disturbances.[48]

Loss of normal function of the hypocretin-orexin neurotransmitter system appears to play a central role in the pathophysiology of narcolepsy. Neurons containing hypocretin-orexin are found in the lateral hypothalamus and project to various parts of the brain that are thought to regulate sleep. In 75% of narcoleptic patients, hypocretin-orexin is undetectable in cerebrospinal fluid.[49] Because narcoleptic patients have deficiencies in hypocretin-orexin–producing neurons,[50] an autoimmune process may be responsible for the destruction of hypocretin-producing cells.[51,52] Onset of disease occurs in adolescence or adulthood, but not at birth, suggesting that environmental influences might also play a role. Molecular studies of HLA have found a high prevalence of the HLA-DR2 and HLA-DQ6/DQB1 haplotypes in narcoleptics.[49] However, the HLA-DR2 haplotype is also common in the nonnarcoleptic population and is not diagnostic.[48] There may also be a genetic component, as 3% of patients have a first-degree relative with the disorder.[48]

TREATMENT

Desired Outcomes

Nonpharmacologic management of narcolepsy includes counseling the patient and family concerning the illness to alleviate misconceptions around the individual's behavior. Good sleep hygiene should be encouraged as well as two or more scheduled daytime naps. Daytime naps lasting 15 minutes each can help the individual with narcolepsy feel refreshed.

7 Pharmacologic management of narcolepsy is focused on two primary areas: treatment of EDS and REM sleep abnormalities. Drug therapy for narcolepsy is summarized in Table 55-4.

Pharmacologic Therapy

Modafinil, a racemic compound unrelated to psychostimulants, is a recognized standard treatment for EDS.[53] Armodafinil is the active R-isomer of modafinil and is also FDA-approved for treatment of EDS in narcolepsy. The precise mechanism of action of modafinil and armodafinil is not fully understood. Common adverse effects are usually mild and include headache, nausea, nervousness, anxiety, and insomnia. The dose of modafinil is between 200 and 400 mg/day, and armodafinil doses are between 150 and 250 mg/day.[54] Although both of these agents are effective in treating EDS, they lack efficacy for the treatment of cataplectic symptoms.[55]

EDS can also be treated with stimulants to improve alertness and to increase daytime performance. Dextroamphetamine and methylphenidate also have FDA approval for the treatment of narcolepsy. Methamphetamine and mixed amphetamine salts have also been used on an off-label basis. Methylphenidate and amphetamines have a fast onset of action and durations of 6 to 10 and 3 to 4 hours, respectively. The dose can range from 5 to 60 mg daily.

Stimulants improve alertness and daytime performance, and they can elevate mood and prevent sleep. Side effects can include insomnia, hypertension, palpitations, and irritability. Tolerance to long-term stimulant therapy can occur, necessitating dosage increases. Amphetamine use is associated with more likelihood of abuse and tolerance, especially when prescribed in high doses. Lisdexamfetamine is a new amphetamine prodrug rapidly absorbed and converted in the body to dextroamphetamine. It has a longer duration of action and less risk of abuse since it is active only when taken orally.

TABLE 55-4 Drugs Used to Treat Narcolepsy

Generic Name	Brand Name	Initial Dose (mg)	Usual Dose (mg)	Comments
Excessive Daytime Somnolence				
Dextroamphetamine	Dexedrine	5–10	5–60	Concurrent use of amphetamines and acidic foods may reduce amphetamine absorption
Dextroamphetamine/amphetamine salts[a]	Adderall	5–20	5–60	See above
Methamphetamine[b]	Desoxyn	5–15	5–15	See above
Lisdexamfetamine	Vyvanse	20–30	20–70	Prodrug of dextroamphetamine
Methylphenidate	Ritalin	10–40	30–80	May increase risk of bleeding with concomitant warfarin therapy
Modafinil	Provigil	100–200	200–400	May reduce effectiveness of hormonal contraceptives
Armodafinil	Nuvigil	150	150–250	May reduce effectiveness of hormonal contraceptives
Sodium oxybate[c]	Xyrem	4.5 g/night	4.5–9 g/night	Do not use with other CNS depressants
Agents for Cataplexy				
Fluoxetine	Prozac	10–20	20–80	Will see cataplexy benefits sooner than antidepressant benefits
Imipramine	Tofranil	50–100	50–250	Anticholinergic side effects
Nortriptyline	Aventyl, Pamelor	50–100	50–200	Anticholinergic side effects
Protriptyline	Vivactil	5–10	5–30	
Venlafaxine	Effexor	37.5	37.5–225	May increase blood pressure
Selegiline	Eldepryl	5–10	20–40	Doses less than 10 mg/day do not require dietary tyramine restrictions

[a]Dextroamphetamine sulfate, dextroamphetamine saccharate, amphetamine aspartate, and amphetamine sulfate.
[b]Not available in some states.
[c]Also is effective at treating cataplexy.

Data from references 52 and 53.

The most effective treatments for cataplexy are TCAs, venlafaxine, and fluoxetine. The mechanism of antidepressants in relieving cataplexy, hypnagogic hallucinations, and sleep paralysis can be mediated through blockade of serotonin and norepinephrine reuptake in the locus coeruleus and raphe and subsequent suppression of REM sleep.[56] Imipramine, protriptyline, clomipramine, fluoxetine, and nortriptyline are effective in approximately 80% of patients. Selegiline improves hypersomnolence and cataplexy through REM suppression and an increase in REM latency. Methylphenidate and amphetamines alone are usually ineffective for complete relief of cataplexy.

Sodium oxybate (γ-hydroxybutyrate, Xyrem) improves symptoms of EDS and decreases episodes of sleep paralysis, cataplexy, and hypnagogic hallucinations. Nightly administration of sodium oxybate changes sleep architecture to resemble normal sleep. It increases slow-wave sleep, decreases nighttime awakenings, and increases REM efficiency.[57] Sodium oxybate is available only as a liquid and is taken as two doses; one is taken at bedtime and the second dose is taken 2.5 to 4 hours later. Sodium oxybate is a potent sedative–hypnotic and should not be used concomitantly with any other sedating medications. The most common side effects include nausea, somnolence, confusion, dizziness, and incontinence.

Clinical **Controversy. . .**

In narcoleptic patients sodium oxybate effectively improves cataplexy and daytime sleepiness. Some practitioners advocate that sodium oxybate can be prescribed as monotherapy to control all narcolepsy symptoms. However, the majority of studies have evaluated the effects of sodium oxybate on daytime sleepiness with concomitant stimulant therapy, and additive benefits are obtained with dual therapy. Many subjects taking sodium oxybate will also require stimulant therapy to optimally control daytime sleepiness. Further study is needed.

Evaluation of Therapeutic Outcomes

The primary objective of pharmacologic treatment of narcolepsy is to reduce symptoms that adversely impact quality of life. The goal is to produce the fullest possible return of normal function for patients at work, school, home, and in social settings. Patients with narcolepsy should keep a diary of the frequency and severity of cataplexy, sleep paralysis, and sleep hallucinations. Patients should be evaluated regularly during medication titrations and then every 6 to 12 months to assess for adverse drug effects (e.g., sleep disturbances, hypertension, and cardiovascular abnormalities). The healthcare provider should consider the benefit-to-risk ratio for the individual patient, the cost of medication, the convenience of administration, and the cost of laboratory tests when selecting narcolepsy therapies.[53] One wake-promoting agent may work better than another in an individual patient. Thus, if one agent is not effective at adequate doses, a trial with another agent should be undertaken.

CIRCADIAN RHYTHM DISORDERS

The sleep–wake cycle is under the circadian control of oscillators and can be disrupted by misalignment between an individual's biologic clock and external demands on the sleep cycle. Circadian rhythm sleep disorders usually present with either insomnia or hypersomnia, depending on the individual's performance requirements. Two commonly occurring circadian rhythm sleep disorders are jet lag and shift work sleep problems.

Jet Lag

Jet lag occurs when a person travels across time zones, and the external environmental time is mismatched with the internal circadian clock. Sleep disturbances typically last for 2 to 3 days but can last as long as 7 to 10 days if the time zone changes are greater than 8 hours. Compared with westward travel, eastward travel is associated with a longer duration of jet lag. Jet lag leads to increased incidence of GI disturbances and a decrease in alertness and performance.

❽ Treatment of jet lag includes nonpharmacologic approaches alone or in combination with drug therapy. Jet lag can be minimized in coast-to-coast travel in the United States if the duration is less than 7 days and the normal sleep–wake cycle is observed. For travel lasting longer than 7 days, jet lag severity can be lessened by 1- to 2-hour adjustments in sleep and wake times prior to departure to the destination time zone. Short-acting BZDRAs, ramelteon, and 0.5 to 5 mg melatonin, taken at appropriate target bedtimes for east or west travel, reduce jet lag and shorten sleep latency.[58]

Shift Work Sleep Disorder

Shift workers comprise approximately 20% of the workforce.[59] Night shift work causes a misalignment in the sleep–wake cycle and circadian rhythm that is associated with a decrease in alertness, performance, and quality of daytime sleep. More than 65% of workers on rotating shifts complain of insomnia, compared with only 20% who work one shift.[60] Shift workers ultimately are at risk of developing shift work sleep disorder (SWSD). SWSD is a complaint of insomnia or excessive sleepiness that occurs because of circadian sleep disruption due to working shifts during normal sleep time.[7,59] Shift workers have a higher injury rate, divorce rate, occurrence of on-the-job sleepiness, and incidence of substance use. They may also be at increased risk of developing peptic ulcers, depression, breast cancer, and sleepiness-related accidents.[59–61] Night shift workers are usually in a state of permanent circadian misalignment because of the tendency to revert to conventional sleep schedules on their days off.[60]

Treatment for shift work sleep problems includes optimizing sleep hygiene, extending daytime sleep by sleeping in the afternoon, scheduling a 2- to 3-hour nap on days off from work, or switching to a day shift job. Short-acting BZDRAs, ramelteon, and melatonin can consolidate sleep during day sleep periods and reduce lost sleep time. Modafinil and armodafinil are FDA-approved to improve wakefulness in patients with EDS associated with SWSD. Scheduled exposure to bright lights at night and darkness in the daytime improves adaptation to night work and daytime sleep.[60]

Restless Legs Syndrome

RLS, or Ekbom's syndrome, is characterized by paresthesias that are usually felt deep in the calf muscles but can also appear in the thighs and arms with the urge to keep limbs in motion. RLS occurs in both males and females, and it occurs more frequently in the elderly. It has been associated with chronic kidney disease, iron deficiency anemia, and pregnancy. Caffeine, stress, alcohol, and fatigue can worsen symptoms. Recent data suggest that RLS can be caused by iron deficiency in the substantia nigra in the CNS.[62] The diagnosis of RLS is based on patient- or partner-reported symptoms and specific diagnostic criteria. Criteria required to diagnose RLS include (a) an urge to move the limbs that is usually associated with uncomfortable and unpleasant sensations, (b) symptoms that begin or worsen during rest or inactivity, (c) symptoms that are exclusively present or worse in the evening or night, and (d) symptoms that are temporarily relieved by movement.[63] The discomfort returns when the person tries to sleep, resulting in insomnia. Practice parameter recommendations for treatment of RLS are shown in Table 55-5.

❾ Dopamine agonists ropinirole, pramipexole, and rotigotine are FDA-approved, are effective for RLS, and are standard treatments.[64] Lower doses of dopamine agonists are used when treating RLS compared with Parkinson's disease. Providers should caution patients that compulsive behaviors (e.g., gambling, shopping, eating, etc.) may emerge during therapy with dopamine agonists.

TABLE 55-5 Evidence-Based Guidelines for Drug Therapy of RLS

Medication Recommendation[a] (Brand Name)	Strength of Recommendation[b]	Body of Evidence Level[c]
Pramipexole (Mirapex)	Standard	High
Ropinirole (Requip)	Standard	High
Levodopa and dopa decarboxylase inhibitor (Sinemet)	Guideline	High
Opioids (e.g., codeine, oxycodone, hydrocodone, methadone)	Guideline	Low
Gabapentin enacarbil (Horizant)	Guideline	High
Gabapentin[d] (Neurontin)	Option	Low
Carbamazepine (Tegretol)	Option	Low
Clonidine (Catapres)	Option	Low
Supplemental iron[e]	Option	Very low

[a]At the time of publishing, rotigotine was not available in the United States, thus, no recommendations were made for rotigotine in the published practice parameters.
[b]"Standard" indicates recommendations for which there is high or moderate quality of evidence where the benefits clearly outweigh the harms; "guideline" indicates low quality of evidence where benefits clearly outweigh the harms, or high or moderate quality of evidence when the benefits are closely balanced with harm/burden or there is uncertainty about the benefits/harms/burdens.
[c]Level of evidence: high—very confident in effect estimate of agent; moderate—moderately confident in effect estimate; low—limited confidence in effect estimate; very low—very little confidence in effect estimate.
[d]Pregabalin is recommended similarly to gabapentin.
[e]In patients with low serum ferritin concentrations.

Data from reference 64.

Levodopa therapy is associated with a high incidence of symptom augmentation and, because of a short half-life, might not provide relief over the entire night. Augmentation is a worsening in symptom severity, increase in symptom distribution, or emergence of symptoms earlier in the evening. Sedative–hypnotic agents can be effective in patients who have frequent awakenings from their RLS symptoms. Clonazepam at doses ranging from 0.5 to 2 mg has been most frequently studied; however, patients may experience carryover sedation because of its long duration of action. Shorter half-life sedative–hypnotics (e.g., zolpidem, zaleplon) can improve sleep and reduce daytime sleepiness without carryover sedation. Opiates such as methadone 5 to 20 mg, codeine 30 to 120 mg, and oxycodone 2.5 mg are effective for patients with painful RLS. The potential for tolerance and dependence on opiate therapy should be considered. Gabapentin 300 to 900 mg near bedtime can also be considered for those with paresthetic or painful RLS symptoms.[65] Gabapentin enacarbil (Horizant) is a gabapentin prodrug that is now FDA-approved for the treatment of RLS at a dose of 600 mg taken at 5 PM. Iron studies should be completed in patients with RLS and iron supplementation initiated in those who are iron deficient. In patients with ferritin concentrations less than 50 to 75 mcg/L (ng/mL), iron supplementation improves RLS symptoms.[66] Patients with RLS or PLMS should be evaluated regularly to monitor for excessive daytime somnolence, tolerance, efficacy, and adverse effects of the medication. Therapy should be monitored for adverse effects found in Table 55-6.

Periodic Leg Movements of Sleep

RLS patients commonly have PLMS, while approximately one third of patients with PLMS have RLS.[64] PLMS are stereotypic, repetitive, periodic movements of the legs that occur during sleep every 20 to 40 seconds and last 10 minutes to several hours.[64] The movements usually involve the big toe, but the ankle, knee, and hip can also flex. They can be terminated by a violent kick or other body movement. Often patients will be unaware of these movements

TABLE 55-6 Monitoring Table for Medications Used to Treat RLS and PLMS

Drug or Drug Class	Adverse Drug Reaction	Monitoring Parameter	Comments
Dopamine agonists	Compulsive behaviors	Frequency and quantity of eating, gambling, shopping, other reward behaviors	May occur at any time during therapy
Levodopa/carbidopa	Symptom augmentation	Location and timing of RLS symptoms	Appearance of symptoms in other areas of body and earlier in day
Gabapentin/pregabalin	Dizziness	Subjective dizziness, falls	—
Sedative–hypnotics (clonazepam, temazepam, zolpidem, etc.)	Carryover sedation	Morning sleepiness, grogginess	More likely to occur with longer-duration agents
Opioids (oxycodone, codeine, hydrocodone, etc.)	Tolerance, constipation	RLS symptoms and response to ongoing therapy	—
Oral iron therapy (ferrous sulfate, etc.)	GI upset, constipation	Monitor for constipation	Prophylactic stool softeners may be necessary to reduce risk of constipation

and only recognize consequent insufficient sleep and morning leg cramps. A bed partner can describe PLMS. PLMS is diagnosed in the sleep laboratory using electromyogram recordings.

PLMS can occur with RLS or alone because of systemic disease (e.g., renal failure) or drug therapy.[67] TCAs, SSRIs, dopaminergic antagonists, xanthines, nicotine, alcohol, and caffeine can all worsen PLMS. The treatment approach for PLMS is similar to that of RLS. If PLMS do not cause disruptions for the patient or bed partner or daytime symptoms, they may not require treatment. Symptomatic or problematic PLMS should be treated with dopaminergic medications to suppress limb movements or sedative–hypnotics to reduce awakenings and consolidate sleep.

PARASOMNIAS

Parasomnias are abnormal behavior or physiologic events that either occur during sleep or are exaggerated by sleep. Many of these disorders are considered to be disorders of partial arousal from various sleep stages. Parasomnias can be categorized as disorders of arousal (sleepwalking, sleep terrors), sleep–wake transition disorders (sleep-talking), rhythmic movement disorder, REM parasomnias (REM behavior disorder, nightmares), and miscellaneous parasomnias (enuresis, bruxism). Sleepwalking, sleep terrors, and sleep-talking predominantly occur during NREM sleep, whereas others (REM behavior disorder) occur during REM sleep.

Sleepwalking and sleep terrors are found normally in children between the ages of 4 and 12 years and usually resolve in adolescence. These disorders are increasingly recognized to also occur in adulthood, and, contrary to previous beliefs, are not related to psychological or psychiatric pathology.[68] Sleep terrors can begin in adults between the ages of 20 and 30 years. Onset of sleepwalking in adults without a childhood history of sleepwalking should prompt a search for a neurologic or substance use condition.[69] Sleepwalking and sleep terror disorder involve intrusions of wakefulness into NREM sleep during the first third of the night. In sleepwalking, individuals become ambulatory, are difficult to awaken, and are amnestic for the event. Sleep terrors involve intense fear and autonomic arousal. Individuals are difficult to awaken, inconsolable, and amnestic for the event.[69] Patients with REM behavior disorder act out their dreams, often in a violent manner, and are at risk for injury.

Treatment of sleepwalking involves protecting the individual from harm by putting safety latches on doors and windows, removing hazardous objects from bedrooms, and covering glass doors with heavy curtains. In adult patients, benzodiazepines, SSRIs, or TCAs can be beneficial therapies for sleepwalking or other NREM disorders of arousal.[68] Benzodiazepines can also be helpful in curtailing sleep terrors in adults.[69] Nightmares are anxiety-provoking dreams characterized by vivid recall. Treatment is directed at reducing stress, anxiety, and sleep deprivation. In extreme cases, low-dose benzodiazepines can be indicated. Clonazepam is the treatment of choice for REM behavior disorder. Melatonin (3 to 12 mg at bedtime) can also be an effective therapy for REM behavior disorder.[70]

PERSONALIZATION OF THERAPY

For the treatment of insomnia, the choice of a particular BZDRA can be based on its pharmacokinetic profile. When used as a single dose, extent of distribution and elimination half-life are important in predicting the duration of action. However, after multiple doses, the elimination half-life and formation of active metabolites determine the extent of drug accumulation and resultant clinical effects.[11] Advanced age, liver dysfunction, and drug interactions can prolong drug effects. The pharmacokinetic profiles of BZDRAs are summarized in Table 55-3. To individualize treatment of narcolepsy many clinicians prescribe both immediate-release and sustained-release stimulants to increase alertness throughout the day. Sustained-release stimulants are prescribed with scheduled administration times, and immediate-release stimulants can be taken as needed when the patient requires alertness (e.g., driving, etc.).

ABBREVIATIONS

ACE	angiotensin-converting enzyme
BZDRA	benzodiazepine receptor agonist
CPAP	continuous positive airway pressure
CSA	central sleep apnea
DSM-IV-TR	*Diagnostic and Statistical Manual of Mental Disorders, Fourth Edition, Text Revision*
EDS	excessive daytime sleepiness
EEG	electroencephalogram
GABA	γ-aminobutyric acid
HLA	human leukocyte antigen
NREM	nonrapid eye movement
OSA	obstructive sleep apnea
PAP	positive airway pressure
PLMS	periodic limb movements of sleep
PSG	polysomnography
RDI	respiratory disturbance index
REM	rapid eye movement
RLS	restless legs syndrome
SWSD	shift work sleep disorder
TCA	tricyclic antidepressant

REFERENCES

1. Walsh JK, Engelhardt CL. The direct economic costs of insomnia in the United States for 1995. Sleep 1999;22: S386–S393.
2. Neylan TC, Reynolds CF III, Kupfer DJ. Sleep disorders. In: Yudofsky SC, Hales RE, eds. American Psychiatric Press Textbook of Neuropsychiatry, 4th ed. Washington, DC: American Psychiatric Press, 2003:975–1000.
3. Benca RM, Cirelli C, Rattenborg NC, Tononi G. Basic science of sleep. In: Sadock BJ, Sadock VA, eds. Kaplan and Sadock's Comprehensive Textbook of Psychiatry, 8th ed. Philadelphia, PA: Lippincott Williams & Wilkins, 2005:280–294.
4. Dagan Y, Abadi J. Sleep–wake disorder disability: A lifelong untreatable pathology of the circadian time structure. Chronobiol Int 2001;18:1019–1027.
5. Franken P. Long-term versus short-term processes regulating REM sleep. J Sleep Res 2002;11:17–28.
6. Stickgold R, Hobson JA, Fosse R, Fosse M. Sleep, learning and dreams: Off-line memory reprocessing. Science 2001; 294:1052–1058.
7. American Academy of Sleep Medicine. The International Classification of Sleep Disorders: Diagnostic and Coding Manual, 2nd ed. Darien, IL: American Academy of Sleep Medicine, 2005.
8. American Psychiatric Association. Sleep disorders. In: Diagnostic and Statistical Manual of Mental Disorders, Fourth Edition, Text Revision. Washington, DC: American Psychiatric Press, 2000:597–644.
9. Schutte-Rodin S, Broch L, Buysse D, et al. Clinical guideline for the evaluation and management of chronic insomnia in adults. J Clin Sleep Med 2008;4:487–504.
10. Chesson AL, Anderson WM, Littner M, et al. Practice parameters for the nonpharmacologic treatment of chronic insomnia. Sleep 1999;8:1–6.
11. Kirkwood CK. Management of insomnia. J Am Pharm Assoc 1999;39:688–696.
12. Sateia MJ, Doghramji K, Hauri PJ, et al. Evaluation of chronic insomnia. Sleep 2000;23:1–39.
13. Lippmann S, Mazour I, Shabab H. Insomnia: Therapeutic approach. South Med J 2001;94:866–874.
14. Vaughn-McCall W. A psychiatric perspective on insomnia. J Clin Psychiatr 2001;62(Suppl 10):27–32.
15. Morgenthaler TI, Kramer M, Alessi C, et al. Practice parameters for the psychological and behavioral treatment of insomnia: An update. An American Academy of Sleep Medicine report. Sleep 2006;29:1415–1419.
16. Sivertsen B, Omvik S, Pallesen S, et al. Cognitive behavioral therapy vs zopiclone for treatment of chronic primary insomnia in older adults: A randomized controlled trial. JAMA 2006;295:2851–2858.
17. Hauri PJ. Insomnia. Clin Chest Med 1998;19:157–168.
18. Jackson CW. Mood disorders. In: Mueller BA, ed. Pharmacotherapy Self Assessment Program (PSAP). Kansas City, MO: American College of Clinical Pharmacy, 2002:203–250.
19. Kryger M, Roth T, Wang-Weigand S, et al. The effects of ramelteon on respiration during sleep in subjects with moderate to severe chronic obstructive pulmonary disease. Sleep Breath 2009;13:79–84.
20. Kryger M, Wang-Weigand S, Roth T. Safety of ramelteon in individuals with mild to moderate obstructive sleep apnea. Sleep Breath 2007;11:159–164.
21. Schulz V, Hansel R, Tyler VE. Rational Phytotherapy: A Physician's Guide to Herbal Medicine. Berlin: Springer, 1998:81.
22. Stone KL, Ensrud KE, Ancoli-Israel S. Sleep, insomnia and falls in elderly patients. Sleep Med 2008;9(Suppl 1): S18–S22.
23. Terzano MG, Rossi M, Palomba V, et al. New drugs for insomnia: Comparative tolerability of zopiclone, zolpidem and zaleplon. Drug Saf 2003;26:261–282.
24. Ambien, zolpidem [product information]. Bridgewater, NJ: Sanofi-Aventis, 2012.
25. Elie R, Ruteher E, Farr IK, et al. Sleep latency is shortened during 4 weeks of treatment with zaleplon, a novel nonbenzodiazepine hypnotic. J Clin Psychiatry 1999;60:536–544.
26. Walsh JK, Fry J, Erwin CS, et al. Efficacy and tolerability of 14-day administration of zaleplon 5 mg and 10 mg for the treatment of primary insomnia. Clin Drug Investig 1998;16:347–354.
27. Walsh JK, Pollack CP, Shark MMB, et al. Lack of residual sedation following middle-of-the-night zaleplon administration in sleep maintenance insomnia. Clin Neuropharmacol 2000;23:17–21.
28. Lunesta, eszopiclone [product information]. Marlborough, MA: Sunovion, 2010.
29. Krystal AD, Walsh JK, Laska E, et al. Sustained efficacy of eszopiclone over 6 months of nightly treatment: Results of a randomized, double-blind, placebo-controlled study in adults with chronic insomnia. Sleep 2003;26:793–797.
30. Jermaine DM. Sleep disorders. In: Carter BL, Angaran DM, Lake KD, Raebel MA, eds. Pharmacotherapy Self-Assessment Program, 2nd ed. Psychiatry Module. Kansas City: American College of Clinical Pharmacy, 1995: 139–154.
31. Young T, Peppard PE, Gottlieb DJ. Epidemiology of obstructive sleep apnea: A population health perspective. Am J Respir Crit Care Med 2002;165:1217–1239.
32. Young T, Palta M, Dempsey J, et al. The occurrence of sleep-disordered breathing among middle-aged adults. N Engl J Med 1993;328:1230–1235.
33. Peppard PE, Szklo-Coxe M, Hla KM, Young T. Longitudinal association of sleep-related breathing disorder and depression. Arch Intern Med 2006;166:1709–1715.
34. Young T, Finn L, Peppard PE, et al. Sleep disordered breathing and mortality: Eighteen-year follow-up of the Wisconsin sleep cohort. Sleep 2008;31:1071–1078.
35. Terán-Santos J, Jimenez-Gomez A, Cordero-Guevara J. The association between sleep apnea and the risk of traffic accidents. N Engl J Med 1999;340:847–851.
36. Somers VK, White DP, Amin R, et al. Sleep apnea and cardiovascular disease: An American Heart Association/ American College of Cardiology Foundation scientific statement from the American Heart Association Council for High Blood Pressure Research Professional Education Committee, Council on Clinical Cardiology, Stroke Council, and Council on Cardiovascular Nursing. J Am Coll Cardiol 2008;52:686–717.
37. Calhoun DA, Jones D, Textor S, et al. Resistant hypertension: Diagnosis, evaluation, and treatment: A scientific statement from the American Heart Association Professional Education Committee of the Council for High Blood Pressure Research. Circulation 2008;117:e510–e526.
38. Marin JM, Agusti A, Villar I, et al. Association between treated and untreated obstructive sleep apnea and risk of hypertension. JAMA 2012;307:2169–2176.
39. Kato M, Roberts-Thomson P, Phillips BG, et al. Impairment of endothelium dependent vasodilation of resistance vessels in patients with obstructive sleep apnea. Circulation 2000;102:2607–2610.

40. Morganthaler TI, Kapen S, Lee-Chiong T, et al. Practice parameters for the medical therapy of obstructive sleep apnea. Sleep 2006;29:1031–1035.
41. Kribbs NB, Pack AJ, Kline LR, et al. Effects of one night without nasal CPAP treatment on sleep and sleepiness in patients with obstructive sleep apnea. Am Rev Respir Dis 2003;147:1162–1168.
42. Peppard PE, Young T, Palta M, et al. Longitudinal study of moderate weight change and sleep-disordered breathing. JAMA 2000;284:3015–3021.
43. Ferguson KA, Cartwright R, Rogers R, et al. Oral appliances for snoring and obstructive sleep apnea: A review. Sleep 2006;29:244–262.
44. Aurora RN, Chowdhuri S, Ramar K, et al. The treatment of central sleep apnea syndromes in adults: Practice parameters with an evidence-based literature review and meta-analyses. Sleep 2012;35:17–40.
45. Javaheri S. Acetazolamide improves central sleep apnea in heart failure: A double-blind, prospective study. Am J Respir Crit Care Med 2006;173:234–237.
46. Javaheri S, Parker TJ, Wexler L, et al. Effect of theophylline on sleep-disordered breathing in heart failure. N Engl J Med 1996;335:562–567.
47. Mitler M, Hayduk R. Benefits and risks of pharmacotherapy for narcolepsy. Drug Saf 2002;25:791–809.
48. Nakayama J, Miura M, Honda M, et al. Linkage of human narcolepsy with HLA association to chromosome 4p-13-q21. Genomics 2000;65:84–86.
49. Nishino S, Ripley B, Overeem S, et al. Low cerebrospinal fluid hypocretin (orexin) and altered energy homeostasis in human narcolepsy. Ann Neurol 2001;50:381–388.
50. Thannicakal TC, Moore RY, Nienhuis R, et al. Reduced number of hypocretin neurons in human narcolepsy. Neuron 2000;27:469–474.
51. Lin L, Hungs M, Mignot E. Narcolepsy and the HLA region. J Neuroimmunol 2001;117:9–20.
52. Mignot E, Thorsby E. Narcolepsy and the HLA system [letter]. N Engl J Med 2001;344:692.
53. Morgenthaler TI, Kapur VK, Brown T, et al. Practice parameters for the treatment of narcolepsy and other hypersomnias of central origin. Sleep 2007;30:1705–1711.
54. Robertson P, Hellriegel ET. Clinical pharmacokinetic profile of modafinil. Clin Pharmacokinet 2003;42:123–127.
55. Feldman N. Narcolepsy. South Med J 2003;96:277–287.
56. Rosenthal MS. Physiology and neurochemistry of sleep. Am J Pharm Educ 1998;62:204–208.
57. Mamelak M, Black J, Montplaisir J, et al. A pilot study of the effects of sodium oxybate on sleep architecture and daytime alertness in narcolepsy. Sleep 2004;27:1327–1334.
58. Herxheimer A, Petrie KJ, Cochrane Depression, Anxiety and Neurosis Group. Melatonin for the prevention and treatment of jet lag [systematic review]. Cochrane Database Syst Rev 2005;2.
59. Drake CL, Roehrs T, Richardson G, et al. Shift work sleep disorder: Prevalence and consequences beyond that of symptomatic day workers. Sleep 2004;27:1453–1462.
60. Garbarino S, Nobili L, Beelke, M, et al. Sleep disorders and daytime sleepiness in state police shiftworkers. Arch Environ Health 2002;57:167–175.
61. Knutsson A. Health disorders of shift workers. Occup Med (Lond) 2003;53:103–108.
62. Connor JR, Boyer PJ, Menzies SL, et al. Neuropathological examination suggests impaired brain iron acquisition in restless legs syndrome. Neurology 2003;61:304–309.
63. Allen RP, Picchietti D, Hening W, et al. Restless legs syndrome: Diagnostic criteria, special considerations and epidemiology: A report from the restless legs syndrome diagnosis and epidemiology workshop at the National Institutes of Health. Sleep Med 2003;4:101–119.
64. Aurora RN, Kristo DA, Bista SR, et al. The treatment of restless legs syndrome and periodic limb movement disorder in adults—An update for 2012: Practice parameters with an evidence-based systematic review and meta-analyses. Sleep 2012;35:1039–1062.
65. Garcia-Borreguero D, Larrosa O, de la Llave Y, et al. Treatment of restless legs syndrome with gabapentin: A double-blind, cross-over study. Neurology 2002;59: 1573–1575.
66. Wang J, O'Reilly B, Venkataraman R, et al. Efficacy of oral iron in patients with restless legs syndrome and low-normal ferritin: A randomized, double-blind, placebo-controlled study. Sleep Med 2009;10:973–975.
67. Montplaisir J, Nicolas A, Denesle R, Gomez-Mancilla B. Restless legs syndrome improved by pramipexole: A double-blind randomized trial. Neurology 1999;52: 938–943.
68. Mahowald MW, Cramer Bornemann MA. NREM arousal parasomnias. In: Kryger MH, Roth T, Dement WC, eds. Principles and Practice of Sleep Medicine, 5th ed. St. Louis: Elsevier Saunders, 2011:1075–1082.
69. Schenck CH, Mahowald MW. Parasomnias managing bizarre sleep-related behavior disorders. Postgrad Med 2000;107:145–156.
70. Mahowald MW, Schenck CH. REM sleep parasomnias. In: Kryger MH, Roth T, Dement WC, eds. Principles and Practice of Sleep Medicine, 5th ed. St. Louis: Elsevier Saunders, 2011:1083–1097.

Disorders Associated with Intellectual Disabilities

56

Nancy C. Brahm, Jerry R. McKee, and Douglas W. Stewart

KEY CONCEPTS

1. Persons diagnosed with Down syndrome (DS) can be at increased risk for medical and psychiatric comorbidities.
2. In persons with DS, a thorough evaluation is needed to differentiate between depression and Alzheimer's disease.
3. Treatment plans for persons with autism focus on increasing social interactions, improving verbal and nonverbal communication, and minimizing the occurrence or impact of ritualistic, repetitive behaviors and other related mood and behavioral problems (e.g., overactivity, irritability, and self-injury).
4. Many purported pharmacologic and nonpharmacologic treatments for autism lack objective evidence-based support.
5. A structured teaching approach focusing on increasing social communication and integration with peers is needed when providing services to persons with autism.
6. Nonpharmacologic interventions for sleep disturbances in children with a diagnosis of autism spectrum disorder should be implemented prior to pharmacotherapy considerations.
7. Psychopharmacologic treatment planning should include monitoring of objective, measurable medication-responsive target behaviors, and assessment of potential adverse effects is of critical importance when treating behavioral symptoms of autism, as the response of individuals to medication therapy is highly variable.
8. The use of FDA-approved medication for off-label indications is an acceptable clinical practice if founded on evidence-based research and informed consent.
9. The four stages of Rett syndrome are associated with developmental regression.

INTRODUCTION

Intellectual disabilities (IDs) can be identified in childhood or adolescence. Current criteria for diagnosis are based on deficiencies in intellectual and adaptive functioning with an onset prior to 18 years of age.[1] This diagnosis is made regardless of the presence or absence of concomitant medical or psychiatric disorders. In the case of mild ID, deficiencies may not be apparent in early life. Problems can be noted when the chronologic age of the child and the developmental milestones achieved by peers with similar backgrounds, cultures, socioeconomic status, and psychosocial settings differ significantly.[1] These gaps between developmental advances widen as the individual ages. Adaptive functioning deficits pose a number of challenges in treating those with an ID.

Whereas it has been estimated that a psychiatric disorder may beset approximately one-fifth of the general population in the United States, the prevalence may be double for persons with an ID.[2] Underrecognition of the need for mental health services may be due to a lack of caregiver awareness regarding psychiatric disorders in persons with IDs and/or insufficient provider training and clinical experience with this population.[2] Additional barriers to accurate diagnosis may arise from deficits in adaptive functioning, a mechanism by which individuals effectively manage commonly encountered life demands and independence compared with nondevelopmentally disabled peers.[1] Communication deficits are a barrier specific to this population. Furthermore, those with an ID often have few social interactions and limited integration into the community. Stimulation and interaction with peers typically shapes behaviors in the general population. A different set of coping skills can develop in their absence. Self-talk is an example of a coping mechanism that can be misinterpreted as a sign of psychosis. Inadequate coping skills may result in a higher risk for the development of adjustment problems.[3] Another potential problem for the clinician assessing persons with an ID is a significant gap between receptive and expressive language skills. If not readily recognized, intellectual capabilities can be overestimated, resulting in incongruent expectations and/or abilities. In the general population, features of psychiatric illnesses are more readily identifiable, and the clinician is able to effectively interview and evaluate the patient. The term "diagnostic overshadowing" has been used to refer to clinician perceptions that behavioral problems are secondary to an ID and not the result of a psychiatric comorbidity.[4]

The term "mental retardation" (MR) is now generally used only with respect to the diagnostic criteria found in the *Diagnostic and Statistical Manual of Mental Disorders, Fourth Edition, Text Revision* (*DSM-IV-TR*).[1] The currently accepted designation is "ID." The American Association on Intellectual and Developmental Disabilities (AAIDD) supports this designation and has a definition on their website.[5] For this chapter, the designation "ID" will be applied to the population of individuals who scored 70 or less on standardized intelligence tests, indicative of some limitations in intellectual functioning and adaptive behavior(s) with onset before 18 years of age. The term MR will be applied sparingly. This chapter focuses on Down syndrome (DS), autistic disorder, and Rett syndrome (RTT).

CLINICAL PRESENTATION Mental Retardation

Diagnostic features

Essential feature: significantly subaverage general intellectual functioning and accompanied by:

Criterion A: significant limitations in adaptive functioning in at least two of the following skill areas:

- Communication
- Self-care
- Home living
- Social/interpersonal skills
- Use of community resources
- Self-direction
- Functional academic skills
- Work, leisure, health, and safety

Criterion B: onset must occur before age 18 years.

Criterion C: MR has many different etiologies and may be seen as a final common pathway of various pathologic processes that affect the functioning of the central nervous system.

Degrees of severity of MR

Mild MR: IQ level 50 to 55 to approximately 70
Moderate retardation: IQ level 35 to 40, to 50 to 55
Severe MR: IQ level 20 to 25, to 35 to 40
Profound MR: IQ level below 20 or 25

Data from reference 1, with permission.

DOWN SYNDROME

1 DS is associated with common dysmorphic features and a wide range of medical and psychiatric concerns, including a number of developmental abnormalities. Congenital heart defects, seizures, orthopedic abnormalities, sensory defects, and disorders of the eye (e.g., cataracts, glaucoma), GI tract, immune system, skin, and thyroid gland are all associated with DS. Persons diagnosed with DS also have a high probability of early onset Alzheimer's disease (AD).[6] This section will focus on DS and the comorbidities of AD and leukemia.

Epidemiology

DS is the most frequently occurring genetically based syndrome associated with an ID.[7] In the United States, the incidence is estimated to be 1 in 732 births, although prevalence rates may be different for specific racial/ethnic populations.[7]

Etiology and Pathophysiology

Chromosomal analysis identified the etiology of DS as the presence of an extra chromosome 21. DS, also referred to as trisomy 21, represents one of the most studied abnormal chromosomal conditions. Nondisjunction of chromosome 21 accounts for the majority of the errors. Chromosomes divide and separate in a process known as disjunction during meiotic division. Failure to fully separate at this stage can result in both chromosomes remaining in the same cell, creating an abnormal number of chromosomes on each strand. The nondisjunction at chromosome 21 is strongly linked to increased maternal age.

For many years, advanced maternal age has been recognized to positively correlate with an increased risk for DS. Consideration has been given to paternal age as a potential risk factor for DS. The possibility of paternally mediated nondisjunction has not been eliminated, but evidence of a link has been inconclusive.[8]

Those with DS are more at risk for congenital heart defects. A retrospective, case–control study that included maternal questionnaire completion and medical records review sought to evaluate use of folic acid supplementation during the periconceptual period and any association between congenital heart defects and DS. Controlling for substance use during pregnancy and demographics, including maternal age at conception, supplementation use was compared between two groups. In the cohort with DS and congenital defects, specifically atrioventricular septal defects, supplement use was less compared with those with DS and no defects.[9]

Clinical Presentation and Diagnosis

The consequences of this chromosomal variance include characteristic facial features, some degree of ID, hypotonia, an increased risk for congenital heart disease, and early onset AD.[6] The characteristic facial features make children with DS more readily identifiable at birth.[10] IDs range from mild to severe.[10]

For the purpose of this chapter, the term *dual diagnosis* refers to an intellectually disabled person with a comorbid psychiatric disorder.[2] The most prevalent psychiatric and/or behavioral disorders in persons with an ID involve attention, mood, personality, and cognitive processing.[11] One population-based study of persons with ID ($n = 1{,}023$) sought to determine the prevalence of psychiatric disorders. Using regression analysis in conjunction with comprehensive individual evaluations, approximately 40% met criteria for needing mental health services.[12] In persons with DS, depression prevalence rates ranged from zero to slightly over 11%.[13] The risk for depression is increased by a number of factors, such as decreased total brain volume; reduced levels of the neurotransmitters, specifically serotonin, γ-aminobutyric acid (GABA), taurine, and dopamine, critical in mood regulation; and decreased cognitive function.[13]

The differential diagnosis for mood disorders in all patients should include an evaluation of thyroid function. The lifetime risk of thyroid disorder as a comorbidity in people with DS is estimated at 3% to 5%.[10] Because clinical signs and symptoms of hypothyroidism can mimic some of the features of depression, thyroid function should be evaluated in patients with DS.

TREATMENT

Desired Outcomes

Treatment goals in DS are to identify medical and psychiatric comorbidities, set realistic goals, and provide effective nonpharmacologic and pharmacologic interventions to improve the quality and length of life.

CLINICAL PRESENTATION Down Syndrome

General

- Individual may have the characteristic physical features described below.

Diagnostic features

- Facial features can suggest DS, but an additional diagnostic evaluation is necessary.
- Degree of ID ranges from mild to profound.
- Growth delays are common.

Common physical characteristics

- Hypotonia can be evident at birth.
- Facial features include flattened, broad facies with upslanted eye folds, and a large, protruding tongue.
- The palate can be narrow and the neck thick and broad.
- Hands are characteristically short and broad.

Other clinical concerns

- An increased risk for congenital heart problems, and a cardiac evaluation is generally done shortly after birth with periodic followup.
- Congenital cataracts and hypothyroidism are common.
- Leukemia is often diagnosed in early childhood.
- Features of AD can present by the third or fourth decade.

Data from references 10 and 14.

General Approach to Treatment

Medical screenings should assess for hypothyroidism, cardiac problems, sensory impairments (including hearing loss secondary to chronic otitis media with effusion or vision defects due to congenital cataracts or glaucoma), and GI problems (including constipation and celiac disease).[10] Guidelines for health supervision and anticipatory guidance in infants, children, and adolescents with DS are available through the American Academy of Pediatrics (AAP).[10] Routine screenings are also recommended throughout the course of life to address psychosocial changes, potential residential or vocational stressors, and the consequences of aging.[10]

Nonpharmacologic Treatments

The use of social supports for both individuals with DS and their family is known to help develop functional adaptive skills and therefore the fulfillment of the potential of the person with DS.[10] Family education and support network development assist caregivers by providing tools and resources necessary to more effectively manage persons with DS, allowing these persons to achieve their full potential. In the treatment of psychiatric disorders, treatment modalities available to the general population also apply to those with DS. Nonpharmacologic options for depression include psychotherapy and electroconvulsive therapy (ECT).[13] Information on the effectiveness of ECT in the DS population is limited to case reports. If communication skills are adequate, psychotherapy may also be an option. Treatment strategies include psychodynamic and cognitive behavior therapy (CBT). A review of the literature found that psychotherapy applicability results can vary with the level of ID. For persons with mild intellectual impairment and depression, this treatment modality may be beneficial. The current behavioral therapy models are more effective in addressing specific problematic behaviors rather than the underlying emotional problems of persons with ID. The extent to which these strategies translate to persons with DS and moderate to severe ID is not known.[13]

Pharmacologic Treatments

Pharmacotherapy for the treatment of depression in patients with DS follows guidelines used in the general population. For more information on the treatment of depression, see Chapter 51.

Features of depression commonly seen in persons with DS, in order of frequency, include apathy, disordered sleep, and changes in weight. Difficulty identifying depression in this population is impacted by the level of cognitive impairment, the ability to express abstract concepts (such as helplessness or hopelessness), and the level of adaptive functioning.[13] Clinical trials focused specifically on this population are few, and most information has been based on small studies or case reports. Efficacy of selective serotonin reuptake inhibitors (SSRIs) and amitriptyline is reported. If psychotic features (e.g., delusions, hallucinations) are present, low-dose antipsychotic augmentation is recommended. In the studies reviewed, treatment duration was 2 to 3 years.[13]

As with treatment of depression in the general population, it is essential to ensure that the medication trial is of appropriate dose and duration of antidepressant or combination antidepressant/antipsychotic. Ruling out comorbid medical conditions that could contribute to depression is essential.

Personalized Pharmacotherapy

In addition to the chromosomal aberration and dysmorphic features associated with DS, certain hematologic malignancies are more common in children with DS, with acute lymphoblastic leukemia (ALL) and the megakaryoblastic form of acute myelogenous leukemia (AML) seen much more frequently than other cancers. Children with DS have anecdotally been observed to have higher rates of methotrexate toxicity during treatment for cancers compared with other children. Speculation concerning causality has focused on alterations in methotrexate metabolism controlled by genes on chromosome 21. Even though mouth ulcers and bone marrow suppression are seen more frequently in children with DS receiving methotrexate, differences in pharmacokinetics do not appear to explain the higher rate of toxicity in patients with DS.[15]

Down Syndrome with Alzheimer's Disease

2 Persons with IDs, including DS, are at greater risk for AD. In adults with DS, more than 25% experience neuropsychiatric symptoms,[16] including aggression, inattention, impulsivity, and

stereotypies. In adults with DS evaluated for AD, it was reported that depressed adults with no discernible reason for sadness were more likely to be positive for dementia.[16]

Assessing changes in functionality and cognition are problematic in this population, particularly in those with greater intellectual impairments. Early studies in this population did not specify the diagnostic criteria used for identification of dementia of Alzheimer's type. A well-delineated diagnosis of AD or dementia, Alzheimer's type, requires a documented decline from baseline cognitive functioning. To meet the diagnostic criteria, the following are needed: baseline functioning data, functionality changes not explained by general aging, and progressive decline.[1] Identification of appropriate assessment scales for use in those with DS has also been problematic. The Dementia Scale for Mentally Retarded Persons (DMR) was used as the primary outcome measure in a medication efficacy trial. It also provided secondary outcome measurement and assessment of cognition, neuropsychiatric features, adaptive behavior, and a global impression.[17]

In persons older than 40 with DS, behavior changes are the primary features of the early stages of dementia. For this older cohort, higher frequencies of irritability, fear, sadness, and suspicion are seen than in a younger population. Violent outbursts have not been identified as a reliable indicator of dementia, but methodologic shortcomings preclude firm conclusions.[16] Furthermore, there is a fivefold greater prevalence of comorbid DS and dementia compared with other IDs and dementia. Gender also is important, as the male-to-female ratio is 3:1 for DS and AD.[18] Selected task skills were found to decline 2 years prior to a diagnosis of AD.[19] In the absence of documentation of change, specific criteria needed for a diagnosis of AD may not be met. Diagnostic criteria for AD include changes in memory, language skills, and activities of daily living (ADLs).[1] Information on the natural progression of cognitive changes in those with DS and AD is limited.

Pathophysiology

Neuritic plaques and neurofibrillary tangles are the hallmarks of AD. A gene for amyloid-β precursor protein is located on chromosome 21.[20] Neuropathic changes associated with AD are typically found in those with DS by middle age.[16] The severity of ID has been theorized to significantly impact the incidence of AD, but study results are inconclusive, and the level of ID may limit evaluation. A study of DS (n = 405) with and without dementia identified specific amyloid-β precursor proteins that might be predictors of dementia in DS regardless of age, gender, and level of ID.[20] A more extensive discussion of the pathophysiology of AD is beyond the scope of this chapter. For more information about AD, see Chapter 38.

TREATMENT

The therapeutic goal is to maintain functioning and quality of life as close to baseline as possible for as long as possible. Approaches to therapy for persons with DS combined with AD include nonpharmacologic and pharmacologic interventions. As with the general population with AD, treatment of AD for those with DS is multimodal and includes currently available treatments and supports in order to maintain functionality as long as possible.[21]

Nonpharmacologic Treatments

Traditionally, this population receives some level of residential living supports in either the family home or a residential facility. Depending on the level of ID, a family member, other caregiver, or residential facility staff may provide information to the clinician regarding functional status.

Pharmacologic Treatments

Pharmacologic treatments neither cure nor stop the pathologic changes associated with AD. The goals of pharmacotherapy in persons with DS and AD, as in the general population of AD patients, are to slow the decline in cognitive function and help preserve ADLs to the greatest extent possible. The use of cholinesterase inhibitors and an *N*-methyl-D-aspartate (NMDA) receptor antagonist in the DS population is being studied.

There is evidence to support the use of cholinesterase inhibitors to enhance learning and memory in persons with DS. The majority of the research in this area has been with donepezil. In a review of the literature, a 24-week, double-blind, placebo-controlled, parallel-group trial (n = 30, 27 completed) used the DMR as the primary outcome measure and the Severe Impairment Battery (SIB), Neuropsychiatric Inventory (NPI), and Adaptive Behavior Scale (ABS) as secondary measures. Findings with the DMR, SIB, and ABS indicated less deterioration for the treatment group versus the control group. The results for the NPI were reversed: the placebo group demonstrated more improvement compared with the treatment group. Dosing was 5 mg daily for the first 4 weeks, and 10 mg daily thereafter. Side effects included diarrhea, insomnia, fatigue, and nausea.[22]

Use of rivastigmine, galantamine, or memantine in those with an ID has not been studied as extensively as donepezil. An assessment of the efficacy of rivastigmine for dementia in AD in the DS population was not statistically significant compared with that in a placebo group from a previous study. Rating scales used were the DMR, NPI, and ABS.[23] Rivastigmine-associated adverse effects included GI upset (e.g., diarrhea, nausea, vomiting), fatigue, and insomnia.[23] For more information about pharmacotherapy treatment guidelines in AD, see Chapter 38.

Preexisting medical comorbidities, such as congenital heart defects, or concomitant pharmacotherapy may limit use of cholinesterase inhibitors in persons with DS. Clinicians are encouraged to monitor patients receiving cholinesterase inhibitors for bradycardia[24] and the potential for drug interactions.

A potential neurologic comorbidity of concern in this population is seizures. Overall, approximately 8% of the DS population has a seizure disorder, and seizure activity increases with age.[25] Distribution of seizure onset is bimodal, with the first peak incidence appearing before 1 year of age. This first peak is predominantly composed of infantile spasms. Seizure patterns in the DS population, in order of prevalence, are partial (47%), infantile spasms (32%), and generalized tonic–clonic (21%).[25] Advanced AD is an independent risk factor for new-onset seizures.[25] Monitoring for new-onset seizure activity and medicating with anticonvulsants as appropriate are essential. For more information about epilepsy and seizure disorders, see Chapter 40.

Evaluation of Therapeutic Outcomes

Baseline functioning must be established early in adult life prior to the onset of AD, which generally occurs during the third or fourth decade of life. This can be particularly crucial in individuals without expressive language skills. Followup evaluations should be performed annually. If cholinesterase inhibitors are used, evaluations every 2 to 4 months (after achieving a maintenance dose) are recommended to monitor for effectiveness if the anticipated gains have not been observed. Monitoring for potential medication-related side effects, including diarrhea, nausea, vomiting, insomnia, and headache, is also essential.[21]

Clinical **Controversy...**

The role of pharmacotherapy for persons 40 years or older with DS and AD is unclear.[22,26] A 52-week prospective, randomized double-blind trial of memantine in persons with DS with and without dementia showed no improvement in cognition or function. In a 24-week, double-blind, placebo-controlled trial of donepezil, three rating scales showed less deterioration in the group taking donepezil than in the placebo group, but differences were not statistically significant.

Down Syndrome and the Immune System

Leukemia is frequently diagnosed in DS children. The relative risk for leukemia is 10 to 20 times greater in persons with DS than in the general population.[27] The two forms more commonly encountered in DS children are ALL and AML. While ALL is the most common form of leukemia in all children, the rate of DS-AML is about equal to DS-ALL in children who are younger than 5 years of age (this ratio is about 1:4 in children without DS). The most commonly identified form of DS-AML is acute megakaryoblastic leukemia (AMKL). The incidence of this disorder in DS has been identified as high as 500 times greater than in the non-DS pediatric population.[28] Another myelodysplastic disorder almost unique to children with DS is transient myeloproliferative disorder (TMD). For TMD, the period prevalence in infants with DS has been estimated to be 10% to 20%.[27] It can spontaneously remit and cannot be clinically differentiated from AML. However, within 4 years following spontaneous remission of TMD, 20% of this population will develop AMKL.[28]

In the DS population, ALL survival rates are lower than in the non-ID pediatric population.[27] Children with DS also experience more chemotherapy-related toxicities (specifically mucositis and infection) compared with non-DS children with ALL.[27]

Chemotherapy-induced cardiotoxicity is of particular concern in children with DS, as 50% may have a congenital heart defect.[10] High rates of cardiomyopathy (17.5%) are reported with treatment with anthracyclines.[27] Children with DS and newly diagnosed with AML ($n = 54$) were enrolled into a standard protocol with daunorubicin and mitoxantrone to evaluate treatment efficacy and toxicities. Researchers reported the treatment protocol effective for remission and survival for the children in the DS-AML arm, but 17.5% of this group developed cardiomyopathy during or shortly after treatment completion, supporting the current practice of dosage reductions.[29] In addition, higher levels of the methotrexate metabolite were found, supporting the link between DS and drug metabolism alterations secondary to alterations on chromosome 21.[27]

Evaluation of Therapeutic Outcomes

Assessment of therapeutic outcomes for those with DS starts with a thorough multidisciplinary evaluation to establish a baseline problem list, identification of clear therapeutic goals, and using valid pharmacotherapeutic rationale to guide medication dosing and adverse drug effect monitoring.

An in-depth list of treatment targets, both subjective and objective, is important in persons with DS to assist in evaluation of medication response. Careful monitoring for emergence of potential side effects should be regularly conducted and documented as part of ongoing assessment of medication effectiveness and to ensure that side effects are not a contributing factor to behavioral changes.

AUTISM

Autistic disorder is one of five behaviorally defined pervasive developmental disorders (PDDs). Others include RTT, Asperger's disorder, childhood disintegrative disorder, and pervasive developmental disorder not otherwise specified (PDD-NOS).[1] These disorders are grouped together and referred to as autism, or autism spectrum disorders (ASDs), by the *DSM-IV-TR*. RTT and childhood disintegrative disorder are rarer, typically more severe in manifestations, and are generally considered separately. This section will focus specifically on autism, which is characterized by severe and sustained impairments in three behavioral domains: (a) reciprocal social interaction (withdrawal or lack of interest in peers), (b) language and communication skills (limitations in the use of speech and nonverbal skills), and (c) range of interests and activities (repetitive, restricted behaviors, stereotyped mannerisms).[1,30] Autism is not a disease but a neurodevelopmental disorder with multiple possible etiologies.[31] The onset is typically younger than 3 years of age and is usually, but not always, associated with some degree of ID.[1] Autism was first described by Leo Kanner in 1943 and has been historically described as early infantile autism, childhood autism, and Kanner's autism.[1]

Epidemiology

There has been a recent sharp increase in the reported prevalence of autism. Newer surveys estimate the prevalence to be 1:88.[32] It is suggested that the reported increased prevalence is primarily related to changing and broadening diagnostic criteria, along with an increased index of suspicion, rather than by an actual increased incidence, as autism is behaviorally identified, and the diagnostic boundaries are not always clear.[33,34] In addition, inclusion of individuals with diagnoses of Asperger's disorder and PDD-NOS in newer studies may contribute to the increase.[34] Some behaviors (e.g., stereotypies) seen in persons with autism can also be seen in nonautistic individuals. One study found children with a history of early institutionalization demonstrated more stereotypical behaviors that markedly decreased following increased interactions postplacement.[35] There is a significant impact of intellectual ability on the expression of symptoms of autism,[36] resulting in a lack of homogeneity in clinical expression of the condition. Autism is between four and five times more prevalent in males.[31] When present, ID ranges from mild to severe. The heterogeneity and early onset represent two methodologic problems for large-scale research studies.[31]

Etiology and Pathophysiology

The etiology of autism is attributed to multiple causal factors, including gene mutations, abnormalities in brain development, and genetic–environment interactions.[30] Autism frequently occurs concomitantly with other developmental disorders that have a known genetic basis such as RTT and fragile X syndrome.[34] Current research primarily focuses on genetics and neuropathology. Although a single genetic mutation or variant leading to autism has yet to be identified, research findings indicate that structural alterations in the genome DNA, known as copy number variations (CNVs), may be involved in ASD. Research identified a number of CNVs associated with ASDs, as this appears to be a highly heritable disorder.[37]

These findings provide support for the heterogeneity of neurodevelopmental disorders, whereby disruption represents a critical period in the development of excitatory and inhibitory neuron development. A combination of genetic and/or environmental factors, in the absence of any compensatory mechanism, may interfere with brain plasticity.[36] A meta-analysis provided some support for the theory that ASD may arise from interference in the excitatory and inhibitory balance expression and/or timing during critical periods.[38] A review of the literature found persons with autism demonstrated what was termed "unusual sensory processing." Additional findings included (a) a diagnosis of autism was associated with greater sensory symptoms than in other developmental disorders, (b) increased age was associated with decreased symptoms, and (c) for children there was a positive correlation between social impairment and sensory symptoms.[39]

Siblings of affected children have a significantly greater risk of having autism (3% to 18.7%) than those in the general population.[40] Results from a national volunteer registry ($n = 2{,}920$ children, 1,235 families, a minimum of 1 child meeting ASD diagnostic criteria, and a minimum of 1 full sibling) found that the sibling concordance rate was 10.9%. Overall an additional 8.9% of the siblings demonstrated language delay with autistic-like speech quality.[41]

Further support for the high heritability of the disorder was shown by additional research in this area. Sibling risk varies based on the gender of the index child: 4% versus 7% for female compared with male. If a second child is diagnosed, the risk for concordance in subsequent siblings increases to between 25% and 30%, higher than previously reported. The risk for a monozygotic twin with autism ranges from 60% to 95% that both twins will be diagnosed with autism.[42]

Parental age has been investigated as a potential risk factor for autism. While results are thus far inconclusive, a number of intriguing results have been found. A case–control study design of a cohort of age- and sex-matched pairs ($n = 68$) found a significant effect linking the age of both parents and a child with a diagnosis of autism. Unadjusted parental ages were higher for both parents (paternal 4 years higher, maternal 4.8 years higher) compared with controls. After adjusting for variables such as educational level and gestational age, the differences widened to 5.9 and 6.5 years, respectively.[43] Shelton et al. found parental age was a risk factor if the mother was less than 30 years old.[44]

Environmental exposures including toxic chemical exposure, teratogens, perinatal insults, prenatal infections,[34] and copper and zinc levels[45] are under investigation. Immunization with measles/mumps/rubella vaccine has been investigated, and no causal association identified.[46]

Autism frequently occurs concomitantly with epilepsy[47] and may be associated with microdeletion gene defects that are also risk factors for schizophrenia and attention-deficit/hyperactivity disorder (ADHD). Examples include the association between autism, ID, schizophrenia, and seizures with microdeletions on the 15q13.3 and 1q21.1 regions.[48] Other sites also may be implicated. The two most common single gene abnormalities associated with autism are fragile X syndrome and tuberous sclerosis.[42]

The neurodevelopmental foundation of autism has sparked significant interest in early morphologic changes in brain development, particularly findings of early brain overgrowth. Head circumference at birth ranges from slightly below normal to within normal limits. This finding changes by 2 to 3 months of age when accelerated head growth occurs. The rate of growth may exceed 2 standard deviations above the average. Approximately 60% of infants diagnosed with autism compared with 6% of normal infants have this rate of accelerated head growth. The increase positively correlates to the increase in ID severity. Following this period of accelerated head growth, during which time the infant brain may achieve the size of the adult brain, deceleration or a complete cessation of head growth is noted.[31]

Accelerated brain growth may predispose the developing brain to increased vulnerability. This is consistent with the concept of plasticity, whereby development of cortical circuitry is established during critical postnatal periods. During this period of development, a balance of excitatory and inhibitory neurofunctionality occurs. It has been theorized that during this critical period if an imbalance occurs, this results in neurodevelopmental disorders, such as autism.[36] This theory is consistent with the diagnostic criteria of onset within the first 3 years, abnormalities in three major areas (socialization, communication, and repetitive behaviors[1]), and disruption in neurocircuitry development.

Dysfunction of virtually all neural systems in the brain has been proposed at some point as a potential basis of autism.[49] The neuropathologic changes noted in persons with autism are suggested to be of prenatal origin, primarily in the first 6 months of gestation.[31] Evidence has been published that suggests that autism affects a functionally diverse and widely distributed set of neural systems, making the disorder far broader in scope than a simple social interaction disorder.[49] Despite these findings, the pattern of brain abnormality appears somewhat discrete. Autism spares many perceptual and cognitive systems. A localized neural deficit can have more widespread neurofunctional implications through its influence on brain development.[49]

There is research to support abnormalities in cholinergic receptors and decreases in the nicotinic receptor binding in the cholinergic system as well as dysfunction in the GABAergic system[47] in persons with autism. Nicotinic receptors enhance cognitive processing (i.e., memory and attention) and open the possibility of therapeutic intervention via cholinergic receptor modulation.[50] Approximately 25% to 60% of children with autism have elevated peripheral platelet concentrations of the neurotransmitter serotonin.[51] Studies of dopamine and catecholamine metabolites have failed to consistently show abnormalities.

Clinical **Controversy. . .**

In the absence of clearly effective drug therapies for the behavioral symptoms of autism, scientifically unsupported complementary and alternative treatments are sometimes used.[52] A study using a naturalistic, case–control design compared the use of micronutrients (vitamins and minerals) with standard medication (e.g., antipsychotics, SSRIs, mood stabilizers, stimulants, clonidine, and bupropion) on rates of self-injurious behavior, aggression, and temper tantrums. Both groups improved on formal assessment measures. The micronutrient group demonstrated significant advantages with less anger, weight gain, and social withdrawal. Frequency remained the same, but the intensity of self-injury was significantly lower in the micronutrient group as well. Despite a desire to assist sometimes desperate families, the clinician should examine the evidence-based support of complementary and alternative medicines prior to recommending or prescribing such treatments. Clearly, more study is needed.

Clinical Presentation and Diagnosis

The differential diagnostic features of autism and nonautistic PDDs are listed in Table 56-1. A multiple-step process has been suggested as a structured approach to differential diagnosis of suspected ASD. As a spectrum disorder, the severity or level of impairment may be highly variable. This structured approach includes a determination of intellectual function and level of language development, followed by assessment of the child's behavior as it relates to chronologic age, mental age, and language age. It is important to identify relevant comorbid medical conditions and the presence of any related contributing psychosocial factors.[53]

Persons with autism are typically normal in physical appearance. Seizure rates are reported for between 5% and 40% of those with an ASD diagnosis.[47] Patients with comorbid seizure

TABLE 56-1 Differential Diagnostic Features of Autism and Nonautistic Pervasive Developmental Disorders

Feature	Autistic Disorder	Asperger's Syndrome	Rett Syndrome	Pervasive Developmental Disorder NOS[a]
Age at recognition (months)	0–36	Usually >36	5–30	Variable
Sex ratio	M > F	M > F	F >> M	M > F
Loss of skills after initial mastery	Variable	Usually not	Marked	Usually not
Social skills	Very poor	Poor	Vary with stage	Variable
Communication skills	Usually poor	Fair	Very poor	Fair to good
Circumscribed interests	Variable (mechanical)	Marked (facts)	NA	Variable
Eye contact	Very poor	Variable	Varies with stage	Variable
Family history of similar problems	Sometimes	Frequent	Not usually	Unknown
Seizure disorder	Common	Uncommon	Frequent	Uncommon
Head growth decelerates	No	No	Yes	No
IQ range	Severe MR to normal	Mild MR to normal	Severe MR	Severe MR to normal
Outcome	Poor to good	Fair to good	Very poor	Fair to good

F, female; IQ, intelligence quotient; M, male; MR, mental retardation; NA, not applicable; NOS, not otherwise specified.

[a]Impairments are not as severe as in autism.

Data from references 1, 34, 57, 59, and 63.

disorders often have greater impairment in intellectual function.[1] Other medical comorbidities commonly reported in this population include sleep disturbances, food intolerances, and GI dysfunction.[54]

The cardinal features of autism are gross and sustained impairment of reciprocal social interaction, sustained abnormalities in verbal and nonverbal communication skills, and restricted, repetitive, and stereotypical patterns of behavior, interests, and activities.[1,53] These are primarily manifested as gaze aversion, little/no interest in making friends, preference for solitary activities, repetition of words/phrases, monotone voice, insistence on sameness, and a lack of awareness of other's feelings.[1,55] In most cases (~75%), there is an associated diagnosis of ID, ranging from mild to profound: approximately 30% of function in the mild to moderate range of ID, whereas 45% to 50% have severe to profound impairment.[53] Epidemiologic data suggest that the risk for development of autism increases as the IQ decreases.[53] A few individuals with autism have unusual abilities called splinter functions or islets of precocity. The most significant of these are evidenced in the autistic savant, in which the individuals can have precocity in mathematic calculations, art, music, or rote memory.[1,53]

In many instances, parents note that they were concerned about the child's lack of interest in social interactions since birth, but were sure at least by 3 years of age.[1] In a controlled setting, use of an integrated model for screening was effective in diagnosing children before 36 months of age.[56] Original findings of behaviors suggesting the need for an intellectual evaluation included lack of babbling, pointing, or other gestures by 12 months, no single-word language development by 16 months, no two-word language development by 24 months of age, and loss of previously held language or social skills at any age.[57] Earlier intervention is recommended when the early signs and symptoms of autism are recognized. It is difficult to determine if autism is present in persons with severe to profound ID. A diagnosis is made in such cases when there are qualitative deficits in social and communicative skills and the specific behaviors characteristic of ASD are present.[1] A central difference is that persons with ID alone typically relate to adults in a manner consistent with their mental age, use their language to communicate with others, and present with a relatively even profile of impairments without splinter functions.[53]

Although there are no definitive biologic markers for identifying individuals with autism, a number of medical evaluations should occur at baseline, to assist in distinguishing the diagnosis as autism and to rule out other disorders. Table 56-2 delineates the parameters to be considered in a medical evaluation for persons suspected of having autism and the rationale for the assessment.

Those individuals with autism and IQs above 70 who use communicative language by ages 5 to 7 have the best prognoses.[53]

TABLE 56-2 Medical Screening for Individuals with Autism

Parameter	Rationale
Medical and developmental history	Perform initial screening or confirm diagnosis; identify underlying cause; assess strengths and weaknesses; identify comorbidities; measure head circumference; identify resources needed
Wood's light exam	Identify depigmented macules associated with tuberous sclerosis
Hearing and vision testing	Profound hearing loss can illicit symptoms mimicking autism (receptive language deficits); most are normal
Heavy metal testing	Perform if there is a history of malnutrition, recurrent vomiting, early onset seizures, dysmorphic features, presence of MR or developmental delays
Genetic testing for karyotype, fragile X, Rett syndrome	Benefits family for genetic counseling purposes; evaluation of siblings, if applicable; review family history for three generations
Test for inborn errors of metabolism/metabolic testing	Indicated in those with a history of lethargy, recurrent vomiting, early seizures, dysmorphic or coarse facial features, MR
CBC, thyroid function testing	CBC if anemia suspected; thyroid function tests to rule out baseline thyroid abnormality that can affect mood/activity level
EEG	Evaluate neurologic findings that cannot be explained by the diagnosis of autism alone or in the presence of developmental regression, particularly language
Neuroimaging	Evaluate neurologic findings that cannot be explained by the diagnosis of autism alone; identify specific neuropathologic changes associated with autism, including brain volume

CBC, complete blood count; EEG, electroencephalograph; MR, mental retardation.

Data from references 45, 57, and 58.

Conversely, low IQ scores and failure to develop communicative language by age 5 years correlate with a poorer long-term prognosis.[58] Outcome studies in persons with autism correlate IQ, particularly verbal IQ, with the ability to be employed and live independently.[49,59] Learning disabilities are an independent risk factor for development of behavioral problems, and 41% of children with mild, moderate, or severe learning difficulties have a significant emotional behavioral disturbance.[59] Studies indicate that high-IQ children with autism can make positive changes in communication and social domains more effectively over time. The areas less likely to improve are those related to ritualistic and repetitive behaviors.[54] Up to 80% of children diagnosed with ASD continued to experience marked impairment in social interactions as adults. Mild to moderate ID was reported for approximately 30%.[60]

In addition to the core symptoms of autism, many persons with this disorder exhibit other significant maladaptive behaviors, such as aggression to self and others. These behavioral issues can interfere with day-to-day activities and are challenging for the individual, families, and caregivers.[61]

Clinical **Controversy. . .**

It has been postulated that thimerosal, an organomercury compound and a preservative previously used in many vaccines, could be causally linked to neurodevelopmental disorders such as autism.[62] Well-conducted case–control, cross-sectional ecologic and cohort studies found no causal association between thimerosal-containing vaccines and the development of autism or deficits in neuropsychological function. Further concerns were posed specific to a postulated link between mercury exposures secondary to dental amalgam restoration (while pregnant) or environmental mercury exposure and autism. A review of the evidence was unclear regarding a causal link between maternal dental exposure and autism. More research is needed to evaluate risk from other environmental exposures. Despite the lack of evidence, the neurotoxic effect of mercury and exposure continue to be a hotly debated issue among many advocates for persons with autism.

TREATMENT

Desired Outcomes

Treatment goals in persons with a diagnosis of ASD are to address deficits in communication and social interaction using a structured approach and minimize the impact of restricted behaviors (e.g., stereotypies or repetition) appropriate to the level of intellectual ability, language development, and chronologic age.

General Approach to Treatment

❸ The multimodal treatment plan should address (a) establishing realistic goals for educational efforts, (b) identifying the presence of behavioral target symptoms for intervention, (c) prioritizing target symptoms and comorbid conditions for intervention, (d) using specific methods of outcome monitoring of functional domains (behavioral, adaptive skills, academic skills, social interaction skills, communication skills), and (e) monitoring for efficacy and potential adverse effects of medication (if used). The National Institutes of Health (NIH) suggests that evidence-based treatment strategies include the use of both psychoeducational therapies and medications.[64] An effective, well-designed, multimodal treatment plan that is consistently executed has the most potential to positively shape the autistic individual's interaction with the environment and improve the quality of life of patients and their families.

After a thorough diagnostic evaluation, treatment planning for the individual with autism is critical to assure consistency and efficacy of interventions. With the often severe nature of the behavioral and adaptive problems, it is not surprising that many potential treatment modalities lacking an evidence basis have been proposed for persons with autism. ❹ The two treatment approaches for autism with evidence-based support and clinical consensus are behavioral/psychoeducational therapies[34,65] and psychoactive medication intervention[30] as appropriate. All stakeholders (family, educators, and clinical professionals) should be involved in the treatment planning process. Treatment decisions should be evidence-based and individualized to the specific identified needs of the individual. The potential for communication deficits often limit self-reporting of psychopathology. A multifaceted approach to information gathering should include direct observation; interviews with patient, parents,

CLINICAL PRESENTATION Autism

General

- Individuals typically present with delays or abnormalities in six or more of the symptoms below with at least two impairments in social interactions and one each in communication and restricted interests or repetitive behaviors.

Diagnostic features

- Significant impairment in nonverbal communications
- Unable to develop peer relationships
- Lack of spontaneous interactions with people or the environment
- Developmental delays in communication
- Inability to use expressive language appropriate to developmental level
- Lack of developmentally appropriate play
- Stereotypical or nonfunctional ritualistic behavior
- Inability to tolerate change
- Stereotypic or repetitive, nonfunctional motor movements
- Limited scope of play or interest

Data from references 1, 57, 61, and 63.

family, caregivers, and teachers; and review of the medical record, including any behavioral rating scale information.

❹ Available evidence suggests that appropriately designed, consistently implemented educational services positively impact the acquisition of social, communicative, self-care, and cognitive skills, each of which facilitates the person's long-term success. Services, such as occupational therapy, physical therapy, and speech pathology, are often integral aspects of an overall educational plan. ❺ Because of the pervasive need for sameness in routine, ongoing and consistent year-round educational programming is more effective than intermittent, episodic interventions. Effective language and communication training can lead to generalized improvements in social skills and repetitive behaviors, and thus positively impact other nonspecific maladaptive behavioral problems such as noncompliance, self-injury, and aggression.[66]

Nonpharmacologic Treatment

Intervention strategies, such as discrete trial training, have demonstrated improvement in challenging behaviors. Educational techniques include structuring the environment, family training, peer role modeling, and sensory integration to optimize environmental interactions.[65]

Pharmacologic Treatment

Many of the studies of psychopharmacologic interventions in persons with ASD have methodologic shortcomings including problems in experimental design and sample size, loose or poorly defined diagnostic criteria, and many clinical outcomes that were limited in duration or of dubious clinical significance.

❹ Among a number of scientifically unsupported treatments for autism is secretin, a polypeptide hormone promoted in the late 1990s as an efficacious therapy. Controlled trials found no reliable evidence of such efficacy.[67] Elimination diets in which casein (from dairy products) and/or gluten (from wheat products) are excluded from the diet also have no scientific basis for efficacy. Other such purported therapies include omega-3 fatty acids and St. John's wort. Only one randomized controlled trial was found regarding use of omega-3 fatty acids for hyperactivity and stereotypic behavior. At this time, safety and efficacy are not established.[68] Modest benefits were reported with St. John's wort for eye contact and expressive language deficits.[69]

Current research on the neurobiologic basis of autism is centered on the serotonergic, peptidergic, dopaminergic, and noradrenergic systems. This research has particular applications for insomnia in children with ASD, as the prevalence of sleep disorders has been reported to range from 44% to 83%.[70] ❻ Parents commonly rate sleep disturbance as a significant clinical issue. As with nonautistic individuals, it is important to determine the underlying etiology of the sleep problem. Behavioral interventions (e.g., improved sleep hygiene, eliminating maladaptive sleep habits, and parental education) should be undertaken prior to implementing pharmacotherapy. No medication has been FDA-approved for pediatric insomnia. While controlled trial data are limited, there is support for the use, safety, and effectiveness of melatonin.[70,71] In a review of the literature for use of melatonin in ASD, doses ranged from 0.75 up to 6 mg of the immediate-release formulation and from 2 up to 15 mg of the controlled-release formulations. Additional studies are needed for safety and effectiveness.[70] In an analysis of 12 studies of potential melatonin-mediated adverse effects, serious side effects were not reported.[71]

Aggression to self and others and severe tantrums are a concern, particularly with adults with ASD. In addition to inclusion of nonpharmacologic interventions, pharmacotherapy is frequently utilized. Despite limited evidence-based support, psychoactive medications have been widely used to minimize the frequency and intensity of these behaviors. ❼ It is important that clinicians identify and carefully monitor specific behavioral target symptom response to avoid the practice of overprescribing psychoactive medications.

An association between dopamine dysregulation and increased aggression, including self-injury, consistent with animal models, has been proposed.[61] Such findings have led to the use of antipsychotic agents that act as dopaminergic antagonists to address aggression and self-injurious behavior. The first-generation antipsychotic agent with the most evidence for short- and long-term safety and efficacy is haloperidol. Target behaviors included impaired learning, anger, mood lability, hyperactivity, and social withdrawal. Although results for improvement in the target behaviors were greater in the antipsychotic treatment compared with the placebo group, the risk for the development of dyskinesias and the introduction of new antipsychotic medications have severely limited haloperidol's use.[30]

As few psychopharmacologic agents have been well studied in this population, and even fewer have received FDA approval, current research is directed primarily toward the second-generation antipsychotics (SGAs). ❽ Off-label use of FDA-approved medications (i.e., use of an approved drug for an unapproved use) is an acceptable clinical practice when there is evidence-based support for the use of the medication and informed consent is obtained; however, there is a relative lack of robust research in this area at the present time.

Aripiprazole and risperidone are currently FDA-approved to treat the behavioral symptoms associated with autism. A review of the literature found both short- and long-term use of orally administered aripiprazole was effective for irritability in pediatric patients with ASD, aged 6 to 17 years. The dosage range was 2 to 15 mg/day. In this range, aripiprazole was well tolerated with moderate side effects that resolved with continued use.[72–75] Weight gain was reported during the first 3 to 6 months, and then it plateaued.[72] Risperidone has the most evidence-based support for treating behavioral problems associated with autism. It is FDA-approved for treatment of the following behaviors in children and adolescents with autism: aggression, self-injury, temper tantrums, and irritability.[30]

The use of olanzapine is supported by limited trial data in children and adolescents with autism. Trial durations were generally short (6 to 8 weeks) with small numbers of participants. Positive results are generally reported in global improvement scale assessment; however, the significant weight gain and sedation noted in olanzapine trials are important considerations in weighing risk versus potential benefit.[30]

At this time there is no FDA-approved medication for the core symptoms of autism. Prior to the inclusion of pharmacotherapy for behavior as a component of the plan, utilization of a multifaceted approach is recommended.[76]

The SGAs are less likely to elicit extrapyramidal side effects than first-generation agents due to more potency at serotonin$_{2A}$ (5-HT$_{2A}$) receptors versus dopamine receptors. However, the SGAs have been implicated in weight gain in some persons with autism.[30] The potential serum prolactin elevation related to risperidone use is of concern. Elevated serum prolactin may lead to amenorrhea, galactorrhea, and osteoporosis in females and gynecomastia and sexual dysfunction in males. The minimum degree of prolactin elevation that is clinically relevant is uncertain as are the implications for long-term use in a pediatric population. If detected, strategies include evaluating the risk–benefit with continued use, reducing doses, or changing to another agent with less impact on prolactin. It is recommended that clinicians monitor for the evidence of potential risperidone-mediated prolactin elevations regardless of whether a prolactin level is obtained.[77] Additional monitoring recommendations for antipsychotic use can be found in Chapter 50.

Serotonin synthesis differs between children diagnosed with ASD and children without this diagnosis. Compared with adults, 5-hydroxytryptamine (5-HT) synthesis may peak at twice the adult level in developmentally normal children by age 5 years, whereas children with ASD have a more gradual developmental arc with a lower peak.[78] The use of SSRIs is often associated with a decrease in some of the core behavioral symptoms such as stereotypies, social withdrawal, and rigid adherence to routine. A review of the literature for citalopram,[79] escitalopram, fluoxetine, and fluvoxamine[78] found limited support for use of SSRIs to address behaviors of ASD.

Psychostimulants have been studied in persons with autism to address hyperactivity, impulsivity, and inattention. Psychostimulants block the reuptake of dopamine and norepinephrine. It is hypothesized that ADHD represents a dysfunction in regulation of these catecholamines.[80] Study design of methylphenidate trials in persons with autism or PDD complicates interpretation of results. Some trials were uncontrolled, and some included children with various diagnoses. The largest and most rigorously controlled trial involved 72 participants, with 74% having a primary diagnosis of autism. In this placebo-controlled trial, methylphenidate was given in divided doses of 0.125, 0.25, and 0.5 mg/kg (morning and noon doses). In an analysis of the 66 youths completing the trial, 16 could not tolerate the 0.5 mg/kg dose phase. All three doses performed better than placebo on improving the core symptoms of ADHD according to parent and teacher ratings. Parent ratings for ADHD were better with the medium dose compared with the low dose. Teacher ratings for inattention were better with the medium dose compared with the low dose.[81] Overall, findings suggest that treatment response to psychostimulants varies and, in general, stimulants do not work as well in this population of children compared with normally developing peers.[82]

The α_2-agonists, clonidine and guanfacine, have been used to treat hyperactivity and agitation in persons with autism because of their effects on inhibition of noradrenergic release and transmission. Both agents have FDA approval for treating symptoms associated with ADHD. However, as with many psychoactive medications used in the population with autism, there is a lack of methodologically sound studies supporting use of these agents. Two trials with guanfacine targeted symptoms that included inattentiveness and hyperactivity. Both reported positive outcomes. In the first ($n = 80$, average age of 7.7 years), guanfacine use was associated with statistically significant improvement in global functioning. In the second trial ($n = 25$, 20 completed), all subjects had not tolerated previous methylphenidate use. Improvement was noted on measures; some reached statistical significance.[82]

Limited data are available on the use of cholinesterase inhibitors for disruptive behaviors, such as hyperactivity and irritability. Use of donepezil for these or the core autism symptoms cannot be supported.[82] No benefit for ADHD or core symptoms was found for galantamine, and results for rivastigmine were unclear. Use of the NMDA receptor antagonist memantine was associated with hyperactivity as both a side effect and a target behavior. Additional study is needed for this agent. Limited support for anticonvulsants for ADHD symptoms in children with ASD was found despite the high comorbidity of seizures in this population.[82]

The current dearth of evidence-based psychopharmacologic and behavioral research in persons with autism is being addressed by a network of NIH-funded research centers, including the Research Units of Pediatric Psychopharmacology, Centers for Programs of Excellence in Autism, and Studies to Advance Autism Research and Treatment. The mission of these units is to foster well-controlled, multicenter, behavioral, and psychopharmacologic intervention studies targeting behavioral symptoms in persons with autism. Additional information can be found at *http://psychmed.osu.edu/*.

Personalized Pharmacotherapy

Aggression to self and others and severe tantrums are a concern, particularly in adults with ASD. In addition to nonpharmacologic interventions, pharmacotherapy is frequently utilized. Despite limited evidence-based support, psychoactive medications have been widely used to minimize the frequency and intensity of these behaviors. Although pharmacogenomics to guide rational and targeted pharmacotherapy would be helpful, at present this information is not available.[83] This may be in part because of the heterogeneity of the ASD population.

Pharmacogenetic research has been limited by lack of sensitive outcome assessment tools to measure the effectiveness of treatments and the presence of multiple confounding factors in studies such as age, sex, medication dosage, and treatment duration, and whether or not the study subjects were drug naive.[84] Studies that have been conducted (primarily with risperidone) are of limited clinical utility due to small sample size, and they need to be replicated in larger populations with more diverse makeup.[84,85] Until more well-conducted, reproducible study results are available to confirm the early work that has been done, using the patient's genotype to algorithmically predict a medication and dose likely to be effective and safe for a given patient with autism remains elusive.

Clinical **Controversy...**

The reported prevalence of autism has increased dramatically in the last 30 years, and evidence suggests that much of the increase is related to improved identification of children with these disorders.[32,33,86,87] Clear diagnostic boundaries are not always apparent, and there is a lack of homogeneity in clinical expression of the condition. The next edition of the *DSM-IV-TR* proposes a different categorization structure for the diagnosis of autism, causing much debate in the psychiatric community. Many families, clinicians, and advocates are concerned that this new diagnostic categorization will have the unintended consequence of eliminating some persons with previously diagnosed high-functioning autism or Asperger's disorder from eligibility for services. The most significant change in criteria is the proposal to combine Asperger's disorder, PDD-NOS, and autistic disorder into a new category of ASD to recognize the essential shared features of the autism spectrum, while attempting to individualize diagnosis through dimensional descriptors.

Evaluation of Therapeutic Outcomes

7 Monitoring the safety, efficacy, and tolerability of psychopharmacologic interventions in persons with autism is imperative to minimize adverse medication-related sequelae and optimize desired therapeutic outcomes. Clinical investigators have used a variety of psychometric assessment instruments in attempts to measure changes in core symptoms.

There are a variety of instruments that have been developed and used in clinical trials to measure symptoms, such as communication impairment, restricted interests, and repetitive behavior. A comprehensive review of many of these instruments is beyond the scope of this chapter. Pharmacotherapy in autism is usually directed toward minimizing maladaptive behaviors, such as irritability, hyperactivity, compulsive, ritualistic, and perseverative behavior, and variants of self-injurious behavior. The Aberrant Behavior Checklist was designed for assessment of behavioral changes in institutionalized individuals enrolled in pharmacotherapy trials; however, a community-based version is also available.[88,89] The Aberrant Behavior Checklist consists of 54 items divided into 5 domains: irritability, hyperactivity, stereotypic behavior, lethargy, and inappropriate speech. The lower the score in each domain, the greater the behavioral improvement. The Children's Yale-Brown Obsessive Compulsive Scale modified for pervasive developmental disorders is a validated scale sensitive to changes in repetitive behavior severity pretreatment and posttreatment.[90]

Intensive medication-related side effects monitoring and assessment is important in this population, as self-reporting can be unreliable. An instrument that is caregiver-rated such as the Monitoring of Side Effects Scale can be useful for this purpose. The Monitoring of Side Effects Scale is a multisystem, quantitative, and qualitative caregiver assessment that rates the presence or absence and severity of a variety of potential medication-related adverse effects for clinician review.[91] Signs and symptoms are written in layperson language and are listed by body area or system. As such, it is a broad-based screening tool that can be enhanced by side effect–specific scales such as those for akathisia (Barnes Akathisia Scale [BAS]), extrapyramidal effects (Simpson-Angus Scale), or tardive dyskinesia (Dyskinesia Identification System: Condensed User Scale [DISCUS]).[92–94]

❼ Use of SGAs has been associated with increased risk of developing metabolic syndrome. Children receiving these agents should be monitored for hyperglycemia, dyslipidemia, and weight gain in a manner consistent with the consensus guidelines suggested by the American Diabetes Association and the American Psychiatric Association.[95] For monitoring guidelines, see Chapter 59.

RETT SYNDROME

Andreas Rett, an Austrian physician, published the first paper describing this disorder in a German language journal in 1966. He documented a sequence of developmental changes affecting young girls who initially achieved normal developmental milestones and then experienced regression. The significance of these findings and the rate of worldwide occurrence were not fully apparent until more formal evaluative and diagnostic criteria were developed.[96] Seizures, scoliosis, and cardiac dysfunction are frequent comorbidities in persons with RTT that can significantly impact the quality of life. The primary goals of treatment are to optimize seizure control and mobility.

Epidemiology

The classical form of RTT[96] affects females almost exclusively. The prevalence of RTT depends on the population surveyed and the diagnostic criteria used. Studies from Sweden and Scotland reported the prevalence to be 1:10,000 to 15,000,[97] whereas more recent estimates varied in the methodology used. Rates from several countries were reported with age ranges for the females. Prevalence for these groups ranged from 0.57 to 0.88:10,000.[98]

Etiology and Pathophysiology

RTT is a neurodevelopmental disorder originating from an X-linked dominant mutation at the Xq28 site involving the methyl-CpG-binding protein 2 (MECP2). This represents the most commonly identified mutation in the majority (95%) of classic cases identified in females.[99] In-depth molecular studies found a variety of mutations on the MECP2 gene that impact the presentation of the clinical phenotype. These mutations may provide an explanation for differences in severity, presentation, and onset.[100]

The etiology of RTT has not been fully identified. Theoretical explanations have extrapolated data from animal models and involve neuronal changes. These include the loss of the MECP2 protein in the dopaminergic pathways in the substantia nigra and the potential impact on alterations in the nigrostriatal pathways. An age-dependent study involving MECP2-altered mice found that mice with dopamine$_2$ (D2) neurons in the substantia nigra region of the brain demonstrated less conductivity as early as 4 weeks of age. Changes preceded symptoms and were lifelong. The authors postulated that D2 dysfunctions in dopamine release could account for motor deficits in symptomatic females.[101]

Clinical Presentation and Diagnosis

Genetic variations have been identified that are thought to moderate the symptoms and progression of RTT, the extent of which is not fully understood. What is known is that females are predominately affected by RTT, and no causal event has been identified. An uneventful pregnancy and birth are followed by seemingly normal development with acquisition of developmentally appropriate milestones. Growth, including head circumference, is within normal limits at birth. Developmental regression appears between 6 and 18 months with the loss of previously acquired skills. Additional developmentally regressive changes have been grouped into a series of stages associated with a range of ages during which these changes occur.[1]

❾ The order of symptom appearance and regressive changes associated with RTT distinguish it from other developmental disorders. The developmental changes for the classical presentation of RTT can be grouped into four stages (Table 56-3). Important features for each stage include the onset of stage I (stagnation) that typically begins at approximately 6 months of age, after initially meeting developmental milestones.[99] The key indicators for the onset of stage 2 (rapid destructive or developmental regression) include lack

TABLE 56-3 Rett Syndrome Stages

Stage	Onset Age	Duration	Suspected Gene Mutation[a]	Characteristics
I	5–18 months, up to 48 months	Months to years	FOXG1	Head growth ceases
			MECP2	Developmental slowing Social withdrawal
			R168X	Purposeful hand movements cease
			168X	Language ceases
II	18 months to 4 years	Weeks to months	FOXG1	Onset of severe to profound MR Breathing irregularities Autistic features appear
			CDKL5	Seizures can appear
III	3–10 years	Years; may stabilize here	CDKL5 R294X	Seizures increase Partial return of language skills Deterioration slows or ceases
			R294X, R168X	Ambulatory ability varies
IV	>10 years old	Decades, if at all		Scoliosis Dystonias Lower limb wasting may be present Seizures may abate

CDKL5, *cyclin-dependent kinase-like 5*; *FOXG1*, forkhead box protein G1; MECP2, methyl-CpG-binding protein 2; MR, mental retardation.

[a]Unless otherwise indicated, specific mutations on the MECP2 gene are associated with developmental tasks acquired and then lost or that never presented.

Data from references 1, 96, 99, 100, and 104.

CLINICAL PRESENTATION Rett Syndrome

General features

- RTT is diagnosed primarily in females.
- Previously acquired skills are lost following apparently normal prenatal and early development.
- There is an increased risk for seizure disorders in the RTT population compared with the general population.

Additional features

- Head growth slows.
- Periods of hyperventilation and apnea may occur.
- Motor skills may vary.
- Stereotypies may occur.
- Unprovoked laughing and/or screaming.
- Intense eye gaze communication.
- Bruxism.

Data from references 1, 96, and 97.

of head growth and features with autistic-like qualities (e.g., stereotypic hand movements and loss of social interactions). The onset of stage 3 (pseudostationary or stationary) varies and previously lost skills may partially reappear. Seizure activity may appear. In one study, the age at which the last seizure occurred ranged from 6 to 15.5 years.[102] Scoliosis may develop and limit ambulation.[103] Stage 4 (late motor deterioration) may last for decades.[99]

Not all RTT presentations fit this classical stage model. Presentations vary in terms of onset and severity. Genetic mutations may be one partial explanation for atypicality.[99] At this time, only the following X-linked gene mutations are recognized as potential moderating influences: cyclin-dependent kinase-like 5 (CDKL5) on early seizure onset, MECP2 for speech preservation, and forkhead box protein G1 (FOXG1) considered responsible for one of the key indicators of the syndrome, small head circumference.[104]

The presence of stereotypic hand movements, social and environmental withdrawal, and irritability (including the inability to be soothed when crying) have given rise to investigating commonalities between RTT and autism.[105] Impairments in communication and environmental interactions, eye contact, and stereotypies are temporary, whereas with autism, these persist.[105]

TREATMENT

Desired Outcomes

Treatment goals in RTT are to identify the characteristic developmental changes of each stage and provide effective nonpharmacologic and pharmacotherapy interventions, as appropriate, to improve quality of life.

General Approach to Treatment

Treatment plans should address the physiologic changes of each stage, optimizing pharmacotherapy, as appropriate. Effective strategies require a systematic approach to (a) address the specific medical needs identified, (b) monitor the medications used as appropriate, and (c) reassess the need for continued pharmacotherapy.

Nonpharmacologic Therapy

Behavioral problems are not commonly encountered with RTT. Other considerations include evaluating for respiratory complications such as obstructive sleep apnea with polysomnography and therapeutic interventions if indicated.[106] Surgical intervention may be indicated to lessen the severity of scoliosis-associated pain, maintain mobility, and decrease respiratory problems. Caregivers provided input on ADL questionnaires related to function and behavior for RTT females who either had surgery ($n = 16$) or did not have surgery ($n = 86$). In the wheelchair-bound surgical intervention group, ADL skills improved. No differences were reported for social interactions, communication skills, or daytime napping presurgical or postsurgical intervention.[107]

Pharmacologic Therapy

Information on pharmacotherapy for comorbidities associated with the RTT population comes from case reports, case series, and small trials. One of the more thoroughly investigated aspects is the treatment of seizures that may appear in stage 2 or 3. Krajnc et al. retrospectively analyzed seizure data on 19 RTT females and found seizure activity present in 84% (16 of 19).[102]

Specific gene mutations may also influence seizure activity, with seizure activity reported in up to 90% of the RTT population. Medication usage was reviewed in two populations with confirmed MECP2 mutations. In the first (n = 162), authors found seizure activity was age-dependent, influenced by the gene mutation, and positively associated with an earlier and more severe regression. The most commonly used medications, either as monotherapy or in combination, were carbamazepine, valproate, and lamotrigine.[108] In a second population (n = 110), carbamazepine (n = 15), sulthiame (n = 15), and valproate (n = 16) were the only medications administered as monotherapy that could be evaluated for analysis. Seizure-free periods were reported with use of all three. Reductions were greatest with carbamazepine, and then sulthiame. Valproate was least effective.[109]

Comorbidities, including seizures and cardiac problems, can impact drug selection. Cardiac mortality is significantly elevated in RTT. There is a 300-fold increase in sudden death from arrhythmias compared with the general population.[110] Causality has not been determined. Electrocardiogram (ECG) findings of QT prolongation and dyssynchronous innervations cannot account for the marked increase in mortality. Concurrent administration of medications that prolong the QT interval should be undertaken with caution and ECG monitoring. Any pharmacotherapy should take into consideration cardiac implications and other potential adverse drug effects.

Personalized Pharmacotherapy

RTT is an X-linked dominant mutation at the Xq28 site. Four mutations on this gene have been identified, CDKL5, FOXG1, R168X, and R294X, that may provide an explanation for differences in severity, onset, and developmental regression. To date, neither pharmacokinetic nor pharmacogenetic considerations have been identified in those with RTT. Continued advances in pharmacogenomics may be identified with CDKL5 and early seizure onset. Monotherapy with carbamazepine has been used,[102] but the extent to which biomarker HLA-B*1502 is involved has not been identified.

Clinical **Controversy. . .**

Although poorly understood, fracture risk in RTT appears to be approximately four times greater than in the general population.[111,112] While the primary genetic mutation site is the X-linked MECP2 gene, phenotype and fracture risk may be mutation-specific. In a 7-year longitudinal study ($n = 233$) adjusted for antiepileptic drug used, mobility, seizure diagnosis, and genotype, use of valproate was associated with a threefold increase in the fracture rate after 1 year.

Evaluation of Therapeutic Outcomes

The most medication-responsive feature of RTT is seizure activity. Seizure frequency changes with age.[108] For more information about epilepsy and seizure disorders, see Chapter 40. Depending on the anticonvulsant used, laboratory monitoring may be needed. Seizure frequency and adverse effects should be monitored when medications are added or doses changed and at regular intervals thereafter. During the late teens and 20s, reassessing the need for continued anticonvulsant treatment is recommended, since seizures have been known to spontaneously abate with age.

ABBREVIATIONS

AADD American Association on Intellectual and Developmental Disabilities
AAP American Academy of Pediatrics
ABS Adaptive Behavior Scale
AD Alzheimer's disease
ADHD attention-deficit/hyperactivity disorder
ADL activity of daily living
ALL acute lymphoblastic leukemia
AMKL acute megakaryoblastic leukemia
AML acute myelogenous leukemia
ASD autism spectrum disorder
BAS Barnes Akathisia Scale
CBT cognitive behavior therapy
CDKL5 cyclin-dependent kinase-like 5
CNV copy number variation
D2 dopamine$_2$
DISCUS Dyskinesia Identification System Condensed User Scale
DMR Dementia Scale for Mentally Retarded Persons
DS Down syndrome
DSM-IV-TR *Diagnostic and Statistical Manual of Mental Disorders, Fourth Edition, Text Revision*
ECG electrocardiogram
ECT electroconvulsive therapy
FOXG1 forkhead box protein G1
GABA γ-aminobutyric acid
5-HT 5-hydroxytryptamine
5-HT$_{2A}$ serotonin$_{2A}$
ID intellectual disability
MECP2 methyl-CpG-binding protein 2
MR mental retardation
NIH National Institutes of Health
NMDA *N*-methyl-D-aspartate
NPI Neuropsychiatric Inventory
PDD pervasive developmental disorder
PDD-NOS pervasive developmental disorder not otherwise specified
RTT Rett syndrome
SGA second-generation antipsychotic
SIB Severe Impairment Battery
SSRI selective serotonin reuptake inhibitor
TMD transient myeloproliferative disorder

REFERENCES

1. American Psychiatric Association. Diagnostic and Statistical Manual of Mental Disorders, Fourth Edition, Text Revision. Washington, DC: American Psychiatric Association, 2000.
2. Werner S, Stawski M. Mental health: Knowledge, attitudes and training of professionals on dual diagnosis of intellectual disability and psychiatric disorder. J Intellect Disabil Res 2012;56:291–304.
3. Bakken TL, Helverschou SB, Eilertsen DE, et al. Psychiatric disorders in adolescents and adults with autism and intellectual disability: A representative study in one county in Norway. Res Dev Disabil 2010;31:1669–1677.
4. Jones S, Howard L, Thornicroft G. 'Diagnostic overshadowing': Worse physical health care for people with mental illness. Acta Psychiatr Scand 2008;118:169–171.
5. American Association on Intellectual and Developmental Disabilities. AAIDD Definition on Intellectual Disability. *http://www.aaidd.org/intellectualdisabilitybook/content_7473.cfm?navID=366.*
6. Abanto J, Ciamponi AL, Francischini E, et al. Medical problems and oral care of patients with Down syndrome: A literature review. Spec Care Dentist 2011;31:197–203.
7. Sherman SL, Allen EG, Bean LH, Freeman SB. Epidemiology of Down syndrome. Ment Retard Dev Disabil Res Rev 2007;13:221–227.
8. Hulten MA, Patel SD, Westgren M, et al. On the paternal origin of trisomy 21 Down syndrome. Mol Cytogenet 2010;3:4.
9. Bean LJ, Allen EG, Tinker SW, et al. Lack of maternal folic acid supplementation is associated with heart defects in Down syndrome: A report from the National Down Syndrome Project. Birth Defects Res A Clin Mol Teratol 2011;91:885–893.
10. American Academy of Pediatrics, Committee on Genetics. American Academy of Pediatrics: Health supervision for children with Down syndrome. Pediatrics 2001;107:442–449.
11. Di Nuovo SF, Buono S. Psychiatric syndromes comorbid with mental retardation: Differences in cognitive and adaptive skills. J Psychiatr Res 2007;41:795–800.
12. Cooper SA, Smiley E, Morrison J, et al. Mental ill-health in adults with intellectual disabilities: Prevalence and associated factors. Br J Psychiatry 2007;190:27–35.
13. Walker JC, Dosen A, Buitelaar JK, Janzing JG. Depression in Down syndrome: A review of the literature. Res Dev Disabil 2011;32:1432–1440.
14. Tyler C, Edman JC. Down syndrome, Turner syndrome, and Klinefelter syndrome: Primary care throughout the life span. Prim Care 2004;31:627–648, x–xi.
15. Buitenkamp TD, Mathot RA, de Haas V, et al. Methotrexate-induced side effects are not due to differences in pharmacokinetics in children with Down syndrome and acute lymphoblastic leukemia. Haematologica 2010;95:1106–1113.

16. Urv TK, Zigman WB, Silverman W. Psychiatric symptoms in adults with Down syndrome and Alzheimer's disease. Am J Intellect Dev Disabil 2010;115:265–276.
17. Prasher VP. Review of donepezil, rivastigmine, galantamine and memantine for the treatment of dementia in Alzheimer's disease in adults with Down syndrome: Implications for the intellectual disability population. Int J Geriatr Psychiatry 2004;19:509–515.
18. Yoo JH, Valdovinos MG, Williams DC. Relevance of donepezil in enhancing learning and memory in special populations: A review of the literature. J Autism Dev Disord 2007;37:1883–1901.
19. Krinsky-McHale SJ, Devenny DA, Kittler P, Silverman W. Selective attention deficits associated with mild cognitive impairment and early stage Alzheimer's disease in adults with Down syndrome. Am J Ment Retard 2008;113:369–386.
20. Coppus AM, Schuur M, Vergeer J, et al. Plasma beta amyloid and the risk of Alzheimer's disease in Down syndrome. Neurobiol Aging 2012;33:1988–1994.
21. Osborn GG, Saunders AV. Current treatments for patients with Alzheimer disease. J Am Osteopath Assoc 2010;110:S16–S26.
22. Prasher VP, Huxley A, Haque MS. A 24-week, double-blind, placebo-controlled trial of donepezil in patients with Down syndrome and Alzheimer's disease—Pilot study. Int J Geriatr Psychiatry 2002;17:270–278.
23. Prasher VP, Fung N, Adams C. Rivastigmine in the treatment of dementia in Alzheimer's disease in adults with Down syndrome. Int J Geriatr Psychiatry 2005;20:496–497.
24. Gill SS, Anderson GM, Fischer HD, et al. Syncope and its consequences in patients with dementia receiving cholinesterase inhibitors: A population-based cohort study. Arch Intern Med 2009;169:867–873.
25. Menendez M. Down syndrome, Alzheimer's disease and seizures. Brain Dev 2005;27:246–252.
26. Hanney M, Prasher V, Williams N, et al. Memantine for dementia in adults older than 40 years with Down's syndrome (MEADOWS): A randomised, double-blind, placebo-controlled trial. Lancet 2012;379:528–536.
27. Rabin KR, Whitlock JA. Malignancy in children with trisomy 21. Oncologist 2009;14:164–173.
28. Malinge S, Izraeli S, Crispino JD. Insights into the manifestations, outcomes, and mechanisms of leukemogenesis in Down syndrome. Blood 2009; 113:2619–2628.
29. O'Brien MM, Taub JW, Chang MN, et al. Cardiomyopathy in children with Down syndrome treated for acute myeloid leukemia: A report from the Children's Oncology Group Study POG 9421. J Clin Oncol 2008;26:414–420.
30. Malone RP, Waheed A. The role of antipsychotics in the management of behavioural symptoms in children and adolescents with autism. Drugs 2009;69:535–548.
31. Polsek D, Jagatic T, Cepanec M, et al. Recent developments in neuropathology of autism spectrum disorders. Transl Neurosci 2011;2:256–264.
32. Autism and Developmental Disablities Monitoring Network Surveillance Year 2008 Principal Investigators, Centers for Disease Control and Prevention. Prevalence of Autism Spectrum Disorders—Autism and Developmental Disabilities Monitoring Network, 14 sites, United States, 2008. MMWR 2012;61:1–19.
33. Muhle R, Trentacoste SV, Rapin I. The genetics of autism. Pediatrics 2004;113:e472–e486.
34. Johnson CP, Myers SM. Identification and evaluation of children with autism spectrum disorders. Pediatrics 2007;120:1183–1215.
35. Bos KJ, Zeanah CH Jr, Smyke AT, et al. Stereotypies in children with a history of early institutional care. Arch Pediatr Adolesc Med 2010;164:406–411.
36. LeBlanc JJ, Fagiolini M. Autism: A "critical period" disorder? Neural Plast 2011;921680.
37. Salyakina D, Cukier HN, Lee JM, et al. Copy number variants in extended autism spectrum disorder families reveal candidates potentially involved in autism risk. PLoS One 2011;6:e26049.
38. Ben-Sasson A, Hen L, Fluss R, et al. A meta-analysis of sensory modulation symptoms in individuals with autism spectrum disorders. J Autism Dev Disorder 2009;39:1–11.
39. Simmons DR, Robertson AE, McKay LS, et al. Vision in autism spectrum disorders. Vision Res 2009;49:2705–2739.
40. Ozonoff S, Young GS, Carter A, et al. Recurrence risk for autism spectrum disorders: A Baby Siblings Research Consortium Study. Pediatrics 2011;128:e488–e495.
41. Constantino JN, Zhang Y, Frazier T, et al. Sibling recurrence and the genetic epidemiology of autism. Am J Psychiatry 2010;167:1349–1356.
42. Dhillon S, Hellings JA, Butler MG. Genetics and mitochondrial abnormalities in autism spectrum disorders: A review. Curr Genomics 2011;12:322–332.
43. Rahbar MH, Samms-Vaughan M, Loveland KA, et al. Maternal and paternal age are jointly associated with childhood autism in Jamaica. J Autism Dev Disord 2012;42:1928–1938.
44. Shelton JF, Tancredi DJ, Hertz-Picciotto I. Independent and dependent contributions of advanced maternal and paternal ages to autism risk. Autism Res 2010;3:30–39.
45. Russo AJ, Devito R. Analysis of copper and zinc plasma concentration and the efficacy of zinc therapy in individuals with Asperger's syndrome, pervasive developmental disorder not otherwise specified (PDD-NOS) and autism. Biomark Insights 2011;6:127–133.
46. Hensley E, Briars L. Closer look at autism and the measles-mumps-rubella vaccine. J Am Pharm Assoc (2003) 2010;50:736–741.
47. Sgado P, Dunleavy M, Genovesi S, et al. The role of GABAergic system in neurodevelopmental disorders: A focus on autism and epilepsy. Int J Physiol Pathophysiol Pharmacol 2011;3:223–235.
48. Mefford HC, Batshaw ML, Hoffman EP. Genomics, intellectual disability, and autism. N Engl J Med 2012;366:733–743.
49. Costa e Silva JA. Autism, a brain developmental disorder: Some new pathophysiologic and genetics findings. Metabolism 2008;57(Suppl 2):S40–S43.
50. Deutsch SI, Urbano MR, Neumann SA, et al. Cholinergic abnormalities in autism: Is there a rationale for selective nicotinic agonist interventions? Clin Neuropharmacol 2010;33:114–120.
51. Kazek B, Huzarska M, Grzybowska-Chlebowczyk U, et al. Platelet and intestinal 5-HT2A receptor mRNA in autistic spectrum disorders—Results of a pilot study. Acta Neurobiol Exp (Warsz) 2010;70:232–238.
52. Mehl-Madrona L, Leung B, Kennedy C, et al. Micronutrients versus standard medication management in autism: A naturalistic case–control study. J Child Adolesc Psychopharmacol 2010;20:95–103.
53. Sadock BJ, Sadock VA. Pervasive developmental disorders. In: Synopsis of Psychiatry, 10th ed. Baltimore, MD: Williams and Wilkins, 2007:1191–1205.
54. Ming X, Brimacombe M, Chaaban J, et al. Autism spectrum disorders: Concurrent clinical disorders. J Child Neurol 2008;23:6–13.

55. Corsello CM. Early intervention in autism. Infants Young Child 2005;18:74–85.
56. Oosterling IJ, Wensing M, Swinkels SH, et al. Advancing early detection of autism spectrum disorder by applying an integrated two-stage screening approach. J Child Psychol Psychiatry 2010;51:250–258.
57. Filipek PA, Accardo PJ, Baranek GT. The screening and diagnosis of autistic spectrum disorders. J Autism Dev Disord 1999;29:439–484.
58. Prater CD, Zylstra RG. Autism: A medical primer. Am Fam Physician 2002;66:1667–1674.
59. Baird G, Cass H, Slonims V. Diagnosis of autism. BMJ 2003;327:488–493.
60. Vanbergeijk E, Klin A, Volkmar F. Supporting more able students on the autism spectrum: College and beyond. J Autism Dev Disord 2008;38:1359–1370.
61. Parikh MS, Kolevzon A, Hollander E. Psychopharmacology of aggression in children and adolescents with autism: A critical review of efficacy and tolerability. J Child Adolesc Psychopharmacol 2008;18:157–178.
62. Schultz ST. Does thimerosal or other mercury exposure increase the risk for autism? A review of current literature. Acta Neurobiol Exp (Warsz) 2010;70:187–195.
63. Chawarska K, Volkmar FR. Autism in infancy and early childhood. In: Volkmar FR, Paul R, Klin A, Cohen DJ, eds. Handbook of Autism and Pervasive Developmental Disorders, 3rd ed. Hoboken, NJ: John Wiley and Sons Inc, 2005:223–246.
64. National Institute of Neurological Disorders and Stroke. National Institute of Health. Autism Fact Sheet. In: NIH Publication No. 06-1877, April 2006. Last updated April 24, 2009.
65. Beversdorf D. Therapeutic interventions in autism: A review for primary care physicians. Mol Med 2008;105:390–395.
66. Bodfish JW. Treating the core features of autism: Are we there yet? Ment Retard Dev Disabil Res Rev 2004;10:318–326.
67. Krishnaswami S, McPheeters ML, Veenstra-Vanderweele J. A systematic review of secretin for children with autism spectrum disorders. Pediatrics 2011;127:e1322–e1325.
68. Bent S, Bertoglio K, Hendren RL. Omega-3 fatty acids for autistic spectrum disorder: A systematic review. J Autism Dev Disord 2009;39:1145–1154.
69. Niederhofer H. St John's wort treating patients with autistic disorder. Phytother Res 2009;23:1521–1523.
70. Miano S, Ferri R. Epidemiology and management of insomnia in children with autistic spectrum disorders. Paediatr Drugs 2010;12:75–84.
71. Rossignol DA, Frye RE. Melatonin in autism spectrum disorders: A systematic review and meta-analysis. Dev Med Child Neurol 2011;53:783–792.
72. Curran MP. Aripiprazole: In the treatment of irritability associated with autistic disorder in pediatric patients. Paediatr Drugs 2011;13:197–204.
73. Aman MG, Kasper W, Manos G, et al. Line-item analysis of the Aberrant Behavior Checklist: Results from two studies of aripiprazole in the treatment of irritability associated with autistic disorder. J Child Adolesc Psychopharmacol 2010;20:415–422.
74. Marcus RN, Owen R, Kamen L, et al. A placebo-controlled, fixed-dose study of aripiprazole in children and adolescents with irritability associated with autistic disorder. J Am Acad Child Adolesc Psychiatry 2009;48:1110–1119.
75. Marcus RN, Owen R, Manos G, et al. Aripiprazole in the treatment of irritability in pediatric patients (aged 6-17 years) with autistic disorder: Results from a 52-week, open-label study. J Am Acad Child Adolesc Psychiatry 2011;21:229–236.
76. Canitano R, Scandurra V. Psychopharmacology in autism: An update. Prog Neuropsychopharmacol Biol Psychiatry 2011;35:18–28.
77. Anderson GM, Scahill L, McCracken JT, et al. Effects of short- and long-term risperidone treatment on prolactin levels in children with autism. Biol Psychiatry 2007;61: 545–550.
78. West L, Brunssen SH, Waldrop J. Review of the evidence for treatment of children with autism with selective serotonin reuptake inhibitors. J Spec Pediatr Nurs 2009;14:183–191.
79. King BH, Hollander E, Sikich L, et al. Lack of efficacy of citalopram in children with autism spectrum disorders and high levels of repetitive behavior: Citalopram ineffective in children with autism. Arch Gen Psychiatry 2009;66: 583–590.
80. Handen BL, Taylor J, Tumuluru R. Psychopharmacological treatment of ADHD symptoms in children with autism spectrum disorder. Int J Adolesc Med Health 2011;23: 167–173.
81. Posey DJ, Aman MG, McCracken JT, et al. Positive effects of methylphenidate on inattention and hyperactivity in pervasive developmental disorders: An analysis of secondary measures. Biol Psychiatry 2007;61:538–544.
82. Aman MG, Farmer CA, Hollway J, Arnold LE. Treatment of inattention, overactivity, and impulsiveness in autism spectrum disorders. Child Adolesc Psychiatr Clin N Am 2008;17:713–738, vii.
83. Hu VW. A systems approach towards an understanding, diagnosis and personalized treatment of autism spectrum disorders. Pharmacogenomics 2011;12:1235–1238.
84. Correia CT, Almeida JP, Santos PE, et al. Pharmacogenetics of risperidone therapy in autism: Association analysis of eight candidate genes with drug efficacy and adverse drug reactions. Pharmacogenomics J 2010;10:418–430.
85. Lit L, Sharp FR, Bertoglio K, et al. Gene expression in blood is associated with risperidone response in children with autism spectrum disorders. Pharmacogenomics J 2012;12:368–371.
86. Willemsen-Swinkels SH, Buitelaar JK. The autistic spectrum: Subgroups, boundaries, and treatment. Psychiatr Clin North Am 2002;25:811–836.
87. Happe F. Criteria, categories, and continua: Autism and related disorders in DSM-5. J Am Acad Child Adolesc Psychiatry 2011;50:540–542.
88. Aman MG, Singh NN, Turbott SH. Reliability of the Aberrant Behavior Checklist and the effect of variations in instructions. Am J Ment Defic 1987;92:237–240.
89. Aman MG, Singh NN. Aberrant Behavior Checklist—Community. Supplemental Manual. East Aurora, NY: Slosson Educational Publications, 1994.
90. Scahill L, McDougle CJ, Williams SK, et al. Children's Yale-Brown Obsessive Compulsive Scale modified for pervasive developmental disorders. J Am Acad Child Adolesc Psychiatry 2006;45:1114–1123.
91. Kalachnik JE. Medication monitoring procedures: Thou shall, here's how. In: Gadow KD, Poling AG, eds. Pharmacotherapy and Mental Retardation. Boston, MA: College-Hill, 1985:231–268.
92. Barnes TR. A rating scale for drug-induced akathisia. Br J Psychiatry 1989;154:672–676.
93. Simpson GM, Angus JW. A rating scale for extrapyramidal side effects. Acta Psychiatr Scand Suppl 1970;212:11–19.
94. Kalachnik JE. Measuring side effects of psychopharmacologic medications in individuals with mental retardation and developmental disabilities. Ment Retard Dev Disabil Res Rev 1999;5:348–359.

95. Morrato EH, Newcomer JW, Kamat S, et al. Metabolic screening after the American Diabetes Association's consensus statement on antipsychotic drugs and diabetes. Diabetes Care 2009;32:1037–1042.
96. Hagberg B. Clinical manifestations and stages of Rett syndrome. Ment Retard Dev Disabil Res Rev 2002;8: 61–65.
97. Dunn HG. Importance of Rett syndrome in child neurology. Brain Dev 2001;23(Suppl 1):S38–S43.
98. Fehr S, Bebbington A, Nassar N, et al. Trends in the diagnosis of Rett syndrome in Australia. Pediatr Res 2011;70:313–319.
99. Chahrour M, Zoghbi HY. The story of Rett syndrome: From clinic to neurobiology. Neuron 2007;56:422–437.
100. Neul J, Fang P, Barrish J, et al. Specific mutations in methyl-CpG-binding protein 2 confer different severity in Rett syndrome. Neurology 2008;70:1313–1321.
101. Gantz SC, Ford CP, Neve KA, Williams JT. Loss of Mecp2 in substantia nigra dopamine neurons compromises the nigrostriatal pathway. J Neurosci 2011;31:12629–12637.
102. Krajnc N, Zupancic N, Orazem J. Epilepsy treatment in Rett syndrome. J Child Neurol 2011;26:1429–1433.
103. Riise R, Brox JI, Sorensen R, Skjeldal OH. Spinal deformity and disability in patients with Rett syndrome. Dev Med Child Neurol 2011;53:653–657.
104. Neul JL, Kaufmann WE, Glaze DG, et al. Rett syndrome: Revised diagnostic criteria and nomenclature. Ann Neurol 2010;68:944–950.
105. Percy AK. Rett syndrome: Exploring the autism link. Arch Neurol 2011;68:985–989.
106. Hagebeuk EE, Bijlmer RP, Koelman JH, Poll-The BT. Respiratory disturbances in Rett syndrome: Don't forget to evaluate upper airway obstruction. J Child Neurol 2012;27:888–892.
107. Downs J, Young D, de Klerk N, et al. Impact of scoliosis surgery on activities of daily living in females with Rett syndrome. J Pediatr Orthop 2009;29:369–374.
108. Jian L, Nagarajan L, de Klerk N, et al. Seizures in Rett syndrome: An overview from a one-year calendar study. Eur J Paediatr Neurol 2007;11:310–317.
109. Huppke P, Kohler K, Brockmann K, et al. Treatment of epilepsy in Rett syndrome. Eur J Paediatr Neurol 2007; 11:10–16.
110. De Felice C, Maffei S, Signorini C, et al. Subclinical myocardial dysfunction in Rett syndrome. Eur Heart J Cardiovasc Imaging 2012;13:339–345.
111. Downs J, Bebbington A, Woodhead H, et al. Early determinants of fractures in Rett syndrome. Pediatrics 2008;121:540–546.
112. Leonard H, Downs J, Jian L, et al. Valproate and risk of fracture in Rett syndrome. Arch Dis Child 2010;95:444–448.

Diabetes Mellitus

57

Curtis L. Triplitt, Thomas Repas, and Carlos A. Alvarez

KEY CONCEPTS

1. Diabetes mellitus (DM) is a group of metabolic disorders of fat, carbohydrate, and protein metabolism that results from defects in insulin secretion, insulin action (sensitivity), or both.
2. The incidence of type 2 DM is increasing. This has been attributed in part to a Western-style diet, increasing obesity, sedentary lifestyle, and an increasing minority population.
3. The two major classifications of DM are type 1 (insulin deficient) and type 2 (combined insulin resistance and relative deficiency in insulin secretion). They differ in clinical presentation, onset, etiology, and progression of disease. Both are associated with microvascular and macrovascular disease complications.
4. Diagnosis of diabetes is made by four criteria: fasting plasma glucose ≥126 mg/dL (≥7 mmol/L), a 2-hour value from a 75-g oral glucose tolerance test ≥200 mg/dL (≥11.1 mmol/L), a casual plasma glucose level of ≥200 mg/dL (≥11.1 mmol/L) with symptoms of diabetes, or a hemoglobin A_{1c} [HbA_{1c}] ≥6.5% (≥0.065; ≥48 mmol/mol Hb). The diagnosis should be confirmed by repeat testing if obvious hyperglycemia is not present.
5. Goals of therapy in DM are directed toward attaining normoglycemia (or appropriate glycemic control based on the patient's comorbidities), reducing the onset and progression of retinopathy, nephropathy, and neuropathy complications, intensive therapy for associated cardiovascular risk factors, and improving quality and quantity of life.
6. Metformin should be included in the therapy for all type 2 DM patients, if tolerated and not contraindicated, as it is the only oral antihyperglycemic medication proven to reduce the risk of total mortality, according to the United Kingdom Prospective Diabetes Study (UKPDS).
7. Intensive glycemic control is paramount for reduction of microvascular complications (neuropathy, retinopathy, and nephropathy) as evidenced by the Diabetes Control and Complications Trial (DCCT) in type 1 DM and the UKPDS in type 2 DM. The UKPDS also reported that control of hypertension in patients with diabetes will not only reduce the risk of retinopathy and nephropathy but also reduce cardiovascular risk.
8. Short-term (3 to 5 years), intensive glycemic control does not lower the risk of macrovascular events as reported by the Action in Diabetes and Vascular Disease, Action to Control Cardiovascular Risk in Diabetes, and Veterans Administration Diabetes Trial trials. Microvascular event reduction may be sustained, and macrovascular events reduced by improved early glycemic control, as evidenced by the UKPDS and DCCT follow-up studies. Significant reductions in macrovascular risk may take 15 to 20 years. This sustained reduction in microvascular risk and new reduction in macrovascular risk has been coined metabolic memory.
9. Knowledge of the patient's quantitative and qualitative meal patterns, activity levels, pharmacokinetics of insulin preparations, and pharmacology of oral and injected antihyperglycemic agents is essential to individualize the treatment plan and optimize blood glucose control while minimizing risks for hypoglycemia and other adverse effects of pharmacologic therapies.
10. Type 1 DM treatment necessitates insulin therapy. Currently, the basal–bolus insulin therapy or pump therapy in motivated individuals often leads to successful glycemic outcomes. Basal–bolus therapy includes a basal insulin for fasting and postabsorptive control, and rapid-acting bolus insulin for mealtime coverage. Addition of mealtime pramlintide in patients with uncontrolled or erratic postprandial glycemia may be warranted.
11. Type 2 DM treatment often necessitates use of multiple therapeutic agents (combination therapy), including oral and/or injected antihyperglycemics and insulin, to obtain glycemic goals due to the persistent reduction in β-cell function over time. Slowing, but not arresting, β-cell failure has been shown with thiazolidinediones and the glucagon-like peptide-1 (GLP-1) agonist class of medications.
12. Aggressive management of cardiovascular disease risk factors in type 2 DM is necessary to reduce the risk for adverse cardiovascular events or death. Smoking cessation, use of antiplatelet therapy as a secondary prevention strategy and in select primary prevention situations, aggressive management of dyslipidemia—primary goal to lower low-density lipoprotein cholesterol (<100 mg/dL [<2.59 mmol/L]) and secondarily to raise high-density

lipoprotein cholesterol to ≥40 mg/dL (≥1.03 mmol/L)—and treatment of hypertension (again often requiring multiple drugs) to <130/80 mm Hg are vital.

13 Prevention strategies for type 1 DM have been unsuccessful. Prevention strategies for type 2 DM are established. Lifestyle changes, dietary restriction of fat, aerobic exercise for 30 minutes five times a week, and weight loss form the backbone of successful prevention. No medication is currently FDA approved for prevention of diabetes, although several, including metformin, acarbose, pioglitazone, and rosiglitazone, have clinical trials demonstrating a delay of diabetes onset.

14 Patient education and ability to demonstrate self-care and adherence to therapeutic lifestyle and pharmacologic interventions are crucial to successful outcomes. Multidisciplinary teams of healthcare professionals including physicians (primary care, endocrinologists, ophthalmologists, and vascular surgeons), podiatrists, dietitians, nurses, pharmacists, social workers, behavioral health specialists, and certified diabetes educators are needed, as appropriate, to optimize these outcomes in persons with DM.

1 Diabetes mellitus (DM) is a heterogeneous group of metabolic disorders characterized by hyperglycemia. It is associated with abnormalities in carbohydrate, fat, and protein metabolism and may result in chronic complications including microvascular, macrovascular, and neuropathic disorders. It is estimated that in 2010, 26 million Americans ≥20 years old have DM, with as many as one fourth of these patients being undiagnosed, and an additional 79 million at high risk for the development of diabetes. The economic burden of DM approximated $218 billion in 2007, for diabetes and prediabetes. This is representative of an annual cost for each citizen of the United States of $700. DM is the leading cause of blindness in adults aged 20 to 74 years and the leading cause of end-stage renal disease in the United States. It also accounts for approximately 65,000 lower extremity amputations annually. Finally, a cardiovascular event is responsible for two thirds of deaths in individuals with type 2 DM and is the leading cause of death in type 1 DM of long duration.[1]

Optimal management of the patient with DM will reduce or prevent complications, decreasing morbidity and mortality while improving quality of life. Research, clinical trials, and drug development efforts over the past several decades have provided valuable information that applies directly to improving outcomes in patients with DM and have expanded the therapeutic armamentarium. Additionally, interventions in an attempt to prevent complications and the onset of diabetes have been reported for type 1 and 2 DM.

EPIDEMIOLOGY

Type 1 DM accounts for 5% to 10% of all cases of DM and is most often due to autoimmune destruction of the pancreatic β cells.[2] Although type 1 DM most frequently develops in childhood or early adulthood, new cases occur at any age.

Type 1 DM is thought to be initiated by the exposure of a genetically susceptible individual to an environmental agent. The development of β-cell autoimmunity occurs in less than 10% of the genetically susceptible population and progresses to type 1 DM in less than 1% of that population.[3] There is a direct relation to the prevalence of β-cell autoimmunity and the incidence of type 1 DM in various populations. The countries of Sweden, Sardinia, and Finland have the highest prevalence of islet cell antibody (ICA; 3% to 4.5%) and are associated with the highest incidence of type 1 DM: 22 to 35 per 100,000.[4] The prevalence of type 1 DM is increasing, but the cause of this increase is not fully understood.

Markers of β-cell autoimmunity are detected in 14% to 33% of persons with adult-onset diabetes. This type of DM is referred to as latent autoimmune diabetes in adults (LADA) and presents with early failure of oral agents and need for insulin therapy.[4]

Idiopathic type 1 DM is a nonautoimmune form of diabetes frequently seen in minorities, especially Africans and Asians, with intermittent insulin requirements.[2]

Secondary forms of DM occur due to a variety of causes.[2] Maturity onset diabetes of youth (MODY) is due to one of six genetic defects. Endocrine disorders such as acromegaly and Cushing's syndrome may also cause diabetes. Any disease of the exocrine pancreas such as cystic fibrosis, pancreatitis, and hereditary hemochromatosis can damage β cells and impair insulin secretion. These unusual causes, however, only cause 1% to 2% of the total cases of DM. Please see Other Specific Types of Diabetes (<5% of Diabetes) below for further discussion.

Type 2 DM accounts for up to 90% of all cases of DM. Overall the prevalence of type 2 DM in the United States is about 11.3% in persons aged 20 or older; this prevalence is increasing. It is estimated that for every four persons who are diagnosed with DM, one person remains undiagnosed.[1]

There are multiple risk factors for the development of type 2 DM, including family history (i.e., parents or siblings with diabetes); obesity (i.e., ≥20% over ideal body weight, or body mass index [BMI] ≥25 kg/m^2); chronic physical inactivity; race or ethnicity (see list below); history of impaired glucose tolerance (IGT), impaired fasting glucose (IFG), or hemoglobin A_{1c} (HbA_{1c}) 5.7% to 6.4% (0.057 to 0.064; 39 to 46 mmol/mol Hb) (see Diagnosis of Diabetes below); hypertension (≥140/90 mm Hg in adults); high-density lipoprotein (HDL) cholesterol (HDL-C) ≤35 mg/dL (≤0.91 mmol/L) and/or a triglyceride level ≥250 mg/dL (≥2.83 mmol/L); history of gestational diabetes mellitus (GDM) (see Classification of Diabetes below) or delivery of a baby weighing >9 lb (>4 kg); history of vascular disease; presence of acanthosis nigricans; and polycystic ovary disease.[5]

2 The prevalence of type 2 DM increases with age and varies widely among various racial and ethnic populations. The prevalence of type 2 DM is especially increased in Native Americans, Hispanic Americans, Asian Americans, African Americans, and Pacific Islanders. While the prevalence of type 2 DM increases with age, the disorder is increasingly being diagnosed in adolescence. Much of the rise in adolescent type 2 DM is related to an increase in overweight/obesity and sedentary lifestyle, in addition to genetic predisposition.[6] Most cases of type 2 DM are polygenetic; the underlying pathophysiology remains uncertain[7] (Figs. 57-1 and 57-2).

GDM complicates approximately 7% of all pregnancies in the United States.[8] Most women become normoglycemic after pregnancy; however, 30% to 50% may develop prediabetes or type 2 DM later in life.

PATHOGENESIS, DIAGNOSIS, AND CLASSIFICATION

Classification of Diabetes

Diabetes is a metabolic disorder characterized by resistance to the action of insulin, insufficient insulin secretion, or both.[2] The clinical manifestation of these disorders is hyperglycemia. The vast majority of diabetic patients are classified into one of two broad

Estimated percentage of people aged 20 years or older with diagnosed and undiagnosed diabetes, by age group, United States, 2005–2008

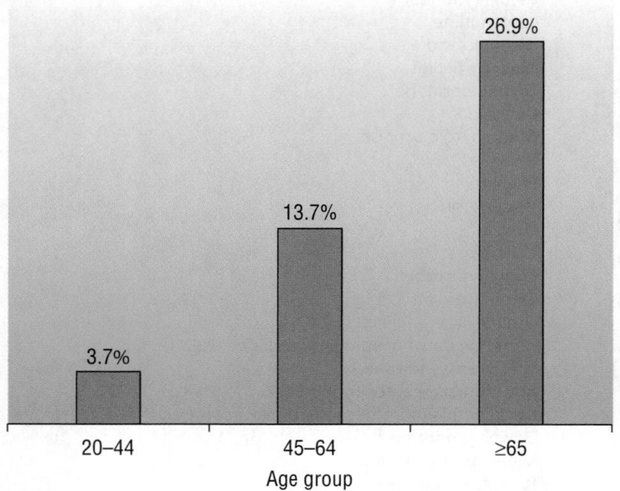

FIGURE 57-1 National Health and Nutrition Evaluation Survey (NHANES) prevalence of diabetes by age among adults ≥20 years of age: United States, 2005–2008. *(Centers for Disease Control and Prevention, 2011 National Diabetes Fact Sheet at http://www.cdc.gov/diabetes/pubs/estimates11.htm.)*

categories: type 1 diabetes caused by an absolute deficiency of insulin or type 2 diabetes defined by the presence of insulin resistance with an inadequate compensatory increase in insulin secretion. Women who develop diabetes due to the stress of pregnancy are classified as having gestational diabetes. Finally, uncommon types of diabetes caused by infections, drugs, endocrinopathies, pancreatic destruction, and known genetic defects are classified separately (Table 57-1).

Type 1 Diabetes

3 This form of diabetes results from autoimmune destruction of the β cells of the pancreas. Evidence of β-cell autoimmunity, including ICAs, antibodies to glutamic acid decarboxylase, islet protein tyrosine phosphatase-like molecule IA2, and/or antibodies to insulin, is present at the time of diagnosis in 90% of individuals. Type 1 diabetes is often thought to most commonly present in children and adolescents; however, it can occur at any age. Younger individuals typically have a more rapid rate of β-cell destruction and often present with ketoacidosis. Adults may maintain sufficient insulin secretion to prevent ketoacidosis for many years; this is referred to as latent autoimmune diabetes in adults.[3,4]

Type 2 Diabetes

3 Type 2 DM is characterized by a combination of some degree of insulin resistance and a relative lack of insulin secretion (being insufficient to normalize plasma glucose levels), with progressively lower insulin secretion over time. Most individuals with type 2 diabetes exhibit abdominal obesity, which itself causes insulin resistance. In addition, hypertension, dyslipidemia (high triglyceride levels and low HDL-C levels), and elevated plasminogen activator inhibitor-1 (PAI-1) levels, which contribute to a hypercoagulable state, are often present in these individuals. Due in part to these factors, patients with type 2 diabetes are at increased risk of developing macrovascular complications in addition to microvascular complications. Type 2 diabetes has a strong genetic predisposition and is more common in all ethnic groups other than those of European ancestry.[4,5]

Gestational Diabetes Mellitus

GDM is defined as glucose intolerance that is first recognized during pregnancy. Hormone changes during pregnancy result in increased insulin resistance, and GDM may ensue when the mother cannot adequately compensate with increased insulin secretion to maintain normoglycemia. In most, glucose intolerance occurs near the

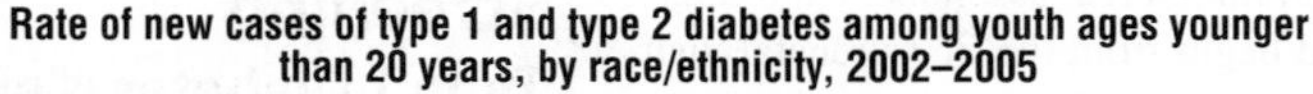

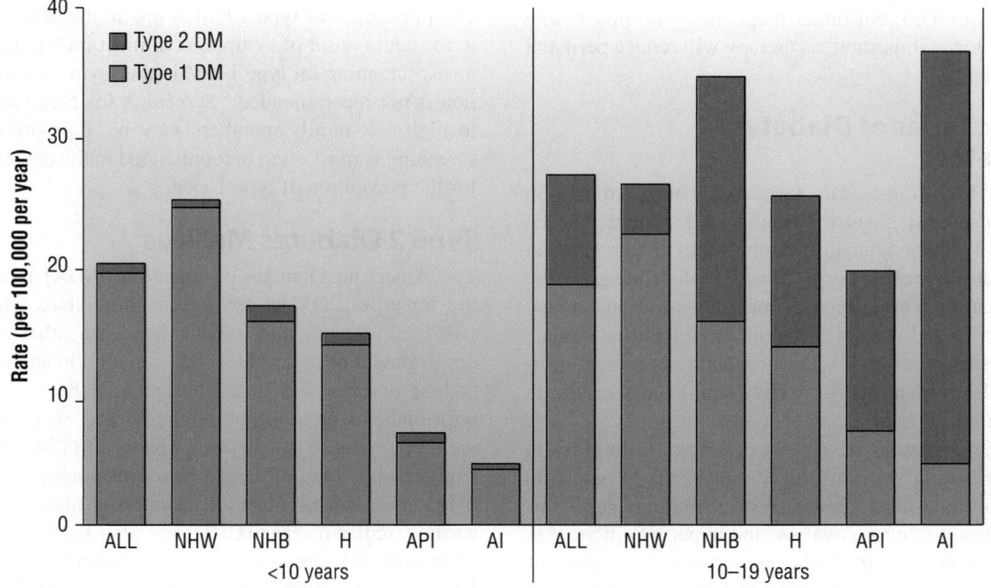

FIGURE 57-2 Rate of new cases of type 1 and type 2 diabetes among youth aged <20 years, by race/ethnicity, 2002–2005. (NHW, non-Hispanic whites; NHB, non-Hispanic blacks; H, Hispanics; API, Asians/Pacific Islanders; AI, American Indians.) *(Centers for Disease Control and Prevention, 2011 National Diabetes Fact Sheet at http://www.cdc.gov/diabetes/pubs/estimates11.htm.)*

TABLE 57-1 Etiologic Classification of Diabetes Mellitus[a]

1. **Type 1 diabetes[b]** (β-cell destruction, usually leading to absolute insulin deficiency)
   - Immune-mediated
   - Idiopathic
2. **Type 2 diabetes[a]** (may range from predominantly insulin resistance with relative insulin deficiency to a predominantly insulin secretory defect with insulin resistance)
3. **Other specific types**
   - Genetic defects of β-cell function
     - Chromosome 20q, HNF-4α (MODY 1)
     - Chromosome 7p, glucokinase (MODY 2)
     - Chromosome 12q, HNF-1α (MODY 3)
     - *Other rare forms*
     - Chromosome 13q, insulin promoter factor-1 (MODY 4)
     - Chromosome 17q, HNF-1β (MODY 5)
     - Chromosome 2q, neurogenic differentiation 1/β-cell e-box transactivator 2 (MODY 6)
     - Chromosome 9q, carboxyl ester lipase (MODY 7)
     - Mitochondrial DNA
   - Genetic defects in insulin action
     - Type A insulin resistance
     - Leprechaunism
     - Rabson-Mendenhall syndrome
     - Lipoatrophic diabetes
   - Diseases of the exocrine pancreas
     - Pancreatitis
     - Trauma/pancreatectomy
     - Neoplasia
     - Cystic fibrosis
     - Hemochromatosis
     - Fibrocalculous pancreatopathy
   - Endocrinopathies
     - Acromegaly
     - Cushing's syndrome
     - Glucagonoma
     - Pheochromocytoma
     - Hyperthyroidism
     - Somatostatinoma
     - Aldosteronoma
   - Drug or chemical induced
     - Vacor (Pyriminil)
     - Pentamidine
     - Nicotinic acid
     - Glucocorticoids
     - Thyroid hormone
     - Diazoxide
     - β-Adrenergic agonists
     - Thiazides
     - Phenytoin
     - γ-Interferon
     - Others
   - Infections
     - Congenital rubella
     - Cytomegalovirus
     - Others
   - Uncommon forms of immune-mediated diabetes
     - "Stiff-man" syndrome
     - Anti-insulin receptor antibodies
   - Other genetic syndromes sometimes associated with diabetes
     - Down's syndrome
     - Klinefelter's syndrome
     - Turner's syndrome
     - Wolfram's syndrome
     - Friedreich's ataxia
     - Huntington's chorea
     - Laurence-Moon-Bieldel syndrome
     - Myotonic dystrophy
     - Porphyria
     - Prader-Willi syndrome
4. **Gestational diabetes mellitus (GDM)**

[a]Other rare forms may exist for all categorizations.
[b]Patients with any form of diabetes may require insulin treatment at some stage of their disease. Such use of insulin does not in itself classify the patient.
Adapted from Diabetes Care 1997;20:1183–1197. Reproduced by permission of the American Diabetes Association.[2]

beginning of the third trimester, although risk assessment and intervention when appropriate should begin from the first prenatal visit due to the risk of undiagnosed diabetes. If DM is diagnosed prior to pregnancy, this is not GDM, but rather pregnancy with preexisting DM. Clinical detection is important, as therapy will reduce perinatal morbidity and mortality.[2]

Other Specific Types of Diabetes (<5% of Diabetes)

Genetic Defects MODY is characterized by impaired insulin secretion in response to a glucose stimulus with minimal or no insulin resistance. Patients typically exhibit mild hyperglycemia at an early age, but diagnosis may be delayed, depending on the severity of presentation. The disease is inherited in an autosomal dominant pattern with at least six different loci identified to date (MODY 2 and 3 are most common). The production of mutant insulin molecules has been identified in a few families and results in mild glucose intolerance.[2]

Several genetic mutations have been described in the insulin receptor and are associated with insulin resistance. Type A insulin resistance refers to the clinical syndrome of acanthosis nigricans, virilization in women, polycystic ovaries, and hyperinsulinemia. In contrast, anti-insulin receptor antibodies may block the binding of insulin. This was referred to in the past as type B insulin resistance. Endocrinopathies, pancreatic exocrine dysfunction, drugs, and infections, among others, may also result in hyperglycemia (Table 57-1).

Screening

Type 1 Diabetes Mellitus

The prevalence of type 1 DM is low in the general population. Due to the acute onset of symptoms in most individuals at time of diagnosis, screening for type 1 DM in the asymptomatic general population is not recommended.[5] Screening for β-cell autoantibody status in high-risk family members may be appropriate; however, such screening is most often recommended in the context of clinical trials for the prevention of type 1 DM.

Type 2 Diabetes Mellitus

The American Diabetes Association (ADA) recommends screening for type 2 DM at any age in individuals who are overweight (BMI ≥25 kg/m^2) and have at least one other risk factor for the development of type 2 DM. Risk factors, in addition to being overweight or obese, include physical inactivity, first-degree relative with diabetes or high-risk ethnicity/race, women who have delivered a baby >9 lb (>4 kg) or a history of GDM, hypertension, high triglycerides, low HDL, women with polycystic ovary syndrome, diagnosed with prediabetes, acanthosis nigricans, or a history of cardiovascular disease (CVD; see also Epidemiology above). The recommended screening test is the fasting plasma glucose (FPG), HbA_{1c}, or 2-hour oral glucose tolerance test (OGTT). Adults without risk factors should be screened starting at age 45 years, as age itself is a risk factor for type 2 DM. The optimal time between screenings is not known, and the index of suspicion for the presence of diabetes should guide the clinician. Repeat testing every 3 to 5 years is cost-effective.[5]

Children and Adolescents

Despite a lack of clinical evidence to support widespread testing of children for type 2 DM, it is clear that more children and adolescents are developing type 2 DM. The ADA, by expert opinion, recommends that overweight (defined as BMI >85th percentile for age and sex, weight for height >85th percentile, or weight >120% of ideal) youths with at least two of the following risk factors: a family history of type 2 diabetes in first- and second-degree relatives; Native Americans, African Americans, Hispanic Americans, and Asians/South Pacific Islanders; those with signs of insulin resistance or conditions associated with insulin resistance (acanthosis nigricans, hypertension, dyslipidemia, polycystic ovary syndrome, or small-for-gestational-age birth weight); or maternal history of diabetes or GDM during the child's gestation be screened. Screening should be done every 3 years starting at 10 years of age or at the onset of puberty if it occurs at a younger age.[5]

Gestational Diabetes

Risk assessment for GDM should occur at the first prenatal visit. Due to the increasing incidence of obesity and undiagnosed DM, it is reasonable to screen women with risk factors for the development of diabetes as soon as feasible. If the initial screening is negative, they should undergo retesting at 24 to 28 weeks' gestation. Screening for GDM is done with a standard 75-g OGTT. The diagnosis of GDM is confirmed when any one plasma glucose value measured at baseline (fasting), 1 hour, or 2 hours meets the diagnostic criteria. These criteria are unique to GDM (Table 57-2).[2,5,8]

Diagnosis of Diabetes

4 The diagnosis of diabetes requires the identification of a glycemic cut point, which discriminates normals from diabetic patients. The cut points are meant to reflect the level of glucose above which microvascular complications have been shown to increase. Cross-sectional studies have shown a consistent increase in the risk of developing retinopathy at a fasting glucose level above 99 to 116 mg/dL (5.5 to 6.4 mmol/L), a 2-hour postprandial level above 125 to 185 mg/dL (6.9 to 10.3 mmol/L), and a HbA_{1c} above 5.9% to 6.0%. (0.059 to 0.060; 41 to 42 mmol/mol Hb). Current diagnostic criteria are slightly above these cut points (Table 57-3).[2]

The HbA_{1c} was not recommended in the past due to many nonstandardized assays. Most laboratories now use a method that is National Glycohemoglobin Standardization Program (NGSP) certified and standardized to the Diabetes Control and Complications Trial (DCCT) assay, which allows for cross-application of their results. If standardized, the HbA_{1c} is logical for the diagnosis of diabetes as it measures glycemic exposure over the past 2 to 3 months, in contrast to a single-day, single-point glucose evaluation. In addition, patients do not have to be fasting and the test is easily monitored. An HbA_{1c} of 6% to 6.4% (0.060 to 0.066; 42 to 46 mmol/mol Hb) denotes a 10-fold increase in risk of diabetes, yet does not consistently identify patients with IFG or IGT. In addition, there are slight race differences in normal HbA_{1c} levels. One-third fewer individuals with diabetes are identified using the A1C ≥6.5% (≥0.065; ≥48 mmol/mol Hb) versus a FPG ≥126 mg/dL (≥7 mmol/L), yet more providers may be more likely to diagnose diabetes from an A1C than from an obviously elevated FPG level. The ADA continues to recommend three other glucose criteria for the diagnosis of DM in nonpregnant adults (Table 57-3). If the patient has obvious hyperglycemia and diabetes, reconfirming the diagnosis by one of the above criteria is not required.[2]

TABLE 57-2 Screening for and Diagnosis of Gestational Diabetes Mellitus with a 75-g Glucose Load[2]

Time	Plasma Glucose
Fasting	≥92 mg/dL (5.1 mmol/L)
1 hour	≥180 mg/dL (10 mmol/L)
2 hours	≥153 mg/dL (8.5 mmol/L)

One abnormal value = diagnostic of GDM. Should be performed at 24–28 weeks' gestation unless the patient has overt diabetes. The test should be done in the morning after an 8- to 14-hour fast.

TABLE 57-3 Criteria for the Diagnosis of Diabetes Mellitus[a]

1. HbA_{1c} ≥6.5% (≥0.065; ≥48 mmol/mol Hb). The test should be performed in a laboratory using a method that is National Glycohemoglobin Standardization Program (NGSP) certified and standardized to the DCCT assay[a]
2. Fasting plasma glucose ≥126 mg/dL (7 mmol/L). Fasting is defined as no caloric intake for at least 8 hours[a]
3. 2-hour plasma glucose ≥200 mg/dL (≥11.1 mmol/L) during an OGTT. The test should be performed as described by the World Health Organization, using a glucose load containing the equivalent of 75-g anhydrous glucose dissolved in water[a]
4. In a patient with classic symptoms of hyperglycemia or hyperglycemic crisis, a random plasma glucose concentration ≥200 mg/dL (≥11.1 mmol/L)

[a]In the absence of unequivocal hyperglycemia, criteria 1–3 should be confirmed by repeat testing.

Increased Risk of Diabetes or Prediabetes

As shown in Table 57-4, the ADA identified a HbA_{1c} value of 5.7% to 6.4% (0.057 to 0.064; 39 to 46 mmol/mol Hb) to define an increased risk for diabetes. The HbA_{1c} lower limit of 5.7% (0.057; 39 mmol/mol Hb) was chosen due to its good specificity, although it has a low sensitivity, to identify patients at increased risk for diabetes. IFG continues to be defined as a plasma glucose of at least 100 mg/dL (5.6 mmol/L) but less than 126 mg/dL (7 mmol/L). IGT is defined as a 2-hour glucose value ≥140 mg/dL (≥7.8 mmol/L), but less than 200 mg/dL (11.1 mmol/L) during a 75-g OGTT.[2,5]

Serial measurements, at clinician-defined intervals, can help to identify patients moving toward diabetes, and those who are stable. Patients who have even minor increases in glucose or HbA_{1c} values

TABLE 57-4 Categorizations of Abnormal Glucose Status

Fasting plasma glucose (FPG)
Impaired fasting glucose (IFG)
- 100–125 mg/dL (5.6–6.9 mmol/L)

Diabetes mellitus[a]
- FPG ≥126 mg/dL (7 mmol/L)

2-hour postload plasma glucose (oral glucose tolerance test)
Impaired glucose tolerance (IGT)
- 2-hour postload glucose 140–199 mg/dL (7.8–11 mmol/L)

Diabetes mellitus[a]
- 2-hour postload glucose ≥200 mg/dL (≥11.1 mmol/L)

HbA_{1c}
Increased risk of diabetes mellitus
- HbA_{1c} 5.7–6.4% (0.057–0.064; 39–46 mmol/mol Hb)

Diabetes mellitus[a]
- HbA_{1c} ≥6.5% (≥0.065; ≥48 mmol/mol Hb)

[a]Diagnosis to be confirmed if not unequivocal hyperglycemia (see Table 57-3).

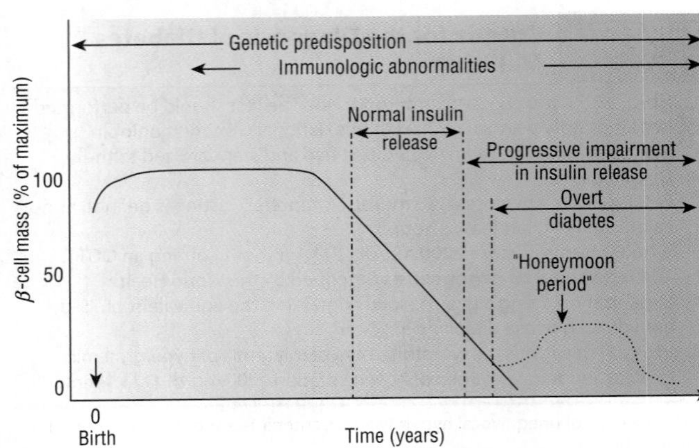

FIGURE 57-3 Scheme of the natural history of the β-cell defect in type 1 diabetes mellitus. *(Copyright © 2008 American Diabetes Association. From Medical Management of Type 1 Diabetes, 5th ed. Reprinted with permission from the American Diabetes Association.)*

over time should be followed closely. Also, the HbA_{1c} measurement can be affected by anemias and several hemoglobinopathies, which necessitates the use of one of the plasma glucose criterion in these individuals.

Pathogenesis

Type 1 Diabetes Mellitus

Type 1 DM results from pancreatic β-cell failure with "absolute" deficiency of insulin secretion. Most often this is due to immune-mediated destruction of pancreatic β cells, but rare unknown or idiopathic processes may also contribute. There often is a long preclinical period of immune-mediated β-cell destruction later followed by onset of hyperglycemia when 80% to 90% of the β cells have been destroyed. Occasionally there is a period of transient remission called the "honeymoon" phase, before established disease develops along with the requirement for lifelong insulin therapy and the potential risk of diabetes-related complications (Fig. 57-3).

It is thought that in order for type 1 DM to develop, there must be a trigger in a genetically susceptible individual. However, it is unknown whether there are one or more inciting factors such as cow's milk (or lack of breast-feeding), or viral, dietary, or other environmental exposures that initiate the autoimmune process.[2,3] Vitamin D deficiency has been observed to be more prevalent in patients who develop type 1 DM; however, further study is needed to confirm a role in causation.[9]

The autoimmune process is mediated by macrophages and T lymphocytes with circulating autoantibodies to various β-cell antigens. The most commonly detected antibody associated with type 1 DM is the ICA. Other autoantibodies include insulin, glutamic acid decarboxylase 65, and zinc transporter 8 (ZnT8). These antibodies are generally considered markers of disease rather than mediators of β-cell destruction. They have been used to identify individuals at risk for type 1 DM and in evaluating disease prevention strategies.[3]

More than 90% of newly diagnosed persons with type 1 DM have one of these antibodies, as will up to 4% of unaffected first-degree relatives. Once insulin autoantibodies are detected, there is an increased risk of development of additional autoantibodies and progression to diabetes. β-Cell autoimmunity may precede the diagnosis of type 1 DM by up to 9 to 13 years. Autoimmunity may remit in some individuals, or can progress to absolute β-cell failure in others. Other autoimmune disorders frequently associated with type 1 DM include Hashimoto's thyroiditis, Graves' disease, Addison's disease, vitiligo, and celiac sprue. The extent of involvement can range from no other associated disorders to autoimmune polyglandular failure.

There are strong genetic linkages to the *DQA* and *B* genes and certain human leukocyte antigens (HLAs). Some are associated with increased risk (*DR3* and *DR4*) while others are protective (*DRB1*04008-DQB1*0302* and *DRB1*0411-DQB1*0302*) on chromosome 6.[10] Additional candidate gene regions have been identified on other chromosomes as well. Because twin studies do not show 100% concordance, environmental factors such as infectious, chemical, and dietary agents likely also contribute to the expression of the disease.

The autoimmune destruction of pancreatic β-cell function results in hyperglycemia due to an absolute deficiency of insulin. Insulin lowers blood glucose (BG) by a variety of mechanisms, including stimulation of tissue glucose uptake, suppression of glucose production by the liver, and suppression of free fatty acid (FFA) release from fat cells.[11] The suppression of FFAs plays an important role in glucose homeostasis. Increased levels of FFAs inhibit the uptake of glucose by muscle and stimulate hepatic gluconeogenesis.[12]

Type 2 Diabetes Mellitus

Normal Metabolism In the fasting state 75% of total body glucose disposal takes place in non–insulin-dependent tissues such as the brain, neurons, and others. Brain glucose uptake occurs at the same rate during fed and fasting periods. The remaining 25% of glucose metabolism takes place in the liver and muscle, which is dependent on insulin. In the fasting state approximately 85% of glucose production is derived from the liver, and the remaining amount is produced by the kidney. Glucagon, produced by pancreatic α cells, is secreted in the fasting state to oppose the action of insulin and stimulate hepatic glucose production and glycogenolysis. Glucagon and insulin secretion are closely linked; one increases while the other decreases to keep plasma glucose levels normal. In the fed state, carbohydrate ingestion increases the plasma glucose concentration and stimulates insulin release from the pancreatic β cells. The resultant hyperinsulinemia (a) suppresses hepatic glucose production, (b) stimulates glucose uptake by peripheral tissues, and (c) suppresses glucagon release (in conjunction with incretin hormones). The majority (~80% to 85%) of glucose is taken up by muscle, with only a small amount (~4% to 5%) being metabolized by adipocytes.[7,13,14]

Although fat tissue is responsible for only a small amount of total body glucose disposal, it plays a very important role in the maintenance of total body glucose homeostasis. Small increments in the plasma insulin concentration exert a potent antilipolytic effect, leading to a marked reduction in the plasma FFA levels. The decline in plasma FFA concentrations results in an increased glucose uptake in muscle and reduces hepatic glucose production indirectly.

Type 2 Diabetes Individuals are characterized by multiple defects including (a) defects in insulin secretion; (b) insulin resistance involving muscle, liver, and the adipocyte; (c) excess glucagon secretion; (d) glucagon-like peptide-1 (GLP-1) deficiency and possibly resistance.[7]

Impaired Insulin Secretion The pancreas in people with a normal-functioning β cell is able to adjust its secretion of insulin to maintain normal plasma glucose levels. In nondiabetic individuals, insulin increases in proportion to the severity of the insulin resistance and plasma glucose remains normal. Impaired insulin secretion is a hallmark finding in T2DM. In early β-cell dysfunction, first-phase insulin release, seen with an IV bolus of glucose, is deficient. First-phase insulin is released if there is stored insulin

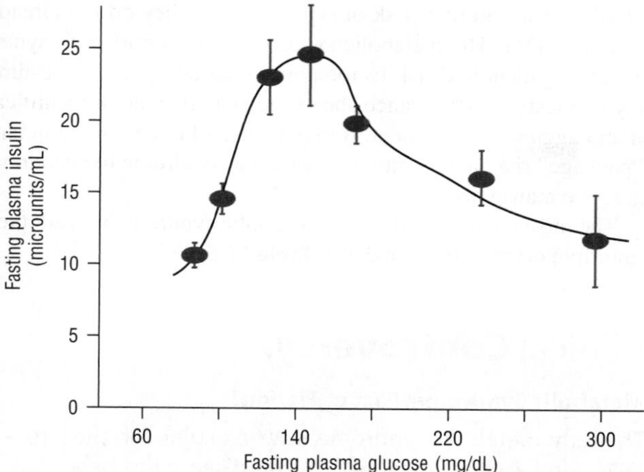

FIGURE 57-4 The relationship between fasting plasma insulin and fasting plasma glucose in 177 normal-weight individuals. Plasma insulin and glucose increase together up to a fasting glucose of 140 mg/dL (7.8 mmol/L). When the fasting glucose exceeds 140 mg/dL (7.8 mmol/L), the β cell makes progressively less insulin, which leads to an overproduction of glucose by the liver and results in a progressive increase in fasting glucose. *(Reprinted from DeFronzo RA. Pathogenesis of type 2 diabetes mellitus. Med Clin N Am 2004;88:787–835, Copyright © 2004, with permission from Elsevier.)*

in the β cell and acts to "prime" the liver to nutrient intake. Absent first-phase insulin necessitates an increase in second-phase insulin to compensate for hyperglycemia. When the insulin released can no longer normalize plasma glucose, dysglycemia, including prediabetes and diabetes, can ensue. Both β-cell mass and function in the pancreas are reduced. β-Cell failure is progressive, and starts years prior to the diagnosis of diabetes. People with T2DM lose ~5% to 7% of β-cell function per year of diabetes. The reasons for this loss are likely multifactorial including (a) glucose toxicity; (b) lipotoxicity; (c) insulin resistance; (d) age; (e) genetics; and (f) incretin deficiency. Age results in declining β-cell responsiveness and possibly mass. β-Cell failure predisposition is also present in high-risk ethnicity/races. Glucotoxicity involves glucose levels chronically exceeding 140 mg/dL (7.8 mmol/L). The β cell is unable to maintain elevated rates of insulin secretion, and releases less insulin as glucose levels increase (Fig. 57-4).[7,13,14]

Incretins In the type 2 diabetic patient, decreased postprandial insulin secretion is due to both impaired pancreatic β-cell function and a reduced stimulus for insulin secretion from gut hormones. The role gut hormones play in insulin secretion is best shown by comparing the insulin response to an oral glucose load versus an isoglycemic IV glucose infusion. In nondiabetic control individuals 73% more insulin is released in response to an oral glucose load compared with reproducing the oral glucose load's plasma glucose curve by giving IV glucose. This increased insulin secretion in response to an oral glucose stimulus is referred to as "the incretin effect" and suggests that gut-derived hormones when stimulated by glucose lead to an increase in pancreatic insulin secretion. In type 2 diabetic patients, this "incretin effect" is blunted, with the increase in insulin secretion only being 50% of that seen in nondiabetic control individuals. It is now known that two hormones, GLP-1 and glucose-dependent insulinotropic polypeptide (GIP), are responsible for over 90% of the increased insulin secretion seen in response to an oral glucose load. Patients with type 2 diabetes remain sensitive to GLP-1 while GIP levels are normal or elevated in T2DM.[7]

GLP-1 is secreted from the L cells, with the highest L-cell concentration in the distal intestinal mucosa, in response to mixed meals. Since GLP-1 levels rise within minutes of food ingestion, neural signals and possibly proximal GI tract receptors stimulate GLP-1 secretion. The insulinotropic action of GLP-1 is glucose dependent, and for GLP-1 to enhance insulin secretion, glucose concentrations must be higher than 90 mg/dL (5 mmol/L). In addition to stimulating insulin secretion, GLP-1 suppresses glucagon secretion, slows gastric emptying, and reduces food intake by increasing satiety. These effects of GLP-1 combine to limit postprandial glucose excursions. GIP is secreted by K cells in the intestine and may have a role with insulin secretion during near-normal glucose levels and may act as an insulin sensitizer in adipocytes. However, GIP has no effect on glucagon secretion, gastric motility, or satiety. The half-lives of GLP-1 and GIP are short (<10 minutes). Both hormones are rapidly inactivated by removal of two N-terminal amino acids by the enzyme dipeptidyl peptidase-4 (DPP-4). GLP-1 levels appear to decrease as glucose values increase from normal to type 2 DM, and it is unlikely to be a primary defect that causes diabetes in the majority of T2DM. Genetically a minority may have the TCF7L2 gene defect, which is associated with a decreased response to GLP-1.[7]

Insulin Resistance

Liver In type 2 diabetic subjects with mild to moderate fasting hyperglycemia (140 to 200 mg/dL, 7.8 to 11.1 mmol/L), basal hepatic glucose production is increased by ~0.5 mg/kg/min. Consequently, during the overnight sleeping hours the liver of an 80-kg diabetic individual with modest fasting hyperglycemia adds an additional 35 g of glucose to the systemic circulation. This increase in fasting hepatic glucose production is the cause of fasting hyperglycemia.[13,14]

Following glucose ingestion, insulin is secreted into the portal vein and carried to the liver, where it reduces hepatic glucose output. T2DM patients also fail to suppress glucagon in response to a meal and may even have a paradoxical rise in glucagon levels. Thus, hepatic insulin resistance and hyperglucagonemia result in continued production of glucose by the liver. Therefore, T2DM patients have two sources of glucose in the postprandial state: one from the diet and one from continued glucose production from the liver. These sources of glucose may result in marked hyperglycemia.

Peripheral (Muscle) Muscle is the major site of postprandial glucose disposal in humans, and approximately 80% of total body glucose uptake occurs in skeletal muscle. In response to a physiologic increase in plasma insulin concentration, muscle glucose uptake increases linearly, reaching a plateau value of 10 mg/kg/min. Even in lean T2DM, the onset of insulin action is delayed for ~40 minutes, and the ability of insulin to stimulate leg glucose uptake is reduced by 50%. Impaired intracellular insulin signaling is a well-established abnormality, with notable impairments at almost every step of activation due to insulin resistance, lipotoxicity, and glucotoxicity. The compensatory hyperinsulinemia required to overcome impaired insulin signaling (insulin resistance) can activate an alternative pathway through MAP kinase, which may be involved in atherosclerosis. Mitochondrial dysfunction may also play a role in muscle insulin resistance. Mitochondrial function and/or density appear to be lower in type 2 DM. This may result in less energy expenditure and an increased risk of dysfunction with high-fat diets (Fig. 57-5).[13,14]

Peripheral (Adipocyte) In obese nondiabetic and T2DM, basal plasma FFA levels are increased and fail to suppress normally after glucose ingestion. FFAs are stored as triglycerides in adipocytes and serve as an important energy source during conditions of fasting. Insulin is a potent inhibitor of lipolysis, and restrains the release of FFAs from the adipocyte by inhibiting the hormone-sensitive lipase enzyme. It is now recognized that chronically elevated plasma FFA concentrations can lead to insulin resistance in muscle and liver, and impair insulin secretion. In addition to FFAs that circulate in plasma in increased amounts, T2DM patients have increased stores

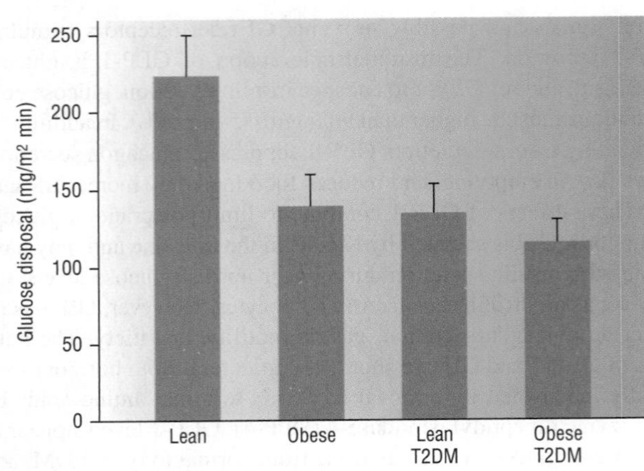

FIGURE 57-5 Whole-body glucose disposal, a measure of insulin resistance, is reduced 40% to 50% in obese nondiabetic and lean type 2 diabetic individuals. Obese diabetic individuals are slightly more resistant than lean diabetic patients. *(From DeFronzo RA. Diabetes Reviews 1977;5:177–269.)*

of intracellular fat products in muscle and liver, and the increased fat content correlates closely with the presence of insulin resistance in these tissues. Excess lipolysis from fat can also contribute to gluconeogenesis indirectly through glycerol and FFAs.[7,13,14]

Cellular Mechanisms of Insulin Resistance

Obesity and Insulin Resistance Weight gain leads to insulin resistance in most, and obese nondiabetic individuals with risk factors often have the same degree of insulin resistance as lean T2DM patients. Subsets of obese, but metabolically normal patients (6% to 30%) do exist, as well as nonobese, but metabolically abnormal patients, so broad categorization of risk for a patient needs to be confirmed by further examination.

The term *visceral adipose tissue* (VAT) refers to fat cells located within the abdominal cavity and includes omental, mesenteric, retroperitoneal, and perinephric adipose tissue. VAT has been shown to correlate with insulin resistance and explain much of the variation in insulin resistance seen. It represents 20% of fat in men and 6% of fat in women. Central obesity can be easily assessed using waist circumference, which is a good surrogate marker for VAT. This fat tissue has been shown to have a higher rate of lipolysis than subcutaneous fat, resulting in an increase in FFA production. These fatty acids are released into the portal circulation and drain into the liver, where they stimulate the production of very-low-density lipoproteins and decrease insulin sensitivity in peripheral tissues.[13,14]

VAT also produces a number of adipocytokines, such as TNF-α, interleukin 6, angiotensinogen, PAI-1, and resistin, which contribute to insulin resistance, hypertension, and hypercoagulability. These factors drain into the portal circulation and reduce insulin sensitivity in peripheral tissues. The fat cell also has the capability of producing at least one adipocytokine that improves insulin sensitivity: adiponectin. This factor is made in decreasing amounts as an individual becomes more obese. In animal models, adiponectin decreases hepatic glucose production and increases fatty acid oxidation in muscle.

The Metabolic Syndrome The metabolic syndrome is a risk indicator, but not an absolute risk indicator, because it does not specifically account for all risk factors, such as age, sex, and low-density lipoprotein cholesterol (LDL-C) levels, or directly measure hypercoagulability of the proinflammatory condition. Patients with metabolic syndrome do have a higher risk for CVD, and at least a fivefold increase in their risk of type 2 DM, if they do not already have type 2 DM. The metabolic syndrome does not identify synergism among identified risk factors, but rather additive risk, leading many to question its relevance above adequate risk factor identification and aggressive treatment. It may be useful to certain clinicians to "package" risk factors into the metabolic syndrome to encourage aggressive management.

The most recent definition of metabolic syndrome was adopted by multiple organizations in 2009 (Table 57-5).[15,16]

Clinical **Controversy. . .**

Metabolic Syndrome: Fact or Fiction?

The term metabolic syndrome was first coined in the late 1970s and associated with CVD. This disease has been studied extensively and also referred to as the "insulin resistance syndrome," "dysmetabolic syndrome," and "syndrome X." In 2001, the National Cholesterol Education Program (NCEP) Adult Treatment Panel (ATP) III formally defined the metabolic syndrome as a clustering of risk factors that include at least three of the following: elevated blood pressure, abdominal obesity, elevated triglycerides, low high-density lipoproteins, and elevated BG.[15] Since the metabolic syndrome was formally defined, several other organizations including the International Diabetes Federation (IDF), American Heart Association (AHA), National Heart, Lung, and Blood Institute (NHLBI), and the World Heart Federation, among others, have released statements to further refine the proposed definition.[16]

It is estimated that 34% of adults in the United States have the metabolic syndrome[17] and are considered to be at high risk of developing CVD and DM.[18] This epidemic has also been described in children and adolescents[19] and is expected to expand as the US obesity rates continue to climb.

However, in 2005 the ADA in conjunction with the European Association for the Study of Diabetes released a joint statement critical of the clinical utility of the metabolic syndrome.[20] They concluded in their statement that there is no doubt that CVD risk factors cluster in certain individuals, although they assert the definition is imprecise and its use as a CVD marker is questionable. They also state that there is critical information missing to warrant its designation as a syndrome. A swift rebuttal from the AHA and NHLBI was released weeks later encouraging the continued use of the metabolic syndrome concept.[21] In their statement, the authors stressed that the metabolic syndrome is not considered a singular entity and that it is a syndrome with no single pathogenesis. The authors of the statement also argue that the distinction of the metabolic syndrome should allow clinicians to approach patients as a whole with an emphasis on intensive lifestyle management. Those in the diabetes community and who authored the ADA/EASD statement contend that there is no additional benefit from identifying these clusters of CVD risk factors over measuring and treating them individually. They maintain the lack of predictive capabilities limits the metabolic syndrome's utility as a CVD marker.

The use of the metabolic syndrome in clinical practice remains a controversy. Clinicians should always take care to individualize therapy for patients who present with high CVD risk. Patient's individual goals, values, and resources should be considered when tailoring a treatment plan.

TABLE 57-5 Defining the Metabolic Syndrome

Defining the Metabolic Syndrome NCEP-ATP III: Five Components of the Metabolic Syndrome (Individuals Having at Least Three Components Meet the Criteria for Diagnosis)

Risk Factor	Defining Level
Abdominal obesity	Waist circumference
Men	>102 cm (>40 in)
Women	>88 cm (>35 in)
Triglycerides	≥150 mg/dL (≥1.70 mmol/L)
High-density lipoprotein C	
Men	<40 mg/dL (<1.03 mmol/L)
Women	<50 mg/dL (<1.29 mmol/L)
Blood pressure	≥130/≥85 mm Hg
Fasting glucose	≥110 mg/dL (≥6.1 mmol/L)

2009 Statement of the International Diabetes Federation Task Force on Epidemiology and Prevention; National Heart, Lung, and Blood Institute; American Heart Association; World Heart Federation; International Atherosclerosis Society; and International Association for the Study of Obesity

Criteria for Clinical Diagnosis of the Metabolic Syndrome (Individuals having at Least Three Components Meet the Criteria for Diagnosis)

Measure	Categorical Cut Points
Elevated waist circumference[a]	Population- and country-specific definitions
Elevated triglycerides (drug treatment for elevated triglycerides is an alternate indicator)[b]	≥150 mg/dL (≥1.7 mmol/L)
Reduced HDL-C (drug treatment for reduced HDL-C is an alternate indicator)[b]	≤40 mg/dL (≤1.03 mmol/L) in males ≤50 mg/dL (≤1.29 mmol/L) in females
Elevated blood pressure: systolic ≥130 mm Hg and/or diastolic ≥80 mm Hg (antihypertensive drug treatment in a patient with a history of hypertension is an alternate indicator)	
Elevated fasting glucose[c] (drug treatment of elevated glucose is an alternate indicator)	≥100 mg/dL (≥2.59 mmol/L)

Current Recommended Waist Circumference Thresholds for Abdominal Obesity by Organization

Population	Organization (Reference)	Men (All values ≥)	Women (All values ≥)
Europid	IDF	94 cm	80 cm
White	WHO	94 cm (increased risk) 102 cm (still higher risk)	80 cm (increased risk) 88 cm (still higher risk)
United States	AHA/NHLBI (ATP III)	102 cm	88 cm
Canada	Health Canada	102 cm	88 cm
European	European CV Societies	102 cm	88 cm
Asia (including Japanese)	IDF	90 cm	80 cm
Asia	WHO	90 cm	80 cm
Japan	Japanese Obesity Society	85 cm	90 cm
China	Cooperative Task Force	85 cm	80 cm
Middle East	Mediterranean IDF	94 cm	80 cm
Sub-Saharan African	IDF	94 cm	80 cm
Central/South American	IDF	90 cm	80 cm

[a]It is recommended that the IDF cut points be used for non-Europeans and either the IDF or AHA/NHLBI cut points used for people of European origin until more data are available.
[b]The most commonly used drugs for elevated triglycerides and reduced HDL-C are fibrates and nicotinic acid. A patient taking one of these drugs can be presumed to have high triglycerides and low HDL-C. High-dose omega-3 fatty acids presume high triglycerides.
[c]Most patients with type 2 diabetes mellitus will have the metabolic syndrome by the proposed criteria.

Reproduced from reference 15. Reprinted with permission from reference 16, © 2009 American Heart Association, Inc.

CLINICAL PRESENTATION

The clinical presentations of type 1 DM and type 2 DM are very different. Autoimmune type 1 DM can occur at any age. Approximately 75% will develop the disorder before age 20 years, but the remaining 25% develop the disease as adults. Individuals with type 1 DM are often thin and are prone to develop diabetic ketoacidosis (DKA) if insulin is withheld, or under conditions of severe stress with an excess of insulin counterregulatory hormones.[2,3,5] Symptoms in patients with type 1 DM such as polyuria, polydipsia, polyphagia, weight loss, and lethargy accompanied by hyperglycemia are the most common initial presentation. In the outpatient setting, many patients initially present with vague complaints such as weight loss and fatigue. Polyuria, polydipsia, and polyphagia may not be apparent unless a comprehensive history is taken. Twenty percent to 40% of patients with type 1 DM present with DKA after several days of polyuria, polydipsia, polyphagia, and weight loss. This presentation is common in patients from a low socioeconomic background. Rarely, type 1 DM patients are diagnosed without multiple symptoms or DKA when they have

CLINICAL PRESENTATION Diabetes Mellitus[a]

Characteristic	Type 1 DM	Type 2 DM
Age	<30 years[b]	>30 years[b]
Onset	Abrupt	Gradual
Body habitus	Lean	Obese or history of obesity
Insulin resistance	Absent	Present
Autoantibodies	Often present	Rarely present
Symptoms	Symptomatic[c]	Often asymptomatic
Ketones at diagnosis	Present	Absent[d]
Need for insulin therapy	Immediate	Years after diagnosis
Acute complications	Diabetic ketoacidosis	Hyperosmolar hyperglycemic state
Microvascular complications at diagnosis	No	Common
Macrovascular complications at or before diagnosis	Rare	Common

[a]Clinical presentation can vary widely.
[b]Age of onset for type 1 DM is generally <20 years of age, but can present at any age. The prevalence of type 2 DM in children, adolescents, and young adults is increasing. This is especially true in ethnic and minority children.
[c]Type 1 may present acutely with symptoms of polyuria, nocturia, polydipsia, polyphagia, and weight loss.
[d]Type 2 children and adolescents are more likely to present with ketones, but after the acute phase may be treated with oral agents. Prolonged fasting can also produce ketones in individuals.

blood tests drawn for other reasons. This rare presentation typically occurs when patients have a first-degree family member with type 1 DM and are closely monitored.

Patients with type 2 DM often present without symptoms, even though complications tell us that they may have been hyperglycemic for several years.[10] Often these patients are diagnosed secondary to unrelated blood testing. Lethargy, polyuria, nocturia, and polydipsia can be seen at diagnosis in type 2 diabetes, but significant weight loss at diagnosis is less common. More often, patients with type 2 DM are overweight or obese. Clinically, DM is a spectrum of diseases ranging from absolute insulin deficiency to relative insulin deficiency, and patients can have normal to grossly abnormal insulin sensitivity. Classical clinical presentation characteristics should be used in conjunction with other definitive laboratory data to properly classify patients (see also Classical Clinical Presentation of Diabetes Mellitus below).

TREATMENT Diabetes Mellitus

Desired Outcome

5 The primary goals of DM management are to reduce the risk for microvascular and macrovascular disease complications, to ameliorate symptoms, to reduce mortality, and to improve quality of life.[5] Early treatment with near-normal glycemia will reduce the risk for development of microvascular disease complications, but aggressive management of traditional cardiovascular risk factors (i.e., smoking cessation, treatment of dyslipidemia, intensive blood pressure control, and antiplatelet therapy) is needed to reduce the likelihood of development of macrovascular disease. Hyperglycemia not only increases the risk for microvascular disease but also contributes to poor wound healing, compromises white blood cell function, alters capillary function, and leads to classic symptoms of DM. DKA and hyperosmolar hyperglycemic state (HHS) are severe manifestations of poor diabetes control, almost always requiring hospitalization. Reducing the potential for microvascular complications is targeted by adherence to therapeutic lifestyle intervention (i.e., diet and exercise programs) and drug therapy regimens, as well as attaining blood pressure goals. Minimizing weight gain and hypoglycemia, especially severe hypoglycemia, and altering the glycemic goal to match the patient's morbidities are necessary. Evidence-based guidelines, as published by the ADA, may help in the attainment of these goals (Table 57-6).[5]

General Approach to Treatment

Appropriate care requires goal setting for glycemia, blood pressure, lipid levels (goals described later in chapter; see also Chaps. 3 and 11), regular monitoring for complications, dietary and exercise modifications, medications, appropriate self-monitoring of blood glucose (SMBG), and laboratory assessment of the aforementioned parameters.[5] Glucose control alone does not sufficiently reduce the risk of macrovascular complications in persons with DM.[22]

Glycemic Goal Setting and Hemoglobin A_{1c}

Controlled clinical trials provide ample evidence that glycemic control is paramount in reducing microvascular complications in both type 1 DM[23] and type 2 DM.[24] HbA_{1c} measurements are the gold standard for following long-term glycemic control for the previous 2 to 3 months.[5] Hemoglobinopathies, anemia, red cell membrane defects, transfusions, and substantial increase or decrease of red blood cell life span in a patient can affect HbA_{1c} measurements. Identification of potential problems and then ensuring the test is performed in a laboratory using a method that is NGSP certified and standardized to the DCCT assay (see *www.ngsp.org*) will minimize issues. Other strategies such as measurement of fructosamine, which measures glycated plasma proteins or glycated albumin, may be necessary to assess diabetes control in patients with altered red blood cell life span, although they are less standardized, and not correlated to risk of complications.

The A1C-Derived Average Glucose study correlated multiple HbA_{1c} and glucose readings to term the phrase estimated average glucose (eAG). The eAG better correlates with HbA_{1c} readings, and

TABLE 57-6 Selected American Diabetes Association Evidence-Based Recommendations[a]

Recommendation Area	Specific Recommendation	Evidence Level[b]
Screening for diabetes	Screen overweight or obese at any age; screen those without risk factors beginning at age 45 years	B
	To screen for diabetes a FPG, 2-hour 75-g OGTT, or HbA_{1c} is appropriate	B
	Interval between screenings should be individualized based on risk, or every 3 years	E
Monitoring	Home blood glucose monitoring is recommended for patients on multidose insulin or pump therapy at least prior to meals and snacks, and before events such as driving	B
	Subjects on other therapeutic interventions, including oral agents, may perform home blood glucose monitoring, but ongoing instruction to patient on how to adjust therapy based on monitoring must be in place	E
	Quarterly HbA_{1c} in individuals not meeting glycemic goals, twice yearly in individuals meeting glycemic goals should be performed	E
	In adults, measure fasting lipid profile at least annually	B
	Perform an annual urine albumin excretion in type 1 diabetes with duration ≥5 years. Type 2 DM from diagnosis	B
	Perform a screen for distal symmetrical polyneuropathy at diagnosis in type 2 DM and after 5 years' duration in type 1 DM; screen at least annually thereafter	B
	A dilated eye examination should be performed within 5 years of diagnosis in type 1 DM, and shortly after diagnosis in type 2 DM, with follow-up every year, or every 2–3 years as recommended by an eye specialist	B
Glycemic goals	HbA_{1c} goal for patients in general is <7% (<0.07; <53 mmol/mol Hb)	B
	HbA_{1c} goal should be individualized, with <6.5% (<0.065; <48 mmol/mol Hb) if achieved without significant hypoglycemia or adverse effects in younger, long life expectancy, and no CVD patient	B
	Less stringent HbA_{1c} goal (<8% [<0.08; <64 mmol/mol Hb]) may be appropriate in patients with a history of severe hypoglycemia, limited life expectancy, advanced microvascular/macrovascular complications or comorbidities, or in difficult to reach goal patients despite adequate therapy	C
	Hospital: Critically ill: 140–180 mg/dL (7.8–10 mmol/L) (A), or more stringent guidelines down to 110–140 mg/dL (6.1–7.8 mmol/L) if without hypoglycemia (C)	See text
	Non–critically ill: No clear evidence but in general premeal BG <140 mg/dL (<7.8 mmol/L) and random BG <180 mg/dL (<10 mmol/L) (E)	
Treatment		
Prevention of type 2 diabetes	Patients with IGT (A), IFG (E), or an A1C of 5.7–6.4% (0.057–0.064; 39–46 mmol/mol Hb) (E) should attempt weight loss (5–10%), increasing physical activity	See text
	Metformin may be considered in obese, <60-year-old patients, and women with prior GDM with IGT (A), IFG (E), or an A1C 5.7–6.4% (0.057–0.064; 39–46 mmol/mol Hb) (E)	See text
Medical nutrition therapy	Weight loss is recommended for all insulin-resistant/overweight or obese individuals. Either low-carbohydrate, low-fat calorie-restricted diets, or Mediterranean diets may work	A
	In patients with known CVD consider ACE inhibitor therapy (C), as well as aspirin and statin therapy (A)	See text
	Saturated fat should be <7% of total calories	B
	Monitoring carbohydrate intake by carbohydrate counting, exchanges, or experienced estimation is recommended to achieve glycemic goals	B
	Routine supplementation with antioxidants, such as vitamins E and C, is not advised due to lack of efficacy	A
Physical activity	150 min/wk of moderate-intensity exercise spread over at least 3 days and with no more than 2 days without exercise	A
	Resistance training of large muscle groups should be ≥2 times per week	A
Blood pressure	Systolic blood pressure should be treated to <140 mm Hg	B
	Diastolic blood pressure should be treated to <80 mm Hg	B
	Initial drug therapy should be with an ACE inhibitor or ARB	C
Nephropathy	In treatment of nonpregnant patients with modest (30–299 mg/day) (C) or higher levels (≥300 mg/day) (A) of urinary albumin excretion, either ACE inhibitors or ARBs are recommended	See text
Dyslipidemia	The primary goal is an LDL <100 mg/dL (<2.59 mmol/L) if without overt CVD	B
	Statin therapy should be added to lifestyle, regardless of baseline lipid levels if patient has CVD, or is >40 years of age and has one other CVD risk factor	A
	In patients with overt CVD, using a statin to achieve a LDL <70 mg/dL (<1.81 mmol/L) is an option	B
	Triglycerides lowered to <150 mg/dL (<1.70 mmol/L) and raising HDL to >40 mg/dL (>1.03 mmol/L) in men and >50 mg/dL (1.29 mmol/L) in women is desirable	C
Antiplatelet	Use aspirin (75–162 mg daily) for secondary cardioprotection	A
	Use aspirin (75–162 mg) for primary prevention in type 1 or 2 DM if the 10-year risk of CVD is >10%, the patient is >50 (men) or >60 (women) with at least one additional risk factor present	C
Hospital	Critically ill: By IV insulin protocol (E); non–critically ill: scheduled subcutaneous insulin with basal, nutritional, and correction coverage (C)	See text

[a]Based on American Diabetes Association practice recommendations. Other evidence-based recommendations available.[8]
[b]Evidence levels: A, clear evidence from well-conducted, generalizable, randomized controlled trials that are adequately powered; B, supportive evidence from well-conducted cohort studies or well-conducted case–control study; C, supportive evidence from poorly controlled or uncontrolled studies or conflicting evidence with weight of evidence supporting intervention; E, expert consensus or clinical experience.

now is regularly reported below HbA_{1c} values on laboratory results. For example, a HbA_{1c} of 6% or 7% (0.060 to 0.070; 42 to 53 mmol/mol Hb) correlates with an average glucose of 126 or 154 mg/dL (7 or 8.5 mmol/L), respectively, and online calculators and graphs are easily found.[25]

Less stringent HbA_{1c} goals (>7% [>0.070; >53 mmol/mol Hb]) may be appropriate in patients with a history of severe hypoglycemia, limited life expectancy, advanced microvascular/macrovascular complications or comorbidities, at-risk elderly, dementia, or in younger children. A HbA_{1c} target of <7% (<0.070; <0.53 mmol/mol Hb) is

TABLE 57-7 Glycemic Goals of Therapy by Organization[8]

Biochemical Index	ADA		ACE and AACE
Hemoglobin A_{1c}	<7% (<0.07; <53 mmol/mol/Hb)[a]		≤6.5% (≤0.065; ≤48 mmol/mol Hb)
Preprandial plasma glucose	70–130 mg/dL (3.9–7.2 mmol/L)		<110 mg/dL (<6.1 mmol/L)
Postprandial plasma glucose	<180 mg/dL[b] (<10 mmol/L)		<140 mg/dL (<7.8 mmol/L)
ADA plasma glucose and HbA_{1c} goals for type 1 DM by age group[c]			
Values by age (years)	Plasma glucose goal		A_{1c}
	Before meals	bedtime/overnight	
Toddlers and preschoolers (0–6)	100–180 (5.6–10 mmol/L)	110–200 (6.1–11.1 mmol/L)	7.5% to 8.5% (<0.085; <69 mmol/mol Hb)
School age (6–12)	90–180 (5–10 mmol/L)	100–180 (5.6–10 mmol/L)	<8% (<0.080; <64 mmol/mol Hb)
Adolescents and young adults (13–19)	90–130 (5–7.2 mmol/L)	90–150 (5–8.3 mmol/L)	<7.5% (<0.075; <58 mmol/mol Hb)

ADA, American Diabetes Association; ACE, American College of Endocrinology; AACE, American Association of Clinical Endocrinologists.

[a]Assay should be National Glycohemoglobin Standardization Program (NGSP)–certified measurement and Diabetes Control and Complications Trial (DCCT) standardized. More stringent glycemic control may be appropriate if accomplished without significant hypoglycemia or adverse effects. Less stringent HbA_{1c} goals may be appropriate in patients with a history of severe hypoglycemia, limited life expectancy, advanced microvascular/macrovascular complications or comorbidities, at-risk elderly, dementia, or in younger children.

[b]Postprandial glucose measurements should be made 1–2 hours after the beginning of the meal, generally the time of peak levels in patients with diabetes.

[c]Vulnerability to hypoglycemia and relatively low risk of complication prior to puberty considered. Adolescents and young adults may have adult goals if without developmental and psychological issues, and if without excessive hypoglycemia.

appropriate for others (Table 57-7), and lower values should be targeted if significant hypoglycemia, weight gain, and other adverse effects can be avoided.[5] Glycemic control recommendations for different age groups of type 1 DM patients are based on the risk of hypoglycemia, the relatively low risk of complications prior to puberty, and psychological and/or developmental issues (Table 57-7).

Initial Evaluation of Diabetes Mellitus

On initial evaluation, a thorough medical history and identification of specific type of diabetes, including duration of diabetes, characteristics of onset (e.g., DKA or asymptomatic), dietary and weight history, education history, medication history including current and past medications for DM, current regimen including medications, diet, physical activity, and adherence, should be performed. Hospitalization history, hypoglycemia (frequency, cause, timing), and diabetes-related complications should be documented. Laboratory evaluation should include at a minimum an A1C, lipid profile, liver function tests, thyroid-stimulating hormone level, serum creatinine and electrolytes, and a urine analysis for microalbuminuria. In type 1 DM, consider screening for celiac disease by measuring tissue transglutaminase or antiendomysial antibodies. The physical examination and pertinent data should include all vital signs, weight and/or BMI, blood pressure assessment, thyroid palpation, cardiovascular and carotid auscultation, skin integrity, assessment for acanthosis nigricans, and a foot examination, including screening for impaired sensation detection with a 10-g force monofilament.[5]

Monitoring for Complications

The ADA recommends initiation of complications monitoring at the time of diagnosis of DM.[8] Current recommendations continue to advocate yearly dilated eye examinations in type 2 DM, and an initial dilated eye examination in the first 3 to 5 years in type 1 DM, and then yearly thereafter. Less frequent testing (every 2 to 3 years) can be implemented on the advice of an eye care specialist. The blood pressure should be assessed at each visit. The feet should be examined at each visit for distal pulses, skin integrity, calluses, and deformities, and yearly screening should be done for loss of protective sensation with a distal polyneuropathy tool, such as the 10-g force Semmes-Weinstein monofilament. A urine test for microalbumin to screen for nephropathy once yearly from diagnosis is appropriate in type 2 DM, and initiated 5 years after diagnosis if the patient has type 1 DM. Yearly testing for lipid abnormalities, and more frequently if needed to achieve lipid goals, is recommended. It is generally accepted that a yearly thyroid-stimulating hormone level may be appropriate in type 1 DM, LADA, and select type 2 DM patients.[5]

Self-Monitored Blood Glucose and Continuous Glucose Monitoring

The advent of SMBG in the early 1980s revolutionized the treatment of DM, enabling patients to know their BG concentration at any moment easily and relatively inexpensively. At its core, SMBG is a tool to provide structure for a change and/or safety: change, in that the patient has an opportunity to intervene when a SMBG value is obtained, and safety, as hypoglycemia and hyperglycemia need to be avoided and/or identified and treated. In general, SMBG frequency should match how complicated the regimen is for glycemic control and minimally allow testing to avoid hypoglycemia.

Frequent SMBG is necessary to achieve near-normal BG concentrations if hypoglycemic agents are used. Assessment for hypoglycemia and hyperglycemia, adjustment of prandial doses of insulin, administration of corrective doses of insulin, change in diet and exercise, and checking accuracy of continuous glucose monitors are but a few of the reasons a patient may need SMBG at a given time. This is particularly true in patients with type 1 DM, as most will be intensively managed with insulin. The more intense the pharmacologic regimen is, the more intense the SMBG needs to be (before meals, at bedtime, occasionally after meals, and middle of sleep cycle in patients on multiple insulin injections or pump therapy whether type 1 or type 2 DM). The optimal frequency of SMBG for patients with type 2 DM on oral agents is unresolved.[26] Frequency of monitoring in type 2 DM should be sufficient to facilitate reaching glucose goals and to test for hypoglycemia. The role of SMBG in improving glycemic control in type 2 DM patients is controversial, but has shown to reduce the HbA_{1c} ~0.4% (~0.004; ~4 mmol/mol Hb) to no improvement. What is clear is that patients must be empowered to change their therapeutic regimen (lifestyle and medications) in response to test results, or no meaningful glycemic improvement is likely to be effected.[5]

Alternate site testing may improve adherence to SMBG recommendations, but only SMBG meters that can "sip" blood onto the strip will accommodate such testing. Alternate site glucose testing is performed on the palm, forearm, or the thigh. These areas tend to have less nerve endings and may be more comfortable for a patient, but several cautions must be observed. Interstitial glucose readings identified with alternative site testing will lag behind fingertip capillary blood, as the capillary flow/density is often less in the alternate testing sites when compared with that in the fingertip. Alternate site testing is discouraged in any situation where immediate action will be needed based on the glucose reading, such as testing for hypoglycemia or in patients with hypoglycemia unawareness, wide fluctuations in SMBG, or when the BG is known to be fluctuating, such as postprandially.

Choosing a meter for your patient depends most importantly on his or her dexterity, eye acuity, strip cost, and features that may be important to him or her. Demonstrate to and then have the patient confirm the monitoring technique to minimize problems. Each meter has specifications on hematocrit, elevation, whole blood versus plasma, and heat/cold tolerance. In addition, acetaminophen, ascorbate, dopamine, mannitol, and sugar-based products may alter testing results. Consult the manufacturer materials for specifics.

Continuous glucose monitoring (CGM) may be useful in select patients. CGM measures interstitial glucose, which lags behind capillary SMBG, and the same cautions as alternate site testing should be followed. CGM can be useful in patients with frequent hypoglycemia or hypoglycemic unawareness, nocturnal hypoglycemia, and for identification of fluctuating glucose patterns and/or previously unknown problems in patients with higher or lower than expected HbA_{1c} results. CGM still needs to be calibrated after insertion of a new sensor and minimally every 12 hours with SMBG readings, alarms need to be properly set, and a new sensor must be placed every 3 to 7 days. The ADA currently recommends that CGM can be considered in type 1 DM adults ≥25 years of age, and those <25 years of age, if adherent to its use, and in others with the above issues noted.[5]

Nonpharmacologic Therapy

Diet

Medical nutrition therapy is recommended for all persons with DM and, along with activity, is a cornerstone of treatment.[5] Paramount for all medical nutrition therapy is the attainment of optimal metabolic outcomes and the prevention and treatment of complications. It is imperative that patients understand the connection between carbohydrate intake, medications, and glucose control. For individuals with type 1 DM, the focus is on physiologically regulating insulin administration with a balanced diet to achieve and maintain a healthy body weight. A healthy meal plan that is moderate in carbohydrates and low in saturated fat (<7% of total calories), with a focus on balanced meals delivering all of the essential vitamins and minerals, is recommended in DM. The amount (grams) and type (via the glycemic index, though controversial) of carbohydrates, whether accounted for by exchanges or carbohydrate counting, should be considered. All foods can be fit into a healthy meal plan, and the days of recommending no sweets are in the past. If a healthy weight and normal glucose goals can be maintained, there is no reason to deny food choices. Overweight/obese patients with type 2 DM often require caloric restriction to promote weight loss, and portion size and frequency are often issues. The specific diet appears to be less important than if the patient will adhere to the diet, although low-fat diet for CVD or avoiding a high-protein diet in nephropathy may be appropriate. Rather than a set diabetic diet, advocate a diet using foods that are within the financial reach and cultural milieu of the patient. Discourage bedtime and between-meal snacks, set realistic goals for changes based on what the patient can/will change, and follow up to see how and if those changes occurred.[27]

Activity

In general, most patients with DM can benefit from increased activity.[28] Aerobic exercise improves insulin sensitivity and modestly improves glycemic control in the majority of individuals, and reduces cardiovascular risk factors, contributes to weight loss or maintenance, and improves well-being. The patient should choose an activity that he or she is likely to continue. Start exercise slowly in previously sedentary patients. It remains unclear which asymptomatic patients should be screened for CVD prior to the beginning of an exercise regimen. Patients with long-standing disease (age >35 years, or >25 years old with DM ≥10 years), patients with multiple cardiovascular risk factors, presence of microvascular disease (especially renal disease), and patients with previous evidence of atherosclerotic disease should have a cardiovascular evaluation, probably including an electrocardiogram, with further workup related to CVD risk. In addition, several complications (uncontrolled hypertension, autonomic neuropathy, insensate feet, and retinopathy) may require restrictions on the activities recommended. Physical activity goals include at least 150 min/wk of moderate (50% to 70% maximal heart rate) intensity exercise spread over at least 3 days a week with no more than 2 days between activity. In addition, resistance/strength training, in patients without retinal contraindications, is recommended to be added into this exercise regimen at least two times a week.[5]

Pharmacologic Therapy

From the late 1970s to 1995, only two options for pharmacologic treatment were available for patients with diabetes: sulfonylureas (for type 2 DM only) and insulin (for type 1 or 2). Since 1995, a number of new oral agents, injectables, and insulins have been introduced in the United States.

The Look Action for Health in Diabetes (Look AHEAD) trial recently reported that no decrease in cardiovascular outcomes from intensive lifestyle changes in type 2 DM subjects was noted after 10 years of follow-up. In addition, intensive lifestyle was not able to obtain intensive glycemic control in the majority of subjects, reiterating the need for early diabetes medication use in conjunction with diet and exercise interventions.

Currently, nine classes of oral agents are approved for the treatment of type 2 diabetes: α-glucosidase inhibitors, biguanides, meglitinides, peroxisome proliferator–activated receptor γ (PPAR-γ) agonists (which are also commonly identified as thiazolidinediones [TZDs] or glitazones), DPP-4 inhibitors, dopamine agonists, bile acid sequestrants, sodium-glucose cotransporter 2 inhibitors, and sulfonylureas. Oral antidiabetic agents are often grouped according to their glucose-lowering mechanism of action. Biguanides and TZDs are often categorized as insulin sensitizers due to their ability to reduce insulin resistance. Sulfonylureas and meglitinides are often categorized as insulin secretagogues because they enhance endogenous insulin release. Three injectable classes, including insulin, GLP-1 receptor agonists, and amylinomimetics, are also available.

Drug Class Information

Insulin

Pharmacology Insulin is an anabolic and anticatabolic hormone. It plays major roles in protein, carbohydrate, and fat metabolism. Endogenously produced insulin is cleaved from the larger proinsulin peptide in the β cell to the active peptide of insulin and inactive C-peptide. All commercially available insulin preparations contain only the active insulin peptide.

Characteristics Characteristics that are commonly used to categorize insulin preparations include source, strength, onset, and duration of action. Additionally, insulin may be characterized as analog,

TABLE 57-8 Available Injectable and Insulin Preparations

Generic Name	Manufacturer	Analog[a]	Administration Options	Room Temperature[b] Expiration
Rapid-acting Insulins				
Humalog (insulin lispro)	Lilly	Yes	Insulin pen 3 mL, vial, or 3-mL pen cartridge	28 days
NovoLog (insulin aspart)	Novo Nordisk	Yes	Insulin pen 3 mL, vial, or 3-mL pen cartridge	28 days
Apidra (insulin glulisine)	Sanofi-Aventis	Yes	Insulin pen 3 mL, vial, or 3-mL pen cartridge	28 days
Short-acting Insulins				
Humulin R (regular) available in U-100 and U-500	Lilly	No	U-100, 10-mL vial U-500, 20-mL vial	28 days
Novolin R (regular)	Novo Nordisk	No	10-mL vial	30 days
Intermediate-acting Insulins				
NPH				
Humulin N	Lilly	No	Vial, 3-mL prefilled pen	Vial: 28 days; pen: 14 days
Novolin N	Novo Nordisk	No	Vial	30 days
Long-acting Insulins				
Lantus (insulin glargine)	Sanofi-Aventis	Yes	Vial, 3-mL pen, 3-mL pen cartridge	28 days
Levemir (insulin detemir)	Novo Nordisk	Yes	Vial, 3-mL prefilled pen	42 days
Premixed Insulins				
Premixed insulin analogs				
Humalog Mix 75/25 (75% neutral protamine lispro, 25% lispro)	Lilly	Yes	Vial, prefilled pen	Vial: 28 days; pen: 10 days
Novolog Mix 70/30 (70% aspart protamine suspension, 30% aspart)	Novo Nordisk	Yes	Vial, 3-mL prefilled pen	Vial: 28 days; others: 14 days
Humalog Mix 50/50 (50% neutral protamine lispro/50% lispro)	Lilly	Yes	Vial, 3-mL pen	Vial: 28 days; pen: 10 days
NPH–regular Combinations				
Humulin 70/30	Lilly	No	Vial, 3-mL prefilled pen	Vial: 28 days; pen: 10 days
Novolin 70/30	Novo Nordisk	No	Vial	30 days
Other Injectables				
Glucagon-like peptide-1 agonists (GLP-1 agonists)				
Byetta (exenatide)	Amylin/BMS	No	5- and 10-mcg pen, ~60 injections (doses)/pen	30 days ≤25°C (≤77°F)
Victoza (liraglutide)	Novo Nordisk	Yes	3-mL pen, delivers 0.6-, 1.2-, or 1.8-mg dose	30 days
Bydureon (exenatide)	Amylin/BMS	No	2-mg vial with separate diluent, single-use system	30 days ≤25°C (≤77°F)
Amylinomimetic				
Symlin (pramlintide)	Amylin	Yes	1.5-mL pen: delivers 15-, 30-, 45-, or 60-mcg dose; 2.7-mL pen: delivers 60- or 120-mcg dose	30 days

[a]All diabetes injectables available in the United States are now made by human recombinant DNA technology. An insulin analog is a modified human insulin molecule that imparts particular pharmacokinetic advantages.
[b]Room temperature defined as 15–30°C (59–86°F). All products are good until expiration date on product if unopened and stored correctly.

defined as insulin preparations that had amino acids within the insulin molecule modified and/or "modifiers" added to impart particular physiochemical and pharmacokinetic advantages. Table 57-8 summarizes available insulin preparations.

U-100 and U-500, 100 and 500 units/mL, respectively, are the strengths of injectable insulin currently available in the United States. U-500 regular insulin is available for individuals who may require large doses of insulin to control their diabetes. In the United States, all other insulin preparations are available only in U-100 strength. For some patients with type 1 diabetes who require extremely low doses of insulin, dilution of U-100 insulin to obtain accurate insulin doses may be necessary. Diluents, instructions on dilution, and empty bottles can be obtained from the manufacturers for dilution.

Historically, insulin came from either beef or pork sources. Manufacturers in the United States have discontinued production of beef and pork source insulin preparations as of December 2003, and now exclusively use recombinant DNA technology to manufacture insulin. Eli Lilly and Sanofi-Aventis currently use a non–disease-producing strain of *Escherichia coli* for synthesis of insulin, whereas Novo Nordisk uses *Saccharomyces cerevisiae*, or bakers' yeast, for synthesis.

Purity of insulin refers to the amount of proinsulin and other impurities present in a given insulin product. Prior to 1980, most insulin contained enough impurities (300 to 10,000 ppm) to cause local reactions on injection, as well as systemic adverse effects from antibody production. Modern technology has provided less expensive techniques to purify insulin. As a result, all insulin products contain ≤10 ppm of proinsulin, with purified preparations (all recombinant DNA human insulin and insulin analogs) containing <1 ppm of proinsulin.

Regular crystalline insulin naturally self-associates into a hexameric (six insulin molecules) structure when injected subcutaneously. Before absorption through a blood capillary can occur, the hexamer must dissociate first to dimers, and then to monomers. This principle is the premise for additives such as protamine and zinc described below, and modification of amino acids for insulin analogs. Lispro, aspart, and glulisine insulin preparations dissociate rapidly to monomers; thus, absorption is rapid. Lispro (B-28 lysine and B-29 proline human insulin; monomeric) insulin with two amino acids transposed, aspart (B-28 aspartic acid human insulin; monomeric and dimeric) insulin with replacement of one amino acid, and glulisine (B-3 lysine and B-29 glutamic acid) are rapidly absorbed, peak faster, and have shorter durations of action when compared with regular insulin. Proteins tend to be insoluble near their isoelectric point, and glargine insulin uses this to prolong absorption. In comparison to human insulin, with an isoelectric point of 5.4, the analog glargine insulin (A-21 glycine, B-30a-arginine, B-30a L-arginine, and B-30b L-arginine human insulin) has an isoelectric point of 6.8. In the bottle, glargine is buffered to a pH of 4, a level at which it is completely soluble, resulting in a clear colorless solution. When injected into the neutral pH of the body, it rapidly forms microprecipitates that slowly dissolve into monomers and dimers that are then subsequently absorbed. The result is a long-acting, approximately 24-hour duration insulin analog. Detemir, in contrast, attaches a C14 fatty acid (a 14-carbon fatty acid) at the B-29 position and removes the B-30 amino acid. This allows the fatty acid side chain to bind to interstitial albumin at the SQ injection site. Also, the formulation allows stronger hexamer self-associations, which prolong absorption. Once detemir dissociates from the interstitial albumin, it is free to enter a capillary, where it is again bound to albumin, which can further prolong action. It then travels to a site of action and interacts, after dissociation from albumin, with insulin receptors.

Insulin analogs are modified human insulin molecules, and safety is paramount for FDA approval. Key factors that should be considered in the approval process include local injection reactions, antigenicity, efficacy compared with human insulin, insulin receptor binding affinity, and insulin-like growth factor 1–receptor affinity (which is compared with that of human insulin to determine mitogenic potential).

Pharmacokinetics Subcutaneous injection kinetics is dependent on onset, peak, and duration of action, and is summarized in Table 57-9. Absorption of insulin from a subcutaneous depot is dependent on several factors, including source of insulin, concentration of insulin, additives to the insulin preparations (e.g., zinc, protamine), blood flow to the area (rubbing of injection area, increased skin temperature, and exercise in muscles near the injection site may enhance absorption), and injection site. Regular or neutral protamine Hagedorn (NPH) insulin is commonly injected in (from most rapid to slowest absorption): abdominal fat, posterior upper arms, lateral thigh area, and superior buttocks area. Insulin analogs, unlike regular or NPH insulin, appear to retain their kinetic profile at all sites of injection. U-500 regular insulin has a delayed onset and peak, and a longer duration of action when compared with U-100 regular insulin; the pharmacokinetic profile of U-500 is more similar to NPH.

Addition of protamine (NPH, NPL, and aspart protamine suspension) or excess zinc (historically lente or ultralente insulin) will delay onset, peak, and duration of the insulin's effect. Variability in absorption, inconsistent suspension of the insulin by the patient or healthcare provider when drawing up a dose, and inherent insulin action based on the pharmacokinetics of the products may all contribute to a labile glucose response. NPH insulin and all suspension-based insulin preparations should be inverted or rolled gently at least 10 times to fully suspend the insulin prior to each use.

As detemir insulin has a unique mechanism to prolong absorption, it should not be surprising that the pharmacokinetics is unique. Detemir insulin reported less intrapatient variability between injections when compared with NPH or glargine insulin. This may be advantageous when variability in the insulin level may make a large difference in glycemic excursions, as in type 1 DM. It should be noted that at low dose (0.2 unit/kg) the duration of action is approximately 14 to 16 hours, while at doses above 0.3 unit/kg, it is close to 24 hours. In type 1 DM, 30% to 50% of patients may require twice-daily use of detemir insulin to cover 24-hour basal insulin needs, but this is unlikely to be an issue in type 2 DM patients, as they tend to use more units per day to attain glycemic goals. Direct comparative data between glargine insulin and detemir insulin are difficult to interpret, as detemir insulin was allowed to be dosed twice daily. Equivalent glycemic control was attained with either insulin. It is possible that glargine insulin in a minority of type 1 DM patients may require twice-daily dosing, but this is poorly documented in the literature.

The half-life of an IV injection of regular insulin is about 9 minutes. Thus, the effective duration of action of a single IV injection is short, and changes in IV insulin rates will reach steady state in approximately 45 minutes. IV pharmacokinetics of other soluble insulin preparations (lispro, aspart, glulisine, and even glargine) is similar to IV regular insulin, but they have no advantages over IV regular insulin and are more expensive. For completeness, aspart, lispro, and glulisine are FDA approved for IV use.

Insulin is degraded in the liver, muscle, and kidney. Liver deactivation is 20% to 50% in a single passage. Approximately 15% to 20% of insulin metabolism occurs in the kidney. This may partially explain the lower insulin dosage requirements in patients with end-stage renal disease.

TABLE 57-9 Pharmacokinetics of Various Insulins Administered Subcutaneously

Type of Insulin	Onset	Peak (Hours)	Duration (Hours)	Maximum Duration (Hours)	Appearance
Rapid Acting					
Aspart	15–30 minutes	1–2	3–5	5–6	Clear
Lispro	15–30 minutes	1–2	3–4	4–6	Clear
Glulisine	15–30 minutes	1–2	3–4	5–6	Clear
Short Acting					
Regular	0.5–1 hours	2–3	4–6	6–8	Clear
Intermediate Acting					
NPH	2–4 hours	4–8	8–12	14–18	Cloudy
Long Acting					
Detemir	2 hours	—[a]	14–24	24	Clear
Glargine	4–5 hours	—[a]	22–24	24	Clear

[a]Glargine is considered "flat" pharmacokinetically, and detemir has a slight peak, but both have exhibited peak effects during comparative testing, and these peak effects may necessitate changing therapy in a minority of type 1 DM patients.

Currently, insulin must be injected to retain its glycemic lowering properties. Alternative absorption pathways, including pulmonary, topical, GI, and even nasal, are being explored. The first inhalation insulin (Exubera) was discontinued due to poor sales and subsequent reports of lung cancer. Technosphere inhaled insulin (Afrezza) was rejected by the FDA due to concerns regarding the redesign of their delivery device. Additional trials are underway to assess the safety of the redesigned delivery device in patients with type 1 and type 2 DM. The onset of action is similar to IV insulin, which is unique.

Microvascular Complications Insulin has been shown to be as efficacious as any oral agent for treating DM. The United Kingdom Prospective Diabetes Study (UKPDS), which used sulfonylureas or insulin, showed equal efficacy in lowering the risk of microvascular events in newly diagnosed type 2 DM.[24] Similarly, in type 1 DM, the DCCT showed efficacy in reducing microvascular complications.[23]

Macrovascular Complications The connection between high insulin levels (hyperinsulinemia), insulin resistance, and cardiovascular events incorrectly leads some clinicians to believe that insulin therapy may cause macrovascular complications. Endogenous hyperinsulinemia in the setting of insulin resistance has been linked to increased cardiovascular events; however, this is not the case with hyperinsulinemia due to exogenous injectable insulin preparations. The UKPDS and DCCT found no differences in macrovascular outcomes with intensive insulin therapy. One study, the Diabetes Mellitus, Insulin Glucose Infusion in Acute Myocardial Infarction study,[29] reported reductions in mortality with insulin therapy. This group assessed the effect of an insulin–glucose infusion in type 2 DM patients who had experienced an acute myocardial infarction (MI). Those randomized to insulin infusion followed by intensive insulin therapy lowered their absolute mortality risk by 11% over a mean follow-up period of approximately 3 years. This was most evident in subjects who were insulin-naïve or had a low cardiovascular risk prior to the acute MI.[29] The importance of glycemic control in hospitalized patients is covered later in the chapter.

Adverse Effects The most common adverse effects reported with insulin are hypoglycemia and weight gain. Hypoglycemia is more common in patients on intensive insulin therapy regimens versus those on less-intensive regimens. Also, patients with type 1 DM tend to have more hypoglycemic events compared with type 2 DM patients. In the UKPDS study, performed over 10 years, the percentage of diabetic patients who needed assistance (third-party or hospitalization) due to a hypoglycemic reaction was 2.3%. The UKPDS reported a rate of 36.5% for risk of any hypoglycemic event, including mild, self-treated events. In the DCCT, tighter control produced a risk three times higher for severe hypoglycemia compared with conventional therapy. Moreover, insulin was associated with 14% of emergency hospitalizations in older Americans using nationally representative public health surveillance data.[30] Glycemic goals should incorporate hypoglycemic risk versus the benefit of lowering the glucose when HbA_{1c} levels are near normal, especially in type 1 DM.

Hypoglycemia Minimization of risk for patients on insulin should include education about the signs and symptoms of hypoglycemia, proper treatment of hypoglycemia, and BG monitoring. BG monitoring is essential for those on insulin, and is particularly of value in patients with hypoglycemia unawareness. Patients with hypoglycemia unawareness do not experience the normal sympathetic symptoms of hypoglycemia (tachycardia, tremulousness, and, often, sweating). Initial hypoglycemia symptoms are neuroglycopenic in nature (confusion, agitation, loss of consciousness, and/or progression to coma). Patients with hypoglycemia unawareness should at least temporarily raise their glycemic goals (requiring a reduction in insulin dose) and check their BG level prior to any activities that may be dangerous with a low blood sugar (e.g., driving and certain sports, among others). Proper treatment of hypoglycemia dictates ingestion of carbohydrates, with glucose being preferred. Unconsciousness is an indication for either IV glucose or glucagon injection, which increases glycogenolysis in the liver. Glucagon use would be appropriate in any situation in which the patient does not have or cannot have ready IV access for glucose administration. Education for reconstitution and injection of glucagon is recommended for close friends and family of a patient who has recurrent neuroglycopenic events. The patient and close contacts should be informed that it can take 10 to 15 minutes for the injection to start raising glucose levels, and patients often vomit during this time. Proper positioning to avoid aspiration should be emphasized.

Weight gain is predominantly from increased truncal fat, and tends to be related to daily dose and plasma insulin levels present. It is undesirable in most type 2 DM patients, but may be seen as beneficial in underweight patients with type 1 DM. Weight gain appears to be related to intensive insulin therapy, and can be somewhat minimized by physiologic replacement of insulin.

Two forms of lipodystrophy, although much less common today in people with diabetes, still occur. Lipohypertrophy is caused by many injections into the same injection site. Due to insulin's anabolic actions, a raised fat mass is present at the injection site with resultant variable insulin absorption. Lipoatrophy, in contrast, is thought to be due to insulin antibodies or allergic-type reactions with destruction of fat at the site of injection. In both cases, injection away from the site with more purified insulin is recommended, although reports of lipoatrophy have been reported with most insulin preparations. Anecdotal evidence has shown that specially formulated cromolyn may help to stabilize the allergic type of reaction.

One large study using administrative data found an association between insulin glargine and cancer. However, several other large database studies and meta-analysis have shown no such association. Glargine in vitro has a higher affinity for IGF-1 than regular human insulin, which could theoretically explain the increased risk of cancer, yet in vivo the metabolite of glargine is mostly present. The metabolite has similar affinity for IGF-1 as regular insulin. However, in the observational retrospective study, confounding by indication, selection, or detection bias in older patients may have played a greater role in the detection of cancer than the insulin glargine therapy. Supporting this premise, when glargine was used in intensive insulin therapy regimens in healthier populations, no such association was seen. Recently, the prospective, randomized Outcome Reduction with Initial Glargine Intervention trial reported no difference in cancer risk or cardiovascular events with low-dose insulin glargine use over approximately 6 years.[31] These data are not definitive, but encouraging.

Drug–Drug Interactions There are no significant drug–drug interactions with injected insulin, although other medications that may affect glucose control can be considered. Detemir does not have albumin binding interactions, as it occupies only a small percent of albumin binding sites. Table 57-10 lists common medications known to affect BG levels.

Dosing and Administration The dose of insulin for any person with altered glucose metabolism must be individualized. In type 1 DM, the average daily requirement for insulin is 0.5 to 0.6 unit/kg, with approximately 50% being delivered as basal insulin, and the remaining 50% dedicated to meal coverage. During the honeymoon phase it may fall to 0.1 to 0.4 unit/kg. During acute illness or with ketosis or states of relative insulin resistance, higher dosages are warranted. In type 2 DM a higher dosage is

TABLE 57-10 Medications that may Affect Glycemic Control[a]

Drug	Effect on Glucose	Mechanism/Comment
Angiotensin-converting enzyme inhibitors	Slight reduction	Improves insulin sensitivity
Alcohol	Reduction	Reduces hepatic glucose production
α-Interferon	Increase	Decreases insulin sensitivity/induces counterregulatory hormones
Atypical antipsychotics	Increase	Decrease insulin sensitivity; weight gain
Calcineurin inhibitors	Increase	Decrease insulin secretion
Diazoxide	Increase	Decreases insulin secretion, decreases peripheral glucose use
Diuretics (thiazides)	Increase	May increase insulin resistance and/or decrease insulin secretion, K^+ change may be in part responsible
Glucocorticoids	Increase	Impairs insulin action
Fluoroquinolones	Increase/decrease	Unclear, potential drug interaction with sulfonylureas or change in insulin secretion
Nicotinic acid	Increase	Impairs insulin action, increases insulin resistance
Oral contraceptives	Increase	Unclear
Pentamidine	Decrease, and then increase	Toxic to β cells; initial release of stored insulin, and then depletion
Phenytoin	Increase	Decreases insulin secretion
Protease inhibitors (PI)	Increase	Worsen insulin resistance/decrease first-phase insulin release or increase lipotoxicity. Dependent on PI
β-Blockers	May increase	Decreases insulin secretion
Ranolazine	Decrease	Improves oxidative glucose disposal
Salicylates	Decrease	Inhibition of IκB kinase-β (IKK-β) (only high doses, e.g., 4–6 g/day)
Sympathomimetics	Slight increase	Increased glycogenolysis and gluconeogenesis

[a]This list is not inclusive of all medications reported to cause glucose changes.

required for those patients with significant insulin resistance. Dosages vary widely depending on underlying insulin resistance and concomitant oral insulin sensitizer use. Strategies on how to initiate and monitor insulin therapy will be described later in Therapeutics below.

U-500 regular insulin is reserved for use in patients with extreme insulin resistance and most often is given two or three times a day. Caution must be used, however, in order to avoid errors in prescribing and dispensing U-500. In the inpatient setting, the prescription of U-500 is often written in volume (mL) and administered using a tuberculin syringe. In an individual prescribed 50 units three times a day before meals, this prescription would be written as follows: "U-500 regular insulin, inject 50 units (0.1 mL) subcutaneously three times daily before meals." In outpatients, however, it is often easier for patients to use U-100 insulin syringes. One unit of U-500 insulin drawn up using the markings of a U-100 equals 5 units of insulin. The same prescription as described above would be written as follows: "U-500 regular insulin: inject 50 units (10 units as measured by the unit markings of a U-100 syringe) subcutaneously three times daily before meals."

Storage It is recommended that unopened injectable insulin be refrigerated (2°C to 8°C [36°F to 46°F]) prior to use. The manufacturer's expiration date printed on the insulin is used for unopened, refrigerated insulin. Once the insulin is in use, the manufacturer-recommended expiration dates will vary based on the insulin and delivery device. Table 57-8 outlines manufacturer-recommended expiration dates for room temperature (15°C to 30°C [59°F to 86°F]) insulin. For financial reasons, patients may attempt to use insulin preparations longer than their expiration dates, but careful attention must be paid to monitoring for glycemic control deterioration and signs of insulin decay (clumping, precipitates, discoloration, etc.) if this is attempted.

Glucagon-Like Peptide-1 Agonists

Exenatide

Pharmacology Exendin 4 is a 39–amino acid peptide isolated from the saliva of the Gila monster (*Heloderma suspectum*) and shares 53% amino acid sequence with human GLP-1. Exenatide is the synthetic version of naturally occurring exendin 4. Exenatide (Byetta, Bydureon) has been shown to bind to GLP-1 receptors in many parts of the body including the brain and pancreas but is more resistant to DPP-4 degradation than endogenous GLP-1. Exenatide and GLP-1 have common glucoregulatory actions. The GLP-1 receptor activity of exenatide is pharmacologic, however, and is approximately three to four times more than the normal peak physiologic GLP-1 activity. Exenatide enhances insulin secretion in a glucose-dependent manner, suppressing inappropriately high postprandial glucagon secretion resulting in decreased hepatic glucose production. It increases satiety, slows gastric emptying, and promotes weight loss.

Pharmacokinetics There are two formulations of exenatide: exenatide injected twice daily (Byetta) and extended-release exenatide injected once weekly (Bydureon).

The concentration of twice-daily exenatide is detectable in plasma within 10 to 15 minutes after subcutaneous injection, and the drug has a t_{max} of ~2 hours and a plasma half life of ~3.3 to 4 hours. Plasma concentrations increase in a dose-dependent manner and concentrations are detectable for up to 10 hours postinjection, although pharmacodynamically, effects last for approximately 6 hours.

Extended-release once-weekly exenatide has a prolonged duration of action due to the exenatide being contained in a suspension of microspheres and gradually released over time. Following a single dose, exenatide is released from the microspheres over approximately 10 weeks. After initiation of once-weekly injections of 2 mg exenatide suspension, there is a gradual increase in plasma exenatide concentration over 6 to 7 weeks, after which steady state is achieved.

Bioavailability of exenatide after injection in the abdomen, upper arm, or the thigh is similar. Elimination of exenatide is primarily by glomerular filtration with subsequent proteolytic degradation. When exenatide is administered to subjects with worsening degrees of renal insufficiency, there is a progressive prolongation of the half-life, and in dialysis patients, plasma clearance of exenatide is markedly reduced. The incidence of GI side effects appears to be increased in individuals with impaired renal function, possibly due to higher plasma levels; thus, caution is advised.

No significant differences in exenatide pharmacokinetics have been observed with obesity, race, gender, or advancing age.

Efficacy The average HbA_{1c} reduction is approximately 0.9% (0.009; 10 mmol/mol Hb) with twice-daily exenatide, similar to oral agents, but HbA_{1c} lowering is dependent on baseline values.

Some patients will have greater or lesser reduction in HbA_{1c}. Similar HbA_{1c} reduction is seen in patients on oral agents. Once-weekly extended-release exenatide resulted in significantly greater changes from baseline compared with twice-daily exenatide in HbA_{1c} (−1.6% vs. −0.9% [−0.016 vs. −0.009; −18 mmol/mol Hb vs. −10 mmol/mol Hb) and FPG (−35 mg/dL vs. −12 mg/dL [−1.9 mmol/L vs. −0.7 mmol/L]).[32]

Exenatide significantly decreases postprandial glucose excursions, but has only a modest effect on FPG values. If a patient has significant elevations in FPG levels, these should be corrected with other agents and then exenatide added later. It is recommended to lower the sulfonylurea dose only if GLP-1 agonists are started with near-normal glucose levels. Sulfonylureas release insulin in a non–glucose-dependent fashion and can cause hypoglycemia.

Exenatide may aid some patients' efforts to lose weight. The average weight loss in controlled trials of twice-daily exenatide was 1 to 2 kg over 30 weeks, without dietary advice being given to the patients. Long-term, open-label follow-up on 10 mcg twice a day shows continued and sustained weight loss for at least 3 years. Approximately 84% of patients on exenatide lost some weight. Exenatide, through decreasing appetite and slowing gastric emptying, may reduce the number of calories a patient eats at a meal. If a patient does not decrease calorie intake, no weight loss is likely to occur, as exenatide does not increase caloric expenditure.

Microvascular Complications Exenatide reduces the HbA_{1c} level, which has been shown to be related to the risk of microvascular complications.

Macrovascular Complications No randomized clinical trials have examined the effect of exenatide on long-term cardiovascular outcomes. However, improvements in several cardiovascular risk factors have been reported. In an open-label study of exenatide 10 mcg twice a day, triglycerides (−37 ± 10 mg/dL [−0.42 ± 0.11 mmol/L]) decreased, and HDL cholesterol (+4.5 ± 0.4 mg/dL [0.12 ± 0.01 mmol/L]) increased. Once-weekly extended-release exenatide resulted in greater reduction in total cholesterol and LDL cholesterol compared with twice-daily exenatide.[33] Nonsignificant reductions in systolic and diastolic blood pressure have been observed; a significant reduction was seen in subjects with above-normal systolic blood pressure. The greatest improvement in cardiovascular risk factors was, in general, seen in subjects who had the greatest weight loss.

Adverse Effects The most common adverse effects associated with exenatide are GI. Nausea is more likely with twice-daily exenatide (>35%) compared with once-weekly extended-release exenatide (~14%). Vomiting or diarrhea occurs in approximately 10% of patients on twice-daily exenatide. As these adverse effects appear to be dose related, the patient on twice-a-day exenatide should be started on 5 mcg twice a day and titrated to 10 mcg twice a day only if the adverse effects have resolved. When the patient is increased to the 10 mcg twice a day dose, these adverse effects may recur for a short period of time. GI adverse effects appear to decrease over time. However, approximately 1 in 20 patients on twice-daily exenatide have prolonged problems with side effects, possibly requiring discontinuation or transition to once-weekly extended-release exenatide.

Many episodes of nausea are better characterized as stomach fullness. Patients should be instructed to eat slowly and stop eating when full, or risk nausea/vomiting. Weight loss does not appear to be related to adverse effects, but rather to a reduction in calories consumed. Exenatide provides glucose-dependent insulin secretion; thus, hypoglycemic rates when combined with metformin or a TZD are not substantially increased. However, when combined with a sulfonylurea or insulin, hypoglycemia may occur. Although exenatide reduces glucagon when the glucose is high, there is no suppression of counterregulatory hormones during hypoglycemia. Exenatide antibodies can occur, but generally decrease over time and usually do not affect glycemic control. In approximately 5% of patients, titers may increase over time, potentially resulting in a deterioration of glycemic control.

Exenatide has been associated with cases of acute pancreatitis, but this has not been shown to be causal. Further study is needed, however, and several important points should be noted: (a) patients with type 2 DM often have risk factors for pancreatitis such as gallstones, hypertriglyceridemia, obesity, and concomitant medication use; (b) GLP-1 agonists could mask initial signs of pancreatitis, including nausea, vomiting, and abdominal pain; and (c) large database studies have not linked exenatide to a higher rate of acute pancreatitis. In a patient with a history of pancreatitis, the benefits of using exenatide must be weighed against potential risks. If a patient with abdominal pain, nausea, and/or vomiting presents, it is best to discontinue exenatide temporarily and confirm that the symptoms are not a sign of a more serious underlying problem. Exenatide given twice daily does not change the risk of thyroid C-cell tumors in rats and does not have a black box warning; no increased risk of C-cell tumors has been reported in humans. Extended-release exenatide has a black box warning in regards to thyroid C-cell tumors due to rat data. The difference appears to be that the extended release continually stimulates the GLP-1 receptor on the thyroid of rodents, increasing the risk of thyroid C-cell tumors. No tumors have been reported in humans.

There have been reports of injection site reactions with extended-release once-weekly exenatide. Nodule injection site reactions are not painful and are often not visible, but can be felt at the injection site, which may have been injected 2 to 4 weeks prior. These nodules are an aggregation of the microspheres subcutaneously, not an immune reaction, and they may last 6 to 8 weeks. Injection site erythema, which can be severe in some cases, is related to exenatide antibody status (potentially worse if very high titers) or may be due to the platform, as this reaction is well described with the poly(D,L-lactide-*co*-glycolide) microsphere material.

Drug Interactions Exenatide delays gastric emptying; if the patient has gastroparesis, exenatide is not recommended. Exenatide can also delay the absorption of other medications. Examples of medications that may be effected include oral pain medications and antibiotics dependent on concentration-dependent efficacy. If rapid absorption of the medication is necessary, it is best to take the mediation 1 hour before, or at least 3 hours after, the injections of twice-daily exenatide. There have been postmarketing reports of increased INR in patients on warfarin on exenatide, sometimes associated with bleeding. It is advised that INR be monitored frequently until stable on initiation of exenatide.

Dosing and Administration Dosing of twice-daily exenatide (Byetta) should begin with 5 mcg twice a day, and titrated to 10 mcg twice a day in 1 month or when tolerability allows and if warranted for glycemic control. Twice-daily exenatide should be injected subcutaneously 0 to 60 minutes before the morning and evening meals. If the patient does not eat breakfast, he or she may take the first injection of the day at lunch. The peak effect of twice-daily exenatide is at approximately 2 hours, so anecdotally the patient may get better appetite suppression if injected an hour prior to the meal.

The dosing of extended-release exenatide (Bydureon) is 2 mg suspension injected subcutaneously every 7 days, at any time of day, with or without meals. Extended-release exenatide is injected immediately after the powder is suspended in the diluent. The process of extended-release once-weekly exenatide injections is more complex than using the twice-daily exenatide pen. Patients must be instructed on self-administration.

Exenatide may be injected in abdomen, thigh, or upper arm region, but patients are advised to use a different injection site when injecting into the same region.

Storage and dosage availability information can be found in Table 57-8.

Liraglutide

Pharmacology Liraglutide (Victoza) is a GLP-1 receptor agonist that has 97% amino acid sequence homology to endogenous GLP-1. The only alteration is an arginine substituted for lysine at position 34. A C-16 fatty acid (palmitic acid) is attached at position 26 (with a glutamic amino acid spacer to optimize GLP-1 receptor interaction) so that liraglutide can bind noncovalently to albumin, prolonging the half-life.

Liraglutide enhances glucose-dependent insulin secretion while suppressing inappropriately high glucagon secretion in the presence of elevated glucose concentrations, resulting in a reduction in hepatic glucose production. Liraglutide reduces food intake, which may result in weight loss, and slows gastric emptying so that the rate of glucose appearance into the plasma better matches the glucose disposition. During hypoglycemia, liraglutide does not stimulate insulin secretion and does not inhibit the release of the counterregulatory hormone glucagon.

Pharmacokinetics After injection of liraglutide, there is self-association into a heptameric structure, binding to albumin first in the interstitial space, then in the blood, and then in the interstitial space around the GLP-1 receptor that prolongs the half-life. In healthy individuals, the half-life is 13 hours, making it suitable for daily administration. Injection into the abdomen, upper arm, and thigh gives clinically similar pharmacokinetics. Maximum concentrations are reached approximately 8 to 12 hours after injection, with steady state reached after approximately 3 days. Liraglutide is extensively plasma protein bound (mostly to albumin as previously stated) with an elimination half-life of 10 to 18 hours. The absolute bioavailability is approximately 50%.

The metabolism of liraglutide appears to be by degradation, similar to other large proteins, and several small minor metabolites (total of 3% to 5% of the dose) may be found. The DPP-4 enzyme in vitro has been shown to slowly metabolize liraglutide, and this may be the case in vivo as well.

The pharmacokinetics of liraglutide does not appear to be affected by age, race, and gender. Severe renal or mild to severe hepatic impairment may actually lower the AUC by approximately 25%, although the clinical significance of this is not known.

Efficacy The average HbA_{1c} reduction is approximately 1.1% (0.0011; 12 mmol/mol Hb) with liraglutide. Similar to other agents, the reduction in HbA_{1c} is dependent on the baseline values. Liraglutide lowers FPG level by approximately 25 to 40 mg/dL (1.4 to 2.2 mmol/L), and postprandial plasma glucose levels are reduced similarly. Due to the longer half-life, liraglutide can suppress glucagon overnight, which improves the FPG. Similar to exenatide, liraglutide-treated patients may lose weight. The average weight loss in controlled trials was 1 to 3 kg over 26 weeks, and weight loss achieved appeared to be sustained through 2 years. Liraglutide, through decreasing appetite and slowing gastric emptying, may reduce the number of calories a patient eats at a meal.

Microvascular Complications Liraglutide reduces the HbA_{1c} level, which has been shown to be related to the risk of microvascular complications.

Macrovascular Complications There are no published clinical trials examining the effect of liraglutide on long-term cardiovascular outcomes; however, no signal of cardiovascular harm was noted on FDA approval.

Adverse Effects The most common adverse effects associated with liraglutide are GI. Nausea occurs in ~11% to 29% of subjects on 1.2 mg, and 14% to 40% of subjects on 1.8 mg daily. Vomiting occurs in approximately 5% of subjects, and diarrhea occurs in approximately 8% to 15% of patients placed on liraglutide. GI adverse effects appear to decrease over time, but approximately 5% to 10% of subjects withdrew due to GI side effects. As these adverse effects appear to be dose related, the patient should be titrated from 0.6 to 1.2 mg, and to 1.8 mg as tolerated. Randomized trials did not allow for individualized titration, and likely had worse tolerability that can be obtained clinically by individualization of titration.

Many episodes of nausea would be better characterized as stomach fullness. To minimize GI side effects, patients should be instructed to eat slowly and stop eating when full, or risk nausea/vomiting. Liraglutide provides glucose-dependent insulin secretion, and hypoglycemic rates when combined with metformin ± a TZD are not substantially increased, but when combined with a sulfonylurea or insulin, significant hypoglycemia may occur. When combined with a sulfonylurea, the rates of hypoglycemia were similar between addition of liraglutide and that of glargine insulin. Liraglutide antibodies can occur (4% to 13%), but the rates are generally low and do not affect glycemic control or risk of side effects.

Liraglutide has been associated with the serious adverse event of acute pancreatitis, but causality has not been proven. Further study is needed, but type 2 DM patients have many risk factors for pancreatitis and the common GI side effects of GLP-1 agonists could mask initial signs of pancreatitis. If a patient with abdominal pain, nausea, and/or vomiting presents, it is best to discontinue liraglutide temporarily and if symptoms persist, evaluate for other potential causes, including pancreatitis. Clinicians must weigh the benefits of liraglutide against the potential risks in a patient with a history of pancreatitis.

A boxed warning about thyroid C-cell tumors (as with extended-release exenatide) is listed in the package insert of liraglutide. Rodent models reported a higher risk of C-cell tumors of the thyroid, including medullary thyroid carcinoma. Rodents may not be the ideal model to study this effect as they express a high number of GLP-1 receptors on thyroid C-cells, whereas in humans the expression of GLP-1 receptors in the thyroid is minimal. Rodents also have a higher baseline prevalence of C-cell tumors compared with humans. In addition, calcitonin, a marker used to screen for C-cell tumors, may increase by a non–clinically significant amount in select patients. No signal for C-cell tumors in humans or nonhuman primates has been noted thus far. As clinical use increases, however, this will continue to be examined. Currently no specific additional monitoring of patients is recommended. Nonetheless, liraglutide is contraindicated in patients with a personal or family history of medullary thyroid cancer, and in those with multiple endocrine neoplasia syndromes.

Drug Interactions Liraglutide delays gastric emptying; thus, it can delay the absorption of other medications. Examples of medications that may be effected include oral pain medications and antibiotics dependent on threshold levels for efficacy. If rapid absorption of the medication is necessary, it is best to take the mediation 1 hour before, or at least 3 hours after, the injection. Liraglutide may worsen gastroparesis and clinically it may not be prudent to use in this patient population.

Dosing and Administration The dosing of liraglutide should begin with 0.6 mg daily for ≥1 week, and then increased to 1.2 mg daily for ≥1 week. Patients may be maintained on the 1.2-mg dose, or increased to the maximum dose of 1.8 mg daily after ≥1 week. The 0.6-mg dose is considered a titration dose, and does not reduce the HbA_{1c} substantially in the majority of patients. This titration is recommended to improve GI tolerability. Titration should be individualized based on side effects and clinical response. Liraglutide is dosed once daily, and may be given independent of meals. As with exenatide, a reduction in insulin secretagogues and insulin may be necessary if the patient is near glycemic goal or hypoglycemia occurs.

Storage and dosage availability information can be found in Table 57-8.

Amylinomimetic

Pramlintide

Pharmacology Pramlintide (Symlin) is an antihyperglycemic agent used in patients currently treated with insulin. Pramlintide is a synthetic analog of amylin (amylinomimetic), a neurohormone cosecreted from the β cells with insulin. Amylin is very low or absent in type 1 DM, and lower than normal in type 2 DM patients requiring insulin therapy. Pramlintide is provided as a 37–amino acid polypeptide, which differs in amino acid sequence from human amylin by replacement positions 25 (alanine), 28 (serine), and 29 (serine) with proline. Pramlintide suppresses inappropriately high postprandial glucagon secretion, increases satiety, which may result in weight loss, and slows gastric emptying so that the rate of glucose appearance into the plasma better matches the glucose disposition.

Pharmacokinetics The absolute bioavailability of pramlintide after subcutaneous injection is 30% to 40%. The t_{max} is approximately 20 minutes, but the C_{max} is dose dependent. The $t_{1/2}$ is approximately 45 minutes; thus, the pharmacodynamic duration of action is about 3 to 4 hours. Pramlintide does not extensively bind to albumin, and should not have significant binding interactions. Metabolism is primarily by the kidneys, and one active metabolite (2-37 pramlintide) has a similar half-life as the parent compound. No accumulation has been seen in renal insufficiency, but caution is advised. Injection into the arm may increase exposure and variability of absorption, so injection into the abdomen or thigh is recommended. Moderate to severe renal insufficiency does not affect exposure.

Efficacy The average HbA_{1c} reduction is approximately 0.6% (0.006; 7 mmol/mol Hb) with pramlintide, although optimization of the insulin and pramlintide doses may result in further drops in HbA_{1c}. If the 120-mcg dose is used in type 2 DM patients on insulin, it may also result in 1.5-kg weight loss. In type 1 DM patients, the average reduction in HbA_{1c} was 0.4% to 0.5% (0.004 to 0.005; 5 to 6 mmol/mol Hb). Prandial pramlintide added versus rapid-acting insulin in type 2 DM subjects uncontrolled on basal insulin reported similar efficacy, but with no weight gain, compared with ~5-kg weight gain with rapid-acting insulin. Pramlintide decreases prandial glucose excursions, but has little effect on the FPG concentration. When pramlintide is injected before the meal, gastric emptying may delay absorption of mealtime nutrients, necessitating delay of rapid-acting insulin. This may be overcome by injecting the mealtime insulin at the conclusion of the meal, or whenever the BG starts to rise. The average weight loss in controlled trials was 1 to 2 kg, without dietary advice being given to the patients. Pramlintide, through decreasing appetite, may reduce the number of calories a patient eats at a meal.

Microvascular Complications Pramlintide reduces the HbA_{1c} level, which has been shown to be related to the risk of microvascular complications.

Macrovascular Complications No published clinical trials have examined the effect of pramlintide on cardiovascular outcomes.

Adverse Effects The most common adverse effects associated with pramlintide are GI in nature. Nausea occurs in ~20% of type 2 DM patients, and vomiting or anorexia occurs in approximately 10% of type 1 or type 2 DM patients. Nausea is more common in type 1 DM, occurring in ~40% to 50% of patients. The higher rates in type 1 DM related to GI adverse effects appear to decrease over time and are dose related; thus, starting at a low dose and slowly titrating as tolerated is recommended. Pramlintide alone does not cause hypoglycemia, but it is indicated for use in patients on insulin; thus, hypoglycemia can occur. The risk of severe hypoglycemia early in therapy is higher in type 1 DM than in type 2 DM patients. A twofold increase in severe hypoglycemic reactions in type 1 DM patients has been reported.

Drug Interactions Pramlintide delays gastric emptying; thus, it can delay the absorption of other medications. Examples of medications that may be effected include oral pain medications and antibiotics dependent on threshold levels for efficacy. If rapid absorption of the medication is necessary, it is best to take the mediation 1 hour before, or at least 3 hours after, the injection of pramlintide.

Dosing and Administration Pramlintide dosing varies in type 1 and type 2 DM. It is imperative that the prandial insulin dose, if used, be reduced 30% to 50% when pramlintide is started to minimize severe hypoglycemic reactions or delayed until postprandial glucose levels rise. Basal insulin may need to be adjusted only if the FPG is close to normal. In type 2 DM, the starting dose is 60 mcg prior to meals, and may be titrated to the maximally recommended 120-mcg dose as tolerated and warranted based on postprandial plasma glucose concentrations. At least one clinical trial started at the 120-mcg dose without significantly more intolerability. In type 1 DM, dosing starts at 15 mcg prior to meals, and can be titrated up in 15-mcg increments to a maximum of 60 mcg prior to each meal if tolerated and warranted. Snacks may or may not need to be covered with pramlintide (recommended if ≥250 kcal [≥1,046 kJ] or ≥30 g of carbohydrate is eaten). Storage information can be found in Table 57-8.

Sulfonylureas

Pharmacology The primary mechanism of action of sulfonylureas is enhancement of insulin secretion. Sulfonylureas bind to a specific sulfonylurea receptor (SUR) on pancreatic β cells. Binding closes an adenosine triphosphate–dependent K^+ channel, leading to decreased potassium efflux and subsequent depolarization of the membrane. Voltage-dependent Ca^{2+} channels open and allow an inward flux of Ca^{2+}. Increases in intracellular Ca^{2+} bind to calmodulin on insulin secretory granules, causing translocation of secretory granules of insulin to the cell surface and resultant exocytosis of the granule of insulin. Elevated secretion of insulin from the pancreas travels via the portal vein and subsequently suppresses hepatic glucose production.

Classification Sulfonylureas are classified as first-generation and second-generation agents. The classification scheme is largely derived from differences in relative potency, potential for selective side effects, and differences in binding to serum proteins (i.e., risk for protein-binding displacement drug interactions). First-generation agents consist of acetohexamide, chlorpropamide, tolazamide, and tolbutamide. Each of these agents is lower in potency relative to the second-generation drugs: glimepiride, glipizide, and glyburide (Table 57-11). It is important to recognize that all sulfonylureas are equally effective at lowering BG when administered in equipotent doses.

Pharmacokinetics All sulfonylureas are metabolized in the liver, some to active and others to inactive metabolites. Glyburide metabolites are active, whereas glipizide and glimepiride do not

TABLE 57-11 Oral Agents for the Treatment of Type 2 Diabetes Mellitus

Drug Name[a]	Brand Name	Dose	Recommended Starting Dosage: Nonelderly	Recommended Starting Dosage: Elderly	Usual/Maximal Dose	Other
Sulfonylureas						
Acetohexamide (Y)	Dymelor	250, 500 mg	250 mg/day	125–250 mg/day	1,500 mg/day	Metabolized in liver; metabolite potency equal to parent compound; renally eliminated
Chlorpropamide (Y)	Diabinese	100, 250 mg	250 mg/day	100 mg/day	500 mg/day	Metabolized in liver; also excreted unchanged renally
Tolazamide (Y)	Tolinase	100, 250, 500 mg	100–250 mg/day	100 mg/day	1,000 mg/day	Metabolized in liver; metabolite less active than parent compound; renally eliminated
Tolbutamide (Y)	Orinase	250, 500 mg	1,000–2,000 mg/day	500–1,000 mg/day	3,000 mg/day	Metabolized in liver to inactive metabolites that are renally excreted
Glipizide (Y)	Glucotrol	5, 10 mg	5 mg/day	2.5–5 mg/day	40 mg/day	Metabolized in liver to inactive metabolites
Glipizide (Y)	Glucotrol XL	2.5, 5, 10, 20 mg	5 mg/day	2.5–5 mg/day	20 mg/day	Slow-release form; do not cut tablet
Glyburide (Y)	DiaBeta, Micronase	1.25, 2.5, 5 mg	5 mg/day	1.25–2.5 mg/day	20 mg/day	Metabolized in liver; elimination one half renal, one half feces. two active metabolites
Glyburide, micronized (Y)	Glynase	1.5, 3, 6 mg	3 mg/day	1.5–3 mg/day	12 mg/day	Better absorption from micronized preparation
Glimepiride (Y)	Amaryl	1, 2, 4 mg	1–2 mg/day	0.5–1 mg/day	8 mg/day	Metabolized in liver to inactive metabolites
Short-acting insulin secretagogues						
Nateglinide (Y)	Starlix	60, 120 mg	120 mg/day with meals	120 mg/day with meals	120 mg three times a day	Metabolized by cytochrome P450 (CYP450) 2C9 and 3A4 to weakly active metabolites; renally eliminated
Repaglinide (N)	Prandin	0.05, 1, 2 mg	0.5–1 mg/day with meals	0.5–1 mg/day with meals	16 mg/day	Caution with gemfibrozil or trimethoprim—potential hypoglycemia
Biguanides						
Metformin (Y)	Glucophage	500, 850, 1,000 mg	500 mg twice a day	Assess renal function	2,550 mg/day	No metabolism; renally secreted and excreted
Metformin ER (Y)	Glucophage XR	500, 750, 1,000 mg	500–1,000 mg with evening meal	Assess renal function	2,550 mg/day	Take full dose with evening meal or may split dose; may consider trial if intolerant to immediate release
Metformin solution	Riomet	500 mg/5 mL	500 mg daily	Assess renal function	2,000 mg/day	Metformin is indicated in children ≥10 years old
Thiazolidinediones						
Pioglitazone (Y)	Actos	15, 30, 45 mg	15 mg/day	15 mg/day	45 mg/day	Metabolized by CYP2C8 and 3A4; two active metabolites have longer half-lives than parent compound
Rosiglitazone (N)	Avandia	2, 4, 8 mg	2–4 mg/day	2 mg/day	8 mg/day or 4 mg twice a day	Limited availability. Continuation of therapy or unable to take pioglitazone. Clinician/patient sign that known risk of MI
α-Glucosidase inhibitors						
Acarbose (Y)	Precose	25, 50, 100 mg	25 mg one to three times a day	25 mg one to three times a day	25–100 mg three times a day	Eliminated in bile. Slow titration key for tolerability. With meals
Miglitol (N)	Glyset	25, 50, 100 mg	25 mg one to three times a day	25 mg one to three times a day	25–100 mg three times a day	Eliminated renally
Dipeptidyl peptidase-4 inhibitors (DPP-4 inhibitors)						
Sitagliptin (N)	Januvia	100, 50, 25 mg	100 mg daily	25–100 mg daily based on renal function	100 mg daily	50 mg daily if estimated creatinine clearance >30 to <50 mL/min (>0.50 to <0.83 mL/s); 25 mg if creatinine clearance <30 mL/min (<0.50 mL/s)

(continued)

TABLE 57-11 Oral Agents for the Treatment of Type 2 Diabetes Mellitus (*Continued*)

			Recommended Starting Dosage			
Drug Name[a]	Brand Name	Dose	Nonelderly	Elderly	Usual/Maximal Dose	Other
Saxagliptin (N)	Onglyza	2.5, 5 mg	5 mg daily	2.5–5 mg daily based on renal function	5 mg daily	2.5 mg daily if creatinine clearance <50 mL/min (<0.83 mL/s) or if on strong inhibitors of CYP3A4/5
Linagliptin (N)	Tradjenta	5 mg	5 mg daily	5 mg daily	5 mg daily	Not substantially eliminated by renal, found in feces. Do not use with strong inducer of CYP3A4/p-glycoprotein
Alogliptin (N)	Nesina	25, 12.5, 6.25 mg	25 mg daily	25 mg	25 mg	~75% eliminated unchanged in urine. 12.5 mg CrCl <60 mL/min (<1 mL/s), 6.25 mg <30–15 mL/min (<0.50–0.25 mL/s)
Bile acid sequestrants						
Colesevelam (N)	Welchol	625-mg tablet 1.875- and 3.75-g oral suspension	6 tablets daily or three tablets twice a day 1.875 g twice a day or 3.75 g daily	6 tablets daily or three tablets twice a day 1.875 g twice a day or 3.75 g daily	3.75 g/day	Constipation may occur. Take with meal. Drug–drug absorption interactions present, may increase triglycerides; contraindicated if TG >500 mg/dL (>5.65 mmol/L)
Dopamine agonist						
Bromocriptine mesylate (N)	Cycloset	0.8-mg tablets	1.6–4.8 mg daily	1.6–4.8 mg daily	4.8 mg daily	Take within 2 hours of rising with food. Significant nausea, other side effects, and drug–drug, drug–disease interactions may occur

[a]Generic version available? Y, yes; N, no.

have active metabolites. Cytochrome P450 (CYP450) 2C9 is involved with the hepatic metabolism of the majority of sulfonylureas. Agents with active metabolites or parent drug that are renally excreted require dosage adjustment or use with caution in patients with compromised renal function. The half-life of the sulfonylurea also relates directly to the risk for hypoglycemia. The hypoglycemic potential is therefore higher with chlorpropamide and glyburide. The long duration of effect of chlorpropamide may be particularly problematic in elderly individuals, whose renal function declines with age, and therefore it has great potential for accumulation, resulting in severe and protracted hypoglycemia. Individuals at high risk for hypoglycemia (e.g., elderly individuals and those with renal insufficiency or advanced liver disease) should be started at a very low dose of a sulfonylurea with a short half-life. Hypoglycemia on low-dose sulfonylureas may dictate a therapy without the risk of hypoglycemia.

Efficacy As mentioned earlier, when given in equipotent doses, all sulfonylureas are equally effective at lowering BG. On average, HbA_{1c} will fall 1.5% to 2% (0.015 to 0.020; 17 to 22 mmol/mol Hb) in drug-naïve patients, with FPG reductions of 60 to 70 mg/dL (3.3 to 3.9 mmol/L), but is dependent on baseline values and duration of diabetes. A majority of patients will not reach glycemic goals with sulfonylurea monotherapy. Patients with inadequate control on a sulfonylurea usually fall into two groups: those with low C-peptide levels and high (>250 mg/dL [>13.9 mmol/L]) FPG levels. These patients are often primary failures on sulfonylureas (<30 mg/dL [<1.7 mmol/L] drop of FPG) and have significant glucose toxicity or LADA. The other group is those with a good initial response (>30 mg/dL [>1.7 mmol/L] drop of FPG), but which is insufficient to reach their glycemic goals. Over 75% of patients fall into the second group. Factors that portend a positive response include newly diagnosed patients with no indicators of type 1 DM, high fasting C-peptide levels, and moderate fasting hyperglycemia (<250 mg/dL [<13.9 mmol/L]).

Microvascular Complications Sulfonylureas showed a reduction of microvascular complications in type 2 DM patients in the UKPDS.[24] A more in-depth discussion follows later in the chapter.

Macrovascular Complications The UKPDS reported no significant benefit or harm in newly diagnosed type 2 DM patients given sulfonylureas over 10 years. The University Group Diabetes Program study documented higher rates of coronary artery disease in type 2 patients given tolbutamide, when compared with patients given insulin or placebo, although this study has been widely criticized.[34] Some sulfonylureas bind to the SUR-2A receptor that is found in cardiac tissue. Binding to the SUR-2A receptor has been implicated in blocking ischemic preconditioning via K^+ channel closure in the heart. Ischemic preconditioning is the premise that prior ischemia in cardiac tissue can provide greater tolerance of subsequent ischemia. Thus, patients with heart disease potentially have one compensatory mechanism to protect the heart from ischemia blocked. Conclusions are controversial, but alternative treatments are available if questioned.

Adverse Effects The most common side effect of sulfonylureas is hypoglycemia. The pretreatment FPG is a strong predictor of hypoglycemic potential. The lower the FPG is on initiation, the higher the potential for hypoglycemia. Also, in addition to the high-risk individuals outlined in Pharmacokinetics below, those who skip meals, exercise vigorously, or lose substantial amounts of weight are also more likely to experience hypoglycemia.

Hyponatremia (serum sodium <129 mEq/L [129 mmol/L]) is reportedly associated with tolbutamide, but it is most common with chlorpropamide and occurs in as many as 5% of individuals treated. An increase in antidiuretic hormone secretion is the mechanism for hyponatremia. Risk factors include age >60 years, female gender, and concomitant use of thiazide diuretics.

Weight gain is common with sulfonylureas. In essence, patients who are no longer glycosuric and who do not reduce caloric intake with improvement of BG will store excess calories. Other notable, although much less common, adverse effects of sulfonylureas are skin rash, hemolytic anemia, GI upset, and cholestasis. Disulfiram-type reactions and flushing have been reported with tolbutamide and chlorpropamide when alcohol is consumed.

Drug Interactions Several drugs are thought to interact with sulfonylureas, most likely through the CYP450 system or altered renal excretion. Protein-binding changes should occur shortly after the interacting medication is given, as the concentration of free (thus active) sulfonylurea will acutely increase. First-generation sulfonylureas, which bind to proteins ionically, are more likely to cause drug–drug interactions than second-generation sulfonylureas, which bind nonionically. The clinical importance of protein-binding interactions has been questioned, as the majority of these drug interactions have been found to be truly due to hepatic metabolism. Drugs that are inducers or inhibitors of CYP450 2C9 should be monitored carefully when used with a sulfonylurea.[35] Additionally, other drugs known to alter BG should be considered (Table 57-10).

Dosing and Administration The usual starting dose and maximum dose of sulfonylureas are summarized in Table 57-11. Lower dosages are recommended for most agents in elderly patients and those with compromised renal or hepatic function. The dosage can be titrated as soon as every 2 weeks based on FPG values (use a longer interval with chlorpropamide) to achieve glycemic goals. This is possible due to the rapid increase of insulin secretion in response to the sulfonylurea. Of note, immediate-release glipizide's maximal dose is 40 mg/day, but its maximal effective dose is about 10 to 15 mg/day. The maximal effective dose of sulfonylureas tends to be about 60% to 75% of their stated maximum dose.

Short-Acting Insulin Secretagogues

Pharmacology Although the binding site is adjacent to the binding site of sulfonylureas, nateglinide and repaglinide stimulate insulin secretion from the β cells of the pancreas, similarly to sulfonylureas. Both repaglinide (a benzoic acid derivative) and nateglinide (a phenylalanine amino acid derivative) require the presence of glucose to stimulate insulin secretion. As glucose levels diminish to normal, stimulated insulin secretion diminishes.

Pharmacokinetics Both nateglinide and repaglinide are rapid-acting insulin secretagogues that are rapidly absorbed (~0.5 to 1 hour) and have a short half-life (1 to 1.5 hours). Nateglinide is highly protein bound, primarily to albumin, but also to α_1-acid glycoprotein. It is predominantly metabolized by CYP2C9 (70%) and CYP3A4 (30%) to less active metabolites. Glucuronide conjugation then allows rapid renal elimination. No dosage adjustment is needed in moderate to severe renal insufficiency. Repaglinide is highly protein bound, and is mainly metabolized by oxidative metabolism and glucuronidation. The CYP3A4 and 2C8 systems have been shown to be involved with metabolism. Approximately 90% of repaglinide is eliminated in the feces, with only 10% found in the urine. Moderate to severe renal insufficiency does not appear to affect repaglinide, but moderate to severe hepatic impairment may prolong exposure.

Efficacy In monotherapy, both significantly reduce postprandial glucose excursions and reduce HbA_{1c} levels. Repaglinide, dosed 4 mg three times a day, when compared with glyburide in diet-treated, drug-naïve patients reduced HbA_{1c} levels less (1% vs. 2.4% [0.01 vs. 0.024; 11 mmol/mol Hb vs. 26 mmol/mol Hb], from baseline, respectively). Nateglinide, dosed 120 mg three times a day, in a similar population reduced HbA_{1c} values by 0.8% (0.008; 9 mmol/mol Hb). The lower efficacy of these agents versus sulfonylureas should be considered when patients are >1% (>0.01; >11 mmol/mol Hb) above their HbA_{1c} goal. These agents can be used to provide increased insulin secretion during meals, when it is needed, in patients close to glycemic goals. Also, it should be noted that addition of either agent to a sulfonylurea will not result in any improvement in glycemic parameters.

Adverse Effects Hypoglycemia is the main side effect noted with both agents. Hypoglycemic risk appears to be less versus sulfonylureas. In part, this is due to the glucose-sensitive release of insulin. If the glucose concentration is normal, less glucose-stimulated release of insulin will occur. In two separate studies, nateglinide rates of hypoglycemia were 3% and repaglinide 15% versus glyburide and glipizide rates of 15% and 19%, respectively. Weight gain of 2 to 3 kg has been noted with repaglinide, whereas weight gain with nateglinide appears to be <1 kg.

Drug Interactions Glycemic control and hypoglycemia should be closely monitored when glucuronidation inhibitors are given with repaglinide. Gemfibrozil more than doubles the half-life of repaglinide and has resulted in prolonged hypoglycemic reactions. It is a potent glucuronidation inhibitor and CYP2C8 inhibitor. Trimethoprim, a CYP2C8 inhibitor, increased repaglinide levels by 60%. Nateglinide appears to be a weak inhibitor of CYP2C9 based on tolbutamide metabolism. Although no significant drug–drug interactions have been reported, caution should be used with strong CYP2C9 and CYP3A4 inhibitors.

Dosing and Administration Nateglinide and repaglinide should be dosed prior to each meal (up to 30 minutes prior). The recommended starting dose for repaglinide is 0.5 mg in subjects with HbA_{1c} <8% (<0.08; <64 mmol/mol Hb) or treatment-naïve patients, increased weekly to a total maximum daily dose of 16 mg (see Table 57-11). The maximal effective dose of repaglinide is likely 2 mg with each meal, as a dose of 1 mg prior to each meal provides approximately 90% of the maximal glucose-lowering effect. Nateglinide should be dosed at 120 mg prior to meals, and does not require titration. A 60-mg dose is available, but the HbA_{1c} decrement is small (0.3% to 0.5% [0.003 to 0.005; 3 to 6 mmol/mol Hb]). If a meal is skipped, the medication can be skipped, and meals extremely low in carbohydrate content may not need a dose. Both agents may be used in patients with renal insufficiency, and may fit into therapy in patients in need of an insulin secretagogue but having hypoglycemia to sulfonylureas, moderate to severe renal insufficiency, and well-controlled diabetes, but with erratic meal schedules.

Biguanides

Pharmacology Metformin is the only biguanide available in the United States. It has been used clinically for more than 50 years, and has been approved in the United States since 1995. Metformin enhances insulin sensitivity of mainly hepatic but also peripheral (muscle) tissues. This allows for an increased uptake of glucose into these insulin-sensitive tissues. All the mechanisms of how metformin accomplishes glucose reduction are still being investigated, although adenosine 5′-monophosphate–activated protein kinase activity, tyrosine kinase activity enhancement, increased adenosine 5′-monophosphate, and partial inhibition of the mitochondrial respiratory chain are involved. Metformin has no direct effect on the β cells, although insulin levels are reduced, reflecting increases in insulin sensitivity.

Pharmacokinetics Metformin has approximately 50% to 60% oral bioavailability, low lipid solubility, and a volume of distribution that approximates body water. It is not metabolized and does not bind to plasma proteins. Metformin is eliminated by renal tubular secretion and glomerular filtration. The average plasma half-life of metformin is 6 hours, although pharmacodynamically, metformin's antihyperglycemic effects last more than 24 hours. Red blood cells are a second compartment of distribution for metformin, delivering an effective half-life of 17 hours.

Efficacy Metformin consistently reduces HbA_{1c} levels by 1.5% to 2% (0.015 to 0.020; 17 to 22 mmol/mol Hb) and FPG levels by 60 to 80 mg/dL (3.3 to 4.4 mmol/L) in drug-naïve patients, and retains the ability to reduce FPG levels when they are extremely high (>300 mg/dL [>16.7 mmol/L]). The sulfonylureas' ability to stimulate insulin release from β cells at extremely high glucose levels is often impaired, a concept commonly referred to as *glucose toxicity*. Metformin also has positive effects on several components of the insulin resistance syndrome. It decreases plasma triglycerides and LDL-C by approximately 8% to 15%, in addition to increasing HDL-C very modestly (2%). Metformin reduces levels of PAI-1 and causes a modest reduction in weight (2 to 3 kg). In preliminary findings, metformin may also lower the risk of pancreatic, colon, and breast cancer in type 2 DM patients. Metformin, potentially through multiple mechanisms including adenosine 5′-monophosphate–activated protein kinase activity, may act as a growth inhibitor in some cancers and help to kill cancer "stem cells" which are resistant to chemotherapy, and liver kinase B1, which is an upstream kinase of adenosine 5′-monophosphate–activated protein kinase. More controlled studies are needed.

Microvascular Complications Metformin (n = 342) was compared with intensive glucose control with insulin or sulfonylureas in the UKPDS. No significant differences were seen between therapies with regard to reducing microvascular complications, but the power of the study is questionable.[36]

❻ ***Macrovascular Complications*** Metformin reduced macrovascular complications in obese subjects in the UKPDS.[36] It significantly reduced all-cause mortality and risk of stroke versus intensive treatment with sulfonylureas or insulin. Metformin also reduced diabetes-related death and MIs versus the conventional treatment arm of the UKPDS. It should be noted that the UKPDS had very few people on lipid-lowering therapy, antihypertensives, or aspirin. Metformin is logical in overweight/obese patients, if tolerated and not contraindicated, as it is the only oral antihyperglycemic medication potentially proven to reduce the risk of total mortality and is generic.

Adverse Effects Metformin causes GI side effects, including abdominal discomfort, stomach upset, and/or diarrhea, in approximately 30% of patients. Anorexia and stomach fullness is likely part of the reason loss of weight is noted with metformin. These side effects are usually mild and can be minimized by slow titration. GI side effects also tend to be transient, lessening in severity over several weeks. If encountered, make sure patients are taking metformin with or right after meals, and reduce the dose to a point at which no GI side effects are encountered. Increases in the dose may be tried again in several weeks. Anecdotally, extended-release metformin (Glucophage XR) may lessen some of the GI side effects. Metallic taste, interference with vitamin B_{12} absorption, and hypoglycemia during intense exercise have been documented, but are clinically uncommon.

Metformin therapy rarely (3 to 9 cases per 100,000 patient-years) causes lactic acidosis. Metformin partially blocks the mitochondrial respiratory chain. In addition, any disease state that may increase lactic acid production or decrease lactic acid removal may predispose to lactic acidosis. Tissue hypoperfusion, such as that due to congestive heart failure, severe lung disease, hypoxic states, shock, or septicemia, via increased production of lactic acid, and severe liver disease or alcohol, via reduced removal of lactic acid in the liver, all increase the risk of lactic acidosis. The clinical presentation of lactic acidosis is often nonspecific flu-like symptoms; thus, the diagnosis is usually made by laboratory confirmation of high lactic acid levels and acidosis. Metformin use in renal insufficiency, defined as a serum creatinine of 1.4 mg/dL (124 μmol/L) in women and 1.5 mg/dL (133 μmol/L) in men or greater, is contraindicated, as it is renally eliminated. Elderly patients, who often have reduced muscle mass, should have their glomerular filtration rate estimated by a 24-hour urine creatinine collection. If the estimated glomerular filtration rate is less than 60 mL/min (1 mL/s), metformin use should be carefully evaluated. Recent evidence has reported that metformin may be fairly safe in moderate renal insufficiency. Metformin use can be modified based on the estimated glomerular filtration rate, at <60, <45 to ≥30, and <30 mL/min/1.73 m^2 (<0.58, <0.43 to ≥0.29, and <0.29 mL/s/m^2); corresponding actions are to monitor renal function every 3 to 6 months, then limit dose to 50% of maximal dose, and then stop metformin, respectively. Due to the risk of acute renal failure during IV dye procedures, metformin therapy should be withheld starting the day of the procedure and resumed in 2 to 3 days, after normal renal function has been documented.

Drug Interactions Cimetidine competes for renal tubular secretion of metformin and concomitant administration leads to higher metformin serum concentrations. At least one case report of lactic acidosis with metformin therapy implicates cimetidine. Theoretically other cationic drugs may interact, but none have been reported to date.

Dosing and Administration Immediate-release metformin is usually dosed 500 mg twice a day with the largest meals to minimize GI side effects. Metformin may be increased by 500 mg as tolerated until glycemic goals or 2,500 mg/day is achieved (see Table 57-11). Metformin 850 mg may be dosed daily, and then increased every 1 to 2 weeks to the maximum dose of 850 mg three times a day (2,550 mg/day). Approximately 80% of the glycemic-lowering effect may be seen at 1,500 mg, and 2,000 mg/day is the maximal effective dose.

Extended-release metformin can be initiated at 500 mg a day with the evening meal and titrated by 500 mg as tolerated to a single evening dose of 2,000 mg/day. Extended-release metformin 750-mg tablets may be titrated as tolerated to the maximum dose of 2,250 mg/day, although, as stated above, 1,500 mg/day provides the majority of the glycemic-lowering effect. Twice-daily to three-times-a-day dosing of extended-release metformin may help to minimize GI side effects and improve glycemic control, but will not change the glycemic reduction.

Thiazolidinediones

Pharmacology TZDs are also referred to as glitazones. Pioglitazone (Actos) and rosiglitazone (Avandia) are the two currently approved TZDs for the treatment of type 2 DM (see Table 57-11). TZDs work by binding to the PPAR-γ, which are primarily located on fat cells and vascular cells. The concentration of these receptors in the muscle is very low, but improvement in mitochondrial function through changes in lipotoxicity, glucotoxicity, and possibly binding of proteins outside the mitochondrial membrane may occur. TZDs enhance insulin sensitivity at muscle, liver, and fat tissues indirectly. They cause preadipocytes to differentiate into mature fat cells in subcutaneous fat stores. Small fat cells are more sensitive to insulin and more able to store FFAs. The result is a flux of FFAs out of the plasma, visceral fat, and liver into subcutaneous fat, a less insulin-resistant storage tissue. Muscle intracellular fat products, which contribute to insulin resistance, also decline. TZDs also affect adipokines (e.g., angiotensinogen, tissue necrosis factor-α, interleukin 6, PAI-1), which can positively affect insulin sensitivity, endothelial function, and inflammation. Of particular note, adiponectin is reduced with obesity and/or diabetes, but is increased with TZD therapy, which improves endothelial function and insulin sensitivity, and has a potent antiinflammatory effect. Lastly, TZDs appear to improve mitochondrial function through a reduction in FFAs. Cyclin-dependent kinase 5 has also recently been purposed as an important activator of PPAR-γ.

Pharmacokinetics Pioglitazone and rosiglitazone are well absorbed with or without food. Both are highly (>99%) bound to albumin. Pioglitazone is primarily metabolized by CYP2C8, to a lesser extent by CYP3A4 (17%), and by hydroxylation/oxidation.

The majority of pioglitazone is eliminated in the feces with 15% to 30% appearing in urine as metabolites. Two active metabolites (M-III and M-IV) are present. Rosiglitazone is metabolized by CYP2C8, and to a lesser extent by CYP2C9, and also by *N*-demethylation and hydroxylation. Two thirds is found in urine and one third in feces. The half-lives of pioglitazone and rosiglitazone are 3 to 7 and 3 to 4 hours, respectively. The two active metabolites of pioglitazone, with longer half-lives, deliver the majority of activity at steady state. Pioglitazone requires no dosage adjustment in moderate to severe renal disease for pharmacokinetic reasons. Interestingly, with pioglitazone the AUC in women is 20% to 60% higher, which is not seen with rosiglitazone, but no dosage adjustment is recommended. Both medications have a duration of antihyperglycemic action of over 24 hours.

Efficacy Pioglitazone and rosiglitazone reduce HbA_{1c} values ~1% to 1.5% (~0.010 to 0.015; 11 to 17 mmol/mol Hb) and reduce FPG levels by ~60 to 70 mg/dL (~3.3 to 3.9 mmol/L) at maximal doses. Glycemic-lowering onset is slow, and maximal glycemic-lowering effects may not be seen until 3 to 4 months of therapy. It is important to inform patients of this fact and that they should not stop therapy even if minimal glucose lowering is initially encountered. The efficacy of both drugs is dependent on sufficient insulinemia. If there is insufficient endogenous insulin production (β-cell function) or exogenous insulin delivery via injections, neither will lower glucose concentrations efficiently. Interestingly, patients who are more obese or who gain weight on either medication tend to have a larger reduction in HbA_{1c} values. Pioglitazone consistently decreases plasma triglyceride levels by 10% to 20%, whereas rosiglitazone tends to have a neutral effect. LDL-C concentrations tend to increase with rosiglitazone 5% to 15%, but do not significantly increase with pioglitazone. Both appear to convert small, dense LDL particles, which have been shown to be highly atherogenic, to large, fluffy LDL particles that are less dense. Large, fluffy LDL particles may be less atherogenic, but any increase in LDL must be of concern. Both drugs increase HDL, although pioglitazone may raise it more than rosiglitazone. TZDs also affect several components of the insulin resistance syndrome. PAI-1 levels are decreased, and many other adipocytokines are affected, endothelial function improves, and blood pressure may decrease slightly.

Microvascular Complications TZDs reduce HbA_{1c} levels, which have been shown to be related to the risk of microvascular complications.

Macrovascular Complications Macrovascular complications with TZDs are controversial. In PROactive, the prospective pioglitazone clinical trial in macrovascular events, pioglitazone 45 mg was added to standard therapy in patients who had experienced a macrovascular event or had peripheral vascular disease.[37] The two groups were well matched at baseline and the reported average observation time period was about 3 years. The primary end point (reduction in death, MI, stroke, acute coronary syndrome, coronary revascularization, leg amputation, and leg revascularization) was reduced 10% ($P = 0.095$). The main secondary end point (all-cause mortality, nonfatal MI, or stroke) was reduced 16% ($P = 0.027$). The seemingly dichotomous results relate to the inclusion of leg revascularization as a primary end point, which were increased in the pioglitazone group. Reasons for the increase are speculative, but may relate to more testing/inspection due to peripheral edema. Also of note, the pioglitazone group had 209 nonadjudicated admissions for heart failure occur versus 153 in the placebo group ($P = 0.007$), although fatal heart failure was not increased. Several published meta-analyses of rosiglitazone reported higher MI rates with rosiglitazone, but none have reported a higher risk of mortality. A hazard ratio (HR) of 1.43 (95% confidence interval [CI], 1.03 to 1.98; $P = 0.03$) for the risk of an MI with rosiglitazone versus other oral agents was reported.[38]

A prospective, multicenter, open-label noninferiority trial in 4,447 patients of rosiglitazone added to background metformin or sulfonylurea versus the active comparator metformin + sulfonylurea was recently reported (Rosiglitazone Evaluated for Cardiovascular Outcomes in Oral Agent Combination Therapy for Type 2 Diabetes [RECORD]). Rosiglitazone was noninferior to the comparator for all CV outcomes except for heart failure. A nonsignificant increase in risk for MI (HR, 1.14; 95% CI, 0.80 to 1.63) as well as a nonsignificant reduction in stroke (HR, 0.72; 95% CI, 0.49 to 1.05) was reported. On subset analysis, previous ischemic heart disease trended toward a higher risk (HR, 1.26; CI, 0.95 to 1.68; $P = 0.055$).[39] Most studies with rosiglitazone trend toward, but do not reach, statistically significant increases in ischemic events. The FDA has placed rosiglitazone under a strict risk evaluation and mitigation program, limiting access to patients and prescribers who acknowledge and consent to knowing its macrovascular risks.

Adverse Effects Troglitazone, the first TZD approved, caused idiosyncratic hepatotoxicity and had deaths from liver failure, which prompted removal from the U.S. market. Newer TZDs do not have the same propensity, but have had postmarketing reports of liver injury. Patients with abnormal alanine aminotransferase (ALT) levels should be started with caution, and if the ALT is >3 times the upper limit of normal, especially if the total bilirubin is also >2 times the upper limit of normal, the medication should be discontinued. Pioglitazone has been shown in one well-designed trial to reduce hepatic steatosis, which may improve abnormal ALT levels in many patients with diabetes.

Retention of fluid leads to many different possible side effects with TZDs. The etiology of the fluid retention has not been fully elucidated, but appears to include peripheral vasodilation and/or improved insulin sensitization at the kidney with a resultant increase in renal sodium and water retention. A reduction in plasma hemoglobin (2% to 4%), attributed to a 10% increase in plasma volume, may result in a dilutional anemia that does not require treatment. Peripheral edema is also commonly (4% to 5% in monotherapy or combination therapy) reported. When a TZD is used in combination with insulin, the incidence of edema (~15%) is increased. TZDs are contraindicated in patients with New York Heart Association Class III and IV heart failure, and great caution should be exercised when given to patients with Class I and II heart failure or other underlying cardiac disease, as pulmonary edema and heart failure have been reported. Edema tends to be dose related and if not severe, a reduction in the dose as well as use of diuretics, anecdotally hydrochlorothiazide with triamterene, amiloride, or spironolactone instead of loop diuretics, will allow the continuation of therapy in the majority of patients. Rarely, TZDs have been reported to worsen macular edema of the eye.

Weight gain, which is also dose related, can be seen with both rosiglitazone and pioglitazone. Mechanistically, both fluid retention and fat accumulation play a part in explaining the weight gain. TZDs, besides stimulating fat cell differentiation, also reduce leptin levels, which stimulate appetite and food intake. Average weight gain varies, but a 1.5- to 4-kg weight gain is not uncommon. Rarely, a patient will gain large amounts of weight in a short period of time, and this may necessitate discontinuation of therapy. Weight gain positively predicts a larger HbA_{1c} reduction, but must be balanced with the well-documented effects of long-term weight gain.

TZDs have also been associated with an increased fracture rate in the upper and lower limbs in women and men, although women appear to have a higher risk. These fractures are not osteoporitic in the classic sense, and do not occur in common osteoporosis fracture sites such as spine or hip. Most occur in wrists, forearms, ankles, or feet. Versus comparative diabetes therapy, TZDs may increase the risk of a fracture by 25%. The underlying pathophysiology is speculative, but may relate to TZD effects on the pluripotent stem cell and shunting of new cells to fat instead of osteocytes as well as altering osteoblasts/osteoclasts. It would be prudent to consider a patient's risk factors for fractures if a TZD is being considered as antidiabetic therapy.

The risk of bladder cancer is slightly increased with pioglitazone, and likely rosiglitazone. Bladder tumors have been noted in rodent models using TZDs. An ongoing 10-year observational study reported an excess of 3 in 10,000 patient-years (from 7 to 10 in 10,000) risk of bladder cancer with pioglitazone at 5 years. Excess risk appears to be mostly in men and smokers, and is dose and duration associated. Mechanisms are speculative, but may involve microcrystals of the drug in the bladder that cause chronic irritation.

As a caution, premenopausal anovulatory patients may resume ovulation on TZDs. Adequate pregnancy and contraception precautions should be explained to all women capable of becoming pregnant, as both agents are pregnancy category C.

Drug Interactions Significant drug interactions that can cause clinical sequelae have not been noted with either medication. Neither pioglitazone nor rosiglitazone appears to be an inhibitor or inducer of CYP3A4/2C8 or CYP2C8/CYP2C9, respectively, although drugs that are strong inhibitors or inducers of these pathways (e.g., gemfibrozil or rifampin) may increase or decrease levels of active drug significantly. The package insert recommends limiting the dose of pioglitazone to 15 mg in combination with gemfibrozil.

Dosing and Administration The recommended starting dosages of pioglitazone and of rosiglitazone are 15 to 30 mg once daily and 2 to 4 mg once daily, respectively. Dosages may be increased slowly based on therapeutic goals and side effects. The maximum dose and maximum effective dose of pioglitazone is 45 mg, and rosiglitazone is 8 mg once daily, although 4 mg twice a day may reduce HbA_{1c} by 0.2% to 0.3% (0.002 to 0.003; 2 to 3 mmol/mol Hb) more versus 8 mg once daily.

Rosiglitazone's availability is limited for now, and an active risk evaluation and mitigation program has been implemented due to the risk of ischemic events. Patients and prescribers must sign up through the rosiglitazone website in order to receive the medication from a central mail-order pharmacy, as local pharmacies no longer carry rosiglitazone. Patients and prescribers must agree either that it is continuation of therapy and the risks versus benefits are known to both or that it is a new prescription and that the patient has been fully informed of the risk, including MI, and of the alternatives available, including pioglitazone. Pioglitazone is not included in this particular risk evaluation and mitigation program.

α-Glucosidase Inhibitors

Pharmacology Currently, there are two α-glucosidase inhibitors available in the United States: acarbose (Precose) and miglitol (Glyset). α-Glucosidase inhibitors competitively inhibit enzymes (maltase, isomaltase, sucrase, and glucoamylase) in the small intestine, delaying the breakdown of sucrose and complex carbohydrates. They do not cause any malabsorption of these nutrients. The net effect from this action is to reduce the postprandial BG rise. GLP-1 may also be increased. Distal intestinal degradation of undigested carbohydrate by the gut flora results in gas (CO_2 and methane) and production of short-chain fatty acids, which may stimulate GLP-1 release from intestinal L cells.

Pharmacokinetics The mechanism of action of α-glucosidase inhibitors is limited to the luminal side of the intestine. Some metabolites of acarbose are systemically absorbed and renally excreted, whereas the majority of miglitol is absorbed and renally excreted unchanged.

Efficacy Postprandial glucose concentrations are reduced (40 to 50 mg/dL [2.2 to 2.8 mmol/L]), while fasting glucose levels are relatively unchanged (~10% reduction). Efficacy on glycemic control is modest (average reductions in HbA_{1c} of 0.3% to 1% [0.003 to 0.010; 3 to 11 mmol/mol Hb]), affecting primarily postprandial glycemic excursions. Thus, patients near target HbA_{1c} levels with near-normal FPG levels, but high postprandial levels, may be candidates for therapy.

Microvascular Complications α-Glucosidase inhibitors modestly reduce HbA_{1c} levels, which has been shown to be related to the risk of microvascular complications.

Macrovascular Complications The STOP-NIDDM study, in subjects with IGT, reported a significant reduction in the risk of cardiovascular events, although the total number of events was very small.[40,41] No large cardiovascular study confirming these preliminary results has been done in prediabetes or diabetes patients.

Adverse Effects The GI side effects, such as flatulence, bloating, abdominal discomfort, and diarrhea, are very common and greatly limit the use of α-glucosidase inhibitors. Mechanistically, these side effects are caused by distal intestinal degradation of undigested carbohydrate by the microflora, which results in gas (CO_2 and methane) production. Microflora convert the carbohydrate to short-chain fatty acids that are mostly absorbed; thus, there is not a large calorie loss. α-Glucosidase inhibitors should be initiated at a low dose and titrated slowly to reduce GI intolerance. Beano, an α-glucosidase enzyme, may help to decrease GI side effects, but may decrease efficacy slightly, and it is better to decrease carbohydrate or the dose of the α-glucosidase inhibitor.

If a patient develops hypoglycemia within several hours of ingesting an α-glucosidase inhibitor, oral glucose is advised because the drug will inhibit the breakdown of more complex sugar molecules. Milk, with lactose sugar, may be used as an alternative when no glucose is available, as acarbose only slightly (10%) inhibits lactase. Fructose may also work, if the others are not available.

Rarely, elevated serum aminotransferase levels have been reported with the highest doses of acarbose. It appeared to be dose and weight related, and is the premise for the weight-based maximum doses.

Dosing and Administration Dosing for both miglitol and acarbose are similar. Initiate with a very low dose (25 mg with one meal a day); increase very gradually (over several months) to a maximum of 50 mg three times a day for patients ≤60 kg or 100 mg three times a day for patients >60 kg (see Table 57-11). Titration speed should be varied based on GI side effects to the target dose. Both α-glucosidase inhibitors should be taken with the first bite of the meal so that drug may be present to inhibit enzyme activity. Only patients consuming a diet high in complex carbohydrates will have significant reductions in glucose levels. α-Glucosidase inhibitors are contraindicated in patients with short-bowel syndrome or inflammatory bowel disease, and neither should be administered in patients with serum creatinine >2 mg/dL (>177 μmol/L), as this population has not been studied.

Dipeptidyl Peptidase-4 Inhibitors Sitagliptin (Januvia), saxagliptin (Onglyza), linagliptin (Tradjenta), and alogliptin (Nesina) are DPP-4 inhibitors currently approved in the United States.

Pharmacology DPP-4 inhibitors prolong the half-life of endogenously produced GLP-1 and GIP that normally is only minutes. GIP levels are normal in type 2 DM, and may contribute a minor amount of insulin secretion but have no effect on glucagon. However, levels of GLP-1 are deficient in type 2 DM. As these agents block nearly 100% of the DPP-4 enzyme activity for at least 12 hours, normal physiologic, nondiabetic GLP-1 levels are achieved. DPP-4 inhibitors significantly reduce the inappropriately elevated glucagon postprandially, although not back to nondiabetic levels, and improve insulin response to hyperglycemia. This results in reduction of glucose levels without increase in hypoglycemia when used as monotherapy. These drugs do not alter gastric emptying and do not have significant satiety effects. DPP-4 inhibitors also appear to be weight neutral.

Pharmacokinetics Sitagliptin has rapid absorption, with a t_{max} of approximately 1.5 hours. Absolute bioavailability after oral intake is approximately 87%. Only ~40% is bound to plasma proteins; the volume of distribution is approximately 200 L. The $t_{1/2}$ of sitagliptin is approximately 12 hours. Seventy-nine percent of the dose of sitagliptin is excreted unchanged in the urine by active tubular secretion; however, the organic anion transporter 3 or p-glycoprotein transport may be involved as well. Sitagliptin exposure is increased by approximately 2.3-, 3.8-, and 4.5-fold relative to healthy subjects for patients with moderate renal insufficiency (creatinine clearance [CL_{cr}] 30 to <50 mL/min [0.50 to <0.83 mL/s]), severe renal insufficiency (CL_{cr} <30 mL/min [<0.50 mL/s]), and ESRD (on dialysis), respectively. This is not a safety or adverse reaction issue; however, reduction of the dose based on renal function is appropriate, as only 100% of the enzyme can be inhibited, and long-term exposure to higher levels in humans has not been extensively studied. Pharmacodynamically, DPP-4 inhibition appeared to mirror directly the plasma concentration of sitagliptin. Doses of 50 mg produce at least 80% inhibition of DPP-4 enzyme activity at 12 hours, and those of 100 mg produce 80% inhibition of DPP-4 enzyme activity at 24 hours. Food has no effect on absorption kinetics of sitagliptin. Hepatic impairment, age, gender, or race has no effect on the pharmacokinetics of sitagliptin.

When saxagliptin is administered with a high-fat meal, the t_{max} increases about 20 minutes and the AUC increases about 27%. However, this is not clinically significant and saxagliptin may be given with or without meals. The oral bioavailability of saxagliptin is approximately 67%. Distribution is similar to the body water compartment. There is negligible protein binding, and one active metabolite, 5-hydroxy saxagliptin, is half as potent a DPP-4 inhibitor as the parent compound, and contributes to activity. Metabolism is by the CYP3A4/5 system, and strong inhibitors or inducers will have an effect on activity. The half-lives of saxagliptin and its active metabolite are 2.5 and 3.1 hours, respectively. Approximately 25% of the dose is found in feces representing unabsorbed drug and bile excretion. Females have ~25% more exposure to 5-hydroxy saxagliptin, and exposure is increased 25% to 50% in elderly, likely due to renal clearance. The majority (75%) of saxagliptin and 5-hydroxy saxagliptin is renally eliminated, and some renal excretion is seen. In moderate (CL_{cr} 30 to 50 mL/min [0.50 to 0.83 mL/s]) or severe (CL_{cr} <30 mL/min [<0.50 mL/s]) renal impairment, saxagliptin and its active metabolite exposure are increased 2.1- and 4.5-fold, respectively.

The peak plasma concentrations of linagliptin occur at approximately 1.5 hours after oral administration of a single 5-mg dose to healthy subjects. The half-life of linagliptin is approximately 12 hours. The absolute bioavailability of linagliptin is approximately 30%. A high-fat meal reduces C_{max} by 15% and increases AUC by 4%. However, this effect is not clinically relevant and linagliptin may be taken with or without food. Linagliptin distributes extensively in tissues and at high concentrations. Seventy percent to 80% is bound to plasma proteins while 20% to 30% is unbound in plasma. Plasma binding is not altered in patients who have renal or hepatic impairment. Following oral administration, metabolism is minimal and about 90% of linagliptin is excreted unchanged. Renal excretion is less than 5% of the administered dose and is not affected by decreased renal function.

Alogliptin has a bioavailability of approximately 100% and can be administered with or without food. It is only 20% bound to plasma proteins and approximately 75% of the dose is found unchanged in the urine. Less than 1% is metabolized to an active metabolite, and <6% to an inactive metabolite.

Efficacy The average reduction in HbA_{1c} is approximately 0.7% to 1% (0.007 to 0.010; 8 to 11 mmol/mol Hb) at maximum dose. The decrease in HbA_{1c} at different baseline values is very small. As these drugs are well tolerated, adjustment in the dose due to adverse effects is unlikely. They tend to have a shallow dose–response curve.

Microvascular and Macrovascular Complications HbA_{1c} levels are reduced, which has been related to a reduction in microvascular complications, but no outcome data are available to date.

Drug–Drug Interactions Significant drug–drug interactions with sitagliptin are unlikely. Sitagliptin is metabolized approximately 20% by CYP450 3A4 with some CYP450 2C8 involvement, but is neither an inhibitor nor an inducer of any CYP450 enzyme system. It is a p-glycoprotein substrate, but had negligible effects on digoxin and cyclosporine A, increasing the AUC by only 30%.

Saxagliptin is metabolized by CYP3A4/5, and is a p-glycoprotein substrate, but is neither an inhibitor nor an inducer. Rifampin, an inducer, can decrease active levels by 50%. However, moderate to strong inhibitors or inducers of CYP3A4/5, such as diltiazem or ketoconazole, can increase the AUC of saxagliptin by approximately twofold, with a corresponding decrease in the formation of the active metabolite 5-hydroxy saxagliptin. In such situations, it is recommended that the dose of saxagliptin be limited to 2.5 mg daily.

Linagliptin is a weak to moderate inhibitor of CYP3A4, and a p-glycoprotein substrate. Thus, efficacy of linagliptin may be reduced when administered in combination with inducers of p-glycoprotein and CYP3A4 (e.g., with rifampin). If patients require the use of such drugs, the use of alternative treatments is recommended. No other significant drug interactions have been reported.

No significant drug–drug interactions with alogliptin have been noted to date.

Adverse Effects DPP-4 inhibitors are very well tolerated, are weight neutral, and do not cause GI side effects. Mild hypoglycemia may occur, but in monotherapy or in combination with medications that have a low incidence of hypoglycemia, DPP-4 inhibitors do not increase the risk of hypoglycemia. Headache and nasopharyngitis, potentially related to the drug, may be slightly more common with DPP-4 inhibitors, but no significant increases in peripheral edema, hypertension, or cardiac outcomes have been noted to date.

Urticaria and/or facial edema may be seen in approximately 1% of patients, and discontinuation is warranted. Rare cases of Stevens-Johnson syndrome have been reported.

In regard to long-term safety, DPP-4 enzymes metabolize a wide variety of peptides (PYY, neuropeptide Y, growth hormone–releasing hormone, vasoactive intestinal polypeptide, and others), potentially affecting other regulatory systems. DPP-4 (also known as CD26) plays an important role for T-cell activation. Theoretically the inhibition of DPP-4 could be associated with adverse immunologic reactions. Saxagliptin results in a dose-related reduction in absolute lymphocyte count in up to 0.5% to 1.5% of patients. In most, recurrence is not observed with reexposure. However, it may recur with rechallenge in some patients. The clinical relevance is not known, but if prolonged infection is encountered, it is logical to measure lymphocyte counts and consider discontinuation.

Dosing and Administration Sitagliptin is dosed orally at 100 mg daily unless renal insufficiency is present. The 50-mg dose is recommended if the CL_{cr} is 30 to <50 mL/min (0.50 to <0.83 mL/s), or 25 mg if <30 mL/min (<0.50 mL/s). Saxagliptin is dosed orally 5 mg daily, unless the CL_{cr} is <50 mL/min (<0.83 mL/s), or strong CYP3A4/5 inhibitors are used; then the recommended daily dose is 2.5 mg. Linagliptin is available only in one dose: 5 mg daily, and does not require dose adjustment in renal insufficiency or related to concomitant drug therapy. Alogliptin, similar to sitagliptin, has a two-step dosing adjustment in renal insufficiency. Alogliptin 25 mg daily should be decreased to 12.5 mg when the CrCl <60 mL/min (<1 mL/s), and 6.25 mg when

<30 mL/min (<0.50 mL/s). Because of their excellent tolerability profile and flat dose–response curve, these drugs should be maximally dosed, unless noted above.

Bile Acid Sequestrants Currently, the only bile acid sequestrant approved for the treatment of type 2 DM is colesevelam (Welchol).

Pharmacology Colesevelam is a bile acid sequestrant that acts in the intestinal lumen to bind bile acid, decreasing the bile acid pool for reabsorption. Whether colesevelam's mechanism of action to lower plasma glucose levels is in the intestinal lumen, a systemic effect due to the intestinal lumen effect or some combination of these two is unknown. Possible mechanisms include effects on the farnesoid X and TGR5 receptors within the intestine as well as effects on farnesoid X receptor within the liver. There is evidence that colesevelam may affect the secretion of GLP-1 and GIP. See also Chapter 11.

Pharmacokinetics Colesevelam is not absorbed from the intestinal lumen; thus, there is no absorption, distribution, or metabolism.

Efficacy HbA_{1c} reductions from baseline (~8% [~0.08; ~64 mmol/mol Hb]) were approximately 0.4% (0.004; 5 mmol/mol Hb) when a dose of 3.8 g/day was added to stable metformin, sulfonylureas, or insulin. The FPG was modestly reduced about 5 to 10 mg/dL (0.3 to 0.6 mmol/L). Colesevelam also reduces LDL-C cholesterol in patients with type 2 DM. A 12% to 16% reduction in LDL-C was reported from baseline LDL-C concentrations of ~105 mg/dL (~2.72 mmol/L). Triglycerides increased when combined with sulfonylureas or insulin, but not with metformin. Colesevelam is weight neutral. Pediatric patients (10 to 17 years of age) have been studied for cholesterol reduction, but not for type 2 DM.

Microvascular Complications Bile acid sequestrants modestly reduce HbA_{1c} levels, which have been shown to be related to the risk of microvascular complications.

Macrovascular Complications Although colesevelam lowers plasma glucose and LDL-C, it has not been proven to prevent cardiovascular morbidity or mortality.

Drug–Drug Interactions There are multiple absorption-related drug–drug interactions with colesevelam. The most important include levothyroxine, glyburide, and oral contraceptives. In addition, phenytoin, warfarin, digoxin, and fat-soluble vitamins have postmarketing reports of altered absorption. It is recommended that medications suspected of an interaction should be moved at least 4 hours prior to dosing the colesevelam. Colesevelam has also been implicated in the malabsorption of fat-soluble vitamins (A, E, D, K). In addition to the obvious fat-soluble vitamin supplementation, this may have implications for associated conditions. Other drugs that are very fat-soluble such as cyclosporine A, drugs that may be affected by a change in fat-soluble vitamin status such as warfarin and vitamin K, or conditions that may be potentially worsened by fat-soluble vitamin status such as some bleeding disorders or dermatologic conditions should be monitored.

Adverse Effects The most common side effects are GI. Constipation (11%) and dyspepsia (8%) are more common with colesevelam than placebo. Because of the constipating effects of colesevelam, it is not recommended in patients with gastroparesis, bowel obstruction, or a history of major GI surgery. It also should not be used in patients with significant swallowing or esophageal issues, as it may worsen the underlying condition or cause obstruction. Colesevelam should be taken with a large amount of water to lower the risk of the above issues. Hypoglycemia rates were low, although caution with insulin or sulfonylureas is prudent.

Colesevelam, similar to all bile acid sequestrants, may raise triglyceride levels. The increase in triglycerides is proportional to baseline triglyceride levels, and colesevelam is contraindicated in patients with a triglyceride >500 mg/dL (>5.65 mmol/L). Close monitoring is recommended if the baseline triglycerides >300 mg/dL (3.39 mmol/L). Colesevelam is contraindicated in patients with a history of triglyceridemia-induced pancreatitis, and prudent clinical judgment should be used in any patient with a history of pancreatitis and elevated triglycerides.

Dosing and Administration Dosing for type 2 DM is six 625-mg tablets daily (total dose/day = 3.75 g), which may be split into three tablets two times a day if desired. A 3.75-g oral suspension packet, dosed daily, or a 1.875-g oral suspension packet dose twice daily is also available. Suspension packets must be diluted in a minimum of one half to one cup of water. Take tablets and suspension with a large amount of water, if possible. All dosage forms should be administered with meals as colesevelam binds to bile released during the meal.

Dopamine Agonists Bromocriptine mesylate (Cycloset) is currently approved for the treatment of type 2 DM.

Pharmacology Bromocriptine is a dopamine agonist, but the exact mechanism of how bromocriptine improves glycemic control is unknown. Low hypothalamic dopamine levels, especially on waking, are augmented, which may decrease sympathetic tone and output. These effects are speculated to improve hepatic insulin sensitivity.

Pharmacokinetics Bioavailability is 65% to 95% after an orally administered dose; bioavailability may be increased ~50% if given with a meal. Peak plasma concentration is about 1 hour if taken without food, but with food it is 90 to 120 minutes. Bromocriptine is highly protein bound, and has a volume of distribution of 61 L. Only ~7% reaches the systemic circulation due to GI-based metabolism and first-pass metabolism. Bromocriptine is extensively metabolized by the CYP3A4 pathway, and the majority (~95%) is excreted in the bile. The half-life is approximately 6 hours. Plasma exposure is increased in females by approximately 18% to 30%, but no dosage adjustment is currently recommended.

Efficacy In clinical trials, bromocriptine mesylate reduced HbA_{1c} by 0.3% to 0.6% (0.003 to 0.006; 3 to 7 mmol/mol Hb) from baseline.

Microvascular and Macrovascular Complications There is no study examining microvascular disease. Macrovascular event reduction has not been proven. In just over 3,000 subjects, bromocriptine decreased a composite cardiovascular outcome over 1 year. The composite outcome occurred in 37 (1.8%) bromocriptine-treated subjects versus 32 (3.2%) subjects not given bromocriptine (HR 0.6 [95% two-sided CI, 0.35 to 0.96]).

Drug–Drug Interactions Bromocriptine is extensively metabolized by CYP3A4 and strong inhibitors or inducers may change bromocriptine levels. As bromocriptine is highly protein bound, it may increase the unbound fraction of other highly protein-bound drugs. Several drug–drug and potential drug–disease interactions are present including antipsychotics in psychotic disorders as they decrease dopamine activity, atypical antipsychotics as they may decrease the effectiveness of bromocriptine, and ergot-based therapy for migraines as bromocriptine may increase migraine and ergot-related nausea and vomiting. There are case reports of hypertension and tachycardia when administered with sympathomimetic drugs in postpartum women, and bromocriptine should not be given to this group of potential patients. The effectiveness in other disease states where dopamine agonism may be indicated is unknown.

Adverse Effects Adverse reactions leading to discontinuation occurred in 24% of bromocriptine patients compared with 9% in the placebo comparator group. Nausea, rhinitis, headache, asthenia, dizziness, constipation, and sinusitis all occurred in over 10% of subjects. Nausea occurred in 25% to 35% of patients, and vomiting, which tended to be more common in women, occurred in 5% to 6% of patients. Nausea, vomiting, fatigue, headache, and dizziness were common adverse events during the titration phase of phase 3 studies, and only 70% of completors could be titrated to the maximum dose. Orthostatic hypotension or syncope occurred in 2.2% and 1.4%, and 0.6% and 0.8% in the bromocriptine and placebo groups, respectively. No predisposing factors were identified, but caution should be exercised in patients with low, normal blood pressure. Somnolence was reported in 4.3% of patients on bromocriptine, compared with 1.3% in the placebo, and response to the drug should be ascertained prior to operating machinery or combining with other sedating medications. Psychiatric disorders including hallucinations and pathologic gambling have been reported with other forms of bromocriptine, but were not seen in phase III trials.

Dosing and Administration Bromocriptine is dosed with 0.8-mg tablets administered within 2 hours of waking from sleep daily with food. From 0.8 mg daily, the dose may be increased weekly based on response by 0.8-mg tablet increments, to a maximum of 4.8 mg daily (0.8 mg × 6 tablets, although it is unclear if another commercial dose could be made available). The minimal effective dose is 1.6 mg daily. It is recommended to be taken with food as this may decrease nausea/vomiting.

Potential Future Medications

Many medications for the treatment of diabetes are currently in late-phase development. No guarantee of FDA approval is given for any agent in development.

Insulin

Insulin degludec is a long-acting basal insulin that appears to be truly peakless. Hypoglycemia in clinical trials has been slightly less to date versus insulin glargine with similar glycemic control.

Incretin Class Medications

Once-daily lixisenatide and several weekly GLP-1 receptor agonist medications are being developed. Closest to market is albiglutide, but also in development is semaglutide.

Selective Sodium-Dependent Glucose Cotransporter-2 Inhibitors (SGLT-2 Inhibitors)

SGLT-2 inhibitors work in the kidney to block the reabsorption of some glucose. Normally, all glucose is reabsorbed back into the systemic circulation from the kidney at normal glucose levels: about 10% through the SGLT-1 receptor, and 90% through the SGLT-2 receptor. Early data have shown approximately 50 to 80 g of glucose per day may be allowed to pass into the urine with SGLT-2 inhibition. This lowers systemic glucose and allows weight loss. Glucose levels may be lowered in both type 1 and type 2 DM by this mechanism of action. Safety data have shown a slightly higher rate of genitourinary yeast infections. SGLT-1 is involved with glucose absorption in the gut, and inhibition of SGLT-1 has been historically thought to cause GI toxicity, but this is unclear and dual inhibitors may be marketed. Canagliflozin (Invokana) is currently the farthest in development, but several are being developed. Dapagliflozin has been rejected by the FDA several times due to concerns about cancer.

Pivotal Trials

Diabetes Control and Complications Trial

7 Much of the last century in diabetes care was dominated by the debate over whether glycemic control actually was causative in complications of DM. Animal studies and some human studies suggested that the worse the glycemia, the greater the risk of complications. But "the glucose hypothesis" was not ultimately accepted as proven until the publication of the DCCT in 1993.[23] In this study, 1,441 patients with type 1 DM were divided into two groups: those without complications (726 subjects, primary prevention) and those with early microvascular complications (715 subjects, secondary prevention). These two groups were then again divided into two groups: one randomized to receive conventional therapy (one or two shots of insulin daily and infrequent SMBG with no attempt to change therapy based on home BG readings) and the other to receive intensive therapy (>3 injections of insulin daily or insulin pump, with frequent SMBG and alteration of insulin therapy based on SMBG results, plus frequent contact with a health professional). After 6.5 years, mean follow-up with a difference in HbA_{1c} between the two groups being ≈2% (≈0.02; 22 mmol/mol Hb) (≈9% vs. ≈7% [≈0.09 vs. ≈0.07; ≈75 mmol/mol Hb vs. ≈53 mmol/mol Hb), retinopathy was decreased by 76% in the primary prevention cohort, with retinopathy progression reduced 54% in the secondary prevention group. Neuropathy was decreased by 60% in both groups combined. Microalbuminuria was decreased 39%, while macroproteinuria was reduced 54% with intensive therapy. Hypoglycemia was more common and weight gain greater with intensive therapy. A nonstatistically significant reduction in coronary events was seen in the intensively treated group as compared with the conventional group. The DCCT revolutionized therapy of DM, demanding that stricter glycemic control be the goal.

United Kingdom Prospective Diabetes Study

7 The UKPDS was a landmark study for the care of patients with type 2 DM, confirming the importance of glycemic control for reducing the risk of microvascular complications.[24] More than 5,000 patients with newly diagnosed type 2 DM were entered into the study. Patients were followed for an average of 10 years. The major portion of the study assessed "conventional therapy" (no drug therapy unless the patient was symptomatic or had FPG >270 mg/dL [>15 mmol/L]), versus intensive therapy starting with either sulfonylureas or insulin, aimed at keeping the FPG <108 mg/dL (6 mmol/L). A subset of obese patients was studied using metformin as the primary therapeutic agent.

Significant findings from the study include the following:

1. Microvascular complications (predominantly the need for laser photocoagulation on retinal lesions) are reduced by 25% when median HbA_{1c} is 7% (0.07; 53 mmol/mol Hb) as compared with 7.9% (0.079; 63 mmol/mol Hb).[24]
2. A continuous relationship exists between glycemia and microvascular complications, with a 35% reduction in risk for each 1% decrement in HbA_{1c} (0.01; 11 mmol/mol Hb). No glycemic threshold for microvascular disease exists.[42]
3. Glycemic control has minimal effect on macrovascular disease risk. Excess macrovascular risk appears to be related to conventional risk factors such as dyslipidemia and hypertension.[43]
4. Sulfonylureas and insulin therapy do not increase macrovascular disease risk.[24]
5. Metformin reduces macrovascular risk in obese patients.[36]
6. Vigorous blood pressure control reduces microvascular and macrovascular events.[43] There was no evidence for a threshold systolic blood pressure above 130 mm Hg for protection against complications. β-Blockers and angiotensin-converting enzyme (ACE) inhibitors appear to be equally efficacious.[44]

Long-Term Follow-up of DCCT (EDIC) and UKPDS

At the conclusion of the DCCT and UKPDS trials, willing subjects continued to be followed over time to ascertain microvascular and macrovascular outcomes. In the follow-up of the DCCT, called the

Epidemiology of Diabetes Interventions and Complications (EDIC), several important points have been discovered. First, HbA_{1c} levels between conventional and intensive groups converged to an HbA_{1c} of approximately 8% (0.08; 64 mmol/mol Hb). Despite similar HbA_{1c} values, continued microvascular and new macrovascular benefit was seen. Microvascular benefits were maintained for 10 to 15 years, and at 17 years of follow-up, a 57% ($P = 0.02$) reduction in death, first occurrence of nonfatal MI, and stroke was seen between the conventional and intensive groups.[45,46]

In the follow-up of the UKPDS, HbA_{1c} (~8% [~0.08; ~64 mmol/mol Hb]) converged and values were not significantly different for the majority of the follow-up. After a mean follow-up of 8.5 years, a 24% ($P = 0.001$) reduction in microvascular complications (during the UKPDS, 25% reduction was reported) and a significant reduction in MI (15%; $P = 0.014$) and all-cause mortality (13%; $P = 0.007$) in the intensively treated group versus the conventional group were reported.[47] Early glycemic control may have long-standing benefits to patients over several decades, despite later glycemic control deterioration. This concept is being called metabolic memory or the legacy effect. These studies lay the framework for why early intensive glycemic control is important not only for short-term but also for long-term prevention of complications.

ACCORD, ADVANCE, and VADT

8 The Action to Control Cardiovascular Risk in Diabetes (ACCORD),[48] Action in Diabetes and Vascular Disease (ADVANCE),[49] and Veterans Affairs Diabetes Trial (VADT)[50] were three trials that reported on the effects of glycemic control and macrovascular disease risk.

ACCORD randomized 10,251 high CVD risk subjects (CVD event or significant risk) with type 2 DM to intensive glycemic control (goal HbA_{1c} <6% [<0.06; <42 mmol/mol Hb]) or standard glycemic control (HbA_{1c} 7% to 7.9% [0.07 to 0.079; 53 to 63 mmol/mol Hb]). Multiple oral agents and/or insulin were allowed to achieve glycemic goals. Baseline HbA_{1c} level was 8.1% (0.081; 65 mmol/mol Hb), and the intensive glycemic group achieved a HbA_{1c} of 6.4% (0.064; 46 mmol/mol Hb), whereas standard glycemic control achieved a HbA_{1c} of 7.5% (0.075; 58 mmol/mol Hb) when the study stopped after a mean follow-up period of 3.5 years. The study was stopped after an interim analysis reported an increased rate of mortality in the intensive arm (1.41%/y vs. 1.14%/y; HR, 1.22; 95% CI, 1.01 to 1.46). Interestingly, the primary end point (myocardial, stroke, or cardiovascular death) was trending down due to a lower risk of nonfatal MI in the intensive therapy group. In addition, on subset analysis, individuals with a baseline HbA_{1c} <8% (<0.08; <64 mmol/mol Hb) or no previous CVD had a significant reduction in the primary outcome. Increased mortality, though substantially increased in the intensive group, could not be associated with a specific medication, hypoglycemia (higher in intensive group), lipid levels, or weight gain. The dichotomous results have been hard to explain, although the ACCORD investigators reported that in the intensive group, it was subjects who could *not* attain intensive glycemic control goals who were at higher risk, not subjects who did achieve the goal. A 20% higher risk of death for each 1% (0.01; 11 mmol/mol Hb) above an HbA_{1c} of 6% (0.06; 42 mmol/mol Hb) was reported.

ADVANCE randomized 11,140 subjects to intensive (≤6.5% HbA_{1c} [≤0.065; ≤48 mmol/mol Hb]) or standard therapy (investigator-driven goals). Extended-release gliclazide, a sulfonylurea available outside of the United States, was used as first-line therapy in the intensive group versus no gliclazide in the standard therapy group, although multiple other agents were needed in both groups. A baseline HbA_{1c} was only 7.5% (0.075; 58 mmol/mol Hb), and at the end of therapy, the intensive group versus standard group HbA_{1c} was ~6.5% versus ~7.2% (~0.065 vs. ~0.072; 48 mmol/mol Hb vs. 55 mmol/mol Hb). ADVANCE reported a significant reduction in renal events, including new or worsening nephropathy (HR, 0.79; 95% CI, 0.66 to 0.93), but no difference in major macrovascular events (HR, 0.94; 95% CI, 0.84 to 1.06) with intensive versus standard therapy.

VADT randomized 1,791 subjects to intensive glycemic control (HbA_{1c} goal <6% [<0.06; <42 mmol/mol Hb], and action required of >6.5% [>0.065; >48 mmol/mol Hb]) versus nonintensive glycemic control (investigator determined). At entry, the HbA_{1c} was the highest of the three trials (9.4% [0.094; 79 mmol/mol Hb]). Multiple medications including insulin were used to achieve glycemic control. The intensive group achieved an HbA_{1c} of 6.9% versus 8.5% (0.069 vs. 0.085; 52 mmol/mol Hb vs. 69 mmol/mol Hb) in the investigator-determined group. The primary end point of nonfatal MI, nonfatal stroke, CVD death, hospitalization for heart failure, and revascularization was not significantly different (HR, 0.88; 95% CI, 0.74 to 1.05) and mortality was unchanged.

These three trials should be viewed as confirmatory that short term (3 to 5 years) of intensive glycemic control does not positively affect the risk of macrovascular risk in type 2 DM. ACCORD reported that a subset of subjects who could not achieve intensive glycemic control may be at higher risk of death, but identifying these patients and implementing this recommendation into clinical practice may prove to be challenging. As previously mentioned in Long-Term Followup of DCCT (EDIC) and UKPDS above, reduction of macrovascular events from improved glycemic control may take over a decade to come to fruition.

Therapeutics

9 Knowledge of the patient's quantitative and qualitative meal patterns, activity levels, pharmacokinetics of insulin preparations and other injectables, and pharmacology of oral and antidiabetic agents for type 2 DM is essential to individualize the treatment plan an optimize BG control while minimizing risks for hypoglycemia and other adverse effects of pharmacologic therapies.

Type 1 Diabetes Mellitus

All patients with type 1 DM require insulin. However, how that insulin is delivered to the patient is a matter of considerable practice difference among patients and clinicians.

Historically, after the discovery of insulin by Banting and Best in 1921, frequent injections of regular insulin (initially the only insulin available) were given. Modifications of insulin led to longer-acting insulin suspensions and the use by many patients of one or two injections of longer-acting insulin each day. Because self-monitored BG and HbA_{1c} testing were not available at that time, patients and practitioners had no idea how well their patients' BG concentrations were controlled, other than a vague sense from an indirect method, measurement of glucose in the urine. While the renal threshold for glucose is relatively predictable in young healthy subjects, it is highly variable in older patients and patients with renal disease. The advent of SMBG and HbA_{1c} testing in the 1980s revolutionized the care of diabetes, enabling patients and practitioners to directly access BG for assessment, and enabling the patient to make instantaneous changes in the insulin regimen if need be. Modern diabetes management would be impossible without these two tools.

Contemporary management of type 1 DM attempts to match carbohydrate intake with glucose-lowering processes, most commonly insulin, as well as with exercise. The goal is to allow the patient to live as normal a life as possible. Understanding the principles of glucose input and glucose egress from the blood allows the practitioner and the patient great latitude in the management of type 1 DM.

Normal secretion of insulin can be divided into a relatively constant background level of insulin ("basal") during the fasting and postabsorptive period, with prandial spikes of insulin after eating ("bolus") (Fig. 57-6).[51] Insulin sensitivity and insulin secretion are not constant throughout the day, however, which renders the concept of stable basal insulin requirements to be inaccurate. However, in

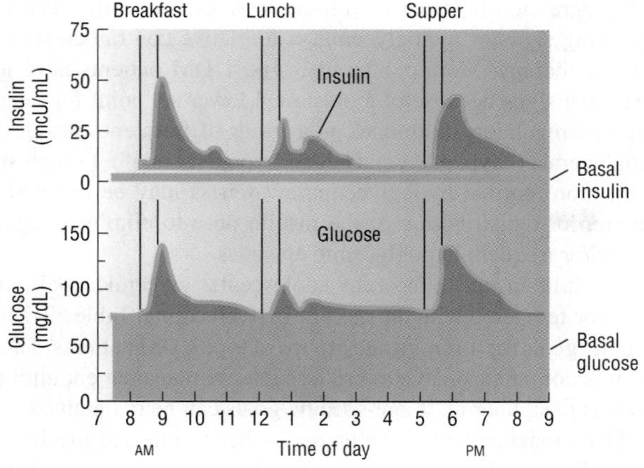

Intensive insulin therapy regimens

	7 AM (meal)	11 AM (meal)	5 PM (meal)	Bedtime
1. 2 doses,[a] R or rapid acting + N	R, L, A, GLU + N		R, L, A, GLU + N	
2. 3 doses, R or rapid acting + N	R, L, A, GLU + N	R, L, A, GLU	R, L, A, GLU + N	
3. 4 doses, R or rapid acting + N	R, L, A, GLU	R, L, A, GLU	R, L, A, GLU	N
4. 4 doses, R or rapid acting + N	R, L, A, GLU + N	R, L, A, GLU	R, L, A, GLU	N
5. 4 doses,[b] R or rapid acting + long acting	R, L, A, GLU	R, L, A, GLU	R, L, A, GLU	G or D[b] (G may be given anytime every 24 hours)
	←	Adjusted basal	→	
6. CS-II pump	Bolus	Bolus	Bolus	
7. 3 prandial doses pramlintide added to regimens above	P	P	P	

[a]Many clinicians may not consider this intensive insulin therapy.
[b]May be given twice a day in type 1 DM = 5 doses.

FIGURE 57-6 Relationship between insulin and glucose over the course of a day and how various insulin and amylinomimetic regimens could be given. (A, aspart; CSII, continuous subcutaneous insulin infusion; D, detemir; G, glargine; GLU, glulisine; L, lispro; P, pramlintide; N, NPH; R, regular.)

most clinical situations, attempting to emulate normal secretion of insulin is a useful paradigm for understanding and applying insulin treatment for the management of type 1 DM. The other basic principle to consider is that the timing of insulin onset, peak, and duration of effect must match meal patterns and exercise schedules to achieve near-normal BG values throughout the day.

Historically, the complexity of insulin regimens was related to the number of injections of insulin administered per day. This was a reasonable classification; however, a single injection of any insulin preparation daily will in no way mimic normal physiology, and therefore is unacceptable. Similarly, two injections of any insulin daily will fail to replicate normal patterns of insulin release.

Injection regimens that begin to approximate physiologic insulin release start with "split-mixed" injections consisting of a morning dose of an intermediate-acting insulin such as NPH and a "bolus" rapid-acting insulin or regular insulin before breakfast, and again before the evening meal. The presumption is made that the morning intermediate-acting insulin gives basal insulin for the day and covers the midday meal, the morning bolus insulin covers breakfast, the evening intermediate-acting insulin gives basal insulin for the rest of the day, and the evening bolus insulin covers the evening meal. If patients are very compulsive about consistency of timing of their injections and meals and intake of carbohydrate, such a strategy may be acceptable. However, the vast majority of patients are not sufficiently predictable in their schedule and food intake to allow "tight" glucose control with such an approach.

A modification that can be made to the above regimen is the movement of the evening NPH to bedtime (now three total injections per day) because the fasting glucose in the morning is too high or there is hypoglycemia in the early hours of sleep. This approach improves glycemic control and may reduce hypoglycemia sufficiently for those patients who decline or are unable to follow more intense regimens. However, most patients with type 1 DM need a more intense approach that also allows greater flexibility in their lifestyle.

10 The basal–bolus concept attempts to replicate normal insulin physiology with a combination of intermediate- or long-acting insulin to provide the basal component, and rapid-acting insulin to provide the bolus or premeal component. Various long-acting insulins have been used to provide the basal insulin component, including once- or twice-daily NPH, detemir, or glargine. Insulin glargine and insulin detemir are the most feasible basal insulins for most patients with type 1 DM.

The bolus or prandial insulin component can be regular insulin, insulin lispro, insulin aspart, or insulin glulisine injected before meals. The rapid onset of action and short time course of rapid-acting insulin analogs more closely replicate normal physiology than does regular insulin. The patient varies the amount of before meal rapid-acting insulin injected, depending on the preprandial BG level, the anticipated activity (upcoming exercise may reduce insulin requirement), and anticipated carbohydrate intake. Many patients start with a prescribed dose of insulin before meals that they vary by use of an "adjusted scale insulin" or "correction factor" to normalize a high premeal plasma glucose reading. Patients on more advanced regimens later may adjust the amount of mealtime insulin based on anticipated carbohydrate intake.

A "correction factor" can be calculated as a starting point to estimate the approximate plasma glucose–lowering effect of 1 unit of short-acting insulin in mg/dL. For regular insulin, one may use a factor of 1,500 (a corresponding factor for calculation of glucose in SI units would require multiplying by 0.0555) divided by the total daily insulin dose in number of units that the patient currently uses. For rapid-acting insulin analogs, a factor of 1,700 is more often used when calculating the correction factor. For example, if a patient is currently taking 40 units of basal insulin and 12 units of rapid-acting insulin at each of three meals, the total daily insulin dose equals 76 units. Using this calculation 1,700 divided by 76 equals 22; thus, each unit of rapid-acting insulin analog will lower the plasma glucose approximately 22 mg/dL (1.2 mmol/L). Review of follow-up BG data permits better individualization of the correction factor.

Carbohydrate counting is a very effective tool for determining the amount of rapid-acting insulin that should be injected preprandially in people with type 1 DM. Instead of using a prescribed or preset dose of rapid-acting insulin before meals, patients can self-adjust their premeal dose based on the estimated grams of carbohydrates that will be consumed. Although general algorithms for carbohydrate counting give rough guidelines, each patient will have to adjust the preprandial insulin dosage based on his or her own individual response to different food items.

One method of calculating how much carbohydrate (grams) 1 unit of rapid-acting insulin will cover is to use 500 divided by the total daily dose of insulin in number of units. Therefore, using the example above with a total daily insulin dose of 76 units, we would use 500 divided by 76, which estimates that 1 unit of rapid-acting insulin will cover approximately 7 g of carbohydrate. Review of follow-up BG data before and 2 hours after meals will enable more precise determination of an individual's insulin-to-carbohydrate ratio.

In type 1 DM, approximately 50% of total daily insulin replacement should be basal insulin, and the other 50% will be bolus insulin, divided into doses before meals. If the patient's ratio is not close to this recommendation, a reassessment of the regimen should be implemented. Empirically, patients may be begun on ≈0.6 unit/kg/day with basal insulin 50% of total dose and prandial insulin 20% of total dose prebreakfast, 15% prelunch, and 15% presupper. Type 1 DM patients generally require between 0.5 and 1 unit/kg/day. The need for significantly higher amounts of insulin suggests the presence of insulin resistance or, less often, of insulin antibodies.

Intensive basal–bolus multi-injection insulin therapy is recommended for all adult patients with type 1 DM at the time of diagnosis to reinforce the importance of glycemic control from the outset rather than change strategies over time because of lack of control. Occasional patients with an extended honeymoon period may need less intense therapy initially, but should later be converted to basal–bolus therapy at the onset of glycemic lability.

For those patients who insist on only two injections daily, intermediate-acting insulin and a rapid-acting insulin or regular insulin (starting at 0.6 unit/kg with two thirds in the morning, two thirds of the morning dose as intermediate-acting insulin, and one half of evening dose as intermediate-acting insulin) is an option; however, most often this approach will not be allowed as an aggressive glycemic control option due to increased risk of hypoglycemia.

Insulin pump therapy (continuous subcutaneous insulin infusion [CSII], generally using a rapid-acting analog insulin) is the most sophisticated form of insulin delivery. In a motivated patient, CSII may be more efficacious in achieving excellent glycemic control than multiple-dose insulin injections. Extensive discussion of this mode of therapy is beyond the scope of this text. Nevertheless, the basic principles for implementation are the same.

One advantage of pump therapy is that the basal insulin dose may be varied, related to changes in basal insulin requirements throughout the day. In selected patients, this feature allows better glycemic control with CSII. However, insulin pumps require even greater attention to detail and frequency of SMBG than does a basal–bolus regimen with four injections daily.[52] In appropriately selected patients willing to pay sufficient attention to detail of SMBG and insulin administration, CSII can be a very effective form of therapy. CSII is only a tool for diabetes control, however. Thus, if the patient is not well controlled and/or unwilling to actively control the diabetes on injections, it is unlikely that the patient will have superior control on a pump. CSII placement and adjustment should be made by an experienced clinician, and only after a discussion with the patient about the reality of CSII, addressing expectations, and proper training on the pump.

Regardless of the insulin regimen chosen, gross adjustments in the total insulin dose are made based on HbA_{1c} measurements and symptoms such as polyuria, polydipsia, and weight gain or loss. Finer insulin adjustments are determined on the basis of the results of frequent BG monitoring, documentation of mealtime carbohydrate intake, physical activity, and other factors that affect glycemic control.

All patients should have extensive education in the recognition and treatment of hypoglycemia. Many patients experiencing hypoglycemia are tempted to overtreat episodes of hypoglycemia resulting in rebound hyperglycemia afterwards. To minimize this, patients are advised to follow the "rule of 15." If hypoglycemia is identified (BG less than 70 mg/dL [3.9 mmol/L]), the patient is instructed to consume 15 g of simple carbohydrate (8 oz [~250 mL] orange juice or four glucose tablets) and then retest his or her BG 15 minutes later. If BG is still less than 70 mg/dL (3.9 mmol/L), the patient may repeat the rule of 15 until his or her BG has normalized.

At each visit, patients with type 1 DM should be questioned about hypoglycemia. The frequency of hypoglycemia, particularly hypoglycemia requiring assistance of another person, a visit to an emergent or urgent care facility, or hospitalization, should be recorded.

In type 1 DM, it is common for patients to develop hypoglycemia unawareness. Hypoglycemic unawareness may result from progression of disease with autonomic neuropathy. The loss of warning signs of hypoglycemia is a relative contraindication to intensive therapy. More commonly, type 1 DM patients have loss of warning signs because of a presumed lower set point for release of counterregulatory hormones as a result of frequent episodes of hypoglycemia ("hypoglycemia begets hypoglycemia"). In such situations, more normal hypoglycemia awareness may be restored by reduction or redistribution of the insulin dose to eliminate significant and/or frequent hypoglycemic episodes.

In children and pubescent adolescents, glycemic goals may need to be tempered with the risks of hypoglycemia. Table 57-7 lists glycemic goals for different age groups of type 1 DM patients. Therefore, it is not unreasonable to use less intense management until the patient is postpubertal, if age-specific goals can be maintained.[5]

Occasional patients develop antibodies to injected insulin, but the significance of the antibodies is usually minimal. Human insulin therapy has not totally eliminated insulin allergies. In most patients local reactions will dissipate over time. If mild reactions at the site of injection occur, reassess the insulin injected. Many times the patient is injecting cold insulin, which may cause compensatory local vasodilation around the injection site in response to the injected cold liquid. Anecdotally, a different type or source of insulin could be tried. If the allergic reaction does not improve or is systemic, insulin desensitization can be carried out. Protocols for desensitization are available from major insulin manufacturers.

While more common in the animal insulin era, lipohypertrophy is still seen in some patients with long-standing type 1 DM. Some patients give their insulin injections in the same site repeatedly to minimize discomfort; over time this can result in lipohypertrophy. Lipohypertrophy can sometimes be visualized on physical examination and also can be identified by palpation of injection sites. Because insulin absorption from an area of lipohypertrophy is unpredictable, it is mandatory to avoid insulin injections into these areas.

There are several common errors in the management of patients with type 1 DM that can cause erratic glucose fluctuations:

1. **Failure to take into account action of insulin:** The timing of meals and/or physical activity must be planned around the peaks of insulin action accordingly.
2. **Choice of insulin injection sites:** There is variability of insulin absorption from site to site such that random selection of insulin injection sites may cause wide glucose swings. The most consistent absorption of insulin is from the abdominal wall. Patients are encouraged to take all their injections in the abdomen. If the patient is unable or unwilling to follow this advice, then systematic site rotation is the next preferable option. The patient should always give the insulin injection in the same region of the body the same time of the day each day. For instance, the arms are always used every morning. Needless to say, the patient should not inject in a limb and then go out and exercise that limb, which could cause increased blood flow and insulin absorption.
3. **Overinsulinization:** The answer to all high BG is not necessarily more insulin. Hyperglycemia could be due to too little insulin or it could be due to "rebounding" from a previous low glucose and treating it with excessive amounts of carbohydrate. Fastidious BG testing, particularly during the night (or selected use of CGM), can assist in sorting this out. Many clinicians do not adequately differentiate type 1 DM from type 2 DM when choosing doses of insulin. Patients with type 1 DM are insulin deficient but have normal insulin sensitivity. Patients with type 2 DM have varying degrees of insulin resistance. Therefore, a small change in the dose of insulin for a patient with type 1 DM can have a dramatic effect on glucose concentrations, whereas in patients with type 2 DM and insulin resistance a change in dose many

times that amount of insulin has little effect on glucose concentrations. Large changes in insulin dose in patients with type 1 DM are not usually indicated unless the patient's BG control is very poor. Widely erratic BGs and/or weight gain may be due to too high a dose of insulin.

4. **Injection technique and BG monitoring:** When in doubt, always reevaluate the patient's technique for insulin dosing, insulin injection, and BG testing. Sometimes simple errors result in unpredictable glycemic control.

Type 1 DM patients who continue to have erratic postprandial control despite implementation of the above strategies may be appropriate for treatment with pramlintide (Symlin). Pramlintide is not recommended to be mixed with insulin; therefore, the patient will need to take an additional injection at each meal. With initiation of pramlintide the doses of prandial insulin (rapid-acting analog or regular insulin) should be reduced by 30% to 50%, to prevent hypoglycemia. Pramlintide should be titrated based on GI adverse effects and postprandial glycemic goals. Injecting pramlintide prior to the meal and the rapid-acting insulin at the time of or after the meal may better match the appearance of the food with the postprandial increase in glucose due to delayed gastric emptying. The patient must be cognizant of the risk of hypoglycemia, GI side effects, and how to reduce both.

Islet cell and whole pancreas transplantation is occasionally used in patients who require immunosuppressive therapy for other reasons, such as renal transplants.[53] Many patients are able to stop insulin and/or only require insulin secretion support therapy with sulfonylureas or GLP-1 agonists. However, within 2 years as many 80% or more will need to reinitiate some form of insulin therapy.

Type 2 Diabetes Mellitus

11 Pharmacotherapy for type 2 DM has changed dramatically in the last few years with the addition of several new drug classes and recommendations to achieve more stringent glycemic control. Symptomatic patients may initially require treatment with insulin or combination oral therapy to reduce glucose toxicity (which may reduce β-cell insulin secretion and worsen insulin resistance). Patients with HbA_{1c} ≈7% (≈0.07; ≈53 mmol/mol Hb) or less are usually treated with therapeutic lifestyle measures and an agent that will not cause hypoglycemia. Those with HbA_{1c} >7% but <8.5% (>0.07 but <0.085; >53 but <69 mmol/mol Hb) could be initially treated with single oral agents, or combination therapy. Patients with higher initial HbA_{1c} may benefit from initial therapy with two oral
12 agents, or insulin. This section addresses management of hyperglycemia; however, this needs to be balanced within a multifactorial risk reduction framework of blood pressure reduction, dyslipidemia and antiplatelet therapy, and smoking cessation. All therapeutic decisions should consider the needs and preferences of the patient, if feasible. Individualization of therapy is necessary for success.

Depending on patient motivation and adherence to therapeutic lifestyle changes, most patients with HbA_{1c} greater than 9% to 10% (0.09 to 0.10; 75 to 86 mmol/mol Hb) will likely require therapy with two or more oral agents to reach glycemic goals. Treatment of type 2 DM often necessitates use of multiple therapeutic agents (combination therapy), to obtain glycemic goals.

The best oral therapy regimen for patients with type 2 DM is widely debated. Based on the results of the UKPDS and safety record, obese patients (>120% ideal body weight) without contraindications should be started on metformin titrated to ≈2,000 mg/day.[5,54] Near-normal-weight patients may be better treated with insulin secretagogues, although metformin will work in this population. Metformin is the only oral antihyperglycemic agent to ever report a reduction in total mortality. Despite this, long-term durability of HbA_{1c} reduction, due to the inability to stop progressive β-cell failure, is suboptimal with metformin, and patients over several years will often need additional therapy. An insulin secretagogue, such as a sulfonylurea, is often added second, although it has clearly been shown that sulfonylureas do not produce durable HbA_{1c} reductions in the majority of patients. Better choices to sustain HbA_{1c} reductions would be a TZD or GLP-1 agonist, but each has limitations as well. Goal-oriented therapy is what we currently strive for, meaning the intervention should be in relation to the distance from the glycemic goal. When initial therapy is no longer keeping the patient at goal, if the HbA_{1c} is close to goal, one additional agent may be appropriate. If >1% to 1.5% (>0.01 to 0.015; >11 to 16 mmol/mol Hb) above goal, it is unlikely any one oral agent will result in reaching the glycemic goal, and multiple oral agents or insulin therapy may be appropriate. TZDs may be substituted in situations in which a patient is intolerant of, or has a contraindication to, metformin, understanding that TZDs should be used with caution in heart failure. Figure 57-7 is a consensus algorithm by the ADA and the European Association for the Study of Diabetes.[54] No algorithm can substitute for good clinical judgment, and algorithms for glycemic control start with the premise that the clinician will identify medication contraindications, adverse reactions, and comorbidities that may be advantageous or harmful if the medication was taken.

We should also treat type 2 DM by matching therapy to the suspected underlying problem. Consider some simple questions to guide therapy: (a) How long has the patient had diabetes? The longer a patient has had diabetes, the more insulinopenic he or she likely is and the more likely that insulin therapy will be needed. (b) Fasting, postprandial, or both plasma glucose readings poorly controlled? Some drugs address postprandial glucose excursions better, whereas some address FPG better. (c) How far do we have to go to goal and what is the goal? Each oral agent has limits on HbA_{1c} reduction, and the reduction is baseline HbA_{1c} dependent. (d) Adverse effect profile? Contraindications, hypoglycemia potential, and tolerability are based on the current status of the patient. (e) Comorbidities? CVD, dementia, life expectancy, depression, osteoporosis, and other conditions where select medications may be poor choices and additionally those comorbidities may drive our HbA_{1c} goal. Based on the ADVANCE, ACCORD, and VADT trials, a HbA_{1c} goal may now be above 7% (0.07; 53 mmol/mol Hb) if certain comorbidities are present. See Figure 57-8 for HbA_{1c} individualization based on comorbidities from the Texas Diabetes Council. Drugs such as metformin, TZDs, sulfonylureas, repaglinide, liraglutide, extended-release exenatide, intermediate-acting insulins given at bedtime, and basal insulins control FPG more effectively. Exenatide, DPP-4 inhibitors, α-glucosidase inhibitors, nateglinide, and regular and rapid-acting insulin better control postprandial glucose excursions. We can also guide therapy based on the risk of hypoglycemia. Metformin, TZDs, liraglutide, exenatide, DPP-4 inhibitors, and α-glucosidase inhibitors have a low risk of hypoglycemia. Combining these agents will allow aggressive targeting of near-normal HbA_{1c} levels while minimizing hypoglycemia and weight gain. Combining these agents early in the diagnosis of type 2 DM is logical to potentially realize the microvascular and macrovascular reduction seen in the long-term follow-up of UKPDS.

Preserving β-cell function, thus arresting the progressive nature of type 2 DM, could be paradigm changing, but to date medications have only shown to slow, not arrest, progression. In the UKPDS, insulin, metformin, or sulfonylureas did not halt β-cell failure. TZDs (out to 5 years with rosiglitazone) and GLP-1 agonists (open-label exenatide has shown durable HbA_{1c} reduction to 3 years and liraglutide to 2 years) may potentially slow β-cell failure. Pathophysiologically treating type 2 DM for potential β-cell preservation is possible, but unproven. It appears unlikely any one drug class will arrest β-cell failure, necessitating combination therapy. TZD and GLP-1 agonist combination is logical as TZDs reduce apoptosis of β cells and GLP-1 agonists augment pancreatic function through insulin secretion in a glucose-dependent manner and reduction of inappropriate glucagon, but long-term data are lacking. β-Cell function is heavily damaged by the time type 2 DM is diagnosed, and it is possible that β-cell failure is inevitable by type 2 DM diagnosis. HbA_{1c}

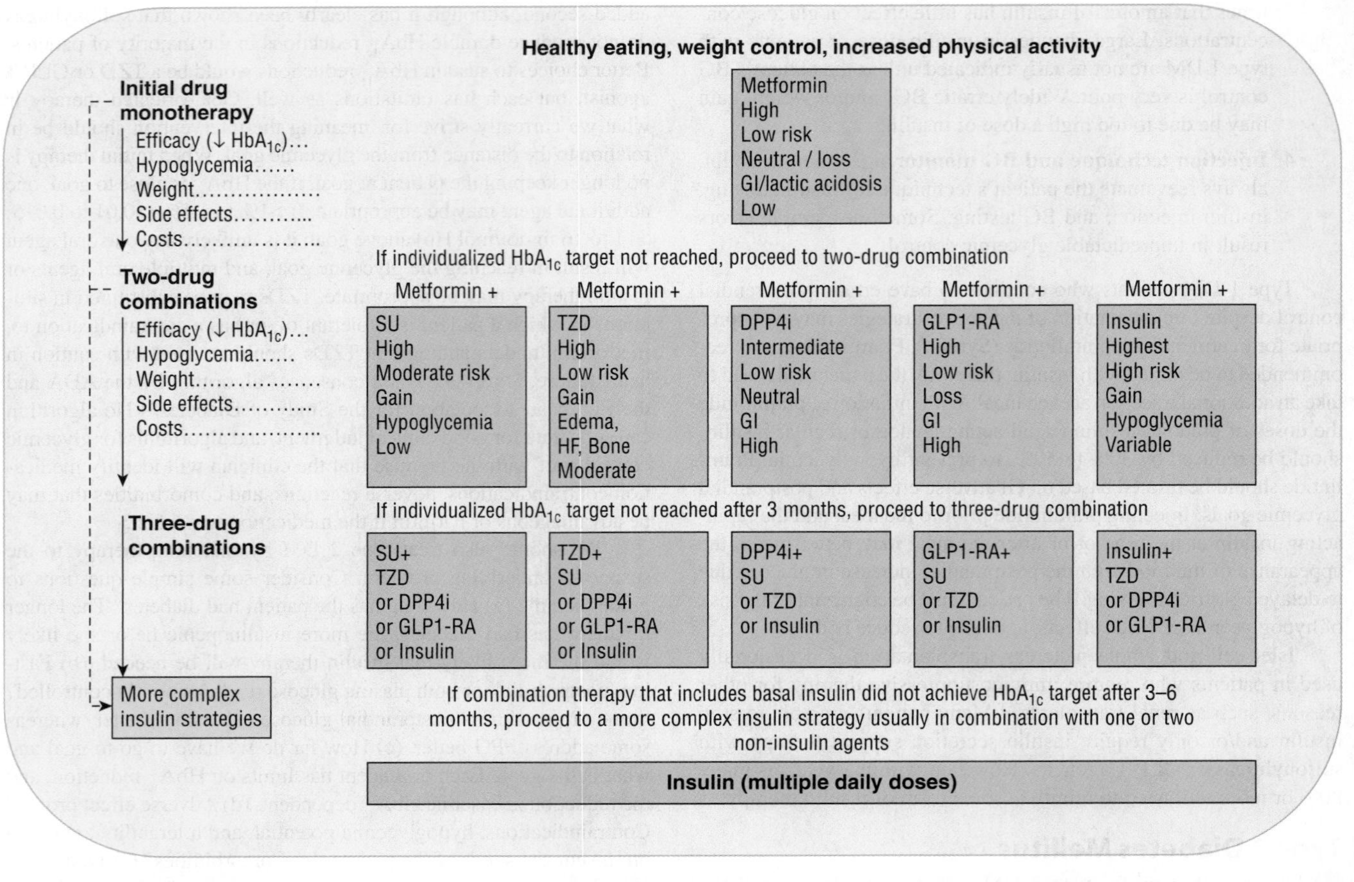

Healthy eating, weight control, increased physical activity

Initial drug monotherapy
Efficacy (↓ HbA_{1c})...
Hypoglycemia......
Weight..................
Side effects...........
Costs....................

Metformin
High
Low risk
Neutral / loss
GI/lactic acidosis
Low

If individualized HbA_{1c} target not reached, proceed to two-drug combination

Two-drug combinations
Efficacy (↓ HbA_{1c})...
Hypoglycemia......
Weight..................
Side effects...........
Costs....................

Metformin +	Metformin +	Metformin +	Metformin +	Metformin +
SU	TZD	DPP4i	GLP1-RA	Insulin
High	High	Intermediate	High	Highest
Moderate risk	Low risk	Low risk	Low risk	High risk
Gain	Gain	Neutral	Loss	Gain
Hypoglycemia	Edema, HF, Bone	GI	GI	Hypoglycemia
Low	Moderate	High	High	Variable

If individualized HbA_{1c} target not reached after 3 months, proceed to three-drug combination

Three-drug combinations

SU+	TZD+	DPP4i+	GLP1-RA+	Insulin+
TZD	SU	SU	SU	TZD
or DPP4i	or DPP4i	or TZD	or TZD	or DPP4i
or GLP1-RA	or GLP1-RA	or Insulin	or Insulin	or GLP1-RA
or Insulin	or Insulin			

More complex insulin strategies

If combination therapy that includes basal insulin did not achieve HbA_{1c} target after 3–6 months, proceed to a more complex insulin strategy usually in combination with one or two non-insulin agents

Insulin (multiple daily doses)

FIGURE 57-7 Position Statement on the Treatment of Type 2 Diabetes Mellitus: American Diabetes Association and European Association for the Study of Diabetes. *(Adapted from reference 54.)*

reduction is dependent on baseline values, with higher reductions seen with higher values, but, again, therapy should be goal oriented. Triple therapy is often with metformin, a sulfonylurea, and a TZD or DPP-4 inhibitor, but a logical alternative is to use metformin, a TZD, and a GLP-1 agonist, which can lower glucose levels and increase satiety, reducing the weight gain potential of a TZD, and still has a low risk of hypoglycemia. A DPP-4 inhibitor may be an alternative, although without weight loss potential, if an injectable product is not preferred. If the HbA_{1c} is >8.5% to 9% (>0.085 to 0.09; >69 to 75 mmol/mol Hb) on multiple therapies, insulin therapy should be considered. Sulfonylureas are often stopped when insulin is added and insulin sensitizers continued. This may be beneficial to decrease hypoglycemia, but continuing the sulfonylurea is permissible until multiple daily injections are started, at which time it should definitely be discontinued. Combination therapy with a TZD and insulin should be closely monitored for excessive weight gain and edema.

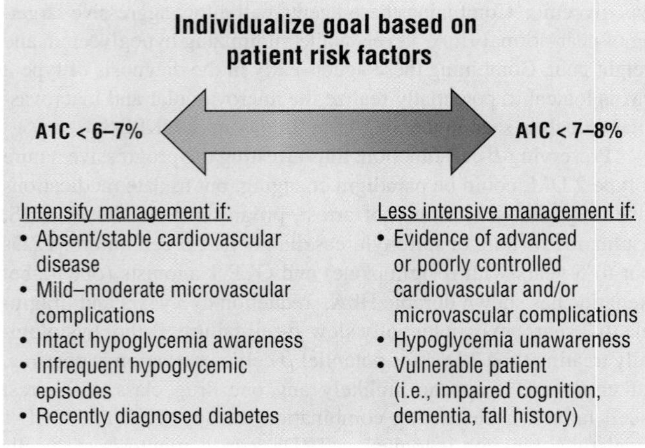

FIGURE 57-8 A1C goals. See *www.texasdiabetescouncil.org* for current algorithms. *(Reprinted with permission from the Texas Diabetes Council.)*

Virtually all patients with type 2 DM ultimately become relatively insulinopenic and will require insulin therapy. Insulin therapy for type 2 DM has changed dramatically in the last few years. Specifically, patients are often "transitioned" to insulin by using a bedtime injection of an intermediate- or long-acting insulin, and using oral agents primarily for control during the day. This strategy leads to less hyperinsulinemia during the day and is associated with less weight gain and has equal efficacy and a lower risk of hypoglycemia for up to 3 years when compared with starting prandial insulin or split-mix twice-daily insulin.[55] Because most patients are insulin resistant, insulin sensitizers are commonly used with insulin therapy. Patients with type 2 DM are usually well buffered against hypoglycemia. Patients should be monitored for hypoglycemia by asking about nocturnal sweating, nightmares (both indicative of nocturnal hypoglycemia), palpitations, tremulousness, and neuroglycopenic symptoms, as well as SMBG. When bedtime insulin plus daytime oral medications fail to achieve glycemic goals, a conventional multiple daily dose insulin regimen while continuing the insulin sensitizers is often tried. This may mean adding an injection of bolus insulin with the largest meal of the day for a total of two injections. If this is unsuccessful, a bolus injection can be given with the second largest meal of the day, for a total of three injections. After this, the standard basal–bolus model is followed. Alternatively, patients may be switched to split-mix insulin such as 70/30 mix insulin, Humalog Mix 75/25, or Novolog Mix 70/30. These are often given twice daily before the first and third meals (see Type 1 Diabetes Mellitus under Therapeutics above for longer explanation), but if inadequate control is seen, a third dose of mix insulin may be given with the third meal of the day. This allows for better prandial coverage, but can also increase the risk of hypoglycemia.[56] Use of GLP-1 agonists or pramlintide for prandial coverage can be considered. GLP-1 agonists, based on chosen drug, can be dosed weekly, daily, or twice daily, whereas pramlintide can be given before each meal. Concerns and problems with insulin administration as addressed in Type 1 Diabetes Mellitus under Therapeutics above generally relate to the therapy of type 2 DM. However, patients with type 2 DM rarely have hypoglycemia unawareness. Also, the variability of insulin resistance means that insulin doses may range from 0.7 to 2.5 units/kg or more. Figure 57-9 is an algorithm for insulin therapy

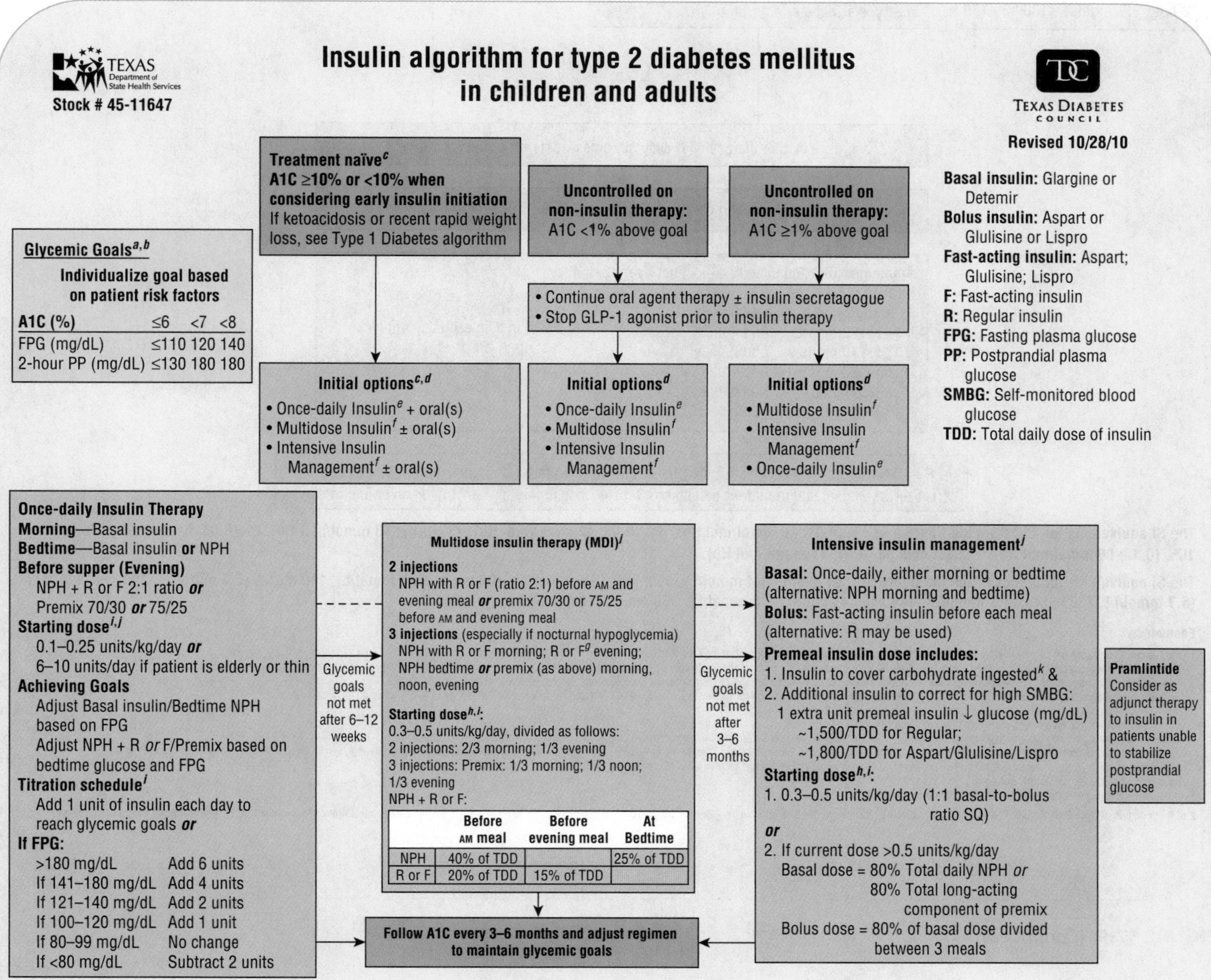

The SI equivalents for A1C from the figure are: 4% (0.04; 20 mmol/mol Hb), 6% (0.06; 42 mmol/mol Hb), 7% (0.07; 53 mmol/mol Hb), 8%(0.08; 64 mmol/mol Hb), 10% (0.10; 86 mmol/mol Hb), and 1% change (0.01; 11 mmol/mol Hb).

The SI equivalents for glucose from the figure are: 80 mg/dL (4.4 mmol/L), 99 mg/dL (5.5 mmol/L), 100 mg/dL (5.6 mmol/L), 110 mg/dL (6.1 mmol/L), 120, and 121 mg/dL (6.7 mmol/L), 130 mg/dL (7.2 mmol/L), 140 and 141 mg/dL (7.8 mmol/L), 180 mg/dL (10 mmol/L).

Footnotes:

[a] **Intensify management if:** Absent/stable cardiovascular disease, mild–moderate microvascular complications, intact hypoglycemia awareness, infrequent hypoglycemic episodes, recently diagnosed diabetes. **Less intensive management if**: Evidence of advanced or poorly controlled cardiovascular and/or microvascular complications, hypoglycemia unawareness, vulnerable patient (i.e., impaired cognition, dementia, fall history). SEE "A1C Goal" treatment strategy for further explanation. A1C is referenced to a nondiabetic range of 4–6% using a DCCT-based assay. (*ADA clinical practice recommendations. Diabetes Care* 2009;32(*suppl 1*)*:S19–S20.*)

[b] Current glucose meters give values corrected to plasma glucose.

[c] May also begin combination oral agent therapy. See *Glycemic Control Algorithm for Type 2 Diabetes Mellitus in Children and Adults.*

[d] Combining metformin with insulin therapy has been shown to result in less weight gain and better glycemic control with lower insulin requirements.

[e] Continue combination oral agent therapy ± sulfonylurea.

[f] Continue metformin (± third oral agent); probably discontinue sulfonylurea.

[g] Fast-acting insulin is given with the start of each meal. Regular insulin to be given 30–60 minutes before meals.

[h] Dosage may differ in children and adolescents; consider referral to pediatric endocrinologist/comprehensive diabetes specialty team.

[i] Start lower and increase slower for thin/elderly/complicated patients.

[j] Consider referral to pediatric/adult endocrinologist/diabetes specialty team (option—insulin pump, Pramlintide).

[k] Typical "carb" bolus = 1 unit bolus insulin covers 500/TDI x g carbohydrate from meal (~10–15 g); **strongly recommend referral to Registered/Licensed Dietitian or Certified Diabetes Educator with experience in diabetes nutrition counseling (see Worksheet D).**

1 of 6—Insulin Algorithm for Type 2 Diabetes Mellitus in Children and Adults—Revised 10/28/10

See disclaimer at www.tdctoolkit.org/algorithms_and_guidelines.asp

FIGURE 57-9 Insulin algorithm for type 2 DM in children and adults. See *www.texasdiabetescouncil.org* for current algorithms. *(Reprinted with permission from the Texas Diabetes Council.)*

TEXAS Department of State Health Services

Stock # 45-11647

Initiation of once-daily insulin therapy for type 2 diabetes mellitus In children and adults

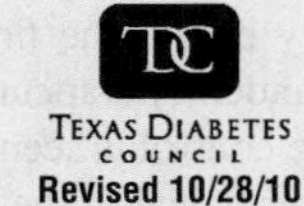

Texas Diabetes Council

Revised 10/28/10

FPG: Fasting plasma glucose
SMBG: Self-monitored blood glucose
PP: Postprandial plasma glucose

Glycemic Goals[b,c]

Individualize goal based on patient risk factors

A1C (%)	≤6	<7	<8
FPG (mg/dL)	≤110	120	140
2-hour PP (mg/dL)	≤130	180	180

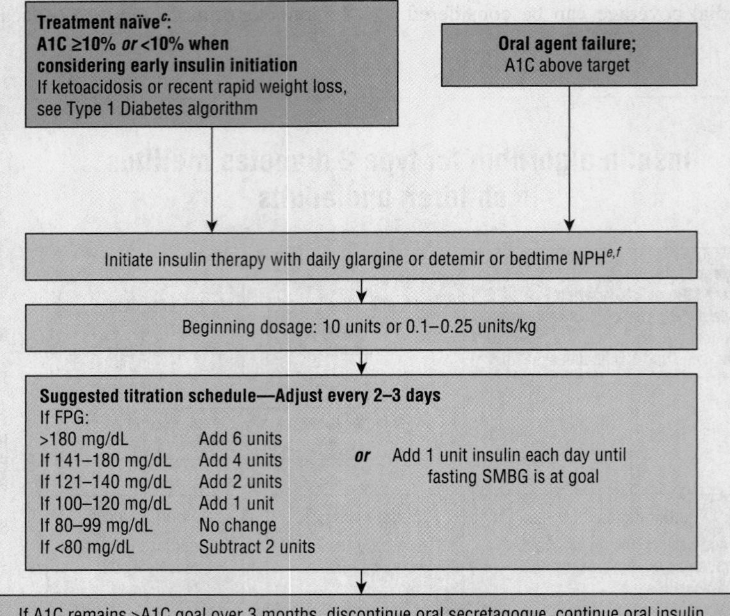

If A1C remains >A1C goal over 3 months, discontinue oral secretagogue, continue oral insulin sensitizer(s), and initiate multidose insulin or intensive insulin therapy[a] or consult an endocrinologist

The SI equivalents for A1C from the figure are: 4% (0.04; 20 mmol/mol Hb), 6% (0.06; 42 mmol/mol Hb), 7% (0.07; 53 mmol/mol Hb), 8%(0.08; 64 mmol/mol Hb), 10% (0.10; 86 mmol/mol Hb), and 1% change (0.01; 11 mmol/mol Hb).

The SI equivalents for glucose from the figure are: 80 mg/dL (4.4 mmol/L), 99 mg/dL (5.5 mmol/L), 100 mg/dL (5.6 mmol/L), 110 mg/dL (6.1 mmol/L), 120, and 121 mg/dL (6.7 mmol/L), 130 mg/dL (7.2 mmol/L), 140 and 141 mg/dL (7.8 mmol/L), 180 mg/dL (10 mmol/L).

Footnotes:

[a] For the complete approach to insulin initiation in Type 2 Diabetes Mellitus, see Insulin Algorithm for Type 2 Diabetes Mellitus in Children and Adults.

[b] **Intensify management if:** Absent/stable cardiovascular disease, mild–moderate microvascular complications, intact hypoglycemia awareness, infrequent hypoglycemic episodes, recently diagnosed diabetes.
Less intensive management if: Evidence of advanced or poorly controlled cardiovascular and/or microvascular complications, hypoglycemia unawareness, vulnerable patient (i.e., impaired cognition, dementia, fall history). See "A1C Goal" treatment strategy for further explanation. A1C is referenced to a nondiabetic range of 4–6% using a DCCT-based assay.
(*ADA clinical practice recommendations. Diabetes Care* 2009;32(*suppl 1*):*S19–S20*.)

[c] Current glucose meters give values corrected to plasma glucose.

[d] Usually with an insulin secretagogue (sulfonylurea, repaglinide, or nateglinide) and sensitizer (metformin, or thiazolidinedione). See Glycemic Control Algorithm.

[e] The pharmacokinetic profile of NPH compared with that of glargine or detemir is less predictable, therefore can result in blood sugar variations and increased nocturnal hypoglycemia. Cost of glargine or detemir is 1.5–2 times that of NPH. Lispro 75/25 or Aspart 70/30 can be considered at presupper adjusting dosage according to HS and fasting SMBG.

[f] ***Important***: See package insert for dosing.

[g] If daytime hypoglycemia develops, contact healthcare professional.

2 of 6 – Initiation of Once Daily Insulin Therapy for Type 2 Diabetes Mellitus in Children and Adults—Revised 10/28/10

FIGURE 57-9 (*Continued*)

options in type 2 diabetes developed by the Texas Diabetes Council. This algorithm gives most options for insulin therapy, but the choice of regimen should be individualized based on the discussion with the patient.

The availability of short-acting insulin secretagogues, rapid-acting insulin analogs, exenatide, DPP-4 inhibitors, and α-glucosidase inhibitors, all of which target postprandial glycemia, has reminded practitioners that glycemic control is a function of fasting, preprandial, and postprandial glycemic excursions. Many clinicians and patients neglect monitoring postprandial glucose. However, postprandial glycemic excursions proportionally contribute more than the FPG to the HbA_{1c} percentage when the HbA_{1c} nears goals, and thus will need to be targeted for optimal glycemic control in many patients. It remains controversial whether targeting after-meal glucose excursions will have more of an effect on complications risk than more conventional strategies.

Special Populations

Children and Adolescents with Type 2 DM

Type 2 DM is increasing in adolescence.[1,6] Obesity and physical inactivity seem to be particular culprits in the pathogenesis of this disease. Given the many years that the patient will have to live with diabetes, and recent evidence that the time frame after diagnosis for microvascular complications may mimic that of older adults, extraordinary efforts should be expended on lifestyle modification measures in an attempt to normalize glucose levels. Failing that strategy, the only labeled oral agent for use in children (10 to 16 years of age) is metformin, although sulfonylureas are also commonly used in therapy. TZDs and DPP-4 inhibitors have not been adequately studied in children, but studies to ascertain safety and efficacy are currently under way. GLP-1 agonist therapy, as it potentially helps the child to lose weight, is attractive, but the long-term effects of this therapeutic modality are unknown. Insulin therapy continues to be the standard therapy after metformin and a sulfonylurea. In adolescent females, the possibility of future pregnancy should be considered in the prescription of any drug regimen. Screening and recommendations for treatment of hypertension, dyslipidemia, nephropathy, retinopathy, hypothyroidism, and celiac disease are available.[6]

Elderly Patients with DM

Elderly patients with newly diagnosed DM (almost always type 2 DM) present a different therapeutic challenge. Consideration of the risks of hypoglycemia, the extent of comorbidities including severe microvascular disease, CVD, dexterity, self-care and social situations, falls risk, mental status, and the probable life span should help determine glycemic goals. If extensive comorbidities, hypoglycemic unawareness, unstable CVD, dementia, high falls risk, or similar diagnosis is made, the clinician may adjust the glycemic goal. Avoidance of hypoglycemia, especially severe hypoglycemia, as well as elevated glucose levels that may exacerbate the comorbidities is necessary (Fig. 57-8). It should also be remembered that elderly may have an altered presentation of hypoglycemia, as they lose adrenergic symptoms due to loss of autonomic nerve function as they age. This may raise the rise of neuroglycopenic symptoms shortly after identification of hypoglycemia. If the patient is newly diagnosed and does not have the above problems, a goal HbA_{1c} <7% (<0.07; <53 mmol/mol Hb) is justified. If the person has significant comorbidities as mentioned above, then a goal <8% (<0.08; <64 mmol/mol Hb) may be reasonable, and if the person has "end-stage" illness, glycemic control should limit symptomatic (polyuria/polydipsia) or mental status issues. If oral agents will work, DPP-4 inhibitors, shorter-acting insulin secretagogues, low-dose sulfonylureas (preferably not long-acting ones), or α-glucosidase inhibitors may be used. The risk for lactic acidosis, which increases with older age and the age-related decline in renal function, makes metformin therapy difficult, but lower doses may be used if not contraindicated. In a patient in whom weight gain or loss may not be unwelcome, TZDs or GLP-1 agonists, respectively, may be considered, but falls risk and fracture risk must be considered with TZDs. DPP-4 inhibitors or α-glucosidase inhibitors are oral medications that may be advantageous due to a low risk of hypoglycemia. Simple insulin regimens such as an injection of basal insulin daily may be appropriate for glycemic control in elderly patients, especially if tight glycemic control is not the goal. The Texas Diabetes Council publishes an algorithm; see *www.tdctoolkit.org*.

Gestational DM and Pregnancy with Preexisting Diabetes

GDM is diagnosed as previously described. The adverse outcomes associated with GDM include birth defects, increased rates of miscarriage, necessity of cesarean section delivery, neonatal hypoglycemia, preeclampsia/eclampsia, preterm delivery, shoulder dystocia/birth injury, and hyperbilirubinemia. Dietary therapy to minimize wide fluctuations in BG is of paramount importance.[5,8] Intensive educational efforts are usually necessary. Pregnant women without DM maintain plasma glucose concentrations between 50 and 130 mg/dL (2.8 and 7.2 mmol/L). Normoglycemia is the goal, and failure to maintain this despite dietary interventions often will necessitate medication use. Goals during therapy are *minimally* a preprandial goal of ≤90 mg/dL (≤5 mmol/L), and either 1-hour postprandial plasma glucose levels ≤120 mg/dL (≤6.7 mmol/L) or 2-hour postprandial plasma glucose levels ≤110 mg/dL (≤6.1 mmol/L), and avoidance of ketones as much as possible. In patients who have preexisting type 1 or type 2 DM and become pregnant, premeal, bedtime, and overnight glucose should be 60 to 90 mg/dL (3.3 to 5 mmol/L), with a peak postprandial of 100 to 120 mg/dL (5.6 to 6.7 mmol/L). HbA_{1c} during pregnancy

Clinical **Controversy...**

Treatment of Type 2 Dm in Older Adults

The U.S. population continues to age. The ACCORD,[48] ADVANCE,[49] and VADT[50] had older individuals who were in their 60s at enrollment. As stated earlier in the chapter, all improved glycemic control but did not reduce the risk of CVD over 3 to 5 years, although more people died in the ACCORD, resulting in termination of the study. ADVANCE reported improvement in nephropathy outcomes, and this did not differ by age, but otherwise these neutral studies did not report improved microvascular outcomes. In addition, one Japanese study had subjects with a mean age of 72 years, and a 6-year follow-up, but changes in glycemia were minimal, thus showing no benefit.[57] This is unfortunate, as up to one in three people in this age category may have type 2 DM. Diabetes in older adults is complicated by clinical and functional heterogeneity. Patients may be relatively healthy, free-living adults all the way to the other end of the spectrum with assistive living, multiple comorbidities, and cognitive issues. Based on this, what is the optimal medication therapy for this group of individuals?

Critical evaluation of most medications in populations over 65 years of age is severely lacking. Many clinicians have decided that insulin, especially basal insulin, is a reasonable choice in this age group, and that minimal orals (maybe metformin if not contraindicated) are reasonable. Yet, in the new ADA guidelines and clinical practice recommendations, a patient-centered approach is stated. It is unlikely that most patients would choose basal insulin as their initial intervention if asked. Also, the cost for basal insulin is not minimal, and one must ask if it is truly more cost-effective than many other interventions. Severe hypoglycemia must be avoided in this population, as it has been associated with a higher risk of death for more than 1 year after the incident. Any of the agents can avoid severe hypoglycemia if used properly, but the risk factors for hypoglycemia are: use of insulin or insulin secretagogues, duration of diabetes, antecedent hypoglycemia, erratic meals, exercise, and renal insufficiency. In addition, self-care, visual acuity, and dexterity issues may be of concern in patients.

Medications that do not cause hypoglycemia may be advantageous. Metformin, if not contraindicated, continues to be an excellent first choice. As metformin may be used in Stage III CKD, with a reduced dose, this may be a reasonable choice. Second-choice agents such as DPP-4 inhibitors, if close to the chosen HbA_{1c} goal, or a GLP-1 receptor agonist, if farther from the chosen goal, may be warranted. Each has its own issues, as both may be cost prohibitive and GLP-1 receptor agonists may be inappropriate for patients with GI issues or gastroparesis, or normal-weight to underweight patients. α-Glucosidase inhibitors, if close to goal and constipation is an issue, may be helped by these agents, although GI tolerability is problematic.

As the care for people with diabetes improves, it is imperative that issues concerning older adults continue to be addressed. It is important for our society that optimal therapy in older adults be properly addressed, as this population will continue to grow, and currently there is no consensus. Several organizations have recommendations in regards to older adults,[58,59] but recommendations on optimal pharmacotherapy are not included.

should be less than 6% (<0.06; <42 mmol/mol Hb), but frequent SMBG is the method of choice for monitoring glycemic control. Titration of insulin and switching to more complicated regimens is guided by SMBG results. Use of basal insulins other than NPH is still debated, but with the ease of use of detemir or glargine insulin, their use in GDM is increasing. In addition, pump therapy for the duration of the pregnancy is often instituted, as it can obtain excellent glycemic control and is quickly adjustable. Both metformin and glyburide have been studied as alternatives to insulin therapy. Glyburide was not detected in the cord serum of any infant in one study, whereas metformin crosses the placenta. Further study is needed prior to routinely recommending them in GDM. Patients with GDM should be evaluated 6 weeks after delivery to ensure that normal glucose tolerance has returned. Because these patients' lifetime risk for the development of type 2 DM is >50%, periodic assessment after that is warranted.

Clinical **Controversy. . .**

Oral Agents in Pregnancy

The use of oral antidiabetic agents for the management of gestational diabetes or type 2 DM during pregnancy is controversial. For those patients who fail to maintain optimal glycemic control during pregnancy with diet and lifestyle modification, traditionally the next step has been to proceed with insulin therapy. More recently, however, some clinicians have begun using oral agents including sulfonylureas and/or metformin in patients with GDM or type 2 DM during pregnancy.

A randomized, open-label, controlled trial evaluated the efficacy of glyburide compared with insulin initiated after 11 weeks' gestation.[60] The control of BG compared with insulin therapy was similar, with less hypoglycemia in the glyburide group. There was not any evidence of significant difference in complications, including cord serum insulin concentrations, incidence of macrosomia (birth weight ≥4,000 g), cesarean delivery, or neonatal hypoglycemia between regimens. Glyburide was not detected in the cord serum of any infant. However, this study limited enrollment to beyond 11 weeks' gestation; therefore, no conclusions can be made regarding teratogenicity from using glyburide in the first trimester.

A more recent retrospective cohort study of 10,682 women with GDM who required medical therapy, however, revealed that babies born to women with GDM who were managed on glyburide were more likely to be macrosomic and to be admitted to the intensive care unit compared with those treated with insulin therapy.[61]

Metformin has also been used in the management of GDM and type 2 DM in pregnancy, and also in polycystic ovarian syndrome to prevent miscarriage. Early studies dating back to the 1980s did not show any differences in perinatal mortality, maternal hypoglycemia, lactic acidosis, or congenital anomalies.[62,63]

However, a more recent cohort study investigating the effects of metformin, sulfonylureas, and insulin in pregnant women with diabetes found a significantly higher rate of preeclampsia in women treated with metformin compared with women treated with sulfonylurea or insulin (32% metformin vs. 7% sulfonylureas vs. 10% insulin). The perinatal mortality was also significantly increased in women treated with metformin in the third trimester compared with women not treated with metformin (11.6% vs. 1.3%).[64]

In contrast, another study of 751 women with GDM randomly assigned subjects at 20 to 33 weeks of gestation to open treatment with metformin (with supplemental insulin if required) or insulin. This study did not find any increased rate of preeclampsia or other perinatal complications compared with insulin.[65]

Subsequently there have also been meta-analyses that also revealed no differences in maternal or neonatal outcomes with the use of glyburide or metformin compared with the use of insulin in women with GDM.[66,67]

The current guidelines of the ADA continue to suggest insulin therapy as the preferred treatment for managing women with gestational diabetes or type 2 DM in pregnancy who fail to achieve optimal control with diet/lifestyle modification alone.[68] Moreover, neither metformin nor glyburide has formal FDA approval for the management of diabetes in pregnancy.

The use of oral antidiabetic agents in pregnancy is becoming more common, but nevertheless remains controversial. Clinicians who prescribe oral agents to manage their patients with diabetes during pregnancy must consider the potential benefits (avoidance of injections, decreased cost, and patient preference) against the potential risk (unknown safety, inconsistent effect on the pregnancy outcomes, and potential liability due to using non–FDA-approved therapy).

Special Situations

Sick Days

Acute self-limited illness rarely presents a major problem for patients with type 2 DM, but can be a significant challenge for insulinopenic type 1 DM patients.[69] While caloric intake generally declines, insulin sensitivity also decreases, meaning that it may take greater amounts of insulin to control BG concentrations. Patients need to be adept at frequent SMBG, checking urine ketones, use of short-acting insulin, and understanding that sugar intake in this situation is not detrimental but may be necessary to balance the glucose levels when extra insulin is needed during illness. Plan to maintain a meal plan containing 120 to 150 g of carbohydrates per day. We encourage patients to continue their usual insulin regimen and to use supplemental rapid-acting insulin based on SMBG results, with additional insulin given if ketonuria develops. Ketone testing should be in type 1 DM patients prone to ketonuria, if two consecutive plasma glucose readings are above 250 mg/dL (13.9 mmol/L), or if vomiting occurs, as it is a possible sign of ketosis. Sugar and electrolyte solutions, can be used to maintain hydration, to provide needed electrolytes if there are significant GI or urinary losses, and to provide sugar to keep the patient from developing hypoglycemia because of the extra insulin that is usually needed. If patients with type 1 DM are consistently hyperglycemic, we suggest they abstain from sugary drinks and increase intake of sugar-free liquids. In contrast, patients with type 2 DM may need to switch to sugar-free drinks if BG levels are continually elevated. Most patients can be taught how to sufficiently manage sick days and avoid hospitalization.

Diabetic Ketoacidosis and Hyperosmolar Hyperglycemic State

DKA and HHS are true diabetic emergencies.[70] A comprehensive discussion of their treatment is beyond the scope of this chapter. In patients with known diabetes, DKA is usually precipitated by insulin omission in type 1 DM, and intercurrent illness, particularly infection, in both type 1 and type 2 DM. However, patients with type 1 or type 2 DM (the latter being usually nonwhites or Hispanics) may present with DKA at initial presentation. It is possible that some of the patients deemed to have type 2 DM actually have type 1 idiopathic DM. Patients with DKA may be alert, stuporous, or comatose at presentation. The hallmark diagnostic laboratory values for DKA include hyperglycemia, anion gap acidosis, and large ketonemia or ketonuria. Diagnostic criteria for HHS are similar with the exception of significantly higher plasma glucose, elevated effective serum osmolality, and little to no ketonuria or ketonemia when compared with DKA. HHS typically evolves over several days to weeks, whereas DKA evolves much quickly. Afflicted patients will have either fluid deficits of several liters or sodium and potassium deficits of several hundred milliequivalents. Restoration of intravascular volume acutely with normal saline, followed by hypotonic saline to replace free water, potassium supplements, and constant infusion of insulin restore the patient's metabolic status relatively quickly. A flow sheet is often helpful in tracking the fluid and insulin therapies and laboratory parameters in these patients. Bicarbonate administration is generally not needed and may be harmful, especially in children. Treatment of the inciting medical condition is also vital. Hourly bedside monitoring of glucose and frequent monitoring (every 2 to 4 hours) of potassium is essential. Metabolic improvement is manifested by an increase in the serum bicarbonate or pH. Serum phosphorus usually starts high and plummets to lower-than-normal levels, although replacing phosphorus, while not unreasonable, is of questionable benefit in most patients. Fluid administration alone will reduce the glucose concentration, so a decrement in glucose values does not necessarily mean that the patient's metabolic status is improving. Rare patients will require larger amounts of insulin than those usually given (5 to 10 units/h). We double the patient's insulin dose if the serum bicarbonate has not improved after the first 4 hours of insulin therapy. Constant infusion of a fixed dose of insulin and the administration of IV glucose when the BG level decreases to <250 mg/dL (<13.9 mmol/L) are preferable to titration of the insulin infusion based on the glucose level. The latter strategy may delay clearance of the ketosis and prolong treatment. The insulin infusion should be continued until the urine ketones clear and the anion gap closes. Long-acting insulin should be given 1 to 3 hours prior to discontinuing the insulin infusion. Intramuscular regular insulin or subcutaneous insulin lispro or aspart given every 1 to 2 hours can be utilized rather than an insulin infusion in patients without hypoperfusion. Patients may develop hyperchloremic metabolic acidosis with treatment if they have been given large volumes of normal saline in the course of their treatment. Such a situation does not require any specific treatment.

HHS usually occurs in older patients with type 2 DM, at times undiagnosed, or in younger patients with prolonged hyperglycemia and dehydration or significant renal insufficiency. Large ketonemia is usually not seen, as residual insulin secretion suppresses lipolysis. Infection or another medical illness is the usual precipitant. Fluid deficits are usually greater and BG concentrations higher (at times >1,000 mg/dL [>55.5 mmol/L]) in these patients than in patients with DKA. BG levels should be lowered very gradually with hypotonic fluids and low-dose insulin infusions (1 to 2 units/h). Rapid correction of the glucose levels, a drop greater than 75 to 100 mg/dL/h (4.2 to 5.6 mmol/L/h), is not recommended, as it can result in cerebral edema. This is especially true for children with DKA. Mortality is high with the HHS.

Hospitalization for Intercurrent Medical Illness

Patients on oral agents may need transient therapy with insulin to achieve adequate glycemic control. In patients requiring insulin, patients should receive scheduled doses of insulin with additional short-acting insulin. "Sliding-scale" insulin is to be discouraged, as it is notorious for not controlling glucose and for sometimes resulting in therapeutic misadventures, with wide amplitudes of glycemic excursions.[71] In-hospital mortality is increased in many hyperglycemic conditions. At least one study documented a reduction in mortality in type 2 diabetes patients with acute MIs[72] who receive constant IV insulin during the acute phase of the event to maintain near-normal glucose concentrations. Similar mortality results have been documented in some intensive care unit settings using IV insulin and tight glucose control.[72,73] The ADA and American Association of Clinical Endocrinologists released a joint consensus statement on inpatient glycemic control stating that glucose control measures should be implemented if the BG is ≥180 mg/dL (≥10 mmol/L), and maintained between 140 and 180 mg/dL (7.8 and 10 mmol/L).[74] The Normoglycemia in Intensive Care Evaluation—Survival Using Glucose Algorithm Regulation trial, and several other negative trials, has resulted in this loosening of inpatient glycemic goals. Critically ill patients had higher 90-day mortality when a goal of 81 to 108 mg/dL (4.5 to 6 mmol/L) was targeted than when BG of ≤180 mg/dL (≤10 mmol/L) (achieved 144 mg/dL [8 mmol/L]) was targeted.[75] For non–critically ill patients there are no established BG goals. Reasonable BG goals for these patients are <140 mg/dL (<7.8 mmol/L) premeal and <180 mg/dL (<10 mmol/L) random.[5] Many protocols for IV insulin infusion are currently available, and implementation for an inpatient setting should use a well-established protocol. It is prudent to stop metformin in all patients who arrive in acute care settings until full elucidation of the reason for presentation can be ascertained, as contraindications to metformin are prevalent in hospitalized patients. Discharge planning is also important, as approximately one third of patients will have newly diagnosed diabetes and another one third will likely have prediabetes, as determined by obtaining an HbA_{1c} on admission (best) or prior to discharge.

Perioperative Management

Surgical patients may experience worsening of glycemia for reasons similar to those listed above for intercurrent medical illness. Therapy should be individualized based on the type of DM, nature of the surgical procedure, previous therapy, and metabolic control prior to the procedure. Patients on oral agents may need transient therapy with insulin to control BG. In patients requiring insulin, scheduled doses of insulin or continuous insulin infusions are preferred. For patients who can eat soon after surgery, the time-honored approach of giving one half of the usual morning NPH insulin dose with dextrose 5% in water IV is acceptable, with resumption of scheduled insulin, perhaps at reduced doses, within the first day. Patients receiving basal/bolus insulin therapy can continue receiving their usual dose of long-acting insulin while holding the premeal bolus doses until the patient can tolerate meals. For patients requiring more prolonged periods without oral nutrition and for major surgery, such as coronary artery bypass grafting and major abdominal surgery, constant infusion of IV insulin is preferred. Use of IV insulin infusion has been shown to reduce deep sternal wound infections in patients after coronary artery bypass grafting, although there is no need to start the infusion during or before the procedure. Metformin should be discontinued temporarily after any major surgery until it is clear that the patient is hemodynamically stable and normal renal function is documented.

Reproductive-Age Women and Preconception Care for Women

An increasing prevalence of DM has been noted in reproductive-age women.[5,76,77] Prepregnancy planning is absolutely mandatory, as organogenesis is largely completed within 8 weeks, so good glycemic control should be obtained prior to conception. Unfortunately, major congenital malformations due to poor glucose control remain the leading cause of mortality and serious morbidity in infants of mothers with type 1 or type 2 DM. For women with DM controlled by lifestyle measures alone, conversion to insulin as soon as the pregnancy is confirmed is appropriate. Patients previously treated with insulin may need intensification of their regimen to achieve therapeutic goals. Normal pregnancy is associated with a decrease in the BG concentration as it is diverted to the fetus.

Human Immunodeficiency Virus (HIV) Patients and Diabetes

Patients living with HIV are at higher risk for the development of type 2 DM.[78] This risk may be related to HIV infection, concomitant infections such as hepatitis C, and concomitant medications often used to treat HIV or comorbidities. Pentamidine, used for *P. carinii* pneumonia, is directly β-cell toxic in some patients; hypoglycemia may be followed by hyperglycemia. Megestrol, used as an appetite stimulant, can have glucocorticoid-like effects in some patients. In addition, protease inhibitors, used to manage HIV, have been shown to potentially worsen insulin sensitivity, decrease the ability of the β cell to secrete insulin, and/or worsen lipotoxicity. Long-term stavudine may also increase the risk of diabetes. Redistribution of fat from medication or HIV infection, with resultant increases in visceral fat and decreases in subcutaneous fat, is not uncommon. Metformin continues to be the first-line therapy choice for HIV patients, as weight gain can be minimized, but additional cautions must be noted. Stavudine, zidovudine, and didanosine may cause lactemia, especially on long-term use, whereas abacavir, lamivudine, and tenofovir have less incidence of lactemia. It may be advisable to check lactate levels in appropriate subjects prior to metformin use. If lactate levels are greater than two times normal, alternative therapy should be considered. If excess visceral adiposity is noted, a TZD, which redistributes fat back to subcutaneous adipose tissue and causes visceral fat apoptosis, may be considered. Significant drug–drug interactions may also be present (refer to specific diabetes drugs in Chap. 103).

Special Topics

Prevention of Diabetes Mellitus

13 Efforts to prevent type 1 DM with niacinamide, injected insulin, or oral insulin therapy have been unsuccessful. Anti-CD3 and anti-CD20 monoclonal antibodies and a GAD vaccine have shown to delay, but not stop, β-cell destruction in type 1 DM. In addition, a 24–amino acid sequence derived from human heat shock protein 60 called DiaPep277® may slow loss of C-peptide secretion in type 1 DM. Future directions include potential combination therapy trials. The Diabetes Prevention Program[79] confirmed that modest weight loss in association with exercise can have a dramatic impact on insulin sensitivity and the conversion from IGT to type 2 diabetes. In this study approximately 2,000 individuals with IGT were randomized to lifestyle changes (diet, exercise, and weight loss) versus usual care. The study, which was originally planned to be ongoing for 5 years, was stopped early after 2.8 years. The usual care group developed diabetes at the rate of 11% each year. The lifestyle arm developed diabetes at a rate of 5% per year, a 58% reduction in the risk of developing diabetes.[79] Surprisingly, a modest amount of diet and exercise yielded impressive results. The exercise program in the lifestyle group was walking 30 minutes 5 days each week. The mean weight loss over the 2.8-year study period was only 8 lb (3.6 kg). In the Diabetes Prevention Program[79] discussed above, approximately 1,000 of the study patients were randomized to metformin therapy. Metformin therapy reduced the risk of developing type 2 DM by 31% compared with usual care and resulted in a 4-lb (1.8-kg) weight loss. Interestingly, young and overweight individuals on metformin had a greater reduction in the risk of developing diabetes than normal-weight and older study patients.[79]

All diabetes medications studied for the prevention of diabetes, when discontinued, do not appear to have residual positive effects on β-cell function. Thus, patients must continue the medication for continued "prevention," although the question arises if this is merely early treatment. Troglitazone, a TZD removed from the market, was able to prevent the development of diabetes in women with a history of gestational diabetes. Total preservation of β-cell function was demonstrated over a 5-year period in women who had near-normal β-cell function at baseline and who initially responded to the drug.[80] The preservation of β-cell function was observed for at least 8 months after the drug had been discontinued. The DREAM trial evaluated rosiglitazone and/or ramipril treatment for the delay or prevention of type 2 DM in impaired glucose-tolerant subjects.[81,82] Rosiglitazone 8 mg daily, over approximately 3 years, reduced the incidence of type 2 diabetes by 60%. In addition, a 37% nonsignificant increase in cardiovascular events was reported. Ramipril 15 mg daily did not significantly prevent the conversion to diabetes. It is possible that longer exposure could have made a difference, but the study was stopped prematurely. In contrast, valsartan, an angiotensin receptor blocker (ARB), administered for 5 years was recently reported to reduce the risk of progression from IGT to type 2 DM by 14%. The ACT Now trial used pioglitazone 45 mg daily in an IGT population and found a 72% reduction in the risk of development of diabetes over 2.4 years.[83] It should be noted that no pharmacologic agents are currently FDA approved or recommended for prevention of type 2 diabetes, although the ADA recommends metformin in conjunction with lifestyle changes if the patient is younger, obese, has a family history of diabetes, dyslipidemia, hypertension, or a HbA_{1c} >6% (>0.06; >42 mmol/mol Hb).[5] The next step is discussions with the FDA to decide how and if medications to prevent diabetes can be approved for this indication.

Patient Education

14 It is not satisfactory to give patients with DM brief instructions with a few pamphlets and expect them to manage their disease adequately.[84] Diabetes education is a lifetime exercise. Successful treatment of DM involves lifestyle changes for the patient (e.g., medical nutrition therapy, physical activity, SMBG and possibly of urine for ketones, recognition of hyperglycemia and hypoglycemia, and taking prescribed medications). The American Association of Diabetes Educators (AADE) has developed the AADE7 self-care behaviors of healthy eating, being active, monitoring, taking medication, problem solving, reducing risk, and healthy coping, which is a good starting framework for patient discussions. The patient must be involved in the decision-making process and must learn as much about the disease and associated complications as possible. Emphasis should be placed on the evidence that indicates that complications can be prevented or minimized with glycemic control and management of risk factors for CVD. Recognition of the need for proper patient education to empower them into self-care has generated programs for certification in diabetes education for pharmacists. Certified diabetes educators (CDEs) must document their patient education hours and sit for a certification examination that assesses the knowledge, tasks, and skills of an educator in order to become certified. An increasing number of nurses, pharmacists, dietitians, and physicians are becoming CDEs to document to the public that they meet a minimum standard for diabetes education, and to fulfill

quality initiatives in meeting guidelines for education recognition. Being a CDE does not guarantee reimbursement of services, and CDEs who are not dietitians will often need to become part of a recognized program to obtain reimbursement. Currently the AADE and ADA have accreditation programs.

Treatment of Concomitant Conditions and Complications

Retinopathy

Patients with established retinopathy should see an ophthalmologist or optometrist trained in diabetic eye disease. A dilated eye examination is required to fully evaluate diabetic eye disease. Early background retinopathy may reverse with improved glycemic control and optimized blood pressure control. More advanced retinopathy will not fully regress with improved glycemia, but caution should be taken on the expediency of glycemia lowering, as aggressive reductions in glycemia may acutely worsen retinopathy. The pathophysiology of retinopathy is better understood to involve inappropriate growth factor increase and microcirculation ischemia. Bevacizumab, used off-label, and ranibizumab, recently FDA approved, are antivascular endothelial growth factor monoclonal antibodies given by intravitreal injection. Although approved for macular edema, use may also apply to other neovascular ocular conditions. A protein kinase C inhibitor has been studied, but results have been modest. Laser photocoagulation has markedly improved sight preservation in diabetic patients. People with diabetes also have a higher rate of cataracts and possibly open-angle glaucoma.

Neuropathy

Neuropathy in diabetes can generally be placed into three categories: peripheral neuropathy, autonomic neuropathy, and focal neuropathy. Distal symmetrical peripheral neuropathy is the most common complication seen in type 2 DM patients in outpatient clinics.[85] Paresthesias, perceived hot or cold, numbness, or pain may be the predominant symptom. The feet are involved far more often than the hands as it affects longer nerves first and progresses proximally. Improved glycemic control is the primary treatment and may alleviate some of the symptoms. If neuropathy is painful, symptomatic pain treatment is indicated, although it will not change the course of the neuropathy nor has one medication been shown to be superior to another. Treatment may be with low-dose tricyclic antidepressants, anticonvulsants (gabapentin, pregabalin, rarely carbamazepine), duloxetine, venlafaxine, topical capsaicin, and various pain medications, including tramadol and nonsteroidal antiinflammatory drugs. Duloxetine and pregabalin have FDA approval for this indication. The numb variant of peripheral neuropathy is not treated with medication, but may lead to pressure areas on the foot and subsequent ulcer in a subset of patients. Clinical manifestations of diabetic autonomic neuropathy include resting tachycardia, exercise intolerance, orthostatic hypotension, constipation, gastroparesis, erectile dysfunction, sudomotor dysfunction (anhidrosis, heat intolerance, gustatory sweating, and/or dry skin), impaired neurovascular function, and hypoglycemic autonomic failure. Gastroparesis can be a severe and debilitating complication of DM. Improved glycemic control, discontinuation of medications that slow gastric motility, and the use of metoclopramide (preferably for only a few weeks at a time) or low-dose erythromycin may be helpful. Gastric pacemakers as therapeutic hardware are rarely used, though available. Cisapride, removed from the market several years ago, is still available for compassionate use and domperidone, available outside of the United States, may be useful. Orthostatic hypotension, after stopping antihypertensives and liberalizing dietary sodium intake, may require pharmacologic management with mineralocorticoids or adrenergic agonist agents. In severe cases, supine hypertension is extreme, mandating that the patient sleep in a sitting or semirecumbent position. Patients with cardiac autonomic neuropathy are at a higher risk for silent MI and sudden cardiac death. The hallmark of diabetic diarrhea is its nocturnal occurrence. Diabetic diarrhea frequently responds to a 10- to 14-day course of an antibiotic such as doxycycline or metronidazole. In more unresponsive cases, octreotide may be useful. Erectile dysfunction is common in diabetes, and initial treatment should include a trial of one of the phosphodiesterase type 5 inhibitors prior to referral. People with diabetes often require the highest doses of these medications to have an adequate response. Sudomotor dysfunction, as earlier defined, results in loss of sweating and resultant dry, cracked skin. Use of hydrating creams and ointments is needed. Hypoglycemic unawareness requires the patient to avoid hypoglycemia, as the body will slowly increase the glycemic level at which it will signal the autonomic signals, although damage may severely lessen the response. Focal neuropathies are uncommon, but occur more often in older, poorly controlled diabetes patients. Diabetic amyotrophy, which is characterized by a proximal thigh muscle pain and weakness, is one of the most debilitating. In addition, cranial nerve III, IV, and VI neuropathies, as well as Bell's palsy, may occur. The presentation can be quite dramatic, but the course is usually self-limited, and partial or full recovery happens in a few weeks to months. Carpal tunnel syndrome, caused by radial nerve entrapment, is also more common in people with diabetes,

Microalbuminuria and Nephropathy

DM, particularly type 2 DM, is the biggest contributor statistically to the development of end-stage renal disease in the United States.[1,5] The ADA recommends a screening urinary analysis for albumin at diagnosis in persons with type 2 DM. Precise onset of type 2 DM can rarely be ascertained, and patients will often present at diagnosis with microvascular complications. In type 1 DM, microalbuminuria rarely occurs with short duration of disease or before puberty. Screening individuals with type 1 DM should begin with puberty and after 5 years' disease duration. There are three methods for assessing microalbuminuria: (a) measurement of the urine albumin-to-creatinine ratio in a random spot collection (preferably the first morning void); (b) 24-hour timed collection; and (c) timed (e.g., 4- or 10-hour overnight) collection. Microalbuminuria on a spot urine specimen is defined as an albumin-to-creatinine ratio of 30 to 300 mg/g (3.4 to 34 mg/mmol creatinine). On timed collections, microalbuminuria is defined as 30 to 300 mg/24 hours or an albumin excretion rate of 20 to 200 mcg/min. Because of day-to-day variability, microalbuminuria should be confirmed on at least two of three samples over 3 to 6 months unless unequivocal. Additionally, when assessing urine protein or albumin, conditions that may cause transient elevations in urinary albumin excretion should be excluded. These conditions include intense exercise, recent urinary tract infections, hypertension, short-term hyperglycemia, heart failure, and acute febrile illness.[5]

In type 2 DM, the presence of microalbuminuria is a strong risk factor for macrovascular disease and is frequently present at the time of diagnosis. Microalbuminuria is a weaker predictor for future end-stage kidney disease in type 2 versus type 1 DM. Glucose and blood pressure control are most important for the prevention of nephropathy, and blood pressure control is the most important for retarding the progression of established nephropathy. ACE inhibitors and ARBs, considered first-line recommended treatment modalities, have shown efficacy in preventing the clinical progression of renal disease in patients with diabetes. Combined renin–angiotensin–aldosterone system blockage (with ACE inhibitors, ARBs, aldosterone receptor blockers, and/or direct renin inhibitors) cannot currently be recommended for routine practice in nephropathy. Diuretics frequently are necessary due to the volume-expanded state of the patient and are recommended second-line therapy. The ADA and the National Kidney Foundation blood pressure goal of <130/80 mm Hg can be difficult to achieve. Three or more antihypertensives are often needed to treat to goal blood pressures (see also Chap. 29).

Peripheral Vascular Disease and Foot Ulcers

Claudication and nonhealing foot ulcers are common in type 2 DM patients.[86] Smoking cessation, correction of lipid abnormalities, and antiplatelet therapy are important strategies in treating claudicants. Cilostazol may be useful for reducing intermittent claudication symptoms in select patients. Revascularization is successful in selected patients, although small vessel disease that cannot be bypassed is common in diabetes. Local débridement and appropriate footwear and foot care are vitally important in the early treatment of foot lesions. In more advanced lesions multiple treatments including grafts, topical wound healing, and even hyperbaric treatments may be necessary. Diabetic foot care is an excellent example of the adage, "an ounce of prevention is worth a pound of cure." Thus, a foot examination at each visit is recommended. A yearly Semmes-Weinstein 5.07/10-g force monofilament test for sensation can be used to identify high-risk patients who need further podiatric evaluation.

Coronary Heart Disease

11 The risk for coronary heart disease (CHD) is two to four times greater in diabetic patients than in nondiabetic individuals. CHD is the major source of mortality in patients with DM. Multiple risk factor intervention (lipids, hypertension, smoking cessation, and antiplatelet therapy)[5] will reduce the burden of excess macrovascular events. The ADA recommends aspirin therapy in all secondary prevention situations, and if allergic to aspirin, consider clopidogrel. Recent evidence in primary prevention studies of antiplatelet therapy in type 2 DM has not shown benefit. The ADA currently recommends that if the 10-year risk of CVD is at least 10%, or the patient is at your judgment high risk, or in women at least 60 years old or men at least 50 years old, primary prevention antiplatelet therapy can be considered. Epidemiologic data suggest that CHD prevention guidelines for type 2 DM apply equally to patients with type 1 DM.[5] β-Blocker therapy supplies an even greater protection from recurrent CHD events in diabetic patients than in nondiabetic subjects. Masking of hypoglycemic symptoms is a greater problem in type 1 DM patients than in patients with type 2 DM, although this risk can be adequately managed with proper glycemic control interventions (see also Chap. 6).

Lipids The Collaborative Atorvastatin Diabetes Study (CARDS) randomized diabetes subjects with no documented CVD to atorvastatin 10 mg daily (n = 1,428) or placebo (n = 1,410). The trial was stopped 2 years early (mean duration of follow-up was 3.9 years) after meeting the primary efficacy end point of major cardiovascular events, which were reduced by 37% (P = 0.001). All-cause death was reduced 27% (P = 0.059), and potentially could have had its significance influenced by the early stoppage of the trial.[87] The Heart Protection Study randomized 5,963 patients aged >40 years with diabetes and total cholesterol >135 mg/dL (>3.49 mmol/L). A significant 22% reduction (95% CI, 13 to 30) in the event rate for major cardiovascular events was seen with simvastatin 40 mg/day. This was evident even at lower LDL levels (<116 mg/dL [<3 mmol/L]), and suggests that ~30% to 40% reduction in LDL levels regardless of starting LDL levels may be appropriate.[88] The ADA recommends statin therapy, regardless of baseline lipid or LDL-C levels in patients with overt CVD or without documented CVD who are over the age of 40 and have CVD risk factors besides diabetes.[5]

TABLE 57-12 Classification of Lipid and Lipoprotein Levels in Adults[5,91,92]

Parameter	Goal	Treatment (In Order of Preference)
LDL cholesterol	<100 mg/dL (<2.59 mmol/L) <70 mg/dL (<1.81 mmol/L)[a]	Lifestyle; HMG-CoA reductase inhibitors; cholesterol absorption inhibitor; niacin or fenofibrate
HDL cholesterol	Men: >40 mg/dL (>1.03 mmol/L) Women: >50 mg/dL (>1.29 mmol/L)	Lifestyle; nicotinic acid; fibric acid derivatives
Triglycerides	<150 mg/dL (<1.70 mmol/L)	Lifestyle; glycemic control; fibric acid derivatives; high-dose statins (in those with high LDL)

HDL, high-density lipoprotein; HMG-CoA, 3-hydroxy-3-methylglutaryl coenzyme A; LDL, low-density lipoprotein.

[a]May be optimal goal in patients with preexisting cardiovascular disease.

The proper use of fibrates in diabetes continues to be controversial. The Fenofibrate Intervention and Event Lowering in Diabetes (FIELD) was conducted in 9,795 subjects (22% with previously documented CVD) with type 2 DM given fenofibrate 200 mg daily or placebo. A relative reduction of 11% (P = 0.16) was seen in any coronary event in conjunction with a slight increase in the risk of all-cause mortality (0.7%; P = 0.18). Reasons for this have been speculated on, including the increased use of statins in the placebo group, but continue to be controversial.[89] On subset analysis, only subjects without CVD had a significant reduction in CVD events. The lipid arm of the ACCORD[90] reported on 5,518 subjects randomized to fenofibrate or placebo given with low-dose simvastatin (~20 mg/day). Fenofibrate addition did not significantly lower cardiovascular events (0.92; 95% CI, 0.79 to 1.08). Niacin in combination with a statin recently failed to improved CVD outcomes as well.

The NCEP-ATP III[15] guidelines classify the presence of DM as a CHD risk equivalent, and therefore recommend that LDL-C be lowered to <100 mg/dL (<2.59 mmol/L). An optional LDL goal in high-risk DM patients, such as those who already have CHD, has been updated to <70 mg/dL (<1.81 mmol/L)[91] (Table 57-12). The primary goal of treatment is to obtain the LDL-C goal. After the LDL-C goal is reached (usually with a statin), via NCEP-ATP, triglycerides are possibly considered for pharmacologic management, assuming unresponsiveness to glycemic control efforts, weight management, and exercise. In such situations, a non–HDL-C goal is established (a surrogate for all apolipoprotein B–containing particles). The non–HDL-C goal for patients with DM is <130 mg/dL (<3.36 mmol/L). Niacin or a fibrate can be added to reach that goal if triglycerides are 201 to 499 mg/dL (2.27 to 5.64 mmol/L), although there is little evidence this will lower CVD. Patients with marked hypertriglyceridemia (≥500 mg/dL [≥5.65 mmol/L]) are at risk for pancreatitis. Efforts to reduce triglycerides with glycemic control, elimination of other secondary causes (including medications), and drug therapy (fibrates, statins, and potentially niacin) are effective treatment strategies. Readers are also referred to the Chapters 3 and 11 for further information.

Hypertension

The role of hypertension in increasing microvascular and macrovascular risk in patients with DM has been confirmed in the UKPDS.[44] The ADA has loosened its goals for blood pressure (<140/80 mm Hg) in patients with DM.[5] The ACCORD blood pressure arm studied type 2 DM patients, with a goal of achieving a systolic blood pressure of either <120 mm Hg (achieved 119 mm Hg) or <140 mm Hg (133 mm Hg achieved).[92] The lower pressure group did not have lower CVD or renal outcomes, but did have a lower risk of stroke. A goal of <130 mm Hg can still be considered in patients at high risk of a stroke or if renal disease is present. ACE inhibitors and ARBs are generally recommended for initial therapy, as they have shown to be cardioprotective, and likely have special renal protection. Many patients require multiple agents, on average three agents, to obtain goals, so diuretics, calcium channel blockers, and β-blockers frequently are useful as second and third agents. African Americans need special consideration. They receive renoprotection from ACE inhibitors or ARBs, but as a population may lower blood pressure slightly less with these agents. It is recommended that combination therapy with a diuretic or calcium channel blocker be considered as first-line therapy. After initial therapy, which agent to add next is still controversial. Blood pressure goals are generally more difficult to achieve than glycemic goals or lipid goals in most diabetic patients. Readers are referred to Chapter 3 for more information.

Transplantation

Whole pancreas and islet cell transplantation are options in patients with type 1 DM; those with end-stage renal disease also receive kidney transplantation. Lifelong immunosuppression is required.

Personalized Pharmacotherapy

Individualization of therapy in DM is based on several factors. There is no optimal regimen in diabetes, and it is mostly based on reaching glycemic goals. In type 1 DM, as insulin must be used, it is to tailor the insulin regimen to the lifestyle of the patient. This almost always involves basal–bolus therapy, individualized based on SMBG readings. In addition, if the patient does not mind being attached to a pump, therapy can be further tailored to the patient. It may in unusual circumstances involve simplification of the regimen to premix insulins, as basal–bolus therapy may not fit into their lifestyle. Elevated glucagon levels in some patients, as the hormone amylin is low or absent, may require glucagon suppression therapy. FDA-approved therapy includes addition of pramlintide, but there is evidence for use of nonapproved medications such as GLP-1 receptor antagonists to act as an alternative to pramlintide, which requires many extra injections per day. In addition, metformin has been used in some type 1 DM patients who are adherent (and thus at low risk of DKA) but have suboptimal control of their FPG readings. Metformin use should not be routine, but in examples such as adolescents who miss injections after frank discussions with patients and parents.

No one regimen in type 2 DM is considered to be optimal for all patients. Common individualization points include mechanism of action, contraindications, side effects, and potential adverse events including hypoglycemia, efficacy (including fasting vs. postprandial control), long-term safety, ease of use, and cost. In addition, "nonglycemic" effects such as weight changes, lipid effects, cardiovascular outcomes, and even perceived β-cell preservation/effects may influence final choices.

EVALUATION OF THERAPEUTIC OUTCOMES

A comprehensive pharmaceutical care plan for the patient with DM will integrate considerations of goals to optimize BG control and protocols to screen for, prevent, or manage microvascular and macrovascular complications. In terms of standards of care for persons with DM, one can review the document published by the ADA that outlines initial and ongoing assessments for patients with DM.[5] The major performance measure by the National Committee for Quality Assurance (NCQA), such as Health Plan Employer Data and Information Set (HEDIS), should assess the ability to meet current standards of care and recognize the minimal treatment goals for glycemia, lipids, and hypertension, and provide targets for monitoring and adjusting pharmacotherapy as discussed in various sections above. Publicly reported quality measures continue to move closer to current guidelines, but lack the ability to differentiate reasons why a patient is not controlled. Glycemic control (tested minimally yearly; HbA_{1c} <8% [<0.08; <64 mmol/mol Hb] is good control and HbA_{1c} >9% [>0.09; >75 mmol/mol Hb] is poor control), lipid (percentage of patients with LDL <100 mg/dL [<2.59 mmol/L]), and hypertension (percentage of patients with blood pressure <130/80 mm Hg, but also with blood pressure <140/90 mm Hg) are NCQA-based measures. Glycemic control is paramount in managing type 1 or type 2 DM, but as readily identified from the above discussion, it requires frequent assessment and adjustment in diet, exercise, and pharmacologic therapies. The ADA also has clinical practice recommendations that are widely cited and followed.[5] Minimally, HbA_{1c} should be measured twice a year in patients meeting treatment goals on a stable therapeutic regimen. Quarterly assessments are recommended for those whose therapy has changed or who are not meeting glycemic goals. Fasting lipid profiles should be obtained as part of an initial assessment and thereafter at each follow-up visit if not at goal, annually if stable and at goal, or every 2 years if the lipid profile suggests low risk. Documenting regular frequency of foot examinations (each visit), urine albumin assessment (annually), dilated ophthalmologic examinations (yearly or more frequently with identified abnormalities), and office visits for follow-up are also important. Assessment for pneumococcal vaccine administration (and one-time revaccination recommended in individuals at least 65 years old), annual administration of influenza vaccine, new recommendations that all people with diabetes receive the hepatitis B vaccine series, and routine assessment for and management of other cardiovascular risks (e.g., smoking and antiplatelet therapy) are components of preventive medicine strategies. The multiplicity of assessments for each patient visit is likely to be better facilitated utilizing an integrative computer program and electronic medical record, standardized progress note forms, or flow sheets, which assist the clinician in identifying whether the patient has met standards of care in the frequency of monitoring and achievement of defined targets of therapy. Adherence continues to be of issue, as with many chronic diseases, and use of frequent education and potential simplification of regimens, if possible through combination medications, may be warranted (Table 57-13). In addition,

TABLE 57-13 Combination Products Available in Type 2 Diabetes Mellitus[a]

Medication	Combined With	Trade Name
Metformin and/or metformin extended release	Pioglitazone	Actosplus Met
	Rosiglitazone	Avandamet
	Sitagliptin	Janumet
	Saxagliptin	Kombiglyze
	Linagliptin	Jentadueto
	Alogliptin	Kazano
	Glyburide	Glucovance
	Glipizide	Metaglip
	Repaglinide	Prandimet
Glimepiride	Pioglitazone	Duetact
	Rosiglitazone	Avandaryl
Pioglitazone	Alogliptin	Oseni

[a]At time chapter written.

TABLE 57-14 Drug Monitoring for Diabetes Mellitus Medications

Medication Class	Adverse Drug Reaction	Monitoring Parameters	Comments
α-Glucosidase inhibitors	GI upset	Gas, bloating, loose stools	Titrate, take in less carbohydrate
Bile acid sequestrants	Constipation	Bowel movement frequency	Do not use if history of bowel obstruction
	Raises triglycerides	Triglycerides	Not recommended TG >500 mg/dL (>5.65 mmol/L)
Biguanides	GI upset	Reflux, nausea, vomiting, stomach upset, loose stools	Take with food and titrate dose; split doses; consider extended release
	Lactic acidosis	Hypoxic states, renal function	Lactate levels usually not measured, but can if suspected toxicity
DPP-4 inhibitors	Hypersensitivity/angioedema and exfoliating dermatologic skin reactions	Skin rash, signs/symptoms of angioedema	Risk factors, such as history of angioedema, possibly ACE inhibitor use, and past history of severe dermal drug reactions, should be explored
	Pancreatitis	Amylase, lipase, abdominal pain with nausea/vomiting	Discontinue; look for underlying causes
Dopamine agonists	Hypotension	Syncopal symptoms	Stop antihypertensives
	Worsening psychiatric issues	Signs/symptoms of underlying mental illness	Avoid use with antipsychotics
	CNS effects	Mental alertness/asthenia/ fatigue/headache	Titrate slowly
	Gastrointestinal side effects	Nausea	Titrate slowly
Thiazolidinediones	Heart failure/pulmonary edema	Signs/symptoms of heart failure, BNP, weight	Discontinue
	Peripheral edema	Peripheral edema measures	Limit dose, consider diuretic (see text), or discontinue
	Weight gain	Weight	Consider if weight is fluid or likely caloric intake
	Peripheral fractures	None except fracture	Avoid use in osteoporosis and osteopenia
Sulfonylureas	Hypoglycemia	Self-monitored blood glucose	
Meglitinides	Hypoglycemia	Self-monitored blood glucose	
GLP-1 receptor agonists	GI	Nausea/vomiting	Titrate slowly; avoid in gastroparesis
	Pancreatitis	Amylase, lipase, abdominal pain with nausea/vomiting	Discontinue; look for underlying causes
	C-cell tumors of thyroid	None recommended, calcitonin	Calcitonin could be measured if suspected, has not occurred in humans to date
Amylinomimetic	GI upset	Nausea/vomiting	Titrate slowly; avoid in gastroparesis
Insulin	Hypoglycemia	Self-monitored blood glucose	

many patients do not take medications because of tolerance, side effects, and perceived risk versus benefit from their clinician or from family, friends, or the Internet (Table 57-14).

ABBREVIATIONS

AADE	American Association of Diabetes Educators
ACCORD	Action to Control Cardiovascular Risk in Diabetes
ACE	angiotensin-converting enzyme
ADA	American Diabetes Association
ADVANCE	Action in Diabetes and Vascular Disease
AHA	American Heart Association
ALT	alanine aminotransferase
ARB	angiotensin receptor blocker
BG	blood glucose
BMI	body mass index
CARDS	Collaborative Atorvastatin Diabetes Study
CDE	certified diabetes educator
CGM	continuous glucose monitoring
CHD	coronary heart disease
CI	confidence interval
CL_{cr}	creatinine clearance
CSII	continuous subcutaneous insulin infusion
CVD	cardiovascular disease
CYP450	cytochrome P450
DCCT	Diabetes Control and Complications Trial
DKA	diabetic ketoacidosis
DM	diabetes mellitus
DPP-4	dipeptidyl peptidase-4
eAG	estimated average glucose
EDIC	Epidemiology of Diabetes Interventions and Complications
FFA	free fatty acid
FIELD	Fenofibrate Intervention and Event Lowering in Diabetes
FPG	fasting plasma glucose
GDM	gestational diabetes mellitus
GIP	glucose-dependent insulinotropic polypeptide
GLP-1	glucagon-like peptide-1
HbA_{1c}	hemoglobin A_{1c}
HDL	high-density lipoprotein
HDL-C	high-density lipoprotein cholesterol
HEDIS	Health Plan Employer Data and Information Set
HHS	hyperosmolar hyperglycemic state
HIV	human immunodeficiency virus
HLA	human leukocyte antigen
HR	hazard ratio
ICA	islet cell antibody
IDF	International Diabetes Federation
IFG	impaired fasting glucose
IGT	impaired glucose tolerance
LADA	latent autoimmune diabetes in adults
LDL-C	low-density lipoprotein cholesterol
Look AHEAD	Look Action for Health in Diabetes
MI	myocardial infarction
MODY	maturity onset diabetes of youth
NCEP-ATP	National Cholesterol Education Program Adult Treatment Panel
NCQA	National Committee for Quality Assurance
NGSP	National Glycohemoglobin Standardization Program

NHLBI	National Heart, Lung, and Blood Institute
NPH	neutral protamine Hagedorn
OGTT	oral glucose tolerance test
PAI-1	plasminogen activator inhibitor-1
PPAR-γ	peroxisome proliferator–activated receptor γ
RECORD	Rosiglitazone Evaluated for Cardiovascular Outcomes in Oral Agent Combination Therapy for Type 2 Diabetes
SGLT-2	sodium-dependent glucose cotransporter-2
SMBG	self-monitoring of blood glucose
SUR	sulfonylurea receptor
TZD	thiazolidinedione
UKPDS	United Kingdom Prospective Diabetes Study
VADT	Veterans Affairs Diabetes Trial
VAT	visceral adipose tissue
ZnT8	zinc transporter 8

REFERENCES

1. Centers for Disease Control and Prevention. National Diabetes Fact Sheet: National Estimates and General Information on Diabetes and Prediabetes in the United States, 2011. Atlanta, GA: U.S. Department of Health and Human Services, Centers for Disease Control and Prevention, 2011.
2. American Diabetes Association. Clinical practice recommendations. Diagnosis and classification of diabetes mellitus. Diabetes Care 2013;36(Suppl 1): S67–S74.
3. Naik R, Lernmark A, Palmer J. Pathophysiology and genetics of type 1 (insulin-dependent) diabetes. In: Porte D Jr, Sherwin RS, Baron A, Ellenberg M, Rifkin H, eds. Ellenberg & Rifkin's Diabetes Mellitus, 6th ed. New York, NY: McGraw-Hill, 2003:301–330.
4. Bennett P, Rewers M, Knowler W. Epidemiology of diabetes mellitus. In: Porte D Jr, Sherwin RS, Baron A, Ellenberg M, Rifkin H, eds. Ellenberg & Rifkin's Diabetes Mellitus, 6th ed. New York, NY: McGraw-Hill, 2003:277–300.
5. American Diabetes Association. Standards for medical care in diabetes—2013. Diabetes Care 2013;36(Suppl 1):S11–S66.
6. American Diabetes Association. Standards of care. Children and adolescents in: Clinical practice recommendations. Diabetes Care 2013;36(Suppl 1):S40–S43.
7. DeFronzo RA. From the triumvirate to the ominous octet: A new paradigm for the treatment of type 2 diabetes mellitus. Diabetes 2009;58:773–795.
8. International Association of Diabetes and Pregnancy Study Groups Consensus Panel, Metzger BE, Gabbe SG, et al. International Association of Diabetes and Pregnancy Study Groups recommendations on the diagnosis and classification of hyperglycemia in pregnancy. Diabetes Care 2010;33: 676–682.
9. Zipitis CS, Akobeng AK. Vitamin D supplementation in early childhood and risk of type 1 diabetes: A systematic review and meta-analysis. Arch Dis Child 2008;93: 512–517.
10. Winter W, Harris N, Schatz M. Immunological markers in the diagnosis and prediction of autoimmune type 1a diabetes. Clin Diabetes 2002;20:183–191.
11. Cherrington AD. Banting Lecture 1997: Control of glucose uptake and release by the liver in vivo. Diabetes 1999;48:1198–1214.
12. McGarry JD. Banting Lecture 2001: Dysregulation of fatty acid metabolism in the etiology of type 2 diabetes. Diabetes 2002;51:7–18.
13. DeFronzo RA. Pathogenesis of type 2 diabetes mellitus: Metabolic and molecular implications for identifying diabetes genes. Diabetes 1997;5:117–269.
14. DeFronzo RA. Pathogenesis of type 2 diabetes mellitus. Med Clin North Am 2004;88:787–835.
15. Expert Panel on Detection, Evaluation, and Treatment of High Blood Cholesterol in Adults. Executive summary of the third report of the National Cholesterol Education Program (NCEP) Expert Panel on Detection, Evaluation, and Treatment of High Blood Cholesterol in Adults (Adult Treatment Panel III). JAMA 2001;285(19):2486–2497.
16. Alberti KGMM, Eckel RH, Grundy SM, et al. Harmonizing the metabolic syndrome. A joint interim statement of the International Diabetes Federation Task Force on Epidemiology and Prevention; National Heart, Lung, and Blood Institute; American Heart Association; World Heart Federation; International Atherosclerosis Society; and International Association for the Study of Obesity. Circulation 2009;120:1640–1645.
17. Ervin RB. Prevalence of Metabolic Syndrome among Adults 20 Years of Age and Over, by Sex, Age, Race and Ethnicity, and Body Mass Index: United States, 2003–2006. National Health Statistics Reports, No. 13. Hyattsville, MD: National Center for Health Statistics, 2009.
18. Alexander CM, Landsman PB, Teutsch SM, et al. NCEP-defined metabolic syndrome, diabetes, and prevalence of coronary heart disease among NHANES III participants age 50 years and older. Diabetes 2003;52(5):1210–1214.
19. Ford ES, Giles WH, Dietz WH. Prevalence of the metabolic syndrome among US adults: Findings from the third National Health and Nutrition Examination Survey. JAMA 2002;287(3):356–359.
20. Kahn R, Buse J, Ferrannini E, Stern M, American Diabetes Association, European Association for the Study of Diabetes. The metabolic syndrome: Time for a critical appraisal: Joint statement from the American Diabetes Association and the European Association for the Study of Diabetes. Diabetes Care 2005;28(9):2289–2304.
21. Grundy SM, Cleeman JI, Daniels SR, et al. Diagnosis and management of the metabolic syndrome: An American Heart Association/National Heart, Lung, and Blood Institute scientific statement. Circulation 2005;112(17): 2735–2752.
22. Gaede P, Vedel P, Larsen N, et al. Multifactorial intervention and cardiovascular disease in patients with type 2 diabetes. N Engl J Med 2003;348:383–393.
23. Diabetes Control and Complications Trial Research Group. The effect of intensive treatment of diabetes on the development and progression of long-term complications in insulin-dependent diabetes mellitus. N Engl J Med 1993; 329:977–986.
24. UK Prospective Diabetes Study Group. Intensive blood-glucose control with sulphonylureas or insulin compared with conventional treatment and risk of complications in patients with type 2 diabetes (UKPDS 33). Lancet 1998; 352:837–853.
25. Nathan DM, Kuenen J, Borg R, et al. Translating the A1C assay into estimated average glucose values. Diabetes Care 2008;31:1473–1478.
26. Malanda UL, Welschen LMC, Riphagen II, et al. Self-monitoring of blood glucose in patients with type 2 diabetes mellitus who are not using insulin. Cochrane Database Syst Rev 2012;(1):CD005060.
27. American Diabetes Association. Nutrition recommendations and interventions for diabetes. Diabetes Care 2008; 31(Suppl 1):S61–S78.

28. American Diabetes Association. Diabetes mellitus and exercise. Diabetes Care 2010;33(Suppl 1):S26–S27.
29. Malmberg K, for the DIGAMI Study Group. Prospective randomised study of intensive insulin treatment on long term survival after acute myocardial infarction in patients with diabetes mellitus. BMJ 1997;314:1512–1515.
30. Budnitz DS, Lovegrove MC, Shehab N, Richards CL. Emergency hospitalizations for adverse drug events in older Americans. N Engl J Med 2011;365:2002–2012.
31. The ORIGIN Trial Investigators. Basal insulin and cardiovascular and other outcomes in dysglycemia. N Engl J Med 2012;367:319–328.
32. Blevins T, Pullman J, Malloy J, et al. DURATION-5. Exenatide once weekly resulted in greater improvements in glycemic control compared to exenatide twice daily in patients with type 2 diabetes. J Clin Endocrinol Metab 2011;96:1301–1310.
33. Drucker DJ, Buse JB, Taylor K, et al. Exenatide once weekly versus twice daily for the treatment of type 2 diabetes: A randomised, open-label, non-inferiority study. Lancet 2008;372:1240–1250.
34. Schor S. The University Group Diabetes Program. A statistician looks at the mortality results. JAMA 1971; 217:1673–1675.
35. Triplitt C. Drug interactions of medications commonly used in diabetes. Diabetes Spectrum 2006;19:202–211.
36. UK Prospective Diabetes Study (UKPDS) Group. Effect of intensive blood-glucose control with metformin on complications in overweight patients with type 2 diabetes (UKPDS 34). Lancet 1998;352:854–865.
37. Dormandy JA, Charbonnel B, Eckland DJA, et al. Secondary prevention of vascular events in patients with type 2 diabetes in the PROactive study prospective pioglitazone clinical trial in macrovascular events: A randomized controlled trial. Lancet 2005;366:1279–1289.
38. Nissen SE, Wolski K. The effect of rosiglitazone on the risk of myocardial infarction and death from cardiovascular causes. N Engl J Med 2007;356:1–15.
39. Home PD, Pocock SJ, Beck-Nielsen H, et al. Rosiglitazone evaluated for cardiovascular outcomes in oral agent combination therapy for type 2 diabetes (RECORD): A multicentre, randomised, open-label trial. Lancet 2009; 373:2125–2135.
40. Chiasson JL, Josse RG, Gomis R, et al. Acarbose for prevention of type 2 diabetes mellitus: The STOP-NIDDM randomized trial. Lancet 2002;359:2072–2077.
41. Chiasson JL, Josse RG, Gomis R, et al. Acarbose treatment and the risk of cardiovascular disease and hypertension in patients with impaired glucose tolerance: The STOP-NIDDM trial. JAMA 2003;290:486–494.
42. Stratton IM, Adler AI, Neil HA. Association of glycaemia with macrovascular and microvascular complications of type 2 diabetes (UKPDS 35): Prospective observational study. BMJ 2000;321:405–412.
43. Adler AI, Stratton IM, Neil HA. Association of systolic blood pressure with macrovascular and microvascular complications of type 2 diabetes (UKPDS 36): Prospective observational study. BMJ 2000;321:412–419.
44. UK Prospective Diabetes Study Group. Efficacy of atenolol and captopril in reducing risk of macrovascular and microvascular complications in type 2 diabetes: UKPDS 39. BMJ 1998;317:713–720.
45. Writing Team for the Diabetes Control and Complications/ Epidemiology of Diabetes Interventions and Complications Research Group. Sustained effect of intensive treatment of type 1 diabetes mellitus on development and progression of diabetic nephropathy: The Epidemiology of Diabetes Interventions and Complications (EDIC) study. JAMA 2003;290:2159–2167.
46. DCCT/EDIC Study Research Group. Intensive diabetes treatment and cardiovascular disease in patients with type 1 diabetes. N Engl J Med 2005;353:2643–2653.
47. Holman RR, Paul SK, Bethel MA, Mathews DR, Neil HAW. 10-Year follow-up of intensive glucose control in type 2 diabetes. N Engl J Med 2008;359:1577–1589.
48. The Action to Control Cardiovascular Risk in Diabetes Study Group. Effects of intensive glucose lowering in type 2 diabetes. N Engl J Med 2008;358:2545–2559.
49. The ADVANCE Collaborative Group. Intensive blood glucose control and vascular outcomes in patients with type 2 diabetes. N Engl J Med 2008;358:2560–2572.
50. Duckworth W, Abraira C, Mortiz T, et al. Glucose control and vascular complications in veterans with type 2 diabetes. N Engl J Med 2009;360:1–11.
51. Strowig S, Raskin P. Intensive management of insulin-dependent diabetes mellitus. In: Porte D Jr, Sherwin RS, eds. Ellenberg & Rifkin's Diabetes Mellitus, 5th ed. Stamford, CT: Appleton & Lange, 1997:709–733.
52. Schade DS, Valentine V. To pump or not to pump. Diabetes Care 2002;25:2100–2102.
53. Kort H, Koning EJ, Rabelink TJ, et al. Islet transplantation in type 1 diabetes. BMJ 2011;342:d247.
54. Inzucchi SE, Bergenstal RM, Buse JB. Management of hyperglycemia in type 2 diabetes: A patient-centered approach: Position statement of the American Diabetes Association (ADA) and the European Association for the Study of Diabetes (EASD). Diabetes Care 2012;35: 1364–1379.
55. Holman RR, Farmer AJ, Davies MJ, et al. Three-year efficacy of complex insulin regimens in type 2 diabetes. N Engl J Med 2009;361:1736–1747.
56. Triplitt CL. How to initiate, titrate, and intensify insulin treatment in type 2 diabetes. US Pharm 2007;32:10–16.
57. Araki A, Iimuro S, Sakurai T, et al. Japanese Elderly Diabetes Intervention Trial Study Group. Long-term multiple risk factor interventions in Japanese elderly diabetic patients: The Japanese Elderly Diabetes Intervention Trial: Study design, baseline characteristics and effects of intervention. Geriatr Gerontol Int 2012;12(Suppl 1):7–17.
58. Kirkman MS, Briscoe VJ, Clark N, et al. Diabetes in older adults. Diabetes Care 2012;35:2650–2664.
59. Sinclair AJ, Paolisso G, Castro M, et al., European Diabetes Working Party for Older People. European Diabetes Working Party for Older People 2011 clinical guidelines for type 2 diabetes mellitus. Executive summary. Diabetes Metab 2011; 37(Suppl 3):S27–S38.
60. Langer O, Conway DL, Berkus MD, Xenakis EM. A comparison of glyburide and insulin in women with gestational diabetes mellitus. N Engl J Med 2000;343: 1134–1138.
61. Cheng YW, Chung JH, Block-Kurbisch I, Inturrisi M, Caughey AB. Treatment of gestational diabetes mellitus: Glyburide compared to subcutaneous insulin therapy and associated perinatal outcomes. J Mater Fetal Neonatal Med 2012;25(4):379–384.
62. Coetzee EJ, Jackson WP. Pregnancy in established non-insulin-dependent diabetics. A five-and-a-half year study at Groote Schuur Hospital. S Afr Med J 1980;58: 795–802.
63. Coetzee EJ, Jackson WP. Oral hypoglycaemics in the first trimester and fetal outcome. S Afr Med J 1984;65: 635–637.

64. Hellmuth E, Damm P, Mølsted-Pedersen L. Oral hypoglycaemic agents in 118 diabetic pregnancies. Diabet Med 2000;17:507–511.
65. Rowan JA, Hague WM, Gao W, Battin MR, Moore MP; MiG Trial Investigators. Metformin versus insulin for the treatment of gestational diabetes. N Engl J Med 2008;358:2003–2015.
66. Nicholson W, Bolen S, Witkop CT, et al. Benefits and risks of oral diabetes agents compared with insulin in women with gestational diabetes: A systematic review. Obstet Gynecol 2009;113:193.
67. Dhulkotia JS, Ola B, Fraser R, Farrell T. Oral hypoglycemic agents vs insulin in management of gestational diabetes: A systematic review and metaanalysis. Am J Obstet Gynecol 2010;203:457.
68. American Diabetes Association. Gestational diabetes mellitus. Diabetes Care 2004;27(1):s88–s90.
69. Laffel L. Sick-day management in type 1 diabetes. Endocrinol Metab Clin North Am 2000;29:707–723.
70. Kitabchi AE, Umpierrez GE, Miles JM, Fisher JN. Hyperglycemic crises in adult patients with diabetes. A consensus statement from the American Diabetes Association. Diabetes Care 2009;32:1335–1343.
71. Hirsch IB. Sliding scale insulin—Time to stop sliding. JAMA 2009;301:213–214.
72. Malmberg K, Norhammar A, Wedel H, Rydén L. Glycometabolic state at admission: Important risk marker of mortality in conventionally treated patients with diabetes mellitus and acute myocardial infarction: Long-term results from the Diabetes and Insulin–Glucose Infusion in Acute Myocardial Infarction (DIGAMI) study. Circulation 1999;99:2626–2632.
73. van den Berghe G, Wouters P, Weekers F, et al. Intensive insulin therapy in the critically ill patients. N Engl J Med 2001;345:1359–1367.
74. Moghissi ES, Korykowski MT, DiNardo M, et al. American Association of Clinical Endocrinologists and American Diabetes Association consensus statement on inpatient glycemic control. Diabetes Care 2009;32:1119–1131.
75. The NICE-SUGAR Study Investigators. Intensive versus conventional glycemic control in critically ill patients. N Engl J Med 2009;360:1283–1297.
76. American Diabetes Association. Preconception care of women with diabetes. Diabetes Care 2004;27(Suppl 1): S76–S78.
77. Mahmud M, Mazza D. Preconception care of women with diabetes: A review of current guideline recommendations. BMC Womens Health 2010;10:5.
78. Spollett G. Hyperglycemia in HIV/AIDS. Diabetes Spectrum 2006;19:163–166.
79. Diabetes Prevention Program Research Group. Reduction in the incidence of type 2 diabetes with lifestyle intervention or metformin. N Engl J Med 2002;346:393–403.
80. Buchanan TA, Xiang AH, Peters RK, et al. Preservation of pancreatic β-cell function and prevention of type 2 diabetes by pharmacological treatment of insulin resistance in high-risk Hispanic women. Diabetes 2002;51:2796–2803.
81. The Dream Trial Investigators. The effect of ramipril on the incidence of diabetes. N Engl J Med 2006;355: 1551–1562.
82. The DREAM Trial Investigators. The effect of rosiglitazone on the frequency of diabetes in patients with impaired glucose tolerance or impaired fasting glucose. A randomised controlled trial. Lancet 2006;368:1096–1105.
83. DeFronzo R, Tripathy D, Schwenke D, et al. Pioglitazone for diabetes prevention in impaired glucose tolerance. N Engl J Med 2011;364:1104–1115.
84. Haas L, Maryniuk M, Beck J, et al. National standards diabetes self-management education. Diabetes Care 2013;36(Suppl 1):S100–S108.
85. Boulton AJ, Malik RA, Arezzo JC, Sosenko JM. Diabetic somatic neuropathies. Diabetes Care 2004;27:1458–1486.
86. Boulton AJM, Armstrong DG, Albert SF, et al. Comprehensive foot exam and risk assessment. Diabetes Care 2008;31:1679–1685.
87. Colhoun HM, Betteridge DJ, Durrington PN, et al. Primary prevention of cardiovascular disease with atorvastatin in type 2 diabetes in the Collaborative Atorvastatin Diabetes Study (CARDS): A multicentre, randomised placebo controlled trial. Lancet 2004;364:685–696.
88. Heart Protection Study Collaborative Group. MRC/BHF Heart Protection Study of cholesterol-lowering with simvastatin in 5963 people with diabetes: A randomised placebo-controlled trial. Lancet 2003;361:2005–2016.
89. The FIELD Study Investigators. Effects of long-term fenofibrate therapy on cardiovascular events in 9795 people with type 2 diabetes mellitus (the FIELD study): Randomised controlled trial. Lancet 2005;366: 1849–1861.
90. The ACCORD Study Group. Effects of combination lipid therapy in type 2 diabetes. N Engl J Med 2010;362: 1563–1574 [erratum 362:1748].
91. Grundy SM, Cleeman JI, Merz CN. Implications of recent clinical trials for the National Cholesterol Education Program Adult Treatment Panel III guidelines. Circulation 2004;110:227–239.
92. The ACCORD Study Group. Effects of intensive blood-pressure control in type 2 diabetes mellitus. N Engl J Med 2010;362:1628–1630.

58

Thyroid Disorders

Jacqueline Jonklaas and Robert L. Talbert

KEY CONCEPTS

1. Advances in the understanding of the structure and metabolism of thyroid hormones, and the molecular biology of thyroid hormone receptors have provided insight into the various abnormalities that give rise to hyperthyroidism and hypothyroidism.
2. Thyrotoxicosis is most commonly caused by Graves' disease, which is an autoimmune disorder in which thyroid-stimulating antibody (TSAb) directed against the thyrotropin receptor elicits the same biologic response as thyroid-stimulating hormone (TSH).
3. Hyperthyroidism may be treated with antithyroid drugs such as methimazole (MMI) or propylthiouracil (PTU), radioactive iodine (RAI: sodium iodide-131 [^{131}I]), or surgical removal of the thyroid gland; selection of the initial treatment approach is based on patient characteristics such as age, concurrent physiology (e.g., pregnancy), comorbidities (e.g., chronic obstructive lung disease), and convenience.
4. MMI and PTU reduce the synthesis of thyroid hormones and are similar in efficacy and overall adverse effects, but their dosing ranges differ by 10-fold.
5. Response to MMI and PTU is seen in 4 to 6 weeks with a maximal response in 4 to 6 months; treatment usually continues for 1 to 2 years, and therapy is monitored by clinical signs and symptoms and by measuring the serum concentrations of TSH and free thyroxine (T_4).
6. Subclinical hyperthyroidism is associated with cardiovascular mortality, especially in the elderly in whom treatment is recommended.
7. Adjunctive therapy with β-blockers controls the adrenergic symptoms of thyrotoxicosis but does not correct the underlying disorder; iodine may also be used adjunctively in preparation for surgery and acutely for thyroid storm.
8. Many patients choose to have ablative therapy with ^{131}I rather than undergo repeated courses of MMI or PTU treatment; most patients receiving RAI eventually become hypothyroid and require thyroid hormone supplementation.
9. Hypothyroidism is most often due to an autoimmune disorder known as *Hashimoto's thyroiditis*.
10. The drug of choice for replacement therapy in hypothyroidism is levothyroxine.
11. Studies of combination therapy with levothyroxine and triiodothyronine have not shown reproducible benefits. This approach to treatment of hypothyroidism requires further study.
12. Monitoring of levothyroxine replacement therapy is achieved by observing clinical signs and symptoms and by measuring the serum TSH. An elevated TSH indicates underreplacement; a suppressed TSH indicates overreplacement.
13. There is controversy about the treatment of mild (subclinical) hypothyroidism. Generally, benefits of treatment are clearest in younger populations.
14. Despite the simplicity of the concept of correction of hypothyroidism with levothyroxine, many treated patients have iatrogenic hyperthyroidism or are underreplaced.
15. Hypothyroidism during pregnancy should be treated to achieve TSH values that are normal, based on reference ranges for TSH derived from the pregnant population.

Thyroid hormones affect the function of virtually every organ system. In a child, thyroid hormone is critical for normal growth and development. In an adult, the major role of thyroid hormone is to maintain metabolic stability. Substantial reservoirs of thyroid hormone in the thyroid gland and blood provide constant thyroid hormone availability. In addition, the hypothalamic–pituitary–thyroid axis is exquisitely sensitive to small changes in circulating thyroid hormone concentrations, and alterations in thyroid hormone secretion maintain peripheral free thyroid hormone levels within a narrow range. Patients seek medical attention for evaluation of symptoms due to abnormal thyroid hormone levels or because of diffuse or nodular thyroid enlargement.

THYROID HORMONE PHYSIOLOGY

Thyroid Hormone Synthesis

1 The thyroid hormones thyroxine (T_4) and triiodothyronine (T_3) (Fig. 58-1) are formed within thyroglobulin (TG), a large glycoprotein synthesized in the thyroid cell. Because of the unique tertiary structure of this glycoprotein, iodinated tyrosine residues present in TG are able to bind together to form active thyroid hormones.[1]

Iodide is actively transported through the basolateral membrane via a Na^+/I^- symporter from the extracellular space into the thyroid follicular cell against an electrochemical gradient, driven by the coupled transport of sodium.[2] Structurally related anions such as thiocyanate (SCN^-), perchlorate (ClO_4^-), and pertechnetate (TcO_4^-) are competitive inhibitors of iodine transport.[3] In addition, bromine, fluorine, and, under certain circumstances, lithium block iodide transport into the thyroid (Table 58-1). Inorganic iodide that enters

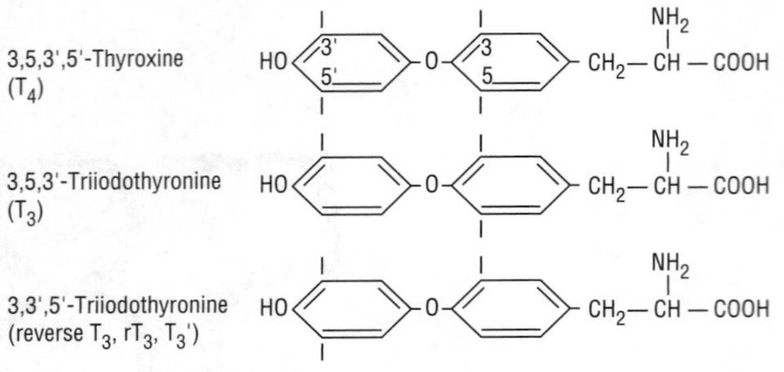

3,5,3',5'-Thyroxine (T_4) — HO–[3',5'-diiodophenyl]–O–[3,5-diiodophenyl]–CH_2–CH(NH_2)–COOH

3,5,3'-Triiodothyronine (T_3) — HO–[iodophenyl]–O–[diiodophenyl]–CH_2–CH(NH_2)–COOH

3,3',5'-Triiodothyronine (reverse T_3, rT_3, T_3') — HO–[diiodophenyl]–O–[iodophenyl]–CH_2–CH(NH_2)–COOH

FIGURE 58-1 Structure of thyroid hormones.

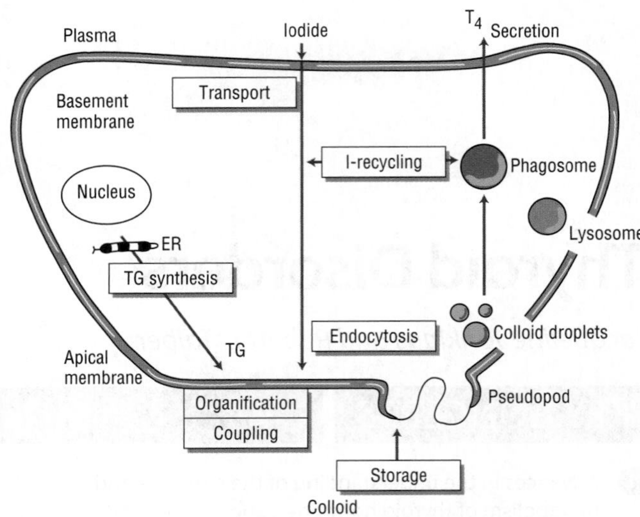

FIGURE 58-2 Thyroid hormone synthesis. Iodide is transported from the plasma, through the cell, to the apical membrane, where it is organified and coupled to the thyroglobulin (TG) synthesized within the thyroid cell. Hormone stored as colloid reenters the cell through endocytosis and moves back toward the basal membrane, where thyroxine (T_4) is secreted.

the thyroid follicular cell is ushered through the cell to the apical membrane, where it is transported into the follicular lumen by pendrin, and possibly other transport proteins.[4,5] Located on the luminal side of the apical membrane, thyroid peroxidase oxidizes iodide and covalently binds the organified iodide to tyrosine residues within TG (Fig. 58-2). It is interesting that although salivary glands and the gastric mucosa are able to actively transport iodide, they are unable to effectively incorporate iodide into proteins given the lack of similar oxidizing machinery.[6] Similarly, when tyrosine molecules are iodinated on proteins other than TG, they lack the proper tertiary structure needed to allow the formation of active thyroid hormones.[7]

The iodinated tyrosine residues monoiodotyrosine (MIT) and diiodotyrosine (DIT) combine to form iodothyronines (Fig. 58-3). Thus, two molecules of DIT combine to form T_4, whereas MIT and DIT constitute T_3. In addition to its role in iodine organification, the hemoprotein thyroid peroxidase also catalyzes the formation of iodothyronines (coupling).

Iodine deficiency causes an increase in the MIT:DIT ratio in TG and leads to a relative increase in the production of T_3.[8] Because T_3 is more potent than T_4, the increase in T_3 production in iodine-deficient areas may be beneficial. The thionamide drugs used to treat hyperthyroidism inhibit thyroid peroxidase and thus block thyroid hormone synthesis.

TG is stored in the follicular lumen and must reenter the cell, where the process of proteolysis liberates thyroid hormone into the bloodstream. Thyroid follicles active in hormone synthesis are identified histologically by columnar epithelial cells lining a follicular lumen, which is depleted of colloid. Inactive follicles are lined by cuboidal epithelial cells and are replete with colloid. Both iodide and lithium block the release of preformed thyroid hormone, through poorly understood mechanisms.

T_4 and T_3 are transported in the bloodstream primarily by three proteins: thyroxine-binding globulin (TBG), transthyretin (TTR), and albumin.[9] It is estimated that 99.96% of circulating T_4 and 99.5% of T_3 are bound to these proteins. However, only the unbound (free) thyroid hormone is able to diffuse into the cell, elicit a biologic effect, and regulate thyroid-stimulating hormone (TSH; also known as *thyrotropin*) secretion from the pituitary. Multiple functions have been ascribed to these transport proteins, including (a) assuring minimal urinary loss of iodide, (b) providing a mechanism for uniform tissue distribution of free hormone, and (c) transport of hormone into the CNS.

Whereas T_4 is secreted solely from the thyroid gland, less than 20% of T_3 is produced in the thyroid. The majority of T_3 is formed from the breakdown of T_4 catalyzed by the 5′-monodeiodinase enzymes found in extrathyroidal peripheral tissues. Because the binding affinity of nuclear thyroid hormone receptors (TRs) is 10 to 15 times

TABLE 58-1 Thyroid Hormone Synthesis and Secretion Inhibitors

Mechanism of Action	Substance
Blocks iodide transport into the thyroid	Bromine Fluorine Lithium (?)
Impairs organification and coupling of thyroid hormones	Thionamides Sulfonylureas Sulfonamide (?) Salicylamide (?) Antipyrine (?)
Inhibits thyroid hormone secretion	Iodide (large doses), lithium

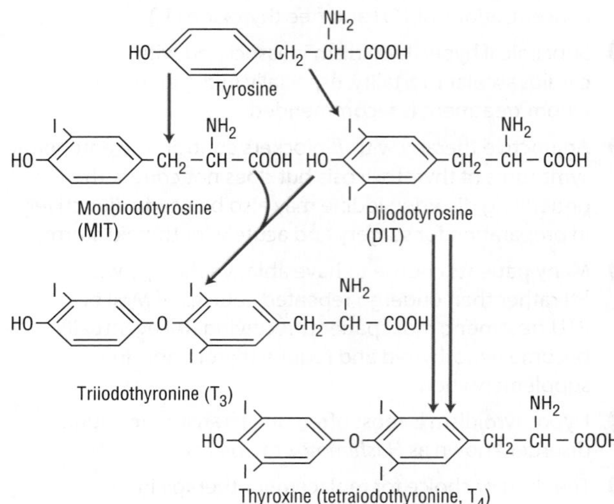

FIGURE 58-3 Scheme of coupling reactions. After tyrosine is iodinated to form monoiodotyrosine (MIT) or diiodotyrosine (DIT) (organification of the iodine), MIT and DIT combine to form triiodothyronine (T_3) or two molecules of DIT combine to form thyroxine T_4.

TABLE 58-2 Properties of Iodothyronine 5′-Deiodinase Isoforms

Property	Type I	Type II	Type III
Susceptibility to propylthiouracil	High	Low	Low
Tissue localization	Thyroid, liver, kidney	Pituitary, thyroid, CNS, brown adipose tissue	Placenta, developing brain, skin
Preferred substrate	rT_3 and T_3	T_4 and rT_3	T_3 and T_4
Physiologic or pathophysiologic role	Clearance of rT_3 and T_3, predominant extrathyroidal source of T_3 in hyperthyroidism	Intracellular T_3 production, especially for brain in hypothyroidism or iodine deficiency, and maintenance of plasma T_3	Clearance of T_3 and T_4
Developmental expression	Expressed latest in development; predominant deiodinase in adult	Expressed second; especially high in brain and brown adipose tissue	Expressed first; high in developing brain; may be important for fetal thyroid hormone metabolism

rT_3, reverse T_3; T_3, triiodothyronine; T_4, thyroxine.

higher for T_3 than for T_4, the deiodinase enzymes play a pivotal role in determining overall metabolic activity. Three different monodeiodinase enzymes are present in the body.[10] Of the enzymes that catalyze 5′-monodeiodination, type I enzymes are present in peripheral tissues such as the liver and kidney, whereas type II enzymes are found in the CNS, pituitary, and thyroid. Type III enzymes, found in the placenta, skin, and developing brain, inactivate T_4 and T_3 by deiodinating the inner ring at the 5 position. The principal characteristics of these enzymes are listed in Table 58-2. T_4 may also be acted on by the enzyme 5′-monodeiodinase to form reverse T_3, but this accounts for a small component of hormone metabolism. Polymorphisms in the deiodinase genes may prove to be of clinical significance. For example, a polymorphism in the type I deiodinase leading to increased activity seems to be associated with an increased circulating ratio of free T_3 to free T_4.[11] Reverse T_3 has no known significant biologic activity. T_3 is removed from the body by deiodinative degradation and through the action of sulfotransferase enzyme systems converting to T_3 sulfate and 3,3-diiodothyronine sulfates, thus facilitating enterohepatic clearance. Thyronamines are derivatives of thyroid hormone that are present in low concentrations in human serum.[12] The most studied thyronamine, 3-iodothyronamine, can theoretically be made from T_4 by decarboxylation and deiodination. Administration of pharmacologic amounts of 3-iodothyronamine to animals has profound effects on temperature regulation and cardiac function, and shifts fuel metabolism from carbohydrates to lipids. However, a possible physiologic role for thyronamines has yet to be determined,[13] although altered levels may be associated with some disease states.[14]

The growth and function of the thyroid are stimulated by activation of the thyrotropin receptor by TSH.[15] The receptor belongs to the family of G-protein–coupled receptors. The thyrotropin receptor is coupled to the α subunit of the stimulatory guanine-nucleotide–binding protein ($G_s\alpha$), activating adenylate cyclase and increasing the accumulation of cyclic adenosine monophosphate. Through this mechanism, TSH stimulates the expression of Na^+/I^- symporter, TG, and thyroid peroxidase genes as well as increases apical iodide efflux. Somatic activating mutations in the receptor are commonly seen in autonomously functioning thyroid nodules.[16] Rarely, germline-activating mutations of the TSH receptor have been reported in kindreds with Leclere's syndrome, and thyrotoxicosis can result from germline-activating mutations in G-protein signaling in McCune-Albright syndrome.[15] Conversely, thyrotropin resistance results from point mutations that prevent TSH binding, leading to abnormalities in the thyrotropin receptor–adenylate cyclase system and congenital hypothyroidism.[17] Individuals with this abnormality have high levels of TSH but decreased TG levels and a normal or small gland.

Thyroid hormone nuclear receptors regulate the transcription of target genes in the presence of physiologic concentrations of T_3.[18] Unlike most other nuclear receptors, TRs also actively regulate gene expression in the absence of hormone, typically resulting in an opposite effect. TRs translocate from the cytoplasm to the nucleus, interact in the nucleus with T_3, and target genes and other proteins required for basal and T_3-dependent gene transcription. TRs exist in several isoforms, including TRβ1, TRβ2, and TRα1. Thyroid hormone has different actions in different tissues based on tissue-specific expression of the different TR isoforms. There is interest in developing thyroid hormone analogs that selectively activate specific TR isoforms. Such agents could theoretically have targeted desirable effects such as stimulating energy expenditure without having adverse effects on other tissues.[19]

The production of thyroid hormone is regulated in two main ways. First, thyroid hormone is regulated by TSH secreted by the anterior pituitary. The secretion of TSH is itself under negative feedback control by the circulating level of free thyroid hormone and the positive influence of hypothalamic thyrotropin-releasing hormone (TRH). Second, extrathyroidal deiodination of T_4 to T_3 is regulated by a variety of factors including nutrition, nonthyroidal hormones, ambient temperatures, drugs, and illness.

THYROTOXICOSIS

Thyrotoxicosis results when tissues are exposed to excessive levels of T_4, T_3, or both.[20] In the National Health and Nutrition Examination Survey III, 0.7% of those surveyed who were not taking thyroid medications and had no history of thyroid disease had subclinical hyperthyroidism (TSH <0.1 milli–international unit/L, and T_4 normal), and 0.5% had "clinically significant" hyperthyroidism (TSH <0.1 milli–international unit/L, and T_4 >13.2 mcg/dL).[21] The prevalence of suppressed TSH values peaked for people aged 20 to 39, declined in those 40 to 79, and increased again in those 80 or older. Abnormal TSH levels were more common among women than among men.

Elderly patients are also more likely to develop atrial fibrillation with thyrotoxicosis than younger patients. The frequency of bowel movements may increase, but frank diarrhea is unusual. For the elderly patient and for the patient with very severe disease, anorexia may be present as well. Palpitations are a prominent and distressing symptom, particularly in the patient with preexisting heart disease. Proximal muscle weakness is common and is noted on climbing stairs or in getting up from a sitting position. Women may note their menses are becoming scanty and irregular. Extremely thyrotoxic patients may have tachycardia, heart failure, psychosis, hyperpyrexia, and coma, a presentation described as thyroid storm.[22]

Differential Diagnosis

If the clinical history and examination do not provide pathognomonic clues to the etiology of the patient's thyrotoxicosis,

CLINICAL PRESENTATION Thyrotoxicosis

General

- Signs and symptoms of hyperthyroidism affect multiple organ systems. Patients may have symptoms for an extended time period before the diagnosis of hyperthyroidism is made.

Symptoms

- The typical clinical manifestations of thyrotoxicosis include nervousness, anxiety, palpitations, emotional lability, easy fatigability, menstrual disturbances, and heat intolerance. A cardinal sign is loss of weight concurrent with an increased appetite.

Signs

- A variety of physical signs may be observed including warm, smooth, moist skin, exophthalmos (in Graves' disease only), pretibial myxedema (in Graves' disease only), and unusually fine hair. Separation of the end of the fingernails from the nail beds (onycholysis) may be noted. Ocular signs that result from thyrotoxicosis include retraction of the eyelids and lagging of the upper lid behind the globe when the patient looks downward (lid lag). Physical signs of a hyperdynamic circulatory state are common and include tachycardia at rest, a widened pulse pressure, and a systolic ejection murmur. Gynecomastia is sometimes noted in men. Neuromuscular examination often reveals a fine tremor of the protruded tongue and outstretched hands. Deep tendon reflexes are generally hyperactive. Thyromegaly is usually present.

Diagnosis

- Low TSH serum concentration. Elevated free and total T_3 and T_4 serum concentrations, particularly in more severe disease.
- Elevated radioactive iodine uptake (RAIU) by the thyroid gland when hormone is being overproduced; suppressed RAIU in thyrotoxicosis due to thyroid inflammation (thyroiditis)

Other Tests

- Thyroid-stimulating antibodies (TSAbs)
- TG
- Thyrotropin receptor antibodies

measurement of the RAIU is critical in the evaluation (Table 58-3). The normal 24-hour RAIU ranges from 10% to 30% with some regional variation that is due to differences in iodine intake. An elevated RAIU indicates endogenous hyperthyroidism, that is, the patient's thyroid gland is actively overproducing T_4, T_3, or both. Conversely, a low RAIU in the absence of iodine excess indicates that high levels of thyroid hormone are not a consequence of thyroid gland hyperfunction but are likely due to thyroiditis or hormone ingestion. The importance of differentiating endogenous hyperthyroidism from other causes of thyrotoxicosis lies in the widely different prognosis and treatment of the diseases in these two categories. Therapy of thyrotoxicosis associated with thyroid hyperfunction is mainly directed at decreasing the rate of thyroid hormone synthesis, secretion, or both. Such measures are ineffective in treating thyrotoxicosis that is not the result of endogenous hyperthyroidism, because hormone synthesis and regulated hormone secretion are already at a minimum.

TABLE 58-3 Differential Diagnosis of Thyrotoxicosis

Increased RAIU[a]	Decreased RAIU
TSH-induced hyperthyroidism	Inflammatory thyroid disease
TSH-secreting tumors	Subacute thyroiditis
Selective pituitary resistance to T_4	Painless thyroiditis
Thyroid stimulators other than TSH	Ectopic thyroid tissue
TSAb (Graves' disease)	Struma ovarii
hCG (trophoblastic diseases)	Metastatic follicular carcinoma
Thyroid autonomy	Exogenous sources of thyroid hormone
Toxic adenoma	Medications containing thyroid hormone or iodine
Multinodular goiter	Food sources containing thyroid gland

hCG, human chorionic gonadotropin; RAIU, radioactive iodine uptake; TSAb, thyroid-stimulating antibody; TSH, thyroid-stimulating hormone.

[a]The RAIU may be decreased if the patient has been recently exposed to excess iodine.

Causes of Thyrotoxicosis Associated with Elevated RAIU

TSH-Induced Hyperthyroidism

To better understand these syndromes, we must first review TSH biosynthesis and secretion. TSH is synthesized in the anterior pituitary as separate α- and β-subunit precursors. The α subunits from luteinizing hormone (LH), follicle-stimulating hormone (FSH), human chorionic gonadotropin (hCG), and TSH are similar, whereas the β subunits are unique and confer immunologic and biologic specificity. Free β subunits are devoid of receptor binding and biologic activity and require combination with an α subunit to express their activity. Criteria for the diagnosis of TSH-induced hyperthyroidism include (a) evidence of peripheral hypermetabolism, (b) diffuse thyroid gland enlargement, (c) elevated free thyroid hormone levels, and (d) elevated or inappropriately "normal" serum immunoreactive TSH concentrations. Because the pituitary gland is extremely sensitive to even minimal elevations of free T_4, a "normal" or elevated TSH level in any thyrotoxic patient indicates the inappropriate production of TSH.

TSH-Secreting Pituitary Adenomas

TSH-secreting pituitary tumors occur sporadically and release biologically active hormone that is unresponsive to normal feedback control.[23] The mean age at diagnosis is around 40 years, with women being diagnosed more than men (8:7). These tumors may cosecrete prolactin or growth hormone; therefore, the patients may present with amenorrhea/galactorrhea or signs of acromegaly. Most patients present with classic symptoms and signs of thyrotoxicosis. Visual field defects may be present due to impingement of the optic chiasm by the tumor. Tumor growth and worsening visual field defects have been reported following antithyroid therapy because lowering of thyroid hormone levels is associated with loss of feedback inhibition from high thyroid hormone levels.

Diagnosis of a TSH-secreting adenoma should be made by demonstrating lack of TSH response to TRH stimulation, inappropriate TSH levels, elevated α-subunit levels, and radiologic imaging; given the lack of routine availability of TRH, the other three criteria are essential. Note that some small tumors are not identified by MRI. Moreover, 10% of "normal" individuals may have incidental pituitary tumors or other benign focal lesions noted on pituitary imaging.

Transsphenoidal pituitary surgery is the treatment of choice for TSH-secreting adenomas. Pituitary gland irradiation is often given following surgery to prevent tumor recurrence. Dopamine agonists and octreotide have been used to treat tumors, especially those that cosecrete prolactin.

Pituitary Resistance to Thyroid Hormone

Resistance to thyroid hormone is a rare condition that can be due to a number of molecular defects, including mutations in the TRβ gene. Pituitary resistance to thyroid hormone (PRTH) refers to selective resistance of the pituitary thyrotrophs to thyroid hormone.[24] As nonpituitary tissues respond normally to thyroid hormone, patients experience the toxic peripheral effects of thyroid hormone excess. About 90% of patients studied have an appropriate increase in TSH in response to TRH; conversely, the TSH will be suppressed by T_3 administration.

Patients with PRTH require treatment to reduce their elevated thyroid hormone levels. Determining the appropriate serum T_4 level is difficult because TSH cannot be used to evaluate adequacy of therapy. Any reduction in thyroid hormone carries the risk of inducing thyrotroph hyperplasia. Ideally, agents that suppress TSH secretion could be used to treat these individuals. Glucocorticoids, dopaminergic drugs, somatostatin and its analogs, and thyroid hormone analogs with reduced metabolic activity have all been tried, but with relatively little benefit. β-Blocker therapy can also be used. Triiodothyroacetic acid (TRIAC), an agent that is devoid of thyromimetic properties on peripheral tissues, but blocks the secretion of TSH, has been used to treat this condition. However, it is not available in the United States. Given the ability of retinoid X receptor ligands to inhibit TSH production, drugs such as bexarotene may have therapeutic benefit in PRTH.[25]

Thyroid Stimulators Other than TSH

Graves' Disease

2 Graves' disease is an autoimmune syndrome that usually includes hyperthyroidism, diffuse thyroid enlargement, exophthalmos, and, less commonly, pretibial myxedema and thyroid acropachy (Fig. 58-4).[20,26] Graves' disease is the most common cause of hyperthyroidism, with a prevalence estimated to be 3 per 1,000 population in the United States. Hyperthyroidism results from the action of TSAbs, which are directed against the thyrotropin receptor on the surface of the thyroid cell.[27] When these immunoglobulins bind to the receptor, they activate downstream G-protein signaling and adenylate cyclase in the same manner as TSH. Autoantibodies that react with orbital muscle and fibroblast tissue in the skin are responsible for the extrathyroidal manifestations of Graves' disease, and these autoantibodies are encoded by the same germline genes that encode for other autoantibodies for striated muscle and thyroid peroxidase.[28] Clinically, the extrathyroidal disorders may not appear at the same time that hyperthyroidism develops.

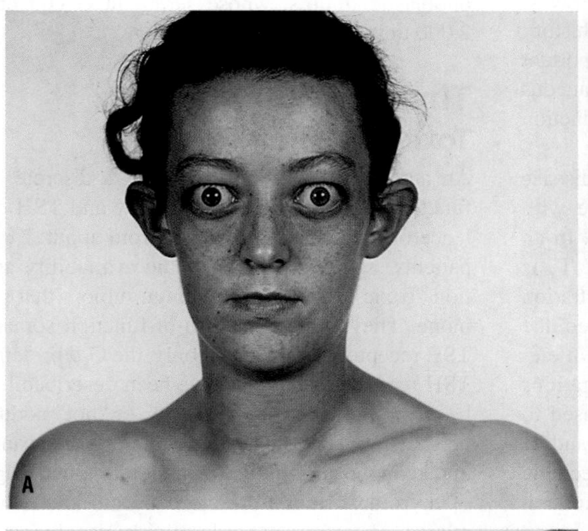

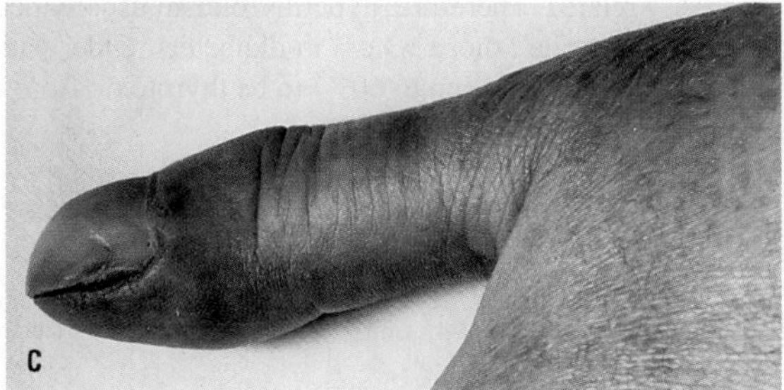

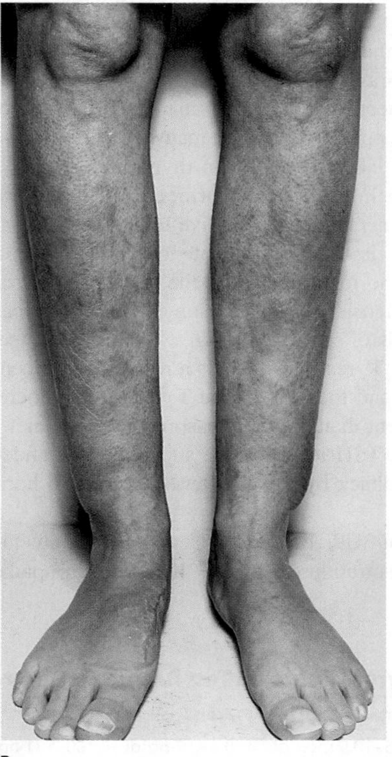

FIGURE 58-4 Features of Graves' disease. *A.* Facial appearance in Graves' disease; lid retraction, periorbital edema, and proptosis are marked. *B.* Thyroid dermopathy over the lateral aspects of the shins. *C.* Thyroid acropachy. *(Reproduced with permission from Fauci AS, Kasper DL, Longo DL, et al., eds. Harrison's Principles of Internal Medicine, 16th ed. New York: McGraw-Hill, 2005:2114.)*

There is now compelling evidence that heredity predisposes the susceptible individual to development of clinically overt autoimmune thyroid disease in the setting of appropriate environmental and hormonal triggers. A role for gender in the emergence of Graves' disease is suggested by the fact that hyperthyroidism is approximately eight times more common in women than in men. Other lines of evidence support a role for heredity. First, there is a well-recognized clustering of Graves' disease within some families. Twin studies in Graves' disease have revealed that a monozygotic twin has a 35% likelihood of ultimately developing the disease compared with a 3% likelihood for a dizygotic twin, resulting in estimation that 79% of the predisposition to Graves' disease is genetic.[29] Second, the occurrence of other autoimmune diseases, including Hashimoto's thyroiditis, is also increased in families of patients with Graves' disease. Third, several studies have demonstrated an increased frequency of certain human leukocyte antigens (HLAs) in patients with Graves' disease. Differing HLA associations have been identified in the various ethnic groups studied. In whites, for example, the relative risk of Graves' disease in carriers of the HLA-DR3 haplotype is between 2.5 and 5, whereas lesser associations have been reported for HLA-B8 and the HLA-DQA*0501 allele.[30] As with other autoimmune conditions, certain polymorphisms of the T-cell immunoregulatory protein CTLA-4 have also been associated with Graves' disease. Despite these statistical associations, however, even detailed molecular genetic linkage studies have failed to identify specific genes responsible for the disease.[31]

The thyroid gland is diffusely enlarged in the majority of patients and is commonly 40 to 60 g (two to three times the normal size). The surface of the gland is either smooth or bosselated, and the consistency varies from soft to firm. For patients with severe disease, a thrill may be felt and a systolic bruit may be heard over the gland, reflecting the increased intraglandular vascularity typical of hyperplasia. Whereas the presence of any of the extrathyroidal manifestations of this syndrome, including exophthalmos, thyroid acropachy, or pretibial myxedema, in a thyrotoxic patient is pathognomonic of Graves' disease, most patients can be diagnosed on the basis of their history and examination of their diffuse goiter (see Fig. 58-4). An important clinical feature of Graves' disease is the occurrence of spontaneous remissions, albeit uncommon. The abnormalities in TSAb production may decrease or disappear over time in many patients.

The results of laboratory tests in thyrotoxic Graves' disease include an increase in the overall hormone production rate with a disproportionate increase in T_3 relative to T_4 (Table 58-4). In an occasional patient, the disproportionate overproduction of T_3 is exaggerated, with the result that only the serum T_3 concentration is increased (T_3 toxicosis). The saturation of TBG is increased due to the elevated levels of serum T_4 and T_3, which is reflected in elevated values for the T_3 resin uptake. As a result, the concentrations of free T_4, free T_3, and the free T_4 and T_3 indices are increased to an even greater extent than are the measured serum total T_4 and T_3 concentrations. The TSH level will be suppressed or undetectable due to negative feedback by elevated levels of thyroid hormone at the pituitary.

For the patient with manifest disease, measurement of the serum free T_4 concentration (or total T_4 and T_3 resin uptake), total T_3, and the TSH value will confirm the diagnosis of thyrotoxicosis. If the patient is not pregnant or lactating, a 24-hour RAIU should be obtained if there is any diagnostic uncertainty, for example, recent onset of symptoms or other factors suggestive of thyroiditis. An increased RAIU documents that the thyroid gland is inappropriately utilizing the iodine to produce more thyroid hormone at a time when the patient is thyrotoxic.

Thyrotoxic periodic paralysis is a rare complication of hyperthyroidism commonly observed in Asian and Hispanic populations.[32] It presents as recurrent proximal muscle flaccidity ranging from mild weakness to total paralysis. The paralysis may be asymmetric and usually involves muscle groups that are strenuously exercised before the attack. Cognition and sensory perception are spared, whereas deep tendon reflexes are markedly diminished commonly. The condition is characterized by hypokalemia and low urinary potassium excretion. Hypokalemia results from a sudden shift of potassium from extracellular to intracellular sites rather than reduced total body potassium. High-carbohydrate loads and exercise provoke the attacks. Treatment includes correcting the hyperthyroid state, potassium administration, spironolactone to conserve potassium, and propranolol to minimize intracellular shifts. Some patients with this condition have a mutation in the inwardly rectifying potassium channel Kir2.6.[33]

Trophoblastic Diseases

hCG is a stimulator of the TSH receptor and may cause hyperthyroidism.[34] The basis for the thyrotropic effect of hCG is the structural similarity of hCG to TSH (similar α subunits and unique β subunits). For patients with hyperthyroidism caused by trophoblastic tumors, serum hCG levels usually exceed 300 units/mL and always exceed 100 units/mL. The mean peak hCG level in normal pregnancy is 50 units/mL. On a molar basis, hCG has only 1/10,000 the activity of pituitary TSH in mouse bioassays. Nevertheless, this thyrotropic activity may be very substantial for patients with trophoblastic tumors, whose serum hCG concentrations may reach 2,000 units/mL.

Thyroid Autonomy

Toxic Adenoma

An autonomous thyroid nodule is a discrete thyroid mass whose function is independent of pituitary and TSH control.[35] The prevalence of toxic adenoma ranges from about 2% to 9% of thyrotoxic patients, and depends on iodine availability and geographic location. Toxic adenomas are benign tumors that produce thyroid hormone. They arise from gain-of-function somatic mutations of the TSH receptor or, less commonly, the $G_s\alpha$ protein; more than a dozen TSH receptor mutations have been described.[16] These nodules may be referred to as *toxic adenomas*, or "hot" nodules, because of their persistent uptake on a radioiodine thyroid scan, despite suppressed uptake in the surrounding nonnodular gland (Fig. 58-5). The amount of thyroid hormone produced by an autonomous nodule is mass related. Therefore, hyperthyroidism usually occurs with larger nodules (i.e., those >3 cm in diameter). Older patients (>60 years) are more likely (up to 60%) to be thyrotoxic from autonomous nodules

TABLE 58-4 Thyroid Function Test Results in Different Thyroid Conditions

	Total T_4	Free T_4	Total T_3	T_3 Resin Uptake	Free Thyroxine Index	TSH
Normal	4.5–10.9 mcg/dL	0.8–2.7 ng/dL	60–181 ng/dL	22–34%	1–4.3 units	0.5–4.7 milli-international units/L
Hyperthyroid	↑↑	↑↑	↑↑↑	↑	↑↑↑	↓↓
Hypothyroid	↓↓	↓↓	↓	↓↓	↓↓↓	↑↑
Increased TBG	↑	Normal	↑	↓	Normal	Normal

TBG, thyroxine-binding globulin; TSH, thyroid-stimulating hormone.

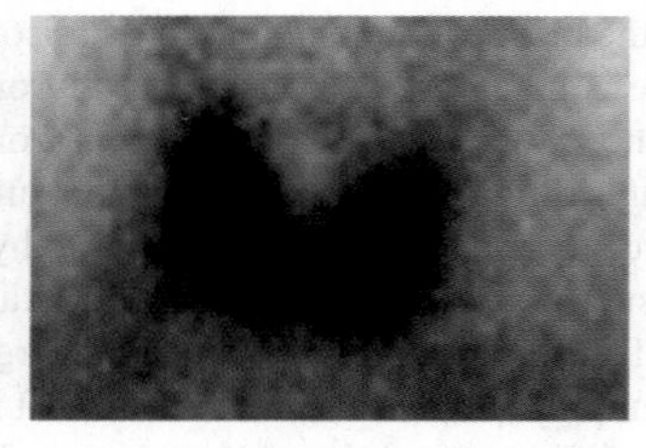

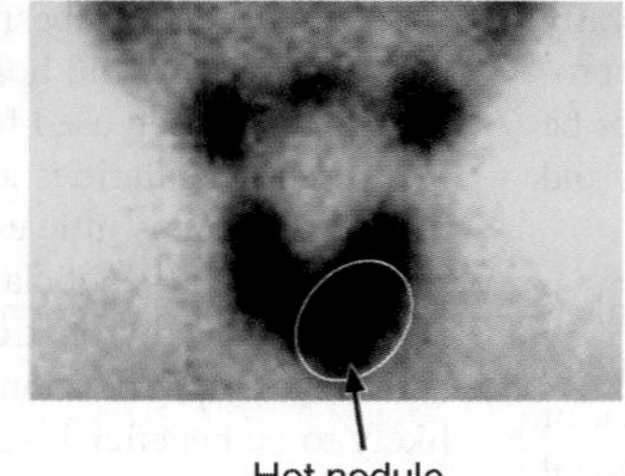

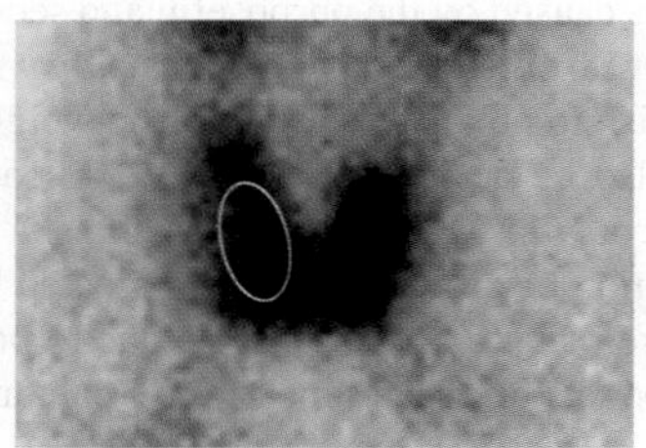

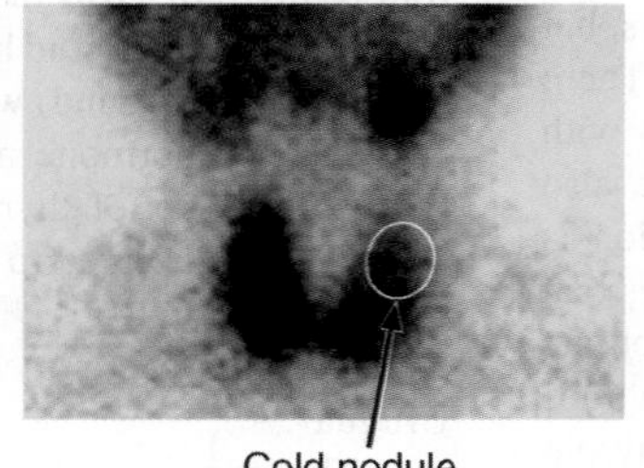

FIGURE 58-5 Radioiodine thyroid scans. *A.* Normal or increased thyroid uptake of iodine-125 (^{125}I). *B.* Thyroid with marked decrease in ^{125}I uptake in a large palpable mass. *C.* Increased ^{125}I uptake isolated to a single nodule, the "hot nodule." *D.* Decreased thyroid ^{125}I uptake in an isolated region, the "cold nodule." *(Reproduced with permission from Molina PE. Endocrine Physiology, 2nd ed. New York: McGraw-Hill, 2006:90. Images courtesy of Dr. Luis Linares, Memorial Medical Center, New Orleans, LA.)*

than are younger patients (12%). There are many reports of isolated elevation of serum T_3 for patients with autonomously functioning nodules. Therefore, if the T_4 level is normal, a T_3 level must be measured to rule out T_3 toxicosis. If autonomous function is suspected but the TSH is normal, the diagnosis can be confirmed by a failure of the autonomous nodule to decrease its iodine uptake during exogenous T_3 administration sufficient to suppress TSH. Surgical resection, thionamides, percutaneous ethanol injection, and radioactive iodine (RAI) ablation are treatment options, but since thionamides do not halt the proliferative process in the nodule, definitive therapies are recommended.[36] Ethanol ablation may be associated with pain and damage to surrounding extrathyroidal tissues, limiting its acceptance in the United States. It has been hypothesized that sublethal radiation doses received by the surrounding nonnodular thyroid tissue during RAI therapy of toxic nodules may lead to induction of thyroid cancer, and excess thyroid cancer mortality has recently been associated with RAI therapy of toxic nodular disease. Thus, an autonomously functioning nodule, if not large enough to cause thyrotoxicosis, can often be observed conservatively without therapy.

Multinodular Goiters

In multinodular goiters (MNGs), follicles with autonomous function coexist with normal or even nonfunctioning follicles. The pathogenesis of MNG is thought to be similar to that of toxic adenoma: diffuse hyperplasia caused by goitrogenic stimuli, leading to mutations and clonal expansion of benign neoplasms.[37] The functional status of the nodule(s) depends on the nature of the underlying mutations, whether activating such as TSH receptor mutations or inhibitory such as ras mutations. Thyrotoxicosis in a MNG occurs when a sufficient mass of autonomous follicles generates enough thyroid hormone to exceed the needs of the patient. It is not surprising that this type of hyperthyroidism develops insidiously over a period of several years and predominantly affects older individuals with long-standing goiters. The patient's complaints of weight loss, depression, anxiety, and insomnia may be attributed to old age. Any unexplained chronic illness in an elderly patient presenting with a MNG calls for the exclusion of hidden thyrotoxicosis.[38] Third-generation TSH assays and T_3 suppression testing may be useful in detecting subclinical hyperthyroidism.

A thyroid scan will show patchy areas of autonomously functioning thyroid tissue intermixed with hypofunctioning areas. When the patient is euthyroid, therapy is based on the need to reduce goiter size due to mass-related symptoms such as dysphagia. Doses of thyroid hormone sufficient to suppress TSH levels may slow goiter growth or cause some degree of shrinkage, but, in general, suppression therapy for nodular disease is inadequate to address mass effect.[39] The preferred treatment for toxic MNG is RAI or surgery. Surgery is usually selected for younger patients and patients in whom large goiters impinge on vital organs. Alternatively, percutaneous injection of 95% ethanol has also been used to destroy single or multinodular adenomas with a 5-year success rate approaching 80%.

Causes of Thyrotoxicosis Associated with Suppressed RAIU

Inflammatory Thyroid Disease

Subacute Thyroiditis Painful subacute (granulomatous or de Quervain) thyroiditis often develops after a viral syndrome, but rarely has a specific virus been identified in thyroid parenchyma.[40] A genetic predisposition exists, with markedly higher risk for developing subacute thyroiditis for patients with HLA-Bw35. Systemic symptoms often accompany the syndrome, including fever, malaise, and myalgia, in addition to those symptoms due to thyrotoxicosis. Typically, patients complain of severe pain in the thyroid region, which often extends to the ear on the affected side.[41] With time, the pain may migrate from one side of the gland to the other. On physical examination, the thyroid gland is firm and exquisitely tender. Signs of thyrotoxicosis are present.

Thyroid function tests typically run a triphasic course. Initially, serum T_4 levels are elevated due to release of preformed thyroid hormone from disrupted follicles. The 24-hour RAIU during this time is less than 2% due to thyroid inflammation and TSH suppression by the elevated T_4 level. As the disease progresses, intrathyroidal hormone stores are depleted, and the patient may become mildly hypothyroid with an appropriately elevated TSH level. During the recovery phase, thyroid hormone stores are replenished, and serum TSH concentration gradually returns to normal. Recovery is generally complete within 2 to 6 months. Most patients remain euthyroid, and recurrences of painful thyroiditis are extremely rare. The patient with painful thyroiditis should be reassured that the disease is self-limited and is unlikely to recur. Thyrotoxic symptoms may be relieved with β-blockers. Aspirin (650 mg orally every 6 hours) will usually relieve the pain. Occasionally, prednisone (20 mg orally three times a day) must be used to suppress the inflammatory process. Antithyroid drugs are not indicated because they will not be effective as they do not decrease the release of preformed thyroid hormone.

Painless Thyroiditis Since its description in 1975, painless (silent, lymphocytic) thyroiditis has been recognized as a common cause of thyrotoxicosis and may represent up to 15% of cases of thyrotoxicosis in North America.[42] In the setting of development of lymphocytic thyroiditis during the first 12 months after the end of pregnancy, the condition is also called *postpartum thyroiditis*.[43] The etiology is not fully understood and may be heterogeneous, but evidence indicates that autoimmunity underlies most cases. There is an increased frequency of HLA-DR3 and DR5 in patients with painless thyroiditis; nonendocrine autoimmune diseases are also more common. Histologically, diffuse lymphocytic infiltration is generally identified. The triphasic course of this illness mimics that of subacute thyroiditis. Most patients present with mild thyrotoxic symptoms. Lid retraction and lid lag are present, but exophthalmos is absent. The thyroid gland may be diffusely enlarged, but thyroid tenderness is absent.

The 24-hour RAIU will typically be suppressed to less than 2% during the thyrotoxic phase of painless thyroiditis. Anti-TG and antithyroid peroxidase antibody (anti-TPOAb) levels are elevated in more than 50% of patients. Patients with mild hyperthyroidism and painless thyroiditis should be reassured that they have a self-limited disease, although patients with postpartum thyroiditis may experience recurrence of the disease with subsequent pregnancies. As with other thyrotoxic syndromes, adrenergic symptoms may be ameliorated with propranolol or metoprolol. Antithyroid drugs, which inhibit new hormone synthesis, are not indicated because they do not decrease the release of preformed thyroid hormone. A small proportion of patients may have recurrent episodes of thyroiditis,[44] or may develop permanent hypothyroidism.[45]

Ectopic Thyroid Tissue

Struma Ovarii Struma ovarii is a teratoma of the ovary that contains differentiated thyroid follicular cells and is capable of making thyroid hormone.[46] This extremely rare cause of thyrotoxicosis is suggested by the absence of thyroid enlargement in a thyrotoxic patient with a suppressed RAIU in the neck and no findings to suggest thyroiditis. The diagnosis is established by localizing functioning thyroid tissue in the ovary with whole-body RAI (sodium iodide-131 [^{131}I]) scanning. Interestingly, struma ovarii without associated hyperthyroidism is much more common than struma ovarii associated with hyperthyroidism. Because the tissue is neoplastic and potentially malignant, combined surgical and radioiodine treatment of malignant struma ovarii for both monitoring and therapy of relapse is the recommended treatment.

Thyroid Cancer In widely metastatic differentiated papillary or follicular carcinomas with relatively well-preserved function, sufficient thyroid hormone can be synthesized and secreted to produce thyrotoxicosis.[47] In most instances, a previous diagnosis of thyroid malignancy has been made. The diagnosis can be confirmed by whole-body ^{131}I scanning. Treatment with ^{131}I is generally effective at ablating functioning thyroid metastases.

Exogenous Sources of Thyroid Hormone or Iodine

Exogenous Thyroid Hormone Thyrotoxicosis factitia was described in the recent American Thyroid Association guidelines on the management of hyperthyroidism as "all causes of hyperthyroidism due to ingestion of thyroid hormone."[48] This category includes hyperthyroidism produced by the intentional ingestion of exogenous thyroid hormone.[49] Obesity is the most common nonthyroidal disorder for which thyroid hormone is inappropriately used, but thyroid hormone has been used for almost every conceivable problem from menstrual irregularities and infertility to hypercholesterolemia and baldness. There is little evidence to suggest that treatment with thyroid hormone is beneficial for such conditions in euthyroid individuals. Obviously, thyrotoxicosis factitia can also occur when too large a dose of thyroid hormone is employed for conditions in which it is likely to be beneficial, such as differentiated thyroid carcinoma. In addition to this iatrogenic cause, accidental ingestion such as may occur with pediatric ingestion or pharmacy error is also possible. Rarely, thyrotoxicosis factitia is caused by the purposeful and secretive ingestion of thyroid hormone by disturbed patients (usually with a medical background) who wish to obtain attention or lose weight.

Thyroid hormone may also be accidentally ingested in food sources. Reports of thyrotoxicosis in Minnesota and Nebraska in 1980s were attributed to ingestion of ground beef contaminated by bovine thyroid glands.[50,51] More recently thyrotoxicosis due to porcine thyroid tissue in meat products has been reported in Spain and Uruguay.[52,53]

Thyrotoxicosis factitia should be suspected in a thyrotoxic patient without evidence of increased hormone production, thyroidal inflammation, or ectopic thyroid tissue. The RAIU uptake is at low levels because the patient's thyroid gland function is suppressed by the exogenous thyroid hormone. Measurement of plasma TG is a valuable laboratory aid in the diagnosis of thyrotoxicosis factitia. TG is normally secreted in small amounts by the thyroid gland; however, when thyroid hormone is taken orally, TG levels tend to be lower than the normal range. In other entities characterized by a low RAIU, such as thyroiditis, leakage of preformed thyroid hormone results in elevated TG levels. If a history of thyroid hormone ingestion is elicited or deduced, exogenous thyroid hormone should be withheld for between 4 and 6 weeks, and thyroid function tests repeated to document that the euthyroid state has been restored. Rarely, thyroid hormone analogs or metabolites may be the drug of abuse, specific detection of which may be difficult with standard thyroid hormone assays. For example, tiratricol (TRIAC), an endogenous metabolite of T_3 that has been used for weight loss and paradoxically by body builders, will suppress TSH at high enough doses and may cross-react in many T_3 immunoassays; thus, thyrotoxicosis factitia due to tiratricol abuse may be misinterpreted as T_3 toxicosis.[54]

Medications Containing Iodine Amiodarone may induce thyrotoxicosis (2% to 3% of patients), overt hypothyroidism (5% of patients), subclinical hypothyroidism (25% of patients), or euthyroid hyperthyroxinema, depending on the underlying thyroid pathology or lack thereof.[55] Because amiodarone contains 37% iodine by weight, approximately 6 mg/day of iodine is released for each 200 mg of amiodarone, 1,000 times greater than the recommended daily amount of iodine of 150 mcg/day. As a result of this iodine overload, iodine-exacerbated thyroid dysfunction commonly occurs among those patients with preexisting thyroid disease: thyrotoxicosis in patients with hyperthyroidism or euthyroid nodular autonomy and hypothyroidism in patients with autoimmune thyroid disease. In contrast to hyperthyroidism with increased synthesis of thyroid hormone induced by amiodarone (type I), destructive thyroiditis with loss of TG and thyroid hormones also occurs (type II), typically among individuals with otherwise normal glands. The two types of amiodarone-induced thyrotoxicosis may be differentiated using color flow Doppler ultrasonography. Such distinction is critically important, given the therapeutic implications of the two syndromes: type I amiodarone-induced hyperthyroidism responds somewhat to thionamides, whereas type II may respond to glucocorticoids or iopanoic acid.[55] Unfortunately, however, the latter agent is no longer available. Obviously, RAI therapy is inappropriate in type

I due to the drug-induced iodine excess, and in type II due to lack of increased hormone synthesis. The manifestations of amiodarone-induced thyrotoxicosis may be atypical symptoms such as ventricular tachycardia and exacerbation of underlying chronic obstructive pulmonary disease, both of which are even more significant given the severe underlying cardiac pathology that led to the use of the drug in the first place. Amiodarone also directly interferes with type I 5′-deiodinase, leading to reduced conversion of T_4 to T_3 and hyperthyroxinemia without thyrotoxicosis.

TREATMENT
Hyperthyroidism

Desired Outcomes

3 Three common treatment modalities are used in the management of hyperthyroidism: surgery, antithyroid medications, and RAI (Table 58-5). The overall therapeutic objectives are to eliminate the excess thyroid hormone and minimize the symptoms and long-term consequences of hyperthyroidism. Therapy must be individualized based on the type and severity of hyperthyroidism, patient age and gender, existence of nonthyroidal conditions, and response to previous therapy.[56,57] Clinical guidelines for the treatment of hyperthyroidism have been published.[48]

Nonpharmacologic Therapy

Surgical removal of the hypersecreting thyroid gland became feasible in 1923 when Plummer discovered that iodine reduced the gland's vascularity, making this definitive procedure possible. Surgery should be considered for patients with a large thyroid gland (>80 g), severe ophthalmopathy, and a lack of remission on antithyroid drug treatment. In case of cosmetic issues or pressure symptoms, the choice in MNG stands between surgery, which is still the first choice, and radioiodine therapy if uptake is adequate (hot). In addition to surgery, the solitary nodule, whether hot or cold, can be treated with percutaneous ethanol injection therapy. If hot, radioiodine is the therapy of choice.[58] Traditional preparation of the patient for thyroidectomy includes methimazole (MMI) or propylthiouracil (PTU) until the patient is biochemically euthyroid (usually 6 to 8 weeks), followed by the addition of iodides (500 mg/day) for 10 to 14 days before surgery to decrease the vascularity of the gland. Iodine supplementation in iodine-deficient areas of the country may lead to a greater reduction in remnant volume in nontoxic goiter.[59] Propranolol for several weeks preoperatively and 7 to 10 days after surgery has also been used to maintain a pulse rate of less than 90 beats/min. Combined pretreatment with propranolol and 10 to 14 days of potassium iodide also has been advocated.

The overall complication rate when surgery is performed for MNG by an experienced endocrine surgeon is low.[60] If subtotal thyroidectomy, or an operation that attempts to maintain euthyroidism, is performed for Graves' disease, there is a risk of recurrence of hyperthyroidism that is directly related to remnant size.[61] Near total thyroidectomy is generally recognized as the procedure of choice for patients with Graves' disease.[48] The complication rates of surgery for Graves' disease are low when surgery is performed by a high-volume thyroid surgeon, and include hypoparathyroidism (up to 2%), and recurrent laryngeal nerve injury (up to 1%). Formal cost-effective analysis indicates that a total thyroidectomy may be the most cost-effective method for managing hyperthyroidism when considering outcomes in quality-adjusted life-years.[62]

Pharmacologic Therapy

Antithyroid Medications

4 **Thiourea Drugs** Two drugs within this category, MMI and PTU, are approved for the treatment of hyperthyroidism in the United States.[63] They are classified as thioureylenes (thionamides), which incorporate an N–C–S=N group into their ring structures.

Mechanism of Action PTU and MMI share several mechanisms to inhibit the biosynthesis of thyroid hormone.[20] These drugs serve as preferential substrates for the iodinating intermediate of thyroid peroxidase and divert iodine away from potential iodination sites in TG. This prevents subsequent incorporation of iodine into iodotyrosines and ultimately iodothyronine ("organification"). Second, they inhibit coupling of MIT and DIT to form T_4 and T_3. The coupling reaction may be more sensitive to these drugs than the iodination reaction. Experimentally, these drugs exhibit immunosuppressive effects, although the clinical relevance of this finding is unclear. For patients with Graves' disease, antithyroid drug treatment has been associated with lower TSAb titers and restoration of normal suppressor T-cell function. However, ClO_4^-, which has a different mechanism of action, also decreases TSAbs, suggesting that normalization of the thyroid hormone level may itself improve the abnormal immune function. PTU inhibits the peripheral conversion of T_4 to T_3. This effect is acutely dose related and occurs within hours of PTU administration. MMI does not have this effect. Over time, depletion of stored hormone and lack of

TABLE 58-5 Treatments for Hyperthyroidism Caused by Graves' Disease

Treatment	Advantages	Disadvantages	Comment
Methimazole (PTU only second-line therapy)	Noninvasive Low initial cost Low risk of permanent hypothyroidism Possible remissions due to immune effects	Low cure rate (30–80%; average 40–50%) Adverse drug reactions Drug compliance	First-line treatment in children, adolescents, and pregnancy Initial treatment in severe cases or preoperative preparation
Radioactive iodine (^{131}I)	Cure of hyperthyroidism Lowest cost, before adjustment for quality of life	Permanent hypothyroidism almost inevitable Might worsen ophthalmopathy Pregnancy must be deferred for 6–12 months; no breast-feeding Small potential risk of exacerbation of hyperthyroidism	Best treatment for toxic nodules and toxic multinodular goiter
Surgery	Rapid, effective treatment, especially in patients with large goiters	Most invasive Least costly in long term after quality-of-life adjustment Permanent hypothyroidism Pain, scar	Potential choice in pregnancy if major side effect from antithyroid drugs Potential complications (recurrent laryngeal nerve damage, hypoparathyroidism) Useful when coexisting suspicious nodule present Option for patients who refuse radioiodine

continuing synthesis of thyroid hormone results in the clinical effects of these drugs.

Pharmacokinetics Both antithyroid drugs are well absorbed (80% to 95%) from the GI tract, with peak serum concentrations about 1 hour after ingestion. The plasma half-life ranges of PTU and MMI are 1 to 2.5 and 6 to 9 hours, respectively, and are not appreciably affected by thyroid status. Urinary excretion is about 35% for PTU and less than 10% for MMI. These drugs are actively concentrated in the thyroid gland, which may account for the disparity between their relatively short plasma half-lives and the effectiveness of once-daily dosing regimens even with PTU. Approximately 60% to 80% of PTU is bound to plasma albumin, whereas MMI is not protein bound. MMI readily crosses the placenta and appears in breast milk. Older studies suggested that PTU crosses the placental membranes only one tenth as well as MMI; however, these studies were done in the course of therapeutic abortion early in pregnancy. Newer studies show little difference between fetal concentrations of PTU and MMI, and both are associated with elevated TSH in about 20% and low T_4 in about 7% of fetuses.[64]

5 ***Dosing and Monitoring*** PTU is available as 50 mg tablets, and MMI as 5 and 10 mg tablets. MMI is approximately 10 times more potent than PTU. Initial therapy with PTU ranges from 300 to 600 mg daily, usually in three or four divided doses. MMI is given in two or three divided doses totaling 30 to 60 mg/day. Although the traditional recommendation is for divided doses, evidence exists that both drugs can be given as single daily doses. Patients with severe hyperthyroidism may require larger initial doses, and some may respond better at these larger doses if the dose is divided. The maximal blocking doses of PTU and MMI are 1,200 and 120 mg daily, respectively. Once the intrathyroidal pool of thyroid hormone is reduced and new hormone synthesis is sufficiently blocked, clinical improvement should ensue. Usually within 4 to 8 weeks of initiating therapy, symptoms will diminish and circulating thyroid hormone levels will return to normal. At this time the tapering regimen can be started. Changes in dose for each drug should be made on a monthly basis, because the endogenously produced T_4 will reach a new steady-state concentration in this interval. Typical ranges of daily maintenance doses for PTU and MMI are 50 to 300 and 5 to 30 mg, respectively.

If the objective of therapy is to induce a long-term remission, the patient should remain on continuous antithyroid drug therapy for 12 to 24 months. Antithyroid drug therapy induces permanent remission rates of 10% to 98%, with an overall average of about 40% to 50%.[65] This is much higher than the remission rate seen with propranolol alone, which is reported to range from 22% to 36%. Patient characteristics for a favorable outcome include older patients (>40 years), low T_4:T_3 ratio (<20), a small goiter (<50 g), short duration of disease (<6 months), no previous history of relapse with antithyroid drugs, duration of therapy 1 to 2 years or longer, and low TSAb titers at baseline or a reduction with treatment.[20] A recent study provides preliminary evidence that a new assay that has better specificity for detection of antibodies that stimulate the TSH receptors, without detecting coexistent blocking antibodies, may be a useful predictor of remission of Graves' disease.[66]

It is important that patients be followed every 6 to 12 months after remission occurs. If a relapse occurs, alternate therapy with RAI is preferred to a second course of antithyroid drugs. Relapses seem to plateau after about 5 years and eventually 5% to 20% of patients will develop spontaneous hypothyroidism. There has been interest in whether concurrent administration of T_4 with thionamide therapy for thyrotoxicosis and subclinical hyperthyroidism can reduce autoantibodies directed toward the thyroid gland and improve remission rate. In a Japanese study, adjunctive treatment with T_4 was associated with a 20-fold reduction in the recurrence rate of Graves' disease compared with the recurrence rate seen for patients treated with antithyroid drugs alone.[67] Attempts to reproduce these results in American and European patients with Graves' disease have failed to show any delay or reduction in the recurrence of Graves' disease with T_4 administration.[68]

6 Subclinical hyperthyroidism is defined as the finding of a serum TSH below the lower limit of the reference range combined with free T_4 and T_3 concentrations that are normal. Subclinical hyperthyroidism is associated with an increased risk of atrial fibrillation, and may be associated with increased all-cause mortality. Some studies show an increased risk of hip fractures in postmenopausal women with subclinical hyperthyroidism. Most practitioners agree that treatment of older patients (greater than 65 years) with TSH values below 0.1 milli–international unit/L is reasonable. In patients who are younger or have TSH values of 0.1 to 0.4 milli–international unit/L a decision whether to treat the patient for mild hyperthyroidism or to monitor thyroid function may depend on his or her cardiovascular risk factors and bone health.[69]

Adverse Effects Minor adverse reactions to MMI and PTU have an overall incidence of 5% to 25% depending on the dose and the drug, whereas major adverse effects occur in 1.5% to 4.6% of patients receiving these drugs.[63] Pruritic maculopapular rashes (sometimes associated with vasculitis based on skin biopsy), arthralgias, and fevers occur in up to 5% of patients and may occur at greater frequency with higher doses and in children. Rashes often disappear spontaneously but, if persistent, may be managed with antihistamines.

Perhaps one of the most common side effects is a benign transient leukopenia characterized by a white blood cell (WBC) count of less than 4,000/mm^3. This condition occurs in up to 12% of adults and 25% of children, and sometimes can be confused with mild leukopenia seen in Graves' disease. This mild leukopenia is not a harbinger of the more serious adverse effect of agranulocytosis, so therapy can usually be continued. If a minor adverse reaction occurs with one antithyroid drug, the alternate thiourea may be tried, but cross-sensitivity occurs for about 50% of patients.[63]

Agranulocytosis is one of the serious adverse effects of thiourea drug therapy and is characterized by fever, malaise, gingivitis, oropharyngeal infection, and a granulocyte count less than 250/mm^3.[63] These drugs are concentrated in granulocytes, and this reaction may represent a direct toxic effect rather than hypersensitivity. This toxic reaction has occurred with both thioureas, and the incidence varies from 0.5% to 6%. It is higher for patients over age 40 receiving a MMI dose greater than 40 mg/day or the equivalent dose of PTU, and is linked to HLA class II genes containing the DRB1*08032 allele.[70] Agranulocytosis usually develops in the first 3 months of therapy. Because the onset is sudden, routine monitoring has not been recommended. Colony-stimulating factors have been used with some success to restore cell counts to normal, but it is unclear how effective this form of therapy is compared with routine supportive care.[71] Peripheral lymphocytes obtained from patients with PTU-induced agranulocytosis undergo transformation in the presence of other thioamides, suggesting that these severe reactions are immunologically mediated and patients should not receive other thionamides. Aplastic anemia has been reported with MMI and may be associated with an inhibitor to colony-forming units. Once antithyroid drugs are discontinued, clinical improvement is seen over several days to weeks. Patients should be counseled to discontinue therapy and contact their physician when flu-like symptoms such as fever, malaise, or sore throat develop.

Arthralgias and a lupus-like syndrome (sometimes in the absence of antinuclear antibodies) have been reported in 4% to 5% of patients. This generally occurs after 6 months of therapy. Uncommonly, polymyositis, presenting as proximal muscle weakness and elevated creatine phosphokinase, has been reported with PTU administration. GI intolerance is also reported to occur in 4% to

5% of patients. Patients receiving interferon products for hepatitis C or other disorders may develop hyperthyroidism or hypothyroidism along with liver enzyme abnormalities.[72] Hypoprothrombinemia is a rare complication of thionamide therapy. Patients who have experienced a major adverse reaction to one thiourea drug should not be converted to the alternate drug because of cross-sensitivity.

Older reports suggested that congenital skin defects (aplasia cutis) may be caused by MMI and carbimazole, although a registry review from the Netherlands could not find an association between maternal use of these drugs and skin defects.[73] However, more recently, several serious congenital malformations including tracheoesophageal fistulas and choanal atresia have been observed with MMI and carbimazole but not PTU use during pregnancy.[74,75] Thus, in the past, PTU was considered the drug of choice throughout pregnancy for women with hyperthyroidism, because of concerns about the possible teratogenic effects of MMI. However, currently heightened concerns about the greater hepatotoxicity of PTU than of MMI have led to the recommendation that PTU no longer be considered a first-line drug, except during the first trimester of pregnancy.

Hepatotoxicity can be seen with both MMI and PTU with a prevalence of approximately 1.3%. In mice, MMI undergoes epoxidation of the C-4,5 double bond by cytochrome P450 enzymes, and after being hydrolyzed, the resulting epoxide is decomposed to form *N*-methylthiourea, a proximate toxicant.[76] At moderate doses, some authors have found that initial enzyme elevations eventually normalize in most patients with continued therapy. PTU-induced subclinical liver injury is common and is usually transient and asymptomatic.[77] Thus, it has generally been thought that therapy with PTU may be continued with caution in the absence of symptoms and hyperbilirubinemia. However, a 1997 literature review documented 49 cases of hepatotoxicity. Twenty-eight cases were associated with PTU use, and 21 cases were associated with MMI use. The hepatotoxicity was associated with seven deaths and three deaths in the PTU and MMI groups, respectively.[78] There did not appear to be a relationship between the dose or duration of thionamide treatment and outcome. During the past 20 years of PTU use in the United States, 22 adults developed severe hepatotoxicity leading to 9 deaths and 5 liver transplants. The risk of this complication was greater in children (1:2,000) than in adults (1:10,000).[79] A recent reanalysis of data reported to the FDA from 1982 to 2008 found that toxicity in children was generally related to higher doses of PTU and that toxicity in both children and adults was associated with therapy lasting more than 4 months in duration.[80] In light of such evidence, it has been recommended by the American Thyroid Association and the FDA that PTU not be considered as first-line therapy in either adults or children.[81] One of three exceptions includes the first trimester of pregnancy, when the risk of MMI-induced embryopathy may exceed that of PTU-induced hepatotoxicity. Other exceptions include intolerance to MMI and thyroid storm.

Iodides Iodide was the first form of drug therapy for Graves' disease. Its mechanism of action is to acutely block thyroid hormone release, inhibit thyroid hormone biosynthesis by interfering with intrathyroidal iodide utilization (the Wolff-Chaikoff effect), and decrease the size and vascularity of the gland. This early inhibitory effect provides symptom improvement within 2 to 7 days of initiating therapy, and serum T_4 and T_3 concentrations may be reduced for a few weeks. Despite the reduced release of T_4 and T_3, thyroid hormone synthesis continues at an accelerated rate, resulting in a gland rich in stored hormones. The normal and hyperfunctioning thyroid soon escapes from this inhibitory effect within 1 to 2 weeks by decreasing the active transfer of iodide into the gland. Iodides are often used as adjunctive therapy to prepare a patient with Graves' disease for surgery, to acutely inhibit thyroid hormone release and quickly attain the euthyroid state in severely thyrotoxic patients with cardiac decompensation, or to inhibit thyroid hormone release following RAI therapy. However, large doses of iodine may exacerbate hyperthyroidism or indeed precipitate hyperthyroidism in some previously euthyroid individuals (Jod-Basedow disease).[82] This Jod-Basedow phenomenon is most common in iodine-deficient areas, particularly for patients with preexisting nontoxic goiter. Iodide is contraindicated in toxic MNG.

Potassium iodide is available either as a saturated solution (SSKI), which contains 38 mg of iodide per drop, or as Lugol's solution, which contains 6.3 mg of iodide per drop. The typical starting dose of SSKI is 3 to 10 drops daily (120 to 400 mg) in water or juice. There is no documented advantage to using doses in excess of 6 to 8 mg/day. When used to prepare a patient for surgery, it should be administered 7 to 14 days preoperatively. As an adjunct to RAI, SSKI should not be used before, but rather 3 to 7 days after RAI treatment, so that the radioactive iodide can concentrate in the thyroid. The most frequent toxic effects with iodide therapy are hypersensitivity reactions (skin rashes, drug fever, rhinitis, and conjunctivitis), salivary gland swelling, "iodism" (metallic taste, burning mouth and throat, sore teeth and gums, symptoms of a head cold, and sometimes stomach upset and diarrhea), and gynecomastia.

Other compounds containing organic iodide have also been used therapeutically for hyperthyroidism. These include various radiologic contrast media that share a triiodoaminobenzene and monoaminobenzene ring with a propionic acid chain (e.g., iopanoic acid and sodium ipodate). The effect of these compounds is a result of the iodine content inhibiting thyroid hormone release as well as competitive inhibition of 5′-monodeiodinase conversion related to their structures, which resemble thyroid analogs. Unfortunately, these extremely useful agents are no longer available in the United States

7 Adrenergic Blockers Because many of the manifestations of hyperthyroidism are mediated by *β*-adrenergic receptors, *β*-blockers (especially propranolol) have been used widely to ameliorate thyrotoxic symptoms such as palpitations, anxiety, tremor, and heat intolerance. Although *β*-blockers are quite effective for symptom control, they have no effect on the urinary excretion of calcium, phosphorus, hydroxyproline, creatinine, or various amino acids, suggesting a lack of effect on peripheral thyrotoxicosis and protein metabolism. Furthermore, *β*-blockers neither reduce TSAb nor prevent thyroid storm. Propranolol and nadolol partially block the conversion of T_4 to T_3, but this contribution to the overall therapeutic effect is small in magnitude. Inhibition of conversion of T_4 to T_3 is mediated by D-propranolol, which is devoid of *β*-blocking activity, and L-propranolol, which is responsible for the antiadrenergic effects, has little effect on the conversion.

β-Blockers are usually used as adjunctive therapy with antithyroid drugs, RAI, or iodides when treating Graves' disease or toxic nodules; in preparation for surgery; or in thyroid storm. The only conditions for which *β*-blockers are primary therapy for thyrotoxicosis are those associated with thyroiditis. The dose of propranolol required to relieve adrenergic symptoms is variable, but an initial dose of 20 to 40 mg four times daily is effective (heart rate <90 beats/min) for most patients. Younger or more severely toxic patients may require as much as 240 to 480 mg/day because there seems to be an increased clearance rate for these patients. *β*-Blockers are contraindicated for patients with decompensated heart failure unless it is caused solely by tachycardia (high output). Nonselective agents and those lacking intrinsic sympathomimetic activity should be used with caution for patients with asthma and bronchospastic chronic obstructive lung disease. *β*-Blockers that are cardioselective and have intrinsic sympathomimetic activity may have a slight margin of safety in these situations. Other patients in whom contraindications exist are those with sinus bradycardia, those receiving monoamine oxidase inhibitors or tricyclic antidepressants, and those with spontaneous hypoglycemia. β-Blockers may also prolong gestation and labor during pregnancy. Other side effects include nausea, vomiting, anxiety, insomnia, light-headedness, bradycardia, and hematologic disturbances.

Antiadrenergic agents such as centrally acting sympatholytics and calcium channel antagonists may have some role in the symptomatic treatment of hyperthyroidism. These drugs might be useful when contraindications to β-blockade exist. When compared with nadolol 40 mg twice daily, clonidine 150 mcg twice daily reduced plasma catecholamines, whereas nadolol increased both epinephrine and norepinephrine after 1 week of treatment. Diltiazem 120 mg given every 8 hours reduced heart rate by 17%; fewer ventricular extrasystoles were noted after 10 days of therapy, and diltiazem has been shown to be comparable to propranolol in lowering heart rate and blood pressure.

8 Radioactive Iodine Although other radioisotopes have been used to ablate thyroid tissue, ^{131}I is considered to be the agent of choice for Graves' disease, toxic autonomous nodules, and toxic MNGs.[83] RAI is administered as a colorless and tasteless liquid that is well absorbed and concentrates in the thyroid. ^{131}I is a β- and γ-emitter with a tissue penetration of 2 mm and a half-life of 8 days. Other organs take up ^{131}I, but the thyroid gland is the only organ in which organification of the absorbed iodine takes place. Initially, RAI disrupts hormone synthesis by incorporating into thyroid hormones and TG. Over a period of weeks, follicles that have taken up RAI and surrounding follicles develop evidence of cellular necrosis, breakdown of follicles, development of bizarre cell forms, nuclear pyknosis, and destruction of small vessels within the gland, leading to edema and fibrosis of the interstitial tissue. Pregnancy is an absolute contraindication to the use of RAI since radiation will be delivered to the fetal tissue, including the fetal thyroid.

β-Blockers may be given any time without compromising RAI therapy, accounting for their role as a mainstay of adjunctive therapy to RAI treatment. If iodides are administered, they should be given 3 to 7 days after RAI to prevent interference with the uptake of RAI in the thyroid gland. Because thyroid hormone levels will transiently increase following RAI treatment due to release of preformed thyroid hormone, patients with cardiac disease and elderly patients are often treated with thionamides prior to RAI ablation. For patients with underlying cardiac disease, it may be necessary to reinstitute antithyroid drug therapy following RAI ablation. The standard practice is to withdraw the thionamide 4 to 6 days prior to RAI treatment and to reinstitute it 4 days after therapy is concluded. Administering antithyroid drug therapy following RAI treatment may result in a higher rate of posttreatment recurrence or persistent hyperthyroidism.[83] Pretreatment with PTU may lead to higher rates of treatment failure, but this does not appear to be the case with MMI pretreatment.[85] Use of lithium, as adjunctive therapy to RAI therapy, has multiple benefits of increasing the cure rate, shortening the time to cure, and preventing posttherapy increase in thyroid hormone levels.[86] Lithium is likely to achieve these effects by increasing RAI retention in the thyroid and inhibiting thyroid hormone release from the gland.

Corticosteroid administration will blunt and delay the rise in antibodies to the TSH receptor, TG, and thyroid peroxidase while reducing T_3 and T_4 concentrations following RAI. Bartalena et al. found no progression in ophthalmopathy for patients receiving prednisone after RAI (0% worsened) compared with 3% worsening in those receiving MMI, and 5% worsening in those receiving RAI alone.[87] Theoretically, if shared thyroidal and orbital antigen is involved in the pathogenesis of Graves' ophthalmopathy, antigen released with RAI treatment could aggravate preexisting eye disease. There is some disagreement as to what degree of ophthalmopathy should be considered a contraindication to RAI. However, in those with moderate or severe orbitopathy it seems reasonable to delay RAI until the patient's eye disease has been stable.

Destruction of the gland attenuates the hyperthyroid state, and hypothyroidism commonly occurs months to years following RAI.[20,88] The goal of therapy is to destroy overactive thyroid cells, and a single dose of 4,000 to 8,000 rad results in a euthyroid state in 60% of patients at 6 months or less. The remaining 40% become euthyroid within 1 year, requiring two or more doses. It is advisable that a second dose of RAI be given 6 months after the first RAI treatment if the patient remains hyperthyroid. Variables that predict an unsuccessful outcome of RAI include gender (men are less likely to develop hypothyroidism), race, the size of the thyroid (euthyroidism is less likely in large glands), severity of disease, and perhaps a higher level of TSAb. In a recent study predictors of successful treatment with RAI included higher ablative dose, female gender, lower free T_4 levels at diagnosis, and absence of a palpable goiter.[84] The acute, short-term side effects of ^{131}I therapy are minimal and include mild thyroidal tenderness and dysphagia. Concern over increased risk of mutations and congenital defects now appears to be unfounded because long-term followup studies have not revealed increased risk for these complications.[89] In studies examining the risk of malignancies after RAI therapy, there seems to be a small but significant increase in the risk of cancer of the small bowel and thyroid.[89] Although RAI is very effective in the treatment of hyperthyroidism, long-term followup from Great Britain suggests that among patients with hyperthyroidism treated with RAI, mortality from all causes and mortality resulting from cardiovascular and cerebrovascular disease and fracture are increased.[90]

A common approach to Graves' hyperthyroidism is to administer a single dose of 5 to 15 mCi (80 to 200 μCi/g of tissue).[83] The optimal method for determining ^{131}I treatment doses for Graves' hyperthyroidism is unknown, and techniques have varied from a fixed dose to more elaborate calculations based on gland size, iodine uptake, and iodine turnover. In a trial of 88 patients with Graves' disease, no difference in outcome was seen among high or low, fixed or adjusted doses.[91] Thyroid glands estimated to weigh >80 g may require larger doses of RAI. Larger doses are likely to induce hypothyroidism and are seldom given outside the United States due to the imposition of stringent safety restrictions. For example, in the United Kingdom, a nursery school teacher is advised to stay out of school for 3 weeks following a 15 mCi dose of ^{131}I.[88]

Evaluation of Therapeutic Outcomes: Hyperthyroidism

After therapy (surgery, thionamides, or RAI) for hyperthyroidism has been initiated, patients should be evaluated on a monthly basis until they reach a euthyroid condition. Clinical signs of continuing thyrotoxicosis (tachycardia, weight loss, and heat intolerance, among others) or the development of hypothyroidism (bradycardia, weight gain, and lethargy, among others) should be noted. β-Blockers may be used to control symptoms of thyrotoxicosis until the definitive treatment has returned the patient to a euthyroid state. Once T_4 replacement is initiated, the goal is to maintain both the free T_4 level and the TSH concentration in the normal range. Once a stable dose of T_4 is identified, the patient may be followed up every 6 to 12 months.

Finally, a common, potentially confusing clinical situation should be mentioned. Why are the TSH concentrations suppressed for some patients who are clinically hypothyroid and who have a low free T_4 level? For patients with long-standing hyperthyroidism, the pituitary thyrotrophs responsible for making TSH become atrophic. The average amount of time required for these cells to resume normal functioning is 6 to 8 weeks.[92] Therefore, if a thyrotoxic patient has his or her free T_4 concentration lowered rapidly, before the thyrotrophs resume normal function, a period of "transient central hypothyroidism" will be observed.

Special Conditions

Graves' Disease and Pregnancy

Inappropriate production of hCG is a cause of abnormal thyroid function tests during the first half of pregnancy, and hCG can cause either subclinical (normal T_4, suppressed TSH) or overt hyperthyroidism.[93,94] This is because the homology of hCG and TSH leads to hCG-mediated stimulation through the TSH receptor. A recent study showed that at hCG concentrations greater than 400 international units/mL, TSH levels were invariably suppressed and free T_4 levels were generally above the normal range. Most patients with hCG greater than 200 international units/mL did not have symptoms of hyperthyroidism.[95] The variability of the thyrotropic potency of hCG is believed to depend on its carbohydrate composition.

Hyperthyroidism during pregnancy is almost solely caused by Graves' disease, with approximately 0.1% to 0.4% of pregnancies affected. Although the increased metabolic rate is usually well tolerated in pregnant women, two symptoms suggestive of hyperthyroidism during pregnancy are failure to gain weight despite good appetite and persistent tachycardia. There is no increase in maternal mortality or morbidity in well-controlled patients; however, postpartum thyroid storm has been reported in about 20% of untreated individuals. Fetal loss is also more common, due to the facts that spontaneous abortion and premature delivery are more common in untreated pregnant women, as are low-birth-weight infants and eclampsia. Transplacental passage of TSAb may occur, causing fetal as well as neonatal hyperthyroidism.[96] An uncommon cause of hyperthyroidism is molar pregnancy; women present with a large-for-dates uterus and evacuation of the uterus is the preferred management approach.[97]

Because RAI is contraindicated in pregnancy and surgery is usually not recommended (especially during the first trimester), antithyroid drug therapy is usually the treatment of choice. MMI readily crosses the placenta and appears in breast milk.

PTU is considered the drug of choice during the first trimester of pregnancy, with the lowest possible doses used to maintain the maternal T_4 level in the high-normal range.[79,81] During this period the risk of MMI-associated embryopathy is believed to outweigh that of PTU-associated hepatotoxicity. To prevent fetal goiter and suppression of fetal thyroid function, PTU is usually prescribed in daily doses of 300 mg or less and tapered to 50 to 150 mg daily after 4 to 6 weeks. PTU doses of less than 200 mg daily are unlikely to produce fetal goiter.[98] During the second and third trimesters, when the critical period of organogenesis is complete, MMI is thought to be the drug of choice because of the greater risk of hepatotoxicity with PTU.[79,81] Thionamide doses should be adjusted to maintain free T_4 within 10% of the upper normal limit of the nonpregnant reference range.[93] During the last trimester, TSAbs fall spontaneously, and some patients will go into remission so that antithyroid drug doses may be reduced. A rebound in maternal hyperthyroidism occurs in about 10% of women postpartum and may require more intensive treatment than in the last trimester of pregnancy.[96] For example, a recent study of patients who were euthyroid after thionamide discontinuation and subsequently became pregnant showed a relative risk of 4.26 for relapse of hyperthyroidism occurring 4 to 8 months after delivery.[99]

Recently, two very comprehensive guidelines have been published by the American Thyroid Association and the Endocrine Society regarding the management of thyroid disease during pregnancy.[100,101]

Neonatal and Pediatric Hyperthyroidism

Following delivery, some babies of hyperthyroid mothers will be hyperthyroid due to placental transfer of TSAbs, which stimulates thyroid hormone production in utero and postpartum.[102] This is likely if the maternal TSAb titers were quite high. The disease is usually expressed 7 to 10 days postpartum and treatment with antithyroid drugs (PTU 5 to 10 mg/kg/day or MMI 0.5 to 1 mg/kg/day) may be needed for as long as 8 to 12 weeks until the antibody is cleared (immunoglobulin G half-life is about 2 weeks). Iodide (potassium iodide one drop per day or Lugol's solution one to three drops per day) and sodium ipodate may be used for the first few days to acutely inhibit hormone release.

Childhood hyperthyroidism has classically been managed with either PTU or MMI. Long-term followup studies suggest that this form of therapy is quite acceptable, with 25% of a cohort experiencing remission every 2 years.[103] Again, current recommendations suggest use of MMI as a first-line agent in both adults and children.

Thyroid Storm

Thyroid storm is a life-threatening medical emergency characterized by decompensated thyrotoxicosis, high fever (often >39.4°C [>103°F]), tachycardia, tachypnea, dehydration, delirium, coma, nausea, vomiting, and diarrhea.[22] Although Graves' disease and less commonly toxic nodular goiter are usually the underlying thyrotoxic pathology,[104] at least two cases of subacute thyroiditis leading to thyroid storm have been reported.[105]

Precipitating factors for thyroid storm include infection, trauma, surgery, RAI treatment, and withdrawal from antithyroid drugs. Although the duration of clinical decompensation lasts for an average duration of 72 hours, symptoms may persist up to 8 days. With aggressive treatment, the mortality rate has been lowered to 20%. The following therapeutic measures should be instituted promptly: (a) suppression of thyroid hormone formation and secretion, (b) antiadrenergic therapy, (c) administration of corticosteroids, and (d) treatment of associated complications or coexisting factors that may have precipitated the storm. Specific agents used in thyroid storm are outlined in Table 58-6. PTU in large doses may be the preferred thionamide because, in addition to interfering with the production of thyroid hormones, it also blocks the peripheral conversion of T_4 to T_3. However, β-blockers and corticosteroids will serve the same purpose. A theoretical advantage of MMI is that it has a longer duration of action. If patients are unable to take medications orally, the tablets can be crushed into suspension and instilled by gastric or rectal tube[106] or given IV.[107] Iodides, which rapidly block the release of preformed thyroid hormone, should be administered after thionamide

TABLE 58-6 Drug Dosages Used in the Management of Thyroid Storm

Drug	Regimen
Propylthiouracil	900–1,200 mg/day orally in four or six divided doses
Methimazole	90–120 mg/day orally in four or six divided doses
Sodium iodide	Up to 2 g/day IV in single or divided doses
Lugol's solution	5–10 drops three times a day in water or juice
Saturated solution of potassium iodide	1–2 drops three times a day in water or juice
Propranolol	40–80 mg every 6 hours
Dexamethasone	5–20 mg/day orally or IV in divided doses
Prednisone	25–100 mg/day orally in divided doses
Methylprednisolone	20–80 mg/day IV in divided doses
Hydrocortisone	100–400 mg/day IV in divided doses

is initiated to inhibit iodide utilization by the overactive gland. If iodide is administered first, it could theoretically provide substrate to produce even higher levels of thyroid hormone.

Antiadrenergic therapy with the short-acting agent esmolol is preferred, both because it may be used in the patient with pulmonary disease or at risk for cardiac failure and because its effects may be rapidly reversed.[108] Corticosteroids are generally recommended, although there is no convincing evidence of adrenocortical insufficiency in thyroid storm, and the benefits derived from steroids may be caused by their antipyretic action and their effect of stabilizing blood pressure.[22] General supportive measures, including acetaminophen as an antipyretic (do not use aspirin or other nonsteroidal antiinflammatory agents because they may displace bound thyroid hormone), fluid and electrolyte replacement, sedatives, digitalis, antiarrhythmics, insulin, and antibiotics, should be given as indicated. Plasmapheresis and peritoneal dialysis have been used to remove excess hormone (and to remove thyroid-stimulating immunoglobulins in Graves' disease) when the patient has not responded to more conservative measures, although these measures do not always work.[109]

A recent analysis was undertaken to identify cases of thyroid storm occurring in Japan during the period 2004 to 2008.[104] The mortality rate was approximately 10% in the group of 282 patients identified. The most common trigger of the thyrotoxicosis was discontinuation or irregular use of antithyroidal agents. The most common cause of death was either multiorgan failure or congestive heart failure.

HYPOTHYROIDISM

Hypothyroidism is defined as the clinical and biochemical syndrome resulting from decreased thyroid hormone production.[110] Overt hypothyroidism occurs in 1.5% to 2% of women and 0.2% of men, and its incidence increases with age. In the Third National Health and Nutrition Examination Survey (NHANES III), levels of serum TSH and total T_4 were measured in a representative sample of adolescents and adults (age 12 or older). Among 16,533 people who neither were taking thyroid medication nor reported histories of thyroid disease, 3.9% had subclinical hypothyroidism (serum TSH >4.5 milli–international units/L, and T_4 normal), and 0.2% had "clinically significant" hypothyroidism (TSH >4.5 milli–international units/L, and T_4 <4.5 mcg/dL).[21] The vast majority of patients have primary hypothyroidism due to thyroid gland failure due to chronic autoimmune thyroiditis. Special populations with higher risk of developing hypothyroidism include postpartum women, individuals with a family history of autoimmune thyroid disorders and patients with previous head and neck or thyroid irradiation or surgery, other autoimmune endocrine conditions (e.g., type 1 diabetes mellitus, adrenal insufficiency, and ovarian failure), some other nonendocrine autoimmune disorders (e.g., celiac disease, vitiligo, pernicious anemia, Sjögren's syndrome, and multiple sclerosis), primary pulmonary hypertension, and Down's and Turner's syndromes. Secondary hypothyroidism due to pituitary failure is uncommon but should be suspected in a patient with decreased levels of T_4 and inappropriately normal or low TSH levels. Most patients with secondary hypothyroidism due to inadequate TSH production will have clinical signs of more generalized pituitary insufficiency, such as abnormal menses and decreased libido, or evidence of a pituitary adenoma, such as visual field defects, galactorrhea, or acromegaloid features, but isolated TSH deficiency can be congenital or acquired as a result of autoimmune hypophysitis.[111] Generalized (peripheral and central) resistance to thyroid hormone is extremely rare.

Thyroid hormone is essential for normal growth and development during embryonic life. Uncorrected thyroid hormone deficiency during fetal and neonatal development results in mental retardation and/or cretinism. There is slowing of physical and mental activity, as well as of cardiovascular, GI, and neuromuscular function.

A rise in the TSH level is the first evidence of primary hypothyroidism. Many patients will have a free T_4 level within the normal range (compensated hypothyroidism) and few, if any, symptoms of hypothyroidism. As the disease progresses, the free T_4 concentration

CLINICAL PRESENTATION Hypothyroidism

General

- Hypothyroidism can lead to a variety of end-organ effects with a wide range of disease severity, from entirely asymptomatic individuals to patients in coma with multisystem failure. In the adult, manifestations of hypothyroidism are varied and nonspecific. In the child, thyroid hormone deficiency may manifest as growth or intellectual retardation.

Symptoms

- Common symptoms of hypothyroidism include dry skin, cold intolerance, weight gain, constipation, and weakness. Complaints of lethargy, depression, fatigue, exercise intolerance, or loss of ambition and energy are also common but are less specific. Muscle cramps, myalgia, and stiffness are frequent complaints of hypothyroid patients. Menorrhagia and infertility may present commonly in women.

Signs

- Objective weakness is common, with proximal muscles being affected more than distal muscles. Slow relaxation of deep tendon reflexes is common. The most common signs of decreased levels of thyroid hormone include coarse skin and hair, cold or dry skin, periorbital puffiness, and bradycardia. Speech is often slow and the voice may be hoarse. Reversible neurologic syndromes such as carpal tunnel syndrome, polyneuropathy, and cerebellar dysfunction may also occur. Galactorrhea may be found in women.

Diagnosis

- In primary hypothyroidism, TSH serum concentration should be elevated. In secondary hypothyroidism, TSH levels may be within or below the reference range; when TSH bioactivity is altered, the levels reported by immunoassay may even be elevated.
- Free and/or total T_4 and T_3 serum concentrations should be low.

Other tests

- TPOAbs and anti-TG antibodies are likely to be elevated in autoimmune thyroiditis.

TABLE 58-7 Causes of Hypothyroidism

Primary hypothyroidism
Hashimoto's disease
Iatrogenic hypothyroidism
Others:
Iodine deficiency
Enzyme defects
Thyroid hypoplasia
Goitrogens
Secondary hypothyroidism
Pituitary disease
Hypothalamic disease

will drop below the normal level. Interestingly, because of TSH stimulation, thyroidal production will shift toward greater amounts of T_3, and thus T_3 concentrations will often be maintained in the normal range in spite of a low T_4. As the hypothyroidism progresses over time, the T_3 concentration will eventually become low too. The RAIU is not a useful test in the evaluation of a hypothyroid patient, as it may be low, normal, or even elevated.

Causes of Hypothyroidism

Table 58-7 outlines the causes of hypothyroidism.

Chronic Autoimmune Thyroiditis

9 Autoimmune thyroiditis (Hashimoto's disease) is the most common cause of spontaneous hypothyroidism in the adult.[110] Patients may present either with goitrous thyroid gland enlargement and mild hypothyroidism or with thyroid gland atrophy and more severe thyroid hormone deficiency. Both forms of autoimmune thyroiditis probably result from cell- and antibody-mediated thyroid injury. The bulk of evidence suggests that the presence of specific defects in suppressor T-lymphocyte function leads to the survival of a randomly mutating clone of helper T lymphocytes, which are directed against normally occurring antigens on the thyroid membrane. Once these T lymphocytes interact with thyroid membrane antigen, B lymphocytes are stimulated to produce thyroid antibodies.[112]

Antithyroid peroxidase (antimicrosomal) antibodies are present in virtually all patients with Hashimoto's thyroiditis and appear to be directed against the enzyme thyroid peroxidase.[113] These antibodies are capable of fixing complement and inducing cytotoxic changes in thyroid cells. Antibodies that are capable of stimulating thyroid growth through interaction with the TSH receptor may occasionally be found particularly in goitrous hypothyroidism; conversely, antibodies that inhibit the trophic effects of TSH may be present in the atrophic type.

Iatrogenic Hypothyroidism

Iatrogenic hypothyroidism follows exposure to destructive amounts of radiation (radioiodine or external radiation) or surgery. Hypothyroidism occurs within 3 months to a year after ^{131}I therapy in most patients treated for Graves' disease. Thereafter, it occurs at a rate of approximately 2.5% each year. External radiation therapy to the region of the thyroid using doses of greater than 2,500 cGy for therapy of neck carcinoma also causes hypothyroidism. This effect is dose dependent, and more than 50% of patients who receive more than 4,000 cGy to the thyroid bed develop hypothyroidism. Total thyroidectomy causes hypothyroidism within 1 month. Excessive doses of thionamides used to treat hyperthyroidism can also cause iatrogenic hypothyroidism.

Other Causes of Primary Hypothyroidism

Iodine deficiency, enzymatic defects within the thyroid gland, thyroid hypoplasia, and maternal ingestion of goitrogens during fetal development may cause cretinism. Early recognition and treatment of the resultant thyroid hormone deficiency is essential for optimal mental development.[114] Large-scale neonatal screening programs in North America, Europe, Japan, and Australia are now in place.[115] The frequency of congenital hypothyroidism in North America and Europe is 1 per 3,500 to 4,000 live births. In the United States, there are racial differences in the incidence of congenital hypothyroidism, with whites being affected seven times as frequently as blacks.

In the adult, hypothyroidism may rarely be caused by iodine deficiency and goitrogens. Rarely, iodine ingestion in the form of expectorants can lead to hypothyroidism. In sensitive persons (particularly those with autoimmune thyroiditis), the iodide blocks the synthesis of thyroid hormone, leading to an increased secretion of TSH and thyroid enlargement. Thus, both iodine excess and iodine deficiency can cause decreased secretion of thyroid hormone. An example of a goitrogen that can induce hypothyroidism is raw bok choy.[116] Several medications can cause hypothyroidism, including lithium, amiodarone, interferon-alfa, interleukin-2, tyrosine kinase inhibitors, and ClO_4^-.

Causes of Secondary Hypothyroidism

Pituitary Disease TSH is required for normal thyroid secretion. Thyroid atrophy and decreased thyroid secretion follow pituitary failure. Pituitary insufficiency may be caused by destruction of thyrotrophs by either functioning or nonfunctioning pituitary tumors, surgical therapy, external pituitary radiation, postpartum pituitary necrosis (Sheehan's syndrome), trauma, and infiltrative processes of the pituitary such as metastatic tumors, tuberculosis, histiocytosis, and autoimmune mechanisms.[117,118] In all these situations, TSH deficiency most often occurs in association with other pituitary hormone deficiencies. The identification of secondary hypothyroidism due to bexarotene use has led to recognition of the role of rexinoids and retinoids to cause dysregulation of TSH production.[25,119]

For most hypothyroid patients with pituitary disease, serum TSH concentrations are generally low or normal. A serum TSH concentration in the normal range is clearly inappropriate if the patient's T_4 is low.

Note that pituitary enlargement in hypothyroidism does not invariably indicate the presence of a primary pituitary tumor. Pituitary enlargement is seen in patients with severe primary hypothyroidism due to compensatory hyperplasia and hypertrophy of the thyrotrophs.[120] With thyroid hormone replacement therapy, serum TSH concentrations decline, indicating that the TSH secretion is not autonomous, and the pituitary resumes a more normal configuration. These patients are easily separated from patients with primary pituitary failure by measuring a TSH level.

Hypothalamic Hypothyroidism TRH deficiency also causes a rare form of central hypothyroidism. In both adults and children it may occur as a result of cranial irradiation, trauma, infiltrative diseases, or neoplastic diseases.

TREATMENT
Hypothyroidism

Pharmacologic Therapy

Desired Outcomes

The goals of therapy are to restore normal thyroid hormone concentrations in tissue, provide symptomatic relief, prevent neurologic deficits in newborns and children, and reverse the biochemical abnormalities of hypothyroidism.

TABLE 58-8 Thyroid Preparations Used in the Treatment of Hypothyroidism

Drug/Dosage Form	Content	Relative Dose	Comments/Equivalency
Thyroid USP Armour Thyroid, Nature-Throid, and Westhroid (T_4:T_3 ratio approximately 4.2:1); Armour, one grain = 60 mg; Nature-Throid and Westhroid, one grain = 65 mg. Doses include 1/4, 1/2, 1, 2, 3, 4, and 5 grain tablets	Desiccated pork thyroid gland	1 grain (equivalent to 74 mcg [~60–100] mcg of T_4)	High T_3:T_4 ratio; inexpensive
Levothyroxine Synthroid, Levothroid, Levoxyl, Thyro-Tabs, Unithroid, and other generics 25, 50, 75, 88, 100, 112, 125, 137, 150, 175, 200, 300 mcg tablets; 200 and 500 mcg per vial injection	Synthetic T_4	100 mcg	Stable; predictable potency; generics may be bioequivalent; when switching from natural thyroid to L-thyroxine, lower dose by one half grain; variable absorption between products; half-life = 7 days, so daily dosing; considered to be drug of choice
Liothyronine Cytomel 5, 25, and 50 mcg tablets	Synthetic T_3	33 mcg (~equivalent to 100 mcg T_4)	Uniform absorption, rapid onset; half-life = 1.5 days, rapid peak and troughs
Liotrix Thyrolar 1/4-, 1/2-, 1-, 2-, and 3-strength tablets	Synthetic T_4:T_3 in 4:1 ratio	Thyrolar 1 = 50 mcg T_4 and 12.5 mcg T_3	Stable; predictable; expensive; lacks therapeutic rationale because T_4 is converted to T_3 peripherally.

General Approach

10 Levothyroxine (L-thyroxine, T_4) is considered to be drug of choice for treatment of hypothyroidism (Table 58-8).[121] Other commercially available thyroid preparations can be obtained but are not considered preferred therapy. Available thyroid preparations are synthetic (L-thyroxine, liothyronine, and liotrix) or natural in origin (i.e., desiccated thyroid and, formerly, TG). The preparations containing both T_4 and T_3 (liotrix, desiccated thyroid) have relatively high proportions of T_3 and tend to be associated with thyrotoxicosis.[122] Liothyronine suffers from being a short-acting preparation that requires dosing multiple times a day in order to achieve stable hormone concentrations.[123] The availability of sensitive and specific assays for total and free hormone levels as well as TSH now allows definitive dose titration to allow adequate replacement without inadvertent overdose. The response of TSH to TRH had been advocated for use by some for "fine-tuning" thyroid replacement, but this is not necessary if the third-generation chemiluminometric assays for TSH, which have detection limits of about 0.01 milli–international unit/L, are used. Moreover, TRH is no longer commercially available. Clinical guidelines for the treatment of hypothyroidism have been published by the American Thyroid Association and the American Association of Clinical Endocrinologists.[121]

Synthetic Thyroid Hormones

L-Thyroxine (T_4) is the drug of choice for thyroid replacement and suppressive therapy because it is chemically stable, relatively inexpensive, and free of antigenicity and has uniform potency. Whereas T_3, and not T_4, is the biologically more active form of thyroid hormone, L-thyroxine administration results in a pool of thyroid hormone that is readily and consistently converted to T_3; in this regard, L-thyroxine may be thought of as a prohormone. The ability of L-thyroxine to achieve normal T_3 concentrations was illustrated in a study of recently athyreotic patients in whom L-thyroxine monotherapy produced similar T_3 levels to those documented prior to the patient's thyroidectomy.[124] Some studies, however, suggest that athyreotic individuals taking T_4 may have low or low-normal T_3 levels.[125] The half-life of L-thyroxine is approximately 7 days. This long half-life is responsible for a stable pool of prohormone and the need for only once-daily dosing with L-thyroxine. Older studies with L-thyroxine suggested that bioavailability was low and erratic; however, this product has been reformulated, and the average bioavailability is now approximately 80%.[126]

Different L-thyroxine preparations contain different excipients such as dyes and fillers. The bioavailabilities of Synthroid, Levoxine, and generic L-thyroxine preparations were compared in a blinded, randomized, four-way crossover trial.[127] The study was sponsored by the manufacturers of Synthroid, who have challenged the authors' conclusions that the L-thyroxine preparations are bioequivalent and should be interchangeable for the majority of patients. However, because the relationship between T_4 concentration and TSH is not linear, very small changes in T_4 concentration can lead to substantial changes in TSH, which is a more accurate reflection of hormone replacement status. Currently, the FDA mandates that L-thyroxine bioequivalency testing be done for normal volunteers (600 mcg in the fasted state) and three baseline free T_4 concentrations be used to correct for endogenous T_4 production. Bioequivalency is based on the area under the curve (AUC) and maximum concentration (C_{max}) of T_4 out to 48 hours. Approximately 70% of the AUC is derived from endogenous production. TSH is not considered, and it is now very clear that T_4 is too insensitive as a measure of bioequivalency.[128,129] To avoid overtreatment and undertreatment, once a product is selected, therapeutic interchange should be discouraged. Currently, there are several L-thyroxine products available, and a number of permutations for interchange are available considering that there are AB1, AB2, AB3, and AB4 products available, and since no reference listed drug is mandated in bioequivalency testing.

The time to maximal absorption of L-thyroxine is about 2 hours and this should be considered when T_4 concentrations are determined. Ingestion of L-thyroxine with food can impair its absorption.[130] This can potentially affect the TSH concentration achieved if L-thyroxine timing with respect to food is varied.[131] Mucosal diseases such as sprue, diabetic diarrhea, and ileal bypass surgery can also reduce absorption. Cholestyramine, calcium carbonate, sucralfate, aluminum hydroxide,[132] ferrous sulfate,[133] soybean formula,[134] dietary fiber supplements,[135] and espresso coffee[136] may also impair the absorption of L-thyroxine from the GI tract. Acid suppression with histamine blockers and proton pump inhibitors may also reduce L-thyroxine absorption.[137] Drugs that increase nondeiodinative T_4 clearance include rifampin, carbamazepine, and possibly phenytoin. Selenium deficiency and amiodarone may block the conversion of T_4 to T_3.

Liothyronine (T_3) is chemically pure with known potency and has a shorter half-life of 1.5 days. Although it can be used diagnostically in the T_3 suppression test, T_3 has some clinical disadvantages, including a higher incidence of cardiac adverse effects, higher cost, and difficulty in monitoring with conventional laboratory tests. If used, T_3 needs to be administered three times a day and it may take a prolonged period of adjustment to achieve stable euthyroidism.[123]

Liotrix is a combination of synthetic T_4 and T_3 in a 4:1 ratio that attempts to mimic natural hormonal secretion. It is chemically stable and pure and has a predictable potency. The major limitations to this product are high cost and lack of therapeutic rationale, because most T_3 is peripherally converted from T_4. In addition, the T_4:T_3 ratio is much higher than the 14:1 molar ratio produced by the thyroid gland in humans.

11 Trials comparing L-thyroxine alone with a combination of L-thyroxine plus partial replacement with liothyronine (T_3) have generally shown that combinations of $T_4 + T_3$ are no better than T_4 alone.[138,139] At least 13 such trials with varying designs have been performed to date. Four of these trials have found that patients expressed a preference for combination therapy. By way of illustration, in one trial of combination therapy, Clyde et al.[139] compared L-thyroxine alone for treatment of primary hypothyroidism with combination therapy using L-thyroxine plus liothyronine. These investigators demonstrated no beneficial changes in body weight, serum lipid levels, hypothyroid symptoms as measured by a health-related quality-of-life questionnaire, and standard measures of cognitive performance.[139] Three meta-analyses and a systematic review have also suggested no benefits.[140–143] However, a recent secondary analysis suggested that individuals harboring a specific deiodinase polymorphism may have a poorer psychological response to L-thyroxine therapy and a better response to combination therapy with both T_4 and T_3.[144] However, no prospective study investigating whether the presence of these polymorphisms affects satisfaction with replacement therapy has yet been reported.

Natural Thyroid Hormones

Desiccated thyroid has historically been derived from pig, beef, or sheep thyroid glands, although pigs are currently the usual source. The *United States Pharmacopeia*, 23rd edition, requires thyroid USP to contain 38 mcg (±15%) of L-thyroxine and 9 mcg (±10%) of liothyronine for each 60 to 65 mg (one grain). Thyroid USP, as an animal protein–derived product, may be antigenic in allergic or sensitive patients. Even though desiccated thyroid is inexpensive, its limitations preclude it from being considered as a drug of choice for hypothyroid patients. TG USP was a purified pig-gland extract, but it had no clinical advantages and is no longer available.

12 **Dosing and Monitoring** Recent studies suggest that the average maintenance dose of L-thyroxine for most adults is about 125 mcg/day.[110] The replacement dose of L-thyroxine is affected by body weight. Estimates of weight-based doses for replacement in hypothyroid patients include 1.6 and 1.7 mcg/kg/day.[145,146] There is, however, a wide range of replacement doses, necessitating individualized therapy and appropriate TSH monitoring to determine an adequate but not excessive dose.

In addition to alleviation of symptoms, the goal of treatment for patients with hypothyroidism is to maintain the patient's TSH within the normal range. Some clinicians are of the opinion that the traditional reference range of approximately 0.5 to 4.5 milli–international units/L includes at its upper end some individuals who have unrecognized thyroid disease.[147] Thus, some believe that the reference range should be modified downwards to 0.5 to 3.5 milli–international units/L or even 0.5 to 2.5 milli–international units/L.[148] If this premise is accepted, both the TSH values that trigger L-thyroxine treatment and the TSH treatment goal could potentially be altered. There are cogent arguments on both sides of the issue. Those who suggest maintaining current reference ranges believe that lowering the upper limit of the reference range could result in treating many individuals with thyroid hormone who would not necessarily benefit from such treatment.[149] Those who favor narrowing the reference range suggest that additional patients would, in fact, derive benefit from thyroid hormone treatment.[148] TSH reference ranges also differ for different populations, such as those who are pregnant, specific ethnic groups, and older individuals.

The required dose of L-thyroxine is dependent on the patient's age[150] and the presence of associated disorders, as well as the severity and duration of hypothyroidism.[151] Most patients will require approximately 1.7 mcg/kg/day once they reach steady state for full replacement. Dose requirement may be better estimated based on ideal body weight, rather than actual body weight.[152] In patients with long-standing disease and older individuals without known cardiac disease, therapy should be initiated with 50 mcg daily of L-thyroxine and increased after 1 month. The recommended initial daily dose for older patients with known cardiac disease is 25 mcg/day titrated upward in increments of 25 mcg at monthly intervals to prevent stress on the cardiovascular system. Some patients may experience an exacerbation of angina with higher doses of thyroid hormone. Although the TSH is an indicator of underreplacement or overreplacement, clinicians often fail to alter the dose based on TSH values clearly outside of the normal range.

13 Patients with subclinical or mild hypothyroidism (seen more commonly in the elderly and women) have no or few signs or symptoms, normal serum T_3 and T_4 concentrations, and an elevated basal TSH concentration.[69] The prevalence of this disorder in the NHANES III study was found to be 4.3%.[21] Untreated individuals with moderate degrees of subclinical hypothyroidism and negative TPOAb may revert to euthyroidism during followup.[153] Increased mortality may be associated with moderate, but not mild subclinical hypothyroidism.[154] Spontaneous recovery of thyroid function and uncertainties about which patient groups may benefit from therapy contribute to the debate about treatment of subclinical hypothyroidism. Although the treatment of subclinical hypothyroidism is controversial, patients presenting with marked elevations in TSH (>10 milli–international units/L) and high titers of TPOAb or prior treatment with ^{131}I may be most likely to benefit from treatment. It should be noted that some studies find that only one of four treated patients experienced improvement. Other patients who may improve with replacement include those with mild symptoms of hypothyroidism and depression. Reduction of events due to ischemic heart disease was only observed in younger patients in one study.[155] If treatment is pursued, reasonable goals in this situation would be to maintain serum T_4 and T_3 levels in the normal range and reduce TSH to a value of 0.5 to 2.5 milli–international units/L in younger patients and 4 to 6 milli–international units/L in older patients.[69]

Once euthyroidism is attained, the daily maintenance dose of L-thyroxine does not fluctuate greatly. As patients age, the dosing requirement may be reduced.[150] Third-generation TSH assays improved the accuracy with which thyroid hormone replacement can be monitored. The TSH concentration is the most sensitive and specific monitoring parameter for adjustment of L-thyroxine dose. Plasma TSH concentrations begin to fall within hours and are usually normalized within 2 weeks, but they may take up to 6 weeks for some patients, depending on the baseline value. Both TSH and T_4 concentrations are used to monitor therapy, and they should be checked every 6 weeks until a euthyroid state is achieved.[121] Laboratory assessment of thyroid function should be performed approximately 6 weeks after L-thyroxine dose initiation or change. This time frame allows achievement of steady state, as the half-life of L-thyroxine is approximately 1 week. Serum T_4 concentrations can be useful in detecting noncompliance, malabsorption, or changes in L-thyroxine product bioequivalence. An elevated TSH concentration indicates insufficient replacement. The appropriate dose maintains the TSH concentration in the normal range. T_4 disposal is accelerated by nephrotic syndrome, other severe systemic illnesses, and several antiseizure medications (phenobarbital, phenytoin, and carbamazepine) and rifampin. Pregnancy increases the T_4 dose requirement for 75% of women, probably because of factors such as increased degradation by the placental deiodinase, increased T_4 pool size, and transfer of T_4 to the fetus. The etiology of hypothyroidism also affects the magnitude of the dosage increase.[156] Initiating postmenopausal hormone replacement therapy increases the dose needed in 35% of women, perhaps due to an increased circulating TBG level. Patient noncompliance with prescribed T_4, the most common cause of inadequate treatment, might be suspected for patients with a dose that is higher than expected, variable thyroid function test results that do not correlate well with prescribed doses, and an elevated serum TSH concentration with serum free T_4 at the upper end of the normal range, which can suggest improved compliance immediately before testing, with a lag in the thyrotropin response.

The metabolism of other pharmacologic agents can be altered for patients with hypothyroidism. The mechanism might be decreased expression of hepatic enzymes involved in drug metabolism, as seen in hypothyroid rats. As a result, increased sensitivity to anesthetic and sedative agents, and higher serum levels of phenytoin have been reported. Hypothyroidism can also cause higher serum digoxin values, an effect attributed to a decreased volume of drug distribution. Conversely, hypothyroidism might decrease sensitivity to warfarin due to slowed metabolism of the vitamin K–dependent clotting factors, and restoration of euthyroidism can then increase the warfarin dose requirement.

For patients with central hypothyroidism caused by hypothalamic or pituitary failure, the serum TSH cannot be used to assess adequacy of replacement. Alleviation of the clinical syndrome and restoration of serum T_4 to the normal range are the only criteria available for estimating the appropriate replacement dose of L-thyroxine. Keeping free T_4 values in the upper part of the normal laboratory reference range is a reasonable approach,[157] with modification of this goal to the middle of the normal range in older patients or patients with comorbidities. Concurrent use of dopamine, dopaminergic agents (bromocriptine), somatostatin or somatostatin analogs (octreotide), and corticosteroids suppresses TSH concentrations in individuals with primary hypothyroidism and may confound the interpretation of this monitoring parameter.[121]

TSH-suppressive L-thyroxine therapy can be given to patients with nodular thyroid disease and diffuse goiter, to patients with a history of thyroid irradiation, and to patients with thyroid cancer. The rationale for suppression therapy is to reduce TSH secretion, which promotes growth and function in abnormal thyroid tissue. However, such management, other than for patients with thyroid cancer or with elevated TSH levels, is quite controversial. Some clinicians rarely recommend or use such therapy; others will recommend a trial of L-thyroxine as suppressive therapy in some patients. The conclusions of three meta-analyses were that suppressive therapy for nodules was associated with a small decrease in nodule growth,[158] a statistically nonsignificant reduction in nodule growth,[159] and a significant reduction in nodule growth that was reduced with longer-term treatment.[39] If suppressive therapy with L-thyroxine is pursued, the age, gender, and menopausal status of the patient need to be considered, along with the risk of cardiac arrhythmias and reduced bone mineral density. L-Thyroxine may be given in nontoxic MNG to suppress the TSH to low-normal levels of 0.5 to 1 milli–international unit/L if the baseline TSH is >1 milli–international unit/L. Goiter size and thyroid volume may be reduced with suppression therapy. Diffuse goiter associated with autoimmune thyroiditis may also be treated with L-thyroxine to reduce goiter size and thyroid volume. L-Thyroxine suppression therapy is of benefit to all but the lowest-risk thyroid cancer patients and is generally used in the management of patients with differentiated thyroid cancer, with the TSH goal being influenced by the patient's thyroid cancer stage and other risk factors.[160] Current guidelines from the American Thyroid Association suggest suppressing the TSH to below 0.1 milli–international unit/L in higher-risk patients, but keeping TSH around the lower limit of normal (0.1 to 0.5 milli–international unit/L) in low-risk patients.[161]

14 Adverse Effects Serious untoward effects are unusual if dosing is appropriate and the patient is carefully monitored during initial treatment. A cross-sectional study showed that of a population of 1,525 individuals taking L-thyroxine, 40% actually had abnormal TSH values.[162] A recent study showed that 57% of individuals 65 years or older receiving thyroid hormone treatment had abnormal TSH values.[163] Both of these studies suggest failure to keep a patient's TSH at goal is common. L-Thyroxine replacement in athyreotic hypothyroid patients restores systolic and diastolic left ventricular performance within 2 weeks, and the use of L-thyroxine may increase the frequency of atrial premature beats but not necessarily ventricular premature beats. Excessive doses of thyroid hormone may lead to heart failure, angina pectoris, and myocardial infarction; rarely, the latter may be caused by coronary artery spasm. Allergic or idiosyncratic reactions can occur with the natural animal–derived products such as desiccated thyroid and TG, but these are extremely rare with the synthetic products used today. The 0.05 mg (50 mcg) Synthroid tablet is the least allergenic (due to a lack of dye and few excipients) and should be tried for the patient suspected to be allergic to thyroid hormone tablets.

Hyperremodeling of cortical and trabecular bone due to hyperthyroidism leads to reduced bone density and may increase the risk of fracture. Compared with normal controls, excess exogenous thyroid hormone results in histomorphometric and biochemical changes similar to those observed in osteoporosis and untreated hyperthyroidism.[164,165] The risk for this complication of therapy seems to be related to the dose of L-thyroxine, patient age, and gender. Markers for bone turnover include urinary *N*-telopeptides, pyridinoline crosslinks of type I collagen, osteocalcin, and bone-specific alkaline phosphatase. When doses of L-thyroxine are used to suppress TSH concentrations to below-normal values (less than 0.3 milli–international unit/L) in postmenopausal women, this adverse effect is more likely to be seen. Cortical bone is affected to a greater degree than trabecular bone at suppressive doses of L-thyroxine. In contrast, it appears to be much less likely in men and in premenopausal women. Maintaining the TSH between 0.7 and 1.5 milli–international units/L does not alter bone mineral density in premenopausal women. Although not all studies have shown consistent results, a recent cohort study suggests that there is no adverse effect on bone density with treatment with L-thyroxine to achieve a normal TSH.[166]

EVALUATION OF THERAPEUTIC OUTCOMES

Hypothyrodism

Patients on optimal thyroid hormone replacement therapy should have TSH and free T_4 serum concentrations in the normal range. Those who are being treated for thyroid cancer should have TSH suppressed to low levels based on their risk stratification,[161] and their TG should be undetectable. Given that the half-life of T_4 is 7 days, the appropriate monitoring interval is no more often than 4 weeks. The signs and symptoms of hypothyroidism should be improved or absent (see Clinical Presentation of Hypothyroidism above), although it may take several months to see improvement.

Special Conditions

Myxedema Coma

Myxedema coma is a rare consequence of decompensated hypothyroidism.[167] Clinical features include hypothermia, advanced stages of hypothyroid symptoms, and altered sensorium ranging from delirium to coma. Mortality rates of 60% to 70% necessitate immediate and aggressive therapy. Traditionally, the initial treatment has been IV bolus L-thyroxine 300 to 500 mcg. However, as deiodinase activity is markedly reduced, impairing T_4 to T_3 conversion, initial treatment with IV T_3, or a combination of both hormones has also been advocated.[167] Glucocorticoid therapy with IV hydrocortisone 100 mg every 8 hours should be given until coexisting adrenal suppression is ruled out. Consciousness, lowered TSH concentrations, and improvement in vital signs are expected within 24 hours. Maintenance doses of L-thyroxine are typically 75 to 100 mcg given IV until the patient stabilizes and oral therapy is begun. Supportive therapy must be instituted to maintain adequate ventilation, blood pressure, and body temperature, and ensure euglycemia. Any underlying disorder, such as sepsis or myocardial infarction, obviously must be diagnosed and treated.

Congenital Hypothyroidism

In congenital hypothyroidism, full maintenance therapy should be instituted early to improve the prognosis for mental and physical development.[168,169] The average maintenance dose in infants and children depends on the age and weight of the child. Several studies demonstrate that aggressive therapy with L-thyroxine is important for normal development, and current recommendations are for initiation of therapy within 45 days of birth at a dose of 10 to 15 mcg/kg/day.[115] This dose is used to keep T_4 concentrations at about 10 mcg/dL within 30 days of starting therapy and is associated with improved IQs in treated infants. The dose is progressively decreased to a typical adult dose as the child ages, the adult dose being given in the age range of 11 to 20 years.

⓯ Hypothyroidism in Pregnancy

Hypothyroidism during pregnancy leads to an increased rate of stillbirths and possibly lower neuropsychological scores in infants born of women who received inadequate replacement during pregnancy.[100,170] Thyroid hormone is necessary for fetal growth and must come from the maternal side during the first 2 months of gestation. Although liothyronine may cross the placental membrane slightly better than L-thyroxine, the latter is considered the drug of choice. The objective of treatment is to decrease TSH to the normal, based on the normal reference range for pregnancy. Recently published guidelines suggest a TSH below 2.5 milli–international units/L during the first trimester and a TSH below 3 milli–international units/L during the remainder of pregnancy.[100,101] Based on elevated TSH levels during pregnancy, it was found in one study that the mean dose of L-thyroxine had to be increased by 48% to decrease TSH into the normal range. However, in individual women the dosage increase needed may vary from approximately 10% to 80%. Increased production of binding proteins, a marginal decrease in free hormone concentration, modification of peripheral thyroid hormone metabolism, and increased T_4 metabolism by the fetal–placental unit all may contribute to increased thyroid hormone demand. As these changes regress after delivery the need for increased L-thyroxine will decline.[94] Up to 60% of women need to have L-thyroxine dose adjustment during pregnancy. Upward adjustment will usually be needed by the eighth week of pregnancy. The etiology of the hypothyroidism affects the magnitude of the required increase in L-thyroxine dose.[156] After delivery the L-thyroxine dose can be reduced based on T_4 concentrations and measurement of TSH, typically about 6 to 8 weeks after delivery.[93] Many patients can return to their prepregnancy dose requirement.

Effects of Hypothyroidism on Selected Medications

Hypothyroidism may affect the metabolism and clinical efficacy of several medications. Digitalis preparations have a decreased volume of distribution in the hypothyroid state, resulting in increased sensitivity to the digitalis effect. Therefore, many hypothyroid patients achieve a therapeutic effect at lower digitalis doses. Insulin degradation may be delayed in hypothyroidism, thereby requiring a lower insulin dose. Hypothyroidism delays the catabolism of clotting factors, and if a patient stabilized on warfarin is made euthyroid with L-thyroxine, the patient may become excessively anticoagulated. Respiratory depressants such as barbiturates, phenothiazines, and opioid analgesics should be avoided, because increased sensitivity may increase carbon dioxide retention and precipitate myxedema coma.

RECOMBINANT TSH IN THYROID CANCER

Patients with previously treated differentiated (papillary, follicular, or their respective variants) thyroid carcinoma require lifelong monitoring for recurrent disease.[171] Two diagnostic tests that play a central role in the followup of these patients—serum TG measurement and radioiodine whole-body scanning—are most accurate during TSH stimulation. Temporary discontinuation of thyroid hormone therapy was previously the sole effective approach for TSH-stimulated testing. However, hormone withdrawal is associated with the morbidity of hypothyroidism and occasional tumor progression. The introduction of recombinant TSH (rTSH)–stimulated testing offers an alternative therapy. Recent clinical trials have shown that the sensitivity of combined rTSH-stimulated radioiodine scanning and serum TG measurement has nearly equivalent sensitivity to testing after thyroid hormone withdrawal.[172] Furthermore, measurement of the rTSH-stimulated TG concentration is a more sensitive way to detect residual thyroid cancer or normal tissue than TG measurement on thyroid hormone therapy. Postthyroidectomy adjuvant radioiodine therapy can also be administered following rTSH, instead of thyroid hormone withdrawal, with equivalent rates of remnant ablation.[173] Patients for whom thyroid hormone withdrawal would be contraindicated may also be successfully treated with radioiodine following rTSH.[174] A recent study reporting short-term followup of 3.7 years on patients receiving their remnant ablation with rTSH showed that rates of residual and recurrent thyroid cancer did not differ between patients prepared for receiving radioiodine using rTSH and those prepared for withdrawal from L-thyroxine.[175] It is not yet known whether use of rTSH stimulation as a means of delivering RAI to patients with metastatic disease is equivalent to preparation by L-thyroxine withdrawal. The studies addressing this issue generally have relatively small numbers of patients and heterogeneous methodology.[176] Recently rTSH has also been used successfully to aid in the treatment of large, compressive goiters in individuals who are not surgical candidates. Radioiodine treatment, delivered following small doses of rTSH, can lead to improved radioiodine uptake and reduced goiter volume,[177] although this is not yet an approved use of rTSH.

NONTHYROIDAL ILLNESS

A wide variety of abnormalities of hypothalamic–pituitary–thyroid function, serum thyroid hormone binding, and extrathyroidal thyroid hormone metabolism occur in patients with nonthyroidal illness.[178] These abnormalities frequently result in decreased serum T_3 concentrations and, with more severe nonthyroidal disease, lead to a decreased serum free T_4 concentration as well. Serum TSH concentrations are initially within the normal range but then tend to decrease with increasing severity of illness. The presence of coexisting primary hypothyroidism can be recognized for patients who have other illnesses by an elevation in the TSH concentration.

The degree and extent of the abnormality in thyroid function generally correlate with the severity of the nonthyroidal illness.

These conditions are frequently referred to as the *euthyroid sick syndrome*. However, it is likely that these changes represent adaptive forms of hypothyroidism that serve to reduce the availability of thyroid hormones to lessen the catabolic impact of the nonthyroidal illness.

Decreased serum T_3 concentrations occur in patients with both acute and chronic illnesses. The fundamental cause of decreased serum T_3 concentrations in these situations is decreased extrathyroidal conversion of T_4 to T_3, normally mediated by T_4-5′-deiodinase. A circulating inhibitor of this enzyme, perhaps interleukin-6, is present in patients with nonthyroidal illness.[179] Serum total and free T_4 concentrations are usually normal in mild illness. The serum reverse T_3 concentration is characteristically high because the same enzyme, 5′-deiodinase, that is necessary to convert T_4 to T_3 is necessary to convert reverse T_3 to its breakdown products.

Low serum T_4 is seen in most critically ill patients.[180,181] This change is caused by diminished serum T_4 synthesis as well as impaired binding to serum transport proteins, resulting either from decreased serum concentrations of TBG, thyroid-binding prealbumin (TBPA), or albumin or from inhibitors of T_4 binding. The free T_4 concentration is generally normal early in critical illness but also declines with more severe disease. This more severe degree of hypothyroidism, which occurs in severely ill patients, produces a greater reduction in thyroid hormone availability. The low serum T_4 concentrations for patients with nonthyroidal illness indicate a grave prognosis. In two studies, more than 60% of hospitalized patients with a low serum free T_4 index died.

Multiple studies have addressed the role of thyroid supplementation in critically ill patients with cardiac disease, sepsis, pulmonary disease (e.g., acute respiratory distress syndrome), or severe infection, or with burn and trauma patients. In spite of a very large number of published studies, it is very difficult to form clear recommendations for treatment with thyroid hormone in the intensive care unit.[180] The few randomized, controlled trials comparing L-thyroxine therapy with no treatment have not shown significant clinical benefit, and have raised some safety concerns. Low doses of T_3 have generally not been linked to harm in clinical trials, but there is nevertheless an absence of data showing significant clinical benefit.[182,183] In summary, although controversial, T_4 or T_3 supplementation has been of no benefit in situations involving the low T_3 syndrome.

To confuse matters, some patients with nonthyroidal illness have elevation of their serum T_4 concentration. Most commonly, this is seen in patients with psychiatric disorders during acute psychotic breaks. Thyroid hormone levels return to normal within 2 weeks after successful treatment of the underlying psychiatric disease. The occurrence of these abnormalities requires that care be taken in diagnosing hypothyroidism or hyperthyroidism for patients who have nonthyroidal illnesses.

GOITROUS THYROID DISEASE

Endemic goiter is the major thyroid disease throughout the world, affecting more than 200 million people. Many goitrous glands contain one or more nodules. The introduction of iodide supplementation has eliminated goiter as a major medical problem in developed countries, although it continues to be a problem in developing countries whose geographic position makes them more susceptible to iodide deficiency. In 1924, Marine postulated that periods of iodide deficiency resulted in cyclic hyperplasia and involution of thyroid follicular cells with eventual development of nodular hyperplasia. This hypothesis is still used to explain goiter formation today. Whatever the specific cause, the final common pathway appears to result from an inadequate thyroid hormone secretion with compensatory TSH secretion and eventual thyroid gland enlargement. Goiters may initially tend to be diffuse, but then become nodular as the cells in some thyroid follicles proliferate more than others. As thyrocytes within the goiter replicate, mutations in the TSH receptor may also favor dysregulated growth.

Sporadic goiter is defined as a goiter occurring in a nonendemic goiter region. Although a number of known goitrogens and errors in thyroid hormone biosynthesis may cause goiter, the majority of cases of sporadic goiter have no known etiology. Genetic factors may be important, as often a family history of goiter exists. There has been an interest in the possibility that growth factors other than TSH play a role in the development of a goiter. Immunoglobulin fractions capable of stimulating thyroid growth have been found in patients with nontoxic goiter and Graves' disease. In these patients, thyroid growth–promoting immunoglobulin titers correlate with goiter size rather than with the thyroid hormone concentration.

Treatment of goiters can include a trial of thyroid hormone suppression in an effort to eliminate TSH as a possible stimulus for continued thyroid growth. Large, long-standing goiters seldom undergo significant reduction in size. If the patient is symptomatic (with dysphagia or dyspnea) or there is a question of malignant thyroid involvement, surgery is recommended.

Clinical **Controversy. . .**

Although the current FDA standards of bioavailability for T_4 products suggest that several products are bioequivalent, the relationship between T_4 serum concentration and TSH response suggests that the products are not truly bioequivalent. New standards of bioequivalency may need to be developed for drug products like T_4.

Combination therapy of $T_4 + T_3$ for hypothyroidism generally offers no objective advantage over monotherapy, although subjective patient improvement or patient preference for combination therapy has been reported in a minority of studies. Although some data suggest that patients with certain deiodinase polymorphisms may, in fact, derive a psychological benefit from combination therapy, studies to specifically test this hypothesis have not yet been performed.

Multiple studies have addressed the role of thyroid supplementation for critically ill patients with cardiac disease, sepsis, pulmonary disease (e.g., acute respiratory distress syndrome), or severe infection or for patients with burn and trauma. In spite of a very large number of published studies, it is very difficult to form clear recommendations for treatment with thyroid hormone in the intensive care unit.

EVALUATION OF THERAPEUTIC OUTCOMES

Patients with idiopathic hypothyroidism and Hashimoto's thyroiditis on optimal thyroid hormone replacement therapy should have TSH and free T_4 serum concentrations in the normal range. Those who are being treated for thyroid cancer should have TSH suppressed to low levels, with the appropriate TSH concentration being determined based on the patient's risk of recurrence or progression, and TG should be undetectable. Given the half-life of T_4 of 7 days, the appropriate monitoring interval is no more often than 4 weeks. The signs and symptoms of hypothyroidism should be improved or absent (see Clinical Presentation of Hypothyroidism above), although it may take several months to the full benefit of therapy to manifest.

ABBREVIATIONS

AUC	area under the curve
C_{max}	maximum concentration
ClO_4^-	perchlorate
DIT	diiodotyrosine
FSH	follicle-stimulating hormone
$G_s\alpha$	the α subunit of the stimulatory guanine-nucleotide–binding protein
hCG	human chorionic gonadotropin
HLA	human leukocyte antigen
^{131}I	sodium iodide-131
L-thyroxine	levothyroxine
LH	luteinizing hormone
MIT	monoiodotyrosine
MMI	methimazole
MNG	multinodular goiter
NHANES III	Third National Health and Nutrition Examination Survey
PRTH	pituitary resistance to thyroid hormone
PTU	propylthiouracil
RAI	radioactive iodine
RAIU	radioactive iodine uptake
rTSH	recombinant thyroid-stimulating hormone
SCN^-	thiocyanate
SSKI	saturated solution of potassium iodide
T_3	triiodothyronine
T_4	thyroxine
TBG	thyroxine-binding globulin
TBPA	thyroid-binding prealbumin
TcO_4^-	pertechnetate
TG	thyroglobulin
TPOAb	thyroid peroxidase antibodies
TR	thyroid hormone receptor
TRH	thyrotropin-releasing hormone
TRIAC	triiodothyroacetic acid
TSAb	thyroid-stimulating antibody
TSH	thyroid-stimulating hormone
TTR	transthyretin
WBC	white blood cell

REFERENCES

1. Nilsson M. Iodide handling by the thyroid epithelial cell. Exp Clin Endocrinol Diabetes 2001;109(1):13–17.
2. Dohan O, De la Vieja A, Paroder V, et al. The sodium/iodide symporter (NIS): Characterization, regulation, and medical significance. Endocr Rev 2003;24(1):48–77.
3. Clewell RA, Merrill EA, Narayanan L, Gearhart JM, Robinson PJ. Evidence for competitive inhibition of iodide uptake by perchlorate and translocation of perchlorate into the thyroid. Int J Toxicol 2004;23(1):17–23.
4. Fong P. Thyroid iodide efflux: A team effort? J Physiol 2011;589(Pt 24):5929–5939.
5. Dunn JT, Dunn AD. Update on intrathyroidal iodine metabolism. Thyroid 2001;11(5):407–414.
6. Riesco-Eizaguirre G, Santisteban P. A perspective view of sodium iodide symporter research and its clinical implications. Eur J Endocrinol 2006;155(4):495–512.
7. Dunn JT, Dunn AD. The importance of thyroglobulin structure for thyroid hormone biosynthesis. Biochimie 1999;81(5):505–509.
8. Obregon MJ, Escobar del Rey F, Morreale de Escobar G. The effects of iodine deficiency on thyroid hormone deiodination. Thyroid 2005;15(8):917–929.
9. Schussler GC. The thyroxine-binding proteins. Thyroid 2000;10(2):141–149.
10. Bianco AC, Kim BW. Deiodinases: Implications of the local control of thyroid hormone action. J Clin Invest 2006;116(10):2571–2579.
11. Panicker V, Cluett C, Shields B, et al. A common variation in deiodinase 1 gene DIO1 is associated with the relative levels of free thyroxine and triiodothyronine. J Clin Endocrinol Metab 2008;93(8):3075–3081.
12. Hoefig CS, Kohrle J, Brabant G, et al. Evidence for extrathyroidal formation of 3-iodothyronamine in humans as provided by a novel monoclonal antibody-based chemiluminescent serum immunoassay. J Clin Endocrinol Metab 2011;96(6):1864–1872.
13. Scanlan TS. Minireview: 3-Iodothyronamine (T1AM): A new player on the thyroid endocrine team? Endocrinology 2009;150(3):1108–1111.
14. Galli E, Marchini M, Saba A, et al. Detection of 3-iodothyronamine in human patients: A preliminary study. J Clin Endocrinol Metab 2012;97(1):E69–E74.
15. Kopp P. The TSH receptor and its role in thyroid disease. Cell Mol Life Sci 2001;58(9):1301–1322.
16. Krohn K, Paschke R. Somatic mutations in thyroid nodular disease. Mol Genet Metab 2002;75(3):202–208.
17. Gillam MP, Kopp P. Genetic regulation of thyroid development. Curr Opin Pediatr 2001;13(4):358–363.
18. Harvey CB, Williams GR. Mechanism of thyroid hormone action. Thyroid 2002;12(6):441–446.
19. Malm J, Farnegardh M, Grover GJ, Ladenson PW. Thyroid hormone antagonists: Potential medical applications and structure activity relationships. Curr Med Chem 2009;16(25):3258–3266.
20. Cooper DS. Hyperthyroidism. Lancet 2003;362(9382):459–468.
21. Hollowell JG, Staehling NW, Flanders WD, et al. Serum TSH, T(4), and thyroid antibodies in the United States population (1988 to 1994): National Health and Nutrition Examination Survey (NHANES III). J Clin Endocrinol Metab 2002;87(2):489–499.
22. Nayak B, Burman K. Thyrotoxicosis and thyroid storm. Endocrinol Metab Clin North Am 2006;35(4):663–686, vii.
23. Socin HV, Chanson P, Delemer B, et al. The changing spectrum of TSH-secreting pituitary adenomas: Diagnosis and management in 43 patients. Eur J Endocrinol 2003;148(4):433–442.
24. Beck-Peccoz P, Persani L, Calebiro D, Bonomi M, Mannavola D, Campi I. Syndromes of hormone resistance in the hypothalamic–pituitary–thyroid axis. Best Pract Res Clin Endocrinol Metab 2006;20(4):529–546.
25. Golden WM, Weber KB, Hernandez TL, Sherman SI, Woodmansee WW, Haugen BR. Single-dose rexinoid rapidly and specifically suppresses serum thyrotropin in normal subjects. J Clin Endocrinol Metab 2007;92(1):124–130.
26. Weetman AP. Controversy in thyroid disease. J R Coll Physicians Lond 2000;34(4):374–380.
27. Davies TF, Ando T, Lin RY, Tomer Y, Latif R. Thyrotropin receptor-associated diseases: From adenomata to Graves disease. J Clin Invest 2005;115(8):1972–1983.
28. Garrity JA, Bahn RS. Pathogenesis of Graves ophthalmopathy: Implications for prediction, prevention, and treatment. Am J Ophthalmol 2006;142(1):147–153.
29. Brix TH, Kyvik KO, Christensen K, Hegedus L. Evidence for a major role of heredity in Graves' disease: A population-based study of two Danish twin cohorts. J Clin Endocrinol Metab 2001;86(2):930–934.

30. Ban Y, Concepcion ES, Villanueva R, Greenberg DA, Davies TF, Tomer Y. Analysis of immune regulatory genes in familial and sporadic Graves' disease. J Clin Endocrinol Metab 2004;89(9):4562–4568.
31. Taylor JC, Gough SC, Hunt PJ, et al. A genome-wide screen in 1119 relative pairs with autoimmune thyroid disease. J Clin Endocrinol Metab 2006;91(2):646–653.
32. Rhee EP, Scott JA, Dighe AS. Case records of the Massachusetts General Hospital. Case 4-2012. A 37-year-old man with muscle pain, weakness, and weight loss. N Engl J Med 2012;366(6):553–560.
33. Ryan DP, da Silva MR, Soong TW, et al. Mutations in potassium channel Kir2.6 cause susceptibility to thyrotoxic hypokalemic periodic paralysis. Cell 2010;140(1):88–98.
34. Rodien P, Jordan N, Lefevre A, et al. Abnormal stimulation of the thyrotrophin receptor during gestation. Hum Reprod Update 2004;10(2):95–105.
35. Siegel RD, Lee SL. Toxic nodular goiter. Toxic adenoma and toxic multinodular goiter. Endocrinol Metab Clin North Am 1998;27(1):151–168.
36. Freitas JE. Therapeutic options in the management of toxic and nontoxic nodular goiter. Semin Nucl Med 2000;30(2):88–97.
37. Krohn K, Fuhrer D, Bayer Y, et al. Molecular pathogenesis of euthyroid and toxic multinodular goiter. Endocr Rev 2005;26(4):504–524.
38. Campbell AJ. Thyroid disorders in the elderly. Difficulties in diagnosis and treatment. Drugs 1986;31(5):455–461.
39. Sdano MT, Falciglia M, Welge JA, Steward DL. Efficacy of thyroid hormone suppression for benign thyroid nodules: Meta-analysis of randomized trials. Otolaryngol Head Neck Surg 2005;133(3):391–396.
40. Luotola K, Hyoty H, Salmi J, Miettinen A, Helin H, Pasternack A. Evaluation of infectious etiology in subacute thyroiditis—Lack of association with coxsackievirus infection. APMIS 1998;106(4):500–504.
41. Fatourechi V, Aniszewski JP, Fatourechi GZ, Atkinson EJ, Jacobsen SJ. Clinical features and outcome of subacute thyroiditis in an incidence cohort: Olmsted County, Minnesota, study. J Clin Endocrinol Metab 2003;88(5):2100–2105.
42. Pearce EN, Farwell AP, Braverman LE. Thyroiditis. N Engl J Med 2003;348(26):2646–2655 [Erratum in N Engl J Med 2003;349(6):620].
43. Stagnaro-Green A. Postpartum thyroiditis. Best Pract Res Clin Endocrinol Metab 2004;18(2):303–316.
44. Mittra ES, McDougall IR. Recurrent silent thyroiditis: A report of four patients and review of the literature. Thyroid 2007;17(7):671–675.
45. Samuels MH. Subacute, silent, and postpartum thyroiditis. Med Clin North Am 2012;96(2):223–233.
46. DeSimone CP, Lele SM, Modesitt SC. Malignant struma ovarii: A case report and analysis of cases reported in the literature with focus on survival and I131 therapy. Gynecol Oncol 2003;89(3):543–548.
47. Als C, Gedeon P, Rosler H, Minder C, Netzer P, Laissue JA. Survival analysis of 19 patients with toxic thyroid carcinoma. J Clin Endocrinol Metab 2002;87(9):4122–4127.
48. Bahn RS, Burch HB, Cooper DS, et al. Hyperthyroidism and other causes of thyrotoxicosis: Management guidelines of the American Thyroid Association and American Association of Clinical Endocrinologists. Endocr Pract 2011;17(3): 456–520.
49. Meurisse M, Gollogly L, Degauque C, Fumal I, Defechereux T, Hamoir E. Iatrogenic thyrotoxicosis: Causal circumstances, pathophysiology, and principles of treatment—Review of the literature. World J Surg 2000;24(11):1377–1385.
50. Hedberg CW, Fishbein DB, Janssen RS, et al. An outbreak of thyrotoxicosis caused by the consumption of bovine thyroid gland in ground beef. N Engl J Med 1987;316(16): 993–998.
51. Kinney JS, Hurwitz ES, Fishbein DB, et al. Community outbreak of thyrotoxicosis: Epidemiology, immunogenetic characteristics, and long-term outcome. Am J Med 1988;84(1):10–18.
52. Conrey EJ, Lindner C, Estivariz C, et al. Thyrotoxicosis outbreak linked to consumption of minced beef and chorizo: Minas, Uruguay, 2003–2004. Public Health 2008;122(11):1264–1274.
53. Megias MC, Iglesias P, Villanueva MG, Diez JJ. Intermittent and recurrent episodes of subclinical hypothyroidism, central hypothyroidism and T3-toxicosis in an elderly woman. BMJ Case Rep 2012;2012 [online case reports].
54. Ferner RE, Burnett A, Rawlins MD. Tri-iodothyroacetic acid abuse in a female body builder [letter]. Lancet 1986;1(8477):383.
55. Basaria S, Cooper DS. Amiodarone and the thyroid. Am J Med 2005;118(7):706–714.
56. Bartalena L, Tanda ML, Bogazzi F, Piantanida E, Lai A, Martino E. An update on the pharmacological management of hyperthyroidism due to Graves' disease. Expert Opin Pharmacother 2005;6(6):851–861.
57. Biondi B, Palmieri EA, Klain M, Schlumberger M, Filetti S, Lombardi G. Subclinical hyperthyroidism: Clinical features and treatment options. Eur J Endocrinol 2005;152(1):1–9.
58. Hegedus L, Bonnema SJ, Bennedbaek FN. Management of simple nodular goiter: Current status and future perspectives. Endocr Rev 2003;24(1):102–132.
59. Carella C, Mazziotti G, Rotondi M, et al. Iodized salt improves the effectiveness of L-thyroxine therapy after surgery for nontoxic goitre: A prospective and randomized study. Clin Endocrinol 2002;57(4):507–513.
60. Zambudio AR, Rodriguez J, Riquelme J, Soria T, Canteras M, Parrilla P. Prospective study of postoperative complications after total thyroidectomy for multinodular goiters by surgeons with experience in endocrine surgery [see comment]. Ann Surg 2004;240(1):18–25.
61. Boger MS, Perrier ND. Advantages and disadvantages of surgical therapy and optimal extent of thyroidectomy for the treatment of hyperthyroidism. Surg Clin North Am 2004;84(3):849–874.
62. In H, Pearce EN, Wong AK, Burgess JF, McAneny DB, Rosen JE. Treatment options for Graves disease: A cost-effectiveness analysis. J Am Coll Surg 2009;209(2): 170–179, e171–e172.
63. Cooper D. Drug therapy: Antithyroid drugs. N Engl J Med 2005;352(9):905–917.
64. Momotani N, Noh JY, Ishikawa N, Ito K. Effects of propylthiouracil and methimazole on fetal thyroid status in mothers with Graves' hyperthyroidism. J Endocrinol Metab 1997;82(11):3633–3636.
65. Raber W, Kmen E, Waldhausl W, Vierhapper H. Medical therapy of Graves' disease: Effect on remission rates of methimazole alone and in combination with triiodothyronine. Eur J Endocrinol 2000;142(2):117–124.
66. Giuliani C, Cerrone D, Harii N, et al. A TSHR-LH/CGR chimera that measures functional thyroid-stimulating autoantibodies (TSAb) can predict remission or recurrence in Graves' patients undergoing antithyroid drug (ATD) treatment. J Clin Endocrinol Metab 2012;97(7): E1080–E1087.

67. Hashizume K, Ichikawa K, Sakurai A, et al. Administration of thyroxine in treated Graves' disease. Effects on the level of antibodies to thyroid-stimulating hormone receptors and on the risk of recurrence of hyperthyroidism. N Engl J Med 1991;324(14):947–953.
68. McIver B, Rae P, Beckett G, Wilkinson E, Gold A, Toft A. Lack of effect of thyroxine in patients with Graves' hyperthyroidism who are treated with an antithyroid drug. N Engl J Med 1996;334(4):220–224.
69. Cooper DS, Biondi B. Subclinical thyroid disease. Lancet 2012;379(9821):1142–1154.
70. Tamai H, Sudo T, Kimura A, et al. Association between the DRB1*08032 histocompatibility antigen and methimazole-induced agranulocytosis in Japanese patients with Graves disease. Ann Intern Med 1996;124(5):490–494.
71. Fukata S, Kuma K, Sugawara M. Granulocyte colony-stimulating factor (G-CSF) does not improve recovery from antithyroid drug-induced agranulocytosis: A prospective study. Thyroid 1999;9(1):29–31.
72. Monzani F, Caraccio N, Dardano A, Ferrannini E. Thyroid autoimmunity and dysfunction associated with type I interferon therapy. Clin Exp Med 2004;3(4): 199–210.
73. Van Dijke CP, Heydendael RJ, De Kleine MJ. Methimazole, carbimazole, and congenital skin defects. Ann Intern Med 1987;106(1):60–61.
74. Foulds N, Walpole I, Elmslie F, Mansour S. Carbimazole embryopathy: An emerging phenotype. Am J Med Genet A 2005;132A(2):130–135.
75. Di Gianantonio E, Schaefer C, Mastroiacovo PP, et al. Adverse effects of prenatal methimazole exposure. Teratology 2001;64(5):262–266.
76. Mizutani T, Yoshida K, Murakami M, Shirai M, Kawazoe S. Evidence for the involvement of *N*-methylthiourea, a ring cleavage metabolite, in the hepatotoxicity of methimazole in glutathione-depleted mice: Structure–toxicity and metabolic studies. Chem Res Toxicol 2000;13(3):170–176.
77. Liaw YF, Huang MJ, Fan KD, Li KL, Wu SS, Chen TJ. Hepatic injury during propylthiouracil therapy in patients with hyperthyroidism. A cohort study. Ann Intern Med 1993;118(6):424–428.
78. Williams KV, Nayak S, Becker D, Reyes J, Burmeister LA. Fifty years of experience with propylthiouracil-associated hepatotoxicity: What have we learned? J Clin Endocrinol Metab 1997;82(6):1727–1733.
79. Bahn RS, Burch HS, Cooper DS, et al. The role of propylthiouracil in the management of Graves' disease in adults: Report of a meeting jointly sponsored by the American Thyroid Association and the Food and Drug Administration. Thyroid 2009;19(7):673–674.
80. Glinoer D, Cooper DS. The propylthiouracil dilemma. Curr Opin Endocrinol Diabetes Obes 2012;19(5):402–407.
81. Cooper DS, Rivkees SA. Putting propylthiouracil in perspective. J Clin Endocrinol Metab 2009;94(6): 1881–1882.
82. Stanbury JB, Ermans AE, Bourdoux P, et al. Iodine-induced hyperthyroidism: Occurrence and epidemiology. Thyroid 1998;8(1):83–100.
83. Kaplan MM, Meier DA, Dworkin HJ. Treatment of hyperthyroidism with radioactive iodine. Endocrinol Metab Clin North Am 1998;27(1):205–223.
84. Boelaert K, Syed AA, Manji N, et al. Prediction of cure and risk of hypothyroidism in patients receiving 131I for hyperthyroidism. Clin Endocrinol 2009;70(1):129–138.
85. Imseis RE, Vanmiddlesworth L, Massie JD, Bush AJ, Vanmiddlesworth NR. Pretreatment with propylthiouracil but not methimazole reduces the therapeutic efficacy of iodine-131 in hyperthyroidism. J Clin Endocrinol Metab 1998;83(2):685–687.
86. Bogazzi F, Giovannetti C, Fessehatsion R, et al. Impact of lithium on efficacy of radioactive iodine therapy for Graves' disease: A cohort study on cure rate, time to cure, and frequency of increased serum thyroxine after antithyroid drug withdrawal. J Clin Endocrinol Metab 2010;95(1): 201–208.
87. Bartalena L, Marcocci C, Bogazzi F, et al. Relation between therapy for hyperthyroidism and the course of Graves' ophthalmopathy. N Engl J Med 1998;338(2):73–78.
88. Franklyn JA. The management of hyperthyroidism. N Engl J Med 1994;330(24):1731–1738.
89. Franklyn JA, Maisonneuve P, Sheppard M, Betteridge J, Boyle P. Cancer incidence and mortality after radioiodine treatment for hyperthyroidism: A population-based cohort study. Lancet 1999;353(9170):2111–2115.
90. Franklyn JA, Maisonneuve P, Sheppard MC, Betteridge J, Boyle P. Mortality after the treatment of hyperthyroidism with radioactive iodine. N Engl J Med 1998;338(11): 712–718.
91. Leslie WD, Ward L, Salamon EA, Ludwig S, Rowe RC, Cowden EA. A randomized comparison of radioiodine doses in Graves' hyperthyroidism. J Clin Endocrinol Metab 2003;88(3):978–983.
92. Uy HL, Reasner CA, Samuels MH. Pattern of recovery of the hypothalamic–pituitary–thyroid axis following radioactive iodine therapy in patients with Graves' disease. Am J Med 1995;99(2):173–179.
93. Chan GW, Mandel SJ. Therapy insight: Management of Graves' disease during pregnancy. Nat Clin Pract Endocrinol Metab 2007;3:470–478.
94. Glinoer D. Management of hypo- and hyperthyroidism during pregnancy. Growth Horm IGF Res 2003;13(Suppl A):S45–S54.
95. Lockwood CM, Grenache DG, Gronowski AM. Serum human chorionic gonadotropin concentrations greater than 400,000 IU/L are invariably associated with suppressed serum thyrotropin concentrations. Thyroid 2009;19(8): 863–868.
96. Momotani N, Noh J, Ishikawa N, Ito K. Relationship between silent thyroiditis and recurrent Graves' disease in the postpartum period. J Clin Endocrinol Metab 1994;79(1):285–289.
97. Coukos G, Makrigiannakis A, Chung J, Randall TC, Rubin SC, Benjamin I. Complete hydatidiform mole. A disease with a changing profile. J Reprod Med 1999;44(8): 698–704.
98. Momotani N, Yamashita R, Makino F, Noh JY, Ishikawa N, Ito K. Thyroid function in wholly breast-feeding infants whose mothers take high doses of propylthiouracil. Clin Endocrinol 2000;53(2):177–181.
99. Rotondi M, Cappelli C, Pirali B, et al. The effect of pregnancy on subsequent relapse from Graves' disease after a successful course of antithyroid drug therapy. J Clin Endocrinol Metab 2008;93(10):3985–3988.
100. Stagnaro-Green A, Abalovich M, Alexander E, et al. Guidelines of the American Thyroid Association for the diagnosis and management of thyroid disease during pregnancy and postpartum. Thyroid 2011;21(10): 1081–1125.
101. De Groot L, Abalovich M, Alexander EK, et al. Management of thyroid dysfunction during pregnancy and postpartum: An Endocrine Society clinical practice guideline. J Clin Endocrinol Metab 2012;97(8):2543–2565.

102. Polak M, Le Gac I, Vuillard E, et al. Fetal and neonatal thyroid function in relation to maternal Graves' disease. Best Pract Res Clin Endocrinol Metab 2004;18(2):289–302.
103. Segni M, Leonardi E, Mazzoncini B, Pucarelli I, Pasquino AM. Special features of Graves' disease in early childhood. Thyroid 1999;9(9):871–877.
104. Akamizu T, Satoh T, Isozaki O, et al. Diagnostic criteria, clinical features, and incidence of thyroid storm based on nationwide surveys. Thyroid 2012;22(7):661–679.
105. Sherman SI, Ladenson PW. Subacute thyroiditis causing thyroid storm. Thyroid 2007;17(3):283.
106. Zweig SB, Schlosser JR, Thomas SA, Levy CJ, Fleckman AM. Rectal administration of propylthiouracil in suppository form in patients with thyrotoxicosis and critical illness: Case report and review of literature. Endocr Pract 2006;12(1): 43–47.
107. Hodak SP, Huang C, Clarke D, Burman KD, Jonklaas J, Janicic-Kharic N. Intravenous methimazole in the treatment of refractory hyperthyroidism. Thyroid 2006;16(7):691–695.
108. Duggal J, Singh S, Kuchinic P, Butler P, Arora R. Utility of esmolol in thyroid crisis. Can J Clin Pharmacol 2006;13(3):e292–e295.
109. Ozbey N, Kalayoglu-Besisik S, Gul N, Bozbora A, Sencer E, Molvalilar S. Therapeutic plasmapheresis in patients with severe hyperthyroidism in whom antithyroid drugs are contraindicated. Int J Clin Pract 2004;58(6):554–558.
110. Roberts CG, Ladenson PW. Hypothyroidism. Lancet 2004;363(9411):793–803.
111. LaFranchi S. Thyroid hormone in hypopituitarism, Graves' disease, congenital hypothyroidism, and maternal thyroid disease during pregnancy. Growth Horm IGF Res 2006;16(Suppl A):S20–S24.
112. Sinclair D. Clinical and laboratory aspects of thyroid autoantibodies. Ann Clin Biochem 2006;43(Pt 3): 173–183.
113. Stassi G, De Maria R. Autoimmune thyroid disease: New models of cell death in autoimmunity. Nat Rev Immunol 2002;2(3):195–204.
114. de Escobar GM, Obregon MJ, del Rey FE. Maternal thyroid hormones early in pregnancy and fetal brain development. Best Pract Res Clin Endocrinol Metab 2004;18(2):225–248.
115. Buyukgebiz A. Newborn screening for congenital hypothyroidism. J Pediatr Endocrinol Metab 2006;19(11):1291–1298.
116. Chu M, Seltzer TF. Myxedema coma induced by ingestion of raw bok choy. N Engl J Med 2010;362(20):1945–1946.
117. Urban RJ. Hypopituitarism after acute brain injury. Growth Horm IGF Res 2006;16(Suppl A):S25–S29.
118. Prabhakar VK, Shalet SM. Aetiology, diagnosis, and management of hypopituitarism in adult life. Postgrad Med J 2006;82(966):259–266.
119. Sherman SI, Gopal J, Haugen BR, et al. Central hypothyroidism associated with retinoid X receptor-selective ligands. N Engl J Med 1999;340(14):1075–1079.
120. Joshi AS, Woolf PD. Pituitary hyperplasia secondary to primary hypothyroidism: A case report and review of the literature. Pituitary 2005;8(2):99–103.
121. Garber JR, Cobin RH, Gharib H, et al. Clinical practice guidelines for hypothyroidism in adults: Cosponsored by the American Association of Clinical Endocrinologists and the American Thyroid Association. Thyroid 2012;22(12): 1200–1235.
122. Lev-Ran A. Part-of-the-day hypertriiodothyroninemia caused by desiccated thyroid. JAMA 1983;250(20):2790–2791.
123. Celi FS, Zemskova M, Linderman JD, et al. The pharmacodynamic equivalence of levothyroxine and liothyronine: A randomized, double blind, cross-over study in thyroidectomized patients. Clin Endocrinol 2010;72(5):709–715.
124. Jonklaas J, Davidson B, Bhagat S, Soldin SJ. Triiodothyronine levels in athyreotic individuals during levothyroxine therapy. JAMA 2008;299(7):769–777.
125. Gullo D, Latina A, Frasca F, Le Moli R, Pellegriti G, Vigneri R. Levothyroxine monotherapy cannot guarantee euthyroidism in all athyreotic patients. PLoS One 2011;6(8):e22552.
126. Berg JA, Mayor GH. A study in normal human volunteers to compare the rate and extent of levothyroxine absorption from Synthroid and Levoxine. J Clin Pharmacol 1992;32(12):1135–1140.
127. Dong BJ, Hauck WW, Gambertoglio JG, et al. Bioequivalence of generic and brand-name levothyroxine products in the treatment of hypothyroidism. JAMA 1997;277(15):1205–1213.
128. Hennessey JV. Levothyroxine dosage and the limitations of current bioequivalence standards. Nat Clin Pract Endocrinol Metab 2006;2(9):474–475.
129. Blakesley V, Awni W, Locke C, Ludden T, Granneman GR, Braverman LE. Are bioequivalence studies of levothyroxine sodium formulations in euthyroid volunteers reliable? Thyroid 2004;14(3):191–200.
130. Wenzel KW. Bioavailability of levothyroxine preparations. Thyroid 2003;13(7):665.
131. Bach-Huynh TG, Nayak B, Loh J, Soldin S, Jonklaas J. Timing of levothyroxine administration affects serum thyrotropin concentration. J Clin Endocrinol Metab 2009;94(10):3905–3912.
132. Liel Y, Sperber AD, Shany S. Nonspecific intestinal adsorption of levothyroxine by aluminum hydroxide. Am J Med 1994;97(4):363–365.
133. Shakir KM, Chute JP, Aprill BS, Lazarus AA. Ferrous sulfate-induced increase in requirement for thyroxine in a patient with primary hypothyroidism. South Med J 1997;90(6):637–639.
134. Jabbar MA, Larrea J, Shaw RA. Abnormal thyroid function tests in infants with congenital hypothyroidism: The influence of soy-based formula. J Am Coll Nutr 1997;16(3):280–282.
135. Liel Y, Harman-Boehm I, Shany S. Evidence for a clinically important adverse effect of fiber-enriched diet on the bioavailability of levothyroxine in adult hypothyroid patients. J Clin Endocrinol Metab 1996;81(2): 857–859.
136. Benvenga S, Bartolone L, Pappalardo MA, et al. Altered intestinal absorption of L-thyroxine caused by coffee. Thyroid 2008;18(3):293–301.
137. Sachmechi I, Reich DM, Aninyei M, Wibowo F, Gupta G, Kim PJ. Effect of proton pump inhibitors on serum thyroid-stimulating hormone level in euthyroid patients treated with levothyroxine for hypothyroidism. Endocr Pract 2007;13(4):345–349.
138. Appelhof BC, Fliers E, Wekking EM, et al. Combined therapy with levothyroxine and liothyronine in two ratios, compared with levothyroxine monotherapy in primary hypothyroidism: A double-blind, randomized, controlled clinical trial. J Clin Endocrinol Metab 2005;90(5): 2666–2674.
139. Clyde PW, Harari AE, Getka EJ, Shakir KM. Combined levothyroxine plus liothyronine compared with levothyroxine alone in primary hypothyroidism: A randomized controlled trial [see comment]. JAMA 2003;290(22):2952–2958.

140. Ma C, Xie J, Huang X, et al. Thyroxine alone or thyroxine plus triiodothyronine replacement therapy for hypothyroidism. Nucl Med Commun 2009;30(8):586–593.
141. Joffe RT, Brimacombe M, Levitt AJ, Stagnaro-Green A. Treatment of clinical hypothyroidism with thyroxine and triiodothyronine: A literature review and metaanalysis. Psychosomatics 2007;48(5):379–384.
142. Grozinsky-Glasberg S, Fraser A, Nahshoni E, Weizman A, Leibovici L. Thyroxine–triiodothyronine combination therapy versus thyroxine monotherapy for clinical hypothyroidism: Meta-analysis of randomized controlled trials. J Clin Endocrinol Metab 2006;91(7):2592–2599.
143. Escobar-Morreale HF, Botella-Carretero JI, Escobar del Rey F, Morreale de Escobar G. REVIEW: Treatment of hypothyroidism with combinations of levothyroxine plus liothyronine. J Clin Endocrinol Metab 2005;90(8): 4946–4954.
144. Panicker V, Saravanan P, Vaidya B, et al. Common variation in the DIO2 gene predicts baseline psychological well-being and response to combination thyroxine plus triiodothyronine therapy in hypothyroid patients. J Clin Endocrinol Metab 2009;94(5):1623–1629.
145. Burmeister LA, Goumaz MO, Mariash CN, Oppenheimer JH. Levothyroxine dose requirements for thyrotropin suppression in the treatment of differentiated thyroid cancer. J Clin Endocrinol Metab 1992;75(2):344–350.
146. Roti E, Minelli R, Gardini E, Braverman LE. The use and misuse of thyroid hormone. Endocr Rev 1993;14(4): 401–423.
147. Spencer CA, Hollowell JG, Kazarosyan M, Braverman LE. National Health and Nutrition Examination Survey III thyroid-stimulating hormone (TSH)–thyroperoxidase antibody relationships demonstrate that TSH upper reference limits may be skewed by occult thyroid dysfunction. J Clin Endocrinol Metab 2007;92(11):4236–4240.
148. Wartofsky L, Dickey RA. The evidence for a narrower thyrotropin reference range is compelling. J Clin Endocrinol Metab 2005;90(9):5483–5488.
149. Surks MI, Goswami G, Daniels GH. The thyrotropin reference range should remain unchanged. J Clin Endocrinol Metab 2005;90(9):5489–5496.
150. Sawin CT, Herman T, Molitch ME, London MH, Kramer SM. Aging and the thyroid. Decreased requirement for thyroid hormone in older hypothyroid patients. Am J Med 1983;75(2):206–209.
151. Kabadi UM. Influence of age on optimal daily levothyroxine dosage in patients with primary hypothyroidism grouped according to etiology. South Med J 1997;90(9):920–924.
152. Santini F, Pinchera A, Marsili A, et al. Lean body mass is a major determinant of levothyroxine dosage in the treatment of thyroid diseases. J Clin Endocrinol Metab 2005;90(1):124–127.
153. Somwaru LL, Rariy CM, Arnold AM, Cappola AR. The natural history of subclinical hypothyroidism in the elderly: The cardiovascular health study. J Clin Endocrinol Metab 2012;97(6):1962–1969.
154. McQuade C, Skugor M, Brennan DM, Hoar B, Stevenson C, Hoogwerf BJ. Hypothyroidism and moderate subclinical hypothyroidism are associated with increased all-cause mortality independent of coronary heart disease risk factors: A PreCIS database study. Thyroid 2011;21(8): 837–843.
155. Razvi S, Weaver JU, Butler TJ, Pearce SH. Levothyroxine treatment of subclinical hypothyroidism, fatal and nonfatal cardiovascular events, and mortality. Arch Intern Med 2012;172:811–817 [epublished].
156. Loh JA, Wartofsky L, Jonklaas J, Burman KD. The magnitude of increased levothyroxine requirements in hypothyroid pregnant women depends upon the etiology of the hypothyroidism. Thyroid 2009;19(3): 269–275.
157. Slawik M, Klawitter B, Meiser E, et al. Thyroid hormone replacement for central hypothyroidism: A randomized controlled trial comparing two doses of thyroxine (T4) with a combination of T4 and triiodothyronine. J Clin Endocrinol Metab 2007;92(11):4115–4122.
158. Zelmanovitz F, Genro S, Gross JL. Suppressive therapy with levothyroxine for solitary thyroid nodules: A double-blind controlled clinical study and cumulative meta-analyses. J Clin Endocrinol Metab 1998;83(11):3881–3885.
159. Castro MR, Caraballo PJ, Morris JC. Effectiveness of thyroid hormone suppressive therapy in benign solitary thyroid nodules: A meta-analysis. J Clin Endocrinol Metab 2002;87(9):4154–4159.
160. Jonklaas J, Sarlis NJ, Litofsky D, et al. Outcomes of patients with differentiated thyroid carcinoma following initial therapy. Thyroid 2006;16(12):1229–1242.
161. Cooper DS, Doherty GM, Haugen BR, et al. Revised American Thyroid Association management guidelines for patients with thyroid nodules and differentiated thyroid cancer. Thyroid 2009;19(11):1167–1214.
162. Canaris GJ, Manowitz NR, Mayor G, Ridgway EC. The Colorado thyroid disease prevalence study. Arch Intern Med 2000;160(4):526–534.
163. Somwaru LL, Arnold AM, Joshi N, Fried LP, Cappola AR. High frequency of and factors associated with thyroid hormone over-replacement and under-replacement in men and women aged 65 and over. J Clin Endocrinol Metab 2009;94(4):1342–1345.
164. Vestergaard P, Mosekilde L. Hyperthyroidism, bone mineral, and fracture risk—A meta-analysis. Thyroid 2003;13(6):585–593.
165. Uzzan B, Campos J, Cucherat M, Nony P, Boissel JP, Perret GY. Effects on bone mass of long term treatment with thyroid hormones: A meta-analysis. J Clin Endocrinol Metab 1996;81(12):4278–4289.
166. Schneider R, Schneider M, Reiners C, Schneider P. Effects of levothyroxine on bone mineral density, muscle force, and bone turnover markers: A cohort study. J Clin Endocrinol Metab 2012;97(11):3926–3934.
167. Wartofsky L. Myxedema coma. Endocrinol Metab Clin North Am 2006;35(4):687–698, vii–viii.
168. Rose SR, Brown RS, Foley T, et al. Update of newborn screening and therapy for congenital hypothyroidism. Pediatrics 2006;117(6):2290–2303.
169. Rovet J, Daneman D. Congenital hypothyroidism: A review of current diagnostic and treatment practices in relation to neuropsychologic outcome. Paediatr Drugs 2003;5(3): 141–149.
170. Haddow JE, Palomaki GE, Allan WC, et al. Maternal thyroid deficiency during pregnancy and subsequent neuropsychological development of the child [see comment]. N Engl J Med 1999;341(8):549–555.
171. Sherman SI. Thyroid carcinoma. Lancet 2003;361(9356): 501–511.
172. Haugen BR, Pacini F, Reiners C, et al. A comparison of recombinant human thyrotropin and thyroid hormone withdrawal for the detection of thyroid remnant or cancer. J Clin Endocrinol Metab 1999;84(11): 3877–3885.
173. Pacini F, Ladenson PW, Schlumberger M, et al. Radioiodine ablation of thyroid remnants after preparation with

recombinant human thyrotropin in differentiated thyroid carcinoma: Results of an international, randomized, controlled study. J Clin Endocrinol Metab 2006;91(3): 926–932.

174. Robbins RJ, Driedger A, Magner J. Recombinant human thyrotropin-assisted radioiodine therapy for patients with metastatic thyroid cancer who could not elevate endogenous thyrotropin or be withdrawn from thyroxine. Thyroid 2006;16(11):1121–1130.

175. Elisei R, Schlumberger M, Driedger A, et al. Follow-up of low-risk differentiated thyroid cancer patients who underwent radioiodine ablation of postsurgical thyroid remnants after either recombinant human thyrotropin or thyroid hormone withdrawal. J Clin Endocrinol Metab 2009;94(11):4171–4179.

176. Klubo-Gwiezdzinska J, Burman KD, Van Nostrand D, Mete M, Jonklaas J, Wartofsky L. Radioiodine treatment of metastatic thyroid cancer: Relative efficacy and side effect profile of preparation by thyroid hormone withdrawal versus recombinant human thyrotropin. Thyroid 2012;22(3): 310–317.

177. Fast S, Nielsen VE, Bonnema SJ, Hegedus L. Time to reconsider nonsurgical therapy of benign non-toxic multinodular goitre: Focus on recombinant human TSH augmented radioiodine therapy. Eur J Endocrinol 2009;160(4):517–528.

178. Peeters RP, Debaveye Y, Fliers E, Visser TJ. Changes within the thyroid axis during critical illness. Crit Care Clin 2006;22(1):41–55, vi.

179. Torpy DJ, Tsigos C, Lotsikas AJ, Defensor R, Chrousos GP, Papanicolaou DA. Acute and delayed effects of a single-dose injection of interleukin-6 on thyroid function in healthy humans. Metabolism 1998;47(10):1289–1293.

180. Stathatos N, Levetan C, Burman KD, Wartofsky L. The controversy of the treatment of critically ill patients with thyroid hormone. Best Pract Res Clin Endocrinol Metab 2001;15(4):465–478.

181. Burman KD, Wartofsky L. Thyroid function in the intensive care unit setting. Crit Care Clin 2001;17(1):43–57.

182. Kaptein EM, Beale E, Chan LS. Thyroid hormone therapy for obesity and nonthyroidal illnesses: A systematic review. J Clin Endocrinol Metab 2009;94(10):3663–3675.

183. Kaptein EM, Sanchez A, Beale E, Chan LS. Clinical review: Thyroid hormone therapy for postoperative nonthyroidal illnesses: A systematic review and synthesis. J Clin Endocrinol Metab 2010;95(10):4526–4534.

59

Adrenal Gland Disorders

Eric Dietrich, Steven M. Smith, and John G. Gums

KEY CONCEPTS

1. Glucocorticoid secretion from the adrenal cortex is stimulated by adrenocorticotropic hormone (ACTH) or corticotropin that is released from the anterior pituitary in response to the hypothalamic-mediated release of corticotropin-releasing hormone (CRH).
2. To ensure the proper treatment of Cushing's syndrome, diagnostic procedures should (a) establish the presence of hypercortisolism and (b) discover the underlying etiology of the disease.
3. The rationale for treating Cushing's syndrome is to reduce the morbidity and mortality resulting from disorders such as diabetes mellitus, cardiovascular disease, and electrolyte abnormalities.
4. The treatment of choice for both ACTH-dependent and ACTH-independent Cushing's syndrome is surgery, whereas pharmacologic agents are reserved for adjunctive therapy, refractory cases, or inoperable disease.
5. Pharmacologic agents that may be used to manage the patient with Cushing's syndrome include steroidogenesis inhibitors, adrenolytic agents, neuromodulators of ACTH release, and glucocorticoid-receptor blocking agents.
6. Spironolactone, a competitive aldosterone receptor antagonist, is the drug of choice in bilateral adrenal hyperplasia (BAH)–dependent hyperaldosteronism.
7. Addison's disease (primary adrenal insufficiency) is a deficiency in cortisol, aldosterone, and various androgens resulting from the loss of function of all regions of the adrenal cortex.
8. Secondary adrenal insufficiency usually results from exogenous steroid use, leading to hypothalamic–pituitary–adrenal (HPA)–axis suppression followed by a decrease in ACTH release, and low levels of androgens and cortisol.
9. Virilism results from the excessive secretion of androgens from the adrenal gland and often manifests as hirsutism in females.

The adrenal glands were first characterized by Eustachius in 1563. After Addison identified a case of adrenal insufficiency in humans, adrenal anatomy and physiology flourished. Most of the work done in the early and mid-1900s centered on the glucocorticoid cortisol. With the discovery of aldosterone by Simpson and Tait in 1952, adrenal pharmacology turned toward the mineralocorticoid. Conn[1] followed with his classical description of primary aldosteronism (PA) in 1955, and numerous clinicians and investigators have continued to explore the variety of disease processes promoted through the adrenal gland.

PHYSIOLOGY, ANATOMY, AND BIOCHEMISTRY

The adrenal glands are located extraperitoneally to the upper poles of each kidney (Fig. 59-1). On average, each adrenal gland weighs 4 g and is 2 to 3 cm in width and 4 to 6 cm in length. The gland is fed by small arteries from the abdominal aorta and renal and phrenic arteries. Drainage of the adrenal gland occurs via the renal vein on the left and the inferior vena cava on the right.

The adrenal medulla occupies 10% of the total gland and is responsible for the secretion of catecholamines. The adrenal cortex accounts for the remaining 90% and is responsible for the secretion of three types of hormones (Fig. 59-2) from three separate zones.

The zona glomerulosa accounts for 15% of the total adrenal cortex and is responsible for mineralocorticoid production, of which aldosterone is the principal end product. Aldosterone maintains electrolyte and volume homeostasis by altering potassium and magnesium secretion and renal tubular sodium reabsorption. The zona fasciculata, the middle zone, makes up 60% of the cortex, is high in cholesterol, and is responsible for basal and stimulated glucocorticoid production. Glucocorticoids, mainly cortisol, are responsible for the regulation of fat, carbohydrate, and protein metabolism. The zona reticularis occupies 25% of the adrenal cortex, and is responsible for adrenal androgen production. The androgens, testosterone and estradiol, are the major end products and influence the reproductive system in addition to modulating primary and secondary sex characteristics.

Hormone Production and Metabolism

Adrenal steroid hormone synthesis begins with the conversion of cholesterol to pregnenolone by cytochrome P450 (CYP) enzymatic side-chain cleavage. Following this rate-limiting step, pregnenolone is converted to various 19- and 21-carbon steroids, depending on the enzymatic capabilities within each zone of the cortex. Androgenic properties predominate in the 19-carbon steroids, whereas mineralocorticoid and glucocorticoid properties manifest in the 21-carbon steroids.

Aldosterone production is initiated by the 21-hydroxylation of progesterone to form deoxycorticosterone. Subsequently, aldosterone synthase converts deoxycorticosterone to aldosterone through the intermediary, corticosterone. The zona glomerulosa preferentially produces aldosterone for three main reasons. First, the zona glomerulosa lacks 17α-hydroxylase activity and therefore can only convert pregnenolone to progesterone. Second, in contrast to the other zones, cells in the zona glomerulosa possess aldosterone synthase activity, which catalyzes the terminal steps in aldosterone synthesis. Lastly, cells of the zona glomerulosa display a greater number of angiotensin II receptors than cells of the other zones.

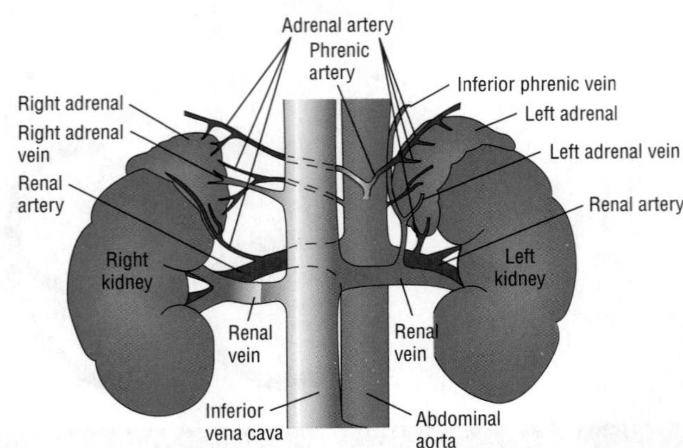

FIGURE 59-1 Anatomy of the adrenal gland.

TABLE 59-1 Rates of Adrenal Production and Plasma Concentrations of Various Steroids

Steroid	24-Hour Secretion (mg)	Plasma Concentration
Aldosterone	0.15	2–9 ng/dL (supine, normal-sodium diet)
Androstenedione	2.2–2.5	50–250 ng/dL
Corticosterone	1–4	2.4 ± 1.5 ng/dL (female) 4.2 ± 2.2 ng/dL (male)
Cortisol	8–25	0–25 mcg/dL
11-Deoxycorticosterone	0.60	2–19 ng/dL
11-Deoxycortisol	0.40	12–158 ng/dL
Progesterone	0	<20 ng/dL (female)[a] 300–2,000 ng/dL (female)[b] <20–140 ng/dL (male)
Testosterone (total)	0.23 (female)	6–86 ng/dL (female) 270–1,070 ng/dL (male)

[a]Follicular phase of menstrual cycle.
[b]Luteal phase of menstrual cycle.

Data from Kratz A, Ferraro M, Sluss PM, Lewandrowski KB. Laboratory reference values. N Engl J Med 2004;351(15):1548–1563. Copyright © 2004 Massachusetts Medical Society. All rights reserved.

Binding of angiotensin II to these receptors provides the stimulus for initiating the aldosterone biosynthesis cascade. Thus, aldosterone synthesis is a unique feature of the zona glomerulosa, explaining why aldosterone is not affected during disease processes limited to the zona fasciculata and/or reticularis.

Cortisol is produced from pregnenolone via four successive hydroxylations. These hydroxylations occur primarily in the zona fasciculata, although the zona reticularis is also capable of producing glucocorticoids.

Androgens, produced primarily in the zona reticularis and less commonly in the zona fasciculata, have a 19-carbon structure and serve as precursors to more potent analogues produced in the periphery. The adrenal gland can synthesize estradiol and estrone from testosterone and androstenedione, respectively; however, these synthesized quantities are extremely small. The rates of production for the various steroids produced by the adrenal gland are listed in Table 59-1.

Glucocorticoid metabolism occurs in the liver and is responsible for converting inactive steroids to active metabolites, as well as modifying active steroids to less active or inactive metabolites. Most pharmaceutical steroid products are active; however, in the case of prednisone and cortisone, metabolism is necessary for conversion to the active prednisolone and cortisol, respectively.

Following metabolic conversion, glomerular filtration is primarily responsible for eliminating endogenously produced glucocorticoids. The half-life of cortisol is 70 to 120 minutes, whereas aldosterone exhibits extremely high intrinsic clearance and a corresponding half-life of only 15 minutes.

Metabolism and conversion of the various steroids can be altered by a variety of disease states and medicinal compounds. Drugs known to enhance steroid clearance include phenytoin, phenobarbital, rifampin, mitotane, and aminoglutethimide. Likewise, diseases such as hyperthyroidism and renal disease (dexamethasone only) can enhance steroid clearance. In contrast, drugs such as estrogens and estrogen-containing oral contraceptives reduce steroid clearance. Similarly, liver disease, age, pregnancy, hypothyroidism, anorexia nervosa, protein–calorie malnutrition, and renal disease (prednisolone only) are associated with reduced steroid clearance.

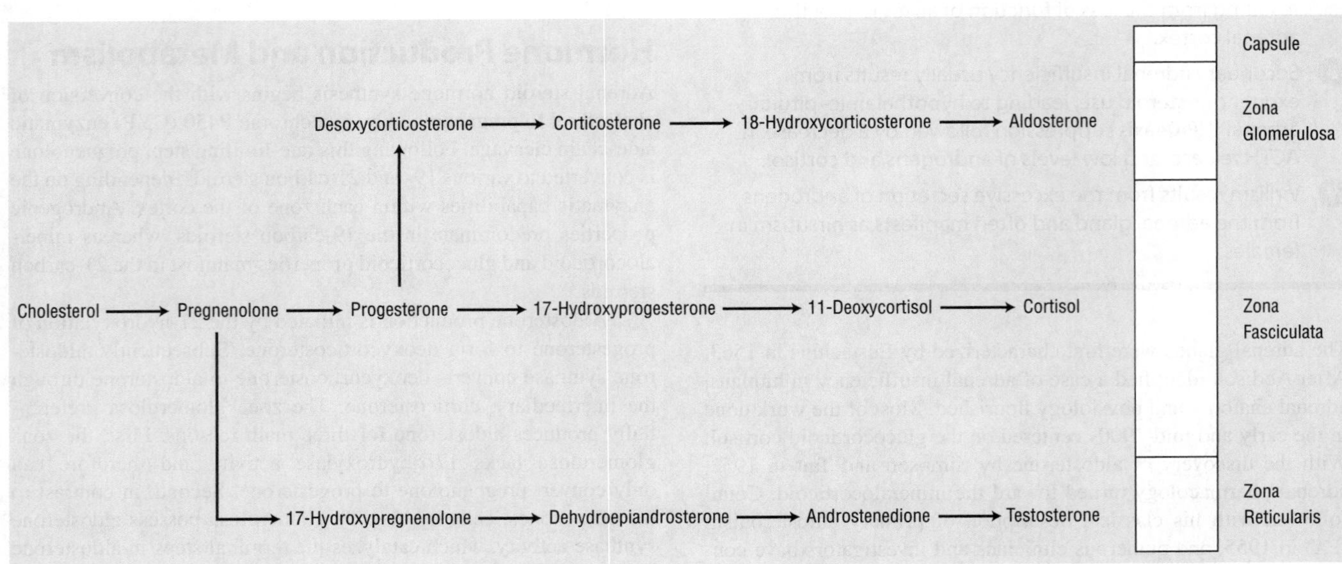

FIGURE 59-2 Hormone synthetic pathways in relation to the zones of the adrenal cortex.

Plasma glucocorticoids are bound to one of three plasma proteins in varying degrees. Corticosteroid-binding globulin (CBG), albumin, and α_1-glycoprotein are capable of binding glucocorticoids, with CBG being the principal binding protein. Steroid binding serves as a reservoir for steroids in their inactive state and ≥95% of cortisol is normally bound in this fashion. This binding prevents glucocorticoid activity at receptor-activating sites. Therefore, a final but important variable in altered plasma concentration of free (active) steroids is concentration of plasma proteins.

Regulation of Hormone Secretion

1 Glucocorticoid secretion is regulated by the pituitary hormone, adrenocorticotropic hormone (ACTH [also known as corticotropin]). Under normal conditions, ACTH is released from the anterior pituitary in response to corticotropin-releasing hormone (CRH), which is secreted by the median eminence of the hypothalamus (Fig. 59-3). Vasopressin and oxytocin have weak ACTH-releasing activity through binding to the inferior V_3 receptor. CRH, in combination with vasopressin and oxytocin, stimulates greater ACTH secretion than each hormone individually.

Additionally, histochemical studies have demonstrated that certain neurotransmitters can stimulate production of CRH or ACTH directly. Specifically, both serotonin and norepinephrine have been shown to increase levels of ACTH. After release, ACTH stimulates the adrenal gland to release cortisol and, to a lesser extent, aldosterone and androgens. The rising cortisol concentration inhibits the secretion of CRH and ACTH through a negative feedback mechanism. In addition, leptin, an adipocyte hormone, can have an inhibitory effect on hypothalamic–pituitary–adrenal (HPA) activity.

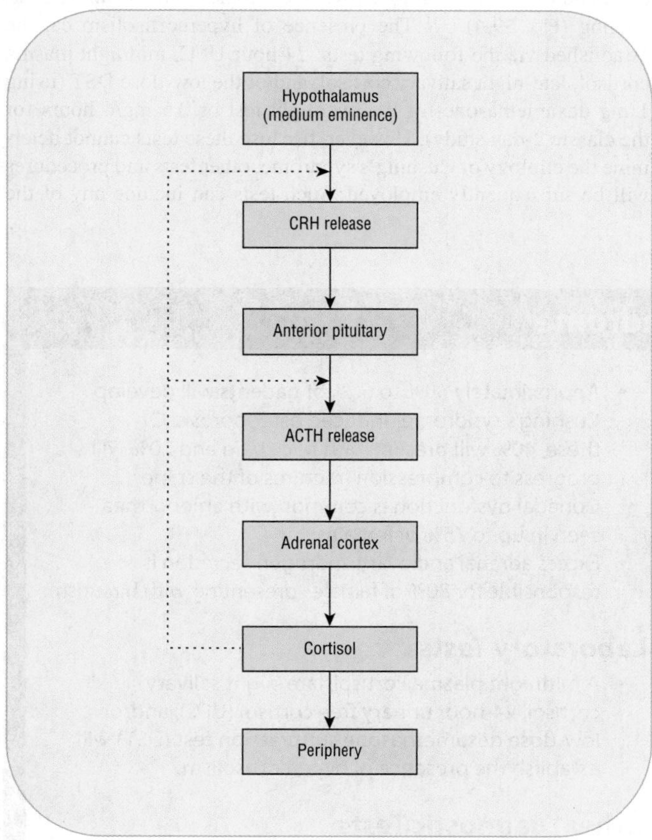

FIGURE 59-3 Negative feedback system involved in the regulation of cortisol secretion under normal conditions. (ACTH, adrenocorticotropic hormone; CRH, corticotropin-releasing hormone.)

Adrenal androgens are regulated in a similar fashion to cortisol. When plasma androgen reaches sufficient concentrations, production is terminated via a negative feedback loop. Androgen release is increased during puberty and in women with hirsutism. Adrenal androgen release decreases with age and in fasting states, including anorexia nervosa.

In contrast to cortisol and adrenal androgens, regulation of aldosterone secretion is considerably more complex. The renin–angiotensin system regulates aldosterone secretion through both intrarenal and extrarenal mechanisms. Renin production and subsequent aldosterone secretion is stimulated by blood pressure lowering (due to volume depletion), erect posture, salt depletion, β-adrenergic stimulation, and CNS excitation (see Chap. 15). Renin production is inhibited by salt loading, angiotensin II, vasopressin, potassium, calcium, blood pressure increases, and a variety of drugs. The renin-mediated production of angiotensin II is the initial stimulus for aldosterone synthesis. Additionally, angiotensin II can be acted on by aminopeptidase and converted to angiotensin III. Both angiotensin II and III are capable of stimulating the zona glomerulosa to secrete aldosterone. Following aldosterone secretion, increases in renal sodium and water retention as well as blood pressure occur, thereby turning off the stimulus for renin release.

HYPERFUNCTION OF THE ADRENAL GLAND

Adrenal disorders can be categorized as hyperfunction or hypofunction of the adrenal gland. Hyperfunction of the adrenal gland generally involves excess production of adrenal hormones, most notably cortisol, resulting in Cushing's syndrome, or aldosterone, resulting in hyperaldosteronism.

Cushing's Syndrome

In 1932, Cushing first described a syndrome of pituitary basophilism that attracted national attention. Until this time, no definitive diagnosis existed for patients with unexplained central obesity, cutaneous striae, osteoporosis, weakness, hypertension, diabetes mellitus, and congestion. Cushing emphasized that the disease was of a pituitary origin. Ten years later, Albright focused his attention on the sugar hormone, which he believed originated from the adrenal cortex.[2]

After the development of a method for measuring urinary steroids, Daughaday discovered elevated steroids in the urine of patients with Cushing's syndrome. Finally, the end product was identified, and Cushing's syndrome was correctly explained as an excess of cortisol in the plasma (hypercortisolism).

Etiology

Cushing's syndrome results from the effects of supraphysiologic levels of glucocorticoids originating either from exogenous administration or, less commonly, from endogenous overproduction by the adrenal glands. Excess glucocorticoids are produced in response to overproduction of ACTH (ACTH-dependent) or by abnormal adrenocortical tissues regardless of ACTH stimulation (ACTH-independent). ACTH-dependent Cushing's syndrome (≈80% of all Cushing's syndrome cases) usually originates from overproduction of ACTH by the pituitary gland, which chronically stimulates the adrenal glands causing bilateral adrenal hyperplasia (BAH). Approximately 85% of these cases are caused by pituitary adenomas (Cushing's disease). Ectopic ACTH-secreting tumors and nonneoplastic corticotropin hypersecretion, possibly secondary to excess CRH production, account for the remainder of ACTH-dependent causes.[3] Ectopic ACTH syndrome refers to excessive ACTH production resulting from an endocrine or nonendocrine tumor, usually

TABLE 59-2 Various Etiologies of Cushing's Syndrome and Their Respective Differences

	Pituitary-Dependent	Ectopic ACTH Syndrome	Adrenal Adenoma	Adrenal Carcinoma
Course	Slow	Rapid	Slow	Rapid
Symptoms	Mild to moderate	Atypical	Mild to moderate	Severe
Dominant sex/age	Female/male	Male	None noted	Children
Virilization	+	+	+	+++
Abdominal mass	0	0	0	++
Plasma ACTH concentration	Slightly elevated	High	0	0
Dexamethasone suppression test	≥50% suppression	No suppression	No suppression	No suppression
Iodocholesterol scan	Bilateral uptake	Bilateral uptake	Unilateral	None

ACTH, adrenocorticotropic hormone.

of the pancreas, thyroid, or lung. Small-cell carcinoma of the lung will lead to ectopic ACTH secretion in 0.5% to 2% of cases, whereas bronchial carcinoid tumors are usually the most common.[4] Distinguishing between the various etiologies requires a careful history and pertinent laboratory work (Table 59-2).

The remaining 20% of Cushing's syndrome cases are ACTH-independent and divided almost equally between adrenal adenomas and adrenal carcinomas, with rare cases caused by macronodular hyperplasia, primary pigmented nodular adrenal disease, and McCune-Albright syndrome.[3,5] The majority of adrenal cortex tumors are benign adenomas. Adrenal carcinoma is found more often in children than in adults with Cushing's syndrome.

Clinical Presentation

Patients with Cushing's syndrome commonly present (>90% of patients) with central obesity and facial rounding. In addition, approximately 50% of patients will exhibit some peripheral obesity and fat accumulation. Fat accumulation in the dorsocervical area (buffalo hump) can be associated with any major weight gain, whereas increased supraclavicular fat pads are more specific for Cushing's syndrome. Striae usually are present along the lower abdomen and take on a red to purple color. Traditionally, hypertensive complications have been major contributors to the morbidity and mortality of Cushing's syndrome. Hypertension is diagnosed in 75% to 85% of patients, with diastolic blood pressures greater than 119 mm Hg noted in over 20% of patients.[6] In addition, glucose intolerance is present in 60% of patients. Thus, many patients meet diagnostic criteria for the metabolic syndrome and have a corresponding increased risk of coronary heart disease (CHD) and stroke. Screening for Cushing's syndrome in this population and in patients with uncontrolled diabetes mellitus has been suggested,[7,8] particularly when these conditions surface at an unusually early age.[9] However, screening all patients with type 2 diabetes is likely not cost-effective.[10]

Diagnosis

2 The diagnosis of Cushing's syndrome involves two steps: (a) establishing the presence of hypercortisolism, which is relatively easy, and (b) differentiating between etiologies, which can be challenging (Fig. 59-4).[5,8,11] The presence of hypercortisolism can be established via the following tests: 24-hour UFC, midnight plasma cortisol, late-night salivary cortisol, and/or the low-dose DST (using 1 mg dexamethasone for the overnight test or 0.5 mg/6 hours for the classic 2-day study). However, because these tests cannot determine the etiology of Cushing's syndrome, other tests and procedures will be subsequently employed. Such tests can include any of the

CLINICAL PRESENTATION Cushing's Syndrome

General

- The most common findings, which are present in 90% of patients, are central obesity and facial rounding.

Symptoms

- Approximately 65% and 58% of patients complain of myopathies and muscular weakness, respectively.

Signs

- Peripheral obesity and fat accumulation is found in 50% of patients.
- Facial plethora is caused by an underlying atrophy of the skin and connective tissue and is seen in approximately 84% of patients.
- Patients often are described as having moon faces with a buffalo hump.
- Hypertension is seen in 75% to 85% of patients.
- Psychiatric changes can occur in as many as 55% of patients.
- Approximately 50% to 60% of patients will develop Cushing's syndrome–induced osteoporosis. Of these, 40% will present with back pain and 20% will progress to compression fractures of the spine.
- Gonadal dysfunction is common with amenorrhea seen in up to 75% of females.
- Excess adrenal and ovary androgen secretion is responsible for 80% of females presenting with hirsutism.

Laboratory Tests

- A midnight plasma cortisol, late-night salivary cortisol, 24-hour urinary free cortisol (UFC), and/or low-dose dexamethasone suppression test (DST) will establish the presence of hypercortisolism.

Other Diagnostic Tests

- The plasma ACTH test, metyrapone stimulation test, CRH stimulation test, or inferior petrosal sinus sampling (IPSS) will help determine the etiology.

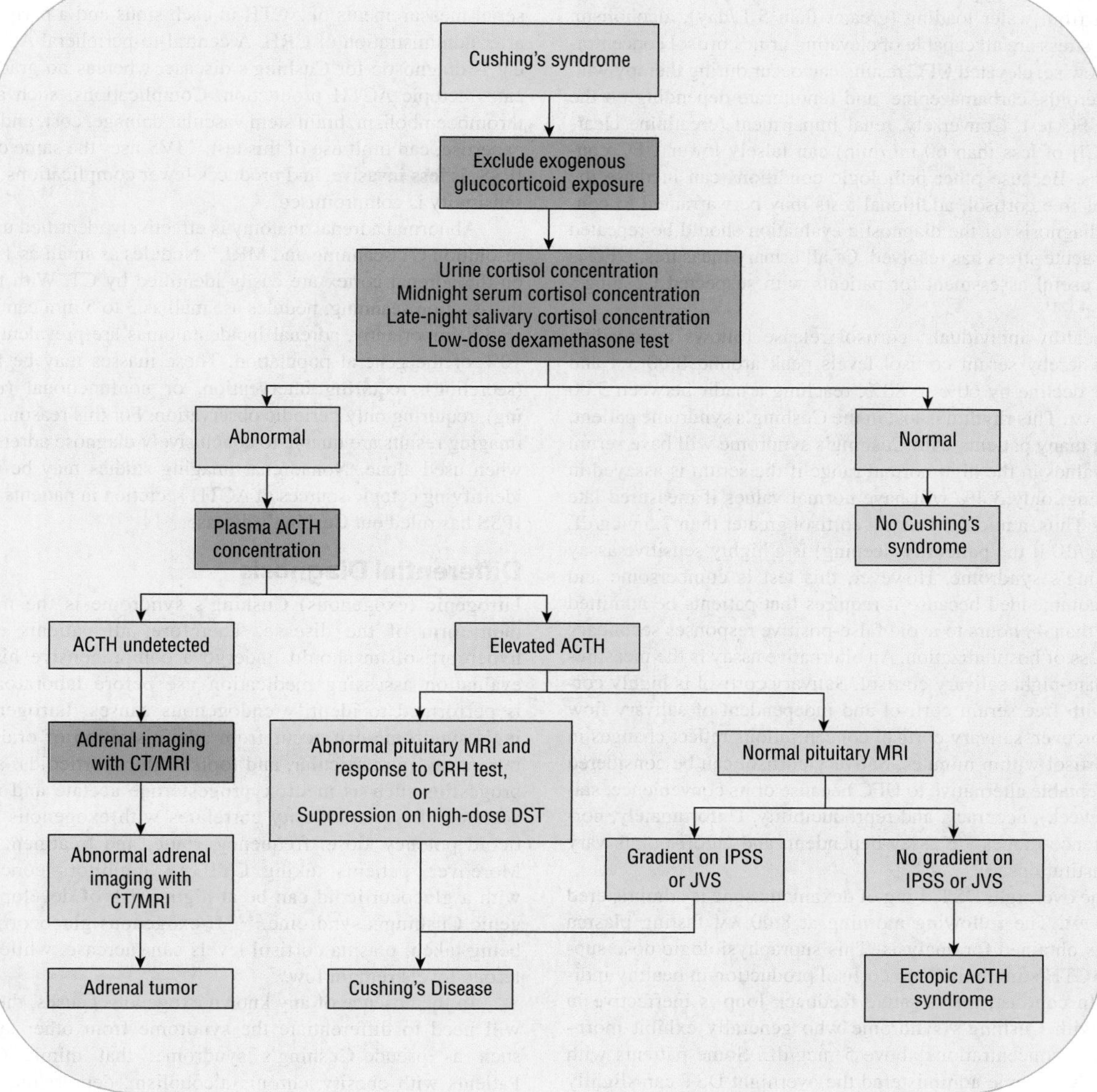

FIGURE 59-4 Algorithm for diagnosing Cushing's syndrome. (ACTH, adrenocorticotropic hormone.)

following: plasma ACTH via immunoradiometric assay (IRMA) or radioimmunoassay (RIA); adrenal vein catheterization; metyrapone stimulation test; adrenal, chest, or abdominal computed tomography (CT); CRH stimulation test; IPSS; jugular venous sampling (JVS); cavernous sinus sampling; and pituitary magnetic resonance imaging (MRI). High-dose DST has been used in the past, but is no longer recommended due to its poor specificity and limited diagnostic value. Other possible tests and procedures include insulin-induced hypoglycemia, somatostatin receptor scintigraphy, the desmopressin stimulation test, the naloxone CRH stimulation test, the loperamide test, the hexarelin stimulation test, and radionuclide imaging.[5,6,8,11–16] Table 59-3 summarizes some of the tests used to diagnose Cushing's syndrome.

Elevated UFC concentrations are highly suggestive of Cushing's syndrome, especially values fourfold greater than the upper limit of normal.[3,13] In contrast to plasma measurements of cortisol, UFC measures only unbound cortisol. Consequently, the UFC test is unaffected by conditions and medications that alter CBG levels. Normal reference values for UFC are 20 to 90 mcg per 24-hour period. A twofold to threefold increase in urine cortisol is not uncommon

TABLE 59-3 Summary of Tests Used to Diagnose Cushing's Syndrome

Test	Normal	Hyperplasia	Adenoma	Carcinoma
Plasma				
Cortisol (mcg/dL, AM/PM)	5–25/5–15	↑/↑↑	↑↑/↑↑	↑↑↑/↑↑↑
After low-dose DST	↓	↔	↔	↔
After high-dose DST	↓	↓/↔	↔	↔
ACTH (pg/mL)	6–76	↑↑	↓	↓
Urine				
Cortisol (mcg/24 hours)	20–90	↑↑	↑↑	↑↑↑
Saliva				
Cortisol (mcg/dL, PM)	Assay-dependent	↑↑	↑↑	↑↑↑

ACTH, adrenocorticotropic hormone; DST, dexamethasone suppression test.

Data from Kratz A, Ferraro M, Sluss PM, Lewandrowski KB. Laboratory reference values. N Engl J Med 2004;351(15):1548–1563. Copyright © 2004 Massachusetts Medical Society. All rights reserved.

in the patient with hyperfunction of the adrenal gland. Starvation, hydration from water loading (greater than 5 L/day), alcoholism, and acute stress are all capable of elevating urine cortisol concentrations. Likewise, elevated UFC results can occur during therapy with topical steroids, carbamazepine, and fenofibrate depending on the type of UFC test. Conversely, renal impairment (creatinine clearance [CrCl] of less than 60 mL/min) can falsely lower UFC concentrations. Because other pathologic conditions can increase the amount of free cortisol, additional tests may be warranted to confirm the diagnosis, or the diagnostic evaluation should be repeated when the acute stress has resolved. Of all urinary measures, UFC is the most useful assessment for patients with suspected Cushing's syndrome.[8,13,15]

In healthy individuals, cortisol release follows a circadian rhythm whereby serum cortisol levels peak around 8:00 AM and thereafter decline by 60% to 80%, reaching a nadir between 3:00 and 4:00 AM. This rhythm is lost in the Cushing's syndrome patient. Although many patients with Cushing's syndrome will have serum cortisol values in the high normal range if the serum is assayed in the morning, only 3.4% will have normal values if measured late at night.[17] Thus, a midnight serum cortisol greater than 7.5 mcg/dL (>1.8 mcg/dL if the patient is sleeping) is a highly sensitive assay for Cushing's syndrome. However, this test is cumbersome and rarely recommended because it requires that patients be admitted for more than 48 hours to avoid false-positive responses secondary to the stress of hospitalization. An alternative assay is the measurement of late-night salivary cortisol. Salivary cortisol is highly correlated with free serum cortisol and independent of salivary flow rates. Moreover, salivary cortisol concentrations reflect changes in serum cortisol within minutes. Salivary cortisol can be considered as an acceptable alternative to UFC because of its convenience, stability (1 week), accuracy, and reproducibility. Unfortunately, normal reference ranges are assay-dependent, and cutoff points vary among institutions.[18,19]

In the overnight DST, 1 mg of dexamethasone is administered at 11:00 PM. The following morning at 8:00 AM fasting plasma cortisol is obtained for analysis. This supraphysiologic dose suppresses ACTH stimulation and cortisol production in healthy individuals. In contrast, the negative feedback loop is ineffective in patients with Cushing's syndrome who generally exhibit morning cortisol concentrations above 5 mcg/dL. Some patients with Cushing's syndrome administered the overnight DST can slightly suppress cortisol and using 1.8 mcg/dL as a cutoff can increase sensitivity, but at the expense of reduced specificity.[20] Therefore, the overnight DST is useful only as a screening tool for Cushing's syndrome. Drugs that induce or inhibit CYP3A4 metabolism can significantly alter dexamethasone levels, increasing the number of false-positive and false-negative DST tests. Concurrent measurements of dexamethasone levels with cortisol may improve the accuracy of testing for patients on CYP3A4-modifying drugs, although dexamethasone assays are not widely available. Also noteworthy, pregnancy and estrogen use (including oral contraceptives) increase CBG levels and frequently elicit false-positive results.[13] Consequently, UFC testing is preferred over DST in these patient populations.

The first test used to determine the etiology of Cushing's syndrome is the plasma ACTH test. Plasma ACTH concentrations can be measured via RIA or IRMA.[12] In ACTH-dependent Cushing's syndrome, ACTH can be normal or elevated. Very high levels of ACTH favor ectopic production. In contrast, ACTH values generally are low (less than 5 pg/mL) in ACTH-independent (adrenal) Cushing's syndrome. Furthermore, ACTH levels can appear artificially low in some ectopic ACTH-producing tumors because ACTH can be secreted as an active prohormone that is not detected by the assay.

IPSS offers the highest sensitivity and specificity of any test in differentiating the etiology of Cushing's syndrome. This technique requires catheterization of both petrosal sinuses with serial measurements of ACTH in each sinus and a peripheral vein after administration of CRH. A central-to-peripheral ACTH gradient is diagnostic for Cushing's disease, whereas no gradient indicates ectopic ACTH production. Complications, such as venous thromboembolism, brain stem vascular damage, cost, and technical expertise, can limit use of this test.[12] JVS uses the same concept as IPSS, is less invasive, and produces fewer complications; however, sensitivity is compromised.

Abnormal adrenal anatomy is effectively identified using high-resolution CT scanning and MRI.[21] Nodules as small as 1 to 1.5 cm on the adrenal cortex are easily identified by CT. With the use of thin-section scanning, nodules as small as 3 to 5 mm can be visualized.[22] Importantly, adrenal incidentalomas are prevalent in 5% to 10% of the general population. These masses may be functional (secreting), requiring intervention, or nonfunctional (nonsecreting), requiring only periodic observation. For this reason, abnormal imaging results are unable to conclusively diagnose adrenal disease when used alone. Nonadrenal imaging studies may be useful for identifying ectopic sources of ACTH secretion in patients for whom IPSS has ruled out Cushing's disease.

Differential Diagnosis

Iatrogenic (exogenous) Cushing's syndrome is the most common form of the disease. Therefore, all patients exhibiting hypercortisolism should undergo a comprehensive history and evaluation assessing medication use before laboratory testing is performed to identify endogenous causes. Iatrogenic Cushing's syndrome can occur from administration of oral, inhaled, intranasal, intraarticular, and topical glucocorticoids, as well as progestins such as medroxyprogesterone acetate and megestrol acetate.[23] Disease severity correlates with exogenous glucocorticoid potency, dose, frequency, route, and treatment duration. Moreover, patients taking CYP3A4 inhibitors concomitantly with a glucocorticoid can be at higher risk of developing iatrogenic Cushing's syndrome.[24,25] If exogenous glucocorticoids are being taken, plasma cortisol levels can increase, while corticosterone levels remain low.[17]

In the absence of any known exogenous causes, the clinician will need to differentiate the syndrome from other syndromes, such as pseudo-Cushing's syndrome, that mimic Cushing's. Patients with obesity, chronic alcoholism, depression, and acute illness of any type can present with certain features of Cushing's syndrome. However, these patients may lack true Cushing's syndrome. For example, depressed patients, although mimicking the urinary steroid abnormalities of Cushing's syndrome, will not resemble a cushingoid patient in appearance. In chronic alcoholics, steroid laboratory panels generally return to baseline after ceasing alcohol intake. And obese patients often will have normal cortisol concentrations on both serum and urinary screening. Thus, identifying true cases of Cushing's syndrome requires a comprehensive history in combination with laboratory and possibly imaging assessment.

TREATMENT

Desired Outcomes

3 If left untreated, Cushing's syndrome is associated with high morbidity and mortality due to associated disorders such as hypertension, diabetes mellitus, cardiovascular disease, and electrolyte abnormalities. These disorders limit the survival of the patient with Cushing's syndrome to 4 to 5 years following initial diagnosis. The desired outcomes of treatment are to limit such detrimental outcomes and return the patient to a normal functional state by

TABLE 59-4 Possible Treatment Options in Cushing's Syndrome Based on Etiology

	Treatment	
Etiology	**Nondrug**	**Drug Name**
Ectopic ACTH syndrome	Surgery, chemotherapy, irradiation	Metyrapone
Pituitary-dependent	Surgery, irradiation	Mitotane Metyrapone Mifepristone Cyproheptadine
Adrenal adenoma	Surgery, postoperative replacement	Ketoconazole
Adrenal carcinoma	Surgery	Mitotane

ACTH, adrenocorticotropic hormone.

removing the source of hypercortisolism while minimizing pituitary or adrenal deficiencies.

❹ The treatment of choice for both ACTH-dependent and ACTH-independent Cushing's syndrome is surgical resection of any offending tumors.[3,11] However, several secondary pharmacologic treatment plans are available, depending on the etiology of the disease (Table 59-4).[26,27] These pharmacologic options are generally used in preoperative patients or as adjunctive therapy in postoperative patients awaiting response. Rarely, monotherapy is used as a palliative treatment when surgery is not indicated.

Pharmacologic Therapy

❺ Pharmacotherapy of Cushing's syndrome (dosing and monitoring parameters can be found in Tables 59-5 and 59-6, respectively)[28] can be divided into four categories based on the anatomic site of action of the agent: (a) steroidogenesis inhibitors, (b) adrenolytic agents, (c) neuromodulators of ACTH release, and (d) glucocorticoid-receptor blocking agents.[26,27]

Steroidogenesis Inhibitors

As their name implies, steroidogenesis inhibitors block the production of cortisol. This class includes metyrapone, ketoconazole, etomidate, and aminoglutethimide. Metyrapone inhibits 11β-hydroxylase, the enzyme responsible for converting 11-deoxycortisol to cortisol. Following administration, a sudden decrease in cortisol levels occurs within hours and prompts a compensatory rise in plasma ACTH concentrations. As ACTH increases and blockage of cortisol synthesis persists, adrenal steroidogenesis efforts are shunted toward androgen production. Consequently, metyrapone is associated with significant androgenic side effects, including hirsutism and increased acne, making it less ideal for females. In addition, metyrapone blocks aldosterone synthesis and causes the accumulation of aldosterone precursors, which exhibit weak mineralocorticoid activity. Blood pressure and electrolyte level variations can ensue, depending on the level of circulating 11-deoxycortisol and the degree of aldosterone inhibition. Additional adverse effects, including nausea, vomiting, vertigo, headache, dizziness, abdominal discomfort, and allergic rash, have been reported following administration, but are often signs of overtreatment.[26,27,29] Metyrapone is currently available through the manufacturer only for compassionate use.

The imidazole derivative antifungal, ketoconazole, effectively inhibits steroidogenesis via multiple mechanisms when used in large doses. In contrast to the quick onset of metyrapone, the benefits of ketoconazole therapy are achieved only after several weeks of therapy. In addition to lowering serum cortisol levels, ketoconazole exhibits antiandrogenic activity attributable to its inhibition of multiple CYP enzymes as well as 11β-hydroxylase and 17α-hydroxylase.[26] This activity may be beneficial in female patients with Cushing's syndrome, but can cause gynecomastia and hypogonadism in males. Sustained therapy with ketoconazole also imparts beneficial effects on serum cholesterol profiles, including lowering total and LDL cholesterol levels. Ketoconazole induces a reversible elevation of hepatic transaminases in approximately 10% of patients.[30] Frequent liver function monitoring is recommended, although progression to serious hepatotoxicity is rare. Additional common adverse effects include GI discomfort and dermatologic reactions.

Ketoconazole may be used concomitantly with metyrapone to achieve synergistic reductions in cortisol levels. Because these drugs differ in their onset of action, coadministration allows for more complete suppression of cortisol synthesis. Moreover, the antiandrogenic actions of ketoconazole therapy may offset the

TABLE 59-5 Drug Dosing in the Treatment of Cushing's Syndrome

Drug	Brand Name	Initial Dose	Usual Range	Special Populations	Comments
Aminoglutethimide	Cytadren®, 250 mg tablets	0.5–1 g/day, divided two to four times a day for 2 weeks	1 g/day, divided every 6 hours		Maximum: 2 g/day
Cyproheptadine	Periactin®, 2 mg/5 mL syrup or 4 mg tablets	4 mg twice daily	24–32 mg/day, divided four times a day	Reduce dose in hepatic impairment	Maximum: 32 mg/day
Ketoconazole	Nizoral®, 200 mg tablets	200 mg once or twice a day	200–1,200 mg/day, divided twice a day	Increased risk of hepatotoxicity in patients with hepatic disease	Maximum: 1,600 mg/day; CYP3A4 substrate and inhibitor (strong)
Metyrapone	Metopirone®, 250 mg tablets	0.5–1 g/day, divided every 4–6 hours	1–2 g/day, divided every 4–6 hours		Maximum: 6 g/day; CYP3A4 inducer
Mifepristone	Korlym®	300 mg once daily, increased by 300 mg/day every 2–4 weeks	600–1,200 mg/day	Do not exceed 600 mg/day in mild to moderate hepatic impairment; avoid in severe hepatic impairment. Do not exceed 600 mg/day in renal impairment	Maximum: 1,200 mg/day not to exceed 20 mg/kg/day
Mitotane	Lysodren®, 500 mg tablets	0.5–1 g/day, increased by 0.5–1 g/day every 1–4 weeks	1–4 g/day		Maximum: 12 g/day. Take with food to decrease GI effects

CYP, cytochrome P450 enzyme.

TABLE 59-6 Drug Monitoring in the Treatment of Cushing's Syndrome

Drug	Adverse Drug Reaction	Monitoring Parameters	Comments
Aminoglutethimide	Drowsiness, morbilliform rash, nausea, vomiting, hirsutism, headache, ataxia		Side effects often limit use
Cyproheptadine	Anticholinergic effects (sedation, weight gain), dizziness, blurred vision		Anticholinergic side effects often limit use
Ketoconazole	GI upset, dermatologic reactions; elevated hepatic transaminases, hepatotoxicity (rare)	Liver function tests	Approximately 10% will experience reversible LFT elevations
Metyrapone	Androgenic effects (hirsutism, acne, etc.), blood pressure and electrolyte abnormalities, nausea, vomiting, vertigo, headache, dizziness, abdominal discomfort, allergic rash	Blood pressure, electrolytes	
Mifepristone	Hypokalemia, nausea, fatigue, headache, peripheral edema, dizziness, endometrial hyperplasia	Serum potassium, pregnancy testing, pelvic ultrasound	Abortifacient; rule out pregnancy in women of childbearing potential
Mitotane	GI upset, nausea, diarrhea, lethargy, somnolence, CNS disturbances	UFC and urinary steroid production, serum potassium	GI upset in up to 80%; GI and CNS effects appear to be dose-dependent

UFC, urinary free cortisol.

androgenic potential of metyrapone, thus attenuating a major limitation of metyrapone therapy.

The anesthetic etomidate is an imidazole derivative similar to ketoconazole that inhibits 11β-hydroxylase.[26] Etomidate is available only in a parenteral formulation and is therefore limited to patients with acute hypercortisolemia requiring emergency treatment.

Initially, aminoglutethimide was used to treat refractory forms of epilepsy, but was later discovered to be a potent inhibitor of adrenal steroid synthesis. Aminoglutethimide inhibits the conversion of cholesterol to pregnenolone early in the steroid biosynthesis pathway, thereby inhibiting the production of cortisol, aldosterone, and androgens. Owing to these broad inhibitory actions, side effects, including severe sedation, nausea, ataxia, and skin rashes, limit the use of aminoglutethimide in many patients.[26,27] Moreover, because other steroidogenesis inhibitors offer greater efficacy combined with fewer side effects, aminoglutethimide has fallen out of favor in the treatment of Cushing's syndrome. If aminoglutethimide is used, it should be coadministered with another steroidogenesis inhibitor, usually metyrapone, secondary to high relapse rates with aminoglutethimide monotherapy.

Adrenolytic Agents

Mitotane is a cytotoxic drug that structurally resembles the insecticide dichlorodiphenyltrichloroethane (DDT). Mitotane inhibits the 11-hydroxylation of 11-desoxycortisol and 11-desoxycorticosterone in the cortex, resulting in a net inhibition of cortisol and corticosterone synthesis. Similar to ketoconazole, mitotane takes weeks to months to exert beneficial effects. Sustained cortisol suppression occurs in most patients and may persist following discontinuation of therapy in up to one third of patients. Because of its cytotoxic nature, mitotane degenerates cells within the zona fasciculata and reticularis, resulting in atrophy of the adrenal cortex. The zona glomerulosa is minimally affected during acute therapy but can become damaged following long-term treatment.[28,31]

Importantly, mitotane can induce significant neurologic and GI side effects and patients should be monitored carefully or hospitalized when initiating therapy. Nausea and diarrhea are common adverse effects that occur at doses greater than 2 g/day and can be avoided by gradually increasing the dose and/or administering the agent with food. Approximately 80% of patients treated with mitotane develop lethargy and somnolence, and other CNS adverse drug reactions occur in approximately 40% of patients. Furthermore, significant but reversible hypercholesterolemia and prolongation of bleeding times can result from mitotane use.[26,27] Mitotane increases production of CBG resulting in artifactually elevated plasma cortisol; thus, UFC and urinary steroid production should be monitored to assess response to therapy.[26] If necessary, steroid replacement therapy can be given. However, because mitotane also increases extraadrenal metabolism of exogenously administered corticosteroids (especially hydrocortisone), higher steroid replacement doses may be required.

Neuromodulatory Agents

Pituitary secretion of ACTH is normally mediated by various neurotransmitters, including serotonin, GABA, acetylcholine, and the catecholamines. Although ACTH-secreting pituitary tumors (Cushing's disease) self-regulate ACTH production to some degree, these neurotransmitters are still capable of promoting pituitary ACTH production. Consequently, agents that target these neurotransmitters have been proposed for the treatment of Cushing's disease. Such agents include cyproheptadine, ritanserin, ketanserin, bromocriptine, cabergoline, valproic acid, octreotide, lanreotide, rosiglitazone, and tretinoin. However, none of these drugs have demonstrated consistent clinical efficacy in the treatment of Cushing's disease.

Cyproheptadine, a nonselective serotonin receptor antagonist and anticholinergic drug, can decrease ACTH secretion in some Cushing's disease patients. However, side effects, including sedation and weight gain, significantly limit the use of this drug. Likewise, selective serotonin type 2 receptor antagonists, including ritanserin and ketanserin, have demonstrated limited efficacy. Owing to their poor efficacy and high relapse rates, these drugs should be avoided except in nonsurgical candidates refractory to more conventional treatments.

Dopamine D_2 receptor agonists, including bromocriptine and cabergoline, initially reduce ACTH secretion in as many as half of all patients with Cushing's disease. This action occurs through activation of inhibitory D_2 receptors that are expressed in approximately 80% of pituitary adenomas.[32] Reductions in ACTH levels are often minor and rarely sustained with long-term bromocriptine therapy. Cabergoline exhibits a higher specificity and affinity for D_2 receptors as well as a prolonged half-life compared with bromocriptine. These differences may explain the greater response rates observed with cabergoline monotherapy; however, a sustained response occurs in only 30% to 40% of patients.[33,34]

The somatostatin analogues, octreotide and lanreotide, generally are ineffective in reducing ACTH secretion in Cushing's disease. These two agents primarily target somatostatin receptor subtype 2 (sst_2), whereas pituitary adenomas predominantly express sst_5. Pasireotide, a recently approved somatostatin analogue, exhibits a high affinity for sst_1, sst_2, sst_3, and, especially, sst_5 receptor subtypes. In a phase 3 study of 162 adults with Cushing's disease and an elevated UFC level, pasireotide administered at 600 or 900 mcg injected subcutaneously twice daily reduced the median UFC by 50% by month 2; levels remained stable for the duration of the 12-month study. Clinical signs and symptoms of Cushing's disease were also improved as were blood pressure, weight, LDL cholesterol, and quality of life. Side effects were mostly GI in nature, although 73% of subjects experienced an adverse event related to hyperglycemia; preexisting diabetes mellitus or impaired glucose tolerance increased the risk for these events. Notably, glycated hemoglobin A1c increased by an average of 1.4%. Gallstones were also rarely seen with six subjects undergoing cholecystectomy.[35]

Glucocorticoid-Receptor Blocking Agents

Mifepristone (RU-486) is a potent progesterone- and glucocorticoid-receptor antagonist that inhibits dexamethasone suppression and increases endogenous cortisol and ACTH levels in normal subjects.[26,29] Clinical experience and trial data in Cushing's syndrome suggest that RU-486 is highly effective in reversing the manifestation of hypercortisolism, including hyperglycemia, hypertension, and weight gain.[36] However, because of its novel site of action, RU-486 induces a compensatory rise in ACTH and cortisol levels. Consequently, efficacy and toxicity monitoring must rely on clinical signs rather than laboratory assessments. Common adverse effects of RU-486 include fatigue, nausea, headache, arthralgia, peripheral edema, endometrial thickening (with or without vaginal bleeding), and significant reductions in serum potassium. Oral potassium supplementation or spironolactone can be effective in mitigating the latter adverse effect, although high doses may be required.[36]

Close monitoring of 24-hour UFC levels and serum cortisol levels is essential to detect treatment-induced adrenal insufficiency. Steroid secretion should be monitored with all of these drugs except RU-486 and steroid replacement given as needed. Whatever the choice, pharmacologic therapy in pituitary-dependent disease is mainly centered around patient stabilization prior to surgery or in patients waiting for potential response to other therapies.

Clinical **Controversy...**

The traditional strategy for suppressing hypercortisolism in Cushing's disease consists of titrating medications to achieve normal cortisol levels. However, some clinicians advocate a "block and replace" strategy, whereby greater doses of medications are used to completely suppress endogenous cortisol production, followed by administration of physiologic doses of glucocorticoids to treat adrenal insufficiency.

Nonpharmacologic Therapy

Surgery

The treatment of choice for Cushing's disease is transsphenoidal resection of the pituitary tumor.[3,11,29,37] The advantages of this procedure include preservation of pituitary function, low complication rate, and high clinical improvement rate. The overall cure rate of histologically proven microadenomas approaches 90%, whereas remission rates for macroadenomas generally do not exceed 65%.

For persistent disease following transsphenoidal surgery or when tumor-specific surgery is not possible, several second-line treatment options are available and should be tailored toward the individual patient. In the case of persistent disease following transsphenoidal surgery, repeat surgery may be performed, although overall remission rates are lower with subsequent procedures. Alternatively, radiotherapy may be preferred for tumors invading the dura or cavernous sinus because these tumors respond poorly to surgical intervention.[38] Radiotherapy provides clinical improvement in approximately 50% of patients within 3 to 5 years, but increases the risk for pituitary-dependent hormone deficiencies (hypopituitarism).

Laparoscopic adrenalectomy is often preferred in patients with unilateral adrenal adenomas for whom transsphenoidal surgery and pituitary radiotherapy have failed or cannot be used.[3,11,29] Bilateral adrenalectomy rapidly reverses hypercortisolism. However, patients can develop Nelson's syndrome, an aggressive pituitary tumor that secretes high quantities of ACTH, which causes hyperpigmentation. Because Nelson's syndrome occurs in as many as 30% of bilateral adrenalectomy cases, patients should undergo regular MRI scans and ACTH level assessments. Additionally, these patients require lifelong glucocorticoid and mineralocorticoid supplementation.

Adrenal Adenoma

Surgical resection of benign adrenal adenoma is associated with relatively few side effects and a high cure rate (95%). The contralateral gland in the patient with adrenal adenoma is usually atrophic; therefore, steroid replacement is needed both perioperatively and postoperatively. Table 59-7 outlines an approach to steroid replacement for three separate routes of hydrocortisone. Therapy should be continued for 6 to 12 months following surgery. Before replacement therapy is discontinued, recovery of the adrenal axis can be assessed by measuring the morning (8 AM) cortisol level. Cortisol levels should exceed 20 mcg/dL before discontinuing exogenous steroids.[23]

Adrenal Carcinoma

Unlike the benign adenoma patient, those with adrenal carcinoma have an unfavorable outcome with surgical resection.[11] Often the complete tumor cannot be excised, leaving the patient with some degree of symptomatology and extraadrenal involvement. Radiotherapy can be used if metastases are discovered. In the patient with adrenal carcinoma who is not a surgical candidate, the focus of treatment is on palliative pharmacologic intervention.

TABLE 59-7 Alternative Steroid Replacement Regimens in the Adrenal Adenoma Patient

	Hydrocortisone Dose (mg)		
Time	IV	IM	PO
Operation day	300	50 before surgery and 50 after surgery	
Postoperative day 1	200	50 every 12 hours	
Postoperative day 2	150	50 every 12 hours	
Postoperative day 3	100	50 every 12 hours	
Postoperative day 4		50 every 12 hours	25 every 6 hours
Postoperative day 5		25 every 12 hours	25 every 6 hours[a]
Postoperative day 7			25 every 6 hours
Postoperative days 8–10			25 every 8 hours
Postoperative days 11–20			25 every 12 hours
Postoperative days 21+			20 at 8 AM 10 at 4 PM

po, orally.

[a]Add fludrocortisone 0.05–2 mg orally once daily starting on postoperative day 5. Adjust dose based on blood pressure, body weight, and serum electrolytes.

Mitotane may be used in inoperable functional and nonfunctional adrenal carcinoma or as adjuvant therapy in surgical patients with a high risk of relapse. However, mitotane induces tumor regression in less than 20% of patients.[39] Metyrapone and ketoconazole can be given to attempt control of steroid hypersecretion; aminoglutethemide is considered a third-line treatment option. 5-Fluorouracil also has been used in combination therapy.

Ectopic ACTH Syndrome

In ectopic ACTH syndrome, ACTH-secreting tumors may exist in a variety of sites, including thymic, pulmonary, appendiceal, pancreatic, and thyroid tissues. Locating these sites is often difficult, but essential for determining an appropriate treatment strategy. Surgical resection is the most effective treatment option for these patients, but only approximately 10% to 30% of patients are cured following surgery due to high rates of metastatic disease or occult tumors. The remaining 70% to 90% receive postoperative medication.

Pharmacologic management with steroidogenesis inhibitors is effective in patients with ectopic ACTH syndrome. Mitotane has been used in this setting; however, its side effect profile generally limits its use. RU-486 and somatostatin analogues also have been reported to reduce the clinical signs of ectopic ACTH syndrome.[40]

Additional tumor-directed therapy can include systemic chemotherapy, interferon α, chemoembolization, radio-frequency ablation, and radiation therapy.[38] If all else fails, bilateral adrenalectomy can prevent the downstream effects (e.g., steroidogenesis) of high levels of tumor ACTH secretion.

Personalized Pharmacotherapy

Unfortunately, several factors limit the ability to personalize pharmacotherapy in patients with Cushing's syndrome. First, few rigorous studies have compared the various pharmacologic options used in Cushing's syndrome. Consequently, data are limited in terms of clinical predictors of disease response to these agents. Second, virtually nothing is known of the pharmacogenomic predictors of individual patient response in these disease states. Finally, because most agents are used off-label, scarce data exist on agent-specific pharmacokinetic parameters in this patient population.

With these limitations in mind, drug selection is determined primarily according to the etiology of Cushing's syndrome, as described previously. Once the etiology has been correctly identified, gender should be considered since some pharmacologic options (steroidogenesis inhibitors in particular) used in Cushing's syndrome affect the sex hormones. Specifically, metyrapone is a clear second choice in women due to a high incidence of hirsutism, whereas ketoconazole may be a secondary choice in men due to drug-induced gynecomastia and hypogonadism. During pregnancy, metyrapone is commonly used, while RU-486 must be avoided. Additionally, women desiring pregnancy within the next 5 years should avoid mitotane as this agent is stored in adipose tissue for up to several years following discontinuation. Preexisting medication profiles should be considered also, since many of the pharmacologic options can inhibit (e.g., ketoconazole) or induce (e.g., metyrapone) important CYP isoenzymes such as 3A4.

Ultimately, pharmacotherapy is guided by patient response and several agents may need to be tried sequentially to elicit a substantial response. Combination therapy may be more effective and better tolerated than monotherapy in some patients, but studies on what constitutes the most appropriate drug regimens are lacking.

Hyperaldosteronism

Excess aldosterone secretion is categorized as either primary or secondary hyperaldosteronism.[41–45] In PA, the stimulation for aldosterone secretion arises from within the adrenal gland. Conversely, extraadrenal stimulation is classified as secondary aldosteronism.

Primary Aldosteronism

Etiology The most common causes of PA include BAH (65%) and aldosterone-producing adenoma (APA; otherwise known as Conn's syndrome) (30%). Other rare causes include unilateral (primary) adrenal hyperplasia, adrenal cortex carcinoma, renin-responsive adrenocortical adenoma, and two forms of familial hyperaldosteronism (FH): FH type 1, also known as glucocorticoid-remediable aldosteronism (GRA), and FH type II.[41,42,44]

Clinical Presentation PA is present in approximately 10% of the general hypertensive population and is the leading cause of secondary hypertension. The disease is more common in women than in men, and diagnosis usually occurs between the third and sixth decades of life. Signs and symptoms can include arterial hypertension, which is often moderate to severe and resistant to pharmacologic intervention, as well as hypokalemia (10% to 40% of PA patients), muscle weakness, fatigue, and headache. These features are nonspecific for PA and many patients are asymptomatic. Historically, hypokalemia was considered a requisite feature for PA diagnosis; however, normokalemia exists frequently in patients and should not obviate concern for PA.

CLINICAL PRESENTATION Primary Aldosteronism

Symptoms

- Patients may complain of muscle weakness, fatigue, paresthesias, and headache.

Signs

- Hypertension
- Tetany/paralysis
- Polydipsia/nocturnal polyuria

Laboratory Tests

- A plasma-aldosterone-concentration–to–plasma-renin-activity (PAC–to–PRA) ratio, or aldosterone-to-renin ratio (ARR) greater than 20 is suggestive of PA.
- Common laboratory findings include suppressed renin activity, elevated plasma aldosterone concentrations (PACs), hypernatremia (>142 mEq/L), hypokalemia, hypomagnesemia, elevated bicarbonate concentration (>31 mEq/L), and glucose intolerance.

Confirmatory Tests

- Oral or IV saline loading, fludrocortisone suppression test (FST), and genetic testing

TABLE 59-8 Differential Diagnosis of Primary Aldosteronism

Disease	Plasma Renin Activity	Plasma Aldosterone Concentration	Blood Pressure
Primary aldosteronism	Low	High	High
Edematous disorders	High	High	Normal
Malignant hypertension	High	High	High
Congenital adrenal hyperplasia	Low	Low	High
Cushing's syndrome	Low to normal	Low to normal	High
Liddle's syndrome	Low	Low	High
Bartter's syndrome	High	High	Low to normal
Licorice ingestion	Low	Low	High
Low-renin essential hypertension	Low	Low to normal	High

Diagnosis Diagnostic confirmation of PA is obtainable through screening, confirmatory tests, and subtype differentiation. As in Cushing's syndrome, discovery of the underlying etiology ensures proper treatment. Table 59-8 lists the various abnormalities that must be ruled out when suspicion of hyperaldosteronism is high.

Initial diagnosis is made through proper screening of patients with suspected PA. Such patients include those with Joint National Committee on Prevention, Detection, Evaluation, and Treatment of High Blood Pressure (JNC) stage two hypertension—appreciating that the prevalence of PA increases with hypertensive severity—and resistant hypertensives. Screening for PA is most often done by using the plasma-aldosterone-concentration–to–plasma-renin-activity (PAC-to-PRA) ratio, otherwise known as the ARR. An elevated ARR is highly suggestive of PA; however, an optimal cutoff level remains undefined because testing conditions (posture, time, current drug therapy, recent dietary salt intake), patient characteristics, and variable levels of specificity and sensitivity among assays can significantly alter test results.[46] ARR cutoffs of 20 to 40 or 20 with an aldosterone level greater than 15 ng/dL are used most often.[43,47,48]

Following a positive ARR screening test, confirmatory testing must be performed to exclude any false-positive cases. Confirmatory tests include the oral sodium loading test, saline infusion test, FST, and the captopril challenge test. Although individual tests can vary in sensitivity, specificity, and reliability, any test can be used depending on patient- and institution-specific considerations. FST generally is considered the most reliable, but requires hospitalization. Prior to performing these tests, potassium levels must be normalized and renin–angiotensin–aldosterone system (RAAS) inhibitors should be temporarily discontinued, if possible. Positive tests indicate autonomous aldosterone secretion under inhibitory pressures and are diagnostic for PA. After diagnosis, patients with confirmed PA before age 20 or with a family history of PA or strokes before age 40 should undergo genetic testing to properly identify GRA.[46]

Differentiating between an APA and BAH is imperative to formulate a proper treatment plan. Most adenomas are singular and small (<1 cm) and occur more often in the left adrenal gland than the right. Patients with APA generally have more severe hypertension, more profound hypokalemia, and higher plasma and urinary aldosterone levels compared with patients with BAH. Adrenal venous sampling (AVS) provides the most accurate means of differentiating unilateral from bilateral forms of PA. However, AVS is expensive, invasive, and frequently unavailable. CT scanning can detect most adenomas, although an incidentaloma can occasionally cause confusion. If CT scanning is inconclusive, AVS is performed to characterize lateralization.[43,49–51]

The underlying abnormality in BAH remains a mystery, but some investigators believe that a hormone factor stimulates the zona glomerulosa, resulting in increased sensitivity to angiotensin II. In contrast to those with an APA, patients with BAH are able to maintain control of the renin–angiotensin system, with little effect following doses of ACTH.

Therapeutic Management

6 *BAH-Dependent Aldosteronism* Aldosterone receptor antagonists are the treatment of choice in bilateral cases of PA (drug dosing and monitoring parameters can be found in Tables 59-9 and 59-10, respectively). Spironolactone, a nonselective aldosterone receptor antagonist, competes with aldosterone for binding at the aldosterone receptor, thus preventing the negative downstream effects of aldosterone receptor activation. Additionally, spironolactone is capable of inhibiting aldosterone synthesis within the adrenal gland; however, the magnitude of this inhibition is relatively small and the effect only occurs at doses above those recommended in the clinical setting.[52] Spironolactone is available in oral form, with most patients responding to doses between 25 and 400 mg/day. The clinician should wait 4 to 8 weeks before reassessing the patient for urinary electrolytes and blood pressure control. Adverse effects of spironolactone are dose-dependent and include GI discomfort, impotence, gynecomastia, menstrual irregularities, and hyperkalemia. Gynecomastia and menstrual irregularities observed with spironolactone therapy arise from activity at androgen and progesterone receptors and inhibition of testosterone biosynthesis. Additionally, because salicylates increase the renal secretion of canrenone, the active metabolite, patients should be advised to avoid concomitant therapy with salicylates. In patients intolerant of spironolactone, alternative options include eplerenone and amiloride.[43,53–55]

Eplerenone is a selective aldosterone receptor antagonist with high affinity for the aldosterone receptor and low affinity for androgen and progesterone receptors. Consequently, eplerenone elicits fewer sex steroid–dependent effects while ostensibly maintaining similar efficacy to spironolactone; however, no significant comparative data exist between these two agents in this setting. Dosing starts at 50 mg daily, with titration to 50 mg twice a day.[53] Titration should occur at 4- to 8-week intervals. In addition, eplerenone is a substrate

TABLE 59-9 Drug Dosing in the Treatment of Hyperaldosteronism

Drug	Brand Name	Initial Dose	Usual Range	Special Populations	Comments
Amiloride	Midamor®, 5 mg tablets	5 mg twice daily	20 mg/day in two divided doses	CrCl 10–50 mL/min: reduce dose by 50%; CrCl <10 mL/min: CI	Maximum: 30 mg/day
Eplerenone	Inspra®, 25 and 50 mg tablets	50 mg once daily	50 mg twice daily; titrate at 4- to 8-week intervals	CrCl <30 mL/min: CI	Maximum: 100 mg/day
Spironolactone	Aldactone®, 25, 50, and 100 mg tablets	25 mg once daily	100–400 mg/day in single or divided doses; titrate at 4- to 8-week intervals	CrCl 10–50 mL/min: extend dosing interval to once daily; CrCl <10 mL/min: CI	Maximum: 400 mg/day

CI, contraindicated; CrCl, creatinine clearance.

TABLE 59-10 Drug Monitoring in the Treatment of Hyperaldosteronism

Drug	Adverse Drug Reaction	Monitoring Parameters	Comments
Amiloride	Electrolyte abnormalities (hyperkalemia), hypotension, nausea, vomiting, diarrhea, headache	Serum creatinine, serum potassium, blood pressure	Electrolyte abnormalities (hyperkalemia) more pronounced with reduced renal function
Eplerenone	Electrolyte abnormalities (hyperkalemia), hypotension, dizziness, headache; gynecomastia and menstrual irregularities are uncommon	Serum creatinine, serum potassium, blood pressure	Electrolyte abnormalities (hyperkalemia) more pronounced with reduced renal function. CYP3A4 substrate; avoid use with potent CYP3A4 inhibitors
Spironolactone	GI discomfort, impotence, gynecomastia, menstrual irregularities, electrolyte abnormalities (hyperkalemia), hypotension	Serum creatinine, serum potassium, blood pressure	Electrolyte abnormalities (hyperkalemia) more pronounced with reduced renal function

CYP, cytochrome P450 enzyme.

of CYP3A4 and should not be taken with potent CYP3A4 inhibitors. Eplerenone has been proven effective in primary essential hypertension; however, its role in the management of hyperaldosteronism has not been established.[56]

Amiloride, a potassium-sparing diuretic, is dosed at 5 mg twice a day up to 30 mg/day if necessary. It is less effective than spironolactone and often requires additional therapy to adequately control blood pressure. Additional second-line options include the calcium channel blockers, ACE inhibitors, and diuretics such as chlorthalidone, although all lack outcome data evaluation in PA.[51,54] However, some agents (e.g., diuretics, calcium channel blockers) can promote a reactive rise in PRA, ultimately leading to increased aldosterone levels and potentially worsening PA. A prudent strategy would be to use these agents only in combination with RAAS inhibitors to mitigate the downstream aldosterone effects of any increase in PRA.

Aldosterone synthase inhibitors, currently under development, may offer additional therapeutic options in the future.

APA-Dependent Aldosteronism The treatment of choice for APA-dependent aldosteronism remains laparoscopic resection of the adenoma.[57] Nearly 100% of patients show blood pressure improvement while 30% to 72% are permanently cured.[55,58] Because APAs are small and often occur in multiples, resection should target the entire adrenal gland. In successful cases, blood pressure control is achieved in 1 to 3 months. Medical management can be efficacious in this population if surgery is contraindicated. However, medical management may be significantly more expensive than unilateral resection.

Glucocorticoid-Remediable Aldosteronism Glucocorticoids are very effective in treating GRA.[42] Low doses are used (0.125 to 0.5 mg/day of dexamethasone or 2.5 to 5 mg/day of prednisone) because complete suppression of ACTH-stimulated aldosterone release is unnecessary. Spironolactone, eplerenone, and amiloride are alternative treatment options.[43]

Summary The diagnosis of PA is made through proper screening of suspected patients followed by confirmatory testing. Subsequent differentiation between the various etiologies ensures appropriate treatment (Fig. 59-5). Patients with APA can be distinguished from patients with BAH by CT scan, but AVS provides increased sensitivity and specificity. Treatment depends on the etiology with surgical resection in adenomas, and spironolactone, eplerenone, or amiloride plus second-line agents in patients with bilateral hyperplasia.

Secondary Aldosteronism

Secondary aldosteronism results from an appropriate response to excessive stimulation of the zona glomerulosa by an extraadrenal factor, usually the renin–angiotensin system. Excessive potassium intake can promote aldosterone secretion, as can oral contraceptive use, pregnancy (aldosterone secretion 10 times normal by the third trimester), and menses. Congestive heart failure, cirrhosis, renal artery stenosis, and Bartter's syndrome also can lead to elevated aldosterone concentrations.

Treatment of secondary aldosteronism is dictated by etiology. Control or correction of the extraadrenal stimulation of aldosterone secretion should resolve the disorder. Medical therapy with spironolactone is the mainstay of treatment until an exact etiology can be located.

HYPOFUNCTION OF THE ADRENAL GLAND

Hypofunction of the adrenal gland can affect any or all adrenal hormones, depending on the etiology of the disorder. However, hypofunction does not always lead to insufficient production of adrenal hormones as might be expected. As described below, some types of adrenal hypofunction can lead to excess production of certain hormones.

Addison's Disease

7 Primary adrenal insufficiency, or Addison's disease, most often involves the destruction of all regions of the adrenal cortex. Deficiencies arise in cortisol, aldosterone, and the various androgens and levels of CRH and ACTH increase in a compensatory manner. In developed countries, autoimmune dysfunction is responsible for most cases (80% to 90%), whereas tuberculosis predominates as the cause in developing countries. Approximately 50% of patients with autoimmune etiologies present with one or more concomitant autoimmune disorders, usually involving other endocrine organs. Autoimmune thyroid disorders (e.g., Hashimoto's thyroiditis or Graves' disease) are the most common, but the ovaries, pancreas, parathyroid gland, and organs of the GI system can also be affected. This polyglandular failure syndrome, termed autoimmune polyendocrine syndrome (APS), is associated with the idiopathic etiology only and has not been seen with adrenal insufficiency associated with tuberculosis or other invasive diseases. Medications that inhibit cortisol synthesis (ketoconazole) or accelerate cortisol metabolism (phenytoin, rifampin, phenobarbital) can also cause primary adrenal insufficiency.[59]

8 Secondary insufficiency is characterized by reduced glucocorticoid production secondary to decreased ACTH levels. Low levels of ACTH most commonly result from exogenous steroid use, leading to suppression of the HPA axis and decreased release of ACTH, resulting in impaired androgen and cortisol production. These effects occur with oral, inhaled, intranasal, and topical glucocorticoid administration.[60–62] Moreover, mirtazapine and progestins, such as medroxyprogesterone acetate and megestrol acetate, have

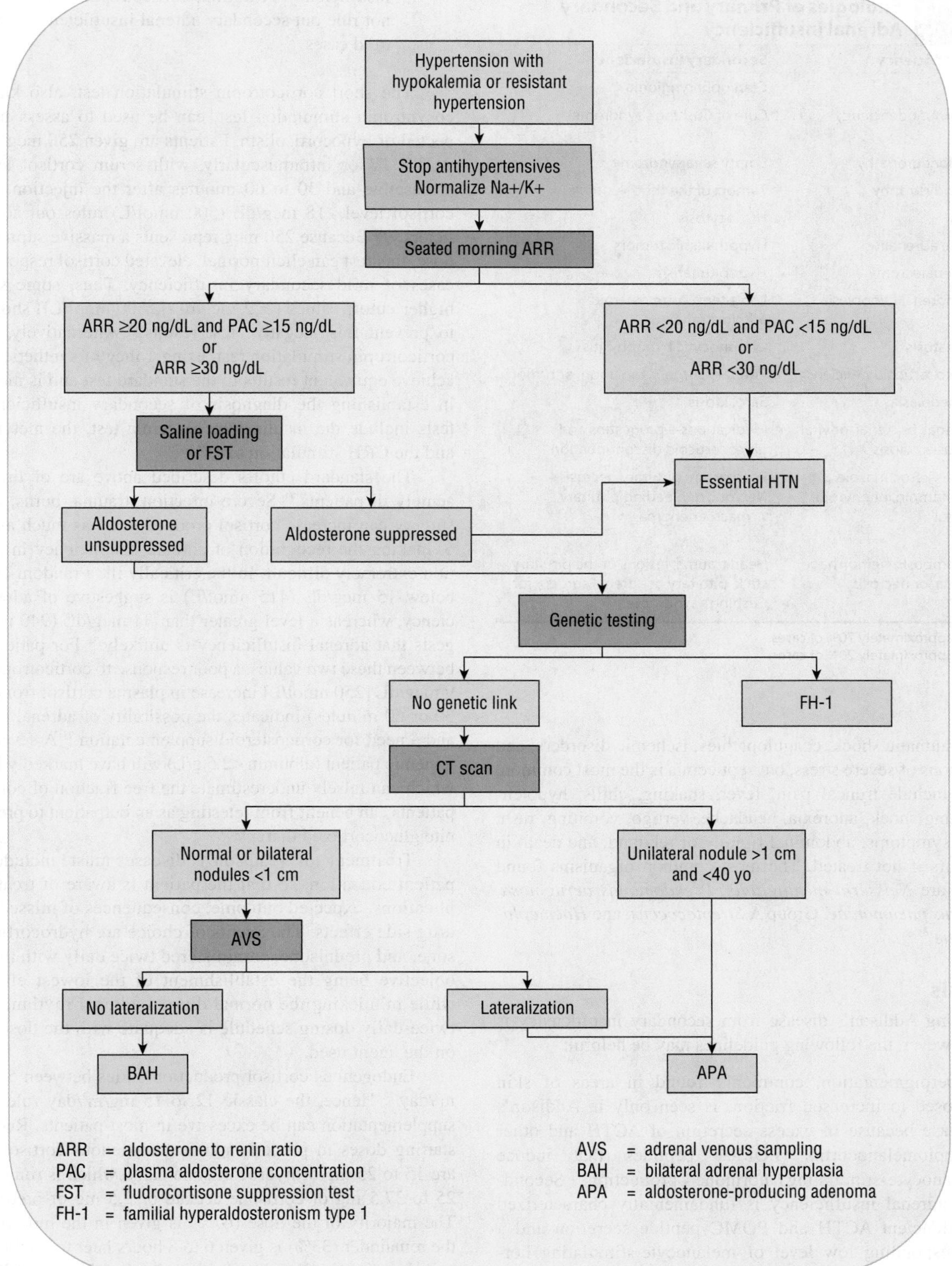

FIGURE 59-5 Algorithm for the diagnosis of primary aldosteronism. (ARR, aldosterone-to-renin ratio; APA, aldosterone-producing adenoma; AVS, adrenal venous sampling; BAH, bilateral adrenal hyperplasia; FH-1, familial hyperaldosteronism type 1; FST, fludrocortisone suppression test; PAC, plasma aldosterone concentration.)

been reported to induce secondary adrenal insufficiency.[63,64] Chronic suppression also can result in atrophy of the anterior pituitary and hypothalamus, impairing recovery of function if the exogenous steroid is reduced. Endogenous secondary insufficiency can occur with tumor development in the hypothalamic–pituitary region. Secondary disease classically presents with normal concentrations of mineralocorticoids since the zona glomerulosa is controlled by the renin–angiotensin system rather than ACTH levels.

Approximately 90% of the adrenal cortex must be destroyed before adrenal insufficiency symptoms will occur.[65] Specific etiologies for both primary and secondary insufficiency are listed in Table 59-11. Adrenal hemorrhage can result from multiple etiologies

TABLE 59-11 Etiologies of Primary and Secondary Adrenal Insufficiency

Primary Insufficiency	Secondary Insufficiency
Slow onset	Craniopharyngioma
Acquired immunodeficiency syndrome	Cure of Cushing's syndrome
Adrenomyeloneuropathy	Empty sella syndrome
Adrenoleukodystrophy	Tumors of the third ventricle
Amyloidosis	Histiocytosis
Autoimmune adrenalitis[a]	Hypothalamic tumors
Bilateral adrenalectomy	Hypopituitarism
Congenital adrenal hypoplasia	Long-term corticosteroid administration
Hemochromatosis	Lymphocytic hypophysitis
Isolated glucocorticoid deficiency	Pituitary surgery, radiation, or tumor
Metastatic neoplasia	Sarcoidosis
Systemic fungal, bacterial, or viral infections, tuberculosis[b]	Medications—progestins and glucocorticoid discontinuation
Medications—ketoconazole, etomidate, rifampin, phenytoin, phenobarbital	Postpartum pituitary necrosis Necrotic or bleeding pituitary macroadenoma
Fast onset	
Adrenal thrombosis, hemorrhage, sepsis, trauma, or necrosis	Head trauma, lesions of the pituitary stalk, pituitary or adrenal surgery for Cushing's syndrome

[a]Accounts for approximately 70% of cases.
[b]Accounts for approximately 20% of cases.

including traumatic shock, coagulopathies, ischemic disorders, and other situations of severe stress, but septicemia is the most common. Symptoms include truncal pain, fever, shaking, chills, hypotension preceding shock, anorexia, headache, vertigo, vomiting, rash, psychiatric symptoms, abdominal rigidity or rebound, and death in 6 to 48 hours if not treated. The most common organisms found on autopsy are *Neisseria meningitidis*, *Pseudomonas aeruginosa*, *Streptococcus pneumoniae*, Group A *Streptococcus*, and *Haemophilus influenzae*.[65,66]

Diagnosis

Distinguishing Addison's disease from secondary insufficiency is difficult; however, the following guidelines may be helpful:

1. Hyperpigmentation, commonly found in areas of skin exposed to increased friction, is seen only in Addison's disease because of excess secretion of ACTH and other proopiomelanocortin (POMC) peptides that induce melanocyte-stimulating hormone production. Secondary adrenal insufficiency is fundamentally characterized by deficient ACTH and POMC peptide secretion and a corresponding low level of melanocyte-stimulating hormone production. In fact, some patients with secondary insufficiency may exhibit pale-colored skin secondary to hypopigmentation.
2. Aldosterone secretion usually is preserved in secondary insufficiency.
3. Weight loss, dehydration, hyponatremia, hyperkalemia, and elevated blood urea nitrogen are common in Addison's disease.
4. Addison's disease will have an abnormal response to the short corticotropin stimulation test. Plasma ACTH levels are usually 400 to 2,000 pg/mL in primary insufficiency, versus low to normal (5 to 50 pg/mL; see Table 59-3) in secondary insufficiency. A normal corticotropin stimulation test does not rule out secondary adrenal insufficiency, particularly in mild cases.

The short corticotropin stimulation test, also known as the cosyntropin stimulation test, can be used to assess patients suspected of hypocortisolism. Patients are given 250 mcg of synthetic ACTH IV or intramuscularly, with serum cortisol levels drawn at baseline and 30 to 60 minutes after the injection. A resulting cortisol level ≥18 mcg/dL (500 nmol/L) rules out adrenal insufficiency.[67] Because 250 mcg represents a massive supraphysiologic dose, this test can elicit normal, elevated cortisol responses in some cases of mild secondary insufficiency. Thus, some suggest that higher cutoff values (≥22 mcg/dL [≥600 nmol/L]) should be used to prevent false-negative test results.[68] Alternatively, a low-dose corticotropin stimulation test, using 1 mcg of synthetic ACTH, can achieve equivalent results to the standard test and is more sensitive in establishing the diagnosis of secondary insufficiency.[69] Other tests include the insulin hypoglycemia test, the metyrapone test, and the CRH stimulation test.[59,67,70]

The standard cutoffs described above are of limited use in acutely ill patients.[71] Severe infection, trauma, burns, illnesses, or surgery can increase cortisol production by as much as a factor of 6, making the recognition of adrenal insufficiency in this population extremely difficult. In the critically ill, a random cortisol level below 15 mcg/dL (415 nmol/L) is suggestive of adrenal insufficiency, whereas a level greater than 34 mcg/dL (940 nmol/L) suggests that adrenal insufficiency is unlikely.[71] For patients who fall between these two values, a poor response to corticotropin (less than 9 mcg/dL [250 nmol/L] increase in plasma cortisol from baseline at 30 or 60 minutes) indicates the possibility of adrenal insufficiency and a need for corticosteroid supplementation.[71] A severe hypoproteinemic patient (albumin <2.5 g/L) will have markedly lower CBG, which can falsely underestimate the free fraction of cortisol. These patients can benefit from retesting as an outpatient to prevent indefinite glucocorticoid therapy.[59]

Treatment of Addison's disease must include adequate patient education, so that the patient is aware of treatment complications, expected outcome, consequences of missed doses, and drug side effects. The agents of choice are hydrocortisone, cortisone, and prednisone, administered twice daily with the treatment objective being the establishment of the lowest effective dose while mimicking the normal diurnal adrenal rhythm.[59] Usually a twice-daily dosing schedule is adequate with the dose depending on the agent used.

Endogenous cortisol production varies between 5 and 10 mg/m^2/day.[72] Hence, the classic 12 to 15 mg/m^2/day rule for cortisol supplementation can be excessive in most patients. Recommended starting doses to properly mimic endogenous cortisol production are 15 to 25 mg of hydrocortisone daily, which is roughly equal to 25 to 37.5 mg of cortisone acetate or 2.5 mg of prednisone.[59,70,72] The majority of the dose (67%) is given in the morning, whereas the remainder (33%) is given 6 to 8 hours later to duplicate the normal circadian rhythm of cortisol production. Since no laboratory test adequately determines the appropriateness of dosing, the patient's symptoms should be monitored every 6 to 8 weeks to assess proper glucocorticoid replacement.

In primary insufficiency, fludrocortisone acetate can be used to supplement mineralocorticoid loss. A dose of 0.05 to 0.2 mg by mouth once a day is adequate. If parenteral therapy is needed, 2 to 5 mg of deoxycorticosterone trimethylacetate in oil intramuscularly every 3 to 4 weeks can be substituted. Mineralocorticoid replacement attenuates the development of hyperkalemia, but may be unnecessary in all primary cases since glucocorticoids also contribute to mineralocorticoid binding. Adverse effects must be monitored closely. Symptoms include gastric upset, edema, hypertension, hypokalemia, insomnia, excitability, and diabetes mellitus. In addition, patient weight, blood pressure, and electrocardiogram should be monitored regularly.[70]

In women, the primary source of dehydroepiandrosterone (DHEA) and androgens is the adrenal cortex, specifically the zona reticularis. DHEA is converted to more potent androgens and estrogens in the periphery. Consequently, women with adrenal insufficiency can have decreased libido. DHEA, available as a dietary supplement, has been advocated as an option for female patients with adrenal insufficiency complaining of decreased libido and low energy.[73] However, clinical trial data for DHEA are conflicting, and a recent meta-analysis suggests no benefit for sexual well-being.[74] Given this limited efficacy and a lack of any standardization among the various commercial products, DHEA should not be used routinely in female patients to improve libido. DHEA may improve mood and well-being in select male and female patients who are already receiving optimal glucocorticoid and mineralocorticoid replacement.

Most adrenal crises occur secondary to glucocorticoid dose reduction or lack of stress-related dose adjustments. Patients receiving corticosteroid replacement therapy should receive an additional 5 to 10 mg of hydrocortisone shortly before strenuous activities such as exercise.[70] Likewise, during times of severe physical stress such as febrile illnesses or injury, patients should be instructed to double their daily dose until recovery.[75,76] For major trauma, surgery, or in critically ill patients, larger doses are required. Parenteral therapy should be used for patients experiencing diarrhea or vomiting. In patients with concomitant, newly diagnosed, or uncontrolled hypothyroidism, thyroid replacement should take place only after adequate glucocorticoid replacement as euthyroidism can trigger an adrenal crisis by accelerating cortisol metabolism.[59]

The end point of therapy is difficult to assess in most patients, but a reduction in excess pigmentation is a good clinical marker. The development of features of Cushing's syndrome indicates excessive replacement. Treatment of secondary adrenal insufficiency is identical to primary disease treatment, except that mineralocorticoid replacement usually is unnecessary. Patient education is paramount with emphasis placed on the medication regimen and adrenal crisis prevention.

Acute Adrenal Insufficiency

Adrenal crisis, or Addisonian crisis, is characterized by an acute adrenocortical insufficiency. It represents a true endocrine emergency. Anything that increases adrenal requirements dramatically can precipitate an adrenal crisis. Stressful situations, surgery, infection, and trauma all are potential triggering events, especially in the patient with some underlying adrenal or pituitary insufficiency. The most common cause of adrenal crisis is HPA-axis suppression brought on by chronic use of exogenous glucocorticoids and abrupt withdrawal.

Treatment of adrenal crisis involves the administration of parenteral glucocorticoids. Hydrocortisone is the agent of choice owing to its combined glucocorticoid and mineralocorticoid activity. Hydrocortisone is initially administered at a dose of 100 mg IV through rapid infusion, followed by a continuous infusion (usually 10 mg/h) or intermittent bolus of 100 to 200 mg every 24 hours.[77] IV administration is continued for 24 to 48 hours, at which time if the patient is stable, oral hydrocortisone can be administered at a dose of 50 mg every 6 to 8 hours, followed by tapering to the individual's chronic replacement needs. Fluid replacement often is required and can be accomplished with dextrose 5% in normal saline solution (D_5NS) at a rate to support blood pressure. During initial treatment for adrenal crisis, mineralocorticoid replacement generally is unnecessary because of hydrocortisone's mineralocorticoid activity (hydrocortisone 50 mg ≈ fludrocortisone 0.1 mg). If hyperkalemia is present after the hydrocortisone maintenance phase, additional mineralocorticoid supplementation can be achieved with 0.1 mg of fludrocortisone acetate daily.

Patients with adrenal insufficiency should be instructed to carry a card or wear a bracelet or necklace, such as MedicAlert, that contains information about their condition. Additionally, patients should have easy access to injectable hydrocortisone or glucocorticoid suppositories in case of an emergency or during times of physical stress, such as febrile illness or injury.[70]

Hypoaldosteronism

Hypoaldosteronism is rare and usually associated with low-renin status (hyporeninemic hypoaldosteronism), diabetes, complete heart block, or severe postural hypotension, or it can occur postoperatively following tumor removal. Hypoaldosteronism can be part of a larger adrenal insufficiency or a stand-alone defect. In nonselective hypoaldosteronism, generalized adrenocortical insufficiency is the most likely etiology (see Addison's Disease above). In selective hypoaldosteronism, insufficient aldosterone levels are precipitated by a specific defect in the stimulation of

CLINICAL PRESENTATION Adrenal Insufficiency

Symptoms

- Patients commonly complain of weakness, weight loss, GI symptoms, craving for salt, headaches, memory impairment, depression, and postural dizziness.
- Early symptoms of acute adrenal insufficiency also include myalgias, malaise, and anorexia. As the situation progresses, vomiting, fever, hypotension, and shock will develop.

Signs

- Increased pigmentation
- Hypotension (postural)
- Fever
- Decreased body hair
- Vitiligo
- Features of hypopituitarism (amenorrhea and cold intolerance)

Laboratory Tests

- The short cosyntropin stimulation test can be used to assess patients suspected of hypercortisolism.

Other Diagnostic Tests

- Other tests include the insulin hypoglycemia test, the metyrapone test, and the CRH stimulation test.

TABLE 59-12 Congenital Adrenal Hyperplasia (CAH)

Enzyme Deficiency (Disorder)	Symptoms	Laboratory Tests	Comments
21-Hydroxylase (nonvirilizing CAH)	Enlarged female genitalia and adrenal gland (caused by cholesterol)	All steroids are low in blood and urine	Poor prognosis for infants
17-Hydroxylase (nonvirilizing CAH)	Hypertension usually present	Low concentrations of cortisol and estrogens	Mineralocorticoid replacement not necessary
21-Hydroxylase (virilizing CAH)	Pubertal irregularities (acne, early pubic hair, voice lowering, and increased muscularity); mature normally with replacement	High progesterone, renin, 17-hydroxyprogesterone, and ACTH; low cortisol, sodium, and aldosterone	Most common form of CAH (90% of total), incidence of 1:10,000; monitor growth velocity, bone age, renin, and 17-hydroxyprogesterone
11-Hydroxylase (virilizing CAH)	Hypertension secondary to high deoxycortisol and virilism from androgen excess; mistaken for Cushing's, but no glucose intolerance	Low plasma cortisone and aldosterone; high ACTH and MSH concentrations	Second most common form of CAH (9% of total), incidence of 1:100,000; final step in biosynthesis of corticosterone and cortisol; found only in adrenal cortex
3-Hydroxysteroid dehydrogenase (mixed CAH)	Both cortisol and aldosterone deficiencies	Decreased aldosterone, cortisol, estrogens, and androgens; increased pregnenolone and cholesterol	Defect affects both adrenals and gonads
18-Hydroxysteroid dehydrogenase (corticosterone methyloxidase deficiency)	Hypotension	Restricted to zona glomerulosa; sole aldosterone defect; hyponatremia, hyperkalemia, increased renin	Mineralocorticoid replacement without glucocorticoid replacement

adrenal aldosterone secretion, with 21-hydroxylase deficiency being most common. Pseudohypoaldosteronism results from a defect in peripheral aldosterone action, whether from increased peripheral resistance or a reduced number of functional aldosterone receptors.

Laboratory analysis reveals hyponatremia, hyperkalemia, or both. Patients often will present with hyperchloremic metabolic acidosis. In most cases, the deficiency is in mineralocorticoid production and replacement with fludrocortisone in a dose of 0.1 to 0.3 mg is usually effective. Patients should be followed for blood pressure response as well as electrolyte status.

Congenital Adrenal Hyperplasia

Because many enzyme systems are needed to complete the complex cholesterol-to-cortisol pathway, enzyme deficiencies can lead to disruptions of the normal cascade of events (see Fig. 59-2). This group of enzyme disorders is collectively referred to as congenital adrenal hyperplasia because of the resultant chronic adrenal gland stimulation that occurs following enzyme deficiency.[78,79] The most frequent cause of congenital adrenal hyperplasia is steroid 21-hydroxylase deficiency, accounting for more than 90% of cases. Any enzyme deficiency is capable of affecting any one or all three of the steroid pathways. Therefore, treatment focuses on replacement of the deficient hormone, psychological support, and surgical repair of the external genitalia in most female patients.[80] Six of the most common enzyme deficiencies are outlined briefly in Table 59-12.

Adrenal Virilism

9 Virilism, excessive secretion of androgens from the adrenal gland, commonly occurs as a result of congenital enzyme defects. Depending on the enzyme deficiency, patients accumulate excess levels of a variety of androgens, most notably testosterone. The condition affects females more often than males, with hirsutism being the dominant feature. Additional coexisting features can include voice deepening, acne, increased muscle mass, menstrual abnormalities, clitoral enlargement, redistribution of body fat and loss of female body contour, breast atrophy, and hair recession and crown balding.[81]

Treatment of virilism centers around suppression of the pituitary–adrenal axis with exogenous glucocorticoids. In adults, the usual steroids used are dexamethasone (0.25 to 0.5 mg), prednisone (2.5 to 5 mg), or hydrocortisone (10 to 20 mg).[82]

Hirsutism

Women presenting with hirsutism exhibit excess terminal hair growth in an androgen-dependent distribution. Such growth has obvious cosmetic consequences, but also can adversely affect quality of life and psychological well-being.[83] Most cases of hirsutism occur in women with some degree of excess androgen production. Androgen excess can be derived from either the ovaries or the adrenal glands, or rarely from pituitary disorders. Polycystic ovarian syndrome (PCOS) is responsible for most cases of ovarian excess and is the most common cause of hirsutism overall.[84] Congenital adrenal hyperplasia accounts for 5% of cases while adrenal and ovarian tumors cause hyperandrogenemia in 0.2% of women.

Cosmetic approaches generally are tried first, with repeated photoepilation offering the greatest long-term success.[84] If these approaches are unsuccessful, subsequent treatment should include pharmacologic intervention. Oral contraceptives are the treatment of choice in most hirsute women, particularly in those requiring concurrent contraception. If oral contraceptives are used, a progestin with low androgen activity (norethindrone, ethynodiol diacetate) or antiandrogenic activity (drospirenone) should be chosen. Other antiandrogens, including spironolactone and finasteride, can supplement or replace oral contraceptive therapy in women who cannot or choose not to conceive. Antiandrogens can take 6 to 12 months to alleviate hirsutism and treatment should be continued for 2 years, followed by a slow dose reduction.[85] Glucocorticoids, such as dexamethasone, can be modestly effective if the androgen source is adrenal, but can induce cushingoid symptoms even in doses of 0.5 mg/day.

Gonadotropin-releasing hormone can be an effective adjunct or alternative to oral contraceptives if the source of androgen is ovarian. However, these products generally are not recommended due to excessive costs, injectable-only routes of administration, and adverse effects resulting from estrogen deficiency. Additionally, insulin sensitizers, such as metformin or thiazolidinediones, can show modest improvement in women with PCOS, but their routine use is not recommended.[84]

TABLE 59-13 Relative Potencies of Glucocorticoids

Glucocorticoid	Antiinflammatory Potency	Equivalent Potency (mg)	Approximate Half-Life (min)	Sodium-Retaining Potency
Cortisone	0.8	25	30	2
Hydrocortisone	1	20	90	2
Prednisone	3.5	5	60	1
Prednisolone	4	5	200	1
Triamcinolone	5	4	300	0
Methylprednisolone	5	4	180	0
Betamethasone	25	0.6	100–300	0
Dexamethasone	30	0.75	100–300	0

Eflornithine hydrochloride, an irreversible ornithine decarboxylase inhibitor, moderately reduces the rate of hair growth but does not remove hair already present. The drug is available as a topical cream that is applied as a thin layer to the affected area twice daily, at least 8 hours apart. Reduction in unwanted hair can be noted within 6 to 8 weeks with a maximal effect at 8 to 24 weeks; therapy must be continued indefinitely to prevent hair regrowth.[82,86] Skin irritation can occur that resolves on discontinuation.

PRINCIPLES OF GLUCOCORTICOID ADMINISTRATION

Originally, the term *glucocorticoid* was given to these agents to describe their glucose-regulating properties. However, carbohydrate metabolism is only one of the myriad effects exhibited by steroids. The activity produced by these drugs is a function of the receptor activated (glucocorticoid vs. mineralocorticoid), the location of the receptor, as well as the agent and dose prescribed.

The mechanism of action of glucocorticoids is complex and not fully known. The glucocorticoid enters the cell through passive diffusion and binds to its specific receptor. Between 5,000 and 100,000 receptors exist in each cell. Steroids exhibit various binding affinities to the vast number of receptors in almost every tissue and therefore elicit a wide variety of biologic effects.

Following receptor binding, a structural change occurs in the receptor, known as *activation*. After activation, the receptor–steroid complex binds to deoxyribonucleic acid sites in the cell called *glucocorticoid response elements* (GREs). This binding alters nearby gene expression and stimulates, or in some cases, inhibits transcription of specific mRNAs. Consequently, the resulting protein, which produces the stimulatory or inhibitory glucocorticoid action, varies according to the tissue and cell type in which the glucocorticoid receptor exists.

Pharmacokinetic properties of the glucocorticoids vary by agent and route of administration. In general, most orally administered steroids are well absorbed. Water-soluble agents are more rapidly absorbed following intramuscular injection than are lipid-soluble agents. IV administration is recommended when a quick onset of action is needed. A summary of these agents is provided in Table 59-13.

In addition to causing iatrogenic Cushing's syndrome, systemic steroids can lead to increased susceptibility to infection, osteoporosis, sodium retention with resultant edema, hypokalemia, hypomagnesemia, cataracts, peptic ulcer disease, seizures, and generalized suppression of the HPA axis. Long-term complications tend to be insidious and less likely to respond to steroid withdrawal.

Suppression of the HPA axis is a major concern whenever systemic steroids are tapered or withdrawn. Single doses of glucocorticoids can prevent the axis from responding to major stressors for several hours. In general, steroid administration at a high dose for long periods of time causes suppression of the axis. However, the possibility of suppression occurs any time the patient is exposed to supraphysiologic doses of a steroid.[23,87] Symptoms of steroid withdrawal resemble those seen in a patient with adrenocortical deficiency.

A variety of recommendations for steroid tapering are available.[23,88–90] In general, patients who have been on long-term steroid therapy will need to be gradually withdrawn toward physiologic doses over months. On average, the normal adult produces approximately 10 to 30 mg of cortisol per day with the peak concentration occurring around 8:00 AM. As the steroid or steroid-equivalent dose approaches the 20- to 30-mg level, the taper should be slowed and the patient checked for axis function. The primary modes to test HPA integrity are the ACTH test, either high or low dose, or a morning (8:00 AM) serum cortisol. A normal morning serum cortisol (>20 mcg/dL) or a normal ACTH test indicates that daily steroid maintenance therapy may be discontinued. If morning serum cortisol is between 3 and 20 mcg/dL, the ACTH or CRH stimulation test can be useful in the assessment of pituitary–adrenal function.[23] A morning cortisol less than 3 mcg/dL indicates axis suppression and the need for continued replacement therapy. Suppression can persist for up to a year in some patients. Caution should be used to prevent disease exacerbation during the steroid taper and to avoid the need for rebolusing the patient with another course of high-dose steroids.

Alternate-day therapy (ADT) regimens have been promoted by some as a means to lessen the impact of prolonged steroid administration.[23,90] ADT theoretically minimizes the hypothalamic–pituitary suppression as well as some of the adverse effects seen with once-daily therapy. This hypothetical advantage may be especially pertinent in treating children and young adults, in whom growth suppression is a major concern. ADT is not recommended for initial management, but rather in the management of the stabilized patient who needs long-term therapy. The patient is exposed to "on" and "off" days, with the "on" day dose gradually increased corresponding with a dose-reduction in the "off" day dose over a period of 14 days. After 2 weeks, no medication is taken on "off" days. Not all patients will have equivalent disease control on ADT, and it should be avoided in certain indications.[23,90]

Clinical **Controversy...**

In an effort to more closely mimic endogenous cortisol secretion, some clinicians advocate thrice-daily dosing of glucocorticoids. Limited comparative data have favored thrice-daily regimens over twice-daily regimens, but serious methodologic flaws make interpretation and application of the study conclusions difficult. If a thrice-daily regimen is selected, the second dose should be administered at noon, followed by a third dose approximately 4 to 6 hours later.

TABLE 59-14 Factors in Successful Glucocorticoid Therapy

Monitoring	Glucose concentrations (serum and urine) Electrolytes (serum and urine) Ophthalmologic examinations Stool tests for occult blood loss Growth and development (children and adolescents)
Counseling	Take with food to minimize GI discomfort Never discontinue medication on your own; check with your physician; gradual dose reduction is usually necessary Carry or wear medical identification indicating that you are on long-term glucocorticoid therapy Dosage increases can be necessary at times of increased stress (surgery or emergency treatments) Be aware of potential side effects (i.e., visual disturbances, bruising, and delayed wound healing) What to do if you miss a dose: If your dosing schedule is: • *Every other day*: Take as soon as possible if remembered that morning. If not remembered until later, skip that day. Take the next morning, and then skip the following day • *Every day*: Take as soon as possible, but skip if almost time for the next dose. Never double doses
Recognizing complications	Early in therapy and essentially unavoidable: insomnia, enhanced appetite, weight gain Common in patients with underlying risk factors: hypertension, diabetes mellitus, peptic ulcer disease Long-term intense treatment: cushingoid habitus, hypothalamic pituitary–adrenal suppression, impaired wound healing Delayed and insidious: cataracts, atherosclerosis Rare and unpredictable: psychosis, glaucoma, pancreatitis

Data from references 91 and 92.

EVALUATION OF THERAPEUTIC OUTCOMES

Successful glucocorticoid therapy involves counseling and monitoring the patient, as well as recognizing complications of therapy (Table 59-14). The risk-to-benefit ratio of glucocorticoid administration should always be considered, especially with concurrent disease states such as hypertension, diabetes mellitus, peptic ulcer disease, and uncontrolled systemic infections.

ABBREVIATIONS

ACTH	adrenocorticotropic hormone
ADT	alternate-day therapy
APA	aldosterone-producing adenoma
APS	autoimmune polyendocrine syndrome
ARR	aldosterone-to-renin ratio
AVS	adrenal venous sampling
BAH	bilateral adrenal hyperplasia
CBG	corticosteroid-binding globulin
CHD	coronary heart disease
CrCl	creatinine clearance
CRH	corticotropin-releasing hormone
CT	computed tomography
CYP	cytochrome P450
D_5NS	dextrose 5% in normal saline solution
DDT	dichlorodiphenyltrichloroethane
DHEA	dehydroepiandrosterone
DST	dexamethasone suppression test
FH	familial hyperaldosteronism
FST	fludrocortisone suppression test
GRA	glucocorticoid-remediable aldosteronism
GRE	glucocorticoid response element
HPA	hypothalamic–pituitary–adrenal
IPSS	inferior petrosal sinus sampling
IRMA	immunoradiometric assay
JNC	Joint National Committee on Prevention, Detection, Evaluation, and Treatment of High Blood Pressure
JVS	jugular venous sampling
MRI	magnetic resonance imaging
PA	primary aldosteronism
PAC	plasma aldosterone concentration
PA-to-PRA	plasma-aldosterone–to–plasma-renin-activity
PAC-to-PRA	plasma-aldosterone-concentration–to–plasma-renin-activity
PCOS	polycystic ovarian syndrome
POMC	proopiomelanocortin
PRA	plasma renin activity
RAAS	renin–angiotensin–aldosterone system
RIA	radioimmunoassay
RU-486	mifepristone
sst_2	somatostatin receptor subtype 2
UFC	urinary free cortisol

REFERENCES

1. Conn JW. Primary aldosteronism, a new clinical syndrome. J Lab Clin Med 1955;45:6–17.
2. Albright F. Cushing syndrome. Harvey Lect 1942–1943;38: 123–186.
3. Newell-Price J, Bertagna X, Grossman AB, Nieman LK. Cushing's syndrome. Lancet 2006;367:1605–1617.
4. Isidori AM, Kaltsas GA, Pozza C, et al. The ectopic adrenocorticotropin syndrome: Clinical features, diagnosis, management, and long-term follow-up. J Clin Endocrinol Metab 2006;91:371–377.
5. Boscaro M, Barzon L, Sonino N. The diagnosis of Cushing's syndrome: Atypical presentations and laboratory shortcomings. Arch Intern Med 2000;160:3045–3053.
6. Williams GH, Dluhy RG. Disorders of the adrenal cortex. In: Fauci AS, Braunwald E, Kasper DL, et al., eds. Harrison's Principles of Internal Medicine, 17th ed. AccessMedicine, 2008, *http://www.accessmedicine.com/content.aspx?aID=2900123* [electronic version].
7. Catargi B, Rigalleau V, Poussin A, et al. Occult Cushing's syndrome in type-2 diabetes. J Clin Endocrinol Metab 2003;88:5808–5813.
8. Findling JW, Raff H. Screening and diagnosis of Cushing's syndrome. Endocrinol Metab Clin North Am 2005;34: 385–402.
9. Nieman LK, Biller BMK, Findling JW, et al. The diagnosis of Cushing's syndrome: An Endocrine Society clinical practice guideline. J Clin Endocrinol Metab 2008;93:1526–1540.
10. Terzolo M, Reimondo G, Chiodini I, et al. Screening of Cushing's syndrome in outpatients with type 2 diabetes: Results of a prospective multicentric study in Italy. J Clin Endocrinol Metab 2012;97:3467–3475. doi:10.1210/jc.2012-1323.
11. Nieman LK, Ilias I. Evaluation and treatment of Cushing's syndrome. Am J Med 2005;118:1340–1346.
12. Lindsay JR, Nieman LK. Differential diagnosis and imaging in Cushing's syndrome. Endocrinol Metab Clin North Am 2005;34:403–421.
13. Arnaldi G, Angeli A, Atkinson AB, et al. Diagnosis and complications of Cushing's syndrome: A consensus statement. J Clin Endocrinol Metab 2003;88:5593–5602.

14. Jackson RV, Hockings GI, Torpy DJ, et al. New diagnostic tests for Cushing's syndrome: Uses of naloxone, vasopressin and alprazolam. Clin Exp Pharmacol Physiol 1996;23: 579–581.
15. Ambrosi B, Bochicchio D, Colombo P, et al. Loperamide to diagnose Cushing's syndrome. JAMA 1993;270: 2301–2302.
16. Arvat E, Giordano R, Ramunni J, et al. Adrenocorticotropin and cortisol hyperresponsiveness to hexarelin in patients with Cushing's disease bearing a pituitary microadenoma, but not in those with macroadenoma. J Clin Endocrinol Metab 1998;83:4207–4211.
17. Newell-Price J, Trainer P, Besser M, Grossman A. The diagnosis and differential diagnosis of Cushing's syndrome and pseudo-Cushing's states. Endocr Rev 1998;19:647–672.
18. Papanicolaou DA, Mullen N, Kyrou I, Nieman LK. Nighttime salivary cortisol: A useful test for the diagnosis of Cushing's syndrome. J Clin Endocrinol Metab 2002;87:4515–4521.
19. Viardot A, Huber P, Puder JJ, et al. Reproducibility of nighttime salivary cortisol and its use in the diagnosis of hypercortisolism compared with urinary free cortisol and overnight dexamethasone suppression test. J Clin Endocrinol Metab 2005;90:5730–5736.
20. Findling JW, Raff H, Aron DC. The low-dose dexamethasone suppression test: A reevaluation in patients with Cushing's syndrome. J Clin Endocrinol Metab 2004;89:1222–1226.
21. Rockall AG, Babar SA, Sohaib SA, et al. CT and MR imaging of the adrenal glands in ACTH-independent Cushing's syndrome. Radiographics 2004;24:435–452.
22. Peppercorn PD, Reznek RH. State-of-the-art CT and MRI of the adrenal gland. Eur Radiol 1997;7:822–836.
23. Hopkins RL, Leinung MC. Exogenous Cushing's syndrome and glucocorticoid withdrawal. Endocrinol Metab Clin North Am 2005;34:371–384.
24. Bolland MJ, Bagg W, Thomas MG, et al. Cushing's syndrome due to interaction between inhaled corticosteroids and itraconazole. Ann Pharmacother 2004;38:46–49.
25. Samaras K, Pett S, Gowers A, et al. Iatrogenic Cushing's syndrome with osteoporosis and secondary adrenal failure in human immunodeficiency virus-infected patients receiving inhaled corticosteroids and ritonavir-boosted protease inhibitors: Six cases. J Clin Endocrinol Metab 2005;90:4394–4398.
26. Nieman LK. Medical therapy of Cushing's disease. Pituitary 2002;5:77–82.
27. Labeur M, Arzt E, Stalla GK, Paez-Pereda M. New perspectives in the treatment of Cushing's syndrome. Curr Drug Targets Immune Endocr Metabol Disord 2004;4: 335–342.
28. McEvoy GK, ed. American Hospital Formulary Service (AHFS) Drug Information. Bethesda, MD: American Society of Health-System Pharmacists, 2005:15–16, 510–516, 1116–1118.
29. Utz AL, Swearingen B, Biller BM. Pituitary surgery and postoperative management in Cushing's disease. Endocrinol Metab Clin North Am 2005;34:459–478.
30. Dang CN, Trainer P. Pharmacological management of Cushing's syndrome: An update. Arq Bras Endocrinol Metabol 2007;51:1339–1348.
31. Sonino N, Boscaro M. Medical therapy for Cushing's disease. Endocrinol Metab Clin North Am 1999;28: 211–222.
32. Pivonello R, Ferone D, de Herder WW, et al. Dopamine receptor expression and function in corticotroph pituitary tumors. J Clin Endocrinol Metab 2004;89:2452–2462.
33. Godbout A, Manavela M, Danilowicz K, et al. Cabergoline monotherapy in the long-term treatment of Cushing's disease. Eur J Endocrinol 2010;163:709–716.
34. Tritos NA, Biller BMK, Swearingen B. Management of Cushing disease. Nat Rev Endocrinol 2011;7:279–289.
35. Colao A, Petersenn S, Newell-Price J, et al. A 12-month phase 3 study of pasireotide in Cushing's disease. N Engl J Med 2012;366:914–924.
36. Fleseriu M, Biller BMK, Findling JW, et al. Mifepristone, a glucocorticoid receptor antagonist, produces clinical and metabolic benefits in patients with Cushing's syndrome. J Clin Endocrinol Metab 2012;97:2039–2049.
37. Semple PL, Vance ML, Findling J, Laws ER. Transsphenoidal surgery for Cushing's disease: Outcome in patients with a normal magnetic resonance imaging scan. Neurosurgery 2000;46:553–558.
38. Biller BMK, Grossman AB, Stewart PM, et al. Treatment of adrenocorticotropin-dependent Cushing's syndrome: A consensus statement. J Clin Endocrinol Metab 2008;93: 2454–2462.
39. Veytsman I, Nieman L, Fojo T. Management of endocrine manifestations and the use of mitotane as a chemotherapeutic agent for adrenocortical carcinoma. J Clin Oncol 2009;27: 4619–4629.
40. Morris D, Grossman A. The medical management of Cushing's syndrome. Ann N Y Acad Sci 2002;970:119–133.
41. Young WF. Minireview: Primary aldosteronism—Changing concepts in diagnosis and treatment. Endocrinology 2003; 144:2208–2213.
42. Stowasser M, Gordon RD. Primary aldosteronism: From genesis to genetics. Trends Endocrinol Metab 2003;14: 310–317.
43. Stowasser M, Gordon RD. Primary aldosteronism. Best Pract Res Clin Endocrinol Metab 2003;17:591–605.
44. Fardella CE, Mosso L. Primary aldosteronism. Clin Lab 2002;48:181–190.
45. Bope ET, Rakel RE, eds. Conn's Current Therapy 2005. Philadelphia, PA: Elsevier Saunders, 2005:745–747.
46. Funder JW, Carey RM, Fardella C, et al. Case detection, diagnosis, and treatment of patients with primary aldosteronism: An Endocrine Society clinical practice guideline. J Clin Endocrinol Metab 2008;93:3266–3281.
47. Schwartz GL, Turner ST. Screening for primary aldosteronism in essential hypertension: Diagnostic accuracy of the ratio of plasma aldosterone concentration to plasma renin activity. Clin Chem 2005;51:386–394.
48. Stowasser M, Gordon RD, Gunasekera TG, et al. High rate of detection of primary aldosteronism, including surgically treatable forms, after "nonselective" screening of hypertensive patients. J Hypertens 2003;21:2149–2157.
49. Mulatero P, Dluhy RG, Giacchetti G, et al. Diagnosis of primary aldosteronism: From screening to subtype differentiation. Trends Endocrinol Metab 2005;16: 114–119.
50. Young WF, Stanson AW, Thompson GB, et al. Role for adrenal venous sampling in primary aldosteronism. Surgery 2004;136:1227–1235.
51. Nwariaku FE, Miller BS, Auchus R, et al. Primary hyperaldosteronism: Effect of adrenal vein sampling on surgical outcome. Arch Surg 2006;141:497–502.
52. Ye P, Yamashita T, Pollock DM, Rainey WE. Contrasting effects of eplerenone and spironolactone on adrenal cell steroidogenesis. Horm Metab Res 2009;41:35–39.
53. Nishizaka MK, Calhoun DA. Primary aldosteronism: Diagnostic and therapeutic considerations. Curr Cardiol Rep 2005;7:412–417.

54. Young WF Jr. Primary aldosteronism: Management issues. Ann N Y Acad Sci 2002;970:61–76.
55. Young WF. Primary aldosteronism—Treatment options. Growth Horm IGF Res 2003;13:S102–S108.
56. Weinberger MH, White WB, Ruilope LM, et al. Effects of eplerenone versus losartan in patients with low-renin hypertension. Am Heart J 2005;150:426–433.
57. Meria P, Kempf BF, Hermieu JF, et al. Laparoscopic management of primary aldosteronism: Clinical experience with 212 cases. J Urol 2003;169:32–35.
58. Meyer A, Brabant G, Behrend M. Long-term follow-up after adrenalectomy for primary aldosteronism. World J Surg 2005;29:155–159.
59. Salvatori R. Adrenal insufficiency. JAMA 2005;294: 2481–2488.
60. Levin C, Maibach HI. Topical corticosteroid-induced adrenocortical insufficiency: Clinical implications. Am J Clin Dermatol 2002;3:141–147.
61. Bello CE, Garrett SD. Therapeutic issues in oral glucocorticoid use. Lippincotts Prim Care Pract 1999; 3:333–341.
62. Sizonenko PC. Effects of inhaled or nasal glucocorticosteroids on adrenal function and growth. J Pediatr Endocrinol Metab 2002;15:5–26.
63. Goodman A, Cagliero E. Megestrol-induced clinical adrenal insufficiency. Eur J Gynaecol Oncol 2000;21:117–118.
64. Schule C, Baghai T, Bidlingmaier M, et al. Endocrinological effects of mirtazapine in healthy volunteers. Prog Neuropsychopharmacol Biol Psychiatry 2002;26:1253–1261.
65. Alevritis EM, Sarubbi FA, Jordan RM, Peiris AN. Infectious cause of adrenal insufficiency. South Med J 2003;96: 888–890.
66. Torrey SP. Recognition and management of adrenal emergencies. Emerg Med Clin North Am 2005;23:687–702.
67. Dorin RI, Qualls CR, Crapo LM. Diagnosis of adrenal insufficiency. Ann Intern Med 2003;139:194–204.
68. Oelkers W. The role of high- and low-dose corticotropin tests in the diagnosis of secondary adrenal insufficiency. Eur J Endocrinol 1998;139:567–570.
69. Magnotti M, Shimshi M. Diagnosing adrenal insufficiency: Which test is best—The 1-mcg or the 250-mcg cosyntropin stimulation test? Endocr Pract 2008;14:233–238.
70. Arlt W, Allolio B. Adrenal insufficiency. Lancet 2003;361:1881–1893.
71. Cooper MS, Stewart PM. Corticosteroid insufficiency in acutely ill patients. N Engl J Med 2003;348:727–734.
72. Crown A, Lightman S. Why is the management of glucocorticoid deficiency still controversial: A review of the literature. Clin Endocrinol (Oxf) 2005;63:483–492.
73. Arlt W. Dehydroepiandrosterone replacement therapy. Semin Reprod Med 2004;22:379–388.
74. Alkatib AA, Cosma M, Elamin MB, et al. A systematic review and meta-analysis of randomized placebo-controlled trials of DHEA treatment effects on quality of life in women with adrenal insufficiency. J Clin Endocrinol Metab 2009;94:3676–3681.
75. Coursin DB, Wood KE. Corticosteroid supplementation for adrenal insufficiency. JAMA 2002;287:236–240.
76. Nieman LK, Turner MC. Addison's disease. Clin Dermatol 2006;24:276–280.
77. Jacobi J. Corticosteroid replacement in critically ill patients. Crit Care Clin 2006;22:245–253.
78. Speiser PW, White PC. Congenital adrenal hyperplasia. N Engl J Med 2003;349:776–788.
79. Forest MG. Recent advances in the diagnosis and management of congenital adrenal hyperplasia due to 21-hydroxylase deficiency. Hum Reprod Update 2004;10:469–485.
80. Merke DP, Bornstein SR. Congenital adrenal hyperplasia. Lancet 2005;365:2125–2136.
81. Yildiz BO. Diagnosis of hyperandrogenism: Clinical criteria. Best Pract Res Clin Endocrinol Metab 2006;20: 167–176.
82. Rosenfield RL. Hirsutism. N Engl J Med 2005;353: 2578–2588.
83. Koulouri O, Conway GS. Management of hirsutism. BMJ 2009;338:823–826.
84. Martin KA, Chang RJ, Ehrmann DA, et al. Evaluation and treatment of hirsutism in premenopausal women: An Endocrine Society clinical practice guideline. J Clin Endocrinol Metab 2008;93:1105–1120.
85. Azziz R. The evaluation and management of hirsutism. Obstet Gynecol 2003;101:995–1007.
86. Moghetti P. Treatment of hirsutism and acne in hyperandrogenism. Best Pract Res Clin Endocrinol Metab 2006;20:221–234.
87. Henzen C, Suter A, Lerch E, et al. Suppression and recovery of adrenal response after short-term, high-dose glucocorticoid treatment. Lancet 2000;355:542–545.
88. Krasner AS. Glucocorticoid-induced adrenal insufficiency. JAMA 1999;282:671–676.
89. Kountz DS, Clark CL. Safely withdrawing patients from chronic glucocorticoid therapy. Am Fam Physician 1997;55:521–552.
90. Baxter JD. Advances in glucocorticoid therapy. Adv Intern Med 2000;45:317–349.
91. United States Pharmacopeial Convention Inc. USPDI. Advice for the Patient: Drug Information in Lay Language, Vol. II, 19th ed. Taunton, MA: Rand-McNally, 1999:612–616.
92. Barlow JE. Complications of therapy. In: Boumpas DT, moderator. Glucocorticoid therapy for immune mediated diseases: Basic and clinical correlates. Ann Intern Med 1993;119:1198–1208.

Pituitary Gland Disorders

Joseph K. Jordan, Amy Heck Sheehan, Jack A. Yanovski, and Karim Anton Calis

60

KEY CONCEPTS

1. Pharmacologic therapy for acromegaly should be considered when surgery and irradiation are contraindicated, when there is poor likelihood of surgical success, when rapid control of symptoms is needed, or when other treatments have failed to normalize growth hormone (GH) and insulin-like growth factor-1 (IGF-1) concentrations.
2. Pharmacotherapy for acromegaly using dopamine agonists provides advantages of oral dosing and reduced cost compared to somatostatin analogs and pegvisomant. However, dopamine agonists effectively normalize IGF-1 concentrations in only 10% of patients. Therefore, somatostatin analogs remain the mainstay of therapy.
3. Blood glucose concentrations should be monitored frequently in the early stages of somatostatin analog therapy in all acromegalic patients.
4. Pegvisomant appears to be the most effective agent for normalizing IGF-1 concentrations. However, further study is needed to determine the long-term safety and efficacy of this agent for the treatment of acromegaly.
5. Recombinant GH is currently considered the mainstay of therapy for treatment of children with growth hormone-deficient (GHD) short stature. Prompt diagnosis of GHD and initiation of replacement therapy with recombinant GH is crucial for optimizing final adult heights.
6. All GH products are generally considered to be equally efficacious. The recommended dose for treatment of GHD short stature in children is 0.3 mg/kg/wk.
7. Pharmacologic agents that antagonize dopamine or increase the release of prolactin can induce hyperprolactinemia. Discontinuation of the offending medication and initiation of an appropriate therapeutic alternative usually normalize serum prolactin concentrations.
8. Cabergoline appears to be more effective than bromocriptine for the medical management of prolactinomas and offers the advantage of less-frequent dosing and fewer adverse effects.
9. Although preliminary data do not suggest cabergoline has significant teratogenic potential, cabergoline is not recommended for use during pregnancy, and patients receiving cabergoline who plan to become pregnant should discontinue the medication as soon as pregnancy is detected.
10. Pharmacologic treatment of panhypopituitarism consists of glucocorticoids, thyroid hormone preparations, sex steroids, and recombinant GH, where appropriate, as lifelong replacement therapy.

INTRODUCTION

In the 1950s, Geoffrey Harris and his colleagues uncovered the physiologic importance of pituitary hormones and proposed the theory of neurohormonal regulation of the pituitary by the hypothalamus.[1] Today the pituitary gland is recognized for its essential role in body homeostasis, and for this reason it is often referred to as the "master gland." The hypothalamus and the pituitary gland are closely connected, and together they provide a means of communication between the brain and many of the body's endocrine organs. The hypothalamus uses nervous input and metabolic signals from the body to control the secretion of pituitary hormones that regulate growth, thyroid function, adrenal activity, reproduction, lactation, and fluid balance.

ANATOMY AND PHYSIOLOGY

The hypothalamus (Fig. 60-1) is a small region at the base of the brain that receives autonomic nervous input from different areas of the body to regulate limbic functions, food and water intake, body temperature, cardiovascular function, respiratory function, and diurnal rhythms. In addition, the hypothalamus controls the release of hormones from the anterior and posterior regions of the pituitary gland. Neurons in the hypothalamus produce vasopressin and oxytocin and make many hormone-releasing factors that

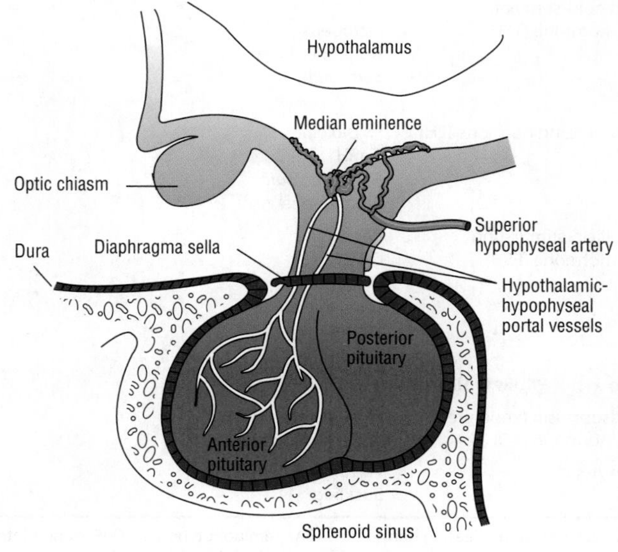

FIGURE 60-1 Pituitary gland.

stimulate or inhibit the release of trophic hormones. At the base of the hypothalamus, a projection known as the *median eminence* is rich with nerve axons and blood vessels and provides both chemical and physical connections between the hypothalamus and the pituitary gland.

The pituitary gland, also referred to as the *hypophysis*, is located at the base of the brain in a cavity of the sphenoid bone known as the *sellaturcica*. The pituitary is separated from the brain by an extension of the dura mater known as the *diaphragma sellae*. The pituitary is a very small gland, weighing between 0.4 and 1 g in adults. It is divided into two distinct regions: the anterior lobe, or adenohypophysis; and the posterior lobe, or the neurohypophysis (see Fig. 60-1).

The posterior pituitary gland secretes two major hormones: oxytocin and vasopressin (antidiuretic hormone) (Table 60-1). Oxytocin release from the posterior pituitary causes contraction of the smooth muscles in the breast during lactation. It also plays a role in uterine contraction during parturition. Vasopressin is essential

TABLE 60-1 Pituitary Hormones

Hormone	Stimulated by	Inhibited by	Physiologic Effects
Anterior Pituitary Hormones			
Growth hormone (GH)	*Physiologic* GH-releasing hormone Ghrelin ADH GABA Norepinephrine Dopamine Serotonin Estrogen Sleep Stress Exercise *Pharmacologic* α-Adrenergic agonists (e.g., clonidine) β-Adrenergic antagonists (e.g., propranolol) Dopamine agonists (e.g., bromocriptine) GABA agonists (e.g., muscimol)	*Physiologic* Somatostatin Elevated IGF-1 Growth hormone Progesterone Glucocorticoids Postprandial hyperglycemia Elevated free fatty acids *Pharmacologic* Dopamine antagonists (e.g., phenothiazines) α-Adrenergic antagonists (e.g., phentolamine) β-Adrenergic agonists (e.g., isoproterenol) Serotonin antagonists (e.g., methysergide)	Stimulates IGF-I production IGF-I and GH promote growth in all body tissues
Prolactin	*Physiologic* TRH VIP Estrogen Serotonin Histamine Endogenous opioids Pregnancy and nursing *Pharmacologic* Dopamine antagonists (e.g., phenothiazines, haloperidol, methyldopa) Opiates Estrogens H_2-antagonists (e.g., cimetidine) MAO inhibitors	*Physiologic* Dopamine GABA *Pharmacologic* Dopamine agonists (e.g., L-dopa, bromocriptine, pergolide, cabergoline)	Lactation
Adrenocorticotropic hormone (ACTH)	CRH	Elevated cortisol	Glucocorticoid effects Pigmentation
Thyroid-stimulating hormone (TSH)	TRH Estrogens Norepinephrine Serotonin	Thyroxine Triiodothyronine Somatostatin Glucocorticoids Dopamine	Iodine uptake and thyroid hormone synthesis
Luteinizing hormone (LH)	*Physiologic* GnRH *Pharmacologic* Clomiphene	Estradiol Testosterone Fasting	Ovulation Maintains corpus luteum
Follicle-stimulating hormone (FSH)	*Physiologic* GnRH Menopause Ovarian disorders *Pharmacologic* Clomiphene	Estradiol Inhibin Fasting	Ovarian follicle development Stimulates estradiol and progesterone
Posterior Pituitary Hormones			
Vasopressin (antidiuretic hormone [ADH])	Hyperosmolality Volume depletion	Hypervolemia Hypoosmolality	Acts on renal collecting ducts to prevent diuresis
Oxytocin	Parturition Suckling		Uterine contraction Milk ejection

CRH, corticotropin-releasing hormone; GABA, γ-aminobutyric acid; GnRH, gonadotropin-releasing hormone; IGF-1, insulin-like growth factor-1; MAO, monoamine oxidase; TRH, thyrotropin-releasing hormone; VIP, vasoactive intestinal peptide.

From Amar and Weiss,[2] Sam and Frohman,[3] and Molitch.[4]

for proper fluid balance and acts on the renal collecting ducts to conserve water. Oxytocin and vasopressin are synthesized in the paraventricular and supraoptic nuclei of the hypothalamus. The posterior pituitary gland contains the terminal nerve endings of these two nuclei as well as specialized secretory granules that release hormones in response to appropriate signals. Loss of anterior pituitary function does not necessarily affect the release of vasopressin or oxytocin because these hormones actually are synthesized in the hypothalamus.

Unlike the posterior pituitary, the release of anterior pituitary hormones is not regulated by direct nervous stimulation but rather is controlled by specific hypothalamic-releasing and inhibitory hormones. The median eminence of the hypothalamus contains a large number of capillaries that converge to form a network of veins known as the *hypothalamic–hypophyseal portal circulation*. Inhibiting and releasing hormones synthesized in the neurons of the hypothalamus reach the anterior pituitary via the hypothalamic–hypophyseal portal vessels to control release of anterior pituitary hormones. Although there is a direct arterial blood supply to the anterior pituitary lobe, the hypothalamic–hypophyseal portal vessels provide the primary blood supply (see Fig. 60-1). In contrast to the posterior pituitary, the anterior pituitary lobe is extremely vascular and has the highest rate of blood flow of all body organs.

The specialized secretory cells of the anterior pituitary lobe secrete six major polypeptide hormones (see Table 60-1). These include growth hormone (GH) or somatotropin, adrenocorticotropic hormone (ACTH) or corticotropin, thyroid-stimulating hormone (TSH) or thyrotropin, prolactin, follicle-stimulating hormone (FSH), and luteinizing hormone (LH). The release of these hormones is regulated primarily by hypothalamic-releasing and inhibiting hormones. Thyrotropin-releasing hormone (TRH) stimulates anterior pituitary release of TSH and prolactin, corticotropin-releasing hormone (CRH) stimulates anterior pituitary release of ACTH, growth hormone-releasing hormone (GHRH) stimulates anterior pituitary release of GH, and gonadotropin-releasing hormone (GnRH) stimulates anterior pituitary release of LH and FSH. Hypothalamic release of somatostatin inhibits release of GH, and hypothalamic release of dopamine (prolactin inhibitory hormone) inhibits the secretion of prolactin. Prolactin differs from the other anterior lobe hormones in that an inhibiting factor, rather than a stimulating factor, is primarily responsible for controlling its secretion. In the absence of hypothalamic input, an excess of prolactin is produced, whereas a deficiency state of other anterior pituitary hormones results. Physiologic regulation and action of anterior and posterior pituitary hormones are summarized in Table 60-1.[2–4]

Destruction of the pituitary gland may result in secondary hypothyroidism, hypogonadism, adrenal insufficiency, GH deficiency, and hypoprolactinemia. The formation of certain types of pituitary tumors may result in pituitary hormone excess. Pituitary tumors may physically compress the pituitary and prevent the release of trophic hypothalamic factors that regulate pituitary hormones. In this chapter, the pathophysiology and role of pharmacotherapy in the treatment of acromegaly, short stature, hyperprolactinemia, and panhypopituitarism are discussed.

GROWTH HORMONE

GH has direct antiinsulin effects on lipid and carbohydrate metabolism. GH decreases utilization of glucose by peripheral tissues, increases lipolysis, and increases muscle mass. GH also stimulates gluconeogenesis in hepatocytes, impairs tissue glucose uptake, decreases insulin-receptor sensitivity, and impairs postreceptor insulin action. The growth-promoting effects of GH are largely mediated by insulin-like growth factors (IGFs) also known as *somatomedins*. GH stimulates the formation of IGF-1 in the liver as well as in other peripheral tissues. This anabolic peptide acts as a direct stimulator of cell proliferation and growth. There are two types of IGFs: IGF-1 and IGF-2. IGF-1 regulates growth to some extent before, and largely after, birth. In contrast, IGF-2 is thought to primarily regulate growth in utero.[5] GH is secreted by the anterior pituitary in a pulsatile fashion, with several short bursts that occur mostly at night. Because of the short half-life of GH in the plasma (~30 minutes), measurements of circulating GH concentrations throughout the waking hours usually are very low or undetectable. Daytime GH pulses are most likely to occur after meals, following exercise, or during periods of stress. The greatest amount of GH secretion occurs during the night within the first 1 to 2 hours of slow-wave sleep (stage III or IV). Secretion of GH is lowest during infancy, increases slightly during childhood, reaches its peak during adolescence, and then begins to gradually decline during the middle-age years.[3]

Growth Hormone Excess

Acromegaly is a pathologic condition characterized by excessive production of GH. This is a rare disorder that affects approximately 50 to 70 adults per million.[6] Gigantism, which is even more rare than acromegaly, is the excess secretion of GH prior to epiphyseal closure in children.[7] Patients diagnosed with acromegaly are reported to have a two- to threefold increase in mortality, usually related to cardiovascular, respiratory, or neoplastic disease.[8–10] Most patients are middle-aged at the time of diagnosis, and this disorder does not appear to affect one sex to a greater extent than the other. The most common cause of excess GH secretion in acromegaly is a GH-secreting pituitary adenoma, accounting for over 90% of all cases.[8] Rarely, acromegaly is caused by ectopic GH-secreting adenomas, GH cell hyperplasia, or excess GHRH secretion, or is one of the manifestations of multiple endocrine neoplasia syndrome type 1, McCune–Albright's syndrome, or the Carney complex, all very rare hypersecretory endocrinopathies.[8]

The clinical signs and symptoms of acromegaly develop gradually over an extended period of time. In fact, because of the subtle and slowly developing changes in physical appearance caused by GH excess, most patients are not definitively diagnosed with acromegaly until 7 to 10 years after the presumed onset of excessive GH secretion.[9] Excessive secretion of GH and IGF-1 adversely affects several organ systems. Almost all acromegalic patients will present with physical signs and symptoms of soft-tissue overgrowth. Table 60-2 summarizes the classic clinical presentation of patients with acromegaly.[8–13] Some patients with acromegaly present with only a few of these classic signs and symptoms, making recognition of this disease extremely difficult.

The diagnosis of acromegaly is based on a combination of diagnostic tests and clinical signs and symptoms. Random measures of plasma GH levels are not usually dependable because of the pulsatile pattern of release. However, some clinicians exclude diagnosis of acromegaly in the presence of a random GH <0.4 mcg/L (<18 pmol/L) and IGF-1 that is normal for age and sex.[8] The oral glucose tolerance test (OGTT) is commonly used as an important diagnostic tool. Postprandial hyperglycemia inhibits the secretion of GH for at least 1 to 2 hours. Therefore, an oral glucose load would be expected to suppress GH concentrations. However, patients with acromegaly continue to secrete GH during the OGTT. Because GH stimulates the production of IGF-1, serum IGF-1 concentrations can also be measured to aid in the diagnosis of acromegaly. Circulating IGF-1 is cleared from the body at a much slower rate than is GH, and measurements can be collected at any time of the day to identify patients with GH excess.[9] Current criteria for the diagnosis of acromegaly include failure of GH suppression <1 mcg/L (<45 pmol/L) following an OGTT in the presence of

TABLE 60-2 Clinical Presentation of Acromegaly

General
The patient will experience slow development of soft-tissue overgrowth affecting many body systems. Signs and symptoms may gradually progress over 7 to 10 years

Symptoms
The patient may complain of symptoms related to local effects of the growth hormone (GH)-secreting tumor, such as headache and visual disturbances. Other symptoms related to elevated GH and insulin-like growth factor-1 (IGF-1) concentrations include excessive sweating, neuropathies, joint pain, and paresthesias

Signs
The patient may exhibit coarsening of facial features, increased hand volume, increased ring size, increased shoe size, an enlarged tongue, and various dermatologic conditions

Laboratory tests
The patient's GH concentration will be >1 mcg/L (>45 pmol/L) following an oral glucose tolerance test (OGTT) and IGF-1 serum concentrations will be elevated. Glucose intolerance may be present in up to 50% of patients

Additional clinical sequelae
- Cardiovascular diseases such as hypertension, coronary heart disease, cardiomyopathy, and left ventricular hypertrophy are common in patients with acromegaly
- Osteoarthritis and joint damage develop in up to 90% of acromegalic patients
- Respiratory disorders and sleep apnea occur in up to 60% of acromegalic patients
- Type 2 diabetes develops in approximately 25% of acromegalic patients
- Patients with acromegaly may have an increased risk for development of esophageal, colon, and stomach cancer

From American Association of Clinical Endocrinologists,[8] Melmed,[9] Attal and Chanson,[11] Lombardi et al.,[12] and Jenkins.[13]

elevated IGF-1 serum concentrations.[8,14] With the development of more sensitive GH and IGF-1 assays, the American Association of Clinical Endocrinologists (AACE) suggests lowering the cutoff for GH suppression to <0.4 mcg/L (<18 pmol/L). Insulin-like growth factor 1 binding protein 3 (IGFBP-3) also can be measured because it is positively regulated by GH and binds to circulating IGF-1 with high affinity. This test may prove useful in the future in monitoring response to therapy but, at present, AACE does not recommend IGFBP-3 measurement for the purpose of clinical management.[8] Computed tomography and magnetic resonance imaging of the pituitary are important diagnostic tests to confirm the presence of a pituitary adenoma.[8,14]

TREATMENT
Acromegaly

The primary treatment goals for patients diagnosed with acromegaly are to reduce GH and IGF-1 concentrations, improve the clinical signs and symptoms of the disease, and decrease mortality.[8,15–17] Many clinicians define biochemical control of acromegaly as suppression of GH concentrations to <1 mcg/L (<45 pmol/L) after a standard OGTT in the presence of normal IGF-1 serum concentrations, although some argue for a lower cutoff GH value of 0.4 mcg/L (18 pmol/L) due to the availability of more sensitive test methods.[16] The treatment of choice for most patients with acromegaly is transsphenoidal surgical resection of the GH-secreting adenoma.[9,15,16] Postsurgical cure rates have been reported to range from 50% to 90%, depending on the type of adenoma and the expertise of the neurosurgeon.[8,16,17] Complications of transsphenoidal surgery are relatively infrequent and include cerebrospinal fluid leak, meningitis, arachnoiditis, diabetes insipidus, and pituitary failure.[8] For patients who are poor surgical candidates, those who have not responded to surgical or medical interventions, or others who refuse surgical or medical treatment, radiation therapy may be considered. Radiation, however, may require several years to relieve the symptoms of acromegaly.

Because neither radiation therapy nor surgery will cure all patients with acromegaly, adjuvant drug therapy is often needed to control symptoms.[9,17,18]

Pharmacologic Therapy

❶ Drug therapy should be considered as primary therapy for acromegalic patients who prefer medical therapy, are poor surgical candidates, or when there is a poor likelihood of surgical success. Drug therapy should be considered as adjunctive therapy in the presence of persistent disease after surgery.[8] Pharmacologic treatment options include dopamine agonists, somatostatin analogs, and the GH receptor antagonist pegvisomant. Dopamine agonists such as bromocriptine and cabergoline are effective in a small subset of patients and provide the advantages of oral dosing and reduced cost. Somatostatin analogs are more effective than dopamine agonists, reducing GH concentrations and normalizing IGF-1 in approximately 50% to 60% of patients. Pegvisomant, a GH receptor antagonist, is highly effective in normalizing IGF-1 concentrations in up to 97% of patients in the first year and in 60% over 5 years.

Dopamine Agonists

❷ In normal healthy adults, dopamine agonists cause an increase in GH production. However, when these agents are given to patients with acromegaly, there is a paradoxical decrease in GH production. Most clinical experience with the use of dopamine agonists in acromegaly is with bromocriptine or cabergoline. Other agents such as pergolide, quinagolide, and lisuride also have been used but are not available in the United States. Bromocriptine and cabergoline are semisynthetic ergot alkaloids that act as dopamine-receptor agonists. Most trials assessing the efficacy of bromocriptine in the treatment of acromegaly were conducted in the 1970s and early 1980s and determined that certain subsets of acromegalic patients with high circulating concentrations of prolactin have a favorable response to drug therapy with bromocriptine.[19] A review evaluating 34 studies concluded that therapy with bromocriptine was effective in suppressing mean serum GH levels to <5 mcg/L (<225 pmol/L) in approximately 20% of patients.[20] While only 10% of patients experience normalization of IGF-1 concentrations with bromocriptine therapy, greater than 50% of patients treated with bromocriptine experience improvement in symptoms of acromegaly.[8,19] According to AACE guidelines, cabergoline appears used more commonly than bromocriptine. A recent meta-analysis of 15 studies concluded that cabergoline as monotherapy was effective in normalizing IGF-1 levels in 34% of patients and resulted normalization of IGF-1 levels in 52% of patients when added to a somatostatin analog in those unresponsive to somatostatin analog monotherapy.[21]

In the United States, bromocriptine is commercially available as 0.8 and 2.5-mg oral tablets and 5-mg oral capsules. The 0.8-mg tablet is indicated as adjunctive therapy in type 2 diabetes mellitus. In acromegalic patients, significant reductions in GH concentrations are observed within 1 to 2 hours of oral dosing. This effect persists for at least 4 to 5 hours. An overall clinical response in acromegalic patients typically occurs after 4 to 8 weeks of continuous bromocriptine therapy. For treatment of acromegaly, bromocriptine is initiated at a dose of 1.25 mg (1/2 of a 2.5-mg tablet) at bedtime and is increased by 1.25-mg increments every 3 to 4 days as needed. Doses as high as 86 mg/day have been used for treatment of acromegaly, but clinical studies have shown that dosages >20 or 30 mg daily do not offer additional benefits in the suppression of GH. When used for treatment of acromegaly, the duration of action of bromocriptine is shorter than that for treatment of hyperprolactinemia. Therefore, the total daily dose of bromocriptine should be divided into three or four doses.

Cabergoline is commercially available as 0.5 mg tablets. Use in acromegaly is considered *off-label*, and dosing is typically initiated at 0.5 mg twice weekly and increased as needed to 0.5 mg every other day. Doses up to 7 mg/wk (0.5 mg twice daily) have been reported in trials.

The most common adverse effects of dopamine agonist therapy include CNS symptoms such as headache, lightheadedness, dizziness, nervousness, and fatigue. GI effects such as nausea, abdominal pain, or diarrhea also are very common. Some patients may need to take dopamine agonists with food to decrease the incidence of adverse GI effects. Most adverse effects are seen early in the course of therapy and tend to decrease with continued treatment.[8,19] Dopamine agonists may cause thickening of bronchial secretions and nasal congestion. Rare cases of psychiatric disturbances, pleural diseases, and an erythromelalgic syndrome (painful paroxysmal dilation of the blood vessels in the skin of the feet and lower extremities) have been reported with dopamine agonist use. These conditions appear to be associated with higher doses and prolonged duration of therapy.[8,19]

Dopamine agonists are not FDA-approved for use during pregnancy. However, surveillance of women who took dopamine agonists throughout pregnancy does not suggest that dopamine agonists are associated with an increased risk for birth defects.[22] If a woman becomes pregnant while taking dopamine agonists, the risks and benefits of therapy should be fully considered. In most cases, the benefits of successful therapy outweigh the risks, and dopamine agonist therapy should be continued if it is effective in improving symptoms and reducing elevated GH concentrations.

Other dopamine agonists that have been used to treat acromegaly include pergolide, lisuride, and quinagolide. Pergolide is no longer commercially available, and lisuride and quinagolide are not commercially available in the United States. Because of the potential cost advantages and convenience of oral administration, dopamine agonists are often considered for treatment of acromegaly prior to initiation of somatostatin analogs. However, the availability of long-acting somatostatin analogs has made these agents more attractive for first-line treatment of acromegaly.

Somatostatin Analogs

Octreotide and lanreotide are long-acting somatostatin analogs that are more potent in inhibiting GH secretion than endogenous somatostatin.[23,24] These agents also suppress the LH response to GnRH; decrease splanchnic blood flow; and inhibit secretion of insulin, vasoactive intestinal peptide (VIP), gastrin, secretin, motilin, serotonin, and pancreatic polypeptide. Pasireotide is a somatostatin analog that has a broader affinity for somatostatin receptor subtypes than octreotide or lanreotide. The binding to additional subtypes of somatostatin receptors may result in greater GH inhibition compared to octreotide or lanreotide and efficacy of pasireotide in the presence of octreotide or lanreotide-resistant adenomas.[23]

Octreotide (Sandostatin) injection is commercially available in the United States for subcutaneous or IV administration. A long-acting intramuscular formulation of octreotide (Sandostatin LAR) is available for monthly administration. In addition to the treatment of acromegaly, octreotide has many other therapeutic uses, including the treatment of carcinoid tumors, vasoactive intestinal peptide-secreting tumors (VIPomas), GI fistulas, variceal bleeding, diarrheal states, and irritable bowel syndrome.

The efficacy of octreotide for treatment of acromegaly has been determined by two major multicenter trials.[25,26] These studies determined that drug therapy with octreotide suppresses mean serum GH concentrations to <5 mcg/L (<225 pmol/L) and normalizes serum IGF-1 concentrations in 50% to 60% of acromegalic patients. Octreotide also is beneficial in reducing the clinical signs and symptoms of acromegaly. In a 6-month multicenter trial, 70% of patients experienced significant relief of headaches.[26] In some patients, relief of headache symptoms occurred within minutes of octreotide administration. In addition, middle-finger circumference was reduced significantly, and 50% to 75% of patients experienced improvement in symptoms of excessive perspiration, fatigue, joint pain, and cystic acne. Long-term follow-up of patients treated with octreotide LAR for up to 9 years showed octreotide therapy to be safe and effective for long-term use in acromegalic patients.[27] Octreotide also has been shown to improve the cardiovascular manifestations of acromegaly and to halt pituitary tumor growth, with some patients experiencing tumor regression.[25–28] Data from more recent studies indicate that shrinkage of pituitary tumor mass during octreotide therapy occurs in approximately 50% of patients.[29]

The pharmacodynamic effects of long-acting octreotide are similar to those of subcutaneously administered octreotide. Single monthly doses of long-acting octreotide have been shown to be at least as effective as daily doses of subcutaneous octreotide administered in divided doses three times daily in normalizing IGF-1 levels and maintaining suppression of mean serum GH concentrations.[30] Trials evaluating the efficacy of long-acting octreotide in acromegalic patients who previously had responded to subcutaneously administered octreotide have reported sustained suppression of GH concentrations to <5 mcg/L (<225 pmol/L) and normalization of IGF-1 in patients following 1 year of therapy.[31]

Response to long-term therapy with octreotide is related to the presence and increased quantity of functioning somatostatin receptors located in the pituitary adenoma. Identification of patients who most likely will respond to octreotide, prior to initiation of therapy, is important when considering the high cost of this medication and the inconvenience of subcutaneous or intramuscular drug administration. Suppression of serum GH concentrations after a single 50-mcg dose of octreotide has been used to predict a favorable long-term response to octreotide therapy.[32,33]

The initial dose of octreotide for treatment of acromegaly is usually 100 mcg administered three times daily followed by either titration to a maximum of 1500 mcg/day or transition to long-acting octreotide.[8,23,24] Some clinicians recommend a starting dose of 50 mcg every 8 hours, then increasing the dose to 100 mcg every 8 hours after 1 week, to improve the patient's tolerance of adverse GI effects. The dose can be increased by increments of 50 mcg every 1 to 2 weeks based on mean serum GH and IGF-1 concentrations. Patients who experience a significant rise in GH prior to the end of the 8-hour dosing interval may benefit from decreasing the dosing interval to every 4 to 6 hours. Although doses as high as 1,500 mcg/day have been used, doses >600 mcg daily generally do not offer additional benefits, and most patients are adequately managed with 100 to 200 mcg three times daily.[8,24] Patients who have been maintained on subcutaneous octreotide for at least 2 weeks and have shown response to therapy can be converted to the long-acting depot form of octreotide. The initial dose of long-acting octreotide is 20 mg administered intramuscularly in the gluteal region every 28 days. Steady-state serum concentrations are not obtained until after 3 months of therapy. Therefore, dosage adjustments for long-acting octreotide should not be considered until after this time. Some patients may require additional subcutaneous injections during the initial dose-titration phase in order to control symptoms. In patients who achieve >50% reduction in GH levels to 30 mg every 4 weeks, some may have added response to a higher-dose regimen of 60 mg every 4 weeks.[34]

A long-acting, intramuscular formulation of lanreotide (lanreotide LA) for twice monthly administration has been available in Europe for many years. In 2007, a new formulation of lanreotide (Somatuline Depot) was approved for use in the United States for monthly deep subcutaneous administration. The efficacy of this preparation of lanreotide for the treatment of acromegaly has been evaluated in several prospective multicenter clinical trials involving treatment-experienced patients who were switched from intramuscular octreotide LAR or intramuscular lanreotide LA to monthly deep subcutaneous lanreotide.[35,36] These studies have determined that deep subcutaneous lanreotide suppresses mean serum GH concentrations to <5 mcg/L (<225 pmol/L) and normalizes serum IGF-1 concentrations in acromegalic patients to a similar extent as octreotide LAR and lanreotide LA. A 4-year follow-up of 23 patients treated with monthly deep subcutaneous lanreotide reported the drug to be well tolerated during long-term therapy with mean serum GH concentrations <5 mcg/L (225 pmol/L) in 62% of patients and normalization of serum IGF-1 concentrations in 43% of patients.[37] Analyses of trials investigating the effects of lanreotide on pituitary tumor mass have shown shrinkage in 66% to 77% of patients.[35] Well-designed trials directly comparing the efficacy of intramuscular octreotide LAR to deep subcutaneous lanreotide are currently lacking. However, these two agents are generally regarded to have comparable efficacy.[8]

Lanreotide (Somatuline Depot) is commercially available in the United States as 60-, 90-, and 120-mg prefilled syringes. In contrast to octreotide LAR, lanreotide injection does not need to be reconstituted prior to administration. The initial recommended dose of lanreotide is 90 mg given by deep subcutaneous injection in the superior external quadrant of the buttock every 28 days. Injection sites should be alternated between the left and right side. The initial dose should be reduced to 60 mg every 28 days for patients with moderate or severe renal or hepatic impairment. After 3 months of therapy, the dose may then be titrated based on serum GH concentrations, serum IGF-1 concentrations, and control of clinical signs and symptoms of acromegaly.[36] Long-acting deep subcutaneous lanreotide injection in doses >120 mg every 28 days has not been studied.

The most common adverse effects of somatostatin analog therapy are GI disturbances such as diarrhea, nausea, abdominal cramps, malabsorption of fat, and flatulence.[16,23] GI adverse effects occur in approximately 75% of patients but usually subside within 10 to 14 days of continued treatment.[23] Octreotide has been reported to cause injection-site pain (4% to 31%), conduction abnormalities and arrhythmias (9%), subclinical hypothyroidism (2% to 12%), biliary tract disorders (4% to 50%), and abnormalities in glucose metabolism (2% to 18%).[20,23] Lanreotide has been reported to cause injection-site reactions (9%), sinus bradycardia (3%), hypertension (5%), biliary tract disorders (20%), and abnormalities in glucose metabolism (7%).[36]

Somatostatin analogs also inhibit cholecystokinin release and gallbladder motility, predisposing patients to the development of cholelithiasis.[23] The development of gallstones is a long-term adverse effect of somatostatin analog therapy and is largely dependent on geographic factors, dietary habits, and length of therapy.[20,24] The incidence of gallstones in acromegalic patients receiving octreotide and lanreotide increases with length of therapy and has been reported to range from 20% to 50%.[24–26] However, most patients are asymptomatic, and the diagnosis of cholelithiasis usually is made following an ultrasonographic study that is not prompted by patient symptoms. It has been estimated that only 1% of patients will develop symptomatic gallstones during 1 year of octreotide treatment.[24] Because somatostatin analog-induced gallstones usually are present without clinical symptoms, prophylactic cholecystectomy or medical therapy with ursodeoxycholic acid for acromegalic patients with asymptomatic gallstones usually is not recommended.[9,16] A small number of studies have suggested that the incidence of gallstone development may be lower with long-acting octreotide compared to subcutaneous octreotide.[30,31] However, further studies are needed to confirm this observation.

❸ The effect of somatostatin analogs on glucose metabolism in patients with acromegaly is multifactorial. Decreases in serum GH concentrations induced by somatostatin analogs should result in decreased hepatic gluconeogenesis and increased insulin-receptor sensitivity. However, somatostatin analogs also decrease insulin secretion and increase IGFBP-1, which is known to inhibit the insulin-like effects of IGF-1. In addition, somatostatin analogs delay the GI absorption of glucose, which may further alter glucose metabolism in acromegalic patients.[38] Small studies conducted in acromegalic patients receiving octreotide have reported improvement in insulin sensitivity as well as impaired insulin secretion.[39] Risk factors associated with worsening glucose tolerance included female sex and elevated baseline insulin values. Although somatostatin analogs appear to have a beneficial effect on glucose tolerance in most patients, glucose determinations should be obtained frequently in the early stages of therapy in all acromegalic patients.

Growth Hormone Receptor Antagonist

❹ Pegvisomant (Somavert) is a genetically engineered GH derivative that binds to, but does not activate, GH receptors and inhibits IGF-1 production. This agent is different from other medications used in the management of acromegaly because it does not inhibit GH production; rather, it blocks the physiologic effects of GH on target tissues. Therefore, GH concentrations remain elevated during therapy, and response to treatment is evidenced by a reduction in IGF-1 concentrations. Unlike somatostatin analogs, the pharmacologic activity of pegvisomant does not depend on the presence and quantity of somatostatin receptors in the pituitary tumor.[40] Studies evaluating the clinical efficacy of pegvisomant in acromegalic patients have reported a dose-dependent normalization of IGF-1 concentrations in 54% to 89% of patients after 12 weeks of therapy and in 97% of patients after 1 year of therapy.[40,41] Significant improvements in the clinical signs and symptoms of acromegaly were reported and persisted throughout the 1-year treatment period.[41] An ongoing, international post-marketing surveillance registry (ACROSTUDY) has recently reported 5-year data in patients treated with pegvisomant. In patients who predominantly had failed prior medical or surgical therapy, IGF-1 normalized in 63%. Investigators note that failure to maintain IGF-1 normalization may reflect suboptimal dosing strategies or more advanced disease than reported in the original studies.[42]

Adverse effects include injection-site pain, GI complaints such as nausea and diarrhea, and flu-like symptoms. Significant elevations in hepatic aminotransferase concentrations, which are generally reversible upon discontinuation of the drug, have been reported in approximately 25% of patients.[43] As a result, hepatic function tests should be monitored very closely during therapy as outlined in the product labeling, and the drug should be used with caution in patients with baseline elevations in hepatic aminotransferase concentrations. GH concentrations may increase significantly during the first 6 months of therapy. Tumor growth has been reported in a small number of patients and there are theoretical concerns that the lack of GH feedback regulation on tumors that lead to persistently elevated GH concentrations may stimulate tumor growth or result in other long-term adverse effects. Interim results of the ongoing ACROSTUDY suggest that the rate of tumor growth of 3.2% is comparable to the background rate in acromegaly, and the incidence of hepatic aminotransferases greater than three times upper limit of normal is low (2.5%).[43]

Pegvisomant is commercially available in the United States for daily subcutaneous use. The first dose should be administered under the supervision of a physician as a 40-mg loading dose. Subsequent doses are self-administered by the patient starting at a dose of 10 mg daily. The dose can be adjusted in 5-mg increments based on serum IGF-1 concentrations every 4 to 6 weeks.[43]

Based on the available data, pegvisomant appears to be among the most effective agents for normalizing IGF-1 serum concentrations. Current guidelines for acromegaly management suggest pegvisomant therapy for patients who have failed to achieve normalization of IGF-1 serum concentrations with other treatments.[8]

Combination Therapy

Several small studies have suggested that combination therapy with somatostatin analogs, dopamine agonists, or pegvisomant may be more beneficial than monotherapy with either drug alone.[8,21,44] Several of these trials have used doses lower than those typically used for monotherapy in order to try to minimize the risk of additive adverse effects. Because of the potential for additive adverse effects, combination therapy should be considered as a therapeutic option only for refractory patients who have not fully responded to monotherapy.[8]

Personalized Pharmacotherapy

The genetics of growth hormone and receptors have been well-studied.[45] At this time, the data are most abundant with pegvisomant. As pegvisomant acts at the growth hormone receptor, researchers have investigated response to GH receptor variants. In patients with exon 3-deleted GH receptors, lower doses and fewer months were needed to obtain IGF-1 normalization.[46] However, recommendations regarding how therapy can be individualized to maximize patient benefit are not yet available.[8]

Clinical **Controversy...**

Some clinicians advocate the use of somatostatin analogs prior to surgery in order to improve comorbidities that may complicate surgery. However, sufficient evidence is lacking.

Conclusions

Acromegaly is a chronic debilitating disease characterized by excess GH secretion most commonly caused by a GH-secreting pituitary adenoma. Transsphenoidal surgical resection of the adenoma is the current treatment of choice for most patients with acromegaly. Patients who are poor surgical candidates may receive radiation therapy or long-term pharmacologic therapy. Drug therapy options within the United States for acromegaly include dopamine agonists, somatostatin analogs, and pegvisomant. Figure 60-2 shows a treatment algorithm for the management of acromegaly.[8,9]

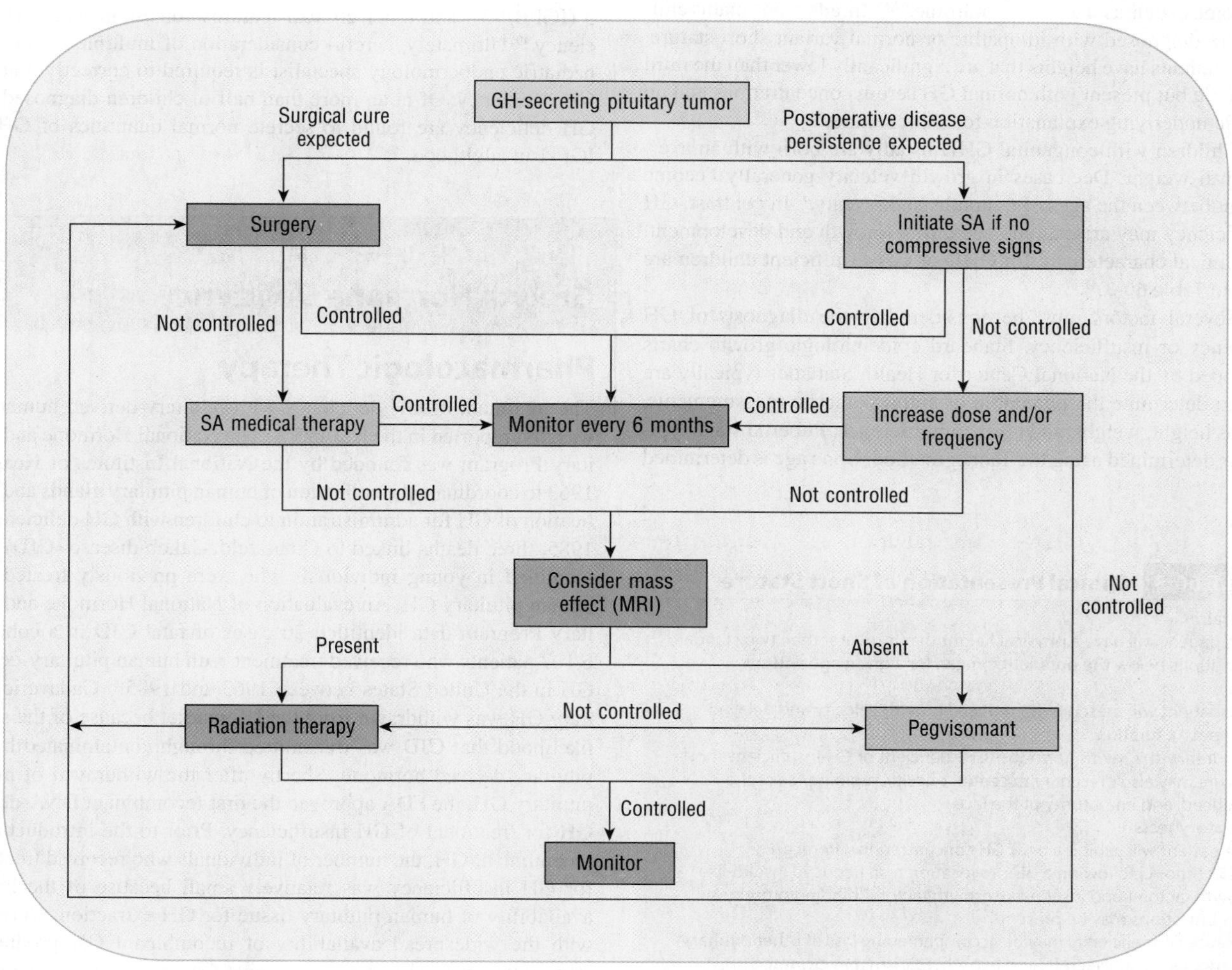

FIGURE 60-2 Treatment algorithm for acromegaly. (SRL, somatostatin analog; MRI, magnetic resonance imaging.) *(Modified from Melmed S, Calao A, Barkan A, et al. Guidelines for acromegaly management: An update. J Clin Endocrinol Metab 2009;94:1509–1517. Copyright 2009, The Endocrine Society.)*

Growth Hormone Deficiency

Short stature is a condition that is commonly defined by a physical height that is more than two standard deviations below the population mean and lower than the third percentile for height in a specific age group.[47] It has been estimated that more than 1.8 million children in the United States can be characterized as having short stature.[47] Short stature is a very broad term describing a condition that may be the result of many different causes. A true lack of GH is among the least common causes and is known as growth hormone-deficient (GHD) short stature. Absolute GH deficiency is a congenital disorder that can result from various genetic abnormalities, such as GHRH deficiency, GH gene deletion, and developmental disorders including pituitary aplasia or hypoplasia.[47] GH insufficiency is an acquired condition that can result from hypothalamic or pituitary tumors (or their neurosurgical treatment), cranial irradiation, head trauma, pituitary infarction, and various types of CNS infections. In addition, psychosocial deprivation, hypothyroidism, poorly controlled diabetes mellitus, treatment of precocious puberty with LH-releasing hormone agonists, and pharmacologic agents such as glucocorticoids, methylphenidate, and dextroamphetamine may induce transient GH insufficiency.[47]

Short stature also occurs with several conditions that are not associated with a true GH deficiency or insufficiency. These conditions include intrauterine growth restriction; constitutional growth delay; malnutrition; malabsorption of nutrients associated with inflammatory bowel disease, celiac disease, and cystic fibrosis; chronic renal failure; skeletal and cartilage dysplasia; and genetic syndromes such as Turner's syndrome.[47,48] In addition, many children are diagnosed with idiopathic or normal variant short stature. These patients have heights that are significantly lower than the third percentile but present with normal GH serum concentrations and no specific underlying explanation for short stature.[48]

Children with congenital GHD usually are born with an average birth weight. Decreases in growth velocity generally become evident between the ages of 6 months and 3 years.[47] In contrast, GH insufficiency may arise at any age during growth and development. The clinical characteristics of GHD or GH-insufficient children are listed in Table 60-3.[47]

Several factors must be considered in the diagnosis of GH deficiency or insufficiency. Standard epidemiologic growth charts developed by the National Center for Health Statistics typically are used to determine the percentile of anthropometric measurements, such as height, weight, and head circumference. Pubertal stage typically is determined using the Tanner method. Bone age is determined according to published standards, and growth velocity is calculated to determine the patient's height velocity percentile using standard growth-velocity charts.[47,48] GH deficiency is rarely seen in the absence of delayed skeletal maturation and decreased growth velocity. In addition, several different provocative stimuli that induce GH secretion may be used diagnostically to determine GH status. Common provocative pharmacologic GH stimuli include insulin-induced hypoglycemia, clonidine, L-dopa, arginine, glucagon, and GHRH.[47] A subnormal GH response during childhood is arbitrarily defined as a peak GH serum concentration <10 mcg/L (<450 pmol/L) during a 2-hour period after administration of one of these agents.[47] However, this maximum may be lower, depending on the specific assay and GH reference product used. For prepubertal and early pubertal patients (Tanner stage less than III), priming with sex hormones to improve the specificity of GH provocation tests is often considered. Some patients exhibit clinical signs of GH deficiency, subnormal growth velocity, and delayed bone age despite GH levels that are within normal limits after provocative testing. This makes diagnosis in this group of patients very difficult. Diagnosis based on GH stimulation tests becomes further complicated because of the paucity of data reporting the normal range of GH concentrations after provocative testing in healthy children and the fact that commercial GH and IGF-1 assays currently available may not be equivalent. Although a gold standard for diagnosis of GHD does not exist, treatment is generally recommended for children who have "idiopathic short stature" and pass GH provocative testing but have most of the following criteria: height greater than 2.25 standard deviations below the mean for age; subnormal growth velocity; delayed bone age; low serum IGF-1 and/or insulin-like growth factor binding protein 3 (IGFBP-3); and other clinical features consistent with GH deficiency.[49] Ultimately, careful consideration of multiple factors by a pediatric endocrinology specialist is required to correctly diagnose GH deficiency. Of note, more than half of children diagnosed with GH deficiency are found to secrete normal quantities of GH and IGF-1 in adulthood.[50]

TABLE 60-3 Clinical Presentation of Short Stature

General
- The patient will have a physical height that is greater than two standard deviations below the population mean for a given age and sex

Signs
- The patient will present with reduced growth velocity and delayed skeletal maturation
- Children with growth hormone (GH)-deficient or GH-insufficient short stature may also present with central obesity, prominence of the forehead, and immaturity of the face

Laboratory tests
- The patient will exhibit a peak GH concentration <10 mcg/L (<450 pmol/L) following a GH provocation test. Reduced insulin-like growth factor-1 and insulin-like growth factor-1 binding protein-3 concentrations may be present
- Because GH deficiency may be accompanied by loss of other pituitary hormones, hypoglycemia, and hypothyroidism may be noted

From American Association of Endocrinologists,[47] and Cohen et al.[48]

TREATMENT
Growth Hormone Deficiency

Pharmacologic Therapy

The treatment of GH deficiency with pituitary-derived human GH was first reported in the late 1950s. The National Hormone and Pituitary Program was founded by the National Institutes of Health in 1963 to coordinate the collection of human pituitary glands and purification of GH for administration to children with GH deficiency. In 1985, three deaths linked to Creutzfeldt–Jakob disease (CJD) were identified in young individuals who were previously treated with human pituitary GH. An evaluation of National Hormone and Pituitary Program data identified 26 cases of fatal CJD in a cohort of 6,107 patients who received treatment with human pituitary-derived GH in the United States between 1963 and 1985.[51] Cadaveric pituitary GH was withdrawn from the US market because of the strong likelihood that CJD was transmitted through contaminated human pituitary-derived hormone. Shortly after the withdrawal of human pituitary GH, the FDA approved the first recombinant DNA-derived GH for treatment of GH insufficiency. Prior to the introduction of recombinant GH, the number of individuals who received treatment for GH insufficiency was relatively small because of the limited availability of human pituitary tissue for GH extraction. Currently, with the widespread availability of recombinant GH products, a large number of children can receive GH replacement therapy at higher doses.

Clinical **Controversy...**

Many pediatric endocrinologists in the United States believe that GH therapy is appropriate treatment in certain patients with non-GHD short stature. However, given the high cost of therapy and small increases in height, use of GH in this patient population remains controversial.

Recombinant Growth Hormone

5 Recombinant GH is currently considered the mainstay of therapy for treatment of GHD short stature. GH replacement therapy in children with documented GHD short stature produces a significant improvement in growth velocity within the first year of therapy and significantly improves final adult height.[52–55] The initial increase in growth velocity often is referred to as *catch-up growth*. Most of the initial studies evaluating the efficacy of GH therapy in GHD children were conducted for short periods of time in small numbers of patients, and, until recently, information about the long-term outcome of GH therapy was limited. Initial data suggested that final adult height is not substantially improved, with an average final adult height reported to be two standard deviations below the population mean.[56–59] Although these results were disappointing, it is important to note that a substantial percentage of patients included in these studies initially had received human pituitary GH in relatively low doses because of its limited availability. In addition, current GH dosing regimens with regard to frequency of administration have changed, making these data difficult to interpret and apply to the patients who are receiving GH replacement therapy today. Recent studies evaluating the adult height of children who received only recombinant GH therapy with currently recommended dosing regimens suggest that current recombinant GH therapy has a greater impact on final adult height than previously reported.[52–55] These studies have reported average final adult heights ranging from 0.5 to 1.7 standard deviations below the population mean. Initiation of therapy at an early chronologic age, prior to the onset of puberty, is associated with a more favorable increase in final height.[47,53,54] Therefore, prompt diagnosis of GH deficiency and early initiation of replacement therapy with recombinant GH are crucial factors in optimizing the final adult height of children with GH deficiency.

Recombinant GH has been shown to increase the short-term growth rate in pediatric patients with chronic renal insufficiency, Turner's syndrome, idiopathic short stature, Prader–Willi syndrome, short stature homeobox gene (SHOX) deficiency, Noonan syndrome, and children born small for gestational age (SGA), and is approved by the FDA for treatment of growth failure associated with these conditions. GH is also FDA approved for treatment of adult GH deficiency, short bowel syndrome in patients receiving specialized nutritional support, and acquired immunodeficiency syndrome wasting syndrome. When used in adult patients, the recommended dosage of recombinant GH is significantly lower than the dosage used in pediatric patients. Adult patients with GH deficiency during childhood must have the diagnosis of GH deficiency confirmed when they are adults. Long-term GH therapy in GHD adults significantly decreases body fat, increases muscle mass, and improves exercise capacity.[50] GH therapy in adults has not been definitively shown to improve the cardiac risk profile or bone mineral density, but it does appear to improve psychological well-being.[60] The Beers Criteria of the American Geriatrics Society recommends avoiding growth hormone therapy except as replacement after pituitary gland removal because the risks in older adults outweigh any potential benefits.[61] Use of GH as an anabolic agent for management of acute catabolism is not recommended.[47]

The majority of short children in the United States do not have an identifiable medical cause for their condition, but with widespread availability of several recombinant GH formulations, many children have received GH therapy regardless of the underlying etiology of their short stature. The use of recombinant GH therapy in children with non-GHD short stature, also referred to as *idiopathic short stature*, has been studied by many investigators and was approved by the FDA in 2003.[48] However, the use of GH therapy in this patient population remains controversial.[62] A meta-analysis of 38 clinical studies evaluating the efficacy of GH treatment in children with idiopathic short stature reported average increases in final adult height of 4 to 5 cm (1.6 to 2 inches) following a mean duration of therapy of 4.7 years.[63] This corresponded to an increase above the predicted final adult height of 0.56 to 0.63 standard deviations of the population mean. A recent systematic review of GH treatment in idiopathic short stature noted that the final adult height gain is usually less than that seen in other FDA-approved conditions associated with growth failure, increasing adult height by about 4 cm. The individual response to therapy is highly variable, and further studies are needed to identify responders.[64]

6 Ten different recombinant GH products currently are available for use in the United States (Genotropin, Humatrope, Norditropin, Nutropin, Nutropin AQ, Omnitrope, Saizen, Serostim, Tev-Tropin, and Zorbtive). Each of these products contains somatropin. Somatropin is composed of the same amino acid sequence as human pituitary GH. Recombinant GH formulations must be administered by intramuscular or subcutaneous injection. Nutropin AQ, Norditropin, and Omnitrope are the only GH products available as liquid formulations. The remaining products are formulated as lyophilized powders for injection, and patients must be instructed regarding proper administration. A needle-free injection device (Tject) is available for use with Tev-Tropin. This device delivers a thin stream of recombinant GH that penetrates the stratum corneum and deposits into the subcutaneous tissue. This product may be particularly useful for patients who experience significant adverse effects from injections. The potency of GH products is expressed as international units per milligram (international units/mg), with 1 mg containing approximately 2.6 international units of GH. Direct comparisons between the different recombinant GH products have not been published. However, all GH products are generally considered to be equally efficacious. The recommended dose for treatment of GHD short stature in children is 0.3 mg/kg/wk.[47,51] Recombinant GH can be administered daily or in equal doses six times per week, depending on the specific GH product used.[47,51] Dosing regimens with greater frequency of administration have been shown to provide more favorable short-term growth responses.[47,51] Recent studies suggest that adjustments in GH replacement can be made based on IGF-1 levels appropriate for age and sex.[65] GH replacement therapy should be initiated as early as possible after diagnosis of GH insufficiency and continued until a desirable height is reached or growth velocity has decreased to <2.5 cm per year after the pubertal growth spurt. However, the suitable time point for discontinuation of therapy with growth-promoting doses remains controversial. Glucocorticoids may inhibit the growth-promoting effects of recombinant GH, and concomitant administration of androgens, estrogens, thyroid hormones, or anabolic steroids may accelerate epiphyseal closure and compromise final height.

Three large databases, the National Cooperative Growth Study, the Kabi International Growth Study, and the Australian and New Zealand growth database (OZGROW), have been developed to collect postmarketing adverse effect data or reports associated with recombinant GH. Development of these databases was prompted by the unexpected and tragic cases of CJD reported in patients treated with human pituitary GH. These databases are maintained by pharmaceutical companies that manufacture GH products.[66,67] Results from the recently released Safety and Appropriateness of Growth Hormone treatments in Europe (SAGhE) study provide additional long-term surveillance data from a noncommercial source.[67] Recombinant GH is generally well tolerated in children, and adverse effects are relatively uncommon.[66,68] A small number of patients may complain of injection-site pain or arthralgias. Idiopathic intracranial hypertension, also known as *pseudotumor cerebri*, has been reported in a very small number of children receiving GH therapy. This condition usually develops within the first 8 to 12 of weeks of treatment and presents with symptoms such as headache, blurred vision, diplopia, nausea, and vomiting.[66,68] The symptoms of idiopathic intracranial hypertension usually resolve after discontinuation of GH therapy, and long-term complications are rare. Cases of slipped capital femoral epiphysis have been reported in children with GH deficiency who are receiving GH therapy.[68] This condition is thought to occur as a result of the increased width of the femoral plate during GH treatment, but it also has been reported in GHD children who are not receiving GH replacement. Patients with this condition typically complain of hip or knee pain. Slipped capital femoral epiphysis can be managed by an orthopedic surgeon, and GH therapy does not need to be withdrawn. Because GH is known to cause decreased insulin sensitivity, hyperglycemia and diabetes mellitus may develop.[68] Patients who have specific predisposing risk factors for diabetes mellitus are at greatest risk for this adverse effect.[66,68] Glycosylated hemoglobin concentrations should be monitored in all patients receiving GH products.[47] GH could theoretically promote the growth of various types of neoplasms and increase tumor recurrence rates in patients with a history of malignancy.[47,66,68] For this reason, GH is not administered to patients with an active malignant tumor or a history of recurrent tumor growth. In 1988, a Japanese report indicated that children receiving GH therapy were twice as likely to develop leukemia as children who were not receiving the hormone. A more recent analysis of all collected reports of leukemia associated with GH therapy determined that these children had other leukemia risk factors (Fanconi's anemia, Bloom's syndrome, or history of cancer).[68] GH therapy in children without these risk factors does not appear to predispose children to develop leukemia.[66,68] Concerns were recently raised based on increased mortality rates seen in adult French subjects (SAGhE) who were treated with GH therapy as children.[69] The interpretation of these results have been questioned by some because of the large number of children (70%) in the study who had normal stature at baseline and also because of the higher doses of GH used in some patients.[70] Another recently published preliminary study from the SAGhE group representing patients from Belgium, The Netherlands, and Sweden did not find similar increases in mortality.[71] However, the observational design of these studies makes interpretation of the findings difficult. It should be noted that some authors have stressed the importance of using growth velocity and provocative testing in deciding whom and when to treat, and at what doses.[70] Finally, recent postmarketing reports suggest an increased risk of death associated with long-term GH treatment in children with Prader–Willi syndrome who are severely obese or have severe respiratory impairment. GH treatment is contraindicated in patients with Prader–Willi syndrome who have any of these risk factors.

Recombinant Insulin-Like Growth Factor-1

Recombinant IGF-1 (mecasermin [Increlex]) is approved by the FDA for the treatment of children with short stature due to severe primary IGF-1 deficiency (defined as children with height standard deviation score ≤–3.0 plus basal IGF-1 standard deviation score ≤–3.0, plus normal or elevated GH concentration) or GH gene deletion with neutralizing antibodies to GH. A combination of IGF-1 with IGFBP-3 (mecasermin rinfabate) was previously approved by FDA but has since been withdrawn from the market. Recombinant IGF-1 products are not intended for use in subjects with secondary forms of IGF-1 deficiency, such as GH deficiency, malnutrition, hypothyroidism, or chronic treatment with pharmacologic doses of antiinflammatory steroids. Recombinant IGF-1 products have been shown to increase growth velocity in children with short stature who have low IGF-1 serum concentrations and resistance to GH.[71–74] However, the efficacy of these agents is less than that reported with GH products in patients with GH deficiency.

The recommended dose of mecasermin is 0.04 to 0.12 mg/kg administered by subcutaneous injection twice daily. Because of the insulin-like effects of these products, patients should be monitored very closely for hypoglycemia, and the drug should be initiated at a dose at the lower end of the dosage range and administered with a meal or snack. Additional adverse effects experienced by patients receiving recombinant IGF-1 products include injection-site reactions, tonsillar/adenoidal hypertrophy, lymphoid hypertrophy, coarsening facial features, anaphylaxis, headache, dizziness, and arthralgia.[72–74] Intracranial hypertension has been reported in a small number of patients.[73] Additional studies are needed to elucidate the exact role of recombinant IGF-1 products in the management of short stature not caused by GH gene deletion or GH receptor defects.

Personalized Pharmacotherapy

Ongoing genetic studies are attempting to predict GH response in subjects. There is some evidence to suggest that patients with exon-3 deleted GH receptors or a specific polymorphism in the IGFBP-3 promoter gene have an enhanced response to GH therapy. However, recommendations regarding how therapy can be tailored to maximize patient benefit based on these findings are not available at this time. The large number of growth hormone deficiency disorders vary in phenotype and in biochemical and molecular characteristics thereby likely contributing to the variability of response reported in trials with GH or IGF-1. Given this variability, and in the absence of specific and well-validated indicators of response, therapy must be carefully individualized.[75]

Evaluation of Therapeutic Outcomes

Appropriate monitoring of therapy for GHD and non-GHD short stature includes regular assessments of height, weight, growth velocity, serum IGF-1 concentrations, and bone age every 6 to 12 months. Additional laboratory tests to monitor for potential adverse effects include serum glucose concentration and thyroid function. The dose of GH will periodically need to be increased as weight increases in growing children.

Conclusions

GH deficiency during childhood results in short stature. Replacement with recombinant GH is considered the mainstay of therapy for patients with GHD short stature, but its use for treatment of non-GHD short stature remains controversial, albeit such treatment is FDA approved. Recombinant GH has proven to be safe for use in children and is associated with few adverse effects. Preparations of IGF-1 may provide benefit for patients with non-GHD short stature. GH regimens can be particularly demanding and inconvenient for pediatric patients because they must be administered by subcutaneous injection. Knowledge of the long-term benefits and risks is critical to the development of rational, cost-effective treatments for patients with short stature.

PROLACTIN

Hyperprolactinemia

Prolactin is secreted in a pulsatile fashion by the lactotroph cells of the anterior pituitary, with the highest peak concentrations observed during sleep.[4] The secretion of prolactin is regulated primarily by tonic hypothalamic inhibitory effects of dopamine. As described earlier in this chapter and in Table 60-1, many factors can affect prolactin secretion. During pregnancy, prolactin serum concentrations rise substantially above normal. All other conditions characterized by excess prolactin serum concentrations, known as *hyperprolactinemia*, are considered pathologic. Hyperprolactinemia is a state of persistent serum prolactin elevation. Prolactin concentrations >20 mcg/L (>870 pmol/L) in women, and >25 mcg/L (>1,090 pmol/L) in men, observed on multiple occasions are generally considered indicative of hyperprolactinemia.[76] Hyperprolactinemia usually affects women of reproductive age.[76–78] The annual incidence of hyperprolactinemia in women between the ages of 24 and 35 years is approximately 24 cases per 1,000 person years.[77]

Hyperprolactinemia has several etiologies. The most common causes are benign prolactin-secreting pituitary tumors, known as *prolactinomas*, and various medications. Prolactinomas are classified according to size. Prolactin-secreting microadenomas are <10 mm in diameter and often do not increase in size.[4] In contrast, macroadenomas are tumors with a diameter >10 mm that continue to grow and can cause invasion of surrounding tissues.[4] In the presence of a prolactinoma, prolactin serum concentrations may remain normal or may be markedly elevated to thousands of micrograms per liter.

7 Any pharmacologic agent that antagonizes dopamine or increases the release of prolactin can induce hyperprolactinemia (Table 60-4).[79] Antipsychotic medications are the most frequently reported agents to cause hyperprolactinemia due to their potent dopamine-receptor blockade. Serotonin is a strong stimulator of prolactin secretion and antidepressants, such as selective serotonin reuptake inhibitors (SSRIs), monoamine oxidase (MAO) inhibitors, and tricyclic and tetracyclic agents, are associated with hyperprolactinemia.[79] More recently, the $5HT_1$ receptor agonist eletriptan has been implicated as a potential cause of hyperprolactinemia.[80] Metoclopramide and domperidone, an antiemetic available in Europe, are potent dopamine-receptor antagonists reported to induce hyperprolactinemia.[79] Hormones such as estrogen and progesterone, commonly prescribed as oral contraceptives, can stimulate lactotroph growth to promote prolactin secretion and have been implicated in drug-induced hyperprolactinemia. Although the exact mechanism of action remains to be determined, the calcium channel-blocking agent verapamil has been associated with cases of hyperprolactinemia.[4,79] Methyldopa and reserpine, although not used frequently in clinical practice today, are antihypertensive agents that can stimulate prolactin secretion.[79] Prolactin concentrations may increase with administration of GnRH analogs such as leuprolide or goserelin.[79] Other medications rarely reported to cause hyperprolactinemia include H_2-receptor blocking agents, benzodiazepines, opioids, and protease inhibitors.[4,79] Prolactin levels do not typically rise to >150 mcg/L (>6,500 pmol/L) in most cases of drug-induced hyperprolactinemia. Measurement of serum prolactin concentrations prior to the initiation of therapy with medications known to cause prolactin elevation may obviate the need for extensive examination of pituitary function and aid with the appropriate diagnosis of drug-induced hyperprolactinemia.

Less common etiologies include CNS lesions that physically compress the pituitary stalk and interrupt tonic hypothalamic dopamine secretion, resulting in hyperprolactinemia.[77] Increased TRH concentrations in hypothyroidism can stimulate prolactin secretion and cause hyperprolactinemia. During conditions of renal or hepatic compromise, the clearance of prolactin is decreased, resulting in elevated prolactin concentrations.[77] Despite vigorous diagnostic effort, the cause of hyperprolactinemia cannot always be determined. This is known as *idiopathic hyperprolactinemia* and most likely is a result of the presence of very small tumors that are not detected by standard imaging techniques.[76] It should be noted that many physiologic factors, such as stress (including the stress of phlebotomy), sleep, exercise, coitus, and eating, also can induce transiently elevated prolactin levels.[4,76] This emphasizes the importance of obtaining multiple prolactin measurements to confirm the diagnosis. Ideally, after an IV line is placed in the patient's arm, the patient should rest in a supine position or in a chair for 2 hours before prolactin samples are collected.

Elevated prolactin serum concentrations inhibit gonadotropin secretion and sex-steroid synthesis.[76] Because prolactin concentrations >60 mcg/L (>2,600 pmol/L) are associated with anovulation, women with hyperprolactinemia typically present with menstrual irregularities such as oligomenorrhea or amenorrhea and infertility.[76,77] In addition, approximately 40% to 80% of women with hyperprolactinemia will have galactorrhea.[76,77] The clinical presentation of patients with hyperprolactinemia is summarized in Table 60-5.[4,76,77]

TABLE 60-4 Drug-Induced Hyperprolactinemia

Dopamine antagonists
Antipsychotics
Phenothiazines
Metoclopramide
Domperidone
Prolactin stimulators
Methyldopa
Reserpine
Selective serotonin reuptake inhibitors (SSRIs)
$5HT_1$ receptor agonists
Estrogens
Progestins
Protease inhibitors
Gonadotropin-releasing hormone analogs
Benzodiazepines
Tricyclic and tetracyclic antidepressants
Monoamine oxidase inhibitors
H_2-Receptor antagonists
Opioids
Cocaine
Other
Verapamil

From Molitch,[4] Melmed,[77] Gillam et al.,[78] Molitch,[79] and Yilmaz et al.[80]

TABLE 60-5 Clinical Presentation of Hyperprolactinemia

General
Hyperprolactinemia most commonly affects women and is very rare in men

Signs and symptoms
- The patient may complain of symptoms related to local effects of the prolactin-secreting tumor, such as headache and visual disturbances, that result from tumor compression of the optic chiasm
- Female patients experience oligomenorrhea, amenorrhea, galactorrhea, infertility, decreased libido, hirsutism, and acne
- Male patients experience decreased libido, erectile dysfunction, infertility, reduced muscle mass, galactorrhea, and gynecomastia

Laboratory tests
Prolactin serum concentrations at rest will be >25 mcg/L (>1,090 pmol/L)

Additional clinical sequelae
- Prolonged suppression of estrogen in premenopausal women with hyperprolactinemia leads to decreased bone mineral density and significant risk for development of osteoporosis
- Risk for ischemic heart disease may be increased with untreated hyperprolactinemia

From Molitch,[4] Schlechte,[76] and Melmed, et al.[77]

The diagnosis of hyperprolactinemia, as defined by a prolactin serum concentration >25 mcg/L (>1,090 pmol/L), is relatively simple.[77] However, identifying the underlying cause of this abnormality may be more challenging. Patients with modest prolactin elevations should have multiple prolactin serum determinations to minimize the potential for detecting only transient increases in prolactin. A careful medication history is essential, and the presence of hypothyroidism, renal failure, or hepatic dysfunction should be evaluated. If the cause of hyperprolactinemia remains ambiguous, a computed tomography scan or magnetic resonance imaging study should be performed to determine the presence of a pituitary tumor.[76,77] If an underlying cause of elevated prolactin serum concentration is not determined, the hyperprolactinemia is considered to be idiopathic.

Clinical **Controversy...**

For patients with antipsychotic-induced hyperprolactinemia in whom it is not feasible to withdraw the offending agent, treatment with dopamine agonists is controversial due to the potential for exacerbation of the underlying psychosis.

TREATMENT
Hyperprolactinemia

The treatment of hyperprolactinemia depends on the underlying cause of the abnormality. In cases of drug-induced hyperprolactinemia, discontinuation of the offending medication and initiation of an appropriate therapeutic alternative usually normalize serum prolactin concentrations.[79] In cases for which an appropriate therapeutic alternative does not exist, medical therapy with dopamine agonists may be carefully considered.[77] Sex-steroid replacement also should be considered.[77] Treatment options for the management of prolactinomas include clinical observation, medical therapy with dopamine agonists, radiation therapy, and transsphenoidal surgical removal of the tumor.[4,76–78] Because prolactin-secreting microadenomas are very small and typically do not increase in size, treatment of these tumors is primarily directed toward alleviating symptoms.[76–78] The goal of therapy is to normalize prolactin serum concentrations and reestablish gonadotropin secretion to restore fertility and reduce the risk of osteoporosis. In patients with asymptomatic elevations in serum prolactin, observation and close follow-up are appropriate.[76–78] For women with amenorrhea who do not wish to become pregnant, dopamine agonist therapy may not be necessary. In these patients, sex-steroid replacement and close follow-up may be sufficient.[76] Treatment goals are more aggressive in patients with prolactin-secreting macroadenomas because these tumors are larger and can cause invasion of local tissues with significant visual defects.[78] Therefore, in addition to normalizing prolactin concentrations, tumor shrinkage and correction of visual defects are primary goals of treatment.

Medical therapy with dopamine agonists usually is more effective than transsphenoidal surgery for both types of pituitary prolactinomas.[4,76–78] Postsurgical cure rates differ depending on tumor type and expertise of the neurosurgeon. Long-term cure rates are reported to be approximately 60% for microprolactinomas and only 25% for macroprolactinomas.[4] Transsphenoidal surgery for removal of prolactinomas usually is reserved for patients who are refractory to or cannot tolerate therapy with dopamine agonists and for patients with very large tumors that cause severe compression of adjacent tissues.[4,76–78] Radiation therapy may require several years for effective tumor shrinkage and reduction in serum prolactin concentrations and usually is used only in conjunction with surgery.[4]

Pharmacologic Therapy

Medical therapy with dopamine agonists has proven to be very effective in normalizing prolactin serum concentrations, restoring gonadal function, and reducing tumor size.[4,77] Cabergoline, a long-acting dopamine agonist that offers the advantage of less-frequent dosing, is the agent of choice for the medical management of prolactinomas because of its superior efficacy in comparison to bromocriptine.[77]

Bromocriptine

Bromocriptine was the first D_2-receptor agonist to be used in the treatment of hyperprolactinemia and had been the mainstay of therapy for over 20 years. It inhibits the release of prolactin by directly stimulating postsynaptic dopamine receptors in the hypothalamus. Hypothalamic release of dopamine (prolactin-inhibitory hormone) inhibits the release of prolactin. Decreases in serum prolactin concentrations occur within 2 hours of oral administration, with maximal suppression occurring after 8 hours and suppressive effects persisting for up to 24 hours. Medical therapy with bromocriptine normalizes prolactin serum concentrations, restores gonadotropin production, and shrinks tumor size in approximately 90% of patients with microprolactinomas and 70% of patients with macroprolactinomas.[78]

For the management of hyperprolactinemia, bromocriptine therapy typically is initiated at a dose of 1.25 to 2.5 mg once daily at bedtime to minimize adverse effects.[76] The dose can be gradually increased by 1.25-mg increments every week to obtain desirable serum prolactin concentrations. Usual therapeutic doses of bromocriptine range from 2.5 to 15 mg/day, although some patients may require doses as high as 40 mg/day.[77] Bromocriptine usually is administered in two or three divided doses, but once-daily dosing has also been shown to be effective.[78]

The most common adverse effects associated with bromocriptine therapy include CNS symptoms such as headache, lightheadedness, dizziness, nervousness, and fatigue. GI effects such as nausea, abdominal pain, and diarrhea also are common. Bromocriptine should be administered with food to decrease the incidence of adverse GI effects. Although most of these adverse effects diminish with continued treatment, approximately 12% of patients will not tolerate the adverse effects associated with bromocriptine therapy.[78] Vaginal preparations of bromocriptine have been studied in an effort to decrease the incidence of adverse effects associated with oral dosage forms.[4,77,81]

Because most patients with hyperprolactinemia are women with a principal complaint of infertility, the safety of bromocriptine in pregnancy must be considered. Greater than 6,000 pregnancies have been reported in women who received bromocriptine throughout gestation, and an increased risk for spontaneous abortion or congenital anomalies has not been detected.[77] Although bromocriptine does not appear to be teratogenic, most clinicians discontinue therapy as soon as pregnancy is detected because the effects of in utero exposure to bromocriptine on gonadal function and fertility of the offspring remain unknown.[4,76–78] In patients with macroprolactinomas undergoing rapid tumor expansion, bromocriptine therapy may need to be continued throughout pregnancy.

Cabergoline

8 Cabergoline is a long-acting dopamine agonist with high selectivity and affinity for dopamine D_2-receptors. This agent is approved for treatment of hyperprolactinemia and has been shown to effectively reduce serum prolactin concentrations and tumor size in patients with both microprolactinomas and macroprolactinomas.[77] A recent systematic review and meta-analysis of four clinical trials comparing the efficacy of cabergoline and bromocriptine reported

that cabergoline was significantly more effective in normalizing serum prolactin concentrations.[82] Cabergoline has also proved effective in patients who are intolerant of or resistant to bromocriptine, and the data suggest that cabergoline is as effective in men as in women with microprolactinomas and macroprolactinomas.[77,83]

Cabergoline is commercially available as 0.5-mg oral tablets. The initial dose of cabergoline for treatment of hyperprolactinemia is 0.25 to 0.5 mg once weekly or in divided doses twice weekly. This dose may be increased by 0.5-mg increments at 4-week intervals based on serum prolactin concentrations.[84] The usual dose is 1 to 2 mg weekly; doses >3 mg per week are infrequently required. However, doses as high as 12 mg weekly have been used safely in patients with treatment-resistant prolactinomas.[85] Following oral administration, peak serum concentrations are obtained within 2 hours, and food does not affect absorption. The elimination of cabergoline from the pituitary appears to be very slow; this rate may explain the long duration of action. Cabergoline is extensively metabolized in the liver by hydrolysis, and the dose should be reduced in patients with severe hepatic failure. This drug is eliminated primarily in the feces, and the elimination half-life ranges from 79 to 155 hours in hyperprolactinemic patients.

The most common adverse effects reported with use of cabergoline are nausea, vomiting, headache, and dizziness.[78,84] These effects are similar to the adverse effects reported with bromocriptine. However, in a large comparative study evaluating bromocriptine and cabergoline, fewer patients receiving cabergoline reported adverse effects than did patients receiving bromocriptine, and only 3% of the patients in the cabergoline group withdrew from the study because of adverse effects versus 12% of patients taking bromocriptine.[86] Other adverse events associated with use of cabergoline include constipation, fatigue, anxiety, depression, and nasal congestion.[77,84] As with other dopamine agonists, adverse events usually occur early in therapy and subside with continued treatment. However, in one study 15% to 20% of patients receiving cabergoline experienced a recurrence of early symptoms or an onset of new symptoms after several weeks of treatment.[86] Mild-to-moderate decreases in blood pressure have been observed in up to 50% of patients taking cabergoline; however, the incidence of symptomatic orthostatic hypotension has not been significant.[84,86] Transient increases in serum alkaline phosphatase, bilirubin, and aminotransferases have been reported in small numbers of patients receiving cabergoline.[86] Pleuropulmonary disease[78] and newly diagnosed cardiac valve regurgitation[87] have been reported with cabergoline use at the larger doses used in the treatment of Parkinson's disease. Although symptomatic cardiac valve abnormalities have not been observed with cabergoline when administered in doses used for the treatment of prolactinomas, some clinicians have recommended routine echocardiography for patients receiving long-term cabergoline treatment for prolactinomas.[88,89]

9 Use of cabergoline in pregnancy has not been extensively studied. However, several case reports of women who received cabergoline therapy during the first and second trimesters of pregnancy have not documented an increased risk of spontaneous abortion, congenital abnormalities, or tubal pregnancy.[90] However, prospective data in large numbers of pregnancies are lacking. Because of the long half-life and limited data on cabergoline use in pregnancy, current guidelines recommend that women receiving cabergoline therapy who plan to become pregnant should discontinue the medication as soon as pregnancy is detected.[77]

Other dopamine agonists that have been used in the treatment of hyperprolactinemia but are not commercially available in the United States include lisuride, terguride, metergoline, dihydroergocristine, and quinagolide.[78] Quinagolide, a D_2-receptor agonist used frequently in Europe, is dosed once daily. Quinagolide has been shown to be as effective as bromocriptine for the management of hyperprolactinemia and may be effective in the treatment of patients who are resistant to or intolerant of bromocriptine.[78]

Personalized Pharmacotherapy

Genetic predisposition to the development of hyperprolactinemia has been reported involving the D_2 receptor and hormone-related genes.[91,92] However, recommendations regarding how therapy can be individualized to maximize patient benefit are not available.

Evaluation of Therapeutic Outcomes

Prolactin serum concentrations should be monitored every 3 to 4 weeks after the initiation of any dopamine-agonist therapy to assess efficacy and appropriately titrate medication dosage.[76] In addition, symptoms such as headache, visual disturbances, menstrual cycles in women, and sexual function in men should be evaluated to assess clinical response to therapy. Once prolactin concentrations have normalized and clinical symptoms of hyperprolactinemia have resolved with dopamine-agonist therapy, prolactin serum concentrations should be monitored every 6 to 12 months. In patients receiving long-term treatment, the dose of the dopamine agonist can be gradually reduced or discontinued in some patients. For patients who have received medical therapy with dopamine agonists for at least 2 years, therapy may be tapered or discontinued if normal serum prolactin concentrations are achieved in the absence of visible tumor.[77] Follow-up of such patients should include prolactin serum concentration measurements every 3 months for the first year (continued annually thereafter), with assessment of MRI findings if prolactin concentrations are elevated.

Conclusions

Hyperprolactinemia is a common disorder that can have a significant impact on fertility. Hyperprolactinemia is most commonly caused by the presence of prolactin-secreting pituitary tumors and various medications that antagonize dopamine or increase the secretion of prolactin. Available treatment options for this disorder include medical therapy with dopamine agonists, radiation therapy, and transsphenoidal surgery. In most cases, medical therapy with dopamine agonists is considered the most effective treatment. Cabergoline is the mainstay of medical therapy because it appears to be better tolerated and more effective.

PANHYPOPITUITARISM

10 Panhypopituitarism is a condition of complete or partial loss of anterior and posterior pituitary function resulting in a complex disorder characterized by multiple pituitary hormone deficiencies. Patients with panhypopituitarism may have ACTH deficiency, gonadotropin deficiency, GH deficiency, hypothyroidism, and hyperprolactinemia. Panhypopituitarism can be classified as either primary or secondary depending on the etiology. Primary panhypopituitarism involves an abnormality within the secretory cells of the pituitary, whereas secondary panhypopituitarism is caused by a lack of proper external stimulation needed for normal release of pituitary hormones. Some of the most common causes of panhypopituitarism include primary pituitary tumors, ischemic necrosis of the pituitary, surgical trauma, irradiation, and various types of CNS infections. Pharmacologic treatment of panhypopituitarism is essential and consists of replacement of specific pituitary hormones after careful assessment of individual deficiencies. Replacement most often consists of glucocorticoids, thyroid hormone preparations, and sex steroids. Administration of recombinant GH also may be necessary. Patients with panhypopituitarism will need lifelong replacement therapy and constant monitoring of multiple homeostatic functions.

ACKNOWLEDGMENT

This research was supported in part by the Intramural Research Program of the National Institute of Child Health and Human Development, National Institutes of Health.

ABBREVIATIONS

ACTH	adrenocorticotropic hormone
CJD	Creutzfeldt–Jakob's disease
CRH	corticotropin-releasing hormone
FSH	follicle-stimulating hormone
GH	growth hormone
GHD	growth hormone-deficient
GHRH	growth hormone-releasing hormone
GnRH	gonadotropin-releasing hormone
IGF	insulin-like growth factor
IGFBP-3	insulin-like growth factor-1 binding protein-3
LH	luteinizing hormone
OGTT	oral glucose tolerance test
SGA	small for gestational age
SHOX	short stature homeobox-containing gene
SSRI	selective serotonin reuptake inhibitor
TRH	thyrotropin-releasing hormone
TSH	thyroid-stimulating hormone
VIP	vasoactive intestinal peptide

REFERENCES

1. Watts AG. Structure and function in the conceptual development of mammalian neuroendocrinology between 1920 and 1965. Brain Res Rev 2011;66:174–204
2. Amar AP, Weiss MH. Pituitary anatomy and physiology. Neurosurg Clin North Am 2003;14:11–23.
3. Sam S, Frohman LA. Normal physiology of hypothalamic pituitary regulation. Endocrinol Metab Clin North Am 2008;37:1–22.
4. Molitch ME. Disorders of prolactin secretion. Endocrinol Metab Clin North Am 2001;30:585–610.
5. Werner H, Weinstein D, Bentov I. Similarities and differences between insulin and IGF-1: Structures, receptors, and signaling pathways. Arch Physiol Biochem 2008;114:17–22.
6. Ribeiro-Oliveira A Jr, Barkan A. The changing face of acromegaly-advances in diagnosis and treatment. Nat Rev Endocrinol 2012;8:605–611.
7. Verge CF, Mowat D. Overgrowth. Arch Dis Child 2010;95:458–463.
8. Katznelson L, Atkinson JL, Cook DM, et al. American Association of Clinical Endocrinologists medical guidelines for clinical practice for the diagnosis and treatment of acromegaly—2011 update. 2011;17(Suppl 4):1–44.
9. Melmed S. Acromegaly. N Engl J Med 2006;355:2558–2573.
10. Dekkers OM, Biermasz NR, Pereira AM, et al. Mortality in acromegaly: A metaanalysis. J Clin Endocrinol Metab 2008;93:61–67.
11. Attal P, Chanson P. Endocrine aspects of obstructive sleep apnea. J Clin Endocrinol Metab 2010;95:483–495.
12. Lombardi G, Galdiero M, Auriemma RS, et al. Acromegaly and the cardiovascular system. Neuroendocrinology 2006;83:211–217.
13. Jenkins PJ. Cancers associated with acromegaly. Neuroendocrinology 2006;83:218–223.
14. Cordero RA, Barkan AL. Current diagnosis of acromegaly. Rev Endocr Metab Disord 2008;9:13–19.
15. Melmed S, Casanueva FF, Klibanski A, et al. A consensus on the diagnosis and treatment of acromegaly complications. Pituitary 2012. doi:10.1007/s11102-012-0420-x.
16. Giustina A, Chanson P, Bronson MD, et al. A consensus on criteria for cure of acromegaly. J Clin Endocrinol Metab 2010;95:3141–3148.
17. Neggers SJ, Biermasz NR, van der Lely AJ. What is active acromegaly and which parameters do we have? Clin Endocrinol 2012;75:609–614.
18. Melmed S. Acromegaly pathogensis and treatment. J Clin Invest 2009;119:3189–3202.
19. Sherlock M, Woods C, Sheppard MC. Medical therapy in acromegaly. Nat Rev Endocrinol 2011;7:291–300.
20. Fleseriu M, Delashaw JB Jr, Cook DM. Acromegaly: A review of current medical therapy and new drugs on the horizon. Neurosurg Focus 2010;29:E15.
21. Sandret L, Maison P, Chanson P. Place of cabergoline in acromegaly: A meta-analysis. J Clin Endocrinol Metab 2011;96:1327–1335.
22. Cheng V, Faiman C, Kennedy L, et al. Pregnancy and acromegaly: A review. Pituitary 2012;15:59–63.
23. Felders RA, Hofland LJ, van Aken MO, et al. Medical therapy of acromegaly: Efficacy and safety of somatostatin analogs. Drugs 2009;69:2207–2226.
24. Fleseriu M. Clinical efficacy and safety results for dose escalation of somatostatin receptor ligands in patients with acromegaly: A literature review. Pituitary 2011;14: 184–193.
25. Vance ML, Harris AG. Long-term treatment of 189 acromegalic patients with the somatostatin analog octreotide. Results of the international multicenter acromegaly study group. Arch Intern Med 1991;151:1573–1578.
26. Ezzat S, Snyder PJ, Young WF, et al. Octreotide treatment of acromegaly: A randomized, multicenter study. Ann Intern Med 1992;117:211–218.
27. Cozzi R, Montini M, Attanasio R, et al. Primary treatment of acromegaly with ocretotide LAR: A long-term (up to nine years) prospective study of its efficacy in the control of disease activity and tumor shrinkage. J Clin Endocrinol Metab 2006;91:1397–1403.
28. Tolis G, Angelopoulos NG, Katounda E, et al. Medical treatment of acromegaly: Comorbidities and their reversibility by somatostatin analogs. Neuroendocrinology 2006;83:249–257.
29. Giustina A, Mazziotti G, Torri V, et al. Meta-analysis on the effects of octreotide on tumor mass in acromegaly. PLoS One 2012;7:e36411
30. Yang LP, Keating GM. Octreotide long-acting release (LAR): A review of its use in the management of acromegaly. Drugs 2010;70:1745–1769.
31. Murray RD, Melmed S. A critical analysis of clinically available somatostatin analog formulations for therapy of acromegaly. J Clin Endocrinol Metab 2008;93: 2957–2968.
32. Gilbert JA, Miell JP, Chambers SM, et al. The nadir growth hormone after an octreotide test dose predicts the long-term efficacy of somatostatin analogue therapy in acromegaly. Clin Endocrinol 2005;62:742–747.
33. Colao A, Auriemma RS, Lombardi G, Pivonello R. Resistance to somatostatin analogs in acromegaly. Endocr Rev 2011;32:247–271.
34. Giustina A, Bonadonna S, Bugari G, et al. High-dose intramuscular octreotide in patients with acromegaly inadequately controlled on conventional somatostatin analogue therapy: A randomized, controlled trial. Eur J Endocrinol 2009;161:331–338.

35. Mazziotti G, Giustina A. Effects of lanreotide SR and Autogel on tumor mass in patients with acromegaly: A systematic review. Pituitary 2010;13:60–67.
36. Croxtall JD, Scott LJ. Lanreotide Autogel: A review of its use in the management of acromegaly. Drugs 2008;68:711–723.
37. Ronchi CL, Boschetti M, Degli Uberti EC, et al. Efficacy of a slow-release formulation of lanreotide (Autogel 120) in patients with acromegaly previously treated with ocretotide long-acting release (LAR): An open, longitudinal, multicenter study. Clin Endocrinol 2007;67:512–519.
38. Mazziotti G, Floriani I, Bonadonna S, et al. Effects of somatostatin analogs on glucose homeostasis: A metaanalysis of acromegaly studies. J Clin Endocrinol Metab 2009;94:1500–1508.
39. Colao A, Auriemma RS, Savastano S, et al. Glucose tolerance and somatostatin analog treatment in acromegaly: A 12-month study. J Clin Endocrinol Metab 2009;94: 2907–2914.
40. van der Lely AJ, Kopchick JJ. Growth hormone receptor antagonists. Neuroendocrinology 2006;83:264–268.
41. Hodish I, Barkan A. Long-term effects of pegvisomant in patients with acromegaly. Nat Clin Pract Endocrinol Metab 2008;4:324–332.
42. van der Lely AJ, Biller BM, Brue T, et al. Long-term safety of pegvisomant in patients with acromegaly: Comprehensive review of 1288 subjects in ACROSTUDY. J Clin Endocrinol Metab 2012;97:1589–1597.
43. Schreiber I, Buchfelder M, Droste M, et al. Treatment of acromegaly with the GH receptor antagonist pegvisomant in clinical practice: Safety and efficacy evaluation from the German Pegvisomant observational study. Eur J Endocrinol 2007;156:75–82.
44. Neggers SJ, van der Lely AJ. Somatostatin analog and pegvisomant combination therapy for acromegaly. Nat Rev Endocrinol 2009;5:546–552.
45. Mullis PE. Genetics of GHRH, GHRH-receptor, GH and GH-receptor: Its impact on pharmacogenetics. Best Pract Res Clin Endocrinol Metab 2011;25:25–41.
46. Bernabeu I, Alvarez-Escola C, Quinteiro C, et al. The exon 3-deleted growth hormone receptor is associated with better response to pegvisomant therapy in acromegaly. J Clin Endocrinol Metab 2010;95:222–229.
47. American Association of Clinical Endocrinologists. Medical guidelines for clinical practice for growth hormone use in adults and children—2003 Update. Endocr Pract 2003;9:64–76.
48. Cohen P, Rogol AD, Deal CL, et al. Consensus statement on the diagnosis and treatment of children with idiopathic short stature: A summary of the Growth Hormone Research Society, the Lawson Wilkins Pediatric Endocrine Society, and the European Society for Pediatric Endocrinology Workshop. J Clin Endocrinol Metab 2008;93:4210–4217.
49. Wilson TA, Rose SR, Cohen P, et al. Update of guidelines for the use of growth hormone in children: The Lawson Wilkins Pediatric Endocrine Society Drug and Therapeutics Committee. J Pediatr 2003;143:415–421.
50. Molitch ME, Clemmons DR, Malozowski S, et al. Evaluation and treatment of adult growth hormone deficiency: An Endocrine Society clinical practice guideline. J Clin Endocrinol Metab. 2011;96:1587–1609.
51. Franklin SL, Geffner ME. Growth hormone: The expansion of available products and indications. Pediatr Clin North Am 2011;58:1141–1165.
52. Blethen SL, Bapitista J, Kuntze J, et al. Adult height in growth hormone (GH)-deficient children treated with biosynthetic GH. J Clin Endocrinol Metab 1997;82:418–420.
53. August GP, Julius JR, Blethen SL. Adult height in children with growth hormone deficiency who are treated with biosynthetic growth hormone: The national cooperative growth study experience. Pediatrics 1998;102:512–516.
54. Frinkik JP, Baptista J. Adult height in growth hormone deficiency: Historical perspective and examples from the national cooperative growth study. Pediatrics 1999;104:1000–1004.
55. Thomas M, Massa G, Bourguignon JP, et al. Final height in children with idiopathic growth hormone deficiency treated with recombinant human growth hormone: The Belgian experience. Horm Res 2001;55:88–94.
56. Rikken B, Massa GG, Wit JM, and the Dutch Growth Hormone Working Group. Final height in a large cohort of Dutch patients with growth hormone deficiency treated with growth hormone. Horm Res 1995;43:136–137.
57. Chipman JJ, Hicks JR, Holcombe JH, Draper MW. Approaching final height in children treated for growth hormone deficiency. Horm Res 1995;43:129–131.
58. Serveri F. Final height in children with growth hormone deficiency. Horm Res 1995;43:138–140.
59. Coste J, Letrait M, Carel JC, et al. Long term results of growth hormone treatment in France in children of short stature: Population, register based study. BMJ 1997;315:708–713.
60. Hazem A, Elamin MB, Bancos I, et al. Body composition and quality of life in adults treated with GH therapy: A systematic review and meta-analysis. Eur J Endocrinol 2012;166:13–20.
61. American Geriatrics Society 2012 Beers Criteria Update Expert Panel. American Geriatrics Society updated Beers Criteria for potentially inappropriate medication use in older adults. J Am Geriatr Soc 2012;60:616–631.
62. Ambler GR, Fairchild J, Wilkinson DJ. Debate: Idiopathic short stature should be treated with growth hormone. J Paediatr Child Health 2013;49:165–169.
63. Finkelstein BS, Imperiale TF, Speroff T, et al. Effect of growth hormone therapy on height in children with idiopathic short stature. Arch Pediatr Adolesc Med 2002; 156:230–240.
64. Deodati A, Cianfarani S. Impact of growth hormone therapy on adult height of children with idiopathic short stature: Systematic review. BMJ 2011;342:c7157.
65. Pawlikowska-Haddal A, Cohen P, Cook DM. How useful are serum IGF-1 measurements for managing GH replacement therapy in adults and children? Pituitary 2012;15:126–134.
66. Bell J, Parker KL, Swinford RD, et al. Long-term safety of recombinant human growth hormone in children. J Clin Endocrinol Metab 2010;95:167–177.
67. Rosenfeld RG, Cohen P, Robison LL, et al. Long-term surveillance of growth hormone therapy. J Clin Endocrinol Metab 2012;97:68–72.
68. Souza FM, Collett-Solberg PF. Adverse effects of growth hormone replacement therapy in children. Arq Bras Endocrinol Metabol 2011;55:559–565.
69. Carel JC, Ecosse E, Landlier F, et al. Long-term mortality after recombinant growth hormone treatment for isolated growth hormone deficiency or childhood short stature: Preliminary report of the French SAGhE study. J Clin Endocrinol Metab 2012;97:416–425.
70. Malozowski S. Reports of increased mortality and GH: Will this affect current clinical practice? J Clin Endocrinol Metab 2012;97:380–383.
71. Savendahl L, Maeas M, Albertsson-Wikland K, et al. Long-term mortality and causes of death in isolated GHD, ISS, and SGA patients treated with recombinant growth hormone

during childhood in Belgium, The Netherlands, and Sweden: Preliminary report of 3 countries participating in the EU SAGhE study. J Clin Endocrinol Metab 2012;97:E213–E217.

72. Collett-Solberg PF, Madhusmita M, the Drug and Therapeutics Committee of the Lawson Wilkins Pediatric Endocrine Society. The role of recombinant human insulin-like growth factor-I in treating children with short stature. J Clin Endocrinol Metab 2008;93:10–18.
73. Chernausek SD, Backeljauw PF, Frane J, et al. Long-term treatment with recombinant insulin-like growth factor (IGF)-1 in children with severe IGF-I deficiency due to growth hormone insensitivity. J Clin Endocrinol Metab 2007;992:902–910.
74. Balhara B, Misra M, Levitsky LL. Recombinant human IGF-1 (Insulin-like growth factor) therapy: Where do we stand today? Indian J Pediatr 2012;79:244–249.
75. Bang P, Ahmed SF, Argente J, et al. Identification and management of poor response to growth-promoting therapy in children with short stature. Clin Endocrinol 2012;77: 169–181.
76. Schlechte JA. Prolactinoma. N Engl J Med 2003;349: 2035–2041.
77. Melmed S, Casanueva FF, Hoffman AR, et al. Diagnosis and treatment of hyperprolactinemia: An Endocrine Society clinical practice guideline. J Clin Endocrinol Metab 2011;96:273–288.
78. Gillam MP, Molitch ME, Lombardi, et al. Advances in the treatment of prolactinomas. Endocr Rev 2006;27:485–534.
79. Molitch ME. Drugs and prolactin. Pituitary 2008;11:209–218.
80. Yilmaz H, Kaya M, Ozbek M, et al. A case of hyperprolactinemia, probably induced by eletriptan. Int J Clin Pharmacol Ther 2012;50:907–908.
81. Darwish AM, Hafez E, El-Gelbali I, et al. Evaluation of a novel vaginal bromocriptine mesylate formulation: A pilot study. Fertil Steril 2005;83:1053–1055.
82. dos Santos Nunes V, El Dib R, Boguszewski CL, et al. Cabergoline versus bromocriptine in the treatment of hyperprolactinemia: A systematic review of randomized controlled trials and meta-analysis. Pituitary 2011;14: 259–265.
83. Colao A, Vitale G, Cappabianca P, et al. Outcome of cabergoline treatment in men with prolactinoma: Effects of a 24-month treatment on prolactin levels, tumor mass, recovery of pituitary function, and semen analysis. J Clin Endocrinol Metab 2004;89:1704–1711.
84. Klibanski A. Prolactinomas. N Engl J Med 2010;362: 1219–1226.
85. Ono M, Miki N, Kawamata T, et al. Prospective study of high-dose cabergoline treatment of prolactinomas in 150 patients. J Clin Endocrinol Metab 2008;93:4721–4727.
86. Webster J, Piscitelli G, Polli A, et al. A comparison of cabergoline and bromocriptine in the treatment of hyperprolactinemic amenorrhea. N Engl J Med 1994;331:904–909.
87. Schade R, Andersohn F, Suissa S, et al. Dopamine agonists and the risk of cardiac-valve regurgitation. N Engl J Med 2007;356:29–38.
88. Herring N, Szmigielski C, Becher H, et al. Valvular heart disease and the use of cabergoline for the treatment of prolactinoma. Clin Endocrinol 2009;70:104–108.
89. Vallette S, Serri K, Rivera J, et al. Long-term cabergoline therapy is not associated with valvular heart disease in patients with prolactinomas. Pituitary 2009;12:153–157.
90. Colao A, Abs R, Barcena DG, et al. Pregnancy outcomes following cabergoline treatment: Extended results from a 12-year observational study. Clin Endocrinol 2008;68: 66–71.
91. Hansen KA, Zhang Y, Colver R, et al. The dopamine receptor D2 genotype is associated with hyperprolactinemia. Fertil Steril 2005;84:711–718.
92. Calarge CA, Elingrod VL, Acion L, et al. Variants of the dopamine D2 receptor and risperidone-induced hyperprolactinemia in children and adolescents. Pharmacogenet Genomics 2009;19:373–382.

Pregnancy and Lactation: Therapeutic Considerations

61

Kristina E. Ward and Barbara M. O'Brien

KEY CONCEPTS

1. Complex physiology surrounds the process of fertilization and pregnancy progression.
2. Drug characteristics and physiologic changes modify drug pharmacokinetics during pregnancy, including changes in absorption, protein binding, distribution, and elimination, requiring individualized drug selection and dosing.
3. Although drug-induced teratogenicity is a serious concern during pregnancy, most drugs required by pregnant women can be used safely. Informed selection of drug therapy is essential.
4. Healthcare practitioners must know where to find and how to evaluate evidence related to the safety of drugs used during pregnancy and lactation.
5. Health issues influenced by pregnancy, such as nausea and vomiting, can be treated safely and effectively with nonpharmacologic treatment or carefully selected drug therapy.
6. Some acute and chronic illnesses pose additional risks during pregnancy, requiring treatment with appropriately selected and monitored drug therapies to avoid harm to the woman and the fetus.
7. Management of the pregnant woman during the peripartum period can encompass uncomplicated pregnancies/deliveries, but can also include a wide variety of potential complications that require use of evidence-based treatments to maximize positive maternal and neonatal outcomes.
8. Understanding the physiology of lactation and pharmacokinetic factors affecting drug distribution, metabolism, and elimination can assist the clinician in selecting safe and effective medications during lactation.

A controversial and emotionally charged subject because of medicolegal and ethical implications, drug use in pregnancy and lactation is a topic often underemphasized in the education of health professionals. Clinicians are responsible for ensuring safe and effective therapy before conception, during pregnancy and parturition, and after delivery. Active patient participation is essential. Optimal treatments of illnesses during pregnancy sometimes differ from those used in the nonpregnant patient.

In many cases, medication dosing recommendations for acute or chronic illnesses in pregnant women are the same as for the general population. However, some cases require different dosing and selection of medications. Principles of drug use during lactation, although similar, are not the same as those applicable during pregnancy.

PHYSIOLOGY OF PREGNANCY

1 Fertilization and progression of pregnancy are complex, resulting in survival of only approximately 50% of embryos.[1] Because most losses occur early, usually in the first 2 weeks after fertilization, many women do not realize they were pregnant. Spontaneous loss of pregnancy later in gestation occurs in about 15% of pregnancies that survive the first 2 weeks after fertilization.[2]

Fertilization occurs when a sperm attaches to the outer protein layer of the egg, the zona pellucida, and renders the egg nonresponsive to other sperm.[3] The attached sperm releases enzymes that allow the sperm to fully penetrate the zona pellucida and contact the egg's cell membrane. The membranes of the sperm and egg then combine to create a new, single cell called a zygote. Male and female chromosomes join in the zygote, fuse to create a single nucleus, and organize for cell division.[4]

Fertilization usually occurs in the fallopian tube.[4] The fertilized egg travels down the fallopian tube over 2 days, with cell division taking place. By day 3, the fertilized egg reaches the uterus. Cell division continues for another 2 to 3 days in the uterine cavity before implantation. Approximately 6 days after fertilization, the cell mass is termed a *blastocyst*. Human chorionic gonadotropin (hCG) now is produced in amounts detectable by commercial laboratories. Implantation begins with the blastocyst sloughing the zona pellucida to rest directly on the endometrium allowing initiation of growth into the endometrial wall. By day 10 postfertilization, the blastocyst is implanted under the endometrial surface and receives nutrition from maternal blood.[4] Now it is called an *embryo*.[5]

After the embryonic period (between weeks 2 and 8 postfertilization), the conceptus is renamed a *fetus*.[6] Most body structures are formed during the embryonic period, and they continue to grow and mature during the fetal period. The fetal period continues until the pregnancy reaches term, approximately 40 weeks after the last menstrual period.[5]

Gravidity is the number of times that a woman is pregnant.[6,7] A multiple birth is counted as a single pregnancy. *Parity* refers to the number of pregnancies exceeding 20 weeks' gestation and relates information regarding the outcome of each pregnancy. In sequence, the numbers reflect (a) term deliveries, (b) premature deliveries,

(c) aborted and/or ectopic pregnancies, and (d) number of living children.[7] A woman who has been pregnant four times; has experienced two term deliveries, one premature delivery, and one ectopic pregnancy; and has three living children would be designated G_4P_{2113}.

Characteristics of Pregnancy

Pregnancy lasts approximately 280 days (about 40 weeks or 9 months); the time period is measured from the first day of the last menstrual period to birth.[6,7] *Gestational age* refers to the age of the embryo or fetus beginning with the first day of the last menstrual period, which is about 2 weeks prior to fertilization. When calculating the estimated due date, add 7 days to the first day of the last menstrual period then subtract 3 months. Pregnancy is divided into three periods of 3 calendar months, each called a *trimester*.

Early symptoms of pregnancy include fatigue and increased frequency of urination. At approximately 6 weeks' gestation, nausea and vomiting can occur. While commonly called *morning sickness*, it can happen at any time of the day. Nausea and vomiting usually resolve at 12 to 18 weeks' gestation. A pregnant woman can feel fetal movement in the lower abdomen at 16 to 20 weeks of gestation. Signs of pregnancy include cessation of menses, change in cervical mucus consistency, bluish discoloration of the vaginal mucosa, increased skin pigmentation, and anatomic breast changes.[6,7]

Pharmacokinetic Changes During Pregnancy

2 Normal physiologic changes that occur during pregnancy may alter medication effects, resulting in the need to more closely monitor and, sometimes, adjust therapy. Physiologic changes begin in the first trimester and peak during the second trimester. For medications that can be monitored by blood or serum concentration measurements, monitoring should occur throughout pregnancy.

During pregnancy, maternal plasma volume, cardiac output, and glomerular filtration increase by 30% to 50% or higher, potentially lowering the concentration of renally cleared drugs.[8,9] As body fat increases during pregnancy, the volume of distribution of fat-soluble drugs may increase. Plasma albumin concentration decreases, which increases the volume of distribution of drugs that are highly protein bound. However, unbound drugs are more rapidly cleared by the liver and kidney during pregnancy, resulting in little change in concentration. Hepatic perfusion increases, which could theoretically increase the hepatic extraction of drugs. Nausea and vomiting, as well as delayed gastric emptying, may alter the absorption of drugs. Likewise, a pregnancy-induced increase in gastric pH may affect the absorption of weak acids and bases. Higher levels of estrogen and progesterone alter liver enzyme activity and increase the elimination of some drugs but result in accumulation of others.[8,9]

Transplacental Drug Transfer

2 Although once thought to be a barrier to drug transfer, the placenta is the organ of exchange for a number of substances, including drugs, between the mother and fetus. Most drugs move from the maternal circulation to the fetal circulation by diffusion.[10] Certain chemical properties, such as lipid solubility, electrical charge, molecular weight, and degree of protein binding of medications, may influence the rate of transfer across the placenta.

Drugs with molecular weights less than 500 Da readily cross the placenta, whereas larger molecules (600 to 1,000 Da) cross more slowly.[10] Drugs with molecular weights greater than 1,000 Da, such as insulin and heparin, do not cross the placenta in significant amounts. Lipophilic drugs, such as opioids and antibiotics, cross the placenta more easily than do water-soluble drugs. Maternal plasma albumin progressively decreases, while fetal albumin increases during the course of pregnancy, which may result in higher concentrations of certain protein-bound drugs in the fetus. Fetal pH is slightly more acidic than maternal pH, permitting weak bases to more easily cross the placenta. Once in the fetal circulation, the molecule becomes more ionized and less likely to diffuse back into the maternal circulation.[10]

DRUG SELECTION DURING PREGNANCY

3 Many misconceptions exist regarding the association of medications and birth defects. Although some drugs have the potential to cause teratogenic effects, most medications required by pregnant women can be used safely.

The baseline risk for congenital malformations is approximately 3% to 6%, with approximately 3% considered severe.[2] Medication exposure is estimated to account for less than 1% of all birth defects. Genetic causes are responsible for 15% to 25%, other environmental issues (e.g., maternal conditions and infections) account for 10%, and the remaining 65% to 75% of congenital malformations result from unknown causes.[2]

Factors such as the stage of pregnancy during exposure, route of administration, and dose can affect outcomes.[2,11] In the first 2 weeks following conception, exposure to a teratogen may result in an "all-or-nothing" effect, which could either destroy the embryo or cause no problems.[11] During organogenesis (18 to 60 days postconception), organ systems are developing, and teratogenic exposures may result in structural anomalies. For the remainder of the pregnancy, exposure to teratogens may result in growth retardation, CNS abnormalities, or death. Examples of medications associated with teratogenic effects in the period of organogenesis include chemotherapy drugs (e.g., methotrexate, cyclophosphamide), sex hormones (e.g., diethylstilbestrol), lithium, retinoids, thalidomide, certain antiepileptic drugs, and coumarin derivatives. Other medications such as nonsteroidal antiinflammatory drugs (NSAIDs) and tetracycline derivatives are more likely to exhibit effects in the second or third trimester.

Medications are necessary during pregnancy for treatment of acute and chronic conditions. Identifying patterns of medication use before conception, eliminating nonessential medications and discouraging self-medication, minimizing exposure to medications known to be harmful, and adjusting medication doses are all strategies to optimize the health of the mother while minimizing the risk to the fetus. In summary, a small number of medications have the potential to cause congenital malformations, and many can be avoided during pregnancy. In situations where a drug may be teratogenic but is necessary for maternal care, considerations related to route of administration, dosage form, and dosing may lessen the risk.

Methods and Resources for Determining Drug Safety in Pregnancy

4 When assessing the safety of using medications during pregnancy, evaluation of the quality of the evidence is important. Ideally, safety data from randomized, controlled trials are most desirable, but pregnant women are not usually eligible for participation in clinical trials. Other types of data commonly used to estimate the risk associated with medication use during pregnancy include animal studies, case reports, case–control studies, prospective cohort studies, historical cohort studies, and voluntary reporting systems.

Animal studies are a required component of drug testing, but extrapolation of the results to humans is not always valid.[12]

Thalidomide was found to be safe in some animal models, but proved to have teratogenic effects in human offspring. The value of case reports is limited because birth defects in the offspring of women who used medication during pregnancy may occur by chance.[12] Case–control studies identify an outcome (congenital anomaly), match subjects with and without that outcome, and report how often exposure to a suspected agent occurred. Recall bias is a concern, as women with an affected pregnancy may be more likely to remember drugs used during the pregnancy than those with a normal outcome.

Cohort studies evaluate the intervention (use of a particular drug) in a group of persons and compare outcomes in a similar group of subjects without the intervention.[12,13] Prospective studies eliminate some of the problems with recall bias, but require time and large numbers of participants. Despite these disadvantages, cohort studies are often used for evaluating the effects of a drug exposure on pregnancy outcomes.

Teratology information services provide pregnant women with information about potential exposures during pregnancy and follow these women throughout the pregnancy to assess the outcomes of the pregnancy.[12] Services may publish pooled data to facilitate information sharing about medications used during pregnancy. Some pharmaceutical companies have organized voluntary reporting systems (also called pregnancy registries) for drugs used during pregnancy.

4 Computerized databases (e.g., *www.motherisk.org*, LactMed [*www.toxnet.nlm.nih.gov*]), tertiary compendia, and textbooks with information from large cohorts of treated women offer valuable assistance. New information regarding drug use in pregnancy and lactation can be obtained from searches of the primary literature for cohort and case–control studies.

The FDA developed risk categories (i.e., A, B, C, D, X, with A considered safe and X considered teratogenic) to guide clinicians regarding medication risk during pregnancy. The FDA ranks very few drugs as safe during pregnancy (category A) because a controlled trial is required to establish safety; this implies that few drugs are safe. Because of multiple limitations of the risk categories, the FDA proposed a new system in 2008 to replace the risk categories with a fetal risk summary and lactation risk summary. Each section discusses clinical considerations and summarizes available data.[14]

In summary, determining drug safety during pregnancy is limited by the quality of data and the types of study designs that can be used. While information from product labeling may provide a rough estimate of risks for medication-related adverse fetal outcomes, careful evaluation of other available information sources is necessary to make decisions about medication use in pregnant women.

PRECONCEPTION PLANNING

Pregnancy outcomes are influenced by maternal health status, lifestyle, and history prior to conception. The goal of preconception care is health promotion, evidence-based screening, and intervention in all women of reproductive age to ensure optimal health and improve pregnancy outcomes.[15] More than 60% of pregnancies in the United States are unintended. Of women who receive prenatal care, 18% seek it after the first trimester.[16] Preconception planning is important, since some behaviors and exposures impart risk to the fetus during the first trimester, often before prenatal care is begun or even before pregnancy is detected.[15] Table 61-1 lists selected preconception risk factors, the potential adverse pregnancy outcomes, and management or prevention options.

The most common major congenital abnormalities are neural tube defects (NTDs), cleft palate and lip, and cardiac anomalies. Each year in the United States approximately 1 in 1,000 infants are born with NTDs.[17] Folic acid supplementation of women substantially reduces the incidence of NTDs in their offspring. This is also true in women who have previously delivered babies with NTDs.[16,17] NTDs occur within the first month of conception because neural tube closure occurs during the first month of pregnancy. Folic acid supplementation with between 0.4 and 0.9 mg daily is recommended throughout a woman's reproductive years, since many pregnancies are unplanned and may not be recognized until after the first month.

TABLE 61-1 Selected Preconception Risk Factors for Adverse Pregnancy Outcomes

Preconception Risk Factor	Potential Adverse Pregnancy Outcomes	Management or Prevention Options
Use of known teratogens		
• Antiepileptic drugs	• Known teratogens; causes craniofacial, cardiac, and limb defects[a] • NTD • Fetal hydantoin syndrome	• Use lowest possible dose to maintain control • Folic acid 4 mg daily
• Isotretinoins	• Miscarriage • Known teratogen; causes CNS, craniofacial, and cardiac defects[a]	• Use effective pregnancy prevention
• Oral anticoagulants	• Fetal warfarin syndrome	• Switch to nonteratogenic anticoagulant (e.g., LMWH) before becoming pregnant
Lifestyle factors		
• Alcohol misuse	• Fetal alcohol syndrome	• Cease alcohol intake before conception
• Obesity	• NTD • Preterm delivery • Diabetes, HTN, VTE • Cesarean section	• Weight loss with appropriate nutritional intake before pregnancy

• Tobacco use	• Preterm birth
	• Low birth weight
	• Spontaneous abortion
	• Increased perinatal mortality
		• Ideally, cease tobacco use before conception
		• Nonpharmacologic therapies (e.g., CBT, counseling, hypnosis)
		• No consensus for NRT product, dosing, or frequency:
		  ▪ Intermittent forms (e.g., gum)
		  ▪ Transdermal patch (limit to 16 hours/day)
		• Bupropion risk may be less than risk posed by smoking; efficacy unclear
		• Varenicline safety unknown

CBT, cognitive behavioral therapy; HTN, hypertension; LMWH, low-molecular weight heparin; NRT, nicotine replacement therapy; NTD, neural tube defect; VTE, venous thromboembolism.

[a]List is not all-inclusive.

Data from references 15 and 19.

Use of alcohol and recreational drugs during pregnancy is associated with birth defects.[15] Of births in the United States in 2003, 10% were to mothers who smoked tobacco during pregnancy.[15] Smoking can cause preterm birth, low birth weight, and other adverse outcomes. In a systematic review of 72 trials of smoking cessation and perinatal outcomes, incidences of low birth weight and preterm birth were reduced, and birth weight increased by 54 g with smoking cessation.[18] Use of nicotine replacement during pregnancy is controversial, since its use is not supported by clinical trial data; however, nicotine replacement theoretically imparts less risk than exposure to the over 4,000 chemicals found in cigarettes.[19]

Clinical **Controversy. . .**

Smoking cessation during pregnancy is highly desirable but challenging. Smoking is known to cause spontaneous abortion, preterm birth, and increased perinatal mortality. Use of nicotine replacement therapy has been advocated by some, but nicotine does cross the placenta and has been shown to impair fetal growth in some animals.[19] Clinical evidence on the use of nicotine replacement during pregnancy is limited as is evidence for other pharmacologic treatment options.

PREGNANCY-INFLUENCED ISSUES

Pregnancy causes or exacerbates conditions that pregnant women commonly experience, including constipation, gastroesophageal reflux, hemorrhoids, and nausea and vomiting. Women with pregnancy-influenced GI issues can be treated safely with lifestyle modification or medications, many of them nonprescription. Gestational diabetes, gestational hypertension, and venous thromboembolism (VTE) have the potential to cause adverse pregnancy consequences. Gestational thyrotoxicosis (GTT) is usually self-limiting.

GI Tract

5 Constipation during pregnancy is prevalent, affecting 25% to 40% of women and may contribute to the development or exacerbation of hemorrhoids; hemorrhoids are more prevalent in pregnant women compared with the general population.[20,21] Light physical exercise and increased intake of dietary fiber and fluid should be instituted first for constipation.[21] If additional treatment is needed, supplemental fiber and/or a stool softener is appropriate.[22] Osmotic laxatives (polyethylene glycol, lactulose, sorbitol, and magnesium and sodium salts) are acceptable for short-term, intermittent use. Some consider polyethylene glycol the ideal laxative for use in pregnancy.[21,22] Senna and bisacodyl can be used occasionally. Castor oil and mineral oil should be avoided because they cause stimulation of uterine contractions and impairment of maternal fat-soluble vitamin absorption, respectively. Data supporting other management options for hemorrhoids during pregnancy are limited. Conservative treatment (i.e., high dietary fiber intake, adequate oral fluid intake, and use of sitz baths) should be tried first. Laxatives and stool softeners can be used if conservative management is inadequate for preventing or treating constipation. Topical anesthetics, skin protectants, and astringents (e.g., witch hazel) can be used for anal irritation and pain. Hydrocortisone may reduce inflammation and pruritis.[20]

Between 40% and 80% of pregnant women experience gastroesophageal reflux disease.[21] An algorithm starting with lifestyle and dietary modifications (e.g., small, frequent meals; alcohol and tobacco avoidance; food avoidance before bedtime; elevation of the head of the bed) should be used. If symptoms are not relieved, antacids (aluminum, calcium, or magnesium preparations) or sucralfate are acceptable; however, sodium bicarbonate and magnesium trisilicate should be avoided. Histamine-2 (H_2) receptor blockers can be used for patients unresponsive to lifestyle changes and antacids; evidence supports the use of ranitidine and cimetidine. Literature evaluating the use of famotidine and nizatidine is limited, but they are likely safe. Less data are available regarding the use of proton pump inhibitors (PPIs) during pregnancy. Although a recent cohort study of 5,082 live births with first trimester exposure to PPIs found no increased risk of major birth defects,[23] use of PPIs should be reserved for women who do not respond to H_2 antagonists.

Nausea and vomiting of pregnancy (NVP) is estimated to affect up to 90% of pregnant women. NVP usually begins during the fifth week of gestation and lasts through week 20; peak symptoms occur between weeks 10 and 16.[21,24] Hyperemesis gravidarum (HG; i.e., unrelenting vomiting causing weight loss of more than 5% prepregnancy weight, dehydration, electrolyte imbalance, and ketonuria) occurs in 0.3% to 2.3% of women.[25] Dietary modifications, such as eating frequent, small, bland meals and avoiding fatty foods, may be helpful. Applying pressure at acupressure point P6 on the volar aspect of the wrist may be beneficial. Pharmacotherapeutic approaches for NVP that have shown efficacy include pyridoxine (vitamin B_6), and antihistamines (including doxylamine).[24] Phenothiazines and metoclopramide are generally considered safe, but sedation and extrapyramidal effects, including dystonia, may limit use.[24] Increasing evidence of safety and efficacy with ondansetron is emerging; ondansetron is better tolerated than older antiemetics.[24] Corticosteroids are effective for HG but are associated with a small increase in the risk of oral clefts when used during the first trimester. Ginger has shown efficacy for hyperemesis in randomized, controlled trials and is probably safe.[21,24]

Gestational Diabetes

5 Gestational diabetes mellitus (GDM) is glucose intolerance of any degree identified during pregnancy, either of new onset or first recognition. It develops in about 7% of pregnant women, although the prevalence ranges from 1% to 14%.[26,27] Risks of GDM are many and include fetal loss, increased risk of major malformations, and fetal macrosomia. Although the U.S. Preventative Services Task Force Independent Expert Panel found a lack of evidence proving that screening for gestational diabetes decreases adverse maternal and fetal outcomes, a consensus panel of the International Association of Diabetes and Pregnancy Study Groups (IADPSG) recommends universal screening of pregnant women not previously diagnosed with diabetes.[26–29] At the first prenatal visit, all women considered high-risk for diabetes (e.g., obesity, glycosuria, strong family history of diabetes) should be screened for overt diabetes using either the A1C, fasting plasma glucose (FPG), or random plasma glucose (RPG).[27,29] Overt diabetes occurs if the A1C is greater than or equal to 6.5% (0.065; 48 mmol/mol Hgb), FPG is greater than or equal to 126 mg/dL (7.0 mmol/L), or RPG is greater than or equal to 200 mg/dL (11.1 mmol/L; requires confirmation with A1C or FPG). If overt diabetes is not diagnosed or for women not at high-risk for diabetes, the IADPSG recommends screening for GDM at weeks 24 to 28 using a 75-g oral glucose tolerance test (OGTT).[27,29] The American College of Obstetricians and Gynecologists (ACOG) recommends screening for gestational diabetes based on clinical risk factors or with the use of a 50 g, 1-hour glucose challenge test followed by a 100 g, 3-hour OGTT to diagnose GDM; this is commonly referred to as the "two-step" method.[30] Screening and diagnosis of GDM using the OGTT is described in the American Diabetes Association practice guidelines.[26,27]

Clinical **Controversy...**

The most common screening test for gestational diabetes in the United States is the 50-g, 1-hour glucose challenge test, that is followed by a 100-g, 3-hour glucose challenge if found to be elevated.[28,30] In 2011, the ACOG upheld this recommendation despite differing with a consensus panel from the IADPSG, with representation from the American Diabetes Association, which recommends universal screening using a 75-g, 2-hour OGTT.[27,29]

Dietary modification is considered first-line therapy for all women who have GDM, with additional caloric restriction for obese women.[31] Daily self-monitoring of blood glucose is required. Drug therapy should be initiated if the following levels are not achieved with dietary modification: FPG concentrations below 90 to 99 mg/dL (5.0 to 5.5 mmol/L), 1-hour postprandial plasma glucose concentration less than or equal to 140 mg/dL (7.8 mmol/L), or 2-hour postprandial plasma glucose concentration below 120 to 127 mg/dL (6.7 to 7.0 mmol/L).[31,32] Traditionally, insulin has been the drug of choice for diabetes management during pregnancy because it does not cross the placenta. Glyburide is an alternative because it minimally crosses the placenta. Increasing data suggest that, although it crosses the placenta, metformin appears to lack teratogenicity making it another alternative to insulin.[31,32]

Evidence supporting dietary modification, self-monitored blood glucose, exercise, and pharmacologic interventions for women with GDM is largely based on one randomized clinical trial that showed reductions in perinatal morbidity (composite of death, nerve palsy, bone fracture, and shoulder dystocia) with nutritional education, blood glucose monitoring, and insulin treatment.[33,34]

Hypertensive Disorders of Pregnancy

❺ Hypertensive disorders of pregnancy (HDP) complicate approximately 10% of pregnancies. Four categories of HDP are established: chronic hypertension (preexisting hypertension or developing before 20 weeks' gestation), gestational hypertension (hypertension without proteinuria developing after 20 weeks' gestation), preeclampsia (hypertension with proteinuria), and preeclampsia superimposed on chronic hypertension.[35] Hypertension in pregnancy is defined as a diastolic blood pressure (dBP) 90 mm Hg or greater based upon the average of two or more measurements from the same arm.[36] Nondrug managements of HDP center on activity restriction, stress reduction, and exercise; however, no evidence indicates that any of these approaches improves pregnancy outcome, and prolonged bed rest may increase the risk of venous thromboembolic disease.[36] Use of supplemental calcium 1 to 2 g/day decreases the relative risk of hypertension by 30% (range, 14% to 43%) and preeclampsia by 48% (range, 31% to 67%).[37] High-risk patients (those with the lowest initial calcium intake) benefited most; however, even women with adequate calcium intake at baseline had a 38% decrease in risk of preeclampsia. Therefore, 1 g/day of supplemental calcium is appropriate for all pregnant women. Antihypertensive drug therapy is discussed under Chronic Illnesses in Pregnancy.

While preeclampsia usually develops after 20 weeks' gestation, up to 30% of chronic and gestational hypertension are complicated by preeclampsia. Preeclampsia is a multisystem syndrome that complicates 2% to 8% of pregnancies and can cause poorer outcomes, including renal failure, maternal morbidity/mortality, preterm delivery, and intrauterine growth restriction.[38,39] Risk factors for development of preeclampsia include primiparity, previous preeclampsia, prepregnancy body mass index above 30 kg/m^2, tobacco use, underlying medical conditions (e.g., diabetes, antiphospholipid antibodies, autoimmune disease, renal disease), multiple gestations (i.e., twins), and ethnicity (black greater than white or Hispanic). Maternal age over 40 years is also a potential risk factor.[39] Signs and symptoms of preeclampsia include blood pressure elevation; proteinuria (300 [or more] mg/24 h); persistent severe headache; persistent new epigastric pain; visual changes; vomiting; hyperreflexia; sudden and severe swelling of hands, face, or feet; HELLP (hemolysis, elevated liver enzymes, low platelets); and increased serum creatinine. Low-dose aspirin (75 to 81 mg/day) in women at risk for preeclampsia decreases the risk of its development by 17%, which corresponds to prevention of one preeclampsia case for every 72 at-risk women treated. Decreased rates of preterm birth (8% reduction) and fetal or neonatal death (14% reduction) also result from low-dose aspirin use.[40] Treatment of hypertension in women with preeclampsia depends upon the blood pressure measurement and follows the same principles discussed under Chronic Illnesses in Pregnancy. The only cure for preeclampsia is delivery of the placenta.[41]

Preeclampsia may progress rapidly to eclampsia, which is the occurrence of seizures superimposed on preeclampsia. Eclampsia is a medical emergency. In high-risk women (i.e., previous severe preeclampsia, renal disease, autoimmune disease, diabetes, and chronic hypertension), use of low-dose aspirin prevents one case of preeclampsia for every 19 women treated.[40] Magnesium sulfate decreases the risk of progression to eclampsia by almost 60%; it is recommended to prevent eclampsia as well as treat eclamptic seizures. The usual dose for magnesium sulfate is 4 to 6 g IV over 15 to 20 minutes followed by a 2 g/h continuous infusion; duration of use varies, but the usual duration is 24 hours. Diazepam and phenytoin should be avoided.[42]

Thyroid Abnormalities

❺ During pregnancy, stimulation of the thyroid gland may occur because of hCG's structural similarity to thyroid-stimulating hormone (TSH; thyrotropin).[43] In 1% to 3% of pregnancies, gestational transient thyrotoxicosis (GTT) may result. Occurrence of GTT is often associated with HG. By 20 weeks' gestation, GTT usually resolves as production of hCG declines. Treatment with antithyroid medication is not usually needed.[43] Nausea and vomiting can be treated as for patients without this pseudohyperthyroid state.

Although not all women experience postpartum thyroiditis (PPT) similarly, the typical presentation is characterized by transient hyperthyroidism during the first 6 months postpartum, a period of transient hypothyroidism, and, finally, euthyroidism within 1 year.[43] The initial hyperthyroid state usually does not require treatment; however, β-blockers (propranolol, starting at 10 to 20 mg daily as needed) can provide symptomatic relief of adrenergic symptoms. Because PTT is from a destructive inflammation process and not overproduction of thyroid hormone, antithyroid drugs are ineffective. Levothyroxine is recommended in the hypothyroid phase of PPT for severe hypothyroid symptoms, duration of hypothyroidism greater than 6 months, breast-feeding women, or if another pregnancy is attempted. Levothyroxine replacement is suggested for a total of 6 to 12 months.[43] Occurrence of permanent hypothyroidism ranges from 2% to 21% of women affected by PPT.

Thromboembolism

❺ The risk of VTE in pregnant women is increased by five- to tenfold over nonpregnant women.[44] Low-molecular-weight heparin (LMWH) is recommended over unfractionated heparin (UFH) and warfarin for treatment of acute thromboembolism during pregnancy. Treatment should be continued throughout pregnancy and for 6 weeks after delivery; the minimum total duration of therapy should not be less than 3 months. Fondaparinux and injectable direct thrombin inhibitors (e.g., lepirudin, bivalirudin) should be avoided unless a severe allergy to heparin (e.g., heparin-induced thrombocytopenia) is present. Dabigatran, rivaroxaban, and apixaban are not recommended.[44] Warfarin is not used because it causes nasal hypoplasia, stippled epiphyses, limb hypoplasia, and eye abnormalities; the risk period appears to be between 6 and 12 weeks' gestation. CNS anomalies are associated with second- and third-trimester exposure.

Recurrent VTE is divided into three categories: low risk, intermediate risk, and high risk of recurrence. Antepartum monitoring is recommended for women with a single episode of VTE who have a low risk of recurrence (i.e., one transient risk factor [e.g., surgery, injury, lengthy travel, or immobility]). For intermediate risk (i.e., hormone-related, pregnancy-related, or unprovoked VTE) and high risk (i.e., more than one unprovoked VTE or continuous risk factors), antipartum prophylaxis with LMWH plus 6-week postpartum prophylaxis with either LMWH or warfarin is recommended. Specific recommendations for thrombophilias (e.g., antiphospholipid antibodies, Factor V Leiden, protein C and S deficiencies) can be found in the American College of Chest Physicians clinical practice guidelines.[44]

Women with prosthetic heart valves should receive LMWH (twice daily) or UFH (every 12 hours) during pregnancy. LMWH should be adjusted to achieve a peak anti-Xa level at 4 hours post-subcutaneous dose, while UFH treatment should target a midinterval aPTT at least twice the control value or an anti-Xa heparin level of 0.35 to 0.7 units/mL.[44] After a discussion of potential risks, LMWH or UFH can be used until week 13 of gestation with subsequent substitution of warfarin until the middle of the third trimester when LMWH or UFH should be resumed. In women considered very high-risk for VTE (e.g., older-generation prosthetic mitral valve, history of thromboembolism), prevention of maternal complications such as valve thrombosis exceeds the risk of fetal malformation; use of warfarin is appropriate until replacement with LMWH or UFH near the end of the third trimester. High-risk women with prosthetic heart valves may also receive low-dose aspirin (75 to 100 mg/day).[44]

ACUTE CARE ISSUES IN PREGNANCY

In some cases, the risks associated with the acute illness are magnified during pregnancy, and early screening and treatment become critical. In other cases, such as during treatment of certain sexually transmitted diseases, the urgency regarding treatment comes from an increased likelihood of infection leading to preterm labor. Occasionally, common acute care issues, such as migraine headache, improve during pregnancy.

Urinary Tract Infection

6 The most common infections in pregnant and nonpregnant women are urinary tract infections (UTIs). Typically, UTIs are characterized as asymptomatic (e.g., asymptomatic bacteriuria) or symptomatic (e.g., lower [cystitis] or upper [pyelonephritis]).[45,46] *Escherichia coli* is the primary cause of infection in 75% to 90% of cases.[46] Other gram-negative rods, such as *Proteus* and *Klebsiella*, as well as Group B *Streptococcus* (GBS) account for some infections. The presence of GBS in the urine indicates heavy colonization of the genitourinary tract, increasing the risk for GBS infection in the newborn.[47]

The incidence of asymptomatic bacteriuria ranges from 2% to 10%. Untreated, bacteriuria progresses to pyelonephritis in approximately 30% of pregnant women.[46,47] While no consensus regarding screening for asymptomatic bacteriuria exists, a urine culture obtained at the first prenatal visit is appropriate; some advocate a urine culture in each trimester. Use of rapid screening tests, such as dipsticks, should be avoided because of poor performance in pregnant women.[47] Acute cystitis occurs in about 1% to 3% of pregnant women. Signs and symptoms of acute cystitis include urgency, frequency, hematuria, pyuria, and dysuria.[46,47]

Treatment of asymptomatic bacteriuria is necessary to prevent pyelonephritis. For asymptomatic bacteriuria, the agents of choice and treatment duration are not well defined. Treatment of acute cystitis is similar to that of asymptomatic bacteriuria. Using outcomes of cure rates, recurrent infection, incidence of preterm delivery or rupture of membranes, admission to neonatal intensive care, need for change of antibiotic, or incidence of prolonged fever, antibiotic treatment has demonstrated effectiveness in treating symptomatic UTIs (including pyelonephritis) in pregnancy. No specific treatment appeared superior to other commonly used treatments.[45,47] Treatment courses for asymptomatic bacteriuria and cystitis of 7 to 14 days are common, but shorter courses of therapy may be sufficient.

The most commonly used antibiotics to treat asymptomatic bacteriuria and cystitis are the β-lactams (including penicillins and cephalosporins) and nitrofurantoin.[45,47] β-Lactams are not known teratogens; however, the incidence of *E. coli* resistance to ampicillin and amoxicillin limits their use as single agents. Nitrofurantoin is not active against *Proteus* species and should not be used after week 37 in patients with glucose-6-phosphate dehydrogenase deficiency because of a theoretical risk for hemolytic anemia in the neonate. Sulfa-containing drugs can contribute to the development of newborn kernicterus; use should be avoided during the last weeks of gestation. Trimethoprim is a folate antagonist and is relatively contraindicated during the first trimester because of associations with cardiovascular malformations. Regionally, increased rates of *E. coli* resistance to trimethoprim-sulfa may limit its use. Fluoroquinolones and tetracyclines are contraindicated because of potential associations with impaired cartilage development and deciduous teeth discoloration (if given after 5 months' gestation), respectively.[47]

Patients with pyelonephritis usually present with bacteriuria and systemic symptoms of costovertebral angle tenderness, dysuria, fever, flank pain, nausea, and vomiting.[46,47] Complications of pyelonephritis include premature delivery, low infant birth weight, hypertension, anemia, bacteremia, and transient renal failure. Hospitalization is the standard of care for pregnant women.[47] Inpatient therapy has included parenteral administration of cephalosporins (e.g., cefazolin, ceftriaxone), ampicillin plus gentamicin, or ampicillin–sulbactam. Switching to oral antibiotics can occur after the woman is afebrile for 48 hours; however, nitrofurantoin should be avoided because it does not achieve therapeutic levels outside of the urine. Outpatient antibiotic therapy can be considered after initial inpatient observation in women who are afebrile and less than 24 weeks' gestation. The total duration of antibiotic therapy for acute pyelonephritis is 10 to 14 days.[47] Suppression therapy with nitrofurantoin can be considered for the remainder of gestation.[46]

Sexually Transmitted Infections

6 Sexually transmitted infections (STIs) in pregnant women range from infections that may be transmitted across the placenta and infect the infant prenatally (e.g., syphilis) to organisms that may be transmitted during birth and cause neonatal infection (e.g., *Chlamydia trachomatis, Neisseria gonorrhoeae*, or herpes simplex virus [HSV]) to infections that pose a threat for preterm labor (e.g., bacterial vaginosis [BV]). Initial screening during the first prenatal visit is recommended for HIV, *C. trachomatis*, and syphilis. Women at high risk for gonorrhea or who live in an area of high prevalence as well as women at high risk for hepatitis C should also be screened during the first prenatal visit. Screening for hepatitis B using the surface antigen should occur during the first trimester. Treatment for selected STIs is summarized in Table 61-2.

TABLE 61-2 Management of Sexually Transmitted Diseases in Pregnancy

STI	Drug Name (Brand Name)	Usual Dose	Monitoring	Comments
Bacterial vaginosis	*Recommended:* Metronidazole (Flagyl) *OR* Clindamycin (Cleocin)	• 500 mg by mouth two times daily × 7 days • 250 mg by mouth three times daily × 7 days • 300 mg by mouth two times daily × 7 days	Follow-up testing not required if symptoms resolve	Vaginal preparations are not recommended because of the risk for subclinical upper-genital tract infection Intravaginal clindamycin during second half of pregnancy has caused low birth weight and neonatal infection
Chancroid	*Recommended:* Azithromycin (Zithromax) *OR* Ceftriaxone (Rocephin) *OR* Erythromycin base (Ery-Tab)	 1 g by mouth × 1 dose 250 mg IM × 1 dose 500 mg by mouth three times daily × 7 days	Re-examine after 3 to 7 days; ulcer improvement should be noticeable by 3 days. Complete healing depends on the ulcer size	Test for HIV when chancroid is diagnosed. If negative, serologic testing for syphilis and HIV should occur 3 months after chancroid diagnosis
Chlamydia	*Recommended:* Azithromycin (Zithromax) *OR* Amoxicillin (Amoxil) *Alternatives*[a]: Erythromycin base Erythromycin ethylsuccinate	 1 g by mouth × 1 dose 500 mg by mouth three times daily × 7 days	Test-of-cure at 3 weeks after therapy completion (except if in first trimester, then retest after 3 months)	Gonorrheal coinfection common; both are treated concurrently Chlamydial infection is asymptomatic in men and women Women below age 25 years and those at high risk (e.g., multiple partners) should be retested in the third trimester
Gonorrhea	*Recommended:* Ceftriaxone (Rocephin) *PLUS* Azithromycin (Zithromax) *Alternative:* Cefixime (Suprax) *PLUS* Azithromycin (Zithromax)	 250 mg IM × 1 dose 1 g by mouth × 1 dose 400 mg by mouth × 1 dose 1 g by mouth × 1 dose	Because of high reinfection rate, repeat testing for gonorrhea 3 months after treatment. For alternative regimen, test-of-cure required in 1 week	Chlamydial coinfection common; both are treated concurrently Use alternative regimen only if ceftriaxone not available
Syphilis[b]				
Primary, secondary, early latent	*Recommended:* Benzathine penicillin G (Bicillin L-A)	2.4 million units IM X 1 dose	Nontreponemal serologic evaluation[c] at 6 and 12 months	For treatment failure or reinfection, use same drug and dose but increase to 3 weekly injections unless neurosyphilis is present
Tertiary, late latent	*Recommended:* Benzathine penicillin G (Bicillin L-A)	2.4 million units IM X 3 doses at 1-week intervals	Nontreponemal serologic evaluation[c] at 6, 12, and 24 months. CSF examination may be required	Use this regimen for late latent or latent syphilis of unknown duration
Neurosyphilis	*Recommended:* Aqueous penicillin G (Pfizerpen) *Alternative:* Procaine penicillin (Wycillin, Pfizerpen-AS) *PLUS* Probenecid	 Three to four million units IV every 4 hours or continuous IV × 10–14 days 2.4 million units IM daily × 10–14 days 500 mg by mouth four times daily × 10–14 days	If initial elevation of leukocytes in CSF, repeat CSF every 6 months until normalization	Consider repeat treatment if CSF leukocytes or protein do not normalize after 2 years Use alternative regimen only if compliance can be ensured
Trichomoniasis	*Recommended:* Metronidazole	 2 g by mouth × 1 dose	Consider rescreening patients at 3 months because of high reinfection rate	While tinidazole is an alternative for nonpregnant women, safe use during pregnancy is not well-studied

CSF, cerebrospinal fluid; IM, intramuscular; STI, sexually transmitted infection.

[a]Refer to reference 47 for specific dosing recommendations.
[b]Pregnant women with history of penicillin allergy should undergo penicillin desensitization as no proven alternatives exist.
[c]Nontreponemal evaluation consists of VDRL (Venereal Disease Research Laboratory) and RPR (rapid plasma regain).

Data from references 48 and 49.

Syphilis

Syphilis is caused by *Treponema pallidum*; complications are many (e.g., mucocutaneous lesions, altered mental status, visual and auditory abnormalities, gumma, cranial nerve palsies). For women who live in areas with a high prevalence of syphilis, are at high risk, have not been previously tested, or had positive serology in the first trimester, additional serologic testing twice during the third trimester (28 to 32 weeks) and at delivery is recommended.[48] With the exception of neurosyphilis, which is treated with aqueous penicillin G, the drug of choice for all stages of syphilis is benzathine penicillin G. Penicillin effectively prevents transmission to the fetus and treats the fetus, if already infected. Treatment during the second half of pregnancy may increase the risk for preterm labor and fetal distress because a Jarisch-Herxheimer reaction may occur; however, treatment should not be withheld or delayed.[48]

Chlamydia and Gonorrhea

Chlamydia is the most commonly reported STI in the United States; complications of *C. trachomatis* include pelvic inflammatory disease (PID), ectopic pregnancy, and infertility. *C. trachomatis* infects the newborn through exposure to the infected cervix during delivery. Perinatal infection most commonly causes conjunctivitis that develops 5 to 12 days postpartum. A subacute, afebrile pneumonia with an onset at ages 1 to 3 months may occur.[48]

Gonorrhea, an STI caused by *N. gonorrhoeae*, is the second-most commonly reported notifiable infection in the United States.[49] In women, recognizable symptoms may be absent initially, but gonorrheal infection can cause PID, a known risk for infertility. Perinatal gonococcal infection results from exposure to the infected cervix during birth. Symptoms usually manifest within 2 to 5 days after delivery. Milder manifestations include rhinitis, vaginitis, and urethritis. More severe presentations include ophthalmia neonatorum and sepsis.[48] Identification and treatment of the infection in neonates is crucial as permanent sequelae such as blindness can occur.

Concerningly, antimicrobial resistance rates among *N. gonorrhoeae* are increasing which has prompted the Centers for Disease Control to remove oral cephalosporins as a preferred treatment option.[49] Coinfection with *C. trachomatis* is common; treatment of most *N. gonorrhoeae* infections includes treatment for *C. trachomatis*.[48,49]

Bacterial Vaginosis and Trichomoniasis

Bacterial vaginosis and trichomoniasis are STIs characterized by vaginal discharge. BV results from the lack of normal vaginal flora (i.e., *Lactobacillus* species) and replacement with anaerobic bacteria, mycoplasmas, and *Gardnerella vaginalis*.[48] It is a risk factor for premature rupture of membranes, preterm labor, preterm birth, intraamniotic infection, and postpartum endometritis. In women at high risk for preterm delivery, data to support routine screening for asymptomatic BV at the first prenatal visit are equivocal.[48] Conflicting data exist with regard to treating women at low risk for preterm labor.

Trichomoniasis is caused by the protozoa, *Trichomonas vaginalis*. Infection with *T. vaginalis* is associated with an increased risk of premature rupture of the membranes, preterm delivery, and low birth weight. Treatment may prevent respiratory or genital infection in the neonate.

Genital Herpes

Genital herpes is a chronic disease most frequently caused by herpes simplex virus-2 (HSV-2), although the number of anogenital herpes infections caused by HSV-1 is increasing. Neonatal herpes often occurs in infants born to women lacking histories of genital herpes. The risk of neonatal transmission is under 1% for women with a history of recurrent herpes at term or those who acquire herpes in the first half of pregnancy, but is 30% to 50% for women who initially acquire genital herpes near term.[48] However, because recurrent herpes occurs more commonly than new acquisition during pregnancy, it remains the cause for most cases of neonatal transmission. Prevention strategies include counseling uninfected women to avoid intercourse during the third trimester with partners having known or suspected genital herpes infection. Women with no history of orolabial herpes should avoid receptive oral sex during the third trimester with partners who have orolabial herpes. Prevention of genital herpes transmission to pregnant women using antiviral agents has not been studied.[48]

All women should be asked about symptoms of genital herpes at the time of delivery and should be examined for lesions. Women who have no symptoms (including prodromal symptoms) or lesions proceed with vaginal childbirth; however, those with evidence of an outbreak undergo cesarean section to decrease the risk of neonatal transmission.[48]

Maternal use of acyclovir during the first trimester has not demonstrated an increased risk for birth defects. Valacyclovir is an alternative, but is more expensive.[50] Safety data with famciclovir are limited. For initial or recurrent episodes, most women receive oral acyclovir therapy; IV acyclovir is reserved for severe infections. In women seropositive for HSV but who have not experienced an outbreak, no data suggest a treatment benefit.[48]

Headache

6 Primary headaches (e.g., tension, migraine) in pregnant and non-pregnant women are the most common types of headache. Secondary headaches can also occur and include those caused by eclampsia, stroke, postdural puncture, cerebral angiopathy, and cerebral venous thrombosis.[51]

Migraine headaches are associated with estrogen fluctuations in women of childbearing age. Between 60% and 70% of pregnant women with a history of migraine headaches experience symptom improvement during pregnancy; 20% experience complete cessation. Improvement is more likely in women who have migraine without aura and in women with a history of menstrual migraine. Women with menstrual migraine are more likely to have postpartum recurrence.[51] Tension headaches are less studied. Most women report no change in the frequency or intensity of tension headaches, and remission is possible.

Relaxation, stress management, and biofeedback are all effective nonpharmacologic treatment methods that should be attempted in pregnant women with migraines and tension headaches because these interventions pose a minimal risk. For tension headache, acetaminophen or ibuprofen can be used if nonpharmacologic treatments fail. While ibuprofen is considered safe, all NSAIDs are contraindicated in the third trimester because of the potential for premature closure of the ductus arteriosus. Aspirin should be avoided in the third trimester because, in addition to its effects on the ductus arteriosis, it can cause maternal and fetal bleeding as well as decreased uterine contractility (hence, prolonged labor). Opioids are rarely used.[51]

Pharmacologic treatment for migraines involves use of analgesics (i.e., acetaminophen, ibuprofen). Opioids have been used, but may contribute to migraine-associated nausea; long-term use near term can cause neonatal withdrawal. For migraines that are not responsive to other treatments, triptans may be used; sumatriptan is the triptan of choice, because other triptans have relatively little information about use in pregnancy. Ergotamine and dihydroergotamine are contraindicated because of effects on uterine tone. Promethazine, prochlorperazine, and metoclopramide can be used for patients who have migraine-associated nausea.[51]

Tension-type headaches do not usually require prophylaxis. Chronic, preventive treatment is reserved for women with severe headaches (usually migraines) that are not responsive to other treatments. The agent of choice is propranolol given at the lowest effective dose. Alternatives include tricyclic antidepressants. Amitriptyline and nortriptyline (each dosed 10 to 25 mg by mouth daily) are preferred over the selective serotonin reuptake inhibitors (SSRI) or serotonin–norepinephrine reuptake inhibitors (SNRI) because data on safe use of these agents during pregnancy are conflicting.[51]

CHRONIC ILLNESSES IN PREGNANCY

For the majority of women and their healthcare providers, pregnancy is a new consideration for a previously diagnosed health condition. Medications used to treat the chronic illness can often be used throughout the pregnancy and during breast-feeding.

Allergic Rhinitis and Asthma

6 Asthma and rhinitis are common chronic illnesses in pregnancy. Asthma affects approximately 8% of pregnancies.[52] During pregnancy, almost equal proportions of patients have symptoms that worsen, improve, or remain unchanged. Diagnosis and staging of asthma during pregnancy is the same as in nonpregnant women, although more frequent follow-up is necessary because of changes in disease severity.[53,54] Health consequences of untreated or poorly treated asthma include preterm labor, preeclampsia, intrauterine growth restriction, premature birth, low birth weight, and stillbirth; therefore, the treatment goal is to achieve and maintain control. Asthma is controlled when there are no daytime symptoms, limitations of activities, nocturnal symptoms, short-acting β_2-agonist use, or exacerbations, and there is normal pulmonary function.[53,54]

The risks of medication use to the fetus are lower than the risks of untreated asthma; therefore, use of medications to achieve and maintain control is warranted. Treatment recommendations are divided into six steps based on symptom control and follow a stepwise approach. Once control is achieved, the goal is maintenance of control at the lowest controlling step. A short-acting β_2-agonist is recommended for all patients with asthma for quick relief of symptoms and is the sole drug therapy recommended for Step 1 (intermittent); albuterol is preferred during pregnancy.[52–54] For persistent asthma (Step 2 and higher), step-appropriate doses (low, medium, high) of inhaled corticosteroids form the foundation of the controller medication regimen. Budesonide is preferred during pregnancy, although other inhaled corticosteroids that were effective before pregnancy can be continued. Long-acting β_2-agonists are considered safe to use during pregnancy because of the similar pharmacologic and safety profiles compared with short-acting agents. Cromolyn, leukotriene receptor antagonists, and theophylline are considered alternative treatments but are not preferred because they are less effective (cromolyn), there is less experience with them (leukotriene receptor antagonists), and there is more potential toxicity (theophylline) than with inhaled corticosteroids. For patients with the most severe disease, addition of systemic corticosteroids is recommended to gain control of symptoms.[52–54]

Approximately 20% of all pregnancies are impacted by allergic rhinitis. Notably, nasal congestion can be caused by pregnancy because of vascular engorgement in the nasal passages and hormonal effects on mucus secretion. Treatment strategies for allergic rhinitis during pregnancy are similar to those used in nonpregnant women and include avoidance of allergens, immunotherapy, and pharmacotherapy. Immunotherapy is not contraindicated in pregnancy, but dose increases during pregnancy are not advised in order to lessen the risk for anaphylaxis.[55]

First-line medications to treat allergic rhinitis during pregnancy include intranasal corticosteroids, nasal cromolyn, and first-generation antihistamines (e.g., chlorpheniramine, hydroxyzine).[56] Intranasal corticosteroids are the most effective treatment and have a low risk of systemic effect; beclomethasone and budesonide have been most widely studied. Second-generation antihistamines (i.e., loratadine and cetirizine) do not appear to increase fetal risk, but are less extensively studied than first-generation products.[55,56] Oral decongestants, such as pseudoephedrine, may be associated with an increased risk for the rare birth defect gastroschisis. Use of an external nasal dilator, short-term topical oxymetazoline, or inhaled corticosteroids may be preferable to use of oral decongestants, especially during early pregnancy.[56]

Diabetes

6 Poorly controlled diabetes can cause fetal malformations, fetal loss, and maternal morbidity. Women with diabetes should use effective contraception until optimal glycemic control is achieved before attempting pregnancy. Additionally, diabetic retinopathy may worsen, hypertension may develop, and renal function may deteriorate during pregnancy, requiring enhanced monitoring for these target-organ problems.[27,57]

Glycemic control can change dramatically during pregnancy; frequent adjustment to management may be needed. Medical nutrition therapy and supervised physical activity programs should continue. Self-monitored blood glucose should occur before and after meals, with occasional early morning (i.e., 2 to 4 am) measurement.[57] For patients with type 1 and type 2 diabetes, insulin is the drug treatment of choice.[57] Women receiving insulin glargine or detemir should be switched to NPH insulin. Glyburide and metformin may be alternatives, but are not recommended by the American Diabetes Association.[31,32,57]

Epilepsy

6 Seizure frequency does not change for most pregnant women with epilepsy. Studies have demonstrated no frequency change in 54% to 80% of women with epilepsy, while decreased frequency ranges between 3% and 24% and increased frequency ranges from 14% to 32%.[58,59] Seizures may become more frequent because of changes in maternal hormones, sleep deprivation, and medication adherence problems (because of perceived teratogenic risk). Another potential cause is changes in free serum concentrations of antiepileptic drugs resulting from increased maternal volume of distribution, decreased protein binding from hypoalbuminemia, increased hepatic drug metabolism, and increased renal drug clearance. A woman's clinical condition and her free serum concentrations of antiepileptic drug should be the basis for dose adjustments.

The risks of untreated epilepsy to the fetus are considered to be greater than those associated with the antiepileptic drugs.[59] Major malformations are two to three times more likely to occur in children born to women taking antiepileptic drugs than to those who do not. Major malformations with valproic acid are dose related and range from 6.2% to 10.7%; use of valproic acid should be avoided if possible during pregnancy to minimize the risk of NTDs (e.g., spina bifida), facial clefts, and cognitive teratogenicity.[60,61] Rates of major malformation for monotherapy with antiepileptic drugs other than valproic acid range between 2.9% and 3.6%. Carbamazepine and lamotrigine appear to be safest based on available data. However, individual antiepileptic drugs are associated with malformations. Phenytoin, lamotrigine, and carbamazepine may cause cleft palate, while phenobarbital is associated with cardiac malformations. Polytherapy with antiepileptic drugs is associated with a greater rate of major malformation than monotherapy.[60,61]

When possible, antiepileptic drug monotherapy is recommended with medication regimen optimization occurring before conception.[60] Medication change solely to minimize teratogenic risk is not recommended. If drug withdrawal is planned, it should be attempted at least 6 months before attempting to conceive.[60] While vitamin K administration during the last month of gestation was previously recommended to decrease the risk of hemorrhagic complications in newborns, evidence to support this practice is lacking. The American Academy of Pediatrics recommends that all neonates receive vitamin K at delivery. All women taking antiepileptic drugs should receive folic acid supplementation: 4 to 5 mg daily starting before pregnancy and continuing through at least the first trimester.[59]

Human Immunodeficiency Virus Infection

6 Pregnant women should receive counseling about HIV, and those infected with the virus should receive treatment with antiretroviral (ARV) therapy to decrease the risk of perinatal transmission of HIV. The treatment regimen should be selected from those suggested for nonpregnant adults, with special consideration given to the teratogenic profile of each drug. Women currently receiving ARV treatment should be continued on their regimen when possible. In a change from past recommendations, women receiving efavirenz as part of ARV therapy should continue treatment since NTDs usually occur through weeks 5 to 6 of gestation, and pregnancy often is not recognized until 4 to 6 weeks' gestation.[62]

For ARV-naïve women, use of a three-drug combination regimen is recommended and usually contains two nucleoside/nucleotide reverse transcriptase inhibitors (NRTIs) with high transplacental passage (preferred: zidovudine, lamivudine; alternatives: emtricitabine, tenofovir, abacavir) along with a protease inhibitor (preferred: atazanavir in combination plus low-dose ritonavir, lopinavir/ritonavir; alternative: darunavir or saquinavir, both with low-dose ritonavir).[62] Nevirapine, a nonnucleoside reverse transcriptase inhibitor (NNRTI), can be used as an alternative to a protease inhibitor but is associated with severe rash that can lead to life-threatening or fatal hepatotoxicity. After discussion of risks and benefits, some women who do not require immediate therapy may choose to delay ARV therapy until after the first trimester to avoid potential teratogenic complications.[62]

For women with HIV, cesarean section before the onset of labor (usually at 39 weeks' gestation) is recommended to reduce the risk of perinatal HIV transmission. If maternal viral load is greater than or equal to 400 copies/mL (400×10^3/L or greater) or not known, IV zidovudine should be initiated with a 1-hour loading dose (2 mg/kg) followed by a continuous infusion (1 mg/kg) for 2 hours (cesarean) or until delivery (for vaginal delivery).[62] Zidovudine IV should still be administered in the presence of resistance to oral zidovudine. Women with a viral load below 400 copies/mL (400×10^3/L or less) near delivery do not require zidovudine IV, but should continue their ARV regimen. Specific recommendations for different clinical scenarios during antepartum, intrapartum, and postpartum are provided in the clinical guidelines.[62]

Hypertension

6 Hypertension occurring before 20 weeks' gestation, the use of antihypertensive medications before pregnancy, or the persistence of hypertension beyond 12 weeks postpartum define chronic hypertension in pregnancy. It is classified as mild/nonsevere (systolic blood pressure [sBP] 140 to 159 mm Hg or dBP 90 to 109 mm Hg) or severe (sBP 160 mm Hg or greater, or dBP 110 mm Hg or greater).[63] Typically, a physiologic decrease in blood pressure occurs during the first part of pregnancy, reaching its lowest point between 16 and 18 weeks' gestation; this decrease may mask undiagnosed hypertension. By the third trimester, blood pressure usually returns to prepregnancy levels.

Severe hypertension (as defined above) can cause maternal complications, hospital admission, and potential premature delivery. Drug therapy is indicated for women with blood pressure of 160/110 mm Hg and above.[63] Blood pressure, as measured by mean arterial pressure, should be lowered by a maximum of 25% in the first minutes to 1 hour with further reduction to below 160/100 mm Hg over a period of hours.[35,38] Initial choice of pharmacologic agent varies, but the most commonly used agents are parenteral labetalol and hydralazine; however, hydralazine is associated with more maternal and fetal adverse effects. Oral nifedipine may also be used.[36,38] Although still commonly used, limited evidence supports the use of magnesium sulfate to lower blood pressure except when being used concomitantly for preeclampsia. Nitroprusside, diazoxide, and nitroglycerin should be reserved for refractory hypertension in an appropriately monitored environment.[36,38]

Treatment of nonsevere hypertension (defined as sBP 140 to 159 mm Hg or dBP 90 to 109 mm Hg) reduces the risk of severe hypertension by 50%, but does not substantially affect fetal outcomes.[35,38] Studies of antihypertensive drug therapy for nonsevere hypertension in pregnancy have not conclusively shown a decrease in the risk of preeclampsia, neonatal death, preterm birth, or small-for-gestational-age babies.[35] No consensus exists on when to initiate treatment of nonsevere hypertension and treatment goals vary. In the United States, recommendations for treatment initiation include blood pressures of 150 to 160/100 to 110 mm Hg, with the goal of treatment to lower blood pressure below 150/100 mm Hg.[63] Treatment of women with blood pressure below 150/100 mm Hg can be withheld and lowering doses or discontinuing therapy can be considered for women already treated for hypertension who achieve blood pressure below 150/100 mm Hg.[63] However, in Canada and the United Kingdom, treatment is suggested for nonsevere hypertension; sBP targets range from 110 to 140 mm Hg while dBP targets range from 80 to 105 mm Hg.[38]

No evidence supports selection of one pharmacologic agent as first-line therapy. Labetalol is increasingly being used to manage hypertension during pregnancy. Other commonly used drugs include methyldopa and calcium channel blockers. With the exception of atenolol, β-adrenoreceptor antagonists can also be used. Atenolol has been associated with fetal growth restriction. Thiazide diuretics, while theoretically lowering the increase in plasma volume during pregnancy, have been successfully used in women who were treated with them before pregnancy. Agents affecting the renin–angiotensin pathway (i.e., angiotensin-converting enzyme inhibitors, angiotensin receptor antagonists, and renin inhibitors) are contraindicated throughout pregnancy.[35,36,38,63]

Mental Health Conditions

6 Psychiatric illness affects approximately 500,000 pregnancies each year.[64] Anxiety disorders, including panic disorder, obsessive–compulsive disorder, generalized anxiety disorder, posttraumatic stress disorder, social anxiety disorder, and phobias, can cause adverse maternal and fetal outcomes such as spontaneous abortion, preterm delivery, prolonged labor, and fetal distress.[64]

Depression occurs in 10% to 16% of pregnant women. Maternal depression is associated with greater risk for premature birth, low birth weight, and fetal growth restriction. In addition to the potential impact of maternal depression on obstetric complications, untreated depression may have long-term implications for normal infant development.[64] Up to 6.4% of Americans have bipolar disorder, with men and women equally affected; the incidence in pregnancy is unclear although perinatal episodes tend toward depressive manifestations.[64] Schizophrenia occurs in 1% to 2% of women; however, the incidence in pregnancy is unknown.[64] Maternal schizophrenia is associated with increased risk of perinatal death, low birth weight, small-for-gestational-age infants, cardiovascular malformations, preterm delivery, stillbirth, and infant death.[64]

Up to 70% of women with mental health conditions discontinue or refuse treatment because of concerns about teratogenicity, or because of paranoid or delusional thinking.[65] Therefore, the risks and benefits of psychotropic medication use during pregnancy must be discussed with the patient. Because most psychotropic medications are used to treat more than one condition, the reader should refer to other sources for information about treatment of specific mental health diagnoses. In general, monotherapy is preferred over polytherapy even if higher doses are required.[64]

Through 2005, the use of SSRIs was considered relatively safe. However, paroxetine may cause a 1.5- to twofold increased risk of cardiac malformations when used during the first trimester use; conflicting data exist regarding first trimester use of other SSRIs.[64,65] Despite this association, SSRIs are not considered major teratogens, as their absolute risk for congenital effects is less than 2 per 1,000 births. Risks with SNRIs are less defined. Use of SSRIs and SNRIs in the latter part of pregnancy is associated with persistent pulmonary hypertension of the newborn and Prenatal Antidepressant Exposure Syndrome (encompasses cardiac, respiratory, neurological, GI, and metabolic complications from drug toxicity or withdrawal of drug therapy).[65] Tricyclic antidepressants were commonly used in pregnancy before the introduction of SSRIs and are not considered major teratogens, although they have also been associated with a neonatal withdrawal syndrome when used late in pregnancy.[64,65] Importantly, women who stop taking antidepressants are more likely to relapse, which can also have implications for the well-being of the infant.

Studies completed over 30 years ago showed an increased risk of oral clefts with diazepam use during pregnancy; these findings were not confirmed in a meta-analysis that found the absolute risk of oral cleft changed from six cases to seven cases per 10,000 exposures (0.01%).[64] Benzodiazepine use in the third trimester can cause infant sedation and withdrawal symptoms (e.g., restlessness, hypertonia, hyperreflexia, tremulousness, apnea, diarrhea, vomiting). "Floppy baby syndrome," consisting of low Apgar scores, hypothermia, poor muscle tone, feeding difficulties, and poor temperature adaptation, has also been described.[64]

Mood stabilizers, such as lithium, lamotrigine, carbamazepine, and valproic acid, are often used to treat bipolar disorder.[64] The reader can find information related to the use of the seizure medications used for mood stabilization in the section on epilepsy. Lithium's place in the treatment of bipolar disorder during pregnancy is controversial because of concerns about cardiovascular anomalies, especially Ebstein's anomaly, in exposed infants.[64] A meta-analysis calculated that the relative risk for cardiac malformations was between 1.2 and 7.7 and for all congenital malformations was between 1.5 and 3. Stated differently, the risk for Ebstein's anomaly after prenatal lithium exposure would rise from 1:20,000 to 1:1,000; it is no longer considered a major human teratogen.[65,66] Other reported neonatal side effects include floppy baby syndrome, nephrogenic diabetes insipidus, hypoglycemia, cardiac arrhythmias, thyroid dysfunction, polyhydramnios, and premature delivery. Lithium may cause lethargy, hypotonia, hypothermia, cyanosis, and changes in electrocardiogram in infants exposed through breast-feeding. If breast-feeding, the infant's lithium levels, thyroid function, and complete blood count should be monitored.[64]

The typical antipsychotics are considered to have minimum toxic or teratogenic potential. Chlorpromazine, haloperidol, and perphenazine have long histories of use during pregnancy, with no reported significant teratogenic effect.[64] Atypical antipsychotics are considered first-line treatment for schizophrenia because of their more favorable side-effect profiles and potential increased efficacy for treating negative symptoms compared with the older agents. However, use of atypical antipsychotics in pregnant women is controversial because of the limited data regarding teratogenic potential. One study found a higher rate (10% vs. 2%) of low-birth-weight infants with olanzapine, clozapine, quetiapine, and risperidone compared with nonexposed infants.[64] Olanzapine is the most commonly used atypical agent during pregnancy; however, olanzapine as well as clozapine and quetiapine can cause weight gain and metabolic syndrome which have implications for poorer obstetric outcomes.[66,67] At present, atypical antipsychotics do not appear to be safer than the typical agents.

Thyroid Disorders

6 Universal screening for thyroid disorders during pregnancy is controversial; some advocate targeted screening of women considered high risk. Hypothyroidism is present in 2% to 3% of pregnancies. Untreated hypothyroidism increases the risk of preeclampsia, premature birth, miscarriage, and growth restriction; impaired neurological development in the fetus may also occur. Causes of hypothyroidism include autoimmune diseases (e.g., Hashimoto's thyroiditis), iodine deficiency (uncommon in the United States), and thyroid dysfunction following surgery or ablative therapy for previous hyperthyroidism. If hypothyroidism is present, thyroid replacement should occur with levothyroxine to attain a TSH of 0.1 to 2.5, 0.2 to 3, and 0.3 to 3 milli-international units per liter in the first, second, and third trimesters, respectively.[43] A reasonable starting dose of levothyroxine is 0.1 mg/day. Women receiving thyroid replacement therapy before pregnancy may have an increased dosage requirement during pregnancy. Laboratory follow-up of TSH should occur every 4 weeks during the first half of pregnancy and at least once between 26 and 32 weeks of pregnancy to allow for dose titration according to TSH levels.[43]

Hyperthyroidism affects approximately 0.4% to 1.7% of pregnancies and is associated with fetal death, low birth weight, intrauterine growth restriction, and preeclampsia. Graves' disease accounts for 85% to 90% of hyperthyroidism in pregnancy.[43] Therapy includes the thioamides (i.e., methimazole, propylthiouracil [PTU]). Dose reductions are possible after becoming euthyroid. Surgery is reserved for the most severe cases. The risks of uncontrolled hyperthyroidism outweigh the risks of the thioamides. However, some support a switch to PTU during the first trimester because of potential risks with methimazole followed by a subsequent switch to methimazole for the second and third trimesters to prevent hepatoxicity from PTU. Iodine-131 is contraindicated because of the risk of thyroid damage in the fetus. The goal of therapy is to attain free thyroxine concentrations near the upper limit of normal to allow for dose minimization and to limit fetal or neonatal hypothyroidism.[43]

LABOR AND DELIVERY

Management of the pregnant woman during the perinatal period often requires drug therapy for pain and for potential complications.

Preterm Labor

7 Preterm labor occurs when there are cervical changes and uterine contractions between 20 and 37 weeks' gestation.[68,69] Preterm birth is the leading cause of infant morbidity and mortality in the world and in the United States, with an incidence of 11% to 18% worldwide and 12% in the United States.[70] Risk factors for preterm delivery include previous preterm delivery, infections, multiple gestation, poverty, nonwhite race, maternal complication factors (e.g., smoking and use of illicit drugs or alcohol), and uterine functional causes (e.g., incompetent cervix); previous history and prior second trimester loss confer a higher risk.[68,69]

No adequate tests are available for monitoring and preventing preterm labor. Monitoring of uterine activity along with intensive surveillance does not minimize risk.[69] The presence of fetal fibronectin, a glycoprotein found in cervicovaginal secretions, indicates a high risk of preterm birth. Cervical shortening is also associated with preterm delivery. Fetal fibronectin determinations and cervical ultrasound have not helped to prevent preterm labor but have been useful for their negative predictive value.[69]

Tocolytic Therapy

The purposes of tocolytic therapy are threefold: (a) postpone delivery long enough to allow for the maximum effect of antenatal steroid administration; (b) allow for transportation of the mother to a facility equipped to deal with high-risk deliveries; and (c) prolongation of pregnancy when there are underlying, self-limited conditions that can cause labor, such as pyelonephritis or abdominal surgery, that are unlikely to cause recurrent preterm labor.[69,71,72] Tocolytics have not reduced the number of premature deliveries. The criteria for starting tocolysis are regular uterine contractions with cervical change. Tocolytic therapy should not be used in cases of intrauterine fetal demise, a lethal fetal anomaly, intrauterine infection, fetal distress, severe preeclampsia, vaginal bleeding, or maternal hemodynamic instability.

Four classes of tocolytics are available in the United States: β-agonists, magnesium, calcium channel blockers, and NSAIDs.[73] All four therapies have similar effectiveness in prolonging pregnancy from 48 hours to 1 week. However, this prolongation of pregnancy was not associated with a statistically significant reduction in overall rates of respiratory distress syndrome or neonatal death.

The β-agonists terbutaline and ritodrine have been used for tocolytic therapy.[71] Ritodrine is no longer available in the United States. Relative to other agents, β-agonists have a higher incidence of maternal side effects, including hyperkalemia, arrhythmias, hyperglycemia, hypotension, and pulmonary edema. Recommended terbutaline doses range from 250 to 500 mcg subcutaneously every 3 to 4 hours.[72]

IV magnesium sulfate has been used for tocolysis; however, a Cochrane review does not support its effectiveness.[74] Heterogeneity of study designs and results along with small treatment arms in the included studies may partially explain this finding; however, its use remains controversial.[71] The incidence of cerebral palsy is increased in premature infants. In one study, IV magnesium use (6 g load followed by 2 g/h continuous infusion) decreased the occurrence of moderate or severe cerebral palsy.[75] Although not the primary end point, the study suggests that women at risk for imminent delivery (up to 34 weeks' gestation) should receive IV magnesium. Maternal side effects are rare but can include pulmonary edema. At toxic levels, hypotension, muscle paralysis, tetany, cardiac arrest, and respiratory depression may occur.[72] Magnesium undergoes renal excretion; dose adjustment is required in women with impaired renal function.

Nifedipine is associated with fewer side effects than magnesium or β-agonist therapy.[71] Several studies have suggested that calcium channel blockers are superior to β-agonists for prolonging labor. One concern with the use of nifedipine is its hypotensive effect and corresponding change in uteroplacental blood flow. However, a meta-analysis showed reduced neonatal morbidity with calcium channel blocker use. With the initial diagnosis of preterm labor, 5 to 10 mg nifedipine can be administered sublingually every 15 to 20 minutes for three doses. After patient stabilization, if no evidence of continuing cervical dilation is seen, 10 to 20 mg nifedipine can be administered orally every 4 to 6 hours for preterm contractions.[72]

NSAIDs such as indomethacin have been used for tocolysis.[71,72] Oral or rectal doses of 50 to 100 mg, followed by an oral dose of 25 to 50 mg every 6 hours, have been used. An increased rate of premature constriction of the ductus arteriosus has been noted in infants with indomethacin use after 32 weeks' gestation and with use exceeding 48 hours.[71] Indomethacin may be used when tocolysis is needed despite treatment with magnesium for neuroprotection because other agents, such as calcium channel blockers, can cause hypotension when administered concurrently with magnesium.

Other Drug Therapies for Preterm Labor Prevention

Infection is a potential cause of preterm labor. Antibiotics have been used, in addition to tocolytics and corticosteroids, to improve the outcome of preterm labor; however, a Cochrane review showed no reduction in the incidence of preterm delivery but a trend toward increased neonatal mortality. Therefore, routine use of antibiotics is not recommended. However, if a patient experiences preterm premature rupture of membranes (PPROM) before 34 weeks' gestation, prophylactic antibiotics should be initiated because a reduction in major morbidities (i.e., death, respiratory distress syndrome, early sepsis, severe intraventricular hemorrhage, and necrotizing enterocolitis) was demonstrated.[76] A 7-day course of antibiotics with reasonable activity against gram negative and anaerobic bacteria should be used with the intent to prolong latency, which is the time from ruptured membranes to delivery. Ampicillin 2 g IV every 6 hours for 48 hours, followed by amoxicillin (500 mg orally three times daily or 875 mg orally twice daily) for 5 days is preferred instead of multiple courses of erythromycin.[76] Cefazolin (1 g every 8 hours) for 48 hours, followed by cephalexin (500 mg four times daily for 5 days) should be used for patients with a penicillin allergy who have a low risk for anaphylaxis to provide coverage for GBS and *E. coli*, the two major causes of neonatal infection. For patients at high risk for anaphylaxis to penicillin, clindamycin 900 mg IV every eight hours for 48 hours plus gentamicin 7 mg/kg (dosed on ideal body weight) for two doses given 24 hours apart, followed by oral clindamycin 300 mg every 8 hours for 5 days is the regimen of choice. For each regimen, one dose of azithromycin (1 g orally) upon admission and a second dose 5 days later also provides coverage for *C. trachomatis*, which can cause neonatal conjunctivitis and pneumonitis.[48]

Progesterone administration in the setting of prior preterm birth is much debated. Two large randomized, controlled trials produced significant findings. First, the administration of intramuscular 17-α-hydroxyprogesterone weekly (250 mg) starting between weeks 16 and 20 and continued through week 36 in high-risk women decreased the incidence of recurrent preterm birth.[77] The second study replicated the findings using vaginal progesterone suppositories (100 mg).[78] However, progesterone supplementation in women whose previous preterm birth occurred beyond 34 weeks produced similar rates of preterm delivery compared with placebo.[79] Currently, ACOG recommends that progesterone supplementation be limited to women with a singleton pregnancy and a previous history of spontaneous preterm birth.[80]

Clinical **Controversy...**

Hydroxyprogesterone (Makena®) was approved in February 2011 for prevention of preterm birth in women with a singleton pregnancy and a history of preterm birth. Prior to its approval, compounding pharmacies were supplying hydroxyprogesterone for this use. The FDA has recommended that when an FDA-approved drug is commercially available, that the commercially available product be used instead of a compounded form. The pricing difference for the FDA-approved product is substantial; many patients continue to use the compounded product.

Antenatal Corticosteroids

Use of antenatal corticosteroids for fetal lung maturation to prevent respiratory distress syndrome, intraventricular hemorrhage, and death in infants delivered prematurely is supported by a Cochrane review.[81] The current clinical recommendation is to administer betamethasone 12 mg intramuscularly every 24 hours for two doses or dexamethasone 6 mg intramuscularly every 12 hours for four doses to pregnant women between 26 and 34 weeks' gestation who are at risk for preterm delivery within the next 7 days. Benefits from antenatal corticosteroids are believed to begin within 24 hours.

Salvage ("rescue") treatment is administered to women who are at risk of delivering within 7 days but who have received a previous course of therapy. The incidence of respiratory distress syndrome was lower with the administration of rescue steroids compared with placebo (41.4% with betamethasone vs. 61.6% with placebo).[82]

Group B *Streptococcus* Infection

7 Maternal infection with GBS is associated with invasive disease in the newborn.[83,84] Women colonized with GBS have an increased risk for pregnancy loss, premature delivery, and transmission of the bacteria to the infant during delivery. Between 10% and 30% of pregnant women are colonized with GBS. The rate of invasive infection (defined as isolation of GBS from blood or other sterile body site excluding urine) in pregnant women is 0.12 per 1,000 live births (range, 0.11 to 0.14 per 1,000 births). The incidence of early-onset disease in neonates, although higher than in pregnant women, has declined steadily from 1.5 per 1,000 live births in 1993 to approximately 0.24 cases per 1,000 live births in 2010. The consequences of neonatal infections include bacteremia, pneumonia, meningitis, and fatality in the newborn.[84] The case-fatality rate is approximately 4%.

Recommendations for prevention of GBS infection were updated in 2010.[84] Universal prenatal screening for GBS colonization is recommended. Antibiotics are given if the woman previously gave birth to an infant with invasive GBS disease or in the presence of GBS bacteriuria. All other pregnant women should have a vaginal/rectal culture at 35 to 37 weeks' gestation. If negative, antibiotics are not indicated. If a woman presents in labor and no screening information is available, antibiotics are given for fever greater than 100.4°F (38°C), membrane rupture at least 18 hours prior, or gestation under 37 weeks.

Penicillin G 5 million units given IV, followed by 2.5 million units given every 4 hours until delivery is the recommended treatment regimen.[84] Alternatively, ampicillin 2 g can be given IV, followed by 1 g every 4 hours. For women with penicillin allergy but not at risk for anaphylaxis, cefazolin 2 g IV, followed by 1 g every 8 hours, is recommended. In women at high risk for anaphylaxis, clindamycin 900 mg IV every 8 hours or erythromycin 500 mg IV every 6 hours is recommended. For penicillin-allergic women, GBS cultures should be sent for sensitivities. If resistant to clindamycin or erythromycin, vancomycin 1 g IV every 12 hours until delivery is appropriate.

Cervical Ripening and Labor Induction

7 Throughout gestation, the cervix is closed and firm. During the last few weeks of pregnancy, the cervix softens and thins to facilitate labor.[85,86] This process is mediated by hormonal changes, including final mediation by prostaglandins E_2 and $F_2\alpha$, which increase collagenase activity in the cervix leading to thinning and dilation.

The rate of pregnancy induction ranges from 9.5% to 33.5%; the most common indications for induction are postdatism (beyond 42 weeks) and pregnancy-induced hypertension, which account for 80% of inductions.[85,86] Other reasons for induction include suspected fetal growth retardation, maternal hypertension, premature rupture of membranes with no active onset of labor, and social factors. Contraindications include placenta previa, oblique or transverse lie, pelvic structure abnormality, prolapsed umbilical cord, and active herpes. Concerns with induction of labor are ineffective labor and side effects, such as uterine hyperstimulation, that may adversely affect the infant and increase the likelihood of cesarean section.

Scoring systems have been used to determine the likelihood of successful labor induction. The Bishop scoring system is most commonly used and is based on five parameters: cervical dilation, cervical effacement (thinning), station of the baby's head, consistency of the cervix, and position of the cervix.[85,86] A Bishop score under six indicates the need for cervical ripening while a score above eight corresponds to a likely successful vaginal delivery.

A number of nonpharmacologic methods are used for cervical ripening. Castor oil, hot baths, sexual intercourse, and nipple stimulation all have been suggested for labor induction.[85] Minimal evidence supports the efficacy of these methods. Use of a Foley catheter placed in an unfavorable cervix for ripening has been found as effective as prostaglandin E_2. Membrane stripping is safe and inexpensive.[85,86]

Prostaglandin E_2 analogs (e.g., dinoprostone [Prepidil gel, Cervidil vaginal insert]) are commonly used for cervical ripening. Prepidil 500 mcg is administered intracervically.[86] The dose may be repeated after 6 hours to a maximum of three doses in 24 hours. After administration, the patient remains supine for 30 minutes. Cervidil contains 10 mg dinoprostone with a slower, more constant release of medication than the gel. The insert is removed when labor begins or after 12 hours. Patients must be attached to a fetal heart rate monitor for the duration of Cervidil use and for 15 minutes after its removal.[85]

Misoprostol, a prostaglandin E_1 analog, is an effective and inexpensive drug for cervical ripening and labor induction.[86] Intravaginal administration of misoprostol is more effective than other prostaglandin agents and results in a shorter time to delivery. Oral misoprostol has been used successfully for cervical ripening and labor induction, but the evidence of safety is more extensive with intravaginal use. The most commonly encountered side effects are uterine hyperstimulation and meconium-stained amniotic fluid. Use of misoprostol is contraindicated in women with a previous uterine scar because of its association with uterine rupture, a catastrophic medical event.

Progesterone inhibits uterine contractions. Preliminary studies show that mifepristone, an antiprogesterone agent, compared with placebo results in a shorter time to delivery and fewer cesarean sections.[87] Limited information on fetal and maternal outcomes is available because of the small sample sizes.

Oxytocin is the most commonly used agent for labor induction after cervical ripening. By the end of pregnancy, the number of oxytocin receptors has increased by 300-fold.[85,86] A solution of 10 milliunits/mL is used for infusion. Oxytocin is effective in both low-dose (physiologic) and high-dose (pharmacologic) regimens.

Labor Analgesia

7 In the first phase of labor, women perceive visceral pain caused by uterine contractions. Pain in the second phase of labor is associated with perineal stretching.[88]

Nonpharmacologic Approaches to Analgesia

Women who receive continuous support from nurses, midwives, childbirth educators, or doulas [lay women trained in labor support], have fewer operative vaginal deliveries, cesarean deliveries, and requests for pain medication.[89] Warm water baths provide temporary pain relief but have not been shown to decrease the use of pharmacologic pain treatments. Intradermal injections of sterile water in the sacral area decrease back pain during labor for 45 to 120 minutes. However, requests for pain medication did not decrease in studies. Acupuncture has also been used for pain relief. Three randomized, controlled trials have shown that acupuncture decreases the need for analgesia, but more methodologically sound studies are needed. Use of audioanalgesia (music or white noise), relaxation and breathing techniques, application of heat and cold, aromatherapy, acupressure, and hypnosis have little to no evidence of effectiveness derived from randomized, controlled trials.

Pharmacologic Approaches to Labor Pain Management

Maternal request alone is a sufficient medical indication for labor analgesia.[90] The two main types of pharmacologic approaches in the United States are parenteral opioids and epidural analgesia.

Parenteral opioids are commonly used to alleviate labor pain.[91] In comparison with epidural analgesia, parenteral opioids have lower rates of oxytocin augmentation, result in shorter stages of labor, and require fewer instrumental deliveries.

Approximately 60% of women in the United States choose an epidural for pain relief during labor and report better pain relief than with other analgesic modalities.[91] With epidural analgesia, a catheter is introduced into the epidural space and an opioid and/or an anesthetic (e.g., fentanyl and/or bupivacaine) is administered. Combined spinal–epidural analgesia consists of injecting a single opioid bolus into the subarachnoid space to provide instant pain relief with additional use of a local anesthetic epidural. Patient-controlled epidural analgesia allows the patient to control the amount and timing of the anesthetic; it results in a lower total dose of local anesthetics used over the course of labor compared with continuous epidural infusions.[92]

Side effects of the regional anesthesia include hypotension, pruritus, and inability to void.[91] Epidural analgesia is associated with prolongation of the first and second stages of labor, higher numbers of instrumental deliveries, and maternal fever. A rare complication of epidural anesthesia is puncture of the subarachnoid space leading to a severe headache, which occurs in approximately 1% of women. Other complications include hypotension, nausea, vomiting, itching, and urinary retention. Low back pain has not been associated with the use of epidural analgesia.

Postpartum Hemorrhage

(7) The placenta is delivered after the delivery of the baby and is referred to as the third stage of labor. Postpartum hemorrhage is an obstetrical emergency and is a major cause of morbidity and mortality.[93] In the United States, the postpartum hemorrhage rate is approximately 1% to 5% for vaginal deliveries.[94] The traditional definition of postpartum hemorrhage is more than 500 mL of blood within 24 hours of a vaginal delivery or 1,000 mL after a cesarean section; however, other definitions have also been suggested. Risk factors include retained placenta, failure to progress during the second stage of labor, placenta previa, placenta accreta, lacerations, instrumental delivery, large for gestational age newborn, hypertensive disorders, labor induction, augmentation of labor with oxytocin, prior history, obesity, and high parity.[95]

A stepwise approach to the treatment of postpartum hemorrhage is advised. After the exclusion of retained products of conception and cervical and vaginal lacerations, attention should be turned to the management of uterine atony if present. The most common cause of postpartum hemorrhage is uterine atony.[93,94] Initial management should include oxytocin. Early clamping and cutting of the umbilical cord as well as controlled traction of the cord also decrease the incidence.[93] Administration of a uterotonic medication (intramuscular oxytocin, ergotamine, or combination) before placental delivery and instituting active management of labor after all uncomplicated vaginal deliveries result in reduced maternal blood loss, fewer cases of postpartum hemorrhage, and less prolongation of the third stage of labor. Other uterotonic agents should be used if an inadequate response is attained with oxytocin alone. Methylergonovine, carboprost, misoprostol, and dinoprostone have all been used; less evidence is available for misoprostol and dinoprostone. If uterotonic drug therapies fail to control the bleeding, uterine artery embolization, intrauterine balloon catheters, or a variety of different surgical techniques can be used.

POSTPARTUM ISSUES

Drug Use During Lactation

(8) A wide variety of benefits (health, nutritional, immunologic, psychological, economic, developmental, and social) are imparted by breast-feeding to infants, mothers, and the family. Women should breastfeed exclusively for 6 months and continue until at least 12 months of age while other foods are introduced.[96] Healthy People 2020 increased targets for breast-feeding to 81.9% of neonates at the time of birth and to 60.5% for infants being breast-fed at 6 months.[96]

Adequate milk removal from the breast by breast-feeding or pumping is necessary to maintain or increase milk production.[97] Relactation is the process of increasing the breast milk supply for women whose milk has not "come in," who have inadequate milk production despite appropriate breast-feeding frequency or pumping, or who have weaned or never breast-fed after delivery. Metoclopramide can be used if nonpharmacologic measures are ineffective because of its stimulation of prolactin secretion. The most common dose is 10 mg orally three times daily for 7 to 14 days.[97] Breast milk production may decrease after metoclopramide therapy is stopped, but production will continue if lactation has been established successfully.

Most drugs transfer into breast milk, but breast-feeding may be continued in most circumstances. Healthcare providers should encourage breast-feeding women who require medications to continue breast-feeding whenever possible. Passive diffusion is the primary mechanism for drug transfer into breast milk, but other drug-related factors influence drug transfer from maternal circulation into breast milk, including (a) degree of protein binding in maternal plasma, (b) molecular weight, (c) lipid solubility (and corresponding fat content of milk), (d) maternal plasma concentration, (e) drug half-life, and (f) drug pH.[98,99] The degree of protein binding to maternal plasma proteins is one of the most significant factors affecting drug transfer to breast milk; highly bound medications transfer in low amounts. Low-molecular-weight drugs passively diffuse into breast milk, but larger molecules are not likely to transfer in large amounts. Higher lipid solubility of drugs also increases the likelihood of transfer. Colostrum is secreted in the first couple of days after birth and has high quantities of immunoglobulins, maternal lymphocytes, and maternal macrophages. Compared with mature milk, colostrum is lower in fat content, so highly lipid-soluble drugs achieve higher concentrations in mature milk. The higher the concentration of drug in the mother's serum, the higher the concentration will be in the breast milk. As the drug is metabolized and excreted by the mother, the mother's serum concentration drops, and the drug in the breast milk may redistribute back into the mother's bloodstream. Maternal plasma pH is 7.4, while the pH of breast milk ranges between 6.8 and 7. Weak bases are not ionized in the maternal circulation and easily transfer to breast milk.[99] In the lower pH of breast milk, molecules become ionized and are less likely to diffuse back into maternal circulation ("ion trapping"). Likewise, drugs with longer half-lives are more likely to maintain higher levels in breast milk, resulting in greater exposure to the infant.

Infant-related factors may also influence the amount of drug ingested through breast-feeding.[98] Both the frequency of feedings and the amount of milk ingested are important considerations. Exclusively breast-fed infants are more likely to ingest larger amounts of drugs than older infants who receive other foods. Drugs unstable in gastric acid (aminoglycosides, omeprazole, heparin, insulin) are less likely to be absorbed by infants. Finally, infants may vary in their ability to metabolize and excrete ingested medication. Premature and full-term infants may not have full renal and liver function.

Strategies for reducing the risk to the infant include selection of medications that would be considered safe for use in the infant.[98] Drugs with shorter half-lives accumulate less, and those that are more protein bound do not cross into breast milk as well as those that are less protein bound. Drugs with lower oral bioavailability and lower lipid solubility are good choices. If the mother is using a once-daily medication, administration before the infant's longest sleep period may be advised to increase the interval to the next feeding. For medications taken multiple times per day, administration immediately after breast-feeding provides the longest interval for back diffusion of drug from the breast milk to the mother's serum. During short-term drug therapy, the mother can pump and discard milk to preserve her milk-producing capability if the medication is not considered compatible with breast-feeding.[99]

Information regarding drug use during breast-feeding is available from expert committees (e.g., American Academy of Pediatrics Committee on Drugs) and evidence-based textbooks or databases (e.g., LactMed [*www.toxnet.nlm.nih.gov*]). All may be of assistance in determining safe and appropriate medications to use during breast-feeding.

Mastitis

8 Mastitis is inflammation in one breast.[100] It can be infectious or noninfectious; the most common cause is milk stasis. About 10% of women in the United States experience mastitis during the first 3 months postpartum. Signs and symptoms include breast tenderness, redness, warmth, and flulike symptoms.[101] Risk factors for developing mastitis include breast engorgement, plugged milk ducts, and cracked nipples.

Staphylococcus aureus is the most common bacterial cause of mastitis; *E. coli* and *Streptococcus* have also been implicated.[100,101] A 10- to 14-day course of antibiotics is usually given for treatment of mastitis; penicillinase-resistant penicillins (e.g., dicloxacillin, oxacillin) and cephalosporins (e.g., cephalexin) are frequently prescribed. Antiinflammatory drugs, such as ibuprofen, may provide some pain relief. Application of heat may also be helpful. Affected women should be counseled to continue breast-feeding from both breasts throughout treatment and to pump if breasts are not emptied completely with feedings.

Postpartum Depression

8 Mood disorders in the postpartum period may include postpartum blues, postpartum depression, and postpartum psychosis.[102] Postpartum blues is common, usually affecting 15% to 85% of new mothers within the first 10 days of delivery, and generally does not require treatment. Symptoms include anxiety, anger, and sadness. Postpartum psychosis is more severe but is rare, affecting less than 1% of new mothers.

Postpartum depression affects up to 15% of women.[102] Symptoms may develop during pregnancy or up to 6 months after delivery, although the strict definition for major depressive disorder after delivery specifies symptom occurrence within 1 month. Psychotherapy, including interpersonal psychotherapy, cognitive behavioral therapy, and group/family therapy, has been shown effective for treatment of postpartum depression.

In cases where pharmacotherapy is warranted, selection of medication with low transfer to breast milk is desirable. Sertraline is generally considered a first-line treatment because of its minimal transfer into breast milk and lack of reported adverse events in infants.[98,102] Paroxetine and nortriptyline are considered second-line.

ABBREVIATIONS

ACOG	American College of Obstetricians and Gynecologists
ARV	antiretroviral
BV	bacterial vaginosis
dBP	diastolic blood pressure
FPG	fasting plasma glucose
GBS	Group B *Streptococcus*
GDM	gestational diabetes mellitus
GTT	gestational thyrotoxicosis
H_2	histamine-2
hCG	human chorionic gonadotropin
HDP	hypertensive disorders of pregnancy
HELLP	hemolysis, elevated liver enzymes, low platelets
HG	hyperemesis gravidarum
HIV	human immunodeficiency virus
HSV	herpes simplex virus
IADPSG	International Association of Diabetes and Pregnancy Study Groups
LMWH	low-molecular-weight heparin
NNRTI	nonnucleoside reverse transcriptase inhibitor
NRTI	nucleoside reverse transcriptase inhibitor
NSAID	nonsteroidal antiinflammatory drug
NTD	neural tube defect
NVP	nausea and vomiting of pregnancy
OGTT	oral glucose tolerance test
PID	pelvic inflammatory disease
PPROM	preterm premature rupture of membranes
PPT	postpartum thyroiditis
PTU	propylthiouracil
RPG	random plasma glucose
sBP	systolic blood pressure
SNRI	serotonin–norepinephrine reuptake inhibitor
SSRI	selective serotonin reuptake inhibitor
STI	sexually transmitted infection
TSH	thyroid-stimulating hormone
UFH	unfractionated heparin
UTI	urinary tract infection
VTE	venous thromboembolism

REFERENCES

1. Ord T. The scourge: Moral implications of natural embryo loss. Am J Bioeth 2008;8:12–19.
2. Brent RL. Environmental causes of human congenital malformations: The pediatrician's role in dealing with these complex clinical problems caused by a multiplicity of environmental and genetic factors. Pediatrics 2004; 113(4 Suppl):957–968.
3. Gupta SK, Bansal P, Ganguly A, Bhandari B, Chakrabarti K. Human zona pellucida glycoproteins: Functional relevance during fertilization. J Reprod Immunol 2009;83:50–55.
4. Cunningham FG, Leveno KJ, Bloom SL, et al. Chap. 3. Implantation, embryogenesis, and placental development. In: Cunningham FG, Leveno KJ, Bloom SL, et al. eds. Williams Obstetrics. 23rd ed. New York: McGraw-Hill; 2010. *http://www.accessmedicine.com/content/aspx?aID=6030341*. Accessed June 14, 2013.

5. Cunningham FG, Leveno KJ, Bloom SL, et al. Chap. 4. Fetal growth and development. In: Cunningham FG, Leveno KJ, Bloom SL, et al. eds. Williams Obstetrics. 23rd ed. New York: McGraw-Hill; 2010. *http://www.accessmedicine.com/content/aspx?aID=6037835.* Accessed June 14, 2013.
6. Bernstein HB, VanBuren G. Chap. 6. Normal pregnancy and prenatal care. In: DeCherney AH, Nathan L, Laufer N, et al. eds. Current Diagnosis and Treatment Obstetrics and Gynecology. 11th ed. New York: McGraw-Hill; 2013. *http://www.accessmedicine.com/content.aspx?aID=5694326.* Accessed June 14, 2013.
7. Cunningham FG, Leveno KJ, Bloom SL, et al. Chap. 8. Prenatal care. In: Cunningham FG, Leveno KJ, Bloom SL, et al. Williams Obstetrics. 23rd ed. New York: McGraw-Hill; 2010. *http://www.accessmedicine.com/content/aspx?aID=6052072.* Accessed June 14, 2013.
8. Feghali MN, Mattison DR. Clinical therapeutics in pregnancy. J Biomed Biotechnol 2011;2011:783528. doi: 10.1155/2011/783528.
9. Flick AA, Kahn DA. Chap. 8. Maternal physiology during pregnancy and fetal and early neonatal physiology. In: DeCherney AH, Nathan L, Laufer N, et al. eds. Current Diagnosis and Treatment Obstetrics and Gynecology. 11th ed. New York: McGraw-Hill; 2013. *http://www.accessmedicine.com/content.aspx?aID=56964738.*
10. Syme MR, Paxton JW, Keelan JA. Drug transfer and metabolism by the human placenta. Clin Pharmacokinet 2004;43:487–514.
11. Polifka JE, Friedman JM. Medical genetics: 1. Clinical teratology in the age of genomics. CMAJ 2002;167: 265–273.
12. Kallen BA. Methodological issues in the epidemiological study of the teratogenicity of drugs. Congenit Anom (Kyoto) 2005;45:44–51.
13. Schaefer C, Ornoy A, Clementi M, et al. Using observational cohort data for studying drug effects on pregnancy outcome—Methodological considerations. Reprod Toxicol 2008;26:36–41.
14. Food and Drug Administration. Content and Format of Labeling for Human Prescription Drug and Biological Products; Requirements for Pregnancy and Lactation Labeling (Proposed Rules). Federal Register 73:104 (May 29, 2008):30831–30868.
15. Johnson K, Posner SF, Biermann J, et al. Recommendations to improve preconception health and health care—United States. A report of the CDC/ATSDR Preconception Care Work Group and the Select Panel on Preconception Care. MMWR Recomm Rep 2006;55(RR-6):1–23.
16. Korenbrot CC, Steinberg A, Bender C, et al. Preconception care: A systematic review. Matern Child Health J 2002;6: 75–88.
17. U.S. Preventive Services Task Force. Folic acid for the prevention of neural tube defects: U.S. Preventive Services Task Force recommendation statement. Ann Intern Med 2009;150:626–631.
18. Lumley J, Chamberlain C, Dowswell T, et al. Interventions for promoting smoking cessation during pregnancy. Cochrane Database Syst Rev 2009(3):CD001055.
19. Rore C, Brace V, Danielian P, et al. Smoking cessation in pregnancy. Expert Opin Drug Saf 2008;7:727–737.
20. Avsar AF, Keskin HL. Haemorrhoids during pregnancy. J Obstet Gynaecol 2010;30:231–237.
21. Keller J, Frederking D, Layer P. The spectrum and treatment of gastrointestinal disorders during pregnancy. Nat Clin Pract Gastroenterol Hepatol 2008;5:430–443.
22. Mahadevan U, Kane S. American Gastroenterological Association Institute Technical Review on the use of gastrointestinal medications in pregnancy. Gastroenterology 2006;131:283–311.
23. Pasternak B, Hviid A. Use of proton–pump inhibitors in early pregnancy and the risk of birth defects. N Engl J Med 2010;363:2114–2123.
24. Lee NM, Saha S. Nausea and vomiting of pregnancy. Gastroenterol Clin North Am 2011;40:309–334.
25. Wegrzyniak LJ, Repke JT, Ural SH. Treatment of hyperemesis gravidarum. Rev Obstet Gynecol 2012;5:78–84.
26. American Diabetes Association. Diagnosis and classification of diabetes mellitus. Diabetes Care 2012;35(Suppl 1):S64–S71.
27. American Diabetes Association. Standards of medical care in diabetes—2012. Diabetes Care 2012;35(Suppl 1):S11–S63.
28. U.S. Preventive Services Task Force. Screening for gestational diabetes mellitus: U.S. Preventive Services Task Force recommendation statement. Ann Intern Med 2008;148:759–765.
29. International Association of Diabetes and Pregnancy Study Groups Consensus Panel, Metzger BE, Gabbe SG, Persson B, et al. International Association of Diabetes and Pregnancy Study Groups recommendations on the diagnosis and classification of hyperglycemia in pregnancy. Diabetes Care 2010;33:676–682.
30. Committee Opinion No. 504: Screening and diagnosis of gestational diabetes mellitus. Obstet Gynecol 2011;118: 751–753.
31. Metzger BE, Buchanan TA, Coustan DR, et al. Summary and recommendations of the Fifth International Workshop-Conference on Gestational Diabetes Mellitus. Diabetes Care 2007;30(Suppl 2):S251–S260.
32. Ballas J, Moore TR, Ramos GA. Management of diabetes in pregnancy. Curr Diab Rep 2012;12:33–42.
33. Crowther CA, Hiller JE, Moss JR, et al. Effect of treatment of gestational diabetes mellitus on pregnancy outcomes. N Engl J Med 2005;352:2477–2486.
34. Alwan N, Tuffnell DJ, West J. Treatments for gestational diabetes. Cochrane Database Syst Rev 2009;(3):CD003395.
35. Mustafa R, Ahmed S, Gupta A, et al. A comprehensive review of hypertension in pregnancy. J Pregnancy 2012; 2012:105918. doi: 10.1155/2012/105918.
36. Magee LA, Helewa M, Moutquin JM, et al. Diagnosis, evaluation, and management of the hypertensive disorders of pregnancy. J Obstet Gynaecol Can 2008;30:S1–S48.
37. Hofmeyr GJ, Duley L, Atallah A. Dietary calcium supplementation for prevention of pre-eclampsia and related problems: A systematic review and commentary. BJOG 2007;114:933–943.
38. Magee LA, Abalos E, von Dadelszen P, et al. How to manage hypertension in pregnancy effectively. Br J Clin Pharmacol 2011;72:394–401.
39. Trogstad L, Magnus P, Stoltenberg C. Pre-eclampsia: Risk factors and causal models. Best Pract Res Clin Obstet Gynaecol 2011;25:329–342.
40. Duley L, Henderson-Smart DJ, Meher S, et al. Antiplatelet agents for preventing pre-eclampsia and its complications. Cochrane Database Syst Rev 2007;(2):CD004659.
41. Payne B, Magee LA, von Dadelszen P. Assessment, surveillance and prognosis in pre-eclampsia. Best Pract Res Clin Obstet Gynaecol 2011;25:449–462.
42. Duley L, Gulmezoglu AM, Henderson-Smart DJ, et al. Magnesium sulphate and other anticonvulsants for women with pre-eclampsia. Cochrane Database Syst Rev 2010;(11):CD000025.

43. Yazbeck CF, Sullivan SD. Thyroid disorders during pregnancy. Med Clin North Am 2012;96:235–256.
44. Bates SM, Greer IA, Middeldorp S, et al. VTE, thrombophilia, antithrombotic therapy, and pregnancy: Antithrombotic therapy and prevention of thrombosis, 9th ed: American College of Chest Physicians Evidence-Based Clinical Practice Guidelines. Chest 2012;141:e691S–e736S.
45. Vazquez JC, Abalos E. Treatments for symptomatic urinary tract infections during pregnancy. Cochrane Database Syst Rev 2011;(1):CD002256.
46. Law H, Fiadjoe P. Urogynaecological problems in pregnancy. J Obstet Gynaecol 2012;32:109–112.
47. Schnarr J, Smaill F. Asymptomatic bacteriuria and symptomatic urinary tract infections in pregnancy. Eur J Clin Invest 2008;38(Suppl 2):50–57.
48. Workowski KA, Berman S; Centers for Disease Control and Prevention (CDC). Sexually transmitted diseases treatment guidelines, 2010. MMWR Recomm Rep 2010;59(RR-12): 1–110.
49. Centers for Disease Control and Prevention (CDC). Update to CDC's Sexually Transmitted Diseases Treatment Guidelines, 2010: Oral cephalosporins no longer a recommended treatment for gonococcal infections. Morb Mortal Wkly Rep 2012;61:590–594.
50. Su CW, McKay B. Treatment of HSV infection in late pregnancy. Am Fam Physician 2012;85:390–393.
51. Macgregor EA. Headache in pregnancy. Neurol Clin 2012;30:835–866.
52. Vatti RR, Teuber SS. Asthma and pregnancy. Clin Rev Allergy Immunol 2012;43:45–56.
53. Expert Panel Report 3 (EPR-3): Guidelines for the Diagnosis and Management of Asthma—Summary Report 2007. J Allergy Clin Immunol 2007;120(5 Suppl):S94–S138.
54. Global Strategy for Asthma Management and Prevention (updated 2011): Global Initiative for Asthma (GINA). *http://www.ginasthma.org*, 2011..
55. Piette V, Daures JP, Demoly P. Treating allergic rhinitis in pregnancy. Curr Allergy Asthma Rep 2006;6:232–238.
56. Gilbert C, Mazzotta P, Loebstein R, et al. Fetal safety of drugs used in the treatment of allergic rhinitis: A critical review. Drug Saf 2005;28:707–719.
57. Kitzmiller JL, Block JM, Brown FM, et al. Managing preexisting diabetes for pregnancy: Summary of evidence and consensus recommendations for care. Diabetes Care 2008;31:1060–1079.
58. Harden CL, Hopp J, Ting TY, et al. Management issues for women with epilepsy-Focus on pregnancy (an evidence-based review): I. Obstetrical complications and change in seizure frequency: Report of the Quality Standards Subcommittee and Therapeutics and Technology Assessment Subcommittee of the American Academy of Neurology and the American Epilepsy Society. Epilepsia 2009;50: 1229–1236.
59. Tomson T, Battino D. Pregnancy and epilepsy: What should we tell our patients? J Neurol 2009;256:856–862.
60. Harden CL, Sethi NK. Epileptic disorders in pregnancy: An overview. Curr Opin Obstet Gynecol 2008;20: 557–562.
61. Harden CL, Meador KJ, Pennell PB, et al. Management issues for women with epilepsy—Focus on pregnancy (an evidence-based review): II. Teratogenesis and perinatal outcomes: Report of the Quality Standards Subcommittee and Therapeutics and Technology Subcommittee of the American Academy of Neurology and the American Epilepsy Society. Epilepsia 2009;50:1237–1246.
62. Panel on treatment of HIV-infected pregnant women and prevention of perinatal transmission. Recommendations for use of antiretroviral drugs in pregnant HIV-1-infected women for maternal health *and* interventions to reduce perinatal HIV transmission in the United States. Available at *http://aidsinfo.nih.gov/contentfiles/lvguidelines/PerinatalGL.pdf.*
63. American College of Obstetricians and Gynecologists. ACOG Practice Bulletin No. 125: Chronic hypertension in pregnancy. Obstet Gynecol 2012;119:396–407.
64. ACOG Practice Bulletin: Clinical Management Guidelines for Obstetrician-Gynecologists No. 92, April 2008 (replaces practice bulletin number 87, November 2007). Use of psychiatric medications during pregnancy and lactation. Obstet Gynecol 2008;111:1001–1020.
65. Gentile S. Drug treatment for mood disorders in pregnancy. Curr Opin Psychiatry 2011;24:34–40.
66. Levey L, Ragan K, Hower-Hartley A, et al. Psychiatric disorders in pregnancy. Neurol Clin 2004;22:863–893.
67. McCauley-Elsom K, Gurvich C, Elsom SJ, et al. Antipsychotics in pregnancy. J Psychiatr Ment Health Nurs 2010;17:97–104.
68. Damus K. Prevention of preterm birth: A renewed national priority. Curr Opin Obstet Gynecol 2008;20:590–596.
69. Chandiramani M, Shennan A. Preterm labour: Update on prediction and prevention strategies. Curr Opin Obstet Gynecol 2006;18:618–624.
70. Hamilton BE, Martin JA, Ventura SJ. Births: Preliminary data for 2010. Natl Vital Stat Rep 2011;60(2):1–6.
71. Giles W, Bisits A. Preterm labour. The present and future of tocolysis. Best Pract Res Clin Obstet Gynaecol 2007;21:857–868.
72. Weismiller DG. Preterm labor. Am Fam Physician 1999;59:593–602.
73. Haas DM, Imperiale TF, Kirkpatrick PR, et al. Tocolytic therapy: A meta-analysis and decision analysis. Obstet Gynecol 2009;113:585–594.
74. Crowther CA, Hiller JE, Doyle LW. Magnesium sulphate for preventing preterm birth in threatened preterm labour. Cochrane Database Syst Rev 2002(4):CD001060.
75. Rouse DJ, Hirtz DG, Thom E, et al. A randomized, controlled trial of magnesium sulfate for the prevention of cerebral palsy. N Engl J Med 2008;359:895–905.
76. ACOG Committee Opinion No. 445. Antibiotics for preterm labor. Obstet Gynecol 2009;114:1159–1160.
77. Meis PJ, Connors N. Progesterone treatment to prevent preterm birth. Clin Obstet Gynecol 2004;47:784–795.
78. da Fonseca EB, Bittar RE, Carvalho MH, et al. Prophylactic administration of progesterone by vaginal suppository to reduce the incidence of spontaneous preterm birth in women at increased risk: A randomized placebo-controlled double-blind study. Am J Obstet Gynecol 2003;188:419–424.
79. Spong CY, Meis PJ, Thom EA, et al. Progesterone for prevention of recurrent preterm birth: Impact of gestational age at previous delivery. Am J Obstet Gynecol 2005;193:1127–1131.
80. ACOG Committee Opinion No. 419, October 2008 (replaces no. 291, November 2003). Use of progesterone to reduce preterm birth. Obstet Gynecol 2008;112:963–965.
81. Roberts D, Dalziel S. Antenatal corticosteroids for accelerating fetal lung maturation for women at risk of preterm birth. Cochrane Database Syst Rev 2006(3);3: CD004454.
82. Garite TJ, Kurtzman J, Maurel K, et al. Impact of a 'rescue course' of antenatal corticosteroids: A multicenter

randomized placebo-controlled trial. Am J Obstet Gynecol 2009;200:248 e1–e9.

83. Phares CR, Lynfield R, Farley MM, et al. Epidemiology of invasive group B streptococcal disease in the United States, 1999–2005. JAMA 2008;299:2056–2065.
84. Verani JR, McGee L, Schrag SJ, et al. Prevention of perinatal group B streptococcal disease—Revised guidelines from CDC, 2010. MMWR Recomm Rep 2010;59(RR-10):1–36.
85. Tenore JL. Methods for cervical ripening and induction of labor. Am Fam Physician 2003;67:2123–2128.
86. Sanchez-Ramos L. Induction of labor. Obstet Gynecol Clin North Am 2005;32:181–200.
87. Hapangama D, Neilson JP. Mifepristone for induction of labour. Cochrane Database Syst Rev 2009;(3): CD002865.
88. Kuczkowski KM. Labor pain and its management with the combined spinal-epidural analgesia: What does an obstetrician need to know? Arch Gynecol Obstet 2007; 275:183–185.
89. Simkin P, Bolding A. Update on nonpharmacologic approaches to relieve labor pain and prevent suffering. J Midwifery Womens Health 2004;49:489–504.
90. ACOG Committee Opinion No. 295: Pain relief during labor. Obstet Gynecol 2004;104:213.
91. Anim-Somuah M, Smyth R, Howell C. Epidural versus non-epidural or no analgesia in labour. Cochrane Database Syst Rev 2005;(4):CD000331.
92. van der Vyver M, Halpern S, Joseph G. Patient-controlled epidural analgesia versus continuous infusion for labour analgesia: A meta-analysis. Br J Anaesth 2002;89: 459–465.
93. Chong YS, Su LL, Arulkumaran S. Current strategies for the prevention of postpartum haemorrhage in the third stage of labour. Curr Opin Obstet Gynecol 2004;16:143–150.
94. Mousa HA, Alfirevic Z. Treatment for primary postpartum haemorrhage. Cochrane Database Syst Rev 2007;(1): CD003249.
95. Sheiner E, Sarid L, Levy A, et al. Obstetric risk factors and outcome of pregnancies complicated with early postpartum hemorrhage: A population-based study. J Matern Fetal Neonatal Med 2005;18:149–154.
96. Section on Breastfeeding. Breastfeeding and the use of human milk. Pediatrics 2012;129:e827–841.
97. Academy Of Breastfeeding Medicine Protocol Committee. ABM Clinical Protocol #9: Use of galactogogues in initiating or augmenting the rate of maternal milk secretion (First Revision January 2011). Breastfeed Med 2011;6:41–49.
98. Ilett KF, Kristensen JH. Drug use and breastfeeding. Expert Opin Drug Saf 2005;4:745–768.
99. Della-Giustina K, Chow G. Medications in pregnancy and lactation. Emerg Med Clin North Am 2003;21:585–613.
100. Jahanfar S, Ng CJ, Teng CL. Antibiotics for mastitis in breastfeeding women. Cochrane Database Syst Rev 2009;(1):CD005458.
101. Walker M. Conquering common breast-feeding problems. J Perinat Neonatal Nurs 2008;22:267–274.
102. Pearlstein T, Howard M, Salisbury A, et al. Postpartum depression. Am J Obstet Gynecol 2009;200:357–364.

62

Contraception

Sarah P. Shrader and Kelly R. Ragucci

KEY CONCEPTS

1. The attitude of the patient and sexual partner toward contraceptive methods, efficacy rate, the reliability of the patient in using the method correctly (which may affect the effectiveness of the method), noncontraceptive benefits, and the patient's ability to pay must be considered when selecting a contraceptive method.
2. Patient-specific factors (e.g., frequency of intercourse, age, smoking status, and concomitant diseases or medications) must be evaluated when selecting a contraceptive method.
3. Adverse effects or difficulties using the chosen method should be monitored carefully and managed in consideration of patient-specific factors.
4. Accurate and timely counseling on the optimal use of the contraceptive method and strategies for minimizing sexually transmitted diseases must be provided to all patients when contraceptives are initiated and on an ongoing basis.
5. Emergency contraception may prevent pregnancy after unprotected intercourse or when regular contraceptive methods have failed.

Unintended pregnancy is a significant public health problem. In the United States, approximately 6 million females become pregnant each year.[1] The most recent data reveal that 37% of pregnancies are unintended, with the highest rates occurring in women aged 20 to 34 years.[1] However, teen pregnancy rates are still an issue and slow to decline; teen births account for 11% of all the births in the United States.[1] About half of all unintended pregnancies end in abortion, and 40% occur in sexually active couples who claim they used some method of contraception.[1] If the goal of contraception—for pregnancies to be planned and desired—is to be realized, education on the use and efficacy of contraceptive methods must be improved.

ETIOLOGY AND PATHOPHYSIOLOGY

Comprehension of the hormonal regulation of the normal menstrual cycle is essential to understanding contraception in women (Fig. 62-1). The cycle of menstruation begins with menarche, usually around age 12 years, and continues to occur in nonpregnant women until menopause, usually around age 50 years. Factors such as race, body weight, medical conditions, and family history can affect the menstrual cycle.[2] The cycle includes the vaginal discharge of sloughed endometrium called *menses*. The menstrual cycle comprises three phases: follicular (or preovulatory), ovulatory, and luteal (or postovulatory).

The Menstrual Cycle

The first day of menses is referred to as *day 1 of the menstrual cycle* and marks the beginning of the follicular phase.[2] The follicular phase continues until ovulation, which typically occurs on day 14. The time after ovulation is referred to as the *luteal phase*, which lasts until the beginning of the next menstrual cycle. The median menstrual cycle length is 28 days, but it can range from 21 to 40 days. Generally, variation in length is greatest in the follicular phase, particularly in the years immediately after menarche and before menopause.[2]

The menstrual cycle is influenced by the hormonal relationships among the hypothalamus, anterior pituitary, and ovaries.[2] The hypothalamus secretes gonadotropin-releasing hormone (GnRH) in a pulsatile fashion.[2] These GnRH bursts stimulate the anterior pituitary to secrete bursts of gonadotropins, follicle-stimulating hormone (FSH), and luteinizing hormone (LH). FSH and LH direct events in the ovarian follicles that result in the production of a fertile ovum.

Follicular Phase

In the first 4 days of the menstrual cycle, FSH levels rise and allow the recruitment of a small group of follicles for continued growth and development (Fig. 62-1).[2] Between days 5 and 7, one follicle becomes dominant and later ruptures, releasing the oocyte. The dominant follicle develops increasing amounts of estradiol and inhibin, which cause a negative feedback on the hypothalamic secretion of GnRH and pituitary secretion of FSH, causing atresia of the remaining follicles recruited during the cycle.

Once the follicle has received FSH stimulation, it must receive continued FSH stimulation or it will die.[2] FSH allows the follicle to enlarge and synthesize estradiol, progesterone, and androgen. Estradiol stops the menstrual flow from the previous cycle, thickening the endometrial lining of the uterus to prepare it for embryonic implantation. Estrogen is responsible for increased production of thin, watery cervical mucus, which will enhance sperm transport during fertilization. FSH regulates the aromatase enzymes that convert androgens to estrogens in the follicle. If a follicle has insufficient aromatase, the follicle will not survive.

Ovulation

When estradiol levels remain elevated for a sustained period of time, the pituitary releases a midcycle LH surge (Fig. 62-1).[2] This LH surge stimulates the final stages of follicular maturation and ovulation (follicular rupture and release of the oocyte). On average, ovulation occurs 24 to 36 hours after the estradiol peak and 10 to 16 hours after the LH peak. The LH surge, which occurs 28 to 32 hours before a follicle ruptures, is the most clinically useful predictor of approaching ovulation. After ovulation, the oocyte is

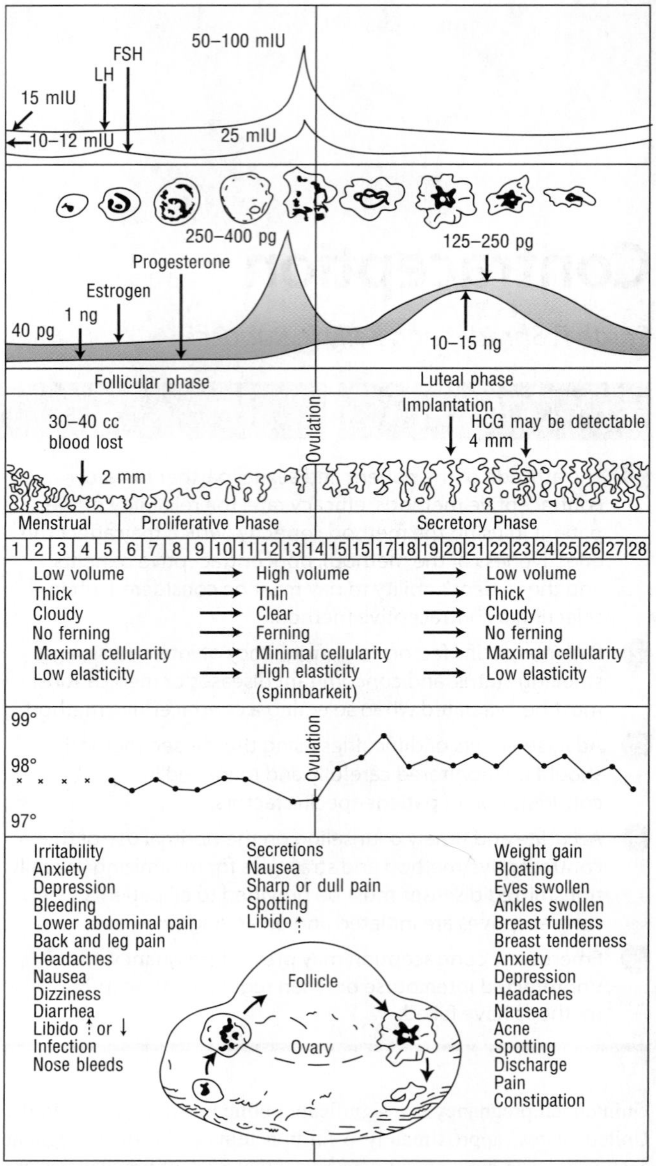

FIGURE 62-1 Menstrual cycle events, idealized 28-day cycle. (FSH, follicle-stimulating hormone; HCG, human chorionic gonadotropin, LH, luteinizing hormone.) LH: 15 milli-international units/mL = 15 international units/L; 50 to 100 milli-international units/mL = 50 to 100 international units/L. FSH: 10 to 12 milli-international units/mL = 10 to 12 international units/L; 25 milli-international units/mL = 25 international units/L. Estrogen: 40 pg/mL = ~150 pmol/L; 250 to 400 pg/mL = ~920 to 1470 pmol/L; 125 to 250 pg/mL = ~460 to 920 pmol/L. Progesterone: 1 ng/mL = 3 nmol/L; 10 to 15 ng/mL = ~30 to 50 nmol/L. Temperatures: 99° F = 37.2° C; 98° F = 36.7° C; 97° F = 36.1° C. *(From Hatcher et al.[2] This figure may be reproduced at no cost to the reader.)*

released and travels to the fallopian tube, where it can be fertilized and transported to the uterus for embryonic implantation. Conception is most successful when intercourse takes place from 2 days before ovulation to the day of ovulation.

Luteal Phase

After rupture of the follicle and release of the ovum, the remaining luteinized follicles become the corpus luteum, which synthesizes androgen, estrogen, and progesterone (Fig. 62-1).[2] Progesterone helps to maintain the endometrial lining, which sustains the implanted embryo and maintains the pregnancy. It also inhibits GnRH and gonadotropin release, preventing the development of new follicles. If pregnancy occurs, human chorionic gonadotropin prevents regression of the corpus luteum and stimulates continued production of estrogen and progesterone secretion to maintain the pregnancy until the placenta is able to fulfill this role.

If fertilization or implantation does not occur, the corpus luteum degenerates, and progesterone production declines.[2] The life span of the corpus luteum depends on the continuous presence of small amounts of LH, and its average duration of function is 9 to 11 days. As progesterone levels decline, endometrial shedding (menstruation) occurs, and a new menstrual cycle begins. At the end of the luteal phase, when estrogen and progesterone levels are low, FSH levels start to rise, and follicular recruitment for the next cycle begins.

EPIDEMIOLOGY

Contraception implies the prevention of pregnancy following sexual intercourse by inhibiting viable sperm from coming into contact with a mature ovum (i.e., methods that act as barriers or prevent ovulation) or by preventing a fertilized ovum from implanting successfully in the endometrium (i.e., mechanisms that create an unfavorable uterine environment). These methods differ in their relative effectiveness, safety, and patient acceptability (Tables 62-1 and 62-2).[2,3]

The actual effectiveness of any contraceptive method is difficult to determine because many factors affect contraceptive failure. A failure in patients who use the contraceptive agent properly is considered a method failure or perfect-use failure. It is also important to consider user failure or typical-use failure rates, which are usually higher because they take into account the user's ability to follow directions correctly and consistently.[2,3]

TABLE 62-1 Comparison of Unintended Pregnancy and Continuation Rates for Pharmacologic Contraceptive Methods

Method	Percent of Women with Pregnancy with Typical Use[a]	Percent of Women with Pregnancy with Perfect Use[a]	Percent of Women Continuing Use[b]
Combined oral contraceptive and progestin-only oral contraceptive	8	0.3	68
Combined hormonal transdermal contraceptive patch	8	0.3	68
Combined hormonal vaginal contraceptive ring	8	0.3	68
Depo-medroxyprogesterone acetate	3	0.3	56
Copper IUD	0.8	0.6	78
Levonorgestrel IUD	0.2	0.2	80
Progestin-only implant	0.05	0.05	84

[a]Failure rates in the United States during first year of use.
[b]Continuation rate in the United States at the end of the first year of use.
Data from Hatcher et al.[2] and Dickey.[3]

CLINICAL PRESENTATION

Most health maintenance annual visits should include assessment of and counseling about reproductive health. Clinicians may use this opportunity to provide contraception and educate patients on prevention of sexually transmitted diseases (STDs). Traditionally, hormonal contraception is provided subsequent to breast and pelvic examinations. However, the need for the physical examination may delay access to contraception and reinforces the incorrect perception that these methods of contraceptives are harmful. Therefore, the American Congress of Obstetrics and Gynecology (ACOG) allow provision of hormonal contraception after a simple medical history and blood pressure measurement.[4] Other preventive measures, such as pelvic and breast examinations, provision of the human papillomavirus vaccine, and screening for cervical neoplasia, can be accomplished during routine annual office visits.[4,5]

TREATMENT

Desired Outcomes

The obvious goal of treatment with all methods of contraception is to prevent pregnancy. However, many health benefits are associated with contraceptive methods, including prevention of STDs (with condoms), improvements in menstrual cycle regularity (with hormonal contraceptives), improvements in certain health conditions (with hormonal contraceptives), and management of perimenopause.[2,6]

Nonpharmacologic Therapy

Periodic Abstinence

❶ ❷ Motivated couples may use the abstinence (rhythm) method of contraception, avoiding sexual intercourse during the days of the menstrual cycle when conception is likely to occur. Physiologic changes, such as basal body temperature and cervical mucus, are used during each cycle to determine the fertile period. The major drawbacks are the relatively high pregnancy rates and avoidance of intercourse for several days during each menstrual cycle.[2]

Barrier Techniques

❶ ❷ The effectiveness of barrier methods depends almost exclusively on motivation to use them consistently and correctly.[2] These methods include condoms, diaphragms, cervical caps, and sponges (Table 62-2). A major disadvantage is higher failure rates than most hormonal contraceptives; thus, provision of counseling and an advanced prescription for emergency contraception (EC) are recommended for all patients using barrier methods as their primary means of contraception.

Male condoms create a mechanical barrier, preventing direct contact of the vagina with semen, genital lesions, and infectious secretions.[2] Most condoms in the United States are made of latex, which is impermeable to viruses. A small proportion are made from lamb intestine, which is not impermeable to viruses. Synthetic condoms manufactured from polyurethane are another option; these condoms are latex-free and do protect against viruses. Condoms are used worldwide as protection from STDs including human immunodeficiency virus (HIV). When condoms are used in conjunction with any other barrier method, their effectiveness theoretically approaches 98%. Spillage of semen or perforation and tearing of the condom can occur, but proper use minimizes these problems. Mineral oil-based vaginal drug formulations (e.g., Cleocin, Premarin, and Monistat), lotions, or lubricants can decrease the barrier strength of latex, thus making water-soluble lubricants (e.g., Astroglide, K-Y Jelly) preferable. Condoms with spermicides are no longer recommended because they provide no additional protection against pregnancy or STDs and may increase vulnerability to HIV.

The female condom is a prelubricated, loose-fitting polyurethane sheath, closed at one end, with flexible rings at both ends.[2] Properly positioned, the ring at the closed end covers the cervix, and the sheath lines the walls of the vagina. The outer ring remains outside the vagina, covering the labia. The pregnancy rate is reported to be higher when compared to male condoms. Male and female condoms should not be used together, as slippage and device displacement may occur.

The diaphragm, a reusable dome-shaped rubber cap with a flexible rim that is inserted vaginally, fits over the cervix in order to decrease access of sperm to the ovum. The diaphragm requires a prescription from a clinician who has fitted the patient for the correct size.[2] Its efficacy is increased when it is used in conjunction with spermicidal cream or jelly. The diaphragm may be inserted up to 6 hours before intercourse and must be left in place for at least 6 hours afterward. However, leaving it in place for more than 24 hours is not recommended due to the potential for toxic shock syndrome (TSS). With subsequent acts of intercourse, the diaphragm should be left in place, and a condom should be used for additional protection.

The cervical cap (FemCap) is a soft, deep cup with a firm round rim that is smaller than a diaphragm and fits over the cervix like a thimble.[2] The cervical cap is available in three sizes and requires a prescription from a clinician who has fitted the patient for the correct size. It should be filled with spermicide prior to insertion. The cervical cap can be inserted 6 hours prior to intercourse and should not be removed for at least 6 hours after intercourse. It can remain in place for multiple episodes of intercourse without adding more spermicide but should not be worn for more than 48 hours at a time

TABLE 62-2 Comparison of Methods of Nonhormonal Contraception

Method	Absolute Contraindications	Advantages	Disadvantages	Percent of Women with Pregnancy[a] Perfect Use	Percent of Women with Pregnancy[a] Typical Use
Condoms, male	Allergy to latex or rubber	Inexpensive STD protection, including HIV (latex only)	High user failure rate Poor acceptance Possibility of breakage Efficacy decreased by oil-based lubricants Possible allergic reactions to latex in either partner	2	15
Condoms, female	Allergy to polyurethane History of TSS	Can be inserted just before intercourse or ahead of time STD protection, including HIV	High user failure rate Dislike ring hanging outside vagina Cumbersome	5	21
Diaphragm with spermicide	Allergy to latex, rubber, or spermicide Recurrent UTIs History of TSS Abnormal gynecologic anatomy	Low cost Decreased incidence of cervical neoplasia Some protection against STDs	High user failure rate Decreased efficacy with increased frequency of intercourse Increased incidence of vaginal yeast UTIs, TSS Efficacy decreased by oil-based lubricants Cervical irritation	6	12
Cervical cap (FemCap)	Allergy to spermicide History of TSS Abnormal gynecologic anatomy Abnormal papanicolaou smear	Low cost Latex-free Some protection against STDs FemCap reusable for up to 2 years	High user failure rate Decreased efficacy with parity Cannot be used during menses	9	16[b]
Spermicides alone	Allergy to spermicide	Inexpensive	High user failure rate Must be reapplied before each act of intercourse May enhance HIV transmission No protection against STDs	18	28
Sponge (Today)	Allergy to spermicide Recurrent UTIs History of TSS Abnormal gynecologic anatomy	Inexpensive	High user failure rate Decreased efficacy with parity Cannot be used during menses No protection against STDs	9[c]	12[d]

HIV, human immunodeficiency virus; STD, sexually transmitted disease; TSS, toxic shock syndrome; UTI, urinary tract infection.

[a]Failure rates in the United States during first year of use.
[b]Failure rate with FemCap reported to be 24% per package insert.
[c]Failure rate with Today sponge reported to be 20% in parous women.
[d]Failure rate with Today sponge reported to be 32% in parous women.

Data from Hatcher et al.[2]

to reduce the risk of TSS. Failure rates are higher than with other methods. Diaphragms and cervical caps do not protect against some STDs including HIV, thus condoms should also be used.

Pharmacologic Therapy

Spermicides

1 2 Spermicides, most of which contain nonoxynol-9, are chemical surfactants that destroy sperm cell walls and act as barriers that prevent sperm from entering the cervical os.[2] They are available as creams, films, foams, gels, suppositories, sponges, and tablets. Spermicides offer no protection against STDs. In fact, when used frequently (more than two times per day), nonoxynol-9 may increase the risk of transmission of HIV by causing small disruptions in the vaginal epithelium.[2,7,8] The World Health Organization (WHO) and the Centers for Disease Control and Prevention (CDC) do not promote products containing nonoxynol-9 for protection against STDs.

Spermicide-Implanted Barrier Techniques

1 2 The vaginal contraceptive sponge (Today) contains 1 g of the spermicide nonoxynol-9.[2] It has a concave dimple on one side to fit over the cervix and a loop on the other side to facilitate removal. After being moistened with water, the sponge is inserted into the vagina up to 6 hours before intercourse. The sponge provides protection for 24 hours, regardless of the frequency of intercourse during this time. After intercourse, the sponge must be left in place for at least 6 hours before removal and should not be left in place for more than 24 to 30 hours to reduce the risk of TSS. Sponges should not be reused; after removal, they should be discarded. The sponge comes in one size and is available over the counter (OTC).

Hormonal Contraception

Hormonal contraceptives contain a combination of estrogen and progestin or a progestin alone. Oral contraceptive (OC) preparations first became available in the 1960s, but options have expanded to include a transdermal patch, a vaginal contraceptive ring, and long-acting injectable, implantable, and intrauterine contraceptives.

Combined hormonal contraceptives (CHCs) contain both estrogen and progestin and work primarily before fertilization to prevent conception. Progestins provide most of the contraceptive effect by thickening cervical mucus to prevent sperm penetration, slowing tubal motility, delaying sperm transport, and inducing endometrial atrophy. Progestins block the LH surge, therefore inhibiting ovulation. Estrogens suppress FSH release from the pituitary, which may contribute to blocking the LH surge and preventing ovulation.

However, the primary role of estrogen in hormonal contraceptives is to stabilize the endometrial lining and provide cycle control.[2,3]

Estrogens Two synthetic estrogens found in hormonal contraceptives available in the United States are ethinyl estradiol (EE) and mestranol. Mestranol must be converted by the liver to EE before it is pharmacologically active and is 50% less potent than EE.[2,3] Most combined OCs, transdermal patch, and vaginal ring contain estrogen at doses of 20 to 50 mcg of EE.[3]

Progestins A variety of progestins are available in the United States, and they vary in their progestational activity and differ with respect to inherent estrogenic, antiestrogenic, and androgenic effects.[2,3] Estrogenic and antiestrogenic properties are secondary to the extent of progestins' metabolism to estrogenic substances. Androgenic activity depends on two variables: the presence of sex hormone (testosterone) binding globulin (SHBG-TBG) and the androgen-to-progesterone activity ratio. If the amount of SHBG-TBG is decreased, free testosterone levels increase, and androgenic side effects are more prominent.[3]

Considerations with Combined Hormonal Contraceptive Use ❶ When selecting a CHC, clinicians are challenged by weighing the benefits and risks associated with the many formulations available. The clinician must determine if the form of contraception is appropriate based upon the patient's lifestyle and potential adherence. A complete medical examination and papanicolaou (Pap) smear are not necessary before a CHC is prescribed. A medical history and blood pressure measurement should be obtained before prescribing a CHC, along with a discussion of the benefits, risks, and adverse effects with each patient.[2,3,9] For example, OCs are associated with noncontraceptive benefits, including relief from menstruation-related problems (e.g., decreased menstrual cramps, decreased ovulatory pain [mittelschmerz], and decreased menstrual blood loss), improvement in menstrual regularity, and decreased iron deficiency anemia.[6] Women who take combination OCs have a reduced risk of ovarian and endometrial cancer. There is a 50% reduction in risk in women who have used OCs for 5 years or more, and protection may persist for more than 10 years post-use. Combination OCs may also reduce the risk of ovarian cysts, ectopic pregnancy, pelvic inflammatory disease, endometriosis, uterine fibroids, and benign breast disease. The CHC transdermal patch and vaginal ring are other combined hormonal options that may be more convenient for women than taking a tablet each day.

❷ ❸ Adverse effects may hinder adherence and therefore efficacy, so they should be discussed prior to initiating a hormonal contraceptive agent.[10] Excessive or deficient amounts of estrogen and progestin are related to the most common adverse effects.[2,3,10] The CHC vaginal ring may be uncomfortable for some women and cause vaginal discharge. The CHC patch may cause irritation and now has information added to product labeling regarding the increased potential for thromboembolism.

An important concern regarding the use of CHCs is the lack of protection against STDs. Because of their high efficacy in preventing pregnancy, patients may choose not to use condoms. In addition to public health awareness, clinicians must encourage patients to use condoms for prevention of STDs. OCs have an extensive history of safety concerns, which traditionally were related to high dose estrogen tablets. To replace the traditional absolute and relative contraindications to the use of OCs, the CDC developed a graded list of precautions for clinicians to consider when initiating CHCs (Table 62-3).[2,9]

In addition to the CDC, the ACOG provides information for clinicians to use when selecting CHCs for women with coexisting medical conditions.[11] Overall, the health risks associated with pregnancy, the specific health risks associated with CHCs, and the noncontraceptive benefits of CHCs should be factored into risk-to-benefit considerations.

Women Older Than 35 Years Use of CHC in women older than 35 is controversial. Older women, especially women in their 40s, retain a level of fertility even in the perimenopausal state and should use contraception to prevent pregnancy. Formulations with lower doses of estrogen (less than 30 mcg) have increased the use of CHCs in these women. In addition to the benefit of pregnancy prevention, they may improve or decrease the chance of developing perimenopausal and menopausal symptoms and increase bone mineral density (BMD). However, the benefits of using CHCs must be weighed against the risks in women older than 35. The increased risk of cardiovascular disease and venous thromboembolism (VTE) should be considered especially in perimenopausal women greater than 40. Older data suggest an increased risk of myocardial infarction (MI) in older women using CHCs, although many women in these studies were current smokers and used older formulations containing higher doses (greater than 50 mcg) of estrogen. More recent data do not support the increased risk of cardiovascular disease when low-dose formulations of CHCs are used in healthy, nonobese women. Other concerns include the increased risk of ischemic stroke in women with migraines and the increased risk of breast cancer in older women.[9,11,12]

The risks and benefits of using CHCs in women greater than 35 must be considered on an individual basis. It is recommended that use of CHCs (with less than 50 mcg of estrogen) may be considered in healthy nonsmoking women. CHCs should not be recommended in women older than 35 years with migraine (with or without aura), uncontrolled hypertension, smoking, or diabetes with vascular disease.[9,11]

Smoking In early studies, OCs with 50 mcg EE or more were associated with MI in women who smoked cigarettes.[2,3,9,11] The United States case–control studies have found that both nonsmoking and smoking women, regardless of age, taking OCs with less than 50 mcg EE did not have an increased risk of MI or stroke. However, these studies included few women older than 35 years who were smokers. European studies, with a higher population of older smoking women, demonstrated an increased risk of MI in this population. Therefore, practitioners should prescribe CHC with caution, if at all, to women older than 35 years who smoke. Smoking 15 or more cigarettes per day by women in this age group is a contraindication to CHC, and the risks generally outweigh the benefits of CHC in those who smoke fewer than 15 cigarettes per day.[9] Progestin-only contraceptive methods should be considered for women in this group.

Hypertension CHCs can cause small increases (i.e., 6 to 8 mm Hg) in blood pressure, regardless of estrogen dosage.[3,9,11] This has been documented in both normotensive and mildly hypertensive women given a 30 mcg EE OC. In case–control studies of women with hypertension, OCs have been associated with an increased risk of MI and stroke. Use of low-dose CHC is acceptable in women younger than 35 years with well-controlled and frequently monitored hypertension. If a CHC-related increase in blood pressure occurs, discontinuing the CHC usually restores blood pressure to pretreatment values within 3 to 6 months.[3] Systolic blood pressure greater than or equal to 160 mm Hg or diastolic blood pressure greater than or equal to 100 mm Hg is considered a contraindication to the use of CHCs. Hypertensive women who have end-organ vascular disease or who smoke should not use CHCs. Women with hypertension who are taking potassium-sparing diuretics, angiotensin-converting enzyme inhibitors, angiotensin-receptor blockers, or aldosterone antagonists may have increased serum potassium concentrations if they are also using an OC-containing drospirenone, which has antialdosterone properties.[3]

TABLE 62-3 U.S. Medical Eligibility Criteria for Contraceptive Use: Classifications for Combined Hormonal Contraceptives

Category 4: Unacceptable health risk (method not to be used)
- Breast-feeding or non-breastfeeding <21 days postpartum
- Current breast cancer
- Severe (decompensated) cirrhosis
- History/risk of or current deep venous thrombosis/pulmonary embolism (not on anticoagulant therapy); thrombogenic mutations
- Major surgery with prolonged immobilization
- Migraines with aura, any age
- Systolic blood pressure ≥160 mm Hg or diastolic ≥100 mm Hg
- Current and history of ischemic heart disease
- Benign hepatocellular adenoma or malignant liver tumor
- Moderately or severely impaired cardiac function; normal or mildly impaired cardiac function <6 months
- Smoking ≥15 cigarettes per day and age ≥35
- Complicated solid organ transplantation
- History of cerebrovascular accident
- SLE; positive or unknown antiphospholipid antibodies
- Complicated valvular heart disease

Category 3: Theoretical or proven risks usually outweigh the advantages
- Breast-feeding 21–30 days postpartum with or without risk factors for VTE
- Breast-feeding 30–42 days postpartum with other risk factors for VTE
- Non-breastfeeding 21–42 days postpartum with other risk factors for VTE
- Past breast cancer and no evidence of disease for 5 years
- History of DVT/PE (not on anticoagulant therapy), but lower risk for recurrent DVT/PE
- Current gallbladder disease, symptomatic and medically treated
- Migraines without aura, age ≥35 (*category 4 with continued use*)
- History of bariatric surgery; malabsorptive procedures
- History of cholestasis, past COC-related
- Hypertension; systolic blood pressure 140–159 mm Hg or diastolic 90–99 mm Hg
- Normal or mildly impaired cardiac function ≥6 months
- Postpartum 21 to 42 days with other risk factors for VTE
- Smoking <15 cigarettes per day and age ≥35
- Use of ritonavir-boosted protease inhibitors
- Use of certain anticonvulsants (phenytoin, carbamazepine, barbiturates, primidone, topiramate, oxcarbazepine, and lamotrigine)
- Use of rifampicin or rifabutin therapy
- Diabetes with vascular disease or >20 years duration (*possibly category 4 depending upon severity*)
- Multiple risk factors for arterial cardiovascular disease (older age, smoking, diabetes, and hypertension) (*possibly category 4 depending on category and severity*)

Category 2: Advantages generally outweigh theoretical or proven risks
- Age ≥40 (in the absence of other comorbid conditions that increase CVD risk)
- Sickle-cell disease
- Undiagnosed breast mass
- Cervical cancer and awaiting treatment; cervical intraepithelial neoplasia
- Family history (first-degree relatives) of DVT/PE
- Major surgery without prolonged immobilization
- Diabetes mellitus (type 1 or type 2)
- Gallbladder disease; symptomatic and treated by cholecystectomy or asymptomatic
- Migraines without aura, age <35 (*category 3 with continued use*)
- History of pregnancy-related cholestasis
- History of high blood pressure during pregnancy
- Benign liver tumors; focal nodular hyperplasia
- Obesity
- Breast-feeding 30–42 days postpartum without risk factors for VTE
- Breast-feeding >42 days postpartum
- Non-breastfeeding 21–42 days postpartum without risk factors for VTE
- Rheumatoid arthritis on or off immunosuppressive therapy
- Smoking and <35 years old
- Uncomplicated sold organ transplantation
- Superficial thrombophlebitis
- SLE and severe thrombocytopenia or immunosuppressive treatment
- Unexplained vaginal bleeding before evaluation
- Uncomplicated valvular heart disease
- Use of nonnucleoside reverse transcriptase inhibitors
- Hyperlipidemia (*possibly category 3 based upon type, severity, and other risk factors*)
- Inflammatory bowel disease (*possibly category 3 for those with increased risk of VTE*)

Category 1: No restriction (method can be used)
- Thalassemia, iron deficiency anemia
- Mild compensated cirrhosis
- Minor surgery without immobilization
- Depression
- Gestational diabetes mellitus
- Endometrial cancer/hyperplasia, endometriosis
- Epilepsy
- Gestational trophoblastic disease
- Nonmigrainous headaches
- History of bariatric surgery; restrictive procedures
- History of pelvic surgery
- HIV infected or high risk
- Malaria
- Ovarian cancer
- Past ectopic pregnancy
- PID
- Postabortion
- Non-breastfeeding >42 days postpartum
- Severe dysmenorrhea
- Sexually transmitted infections
- Varicose veins
- Thyroid disorders
- Tuberculosis
- Uterine fibroids
- Use of nucleoside reverse transcriptase inhibitors
- Use of broad-spectrum antibiotics, antifungals, and antiparasitics

CHC, combined hormonal contraception; HIV, human immunodeficiency virus; VTE, venous thromboembolism; PE, pulmonary embolism; CVD, cardiovascular disease; PID, pelvic inflammatory disease.

Data from CDC.[9,25]

Dyslipidemia Generally, synthetic progestins adversely affect lipid metabolism by decreasing high-density lipoprotein (HDL) and increasing low-density lipoprotein (LDL).[3,11] Estrogens tend to have more beneficial effects by enhancing removal of LDL and increasing HDL levels. Estrogens may moderately increase triglycerides. As a net result, most low-dose CHCs have no significant impact on HDL, LDL, triglycerides, or total cholesterol. CHCs containing more androgenic progestins (e.g., levonorgestrel) may result in lower HDL levels in some patients. Although the lipid effects of CHCs theoretically can influence cardiovascular risk, the mechanism of increased cardiovascular disease in CHC users is believed to be due to thromboembolic and thrombotic changes, not atherosclerosis. Women with controlled dyslipidemia can use low-dose CHCs, although periodic fasting lipid profiles are recommended. Women with uncontrolled dyslipidemia (LDL greater than 160 mg/dL [4.14 mmol/L], HDL less than 35 mg/dL [0.91 mmol/L], triglycerides greater than 250 mg/dL [2.83 mmol/L]) and additional risk factors (e.g., coronary artery disease, diabetes, hypertension, smoking, or positive family history) should consider an alternative method of contraception.

Diabetes Any effect of CHCs on carbohydrate metabolism is thought to be due to the progestin component.[3,11] However, with the exception of some levonorgestrel-containing products, formulations containing low doses of progestins do not significantly alter insulin, glucose, or glucagon release after a glucose load in healthy women or in those with a history of gestational diabetes. The new progestins are believed to have little, if any, effect on carbohydrate metabolism. CHCs do not appear to alter the hemoglobin A_{1c} values or accelerate the development of microvascular complications in women with diabetes. Therefore, nonsmoking women younger than 35 years with diabetes but no associated vascular disease can safely use CHCs. Diabetic women with vascular disease (e.g., nephropathy, retinopathy, neuropathy, or other vascular disease) or diabetes of more than 20 years' duration should not use CHCs.[9]

Migraine Headaches Women with migraine headaches may experience a decreased or an increased frequency of migraine headaches when using CHCs.[3,9,11,13] Studies have demonstrated a higher risk of stroke in women experiencing migraine with aura compared to women with simple migraine. In population-based studies, the risk of stroke in women with migraines has been elevated twofold to threefold. However, given the low absolute risk of stroke in young women (age less than 35 years), the ACOG recommends considering CHCs in healthy, nonsmoking women with migraine headaches without aura.[11] Women of any age who have migraine with aura and women over the age of 35 with any type of migraine should not use CHC. Women who develop migraines (with or without aura) while receiving CHC should discontinue use and consider a progestin-only option.

Breast Cancer Worldwide epidemiologic data from 54 studies in 25 countries (many of which studied high dose OCs) were collected to assess the relationship between OCs and breast cancer.[11] Overall, investigators noted a small increased risk of breast cancer associated with current or recent use, but OCs did not further increase risk in women with a history of benign breast disease or a family history of breast cancer. A more recent U.S.-based case–control study found no association between overall breast cancer and current or past OC use.[11] This study also found no association between depo-medroxyprogesterone acetate (DMPA) and breast cancer. Although some studies have found differences in risk of breast cancer based on the presence of *BRCA1* and *BRCA2* mutations, the most recent cohort study found no association with low-dose OCs and the presence of either mutation. The choice to use CHCs should not be affected by the presence of benign breast disease or a family history of breast cancer with either mutation. Women with current or past history of breast cancer should not use CHCs.[2,9]

Thromboembolism Estrogens increase hepatic production of factor VII, factor X, and fibrinogen in the coagulation cascade, therefore increasing the risk of thromboembolic events (deep vein thrombosis, pulmonary embolism). These risks are increased in women who have underlying hypercoagulable states (e.g., deficiencies in antithrombin III, protein C, and protein S; factor V Leiden mutations, prothrombin G2010 A mutations) or who have acquired conditions (e.g., obesity, pregnancy, immobility, trauma, surgery, and certain malignancies) that predispose them to coagulation abnormalities.[3,9,11] In the U.S. case–control studies, the risk of VTE in women currently using low-dose OCs (less than 50 mcg EE) was four times the risk in nonusers.[3,11] However, this risk is less than the risk of VTE incurred during pregnancy. OCs containing newer progestins such as drosperinone, desogestrel, and norgestimate are associated with a slightly increased risk of thrombosis.[2] Although the mechanism for this increased risk is unclear, it is thought that third- and fourth-generation progestins have a greater effect on the procoagulant, anticoagulant, and fibrinolytic pathways.[2,14,15] These progestins may also be associated with increased resistance to protein C and may increase levels of sex hormone-binding globulin.[2,14] It is thought that continuous, higher exposure to estrogen seen with the transdermal patch or vaginal ring is the reason for an increased thromboembolic risk with these agents as well. An advisory committee to the FDA decided to change the product labeling of the transdermal patch as well as products containing drosperinone to include additional information about the increased risk of thromboembolism.[16,17] Therefore, for women who are at an increased risk of thromboembolism (e.g., older than 35 years, obesity, smoking, personal or family history of venous thrombosis, prolonged immobilization), it would be prudent to first consider low-dose oral estrogen contraceptives containing older progestins or progestin-only contraceptive methods. It is important to note that EC has not been associated with an increased risk of thromboembolic events.

Clinical **Controversy...**

Weighing the risk versus benefit of using CHCs containing third- and fourth-generation progestins, and determining their place in therapy is controversial. Third-generation progestins (desogestrel, norgestimate) and a fourth-generation progestin (drosperinone) have been associated with a higher risk of thromboembolism. Mechanisms underlying this increased risk may include: (a) a greater effect on the procoagulant, anticoagulant, and fibrinolytic pathways than earlier generation progestins; (b) increased resistance to the anticoagulant effect of activated protein C; (c) increased levels of sex hormone-binding globulin; and (d) antiandrogenic effects of drosperinone make the CHC more estrogenic. The overall risk of VTE with older low-dose agents is 6 per 10,000 women per year (compared with 2 to 3 per 10,000 in nonusers). The risk increases to 10 to 15 per 10,000 women per year with drosperinone-containing OCs. Risk of VTE is also higher with the transdermal patch (10 to 15 per 10,000 women per year) and possibly with the vaginal ring (8 per 10,000 women per year). It is thought that continuous, higher exposure to estrogen seen with these formulations may be the cause of this increased risk. It is important to remember that regardless of contraceptive product, the risk is still lower than the risk of thromboembolism during pregnancy (17 per 10,000 women per year).

Obesity The prevalence of obesity continues to rise each year among all age groups including women of childbearing age. It has been hypothesized that women with increased body weight have increased basal metabolic rates and induction of hepatic enzymes, leading to increased hormonal clearance and decreased serum concentrations of hormonal contraceptives. In addition, women who are obese have more adipose tissue, increasing hormonal sequestration, and decreased free hormone serum concentrations resulting in lower efficacy.[2,3,11] It is estimated that there is an additional two to four pregnancies per 100 woman-years of use in overweight or obese users.[18] This decreased efficacy may be a particular issue with the low-dose OCs. Along these same lines, ACOG recommends that the transdermal contraceptive patch should not be used as a first-line option in women weighing greater than 90 kg.[11,17] Increased pregnancy rates have not been demonstrated in obese women using DMPA or the levonorgestrel intrauterine device (IUD). It is important to note that the CDC recommends that the benefit outweighs the potential risk of decreased efficacy in obese women.[9]

Obese women are also at risk of VTE, although studies evaluating the incidence of thromboembolism in obese women taking hormonal contraceptives have produced conflicting results. ACOG suggests that progestin-only hormonal contraception may be more appropriate for obese women over the age of 35 years, and women should be counseled on the risk and consider alternative contraceptive methods on an individual basis.[11] Again, it should be noted that the risk of thromboembolism during pregnancy and in the peripartum period is significantly greater than the risk with any hormonal contraceptive agent.

Systemic Lupus Erythematosus Contraception is important in women with systemic lupus erythematosus (SLE) because the risks associated with pregnancy are high in this population. Historically, clinicians have thought that CHCs exacerbated the symptoms of SLE.[3,11] However, trials have shown that OCs do not increase the risk of flare among women with stable SLE and without antiphospholipid/anticardiolipin antibodies. Because 25% of women with SLE who become pregnant choose to terminate the pregnancy, effective contraception is essential for these patients. CHCs should be avoided in women with SLE and antiphospholipid antibodies or vascular complications; progestin-only contraceptives can be used in this situation.[9]

Sickle-Cell Disease Advantages of CHC generally outweigh the theoretical or proven risks in those with sickle-cell disease.[9] Theoretical concerns about the effects of CHCs on platelet activation and red cell deformity, for example, led clinicians to avoid their use in women with sickle-cell disease. However, this concern has been largely disproven. In addition, two-controlled trials have actually demonstrated a reduction in risk of vasoocclusive crises in women with sickle-cell disease using DMPA as the method of contraception.[11] Therefore, many clinicians prefer to use DMPA in this patient population.

Oral Contraceptives ❶ ❷ With perfect-use OCs have a 99% efficacy rate, but with typical-use up to 8% of users may become pregnant (Table 62-1).[2,3] The OCs currently available are modifications of the original products introduced in the 1960s and contain significantly less estrogen and progestin. High-dose formulations were associated with vascular and embolic events, cancers, and significant side effects, but reductions in hormone doses have been associated with fewer complications.

Monophasic OCs contain the same amounts of estrogen and progestin for 21 days, followed by 7-day placebo phase. Multiphasic pills contain variable amounts of estrogen and progestin for 21 days, also followed by a 7-day placebo phase. There are no published data demonstrating increased safety or efficacy with the multiphasic tablets compared to monophasic tablets.[2,19,20] Extended-cycle tablets and continuous combination regimens may offer some benefits for patients in terms of side effects and convenience. One particular extended-cycle OC increases the number of hormone-containing pills from 21 to 84 days, followed by a 7-day placebo phase, resulting in four menstrual cycles per year.[21] Another product provides hormone-containing tablets daily throughout the year.[22] Women taking extended-cycle and continuous-cycle tablets tend to have a decreased amount of bleeding over time, often leading to amenorrhea. Continuous combination regimens provide OCs for 21 days, then very low dose estrogen and progestin for an additional 4 to 7 days (during the traditional placebo phase).[16,23]

Table 62-4 lists available OC products by brand name and specifies hormonal composition. Progestin-only "minipills" (28 days of active hormone per cycle) are also available options.[2,3] Progestin-only OCs are less effective than combination OCs and are associated with irregular and unpredictable menstrual bleeding.[2,3] Minipills must be taken every day of the menstrual cycle at approximately the same time to maintain contraceptive efficacy. If a progestin-only OC is taken more than 3 hours late, patients should use a backup method of contraception for 48 hours.[3] Minipills may not block ovulation (nearly 40% of women continue to ovulate normally), so the risk of ectopic pregnancy is higher with their use than with other hormonal contraceptives.

Initiating an Oral Contraceptive ❹ OCs may be initiated by several different methods, including on the first day of bleeding during the menstrual cycle, on the first Sunday after the menstrual cycle begins or on the fifth day after the menstrual cycle begins. The most popular "Sunday start" method is to begin pills on the first Sunday after the menstrual cycle begins, as this may provide for weekends free of menstrual periods.[2,3,24] Women should be instructed to use a second method of contraception for at least 7 days after initiation for maximum effectiveness. It may be preferable to have women use additional contraception for the entire first cycle, due to user failure in the first month. In the "quick start" method for initiating OCs, the patient takes the first tablet on the day of her office visit. Women should be instructed to use a second method of contraception for at least 7 days and informed that the menstrual period will be delayed until completion of the active tablets in the current OC pack. This method has been shown to be more successful in getting women to start OCs and to continue using OCs through the third cycle of use.

Postpartum Use of CHCs In the postpartum phase, there is concern about use of CHCs because of the mother's hypercoagulability and the effects on lactation. In the first 21 days postpartum (when the risk of thrombosis is higher), estrogen-containing hormonal contraceptives should be avoided (Table 62-3).[9,25] If contraception is required during this period, progestin-only contraceptive methods may be acceptable alternatives. It is recommended that women who are breast-feeding avoid CHCs for the first 42 days postpartum in those with risk factors for VTE and for 30 days in those without risk factors. In those women who are not breast-feeding, CHCs should be avoided for up to 42 days postpartum in those with risk factors for VTE.[25] After 42 days postpartum, there is no restriction to the use of CHCs.

Choice of Oral Contraceptive ❶ ❷ Because all combined OCs are similarly effective in preventing pregnancy (Table 62-1), the initial choice is based on the hormonal content and dose, preferred formulation, and coexisting medical conditions (Table 62-3).[9] In women without coexisting medical conditions, an OC containing 35 mcg or less of EE and less than 0.5 mg of norethindrone is recommended (Table 62-4).[3] This strategy is based on evidence that complications and side effects from CHC (i.e., VTE, stroke, or MI) result from excessive hormonal content. Adolescents, underweight women (less than 50 kg [110 lb]), women older than 35 years, and those who are perimenopausal may have fewer side effects with OCs containing 20 to 25 mcg of EE. With nonadherence to OCs, the risk of pregnancy may be greater in women taking OCs containing less than 35 mcg of EE. Overweight and obese women may have higher contraceptive failure rates with low-dose OCs and may benefit from pills containing at least 35 mcg of EE. Women with oily skin, acne, or hirsutism should be given low androgenic OCs.[3] Choice of agent based upon coexisting medical conditions have been previously addressed (Table 62-3).[9,11]

Conventional regimens (21 days of active pills, 7 days of placebo) provide predictable menses. Because monophasic OCs may be easier to take, easier to identify/manage side effects, and easier to manipulate to alter the timing of the menstrual cycle, they are preferred over multiphasic OCs.[2,3] Extended-cycle OCs either eliminate or reduce the number of menstrual cycles per year, leading to less premenstrual symptoms and dysmenorrhea. Commercially available extended-cycle OCs are available, or monophasic 28 day OCs can be cycled by skipping the 7-day placebo phase. With continued use of extended-cycle OCs for 1 year, no significant changes in adverse effects have been noted. However, long-term studies have not been performed to assess the risk of cancer, VTE, or changes in fertility. Continuous combination regimens provide a shortened pill-free interval, from the traditional 7 days to 2 to 4 days. These regimens may be beneficial for women with symptoms such as dysmenorrhea or menstrual migraines.

Managing Oral Contraceptive Side Effects ❸ Many symptoms occurring with early OC use (e.g., nausea, bloating, breakthrough bleeding) improve spontaneously by the third cycle of use after adjusting to the altered hormone levels.[2,3] Women should be counseled to continue their OC for 2 to 3 months before a change

TABLE 62-4 Composition of Commonly Prescribed Oral Contraceptives[a]

Product	Estrogen	Micrograms[b]	Progestin	Milligrams[b]	Spotting and Breakthrough Bleeding
50 mcg Estrogen					
Necon 1/50, Norinyl 1+50	Mestranol	50	Norethindrone	1	10.6
Ovcon 50	Ethinyl estradiol	50	Norethindrone	1	11.9
Ogestrel 0.5/50	Ethinyl estradiol	50	Norgestrel	0.5	4.5
Zovia 1/50	Ethinyl estradiol	50	Ethynodiol diacetate	1	13.9
Sub-50 mcg Estrogen Monophasic					
Aviane, Falmina, Lessina, Levlite, Lutera, Orsythia, Sronyx	Ethinyl estradiol	20	Levonorgestrel	0.1	26.5
Brevicon, Modicon, Necon 0.5/35, Nortrel 0.5/35 Wera	Ethinyl estradiol	35	Norethindrone	0.5	24.6
Zovia 1/35, Kelnor	Ethinyl estradiol	37.4	Ethynodiol diacetate	1	37.4
Apri, Desogen, Emoquette, Ortho-Cept, Reclipsen, Solia	Ethinyl estradiol	30	Desogestrel	0.15	13.1
Levora, Nordette, Portia, Altavera, Kurvelo, Marlissa	Ethinyl estradiol	30	Levonorgestrel	0.15	14
Gildess Fe 1/20, Junel 1/20, Junel Fe 1/20, Loestrin 1/20; Fe 1/20, Microgestin 1/20; Fe 1/20	Ethinyl estradiol	20	Norethindrone 1mg	1	26.5
Gildess Fe 1.5/30, Junel 1.5/30, Junel Fe 1.5/30, Loestrin Fe 1.5/30, Microgestin 1.5/30, Microgestin Fe 1.5/30	Ethinyl estradiol	30	Norethindrone acetate	1.5	25.2
Cryselle, Elinest, Lo-Ovral, Low-Ogestrel	Ethinyl estradiol	30	Norgestrel	0.3	9.6
Necon 1/35, Norinyl 1+35, Nortrel 1/35, Ortho-Novum 1/35, Alyacen 1/35, Cyclafem 1/35, Dasetta 1/35	Ethinyl estradiol	35	Norethindrone	1	14.7
Ortho-Cyclen, Mononessa, Mono-Linyah, Previfem, Sprintec	Ethinyl estradiol	35	Norgestimate	0.25	14.3
Ovcon-35, Balziva, Femcon Fe chewable, Zenchent, Briellyn, Gildagia, Philith, Zeosa chewable	Ethinyl estradiol	35	Norethindrone	0.4	11
Yasmin, Ocella, Safyral, Syeda, Zarah	Ethinyl estradiol	30	Drospirenone	3	14.5
Sub-50 mcg Estrogen Monophasic Extended Cycle					
Loestrin-24 FE[c]	Ethinyl estradiol	20	Norethindrone	1	50[e]
Lybrel, Amethyst	Ethinyl estradiol	20	Levonorgestrel	0.09	52[e]
Introvale, Seasonale, Jolessa, Quasense[d]	Ethinyl estradiol	30	Levonorgestrel	0.15	58.5[e]
Beyaz, Gianvi, Loryna, Vestura, Yaz[c]	Ethinyl estradiol	20	Drospirenone	3	52.5[e]
Sub-50 mcg Estrogen Multiphasic					
Caziant, Cyclessa, Cesia, Velivet	Ethinyl estradiol	25 (7) 25 (7) 25 (7)	Desogestrel	0.1 (7) 0.125 (7) 0.15 (7)	11.1
Estrostep Fe, Tilia Fe, Tri-Legest Fe	Ethinyl estradiol Ethinyl estradiol Ethinyl estradiol	20 (5) 30 (7) 35 (9)	Norethindrone acetate Norethindrone acetate Norethindrone acetate	1 (5) 1 (7) 1 (9)	21.7
Kariva, Mircette, Azurette, Viorele	Ethinyl estradiol Ethinyl estradiol	20 (21) 10 (5)	Desogestrel Desogestrel	0.15 (21)	19.7
Necon 10/11	Ethinyl estradiol Ethinyl estradiol	35 (10) 35 (11)	Norethindrone Norethindrone	0.5 (10) 1 (11)	17.6
Ortho-Novum 7/7/7, Nortrel 7/7/7, Necon 7/7/7, Alyacen 7/7/7, Cyclafem 7/7/7, Dasetta 7/7/7	Ethinyl estradiol Ethinyl estradiol Ethinyl estradiol	35 (7) 35 (7) 35 (7)	Norethindrone Norethindrone Norethindrone	0.5 (7) 0.75 (7) 1 (7)	14.5
Ortho Tri-Cyclen, Trinessa, Tri-Previfem, Tri-Sprintec, Tri-Estarylla, Tri-Linyah	Ethinyl estradiol Ethinyl estradiol Ethinyl estradiol	35 (7) 35 (7) 35 (7)	Norgestimate Norgestimate Norgestimate	0.18 (7) 0.215 (7) 0.25 (7)	17.7
Ortho Tri-Cyclen Lo, Tri Lo Sprintec	Ethinyl estradiol Ethinyl estradiol Ethinyl estradiol	25 (7) 25 (7) 25 (7)	Norgestimate Norgestimate Norgestimate	0.18 (7) 0.215 (7) 0.25 (7)	11.5
Aranelle, Leena, Tri-Norinyl	Ethinyl estradiol Ethinyl estradiol Ethinyl estradiol	35 (7) 35 (9) 35 (5)	Norethindrone Norethindrone Norethindrone	0.5 (7) 1 (9) 0.5 (5)	25.5
Enpresse, Trivora, Levonest Myzilra	Ethinyl estradiol Ethinyl estradiol Ethinyl estradiol	30 (6) 40 (5) 30 (10)	Levonorgestrel Levonorgestrel Levonorgestrel	0.05 (6) 0.075 (5) 0.125 (10)	
Natazia	Estradiol valerate	3 (2) 2 (22) 1 (2)	Dienogest	0 (2) 2 (5) 3 (17) 0 (4)	

(continued)

TABLE 62-4 Composition of Commonly Prescribed Oral Contraceptives[a] (*Continued*)

Product	Estrogen	Micrograms[b]	Progestin	Milligrams[b]	Spotting and Breakthrough Bleeding
Sub-50 mcg Estrogen Multiphasic Extended Cycle					
Amethia, Seasonique	Ethinyl estradiol Ethinyl estradiol	30 (84) 10 (7)	Levonorgestrel Levonorgestrel	0.15 (84) 0.15 (7)	42.5[e]
Progestin Only					
Camila, Errin, Heather, Jolivette, Micronor, Nor-QD, Nora-BE	Ethinyl estradiol	–	Norethindrone	0.35	42.3

[a]28-day regimens (21-day active pills, then 7-day pill-free interval) unless otherwise noted.
[b]Number in parentheses refers to the number of days the dose is received in multiphasic oral contraceptives.
[c]28-day regimen (24-day active pills, then 4-day pill-free interval).
[d]91-day regimen (84-day active pills, then 7-day pill-free interval).
[e]Percent reporting after 6 to 12 months of use.

Data from Hatcher et al.[2] and Dickey.[3]

is made to adjust the hormonal content. However, a large majority of women who discontinue OCs do so because of the side effects. Patient education and early reevaluation within 3 to 6 months are necessary to identify and manage adverse effects, in an effort to improve adherence. Serious adverse effects that may occur with the use of CHCs are listed in Table 62-5, and common side effects and recommended monitoring are reviewed in Table 62-6.[2,3,10] Patients should be instructed to immediately discontinue CHCs if they experience warning signs, described as ACHES (abdominal pain, chest pain, headaches, eye problems, and severe leg pain).[3]

Managing Oral Contraceptive Drug Interactions 3 The effectiveness of an OC is sometimes limited by drug interactions that interfere with GI absorption, increase intestinal motility by altering gut bacteriologic flora, and alter the metabolism, excretion, or binding of the OC.[2,11] The lower the dose of hormone in the OC, the greater the risk that a drug interaction will compromise its efficacy. Women should be instructed to use an additional method of contraception if there is a possibility of a drug interaction altering the efficacy of the OC.[3] Although less well documented, these recommendations generally apply to patients receiving transdermal and vaginal CHC products.

Of all antibiotics, rifampin is the one with a true documented pharmacokinetic interaction. Pharmacokinetic studies of other antibiotics have not shown any consistent interaction, but case reports of individual patients have shown a reduction in EE levels when OCs are taken with tetracyclines and penicillin derivatives. The ACOG states that ampicillin, doxycycline, fluconazole, metronidazole, miconazole, fluoroquinolones, and tetracyclines do not decrease steroid levels in women taking OCs.[11] The Council on Scientific Affairs at the American Medical Association recommends that women taking rifampin should be counseled about the risk of OC failure and advised to use an additional nonhormonal contraceptive agent during the course of rifampin therapy (Table 62-3). The council also recommends that women be informed about the small risk of interactions with other antibiotics, and, if desired, appropriate additional nonhormonal contraceptive agents should be considered. In addition, women who develop breakthrough bleeding during concomitant use of antibiotics and OCs (and other CHCs) should be advised to use an alternate method of contraception during the period of concomitant use.

Women receiving certain anticonvulsants for a seizure disorder should be offered another form of contraception such as DMPA or IUDs (Table 62-3).[9] Some anticonvulsants (mainly phenobarbital, carbamazepine, phenytoin) induce the metabolism of estrogen and progestin, inducing breakthrough bleeding and potentially reducing contraceptive efficacy. In addition, some anticonvulsants (e.g., phenytoin) are known teratogens.

Patient Instructions with Oral Contraceptives 4 Many women who take OCs are not educated properly on the appropriate use of these medications. Women should be given the package insert that accompanies all estrogen products and instructed to read it. The written patient information should be supplemented with verbal information describing the mechanism of the medication, both common and serious side effects, and management of these side effects. Although several transient self-limiting side effects often occur, the patient should be aware of the danger signals that require immediate medical attention (Table 62-5). The benefits and risks should be discussed, including the fact that OCs provide no physical barrier to the transmission of STDs, including HIV. Detailed instructions on when to start taking the OC should be provided. Patients should be told the importance of routine daily administration to ensure consistent plasma concentrations and improve adherence and specific instructions should be given regarding what to do if a tablet is missed. The WHO Selected Practice Recommendations for Contraceptive Use have guidelines for managing missed oral contraceptives.[26] In addition to when the tablet(s) is missed and how many are missed, the guidelines take into consideration whether the OC contains less than 30 mcg of EE. Limited evidence suggests that the risk of pregnancy is greater when 20 mcg tablets are missed than when 30 to 35 mcg tablets are missed. For instance, if a woman is taking a tablet containing 20 mcg EE and misses one dose or starts a pack 1 day late, she should take a tablet as soon as possible (two tablets on the

TABLE 62-5 Serious Symptoms That May Be Associated with Combined Hormonal Contraception

Serious Symptoms	Possible Underlying Problem
Blurred vision, diplopia, flashing lights, blindness, papilledema	Stroke, hypertension, temporary vascular problem of many possible sites, retinal artery thrombosis
Numbness, weakness, tingling in extremities, slurred speech	Hemorrhagic or thrombotic stroke
Migraine headaches	Vascular spasm, stroke
Breast mass, pain, or swelling	Breast cancer
Chest pain (radiating to left arm or neck), shortness of breath, coughing up blood	Pulmonary embolism, myocardial infarction
Abdominal pain, hepatic mass or tenderness, jaundice, pruritus	Gallbladder disease, hepatic adenoma, pancreatitis, thrombosis of abdominal artery or vein
Excessive spotting, breakthrough bleeding	Endometrial, cervical, or vaginal cancer
Severe leg pain (calf, thigh), tenderness, swelling, warmth	Deep-vein thrombosis

Data from Hatcher et al.[2] and Dickey.[3]

TABLE 62-6 Drug Monitoring Table for Hormonal Contraception

Drug (or Drug Class)	Adverse Drug Reactions	Monitoring Parameter	Comments
Combined hormonal contraception	Nausea/vomiting	Patient symptoms	Typically improves after two to three cycles; consider changing to lower estrogenic
	Breast tenderness	Patient symptoms	
	Weight gain	Weight	
	Acne, oily skin	Visual inspection	Consider changing to lower androgenic
	Depression, fatigue	Depression screening	Data are limited and conflicting
	Breakthrough bleeding/spotting	Menstrual symptoms	Consider changing to higher estrogenic
	Application site reaction (transdermal)	Visual inspection	
	Vaginal irritation (vaginal ring)	Patient symptoms	
Depo-medroxyprogesterone acetate	Menstrual irregularities	Menstrual symptoms	
	Weight gain	Weight	
	Acne	Visual inspection	
	Hirsutism	Visual inspection	
	Depression	Depression screening	Data are limited and conflicting
	Decreased bone density	BMD	Do not routinely screen with DXA
Levonorgestrel IUD	Menstrual irregularities	Menstrual symptoms	Typically spotting, amenorrhea
	Insertion-related complications	Cramping, pain	Prophylactic NSAIDs or local anesthetic may reduce occurrence
	Expulsion	Cramping, pain, spotting, dyspareunia, missing strings	IUD strings should be checked regularly by women to ensure IUD properly placed
	Pelvic inflammatory disease	Lower abdominal pain, unusual vaginal discharge, fever	Overall risk of developing is rare, but counseling on STD prevention is important
Copper IUD	See levonorgestrel IUD above	See levonorgestrel IUD above	Menstrual irregularities are typically heavier menses with copper IUD
Progestin-only implant	Menstrual irregularities	Menstrual symptoms	
	Insertion-site reactions	Pain, bruising, skin irritation, erythema, pus, fever	Typically well-tolerated and resolve without treatment, infection is rare

Data from Hatcher et al.[2] and Barr.[10]

same day) and then continue taking the rest of the tablets daily. No additional contraceptive protection is necessary. If, however, two or more tablets are missed or the pack is started two or more days late, the woman should follow the same instructions, but condoms should be used or she should abstain from sexual intercourse until she has taken active tablets for 7 days in a row. If missed tablets occur in the third week, she should finish the active tablets in the current pack and start a new pack the next day. She should not take the seven inactive tablets. If the missed doses occur in the first week and unprotected intercourse has occurred, she should consider the use of EC. Instructions are similar for the 30 to 35 mcg tablets; however, no additional contraceptive protection is necessary unless three or more active tablets are missed or the woman starts a pack 3 or more days late. It should be noted that the Society of Obstetricians and Gynecologists of Canada also published guidelines in 2008 for missed doses.[26] These guidelines differ slightly and do not account for the estrogen content of the tablet. Instructions also may vary in package inserts, which can make for increased confusion with patients and clinicians. It may be prudent, when differing instructions exist, to recommend the more conservative of approaches when dealing with individual patient situations.

Discontinuing Oral Contraceptives and Return of Fertility The ACOG states that there is no evidence that OC use decreases subsequent fertility. The transdermal patch and vaginal ring CHCs also have similar effects on fertility. The average delay in ovulation after discontinuing OCs is 1 to 2 weeks; however, delayed ovulation is more common in women with a history of irregular menses. If amenorrhea does continue beyond 6 months, women should be counseled to see a gynecologist for further fertility work-up.[2,3,11] In the past, women were counseled to allow two to three normal menstrual periods before becoming pregnant to permit the reestablishment of menses and ovulation. However, in several large cohort and case–control studies, infants conceived in the first month after discontinuation of an OC had no greater chance of miscarriage or being born with a birth defect than those born in the general population.

Transdermal Contraceptives ❶ ❷ A CHC is available as a transdermal patch (Ortho Evra), which includes 0.75 mg of EE and 6 mg of norelgestromin, the active metabolite of norgestimate.[2,3] Comparative trials have shown the transdermal patch to be as effective as combined OCs in patients weighing less than 90 kg. Of the 15 pregnancies reported in the clinical trials, five were among women weighing more than 90 kg; therefore, this product is not recommended as a first-line option for these women.[2,3,17] ❸ Some patients experience application-site reactions, but other side effects are similar to those experienced with OCs (e.g., breast discomfort, headache, and nausea).[3] A warning from the manufacturer states that women using the patch are exposed to approximately 60% more estrogen than from a typical OC containing 35 mcg of EE. Evidence suggests that higher exposure to estrogen may lead to increased thromboembolic risk, and the labeling for the contraceptive patch now contains a warning of this risk.[17] The patch should be applied to the abdomen, buttocks, upper torso, or upper arm at the beginning of the menstrual cycle and replaced every week for 3 weeks (the fourth week is patch-free).[2,3] The patch releases estrogen and progestin for 9 days. If the woman forgets to change her patch or restarts the active patches after the ninth day, a backup method should be used for 7 days. Approximately 5% of patches will need to be replaced because they become partly detached or fall off altogether, so single replacements are available. If the patch is detached for more than 24 hours, a new 4-week cycle should be restarted and a backup method used for 7 days.[2,3] Users have demonstrated greater adherence with the patch than with an OC, but whether this results in reduced pregnancy rates remains to be seen. The benefits of adherence must be weighed against of the risk of increased estrogen exposure and possibility of VTE.

Vaginal Rings ❶ ❷ The vaginal contraceptive ring contains EE and etonogestrel (NuvaRing).[27] It is a 54 mm flexible ring, 4 mm in thickness. Over a 3-week period, the ring releases approximately 15 mcg/day of EE and 120 mcg/day of etonogestrel. Comparative trials have shown the vaginal ring to be as effective as combined

OCs. On the first cycle of use, the ring should be inserted on or before the fifth day of the menstrual cycle, remain in place for 3 weeks, then removed for 1 week to allow for withdrawal bleeding. The new ring should be inserted on the same day of the week as it was during the last cycle, similar to starting a new OC pack on the same day of the week. A second method of contraception should be used if the ring has been expelled accidentally for more than 3 hours; if less than 3 hours, it should be washed and reinserted.[2,3,27]

❸ Side effects, precautions, and contraindications for use of the hormonal ring are similar to those for all CHCs. The most commonly reported reasons for discontinuation of use were device-related issues, such as foreign-body sensation, device expulsion, and vaginal symptoms.[27] Cycle control with the vaginal ring appears to be equal or better than with combined OCs, with a low incidence of breakthrough bleeding and spotting after the second cycle of use. Patient acceptability of the delivery system has been studied, and the majority of women do not complain of discomfort in general or during intercourse.[3] A potential concern is the possibility of increased VTE (eight cases per 10,000 per year vs. six cases with most CHCs) since etonogestrel is a metabolite of desogestrel which may be associated with increased risk.[28] The ring should be inserted vaginally. In contrast to diaphragms and cervical caps, precise placement is not an issue because the hormones are absorbed anywhere in the vagina. Women should be in a comfortable position, and compress the ring between the thumb and index finger and push it into the vagina. There is no danger of inserting the ring too far because the cervix will prevent it from traveling up the genital tract. Removal of the ring is performed in a similar manner; pulling it out and discarding into the foil patch (the ring should not be flushed down the toilet).[27] Patients should be discouraged from douching, but other vaginal products, including antifungal creams and spermicides, can be used.[3,27]

Injectable Progestins Steroid hormones provide longer-term contraception when injected into the skin. Sustained progestin exposure blocks the LH surge, thus inhibiting ovulation. Should ovulation occur, progestins reduce ovum motility in the fallopian tubes. Even if fertilization occurs, progestins thin the endometrium, reducing the chance of implantation. Progestins also thicken the cervical mucus, producing a barrier to sperm penetration. This method of contraception does not provide any protection from STDs.[2,9]

❶ ❷ Women who may benefit from injectable progestins are those who are breast-feeding, those who are intolerant to estrogens (i.e., have a history of estrogen-related headache, breast tenderness, or nausea) or those with concomitant medical conditions in which estrogen is not recommended (Table 62-3). Additionally, injectable progestins are beneficial for women with adherence issues; they have lower failure rates than combined hormonal contraceptive methods (Table 62-1).[2,9]

Depo-Medroxyprogesterone Acetate ❶ ❷ Medroxyprogesterone acetate is similar in structure to naturally occurring progesterone. DMPA (Depo-Provera) is administered every 3 months either by deep intramuscular injection in the gluteal or deltoid muscle or subcutaneously in the abdomen or thigh within 5 days of onset of menstrual bleeding.[29,30] With perfect use, the efficacy of DMPA is more than 99%; however, with typical use, 3% of women experience unintended pregnancy.[2] Although these injections may inhibit ovulation for up to 14 weeks, the dose should be repeated every 3 months (12 weeks) to ensure continuous contraception. The manufacturer recommends excluding pregnancy in women with a lapse of 13 or more weeks between injections for the intramuscular formulation or 14 or more weeks between injections for the subcutaneous formulation. Depo-Provera is available as a 150 mg/mL injection vial or prefilled syringe for IM injection and Depo-SubQ Provera 104 is available as a prefilled syringe.[29,30] Administration of both formulations of DMPA requires a medical office visit; however, pilot studies of patient self-administration of subcutaneous DMPA have demonstrated positive results.[31]

Although no adverse effects have been documented in infants exposed to DMPA through breast milk, the manufacturer recommends not initiating DMPA until 6 weeks postpartum in breast-feeding women.[29,30] However, the CDC cites a lack of evidence supporting this claim and classifies DMPA use during this timeframe as a category 2 suggesting that the benefit may outweigh the theoretical risk.[9] Women who are not breast-feeding but require contraception can receive DMPA immediately postpartum.[9,29,30] Women with sickle-cell disease are good candidates for DMPA, as studies have demonstrated a reduction in sickle cell pain crises in women using DMPA.[9] In addition, women with seizure disorders may experience fewer seizures when taking DMPA for contraception, and there is not a concern with anticonvulsants reducing the contraceptive efficacy of DMPA.[2,9] Because return of fertility may be delayed after discontinuation of DMPA, it should not be recommended to women desiring pregnancy in the near future. The median time to conception from the first omitted dose is 10 months. Sixty-eight percent of women will be able to conceive within 12 months, 83% within 15 months, and 93% within 18 months of the last injection.[2,29,30]

❸ Menstrual irregularities are the most frequent adverse effects of both formulations of DMPA. Women who cannot tolerate prolonged bleeding may benefit from a short course of estrogen (e.g., 7 days of 2 mg estradiol or 1.25-mg conjugated estrogen given orally), but this will not help reduce the incidence in the long-term.[2,10] The incidence of irregular bleeding decreases from 30% in the first year to 10% thereafter. After 12 months of therapy, 55% of women report amenorrhea, with the incidence increasing to 68% after 2 years.[10,29,30]

Other adverse effects, including breast tenderness and depression, occur less commonly. Weight gain is a concern for many women using DMPA, and the incidence and amount gained vary widely. It has been reported that weight gain averages 1 kg annually and may not resolve until 6 to 8 months after the last injection or patients gain 12 kg on average after using DMPA for 3 years.[10,29,30]

DMPA has been associated with short-term bone loss in younger women of reproductive age. This potential side effect may be due to lower ovarian estrogen production that occurs when gonadotropin secretion is suppressed.[29,30,32] Because longitudinal studies demonstrated effects on BMD, the FDA issued a black box warning for DMPA in 2004.[29,30] It states that DMPA should be continued for more than 2 years only if other contraceptive methods are inadequate. It also states that the loss of BMD seems to be greater with increasing duration of use and may not be completely reversible. However, the majority of clinicians view the effects of DMPA on BMD (which in the majority of cases is reversible) as a surrogate marker and there are no clear data that demonstrate the effects of DMPA on fracture risk.[32,33] The ACOG and CDC continue to recommend that for most patients the benefits of DMPA outweigh the risks even when used beyond 2 years of use.[9,32] ACOG does not recommend the routine screening of BMD in most patients.[32] A discussion regarding the risks and benefits of this contraceptive option is recommended prior to initiation and with prolonged use.

Long-acting Reversible Contraception Long-acting reversible contraception (LARC) refers to a category of hormonal and nonhormonal contraceptives that include IUDs and implants. This type of contraception is highly efficacious in preventing pregnancy, but the effects are quickly reversible upon removal.[34] LARC does not require effort or adherence by the patient once they are inserted. Therefore, both perfect-use and typical-use efficacy rates do not differ, and they are similar to surgical options such as tubal ligation (Table 62-1).[2,34] When compared to other methods of hormonal contraception, especially OCs, LARC methods are not used as frequently in the United States.[35] All women should be considered potential candidates for this method. In the past, many clinicians offered LARC only when adherence was an issue or in women with contraindications to estrogen. However, with increasing education and ongoing studies, their use is slowly increasing, and many women are choosing them as their first-line contraceptive method.[36] Due to the high efficacy rates of LARC methods, many advocates propose that increased use may decrease unintended pregnancy rates.[1,34]

Subdermal Progestin Implants ❶ ❷ Nexplanon (formerly called Implanon in the United States) is a single 4-cm-long implant, containing 68 mg of etonogestrel that is placed under the skin of the upper arm using a preloaded inserter.[2,37] Clinicians must receive training from the manufacturer prior to insertion or removal of the device. Implanon releases etonogestrel at a rate of 60 mcg daily for the first month, then decreases to an average of 30 mcg daily at the end of the 3 years of recommended use. The primary mechanism of action is suppression of ovulation. When ovulation is not suppressed, etonogestrel still is effective as the progestin thickens the cervical mucus and produces an atrophic endometrium. With both perfect and typical use, the efficacy rate is over 99%.[34,37] However, in overweight and obese women weighing more than 130% of their ideal body weight, there is a precaution from the manufacturer of the possibility of decreased efficacy especially over time.[37]

❹ The etonogestrel implant should be inserted between days 1 and 5 of the menstrual cycle in women who have not previously used hormonal contraception.[37] If it is inserted at any other time of the menstrual cycle, then it is recommended to use a barrier backup method for 7 days. Women currently taking OCs can have the implant inserted within 7 days after taking the last active OC tablet. Women currently taking progestin-only OCs should have the implant inserted without skipping any days, on the same day that the progestin-only IUD is removed, or on the day that the DMPA injection is due. After removal, fertility returns within 30 days.

❸ The major adverse effect associated with Nexplanon is irregular menstrual bleeding, which led to discontinuation of the implant in 11% of patients in clinical trials.[34,37] Women should be counseled about the risk of irregular bleeding patterns so that patients will not request early removal of Nexplanon. Some women (22%) became amenorrheic with continued use, but many continued to have prolonged bleeding and spotting (18% and 34%, respectively) and frequent bleeding (7%). Insertion and removal complications are rare (less than 2%).[34,37] Information from the manufacturer suggests using precaution when there is potential for drug interactions in the presence of potent CYP450 inducers (e.g., rifampin, phenytoin, carbamazepine).[37] This information conflicts with CDC recommendations; those recommendations classify combining those medications with Implanon as a category 2, suggesting that the benefits typically outweigh the theoretical risks.[9] Clinicians should counsel their patients about the benefits and risks if the there is a possibility of a drug interaction.

Intrauterine Devices ❶ ❷ There are currently three IUDs available, all are T-shaped and are medicated, one with copper (ParaGard) and two with levonorgestrel (Mirena and Skyla). Clinicians must receive training from the manufacturer prior to insertion or removal of the IUDs. These IUDs have several possible mechanisms of action including inhibition of sperm migration, damaging ovum or disrupting transport, and possibly damaging the fertilized ovum. Due to the presence of local progestin, the Mirena and Skyla IUDs have additional mechanisms of endometrial suppression and thickening cervical mucus. The most recent evidence regarding the mechanisms of action demonstrate that the contraceptive activity of IUDs occurs before implanatation.[2,34] Efficacy rates with IUDs are greater than 99% with both perfect and typical use.[2,34,38,39] IUDs should not be used in the presence of current pregnancy, current pelvic inflammatory disease, current STD, puerperal or postabortion sepsis, purulent cervicitis, undiagnosed abnormal vaginal bleeding, malignancy of genital tract, uterine anomalies or fibroids distorting uterine cavity, allergy to IUD component, or Wilson's disease (for copper IUD).[38,39] The risk of pelvic inflammatory disease among IUD users is low and ranges from 1% to 2.5%. Because the increased risk of infection appears to be related to introduction of bacteria into the genital tract during IUD insertion, the risk is highest during the first 20 days after the procedure.[34,40]

❸ ParaGard is a highly effective IUD that can be left in place for 10 years.[2,38] A disadvantage of ParaGard is increased menstrual blood flow and dysmenorrhea; average monthly blood loss among users increased by 35% in clinical trials. Mirena is the more recently approved IUD in the United States, and its use is increasing.[35] It is also a highly effective IUD, and it can be left in place for 5 years.[34,39] Mirena releases 20 mcg of levonorgestrel daily, but release decreases to 10 mcg daily over the 5 years of use.[2,34] Skyla is the most recent IUD to be approved. It releases 14 mcg of levonorgestrel daily and can be left in place for 3 years.[41] Systemically absorbed levonorgestrel is minimal and considerably less than with OCs. The levonorgestrel IUD produces its effects locally via suppression of the endometrium, causing a reduction in menstrual blood loss. In contrast to the copper IUD, menstrual flow in users of the levonorgestrel IUD is decreased, and development of amenorrhea has been observed in 20% of users in the first year and 60% in the fifth year. A disadvantage of the levonorgestrel IUD is increased spotting in the first 6 months of use; women should be counseled that the spotting will decline gradually over time.[2,39]

Due to the local effects on the endometrium and decrease in blood loss, Mirena has an additional indication for treatment of heavy menstrual bleeding (menorrhagia).[34,42,43] Return to fertility is rapid and typically occurs within 30 days after removal of the IUD.[34,39] Historically, use in nulliparous and adolescent women was considered a precaution to use of an IUD. However, recent evidence, clinical experience, and expert opinion do not preclude use in these populations. Risk versus benefits should be considered, and the woman must be counseled on the IUD.[34,44] Strong consideration of an IUD is appropriate in this population due to high efficacy rates.[44] In addition, Skyla does not include nulliparous women as a precaution and included about 40% of patients in this population in the clinical trials.[41] The influence of drug interactions on the efficacy of IUDs is not a primary concern based on manufacturer recommendations.[39,43] In addition, the CDC classifies the potential drug interactions with potent CYP450 inducers as a category 2, determining that the benefits typically outweigh any of the theoretical risks.[9]

Clinical **Controversy. . .**

Ulipristal is a selective receptor modulator with mixed progesterone agonist and antagonist activities, and limited data on its mechanism of action are available in humans. Controversy exists because the chemical structure of ulipristal is similar to mifepristone, which given in higher doses is used for medical termination of pregnancy. Limited, small animal study models have demonstrated that ulipristal may inhibit implantation, but it does not terminate pregnancy. It is important to note that pregnancy is defined as the period from implantation to delivery, so prevention of implantation would be an additional contraceptive mechanism. Despite the controversy, there is no clear evidence in humans that ulipristal inhibits implantation or terminates a pregnancy, but clear evidence exist that it is a highly effective formulation of EC.

Emergency Contraception

5 EC is used to prevent unwanted pregnancy after unprotected or inadequately protected sexual intercourse (e.g., no contraception, condom breakage, OC nonadherence, sexual assault). Pregnancy occurs when the fertilized egg is implanted into the endometrial lining. After intercourse, implantation of the fertilized egg typically takes approximately 5 days.[45] Progestin-only and progesterone receptor modulator products are approved by the FDA and recommended as first-line EC options.[2,3,45] Insertion of the copper IUD or prescribing higher doses of combined OCs (containing estrogen and progestin) are other options but are not widely used.

Currently, the progestin-only formulation containing levonorgestrel (currently marketed as Plan B One-Step and Next Choice) is approved specifically for EC in the United States.[46,47] Recent studies support that the primary mechanism of action of progestin-only EC is inhibiting or delaying ovulation. Additional evidence suggests it may impair sperm transport and corpus luteum function, therefore inhibiting fertilization. The most recent data do not support that it may prevent the fertilized egg from implanting into the endometrium.[45,48,49] Oral EC will not disrupt the fertilized egg after implantation has occurred.[45,48] The levonorgestrel-containing EC formulation is the regimen of choice due to availability, improved tolerability, and potentially increased efficacy rates. Next choice, a two-dose formulation, contains two tablets each containing 0.75 mg of levonorgestrel. The first dose is taken within 72 hours of unprotected intercourse (although the sooner, the more effective); the second dose is taken 12 hours later (the second dose taken 24 hours after the first dose is also efficacious).[45,47] A one-dose formulation, Plan B One-Step, containing one tablet of 1.5 mg of levonorgestrel taken within 72 hours of unprotected intercourse is equally effective as the older two-dose formulation.[45,46] Evidence does support that the levonorgestrel-containing EC products can be moderately effective in preventing pregnancy up to 120 hours after unprotected intercourse.[45] Levonorgestrel-containing EC is now available without a prescription to women and girls of all ages in the United States.[45]

5 Ulipristal (Ella) is the newest EC product and was approved for use by the FDA in 2010.[50] Ulipristal is a selective progesterone receptor modulator with mixed progesterone agonist and antagonist properties.[50–52] Its mechanism of action depends on the timing of administration relative to the woman's menstrual cycle. The primary mechanism of action appears to delay ovulation. Ulipristal is available by prescription only and is available as a single dose of 30 mg taken within 120 hours after unprotected intercourse. Evidence supports that it maintains efficacy for the full 120-hour window.[51,53] Data exist to support noninferiority of ulipristal compared to levonorgestrel-containing EC; additionally a meta-analysis concluded that pregnancy rates were significantly lower in women taking ulipristal compared to levonorgestrel-containing EC methods.[54,55]

5 Despite the availability of progestin-only and progesterone receptor modulator EC formulations, use of higher doses of regular combined OCs for EC (Yuzpe method) still is permissible, although studies suggest that they may not be as effective and may be associated with more adverse effects (especially nausea and vomiting).[2,3,45] Patients should be counseled to take the appropriate number of tablets within 72 hours and as soon as possible after unprotected sexual intercourse and to repeat the dose in 12 hours. Taking all the tablets at once as a single dose is not recommended when using combination OCs.

Determining the exact effectiveness rate of EC is difficult; however, the range has been reported to be between 59% and 94%.[45] Evidence reported that EC may prevent an average of 75% of expected pregnancies when taken appropriately. It is recommended that women have an advanced prescription on hand or access to an OTC formulation to maximize the effectiveness of EC.

3 Common adverse effects include nausea, vomiting, and irregular bleeding.[45] Nausea and vomiting occur significantly less when progestin-only and progesterone receptor modulator EC is administered. If the Yuzpe method is prescribed, antiemetics given 1 hour before the dose is taken may be warranted to prevent the increased amount of estrogen-induced GI adverse effects. Many women will experience irregular bleeding regardless of which EC method is used, with the menstrual period usually occurring 1 week before or after the expected time. Routine screening prior to or after receiving progestin-only and progesterone receptor modulator EC is not recommended. If a pregnancy already exists, the EC will not disrupt or harm the embryo. Additionally, there are no contraindications to the use of these methods of EC (for the Yuzpe and copper IUD methods clinicians must adhere to their contraindications and precautions). No current data regarding the safety of repeated use EC are available, but current consensus suggests that the risks are low, and women can receive multiple regimens if warranted. Appropriate counseling should be provided regarding timing of the dose, common adverse effects, and use of a regular contraceptive method (backup barrier methods should be used after EC for at least 7 days).

Personalized Pharmacotherapy

Selecting a contraceptive method should involve the patient and clinician using a shared-decision making model. Contraceptive pharmacotherapy should be personalized for each patient, taking into account desired outcomes from a contraceptive and noncontraceptive perspective. Factors to consider include efficacy, presence of coexisting medical conditions or medications, safety, adverse effects, cost, and patient preference of the contraceptive method (e.g., long-acting, short-acting, hormonal, oral, nonoral, barrier).

EVALUATION OF THERAPEUTIC OUTCOMES

4 Patients should receive both verbal and written instructions on the chosen method of contraception. Followup appointments can increase adherence and provide opportunities to address other health maintenance issues. The contraceptive outcome of pregnancy prevention can be assessed when needed by obtaining a serum or urine pregnancy test.

Monitoring of the Pharmaceutical Care Plan

Contraceptive users should receive cytologic screening as well as annual pelvic and breast examination and a well-woman consultation for routine health maintenance screening and to assess for clinical problems or adverse effects related to contraception (Table 62-6). It is important to note that these annual screenings do not have to occur prior to prescribing hormonal contraception.

Annual blood pressure monitoring is recommended for all users of CHC. When a patient with a history of glucose intolerance or diabetes mellitus begins or discontinues the use of hormonal contraception, glucose levels must be monitored. Monitoring for the presence of adverse effects related to hormonal content or the presence of coexisting medical conditions is recommended for women using CHCs. Women using Implanon should be monitored annually for menstrual cycle disturbances, weight gain, local inflammation, or infection at the implant site, acne, breast tenderness, headaches, and hair loss. Women using DMPA should be asked at 3-month followup visits about weight gain, menstrual cycle disturbances, and fractures. Women using IUDs should be asked at 1- to 3-month follow-up visits about IUD placement (checking for IUD strings to assure the IUD is still in the proper position), changes in menstrual bleeding patterns, and symptoms and protection against STDs.

Clinicians should check for proper IUD positioning and symptoms of upper genital tract infection.

Finally, clinicians should monitor and when indicated screen for HIV and STDs. All women should receive counseling about healthy sexual practices including the use of condoms to prevent the transmission of STDs when necessary.

ABBREVIATIONS

ACOG	American Congress of Obstetrics and Gynecology
BMD	bone mineral density
CDC	Centers for Disease Control and Prevention
CHC	combined hormonal contraceptive
DMPA	depo-medroxyprogesterone acetate
EC	emergency contraception
EE	ethinyl estradiol
FSH	follicle-stimulating hormone
GnRH	gonadotropin-releasing hormone
HDL	high-density lipoprotein
HIV	human immunodeficiency virus
IUD	intrauterine device
LARC	long-acting reversible contraception
LDL	low-density lipoprotein
LH	luteinizing hormone
MI	myocardial infarction
OC	oral contraceptive
OTC	over the counter
Pap	papanicolaou (smear)
SHBG-TBG	sex hormone (testosterone) binding globulin
SLE	systemic lupus erythematosus
STD	sexually transmitted disease
TSS	toxic shock syndrome
VTE	venous thromboembolism
WHO	World Health Organization

REFERENCES

1. Mosher WD, Jones J, Abma JC. Intended and unintended births in the United States: 1982–2010. National Health Statistics Reports, No. 55. Hyattsville, MD: National Center for Health Statistics, 2012.
2. Hatcher RA, Trussell J, Nelson AL, et al. Contraceptive Technology, 20th ed. New York: Bridging the Gap Communications, 2011.
3. Dickey RP. Managing Contraceptive Pill Patients, 14th ed. Durant: EMIS Inc., 2010.
4. American College of Obstetricians and Gynecologists. Cervical cytology screening. Practice Bulletin No. 109. Obstet Gynecol 2009;114:1409–1420.
5. Leeman L. Medical barriers to effective contraception. Obstet Gynecol Clin North Am 2007;34:19–29.
6. American College of Obstetricians and Gynecologists. Noncontraceptive uses of hormonal contraceptives. Practice Bulletin No. 110. Obstet Gynecol 2010;115:206–218.
7. Roddy RE, Zekeng L, Ryan KA, et al. A controlled trial of nonoxynol 9 film to reduce male-to-female transmission of sexually transmitted diseases. N Engl J Med 1998;339:504–510.
8. Van Damme L, Ramjee G, Alary M, et al. Effectiveness of COL-1492, a nonoxynol-9 vaginal gel, on HIV-1 transmission in female sex workers: A randomised controlled trial. Lancet 2002;360:971–977.
9. Centers for Disease Control and Prevention. U.S. Medical Eligibility Criteria for Contraceptive Use, 2010. MMWR Early Release 2010;59 [May 28]:1–86.
10. Barr NG. Managing adverse effects of hormonal contraceptives. Am Fam Physician 2010;82:1499–1506.
11. American College of Obstetricians and Gynecologists. Use of hormonal contraception in women with coexisting medical conditions. ACOG Practice Bulletin No 73. Obstet Gynecol 2006;107:1453–1472.
12. Bhathena RK, Guillebauld J. Contraception for the older woman: An update. Climacteric 2006;9:264–276.
13. Curtis KM, Mohllajee AP, Peterson HB. Use of combined oral contraceptives among women with migraine and nonmigrainous headaches: A systematic review. Contraception 2006;73:189–194.
14. Lidegaard OM, Nielsen LH, Skovlund CW, Lokkegaard E. Venous thromboembolism in users of non-oral hormonal contraception: Follow-up study, Denmark 2001–2010. BMJ 2012. Published on-line ahead of print, May 10, 2012. doi:10.1136/bmj.e2990.
15. Jick SS, Hernandez RK. Risk of non-fatal thromboembolism in women using oral contraceptives containing drospirenone compared with women using oral contraceptives containing levonorgestrel: Case-control study using United States claims data. BMJ 2011;342:d2151.
16. Yasmin/Yaz Package Insert, 2012. *http://www.accessdata.fda.gov/drugsatfda_docs/label/2012/021098s019lbl.pdf.*
17. Ortho Evra Package Insert, 2012. *http://www.myortho360.com/myortho360/shared/pi/OrthoEvraPI.pdf#zoom=100.*
18. Holt VL, Scholes D, Wicklund KG, et al. Body mass index, weight, and oral contraceptive failure risk. Obstet Gynecol 2005;105:46–52.
19. Van Vliet HAAM, Grimes DA, Helmerhorst FM, Schulz KF. Biphasic versus monophasic oral contraceptives for contraception. Cochrane Database Syst Rev 2006;3:CD002032.
20. Van Vliet HAAM, Grimes DA, Helmerhorst FM, Schulz KF. Biphasic versus triphasic oral contraceptives for contraception. Cochrane Database Syst Rev 2006;3:CD003283.
21. Seasonique Package Insert, 2006. *https://www.seasonique.com/docs/prescribing-information.pdf.*
22. Lybrel Package Insert, 2010. *http://labeling.pfizer.com/showlabeling.aspx?id=489.*
23. Loestrin 24 Fe Package Insert, 2012. *http://www.loestrin24.com/loestrin/pdf/pi_loestrin24_fe.pdf#page=1.*
24. Lesnewski R, Prine L. Initiating hormonal contraception. Am Fam Physician 2006;71:105–112.
25. Centers for Disease Control and Prevention. Update to CDC's U.S. Medical Eligibility Criteria for Contraceptive Use, 2010: Revised Recommendations for the Use of Contraceptive Methods During the Postpartum Period. MMWR 2011;60: 878–883.
26. Guilbert E, Black A, Dunn S, et al. Missed hormonal contraceptives: New recommendations. J Obstet Gynecol 2008;30:1050–1062.
27. NuvaRing Package Insert, 2012. *http://www.spfiles.com/pinuvaring.pdf.*
28. PL Detailed Document, Hormonal Contraceptives and the Risk of Thrombosis. Pharmacist's Letter/Prescriber's Letter, 2012.
29. Depo-Provera Package Insert, 2002. *http://www.accessdata.fda.gov/drugsatfda_docs/label/2003/20246scs019_Depo-provera_lbl.pdf.*
30. Depo-SubQ Provera 104 Package Insert, 2005. *http://www.deposubqprovera104.com.*
31. Cameron ST, Glasier A, Johnstone A. Pilot study of home self administration of subcutaneous depo-medroxyprogesterone acetate for contraception. Contraception 2012;85:458–464.

32. American College of Obstetricians and Gynecologists. Depot medroxyprogesterone acetate and bone effects. ACOG Committee Opinion No. 415. Obstet Gynecol 2008;112:727–730.
33. Lopez LM, Chen M, Mullins S, et al. Steroidal contraceptives and bone fractures in women: Evidence from observational studies. Cochrane Database of Systematic Reviews 2012;8:CD009849. doi: 10.1002/14651858. CD009849.pub2.
34. American College of Obstetricians and Gynecologists. Long-acting reversible contraception: Implants and intrauterine devices. Practice Bulletin No. 121.Obstet Gynecol 2011;118:184–196.
35. Mosher WD, Jones J. Use of contraception in the United States: 1982–2008. Vital Health Stat 23 2010;(29):1–44.
36. Peipert JF, Zhao Q, Allsworth JE, et al. Continuation and satisfaction of reversible contraception. Obstet Gynecol 2011;117:1105–1113.
37. Nexplanon Package Insert, 2012. *http://www.nexplanon-usa.com/en/consumer/main/prescribing-information.asp*.
38. ParaGard package insert, 2012. *http://hcp.paragard.com/global/pdf/ParaGard_info.pdf*.
39. Mirena: An intrauterine system. Product Monograph. Bayer Schering Pharma, September 2011.
40. Mohllajee AP, Curtis KM, Peterson HB. Does insertion and use of intrauterine device increase the risk of pelvic inflammatory disease among women with sexually transmitted infection? A systematic review. Contraception 2006;73:145–153.
41. Skyla Package Insert, 2013. *http://hcp.skyla-us.com/index.php*.
42. Kaunitz AM, Meredith S, Inki P, et al. Levonorgestrel-releasing intrauterine system and endometrial ablation in heavy menstrual bleeding: A systematic review and meta-analysis. Obstet Gynecol 2009;113:1104–1116.
43. Mirena Extended CCDS 2011. Bayer HealthCare Pharmaceuticals, Berlin, Germany, 22nd March 2011.
44. American College of Obstetricians and Gynecologists. Intrauterine device and adolescents. ACOG Committee Opinion No. 392. Obstet Gynecol 2007;110: 1493–1495.
45. American College of Obstetricians and Gynecologists. Emergency contraception. Practice Bulletin No. 112. Obstet Gynecol 2010;115:1100–1109.
46. Plan B One-Step Package Insert, 2009. *http://www.planbonestep.com/pdf/PlanBOneStepFullProductInformation.pdf*.
47. Next Choice Package Insert, 2012. *http://www.mynextchoice.com/pi.asp*.
48. International Consortium for Emergency Contraception, 2008. *www.cecinfo.org/publications/policy.htm*
49. Novikova N, Weisberg E, Stanczyk FZ, et al. Effectiveness of levonorgestrel emergency contraception given before or after ovulation—A pilot study. Contraception 2007;75: 112–118.
50. Ella Package Insert, 2010. *http://pi.watson.com/data_stream.asp?product_group=1699&p=pi&language=E*.
51. Shrader SP, Hall LN, Ragucci KR, Rafie S. Updates in hormonal emergency contraception. Pharmacotherapy 2011;31:887–895.
52. Brache V, Cochon L, Jesam C, et al. Immediate pre-ovulatory administration of 30 mg ulipristal acetate significantly delays follicular rupture. Hum Reprod 2010;25:2256–2263.
53. Paul F, Mathe H, Ginde S, et al. Ulipristal acetate taken 48–120 hours after intercourse for emergency contraception. Obstet Gynecol 2010:115:257–263.
54. Glasier AF, Cameron ST, Fine PM, et al. Ulipristal acetate versus levonorgestrel for emergency contraception: A randomized non-inferiority trial and meta-analysis. Lancet 2010;375:555–562.
55. Creinin MD, Schlaff W, Archer DF, et al. Progesterone receptor modulator for emergency contraception: A randomized controlled trial. Obstet Gynecol 2006; 108:1089.

Menstruation-Related Disorders

Elena M. Umland and Jacqueline Klootwyk

63

KEY CONCEPTS

1. Unrecognized pregnancy is the most common cause of amenorrhea. A urine pregnancy test should be one of the first steps in evaluating this disorder.
2. For hypoestrogenic conditions associated with primary and secondary amenorrhea, estrogen (with a progestin) is provided.
3. Causes of menorrhagia are either systemic disorders or specific uterine abnormalities.
4. Pregnancy, including intrauterine pregnancy, ectopic pregnancy, and miscarriage, must be at the top of the differential diagnosis for any woman presenting with heavy menses.
5. The reduction in menorrhagia-related blood loss with use of nonsteroidal antiinflammatory drugs and oral contraceptives is directly proportional to the amount of pretreatment blood loss.
6. Intrauterine devices (IUDs) are considered therapeutic options in a variety of menstruation-related disorders. Guidelines from the American College of Obstetricians and Gynecologists indicate that both nulliparous and multiparous women at low risk of sexually transmitted diseases are good candidates for IUD use.
7. Anovulatory bleeding is the standard terminology used to describe bleeding from the uterine endometrium as a result of a dysfunctioning menstrual system, specifically excluding an anatomic lesion of the uterus.
8. Polycystic ovary syndrome (PCOS) can present as a variety of menstruation disorders, including amenorrhea, menorrhagia, and anovulatory bleeding. Although its definition continues to evolve, it is generally considered a disorder of androgen excess that often includes polycystic ovarian morphology and ovulatory dysfunction.
9. Metformin and thiazolidinedione use for anovulatory bleeding associated with PCOS is beneficial not only for anovulatory bleeding and fertility but also for improving glucose tolerance and other metabolic parameters that contribute to cardiovascular risk.
10. The selective serotonin reuptake inhibitors are first-line pharmacologic treatment options for premenstrual dysphoric disorder.

Problems related to the menstrual cycle are exceedingly common in women of reproductive age. This chapter discusses the most frequently encountered menstruation-related difficulties: amenorrhea, menorrhagia, anovulatory bleeding (including polycystic ovary syndrome, PCOS), dysmenorrhea, premenstrual syndrome (PMS), and premenstrual dysphoric disorder (PMDD). The need for effective treatments of these disorders stems from their negative impact on any or all of the following: quality of life, reproductive health, and long-term detrimental health effects, such as increased risk of osteoporosis with amenorrhea and cardiovascular disease with PCOS.

AMENORRHEA

Amenorrhea is described as either primary or secondary in nature. Primary amenorrhea is the absence of menses by age 16 years in the presence of normal secondary sexual development or the absence of menses by age 14 in the absence of normal secondary sexual development. Secondary amenorrhea is the absence of menses for three cycles or for 6 months in a previously menstruating woman. There is a significant amount of overlap between the two. The initial evaluation of amenorrhea often is the same, regardless of age of onset, except in unusual clinical situations.[1]

Epidemiology

Primary amenorrhea occurs in less than 0.1% of the general population. Secondary amenorrhea, in comparison, has an incidence of 0.7% to 5% in the general population and occurs more frequently in women younger than 25 years with a history of menstrual irregularities and in those involved in competitive athletics.[2]

Etiology

1 Unrecognized pregnancy is the most common cause of amenorrhea. A urine pregnancy test should be one of the first steps in evaluating this disorder. In organizing an approach to diagnosis and treatment, it is helpful to consider the organs involved in the menstrual cycle, which include the uterus, ovaries, anterior pituitary, and hypothalamus.

After excluding pregnancy, the most common causes of secondary amenorrhea are hypothalamic suppression, chronic anovulation, hyperprolactinemia, ovarian failure, and uterine disorders.[3]

Pathophysiology

Each organ in the hypothalamic–pituitary–ovarian–uterine axis is of importance in determining amenorrhea's etiology and pathophysiology. Beginning with the uterus/outflow tract and progressing caudally will result in a comprehensive differential diagnosis. Table 63-1 lists the pathophysiology of amenorrhea relative to the organ system(s) involved and the specific condition(s) that results in amenorrhea.

TABLE 63-1 Pathophysiology of Selected Menstrual Bleeding Disorders

Organ System	Condition	Pathophysiology/Laboratory Findings
Amenorrhea		
Uterus	Asherman's syndrome	Postcurettage/postsurgical uterine adhesions
	Congenital uterine abnormalities	Abnormal uterine development
Ovaries	Turner's syndrome	Lack of ovarian follicles
	Gonadal dysgenesis	Other genetic abnormalities
	Premature ovarian failure	Early loss of follicles
	Chemotherapy/radiation	Gonadal toxins
Anterior pituitary	Pituitary prolactin-secreting adenoma	↑ Prolactin suppresses the HPO axis
	Hypothyroidism	TRH causes ↑ prolactin, other abnormalities
	Medication (antipsychotics, verapamil)	↑ Prolactin suppresses the HPO axis
Hypothalamus	"Functional" hypothalamic amenorrhea	↓ Pulsatile GnRH secretion in the absence of other abnormalities
	Eating disorder	↓ Pulsatile GnRH secretion, ↓ FSH and LH secondary to weight loss
	Exercise	↓ Pulsatile GnRH secretion, ↓ FSH and LH secondary to low body fat
	Anovulation/PCOS	Asynchronous gonadotropin and estrogen production, abnormal endometrial growth
Anovulatory Bleeding		
Physiologic causes	Adolescence	Immaturity of the HPO axis: no LH surge
	Perimenopause	Declining ovarian function
Pathologic causes	Hyperandrogenic anovulation (PCOS)	Hyperandrogenism: high testosterone, high LH, hyperinsulinemia, and insulin resistance
	Hypothalamic dysfunction (physical or emotional stress, exercise, weight loss)	Suppression of pulsatile GnRH secretion and estrogen deficiency: low LH, low FSH
	Hyperprolactinemia (pituitary gland tumor, psychiatric medications)	High prolactin
	Hypothyroidism	High TSH
	Premature ovarian failure	High FSH
Menorrhagia		
Hematologic	von Willebrand's disease	Factor VII defect causing impaired platelet adhesion and increased bleeding time
	Idiopathic thrombocytopenic purpura	Decrease in circulating platelets, can be acute or chronic
Hepatic	Cirrhosis	Decreased estrogen metabolism, underlying coagulopathy
Endocrine	Hypothyroidism	Alterations in the HPO axis
Uterine	Fibroids	Alteration of endometrium, changes in uterine contractility
	Adenomyosis	Alteration of endometrium, changes in uterine contractility
	Endometrial polyps	Alteration of endometrium
	Gynecologic cancers	Various dysplastic alterations of endometrium, uterus, cervix

FSH, follicle-stimulating hormone; GnRH, gonadotropin-releasing hormone; HPO, hypothalamic–pituitary–ovarian axis; LH, luteinizing hormone; PCOS, polycystic ovary syndrome; TSH, thyroid-stimulating hormone; TRH, thyrotropin-releasing hormone.

Data from references 1–6.

Uterus/Outflow Tract

For menstruation to occur, a uterus, functional endometrium, and patent vagina must be present. Several anatomic abnormalities may cause amenorrhea. If primary amenorrhea is the presenting symptom, a congenital anomaly such as imperforate hymen or uterine agenesis may be present and often discovered by physical examination. An acquired condition of the genital tract, such as Asherman's syndrome or cervical stenosis, is more likely in secondary amenorrhea.

Ovaries

Normal ovarian function is critical for menstruation to occur. The ovaries must respond appropriately to follicle-stimulating hormone (FSH) and luteinizing hormone (LH) by secreting estrogen and progesterone in proper sequence to influence endometrial growth and shedding (Fig. 63-1).

Premature ovarian failure occurs when no viable follicles remain in the ovaries. This is because estrogen production is insufficient to stimulate endometrial growth in the absence of follicles. In a woman younger than 30 years, amenorrhea due to premature ovarian failure may be the result of genetic anomalies.[1]

The ovaries may play a role in amenorrhea through anovulation. Ovulation is required for the follicle (an estrogen-secreting body) to become a corpus luteum (a progesterone-secreting body). Without ovulation, the proper sequence of estrogen production, progesterone production, and estrogen/progesterone withdrawal will not occur. This can result in amenorrhea. Anovulation can occur secondary to thyroid disease, androgen excess (as in PCOS), or chronic illness.

Pituitary Gland

The anterior pituitary gland secretes FSH and LH in sequential fashion in response to hypothalamic stimulation and a complex ovarian feedback mechanism. Normal secretion of FSH and LH is altered by several endocrinologic and iatrogenic conditions, including thyroid disease, hyperprolactinemia, and dopaminergic drug administration.

Hypothalamus

The hypothalamus secretes cyclic gonadotropin-releasing hormone (GnRH), which causes the pituitary to produce FSH and LH. Disrupting this cyclic process will interrupt the hormonal cascade that results in normal menstruation. Anorexia nervosa, bulimia, intense exercise, and stress may cause hypothalamic amenorrhea.

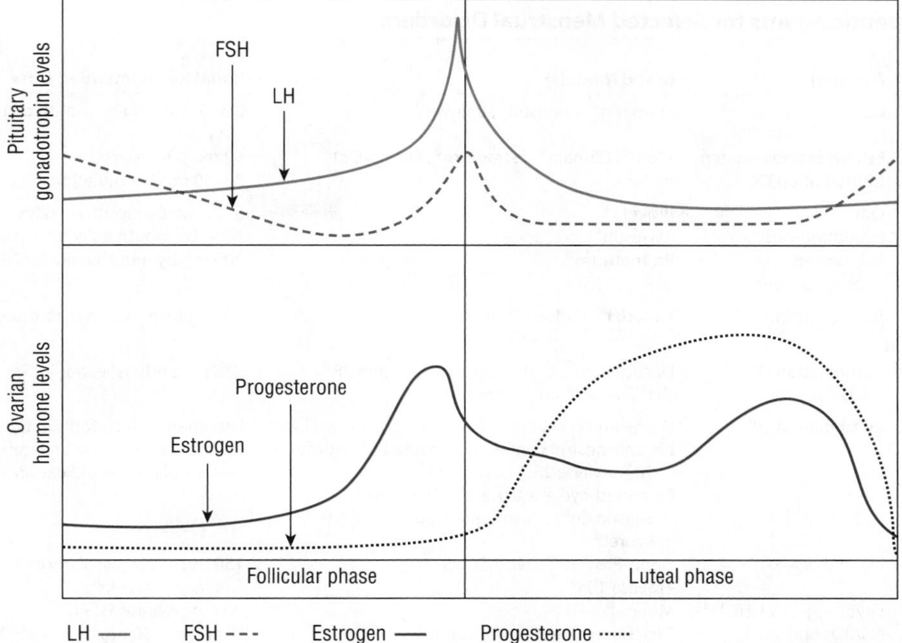

FIGURE 63-1 Hormonal fluctuations with the normal menstrual cycle. (FSH, follicle-stimulating hormone; LH, luteinizing hormone.) *(Courtesy of Hatcher RA, Nelson AL, Zieman M, et al. A Pocket Guide to Managing Contraception. Tiger GA: Bridging the Gap Foundation, 2003;1–146.)*

TREATMENT

The treatment options for amenorrhea are as varied as its causes.

Desired Outcome

Therapeutic modalities for amenorrhea should ensure the occurrence of normal puberty and restore the menstrual cycle. Treatment goals include bone density preservation, bone loss prevention, and ovulation restoration, improving fertility as desired.

Amenorrhea from hypoestrogenism may affect quality of life via hot flash induction (premature ovarian failure), dyspareunia, and, in prepubertal females, lack of secondary sexual characteristics and absence of menarche. Treatment is targeted at reversing these effects.

General Approach to Treatment

The overall success of any intervention to treat amenorrhea depends on proper identification of the disorder's underlying cause(s). Once the cause is identified, the appropriate intervention(s) can be made.

CLINICAL PRESENTATION Amenorrhea

General

- Although patients may be concerned about cessation of menses and implications for fertility, patients are generally not in acute distress

Symptoms

- Patients will note cessation of menses
- Patients may complain of infertility, vaginal dryness, or decreased libido

Signs

- Cessation of menses for more than 6 months in women with established menstruation, absence of menses by age 16 in the presence of normal secondary sexual development, or absence of menses by age 14 in the absence of normal secondary sexual development
- Recent significant weight loss or weight gain
- Presence of acne, hirsutism, hair loss, or acanthosis nigrans may suggest androgen excess

Laboratory Tests

- Pregnancy test
- Thyroid-stimulating hormone
- Prolactin
- If PCOS is suspected, consider free or total testosterone, 17-hydroxyprogesterone, fasting glucose, fasting lipid panel
- If suspect premature ovarian failure, consider FSH and LH

Other Diagnostic Tests

- Progesterone challenge
- Pelvic ultrasound to evaluate for polycystic ovaries

TABLE 63-2 Therapeutic Agents for Selected Menstrual Disorders

Specific Menstrual Disorder(s)	Agent(s)	Brand Name(s)	Usual Recommended Dose
Amenorrhea (primary or secondary)	CEE	Premarin®, Cenestin®, Enjuvia®	0.625–1.25 mg by mouth daily on days 1–25 of the cycle[8]
	Ethinyl estradiol patch	Alora®, Climara®, Estraderm®, Vivelle-Dot®	50 mcg/24 hours[8]
	Combination OC	Various	30–40 mcg formulations[8]
Amenorrhea (secondary)	Oral MPA	Provera®	5–10 mg by mouth on days 14–25 of the cycle[9]
	Norethindrone	Aygestin®	5 mg by mouth daily for 7–10 days[9]
	Micronized progesterone	Prometrium®	400 mg by mouth daily for 7–10 days[9]
Amenorrhea related to hyperprolactinemia	Bromocriptine[3,8,10]	Parlodel®, Parlodel® SnapTabs	2.5 mg by mouth two to three times daily
Anovulatory bleeding	Combination OC	Desogen 28®, Ortho-Cept 28®, Yasmin 28®, Yaz®, Beyaz®, and others	≤35 mcg ethinyl estradiol
Dysmenorrhea	Combination OC	Norgestrel containing: Cryselle 28®, Lo/Ovral 28® Levonorgestrel containing: Levora 28®, Nordette 28®, Aviane 28®, Lessina 28® Extended-cycle: Introvale®, Quasense®, Seasonale®, Seasonique®, LoSeasonique®, Lybrel®	Less than 35 mcg formulations + norgestrel or levonorgestrel[11]; use of extended-cycle formulations is beneficial for this indication
	Injectable MPA[11]	Depo-Provera®, Depo-SubQ Provera 104®	150 mg intramuscularly or 104 mg subcutaneously every 12 weeks
	Levonorgestrel IUD[11–13]	Mirena®	20 mcg released daily
	NSAIDs (any are acceptable); the most commonly studied/cited are included in this table	Diclofenac (Cataflam®); ibuprofen (Motrin®, Advil®), mefenamic acid (Ponstel®)	Diclofenac 50 mg by mouth three times daily; ibuprofen 800 mg by mouth three times daily; mefenamic acid 500 mg by mouth as a loading dose, then 250 mg by mouth up to four times daily as needed[14]
		Naproxen (Naprosyn®)	Naproxen 550-mg loading dose by mouth started 1–2 days prior to menses followed by 275 mg by mouth every 6–12 hours as needed[11]
	Celecoxib[11,12,15]	Celebrex®	400 mg by mouth followed by 200 mg by mouth every 12 hours as needed during menses
Menorrhagia	Combination OC[16]	Various	Optimal dose unknown
	Levonorgestrel IUD[16–18]	Mirena®	20 mcg released daily
	Oral MPA	Provera®	5–10 mg by mouth on days 5–26 of the cycle or during the luteal phase[13,17]
	NSAIDs[17]	As above for dysmenorrhea	Doses as recommended for dysmenorrhea may be used; therapy should be initiated with the onset of menses[13]
	Tranexamic acid[17,19]	Lysteda®	1,300 mg by mouth every 8 hours once heavy bleeding begins; dose for 4–7 days as needed per cycle
PCOS-related amenorrhea and/or anovulatory bleeding	Injectable MPA	Depo-Provera®, Depo-SubQ Provera 104®	150 mg intramuscularly or 104 mg subcutaneously every 12 weeks
	Combination OC[20,21]	Desogestrel containing: Desogen 28®, Ortho-Cept 28® Norgestimate containing: OrthoTri-Cyclen Lo® Drospirenone containing: Yasmin 28®, Yaz®, Beyaz®	≤30 mcg ethinyl estradiol with either desogestrel, norgestimate or drospirenone
	Oral MPA	Provera®	10 mg by mouth for 10 days[5]
	Metformin[5,21]	Glucophage®, Fortamet®, Glucophage XR®, Glumetza®	1,500–2,000 mg by mouth daily[21]
	Pioglitazone, rosiglitazone[5,21]	Pioglitazone = Actose®, rosiglitazone = Avandia®	Pioglitazone 15–45 mg by mouth daily; rosiglitazone 4–8 mg by mouth daily
PMDD	Clomipramine[22]	Anafranil®	25–75 mg by mouth daily taken either continuously or only during the luteal phase
	Drospirenone	Yasmin 28®, Yaz®, Beyaz®	3 mg (+ ≤30 mcg ethinyl estradiol) by mouth on days 1–21 of the menstrual cycle[23]
	Leuprolide	Lupron Depot®	3.75 mg intramuscularly[22]
	SSRIs[25]	Citalopram = Celexa®; escitalopram = Lexapro®; fluoxetine = Prozac®, Sarafem®; paroxetine = Paxil®; sertraline = Zoloft®	Citalopram 10–30 mg; escitalopram 10–20 mg[24]; fluoxetine 10–20 mg; fluvoxamine 50 mg; paroxetine 10–30 mg; sertraline 25–150 mg; all agents are given by mouth daily and can be dosed either continuously or during the luteal phase only[22]

CEE, conjugated equine estrogen; IUD, intrauterine device; MPA, medroxyprogesterone acetate; NSAID, nonsteroidal antiinflammatory drug; OC, oral contraceptive; PCOS, polycystic ovary syndrome; PMDD, premenstrual dysphoric disorder; SSRI, selective serotonin reuptake inhibitors.

Data from references 3, 8–13, and 14–24.

For patients experiencing amenorrhea secondary to hypoestrogenic states, a diet rich in calcium and vitamin D is essential to minimize negative impact on bone health.

Nonpharmacologic Therapy

Nonpharmacologic therapy for amenorrhea varies depending upon the underlying cause. Amenorrhea secondary to anorexia may respond to weight gain. In young women for whom excessive exercise is an underlying cause, reduction of exercise quantity and intensity are important.

Pharmacologic Therapy

❷ For hypoestrogenic conditions associated with primary or secondary amenorrhea, estrogen (with a progestin) is provided. It can be administered as an oral contraceptive (OC), conjugated equine estrogen, or estradiol patch. Estrogen therapy in this patient population reduces osteoporosis risk[7] and improves quality of life. Table 63-2 lists therapeutic agents for amenorrhea treatment, including recommended doses. Figure 63-2 illustrates a treatment algorithm for management of amenorrhea.

When hyperprolactinemia is the cause of amenorrhea, dopamine agonists such as bromocriptine aid in reducing prolactin concentrations and the resumption of menses. Bromocriptine normalizes prolactin levels in 90% of affected women, and fertility is restored in 80% of treated women.[10]

Amenorrhea related to PCOS-induced anovulation may respond to agents that reduce insulin resistance. Metformin and the thiazolidinediones for this purpose are discussed in the "Anovulatory bleeding" section.

Progestins induce withdrawal bleeding in women with secondary amenorrhea. Several factors predict progesterone's efficacy for this purpose.[9] These factors include estrogen concentrations greater than or equal to 35 pg/mL (128 pmol/L) and endometrial thickness (greater initial thickness resulting in more withdrawal bleeding).

Progestin efficacy for secondary amenorrhea varies by formulation used. Progesterone in oil administered intramuscularly results in withdrawal bleeding in 70% of treated patients, whereas oral medroxyprogesterone acetate (MPA) induces withdrawal bleeding in 95% of treated patients.[9] Table 63-2 identifies the types and doses of progestins used for secondary amenorrhea treatment. Figure 63-2 illustrates when to consider progestin use for amenorrhea treatment.

Special Populations

Amenorrhea in the adolescent population is of concern because this is the developmental time when peak bone mass is achieved. The cause of amenorrhea, whether primary or secondary, must be promptly identified in this population, as amenorrhea and its related hypoestrogenism negatively affect bone development. In addition to treating or eliminating amenorrhea's underlying cause, ensuring that the patient is receiving adequate amounts of calcium and vitamin D is imperative. Estrogen replacement, typically via an OC, is important.

Drug Class Information

Table 63-3 identifies the significant pharmacologic properties requiring monitoring of the agents used for amenorrhea management.

Evaluation of Therapeutic Outcomes

Table 63-3 lists the expected outcomes and specific monitoring parameters for treatment modalities used in amenorrhea management.

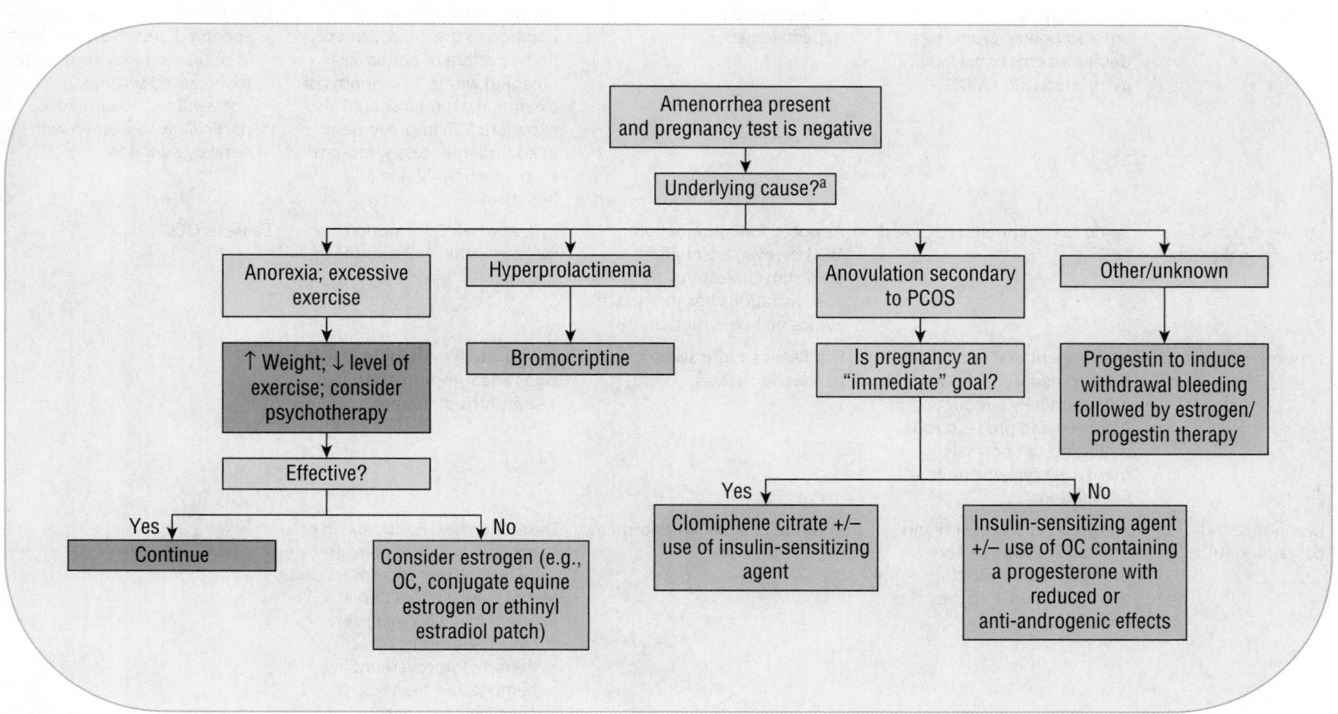

FIGURE 63-2 Treatment algorithm for amenorrhea. [a]Regardless of cause, adequate calcium and vitamin D intake must be ensured. (OC, oral contraceptive; PCOS, polycystic ovary syndrome.)

TABLE 63-3 Pharmacologic Properties and Monitoring Parameters for Agents Used in the Management of Menstrual Disorders

Therapeutic Agent/ Drug Class	Mechanism of Action/Role in Particular Menstrual Disorders	Adverse Drug Reactions	Monitoring for Expected Outcomes of Specific Menstrual Disorders	Comments
Clomipramine	PMDD: Exact mechanism unknown	Dry mouth, constipation, fatigue, vertigo, sweating	Reduction in or absence of initial symptoms and improved quality of life within 1–3 menstrual cycles of therapy	
Combination OCs	Exogenous estrogen and progesterone that suppresses FSH and LH production and thus inhibits ovulation Can be used to reduce menstrual flow (menorrhagia, dysmenorrhea), and control menstrual cycle (anovulatory bleeding secondary to hypoestrogenism)	Thromboembolism, breast enlargement, breast tenderness, bloating, nausea, GI upset, headache, peripheral edema	Amenorrhea: Resumption of menses within 1–2 months of therapy Anovulatory bleeding: Improvement in pattern of abnormal bleeding within 1–2 months of therapy Dysmenorrhea: Reduction in or absence of pelvic pain within 1–2 months of therapy Menorrhagia: Reduction in blood loss with menses over 1–2 months of therapy. Improvement in hemoglobin/hematocrit after 3 months of therapy compared to baseline	St. John's Wort contributes to altered menstrual bleeding Rifampin induces estrogen metabolism, possibly contributing to treatment failure Sulfa-containing drugs may contribute to increased photosensitivity
CEE	Estrogen replacement for hypoestrogenic states leading to anovulatory bleeding	As noted for combination OC	Anovulatory bleeding: Improvement in pattern of abnormal bleeding within 1–2 months of therapy	Same as OCs
Bromocriptine	Dopamine agonist that suppresses prolactin production from pituitary tumors such that resumption of normal FSH and LH production occurs	Hypotension, nausea, constipation, anorexia, Raynaud's phenomenon	Amenorrhea related to hyperprolactinemia: Baseline and weekly prolactin levels should be measured with dosage increases until resumption of menses is observed. Continue therapy discontinuation after 6–12 months of menses and continued normalization of serum prolactin levels	Inhibits CYP3A4 and is metabolized by CYP3A4 St. John's Wort induces CP3A4; coadministration may lead to treatment failure
Drospirenone-containing OCs	Progesterone with antimineralocorticoid and antiandrogenic properties; decreases emotional lability associated with PMDD	As noted for combination OC; increased risk of hyperkalemia	PCOS-related amenorrhea or anovulatory bleeding: In addition to the improvement in the pattern of abnormal bleeding within 1–2 months of treatment, women should also experience an improvement in androgen-excess symptoms such as acne/oily skin and hirsutism	Same as OCs Coadministration of potassium-sparing diuretics or diets high in potassium may contribute to increased serum potassium concentrations, particularly in women with renal dysfunction
Ethinyl estradiol transdermal patch	Same as combination OCs and CEE	As noted for combination OC; however, lesser effects on serum cholesterol concentrations because patch avoids first-pass metabolism	Amenorrhea: Resumption of menses within 1–2 months of therapy	Same as OCs
Leuprolide	GnRH agent that contributes to suppression of FSH and LH and ultimately a reduction in estrogen and progesterone, inhibiting the normal menstrual cycle/hormonal fluctuations	Hot flashes, night sweats, headache, nausea	PMDD: Improvement in PMDD signs and symptoms within 1–2 months of therapy	
Levonorgestrel-containing IUD	Suppresses FSH and LH and ultimately estrogen and progesterone, inhibiting the usual growth of the endometrium	Irregular menses, amenorrhea	Dysmenorrhea: Reduction in or absence of pelvic pain after 1–2 months of therapy Menorrhagia: Reduction in blood loss with menses over 1–2 months of therapy. Improvement in hemoglobin/hematocrit after 3 months of therapy compared to baseline	

(continued)

TABLE 63-3 Pharmacologic Properties and Monitoring Parameters for Agents Used in the Management of Menstrual Disorders (*Continued*)

Therapeutic Agent/ Drug Class	Mechanism of Action/Role in Particular Menstrual Disorders	Adverse Drug Reactions	Monitoring for Expected Outcomes of Specific Menstrual Disorders	Comments
MPA (oral and injectable)	Suppresses FSH and LH and ultimately estrogen and progesterone, inhibiting the usual growth of the endometrium	Edema, anorexia, depression, insomnia, weight gain or loss, increase in serum total and LDL cholesterol, may reduce HDL cholesterol	Dysmenorrhea: Reduction in or absence of pelvic pain after 1–2 months of therapy Menorrhagia: Reduction in blood loss with menses over 1–2 months of therapy. Improvement in hemoglobin/hematocrit after 3 months of therapy compared to baseline PCOS-related amenorrhea and/or anovulatory bleeding: Resumption of menses over 1–2 courses of therapy	
Metformin	Inhibits hepatic glucose production and increases sensitivity of tissues to insulin, thus reducing insulin resistance	Anorexia, nausea, vomiting, diarrhea, flatulence, lactic acidosis (rare)	PCOS-related amenorrhea and/or anovulatory bleeding: If desired, monitor for ovulation after 3–6 months of therapy	IV contrast dye may increase the risk of lactic acidosis; stop metformin 1 day prior and restart when renal function is normal and stabilized following the IV dye
NSAIDs	Inhibits prostaglandin release that occurs with menses, thus reducing inflammatory response contributing to dysmenorrhea	GI upset, stomach ulcer, nausea, vomiting, heartburn, indigestion, rash, dizziness	Dysmenorrhea: Reduction in or absence of pelvic pain within hours of initiating. Menorrhagia: Reduction in blood loss with menses over 1–2 months of therapy	
SSRIs	Exact mechanism in PMDD unknown	Sexual dysfunction (reduced libido, anorgasmia), insomnia, sedation, hypersomnia, nausea, diarrhea	Improvement in PMDD signs and symptoms observed within 1–3 months of therapy	
Thiazolidinediones	Increases peripheral tissue sensitivity to insulin, thus reducing insulin resistance	Weight gain; increase in total, LDL, and HDL cholesterol; edema; headache; fatigue; hepatic injury (rare)	PCOS-related amenorrhea and/or anovulatory bleeding: If desired, monitor for ovulation after 3–6 months of therapy	
Tranexamic acid	Antifibrinolytic effects by reversibly blocking lysine binding sites on plasminogen, preventing fibrin degradation and a reduction in menstrual blood loss	Nausea, vomiting, diarrhea, dyspepsia	Menorrhagia: Reduction in blood loss with menses should be noticeable with the first month of therapy. Improvement in hemoglobin/hematocrit after 3 months of therapy compared to baseline	
Venlafaxine	Exact mechanism in PMDD unknown		Improvement in PMDD signs and symptoms observed within 1–3 months of therapy	

CEE, conjugated equine estrogen; FSH, follicle-stimulating hormone; GnRH, gonadotropin-releasing hormone; HDL, high-density lipoprotein; IUD, intrauterine device; LDL, low-density lipoprotein; LH, luteinizing hormone; MPA, medroxyprogesterone acetate; NSAID, nonsteroidal antiinflammatory drug; OC, oral contraceptive; PMDD, premenstrual dysphoric disorder; SSRI, selective serotonin reuptake inhibitor.

Data from references 4, 5, 7, 10, 13, 14, 19, 22, and 25–32.

MENORRHAGIA

Menorrhagia is the term used to describe heavy menstrual blood loss (greater than 80 mL per cycle) or prolonged menstrual bleeding (menses for greater than 7 days).[1,4] This definition has been questioned because of several factors, including difficulty quantifying menstrual loss in clinical practice. Additionally, many women with "heavy menses" but blood loss less than 80 mL merit treatment consideration because of flow containment issues, unpredictably heavy flow days, or other associated symptoms.[28,32,33]

Epidemiology

Menorrhagia rates in healthy women range from 9% to 14%.[4] In women with coagulation disorders such as von Willebrand's disease or platelet dysfunction, the rates of menorrhagia are as high as 100% and 98%, respectively.[6,33]

Etiology

❸ Causes of menorrhagia are either systemic disorders or specific uterine abnormalities. ❹ Pregnancy, including intrauterine pregnancy, ectopic pregnancy, and miscarriage, must be at the top of the differential diagnosis list for any woman presenting with heavy menses. In several studies of adolescents with acute menorrhagia, underlying bleeding disorders accounted for 3% to 13% of emergency room presentations. For example, von Willebrand's disease has an incidence of 1% in the general population;[34] its prevalence in women with menorrhagia may be as high as 20%.[35] Menorrhagia initially may present as heavy menses in the adolescent.[34] Hypothyroidism also may be associated with heavy menses. Specific uterine causes of menorrhagia are more common in older childbearing women and include fibroids, adenomyosis, endometrial polyps, and gynecologic malignancies.

CLINICAL PRESENTATION Menorrhagia

General

- Patients may or may not be in acute distress

Symptoms

- Patients may complain of heavy/prolonged menstrual flow. They also may have signs of fatigue and lightheadedness in cases of severe blood loss. These symptoms may or may not occur with dysmenorrhea

Signs

- Orthostasis, tachycardia, and pallor may be noted, especially in cases of significant acute blood loss

Laboratory Tests

- Complete blood count and ferritin levels; hemoglobin and hematocrit results may be low
- If the history dictates, testing may be performed to identify coagulation disorder(s) as a cause

Other Diagnostic Tests

- Pelvic ultrasound
- Pelvic magnetic resonance imaging
- Papanicolaou (Pap) smear
- Endometrial biopsy
- Hysteroscopy
- Sonohysterogram

Pathophysiology

Table 63-1 lists the pathophysiology of menorrhagia relative to the organ system(s) involved and the specific conditions that result in menorrhagia.

TREATMENT

Initial treatment choice for menorrhagia is influenced by whether or not the woman desires to become pregnant.

Desired Outcome

Menorrhagia therapy should reduce menstrual blood flow, improve the patient's quality of life, and defer the need for surgical intervention. Table 63-2 lists the agents and their recommended dosing for menorrhagia management. Figure 63-3 presents an algorithm for menorrhagia treatment.

General Approach to Treatment

Several treatment options exist for menorrhagia. Initial and subsequent treatment options should be thoughtfully chosen in an effort to avoid surgery.

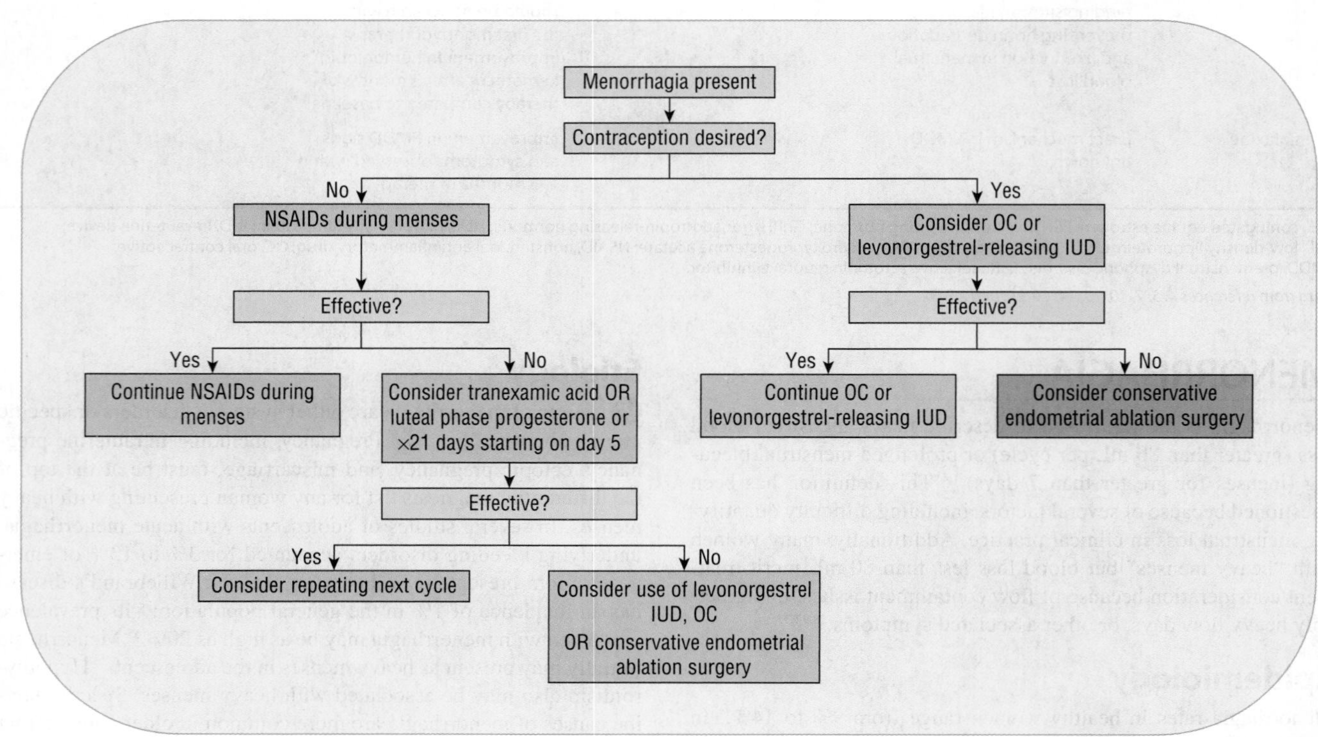

FIGURE 63-3 Treatment algorithm for menorrhagia. (IUD, intrauterine device; NSAIDs, nonsteroidal antiinflammatory drugs; OC, oral contraceptive.)

Nonpharmacologic Therapy

Nonpharmacologic interventions for menorrhagia include surgical procedures that are generally reserved for patients not responding to pharmacologic treatment. These interventions vary from conservative endometrial ablation to hysterectomy.[36]

Pharmacologic Therapy

Among the agents used to treat menorrhagia, the nonsteroidal anti-inflammatory drugs (NSAIDs) have the advantage of administration only during menses. NSAID use is associated with a 20% to 50% reduction in blood loss in 75% of treated women.[13,32] In some patients, as much as an 80% reduction in blood loss has been observed.[13]

For women desiring to avoid pregnancy, OC use is beneficial for menorrhagia and should be considered. A 40% to 50% reduction in menstrual blood loss has been observed in patients treated with cyclic combined OCs.[37] **5** The reduction in menorrhagia-related blood loss with use of NSAIDs and OCs is directly proportional to the amount of pretreatment blood loss.[13]

Another menorrhagia treatment option is the levonorgestrel-releasing intrauterine device (IUD). This is a very effective treatment to reduce menstrual flow.[38] In particular, a 79% to 97% reduction in blood loss has been observed with its use.[38] Its use has also resulted in postponing or cancelling scheduled endometrial ablation surgery or hysterectomy. Sixty percent of treated patients avoided hysterectomy when employing this treatment option,[39] and its therapeutic efficacy is similar to endometrial ablation up to 2 years following treatment.[18]

Progesterone therapy either during the luteal phase of the menstrual cycle or for 21 days, starting on day 5 after onset of menses, results in a 32% to 50% reduction in menstrual blood loss.[13] However, progesterone use is not superior to other medical treatments, including the NSAIDs.[13]

Tranexamic acid was recently approved in the United States for primary menorrhagia treatment. Its use is associated with a significant 26% to 60% reduction in menstrual blood loss.[40]

Drug Treatments of First Choice

For women who have menorrhagia associated with ovulatory cycles and do not desire hormonal therapy and/or contraception, NSAIDs during menses is a reasonable choice in the absence of any contraindications or GI illnesses such as peptic ulcer disease or gastroesophageal reflux disease. This choice is convenient (only taken during menses) and comparatively inexpensive. For women desiring contraception, it is reasonable to start with either an OC or the levonorgestrel-releasing IUD. Either choice is acceptable for both nulligravid and multiparous women who desire a long-term reversible form of contraception.[37,38] Given cost-effectiveness data, the levonorgestrel-releasing IUD is the best first-line choice for women desiring contraception.[41] Clinical trial data illustrate a higher failure rate with the OCs (62.5%) compared to the levonorgestrel-releasing IUD (34%) as the primary treatment method.[41]

Alternative Drug Treatments

Given their side effects, reduced efficacy compared to the first-line agents, and/or cost, use of oral progesterone and depot MPA should be reserved. Tranexamic acid is another treatment option. In comparison to luteal phase oral progesterone, tranexamic acid results in a significantly greater reduction in menstrual blood loss and greater relief of patient-reported symptoms.[13] Its use has been associated with a significant improvement in quality of life and high patient satisfaction following three cycles of use.[19,42]

Special Populations

Although historically it was believed that IUD use should be avoided in nulliparous women, **6** guidelines from the American College of Obstetricians and Gynecologists (ACOG) indicate that both nulliparous and multiparous women at low risk of sexually transmitted diseases are good candidates for IUD use.[38] Therefore, any of the treatments discussed are options in any female presenting with menorrhagia. Dosage adjustment for tranexamic acid is recommended for reduced renal function. Women with serum creatinine between 1.4 and 2.8 mg/dL (124 and 248 μmol/L) should receive only 1,300 mg by mouth twice daily; women with serum creatinine between 2.9 and 5.7 mg/dL (256 and 504 μmol/L) should receive 1,300 mg by mouth once daily; those with serum creatinine above 5.7 mg/dL (504 μmol/L) should receive 650 mg by mouth once daily.

Drug Class Information

Table 63-3 identifies the significant pharmacologic properties that require monitoring for the agents used to manage menorrhagia.

Evaluation of Therapeutic Outcomes

Table 63-3 illustrates the expected outcomes and specific monitoring parameters for the treatment modalities used in menorrhagia management.

ANOVULATORY BLEEDING

7 Anovulatory bleeding is the standard terminology used to describe bleeding from the uterine endometrium as a result of a dysfunctioning menstrual system, specifically excluding an anatomic lesion of the uterus.[1,29] Anovulatory bleeding is also referred to as dysfunctional or irregular uterine bleeding.

Epidemiology

Anovulatory bleeding is the most common form of noncyclic uterine bleeding.[4] The most common cause is PCOS, for which the prevalence rates range from 6% to 8%.[43–45] In fact, PCOS is the most common endocrine abnormality among U.S. women of reproductive age.[45] **8** PCOS can present as a variety of menstruation disorders, including amenorrhea, menorrhagia, and/or anovulatory bleeding. Although its exact definition continues to evolve, it is a disorder of androgen excess that often includes polycystic ovarian morphology and ovulatory dysfunction. It is a significant risk factor for the metabolic syndrome, type 2 diabetes, dyslipidemia, hypertension, and possibly cardiovascular disease.[21,46,47] PCOS is a common cause of ovulation dysfunction in adult women.[21] Other common causes in adult women include hyperprolactinemia, hypothalamic amenorrhea, also known as hypogonadotropichypogonadism, premature ovarian failure, and thyroid dysfunction.[1,29]

Etiology

When considering the etiology of anovulatory bleeding, the patient's age must be considered. All patients presenting with abnormal bleeding should be evaluated for pregnancy. Most adolescents will experience physiologic anovulatory cycles in the first few years following menarche because their hypothalamic–pituitary–gonadal axis is still maturing. However, if an adolescent has not developed regular menstrual cycles within 5 years of menarche, further evaluation for the cause, such as PCOS, should be considered.[48] Anovulatory cycles may "unmask" an underlying bleeding disorder. When irregular menses is associated with significant bleeding, an inherited bleeding disorder should be a considered cause, especially in adolescence.[6,29] Women experiencing anovulation in their reproductive years should be evaluated for pathologic causes, including PCOS, thyroid dysfunction, hyperprolactinemia, primary pituitary disease, premature ovarian failure, hypothalamic dysfunction, disordered eating, adrenal disease, and androgen-producing tumors. Women in their perimenopausal years may experience "physiologic" anovulatory cycles because of intermittently declining estrogen levels. Regardless of age, evaluation for endometrial hyperplasia and/or endometrial cancer should be considered when a woman experiences excessive bleeding with anovulatory cycles. When considering the etiology of anovulation, it is common for several conditions to coexist (e.g., PCOS and hypothyroidism), each contributing to the woman's constellation of symptoms. All common etiologies should be considered when beginning to evaluate anovulation.[1]

Pathophysiology

Normal menstrual cycles occur through a complex interaction of the hypothalamus, pituitary gland, ovaries, and endometrium (Fig. 63-1). In an ovulatory cycle, the ovary produces a mature, estrogen-secreting follicle in response to FSH release from the pituitary. The endometrium proliferates under the influence of this estrogen production. At a critical level of estrogen concentration, the pituitary responds by producing an "LH surge," which creates a cascade of ovarian events, culminating in ovulation. Upon oocyte release, the follicle becomes a progesterone-producing corpus luteum. The endometrium "organizes" into secretory endometrium in the presence of adequate progesterone. If conception and implantation do not occur, corpus luteum involution causes a decline in estrogen and progesterone leading to predictable, organized menstrual flow as the endometrium sloughs.

If ovulation does not occur, progesterone is not produced, and the endometrium will continue to proliferate in an "unorganized" fashion under the influence of continued estrogen production. Eventually the endometrium will become so thick that it can no longer be supported by continued estrogen production. This results in unorganized, sporadic sloughing of the endometrium, characteristic of the unpredictable and heavy bleeding of anovulation. Anovulation has several etiologies. In adolescence, hypothalamic–pituitary axis immaturity contributes to the absence of the LH surge required for ovulation. In the anorexic patient, the hypothalamus loses much of its pulsatile GnRH release, leading to low levels of FSH and LH, enough for estrogen production but not enough to induce ovulation.

TREATMENT

Optimizing anovulatory bleeding therapy depends on accurate identification of the disorder's cause(s). The treatment options for anovulatory bleeding are wide and varied.

Desired Outcome

Control of excessive bleeding in the short-term is paramount. Longer-term goals of therapy include restoring the natural cycle of orderly endometrial growth and shedding,[29,49] decreasing anovulation complications (e.g., osteopenia, infertility), and improving overall quality of life. Table 63-2 identifies the agents used to manage anovulatory bleeding and their recommended doses.

General Approach to Treatment

Although the appropriate primary treatment choice for anovulatory bleeding depends on the accurate diagnosis of its cause and identification of desired outcomes, additional treatment may be necessary to manage other signs and symptoms. Treatment to resolve anovulatory bleeding should be initiated and any underlying menorrhagia should be managed.

Nonpharmacologic Therapy

Nonpharmacologic treatment options for anovulatory bleeding depend on the underlying cause. In a woman of reproductive age with PCOS, moderate weight loss of 2% to 5% may result in improved menstrual regularity and ovulatory function, reduced hirsutism, increased insulin sensitivity, and improved response to fertility treatments.[21] In women who have completed childbearing or who have not responded to medical management, endometrial ablation or resection and hysterectomy are surgical options. Procedure choice involves shared decision making with the patient. In the short term, ablation results in less morbidity and shorter recovery periods. However, a significant number of women eventually undergo hysterectomy in the subsequent 5 years.[29]

Pharmacologic Therapy

Estrogen is the recommended treatment for managing acute severe bleeding episodes because it promotes endometrial stabilization.[49] Following its initial use to control acute bleeding episodes, therapy continuation may be necessary to prevent future occurrences. OC use fulfills this role and contributes to predictable menstrual cycles.

OCs prevent recurrent anovulatory bleeding by providing a progestin and suppressing ovarian hormones and adrenal androgen production. They also, indirectly, increase sex hormone-binding globulin (SHBG). SHBG binds androgens and reduces their circulating free concentrations. For women with high androgen levels and its related signs such as hirsutism (e.g., those with PCOS) OCs containing less than or equal to 35 mcg of ethinyl estradiol and a progesterone that exhibits minimal androgenic

CLINICAL PRESENTATION Anovulatory Bleeding

General

- Patients may or may not be in acute distress

Symptoms

- Irregular, heavy, or prolonged vaginal bleeding, perimenopausal symptoms (hot flashes, nights sweats, vaginal dryness)

Signs

- Acne, hirsutism, obesity

Laboratory Tests

- If PCOS is suspected, consider free or total testosterone, fasting glucose, fasting lipid panel
- If perimenopause is suspected, measure FSH
- Thyroid-stimulating hormone

Other Diagnostic Tests

- If the patient is older than 35 years, endometrial biopsy
- Pelvic ultrasound to evaluate for polycystic ovaries
- If perimenopause is suspected, measure FSH

side effects (e.g., norgestimate and desogestrel) or with antiandrogenic effects (e.g., drospirenone) may be desirable.[20]

Clinical **Controversy. . .**

OCs containing antiandrogenic progesterones are very effective for managing the acne and hirsutism that accompany PCOS; they also suppress ovarian androgen production and increase sex hormone-binding globulin, thus reducing free testosterone concentrations. Controversy regarding their use in PCOS exists secondary to their potential adverse effects on insulin resistance, glucose tolerance, vascular reactivity, and coagulability.[20] An increase in high-sensitivity C-reactive protein (a predictor of cardiovascular disease) and an increase in homocysteine levels (indicating an increased risk of cardiovascular disease) have been observed with the use of such OCs.[50] Another trial found a reduction in brachial artery flow-mediated dilatation and an increase in carotid intima-media thickness, both indicators of endothelial dysfunction, following therapy with OCs containing ethinyl estradiol and cyproterone acetate.[51] Additional, longer-term clinical trials will clarify whether the benefits of these agents outweigh the risks. It has been suggested that cardiovascular risk calculators be employed as an adjunct to guidelines suggesting the use of OCs in this patient population.[52]

In women with contraindication(s) to estrogen or in whom the side effects are unacceptable, progesterone-only products are an option. They should be strongly considered for women experiencing menorrhagia associated with anovulatory bleeding.[53] In women with PCOS, depot and intermittent oral MPA provide endometrial protection through endometrial shedding.[5] If pregnancy is not a desired outcome of treatment, another progesterone option is placement of a levonorgestrel-containing IUD.[29,53]

Metformin and the thiazolidinediones, including pioglitazone and rosiglitazone, improve insulin sensitivity. In patients with PCOS, this contributes to reduced circulating androgen concentrations, increased ovulation rates,[5,54,55] and improved glucose tolerance.[5,21] These improvements occur due to the SHBG increase that occurs via increased insulin sensitivity. **9** Metformin and thiazolidinedione use for anovulatory bleeding associated with PCOS is beneficial not only for anovulatory bleeding and fertility but also for improving glucose tolerance and other metabolic parameters that contribute to cardiovascular risk.[5,21,56] For women desiring pregnancy, metformin is pregnancy category B, and pioglitazone and rosiglitazone are category C.

Clinical **Controversy. . .**

The overall role of metformin in treating PCOS and its duration of therapy remain controversial. For ovulation induction, data show that metformin is highly effective in both clomiphene citrate-resistant patients and patients using it as initial therapy.[54,55] Its use throughout pregnancy has been associated with a reduction in early pregnancy loss rates.[57] The presence of dyslipidemia and hyperinsulinemia increases the long-term risk for developing cardiovascular disease in PCOS patients. Current research indicates that metformin should be considered to reduce cardiovascular risk in these women.[56] More research is needed to definitively identify the role(s) of metformin in PCOS, particularly as it relates to ovulation induction.

If the treatment goal is improved fertility via ovulation induction, clomiphene citrate is an option. Treatment with 50 mg/day for 5 days can be initiated between menstrual cycle days 3 and 5. This often occurs after inducing withdrawal bleeding with a progesterone such as MPA 10 mg daily orally for 10 days. If ovulation does not occur with this dose of clomiphene, a dose of 100 mg/day is warranted. In rare instances, it may be increased by 50 mg increments up to 250 mg/day.

Drug Treatments of First Choice

As with many menstruation-related disorders, there is not one universal treatment option of first choice for anovulatory bleeding. Rather, the treatment(s) chosen depends on accurate etiologic diagnosis as well as identification of the desired treatment outcome(s).

OCs are the first-choice treatment in women with anovulatory bleeding who do not desire pregnancy.[22] The use of OCs containing ethinyl estradiol and a progesterone with minimal androgenic or antiandrogenic effects is effective for cycle control and minimizing the androgenic signs and symptoms of PCOS.[20,47,49]

Relative to anovulation in women with PCOS, insulin-sensitizing agents including metformin and the thiazolidinediones improve ovulatory frequency and metabolic parameters. Clomiphene use may further assist in achieving ovulation induction.

More recent data support even further metformin's use compared to clomiphene for ovulation induction.[54,55] Metformin for ovulation induction[54] as well as its use throughout pregnancy[57] in women with PCOS has been associated with reduced miscarriage rates in this patient population.

Special Populations

Anovulatory cycles are fairly common in the perimenarchal reproductive years. Ovulation typically is established 1 year or more following menarche. Anovulatory bleeding occurring in this population may be excessive. If excessive bleeding occurs, the patient should be evaluated for bleeding disorders. The prevalence of bleeding disorders, including von Willebrand's disease, prothrombin deficiency, and idiopathic thrombocytopenia purpura, in this population ranges from 5% to 24%.[6]

If identified, the specific bleeding disorders should be treated. Acute severe bleeding can be managed with high-dose estrogen. OCs containing less than or equal to 35 mcg of ethinyl estradiol is a first-line treatment in adolescents with chronic anovulation.[49]

Drug Class Information

Table 63-3 identifies the significant pharmacologic properties that require monitoring for the agents used to treat anovulatory bleeding.

Personalized Pharmacotherapy

While not typically an issue among the relatively young population of patients treated with metformin for PCOS, one must be cognizant of the risk of lactic acidosis in metformin users with renal impairment. As such, this drug should be avoided in women with serum creatinine >1.4 mg/dL (124 μmol/L).

Evaluation of Therapeutic Outcomes

Table 63-3 lists the expected outcomes and specific monitoring parameters for the treatment modalities used to manage anovulatory bleeding.

DYSMENORRHEA

Dysmenorrhea is one of the most commonly encountered gynecologic complaints. It is defined as crampy pelvic pain occurring with or just prior to menses. Primary dysmenorrhea implies pain in the

CLINICAL PRESENTATION Dysmenorrhea

General

- Patients may or may not be in acute distress, depending on the level of menstrual pain experienced

Symptoms

- Patients complain of crampy pelvic pain beginning shortly before or at the onset of menses. Symptoms typically last from 1 to 3 days

Laboratory Tests

- Pelvic examination should be performed to screen for sexually transmitted diseases as a cause of the pain in sexually active females
- Gonorrhea, Chlamydia cultures or polymerase chain reaction, wet mount

Other Diagnostic Tests

- Pelvic ultrasound can be used to identify potential anatomic abnormalities such as masses/lesions or to detect ovarian cysts and endometriomas

setting of normal pelvic anatomy and physiology. Secondary dysmenorrhea is associated with underlying pelvic pathology.[14]

Epidemiology

Dysmenorrhea prevalence rates range from 16% to 90%.[30,31] Its presence may be associated with significant interference in work and school attendance. Risk factors include young age, heavy menses, nulliparity, early menarche, and cigarette smoking.[9,11]

Etiology

For most patients, dysmenorrhea is associated with normal ovulatory cycles and normal pelvic anatomy. This is referred to as primary, or functional, dysmenorrhea. However, in approximately 10% of the adolescents and young adults presenting with painful menses, an underlying anatomic or physiologic cause exists.[11]

Pathophysiology

The most significant mechanism for primary dysmenorrhea is the release of prostaglandins and leukotrienes into the menstrual fluid, initiating an inflammatory response and possibly vasopressin-mediated vasoconstriction.[9,11,34] Causes of secondary dysmenorrhea include cervical stenosis, endometriosis, pelvic infections, pelvic congestion syndrome, uterine or cervical polyps, uterine fibroids, genital outflow tract obstructions, and pelvic adhesions.[11,31] Pregnancy and miscarriage must be considered in new onset dysmenorrhea.

TREATMENT

Initial treatment choice is influenced by whether or not the woman desires pregnancy. Nonpharmacologic options have been studied and observed to be as effective as some existing pharmacologic options.

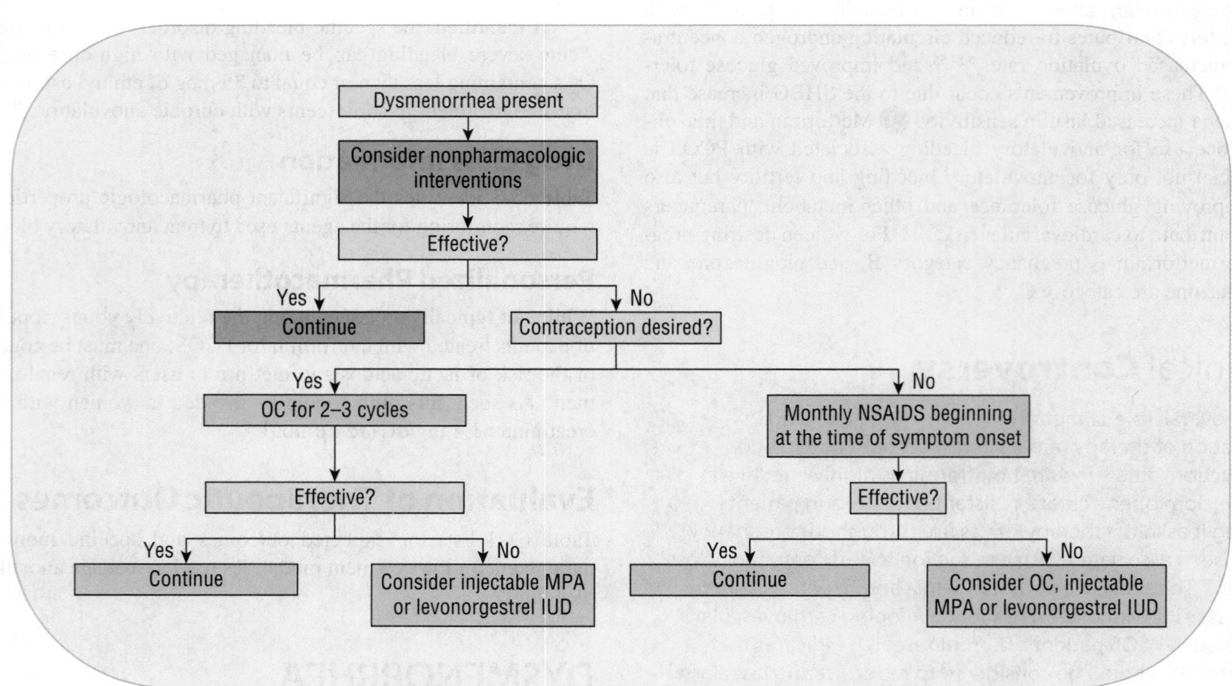

FIGURE 63-4 Treatment algorithm for dysmenorrhea. (IUD, intrauterine device; MPA, medroxyprogesterone acetate; NSAIDs, nonsteroidal antiinflammatory drugs; OC, oral contraceptive.)

Desired Outcome

Medical management of dysmenorrhea should relieve the pelvic pain and result in reducing lost school and work days. Table 63-2 identifies the agents used to manage dysmenorrhea and their recommended doses. Figure 63-4 shows a treatment algorithm for dysmenorrhea management.

General Approach to Treatment

A variety of effective treatment options for dysmenorrhea are available, including nonhormonal and hormonal pharmacologic options and noninvasive nonpharmacologic options. Treatment choice is influenced by the desire for contraception, the patient's level of sexual activity, potential for adverse effects, and cost.

Nonpharmacologic Therapy

Several nonpharmacologic interventions are used for managing dysmenorrhea. Among these, topical heat therapy, exercise, and a low-fat vegetarian diet have been shown to reduce dysmenorrhea intensity.[11,12,14,30] Dietary changes may shorten dysmenorrhea duration. Topical heat application via an abdominal patch is as effective as 400 mg of ibuprofen dosed three times daily.[58] Because topical heat, exercise, and dietary changes do not impart systemic effects, they are associated with little to no risk compared to the pharmacologic options. Nonpharmacologic options that are reserved for use following a failed trial of pharmacologic interventions include transcutaneous electric nerve stimulation, acupressure, and acupuncture.[14,30]

Pharmacologic Therapy

Given the role of prostaglandins in dysmenorrhea pathophysiology, NSAIDs are the initial treatment of choice. These agents do not differ in efficacy. The most commonly used agents are naproxen and ibuprofen.

All NSAIDs have a propensity for causing GI distress and ulceration; their administration with food or milk minimizes these effects. In women who have a history of NSAID-induced gastric effects, the use of celecoxib, a cyclo-oxygenase-2 (COX-2) inhibitor, is an alternative.[11,15] Choice of one agent over another may be based on cost, convenience, and patient preference.[14] Some research suggests that NSAID therapy should begin at the onset of menses or perhaps even the day before and continued around the clock instead of waiting until symptom onset. The data substantiating this are weak.[30] If an NSAID or celecoxib use is contraindicated or not desired, hormonal agents should be considered. Acetaminophen is inferior to NSAID in treatment of this disorder.[14,30]

OCs improve dysmenorrhea by inhibiting endometrial tissue proliferation which reduces endometrial-derived prostaglandins that cause the pelvic pain.[11,12,30] Significant improvements in mild, moderate, and severe dysmenorrhea have been noted with OCs. Evidence supporting monophasic versus multiphase OC regimens, however, is lacking. And while the use of extended-cycle OCs would be desirable for this purpose, data illustrating their superiority over traditional monthly OCs do not currently exist.

Depot MPA can be considered for dysmenorrhea treatment. Its efficacy is secondary to its ability to render most patients amenorrheic within 6 to 12 months of use.[14,30] Because the pelvic pain of dysmenorrhea is related to the prostaglandins released during menses, in the setting of amenorrhea the underlying cause of dysmenorrhea is removed.

Another progesterone product used for dysmenorrhea management is the levonorgestrel-releasing IUD. Observational data indicate its ability to reduce dysmenorrhea from 60% to 29% after 3 years of use.[11,14] As observed with depot MPA, this reduction likely is secondary to its effect in reducing menstrual flow.

Drug Treatments of First Choice

Several factors influence the choice of first-line treatment for dysmenorrhea. If contraception is desired, then a hormonal option may be considered taking into account cost, adherence issues, and side effects. If contraception is not desired, then NSAID use would be desirable from cost and convenience standpoints. If NSAIDs are not tolerated, celecoxib could be recommended. In patients for whom OCs, NSAIDs, or celecoxib is not an option, topical heat should be considered.

Special Populations

Dysmenorrhea is common in adolescent females. The treatment measures used for adult patients are also appropriate for adolescents. Although NSAIDs, topical heat, and OCs are among the top choices, use of the levonorgestrel IUD is also an option.[38]

Drug Class Information

Table 63-3 identifies the significant pharmacologic properties requiring monitoring for the agents used to treat dysmenorrhea.

Evaluation of Therapeutic Outcomes

Table 63-3 lists the expected outcomes and specific monitoring parameters for the treatment modalities used in the management of dysmenorrhea.

CLINICAL PRESENTATION PMDD

A summary of the American Psychiatric Association's criteria for PMDD is as follows[1,62]:

- Symptoms are temporally associated with the last week of the luteal phase and remit with onset of menses
- At least five of the following symptoms are present: markedly depressed mood, marked anxiety, marked affective lability, marked anger or irritability, decreased interest in activities, fatigue, difficulty concentrating, changes in appetite, sleep disturbance, feelings of being overwhelmed, and physical symptoms, such as breast tenderness or bloating
- One of the symptoms must be markedly depressed mood, anxiety, irritability, or affective lability
- Symptoms interfere significantly with work and/or social relationships
- Symptoms are not an exacerbation of another underlying psychiatric disorder
- The criteria are confirmed prospectively by daily ratings over two menstrual cycles

PREMENSTRUAL SYNDROME AND PREMENSTRUAL DYSPHORIC DISORDER

PMS is a constellation of symptoms including mild mood disturbances and physical symptoms occurring prior to menses and resolving with menses initiation. It is distinct from PMDD.

Epidemiology

Up to 75% of menstruating women experience PMS symptoms.[59] However, a spectrum of premenstrual mood disturbances exists, and PMDD is the most severe. Approximately 3% to 8% of women have PMDD.[59–61]

Etiology and Pathophysiology

PMDD is a complex psychiatric disorder with multiple biological, psychological, and sociocultural determinants.[62] Although cyclic hormonal changes are in some way related to PMS and PMDD, the association is neither linear nor simple. When ovulation is suppressed medically or surgically, symptoms improve. Some evidence suggests that PMS and PMDD symptoms are related to low levels of the centrally active progesterone metabolite allopregnanolone in the luteal phase and/or lower cortical γ-aminobutyric acid levels in the follicular phase.[62] A number of studies suggest a link between PMS and PMDD and low serotonin levels.[62] Despite similar affective symptoms, hypothalamic–pituitary–adrenal (HPA) axis function in PMS and PMDD is distinct from that seen in major depressive disorder. Specifically, women with PMS show a decrease in stimulated HPA axis response, whereas this response is increased in women with major depressive disorder.[63] Although several cross-cultural studies suggest that PMS physical symptoms are consistent across cultures, the negative affective symptoms are part of the negative "menstrual socialization" in western culture.[1,62]

TREATMENT

Women experiencing PMS and PMDD symptoms miss significantly more work and school than do controls. They also report significant impairment of their ability to participate in social activities and hobbies and in their relationships with others.[61] Given this, the need for effective treatment modalities is clear.

Desired Outcome

PMS and PMDD interventions should alleviate the presenting symptoms and subsequently improve quality of life. Table 63-2 lists the various agents used in the managing PMS and PMDD and their recommended dosing.

General Approach to Treatment

A treatment modality that is minimally invasive or without systemic effects is desired for initial therapy. Key to the successful choice of pharmacologic therapy for PMS and PMDD is having the patient chart her specific symptoms for at least 2 months.

Nonpharmacologic Therapy

Lifestyle interventions should be started and followed for 2 months while the patient charts her symptoms. Although these interventions lack significant supporting clinical trial data, anecdotal reports of efficacy exist. Some lifestyle changes for women with mild-to-moderate premenstrual symptoms include minimizing intake of caffeine, refined sugar, and sodium and increasing exercise.[22,59,64] Vitamin and mineral supplements, such as vitamin B_6 (50–100 mg daily) and calcium carbonate (1,200 mg daily), may help reduce the physical symptoms associated with PMS.[22,60] A clinical trial review concludes that the following options lack efficacy and safety data and should not be recommended: herbal medicines, homeopathic remedies, dietary supplements, relaxation, massage therapy, reflexology, chiropractic treatments, and biofeedback.[65,66]

Pharmacologic Therapy

If symptoms persist after 2 months of symptom charting and lifestyle modifications, pharmacologic therapy for PMDD management is warranted. Over the past decade, the selective serotonin reuptake inhibitors (SSRIs) have been studied significantly for this disorder.[24,67–69] Studies have revealed very positive results relative to most symptoms associated with PMDD. Other agents that have been studied and are alternatives include the selective serotonin–norepinephrine reuptake inhibitor venlafaxine, as well as OCs, tricyclic antidepressants, and GnRH agonists.

Drug Treatments of First Choice

10 The first-line pharmacologic treatment options for PMDD are the SSRIs.[22,59] Among this class of agents, data support the use of citalopram, escitalopram, fluoxetine, fluvoxamine, paroxetine, and sertraline. Whether to dose these agents continuously or only during the luteal phase[67] and the optimal duration of treatment[70] are still not evident. The use of paroxetine, in particular, may be questioned, as this agent has been associated with an increased risk of congenital abnormalities when taken during the first trimester of pregnancy.[22] Paroxetine is pregnancy category D; its use should be avoided in women of childbearing age who do not use a reliable form of contraception.

> **Clinical Controversy...**
>
> Current evidence supports SSRIs as first-line PMDD treatment, either dosed continuously or during the luteal phase alone. Some evidence suggests that SSRI dosing at symptom onset also may be effective.[71] The bulk of studies include women over age 18 and with treatment durations not longer than 3 to 6 months.[59] Contrary to the excitement surrounding luteal phase dosing, a meta-analysis found in favor of the continuous dosing regimen for efficacy.[69] Relapse rates appear to be higher with shorter-duration treatment (4 months vs. 12 months).[70] The most effective dosing strategy[67] (continuous, luteal phase, or symptom onset), most efficacious treatments in the adolescent versus perimenopausal populations, and the optimal treatment duration[70] are not evident at this time and warrant further investigation.

The SSRIs are efficacious in more than half of the treated patients compared to less than 30% of those receiving placebo.[22,68,71] A meta-analysis reports 50% or greater symptom reduction with SSRI treatment compared to baseline.[69] Improvement often occurs during the first cycle of use.[22]

Alternative Drug Treatments

The serotonin–norepinephrine reuptake inhibitor (SNRI), venlafaxine, has been studied dosed on a continuous daily basis[22,72] and dosed during the luteal phase only.[73] Both regimens resulted in significant symptom improvement (compared to placebo) in more than 60% of treated women.

The use of a monophasic OC containing 20 mcg of ethinyl estradiol and 3 mg of drospirenone, a progesterone with antiandrogenic effects, improves premenstrual symptoms in women with PMDD.[23] The continuous cycle OC regimen delivering 90 mcg of levonorgestrel and 20 mcg of ethinyl estradiol daily has also been studied in controlled trials resulting in a 30% to 59% improvement in symptoms.[74] As with the SSRI and SNRI agents, optimal treatment duration is unknown, and superiority of one OC relative to another OC has not been established.

If treatment with the above options is unsuccessful, hormonal treatment with a GnRH agonist, such as leuprolide, can be considered.[22] Leuprolide improves premenstrual emotional symptoms as well as some physical symptoms, such as bloating and breast tenderness. However, its cost, the need for intramuscular administration, and its hypoestrogenism side effects (e.g., vaginal dryness, hot flashes, and bone demineralization) severely limit its use.

Drug Class Information

Table 63-3 lists the significant pharmacologic properties that require monitoring for the agents used to treat PMDD.

Personalized Pharmacotherapy

It is important that concomitant drug therapy of women prescribed any of the SSRIs or venlafaxine be evaluated closely for pharmacokinetic drug–drug interactions given the interface of these drugs with cytochrome P450 isoenzyme systems.

Evaluation of Therapeutic Outcomes

Table 63-3 lists the expected outcomes and specific monitoring parameters for the treatment modalities used in PMDD management.

ABBREVIATIONS

COX-2 cyclo-oxygenase-2
FSH follicle-stimulating hormone
GnRH gonadotropin-releasing hormone
HPA hypothalamic–pituitary–adrenal
IUD intrauterine device
LH luteinizing hormone
MPA medroxyprogesterone acetate
NSAID nonsteroidal antiinflammatory drug
OC oral contraceptive
PCOS polycystic ovary syndrome
PMDD premenstrual dysphoric disorder
PMS premenstrual syndrome
SHBG sex hormone-binding globulin
SNRI serotonin–norepinephrine reuptake inhibitor
SSRI selective serotonin reuptake inhibitor

REFERENCES

1. Fritz MA, Speroff L. Clinical Gynecologic Endocrinology and Infertility, 8th ed. Philadelphia: Lippincott Williams & Wilkins, 2010:435–493, 591–619.
2. Lobo RA. Primary and secondary amenorrhea and precocious puberty: Etiology, diagnostic evaluation, management. In: Katz VL, ed. Comprehensive Gynecology, 5th ed. Philadelphia, PA: Mosby Elsevier, 2007:933–962.
3. Heiman DL. Amenorrhea. Prim Care Clin Office Pract 2009;36:1–17.
4. Lobo RA. Abnormal Uterine Bleeding: Ovulatory and Anovulatory Dysfunctional Uterine Bleeding, Management of Acute and Chronic Excessive Bleeding. In: Katz VL, ed. Comprehensive Gynecology, 5th ed. Philadelphia, PA: Mosby Elsevier, 2007:915–932.
5. Setji TL, Brown AJ. Polycystic ovarian syndrome: Diagnosis and treatment. Am J Med 2007;120:128–132.
6. James AH, Kouides PA, Abdul-Kadir R, et al. Von Willebrand disease and other bleeding disorders in women: Consensus on diagnosis and management from an international expert panel. Am J Obstet Gynecol 2009;201:12.e1–e8.
7. Tolaymat LL, Kaunitz AM. Use of hormonal contraception in adolescents: Skeletal health issues. Curr Opin Obstet Gynecol 2009;21(5):396–401.
8. Master-Hunter T, Heiman DL. Amenorrhea: Evaluation and treatment. Am Fam Physician 2006;73(8):1374–1382.
9. Simon JA. Progestogens in the treatment of secondary amenorrhea. J Reprod Med 1999;44(2 Suppl):185–189.
10. Lobo RA. Hyperprolactinemia, galactorrhea, and pituitary adenomas: Etiology, differential diagnosis, natural history, management. In: Katz VL, ed. Comprehensive Gynecology, 5th ed. Philadelphia, PA: Mosby Elsevier, 2007;963–978.
11. Harel Z. Dysmenorrhea in adolescents and young adults. J Pediatr Adolesc Gynecol 2006;19:363–371.
12. French L. Dysmenorrhea in adolescents—Diagnosis and treatment. Pediatr Drugs 2008;10(1):1–7.
13. Roy SN, Bhattacharya S. Benefits and risks of pharmacological agents used for the treatment of menorrhagia. Drug Safety 2004;27:75–90.
14. French L. Dysmenorrhea. Am Fam Physician 2005;71: 285–291.
15. Daniels S, Robbins J, West CR, Nemeth MA. Celecoxib in the treatment of primary dysmenorrhea: Results from two randomized, double-blind, active- and placebo-controlled, crossover studies. Clin Ther 2009;31(6):1192–1208.
16. Tasci Y, Caglar GS, Kayikcioglu F, et al. Treatment of menorrhagia with levonorgestrel releasing intrauterine system: Effects on ovarian function and uterus. Arch Gynecol Obstet 2009;280:39–42.
17. Desai RM. Efficacy of levonorgestrel releasing intrauterine system for the treatment of menorrhagia due to benign uterine lesions in perimenopausal women. J Midlife Health 2012;3(1):20–23.
18. Kaunitz AM, Meredith S, Inki P, et al. Levonorgestrel-releasing intrauterine system and endometrial ablation in heavy menstrual bleeding: A systematic review and meta-analysis. Obstet Gynecol 2009;113:1104–1116.
19. Naoulou B, Tsai MC. Efficacy of tranexamic acid in the treatment of idiopathic and non-functional heavy menstrual bleeding: A systematic review. Acta Obstet Gynecol Scand 2012;91(5):529–537.
20. Mathur R, Levin O, Azziz R. Use of ethinyl estradiol/drospirenone combination in patients with polycystic ovary syndrome. Therapeutics and clinical risk management 2008;4(2):487–492.
21. Du Q, Yang S, Wang Y, et al. Effects of thiazolidinediones on polycystic ovary syndrome: A meta-analysis of randomized placebo-controlled trials. Adv Ther 2012;29(9): 763–774.
22. Biggs WS, Demuth RH. Premenstrual syndrome and premenstrual dysphoric disorder. Am Fam Physician 2011;84(8):918–924.
23. Lopez LM, Kaptein AA, Helmerhorst FM. Oral contraceptives containing drospirenone for premenstrual syndrome. Cochrane Database Syst Rev 2012(2): CD006586. DOI: 10.1002/14651858. CD006586.pub4.

24. Eriksson E, Ekman A, Sinclair S, et al. Escitalopram administered in the luteal phase exerts a marked and dose-dependent effect in premenstrual dysphoric disorder. J Clin Psychopharmacol 2008;28(2):195–202.
25. Kvernmo T, Hartter S, Burger E. A review of the receptor-binding and pharmacokinetic properties of dopamine agonists. Clin Ther 2006;28:1065–1078.
26. Eng PM, Seeger JD, Loughlin J, et al. Serum potassium monitoring for users of ethinyl estradiol/drospirenone taking medications predisposing to hyperkalemia: Physician compliance and survey of knowledge and attitudes. Contraception 2007;75:101–107.
27. Schurmann R, Blode H, Benda N, et al. Effect of drospirenone on serum potassium and drospirenone pharmacokinetics in women with normal or impaired renal function. J Clin Pharmacol 2006;46:867–875.
28. Warner PE, Critchley HO, Lumsden MA, et al. Menorrhagia I. Measured blood loss, clinical features, and outcome in women with heavy periods: A survey with follow-up data. Am J Obstet Gynecol 2004;190:1216–1223.
29. Casablanca Y. Management of dysfunctional uterine bleeding. Obstet Gynecol Clin N Am 2008;35(2): 219–234.
30. Morrow C, Naumburg EH. Dysmenorrhea. Prim Care 2009;36(1):19–32.
31. Lentz GM. Primary and secondary dysmenorrhea, premenstrual syndrome, and premenstrual dysphoric disorder: Etiology, diagnosis, management. In: Katz VL, ed. Comprehensive Gynecology, 5th ed. Philadelpha, PA: Mosby Elsevier, 2007:900–914.
32. Warner PE, Critchley HO, Lumsden MA, et al. Menorrhagia II. Is the 80-mL blood loss criterion useful in management of complaint of menorrhagia? Am J Obstet Gynecol 2004;190:1224–1229.
33. Von Mackensen S. Quality of life in women with bleeding disorders. Haemophilia 2011;17(Suppl 1):33–37.
34. Adams Hillard PJ, Deitch HR. Menstrual disorders in the college age female. Pediatr Clin North Am 2005;52: 179–197.
35. James AH, Ragni MV, Picozzi VJ. Bleeding disorders in premenopausal women: (Another) public health crisis for hematology? Hematol Am Soc Hematol Educ Prog 2006;2006(1):474–485.
36. Battacharya S, Middleton SJ, Tsourapas A, et al. Hysterectomy, endometrial ablation and Mirena® for heavy menstrual bleeding: A systematic review of clinical effectiveness and cost effectiveness analysis. Health Technol Assess 2011;15(9):iii–xvi, 1–252.
37. The American College of Obstetricians and Gynecologists. ACOG Practice Bulletin No. 110. Noncontraceptive uses of hormonal contraceptives. Obstet Gynecol 2010;115(1): 206–219.
38. The American College of Obstetricians and Gynecologists. ACOG Practice Bulletin No. 121. Long-acting reversible contraception: Implants and intrauterine devices. Obstet Gynecol 2011;118:184–196.
39. Hurskainen R, Teperi J, Rissanen P, et al. Clinical outcomes and costs with the levonorgestrel-releasing intrauterine system or hysterectomy for treatment of menorrhagia: Randomized trial 5-year follow-up. JAMA 2004;291: 1456–1463.
40. Leminen H, Hurskainen R. Tranexamic acid for the treatment of heavy menstrual bleeding: Efficacy and safety. Int J Womens Health 2012;4:413–421.
41. Blumenthal PD, Trussell J, Singh RH, et al. Cost-effectiveness of treatments for dysfunctional uterine bleeding in women who need contraception. Contraception 2006;74:249–258.
42. Kadir RA. Menorrhagia: Treatment options. Thromb Res 2009;123(Suppl 2):S21–S29.
43. The American College of Obstetricians and Gynecologists. ACOG Practice Bulletin No. 108. Polycystic ovary syndrome. Obstet Gynecol 2009;114(4):936–949.
44. Carmina E, Azziz R. Diagnosis, phenotype and prevalence of polycystic ovary syndrome. Fertil Steril 2006;86(Suppl 1): S7–S8.
45. Azziz R, Carmina E, Dewailley D, et al. Task force on the phenotype of the polycystic ovary syndrome of the androgen excess and PCOS society criteria for the polycystic ovary syndrome: The complete task force report. Fertil Steril 2009;91:456–488.
46. Azziz R, Carmina E, Dewailley D, et al. Position statement: Criteria for defining polycystic ovarian syndrome: An Androgen Excess Society Guideline. J Clin Endocrinol Metab 2006;91:4237–4245.
47. Costello MF, Shrestha B, Eden J, et al. Metformin versus oral contraceptive pills in polycystic ovary syndrome: A Cochran review. Hum Reprod 2007;22(5):1200–1209.
48. Matytsina LA, Zoloto EV, Sinenko LV, et al. Dysfunctional uterine bleeding in adolescents: Concept of pathophysiology and management. Prim Care 2006;33:503–515.
49. Sweet MG, Schmidt-Dalton TA, Weiss PM, Madsen KP. Evaluation and management of abnormal uterine bleeding in premenopausal women. Am Fam Phys 2012;85(1):35–43.
50. Harmanci A, Cinar N, Bayraktar M, Yildiz BO. Oral contraceptive plus antiandrogen therapy and cardiometabolic risk in polycystic ovary syndrome. Clin Endocrinol 2013;78:120–125.
51. Gode F, Karagoz C, Posaci C, et al. Alteration of cardiovascular risk parameters in women with polycystic ovary syndrome who were prescribed ethinyl estradiol-cyproterone acetate. Arch Gynecol Obstet 2011;284:923–929.
52. Beller JP, McCartney CR. Cardiovascular risk and combined oral contraceptives: Clinical decisions in settings of uncertainty. Am J Obstet Gynecol 2013;208(1):39–41.
53. Ely JW, Kennedy CM, Clark EC, et al. Abnormal uterine bleeding: A management algorithm. J Am Board Fam Med 2006;19:590–602.
54. Palomba S, Pasquali R, Orio F, Nestler JE. Clomiphene citrate, metformin or both as first-step approaches in treating anovulatory infertile patients with polycystic ovary syndrome (PCOS): A systematic review of head-to-head randomized controlled studies and meta-analysis. Clin Endocrinol 2009;70(2):311–321.
55. Siebert TI, Kruger TF, Steyn DW, et al. Is the addition of metformin efficacious in the treatment of clomiphene citrate-resistant patients with polycystic ovary syndrome? A structured literature review. Fertil Steril 2006;86:1432–1437.
56. Banaszewska B, Duleba AJ, Spaczynski RZ, et al. Lipids in polycystic ovary syndrome: Role of hyperinsulinemia and effects of metformin. Am J Obstet Gynecol 2006;194: 1266–1272.
57. Khattab S, Mohsen IA, Foutouh IA, et al. Metformin reduces abortion in pregnant women with polycystic ovary syndrome. Gynecol Endocrinol 2006;22:680–684.
58. Navvabi-Rigi S, Kermansaravi F, Navidian A, et al. Comparing the analgesic effect of heat patch containing iron chip and ibuprofen for primary dysmenorrhea: A randomized clinical trial. BMC Women's Health 2012;12:25–31.
59. Steiner M, Pearlstein T, Cohen LS, et al. Expert guidelines for the treatment of severe PMS, PMDD, and comorbidities: The role of SSRIs. J Womens Health 2006;15:57–69.

60. Yonkers KA, O'Brien PMS, Eriksson E. Premenstrual syndrome. Lancet 2008;371:1200–1210.
61. Dennerstein L, Lehert P, Heinemann K. Epidemiology of premenstrual symptoms and disorders. Menopause Int 2012;18(2):48–51.
62. Matsumoto T, Asakura H, Hayashi T. Biopsychosocial aspects of premenstrual syndrome and premenstrual dysphoric disorder. Gynecol Endocrinol 2013;29(1): 67–73.
63. Roca CA, Schmidt PJ, Altemus M, et al. Differential menstrual cycle regulation of hypothalamic–pituitary–adrenal axis in women with premenstrual syndrome and controls. J Clin Endocrinol Metab 2003;88:3057–3063.
64. Jarvis CI, Lynch AM, Morin AK. Management strategies for premenstrual syndrome/premenstrual dysphoric disorder. Ann Pharmacother 2008;42:967–978.
65. Deligiannidis KM, Freeman MP. Complementary and alternative medicine for the treatment of depressive disorders in women. Psychiatr Clin North Am 2010;33(2):441–463.
66. Dante G, Facchinetti F. Herbal treatments for alleviating premenstrual symptoms: A systematic review. J Psychosom Obstet Gynecol 2011;32(10):42–51.
67. Steiner M, Ravindran AV, LeMelledo JM, et al. Luteal phase administration of paroxetine for the treatment of premenstrual dysphoric disorder: A randomized, double-blind, placebo-controlled trial in Canadian women. J Clin Psychiatry 2008;69(6):991–998.
68. Yonkers KA, Holthausen GA, Poschman K, et al. Symptom-onset treatment for women with premenstrual dysphoric disorder. J Clin Psychopharmacol 2006;26:198–202.
69. Shah NR, Jones JB, Aperi J, et al. Selective serotonin reuptake inhibitors for premenstrual syndrome and premenstrual dysphoric disorder—A meta-analysis. Obstet Gynecol 2008;111:1175–1182.
70. Freeman EW, Rickels K, Sammel MD, et al. Time to relapse after short- or long-term treatment of severe premenstrual syndrome with sertraline. Arch Gen Psychiatry 2009;66(5):537–544.
71. Kornstein SG, Pearlstein TB, Fayyad R, et al. Low-dose sertraline in the treatment of moderate-to-severe premenstrual syndrome: Efficacy of 3, dosing strategies. J Clin Psychiatry 2006;67:124–132.
72. Freeman EW, Rickels K, Yonkers KA, et al. Venlafaxine in the treatment of premenstrual dysphoric disorder. Obstet Gynecol 2001;98(5 Pt 1):737–744.
73. Cohen LS, Soares CN, Lyster A, et al. Efficacy and tolerability of premenstrual use of venlafaxine (flexible dose) in the treatment of premenstrual dysphoric disorder. J Clin Psychopharmacol 2004;24:540–543.
74. Freeman EW, Hallbreich U, Grubb GS, et al. An overview of four studies of a continuous oral contraceptive (levonorgestrel 90 mcg/ethinyl estradiol 20 mcg) on premenstrual dysphporic disorder and premenstrual syndrome. Contraception 2012;85(5):437–445.

64

Endometriosis

Deborah A. Sturpe and Kathleen J. Pincus

KEY CONCEPTS

1. Endometriosis should be suspected in any woman of reproductive age with recurring cyclic or acyclic pelvic pain and/or subfertility, especially if pain does not improve with nonsteroidal antiinflammatory drugs and hormonal contraceptives.
2. The etiology of endometriosis is likely multifactorial and requires a genetic or immunologic predisposition. Retrograde menstruation is the most widely accepted theory to account for displacement of endometrial tissue, although alternative theories have been proposed.
3. Treatment goals include improvement of painful symptoms and maintenance or improvement of fertility. Therapy is considered successful based on resolution of the patient's symptoms or achievement of pregnancy.
4. Both drug therapy and surgery may treat endometriosis-related pain, but infertility can only be treated with surgery or assisted reproductive techniques.
5. No medical therapy has been proven to be more effective than another; thus, the choice among agents is determined primarily by side effect profile, cost, and individual patient response.
6. For endometriosis pain, surgical therapy is typically reserved for medical therapy failure.
7. Diagnosis of endometriosis can be made only via surgical visualization of lesions, not by physical examination or laboratory testing. Empiric treatment without confirmation of diagnosis is acceptable in most cases.
8. To help avoid loss of bone mineral density, add-back therapy should be strongly considered in any woman receiving a gonadotropin-releasing hormone agonist.

INTRODUCTION

❶ Endometriosis causes secondary dysmenorrhea and is associated with infertility. Presence of endometrial tissue outside the uterus is chronic and relapsing. Endometriosis treatment targets pain relief and fertility improvement.

EPIDEMIOLOGY

The prevalence of endometriosis is estimated at 5% to 10% of the general female population.[1–4] Four percent of premenopausal women presenting to primary care for nongynecologic problems have endometriosis, and up to 80% of adult women and 50% of adolescents with chronic pelvic pain are diagnosed with the disorder.[1,4–8] The incidence is 10-fold higher in women with infertility (20% to 50%) compared with that in fertile women (0.5% to 5%).[1,4–7,9] A genetic predisposition for endometriosis has also been noted.[2]

ETIOLOGY

Endometriosis is characterized by findings of endometrial tissue outside of the normal uterine cavity. It may be diagnosed at any age, but is most commonly found during the reproductive years (range 12 to 80 years old, average 28 years).[1,7] Risk of developing endometriosis increases with early menarche (≤11 years), shorter menstrual cycles (<27 days), and heavy, prolonged menstruation.[4,7] Taller, thinner women are more likely to develop endometriosis than patients with higher body weights, body mass indexes, or waist-to-hip ratios potentially due to higher follicular-phase estradiol levels.[7] Altered pelvic anatomy, such as Müllerian duct anomalies and cervical or vaginal outlet obstruction, also increases risk of developing endometriosis, as does in utero exposure to environmental toxins or potent estrogens.[2,3,7] Conversely, higher parity, increased duration of lactation, regular exercise (>4 h/wk), greater birth weight, and breast-feeding decrease the risk of endometriosis.[4,7]

Gene mutation studies suggest genes regulating inflammation, sex steroid regulation, metabolism, biosynthesis, detoxification, vascular function, and tissue remodeling may contribute to endometriosis, but no validated associations have been confirmed.[10] Alterations on chromosomes 7 and 10 have been identified in clusters of women with endometriosis.[2] It is most likely that a multitude of genetic mutations are involved with the development of endometriosis.

PATHOPHYSIOLOGY

❷ Multiple theories exist to explain why endometrial tissue is present outside the uterine cavity, and the true pathophysiology is likely multifactorial.[1–3,5] The most widely accepted theory proposes that endometrial tissue is deposited in the peritoneal cavity by retrograde menstruation through the fallopian tubes.[3] However, retrograde menstruation occurs in up to 90% of women while only 10% to 15% develop endometriosis, indicating that additional factors are necessary for endometrial lesions to attach, survive, and proliferate.[1,2,4] Alternative theories include the inappropriate differentiation of mesothelial cells into endometrium-like tissue (coelomic metaplasia), the differentiation of stem cells from either bone marrow or the endometrial basalis layer into endometrial-like tissues (stem cell theory), and the spread of menstrual tissue to distant sites through veins or lymphatic vessels (lymphatic or hematogenous spread).[2,3]

Endometriosis is a chronic inflammatory disorder that exhibits cellular proliferation, cellular invasion, and angiogenesis not unlike

CLINICAL PRESENTATION

Symptoms

- Most common are dysmenorrhea and infertility.
- Other symptoms include dyspareunia, menorrhagia, chronic pelvic pain (cyclic or acyclic), ovulation pain, sacral back pain, cyclic or perimenstrual bowel and bladder complaints (e.g., GI disturbances, painful defecation, tenesmus dysuria, and/or hematuria), chronic fatigue, or rarely neuropathic pain.
- Some patients may be asymptomatic.

Signs

- Findings on physical examination are best observed during menstruation and may include pelvic tenderness, tender uterosacral ligaments, enlarged ovaries, pelvic masses or nodules, or a fixed, retroverted uterus.
- Findings on laparoscopic examination may range from a few small lesions located on the ovaries, serosal surfaces, or peritoneum to large cysts called endometriomas. Lesions are often described as: "powder burn" or "gunshot" lesions; dark brown, black, or blue lesions, nodules, and cysts; and "chocolate cysts" (endometriomas containing blood).

Diagnosis

- Definitive diagnosis can be made only by direct surgical visualization of endometrial lesions; however, treatment guidelines allow for nondefinitive diagnosis in patients presenting with chronic pelvic pain provided that other causes of pain are ruled out and that pain responds to empiric therapies.
- Ultrasonography, magnetic resonance imaging, and computed tomography have much lower sensitivity for endometrial lesions, but have utility in assessing for pelvic or adnexal masses.

Disease Staging

- Severity of disease can be classified according to the American Society of Reproductive Medicine staging system (stage I [mild] to stage IV [severe]), but clinical utility of this staging system is limited because findings do not correlate with painful symptoms, nor does the staging system predict pregnancy rates. Staging may be useful in guiding decisions regarding prognosis and treatment for infertility.

Data from references 4 and 20.

solid tumor malignancies.[11] Genetic alterations may predispose endometrial lesion survival in certain women, and immunologic abnormalities may decrease the clearance of displaced endometrial tissue.[1,2,4] Findings of abnormal B- and T-cell function, decreased apoptosis, and altered levels of prostanoids, cytokines, growth factors, interleukins, and aromatase in endometrial lesions and peritoneal fluid of affected women support this theory.[1,2,12]

Pain associated with endometriosis results from increased concentrations of inflammatory markers, including prostaglandins, and increased nerve density at lesion sites. Proinflammatory cytokines found in endometrial lesions, including tumor necrosis factor-α and interleukins 1, 6, and 8, promote lesion formation, adhesion, and infiltration and induce pain through pelvic nerve stimulation.[2,4] Prostaglandin $F_{2\alpha}$ induces vasoconstriction and can cause uterine contractions, a component of dysmenorrhea, while prostaglandin E_2 can induce pain through direct actions on nerves.[2] Increased density of sensory, cholinergic, and adrenergic nerves and an overexpression of nerve growth factors near lesions in endometrial tissue also cause pain.[3] Researchers have demonstrated that these nerve fibers are found significantly more often in patients with endometriosis than in those without endometriosis, in greater density in patients with higher pain scores (≥3 vs. ≤20), and in greater density in patients with deep infiltrating lesions.[11,13–15] The interplay between increased density of nerve fibers in endometrial lesions and increased concentrations of cytokines and prostaglandins in peritoneal fluid combines to confer significant pelvic pain in many patients.

The pathophysiology for infertility in endometriosis is less well defined, especially in mild disease. In advanced endometriosis, inflammation and anatomic abnormalities such as ovarian cysts and adhesions may physically block fallopian tubes and decrease receptivity of the endometrium, thus hindering oocyte and embryo development.[2,4] The same inflammatory cytokines that lead to pain also create a hostile peritoneal environment leading to damage of sperm DNA and cell membranes.[16] Hormonal dysregulation resulting from the disease also leads to decreased ovarian reserve, altered follicular morphology, oocyte dysfunction, and decreased efficacy of fertility treatments.[17]

TREATMENT

Endometriosis is a chronic, relapsing disease. Lifelong treatment plans must consider individual patient symptoms, goals for fertility, and impact on quality of life.[18] Various organizations, including the American Congress of Obstetricians and Gynecologists, the American Society for Reproductive Medicine, the Society of Obstetricians and Gynaecologists of Canada, and the European Society of Human Reproduction and Embryology, have published recent evidence-based and/or expert opinion-based guidelines for treating endometriosis.[4,6,18–20] These guidelines should be used to help inform treatment choice.

Desired Outcomes

Identification of endometriosis treatment goals depends on individual patient presentation and needs. 3 4 Typical outcomes include minimization of associated pain, improved quality of life, and correction of associated infertility. The first two outcomes can often be achieved through use of pharmacologic therapy and surgery.[4,6,18] Infertility is nonresponsive to medical therapies; thus, surgical intervention to remove endometrial lesions coupled with various assisted reproductive techniques must be employed.[4,19] Even with such efforts, not all women with endometriosis will be able to conceive, and exact success rates are unknown due to a paucity of well-designed clinical studies.

General Approach to Treatment

Treatment of the asymptomatic patient consists of expectant management (watchful waiting). For symptomatic patients, the foundation of therapy includes medical treatment, surgical treatment, or both. To date, no studies have directly compared medical and surgical treatment as first-line therapy. Furthermore, determining the optimal medical or surgical approach is difficult secondary to a paucity of well-designed, randomized controlled trials comparing options. 5 All commonly prescribed medical therapies relieve endometriosis-related pain by regressing lesions via induction of a pseudopregnancy or pseudomenopausal state, but medications do not eradicate lesions or improve fertility. The choice of initial therapy depends on factors such as the patient's primary complaint, the location and extent of disease, desire for future fertility, cost of therapy, contraindications to therapy, and potential side effects.[4,6,18,20] Information regarding drugs commonly prescribed for endometriosis, their dosing, side effects, and special monitoring parameters are listed in Tables 64-1 and 64-2. No endometriosis treatments are guaranteed to provide full relief of symptoms; consequently, analgesics such as nonsteroidal antiinflammatory drugs or opioids are often used as adjunctive therapy for pain relief.

Nonpharmacologic Therapy

Surgery, generally performed via laparoscopy, is used in endometriosis as both a diagnostic and a therapeutic tool.[19,20] 4 6 Due to lack of data supporting superiority of surgery over medical therapies in relieving endometriosis pain, surgical therapy is typically reserved for patients experiencing medication failure or who suffer from infertility. Women with continuing pain symptoms who do not desire pregnancy may be offered the option of hysterectomy with or without oophorectomy. In one long-term followup study conducted at the Cleveland Clinic, surgery-free rates 7 years after initial

TABLE 64-1 Dosing of Drugs Used in Treatment of Endometriosis

Drug	Brand Name	Initial Dose	Usual Range	Other
Combined Hormonal Contraceptives				
Combined oral contraceptive pill	Various (see Chap. 62)	One pill orally daily	One pill orally daily	Continuous dosing may improve efficacy
Etonogestrel/ethinyl estradiol (vaginal ring)	NuvaRing	Insert one ring monthly	Insert one ring monthly	Continuous dosing may improve efficacy
Norelgestromin/ethinyl estradiol (transdermal)	Ortho Evra	Apply one patch weekly	Apply one patch weekly	Continuous dosing may improve efficacy
Progestins				
Depot medroxyprogesterone (IM or Sub-Q)	Depo-Provera Depo-SubQ Provera	150 mg IM every 13 weeks 104 mg Sub-Q every 12–14 weeks	150 mg IM every 13 weeks 104 mg Sub-Q every 12–14 weeks	
Dienogest	Visanne	2 mg orally daily	2 mg orally daily	Not available in the United States
Levonorgestrel intrauterine system	Mirena	Single insertion for up to 5 years	Single insertion for up to 5 years	
Norethindrone	Aygestin	5 mg orally daily	Titrate as needed to maximum dose 20 mg orally daily	
Gonadotropin-releasing Hormone Agonists				
Goserelin	Zoladex	3.6 mg monthly Sub-Q implant	3.6 mg monthly Sub-Q implant	Use add-back therapy
Leuprolide	Lupron Depot	3.75 mg IM monthly or 11.25 mg IM every 3 months	3.75 mg IM monthly or 11.25 mg IM every 3 months	Use add-back therapy
Nafarelin	Synarel	400 mcg intranasally daily, dosed as one spray in one nostril AM and one spray in opposite nostril PM	May titrate to maximum 800 mcg intranasally daily, dosed as one spray in each nostril twice daily	Use add-back therapy
Triptorelin	Trelstar Depot	3.75 mg IM monthly	3.75 mg IM monthly	Use add-back therapy. Not FDA approved for endometriosis
Androgens				
Danazol	Danocrine	100–200 mg orally twice daily	Titrate as needed to maximum 400 mg orally twice daily	
Aromatase Inhibitors				
Anastrozole	Arimidex	1 mg orally daily	1 mg orally daily	Not FDA approved for endometriosis Consider add-back therapy
Letrozole	Femara	2.5 mg orally daily	2.5 mg orally daily	Not FDA approved for endometriosis Consider add-back therapy

IM, intramuscular; Sub-Q, subcutaneous.

TABLE 64-2 Monitoring Drug Therapy for Endometriosis

Drug	Adverse Drug Reactions	Monitoring Parameters	Comments
Combined oral contraceptive pills	Nausea, vomiting, breast tenderness, weight gain, acne, oily skin, depression, fatigue, breakthrough bleeding or spotting, elevated blood pressure	Blood pressure within 3 months of starting new method	Many symptoms improve after two to three cycles of use
Etonogestrel/ethinyl estradiol (vaginal ring)	Nausea, vomiting, breast tenderness, weight gain, acne, oily skin, depression, fatigue, breakthrough bleeding or spotting, vaginal irritation, elevated blood pressure	Blood pressure within 3 months of starting new method	Many symptoms improve after two to three cycles of use
Norelgestromin/ethinyl estradiol (transdermal)	Nausea, vomiting, breast tenderness, weight gain, acne, oily skin, depression, fatigue, breakthrough bleeding or spotting, application site reaction, elevated blood pressure	Blood pressure within 3 months of starting new method	Many symptoms improve after two to three cycles of use
Depot medroxyprogesterone (IM or Sub-Q)	Menstrual irregularities, weight gain, acne, hirsutism, depression, decreased bone mineral density	None	Bone mineral density testing specifically not recommended at this time
Levonorgestrel intrauterine system	Menstrual irregularities, insertion-related complications, expulsion, pelvic inflammatory disease	None	Counsel on sexually transmitted infection prevention
Norethindrone	Breast tenderness, nausea, peripheral edema Venous thromboembolism	None	
Goserelin	Acne, depression, hot flashes, mood swings, peripheral edema, vaginitis Bone mineral density loss	May consider bone mineral density testing every 1–2 years and serum lipid levels every 6 months if treatment extended beyond 12 months	Add-back therapy prevents many adverse reactions
Leuprolide	Acne, depression, dizziness, headache, hot flashes, mood swings, nausea/vomiting, triglyceride elevation, vaginitis Anaphylaxis, bone mineral density loss, venous thromboembolism	May consider bone mineral density testing every 1–2 years and serum lipid levels every 6 months if treatment extended beyond 12 months	Add-back therapy prevents many adverse reactions
Nafarelin	Acne, headache, hot flashes, mood swings, vaginal dryness Bone mineral density loss, venous thromboembolism	May consider bone mineral density testing every 1–2 years and serum lipid levels every 6 months if treatment extended beyond 12 months	Add-back therapy prevents many adverse reactions
Triptorelin	Headache, high blood pressure, hot flashes Anaphylaxis, angioedema	May consider bone mineral density testing every 1–2 years and serum lipid levels every 6 months if treatment extended beyond 12 months	Add-back therapy prevents many adverse reactions
Danazol	Acne, peripheral edema, hirsutism, lipid abnormalities, weight gain Hepatic dysfunction	Liver function tests and serum cholesterol every 3–6 months	
Anastrozole	Arthralgias, hot flashes, myalgias Decreased bone mineral density	May consider bone mineral density testing every 1–2 years if treatment extended beyond 12 months	Limited adverse reaction data in premenopausal women with endometriosis
Letrozole	Arthralgias, hot flashes, myalgias Decreased bone mineral density	May consider bone mineral density testing every 1–2 years if treatment extended beyond 12 months	Limited adverse reaction data in premenopausal women with endometriosis

surgery were lower with laparotomy alone versus hysterectomy (45.7% vs. 84.6% surgery free).[21] In both groups, ovary removal did not improve surgery-free rates regardless of baseline ovarian disease involvement.[21]

Clinical **Controversy. . .**

The optimal use of medical therapy after laparoscopy or hysterectomy remains ill-defined. It is known that pain recurrence after surgery is high, yet the optimal dose and duration for postoperative medications are unknown. Some experts advocate avoidance of drug therapy unless pain symptoms recur, while others recommend immediate use of medications in order to extend the pain-free interval. Medications studied for these indications include combined oral contraceptives (both continuous and cyclic dosing), GnRH agonists, and the levonorgestrel intrauterine system.

Other nonpharmacologic methods that have been investigated in the treatment of endometriosis pain include acupuncture and dietary therapy, but data for both are sparse.

Effectiveness of acupuncture has been investigated in a small, crossover study that compared targeted site acupuncture (treatment arm that was specific for the pelvic region) with nontargeted acupuncture (control arm that was for generalized pain conditions).[22] Despite the inclusion of this potentially effective control arm, a significant decrease in endometriosis pain was noted by all patients when receiving the targeted site acupuncture as compared with nontargeted treatments.

Interest in using dietary therapy to treat endometriosis stems from the observation that supplements may be able to modify some of the inflammatory processes that lead to dysmenorrhea.[23] In a randomized, placebo-controlled trial, women with severe endometriosis were randomized to 6 months of postsurgical treatment with one of the following three treatments: hormone therapy (combined oral contraceptive or gonadotropin-releasing hormone [GnRH] agonist); dietary therapy consisting of vitamins (B_6, A, C, E), mineral salts (calcium, magnesium, selenium, zinc, and iron), lactic ferments, and omega-3 and omega-6 fatty acids; or placebo.[24] Results revealed statistically significant decreases in dysmenorrhea and nonmenstrual pelvic pain in all active groups compared with placebo. Although the results of this study must still be confirmed by additional research, the relative safety of such dietary supplementation makes its use intriguing.

Pharmacologic Therapy

6 Pharmacologic therapy is typically the first choice for treatment of endometriosis-related pain to minimize risks from multiple surgeries such as scarring and tissue adhesions (see Fig. 64-1).

Drug Treatments of First Choice

First-line therapy for endometriosis-associated pain includes oral, transdermal, or vaginal combined hormonal contraception (CHC) or progestins (norethindrone or depot medroxyprogesterone) since both drug classes are as effective as, but less costly and toxic than, other pharmacologic options.[4,6,18,20] Choice among these agents depends on patient characteristics such as the desire for contraception, pain patterns, and contraindications as no direct comparisons are available in the literature. Long-term maintenance therapy with these agents should be considered for women achieving a good therapeutic response.[4] 7 These drugs may be used empirically for suspected endometriosis prior to laparoscopy in patients of any age.[4,6,18,20]

Alternative Drug Treatments

Patients whose endometriosis pain does not respond to CHCs or progestins may next be empirically treated with GnRH agonists or the levonorgestrel intrauterine system provided the patient is older than 16 years.[4,18,20,25] 7 Selection is again driven primarily by side effect profile, available dosage forms, and medication costs, since no method has been proven superior to another.[4,6,18] Unlike the first-line agents, the safety of long-term use of these options is unknown. Most clinical trials have only examined use of GnRH agonists for up to 6 months duration, yet recurrence of painful symptoms after drug cessation is high, thus necessitating off-label extended treatment or retreatment.[1,6] One of the biggest concerns with such extension of therapy is bone mineral density loss, but add-back therapy with a progestin and/or estrogen and progestin combination minimizes this loss along with mitigation of other bothersome side effects.[26] 8 Consequently, practice guidelines now recommend use of add-back therapy on immediate initiation of GnRH agonist treatments.[4,18]

Pharmacologic options for endometriosis pain refractory to the aforementioned drug and nondrug methods include danazol or the aromatase inhibitors. Danazol was once the mainstay of endometriosis treatment, but its side effect profile has caused the drug to fall out of favor for most clinicians.[4,6,18] Data on use of aromatase inhibitors for endometriosis pain are still sparse enough that these medications are not yet recommended within practice guidelines, but this class of medications is often the focus of current research efforts.

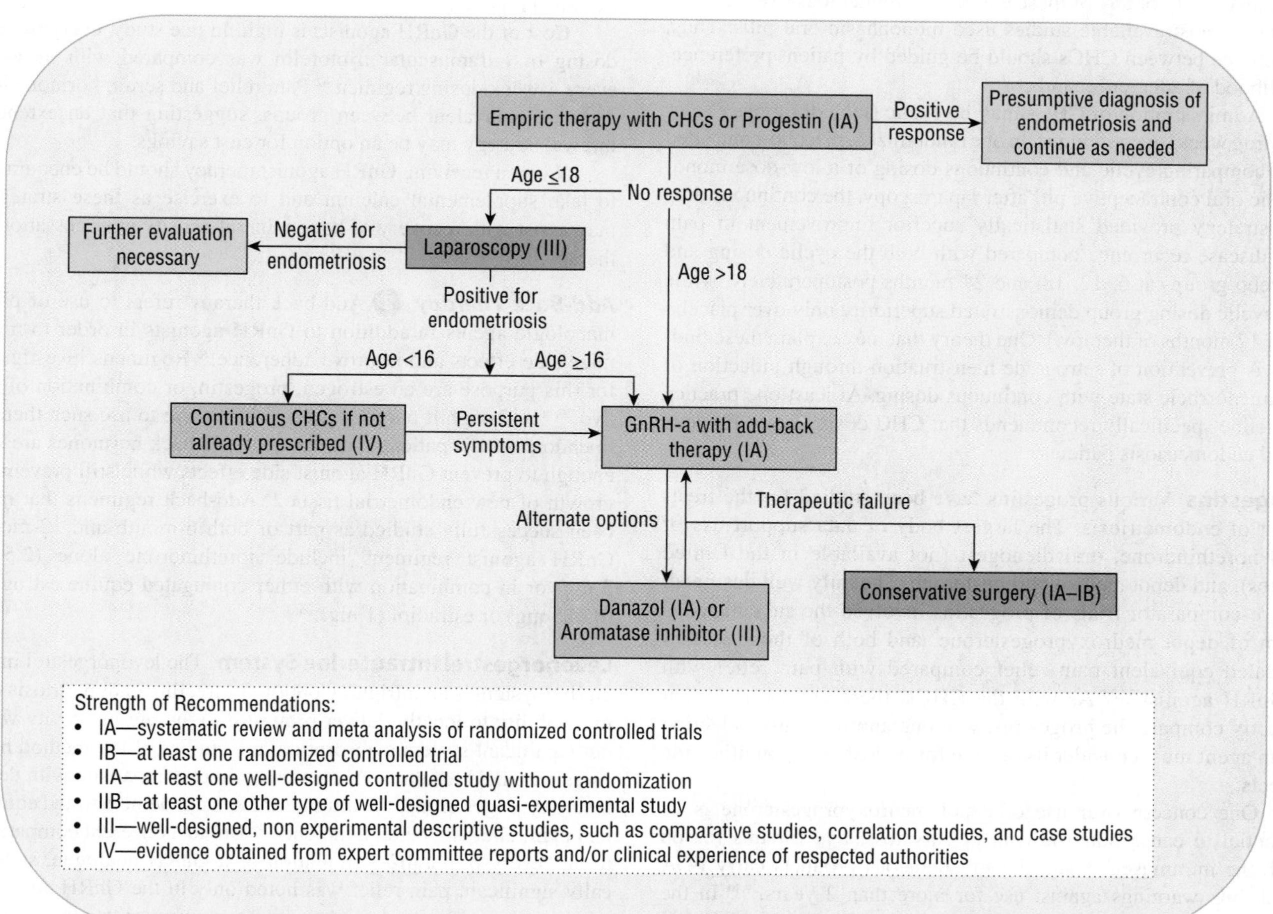

FIGURE 64-1 Treatment algorithm for chronic pelvic pain and suspected endometriosis. (CHC, combined hormonal contraceptive; GnRH-a, gonadotropin-releasing hormone agonist.) *(Data from references 4, 6, 18, and 20.)*

Special Populations

Treatment of the adolescent patient with endometriosis presents a unique challenge, as these patients often present with normal physical findings and laparoscopic findings that are atypical for endometriosis; thus, endometriosis must be strongly suspected in any patient whose dysmenorrhea fails to respond to first-line agents.[18] Treatment algorithms for such patients are extrapolated from adult recommendations and expert opinion, but generally follow the same recommendations as for adult patients.[18,25] Pertinent differences include less aggressive use of GnRH agonist therapy prior to laparoscopy in patients younger than age 18 and avoidance (if possible) of this medication class in patients younger than age 16 due to concerns over the potential long-term detrimental effects of bone loss.[18,25] Despite these limitations, early recognition and treatment of endometriosis in the adolescent population may be critical for maintenance of quality of life in this age group.[27]

Drug Class Information

No single drug therapy has been shown to be superior to another for the treatment of endometriosis pain. Therefore, the choice of drug between and within classes is often dependent on patient factors and clinician experience.

Combined Hormonal Contraception Effectiveness of oral CHCs in treating endometriosis pain has been demonstrated in numerous observational, placebo-controlled, and active-comparator trials.[28–34] More recently, effectiveness of the CHC patch and vaginal ring has also been demonstrated.[35] There is no evidence to suggest superiority of any of these contraceptive methods over another, although most available studies used monophasic oral pills. Thus, the choice between CHCs should be guided by patient preference, likelihood of adherence, and cost.

Administration of CHCs may be cyclic (includes a placebo or nondrug week) or continuous. In one randomized, placebo-controlled trial comparing cyclic and continuous dosing of a low-dose monophasic oral contraceptive pill after laparoscopy, the continuous dosing strategy provided statistically superior improvement in pain and disease recurrence compared with both the cyclic dosing and placebo groups at 6, 12, 18, and 24 months postoperatively, while the cyclic dosing group demonstrated superiority only over placebo after 12 months of therapy.[36] One theory that may explain these findings is prevention of retrograde menstruation through induction of an amenorrheic state with continuous dosing. At least one practice guideline specifically recommends that CHC dosing be continuous in all endometriosis patients.[18]

Progestins Various progestins have been studied for the treatment of endometriosis. The largest body of data support use of oral norethindrone, oral dienogest (not available in the United States), and depot medroxyprogesterone. The only well designed, active-comparator trials of progestins involved the subcutaneous form of depot medroxyprogesterone, and both of those studies revealed equivalent pain relief compared with pain relief with a GnRH agonist.[37,38] As with the CHCs, there are no trials that directly compare the progestins with one another; thus, selection of an agent must consider its dosage form, cost, and potential side effects.

One concern over use of depot medroxyprogesterone is its potential to cause bone mineral density loss, and for this reason both the intramuscular and the subcutaneous products carry FDA black box warnings against use for more than 2 years.[39,40] In the two comparator studies of depot medroxyprogesterone and GnRH agonist, the extent and degree of bone loss was less severe with the progestin.[37,38] One limitation to these findings, however, is that add-back therapy was not used with the GnRH agonist. Prolonged delays in return to ovulation after cessation of therapy is also concerning; thus, depot medroxyprogesterone may not be optimal for use in women desiring future pregnancy.[18]

Gonadotropin-Releasing Hormone Agonists GnRH agonists create a functional oophorectomy via inhibition of follicle-stimulating hormone and luteinizing hormone secretion. When first initiated, GnRH agonists create a gonadotropin flare prior to receptor downregulation that may cause a temporary increase in pain. Initiating therapy during the mid-luteal phase may minimize such effects, and use of analgesics during this time frame is also critical. Of the four agents available for use in the United States (goserelin, leuprolide, nafarelin, and triptorelin), route of administration and cost is the primary distinguishing factor that determines choice of drug.

Pain relief with GnRH agonists is superior to placebo and comparable to other therapies such as danazol, CHCs, depot medroxyprogesterone, and intrauterine progestins.[41] Although typically used for only a 6-month treatment duration, recurrence of pain is high after cessation of therapy.[6] Thus, therapy may be extended beyond 6 months to maintain efficacy, although data regarding such extended usage are limited.

Side effects are the primary limitation of GnRH agonist use. The pharmacologically induced hypoestrogenic environment results in bone mineral density loss and vasomotor symptoms such as hot flashes, vaginal dryness, and insomnia. Loss of bone mineral density is estimated at 4% to 6% over a 6-month treatment course, but this loss is partially to fully recoverable on cessation of the drug.[1] Extended use up to 12 months duration results in continuing and progressive loss that is not fully reversed on drug cessation; thus, add-back therapy is especially critical when these drugs are used as extended regimens.[26]

Cost of the GnRH agonists is high. In one study, every 6-week dosing of intramuscular triptorelin was compared with its usual every 4-week dosing regimen.[42] Pain relief and serum hormone levels were equivalent between groups, suggesting that an extended interval strategy may be an option for cost savings.

Women receiving GnRH agonist therapy should be encouraged to take supplemental calcium and to exercise as these strategies may assist with recovery of bone mineral density after cessation of therapy.[43]

Add-Back Therapy (8) Add-back therapy refers to use of pharmacologic agents in addition to GnRH agonists in order to minimize side effects and improve adherence.[26] Regimens investigated for this purpose are an estrogen, progestin, or combination of the two.[26,44] Although it may seem counterintuitive to use such therapy in endometriosis patients, the doses of add-back hormones are low enough to prevent GnRH agonist side effects while still preventing growth of new endometrial tissue.[18] Add-back regimens that have been successfully studied as part of both 6-month and 12-month GnRH agonist regimens include norethindrone alone (2.5 to 5 mg) or in combination with either conjugated equine estrogens (0.625 mg) or estradiol (1 mg).[26]

Levonorgestrel Intrauterine System The levonorgestrel intrauterine system is an intriguing option for treating endometriosis due to its ability to locally deliver progestin to the uterine cavity without significant systemic absorption, but studies of the method have revealed mixed results.[45–48] In a small, direct comparison with depot medroxyprogesterone, the intrauterine system demonstrated equivalent pain relief and better adherence.[46] But in a different comparison to an "every 6-month" formulation of a GnRH analogue, statistically significant pain relief was noted only in the GnRH analogue group, and intrauterine system users reported lower satisfaction with treatment.[47]

Disadvantages of the levonorgestrel intrauterine system include potential difficulty of inserting the device into nulliparous women, a

5% expulsion rate, and the potential for growth of ovarian endometriomas since the method does not inhibit ovulation.[18]

Danazol Danazol has been shown to be effective both empirically and after surgery compared with placebo.[49] Formerly the "gold standard" of endometriosis treatment, the popularity of danazol has decreased with the development of agents with more favorable side effect profiles. Danazol should not be initiated in women with hyperlipidemia or liver disease. It is teratogenic; thus, barrier forms of contraception must be used.

In an effort to diminish the high rate of androgenic side effects noted with danazol while maintaining effectiveness, vaginal danazol formulations (100 to 200 mg/day) have been investigated in three small studies.[50–52] Each study was a nonrandomized, prospective trial in women who had failed other therapies such as surgery, GnRH agonists, and the levonorgestrel intrauterine system. In each, improvements in dysmenorrhea, deep dyspareunia, and pelvic pain were noted without incidence of systemic side effects; thus, vaginal delivery of this drug may prove to be a viable method. Unfortunately, a vaginal formulation is not yet available in the United States.

Aromatase Inhibitors Although practice guidelines currently make no specific recommendations for the use of aromatase inhibitors to treat endometriosis, the body of literature supporting use of these agents is growing. Numerous case reports and retrospective, nonrandomized and noncomparative, as well as randomized comparative studies support the effectiveness of both letrozole and anastrozole in decreasing pain, improving quality of life, and reducing postoperative recurrence of disease.[53–58] In all cases, the aromatase inhibitor was used in combination with a progestin, a combined oral contraceptive, or a GnRH agonist. Because most safety information for the aromatase inhibitors is derived from use in postmenopausal women with cancer, it is unknown if similar issues will be experienced by premenopausal women using these agents for endometriosis. Based on available data, it does appear that use of progestins and combined oral contraceptives in combination with the aromatase inhibitors helps to limit side effects and bone mineral density loss.[55]

Personalized Pharmacotherapy

At this point in time, no evidence exists to suggest how to select or dose therapy for endometriosis based on pharmacogenomic, pharmacogenetic, or pharmacokinetic differences between patients. As additional understanding of the pathogenesis of endometriosis emerges, such personalized pharmacotherapy options might be realized.

Evaluation of Therapeutic Outcomes

Size, number, and distribution of endometrial lesions do not correlate with pain symptoms or fertility potential; thus, therapeutic outcome monitoring should focus solely on subjective relief of symptoms.[4] Although traditional measures such as visual pain scales and symptom diaries have been utilized to measure treatment effectiveness, such measures do not capture overall patient satisfaction with treatment, a factor which has been correlated to treatment adherence.[59] Recently, a patient-reported outcome instrument, the Endometriosis Treatment Satisfaction Questionnaire, has been developed and validated.[59] The tool includes six items (pain before and/or during periods, pain during and/or after sex, endometriosis pain, bleeding/spotting, tolerability, overall satisfaction) that are rated by patients on a 7-point Likert scale.[59]

❸ Endometriosis-related pain should be relieved within 2 months of initiating medical therapy. If symptoms persist, consideration should be given to different medical and/or surgical therapy. For endometriosis-related infertility, most experts recommend 6 months of watchful waiting after surgical intervention. If pregnancy is not achieved within that time, assisted reproductive techniques can be considered.

Clinical **Controversy. . .**

Numerous medications used to treat endometriosis are known to diminish bone mineral density, yet the optimal method for monitoring this effect is unknown. Although some clinicians may select to routinely measure bone mineral density through dual-energy x-ray absorptiometry before, during, or after treatment, no data exist to support this practice. What is known is that add-back therapy effectively mitigates most bone mineral density loss and that any loss is generally recovered on cessation of therapy. Consequently, use of bone mineral density testing may be best reserved for the clinical trial environment until more information is known about the predictive utility of such testing in routine practice.

ABBREVIATIONS

CHC	combined hormonal contraceptive
GnRH	gonadotropin-releasing hormone

REFERENCES

1. Olive DL. Gonadotropin-releasing hormone agonists for endometriosis. N Engl J Med 2008;359(11):1136–1142.
2. Bulun SE. Endometriosis. N Engl J Med 2009;360(3):268–279.
3. Sasson IE, Taylor HS. Stem cells and the pathogenesis of endometriosis. Ann N Y Acad Sci 2008;1127:106–115.
4. Committee on Gynecologic Practice. Management of endometriosis. Obstet Gynecol 2010;116(1):223–236.
5. Farquhar C. Endometriosis. BMJ 2007;334(7587):249–253.
6. Practice Committee of American Society for Reproductive Medicine. Treatment of pelvic pain associated with endometriosis. Fertil Steril 2008;90(5 Suppl):S260–S269.
7. Ozkan S, Murk W, Arici A. Endometriosis and infertility: Epidemiology and evidence-based treatments. Ann N Y Acad Sci 2008;1127:92–100.
8. Ferrero S, Arena E, Morando A, Remorgida V. Prevalence of newly diagnosed endometriosis in women attending the general practitioner. Int J Gynaecol Obstet 2010;110(3):203–207.
9. Meuleman C, Vandenabeele B, Fieuws S, et al. High prevalence of endometriosis in infertile women with normal ovulation and normospermic partners. Fertil Steril 2009;92(1):68–74.
10. Tempfer CB, Simoni M, Destenaves B, Fauser BC. Functional genetic polymorphisms and female reproductive disorders: Part II—Endometriosis. Hum Reprod Update 2009;15(1):97–118.
11. Tokushige N, Markham R, Russell P, Fraser IS. Nerve fibres in peritoneal endometriosis. Hum Reprod 2006;21(11):3001–3007.
12. Committee on Gynecologic Practice. Aromatase inhibitors in gynecologic practice. Obstet Gynecol 2008;112(2):405–407.
13. Tokushige N, Markham R, Russell P, Fraser IS. High density of small nerve fibres in the functional layer of the endometrium in women with endometriosis. Hum Reprod 2006;21(3):782–787.

14. Wang G, Tokushige N, Markham R, Fraser IS. Rich innervation of deep infiltrating endometriosis. Hum Reprod 2009;24(4):827–834.
15. Mechsner S, Kaiser A, Kopf A, et al. A pilot study to evaluate the clinical relevance of endometriosis-associated nerve fibers in peritoneal endometriotic lesions. Fertil Steril 2009;92(6):1856–1861.
16. Mansour G, Aziz N, Sharma R, et al. The impact of peritoneal fluid from healthy women and from women with endometriosis on sperm DNA and its relationship to the sperm deformity index. Fertil Steril 2009;92(1):61–67.
17. Lemos NA, Arbo E, Scalco R, et al. Decreased anti-mullerian hormone and altered ovarian follicular cohort in infertile patients with mild/minimal endometriosis. Fertil Steril 2008;89(5):1064–1068.
18. Leyland N, Casper R, Laberge P, Singh SS. Endometriosis: Diagnosis and management. J Obstet Gynaecol Can 2010; 32(7 Suppl 2):S1–S32.
19. Practice Committee of the American Society for Reproductive Medicine. Endometriosis and infertility. Fertil Steril 2006;86(5 Suppl):S156–S160.
20. ESHRE Guideline for the Diagnosis and Treatment of Endometriosis. 2007, *http://guidelines.endometriosis.org/index.html*.
21. Shakiba K, Bena JF, McGill KM, et al. Surgical treatment of endometriosis: A 7-year follow-up on the requirement for further surgery. Obstet Gynecol 2008;111(6): 1285–1292.
22. Rubi-Klein K, Kucera-Sliutz E, Nissel H, et al. Is acupuncture in addition to conventional medicine effective as pain treatment for endometriosis? A randomised controlled cross-over trial. Eur J Obstet Gynecol Reprod Biol 2010;153(1):90–93.
23. Proctor M, Murphy PA. Herbal and dietary therapies for primary and secondary dysmenorrhoea. Cochrane Database Syst Rev 2001;(3):CD002124.
24. Sesti F, Pietropolli A, Capozzolo T, et al. Hormonal suppression treatment or dietary therapy versus placebo in the control of painful symptoms after conservative surgery for endometriosis stage III-IV. A randomized comparative trial. Fertil Steril 2007;88(6):1541–1547.
25. Dovey S, Sanfilippo J. Endometriosis and the adolescent. Clin Obstet Gynecol 2010;53(2):420–428.
26. Surrey ES. Gonadotropin-releasing hormone agonist and add-back therapy: What do the data show? Curr Opin Obstet Gynecol 2010;22(4):283–288.
27. Ballweg ML. Treating endometriosis in adolescents: Does it matter? J Pediatr Adolesc Gynecol 2011;24(5 Suppl):S2–S6.
28. Hughes E, Brown J, Collins JJ, et al. Ovulation suppression for endometriosis. Cochrane Database Syst Rev 2007;(3): CD000155.
29. Guzick DS, Huang LS, Broadman BA, et al. Randomized trial of leuprolide versus continuous oral contraceptives in the treatment of endometriosis-associated pelvic pain. Fertil Steril 2011;95(5):1568–1573.
30. Mabrouk M, Frasca C, Geraci E, et al. Combined oral contraceptive therapy in women with posterior deep infiltrating endometriosis. J Minim Invasive Gynecol 2011;18(4):470–474.
31. Roman H. Oral contraceptives and endometriosis. Hum Reprod 2011;26(6):1600–1601.
32. Fedele L, Bianchi S, Montefusco S, et al. A gonadotropin-releasing hormone agonist versus a continuous oral contraceptive pill in the treatment of bladder endometriosis. Fertil Steril 2008;90(1):183–184.
33. Harada T, Momoeda M, Taketani Y, et al. Low-dose oral contraceptive pill for dysmenorrhea associated with endometriosis: A placebo-controlled, double-blind, randomized trial. Fertil Steril 2008;90(5):1583–1588.
34. Vercellini P, Trespidi L, Colombo A, et al. A gonadotropin-releasing hormone agonist versus a low-dose oral contraceptive for pelvic pain associated with endometriosis. Fertil Steril 1993;60(1):75–79.
35. Vercellini P, Barbara G, Somigliana E, et al. Comparison of contraceptive ring and patch for the treatment of symptomatic endometriosis. Fertil Steril 2010;93(7):2150–2161.
36. Seracchioli R, Mabrouk M, Frasca C, et al. Long-term oral contraceptive pills and postoperative pain management after laparoscopic excision of ovarian endometrioma: A randomized controlled trial. Fertil Steril 2010;94(2):464–471.
37. Schlaff WD, Carson SA, Luciano A, et al. Subcutaneous injection of depot medroxyprogesterone acetate compared with leuprolide acetate in the treatment of endometriosis-associated pain. Fertil Steril 2006;85(2):314–325.
38. Crosignani PG, Luciano A, Ray A, Bergqvist A. Subcutaneous depot medroxyprogesterone acetate versus leuprolide acetate in the treatment of endometriosis-associated pain. Hum Reprod 2006;21(1):248–256.
39. Depo-Provera Prescribing Information. 2011, *http://www.accessdata.fda.gov/drugsatfda_docs/label/2011/020246s035lbl.pdf*.
40. Depo-SubQ Provera 104 Prescribing Information. 2009, *http://www.accessdata.fda.gov/drugsatfda_docs/label/2009/021583s011lbl.pdf*.
41. Brown J, Pan A, Hart RJ. Gonadotropin hormone releasing analogues for pain associated with endometriosis. Cochrane Database Syst Rev 2010;(12):CD008475.
42. Kang JL, Wang XX, Nie ML, Huang XH. Efficacy of gonadotropin-releasing hormone agonist and an extended-interval dosing regimen in the treatment of patients with adenomyosis and endometriosis. Gynecol Obstet Invest 2010;69(2):73–77.
43. Bergstrom I, Freyschuss B, Jacobsson H, Landgren B. The effect of physical training on bone mineral density in women with endometriosis treated with GnRH analogs: A pilot study. Acta Obstet Gynecol Scand 2005;84(4):380–383.
44. Kim NY, Ryoo U, Lee DY, et al. The efficacy and tolerability of short-term low-dose estrogen-only add-back therapy during post-operative GnRH agonist treatment for endometriosis. Eur J Obstet Gynecol Reprod Biol 2011;154(1):85–89.
45. Petta CA, Ferriani RA, Abrao MS, et al. Randomized clinical trial of a levonorgestrel-releasing intrauterine system and a depot GnRH analogue for the treatment of chronic pelvic pain in women with endometriosis. Hum Reprod 2005;20(7):1993–1998.
46. Wong AY, Tang LC, Chin RK. Levonorgestrel-releasing intrauterine system (Mirena) and depot medroxyprogesterone acetate (Depo-Provera) as long-term maintenance therapy for patients with moderate and severe endometriosis: A randomised controlled trial. Aust N Z J Obstet Gynaecol 2010;50(3):273–279.
47. Bayoglu Tekin Y, Dilbaz B, Altinbas SK, Dilbaz S. Postoperative medical treatment of chronic pelvic pain related to severe endometriosis: Levonorgestrel-releasing intrauterine system versus gonadotropin-releasing hormone analogue. Fertil Steril 2011;95(2):492–496.
48. Abou-Setta AM, Al-Inany HG, Farquhar C. Levonorgestrel-releasing intrauterine device (LNG-IUD) for symptomatic

endometriosis following surgery. Cochrane Database Syst Rev 2013;(1):CD005072.
49. Selak V, Farquhar C, Prentice A, Singla AA. Danazol for pelvic pain associated with endometriosis. Cochrane Database Syst Rev 2007;(4):CD000068.
50. Razzi S, Luisi S, Calonaci F, et al. Efficacy of vaginal danazol treatment in women with recurrent deeply infiltrating endometriosis. Fertil Steril 2007;88(4):789–794.
51. Bhattacharya SM, Tolasaria A, Khan B. Vaginal danazol for the treatment of endometriosis-related pelvic pain. Int J Gynaecol Obstet 2011;115(3):294–295.
52. Ferrero S, Tramalloni D, Venturini PL, Remorgida V. Vaginal danazol for women with rectovaginal endometriosis and pain symptoms persisting after insertion of a levonorgestrel-releasing intrauterine device. Int J Gynaecol Obstet 2011;113(2):116–119.
53. Abushahin F, Goldman KN, Barbieri E, et al. Aromatase inhibition for refractory endometriosis-related chronic pelvic pain. Fertil Steril 2011;96(4):939–942.
54. Colette S, Donnez J. Are aromatase inhibitors effective in endometriosis treatment? Expert Opin Investig Drugs 2011;20(7):917–931.
55. Ferrero S, Gillott DJ, Venturini PL, Remorgida V. Use of aromatase inhibitors to treat endometriosis-related pain symptoms: A systematic review. Reprod Biol Endocrinol 2011;9:89.
56. Nothnick WB. The emerging use of aromatase inhibitors for endometriosis treatment. Reprod Biol Endocrinol 2011;9:87.
57. Nawathe A, Patwardhan S, Yates D, et al. Systematic review of the effects of aromatase inhibitors on pain associated with endometriosis. BJOG 2008;115(7):818–822.
58. Alborzi S, Hamedi B, Omidvar A, et al. A comparison of the effect of short-term aromatase inhibitor (letrozole) and GnRH agonist (triptorelin) versus case control on pregnancy rate and symptom and sign recurrence after laparoscopic treatment of endometriosis. Arch Gynecol Obstet 2011;284(1):105–110.
59. Deal LS, Williams VS, DiBenedetti DB, Fehnel SE. Development and psychometric evaluation of the endometriosis treatment satisfaction questionnaire. Qual Life Res 2010;19(6):899–905.

65

Hormone Therapy in Women

Sophia N. Kalantaridou, Devra K. Dang, and Karim Anton Calis

KEY CONCEPTS

1. The decision to use perimenopausal or postmenopausal hormone therapy must be individualized and based on several parameters, including menopausal symptoms, osteoporosis fracture risk, cardiovascular disease risk, breast cancer risk, and thromboembolic risk.
2. Hormone therapy is the most effective treatment option for alleviating vasomotor and vaginal symptoms of menopause.
3. Osteoporotic fracture prevention is an indication for use of systemic estrogen products when alternate therapies are contraindicated or cause adverse effects.
4. Hormone therapy may improve depressive symptoms in symptomatic menopausal women.
5. Cardiovascular disease, including coronary artery disease, stroke, and peripheral vascular disease, is the leading cause of death among women. Postmenopausal hormone therapy should not be used for reducing the risk of cardiovascular disease.
6. Because of the increased risk of endometrial hyperplasia and endometrial cancer with estrogen monotherapy (i.e., unopposed estrogen), hormone therapy in women who have not undergone hysterectomy should include a progestogen in addition to the estrogen.
7. Use of hormone therapy at doses lower than those prescribed historically (i.e., prior to the Women's Health Initiative study) is effective in the management of menopausal symptoms.
8. Results from randomized trials of hormone therapy in postmenopausal women cannot be extrapolated to premenopausal women with ovarian dysfunction. Women with primary ovarian insufficiency need exogenous sex steroids to compensate for decreased production by their ovaries.

MENOPAUSE AND PERIMENOPAUSAL AND POSTMENOPAUSAL HORMONE THERAPY

Epidemiology

Menopause is the permanent cessation of menses following the loss of ovarian follicular activity. The median age at the onset of menopause in the United States is 51 years. By definition, it is a physiologic event that occurs after 12 consecutive months of amenorrhea, so the time of the final menses is determined retrospectively. Women who have undergone hysterectomy must rely on their symptoms to estimate the actual time of menopause.

Etiology

Menopause refers to loss of ovarian function and subsequent hormonal deficiency. This can be due to the normal process of aging (i.e., natural menopause), ovarian surgery (bilateral oophorectomy), medications (e.g., cancer chemotherapy), or pelvic irradiation.

Pathophysiology

A woman is born with approximately two million primordial follicles in her ovaries. During a normal reproductive life span, she ovulates fewer than 500 times. The vast majority of follicles undergo atresia.

The hypothalamic–pituitary–ovarian axis dynamically controls reproductive physiology throughout the reproductive years. The pituitary is regulated by pulsatile secretion of gonadotropin-releasing hormone (GnRH) from the hypothalamus. Follicle-stimulating hormone (FSH) and luteinizing hormone (LH), produced by the pituitary in response to GnRH, regulate ovarian function. These gonadotropins also are influenced by negative feedback from estradiol and progesterone. Ovarian follicular activity is reflected by the circulating concentrations of sex steroids and by peptide hormones including inhibin, activin, and anti-Mullerian hormone (AMH). AMH is a product of growing ovarian follicles, which appears to be independent of the hypothalamic–pituitary–gonadal axis. It is a principal regulator of early follicular recruitment from the primordial pool such that the concentration of AMH in blood may also reflect the nongrowing follicle population. AMH concentrations decline with age. For women without any menstrual cycle disorder, AMH levels predicted the median time to menopause.[1] The sex steroids include estradiol, produced by the dominant follicle; progesterone, produced by the corpus luteum after maturation of the dominant ovarian follicle; and androgens, primarily testosterone and androstenedione, secreted by the ovarian stroma. Sex steroids are important for the healthy functioning of many organs, including the bones, brain, skin, and reproductive and urogenital tracts. They act primarily by regulating gene expression.

Pathophysiologic changes associated with menopause are caused by loss of ovarian follicular activity. Ovarian primordial follicle numbers decrease with advancing age, and at the time of the menopause, few follicles remain in the ovary. Hence, the postmenopausal ovary is no longer the primary site of estradiol or progesterone synthesis. The postmenopausal ovary secretes primarily androstenedione. In contrast to the acute fall in circulating estrogen at the time of menopause, the decline in circulating androgens commences in the decade leading up to the average age of natural menopause and closely parallels increasing age.[2] Whether the ovary continues to secrete testosterone after menopause remains controversial.[3]

Hypertrophy of the ovarian stroma may develop after menopause, probably secondary to high LH concentrations, thereby resulting in increased ovarian testosterone production. Alternatively, the ovaries may become fibrotic and a poor source of sex steroids. No endocrine event clearly signals the time just prior to final menses.[4]

As women age, a progressive rise in circulating FSH and a concomitant decline in ovarian inhibin-B and AMH are observed. In women who continue to experience menstrual bleeding, FSH determinations on day 2 or 3 of the menstrual cycle are considered elevated when concentrations exceed 10 to 12 international units/L (10 to 12 IU/L), an indication of diminished ovarian reserve. Alternatively AMH measured at any time in the cycle predicts diminishing ovarian reserve.[2] Clear elevations in serum FSH are seen in women approximately at age 40 years.[4] When ovarian function has ceased, serum FSH concentrations are greater than 40 international units/L (40 IU/L). Menopause is characterized by a 10- to 15-fold increase in circulating FSH concentrations compared with concentrations of FSH in the follicular phase of the cycle, a fourfold to fivefold increase in LH, and a greater than 90% decrease in circulating estradiol concentrations.[4] During the perimenopause, FSH concentrations may rise to the postmenopausal range during some cycles but return to premenopausal levels during subsequent cycles. Thus, high concentrations of FSH should not be used to diagnose menopause in perimenopausal women.

Clinical Presentation

The perimenopause commences with the onset of menstrual irregularity and ends 12 months after the last menstrual period.[5] The menstrual cycle irregularity is caused by the increased frequency of anovulatory cycles. Women commonly experience symptoms during the perimenopause, which substantially impact their health and daily function. Research has shown that 25% of women experience severe vasomotor symptoms (e.g., hot flushes and night sweats), 30% experience severe psychological symptoms (e.g., depression, anxiety), and 50% report moderate to severe symptoms of sleep disturbance, joint pain, or headache, and at least one in four women have sexual dysfunction.[6,7]

Women who experience severe symptoms, either from early in the menopause transition or from their final menstrual period, are likely to continue to experience severe symptoms for several years.[6] The perimenopause is associated with a higher vulnerability to depression with the risk increasing from early to late perimenopause and decreasing during postmenopause.[8] Women with a history of depression are nearly five times as likely to be diagnosed with depression during the perimenopause, whereas women with no history of depression are two to four times more likely to have a diagnosis compared with premenopausal women.[8]

In addition to the symptoms of menopause, loss of estrogen production results in significant metabolic changes including effects on body composition, lipids, vascular function, and bone metabolism. The menopause transition is associated with a significant increase in central abdominal fat, which may occur without commensurate change in body weight.[9]

Symptoms in perimenopausal women may require treatment despite the presence of menstrual bleeding. Although other conditions that may cause similar symptomatology should be first excluded, there is no condition that mimics classic menopausal vasomotor symptomatology.

Dysfunctional uterine bleeding may occur during the perimenopausal years because of anovulatory cycles; however, abnormal uterine bleeding always merits investigation when it cannot be simply explained by menopausal cyclical irregularity. Treatment options for dysfunctional uterine bleeding include insertion of an intrauterine progestin-impregnated device, systemic progestogen therapy, or the combined oral contraceptive pill.

TREATMENT

Nonpharmacological options may alleviate mild symptoms but are unlikely to be effective for severely symptomatic women.

Desired Outcomes

Menopause is a natural life event, not a disease. The primary goals of therapy for menopause are to relieve symptoms and improve quality of life while minimizing adverse effects.

General Approach to Treatment

In women with mild vasomotor and/or vaginal symptoms, nonpharmacologic therapy can be considered. However, for some women these are not effective. Figure 65-1 outlines a treatment algorithm for women requiring pharmacologic therapy. In the absence of contraindications, hormone therapy is appropriate for women with hot flushes and vulvar or vaginal atrophy (Table 65-1).

❶ The decision to use hormone therapy and the type of formulation used must be individualized and based on several parameters, including the woman's assessment of the severity of her menopausal symptoms and her wishes, the risk of osteoporosis fracture, cardiovascular disease, breast cancer, and venous thromboembolic events

CLINICAL PRESENTATION AND DIAGNOSIS — Perimenopause and Menopause

Symptoms

- Vasomotor symptoms (hot flushes and night sweats)
- Sleep disturbances
- Mood changes
- Problems with concentration and memory
- Vaginal dryness and dyspareunia
- Arthralgia

Signs

- Perimenopause: dysfunctional uterine bleeding as a result of anovulatory cycles (other gynecologic disorders should be excluded)
- Menopause: signs of urogenital atrophy

Laboratory Tests

- Perimenopause: FSH on day 2 or 3 of the menstrual cycle greater than 10–12 international units/L (10–12 IU/L)
- Menopause: FSH greater than 40 international units/L (40 IU/L)

Other Relevant Diagnostic Tests

- Thyroid function tests
- Iron stores
- Lipid profile

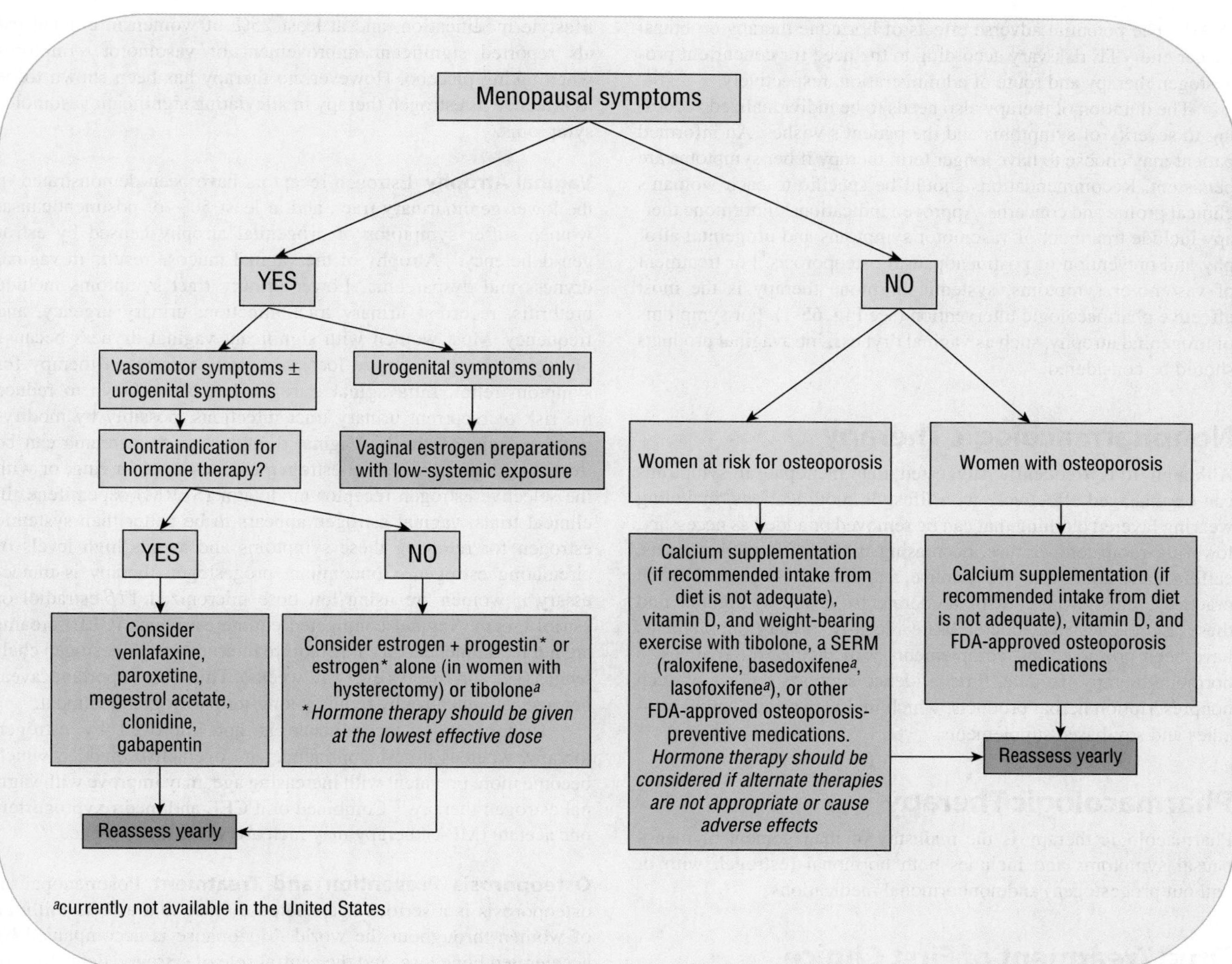

FIGURE 65-1 Algorithm for pharmacologic management of menopausal symptoms.

TABLE 65-1 FDA Indications and Contraindications for Menopausal Hormone Therapy with Estrogens and Progestins

Indications	
For systemic use	Treatment of moderate to severe vasomotor symptoms (i.e., moderate to severe hot flushes)
For intravaginal use (low systemic exposure)	Treatment of moderate to severe symptoms of vulvar and vaginal atrophy (i.e., moderate to severe vaginal dryness, dyspareunia, and atrophic vaginitis)
Contraindications	
Absolute contraindications	Undiagnosed abnormal genital bleeding Known, suspected, or history of cancer of the breast Known or suspected estrogen- or progesterone-dependent neoplasia Active deep vein thrombosis, pulmonary embolism, or a history of these conditions Active or recent (e.g., within the past year) arterial thromboembolic disease (e.g., stroke, myocardial infarction) Liver dysfunction or disease
Relative contraindications	Elevated blood pressure Hypertriglyceridemia Impaired liver function and past history of cholestatic jaundice Hypothyrodism Fluid retention Severe hypocalcemia Ovarian cancer Exacerbation of endometriosis Exacerbation of asthma, diabetes mellitus, migraine, systemic lupus erythematosus, epilepsy, porphyria, and hepatic hemangioma

Data from reference 148.

(VTE). The potential adverse effects of hormone therapy on breast cancer and VTE risk vary according to the need for concurrent progestogen therapy and route of administration, respectively.

The duration of therapy also needs to be individualized according to severity of symptoms and the patient's wishes. An informed patient may choose to have longer term therapy if her symptoms are persistent. Recommendations should be specific to each woman's clinical profile and concerns. Approved indications of hormone therapy include treatment of vasomotor symptoms and urogenital atrophy and prevention of postmenopausal osteoporosis. For treatment of vasomotor symptoms, systemic hormone therapy is the most effective pharmacologic intervention (see Fig. 65-1). For symptoms of urogenital atrophy, such as vaginal dryness, intravaginal products should be considered.

Nonpharmacologic Therapy

Although it is frequently suggested that menopausal symptoms can be managed effectively with lifestyle modifications, including wearing layered clothing that can be removed or added as necessary, lowering room temperature, decreasing intake of hot spicy foods, caffeine, and hot beverages, exercise, and other good general health practices, most women with moderate to severe symptoms find these approaches inadequate. More recently, dietary supplements have been promoted as "complementary medicine" alternatives to hormone therapy. To date, little evidence supports the use of such nonprescription herbal products, which include various herbal remedies and soy-based supplements.

Pharmacologic Therapy

Pharmacologic therapy is the mainstay of management of menopausal symptoms and includes both hormonal (estrogen with or without progestogen) and nonhormonal medications.

Drug Treatment of First Choice

2 Hormone therapy is the most effective treatment option for alleviating moderate and severe vasomotor and vaginal symptoms. In women with an intact uterus, hormone therapy consists of an estrogen plus a progestogen to prevent endometrial hyperplasia. In women who have undergone hysterectomy, estrogen therapy is given unopposed by a progestogen.

Published Guidelines

A number of national and international guidelines and consensus statements on the management of menopause are available.[10–14] The United States Preventive Services Task Force also provides a recommendation statement on the use of hormone therapy for the prevention of chronic medical conditions in postmenopausal women.[15]

Hormone Therapy for Vasomotor Symptoms and Vaginal Atrophy

Hormone therapy remains the most effective treatment for moderate and severe vasomotor symptoms, impaired sleep quality, and urogenital symptoms of menopause.

Vasomotor Symptoms The major indication for postmenopausal hormone therapy is management of vasomotor symptoms. Most women with vasomotor symptoms require hormone treatment for fewer than 5 years, so the risks of therapy appear to be small.

Fewer than 25% of women experience a menopausal transition without symptoms, whereas more than 25% suffer severe menopausal symptoms, most commonly hot flushes and night sweats. Women with mild vasomotor symptoms can experience relief by lifestyle modification, and at least 25% of women in clinical trials reported significant improvement of vasomotor symptoms when taking placebo. However, no therapy has been shown to be as effective as estrogen therapy in alleviating significant vasomotor symptoms.

Vaginal Atrophy Estrogen receptors have been demonstrated in the lower genitourinary tract, and at least 50% of postmenopausal women suffer symptoms of urogenital atrophy caused by estrogen deficiency.[16] Atrophy of the vaginal mucosa results in vaginal dryness and dyspareunia. Lower urinary tract symptoms include urethritis, recurrent urinary tract infection, urinary urgency, and frequency. Most women with significant vaginal dryness because of vaginal atrophy require local or systemic estrogen therapy for symptom relief. Intravaginal estrogen has been shown to reduce the risk of recurrent urinary tract infections, possibly by modifying the vaginal flora.[13,17] Vaginal dryness and dyspareunia can be treated with an intravaginal estrogen cream, tablet, or ring; or with the selective estrogen receptor modulator (SERM) ospemifene. In clinical trials, vaginal estrogen appears to be better than systemic estrogen for relieving these symptoms and avoids high levels of circulating estrogen. Concomitant progestogen therapy is unnecessary if women are using low-dose micronized 17β-estradiol or estriol cream. Vaginal conjugated equine estrogens (CEE) creams are not recommended, as they require intermittent progestogen challenges (i.e., for 10 days every 12 weeks). This is an important caveat because vaginal atrophy requires long-term estrogen treatment.[17]

Urinary stress incontinence is not improved by estrogen therapy, whereas urge incontinence and overactive bladder, which become more prevalent with increasing age, may improve with vaginal estrogen therapy.[18] Combined oral CEE and medroxyprogesterone acetate (MPA) therapy may increase stress incontinence.[19]

Osteoporosis Prevention and Treatment Postmenopausal osteoporosis is a serious age-related disease that affects millions of women throughout the world. Menopause is accompanied by accelerated bone loss, and the central role of estrogen deficiency in postmenopausal osteoporosis is well established. Osteoporosis is characterized by reduced bone mass associated with architectural deterioration of the skeleton and increased risk for fracture. Estrogen deficiency results in bone loss through its actions in accelerating bone turnover and uncoupling bone formation from resorption. It is important to recognize that bone loss commences 2 years before the final menstrual period.[20] Throughout menopause, the average loss of bone mineral density (BMD) is around 6.4% at the lumbar spine and 4% to 5% at the femoral neck, with obese women experiencing less bone loss than nonobese women.[20] An observational study of more than 9,000 postmenopausal women examined the relationship between endogenous estrogens and BMD, bone loss, fractures, and breast cancer.[21–24] Women with detectable serum estradiol concentrations (5 to 25 pg/mL [18 to 92 pmol/L]) had a 6% to 7% higher BMD at the total hip and spine compared with women with undetectable levels (less than 5 pg/mL [18 pmol/L]).[23] They also had significantly less bone loss at the hip than women with undetectable levels.[22] Women with undetectable serum estradiol concentrations had a relative risk of 2.5 for subsequent hip and vertebral fractures.[24] However, women with the highest estradiol serum concentrations had the greatest risk of developing breast cancer.[21]

The Women's Health Initiative (WHI), a landmark controlled clinical trial evaluating the benefits and risks of postmenopausal hormone therapy, was the first randomized trial to demonstrate that hormone therapy reduces the risk of fractures at the hip, spine, and wrist.[25,26] These findings are in agreement with observational data and several meta-analyses of the efficacy of hormone therapy for reducing fractures in postmenopausal women.[27] Estrogen therapy reduces bone turnover and increases bone density in postmenopausal women of all ages. The protective effect persists as long as the treatment is maintained. With cessation of therapy, postmenopausal bone loss resumes at the same rate as in untreated women.[28,29] The standard bone-sparing daily estrogen dose is equivalent to 0.625 mg CEE.[30] However, lower doses of estrogen have been shown to increase bone mass to the same extent as standard-dose estrogen therapy.[31]

3 Systemic estrogen therapy is indicated for the prevention of osteoporotic fracture in postmenopausal women younger than 60 years of age who are at increased fracture risk when alternate therapies are contraindicated or cause adverse effects. Indeed estrogen is one of the few treatments shown to prevent fragility fractures in osteopenic women.

General protective measures, such as regular weight-bearing exercise and avoidance of detrimental lifestyle habits such as smoking and alcohol abuse, are appropriate for all women. Some women require calcium supplementation to their dietary intake. Adequate vitamin D intake and/or supplementation is also needed. See Chapter 73 for a full discussion of osteoporosis prevention and treatment.

Colon Cancer Risk Reduction

Colorectal cancer is the fourth most common cancer and the second leading cause of cancer death in the United States (see Chap. 107). The estrogen–progestogen arm of the WHI study showed that combined estrogen–progestogen therapy may reduce colon cancer risk.[25] In the postintervention follow-up period, the reduction in colorectal cancer risk disappeared.[28]

Quality of Life, Mood, Cognition, and Dementia

4 Hormone therapy improves depressive symptoms in symptomatic menopausal women, most probably by relieving flushing and improving sleep.[32] Women with vasomotor symptoms receiving hormone therapy have improved mental health and fewer depressive symptoms compared with women receiving placebo; however, hormone therapy may worsen quality of life in women without flushes.[33]

There is no evidence that hormone therapy improves quality of life or cognition in older, asymptomatic women.[32–36]

Clinical **Controversy...**

Some clinicians believe that hormone therapy can improve well-being and quality of life of early menopausal women, whereas others believe that hormone therapy, at best, has no effect in this population.

More than 33% of women 65 years and older will develop dementia during their lifetime.[37] Several observational studies have suggested that estrogen therapy may be protective against Alzheimer's disease (see Chap. 38). The WHI Memory Study (WHIMS, an ancillary study of the WHI trial) evaluated the effect of combined hormone therapy on dementia and cognition in 4,532 women 65 to 79 years old.[35] The study found that postmenopausal women 65 years and older taking estrogen plus progestogen therapy had twice the rate of dementia, including Alzheimer's disease, than women taking placebo (HR 2.05, 95% CI: 1.21 to 3.48).[35] In addition, estrogen plus progestogen therapy in these women did not prevent mild cognitive impairment, a cognitive and functional state between normal aging and dementia that frequently progresses to dementia.[35] The estrogen alone arm of the WHI trial showed similar findings.[38,39]

In contrast, the Women's Health Initiative Memory Study of Younger Women (WHIMSY) found that neither estrogen plus progestogen or estrogen therapy alone confer any risk or benefit to cognitive function when taken by postmenopausal women aged 50 to 55 years old.[40]

Other Potential Effects

Diabetes In healthy postmenopausal women, hormone therapy appears to have a beneficial effect on fasting glucose levels in women with elevated fasting insulin concentrations.[41] Also, in women with coronary artery disease, hormone therapy reduces the incidence of diabetes by 35%.[42] These findings provide important insights into the metabolic effects of hormone therapy but are insufficient to recommend the long-term use of hormone therapy in women with diabetes.

Body Weight A meta-analysis of randomized controlled trials showed that unopposed estrogen or estrogen combined with a progestogen has no effect on body weight, suggesting that hormone therapy does not cause weight gain in excess of that normally observed at the time of menopause.[43]

Risks of Hormone Therapy

The potential risks of hormone therapy include ovarian cancer, endometrial cancer, breast cancer, venous thromboembolism, gallbladder disease, and possibly cardiovascular disease and lung cancer in older women. The level of risk may depend on the hormonal regimen used (estrogen only vs. estrogen plus progestogen), the route of administration, dose, duration of therapy, age at treatment initiation, and the patient's other risk factors. Data on potential risks of hormone therapy remain limited.

Cardiovascular Disease

5 Cardiovascular disease, including coronary artery disease, stroke, and peripheral vascular disease, is the leading cause of death among women. Menopause is associated with the development of a more adverse lipid profile, increasing the risk for cardiovascular disease.[44]

In the decade prior to the publication of the WHI results in 2002, an expectation of coronary benefit had been a major reason for use of postmenopausal hormones because observational studies indicated that women who use hormone therapy have a 35% to 50% lower risk of coronary heart disease (CHD) than nonusers.[45] In addition, previous studies have shown that estrogen exerts protective effects on the cardiovascular system, including lipid-lowering,[46] antioxidant,[47] and vasodilating effects.[47] However, in the 2000s, published results of several randomized clinical trials provided no evidence of cardiovascular disease protection and even some evidence of harm with hormone therapy.[25,48–51]

The primary findings of the estrogen plus progestogen arm of the WHI trial showed an overall increase in the risk of CHD (HR 1.29, 95% CI 1.02–1.63) among healthy postmenopausal women 50 to 79 years old receiving combined estrogen–progestogen hormone therapy compared with those receiving placebo.[25] The primary findings of the estrogen-only arm of the WHI trial show no effect (either increase or decrease) on the risk of coronary heart disease in women taking estrogen alone.[52] Subgroup analyses performed in the years after the WHI was first published in 2002 revealed that women who initiated hormone therapy 10 or more years after the time of menopause tended to have increased CHD risk compared with women who initiated therapy within 10 years of menopause.[53,54] Neither estrogen alone nor estrogen plus progestogen was associated with a statistically significant effect on CHD in women aged 50–59 years, and hormone therapy was associated with reduced overall mortality, although this decrease was not statistically significant.[53] More recently, subgroup analyses from the WHI that included only adherent study participants found that the risk of CHD with estrogen plus progestogen use is increased in the first 2 years of treatment, even in women aged 50–59 years at study entry. However, the risk of CHD in women who initiated therapy within 10 years of menopause appears to decrease after 6 years of treatment.[54] Most women who commence estrogen or estrogen plus progestogen therapy do so within the first few years of becoming menopausal.

A randomized controlled study of 1,006 recently menopausal women revealed that 10-year hormone therapy was associated with a significantly reduced risk of cardiovascular disease.[55] In addition, studies of recently menopausal women showed that the presence and severity of hot flushes are associated with vascular endothelial dysfunction and vascular inflammation (markers of increased risk for CHD); hormone therapy improved both parameters.[56–58] Randomized controlled studies of low-dose hormone therapy started around the time of menopause are awaited.

Clinical **Controversy. . .**

Although some clinicians believe that early menopausal women using hormone therapy are at increased risk for cardiovascular disease, others believe that hormone therapy use early in menopause may be associated with a reduced cardiovascular disease risk.

Hormone therapy should not be initiated or continued solely for the prevention of cardiovascular disease. Adherence to a healthful lifestyle (cessation of smoking, regular exercise, healthy diet, and body mass index less than 25 kg/m^2) may prevent the onset of cardiovascular disease in postmenopausal women.

In the estrogen plus progestogen arm of the WHI study, the increased risk for stroke and venous thromboembolism continued throughout the 5 years of therapy.[25] Increased risk was observed only for ischemic stroke and not for hemorrhagic stroke.[59] In the estrogen-alone arm of the study, a similar increased risk for stroke was observed.[52] After the cessation of treatment, there is no increased risk for stroke.[28,29]

Breast Cancer

The WHI trial found that combined estrogen plus progestogen oral therapy has an increased risk of invasive breast cancer (HR 1.26, 95% CI: 1.0 to 1.59) and a trend toward increasing risk with increasing duration of therapy.[25] This risk does not persist after discontinuation of hormone treatment.[28] The estrogen-only arm of the WHI trial found a decreased risk for breast cancer during the 7-year follow-up period,[52] which persisted after discontinuation of treatment.[29]

In the estrogen plus progestogen arm, the increased breast cancer risk did not appear until after 3 years of study participation.[25] The risk was seen only in women who initiated therapy within 5 years of the start of menopause but not in those who started therapy more than 5 years after menopause.[60] The breast cancers diagnosed in women in the hormone therapy group had similar histology and grade but were more likely to be in an advanced stage compared with women in the placebo group.[61] The risk of breast cancer returns to baseline rapidly after discontinuation of hormone therapy.[28,62] In an unselected postmenopausal population, the Million Women Study found that current use of hormone therapy increased breast cancer risk and breast cancer mortality (relative risk 1.66 and 1.22, respectively). Increased incidence was observed for estrogen-only use (relative risk 1.30), for estrogen plus progestogen (relative risk 2), and for tibolone (relative risk 1.45).[63] The risk for estrogen only and estrogen plus progestin therapy were higher for those who initiated treatment within 5 years of menopause compared to those who started therapy 5 or more years after menopause.[64]

For women in the United States, the lifetime risk of developing breast cancer is approximately one in eight,[65] and the greatest incidence occurs in women older than 60 years (see Chap. 105). In a collaborative re-analysis of data from 51 studies evaluating 52,705 women with breast cancer and 108,411 controls, less than 5 years of combined estrogen–progestogen therapy was associated with a 15% increase in breast cancer risk, and the risk increased with longer duration (relative risk 1.35 with 5 or more years of use).[66] However, 5 years after discontinuation of hormone therapy, the risk of breast cancer was no longer increased.[66]

Addition of progestogens to estrogen may increase breast cancer risk beyond that observed with estrogen alone.[67]

Sex-steroid deficiency during the menopause results in lipomatous involution of the breast, which is seen as decreased mammographic breast density and markedly improved radiotransparency of breast tissue. Thus, mammographic changes indicating breast cancer can be recognized more easily and earlier after the menopause. Conversely, combination hormone therapy results in increased mammographic breast density, and increased density on mammography has been associated with higher breast cancer risk.[68–70]

Endometrial Cancer

The WHI trial suggests that combined oral hormone therapy does not increase endometrial cancer risk compared with placebo (HR 0.81, 95% CI: 0.48 to 1.36).[71] However, estrogen alone given to women with an intact uterus significantly increases uterine cancer risk.[72] The excess risk increases with dose and duration of estrogen (10 years of unopposed estrogen increases the risk 10-fold), is apparent within 2 years of the start of treatment, and persists for many years after estrogen replacement is discontinued.[72] Estrogen-induced endometrial cancer usually is of a low stage and grade at the time of diagnosis,[55] and it can be prevented almost entirely by progestogen coadministration. The sequential addition of progestogen to estrogen for at least 10 days of the treatment cycle or continuous combined estrogen–progestogen does not increase the risk of endometrial cancer.[73]

Lower doses of estrogen may be associated with a lower risk of endometrial hyperplasia.[74] SERMs do not result in endometrial hyperplasia.[75] A 4-year trial of raloxifene in women with osteoporosis showed no increased risk of endometrial cancer.[76]

Ovarian Cancer

Lifetime risk of ovarian cancer is low (1.7%). The WHI trial suggested that orally administered combined hormone therapy does not increase the risk of ovarian cancer (HR 1.58, 95% CI: 0.77 to 3.24).[71] An observational study reported an increased risk of ovarian cancer in women taking postmenopausal estrogen-only therapy for more than 10 years (relative risk 1.8, 95% CI: 1.1 to 3.0 and 3.2, 95% CI: 1.7 to 5.7 for 10 to 19 years and 20 or more years, respectively), but no increased risk of ovarian cancer among women receiving combination estrogen–progestogen therapy.[77]

Lung Cancer

The WHI trial found that combined oral estrogen–progestogen therapy did not increase lung cancer incidence, but significantly increased deaths from lung cancer, mainly from nonsmall cell lung cancers (HR 1.87, 95% CI: 1.22–2.88).[78] The estrogen-only arm of the WHI trial found no increased risk for lung cancer death.[79]

It should be noted that the WHI was not designed to assess lung cancer.[13]

Venous Thromboembolism

Venous thromboembolism, including thrombosis of the deep veins of the legs and embolism to the pulmonary arteries, is uncommon in the general population. Women taking oral estrogen therapy have a twofold increased risk for thromboembolic events, with the highest risk occurring in the first year of use.[25,52] However, women with certain risk factors for venous thromboembolism including those with a Factor V Leiden mutation, obesity, and history of previous thromboembolic events, are at increased risk with hormone therapy.[13] Lower doses of estrogen are associated with a decreased risk for thromboembolism as compared with higher doses.[80] Oral administration of estrogen increases the risk of venous thromboembolism compared to the transdermal route.[81] In addition, the norpregnane progestogens, unlike micronized progesterone, appear to be thrombogenic.

Currently, there is no indication for thrombophilia screening before initiating hormone therapy. However, hormone therapy should be avoided in women at high risk for thromboembolic events.

Gallbladder Disease

Gallbladder disease is a commonly cited complication of oral estrogen use. The WHI studies reported an increased risk for cholecystitis, cholelithiasis, and cholecystectomy among women taking oral estrogen or estrogen–progestogen therapy.[82] Transdermal estrogen is an alternative to oral therapy for women at high risk for cholelithiasis.

Estrogens

Estrogens are naturally occurring hormones or synthetic steroidal or nonsteroidal compounds with estrogenic activity. The primary indication for systemic estrogen-based hormone therapy is the relief of moderate and severe vasomotor symptoms, and the initial dose should be the lowest effective dose for symptom control.

Adverse Effects Common adverse effects of estrogen include nausea, headache, breast tenderness, and heavy bleeding. More serious adverse effects include increased risk for CHD, stroke, venous thromboembolism, breast cancer, and gallbladder disease. Transdermal estradiol is associated with a lower incidence of breast tenderness and deep vein thrombosis than is oral estrogen.[55,83,84]

Dose and Administration Various systemically administered estrogens (typically oral and transdermal) are suitable for replacement therapy (Table 65-2). Estrogens can be administered orally, percutaneously (transdermal patches and topical products), intravaginally (creams, tablets, or rings), intramuscularly, and even subcutaneously in the form of implanted pellets. The choice of estrogen delivery (product, route, and method) should be determined in consultation with the patient to ensure acceptability and enhance adherence. In general, the oral and transdermal routes are used most frequently. No evidence indicates that one estrogen compound is more effective than another in relieving menopausal symptoms or preventing osteoporosis.

Oral Estrogen Oral CEE has been available for more than 50 years. CEE is prepared from the urine of pregnant mares and is composed of estrone sulfate (50% to 60%) and multiple other equine estrogens such as equilin and 17α-dihydroequilin.[85]

Estradiol is the predominant and most active form of endogenous estrogens. A micronized form of estradiol (produced by a technique that yields extremely small particles of the pure hormone) is readily absorbed from the small intestines.[85] When given orally, estradiol is metabolized by the intestinal mucosa and the liver during the first hepatic passage, and only 10% reaches circulation as free estradiol. Metabolism of estrogen is partly mediated by the cytochrome P450 3A4 isoenzyme. Gut and liver metabolism converts a large proportion of estradiol to the less potent estrone. Thus, measurement of serum estradiol is not useful for monitoring oral estrogen replacement. The principal metabolites of micronized estradiol are estrone and estrone sulfate. Administration of estradiol via the oral route results in estrone concentrations that are three to six times those of estradiol. Ethinyl estradiol is a highly potent semisynthetic estrogen that has similar activity following administration by the oral or nonoral route.

Orally administered estrogens stimulate the synthesis of hepatic proteins and increase the circulating concentrations of sex hormone-binding globulin, which, in turn, may compromise the bioavailability of androgens and estrogens.

Other Routes Nonoral forms of estrogens bypass the GI tract and thereby avoid first-pass liver metabolism. These routes of estradiol delivery result in a more physiologic estradiol-to-estrone ratio (estradiol concentrations greater than estrone concentrations), as seen in the normal premenopausal state. Transdermal estrogen therapy also is less likely to affect sex hormone-binding globulin compared with oral therapy. These regimens produce little or no change in circulating lipids, coagulation parameters, or C-reactive protein levels.[86]

Transdermal estrogen patches share the advantages of other nonoral estrogen routes and have the added advantage of delivering estradiol to the general venous circulation at a continuous rate. The matrix transdermal systems (estrogen in adhesive) generally are well tolerated, and fewer than 5% of women experience skin reactions.[87] The incidence of skin irritation diminishes when the application site is rotated. Topical antiinflammatory products (e.g., hydrocortisone cream) can be applied for managing the rashes, and switching to another transdermal patch is often a viable option.

Topical gels, sprays, and emulsions are convenient, but variability in drug absorption has been noted with some formulations. These forms of estrogen are also used for systemic therapy.

Estradiol pellets (implants) containing pure crystalline 17β-estradiol have been available for more than 50 years. They are inserted subcutaneously into the anterior abdominal wall or buttock. Pellets are difficult to remove and may continue to release estradiol for a long time after insertion. Implantation should not be repeated until serum estradiol concentrations have fallen to values similar to those at the midfollicular phase of the menstrual cycle. Estradiol pellets are not available in the United States.

Intravaginal creams, tablets, and rings are used for treatment of urogenital (vulvar and vaginal) atrophy. However, this route of administration can have more than just a local effect. Systemic estrogen absorption is lower with vaginal tablets and rings (specifically Estring) compared with vaginal creams. Nonetheless, local application of the cream at low doses can reverse atrophic vaginal changes and avoid significant systemic exposure. Nonestrogen vaginal moisturizers and lubricants also may provide local symptom relief. These products can be used alone or in combination with locally acting intravaginal estrogens. Intravaginal rings are a sustained-release delivery system composed of a biologically inert liquid polymer matrix with pure crystalline estradiol that can maintain adequate estradiol concentrations. One such intravaginal ring product (Femring) is designed to achieve systemic concentrations of estrogen and is indicated for treatment of moderate to severe vasomotor symptoms.

Progestogens

6 Because of the increased risk of endometrial hyperplasia and endometrial cancer with estrogen monotherapy (unopposed estrogen), women who have not undergone hysterectomy should be treated concurrently with a progestogen in addition to the estrogen.[88]

TABLE 65-2 Estrogen Products for Hormone Therapy

Drug	Brand Name[a]	Initial Dose/ Low Dose	Usual Dose Range	Comments
Systemic Estrogen Products (for the treatment of moderate and severe vasomotor symptoms ± urogenital symptoms)				
Oral estrogens[b]				
Conjugated equine estrogens	Premarin (once daily)	0.3 or 0.45 mg	0.3–1.25 mg	Dosage form available as 0.3, 0.45, 0.625, 0.9, 1.25 mg
Synthetic conjugated estrogens	Cenestin, Enjuvia (once daily)	0.3 mg	0.3–1.25 mg	Dosage form available as 0.3, 0.45, 0.625, 0.9, 1.25 mg
Esterified estrogens (75–85% estrone + 6–15% equilin)	Menest (once daily)	0.3 mg	0.3–2.5 mg	Administer 3 weeks on and 1 week off Dosage form available as 0.3, 0.625, 1.25, 2.5 mg
Estropipate (piperazine estrone sulfate)	Ogen, Ortho-Est, Generics (once daily)	0.75 mg	0.75–6 mg	Dosage form available as 0.75, 1, 5, 3, 6 mg
Estradiol acetate	Femtrace (once daily)	0.45 mg	0.45–1.8 mg	Dosage form available as 0.45, 0.9, 1.8 mg
Micronized 17β-estradiol	Estrace Generics (once daily)	1 mg	1 or 2 mg	Administer 3 weeks on and 1 week off Dosage form available as 1, 2 mg
Transdermal estrogens patches				
17β-estradiol	Alora (patch applied twice weekly)[c]	0.025 mg/day	0.025–0.1 mg/day	Dosage form available as 0.025, 0.05, 0.075, 0.1 mg/day
	Climara (patch applied once weekly)[c]	0.025 mg/day	0.025–0.1 mg/day	Dosage form available as 0.025, 0.0375, 0.05, 0.06, 0.075, 0.1 mg/day
	Menostar (patch applied once weekly)[c,d]	0.014 mg/day	0.014 mg/day	
	Estraderm (patch applied twice weekly)[c]	–	0.05 or 0.1 mg/day	Dosage form available as 0.05, 0.1 mg/day
	Vivelle, Vivelle Dot (patch applied twice weekly)[c]	0.025 mg/day	0.025–0.1 mg/day, 0.05 is standard dose	Dosage form available as 0.025, 0.0375, 0.05 (standard dose), 0.075, 0.1 mg/day
Other topical forms of estrogen				
17β-estradiol topical emulsion	Estrasorb 0.25% emulsion (topical once daily)	–	Two pouches (which delivers 0.05 mg of estradiol per day)	Apply to legs
17β-estradiol topical gel	EstroGel 0.06% metered-dose pump (topical once daily)	–	1.25 g/day (contains 0.75 mg estradiol)	Apply from wrist to shoulder
	Elestrin 0.06% metered-dose pump (topical once daily)		1–2 unit doses (1 unit dose: 0.87 g, which contains 0.52 mg estradiol)	Apply to upper arm
	Divigel 0.1% (topical once daily)	0.25 g	0.25–1 g (provides 0.25–1 mg of estradiol)	Apply to upper thigh. Dosage form available as 0.25, 0.5, 1 g
17β-estradiol transdermal spray	Evamist (topical once daily)	1 spray	2–3 sprays (1.53 mg of estradiol per spray)	Apply to inner surface of forearm
Implanted estrogens[e]				
Implanted 17β-estradiol	Estradiol pellets implanted subcutaneously every 6 months	25 mg	50–100 mg	
Vaginal estrogens				
Estradiol acetate vaginal ring	Femring (intravaginally; replaced every 3 months)	12.4 mg ring	12.4, 24.8 mg ring (delivers 0.05 or 0.1 mg estradiol/day)	
Intravaginal Estrogen Products (for the treatment of urogenital symptoms only/low systemic exposure)				
Conjugated equine estrogens (CEE) vaginal cream	Premarin		0.5–2 g/day (contains 0.625 mg CEE per g)	
17β-estradiol vaginal cream	Estrace		1 g/day (contains 0.1 mg estradiol per g)	
17β-estradiol vaginal ring	Estring (intravaginally; replaced every 90 days)		2 mg ring (delivers 0.0075 mg/day)	
Estradiol hemihydrate vaginal tablet	Vagifem (intravaginally; twice weekly)	10 mcg	10 or 25 mcg	

[a]United States brand names.
[b]Orally administered estrogens stimulate synthesis of hepatic proteins and increase circulating concentrations of sex hormone-binding globulin, which in turn may compromise the bioavailability of androgens and estrogens. Women with elevated triglyceride concentrations or significant liver function abnormalities are candidates for nonoral estrogen therapy.
[c]Do not apply estrogen patches on or near breasts. Avoid waistline as patch may rub off with tight-fitting clothing.
[d]FDA-approved for prevention of postmenopausal osteoporosis only.
[e]Not available in the United States.

Progestogens reduce nuclear estradiol receptor concentrations, suppress DNA synthesis, and decrease estrogen bioavailability by increasing the activity of endometrial 17-hydroxysteroid dehydrogenase, an enzyme responsible for converting estradiol to estrone.[72]

The first generation of progestogens included the C-19 androgenic progestogens norethindrone (also known as norethisterone), norgestrel, and levonorgestrel. More recent preparations have included the C-21 progestogens dydrogesterone and MPA, which are less androgenic. Drospirenone, a synthetic progestogen analog of the potassium-sparing diuretic spironolactone, has both antiandrogenic and antialdosterone properties. Micronized progesterone also has become available for use in postmenopausal women. The most commonly used oral progestogens are MPA, micronized progesterone, and norethindrone acetate. The latter can be administered transdermally in the form of a combined estrogen–progestogen patch.

Adverse Effects Common adverse effects of progestogens include irritability, weight gain, bloating, and headache. Changing from a cyclic to a continuous-combined regimen or changing from one progestogen to another may decrease the incidence or severity of untoward effects. Adverse effects of progestogens are difficult to evaluate and can vary with the agent administered. Some women experience "premenstrual-like" symptoms, such as mood swings, bloating, fluid retention, and sleep disturbance. Newer methods and routes of progestogen delivery (e.g., locally by an intrauterine device that releases levonorgestrel or a progesterone-containing bioadhesive vaginal gel) may be associated with fewer adverse effects.

Dose and Administration Several progestogen regimens designed to prevent endometrial hyperplasia are available (Table 65-3). Progestogens must be taken for a sufficient period of time during each cycle. A minimum of 12 to 14 days of progestogen therapy each month is required for complete protection against estrogen-induced endometrial hyperplasia.[89] Of note, use of even low-dose estrogen, including some intravaginal preparations, requires progestogen coadministration for endometrial protection in women with an intact uterus.[90] However, rarely is progestogen administration needed in women who have undergone hysterectomy (i.e., women with hysterectomy and a past history of endometriosis).

Methods of Combined Estrogen and Progestogen Administration

Four combination estrogen and progestogen regimens currently in use are continuous cyclic (sequential), continuous combined, continuous long-cycle (or cyclic withdrawal), and intermittent combined (or continuous-pulsed) hormone therapy.[91] Various hormone therapy regimens that combine an estrogen and a progestogen are available (Table 65-4).

TABLE 65-3 Progestogen Doses for Endometrial Protection (Oral Cyclic Administration)

Progestogen	Brand Name	Dosage
Dydrogesterone[a]	Duphaston	10–20 mg/day for 12–14 days per calendar month (oral dosage form available as 10 mg tablets)
Medroxyprogesterone acetate	Provera	5–10 mg/day for 12–14 days per calendar month (oral dosage form available as 2.5, 5, 10 mg tablets)
Micronized progesterone	Prometrium	200 mg/day for 12–14 days per calendar month (oral dosage form available as 100 and 200 mg tablets)
Norethindrone acetate	Aygestin[b]	5 mg/day for 12–14 days per calendar month (oral dosage form available as 2.5, 5 mg tablets)

[a]Not available in the United States.
[b]Not approved for postmenopausal hormone therapy in the United States.

TABLE 65-4 Common Combination Postmenopausal Hormone Therapy Regimens

Regimen	Brand name	Dosage
Oral Regimens		
Conjugated equine estrogen (CEE) + medroxyprogesterone acetate (MPA)	Prempro (continuous)	0.625 mg/2.5 MPA, 0.625 mg/5 mg daily Low dose: 0.3 mg/1.5 mg, 0.45 mg/1.5 mg daily
	Premphase (continuous sequential)	0.625 mg CEE daily only in the first 2 weeks of a 4-week cycle then 0.625 mg daily CEE + 5 mg MPA daily in the last 2 weeks of a 4-week cycle
Ethinyl estradiol (EE) + norethindrone acetate (NETA)	Generic, Femhrt (continuous)	5 mcg EE/1 mg NETA daily Low dose (Femhrt only): 2.5 mcg EE/0.5 mg NETA daily
Estradiol (E) + drospirenone (DRSP)	Angeliq (continuous)	1 mg E/5 mg DRSP daily Low dose: 0.5 mg E/0.25 mg DRSP daily
Estradiol (E) + norgestimate	Prefest (estrogen/intermittent progestogen)	1 mg E daily for first 3 days then 1 mg E/0.09 mg norgestimate daily for next 3 days; this pattern is repeated continuously
Estradiol (E) + norethindrone acetate (NETA)	Activella (continuous)	1 mg E/0.5 mg NETA daily Low-dose: 0.5 mg E/0.1 mg NETA daily
	Mimvey (continuous)	1 mg E/0.5 mg NETA daily
Transdermal Regimens		
Estradiol + norethindrone acetate patch	CombiPatch (continuous)	Continuous: 0.05/0.14 mg, 0.05/0.25 mg (apply 1 patch twice weekly)
	CombiPatch (continuous sequential)	Continuous sequential: 0.05 mg of an estradiol only patch (apply 1 patch twice weekly) in the first 2 weeks of a 4-week cycle then either dose of the CombiPatch (apply 1 patch twice weekly) in the last 2 weeks of a 4-week cycle
Estradiol (E) + levonorgestrel patch	Climara Pro (continuous)	0.045 mg E/0.015 mg/day (apply 1 patch once weekly)

CEE, conjugated equine estrogen; DRSP, drospirenone; E, estradiol; EE, ethinyl estradiol; NETA, norethindrone acetate; MPA, medroxyprogesterone acetate.

Continuous Cyclic Estrogen–Progestogen (Sequential) Treatment Estrogen typically is administered continuously (daily). A progestogen is coadministered with the estrogen for at least 12 to 14 days of a 28-day cycle.[89] The progestogen causes scheduled withdrawal bleeding in approximately 90% of women. With this regimen, bleeding usually begins 1 to 2 days after the last progestogen dose. Occasionally, bleeding begins during the latter phase of progestogen administration.

Continuous Combined Estrogen–Progestogen Treatment Continuous combined estrogen–progestogen administration results in endometrial atrophy and the absence of vaginal bleeding. Continuous combined hormone therapy is more acceptable than traditional cyclic therapy. This method of treatment can be achieved by using either commercially available oral and transdermal preparations or by administering systemic oral or nonoral estrogen along with the use of the levonorgestrel-releasing intrauterine system.

Continuous Long-Cycle Estrogen–Progestogen Treatment

This modified sequential regimen was developed to decrease the incidence of uterine bleeding.[91] In the continuous long-cycle (or cyclic withdrawal) estrogen–progestogen regimen, estrogen is given daily, and progestogen is given six times per year, every other month for 12 to 14 days, resulting in six periods per year. Bleeding episodes may be heavier and last for more days than withdrawal bleeding with continuous cyclic regimens. The effect of continuous long-cycle estrogen–progestogen treatment on endometrial protection is unclear.

Intermittent Combined Estrogen–Progestogen Treatment

The intermittent combined estrogen–progestogen regimen, also called *continuous-pulsed estrogen–progestogen* or *pulsed-progestogen*, consists of 3 days of estrogen therapy alone, followed by 3 days of combined estrogen and progestogen, which is then repeated without interruption.[91] This regimen is designed to lower the incidence of uterine bleeding. It is based on the assumption that pulsed-progestogen administration will prevent downregulation of progesterone receptors that can be produced by continuous combined regimens. The lower progestogen dose induces fewer side effects and can be better tolerated. The long-term effect of intermittent combined regimens in endometrial protection is undetermined.

Low-Dose Hormone Therapy

7 Increasingly, it has become recognized that use of hormone therapy at doses lower than those prescribed historically (i.e., prior to the WHI study) may be effective in the management of menopausal symptoms (Table 65-2). Low-dose estrogen regimens include 0.3 to 0.45 mg conjugated estrogens, 0.5 mg micronized 17β-estradiol, and 0.014 to 0.0375 mg transdermal 17β-estradiol patch.[13] The standard dose of estrogen previously believed to be effective in alleviating vasomotor symptoms is equivalent to 0.625 mg CEE,[30] but new evidence indicates that lower doses of estrogen also are effective in controlling postmenopausal symptoms and reducing bone loss.[92–95] The Women's Health, Osteoporosis, Progestin, Estrogen (HOPE) trial demonstrated equivalent symptom relief and bone density preservation without an increase in endometrial hyperplasia using lower doses of hormone therapy (CEE 0.45 mg/day and MPA 1.5 mg/day).[93–95] Even ultralow doses of 17β-estradiol delivered by a vaginal ring (Estring) improved serum lipid profiles and prevented bone loss in elderly women.[96] Whether lower doses of estrogen will be safer (lower incidence of venous thromboembolism and breast cancer) remains to be proven.

Compounded Hormones Compounded "bioidentical" hormone therapy has received much attention by patients, health care professionals, and the media since the initial publication of the WHI results. Advocates of this practice tout the benefits of natural rather than synthetic formulations of sex hormones. Often, these hormones are compounded in pharmacies to make a variety of formulations, in theory, to individualize hormone therapy based on each patient's specific physiologic hormone milieu as measured via salivary hormone concentrations. This strategy is thought to reduce the risk of adverse effects. However, there is a paucity of evidence regarding both their efficacy and safety.[97] Bioidentical hormones appear to carry the same risks as traditional hormone therapy. Several major medical organizations, along with the FDA, have released statements that dissuade against the use of this treatment approach.[98,99]

Other Treatments

In women who have contraindications to estrogen and progestogen use, prefer not to take estrogen and/or progestogen, or cannot tolerate estrogen and/or progestogen administration, a number of other medications may be considered, depending on the goals of therapy. These include the prescription medications testosterone, SERMs (only raloxifene is currently available in the United States), and tibolone (not currently available in the United States) as well as nonhormonal prescription medications (e.g., selective serotonin reuptake inhibitors). Some women prefer to use herbals and other natural therapies, but the efficacy and safety of these methods have not been definitively established.

Alternatives to estrogen for treatment of hot flushes include tibolone, selective serotonin reuptake inhibitors (e.g., paroxetine, fluoxetine), dual serotonin and norepinephrine reuptake inhibitors (e.g., venlafaxine), MPA, megestrol acetate, clonidine, and gabapentin (Table 65-5).[100] Progestogens alone may be an option for some women (e.g., those with a history of venous thrombosis), but weight gain, vaginal bleeding, and other adverse effects often limit their use. Tibolone and progestogens cannot be considered nonhormonal agents for treatment of hot flushes in women for whom hormone therapy is contraindicated. For this group of patients, selective serotonin reuptake inhibitors and venlafaxine are considered by some to be a first-line therapy.[100,101] However, the efficacy of venlafaxine for treatment of hot flushes has not been shown to extend beyond 12 weeks.[102] Furthermore, in breast cancer patients, evidence suggests that selective serotonin reuptake inhibitors could interfere with metabolism of endocrine therapies, such as tamoxifen via cytochrome P450 2D6 inhibition.[103] Clonidine is often effective for symptom control, but its side effects (e.g., sedation, dry mouth, hypotension) are not always well tolerated by women.

Androgens

Pathophysiologic states affecting ovarian and adrenal function, along with aging, have been associated with androgen deficiency in women.[104] The therapeutic use of testosterone in women, although controversial, is becoming more widespread despite the lack of accurate clinical or biochemical findings of androgen deficiency.[104] Androgens have important biologic effects in women, acting both directly via androgen receptors in tissues, such as bone, skin fibroblasts, hair follicles, and sebaceous glands, and indirectly via the aromatization of testosterone to estrogen in the ovaries, bone, brain, adipose tissue, and other tissues.

Efficacy A cluster of symptoms that characterizes androgen insufficiency in women, manifested as diminished sense of well-being, persistent or unexplained fatigue, and sexual function changes such as decreased libido, decreased sexual receptivity, and decreased pleasure has been reported.[104] However, studies designed to evaluate this have shown no relationships between serum total and free testosterone levels and either sexual function[105] or well-being[106] in women. Thus, as data supporting an androgen deficiency syndrome are lacking, in 2006 the American Endocrine Society recommended against making a diagnosis of androgen deficiency in women at the present time.[105] Several large randomized placebo-controlled clinical trials involving naturally[107,108] and surgically[109] postmenopausal women presenting with low libido demonstrate that testosterone therapy, with and without concurrent estrogen therapy, improves the quality of the sexual experience, with preliminary data that this may also apply to premenopausal women.[110]

Adverse Effects Absolute contraindications to androgen therapy include pregnancy or lactation and known or suspected androgen-dependent neoplasia. Relative contraindications include concurrent use of CEEs (for systemic testosterone therapy), low sex hormone-binding globulin level (below the normal range for women) moderate to severe acne, clinical hirsutism, and androgenic alopecia.

Adverse effects from excessive dosage include virilization, fluid retention, and potentially adverse lipoprotein lipid effects, which are more likely with oral administration. There is no evidence that systemic transdermal testosterone is associated with increased cardiovascular morbidity or mortality[111] or of a significant change in the risk of invasive breast cancer.[112,113] However, further

TABLE 65-5 Alternatives to Estrogen for Treatment of Hot Flushes[a]

Drug	Brand Name[b]	Initial Dose	Usual Dose Range	Comments
Tibolone[c]	Livial (not available in the United States)	2.5 mg	2.5 mg/day	Tibolone is not recommended during the perimenopause period because it may cause irregular bleeding
Venlafaxine	Effexor, Effexor XR	37.5 mg	37.5–150 mg/day	Adverse effects include nausea, headache, somnolence, dizziness, insomnia, nervousness, xerostomia, anorexia, constipation, diaphoresis, weakness, and hypertension
Desvenlafaxine	Pristiq	100–150 mg	100–150 mg/day	Adverse effects include nausea, headache, somnolence, dizziness, insomnia, xerostomia, anorexia, constipation, diaphoresis, and weakness
Paroxetine, paroxetine CR[d]	Brisdelle,[e] Paxil, Paxil CR, Pexeva	17.5 mg/day (paroxetine),[e] 10 mg/day (paroxetine), or 12.5 mg/day (paroxetine CR)	7.5 mg/day,[e] 10–20 mg/day or 12.5–25 mg/day	Adverse effects include nausea, somnolence, insomnia, headache, dizziness, xerostomia, constipation, diarrhea, weakness, and diaphoresis
Megestrol acetate	Megace	20 mg/day	20–40 mg/day	Progesterone may be linked to breast cancer etiology; also, there is concern regarding the safety of progestational agents in women with preexisting breast cancer
Clonidine	Catapres and generic tablets (oral) Catapres-TTS (transdermal) Kapvay tablets (extended release; oral)	0.1 mg/day	0.1 mg/day	Adverse effects include drowsiness, dizziness, hypotension, and dry mouth, especially with higher doses
Gabapentin	Gralise, Neurontin	300 mg at bedtime	900 mg/day (divided in three daily doses), doses up to 2,400 mg/day (divided in three daily doses) have been studied	Adverse effects include somnolence and dizziness; these symptoms often can be obviated with a gradual increase in dosing

CR, controlled release.

[a]Treatment of postmenopausal hot flushes is an off-label indication in the United States for all medications listed except for one formulation of paroxetine.
[b]United States brand names.
[c]Not available in the United States.
[d]Other selective serotonin reuptake inhibitors (e.g., citalopram, escitalopram, fluoxetine, and sertraline) have also been studied may also be used for the treatment of hot flushes.
[e]The brand Brisdelle contains 7.5 mg of paroxetine and is FDA-approved to treat moderate to severe vasomotor symptoms of menopause. This specific product is not FDA-approved for treating psychiatric conditions.

Data from references 149–151.

studies are required to determine the long-term safety of testosterone in women.

Dose and Administration Testosterone is available as oral methyltestosterone in the United States. Methyltestosterone in combination with esterified estrogen (either 0.625 mg esterified estrogen plus 1.25 mg methyltestosterone or 1.25 mg esterified estrogen plus 2.5 mg methyltestosterone) is the most widely studied.

Testosterone replacement for women is available in a variety of formulations (Table 65-6). Most of the earlier studies showing clinical improvement with testosterone therapy reported supraphysiologic levels. More recent studies using transdermal patch therapy have shown efficacy with free testosterone levels in the upper normal range for young women. The availability of testosterone regimens specifically designed for women has the potential to maintain testosterone levels within the normal range and help to clarify whether the apparent beneficial effects of testosterone therapy are physiologic or pharmacologic.[109,114] In general, testosterone treatment can be administered to postmenopausal women with and without concurrent estrogen therapy. At present, generalized use of testosterone is not recommended because the indications are inadequate, and evidence from long-term studies evaluating safety is lacking.[115]

Selective Estrogen Receptor Modulators

SERMs are a group of nonsteroidal compounds that are chemically distinct from estradiol. They act as estrogen agonists in some tissues, such as bone, and as estrogen antagonists in other tissues, such as breast, through specific, high-affinity binding to the estrogen receptor.

Efficacy The ideal SERM would protect against osteoporosis and decrease the incidence of breast, endometrial, and colorectal cancer and CHD without exacerbating menopausal symptoms or increasing the risk of venous thromboembolism or gallbladder disease. To date, no SERM meets these ideals. Tamoxifen, the first-generation SERM (a nonsteroidal triphenylethylene derivative), has estrogen

TABLE 65-6 Androgen Regimens Used for Women

Regimen	Brand Name	Usual Dose	Frequency	Comments
Methyltestosterone in combination with esterified estrogens	Covaryx	2.5 mg methyltestosterone + 1.25 mg esterified estrogens daily	Daily	Oral
	Covaryx HS	1.25 mg methyltestosterone + 0.625 mg esterified estrogens daily Both regimens given 3 weeks on and 1 week off		
Testosterone pellets[b]	Testopel	50 mg[c]	Every 6 months	Subcutaneous (implanted)
Transdermal testosterone system[a]	Intrinsa	150 or 300 mcg/day	Every 3–4 days	Transdermal patch

[a]Not available in the United States.
[b]Not approved for use in women in the United States.
[c]Only 75 mg pellets available in the United States.

antagonist activity on the breast and estrogen-like agonist activity on bone and endometrium. The second-generation SERM raloxifene, a nonsteroidal benzothiophene derivative, is used to reduce the risk of postmenopausal osteoporosis and invasive breast cancer, and also for treatment of postmenopausal osteoporosis. The third generation of SERMs, bazedoxifene and lasofoxifene, have similar efficacy and adverse effect profile compared to raloxifene.[75] These new SERMs are approved only in Europe. SERMs do not alleviate, or may even exacerbate, vasomotor symptoms, and increase the risk for venous thromboembolism.[75]

Raloxifene increases BMD in the spine and femoral neck and reduces the risk of vertebral fractures.[116] It has not been shown to decrease the risk of hip fractures. Raloxifene decreases bone loss in recently menopausal women without affecting the endometrium and has estrogen-like actions on lipid metabolism.[116] Lasofoxifene and bazedoxifene have shown similar effects.[117,118] Raloxifene use is associated with a significantly lower incidence of breast cancer compared with placebo.[76,119] This benefit is primarily due to a reduced risk of estrogen receptor-positive invasive breast cancers.[76,119] A prospective randomized double-blinded trial of 19,747 women at high risk for breast cancer (Study of Tamoxifen and Raloxifene [STAR]) showed that raloxifene is as effective as tamoxifen in reducing the risk of invasive breast cancer and has a lower risk of thromboembolic events.[120] The tissue-selective estrogen complex (TSEC), a novel regimen pairing a SERM with one estrogen, is currently under investigation aiming to treat both menopausal symptoms and bone loss.

Ospemifene is an orally administered SERM approved by the FDA in the first quarter of 2013 for the treatment of moderate-to-severe dyspareunia from menopausal vulvar and vaginal atrophy. Ospemifene's labeling carries a boxed warning about its estrogenic effect on the endometrium: there is an increased risk of endometrial hyperplasia and endometrial cancer in a woman with a uterus who takes unopposed estrogen therapy. Ospemifene also has a boxed warning about the possible risk of stroke and venous thromboembolism. At the time of writing, safety data longer than 1 year have not been published.

Adverse Effects SERMs are commonly associated with hot flushes and less often with leg cramps. SERMs increase the risk of venous thromboembolism[76,116–118] and fatal stroke[76] to a degree similar to that of oral estrogen.

Dose and Administration Raloxifene is FDA-approved for the treatment and prevention of postmenopausal osteoporosis and for the reduction of the risk of invasive breast cancer in postmenopausal women with osteoporosis as well as postmenopausal women at high risk for invasive breast cancer. The dose is 60 mg orally once daily.

Tibolone

Tibolone is a gonadomimetic synthetic steroid in the norpregnane family with combined estrogenic, progestogenic, and androgenic activity.[121] Tibolone has been used for three decades in Europe for treatment of menopausal symptoms and prevention of osteoporosis but is currently not available in the United States. The hormonal effects of this synthetic steroid depend on its metabolism and activation in peripheral tissues. The parent compound has been described as a prodrug that is metabolized quickly in the GI tract. It has several active metabolites, including a $\Delta 4$-isomer and 3α-OH and 3β-OH compounds.[121] The $\Delta 4$-isomer metabolite confers significant progestogenic and androgenic properties.

Efficacy Tibolone has beneficial effects on mood and libido and improves menopausal symptoms and vaginal atrophy. Tibolone protects against bone loss and significantly reduces the risk of vertebral fractures in postmenopausal women with osteoporosis.[122] It has also been shown to decrease the risk of breast cancer and colon cancer in healthy women aged 60 to 85 years.[122] It is also more effective than conventional hormone therapy for management of sexual dysfunction.[123]

Adverse Effects Tibolone use in elderly women has been reported to be associated with an increased risk of stroke.[122] Tibolone use is associated with breast cancer recurrence in breast cancer patients with vasomotor symptoms.[124] Tibolone lowers concentrations of total cholesterol, triglycerides, and lipoprotein (a) but may decrease high-density lipoprotein (HDL) cholesterol.[85] The Million Women Study, an observational cohort study, found a greater risk of endometrial cancer (adjusted relative risk 1.79, 95% CI: 1.43 to 2.25).[125] However, other randomized placebo-controlled studies have not shown an increased risk of endometrial cancer with tibolone and suggest that tibolone has an endometrial safety profile similar to continuous combined CEE and MPA.[126]

The most commonly reported adverse effects of tibolone include weight gain and bloating.

Complementary and Alternative Medicine

Some women prefer to use natural remedies due to a belief that they are safer. Randomized, placebo-controlled trials of complementary and alternative therapies have been equivocal and have not established the safety and efficacy of herbal remedies, homeopathic treatments, or acupuncture for the prevention or treatment of hot flushes.

Phytoestrogens Phytoestrogens have physiologic effects in humans.[127] They are plant compounds with estrogen-like biologic activity and relatively weak estrogen receptor-binding properties. Epidemiologic studies suggest that consumption of a phytoestrogen-rich diet, which is common in traditional Asian societies, is associated with a lower risk of breast cancer.[127]

The biologic potencies of phytoestrogens vary. Most of these compounds are nonsteroidal and are less potent than synthetic estrogens. The three main classes of phytoestrogens are isoflavones, lignans, and coumestans, all of which are found in plants or their seeds.[127] The most commonly studied phytoestrogen is the isoflavone class. Genistein and daidzein are the most abundant active components of isoflavones. The concentration of isoflavones per gram of soy protein varies considerably among preparations. Also, a single plant often contains more than one class of phytoestrogen. Common food sources of phytoestrogens include soybeans (isoflavones), cereals, oilseeds such as flaxseed (lignans), and alfalfa sprouts (coumestans).

Mild estrogenic effects have been seen in postmenopausal women,[127] but current data suggest that phytoestrogen supplementation is no more effective than placebo in relieving hot flushes or other symptoms of menopause in postmenopausal women.[128]

Phytoestrogens decrease low-density lipoprotein (LDL) cholesterol and triglyceride concentrations with no significant change in HDL cholesterol concentrations.[129] Furthermore, phytoestrogens have the ability to inhibit LDL oxidation and normalize vascular reactivity in estrogen-deprived primates.[129] In addition, BMD may be improved by phytoestrogens.[127] Common adverse effects include constipation, bloating, and nausea.[130]

A recent meta-analysis reported that phytoestrogen use is not associated with increased rates of endometrial cancer, vaginal bleeding, and breast cancer.[130] Large, long-term studies are needed to further document the effects of phytoestrogens on the breast, bone, and endometrium. Furthermore, differences among classes of phytoestrogens must be identified clearly, including dosing and biologic activity, before phytoestrogens can be considered an alternative to conventional hormone therapy in postmenopausal women.

Other Herbal Products Black cohosh (*Cimicifuga racemosa* or *Actaea racemosa*), a widely used herbal supplement, may not offer substantial benefits for relief of vasomotor symptoms as suggested by earlier trials.[131] This substance does not appear to have strong intrinsic estrogenic properties but may act through the serotonergic system. Black cohosh appears to be generally well tolerated, although hepatotoxicity has been reported. It is unclear if this is due to the herb itself or adulterations of commercially available products.[132] The long-term effects of black cohosh are unknown. Other herbals and alternative treatments that may be used by women include dong quai, red clover leaf (contains phytoestrogens), kava, and dehydroepiandrosterone. These have not been shown to be effective in the treatment of menopausal symptoms and may carry the risk of adverse events.[133] Complementary and alternative therapies should not be recommended to treat menopausal symptoms.

Personalized Pharmacotherapy

The severity of menopausal symptoms varies widely from woman to woman. The decision to use menopausal hormone therapy must be individualized and based on several parameters, including vasomotor and urogenital symptoms, osteoporosis risk, cardiovascular disease risk, breast cancer risk, and thromboembolism risk. Hormone therapy is not indicated for prevention of chronic diseases of aging.

Moderate and severe menopausal symptoms likely require pharmacologic therapy, after the exclusion of possible contraindications for hormone therapy (Table 65-1). Estrogen therapy is the most effective treatment for moderate and severe vasomotor symptoms, impaired sleep quality, and urogenital symptoms of menopause (Fig. 65-1). A thorough discussion of the risks and benefits of hormone therapy should be completed with the patient so that she can weigh the risks and benefits versus alternatives and make a rational decision about whether to use hormone therapy. For a healthy recently menopausal woman who has vasomotor symptoms, the benefits of hormonal therapy outweigh the risks. The risk primary involves the venous thromboembolism risk. The benefits include the control of vasomotor symptoms, treatment of urogenital atrophy, and prevention of postmenopausal bone loss.

Hormone therapy should be tailored for optimal formulation, dose, route of delivery, and counseling should be based on age, years since menopause, and hysterectomy status. Women who have undergone hysterectomy use hormone therapy more frequently than do women with an intact uterus (58.7% vs. 19.6%).[134]

Estrogens diminish hot flushes in most women, and all types and routes of administration of estrogen are equally effective.[13] A dose-dependent relationship between estrogen administration and suppression of hot flushes is well established. Some women, especially younger women, may require a higher than average dose of estrogen to suppress symptoms. On the other hand, many women with hot flushes at the time of menopause require lower doses of estrogen.[135] Initiating therapy with low doses of estrogen often will minimize adverse effects, such as breast tenderness and unscheduled bleeding. Transdermal estradiol is less likely than oral estrogen to cause nausea and headache. In many cases changing from one estrogen regimen to another can alleviate certain adverse effects.

Prior to initiating pharmacologic therapy, a complete medical history and physical examination should be performed. Medical history should include a personal and family history of cardiovascular disease and thrombotic problems. The physical examination should include a complete cardiovascular examination, clinical assessment of thyroid status, and breast and pelvic examinations. Papanicolaou cervical cytologic examination and screening mammography negative for malignancy are required before initiating hormone therapy. Thyroid function tests and lipoprotein lipid profile also are performed at the discretion of the clinician. Oral estrogen should be avoided in women with hypertriglyceridemia, liver disease, and gallbladder disease. For these women, transdermal administration is a safer approach. Sequential estrogen/progestogen therapy results in scheduled vaginal withdrawal bleeding but often is scant or completely absent in older women. For many women, scheduled withdrawal bleeding is one of the main reasons for avoiding or discontinuing hormone therapy. Because there is no physiologic need for bleeding, new hormone therapy regimens that reduce monthly bleeding (e.g., continuous long-cycle regimens) or prevent monthly bleeding (e.g., continuous combined and intermittent combined regimens) were developed. Continuous combined estrogen–progestogen administration results in endometrial atrophy and the absence of vaginal bleeding. Initially, it causes unpredictable spotting or bleeding, which usually resolves within 6 to 12 months. Decreasing the estrogen dose or increasing the progestogen dose usually decreases or stops the spotting. Occasionally, a drug-free period of 1 or 2 weeks is useful to stop the bleeding. Women who recently have undergone menopause have a higher risk for excessive, unpredictable bleeding while receiving continuous therapy; thus, this regimen is best reserved for women who are at least 2 years postmenopause.

If hormone therapy is to be initiated, the selection of the drug should also take into account the potential for drug interactions, including those involving the cytochrome P450 (CYP450) microsomal enzyme system. Estrogen is metabolized partly by the CYP 450 isoenzymes 1A2 and 3A4, and the progestin medroxyprogesterone is metabolized by CYP450 3A4. Inducers or inhibitors of these enzymes may either decrease or increase, respectively, the therapeutic effects or result in side effects. Similarly, selection of nonhormonal drug therapy options should take into account the potential for interactions with other prescription and nonprescription medications the patient may be taking. Selective serotonin reuptake inhibitors and serotonin norepinephrine reuptake inhibitors can have major interactions with other drugs also affecting CYP450 2D6 and 3A4 (Chap. 51). Patients using vaginal estrogen creams or nonestrogen vaginal moisturizers should be warned that products with oil-based lubricants or vehicles can weaken latex condoms, which can decrease protection against sexually transmitted infections. Pharmacodynamic drug interactions (e.g., additive side effects) should also be considered.

Evaluation of Therapeutic Outcomes

Even before publication of the WHI trial findings, only a fraction of women filled their hormone therapy prescriptions, and only 25% to 40% continued to take postmenopausal hormone therapy for more than 1 year.[136] Hormone therapy use in the United States declined substantially after dissemination of the WHI trial results.[137]

The main reasons for discontinuing hormone therapy are side effects such as bleeding, breast tenderness, bloating, and "premenstrual-like symptoms." Reducing the dose or changing the regimen or the route of administration can minimize these effects. Alternatively, if vasomotor symptoms are not controlled adequately with a lower-dose regimen, increasing the estrogen dose may be a reasonable option. Therefore, after the menopausal woman begins hormone therapy, a brief follow-up visit 6 weeks later may be useful to discuss patient concerns about hormone therapy and to evaluate the patient for symptom relief, adverse effects, and patterns of withdrawal bleeding (Table 65-7). Women receiving hormone therapy should be seen by the clinician for annual monitoring (Table 65-7).

The main indication for hormone therapy is relief of menopausal symptoms. If combined estrogen/progestogen treatment is stopped within 5 years, no evidence of increased risk of breast cancer is observed.[25] Estrogen-only treatment is not associated with an increased risk of breast cancer.[52]

Many women have no difficulty abruptly stopping hormone therapy; others develop vasomotor symptoms after discontinuation. Although these symptoms may be mild and resolve over a few months, in some women the symptoms are severe and intolerable. There is no evidence that gradual discontinuation of hormone therapy reduces the recurrence of hot flushes compared with sudden discontinuation.[138]

TABLE 65-7 Monitoring Patients Taking Hormone Therapy Regimens

Drug	Adverse Drug Reaction	Monitoring Parameter	Suggested Change
Initiation of Hormone Therapy Hormone therapy should be used only as long as symptom control is necessary (typically 2–3 years)			
6-Week Follow-up Visit • To discuss patient concerns about hormone therapy • To evaluate the patient for symptom relief, adverse effects, and patterns of withdrawal bleeding (if continuous sequential hormone therapy is given)			
Estrogen		Persistence of hot flushes	Increase estrogen dose
Estrogen	Breast tenderness		Reduce estrogen dose; switch to a transdermal regimen
Progestogen	Bloating Premenstrual-like symptoms		Switch to another progestogen
Annual Follow-up Visit			
Annual monitoring: medical history, physical examination, pelvic examination, blood pressure measurement, and routine endometrial cancer surveillance (as indicated). Additional follow-up is determined based on the patient's initial response to therapy and the need for any modification of the regimen **Breast examinations:** perform monthly breast self-examinations, and receive periodic mammograms (scheduled based on patient's age and risk factors) **Osteoporosis prevention:** BMD should be measured in women 65 years and older and in women younger than 65 years with risk factors for osteoporosis. Although bone densitometry has been shown to predict fractures, at present there are no guidelines for follow-up BMD testing. However, in women with significant bone loss, repeat testing should be performed as clinically indicated			
In women taking sequential hormone therapy	Transvaginal ultrasound, and where indicated an endometrial biopsy should be performed if vaginal bleeding occurs at any time other than the expected time of withdrawal bleeding or when heavier or more prolonged withdrawal bleeding occurs (if endometrial pathology cannot be excluded by endovaginal ultrasonography, further evaluation may be required, such as hysteroscopy)		
In women taking continuous combined hormone therapy	Endometrial evaluation should be considered when irregular bleeding persists for more than 6 months after initiating therapy		

BMD, bone mineral density.

TABLE 65-8 Evidence-Based Hormone Therapy Guidelines for Menopausal Symptom Management

Recommendation	Recommendation Grade[a]
In the absence of contraindications, estrogen-based postmenopausal hormone therapy should be used for treatment of moderate to severe vasomotor symptoms	A1
Systemic or vaginal estrogen therapy should be used for treatment of urogenital symptoms and vaginal atrophy	A1
Postmenopausal women taking estrogen-based therapy should be followed up every year, taking into account findings from new clinical trials	A1
Postmenopausal women taking estrogen-based therapy should be informed about potential risks	A1
Safety and tolerability may vary substantially with the type and regimen of hormone therapy	B2
Breast cancer risk increases after use of continuous combined hormone therapy for longer than 5 years	A1
Breast cancer risk does not increase after long-term estrogen-only therapy (6.8 years) in postmenopausal women with hysterectomy	A1
Hormone therapy should not be used for primary or secondary prevention of coronary heart disease	A1
Oral hormone therapy increases risk of venous thromboembolism	A1
Nonoral hormone therapy may be safer for postmenopausal women at risk for venous thromboembolism who choose to take hormone therapy	B2
Oral hormone therapy increases risk of ischemic stroke	A1
Although hormone therapy decreases risk of osteoporotic fractures, it cannot be recommended as a first-line therapy for the treatment of osteoporosis	A1
Potential harm (cardiovascular disease, breast cancer, and thromboembolism) from long-term hormone therapy (use greater than 5 years) outweighs potential benefits	A1
Young women with primary ovarian insufficiency have severe menopausal symptoms and increased risk for osteoporosis and cardiovascular disease. Decisions on whether and how these young women must be treated should not be based on studies of hormone therapy in women older than 50 years	B3

Quality of evidence: 1, evidence from more than one properly randomized controlled trial; 2, evidence from more than one well-designed clinical trial with randomization from cohort or case-controlled analytic studies or multiple time series, or dramatic results from uncontrolled experiments; 3, evidence from opinions of respected authorities based on clinical experience, descriptive studies, or reports of expert communities.

[a]*Strength of recommendations*: A, good evidence to support recommendation; B, moderate evidence to support recommendation; C, poor evidence to support recommendation.

Conclusions

Menopause is a natural life event, not a disease. Therefore, the decision to use hormone therapy must be individualized based on the severity of menopausal symptoms, risk of osteoporosis fracture, and consideration of factors such as cardiovascular disease, breast cancer, and thromboembolism (Table 65-8).

The WHI trial reported increased risk of cardiovascular disease, breast cancer, stroke, and thromboembolic disease among women using continuous combined therapy with CEE plus MPA compared with placebo. In the estrogen-alone arm of the study, CEE had no effect on cardiovascular disease or breast cancer risk compared to placebo, but an increased risk of stroke and thromboembolic disease was noted in those who received estrogen. The WHI trial also demonstrated that quality of life and cognition were no better in the group receiving hormone therapy than in the placebo group, and that hormone therapy increases dementia risk in women 65 years or older.

In the absence of contraindications, hormone therapy is the most effective treatment for managing postmenopausal symptoms, such as hot flushes, night sweats, and vaginal dryness. For short-term use of hormone therapy for relief of menopausal symptoms, the benefits for many women outweigh the risks. For symptoms of genital atrophy alone, local estrogen, nonhormonal lubricants, or ospemifene should be considered.

Long-term use of hormone therapy cannot be recommended routinely for osteoporosis prevention given the availability of alternative therapies, such as bisphosphonates and raloxifene. For long-term hormone therapy use, the potential harm (cardiovascular disease, breast cancer, and thromboembolism) outweighs the potential benefits. Hormone therapy should not be used for prevention of CHD. Women with cardiovascular risk factors (e.g., hypertension, lipid abnormalities) can benefit from reduction of these risk factors through interventions such as weight loss, lipid-lowering therapy, use of aspirin, and physical activity.

PRIMARY OVARIAN INSUFFICIENCY AND PREMENOPAUSAL HORMONE REPLACEMENT THERAPY

Primary ovarian insufficiency is a condition characterized by sex-steroid deficiency, amenorrhea, and infertility in women younger than 40 years.[139] Primary ovarian insufficiency was once considered irreversible and was described as "premature menopause," and the condition is still referred to as *premature ovarian failure*. However, primary ovarian insufficiency is not an early, natural menopause. Normal menopause results from ovarian follicle depletion, whereas primary ovarian insufficiency is characterized by intermittent ovarian function in half of affected women.[139] These women produce estrogen intermittently and may ovulate despite the presence of high gonadotropin concentrations. Pregnancies have occurred in 5% to 10% of women after the diagnosis of premature ovarian failure, even in women with no follicles observed on ovarian biopsy.

TABLE 65-9 Etiology of Primary Ovarian Insufficiency

Idiopathic or karyotypically normal spontaneous primary ovarian insufficiency
Autoimmunity: (A) Isolated autoimmune primary ovarian insufficiency (B) As a component of an autoimmune polyglandular syndrome in association with Addison's disease, hypothyroidism, hypoparathyroidism, or mucocutaneous candidiasis (*AIRE* gene mutations; 21q22.3)
Ovarian insufficiency due to chemotherapy, radiation, and extensive ovarian surgery
Chromosomal abnormalities: (A) X-chromosome defects (X-monosomy; X-mosaicism; X-chromosome translocations or partial deletions; *FMR1* gene permutations, Xq27,3; *FMR2* gene permutations, Xq28; *BMP15* gene mutation, Xp11.2) (B) Autosomal chromosome abnormalities
Gonadotropin-receptor abnormalities affecting ovarian function (FSH-receptor gene mutations, 2p21-p16; LH-receptor gene mutations, 2p21)
Enzyme deficiencies affecting ovarian function (A) Cholesterol desmolase deficiency (B) 17α-hydroxylase deficiency (C) 17–20 desmolase deficiency
Galactosemia (galactose-1-phosphate uridyl transferase, *GALT* gene mutations, 9p13)
Blepharophimosis, ptosis, and epicanthus in versus syndrome type 1 (autosomal dominant syndrome, in which primary ovarian insufficiency is the predominant syndrome)
Perrault's syndrome (familial autosomal recessive primary ovarian insufficiency in association with deafness)

Epidemiology

The prevalence of primary ovarian insufficiency increases with increasing age, reaching approximately 1% of women by age 40 years.[140]

Etiology

A number of physiologic or metabolic abnormalities can lead to primary ovarian insufficiency (Table 65-9). In most cases, the etiology cannot be identified.

Pathophysiology

Primary ovarian insufficiency may occur as a result of ovarian follicle dysfunction or ovarian follicle depletion and may present as either primary amenorrhea (absence of menses in a girl who has reached age 16 years) or secondary amenorrhea (cessation of menses in a woman previously menstruating for at least 6 months). Approximately 50% of women with primary ovarian insufficiency have documented ovarian follicle function.[139]

Clinical Presentation

No characteristic menstrual pattern or history precedes primary ovarian insufficiency. Approximately 50% of patients with this condition have a history of oligomenorrhea or dysfunctional uterine bleeding (prodromal premature ovarian failure), and approximately 25% develop amenorrhea acutely. Some patients develop amenorrhea postpartum, whereas others experience amenorrhea after discontinuing oral contraceptives. Primary amenorrhea is not associated with symptoms of estrogen deficiency. In cases of secondary amenorrhea, symptoms may include hot flushes, night sweats, fatigue, and mood changes. Prodromal primary ovarian insufficiency may present with hot flushes even in women who menstruate regularly. Incomplete development of secondary sex characteristics may occur

CLINICAL PRESENTATION AND DIAGNOSIS Primary Ovarian Insufficiency

Symptoms

- Primary amenorrhea: no symptoms of estrogen deficiency
- Secondary amenorrhea: vasomotor symptoms (hot flushes and night sweats), sleep disturbances, mood changes, sexual dysfunction, problems with concentration and memory, vaginal dryness, and dyspareunia

Signs

- Primary amenorrhea: incomplete development of secondary sex characteristics
- Secondary amenorrhea: normal development of secondary sex characteristics, signs of urogenital atrophy

Laboratory Tests

- FSH greater than 40 international units/L (40 IU/L)
- Other relevant diagnostic tests (e.g., bone mineral density, ultrasound of the ovaries)
- Thyroid function tests, fasting glucose level, and adrenocorticotropic hormone stimulation test

in women with primary amenorrhea, whereas these characteristics typically are normal in women with secondary amenorrhea. In general, women with primary ovarian insufficiency have normal fertility before the disorder develops.

Primary ovarian insufficiency is defined by the presence of at least 4 months of amenorrhea and at least two serum FSH concentrations measuring greater than 40 international units/L (40 IU/L) (obtained at least 1 month apart) in women younger than 40 years. A complete history should be taken, considering other factors that can affect ovarian function such as prior ovarian surgery, chemotherapy, radiation, and autoimmune disorders. In patients with primary amenorrhea, particular attention should be paid to breast and pubic hair development according to Tanner stages. Short stature, stigmata of Turner syndrome, and other dysmorphic features of gonadal dysgenesis should be considered. Ideally, a pelvic examination is performed but is not always clinically appropriate. Alternatively, transabdominal ultrasonography can be performed in patients with primary amenorrhea to confirm the presence of normal anatomic structures. In the majority of cases, physical examination is completely normal. A karyotype should be performed in all patients experiencing primary ovarian insufficiency. Women with ovarian insufficiency and a karyotype containing a Y chromosome should undergo bilateral gonadectomy because of substantial risk for gonadal germ cell neoplasia.[139] Ovarian biopsy and antiovarian antibody testing are investigational procedures with no proven clinical benefit in primary ovarian insufficiency. As clinically indicated, the workup should include tests for the diagnosis of other possible associated autoimmune disorders, such as hypothyroidism, diabetes mellitus, and Addison's disease.

In the majority of patients, ovarian insufficiency develops after the establishment of regular menses. Young women with primary ovarian insufficiency who develop ovarian dysfunction before they achieve peak adult bone mass sustain sex steroid deficiency for more years than do naturally menopausal women. This deficiency can result in a significantly higher risk for osteoporosis[141] and cardiovascular disease.[142,143] Importantly, a survey of more than 19,000 women between the ages of 25 and 100 years suggests that ovarian insufficiency occurring before age 40 years is associated with significantly increased mortality, with an age-adjusted odds ratio for all-cause mortality of 2.14 (95% CI: 1.15 to 3.99).[144]

Young women find the diagnosis of primary ovarian insufficiency particularly traumatic and frequently need extensive emotional and psychological support. Although most of these women will, in fact, be infertile, it is important to emphasize that primary ovarian insufficiency can be transient and that spontaneous pregnancies have occurred even years after diagnosis.

TREATMENT

8 Results from randomized trials of hormone therapy in postmenopausal women cannot be extrapolated to premenopausal women with ovarian dysfunction. Postmenopausal women who take hormone therapy prolong their exposure to estrogen beyond the average age of completion of their reproductive phase. In contrast, women with primary ovarian insufficiency need exogenous sex steroids to compensate for the decreased production by their ovaries. Importantly, 47% of young women with primary ovarian insufficiency have significantly reduced BMD within 1.5 years of their diagnosis despite taking standard hormone therapy.[141]

Desired Outcome

The goal of therapy in young women with primary ovarian insufficiency is to provide a hormone replacement regimen that maintains sex steroid status as effectively as the normal, functioning ovary.

General Approach to Treatment

Hormone therapy with estrogen, progestogen, and testosterone is used and generally should be continued until the average age of natural menopause.

Personalized Pharmacotherapy

Optimal hormone therapy depends on whether the patient has primary or secondary amenorrhea. Young women with primary amenorrhea in whom secondary sex characteristics have failed to develop initially should be given very low doses of estrogen in an attempt to mimic the gradual pubertal maturation process. A typical regimen is 0.3 mg CEE unopposed (i.e., no progestogen) daily for 6 months, with incremental dose increases at 6-month intervals until the required maintenance dose is achieved. Gradual dose escalation often results in optimal breast development and allows time for the young woman to adjust psychologically to her physical maturation. Cyclic progestogen therapy, given 12 to 14 days per month, should be instituted toward the end of the second year of treatment.

Women with secondary amenorrhea who have been estrogen deficient for 12 months or longer also should be given low-dose estrogen replacement initially to avoid adverse effects such as mastalgia and nausea. However, the dose can be titrated up to maintenance levels over a 6-month period, and progestogen therapy can be instituted with the initiation of estrogen therapy. Women with a brief history of secondary amenorrhea are less likely to experience undesired effects from hormone therapy if they are given a reduced dose for the first month of therapy, followed by a full dose from the second month onward.

An estrogen dose equivalent to at least 1.25 mg CEE (or 100 mcg transdermal estradiol) is needed to achieve adequate estrogen replacement in young women. A progestogen should be given for 12 to 14 days per calendar month to prevent endometrial hyperplasia (Table 65-10). Estrogens given in usual replacement doses do not suppress spontaneous follicular activity or ovulation. Because women with primary ovarian insufficiency can have spontaneous pregnancies, hormone therapy should produce regular, predictable menstrual flow patterns (i.e., only cyclic regimens should be used). Patients who miss an expected menses should be tested for pregnancy and should discontinue hormone therapy. Because most young women negatively associate hormone therapy with menopause in older women, some clinicians prefer to prescribe oral contraceptives for hormone replacement in premenopausal women with hypogonadism. However, oral contraceptives may not inhibit ovulation or effectively prevent pregnancy in young women with elevated gonadotropin levels.

Women with primary ovarian insufficiency have testosterone deficiency.[145] In these young women, testosterone replacement, in addition to estrogen, may be important.[114] However, preliminary analysis of a prospective study at the National Institutes of Health suggests that long-term "physiologic" testosterone supplementation (150 mcg/day), in addition to standard hormone replacement, did not significantly improve BMD and sexual function in these young women.[146,147]

Importantly, all women with primary ovarian insufficiency should understand that hormone therapy generally should be continued until the average age of natural menopause and that long-term follow-up is necessary.

Evaluation of Therapeutic Outcomes

Similar to the treatment of menopause, an assessment of the efficacy of hormone therapy, and its accompanying risks, should be performed on a regular basis. Young women with primary ovarian insufficiency should be monitored annually for their response to treatment, and their adherence with hormone therapy should be

TABLE 65-10 Premenopausal Hormone Replacement Therapy for Young Women with Primary Ovarian Insufficiency (Continuous Sequential Therapy)

Regimen[a]	Brand Name	Dosage
Estrogen Therapy		
Conjugated equine estrogens	Premarin	1.25 mg (oral; daily)
Estropipate (piperazine estrone sulfate)	Ogen Ortho-Est	2.5 mg (oral; daily)
Micronized 17β-estradiol	Estrace	4 mg (oral; daily)
Transdermal estrogen system (estradiol)	Alora Climara Vivelle, Vivelle Dot	0.1 mg, apply patch twice weekly 0.1 mg, apply patch twice weekly 0.1 mg, apply patch twice weekly
Progestogen Therapy		
Dydrogesterone[b]	Duphaston	10–20 mg/day for 12–14 days per calendar month (oral dosage form available as 10 mg tablets)
Medroxyprogesterone acetate	Provera Generic MPA	5–10 mg/day for 12–14 days per calendar month (oral dosage form available as 2.5, 5, 10 mg tablets)
Micronized progesterone	Prometrium	200 mg/day for 12–14 days per calendar month (oral dosage form available as 100 and 200 mg tablets)
Norethindrone acetate	Norethindrone acetate	5 mg/day for 12–14 days per calendar month (oral dosage form available as 5 mg tablets)
	Aygestin	5 mg/day for 12–14 days per calendar month (oral dosage form available as 2.5, 5 mg tablets)

[a]Off-label indication in the United States.
[b]Not available in the United States.

assessed regularly. Patients should be evaluated continuously for the presence of signs and symptoms of associated autoimmune endocrine disorders, such as hypothyroidism, adrenal insufficiency, and diabetes mellitus. Baseline BMD testing should be performed in all women with primary ovarian insufficiency. Mammography should be performed annually after age 40 years in accordance with accepted guidelines. Additional mammography screening in premenopausal women younger than 40 years who are receiving physiologic hormone therapy is not warranted. Other tests should be performed as clinically indicated.

Conclusions

Approximately 1% of women spontaneously develop ovarian insufficiency before age 40 years. Primary ovarian insufficiency is not an early natural menopause. Most affected women produce estrogen intermittently and may ovulate despite the presence of high gonadotropin concentrations. However, these women sustain sex steroid deficiency for more years than do naturally menopausal women, resulting in a significantly higher risk for osteoporosis and cardiovascular disease.

Women with primary ovarian insufficiency need exogenous sex steroids to compensate for the decreased production by their ovaries. Thus, premenopausal hormone therapy is required at least until these women reach the age of natural menopause.

The goal of therapy is to provide a hormone replacement regimen that maintains sex steroid status as effectively as the normal, functioning ovary. This usually requires the administration of estrogen at a dose greater than the standard dose given to older women experiencing natural menopause.

Because women with primary ovarian insufficiency can have spontaneous pregnancies, hormone therapy should produce regular, predictable menstrual flow patterns. Patients who miss an expected menses should be tested for pregnancy and, if positive, the hormone therapy should be promptly discontinued.

Annual follow-up should include assessment of adherence with the prescribed hormone therapy regimen and evaluation for signs and symptoms of associated endocrine disorders.

ACKNOWLEDGMENT

This research was supported in part by the Intramural Research Program of the National Institute of Child Health and Human Development, National Institutes of Health.

ABBREVIATIONS

AMH	anti-Mullerian hormone
BMD	bone mineral density
CEE	conjugated equine estrogens
CHD	coronary heart disease
FSH	follicle-stimulating hormone
GnRH	gonadotropin-releasing hormone
HDL	high-density lipoprotein
HR	hazard ratio
LDL	low-density lipoprotein
LH	luteinizing hormone
MPA	medroxyprogesterone acetate
NETA	norethindrone acetate
SERM	selective estrogen receptor modulator
STAR	Study of Tamoxifen and Raloxifene
TSEC	tissue-selective estrogen complex
VTE	venous thromboembolism
WHI	Women's Health Initiative

REFERENCES

1. Freeman EW, Sammel MD, Lin H, Gracia CR. Anti-Mullerian hormone as a predictor of time to menopause in late reproductive age women. J Clin Endocrinol Metab 2012;97:1673–1680.
2. Zumoff B, Strain GW, Miller LK, Rosner W. Twenty-four-hour mean plasma testosterone concentration declines with age in normal premenopausal women. J Clin Endocrinol Metab 1995;80:1429–1430.

3. Fogle RH, Stanczyk FZ, Zhang X, Paulson RJ. Ovarian androgen production in postmenopausal women. J Clin Endocrinol Metab 2007;92:3040–3043.
4. Burger HG. The endocrinology of the menopause. J Steroid Biochem Mol Biol 1999;69:31–35.
5. Harlow SD, Gass M, Hall JE, et al. Executive summary of the stages of reproductive aging workshop +10: Addressing the unfinished agenda of staging reproductive aging. J Clin Endocrinol Metab 2012;97:1159–1168.
6. Mishra GD, Kuh D. Health symptoms during midlife in relation to menopausal transition: British prospective cohort study. BMJ 2012;344:e402.
7. Avis NE, Brockwell S, Randolph JF, et al. Longitudinal changes in sexual functioning as women transition through menopause: Results from the Study of Women's Health Across the Nation. Menopause 2009;16:442–452.
8. Freeman EW, Sammel MD, Lin H. Temporal associations of hot flashes and depression in the transition to menopause. Menopause 2009;16:728–734.
9. Davis SR, Castelo-Branco C, Chedraui P, et al. Understanding weight gain at menopause. Climacteric 2012;15:419–429.
10. Santen RJ, Allred DC, Ardoin SP, Endocrine Society scientific statement: Postmenopausal hormone therapy. J Clin Endocrinol Metab 2010;95(Suppl 1):S1–S66.
11. Management of osteoporosis in postmenopausal women: 2010 position statement of The North American Menopause Society. Menopause 2010;17:25–54;quiz:55–56.
12. The role of local vaginal estrogen for treatment of vaginal atrophy in postmenopausal women: 2007 position statement of The North American Menopause Society. Menopause 2007;14:355–369;quiz 370–371.
13. The 2012 hormone therapy position statement of the North American Menopause Society. Menopause 2012;19: 257–271.
14. National Institutes of Health State-of-the-Science Conference statement: Management of menopause-related symptoms. Ann Intern Med 2005;142:1003–1013.
15. Moyer VA. U.S. Preventive Services Task Force. Menopausal hormone therapy for the primary prevention of chronic conditions: U.S. Preventive Services Task Force recommendation statement. Ann Intern Med 2013;158: 47–54.
16. Bachmann G. A new option for managing urogenital atrophy in postmenopausal women. Cont Obstet Gynecol 1997;42:13–28.
17. Davis S. Hormone replacement therapy. Indications, benefits and risk. Aust Fam Physician 1999;28:437–445.
18. Cardoso L, Lose G, McClish D, Versi E. A systematic review of the effects of estrogens for symptoms suggestive of overactive bladder. Acta Obstet Gynecol Scand 2004;83:892–897.
19. Grady D, Brown JS, Vittinghoff E, et al. Postmenopausal hormones and incontinence: The Heart and Estrogen/ Progestin Replacement Study. Obstet Gynecol 2001;97: 116–120.
20. Sowers MR, Zheng H, Jannausch ML, et al. Amount of bone loss in relation to time around the final menstrual period and follicle-stimulating hormone staging of the transmenopause. J Clin Endocrinol Metab 2010;95:2155–2162.
21. Cauley JA, Lucas FL, Kuller LH, et al. Elevated serum estradiol and testosterone concentrations are associated with a high risk for breast cancer. Study of Osteoporotic Fractures Research Group. Ann Intern Med 1999;130:270–277.
22. Stone K, Bauer DC, Black DM, et al. Hormonal predictors of bone loss in elderly women: A prospective study. The Study of Osteoporotic Fractures Research Group. J Bone Miner Res 1998;13:1167–1174.
23. Ettinger B, Pressman A, Sklarin P, et al. Associations between low levels of serum estradiol, bone density, and fractures among elderly women: The study of osteoporotic fractures. J Clin Endocrinol Metab 1998;83: 2239–2243.
24. Cummings SR, Browner WS, Bauer D, et al. Endogenous hormones and the risk of hip and vertebral fractures among older women. Study of Osteoporotic Fractures Research Group. N Engl J Med 1998;339:733–738.
25. Rossouw JE, Anderson GL, Prentice RL, et al. Risks and benefits of estrogen plus progestin in healthy postmenopausal women: Principal results from the Women's Health Initiative randomized controlled trial. JAMA 2002;288:321–333.
26. Cauley JA, Robbins J, Chen Z, et al. Effects of estrogen plus progestin on risk of fracture and bone mineral density: The Women's Health Initiative randomized trial. JAMA 2003;290:1729–1738.
27. Wells G, Tugwell P, Shea B, et al. Meta-analyses of therapies for postmenopausal osteoporosis. V. Meta-analysis of the efficacy of hormone replacement therapy in treating and preventing osteoporosis in postmenopausal women. Endocr Rev 2002;23:529–539.
28. Heiss G, Wallace R, Anderson GL, et al. Health risks and benefits 3 years after stopping randomized treatment with estrogen and progestin. JAMA 2008;299:1036–1045.
29. LaCroix AZ, Chlebowski RT, Manson JE, et al. Health outcomes after stopping conjugated equine estrogens among postmenopausal women with prior hysterectomy. A randomized controlled trial. JAMA 2011;305: 1305–1314.
30. Lindsay R, Hart DM, Clark DM. The minimum effective dose of estrogen for prevention of postmenopausal bone loss. Obstet Gynecol 1984;63:759–763.
31. Langer RD. Efficacy, safety, and tolerability of low-dose hormone therapy in managing menopausal symptoms. J Am Board Fam Med 2009;22:563–573.
32. Schmidt PJ, Nieman L, Danaceau MA, et al. Estrogen replacement in perimenopause-related depression: A preliminary report. Am J Obstet Gynecol 2000;183: 414–420.
33. Hlatky MA, Boothroyd D, Vittinghoff E, et al. Quality-of-life and depressive symptoms in postmenopausal women after receiving hormone therapy: Results from the Heart and Estrogen/Progestin Replacement Study (HERS) trial. JAMA 2002;287:591–597.
34. Shumaker SA, Legault C, Rapp SR, et al. Estrogen plus progestin and the incidence of dementia and mild cognitive impairment in postmenopausal women: The Women's Health Initiative Memory Study: A randomized controlled trial. JAMA 2003;289:2651–2662.
35. Rapp SR, Espeland MA, Shumaker SA, et al. Effect of estrogen plus progestin on global cognitive function in postmenopausal women: The Women's Health Initiative Memory Study: A randomized controlled trial. JAMA 2003;289:2663–2672.
36. Hays J, Ockene JK, Brunner RL, et al. Effects of estrogen plus progestin on health-related quality of life. N Engl J Med 2003;348:1839–1854.
37. Ott A, Breteler MM, van Harskamp F, et al. Incidence and risk of dementia. The Rotterdam Study. Am J Epidemiol 1998;147:574–580.
38. Shumaker SA, Legault C, Kuller L, et al. Conjugated equine estrogens and incidence of probable dementia and mild

cognitive impairment in postmenopausal women: Women's Health Initiative Memory Study. JAMA 2004;291: 2947–2958.
39. Espeland MA, Rapp SR, Shumaker SA, et al. Conjugated equine estrogens and global cognitive function in postmenopausal women: Women's Health Initiative Memory Study. JAMA 2004;291:2959–968.
40. Espeland MA, Shumaker SA, Leng I, et al. Long-term effects on cognitive function of postmenopausal hormone therapy prescribed to women aged 50 to 55 years. JAMA Intern Med 2013;24:1–8. [Epub ahead of print]
41. Espeland MA, Hogan PE, Fineberg SE, et al. Effect of postmenopausal hormone therapy on glucose and insulin concentrations. PEPI Investigators. Postmenopausal Estrogen/Progestin Interventions. Diabetes Care 1998;21:1589–1595.
42. Kanaya AM, Herrington D, Vittinghoff E, et al. Glycemic effects of postmenopausal hormone therapy: The Heart and Estrogen/progestin Replacement Study. A randomized, double-blind, placebo-controlled trial. Ann Intern Med 2003;138:1–9.
43. Norman RJ, Flight IH, Rees MC. Oestrogen and progestogen hormone replacement therapy for peri-menopausal and post-menopausal women: Weight and body fat distribution. Cochrane Database Syst Rev 2000:CD001018.
44. Matthews KA, Crawford SL, Chae CU, et al. Are changes in cardiovascular disease risk factors in midlife women due to chronological age or to the menopausal transition? J Am Coll Cardiol 2009;54:2366–2373.
45. Grodstein F, Manson JE, Colditz GA, et al. A prospective, observational study of postmenopausal hormone therapy and primary prevention of cardiovascular disease. Ann Intern Med 2000;133:933–941.
46. Sack MN, Rader DJ, Cannon RO 3rd. Oestrogen and inhibition of oxidation of low-density lipoproteins in postmenopausal women. Lancet 1994;343:269–270.
47. Koh KK, Jin DK, Yang SH, et al. Vascular effects of synthetic or natural progestagen combined with conjugated equine estrogen in healthy postmenopausal women. Circulation 2001;103:1961–1966.
48. Vickers MR, MacLennan AH, Lawton B, et al. Main morbidities recorded in the Women's international study of long duration oestrogen after menopause (WISDOM): A randomised controlled trial of hormone replacement therapy in postmenopausal women. BMJ 2007;335:239.
49. Viscoli CM, Brass LM, Kernan WN, et al. A clinical trial of estrogen-replacement therapy after ischemic stroke. N Engl J Med 2001;345:1243–1249.
50. Herrington DM, Reboussin DM, Brosnihan KB, et al. Effects of estrogen replacement on the progression of coronary-artery atherosclerosis. N Engl J Med 2000;343: 522–529.
51. Hulley S, Grady D, Bush T, et al. Randomized trial of estrogen plus progestin for secondary prevention of coronary heart disease in postmenopausal women. Heart and Estrogen/progestin Replacement Study (HERS) Research Group. JAMA 1998;280:605–613.
52. Anderson GL, Limacher M, Assaf AR, et al. Effects of conjugated equine estrogen in postmenopausal women with hysterectomy: The Women's Health Initiative randomized controlled trial. JAMA 2004;291:1701–1712.
53. Rossouw JE, Prentice RL, Manson JE, et al. Postmenopausal hormone therapy and risk of cardiovascular disease by age and years since menopause. JAMA 2007;297:1465–1477.
54. Toh S, Hernandez-Diaz S, Logan R, et al. Coronary heart disease in postmenopausal recipients of estrogen plus progestin therapy: Does the increased risk ever disappear? A randomized trial. Ann Intern Med 2010;152:211–217.
55. Schierbeck LL, Rejnmark L, Tofteng CL, et al. Effect of hormone replacement therapy on cardiovascular events in recently postmenopausal women: Randomized trial. BMJ 2012;345:e6409.
56. Bechlioulis A, Kalantaridou SN, Naka KK, et al. Endothelial function, but not carotid intima-media thickness, is affected early in menopause and is associated with severity of hot flushes. J Clin Endocrinol Metab 2010;95:1199–1206.
57. Bechlioulis A, Naka KK, Kalantaridou SN, et al. Increased vascular inflammation in early menopausal women is associated with hot flush severity. J Clin Endocrinol Metab 2012;97:E760–E764.
58. Bechlioulis A, Naka KK, Kalantaridou SN, et al. Short-term hormone therapy improves sCD40L and endothelial function in early menopausal women: Potential role of estrogen receptor polymorphisms. Maturitas 2012;71:389–395.
59. Wassertheil-Smoller S, Hendrix SL, Limacher M, et al. Effect of estrogen plus progestin on stroke in postmenopausal women: The Women's Health Initiative: A randomized trial. JAMA 2003;289:2673–2684.
60. Prentice RL, Chlebowski RT, Stefanick ML, et al. Estrogen plus progestin therapy and breast cancer in recently postmenopausal women. Am J Epidemiol 2008;167:1207–1216.
61. Chlebowski RT, Hendrix SL, Langer RD, et al. Influence of estrogen plus progestin on breast cancer and mammography in healthy postmenopausal women: The Women's Health Initiative Randomized Trial. JAMA 2003;289:3243–3253.
62. Chlebowski RT, Kuller LH, Prentice RL, et al. Breast cancer after use of estrogen plus progestin in postmenopausal women. N Engl J Med 2009;360:573–587.
63. Beral V. Breast cancer and hormone-replacement therapy in the Million Women Study. Lancet 2003;362:419–427.
64. Beral V, Reeves G, Bull D, Green J; Million Women Study Collaborators. Breast cancer risk in relation to the interval between menopause and starting hormone therapy. J Natl Cancer Inst 2011;103:296–305.
65. Swanson GM. Breast cancer risk estimation: A translational statistic for communication to the public. J Natl Cancer Inst 1993;85:848–849.
66. Breast cancer and hormone replacement therapy: Collaborative reanalysis of data from 51 epidemiological studies of 52,705 women with breast cancer and 108,411 women without breast cancer. Collaborative Group on Hormonal Factors in Breast Cancer. Lancet 1997;350: 1047–1059.
67. Schairer C, Lubin J, Troisi R, et al. Menopausal estrogen and estrogen–progestin replacement therapy and breast cancer risk. JAMA 2000;283:485–491.
68. Freedman M, San Martin J, O'Gorman J, et al. Digitized mammography: A clinical trial of postmenopausal women randomly assigned to receive raloxifene, estrogen, or placebo. J Natl Cancer Inst 2001;93:51–56.
69. Greendale GA, Reboussin BA, Slone S, et al. Postmenopausal hormone therapy and change in mammographic density. J Natl Cancer Inst 2003;95:30–37.
70. McTiernan A, Martin CF, Peck JD, et al. Estrogen-plus-progestin use and mammographic density in postmenopausal women: Women's Health Initiative randomized trial. J Natl Cancer Inst 2005;97: 1366–1376.
71. Anderson GL, Judd HL, Kaunitz AM, et al. Effects of estrogen plus progestin on gynecologic cancers and

associated diagnostic procedures: The Women's Health Initiative randomized trial. JAMA 2003;290:1739–1748.
72. Casper RF. Estrogen with interrupted progestin HRT: A review of experimental and clinical studies. Maturitas 2000;34:97–108.
73. Pike MC, Peters RK, Cozen W, et al. Estrogen–progestin replacement therapy and endometrial cancer. J Natl Cancer Inst 1997;89:1110–1116.
74. Genant HK, Lucas J, Weiss S, et al. Low-dose esterified estrogen therapy: Effects on bone, plasma estradiol concentrations, endometrium, and lipid levels. Estratab/Osteoporosis Study Group. Arch Intern Med 1997;157: 2609–2615.
75. Hadji P. The evolution of selective estrogen receptor modulators in osteoporosis therapy. Climacteric 2012:15:513–523. Epub 2012 Aug 1.
76. Barrett-Connor E, Mosca L, Collins P, et al. Effects of raloxifene on cardiovascular events and breast cancer in postmenopausal women. N Engl J Med 2006;355: 125–137.
77. Lacey JV Jr, Mink PJ, Lubin JH, et al. Menopausal hormone replacement therapy and risk of ovarian cancer. JAMA 2002;288:334–341.
78. Chlebowski RT, Schwartz AG, Wakelee H, et al. Estrogen plus progestin and lung cancer in postmenopausal women. Lancet 2009;374:1243–1251.
79. Chlebowski RT, Anderson GL, Manson JE, et al. Lung cancer among postmenopausal women treated with estrogen alone in the Women's Health Initiative Randomized Trial. J Natl Cancer Inst 2010;102:1413–1421.
80. Jick H, Derby LE, Myers MW, et al. Risk of hospital admission for idiopathic venous thromboembolism among users of postmenopausal oestrogens. Lancet 1996;348: 981–983.
81. Canonico M, Oger E, Plu-Bureau G, et al. Hormone therapy and venous thromboembolism among postmenopausal women: Impact of the route of estrogen administration and progestogens: The ESTHER study. Circulation 2007;115:840–845.
82. Cirillo DJ, Wallace RB, Rodabough RJ, et al. Effect of estrogen therapy on gallbladder disease. JAMA 2005;293:330–339.
83. Canonico M, Plu-Bureau G, Lowe GD, Scarabin PY. Hormone replacement therapy and risk of venous thromboembolism in postmenopausal women: Systematic review and meta-analysis. BMJ 2008;336:1227–1231.
84. Scarabin PY, Oger E, Plu-Bureau G. Differential association of oral and transdermal oestrogen-replacement therapy with venous thromboembolism risk. Lancet 2003;362: 428–432.
85. Sturdee DW. Newer HRT regimens. Br J Obstet Gynaecol 1997;104:1109–1115.
86. Lowe GD, Upton MN, Rumley A, et al. Different effects of oral and transdermal hormone replacement therapies on factor IX, APC resistance, t-PA, PAI and C-reactive protein—A cross-sectional population survey. Thromb Haemost 2001;86:550–556.
87. Greendale GA, Lee NP, Arriola ER. The menopause. Lancet 1999;353:571–580.
88. Lethaby A, Farquhar C, Sarkis A, et al. Hormone replacement therapy in postmenopausal women: Endometrial hyperplasia and irregular bleeding. Cochrane Database Syst Rev 2000:CD000402.
89. Judd HL, Mebane-Sims I, Legault C. Effects of hormone replacement therapy on endometrial histology in postmenopausal women. The Postmenopausal Estrogen/Progestin Interventions (PEPI) Trial. The Writing Group for the PEPI Trial. JAMA 1996;275:370–375.
90. Cushing KL, Weiss NS, Voigt LF, et al. Risk of endometrial cancer in relation to use of low-dose, unopposed estrogens. Obstet Gynecol 1998;91:35–39.
91. Role of progestogen in hormone therapy for postmenopausal women: Position statement of The North American Menopause Society. Menopause 2003;10:113–132.
92. Bachmann GA, Schaefers M, Uddin A, Utian WH. Lowest effective transdermal 17beta-estradiol dose for relief of hot flushes in postmenopausal women: A randomized controlled trial. Obstet Gynecol 2007;110:771–779.
93. Lindsay R, Gallagher JC, Kleerekoper M, Pickar JH. Effect of lower doses of conjugated equine estrogens with and without medroxyprogesterone acetate on bone in early postmenopausal women. JAMA 2002;287:2 668–2676.
94. Utian WH, Shoupe D, Bachmann G, et al. Relief of vasomotor symptoms and vaginal atrophy with lower doses of conjugated equine estrogens and medroxyprogesterone acetate. Fertil Steril 2001;75:1065–1079.
95. Pickar JH, Yeh I, Wheeler JE, et al. Endometrial effects of lower doses of conjugated equine estrogens and medroxyprogesterone acetate. Fertil Steril 2001;76:25–31.
96. Naessen T, Rodriguez-Macias K, Lithell H. Serum lipid profile improved by ultra-low doses of 17beta-estradiol in elderly women. J Clin Endocrinol Metab 2001;86: 2757–2762.
97. Files JA, Ko MG, Pruthi S. Bioidentical hormone therapy. Mayo Clin Proc 2011;86:673–680.
98. Food and Drug Administration. Bio-identicals: Sorting myths from facts. 2008, *http://www.fda.gov/ForConsumers/ConsumerUpdates/ucm049311.htm*.
99. American College of Obstetricians and Gynecologists Committee on Gynecologic Practice and American Society for Reproductive Medicine Practice Committee. Compounded bioidentical menopausal hormone therapy. Fertil Steril 2012:98:308–312.
100. Hickey M, Davis SR, Sturdee DW. Treatment of menopausal symptoms: What shall we do now? Lancet 2005;366: 409–421.
101. Loprinzi CL, Kugler JW, Sloan JA, et al. Venlafaxine in management of hot flashes in survivors of breast cancer: A randomised controlled trial. Lancet 2000;356:2059–2063.
102. Evans ML, Pritts E, Vittinghoff E, et al. Management of postmenopausal hot flushes with venlafaxine hydrochloride: A randomized, controlled trial. Obstet Gynecol 2005;105:161–166.
103. Stearns V, Johnson MD, Rae JM, et al. Active tamoxifen metabolite plasma concentrations after coadministration of tamoxifen and the selective serotonin reuptake inhibitor paroxetine. J Natl Cancer Inst 2003;95:1758–1764.
104. The role of testosterone therapy in postmenopausal women: Position statement of The North American Menopause Society. Menopause 2005;12:496–511;quiz 649.
105. Davis SR, Davison SL, Donath S, Bell RJ. Circulating androgen levels and self-reported sexual function in women. JAMA 2005;294:91–96.
106. Bell RJ, Donath S, Davison SL, Davis SR. Endogenous androgen levels and well-being: differences between premenopausal and postmenopausal women. Menopause 2006;13:65–71.
107. Shifren JL, Davis SR, Moreau M, et al. Testosterone patch for the treatment of hypoactive sexual desire disorder in naturally menopausal women: Results from the INTIMATE NM1 Study. Menopause 2006;13:770–779.

108. Davis SR, Moreau M, Kroll R, et al. Testosterone for low libido in postmenopausal women not taking estrogen. N Engl J Med 2008;359:2005–2017.
109. Shifren JL, Braunstein GD, Simon JA, et al. Transdermal testosterone treatment in women with impaired sexual function after oophorectomy. N Engl J Med 2000;343: 682–688.
110. Davis S, Papalia MA, Norman RJ, et al. Safety and efficacy of a testosterone metered-dose transdermal spray for treating decreased sexual satisfaction in premenopausal women: A randomized trial. Ann Intern Med 2008;148: 569–577.
111. van Staa TP, Sprafka JM. Study of adverse outcomes in women using testosterone therapy. Maturitas 2009;62: 76–80.
112. Jick SS, Hagberg KW, Kaye JA, Jick H. Postmenopausal estrogen-containing hormone therapy and the risk of breast cancer. Obstet Gynecol 2009;113:74–80.
113. Davis SR, Wolfe R, Farrugia H, et al. The incidence of invasive breast cancer among women prescribed testosterone for low libido. J Sex Med 2009;6:1850–1856.
114. Kalantaridou SN, Calis KA, Mazer NA, et al. A pilot study of an investigational testosterone transdermal patch system in young women with spontaneous premature ovarian failure. J Clin Endocrinol Metab 2005;90:6549–6552.
115. Wierman ME, Basson R, Davis SR, et al. Androgen therapy in women: An Endocrine Society Clinical Practice Guideline. J Clin Endocrinol Metab 2006;91:3697–3710.
116. Ettinger B, Black DM, Mitlak BH, et al. Reduction of vertebral fracture risk in postmenopausal women with osteoporosis treated with raloxifene: Results from a 3-year randomized clinical trial. Multiple Outcomes of Raloxifene Evaluation (MORE) Investigators. JAMA 1999;282: 637–645.
117. Cummings SR, Ensrud K, Delmas PD, et al. Lasofoxifene in postmenopausal women with osteoporosis. N Engl J Med 2010;362:686–696.
118. Silverman SL, Chines AA, Kendler DL, et al. Sustained efficacy and safety of bazedoxifene in preventing fractures in postmenopausal women with osteoporosis: Results of a 5-year, randomized, placebo-controlled study. Osteoporos Int 2012;23:351–363.
119. Martino S, Cauley JA, Barrett-Connor E, et al. Continuing outcomes relevant to Evista: Breast cancer incidence in postmenopausal osteoporotic women in a randomized trial of raloxifene. J Natl Cancer Inst 2004;96:1751–1761.
120. Vogel VG, Costantino JP, Wickerham DL, et al. Effects of tamoxifen vs raloxifene on the risk of developing invasive breast cancer and other disease outcomes: The NSABP Study of Tamoxifen and Raloxifene (STAR) P-2 trial. JAMA 2006;295:2727–2741.
121. Kenemans P, Speroff L. Tibolone: Clinical recommendations and practical guidelines. A report of the International Tibolone Consensus Group. Maturitas 2005;51:21–28.
122. Cummings SR, Ettinger B, Delmas PD, et al. The effects of tibolone in older postmenopausal women. N Engl J Med 2008;359:697–708.
123. Nijland EA, Weijmar Schultz WC, Nathorst-Boos J, et al. Tibolone and transdermal E2/NETA for the treatment of female sexual dysfunction in naturally menopausal women: Results of a randomized active-controlled trial. J Sex Med 2008;5:646–656.
124. Kenemans P, Bundred NJ, Foidart JM, et al. Safety and efficacy of tibolone in breast-cancer patients with vasomotor symptoms: A double-blind, randomized, non-inferiority trial. Lancet Oncol 2009;10:135–146.
125. Beral V, Bull D, Reeves G. Endometrial cancer and hormone-replacement therapy in the Million Women Study. Lancet 2005;365:1543–1551.
126. Langer RD, Landgren BM, Rymer J, Helmond FA. Effects of tibolone and continuous combined conjugated equine estrogen/medroxyprogesterone acetate on the endometrium and vaginal bleeding: Results of the OPAL study. Am J Obstet Gynecol 2006;195:1320–1327.
127. Murkies AL, Wilcox G, Davis SR. Clinical review 92: Phytoestrogens. J Clin Endocrinol Metab 1998;83:297–303.
128. Tice JA, Ettinger B, Ensrud K, et al. Phytoestrogen supplements for the treatment of hot flashes: The Isoflavone Clover Extract (ICE) Study: A randomized controlled trial. JAMA 2003;290:207–214.
129. Lissin LW, Cooke JP. Phytoestrogens and cardiovascular health. J Am Coll Cardiol 2000;35:1403–1410.
130. Tempfer CB, Froese G, Heinze G, et al. Side effects of phytoestrogens: A meta-analysis of randomized trials. Am J Med 2009;122:939–946.e9.
131. Newton KM, Reed SD, LaCroix AZ, et al. Treatment of vasomotor symptoms of menopause with black cohosh, multibotanicals, soy, hormone therapy, or placebo: A randomized trial. Ann Intern Med 2006;145:869–879.
132. National Institutes of Health Office of Dietary Supplements. Dietary supplements fact sheet: Black cohosh. 2008, *http://ods.od.nih.gov/factsheets/BlackCohosh_pf.asp*.
133. Nedrow A, Miller J, Walker M, et al. Complementary and alternative therapies for the management of menopause-related symptoms: A systematic evidence review. Arch Intern Med 2006;166:1453–1465.
134. American College of Obstetricians and Gynecologists Women's Health Care Physicians. Executive summary. Hormone therapy. Obstet Gynecol 2004;104:1S–4S.
135. Ettinger B. Vasomotor symptom relief versus unwanted effects: Role of estrogen dosage. Am J Med 2005;118 (Suppl 12B):74–78.
136. Ettinger B, Pressman A. Continuation of postmenopausal hormone replacement therapy in a large health maintenance organization: Transdermal matrix patch versus oral estrogen therapy. Am J Manag Care 1999;5:779–785.
137. Majumdar SR, Almasi EA, Stafford RS. Promotion and prescribing of hormone therapy after report of harm by the Women's Health Initiative. JAMA 2004;292:1983–1988.
138. Cunha EP, Azevedo LH, Pompei LM, et al. Effect of abrupt discontinuation versus gradual dose reduction of postmenopausal hormone therapy on hot flushes. Climacteric 2010;13:362–367.
139. Kalantaridou SN, Davis SR, Nelson LM. Premature ovarian failure. Endocrinol Metab Clin North Am 1998;27: 989–1006.
140. Coulam CB, Adamson SC, Annegers JF. Incidence of premature ovarian failure. Obstet Gynecol 1986;67: 604–606.
141. Anasti JN, Kalantaridou SN, Kimzey LM, et al. Bone loss in young women with karyotypically normal spontaneous premature ovarian failure. Obstet Gynecol 1998;91:12–15.
142. Kalantaridou SN, Naka KK, Papanikolaou E, et al. Impaired endothelial function in young women with premature ovarian failure: Normalization with hormone therapy. J Clin Endocrinol Metab 2004;89:3907–3913.
143. van der Schouw YT, van der Graaf Y, Steyerberg EW, et al. Age at menopause as a risk factor for cardiovascular mortality. Lancet 1996;347:714–718.
144. Snowdon DA, Kane RL, Beeson WL, et al. Is early natural menopause a biologic marker of health and aging? Am J Public Health 1989;79:709–714.

145. Kalantaridou SN, Calis KA, Vanderhoof VH, et al. Testosterone deficiency in young women with 46,XX spontaneous premature ovarian failure. Fertil Steril 2006;86:1475–1482.
146. Popat VB, Kalantaridou SN, Vanderhoof VH, et al. Effect of long-term physiologic transdermal testosterone (150 mcg/day) replacement therapy on femoral neck bone density in women with spontaneous premature ovarian failure: Results of a 3-year double-blind placebo-controlled clinical trial, P1–349. Abstract presented at the Annual Meeting of the Endocrine Society, June 2–5, 2007, Toronto, Canada.
147. Kalantaridou SN, Vanderhoof VH, Calis KA, et al. Physiologic transdermal testosterone replacement (150 mcg/day) does not significantly improve sexual function in women with 46,XX spontaneous premature ovarian failure: A placebo-controlled randomized study, OR27-4. Abstract presented at the Annual Meeting of the Endocrine Society, June 2–5, 2007, Toronto, Canada.
148. US Department of Health and Human Services, Food and Drug Administration, Center for Drug Evaluation and Research. Guidance for Industry: Noncontraceptive Estrogen Drug Products for the Treatment of Vasomotor Symptoms and Vulvar and Vaginal Atrophy Symptoms—Recommended Prescribing Information for Health Care Providers and Patient Labeling, *http://www.fda.gov/downloads/Drugs/DrugSafety/InformationbyDrugClass/UCM135336.pdf*.
149. Sturdee DW, Pines A, International Menopause Society Writing Group, et al. Updated IMS recommendations on postmenopausal hormone therapy and preventive strategies for midlife health. Climacteric 2011;14: 302–320.
150. Umland EM, Falconieri L. Treatment options for vasomotor symptoms in menopause: Focus on desvenlafaxine. Int J Womens Health 2012;4:305–319.
151. Carroll DG, Kelley KW. Use of antidepressants for management of hot flashes. Pharmacotherapy 2009;29: 1357–1374.

66 Erectile Dysfunction

Mary Lee

KEY CONCEPTS

1. The incidence of erectile dysfunction is low in men younger than 40 years of age. The incidence increases as men age, likely as a result of concurrent medical conditions that impair the vascular, neurologic, psychogenic, and hormonal systems necessary for a normal penile erection.
2. Many commonly used drugs have sympatholytic, anticholinergic, sedative, or antiandrogenic effects that may exacerbate or contribute to the development of erectile dysfunction. Clinicians should be familiar with these agents and be prepared to make adjustments in drug regimens to minimize adverse effects of these drugs on a patient's erectile function.
3. The first step in clinical management of erectile dysfunction is to identify and, if possible, reverse the underlying causes. Risk factors for erectile dysfunction, including hypertension, diabetes mellitus, smoking, and chronic ethanol abuse, should be addressed and minimized.
4. Specific treatments for erectile dysfunction include vacuum erection devices (VEDs), pharmacologic treatments, psychotherapy, and surgery. Of these, phosphodiesterase inhibitors are the medications of first choice.
5. The ideal treatment of erectile dysfunction should have a fast onset, be effective, be convenient to administer, be cost effective, have a low incidence of serious adverse effects, and be free of serious drug interactions.
6. Specific treatment is first initiated with the least invasive forms of treatment, including VEDs or oral phosphodiesterase inhibitors, followed by intracavernosal injections or intraurethral inserts, and finally by surgical insertion of a penile prosthesis.
7. VEDs can have a slow onset of action (30 minutes) and are not discreet; therefore, they are most effective for a couple in a stable relationship.
8. Although phosphodiesterase inhibitors are convenient and effective regardless of the etiology of erectile dysfunction, they fail in 30% to 40% of patients. Also, phosphodiesterase inhibitors are contraindicated in patients taking any dosage formulation of nitrate.
9. Testosterone supplementation should be reserved for patients with primary or secondary hypogonadism who have erectile dysfunction as a consequence of a decreased libido. Testosterone supplementation should not be used by patients with erectile dysfunction who have normal serum testosterone levels.
10. Although intracavernosal injections and intraurethral pellets of alprostadil are effective independent of the etiology of erectile dysfunction, they fail in one third of patients. To self-administer medication by these routes, patients require training to minimize administration-related adverse effects.

The National Institutes of Health Consensus Development Panel on Impotence defines erectile dysfunction as the persistent failure to achieve a penile erection to allow for satisfactory sexual intercourse.[1] A persistent failure refers to erectile dysfunction for a minimum of 3 months.[2] Patients may refer to it as impotence.

Erectile dysfunction must be distinguished from disorders of libido, ejaculatory disorders, and infertility, which are caused by different pathophysiologic mechanisms and are treated with alternative agents (Table 66-1). A patient may suffer from one or more disorders of sexual dysfunction. For example, an elderly man with primary hypogonadism may suffer from decreased libido and erectile dysfunction. Diagnosis of the type of sexual disorder that a patient has is a key to initiating the most appropriate treatment.

EPIDEMIOLOGY

1 The incidence of erectile dysfunction is low in men younger than 40 years of age but increases as men age.[3–5] The Massachusetts Male Aging Study, a cross-sectional survey of a random sample of 1,290 men in the Boston area, was conducted during the period from 1987 to 1989. The study reported an overall prevalence of 52% for any degree of erectile dysfunction in men aged 40 to 70 years, with an age-related increase in incidence ranging from 12.4% in men aged 40 to 49 years, up to 46.4% in men aged 60 to 69 years.[1,3] In the more recent Health Professional Follow-Up Study of more than 31,000 male health professionals aged 53 to 90 years, the prevalence of erectile dysfunction was 33%.[4] Interestingly, although the prevalence of erectile dysfunction increases with patient age, many patients fail to seek medical treatment.[5]

TABLE 66-1 Types of Sexual Dysfunction in Men

Type of Dysfunction	Definition
Decreased libido	Decreased sexual drive or desire
Increased libido	Inappropriate and excessive sexual drive or desire
Erectile dysfunction (impotence)	Failure to achieve a penile erection suitable for satisfactory sexual intercourse
Delayed ejaculation	Commonly referred to as "dry sex"; ejaculation is delayed or absent
Retrograde ejaculation	Ejaculate passes retrograde into the bladder, instead of toward the anterior urethra (antegrade) and out of the penis
Infertility	Sperm are insufficient in number, have abnormal morphology, or have inadequate motility, and fail to fertilize the ovum

Erectile dysfunction is sometimes assumed to be a symptom of the aging process in men. However, more likely it results from concurrent medical conditions of the patient (e.g., hypertension, arteriosclerosis, hyperlipidemia, diabetes mellitus, or psychiatric disorders) or from medications that patients may be taking for these diseases.[6,7] For example, up to 50% of patients with diabetes mellitus develop erectile dysfunction, and medications such as β-blockers are associated with a high incidence of erectile dysfunction.

PHYSIOLOGY OF A NORMAL PENILE ERECTION

A normal penile erection requires full functioning of several physiologic systems: vascular, nervous, and hormonal. The patient also must be psychologically receptive to sexual stimuli.[8,9]

Vascular System

The penis comprises two corpora cavernosa on the dorsal side and one corpus spongiosum on the ventral side. The corpus spongiosum surrounds the urethra and forms the glans penis. The corpora are composed of multiple interconnected sinuses, which can fill with blood to produce an erection. The corpora cavernosa are encased by the tunica albuginea, a fibrous tissue membrane, which has limited distensibility. In the flaccid state, arterial flow into and venous outflow from the corpora are balanced. During the erectile phase, arterial blood flow increases and blood fills the sinusoids within the corpora, which causes penile swelling and elongation. The erection is prolonged by a decrease in venous outflow from the corpora, which is caused by compression of subtunical venules against the tunica albuginea by the swollen corpora (Fig. 66-1).

Arterial flow into the corpora is enhanced by acetylcholine-mediated vasodilation. Acetylcholine indirectly enhances arterial flow to the corpora and increases sinusoidal filling of the corporal tissue. That is, acetylcholine is a coneurotransmitter, which works along with other nonpeptidergic intracellular

Penile arteries and veins
Corpus cavernosum
Skin
Tunica albuginea
Erectile tissue
Corpus spongiosum
A
Urethra

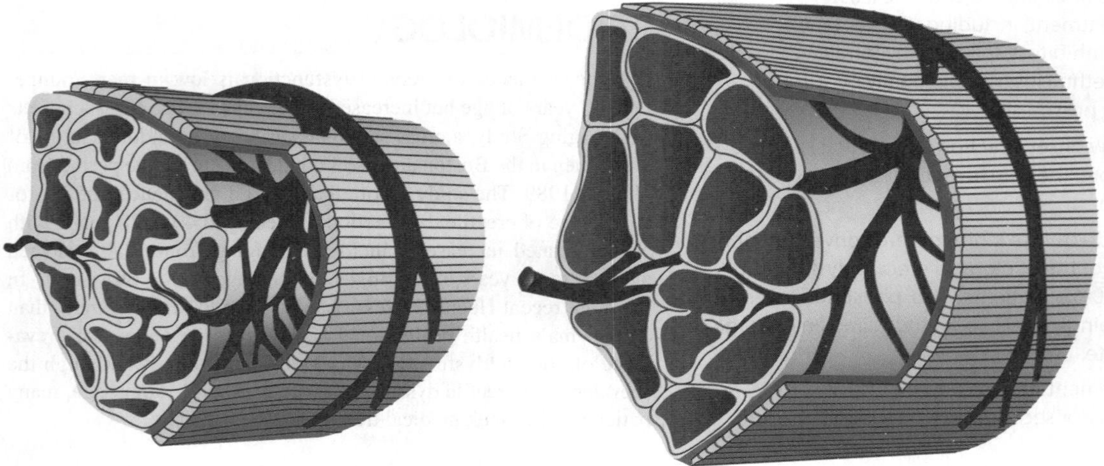

B
Flaccid State
Erectile Phase

FIGURE 66-1 Microanatomy of and vascular changes in the penis in flaccid and erect states. In the flaccid state, arterial flow into and venous outflow from the corpora are balanced. During the erectile phase, arterial blood flow increases and blood fills the sinusoids within the corpora, causing penile swelling and elongation. The erection is prolonged by a decrease in venous outflow from the corpora, which is caused by compression of subtunical venules by the swollen corpora. *(From Walsh PC, ed. Campbell's Urology, 8th ed. Philadelphia, PA: WB Saunders; 2002:1595, 1697.)*

neurotransmitters—including cyclic guanosine monophosphate (cGMP), cyclic adenosine monophosphate (cAMP), or vasoactive intestinal polypeptide—to produce vasodilation. In effect, cGMP and cAMP are secondary messengers that direct desired effects in target tissues.

Specifically, acetylcholine produces an erection probably through two different pathways. Through one pathway, in the presence of sexual stimulation to genital tissue, acetylcholine enhances the production of nitric oxide by endothelial cells and nonadrenergic–noncholinergic neurons. Nitric oxide enhances the activity of guanylate cyclase, which increases the conversion of cyclic guanosine triphosphate to cGMP. cGMP decreases intracellular calcium concentrations in smooth muscle cells of penile arteries and cavernosal sinuses. As a result, smooth muscle relaxation occurs, which enhances arterial blood flow to and blood filling of the corpora.[9] An erection results.

In an alternative pathway, acetylcholine or prostaglandin E enhances the activity of adenyl cyclase, which increases the conversion of cyclic adenosine triphosphate to cAMP, a potent muscle relaxant. Similar to cGMP, cAMP decreases intracellular calcium concentrations to produce smooth muscle relaxation in cells of the arteries and cavernosal sinuses. Arterial blood flow to and blood filling of the corpora are enhanced, and a penile erection results.[9]

Nervous System and Psychogenic Stimuli

Some erections are mediated by a sacral nerve reflex arc (e.g., erections can occur while the patient is sleeping). However, in the conscious patient, sensory sexual stimulation mediates erections via the CNS. That is, when a patient sees an attractive partner, hears sweet words, smells a particular scent, or tastes or touches a pleasant object, these situations can result in an erection. In this case, the patient's brain processes this information and the nervous impulse is carried down the spinal cord to peripheral cholinergic nerves that innervate the vascular supply to the corpora, resulting in an erection.

The medial preoptic area of the hypothalamus is thought to be that portion of the brain responsible for integrating external stimuli. Here dopamine exerts a proerectogenic effect, whereas, α_2-adrenergic stimulation causes the penis to become and/or remain flaccid. After moving down the spinal cord, stimulatory nerve impulses travel to the penis by efferent peripheral nerves, including inhibitory sympathetic neurons (T11–L2), proerectogenic parasympathetic neurons (S2–S4), and proerectogenic somatic neurons (S2–S4).

In summary, acetylcholine produces an erection by working along with other coneurotransmitters, including cGMP and cAMP. Thus, an erection is mediated neurologically, maintained by arterial blood filling of the corpora, and sustained by occlusion of venous outflow from the corpora.

Detumescence, or the progression of an erect penis to a flaccid state, results from the actions of norepinephrine, which contracts vascular smooth muscle to decrease arterial inflow to the corpora and contracts sinusoidal tissue in the corpora. As a result, venous outflow from the corpora increases.

Hormonal System

Testosterone is principally produced by the testes at a daily rate of 4 to 8 mg. Production follows a circadian pattern with highest blood levels in the morning and lowest levels in the evening. Physiologically active (free) testosterone comprises only 2% of circulating blood levels. About 50% to 60% of testosterone in the bloodstream is tightly bound to sex hormone-binding globulin and is inactive. The rest of circulating testosterone is reversibly bound to albumin; this portion of testosterone is in equilibrium with the free fraction.

Testosterone stimulates libido (sexual drive) and increases muscle mass in males. In some target cells with 5-α reductase, testosterone is activated to dihydrotestosterone. Dihydrotestosterone, which is more potent than testosterone, stimulates prostate gland growth, increases facial and body hair, induces baldness, and causes acne. In adipose tissue, a small portion of testosterone is converted to estradiol which can lead to gynecomastia.

Beginning at age 40 years, men experience a gradual decrease in testicular production of testosterone, with an associated decrease in muscle mass and sexual function.[10] The Massachusetts Male Aging Study reported that 6% to 12% of elderly males had symptoms of hypogonadism.[11]

Within the normal physiologic serum total testosterone concentration range (normal, 300–1,100 ng/dL; 10.4–38.2 nmol/L), sexual drive is usually normal. However, because of variability in circulating levels of sex hormone-binding globulin, a patient's serum concentration of testosterone should always be interpreted in the context of the patient's symptoms and physical exam findings. To confirm hypogonadism when the serum total testosterone concentration is equivocal, the clinician should obtain a serum-free (bioavailable) testosterone level.

The relationship between erectile dysfunction and serum testosterone levels is complicated. Patients with normal serum testosterone levels may have erectile dysfunction, and patients with subnormal serum testosterone levels may have normal sexual function.[5] When a patient has hypogonadism and libido is decreased, a patient may not develop erections. In this case, erectile dysfunction is considered secondary to a decreased libido.

PATHOPHYSIOLOGY

Erectile dysfunction can result from any single abnormality or combination of abnormalities of the four systems necessary for a normal penile erection. Vascular, neurologic, or hormonal etiologies of erectile dysfunction are collectively referred to as *organic erectile dysfunction*. Approximately 80% of patients with erectile dysfunction have the organic type. Patients who do not respond to psychogenic stimuli and have no organic cause for dysfunction have *psychogenic erectile dysfunction*.

Diseases that compromise vascular flow to the corpora cavernosum (e.g., peripheral vascular disease, arteriosclerosis, and essential hypertension) are associated with an increased incidence of erectile dysfunction. Diseases that impair nerve conduction to the brain (e.g., spinal cord injury or stroke) or conditions that impair peripheral nerve conduction to the penile vasculature (e.g., diabetes mellitus) can result in erectile dysfunction.[7]

Diseases associated with hypogonadism, primary or secondary, result in subphysiologic levels of testosterone, which cause diminished sexual drive (decreased libido) and secondary erectile dysfunction. Primary hypogonadism can be associated with the normal aging process in men or surgical removal of the testes for treatment of prostate or testicular cancer. Secondary hypogonadism may result from hypothalamic or pituitary disorders of luteinizing hormone–releasing hormone or luteinizing hormone, respectively; or elevated prolactin levels, which can be associated with pituitary tumors or can occur in patients with chronic renal failure.

Patients must be in the proper mental frame of mind to be receptive to sexual stimuli. Patients who suffer from malaise, have reactive depression or performance anxiety, are sedated, have Alzheimer's disease, have hypothyroidism, or have mental disorders commonly complain of erectile dysfunction. In most studies, patients with psychogenic erectile dysfunction generally exhibit a higher response rate to various interventions than do patients with organic erectile dysfunction because the former have less severe disease.

Social habits of patients have been linked to erectile dysfunction. The vasoconstrictor effect of cigarette smoking may

TABLE 66-2 Medication Classes That Can Cause Erectile Dysfunction

Drug Class	Proposed Mechanism by Which Drug Causes Erectile Dysfunction	Special Notes
Anticholinergic agents (antihistamines, antiparkinsonian agents, tricyclic antidepressants, phenothiazines)	Anticholinergic activity	• Second-generation nonsedating antihistamines (e.g., loratadine, fexofenadine, or cetirizine) are associated with less erectile dysfunction than first-generation agents • Selective serotonin reuptake inhibitor (SSRI) and multiple receptor reuptake inhibitor antidepressants cause less erectile dysfunction than tricyclic antidepressants. Of the SSRIs, paroxetine, sertraline, fluvoxamine, and fluoxetine cause erectile dysfunction more commonly than venlafaxine, nefazodone, trazodone, bupropion, duloxetine, or mirtazapine • Phenothiazines with less anticholinergic effect (e.g., chlorpromazine) can be substituted in some patients if erectile dysfunction is a problem
Dopamine antagonists (e.g., metoclopramide, phenothiazines)	Inhibit prolactin inhibitory factor, thereby increasing prolactin levels	• Increased prolactin levels inhibit testicular testosterone production; depressed libido results
Estrogens, antiandrogens (e.g., luteinizing hormone-releasing hormone superagonists, digoxin, spironolactone, ketoconazole, cimetidine)	Suppress testosterone-mediated stimulation of libido	• In the face of a decreased libido, a secondary erectile dysfunction develops because of diminished sexual drive
CNS depressants (e.g., barbiturates, narcotics, benzodiazepines, short-term use of large doses of alcohol, anticonvulsants)	Suppress perception of psychogenic stimuli	
Agents that decrease penile blood flow (e.g., diuretics, peripheral β-adrenergic antagonists, or central sympatholytics [methyldopa, clonidine, guanethidine])	Reduce arteriolar flow to corpora	• Any diuretic that produces a significant decrease in intravascular volume can decrease penile arteriolar flow • Safer antihypertensives include angiotensin-converting enzyme inhibitors, postsynaptic α_1-adrenergic antagonists (terazosin, doxazosin), calcium channel blockers, and angiotensin II receptor antagonists[9]
Miscellaneous • Finsteride, dutasteride • Lithium carbonate • Gemfibrozil • Interferon • Clofibrate • Monoamine oxidase inhibitors • Opiates	Unknown mechanism	

From Handler,[12] Lee and Sharifi,[13] and Kennedy.[14]

compromise blood flow to the corpora and decrease cavernosal filling. Excessive ethanol intake may lead to androgen deficiency, peripheral neuropathy, or chronic liver disease, all of which can contribute to erectile dysfunction.

❷ Medications may cause erectile dysfunction through similar pathophysiologic mechanisms (Table 66-2).[12–14] Medications are estimated to be responsible for approximately 10% to 25% of cases of erectile dysfunction.

DIAGNOSIS

With the availability in the late 1990s of effective medications for erectile dysfunction independent of the etiology, diagnostic evaluation of erectile dysfunction became streamlined. Key assessments include a description of the severity of erectile dysfunction, complete medical, psychosocial, and surgical histories, review of concurrent medications, physical examination, and selected clinical laboratory tests.[8,15]

To assess the severity of erectile dysfunction, the patient should be asked about the quality of sexual intercourse for the past 4 weeks to 6 months. A self-administered standardized questionnaire, such as the International Index of Erectile Dysfunction (IIEF), is often used. It is administered before initiation of any treatment and repeated at regular intervals during treatment. It includes 15 questions about the quality of sexual function and satisfactoriness of sexual intercourse.[16] Questions include the following: How often were you able to maintain an erection? How difficult was it to sustain an erection? How satisfied are you with your sexual life? The physician should carefully assess the expectations for erectile function of the patient and the partner to ensure that expectations are reasonable. Shorter versions of the IIEF and other self-reporting questionnaires are also used in clinical practice. For example, the IIEF-EF comprises the six questions from the IIEF that focus on erectile function. The patient responds to each question, each response is scored on a range of 1 to 5. A score of 26 to 30 is considered normal function, 22 to 25 is mild erectile dysfunction, 17 to 21 is mild-to-moderate erectile dysfunction, 11 to 16 is moderate erectile dysfunction, and 10 or less is severe erectile dysfunction.

A medical history should be obtained to identify concurrent medical illnesses (e.g., hypertension, atherosclerosis, hyperlipidemia, diabetes mellitus, and depression) or surgical procedures (e.g., perineal or pelvic) that are risk factors for or are associated with organic or psychogenic erectile dysfunction. Underlying diseases that do not optimally respond to treatment should be addressed before specific treatment for erectile dysfunction is initiated. If the patient smokes cigarettes, drinks excessive amounts of ethanol, or uses recreational drugs, these social habits should be discontinued before specific treatment for erectile dysfunction is started.

CLINICAL PRESENTATION Erectile Dysfunction

General

- Men are affected emotionally in many different ways
- Depression
- Performance anxiety
- Marital difficulties and avoidance of sexual intimacy (patients are often brought to a physician by their partners)
- Nonadherence to medications patient believes are causing erectile dysfunction

Symptoms

- Erectile dysfunction or inability to have sexual intercourse

Signs

- If completing an International Index of Erectile Dysfunction survey, results are consistent with low satisfaction with the quality of erectile function
- Medical history may identify concurrent medical illnesses, past surgical procedures that interfere with good vascular flow to the penis or damage nerve function to the corpora, or mental disorders associated with decreased reception of sexual stimuli
- Medication history may reveal prescription or nonprescription medications that could cause erectile dysfunction
- Physical examination may reveal signs of hypogonadism (e.g., gynecomastia, small testicles, decreased body hair or beard, and decreased muscle mass), which may contribute to erectile dysfunction. The patient may have an abnormally curved penis when erect, decreased pulses in the pelvic region (suggesting impaired vascular flow to the penis), or decreased anal sphincter tone (suggesting impaired nerve function to the corpora). Men older than 50 years should undergo a digital rectal examination to determine whether an enlarged prostate is contributing to the patient's erectile dysfunction

Laboratory Tests

- If the patient has signs of hypogonadism and complains of decreased libido, a serum testosterone concentration may be below the normal range, which would be consistent with a hormonal cause of erectile dysfunction
- If the patient has an enlarged prostate noted on digital rectal examination, a blood sample for prostate-specific antigen should be obtained. If elevated, the patient should be evaluated for a prostate disorder, which could contribute to erectile dysfunction

A complete listing of the patient's prescription and nonprescription medications and dietary supplements should be reviewed by the clinician, who should identify drugs that may be contributing to erectile dysfunction. If possible, causative agents should be discontinued or the dose should be reduced.

A physical examination of the patient should include a check for hypogonadism (i.e., signs of gynecomastia, small testicles, and decreased beard or body hair). The penis should be evaluated for diseases associated with abnormal penile curvature (e.g., Peyronie's disease), which are associated with erectile dysfunction. Femoral and lower extremity pulses should be assessed to provide an indication of vascular supply to the genitals. Anal sphincter tone and other genital reflexes should be checked for the integrity of the nerve supply to the penis. A digital rectal examination in patients 50 years or older is needed to rule out benign prostatic hyperplasia, which may contribute to erectile dysfunction.

Selected laboratory tests should be obtained to identify the presence of underlying diseases that could cause erectile dysfunction. They include a fasting serum blood glucose and lipid profile. Serum testosterone levels should be checked in patients older than 50 years and in younger patients who complain of decreased libido and erectile dysfunction. At least two early morning serum testosterone levels on different days are needed to confirm the presence of hypogonadism.[17]

Finally, erectile dysfunction is a potential marker for arteriosclerosis. Therefore, older patients and those at intermediate and high risk for cardiovascular disease should undergo a cardiovascular risk assessment before starting on drug treatment for erectile dysfunction. By doing so, patients will be categorized into low-, intermediate-, or high-risk groups for cardiovascular morbidity related to sexual intercourse. Patients in the intermediate-risk group should undergo additional testing to reclassify them into the low- or high-risk group. The high-risk group should defer sexual activity. Patients in the low-risk group may start specific treatment for erectile dysfunction.[8,18–20]

TREATMENT
Erectile Dysfunction

Desired Outcomes

The goal of treatment is improvement in the quantity and quality of penile erections suitable for intercourse and considered satisfactory by the patient and his partner. Simple as this may sound, healthcare providers must ensure that patients and their partners have reasonable expectations for any therapies that are initiated. Furthermore, only patients with erectile dysfunction should be treated. Patients who have normal sexual function should not seek—or be encouraged to seek—treatment in an effort to enhance sexual function or enable increased activity. In addition, treatment should be well tolerated and be of reasonable cost.

General Approach to Treatment

❸ The Third Princeton Consensus Conference is a widely accepted multidisciplinary approach to managing erectile dysfunction that maps out a stepwise treatment plan.[20–22] The first step in clinical management of erectile dysfunction is to identify and, if possible, reverse underlying causes. Risk factors for erectile dysfunction, including hypertension, coronary artery disease, dyslipidemia, diabetes mellitus, smoking, or chronic ethanol abuse, should be addressed and minimized. Patients should follow a heart-healthy lifestyle, which includes physical fitness, weight loss to achieve a normal body mass index, low cholesterol diets, no excessive ethanol intake, and no smoking.[23] In some cases, these types of interventions are sufficient to restore erectile function.[24] However, if erectile dysfunction does not respond to these measures, specific treatment is indicated.

For patients with psychogenic erectile dysfunction, psychotherapy can be used as monotherapy or as an adjunct to specific treatments for the disorder. To enhance the relevance of psychotherapy, both the patient and the partner should be included in the counseling sessions. Treatment should be individualized and should address immediate factors that may be causing performance anxiety or depression. The effectiveness of psychotherapy is generally low, and long-term psychotherapy is often necessary.

4 5 6 Specific treatments of erectile dysfunction include vacuum erection devices (VEDs), pharmacologic treatments, and surgery. The ideal treatment of this disorder should have a fast onset, be effective, be convenient to administer, be cost-effective, have a low incidence of serious adverse effects, and be free of serious drug interactions (Table 66-3). Generally, when choosing from among treatment approaches, those that are least invasive are selected first; more invasive therapies are reserved for patients who do not respond to first-line agents.

The American Urological Association Guideline on the Management of Erectile Dysfunction,[15] the 2009 International Consultation of Sexual Medicine,[25] and the American College of Physicians[2] clearly identify oral phosphodiesterase inhibitors for first-line treatment. VEDs, intracavernosal injection of erectogenic agents, or intraurethral prostaglandin inserts are second-line treatments; prescribing of a particular agent for a patient should be individualized. Surgical intervention should be reserved for patients who fail to respond to first- and second-line treatments. A sample algorithm that guides selection of treatment is shown in Figure 66-2.

Vacuum Erection Device

A VED has two parts: a pump, which generates a negative vacuum pressure; and a cylinder, which is closed at one end and into which the penis is inserted. The patient inserts his penis into the open end of the cylinder, which is then pushed up flush against his lower abdomen to create a vacuum chamber. Then the patient activates the pump to produce a vacuum pressure, which draws arteriolar blood into the corpora cavernosa. To prolong the erection, the patient can use constriction bands or tension rings, which are placed at the base of the penis, to keep the arteriolar blood in and reduce venous outflow from the penis. With the assistance of loading cones to protect the glans, these bands or rings can be rolled over the glans penis and up the erect penile shaft. Alternatively, they can be first threaded onto the plastic cylinder before the penis is inserted. Once the penis is erect, the band or ring can be rolled off the cylinder onto the base of the penis (Fig. 66-3). However, some patients prefer to apply the band or ring before the penis is erect.[26,27]

7 The onset of action of the VED is 3 to 20 minutes. VEDs are not discreet. That is, a patient's use of a VED is evident to the partner. For this reason, VEDs appear to work best in older patients who are married or who have stable sexual relationships. In this group, VEDs could be considered first-line therapy, and the overall satisfaction rate can be as high as 60% to 80% (range, 27–94%).[26,27] VEDs may be used as second-line therapy in patients who do not respond to oral phosphodiesterase inhibitors, which includes patients who have had radical prostatectomy[26] or those who do not respond to injectable drug treatments for erectile dysfunction. The combination of a VED with intracavernosal or intraurethral alprostadil[26] or a phosphodiesterase inhibitor[28] is associated with a higher efficacy rate than use of the VED alone. As a result, combination therapy sometimes is attempted before penile prosthesis surgery is considered in the patient who fails VED monotherapy.

Patients may discontinue using VEDs because they are inconvenient and or not discreet. It has been reported that 20% to 50% and 50% to 64% of initial users continue with VEDs after 1 year and 5 years, respectively.[26,29] Also, 6% to 11% of partners complain that the penis is cool to the touch or is discolored (bluish) in appearance, particularly when constriction bands are used.

VEDs are available with battery-operated pumps, which offer convenience, particularly in patients with arthritis of the hands. The American Urological Association recommends the use of commercially available VEDs by prescription only. These have safety mechanisms that minimize the likelihood of excessively high vacuum pressures which can cause penile discomfort and injury.[15]

Pain or injury from VEDs most often is caused by the constriction bands used to sustain an erection. Because these rings trap blood in the corpora and reduce arteriolar flow into the penis, the penile shaft may feel cold and numb. If the constriction bands are applied for longer than 30 minutes, the penile shaft may turn blue and hurt. Patients may complain that a hinge-like erection is produced in that the penis pivots on the rubber ring or tension band. Patients sometimes fail to ejaculate.

VEDs are contraindicated in patients with sickle cell disease. These patients are prone to priapism, which can be exacerbated by the use of constriction bands with VEDs. The devices also should be used cautiously by patients taking oral anticoagulants because warfarin, through a poorly understood and idiosyncratic mechanism, can cause priapism.

Phosphodiesterase Inhibitors

Mechanism

In the presence of sexual stimulation, nitric oxide is released by neurons and endothelial cells in cavernosal tissue, thereby enhancing the activity of guanylate cyclase, the enzyme responsible for conversion of guanylate triphosphate to cGMP (Fig. 66-4).[30] cGMP is a vasodilatory secondary messenger that upregulates the response to nitric oxide by activating protein kinase G. This decreases intracellular calcium levels, resulting in smooth muscle relaxation, enhanced arterial flow to the corpora cavernosa, and enhanced blood filling of cavernosal sinuses.[30] Catabolism of cGMP in cavernosal tissue is mediated by phosphodiesterase isoenzyme type 5.

Four competitive, reversible inhibitors of the phosphodiesterase isoenzyme type 5 found in genital tissue are marketed for erectile dysfunction in the United States (Table 66-4). Chemically, they are nonhydrolyzable analogs of cGMP and they act by decreasing catabolism of cGMP. However, phosphodiesterase isoenzyme type 5 is also found in peripheral vascular tissue, tracheal smooth muscle, and platelets. Inhibition of phosphodiesterase in these nongenital tissues can produce unwanted effects.[30]

The four marketed phosphodiesterase inhibitors differ in their degree of selectivity in inhibiting phosphodiesterase isoenzyme type 5 and other phosphodiesterase isoenzymes, pharmacokinetic profiles, drug–food interactions, and adverse effects (see Table 66-4).

Efficacy

Because of their apparent effectiveness, convenient route of administration, and comparatively low incidence of serious adverse effects, phosphodiesterase inhibitors are considered first-line therapy for erectile dysfunction, particularly in younger patients. They allow for discreet use. Although not based on direct comparison trials, all four commercially available phosphodiesterase inhibitors are considered to be equally effective.[31,32] Patient preference studies show that some patients may prefer one agent over another based on the preferences of the patient or partner; or the onset, duration, or

TABLE 66-3 Dosing Regimens for Selected Drug Treatments for Erectile Dysfunction

Drug	Brand Name	Initial Dose	Usual Range	Special Population Dose	Other
Phosphodiesterase Inhibitor					
Sildenafil	Viagra	50 mg orally 1 hour before intercourse	25–100 mg 1 hour before intercourse. Limit to one dose per day	In patients age 65 years and older, start with 25 mg dose. In patients with creatinine clearance less than 30 mL/minute or severe hepatic impairment, limit starting dose to 25 mg. In patients taking potent P450 CYP3A4 inhibitors, limit starting dose to 25 mg	Titrate dose so that erection lasts no more than 1 hour. Food decreases absorption by 1 hour. Contraindicated with nitrates by any route of administration
Vardenafil	Levitra	5–10 mg orally 1 hour before intercourse	5–20 mg 1 hour before intercourse. Limit to one dose per day	In patients age 65 years and older, start with 5 mg Levitra. In patients with moderate hepatic impairment, start with 5 mg Levitra. In patients taking potent P450 CYP3A4 inhibitors, limit starting dose to 2.5–5 mg every 24–72 hours	Titrate dose so that erection lasts no more than 1 hour. Food decreases absorption by 1 hour. Contraindicated with nitrates by any route of administration
	Staxyn	10 mg tablet to dissolve on the tongue 1 hour before intercourse	10 mg tablet to dissolve on the tongue 1 hour before intercourse. Limit to one dose per day.	Dose of Staxyn requires no adjustment in patients 65 years or older or in patients with creatinine clearance less than 30 mL/minute. Do not use in patients with severe hepatic impairment or those taking potent P450 CYP3A4 inhibitors. Do not initiate Staxyn in patients taking α-adrenergic antagonists	Staxyn should be taken without any liquid or food. The tablet should be placed on the tongue where it will dissolve. No uptitration of dose is recommended
Tadalafil	Cialis	5–10 mg orally before intercourse OR 2.5–5 mg orally once daily	10–20 mg before intercourse. Limit to one dose per day; the drug improves erectile function for up to 36 hours 2.5–5 mg once daily. Limit to one dose per day	Dose of tadalafil requires no dosage adjustment in patients 65 years or older. In patients with creatinine clearance of 30–50 mL/min, limit starting dose to 10 mg every 48 hours; if less than 30 mL/min, limit starting dose to 5 mg every 72 hours. In patients with mild-moderate hepatic impairment, limit starting dose to 10 mg every 24 hours. Do not use in patients with severe hepatic impairment. In patients taking potent P450 CYP3A4 inhibitors, limit starting dose to 10 mg every 72 hours	Titrate dose so that erection lasts not more than 1 hour. Food does not affect rate or extent of drug absorption. Contraindicated with nitrates by any route of administration. When taken with large amounts of ethanol, tadalafil may cause orthostatic hypotension
Avanafil	Stendra	100 mg orally 30 minutes before intercourse	50–200 mg orally 30 minutes before intercourse	In patients with creatinine clearance of 30–89 mL/min, no dosage adjustment is needed. Do not use if creatinine clearance is less than 30 mL/min, if the patient has severe hepatic disease, or if the patient is taking P450 CYP3A4 inhibitors	May be taken with food. When taken with large amounts of ethanol, avanafil may cause orthostatic hypotension
Prostaglandin E1					
Alprostadil intracavernosal injection	Caverject, Edex	2.5 mcg intracavernosally 5–10 minutes before intercourse	10–20 mcg 5–10 minutes before intercourse. Maximum recommended dose is 60 mcg. Limit to not more than one injection per day and not more than three injections per week	Titrate dose to achieve an erection that lasts 1 hour	Patient will require training on an aseptic intracavernosal injection technique. Avoid intracavernosal injections in patients with sickle cell anemia, multiple myeloma, leukemia, severe coagulopathy, schizophrenia, poor manual dexterity, severe venous incompetence, or severe cardiovascular disease
Alprostadil intraurethral pellet	Muse	125–250 mcg intraurethrally 5–10 minutes before intercourse	250–1,000 mcg just before intercourse. Limit to not more than two doses per day		Patient will require training on proper intraurethral administration techniques Use applicator provided to administer medications to avoid urethral injury
Testosterone Supplements					
Methyltestosterone	Android, Testred, Methitest	10 mg once daily	10–50 mg once daily		Not recommended for use due to extensive first-pass hepatic catabolism and because it is associated with hepatotoxicity
Fluoxymesterone	Androxy	5 mg once daily	5–20 mg once daily	Contraindicated in patients with severe renal or hepatic impairment	Not recommended because it is associated with hepatotoxicity. This is a 17α-alkylated androgen

(*continued*)

TABLE 66-3 Dosing Regimens for Selected Drug Treatments for Erectile Dysfunction (*Continued*)

Drug	Brand Name	Initial Dose	Usual Range	Special Population Dose	Other
Testosterone buccal system	Striant	30 mg every 12 hours, morning and evening	30 mg every 12 hours, morning and evening		Place buccal system just above incisor tooth on both sides of the mouth. To remove, slide buccal system down toward the tooth. Buccal tablet may become detached during eating. If this occurs, discard and replace with new buccal system. Do not chew or swallow buccal system
Testosterone cypionate intramuscular injection	Depo-Testosterone	200–400 mg every 2–4 weeks	200–400 mg every 2–4 weeks	Contraindicated in patients with severe hepatic or renal impairment	During the dosing interval, supraphysiologic serum concentrations of testosterone are produced during a portion of the dosing interval. This has been linked to mood swings
Testosterone enanthate	Delatestryl	200–400 mg every 2–4 weeks	200–400 mg every 2–4 weeks	Although not so labeled, it should probably not be used in patients with severe hepatic or renal impairment	During the dosing interval, supraphysiologic serum concentrations of testosterone are produced during a portion of the dosing interval. This has been linked to mood swings
Testosterone transdermal patch	Androderm	4 mg as a single dose at bedtime	2–6 mg as a single dose at bedtime	Safety in patients with hepatic or renal dysfunction has not been evaluated	When administered at bedtime, serum concentrations of testosterone in the usual circadian pattern are produced. Apply to those sites recommended in the package labeling: upper arm, back, abdomen, and thigh. Rotate application sites. Avoid swimming, showering, or washing administration site for 3 hours after patch application
Testosterone gel	Androgel 1%, Testim 1%	5–10 g (equivalent to 50–100 mg testosterone, respectively) gel as a single dose in the morning	5–10 g (equivalent to 50–100 mg testosterone, respectively) gel as a single dose in the morning. Titrate dose up at 14-day intervals		Cover application site to avoid inadvertent transfer to others. Avoid swimming, showering, or washing administration site for 2 hours after gel application. Apply to those sites recommended in the product labeling: shoulders, upper arms, abdomen. Children and women should avoid contact with unclothed or unwashed application sites. Patients should wash hands with soap and water after administration of transdermal testosterone product
Testosterone transdermal spray	Fortesta	Four sprays (equivalent to 40 mg testosterone) once daily	Four to seven sprays (equivalent to 40–70 mg testosterone) once daily. Titrate dose up at 14- to 35-day intervals.		Cover application site to avoid inadvertent transfer to others. Avoid swimming, showering, or washing administration site for 2 hours after spray application. Apply to those sites recommended in the product labeling: front and inner thighs. Children and women should avoid contact with unclothed or unwashed application sites. Patients should wash hands with soap and water after administration of transdermal testosterone product
Testosterone transdermal solution	Axiron	One to four (30–90 mg, respectively) pump sprays to left or right axilla daily	One to four (30–120 mg, respectively) pump sprays to left or right axilla daily. Titrate dose up at 14- to 35-day intervals		Limit application to axilla. Apply antiperspirant or deodorant before Axiron
Testosterone subcutaneous implant pellet	Testopel	150–450 mg as a single dose every 3–6 months. Administration of the dose requires a forearm incision and subcutaneous dose implant under local anesthesia	150–450 mg as a single dose every 3–6 months		Trained health professional is required to administer the dose. Should use sterile implanter kit. Clinical onset is delayed for 3–4 months after initial dose

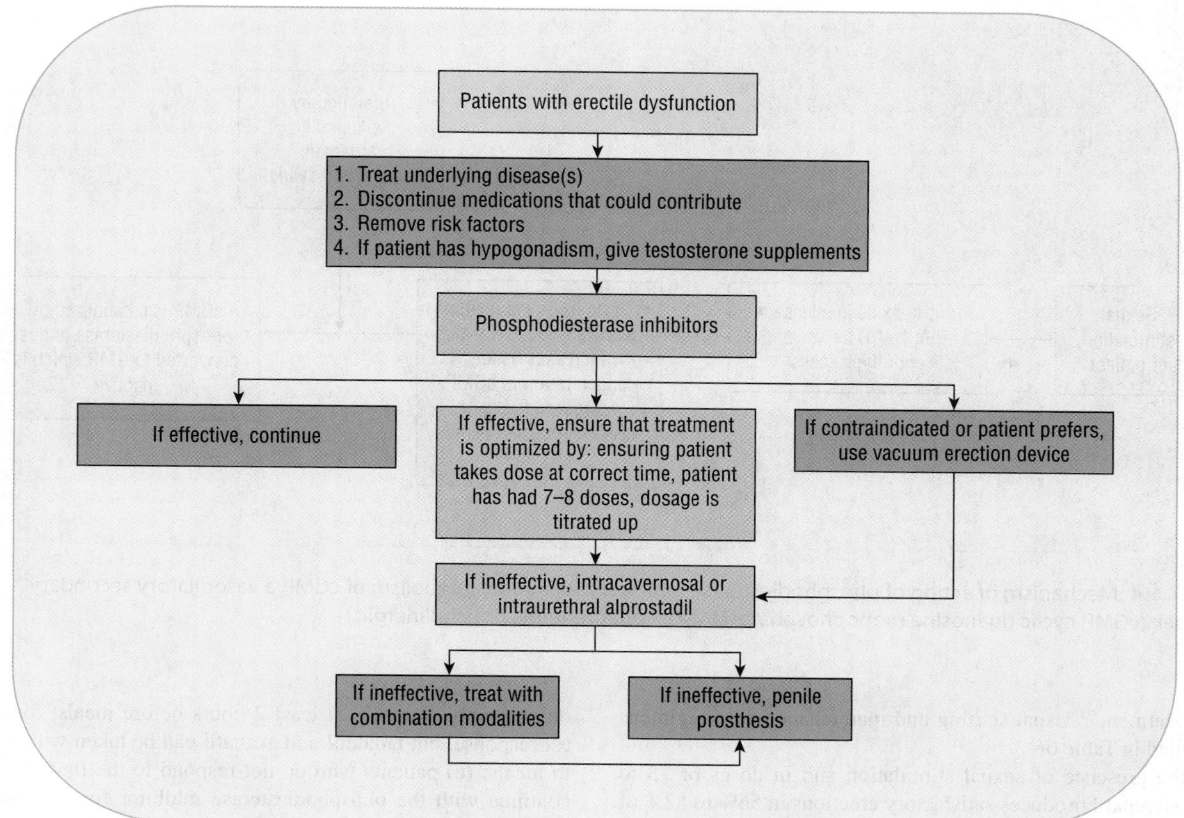

FIGURE 66-2 Algorithm for selecting treatment for erectile dysfunction.

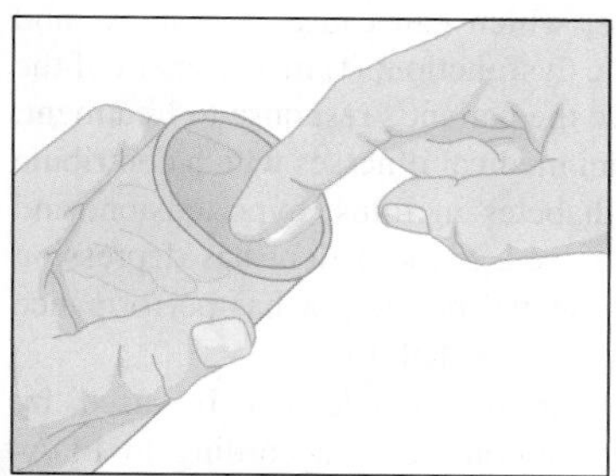

Assemble your system according to the two-step procedure.

Step 1

Apply Osbon Personal Lubricant™ to the following:

1. two inches inside the open end of the cylinder;

2. the rim of the cylinder that meets the body to form the vacuum seal; and

3. the entire head of the penis.

Applying lubricant properly will help you achieve the best erection possible.

Tip: Trimming the pubic hair around the base of the penis with a pair of scissors may also prove helpful in creating an airtight seal.

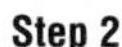

Step 2

It is recommended that you stand for this step (the system can also be used when you are sitting or lying down).

Place the lubricated penis inside the cylinder with the label on the cylinder facing up. With one hand, hold the cylinder at a downward 45° angle with the open end snugly against the body.

Tip: Rotate cylinder slightly back and forth to make an airtight seal against the body, make sure the testicles are not drawn into the cylinder.

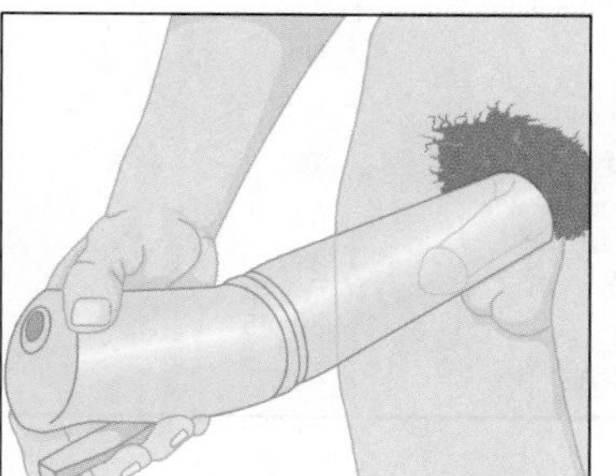

FIGURE 66-3 Technique for using a vacuum erection device. *(From Osbon Erec Aid Esteem Vacuum Therapy System User Guide. Eden Prairie, MN: TIMM Medical Technologies, http://www.timmmedical.com/_l/pdf/timm-brochure-2012.pdf. Reprinted with permission.)*

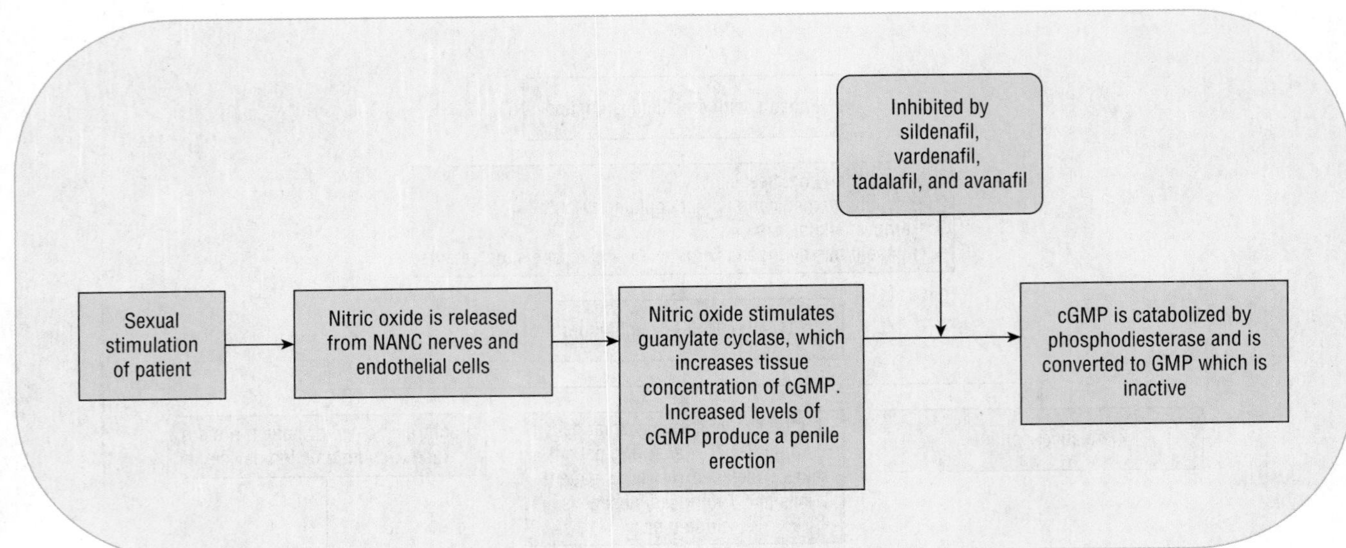

FIGURE 66-4 Mechanism of action of phosphodiesterase inhibitors. All inhibit catabolism of cGMP, a vasodilatory secondary messenger. (cGMP, cyclic guanosine monophosphate; NANC, nonadrenergic noncholinergic.)

cost of treatment.[33] Usual starting and maintenance dose regimens are included in Table 66-3.

In the presence of sexual stimulation and in doses of 25 to 100 mg, sildenafil produces satisfactory erections in 56% to 82% of patients, independent of the etiology of erectile dysfunction. Similar results are documented in the product labeling for the other agents in this class (65–80% for vardenafil, 62–77% for tadalafil, and 50–55% for avanafil). Response rates in the lower range for phosphodiesterase inhibitors have been documented in patients with diabetes mellitus or after radical prostatectomy, or those with severe vascular disease, probably due to neuropathy or surgery-related nerve damage, respectively, in which nitric oxide availability is compromised.[6,15,34] The effectiveness of the drugs appears to be dose related.

8 Approximately 30% to 40% of patients do not respond to phosphodiesterase inhibitors.[15] At least half of nonresponders can benefit from education on proper use of the drugs.[34,35] Therefore, follow-up is always recommended after a phosphodiesterase inhibitor is initiated. Education of patients should include the following points: (a) patients must engage in sexual stimulation (foreplay) for the best response; (b) sildenafil and vardenafil should be taken on an empty stomach, at least 2 hours before meals, for the fastest response, but tadalafil and avanafil can be taken without regard to meals; (c) patients who do not respond to the first dose should continue with the phosphodiesterase inhibitor for at least five to eight doses before failure is declared, as increasing success rates are reported with sequential dose administration; (d) some patients require dosage titration up to 100 mg sildenafil, 20 mg vardenafil, 20 mg tadalafil, or 200 mg avanafil for a response; (e) patients should avoid excessive alcohol intake, which can cause drowsiness and hypotension and worsen erectile dysfunction; (f) involvement of the sexual partner can help improve the patient's response to treatment; and (g) treatment of concomitant medical illnesses which contribute to erectile dysfunction (e.g., diabetes mellitus, hypertension, and hypogonadism) should be optimized. If the patient has depression because of divorce or loss of a sexual partner, or has performance anxiety, psychologic counseling may be helpful.[21]

The phosphodiesterase inhibitors should not be used by patients with normal erectile function. Also, according to FDA-approved labeling, the drugs should not be used in combination with other forms of therapy for erectile dysfunction because prolonged

TABLE 66-4 Pharmacodynamics and Pharmacokinetics of Phosphodiesterase Inhibitors

	Sildenafil (Viagra)	Vardenafil (Levitra/Staxyn)	Tadalafil (Cialis)	Avanafil (Stendra)
Inhibits PDE-5	Yes	Yes	Yes	Yes
Inhibits PDE-6	Yes	Minimally	No	Minimally
Inhibits PDE-11	No	No	Yes	Minimally
Time to peak plasma level (hours)	0.5–1	0.7–0.9/1.5	2	0.5–0.8
Oral bioavailability (%)	40	15/21–44	Not determined	15
Fatty meal decreases rate of oral absorption?	Yes	Yes/No[a]	No	No
Mean plasma half-life (hours)	3.7	4.4–4.8/4–6	18	4–5
Active metabolite	Yes	Yes/Yes	No	Yes
Percentage of dose excreted in feces	80	91–95/91–95	61	62
Percentage of dose excreted in urine	13	2–6/2–6	36	21
Onset (minutes)	30	30/60	45	30–45
Duration (hours)	4	4–5/4–6	24–36	4–5

PDE, phosphodiesterase.

[a]When Staxyn is taken with water, the area under the curve decreases by 29%.

erections (which may lead to priapism) may result.[15,36] Also, phosphodiesterase inhibitors should be avoided in patients predisposed to developing priapism, including men with sickle cell anemia, leukemia, or multiple myeloma.

Long-term use of phosphodiesterase inhibitors for five to six consecutive years continues to be effective and is not associated with tachyphylaxis. The voluntary discontinuation rate among patients who respond to phosphodiesterase inhibitors is less than 2% per year.[36–38]

Clinical **Controversy...**

Whether tachyphylaxis develops with long-term use of phosphodiesterase inhibitors is unclear. Some patients continue to respond to the medication even after many years of regular use. Other patients eventually become nonresponsive to treatment. This lack of response could be due to tachyphylaxis, or it could be due to worsening erectile dysfunction.

Despite the initial effectiveness of phosphodiesterase inhibitors and the measures to salvage patients with re-education, some patients will show minimal or no response to maximum doses of a phosphodiesterase inhibitor. Various strategies have been attempted in this subgroup of patients, including the following:

1. The effectiveness of switching from one phosphodiesterase inhibitor to another when the patient does not respond to an initial agent is controversial. In one study, vardenafil was beneficial in patients who did not respond to sildenafil.[39] However, less than 5% of patients who fail to respond to a phosphodiesterase inhibitor experience benefit from switching to another phosphodiesterase inhibitor.[34] Controlled clinical trials in larger patient groups are needed before this strategy is used as routine treatment.
2. High-dose phosphodiesterase inhibitor treatment (e.g., sildenafil 200 mg) has been used anecdotally. However, such doses are also associated with a higher frequency of adverse effects.[40]
3. In patients with primary hypogonadism and erectile dysfunction, correcting the former with testosterone supplementation improves the response to a phosphodiesterase inhibitor.[41]
4. Phosphodiesterase inhibitors have been combined with intracavernosal or intraurethral alprostadil in selected patients.[42,43]

Clinical **Controversy...**

For patients who fail to respond to a particular phosphodiesterase inhibitor, a common strategy employed is to switch the patient to another phosphodiesterase inhibitor. Although a low percentage of patients respond to the switch, most patients do not. The benefit of switching from one agent to another is controversial.

Selectivity of Other Phosphodiesterase Isoenzymes

More than 25 different phosphodiesterase isoenzymes have been identified; however, the physiologic effects of stimulation and inhibition of some of these isoenzymes remain to be elucidated. Of note, phosphodiesterase isoenzyme type 6 is localized to the rods and cones of the eye. Inhibition of this isoenzyme has been associated with blurred vision and cyanopsia. Sildenafil is the most potent inhibitor of phosphodiesterase isoenzyme type 6, vardenafil and avanafil are intermediate inhibitors, and tadalafil is the least potent inhibitor.[32] Likewise, phosphodiesterase isoenzyme type 11 is localized to striated muscle. Inhibition of this isoenzyme has been associated with myalgia and muscle pain. Tadalafil exerts the greatest inhibitory activity against phosphodiesterase type 11.[9]

Pharmacokinetics and Drug–Food Interactions

Pharmacokinetic parameters of the phosphodiesterase inhibitors are listed in Table 66-4.

Sildenafil and the conventional oral formulation of vardenafil have similar pharmacokinetic profiles. Both drugs have a 1-hour onset of action and short duration of action. Oral absorption is significantly delayed by 1 hour when either drug is taken within 2 hours of a fatty meal. In contrast, tadalafil has a slower onset of action of 2 hours, has a prolonged duration of action up to 36 hours, and food does not affect its rate of absorption. Thus, tadalafil offers greater spontaneity for patients, as one dose can last through an entire weekend and allows for multiple acts of sexual intercourse over multiple days with a single dose.[31,32] An oral disintegrating tablet formulation of vardenafil, which dissolves on the tongue, has 1.2- to 1.4-fold higher bioavailability than the conventional oral tablet. The oral disintegrating tablet formulation is not susceptible to the drug–food interaction of the conventional oral tablet, which is an advantage for some patients.[44] Avanafil has an onset and duration similar to sildenafil and vardenafil, but food does not significantly affect its rate or extent of absorption.

The onset of action of these agents has undergone reexamination to assess how soon after drug administration patients can expect to have an erection suitable for intercourse. Although up to 50% of patients may develop an erection within 20 to 30 minutes of sildenafil 100 mg, vardenafil 20 mg, tadalafil 20 mg, or avanafil 200 mg, the rest of the patients may require a full hour to achieve an adequate erectile response.[45] Therefore, patients should be instructed to allow adequate time for the drug to work. In addition, sildenafil and vardenafil have been reported to be effective in some patients up to 12 hours after dosing, which is long after plasma concentrations have declined. It has been hypothesized that this may be due to the continued intracellular action of the phosphodiesterase inhibitor.[46–49]

Concomitant ingestion of ethanol with phosphodiesterase inhibitors can result in orthostatic hypotension and drowsiness. Therefore, the manufacturer recommends that patients avoid ethanol when taking these medications.

All four phosphodiesterase inhibitors are hepatically catabolized principally by the cytochrome P450 3A4 microsomal isoenzyme and by other P450 isoenzymes (minor routes) and/or other hepatic enzymes (Table 66-4). Sildenafil has an active metabolite, which is excreted primarily in the urine. Tadalafil has a clinically insignificant active metabolite; however, 36% of the parent drug is renally eliminated. Thus, both sildenafil and tadalafil doses should be reduced in patients with significant renal impairment. Vardenafil and avanafil have active metabolites that are largely excreted in feces; no dosage reduction of vardenafil is required in patients with renal impairment (see Table 66-3).

Dosing

The usual oral doses of the phosphodiesterase inhibitors are listed in Table 66-3. Sildenafil, vardenafil, and avanafil should be taken on demand at least 30 to 60 minutes before sexual intercourse. Tadalafil should be taken at least 2 hours before sexual intercourse. The durations of action for sildenafil, vardenafil, and avanafil are 4 to 5 hours, whereas the effects of tadalafil last for 36 hours. The agents vary as to whether doses must be adjusted for patients 65 years and older and those with compromised hepatic or renal function. Patients should be advised to take not more than the amount prescribed and to use only one dose per day (or less often in the case of most patients taking tadalafil). Doses higher than those recommended have been described in the published literature (e.g., sildenafil 200 mg[40]); however, such dosing regimens have not consistently produced improved erectile responses.

For patients who do not respond to an adequate course of on-demand phosphodiesterase inhibitors for erectile dysfunction, daily low dosing of these agents may improve endothelial function in cavernosal tissue. That is, regular use of phosphodiesterase inhibitors may activate endothelial nitric oxide synthase, increase local concentrations of cGMP, which may lead to increased oxygen tension, improved blood flow, and reduced endothelial damage and cavernosal fibrosis. A preliminary clinical trial of daily use of tadalafil 2.5 or 5 mg showed a 58% frequency of successful sexual intercourse compared with conventional on-demand use of tadalafil 5 to 20 mg, which produced a 21% frequency of success.[48,50] Other potential advantages of daily low dosing regimens include a lower potential for dose-related adverse effects, lower cost, and increased spontaneity of sexual intercourse.[51] However, a disadvantage of the daily low-dose regimen is that patients with more severe erectile dysfunction, who may require higher doses of a phosphodiesterase inhibitor, may not respond.[51] Although clinical trials of daily dosing of tadalafil 10 and 20 mg,[51] and sildenafil 50 and 100 mg[52,53] have been published, the only FDA-approved labeling is for daily dosing of tadalafil 2.5 or 5 mg.

Adverse Effects

Most adverse effects of the phosphodiesterase inhibitors are mild or moderate and are self-limited, and patients often become tolerant to them with continued use.[54,55] The rates of drug discontinuation caused by adverse effects are low, ranging from 2.1% to 25%, and are similar for all four agents. In usual doses, the most common adverse effects are headache (11%), facial flushing (12%), dyspepsia (5%), nasal congestion (3.4%), and dizziness (3%),[56] all of which are dose-related and result from vasodilation or smooth muscle relaxation secondary to inhibition of phosphodiesterase isoenzyme type 5 in extragenital tissues.

Sildenafil and vardenafil produce an 8- to 10-mm Hg decrease in systolic and a 5- to 6-mm Hg decrease in diastolic blood pressure starting approximately 1 hour after a dose is taken and lasting for 4 hours. Most patients are asymptomatic as a result of these blood pressure changes, but some patients, particularly those taking multiple antihypertensives or nitrates or those with baseline hypotension, may develop clinical symptoms as a consequence of these peripheral vascular effects. Avanafil can produce similar decreases in blood pressure, especially when used along with other antihypertensives or α-adrenergic antagonists. Tadalafil does not produce decreases in blood pressure, but it must be used with caution in patients with cardiovascular disease because of the cardiac risk inherent to sexual activity. A management approach for such patients, developed based on an analysis of deaths in men who were using sildenafil and commonly referred to as the recommendations of the Princeton Consensus Guideline Conference III,[20] should be applied to all the phosphodiesterase inhibitors (Table 66-5).

Sildenafil, vardenafil, and avanafil cause increased sensitivity to light, blurred vision, or loss of blue–green color discrimination in 2% to 3% of patients. The adverse effect is dose-related with the incidence increasing to 40% to 50% in patients taking sildenafil 200 mg.[57] These effects result from inhibition of phosphodiesterase type 6 in the photoreceptor cells of in retinal rods and cones. Visual adverse effects commonly occur at the time of peak serum concentrations. Although visual adverse effects are mild and reversible, caution regarding use is recommended for airplane pilots, who rely on green and blue lights for landing planes. Avanafil has moderate and tadalafil has minimal to no inhibitory activity against type 6 phosphodiesterase, and a lower incidence of visual adverse effects (less than 1%) has been reported.[31,58] Nevertheless, according to current product labeling, all phosphodiesterase inhibitors should be used cautiously in patients at risk for retinitis pigmentosa, a genetic disease associated with retinal phosphodiesterase deficiency.

Nonarteritic anterior ischemic optic neuropathy (NAION) is a sudden, unilateral, painless blindness, which may be irreversible. Isolated cases of NAION have been associated with phosphodiesterase inhibitor use.[58] NAION has developed at variable and unpredictable times after starting a phosphodiesterase inhibitor, ranging from 6 hours to months or years after the first dose.[57] Although a cause-and-effect relationship has not been definitively established, the blood pressure-lowering effects of these medications may decrease blood flow to the optic nerve and lead to a sudden unilateral decrease in vision.[58] Because NAION may lead to permanent vision loss,

TABLE 66-5 Recommendations of the Third Princeton Consensus Conference for Cardiovascular Risk Stratification of Patients Being Considered for Phosphodiesterase Inhibitor Therapy

Risk Category	Description of Patient's Condition	Management Approach
Low risk	Has asymptomatic cardiovascular disease with <3 risk factors for cardiovascular disease Has well-controlled hypertension Has mild congestive heart failure (NYHA class I or II) Has mild valvular heart disease Had a myocardial infarction >8 weeks ago	Patient can be started on phosphodiesterase inhibitor
Intermediate risk	Has ≥3 risk factors for cardiovascular disease Has mild or moderate, stable angina Had a recent myocardial infarction or stroke within the past 2–8 weeks Has moderate congestive heart failure (NYHA class III) History of stroke, transient ischemic attack, or peripheral artery disease	Patient should undergo complete cardiovascular workup and treadmill stress test to determine tolerance to increased myocardial energy consumption associated with increased sexual activity. Reclassify in low or high risk category
High risk	Has unstable or refractory angina, despite treatment Has uncontrolled hypertension Has severe congestive heart failure (NYHA class IV) Had a recent myocardial infarction or stroke within past 2 weeks Has moderate or severe valvular heart disease Has high-risk cardiac arrhythmias Has obstructive hypertrophic cardiomyopathy	Phosphodiesterase inhibitor is contraindicated; sexual intercourse should be deferred

NYHA, New York Heart Association.

From Nehra et al.,[20] Rosen et al.,[21] and Nehra et al.[22]

the FDA has required inclusion of warnings on the product labeling of phosphodiesterase inhibitors. Specifically, before receiving these agents, patients at risk for NAION should be evaluated by an ophthalmologist, risk factors for NAION should be addressed, and the patient should be cautioned against using a phosphodiesterase inhibitor.

Patients at risk include a wide variety of patients: those with glaucoma, macular degeneration, diabetic retinopathy or hypertension, those who have undergone eye surgery or have experienced eye trauma, patients who are age 50 years or more, or smokers. A patient who experiences sudden vision loss in one eye while taking a phosphodiesterase inhibitor should be evaluated for NAION before continuing treatment. If NAION is present, the phosphodiesterase inhibitor should be discontinued as there is a 15% to 25% risk of developing NAION in the other eye in the ensuing 5 to 10 years.[57,58]

Tadalafil produces lower back and limb muscle pain, which occur in a dose-related fashion in 7% to 30% of patients treated with doses of 10 to 100 mg.[31] The mechanism for this is not known. It may be linked to inhibition of type 11 phosphodiesterase, a unique characteristic of tadalafil.

Vardenafil can cause prolongation of the QT interval. Therefore, it should be used cautiously in patients with this anomaly or in patients who are taking class IA or III antiarrhythmic medications that prolong the QT interval (e.g., quinidine, procainamide, amiodarone, and sotalol).

Acute unilateral hearing loss has also been reported after use of a phosphodiesterase inhibitor. A cause–effect relationship has not been established. In the cases reported, the hearing loss occurred within 1 day of starting treatment; it was variably accompanied by tinnitus or vertigo, and often resulted in residual hearing loss despite discontinuation of the phosphodiesterase inhibitor.[59,60]

Priapism is a rare adverse effect of phosphodiesterase inhibitors, particularly sildenafil and vardenafil, which have shorter plasma half-lives than tadalafil. Priapism has been associated with excessive doses of the phosphodiesterase inhibitor or concomitant use with other erectogenic drugs.

Recommendations for adverse effect monitoring are included in Table 66-6.

Drug Interactions

Patients taking organic nitrates may develop severe hypotension if they are taken with phosphodiesterase inhibitors as a result of two major factors: (a) organic nitrates on their own produce hypotension, and (b) organic nitrates are nitric oxide donors, which can stimulate the activity of guanylate cyclase and increase tissue levels of cGMP. For this reason, use of phosphodiesterase inhibitors is contraindicated in patients taking nitrates given by any route at scheduled times or intermittently.[20,61] Furthermore, nitrates should be withheld for 24 hours after sildenafil or vardenafil administration and for 48 hours after tadalafil administration.[20,61] Finally, if a patient who has taken a phosphodiesterase inhibitor requires medical treatment of angina, non–nitrate-containing agents (e.g., calcium channel blocker, β-adrenergic antagonist, and morphine) should be used.

If severe hypotension occurs after exposure to nitrates and a phosphodiesterase inhibitor, the patient should be placed in a Trendelenburg position and aggressive fluid administration initiated. If severe hypotension continues, parenteral β-adrenergic agonists (e.g., dopamine) should be administered cautiously.

Interestingly, dietary sources of nitrates, nitrites, or L-arginine (a precursor for nitrates) do not interact with phosphodiesterase inhibitors. This is because dietary sources do not increase circulating levels of nitric oxide in humans.

The phosphodiesterase inhibitors have a low potential to interact with antihypertensive medications.[62] In retrospective analyses of patients taking sildenafil in combination with α-adrenergic antagonists, β-adrenergic antagonists, diuretics, angiotensin-converting enzyme inhibitors, angiotensin receptor blockers, or calcium channel blockers, the incidence of hypotension was similar to that reported in patients taking sildenafil alone.[63] This finding was confirmed by a retrospective analysis of pooled data on more than 4,800 patients in 35 clinical trials.[64]

Small decreases in blood pressure with clinically symptomatic hypotension have been described in some patients taking phosphodiesterase inhibitors and α-adrenergic antagonists. The degree of hypotension that develops is dependent on several factors: (a) stability of patient's blood pressure prior to taking both drugs; (b) dose of the α-adrenergic antagonist used; (c) particular α-adrenergic antagonist used; (d) particular phosphodiesterase inhibitor used; and (e) timing of administration of both drugs. The drug interaction produces less hypotension when the patient has stable blood pressure prior to taking both drugs; a low dose of α-adrenergic antagonist is taken; a uroselective (e.g., tamsulosin or silodosin) or extended-release formulation of α-adrenergic antagonist (e.g., alfuzosin, or modified-release doxazosin) is used; tadalafil is preferentially prescribed over sildenafil, vardenafil, or avanafil; and when there is an interval of 4 to 6 hours between the dosing of the α-adrenergic antagonist and phosphodiesterase inhibitor.[62,64–67]

Hepatic metabolism of all three phosphodiesterase inhibitors can be inhibited by enzyme inhibitors of CYP 3A4, including cimetidine, erythromycin, clarithromycin, ketoconazole, itraconazole, ritonavir, saquinavir, and grapefruit juice.[64] Lower starting doses should be used in these patients to minimize dose-related adverse effects, including cyanopsia, hypotension, flushing, nasal congestion, and priapism (see Table 66-4).

Testosterone Replacement Regimens

Mechanism

9 Testosterone replacement regimens supply exogenous testosterone and restore serum testosterone levels to the normal range (300 to 1,100 ng/dL; 10.4 to 38.2 nmol/L). In so doing, testosterone replacement regimens correct symptoms of hypogonadism, which include malaise, loss of muscle strength, depressed mood, and decreased libido. Testosterone can directly stimulate androgen receptors in the CNS and is thought to be responsible for maintaining normal sexual drive. In addition, testosterone may stimulate nitric oxide synthase, thereby increasing cavernosal concentrations of nitric oxide, and enhancing the effects of phosphodiesterase type 5 in cavernosal tissue.[68]

Indications

Testosterone replacement regimens are indicated in symptomatic patients with primary or secondary hypogonadism, as confirmed by both the presence of a decreased libido and low serum concentrations of testosterone.[2] Primary hypogonadism can be a characteristic of aging men who undergo andropause, in which the Leydig cells of the testes slowly and progressively decrease testosterone production.[69] This is often referred to as late-onset hypogonadism, symptomatic late-onset hypogonadism andropause, or the male menopause. Symptoms include decreased libido, erectile dysfunction, gynecomastia, small testes, reduced growth of body hair and beard, decreased muscle mass, and increased body fat. If left untreated, patients develop anemia and osteoporosis.

Serum testosterone concentrations typically are measured in the early morning (approximately 8 am) because the secretion pattern of this hormone follows a circadian pattern, with highest serum concentrations in the morning hours and the lowest level at night (approximately 10 pm). A low measured serum testosterone level is confirmed with a repeat measurement on a separate day. Simultaneous serum luteinizing hormone levels help to distinguish patients with primary hypogonadism, who have elevated luteinizing

TABLE 66-6 Drug Monitoring Table

Drug	Adverse Drug Reaction	Monitoring Parameter	Comments
Phosphodiesterase Inhibitor			
Sildenafil	Headache Flushing Gastroesophageal reflux Nasal congestion Cyanopsia NAION Hypotension Priapism	Clinical symptoms Visual complaints, loss of vision Blood pressure Pulse	Discontinue sildenafil if the patient has any visual loss and refer the patient to a physician If the patient is taking any antihypertensives, stabilize the blood pressure before starting sildenafil If the patient develops priapism, he should proceed to the emergency department
Vardenafil	Headache Flushing Gastroesophageal reflux Nasal congestion Cyanopsia NAION Hypotension QT interval prolongation on EKG Priapism	Clinical symptoms Visual complaints, loss of vision Blood pressure Pulse Palpitations or dizziness	Discontinue vardenafil if the patient has any visual loss and refer the patient to a physician If the patient is taking any antihypertensives, stabilize their blood pressure before starting vardenafil If the patient has palpitations or dizziness, check EKG. If QT prolongation is present, refer the patient for appropriate medical care If the patient develops priapism, he should proceed to the emergency department
Tadalafil	Headache Flushing Gastroesophageal reflux Nasal congestion Cyanopsia Hearing loss NAION Hypotension Low back or muscle pain QT interval prolongation on EKG Priapism	Clinical symptoms Visual complaints, loss of vision Blood pressure Pulse Palpitations or dizziness Hearing loss	Discontinue tadalafil if the patient has any visual or hearing loss and refer the patient to a physician If the patient is taking any antihypertensives, stabilize their blood pressure before starting tadalafil If the patient develops priapism, he should proceed to the emergency department If the patient has palpitations or dizziness, check EKG. If QT prolongation is present, refer the patient for appropriate medical care
Avanafil	Headache Flushing Gastroesophageal reflux Nasal congestion Cyanopsia Hearing loss NAION Hypotension Low back or muscle pain QT interval prolongation on EKG Priapism	Clinical symptoms Visual complaints, loss of vision Blood pressure Pulse Palpitations or dizziness Hearing loss	Discontinue avanafil if the patient has any visual or hearing loss and refer the patient to a physician If the patient is taking any antihypertensives, stabilize their blood pressure before starting avanafil If the patient develops priapism, he should proceed to the emergency department If the patient has palpitations or dizziness, check EKG. If QT prolongation is present, refer the patient for appropriate medical care
Prostaglandin E_1			
Alprostadil, intracavernosal	Penile pain Hematoma at injection site Priapism Hypotension Fibrotic nodules along penile shaft Decreased blood pressure Dizziness	Clinical symptoms Presence of hematoma or fibrotic nodules Blood pressure Pulse	Penile pain responds to acetaminophen To avoid hematoma, apply pressure to injection site for 5–10 minutes after injection If the patient develops priapism, he should proceed to the emergency department Fibrotic nodules are rare but may occur after repeated injections. These may cause curvature of the penis during an erection and this requires assessment by a urologist Hypotension and dizziness are uncommon and are associated with inadvertent venous injection of the drug
Alprostadil, intraurethral	Aching pain in penis, testicles, legs, and perineum Urethral burning, bleeding, or tearing Decreased blood pressure Dizziness Female partner may experience vaginal pain and burning sensation	Clinical symptoms Urethral injury as evidenced by pain, bleeding, or tissue damage Blood pressure Pulse	Burning pain usually resolves spontaneously. If urethral injury is suspected, this requires assessment by a urologist. Pain experienced by the female partner is due to leakage of medication from male urethra into vagina. Pain will usually resolve spontaneously If the patient develops priapism, he should proceed to the emergency department Hypotension and dizziness are uncommon, occurring in only 3% of patients, and are associated with systemic absorption of the drugs Alprostadil is embryotoxic and contact should be avoided if the female sex partner is pregnant
Testosterone Supplements			
Methyltestosterone	Sodium and water retention Hyperlipidemia Increased hematocrit Gynecomastia Sleep apnea Increased libido Mood swings Oligospermia Hepatotoxicity Prostate enlargement	Physical exam for edema Blood pressure Serum lipids, hematocrit, hepatic transaminases, prostate specific antigen	Discontinue if the patient has signs of hepatoxicity. If hematocrit exceeds 55%, methyltestosterone should be discontinued. Testosterone supplements may worsen LUTS in patients with BPH. It is contraindicated in patients with untreated prostate cancer or men with breast cancer

(continued)

TABLE 66-6 Drug Monitoring Table (*Continued*)

Drug	Adverse Drug Reaction	Monitoring Parameter	Comments
Fluoxymesterone	Sodium and water retention Hyperlipidemia Increased hematocrit Gynecomastia Sleep apnea Increased libido Mood swings Oligospermia Hepatotoxicity Prostate enlargement	Physical exam for edema Blood pressure Serum lipids, hematocrit, hepatic transaminases, prostate-specific antigen	Discontinue if the patient has signs of hepatoxicity. If hematocrit exceeds 55%, fluoxymesterone should be discontinued. Testosterone supplements may worsen LUTS in patients with BPH. It is contraindicated in patients with untreated prostate cancer or men with breast cancer
Testosterone buccal system	Sodium and water retention Hyperlipidemia Increased hematocrit Gynecomastia Sleep apnea Increased libido Mood swings Oligospermia Hepatotoxicity Gum irritation Bitter taste Prostate enlargement	Physical exam for edema Blood pressure Serum lipids, hematocrit, hepatic transaminases, prostate-specific antigen	Discontinue if the patient has signs of hepatoxicity. If hematocrit exceeds 55%, testosterone buccal system should be discontinued. Testosterone supplements may worsen LUTS in patients with BPH. It is contraindicated in patients with untreated prostate cancer or men with breast cancer
Testosterone cypionate or enanthate	Sodium and water retention Hyperlipidemia Increased hematocrit Gynecomastia Sleep apnea Increased libido Oligospermia Mood swings Hepatotoxicity Prostate enlargement	Clinical symptoms Physical exam for edema Blood pressure Serum lipids, hematocrit, hepatic transaminases, prostate-specific antigen	Discontinue if the patient has signs of hepatoxicity. If hematocrit exceeds 55%, testosterone supplement should be discontinued. Testosterone supplements may worsen LUTS in patients with BPH. It is contraindicated in patients with untreated prostate cancer or men with breast cancer. These formulations produce supraphysiologic serum concentrations of testosterone. Mood swings have been reported with these agents
Testosterone patch	Sodium and water retention Hyperlipidemia Increased hematocrit Gynecomastia Sleep apnea Increased libido Mood swings Oligospermia Hepatotoxicity Contact dermatitis Erythema Pruritus Prostate enlargement	Clinical symptoms Physical exam for edema Blood pressure Serum lipids, hematocrit, hepatic transaminases, prostate-specific antigen	If hematocrit exceeds 55%, testosterone supplement should be discontinued. Testosterone supplements may worsen LUTS in patients with BPH. It is contraindicated in patients with untreated prostate cancer or men with breast cancer. Contact dermatitis has been associated with the alcohol-based agent used to enhance transdermal drug absorption. It responds to topical corticosteroids. Of significance, hepatotoxicity has not been reported with transdermal patches
Testosterone gel/spray/axillary solution	Sodium and water retention Hyperlipidemia Increased hematocrit Gynecomastia Sleep apnea Increased libido Mood swings Oligospermia Hepatotoxicity Dermatitis Erythema Pruritis Prostate enlargement	Clinical symptoms Physical exam for edema Blood pressure Serum lipids, hematocrit, hepatic transaminases, prostate specific antigen	If hematocrit exceeds 55%, testosterone supplement should be discontinued. Testosterone supplements may worsen LUTS in patients with BPH. It is contraindicated in patients with untreated prostate cancer or men with breast cancer
Testosterone subcutaneous implant	Sodium and water retention Hyperlipidemia Increased hematocrit Gynecomastia Sleep apnea Increased libido Mood swings Oligospermia Hepatotoxicity Prostate enlargement Infection at the implant site	Clinical symptoms Physical exam for edema Blood pressure Serum lipids	Subcutaneous implant pellet may be extruded with loss of the dose. Androgen-related adverse effects may persist for a long time after drug administration unless the implant is removed. If hematocrit exceeds 55%, testosterone supplement should be discontinued. Testosterone supplements may worsen LUTS in patients with BPH. It is contraindicated in patients with untreated prostate cancer or men with breast cancer

LUTS, lower urinary tract symptoms.

TABLE 66-7 Comparison of Testosterone Replacement Regimens and Ideal Testosterone Replacement Regimen

	Achieves Serum Testosterone Concentrations in Normal Range?	Produces Normal Circadian Pattern of Serum Testosterone Concentrations?	Produces Normal Pattern of Serum Concentrations of Androgen Metabolites?	Adverse Effects
Oral testosterone	No	No	No	Hyperlipidemia Sodium retention
Oral alkylated androgens	Yes	No	No	Hyperlipidemia Sodium retention Hepatotoxicity
Intramuscular testosterone cypionate or enanthate	Yes	No; produces supraphysiologic serum concentrations for several days after injection	No, excess testosterone is converted to estradiol	Mood swings Gynecomastia Polycythemia Hyperlipidemia
Transdermal nonscrotal skin patch	Yes	Yes, provided the patch is placed at night	Yes	Dermatitis due to permeation enhancers in formulation
Transdermal gel	Yes	Yes	Yes	May be inadvertently transferred to others who rub up against the patient's skin treated area
Testosterone subcutaneous implant	Yes	No	No; produces elevated concentrations of dihydrotestosterone	Pellet may be extruded accidentally, resulting in loss of drug effect
Buccal system	Yes	No	No	Gum irritation, bitter taste

hormone levels, from those with secondary hypogonadism, who have decreased luteinizing hormone levels.[2,69]

Testosterone replacement regimens should never be administered to men with normal serum testosterone levels, or in patients with isolated erectile dysfunction as the only sign of hypogonadism.[2,68–70]

Efficacy

Testosterone replacement regimens restore muscle strength and sexual drive and improve mood in patients with hypogonadism. Improvements are generally observed within days or weeks of the start of testosterone replacement. Administration of testosterone will correct the serum testosterone level to the normal range. No additional benefit has been demonstrated for large doses of testosterone, which increase the serum testosterone level from the low end to the upper end of the normal range or to the above-normal range.[70] Testosterone replacement regimens do not directly correct erectile dysfunction; instead, they improve libido, thereby correcting secondary erectile dysfunction.[70]

Testosterone replacement regimens can be administered orally, bucally, parenterally, or transdermally (Tables 66-3 and 66-7). Injectable testosterone replacement regimens are the preferred treatment for symptomatic patients with primary or secondary hypogonadism because they are effective, inexpensive, and not associated with the bioavailability problems or hepatotoxic adverse effects of oral androgens.[2,68–70] Although convenient for the patient, testosterone patches, gels, and sprays are much more expensive than other forms of androgen replacement; therefore, they should be reserved for patients who refuse injectable testosterone.

In the ideal testosterone replacement regimen, the medication would mimic the normal circadian pattern of serum testosterone concentrations such that peak and trough concentrations occur in the early morning and late afternoon, respectively; produce serum concentrations in the normal range; produce serum concentrations of dihydrotestosterone and estradiol, which are metabolites of testosterone that mimic the normal physiologic pattern; and produce minimal adverse effects.[70] Table 66-7 compares commercially available testosterone replacement regimens for these characteristics and shows that an ideal regimen has yet to be identified.

Pharmacokinetics

Natural testosterone has poor oral bioavailability because of extensive first-pass hepatic metabolism; therefore, large doses must be taken. To improve oral bioavailability, alkylated derivatives were formulated. Of these derivatives, methyltestosterone and fluoxymesterone are more resistant to hepatic catabolism and can be taken in smaller daily doses, which are potentially safer. However, oral alkylated derivatives of testosterone are not metabolized to dihydrotestosterone or estradiol, are associated with a higher incidence of serious hepatotoxicity, and therefore are not preferred for management of hypogonadism.

An alternative to oral administration is the testosterone buccal system (Striant), which is applied to the gum above the upper incisor teeth twice per day. Over time it forms a gel from which testosterone is absorbed. One advantage of this route of administration is that the drug bypasses first-pass hepatic catabolism, which allows for increased bioavailability of testosterone. Serum testosterone levels are maintained in the normal range for approximately 80% of the day.[71]

Several testosterone esters have been formulated for intramuscular injection, with different durations of action (see Table 66-3). The shorter-acting testosterone propionate, which requires dosing three times per week, has been replaced with testosterone cypionate or enanthate, which can be dosed every 2, 4, or 6 weeks in most patients. These testosterone formulations produce suprapharmacologic patterns of serum testosterone during the dosing interval, which have been linked to mood swings in some patients. An even longer-acting parenteral testosterone is available as a subcutaneous implant for dosing every 3 to 6 months. Although this schedule minimizes repeat visits to the clinician's office for dosing, the implant must be administered by a physician, and the implanted pellet may be extruded after administration. This extrusion has been reported in up to 8.5% of treated patients and results in loss of drug effect.

Topical testosterone replacement regimens can be delivered as once-daily patches or gel. Testosterone patches increase serum testosterone levels into the normal range in 2 to 6 hours. Serum testosterone levels return to baseline 24 hours after patch administration. However, unlike oral or injectable supplements, transdermal testosterone patches applied at bedtime or testosterone gel applied each morning produce physiologic patterns of serum testosterone levels throughout the day. The clinical importance of this biochemical effect is unknown.[68,72]

The original Testoderm brand patch was formulated for scrotal application. Scrotal skin is thinner and has a richer vascular supply than does the skin on the arms or thighs. Therefore, application of

Testoderm patches produced excellent absorption of the hormone. However, the patch could detach when the scrotum became damp or moist, when the patient exercised, or if the scrotum was excessively hairy.[72]

For improved convenience, Androderm patches were formulated for application to the upper arms, back, abdomen, or thighs. The addition of absorption enhancers and different adhesives has been linked to a higher incidence of contact dermatitis with Androderm patches compared with the original Testoderm scrotal patch.[72]

Testosterone gel 1% formulation (AndroGel) is applied in much larger doses (5 or 10 g each day) to the skin of the shoulders, upper arms, or abdomen. The hormone is absorbed quickly, within 30 minutes, but several hours may be required for complete absorption of the dose. For this reason, the patient should be reminded to wait at least 2 hours after application before showering. To prevent inadvertent transfer of testosterone gel to others, the patient should thoroughly wash his hands with soap and water after administration of a dose, allow the application site to dry undisturbed for several minutes before dressing or covering it, and ensure that there is no contact with clothing contaminated with the gel by children and female members of the household.

Dosing

Table 66-3 lists the usual doses for testosterone replacement regimens. Two to three months is considered an adequate treatment trial with a particular dose. Thus, a dose should not be increased until the patient has used one particular dose for at least this time period.[69] The serum testosterone level should return to the normal range and symptoms of androgen deficiency should be relieved with appropriate dosing. After starting treatment, the patients should be reassessed in 1 to 3 months. If the patient is responding to treatment and serum testosterone levels have returned to normal, then the patient can be followed up annually. At each visit, the use of a validated self-assessment tool (e.g., Androgen Deficiency in Aging Men Questionnaire) can assist the physician in gauging the patient's response to treatment.[73]

Before initiating any testosterone replacement regimen in patients 40 years and older, patients should be screened for breast cancer, benign prostatic hyperplasia, and prostate cancer. All are testosterone-dependent conditions and theoretically could be worsened by exogenous administration of testosterone. Untreated prostate cancer is a contraindication to androgen supplementation. To screen for prostate disorders, a prostate-specific antigen serum concentration should be obtained and a digital rectal examination of the prostate performed. These tests are generally repeated at 1-year intervals after treatment is started.[68–70]

Adverse Effects

Testosterone replacement regimens can cause sodium retention, which can cause weight gain, or exacerbate hypertension, congestive heart failure, and edema. Gynecomastia can occur as a result of conversion of testosterone to estrogen in peripheral tissues. This has been reported most often in patients with liver cirrhosis.

Although serum lipoprotein perturbations may occur, testosterone replacement regimens have a neutral effect in that they decrease both total cholesterol and high-density lipoprotein cholesterol levels. No cases of cardiovascular disease have been reported with testosterone replacement regimens.

Large doses of parenteral testosterone can produce adverse metabolic effects. Thus, patients on long-term testosterone replacement regimens must undergo clinical laboratory testing for a serum testosterone level and hematocrit before starting treatment and every 6 to 12 months during treatment.[70] Repeated serum testosterone levels that exceed the normal range require a dosage reduction or increased interval between drug doses. If the hematocrit exceeds 55% (0.55), the testosterone replacement regimen should be withheld to avoid polycythemia and its consequences.

Oral alkylated testosterone replacement regimens have caused hepatotoxicity, ranging from mild elevations of hepatic transaminases to serious liver diseases, including peliosis hepatis (hemorrhagic liver cysts), hepatocellular and intrahepatic cholestasis, and benign or malignant tumors. For this reason, parenteral testosterone replacement regimens are preferred.

Topical testosterone patches may cause contact dermatitis, which responds well to topical corticosteroids. This adverse effect has been associated with the presence of permeation enhancers, which are added to patch formulations. If the dermatitis becomes problematic, an alternative is testosterone gel formulations, which are associated with a lower incidence of contact dermatitis compared with patches.

Alprostadil

Mechanism

Alprostadil, also known as prostaglandin E_1, stimulates adenyl cyclase, resulting in increased production of cAMP, a secondary messenger that decreases the intracellular calcium concentration and causes smooth muscle relaxation of the arterial blood vessels and sinusoidal tissues in the corpora. This results in enhanced blood flow to and blood filling of the corpora. Because it does not require nitric oxide to produce its clinical effects, patients with erectile dysfunction due to diseases that are associated with an impaired nitric oxide pathway (e.g., diabetes mellitus, postradical prostatectomy, and who have failed phosphodiesterase treatment) may respond to alprostadil.[74] In one study, 88% of men who failed to respond to sildenafil responded to intracavernosal alprostadil.[75]

Alprostadil is commercially available as an intracavernosal injection (Caverject and Edex) and as an intraurethral insert (medicated urethral system for erection [MUSE]).

Indications

Both commercially available formulations of alprostadil are FDA approved as monotherapy for management of erectile dysfunction. Alprostadil is more effective by the intracavernosal route than the intraurethral route.

The enhanced efficacy of the intracavernosal injection may be related to the excellent bioavailability of the drug when injected directly into the corpora cavernosum. In contrast, intraurethral alprostadil doses generally are several hundred times larger than intracavernosal doses. This is because intraurethral alprostadil must be absorbed from the urethra, through the corpus spongiosum, and into the corpus cavernosum, where it exerts its full proerectogenic effect.

Although several other agents, including papaverine, phentolamine, and atropine, have been used off-label for intracavernosal therapy, alprostadil is preferentially prescribed. This is because intracavernosal alprostadil has been FDA approved for erectile dysfunction, it does not require extemporaneous compounding, and it has a low potential for causing prolonged erections and priapism.

Both formulations of alprostadil are considered more invasive than VEDs or phosphodiesterase inhibitors. For this reason, intracavernosal alprostadil is generally prescribed after patients do not respond to or cannot use less invasive interventions. Intracavernosal alprostadil is preferred over intraurethral alprostadil because of its greater effectiveness. Intracavernosal alprostadil may be preferred in patients with diabetes mellitus, who are accustomed to injectable drug therapy and may have peripheral neuropathies, which decrease the patient's perception of pain upon injection. Intraurethral alprostadil is generally reserved as a treatment of last resort for patients who do not respond to other less invasive and more effective forms of therapy, and who refuse surgery.

Intracavernosal Alprostadil

Efficacy The overall efficacy of intracavernosal alprostadil is 70% to 90%.[6–8,76] Three characteristics of intracavernosal alprostadil include the following:

1. The effectiveness of alprostadil is dose related over the range of 2.5 to 20 mcg. The mean duration of erection is directly related to the dose of alprostadil administered and ranges from 12 to 44 minutes.
2. A higher percentage of patients with psychogenic and neurogenic erectile dysfunction respond to alprostadil at a lower dose compared to patients with vasculogenic erectile dysfunction.
3. Tolerance does not appear to develop with continued use of intracavernosal alprostadil at home.

(10) Although 70% to 75% of patients respond to intracavernosal alprostadil, a high proportion of patients elect to discontinue its use over time. Depending on the study and the length of observation, 30% to 50% of patients voluntarily discontinue therapy, usually during the first 6 to 12 months. Common reasons for discontinuation include lack of perceived effectiveness; inconvenience of administration; an unnatural, nonspontaneous erection; needle phobia; loss of interest; and cost of therapy.[15,76–78]

Approximately one third of patients do not respond to usual doses of intracavernosal alprostadil. In these patients, intracavernosal alprostadil has been used successfully along with VEDs. Such combination therapy can be attempted by patients before transitioning to more invasive surgical procedures.[76,78] Alternatively, intracavernosal injections of synergistic combinations of vasoactive agents that act by different mechanisms have been used.[77] Intracavernosal drug combinations typically produce an erection that lasts longer than an erection produced by any one of the agents in the mixture. In addition, because of the low dosage of each agent in the combination, fewer systemic and local fibrotic adverse effects develop compared with high-dose monotherapy. For example, when used in low-dose combination regimens, papaverine is less likely to induce hypotension and liver dysfunction, and phentolamine is less likely to induce tachycardia and hypotension.[76] However, as previously mentioned, such intracavernosal drug combinations are not commercially available and must be extemporaneously compounded.

Pharmacokinetics Intracavernosal injection should be administered into only one corpus cavernosum. From this injection site, the drug will reach the other corpus cavernosum through vascular communications between the two corpora. Alprostadil acts rapidly, with an onset of 5 to 15 minutes. The duration is directly related to the dose. Within the usual dosage range of 2.5 to 20 mcg, the duration of erection is not more than 1 hour. Higher doses are expected to exhibit a longer duration of action. Local enzymes in the corpora cavernosum quickly metabolize alprostadil. Any alprostadil that escapes into the systemic circulation is deactivated on first pass through the lungs.[76] Hence, the plasma half-life of alprostadil is approximately 1 minute, and the potential for systemic adverse effects is negligible. Dose modification is not necessary in patients with renal or hepatic disease.

Dosing The usual dose of intracavernosal alprostadil is 10 to 20 mcg, with a maximum recommended dose of 60 mcg. Doses greater than 60 mcg have not produced any greater improvement in penile erection but may cause hypotension or prolonged erections lasting more than 1 hour.[78] The dose should be administered 5 to 10 minutes before intercourse. The manufacturer recommends that patients be slowly titrated up to the minimally effective dosage to minimize the likelihood of hypotension. Under a physician's supervision, patients should be started with a 1.25-mcg dose, which can be increased in increments of 1.25 to 2.50 mcg at 30-minute intervals up to the lowest dose that produces a firm erection for 1 hour and does not produce adverse effects. In clinical practice, this process is rarely done because it is time consuming. Thus, many physicians start the patient on 10 mcg and move quickly up the dosage range to identify the best dose for the patient. To avoid adverse effects, patients should receive not more than one injection per day and not more than three injections per week (Table 66-3).

Intracavernosal injections should be performed using a 0.5-inch, 27- or 30-gauge needle. A tuberculin syringe or a syringe prefilled with diluent as supplied by the manufacturer should be used to ensure precise measurement of doses. Patients with needle phobia, poor vision, or poor manual dexterity can use commercially available autoinjectors (e.g., PenInject) to facilitate administration of intracavernosal alprostadil.

Intracavernosal injections require that the patient or the sexual partner practice good aseptic techniques (to avoid infection), have good manual skills and visual ability, and be comfortable with injection techniques. When practicing self-injection, the patient should use one hand to firmly hold the glans penis against his thigh to expose the lateral surface of the shaft. The injection should be made at right angles into one of the lateral surfaces of the proximal third of the penis. The injection should never be made into the dorsal or ventral surface of the penis. This will prevent inadvertent injection of the drug into arteries on the dorsal surface or the urethra on the ventral surface. After the injection, the penis should be massaged to help distribute the drug into the opposite corpus cavernosum. Injection sites should be rotated with each dose. Finally, manual pressure should be applied to the injection site for 5 minutes to reduce the likelihood of hematoma formation (Fig. 66-5).

Once the optimal dosage of intracavernosal alprostadil is established, the patient should return for routine medical follow-up every 3 to 6 months. Some patients subsequently require dosage adjustment, largely attributed to worsening of the underlying disease that is contributing to the erectile dysfunction.

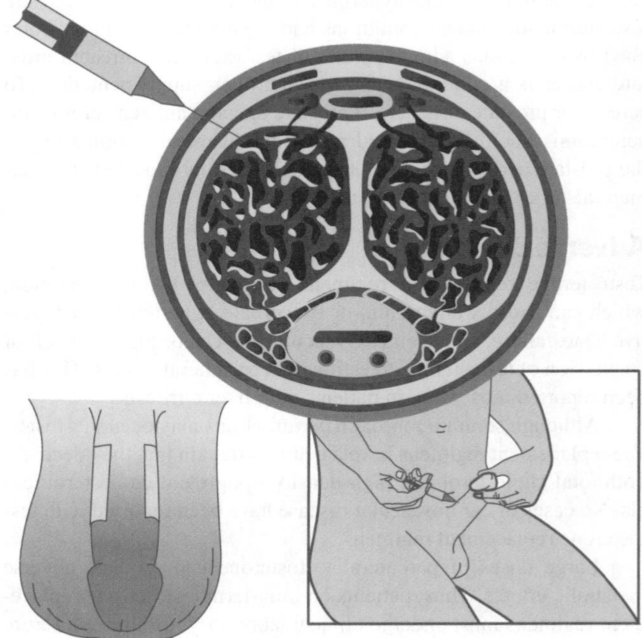

FIGURE 66-5 Technique for administration of intracavernosal injections. *(From Caverject [package insert]. New York, NY: Pfizer Inc.; 1999. Data from http://media.pfizer.com/files/products/uspi_caverject_powder.pdf.)*

Adverse Effects Intracavernosal alprostadil is most commonly associated with local adverse effects, which occur most often during the first year of therapy. However, an improved administration technique with continued use is believed to account for the lower frequency of adverse effects during subsequent treatment periods.

Intracavernosal injections are associated with several local adverse effects. Cavernosal plaques or areas of fibrosis at injection sites form in approximately 2% to 12% of patients. When they occur, the patient should suspend further injections until the plaques resolve. These plaques may cause penile curvature, similar to Peyronie's disease, which makes sexual intercourse difficult or impossible. The cause of corporal fibrosis and plaque formation is unknown. This adverse effect may be caused by poor injection technique or by alprostadil itself. Although patients have developed corporal fibrosis, alprostadil may be less likely to cause this adverse effect compared to other intracavernosal drug combinations, such as phentolamine or papaverine. Unlike cavernosal fibrosis associated with large doses and repeated administration of papaverine, penile scarring secondary to alprostadil appears to be unpredictable.

Alprostadil causes penile pain in approximately 10% to 44% of patients. The pain has been described as a burning discomfort or dull pain near the injection site or during the erection, which generally does not persist after the penis becomes flaccid. The pain usually is mild, generally does not require discontinuation of therapy, and often abates even with continued treatment. However, 2% to 5% of patients discontinue taking alprostadil because of severe pain. The pain can be managed by oral analgesics (e.g., acetaminophen), if necessary. One investigator has recommended adding procaine to intracavernosal alprostadil, but this may mask the signs of more serious adverse effects of the drug or of penile injury during intercourse and is not recommended.[79] The mechanism of this adverse reaction is poorly understood. Alprostadil may intrinsically produce pain. In addition, the pain may be a result of the pH of the parenteral solution. Alprostadil is acidic, and the commercially available Caverject formulation is buffered with sodium citrate, a weak base, to reduce pain on injection.

Priapism, a prolonged, painful erection lasting more than 1 hour, occurs in 1% to 15% of treated patients. It occurs most often during the dose titration period and is rare thereafter. Blood sludging in the corpora can lead to tissue hypoxia and cavernosal fibrosis and scarring. The risk for this complication is greatest for erections that persist beyond 4 hours. Patients are advised to seek medical attention immediately when drug-induced erections last more than 1 hour, as this is considered a urologic emergency. Its management includes supportive care, including analgesics for pain and sedatives for anxiety. In addition, needle aspiration of sludged blood in the corpora or intracavernosal injection of α-adrenergic agonists (e.g., phenylephrine) has been used. These procedures facilitate venous drainage of the corpora, allowing venous outflow to "catch up" with arterial inflow.

The likelihood of prolonged erections with intracavernosal alprostadil is dose related. Therefore, to prevent this adverse effect, the lowest effective dose should be used, and the dose should be titrated to ensure that the duration of the erection is not more than 1 hour.

Other local adverse effects include injection site hematomas and bruising. These effects are largely the result of poor injection technique. To minimize the risk of injection site hematomas, patients should be advised to apply pressure to the injection site for 5 minutes after each dose. Similarly, infection at the injection site has been reported. Meticulous aseptic technique is necessary to prevent this complication.

Intracavernosal alprostadil rarely causes systemic adverse effects, owing to the agent's local catabolism in cavernosal tissue and rapid deactivation in pulmonary tissue (if any of the drug escapes into the systemic circulation). However, large doses greater than 20 mcg are associated with dizziness and hypotension in some patients and is one reason why such large doses are not commonly used.

Intracavernosal injection therapy should be used cautiously by patients at risk for priapism, including patients with sickle cell disease, leukemia, or multiple myeloma. It should be used cautiously by patients who may develop bleeding complications secondary to injections, including patients with thrombocytopenia or those taking anticoagulants. It also should be used cautiously by patients who use poor-quality injection technique, including patients with psychiatric disorders, obese patients (who may not be able to reach or see the penile injection site), patients who are blind, and patients with severe arthritis.

Intraurethral Alprostadil

Efficacy (10) Intraurethral alprostadil inserts are marketed as MUSE, which contains a medication pellet inside a prefilled urethral applicator. Multiple studies show this product has an overall effectiveness rate of 43% to 65%[78] compared with 70% to 90% for intracavernosal alprostadil. Its decreased effectiveness and inconvenient administration method have resulted in this product being considered a third-line treatment option for patients with erectile dysfunction. However, some patients have responded to intraurethral alprostadil even though they did not respond to intracavernosal alprostadil[80] or sildenafil.[81]

Intraurethral alprostadil has been combined with an adjustable penile constriction band to improve treatment response.[81]

Pharmacokinetics Following intraurethral instillation, alprostadil is absorbed quickly through the urethra, into the corpus spongiosum, and then into the corpora cavernosum. As much as 90% of each dose is absorbed by the urethra and corpus spongiosum in less than 10 minutes, with peak absorption occurring in 20 to 25 minutes. An estimated 20% of each dose is delivered to the corpora cavernosum. As with intracavernosal injections of alprostadil, any drug absorbed into the systemic circulation is rapidly metabolized on first pass through the lungs.

The onset after intraurethral insertion is similar to that of intracavernosal injection, 5 to 10 minutes.

Dosing The usual dose of intraurethral alprostadil is 125 to 1,000 mcg. The dose should be administered 5 to 10 minutes before sexual intercourse. Not more than two doses per day are recommended. Before administration, the patient should be advised to empty his bladder, voiding completely (Table 66-3).

Similar to intracavernosal injection treatments, intraurethral insertion of alprostadil requires good manual and visual skills to minimize the risk of urethral injuries. Intraurethral alprostadil is supplied in a prefilled intraurethral applicator. The patient should void first. With one hand the patient holds the glans penis, and with the other hand the patient inserts the intraurethral applicator 0.5 inch (1.3 cm) into the urethra. The drug pellet is then pushed into the urethra. The penis should be massaged to enhance drug dissolution in the urethral fluids and drug absorption (Fig. 66-6).

Adverse Effects The urethra can be injured because of an improper administration technique. Injuries can lead to urethral stricture and difficulty voiding. Patients should receive complete education about optimal administration procedures before starting treatment.

Urethral pain has been reported in 24% to 32% of patients. Usually it is mild and does not require discontinuation of treatment. Female sexual partners may experience vaginal burning, itching, or pain, which probably is related to transfer of alprostadil from the man's urethra to the woman's vagina during intercourse.

Prolonged painful erections (priapism) have been rarely reported. Syncope and dizziness have been reported rarely (only 2–3% of patients) and likely are related to use of excessively large doses.

Intraurethral alprostadil should be avoided in patients with urethral stricture or urethritis.

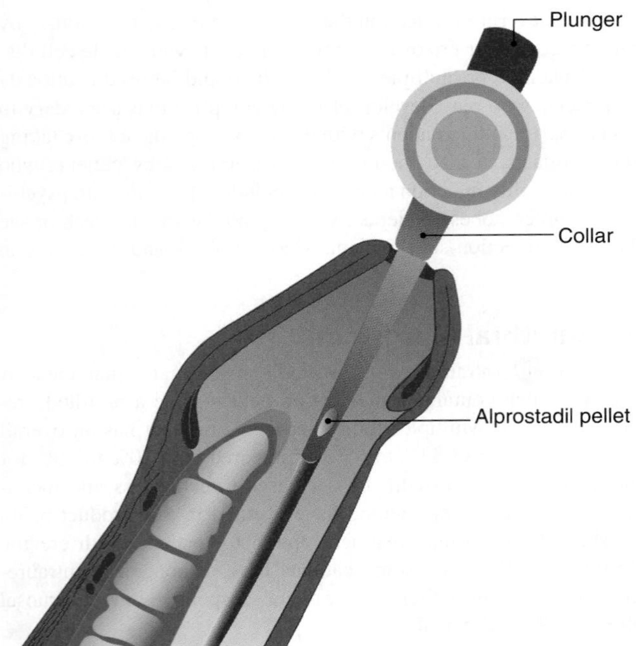

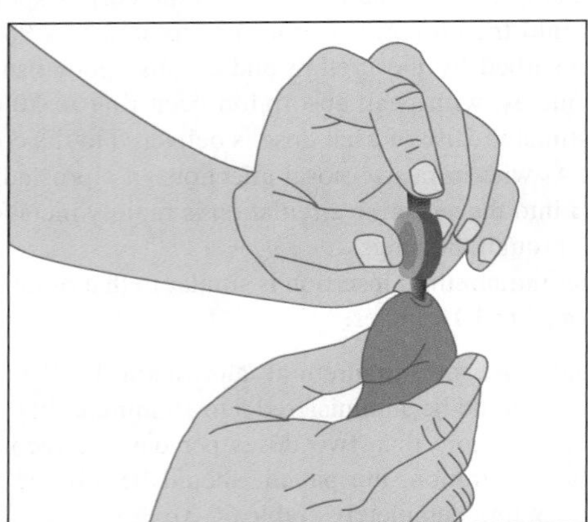

FIGURE 66-6 Technique for administration of intraurethral alprostadil with a medicated urethral system for erection applicator. *(From Muse [package insert]. Mountain View, CA: Vivus, Inc.; 2003. Data from http://www.vivus.com.)*

Clinical **Controversy. . .**

Although not recommended by the manufacturer, combinations of erectogenic medications or use of erectogenic medications with VEDs is a common practice. Published clinical trials of good research design are often lacking. Use of such combinations must take into consideration the published data available to support the use, potential adverse effects of the combination, and cost.

Unapproved Agents

A variety of other commercially available and investigational agents have been used for management of erectile dysfunction. Although it is beyond the scope of this chapter to discuss all of them, some of the more commonly used agents are discussed here.

Trazodone

The mechanism by which trazodone produces an erection is not clear. It likely acts peripherally to antagonize α-adrenergic receptors. As a result, a predominant cholinergic effect results, which causes peripheral arteriolar vasodilation and relaxation of cavernosal tissues, enhancing blood filling of the corpora. Intracavernosal injection of trazodone in experimental studies supports this likely mechanism.[82]

Although some clinical trials suggested that trazodone 50 to 200 mg daily by mouth might be effective in the management of erectile dysfunction, these trials were generally poorly controlled, were nonrandomized, included small samples treated for short time periods, and did not include validated objective parameters of response.[82,83]

The adverse effects of trazodone, when used for erectile dysfunction, are similar to those reported with trazodone when used to treat depression and include dry mouth, sedation, and dizziness.

Yohimbine

Yohimbine, a tree-bark derivative also known as *yohimbe*, is widely used as an aphrodisiac. Yohimbine is a central α_2-adrenergic antagonistic that increases catecholamines and improves mood. Some investigators believe that yohimbine has peripheral proerectogenic effects. Yohimbine may reduce peripheral α-adrenergic tone, thereby permitting a predominant cholinergic tone, which could result in a vasodilatory response.[76,78] The usual oral dose is 5.4 mg three times per day.

A controlled clinical trial has shown that high-dose yohimbine (100 mg daily) is not more effective than placebo.[84] Based on a meta-analysis of published studies that came to the same conclusion, the American Urological Association has cautioned against the use of yohimbine.[15] In addition, yohimbine can cause many systemic adverse effects, including anxiety, insomnia, tachycardia, and hypertension.

Papaverine

Papaverine is a nonspecific phosphodiesterase inhibitor that decreases metabolic catabolism of cAMP in cavernosal tissue. As a result of enhanced tissue levels of cAMP, smooth muscle relaxation occurs. Cavernosal sinusoids fill with blood, and a penile erection results.

Papaverine is not FDA approved for erectile dysfunction. Intracavernosal papaverine alone is not commonly used for management of erectile dysfunction because the large doses required produce dose-related adverse effects, such as priapism, corporal fibrosis, hypotension, and hepatotoxicity.[76,85] Papaverine is more often administered in lower doses combined with phentolamine and/or alprostadil. A variety of formulas have been used, but no one mixture has been proven better than other mixtures. Combination formulations are considered safer and are associated with the potential for fewer serious adverse effects than high doses of any one of these agents.

A portion of each papaverine dose is systemically absorbed, and its prolonged plasma half-life of 1 hour contributes to adverse effects. The usual dose of papaverine is 7.5 to 60 mg when used as a single agent for intracavernosal injection. When used in combination, the dose decreases to 0.5 to 20 mg.

If treated with papaverine, patients with a history of underlying liver disease or alcohol abuse should undergo liver function testing at baseline and every 6 to 12 months during continued treatment.

Phentolamine

Phentolamine is a competitive nonselective α-adrenergic blocking agent. It reduces peripheral adrenergic tone and enhances cholinergic tone. As a result, it improves cavernosal filling and is proerectogenic.

Phentolamine has most often been administered as an intracavernosal injection. Monotherapy is avoided because large doses are required for an erection, and at these large doses systemic hypotensive adverse effects would be prevalent. Most often, phentolamine has been used in combination with other vasoactive agents for intracavernosal administration. A ratio of 30 mg papaverine to 0.5 to 1 mg phentolamine is typical, and the usual dose ranges from 0.1 to 1 mL of the mixture. Such a mixture promotes local effects of phentolamine and minimizes systemic hypotensive adverse effects.

Hypotension is the most common adverse effect of intracavernosal phentolamine. It is more common and more severe with large doses or in patients with a poor injection technique who have injected into a vein (rather than the cavernosa). Prolonged erections have been reported in patients who used excessive doses of intracavernosal medications in combination.

Penile Prostheses

Surgical insertion of a penile prosthesis is the most invasive treatment of erectile dysfunction. It is reserved for patients who do not respond to or who are not candidates for less invasive oral or injectable treatments.

Prosthesis insertion requires anesthesia and skilled urologists. Two prostheses are widely used: malleable and inflatable. Malleable or semirigid prostheses consist of two bendable rods that are inserted into the corpora cavernosa. The patient appears to have a permanent erection after the procedure; the patient is able to bend the penis into position at the time of intercourse.

The inflatable prosthesis has several mechanical parts. The inflatable prosthesis produces a more natural erection. The patient develops an erection only when the device is activated. Some newer advances in inflatable prosthesis technology have resulted in devices with fewer mechanical parts. These devices can be placed during shorter surgical procedures and have a low 5-year mechanical failure rate (6% to 10%) as compared with the original inflatable prostheses (Fig. 66-7).[15,76,86]

Penile prostheses provide penile rigidity suitable for vaginal intercourse and are associated with a greater than 90% patient satisfaction rate, which is generally higher than that observed with any other drug treatment or VED.[87] The surgical success rate after insertion is 82% to 98%.[76]

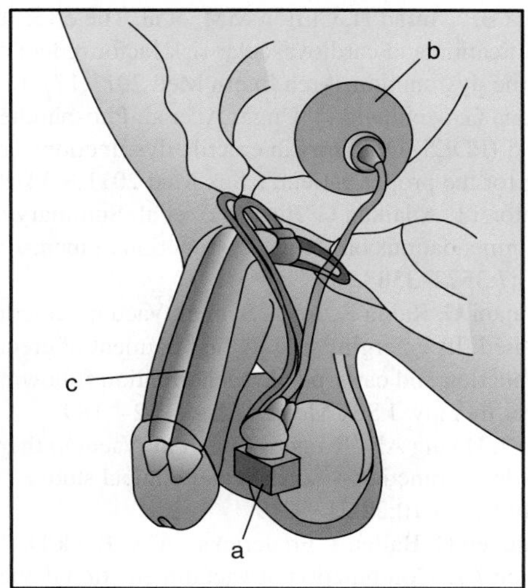

FIGURE 66-7 Example of surgically implanted penile prosthesis. (a, activation mechanism; b, reservoir with fluid for inflating prosthesis; c, inflatable rods in corpora.) *(From http://kidney.niddk.nih.gov/kudiseases/pubs/impotence.)*

Adverse effects of prosthesis insertion can occur early or late after the surgical procedure. The most common early complication is infection. Late complications include mechanical failure of the prosthesis, particularly when an inflatable prosthesis has been inserted. With improved technology, the mechanical failure rate has decreased to 5%.[76] Other late complications include erosion of the rods through the penis or late-onset infection. Although some salvage procedures have been devised, in many cases the prosthesis requires removal.

Personalized Pharmacotherapy

For the management of erectile dysfunction, treatment selection must be individualized based on the patient's preferences for and perception of the effectiveness of various treatment options and potential adverse effects.

In general, patients prefer a discreet form of treatment that is not obvious to the sexual partner and that does not require careful attention to timing of administration relative to sexual intercourse. Because treatment for erectile dysfunction is not included as a covered item on many insurance plans, the cost of treatment is likely to be a consideration for most patients.

For patients with both moderately symptomatic benign prostatic hyperplasia and erectile dysfunction, a reasonable approach is the use of daily tadalafil, which should be effective for both conditions.

For patients who fail treatment with a single medication, a VED, a combination drug regimen, or surgical intervention are options.

EVALUATION OF THERAPEUTIC OUTCOMES

The primary therapeutic outcomes of specific treatments for erectile dysfunction include (a) improvement in the quantity and quality of penile erections suitable for intercourse and (b) avoidance of adverse drug reactions and drug interactions.

At baseline and after the patient has completed a clinical trial period of 1 to 3 weeks with a specific treatment for erectile dysfunction, the physician should conduct assessments to determine whether the quality and quantity of penile erections has improved. A patient's level of satisfaction is highly individualized, depending on his lifestyle and expectations. Therefore, a patient who has successful intercourse once per week might be completely satisfied, whereas another patient might judge this to be unsatisfactory. Patients with unrealistic expectations in this regard must be identified and counseled by clinicians to avoid adverse effects of excessive use of erectogenic agents.

Failure to improve the quality and quantity of penile erections suitable for intercourse after an appropriate clinical trial period with a specific treatment for erectile dysfunction occurs in a significant percentage of patients. In this case, physicians generally take the following steps in order:

1. Ensure that the patient has been prescribed a maximum tolerated dose and has an adequate clinical trial of a specific treatment before discarding it as ineffective.
2. Switch to another drug (see Fig. 66-2).
3. Reserve surgical treatment for patients who do not respond to drug treatment.

CONCLUSIONS

Erectile dysfunction is a common disorder of aging men. Its incidence is higher in patients with underlying medical disorders that compromise the vascular, neurologic, hormonal, or psychogenic systems necessary for a normal penile erection. Medications are common causes of erectile dysfunction. By correcting the underlying etiology, erectile dysfunction can often be reversed without the use of specific treatments.

When treatments of erectile dysfunction are needed, the least invasive forms of treatment should be used first because they produce the lowest incidence of serious adverse effects. VEDs or phosphodiesterase inhibitors are considered first-line treatments. If these treatments fail, intracavernosal alprostadil injection therapy can be initiated. If this treatment fails, the patient can attempt a combination of intracavernosal alprostadil plus VED, combination intracavernosal therapy, or intraurethral alprostadil. If this treatment fails, the patient may require insertion of a penile prosthesis.

Some insurance companies do not reimburse for drug treatments for erectile dysfunction, so cost is an important issue for some patients.

Clinicians should provide clear and simple advice. Patient confidentiality and privacy, which are extremely important to men with erectile dysfunction, should be maintained at all times.

ABBREVIATIONS

cAMP cyclic adenosine monophosphate
cGMP cyclic guanosine monophosphate
CNS central nervous system
IIEF International Index of Erectile Dysfunction
LUTS lower urinary tract symptoms
NAION nonarteritic anterior ischemic optic neuropathy
VED vacuum erection device

REFERENCES

1. NIH Consensus Conference. NIH Consensus Development Panel on Impotence. Impotence. JAMA 1993;270:83–90.
2. Qaseem A, Snow V, Denberg TD, et al. Clinical efficacy assessment subcommittee of the American College of Physicians: Hormonal testing and pharmacologic treatment of erectile dysfunction: A clinical practice guideline from the American College of Physicians. Ann Intern Med 2009;151:639–649.
3. Johannes CB, Aranjo AB, Feldman HA, et al. Incidence of erectile dysfunction in men 40–69 years old: Longitudinal results from the Massachusetts Male Aging Study. J Urol 2000;163:460–463.
4. Bacon CG, Mittleman MA, Kawach I, et al. Sexual function in men older than 50 years of age: Results from the Health Professionals Follow-up Study. Ann Intern Med 2003;139:161–168.
5. Lindau ST, Schumm LP, Laumann EO, et al. A study of sexuality and health among older adults in the United States. N Engl J Med 2007;357:762–774.
6. Albersen M, Orabi H, Lue TF. Evaluation and treatment of erectile dysfunction in the aging male: A mini-review. Gerontology 2012;58:3–14.
7. Berookhim BM, Bar-Chama N. Medical implications of erectile dysfunction. Med Clin N Am 2011;95:213–221.
8. Albersen M, Mwamukonda KB, Shindel AW, Lue TF. Evaluation and treatment of erectile dysfunction. Med Clin N Am 2011;95:201–212.
9. Andersson KE. Mechanisms of penile erection and basis for pharmacological treatment of erectile dysfunction. Pharmacol Rev 2011;63(4):811–859.
10. Araujo AB, Esche GR, Kupelian V, et al. Prevalence of symptomatic androgen deficiency in men. J Clin Endocrinol Metab 2007;92:4241–4247.
11. Travison TG, Araujo AB, O'Donnell AB, et al. A population-level decline in serum testosterone levels in American men. J Clin Endocrinol Metab 2007;92:196–202.
12. Handler J. Managing erectile dysfunction in hypertensive patients. J Clin Hypertens 2011;13:450–454.
13. Lee M, Sharifi R. Sexual dysfunction in males. In: Tisdale JE, Miller DA, eds. Drug-Induced Diseases: Prevention, Detection, and Management, 2nd ed. Bethesda, MD: ASHP, 2010:686–701.
14. Kennedy SH, Rizvi S. Sexual dysfunction, depression, and the impact of antidepressants. J Clin Psychopharmacol 2009;29(2):157–164.
15. American Urological Association Guideline on the Management of Erectile Dysfunction: Diagnosis and Treatment Recommendations; updated 2006. *http://www.auanet.org/content/guidelines-and-quality-care/clinical-guidelines.cfm?sub=ed.*
16. Rosen RC, Riley A, Wagner G, et al. The International Index of Erectile Function (IIEF): A multidimensional scale for assessment of erectile dysfunction. Urology 1997;49: 822–830.
17. Zitzman M, Faber S, Nieschlag E. Association of specific symptoms and metabolic risks with serum testosterone in older men. J Clin Endocrinol Metab 2006;91:4335–4345.
18. Inman BA, St. Souver JL, Jacobson DJ, et al. A population-based longitudinal study of erectile dysfunction and future coronary artery disease. Mayo Clin Proceed 2009;84: 108–113.
19. Nehra A. Erectile dysfunction and cardiovascular disease: Efficacy and safety of phosphodiesterase type 5 inhibitors in men with both conditions. Mayo Clin Proceed 2009;84: 139–148.
20. Nehra A, Jackson G, Miner M, et al. The Princeton III Consensus Recommendations for the Management of Erectile Dysfunction and Cardiovascular Disease. Mayo Clin Proc 2012;87(8):766–778.
21. Rosen RC, Friedman M, Kostis JB. Lifestyle management of erectile dysfunction: The role of cardiovascular and concomitant risk factors. Am J Cardiol 2005;96(Suppl): 76M–79M.
22. Nehra A, Jolly N, Rybak J. Review of erectile dysfunction and cardiovascular risk. Minerva Urol Nefrol 2013;65(2): 109–115.
23. Gupta BP, Murad H, Clifton MM, et al. The effect of lifestyle modification and cardiovascular risk factor reduction on erectile dysfunction. Arch Intern Med 2011;171:1797–1803.
24. Corona G, Mondaini N, Ungar A, et al. Phosphodiesterase type 5 (PDE5) inhibitors in erectile dysfunction: The proper drug for the proper patient. J Sex Med 2011;8:3418–3432.
25. Montorsi F, Adaikan G, Becher E, et al. Summary of the recommendations on sexual dysfunction in men. J Sex Med 2010;7:3572–3588.
26. Pahlajani G, Raina R, Jones S, et al. Vacuum erection devices revisited: Its emerging role in the treatment of erectile dysfunction and early penile rehabilitation following prostate cancer therapy. J Sex Med 2012;9:1182–1189.
27. Yuan J, Hoang AN, Romero CA, et al. Vacuum therapy in erectile dysfunction—Science and clinical studies. Int J Impot Res 2010;22:211–219.
28. Canguven O, Bailen J, Fredericksson W, Bock D, Burnett AL. Combination of vacuum erection device and PDE5 inhibitors as salvage therapy in PDE5 inhibitor nonresponders with erectile dysfunction. J Sex Med 2009;6(9):2561–2567.
29. Raina R, Pahlajani RR, Agarwal A, Jones S, Zippe C. Long term potency after early use of a vacuum

erection device following radical prostatectomy. BJU Int 2010;106(11):1719–1722.

30. Ravipati G, McClung JA, Aronow WS, et al. Type 5 phosphodiesterase inhibitors in the treatment of erectile dysfunction and cardiovascular disease. Card Rev 2007;15:76–86.
31. Carson CC. Phosphodiesterase type 5 inhibitors: State of the therapeutic class. Urol Clin North Am 2007;34: 507–515.
32. Tsertsvadze A, Fink HA, Yazdi F, et al. Oral phosphodiesterase-5 inhibitors and hormonal treatments for erectile dysfunction: A systematic review and meta-analysis. Ann Intern Med 2009;151:650–661.
33. Mirone V, Fusco F, Rossi A, et al. Tadalafil and vardenafil vs sildenafil: A review of patient preference studies. BJU Int 2009;103:1212–1217.
34. Hatzichristou D, Moysidis K, Apostolidis A, et al. Sildenafil failures may be due to inadequate patient instructions and follow-up: A study of 100 non-responders. Eur Urol 2005;47:518–523.
35. Lau DH, Kommu S, Mumtaz FH, et al. The management of phosphodiesterase 5 (PDE5) inhibitor failure. Curr Vasc Pharmacol 2006;4:89–93.
36. Padma-Nathan H, Eardley I, Kloner RA, et al. A 4-year update on the safety of sildenafil citrate (Viagra). Urology 2002;60(Suppl 2B):67–90.
37. Carson CC. Long-term use of sildenafil. Expert Opin Pharmacother 2003;4:397–405.
38. Lombardi G, Macchiarella A, Cecconi F, Del Popolo G. Ten-year follow-up of sildenafil use in spinal cord-injured patients with erectile dysfunction. J Sex Med 2009;6(12):3449–3457.
39. Brisson TE, Broderick GA, Thiel DD, et al. Vardenafil rescue rates of sildenafil nonresponders: Objective assessment of 327 patients with erectile dysfunction. Urology 2006;68:397–401.
40. McMahon CG. High dose sildenafil as a salvage therapy for severe erectile dysfunction. Int J Impot Res 2002;14: 533–538.
41. Buvat J, Montorsi F, Maggi M, et al. Hypogonadal men nonresponders to the PDE5 inhibitor tadalafil benefit from normalization of testosterone levels with a 1% hydroalcoholic testosterone gel in the treatment of erectile dysfunction (TADTEST) study. J Sex Med 2011;8(1): 284–293.
42. Dhir RR, Lin H-C, Canfield SE, Wang R. Combination therapy for erectile dysfunction: An update review. Asian J Androl 2011;13:382–390.
43. Mydlo JH, Viterbo R, Crispen P. Use of combined intracorporal injection and a phosphodiesterase-5 inhibitor therapy for men with a suboptimal response to sildenafil and/or vardenafil monotherapy after radical retropubic prostatectomy. BJU Int 2005;95:843–846.
44. Sperling H, Gittelman M, Norenberg C, et al. Efficacy and safety of an orodispersible vardenafil formulation for the treatment of erectile dysfunction in elderly men and those with underlying conditions: An integrated analysis of two pivotal trials. J Sex Med 2011;8:261–271.
45. Shabsigh R, Seftel AD, Rosen RC, et al. Review of time of onset and duration of clinical efficacy of phosphodiesterase type 5 inhibitors in treatment of erectile dysfunction. Urology 2006;68:689–696.
46. Hatzimouratidis K, Hatzichristou D. Phosphodiesterase type 5 inhibitors: The day after. Eur Urol 2007;51:75–89.
47. McCullough AR, Steidle CP, Klee B, Tseng L-J. Randomized, double-blind, crossover trial of sildenafil in men with mild to moderate erectile dysfunction: Efficacy at 8 and 12 hours postdose. Urology 2008;71:686–692.
48. Washington SL, Shindel AW. A once-daily dose of tadalafil for erectile dysfunction: Compliance and efficacy. Drug Design Devel Ther 2010;4:159–171.
49. Wright PJ. Comparison of phosphodiesterase type 5 inhibitors. Int J Clin Pract 2006;60:967–975.
50. Porst H, Giuliano F, Glina S, et al. Evaluation of the efficacy and safety of once-a-day dosing of tadalafil 5 mg and 10 mg in the treatment of erectile dysfunction: Results of a multicenter, randomized, double-blind, placebo-controlled trial. Eur Urol 2006;50:351–359.
51. Fusco F, Razzoli F, Imbimbo C, et al. A new era in the treatment of erectile dysfunction: Chronic phosphodiesterase type 5 inhibition. BJU Int 2010:105:1634–1639.
52. Porst H, Hell-Momeni K, Buttner H. Chronic PDE-5 inhibition in patients with erectile dysfunction—A treatment approach using tadalafil once-daily. Expert Opin Pharmacother 2012;13(10):1481–1494.
53. El-Sakka AI. Alleviation of post-radical prostatectomy cavernosal fibrosis: Future directions and potential utility for PDE5 inhibitors. Expert Opin Investig Drugs 2011;20(1):1305–1309.
54. Taylor J, Baldo OB, Storey A, et al. Differences in side effect, duration and related bother levels between phosphodiesterase type 5 inhibitors. BJU Int 2009;103: 1392–1395.
55. Giuliano F, Jackson G, Montorsi F, et al. Safety of sildenafil citrate: Review of 67 double-blind placebo-controlled trials and the postmarketing safety database. Int J Clin Pract 2010;64:240–255.
56. Jannini EA, Isidori AM, Gravina GL, et al. The Endotrial Study: A spontaneous, open label, randomized, multicenter cross-over study on the efficacy of sildenafil, tadalafil, and vardenafil in the treatment of erectile dysfunction. J Sex Med 2009;6:2547–2560.
57. Laties A. Vision disorders and phosphodiesterase type 5 inhibitors. Drug Safety 2009;32:1–18.
58. Dundar SO. Visual loss associated with erectile dysfunction drugs. Can J Ophthalmol 2007;42:10–12.
59. Maddox Pt, Saunders J, Chandrasekhar SS. Sudden hearing loss from PDE-5 inhibitors: A possible cellular stress etiology. Laryngoscope 2009;119:1586–1589.
60. Okuyucu S, Guven OE, Akoglu E, et al. Effect of phosphodiesterase-5 inhibitor on hearing. J Laryngol Otol 2009;123:718–722.
61. Kloner RA, Hutter AM, Emmick JT. Time course of the interaction between tadalafil and nitrates. J Am Coll Cardiol 2003;42:1855–1860.
62. Reffelmann T, Kieback A, Kloner RA. The cardiovascular safety of tadalafil. Expert Opin Drug Saf 2008;7:43–52.
63. Kloner RA. Pharmacology and drug interaction effects of the phosphodiesterase 5 inhibitors: Focus on α blocker interactions. Am J Cardiol 2005;96(Suppl):42M–46M.
64. Schwartz BG, Kloner RA. Drug interactions with phosphodiesterase-5 inhibitors used for the treatment of erectile dysfunction or pulmonary hypertension. Circulation 2010;122(1):88–95.
65. Giuliano F, Kaplan SA, Cabanis MJ, Astruc B. Hemodynamic interaction study between the $alpha_1$ blocker alfuzosin and the phosphodiesterase-5 inhibitor tadalafil in middle-aged healthy male subjects. Urology 2006;67: 1199–1204.
66. Ng C-F, Wong A, Cheng C-W, et al. Effect of vardenafil on blood pressure profile of patients with erectile dysfunction concomitantly treated with doxazosin gastrointestinal

therapeutic system for benign prostatic hyperplasia. J Urol 2008;180:1042–1046.
67. Corona G, Razzoli E, Forti G, Maggi M. The use of phosphodiesterase 5 inhibitors with concomitant medications. J Endocrinol Invest 2008;31(9):799–808.
68. Barkin J. Erectile dysfunction and hypogonadism. Can J Urol 2011;18(Suppl 1):2–7.
69. Gore JL, Swerdloff RS, Rajfer J. Androgen deficiency in the etiology and treatment of erectile dysfunction. Urol Clin North Am 2005;32:457–468.
70. Bolona ER, Uraga MV, Haddad RM, et al. Testosterone use in men with sexual dysfunction: A systematic review and meta-analysis of randomized placebo-controlled trials. Mayo Clin Proceed 2007;82:20–28.
71. Wang C, Swerdloff R, Kipnes M, et al. New testosterone buccal system (Striant) delivers physiological testosterone levels: Pharmacokinetics study in hypogonadal men. J Clin Endocrinol Metab 2004;89:3821–3829.
72. Jordan WP. Allergy and topical irritation associated with transdermal testosterone administration: A comparison of scrotal and nonscrotal transdermal systems. Am J Contact Dermatol 1997;8:108–113.
73. Morely JE, Charlton E, Patrick P, et al. Validation of a screening questionnaire for androgen deficiency in aging males. Metabolism 2000;49:1239–1242.
74. Kendirci M, Tanriverdi O, Trost L, et al. Management of sildenafil treatment failures. Curr Opin Urol 2006;16: 449–459.
75. Shabsigh R, Padma-Nathan H, Gittleman M, et al. Intracavernous alprostadil alfadex (Edex/Viridal) is effective and safe in patients with erectile dysfunction after failing sildenafil (Viagra). Urology 2000;55:477–480.
76. McVary KT. Erectile dysfunction. N Engl J Med 2007;357:2472–2481.
77. Chen Y, Dai Y, Wang R. Treatment strategies for diabetic patients suffering from erectile dysfunction. Expert Opin Pharmacother 2008;9:257–260.
78. Nehra A. Oral and non-oral combination therapy for erectile dysfunction. Rev Urol 2007;9:99–105.
79. Albaugh J, Ferrans CE. Patient reported pain with initial intracavernosal injection. J Sex Med 2009;6: 513–519
80. Engel JD, McVary KT. Transurethral alprostadil as therapy for patients who withdrew from or failed prior intracavernous injection therapy. Urology 1998;51:687–692.
81. Jaffe JS, Antell MR, Greenstein M, et al. Use of intraurethral alprostadil in patients not responding to sildenafil citrate. Urology 2004;63:951–954.
82. Fink HA, MacDonald R, Rutks IR, Wilt TJ. Trazodone for erectile dysfunction: A systematic review and meta-analysis. BJU Int 2003;92:441–446.
83. Vitezic D, Pelcic JM. Erectile dysfunction: Oral pharmacotherapy options. Int J Clin Pharmacol Ther 2002;40:393–403.
84. Teloken C, Rhoden EL, Sogari P, et al. Therapeutic effects of high-dose yohimbine hydrochloride on organic erectile dysfunction. J Urol 1998;159:122–124.
85. Brown SL, Haas CA, Koehler M, et al. Hepatotoxicity related to intracavernous pharmacotherapy with papaverine. Urology 1998;52:844–847.
86. Henry GD, Wilson SK. Updates in inflatable penile prosthesis. Urol Clin North Am 2007;34:535–547.
87. Rajpurkar A, Dhabuwala CB. Comparison of satisfaction rates and erectile function in patients treated with sildenafil, intracavernous prostaglandin E1 and penile implant surgery for erectile dysfunction in urology practice. J Urol 2003;170:159–163.

67 Benign Prostatic Hyperplasia

Mary Lee

KEY CONCEPTS

1. Although symptomatic benign prostatic hyperplasia (BPH) is rare in men younger than 50 years of age, it is very common in men 60 years and older because of androgen-driven growth in the size of the prostate. Symptoms commonly result from both static and dynamic factors.
2. BPH symptoms may be exacerbated by medications, including antihistamines, phenothiazines, tricyclic antidepressants, and anticholinergic agents. In these cases, discontinuing the causative agent can relieve symptoms.
3. Specific treatments for BPH include watchful waiting, drug therapy, and surgery.
4. For patients with mild disease who are asymptomatic or have mildly bothersome symptoms and no complications of BPH disease, no specific treatment is indicated. These patients can be managed with watchful waiting. Watchful waiting includes behavior modification and return visits to the physician at 6- or 12-month intervals for assessment of worsening symptoms or signs of BPH.
5. If symptoms progress to a moderate or severe level, drug therapy or surgery is indicated. Drug therapy with an α_1-adrenergic antagonist is an interim measure that relieves voiding symptoms. In select patients with prostates of at least 40 g, 5α-reductase inhibitors delay symptom progression and reduce the incidence of BPH-related complications.
6. All α_1-adrenergic antagonists are equally effective in relieving BPH symptoms, but do not halt disease progression or delay surgical intervention. Older second-generation immediate-release formulations of α_1-adrenergic antagonists (e.g., terazosin, doxazosin) can cause adverse cardiovascular effects, mainly first-dose syncope, orthostatic hypotension, and dizziness. For patients who cannot tolerate hypotensive effects of the second-generation agents, the third-generation, pharmacologically uroselective agents (e.g., tamsulosin, silodosin) are good alternatives. An extended-release formulation of alfuzosin, a second-generation, functionally uroselective agent, and third-generation pharmacologically uroselective agents have fewer cardiovascular adverse effects than immediate-release formulations of terazosin or doxazosin. Generic formulations are less expensive than single-source agents and should be preferentially prescribed in patients with limited financial resources.
7. 5α-Reductase inhibitors are useful primarily for patients with large prostates greater than 40 g who wish to avoid surgery and cannot tolerate the side effects of α_1-adrenergic antagonists. 5α-Reductase inhibitors have a slow onset of action, taking up to 6 months to exert maximal clinical effects, which is a disadvantage of their use. In addition, decreased libido, erectile dysfunction, and ejaculation disorders are common adverse effects, which may be troublesome problems in sexually active patients.
8. Phosphodiesterase inhibitors are indicated in patients with moderate-severe BPH and erectile dysfunction. They improve lower urinary tract symptoms (LUTS), but do not increase urinary flow rate or reduce postvoid residual (PVR) urine volume. For these reasons, phosphodiesterase monotherapy is considered less effective than an α-adrenergic antagonist for BPH. A phosphodiesterase inhibitor may be used alone or along with an α-adrenergic antagonist.
9. Anticholinergic agents are indicated in patients with moderate to severe LUTS with a predominance of irritative voiding symptoms. Because older patients are at high risk of systemic anticholinergic adverse effects, uroselective anticholinergic agents may be preferentially prescribed. To minimize the risk of acute urinary retention, a patient's PVR urine volume should be less than 250 mL before initiating treatment with an anticholinergic agent.
10. Surgery is indicated for moderate to severe symptoms of BPH for patients who do not respond to or do not tolerate drug therapy or for patients with complications of BPH. It is the most effective mode of treatment in that it relieves symptoms in the greatest number of men with BPH. However, the two most widely used techniques, transurethral resection of the prostate and open prostatectomy, are associated with the highest rates of complications, including retrograde ejaculation and erectile dysfunction. Therefore, minimally invasive surgical procedures are often desired by patients. These relieve symptoms and are associated with a lower rate of adverse effects, but they have higher reoperation rates than the gold standard procedures.

Benign prostatic hyperplasia (BPH) is the most common benign neoplasm of American men. A nearly ubiquitous condition among elderly men, BPH is of major societal concern, given the large number of men affected, the progressive nature of the condition, and the healthcare costs associated with it.

This chapter discusses BPH and its available treatments: watchful waiting, α_1-adrenergic antagonists, 5α-reductase inhibitors, phosphodiesterase inhibitors, anticholinergic agents, and surgery. The limitations of phytotherapy are described.

EPIDEMIOLOGY

1 According to the results of autopsy studies, approximately 80% of elderly men develop microscopic evidence of BPH. About half of the patients with microscopic changes develop an enlarged prostate gland, and as a result, they develop symptoms including difficulty emptying urine from the urinary bladder. Approximately half of symptomatic patients eventually require treatment.

The peak incidence of clinical BPH occurs at 63 to 65 years of age. Symptomatic disease is uncommon in men younger than 50 years, but some urinary voiding symptoms are present by the time men turn 60 years of age. The Boston Area Normative Aging Study estimated that the cumulative incidence of clinical BPH was 78% for patients at age 80 years.[1] Similarly, the Baltimore Longitudinal Study of Aging projected that approximately 60% of men at least 60 years old develop clinical BPH.[2]

NORMAL PROSTATE PHYSIOLOGY

Located anterior to the rectum, the prostate is a small heart-shaped, chestnut-sized gland located below the urinary bladder. It surrounds the proximal urethra like a doughnut.

Soft, symmetric, and mobile on palpation, a normal prostate gland in an adult man weighs 15 to 20 g. Physical examination of the prostate must be done by digital rectal examination (i.e., the prostate is manually palpated by inserting a finger into the rectum). Thus, the prostate is examined through the rectal mucosa.

The prostate has two major functions: (a) to secrete fluids that make up a portion (20–40%) of the ejaculate volume and (b) to provide secretions with antibacterial effect possibly related to its high concentration of zinc.[2]

At birth, the prostate is the size of a pea and weighs approximately 1 g. The prostate remains that size until the boy reaches puberty. At that time, the prostate undergoes its first growth spurt, growing to its normal adult size of 15 to 20 g by the time the young man is 25 to 30 years of age. The prostate remains this size until the patient reaches age 40 years, when a second growth spurt begins and continues for the rest of his lifetime. During this period, the prostate can quadruple in size or grow even larger.

The prostate gland comprises three types of tissue: epithelial tissue, stromal tissue, and the capsule. Epithelial tissue, also known as *glandular tissue*, produces prostatic secretions. These secretions are delivered into the urethra during ejaculation and contribute to the total ejaculate volume. Androgens stimulate epithelial tissue growth. Stromal tissue, also known as *smooth muscle tissue*, is embedded with α_1-adrenergic receptors. Stimulation of these receptors by norepinephrine causes smooth muscle contraction, which results in an extrinsic compression of the urethra, reduction of the urethral lumen, and decreased urinary bladder emptying. The normal prostate is composed of a higher amount of stromal tissue than epithelial tissue, as reflected by a stromal-to-epithelial tissue ratio of 2:1. This ratio is exaggerated to 5:1 for patients with BPH, which explains why α_1-adrenergic antagonists are quickly effective in symptomatic management and why 5α-reductase inhibitors reduce an enlarged prostate gland by only 25%.[2,3] The capsule, or outer shell of the prostate, is composed of fibrous connective tissue and smooth muscle, which also is embedded with α_1-adrenergic receptors. When stimulated with norepinephrine, the capsule contracts around the urethra (Fig. 67-1).

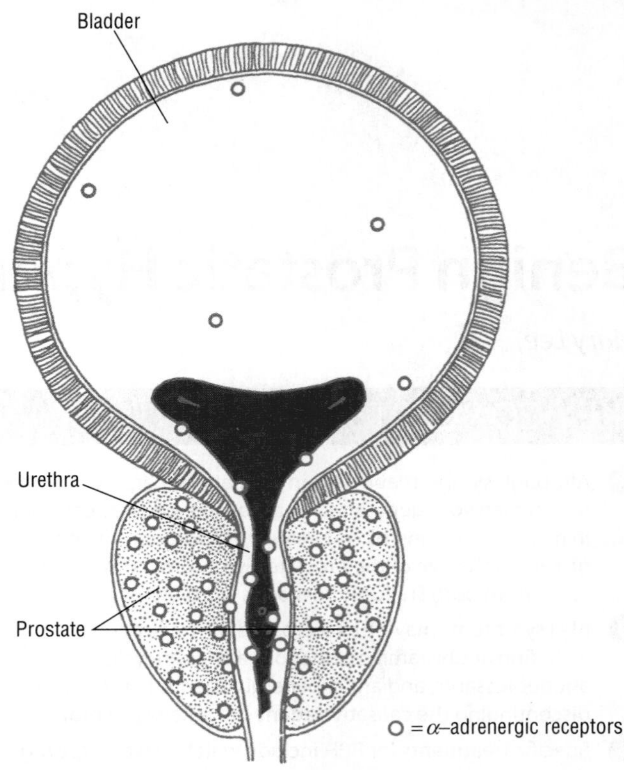

FIGURE 67-1 Representation of the anatomy of and α-adrenergic receptor distribution in the prostate, urethra, and bladder. *(Western J Med 1994;161:501. Reproduced with permission from the BMJ Publishing Group.)*

Testosterone is the principal testicular androgen in males, whereas androstenedione is the principal adrenal androgen. These two hormones are responsible for penile and scrotal enlargement, increased muscle mass, and maintenance of the normal male libido. These androgens are converted by 5α-reductase in target cells to dihydrotestosterone (DHT), an active metabolite. Two types of 5α-reductase exist. Type I enzyme is localized to sebaceous glands in the frontal scalp, liver, and skin, although a small amount is in the prostate. DHT produced at these target tissues causes acne and increased body and facial hair. Type II enzyme is localized to the prostate, genital tissue, and hair follicles of the scalp. In the prostate, DHT induces growth and enlargement of the gland.[3]

In prostate cells, DHT has greater affinity for intraprostatic androgen receptors than testosterone, and DHT forms a more stable complex with the androgen receptor. Thus, DHT is considered a more potent androgen than testosterone in the prostate. Of note, despite the decrease in testicular androgen production in the aging male, intracellular DHT levels in the prostate remain normal, probably due to increased activity of intraprostatic 5α-reductase.[3]

Estrogen, a product of peripheral metabolism of androgens, is believed to stimulate the growth of the stromal portion of the prostate gland. Estrogens are produced when testosterone and androstenedione are converted by aromatase enzymes in peripheral adipose tissues. In addition, estrogens may induce the androgen receptor.[2] As men age, the ratio of serum levels of testosterone to estrogen decreases as a result of a decline in testosterone production by the testes and increased adipose tissue conversion of androgen to estrogen.

PATHOPHYSIOLOGY

Although the precise pathophysiologic mechanisms causing BPH remain unclear, the role of intraprostatic DHT and type II 5α-reductase in the development of BPH is evidenced by several observations:

1. BPH does not develop in men who are castrated before puberty.
2. Patients with type II 5α-reductase enzyme deficiency do not develop BPH.

3. Castration causes an enlarged prostate to shrink.
4. Administration of testosterone to orchiectomized dogs of advanced age produces BPH.

The pathogenesis of BPH is often described as resulting from both static and dynamic factors. Static factors relate to anatomic enlargement of the prostate gland, which produces a physical block at the bladder neck and thereby obstructs urinary outflow. Enlargement of the gland depends on androgen stimulation of epithelial tissue and estrogen stimulation of stromal tissue in the prostate. Dynamic factors relate to excessive α-adrenergic tone of the stromal component of the prostate gland, bladder neck, and posterior urethra, which results in contraction of the prostate gland around the urethra and narrowing of the urethral lumen.

Symptoms of BPH disease may result from static and/or dynamic factors, and this must be recognized when drug therapy is considered. For instance, some patients may present with obstructive voiding symptoms but have prostates of normal size. In these patients, dynamic factors likely are responsible for the symptoms. However, for patients with enlarged prostate glands, static and dynamic factors likely are working in concert to produce the observed symptoms. Moreover, the likelihood of developing moderate to severe voiding symptoms is directly related to the increasing size of the prostate gland.[4]

Static factors may be accentuated if the patient becomes stressed or is in pain. In these situations, increased α-adrenergic tone may precipitate excessive contraction of prostatic stromal tissue. When the stressful event resolves, voiding symptoms often improve.[2]

MEDICATION-RELATED SYMPTOMS

2 Medications in several pharmacologic categories should be avoided for patients with BPH because they may exacerbate symptoms.[5] Testosterone replacement regimens, used to treat primary or secondary hypogonadism, deliver additional substrate that can be metabolized to DHT by the prostate. Although no cases of BPH have been reported because of exogenous testosterone administration, cautious use is advised for patients with prostatic enlargement. α-Adrenergic agonists, used as oral or intranasal decongestants (e.g., pseudoephedrine, ephedrine, or phenylephrine), can stimulate α-adrenergic receptors in the prostate, resulting in muscle contraction. By decreasing the caliber of the urethral lumen, bladder emptying may be compromised. β-Adrenergic agonists (e.g., terbutaline) may cause relaxation of the bladder detrusor muscle, which prevents bladder emptying.[6] Drugs with significant anticholinergic adverse effects (e.g., antihistamines, phenothiazines, tricyclic antidepressants, or anticholinergic drugs used as antispasmodics or to treat Parkinson's disease) may decrease contractility of the urinary bladder detrusor muscle. For patients with BPH who have a narrowed urethral lumen, loss of effective detrusor contraction could result in acute urinary retention, particularly for patients with significantly enlarged prostate glands. Diuretics, particularly in large doses, can produce polyuria, which may present as urinary frequency, similar to that experienced by patients with BPH.

CLINICAL PRESENTATION

Patients with BPH can present with a variety of symptoms and signs of disease. All symptoms of BPH can be divided into two categories: obstructive and irritative.

Obstructive symptoms, also known as *prostatism* or *bladder outlet obstruction*, result when dynamic and/or static factors reduce bladder emptying. The force of the urinary stream becomes diminished, urinary flow rate decreases, and bladder emptying is incomplete and slow. Patients report urinary hesitancy and straining and a weak urine stream. Urine dribbles out of the penis, and the urinary bladder always feels full, even after patients have voided. Some patients state that they need to press on their bladder to force out the urine. In severe cases, patients may go into urinary retention when bladder emptying is not possible. In these cases, suprapubic pain can result from bladder overdistension.

Approximately 50% to 80% of patients have irritative voiding symptoms, which typically occur late in the disease course. Irritative voiding symptoms result from long-standing obstruction at the bladder neck. To compensate, the bladder muscle undergoes hypertrophy so that it can generate a greater contractile force to empty urine past the anatomic obstruction at the bladder neck. Although initially helpful, decompensation eventually occurs, and the hypertrophied bladder muscle is no longer able to generate adequate contractile force as it becomes hypersensitive and ineffective in storing urine. As a result, small amounts of urine irritate the bladder and initiate a bladder emptying response. Patients complain of urinary frequency and urgency. Bedwetting or clothes wetting occurs. Patients report waking up every 1 to 2 hours at night to void (nocturia), which significantly reduces quality of life.

Symptoms of BPH vary over time. Symptoms may improve, remain stable, or worsen spontaneously. Thus, BPH is not necessarily a progressive disease; in fact, some patients experience symptom regression. Between one and two thirds of men with mild disease

CLINICAL PRESENTATION Benign Prostatic Hyperplasia

General

- A patient is in no acute distress unless he has moderate to severe symptoms or complications of BPH

Symptoms

- Urinary frequency, urgency, intermittency, nocturia, decreased force of stream, hesitancy, and straining

Signs

- Digital rectal examination reveals an enlarged prostate (>20 g) with no nodules or indurations; prostate is soft, symmetric, and mobile

Laboratory Tests

- Increased blood urea nitrogen (BUN) and serum creatinine with long-standing, untreated bladder outlet obstruction, elevated PSA level

Other Diagnostic Tests

- Increased American Urological Association (AUA) Symptom Score, decreased urinary flow rate (<10 mL/s), and increased postvoid residual (PVR) urine volume stabilize or improve without treatment over 2.5 to 5 years.[2,4] However, other patients experience a slow progression of disease.

Collectively, obstructive and irritative voiding symptoms and their impact on a patient's quality of life are referred to as *lower urinary tract symptoms* (LUTS). However, LUTS is not pathognomonic for BPH and may be caused by other diseases, such as neurogenic bladder and urinary tract infection.[2]

Another presentation of BPH is silent prostatism. Patients have obstructive or irritative voiding symptoms, but adapt to them and do not voluntarily complain about them. Such patients do not present for medical treatment until complications of BPH disease arise or a spouse brings in the symptomatic patient for medical care.

BPH can be a progressive disease, although the rate of progression is variable among patients.[2,5] When BPH progresses, it can produce complications that include the following:

1. Acute, painful urinary retention, which can lead to acute renal failure
2. Persistent gross hematuria when tissue growth exceeds its blood supply
3. Overflow urinary incontinence or unstable bladder
4. Recurrent urinary tract infection that results from urinary stasis
5. Bladder diverticula
6. Bladder stones
7. Chronic renal failure from long-standing bladder outlet obstruction

Approximately 17% to 20% of patients with symptomatic BPH require treatment because of disease complications.[7] Older men greater than 70 years of age with large prostates greater than 40 g and a postvoid residual (PVR) urine volume greater than 100 mL are three times more likely to have severe symptoms or suffer from acute urinary retention and to require prostatectomy than patients with smaller prostates.[8–10] Thus, a serum prostate-specific antigen (PSA) level of 1.4 ng/mL (1.4 mcg/L) has been used as a surrogate marker for an enlarged prostate gland to identify patients at risk for developing complications of BPH disease[6,10] and has been used to guide selection of the most appropriate treatment modality in some patients.[11,12]

DIAGNOSTIC EVALUATION

Because the obstructive and irritative voiding symptoms associated with BPH are not unique to the disease and can be presenting symptoms of other genitourinary tract disorders, including prostate or bladder cancer, neurogenic bladder, prostatic calculi, or urinary tract infection, the patient presenting with signs and symptoms of BPH must be thoroughly evaluated.

A careful medical history should be taken to ensure that a complete listing of symptoms is collected as well as to identify concomitant disorders that may be contributing to voiding symptoms. The medical history should be followed by a thorough medication history, including all prescription and nonprescription medications and dietary supplements that the patient is taking. Any drugs that could be causing or exacerbating the patient's symptoms should be identified. If possible, the suspected drugs should be discontinued or the dosing regimen modified to ameliorate the voiding symptoms.

The patient should undergo a physical examination, including a digital rectal examination, although the size of the prostate gland may not correspond to symptoms. BPH usually presents as an enlarged, soft, smooth, symmetric gland, greater than 20 g in size. Some patients have only a slightly enlarged gland and yet have bothersome or even serious voiding difficulties. Other patients have intravesical enlargement of the prostate gland (i.e., the gland grows into the urinary bladder and produces a ball-valve blockage of the bladder neck). This type of prostate enlargement is not palpable on digital examination.

TABLE 67-1 Categories of BPH Disease Severity Based on Symptoms and Signs

Disease Severity	AUA Symptom Score	Typical Symptoms and Signs
Mild	≤7	Asymptomatic Peak urinary flow rate <10 mL/s PVR urine volume >25–50 mL
Moderate	8–19	All of the above signs plus obstructive voiding symptoms and irritative voiding symptoms (signs of detrusor instability)
Severe	≥20	All of the above plus one or more complications of BPH

AUA, American Urological Association; BPH, benign prostatic hyperplasia; BUN, blood urea nitrogen; PVR, postvoid residual.

The patient's perception of the severity of BPH symptoms guides selection of a particular treatment modality in a patient. To evaluate the patient's perceptions objectively, validated instruments, such as the AUA Symptom Score (Table 67-1), are commonly used. Using the AUA Symptom Score, the patient rates the "bothersomeness" of seven obstructive and irritative voiding symptoms.[2,13] Each item is rated for severity on a scale from 0 to 5, such that 35 is the maximum score and is consistent with the most severe symptoms. Patients usually are stratified into the three groups shown in the table based on disease severity for the purposes of deciding a treatment approach.

In addition, the patient can complete a voiding diary in which he records the number of voids, the volume of each void, and voiding symptoms for several days. This information is used to evaluate symptom severity and tailor recommendations for lifestyle modifications that may ameliorate symptoms.

The only clinical laboratory test that must be performed is a urinalysis. Because many of the voiding symptoms of BPH could be caused by other urologic disorders, a urinalysis can help screen for bladder cancer, stones, and infection. To screen for prostate cancer, another common cause of glandular enlargement, a PSA test should be performed for patients aged 40 years or more, with at least a 10-year life expectancy in whom the cost of the test will be outweighed by the potential benefit of diagnosing the disorder.[13,14]

Additional objective measures of bladder emptying should be performed if surgical treatment is being considered. Measures include peak and average urinary flow rate (normal is at least 10 mL/s). These measures are determined using an uroflowmeter, which checks the rate of urine flow out of the bladder. This is a quick noninvasive outpatient procedure in which the patient is instructed to drink water until his bladder feels full and then the patient's urinary flow is clocked during voiding. A low urinary flow rate (<10 to 12 mL/s) implies failure of bladder emptying or a functional disorder of the detrusor muscle. Thus, the degree of bladder outlet obstruction may not correlate with peak urinary flow rate.[13]

Another objective measure is PVR urine volume (normal is 0 mL), which is assessed using a transabdominal ultrasound. A high PVR urine volume (>25 to 30 mL) implies failure of bladder emptying and a predisposition for urinary tract infections. Because of a weak correlation among voiding symptoms, prostate size, and urinary flow rate, most physicians use a combination of measures, including the patient's assessment of symptoms along with objective evaluation of urinary outflow and presence of complications of BPH to determine the need for treatment.

Many other tests can be performed if additional information is needed to assess the severity of BPH disease and its complications, to assist in the preoperative assessment of the patient, or to distinguish prostate enlargement due to BPH from that caused by prostate cancer. Tests include a serum blood urea nitrogen (BUN) and creatinine, voiding cystometrogram, transrectal ultrasound of the prostate, IV pyelogram, renal ultrasound, and prostate biopsy.

TREATMENT
Benign Prostatic Hyperplasia

The goals of treatment are to control symptoms, as evidenced by a minimum of a 3-point decrease in the AUA symptom index, prevent progression of complications of BPH disease, and delay the need for surgical intervention for BPH.

As a disease of symptoms, BPH is treated by relieving bothersome symptoms. However, selection of a single best treatment for a patient must consider the variable costs and adverse effects of treatment options, the inability to clearly distinguish patients who experience spontaneous regression or disease stabilization from those in whom symptoms progress, and the potential benefit that may occur in a comparatively small number of treated patients.

The AUA Guidelines on Management of Benign Prostatic Hyperplasia is the principal tool used in the United States,[13] and the AUA recommendations are similar to the European[15] and Canadian Practice Guidelines (Fig. 67-2).[16]

3 All patients should be encouraged to initiate and maintain a heart healthy lifestyle, including a low-fat diet, high intake of plenty of fresh fruits and vegetables, regular physical exercise, and no smoking.[17] Specific treatment options include watchful waiting, pharmacologic therapy, and surgical intervention. Although phytotherapy is used by some patients alone or along with conventional medications for BPH, head-to-head comparisons with FDA-approved treatments are lacking; consequently, such herbals cannot be recommended at this time.

4 Patients with mild disease are asymptomatic or have mildly bothersome symptoms and have no complications of BPH disease. For these patients, no specific treatment is indicated. These patients can be managed with watchful waiting, which entails having the patient return for reassessment at intervals of 6 to 12 months. At each return visit, the patient should complete a standardized, validated survey tool to assess severity of symptoms. Watchful waiting should be accompanied by patient education about the disease and behavior modification to avoid practices that exacerbate voiding symptoms. Behavior modification includes restricting fluids close to bedtime, minimizing caffeine and alcohol intake, frequent emptying of the bladder during waking hours (to avoid overflow incontinence and urgency), and avoiding drugs that could exacerbate voiding symptoms.[18] At each visit, physicians should assess the patient's risk of developing acute urinary retention by evaluating the patient's prostate size or using PSA as a surrogate marker of prostate enlargement.[13]

5 If symptoms progress to the moderate or severe level, or the patient perceives his symptoms to be bothersome, the patient should be offered specific treatment. In these patients, watchful waiting delays—but does not decrease—the need for prostatectomy. In symptomatic patients, watchful waiting can lead to intractable urinary retention, increased PVR urine volumes, and significant voiding symptoms.[18,19] Recommended treatment options include drug therapy with an α_1-adrenergic antagonist or 5α-reductase inhibitor, a combination of an α_1-adrenergic antagonist and a 5α-reductase inhibitor, a phosphodiesterase inhibitor or an anticholinergic agent; or surgery.

Patients with serious complications of BPH should be offered surgical correction (transurethral or open prostatectomy, or a minimally invasive surgical procedure). Drug therapy is considered an interim measure for such patients because it only delays worsening of complications and the need for surgical intervention.[13,18,19]

Desired Outcomes

The desired outcomes of treatment include reducing LUTS as evidenced by an improvement of AUA Symptom Score by at least three points, an increase in the peak urinary flow rate, and a normalization of PVR to less than 50 mL. In addition, treatment should prevent the development of disease complications and reduce the need for surgical intervention. Treatment should be well tolerated and be cost-effective.

Personalized Pharmacotherapy

In selecting the most appropriate treatment for an individual patient, consideration should be given to the severity and quality of the patient's LUTS, the likelihood of developing complications of BPH

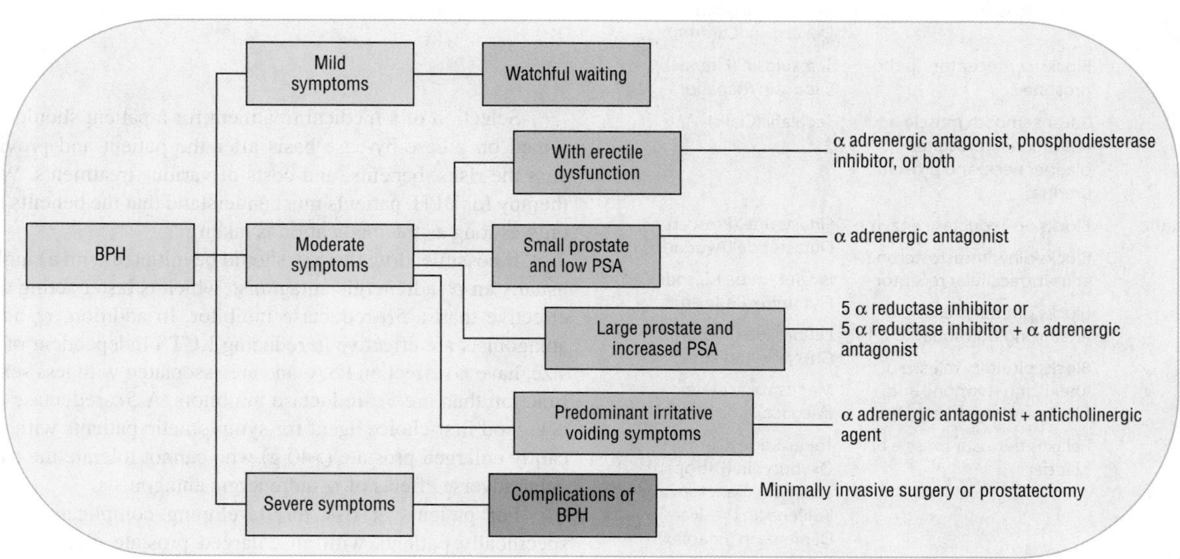

FIGURE 67-2 Management algorithm for benign prostatic hyperplasia (BPH).

(based on size of the patient's prostate gland), and the patient's preference for medical versus surgical intervention.

Concurrent medical illnesses of the patient should also be considered. For example, if the patient has erectile dysfunction and moderate BPH, then a phosphodiesterase inhibitor might be preferred over a 5α-reductase inhibitor. If medical treatment is initiated, the patient's level of renal function should be assessed, as the daily dose of some α-adrenergic antagonists and some anticholinergics require modification to avoid accumulation.

Pharmacologic Therapy

Drug therapy for BPH can be categorized into three types: agents that relax prostatic smooth muscle (reducing the dynamic factor), agents that interfere with testosterone's stimulatory effect on prostate gland enlargement (reducing the static factor), and agents that relax bladder detrusor muscle (Tables 67-2 and 67-3). Of the agents that relax prostatic smooth muscle, second- and third-generation α_1-adrenergic antagonists have been most widely used. These agents relax the intrinsic urethral sphincter and prostatic smooth muscle, thereby enhancing urinary outflow from the bladder. Phosphodiesterase inhibitors also relax bladder neck and prostatic smooth muscle. α_1-Adrenergic antagonists and phosphodiesterase inhibitors do not reduce prostate size. Of the agents that interfere with testosterone's stimulatory effect on prostate gland size, the only agents approved by the FDA are 5α-reductase inhibitors (e.g., finasteride, dutasteride). Other agents that interfere with androgen stimulation of the prostate have not been popular in the United States because of the many adverse effects associated with their use. The luteinizing hormone-releasing hormone superagonists leuprolide and goserelin decrease libido and can cause erectile dysfunction, gynecomastia, and hot flashes. Antiandrogens (e.g., bicalutamide, flutamide) produce nausea, diarrhea, and hepatotoxicity. Finally, antimuscarinic agents relax detrusor muscle contraction, which reduces irritable voiding symptoms in some patients with BPH.

TABLE 67-2 Medical Treatment Options for Benign Prostatic Hyperplasia

Category	Mechanism	Drug (Brand Name)
Reduces dynamic factor	Blocks α_1-adrenergic receptors in prostatic stromal tissue	Prazosin (Minipress) Alfuzosin (Uroxatral) Terazosin (Hytrin) Doxazosin (Cardura)
	Blocks α_{1A}-receptors in the prostate	Tamsulosin (Flomax) Silodosin (Rapaflo)
	Causes smooth muscle relaxation of prostate, bladder neck, and prostatic urethra	Tadalafil (Cialis)
Reduce static factor	Blocks 5α-reductase enzyme	Finasteride (Proscar) Dutasteride (Avodart)
	Blocks dihydrotestosterone at its intracellular receptor	Bicalutamide (Casodex)[a] Flutamide (Eulexin)[a]
	Blocks pituitary release of luteinizing hormone	Leuprolide (Lupron)[a] Goserelin (Zoladex)[a]
	Blocks pituitary release of luteinizing hormone and blocks androgen receptor	Megestrol acetate (Megace)[a]
Other	Relaxes detrusor muscle of bladder	Tolterodine (Detrol) Oxybutynin (Ditropan) Trospium (Sanctura) Solifenacin (Vesicare) Darifenacin (Enablex) Fesoterodine (Toviaz)

[a]Not FDA approved for treatment of benign prostatic hyperplasia.

TABLE 67-3 Comparison of α_1-Adrenergic Antagonists, 5α-Reductase Inhibitors, Phosphodiesterase Inhibitors, and Anticholinergic Agents for BPH

	α_1-Adrenergic Antagonists	5α-Reductase Inhibitors
Relaxes prostatic smooth muscle	Yes	No
Decreases prostate size	No	Yes
Halts disease progression	No	Yes
Peak onset	1–6 weeks	3–6 months
Efficacy in relieving BOO	++	++ (for patients with enlarged prostates)
Frequency of dosing	One to two times per day, depending on the agent and dosage formulation	Once per day
Decreases prostate-specific antigen (PSA)	No	Yes
Sexual dysfunction adverse effects	EJD	Decreased libido, ED, EJD
Cardiovascular adverse effects	Yes	No
	Phosphodiesterase Inhibitors	**Anticholinergic Agents**
Relaxes prostatic smooth muscle	Yes	No
Decreases prostate size	No	No
Halts disease progression	No	No
Peak onset	4 weeks	1–2 weeks
Efficacy in relieving BOO	+	0 (irritative symptoms only)
Frequency of dosing	Once per day	Once per day
Decreases prostate-specific antigen	No	No
Sexual dysfunction adverse effects	No	ED
Cardiovascular adverse effects	Yes (mild hypotension)	Yes (tachycardia)

ED, erectile dysfunction; EJD, ejaculation disorder.

+ Notation is a quantitative assessment.

Selection of a medical treatment for a patient should be determined on a case-by-case basis after the patient and provider discuss the risks, benefits, and costs of various treatments. With drug therapy for BPH, patients must understand that the benefits continue only as long as the medication is taken.

If possible, drug therapy should be initiated with a single agent, usually an α_1-adrenergic antagonist, which is faster acting and more effective than a 5α-reductase inhibitor. In addition, α_1-adrenergic antagonists are effective in reducing LUTS independent of prostate size, have no effect on PSA, and are associated with less sexual dysfunction than are 5α-reductase inhibitors. A 5α-reductase inhibitor is a good first-choice agent for symptomatic patients with a significantly enlarged prostate (>40 g) who cannot tolerate the cardiovascular adverse effects of α_1-adrenergic antagonists.

For patients at risk for developing complications of BPH, specifically patients with an enlarged prostate gland greater than 40 g[7] and an elevated PSA ≥1.4 ng/mL (1.4 mcg/L), combination drug therapy with an α_1-adrenergic antagonist and a 5α-reductase inhibitor is more beneficial than single drug therapy. The pharmacologic rationale for such a combination is that using two drugs with different mechanisms of action can be more effective than either drug alone. The clinical benefit of combination therapy is that it quickly relieves symptoms, delays disease progression, and reduces the need for surgical intervention.

For patients with both erectile dysfunction and BPH, a phosphodiesterase inhibitor alone or in combination with an α-adrenergic antagonist may be used. However, it should be noted that a phosphodiesterase inhibitor alone will only relieve LUTS and will not improve urinary flow rate or decrease postvoid urine volume. Therefore, a phosphodiesterase inhibitor is generally considered less effective than an α-adrenergic antagonist.

For patients with LUTS with a predominance of irritative voiding symptoms, an anticholinergic agent could be added to an existing drug regimen for BPH. To reduce the risk of developing systemic anticholinergic adverse effects, an uroselective anticholinergic agent may be preferentially prescribed. To avoid the risk of developing acute urinary retention, the patient's PVR volume should be less than 250 mL before starting an anticholinergic agent.

α-Adrenergic Antagonists

Three generations of α-adrenergic antagonists have been used to treat BPH. They all relax smooth muscle in the prostate and bladder neck. Because of their antagonism of presynaptic α_2-adrenergic receptors that results in tachycardia and arrhythmias, first-generation agents such as phenoxybenzamine have been replaced by the second-generation postsynaptic α_1-adrenergic antagonists and third-generation uroselective postsynaptic α_{1A}-adrenergic antagonists.

6 The second- and third-generation α_1-adrenergic antagonists are considered equally effective for treatment of BPH.[13,20,21] These agents generally improve the AUA Symptom Score by 30% to 40%, decreasing the AUA Symptom Index by three to six points, within 2 to 6 weeks, depending on the need for up dose titration; increase urinary flow rate by 2 to 3 mL/s in 60% to 70% of treated patients; and reduce PVR urine volume. With continued use, durable clinical benefit has been demonstrated for years.[21] They have no effect on prostate volume. α_1-Adrenergic antagonists do not reduce PSA levels, preserving the utility of this prostate cancer marker in this high-risk population.[13]

Adrenergic agents differ in their causation of hypotensive adverse effects and ejaculation disorders. Modified- or extended-release formulations and third-generation α-adrenergic$_{1A}$ antagonists produce a lower prevalence of hypotension than immediate-release, second-generation agents. In addition, older, immediate-release, second-generation α-adrenergic antagonists are available as inexpensive generic formulations, which may be desirable in selected patients.[13]

Second-generation agents include prazosin, terazosin, doxazosin, and alfuzosin. At the usual doses used to treat BPH, prazosin, terazosin, and doxazosin antagonize peripheral vascular α_1-adrenergic receptors in addition to those in the prostate. As a result, first-dose syncope, orthostatic hypotension, and dizziness are characteristic adverse effects. To improve tolerance to these adverse effects, therapy should start with a low dose of 1 mg daily and then should be slowly titrated up to a full therapeutic dose over several weeks.[20,22] Additive blood-pressure-lowering effects commonly occur when these agents are used with antihypertensive agents, which limit the use of these agents for some patients.[13] These agents differ in terms of duration of action and dosage formulation. Whereas prazosin requires dosing two to three times per day, terazosin, doxazosin, and alfuzosin offer more convenient once-daily dosing. Because prazosin requires twice- to thrice-daily dosing and has significant cardiovascular adverse effects, it is not recommended in the current AUA guidelines for treatment of BPH.[13] Extended-release dosage formulations are available for doxazosin and alfuzosin. These offer the convenience of once-daily dosing, treatment initiation with a full therapeutic dose, and decreased dose-related hypotension as the formulation produces lower peak serum concentrations than immediate-release products.[23,24] An α_1-adrenergic antagonist is not preferred as single-drug therapy for treatment of both BPH and hypertension in a patient. In the Antihypertensive and Lipid-Lowering Treatment to Prevent Heart Attack Trial (ALLHAT) of 24,000 patients with hypertension, doxazosin produced more congestive heart failure than amlodipine, lisinopril, or chlorthalidone.[25] Thus, both the AUA and the Joint National Committee on Prevention, Detection, Evaluation and Treatment of High Blood Pressure[13,26] recommend that patients with BPH and hypertension be treated with separate and appropriate drug treatment for each medical condition.[27]

Alfuzosin is considered functionally and clinically uroselective in that usual doses used to treat BPH are less likely than other second-generation agents to cause cardiovascular adverse effects in animal or human models.[23] This clinical observation has been observed more often with the once-daily, extended-release formulation of alfuzosin, which is the only commercially available formulation in the United States, as compared with the immediate-release formulation that is dosed three times per day, which is available in Europe.[28] Its clinical uroselectivity has been postulated to be due to higher concentrations of alfuzosin achieved in the prostate versus serum after usual doses,[29] decreased blood–brain barrier penetration of alfuzosin,[30] absence of high peak serum levels with the extended-release formulation,[31] and the fixed dosing schedule of the extended-release formulation. The extended-release alfuzosin dosing is FDA approved for 10 mg daily, with no dose titration increase. This formulation is particularly convenient for physician prescribers and patients who are starting to take the medication.

Tamsulosin and silodosin are the only third-generation α_1-adrenergic antagonists available in the United States. They are an advance over second-generation agents in that they are pharmacologically selective for prostatic α_{1A}-adrenergic receptors, which comprise approximately 70% to 75% of the adrenergic receptors in the prostate gland, prostatic urethra, and bladder neck.[32,33] Blockade of these receptors results in smooth muscle relaxation of the prostate and bladder neck without causing peripheral vascular smooth muscle relaxation. Tamsulosin and silodosin have low affinity for vascular α_{1B}-adrenergic receptors, which explains why hypotension is not a common adverse effect.[34]

Uroselectivity of these drugs for α_{1A}-adrenergic receptors has multiple implications. Dose titration is minimal; therefore, patients can begin tamsulosin with the lowest effective maintenance dose. Patients can be instructed to take the dose anytime during the day, unlike immediate-release formulations of terazosin and doxazosin, which should be taken at bedtime so that patients can sleep through the time when peak cardiovascular adverse effects are most likely to occur. However, for best oral absorption, tamsulosin should be taken on an empty stomach because food decreases the drug's bioavailability and reduces the peak serum concentration of the drug after dosing. The onset of peak action is quick, in the range of 1 week, and only a minority of patients will require uptitration to a higher daily dose. No decreases in blood pressure or increases in heart rate have been reported in normotensive patients, the elderly, subgroups of patients with well-controlled hypertension, or those with uncontrolled hypertension.[35] Thus, tamsulosin allows initiation of treatment with a therapeutic dose that is not limited by cardiovascular adverse effects, unlike immediate-release formulations of terazosin and doxazosin.[34] Finally, the addition of tamsulosin to select antihypertensive regimens of patients does not result in potentiation of the hypotensive effect of furosemide, enalapril, nifedipine, and atenolol.[36,37] Therefore, tamsulosin is a good choice, particularly for patients who cannot tolerate hypotension; have severe coronary artery disease, volume depletion, cardiac arrhythmias, severe orthostasis, or liver failure; are taking multiple antihypertensives; or when the titration would be too complicated for the patient or produce an unacceptable delay in onset for a particular patient.

As compared with tamsulosin, silodosin requires dosage modification in patients with hepatic impairment and renal impairment (creatinine clearance less than 30 mL/min [0.5 mL/s]), and has the potential for more drug interactions with inhibitors of CYP 3A4 (e.g., clarithromycin, itraconazole, ketoconazole, ritonavir) and P-glycoprotein (e.g., cyclosporine). In addition, silodosin's safety in patients with cardiovascular disease has been documented in fewer studies when compared with tamsulosin.[33] Finally, silodosin is commercially available from only one source, whereas tamsulosin is available as a generic formulation. For these reasons, tamsulosin is the preferred third-generation α_1-adrenergic antagonist in clinical practice.[20,33,38]

The usual doses of α_1-adrenergic antagonists are summarized in Table 67-4.

When using immediate-release formulations of the second-generation α_1-adrenergic antagonists terazosin and doxazosin, slow titration up to a therapeutic maintenance dose is necessary to minimize orthostatic hypotension and first-dose syncope. Conservatively, dosages should be increased in an orderly stepwise process, at 2- to 7-day intervals, depending on the patient's response to the medication. A faster titration schedule can be used as long as the patient does not develop orthostatic hypotension or dizziness. Two sample titration schedules for terazosin are as follows:

- *Schedule 1: Slow titration*
  Days 4 to 14: 2 mg at bedtime
  Weeks 2 to 6: 5 mg at bedtime
  Weeks 7 and on: 10 mg at bedtime
- *Schedule 2: Quicker titration*
  Days 1 to 3: 1 mg at bedtime
  Days 4 to 14: 2 mg at bedtime
  Weeks 2 to 3: 5 mg at bedtime
  Weeks 4 and on: 10 mg at bedtime

Patients should continue taking the drug as long as they continue to respond to it. Durable responses for 6 and 10 years have been reported for tamsulosin[39] and doxazosin,[40] respectively. If BPH symptoms worsen despite maximum tolerable drug doses, surgery should be considered.

With the exception of silodosin, no dosage adjustments are recommended for α_1-adrenergic antagonists for patients with renal failure. Because these drugs are hepatically catabolized, the lowest effective dose should be used for patients with hepatic dysfunction, and patients should be monitored carefully for adverse effects. With the exception of silodosin, no specific dosing guidelines for this patient population are available. For silodosin, a reduced daily dose of 4 mg is recommended for patients with moderate renal impairment or those with hepatic dysfunction.

Approximately 10% to 12% of patients discontinue taking second-generation α_1-adrenergic antagonists because of adverse effects, especially those that affect the cardiovascular system (e.g., syncope, dizziness, hypotension).[41] Patients who tolerate hypotension poorly should avoid second-generation α_1-adrenergic antagonists.[42] This includes patients with poorly controlled angina, serious cardiac arrhythmias, patients with reduced circulating volume, patients with untreated hypertension, and patients taking multiple antihypertensives.[22,41] These patients are candidates for a third-generation α_1-adrenergic antagonist or finasteride, if drug therapy is deemed necessary. Whether extended-release alfuzosin or silodosin is a good choice remains to be elucidated in controlled comparison trials with tamsulosin.[43,44]

Tiredness and asthenia, anejaculation, flu-like symptoms, and nasal congestion are the most common dose-related adverse effects of tamsulosin and silodosin.[45] These adverse effects are extensions of their α-adrenergic antagonist activity and are unavoidable, but with proper education patients likely will not discontinue treatment.

Floppy iris syndrome has been associated with doxazosin, silodosin, and tamsulosin use, although the number of reported cases is highest with tamsulosin.[46] The mechanism for this adverse reaction is related to blockade of α_{1A}-adrenergic receptors in iris dilator muscles. As a result, during cataract surgery, pupillary constriction occurs and the iris billows out (floppy iris), both of which complicate the procedure or can increase the likelihood of postoperative complications, including posterior capsular rupture, retinal detachment, residual retained lens material, or endophthalmitis.[46–48] Permanent loss of vision can result.

Patients who are taking α_1-adrenergic antagonists and who plan to undergo cataract surgery should inform their ophthalmologist that they are taking this medication so that appropriate measures can be taken during eye surgery, for example, use of iris retractors, pupillary expansion rings, or potent mydriatic agents.[46–48] No benefit has been demonstrated with holding the α_1-adrenergic antagonist preoperatively.

For patients who are scheduled to have cataract surgery, and who have not yet started an α_1-adrenergic antagonist, they should be advised to delay the start of the α_1-adrenergic antagonist until surgery has been completed.[46–48]

Patients with severe sulfa allergy should avoid tamsulosin.

Caution is needed when CYP 3A4 inhibitors, for example cimetidine and diltiazem, are used with α_1-adrenergic antagonists because a drug–drug interaction could lead to decreased metabolism of the latter agents. In contrast, concurrent use of potent CYP 3A4 stimulators, for example carbamazepine and phenytoin, may increase hepatic catabolism of α_1-adrenergic antagonists.

Phosphodiesterase inhibitors (e.g., sildenafil, vardenafil, tadalafil) may produce hypotension if used in large doses along with α_1-adrenergic antagonists. The mechanisms for this interaction are related to the intrinsic vasodilatory effects of phosphodiesterase inhibitors and the higher susceptibility of elderly patients to venous pooling because of autonomic incompetence.[28,49,50] The prevalence of hypotension depends on the specific phosphodiesterase inhibitor and α_1-adrenergic antagonist agent, specifically the combination of tadalafil and tamsulosin is least likely to produce a clinically significant drug interaction, as compared with other combinations.[50] Therefore, a patient's blood pressure should be stabilized on the α_1-adrenergic antagonist before starting a phosphodiesterase inhibitor. In addition, patients who are taking phosphodiesterase inhibitors with α_1-adrenergic antagonists should have their blood pressure monitored closely when initiating combined drug use.

Clinical **Controversy. . .**

Among the α-adrenergic antagonists, agents that are uroselective appear to have a lower potential to cause hypotension than nonuroselective agents. However, it is unclear if there is any distinct advantage of using silodosin or alfuzosin, as opposed to tamsulosin.

5α-Reductase Inhibitors

7 Finasteride competitively inhibits type II 5α-reductase, the predominant isoform of the enzyme in the prostate, suppresses intraprostatic DHT by 80% to 90%, and decreases serum DHT levels by 70%.[11] Dutasteride is a nonselective inhibitor of type I and II 5α-reductase. It more quickly and completely suppresses intraprostatic DHT production and decreases serum DHT levels by 90%.[51] However, direct comparison clinical trials show no advantages of

TABLE 67-4 Dosing of Drugs Used in Treatment of Benign Prostatic Hyperplasia

Drug	Brand Name	Initial Dose	Usual Dose	Special Population Dose
α-Adrenergic Antagonists				
Prazosin	Minipress	0.5 mg twice a day orally	1–5 mg twice a day orally	For uptitrating the dose, double the dose every 2 weeks
Terazosin	Hytrin	1 mg at bedtime orally	10–20 mg daily orally	For uptitrating the dose, increase slowly to 2 mg, 5 mg, and then 10 mg daily in a stepwise fashion. Take extra care if the patient is taking other drugs that lower blood pressure
Doxazosin	Cardura Cardura XL	1 mg daily orally 4 mg daily orally	8 mg daily orally 4–8 mg daily	For the immediate-release formulation, doses of 16 mg daily have been used for hypertension. For the XL formulation, increase from 4 to 8 mg daily after a 3- to 4-week interval. When switching from the immediate- to the extended-release formulation, start at 4 mg of the extended-release formulation no matter what maintenance dose of immediate-release doxazosin the patient is taking
Alfuzosin	Uroxatral	10 mg daily orally	10 mg daily orally	This is an extended-release formulation, and it should not be chewed or crushed. The drug should be taken after meals and used cautiously in patients with impaired renal function
Tamsulosin	Flomax	0.4 mg daily orally	0.4–0.8 mg daily orally	This is an extended-release formulation, and it should not be chewed or crushed. The drug should be taken after meals. No dosage adjustment is needed in patients with renal or liver dysfunction. Allow several weeks after starting a dose before increasing to a higher dose
Silodosin	Rapaflo	8 mg daily orally	8 mg daily orally	This drug is contraindicated when creatinine clearance is less than 30 mL/min (0.5 mL/s). If creatinine clearance is 30–50 mL/min (0.5–0.83 mL/s), use 4 mg daily orally. The drug should be taken with meals
5α-Reductase Inhibitors				
Finasteride	Proscar	5 mg daily orally	5 mg daily orally	No dosage adjustment in patients with renal impairment. Use cautiously in patients with hepatic impairment
Dutasteride	Avodart	0.5 mg daily orally	0.5 mg daily orally	No dosage adjustment in patients with renal impairment. Use cautiously in patients with hepatic impairment
Phosphodiesterase Inhibitor				
Tadalafil	Cialis	5 mg daily orally	5 mg daily orally	If creatinine clearance is 30–50 mL/min (0.5–0.83 mL/s), use 2.5 mg daily orally. Do not use if creatinine clearance is less than 30 mL/min (0.5 mL/s)
Anticholinergic Agents				
Darifenacin	Enablex	7.5 mg daily orally	7.5–15 mg daily orally	For uptitrating the dose, double the dose after 2 weeks. If the patient is taking a potent CYP3A4 inhibitor (e.g., ketoconazole, itraconazole, ritonavir, nelfinavir, and clarithromycin), do not exceed 7.5 mg daily orally
Fesoterodine	Toviaz	4 mg daily orally	4–8 mg daily orally	This is an extended-release formulation, and it should not be chewed or crushed. If the patient is taking a potent CYP3A4 inhibitor (e.g., ketoconazole, itraconazole, ritonavir, nelfinavir, and clarithromycin), do not exceed 4 mg daily orally. If the creatinine clearance is less than 30 mL/min (0.5 mL/s), do not exceed 4 mg daily orally
Oxybutynin	Ditropan	5 mg two to three times a day orally	5-10 mg two to three times a day orally	Increase daily dose at 5-mg increments at weekly intervals
	Ditropan XL	5 mg daily orally	5–30 mg daily orally	This is an extended release formulation, and it should not be crushed or chewed. Increase daily dose at 5-mg increments at weekly intervals
Solifenacin	Vesicare	5 mg daily orally	5–10 mg daily orally	If the creatinine clearance is less than 30 mL/min (0.5 mL/s) or the patient has moderate hepatic impairment, do not exceed 5 mg daily orally. If the patient is taking a potent CYP3A4 inhibitor (e.g., ketoconazole, itraconazole, ritonavir, nelfinavir, and clarithromycin), do not exceed 5 mg daily orally
Tolterodine	Detrol	2 mg twice daily orally	2 mg twice daily orally	If the patient has significant renal impairment, limit dose to 1 mg twice a day
	Detrol LA	4 mg daily orally	4 mg daily orally	The LA formulation is an extended-release formulation, and it should not be chewed or crushed. If the creatinine clearance is 10–30 mL/min (0.17–0.5 mL/s) or the patient has mild/moderate hepatic impairment, do not exceed 2 mg daily orally. If the creatinine clearance is less than 10 mL/min (0.17 mL/s), do not use Detrol LA
Trospium	Sanctura	20 mg twice daily orally	20 mg twice daily orally	Avoid alcohol ingestion for 2 hours after a dose. Use cautiously in patients with moderate or severe hepatic impairment. In patients older than 75 years, use the immediate-release formulation and start with 20 mg daily orally. If the creatinine clearance is less than 30 mL/min (0.5 mL/s), use 20-mg immediate-release formulation
	Sanctura XR	60 mg daily orally	60 mg daily orally	The XR is an extended-release formulation, and it should not be chewed or crushed. Product not recommended in patients with creatinine clearance less than 30 mL/min (0.5 mL/s)

these pharmacodynamic actions of dutasteride when compared with finasteride.[52] These agents are indicated for management of moderate to severe BPH disease for patients with enlarged prostate glands of at least 40 g.[52] For such patients, 5α-reductase inhibitors may slow disease progression and decrease the risk of disease complications, thereby decreasing the ultimate need for surgical intervention. When taken continuously for 4 years or 6 years, dutasteride or finasteride, respectively, has been shown to decrease the risk of acute urinary retention and prostatectomy.[53,54] For patients with severe disease, these agents generally can be used with a 6-month short course of an α_1-adrenergic antagonist, which will provide fast symptom relief until the 5α-reductase inhibitor starts to work. 5α-Reductase inhibitors may be preferred for patients with BPH and an enlarged prostate gland who have uncontrolled arrhythmias, have poorly controlled angina, are taking multiple antihypertensive agents, or are unable to tolerate hypotensive adverse effects of α_1-adrenergic antagonists.

5α-Reductase inhibitors reduce prostate size by 25%, increase peak urinary flow rate by 1.6 to 2.0 mL/s, improve voiding symptoms in approximately 30% of treated patients, and produce few serious adverse effects. Compared with α_1-adrenergic antagonists, 5α-reductase inhibitors have several disadvantages. 5α-Reductase inhibitors have a delayed peak onset of clinical effect, which is undesirable for patients with bothersome symptoms, and an adequate clinical trial is 6 to 12 months. In addition, patients experience less objective improvement of the AUA Symptom Score and urinary flow rate with 5α-reductase inhibitors than with α_1-adrenergic antagonists.[13] 5α-Reductase inhibitors cause more sexual dysfunction than α_1-adrenergic receptor antagonists; therefore, physicians consider 5α-reductase inhibitors to be the second-line agents for treatment of BPH in sexually active males (Tables 67-3 and 67-5).[13]

Patients with BPH who have large prostate glands, PSA level less than 3 ng/mL (3 mcg/L) and are concerned about developing prostate cancer can be prescribed finasteride 5 mg daily for up to 7 years. In the Prostate Cancer Prevention Trial, finasteride reduced the 7-year prevalence of prostate cancer by 25%.[55] However, in this study, finasteride was associated with a 27% increase in the number of patients who developed high-grade prostate cancer, which has a potential for invasiveness. Although originally thought to be an disadvantage of finasteride use, it is now thought that the higher incidence of prostate cancer is due to biopsy sampling bias. That is, since finasteride reduces the size of the prostate gland, this results in increased sensitivity of sampling biopsies to detect prostate cancer.

Another clinical trial produced similar results. The Reduction by Dutasteride in Prostate Cancer Events (REDUCE) study compared the effect of 4 years of continuous use of dutasteride versus placebo on reducing the incidence of prostate cancer in more than 6,700 men at high risk for developing prostate cancer. At the end of the study, dutasteride-treated patients had a 22.8% decreased relative risk of prostate cancer. Of the patients with biopsy-positive prostate cancer, a similar number of patients in each treatment group developed high grade tumors of Gleason grade 7 to 10 with no statistical difference between the groups.[56]

Thus, when finasteride is administered to patients with BPH and is also being continued to prevent prostate cancer, it should be reserved for patients with a family history of prostate cancer or in men of African descent who have an increased risk of developing prostate cancer. The possibility of developing a high-grade prostate cancer should be discussed with the patient before he initiates treatment with a 5α-reductase inhibitor for prevention of prostate cancer.[55]

Finasteride is well absorbed from the GI tract (95%), and its absorption is unaffected by food. Peak serum concentrations are

TABLE 67-5 Monitoring of Drugs Used in Treatment of Benign Prostatic Hyperplasia

Drug	Adverse Reaction	Monitoring Parameter	Comment
α-Adrenergic antagonists	Syncope Lightheadedness Orthostatic hypotension Tachycardia Nasal congestion Ejaculatory dysfunction Priapism Floppy iris syndrome	Blood pressure Heart rate	If prescribing an immediate-release formulation, start the patient on the lowest possible dose and instruct the patient to take the first dose at bedtime. Slowly uptitrate the dose over several weeks. Stabilize the patient's blood pressure on the α-adrenergic antagonist before adding any other hypotensive agent. If the patient needs cataract surgery, instruct the patient to inform the ophthalmologist so that appropriate measures can be taken during the procedure to prevent intraoperative complications. If the patient has a painful erection lasting longer than 4 hours, the patient should seek immediate medical attention
5α-Reductase inhibitors	Erectile dysfunction Decreased libido Ejaculatory dysfunction Gynecomastia	Prostate-specific antigen (PSA)	The patient's PSA level should decrease by 50% if he is adherent to therapy
Phosphodiesterase inhibitor	Headache Dizziness Nasal congestion Dyspepsia Back pain Myalgia Hearing loss	Blood pressure Pulse Hearing loss	If the patient experiences hearing loss, discontinue tadalafil
Anticholinergic agents	Dry mouth Constipation Headache Tachycardia Blurry vision Acute urinary retention Drowsiness Confusion Angioedema Anaphylaxis Erectile dysfunction	Mental status Bowel habits Ability to urinate	Adverse effects are dose-related and generally reversible. Patients with signs of severe allergic reaction need immediate medical attention

reached 1 to 2 hours after the dose. Finasteride is highly protein bound. The liver extensively metabolizes finasteride to inactive metabolites, which are largely excreted in stool. The plasma half-life is 4.7 to 7.1 hours, but its biologic half-life probably is longer, as decreased serum DHT levels persist for up to 2 weeks after finasteride dosing is stopped.

For BPH, finasteride is given in doses of 5 mg by mouth daily. The dose can be taken with meals or on an empty stomach. No dosage adjustment is needed for patients with renal dysfunction. Although no dosage reduction is recommended for patients with hepatic insufficiency, patients should be monitored carefully. Maximal reductions in prostate volume or symptom improvement may not be evident for 12 months, but noticeable changes from baseline should occur after 6 months of continuous treatment. No clinically relevant drug interactions have been reported with 5α-reductase inhibitors.

Patients must continue to take 5α-reductase inhibitors as long as they respond. Durable responses to finasteride and dutasteride have been reported with continued treatment for 6 years[54] and 4 years,[52] respectively. Upon discontinuation of the drug, prostate size and voiding symptoms generally return to baseline.

5α-Reductase inhibitors can produce sexual dysfunction, and this has led to discontinuation of therapy in up to 12% of treated patients in one pooled analysis.[52] Ejaculation disorders (dry sex or delayed ejaculation) have been reported in 3% to 8% of treated patients.[57] These disorders, which are possible results of decreased prostatic secretion, are reversible with drug discontinuation.

Erectile dysfunction has been reported for 3% to 16% of patients.[52] It may be secondary to ejaculation disorders or may be due to drug-induced inhibition of nitric oxide synthase (which is needed to produce nitric oxide, a vasodilatory substance) in cavernosal tissue.[58] The role of 5α-reductase inhibitors in causing erectile dysfunction is not clear, as elderly men with BPH commonly develop erectile dysfunction as they age or have concurrent medical illnesses or concomitant drug therapies that may predispose to the development of sexual dysfunction. Decreased libido has been reported in 2% to 10% of treated patients.[52]

Other minor adverse effects include nausea, abdominal pain, asthenia, dizziness, flatulence, headache, rash, muscle weakness, and gynecomastia.

5α-Reductase inhibitors are in FDA pregnancy category X, which means that they are contraindicated in pregnant females. Exposure of the male fetus to finasteride may produce pseudohermaphroditic offspring with ambiguous genitalia, similar to those of patients with a rare genetic deficiency of type II 5α-reductase. Because of this teratogenic effect, women who are pregnant or seeking to become pregnant should not handle 5α-reductase inhibitor tablets and should not have contact with semen from men being treated with 5α-reductase inhibitors. Women health professionals of childbearing age should handle this product with rubber gloves if there is any chance that they are pregnant.

Usual doses of 5α-reductase inhibitors produce a median reduction of serum PSA levels by 50% at months 6 to 12 after the start of treatment. For this reason, PSA levels must be measured before treatment begins, and the patient should have a digital rectal examination. After 6 months of therapy, the patient should have a repeat PSA. If the level does not decline by 50% and the patient has been adherent to the 5α-reductase inhibitor regimen, he should be evaluated for prostate cancer. Annually thereafter, the patient should have a PSA assay and digital rectal examination. Patients with an increase in PSA level of 0.3 ng/L or more above the baseline nadir level should be evaluated for prostate cancer[59] or noncompliance to the prescribed regimen. To interpret a PSA level in a patient being treated with a 5α-reductase inhibitor, it is generally recommended that the actual measured level be doubled to get an estimate of the true level.[13,59]

Clinical **Controversy...**

Dutasteride is a nonselective 5α-reductase inhibitor that more quickly and effectively lowers intraprostatic DHT production and lowers plasma DHE levels than finasteride. Whether these hormonal changes result in clinical advantages over finasteride remains to be elucidated.

Combination Therapy of 5α-Reductase Inhibitor and α-Adrenergic Antagonist

Combination therapy with an α_1-adrenergic antagonist and a 5α-reductase inhibitor is ideal for patients with severe symptoms, who also have an enlarged prostate gland of at least 40 g and PSA of at least 1.4 ng/mL (1.4 μg/L), a surrogate marker for an enlarged prostate gland.[7,13,60] Such patients appear to be at high risk for disease progression, as evidenced by symptom worsening and development of disease complications, including acute urinary retention, recurrent urinary tract infection, or need for surgical intervention.[7]

In the landmark Multiple Treatment of Prostate Symptoms Study (MTOPS), a regimen of finasteride and doxazosin for 5 years was shown to prevent symptom progression by 66%, decrease the risk of developing acute urinary retention by 81%, and decrease the need for prostate surgery by 67%. Moreover, urinary symptom improvement and higher urinary flow rates at 15–18 months were observed in patients treated with combination therapy, as compared with monotherapy with finasteride alone or doxazosin alone.[7] In another key clinical trial, the Combination of Avodart and Tamsulosin (COMBAT) study, dutasteride versus tamsulosin versus a combination of dutasteride and tamsulosin were evaluated in patients with large prostate glands (i.e., mean prostate volume of 55 ± 23 cc [55 ± 23 mL] and a mean PSA of 4 ng/mL [4 mcg/L]). The combination regimen was more effective in reducing symptoms 9 months after the start of treatment than dutasteride alone or tamsulosin alone. Whether the combination of dutasteride and tamsulosin prevents disease progression after 4 years awaits long-term study results, although preliminary subgroup analysis has shown that combination therapy reduces the percentage of patients who develop disease progression.[61,62]

Although not proven by direct comparison trials, any combination of 5α-reductase inhibitor and α_1-adrenergic antagonist probably is similarly effective for patients with the aforementioned characteristics.[13] The disadvantages of a combination regimen include increased medication cost to the patient and an increased incidence of adverse drug effects (i.e., 18% to 27% of patients discontinued treatment due to hypotension).

Clinical **Controversy...**

The combination of an α_1-adrenergic antagonist and 5α-reductase inhibitor can relieve LUTS, slow progression of BPH, and reduce the need for prostate surgery for patients with moderate to severe symptoms and a prostate of 40 g or larger. It may be possible to discontinue the α_1-adrenergic antagonist after the first several months; however, this potentially cost-saving measure requires further clinical study.

Phosphodiesterase Inhibitors

8 Several observations led to the use of phosphodiesterase inhibitors for management of BPH. BPH and erectile dysfunction are often present concurrently in the same patient.[63] Adverse effects of

α-adrenergic antagonists and 5α-reductase inhibitors include erectile dysfunction, which is likely to respond to a phosphodiesterase inhibitor.[64] The pathophysiology of BPH and erectile dysfunction may be common in so far as both disorders may be associated with increased vascular smooth muscle tone and pelvic atherosclerosis.

Phosphodiesterase inhibitors are thought to relax smooth muscle in the prostate and bladder neck, probably by increasing cyclic GMP. By so doing, phosphodiesterase inhibitors inactivate the rho-kinase pathway, which normally regulates smooth muscle contraction mediated by endothelin and α-adrenergic stimulation and contributes to the presence of obstructive voiding symptoms.[64–66] In addition, phosphodiesterase inhibitors may cause direction relaxation of the detrusor muscle of the bladder, which could reduce irritative voiding symptoms.[67]

In multiple clinical trials of patients with moderate LUTS, tadalafil caused significant improvements in voiding symptoms as measured by the AUA Symptom Index score or IPSS, with the level of improvement similar to that observed with α-adrenergic antagonists.[66,68] However, no increase in urinary flow rate or reduction in PVR urine volume occurred with tadalafil alone.[69,70] Tadalafil 2.5 mg was inferior to 5 mg, and doses of 10 mg or 20 mg were not superior to 5 mg.[65,71] This is the basis of the current product labeling dose of tadalafil 5 mg daily for BPH. The most common adverse effects observed are headache, flushing, gastroesophageal reflux, sinusitis, and back pain, which are generally reversible and do not require discontinuation of therapy. When tadalafil was combined with an α-adrenergic antagonist, patients experienced significant improvements in LUTS, increased urinary flow rates, and decreased PVR volume.[70]

A few other studies have included sildenafil 50 mg or 100 mg daily or vardenafil 10 mg twice a day.[65,72] Most of the clinical trials have evaluated tadalafil for treatment of BPH. This is probably because BPH is viewed as a chronic disease and tadalafil has been FDA-approved for once-daily dosing, and has the longest half-life and duration of action among the phosphodiesterase inhibitors. The recommended tadalafil dose is 5 mg daily.

Based on the limited benefit, cost, and potential adverse effects of tadalafil, it would be prudent to reserve its use for patients with both BPH and erectile dysfunction.[69,70,73] If used in combination with an α-adrenergic antagonist, precautions should be taken to minimize hypotension, specifically, stabilize the patient's blood pressure on the α-adrenergic antagonist before adding tadalafil.

Anticholinergic Agents

9 Treatment with an α_1-adrenergic antagonist, 5α-reductase inhibitor, or surgery may improve urinary flow rate and bladder emptying; however, the patient may still complain of irritative voiding symptoms (e.g., urinary frequency, urgency, and nocturia), which mimic those of overactive bladder syndrome. A variety of anticholinergic agents, including oxybutynin and tolterodine, have been added to α-adrenergic antagonist regimens to relieve these symptoms.[74–76]

By blocking muscarinic receptors in the detrusor muscle, anticholinergic agents can reduce uninhibited detrusor contractions, a sequela of prolonged bladder outlet obstruction from BPH. Thus, they can reduce urinary frequency and urgency. Because older patients are sensitive to the drugs' CNS adverse effects and dry mouth, patients should be started on the lowest effective dose and then slowly titrated up.[74–76]

Uroselective anticholinergic agents, which preferentially inhibit M_3 receptors (e.g., darifenacin or solifenacin), or transdermal (oxybutynin) or extended-release formulations of anticholinergic agents (e.g., tolterodine) are recommended for patients who poorly tolerate systemic anticholinergic adverse effects. In the presence of BPH, anticholinergic agents can rarely cause acute urinary retention. Therefore, before prescribing an anticholinergic agent, a PVR urine volume should be measured and should be less than 250 mL.[13]

Surgical Intervention

10 The gold standard for treatment of patients with complications of BPH is prostatectomy performed either transurethrally or as an open surgical procedure.[13,18] Surgical intervention is also used for patients with moderate to severe symptoms, who are not responsive to drug therapy, who are noncompliant with drug therapy, or who prefer surgical intervention. Surgical intervention is always indicated for patients with complications of BPH, including acute urinary retention not responsive to drug treatment, chronic urinary retention associated with decreased renal function or overflow urinary incontinence, urolithiasis, or recurrent hematuria.[77] Surgical removal of the prostate offers the highest rate of symptom improvement, but it also has the highest complication rate.

With transurethral resection of the prostate (TURP), an endoscopic resectoscope inserted through the urethra is used to remove the inside core of the prostate. This enlarges the urethral opening at the bladder neck. Often performed as outpatient surgery, this procedure produces on average a peak urinary flow rate increase of 125% and improvement of voiding symptoms by almost 90% in approximately 90% of patients.[18] A common complication of TURP is retrograde ejaculation, occurring in up to 75% of patients. Significant bleeding, urinary incontinence, and erectile dysfunction occur in smaller, but significant numbers of patients (2% to 15%).[78] Approximately 2% to 10% and 12% to 15% of patients require second surgeries within 5 and 8 years, respectively.[78]

Alternatively, an open surgical procedure (open prostatectomy) can be performed retropubically or suprapubically. This necessitates hospitalization for at least a few days, anesthesia, and a longer recuperation time. Adverse effects of open prostatectomy include bleeding, urinary and soft-tissue infection, retrograde ejaculation in 77% of patients, erectile dysfunction in 16% to 33% of patients, and urinary incontinence in 2% of patients. The reoperation rate is 3% to 5% at 10 years.[13]

Transurethral incision of the prostate (TUIP) is an alternative surgical procedure for patients with moderate to severe voiding symptoms who have an enlarged prostate gland less than 30 g in size. In the short term TUIP is as effective as TURP but requires less operation time, causes less blood loss, and produces fewer adverse effects.[13] TUIP involves using an endoscopic resectoscope to make two or three incisions at the bladder neck to widen the opening. In limited long-term studies, the reoperation rate for TUIP is slightly higher than with TURP.

Minimally invasive surgical procedures are highly desirable by patients. The procedures are short (lasting minutes), have a lower potential to produce adverse effects, are less expensive than continuous drug therapy regimens lasting years, and they may be particularly useful in debilitated patients who are poor surgical candidates. The ideal candidates have moderate to severe voiding symptoms with smaller sized prostate glands. These procedures typically use heat energy from microwaves, water, or laser to destroy prostate tissue.[13] Commonly used procedures include transurethral needle ablation of the prostate and transurethral microwave thermotherapy of the prostate.[79,80] A disadvantage of all minimally invasive surgical procedures is the high percentage of patients who may develop acute urinary retention in the immediate postoperative period. In addition, patients who undergo minimally invasive procedures generally experience smaller improvements in voiding symptoms and urinary flow rates, and are more likely to require reoperation after an initial improvement in symptoms than patients who undergo TURP or open prostatectomy.[81,82]

Phytotherapy

Although phytotherapy is widely used in Europe for the management of BPH, the published data on herbal agents are largely inconclusive and conflicting. Studies often lack placebo controls, which are essential for assessing treatments of BPH because spontaneous regression of symptoms can occur. Furthermore, because these agents are marketed under the Dietary Supplements Health and Education Act, their efficacy, safety, and quality are not regulated by the FDA. For these reasons, herbal products—including saw palmetto berry (*Serenoa repens*), stinging nettle (*Urtica dioica*), South African star grass (*Hypoxis rooperi*), pumpkin seed (*Cucurbita pepo*), and African plum (*Pygeum africanum*)—are not recommended for treatment of BPH.[13,83] An excellent review on phytotherapy for BPH has been published.[84]

EVALUATION OF THERAPEUTIC OUTCOMES

The primary therapeutic outcome of BPH therapy is improvement of voiding symptoms with minimal treatment-related adverse effects. As a disease for which therapy is directed at the voiding symptoms that the patient finds most bothersome, assessment of outcomes depends on the patient's perceptions of the effectiveness of therapy. Use of a validated, standardized instrument, such as the AUA Symptom Score, for assessing patient's voiding symptoms is important in this process.[13]

For patients being considered for surgical treatment, objective measures of bladder emptying are useful and include the urinary flow rate and PVR urine volume (see Diagnostic Evaluation above).

Because this patient population is at high risk for prostate cancer, PSA should be measured and a digital rectal examination performed annually if the patient has a life expectancy of at least 10 years. For patients taking 5α-reductase inhibitors, a second PSA taken after 6 months of treatment should be compared with baseline measurements. If the patient is suspected of having developed renal impairment as a consequence of long-standing bladder outlet obstruction, then BUN and serum creatinine should be evaluated at regular intervals.

SUMMARY

A ubiquitous disease of aging men, symptomatic BPH requires medical attention to preserve the patient's quality of life and to prevent disease complications, many of which can be life threatening in this patient population. In men who have no or mildly bothersome symptoms, watchful waiting and behavior modification are the best treatment approach, as BPH remains stable or even regresses in approximately half of these men.

For patients with voiding symptoms that are moderate to severely bothersome, pharmacotherapy is indicated. An α_1-adrenergic antagonist is the agent of first choice. Second-generation agents include terazosin, doxazosin, and alfuzosin, and third-generation agents include tamsulosin and silodosin. Immediate-release formulations of terazosin and doxazosin cause more cardiovascular adverse effects than do extended-release formulations (e.g., doxazosin or alfuzosin), or uroselective α_{1A}–adrenergic agents (e.g., tamsulosin or silodosin). 5α-Reductase inhibitors are preferred drug treatment for patients with enlarged prostates who poorly tolerate the hypotensive adverse effects of α_1-adrenergic antagonists. However, 5α-reductase inhibitors have a slow onset of action. For patients who do not respond to monotherapy, combination drug therapy could be attempted. Such regimens have been found to be most effective for patients with enlarged prostates greater than 40 g. Alternatively, surgery is an option.

For patients with both moderate-severe BPH and erectile dysfunction, a phosphodiesterase inhibitor alone or combined with an α-adrenergic antagonist may be prescribed. For patients with moderate to severe BPH with a predominance of irritative voiding symptoms, an anticholinergic agent may be added to an existing drug treatment regimen for BPH provided that the patient has a PVR urine volume less than 250 mL.

For patients who have complications of BPH, surgery is required. Although it has more adverse complications than does pharmacotherapy or watchful waiting, TURP is considered the gold standard.

ABBREVIATIONS

AUA	American Urological Association
BPH	benign prostatic hyperplasia
BUN	blood urea nitrogen
COMBAT	Combination of Avodart and Tamsulosin (Study)
CYP	cytochrome P-450
DHT	dihydrotestosterone
IPSS	International Prostate Symptom Score
LUTS	lower urinary tract symptoms
MTOPS	Multiple Treatment of Prostate Symptoms (Study)
PSA	prostate-specific antigen
PVR	postvoid residual (pertains to urine volume)
TURP	transurethral resection of the prostate
TUIP	transurethral incision of the prostate

REFERENCES

1. Glynn RJ, Campion EW, Bouchard GR, Silbert JE. The development of benign prostatic hyperplasia among volunteers in the normative aging study. Am J Epidemiol 1985;131:79–90.
2. Thorpe A, Neal D. Benign prostatic hyperplasia. Lancet 2003;361:1359–1367.
3. Roehrborn CG. Pathology of benign prostatic hyperplasia. Int J Imp Res 2008;20:S11–S18.
4. St. Sauver JL, Jacobson DJ, Girman CJ, et al. Tracking of longitudinal changes in measures of benign prostatic hyperplasia in a population based cohort. J Urol 2006;175:1918–1922.
5. Selius BA, Subedi R. Urinary retention in adults: Diagnosis and initial management. Am Fam Physician 2008;77:643–650.
6. Wuerstle MC, Van Den Eede SK, Poon KT, et al. for the Urologic Diseases in American Project. Contribution of common medications to lower urinary tract symptoms in men. Arch Intern Med 2011;171:1680–1682.
7. McConnell JD, Roehrborn CG, Bautista OM, et al. The long term effect of doxazosin, finasteride, and combination therapy on the clinical progression of benign prostatic hyperplasia. N Engl J Med 2003;349:2387–2398.
8. Marks LS, Roehrborn CG, Andriole GL. Prevention of benign prostatic hyperplasia disease. J Urol 2006;176:1299–1306.
9. Patel AK, Chapple CR. Benign prostatic hyperplasia: Treatment in primary care. BMJ 2006;333:535–539.
10. Roehrborn CG. Male lower urinary tract symptoms (LUTS) and benign prostatic hyperplasia (BPH). Med Clin North Am 2011;95:87–100.
11. Marks LS. Use of 5-α reductase inhibitors to prevent benign prostatic hyperplasia disease. Curr Urol Rep 2006;4: 293–303.
12. Crawford ED. Management of lower urinary tract symptoms suggestive of benign prostatic hyperplasia: The central role of the patient risk profile. BJU Int 2005;95(Suppl 4):1–5.
13. McVary KT, Roehrborn CG, Avins AL, et al. Update on AUA guideline on the management of benign prostatic hyperplasia. J Urol 2011;185:1767–803.
14. Wilt TJ, Dow JN. Benign prostatic hyperplasia. Part 1—Diagnosis. BMJ 2009:336:146–149.

15. Herout R, Farr A, Sevcenco S, et al. New findings in benign prostatic hyperplasia and incontinence: Highlights from the 26th Annual Congress of the European Association of Urology, March 18–22, 2011, Vienna, Austria. Rev Urol 2011;13:112–117.
16. Nickel JC, Herschorn S, Corcos J, et al. Canadian guidelines for the management of benign prostatic hyperplasia. Can J Urol 2005;12:2677–2683.
17. Parsons JK. Lifestyle factors, benign prostatic hyperplasia, and lower urinary tract symptoms. Curr Opin Urol 2011;21:1–4.
18. Wasson JH, Reda DJ, Bruskewitz RC, et al. for the Veterans Affairs Cooperative Study Group on Transurethral Resection of the Prostate. A comparison of transurethral surgery with watchful waiting for moderate symptoms of benign prostatic hyperplasia. N Engl J Med 1995;332:75–79.
19. Sarma AV, Wei JT. Benign prostatic hyperplasia and lower urinary tract symptoms. N Engl J Med 2012;367:248–257.
20. Auffenberg GB, Helfand BT, McVary KT. Established medical therapy for benign prostatic hyperplasia. Urol Clin N Am 2009;36:443–459.
21. Roehrborn CG. Efficacy of α-adrenergic receptor blockers in the treatment of male lower urinary tract symptoms. Rev Urol 2009;11(Suppl 1):S1–S8.
22. Nickel JC, Sander S, Moon TD. A meta-analysis of the vascular-related safety profile and efficacy of alpha-adrenergic blockers for symptoms related to benign prostatic hyperplasia. Int J Clin Pract 2008;62:1547–1559.
23. MacDonald R, Wilt TJ. Alfuzosin for treatment of lower urinary tract symptoms compatible with benign prostatic hyperplasia: A systematic review of efficacy and adverse effects. Urology 2005;66:780–788.
24. Goldsmith DR, Plosker GL. Doxazosin gastrointestinal therapeutic system. Drugs 2006;65:2037–2047.
25. ALLHAT Collaborative Research Group. Major cardiovascular events in hypertensive patients randomized to doxazosin vs chlorthalidone: The Antihypertensive and Lipid-Lowering Treatment to Prevent Heart Attack Trial (ALLHAT) [erratum appear in JAMA 2002;288:2976]. JAMA 2000;283:1967–1975.
26. U.S. Department of Health and Human Services, National Institutes of Health, National Heart, Lung, and Blood Institute. 7th Report of the Joint National Committee on Prevention, Detection, Evaluation, and Treatment of High Blood Pressure. 2004, *http://www.nhlbi.nih.gov/guidelines/hypertensionb/jnc7full.pdf*.
27. White WB, Moon T. Treatment of benign prostatic hyperplasia in hypertensive men. J Clin Hypertens 2005;7:212–217.
28. Elhilali MM. Alfuzosin: An α_1 receptor blocker for the treatment of lower urinary tract symptoms associated with benign prostatic hyperplasia. Expert Opin Pharmacother 2006;7:583–596.
29. Mottet N, Bressolle F, Delmas V, et al. Prostatic tissue distribution of alfuzosin in patients with benign prostatic hyperplasia following repeated oral administration. Eur Urol 2003;44:101–105.
30. Rossi M, Roumeguere T. Silodosin in the treatment of benign prostatic hyperplasia. Drug Des Devel Ther 2010;4:291–297.
31. Roehrborn CG for the ALFUS Study Group. Efficacy and safety of once daily alfuzosin in the treatment of lower urinary tract symptoms and clinical benign prostatic hyperplasia: A randomized, placebo-controlled trial. Urology 2001;58:953–959.
32. Lepor H, Kazzazi A, Djavan B. α-Blockers for benign prostatic hyperplasia: The new era. Curr Opin Urol 2012;22:7–15.
33. Curran MP. Silodosin. Drugs 2011;71:897–907.
34. Lepor H, Hill LA. Silodosin for the treatment of benign prostatic hyperplasia: Pharmacology and cardiovascular tolerability. Pharmacotherapy 2010:30:1303–1312.
35. Chapple CR, Baert L, Thind P, et al. Tamsulosin 0.4 mg once daily: Tolerability in older and young patients with lower urinary tract symptoms suggestive of benign prostatic obstruction. The Europ Tamsulosin Study Group. Eur Urol 1997;32:462–470.
36. Lowe FC. Coadministration of tamsulosin and three antihypertensive agents in patients with benign prostatic hyperplasia: Pharmacodynamic effect. Clin Ther 1997;19: 730–742.
37. De Mey C. Cardiovascular effects of alpha blockers used for the treatment of symptomatic BPH. Impact on safety and well being. Eur Urol 1998;34(Suppl 2):18–28.
38. Djavan B, Margreiter M, Dianat SS. An algorithm for medical management in male lower urinary tract symptoms. Curr Opin Urol 2011;21:5–12.
39. Narayan P, Evans CP, Moon T. Long-term safety and efficacy of tamsulosin for the treatment of lower urinary tract symptoms associated with benign prostatic hyperplasia. J Urol 2003;170:498–502.
40. Dutkiewicz S. Long term treatment with doxazosin in men with benign prostatic hyperplasia: 10 year follow-up. Int Urol Nephrol 2004;36:169–173.
41. Michel MC. The forefront for novel therapeutic agents based on the pathophysiology of lower urinary tract dysfunction: alpha-blockers in the treatment of male voiding dysfunction—how do they work and why do they differ in tolerability? J Pharmacol Sci 2010;112(2):151–157. Epub 2010 Feb 4. Review. PubMed PMID: 20134112.
42. Kaplan SA, Neutel J. Vasodilatory factors in treatment of older men with symptomatic benign prostatic hyperplasia. Urology 2006;67:225–231.
43. Hartung R, Matzkin H, Alcarez A, et al. Age, comorbidity and hypertensive co-medication do not affect cardiovascular tolerability of 10 mg alfuzosin once daily. J Urol 2006;175: 624–628.
44. Michel MC, Chapple CR. Comparison of the cardiovascular effects of tamsulosin oral controlled absorption system (OCAS) and alfuzosin prolonged release (XL). Eur Urol 2006;49:501–508.
45. Hellstrom WJG, Sikka SC. Effects of acute treatment with tamsulosin versus alfuzosin on ejaculatory function in normal volunteers. J Urol 2006;176:1529–1533.
46. Friedman AH. Tamsulosin and the intraoperative floppy iris syndrome. JAMA 2009;301:2044–2045.
47. Bell CM, Hatch WV, Fischer HD, et al. Association between tamsulosin and serious ophthalmic adverse events in older men following cataract surgery. JAMA 2009;301:1991–1996.
48. Yaycioglu O, Altan-Yaycioglu RA. Intraoperative floppy iris syndrome: Facts for the urologist. Urology 2010;76:272–276.
49. Nieminen T, Tammela TLJ, Koobi T, Kahonen M. The effects of tamsulosin and sildenafil in separate and combined regimens on detailed hemodynamics in patients with benign prostatic hyperplasia. J Urol 2006;175:2551–2556.
50. Goldfischer E, Kowalczyk JJ, Clark WR, et al. Hemodynamic effects of once-daily tadalafil in men with signs and symptoms of benign prostatic hyperplasia on concomitant α_1-adrenergic antagonist therapy: Results of a multicenter randomized, double-blind, placebo-controlled trial. Urology 2012;79:875–882.
51. Anonymous. Dutasteride (Avodart) for benign prostatic hyperplasia. Med Lett Drugs Ther 2002;44:109–110.
52. Nickel JC, Gilling P, Tammela TL, et al. Comparison of dutasteride and finasteride for treating benign prostatic

hyperplasia: The Enlarged Prostate International Comparator Study (EPICS). BJU Int 2011;108:388–394.

53. Roehrborn CG, Nickel JC, Andriole GL, et al. Dutasteride improves outcomes of benign prostatic hyperplasia when evaluated for prostate cancer risk reduction: Secondary analysis of the Reduction by Dutasteride of Prostate Cancer Events (REDUCE) trial. Urology 2011;78:641–647.
54. Roehrborn CG, Bruskewitz R, Nickel JC, et al. Sustained decrease in incidence of acute urinary retention and surgery with finasteride for 6 years in men with benign prostatic hyperplasia. J Urol 2004;171:1194–1198.
55. Kramer BS, Hagerty KL, Justman S, et al. Use of 5α-reductase inhibitors for prostate cancer chemoprevention. American Society of Clinical Oncology/American Cancer Society 2008 Clinical Practice Guideline. J Urol 2009;181:1642–1657.
56. Andriole GL, Bostwick DG, Brawley OW, et al. for the REDUCE Study Group. Effect of dutasteride on the risk of prostate cancer. N Engl J Med 2010;362:1192–1202.
57. Rosen R, O'Leary M, Altwein J, et al. Ejaculatory disorders are frequent and bothersome in aging males with LUTS. A worldwide survey (MSAM-7) [abstract]. J Urol 2003;169(Suppl 1):365.
58. Park KH, Kim SW, Kim KD, et al. Effects of androgens on the expression of nitric oxide synthase mRNA in rat corpus cavernosum. BJU Int 1999;83:327–333.
59. Stavros G, Oelke M. Current status of 5α-reductase inhibitors in the management of lower urinary tract symptoms and BPH. World J Urol 2010;28:9–15.
60. McVary KT. A review of combination therapy in patients with benign prostatic hyperplasia. Clin Ther 2007;29:387–398.
61. Roehrborn CG, Siami P, Barkin J, et al. for CombAT Study Group. The effects of combination therapy with dutasteride and tamsulosinon clinical outcomes in men with symptomatic benign prostatic hyperplasia: 4 year results from the COMBAT study. Eur Urol 2010;57:123–131.
62. Haillot O, Fraga Am, Maciukiewicz P, et al. The effects of combination therapy with dutasteride plus tamsulosin on clinical outcomes in men with symptomatic BPH: 4 year post hoc analysis of European men in the CombAT study. Prostate Cancer Prostatic Dis 2011;14:302–306.
63. Sciarra A. Lower urinary tract symptoms (LUTS) and sexual dysfunction (SD): New targets for new combination therapies? Eur Urol 2007;51:1485–1487.
64. Mirone V, Sessa A, Giuliano F, et al. Current benign prostatic hyperplasia treatment: Impact on sexual function and management of related sexual adverse events. Int J Clin Pract 2011;65:1005–1013.
65. Laydner HK, Oliveira P, Oliveira RA, et al. Phosphodiesterase 5 inhibitors for lower urinary tract symptoms secondary to benign prostatic hyperplasia: A systematic review. BJU Int 2010;107:1104–1109.
66. Porst H, Dim ED, Casabe AR, et al. for the LVHJ study team. Efficacy and safety of tadalafil once daily in the treatment of men with lower urinary tract symptoms suggestive of benign prostatic hyperplasia: Results of an international randomized, double-blind, placebo-controlled trial. Eur Urol 2011;60:1105–1113.
67. Tinel H, Stelte-Ludwig B, Hutter J, et al. Preclinical evidence for the use of phosphodiesterase-5 inhibitors for treating benign prostatic hyperplasia and lower urinary tract symptoms. BJU Int 2006;98:1259–1263.
68. Oelke M, Giuliano F, Mirone V, et al. Monotherapy with tadalafil or tamsulosin similarly improved lower urinary tract symptoms suggestive of benign prostatic hyperplasia in an international, randomized, parallel, placebo-controlled clinical trial. Eur Urol 2012;61:917–925.
69. Liu L, Zheng S, Han P, Wei Q. Phosphodiesterase-5 inhibitors for lower urinary tract symptoms secondary to benign prostatic hyperplasia: A systematic review and meta-analysis. Urology 2011;77:123–130.
70. Gacci M, Corona G, Salvi M, et al. A systematic review and meta-analysis on the use of phosphodiesterase 5 inhibitors alone or in combination with α-blockers for lower urinary tract symptoms due to benign prostatic hyperplasia. Eur Urol 2012;61:994–1003.
71. Egerdie RB, Auerbach S, Roehrborn CG, et al. Tadalafil 2.5 mg or 5 mg administered once daily for 12 weeks in men with both erectile dysfunction and signs and symptoms of benign prostatic hyperplasia: Results of a randomized, placebo-controlled, double-blind study. J Sex Med 2012;9:271–281.
72. Kaplan SA, Gonzalez RR, Te AE. Combination of alfuzosin and sildenafil is superior to monotherapy in treating lower urinary tract symptoms and erectile dysfunction. Eur Urol 2007;51:1717–1723.
73. Anonymous. Tadalafil (Cialis) for signs and symptoms of benign prostatic hyperplasia. Med Lett Drugs Ther 2011;53:89–90.
74. Kaplan SA, Roehrborn CG, Abrams P, et al. Antimuscarinics for treatment of storage lower urinary tract symptoms in men: A systematic review. Int J Clin Pract 2011;65:487–507.
75. Rover ES, Kreder K, Sussman DO, et al. Effect of tolterodine extended release with or without tamsulosin on measures of urgency and patient reported outcomes in men with lower urinary tract symptoms. J Urol 2008;180:1034–1041.
76. Chung DE, Te AE, Staskin DR, Kaplan SA. Efficacy and safety of tolterodine extended release and dutasteride in male overactive bladder patients with prostates >30 grams. Urology 2010;75:1144–1148.
77. Djavan B, Eckersberger E, Finkelstein J, et al. Benign prostatic hyperplasia: Current clinical practice. Prim Care Clin Office Pract 2010;37:583–597.
78. Rassweiler J, Teber D, Kuntz R, Hofmann R. Complications of transurethral resection of the prostate (TURP): Incidence, management, and prevention. Eur Urol 2006;50:969–980.
79. Malaeb BS, Yu X, McBean AM, Elliott SP. National trends in surgical therapy for benign prostatic hyperplasia in the United States (2000–2008). Urology 2012;79:1111–1117.
80. Lourenco T, Pickard R, Vale L, et al. Minimally invasive treatments for benign prostatic enlargement: Systematic review of randomized controlled trials. Br Med J 2009;2008:337. doi:10.1136/bmj.a1662.
81. Djavan B, Eckersberger E, Handl MJ, et al. Durability and retreatment rates of minimal invasive treatments of benign prostatic hyperplasia: A cross-analysis of the literature. Can J Urol 2010;17:5249–5254.
82. Lourenco T, Armstrong N, N'Dow J, et al. Systematic review and economic modeling of effectiveness and cost utility of surgical treatments for men with benign prostatic enlargement. Health Tech Assessment 2008;12:1–167.
83. MacDonald R, Tacklind JW, Rutks I, Wilt TJ. Serenoa Repens monotherapy for benign prostatic hyperplasia (BPH): An updated Cochrane systematic review. BJU Int 2012;109(12):1756–1761.
84. Kim TH, Lim HJ, Kim MS, Lee MS. Dietary supplements for benign prostatic hyperplasia: An overview of systematic reviews. Maturitas 2012;73(3):180–185.

68

Urinary Incontinence

Eric S. Rovner, Jean Wyman, and Sum Lam

KEY CONCEPTS

1. In evaluating urinary incontinence (UI), drug-induced or drug-aggravated etiologies must be ruled out.
2. Accurate diagnosis and classification of UI type are critical to the selection of appropriate pharmacotherapy.
3. Goals of treatment for UI are reduction of symptoms, minimization of adverse effects, and improvement in quality of life.
4. Nonpharmacologic, nonsurgical treatment is the first-line therapy for several types of UI, and should be continued even when drug therapy is initiated.
5. Anticholinergic/antimuscarinic agents are first-line therapies for urge incontinence. Choice of agent should be based on patient characteristics (e.g., age, comorbidities, concurrent medications, and ability to adhere to the prescribed regimen).
6. Mirabegron, a β_3-adrenergic agonist, can be considered as an alternative in patients who failed to achieve optimal efficacy or cannot tolerate adverse effects of anticholinergics.
7. Duloxetine (approved in Europe only), α-adrenergic receptor agonists, and topical (vaginal) estrogens (alone or together) are the drugs of choice for urethral underactivity (stress incontinence).
8. Assessment of patient outcomes should include efficacy, adverse effects, adherence, and quality of life.
9. Management of UI should target individualized goals, which may change over time. If therapeutic goals are not achieved with a given agent at optimal dosage for an adequate duration of trial, consider switching to an alternative agent.

Urinary incontinence (UI) is defined as involuntary leakage of urine.[1] It is frequently accompanied by other bothersome lower urinary tract symptoms, such as urgency, increased daytime frequency, and nocturia. It is a common yet underdetected and underreported health problem that can significantly affect quality of life. Patients with UI may have depression as a result of the perceived lack of self-control, loss of independence, and lack of self-esteem, and they often curtail their activities for fear of an "accident." UI may also have serious medical and economic ramifications for untreated or undertreated patients, including perineal dermatitis, worsening of pressure ulcers, urinary tract infections, and falls.

This chapter highlights the epidemiology, etiology, pathophysiology, and treatment of stress, urge, mixed, and overflow UI in men and women.

EPIDEMIOLOGY

UI is highly prevalent, and the impact of this condition is substantial, crossing all racial, ethnic, and geographic boundaries. In addition, associated lower urinary tract symptoms such as overactive bladder (OAB) are also quite debilitating.[2] Several studies have objectively shown that UI is associated with reduced levels of social and personal activities, increased psychological distress, and overall decreased quality of life as measured by numerous indices.[3] The condition can affect people of all age groups, but the peak incidence of UI, at least in women, appears to occur around the age of menopause, with a slight decrease in the age group 55 to 60 years, and then a steadily increasing prevalence after age 65 years.

Determining the true prevalence of UI is difficult because of problems with definition, reporting bias, and other methodologic issues.[4] The Medical, Epidemiologic, and Social Aspects of Aging survey found that the prevalence of UI in noninstitutionalized women 60 years of age and older was approximately 38%. Almost one third of those surveyed noted urine loss at least once weekly, and 16% noted UI daily. A publication from a National Institutes of Health working group conference estimated the median level of UI prevalence to be approximately 20% to 30% during young adult life, with a broad peak around middle age (30% to 40% prevalence) and an increase in the elderly (30% to 50% prevalence).[5]

In the United States, chronic UI is one of the most common reasons cited for institutionalization of the elderly, and the condition is frequently encountered in the nursing home setting. Little is known about the basic differences in clinical and epidemiologic characteristics of incontinence across racial or ethnic groups. Some studies report a higher incidence of UI overall in white populations as compared with African Americans, but differences in access to healthcare as well as cultural attitudes and mores may contribute to these differences.[6,7]

Consistent across all studies of unselected, noninstitutionalized populations is that UI is at least half as common in men as in women.[8] Overall, the prevalence of UI in men has been estimated to be approximately 9%.[10] Unlike in women, the prevalence of UI in men increases steadily with age across most studies, with the highest prevalence recorded in the oldest patient cohorts.[9]

ETIOLOGY AND PATHOPHYSIOLOGY

Anatomy

The lower urinary tract consists of the bladder, urethra, urinary or urethral sphincter, and surrounding musculofascial structures, including connective tissue, nerves, and blood vessels. The urinary bladder is a hollow organ composed of smooth muscle and connective tissue located deep in the bony pelvis in men and women. The urethra is a hollow tube that acts as a conduit for urine flow out of the bladder. An epithelial cell layer termed the urothelium, which is in constant contact with urine, lines the interior surface of both the bladder and the urethra. Previously considered inert and inactive, the urothelium may play an active role in the pathophysiology of many lower urinary tract disorders, including interstitial cystitis and UI[10] and may be a targeted location for future pharmacologic therapeutic interventions for some types of lower urinary tract dysfunction.[11] The urinary or urethral sphincter is a combination of smooth and striated muscle within and surrounding the proximal portion of the urethra adjacent to the bladder. In the male, the prostate gland lies just beyond the bladder outlet and is intimately associated with the urethral sphincter. Its location accounts for both the favorable effects of pharmacological manipulation on male lower symptoms as well as the risk of UI in males following some types of prostate surgery.

To understand the principles of pharmacotherapy for UI, an understanding of the neuroanatomy and neurophysiology of the bladder and urethra is needed. The primary motor (efferent) input to the detrusor muscle of the bladder is parasympathetic and travels along the pelvic nerves emanating from spinal cord segments S2 to S4. Acetylcholine appears to be the primary neurotransmitter at the neuromuscular junction in the human lower urinary tract. Both volitional and involuntary detrusor contractions are mediated by activation of postsynaptic muscarinic receptors by acetylcholine. Of the five known subtypes of muscarinic receptors, the majority of bladder smooth muscle cholinergic receptors are of the M_2 variety. In humans, the ratio of M_2/M_3 receptor numbers is approximately 3:1. However, M_3 receptors are the subtype responsible for both emptying contractions of normal micturition as well as involuntary bladder contractions that may result in UI.[10] Thus, most pharmacologic antimuscarinic therapy is primarily anti-M_3 based.

Urinary Continence

To prevent incontinence during the bladder filling and storage phase of the micturition cycle, the urethra, or more accurately the urethral sphincter, must maintain adequate closure in order to resist the flow of urine from the bladder at all times until voluntary voiding is initiated. Urethral closure or resistance to flow is maintained to a large degree by the proximal (under involuntary control) and distal (under both voluntary and involuntary control) urinary sphincters. Variable contributions to urethral closure may also come from the urethral mucosa, submucosal spongy tissue, and the overall length of the urethra. During bladder filling and urinary storage, the bladder accommodates to increasing volumes of urine flowing in from the upper urinary tract without a significant increase in bladder (intravesical) pressure. The maintenance of a low intravesical pressure despite increasing volumes of urine is a unique property of the bladder and is termed *compliance*. In addition, bladder or detrusor smooth muscle activity is normally suppressed during the filling phase by centrally mediated neural reflexes. Normal bladder emptying occurs with opening of the urethral sphincters concomitant with a volitional bladder contraction. Bladder contraction occurs in a coordinated fashion, resulting in a rise in intravesical pressure. The rise in intravesical pressure is ideally of adequate magnitude and duration to empty the bladder to completion. Opening and funneling of the bladder outlet results in urine flow into the urethra until the bladder is emptied to near completion.

The bladder and urethra normally operate in unison during the bladder filling and storage phase, as well as the bladder emptying phase of the micturition cycle. The smooth and striated muscles of the bladder and urethra are organized during the micturition cycle by a number of reflexes coordinated at the pontine micturition center in the midbrain. Disturbances in the neural regulation of micturition at any level (brain, spinal cord, or pelvic nerves) often lead to characteristic changes in lower urinary tract function that may result in UI.[12,13]

Mechanisms of Urinary Incontinence

Simply stated, UI may occur as a result of abnormalities of only the urethra (including the bladder outlet and urinary sphincter) or only the bladder or as a combination of abnormalities in both. Abnormalities may result in either overfunction or underfunction of the bladder and/or urethra, with resulting development of UI. Although this simple classification scheme excludes extremely rare causes of UI such as congenital ectopic ureters and urinary fistulas, it is useful for gaining a working understanding of the condition and understanding the basis for therapeutic intervention including pharmacotherapy of various lower urinary tract disorders.

Urethral Underactivity (Stress Urinary Incontinence) This type of incontinence is characterized by brief bursts of UI concomitant with exertional activities such as exercise, running, lifting, coughing, and sneezing. The pathophysiology of *stress urinary incontinence* (SUI) is related to decreased or inadequate urethral closure forces. In individuals with SUI, the muscular tissues surrounding the urethra that form the urethral sphincter are compromised and thus not able to resist the expulsive forces resulting from transient increases in intraabdominal pressure during physical activity. Such forces are transmitted to the bladder (an intraabdominal organ), compressing it to such an extent as to cause the egress of urine through the urethra. SUI is characterized by episodic, usually low volume urinary leakage but is clearly proportional to the amount of physical exertion or other increases in abdominal pressure such as that related to coughing and sneezing.

Risk factors for SUI in the female include pregnancy, childbirth, menopause, cognitive impairment, obesity, and aging.[14,15] In males, SUI is most commonly the result of prior lower urinary tract surgery and injury to the sphincter mechanism within and external to the urethra. Radical prostatectomy for treatment of adenocarcinoma of the prostate and transurethral resection of the prostate (TURP) are probably the most common proximate causes of SUI in the male. Notably, compared with its prevalence in females, SUI in males is actually quite rare.

SUI may be caused or aggravated by some pharmacologic agents such as α-antagonists and angiotensin-converting enzyme (ACE) inhibitors.[16] α-Antagonists may relax the smooth muscle at the level of the urethral sphincter, resulting in a weakened closure mechanism and the onset of SUI. An adverse effect of some ACE inhibitors is chronic cough, which can also aggravate existing SUI.

Bladder Overactivity (Urge Urinary Incontinence) Urge incontinence is defined as the leakage of urine associated with urgency, a compelling desire to void.[1] This is most often related to detrusor (bladder) overactivity due to involuntary bladder contractions. Bladder overactivity describes the condition in which the detrusor muscle contracts inappropriately during urinary storage that, in the neurologically normal individual, results in a sense of urinary urgency. The terms *overactive bladder* and *detrusor (bladder) overactivity* are distinct and should not be used interchangeably.

The International Continence Society defines OAB as a symptom syndrome characterized by urinary urgency, with frequency and nocturia, with/without associated UI in the absence of a known pathologic condition that may result in similar symptoms (e.g., urinary tract infection, bladder cancer).[1] *Frequency* is defined as micturition more than eight times per day. *Urgency* is described as a sudden compelling desire to urinate that is difficult to delay.[1] People suffering from OAB typically have to empty their bladder frequently, and, when they experience a sensation of urgency, they may leak urine if they are unable to reach the toilet quickly. Many patients have associated nocturia (>1 micturition per night) and/or nocturnal incontinence (enuresis). Patients with urge urinary incontinence (UUI) often experience high-volume urine leakage when it occurs. Although detrusor overactivity may be related to OAB, the former diagnosis requires urodynamic testing while the latter is symptomatically defined.

Most patients with OAB and UUI have no identifiable underlying etiology and thus are classified as "idiopathic." Patients with a relevant neurologic condition and with UI related to involuntary bladder contractions demonstrated on urodynamic testing are classified as having neurogenic detrusor overactivity. Clearly identifiable risk factors for UUI include normal aging, neurologic disease (including stroke, Parkinson's disease, multiple sclerosis, and spinal cord injury), and bladder outlet obstruction (e.g., due to benign prostatic hyperplasia [BPH] or prostate cancer).

The pathophysiology of OAB and UUI is not well understood but is likely related to either neurogenic or myogenic factors or combination of both.[17] A full discussion of these differences is complex and beyond the scope of this chapter. However, in practice, although the cause of UUI is difficult to define, the treatment is identical regardless of etiology and pathophysiology.

Some pharmacologic agents may cause or aggravate UUI. Diuretics will cause the rapid accumulation of urine in the bladder with resulting urinary urgency and frequency that can result in UUI. Alcohol will have similar effects. Anticholinesterase inhibitors may also produce urgency and frequency.

Urethral Overactivity and/or Bladder Underactivity (Overflow Incontinence) Overflow incontinence is urinary leakage resulting from an overfilled and distended bladder that is unable to empty. This type of UI occurs when the bladder is filled to capacity at all times but is unable to empty, causing urine to leak from a distended bladder past a normal or even overactive sphincter. Another term related to overflow incontinence is chronic urinary retention.

Overflow incontinence is the result of urethral overactivity, bladder underactivity, or a variable combination of both. Clinically and practically, the most common causes of urethral overactivity in men are anatomic urethral obstruction, including that due to BPH and prostate cancer. In women, urethral overactivity is rare but may result from cystocele formation (with resultant kinking or obstruction of the urethra) or surgical overcorrection following surgery for the repair of SUI (iatrogenic obstruction). In both men and women, overflow UI may be associated with systemic neurologic dysfunction or diseases, such as spinal cord injury or multiple sclerosis.

Bladder underactivity occurs as a result of the detrusor muscle of the bladder becoming progressively weakened and eventually losing the ability to voluntarily contract and expel urine during voiding. In the absence of adequate contractility, the bladder is unable to empty completely, and large volumes of residual urine are left after voiding. Both myogenic and neurogenic factors have been implicated in producing the impaired contractility seen in this condition. Clinically, overflow incontinence is most commonly seen in the setting of long-term chronic bladder outlet obstruction in men, such as that due to BPH or prostate cancer, diabetes mellitus, or denervation due to radical pelvic surgery, such as abdominopelvic resection or radical hysterectomy.

There are numerous pharmacologic agents that can result in urinary retention and overflow incontinence. Agents that increase urethral resistance or closure pressure include α-agonists and tricyclic antidepressants. Over-the-counter cold and cough remedies as well as diet pills may contain agents with α-adrenergic properties and/or antihistaminic properties that can result in voiding dysfunction and urinary retentions. Agents that can decrease bladder contractility include anticholinergics, tricyclic antidepressants, calcium channel blockers, narcotic analgesics, and antipsychotics.

Mixed Incontinence and Other Types of Urinary Incontinence Various types of UI may coexist in the same patient. The combination of bladder overactivity and urethral underactivity is termed *mixed incontinence*. The diagnosis is often difficult because of the confusing array of presenting symptoms. Bladder overactivity may also coexist with impaired bladder contractility. This occurs most commonly in the elderly and is termed *detrusor hyperactivity with impaired contractility*.[18]

Functional incontinence is not caused by bladder- or urethra-specific factors. Rather, in patients with conditions such as dementia or cognitive or mobility deficits, the UI is linked to the primary disease process more than any extrinsic or intrinsic deficit of the lower urinary tract. An example of functional incontinence occurs in the postoperative orthopedic surgery patient. Following extensive orthopedic reconstructions such as total hip arthroplasty, patients are often immobile secondary to pain or traction. Therefore, patients may be unable to access toileting facilities in a reasonable amount of time and may become incontinent as a result. Treatment of this type of UI may involve simple interventions such as placing a urinal or commode at the bedside that allows for uncomplicated access to toileting. Pharmacologically, functional incontinence can be induced by sedative-hypnotics, narcotic analgesics, and other medications with cognitive adverse effects.

Many localized or systemic illnesses may result in UI because of their effects on the lower urinary tract or the surrounding structures:

1. Dementia/delirium
2. Depression
3. Urinary tract infection (cystitis)
4. Postmenopausal atrophic urethritis or vaginitis
5. Diabetes mellitus
6. Neurologic disease (e.g., stroke, Parkinson's disease, multiple sclerosis, spinal cord injury)
7. Pelvic malignancy
8. Constipation
9. Congenital malformations of the urinary tract

(1) As noted above, many commonly used medications may precipitate or aggravate existing voiding dysfunction and UI (Table 68-1).[19]

TABLE 68-1 Medications That Influence Lower Urinary Tract Function

Medication	Effect
Diuretics, acetylcholinesterase inhibitors	Polyuria, frequency, urgency
α-Receptor antagonists	Urethral relaxation and stress urinary incontinence in women
α-Receptor agonists	Urethral constriction and urinary retention in men
Calcium channel blockers	Urinary retention
Narcotic analgesics	Urinary retention from impaired contractility
Sedative hypnotics	Functional incontinence caused by delirium, immobility
Antipsychotic agents	Anticholinergic effects and urinary retention
Anticholinergics	Urinary retention
Antidepressants, tricyclic	Anticholinergic effects, α-antagonist effects
Alcohol	Polyuria, frequency, urgency, sedation, delirium
ACEIs	Cough as a result of ACEIs may aggravate stress urinary incontinence by increasing intraabdominal pressure

ACEIs, angiotensin-converting enzyme inhibitors.

CLINICAL PRESENTATION Urinary Incontinence Related to Urethral Underactivity

General

- The patient usually notes UI during activities such as exercise, running, lifting, coughing, and sneezing. Occurs much more commonly in women (seen only in men with lower urinary tract surgery or injury compromising the sphincter)

Symptoms

- Urine leakage with physical activity (volume is proportional to activity level). No UI with physical inactivity, especially when supine (no nocturia). May develop urgency and frequency as a compensatory mechanism (or as a separate component of bladder overactivity)

Diagnostic Tests

- Observation of urethral meatus while patient coughs or strains

Generally, SUI is considered the most common type of UI and probably accounts for at least a portion of UI in more than half of all incontinent women. Some studies have found that mixed UI (SUI plus UUI) is the most common type of UI. However, the proportions of SUI, UUI, and mixed UI vary considerably with age group and gender of patients studied, study methodology, and a variety of other factors.

CLINICAL PRESENTATION

❷ UI may present in a number of ways, depending on the underlying pathophysiology. A complete medical and medication history, including an assessment of symptoms and a physical examination, is essential for correctly classifying the type of incontinence and thereby assuring appropriate therapy.

Urine Leakage

UI represents a spectrum of severity in terms of both volume of leakage and degree of bother to the patient. It is important to carefully consider the level of patient discomfort and bother when discussing urine leakage as each individual may or may not desire therapy. A careful and complete history during the patient interview is essential to accurately determine the precise nature of the problem. The onset, nature, timing, and volume of incontinence are recorded as is the use of pads. Use of absorbent products, such as panty liners, pads, or briefs, is an important point of discussion, but the clinician must keep in mind that use of these products varies among patients. The number and type of pads may not relate to the amount or type of incontinence, as their use is a function of personal preference and hygiene. A high number of absorbent pads may be used every day by a patient with severe, high-volume UI or, alternatively, by a fastidiously hygienic patient with low-volume leakage who simply changes pads often to prevent wetness or odor. Nevertheless, a large number of pads that are described by the patient as "soaked" is indicative of high-volume urine loss.

Regardless of the volume of urine loss, the desire to seek evaluation for UI in the majority of patients is most commonly elective and therapy is often contingent on the degree of bother to the individual patient. As with the use of absorbent products, patients differ with regard to the amount of urine loss they will tolerate before considering the condition bothersome enough to seek assistance. However, it is critically important that in some individuals new-onset UI may be the first manifestation of an undiagnosed illness, or may occur as a result of treatment or drug therapy of an unrelated condition. It is these individuals who mandate a full evaluation and treatment.

Symptoms

Under the best of circumstances, UI is difficult to categorize based on symptoms alone (Table 68-2).[20] In a study of patients who appeared to have SUI based on symptoms and patient history, urodynamics showed that only 72% of patients had SUI as the sole cause of incontinence.[21]

Patients with SUI characteristically complain of urinary leakage with physical activity. Volume of leakage is proportional to the level of activity. They will often leak urine during periods of exercise, coughing, sneezing, lifting, or even when rising from a seated to a standing position. Patients with pure SUI will not have leakage when physically inactive, especially when they are supine. Often they will have little or no UI at night, will not awaken to void during the night (nocturia), will not wet the bed, and often do not even wear absorbent products during the night. Urinary urgency and frequency may be associated with SUI, either as a separate component caused by bladder overactivity (mixed incontinence) or as a compensatory mechanism wherein the patient with SUI learns to toilet frequently to prevent large-volume urine loss during physical activity.

CLINICAL PRESENTATION Urinary Incontinence Related to Bladder Overactivity

General

- Can have bladder overactivity and UI without urgency if sensory input from the lower urinary tract is absent

Symptoms

- Urinary frequency (>8 micturitions per day), urgency with or without urge incontinence; nocturia (≥1 micturition per night) and enuresis may be present

Diagnostic Tests

- Urodynamic studies are the gold standard for diagnosis. Urinalysis and urine culture should be negative (rule out urinary tract infection as the cause of frequency)

CLINICAL PRESENTATION Overflow Incontinence (Chronic Urinary Retention)

General

- Important but rare type of UI in both men and women. Urethral overactivity is usually due to prostatic enlargement (males) or cystocele formation or surgical overcorrection following stress incontinence surgery in women

Symptoms

- Lower abdominal fullness, hesitancy, straining to void, decreased force of stream, interrupted stream, sense of incomplete bladder emptying. May have urinary frequency and urgency. Abdominal pain if acute urinary retention is present

Signs

- Increased postvoid residual urine volume

Diagnostic Tests

- Digital rectal examination or transrectal ultrasound to rule out prostatic enlargement. Renal function tests to rule out renal failure due to acute urinary retention

Typical symptoms of UUI and bladder overactivity include frequency, urgency, and high-volume incontinence. Nocturia and nocturnal incontinence are often present. Urine leakage is unpredictable, and the volume loss may be quite large. Patients often wear protection both day and night. Urinary frequency can be affected by a number of factors unrelated to bladder overactivity, including excessive fluid intake (polydipsia) and bladder hypersensitivity states such as interstitial cystitis and urinary tract infection. In some patients, bladder overactivity manifests as UI without awareness in the absence of a sense of urinary urgency or frequency. *Urinary urgency*, a sensation of impending micturition, requires intact sensory input from the lower urinary tract. In patients with spinal cord injury, sensory neuropathies, and other neurologic diseases, a diminished ability to perceive or process sensory input from the lower urinary tract may result in bladder overactivity and UI without urgency or urinary frequency. When bladder contraction occurs without warning and sensation is absent, the condition is referred to as *reflex incontinence*.

Patients with overflow incontinence may present with lower abdominal fullness as well as considerable obstructive urinary symptoms, including hesitancy, straining to void, decreased force of urinary stream, interrupted stream, and a vague sense of incomplete bladder emptying. These patients may also have a significant component of urinary frequency and urgency. In patients with acute urinary retention and overflow incontinence, lower abdominal pain may be present. Although these symptoms are not specific for overflow incontinence, they may warrant further investigation, including an assessment of postvoid residual urine volume.

TABLE 68-2 Differentiating Bladder Overactivity from Urethral Underactivity-Related UI

Symptoms	Bladder Overactivity (UUI)	Urethral Underactivity (SUI)
Urgency (strong, sudden desire to void)	Yes	Sometimes
Frequency with urgency	Yes	Rarely
Leaking during physical activity (e.g., coughing, sneezing, lifting)	No	Yes
Amount of urinary leakage with each episode of incontinence	Large if present	Usually small
Ability to reach the toilet in time following an urge to void	No or just barely	Yes
Nocturnal incontinence (presence of wet pads or undergarments in bed)	Yes	Rare
Nocturia (waking to pass urine at night)	Usually	Seldom

Signs

A presenting complaint of UI mandates a directed physical examination and a brief neurologic assessment. The workup ideally includes an abdominal examination to exclude a distended bladder, neurologic assessment of the perineum and lower extremities, pelvic examination in women (looking especially for evidence of prolapse or hormonal deficiency), and genital and prostate examination in men. Perineal skin maceration, erythema, breakdown, and ulceration may be indicative of chronic, severe UI. Patients with chronic incontinence may also manifest fungal infections of the skin of the perineum and upper thighs.

SUI can usually be objectively demonstrated by having the patient cough or strain during the examination and observing the urethral meatus for a sudden spurt of urine. In women, SUI may be associated with varying degrees of vaginal prolapse, including cystourethrocele (bladder and urethral prolapse).

In both men and women, digital rectal examination provides an opportunity to check ambient rectal tone and the integrity of the sacral reflex arc (e.g., anal wink) as well as assess the patient's ability to perform a voluntary pelvic floor muscle contraction (i.e., Kegel exercise), which may be an important factor in deciding on appropriate therapy. In men, a digital examination of the prostate assesses for the presence of prostate cancer, inflammation, and BPH.

A targeted neurologic examination includes assessment of reflexes, rectal tone, and sensory or motor deficits in the lower extremities, which might be indicative of systemic or localized neurologic disease. Neurologic diseases have the potential to affect bladder and sphincter function and thus may have significant implications in the incontinent patient.

Prior Medical or Surgical Illness

UI may present in the setting of concurrent, seemingly unrelated illnesses. New-onset UI may be the initial manifestation of systemic illnesses such as diabetes mellitus, metastatic malignancies, and neurologic diseases such as Parkinson's disease, brain tumors, and multiple sclerosis. CNS disease, or injury above the level of the pons, generally results in symptoms of bladder overactivity and UUI. Spinal cord injury or disease may manifest as bladder overactivity and UUI or as overflow incontinence, depending on the spinal level and completeness of the injury or disease.

Medications may have wide-ranging effects on lower urinary tract function (see Table 68-1). A thorough inquiry into the use of new medications in the setting of recent-onset UI may show a relationship.

Acute UI manifesting in the immediate postoperative setting may be secondary to a number of factors, including surgical manipulation and immobility, and to a number of medications, especially opioid analgesics and sedative-hypnotics.

Prior surgery may have effects on lower urinary tract function. UI following prostate surgery in men is highly suggestive of injury to the sphincter and resultant SUI. Pelvic surgery for benign and malignant conditions may result in denervation or injury to the lower urinary tract. This includes bowel surgery and gynecologic procedures. For example, new-onset total UI following gynecologic surgery suggests intraoperative bladder injury and subsequent development of a postoperative vesicovaginal fistula. Radiation therapy to the pelvis for malignant disease (e.g., prostate cancer or cervical cancer) may result in injury to the bladder or urethra and subsequent UI.

In women, UI may be related to several gynecologic factors, including childbirth, hormonal status, and prior gynecologic surgery although recently the relationship of some of these factors to UI has come under debate.[22] Pregnancy and childbirth, particularly vaginal delivery, are associated with SUI and pelvic prolapse. Significant SUI in the nulliparous woman is uncommon. UI that becomes progressive at or around menopause suggests a hormonal component that may be responsive to estrogen or hormone replacement therapy.

UI may present in the setting of other significant pelvic floor disorders, signs, and symptoms. Constipation, diarrhea, fecal incontinence, dyspareunia, sexual dysfunction, and pelvic pain may be related to UI. A history of gross hematuria in the setting of UI mandates further urologic investigation, including radiologic imaging of the upper urinary tract and cystoscopy. Acute dysuria with or without hematuria in the setting of UI suggests cystitis. Urinalysis and urine culture should be performed in these patients.

TREATMENT

Desired Outcomes

3 The efficacy goals for the management of UI include restoration of continence, reduction of the number of UI episodes, and prevention of complications (pressure ulcers, nursing home placement, etc.). Other desired outcomes are minimization of adverse treatment consequences and cost, as well as improvement in patient's quality of life.

General Approach to Treatment

Nonsurgical, nonpharmacologic intervention is the first-line treatment for UI. Drug therapy may be considered in patients whose UI is not adequately controlled by nonpharmacologic therapies and in those who have no major contraindications to drug treatment. In general, pharmacotherapy provides better response when combined with nonpharmacologic interventions. Selection of agent should be based on the type of UI, and patient characteristics (e.g., age, comorbidities, concurrent drug therapies, ability to maintain medication adherence). Surgery can be considered when the degree of bother or lifestyle compromise is sufficient and other nonsurgical interventions are undesired or ineffective.

Antimuscarinic agents have been the mainstay of pharmacotherapy for OAB and UUI. According to American Urological Association (AUA) guideline, clinicians should avoid antimuscarinic agents in patients with narrow-angle glaucoma unless approved by the treating ophthalmologist. Antimuscarinic agents should be cautiously used in patients with frailty, impaired gastric emptying or a history of urinary retention, or in those who are taking other drugs with anticholinergic properties. When one agent offers inadequate symptom control and/or unacceptable adverse drug events, consider a dose modification or switching to another agent. Before abandoning effective antimuscarinic therapy, clinicians should manage constipation and dry mouth (bowel regimen, fluid management, dose modification or alternative antimuscarinics).[23]

Nonpharmacologic Therapy

Nonsurgical Treatment

4 Nonpharmacologic, nonsurgical treatment of UI is recommended as the first-line therapy at a primary care level. It is the only option for patients in whom pharmacologic and/or surgical management is inappropriate or undesired. Examples of patients who fulfill these criteria for nonpharmacologic treatment include those who with mild to moderate symptoms who do not want to take medication; those with comorbid conditions that place them at high risk for adverse effects from drug therapy; those who are not medically fit for surgery; those who plan future pregnancies (which may adversely affect long-term surgical outcomes); those with overflow incontinence whose condition is not amenable to surgery or drug therapy; and those who are delaying surgery or do not want to undergo surgery.[24,25]

Nondrug interventions for UI include behavioral interventions, external neuromodulation, alternative medicine therapy, antiincontinence devices, and supportive interventions (Table 68-3).[24,25] Behavioral interventions are generally the first-line of treatment for SUI, UUI, and mixed UI. Interventions include lifestyle modifications, toilet scheduling regimens, and pelvic floor muscle rehabilitation. Because the key to success with any type of behavioral intervention is motivation of patients or caregivers, these individuals must be active participants in developing a treatment plan. Regular follow-up is needed to help motivate patients and caregivers, provide reassurance and support, and monitor treatment outcomes.

External neuromodulation may include nonimplantable electrical stimulation, percutaneous tibial nerve stimulation, or extracorporeal magnetic stimulation. This treatment option is typically prescribed when traditional pelvic floor muscle rehabilitation has failed. Antiincontinence devices such bed alarms, catheters, pessaries, and penile clamps and external collection devices are reserved for special situations depending on patients' UI symptoms, cognitive and mobility status, and overall health status. Supportive interventions such as physical therapy may be beneficial for patients with muscle weakness and slow gait to reach the toilet in a timelier manner, and absorbent products will provide greater confidence in dealing with unpredictable urine loss.

Surgical Treatment

Only rarely does surgery play a role in the initial management of UI.[26] In the absence of secondary complications from UI (e.g., skin breakdown or infection), the decision to surgically treat symptomatic UI should be based on the premise that the degree of bother or lifestyle compromise to the patient is great enough to warrant an elective operation, and that nonsurgical therapy either is undesired or has been ineffective.

Successful application of surgery depends mostly on defining the underlying abnormalities responsible for UI (bladder vs. urethra, underactivity vs. overactivity). Once the underlying factors are determined, other considerations include renal function, sexual function, severity of leakage, history of abdominal or pelvic surgery, presence of concurrent abdominal or pelvic pathology requiring surgical correction, and finally the patient's suitability for the procedure and willingness to accept the risks of surgery.

If patients with uncomplicated SUI become dissatisfied with the initial management approaches of pelvic floor exercises, medications, and/or behavioral modification, surgical treatment assumes the primary role.[26]

Surgical correction of female SUI (urethral underactivity) is directed toward either (a) repositioning the urethra and/or creating a backboard of support, or otherwise stabilizing the urethra and bladder neck in a well-supported retropubic (intraabdominal)

TABLE 68-3 Nonpharmacologic Management of Urinary Incontinence

Intervention	Description	Patient Characteristics
Lifestyle Modifications		
	Self-management strategies targeted toward reducing or eliminating risk factors that cause or exacerbate UI	Smoking cessation, weight reduction for obese patients with stress and urgency incontinence, constipation prevention, caffeine reduction, fluid modification only for those with abnormally high fluid intake
Scheduling Regimens		
Timed voiding	Toileting on a fixed schedule where interval does not change, typically every 2 hours during waking hours	Used for patients with cognitive or physical impairments
Habit retraining	Scheduled toiletings with adjustments of voiding intervals (longer or shorter) based on patient's voiding pattern	Used for institutionalized or homebound patients with cognitive or physical impairments
Prompted voiding	Scheduled toiletings that require prompts to void from a caregiver, typically every 2 hours; patient assisted in toileting only if response is positive; used in conjunction with operant conditioning techniques for rewarding patients for maintaining continence and appropriate toileting	Used for patients who are functionally able to use toilet or toilet substitute, able to feel urge sensation, and able to request toileting assistance appropriately; primarily used in institutional settings or in homebound patients with an available caregiver
Bladder training	Scheduled toiletings with progressive voiding intervals; includes teaching urgency suppression strategies using relaxation and distraction techniques, self-monitoring, and use of reinforcement techniques; sometimes combined with drug therapy	Used for stress, urgency, and mixed incontinence in patients who are cognitively intact, able to toilet, and motivated to comply with training program
Pelvic Floor Muscle Rehabilitation		
Pelvic floor muscle exercises (e.g., Kegel exercises)	Regular practice of pelvic floor muscle contractions; may involve use of pelvic floor muscle contraction for prevention of stress leakage and urge inhibition	Used for stress, urgency, and mixed incontinence in patients who can isolate and correctly contract pelvic floor muscles; requires cognitively intact and highly motivated patient
Biofeedback	Use of electronic or mechanical instruments to display visual or auditory information about neuromuscular or bladder activity; used to teach correct pelvic floor muscle contraction or urge inhibition; home trainers available	Used for stress, urgency, and mixed incontinence in patients who have the capability to learn voluntary control through observation and are motivated; used in conjunction with pelvic floor muscle exercises
Vaginal weight training	Active retention of increasing vaginal weights; typically used in combination with pelvic floor muscle exercises at least twice per day	Women with stress incontinence who are cognitively intact, can correctly contract pelvic floor muscles, able to stand, and have sufficient vaginal vault and introitus to retain cone, and are highly motivated; contraindicated in patients with moderate to severe pelvic organ prolapse
External Neuromodulation		
Nonimplantable electrical stimulation	Application of electrical current through vaginal, anal, surface, or fine needle electrodes; used to inhibit bladder overactivity and improve awareness, contractility, and efficacy of pelvic floor muscle contraction; handheld stimulators for home use are available	Used for stress, urgency, and mixed incontinence in patients who are highly motivated; contraindicated in patients with diminished sensory perception; urinary retention, history of cardiac arrhythmia, cardiac pacemakers, implantable defibrillators, pregnant or attempting pregnancy; vaginal or anal electrodes are contraindicated in moderate or severe pelvic organ prolapse
Percutaneous tibial nerve stimulation	Application of a pulsed electrical current through a fine needle electrode placed externally near the tibial nerve	Used for treatment of overactive bladder with urinary urgency, frequency, and urgency incontinence; contraindicated in patients with pacemakers or implantable defibrillators, prone to excessive bleeding, or women who are pregnant
Extracorporeal magnetic electrical stimulation	Pulsed magnetic stimulation to pelvic floor musculature causing depolarization of motor neurons, thus inducing pelvic floor muscle contraction; stimulation is provided through a specially designed chair that contains a device for producing a pulsing magnetic field	Used for treatment of stress, urgency, and mixed incontinence; contraindicated in patients with demand cardiac pacemakers or metallic joint replacements; may be useful treatment option when other approaches fail or are not feasible
Alternative Medicine Therapies		
Acupuncture	Involves insertion of disposable sterile fine stainless steel needles into points on the skin that are thought to suppress or stimulate spinal and/or supraspinal reflexes to the bladder and/or urethra	Used for stress, urgency, and mixed incontinence and UI due to spinal cord injury
Antiincontinence Devices		
Bed or pant alarms	Sensor devices that respond to wetness; used to awaken or alert individuals via noise or vibrating mechanism	Primarily used for nocturnal enuresis in children; system available for monitoring incontinence in home care and institutional environments
Pessaries	Intravaginal devices designed to support the bladder neck, relieve minor to moderate pelvic organ prolapse, and change pressure transmission to the urethra	Used for female stress incontinence and mild to moderate pelvic organ prolapse; in postmenopausal women, topical estrogen therapy is typically prescribed to prevent ulceration and breakdown of vaginal tissue; requires good manual dexterity to manipulate device
Urethral insert (women only)	Intraurethral device	Used in female stress incontinence with stress incontinence who are cognitively intact and have good manual dexterity
Urethral compression device (men only)	Penile clamp	Used in men patients with stress incontinence who are cognitively intact and have good manual dexterity
External collection devices (men only)	Condom catheter with leg bag	Used in men with urgency, stress, and overflow incontinence and in those with functional impairments

(continued)

TABLE 68-3 Nonpharmacologic Management of Urinary Incontinence *(Continued)*

Intervention	Description	Patient Characteristics
Catheters	Disposable, intermittent urethral catheters and indwelling urethral and suprapubic catheters	Used for overflow incontinence; used in patients who are bed-bound or with significant mobility impairments and severe incontinence; those with terminal illness; those with sacral pressure ulcers until healing occurs
Supportive Interventions		
Toileting substitutes and other environmental modifications	Female and male urinals, bedside commodes, elevated toilet seats	Used for patients with mobility impairments that make reaching toilet in timely fashion difficult
Absorbent products	Variety of reusable and disposable liners, pads, male drip collectors, male guard, collector undergarment, fitted brief, and pant systems; some products contain a polymer that absorbs and wicks urine away from the body	Used for all types of incontinence
Physical therapy	Gait and/or strength training	Used for older patients with mobility impairments that make reaching a toilet in timely fashion difficult

position that is receptive to changes in intraabdominal pressure; or (b) improving the sealing mechanism and/or creating compression or otherwise augmenting the urethral resistance provided by the intrinsic sphincteric unit, with (i.e., sling) or without (i.e., periurethral injectable bulking agents) urethral and bladder neck support.

Bulking agents are injected into the urethra at the level of the urinary sphincter as an office-based procedure and are generally considered quite safe. However, their durability and efficacy are likely inferior to other options.[27]

Midurethral synthetic slings have become the most common approach to the treatment of SUI in women in the United States.[28] These can be inserted as outpatient procedures that have shorter convalescence periods and allow faster return to usual activities compared with many of the older procedures. These procedures are generally felt to be highly durable and efficacious. However, safety concerns have been recently expressed regarding the implantation of surgical mesh in some patients, the implications of which are yet to be fully clarified.[29]

SUI in men is very rare in the absence of prior pelvic surgery, injury, or neurologic disease. When it occurs, SUI in men can be treated in a number of ways.[30] Bulking agents can be injected periurethrally and submucosally into the region of the external urinary sphincter. This approach is less effective and far less durable than alternative surgical procedures, although it can be performed in the office setting without the need for general anesthesia.

The artificial urinary sphincter is generally considered to be the gold standard for treatment of male SUI.[30] Placement of this manually operated silicone device has been associated with very high long-term success and satisfaction rates.[31] Male slings placed through a perineal incision are a newer alternative to the artificial urinary sphincter. However, long-term efficacy and safety data are lacking.[32]

Most patients with UUI are managed nonsurgically with a combination of behavioral modification, pelvic floor exercises, and pharmacologic therapy. However, for patients refractory to such measures, invasive therapy can beneficial. Posterior tibial nerve stimulation is an office-based percutaneous treatment for UUI or OAB. Therapy consists of weekly 30-minute treatments with a needle placed posteriorly to the medial malleolus of the ankle for 3 months. Efficacy appears similar to or slightly better than oral pharmacotherapy.[33] However, long-term efficacy and safety data are lacking.[34]

Surgery for the treatment of UUI generally consists of implantation of a sacral nerve stimulator (neuromodulation) or endoscopic office-based injection of botulinum toxin directly into the detrusor muscle.[35,36] Neuromodulation is a staged surgical procedure in which a neurostimulator lead is placed transforaminally at the level of sacral spinal cord root S3. Its exact mechanism is unknown, but the device may exert its favorable effects on urination and UUI by rebalancing the afferent and efferent nerve impulses to the lower urinary tract and pelvic floor. The injection of botulinum toxin is performed in the office generally with local anesthesia. The toxin is taken up by the efferent nerve terminals and prevents the release of acetylcholine into the synapse at the neuromuscular junction, thus inducing paralysis of the affected detrusor muscle. The duration of effect of the toxin is about 4 to 8 months, after which repeat injection is necessary to maintain effect. The therapeutic algorithm involving these two choices for treatment of refractory UUI is evolving and is determined largely by patient preference.[37]

Few surgical treatments for bladder underactivity are effective. After an appropriate evaluation for reversible causes, the most effective management of this condition is intermittent self-catheterization performed by the patient or a caregiver three or four times per day. Sacral nerve stimulation (neuromodulation) has shown some efficacy in this patient population, but success rates for detrusor underactivity (nonobstructive urinary retention) are inferior to those seen with urinary frequency and urgency.[38] Proper patient selection for this therapy remains poorly defined. Alternative methods of management that are less satisfactory or more invasive include indwelling urethral or suprapubic catheters and urinary diversion.

Urethral overactivity is most commonly caused by anatomic obstruction. Anatomic obstruction in men is most often caused by benign prostatic enlargement. Treatments may include transurethral surgical resection of the prostate (see Chap. 67).

Rarely, bladder outlet obstruction is caused by a functional obstruction at the level of the bladder neck or external sphincter. Hypertrophy of the smooth muscle fibers at the level of the bladder neck in men and women may result in obstruction to the flow of urine. In patients who do not respond to pharmacologic therapy with α-adrenergic receptor antagonists, endoscopic incision using the cystoscope is highly effective in treating this very uncommon condition.

Pharmacologic Therapy

Urge Urinary Incontinence

5 Anticholinergic/antimuscarinic agents are the first-line drug therapy for relieving UUI symptoms and preventing its complications. Table 68-4 summarizes AUA recommendations for treating OAB in adults.[23] Mirabegron, a β_3-adrenergic agonist, was approved in 2012 for OAB or UUI. While the guideline does not discuss its role in comparison to other existing drug options, it may be considered as first-line therapy or in patients who do not adequately respond to or cannot tolerate anticholinergic/antimuscarinic drugs. Table 68-5 lists the usual dosage for approved agents for OAB or UUI. Table 68-6 suggests common monitoring parameters for these agents.

TABLE 68-4 AUA Guideline for Treatment of Overactive Bladder in Adults

Recommendation	Evidence Strength Grade[c]
First-Line Treatments	
Behavioral therapies (e.g., bladder training, bladder control strategies, pelvic floor muscle training, fluid management)	B
Behavioral therapies may be combined with antimuscarinic therapies	C
Second-Line Treatments	
Oral antimuscarinics including darifenacin, fesoterodine, oxybutynin, solifenacin, tolterodine, or trospium as second-line therapy[a]	B
If an IR and an ER formulation are available, prefer ER formulations because of lower rates of dry mouth	B
Transdermal oxybutynin (patch or gel) may be offered	C
Third-Line Treatments	
Sacral neuromodulation in carefully selected patients with severe refractory OAB symptoms or in those who are not candidates for second-line therapy and are willing to undergo a surgical procedure	C
Peripheral tibial nerve stimulation in a carefully selected patient population	C
Intradetrusor onabotulinum toxin A (not FDA approved) in carefully selected patients who have been refractory to first- and second-line OAB treatments[b]	C

AUA, American Urological Association; IR, immediate-release; ER, extended-release; OAB, overactive bladder.

[a]Drugs listed in alphabetical order; no hierarchy is implied.

[b]The patient must be able and willing to return for frequent postvoid residual evaluation and able and willing to perform self-catheterization if necessary.

[c]When sufficient evidence existed, the body of evidence for a particular treatment was assigned a strength rating of A (high), B (moderate), or C (low). Both B and C indicate that benefits outweigh risks/burdens.

TABLE 68-5 Dosing of Medications Approved for OAB or UUI

Drug	Brand Name	Initial Dose	Usual Range	Special Population Dose	Comments
Anticholinergics/Antimuscarinics					
Oxybutynin IR	Ditropan	2.5 mg twice daily	2.5–5 mg two to four times daily		Titrate in increments of 2.5 mg/day every 1–2 months; available in oral solution
Oxybutynin XL	Ditropan XL	5–10 mg once daily	5–30 mg once daily		Adjust dose in 5-mg increments at weekly interval; swallow whole
Oxybutynin TDS	Oxytrol		3.9 mg/day apply one patch twice weekly		Apply every 3 to 4 days; rotate application site
Oxybutynin gel 10%	Gelnique		One sachet (100 mg) topically daily		Apply to clean and dry, intact skin on abdomen, thighs or upper arms/shoulders; contains alcohol
Oxybutynin gel 3%	Gelnique 3%		Three pumps (84 mg) topically daily		Same as above
Tolterodine IR	Detrol		1–2 mg twice daily	1 mg twice daily if patient is taking CYP3A4 inhibitors, or with renal/hepatic impairment	
Tolterodine LA	Detrol LA		2–4 mg once daily	2 mg once daily in those who are taking CYP3A4 inhibitors or with renal/hepatic impairment	Swallow whole; avoid in patients with creatinine clearance ≤10 mL/min (0.17 mL/s)
Trospium chloride IR	Sanctura		20 mg twice daily	20 mg once daily in patient age ≥75 years or creatinine clearance ≤30 mL/min (0.5 mL/s)	Take 1 hour before meals or on empty stomach; patient age ≥75 years should take at bedtime
Trospium chloride ER	Sanctura XR		60 mg once daily	Avoid in patient age ≥75 years or creatinine clearance ≤30 mL/min (0.5 mL/s)	Take 1 hour before meals or on empty stomach; swallow whole
Solifenacin	VESIcare	5 mg daily	5–10 mg once daily	5 mg daily if patient is taking CYP3A4 inhibitors or with creatinine clearance ≤30 mL/min (0.5 mL/s) or moderate hepatic impairment; avoid in severe hepatic impairment	Swallow whole
Darifenacin ER	Enablex	7.5 mg once daily	7.5–15 mg once daily	7.5 mg daily if patient is taking potent CYP3A4 inhibitors or with moderate hepatic impairment; avoid in severe hepatic impairment	Titrate dose after at least 2 weeks; swallow whole
Fesoterodine ER	Toviaz	4 mg once daily	4–8 mg once daily	4 mg daily if patient is taking potent CYP3A4 inhibitors or with creatinine clearance ≤30 mL/min (0.5 mL/s); avoid in severe hepatic impairment	Prodrug (metabolized to 5-hydroxymethyl tolterodine); swallow whole
β_3-Adrenergic Agonist					
Mirabegron ER	Myrbetriq	25 mg once daily	25–50 mg once daily	25 mg once daily if creatinine clearance 15–29 mL/min (0.25–0.49 mL/s); avoid in patients with ESRD or severe hepatic impairment	Swallow whole

OAB, overactive bladder; UUI, urge urinary incontinence; IR, immediate-release; LA, long-acting; TDS, transdermal system; XL, extended-release; ER, extended-release; ESRD, end stage renal disease; CYP, cytochrome P450 enzyme.

TABLE 68-6 Monitoring of Medications Approved for OAB or UUI

Drug	Adverse Drug Reaction	Monitoring Parameters	Comments
Anticholinergic/Antimuscarinic			
Oxybutynin IR Oxybutynin XL Oxybutynin TDS Oxybutynin gel 10% Oxybutynin gel 3% Tolterodine IR Tolterodine LA Trospium chloride IR Trospium chloride ER Solifenacin Darifenacin ER Fesoterodine ER	Anticholinergic adverse effects: dry mouth, constipation, headache, dyspepsia, dry eyes, blurred vision, cognitive impairment, tachycardia, sedation, orthostatic hypotension Application site reactions (topical agents): pruritus, erythema	Contraindications and precautions: urinary retention, gastric retention, severely decreased GI motility, angioedema, myasthenia gravis, uncontrolled narrow-angle glaucoma Worsening of renal/hepatic condition or concomitant drug therapy, which may necessitate dosage reduction or drug cessation Mental status change or risk for falls in elderly or frail patients	In general, ER, LA, XL, and topical products are associated with fewer anticholinergic adverse effects, particularly dry mouth Possible transference of drug from topical application Avoid open fire or smoke until alcohol-based gel has dried
β_3-Adrenergic Agonist			
Mirabegron ER	Hypertension, nasopharyngitis, urinary tract infection, headache	Precautions: urinary retention, severe uncontrolled hypertension Worsening of renal/hepatic condition, which may necessitate dosage reduction or drug cessation Increased effect of narrow therapeutic index drugs that are CYP2D6 substrates	Mirabegron is a CYP2D6 inhibitor

OAB, overactive bladder; UUI, urge urinary incontinence; IR, immediate-release; LA, long-acting; TDS, transdermal system; XL, extended-release; ER, extended-release; CYP, cytochrome P450 enzyme.

Anticholinergic/antimuscarinic agents (oxybutynin, tolterodine, trospium, solifenacin, darifenacin, and fesoterodine) antagonize muscarinic receptors and suppress premature detrusor contractions, thereby enhance bladder storage. They have similar contraindications, precautions, and side effect profiles with incidence/severity varies with each individual agent.[39] Choice of therapy should be based on patient characteristics (e.g., age, comorbidities, concurrent medications, and ability to adhere to the prescribed regimen). These agents have been demonstrated to improve quality of life in patients with UUI, and are considered equally effective based on statistical superiority over placebo or active controls. In clinical trials, major efficacy outcomes for these agents in the management of UI are reduction of the mean number of UI episodes, decrease in the number of micturitions per day, and increase of urine volume voided per micturition.[40]

Oxybutynin IR Oxybutynin IR is the oldest treatment for UUI and the gold standard against which other drugs are compared. It has the disadvantages of giving substantial nonurinary antimuscarinic effects, and these may lead to therapy cessation. Besides antimuscarinic effects, oxybutynin IR also causes orthostatic hypotension, and sedation/weight gain, due to the blockage of α-adrenergic-, and histamine H_1-receptors, respectively.[41] Overall, significant adverse effects of this agent jeopardize medication adherence and can prevent dose escalation to achieve optimal benefit. Its multiple daily dosing may be too complicated for patients with cognitive impairment or those who are taking multiple medications. It is available in oral solution formulation, which may be easier to administer to patients who have difficulty in swallowing. It is also available generically and thus less costly.

The high incidence of adverse effects, especially dry mouth, with use of oxybutynin IR is largely due to it active metabolite *N*-desethyloxybutynin (DEO), which is generated during extensive first-pass metabolism in the liver and upper GI tract.[41] The lower DEO plasma concentrations seen with long-acting (LA) forms of oxybutynin (due to reduced first-pass metabolism) compared with those of oxybutynin IR may explain the lesser propensity of the LA formulations to cause dry mouth and other anticholinergic adverse effects.[42] Another factor associated with the adverse effects of oxybutynin IR, especially in older patients, is the transient high peak serum oxybutynin plasma concentrations.

To optimize tolerability, initiate dose at no more than 2.5 mg twice daily, increase to 2.5 mg three times daily after 1 month, then titrate in increments of 2.5 mg/day every 1 to 2 months until the desired response or the maximum recommended or tolerated dose is attained. The optimal response usually requires no more than 5 mg three times daily. Side effects may be managed by dose reduction. Also, dry mouth may be relieved by use of sugarless hard candy, gum, or a saliva substitute. Constipation can be minimized by increasing the intake of water, dietary fiber, physical activity, or laxative therapy.

Oxybutynin Extended-Release An extended-release (XL) formulation of oxybutynin can be considered an alternative therapy in patients who cannot tolerate IR formulation. These have been shown to be more effective than placebo and are as effective as oxybutynin IR in efficacy outcomes.[42]

The XL product delivers a controlled amount of oxybutynin over a 24-hour period, reducing first-pass metabolism by cytochrome P450 (CYP) isoenzyme 3A4. This explains the lower dry mouth incidence associated with the XL product. In short-term studies of up to 12 weeks' duration, oxybutynin XL was better tolerated than oxybutynin IR, with approximately 7% of patients discontinuing treatment because of adverse effects (compared with approximately 27% of those taking oxybutynin IR). The rate and severity of adverse effects did not differ significantly between elderly persons (≥65 years old) and younger adults.[42]

In a 12-week study, oxybutynin XL was more effective than tolterodine IR in reducing the mean number of weekly incontinence episodes and micturitions. In another study, it was as effective as tolterodine LA in decreasing the mean number of incontinence episodes, but oxybutynin XL was superior in reducing weekly micturition frequency and achieving total dryness. Pooled results of two open-label studies suggested that oxybutynin XL was inferior in patient-perceived improvement in bladder control and adverse effects profile to tolterodine LA. However, both agents provided similar patients' or physicians' perception of benefit over baseline and proportions of withdrawals due to lack of efficacy. A major limitation of this study was lack of blinding, which may lead to patient and observer bias.[39]

Oxybutynin XL should be administered once daily, and should not be crushed or chewed. Elderly patients should start with a dose of 5 mg once daily and titrate gradually to desired effects, which may take at least 4 weeks after dose initiation or escalation. Drug interactions may occur when oxybutynin is used with other anticholinergic drugs, potent CYP3A4 inhibitors (e.g., itraconazole, miconazole, erythromycin, and clarithromycin), and acetylcholinesterase inhibitors via pharmacodynamic antagonism. Elimination of oxybutynin XL is not altered in patients with renal or hepatic impairment or in geriatric patients (up to age 78 years).[42]

Transdermal Oxybutynin The oxybutynin transdermal system (TDS) is another option for patients who cannot tolerate IR oxybutynin or who prefer topical drug delivery route. The patch allows oxybutynin to bypass first-pass hepatic and gut metabolism, and gives a more tolerable adverse effect profile compare with oral formulations.[43] It is superior to placebo in efficacy outcomes, and similar to oxybutynin IR in reducing the frequency of UUI episodes and improving patient-perceived urinary leakage.[43,44] Compared with tolterodine LA, oxybutynin TDS provided similar efficacy outcomes, including attaining complete continence and improving quality of life.[39] A large multicenter trial (n = 2,878) reported improved quality of life and good tolerability in patients 65 years or older; increase in work productivity was noted among younger patients.[45,46]

Patients should apply oxybutynin TDS to dry, intact skin on the abdomen, hip, or buttocks every 3 to 4 days (twice weekly). Rotating application site at least weekly may help to minimize local side effects. The most common adverse effects are pruritus (14% to 17%) and erythema (6% to 9%) at the application site, dry mouth (5% to 10%), constipation (3%), and abnormal vision (2.5%), which occur similarly among older and younger populations.[43]

Oxybutynin Topical Gel Another option for topical application of oxybutynin is gel formulation (available in 10% or in 3%).[47,48] It has the same effects on oxybutynin and DEO plasma concentrations as with the patch formulation.[49] It causes significantly less dry mouth than oxybutynin (6.1% vs. 73.1%).[50] In 12-week, randomized, placebo-controlled studies, oxybutynin topical gel has been superior to placebo in efficacy outcomes with common adverse effects being dry mouth and application site reactions.[51] Use of this product for 1 week did not cause cognitive impairment in healthy older adults aged 60 to 79 years.[52] However, clinicians should monitor for anticholinergic effects during long-term therapy, particularly in frail patients with baseline susceptibility to these adverse effects.

The most common adverse events include dry mouth (8% to 12%), application site reactions (5% to 11%), and dizziness (3%).[47,48] Clinicians should counsel patients to avoid applying sunscreen within half an hour before or after application and to avoid showering within 1 hour after application. The transfer of gel between individuals may occur if vigorous skin contact is made at the application site; patients should avoid open fires or exposure to smoking until this alcohol-based gel has dried.[47,48]

Tolterodine Immediate Release Tolterodine is a competitive muscarinic receptor antagonist that can be considered first-line therapy for UI in patients with symptoms of urinary frequency, urgency, or urge incontinence. It is as effective as oxybutynin IR in efficacy outcomes, and is associated with lower drug discontinuation rates (8% vs. 27% oxybutynin IR).[39,53] A retrospective 2-year cohort study suggested that tolterodine was associated with better medication adherence than oxybutynin due to better tolerability among older patients.[54]

Tolterodine is predominantly eliminated by hepatic metabolism, which is partially under the control of genetic polymorphism.[53] The principal metabolic pathway in extensive metabolizers involves oxidation of the parent drug by CYP isoenzyme 2D6 to the active 5-hydroxymethyl metabolite (DD01), followed by further oxidation and dealkylation. In poor metabolizers who lack the CYP2D6 (approximately 7% of the U.S. population), the principal metabolic pathway involves CYP3A4, with dealkylation of the amino group, oxidation to a dealkylated hydroxy metabolite, and further oxidation to a dealkylated acid metabolite that undergoes glucuronidation. Because tolterodine is principally metabolized by CYP3A4 in this case, its elimination may be impaired by inhibitors of this isoenzyme (e.g., fluoxetine, sertraline, fluvoxamine, macrolide antibiotics, azole antifungals, and grapefruit juice). For example, fluoxetine, an inhibitor of CYP2D6 and 3A4, decreases the metabolism of tolterodine to DD01. The result is a mean 4.8-fold increase in the tolterodine area under the plasma concentration-versus-time curve (AUC), mean 52% decrease in peak plasma concentration, and mean 20% decrease in the AUC of DD01.[53] Whether tolterodine significantly alters the pharmacokinetics of drugs metabolized by CYP2D6 is unknown, so caution is advised with concurrent use with agents metabolized by CYP2D6.

A pharmacokinetic study demonstrated that tolterodine pharmacokinetics did not differ significantly in healthy elderly volunteers (age 64 to 80 years) and younger healthy volunteers who were below 40 years of age. However, in another phase I study, the mean serum concentrations of tolterodine and DD01 were 20% and 50% greater in elderly volunteers than in young healthy volunteers, respectively. Despite possibly altered pharmacokinetics in elderly individuals, no differences in the incidences and severity of adverse events between these age groups have been noted in clinical trials, so no dosage adjustment is recommended on the basis of age alone.[53]

Tolterodine IR can be given 1 to 2 mg twice daily with or without food. It is not recommended in patients with creatinine clearance <10 mL/min (<0.17 mL/s) or severe hepatic impairment. The dose should be reduced to 2 mg in patients with mild to moderate hepatic impairment, or creatinine clearance 10 to 30 mL/min (0.17 to 0.5 mL/s), or in those taking potent CYP3A4 inhibitors. The maximum benefit from tolterodine may take up to 8 weeks after therapy initiation or dose escalation.[53]

The most common adverse effects of tolterodine are dry mouth, dyspepsia, headache, constipation, and dry eyes. Of note, patients who have known hypersensitivity to fesoterodine fumarate should not receive tolterodine because both agents are metabolized to DD01. Monitoring QT prolongation in patients who are also taking Class IA (e.g., quinidine, procainamide) or Class III (e.g., amiodarone, sotalol) antiarrhythmic medications.[53]

Tolterodine Long Acting Tolterodine LA offers a convenient once-daily dosing, and is a preferred agent in patients who are bothered by dry mouth while taking IR products. It is better than placebo in efficacy outcomes, including ability to complete tasks before voiding and patient perception of benefit.[55] It also improves OAB symptoms in men who were taking α-adrenergic blockers.[56]

Tolterodine LA should be given once daily, and should not be crushed or chewed. The dose should be limited to 2 mg once daily in patients with mild to moderate hepatic impairment (Child-Pugh class A or B), severe renal impairment creatinine clearance 10 to 30 mL/min (0.17 to 0.50 mL/s), or taking drugs that are potent CYP3A4 inhibitors (ketoconazole, itraconazole, clarithromycin, or ritonavir). Patients with creatinine clearance less than <10 mL/min (<0.17 mL/s) or severe hepatic impairment (Child-Pugh Class C) should avoid taking the drug. Patients should be counseled that it takes up to 8 weeks to see maximum benefit after starting therapy or dose escalation. Common adverse effects and monitoring parameters for tolterodine LA are similar to its IR product.[55]

Fesoterodine Fumarate Fesoterodine fumarate is also indicated for symptoms of urinary frequency, urgency, or urge incontinence. It is a prodrug that is metabolized to its active metabolite,

5-hydroxymethyl tolterodine (also a metabolite of tolterodine), by nonspecific plasma esterases.[57]

In a large 12-week, randomized, double-blind, placebo-controlled study, fesoterodine was better than tolterodine ER 4 mg and placebo on reducing UUI episodes, micturitions, urgency and improving health-related quality of life. However, fesoterodine caused more dry mouth (28% vs. 13%), and constipation (4% vs. 3%) than tolterodine ER. It has been associated with higher discontinuation rates due to adverse events (5% vs. 3%).[58]

The usual starting dose is 4 mg daily, increasing to 8 mg daily, as needed and tolerated. The dose of fesoterodine should not exceed 4 mg daily in the presence of severe renal impairment (creatinine clearance <30 mL/min [0.50 mL/s]) or in patients also taking potent CYP3A4 inhibitors. Fesoterodine is not recommended in patients with severe hepatic impairment. It is available in extended-release tablets, which should be swallowed whole; patients should not chew, crush, or divide the product.[57]

The most common adverse effects of fesoterodine are dry mouth (27%), constipation (5.1%), dyspepsia (2%), and dry eyes (1.6%). Anticholinergic adverse effects associated with fesoterodine are dose related.[57]

Trospium Chloride Immediate Release Trospium chloride, a quaternary ammonium anticholinergic, is a second-generation antimuscarinic agent for UUI. Trospium chloride is poorly absorbed after oral administration (<10%), and food reduces bioavailability by 70% to 80%. It is principally cleared by the renal route (60%). Metabolites account for approximately 40% of the excreted dose following oral administration. The major metabolic pathway is hypothesized as ester hydrolysis with subsequent conjugation of benzylic acid to form azoniaspironortropanol with glucuronic acid. CYP is not expected to contribute significantly to the elimination of trospium. The plasma half-life is approximately 20 hours, with renal clearance about 30 L/h. Active tubular secretion is a major route of elimination for trospium, which explains its drug interaction profile. Advancing age and mild to moderate hepatic impairment do not affect trospium chloride pharmacokinetics to a clinically significant degree. In contrast, renal impairment does significantly reduce drug clearance. When creatinine clearance is less than 30 mL/min (0.50 mL/s), AUC is increased by a mean of 4.5-fold, peak plasma concentration by a mean of twofold, and terminal disposition half-life by a mean of two- to threefold.[59]

In a study involving a large proportion of elders (mean age, 63 years), trospium chloride was better than placebo in efficacy outcomes of UUI.[60] In a 12-week, controlled study, trospium chloride IR was noninferior to oxybutynin IR in managing UUI, but was associated with less dry mouth.[61]

The frequency of anticholinergic side effects of trospium was higher in patients 75 years and older than younger subjects. This occurrence is believed to be pharmacodynamic (i.e., increased sensitivity) and not pharmacokinetic in nature. No data at present support the hypothesis that trospium chloride is less neurotoxic than nonquaternary ammonium anticholinergics (based on the hypothesis of reduced transit across the blood–brain barrier of trospium chloride due to its positive electrical charge on the quaternary nitrogen). Trospium may interact with other drugs that are eliminated by active tubular secretion via competition (e.g., procainamide, pancuronium, morphine, vancomycin, and tenofovir).[59] Thus, clinicians should monitor the clinical effects of these agents when used concomitantly.

The usual dosage of trospium IR is 20 mg twice daily. The drug should be taken on an empty stomach. Dosage reduction (by 50% of the daily dose) is recommended when creatinine clearance is less than 30 mL/min (0.50 mL/s). In patients age 75 years and older, dose reduction to 20 mg once daily should be considered based upon tolerability.[59]

Trospium Chloride Extended-Release Trospium chloride ER offers once-daily dosing. Its efficacy and safety have been demonstrated in patients with OAB, including those who are older and taking multiple medications.[62–64]

Trospium is eliminated primarily unchanged in the urine. It is not recommended in patients with severe renal impairment (creatinine clearance <30 mL/min [0.50 mL/s]).

Alcohol should not be consumed within 2 hours of trospium ER administration. Coadministration with antacid may increase or decrease trospium exposure, but the clinical relevance of these findings is unknown. In addition, coadministration of immediate-release (IR) metformin 500 mg twice daily reduced the steady-state systemic exposure of trospium by approximately 29% and peak concentration by 34%.[63]

The usual dosage of trospium ER is 60 mg daily. Because food decreases the bioavailability by 35% to 60%, extended-release trospium chloride must be taken on an empty stomach (1 hour before or 2 hours after meals).[63] Common adverse effects with trospium chloride ER have been dry mouth (11%), constipation (9%), dizziness (2%), dry eyes (1.6%), flatulence (1.6%), nausea (1.4%), and abdominal pain (1.4%). Patients should be informed that alcohol may enhance the drowsiness caused by anticholinergic agents.[63]

Solifenacin Succinate Solifenacin succinate is a second-generation antimuscarinic agent indicated for the treatment of OAB with urge incontinence, urgency, and urinary frequency. Solifenacin was better than tolterodine ER in terms of reducing the number of UUI episodes and pad usage and in improving patients' perception of their bladder condition.[65] An analysis of pooled data from two phase III studies showed that solifenacin recipients had significant improvement in 5 of 10 quality-of-life domains from baseline compared with placebo recipients.[66] Compared with oxybutynin IR, solifenacin was associated with fewer episodes (35% vs. 83%) and lower severity of dry mouth.[67,68]

Solifenacin is well absorbed (mean absolute bioavailability, 88%), and food has no clinically relevant effect on absorption. It is principally eliminated via metabolism and renal excretion of metabolites, with renal excretion of parent compound less than 10% of the dose. With a mean terminal disposition half-life of 50 to 60 hours, the drug can be dosed once daily.[64] The primary pathway for elimination of solifenacin is via CYP3A4. Adverse effects, including dry mouth, occurred similarly between younger and older patients.[67]

The recommended dose of solifenacin is 5 mg once daily. If the drug is well tolerated but the effectiveness is not optimal, the dose can be increased to 10 mg once daily. Little additional benefit is generally achieved with doses exceeding 5 mg daily. Solifenacin can be administered with or without food. For patients with creatinine clearance rates less than 30 mL/min (0.50 mL/s) or with moderate hepatic impairment (Child-Pugh class B), the daily dosage should not exceed 5 mg. Patients who have severe hepatic impairment (Child-Pugh class C) should avoid using this drug. If the patient is receiving concurrent therapy with one or more potent CYP3A4 inhibitors, the daily dose should not exceed 5 mg.

The most common adverse reactions of solifenacin are dry mouth (11% to 28%), constipation (5% to 13%), urinary tract infection (4% to 5%) and blurred vision (3% to 5%). It interacts with CYP3A4 inhibitors and inducers; close patient monitoring is required. Prolonged corrected QT intervals have been reported with high-dose solifenacin, thus its use should be cautioned in at-risk patients.[64]

Darifenacin Darifenacin is another second-generation antimuscarinics for the management of OAB or UUI. It has demonstrated efficacy outcomes, including improving quality of life.[69,70] It may be considered in patients who are dissatisfied with previous antimuscarinic treatments.[71]

The mean absolute bioavailabilities of the 7.5-, 15-, and 30-mg extended-release (ER) formulations are 15%, 19%, and 25%, respectively. Bioavailability is affected by formulation, CYP2D6 genotype, dose, and race. Bioavailability is enhanced using an ER formulation (70% to 110% higher than IR), in heterozygous CYP2D6 extensive metabolizers and poor metabolizers (40% to 90% higher than homozygous extensive metabolizers), and white race (56% higher than Japanese). Darifenacin is extensively metabolized, with cumulative urinary excretion of the parent compound less than 10%. The 2D6 and 3A4 isoenzymes of CYP are responsible for darifenacin metabolism. With a mean terminal disposition half-life of 3 to 5 hours (depending on CYP2D6 metabolizer status), an ER formulation is needed to allow once-daily dosing.[72]

Darifenacin ER should be initiated at 7.5 mg once daily, and may be increased to 15 mg once daily after 2 weeks to target clinical response. The dosage should be limited to 7.5 mg daily in patients with moderate hepatic impairment (Child-Pugh B), taking potent CYP3A4 inhibitors. It should be avoided in patients with severe hepatic impairment (Child-Pugh C). It must be swallowed whole without chewing, dividing, or crushing. The most frequently reported adverse reactions are constipation (21%), dry mouth (19%), headache (7%), dyspepsia (5%), and nausea (4%). Darifenacin may interact with substrates of CYP2D6 (flecainide, thioridazine, and tricyclic antidepressants), thus clinical effects of these drugs should be closely monitored.[72]

Clinical **Controversy. . .**

Should antimuscarinic pharmacotherapy be used to treat UUI in patients with mild cognitive impairment or dementia? Antimuscarinic agents may worsen cognitive function, especially in older adults. Caution should be exercise as these agents may antagonize the therapeutic effects of acetylcholine esterase inhibitors indicated for dementia.

Mirabegron Mirabegron is a β_3-adrenergic agonist approved by FDA in June 2012 for the treatment of OAB with symptoms of UUI, urgency, and urinary frequency.

6 Mirabegron is an alternative to anticholinergics/antimuscarinic drugs for managing UUI. Similar to other previously approved agents, it is only modestly effective and reduces urinary frequency and incontinence episodes by less than one per day. It increases bladder capacity by relaxing the detrusor smooth muscle during the storage phase of the urinary bladder fill-void cycle by the activation of β_3-adrenergic receptors.[73]

The efficacy and safety of mirabegron have been demonstrated in three 12-week, multicenter, double-blind, randomized, placebo-controlled trials. The majority of patients were female Caucasians with a mean age of 59 years (range, 18 to 95 years). About half the study subjects had prior antimuscarinic pharmacotherapy for OAB. Overall, mirabegron reduced mean number of incontinence episodes per 24 hours, mean number of micturitions per 24 hours, and increased mean volume voided per micturition. The efficacy was seen during 4 to 8 weeks of therapy, and was maintained through the 12-week treatment period.[73]

Mirabegron reaches its peak plasma concentrations at approximately 3.5 hours, with an oral bioavailability of 29% to 35% with approved doses. It achieves steady state within 7 days of therapy. Coadministration with high-fat meals reduced its peak concentration and drug exposure by 45% and 17%, respectively. In contrast, low-fat meals decreased these parameters by 75% and 51%, respectively. Nevertheless, mirabegron can be taken with or without food.

Mirabegron is extensively distributed in the body, with a volume of distribution of approximately 1,670 L. It has protein binding of approximately 71% to both albumin and α_1 acid glycoprotein. Mirabegron is metabolized via multiple pathways involving dealkylation, oxidation, glucuronidation, and amide hydrolysis. It has two inactive metabolites (16% and 11% of total exposure), respectively. Isoenzymes CYP2D6 and 3A4 play a limited role in its elimination. Poor metabolizers of CYP2D6 had an increased mean peak concentration and drug exposure compared to extensive metabolizers of CYP2D6 (16% and 17%, respectively). Other enzymes that are involved in mirabegron metabolism include butylcholinesterase, uridine diphospho-glucuronosyltransferases (UGT) and possibly alcohol dehydrogenase.

Total body clearance of mirabegron is about 57 L/h, with a terminal elimination half-life of 50 hours. Renal clearance equals approximately 13 L/h, primarily through active tubular secretion along with glomerular filtration. The urinary elimination of unchanged mirabegron is dose-dependent and ranges from 6% to 12% after a daily dose of 25 to 100 mg.[73]

Mirabegron should be initiated at 25 mg once daily, and may titrate upward to 50 mg once daily after 8 weeks, based on individual efficacy and tolerability; limit dose to 25 mg once daily in patients with severe renal impairment or moderate hepatic disease. Mirabegron is available in extended-release tablets, and should be swallowed whole with water without chewing, dividing, or crushing. It should be avoided in patients with end-stage renal disease, severe hepatic impairment, or severe uncontrolled hypertension (≥180/110 mm Hg). Most commonly reported adverse reactions were hypertension (7% to 11%), nasopharyngitis (4%), urinary tract infection (3% to 6%), and headache (3% to 4%). Patient should be monitored for increased blood pressure and urinary retention, particularly in patients with bladder outlet obstruction or those who are taking anticholinergic drugs.[73]

Mirabegron is a moderate inhibitor of CYP2D6, and may affect the dosage requirement for some 2D6 substrates (e.g., metoprolol and desipramine). Thus, drug level monitoring for certain medications with a narrow therapeutic range, such as thioridazine, flecainide, and propafenone, is advised. When initiating a combination of mirabegron and digoxin, start with the lowest possible dose of digoxin and titrate based drug level and clinical effect.[73]

Other Anticholinergics and Antimuscarinics Other drugs for treatment of UUI are less effective, are no safer, or have not been adequately studied.[24] Thus their use is not recommended. Tricyclic antidepressants are generally no more effective than oxybutynin IR, and they exhibit a high incidence of bothersome and potentially serious adverse effects (e.g., orthostatic hypotension, cardiac conduction abnormalities, dizziness, and confusion). They are also potentially life threatening in overdose. Therefore, their use should be limited to individuals who have one or more additional medical indications for these agents (e.g., depression or neuropathic pain); patients with mixed UI (because of their effect of decreasing bladder contractility and increasing outlet resistance); and possibly those with nocturnal incontinence associated with altered sleep patterns.[74–76] Because of the lower incidence of adverse effects, desipramine and nortriptyline may be preferred over imipramine and doxepin. However, due to their lower anticholinergic activity, they may not be as effective.

Propantheline, a quaternary ammonium anticholinergic and potential treatment, produces a high incidence of adverse effects and is only modestly effective for UUI. When used, propantheline appears to be best tolerated at a dose no more than 15 mg three times daily plus 60 mg at bedtime.[77]

Flavoxate is a tertiary amine that relaxes smooth muscle in vitro. Four controlled trials revealed that flavoxate is no more effective than placebo for treatment of UUI; therefore, flavoxate is not recommended.[24]

Dicyclomine hydrochloride, an anticholinergic agent that relaxes smooth muscle, produced minimal benefit as well as bothersome adverse effects in two small studies.[78]

Hyoscyamine, an anticholinergic and antispasmodic drug related to atropine, has been suggested for treatment of UUI, but data recommending its use are insufficient.[24]

Clinical **Controversy...**

Which approved agent should be used as first-line pharmacotherapy of UUI (oxybutynin, tolterodine, trospium chloride, solifenacin, darifenacin, fesoterodine, or mirabegron)? Financial considerations currently favor generic oxybutynin IR. Choice of an initial agent should be individualized based on tolerability, affordability, and adherence issues. Patient comorbidities may favor the use of more expensive branded agents.

Comparative Data In a meta-analysis, 50 randomized, controlled trials and three pooled analyses were examined for significant difference among anticholinergic agents. Adverse events, particularly dry mouth, were seen less frequently with use of LA products, as compared with IR formulations (oxybutynin and tolterodine). Of interest, the incidence of headache was higher with the use of LA versus IR formulations of tolterodine although LA tolterodine was more effective in the parameters of number of micturitions and volume voided per micturition.[79]

For tolterodine IR, efficacy was similar for the 2 and 4 mg daily doses, while only dry mouth occurred more frequently with 4 mg daily dose. The IR products of oxybutynin and tolterodine were similar in efficacy. Oxybutynin IR was associated with lower tolerability, particularly dry mouth, than tolterodine IR or LA. Oxybutynin IR, TDS (patch), and tolterodine LA produced similar reductions in the number of incontinence episodes. However, the oral agents were associated with higher frequencies of dry mouth and constipation. In contrast, the patch formulation was associated with higher frequencies of local (application site) reactions.[79]

Solifenacin 10 mg daily dose achieved better percentage of patients with a 50% or greater reduction in incontinence episode frequency than 5 mg daily dose, but with higher study withdrawal rates due to adverse events, dry mouth, and constipation. Similarly, darifenacin 15 mg daily dose was associated with higher study withdrawal rates due to dry mouth and constipation than 7.5 mg daily dose.[79]

In a systematic literature review, 94 randomized controlled trials involving drugs for UUI were examined. Overall, drugs for UUI showed similar small benefits.[40] Per 1,000 treated women, continence was restored in this decreasing order: fesoterodine, oxybutynin or trospium, solifenacin, and tolterodine. Rates of treatment discontinuation due to adverse effects in this decreasing order: oxybutynin, fesoterodine, trospium, and solifenacin.[40] Tolterodine was found to be better tolerated than fesoterodine or oxybutynin. More data are needed to assess long-term adherence and drug safety, quality-of-life improvements, and comparative effectiveness among drugs.[40]

Currently, there is no direct comparison between antimuscarinics and mirabegron. Selection of an initial drug therapy most likely depends on side effect profile, comorbidities, concurrent drug therapy and patient preference in drug delivery methods. Table 68-7 lists the adverse event frequencies for the most common events for oxybutynin, tolterodine, trospium chloride, solifenacin, darifenacin, fesoterodine, and mirabegron based on manufacturers' product information.

TABLE 68-7 Adverse Event Incidence Rates with Approved Drugs for Bladder Overactivity[a]

Drug	Dry Mouth	Constipation	Dizziness	Vision Disturbance
Oxybutynin IR	71	15	17	10
Oxybutynin XL	61	13	6	14
Oxybutynin TDS	7	3	NR	3
Oxybutynin gel	10	1	3	3
Tolterodine	35	7	5	3
Tolterodine LA	23	6	2	4
Trospium chloride IR	20	10	NR	1
Trospium chloride XR	11	9	NR	2
Solifenacin	20	9	2	5
Darifenacin ER	24	18	2	2
Fesoterodine ER	27	5	NR	3
Mirabegron ER	3	3	3	NR

IR, immediate-release; LA, long-acting; TDS, transdermal system; XL, extended-release; XR/ER, extended-release; NR, not reported.

[a]All values constitute mean data, predominantly using product information from the manufacturers.

Botulinum Toxin A Enthusiasm is considerable for the application of botulinum toxin A for treatment of voiding dysfunction. Botulinum toxin is a naturally occurring powerful muscle relaxant produced by *Clostridium botulinum*.

Injected into smooth or striated muscle, botulinum toxin acts as a neurotoxin by temporarily paralyzing the muscle. The mechanism of action of the paralytic effect is generally ascribed to prevention of the release of the neurotransmitter acetylcholine into the synapse at the neuromuscular junction, although other pathways in neurotransduction may also be affected.

This compound is commercially produced for medical use in a number of conditions such as muscle spasticity, hyperhidrosis, and cosmetic reduction of skin wrinkles. It is currently indicated for the treatment of refractory UUI associated with neurogenic detrusor overactivity. However, outside of this indication in neurogenic bladder patients, botulinum toxin does not carry an FDA-approved indication in any other lower urinary tract disorders. Nevertheless, it has been used for the "off label" treatment of OAB and nonneurogenic (idiopathic) urge incontinence.[80–82] Despite this lack of a current OAB indication, botulinum toxin is recommended by AUA as the third-line agent in adult patients with idiopathic OAB.[23] In the lower urinary tract, it has also been used to treat external urethral sphincter spasticity by direct injection into the external urethral sphincter.

Botulinum toxin is delivered into the detrusor muscle (intravesical injection) using a cystoscope equipped with a needle. The usual dosage is between 100 and 300 units per session. It is injected through the needle directly into the bladder muscle in 10 to 30 injections spaced over 5 to 10 minutes. The procedure is carried out as an outpatient procedure without general anesthesia. The duration of therapeutic effect varies, lasting usually from 4 to 8 months. Repeat injections are necessary to maintain the beneficial effects.[82]

The adverse effects of botulinum toxin A when used in the urinary tract most frequently include dysuria, hematuria, urinary tract infection, and urinary retention. Urinary retention occurs in up to 20% of treated individuals and persists until the paralytic effects have worn off (up to 6 to 8 months). Therapeutic and adverse effects may not become evident for 3 to 7 days, presumably because this period of time is required for uptake of the toxin following injection.[81,82]

Intravesical (i.e., bladder) injection of botulinum toxin A in patients with refractory OAB resulted in increased bladder capacity, increased bladder compliance, and improved quality of life.[81,82] Adverse effects include urinary tract infection and urinary retention.[81] Comparative data with placebo and other interventions, long-term safety and efficacy outcomes, and data regarding the optimal dose of botulinum toxin for idiopathic OAB are needed.

An alternative mechanism of delivery other than intravesical injection would greatly improve the appeal of this agent as needle injection can be painful in some individuals. Results of an open-label trial of intravesical botulinum toxin A in dimethylsulfoxide in 21 women with refractory idiopathic detrusor overactivity demonstrated a significant reduction in the frequency of incontinence episodes without any effect on postvoid residual urine volumes.[83] Further studies are needed in this regard.

Catheterization Combined with Medications Patients with UUI and an elevated postvoid residual urine volume due to retention may require intermittent self-catheterization along with frequent voiding between catheterizations.

If intermittent catheterization is not possible, surgical placement of a suprapubic catheter may be necessary. Use of a chronic indwelling catheter should be avoided because of the increased occurrence of urinary tract infections and nephrolithiasis.

Regardless of catheterization status, patients may experience symptom relief with oxybutynin (IR, XL, or TDS formulations), tolterodine (IR or LA formulations), trospium chloride, solifenacin, fesoterodine, darifenacin, or mirabegron, as these agents relax the detrusor muscle and enhance bladder storage. Patients with UUI and symptoms of retention may also benefit from an α-adrenergic receptor antagonist that relaxes the internal bladder sphincter (e.g., prazosin, terazosin, doxazosin, tamsulosin, silodosin, and alfuzosin). Although theoretically of benefit, bethanechol, a cholinergic agonist, has not been demonstrated effective in improving bladder emptying in well-done trials. In addition, it causes numerous bothersome (e.g., muscle and abdominal cramping and diarrhea) and potentially life-threatening adverse effects and should not be used in patients with asthma or heart disease.[24]

Urethral Underactivity

7 Urethral underactivity, or SUI, may be aggravated by agents with α-adrenergic receptor blocking activity, including prazosin, terazosin, doxazosin, tamsulosin, alfuzosin, silodosin, methyldopa, clonidine, guanfacine, guanadrel, and labetalol. The goal of therapy for SUI is to improve the urethral closure mechanism by stimulating α-adrenergic receptors in the smooth muscle of the bladder neck and proximal urethra, enhancing the supportive structures underlying the urethral epithelium, or enhancing the positive effects of serotonin and norepinephrine in the afferent and efferent pathways of the micturition reflex.[84]

Estrogens Local and systemic estrogens have been used extensively for the pharmacologic management of SUI since the 1940s. Estrogens are believed to work via several mechanisms, including enhancement of the proliferation of urethral epithelium, local circulation, and numbers and/or sensitivity of urogenital α-adrenergic receptors. However, a trial has questioned whether estrogens exert a stimulatory effect on vaginal collagen production, at least over the short term.[85]

Open trials support the use of a variety of estrogens in the management of SUI: transdermal estradiol, conjugated estrogen vaginal cream, Estring, oral conjugated estrogen, oral quinestradol, oral estriol, intramuscular estrogens, estriol vaginal suppositories, and oral estradiol.[86] Variable effects of estrogen treatment on urodynamic parameters, such as maximum urethral closure pressure, functional urethral length, and pressure transmission ratio, have been noted in these studies. Progestogens have an antagonistic effect compared with estrogens, by reducing genitourinary tract muscle tone.

Results of four placebo-controlled comparative trials have not been as favorable, finding no significant clinical or urodynamic effects for oral estrogen compared with placebo.[87] In fact, observational studies have documented that oral or systemic estrogen use is associated with an increased risk of UI compared with that in nonusers.[88] Systemic estrogen therapy is associated with numerous adverse effects, including mastodynia, uterine bleeding, nausea, thromboembolism, cardiac and cerebrovascular ischemic events, and enhancement of the risk of certain cancers.[88] If estrogens are to be used for treatment of SUI, only topical products should be administered. Estrogen use is best justified when SUI exists with urethritis or vaginitis due to estrogen deficiency.

α-Adrenergic Receptor Agonists Numerous open trials have supported the use of a variety of α-adrenergic receptor agonists in SUI, including ephedrine, norfenefrine, phenylpropanolamine, and midodrine.[86] Phenylpropanolamine was withdrawn from the U.S. market in 2000 because of a risk for stroke in women using the agent.[89] Some patients may have left over supplies of this agent or may obtain it from international sources. If so, individuals with the contraindications listed later in the chapter (especially coronary artery disease and/or cardiac arrhythmias) should be warned against self-treatment with this or other α-adrenergic receptor agonists.

Placebo-controlled comparative trials with phenylpropanolamine, norfenefrine, and norephedrine support the modest efficacy of these agents for treatment of mild or moderate SUI.[86,89] These agents have been found to variably affect maximum urethral closure pressure and functional urethral length.

Adverse effects include hypertension, headache, dry mouth, nausea, insomnia, and restlessness. Contraindications to the use of these agents include the presence of hypertension, tachyarrhythmias, coronary artery disease, myocardial infarction, cor pulmonale, hyperthyroidism, renal failure, and narrow-angle glaucoma.

Several studies have evaluated whether the clinical and urodynamic effects of a combination of estrogen and an α-adrenergic receptor agonist exceed those of the individual therapies in SUI.[90] In general, combination therapy has resulted in somewhat superior clinical and urodynamic responses compared with monotherapy, including severity of complaints, amount of urine lost per episode, number of daily voluntary micturitions, number of leakage episodes per day, patient preference, pad use, maximum urethral closure pressure, functional urethral length, and pressure transmission ratio.

Duloxetine Duloxetine, a dual inhibitor of serotonin and norepinephrine reuptake (SNRI), was approved in 2004 for treatment of depression and painful diabetic neuropathy in the United States.[91] It is approved for SUI in Europe only. It is believed to affect central serotoninergic and noradrenergic regions, which are involved in ascending and descending control of urethral smooth muscle and the external urethral sphincter. These mechanisms facilitate the bladder-to-sympathetic reflex pathway, increasing urethral and external urethral sphincter muscle tone during the storage phase.

The mean terminal disposition half-life, clearance, and volume of distribution of duloxetine in healthy volunteers are 10 to 12 hours, 114 to 119 L/h, and 1,787 to 1,943 L, respectively. The drug is extensively metabolized to inactive metabolites via oxidation and eliminated in the urine as conjugated metabolites. Duloxetine is involved with CYP2D6 and 1A2 enzymes. Duloxetine increased the peak plasma concentration, AUC, and terminal disposition half-life of desipramine, a CYP2D6 substrate, by 1.7-, 2.9-, and 1.9-fold, respectively. Paroxetine, a CYP2D6 inhibitor, increased the peak plasma concentration, AUC, and terminal disposition half-life of duloxetine by 1.6-, 1.6-, and 1.3-fold, respectively. Fluvoxamine, a CYP1A2 inhibitor, increased the peak plasma concentration, AUC, and terminal disposition half-life of duloxetine by over fivefold, 2.5-fold, and threefold, respectively. Thus clinicians must be careful when prescribing duloxetine concurrently with CYP2D6 and 1A2 substrates or inhibitors.[91]

The effect of advancing age on duloxetine pharmacokinetics is not clinically significant. Moderate hepatic dysfunction (Child-Pugh class B) significantly affects duloxetine disposition, increasing mean AUC and terminal disposition half-life by fivefold and threefold, respectively, and reducing clearance 85% compared with controls. Mild or moderate renal impairment (creatinine clearance 30 to 80 mL/min [0.50 to 1.34 mL/s]) does not affect drug disposition. In severe renal impairment (hemodialysis patients), mean peak plasma concentration and AUC are both increased 100%, whereas metabolite concentrations are increased up to 900%.[91]

Results of six large clinical trials with duloxetine in SUI have been published. All were double-blinded, randomized, placebo-controlled, and parallel group in design. Compared with placebo, duloxetine therapy produced significant reductions in incontinence episode frequency and number of micturitions per day, improvement in incontinence quality-of-life questionnaire scores and patient self-assessment, and increase in mean micturition interval. Results were independent of baseline UI severity (severity based on incontinent episode frequency). Significant intergroup differences were seen by week 4. However, cure rates were generally not improved by duloxetine. When evaluating the absolute differences between treatments, the actual benefit of duloxetine was generally quite modest.[91] Duloxetine also reduced incontinence episodes and improved quality of life in men with SUI after radical prostatectomy.[92]

A randomized, placebo-controlled clinical trial evaluated the effects of duloxetine (80 mg daily), pelvic floor muscle training (PFMT), and the combination of both modalities on incontinent episode frequency, incontinence-related quality of life, pad use, and patient global impression of change. Sham PFMT was used in the placebo group. Results indicated that duloxetine plus PFMT were probably additive in effect and that combination therapy afforded greater improvement than either monotherapy.[93]

The adverse events associated with duloxetine may make adherence problematic. In the SUI trials, treatment-emergent adverse events occurred in 68% to 93% of duloxetine and 50% to 72% of placebo recipients. Premature study withdrawal rates (due to adverse events) were as high as up to 33%. The most common adverse events reported with duloxetine were nausea (≤46%), headache (≤27%), constipation (≤27%), dry mouth (≤22%), and insomnia (≤14%). Of interest, the drug may be associated with small increases in blood pressure (like venlafaxine, another dual reuptake inhibitor) and withdrawal symptoms (sleep disturbances). Unfortunately, adherence to long-term therapy is quite poor due to a combination of adverse events and lack of efficacy.[94]

Despite these negatives, duloxetine is the first drug approved by a regulatory agency for treating SUI in Europe. Based on studies conducted to date, a dosage regimen of 40 to 80 mg/day (in one or two doses) appears reasonable. Gradual dose titration (40 mg daily for 2 weeks, then 80 mg daily) helps to reduce the risks of nausea, dizziness, and premature drug discontinuation. If cessation of duloxetine is desired, consider tapering the dosage by 50% for 2 weeks before discontinuation to avoid withdrawal symptoms.

Venlafaxine Venalfaxine is another SNRI. A double-blind, randomized, placebo-controlled clinical trial has demonstrated the benefit of venlafaxine 75 mg once daily for 12 weeks over placebo in terms of incontinence episode frequency, voiding interval, quality of life, and patient global impression of improvement. Nausea occurred in 40% of the venlafaxine group compared with 15% of the placebo group.[95]

Overflow Incontinence

Overflow incontinence secondary to benign or malignant prostatic hyperplasia may be amenable to pharmacotherapy. For management of malignant prostatic disease, see Chapter 108. The pharmacotherapy of BPH is discussed in Chapter 67.

Clinical **Controversy...**

The optimal approach to pharmacotherapy of SUI is unclear. Although not supported by evidence-based medicine, many clinicians initiate a trial of topical estrogen, followed by addition of an α-adrenergic receptor agonist in estrogen nonresponders unless contraindicated. No drugs, except duloxetine in Europe, have been approved for the management of SUI. However, long-term tolerability issues may hinder chronic use.

PERSONALIZED PHARMACOTHERAPY

Patient factors (age, comorbidities, concurrent drug therapies, ability to adhere to prescribe regimen, etc.) should be considered when selecting pharmacotherapy for patients with UI.

All anticholinergic/antimuscarinic drugs have similar contraindications and precautions, including urinary retention, gastric retention, uncontrolled narrow-angle glaucoma, CNS effects, angioedema, and myasthenia gravis. IR formulations of older agents (oxybutynin and tolterodine) have been associated with higher rates of anticholinergic adverse effects (dry mouth, constipation, headache, dyspepsia, dry eyes, cognitive impairment, tachycardia, and urinary retention). Older patients are particularly susceptible to these adverse events, thus requires close monitoring of adverse effects. Significant dry mouth may lead to dental caries, ill-fitting dentures, and swallowing difficulty. Orthostatic hypotension and sedation may lead to falls in patients with baseline cognitive or cardiac conditions. Constipation is prevalent among the older patients because of polypharmacy and age-related physiologic changes.

All patients on anticholinergics should be warned about risk of somnolence and advised not to drive or operate heavy machinery until they know how the drugs affect them. Women with mixed UI or UUI plus urethritis or vaginitis may benefit from a topical estrogen (alone or in combination with an anticholinergic drug). Men with irritative symptoms of BPH that are nonresponsive to drug therapy may benefit from anticholinergic therapy while being closely monitored for the risk of precipitating acute urinary retention.

Anticholinergic drugs should be considered for the management of UUI as monotherapy or in combination with nonpharmacologic interventions. None of the currently available anticholinergic agents appears to have a clear advantage in efficacy over others. Selection of an agent should be based on drug tolerability, dosing convenience, cost considerations, and patient preference. In general, LA or ER products given once daily are preferable over IR ones because of better tolerability. Dose escalation of IR formulations may result in improved efficacy, albeit limited, at the cost of an increase in adverse event frequency and severity. Trospium chloride with its quaternary amine structure and reduced penetration of the brain may be a good choice for patients who are intolerable of CNS adverse effects. Topical formulations, such as oxybutynin TDS or gel, may offer favorable systemic adverse effect profiles and convenient dosing. Selection of an agent should also be based on patient factors, such as renal/hepatic function, concomitant diseases, and concurrent drug therapy. It is advisable to review concomitant medications for any possibility of additive, synergistic, antagonistic drug interactions in cholinergic system and liver enzymes (CYP3A4 and 2D6).

EVALUATION OF THERAPEUTIC OUTCOMES

8 Assessment of patient outcomes should include efficacy, side effects, adherence, and quality of life. During long-term management of UI, patient-specific clinical signs and symptoms of most distress ("bother") to the individual must be monitored. A daily diary may be useful in this regard. Some of the short-form instruments used in incontinence research for measuring symptom impact and condition-specific quality of life can be used in clinical monitoring. In addition, quantitating the use of ancillary supplies, such as pads, may be useful.

9 The main goal of therapy is to minimize the signs and symptoms most bothersome to the patient, as well as the use of pads and other ancillary supplies or devices. Total elimination of UI signs and symptoms may not be possible, and patients and practitioners need to mutually establish realistic goals of therapy. Because the therapies for UI frequently have nuisance adverse effects (e.g., anticholinergic effects such as dry mouth, constipation, sedation, etc.) that may compromise regimen adherence, the presence and severity of adverse effects must be carefully elicited at each visit to the healthcare practitioner. Queries of the patient and caregiver regarding CNS effects are important in elderly or frail patient as these effects can be severe enough to cause loss of independent living skills. Emergence of adverse effects may necessitate drug dosage adjustment or use of alternative strategies (e.g., chewing sugarless gum, sucking on hard sugarless candy, or use of saliva substitutes in xerostomia) or even drug discontinuation. Patient should be encouraged to persist with a particular treatment for 4 to 8 weeks before declaring treatment failure. Nonresponders to an antimuscarinic should be offered at least one other antimuscarinic and/or dose modification attempted to obtain a better balance between efficacy and side effects.

ABBREVIATIONS

AUA	American Urological Association
AUC	area under the plasma or serum concentration-versus-time curve
BPH	benign prostatic hyperplasia
CYP	cytochrome P450
DD01	5-hydroxymethyl metabolite
DEO	*N*-desethyloxybutynin
ER	extended-release
IR	immediate-release
LA	long acting
OAB	overactive bladder
PFMT	pelvic floor muscle training
SUI	stress urinary incontinence
TDS	transdermal system
UI	urinary incontinence
UUI	urge urinary incontinence
XL	extended-release

REFERENCES

1. Abrams P, Cardozo L, Fall M, et al. The standardization of terminology of lower urinary tract function: Report from the standardization subcommittee of the International Continence Society. Neurourol Urodyn 2002;21:167–178.
2. Milsom I, Kaplan SA, Coyne KS, et al. Effect of bothersome overactive bladder symptoms on health-related quality of life, anxiety, depression, and treatment seeking in the United States: results from EpiLUTS. Urology 2012;80(1):90–96.
3. Simeonova Z, Milsom I, Kullendorff AM, et al. The prevalence of urinary incontinence and its influence on the quality of life in women from an urban Swedish population. Acta Obstet Gynecol Scand 1999;78:546–551.
4. Arnold EP, Burgio K, Diokno AC, et al. Epidemiology and natural history of urinary incontinence (UI). In: Abrams P, Khoury S, Wein AJ, eds. Incontinence. Plymouth, UK: Plymbridge Distributors, 1999:199–226.
5. Brown JS, Nyberg LM, Kusek JW, et al. Proceedings of the National Institute of Diabetes, Digestive and Kidney Diseases International Symposium on epidemiologic issues in urinary incontinence in women. Am J Obstet Gynecol 2003;188:S77–S88.
6. Bump RC. Racial comparisons and contrasts in urinary incontinence and pelvic organ prolapse. Obstet Gynecol 1993;81:421–425.
7. Burgio KL, Matthews KA, Engel BT. Prevalence, incidence and correlates of urinary incontinence in healthy, middle-aged women. J Urol 1991;146:1255–1259.
8. Breakwell SL, Walker SN. Differences in physical health, social interaction and personal adjustment between continent and incontinent homebound aged women. J Community Health Nurs 1988;5:19–31.
9. Malmsten UG, Milsom I, Molander U, Norlen LJ. Urinary incontinence and lower urinary tract symptoms: An epidemiological study of men aged 45–99 years. J Urol 1997;158:1733–1737.
10. Andersson K-E, Wein AJ. Pharmacology of the lower urinary tract: Basis for current and future treatments of urinary incontinence. Pharmacol Rev 2004;56:581–631.
11. Kanai A, Wyndaele JJ, Andersson KE, et al. Researching bladder afferents-determining the effects of $\beta(3)$-adrenergic receptor agonists and botulinum toxin type-A. Neurourol Urodyn 2011;30(5):684–691.
12. Fowler C. Integrated control of the lower urinary tract—Clinical perspective. Br J Pharmacol 2006;147(Suppl 2):s14–s24.
13. Blok BF. Brain control of the lower urinary tract. Scand J Urol Nephrol Suppl. 2002;(210):11–15.
14. Kuh D, Cardozo L, Hardy R. Urinary incontinence in middle-aged women: Childhood enuresis and other lifetime risk factors in a British prospective cohort. J Epidemiol Community Health 1999;53:453–458.
15. Groutz A, Gordon D, Keidar R, et al. Stress urinary incontinence: Prevalence among nulliparous compared with primiparous and grand multiparous premenopausal women. Neurourol Urodyn 1999;18:419–425.
16. Ruby CM, Hanlon JT, Boudreau RM, et al. Health, aging and body composition study. The effect of medication use on urinary incontinence in community-dwelling elderly women. J Am Geriatr Soc 2010;58(9):1715–1720.
17. Steers W. Pathophysiology of overactive bladder and urge urinary incontinence. Rev Urol 2002;4(Suppl):S7–S18.

18. Resnick NM, Yalla S. Detrusor hyperactivity with impaired contractile function. An unrecognized but common cause of incontinence in the elderly patient. JAMA 1987;257: 3076–3081.
19. Hall SA, YangM, Gates MA, et al. Associations of commonly used medications with urinary incontinence in a community based sample. J Urol 2012;188(1):183–189.
20. Rovner ES, Wein AJ. Today's treatment of overactive bladder and urge incontinence. Womens Health Prim Care 2000;3: 179–192.
21. James M, Jackson S, Shepard A, Abrams P. Pure stress leakage symptomatology: Is it safe to discount detrusor instability? Br J Obstet Gynaecol 1999;106:1255–1258.
22. Fritel X, Ringa V, Quiboeuf E, Fauconnier A. Female urinary incontinence, from pregnancy to menopause: A review of epidemiological and pathophysiological findings. Acta Obstet Gynecol Scand. 2012;91(8): 901–910.
23. Gormley EA, Lightner DJ, Burgio KL, et al. Diagnosis and treatment of overactive bladder (non-neurogenic) in adults: AUA/SUFU guideline. J Urol 2012;188(6 Suppl): 2455–2463.
24. Cottenden A, Bliss DZ, Buckley B, et al. Management using continence products. In: Abrams P, Cardozo L, Khoury S. Wein A, eds. Incontinence, 4th ed. Paris, France: Health Publications, Ltd. 2009:1519–1642.
25. Shamliyan T, Wyman J, Bliss DZ, Kane RL, Wilt TJ. Prevention of Urinary and Fecal Incontinence. Prepared by the Minnesota Evidence-based Practice Center under Contract 290-02-0009. Publication No. 08-E003. Rockville, MD: Agency for Healthcare Policy and Research, 2007.
26. Urinary Incontinence Guideline Panel. Urinary Incontinence in Adults: Clinical Practice Guideline. AHCPR Pub. No. 92-0038. Rockville, MD: Agency for Health Care Policy and Research, Public Health Service, U.S. Department of Health and Human Services, 1992.
27. Kirchin V, Page T, Keegan PE, Atiemo K, Cody JD, McClinton S. Urethral injection therapy for urinary incontinence in women. Cochrane Database Syst Rev 201215;2:CD003881.
28. Suskind AM, Kaufman SR, Dunn RL, Stoffel JT, Clemens JQ, Hollenbeck BK. Population-based trends in ambulatory surgery for urinary incontinence. Int Urogynecol J 2012, Epub ahead of print.
29. Winters JC. Vaginal mesh update: a look at the issues. Curr Opin Urol 2012;22(4):263–264.
30. Sandhu JS. Treatment options for male stress urinary incontinence. Nat Rev Urol 2010;7(4):222–228.
31. Wilson LC, Gilling PJ. Post-prostatectomy urinary incontinence: A review of surgical treatment options. BJU Int 2011;107(Suppl3):7–10.
32. Welk BK, Herschorn S. The male sling for post-prostatectomy urinary incontinence: A review of contemporary sling designs and outcomes. BJU Int 2012;109(3):328–344.
33. Peters KM, Macdiarmid SA, Wooldridge LS, et al. Randomized trial of percutaneous tibial nerve stimulation versus extended-release tolterodine: Results from the overactive bladder innovative therapy trial. J Urol 2009; 182(3):1055–1061.
34. Abrams P, Cardozo L, Khoury S, Wein A, eds. Recommendations of the International Scientific Committee: Evaluation and treatment of urinary incontinence, pelvic organ prolapse, and faecal incontinence. In: Incontinence, 3rd ed. Plymouth, UK: Health Publications Ltd., 2005: 1589–1630.
35. Van Kerrebroeck PE, Marcelissen TA. Sacral neuromodulation for lower urinary tract dysfunction. World J Urol 2012;30(4):445–450.
36. Rovner E, Kennelly M, Schulte-Baukloh H, et al. Urodynamic results and clinical outcomes with intradetrusor injections of onabotulinum toxin A in a randomized, placebo-controlled dose-finding study in idiopathic overactive bladder. Neurourol Urodyn 2011;30(4): 556–562.
37. Shepherd JP, Lowder JL, Leng WW, Smith KJ. InterStim sacral neuromodulation and botox botulinum-A toxin intradetrusor injections for refractory urge urinary incontinence: A decision analysis comparing outcomes including efficacy and complications. Female Pelvic Med Reconstr Surg 2011;17(4):199–203.
38. van Kerrebroeck PE, van Voskuilen AC, Heesakkers JP, et al. Results of sacral neuromodulation therapy for urinary voiding dysfunction: Outcomes of a prospective, worldwide clinical study. J Urol 2007;178(5):2029–2034.
39. Lam S, Hilas O. Pharmacologic management of overactive bladder. Clin Intervent Aging 2007;2:337–345.
40. Shamliyan T, Wyman JF, Ramakrishnan R, Sainfort F, Kane RL. Benefits and harms of pharmacologic treatment for urinary incontinence in women: A systematic review. Ann Intern Med 2012;156(12):861–874, W301–W310.
41. Ortho-McNeil-Janssen Pharmaceuticals. Ditropan (Oxybutynin) Package Insert. Raritan, NJ: Ortho-McNeil-Janssen, 2012.
42. Ortho-McNeil Pharmaceuticals. Ditropan XL (Oxybutynin Chloride) Extended-Release Tablets Package Insert. Raritan, NJ: Ortho-McNeil Pharmaceuticals, 2012.
43. Watson Pharma. Oxytrol (Oxybutynin Transdermal System) Package Insert. Parsippany, NJ: Watson Pharma, 2012.
44. Cartwright R, Srikrishna S, Cardozo L, Robinson D. Patient-selected goals in overactive bladder: A placebo controlled randomized double-blind trial of transdermal oxybutynin for the treatment of urgency and urge incontinence. BJU Int 2011;107(1):70–76.
45. Pizzi LT, Talati A, Gemmen E, et al. Impact of transdermal oxybutynin on work productivity in patients with overactive bladder: Results from the MATRIX study. Pharmacoeconomics 2009;27(4):329–339.
46. Newman DK. The MATRIX study: Evaluating the data in older adults. Director 2008;16(2):21–24.
47. Watson Pharma. Gelnique 3% (Oxybutynin Chloride 3% Gel) Package Insert. Parsippany, NJ: Watson Pharma, 2012.
48. Watson Pharma. Gelnique (Oxybutynin Chloride 10% Gel) Package Insert. Corona, CA: Watson Pharma, 2012.
49. Gomelsky A, Dmochowski RR. Oxybutynin gel for the treatment of overactive bladder. Expert Opin Pharmacother 2012;13:1337–1343.
50. Sand PK, Davila GW, Lucente VR, et al. Efficacy and safety of oxybutynin chloride topical gel for women with overactive bladder syndrome. Am J Obstet Gynecol 2012;206(2): 168.e1–e6.
51. Staskin DR, Dmochowski RR, Sand PK, et al. Efficacy and safety of oxybutynin chloride topical gel for overactive bladder: A randomized, double-blind, placebo controlled, multicenter study. J Urol 2009;181:1764–1772.
52. Kay GG, Staskin DR, MacDiarmid S, et al. Cognitive effects of oxybutynin chloride topical gel in older healthy subjects: A 1-week, randomized, double-blind, placebo- and active-controlled study. Clin Drug Investig 2012;32(10): 707–714.
53. Pharmacia & Upjohn. Detrol (Tolterodine) Package Insert. New York, NY: Pharmacia & Upjohn, 2008.

54. Gomes T, Juurlink DN, Mamdani MM. Comparative adherence to oxybutynin or tolterodine among older patients. Eur J Clin Pharmacol 2012;68(1):97–99.
55. Pharmacia & Upjohn. Detrol LA (Tolterodine Tartrate Extended Release Capsule). New York, NY: Pharmacia & Upjohn, 2011.
56. Chapple CR, Herschorn S, Abrams P, et al. Efficacy and safety of tolterodine extended-release in men with overactive bladder symptoms treated with an α-blocker: effect of baseline prostate-specific antigen concentration. BJU Int 2010;106(9):1332–1338.
57. Pfizer Laboratories, Toviaz (Fesoterodine Fumarate Extended-Release Tablets) Package Insert. New York, NY: Pfizer, 2012.
58. Kaplan SA, Schneider T, Foote JE, et al. Superior efficacy of fesoterodine over tolterodine extended release with rapid onset: A prospective, head-to-head, placebo-controlled trial. BJU Int 2011;107(9):1432–1440.
59. Allergan. Sanctura (Trospium Chloride) Tablets Package Insert. Irvine, CA: Allergan, 2012.
60. Junemann KP, Al-Shukri S. Efficacy and tolerability of trospium chloride and tolterodine in 234 patients with urge-syndrome: A double-blind, placebo-controlled, multicentre clinical trial. Neurourol Urodyn 2000;19: 488–490.
61. Zellner M, Madersbacher H, Palmtag H, et al. Trospium chloride and oxybutynin hydrochloride in a german study of adults with urinary urge incontinence: Results of a 12-week, multicenter, randomized, double-blind, parallel-group, flexible-dose noninferiority trial. Clin Ther 2009;31(11):2519–2539.
62. Sand PK, Rovner ES, Watanabe JH, Oefelein MG. Once-daily trospium chloride 60 mg extended release in subjects with overactive bladder syndrome who use multiple concomitant medications: Post hoc analysis of pooled data from two randomized, placebo-controlled trials. Drugs Aging 2011;28(2):151–160.
63. Allergan, Sanctura XR (Trospium Chloride Extended-Release Capsules) Package Insert. Irvine, CA: Allergan, 2012.
64. Astellas Pharma Technologies. Vesicare (Solifenacin Succinate) Package Insert. Norman, Oklahoma: Stellas Pharma Technologies, 2012.
65. Chapple CR, Martinez-Garcia R, Selvaggi L, et al. A comparison of the efficacy and tolerability of solifenacin succinate and extended release tolterodine at treating overactive bladder syndrome: Results of the STAR trial. Eur Urol 2005;48:464–470.
66. Kelleher CJ, Cardozo L, Chapple CR, Haab F, Ridder AM. Improved quality of life in patients with overactive bladder symptoms treated with solifenacin. BJU Int 2005;95: 81–85.
67. Herschorn S, Pommerville P, Stothers L, et al. Tolerability of solifenacin and oxybutynin immediate release in older (>65 years) and younger (≤65 years) patients with overactive bladder: Sub-analysis from a Canadian, randomized, double-blind study. Curr Med Res Opin 2011;27(2): 375–382.
68. Herschorn S, Stothers L, Carlson K, et al. Tolerability of 5 mg solifenacin once daily versus 5 mg oxybutynin immediate release 3 times daily: Results of the VECTOR trial. J Urol. 2010 May;183(5):1892–1898.
69. Dwyer P, Kelleher C, Young J, et al. Long-term benefits of darifenacin treatment for patient quality of life: Results from a 2-year extension study. Neurourol Urodyn 2008;27(6): 540–547.
70. Abrams P, Kelleher C, Huels J, et al. Clinical relevance of health-related quality of life outcomes with darifenacin. BJU Int 2008;102(2):208–213.
71. Zinner N, Tuttle J, Marks L. Efficacy and tolerability of darifenacin, a muscarinic M3 selective receptor antagonist (M3SRA), compared with oxybutynin in the treatment of overactive bladder (OAB). World J Urol 2005;23: 248–252.
72. Warner Chilcott. Enablex (Darifenacin Extended Release) Package Insert. Rockaway, NJ: Warner Chilcott, 2012.
73. Astellas Pharma Technologies. Myrbetriq (Mirabegron) Package Insert. Norman, OK: Astellas Pharma Technologies, 2012.
74. Milner G, Hills NF. A double-blind assessment of antidepressants in the treatment of 212 enuretic patients. Med J Aust 1968;1:943–947.
75. Castleden CM, George CF, Renwick AG, Asher MJ. Imipramine—A possible alternative to current therapy for urinary incontinence in the elderly. J Urol 1981;125: 318–320.
76. Lose G, Jorgenson L, Thuriedborg P. Doxepin in the treatment of female detrusor overactivity: A randomized double-blind crossover study. J Urol 1989;142: 1024–1026.
77. Thuroff JW, Bunke B, Ebner A, et al. Randomized, double-blind, multicentre trial on treatment of frequency, urgency and incontinence related to detrusor hyperactivity: Oxybutynin versus propantheline versus placebo. J Urol 1991;145:813–817.
78. Castleden CM, Duffin HM, Millar AW. Dicyclomine hydrochloride in detrusor instability: A controlled clinical pilot study. J Clin Exp Gerontol 1987;9:265–270.
79. Novara G, Galfano A, Secco S, et al. A systematic review and meta-analysis of randomized controlled trials with antimuscarinic drugs for overactive bladder. Eur Urol 2008;54:740–764.
80. Anger JT, Weinberg A, Suttorp MJ, et al. Outcomes of intravesical botulinum toxin for idiopathic overactive bladder symptoms: A systematic review of the literature. J Urol 2010;183(6):2258–2264.
81. Dmochowski R, Chapple C, Nitti VW, et al. Efficacy and safety of onabotulinum toxin A for idiopathic overactive bladder: A double-blind, placebo controlled, randomized, dose ranging trial. J Urol 2010;184(6):2416–2422.
82. Duthie JB, Vincent M, Herbison GP, Wilson DI, Wilson D. Botulinum toxin injections for adults with overactive bladder syndrome. Cochrane Database Syst Rev. 2011;(12): CD005493.
83. Petrou SP, Parker AS, Crook JE, et al. Botulinum A toxin/ dimethylsulfoxide bladder instillations for women with refractory idiopathic detrusor overactivity: A phase I/II study. Mayo Clin Proc 2009;84:702–706.
84. Tsakiris P, de la Rosette JJ, Michel MC, et al. Pharmacologic treatment of male stress urinary incontinence: Systematic review of the literature and levels of evidence. Eur Urol 2008;53:53–59.
85. Jackson S, James M, Abrams P. The effect of oestradiol on vaginal collagen metabolism in postmenopausal women with genuine stress incontinence. BJOG 2002;109: 339–344.
86. Guay DRP. Incontinence. Clin Trends Pharm Pract 2002;(June):entire issue.
87. Jackson S, Shepherd A, Brookes S, Abrams P. The effect of oestrogen supplementation on post-menopausal urinary stress incontinence: A double-blind placebo-controlled trial. Br J Obstet Gynaecol 1999;106:711–718.

88. Grady D, Brown JS, Vittinghoff E, et al. Postmenopausal hormones and incontinence: The Heart & Estrogen/Progestin Replacement Study. Obstet Gynecol 2001;97:116–120.
89. Kernan WN, Viscoli CM, Brass LM, et al. Phenylpropanolamine and the risk of hemorrhagic stroke. N Engl J Med 2000:343:1826–1832.
90. Alhasso A, Glazener CM, Pickard R, N'dow J. Adrenergic drugs for urinary incontinence in adults. Cochrane Database Syst Rev 2005;3:CD001842.
91. Guay DRP. Duloxetine in the management of stress urinary incontinence. Am J Geriatr Pharmacother 2005;3:25–38.
92. Cornu JN, Merlet B, Ciofu C, et al. Duloxetine for mild to moderate postprostatectomy incontinence: Preliminary results of a randomised, placebo-controlled trial. Eur Urol 2011;59(1):148–154.
93. Ghoneim GM, VanLeeuwen JS, Elser DM, et al. A randomized controlled trial of duloxetine alone, pelvic floor muscle training alone, combined treatment and no active treatment in women with stress urinary incontinence. J Urol 2005;173:1647–1653.
94. Bump RC, Voss S, Beardsworth A, et al. Long-term efficacy of duloxetine in women with stress urinary incontinence. Br J Urol Int 2008;102:214–218.
95. Erdinc B, Gurates B, Celik H, et al. The efficacy of venlafaxine in the treatment of women with stress urinary incontinence. Arch Gynecol Obstet 2009;279:343–348.

69 Systemic Lupus Erythematosus

Beth H. Resman-Targoff

KEY CONCEPTS

1. Systemic lupus erythematosus (SLE) is considered a disease primarily of young women, but can occur in anyone. The prevalence and severity vary with sex, race, ethnicity, and socioeconomic factors.
2. Understanding the etiology of SLE and environmental factors that can initiate or exacerbate the disease may make it possible to avoid those triggers.
3. SLE is an autoimmune disease characterized by the presence of autoantibodies, some of which may play a role in the pathogenesis of the disease. An understanding of disease mechanisms can lead to targeted drug therapy.
4. SLE is a multisystem disease that can involve almost any organ and may present in many different ways. Therapy is determined by the manifestations in each patient. These may change and fluctuate in severity over time.
5. Lifestyle changes can modify risk factors for SLE flares and complications.
6. The overall goals of therapy are to prevent disease flares and involvement of other organs, decrease disease activity and prevent damage, maintain remission, reduce use of corticosteroids, and improve quality of life, while minimizing adverse effects and costs. Most patients with SLE should receive hydroxychloroquine alone or in combination with other therapy appropriate for the disease manifestations.
7. Pregnancy planning is essential for good outcomes. Pregnancy outcomes are best when the disease is controlled before conception. Drugs used to treat SLE may adversely affect fertility and the fetus.
8. Antiphospholipid antibodies are associated with arterial and venous thrombosis and obstetric complications.
9. Many drugs can induce a lupus-like syndrome. The manifestations and laboratory findings may be different between the traditional drug-induced lupus and that seen with use of tumor necrosis factor-alpha inhibitors.
10. Since SLE can present in many different ways, it is difficult to design standard response criteria. Development of appropriate criteria is essential for getting new drugs approved.

Systemic lupus erythematosus (SLE) is an autoimmune disease associated with autoantibody production. The term "lupus" was first used to describe a skin disease in medieval times. The name may have been selected since the lesions looked like skin that had been gnawed by a wolf. In the mid-1800s, it was recognized that other organs may be affected and we now know that SLE is a multisystem disease. The common finding in SLE is production of antibodies to self-constituents.[1] This is an exciting time in the management of SLE because better understanding of disease mechanisms has led to the development of new drugs. In addition, new response criteria are being developed to show efficacy of drugs, even with the background of standard therapy. This has led to the first approval of a drug for treatment of SLE in over 50 years. Despite these advances, management of this disease remains a challenge. It has a myriad of manifestations and many of the drugs used to treat it are not approved for this indication. As a result, there is no standard dosing for many of the drugs considered to be standard-of-care therapy.

EPIDEMIOLOGY

1 SLE is generally considered to occur most frequently in women of reproductive age in their late teens to early 40s.[2] This is especially characteristic of the disease in nonwhite women. Statistics regarding SLE depend on the population studied and sampling and recruitment criteria. These have profound effects on estimates of incidence and prevalence, disease activity and severity, and mortality. The incidence is 1 to 10 per 100,000 person-years and the prevalence is 20 to 70 per 100,000 persons. Rates are 10 times higher in women than in men so overall population statistics can be rather misleading. It is affected by ethnicity, which includes genetic, geographic, cultural, social, and other aspects within a group. Rates are two to three times higher in people of African or Asian background than in the white population.[3] It is also more common in Hispanics and Native Americans (called First Nations in Canada) than in whites.[3,4] Most people are of mixed race, so race by itself can be difficult to analyze. Nonwhites tend to have an earlier onset, more severe disease, and a higher mortality rate, but it can be difficult to separate out the influence of socioeconomic factors and access to medical care.[5] The disease tends to be more severe in men, children, and those with onset at a later age (over 50 years).[3]

Survival rates have improved in recent years with better therapy and earlier diagnosis and initiation of treatment. Overall SLE survival is 95% at 5 years and 92% at 10 years after diagnosis. This is reduced to about 88% at 10 years with lupus nephritis and even less than that in African Americans with lupus nephritis.[6] The survival rate may be lower in men, but the small number of males in most studies makes this difficult to determine.[3]

ETIOLOGY

2 The exact etiology for SLE is unknown but many abnormal factors have been identified that appear to play a role in the disease. Some are predisposing factors and others are involved in the disease mechanisms. Categories of these elements include genetic influences, epigenetic regulation of gene expression, environmental factors, hormones, and abnormalities in immune cells and cytokines.[4]

The incidence of SLE is increased in affected families. Siblings of patients with SLE are 20 times more likely to develop the disease than those in a general population. Ten percent of patients with SLE have relatives with the disease.[7] The concordance rate is 25% for identical twins and 2% for fraternal twins.[8] The genetic predisposition to SLE is a result of the interplay of a combination of genes. In rare cases, it is thought to result primarily from a single abnormal gene.[4] The major histocompatibility complex (MHC) class II alleles HLA-DR2 and HLA-DR3 are known to be linked to SLE.[7] An increasing number of other gene loci are being identified as having associations with the disease.[9] Gene expression is regulated by DNA methylation and histone modifications. These epigenetic changes can cause alterations that may influence SLE. Interestingly, hydralazine and procainamide, two drugs that may induce lupus, inhibit DNA methylation.[4]

In a genetically susceptible individual, environmental triggers can initiate the disease. It is possible that the type of trigger may influence the specific organ involvement. Cigarette smoke has many components, such as hydrazine, that may affect the immune system. Chronic smokers and former smokers are more likely to have elevated titers of anti-double-stranded DNA (anti-dsDNA) antibodies. Cigarette smoking is phototoxic and associated with cutaneous lupus.[10] Ultraviolet light can cause keratinocytes in the skin to release nuclear material that can further stimulate the immune system and autoantibody production by B cells.[4,10] Viruses may trigger SLE. Several studies have suggested a potential role for the Epstein–Barr virus.[4] Other implicated triggers include infections, medications (including vaccines and biologics), psychological stress, silica dust, hydrazines, petroleum, solvents (such as nail polish and metal cleaners), dyes, and pesticides.[10]

The greater prevalence in women suggests that hormones such as estrogens and progesterones may play a role in SLE, but the presence of the X chromosome may also contribute.[4] The incidence of SLE is increased in men with Klinefelter's (XXY) syndrome and decreased in women with Turner's (XO) syndrome.[11]

PATHOPHYSIOLOGY

3 SLE is a multisystem disease characterized by disorders of the immune system (Fig. 69-1). T and B lymphocyte activation and signaling are altered in SLE and there is abnormal clearance of apoptotic cells.[8] The number of plasma cells is increased in active SLE and these cells produce autoantibodies, which can cause tissue damage.[4] Antibodies directed at dsDNA are seen in about 70% of patients with SLE and only 0.5% of patients without the disease.[8] The titers of anti-dsDNA may fluctuate with disease activity. Some autoantibodies may play a role in the pathogenesis of clinical features of SLE; these autoantibodies may target Ro/SSA (antigen

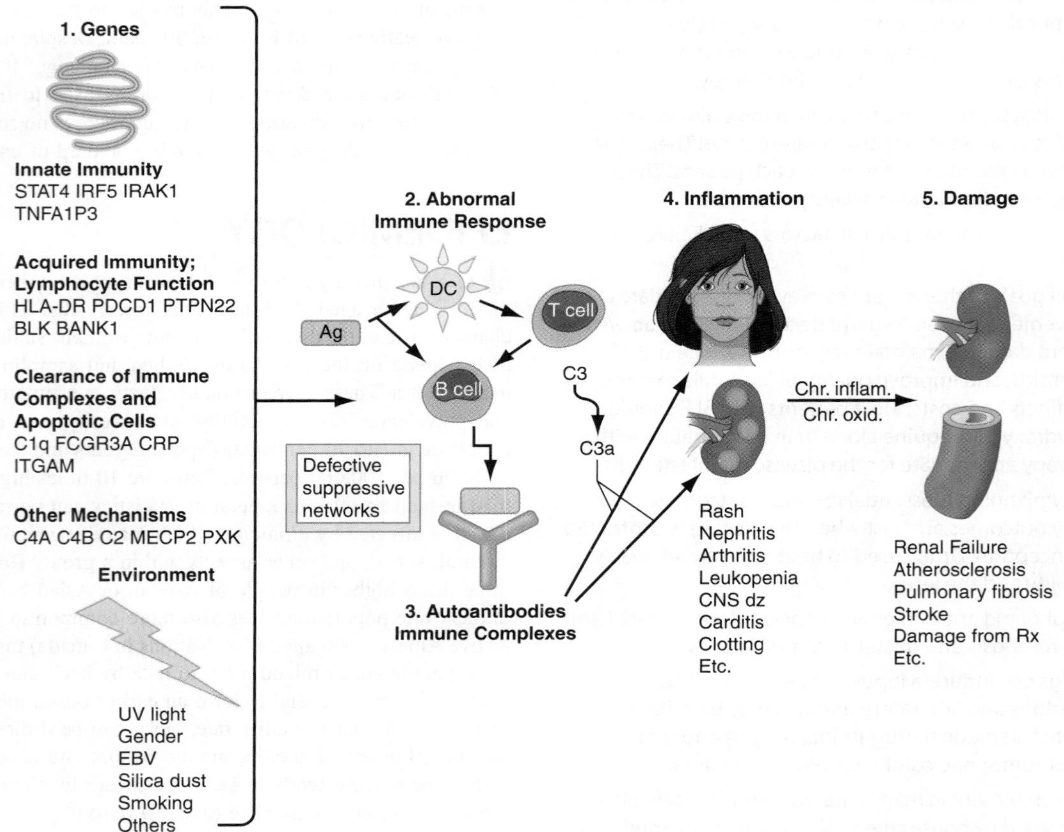

FIGURE 69-1 Pathogenesis of SLE. Listed genes increase susceptibility to SLE or lupus nephritis. Gene–environment interactions result in abnormal immune responses that generate pathogenic autoantibodies and immune complexes that deposit in tissue, activate complement, cause inflammation, and lead to irreversible organ damage. Ag, antigen; C1q, complement system; C3, complement component; DC, dendritic cell; EBV, Epstein–Barr virus; HLA, human leukocyte antigen; FcR, immunoglobulin Fc-binding receptor; IL, interleukin; MCP, monocyte chemotactic protein; PTPN, phosphotyrosine phosphatase; UV, ultraviolet light. *(From Hahn BH. Systemic lupus erythematosus. In: Longo DL, Fauci AS, Kasper DL, et al., eds. Harrison's Principles of Internal Medicine. 18th ed. [electronic version]. 2012, Access Medicine. Chapter 319.)*

Ro/Sjögren's syndrome A, ribonucleoprotein complex), La/SSB (antigen La/Sjögren's syndrome antigen B, RNA-binding protein), C1q (subunit of the C1 complement component), Sm (nuclear particles), *N*-methyl-D-aspartate (NMDA) receptor (amino acid released by neurons), phospholipids, nucleosomes (from apoptosis cellular debris), and histones (protein core of nucleosome). The autoantibodies can be present for many years before SLE is clinically apparent and they may be associated with specific organ involvement, such as anti-dsDNA with lupus nephritis.[2,8]

Immune complexes form when antinuclear antibodies (ANA) bind to nuclear material in blood and tissues, and they can accumulate in the kidneys, skin, CNS, and other sites. They activate the complement cascade, leading to an influx of inflammatory cells and tissue injury. Antibodies to blood cells can cause cytopenias. Antibodies against phospholipids can lead to thrombosis and fetal loss. These antiphospholipid antibodies interfere with protein C and endothelial cell function, inducing tissue factor that leads to thrombus formation. They also cause platelet aggregation. The antiphospholipid antibodies bind to placental trophoblast cells and activate complement, which can lead to fetal loss.[4]

Antigens can interact with MHC molecules on the surface of antigen-presenting cells, such as B cells, macrophages, and dendritic cells. T cells respond to these antigens along with other receptors on the antigen-presenting cells and become activated. Examples of these paired receptors are the CD40-CD40 ligand and CD28-B7. Cytokines produced by activated T cells can stimulate B cells.[8]

Cytokines play multiple roles in SLE. Anti-T-cell antibodies decrease interleukin-2 production, which can increase the risk for infections by decreasing the activity of cytotoxic T cells and increasing the lifespan of autoreactive T cells. Increased T cell production of interkeukin-17 and expression of adhesion molecule CD44 may contribute to kidney and other organ damage. Plasmacytoid dendritic cells accumulate in skin and kidneys and secrete interferon-α. B-lymphocyte stimulator (BLyS), also known as BAFF or B cell activating factor of the TNF family, increases survival of B cells. Interleukin-6 promotes production of antibodies.[4] The role of tumor necrosis factor-alpha (TNF-α) in SLE is unclear. In some patients it appears to be harmful, and in others, protective.[12]

CLINICAL PRESENTATION

❹ SLE is an autoimmune disease that can involve almost any organ and may present in many different ways. This can make it difficult to establish a diagnosis and an extensive work-up may be needed to determine the full extent of involvement and to exclude other possible etiologies for the manifestations. More common features include involvement of the skin and mucus membranes, joints, kidneys, CNS, serous membranes, cardiovascular system, and hematologic cell lines. Fatigue and depression are frequent symptoms and can adversely affect quality of life.[13] Arthritis or arthralgias are experienced by 83% to 95% of patients with SLE.[7] SLE may present differently in men and women. For example, men tend to get SLE at an older age and are more likely to have renal and hematologic involvement, but have fewer dermatologic features. Race and ethnicity may also affect the specific manifestations.[14]

Disease manifestations fluctuate with periods of remission, flares, and progression.[7] The presence of ANA may be used as a screening test for SLE. Most patients with SLE have these antibodies, but they are not specific for the disease.[15]

An international group of SLE researchers developed and validated new criteria for classification of SLE in 2012. These are referred to as the Systemic Lupus International Collaborating Clinics (SLICC) classification criteria and were developed to identify patients with the disease for clinical studies. They are not intended for establishing a diagnosis in an individual patient, but may be helpful in assessing the likelihood that a patient has SLE. The widely used American College of Rheumatology (ACR) criteria were developed in 1982 and revised in 1997. The 1997 version was not validated. The SLICC criteria are more clinically relevant and sensitive than the ACR criteria. When validated, the SLICC criteria had a sensitivity of 97% and specificity of 84% compared to 83% and 96% for the ACR criteria. The number of criteria was expanded from 11 to 17 and, unlike the ACR criteria, they are divided into clinical and immunologic parameters. The ACR criteria required 4 of the 11 elements to be present, serially or simultaneously. To satisfy the SLICC criteria, a patient must still meet at least four of the elements, but now these must include at least one clinical and one immunologic criterion or the patient must have biopsy-proven lupus nephritis with positive ANA or anti-dsDNA antibodies. An abbreviated version of the SLICC criteria, with comparison to the ACR criteria, is shown in Table 69-1.[15–17]

An international working group of SLE experts devised a consensus definition of SLE flare: "A flare is a measurable increase in disease activity in one or more organ systems involving new or worse clinical signs and symptoms and/or laboratory measurements. It must be considered clinically significant by the assessor and usually there would be at least consideration of a change or an increase in treatment."[18]

Some skin involvement is seen in 70% to 85% of patients with SLE.[19] This can be disfiguring and affect a patient's feelings of self-esteem.[10] Three main types of cutaneous lupus erythematosus have been observed. Acute cutaneous lupus erythematosus is typically seen in patients with SLE and is characterized by a malar rash over the cheeks and nose with sparing of the nasolabial folds. The arms and trunk may be involved. The manifestations usually wax and wane without scarring. Severe SLE is less common with the other forms of cutaneous lupus. Subacute cutaneous lupus erythematosus is usually photosensitive and is manifested by annular or psoriasiform plaques that usually heal without scarring. It can be accompanied by musculoskeletal complaints and patients usually

CLINICAL PRESENTATION

Symptoms

- Fatigue, depression, photosensitivity, joint pain, headache, weight loss, nausea/abdominal pain

Signs

- Rash, alopecia, fever, oral and nasal ulcers, arthritis, renal dysfunction, seizure, psychosis, pleuritis, pleural effusion, cardiovascular disease, pericarditis/myocarditis, heart murmur, hypertension, anemia, leukopenia, thrombocytopenia, lymphadenopathy, Raynaud's phenomenon, vasculitis

Diagnostic Tests

- Serology: autoantibodies, antiphospholipid antibodies, complement; inflammatory markers: C-reactive protein, erythrocyte sedimentation rate; blood chemistries; complete blood count; urinalysis; lumbar puncture; renal biopsy

TABLE 69-1 2012 Systemic Lupus International Collaborating Clinics (SLICC) Classification Criteria for Systemic Lupus Erythematosus

Clinical Criteria
1. Acute/subacute cutaneous lupus/malar rash[a]/photosensitive rash[a]
2. Chronic cutaneous lupus/discoid rash
3. Oral *or* nasal ulcers
4. Nonscarring alopecia
5. Arthritis/synovitis *or* tenderness
6. Serositis (pleuritis, pericarditis)
7. Renal (urine protein-to-creatinine ratio [or 24-hour urine protein] representing 500 mg protein/24 h *or* red blood cell casts)
8. Neurologic (seizure, psychosis, mononeuritis multiplex, myelitis, peripheral or cranial neuropathy, acute confusional state)
9. Hemolytic anemia[b]
10. Leukopenia (<4000/mm^3 [4 × 10^9/L]) *or* lymphopenia (<1000/mm^3 [1 × 10^9/L])[b]
11. Thrombocytopenia (<100,000/mm^3 [100 × 10^9/L])[b]
Immunologic Criteria
1. Antinuclear antibody (ANA)
2. Anti-double-stranded DNA (anti-dsDNA)[c]
3. Anti-Sm[c]
4. Antiphospholipid antibody (lupus anticoagulant, anticardiolipin, anti-β_2-glycoprotein I, false-positive rapid plasma reagin test for syphilis)[c]
5. Low complement (C3, C4, and CH50)
6. Direct Coomb's test (without hemolytic anemia)

At least four criteria, including at least one clinical and one immunologic criterion *or* biopsy-proven lupus nephritis with positive ANA or anti-dsDNA required for diagnosis.

[a]In the ACR criteria, malar rash and photosensitivity are two separate criteria.
[b]In the ACR criteria, hemolytic anemia, leukopenia, lymphopenia, and thrombocytopenia count as one criterion.
[c]In the ACR criteria, anti-dsDNA, anti-Sm, and antiphospholipid antibody count as one criterion

Data from Petri M, Orbai AM, Alarcón GS, et al. Derivation and validation of the Systemic Lupus International Collaborating Clinics classification criteria for systemic lupus erythematosus. Arthritis Rheum 2012;64:2677–2686; Tan EM, Cohen AS, Fries JF, et al. The 1982 revised criteria for the classification of systemic lupus erythematosus. Arthritis Rheum 1982;25:1271–1277; and Hochberg MC. Updating the American College of Rheumatology revised criteria for the classification of systemic lupus erythematosus. Arthritis Rheum 1997;40:1725.

have anti-Ro/SSA autoantibodies. Many subtypes of chronic cutaneous lupus erythematosus have been identified. The most common is discoid lupus, which is confined to the head and neck in about two-thirds of patients, but it can be generalized.[20,21] Chronic discoid lupus is the first manifestation of SLE in up to 10% of cases. Discoid lupus progresses to SLE in about 5% to 10% of patients. It is more common in smokers and African Americans. It may be associated with scarring, scarring alopecia, malar rash, photosensitivity, oral ulcers, leukopenia, vasculitis, and chronic seizures. Chronic discoid lupus is associated with a lower incidence of arthritis, end-stage renal disease, and immunologic markers such as ANA, anti-dsDNA, and antiphospholipid antibodies.[19]

Lupus nephritis is present at the time of SLE diagnosis in about 35% of adult patients and 50% to 60% of patients develop it by 10 years. It is more common in African American and Hispanic patients than in whites and more prevalent in men than in women. The International Society of Nephrology/Renal Pathology Society devised a classification system for lupus nephritis based on histologic findings: Class I: minimal mesangial, Class II: mesangial proliferative; Class III: focal (less than 50% of glomeruli involved); Class IV: diffuse (50% or more of glomeruli involved); Class V: membranous; and Class VI: advanced sclerosing (at least 90% globally sclerosed glomeruli without residual activity). Patients with nephritis may also have hypertension and atherosclerosis.[6]

The central and peripheral nervous systems can be involved in SLE. The frequency of this involvement is around 30% to 40%, but depends on the population studied and methods for detecting the occurrence. About 50% to 60% of neuropsychiatric events appear within the first year after the diagnosis of SLE, usually during times of generalized disease activity. Mild nonspecific neuropsychiatric findings such as headache, mood disorders, anxiety, and mild cognitive dysfunction are common in SLE but may not reflect overt CNS disease activity. Findings more indicative of neuropsychiatric lupus include cerebrovascular disease (ischemic stroke and/or transient ischemic attack) and seizures in 5% to 15% of patients; severe cognitive dysfunction, major depression, acute confusional state, and peripheral nervous disorders (e.g., polyneuropathy, mononeuropathy) in 1% to 5%; and psychosis, myelitis, chorea, cranial neuropathies, and aseptic meningitis in <1% of patients. Risk factors include general SLE disease activity, prior neuropsychiatric events, and presence of moderate-to-high titers of antiphospholipid antibodies. It is important to assess contributing factors and to rule out other possible etiologies of these manifestations. The diagnostic approach will vary depending on the clinical presentation and preliminary findings, but can include a thorough history and physical, lumbar puncture with cerebrospinal fluid analysis (mostly to exclude infection), electroencephalogram, serology, complete blood count, blood chemistries, neuropsychological assessment of cognitive function, nerve conduction studies, and magnetic resonance imaging.[22]

Not only are there cardiac manifestations of SLE, such as pericarditis and myocarditis, but patients with SLE are also at increased risk for cardiovascular disease with accelerated atherosclerosis. This is probably related to the chronic inflammation associated with the disease and adverse effects of the drugs (e.g., high-dose corticosteroids) used to treat it.[2]

TREATMENT
Systemic Lupus Erythematosus

Treatment of SLE is determined by the patient's symptoms and organ involvement.

Desired Outcomes

The overall goals of therapy are to prevent disease flares and involvement of other organs, decrease disease activity and prevent damage, maintain remission, reduce use of corticosteroids, and improve quality of life, while minimizing adverse effects and costs. Success in achieving these outcomes depends on disease severity and the type and extent of organ impairment. In general, the prognosis is better if lupus is limited to skin and musculoskeletal findings. The worst prognosis is seen with renal or CNS involvement.[7] Many of the desired outcomes have been observed with antimalarials, although most patients require additional therapy.[23] Survival and quality of life have improved with better understanding of disease mechanisms and new therapeutic options. Mortality is affected by SLE disease activity, cardiovascular risks, and infections.

General Approach

Patients with SLE should be counseled about the importance of lifestyle modifications such as protection from the sun, smoking cessation, exercise, and weight control. The need for immunizations should be assessed with consideration of appropriate timing with respect to immunosuppressive use. The effects of disease activity and treatment on pregnancy outcomes should be discussed. Patients should be evaluated and treated for any comorbidities such as hypertension, hyperlipidemia, and depression. Mild symptoms can be managed with nonsteroidal antiinflammatory drugs (NSAIDs) or acetaminophen.[24] Antimalarial drugs have numerous beneficial effects in SLE and many experts feel that most patients with the disease should always receive one of these drugs.[23] Corticosteroids are used to treat most forms of SLE and up to 80% of patients receive low doses indefinitely as maintenance therapy. The need for osteoporosis prevention should be assessed.[25] If the above therapy is ineffective or major organs are involved, immunosuppressive or immunomodulatory drugs are added.[24] The specific treatment is determined by the organs involved and severity of the disease.

Nonpharmacologic Therapy

❺ Patient perceptions of well-being and quality of life are affected not only by disease activity, but also by social support, coping mechanisms, feelings of helplessness, and abnormal illness-related behaviors.[3] Good social support can improve outcomes, in part by making it easier for patients and their families to navigate the health-care system and utilize resources. Counseling and support groups may help patients' mental well-being and coping mechanisms, but do not affect SLE disease activity. Aerobic cardiovascular exercise may help decrease patients' risk for cardiovascular events and osteoporosis and may also improve fatigue and sleep disturbances, which are frequently experienced in SLE.[26]

Since photosensitivity is common in SLE, patients should protect themselves from the sun by wearing protective clothing and hats and using sunscreens. They should avoid tanning salons.[20] The FDA issued new regulations for testing and labeling of sunscreens that took effect in 2012. Sunscreens labeled as broad spectrum protect against ultraviolet A and B radiation. They have sun protection factors (SPFs) of 15 to 50+.[27] Patients with SLE should use sunscreens with high SPF values and apply them every 2 hours while in the sun.[20]

Patients should be counseled to stop smoking. Smoking cessation is important, not only because it decreases cardiovascular risk, but because smoking can exacerbate SLE and diminish the effectiveness of antimalarials.[28] Smokers also have a higher incidence of active rashes with skin damage and scarring.[29]

Pharmacologic Therapy

❻ Treatment is determined by the manifestations of SLE in the individual patient. It consists of a combination of immunosuppression and symptomatic and supportive therapies. The only drugs approved by the FDA for treatment of SLE are aspirin, prednisone, hydroxychloroquine, and belimumab. The use of other drugs for SLE, even those considered "standard of care," is considered to be "off-label" use. For many of these drugs, the optimal doses and duration of therapy for induction and maintenance of response in SLE have not been determined.

Organization or expert task force treatment recommendations have been published for lupus nephritis, neuropsychiatric lupus, and antiphospholipid antibody carriers.[6,22,30] A committee of the ACR developed guidelines for screening, treatment, and management of lupus nephritis. All patients with nephritis should receive hydroxychloroquine to reduce damage and flares. An angiotensin-converting enzyme inhibitor or angiotensin receptor blocker can reduce proteinuria by about 30% in those with proteinuria of 0.5 g/day or more, and delay progression of renal disease. Blood pressure should be maintained at no more than 130/80 mm Hg. Patients with a low-density lipoprotein cholesterol greater than 100 mg/dL (2.59 mmol/L) should receive a statin to prevent accelerated atherosclerosis. More specific treatment is based on the type of nephritis. The first two classes, minimal mesangial and mesangial proliferative lupus nephritis do not usually need immunosuppressive therapy. Focal and diffuse lupus nephritis (Classes III and IV) are treated similarly with aggressive use of glucocorticoids and immunosuppressive therapy. Figure 69-2 shows the induction regimens for these patients and the levels of evidence to support the recommendations. Patients with a combination of Class V with III or IV would be treated similarly to those with only III or IV. The initial cyclophosphamide or mycophenolate mofetil therapy should be continued for 6 months unless proteinuria or serum creatinine worsens by 50% or more at 3 months (Level A evidence). After 6 months of induction therapy, patients who have improved can be maintained on mycophenolate mofetil or azathioprine, with low doses of corticosteroids if needed. Patients with pure Class V, membranous lupus nephritis, and nephrotic range proteinuria of more than 3 g/day should receive induction therapy with mycophenolate mofetil 2 to 3 g/day with prednisone 0.5 mg/kg/day for 6 months (Level A evidence). Those who improve can be maintained on mycophenolate mofetil 1 to 2 g/day or azathioprine 2 mg/kg/day. Patients who do not respond should be treated with cyclophosphamide 500 to 1000 mg/m^2/month for 6 months with IV pulse glucocorticoids, followed by prednisone 0.5 to 1 mg/kg/day. Patients with advanced sclerosing lupus nephritis (Class VI) should be considered for renal replacement therapy.[6]

A task force of the European League Against Rheumatism (EULAR) devised recommendations for the management of neuropsychiatric lupus. Treatment depends on the manifestations. Symptomatic therapy (e.g., anticonvulsants, antidepressants) should be given as needed. More specific treatment depends on whether the problem is determined to be inflammatory or thrombotic or both. If there is inflammation or neurotoxic damage in the presence of generalized SLE activity, glucocorticoids alone or in conjunction with immunosuppressive drugs such as azathioprine or cyclophosphamide should be given (Strong evidence). If the condition does not respond, other treatments such as plasma exchange, IV immunoglobulin, or rituximab can be tried. If the problem is related to moderate-to-high titers of antiphospholipid antibodies and/or thrombosis, anticoagulants and/or inhibitors of platelet aggregation should be used (Sufficient evidence).[22]

For patients with intermittent joint pain associated with SLE, NSAIDs are good initial therapy. If the pain is more severe or persistent, prednisone in a dose of 10 mg/day or less in combination with hydroxychloroquine should be instituted. Intraarticular corticosteroid injections can be used for localized joint pain. If this therapy is inadequate, methotrexate can be added to hydroxychloroquine therapy. For patients who fail or are intolerant of these therapies, mycophenolate mofetil or azathioprine can be tried. If alternative treatment is needed, leflunomide, belimumab, rituximab, abatacept, or TNF-α inhibitors may be considered.[31]

The first step in management of cutaneous lupus erythematosus is counseling patients to protect themselves from ultraviolet light as described above.[20] Choice of drug treatment is based on the extent and severity of involvement. Topical corticosteroids are commonly used and may relieve symptoms such as itching or burning, but may not provide adequate clearing of lesions when used alone.[20] The choice of corticosteroid depends on the location of application. Low potency corticosteroids (e.g., fluocinolone acetonide 0.01% and hydrocortisone butyrate 1%) should be used on areas with thin skin such as the face, mid-potency (e.g., triamcinolone acetonide and betamethasone valerate) for trunk and extremities, and high potency (e.g., clobetasol propionate) for thick-skin areas such as scalp, soles, and palms. Creams or ointments are used on the body, and foams or solutions on the scalp.[21] Intralesional corticosteroids may be used in discoid lupus, but should not be repeated more often than every 4 to 6 weeks.[20] To avoid the adverse effects of topical corticosteroids, such as skin atrophy, telangiectasias, and rosacea, the duration of therapy should be limited. Alternatively, topical calcineurin inhibitors may be used instead. Pimecrolimus is more lipophilic than tacrolimus and has greater affinity to the skin.[20] Antimalarials have photoprotective effects and are commonly used in the management of cutaneous lupus. If hydroxychloroquine alone is ineffective, quinacrine, available from compounding pharmacies, may be added.

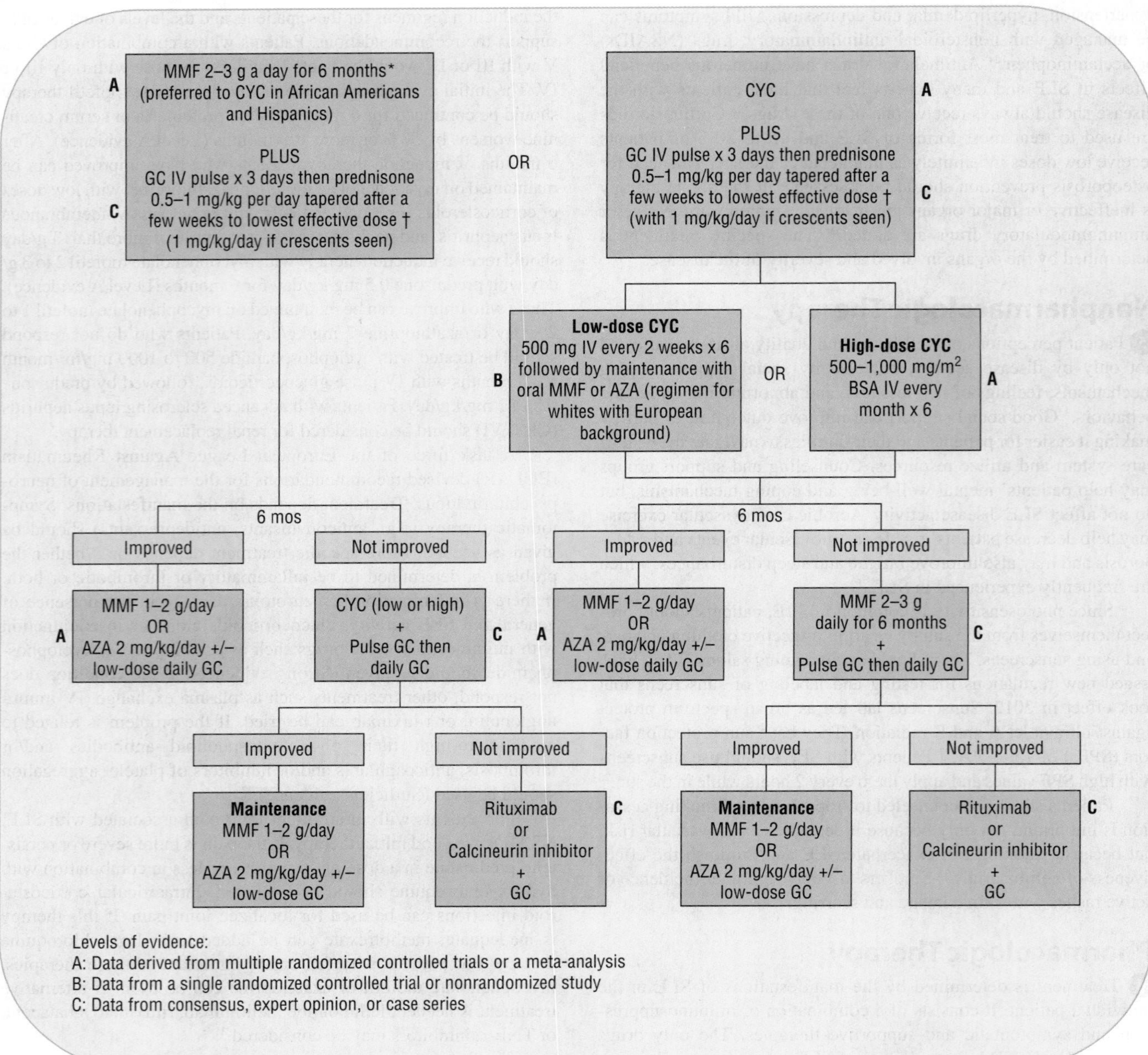

FIGURE 69-2 American College of Rheumatology guidelines for therapy for Class III/IV lupus nephritis. (AZA, azathioprine; BSA, body surface area; GC, glucocorticoids; MMF, mycophenolate mofetil; *, preference of MMF over cyclophosphamide (CYC) in patients who desire to preserve fertility; †, recommended background therapies discussed in text.) *(Modified from Hahn BH, McMahon MA, Wilkinson A, et al. American College of Rheumatology guidelines for screening, treatment, and management of lupus nephritis. Arthritis Care Res [Hoboken] 2012;64:797–808. Figure 2, Page 800.)*

For refractory disease, systemic immunosuppressive (e.g., corticosteroids, methotrexate, mycophenolate mofetil, or azathioprine) or immunomodulatory drugs (e.g., dapsone or thalidomide) may be added. The evidence to support their use in management of cutaneous lupus is mainly on case reports rather than controlled studies. The choice of agents may be guided by other organ involvement.[21]

Specific Drug Classes

Dosing information for selected drugs is shown in Table 69-2. Since most of the drugs used to treat SLE are not FDA-approved for that indication, the doses given are based on other uses for those drugs. Table 69-3 lists adverse effects and drug monitoring parameters. Selected issues concerning the drugs are discussed below.

Nonsteroidal Antiinflammatory Drugs NSAIDs are used as first-line treatment for arthritis, musculoskeletal complaints, fever, and serositis.[32] Low-dose aspirin is used in patients with antiphospholipid antibodies.[30] One concern with use of NSAIDs is that they can decrease renal function, which can complicate evaluation of lupus nephritis. They have the potential to increase cardiac events in patients who already are at elevated risk. Other adverse effects include hepatotoxicity, GI bleeding, and aseptic meningitis.[32]

Corticosteroids Corticosteroids as monotherapy or as adjuncts to other treatment can control flares and maintain low disease activity in SLE. Their effects have a rapid onset, whereas other therapies may take months or over a year to achieve their maximum benefits. The corticosteroids can be used topically or systemically. Although corticosteroids have been used in the management of SLE since the 1950s, optimal doses have not been determined. High doses given in a pulse IV administration regimen are used to treat flares and quickly reduce inflammation. Doses should slowly be tapered down

TABLE 69-2 Dosing of Drugs Used to Treat Systemic Lupus Erythematosus

Drug	Brand Name	Initial or Starting Dose	Usual Range or Maintenance Dose	Special Population Doses	Comments (Adverse Drug Reactions, Special Populations)
NSAIDs/Salicylates	Various drugs				Caution in patients with renal insufficiency, cardiovascular disease, GI problems
Glucocorticoids	Deltasone (prednisone) Medrol (prednisolone)	0.1–1.5 mg/kg/day PO	Prefer <10 mg PO daily		Dose depends on organ involvement and severity; initial dose may be given for 4–6 weeks, then tapered down for maintenance; no standard dose
	Solu-Medrol (methylprednisolone)	100–1000 mg IV daily × 3			Severe disease; later, dose tapered and changed to PO
Hydroxychloroquine	Plaquenil	400 mg PO daily or twice daily	200–400 mg PO daily	Dosing adjustment may be needed with renal or hepatic dysfunction	Dose should not exceed 6.5 mg/kg/day to minimize retinopathy risk
Belimumab	Benlysta	10 mg/kg IV every 2 weeks × 3	10 mg/kg IV every 4 weeks	Use with caution in African Americans; no data on use in hepatic impairment; no adjustment for renal impairment if CrCl ≥15 mL/min; pregnancy category C; no studies in pregnant or breastfeeding women	IV infusion over 1 h; consider premedication to prevent infusion and hypersensitivity reactions; hypersensitivity reactions up to 4 h after administration; most common with first two infusions
Cyclophosphamide	Cytoxan	500–1000 mg/m² BSA IV every month × 6 or 500 mg IV every two weeks × 6		Dosing adjustment might be needed with renal dysfunction; low and high doses may have equivalent efficacy in white patients with European background	Infertility in women and men, teratogenicity of concern
Mycophenolate mofetil	Cellcept Myfortic (enteric-coated mycophenolate sodium)	2–3 g/day PO	0.5–3 g/day PO	Lower doses may be needed in Asians than non-Asians; may be more effective than cyclophosphamide in African Americans and Hispanics	Contraindicated in pregnancy
Azathioprine	Imuran	2 mg/kg/day PO	1.5–2 mg/kg/day PO		Lower dose if thiopurine methyltransferase (TPMT) deficient
Methotrexate	Rheumatrex, Trexall		15–25 mg PO or SC weekly		Decrease toxicity by giving with folic acid
Rituximab	Rituxan	375 mg/m² BSA IV weekly × 4 or 500–1000 mg IV on days 1 and 15		Variable doses have been used	Alternative for patients refractory to other treatments; may be more effective in African Americans

BSA, body surface area; CrCl, creatinine clearance; NSAIDs, nonsteroidal antiinflammatory drugs; PO, orally.

to the lowest effective dose. Corticosteroids are the foundation for treatment of most forms of SLE.[25]

High doses of systemic corticosteroids are associated with infections, myopathy, psychological disturbances, osteonecrosis, and stroke.[25] Psychiatric disease, mostly mood disorder, occurs in 10% of patients receiving prednisone doses of 1 mg/kg or higher.[22] Common side effects of low (less than 7.5 mg prednisone/day) to moderate (7.5 to 30 mg/day) doses are shown in Table 69-3. Although higher doses may be divided, single morning doses may be associated with fewer adverse effects and less adrenal suppression. Chronic use of any dose is associated with coronary artery disease, cataracts, and osteoporosis.[25] Corticosteroids increase catabolism of 25(OH) vitamin D and 1,25$(OH)_2$ vitamin D. Osteoporosis prophylaxis is often found to be inadequate.[33] To avoid adrenal insufficiency, patients on chronic corticosteroid therapy should not have treatment stopped abruptly and they may need increased doses at times of stress such as surgery. Prolonged use of topical corticosteroids can lead to atrophy of the skin and telangiectasias (small dilated blood vessels).[25]

Antimalarials The antimalarials chloroquine and hydroxychloroquine have long been used in rheumatology practice. Hydroxychloroquine is thought to have fewer adverse reactions and is the preferred drug. In the past, hydroxychloroquine was mainly used for skin and joint manifestations of SLE, but now many believe that all patients with SLE should receive hydroxychloroquine. There is high quality evidence that it decreases disease activity and improves survival; moderate quality evidence that it increases bone mineral density and has protective effects against thrombosis and irreversible organ damage; and low quality evidence that it reduces severe flares, enhances the response to other drugs in patients with nephritis, has a beneficial effect on lipids, and protects against cancer. It can allow corticosteroid doses to be decreased. When given to patients with some findings consistent with SLE, it can delay the time for them to fully meet criteria for the disease.[23] Patients receiving hydroxychloroquine often have disease flares when the drug is discontinued.

Hydroxychloroquine has antiinflammatory, immunomodulatory, and antithrombotic effects. It reduces concentrations of inflammatory cytokines such as interleukins 1, 2, and 6 and TNF-α. It inhibits antigen processing and presentation, and T cell signaling. In addition, it decreases activation of toll-like receptors, which are important in the pathogenesis of antiphospholipid syndrome (APS). It reduces red blood cell sludging, blood viscosity, and platelet aggregation.[34] It also delays ultraviolet light absorption and may decrease the number of skin antigen-presenting cells.[35] Finally, it may reduce

TABLE 69-3 Monitoring of Drugs Used to Treat Systemic Lupus Erythematosus

Drug	Adverse Drug Reaction	Monitoring Parameter	Comments
NSAIDs/Salicylates	GI bleeding, hepatic toxicity, renal toxicity, hypertension, cardiovascular events, aseptic meningitis	CBC,[a] platelets,[a] creatinine,[a] urinalysis, AST/ALT,[a] blood pressure[a]	Antihypertensive effects of calcium channel blockers affected less than other classes
Glucocorticoids, systemic	Osteoporosis, cataracts, glaucoma, hyperglycemia/diabetes, hypertension, dyslipidemia, thinning of the skin, weight gain, fat redistribution	Blood pressure,[a] serum glucose,[a] lipid panel,[a] bone densitometry, ophthalmic exams	Patients should receive osteoporosis preventive therapy; high doses of systemic corticosteroids are associated with infections, myopathy, psychological disturbances, osteonecrosis, and stroke
Glucocorticoids, topical	Skin atrophy, telangiectasias	Skin appearance	Avoid prolonged use, especially of high-potency steroids
Hydroxychloroquine	Retinal toxicity	Funduscopic and visual field exams (frequency depends on level of risk), CBC, AST/ALT, albumin, chemistry panel, creatinine	Risk for retinal toxicity increased with doses greater than 6.5 mg/kg/day ideal body weight, more than 5 years therapy, or age over 60 years
Belimumab	Infusion reactions, hypersensitivity, nausea, diarrhea, fever, nasopharyngitis, bronchitis, insomnia, pain in extremity, depression, migraine	Monitor for serious infections, hypersensitivity/infusion reactions, worsening depression, mood changes, or suicidal thoughts	No live vaccines 30 days before or during belimumab therapy; not recommended with other biologics or IV cyclophosphamide; consider premedication with acetaminophen and diphenhydramine
Cyclophosphamide	Myelosuppression, opportunistic infections, hemorrhagic cystitis, bladder malignancy, infertility	CBC,[b] platelets,[b] creatinine, AST/ALT, urinalysis,[b] urine cytology,[a] PAP test[a]	Greater risk for cystitis with oral form than IV; decrease with hydration and mesna
Mycophenolate mofetil	Myelosuppression, nausea, vomiting, diarrhea	CBC,[c] platelets,[c] creatinine, chemistry panel, AST/ALT, chest X-ray	GI side effects may limit use and compliance; these symptoms may be less with use of an enteric-coated form
Azathioprine	Myelosuppression, hepatotoxicity	CBC,[c,d] platelets,[c,d] creatinine,[e] AST/ALT,[c,f] chemistry panel,[e] albumin, TPMT assay, PAP test	Test thiopurine methyltransferase (TPMT) before starting; toxicity greatly increased if deficient
Methotrexate	Hepatic, hematologic, pulmonary toxicity; stomatitis	CBC,[c,g] platelets,[c,g] creatinine,[c,g] AST/ALT,[c,g] albumin,[c] bilirubin, chemistry panel,[h] alkaline phosphatase,[c] chest X-ray	Check hepatitis B and C serologies before starting if at risk
Rituximab	Infusion reactions, infections, neutropenia, mucocutaneous reactions, fever, fatigue, progressive multifocal leukoencephalopathy	CBC,[i] platelets,[i] creatinine, vital signs, human antichimeric antibody (HACA) titers	Consider pretreatment with acetaminophen, diphenhydramine, corticosteroid to decrease infusion reactions

ALT, alanine aminotransferase; AST, aspartate aminotransferase; CBC, complete blood count; PAP, pulmonary arterial pressure.

Monitoring parameters should be checked at baseline and at interval noted: [a]52 weeks, [b]4 weeks, [c]12 weeks, [d]every 1 to 2 weeks after dose change, [e]26 weeks, [f]every 2 weeks after dose change, [g]2 to 4 weeks during 3 months after dose change, [h]8 weeks, and [i]8 to 16 weeks.

Data from Schmajuk G, Yazdany J. Drug monitoring in systemic lupus erythematosus: A systematic review. Semin Arthritis Rheum 2011;40:559–575; Yazdany J, Panopalis P, Gillis JZ, et al. Systemic Lupus Erythematosus Quality Indicators Project Expert Panels. A quality indicator set for systemic lupus erythematosus. Arthritis Rheum 2009;61:370–377; Dennis GJ. Belimumab: A BLyS-specific inhibitor for the treatment of systemic lupus erythematosus. Clin Pharmacol Ther 2012;91:143–149; online.lexi.com. Last accessed February 12, 2013.

cardiovascular risk factors such as hyperlipidemia and diabetes mellitus.[34] The LUMINA (LUpus in MInorities, NAture versus nurture) database was initiated in 1994 to look at differences in SLE outcomes based on ethnic backgrounds. It included African Americans, Hispanics, and Caucasians. Some findings based on study of this cohort are that hydroxychloroquine may delay the occurrence of integument damage (severe skin damage including scarring, ulcers, and scarring alopecia), decrease accrual of damage, and improve survival.[35,36]

Hydroxychloroquine activity correlates with blood concentrations over 1000 ng/mL, but this is not routinely monitored.[37] The drug has a very long elimination half-life that exceeds 40 days.[38] Smoking may interfere with the metabolism of hydroxychloroquine by inducing cytochrome P450 enzymes and thus decrease its effectiveness.[35]

The frequency of adverse effects with hydroxychloroquine is low and they are usually mild. Most common are GI and skin reactions. The main concern is retinal toxicity, but the incidence is low and less than that seen with chloroquine.[21,23] The incidence increases to 1% in patients receiving the drug for more than 5 years or who have received a cumulative dose of 1000 g. Other risk factors are daily doses more than 400 mg or 6.5 mg/kg ideal body weight, advanced age, or patients with kidney or liver dysfunction or preexisting retinal or macular disease. The retinal damage has a characteristic bull's-eye appearance on funduscopic exam and is irreversible. Early recognition of damage may minimize vision loss. The current monitoring recommendations are to have several baseline screening tests including visual fields, then after 5 years, begin annual exams unless the patient is considered to be at high risk, in which case yearly testing would not be postponed. If there are changes suspicious for toxicity, the drug should be stopped, or, after consultation with the patient about risks of blindness, exams should be repeated every 3 to 6 months until the diagnosis is confirmed.[37]

Clinical **Controversy. . .**

Belimumab is an exciting new drug for the treatment of SLE, but its approval trials excluded patients with severe active lupus nephritis or CNS lupus. Results also suggested that the drug may not be beneficial for African Americans with SLE. More evidence is needed to determine the role of belimumab in treatment of these patients.

Biologic Agents Since autoantibody formation is an important feature of SLE, B cells make a logical target for SLE therapy. BLyS, or B-lymphocyte stimulator, is a cytokine that is important for B cell survival, maturation, and differentiation. Belimumab is a fully human IgG1-λ monoclonal antibody that binds to soluble BLyS, which prevents BLyS from binding to receptors on B cells and promotes apoptosis of B lymphocytes. Belimumab is FDA-approved for treatment of autoantibody-positive active SLE in addition to standard therapy. It is the first drug approved by the FDA in over 50 years for management of SLE.[39] Approval of belimumab was based on two international phase III trials: BLISS-76, conducted primarily in Western Europe and North America, and BLISS-52, which was carried out in Eastern Europe, Latin America, and the Asia-Pacific region. These trials had strict entry criteria and used the new SLE Responder Index (SRI) assessment criteria. For both studies, the primary efficacy endpoint was the SRI at 52 weeks. Entry requirements included age ≥18 years old, positive ANA or anti-dsDNA, and active SLE (SELENA-SLEDAI [measure of disease activity] score ≥6) while receiving standard treatment (prednisone, NSAIDs, antimalarials, and/or immunosuppressives [but not cyclophosphamide or other biologics]). Patients had to be on stable therapy for at least 30 days. The most common organ systems involved were musculoskeletal and mucocutaneous. Patients with severe active lupus nephritis or CNS lupus were excluded. Patients received belimumab 1 mg/kg, 10 mg/kg, or placebo by IV infusion every 2 weeks for two doses, then every 4 weeks, in addition to their standard therapy. There were restrictions on concomitant medications, and those became stricter as the studies progressed. The response rate was significantly higher in the group receiving belimumab 10 mg/kg as compared to placebo in both studies.[39] A post-hoc analysis of SRI response in patients of African descent showed that they did not benefit from belimumab and actually had lower SRI scores than those receiving placebo.[40]

Clinical **Controversy...**

There is conflicting evidence regarding the use of rituximab for SLE treatment. Although many believe it is effective, trials have not proven this. The discrepancy may be due to inadequate assessment criteria, selection of study population, differences in efficacy across patient subgroups, or other problems with study designs.

Rituximab is a chimeric monoclonal antibody directed at the CD20 antigen on B cells.[41] Although many case reports and open-label trials have shown benefits of rituximab in treatment of SLE, randomized, placebo-controlled trials have not. The largest of these were the EXPLORER (Efficacy and Safety of Rituximab in Moderately-to-Severely Active Systemic Lupus Erythematosus) trial which evaluated patients with extrarenal involvement treated with rituximab and immunosuppressives and the LUNAR (LUpus Nephritis Assessment with Rituximab) trial that examined use of rituximab with mycophenolate mofetil and corticosteroids in patients with lupus nephritis. Failure to show significant benefit could be due to the short duration of the trials or the choice of endpoints. Further improvement has been observed in the second year of therapy. Exploratory analyses of specific patient subgroups or use of different response criteria suggested some benefit. Rituximab may be more effective in patients of African descent with lupus nephritis than those of other races, or in combination with cyclophosphamide instead of mycophenolate mofetil. It may serve as an alternative therapy in treatment of refractory lupus nephritis, severe hematological lupus, and some CNS manifestations of the disease.[41,42]

Other drugs targeting B cells are being investigated in SLE. Examples of these are epratuzumab, which targets the CD22 cell surface marker on mature B cells, and atacicept which blocks both BLyS- and APRIL (a proliferation-inducing ligand)-mediated B cell stimulation.[43] Other biologic agents have been tried in SLE with varying degrees of success, such as tocilizumab, which inhibits interleukin-6, and abatacept, which inhibits T cell costimulation.[32] The observed efficacy of drugs may depend on the definition of response used. Interestingly, a study of abatacept for lupus nephritis failed to show efficacy, but when other investigators applied endpoint criteria used in different studies of the disease to that data, very different results were observed.[44]

As discussed later, there is concern about TNF-α inhibitors inducing lupus. However, induction therapy with infliximab may confer long-lasting benefits in patients with lupus nephritis. When TNF-α inhibitors are used to treat lupus arthritis, patients respond but relapse within a few months after the drug is stopped.[45] Biologic drugs should not be combined.

Immunosuppressive Drugs Cyclophosphamide has long been used to treat severe organ involvement in SLE such as lupus nephritis, CNS lupus, lung disease, and severe systemic vasculitis.[32,46] Its role in therapy is being redefined because of the availability of newer drugs, as discussed elsewhere in this chapter. Response rate and dosing requirements may vary with patient race. Cyclophosphamide is an alkylating agent that causes crosslinkage of DNA leading to cell death. It may also suppress B cells and IgG production, and decrease production of adhesion molecules and cytokines. Cyclophosphamide has an oral bioavailability of 75% to 100%. It is a prodrug that is metabolized to active and inactive metabolites via the cytochrome P450 enzyme system. Cyclophosphamide is primarily cleared by the liver, but its active metabolites may persist in renal failure.[47]

With cyclophosphamide, there are concerns about the potential for hemorrhagic cystitis and bladder cancer due to acrolein, a metabolite of the drug that concentrates in the bladder. It is thought that the risk is greater with oral administration, higher cumulative doses, and in smokers. The association with intermittent pulse IV doses in SLE patients is less clear. One approach to decreasing these adverse effects is hydration and frequent voiding. With oral administration, patients are advised to take the drug in the morning and to drink fluids for several hours. Adherence is not good with this regimen. With IV administration, IV fluids are begun before administration of the cyclophosphamide and continued for several hours after. Patients are encouraged to maintain oral hydration for 72 hours. Another method to decrease bladder toxicity is to use sodium-2-mercaptoethane sulfonate (mesna), which binds acrolein and prevents its harmful effects on the bladder. Although mesna is sometimes used with high-dose cyclophosphamide, it is only FDA-approved for use with ifosfamide. Use of mesna with daily oral cyclophosphamide is expensive and awkward based on available dosage forms. The recommended mesna regimen with IV pulse doses of cyclophosphamide is to give IV doses, each equivalent to 20% of the cyclophosphamide dose, 15 to 30 minutes before the cyclophosphamide, then 4 and 8 hours after. Since oral mesna is about 50% bioavailable, the 4- and 8-hour mesna doses after cyclophosphamide may be given orally, each in doses equivalent to 40% of the administered dose of cyclophosphamide.[47] In practice, a variety of mesna regimens are used.

Mycophenolic acid (MPA) reversibly inhibits the enzyme inosine 5-monophosphate dehydrogenase (IMPDH), which is important for de novo synthesis of purine (guanosine) nucleotides. This inhibits proliferation and differentiation of lymphocytes. The drug also has other immunomodulating effects such as induction of activated T cell apoptosis, inhibition of adhesion molecule expression, and antifibrotic and antiproliferative effects on cells such as fibroblasts, dendritic cells, and vascular smooth muscle cells.[48]

Mycophenolate mofetil is hydrolyzed to MPA, its active form. The mofetil salt has greater bioavailability. MPA is bound to albumin, so unbound drug concentrations can be affected by changes in albumin. MPA is glucuronidated in the liver to an inactive metabolite, mycophenolic glucuronide. The metabolite undergoes enterohepatic recycling, with conversion back to the active form.[48]

Mycophenolate mofetil has been most studied in treatment of lupus nephritis. It has been shown to be at least as effective as cyclophosphamide for induction therapy and as azathioprine for maintenance treatment. The Aspreva Lupus Management Study (ALMS) was a multinational study of lupus nephritis in 370 patients. The 6-month induction phase showed mycophenolate mofetil to be equivalent in efficacy to monthly IV pulse doses of cyclophosphamide, including in a small group of patients with an estimated glomerular filtration rate (eGFR) less than 30 mL/min (0.5 mL/s).[48] The response to therapy at 6 months correlated with the baseline complement C4 concentration, time since diagnosis of lupus nephritis, and eGFR. Normalization of complement C3 and/or C4 and reduction in proteinuria of at least 25% at 8 weeks also predicted renal improvement at 6 months.[49] In the 36-month maintenance phase, mycophenolate mofetil was superior to azathioprine in maintaining renal response to treatment and preventing disease relapse. Although adverse events occurred in more than 97% of patients in both groups, more patients receiving azathioprine withdrew from the study due to toxicity than those receiving mycophenolate mofetil.[50] The MAINTAIN trial did not find a difference in the rate of renal flare with mycophenolate mofetil compared to azathioprine 5 years after induction with IV cyclophosphamide. The difference in these results compared to the ALMS trial may be due to the difference in populations studied. The MAINTAIN trial studied 105 predominantly white European patients, whereas the larger ALMS trial included a more racially diverse population.[48]

Mycophenolate mofetil may also be useful for other manifestations of SLE such as arthritis, cutaneous lupus, and hematologic involvement, including hemolytic anemia and thrombocytopenia.[48]

The most common adverse effects observed with mycophenolate mofetil are GI, including nausea, vomiting, and diarrhea. These may be severe enough to require discontinuation of therapy. Hematologic effects such as red cell aplasia may also be seen. The side effects may be diminished with a reduction in dose. Use of an enteric-coated form may decrease GI symptoms. Numerous congenital malformations have been reported with mycophenolate mofetil and it is contraindicated in pregnancy.[48]

Azathioprine is a purine analog that is metabolized to mercaptopurine. It inhibits DNA synthesis and prevents immune cell proliferation. Mercaptopurine is inactivated by thiopurine methyltransferase (TPMT). If activity of that enzyme is low, patients may experience severe toxicity such as myelosuppression and hepatotoxicity. The metabolism of azathioprine and mercaptopurine is also inhibited by allopurinol and febuxostat. If the combination of these drugs is to be used, a reduction in dose is required.[51] Azathioprine is less effective than cyclophosphamide for induction therapy in lupus nephritis, but it can be useful as an alternative to mycophenolate mofetil for maintenance treatment.[6] Azathioprine may also be used for SLE-related arthritis, serositis, mucocutaneous manifestations, and for hematologic involvement. It has steroid-sparing effects, allowing use of lower doses of corticosteroids.[32,46]

Methotrexate is an inhibitor of folic acid reductase, which is needed for DNA synthesis and cell growth. Its toxicities are reduced by administration of folic acid. It is important to note that it is dosed once weekly in the management of SLE. It is used for arthritis and skin disease and as a steroid-sparing drug.[32]

Numerous other immunosuppressive drugs have been used in SLE, especially in patients who have contraindications to use of the agents already discussed or who cannot tolerate them, or those whose disease is refractory to conventional treatment.

Alternative Treatments

Studies have shown that SLE patients receiving conventional treatment frequently feel they have unmet needs. Often these are psychosocial and may include anxiety or depression. These needs can lead patients to try alternative therapies. It is important for healthcare providers to have an open dialogue with patients about these therapies so that patients will report them. This allows practitioners to monitor for interactions with other treatments and to guide patients to therapies with greater potential for benefit and less for harm.[26]

The ACR has defined complementary and alternative medicine as treatments, products, and practices that are outside the realm of traditional allopathic medicine. In general, these have not been evaluated in randomized controlled trials involving SLE patients.[26]

Concentrations of dehydroepiandrosterone (DHEA), a weak androgen, are typically decreased in SLE. Some small studies have suggested that DHEA supplementation may offer some limited benefit for health-related quality of life (HRQoL) in SLE.[26]

Clinical **Controversy...**

Vitamin D promotes bone and heart health and contributes to immune response; deficiency may be associated with greater SLE disease activity, flares, and fatigue. Concentrations of vitamin D are commonly decreased in SLE, and it has been suggested that all patients with the disease should receive vitamin D supplementation. However, not all experts agree and appropriate target vitamin D concentrations are yet to be determined.

Vitamin D concentrations are decreased in SLE, especially in patients with high disease activity and those with darker skin pigmentation (e.g., African Americans). A contributing factor to the deficiency is that patients are told to protect themselves from sunlight because of the photosensitivity that accompanies SLE.[33] This can not only affect bone health, but there are some data showing that low concentrations of vitamin D may also be associated with greater SLE disease activity, flares, and fatigue.[52–54] Vitamin D plays a role in the immune response, including suppression of T lymphocyte proliferation, inhibition of immunoglobulin production by B cells, and effects on dendritic cells, which affect protective immunity and self-tolerance. Vitamin D also has cardioprotective effects and may decrease cancer risks.[33] Some experts suggest that most patients with SLE should receive vitamin D supplements of at least 400 IU/day of vitamin D3.[20] One recommendation is to check a baseline 25(OH) vitamin D concentration with a current goal of 30 ng/mL (75 nmol/L). An optimal goal has not yet been determined. The concentration should be rechecked 3 months after a change in vitamin D dosing since that is the time required to reach steady state.[33]

Special Populations

Pregnancy and Contraception ❼ Pregnancy planning with assessment of risk factors is key for achieving good outcomes for women with SLE and healthy babies. Timing of pregnancies with respect to disease activity and use of teratogenic medications make contraception counseling very important. Cyclophosphamide therapy is associated with ovarian failure and infertility. This is especially of concern in older women who wish to conceive. Estrogen-containing oral contraceptives are associated with SLE flares and thrombosis. Although recent studies did not show an association with disease exacerbation, the results may be influenced by study inclusion and exclusion criteria.[55] Estrogen replacement may increase the risk of thrombosis in postmenopausal women.[10] Progesterone-only contraceptives may be used but the risk of osteoporosis increases after 2 years of use. Intrauterine devices or barrier methods with spermicides may be better choices for contraception.[55]

Pregnancy during SLE is considered to be high risk. The risk of maternal mortality, cesarean delivery, preterm labor, and preeclampsia and the risk of thrombotic, infectious, and hematologic complications are increased. Fetal loss and growth retardation may relate to placental pathology with vascular changes and thrombi, even in the absence of antiphospholipid antibodies. Complement activation may contribute to these occurrences. Preeclampsia occurs in 10% to 25% of women with SLE and is defined as hypertension (BP >140/90) and proteinuria (>300 mg/24 h) that develop for the first time after 20 weeks of gestation. This can be difficult to distinguish from lupus nephritis. The risk for preeclampsia and fetal loss may be decreased with daily use of low-dose aspirin.[56] Flares during pregnancy may be difficult to identify since they may share characteristics of a normal pregnancy. The complications are more likely in patients with active disease, especially lupus nephritis. If the mother has anti-Ro/SSA or anti-La/SSB antibodies, the fetus is at risk for neonatal lupus with rash and cardiac abnormalities including heart block. Treatment of pregnant women with antiphospholipid antibodies is discussed below. Pregnancy should be discouraged in patients with severe pulmonary hypertension, advanced renal insufficiency, severe restrictive lung disease, heart failure, or a history of severe preeclampsia. It also is not advised within 6 months of a severe SLE flare, active lupus nephritis, or a stroke. The best pregnancy outcomes are observed in patients who have had inactive disease for at least 6 months prior to the pregnancy. Drugs used to control the SLE should be those such as hydroxychloroquine, which can be continued throughout the pregnancy and may decrease the incidence of flares. Any potentially teratogenic drugs (e.g., methotrexate, leflunomide, mycophenolate, cyclophosphamide, and thalidomide) should be stopped at least 3 months before attempting pregnancy. Leflunomide should be removed through the oral cholestyramine elimination procedure (8 g three times a day for 11 days with confirmation of undetectable serum concentrations) prior to conception. Close monitoring and disease management of the mothers and fetuses are essential during pregnancy. The risks of drug use and harmful effects of disease flare both need to be considered. If a flare occurs and an immunosuppressive drug is required during the pregnancy, azathioprine may be considered, since the fetal liver is unable to metabolize it to its active form.[55] The dose should not exceed 2 mg/kg/day.[6] If corticosteroids are needed, maintenance doses should be kept at the equivalent of prednisone 10 mg daily or less to decrease the risk of gestational diabetes mellitus, infections, and premature rupture of membranes.[25,55] Fluorinated corticosteroids (such as dexamethasone or betamethasone) should be avoided unless they are being used to treat the fetus, since they cross the placenta. Cyclophosphamide should only be used during pregnancy if alternatives failed and the mother's life is in danger. If treatment of hypertension is needed, methyldopa and labetalol are preferred with nifedipine considered as an alternative. Angiotensin-converting enzyme inhibitors and angiotensin receptor blockers may damage the fetal kidneys and cause fetal loss. Diuretics are generally avoided but if one is needed, furosemide is preferred.[55]

SLE–Antiphospholipid Syndrome Overlap 8 The antiphospholipid antibodies consist of anticardiolipin, anti-β-2-glycoprotein I, and lupus anticoagulant and they can promote clotting and inflammation.[57] The diagnosis of APS requires clinical and laboratory features. The clinical aspects are vascular events such as venous or arterial thrombi and/or obstetric complications. The obstetric complications meeting the criteria are three or more unexplained consecutive miscarriages before the tenth week of gestation, one or more unexplained deaths of fetuses at or beyond the tenth week of gestation, and one or more births of infants before the 34th week of gestation associated with eclampsia or severe preeclampsia.[57] Adverse pregnancy outcomes after 12 weeks of gestation are especially associated with the presence of lupus anticoagulant.[58] Laboratory criteria are the presence of antiphospholipid antibodies on two separate occasions, 12 weeks apart.[59] Antiphospholipid antibodies are found in about 40% of patients with SLE, but less than 40% of those experience thrombotic events.[57] Patients with lupus anticoagulant or persistently positive anticardiolipin at medium-high titers are at high risk for thrombosis, and those with all three antibodies (triple positivity) are at highest risk. Patients with isolated, intermittently positive anticardiolipin or anti-β_2-glycoprotein I at low-medium titers are considered to be at low risk. Patients with thrombosis often have other cardiovascular risk factors (such as hypertension, hyperlipidemia, smoking, or use of estrogen-containing medications) or an underlying autoimmune disease such as SLE. It is recommended that any modifiable factors be controlled. In deciding choice, intensity, and duration of treatment, the clinician should balance benefits with the patient's risk of bleeding. Consideration should also be given to whether thrombotic events are associated with identified transient precipitating factors. An international group of physicians who had clinical and research experience with APS reviewed the literature and developed consensus guidelines for management of thrombosis in patients with antiphospholipid antibodies (Table 69-4).[30]

TABLE 69-4 Recommendations for Thromboprophylaxis in Patients with Systemic Lupus Erythematosus and Antiphospholipid Antibodies

Recommendation	Grade of Recommendation
1. General measures for aPL carriers	
Control cardiovascular risk factors if high risk aPL profile	Nongraded
Thromboprophylaxis with low-molecular-weight heparin in high-risk situations such as surgery, prolonged immobilization, and after childbirth	1C
2. Primary thromboprophylaxis	
Regularly assess patients for presence of aPL	Nongraded
Thromboprophylaxis with hydroxychloroquine (1) and low-dose aspirin (2) for patients with positive LA or persistent aCL at medium-high titers	1B (1) 2B (2)
3. Secondary thromboprophylaxis	
Treat patients with arterial or venous thrombosis and aPL who do not meet APS criteria with standard thrombosis treatment	1C
Treat patients with definite APS and first venous event with warfarin to target INR 2–3	1B
Treat patients with definite APS and arterial thrombosis with warfarin at INR greater than 3 or combined antiaggregant-warfarin (INR 2–3) therapy	Nongraded
Assess bleeding risk before high-intensity warfarin or combined antiaggregant-warfarin therapy	Nongraded
4. Duration of treatment	
Indefinite antithrombotic therapy in patients with definite APS and thrombosis	1C
For the first venous event, low-risk APS profile and known transient precipitating factor, anticoagulate for 3–6 months	Nongraded
5. Refractory and difficult cases	
If recurrent thrombosis, fluctuating INR, major bleeding or high risk for major bleeding, consider alternative such as low-molecular-weight heparin, hydroxychloroquine, or statins	Nongraded

aPL, antiphospholipid; LA, lupus anticoagulant; aCL, anticardiolipin; APS, antiphospholipid syndrome; INR, international normalized ratio.

Grades of recommendation: 1B: Strong recommendation, moderate quality evidence; 1C: Strong recommendation, low or very low-quality evidence; 2B: Weak recommendation, moderate quality evidence; and 2C: Weak recommendation, low or very low-quality evidence.

Adapted from Ruiz-Irastorza G, Cuadrado MJ, Ruiz-Arruza I, et al. Evidence-based recommendations for the prevention and long-term management of thrombosis in antiphospholipid antibody-positive patients: Report of a Task Force at the 13th International Congress on Antiphospholipid Antibodies. Lupus 2011;20:206–218, Table 6, page 215. Reprinted by permission of SAGE.

Patients with antiphospholipid antibodies may also have a false-positive test for syphilis (rapid plasma reagin).[15] Other common manifestations of APS are cognitive impairment, thrombocytopenia, stroke or transient ischemic attack, migraine, and livedo reticularis.[57]

It is not clear how to treat pregnant women with antiphospholipid antibodies. Those with no history of thrombosis who have experienced early fetal loss may be treated with low-dose aspirin (81 mg) alone or in combination with prophylactic doses of heparin or low-molecular-weight heparin.[57] Not only does heparin have anticoagulant effects, but it also can inhibit complement activation.[4] Those without thrombosis who have had later miscarriages or premature births associated with eclampsia or preeclampsia may receive low dose aspirin plus prophylactic or intermediate doses of heparin or prophylactic doses of low-molecular-weight heparin. Pregnant patients with APS and a history of thrombosis should receive low-dose aspirin with therapeutic doses of heparin or low-molecular-weight heparin. Warfarin should be avoided during pregnancy; it is teratogenic between 6 and 12 weeks gestation and increases the risk of fetal bleeding after 12 weeks.[57] If low-molecular-weight heparin is used, it should be switched to unfractionated heparin 4 weeks before the anticipated delivery date. The heparin should be stopped at the start of labor or 8 hours before a planned cesarean delivery.[55] All women with APS should receive anticoagulation with prophylactic doses of heparin, low-molecular-weight heparin, or warfarin for 4 to 6 weeks postpartum. Both heparin and warfarin are safe during breastfeeding.[57]

For patients who do not respond to conventional APS therapy or for whom it is contraindicated, alternative therapies include other platelet inhibitors, new oral anticoagulants, hydroxychloroquine, statins, and rituximab.[57]

The most severe form of APS is called catastrophic and is associated with widespread thrombosis, multiorgan failure, and greater than 50% mortality.[57]

Drug-Induced Lupus 9 About 10% of cases of SLE can be attributed to drugs. These are idiosyncratic reactions precipitated by the interplay of genetic predisposition, concurrent illnesses, environmental factors, and other drugs or foods. Various pathophysiologic mechanisms have been proposed for different drugs in inducing lupus. Most drugs are small molecules that can induce an immune response by binding to larger molecules such as proteins, a process called haptenization. Another proposed mechanism is interfering with macrophage uptake of apoptotic or necrotic cells, leading to accumulation of nucleosomes that can be targets for anti-DNA antibodies.[60]

Because drug-induced lupus can be so diverse in its manifestations, there are no standard diagnostic criteria. The diagnosis is based on lupus-like findings in a patient with no history of the disease and the temporal relationship with the drug, including onset after initiation and loss of manifestations within weeks to months after the drug is discontinued. The time-frame, however, can be variable.[60]

Many drugs of varied classes have been implicated. The drugs considered to have the highest risk for inducing traditional drug-induced lupus are procainamide (20%) and hydralazine (5–8%), especially with hydralazine doses over 200 mg per day. Common manifestations include arthralgias, arthritis, and myalgias. Constitutional symptoms such as fever, fatigue, and weight loss are common, but the incidence is about one-half that seen with idiopathic SLE. Other clinical features include rash, serositis (pleuritis, pericarditis), hematologic abnormalities, and hepatosplenomegaly. Glomerulonephritis and neuropsychiatric symptoms are rare in drug-induced lupus. The incidence and types of reactions vary depending on the offending drug. Laboratory abnormalities associated with drug-induced lupus include positive ANA (99%) and antibodies to histones (96%). Other antibodies such as anticardiolipin (5 to 20%), anti-dsDNA (less than 5%), and antineutrophil cytoplasmic antibodies (ANCA) may be seen with some drugs. A drug with moderate risk for lupus is quinidine. The incidence of quinidine- and procainamide-induced lupus is declining because of decreased prescribing of the drugs and use of lower doses. The other almost 100 drugs of many different classes that have been implicated are considered to be of low risk. One that affects younger patients, including children, is minocycline.[60] Other drugs with well-established links to lupus are isoniazid, methyldopa, and chlorpromazine.[10] A variant of the syndrome is drug-induced subacute cutaneous lupus, which has been associated with calcium channel antagonists, thiazide diuretics, angiotensin-converting enzyme inhibitors, and terbinafine. The mean age for this syndrome is 58 years; most patients are white women, and 80% have anti-Ro/SSA antibodies. It may occur after weeks to years of therapy.[61] Chronic cutaneous lupus has been reported with fluorouracil and NSAIDs.[60] It can take months for skin lesions to resolve after the offending drug has been stopped.[10]

A separate category of drug-induced lupus is that involving TNF-α inhibitors, such as adalimumab, etanercept, and infliximab. These are known to induce autoantibodies. Other theories explaining the mechanism for TNF-α inhibitor-induced lupus are that they cause a shift into other pathways of cytokine production or that they interfere with apoptosis.[60] It is common for patients receiving these drugs to develop positive ANAs and anti-dsDNA. Antihistone antibodies are less commonly seen than with other drug-induced lupus (17% to 57%).[62] As with traditional drug-induced lupus, the incidence of clinical lupus is low compared to the numbers that develop autoantibodies. Rashes, hypocomplementemia, leukopenia, and thrombocytopenia are more common features with TNF-α inhibitors than traditional drug-induced lupus, and arthralgias, arthritis, and myalgias are less common. The underlying diseases being treated with these drugs may be a factor in development of the observed reactions. Autoimmune diseases have also been reported following use of interferon therapy.[60]

The primary treatment for drug-induced lupus is stopping the implicated drug. Some patients require treatment with topical or systemic corticosteroids and supportive care, and a few may require immunosuppressive therapy.[60,62]

Immunizations

Patients with SLE are at increased risk for infections because of immune dysfunction caused by the disease itself and the immunosuppressive therapy the patients receive. It is important to try to protect patients against these infections, but there are areas of concern regarding the safety and efficacy of vaccines in patients with SLE. SLE cases developing or flaring after vaccine administration have been reported; the actual risk appears low when considering how many people receive immunizations. Another concern is that immunosuppressed patients may have an impaired response to vaccines as compared with healthy individuals. This can be assessed by checking titers after immunization. In some cases revaccination may be needed. Whenever possible, to achieve the best response, vaccines should be administered prior to initiating immunosuppressive medications. Killed vaccines are considered safe in immunosuppressed patients. It is recommended that SLE patients receive pneumococcal vaccine, since they are particularly susceptible to *Streptococcus pneumoniae* infections. They should also receive annual influenza vaccines, and, if considered to be at risk, hepatitis B vaccine. Live-attenuated virus vaccines, such as measles–mumps–rubella, varicella, zoster, intranasal influenza, and yellow fever, are contraindicated in patients receiving biologic agents.[63] They should be avoided with consideration of risks versus benefits in patients taking high doses of other immunosuppressive drugs.[64,65] Doses of corticosteroids equivalent to prednisone 20 mg/day or more given for at least 2 weeks are considered immunosuppressive.[63] Live vaccines should be given at least 2 to 4 weeks before starting immunosuppressive drugs or 3 months after stopping them.[63,66]

PERSONALIZED PHARMACOTHERAPY

Pharmacotherapy is determined by disease manifestations and patient-specific factors. Hydroxychloroquine should be considered for all patients with SLE. Comorbidities and organ function should be considered in selection of therapy, as previously discussed.

Race appears to influence response to treatment, but many people are of mixed race. Genetic testing may provide a better guide in the future. In studies of lupus nephritis, whites with Western or Southern European backgrounds respond as well to low-dose IV cyclophosphamide ("Euro-Lupus" regimen of 500 mg every 2 weeks for six doses) as to high-dose regimens (500 to 1000 mg/m^2 body surface area once a month for six doses) (Level B evidence). African Americans and Hispanics respond less well to IV cyclophosphamide than do whites or Asians. Patients of African or Hispanic origin may respond better to mycophenolate mofetil than to cyclophosphamide. Asians require lower doses of mycophenolate mofetil (Level C evidence).[6] African Americans with lupus nephritis may respond to rituximab better than whites.[42] Patients of African descent did not respond to belimumab in the BLISS studies.[40]

Blood concentrations of drugs are not usually measured in SLE management, even for drugs that are monitored that way when used for other diseases. Hydroxychloroquine blood concentrations appear to correlate with efficacy, but they are not routinely monitored.[37] Although therapeutic mycophenolate drug concentration monitoring is used in transplant patients, it is not yet common practice in SLE patients. Preliminary studies have shown that MPA area under the plasma concentration–time curve appears to correlate with SLE disease activity but not adverse effects or daily doses.[48] Patients should have TPMT testing before receiving azathioprine[51] and be screened for glucose-6-phosphate dehydrogenase (G6PD) deficiency before getting dapsone.[21]

Pregnancy plans should be considered in choosing therapy. Attention must be given to the effects of drugs on fertility and on the fetus, as well as the adverse effects of active disease on pregnancy outcomes.

EVALUATION OF THERAPEUTIC OUTCOMES

Patients must be assessed for the activity and extent of lupus and monitored for adverse drug effects. Monitoring for specific drugs is listed in Table 69-3. **10** Many instruments have been developed and modified over the years to assess SLE therapy in trials. It is difficult to assess SLE therapy because milder forms of the disease may fluctuate, regardless of therapy. Examples of measures of disease activity include the Safety of Estrogens in Lupus Erythematosus National Assessment-Systemic Lupus Erythematosus Disease Activity Index (SELENA-SLEDAI), and British Isles Lupus Assessment Group (BILAG). The SELENA-SLEDAI is a measure of disease activity that considers 24 manifestations. BILAG measures clinical disease activity in eight organ systems compared to the prior month, considering 86 disease manifestations. The organ domains are given scores based on severity: A (severe disease activity flare that requires additional treatment), B (moderate flare), C (mild, stable disease), D (previously affected but no current disease activity), and E (never been involved). Other instruments used in studies are the Systemic Lupus Activity Measure (SLAM) and European Consensus Lupus Activity Measurement (ECLAM).[67] Individually, these indices were inadequate for showing superiority of new drugs over standard therapy. To overcome this problem, belimumab investigators developed the SRI assessment criteria. The SRI has three components: (a) Reduction in disease activity by SELENA-SLEDAI ≥4 points; (b) No worsening of disease activity (BILAG A) and no more than one new BILAG B score; and (c) <0.3 point increase (worsening) in physician global assessment (PGA). The PGA assesses patients' general health status on a scale of 0 (no disease activity) to 3 (severe).[40] Another important assessment of therapy is HRQoL, which may use a tool such as the generic Medical Outcomes Survey Short Form-36 (SF-36).[67]

A EULAR panel developed recommendations for the monitoring of patients with SLE in clinical practice and observational studies. Patients should be evaluated for SLE disease activity and organ involvement, cardiovascular risk factors, comorbidities, and risk for infection. Clinical and laboratory assessments should be performed every 6 to 12 months in patients with inactive disease and no organ damage, and more frequently if abnormalities are found.[68]

The Revised Cutaneous Lupus Erythematosus Disease Area and Severity Index (RCLASI) may be used to assess the extent and severity of cutaneous lupus erythematosus and response to therapy.[69]

ABBREVIATIONS

ACR	American College of Rheumatology
ANA	antinuclear antibody
Anti-dsDNA	anti-double-stranded DNA
ANCA	antineutrophil cytoplasmic antibodies
APRIL	a proliferation-inducing ligand
APS	antiphospholipid syndrome
BAFF	B cell activating factor of the TNF family
BILAG	British Isles Lupus Assessment Group
BLyS	B-lymphocyte stimulator
DHEA	dehydroepiandrosterone
DNA	deoxyribonucleic acid
ECLAM	European Consensus Lupus Activity Measurement
eGFR	estimated glomerular filtration rate
EULAR	European League Against Rheumatism
HRQoL	health-related quality of life
IMPDH	inosine 5-monophosphate dehydrogenase
La/SSB	antigen La/Sjögren's syndrome antigen B
Mesna	sodium-2-mercaptoethane sulfonate
MHC	major histocompatibility complex
MPA	mycophenolic acid
NSAID	nonsteroidal antiinflammatory drug
PGA	physician global assessment
Ro/SSA	antigen Ro/Sjögren's syndrome A
SELENA-SLEDAI	Safety of Estrogens in Lupus Erythematosus: National Assessment-Systemic Lupus Erythematosus Disease Activity Index
SF-36	Medical Outcomes Survey Short Form-36
SLAM	Systemic Lupus Activity Measure
SLE	systemic lupus erythematosus
SPF	sun protection factor
SRI	SLE Responder Index

REFERENCES

1. Scofield RH, Oates J. The place of William Osler in the description of systemic lupus erythematosus. Am J Med Sci 2009;338:409–412.
2. D'Cruz DP, Khamashta MA, Hughes GR. Systemic lupus erythematosus. Lancet 2007;369:587–596.

3. Pons-Estel GJ, Alarcón GS, Scofield L, et al. Understanding the epidemiology and progression of systemic lupus erythematosus. Semin Arthritis Rheum 2010;39:257–268.
4. Tsokos GC. Systemic lupus erythematosus. N Engl J Med 2011;365:2110–2121.
5. Sánchez E, Rasmussen A, Riba L, et al. Impact of genetic ancestry and sociodemographic status on the clinical expression of systemic lupus erythematosus in American Indian–European populations. Arthritis Rheum 2012;64:3687–3694.
6. Hahn BH, McMahon MA, Wilkinson A, et al. American College of Rheumatology guidelines for screening, treatment, and management of lupus nephritis. Arthritis Care Res (Hoboken) 2012;64:797–808.
7. Robinson M, Cook SS, Currie LM. Systemic lupus erythematosus: A genetic review for advanced practice nurses. J Am Acad Nurse Pract 2011;23:629–637.
8. Rahman A, Isenberg DA. Systemic lupus erythematosus. N Engl J Med 2008;358:929–939.
9. Lessard CJ, Adrianto I, Ice JA, et al. Identification of IRF8, TMEM39A, and IKZF3-ZPBP2 as susceptibility loci for systemic lupus erythematosus in a large-scale multiracial replication study. Am J Hum Genet 2012;90:648–660.
10. Zandman-Goddard G, Solomon M, Rosman Z, et al. Environment and lupus-related diseases. Lupus 2012;21:241–250.
11. Sawalha AH, Harley JB, Scofield RH. Autoimmunity and Klinefelter's syndrome: When men have two X chromosomes. J Autoimmun 2009;33:31–34.
12. Jacob N, Jacob CO. On anti-tumor necrosis factor-induced systemic lupus erythematosus. J Rheumatol 2010;37:3–5.
13. Choi ST, Kang JI, Park IH, et al. Subscale analysis of quality of life in patients with systemic lupus erythematosus: Association with depression, fatigue, disease activity and damage. Clin Exp Rheumatol 2012;30:665–672.
14. Tan TC, Fang H, Magder LS, Petri MA. Differences between male and female systemic lupus erythematosus in a multiethnic population. J Rheumatol 2012;39:759–769.
15. Petri M, Orbai AM, Alarcón GS, et al. Derivation and validation of the Systemic Lupus International Collaborating Clinics classification criteria for systemic lupus erythematosus. Arthritis Rheum 2012;64:2677–2686.
16. Tan EM, Cohen AS, Fries JF, et al. The 1982 revised criteria for the classification of systemic lupus erythematosus. Arthritis Rheum 1982;25:1271–1277.
17. Hochberg MC. Updating the American College of Rheumatology revised criteria for the classification of systemic lupus erythematosus. Arthritis Rheum 1997;40:1725.
18. Ruperto N, Hanrahan LM, Alarcón GS, et al. International consensus for a definition of disease flare in lupus. Lupus 2011;20:453–462.
19. Santiago-Casas Y, Vilá LM, McGwin G Jr, et al. Association of discoid lupus erythematosus with clinical manifestations and damage accrual in a multiethnic lupus cohort. Arthritis Care Res (Hoboken) 2012;64:704–712.
20. Hansen CB, Dahle KW. Cutaneous lupus erythematosus. Dermatol Ther 2012;25:99–111.
21. Chang AY, Werth VP. Treatment of cutaneous lupus. Curr Rheumatol Rep 2011;13:300–307.
22. Bertsias GK, Ioannidis JP, Aringer M, et al. EULAR recommendations for the management of systemic lupus erythematosus with neuropsychiatric manifestations: Report of a task force of the EULAR standing committee for clinical affairs. Ann Rheum Dis 2010;69:2074–2082.
23. Ruiz-Irastorza G, Ramos-Casals M, Brito-Zeron P, Khamashta MA. Clinical efficacy and side effects of antimalarials in systemic lupus erythematosus: A systematic review. Ann Rheum Dis 2010;69:20–28.
24. Drug Therapeutics Bulletin. Systemic lupus erythematosus—An update. Drug Ther Bull 2011;49:81–84.
25. Mosca M, Tani C, Carli L, Bombardieri S. Glucocorticoids in systemic lupus erythematosus. Clin Exp Rheumatol 2011;29:S126–S129.
26. Haija AJ, Schulz SW. The role and effect of complementary and alternative medicine in systemic lupus erythematosus. Rheum Dis Clin North Am 2011;37:47–62.
27. Food and Drug Administration. HHS. Labeling and effectiveness testing; sunscreen drug products for over-the-counter human use. Final rule. Fed Regist 2011;76: 35620–35665.
28. Ezra N, Jorizzo J. Hydroxychloroquine and smoking in patients with cutaneous lupus erythematosus. Clin Exp Dermatol 2012;37:327–334.
29. Turchin I, Bernatsky S, Clarke AE, et al. Cigarette smoking and cutaneous damage in systemic lupus erythematosus. J Rheumatol 2009;36:2691–2693.
30. Ruiz-Irastorza G, Cuadrado MJ, Ruiz-Arruza I, et al. Evidence-based recommendations for the prevention and long-term management of thrombosis in antiphospholipid antibody-positive patients: Report of a Task Force at the 13th International Congress on Antiphospholipid Antibodies. Lupus 2011;20:206–218.
31. Artifoni M, Puechal X. How to treat refractory arthritis in lupus? Joint Bone Spine 2012;79:347–350.
32. Elbirt D, Sthoeger D, Asher I, Sthoeger ZM. The management of systemic lupus erythematosus: Facts and controversies. Clin Dermatol 2010;28:330–336.
33. Kamen DL. Vitamin D in lupus—New kid on the block? Bull NYU Hosp Jt Dis 2010;68:218–222.
34. Petri M. Use of hydroxychloroquine to prevent thrombosis in systemic lupus erythematosus and in antiphospholipid antibody-positive patients. Curr Rheumatol Rep 2011;13:77–80.
35. Pons-Estel GJ, Alarcón GS, González LA, et al. Possible protective effect of hydroxychloroquine on delaying the occurrence of integument damage in lupus: LXXI, data from a multiethnic cohort. Arthritis Care Res (Hoboken) 2010;62:393–400.
36. Alarcón GS, McGwin G, Bertoli AM, et al. Effect of hydroxychloroquine on the survival of patients with systemic lupus erythematosus: Data from LUMINA, a multiethnic US cohort (LUMINA L). Ann Rheum Dis 2007;66:1168–1172.
37. Marmor MF, Kellner U, Lai TY, et al. Revised recommendations on screening for chloroquine and hydroxychloroquine retinopathy. Ophthalmology 2011;118:415–422.
38. Costedoat-Chalumeau N, Leroux G, Piette JC, Amoura Z. Why all systemic lupus erythematosus patients should be given hydroxychloroquine treatment? Joint Bone Spine 2010;77:4–5.
39. Dennis GJ. Belimumab: A BLyS-specific inhibitor for the treatment of systemic lupus erythematosus. Clin Pharmacol Ther 2012;91:143–149.
40. Burness CB, McCormack PL. Belimumab: In systemic lupus erythematosus. Drugs 2011;71:2435–2444.
41. van Vollenhoven RF. Rituximab—Shadow, illusion or light? Autoimmun Rev 2012;11:563–567.
42. Coca A, Sanz I. Updates on B-cell immunotherapies for systemic lupus erythematosus and Sjogren's syndrome. Curr Opin Rheumatol 2012;24:451–456.
43. Dall'Era M, Chakravarty EF. Treatment of mild, moderate, and severe lupus erythematosus: Focus on new therapies. Curr Rheumatol Rep 2011;13:308–316.

44. Wofsy D, Hillson JL, Diamond B. Abatacept for lupus nephritis: Alternative definitions of complete response support conflicting conclusions. Arthritis Rheum 2012;64:3660–3665.
45. Aringer M, Smolen JS. TNF inhibition in SLE: Where do we stand? Lupus 2009;18:5–8.
46. Aringer M, Burkhardt H, Burmester GR, et al. Current state of evidence on 'off-label' therapeutic options for systemic lupus erythematosus, including biological immunosuppressive agents, in Germany, Austria and Switzerland—A consensus report. Lupus 2012;21:386–401.
47. Monach PA, Arnold LM, Merkel PA. Incidence and prevention of bladder toxicity from cyclophosphamide in the treatment of rheumatic diseases: A data-driven review. Arthritis Rheum 2010;62:9–21.
48. Dall'Era M. Mycophenolate mofetil in the treatment of systemic lupus erythematosus. Curr Opin Rheumatol 2011;23:454–458.
49. Dall'Era M, Stone D, Levesque V, et al. Identification of biomarkers that predict response to treatment of lupus nephritis with mycophenolate mofetil or pulse cyclophosphamide. Arthritis Care Res (Hoboken) 2011;63:351–357.
50. Dooley MA, Jayne D, Ginzler EM, et al. Mycophenolate versus azathioprine as maintenance therapy for lupus nephritis. N Engl J Med 2011;365:1886–1895.
51. Schmajuk G, Yazdany J. Drug monitoring in systemic lupus erythematosus: A systematic review. Semin Arthritis Rheum 2011;40:559–575.
52. Amital H, Szekanecz Z, Szucs G, et al. Serum concentrations of 25-OH vitamin D in patients with systemic lupus erythematosus (SLE) are inversely related to disease activity: Is it time to routinely supplement patients with SLE with vitamin D? Ann Rheum Dis 2010;69:1155–1157.
53. Birmingham DJ, Hebert LA, Song H, et al. Evidence that abnormally large seasonal declines in vitamin D status may trigger SLE flare in non-African Americans. Lupus 2012;21:855–864.
54. Ruiz-Irastorza G, Gordo S, Olivares N, et al. Changes in vitamin D levels in patients with systemic lupus erythematosus: Effects on fatigue, disease activity, and damage. Arthritis Care Res (Hoboken) 2010;62:1160–1165.
55. Baer AN, Witter FR, Petri M. Lupus and pregnancy. Obstet Gynecol Surv 2011;66:639–653.
56. Clowse ME. Managing contraception and pregnancy in the rheumatologic diseases. Baillieres Best Pract Res Clin Rheumatol 2010;24:373–385.
57. Ruiz-Irastorza G, Crowther M, Branch W, Khamashta MA. Antiphospholipid syndrome. Lancet 2010;376:1498–1509.
58. Lockshin MD, Kim M, Laskin CA, et al. Prediction of adverse pregnancy outcome by the presence of lupus anticoagulant, but not anticardiolipin antibody, in patients with antiphospholipid antibodies. Arthritis Rheum 2012;64:2311–2318.
59. Wijetilleka S, Scoble T, Khamashta M. Novel insights into pathogenesis, diagnosis and treatment of antiphospholipid syndrome. Curr Opin Rheumatol 2012;24:473–481.
60. Chang C, Gershwin ME. Drug-induced lupus erythematosus: Incidence, management and prevention. Drug Saf 2011;34:357–374.
61. Lowe G, Henderson CL, Grau RH, et al. A systematic review of drug-induced subacute cutaneous lupus erythematosus. Br J Dermatol 2011;164:465–472.
62. Williams VL, Cohen PR. TNF alpha antagonist-induced lupus-like syndrome: Report and review of the literature with implications for treatment with alternative TNF alpha antagonists. Int J Dermatol 2011;50:619–625.
63. Millet A, Decaux O, Perlat A, et al. Systemic lupus erythematosus and vaccination. Eur J Intern Med 2009;20:236–241.
64. Heijstek MW, Ott de Bruin LM, Bijl M, et al. EULAR recommendations for vaccination in paediatric patients with rheumatic diseases. Ann Rheum Dis 2011;70:1704–1712.
65. Anonymous. Recommended adult immunization schedule—United States, 2012. JAMA 2012;308:22–28.
66. O'Neill SG, Isenberg DA. Immunizing patients with systemic lupus erythematosus: A review of effectiveness and safety. Lupus 2006;15:778–783.
67. Strand V, Chu AD. Measuring outcomes in systemic lupus erythematosus clinical trials. Expert Rev Pharmacoecon Outcomes Res 2011;11:455–468.
68. Mosca M, Tani C, Aringer M, et al. European League Against Rheumatism recommendations for monitoring patients with systemic lupus erythematosus in clinical practice and in observational studies. Ann Rheum Dis 2010;69:1269–1274.
69. Kuhn A, Meuth AM, Bein D, et al. Revised Cutaneous Lupus Erythematosus Disease Area and Severity Index (RCLASI): A modified outcome instrument for cutaneous lupus erythematosus. Br J Dermatol 2010;163:83–92.

70

Solid-Organ Transplantation

Kristine S. Schonder and Heather J. Johnson

KEY CONCEPTS

1. A combination of two to four immunosuppressive drugs is used to target different levels of the immune cascade to prevent allograft rejection and allow lower doses of the individual agents to minimize their toxicity.
2. Calcineurin inhibitors (CNIs), such as cyclosporine and tacrolimus, which inhibit interleukin (IL)-2 and thus block T-cell activation are the backbone of immunosuppressive regimens. However, they are associated with significant adverse effects, namely, nephrotoxicity and neurotoxicity.
3. CNI-induced nephrotoxicity is one of the most common side effects observed in transplant recipients and is the leading cause of renal dysfunction in nonrenal transplant patients. Therapeutic drug monitoring is used in an attempt to optimize the use of CNIs.
4. Corticosteroids are a key component of immunosuppressive regimens because they block the initial steps in allograft rejection. However, the adverse effects associated with their long-term use have prompted the investigation of corticosteroid-free immunosuppressive protocols. Corticosteroids remain the cornerstone of the treatment of allograft rejection.
5. Antimetabolites agents such as azathioprine and mycophenolate inhibit T-cell proliferation by altering purine synthesis to prevent acute rejection. Bone marrow suppression is the most significant adverse effect associated with these agents.
6. The proliferation signal inhibitors (PSI) sirolimus and everolimus exert their activity by inhibiting the mammalian target of rapamycin (mTOR) receptor, which alters T-cell response to IL-2. The adverse effects associated with sirolimus include thrombocytopenia, anemia, and hyperlipidemia.
7. Antibody preparations that target specific receptors on T cells are classified as depleting or nondepleting. Most lymphocyte-depleting antibodies are associated with significant infusion-related reactions.
8. Long-term allograft and patient survival is limited by chronic rejection, cardiovascular disease, and long-term immunosuppressive complications such as malignancy.

INTRODUCTION

Solid-organ transplantation provides a lifesaving treatment for patients with end-stage cardiac, kidney, liver, lung, and intestinal disease. Over 300 U.S. hospitals offer transplant services, and pharmacists are often an integral part of the transplant team. The Centers for Medicare and Medicaid Services regulations require that transplant programs have a multidisciplinary team including individuals with experience in pharmacology. While the regulations do not specifically state that each center must have a pharmacist, a pharmacist would certainly provide the desired expertise in transplant pharmacotherapy that the regulations mandate.[1]

With the success of transplantation, an increasing number of transplant recipients are in our communities. By the end of 2009 there were nearly 200,000 people living with a solid-organ transplant in the United States, which has doubled over the previous decade.[1] In 2011, 28,537 solid-organ transplants were performed. Kidney transplants remain the most common; 11,043 were from cadaveric donors and 5,770 from living donors. The next most frequently transplanted organ was the liver, with 6,095 from cadaveric donors and 247 from living donors. Heart and pancreas (or combined kidney–pancreas) transplants account for over 2,300 and almost 1,100 transplants, respectively; over 1,800 lung transplants were performed as well.[1] While the demand for transplantation continues to grow, the number of cadaveric donors has remained relatively stable during the last decade. In 2012, more than 115,000 persons in the United States were waiting for a transplant (over 93,000 people were awaiting a kidney, 16,000 a liver, and 3,000 were on the list for a heart transplant). Median waiting time for a cadaveric kidney is more than 3.5 years. For liver transplantation the median time to transplant is about 1 year, whereas for heart transplantation it is approximately 6 months. For heart, liver, and lung transplantation clinical status is an important factor affecting waiting times, with the sickest patients receiving priority for available organs.[1]

To increase the number of organs available for transplantation, several strategies have been employed in the last several years. The use of living donors for renal transplantation represents over one third of all kidney transplants, more than any other organ. Living-donor transplantation is also becoming increasingly important for those with end-stage liver and lung disease. Efforts to expand the cadaveric donor pool have included relaxation of age restrictions, development of better preservation solutions, use of "extended-criteria" and non–heart-beating donors, and, in the case of liver transplants, the transplantation of one liver to more than one recipient or implantation of only a segment of a liver. Although very controversial, others advocate the creation of a regulated system for compensating individuals in a monetary fashion for the "donation" of a kidney.

Clinical **Controversy...**

Several strategies have been used to increase the number of available organs for transplant. Some centers will use extended-criteria deceased donors, including older donors, donors with less than perfect organ function, and donors whose hearts have stopped beating for a period of time before organ harvest, all of which may increase the potential for delayed graft function. Strategies to increase the living donor pool include using plasmapheresis before transplant to remove antibodies to allow for transplanting organs that are not ABO-compatible with the recipient or organs into recipients with donor-specific antibodies.

Despite all these efforts, patients continue to die awaiting transplantation. In 2009, more than 7,000 people who were on transplantation waiting lists died. In all areas, efforts have been made to improve organ allocation by moving toward allocation based primarily on "medical necessity" versus time on the waiting list. Although dialysis can be used for an extended period of time to partially replace the function of the kidneys, such options are not readily available for most liver and heart transplantation candidates. Left ventricular assist devices are now used commonly as a bridge to transplantation for many heart transplantation candidates; however, hepatocyte transplantation and artificial liver support remain investigational alternatives or bridges to liver transplantation.[2]

Patient and graft survival rates following transplantation have improved significantly over the past 30 years as a result of advances in pharmacotherapy, surgical techniques, organ preservation, and the postoperative management of patients (Table 70-1). The half-life of transplanted kidneys has also continued to improve, but is lower for kidneys from deceased donors compared to living donors, 14.7 years and 26.6 years, respectively. Similarly, the half-life of the transplanted livers and hearts has improved to 10 years for livers from deceased donors and 14.9 years for hearts.[1] In this chapter, the epidemiology of end-stage kidney, liver, and heart disease is briefly reviewed, the pathophysiology of organ rejection is reviewed, the pharmacotherapeutic options for individualized immunosuppressive regimens are critiqued, and the unique complications of these regimens along with the therapeutic challenges they present are discussed.

EPIDEMIOLOGY AND ETIOLOGY

The epidemiology and etiology associated with solid-organ transplant is specific to the type of organ transplant.

TABLE 70-1 Organ-Specific Patient and Graft Survival Rates[1]

	Patient Survival (%)		Graft Survival (%)	
Organ	**1 Year**	**5 Years**	**1 Year**	**5 Years**
Kidney				
Living donor	98.6	91.6	96.5	82.8
Deceased donor	96	82.7	91.7	70.8
Liver				
Living donor	92	80.8	88.2	74.6
Deceased donor	88.9	73.6	85.2	68.5
Heart	88.9	75	88.3	73.9

Kidney

Renal transplantation is the preferred long-term therapeutic option for most patients with end-stage renal disease (ESRD) because it provides patients with the greatest potential improvement in quality of life. Dialysis catheter-related infections, peritoneal dialysis-associated peritonitis, and scheduled dialysis treatments are avoided, and dietary restrictions are fewer. Patients who receive a renal transplant before the initiation of dialysis have markedly improved quality of life and prolonged life expectancy.[3] The use of living-donor transplantation has made this increasingly possible. Although the analysis of quality of life is complex, patients generally report improved quality of life following transplantation as compared with patients on maintenance dialysis.[4]

Diabetes mellitus, hypertension, and glomerulonephritis are the three leading causes of ESRD leading to kidney transplantation and account for more than 70% of patients (see Chap. 29).[5] Patients with medical conditions such as unstable cardiac disease or recently diagnosed malignancy, for whom the risk of surgery or chronic immunosuppression would be greater than the risks associated with chronic dialysis, are generally excluded from consideration for transplantation.

Liver

Noncholestatic cirrhosis (hepatitis C, alcoholic cirrhosis, hepatitis B, nonalcoholic steatohepatitis, and autoimmune hepatitis) is the primary cause of end-stage liver disease and more than 70% of liver transplant recipients have been diagnosed with one of these conditions.[1] Livers are allocated based on a United Network for Organ Sharing-adapted, Model for End-stage Liver Disease (MELD) score.[6] This score, based on serum creatinine concentration, total serum bilirubin concentration, international normalized ratio, and etiology of cirrhosis, has been demonstrated to be a useful tool to predict impending mortality.

The few absolute contraindications to liver transplantation are active alcohol or substance abuse. Although hepatitis B and C can recur in the transplanted liver, these are not absolute contraindications to liver transplantation.[2,7]

Heart

Cardiac transplant candidates are typically patients with end-stage heart failure who have New York Heart Association class III or IV symptoms despite maximal medical management and have an expected 1-year mortality risk of 50% or greater without a transplant.[8] Idiopathic cardiomyopathy and ischemic heart disease account for heart failure in more than 90% of heart transplantation recipients.[1] Other etiologies include valvular disease, retransplantation for graft atherosclerosis or dysfunction, and congenital heart disease. The role of heart transplantation as a therapeutic option for patients with heart failure is discussed in Chapter 4.

Absolute contraindications to orthotopic cardiac transplantation include the presence of an active infection (except in the case of an infected ventricular assist device, which is an indication for urgent transplantation) or the presence of other diseases (e.g., malignancy) that may limit survival and/or rehabilitation and severe, irreversible pulmonary hypertension.

PHYSIOLOGIC CONSEQUENCES OF TRANSPLANTATION

Transplantation is truly lifesaving for heart, liver, and lung transplantation recipients, whereas renal transplantation is associated with improved quality of life and survival when compared with dialysis.[9]

Most heart transplantation patients return to New York Heart Association functional class I following transplantation. Although not all return to work, 89.9% of patients consider themselves to have no activity limitations at 1-year follow-up.[10] The specific physiologic consequences of kidney, liver, and heart transplantation are discussed below.

Kidney Transplantation

The glomerular filtration rate (GFR) of a successfully transplanted kidney may be near normal almost immediately after transplantation. In some patients, however, the concentration of standard biochemical indicators of renal function, such as serum creatinine and blood urea nitrogen, may remain elevated for several days. Standard formulas used to predict drug dosing rely on a stable serum creatinine and may be inaccurate immediately following transplantation (see eChap. 18 and Chap. 33).

Although the allograft is able to remove uremic toxins from the body, it may take several weeks for other physiologic complications of ESRD, such as anemia, calcium and phosphate imbalance, and altered lipid profiles, to resolve. The renal production of erythropoietin and 1-hydroxylation of vitamin D may return toward normal early in the postoperative period. Because the onset of physiologic effects may be delayed, continuation of the patient's pretransplantation vitamin D, calcium supplementation, and/or phosphate binders may be warranted. The duration of therapy will depend on how rapidly kidney function improves. Patients should be monitored for hypophosphatemia and hypercalcemia for the first few days to weeks after kidney transplantation.

Primary nonfunction of a renal allograft or delayed graft function (DGF) is characterized by the need for dialysis in the first postop week or the failure of the serum creatinine to fall by 30% of the pretransplantation value. The incidence of DGF in cadaveric renal transplantation ranges from 8% to 50% and results in a slower return of the kidney's excretory, metabolic, and synthetic functions. DGF is associated with prolonged hospital stays, higher costs, difficult management of immunosuppressive therapy, slower patient rehabilitation, and poor graft survival. Other early causes of renal dysfunction such as urethral obstruction or arterial or venous stenosis or thrombosis should be distinguished from DGF.

The primary cause of DGF is acute tubular necrosis (ATN). The incidence of ATN is higher when kidneys are harvested from donors who recently experienced a cardiac arrest, those who were hypotensive or on vasopressors, or older donors (age >55 years). While cyclosporine and tacrolimus have been implicated in the prolongation of ATN, a clear cause-and-effect relationship has not been established. Nonetheless, most clinicians will decrease calcineurin inhibitor (CNI) doses in patients with ATN. DGF predisposes patients to acute rejection, possibly as a consequence of decreased CNI levels and a resultant reduction in the level of immunosuppression.

Clinical **Controversy...**

Some clinicians feel that deceased donor kidney allografts should be allocated such that younger recipients receive organs from younger donors, while older recipients receive organs from older donors or kidneys with less than optimal function. Other clinicians feel that kidneys should be allocated based solely on waiting time, such that the recipient who has waited on the list the longest receives the first available kidney allograft, regardless of recipient or donor age or the function of the kidney.

Liver Transplantation

The physiologic consequences of liver transplantation are complex, involving changes in both metabolic and synthetic function. Postoperatively, the liver transplant recipient will likely have many fluid, electrolyte, and nutritional abnormalities. Biliary tract dysfunction may alter the absorption of fats and fat-soluble drugs.[11] Poor absorption of the lipid-soluble drug cyclosporine improves after successful liver transplantation and reestablishment of bile flow. Vitamin E deficiency and its neurologic complications in liver failure patients are reversed after successful liver transplantation. In stable adult liver transplant patients, the concentrations of retinol and tocopherol are similar to those seen in normal healthy subjects, indicating recovery of transplanted liver production and excretion of bile salts needed for fat-soluble vitamin absorption. Table 70-2 summarizes the effects of liver transplantation on metabolism and renal elimination that are seen in the immediate postoperative period. Most of these changes resolve as liver function normalizes.

The newly transplanted liver fails to function in 10% to 15% of recipients as the result of several different mechanisms. Early graft failure can result from preexisting disease in the donor, and even coagulation defects have been acquired through donor organs. The technical complexity of the operation can produce flaws in revascularization that also lead to graft nonfunction. Surgical complications include portal vein or hepatic artery thrombosis and bile duct leaks. Ischemic injury can also result in early graft dysfunction. While hyperacute rejection in liver transplantation rarely occurs, graft failure in the first two postoperative weeks may indicate antibody-mediated graft destruction.

TABLE 70-2 Perioperative Changes in Drug Disposition and Elimination Following Liver Transplantation

	Result	Comment
Serum proteins		
↓ Albumin	↑ Free fraction of drugs usually bound to albumin	Diazepam, salicylic acid binding greater in liver transplant than chronic liver disease because of endogenous binding inhibitors (up to 45 days posttransplant)
↑ Alpha-1-Acid glycoprotein	Lower free fraction of drugs	Lidocaine
Metabolism/elimination		
Microsomal enzymes	↑ CYP2E1 activity	Increased drug metabolism (induction)
	↔ CYP2D6	Unaffected
	↓ CYP activity	Decreased drug elimination (inhibition)
Oxidation	Stable	
Conjugation	Normalizes after transplant	
Biliary function	↓ Absorption of lipophilic compounds	
	↑ Cyclosporine metabolites in blood	
Renal elimination	Elimination of gentamicin, vancomycin, cephalosporins less than predicted by serum creatinine	Renal elimination of metabolites limited

Adapted from reference 11.

TABLE 70-3 Altered Responses to Cardiac Drugs in the Denervated Transplanted Heart

Drug	Effect	Mechanism	Comment
Digitalis	Normal inotropic effect; minimal effect on AV node	Direct myocardial effect; denervation	
Atropine	No effect on AV node	Denervation	
Adrenaline/noradrenaline	Increased contractility; increased chronotropy	Denervation; hypersensitivity	Increased cardiac output mediated by increased heart rate
Isoproterenol	Normal increase in contractility; normal increase in chronotropy	No neuronal uptake	
Quinidine	No vagolytic effect	Denervation	
Verapamil	AV block	Direct effect	
Nifedipine	No reflex tachycardia	Denervation	
Hydralazine	No reflex tachycardia	Denervation	
β-Blocker	Increased antagonist effect	Denervation	Impaired heart rate response, use sparingly
Adenosine	Negative chronotropic effect	Hypersensitivity; effect on sinus node of denervated heart	Life-threatening asystole (>0.5 min) may occur if used to treat supraventricular arrhythmia or stress testing
Acetylcholine	Negative chronotropic effect	Hypersensitivity; effect on sinus node of denervated heart	

AV, atrioventricular.

Reproduced from Deng MC. Heart failure: Cardiac transplantation. Heart 2002;87:177–184 with permission from the BMJ Publishing Group Ltd.

Heart Transplantation

The orthotopically transplanted heart is denervated and no longer responds to physiologic stimuli and pharmacologic agents in a normal manner (Table 70-3).[9] In situations requiring an increased heart rate such as exercise or hypotension, the denervated heart is unable to acutely increase heart rate but instead relies on increasing the stroke volume. Later in the course of exercise or hypotension, heart rate increases in response to circulating catecholamines. While the maximum exercise capacity of heart transplant recipients is below normal, most patients are able to resume normal lifestyles and reasonably vigorous activity levels. Partial reinnervation may occur over time, thereby facilitating more normal physiologic and pharmacologic responses and better exercise capacity.[10]

A number of autoregulatory, anatomic, and physiologic responses present in the normal heart are interrupted or blunted for the first 6 weeks after transplantation. The donor sinus node function may be impaired by preservation injury, direct surgical trauma at excision, the presence of long-acting antiarrhythmics (e.g., amiodarone) taken prior to transplant by the recipient, and a lack of "conditioning" responsiveness to catecholamines.[10] Consequently, the transplanted heart generally requires chronotropic support with either milrinone or pacing in the perioperative period to maintain a heart rate of 90 to 110 beats per minute and satisfactory hemodynamics (i.e., blood pressure, urine output, and tissue perfusion). Approximately 10% to 20% of transplant patients will have persistent chronotropic incompetence requiring either short courses of medications, such as terbutaline or theophylline, or permanent cardiac pacing.

Right ventricular function is frequently impaired, presumably as a result of preservation injury and elevated pulmonary vascular resistance. A "restrictive" hemodynamic pattern may be present initially but usually improves in 6 weeks following transplantation. Donor–recipient size mismatch may contribute to early posttransplantation hemodynamic abnormalities characterized by higher right and left ventricular end-diastolic pressures. Supraventricular arrhythmias are usually transient and may result from over vigorous use of catecholamines or milrinone. If this type of arrhythmia occurs after the perioperative period, the astute clinician should consider the possibility of acute rejection.

Myocardial depression frequently occurs and generally requires inotropic support with agents such as dobutamine, milrinone, and epinephrine. On occasion, intra- or postoperative administration of vasodilators, including nitric oxide, and inotropic agents may be necessary to treat right-sided failure in the transplant patient; milrinone and isoproterenol are preferred in this setting.

Persistent abnormalities of diastolic function are often noted in the transplanted heart such that intracardiac pressures increase in an exaggerated fashion in response to exercise and/or volume infusion.[10] These abnormalities are due in part to denervation, but also to acute rejection or to the scarring secondary to previously treated rejection episodes, hypertension, or cardiac allograft vasculopathy.

Hypertension may occur following surgery secondary to the effect of elevated catecholamine levels and systemic vascular resistance as the residual effects of end-stage heart failure on the healthy heart. Systolic blood pressure should be maintained at 110 to 120 mm Hg to enhance cardiac function. In the acute posttransplantation period, IV nitroprusside or nitroglycerin may be needed, whereas oral angiotensin-converting enzyme inhibitors (ACEIs) and/or amlodipine are commonly used once the patient can ingest oral medications.

PATHOPHYSIOLOGY OF REJECTION

Rejection of the transplanted tissue can take place at any time following surgery and is classified clinically as hyperacute rejection, acute cellular rejection (ACR), humoral rejection, and chronic rejection.

General Concepts

Rejection of any transplanted organ is primarily mediated by activation of alloreactive T cells and antigen-presenting cells such as B lymphocytes, macrophages, and dendritic cells. Acute allograft rejection is caused primarily by the infiltration of T cells into the allograft, which triggers inflammatory and cytotoxic effects on the graft. Complex interactions between the allograft and cellular cytokines, cell-to-cell interactions, CD4+ and CD8+ T cells, and B cells ultimately lead to chronic rejection and graft loss if adequate immunosuppression is not maintained.[12]

The sequence of events that underlies graft rejection is recognition, via major histocompatibility complex (MHC) class I and II antigens, of the donor's histocompatibility differences by the recipient's immune system, recruitment of activated lymphocytes,

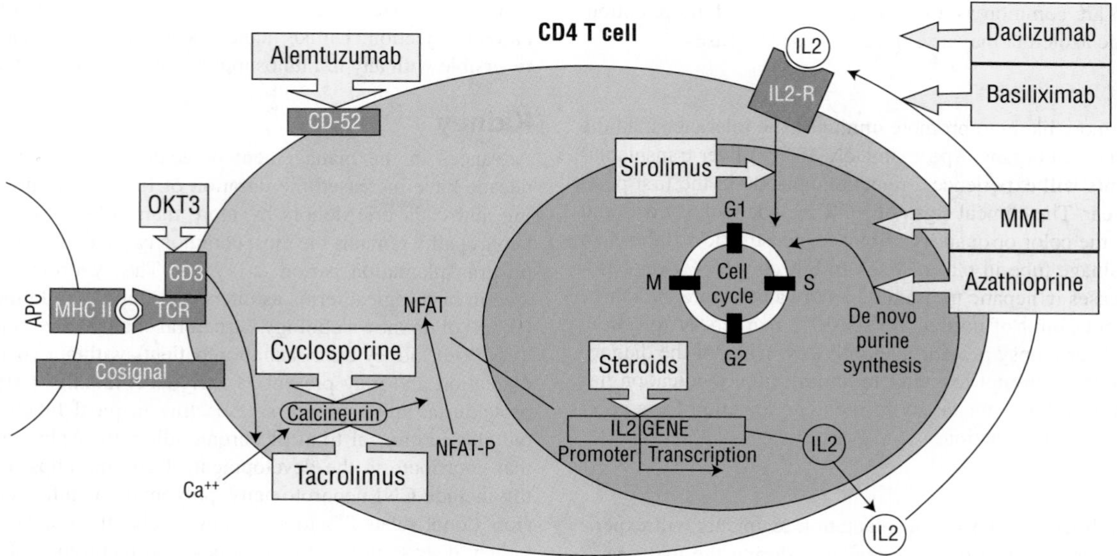

FIGURE 70-1 Stages of CD4 T-cell activation and cytokine production with identification of the sites of action of different immunosuppressive agents. Antigen major histocompatibility complex (MHC) II molecule complexes are responsible for initiating the activation of CD4 T cells. These MHC–peptide complexes are recognized by the T-cell recognition complex (TCR). A costimulatory signal initiates signal transduction with activation of second messengers, one of which is calcineurin. Calcineurin removes phosphates from the nuclear factors (NFAT-P) allowing them to enter the nucleus. These nuclear factors specifically bind to an interleukin (IL)-2 promoter gene facilitating IL-2 gene transcription. Interaction of IL-2 with the IL-2 receptor (IL-2R) on the cell membrane surface induces cell proliferation and production of cytokines specific to the T cell. (APC, antigen-presenting cells; MMF, mycophenolate mofetil.) *(Reprinted from Mueller XM. Drug immunosuppressive therapy for adult heart transplantation. Part I. Immune response to allograft and mechanism of action of immunosuppressants. Ann Thorac Surg 2004;77:354–362, Copyright © 2004, with permission from Elsevier.)*

initiation of immune effector mechanisms, and finally graft destruction. The specifics of this immune cascade of organ rejection are discussed in eChapter 20. The complex nature of cytokine interactions makes it very difficult to design drugs with exclusive actions (Fig. 70-1).

Efforts are made to allocate well-matched kidneys, according to human leukocyte antigens (HLA)-A, -B, and -DR, to minimize rejection and enhance survival. However, the benefit of having no recipient donor mismatches may be negated by excessive cold ischemia time (>36 hours) and donor age older than 60 years. HLA tissue matching is not performed routinely before transplantation for livers and hearts because organ availability is more limited and the optimal cold ischemia time is shorter. However, if the potential recipient's blood is reactive against a panel of random donor blood samples (i.e., panel reactive antibody [PRA] >10% to 20%), a negative T-cell crossmatch is required prior to transplantation. Transplanted organs must be matched for ABO blood group compatibility with the recipient as ABO mismatching will result. Liver transplantation may be carried out in emergency situations across ABO blood groups, but survival is lower.

Hyperacute Rejection

Hyperacute rejection may be evident within minutes of the transplantation procedure when preformed donor-specific antibodies are present in the recipient at the time of the transplant. Hyperacute rejection can also be induced by immunoglobulin G antibodies that bind to antigens on the vascular endothelium, such as class I MHC, ABO, and vascular endothelial cell antigens. Tissue damage can be mediated through antibody-dependent, cell-mediated cytotoxicity, or through activation of the complement cascade. The ischemic damage to the microvasculature rapidly results in tissue necrosis.

Hyperacute rejection has become uncommon in kidney and heart transplants. A positive crossmatch presents a serious risk for graft failure even if hyperacute rejection does not occur. A negative lymphocytotoxicity crossmatch does not entirely rule out the possibility of hyperacute rejection because non-MHC antigens on the vascular endothelium can serve as targets of donor-specific antibodies. Early graft dysfunction is treated with supportive care and retransplantation if possible. The reason for the rarity of hyperacute rejection in liver transplantation is not fully understood, but the local release of cytokines may alter the immunologic reaction in the liver.

Acute Cellular Rejection

Acute rejection is most common in the first few months following transplantation but can occur at any time during the life of the allograft. ACR is mediated by alloreactive T-lymphocytes that appear in the circulation and infiltrate the allograft through the vascular endothelium. After the graft is infiltrated by lymphocytes, the cytotoxic cells specifically target and kill the functioning cells in the allograft. At the same time, local release of lymphokines attracts and stimulates macrophages to produce tissue damage through a delayed hypersensitivity-like mechanism. These immunologic and inflammatory events lead to nonspecific signs and symptoms including pain and tenderness over the graft site, fever, and lethargy.

Kidney

Acute rejection, which may affect up to 20% of patients during the first 6 months following transplantation, is evidenced by an abrupt rise in serum creatinine concentration of ≥30% over baseline. A specific histologic diagnosis can be obtained via biopsy of the allograft and is often used to guide therapy for rejection. A biopsy specimen with a diffuse lymphocytic infiltrate is consistent with ACR. After the diagnosis of rejection has been confirmed, the potential risks and benefits of specific antirejection therapies must be evaluated. Hypertension often worsens during an episode of rejection, and edema and weight gain are common as a result of sodium and fluid retention. Symptomatic azotemia may also develop in severe cases.

Liver

The liver is more likely to promote immunologic tolerance than the other vascularized organs. Approximately 18% of liver transplantation recipients will experience a rejection episode in the first posttransplant year. The clinical signs of ACR include leukocytosis and a change in the color or quantity of bile for those who still have an external drainage tube in place. A serum bilirubin 50% over baseline or increases in hepatic transaminases to values more than three times the upper limit of normal are sensitive markers of rejection. Although a liver biopsy provides definitive evidence of the diagnosis of rejection, a prompt response to antirejection medication has also proven useful as a means to differentiate rejection from other causes of hepatic dysfunction.

Heart

Approximately 16% of heart transplantation recipients will experience at least one episode of acute rejection during the first year.[13] Because rejection of the cardiac allograft is not necessarily accompanied by overt clinical signs or symptoms and because the incidence of acute rejection is highest during the first year posttransplant, endomyocardial biopsies are often performed at regularly scheduled intervals following transplantation.[14] A typical biopsy schedule would be weekly for the first postoperative month, biweekly for the next 2 months, and monthly to bimonthly through the remainder of the first posttransplant year. Nonspecific symptoms, including low-grade fever, malaise, mild reduction in exercise capacity, heart failure, or atrial arrhythmias may also be evident and if present are reflective of a more severe rejection episode.

Antibody-Mediated Rejection

Antibody-mediated rejection (AMR), sometimes referred to as vascular or humoral rejection, is characterized by the presence of antibodies directed against HLA antigens present on the donor vascular endothelium. The antibodies activate complement, which creates a membrane attack complex that directly damages the organ tissue and further attracts inflammatory cells to the allograft. The resultant damage is histologically distinct from cellular rejection that involves microvascular injury, often to the peritubular capillaries.[15] Definitive diagnosis of AMR is based on the presence of three criteria: presence of donor-specific antibodies, immunofluorescence staining of C4d deposits in the peritubular capillaries, and evidence of allograft dysfunction.[16] Circulating immune complexes often precede humoral rejection. This form of rejection is less common than cellular rejection and generally occurs in the first 3 months after transplantation. It is associated with an increased fatality rate and appears to be more common when antilymphocyte antibodies are used for rejection prophylaxis. An increased risk of humoral rejection is associated with female gender, elevated PRA, cytomegalovirus (CMV) seropositivity, a positive crossmatch, and prior sensitization to OKT3 (muromonab-CD3).[17] Strategies to reverse humoral rejection include plasmapheresis, often in combination with IV immunoglobulin, high-dose IV corticosteroids, antithymocyte globulin (ATG), cyclophosphamide, rituximab, and mycophenolate mofetil.

Chronic Rejection

Chronic rejection is a major cause of graft loss. It presents as a slow and indolent form of ACR, in which the involvement of the humoral immune system and antibodies against the vascular endothelium appear to play a role. Persistent perivascular and interstitial inflammation is a common finding in kidney, liver, and heart transplantation. As a result of the complex interaction of multiple drugs and diseases over time, it is difficult to delineate the true nature of chronic rejection. Unlike acute rejection, chronic rejection is not reversible with any immunosuppressive agents currently available.

Kidney

Advances in the management of acute rejection during the last decade have increased the duration of functioning grafts from living and cadaveric donors by more than 70%.[18] Chronic allograft nephropathy remains the most common cause of graft loss in the late posttransplantation period (>1 year). The syndrome is characterized in histological terms as interstitial fibrosis and tubular atrophy (IFTA) of unknown etiology. Structural changes are seen in as many as 50% of kidney transplantation patients within a year after transplantation and may present as early as 3 months.[19] Hypertension, proteinuria, and a progressive decline in renal function represent the classic clinical triad of chronic allograft nephropathy. Factors that contribute to the development of chronic allograft nephropathy include CNI nephrotoxicity, polyomavirus infection, hypertension, donor-related factors including ischemia time and undetected kidney disease in the donor kidney, and recurrence of the primary kidney disease in the recipient.

Liver

Approximately 3% to 5% of transplant livers are affected by chronic rejection, which is characterized by an obliterative arteriopathy and the gradual loss of bile ducts, often referred to as the vanishing bile duct syndrome. Initially patients experience an asymptomatic rise in the alkaline phosphatase and γ-glutamyl transpeptidase. As levels of bilirubin increase, patients become jaundiced and may experience itching.

Heart

Cardiac allograft vasculopathy, characterized by accelerated intimal thickening or development of atherosclerotic plaques, is the leading cause of graft failure and death in heart transplant recipients.[20] Endothelial injury, caused by both cell-mediated and humoral responses, is the first step in the process. Vasculopathy is restricted to the transplanted allograft. Routine surveillance with coronary angiography, intravascular ultrasound, or other procedures can aid in the diagnosis of vasculopathy. Evidence of cardiac allograft vasculopathy can be seen in as many as 14% of patients within 1 year of transplantation and in as many as 50% of patients within 5 years.[20] While chronic rejection of the kidney or liver allograft is generally not amenable to treatment, 3-hydroxy-3-methylglutaryl-coenzyme A (HMGCoA) reductase inhibitors and ACEIs have been used to decrease the incidence of vasculopathy in the heart allograft.[20] More recently, sirolimus and everolimus have been shown to reduce the incidence and slow progression of cardiac allograft vasculopathy.[20] Percutaneous transluminal coronary angioplasty and coronary artery bypass grafting have been used in severe cases of vasculopathy; these procedures, however, are limited by significantly increased mortality compared with the general population.[20]

TREATMENT

Immunosuppresion can be achieved with a variety of agents and the accepted regimens for most solid organs are usually comprised of two or more agents.

Desired Outcomes

Immediately following surgery, the primary goal of therapy is to prevent hyperacute and acute rejection. The high doses of immunosuppressants required to achieve this goal, if maintained long term, may result in serious complications such as nephrotoxicity, infection, thrombocytopenia, and drug-induced diabetes. Therefore, rapid dosage reductions are frequently used to minimize these effects. Transplant immunosuppression must be balanced to optimize both graft and patient survival.

General Approach to Treatment

1 A multidrug approach is rational from an immunomechanistic viewpoint because the many agents have overlapping and potentially synergistic mechanisms of action. Furthermore, the use of a multidrug immunosuppression regimen may allow the use of lower doses of individual agents, thus reducing the severity of dose-related adverse effects (Fig. 70-2). The protocols and individual drug regimens tend to be medical center specific. Although induction therapy may not be uniformly used, in almost every setting, patients receive IV methylprednisolone intraoperatively. Patients may also receive a descending dose of methylprednisolone over the first 5 to 7 postoperative days before beginning oral prednisone. Protocols generally combine a drug from two or three of the following classes: calcineurin inhibitors (CNIs), antimetabolites or proliferation signal inhibitors (PSIs), and corticosteroids.

If rejection is suspected, a biopsy can be done for definitive diagnosis or the patient may be empirically treated for rejection. Empiric treatment generally involves administration of high-dose corticosteroids, usually 500 to 1,000 mg of methylprednisolone IV for one to three doses. If signs and symptoms of rejection are resolved with empiric therapy, the maintenance immunosuppressive regimen

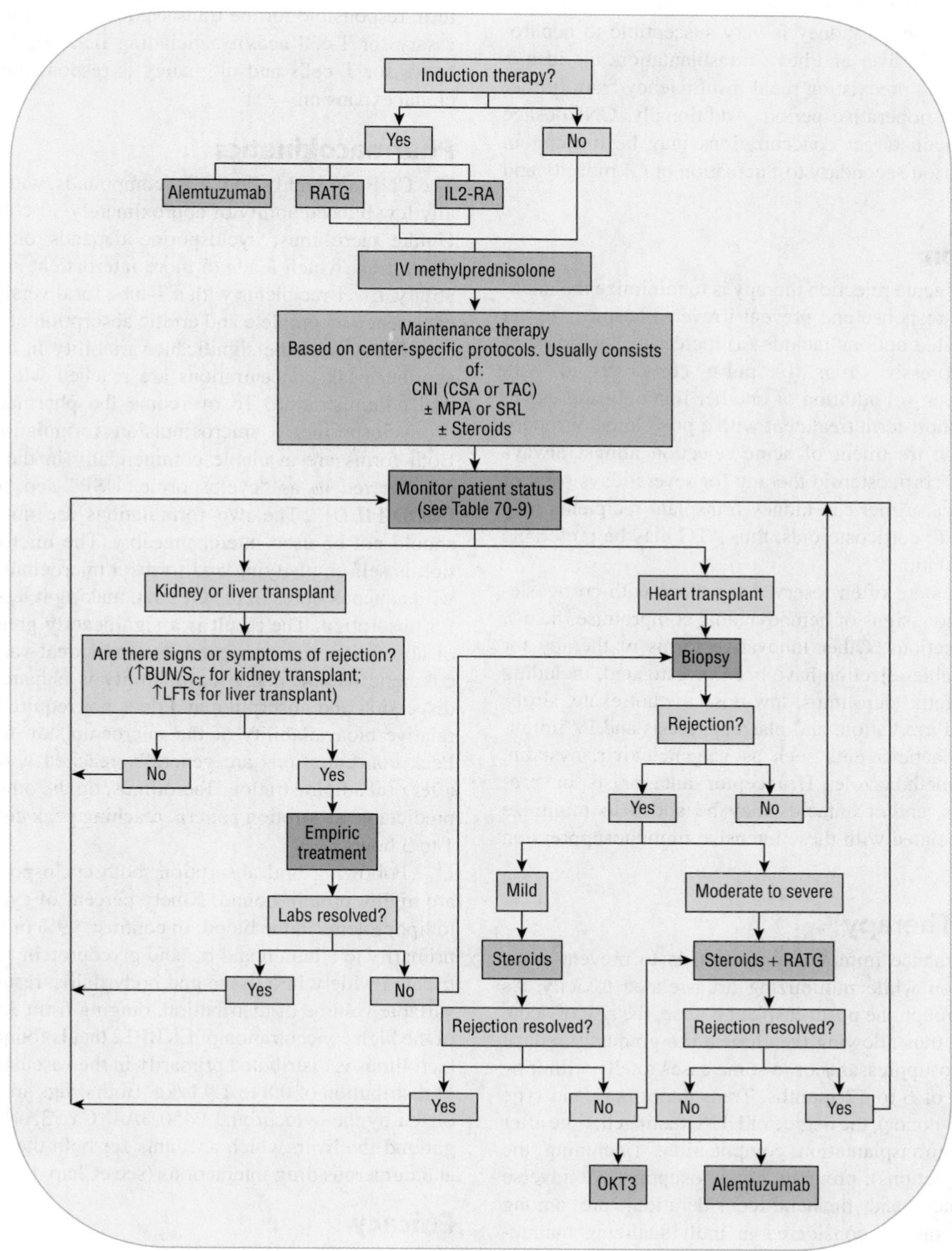

FIGURE 70-2 General approach to solid-organ transplant immunosuppression. (BUN, blood urea nitrogen; CNI, calcineurin inhibitor; CSA, cyclosporine; IL2RA, interleukin-2 receptor antagonist; LFTs, liver function tests; MPA, mycophenolic acid; OKT3, muromonab-CD3; RATG, rabbit antithymocyte immunoglobulin; Scr, serum creatinine; SRL, sirolimus; TAC, tacrolimus.)

is generally modified to provide a greater level of overall immunosuppression. If rejection is confirmed by biopsy, treatment may be based on the severity of rejection with polyclonal and monoclonal antibodies being reserved for moderate-to-severe rejections or those that have not responded to a course of corticosteroids.

Induction Therapy

Induction therapy provides a high level of immunosuppression, at the time of transplantation, with or without the immediate introduction of cyclosporine or tacrolimus (see Fig. 70-2). Two perioperative immunosuppressive strategies have been predominantly utilized to achieve this goal: (a) the provision of a highly intense immunosuppression, often on the basis of patient-specific risk factors such as age and race, or (b) the use of antibody therapy to provide enough immunosuppression to delay the initiation of therapy with the nephrotoxic CNIs. The rationale for delayed CNI administration varies slightly depending on the type of transplant. In renal transplantation, the newly transplanted kidney is very susceptible to nephrotoxic injury, whereas in liver and heart transplantation, the idea is to protect patients with preexisting renal insufficiency from further insults during the perioperative period. Additionally, CNI dosage adjustment to maintain target concentrations may be difficult in the perioperative period secondary to fluctuation of GI motility and enteral intake.

Acute Rejection

The primary goal of acute rejection therapy is to minimize the intensity of the immune response and prevent irreversible injury to the allograft. The available options include (a) increasing the doses of current immunosuppressive drugs, (b) "pulse" corticosteroids with subsequent dose taper, (c) addition of another immunosuppressant indefinitely, or (d) short-term treatment with a polyclonal or monoclonal antibody. The treatment of acute rejection almost always begins with "pulse" corticosteroid therapy for several days (oral or IV). However, African American kidney transplant recipients may not respond as well to corticosteroids; thus ATG may be preferable for this patient population.[21]

Cytolytic agents are often reserved for those with corticosteroid-resistant rejection, signs of hemodynamic compromise (heart), or more severe rejections. Other innovative forms of therapy for persistent or intractable rejection have been investigated, including mycophenolate mofetil, tacrolimus, low-dose methotrexate, sirolimus, total lymphoid irradiation, and plasmapheresis and IV immunoglobulin. Prophylactic agents such as valganciclovir, nystatin, trimethoprim–sulfamethoxazole, H_2-receptor antagonists or proton-pump inhibitors, and/or antacids may be added to minimize adverse effects associated with these intensive immunosuppression regimens.

Maintenance Therapy

The goal of maintenance immunosuppression is to prevent acute and chronic rejection while minimizing drug-related toxicity. As patients progress through the posttransplant course, the risk of acute rejection decreases, thus allowing the clinician to gradually reduce the doses of immunosuppressants or in some cases totally withdraw them over a period of 6 to 12 months. Transplant organ and type (cadaveric vs. living-donor), the degree of HLA mismatch, time after transplantation, posttransplantation complications (including the number of acute rejections), previous immunosuppressive adverse reactions, compliance, and financial considerations are among the patient-specific factors considered in individualizing maintenance immunosuppression. CNIs are generally a central component in most maintenance regimens, although CNI-free immunosuppression remains a future goal because of the significant nephrotoxicity associated with these agents. Ideally, immunosuppression should be optimized to prevent acute rejection episodes, minimize the occurrence of chronic rejection, and prevent long-term toxicities.

Calcineurin Inhibitors

❷ Cyclosporine and tacrolimus are the two CNIs currently used for most solid-organ transplant recipients. With the exception of heart transplant recipients (69%), more than 80% of transplant recipients receive tacrolimus as part of their immunosuppressive regimen.[1]

Pharmacology/Mechanism of Action

CNIs block T-cell proliferation by inhibiting the production of IL-2 and other cytokines by T cells (see Fig. 70-1). Cyclosporine and tacrolimus bind to unique cytoplasmic immunophilins cyclophilin and FK-binding protein-12 (FKBP12), respectively. The drug–immunophilin complex inhibits the action of calcineurin, an enzyme that activates the nuclear factor of activated T cells, which is, in turn, responsible for the transcription of several key cytokines necessary for T-cell activity, including IL-2. IL-2 is a potent growth factor for T cells and ultimately is responsible for activation and clonal expansion.

Pharmacokinetics

The CNIs are highly lipophilic compounds, with variable but generally low bioavailability of approximately 30% (range, 5% to 60%). Unlike tacrolimus, cyclosporine depends on bile for intestinal absorption, which lends to more interpatient and intrapatient variability. Liver recipients with a T-tube for diversion of bile may thus experience incomplete and erratic absorption of cyclosporine.

Because of the significant variability in absorption of cyclosporine, peak concentrations are reached within 2 to 6 hours of oral administration. To overcome the pharmacokinetic problems of cyclosporine, a microemulsion formulation was developed. Both forms are available commercially in the United States and are referred to as "cyclosporine, USP" and "cyclosporine, USP [MODIFIED]." The two formulations are not bioequivalent and should not be used interchangeably. The microemulsion formulation is self-emulsifying and forms a microemulsion spontaneously with aqueous fluids in the GI tract, making it less dependent on bile for absorption. The result is a significantly greater rate and extent of absorption and decreased intraindividual variability in pharmacokinetic parameters. Bioavailability is enhanced owing to better dispersion and absorption and does not require bile excretion. The relative bioavailability of the microemulsion formulation is 60%. Peak concentrations are generally reached within 1.5 to 2 hours after oral administration. Tacrolimus, on the other hand, has a more predictable absorption pattern, reaching peak concentrations within 1 to 3 hours.

Following oral absorption, both cyclosporine and tacrolimus are highly protein bound. Ninety percent of cyclosporine is bound to lipoproteins in the blood. In contrast, 99% of tacrolimus is bound primarily to albumin and α_1-acid glycoprotein. Cyclosporine is distributed widely into tissue and body fluids, resulting in a large and variable volume of distribution, ranging from 3 to 5 L/kg. Because of the high concentration of FKBP12 that is found in red blood cells, tacrolimus is distributed primarily in the vasculature, with a volume of distribution of 0.8 to 1.9 L/kg. Both drugs are extensively metabolized by the cytochrome P450 3A4 (CYP3A4) system in both the gut and the liver, which accounts for both the poor bioavailability and numerous drug interactions (see eChap. 6).

Efficacy

The introduction of the CNIs significantly improved the outcomes of solid-organ transplantation in terms of patient and graft survival, with 1-year graft survival improving from 75% to 87% for cadaveric grafts.[18] Both cyclosporine and tacrolimus are currently approved

TABLE 70-4 Comparison of Common Adverse Effects of Maintenance Immunosuppressants

AZA	MMF	SIR/EVR	Steroids	CSA	TAC	Bela
Nausea, vomiting Thrombocytopenia Leukopenia	Diarrhea, nausea Leukopenia Thromobocytopenia	Hyperlipidemia Thrombocytopenia Leukopenia	GI bleeding Hyperlipidemia Leukocytosis Hypertension Hyperglycemia Weight gain Mood changes	Hyperlipidemia Nephrotoxicity Tremor Hypertension Hyperglycemia Gingival hyperplasia Hirsutism	Diarrhea, nausea Hepatotoxicity Nephrotoxicity Tremor, headache Hypertension Hyperglycemia Hyperkalemia, hypomagnesemia	Diarrhea Neutropenia Anemia Peripheral edema Urinary tract infection

AZA, azathioprine; Bela, belatacept; CSA, cyclosporine; EVR, everolimus; MMF, mycophenolate mofetil; SIR, sirolimus; TAC, tacrolimus.

for prophylaxis of organ rejection in kidney, liver, and heart transplantations. When compared with the standard formulation, the microemulsion formulation of cyclosporine has demonstrated equivalent or superior efficacy in kidney, liver, and heart transplantation recipients. Studies comparing tacrolimus with either formulation of cyclosporine as primary immunosuppression demonstrate equivalent efficacy between the two agents in all transplantation situations.

Monotherapy with CNIs has been described.[22] The avoidance of long-term corticosteroids is the primary advantage of CNI monotherapy, whereas the primary disadvantage is the higher incidence of rejection. As a result, CNIs are rarely used as monotherapy.

Adverse Effects

Table 70-4 summarizes the adverse effects of CNIs, cyclosporine and tacrolimus, and other immunosuppressants. The nephrotoxic potential of both drugs is equal and is often related to the dose and duration of exposure. Neurotoxicity typically manifests as tremors, headache, and peripheral neuropathy; occasionally, however, seizures have been observed. Tacrolimus may be associated with an increased occurrence of neurologic complications compared with cyclosporine.

Cyclosporine appears to have a greater propensity to cause or worsen hypertension and hyperlipidemia compared with tacrolimus.[23–26] On the other hand, hyperglycemia is more common with tacrolimus than with cyclosporine but is often reversible when doses of tacrolimus and/or corticosteroids are reduced.[24] Cyclosporine is associated with cosmetic effects, such as hirsutism and gingival hyperplasia, which may be managed by converting from cyclosporine to tacrolimus or by proper hygiene in patients who cannot be switched to tacrolimus. Tacrolimus, in contrast, has been reported to cause alopecia, which is usually self-limiting and reversible.

Calcineurin Inhibitor Nephrotoxicity 3 Two types of nephrotoxicity can occur with CNIs. Acute nephrotoxicity is frequently seen early and is dose-dependent and reversible, but chronic nephropathy is more common. Clinical manifestations of CNI nephrotoxicity include elevated serum creatinine and blood urea nitrogen levels, hyperkalemia, hyperuricemia, mild proteinuria, and a decreased fractional excretion of sodium. CNI nephrotoxicity is recognized as the leading cause of renal dysfunction following nonrenal solid-organ transplant.

The predominant mechanism for CNI nephrotoxicity is renal vasoconstriction, primarily of the afferent arteriole, resulting in increased renal vascular resistance, decreased renal blood flow by up to 40%, reduced GFR by up to 30%, and increased proximal tubular sodium reabsorption with a reduction in urinary sodium and potassium excretion. A number of other mechanisms have been implicated, including changes in the renin–angiotensin–aldosterone system, prostaglandin synthesis, nitrous oxide production, sympathetic nervous system activation, and calcium handling.[27]

Measures to reduce CNI nephrotoxicity include delaying administration immediately postoperatively in patients at high risk for nephrotoxicity (using alternative induction protocols including an IL-2 receptor antagonist or antilymphocyte globulin), monitoring CNI trough blood levels and reducing the CNI dosage if the vasoconstrictive effects are problematic, and avoiding other nephrotoxins (e.g., aminoglycosides, amphotericin B, and nonsteroidal antiinflammatory agents) when possible. Currently, no proven therapies consistently prevent or reverse the nephrotoxic effects of CNIs.

In patients who have received a kidney transplant, it is often difficult to differentiate CNI nephrotoxicity from renal allograft rejection. Because the clinical features of acute renal allograft rejection and CNI nephrotoxicity may overlap considerably, a renal biopsy is necessary to differentiate the two (Table 70-5). However, differentiating between chronic renal allograft rejection and CNI nephrotoxicity may be more difficult because, in addition to clinical signs and symptoms, biopsy findings may also be similar.

Drug–Drug and Drug–Food Interactions

Drug interactions occur frequently with the CNIs because they are substrates for CYP3A4 and P-glycoprotein.[28,29] The most commonly administered drugs that are known to significantly alter cyclosporine and tacrolimus levels are highlighted in Table 70-6. Inhibitors of CYP3A4, such as diltiazem or erythromycin, can increase drug concentrations up to 82%, whereas drugs that induce CYP3A4 activity, such as phenytoin or rifampin, can decrease drug concentrations by 50%.[43] Some have taken advantage of these interactions by

TABLE 70-5 Differential Diagnosis of Acute Rejection and Cyclosporine or Tacrolimus Nephrotoxicity

	Nephrotoxicity in Renal Transplant Recipients	
	Acute Rejection	**CSA or TAC Nephrotoxicity**
History	Often <4 weeks postoperatively	Often >6 weeks postoperatively
Clinical presentation	Fever	Afebrile
	Hypertension	Hypertension
	Weight gain	Graft nontender
	Graft swelling/tenderness	Good urine output
	Decreased daily urine volume	
Laboratory biopsy	Rapid rise in serum Cr (0.3 mg/dL/day [27 μmol/L/day])	Gradual rise in serum Cr (>0.15 mg/dL/day [>13 μmol/L/day])
	Normal CSA or TAC concentration	Elevated CSA or TAC concentration
	Interstitial lymphocytic infiltrates	Interstitial fibrosis, tubular atrophy, glomerular thrombosis, arterial inflammation

Cr, creatinine; CSA, cyclosporine; TAC, tacrolimus.

TABLE 70-6 Effect of Concomitant Drug Administration on Cyclosporine, Tacrolimus, Sirolimus, and Everolimus

Cyclosporine Levels		Tacrolimus Levels		Sirolimus and Everolimus Levels	
Increase	**Decrease**	**Increase**	**Decrease**	**Increase**	**Decrease**
Ketoconazole	Rifampicin	Ketoconazole	Rifampin	Ketoconazole	Rifampin
Fluconazole	Phenytoin	Fluconazole	Dexamethasone	Fluconazole	Phenytoin
Itraconazole	Phenobarbital	Itraconazole	Phenytoin	Itraconazole	
Voriconazole	Carbamazepine	Voriconazole		Voriconazole	
Erythromycin	Sulfadimidine	Erythromycin		Erythromycin	
Levofloxacin	Trimethoprim	Levofloxacin		Clarithromycin	
Diltiazem	Mycophenolic Acid (vs. TAC)	Diltiazem		Diltiazem	
Verapamil		Verapamil		Verapamil	
Danazol		Danazol		Atorvastatin	
Nicardipine		Cimetidine		Cyclosporine	
Metoclopramide		Omeprazole		Protease inhibitors (HIV and HCV)	
Methylprednisolone		Clotrimazole			
Norethisterone		Nefazodone			
Sirolimus		Corticosteroids			
Tacrolimus		Cyclosporine			
Protease inhibitors (HIV and HCV)		Basiliximab			
		Protease inhibitors (HIV and HCV)			

HIV, human immunodeficiency virus; HCV, hepatitis C virus.
Data from references 28, 42, and 57.

routinely prescribing CYP3A4 inhibitors to reduce the dosage and cost of CNI therapy while maintaining the same therapeutic concentrations. This strategy seems more beneficial with cyclosporine than with tacrolimus.[29–31] While in vitro data suggest that drugs that increase the pH of the GI tract, such as magnesium-, aluminum-, or calcium-containing antacids, sodium bicarbonate, and magnesium oxide, can cause a pH-mediated degradation of tacrolimus by physically adsorbing tacrolimus in the GI tract, this has not been borne out in clinical studies.[32] Some clinicians suggest separating such compounds from tacrolimus administration by at least 2 hours to avoid any potential interaction.

Cyclosporine, and to a lesser extent, tacrolimus, are inhibitors of CYP3A4 and P-glycoprotein.[33] The inhibitory effects of cyclosporine and tacrolimus on CYP3A4 can be seen with weaker substrates, such as the HMG-CoA reductase inhibitors ("statins"). Concomitant administration of a CNI with an HMG-CoA reductase inhibitor results in an increase in the HMG-CoA reductase inhibitor levels, which increases the risk of HMG-CoA reductase inhibitor adverse effects, most notably myopathy.[34,35] Patients should be monitored for clinical signs of myopathy when receiving HMG-CoA reductase inhibitors in combination with cyclosporine and tacrolimus. The interaction appears to be more pronounced between cyclosporine and HMG-CoA reductase inhibitors due to inhibition of organic anion-transporter proteins (OATP) by cyclosporine.[36]

Consistency in administration of the CNIs with regard to meals and food intake is important to sustain an effective concentration time profile. High-fat meals can enhance both plasma clearance and the volume of distribution of cyclosporine by more than 60%.[37] Food reduces the rate and extent of tacrolimus absorption, and a high-fat meal may further delay gastric emptying and reduce the maximum achieved serum concentration (C_{max}), and the area under the concentration–time curve (AUC).[30] Furocoumarins, such as quercetin, naringin, and bergamottin, found in grapefruit juice, are potent inhibitors of CYP3A4 and have been reported to increase both cyclosporine and tacrolimus concentrations significantly. The AUC and C_{max} of cyclosporine have been reported to be increased by more than 55% and 35%, respectively.[38]

Dosing and Administration

Initial oral cyclosporine doses range from 8 to 18 mg/kg per day administered every 12 hours. Higher doses of cyclosporine are used more commonly in two-drug regimens, whereas lower doses are part of triple-drug regimens. Oral tacrolimus doses usually are in the range of 0.1 to 0.3 mg/kg per day given every 12 hours. Children require higher doses to maintain therapeutic drug concentrations, up to 14 to 18 mg/kg per day for cyclosporine and 0.3 mg/kg per day for tacrolimus. A once-daily formulation of tacrolimus was recently approved in the United States. After mg:mg conversion based on total daily dose, about one-third of patients required downward dose adjustments on the basis of 24-trough concentrations.[39] If oral administration is not possible, both drugs can be administered IV at one third the oral dosage, since administration by this route avoids first-pass metabolism. The usual IV dose of cyclosporine is 2 to 5 mg/kg per day, given as a continuous infusion or as single or twice-daily injection. IV tacrolimus doses range from 0.05 to 0.1 mg/kg per day and must be administered by continuous infusion.

Therapeutic Drug Monitoring

CNI serum concentrations are measured routinely in an attempt to optimize therapy (Table 70-7). The most common and practical method for monitoring CNIs is by measuring trough blood concentrations. Tacrolimus concentrations are most commonly measured by microparticle enzyme immunoassays or enzyme-linked immunoassays. Both drugs can be measured by high-performance

TABLE 70-7 Therapeutic Concentrations of Immunosuppressants by Various Methods

		Concentrations (ng/mL or mcg/L [μmol/L])	
Drug	**Sampling Medium**	**HPLC**	**RIA**
Cyclosporine	Whole blood	100–300 [83-250]	100–500 [83–416]
	Plasma	75–100 [62–83]	150–250 [125–208]
Tacrolimus	Whole blood	8–13 [10–16]	5–20 [6–25]
	Plasma		0.2–0.8 [0.25–1]
Sirolimus (with CNIs)	Whole blood	10–15 [11–16]	15–20 [16–22]
Sirolimus (without CNIs)	Whole blood	15–25 [16–27]	20–30 [22–33]
Everolimus (with CNIs)	Whole blood	3–8 [3–8]	

CNIs, calcineurin inhibitors; HPLC, high-performance liquid chromatography; RIA, radioimmunoassay.

liquid chromatography (HPLC), which is recognized as the reference procedure.[37] Therapeutic target ranges are assay specific because some quantitate parent plus metabolite concentration, while others only measure the parent compound. Thus, the target concentrations will be lower for the specific assays (HPLC) compared with nonspecific assays (radioimmunoassay [RIA] and microparticle enzyme immunoassays) by approximately 20% to 25%. The specific goal level for both drugs is dependent on transplant type, time after transplantation, concomitant immunosuppression, and transplantation center. One review of the role of tacrolimus in renal transplantation suggests that target 12-hour whole blood concentrations for tacrolimus are 15 to 20 ng/mL (15 to 20 mcg/L; 18.6 to 24.8 nmol/L) (0 to 1 month after transplantation), 10 to 15 ng/mL (10 to 15 mcg/L; 12.4 to 18.6 nmol/L) (1 to 3 months after transplantation), and 5 to 12 ng/mL (5 to 12 mcg/L; 6.2 to 14.9 nmol/L) (>3 months after transplantation).[24] Serum drug concentrations should be measured frequently (daily or three times per week) following initiation of the drug and during the stabilization period after transplantation. As the time increases after transplantation, serum concentrations are measured less frequently, usually monthly.

Studies have revealed lack of predictive value of trough cyclosporine concentrations and rejection.[40] Alternative strategies, including AUC and peak concentration, have been suggested to better correlate with rejection.[37,40] Limited sampling techniques using two to five blood samples within the first 4 hours after an oral dose have been used to determine AUC and it was observed that AUC levels >4,400 mcg/L (>3,361 nmol/L) per hour correlated with a reduction in rejection.[37,40] Cyclosporine peak concentration (C_2) has also been found to correlate with rejection and toxicity. Some transplantation centers have adopted this strategy to manage cyclosporine concentrations because of the convenience and reduced cost associated with the measurement of a single blood concentration. The suggested therapeutic range for C_2 cyclosporine levels is 1,500 to 2,000 ng/mL (1,500 to 2,000 mcg/L; 1,248 to 1,664 nmol/L) for the first few months after transplant and 700 to 900 ng/mL (700 to 900 mcg/L; 582 to 749 nmol/L) after 6 to 12 months.[40]

Corticosteroids

4 Corticosteroids have been used since the beginning of the modern transplantation era. Despite their many adverse events, they continue to be a cornerstone of immunosuppression regimens in many transplant centers, with 30% and 60% of liver and kidney transplant patients, respectively, receiving corticosteroids for at least the first year after transplantation.[1] The most commonly used corticosteroids are methylprednisolone and prednisone.

Pharmacology/Mechanism of Action

Corticosteroids block cytokine activation by binding to corticosteroid response elements, thereby inhibiting IL-1, IL-2, IL-3, IL-6, γ-interferon, and tumor necrosis factor-α synthesis (see Fig. 70-1). Additionally, corticosteroids interfere with cell migration, recognition, and cytotoxic effector mechanisms.[41]

Pharmacokinetics

Prednisone is converted to active prednisolone in the body and has multiple effects on the immune system. Prednisone is very well absorbed from the GI tract and has a long biologic half-life, permitting daily administration.

Efficacy

Corticosteroids became a part of the immunosuppressive regimens used in the first human transplantations[42] and continue to be used today. Their efficacy is irrefutable based on the decades of clinical experience. Systematic studies comparing corticosteroid-free immunosuppressive agent combinations with conventional therapy are difficult to perform because of the hundreds of potential combinations that now exist. However, recent studies of corticosteroid-free immunosuppressive agent combinations with newer, more specific immunosuppressants suggest that corticosteroids may in the future have less of a role in maintenance immunosuppression.[42,43]

Adverse Effects

Adverse effects of prednisone that occur in more than 10% of patients include increased appetite, insomnia, indigestion (bitter taste), and mood changes. Side effects that occur less often but which are seen with high doses or prolonged therapy include cataracts, hyperglycemia, hirsutism, bruising, acne, sodium and water retention, hypertension, bone growth suppression, and ulcerative esophagitis. The adverse effects of corticosteroids are summarized in Table 70-4.

Drug–Drug and Drug–Food Interactions

Barbiturates, phenytoin, and rifampin induce hepatic metabolism of prednisone and thus decrease the effectiveness of prednisone. Prednisone decreases the effectiveness of vaccines and toxoids.[41]

Dosing and Administration

An IV corticosteroid, commonly high-dose methylprednisolone, is given at the time of transplantation. The dose of methylprednisolone is tapered rapidly and discontinued within days, and oral prednisone is initiated. Prednisone doses are tapered progressively over time, depending on the type of additional immunosuppression and organ function. It is preferable to administer corticosteroids between 7 AM and 8 AM to mimic the body's diurnal release of cortisol. While conversion to alternate-day regimens or complete withdrawal of prednisone in patients with stable posttransplantation courses has been used with success in some transplantation centers, corticosteroids are often continued for the entire life of the functional graft.

The first-line therapy for the treatment of acute graft rejection is high-dose IV methylprednisolone (250 to 1,000 mg) daily for 3 days or oral prednisone (200 mg). Doses of oral prednisone are then tapered over 5 days to 20 mg/day. Prednisone should be taken with food to minimize GI upset. It is becoming a frequent practice to taper prednisone, with the goal of discontinuation over a period of months. Corticosteroids should never be discontinued abruptly; tapering should be gradual because of suppression of the hypothalamic–pituitary–adrenal axis. Corticosteroids slow the growth rates in children, prompting clinicians to use alternate-day dosing or to withhold corticosteroids until rejection occurs.

Antimetabolites

5 Antimetabolites have been used since the early days of transplantation because they prevent proliferation of lymphocytes. Azathioprine, long considered a part of the "gold standard" regimen with cyclosporine and corticosteroids, has largely been supplanted by mycophenolic acid (MPA) derivatives as they are more specific in their effects on lymphocytes and have fewer side effects.

Mycophenolic Acid Derivatives

MPA was first isolated from the *Penicillium glaucum* mold. Two formulations of MPA are currently available in the United States: mycophenolate mofetil is the morpholinoethyl ester of MPA, whereas mycophenolate sodium is available as an enteric-coated formulation of the sodium salt of MPA.

Pharmacology/Mechanism of Action The immunosuppressive effect of MPA is exerted through noncompetitive binding to inosine monophosphate dehydrogenase (IMPDH), the key enzyme responsible for guanosine nucleotide synthesis via the de novo pathway. Inhibition of IMPDH results in decreased nucleotide synthesis and diminished DNA polymerase activity, ultimately reducing lymphocyte proliferation.[44] Although MPA inhibits both types of IMPDH: IMPDH I, expressed by all cells in the body, and IMPDH II, which is expressed only in T and B lymphocytes, it is more specific for IMPDH II.[44] In addition to this, T and B lymphocytes only use the de novo pathway for nucleotide synthesis (see Fig. 70-1), making MPA very specific for these cells. Other cells within the body have a salvage pathway by which they can synthesize nucleotides, making them less susceptible to the actions of MPA and thereby reducing, but not eliminating, the potential for the hematologic adverse effects seen with azathioprine. In addition to decreasing lymphocyte proliferation, MPA may also downregulate activation of lymphocytes.[45]

Pharmacokinetics Because MPA is unstable in an acidic environment, mycophenolate mofetil acts as a prodrug that is readily absorbed from the GI tract, after which it is rapidly and completely converted to MPA by first-pass metabolism. The enteric coating of mycophenolate sodium protects MPA from the acidic gastric pH and allows for MPA to be released directly into the small intestine for absorption. The absolute bioavailability of MPA when delivered from mycophenolate mofetil and mycophenolate sodium is 94% and 72%, respectively. Peak concentrations of mycophenolate mofetil are reached within 1 to 2 hours following oral administration, while the enteric coating of mycophenolate sodium delays absorption and peak concentrations are not reached until 4 hours after administration.[45]

MPA is extensively bound (97%) to albumin in the blood. It is eliminated by the kidney and also undergoes glucuronidation in the liver to an inactive glucuronide metabolite (MPAG) that is excreted in the bile and urine. Enterohepatic cycling of MPAG can lead to deconjugation, thereby recirculating MPA into the bloodstream. This can account for 10% to 60% of total MPA exposure and results in a second peak 6 to 12 hours after oral administration.[45] The half-life of MPA is 18 hours.

Efficacy Currently, mycophenolate mofetil is approved for use in kidney, liver, and heart transplantations. Mycophenolate sodium was approved in 2004 for use in kidney transplantations only. Early studies comparing mycophenolate to azathioprine in patients receiving cyclosporine and corticosteroids demonstrated a statistically significant improvement in patient and graft survival at 1 and 3 years.[46] Subsequent studies have confirmed the efficacy of mycophenolate combined with tacrolimus. Mycophenolate has also demonstrated efficacy in the treatment of acute rejection.[47]

MPA derivatives are a key component of CNI-sparing protocols. Although MPA monotherapy has been investigated, patients experienced an unacceptable increase in rejection. Combination of MPA with sirolimus, on the other hand, resulted in improved renal function with no change in acute rejection and patient and graft survival.[46]

Adverse Effects Unlike cyclosporine and tacrolimus, MPA is not associated with nephrotoxicity, neurotoxicity, or hypertension. The most common side effects are related to the GI tract, including nausea, vomiting, diarrhea, and abdominal pain (see Table 70-4), which occur with similar frequency during IV and oral therapy. Strategies to reduce GI symptoms include dose reduction, division of the total daily dose into three or four doses, administration with food, or titration upward from lower doses during initial therapy. MPA also has hematologic effects, such as leukopenia and anemia, particularly with higher doses. Recently, the rare but serious adverse events of progressive multifocal leukoencephalopathy (PML) and pure red cell aplasia have been reported. Because peripheral IV mycophenolate administration is associated with local edema and inflammation, central venous administration may be the preferred route.

Drug–Drug and Drug–Food Interactions Food has no effect on MPA AUC, but it delays the absorption and decreases MPA C_{max} by 40% and 33% when mycophenolate mofetil and mycophenolate sodium, respectively, are administered. Administration with aluminum- and magnesium-containing antacids or cholestyramine significantly decreases the AUC of MPA and should be avoided.[48] It has been suggested that administration of iron may produce similar results, but this has not been tested. Concomitant administration of mycophenolate mofetil with pantoprazole has been reported to decrease MPA levels by 57% and AUC by 12% in healthy volunteers. The same effect was not observed with mycophenolate sodium.[49]

Acyclovir, commonly used in renal transplant recipients for the treatment and prevention of viral infections, competes with MPAG for renal tubular secretion. AUCs of both entities are increased with concomitant acyclovir and MPA administration. No pharmacokinetic interaction with other antiviral agents has been demonstrated. However, there is potential for additive pharmacodynamic effects such as bone marrow suppression.

Decreased MPA trough concentrations have been reported when MPA is administered with cyclosporine compared with those achieved when MPA is given with tacrolimus or sirolimus. This interaction is most likely a result of cyclosporine inhibition of multidrug-resistance-associated protein 2 (MRP2), which inhibits the enterohepatic recycling of MPAG, resulting in decreased MPA concentrations.[45] Cyclosporine decreases MPA levels by approximately 40% to 50% compared to tacrolimus.[24] To achieve equivalent MPA and MPAG serum concentrations, it may be necessary to administer higher doses of MPA with cyclosporine compared to tacrolimus. Antibiotics may also interfere with enterohepatic recycling of MPAG by decreasing bacterial-mediated deglucuronidation in the colon.[45]

Dosing and Administration Mycophenolate mofetil is currently available in both oral and IV formulations. Although IV administration of equal doses closely mimics oral administration, the two cannot be considered bioequivalent. Mycophenolate sodium is only available as an oral formulation. To optimize immunosuppression and minimize adverse effects, MPA is administered in two divided doses given every 12 hours. The total daily dose for kidney and liver transplants is typically 2 g/day for mycophenolate mofetil and 1.44 g/day for mycophenolate sodium. A higher level of immunosuppression is required for heart transplants; thus for these patients a total daily dose of 3 g/day for mycophenolate mofetil and 2.16 g/day for mycophenolate sodium is recommended. The recommended pediatric dose is 600 mg/m^2 for mycophenolate mofetil and 400 mg/m^2 for mycophenolate sodium, in two divided doses.

While an increasing body of literature exists, the routine therapeutic drug monitoring of MPA remains controversial. Plasma appears to be the most appropriate medium in which to measure MPA for therapeutic drug monitoring. Numerous studies have demonstrated a relationship between plasma MPA concentrations and improved clinical outcomes in patients receiving concomitant CNIs and corticosteroids. Patients with trough MPA levels between 1 and 3.5 mcg/mL (1 to 3.5 mg/L; 3.1 to 10.9 μmol/L) experienced fewer significant complications. Free (fMPA) concentrations as opposed to total MPA concentrations have been suggested as the relevant measure, especially in patients with liver disease, hypoalbuminemia, and severe infection.[50] Trough concentrations may not be accurate in predicting total drug exposure during a 12-hour interval and thus AUC monitoring has been proposed as the most appropriate measure of MPA drug exposure to predict therapeutic outcomes.[50] Better outcomes are associated with MPA AUC levels of greater than 42.8 mcg/mL (42.8 mg/L; 134 μmol/L) per hour (by HPLC),[51] although a reference range of 30 to 60 mcg/mL (30 to 60 mg/L; 94 to 188 μmol/L) has been proposed. The correlation between MPA AUC levels and adverse effects is low. Further studies are required to determine the best means to evaluate MPA levels, the acceptable targets for each, and the appropriate strategy to monitor MPA levels.[51]

Azathioprine

Azathioprine, a prodrug for 6-mercaptopurine (6-MP), has been used as an immunosuppressant in combination with corticosteroids since the earliest days of the modern transplantation era. It is associated with substantial toxicities, however, and its use has dramatically declined with the availability of newer immunosuppressants.

Pharmacology/Mechanism of Action Azathioprine is an inactive compound that is converted rapidly to 6-MP in the blood and is subsequently metabolized by three different enzymes. Xanthine oxidase, found in the liver and GI tract, converts 6-MP to the inactive final end product, 6-thiouric acid. Thiopurine *S*-methyltransferase (TPMT), found in hematopoietic tissues and red blood cells, methylates 6-MP to an inactive product, 6-methylmercaptopurine. Finally, hypoxanthine-guanine phosphoribosyltransferase is the first step responsible for converting 6-MP to 6-thioguanine nucleotides (6-TGNs), the active metabolites, which are incorporated into nucleic acids, ultimately disrupting both the salvage and de novo pathways of DNA, RNA, and protein synthesis. This process is toxic to the cell and renders the cell unable to proliferate (see Fig. 70-1). Eventually, 6-TGNs are catabolized by xanthine oxidase and thiopurine *S*-methyltransferase to inactive products.[52]

Pharmacokinetics Oral bioavailability of azathioprine is approximately 40%. Metabolism of 6-MP is primarily by xanthine oxidase to inactive metabolites, which are excreted by the kidneys. The half-life of azathioprine, the parent compound, is very short, approximately 12 minutes. The half-life of 6-MP is longer, ranging from 0.7 to 3 hours. However, it is the activity of the 6-TGNs that determines the pharmacodynamic half-life of the drug. The half-life of 6-TGNs has been estimated to be 9 days.[52]

Adverse Effects Dose-limiting adverse effects of azathioprine are often hematologic (see Table 70-4). Leukopenia, anemia, and thrombocytopenia can occur within the first few weeks of therapy and can be managed by dose reduction or discontinuation of azathioprine. Other common adverse effects include nausea and vomiting, which can be minimized by taking azathioprine with food. Alopecia, hepatotoxicity, and pancreatitis are less common adverse effects of azathioprine and are reversible on dose reduction or discontinuation. Activity of TPMT can affect the occurrence of adverse effects with azathioprine. Approximately 10% of the population has intermediate TPMT activity and 0.3% has low activity of the enzyme. In both scenarios, the incidence of leukopenia and hepatotoxicity is increased. As a result, TPMT genotyping may be useful to guide dosing of azathioprine to minimize adverse effects.[53]

Drug–Drug and Drug–Food Interactions The xanthine oxidase inhibitors allopurinol and febuxostat can increase azathioprine and 6-MP concentrations by as much as fourfold.[54] The metabolic pathways shift to favor production of 6-TGNs, which ultimately results in increased bone marrow suppression and pancytopenia. Doses of azathioprine should be reduced by 50% to 75% when allopurinol is added.

Dosing and Administration Initial doses of azathioprine are 3 to 5 mg/kg per day IV or orally. Individualization to maintain the white blood cell count between 3,500 and 6,000 cells/mm^3 (3.5×10^9 and 6.0×10^9/L) may be accomplished in some with doses as low as 0.25 mg/kg per day. Patients are often instructed to take azathioprine in the evening when initiating or titrating therapy to allow for dose adjustments based on morning determinations of their white blood cell count.

Proliferation Signal Inhibitors

6 Two PSIs have been approved in the United States for use in transplantation. Sirolimus, also known as rapamycin, is an immunosuppressive macrolide antibiotic that is structurally similar to tacrolimus, and is effective in reducing the risk of acute rejection. Sirolimus is thought to have potential to reduce chronic rejection, but this remains to be proven. Everolimus, a derivative of sirolimus, was approved in the United States in 2009 and was developed to improve the pharmacokinetics of sirolimus. Everolimus has a significantly shorter half-life than sirolimus.

Sirolimus and Everolimus

Pharmacology/Mechanism of Action Sirolimus and everolimus both bind to FKBP12, forming a complex that binds to the mammalian target of rapamycin (mTOR), which inhibits the response to cytokines (see Fig. 70-1). As such, the drugs are commonly referred to as mTOR inhibitors. IL-2 stimulates mTOR to activate kinases that ultimately advance the cell cycle from G1 to the S phase. Thus these drugs reduce T-cell proliferation by inhibiting the cellular response to IL-2 and progression of the cell cycle.[55,56]

Pharmacokinetics Bioavailability after oral administration is low for both, only 15% to 16%, with peak concentrations being reached within 1 to 2 hours for sirolimus and 0.5 to 4 hours for everolimus.[55,56] Both have large volumes of distribution, 5.6 to 16.7 L/kg for sirolimus and approximately 110 L for everolimus. Both are metabolized primarily by CYP3A4 both in the gut and in the liver. Likewise, both are also substrates for P-glycoprotein. The half-life for sirolimus is reported to be 60 hours but can be as long as 110 hours in patients with liver dysfunction, while that of everolimus is much shorter, 18 to 35 hours.[55,56]

Efficacy Sirolimus is only approved for the prevention of rejection in kidney transplant recipients when given in combination with corticosteroids and cyclosporine or after withdrawal of cyclosporine in patients with low-to-moderate immunologic risk. Because of the risks of delayed wound healing sirolimus is usually not started until 3 months after transplantation or later, once the surgical wound has healed. Sirolimus has also been demonstrated to be effective in combination with tacrolimus or mycophenolate in kidney transplants, with patient survival rates >99% and graft survival rates >96%.[55] Combination therapy with sirolimus and mycophenolate can be used to avoid the use of CNIs and decrease the risk of nephrotoxicity. Everolimus is approved for use in renal transplantation in combination with basiliximab, cyclosporine, and corticosteroids and for use in liver transplantation in combination with tacrolimus and corticosteroids. Everolimus has also been used with tacrolimus in kidney transplantation with similar results as sirolimus.[57] Everolimus appears to have less of an effect on wound healing and thus may potentially be used earlier after transplantation.

Early cyclosporine withdrawal has been studied in patients receiving sirolimus-based immunosuppressive protocols. Ideal candidates are patients who have not had a recent or severe rejection episode and adequate renal function 3 months after transplant. Rejection occurred in 5.6% of patients after discontinuation of cyclosporine, with no difference in graft survival. Long-term follow-up (2 years) showed improved renal function and blood pressure without an increase in acute rejection or graft loss in patients who discontinued cyclosporine.[55] Similar results have been demonstrated with everolimus.[57]

PSIs have demonstrated efficacy to reduce CNI use and nephrotoxicity in liver,[58] heart,[55] and lung transplant.[56] PSIs are also being investigated in liver transplant patients as a means to reduce the recurrence of hepatitis C and hepatocellular carcinoma.[58] They may also slow the progression of vaculopathy, which may reduce the incidence of chronic rejection and prolong long-term patient survival after heart transplantation.[20] However, the same effects have not been seen with lung transplantation.[59]

Clinical **Controversy. . .**

The benefits of PSIs after liver and lung transplant include decreased CNI-induced nephrotoxicity, anticancer properties, and anti-CMV and anti-HCV activity. Early introduction in these patients has demonstrated increased hepatic artery thrombosis and bronchial anastomotic dehiscence. The optimal timing of initiation of PSIs in these populations is controversial to minimize potential benefits while minimizing serious complications.

Adverse Effects Both everolimus and sirolimus are associated with dose-related myelosuppression. Thrombocytopenia is usually seen within the first 2 weeks of sirolimus therapy but generally improves with continued treatment; leukopenia and anemia are also typically transient.[55,56] Sirolimus trough serum concentrations greater than 15 ng/mL (15 mcg/L; 16 µmol/L) have been correlated with thrombocytopenia and leukopenia.[55] Hypercholesterolemia and hypertriglyceridemia are also common in patients receiving everolimus or sirolimus. It is postulated that the mechanism of this adverse effect is related to an overproduction of lipoproteins or inhibition of lipoprotein lipase. Peak cholesterol and triglyceride levels are often seen within 3 months of sirolimus initiation but usually decrease after 1 year of therapy and can be managed by reducing the dose, discontinuing sirolimus, or initiating therapy with an HMG-CoA reductase inhibitor or a fibric acid derivative. One study suggests that the dyslipidemia associated with sirolimus is not a major risk factor for early cardiovascular complications following kidney transplantation.[55] Delayed wound healing and dehiscence could be a result of inhibition of smooth muscle proliferation and intimal thickening.[55] Mouth ulcers are reported in as many as 60% of patients treated with sirolimus and appears to be dose-related.[55] Reversible interstitial pneumonitis has been described in kidney, liver, and heart–lung transplantation recipients.[55] Other adverse effects reported with sirolimus include increased liver enzymes, hypertension, rash, acne, diarrhea, and arthralgia (see Table 70-4).

Drug–Drug and Drug–Food Interactions The major metabolic pathway for everolimus and sirolimus is CYP3A4; thus, the drug interactions mediated by induction or inhibition of the CYP3A4 enzyme system are similar to those seen with cyclosporine and tacrolimus (see Table 70-5). Administration of the microemulsion formulation of cyclosporine with sirolimus significantly increases the AUC and trough sirolimus levels. The same is not seen with the standard formulation of cyclosporine. Conversely, cyclosporine concentrations and AUC are also increased when it is given concomitantly with sirolimus. The mechanism is proposed to be competitive binding to CYP3A4 and P-glycoprotein.[55,56] It is recommended that patients separate the dose of sirolimus and cyclosporine by 4 hours to minimize the interaction.[55] Concomitant administration of tacrolimus does not affect sirolimus levels.[55] Although everolimus AUC was increased by the administration of a single dose of cyclosporine modified, no specific recommendations for dose timing are given. It should be expected, however, that any changes in CSA dose may also necessitate a modification of everolimus dose and increased therapeutic drug monitoring is indicated.[56]

As with cyclosporine and tacrolimus, grapefruit juice increases sirolimus levels. Administration of sirolimus with a high-fat meal is associated with a delayed rate of absorption, decreased C_{max}, and increased AUC, indicating an increased drug exposure, whereas the half-life remains unchanged.[55] Conversely, administration of everolimus with a high-fat meal decreases both C_{max} and AUC.[56]

Dosing and Administration A fixed sirolimus dosing regimen is approved for concomitant use with cyclosporine that includes a loading dose of 6 or 15 mg followed by 2 or 5 mg daily, respectively. Therapeutic monitoring of sirolimus is advocated using whole-blood concentrations measured by HPLC, which is specific for the parent compound (see Table 70-7). For everolimus a starting dose of 0.75 mg twice daily is indicated in regimens that contain cyclosporine, corticosteroids, and basiliximab. Target concentrations are 3 to 8 ng/mL (3 to 8 mcg/L; 3 to 8 µmol/L).

Costimulatory Signal Inhibitor

Belatacept, derived from abatacept, is the only drug currently approved in the newest class of immunosuppressive agents. Belatacept may replace CNIs in the immunosuppressive regimen, which may abate toxicities associated with CNIs, namely, nephrotoxicity.[60] Currently, belatacept is only approved for kidney transplantation.

Belatacept

Pharmacology/Mechanism of Action Belatacept is a selective costimulation blocker that binds costimulatory ligands (CD80 and CD86) on antigen presenting cells, preventing interaction with CD28 on T cells. The interaction of CD80 and CD86 with CD28 is required for the initiation of "signal 2", the costimulatory signal that produces calcineurin, protein kinases, and nuclear factor-$\kappa\beta$ that lead to activation and proliferation of T-cells. Thus, blockade of CD80 and CD86 prevents T-cell activation.[60]

Pharmacokinetics Belatacept, which is only available as an IV solution, has a volume of distribution of 0.11 L/kg. The half-life of belatacept is approximately 11 days and is not affected by kidney or liver function.[60]

Efficacy A phase III clinical trial comparing belatacept to cyclosporine in first time kidney transplants demonstrated similar efficacy in terms of both patient and graft survival. In the trial, the cyclosporine group experienced more chronic allograft nephropathy at month 12. However, the belatacept group experienced more frequent and more severe ACR. Despite this, the measured GFR was 13 to 15 mL/min (0.22 to 0.25 mL/s) higher in the belatacept group compared to the cyclosporine group, a trend that persisted for 5 years.[60]

Studies have also evaluated conversion from CNI-based regimens to belatacept in kidney transplant recipients with stable kidney function. The results show improved GFR from baseline in those converted to belatacept compared to patients who remained on CNIs. However, the difference was not statistically significant as the study was not adequately powered.[61] Acute rejection occurred more frequently in patients who switched to belatacept, compared with no acute rejection in the patients who remained on CNIs.[60]

Early studies with belatacept in liver transplant resulted in increased graft loss and death.[62] Therefore, belatacept is not indicated for use in liver transplantation.

Adverse Effects The most common adverse effects of belatacept include anemia, neutropenia, diarrhea, urinary tract infections, headache, and peripheral edema.[60] Infusion-related reactions are rare with belatacept. In the clinical trials, patients who were Epstein–Barr virus (EBV) naïve experienced a significantly higher incidence of posttransplant lymphoproliferative disease (PTLD). Most of the cases of PTLD occurred within the first 18 months of treatment and the majority occurred in the CNS. There was no increase in incidence of PTLD in patients who were EBV-seropositive. As a result, belatacept carries a black box warning for PTLD and is contraindicated in patients who are EBV-seronegative. PML was also reported with belatacept.[60]

Drug–Drug and Drug–Food Interactions No drug or food interactions have been reported with belatacept.

Dosing and Administration Patients for whom belatacept is being considered must first be screened for EBV-serostatus prior to initiation of therapy. Only patients who are EBV-seropositive may receive belatacept due to the increased risk of PTLD in EBV-seronegative patients. The risk evaluation and mitigation strategy (REMS) for belatacept involves screening for symptoms of PTLD and PML with counseling and education related to each prior to each dose of belatacept. As a primary immunosuppressant for first time kidney transplant, belatacept is administered as 10 mg/kg IV over 30 minutes on days 0, 4, 14, 28, and at the end of weeks 8 and 12. Thereafter, the dose is reduced to the maintenance dose of 5 mg/kg administered IV over 30 minutes every 4 weeks beginning at week 16.

When converting to belatacept from a CNI-based regimen, the proposed dosing schedule is 5 mg/kg IV administered every 2 weeks for 5 doses on days 0, 14, 28, 42, and 56, then every 4 weeks thereafter. The CNI dose should be decreased by 50% after the second dose of belatacept, then discontinued after the fourth dose.[60]

Antibody Agents

7 Both polyclonal and monoclonal antibody preparations are used in transplantation. These agents can also be differentiated by their level of specificity, that is, particular receptor(s), or their downstream affects. In the following text, the agents are discussed as those that deplete lymphocytic cell lines (depleting antibodies) and those that generally bind to specific receptors but do not result in depletion of the cell to which they bind.

Depleting Antibodies

Antithymocyte Globulin Two antithymocyte globulins are available in the United States: ATG (Atgam, Pfizer, New York, NY), an equine polyclonal antibody, and RATG (Thymoglobulin, Genzyme, Cambridge, MA), a rabbit polyclonal antibody. The rabbit preparation is less immunogenic and may have other advantages over the equine preparation. Both ATG and RATG are often used as induction therapy to prevent acute rejection. In 2009, over 50% of kidney transplant recipients received RATG induction.[1]

Pharmacology/Mechanism of Action Because of their polyclonal antibody nature, both ATG and RATG exert their immunosuppressive effect by binding to a wide array of lymphocyte receptors (CD2, CD3, CD4, CD8, CD25, CD45, and others). Binding of ATG or RATG to the various receptors results in complement-mediated lysis and subsequent lymphocyte depletion. While T cells are the major lymphocytic target for the compounds, other blood cell components such as B cells and other leukocytes are also affected (see Fig. 70-1). Damaged T cells are subsequently removed by the spleen, liver, and lungs.

Pharmacokinetics ATG is poorly distributed into lymphoid tissue and binds primarily to circulating lymphocytes, granulocytes, and platelets. The terminal half-life of ATG is 5.7 days. RATG has a volume of distribution of 0.12 L/kg, and its terminal half-life in renal transplant recipients is significantly longer than ATG at 30 days.[63] Peak plasma concentrations are reached after 5 to 7 days of ATG or RATG infusions. Antiequine antibodies can form in up to 78% of patients who are receiving ATG therapy. Similarly, antirabbit antibodies have been reported in up to 68% of patients who are receiving RATG therapy. The effects of preformed antibodies on the efficacy and safety of these preparations have not been studied adequately.

Efficacy ATG and RATG are used most commonly for the treatment of acute allograft rejection or as induction therapy to prevent acute rejection. ATG is currently approved for both indications in kidney transplants. RATG is approved only for the treatment of acute allograft rejection in kidney transplantations. Both drugs have been studied extensively for both indications.

Use of RATG as part of quadruple therapy in liver transplantation is associated with similar rates of patient and graft survival and acute rejection compared with dual therapy. In kidney transplant RATG was associated with improved graft survival at 5 years as compared with equine ATG. Quadruple-drug therapy results in similar rates of patient and graft survival and malignancy in heart transplantations, but a significantly lower rate of acute rejection and infection episodes is seen at 1 year compared with triple-drug therapy. CMV is an adverse effect of this strategy, but recent data indicate that routine prophylaxis is successful in this setting.[64]

Adverse Effects Most adverse effects reported with ATG and RATG are related to the lack of specificity for T cells owing to their polyclonal nature. Dose-limiting myelosuppression (leukopenia, anemia, and thrombocytopenia) occurs frequently. Other adverse effects include anaphylaxis, hypotension, hypertension, tachycardia, dyspnea, urticaria, and rash. Serum sickness is seen more frequently with ATG than with RATG. Nephrotoxicity has been reported but is rare in the absence of serum sickness. Infusion-related febrile reactions are most common with the first few doses and can be managed by premedicating the patient with acetaminophen, diphenhydramine, and corticosteroids. Finally, as with any immunosuppressive agent, ATG and RATG are associated with an increased risk of infections, particularly viral infections, and malignancy.

Drug–Drug and Drug–Food Interactions No drug or food interactions have been reported with ATG or RATG.

Dosing and Administration ATG doses range from 10 to 30 mg/kg per day as a single dose for 7 to 14 days. RATG is a more potent compound and is administered at doses of 1 to 1.5 mg/kg per day as a single dose for 7 to 14 days for acute rejection or for 5 to 10 days for induction of immunosuppression. It is recommended that both ATG and RATG be administered through a central line or through a high-flow vein with an in-line 0.22-micron filter over at least 4 hours to minimize phlebitis and thrombosis whenever possible.[64,65] Literature supports peripheral administration of both agents. However, heparin and hydrocortisone are commonly added to the infusion to minimize phlebitis and thrombosis.[66]

Alemtuzumab

Alemtuzumab is approved for use in B-cell chronic lymphocytic leukemia. However, its effects on depleting both T and B lymphocytes make it useful in solid-organ transplants. While alemtuzumab is not FDA approved for solid-organ transplantation, it is increasingly recognized as a viable therapeutic option. In 2009, 10% of kidney transplant patients received alemtuzumab at the time of transplant.[1] However, in 2012, commercial distribution of alemtuzumab ceased for transplantation and leukemia, requiring centers to enroll in the manufacturer's distribution program for these indications.

Pharmacology/Mechanism of Action Alemtuzumab is a humanized monoclonal antibody against the CD52 surface antigen found on both T and B lymphocytes, as well as macrophages, monocytes, eosinophils, and natural killer cells. When alemtuzumab binds to the CD52 surface antigen, antibody-dependent lysis occurs, which removes both T and B lymphocytes from the blood, bone marrow, and organs, resulting in complete lymphocyte depletion.[67]

Pharmacokinetics The pharmacokinetics of alemtuzumab in solid-organ transplantation patients have not been investigated. Data from patients with B-cell chronic lymphocytic leukemia indicate that the volume of distribution of alemtuzumab after repeated dosing is 0.18 L/kg. The mean half-life after the first 30 mg dose was 11 hours, but increased to 6 days after 12 weeks of therapy. The extrapolation of these data to solid-organ transplantation is difficult because of the differences in dosing strategies (single or double doses in solid-organ transplantation vs. weekly to thrice weekly dosing in B-cell chronic lymphocytic leukemia). One or two doses of alemtuzumab result in complete and prolonged lymphocyte depletion. Following administration, B-lymphocyte counts return to normal within 3 to 12 months. T lymphocytes, however, remain depressed for as long as 3 years following administration.[67,68]

Efficacy Alemtuzumab is effective as induction therapy for the prevention of acute rejection in kidney, liver, pancreas, intestinal, and lung transplants.[67] Additionally, alemtuzumab has been used to successfully treat acute rejection following transplantation and is effective for corticosteroid- and antibody-resistant rejection.[68,69]

Adverse Effects Adverse effects of alemtuzumab are primarily infusion related, hematologic, and infectious. Because alemtuzumab causes complete lymphocyte depletion and associated cytokine release, infusion-related reactions include rigors, hypotension, fever, shortness of breath, bronchospasms, and chills. The potential for developing these reactions can be reduced by administering premedications such as acetaminophen, corticosteroids, and diphenhydramine or by administering smaller doses and escalating the dose gradually. Hematologic effects include pancytopenia, neutropenia, thrombocytopenia, and lymphopenia.

Drug–Drug and Drug–Food Interactions No drug or food interactions have been reported with alemtuzumab.

Dosing and Administration Several dosing regimens have been proposed for alemtuzumab in solid-organ transplantation. The most common dosing strategy for alemtuzumab is 30 mg as a single dose; some centers administer a second dose 1 to 5 days after transplantation.[67] Other studied dosing strategies include 0.3 mg/kg per dose, as a single- or multiple-dose regimen, and, finally, two 20-mg doses given on the day of transplantation and the first postoperative day.[69]

Nondepleting Antibodies

Interleukin-2 Receptor Antagonists Basiliximab, a chimeric monoclonal antibody (25% murine), is the only available IL-2 receptor antagonist in the United States. It is approved for use in kidney transplantation, but is also extensively used in other organ transplants as well.[71]

Pharmacology/Mechanism of Action Basiliximab exerts its immunosuppressive effect by specifically binding with high affinity to the α-chain (CD25) on the surface of activated T lymphocytes (see Fig. 70-1). Binding of basiliximab to the IL-2 receptor prevents IL-2-mediated activation and proliferation of T cells, a critical step in clonal expansion of T cells and the development of allograft rejection. Saturation of the IL-2 receptor occurs rapidly and confers an immunosuppressive effect that lasts for 4 to 6 weeks after administration.[70]

Pharmacokinetics Most of the pharmacokinetic data available for basiliximab is in renal transplantation patients. Caution must be used when extrapolating these data to nonrenal transplantation recipients. The volume of distribution is approximately 8 L for basiliximab. Basiliximab saturates CD25 in vivo at serum concentrations of 0.2. Basiliximab has a half-life of approximately 7 days in renal transplant recipients. Clearance of basiliximab is increased in patients who have received a liver transplant, primarily as a consequence of drainage of ascites. It is recommended that patients with greater than 10 L of ascites receive an additional dose of basiliximab on postoperative day 8.[71]

Efficacy Basiliximab is approved for use in kidney transplantation in combination with cyclosporine and corticosteroids, although induction therapy has also been studied extensively in liver and heart transplantation recipients. In 2009 29.6% of kidney and heart transplant recipients received an IL-2 receptor antagonist at the time of transplant.[1] A meta-analysis of basiliximab in renal transplantation concluded that IL-2 receptor antagonists reduced the risk of rejection significantly with no increases in graft loss, infectious complications, malignancy, or death.[70] Similar results were seen in liver and heart transplantation.[71]

IL-2 receptor antagonists offer a reasonable addition to CNI- or corticosteroid-sparing protocols. While CNI therapy cannot be completely avoided in most cases, IL-2 receptor antagonists allow for delayed use or reduced doses of CNIs, thus minimizing the risk of nephrotoxicity in the early posttransplantation period. Similar rates of rejection and corticosteroid-resistant rejection were seen in patients with DGF who received an IL-2 receptor antagonist in conjunction with lower tacrolimus doses compared with patients without DGF who received standard tacrolimus doses and no IL-2 receptor inhibitor induction.[70]

Adverse Effects Few adverse effects have been reported with basiliximab. In contrast to lymphocyte-depleting agents, basiliximab has not been associated with infusion-related reactions. However, since the marketing of basiliximab, an increased number of hypersensitivity reactions have been reported. Of note, only one patient developed antiidiotypic antibodies to the murine portion during clinical trials.[71] The manufacturer of basiliximab reported an increase in mortality in a placebo-controlled trial, which was associated with an increase in severe infections. No increased risk of malignancy has been reported.

Drug–Drug and Drug–Food Interactions Reports of increased cyclosporine and tacrolimus levels in patients receiving concomitant basiliximab were recently published.[70] Both authors hypothesized a potential interaction with the cytochrome P450.

Dosing and Administration Basiliximab is administered as two 20-mg IV doses, intraoperatively and again on postoperative day 4. Basiliximab is compatible with both 0.9% sodium chloride and 5% dextrose and can be administered either centrally or peripherally over 20 to 30 minutes in a volume of 50 mL. This regimen results in saturation of the IL-2 receptor for 30 to 45 days.

Investigational Agents

Rituximab

Rituximab is a chimeric monoclonal antibody against the CD20 receptor found on B cells. While it is FDA approved for non-Hodgkin lymphoma and rheumatoid arthritis, it has also been used in various aspects of transplant medicine, including treatment of AMR, suppression of alloantibodies prior to transplantation, and PTLD.[72] Rituximab has been shown to improve graft survival in combination with plasmapheresis and IVIG in patients with AMR.[16] In highly sensitized patients, rituximab administration prior to transplantation has been shown to suppress alloantibodies and even allow transplantation across ABO-incompatibility.[72] In PTLD, rituximab is most effective in patients with CD20-positive malignancies.[72] The optimal dose of rituximab in transplantation has not been defined.

Bortezomib

Bortezomib, a proteosomal inhibitor that is FDA approved for the treatment of multiple myeloma, has been used in the treatment of AMR. In one series, 20 patients with AMR received four doses of bortezomib 1.3 mg/m^2 on days 1, 4, 7, and 11 with plasmapheresis. Bortezomib was effective in lowering donor-specific antibodies by 50%.[16] Another series showed benefit of bortezomib over rituximab.[16] However, bortezomib is associated with significant side effects, namely diarrhea that leads to dehydration, nausea, edema, vomiting, and infections. Side effects led to hospitalizations in one-third of patients in one series.[16]

Janus Kinase Inhibitors

Janus kinases are important for transduction of intracellular signals in lymphocytes to stimulate proliferation and lymphocyte activity. Tofacitinib is a Janus Kinase 3 (JAK3) inhibitor that has been compared to cyclosporine in combination with mycophenolate mofetil and steroids. Tofacitinib showed similar efficacy to cyclosporine, but was associated with an increased incidence of CMV and BK virus infections.[73] Clinical trials continue to evaluate long-term efficacy and safety of JAK3 inhibitors.

EVALUATION OF THERAPEUTIC OUTCOMES

8 The success of transplantation can be measured in terms of length of graft and patient survival or quality of life. Several donor and recipient factors that have an impact on graft and patient survival have been identified (Table 70-8). The greatest risk to short-term graft survival is acute rejection. Routine surveillance of appropriate biochemical markers and serum drug concentrations are essential to minimize the potential for acute rejection. These parameters should be assessed daily to weekly for the first 1 to 3 months after transplantation. Monitoring should include complete blood counts, serum electrolyte concentrations, serum creatinine and blood urea nitrogen concentrations, and the appropriate serum drug concentrations. Liver function tests should also be evaluated using the same schedule in liver transplantation recipients. Routine biopsies are necessary to monitor for acute rejection in heart transplantation recipients. As the time after transplantation increases, the frequency of monitoring decreases. Once 3 months have elapsed after transplantation, monitoring of these parameters can be reduced to biweekly or monthly for most patients.

Long-term graft survival is limited by chronic rejection. Overall survival rates for solid-organ transplantations are described in terms of half-life, or the time after transplantation at which only 50% of transplanted organs are still functioning. Estimated half-lives for kidneys are 26.9 years for HLA-identical grafts and 12.2 and 10.8 years, respectively, for grafts from a sibling or parent who are 1-haplotype matches. The estimated half-life for HLA-matched grafts was 17.3 years while a markedly lower value of 7.8 years has been noted with mismatched kidneys.[18] The overall median patient survival time for heart transplantation recipients is 9.8 years, but in these patients surviving the first year after transplantation, the median survival increases to 12 years.[1] The highest rate of mortality occurs within the first year after liver transplantation due to the risks of surgery and early postoperative complications. Table 70-9 depicts a typical posttransplantation laboratory monitoring plan.

TABLE 70-8 Factors Negatively Affecting Allograft and Patient Survival

	Kidney	Liver	Heart
Donor factors	Decreased HLA matching Increased age Increased serum creatine Cardiac instability Prolonged ischemia time History of hypertension	Size mismatch Age (youngest, oldest)	Size mismatch Increased age Prolonged ischemia time
Recipient factors	Age <15, >50 years Retransplantation African race Elevated PRA Multiparous women Poor drug compliance	Increased age Retransplantation African race ICU pretransplant ABO blood type Poor drug compliance	Age <5, >60 years ICU pretransplant Mechanical ventilation LVAD IABP Poor drug compliance

HLA, human leukocyte antigens; IABP, intraaortic balloon pump; LVAD, left ventricular assist device; PRA, panel of reactive antibodies.

PERSONALIZED PHARMACOTHERAPY

Individualization of immunosuppression therapy starts with identifying the patient's risk of rejection prior to transplantation. Most clinicians will use induction therapy with a lymphocyte depleting agent for patients at high risk of rejection, including those patients who are sensitized to more HLA antigens due to previous exposure to blood products or previous transplant, younger patients and African Americans. Similarly, organs associated with a higher risk of rejection, including heart and lung transplants, require higher doses of immunosuppressants as maintenance therapy.

Therapeutic drug monitoring is a key component of individualizing the immunosuppressant regimen to ensure adequate immunosuppression is achieved while minimizing drug-related toxicities. Blood concentrations are routinely monitored for CNIs and PSIs

TABLE 70-9 Laboratory Monitoring after Transplantation as a Function of Time Posttransplant

	1–2 Weeks	1 Month	2–4 Months	4–12 Months	>12 Months
SCr/BUN	Daily	1–2 times per week	Every 1–2 weeks	Monthly	Every 1–2 months
Chemistries[a]	Daily	1–2 times per week	Every 1–2 weeks	Monthly	Every 1–2 months
Liver function tests[b]					
Kidney or heart recipient	Once	Once	Monthly	Every 1–3 months	Every 1–3 months
Liver recipient	Daily	1–3 times per week	Every 1–2 weeks	Monthly	Every 1–2 months
Immunosuppressant level	Daily	1–2 times per week	Every 1–2 weeks	Monthly	Every 1–2 months
Complete blood count[c]	Daily	1–2 times per week	Every 1–2 weeks	Monthly	Every 1–2 months
Lipid panel[d]	Once	Every 3 months	Every 3 months	Every 3 months	Every 3 months
HbA_{1c}	Once	Every 3 months	Every 3 months	Every 3 months	Every 3 months

BUN, blood urea nitrogen; HbA_{1c}, hemoglobin A1c; SCr infusion, serum creatinine.

[a]Chemistries include sodium, potassium, chloride, CO_2 content, magnesium, calcium, phosphorus, and blood glucose.
[b]Liver function tests include total bilirubin, aspartate transaminase (AST), alanine transaminase (ALT), gamma glutamyl transpeptidase (GGTP), and alkaline phosphatase.
[c]Complete blood count includes white blood cells (WBC), red blood cells (RBC), platelets, and/or differential.
[d]Lipid panel includes total cholesterol, low-density lipoprotein (LDL), high-density lipoprotein (HDL), triglyceride, and/or very low-density lipoprotein (VLDL).

throughout the duration of therapy. Studies are ongoing to determine the correlation between blood concentrations and MPA. Consensus guidelines suggest that MPA monitoring may be warranted when MPA is used as the primary immunosuppressant, CNI doses are reduced or discontinued, the patient has altered liver or kidney function, or medications that interact with MPA are administered concomitantly.[51] One study suggests that African Americans may require monitoring of MPA levels due to more rapid clearance of MPA compared to Caucasians.[74]

Research is ongoing for pharmacogenetic monitoring of immunosuppressive therapies. Cytochrome P450 genetic polymorphisms are important for CNI metabolism. Both cyclosporine and tacrolimus are metabolized by CYP3A5, which contributes to the interpatient variability associated with CNIs. It is estimated that 30% of Caucasians and 50% of African Americans express high levels of CYP3A5 enzymes. Patients who express CYP3A5 require significantly higher doses of CNIs to achieve therapeutic levels.[75] CYP3A5 genotyping may help to identify patients who require higher doses of CNIs to optimize immunosuppressive therapy earlier after transplantation and potentially decrease the risk of rejection. However, larger studies are needed to determine the effectiveness of this strategy.

Pharmacodynamic monitoring of immunosuppressants is currently being explored. This involves monitoring the specific targets of immunosuppressants rather than blood concentrations. Research is ongoing to determine the value of monitoring calcineurin activity for CNIs[76] and IMPDH activity for MPA.[45]

Generic Substitution

In recent years, a number of generic versions of immunosuppressants have entered the market. While generic versions of corticosteroids and azathioprine have long been in the marketplace, there are now generic versions of cyclosporine, USP [MODIFIED], tacrolimus, and mycophenolate mofetil, the latter being considered narrow therapeutic index drugs. While these formulations have demonstrated bioequivalence to the innovator product in healthy individuals, bioequivalence testing in transplant patients is not required for approval.[77]

Although there would be no differences in the action of the molecule once absorbed into the systemic circulation, several potential differences in absorption could result in variability not seen in healthy volunteers. The presence of diabetes may delay gastric emptying, whereas cystic fibrosis may lead to differences in tacrolimus or cyclosporine secondary to fat malabsorption. None of these generic formulations have been studied in pediatric patients.[78]

As generic medications may offer a significant cost advantage compared with the innovator product, their use will increase over time. Much of the concern with generic substitution for immunosuppressant and other narrow therapeutic index medications relates to the potential for unmonitored changes in formulations. Systems that alert patients and prescribers to changes in formulation (e.g., labels on medications, direct notification to physicians) could trigger clinicians to more closely monitor patients for efficacy and toxicity as well as heightened therapeutic drug monitoring during a switch. However, the extent to which increased monitoring could offset cost savings associated with generic substitution has not been fully delineated.

IMMUNOSUPPRESSION-RELATED COMPLICATIONS

Comorbidities such as cardiovascular disease and malignancy, recurrent disease, drug toxicities (namely nephrotoxicity), and chronic rejection are the primary causes of mortality in patients who have a functioning graft 5 or more years after transplantation.[1]

Cardiovascular Disease

Cardiovascular disease is a leading cause of morbidity and mortality in transplant patients.[79] Preexisting cardiovascular disease, which is common in end-stage organ failure, is not reversed with transplantation. Additionally, hypertension, hyperlipidemia, and diabetes are common complications in transplantation recipients and are independent risk factors that contribute significantly to cardiovascular disease. Chronic rejection has been linked to hypertension[80] and hyperlipidemia.[81]

Hypertension

Corticosteroids, cyclosporine, tacrolimus, and impaired kidney graft function may cause posttransplantation hypertension. The primary mechanism of CNI-associated hypertension in heart transplantation recipients may be related to the CNI-induced stimulation of intact renal sympathetic nerves and the absence of reflex cardiac inhibition of the sympathetic nervous system, but a number of other mechanisms, including decreased prostacyclin and nitric oxide production, have also been proposed.[40,82] In addition to the propensity to cause peripheral vasoconstriction, CNIs promote sodium retention, resulting in extracellular fluid volume expansion. Tacrolimus appears to have less potential to induce hypertension following transplantation than cyclosporine.[83]

Calcium channel blockers have traditionally been the first-line agents to treat hypertension after transplantation.[84] Calcium channel blockers may ameliorate the nephrotoxic effects of cyclosporine, improve renal hemodynamics, decrease the incidence of DGF and the development of allograft atherosclerosis, and provide some immunosuppression. Calcium channel blockers, however, may also contribute to gingival hyperplasia that is often associated with cyclosporine-based immunosuppression.

ACEIs and angiotensin II receptor blockers have traditionally been avoided in kidney transplantation recipients, especially in the perioperative phase, because of the potential for hyperkalemia and their potentially negative influence on GFR. ACEIs and angiotensin II receptor blockers are now considered to be an equivalent alternative to calcium channel blockers for the treatment of hypertension in all transplant recipients, and are preferred in patients with proteinuria.[84] When ACEIs or angiotensin II receptor blockers are used in patients after transplantation, serum creatinine and potassium levels should be monitored closely. If the increase in serum creatinine is greater than 30% within 1 to 2 weeks after initiating ACEIs or angiotensin II receptor blockers, other alternatives must be considered (see Chap. 3).

Multiple antihypertensive agents are usually necessary to achieve the goal blood pressure in transplant recipients; consequently, the addition of a β-blocker, diuretic, or centrally acting antihypertensive is usually necessary. β-blockers are generally considered to be second-line therapy in solid-organ transplantation recipients because of the potential to worsen metabolic disturbances caused by immunosuppressants, such as hyperkalemia and dyslipidemia. CNI-induced hypertension is often salt-sensitive, making it very responsive to diuretics. Central-acting agents (e.g., clonidine) are used often as adjunctive therapy in transplantation recipients who are unable to achieve blood pressure control with calcium channel blockers or ACEIs.

Hyperlipidemia

Hyperlipidemia may be exacerbated by corticosteroids, CNIs, PSIs, diuretics, and β-blockers.[81,84] Corticosteroids promote insulin resistance and a decrease in lipoprotein lipase activity, as well as excessive triglyceride production. The mechanism of CNI-induced hyperlipidemia is not well understood. CNIs may decrease the activity of the low-density lipoprotein (LDL) receptor or lipoprotein lipase, altering LDL catabolism.[81] Tacrolimus appears to have less potential than cyclosporine to induce hyperlipidemia.[24,26,35,43,81] It is controversial whether the management of hyperlipidemia in transplant recipients should be more aggressive than the current guidelines for the general population established by the National Cholesterol Education Program.[84] Aggressive lipid lowering may not only arrest the progress or prevent the complications of atherosclerosis but also promote graft survival in the kidney and heart transplant recipients. Current recommendations suggest monitoring lipid panels 2 to 3 months after transplantation and annually thereafter.[84]

For most patients, the combination of dietary intervention and an HMG-CoA reductase inhibitor should be considered the treatment of choice. HMG-CoA reductase inhibitors are highly effective in the treatment of hyperlipidemia, especially increased LDL, in transplantation patients. HMG-CoA reductase inhibitors as a class also have immunomodulatory effects on MHC expression and T-cell activation and reduce cardiac allograft rejection.[34,35,81]

HMG-CoA reductase inhibitors should be used with caution in transplantation recipients because of several reports of rhabdomyolysis when these agents are combined with CNIs.[34] Safety measures include using low HMG-CoA reductase inhibitor doses and avoiding inappropriately high cyclosporine or tacrolimus concentrations. Concurrent use of simvastatin and cyclosporine is contraindicated; due to the increased risk of rhabdomyolysis.[85] The concurrent use of medications known to increase the risk of myopathy (such as gemfibrozil) should be avoided.[81] Patients should be informed of the signs and symptoms of rhabdomyolysis. Baseline and follow-up creatine phosphokinase measurements (every 6 months) have been used to identify patients who develop subclinical rhabdomyolysis when cholesterol-lowering therapy is used. Pravastatin may be preferred as a result of its lower interactive potential with CNIs because it is not metabolized by CYP3A4. The potential for hepatotoxicity from HMG-CoA reductase inhibitors warrants close monitoring of liver function in all transplantation recipients.[84]

Bile acid-binding resins may be used to lower cholesterol in transplant patients, but adequate doses are difficult to achieve without the development of GI adverse effects. Because the absorption of cyclosporine is dependent on the presence of bile in the GI tract, patients should be instructed to separate dosing of bile acid-binding resins and cyclosporine by at least 2 hours. Bile acid-binding resins should also be separated from other immunosuppressants by at least 2 hours to avoid physical adsorption in the GI tract. For transplant patients who have hypertriglyceridemia refractory to dietary intervention, fish oil and fibric acid derivatives are well-tolerated, effective alternatives (see Chap. 11). Fibric acid derivatives are most effective in lowering serum triglyceride concentrations.

New-Onset Diabetes after Transplantation

Corticosteroids and CNIs can impair glucose control in previously diabetic patients, as well as cause new-onset diabetes after transplantation (NODAT) in 4% to 20% of patients. Corticosteroids induce insulin resistance and impair peripheral glucose uptake, whereas CNIs appear to inhibit insulin production.[81] Tacrolimus seems to be more diabetogenic than cyclosporine, although recent studies have failed to show a statistical difference.[43] Other possible risk factors that have been identified for NODAT include African American or Hispanic ethnicity, age >40 years, family history, and weight, as well as CMV and hepatitis C virus (HCV) infection.[81]

Up to 40% of patients with NODAT will require insulin therapy.[80] In diabetic patients who can be managed with an oral hypoglycemic agent, glipizide, which is metabolized extensively by the liver, may be preferred over renally eliminated agents such as glyburide. Metformin should be used with extreme caution because of the risk of accumulation and lactic acidosis in those with moderate renal impairment. Regardless of therapy, frequent blood glucose monitoring is imperative in the early postoperative phase both to improve glucose control and to identify those with NODAT. Changes in renal function secondary to CNI nephrotoxicity or DGF or acute rejection in kidney transplant recipients affect the elimination of many hypoglycemic agents, including insulin, and may result in hyper- or hypoglycemia. Dose changes of immunosuppressant drugs also affect glycemic control. Tapering of immunosuppressive medications may result in reduced insulin requirements, whereas corticosteroid pulses for the treatment of rejection may result in increased insulin requirements.

Infection

Increased risk of infection is a natural consequence of therapeutic immunosuppression. Many infections, including CMV and fungal infections, in solid-organ transplant recipients are reviewed in Chapter 100.[86]

Polyomavirus-associated nephropathy (PVAN) is an important cause of renal dysfunction in kidney transplant recipients. The specific polyomavirus that infects kidney allografts is the BK virus. Primary infection with BK virus occurs in childhood as an asymptomatic infection in 50% to 90% of the general population. The precise mechanism of transmission is not clear but is suspected to be via the oral or respiratory routes. The virus then remains latent primarily in the genitourinary tract. Reactivation of BK virus is limited to people with compromised immune function and is most common in kidney transplant recipients. Reactivation can be detected as the presence of BK virus in the urine of approximately 30% to 40% of kidney transplant recipients, although it does not progress to nephropathy in the majority of patients. However, BK viremia if it develops has been noted to progress to allograft nephropathy in 50% of patients.[87] The development of BK virus nephropathy results in graft loss in about 46% of affected patients.[87]

It has been recommended that all kidney transplant recipients be screened for urinary BK virus replication monthly for the first 3 to 6 months after transplant and every 3 months thereafter for the first year. Screening for BK virus should also occur any time the serum creatinine is elevated without known cause and after treatment of acute rejection.[84] Treatment of BK virus should be initiated when plasma concentrations persist above 10,000 copies/mL (10×10^6/L).[84] The first line of treatment is to reduce immunosuppressive medications. Other treatment strategies include cidofovir, leflunomide, and fluoroquinolones, although studies with these agents are limited.[88]

HCV recurs almost universally following liver transplantation and the course of the disease is accelerated. Within 5 years, 10% to 20% of liver transplant recipients with HCV recurrence will progress to cirrhosis requiring retransplantation, compared to the general population where 20% to 30% will develop cirrhosis over 20 to 30 years. Liver donor age over 40 years has been shown to be the primary risk factor for HCV recurrence. Females with HCV recurrence develop more severe disease than the general population. Standard treatment for HCV recurrence includes interferon alfa-2b in combination with ribavirin. However, the virologic response is reduced after liver transplantation compared to the general population. The therapy is further complicated by significant side effects, namely leukopenia and anemia. Administration of hematopoietic growth factors may be needed to allow administration of adequate doses of interferons and ribavirin. Interferon alone shows minimal effect against HCV recurrence after liver transplantation.[89] There is no data on the use of the HCV protease inhibitors, boceprevir and telaprevir, after liver transplantation. The potent CYP3A4 inhibition of these drugs, however, will have significant effects on CNI and PSI dosing. One study in healthy volunteers reported telaprevir increased the AUC of cyclosporine by 4.6-fold and tacrolimus by 70-fold.[90] The role of these agents after transplantation is currently being investigated to determine the optimal dose adjustments needed for CNIs.[89]

In the absence of preventative therapy, hepatitis B recurs in approximately 80% of patients after transplantation. Initial studies with short-term IV administration of hepatitis B immunoglobulin (HBIg) showed equally high rates of recurrence upon discontinuation of therapy. However, strategies that employ the long-term administration of HBIg with or without antiviral therapy report much lower recurrence rates, 15% to 30% and 20% to 40%, for nonreplicative and replicative hepatitis B virus, respectively. Common strategies include IV HBIg 10,000 units during the anhepatic phase followed by 10,000 units daily for 6 days. Antihepatitis B surface titer should be monitored weekly to ensure adequate levels for protection as well as to optimize HBIg use. HBIg has been typically dosed to maintain titers >100 to 500 international units/L. Long-term HBIg therapy is extremely costly, estimated at $100,000 for the first postoperative year and $50,000 for each subsequent year. Combination therapy with antiviral agents appears to be synergistic and is the current standard. Lamivudine resistance is a concern with long-term utilization both pre- and posttransplant. The role of newer antiviral agents, including adefovir, entecavir, and tenofovir, remains to be defined. Other strategies that have been investigated and show promise include pretransplant viral load reduction and reduced-dose HBIg. Treatment for active hepatitis B virus graft infection should include HBIg, antiviral therapy, and concomitant reduction in immunosuppression.[91]

Malignancy

Although advances in immunosuppression have decreased the incidence of acute rejection and increased patient survival, they have also increased the patient's lifetime exposure to immunosuppression. While the precise mechanism is unclear, posttransplantation malignancy seems to be related to the overall level of immunosuppression, as evidenced by a difference in the rates of malignancy associated with quadruple versus triple versus dual immunosuppressant regimens. The risk of de novo malignancy in transplantation recipients is increased three- to fivefold over the general population. The age-adjusted incidence of lung, breast, colon, and prostate cancers was doubled in renal transplant recipients. A number of cancers that are uncommon in the general population occur with much higher prevalence in transplantation recipients: posttransplantation lymphomas and lymphoproliferative disorders (PTLDs), Kaposi's sarcoma, renal carcinoma, in situ carcinomas of the uterine cervix, hepatobiliary tumors, and anogenital carcinomas. Skin cancers are the most common tumors. Factors that may predispose transplant recipients to skin cancers include copious sun exposure and therapy with azathioprine.[92] While too early to definitively assess the impact of MPA derivatives on malignancy, one analysis showed a lower risk of PTLD with MMF compared with AZA. PSIs have a theoretical benefit in terms of the development of malignancy. In addition to immunosuppressive properties, PSIs also have antiproliferative effects. In fact, a decreased incidence of malignancy was reported in patients receiving PSIs versus CNIs, and conversion to PSIs from CNIs can result in regression of Kaposi's sarcoma.[92]

PTLD encompasses a broad spectrum of disorders, ranging from benign polyclonal hyperplasias to malignant monoclonal lymphomas. Factors that predispose patients to PTLD include EBV seronegativity at transplantation and intense immunosuppression, particularly with lymphocyte-depleting agents. Nonrenal transplantation recipients are more likely to develop PTLD secondary to the heavy immunosuppression used to reverse rejection. Administration of ganciclovir or acyclovir preemptively during antilymphocyte therapy may decrease the risk of EBV seroconversion and infection, reducing the eventual risk of PTLD. Treatment of life-threatening PTLD generally includes severe reduction or cessation of immunosuppression. Other options include systemic chemotherapy or rituximab.[72]

Posttransplantation malignancies appear an average of 5 years after transplantation and increase with the length of follow-up: as many as 72% of patients surviving greater than 20 years may be affected. Malignancy accounts for 11.8% of deaths after cardiac transplantation and is the single most common cause of death in the sixth to the tenth posttransplant years.[92]

CLINICAL BOTTOM LINE

Transplantation is a lifesaving therapy for several types of end-organ failure. Advances in the understanding of transplant immunology have produced an unprecedented number of choices in terms of immunosuppression. The increasing number of effective immunosuppressive medications and therapies offers clinicians diverse ways to prevent allograft rejection in a patient-specific manner. However, the vast array and efficacy of currently available immunosuppressive agents make it increasingly difficult to evaluate their long-term efficacy. Clinicians must be keenly aware of the adverse effects of immunosuppressive medications and their treatment in order to optimize the care of the transplanted patient.

ABBREVIATIONS

ACEI	angiotensin-converting enzyme inhibitor
ACR	acute cellular rejection
AMR	antibody-mediated rejection
ATG	antithymocyte globulin
ATN	acute tubular necrosis
AUC	area under the concentration–time curve
C_2	concentration 2 hours after dose
C_{max}	peak concentration
CMV	cytomegalovirus
CYP	cytochrome P450 liver enzyme system
DGF	delayed graft function
FKBP	FK-binding protein
HBIg	hepatitis B immunoglobulin
HLA	human leukocyte antigen
HPLC	high-performance liquid chromatography
IL	interleukin
IMPDH	inosine monophosphate dehydrogenase
LDL	low-density lipoprotein
MELD	model for end-stage liver disease
MHC	major histocompatibility complex
MPA	mycophenolic acid
MPAG	mycophenolic acid glucuronide
mTOR	mammalian target of rapamycin
NODAT	new-onset diabetes after transplantation
OKT3	muromonab-CD3
PML	progressive multifocal leukoencephalopathy
PRA	panel of reactive antibody
PSI	proliferation signal inhibitor
PTLD	post-transplantation lymphoproliferative disorder
PVAN	polyomavirus-associated nephropathy
RIA	radioimmunoassay
6-MP	6-mercaptopurine

REFERENCES

1. Organ Procurement and Transplantation Network (OPTN) and Scientific Registry of Transplant Recipients (SRTR). OPTN/SRTR 2010 Annual Data Report. Rockville, MD: Department of Health and Human Services, Health Resources and Services Administration, Healthcare Systems Bureau, Division of Transplantation, 2011.
2. Wolfe RA, Ashby VB, Milford EL, et al. Comparison of mortality in all patients on dialysis, patients on dialysis awaiting transplantation and recipients of a first cadaveric transplant. N Engl J Med 1999;341:1725–1730.
3. Kovacs AZ, Molnar MZ, Szeifert L, et al. Sleep disorders, depressive symptoms and health-related quality of life—a cross-sectional comparison between kidney transplant recipients and waitlisted patients on maintenance dialysis. Nephrol Dial Transplant 2011;26:1058–1065.
4. U.S. Renal Data System, USRDS 2012 Annual Data Report: Atlas of Chronic Kidney Disease and End-Stage Renal Disease in the United States. Bethesda, MD: National Institutes of Health, National Institute of Diabetes and Digestive and Kidney Diseases, 2012.
5. Tritto G, Davies NA, Jalan R. Liver replacement therapy. Semin Respir Crit Care Med 2012;33(1):70–79.
6. Quante M, Benckert C, Thelen A, Jonas S. Experience since MELD implementation: How does the new system deliver? Int J Hepatol 2012;2012:264015. PubMed PMID: 23091734.
7. Sheiner P, Rochon C. Recurrent hepatitis C after liver transplantation. Mt Sinai J Med 2012;79:190–198.
8. McCalmont V, Ohler L. Cardiac transplantation: candidate identification, evaluation, and management. Crit Care Nurs 2008;31(3):216–229.
9. Deng MC. Heart failure: Cardiac transplantation. Heart 2002;87:177–184.
10. Braith RW, Edwards DG. Exercise following heart transplantation. Sports Med 2000;30:171–192.
11. Venkataramanan R, Habucky K, Burckart GJ, et al. Clinical pharmacokinetics in organ transplant patients. Clin Pharmacokinet 1989;16:134–161.
12. Ingulli E. Mechanism of cellular rejection in transplantation. Pediatr Nephrol 2010;25(1):61–74.
13. Stehlik J, Edwards LB, Kucheryavaya AY, et al. Registry of the international society for heart and lung transplantation: 29th official adult heart transplant report—2012. J Heart Lung Transplant 2012;31(10):1052–1064.
14. Costanzo MR, Dipchand A, Starling R, et al. The International Society of Heart and Lung Transplantation guidelines for the care of heart transplant recipients. J Heart Lung Transplant 2010;29(8):914–956.
15. Haas M. Pathologic features of antibody-mediated rejection in renal allografts: An expanding spectrum. Curr Opin Nephrol Hypertens 2012;21(3):264–271.
16. Fehr T, Gaspert A. Antibody-mediated kidney allograft rejection: Therapeutic options and their experimental rationale. Transplant Int 2012;25:623–632.
17. Michaels PJ, Espejo ML, Kobashigawa J, et al. Humoral rejection in cardiac transplantation: Risk factors, hemodynamic consequences and relationship to transplant coronary artery disease. J Heart Lung Transplant 2003;22:58–69.
18. Hariharan S, Johnson CP, Bresnahan BA, et al. Improved graft survival after renal transplantation in the U.S., 1988 to 1996. N Engl J Med 2000;342:605–612.
19. Merville P. Combating chronic renal allograft dysfunction: Optimizing immunosuppressive regimens. Drugs 2005;65: 615–631.
20. Schmauss D, Weis M. Cardiac allograft vasculopathy: Recent developments. Circulation 2008;117;2131–2141.
21. Malat GE, Culkin C, Palya A, Panganna K, Anil Kumar MS. African American kidney transplantation survival: The ability of immunosuppression to balance the inherent pre- and post-transplant risk factors. Drugs 2009;69(15):2045–2062.
22. Augustine JJ, Hricik DE. Steroid sparing in kidney transplantation: Changing paradigms, improving outcomes, and remaining questions. Clin J Am Soc Nephrol 2006;1:1080–1089.
23. Scott LJ, McKeage K, Keam SJ, Plosker GL. Tacrolimus: A further update of its use in the management of organ transplantation. Drugs 2003;63:1247–1297.
24. Bowman LJ, Brennan DC. The role of tacrolimus in renal transplantation. Expert Opin Pharmacother 2008;9: 635–643.
25. Keogh A. Calcineurin inhibitors in heart transplantation. J Heart Lung Transplant 2004;23:S203–S206.
26. Jose M. Calcineurin inhibitors in renal transplantation: Adverse effects. Nephrology 2007;12:S66–S74.
27. Bobadilla MA, Gamba G. New insights into the pathophysiology of cyclosporine nephrotoxicity: A role of aldosterone. Am J Physiol Renal Physiol 2007;293:F2–F9.
28. Spriet I, Meersseman W, deHoon J, von Winckelmann S, Wilmer A, Willems L. Mini-series, II: Clinical aspects. Clinically relevant CYP450-mediated drug interactions in the ICU. Intensive Care Med 2009;35:603–612.
29. Jones TE. The use of other drugs to allow a lower dosage of cyclosporine to be used: Therapeutic and pharmacoeconomic considerations. Clin Pharmacokinet 1999;32:357–367.
30. Kothari J, Nash M, Zaltzman J, et al. Diltiazem use in tacrolimus-treated renal transplant recipients. J Clin Pharm Therap 2004;29:425–430.
31. Kumana CR, Tong MKL, Li CS, et al. Diltiazem co-treatment in renal transplant patients receiving microemulsion cyclosporin. Br J Clin Pharmacol 2003;56:670–678.
32. Chisholm MA, Mulloy LL, Jagadeesan M, et al. Coadministration of tacrolimus with anti-acid drugs. Transplantation 2003;76:665–666.
33. Amundsen R, Asberg A, Ohm IK, Christensen H. Cyclosporine A- and tacrolimus-mediated inhibition of CYP3A4 and CYP3A5 in vitro. Drug Metab and Disp 2012;40(4):665–661.
34. Gazi IF, Liperopoulous EN, Athyros VG, et al. Statins and solid organ transplantation. Current Pharm Des 2006;12:4771–4783.
35. Olyaei A, Greer E, Santos RD, Rueda J. The efficacy and safety of 3-hydroxy-3-methylglutaryl-CoA reductase inhibitors in chronic kidney disease, dialysis, and transplant patients. Clin J Am Soc Nephrol 2011;6(3):664–678.
36. Amundsen R, Christensen H, Zagihyan B, Åsberg A. Cyclosporine A, but not tacrolimus, shows relevant inhibition of organic anion-transporting protein 1B1-mediated transport of atorvastatin. Drug Metab Disp 2010;38(9):1499–1504.
37. Schiff J, Cole E, Cantarovich M. Therapeutic monitoring of calcineurin inhibitors for the nephrologist. Clin J Am Soc Nephrol 2007;2:374–384.
38. Nowack R. Cytochrome P450 enzyme, and transport protein mediated herb–drug interactions in renal transplant patients: Grapefruit juice, St. John's Wort—and beyond! Nephrology 2008;13:337–347.
39. Cross SA, Perry CM. Tacrolimus once-daily formulation: In the prophylaxis of transplant rejection in renal or liver allograft recipients. Drugs 2007;67:1931–1943.

40. Kuypers DRJ. Immunosuppressive drug monitoring—What to use in clinical practice today to improve renal graft outcome. Transpl Int 2005;18:140–150.
41. Bush WW. Overview of transplantation immunology and the pharmacotherapy of adult solid organ transplant recipients: Focus on immunosuppression. AACN Clin Issues 1999;10:253–269.
42. Halloran PF. Immunosuppressive drugs for kidney transplantation. N Engl J Med 2004;351:2715–2729.
43. Pascual J, Rouuela A, Galeano C, Crespo M, Zamora J. Very early steroid withdrawal or complete avoidance for kidney transplant recipients: A systematic review. Nephrol Dial Transplant 2012;27:825–832.
44. de Jonge H, Naesense M, Kuypers DRJ. New insights into the pharmacokinetics and pharmacodynamics of the calcineurin inhibitors and mycophenolic acid: Possible consequences for therapeutic drug monitoring in solid organ transplantation. Ther Drug Monit 2009;31(4):416–435.
45. Weigel G, Griesmacher A, Karimi A, et al. Effect of mycophenolate mofetil therapy on lymphocyte activation in heart transplant recipients. J Heart Lung Transplant 2002;21:1074–1079.
46. Ciancio G, Miller J, Gonwa TJ. Review of major clinical trials with mycophenolate mofetil in renal transplantation. Transplantation 2005;80(2S):S191–S200.
47. Shah S, Collett D, Johnson R, et al. Long-term graft outcome with mycophenolate mofetil and azathioprine: A paired kidney analysis. Transplantation 2006;82:1634–1639.
48. Shaw LM, Figurski M, Milone MC, et al. Therapeutic drug monitoring of mycophenolic acid. Clin J Am Soc Nephrol 2007;2:1062–1072.
49. Rupprecht K, Schmidt C, Raspe A, et al. Bioavailability of mycophenolate mofetil and enteric-coated mycophenolate sodium is differently affected by pantoprazole in healthy volunteers. J Clin Pharmacol 2009;49(10):1196–1201.
50. Elbarbary FA, Shoker AS. Therapeutic drug measurement of mycophenolic acid derivatives in transplant patients. Clin Biochem 2007;40:752–764.
51. Kuypers DRJ, Le Meur Y, Cantarovich M, et al. Consensus report on therapeutic drug monitoring of mycophenolic acid in solid organ transplantation. Clin J Am Soc Nephrol 2010;5:341–358.
52. Lancaster DL, Patel N, Lennard L, Lilleyman JS. 6-Thioguanine in children with acute lymphoblastic leukemia: Influence of food on parent drug pharmacokinetics and 6-thioquanine nucleotide concentrations. Br J Clin Pharmacol 2001;51:531–539.
53. Kurzawski M, Dziewanowski K, Gawrońska-Szklarz B, Domański L, Droździk M. The impact of thiopurine *S*-methyltransferase polymorphism on azathioprine-induced myelotoxicity in renal transplant recipients. Ther Drug Monit 2005;27(4):435–441.
54. Imuran® (azathioprine) [product information]. San Diego, CA: Prometheus Laboratories Inc, 2011.
55. Augustine JJ, Bodziak KA, Hricik DE. Use of sirolimus in solid organ transplantation. Drugs 2007;67:369–391.
56. Monchaud C, Marquet P. Pharmacokinetic optimization of immunosuppressive therapy in thoracic transplantation: Part II. Clin Pharmacokinet 2009;48:489–516.
57. Gabardi S, Baroletti SA. Everolimus: a proliferation signla inhibitor with clinical applications in organ transplantation, oncology, and cardiology. Pharmacotherapy 2010;30(10):1044–1056.
58. Kawahara T, Asthana S, Kneteman NM. m-TOR inhibitors: What role in liver transplantation? J Hepatol 2011;55: 1441–1451.
59. Hopkins PM, McNeil K. Evidence for immunosuppression in lung transplantation. Curr Opin Organ Transplant 2008;13:477–483.
60. Victoria CH, Harrison J, Rogers C, Ensom MHH. Belatacept: A new biologic and its role in kidney transplantation. Ann Pharmacother 2012;46(1):57–67.
61. Rostaing L, Massari P, Garcia VD, et al. Switching from calcineurin inhibitor-based regimens to a belatacept-based regimen in renal transplant recipients: A randomized phase II study. Clin J Am Soc Nephrol 2011;6:430–439.
62. Nulojix® (belatacept) [product information]. Princeton, NJ: Bristol-Myers Squibb Company, 2011.
63. Bunn D, Lea CK, Bevan DJ, et al. The pharmacokinetics of anti-thymocyte globulin (ATG) following intravenous infusion in man. Clin Nephrol 1996;45:29–32.
64. Webster AC, Pankhurst T, Rinaldi F, Chapman JR, Craig JC. Monoclonal and polyclonal antibody therapy for treating acute rejection in kidney transplant recipients: A systematic review of randomized trial data. Transplantation 2006;81:953–965.
65. Hardinger KL. Rabbit antithymocyte globulin induction therapy in adult renal transplantation. Pharmacotherapy 2006;26:1771–1783.
66. Erickson AL, Roberts K, Malek SK, Chandraker AK, Tullius SG, Gabardi S. Analysis of infusion-site reactions in renal transplant recipients receiving peripherally administered rabbit antithymocyte globulin as compared with basiliximab. Transplant Int 2010;23(6):636–640.
67. Morris PJ, Russell NK. Alemtuzumab (Campath-1H): A systematic review in organ transplantation. Transplantation 2006;81:1361–1367.
68. Bloom DD, Hu H, Fechner JH, Knechtle SJ. T-lymphocyte alloresponses of Campath-1H-treated kidney transplant patients. Transplantation 2006;81:81–87.
69. Tan HP, Smaldone MC, Shapiro R. Immunosuppressive preconditioning or induction regimens: Evidence to date. Drugs 2006;66:1535–1545.
70. McKeage K, McCormack PL. Basiliximab: A review of its use as induction therapy in renal transplantation. Drugs 2010;24(1):55–76.
71. Ramirez CB, Marino IR. The role of basiliximab induction therapy in organ transplantation. Exper Opin Biol Ther 2007;7:137–148.
72. Ramanath V, Nistala R, Chaudhary K. Update on the role of rituximab in kidney diseases and transplant. Expert Opin Biol Ther 2012;12(2):223–233.
73. Wojciechowski D, Vincenti F. Targeting JAK3 in kidney transplantation: Current status and future options. Curr Opin Organ Transplant 2011;16:614–619.
74. Tornatore KM, Sudchada P, Dole K, et al. Mycophenolic acid pharmacokinetics during maintenance immmunosuprpession in African American and Caucasian renal transplant patients. J Clin Pharmacol 2011;51:1213–1222.
75. Barry A, Levine M. A systematic review of the effect of CYP3A5 genotype on the apparent oral clearance of tacrolimus in renal transplant recipients. Ther Drug Monit 2010;32(6):708–714.
76. van Rossum HH, de Fijter JW, van Pelt J. Pharmacodynamic monitoring of calcineurin inhibition therapy: Principles, performance, and perspectives. Ther Drug Monit 2010;32(1):3–10.
77. Christians U, Klawitter J, Clavijo CF. Bioequivalence testing of immunosuppressants: Concepts and misconceptions. Kidney Int 2010;77:S1–S7.
78. Uber PA, Ross HJ, Zuckermann AO, et al. Generic drug immunosuppression in thoracic transplantation: An

ISHLT educational advisory. J Heart Lung Transplant 2009;28:655–660.
79. Bostom AD, Brown RS, Chavers BM, et al. Prevention of post-transplant cardiovascular disease: Report and recommendations of an ad hoc group. Am J Transplant 2002;2:491–500.
80. Zhang R, Leslie B, Boudreaux P, et al. Hypertension after kidney transplantation: Impact, pathogenesis and therapy. Am J Med Sci 2003;325:202–208.
81. Subramanian S, Trence DL. Immunosuppressive agents: Effects on glucose and lipid metabolism. Endocrinol Metab Clin N Am 2007;36:891–905.
82. Ventura HO, Malik FS, Mehra MR, et al. Mechanisms of hypertension in cardiac transplantation and the role of cyclosporine. Curr Opin Cardiol 1997;12:375–381.
83. Chobanian AV, Bakris GL, Black HR, et al. The seventh report of the Joint National Committee on Prevention, Detection, Evaluation, and Treatment of High Blood Pressure: The JNC 7 report. JAMA 2003:289;2560–2572.
84. Kasiske BL, Zeier MG, Chapman JR, et al. KDIGO clinical practice guideline for the care of kidney transplant recipients. Kidney Int 2009;9(Suppl 3):S1–S155.
85. Florentin M, Elisaf MS. Simvastatin interactions with other drugs. Expert Opin Drug Safety 2012;11(3):439–444.
86. Fishman JA. Infection in solid-organ transplant recipients. N Eng J Med 2007;357:2601–2614.
87. Hirsch HH, Brennan DC, Drachenberg CB, et al. Polyomavirus-associated nephropathy in renal transplantation: Interdisciplinary analyses and recommendations. Transplantation 2005;79:1277–1286.
88. Dharnidharka VR, Abdulnour HA, Araya CE. The BK virus in renal transplant recipients—Review of pathogenesis, diagnosis, and treatment. Pediatr Nephrol 2011;26:1763–1774.
89. Sheiner P, Rochon C. Recurrent hepatitis C after liver transplantation. Mt Sinai J Med 2012;79(2):190–198.
90. Garg V, von Heeswijk R, Lee JE, Alves K, Nadkarni P, Lou X. Effect of telaprevir on the pharmacokinetics of cyclosporine and tacrolimus. Hepatology 2001;54(1): 20–27.
91. Cholangitas E, Goulis J, Akriviadis E, Papatheodoridis GV. Hepatitis B immunoglobulin and/or nucleos(t)ide analogues for prophylaxis against hepatitis b virus recurrence after liver transplantation: A systematic review. Liver Transplant 2011;17(10):1176–1190.
92. Dantal J, Pohanka E. Malignancies in renal transplantation: An unmet medical need. Nephrol Dial Transplant 2007;22:i4–i10.

71

Osteoarthritis

Lucinda M. Buys and Mary Elizabeth Elliott

KEY CONCEPTS

1. Millions of Americans have osteoarthritis (OA). OA prevalence increases with age, with women more commonly affected than men.
2. Contributors to OA are systemic (age, genetics, hormonal status, obesity, occupational, or recreational activity) and/or local (injury, overloading of joints, muscle weakness, or joint deformity).
3. OA is primarily a disease of cartilage that reflects a failure of the chondrocyte to maintain proper balance between cartilage formation and destruction. This leads to loss of cartilage in the joint, local inflammation, pathologic changes in underlying bone, and further damage to cartilage triggered by the affected bone.
4. Manifestations of OA are local, affecting one or a few joints; the knees are most commonly affected, as well as the hips and hands. Osteophytes (bony proliferation of affected joints) are often found, in contrast to the soft tissue swelling of rheumatoid arthritis.
5. Nonpharmacologic therapy is the foundation of the treatment plan for all patients with OA. Nonpharmacologic therapy should be initiated before or concurrently with pharmacologic therapy.
6. The most common symptom associated with OA is pain, which leads to decreased function and motion. Pain relief is the primary objective of medication therapy.
7. Based on efficacy, safety, and cost considerations, scheduled acetaminophen, up to 4 g/day in divided doses, should be tried initially for pain relief in knee and hip OA. If this fails, topical or oral nonsteroidal antiinflammatory drugs (NSAIDs) are recommended, if there are no contraindications.
8. Strategies to reduce NSAID-induced GI toxicity include the use of nonacetylated salicylates, COX-2 selective inhibitors, or the addition of misoprostol or a proton-pump inhibitor. COX-2 selective inhibitors vary in their ability to prevent GI toxicity, and concomitant use of aspirin largely negates their gastroprotective effects.
9. COX-2 selective inhibitors can increase the risk of cardiovascular events. This may be a class effect, but the extent of this risk varies among COX-2 selective inhibitors, and traditional NSAIDs may also pose risks. This hazard, in addition to the GI toxicity possible with all NSAIDs, underscores the importance of using NSAIDs only as needed and after assessing the individual patient's risk.
10. NSAIDs are associated with GI, renal, cardiovascular, liver, and CNS toxicity. Monitoring with complete blood count, serum creatinine, and hepatic transaminase levels can be valuable in detecting potential toxicity.
11. Topical NSAIDs are recommended for patients older than 75 years to decrease the risks of systemic toxicity.
12. Other agents useful in treating knee OA include tramadol, intraarticular injections of corticosteroids, and duloxetine.

Osteoarthritis (OA) is the most common joint disease and is one of the leading causes of disability in the United States.[1–3] Knee OA alone is as important a contributor to disability as cardiovascular disease and more important than other comorbidities in this respect. In 2009, OA was ranked fourth as a cause for hospitalization in the United States.[3]

The progressive destruction of articular cartilage has long been appreciated in OA, but OA involves the entire diarthrodial joint, including articular cartilage, synovium, capsule, and subchondral bone, with surrounding ligaments and muscles also playing important roles. Changes in structure and function of these tissues produce clinical OA, characterized by joint pain and tenderness, with decreased range of motion, weakness, joint instability, and disability.

This chapter will review the epidemiology, etiology, pathogenesis, and diagnosis of OA. It then will focus on nonpharmacologic and pharmacologic treatments for OA, as well as investigational agents. Because millions of persons take medications for OA, the overall risks posed by these medications require serious consideration, particularly by clinicians who treat or advise patients on drug therapy for OA. This chapter examines the risks and benefits of OA treatments, with emphasis on those individuals who have the highest risk for adverse events, to help clinicians maximize benefits and reduce risks to their patients with OA.

EPIDEMIOLOGY

1 Twenty-seven million adults in the United States were estimated to have clinical OA in 2005, which represented an increase from 21 million in 1995.[4] Prevalence of arthritis-related disability is expected to increase to 11.6 million in the United States by 2020, and an estimated 67 million persons will have OA by 2030.[3,5]

OA imposes a tremendous cost burden, with total medical costs for OA approximately $336 billion in 2004.[6] For 2005, out-of-pocket and insurer expenditures were $36 billion and $149 billion, respectively.[7] In 2009, more than 900,000 knee and hip replacements were carried out, at a cost of $42 billion, with most of these surgeries necessitated by OA.[3]

Prevalence by Age, Sex, and Race

Prevalence estimates for OA vary depending on the age group of interest, gender, ethnic group, and the specific joint involved. Estimates also depend on the specific means by which OA is assessed and documented. Clinical OA is based on physical exam and patient history, whereas radiographic OA is determined by X-ray or other imaging, and symptomatic OA is based on history and physical plus X-ray.[1,3,5]

OA is more prevalent with increasing age. In the United States, prevalence of radiographic knee OA was estimated as 13.8% for all persons over age 25, but 37.4% for persons age 60 and older.[4] Prevalence for symptomatic knee OA was estimated as 4.9% for all persons over age 25, but 12.1% for persons age 60 and older.[4] Radiologically confirmed hip OA shows clear trends through all age groups, affecting 1.6% of those between ages 30 and 39, up to a prevalence of 14% in those over 85 years of age.[8] Radiographic hand OA is found in 5% of those age 40, but in 65% of those over 80 years of age.[9]

Prevalence of hip OA is 9% in white populations, but is only 4% for Asian, black, and Indian populations. Before age 50, men are more likely to have OA than women, attributed to higher rates of sports and other injuries.[10] Women exhibit a higher prevalence of hip and knee OA than men, and are at especially greater risk for hand OA, with 26% of women and 12% of men over age 70 affected.[9] Women are also more likely to have inflammatory OA of the proximal and distal interphalangeal joints of the hands, giving rise to the formation of Bouchard's and Heberden's nodes, respectively (Fig. 71-1).

Incidence

The incidence of symptomatic OA determined in a large managed care organization was 100 per 100,000 patient-years for hand OA, 88 per 100,000 patient-years for hip OA, and 240 per 100,000 patient-years for knee OA.[8] Using a population database of approximately 4 million persons, a recent Canadian study estimated the annual incidence rate of physician-diagnosed OA in men to be 11.6 per 1000 in the period 2003 to 2004, similar to the rate of 11.3 per 1000 estimated for 1996 to 1997.[11] For women, the incidence rate significantly increased from 14.7 to 16.7 per 1000 from the period 1996 to 1997 to the period 2003 to 2004. Some of the increase observed for women could have resulted from the aging of the population and women's longer life expectancy.

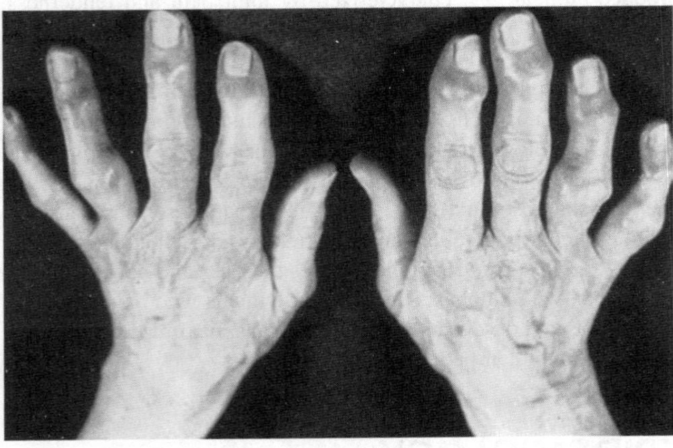

FIGURE 71-1 Heberden's nodes (distal interphalangeal joint) noted on all fingers and Bouchard's nodes (proximal interphalangeal joint) noted on most fingers. *(From Johnson BE. Arthritis: Osteoarthritis, Gout and Rheumatoid Arthritis. In: South-Paul JE, Matheny SC, Lewis EL, eds. Current Diagnosis and Treatment in Family Medicine. New York: McGraw-Hill, 2004:266, 267.)*

ETIOLOGY

❷ The etiology of OA is multifactorial and complex, with development of OA depending on interplay between factors such as genetic predisposition and joint injury.[1] Many patients have more than one risk factor for the development of OA. The most common risk factors for the development of OA include age, obesity, gender, occupation, participation in certain sports, history of joint injury or surgery, and genetic predisposition.

Obesity

Obesity is the most important preventable risk factor for OA. This linkage is strongest for knee OA, although hip OA may also be linked with weight. Hand OA does not appear to be linked. As the epidemic of obesity spreads in the United States and in other developed countries, so will the burdens imposed by OA.[5] Obesity often precedes OA and contributes to its development, rather than occurring as a result of inactivity from joint pain.[12] In an 11-year study of approximately 30,000 Norwegian men and women, obesity significantly increased the risk of developing OA.[13] Men who were obese at baseline had a 2.8-fold increased risk of developing knee OA compared with nonobese men, whereas women who were obese at baseline had a 4.4-fold increased risk of developing knee OA compared with nonobese women. Also, there was an increased risk for severe knee OA in obese subjects.

In addition to being a risk factor for OA, obesity is also a predictor for eventual prosthetic joint replacement. In a US study, women who were obese at age 18 were at increased risk of undergoing hip replacement surgery in later life.[3] The risk of developing OA increases by approximately 10% with each additional kilogram of weight, and in obese persons without OA, weight loss of even 5 kg (11 pounds) decreases the risk of future knee OA by half.[12]

Occupation, Sports, and Trauma

OA risk is increased for people in occupations involving excessive mechanical stress. Work that involves prolonged standing, kneeling, squatting, lifting, or moving of heavy objects increases risk of OA. Such occupations include construction, mining, health care assistance, factory work, carpentry, and farming.[1,3,14] Repetitive motion also contributes to hand OA, with the dominant hand usually affected.[9] Risk for OA depends on the type and intensity of physical activity and whether injury is incurred in the activity. Increased risk of OA is associated with participation in activities such as wrestling, boxing, baseball pitching, cycling, and football, although recreational participants do not have the increased risk seen in the professional athlete.[1,3] In the above-referenced study of 30,000 Norwegians, exercise intensity was not associated with any increased risk in the obese subjects compared with those of normal weight.[13]

Traumatic injury to articular cartilage during sports and other activities or in accidents greatly increases OA risk.[1,3,14] Meniscal damage increases the risk of knee OA because of the loss of proper load bearing and shock absorption, increased focal load on cartilage and on subchondral bone. Knee injury in young persons is also an important risk factor for knee OA in old age.[1] Quadriceps muscle weakness is also recognized to increase the risk for knee OA, as these muscles are important in maintaining joint stability.[10,12] Whether knee malalignment increases risk of developing

OA remains unsettled.[1] In the person who already has OA, knee malalignment is strongly associated with faster progression of OA.[1]

Genetic Factors

OA is a complex, polygenic disease. Identification of the genes involved may promote development of agents to prevent OA or to slow or halt its progression.

Genetic influences on OA have been appreciated for many years. Heberden's nodes are 10 times more prevalent in women than in men, for example, with a twofold higher risk if the woman's mother had them. Genetic links have been shown with OA of the first metatarsophalangeal joint and with generalized OA. Twin studies indicate that OA can be attributed substantially to genetic factors (39% to 65%, 60%, and 70% for hand, hip, and spine OA, respectively).[15] In other twin studies of OA progression, radiographic measurements over 2 years showed that the increased risk for a sibling having radiographic progression if the proband had progression that was threefold for joint space narrowing and 1.5-fold for osteophyte progression.[16]

One approach OA researchers have used is the candidate gene approach. This hypothesis is based and focuses on genes with known function that could be plausibly linked with the disease. Genome-wide association studies (GWAS) (associating OA with a specific region out of the total human genome, using cases versus controls, offers a powerful approach in seeking the genetic basis for OA.[17,18] Using GWAS and candidate gene approaches, possible genetic associations to OA have been found, and some of these appear to code for known proteins that have intriguing connections.[18–20] These genes include Col11A1 (extracellular matrix), Chrom 19 (cartilage morphogenesis), MCFL (pain perception), CHST11 (cartilage morphogenesis), GDF5 (TGF-β signaling), and Chrom7Q22. A meta-analysis of GWAS with 6,709 knee OA cases and 44,439 controls revealed that the Chrom7Q22 locus was very highly significantly associated with knee OA. The locus also included six genes that code for proteins known to be expressed in joint tissues.[19]

For most genes that appear to be linked to OA, the associations have been weak or modest, even if replicable.[17] It is quite likely that the genetic risk of developing OA, like many other diseases, may be substantially determined by a combination of modest genetic differences, and this underscores the point that understanding of the genetics and pathology of OA is in its infancy.

PATHOPHYSIOLOGY

OA falls into two major etiologic classes. *Primary (idiopathic) OA*, the more common type, has no identifiable cause. *Secondary OA* is that associated with a known cause such as rheumatoid or another inflammatory arthritis, trauma, metabolic or endocrine disorders, and congenital factors.[10]

The old view of OA as a "wear-and-tear" or degenerative disease, largely focused on joint cartilage, has long been superseded by an appreciation of the dynamic nature of OA and that it represents a failure of the joint and surrounding tissues.[21] Some changes in the OA joint may reflect compensatory processes to maintain function in the face of ongoing joint destruction. Not only biomechanical forces but also inflammatory, biochemical, and immunologic factors are involved. An appreciation of the biology and function of normal cartilage can aid in understanding osteoarthritic cartilage and is summarized below.

Normal Cartilage

Function, Structure, and Composition of Cartilage

Articular cartilage possesses viscoelastic properties that provide lubrication with motion, shock absorbency during rapid movements, and load support. In synovial joints, articular cartilage is found between the synovial cavity on one side and a narrow layer of calcified tissue overlying subchondral bone on the other side (Fig. 71-2).[22] The layer of cartilage is narrow, with human medial femoral articular cartilage being approximately 2 to 3 mm thick. Despite this, healthy articular cartilage in weight-bearing joints withstands millions of cycles of loading and unloading each year. Cartilage is easily compressed, losing up to 40% of its original height when a load is applied. Compression increases the area of contact and disperses force more evenly to underlying bone, tendons, ligaments, and muscles. In addition, cartilage is almost frictionless, and together with its compressibility, this enables smooth movement in the joint, distributes load across joint tissues to prevent damage, and stabilizes the joint.

Strength, a low coefficient of friction, and compressibility of cartilage derive from its unique structure. Cartilage is a complex, hydrophilic, extracellular matrix (ECM). It is approximately 75% to 85% water and contains 2% to 5% chondrocytes collagen and other proteins, proteoglycans, and long hyaluronic acid (HA) molecules.[22] The two major structural components in articular cartilage are type II collagen and aggrecans.[23] Type II collagen has a tightly woven triple helical structure, which provides the tensile strength of cartilage. Aggrecan is a proteoglycan linked with HA, providing the long aggrecan molecules a high negative charge. These are squeezed together by surrounding fibrils of type II collagen. The strong electrostatic repulsion of proteoglycans held in close proximity gives cartilage the ability to withstand further compression. Within the cartilage ECM are the chondrocytes, the only cells in cartilage, responsible for laying down all the components of cartilage.

Normal cartilage turnover helps repair and restore cartilage in response to demands of joint loading and during physical activity. In adults, cartilage chondrocyte metabolism is slow and is regulated by growth factors, including bone morphogenetic protein 2, insulin-like growth factor-1, and transforming growth factor, and by catabolism and proteolysis stimulated by matrix metalloproteinases (MMPs), tumor

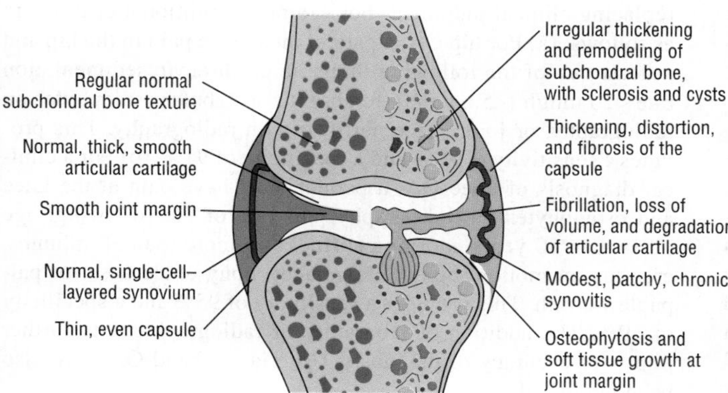

FIGURE 71-2 Characteristics of osteoarthritis in the diarthrodial joint. *(Courtesy of Dr. D. Gotlieb.)*

necrosis factor-α (TNF-α), interleukin-1, and other cytokines. Tissue inhibitors of metalloproteinase (TIMP) also contribute to the balance by restraining the catabolic actions of MMPs. If cartilage is injured, chondrocytes react by removing the damaged areas and increasing synthesis of matrix constituents to repair and restore cartilage.[23,24]

Another component supporting healthy joints are the joint protective mechanisms, such as muscles bridging the joint, sensory receptors in feedback loops to regulate muscle and tendon function, supporting ligaments, and subchondral bone that has shock-absorbent properties.

Finally, it is important to note that adult articular cartilage is avascular, with chondrocytes nourished by synovial fluid. With movement and cyclic loading and unloading of joints, nutrients flow into the cartilage, whereas immobilization reduces nutrient supply. This is one of the reasons that normal physical activity is beneficial for joint health.

Osteoarthritic Cartilage

3 Important contributors to the development of OA are local mechanical influences, genetic factors, inflammation, and aberrant chondrocyte function leading to loss of articular cartilage.[23,24] At a molecular level, OA pathophysiology involves the interplay of dozens, if not hundreds, of extracellular and intracellular molecules with roles including chondrocyte regulation, phenotypic changes, proteolytic degradation of cartilage components, and interactions between articular cartilage, underlying subchondral bone, and the joint synovium.[2,5,23–27]

OA most commonly begins with damage to articular cartilage, through trauma or other injury, excess joint loading from obesity or other reasons, or instability or injury of the joint that causes abnormal loading. In response to cartilage damage, chondrocyte activity increases in an attempt to remove and repair the damage. Depending on the degree of damage, the balance between breakdown and resynthesis of cartilage can be lost, and a vicious cycle of increasing breakdown can lead to further cartilage loss and apoptosis of chondrocytes.[2,5,23–27] Recent studies have revealed several respects of the very complex nature of OA. For example, expression of hundreds of specific genes are affected by acute experimental injury of human cartilage tissue, that is, injury alters the chondrocyte phenotype.[28] Researchers have also shown that within different regions of human OA cartilage obtained at surgery, chondrocyte gene expression from the most damaged areas of cartilage is different from that from less damaged or normal areas.[29] Another exciting discovery is that comparative proteomics of articular cartilage from normal persons compared with cartilage from those with OA showed different expression.[30]

There is increased appreciation of the role of tissues beyond cartilage, within the joint and surrounding it, subchondral bone.[24] Subchondral bone undergoes pathologic changes that may precede, coincide with, or follow damage to the articular cartilage. In OA, subchondral bone releases vasoactive peptides and MMPs, and damage to subchondral bone may trigger further damage to articular cartilage.[31] Neovascularization and subsequent increased permeability of the adjacent cartilage occur and contributes further to cartilage loss.

Joint space narrowing results from loss of cartilage, which can lead to a painful, deformed joint (Fig. 71-3). Remaining cartilage softens and develops fibrillations (vertical clefts into the cartilage), followed by splitting off of more cartilage and exposure of underlying bone.[32] During this time, adjacent subchondral bone undergoes further pathologic changes; cartilage is eroded completely, leaving denuded subchondral bone, which becomes dense, smooth, and glistening (eburnation). A more brittle, stiffer bone results, with decreased weight-bearing ability and development of sclerosis and microfractures. New bone formations, or osteophytes, also appear at joint margins distant from cartilage destruction and are thought to arise from local and humoral factors. There is direct evidence that osteophytes can help stabilize osteoarthritic joints.[33]

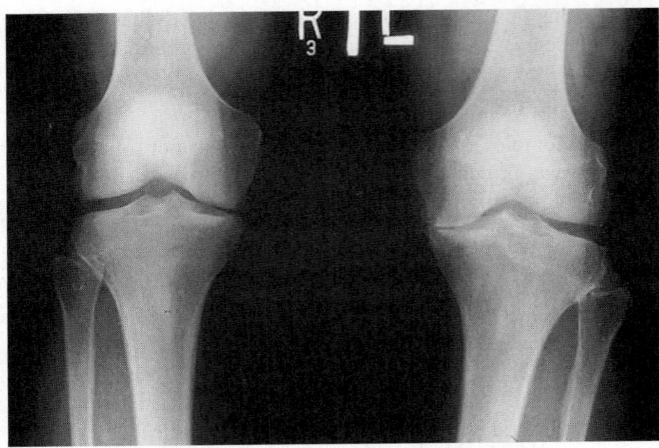

FIGURE 71-3 Plain x-ray films of the knee demonstrating joint space narrowing. *(From Johnson BE. Arthritis: Osteoarthritis, Gout and Rheumatoid Arthritis. In: South-Paul JE, Matheny SC, Lewis EL, eds. Current Diagnosis and Treatment in Family Medicine. New York: McGraw-Hill, 2004:267.)*

In the joint capsule and synovium, inflammatory changes and pathologic changes can occur.[2,22,24–27] Contributors to inflammation may include crystals or cartilage shards in synovial fluid. Other possible players are interleukin-1, prostaglandin E_2, TNF-α, and nitric oxide, which are found in synovial fluid. With inflammatory changes in the synovium, effusions and synovial thickening occur.

The pain of OA is not related to the destruction of cartilage but arises from the activation of nociceptive nerve endings within the joint by mechanical and chemical irritants.[5] OA pain may result from distension of the synovial capsule by increased joint fluid, microfracture, periosteal irritation, or damage to ligaments, synovium, or the meniscus.

CLINICAL PRESENTATION

Diagnosis

4 The diagnosis of OA is made through history, physical examination, characteristic radiographic findings, and laboratory testing.[10,34,35] The major diagnostic goals are (a) to discriminate between primary and secondary OA and (b) to clarify the joints involved, severity of joint involvement, and response to prior therapies, providing a basis for a treatment plan. The American College of Rheumatology has published traditional diagnostic criteria and "decision trees" for OA diagnosis.[35] As with all guidelines, the authors stress these are for assisting the clinician rather than replacing clinical judgment. For example, traditional criteria are as follows: (a) For hip OA, a patient must have pain in the hip and at least two of the following three: an erythrocyte sedimentation rate <20 mm/h (<5.6 μm/s), femoral or acetabular osteophytes on radiography, or joint space narrowing on radiography. This provides a sensitivity of 89% and a specificity of 91%. (b) For a clinical diagnosis of knee OA, a patient must have pain at the knee and osteophytes on radiography plus one of the following: age older than 50 years, morning stiffness no more than 30 minutes, crepitus on motion, bony enlargement, bony tenderness, or palpable warmth. This provides a sensitivity of 95% and a specificity of 69%. The addition of laboratory or radiographic data further improves accuracy of diagnosis. Criteria for hand OA have also been published.[36]

CLINICAL PRESENTATION Osteoarthritis

Age

- Usually elderly

Gender

- Age <45 more common in men
- Age >45 more common in women

Symptoms

- Pain
- Deep, aching character
- Pain on motion
- Stiffness in affected joints
- Resolves with motion, recurs with rest ("gelling phenomenon")
- Usually duration <30 minutes
- Often related to weather
- Limited joint motion
- May result in limitations of activities of daily living
- Instability of weight-bearing joints

Signs, History, and Physical Examination

- Monoarticular or oligoarticular, asymmetrical involvement
- Hands
  - Distal interphalangeal joints
    - Heberden's nodes (osteophytes or bony enlargements) (Fig. 71-1)
  - Proximal interphalangeal joints
    - Bouchard's nodes (osteophytes)
  - First metacarpal joint
    - Osteophytes give characteristic square appearance to hands
- Knee
  - Pain related to climbing stairs
  - Transient joint effusion
  - Genu varum ("bow-legged")
- Hips
  - Groin pain during weight-bearing exercises
  - Stiffness, especially after activity
  - Limited joint movement
- Spine
  - Lumbar involvement is most common at L3 and L4
  - Paraesthesias
  - Loss of reflexes
- Feet
  - Typically involves the first metatarsophalangeal joint
  - Shoulder, elbow, acromioclavicular, sternoclavicular, and temporomandibular joints may also be affected
- Observation on joint examination
  - Bony proliferation or occasional synovitis
  - Local tenderness
  - Crepitus
  - Limited motion with passive/active movement
  - Deformity
- Radiologic evaluation
  - Early mild OA
    - Radiographic changes often absent
  - Progressive OA
  - Joint space narrowing (Fig. 71-3)
  - Subchondral bone sclerosis
  - Marginal osteophytes
- Late OA
  - Abnormal alignment of joints
  - Effusions

Prognosis

The prognosis for patients with primary OA is variable and depends on the joint involved. If a weight-bearing joint or the spine is involved, considerable morbidity and disability are possible. In the case of secondary OA, the prognosis depends on the underlying cause. Treatment of OA may relieve pain or improve function but does not reverse preexisting damage to the joint.

TREATMENT

Desired Outcome

Management of the patient with OA begins with a diagnosis based on a careful history, physical examination, radiographic findings, and an assessment of the extent of joint involvement. Treatment should be tailored to each individual. Goals are (a) to educate the patient, family members, and caregivers; (b) to relieve pain and stiffness; (c) to maintain or improve joint mobility; (d) to limit functional impairment; and (e) to maintain or improve quality of life.[37–39]

General Approach to Treatment

Treatment for each OA patient depends on the distribution and severity of joint involvement, comorbid disease states, concomitant medications, and allergies. Management for all individuals with OA should begin with both oral and written patient education, a customized activity and exercise program, and weight loss, if the patient is overweight or obese.[37–39]

The primary objective of medication is to alleviate pain.[37–39] Scheduled acetaminophen, up to 4 g/day in divided doses, should be tried initially (knee, hip), if contraindications are not present. Application of topical NSAIDs over specific joints (knee, hands) and topical capsaicin (hands) are recommended as initial therapy. Nonsteroidal antiinflammatory drugs (NSAIDs) or possibly a cyclooxygenase-2 (COX-2)–selective inhibitor (celecoxib) can be prescribed after careful risk assessment if additional pain control is needed. Intraarticular corticosteroid injections (knee or hip) can relieve pain and are offered concomitantly with oral analgesics or after failed trials of first-line medications, depending on the practitioner's preference. With centrally acting serotonin reuptake inhibition and analgesic properties, tramadol can also be considered if acetaminophen or topical treatment is ineffective or not tolerated.

Opioid analgesics may be considered if first-line medications are ineffective or pose significant safety concerns in an individual patient. Consideration can also be given to duloxetine or less frequently, HA injections when additional pain control is needed for knee OA. When symptoms are intractable or there is significant loss of function, joint replacement can be appropriate if the patient is a surgical candidate.

There is general agreement that glucosamine and/or chondroitin and topical rubefacients lack uniform efficacy in the treatment of hip and knee OA pain and are not preferred treatment options.

Nonpharmacologic Therapy

5 Nonpharmacologic therapy is an integral part of the treatment plan for all patients with OA.[37–39] Nonpharmacologic therapy is the only available treatment that has been shown to delay the progression of OA.[40] Delaying the progression of OA through active use of nonpharmacologic therapy is critical to prevent future functional impairment. Patient-specific characteristics such as the number and location of affected joints, degree of functional impairment, body mass index, motivation, and overall health status determine which nonpharmacologic therapies should be offered. Nonpharmacologic therapy should be ongoing treatment for all patients, even those who require pharmacologic therapy for pain control (Table 71-1).

Patient Education

The first step in OA treatment is patient education about the disease process, the extent of OA, the prognosis, and treatment options. Education is paramount in that OA is often seen as a wear-and-tear disease, an inevitable consequence of aging for which nothing helps. Even worse, patients may resort to the use of alternative but unproven medications or quackery. Organizations such as the Arthritis Foundation provide a wealth of educational information for patients regarding OA, OA medications, local clinics, and agencies offering physical and economic assistance. Exercise, weight loss, and nutritional information are also available. Most educational information is readily available online for patient use.

The benefits of patient education have been documented in a variety of programs.[41] These programs are provided across a wide spectrum of delivery methods: from trained volunteers using telephone calls to group sessions for patient support to one-on-one educational sessions with physical therapists or nurse educators. While nearly all of these delivery methods are effective, cost of delivery is highly variable. Long-term cost-effectiveness is very important for sustainability of these patient education programs.

Weight Loss

Excess weight increases the biomechanical load on weight-bearing joints and is the single best predictor of need for eventual joint replacement.[42,43] Weight loss of amounts as small as 4% of body weight can lessen OA pain in the knee.[44] Greater amounts of weight loss, especially when associated with regular exercise, improve joint function and substantially lessen pain.[42,45] At least one randomized controlled trial has demonstrated improvement in pain and self-reported physical function using a combination of modest weight loss (5%) and exercise.[46] Patients with appropriate indications for bariatric surgery have significant improvement in joint function and pain associated with the subsequent weight loss.[47] A large weight-loss and activity trial is under way, and the Intensive Diet and Exercise for Arthritis trial (IDEA) will address weight-related joint loading and inflammatory biomarkers.[48] Weight loss requires a motivated patient, but it should be encouraged and supported for all obese and overweight patients with OA. Effective behavior change strategies should be employed to promote weight loss in patients with OA.[40]

TABLE 71-1 Nonpharmacologic Interventions in the Treatment of OA[37–39]

Type of Nonpharmacologic Intervention	Strength of Recommendation
Exercise	Strong
Weight loss (if overweight)	Strong
Patient education	Strong
Use of assistive device (i.e., cane)	Moderate
Use of shoe insoles	Moderate
Application of heat	Moderate
Use of fitted knee braces	Minimal
Lateral patellar taping	Minimal
Passive exercise alone	Minimal

Strength of recommendation: Strong—fully supported by evidence-based guidelines, moderate—supported by evidence-based guidelines, minimal—little support by evidence-based guidelines.

Exercise

Exercise programs can improve joint function and can decrease disability, pain, and analgesic use by OA patients.[40,44,46] Isometric exercise is preferred over isotonic exercise because the latter can aggravate affected joints. Exercises can be taught and then observed before the patient exercises at home. The frequency, types of exercise, and setting of exercise are still uncertain, but patients who exercise at least two to three times per week with a variety of exercises (>8 types) have improved outcomes.[49] The patient should be instructed to decrease the number of repetitions if severe pain develops with exercise.

Some regular exercise should be encouraged for all patients with OA.[39] With weak or deconditioned muscles, the load is transmitted excessively to the joints; weight-bearing activities can exacerbate symptoms. Many patients fear that exercise will promote further joint damage and avoid exercise as a means to protect the joint. However, avoidance of regular exercise by those with hip or knee OA leads to further deconditioning and/or weight gain. This leads to more pain and impaired joint function, promoting a downward spiral of disability. Current research regarding exercise revolves around effective strategies to promote sustained behavior change in patients.[40] A program of patient education, muscle stretching and strengthening, and supervised walking can improve physical function and decrease pain for patients with knee OA.[46]

Referral to the physical and/or occupational therapist is especially helpful for developing a customized exercise plan for patients with functional disabilities. The therapist can assess muscle strength and joint stability and recommend exercises and assistive and orthotic devices, such as canes, walkers, braces, heel cups, splints, or insoles for use during exercise or daily activities. Heat or cold treatments help to maintain and restore joint range of motion and to reduce pain and muscle spasms. Warm baths or warm water soaks may decrease pain and stiffness. Heating pads should be used with caution, especially in the elderly. Patients should be warned not to fall asleep on the heat source or to lie on it for more than brief periods to avoid burns.

Surgery

Surgery can be recommended for OA patients with functional disability and/or severe pain unresponsive to conservative therapy. Criteria for total joint replacement (arthroplasty) of the knee and hip have been developed, although there is substantial overlap in eligibility criteria.[50,51]

Few randomized, controlled trials are available comparing total joint arthroplasty with other treatment modalities. Although total knee arthroplasty can decrease pain and improve function for many patients, about 20% experience little or no improvement in pain, disability, and/or quality of life.[52] These findings coupled with overlapping indications for the procedure and the expected increase in the number of patients with OA lend some urgency to the need for controlled trials to evaluate the outcome of joint replacement with other treatment modalities.

The MEDIC-study of total knee replacement plus physical and medical therapy or treatment with physical and medical therapy alone is currently enrolling patients in hopes of answering some of these important questions about the role of surgery in the treatment of knee OA.[52]

Total joint arthroplasty is responsible for a large portion of the direct medical costs associated with OA in the United States. The cost-effectiveness of total knee arthroplasty has been evaluated for a Medicare-age population.[53] Calculations were based on Medicare claims data and costs and outcomes data. Cost projections were calculated for lifetime costs as well as quality-adjusted life expectancy (QALE) for different risk populations and across low-volume to high-volume hospitals. Although total knee arthroplasty was found to be cost-effective across hospital settings and patient risk categories, the procedure was found to be most cost-effective when performed in high-volume centers.

Other surgical options are also available. Arthrodesis (joint fusion) can reduce pain but will restrict motion and may be appropriate for smaller joints that are causing intractable pain. For patients with mild knee OA, an osteotomy (removal of bony tissue) may correct the misalignment of genu varum ("bowlegged" knees) or genu valgum ("knock-knees"). In addition, osteotomies of the pelvis or femur can ameliorate joint misalignment in hip OA, subsequently slowing progression of disease. Knee arthroscopy or lavage appear to be equivalent to sham surgery and are not recommended.[37] Experimental but potentially restorative approaches involve soft-tissue grafts, chondrocyte transplantation, gene therapy, and use of growth factors or artificial matrices.[54] Cartilage-restoration approaches are investigational, and results regarding pain control and joint function have been mixed.

Pharmacologic Therapy

6 Drug therapy in OA is targeted at relief of pain. OA is commonly seen in older individuals who have other medical conditions, and OA treatment is often long term. As such, a conservative approach to drug treatment, focusing on the needs of the individual patient, is warranted (see Figs. 71-4 and 71-5).[37–39] Even when pharmacologic therapy is initiated, appropriate nondrug therapies should be continued and reinforced. Specific drug therapy recommendations depend on which joint(s) are affected, response to previous trials of medication, and patient comorbidities.

Knee and Hip OA

First-Line Treatments

Acetaminophen 7 The American College of Rheumatology, as well as others, recommend acetaminophen as a first-line treatment for knee and hip OA.[37,39,55] Acetaminophen has been extensively studied in the treatment of knee and hip OA and is more effective than placebo in controlling OA pain.[55,56] Compared with oral NSAIDs, acetaminophen may be modestly less effective, but it has a lower risk of serious GI and cardiovascular adverse events and as a consequence is preferred over oral NSAIDs as first-line treatment.[55] The significantly lower risks of both minor and major adverse events associated with acetaminophen in the treatment of knee and hip OA favors a trial of acetaminophen in all patients without underlying liver disease.[55,56]

Oral NSAIDs The American College of Rheumatology and other key groups recommend nonspecific or COX-2 selective NSAIDs, depending on patient risk factors, as a first-line option for knee and hip OA if the patient fails acetaminophen.[37,39,55] NSAIDs have a consistent record of providing superior pain relief in comparison to acetaminophen, but no NSAID has proven superior to another.[55,56] Nonselective and COX-2–selective NSAIDs pose higher risks for GI, renal, and cardiovascular adverse events compared with acetaminophen. COX-2 inhibitors carry less risk for both minor and serious GI adverse events in comparison to nonselective NSAIDs (with the exception of diclofenac). It is unclear whether the reduced GI risk seen with COX-2 selectivity persists past 3 to 6 months, and this advantage is substantially diminished for patients taking aspirin.[55] Proton-pump inhibitors (PPIs) and misoprostol significantly reduce the occurrence of GI adverse events in those taking NSAIDs.[55]

Topical NSAIDs—Knee Only The American College of Rheumatology and other authoritative organizations recommend topical

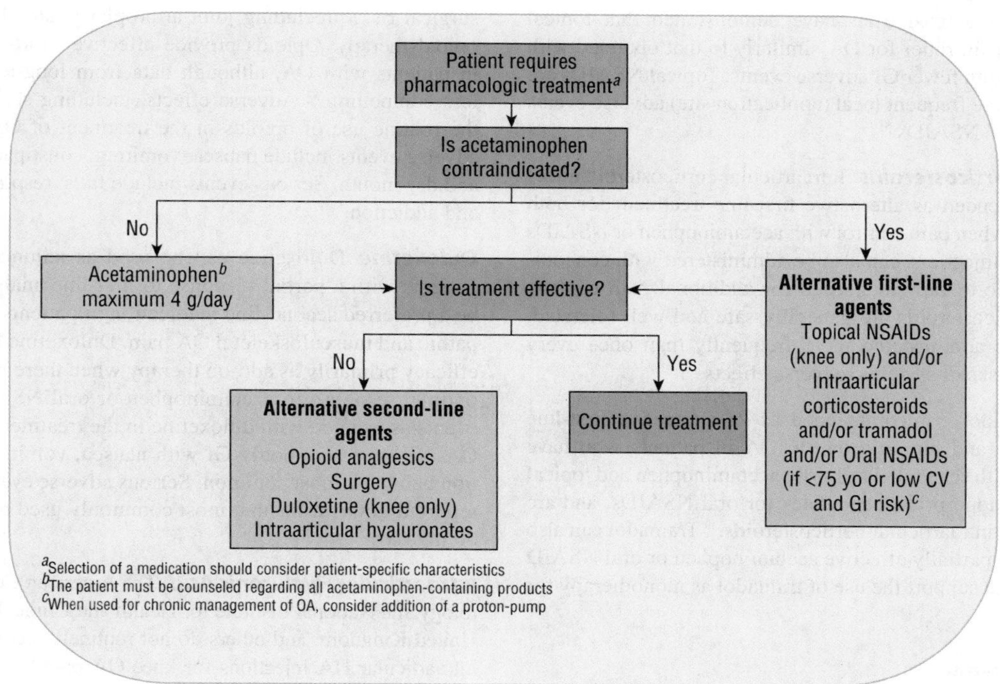

FIGURE 71-4 Treatment recommendations for knee and hip osteoarthritis.[37–39] (CV, cardiovascular; NSAID, nonsteroidal antiinflammatory drug.)

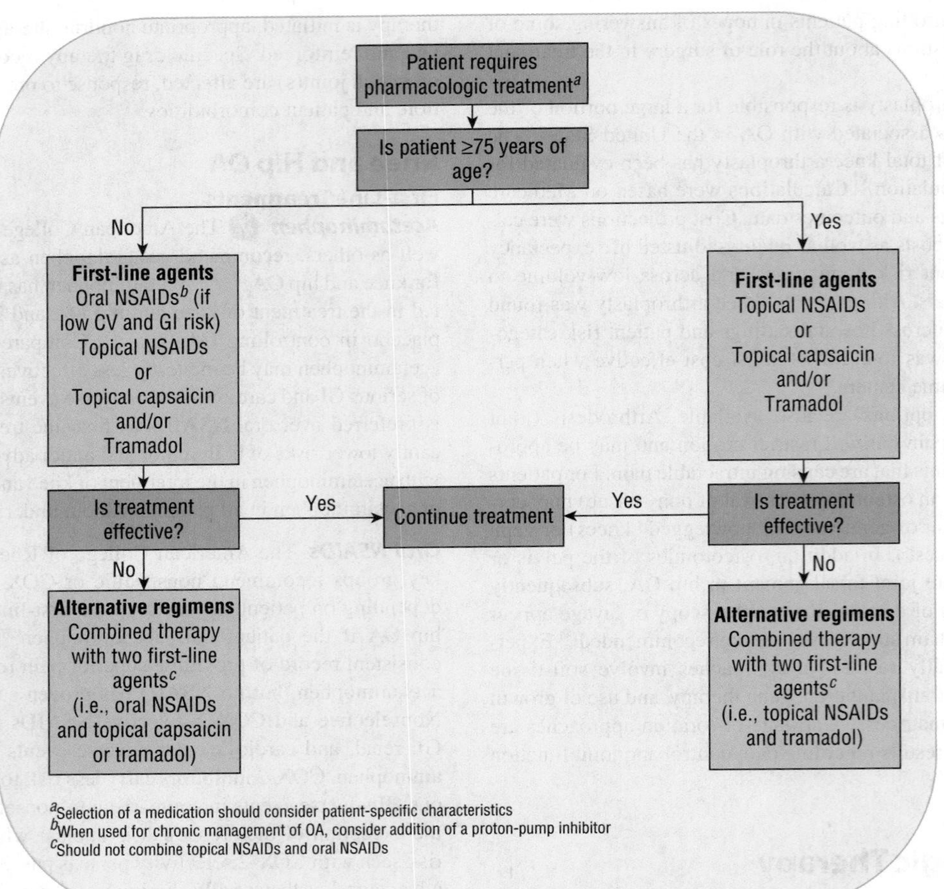

FIGURE 71-5 Treatment recommendations for hand osteoarthritis.[37–39] (NSAID, nonsteroidal antiinflammatory drug.)

NSAIDs as a first-line option for knee OA if the patient fails acetaminophen, and is preferred over oral NSAIDs for those older than 75.[37,39,55] Randomized trials have demonstrated that topical NSAIDs provide pain relief for OA similarly to that obtained with oral NSAIDs but with fewer GI adverse events. Topical NSAIDs are associated with more frequent local (application site) adverse events compared with oral NSAIDs.[55]

Intraarticular Corticosteroids Intraarticular corticosteroid injections are recommended as alternative first-line treatment for both knee and hip OA when pain control with acetaminophen or NSAIDs is suboptimal.[37,39] Injections can also be administered with concomitant oral analgesic therapy as needed for additional pain control. Intraarticular corticosteroids are generally safe and well tolerated, but should not be administered more frequently than once every 3 months due to risks of systemic adverse effects.

Tramadol Tramadol is recommended as an alternative first-line treatment of knee and hip pain due to OA in patients who have failed treatment with scheduled full-dose acetaminophen and topical NSAIDs, are not appropriate candidates for oral NSAIDs, and are not able to receive intraarticular corticosteroids.[39] Tramadol can also safely be added to partially effective acetaminophen or oral NSAID therapy. Fewer data support the use of tramadol as monotherapy for OA pain.

Second-Line Treatments

Opioid Analgesics The American College of Rheumatology recommends opioid analgesics as the primary second-line medication for both knee and hip OA.[39] Opioids should be considered in patients who have not had an adequate response to both nonpharmacologic and first-line pharmacologic therapies. Patients who are at high surgical risk, precluding joint arthroplasty, are also candidates for opioid therapy. Opioids provide effective short-term pain control in patients with OA, although data from long-term use trials are less compelling.[57] Adverse effects, including serious events, limit the routine use of opioids in the treatment of OA pain. Common adverse events include nausea, vomiting, constipation, somnolence, and dry mouth. Serious events include falls, respiratory depression, and addiction.[57]

Duloxetine Duloxetine can be used as adjunctive treatment in patients with a partial response to first-line analgesics.[37,39] It may be a preferred second-line medication in patients with both neuropathic and musculoskeletal OA pain. Duloxetine has demonstrated efficacy primarily as add-on therapy when there has been less than optimal response to acetaminophen or oral NSAIDs.[58,59] Adverse events associated with duloxetine in the treatment of knee and hip OA are most commonly GI with nausea, vomiting, and constipation being the most common. Serious adverse events have not been reported in OA trials that most commonly used moderate doses of 60 mg/day.

Intraarticular Hyaluronic Acid The American College of Rheumatology, the National Institute for Health and Clinical Excellence in the United Kingdom, and others do not routinely recommend the use of intraarticular HA injections for knee OA pain.[37–39] HA injections do not appear to provide clinically meaningful improvement in pain and/or function scores, although some studies may report statistical differences in scores. These agents may be associated with serious adverse events such as increased pain, joint swelling, and stiffness. Limited efficacy and risks of serious events limit the routine use of these agents.

Hand OA

First-Line Treatments

NSAIDs The American College of Rheumatology and the U.K. National Institute for Health and Clinical Excellence (NICE) recommend topical NSAIDs as a first-line option for hand OA.[38,39] Application of diclofenac gel compared with vehicle for hand OA provided significant relief, with mild application-site paresthesia as the only treatment-related adverse effect.[60] Topical diclofenac showed similar efficacy as oral ibuprofen as well as oral diclofenac, but with fewer GI adverse events.[61,62] Topical diclofenac use was associated with more frequent local (application site) events compared with oral NSAIDs. In all of these studies, topical diclofenac produced fewer GI adverse events.[55,61,62]

Oral NSAIDs are recommended as an alternative first-line treatment for hand OA by the American College of Rheumatology and as second-line therapy in the NICE guidelines.[38,39] For hand OA, there has long been a focus toward topical treatment, perhaps due to reluctance to undergo systemic exposure to strong treatment in patients without pain in a weight-bearing joint.[62] Ibuprofen, lumiracoxib, and meclofenamate each provided improvement in hand pain and other symptoms when compared with placebo.[61] Active comparator studies for hand OA compared rofecoxib with naproxen and compared lumiracoxib with celecoxib. Efficacy was similar for the comparator NSAIDs in each study, with similar percentages of patients discontinuing due to side effects. For the person who cannot tolerate local skin reactions or who received inadequate relief from topical NSAIDs, oral NSAIDs can offer relief, but the patient then faces increased risk for GI and cardiovascular adverse events.

Topical Capsaicin Capsaicin cream is recommended as an alternative first-line treatment for hand OA.[39] Clinical trial data supporting the use of capsaicin for the treatment of hand OA is limited to small studies, but the agent demonstrates modest benefits in improvement of pain scores.[61] Adverse effects associated with capsaicin are primarily skin irritation and burning; therefore, it is a reasonable therapeutic alternative for patients not able to take oral NSAIDs.

Tramadol Tramadol is recommended by the American College of Rheumatology as an alternative first-line treatment for OA of the hand.[39] In clinical practice, tramadol is a therapeutic option for patients who do not respond to topical therapy and are not candidates for oral NSAID treatment due to high GI, cardiovascular, or renal risks. Tramadol may also be used in combination with partially effective acetaminophen, topical therapy, or oral NSAIDs.

DRUG CLASS INFORMATION

Highlighted drug information will be reviewed below. This section is not intended to be all inclusive, but aims to provide pertinent drug information to facilitate the safe and effective use of these medications in patients with OA.

First-Line Treatments

Acetaminophen

Pharmacology and Mechanism of Action Acetaminophen is understood to act within the CNS by inhibiting synthesis of prostaglandins, agents that enhance pain sensations. Acetaminophen prevents prostaglandin synthesis by blocking the action of central cyclooxygenase (COX). Acetaminophen is well absorbed after oral administration, with a bioavailability of 60% to 98%. It achieves peak concentrations within 1 to 2 hours, it is inactivated in the liver by conjugation with sulfate or glucuronide, and its metabolites are renally excreted.

Adverse Effects Although acetaminophen is one of the safest analgesics, its use carries some risks, primarily hepatotoxicity and possibly renal toxicity with long-term use.[63,64] Serious hepatotoxicity, including fatalities, have been well documented with acetaminophen overdose (see eChap. 10, Clinical Toxicology, for information on treatment of acetaminophen overdose). Continued reports of serious hepatotoxicity, including fatalities from unintentional overdose, have led to labeling revisions of all nonprescription acetaminophen-containing analgesics.[65] Unintentional overdoses of acetaminophen are due to a variety of circumstances including narrow therapeutic window at the maximum dose (4 g/day), interpatient differences in sensitivity to liver injury from acetaminophen, a wide array of nonprescription and prescription products that contain acetaminophen and the difficulty of identifying the agent on product labels, and consumers' lack knowledge about the association of acetaminophen and serious liver injury.

In a study of normal, healthy volunteers administered acetaminophen 4 g/day (1 g every 6 hours), alone or with concomitant opioid therapy, for 14 days, elevations of alanine aminotransferase at levels above three times the upper limits of normal were found in 31% to 44% of patients, depending on the treatment group.[66] None of these participants had clinical symptoms of acute liver disease. Although the results of this study are not robust enough to alter the current standard dosing recommendations, it serves as an important reminder that the maximum dose of acetaminophen should be not be exceeded in any patient population and that long-term use of the maximum daily dose of 4 g/day can affect the liver.

Acetaminophen should be used cautiously in patients with liver disease or in those who abuse alcohol. Acute liver failure has been reported in patients taking less than 4 g/daily.[67] The most common risk factor for liver failure for these patients was chronic alcohol intake. The FDA has recommended that chronic alcohol users (three or more drinks daily) avoid acetaminophen intake as it increases the risk of liver damage or GI bleeding. Other individuals do not appear to be at increased risk of GI bleeding.

The National Kidney Foundation strongly discourages the use of nonprescription combination analgesic products (e.g., acetaminophen and NSAIDs) because this is associated with an increased prevalence of renal failure.[63] A recent large cohort study of patients with chronic kidney disease found acetaminophen, aspirin, and NSAID use to associated with an increased risk of end-stage renal disease (ESRD).[64] In addition, the increased risk of ESRD was dose-dependent.

Clinical **Controversy...**

Is regular use of acetaminophen with an NSAID safe for the kidney?

ESRD caused by phenacetin was recognized more than 20 years ago when the drug was in use, often in combination with an NSAID. The Ad Hoc Review Committee of the International Study Group on Analgesics and Nephropathy studied whether the newer, nonphenacetin-containing combined analgesics were associated with renal disease. The Committee concluded in 2000 that there was not enough evidence to associate nonphenacetin-combined analgesics with nephropathy and that new studies should be done to help resolve the question.

Uncertainty remains about this issue. Most recent OA guidelines do not specifically address the issue of acetaminophen in combination with an NSAID if the patient fails acetaminophen. Some experts recommended that addition of an NSAID to an acetaminophen regimen is reasonable, and some patients take both regularly.

Drug–Drug Interactions and Drug–Food Interactions Drug interactions with acetaminophen can occur; for example, isoniazid can increase the risk of hepatotoxicity. Chronic ingestion of maximal doses of acetaminophen may intensify the anticoagulant effect for patients taking warfarin; such individuals may need closer monitoring.

Although food decreases the maximum serum concentration of acetaminophen by approximately half, the overall efficacy is unchanged.

Dosing and Administration When used for chronic OA, acetaminophen should be administered in a scheduled manner. It may be taken with or without food. Acetaminophen can be taken at 325 to 650 mg every 4 to 6 hours, but the total dose must not exceed 4 g/day (see Adverse Effects above). FDA labeling requirements warn patients about potential liver toxicity if they inadvertently ingest more than the recommended dose when using multiple products containing acetaminophen. Additionally, FDA has also requested that all manufacturers of prescription analgesics containing acetaminophen limit the drug content to 325 mg per tablet or capsule to further decrease the possibility of inadvertent overdoses. Acetaminophen should be avoided in the setting of chronic alcohol intake or in those with underlying liver disease.

Oral Nonsteroidal Antiinflammatory Drugs

Pharmacology and Mechanism of Action NSAIDs reduce pain, inflammation, and fever by preventing synthesis of tissue prostaglandins and related prostanoids, which play a role in triggering these symptoms. All NSAID drugs bind reversibly to the COX-2 enzyme, blocking its action and thus prostanoid production. Blockade of prostaglandin synthesis by inhibiting COX enzymes (mainly COX-2) is thought to account for NSAIDs' ability to relieve pain and inflammation (Fig. 71-6).[68,69] Nonselective NSAIDs were developed before extensive knowledge of COX enzymes was available, but in fact they block both COX-2 and COX-1. COX-1 has required "housekeeping" functions such as gastroprotection. COX-2 inhibitors selectively block COX-2 and have no COX-1 activity.

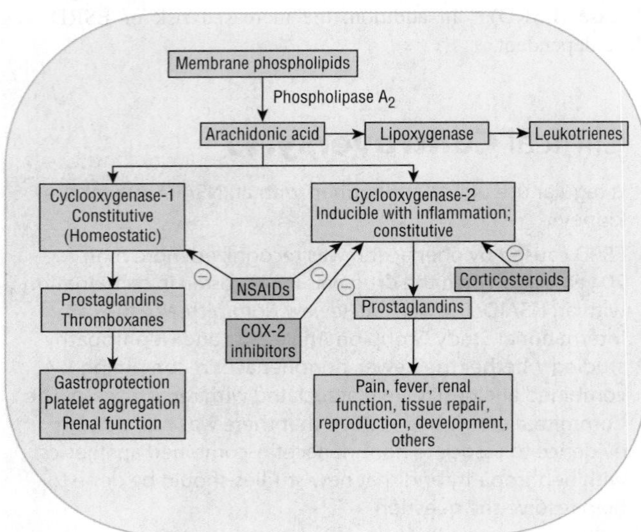

FIGURE 71-6 Pathway of synthesis for prostaglandins and leukotrienes. COX-1 and COX-2 are cyclooxygenase-1 and cyclooxygenase-2 enzymes, respectively. The minus (–) sign indicates inhibitory influence. Prostaglandins include PGE_2 and PGI_2; the latter is also known as prostacyclin.

The various NSAIDs exhibit several pharmacokinetic similarities, including high oral availability, high protein binding, and absorption as active drugs (except for sulindac and nabumetone, which require hepatic conversion for activity). There is a broad range of serum half-lives for different NSAIDs, which influence dosing frequency, and potentially, compliance with therapy.[70] Elimination of NSAIDs largely depends on hepatic inactivation, with a small fraction of active drug being renally excreted. NSAIDs penetrate joint fluid, reaching approximately 60% of blood levels.

Adverse Effects

Gastrointestinal Effects of Nonselective NSAIDs 8 The most common adverse effects of NSAIDs involve the GI tract, contributing to many treatment failures.[71–73] Minor complaints—nausea, dyspepsia, anorexia, abdominal pain, flatulence, and diarrhea—affect 10% to 60% of patients. All NSAIDs increase ulcer risk, but the serious GI complications associated with NSAIDs include perforations, gastric outlet obstruction, and bleeding. These important GI complications occur in 1.5% to 4% of patients per year. NSAIDs are so widely used that these small percentages translate into substantial morbidity and mortality. Moreover, the risk increases substantially for patients with risk factors including a history of complicated ulcer, concomitant use of multiple NSAIDs (including aspirin) or anticoagulant medications, use of high-dose NSAIDs, and age older than 70 years.[74] Consequently, about 16,500 deaths and 103,000 hospitalizations in the United States are associated annually with NSAID use in rheumatoid arthritis or OA patients.

Several options are available for reducing the GI risk of traditional NSAIDs:

1. Take the lowest dose of the NSAID possible, and take only when needed.
2. With the NSAID, take the prostaglandin analog misoprostol four times daily. It reduces the rate of ulcers and serious GI complications. However, many patients cannot tolerate the GI adverse events of misoprostol, especially diarrhea.
3. With the NSAID, take a PPI daily.[75]
4. With the NSAID, take a full-dose histamine H_2 blocker daily. The PPI and the H_2 blocker reduce minor GI complaints and the risk of ulcers, but they are not rigorously proven to cut down on the serious complications, possibly because of lack of power to detect rare events in clinical trials.

Another choice that is available to reduce risk of GI events with an NSAID is to take a COX-2 selective inhibitor ("coxib").[68–74] Celecoxib is the only coxib available in the United States. Because this drug does not block the "housekeeping" gene, it may not have the same GI risks as nonselective NSAIDs. The Celecoxib Long-Term Arthritis Safety Study (CLASS) study demonstrated a reduced risk of ulcer complications and symptomatic ulcers for celecoxib 400 mg daily compared with nonselective NSAID combined at the 6-month point. Celecoxib was approved and has been used extensively because of the advantages shown in this study, as well as its effectiveness, and other studies have demonstrated that it has GI advantages over nonselective NSAIDs.[68]

However, there remains concern that the GI protective effects of celecoxib may not be maintained long term and that it was not shown to consistently decrease the risk of serious complications (perforation, obstruction, or bleeding) as an independent endpoint. Another concern is that there is little or no gastroprotection afforded by celecoxib in those patients taking aspirin.[68]

Clinical **Controversy...**

Which is safer in OA:celecoxib alone or a nonselective NSAID with a PPI?

Celecoxib is associated with reduced risk for GI ulcers and their complications compared with nonselective NSAIDs, although this benefit is less certain with long-term use of celecoxib or for those taking aspirin. Use of PPIs with nonselective NSAIDs offers protection against development of GI ulcers, but head-to-head studies between this regimen and celecoxib are not definitive. For very high GI risk patients, the combination of celecoxib with a PPI is appealing. However, celecoxib appears to increase the risk of MI, although less so than other coxibs. Naproxen appears to be the safest NSAID to use with respect to the heart, so a difficult choice remains for the patient with high GI and cardiovascular risks.

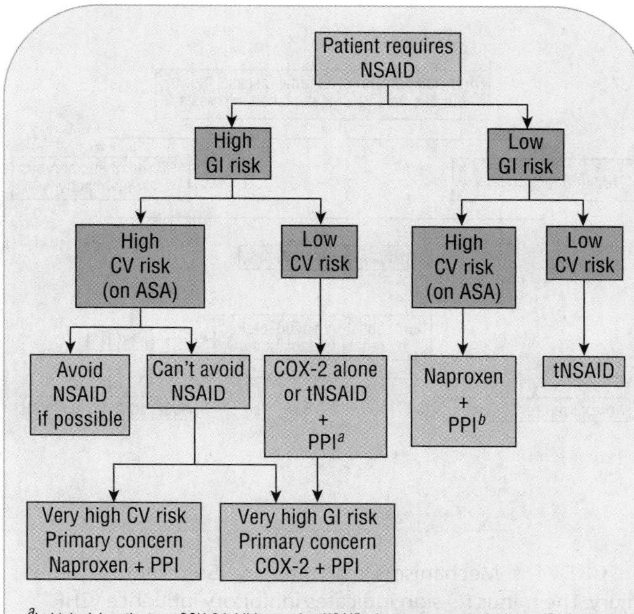

FIGURE 71-7 Algorithm for the use of long-term NSAID therapy and gastroprotective agents according to a patient's GI and cardiovascular risk. *(Rostom A, Moayyedi P, Hunt R; Canadian Association of Gastroenterology Consensus Group. Canadian Consensus Guidelines on long-term nonsteroidal anti-inflammatory drug therapy and the need for gastroprotection: Benefits versus risks. Aliment Pharmacol Ther 2009;29(5):481. Wiley-Blackwell Publishers.)*

❾ ***Cardiovascular Risk of COX-2 Inhibitors and Traditional NSAIDs*** In 2004, rofecoxib was withdrawn from the market after analysis of the Adenomatous Polyp Prevention on Vioxx (APPROVe) trial, where rofecoxib doubled the risk of cardiovascular events compared with placebo.[76] Celecoxib use in the Adenoma Prevention with Celecoxib (APC) trial (up to 800 mg/day) also increased cardiovascular risk.[77] This prompted evaluation of all NSAIDs for possible cardiovascular risks.[78] The same evaluation included meta-analyses of NSAIDs compared with placebo. Diclofenac had a significantly increased risk of cardiovascular events [RR = 1.63 (1.12 to 2.37)], while the increase seen with ibuprofen did not reach significance [RR = 1.51 (0.96 to 2.37)]. No increased risk was seen with naproxen. A drawback in this work was the small number of cardiovascular events in the meta-analyses, making it impossible to statistically differentiate the risk of one coxib compared with another.

Data from controlled trials and observational studies confirm the increased cardiovascular risk seen with rofecoxib. Celecoxib 200 mg/day or even 400 mg/day does not appear to increase risk, but cardiovascular risk is likely increased with doses above 400 mg/day. In addition, the risk of taking higher doses of celecoxib is greater for those with high cardiovascular risk than for those with low cardiovascular risk. The balance of the evidence also suggests that for the traditional NSAIDs that have been examined, with the exception of diclofenac, there is no significant or substantial increase in risk.

In a 2012 Danish study, national hospitalization records and pharmacy records of approximately 100,000 first-time MI patients revealed increased risks associated with use of any NSAID after MI. NSAID use was associated with a 1.59-fold increased risk of death (95% CI, 1.49 to 1.69) within 1 year of MI and 1.63-fold increased risk (95% CI, 1.52 to 1.74) after 5 years.[79] Moreover, there was a 1.30-fold increased risk of coronary death or nonfatal recurrent MI (95% CI, 1.22 to 1.39) within 1 year of MI and 1.41-fold increased risk (95% CI, 1.28 to 1.55) after 5 years. Increased risk with NSAID use after MI was lowest with naproxen and highest with diclofenac.

Considerations for Patients at Risk for Both GI and Cardiovascular Events ❿ Recently, Canadian consensus guidelines were developed to recommend gastroprotection for those on NSAID therapy.[73] A multidisciplinary group focused on four areas: benefits of traditional NSAIDs, aspirin, and COX-2 inhibitors; harms of traditional NSAIDs, aspirin, and COX-2 inhibitors; reducing harms of traditional NSAIDs, aspirin, and COX-2 inhibitors; and economic considerations. Recommendations were made for patients at low GI and cardiovascular risk, low GI risk and high cardiovascular risk, high GI risk and low cardiovascular risk, and for those with high GI and cardiovascular risk (Fig. 71-7).

Other Toxicities Associated with NSAIDs ❿ NSAIDs may cause kidney diseases, including acute renal insufficiency, tubulointerstitial nephropathy, hyperkalemia, and renal papillary necrosis.[80] Clinical features of these NSAID-induced renal syndromes include increased serum creatinine and blood urea nitrogen, hyperkalemia, elevated blood pressure, peripheral edema, and weight gain. Patients at high risk are those with conditions associated with decreased renal blood flow or taking certain medications. Examples are those with chronic renal insufficiency, congestive heart failure, severe hepatic disease, and nephrotic syndrome, those of advanced age, or those taking diuretics, angiotensin-converting enzyme inhibitors, cyclosporine, or aminoglycosides (Fig. 71-8).

Close monitoring is advisable for high-risk patients taking an NSAID, with monitoring of serum creatinine at baseline and within 3 to 7 days of drug initiation. For those with impaired renal function, the National Kidney Foundation recommends acetaminophen over NSAIDs, although acetaminophen may pose risks, as discussed above.

Coxibs and NSAIDs uncommonly cause drug-induced hepatitis; the two NSAIDs most frequently implicated are diclofenac and sulindac. Patient monitoring should include periodic liver enzymes (aspartate aminotransferase and alanine aminotransferase), with cessation of therapy if these values exceed two to three times the upper limit of normal. In a pooled analysis of 41 studies including

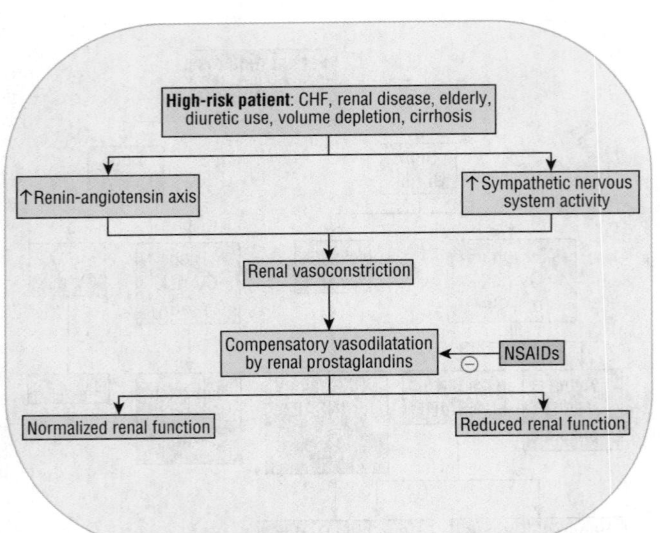

FIGURE 71-8 Mechanisms implicated in NSAID-induced renal injury. The minus (–) sign indicates inhibitory influence (CHF, congestive heart failure; NSAIDs, nonsteroidal antiinflammatory drugs.)

celecoxib, there was a low rate of serious, hepatic-related adverse events with celecoxib (1.11%), with no significant difference from naproxen or ibuprofen, but a significantly higher incidence with diclofenac (4.24%).[81]

Other toxic effects of NSAIDs include hypersensitivity reactions, rash, and CNS complaints of drowsiness, dizziness, headaches, depression, confusion, and tinnitus.[70] It is also recommended that NSAIDs be avoided for patients with asthma who are aspirin-intolerant.

All nonspecific NSAIDs inhibit COX-1–dependent thromboxane production in platelets and thus increase bleeding risk. Unlike aspirin, celecoxib and nonspecific NSAIDs inhibit thromboxane formation reversibly, with normalization of platelet function 1 to 3 days after the drug is stopped. Warfarin and celecoxib are metabolized by the cytochrome P450 isoenzyme CYP2C9; patients receiving warfarin and COX-2 inhibitors should be followed closely.

Finally, NSAIDs should be used only with great caution and only if definitely necessary during pregnancy because of the risk to the fetus posed by the bleeding problems. In late pregnancy, all NSAIDs should be avoided.

Finally, if misoprostol is taken for GI protection, great care is indicated. Because of its abortifacient properties, misoprostol is contraindicated in pregnancy and in women of childbearing age who are not maintaining adequate contraception. It must be dispensed in its original container, which carries a warning for these individuals. Misoprostol is also available in a combination product with diclofenac, which bears the same restrictions as misoprostol alone.

Drug–Drug and Drug–Food Interactions Avoidance of concomitant use, or anticipation and careful monitoring can often prevent serious events when concomitant therapy with NSAIDs and potentially interacting drugs is being considered. The most potentially serious interactions include the use of NSAIDs with lithium, warfarin, other agents that increase bleeding risk, oral hypoglycemics, methotrexate, antihypertensives, angiotensin-converting enzyme inhibitors, β-blockers, and diuretics.[70] In addition, there are probable drug interactions with tacrolimus for ibuprofen, naproxen, diclofenac, and possibly other NSAIDs.

Specific drug interactions are also seen with celecoxib.[82] Celecoxib metabolism is primarily via CYP2C9.[82] Cytochrome P450 inducers such as rifampin, carbamazepine, and phenytoin have the potential to reduce celecoxib levels. Concomitant administration of celecoxib with fluconazole can increase plasma concentrations of celecoxib, due to fluconazole inhibition of the CYP2C9 isoenzyme. Because warfarin and celecoxib are both metabolized by CYP2C9, patients receiving warfarin and COX-2 inhibitors should be followed closely. Celecoxib inhibits CYP2D6, and this may increase concentrations of a variety of agents, including antidepressants. Celecoxib is a sulfonamide and is thus contraindicated for those with sulfa allergies.[82]

Another drug interaction has been noted for those taking some NSAIDs and cardioprotective doses of aspirin. Ibuprofen at doses of 400 mg or more may block aspirin's antiplatelet effect if it is taken first. Patients taking ibuprofen have been advised to take a single dose of ibuprofen at least 30 minutes after taking aspirin, or to take their aspirin at least 8 hours after taking ibuprofen. Other nonselective NSAIDs, such as naproxen, also may cause such interactions. Currently, the ACR recommends that patients who need an oral NSAID for OA choose an NSAID other than ibuprofen or COX-2 selective inhibitors.[39]

Acetaminophen does not appear to interfere with the antiplatelet effect of aspirin.

Dosing and Administration Administration of NSAIDs must be tailored to the individual patient with OA. Selection of an NSAID depends on the prescriber's experience, medication cost, patient preference, allergies, toxicities, and adherence issues. Individual patient response differs among NSAIDs (see Table 71-2), so if an inadequate response is obtained with one NSAID, another NSAID may yet provide benefit.[37–39]

Topical NSAIDs

Pharmacology and Mechanism of Action 11 The mechanism of action of topical NSAIDs is considered to be through inhibition of the COX-2 enzyme in tissues near the site of application. Studies show significant placebo effects that could result from rubbing the product into the skin, which may have a counterirritant effect. Topical NSAIDs are significantly more efficacious compared with placebo vehicle in reducing pain due to musculoskeletal conditions, including OA. Topical ketoprofen is efficacious, as well as topical ibuprofen to a certain extent, but diclofenac is the best studied and most effective topical agent. Most trials have shown topical diclofenac to be as effective as oral NSAIDs, including both oral diclofenac and other comparators.[55,62,83] Diclofenac 1% gel as well as the newer diclofenac liquid drops and diclofenac patches are currently approved in the United States for OA.

Adverse Effects Compared with oral NSAIDs, topical NSAIDs are associated with many fewer GI adverse events and fewer adverse events overall, except for local application site reactions (Table 71-3).

Topical NSAIDs produce local adverse events, most often mild skin reactions such as itching or rash, but very few serious adverse effects. In a comparison of oral (n = 311) and topical diclofenac (n = 311), significantly more persons receiving topical diclofenac developed dry skin, rash, and itching, though none was considered serious. However, significantly more persons receiving oral diclofenac had severe GI effects, asthma, dizziness, dyspnea, change from normal to abnormal hemoglobin, ALT increase to more than three times upper limit of normal, and creatinine clearance changing from normal to abnormal.[55]

Case–control studies revealed that hospital admissions for upper GI bleeding and perforation in those who had used topical NSAIDs in the prior 45 days, when adjusted for oral NSAID use and ulcer healing drugs, was not significantly increased relative to either community or hospital controls. The relative risk for those who had received oral NSAIDs was significantly increased by 2.6-fold and 2.0-fold using community or hospital controls, respectively.[55] A nested case–control

TABLE 71-2 Drug Dosing Table

Drug	Brand Name	Starting Dose	Usual Range	Special Population Dose	Other
Oral Analgesics					
Acetaminophen	Tylenol	325–500 mg three times a day	325–650 mg every 4–6 hours or 1 g three to four times a day	Chronic alcohol intake, hepatic disease	Contained in many combination analgesics
Tramadol	Ultram	25 mg in the morning	Titrate dose in 25 mg increments to reach a maintenance dose of 50–100 mg three times a day.	CrCl <30 mL/min—maximum dose is 200 mg daily	May need to taper dose upon discontinuation to prevent withdrawal symptoms
Tramadol ER	Ultram ER	100 mg daily	Titrate to 200 to 300 mg daily	Do not use if CrCl <30 mL/min	
Hydrocodone/acetaminophen	Lortab, Vicodin	5 mg/325 mg three times daily	2.5–10 mg/325–650 mg three to five times daily	Titrate dose slowly in elderly patients	Maximum dose limited by total daily dose of acetaminophen
Oxycodone/acetaminophen	Percocet	5 mg/325 mg three times daily	2.5–10 mg/325–650 mg three to five times daily	Titrate dose slowly in elderly patients	Maximum dose limited by total daily dose of acetaminophen
Topical Analgesics					
Capsaicin 0.025% or 0.075%	Capzasin-HP		Apply to affected joint three to four times per day		—
Diclofenac 1% gel	Voltaren		Apply 2 or 4 g per site as prescribed, four times daily		
Diclofenac 1.3% patch	Flector		Apply one patch twice daily to the site to be treated, as directed. Apply 40 drops to the affected knee, applying and rubbing in 10 drops		
Diclofenac 1.5% solution	Pennsaid		Apply 40 drops to the affected knee, applying and rubbing in 10 drops at a time. Repeat for a total of four times daily		
Intraarticular Corticosteroids					
Triamcinolone	Kenalog	5–15 mg per joint	10–40 mg per large joint (knee, hip, shoulder)	If multiple joints injected, maximum total dose is usually 80 mg	Often administered concomitantly with a local anesthetic
Methylprednisolone acetate	Depo-Medrol	10–20 mg per joint	20–80 mg per large joint (knee, hip, shoulder)	10–40 mg for medium joints (elbows, wrists)	
Nonsteroidal Antiinflammatory Drugs (NSAIDs)					
Aspirin, plain, buffered, or enteric-coated	Bayer, Ecotrin, Bufferin	325 mg three times a day	325–650 mg four times a day		Doses of 3,600 mg/day are needed for antiinflammatory activity
Celecoxib	Celebrex	100 mg daily	100 mg twice daily or 200 mg daily		
Diclofenac XR	Voltaren-XR	100 mg daily	100–200 mg daily		
Diclofenac IR	CataflCCataflam	50 mg twice a day	50–75 mg twice a day		
Diflunisal	Dolobid	250 mg twice a day	500–750 mg twice a day		
Etodolac	Lodine	300 mg twice a day	400 to 500 mg twice a day		
Fenoprofen	Nalfon	400 mg three times a day	400–600 mg three to four times a day		
Flurbiprofen	Ansaid	100 mg twice a day	200–300 mg/day in two to four divided doses		
Ibuprofen	Motrin, Advil	200 mg three times a day	1200–3,200 mg/day in three to four divided doses		Available OTC and Rx
Indomethacin	Indocin	25 mg twice a day	Titrate dose by 25–50 mg/day until pain controlled or maximum dose of 50 mg three times a day		
Indomethacin SR	Indocin SR	75 mg SR once daily	Can titrate to 75 mg SR twice daily if needed		
Ketoprofen	Orudis	50 mg three times a day	50–75 mg three to four times a day		
Meclofenamate	Meclomen	50 mg three times a day	50–100 mg three to four times a day		
Mefenamic acid	Ponstel	250 mg three times a day	250 mg four times a day		FDA approval for 1 week of therapy
Meloxicam	Mobic	7.5 mg daily	15 mg daily		
Nabumetone	Relafen	500 mg daily	500–1000 mg one to two times a day		
Naproxen	Naprosyn	250 mg twice a day	500 mg twice a day		Available OTC and Rx
Naproxen sodium	Anaprox, Aleve	220 mg twice a day	220–550 mg twice a day		
Naproxen sodium XR	Naprelan		375–750 mg twice a day		
Oxaprozin	Daypro	600 mg daily	600–1200 mg daily		
Piroxicam	Feldene	10 mg daily	20 mg daily		
Salsalate	Disalcid	500 mg twice a day	500–1000 mg two to three times a day		

TABLE 71-3 Drug Monitoring Table

Drug	Adverse Drug Reactions	Monitoring Parameters	Comments
Oral Analgesics			
Acetaminophen	Hepatotoxicity	Total daily dose limits	Use caution with multiple acetaminophen-containing products—total 4 g limit
Tramadol	Nausea, vomiting, somnolence	No routine labs recommended	Drug–drug interaction with other serotonergic medications
Opioids	Sedation, constipation, nausea, dry mouth, hormonal changes	No routine labs recommended	Risks of addiction, dependence, and drug diversion
NSAIDs	Dyspepsia, CV events, GI bleeding, renal impairment	BUN/creatinine, Hgb/Hct, blood pressure	Risks higher in those over 75 years of age
Topical Analgesics			
Capsaicin	Skin irritation and burning	Inspection of areas of application	Wash hands thoroughly after application
NSAIDs	Skin itching, rash, irritation, dyspepsia, CV events, GI bleeding, renal impairment	Inspection of areas of application As needed: BUN/creatinine, Hgb/Hct, blood pressure	Wash hands thoroughly after application. Avoid oral NSAID or aspirin other than cardioprotective dose. Ensure patient applying gel, solution, or patch correctly
Injectable Drugs			
Intraarticular corticosteroids	Hypertension, hyperglycemia	Glucose, blood pressure	HPA axis suppression if used too frequently
Intraarticular hyaluronates	Local joint swelling, stiffness, pain	No routine labs recommended	Less effective than intraarticular corticosteroids; expensive

study from the United Kingdom revealed no significant association between topical NSAID use and renal failure, whereas oral NSAID use was significantly associated with a doubling of risk.[55]

An estimated 1% to 15% of topical NSAID enters the systemic circulation (usually less than 5%), and this contributes to its favorable safety profile.[38,83]

Drug–Drug Interactions Interactions listed for topical diclofenac are the same as those listed above for oral NSAIDs. The most potentially serious interactions include the use of NSAIDs with lithium, warfarin, and other agents that increase bleeding risk, oral hypoglycemics, methotrexate, antihypertensives, angiotensin-converting enzyme inhibitors, β-blockers, and diuretics. Other topical agents have not been studied with topical diclofenac, and changes in tolerability and absorption are possible.

For all of these interactions, as there is only a small percentage of diclofenac absorbed, the risks are likely significantly less than with oral drug, but the patient and provider would be wise to monitor appropriately for these interactions for any of these drugs the patient is taking.

Patients should avoid oral NSAIDs while using topical products to minimize potential for additive adverse effects. Care should be taken to avoid contact with the eyes or open wounds and to wash hands after application (except when treating hand OA).

Dosing and Administration Diclofenac 1% gel (Voltaren) can be used for hand or knee OA or other joints amenable to topical application (not the hip). The gel is applied four times daily using the dose measuring cards provided by the manufacturer. For application to the affected area in the lower limbs, the recommended dose is 4 g four times daily. For upper extremities, the recommended dose is 2 g four times daily.

Diclofenac drops (Pennsaid), only approved for knee OA, are provided in a 1.5% solution in dimethylsulfoxide, and 40 drops are applied four times a day for each knee to be treated. The solution should be applied to the back, front, and sides of the knee. For each dose, the patient places 10 drops at a time directly onto the painful knee (or first into the hands and then immediately onto the knee) and rubs the solution in. The patient then repeats this process three more times until 40 drops have been applied to the painful knee for that particular dose.

The diclofenac patch (diclofenac epolamine 180 mg) is applied twice daily. If the patch does not stick well, the patient can tape edges with first-aid bandages. Patient counseling is important to carefully explain how to apply the topical products and how long to wait before dressing, putting on gloves, showering, and so forth.

Intraarticular Corticosteroids

⓬ **Pharmacology and Mechanism of Action** The antiinflammatory properties of corticosteroids as a class are the primary mechanism of pain relief in the treatment of OA. These properties decrease the formation and release of prostaglandins, kinins, liposomal enzymes, and histamine. Intraarticular corticosteroid injections can provide excellent pain relief, particularly when a joint effusion is present.[39,84]

Aspiration of the effusion and injection of glucocorticoid are carried out aseptically, with examination of the aspirate recommended to exclude crystalline arthritis or infection. The incidence of infection is low, however—approximately 1 in 50,000 procedures.

Several randomized, placebo-controlled, double-blind studies have shown that intraarticular corticosteroids are superior to placebo in alleviating knee pain and stiffness caused by OA.[84] The branched esters of triamcinolone and methylprednisolone are preferred by practitioners because of the reduced solubility that allows the agents to remain in the joint space longer. There is no evidence of a clinically superior corticosteroid for intraarticular use, with equipotent doses of methylprednisolone acetate and triamcinolone hexacetonide having similar efficacy.[85]

Adverse Events Adverse events associated with intraarticular injection of corticosteroids can be local or systemic in nature.

Systemic adverse events are the same as with any other systemic corticosteroid and can include hyperglycemia, edema, elevated blood pressure, flushing, dyspepsia, and adrenal suppression. Multiple injections over longer periods of time (up to 10 years) are more likely to lead to adrenal suppression as recovery time to baseline adrenal function is longer with repeated injections.[86] Hyperglycemia may occur in patients with stable diabetes mellitus as well as those without history of abnormal glycemic control.[86] Hyperglycemia can occur within 24 hours of injection and last for up to 2 weeks.

Local adverse effects can include infection in the affected joint, osteonecrosis, tendon rupture, and skin atrophy at the injection site.

It has long been thought that intraarticular corticosteroids can hasten cartilage loss, but the potential risk of cartilage destruction with steroid injections has not been substantiated. Systemic corticosteroid therapy is not recommended in OA, given the lack of proven benefit and the well-known adverse effects with long-term use.

Dosing and Administration Average doses for injection of large joints in adults are 10 to 20 mg of triamcinolone hexacetonide or 20 to 40 mg of methylprednisolone acetate. This therapy is generally limited to three or four injections per year due to the potential systemic effects of corticosteroids and because the need for more frequent injections indicates little response to the therapy.

After injection, the patient should minimize activity and stress on the joint for several days. Initial pain relief may be seen within 24 to 72 hours after injection, with peak pain relief about 7 to 10 days after injection and lasting up to 4 to 8 weeks.

Capsaicin

Pharmacology and Mechanism of Action Capsaicin, isolated from hot peppers, releases and ultimately depletes substance P from afferent nociceptive nerve fibers. Substance P has been implicated in the transmission of pain in arthritis, and capsaicin cream has been shown in four placebo-controlled studies to provide pain relief in knee and hand OA when applied over affected joints.[62] Due to the larger surface area and distance from the site of application to the joint, it is not expected that application of capsaicin would provide efficacy in the treatment of hip OA.

Adverse Effects Adverse events associated with capsaicin are primarily local, with one in three patients experiencing burning, stinging, and/or erythema that usually subsides with repeated application. FDA has recently issued a public drug safety communication notifying consumers that rare cases of severe burns have been reported.[87] Some patients may experience coughing associated with application.

Dosing and Administration To be effective, capsaicin must be used regularly, and it may take up to 2 weeks to take effect. Although use is recommended four times a day, a twice-daily application may enhance long-term adherence and still provide adequate pain relief.[62] Patients should be counseled not to get the cream in their eyes or mouth. Patients should also notify their healthcare provider immediately if they experience pain, swelling, or blistering skin at the site of application.

When patients were queried using an electronic questionnaire that considered possible toxicities of treatments, as well as route of administration and cost, capsaicin was the most preferred by patients, even when it was portrayed as being less effective than NSAIDs.[88]

Capsaicin is a nonprescription product available as a cream, gel, or lotion in concentrations ranging from 0.025% to 0.075%.

Tramadol

Pharmacology and Mechanism of Action Tramadol, an analgesic with affinity for the μ-opioid receptor, as well as weak inhibition of the reuptake of norepinephrine and serotonin neurotransmitter, has modest analgesic effects (with or without acetaminophen) for patients with OA when compared with placebo.[89] Tramadol is also modestly effective as add-on therapy for patients taking concomitant acetaminophen, NSAIDs or COX-2–selective inhibitors. Tramadol may be helpful for patients who cannot take NSAIDs or COX-2–selective inhibitors.

Adverse events Opioid-like adverse effects such as nausea, vomiting, dizziness, constipation, headache, and somnolence are common with tramadol. These occur in 60% to 70% of treated patients, and 40% discontinue tramadol because of an adverse effect.[89] Although the frequency of adverse effects is high, the severity of adverse effects is less than with NSAIDs, as tramadol use is not associated with life-threatening GI bleeding, cardiovascular events, or renal failure. The most notable serious adverse event associated with tramadol use is seizures. Tramadol is not classified as a controlled substance, but there are numerous reports of patients displaying drug-seeking behaviors similar to those displayed by patients who are dependent and/or addicted to opioid analgesics.[39]

Drug–Drug Interaction Medications that lower the seizure threshold should be used with caution in patients taking tramadol. These include tricyclic antidepressants, first-generation antipsychotic medications and cyclobenzaprine, as well as others. There is also an increased risk of serotonin syndrome (see eChap. 10, Clinical Toxicology, for description and management of this condition) when tramadol is used concomitantly with other serotonergic medications, including duloxetine.

Dosing and Administration Tramadol should be initiated at a lower dose (100 mg per day) and may be titrated as needed for pain control to a dose of 200 mg per day.

Tramadol is available in a combination tablet with acetaminophen and as a sustained-release (SR) tablet.

Second-Line Treatments

Opioid Analgesics

Opioid analgesics can be useful for patients who experience limited pain relief with acetaminophen, oral NSAIDs, intraarticular injections, or topical therapy.[90] For patients with underlying conditions that limit the use of first-line analgesics, opioid analgesics can effectively relieve acute OA pain. A common clinical scenario may include the patient who cannot take oral NSAIDs because of renal failure or cardiovascular disease. Patients in whom all other treatment options have failed and who are at high surgical risk, precluding joint arthroplasty are also candidates for opioid therapy. As many patients with OA are elderly, it is important to carefully use opioids to promote safety. The following recommendations have been suggested to optimize opioid therapy: (a) use the least invasive route of administration, (b) initiate one agent at a time, at a low dose, (c) allow a sufficiently long interval between dose increases to allow an assessment of efficacy and safety, (d) use a long-acting preparation, (e) therapy should be constantly monitored and adjusted if necessary, (f) changing opioids may be necessary.[90]

SR compounds usually offer better pain control throughout the day, and are used when immediate-release (IR) opioids do not provide a sufficient duration of pain control. A variety of IR and SR opioid compounds have been studied including oxycodone IR and SR, morphine IR and SR, hydromorphone, and fentanyl transdermal patch.[57]

Adverse effects are common in opioid-treated OA patients. More than 75% of patients in clinical trials experience at least one typical opioid-related (i.e. nausea, somnolence, constipation, dry mouth, and dizziness) adverse effect. Although this is not an unexpected finding, it serves as a reminder to use opioids cautiously in elderly patients who may be more susceptible to adverse effects.

Opioid dependence, addiction, tolerance, hyperalgesia, and issues surrounding drug diversion are more serious adverse effects associated with long-term treatment. Prescription opioid misuse/abuse/addiction is a major public health concern with the CDC reporting almost 15,000 deaths in 2008.[91] In 2009, there were 475,000 emergency room visits attributed to the misuse and abuse of prescription opioids.[91] To address this growing safety issue, the American Pain Society/American Academy of Pain Medicine has published recommendations on the use of opioids in the management of chronic noncancer pain.[92]

If pain is intolerable and limits activities of daily living, and the patient has sufficiently good cardiopulmonary health to undergo major surgery, joint replacement may be preferable to continued reliance on opioids.

Duloxetine

Duloxetine is a centrally acting dual-reuptake inhibitor of both serotonin and norepinephrine, although norepinephrine reuptake inhibition does not occur until doses reach 60 mg/day. While the most common pain target in OA is peripheral nociceptive pain, there is some evidence that chronic nociceptive pain leads to central pain sensitization, thereby lowering the pain threshold.[59] Duloxetine provides pain relief through blockade of central pain transmitters, including serotonin and norepinephrine.

Adverse effects commonly associated with duloxetine therapy include nausea, dry mouth, constipation, and anorexia. Expected neurologic adverse effects include fatigue, somnolence, and dizziness. Rare but serious adverse events associated with duloxetine include Stevens–Johnson syndrome and liver failure. Patients should contact their healthcare provider immediately if they develop a rash while taking duloxetine.

Particular care should be taken to avoid the use of duloxetine with other serotonergic medications, including tramadol. As tramadol is a first-line treatment recommendation for OA, the likelihood of encountering this combination is high. Concomitant use of duloxetine with other medications that increase serotonin concentrations increases the risk of serotonin syndrome (see eChap. 10, Clinical Toxicology).

Hyaluronic Acid Injections

Agents containing HA (sodium hyaluronate) are available for intraarticular injection for treatment of knee OA.[93]

High-molecular-weight HA is an important constituent of synovial fluid. Endogenous HA may also have antiinflammatory effects. Because the concentration and molecular size of synovial HA decreases in OA, administration of exogenous HA products have been studied, with the theory that this could reconstitute synovial fluid and reduce symptoms. In fact, HA injections temporarily and modestly increase viscosity. When evaluating pain score improvements, it is essential to determine if score improvement corresponds to clinically meaningful improvement for patients. Extensive evaluation of the literature has revealed potential publication bias of HA studies including bias related to high levels of industry sponsorship as well as a substantial number of studies with unpublished data.[94]

Most HA products are injected once weekly for either 3 or 5 weeks, depending on the specific agent administered. Injections are generally well tolerated, although acute joint swelling, effusion, and stiffness can occur as well as local skin reactions, including rash, ecchymoses, and pruritus have been reported. Rarely, systemic adverse events including hypersensitivity reactions have occurred.

HA injections have limited beneficial effects for patients with knee OA. HA products have not been shown to benefit patients with hip OA.[95] These agents are expensive because the treatment includes both drug costs and administration costs.

Glucosamine and Chondroitin

Interest in chondroitin and glucosamine was spurred initially by anecdotal reports of benefit in animals and humans and by the ability of these substances to stimulate proteoglycan synthesis from articular cartilage in vitro. Over the last decade, enthusiasm for these agents has waned as additional efficacy data have become available to the point that the American College of Rheumatology conditionally recommends against the use of glucosamine and chondroitin.[39] Glucosamine, alone or in combination, has not been shown to provide uniform improvements in pain control or functional status in patients with OA of the knee or hip.[96]

Numerous trials have been conducted with suboptimal study designs, and this has led to a variable response to glucosamine and/or chondroitin.[94] In contrast to the early reports of suboptimally designed studies, a large, well-controlled National Institutes of Health-sponsored study demonstrated no significant clinical response to glucosamine therapy alone, chondroitin therapy alone, or combination glucosamine–chondroitin therapy when compared with placebo across all patients.[97] This trial provided high-quality evidence on the use of glucosamine and chondroitin in OA and demonstrated that the safety and efficacy glucosamine and chondroitin therapy was similar to placebo.

Because glucosamine and chondroitin are marketed in the United States as dietary supplements, neither the products nor their purity is adequately regulated by the FDA. The potential consequences related to the lack of regulatory oversight for these products can affect both efficacy and safety. Products containing less than labeled doses can compromise efficacy, while those containing ingredients not included on the labeling can compromise safety. A variety of brand name and generic products are available.

Considerations for Future Therapeutic Options

Strategies aimed at expanding therapeutic options for OA include an array of disease-modifying drugs, new drug classes to provide symptomatic relief of OA pain, and behavior modification strategies to improve patient participation in nonpharmacologic therapies.[98]

Disease-modifying drugs are targeted at preventing, retarding, or reversing damage to articular cartilage. Currently, OA is a progressive disease. Current approaches to slow progression of OA are directed at three different tissue-specific targets: (a) cartilage, (b) synovial membrane and associated inflammation, and (c) subchondral bone. Therapies directed at preserving cartilage include enzyme inhibitors of MMPs, inhibitors of inducible nitric oxide synthase, cathepsin K inhibitors, and nerve growth factor inhibitors.[98] Several of these investigational agents are in Phase I and Phase II clinical trials in humans. Doxycycline, as a TIMP, potentially decreases cartilage destruction. In knee OA, doxycycline has been shown to delay loss of articular cartilage (joint space narrowing) in humans when compared with placebo, although the clinical impact of this finding is unclear.[99]

Several antiinflammatory agents targeting symptom improvement as well as structure-modifying properties at the synovial membrane are in clinical trials. The agents include interleukin-1 inhibitors, the antitumor necrosis factor inhibitor adalimumab, and adenosine A2 and A3 receptor agonists.[98] Current animal research supports these receptor targets to prevent ongoing joint destruction, and early results for some of these agents, particularly adalimumab, are encouraging.

Ongoing phase III clinical trials with licofelone, a lipoxygenase/cyclooxygenase inhibitor (LOX/COX), has demonstrated some preliminary data in treatment of OA pain. The efficacy of licofelone may be similar to that of NSAIDs, but adverse event advantages are still being investigated.[100] Combined LOX/COX inhibition may decrease the production of proinflammatory leukotrienes associated with the progression of OA.

Slowing the progression of OA may also be achieved by attempts to modify or repair bony changes associated with OA. Current strategies being evaluated in humans include the use of bisphosphonates, calcitonin, cholecalciferol, selective estrogen receptor modulators, parathyroid hormone, strontium, and MMP-13 inhibitors. The definitive role of these agents in modifying bone resorption as a strategy to delay the progression of bone damage associated with OA is yet to be determined.

Additionally, new agents and methods to treat symptoms of OA are being studied. These approaches include nerve growth factor inhibitors, cannabinoid receptor agonists, bradykinin receptor antagonists, kainate receptor antagonists, and transient receptor potential ion channel agonists (TRVP-1).[98]

Of these agents, the nerve growth inhibitor tanezumab has undergone the most extensive evaluation. Unfortunately, Phase III study results with tanezumab have revealed potential safety issues with treatment, and it appears unlikely to become a viable treatment for OA pain.[101]

Several other compounds targeted toward the described receptors are under active investigation. Although many of these compounds are years away from potential market approval, the extensive nature of the work is encouraging.

In addition to pharmacologic agents, acupuncture has been examined in OA. In a systematic analysis of 18 randomized, controlled trials of manual or electroacupuncture, 10 showed positive effects for acupuncture.[102] However, in a recent, large, randomized, and well-controlled study, acupuncture was not seen to be any more effective than sham controls.[103]

PERSONALIZED PHARMACOTHERAPY

OA has substantial negative impact on the quality of life for individual patients. OA is also associated with a negative impact on society as the disease is extremely common, and OA ranks second in causes of disability in the United States.[39]

Most OA patients use a multidisciplinary approach to their treatment.[39,104] Treatments include nonpharmacologic and pharmacologic therapy, in addition to surgical options in some patients. Unfortunately, many patients have less than optimal response to treatment and commonly require a change in therapy or augmentation of partially effective therapy. Achieving adequate pain control and minimizing functional impairment in OA patients require careful assessment of comorbid conditions in each patient to safely provide effective pharmacotherapy treatments. Nonpharmacologic interventions may also require regular reinforcement and modifications.

A multidisciplinary intervention for knee OA initiated by pharmacists has been shown to improve adherence to OA guideline recommendations, decrease pain scores, and improve functional assessment scores.[105] These types of multidisciplinary disease management programs that implement strategies to provide comprehensive care should be offered to all OA patients to maximize outcomes.

Total indirect and direct medical costs for OA patients are high.[104] The highest costs associated with the pharmacotherapy of OA are hospitalization for treatment of NSAID-related complications, particularly serious GI adverse events. Historically, gastroprotective therapy or the use of COX-2–selective inhibitors for low-risk patients has not been cost-effective because of the large number needed to treat to prevent serious events, but current data suggest that concomitant PPI therapy in low-risk patients is cost-effective if the agent selected is a generic, multisource product.[106] The use of COX-2–selective inhibitors to protect gastric mucosa in aspirin users is not cost-effective, because aspirin negates most, if not all, of the gastroprotective effects of these agents.[107] Pharmacoeconomic considerations for OA involve the proper selection of therapy for the initial treatment of each patient with OA. Use of the nonprescription analgesic acetaminophen as initial therapy has greatly reduced medication costs in comparison with the use of NSAIDs, many of which are by prescription only. Oral NSAID costs vary considerably, depending on the medication, daily dose, and regimen selected. As oral NSAIDs as a class are therapeutically similar, the use of a less-expensive agent such as nonprescription ibuprofen or naproxen or a multisource generic product may minimize the cost. More-expensive NSAIDs can be prescribed if neither of these offers benefit after a 2-week trial at sufficient doses. Topical NSAIDs are significantly more costly than oral agents, although may still be cost-effective in patients at high-risk for costly complications associated with oral NSAID therapy.

EVALUATION OF THERAPEUTIC OUTCOMES

For the person with OA, treatment decisions and pharmacotherapy monitoring is patient specific. The patient's situation and individual needs should be considered when devising a treatment plan. Is the patient bothered primarily by pain, by limitations in activity, or with concerns about side effects from medications? Does the patient understand what OA is and why certain treatments are useful?

When the patient is first being assessed for the possibility of OA, the diagnosis is often straightforward, including history and physical exam, plain films of the affected joint(s), and laboratory tests. The older patient with unilateral knee pain, limited range of motion, no palpable warmth, crepitus, without prolonged morning stiffness, and without other suspicious findings is highly likely to have knee OA. It is still reasonable to obtain x-ray films, which may help follow disease over time (although joint space narrowing often does not correlate with the extent of pain or difficulty walking). Basic laboratory tests can shed light on what pharmacologic therapy is possible (e.g., in a patient with poor renal function, NSAIDs should be avoided). Pain can be assessed using a visual analog scale, and physical examination is helpful to determine range of motion for affected joints. Additional tests of OA severity may include measurement of grip strength, 50 ft walking time, patient and physician global assessment of OA severity, and assessment of ability to perform activities of daily living. Once the patient is assessed and diagnosed, patient and family education is essential. Nondrug therapy may include a referral for physical and/or occupational therapy services, where the therapists can help to maintain and improve range of motion, decrease pain modestly, lose weight if necessary, and become more active once the OA symptoms are better controlled.

Setting the stage for pharmacotherapy with the above is important but in the meantime, the patient needs pain relief. A few years ago, acetaminophen would be the only "first choice" for pain relief. Adverse events with acetaminophen are uncommon, although it is crucial that the patient understand the maximum daily dose limits and realize that many products contain acetaminophen. Although some patients do well on acetaminophen, many do not achieve sufficient pain relief.

A step up to oral NSAIDs or opioid therapy might be necessary, but this poses significant risks beyond acetaminophen. A switch to NSAIDs requires careful consideration of the patient's age and comorbidities, renal function, history of GI problems, hypertension, and cardiovascular health. Periodic monitoring would include open-ended questions followed by direct questions relating to the commonest adverse effects associated with the respective medication. For an oral NSAID, symptoms of abdominal pain, heartburn, nausea, or change in stool color provide valuable clues to the presence of GI complications, although serious GI complications can occur without warning. Patients should be monitored for the development of hypertension, weight gain, edema, skin rash, and CNS adverse effects such as headaches and drowsiness. Baseline serum creatinine, complete blood count, and serum transaminases are repeated at 6- to 12-month intervals to identify GI, renal, and hepatic toxicities.

Topical NSAIDs are now known to have efficacy in OA of the hand and knee and are as effective as oral NSAIDs. Although they carry the same cardiovascular, renal, and GI warnings, the amount of a typical dose absorbed into the bloodstream is only a few percent of that from an equivalent dose of oral NSAID (as measured by areas under serum concentration–time curves). Topical NSAIDs' most common adverse effects are local, with irritated skin, rash, or itching, usually mild, and with many fewer adverse effects of cardiovascular, GI, or renal nature. These agents are a welcome addition to the limited treatment modalities for the very common, costly, painful, and often disabling disease of OA. It is important that the patient apply the topical products appropriately to achieve maximum benefit and avoiding adverse events.

For patients receiving intraarticular corticosteroids, improvement should begin within 2 to 3 days and last 4 to 8 weeks. Patients should be advised about possible injection site reactions, as well as possible systemic effects, especially for those with hypertension or diabetes, as there is a potential for increased blood pressure or blood glucose. For patients receiving opioids or tramadol, relief from pain should occur rapidly. Frail or elderly patients should be monitored carefully and cautioned about sedation, dysphoria, nausea, risk of falls, and constipation. Additional monitoring should include strategies to assess development of opioid tolerance and addiction.

CONCLUSION

OA is a very common, slowly progressive disorder that affects diarthrodial joints and is characterized by progressive deterioration of articular cartilage, subchondral sclerosis, and osteophyte production. Clinical manifestations include gradual onset of joint pain, stiffness, and limitation of motion. The primary treatment goals are to reduce pain, maintain function, and prevent further destruction. An individualized approach based on education, rest, exercise, weight loss as needed, and analgesic medication can succeed in meeting these goals. Recommended drug treatment starts with acetaminophen ≤4 g/day and topical analgesics as needed. If acetaminophen is ineffective, oral NSAIDs may be used in appropriately selected patients, often providing satisfactory relief of pain and stiffness. Individuals at increased risk for toxicity from NSAIDs, especially for GI, cardiovascular, or renal events, deserve special attention. Celecoxib may have safety advantages in some OA patients, but its safety relative to other NSAIDs and its role in OA remains poorly defined. Adjunctive therapy with tramadol, intraarticular corticosteroids, and opioid analgesics may be helpful in patients with poorly controlled pain. Experimental therapy aimed at preventing the progression of OA requires further clinical investigation before entering widespread clinical use.

ABBREVIATIONS

APC Adenoma Prevention with Celecoxib
APPROVe Adenomatous Polyp Prevention on Vioxx
CLASS Celecoxib Long-Term Arthritis Safety Study
COX cyclooxygenase
ECM extracellular matrix
FDA Food and Drug Administration
GWAS genome-wide association studies
HA hyaluronic acid
IDEA Intensive Diet and Exercise for Arthritis
IR immediate-release
LOX lipoxygenase
MMP matrix metalloproteinase
NICE National Institute for Health and Clinical Excellence
NSAID nonsteroidal antiinflammatory drug
OA osteoarthritis
PPI proton-pump inhibitor
QALE quality-adjusted life expectancy
SR sustained-release
TIMP tissue inhibitors of metalloproteinase
TNF tumor necrosis factor

REFERENCES

1. Zhang Y, Jordan JM. Epidemiology of osteoarthritis. Clin Geriatr Med 2010;26(3):355–369.
2. Bijlsma JW, Berenbaum F, Lafeber FP. Osteoarthritis: An update with relevance for clinical practice. Lancet 2011;377(9783):2115–2126.
3. Murphy L, Helmick CG. The impact of osteoarthritis in the United States: A population-health perspective. Am J Nurs 2012;112(3 Suppl 1):S13–S19.
4. Lawrence RC, Felson DT, Helmick CG, et al. Estimates of the prevalence of arthritis and other rheumatic conditions in the United States. Part II. Arthritis Rheum 2008;58(1):26–35.
5. Hunter DJ. Insights from imaging on the epidemiology and pathophysiology of osteoarthritis. Radiol Clin North Am 2009;47(4):539–551.
6. Chu CR, Williams AA, Coyle CH, Bowers ME. Early diagnosis to enable early treatment of pre-osteoarthritis. Arthritis Res Ther 2012;14(3):212.
7. Kotlarz H, Gunnarsson CL, Fang H, Rizzo JA. Osteoarthritis and absenteeism costs: Evidence from US national survey data. J Occup Environ Med 2010;52(3):263–268.
8. Dagenais S, Garbedian S, Wai EK. Systematic review of the prevalence of radiographic primary hip osteoarthritis. Clin Orthop Relat Res 2009;467(3):623–637.
9. Feydy A, Pluot E, Guerini H, Drape JL. Osteoarthritis of the wrist and hand, and spine. Radiol Clin North Am 2009;47(4):723–759.
10. Hunter DJ. In the clinic: Osteoarthritis. Ann Intern Med 2007;147(3):ITC8-1–ITC8-16.
11. Kopec JA, Rahman MM, Sayre EC, et al. Trends in physician-diagnosed osteoarthritis incidence in an administrative database in British Columbia, Canada, 1996–1997 through 2003–2004. Arthritis Rheum 2008;59(7):929–934.
12. Garstang SV, Stitik TP. Osteoarthritis: Epidemiology, risk factors, and pathophysiology. Am J Phys Med Rehabil 2006;85(11 Suppl):S2–11; quiz S12–S14.
13. Mork PJ, Holtermann A, Nilsen TI. Effect of body mass index and physical exercise on risk of knee and hip osteoarthritis: Longitudinal data from the Norwegian HUNT study. J Epidemiol Community Health 2012;66(8):678–683.
14. Andersen S, Thygesen LC, Davidsen M, Helweg-Larsen K. Cumulative years in occupation and the risk of hip or knee osteoarthritis in men and women: A register-based follow-up study. Occup Environ Med 2012;69(5):325–330.
15. Sun BH, Wu CW, Kalunian KC. New developments in osteoarthritis. Rheum Dis Clin North Am 2007;33(1):135–148.
16. Botha-Scheepers SA, Watt I, Slagboom E, et al. Influence of familial factors on radiologic disease progression over two years in siblings with osteoarthritis at multiple sites: A prospective longitudinal cohort study. Arthritis Rheum 2007;57(4):626–632.
17. Valdes AM, Spector TD. The contribution of genes to osteoarthritis. Med Clin North Am 2009;93(1):45–66, x.
18. Valdes AM, Spector TD. Genetic epidemiology of hip and knee osteoarthritis. Nat Rev Rheumatol 2011;7(1):23–32.
19. Evangelou E, Valdes AM, Kerkhof HJ, et al. Meta-analysis of genome-wide association studies confirms a susceptibility locus for knee osteoarthritis on chromosome 7q22. Ann Rheum Dis 2011;70(2):349–355.
20. Meulenbelt I. Osteoarthritis year 2011 in review: Genetics. Osteoarthritis Cartilage 2012;20(3):218–222.
21. Dieppe P. Developments in osteoarthritis. Rheumatology (Oxford) 2011;50(2):245–247.
22. Sandell LJ, Heinegard D, Hering TH. Cell biology, biochemistry, and molecular biology of articular cartilage

in osteoarthritis. In: Moscowitz RW, Altman RD, Hochberg MC, Buckwalter JA, Goldberg VM, eds. Osteoarthritis: Diagnosis and Medical/Surgical Management, 4th ed. Philadelphia: Lippincott, Williams, & Wilkins, 2007:73–106.
23. Felson DT. Osteoarthritis. In: Fauci AS, Braunwald E, Kaspar DL, Hauser DL, Longo DLJ, Loscalzo J, eds. Harrison's Principles of Internal Medicine. New York, NY: McGraw-Hill, 2009:2158–2165.
24. Loeser RF, Goldring SR, Scanzello CR, Goldring MB. Osteoarthritis: A disease of the joint as an organ. Arthritis Rheum 2012;64(6):1697–1707.
25. Goldring SR, Goldring MB. The role of cytokines in cartilage matrix degeneration in osteoarthritis. Clin Orthop Relat Res 2004;(427 Suppl):S27–S36.
26. Vincent TL, Saklatvala J. Is the response of cartilage to injury relevant to osteoarthritis? Arthritis Rheum 2008;58(5):1207–1210.
27. Goldring MB, Marcu KB. Cartilage homeostasis in health and rheumatic diseases. Arthritis Res Ther 2009;11(3):224.
28. Dell'accio F, De Bari C, Eltawil NM, Vanhummelen P, Pitzalis C. Identification of the molecular response of articular cartilage to injury, by microarray screening: Wnt-16 expression and signaling after injury and in osteoarthritis. Arthritis Rheum 2008;58(5):1410–1421.
29. Fukui N, Ikeda Y, Ohnuki T, et al. Regional differences in chondrocyte metabolism in osteoarthritis: A detailed analysis by laser capture microdissection. Arthritis Rheum 2008;58(1):154–163.
30. Wu J, Liu W, Bemis A, et al. Comparative proteomic characterization of articular cartilage tissue from normal donors and patients with osteoarthritis. Arthritis Rheum 2007;56(11):3675–3684.
31. Karsdal MA, Leeming DJ, Dam EB, et al. Should subchondral bone turnover be targeted when treating osteoarthritis? Osteoarthritis Cartilage 2008;16(6):638–646.
32. Rosenberg AE. Bones, joints and soft tissue tumors. In: Kumar V, Abbas AK, Fausto N, Aster J, eds. Robbins and Cotran Pathologic Basis of Disease, Professional Edition, 8th ed. Philadelphia, PA: W.B. Saunders, 2009:1235–1236.
33. Altman RD. Laboratory diagnosis of osteoarthritis. In: Moscowitz RW, Altman RD, Hochberg MC, Buckwalter JA, Goldberg VM, eds. Osteoarthritis: Diagnosis and Medical/Surgical Management, 4th ed. Philadelphia: Lippincott, Williams, & Wilkins, 2007:201–214.
34. Lane NE. Clinical practice. Osteoarthritis of the hip. N Engl J Med 2007;357(14):1413–1421.
35. *http://www.rheumatology.org/publications/*.
36. Zhang W, Doherty M, Leeb BF, et al. EULAR evidence based recommendations for the management of hand osteoarthritis: Report of a task force of the EULAR standing committee for international clinical studies including therapeutics (ESCISIT). Ann Rheum Dis 2007;66(3):377–388.
37. Bennell KL, Hunter DJ, Hinman RS. Management of osteoarthritis of the knee. BMJ 2012;345:e4934.
38. Conaghan PG, Dickson J, Grant RL, Guideline Development Group. Care and management of osteoarthritis in adults: Summary of NICE guidance. BMJ 2008;336(7642):502–503.
39. Hochberg MC, Altman RD, April KT, et al. American college of rheumatology 2012 recommendations for the use of nonpharmacologic and pharmacologic therapies in osteoarthritis of the hand, hip, and knee. Arthritis Care Res (Hoboken) 2012;64(4):455–474.
40. Knittle K, De Gucht V, Maes S. Lifestyle- and behaviour-change interventions in musculoskeletal conditions. Best Pract Res Clin Rheumatol 2012;26(3):293–304.
41. Hawker GA, Mian S, Bednis K, Stanaitis I. Osteoarthritis year 2010 in review: Non-pharmacologic therapy. Osteoarthritis Cartilage 2011;19(4):366–374.
42. Christensen R, Bartels EM, Astrup A, Bliddal H. Effect of weight reduction in obese patients diagnosed with knee osteoarthritis: A systematic review and meta-analysis. Ann Rheum Dis 2007;66(4):433–439.
43. Reijman M, Pols HA, Bergink AP, et al. Body mass index associated with onset and progression of osteoarthritis of the knee but not of the hip: The Rotterdam study. Ann Rheum Dis 2007;66(2):158–162.
44. Vincent HK, DeJong G, Mascarenas D, Vincent KR. The effect of body mass index and hip abductor brace use on inpatient rehabilitation outcomes after total hip arthroplasty. Am J Phys Med Rehabil 2009;88(3):201–209.
45. Messier SP. Diet and exercise for obese adults with knee osteoarthritis. Clin Geriatr Med 2010;26(3):461–477.
46. Jenkinson CM, Doherty M, Avery AJ, et al. Effects of dietary intervention and quadriceps strengthening exercises on pain and function in overweight people with knee pain: Randomised controlled trial. BMJ 2009;339:b3170.
47. Josbeno DA, Kalarchian M, Sparto PJ, Otto AD, Jakicic JM. Physical activity and physical function in individuals post-bariatric surgery. Obes Surg 2011;21(8):1243–1249.
48. Messier SP, Legault C, Mihalko S, et al. The intensive diet and exercise for arthritis (IDEA) trial: Design and rationale. BMC Musculoskelet Disord 2009;10:93.
49. Fernandes L, Storheim K, Nordsletten L, Risberg MA. Development of a therapeutic exercise program for patients with osteoarthritis of the hip. Phys Ther 2010;90(4):592–601.
50. Fitzpatrick R, Shortall E, Sculpher M, et al. Primary total hip replacement surgery: A systematic review of outcomes and modelling of cost-effectiveness associated with different prostheses. Health Technol Assess 1998;2(20):1–64.
51. Gossec L, Paternotte S, Maillefert JF, et al. The role of pain and functional impairment in the decision to recommend total joint replacement in hip and knee osteoarthritis: An international cross-sectional study of 1909 patients. Report of the OARSI-OMERACT task force on total joint replacement. Osteoarthritis Cartilage 2011;19(2):147–154.
52. Skou ST, Roos EM, Laursen MB, et al. Total knee replacement plus physical and medical therapy or treatment with physical and medical therapy alone: A randomised controlled trial in patients with knee osteoarthritis (the MEDIC-study). BMC Musculoskelet Disord 2012;13:67.
53. Losina E, Walensky RP, Kessler CL, et al. Cost-effectiveness of total knee arthroplasty in the United States: Patient risk and hospital volume. Arch Intern Med 2009;169(12):1113–1121; discussion 1121–1122.
54. Kuo CK, Li WJ, Mauck RL, Tuan RS. Cartilage tissue engineering: Its potential and uses. Curr Opin Rheumatol 2006;18(1):64–73.
55. Chou R, McDonagh MS, Nakamoto E, Griffin J. Analgesics for Osteoarthritis: An Update of the 2006 Comparative Effectiveness Review. Comparative Effectiveness Review No. 38 (Prepared by the Oregon Evidence-based Practice Center under Contract HHSA 290 2007 10057 I) AHRQ Publication No. 11(12)-EHC076-EF. Rockville, MD: Agency for Healthcare Research and Quality, October 2011.
56. Towheed TE, Maxwell L, Judd MG, Catton M, Hochberg MC, Wells G. Acetaminophen for osteoarthritis. Cochrane Database Syst Rev 2006;(1):CD004257.
57. Nuesch E, Rutjes AW, Husni E, Welch V, Juni P. Oral or transdermal opioids for osteoarthritis of the knee or hip. Cochrane Database Syst Rev 2009;(4):CD003115.

58. Frakes EP, Risser RC, Ball TD, Hochberg MC, Wohlreich MM. Duloxetine added to oral nonsteroidal anti-inflammatory drugs for treatment of knee pain due to osteoarthritis: Results of a randomized, double-blind, placebo-controlled trial. Curr Med Res Opin 2011;27(12):2361–2372.
59. Hochberg MC, Wohlreich M, Gaynor P, Hanna S, Risser R. Clinically relevant outcomes based on analysis of pooled data from 2 trials of duloxetine in patients with knee osteoarthritis. J Rheumatol 2012;39(2):352–358.
60. Altman RD, Dreiser RL, Fisher CL, Chase WF, Dreher DS, Zacher J. Diclofenac sodium gel in patients with primary hand osteoarthritis: A randomized, double-blind, placebo-controlled trial. J Rheumatol 2009;36(9):1991–1999.
61. Altman RD. Pharmacological therapies for osteoarthritis of the hand: A review of the evidence. Drugs Aging 2010;27(9):729–745.
62. Altman RD, Barthel HR. Topical therapies for osteoarthritis. Drugs 2011;71(10):1259–1279.
63. Henrich WL, Agodoa LE, Barrett B, et al. Analgesics and the kidney: Summary and recommendations to the scientific advisory board of the national kidney foundation from an ad hoc committee of the National Kidney Foundation. Am J Kidney Dis 1996;27(1):162–165.
64. Kuo HW, Tsai SS, Tiao MM, Liu YC, Lee IM, Yang CY. Analgesic use and the risk for progression of chronic kidney disease. Pharmacoepidemiol Drug Saf 2010;19(7):745–751.
65. Federal Register. Rockville, MD: Department of Health and Human Services Vol. 74, No. 81, 2009.
66. Watkins PB, Kaplowitz N, Slattery JT, et al. Aminotransferase elevations in healthy adults receiving 4 grams of acetaminophen daily: A randomized controlled trial. JAMA 2006;296(1):87–93.
67. Larson AM, Polson J, Fontana RJ, et al. Acetaminophen-induced acute liver failure: Results of a United States multicenter, prospective study. Hepatology 2005;42(6):1364–1372.
68. Laine L, White WB, Rostom A, Hochberg M. COX-2 selective inhibitors in the treatment of osteoarthritis. Semin Arthritis Rheum 2008;38(3):165–187.
69. Grosser T. The pharmacology of selective inhibition of COX-2. Thromb Haemost 2006;96(4):393–400.
70. McEvoy GK, ed. AHFS Drug Information®. Bethesda, MD: American Society of Health-System Pharmacists, Inc. ISBN 978-1-58528-247-0. ISSN 8756-6028. STAT!Ref Online Electronic Medical Library, *http://online.statref.com*, 2012.
71. Lanas A. Nonsteroidal antiinflammatory drugs and cyclooxygenase inhibition in the gastrointestinal tract: A trip from peptic ulcer to colon cancer. Am J Med Sci 2009;338(2):96–106.
72. Lazzaroni M, Porro GB. Management of NSAID-induced gastrointestinal toxicity: Focus on proton pump inhibitors. Drugs 2009;69(1):51–69.
73. Rostom A, Moayyedi P, Hunt R, Canadian Association of Gastroenterology Consensus Group. Canadian Consensus Guidelines on long-term nonsteroidal anti-inflammatory drug therapy and the need for gastroprotection: Benefits versus risks. Aliment Pharmacol Ther 2009;29(5):481–496.
74. Tannenbaum H, Bombardier C, Davis P, Russell AS, Third Canadian Consensus Conference Group. An evidence-based approach to prescribing nonsteroidal antiinflammatory drugs: Third Canadian Consensus Conference. J Rheumatol 2006;33(1):140–157.
75. Chan FK, Hung LC, Suen BY, et al. Celecoxib versus diclofenac and omeprazole in reducing the risk of recurrent ulcer bleeding in patients with arthritis. N Engl J Med 2002;347(26):2104–2110.
76. Bresalier RS, Sandler RS, Quan H, et al. Cardiovascular events associated with rofecoxib in a colorectal adenoma chemoprevention trial. N Engl J Med 2005;352(11):1092–1102.
77. Solomon SD, McMurray JJ, Pfeffer MA, et al. Cardiovascular risk associated with celecoxib in a clinical trial for colorectal adenoma prevention. N Engl J Med 2005;352(11):1071–1080.
78. Kearney PM, Baigent C, Godwin J, Halls H, Emberson JR, Patrono C. Do selective cyclooxygenase-2 inhibitors and traditional non-steroidal anti-inflammatory drugs increase the risk of atherothrombosis? Meta-analysis of randomised trials. BMJ 2006;332(7553):1302–1308.
79. Olsen AM, Fosbol EL, Lindhardsen J, et al. Long-term cardiovascular risk of nonsteroidal anti-inflammatory drug use according to time passed after first-time myocardial infarction: A nationwide cohort study. Circulation 2012;126(16):1955–1963.
80. Zhang J, Ding EL, Song Y. Adverse effects of cyclooxygenase 2 inhibitors on renal and arrhythmia events: Meta-analysis of randomized trials. JAMA 2006;296(13):1619–1632.
81. Soni P, Shell B, Cawkwell G, Li C, Ma H. The hepatic safety and tolerability of the cyclooxygenase-2 selective NSAID celecoxib: Pooled analysis of 41 randomized controlled trials. Curr Med Res Opin 2009;25(8):1841–1851.
82. Celebrex [package insert]. Pfizer, Inc., Mission, KS, 2012. *http://www.celebrex.com/about-celebrex.aspx?source=google&HBX_PK=s_celebrex&o=23040695|165564013|0&skwid=43700003360426290*
83. Derry S, Moore RA, Rabbie R. Topical NSAIDs for chronic musculoskeletal pain in adults. Cochrane Database Syst Rev 2012;9:CD007400.
84. Bellamy N, Campbell J, Robinson V, Gee T, Bourne R, Wells G. Intraarticular corticosteroid for treatment of osteoarthritis of the knee. Cochrane Database Syst Rev 2006;(2):CD005328.
85. Pyne D, Ioannou Y, Mootoo R, Bhanji A. Intra-articular steroids in knee osteoarthritis: A comparative study of triamcinolone hexacetonide and methylprednisolone acetate. Clin Rheumatol 2004;23(2):116–120.
86. Habib GS, Bashir M, Jabbour A. Increased blood glucose levels following intra-articular injection of methylprednisolone acetate in patients with controlled diabetes and symptomatic osteoarthritis of the knee. Ann Rheum Dis 2008;67(12):1790–1791.
87. *http://www.fda.gov/Drugs/DrugSafety/ucm318858.htm*—capsaicin warning.
88. Fraenkel L, Bogardus ST, Jr, Concato J, Wittink DR. Treatment options in knee osteoarthritis: The patient's perspective. Arch Intern Med 2004;164(12):1299–1304.
89. Cepeda MS, Camargo F, Zea C, Valencia L. Tramadol for osteoarthritis: A systematic review and metaanalysis. J Rheumatol 2007;34(3):543–555.
90. Pergolizzi J, Boger RH, Budd K, et al. Opioids and the management of chronic severe pain in the elderly: Consensus statement of an international expert panel with focus on the six clinically most often used world health organization step III opioids (buprenorphine, fentanyl, hydromorphone, methadone, morphine, oxycodone). Pain Pract 2008;8(4):287–313.
91. *http://www.cdc.gov/homeandrecreationalsafety/rxbrief/*
92. Chou R. 2009 Clinical Guidelines from the American Pain Society and the American Academy of pain medicine on the use of chronic opioid therapy in chronic noncancer pain: What are the key messages for clinical practice? Pol Arch Med Wewn 2009;119(7–8):469–477.

93. Bellamy N, Campbell J, Robinson V, Gee T, Bourne R, Wells G. Visco supplementation for the treatment of osteoarthritis of the knee. Cochrane Database Syst Rev 2006;(2):CD005321.
94. Samson DJ, Grant MD, Ratko TA, Bonnell CJ, Ziegler KM, Aronson N. Treatment of primary and secondary osteoarthritis of the knee. Evid Rep Technol Assess (Full Rep) 2007;(157):1–157.
95. Hunter DJ. Osteoarthritis: Hyaluronic acid is not effective in symptomatic hip OA. Nat Rev Rheumatol 2009;5(7):359–360.
96. Wandel S, Juni P, Tendal B, et al. Effects of glucosamine, chondroitin, or placebo in patients with osteoarthritis of hip or knee: Network meta-analysis. BMJ 2010;341:c4675.
97. Clegg DO, Reda DJ, Harris CL, et al. Glucosamine, chondroitin sulfate, and the two in combination for painful knee osteoarthritis. N Engl J Med 2006;354(8):795–808.
98. Berenbaum F. Targeted therapies in osteoarthritis: A systematic review of the trials on *www.clinicaltrials.gov*. Best Pract Res Clin Rheumatol 2010;24(1):107–119.
99. Brandt KD, Mazzuca SA, Katz BP, et al. Effects of doxycycline on progression of osteoarthritis: Results of a randomized, placebo-controlled, double-blind trial. Arthritis Rheum 2005;52(7):2015–2025.
100. Kulkarni SK, Singh VP. Licofelone: The answer to unmet needs in osteoarthritis therapy? Curr Rheumatol Rep 2008;10(1):43–48.
101. Lane NE, Schnitzer TJ, Birbara CA, et al. Tanezumab for the treatment of pain from osteoarthritis of the knee. N Engl J Med 2010;363(16):1521–1531.
102. Kwon YD, Pittler MH, Ernst E. Acupuncture for peripheral joint osteoarthritis: A systematic review and meta-analysis. Rheumatology (Oxford) 2006;45(11):1331–1337.
103. Scharf HP, Mansmann U, Streitberger K, et al. Acupuncture and knee osteoarthritis: A three-armed randomized trial. Ann Intern Med 2006;145(1):12–20.
104. White AG, Birnbaum HG, Janagap C, Buteau S, Schein J. Direct and indirect costs of pain therapy for osteoarthritis in an insured population in the united states. J Occup Environ Med 2008;50(9):998–1005.
105. Marra C, Cibere J, Grubisic M, et al. Pharmacist initiated intervention trial in osteoarthritis (PhIT-OA): A multidisciplinary intervention for knee osteoarthritis. Arthritis Care Res (Hoboken) 2012;64(12):1837–1845.
106. Latimer N, Lord J, Grant RL, et al. Cost effectiveness of COX 2 selective inhibitors and traditional NSAIDs alone or in combination with a proton pump inhibitor for people with osteoarthritis. BMJ 2009;339:b2538.
107. Hur C, Chan AT, Tramontano AC, Gazelle GS. Coxibs versus combination NSAID and PPI therapy for chronic pain: An exploration of the risks, benefits, and costs. Ann Pharmacother 2006;40(6):1052–1063.

72

Rheumatoid Arthritis

Kimberly Wahl and Arthur A. Schuna

KEY CONCEPTS

1. Rheumatoid arthritis (RA) is a systemic disease characterized by symmetrical inflammation of joints, yet may involve other organ systems.
2. Control of inflammation is the key to slowing or preventing disease progression as well as managing symptoms.
3. Drug therapy should be only part of a comprehensive program for patient management, which would also include physical therapy, exercise, and rest. Assistive devices and orthopedic surgery may be necessary in some patients.
4. Disease-modifying antirheumatic drugs (DMARDs) or biologic agents should be started early in the course of the disease and shortly after diagnosis of RA.
5. Nonsteroidal antiinflammatory drugs and/or corticosteroids should be considered adjunctive therapy early in the course of treatment and as needed if symptoms are not adequately controlled with DMARDs.
6. When DMARDs used singly are ineffective or not adequately effective, combination therapy with two or more DMARDs or a DMARD plus biologic agent may be used to induce a response.
7. Patients require careful monitoring for toxicity and therapeutic benefit for the duration of treatment.

Rheumatoid arthritis (RA) is the most common systemic inflammatory disease characterized by symmetrical joint involvement. Extraarticular involvement, including rheumatoid nodules, vasculitis, eye inflammation, neurologic dysfunction, cardiopulmonary disease, lymphadenopathy, and splenomegaly, can be manifestations of the disease. Although the usual disease course is chronic, some patients will enter a remission spontaneously.

EPIDEMIOLOGY

RA is estimated to have a prevalence of 1% and does not have any racial predilections. It can occur at any age, with increasing prevalence up to the seventh decade of life. The disease is three times more common in women. In people ages 15 to 45 years, women predominate by a ratio of 6:1; the sex ratio is approximately equal among patients in the first decade of life and in those older than age 60 years.

Epidemiologic data suggest that a genetic predisposition and exposure to unknown environmental factors may be necessary for expression of the disease. The major histocompatibility complex molecules, located on T lymphocytes, appear to have an important role in most patients with RA. These molecules can be characterized using human lymphocyte antigen (HLA) typing. A majority of patients with RA have HLA-DR4, HLA-DR1, or both antigens in the major histocompatibility complex region. Patients with HLA-DR4 antigen are 3.5 times more likely to develop RA than those patients who have other HLA-DR antigens.[1] Although the major histocompatibility complex region is important, it is not the sole determinant as patients can have the disease without these HLA types. RA is six times more common among dizygotic twins and nontwin children of parents with rheumatoid factor-positive, erosive RA when compared with children whose parents do not have the disease. If one of a pair of monozygotic twins is affected, the other twin has a 30 times greater risk of developing the disease.[2,3]

PATHOPHYSIOLOGY

1 Chronic inflammation of the synovial tissue lining the joint capsule results in the proliferation of this tissue. The inflamed, proliferating synovium characteristic of RA is called *pannus*. This pannus invades the cartilage and eventually the bone surface, producing erosions of bone and cartilage and leading to destruction of the joint. The factors that initiate the inflammatory process are unknown.

The immune system is a complex network of checks and balances designed to discriminate self from nonself (foreign) tissues. It helps rid the body of infectious agents, tumor cells, and products associated with the breakdown of cells. In RA, this system is no longer able to differentiate self from nonself tissues and attacks the synovial and other connective tissues.

In addition to the genetic factors mentioned above, environmental factors play a role. It is known that smoking and pulmonary disease may increase risk. Infectious agents (e.g., Epstein-Barr virus, *Escherichia coli*) and periodontal disease (*Porphyromonas gingivalis*) have been associated with RA.

The immune system has both humoral and cell-mediated functions (Fig. 72-1). The humoral component is necessary for the formation of antibodies. These antibodies are produced by plasma cells, which are derived from B lymphocytes. Most patients with RA form antibodies called *rheumatoid factors*. Rheumatoid factors have not been identified as pathogenic, nor does the quantity of these circulating antibodies always correlate with disease activity. Seropositive patients tend to have a more aggressive course of their illness than do seronegative patients. Anticitrullinated protein antibody (ACPA) is another antibody identified, which is produced in most patients with RA and has become an important diagnostic tool. Patients may develop ACPA long before they develop symptoms of RA, and those with positive antibodies have a poorer prognosis than those without.

The invasion of the synovium and joint by leukocytes results in synovitis. These leukocytes migrate to the region directed by chemokines and adhesion molecules. Early in the inflammatory process, increased vascularity aids in cell trafficking. The synovium proliferates and fibroblasts are activated, and this promotes bone and connective tissue destruction.

Immunoglobulins can activate the complement system. The complement system amplifies the immune response by encouraging chemotaxis, phagocytosis, and the release of lymphokines by

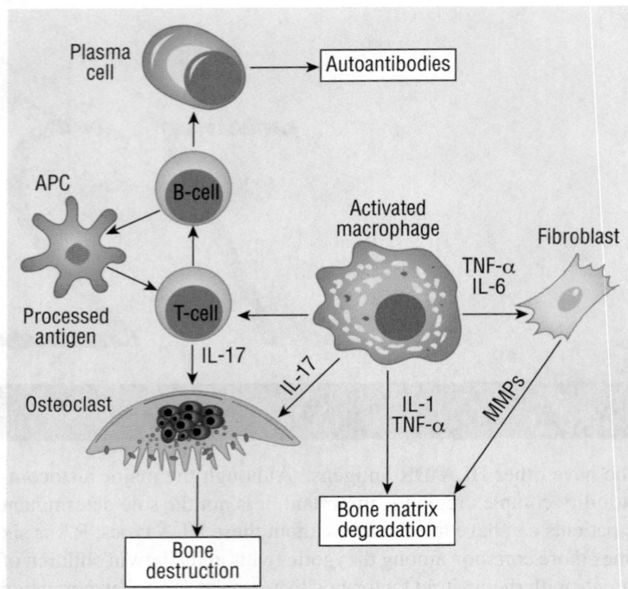

FIGURE 72-1 Pathogenesis of the inflammatory response. Antigen-presenting cells process and present antigens to T cells, which may stimulate B cells to produce antibodies and osteoclasts to destroy and remove bone. Macrophages stimulated by the immune response can stimulate T cells and osteoclasts to promote inflammation. They also can stimulate fibroblasts, which produce matrix metalloproteinases to degrade the bone matrix and produce proinflammatory cytokines. Activated T cells and macrophages release factors that promote tissue destruction, increase blood flow, and result in cellular invasion of synovial tissue and joint fluid. (APC, antigen-presenting cell; IL, interleukin; MMP, matrix metalloproteinase; TNF-α, tumor necrosis factor α.)

mononuclear cells, which are then presented to T lymphocytes. The processed antigen is recognized by major histocompatibility complex proteins on the lymphocyte, which activates it to stimulate the production of T and B cells. The proinflammatory cytokines tumor necrosis factor (TNF), interleukin (IL)-1 and IL-6 are key substances in the initiation and continuance of rheumatoid inflammation. IL-17 can induce proinflammatory cytokines in fibroblasts and synoviocytes and stimulate the release of matrix metalloproteinases and other cytotoxic substances, which leads to cartilage destruction. Activated T cells produce cytotoxins, which are directly toxic to tissues, and cytokines, which stimulate further activation of inflammatory processes and attract cells to areas of inflammation. Macrophages are stimulated to release prostaglandins and cytotoxins.[4–6] T-cell activation requires both stimulation by proinflammatory cytokines as well as interaction between cell surface receptors, called *costimulation*. One of these costimulation interactions is between CD28 and CD80/86. The binding of the CD80/86 receptor by the drug abatacept has proved to be an effective treatment for RA by preventing costimulation interactions between T cells.[7]

Although it has been suggested that T cells play a key role in the pathogenesis of RA, B cells clearly have an equally important role. Evidence for this importance may be found in the effectiveness of B-cell depletion using the drug rituximab in controlling rheumatoid inflammation. Activated B cells produce plasma cells, which form antibodies. These antibodies in combination with the complement system result in the accumulation of polymorphonuclear leukocytes, which release cytotoxins, oxygen-free radicals, and hydroxyl radicals that promote cellular damage to synovium and bone. The benefits of B-cell depletion occur even though antibody formation is not suppressed with rituximab therapy; this suggests that other mechanisms play a role in reducing RA activity. B cells produce cytokines that may alter the function of other immune cells, and they also have the ability to process antigens and act as antigen-presenting cells, which interact with T cells to activate the immune process.[8–11]

In the synovial membrane, $CD4^+$ T cells are abundant and communicate with macrophages, osteoclasts, fibroblasts, and chondrocytes either through direct cell–cell interactions using cell surface receptors or through proinflammatory cytokines such as TNF-α, IL-1, and IL-6. These cells produce metalloproteinases and other cytotoxic substances, which lead to the erosion of bone and cartilage. They also release substances promoting growth of blood vessels and adhesion molecules, which assists in proinflammatory cell trafficking and attachment of fibroblasts to cartilage and eventual synovial invasion and destruction.[12–15] TNF inhibitors are widely used to treat RA. Although anakinra inhibits IL-1 by attaching to receptors on cell surface, the benefits of this approach have not been as great as expected. Tocilizumab has proven effective as an inhibitor of IL-6 activity.

There are also a number of signaling molecules that are important for activating and maintaining inflammation. One of these is Janus kinase (JAK), which is a tyrosine kinase responsible for regulating leukocyte maturation and activation. JAK also has effects on the production of cytokines and immunoglobulins.

CLINICAL PRESENTATION Rheumatoid Arthritis

Symptoms

- Joint pain and stiffness of more than 6 weeks' duration. May also experience fatigue, weakness, low-grade fever, loss of appetite. Muscle pain and afternoon fatigue may also be present. Joint deformity is generally seen late in the disease.

Signs

- Tenderness with warmth and swelling over affected joints usually involving hands and feet. Distribution of joint involvement is frequently symmetrical. Rheumatoid nodules may also be present.

Laboratory Tests

- Rheumatoid factor (RF) detectable in 60% to 70%.
- Anticyclic citrullinated peptide (anti-CCP) antibodies have similar sensitivity to RF (50% to 85%) but are more specific (90% to 95%) and are present earlier in the disease.
- Elevated erythrocyte sedimentation rate and C-reactive protein are markers for inflammation.
- Normocytic normochromic anemia is common as is thrombocytosis.

Other Diagnostic Tests

- Joint fluid aspiration may show increased white blood cell counts without infection, crystals.
- Joint radiographs may show periarticular osteoporosis, joint space narrowing, or erosions.

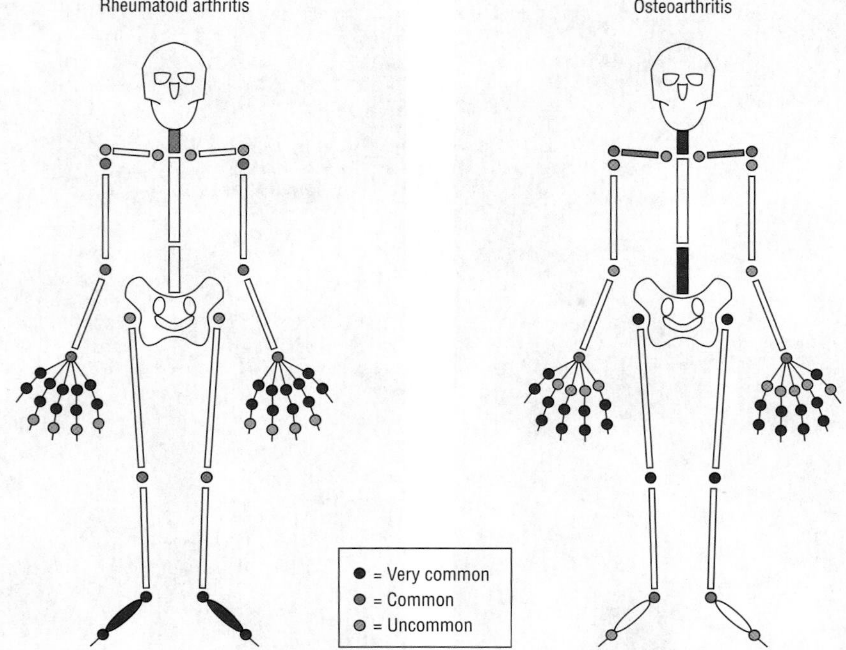

FIGURE 72-2 Patterns of joint involvement in rheumatoid arthritis and osteoarthritis.

Tofacitinib, an oral JAK inhibiting drug, has proven to be very effective in RA and appears to inhibit IL-6 activity as the major mechanism of action.

Vasoactive substances also play a role in the inflammatory process. Histamine, kinins, and prostaglandins are released at the site of inflammation. These substances increase both blood flow to the site of inflammation and the permeability of blood vessels. These substances cause the edema, warmth, erythema, and pain associated with joint inflammation and make it easier for granulocytes to pass from blood vessels to the site of inflammation.

The end results of the chronic inflammatory changes are variable. Loss of cartilage may result in a loss of the joint space. The formation of chronic granulation or scar tissue can lead to loss of joint motion or bony fusion (called *ankylosis*). Laxity of tendon structures can result in a loss of support to the affected joint, leading to instability or subluxation. Tendon contractures also may occur, leading to chronic deformity.[12,16]

The symptoms of RA usually develop insidiously over the course of several weeks to months. Prodromal symptoms include fatigue, weakness, low-grade fever, loss of appetite, and joint pain. Stiffness and muscle aches (myalgias) may precede the development of joint swelling (synovitis). Fatigue may be more of a problem in the afternoon. During disease flares, the onset of fatigue begins earlier in the day and subsides as disease activity lessens. Most commonly, joint involvement tends to be symmetrical; however, early in the disease some patients present with an asymmetrical pattern involving one or a few joints that eventually develops into the more classic presentation. Approximately 20% of patients develop an abrupt onset of their illness with fevers, polyarthritis, and constitutional symptoms (e.g., depression, anxiety, fatigue, anorexia, and weight loss).[2,3]

No single test or physical finding can be used to make the diagnosis of RA. In early disease, the diagnosis can be particularly challenging given that radiographic findings are usually absent and rheumatoid factor test can be undetectable. Duration of joint pain and swelling, morning stiffness lasting more than 1 hour, and involvement of three or more joints are important early predictors of the development of persistent erosive RA.[17]

JOINT INVOLVEMENT

The joints affected most frequently by RA are the small joints of the hands, wrists, and feet (Fig. 72-2). In addition, elbows, shoulders, hips, knees, and ankles may be involved. Patients usually experience joint stiffness that typically is worse in the morning. The duration of stiffness tends to be correlated directly with disease activity, usually exceeds 30 minutes, and may persist all day. Chronic inflammation with lack of an adequate exercise program results in loss of range of motion, atrophy of muscles, weakness, and deformity (Figs. 72-3 and 72-4).

On examination, the swelling of the joints may be visible or may be apparent only by palpation. The swelling feels soft and spongy because it is caused by proliferation of soft tissues or fluid accumulation within the joint capsule. The swollen joint may appear erythematous and feel warmer than nearby skin surfaces, especially early in the course of the disease. In contrast, the swelling associated

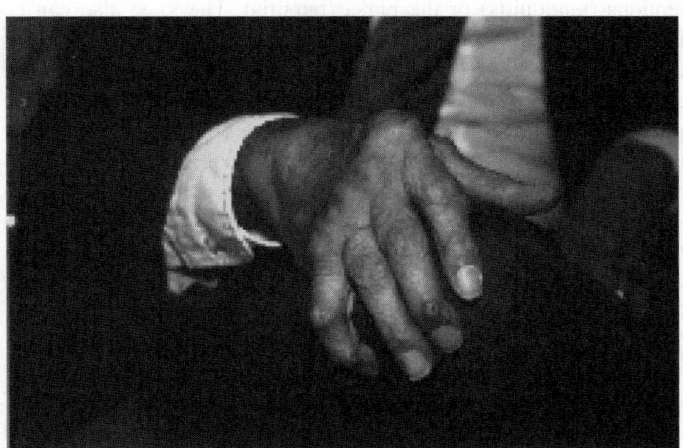

FIGURE 72-3 Deformities of rheumatoid arthritis, with marked ulnar deviation, swan-neck deformity, active synovitis, and nodules. *(Reproduced with permission from Brunicardi FC, Anderson DK, Billiar TR, et al. Schwartz's Principles of Surgery, 8th ed. New York: McGraw-Hill, 2005.)*

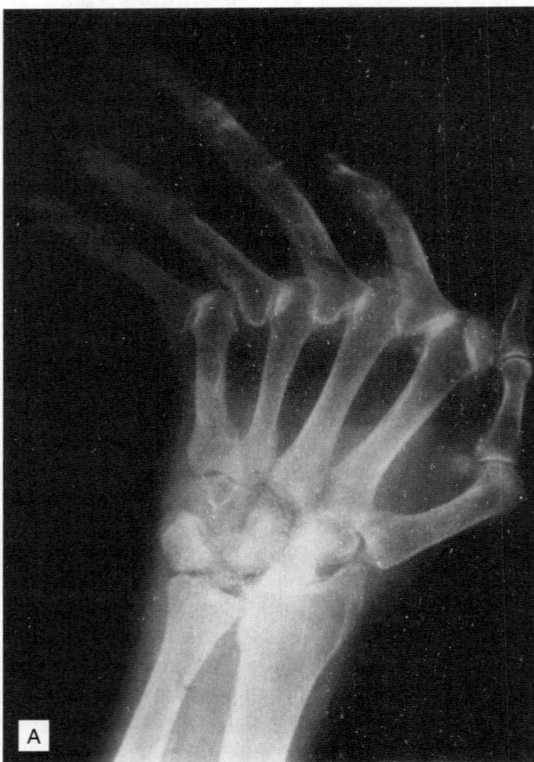

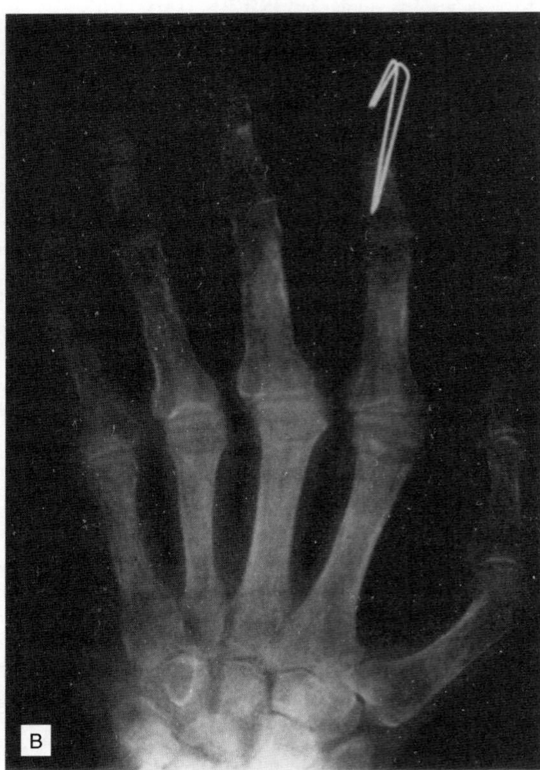

FIGURE 72-4 *A.* Preoperative view of metacarpophalangeal joints in rheumatoid arthritis. *B.* Following resection arthroplasty. *(Reproduced with permission from Skinner H., ed. Current Diagnosis & Treatment in Orthopedics, 4th ed. New York: McGraw-Hill, 2006:592.)*

with osteoarthritis usually is bony (caused by osteophytes) and infrequently is associated with signs of inflammation.

Involvement of the hands and wrists is common in RA. Hand involvement is manifested by pain, swelling, tenderness, and grip weakness during the acute phase and by subluxation, instability, deformity, and muscle atrophy in the chronic phase of the disease. Functional difficulties with clasp, grasp, and pinch alter both strength and fine motor movement.

Deformity of the hand may be seen with chronic inflammation. These changes may alter the mechanics of hand function, reducing grip strength and making it difficult to perform usual daily activity.

Pain in the elbow and shoulder may be the result of true joint inflammation or inflammation of soft-tissue structures such as tendons (tendonitis) or the bursa (bursitis). The knee also can be involved, with loss of cartilage, instability, and joint pain. Synovitis of the knee may cause the formation of a cyst behind the knee called a *popliteal* or *Baker's cyst*. These cysts may become painful as they get tense, or they may rupture, producing a clinical picture similar to thrombophlebitis secondary to the release of inflammatory components into the area of the calf muscle (pseudothrombophlebitis syndrome). Chronic joint pain leads to muscle atrophy, which can result in a laxity of the ligamentous structures that support the knee, causing instability. Maintenance of an adequate range of motion of the knee is essential to normal gait.

Foot and ankle involvement in RA is common. The metatarsophalangeal joints are involved frequently in RA, making walking difficult. Subluxation of the metatarsal heads leads to "cock-up" or hammer toe deformities. Subluxation also may cause a flexion deformity at the proximal interphalangeal joint of the toe, leading to pressure necrosis of the skin over the joint secondary to irritation caused by shoes. Hallux valgus (lateral deviation of the digit) and bunion or callus formation may occur at the great toe. A widening of the foot occurs commonly with long-standing disease.

Involvement of the spine usually occurs in the cervical vertebrae; lumbar vertebral involvement is rare. Involvement of the first and second cervical vertebrae (C1 to C2) can lead to instability of this joint. Patients with this problem are at a greater risk for spinal cord compression, although this complication is rare.

The temporomandibular joint (jaw) can be affected, resulting in malocclusion and difficulty in chewing food. Inflammation of cartilage in the chest can lead to chest wall pain. Hip pain may occur as a result of destructive changes in the hip joint, soft-tissue inflammation (e.g., bursitis), or referred pain from nerve entrapment at the lumbar vertebrae.

EXTRAARTICULAR INVOLVEMENT

Although joint involvement in RA is a hallmark finding in RA, it is important to recognize that, as a systemic disease, other organ systems are often involved.

Rheumatoid Nodules

Rheumatoid nodules occur in 20% of patients with RA. These nodules are seen most commonly on the extensor surfaces of the elbows, forearms, and hands but also may be seen on the feet and at other pressure points. They also may develop in the lung or pleural lining of the lung and, rarely, in the meninges. Rheumatoid nodules usually are asymptomatic and do not require any special intervention. Nodules are observed more commonly in patients with erosive disease.[18]

Vasculitis

Vasculitis usually is seen in patients with long-standing RA. Vasculitis may result in a wide variety of clinical presentations. Invasion of blood vessel walls by inflammatory cells results in an obliteration of the vessel, producing infarction of tissue distal to the area of involvement. Most commonly, small-vessel vasculitis produces infarcts near the ends of the fingers or toes, especially around the nail beds. These infarcts are usually of little consequence.

Vasculitis also may cause the breakdown of skin, especially in the lower extremities, producing ulcers that may be indistinguishable in appearance from stasis ulcers. However, these ulcers do not heal with the usual modes of treatment used for stasis ulcers. Involvement of larger vessels with vasculitis can result in life-threatening complications. Infarction of vessels supplying blood to nerves can cause irreversible motor deficits. Involvement of vessels supplying other organ systems can lead to visceral involvement and a polyarteritis nodosa-like illness. Aggressive treatment of the inflammatory process is necessary in these patients. Fortunately, vasculitis has become much less frequently seen since the advent of methotrexate and biologic therapy.

Pulmonary Complications

RA may involve the pleura of the lung, which is often asymptomatic, although pleural effusions may result. Pulmonary fibrosis also may develop as a result of rheumatoid involvement; smoking appears to increase the risk of this complication. Rheumatoid nodules may develop in lung tissue and appear similar to neoplasms on chest radiographs. Interstitial pneumonitis and arteritis are rare, potentially life-threatening complications of RA.

Ocular Manifestations

Ocular manifestations include keratoconjunctivitis sicca and inflammation of the sclera, episclera, and cornea. Atrophy of the lacrimal duct may result in a decrease in tear formation, causing dry and itchy eyes, termed *keratoconjunctivitis sicca*. When this is observed in association with RA, it is referred to as *Sjögren's syndrome*. Artificial tears may be used to relieve symptoms. The salivary glands may also be involved in Sjögren's syndrome, resulting in dry mouth (xerostomia). Inflammation of the superficial layers of the sclera (episcleritis) is generally self-limiting. Involvement of deeper tissues (scleritis) usually results in a more serious, painful, and chronic inflammation. Rheumatoid nodules may develop on the sclera.

Cardiac Involvement

The heart is sometimes affected by RA. RA is associated with an increased risk of cardiovascular mortality. This risk appears to be higher in those with more active inflammation and is reduced with treatment, particularly with methotrexate.[19,20] Pericarditis may occur, resulting in the accumulation of fluid. Although many patients show evidence of previous pericarditis at autopsy, the development of clinically evident pericarditis with tamponade is a rare complication. Cardiac conduction abnormalities and aortic valve incompetence, caused by aortic root dilation, may occur. Myocarditis is a rare complication of RA.

Felty's Syndrome

RA in association with splenomegaly and neutropenia is known as *Felty's syndrome*. Thrombocytopenia also may be a manifestation of the syndrome. Patients with Felty's syndrome and severe leukopenia are more susceptible to infection. The decrease in granulocytes appears to be mediated by the immune system because splenectomy does not result in improvement of the patient.[18]

Other Complications

Lymphadenopathy may occur in patients with RA, particularly in nodes proximal to more actively involved joints. Renal involvement is rare but can be associated with treatment, including nonsteroidal antiinflammatory drugs (NSAIDs), gold salts, and penicillamine. Amyloidosis is a rare complication of longstanding RA. It appears to be more common in Europe than in the United States.

LABORATORY FINDINGS

Hematologic tests often reveal a mild-to-moderate anemia with normocytic, normochromic indices. The hematocrit may fall as low as 30%. The anemia is usually inversely related to inflammatory disease activity and is referred to as an *anemia of chronic disease*. This type of anemia does not respond to iron therapy and can present a diagnostic dilemma because NSAIDs may induce gastritis and chronic blood loss, leading to iron-deficiency anemia. Laboratory tests useful in differentiating these anemias include stool guaiac (or other stool tests for occult blood), serum iron-to-iron-binding capacity ratio (decreased in iron deficiency), ferritin (decreased in iron deficiency), and mean corpuscular volume (more likely to be decreased in iron deficiency). Other causes of anemia also must be considered in the differential diagnosis (see Chaps. 80 and 82).

Thrombocytosis is another common hematologic finding with active RA. Platelet counts rise and fall in direct correlation with disease activity in many patients. Thrombocytopenia may result from toxicity of immunosuppressive therapy. Thrombocytopenia also may be observed in Felty's syndrome or vasculitis.

Although leukopenia is associated with Felty's syndrome, it also may result from toxicity of methotrexate, gold, sulfasalazine, penicillamine, and immunosuppressive drugs. Leukocytosis is seen commonly as a result of corticosteroid treatment.

The erythrocyte sedimentation rate (ESR) is usually elevated in patients with RA and other inflammatory diseases. This test is very nonspecific, and although the ESR usually falls as patients respond to therapy, there is a large variability among patients in response to treatment. C-reactive protein (CRP) is another nonspecific marker for inflammatory arthritis when it is elevated. This protein is produced by the liver in response to certain cytokines.

Rheumatoid factor (RF) is present in 60% to 70% of patients with RA. The usual laboratory test for RF is an antibody specific for immunoglobulin (Ig)M RF. Patients with RA and a negative test for RF may have IgG or IgA RFs, but tests for these are not routinely available. RF tests may be reported positive at a specific serum dilution. Serum is diluted to a standard series of dilutions; the greatest dilution that yields a positive test result will be reported (e.g., RF positive at 1:640). Some laboratories quantify RF rather than using titers. Higher dilutional titers or serum concentrations of RFs usually indicate a more severe disease, but like the ESR, the large interpatient variability makes this test unreliable as a means of assessing patient progress. RF may be positive in patients without RA (Table 72-1).

ACPA has similar sensitivity for RA, being found in 50% to 85% of patients with the disease, but is more specific (90% to 95%) and is detectable very early in the disease. Many rheumatologists will do both tests in evaluating new patients.

Antinuclear antibodies (ANAs) are detected in 25% of patients with RA. These antibodies usually have a diffuse pattern of immunofluorescence. Tests for antibodies to double-stranded DNA (usually positive in systemic lupus erythematosus) are negative. Serum complement is usually normal, although complement concentrations of joint fluid often are depressed from consumption secondary to the inflammatory process. In patients with vasculitis, serum complement concentrations may be low.[21,22]

Synovial fluid usually is turbid because of the large number of leukocytes in inflammatory fluid. White cell counts of 5,000 to 50,000/mm^3 (5×10^9 to 50×10^9/L) are not uncommon in inflamed joints. The fluid is usually less viscous than that in normal joints or fluid associated with osteoarthritis. Glucose concentrations of

TABLE 72-1 Diseases Associated with a Positive Rheumatoid Factor

Rheumatic diseases
Rheumatoid arthritis
Sjögren's syndrome (with or without arthritis)
Systemic lupus erythematosus
Progressive systemic sclerosis
Polymyositis/dermatomyositis
Infectious diseases
Bacterial endocarditis
Tuberculosis
Syphilis
Infectious mononucleosis
Infectious hepatitis
Leprosy
Other causes
Aging
Interstitial pulmonary fibrosis
Cirrhosis of the liver
Chronic active hepatitis
Sarcoidosis

joint fluid are normal or low compared with those in serum drawn at the same time as synovial aspirates. The decrease is not as profound as the decrease associated with joint infection or systemic lupus erythematosus.

Early radiographic manifestations of RA include soft-tissue swelling and osteoporosis near the joint (periarticular osteoporosis). Joint space narrowing occurs as a result of cartilage degradation. Erosions tend to occur later in the course of the disease and usually are seen first in the metacarpophalangeal and proximal interphalangeal joints of the hands and the metatarsophalangeal joints of the feet. Periodic joint radiographs are a useful way of evaluating disease progression.

Diagnostic Criteria

The American College of Rheumatology and European League Against Rheumatism (ACR/EULAR) revised criteria for the diagnosis of RA.[23] These criteria were developed to be used for patients early in their disease; they, therefore, emphasize early manifestations of the disease. Late manifestations of RA such as erosive disease or nodules are no longer in the diagnostic criteria, but these patients would have previously met these criteria based on retrospective data.

Patients with synovitis of at least one joint and no other explanation for the finding are candidates for these criteria. The criteria use a scoring system with a score of >6 out of a possible total score of 10 as being diagnostic for RA. More points are given for patients presenting with more actively involved joints. Positive laboratory tests including RF, ACPA, CRP, and ESR result in additional points.

Duration of symptoms ≥6 weeks results in an additional point. It is important to note that not all patients with RA may have a score >6 initially, particularly if seen very early in their disease but may evolve to higher scores over time. Reassessment should be considered for those with ongoing symptoms.

Seronegative Inflammatory Arthritis

Although RA may have a negative RF titer, a number of other systemic inflammatory arthritic conditions exist including psoriatic arthritis, reactive arthritis, ankylosing spondylitis, and arthritis associated with inflammatory bowel disease. These conditions often tend to be less aggressive than what is typically seen with RA. Detailed discussion about these conditions is beyond the scope of this chapter, but further information may be found elsewhere.[2] Management principles are similar to those for RA.

TREATMENT
Rheumatoid Arthritis

Desired Outcome

❷ The primary objective in the treatment of RA is to improve or maintain functional status, thereby improving quality of life. The ultimate goal is to achieve complete disease remission or low disease activity, although this goal may not be possible to achieve in some patients. Additional goals of treatment include controlling disease activity and joint pain, maintaining the ability to function in daily activities or work, slowing destructive joint changes, and delaying disability.

General Approach to Treatment

The multifaceted treatment approach includes pharmacologic and nonpharmacologic therapies with recent emphasis being placed on aggressive treatment early in the disease course. Early aggressive treatment may prevent irreversible joint damage and disability. As many pharmacologic agents are available for the treatment of RA, the recommended drug therapy is based on disease duration, activity, and prognosis.[24,25] In general, patients with less active disease and good prognostic indicators may be treated with oral agents as monotherapy. Those with high disease activity and/or poor prognostic features are candidates for combination therapy and biologics to suppress inflammation. Controlling inflammation with therapeutic interventions improves symptoms, slows the disease course, and prevents disease progression.

Nonpharmacologic Therapy

❸ Rest, occupational therapy, physical therapy, use of assistive devices, weight reduction, and surgery are the most useful types of nonpharmacologic therapy used in patients with RA. Rest is an essential component of a nonpharmacologic treatment plan. It relieves stress on inflamed joints and prevents further joint destruction. Rest also aids in alleviation of pain. Too much rest and immobility, however, may lead to decreased range of motion and, ultimately, muscle atrophy, and contractures.

Occupational and physical therapy can provide the patient with skills and exercises necessary to increase or maintain mobility. These disciplines may also supply patients with supportive and adaptive devices such as canes, walkers, and splints.

Other nonpharmacologic therapeutic options include weight loss and surgery. Weight reduction helps to alleviate stress on inflamed joints. This should be instituted and monitored with close supervision of a healthcare professional. Tenosynovectomy, tendon repair, and joint replacements are surgical options for patients with RA. Such management is reserved for patients with severe disease.[26–27]

Pharmacologic Therapy

❹ ❺ Pharmacologic agents that reduce RA symptoms and impede radiographic joint damage can be categorized as either nonbiologic disease-modifying antirheumatic drugs (DMARDs) or biologic DMARDs, which include TNF-α inhibitor biologics or non-TNF biologics. DMARDs are a treatment cornerstone and should be started as soon as possible after disease onset as early introduction results in more favorable outcomes[28–30] and reduces mortality rates comparable to patients without the disease.[19,31] NSAIDs and/or corticosteroids may be used for symptomatic relief if needed. They provide relatively rapid improvement in symptoms compared with DMARDs, which may take weeks to months before benefit is seen; however,

NSAIDs have no impact on disease progression and the long-term complication risks of corticosteroids make them less desirable.[28]

DMARDs and biologic agents slow RA disease progression. DMARDs commonly used include methotrexate, hydroxychloroquine, sulfasalazine, and leflunomide. The biologic agents with disease-modifying activity include the anti-TNF drugs (etanercept, infliximab, adalimumab, certolizumab, golimumab, tofacitinib), the costimulation modulator abatacept, the IL-6 receptor antagonist tocilizumab, and rituximab, which depletes peripheral B cells. Agents less frequently used because of reduced efficacy, greater toxicity, or both include the IL-1 receptor antagonist anakinra, azathioprine, D-penicillamine, gold (including auranofin), minocycline, cyclosporine, and cyclophosphamide.

DMARDs, either as monotherapy or in combination, are first-line agents for most patients with RA. The order in which these agents are used is not clearly defined, although methotrexate is often chosen because long-term data suggest superior outcomes with methotrexate than with other DMARDs. There is also good documentation for better outcomes with methotrexate in combination therapy if methotrexate monotherapy does not achieve an adequate response. Leflunomide appears to have similar long-term efficacy as that of methotrexate.[32]

6 Combination therapy with two or more DMARDs may be effective when single-DMARD treatment is unsuccessful.[29,33–35] One study suggests that initial combination therapy with either methotrexate, sulfasalazine plus prednisone, or infliximab plus methotrexate was superior to more conventional sequential monotherapy or step-up combinations of DMARDs in early RA.[33] For patients with moderate-to-high disease activity, ACR recommends dual DMARD combinations of methotrexate plus hydroxychloroquine, methotrexate plus leflunomide, or methotrexate plus sulfasalazine. They also recommend the triple combination of sulfasalazine, hydroxychloroquine, and methotrexate.[24]

The anti-TNF and non-TNF biologic agents have proven effective for patients who fail treatment with other DMARDs and were previously reserved for this population subset, partly due to cost. However, ACR now endorses the use of anti-TNF biologics in patients with early disease of high activity and presence of poor prognostic factors, regardless of previous DMARD use.[24] Features of poor prognosis include functional limitation, extraarticular disease (e.g., rheumatoid nodules, vasculitis), positive RF or ACPA, or bone erosions. Anti-TNF biologics can be used as either monotherapy or in combination with other DMARDs.[25] Use of biologics in combination with methotrexate is more effective than biologic monotherapy and the combination is frequently used. Infliximab, specifically, should be given in combination with methotrexate to prevent development of antibodies that may reduce drug efficacy or induce allergic reactions.[24]

ACR published recommendations for use of nonbiologic and biologic DMARDs in 2008 and updated them in 2012. These recommendations are not intended to be prescriptive but provide guidance for treatment choice. Recommendations are given based on disease duration, degree of disease activity, and likely prognosis. The recommendations take into account barriers to treatment, including cost and insurance restrictions, by suggesting treatment options with and without expensive biologic agents. Simplified algorithms summarizing these treatment recommendations are provided in Figures 72-5 and 72-6. For more details, see the published recommendations.[24,25]

Corticosteroids can be used in various ways in the treatment of RA but should not be used as monotherapy. Corticosteroids are valuable in controlling symptoms before DMARDs take effect and are used in acute RA flares as burst therapy. Additionally, continuous low doses of corticosteroids may be used as adjunct therapy when DMARDs do not provide adequate disease control. Corticosteroids may be injected into joints and soft tissues to control local inflammation. There are data to suggest they have disease-modifying activity;[33,34,36] however, it is preferable to avoid chronic use when possible to avoid long-term complications. NSAIDs and DMARDs have steroid-sparing properties that permit corticosteroid dose reductions.

As immunosuppression may reduce the ability to mount an antibody response, the need for immunizations should be assessed, and these should be administered if needed before nonbiologic or biologic DMARDs are started.[25] Postvaccination antibody titers seem to be only minimally affected by conventional DMARDs and TNF antagonists. Rituximab and abatacept seem to reduce the

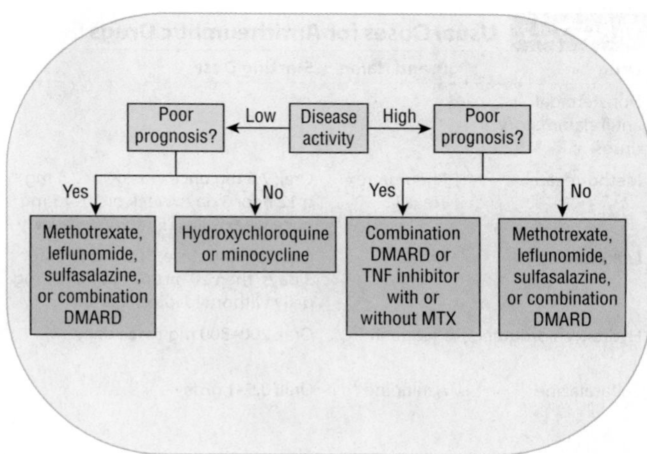

FIGURE 72-5 Algorithm for treatment of rheumatoid arthritis (RA) in early RA (<6 months). Poor prognosis is defined as limitation in function, extraarticular findings (rheumatoid nodules, vasculitis, Felty's syndrome, Sjögren's syndrome, rheumatoid lung findings, erosions on radiograph), bone erosions, and positive rheumatoid factor or anticitrullinated protein antibody. (DMARD, disease-modifying antirheumatic drug; MTX, methotrexate; NSAID, nonsteroidal antiinflammatory drug.)

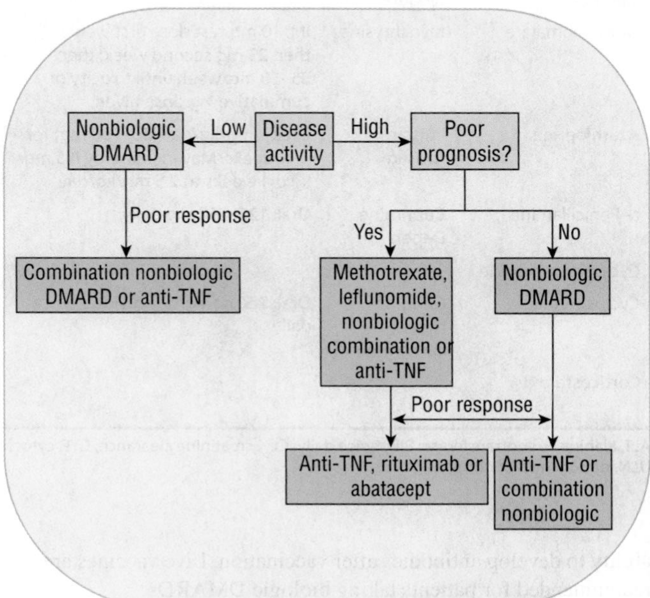

FIGURE 72-6 Algorithm for treatment of rheumatoid arthritis (RA) in established RA (>6 months). Poor response is defined as a deterioration of disease activity or the patient continues with moderate to high disease activity after 3 months of therapy.

TABLE 72-2 Usual Doses for Antirheumatic Drugs

Drug	Brand Name	Starting Dose	Usual Range or Maintenance Dose	Comments
Nonsteroidal antiinflammatory drugs			See Table 71-2 in Chapter 71	
Methotrexate	Rheumatrex Trexall	Oral: 7.5 mg once weekly or 2.5 mg q 12 h for 3 days/week or 10–15 mg once weekly IM: 15 mg once weekly	Oral or IM: 7.5–15 mg q wk	May be given with folic acid 1–5 mg/week to reduce adverse reactions
Leflunomide	Arava	Oral: loading dose: 100 mg daily for 3 days, then 20 mg/day or 10–20 mg daily without loading dose	Oral: 10–20 mg daily	Not recommended in liver disease (ALT > 2 times ULN)
Hydroxychloroquine	Plaquenil	Oral: 200–300 mg twice daily	Oral: After 1–2 mo may decrease to 200 mg daily or 200 mg BID	Take with food or milk; use with caution in renal or hepatic impairment
Sulfasalazine	Azulfidine	Oral: 0.5–1 g/day	Oral: Increase weekly to 1 g bid (max. dose is 3 g/day if inadequate response after 12 weeks of 2 g/day)	Not recommended in renal of hepatic impairment
Minocycline	Dynacin Minocin		Oral 100–200 mg daily	Use with caution in renal impairment
Etanercept	Enbrel		50 mg SubQ once weekly or 25 mg twice weekly	
Infliximab	Remicade	3 mg/kg IV at 0, 2, 6 weeks then 3 q 8 weeks	3–10 mg/kg IV q 4–8 weeks	Given in combination with methotrexate therapy
Adalimumab	Humira		40 mg SubQ q 2 weeks (may increase to 40 mg once weekly if not taking methotrexate)	
Certolizumab	Cimzia	400 mg SubQ at 0, 2, 4 weeks	200 mg SubQ every other week	
Golimumab	Simponi		50 mg SubQ once monthly	
Rituximab	Rituxan	1,000 mg IV twice, 2 weeks apart	Initial dose may be repeated every 16–24 weeks based on response	
Abatacept	Orencia	IV: <60 kg: 500 mg 60–100 kg: 750 mg >100 kg: 1000 mg at 0, 2, and 4 weeks or initial IV dose followed by 125 mg SubQ within 24 hours	IV: dose based on weight q 4 weeks SubQ: 125 mg once weekly	
Tocilizumab	Actemra	4 mg/kg IV q 4 weeks	4–8 mg/kg q 4 weeks (max 800 mg/infusion)	
Anakinra	Kineret		100 mg SubQ once daily	
Tofacitinib	Xeljanz		5 mg BID	5 mg once daily in moderate-to-severe renal insufficiency, moderate hepatic impairment, or concomitant CYP3A4 or CYP2C19 inhibitors
Auranofin	Ridaura		Oral: 3 mg daily to bid	
Gold thiomalate	Myochrysine	IM: 10 mg test dose first week, then 25 mg second week; then 25–50 mg/week until toxicity or cumulative 1 g dose given	IM: 25–50 mg every other week for 2–20 weeks then every 3–4 weeks	CL_{cr} 50–80 mL/min (0.83–1.34 mL/s): give 50% recommended dose; CL_{cr} <50 mL/min (<0.83 mL/s) avoid use
Azathioprine	Imuran Azasan	Oral: 1 mg/kg/day (50–100 mg) for 6–8 weeks. May increase by 0.5 mg/kg q 4 weeks to 2.5 mg/kg/day	Oral: 50–150 mg daily	
D-Penicillamine	Cuprimine Depen	Oral: 125–250 mg daily,	Oral: may ↑ by 125–250 mg q 1–2 months, max. 750 mg daily	Caution with renal impairment
Cyclophosphamide			Oral: 1–2 mg/kg/day	
Cyclosporine	Gengraf Neoral Sandimmune	Oral: 2.5 mg/kg/day divided twice daily	Oral: may ↑ by 0.5–0.75 mg/kg/day at 8 and 12 weeks to max dose 4 mg/kg/day	
Corticosteroids			Oral, IV, IM, IA, and soft-tissue injections: variable	

ALT, alanine aminotransferase; BID, twice daily; CL_{cr}, creatinine clearance; CYP, cytochrome P450; IA, intraarticular; IM, intramuscular; q, every; SubQ, subcutaneous; ULN, upper limits of normal.

ability to develop antibodies after vaccination. Live vaccines are not recommended for patients taking biologic DMARDs.[37]

Some biologic agents are contraindicated in the setting of hepatitis or malignancies because of immunosuppression. Etanercept, an anti-TNF biologic, is the only agent recommended for possible treatment of RA in patients with hepatitis C. No biologic agent should be used in patients with untreated hepatitis B or treated hepatitis B with liver dysfunction (Child-Pugh class B or higher). Rituximab is preferred in patients with previously treated solid malignancies, skin cancers, or lymphoproliferative malignancies. For patients with solid or nonmelanoma skin cancers treated more than 5 years ago, any biologic agent can be initiated or restarted.[24]

❼ Tables 72-2, 72-3, and 72-4 provide monitoring parameters and dosing guidelines for DMARDs and NSAIDs used in RA.

TABLE 72-3 Clinical Monitoring of Drug Therapy in Rheumatoid Arthritis

Drug	Adverse Drug Reaction	Initial Monitoring	Maintenance Monitoring	Symptoms to Inquire About[a]
NSAIDs and salicylates	GI ulceration and bleeding, renal damage	S_{cr} or BUN, CBC q 2–4 wk p starting therapy × 1–2 mo salicylates: serum salicylate levels if therapeutic dose and no response	Same as initial plus stool guaiac q 6–12 mo	Blood in stool, black stool, dyspepsia, nausea/vomiting, weakness, dizziness, abdominal pain, edema, weight gain, SOB
Corticosteroids	Hypertension, hyperglycemia, osteoporosis[b]	Glucose, blood pressure q 3–6 months	Same as initial	Blood pressure if available, polyuria, polydipsia, edema, SOB, visual changes, weight gain, headaches, broken bones or bone pain
Gold (intramuscular or oral)	Myelosuppression, proteinuria, rash, stomatitis	Baseline & until stable: UA, CBC w/plt preinjection	Same as initial—every other dose	Symptoms of myelosuppression, edema, rash, oral ulcers, diarrhea
Hydroxychloroquine	Macular damage, rash, diarrhea	Baseline: color fundus photography and automated central perimetric analysis	Ophthalmoscopy q 9–12 mo and Amsler grid at home q 2 wk	Visual changes including a decrease in night or peripheral vision, rash, diarrhea
Methotrexate	Myelosuppression, hepatic fibrosis, cirrhosis, pulmonary infiltrates or fibrosis, stomatitis, rash	Baseline: AST, ALT, alk phos, alb, t. bili, hep B & C studies, CBC w/plt, S_{cr}	CBC w/plt, AST, alb q 1–2 mo	Symptoms of myelosuppression, SOB, nausea/vomiting, lymph node swelling, coughing, mouth sores, diarrhea, jaundice
Leflunomide	Hepatitis, GI distress, alopecia	Baseline: ALT, CBC with platelets	CBC with platelets and ALT monthly initially and then every 6–8 wk	Nausea/vomiting, gastritis, diarrhea, hair loss, jaundice
Penicillamine	Myelosuppression, proteinuria, stomatitis, rash, dysgeusia	Baseline: UA, CBC w/plt, then q week × 1 month	Same as initial—q 1–2 mo, but q 2 wk if dose change	Symptoms of myelosuppression, edema, rash, diarrhea, altered taste perception, oral ulcers
Cyclophosphamide	Alopecia, infertility, GI distress, hemorrhagic cystitis, myelosuppression, nephrotoxicity, cardiotoxicity	UA, CBC w/plt q week × 1 month	Same as initial—q 2–4 wk	Nausea/vomiting, gastritis, diarrhea, hair loss, urination difficulties, chest pain, rash, respiratory difficulties
Cyclosporine	Hepatotoxicity, nephrotoxicity, hypertension, headache, malignancy, infections, GI distress	S_{cr}, blood pressure q month	Same as initial	Nausea/vomiting, diarrhea, symptoms of infection, symptoms of elevated blood pressure
Sulfasalazine	Myelosuppression, rash	Baseline: CBC w/plt, then q week × 1 month	Same as initial—q 1–2 mo	Symptoms of myelosuppression, photosensitivity, rash, nausea/vomiting
Tocilizumab	Local injection-site reactions, infection	AST/ALT, CBC w/plt, lipids	AST/ALT, CBC w/plt, lipids q 4–8 weeks	Symptoms of infection
Anakinra	Local injection-site reactions, infection	Neutrophil count	Neutrophil count monthly for 3 months then quarterly up to 1 year	Symptoms of infection
Etanercept, adalimumab, golimumab, certolizumab	Local injection-site reactions, infection	Tuberculin skin test hepatitis B and C screening	None	Symptoms of infection
Infliximab, rituximab, abatacept	Immune reactions, infection	Tuberculin skin test hepatitis B and C screening	None	Postinfusion reactions, symptoms of infection
Tofacitinib	Infection, malignancy, GI perforations, upper respiratory tract infections, headache, diarrhea, nasopharyngitis	Tuberculin skin test, hepatitis B and C screening, neutrophil count, lymphocytes, Hgb, AST/ALT	Neutrophils, Hgb, FLP at 4–8 weeks after treatment start, then lymphocytes, neutrophils, and Hgb q 3 months	Symptoms of infection or myelosuppression, SOB, blood in stool, black stool, dyspepsia

Alb, albumin; alk phos, alkaline phosphatase; ALT, alanine aminotransferase; AST, aspartate aminotransferase; BUN, blood urea nitrogen; CBC, complete blood count; FLP, fasting lipid panel; hep, hepatitis; Hgb, hemoglobin; IA, intraarticular; IM, intramuscular; p, after; plt, platelet; q, every; S_{cr}, serum creatinine; t. bili, total bilirubin; UA, urinalysis; GI, gastrointestinal; NSAIDs, nonsteroidal antiinflammatory drugs; SOB, shortness of breath.

[a]Altered immune function increases infection; this should be considered particularly in those patients taking azathioprine, methotrexate, and corticosteroids or other drugs as a symptom of myelosuppression.

[b]Osteoporosis is unlikely to manifest itself early in treatment, but all patients should be taking appropriate steps to prevent bone loss.

Nonsteroidal Antiinflammatory Drugs

NSAIDs should seldom be used as monotherapy for RA because they do not alter the course of the disease; instead, they should be viewed as adjuncts to DMARD treatment. NSAIDs possess both analgesic and antiinflammatory properties and reduce stiffness associated with RA. These agents mainly inhibit prostaglandin synthesis, which is only a small portion of the inflammatory cascade. For details on these agents see Chapter 71, Osteoarthritis.

Methotrexate

Methotrexate is now considered the nonbiologic DMARD of choice by many rheumatologists for treating RA. It inhibits cytokine production, inhibits purine biosynthesis, and may stimulate release of

TABLE 72-4 Dosage Regimens for Nonsteroidal Antiinflammatory Drugs

	Recommended Antiinflammatory Total Daily Dosage		
Drug	**Adult**	**Children**	**Dosing Schedule**
Aspirin	2.6–5.2 g	60–100 mg/kg	Four times daily
Celecoxib	200–400 mg	—	Daily to twice daily
Diclofenac	150–200 mg		Three times per day to four times daily Extended release twice daily
Diflunisal	0.5–1.5 g	—	Twice daily
Etodolac	0.2–1.2 g (max. 20 mg/kg)	—	Twice daily to four times daily
Fenoprofen	0.9–3.0 g	—	Four times daily
Flurbiprofen	200–300 mg	—	Twice daily to four times daily
Ibuprofen	1.2–3.2 g	20–40 mg/kg	Three times per day to four times daily
Indomethacin	50–200 mg	2–4 mg/kg (max. 200 mg)	Twice daily to four times daily Extended release daily
Meclofenamate	200–400 mg	—	Three times per day to four times per day
Meloxicam	7.5–15 mg	—	Daily
Nabumetone	1–2 g	—	Daily to twice daily
Naproxen	0.5–1.0 g	10 mg/kg	Twice daily Extended release–daily
Naproxen sodium	0.55–1.1 g	—	Twice daily
Nonacetylated salicylates	1.2–4.8 g	—	Twice daily to six times per day
Oxaprozin	0.6–1.8 g (max. 26 mg/kg)	—	Daily to three times a day
Piroxicam	10–20 mg	—	Daily
Sulindac	300–400 mg	—	Twice daily
Tolmetin	0.6–1.8 g	15–30 mg/kg	Twice daily to four times daily

adenosine, all of which may lead to its antiinflammatory properties. The drug has a fairly rapid onset of action; results may be seen as early as 2 to 3 weeks after starting therapy. Some 45% to 67% of patients remain on methotrexate therapy in studies ranging from 5 to 7 years.[38]

Absorption of methotrexate is variable and averages approximately 70% of an oral dose. Methotrexate is 35% to 50% bound to albumin; it may be displaced by highly protein-bound drugs such as NSAIDs, but the clinical importance of this interaction in the relatively low doses of methotrexate used in RA is unknown. Methotrexate is extensively metabolized intracellularly to polyglutamated derivatives. It is excreted by the kidney, 80% unchanged, by glomerular filtration and active transport. Some methotrexate may be reabsorbed, but this transport process may be saturated even with low doses, resulting in increased renal clearance.

Methotrexate is contraindicated in pregnant and nursing women as it is teratogenic. Patients should use contraception to avoid pregnancy and discontinue the drug if conception is planned. It is also contraindicated in patients with chronic liver disease, immunodeficiency, pleural or peritoneal effusions, leukopenia, thrombocytopenia, preexisting blood disorders, and a creatinine clearance of less than 40 mL/min (0.67 mL/s).

The toxicities of methotrexate therapy are mainly gastrointestinal, hematologic, pulmonary, and hepatic. Stomatitis occurs in 3% to 10% of patients and may be painful or painless. Diarrhea, nausea, and vomiting may occur in up to 10% of patients. The most common hematologic toxicity is thrombocytopenia in 1% to 3% of patients. Leukopenia also may occur, but in a smaller number of patients. Although pulmonary fibrosis and pneumonitis can be severe adverse effects, they are rare.

Elevated liver enzymes may occur in up to 15% of patients; cirrhosis is rare. Liver function tests, aspartate aminotransferase or alanine aminotransferase, should be performed periodically. Methotrexate should be discontinued if these test values show sustained results greater than twice the upper limits of normal. Albumin should also be checked periodically as a sign of liver toxicity because some patients may not have liver inflammation manifested by aspartate aminotransferase or alanine aminotransferase elevation. Liver biopsy is now recommended before beginning methotrexate therapy only for patients with a history of excessive alcohol use, ongoing hepatitis B or C infection, or recurring elevation of aspartate aminotransferase. Biopsies during methotrexate therapy are recommended only for patients who develop consistently abnormal liver function tests.[26]

Because it is a folic acid antagonist, methotrexate can induce a folic acid deficiency. This deficiency is thought to be partly responsible for methotrexate toxicity, and supplementation with folic acid does alleviate some adverse effects. Addition of folic acid to a methotrexate regimen for RA does not compromise drug efficacy.[26,24,39]

Methotrexate may be given intramuscularly, subcutaneously, or orally. Doses greater than 15 mg per week generally are given parenterally because of decreased oral bioavailability of larger doses.

Leflunomide

Leflunomide is a DMARD that inhibits pyrimidine synthesis, leading to a decrease in lymphocyte proliferation and modulation of inflammation. It has efficacy similar to methotrexate for treating RA. The drug may cause liver toxicity and is contraindicated in patients with preexisting liver disease. Patients taking the drug should have alanine aminotransferase monitored monthly initially and periodically thereafter as long as they continue treatment. Leflunomide may cause bone marrow toxicity and complete blood count with platelets is recommended monthly for 6 months and then every 6 to 8 weeks thereafter.

The drug is teratogenic, and appropriate contraceptive measures are recommended to avoid pregnancy for all sexually active male and female patients who are taking leflunomide. If conception is desired, leflunomide must be discontinued. Because leflunomide undergoes enterohepatic circulation, the drug takes many months to drop to a plasma concentration considered safe during pregnancy (<0.02 μg/mL [<0.02 mg/L; 74 nmol/L]). Cholestyramine may be used to rapidly clear the drug from plasma. In addition to pregnancy, cholestyramine use may be warranted to rapidly clear the drug in the event of severe toxicity.

Leflunomide may be given as a loading dose of 100 mg daily for 3 days, followed by a maintenance dose of 20 mg daily. Lower doses may be used if patients have gastrointestinal intolerance, complain of hair loss, or have other signs of dose-related toxicity. The loading dose allows the patient to achieve a more rapid therapeutic response, usually within the first month. The long elimination half-life of the drug (14 to 16 days) would require the patient to take the drug for several months to achieve steady state without a loading dose. Some rheumatologists prefer to begin with maintenance dosing as the loading dose may put the patient at increased risk for toxicity.[32,40,41]

Hydroxychloroquine

Hydroxychloroquine is often used in mild RA or as an adjuvant in combination DMARD therapy in more progressive disease. The pharmacokinetics and mechanism of action of this drug are poorly understood, but it is thought to dampen antigen–antibody reactions at sites of inflammation.[27] It is well absorbed orally and widely distributed to body tissues. Hydroxychloroquine is partially metabolized in the liver and is excreted by the kidney. The onset of action of hydroxychloroquine may be delayed up to 6 weeks, but the drug is considered a therapeutic failure only when 6 months of therapy without a response has elapsed.

The main advantage of hydroxychloroquine is the lack of myelosuppressive, hepatic, and renal toxicities that may be seen with other DMARDs, which simplifies monitoring. Short-term toxicities of hydroxychloroquine include gastrointestinal effects such as nausea, vomiting, and diarrhea, which can be managed by taking doses with food. Ocular toxicity includes accommodation defects, benign corneal deposits, blurred vision, scotomas (small areas of decreased or absent vision in the visual field), and night blindness. Although the risk of true retinopathy with hydroxychloroquine approaches zero, preretinopathy may occur in 2.7% of patients. All patients must understand the importance of adhering to hydroxychloroquine monitoring guidelines, as delineated in Table 72-2. Any visual change must be reported immediately. Dermatologic toxicities include rash, alopecia, and increased skin pigmentation; neurologic adverse effects such as headache, vertigo, and insomnia usually are mild.[35,42,43]

Sulfasalazine

Sulfasalazine, a prodrug, is cleaved by bacteria in the colon into sulfapyridine and 5-aminosalicylic acid. It is believed that the sulfapyridine moiety is responsible for the agent's antirheumatic properties, although the exact mechanism of action is unknown. Once the colonic bacteria have cleaved sulfasalazine, sulfapyridine and 5-aminosalicylic acid are absorbed rapidly from the gastrointestinal tract. Sulfapyridine distributes rapidly throughout the body, but higher concentrations are found in certain tissues such as serous fluid, liver, and intestines. Both sulfasalazine and its metabolites are excreted in the urine. Antirheumatic effects should be seen in 2 months.

Use of sulfasalazine is often limited by its adverse effects. Gastrointestinal adverse effects such as nausea, vomiting, diarrhea, and anorexia are the most common. These can be minimized by initiating therapy with low doses and titrating gradually to higher doses, dividing the dose more evenly throughout the day, or using enteric-coated preparations. Rash, urticaria, and serum sickness-like reactions can be managed with antihistamines and, if indicated, corticosteroids. If a hypersensitivity reaction occurs, therapy should be stopped immediately and another DMARD substituted. Sulfasalazine is associated with leukopenia, alopecia, stomatitis, and elevated hepatic enzymes. It also may cause the patient's urine and skin to turn a yellow-orange color, which is of no clinical consequence however; patients should be educated about this to avoid premature discontinuance.

Sulfasalazine's absorption can be decreased when antibiotics are used that destroy the colonic bacteria. Sulfasalazine also binds iron supplements in the gastrointestinal tract that can lead to a decreased absorption of sulfasalazine. The administration of these two agents should be separated temporally to avoid this interaction. Sulfasalazine can potentiate warfarin's effects by displacing it from protein-binding sites. Close monitoring of the patient's international normalized ratio is indicated.[44,45]

Minocycline

The tetracycline derivative minocycline has been suggested as a treatment alternative for patients with mild disease and without features of poor prognosis. While the mechanism of action is not completely understood, inhibition of metalloproteinases active in damaging articular cartilage is thought to play a role.[27] A meta-analysis of 10 clinical trials using tetracyclines for more than 3 months found mild reductions in tender and swollen joint counts and ESR but no effect on erosion progression; however, the number of patients and treatment duration in the two trials that looked at erosions were limited. The dose of minocycline for RA treatment is 100 to 200 mg daily. Adverse effects are uncommon and were reported no more frequently than placebo control groups.[46]

Tofacitinib

Tofacitinib (Xeljanz) is a JAK inhibitor for use in patients with moderate to severe RA who have failed, or have intolerance to methotrexate.

JAK is a tyrosine kinase, which mediates signal transduction from cytokines responsible for leukocyte functioning. Thus, inhibition of JAK results in modulation and suppression of the immune system through cytokine signal reduction.

In clinical trials, oral doses of tofacitinib 5 mg twice daily resulted in 55% to 59% of patients achieving at least a 20% improvement in RA symptoms at 3 months. An improvement in symptoms of 50% occurred in approximately 30% of patients.[47,48] The FDA-approved dosing of tofacitinib is 5 mg twice daily as monotherapy or in combination with other nonbiologic DMARDs.

Risks, for which black box warnings exist, include serious infections, lymphomas, and other malignancies. Patients should be tested and treated for latent tuberculosis before therapy with tofacitinib. Monitoring for reductions in lymphocytes, neutrophils, and hemoglobin should be completed at baseline and periodically throughout therapy at 4 to 8 weeks postinitiation and every 3 months thereafter.

Tofacitinib therapy has been associated with elevated plasma liver enzymes and lipids. Live vaccinations should not be given during treatment. Further data assessing long-term safety and impact on radiographic joint damage are needed before tofacitinib's place in the treatment of RA will be clear.

Other Disease-Modifying Antirheumatic Drugs

Gold salts, azathioprine, D-penicillamine, cyclosporine, and cyclophosphamide have all been used to treat RA. Although these drugs can be effective and they may be of value in certain clinical settings, they are used less frequently today because of toxicity, lack of long-term benefit, or both. Tables 72-2 and 72-3 provide dosing information and toxicity information.

Biologic Agents

Biologic agents are genetically engineered protein molecules that block the proinflammatory cytokines TNF-α (infliximab, etanercept, adalimumab, golimumab, and certolizumab), IL-1 (anakinra), and IL-6 (tocilizumab), deplete peripheral B cells (rituximab), or bind to CD80/86 on T cells to prevent the costimulation needed to fully activate T cells (abatacept). These drugs may be effective when nonbiologic DMARDs fail to achieve adequate responses but are considerably more expensive to use. Other than anakinra and tocilizumab, these agents have no toxicities requiring laboratory monitoring, but they do carry a small increased risk for infection. There is an increased incidence of tuberculosis in patients treated with these agents. Tuberculin skin testing is recommended prior to treatment with biologic agents so that latent tuberculosis can be detected.[25] Patients with a history of significant tuberculosis exposure or recurrent infection may not be good candidates for these drugs. Those who develop infections while on biologic agents should at least temporarily discontinue them until the infection is cured. Live vaccines should not be given to patients taking biologic agents.

TNF-α Inhibitors

While the anti-TNF biologics have differing structures, pharmacokinetics, and dosing, their side effects and contraindications are similar in that they all block TNF. Chronic heart failure (CHF) is a relative contraindication for anti-TNF agents. Increased cardiac mortality has been seen in patients treated with infliximab and etanercept-associated heart failure exacerbations have been documented.[41,49] Patients with New York Heart Association class III or IV and an ejection fraction of 50% or less should not use anti–TNF-α therapy. Patients whose CHF worsens while taking anti–TNF-α therapy should discontinue the drug.[24]

Anti–TNF-α therapy has also been reported to induce a multiple sclerosis-like illness or exacerbate multiple sclerosis in patients with the disease. Patients with neurologic symptoms suggestive of multiple sclerosis should discontinue therapy. TNF inhibitors may predispose patients to increased cancer risk, especially lymphoproliferative cancer, as TNF plays a role in ridding the body of cancer cells. The U.S. Food and Drug Administration (FDA) added a black box warning to product labeling for anti-TNF drugs alerting prescribers of increased lymphoproliferative and other cancers in children and adolescents treated with these drugs.[50]

Etanercept Etanercept is a fusion protein consisting of two p75-soluble TNF receptors linked to an Fc fragment of human IgG_1. The drug binds to TNF, making it biologically inactive and preventing it from interacting with the cell-surface TNF receptors that would lead to cell activation.

The drug is given by subcutaneous injection, 50 mg once weekly or 25 mg twice weekly, usually through self-injections or administration by a caregiver. Aside from local injection-site reactions, adverse effects are rare. There are case reports of pancytopenia and neurologic demyelinating syndromes like multiple sclerosis associated with use of etanercept, but these are rare. No laboratory monitoring is required. Clinical trials have used etanercept in patients who failed DMARDs. Response was seen in 60% to 75% of patients. The drug has also been FDA approved for the treatment of juvenile RA, ankylosing spondylitis, psoriatic arthritis, and moderate-to-severe psoriasis. Clinical trials have shown that it slows erosive disease progression to a greater degree than oral methotrexate therapy.[51–53]

Infliximab Infliximab is a chimeric antibody combining portions of mouse and human IgG_1. Approximately 25% of the antibody is derived from mouse amino acids. This antibody, when injected in humans, binds to TNF and prevents its interaction with TNF receptors on inflammatory cells.

Infliximab is given by IV infusion at a dose of 3 mg/kg at 0, 2, and 6 weeks and then every 8 weeks. To prevent the formation of an antibody response to this foreign protein, oral methotrexate should be given concurrently in doses typically used to treat RA for as long as the patient continues on infliximab. Antibodies develop in 14% to 40% of patients, which leads to a greater risk of infusion reactions and also may reduce the efficacy of the drug. Loss of response may be seen in patients with RA who have good initial response requiring increased doses or shorter intervals between doses to maintain response. Infusion reactions may occur in any patient treated with the drug. Both acute (within 24 hours of infusion) and delayed (24 hours to 14 days) reactions following infusion have been identified. An acute infusion reaction with symptoms including fever, chills, pruritus, and rash may occur during infusion or within 1 to 2 hours after giving the drug. Treatment includes slowing infusion rates and administering acetaminophen, diphenhydramine, or corticosteroids, depending on the severity of symptoms. Fortunately these reactions are rarely severe or anaphylactic in nature.[54] The drug may increase the risk of infection. Autoantibodies and lupus-like syndrome also have been reported. In addition to RA, infliximab is indicated for the treatment of psoriatic arthritis and ankylosing spondylitis.[55–56]

Adalimumab Adalimumab is a human IgG_1 antibody to TNF. Because it has no foreign protein components, it is less antigenic than infliximab. The drug is provided as either premixed syringes or injection pens containing 40 mg, which is administered by subcutaneous injection every 14 days. It has similar response rates to those seen with the other TNF inhibitors. Local injection-site reactions were the most common adverse reactions noted in clinical trials. It has the same precautions regarding tuberculosis and other infections as the other biologics.[57–59]

Golimumab Golimumab is a human antibody to TNF-α. In addition to RA, this agent is also indicated for treatment of psoriatic arthritis and ankylosing spondylitis. The drug is available as an injection pen, through which a dose of 50 mg is given monthly by subcutaneous injection. Precautions are similar to other TNF-α inhibitors.[60]

Certolizumab Certolizumab is a humanized antibody specific for human TNF-α. For RA, dosing recommendations are for 400 mg (2 doses of 200 mg) given by subcutaneous injection at weeks 0, 2, and 4 followed by 200 mg every 2 weeks. Precautions and side effects are similar to other TNF-α inhibitors.[61]

Non-TNF Biologics

Abatacept Abatacept is a costimulation modulator approved for the treatment of RA in patients with moderate to severe disease who fail to achieve an adequate response from one or more DMARDs. By binding to CD80/CD86 receptors on antigen-presenting cells, abatacept inhibits interactions between the antigen-presenting cells and T cells. This prevents T-cell activation to promote the inflammatory process, thus resulting in reductions in cytokines, T-cell proliferation, and other consequences of T-cell activation.

Abatacept is a fusion protein made using the extracellular domain of human cytotoxic T lymphocyte antigen 4 (the binding portion of the drug) and a fragment of the Fc domain of human IgG modified to prevent complement fixation. The drug is given by IV infusion based on patient weight (<60 kg [<132 lb]: 500 mg; 60 to 100 kg [132 to 220 lb]: 750 mg; >100 kg [>220 lb]: 1,000 mg) every 2 weeks for two doses after the initial dose and then every 4 weeks. Alternatively, the drug may be given by subcutaneous injection with the first dose of 125 mg given within 24 hours of a single IV infusion and every 7 days after that. Abatacept may be used as monotherapy or in combination with nonbiologic DMARDs.

The adverse effects include headache, nasopharyngitis, dizziness, cough, back pain, hypertension, dyspepsia, urinary tract infection, rash, and extremity pain reported more frequently than placebo in clinical trials. Infusion reactions were 50% more likely with abatacept than with placebo and there was a slightly higher rate of serious infections with active treatment.[62–64] In patients who failed to achieve adequate responses with TNF-α inhibitors, half had a clinical response to abatacept.[84] Live vaccines should not be given to patients during and for 3 months after the completion of abatacept therapy.[65]

Rituximab Rituximab is a monoclonal chimeric antibody consisting of mostly human protein with the antigen-binding region derived from a mouse antibody to CD20 protein found on the cell surface of mature B lymphocytes. The binding of rituximab to B cells results in nearly complete depletion of peripheral B cells. Although its mechanism of action in RA is not completely known, it is thought that this depletion in B cells decreases antigen presentation to T cells, thus decreasing symptoms and delaying structural damage. After administration of rituximab, it takes several months for B cell recovery. This prolonged effect on B cells results in a variable duration of action that allows for intermittent therapy based on reactivation of arthritis symptoms.

Rituximab is useful in patients who failed methotrexate or TNF inhibitors.[66–70] Two infusions of 1,000 mg are given 2 weeks apart. Methylprednisolone 100 mg should be given 30 minutes prior to rituximab to reduce the incidence and severity of infusion reactions. Acetaminophen and antihistamines may also be of benefit in patients who have a history of reactions. Methotrexate should be given concurrently in the usual doses used for RA, as the combination has proved to provide the best therapeutic outcomes. Duration of benefit is variable after a course of rituximab and patients will need retreatment with reactivation of their disease. Live vaccines should not be given to patients given rituximab.

Tocilizumab IL-6 is a major cytokine believed to have a role in promoting inflammation in RA. Tocilizumab is a humanized monoclonal antibody that attaches to IL-6 receptors, preventing the cytokine from interacting with the IL-6 receptor. It is approved for use in adults with moderately to severely active RA who have failed to respond to one or more anti-TNF biologic agents. It is used as either monotherapy or in combination with methotrexate or another DMARD. The initial starting dose is 4 mg/kg given IV every 4 weeks with dose escalation to 8 mg/kg IV every 4 weeks based on clinical response and tolerance.

The rates of adverse events are generally low but higher with combination therapy as compared to monotherapy. The most serious adverse effects reported include infusion reactions, increased infection risk, elevated plasma lipids, elevated liver enzymes, and gastrointestinal perforation. Tocilizumab use may also lead to increased metabolism of concomitant cytochrome P450 (CYP)3A4 substrate medications. It is recommended to monitor agents with narrow therapeutic window such as warfarin. Oral contraceptives and CYP3A4 statins may also be affected.[71]

Anakinra Anakinra is a naturally occurring IL-1 receptor antagonist. Results of clinical trials suggest it to be less effective than other biologic DMARDs.[72] The ACR did not include anakinra in their RA treatment recommendations because of limited use of this drug, but select patients with refractory disease could benefit from treatment with this drug.[24]

Clinical **Controversy...**

The order of DMARD or biologic agent choice is not clearly defined. No direct comparative studies exist for biologics to guide in the determination of optimal treatment order.

Treatment Strategies for Patients with Suboptimal Response to Biologics

TNF-α antagonists are generally the first biologic agents chosen for use in patients with RA. Approximately 30% of patients discontinue treatment with these drugs because of lack of efficacy or adverse effects. Lack of efficacy can further be defined as a primary failure (failure to see a treatment response 3 to 6 months after therapy initiation) or secondary failure (loss of response after an initial improvement is observed).

In such situations, addition of a nonbiologic DMARD may be beneficial if the patient is not already taking one. Dose escalation or decreased interval between infusions may be useful for those patients taking infliximab; higher doses of other TNF-α inhibitors have not been demonstrated to be effective. Choosing an alternative TNF-α inhibitor after failure of the initial anti-TNF agent may be beneficial for some patients; however, no randomized controlled trials have compared the effectiveness of cycling among agents in this class. One observational study found both decreased response and persistence rates with a second anti-TNF agent compared with the first TNF-agent.[73] Treatment with rituximab, abatacept, or tocilizumab may also prove to be effective in TNF-α treatment failures.[64,66] Combination biologic DMARD therapy is not recommended because of the increased risk for infection.[74]

Clinical **Controversy...**

After failure of an initial anti-tumor necrosis factor (TNF) agent, subsequent treatment may include trialing an alternative anti-TNF agent or changing to a non-TNF biologic. Is more benefit seen with a second anti-TNF agent based on the reason for discontinuation of the original anti-TNF agent?

Corticosteroids

Corticosteroids are used in RA for their antiinflammatory and immunosuppressive properties. They interfere with antigen presentation to T lymphocytes, inhibit prostaglandin and leukotriene synthesis, and inhibit neutrophil and monocyte superoxide radical generation. Corticosteroids also impair cell migration and cause redistribution of monocytes, lymphocytes, and neutrophils, thus blunting the inflammatory and autoimmune responses.

Oral corticosteroids are absorbed rapidly and completely from the gastrointestinal tract. They are metabolized and inactivated primarily by the liver and excreted in the urine. The elimination half-life of most corticosteroids is sufficiently long that once-daily dosing is possible.

Oral corticosteroids can be used in several ways. They can be used in bridging therapy, continuous low-dose therapy, and short-term, high-dose bursts to control flares. Oral steroids (e.g., prednisone, methylprednisolone) can be used to control pain and synovitis while DMARDs are taking effect. This is termed *bridging therapy* and is often used in patients with debilitating symptoms when DMARD therapy is initiated. Patients with difficult-to-control disease may be placed on low-dose, long-term corticosteroid therapy to control their symptoms. Prednisone doses below 7.5 mg daily are well tolerated but are not devoid of the long-term adverse effects associated with corticosteroids. The lowest dose of corticosteroid that controls symptoms should be used to reduce adverse effects. Alternate-day dosing of low-dose oral corticosteroids usually is ineffective in RA; symptoms usually flare on days without medication. High-dose corticosteroid bursts often are used to suppress disease flares. High doses are sustained for several days until symptoms are controlled, followed by a taper to the lowest effective dose.

Corticosteroids also may be delivered by injection. The intramuscular route may be preferable in patients with adherence problems for short-term therapy. Long-acting depot forms of corticosteroids include triamcinolone acetonide, triamcinolone hexacetonide, and methylprednisolone acetate. This provides the patient with 2 to 6 weeks of symptomatic control. The depot effect provides a physiologic taper, avoiding withdrawal reaction associated with hypothalamic–pituitary axis suppression. IV corticosteroids may be used to provide the patient with large amounts of drug during a steroid burst to control severe symptoms. Intraarticular injections of depot forms of corticosteroids can be useful in treating synovitis and pain when a small number of joints are affected. The onset and duration of symptomatic relief are similar to those of intramuscular injection. The intraarticular route often is preferred because it is associated with the fewest number of systemic adverse effects. If efficacious, intraarticular injections may be repeated every 3 months. No one joint should be injected more than two to three times per year because of the risk of accelerated joint destruction and atrophy of tendons. Soft tissues such as tendons and bursae also may be injected. This may help control the pain and inflammation associated with these structures. The onset and duration of symptomatic relief are similar to those of intramuscular and intraarticular injections.

The major limitation to the long-term use of corticosteroids is adverse effects. They include hypothalamic-pituitary–adrenal suppression, Cushing's syndrome, osteoporosis, myopathies, glaucoma, cataracts, gastritis, hypertension, hirsutism, electrolyte imbalances, glucose intolerance, skin atrophy, and increased susceptibility to infections. To minimize these effects, use the lowest effective corticosteroid dose and limit the duration of use. Prednisolone 7.5 mg daily results in an average of 9.5% loss of bone density from the spine. Corticosteroids double the risk for osteoporosis in patients.[75] Patients on long-term therapy should be given calcium and vitamin D to minimize bone loss. Alendronate is effective in preventing bone loss in corticosteroid-treated patients and should be considered prophylactically for patients when long-term corticosteroid therapy is anticipated, particularly for patients who are at high risk of bone loss (e.g., postmenopausal women, elderly).[76–79] There is no evidence that corticosteroids alone increase the risk of gastrointestinal ulcerations, although they often have been implicated. Consequently, gastrointestinal protective measures usually are not indicated.[80–82]

TABLE 72-5 Rheumatoid Arthritis Therapy Recommendations Based on Comorbidity

Comorbidity	Recommended	Not Recommended
Tuberculosis (latent or active prior to antitubercular therapy)		Any biologic Methotrexate Leflunomide Tofacitinib
Pregnant/Breastfeeding		Methotrexate Leflunomide Minocycline
CHF (NYHA class III/IV with LVEF ≤50%)		Anti-TNF biologic
Malignancy		
• Treated solid malignancies, skin cancers, or lymphoproliferative malignancies	Rituximab	
• Solid or non-melanoma skin cancers treated more than 5 years ago	Any biologic	
Liver		
• Transaminase elevated 2× ULN		Methotrexate Leflunomide Sulfasalazine
• Hepatitis C virus	Etanercept	Methotrexate Leflunomide Sulfasalazine[a] Minocycline[a] Hydroxychloroquine[b]
• Hepatitis B virus (untreated or treated but with Child-Pugh class B or higher)		Any biologic Methotrexate Leflunomide Sulfasalazine[a] Minocycline[a] Hydroxychloroquine[b]

CHF, chronic heart failure; LVEF, left ventricular ejection fraction; NYHA, New York Heart Association; TB, tuberculosis; ULN, upper limit of normal.

[a]Contraindicated in patients with Child-Pugh class C liver failure.
[b]Contraindicated in patients with Child-Pugh class C liver failure or if patient is not receiving treatment for hepatitis.

Clinical **Controversy. . .**

Even the best therapy available today does not completely eliminate all the signs, symptoms, or progression of disease for most patients. How much treatment is enough?

PERSONALIZED PHARMACOTHERAPY

With various pathways involved leading to inflammation in RA and an increasing number of agents available, it is important to consider patient-specific factors when making therapeutic decisions. Disease activity and the presence of poor prognostic (see Fig. 72-5 for explanation of poor prognostic feature) features may help guide treatment and lead to early aggressive therapy in patients with more severe disease.

Therapy must be tailored for various comorbidities the patient may have (Table 72-5). Hepatitis and other liver diseases, heart failure, renal failure, and history of cancer are among the comorbidities that influence treatment choice. Individual patients may also significantly differ in their response to a specific agent; currently, there are no clear predictors of response to therapeutic interventions.

Pharmacokinetic parameters should be taken into consideration when determining therapeutic options for specific patients. NSAIDs should be avoided in patients with renal impairment or in patients at high risk for NSAID-induced renal injury including the elderly, those with congestive heart failure or cirrhosis, or patients at risk for volume depletion such as those using diuretics.[83] Dose adjustments are recommended in patients with renal dysfunction for methotrexate and anakinra. Dose reductions are also recommended with tofacitinib in patients with moderate or severe renal impairment, moderate hepatic dysfunction, or patients treated concomitantly with CYP3A4 inhibitors.

While azathioprine is now used less frequently for RA, genetic testing for null or decreased thiopurine *S*-methyltransferase (TPMT) activity is available to help predict those patients with a higher risk of myelosuppression due to reduced metabolism of the drug, and dosage reductions may be made in those patients.[84]

EVALUATION OF THERAPEUTIC OUTCOMES

The evaluation of therapeutic outcomes is based primarily on improvements of clinical signs and symptoms of RA. Clinical signs of improvement include a reduction in joint swelling, decreased warmth over actively involved joints, and decreased tenderness to joint palpation. Improvement in RA symptoms includes reduction in perceived joint pain and morning stiffness, longer time to onset of afternoon fatigue, and improvement in ability to perform activities of daily living. Improvement of activities of daily living may be assessed objectively using a health assessment questionnaire score. Joint radiographs may be of some benefit in assessing the progression of the disease and should show little or no evidence of disease progression if treatment is effective.

Laboratory monitoring is of little value in monitoring individual patient response to therapy. Tables 72-2 and 72-3 provide monitoring of drug toxicity information. Routine monitoring of patients is essential to the safe use of these drugs. In addition, patients should be questioned about symptoms of the adverse effects outlined in the drug section of this chapter.

CONCLUSIONS

RA is the most common inflammatory arthritis, affecting approximately 1% of the population. The disease is characterized by symmetrical swelling and stiffness of the involved joints. The stiffness is usually more prominent in the morning. Extraarticular features of RA include rheumatoid nodules, vasculitis, and ocular, cardiac, and pulmonary complications. The course of the disease is highly variable. Treatment is aimed at relieving pain and inflammation and maintaining and preserving joint function. Nondrug therapy, including exercise and adequate rest periods, should also be used early in the course of treatment. Early use of a DMARD or biologic agent results in better patient outcomes. Methotrexate, sulfasalazine, and hydroxychloroquine are often considered for initial therapy. Biologics have also been shown to be effective in these patients but may be considered second choice because of cost considerations; however, they are effective in patients who fail to achieve adequate response from nonbiologic DMARDs. Combination DMARDs or biologics may be considered in those who fail adequate trials of single-agent therapy. Corticosteroids and NSAIDs may be useful adjuncts for treatment, but because of adverse effects and limited impact on long-term outcomes, they should not be considered as sole treatment for most patients.

ABBREVIATIONS

ACPA	anticitrullinated protein antibody
ACR	American College of Rheumatology
ANA	antinuclear antibody
CHF	chronic heart failure
CRP	C-reactive protein
CYP	cytochrome P450
DMARD	disease-modifying antirheumatic drug
ESR	erythrocyte sedimentation rate
EULAR	European League Against Rheumatism
FDA	Food and Drug Administration
HLA	human lymphocyte antigen
Ig	immunoglobulin
IL	interleukin
JAK	Janus kinase
NSAID	nonsteroidal antiinflammatory drug
RA	rheumatoid arthritis
RF	rheumatoid factor
TNF	tumor necrosis factor
TPMT	thiopurine *S*-methyltransferase

REFERENCES

1. Smith JB, Haynes MK. Rheumatoid arthritis—A molecular understanding. Ann Intern Med 2002;136(12):908–922.
2. Klippel JH CL, Stone JH, Crofford LJ, White PH, eds. Primer on the Rheumatic Diseases, 13th ed. Atlanta, GA: Arthritis Foundation, 2008.
3. Harris ED, Firestein GS. The clinical features of rheumatoid arthritis. In: Firestein GS, Budd RC, Harris ED, et al., eds. Kelley's Textbook of Rheumatology, 8th ed. St. Louis, MO: Saunders, 2008. *http://www.mdconsult.com.*
4. Jiang H, Chess L. Regulation of immune response by T cells. N Engl J Med 2006;354:1166–1176.
5. Brennan FM, McInnes IB. Evidence that cytokines play a role in rheumatoid arthritis. J Clin Invest 2008;118: 3537–3545.
6. Moissec P, Korn T, Kuchroo VK. Interleukin-17 and type 17 helper T cells. N Engl J Med 2009;361:888–898.
7. Isaacs JD. Therapeutic T-cell manipulation in rheumatoid arthritis: Past, present and future. Rheumatology 2008;49: 1461–1468.
8. Tsokos GC. B cells, be gone—B-cell depletion in the treatment of rheumatoid arthritis. N Engl J Med 2004;350(25):2546–2548.
9. Weinstein E, Peeva E, Putterman C, Diamond B. B-cell biology. Rheum Dis Clin North Am 2004;30(1):159–174.
10. Carter RH. B cells in health and disease. Mayo Clin Proc 2006;81:377–384.
11. Youinou P, Taher TE, Pers J-O, Mageed RA, Renaudineau Y. B lymphocyte cytokines and rheumatoid autoimmune disease. Arthritis Rheum 2009;60:1873–1880.
12. Choy EH, Panayi GS. Cytokine pathways and joint inflammation in rheumatoid arthritis. N Engl J Med 2001;344(12):907–916.
13. McInnes IB, Schett G. The pathogenesis of rheumatoid arthritis. N Engl J Med 2011;365:2205–2219.
14. Arend WP. Physiology of cytokine pathways in rheumatoid arthritis. Arthritis Care Res 2001;45:101–106.
15. Huber LC, Distler O, Tarner I, Gay RE, Gay S, Pap T. Synovial fibroblasts: Key players in rheumatoid arthritis. Rheumatology 2006;45:669–675.
16. Firestein GS. Etiology and pathogenesis of rheumatoid arthritis. In: Firestein GS, Budd RC, Harris ED, et al., eds. Kelley's Textbook of Rheumatology, 8th ed. St. Louis, MO: Saunders, 2008. *http://www.mdconsult.com.*
17. Visser H. Early diagnosis of rheumatoid arthritis. Best Pract Res Clin Rheumatol 2005;19(1):55–72.
18. Hard ER. Extraarticular manifestations of rheumatoid arthritis. Semin Arthritis Rheum 1979;8:151–176.
19. Choi HK, Hernan MA, Seeger JD, et al. Methotrexate and mortality in patients with rheumatoid arthritis: A prospective study. Lancet 2002;359:1173–1177.
20. Wallberg-Jonsson S, Johansson H, Ohman ML, Rantapaa-Dahlqvist S. Extent of inflammation predicts cardiovascular disease and overall mortality in seropositive rheumatoid arthritis. A retrospective cohort study from disease onset. J Rheumatol 1999;26(12):2562–2571.
21. Colglazier CL, Sutej PG. Laboratory testing in rheumatic diseases: A practical review. South Med J 2005;98(2): 185–191.
22. Shmerling RH. Diagnostic tests for rheumatic disease: Clinical utility revisited. South Med J 2005;98(7): 704–711.
23. Aletaha D, Neogi T, Silman AJ, Fuovits J, et al. 2010 Rheumatoid arthritis classification criteria: An American College of Rheumatology/European League Against Rheumatism collaborative initiative. Arthritis Rheum 2010;62:2569–2581.
24. Saag KG, Teng GG, Patkar NM, Anuntiyo J, et al. American College of Rheumatology 2008 recommendations for the use of nonbiologic and biologic disease-modifying antirheumatic drugs in rheumatoid arthritis. Arthritis Rheum 2008;59:762–784.

25. Singh JA, Furst DE, Bharat A, et al. 2012 Update of the 2008 American College of Rheumatology recommendations for the use of disease-modifying antirheumatic drugs and biologic agents in the treatment of rheumatoid arthritis. Arthritis Care Res 2012;64(5):625–639.
26. American College of Rheumatology Subcommittee on Rheumatoid Arthritis G. Guidelines for the management of rheumatoid arthritis: 2002 Update. Arthritis Rheum 2002;46(2):328–346.
27. Genovese MC. The treatment of rheumatoid arthritis. In: Firestein GS, Budd RC, Harris ED, et al., eds. Kelley's Textbook of Rheumatology, 8th ed. St. Louis, MO: Saunders, 2008. *http://www.mdconsult.com.*
28. Mottonen T, Hannonen P, Korpela M, et al. Delay to institution of therapy and induction of remission using single-drug or combination-disease-modifying antirheumatic drug therapy in early rheumatoid arthritis. Arthritis Rheum 2002;46(4):894–898.
29. Goldbach-Mansky R, Lipsky PE. New concepts in the treatment of rheumatoid arthritis. Annu Rev Med 2003;54:197–216.
30. O'Dell JR. Therapeutic strategies for rheumatoid arthritis. N Engl J Med 2004;350(25):2591–2602.
31. Kroot EJ, VanLeeuwen MA, VanRijswijk MH, et al. No increased mortality in patients with rheumatoid arthritis: Up to 10 years of follow up from disease onset. Ann Rheum Dis 2000;59:954–958.
32. Kalden JR, Schattenkirchner M, Sorensen H, et al. The efficacy and safety of leflunomide in patients with active rheumatoid arthritis: A five-year followup study. Arthritis Rheum 2003;48(6):1513–1520.
33. Goekoop-Reuterman YP, deVries-Bouwstra JK, Allaart CF, et al. Comparison of treatment strategies in early rheumatoid arthritis: A randomized trial. Ann Intern Med 2007;146: 406–415.
34. O'Dell JR. Combinations of conventional disease-modifying antirheumatic drugs. Rheum Dis Clin North Am 2001;27(2): 415–426, x.
35. Kremer JM. Rational use of new and existing disease-modifying agents in rheumatoid arthritis. Ann Intern Med 2001;134(8):695–706.
36. Bijlsma JW, Van Everdingen AA, Huisman M, De Nijs RN, Jacobs JW. Glucocorticoids in rheumatoid arthritis: Effects on erosions and bone. Ann N Y Acad Sci 2002;966:82–90.
37. Glick T, Müller-Ladner U. Vaccination in patients with chronic rheumatic or autoimmune diseases. Clin Infect Dis 2008;46:1459–1465.
38. Pincus T, Ferraccioli G, Sokka T, et al. Evidence from clinical trials and long-term observational studies that disease-modifying anti-rheumatic drugs slow radiographic progression in rheumatoid arthritis: Updating a 1983 review. Rheumatology 2002;41(12):1346–1356.
39. Borchers AT, Keen CL, Cheema GS, Gershwin ME. The use of methotrexate in rheumatoid arthritis. Semin Arthritis Rheum 2004;34(1):465–483.
40. Osiri M, Shea BJ, Robinson V, et al. Leflunomide for treating rheumatoid arthritis. Cochrane Database Syst Rev 2003(1): CD002047.
41. Cush JJ. Safety overview of new disease-modifying antirheumatic drugs. Rheum Dis Clin North Am 2004;30(2): 237–255, v.
42. Maturi RK, Folk JC, Nichols B, Oetting TT, Kardon RH. Hydroxy-chloroquine retinopathy. Arch Ophthalmol 1999;117(9):1262–1263.
43. Suarez-Almazor ME, Belseck E, Shea B, Homik J, Wells G, Tugwell P. Antimalarials for treating rheumatoid arthritis. Cochrane Database Syst Rev 2000(4):CD000959.
44. Weinblatt ME, Reda D, Henderson W, et al. Sulfasalazine treatment for rheumatoid arthritis: A meta-analysis of 15 randomized trials. J Rheumatol 1999;26(10):2123–2130.
45. Rains CP, Noble S, Faulds D. Sulfasalazine: A review of its pharmacological properties and therapeutic efficacy in the treatment of rheumatoid arthritis. Drugs 1995;50:137–156.
46. Stone M, Fortin PR, Pacheco-Tena C, Inman RD. Should tetracycline treatment be used more extensively for rheumatoid arthritis? Meta-analysis demonstrates clinical benefit with reduction in disease activity. J Rheumatol 2003;30:2112–2122.
47. van Vollenhoven RF, Fleischmann R, Cohen S, et al. Tofacitinib or adalimumab versus placebo in rheumatoid arthritis. N Engl J Med 2012;367(6):508–519.
48. Fleischmann R, Kremer J, Cush J, et al. Placebo-controlled trial of tofacitinib monotherapy in rheumatoid arthritis. N Engl J Med 2012;367(6):495–507.
49. Scott DL, Kingsley MB. Tumor necrosis factor inhibitors for rheumatoid arthritis. N Engl J Med 2006;355:704–712.
50. Food and Drug Administration. Information for Healthcare Professionals: Tumor Necrosis Factor (TNF) Blockers (marketed as Remicade, Enbrel, Humira, Cimzia, and Simponi). FDA Alert August 4, 2009, *http://www.fda.gov/Drugs/DrugSafety/PostmarketDrugSafetyInformationforPatientsandProviders/DrugSafetyInformationforHeathcareProfessionals/ucm174474.htm.*
51. Genovese MC, Kremer JM. Treatment of rheumatoid arthritis with etanercept. Rheum Dis Clin North Am 2004;30(2):311–328, vi–vii.
52. Nanda S, Bathon JM. Etanercept: A clinical review of current and emerging indications. Expert Opin Pharmacother 2004;5(5):1175–1186.
53. Blumenauer B, Judd MG, Cranney A, et al. Etanercept for the treatment of rheumatoid arthritis. Cochrane Database Syst Rev 2003(3):CD004525.
54. Cheifitz A, Mayer L. Monoclonal antibodies, immunogenicity, and associated infusion reactions. Mt Sinai J Med 2005;72:250–256.
55. Blumenauer B, Judd M, Wells G, et al. Infliximab for the treatment of rheumatoid arthritis. Cochrane Database Syst Rev 2002(3):CD003785.
56. Maini SR. Infliximab treatment of rheumatoid arthritis. Rheum Dis Clin North Am 2004;30(2):329–347, vii.
57. Navarro-Sarabia F, Ariza-Ariza R, Hernandez-Cruz B, Villanueva I. Adalimumab for treating rheumatoid arthritis. J Rheumatol 2006;(6):1075–1081.
58. den Broeder A, van de Putte L, Rau R, et al. A single dose, placebo controlled study of the fully human anti-tumor necrosis factor-alpha antibody adalimumab (D2E7) in patients with rheumatoid arthritis. J Rheumatol 2002;29(11):2288–2298.
59. Keystone E, Haraoui B. Adalimumab therapy in rheumatoid arthritis. Rheum Dis Clin North Am 2004;30(2):349–364, vii.
60. Singh JA, Noorbaloochi S, Singh G. Golimumab for rheumatoid arthritis. Cochrane Database Syst Rev 2010(1):CD008341.
61. Mease PJ. Certolizumab pegol in the treatment of rheumatoid arthritis: a comprehensive review of its clinical efficacy and safety. Rheumatology (Oxford) 2011;50(2):261–270.
62. Maxwell L, Singh JA. Abatacept for rheumatoid arthritis. Cochrane Database Syst Rev 2009(4):CD007277.
63. Hervey PS, Keam SJ. Abatacept. BioDrugs 2006;20(1):53–61; discussion 62.
64. Genovese MC, Becker JC, Schiff M, et al. Abatacept for rheumatoid arthritis refractory to tumor necrosis factor alpha inhibition. N Engl J Med 2005;353(11):1114–1123.

65. Orencia [package insert]. Princeton, NJ: Bristol-Meyers Squibb. August 2009, *http://packageinserts.bms.com/pi/pi_orencia.pdf.*
66. Cohen SB, Emery P, Greenwald MW, et al. Rituximab for rheumatoid arthritis refractory to anti-tumor necrosis factor therapy: Results of a multicenter, randomized, double-blind, placebo-controlled, phase III trial evaluating primary efficacy and safety at twenty-four weeks. Arthritis Rheum 2006;54(9):2793–2806.
67. De Vita S, Quartuccio L. Treatment of rheumatoid arthritis with rituximab: An update and possible indications. Autoimmun Rev 2006;5(7):443–448.
68. Emery P, Fleischmann R, Filipowicz-Sosnowska A, et al. The efficacy and safety of rituximab in patients with active rheumatoid arthritis despite methotrexate treatment: Results of a phase IIB randomized, double-blind, placebo-controlled, dose-ranging trial. Arthritis Rheum 2006;54(5):1390–1400.
69. Smolen JS, Emery P, Keystone EC, et al. Consensus statement on the use of rituximab in patients with rheumatoid arthritis. Ann Rheum Dis 2007;66:143–150.
70. Schuna, AA. Rituximab for the treatment of rheumatoid arthritis. Pharmacotherapy 2007;27:1702–1710.
71. Navarro-Millan I, Singh JA, Curtis JR. Systematic review of tocilizumab for rheumatoid arthritis: A new biologic agent targeting the interleukin-6 receptor. Clin Ther 2012;34(4):788–802.
72. Mertens M, Singh JA. Anakinra for rheumatoid arthritis. Cochrane Database Syst Rev 2009(1):CD005121.
73. Greenberg JD, Reed G, Decktor D, et al. A comparative effectiveness study of adalimumab, etanercept and infliximab in biologically naïve and switched rheumatoid arthritis patients: Results from the US CORROA registry. Ann Rheum Dis 2012;71(7):1134–1142.
74. Lutt JR, Deodhar A. Rheumatoid arthritis: Strategies in the management of patients showing an inadequate response to TNFα antagonists. Drugs 2008;68:591–606.
75. DaSilva JAP, Jacogs JWG, Kirwan JR, et al. Safety of low dose glucocorticoid treatment in rheumatoid arthritis: Published evidence and prospective trial data. Ann Rheum Dis 2006;65:285–293.
76. Adachi JD, Saag KG, Delmas PD, et al. Two-year effects of alendronate on bone mineral density and vertebral fracture in patients receiving glucocorticoids: A randomized, double-blind, placebo-controlled extension trial. Arthritis Rheum 2001;44(1):202–211.
77. McIlwain HH. Glucocorticoid-induced osteoporosis: Pathogenesis, diagnosis, and management. Prev Med 2003;36(2):243–249.
78. da Silva JAP, Jacobs JWG, Kirwan JR, Boers M, et al. Safety of low dose glucocorticoid treatment in rheumatoid arthritis: published evidence and prospective trial data. Ann Rheum Dis 2006;65:285–293.
79. American College of Rheumatology Ad Hoc Committee on Glucocorticoid-Induced Osteoporosis. Recommendations for the prevention and treatment of glucocorticoid-induced osteoporosis. Arthritis Rheum 2001;44:1496–1503.
80. Morand EF. Corticosteroids in the treatment of rheumatologic diseases. Curr Opin Rheumatol 1998;10(3):179–183.
81. Bijlsma JWJ, Saag KG, Buttgereit F, da Silva JAP. Developments in glucocorticoid therapy. Rheum Dis Clin North Am 2005;31:1–17.
82. Criswell LA, Saag KG, Sems KM, et al. Moderate-term, low-dose corticosteroids for rheumatoid arthritis. Cochrane Database Syst Rev 1998(3):CD001158.
83. Epstein M. Non-steroidal anti-inflammatory drugs and the continuum of renal dysfunction. J Hypertens 2002; 20(suppl):S17–S23.
84. Ford LT, Berg JD. Thiopurine S-methyltransferase (TPMT) assessment prior to starting thiopurine drug treatment; a pharmacogenetic test whose time has come. J Clin Pathol 2010;63(4):288–295.

Osteoporosis and Other Metabolic Bone Diseases

Mary Beth O'Connell and Jill S. Borchert

73

KEY CONCEPTS

1. Osteoporosis is a public health epidemic that affects all ages, genders, races, and ethnicities. Lifestyle behaviors, diseases, and medications should be reviewed to identify risk factors for developing osteoporosis and osteoporotic fractures. Healthcare practitioners should identify and resolve reversible risks. Patients with early onset or severe osteoporosis should be evaluated for secondary causes of bone loss.
2. Bone physiology and pathophysiology are complex, involving many different cell lines, pathways, and biofeedback systems. As these processes become more delineated, opportunities for additional drug targets exist creating new classes of investigational agents.
3. An adult's 10-year probability of developing an osteoporotic fracture can be estimated with the World Health Organization fracture risk assessment (FRAX) tool. Central bone densitometry can determine bone mass, predict fracture risk, and influence patient and provider treatment decisions. Portable equipment can be used for osteoporosis screening in the community to determine the need for further testing.
4. All people throughout their life spans should incorporate a bone-healthy lifestyle, which emphasizes regular exercise, nutritious diet, tobacco avoidance, minimal alcohol use, and fall prevention to prevent and treat osteoporosis.
5. Treatment should be considered for men or women older than age 50 years who have a hip or vertebral fracture, T-score ≤ −2.5 at the femoral neck or spine or those who have low bone mass (T-score between −1.0 and −2.5) at the femoral neck or spine and a 10-year probability of major osteoporotic fracture of ≥20% or hip fracture of ≥3% based on FRAX.
6. The recommended dietary allowance for calcium in American adults is 1,000 to 1,200 mg of elemental calcium daily with diet as the preferred source. Supplements are only added when diet is insufficient.
7. The recommended dietary allowance for vitamin D for American adults is 600 units and for older adults 800 units daily, with some organizations and guidelines recommending higher doses of at least 800 to 1000 units daily. The daily target is achieved through sun exposure, fortified foods, and supplements. Vitamin D insufficiency, usually defined as 25-hydroxy vitamin D concentrations of <30 ng/mL (<75 nmol/L), is common in Americans.
8. Alendronate, risedronate, zoledronic acid, and denosumab decrease vertebral, hip, and nonvertebral fractures and are considered first-line osteoporosis treatments. Ibandronate and raloxifene are alternatives, and calcitonin is a last-line agent. Teriparatide is reserved for severe osteoporosis or for those intolerant to other medications.
9. Adherence with osteoporosis medications is frequently suboptimal, and poor adherence is associated with less fracture prevention. Healthcare providers have an important role in prevention and treatment of osteoporosis by assessing medication administration and adherence and by providing additional medication and disease education.
10. Patients taking long-term oral glucocorticoids and certain chemotherapeutic agents need to be identified and started on a bone-healthy lifestyle and usually should receive a bisphosphonate, denosumab, or teriparatide therapy to prevent or treat drug-induced osteoporosis.

1 Osteoporosis is a bone disorder characterized by low bone density, impaired bone architecture, and compromised bone strength that predisposes a person to increased fracture risk.[1] Osteoporosis is a major public health threat, especially with 55% of the Americans 50 years of age and older expected to have this disease.[2] In the United States, 8 million women and 2 million men are estimated to have osteoporosis. The at-risk population is also large, with low bone density (osteopenia) estimates of 34 million Americans[2] and 37% to 50% of white women.[1]

Attention to bone health is needed in people of all ages. The development of osteoporosis and osteoporotic fractures is multifactorial, beginning at birth with genetics and then throughout life as a result of health behaviors that influence bone growth and maintenance, skeletal factors that lead to compromised bone strength, and nonskeletal factors that lead to falls (Fig. 73-1). Therefore all healthcare providers should educate everyone about prevention, especially providing encouragement to practice a bone-healthy lifestyle, monitor bone health in patients at risk, and provide optimal treatment for patients with osteoporosis.

EPIDEMIOLOGY

1 Low bone density, osteoporosis, and osteoporotic fractures are very common and affect all ethnic groups. Low bone density is estimated to occur in 52% of white and Asian, 49% of Hispanic, and 35% of black women age 50 and older.[2] Osteoporosis affects 20% of white and Asian, 10% of Hispanic, and 5% of black women age 50 and older. Disease prevalence greatly increases with age; from 4% in women 50 to 59 years of age to 44% to 52% in women 80 years of age and older.[1] White and Hispanic women have the highest fragility fracture (those occurring after falls from no more than a standing height and with minimal or no trauma) rate followed by Native American, African American, and Asian women when the data are adjusted for weight, bone mineral density (BMD), and other factors. Approximately 20% to 27% of men aged 50 years and older

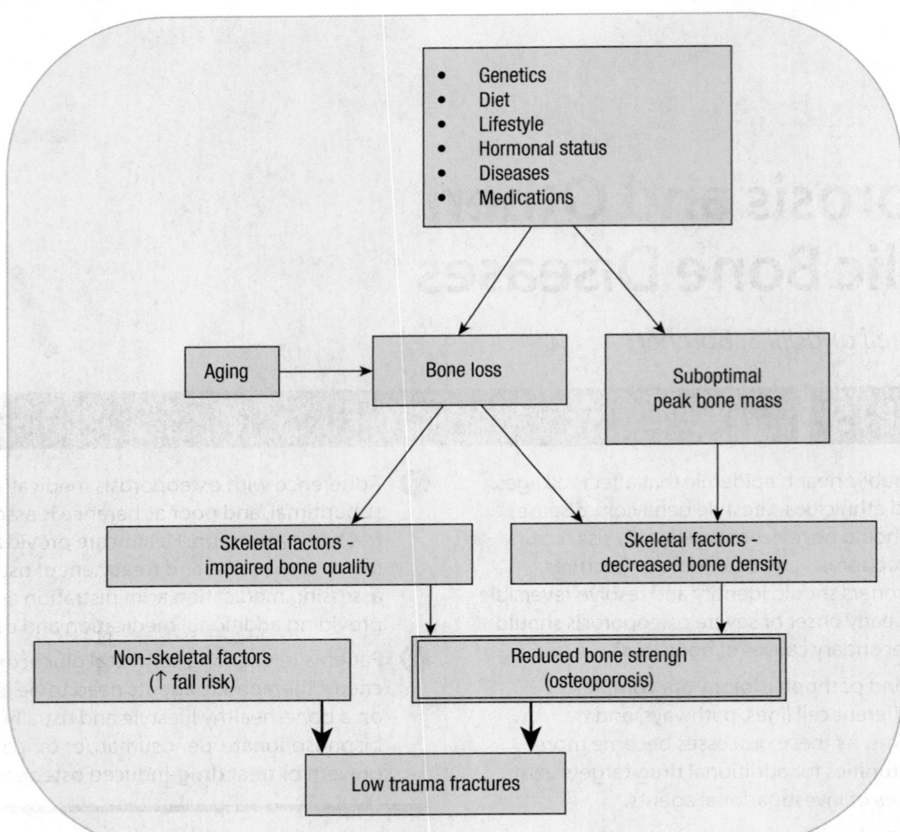

FIGURE 73-1 Etiology of osteoporosis and osteoporotic fractures.

have low bone density rising to 49% in men 80 years and older.[3] Osteoporosis prevalence in non-Hispanic white men is 4% to 5%, non-Hispanic black men is 3%, and Hispanic men is 2%. Osteoporosis prevalence rises to 17% in men 80 years and older. Although osteoporosis is a common finding in older adults with fractures, up to 50% of fragility fractures occur in patients with normal or low bone mass.[1]

Fragility wrist and vertebral fractures are common throughout adulthood, and hip fractures are more common in older adults. Fracture incidence has been estimated at 2 million (71% in women, 29% in men) in 2005, with an estimated total medical cost of $17 billion.[4] Fractures in women accounted for 75% of the costs and in older adults 87% of the costs. Hip fractures represented 72% of these costs. Forecasting predicts 3 million fractures at a cost of $25 billion in 2025. The incidences of hip fracture and associated mortality are decreasing for both genders,[5] with the hypothesis related to better efforts at osteoporosis prevention (e.g., bone-healthy lifestyle) and use of bisphosphonates. In a woman's lifetime, she has a 17% likelihood of a hip fracture, 15.6% likelihood of a vertebral fracture, and 16% likelihood of a forearm fracture.[1] In a man's lifetime, osteoporotic fracture risk is 13% to 30%. However, rates in the United States remain higher than those in other countries, and comorbidities are increasing,[5] suggesting a need for continued focus on bone health.

ETIOLOGY

1 Figure 73-1 depicts a model describing the etiology of osteoporosis and fractures. Table 73-1[1,6–9] lists risk factors for osteoporosis, and Tables 73-2[1,6,8,10–13] and 73-3[10,14,15] list secondary causes of this condition.

TABLE 73-1 Risk Factors for Osteoporosis and Osteoporotic Fractures

Low bone mineral density[a]
Female sex[a]
Advanced age[a]
Race/ethnicity[a]
History of a previous fragility fracture as an adult[a] (especially clinical vertebral fracture or hip fracture)
Osteoporotic fracture in a first-degree relative (especially parental hip fracture[a])
Low body weight or body mass index[a]
Premature menopause (<45 years old)
Secondary osteoporosis[b] (especially rheumatoid arthritis[a])
Past or present systemic oral glucocorticoid therapy[a,c]
Cigarette smoking[a,c]
Alcohol intake of 3 or more drinks/day[a,c]
Low calcium intake
Low physical activity or immobilization
Vitamin D insufficiency
Recent falls
Cognitive impairment
Impaired vision

[a]Factors included in World Health Organization fracture risk assessment tool (FRAX).

[b]Secondary causes included in the FRAX tool are diabetes type 1, osteogenesis imperfecta as an adult, long-standing untreated hyperthyroidism, hypogonadism, premature menopause (<45 years old), chronic malnutrition, malabsorption, and chronic liver disease.

[c]Risk is larger with greater exposure.

Data from references 1 and 6–8.

TABLE 73-2 Select Medical Conditions Associated with Osteoporosis in Children and Adults

Endocrine/Hormonal
Primary or secondary ovarian failure
Testosterone deficiency
Hyperthyroidism
Cushing's syndrome
Growth hormone deficiency (in children)
Primary hyperparathyroidism
Diabetes, types 1 and 2
Gastrointestinal
Nutritional disorders (e.g., anorexia nervosa)
Malabsorptive states (Crohn's or celiac disease, chronic pancreatitis, gastric bypass, gastrectomy, bariatric surgery)
Chronic liver disease (e.g., primary biliary cirrhosis)
Billroth I
Inflammatory Disorders
Rheumatoid arthritis
Ankylosing spondylitis
Systemic lupus erythematosus
Chronic obstructive pulmonary disease
Chronic Illness
Chronic kidney disease
Malignancies (multiple myeloma, lymphoma, leukemia)
Human immunodeficiency virus infection/acquired immunodeficiency syndrome
Organ transplant
Disuse/Immobility
Muscular dystrophy
Multiple sclerosis
Stroke/cerebrovascular accident
Genetic
Osteogenesis imperfecta
Turner's syndrome
Down's syndrome
Marfan's syndrome
Klinefelter's syndrome
Cystic fibrosis
Hemochromatosis
Hypophosphatasia

Data from references 1, 6, 8, and 10–13.

TABLE 73-3 Selected Medications Associated with Increased Bone Loss and/or Fracture Risk

Medications	Comments
Anticonvulsant therapy (phenytoin, carbamazepine, phenobarbital, valproic acid)	↓ BMD and ↑ fracture risk; increased vitamin D metabolism leading to low 25(OH) vitamin D concentrations
Aromatase inhibitors (e.g., letrozole, anastrozole)	↓ BMD and ↑ fracture risk; reduced estrogen concentrations
Furosemide	↑ Fracture risk; increased calcium renal elimination
Glucocorticoids (chronic oral therapy)	↓ BMD and ↑ fracture risk; dose and duration dependent; see special populations section
Gonadotropin-releasing hormone agonists or analogs (e.g., leuprolide, goserelin)	↓ BMD and ↑ fracture risk; decreased sex hormone production
Heparin (unfractionated) or low-molecular-weight heparin	↓ BMD and ↑ fracture risk (unfractionated >>> low molecular weight) with long-term use (e.g., >6 mo); decreased osteoblast function and increased osteoclast function
HIV medications Nucleoside reverse transcriptase inhibitors (antiretroviral therapy) (zidovudine, didanosine, lamivudine) Protease inhibitors (nelfinavir, indinavir, saquinavir, ritonavir, lopinavir)	↓ BMD (ART > PI), no fracture data; increased osteoclast activity and decreased osteoblast activity
Medroxyprogesterone acetate depot administration	↓ BMD, no fracture data; possible BMD recovery with discontinuation; central DXA monitoring of BMD recommended with ≥2 years of use; decreased estrogen concentrations
Proton pump inhibitor therapy (long-term therapy)	↑ Vertebral and hip fracture risk; possible calcium malabsorption secondary to acid suppression for carbonate salts
Selective serotonin reuptake inhibitors	↑ Hip fracture risk; decreased osteoblast activity
Thiazolidinediones (pioglitazone, rosiglitazone)	↓ BMD and ↑ fracture risk; risk may be greater in women than men; decreased osteoblast function
Thyroid hormone: excessive supplementation	↓ BMD and ↑ fracture risk (> in men); risk increases with TSH concentration <0.1 mIU/L; possible increase in bone resorption
Vitamin A: excessive intake (≥1.5 mg of retinol form)	↓ BMD and ↑ fracture risk; decreased osteoblast activity and increased osteoclast activity

ART, antiretroviral therapy; BMD, bone mineral density; DXA, dual-energy x-ray absorptiometry; HIV, human immunodeficiency virus; PI, protease inhibitors; TSH, thyroid stimulating hormone.

Data from references 10, 14, and 15.

Low Bone Density

BMD is a major predictor of fracture risk. Every standard deviation decrease in BMD in women represents a 10% to 12% decrease in bone mass and a 1.5- to 2.6-fold increase in fracture risk.[2] Low BMD can occur as a result of failure to reach a normal peak bone mass or bone loss. Bone loss occurs when bone resorption exceeds bone formation, usually from high bone turnover; when the number or depth of bone resorption sites greatly exceeds the rate and ability of osteoblasts to form new bone. Women and men begin to lose a small amount of bone mass starting in the third to fourth decade of life as a consequence of a slight reduction in bone formation.[16] During perimenopause and menopause, bone loss occurs predominantly due to increases in bone resorption secondary to estrogen deficiency. Older adults steadily lose bone mass as a consequence of an accelerated rate of bone remodeling combined with reduced bone formation.

The major risk factors (see Tables 73-1, 73-2, and 73-3) influencing bone loss are hormonal status, exercise, aging, nutrition, lifestyle, disease states, medications, and some genetic influences. Nonhormonal risk factors are similar between women and men.

Impaired Bone Quality

In addition to BMD, the strength of bone is highly affected by the quality of the bone's composition and its structure.[16] For example, besides decreasing bone mass, accelerated bone turnover can also impair bone quality and the structural integrity of bone by increasing the quantity of immature bone that is not yet adequately mineralized. In men, the bone loss that results from thinning of trabeculae with aging is less damaging to the quality and strength of bone structure than bone loss in women where damage to trabecular crosslinks is seen. Bone quality assessment is important because changes in bone quality affect bone strength much more than bone mass changes. Future osteoporosis diagnostic testing will assess both bone quality and density.

Falls

Although up to 50% of vertebral fractures can occur spontaneously with minimal to no trauma, most wrist fractures and greater than 90% of hip fractures result from a fall from standing height or less.[2] One-third to one-half of all older adults fall each year, and 50% fall more than once. Up to 5% of all falls will result in a fracture. According to 2006 statistics, 2.1 million older adults were treated in the emergency department and 600,000 hospitalized for fall-related injuries, incurring costs of about $20 billion.[17] Close to 17,000 older adults died in 2006 due to a fall-related injury.[18]

PATHOPHYSIOLOGY

Bone Physiology

The skeleton has two types of bone.[19] Cortical bone makes up the majority of the skeleton (80%) and is found mostly in the long bones (e.g., forearm and hip). Trabecular bone is found mostly in the vertebrae and ends of long bones. This bone type is 10 times more metabolically active compared with cortical bone due to a much higher bone turnover rate because of its large surface area and honeycomb-like shape.

Bone is made of collagen and mineral components.[19] The collagen component gives bone its flexibility and energy-absorbing capability. The mineral component gives bone its stiffness and strength. The correct balance of these substances is needed for bone to adequately accommodate stress and strain and resist fractures. Imbalances can impair bone quality and lead to reduced bone strength.

Bone strength reflects the integration of bone mass and bone quality (composition and microarchitecture).[19] Bone mass increases rapidly throughout childhood and adolescence. Peak bone mass is attained by age 18 to 21 years.[6,20] Peak bone mass is highly dependent on genetic factors that account for approximately 60% to 80% of the variability.[8] The remaining 20% to 40% is influenced by modifiable factors such as nutritional intake (e.g., calcium, vitamin D, and protein), exercise, adverse lifestyle practices (e.g., smoking), hormonal status, and certain diseases and medications. Optimizing peak bone mass is important for preventing osteoporosis. The higher the peak bone mass, the more bone one can lose before being at an increased fracture risk. As the microarchitecture of bone deteriorates, the bone strength greatly decreases. Women loose more bone structure than men.[6]

2 Bone remodeling is a dynamic process that occurs continuously throughout life Figure 73-2A–C.[19,21–26] One to two million tiny sections of bone are in the process of remodeling at any given time. Many cytokines, growth factors, and hormones influence each remodeling step. The complete physiology of bone remodeling is not fully known but appears to begin with signals from lining cells or osteocytes (bone communication cells) that are triggered by stress, microfractures, biofeedback systems responsive to cytokines and growth factors, and potentially certain diseases and medications (see Fig. 73-2B, step 1). A major stimulus for hematopoietic stem cell (monocyte–macrophage lineage) differentiation to become mature osteoclasts (bone-resorbing cells) is the receptor activator of nuclear factor kappa B ligand (RANKL), which is emitted from

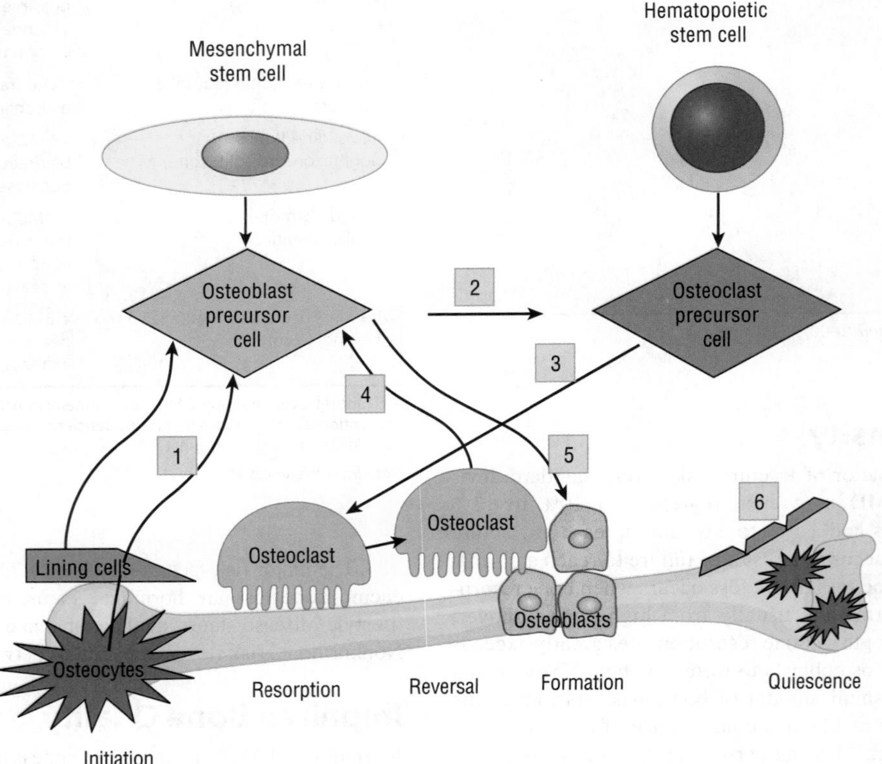

FIGURE 73-2 Bone remodeling cycle.[19,21–26] *A*. Overview of remodeling process: step 1, initiation; steps 2 and 3, resorption; step 4, reversal; step 5, formation; and step 6, quiescence.

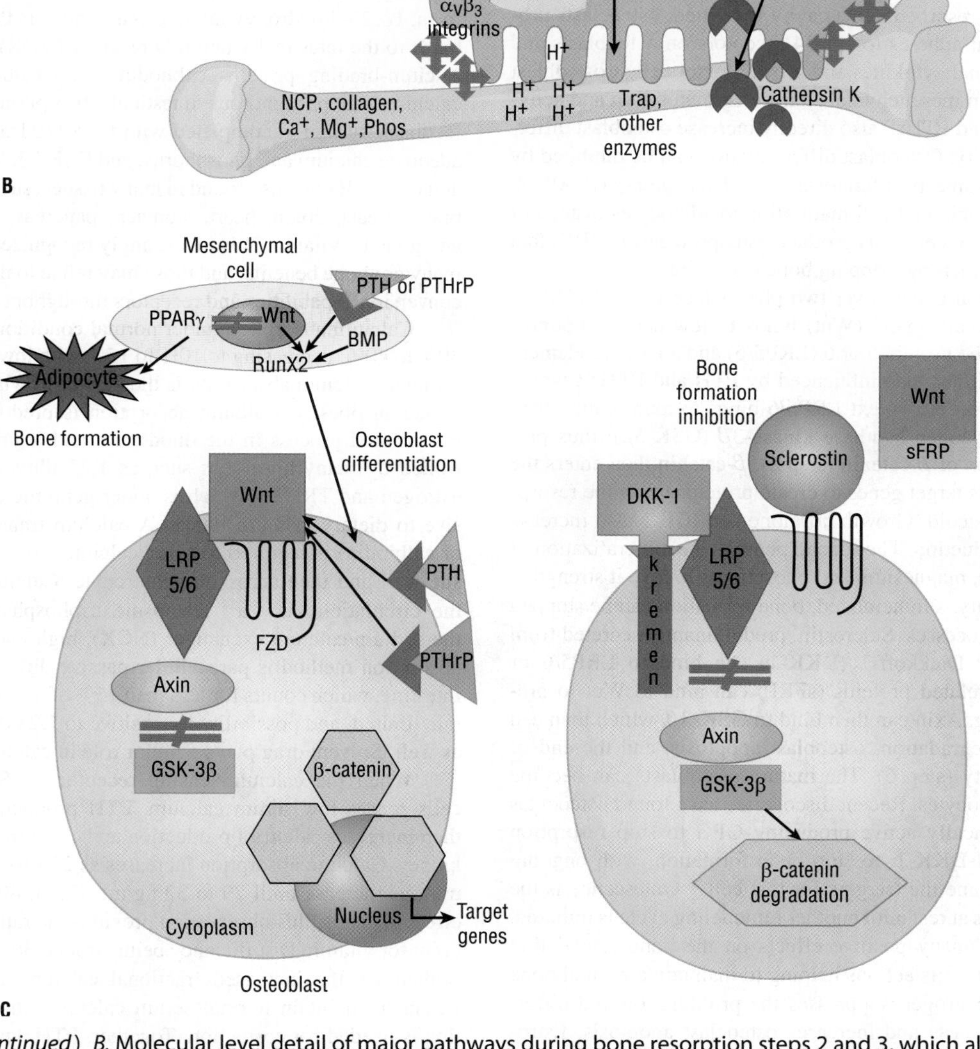

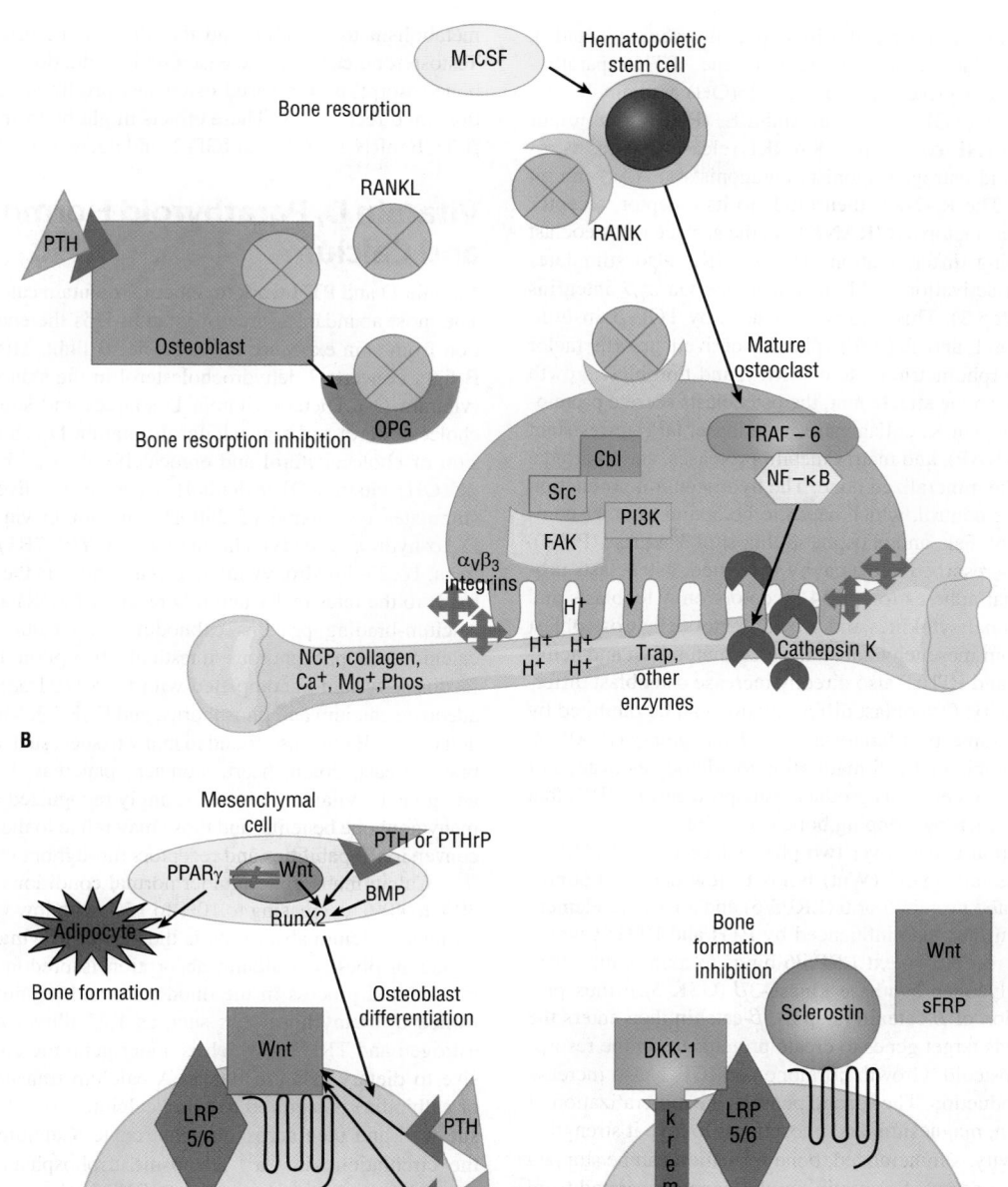

FIGURE 73-2 (*Continued*) *B*. Molecular level detail of major pathways during bone resorption steps 2 and 3, which also showcase drug targets for approved and investigational agents. (Ca^+, calcium ion; Cbl, a ubiquitin ligase; FAK, focal adhesion kinase; H^+, hydrogen ion; M-CSF, macrophage colony-stimulating factor; Mg^+, magnesium ion; NCP, noncollagenous protein; NF-κB, nuclear factor kappa B; OPG, osteoprotegerin; PI3K, phosphatidylinositol 3′-kinase; Phos, phosphorus; PTH, parathyroid hormone; RANK, receptor activator of nuclear factor-κB; RANKL, receptor activator of nuclear factor-κB ligand; src, tyrosine-protein kinase; TRAF-6, tumor necrosis factor receptor associated factor 6; Trap, tartrate-resistant acid phosphate.) *C*. Molecular level detail of major pathways during bone formation steps 4 and 5, which also showcase drug targets for approved and investigational agents. (BMP, bone morphogenetic protein; DKK-1, Dickkoff-1; FZD, frizzled element; GSK-3β, glycogen synthase kinase-3β; LRP5/6, lipoprotein receptor-related protein 5 or 6; PPAR-γ, peroxisome proliferator-activated receptor-γ; PTH, parathyroid hormone; PTHrP, parathyroid hormone-related protein; runX2, runt-related transcription factor; sFRP, secreted frizzled related protein; Wnt, wingless tail ligand.)

the osteoblast (bone-forming cells) in step 2. Interleukin 1 and 6, colony-stimulating factor, parathyroid hormone (PTH), parathyroid hormone-related protein (PTHrP), 1,25(OH) vitamin D, tissue growth factor-β (TGF-β), prostaglandin E_2 (PGE_2), and tumor necrosis factor-α (TNF-α) stimulate RANKL release whereas estrogen, calcitonin, and estrogen agonists antagonists (EAAs) inhibit RANKL release. The RANKL then binds to its receptor, receptor activator of nuclear factor-κB (RANK), on the surface of osteoclast precursors initiating differentiation. The RANKL also stimulates mature osteoclast activation and bone adherence via $\alpha_v\beta_3$ integrins to resorb bone (step 3). This step is influenced by TGF-β, insulin-like growth factor-1 and 2 (IGF), platelet derived growth factor (PDGF), bone morphometric protein (BMP), and fibroblast growth factor (FGF). After bone attachment, the osteoclasts secrete proteinases, such as cathepsin K, collagenase, gelatinase, tartrate-resistant acid phosphate (TRAP), and matrix metalloproteases, and hydrogen ions to dissolve the mineralized bone. The hydrogen ion production is under src kinase control, which needs to be bound to other compounds such as Cbl, Fak, and phosphatidylinositol 3′-kinase (P13K).

After bone is resorbed and a cavity is created, osteoclasts produce ephrinB2 that adheres to ephB4 receptors on osteoblasts and along with additional cytokines and growth factors elicit osteoblast differentiation from mesenchymal stem cells, maturation and activity (step 4). PTH and PTHrP also directly increase osteoblast differentiation and activity. Osteoblast differentiation can be inhibited by leptin and peroxisome proliferator-activated receptor-γ (PPAR-γ), which direct mesenchymal cell maturation to adipocytes instead of osteoblasts. Mature osteoblasts produce osteoprotegerin (OPG) that binds to RANKL, thereby stopping bone resorption.

Bone formation occurs over two phases (see Fig. 73-2C).[22–25] First the wingless tail ligand (Wnt) binds to low-density lipoprotein receptor–related protein 5 or 6 (LRP5/6) and a frizzled element (FZD). Wnt function is also influenced by PTH and PTHrP, which fit into the same receptor. Next LRP5/6 binds to axin, which then cannot bind to glycogen synthase kinase-3β (GSK-3β), thus preventing degradation of β-catenin (step 5). β-catenin then enters the nucleus and signals target genes to create proteins to fill the resorption cavity with osteoid. Growth hormone and IGF-1 also increase bone collagen production. The second phase is the mineralization of bone with calcium, magnesium and phosphorus to give it strength.

Once the cavity is mineralized, bone formation can be stopped by at least three processes. Sclerostin, predominantly secreted from osteocytes, and/or Dickkoff-1 (DKK-1) can bind to LRP5/6 or secreted frizzled related proteins (sFRP) can bind to Wnt to prevent Wnt signaling. Axin can then bind to GSK-3β, which then can cause β-catenin degradation, osteoblast apoptosis, and the end of osteoblastic activity (step 6). The mature osteoblasts can become lining cells or osteocytes. Recent discoveries have found osteocytes to be very biologically active producing OPG to stop resorption and sclerostin and DKK-1, to stop bone formation, with ongoing research to determine the triggers for this cell.[25] Quiescence is the phase when bone is at rest until another remodeling cycle is initiated.

Estrogen has many positive effects on the bone remodeling process, with most of its actions helping to maintain a normal bone resorption rate.[21] Estrogen suppresses the proliferation and differentiation of osteoclasts and increases osteoclast apoptosis. Estrogen decreases the production of several cytokines that are potent stimulators of osteoclasts, including interleukins (ILs) 1 and 6, TNF-α, and macrophage colony-stimulating factor (M-CSF), and increases TGF-α, which increases osteoclast apoptosis. Estrogen also decreases the production of RANKL, increases the production of OPG and TGF-α, which reduce osteoclastogenesis. Osteoclast apoptosis increases by activating Fas/FasL signaling.

Testosterone's role in bone health is becoming more apparent with recent identification of some direct effects on bone resorption and osteoblasts.[21] Most of testosterone's bone effects relate to its metabolism to estradiol and the above bone effects of estrogens. Testosterone can also increase OPG production, which will inhibit bone resorption. Increased osteoblast proliferation and differentiation are direct effects. These effects might be from increasing TGF-β, TGF mRNA, FGF, and IGF-2, and decreasing IL-6.

Vitamin D, Parathyroid Hormone, and Calcium

Vitamin D and PTH work together to maintain calcium homeostasis. The most abundant source of vitamin D is the endogenous production from skin exposure to ultraviolet B light. The sun's ultraviolet B light converts 7-dehydrocholesterol in the skin to cholecalciferol (vitamin D_3). Dietary vitamin D sources and supplements include cholecalciferol and ergocalciferol (vitamin D_2). Subsequent conversion of cholecalciferol and ergocalciferol to 25-hydroxyvitamin D [25(OH) vitamin D] (calcidiol) occurs in the liver, and then PTH stimulates conversion of 25(OH) vitamin D via 25(OH) vitamin D-1α-hydroxylase (cytochrome P450 [CYP]27B1) to its final active form, 1α,25-dihydroxyvitamin D (calcitriol), in the kidney. Calcitriol binds to the intestinal vitamin D receptor (VDR) and then increases calcium-binding proteins calmodulin and calbindin. As a result, calcium and phosphorous intestinal absorption is increased. The feedback system is completed with CYP27B1 activity inhibited by adequate calcium and phosphorus, and FGF-23. Vitamin D receptors and CYP27B1 are also found in many tissues, such as bone, intestine, brain, breast, colon, heart, stomach, pancreas, lymphocytes, skin, and gonads. Vitamin D is increasingly recognized as contributing to many nonbone benefits, and those may relate to the presence of these conversion capabilities and receptors throughout the body.

Calcium absorption under normal conditions is approximately 30% to 40%, decreasing to 10% to 15% with low vitamin D concentrations. Calcium absorption is thus lower in winter and is reported higher in obesity. Calcium absorption is predominantly an active rate-limited process in the duodenum and jejunum, which is controlled by many hormones such as 1,25 dihydroxyvitamin D and estrogen and TRPV6, which is under genomic control and responsive to dietary calcium intake. A calcium transporter (calmodulin or calbindin) is required to bring calcium from the gut into the tissue wall and then across the enterocyte. Calcium is extruded into the circulation via Ca^{2+} adenosine triphosphatase (ATPase) and the sodium/calcium exchanger (NCX), high energy steps. Another absorption method is paracellular passive diffusion throughout the intestine, which counts for less than 15% of absorbed calcium, is not rate limited, and possibility is sensitive to 1,25 dihydroxyvitamin D as well. Solvent drag plays a minor role in calcium absorption.

When the calcium-sensing receptor (CaSR) on parathyroid cells senses low serum calcium, PTH production increases. PTH then increases calcitriol production and calcium reabsorption by the kidney. Calcium absorption increases as 25(OH) vitamin D concentrations increase until 29 to 32 ng/mL (72 to 80 nmol/L) when the effect plateaus; this observation provides the rationale for the cutoff point for vitamin D sufficiency being around 30 ng/mL (75 nmol/L). Sometimes the increased fractional calcium absorption is insufficient to maintain normal serum calcium, and thus bone resorption is needed for correction. Together, PTH and calcitriol increase RANKL and osteoclast activity, thereby releasing calcium from bone to restore calcium homeostasis.

Osteoporosis pathophysiology depends on sex, age, diet, genetics, and presence of secondary causes.

Postmenopausal Osteoporosis

Estrogen deficiency causes significant bone density loss and compromises bone architecture. Estrogen deficiency increases proliferation, differentiation, and activation of new osteoclasts and prolongs survival of mature osteoclasts.[21] Interleukins, prostaglandin E_2, TNF-α, and interferon γ also increase resulting in more RANKL and less OPG. Loss of estrogen also increases calcium excretion and decreases calcium gut absorption through decreases in TRPV6 activity and 1,25 dihydroxyvitamin D binding proteins.[27] The results of this deficiency can also be seen in other settings such as anorexia nervosa and during lactation, and with medications such as prolonged depot medroxyprogesterone acetate implants, aromatase inhibitors and gonadotropin releasing hormone agonists.[14,21]

During menopause, trabecular bone is most susceptible, leading to vertebral and wrist fractures. Accelerated bone loss begins during perimenopause and continues for 3 to 4 years after menopause from bone resorption exceeding formation.[1,20] During this time annual bone loss can be as high as 2%, with total BMD loss due to menopause approximately 6% to 7%.[1,20] The number of remodeling sites increases, and resorption pits are deeper and inadequately filled by normal osteoblastic function.

Male Osteoporosis

Male bone also decreases with decreased testosterone.[3,6,21,28,29] Men do not undergo a period of accelerated bone resorption similar to menopause, but slowly decreasing testosterone concentrations with aging and or conditions or medications causing hypogonadism cause bone loss. Although the major effect of low testosterone is the loss of metabolism to estradiol, some direct positive bone effects are loss as well. Men are at a lower risk for developing osteoporosis and osteoporotic fractures because of larger bone size, greater peak bone mass, increase in bone width with aging, fewer falls, and shorter life expectancy. However, mortality rate after a fracture is greater for men than women.

The etiology of male osteoporosis tends to be multifactorial (see Tables 73-2 and 73-3). Most common risk factors for men are smoking, low body weight, weight loss, age, long-term glucocorticoid use, androgen deprivation therapy, and low testosterone concentrations.[3]

Age-Related Osteoporosis

Age-related osteoporosis occurs in older adults because of accelerated bone turnover rate and reduced osteoblast bone formation.[30] These bone changes result from hormone,[31] calcium,[27] and vitamin D[27] deficiencies and/or changes in their absorption and metabolism, decreased production or function of cytokines or other bone biochemicals, increases in redox status and free radical formation, increases in adipocytes, telomere shortening, and less exercise. Approximately 0.5% BMD is loss each year after age 60 years.[8] Fracture risk for a given BMD value increases with aging. Hip fracture risk rises dramatically in older adults as a consequence of the cumulative loss of cortical and trabecular bone and an increased risk for falls. Aging is associated with muscle changes as well, resulting in weakness, balance instability, and greater likelihood of falls.[31]

Secondary Causes of Osteoporosis

❶ Osteoporosis often has secondary causes (see Tables 73-2 and 73-3).[1,6,8,10–15] Symptoms, initial screening laboratory test results, medication profile review, and or an elevated Z-score from a dual-energy absorptiometry (DXA) test can suggest a secondary cause could be present, warranting more comprehensive workups.

CLINICAL PRESENTATION

Osteoporosis is diagnosed by BMD measurement or presence of a fragility fracture. Many vertebral fractures are asymptomatic, with patients sometimes attributing mild lower back pain to "old age."

CLINICAL PRESENTATION

General

- Many patients are unaware they have osteoporosis until testing for a fracture.
- Fractures can occur after bending, lifting, or falling, or independent of any activity.

Symptoms

- Frequently asymptomatic
- Pain
- Immobility
- Depression, fear, and low self-esteem from physical limitations and deformities

Signs

- Shortened stature (>1.5-inch [3.81-cm] loss), kyphosis, or lordosis
- Atraumatic vertebral, hip, wrist, or forearm fracture

Laboratory Tests

- Routine tests: complete blood count, metabolic profile, creatinine, calcium, phosphorous, electrolytes, alkaline phosphatase, albumin, 25(OH) vitamin D, thyroid-stimulating hormone, total testosterone (for men), and 24-hour urine concentrations of calcium and creatinine. Twenty-four hour urine concentrations of phosphorous and protein are sometimes assessed.
- Bone turnover markers (e.g., urinary or serum NTX, serum CTX, serum P1NP) are sometimes used, especially to determine if high bone turnover exists.
- Additional testing if the patient's history, physical examination, or initial laboratory and or diagnostic tests suggest a specific secondary cause (e.g., intact parathyroid hormone, free testosterone, serum protein electrophoresis, serum parathyroid, celiac panel).

Other Diagnostic Tests

- Spine and hip bone-density measurement using central dual-energy x-ray absorptiometry (DXA)
- Vertebral fracture assessment (VFA) with DXA technology
- Radiograph ordered for other reasons that shows low bone density
- Radiograph to confirm fracture
- Balance and mobility tests

CTX, C-terminal crosslinking telopeptide of type 1 collagen; NTX, N-terminal crosslinking telopeptide of type 1 collagen; P1NP, procollagen type 1 N-terminal propeptide.

From references 1, 6, 8, 10, 20, 37, and 38.

Some fractures present with moderate-to-severe back pain that radiates down the leg after a new vertebral fracture. The pain usually subsides significantly after 2 to 4 weeks; however, residual chronic lower back pain can persist. Multiple vertebral fractures decrease height and sometimes curve the spine (kyphosis or lordosis) with or without significant back pain. Patients who have experienced a nonvertebral fracture frequently present with severe pain, swelling, and reduced function and mobility at the fracture site.

Consequences of Osteoporosis

A fragility fracture is defined as one that occurs as a result of a fall from standing height or less or with minimal to no trauma, sometimes referred to as atraumatic fracture. Fractures of the vertebrae, hip, forearm, or humerus are considered major osteoporotic fractures. Fractures of the face, skull, fingers, and toes are typically not considered osteoporosis-related. Osteoporotic fractures can lead to increased morbidity and mortality and decreased quality of life. Depression is common because of fear, pain, loss of self-esteem from physical deformity, and loss of independence and mobility.

Symptomatic vertebral fractures can cause significant pain, physical deformity, and adverse health consequences. Patients with severe kyphosis can experience respiratory problems as a result of compression of the thoracic region and gastrointestinal complications, such as poor nutrition, from intraabdominal compression. Women and men who suffer a symptomatic vertebral fracture have a lower survival rate compared with those without a fracture history.[7]

Wrist fractures occur more commonly in younger postmenopausal women and are frequently a result of a fall on an outstretched hand. Negative outcomes include prolonged pain and weakness, and decreased instrumental, (advanced) activities of daily living (such as cooking and shopping).

Hip fractures are associated with the greatest increase in morbidity and mortality. In 2007, hip fractures resulted in approximately 281,000 hospital admissions in those age 65 and older.[32] After a hip fracture, only 50% of patients regain their ability to perform basic activities of daily living, while 20% become nonambulatory.[33] Of patients age 50 and over, almost one-quarter die within 1 year either from complications of the hip fracture or other comorbid disease processes.[2] Men have a twofold higher 1-year mortality rate after hip fracture than women.

Once a low-trauma fracture has occurred, the risk for subsequent fractures goes up exponentially. Peri- or post-menopausal women with a history of fracture have double the risk of a subsequent fracture compared to women without a fracture history.[1] In older women with two or more vertebral fractures, the risk of a new fracture is 12-fold higher, than for subjects who did not have baseline fractures.

PATIENT ASSESSMENT

Bone pain, postural changes (i.e., kyphosis), and loss of height are simple useful physical examination findings. A height loss greater than 1.5 inches (3.8 cm) from the tallest mature height is considered significant and warrants further investigation.[34,35] Height should be routinely measured using a wall-mounted stadiometer. Proper technique is essential; height is frequently measured incorrectly.[36] A spine radiograph can be obtained to confirm the presence of vertebral fractures. Low bone density or osteopenia reported on routine radiographs is a sign of significant bone loss and requires further evaluation for osteoporosis. In addition to physical examination and laboratory studies (see Clinical Presentation),[1,6,8,10,20,37,38] patients can be assessed with risk factor assessments, osteoporosis questionnaires, peripheral and central DXA or ultrasonography, and bone turnover biomarkers.[5]

Risk Factor Assessment

The aim of an initial osteoporosis risk assessment (see Table 73-1) is to identify those patients who are at highest risk for low bone density and who would benefit from further evaluation. Many risk factors for osteoporosis have been identified and are similar for both sexes. The majority of risk factors are predictors of either low BMD (e.g., female sex, ethnicity) or an increased fracture and fall risk (e.g., cognitive impairment, previous falls). The most important risk factors are those associated with fracture risk independent of BMD and fall risk. These major risk factors, in combination with BMD, are used to determine which patients are at greatest risk for fracturing and would benefit most from pharmacologic intervention.

❸ A fracture prediction model used for treatment risk stratification was developed for the World Health Organization (WHO).[9,39] The WHO model for the United States uses the following risk factors: age, race/ethnicity, sex, previous fragility fracture, parent history of hip fracture, body mass index, glucocorticoid use (current or past use for 3 or more months of prednisolone 5 mg daily or equivalent doses of other glucocorticoids), current smoking, alcohol use of three or more drinks per day, rheumatoid arthritis, and select secondary causes with femoral neck BMD data optional to predict an individual's percent probability of fracturing in the next 10 years. The WHO fracture risk assessment (FRAX) tool can be used to help predict fracture risk in patients who do not have access to DXA. The FRAX model should not be used to predict fracture risk in patients already on therapy for osteoporosis although under investigation. Some risk factors for fracture are not accommodated in the FRAX model.[9] For example, falls are a risk factor for fracture, but at this time researchers are unable to quantify the risk to add it to the model. Therefore, clinicians should use the FRAX model but also continue to assess all risk factors in an osteoporosis risk assessment.

Screening Using Peripheral Bone Mineral Density Devices

Peripheral bone density devices that use DXA (pDXA) or quantitative ultrasonography are helpful as screening tools to determine which patients require further evaluation with central DXA or for decision making if central DXA testing is not available.[34,35] pDXA of the forearm, heel, and finger uses a low amount of radiation and requires personnel with special training. Heel quantitative ultrasonography uses sound waves without radiation or need for special training. Heel ultrasonography has better fracture predictive value than pDXA. The specific peripheral T-score threshold for referral is not universally defined and varies by device. These tests should not be used for diagnosis or for monitoring response to therapy.

Because peripheral devices are considerably less expensive than central DXA, easy to use, portable, fast (<5 minutes), and can predict general fracture risk, they are very popular for screening patients at health fairs, community pharmacies, and clinics. No guidelines specifically address screenings, but it is reasonable to limit use to postmenopausal women and men 65 years and older for whom results are predictive of future fracture risk.[7,35] Healthy premenopausal women generally should not be screened. Patients already identified as being at high risk for osteoporosis based on risk factors, fragility fracture, or secondary causes for osteoporosis should not be screened but rather referred to a physician for central DXA testing.

Central Dual-Energy X-ray Absorptiometry

❸ BMD measurements at the hip or spine (or radius if these bones cannot be scanned) can be used to assess fracture risk, establish the diagnosis and severity of osteoporosis, and sometimes confirm osteoporosis as causative for low-trauma fractures.[1,6–8,35] Central DXA is considered the gold standard for measuring BMD because of its high precision, short scan times, low radiation dose (comparable to the average daily dose from natural background), and stable calibration. Measurement of lumbar spine, proximal femur, and total hip BMD is recommended with the lowest BMD value used for diagnosis. Newer methods, such as micromagnetic resonance imaging, are undergoing investigation to provide measurements of bone quality in addition to bone density.

Several consensus guidelines or position statements are consistent in recommending central BMD testing for all women aged 65 years or older, men aged 70 years or older, postmenopausal women younger than 65 years of age and men 50 to 69 years old with risk factors for fracture, and patients with an identified secondary cause for bone loss. The United States Preventive Services Task Force agrees with respect to women 65 years and older, but for women between 50 to 65 years old, the task force recommends getting a DXA only for those women with a FRAX major osteoporotic fracture score ≥9.3%.[40] They feel data are inadequate to make recommendations for men. Patients with a fragility fracture do not need a DXA for an osteoporosis diagnosis, but the results are helpful for determining disease severity and as a baseline for monitoring therapy effects. The DXA results can help patients make decisions about the need for lifestyle changes and prescription osteoporosis medications. In the absence of a suspected or known secondary cause for osteoporosis or a history of a low-trauma fracture, central BMD testing is not recommended for children, premenopausal women, or men younger than 50 years of age.

A central DXA BMD report provides the actual bone density value, T-score, and Z-score.[34,35] The actual bone density value (g/cm^2) is most useful for serial monitoring of therapy response, which is typically performed 1 to 2 years after medication initiation. The T-score is used for diagnosis and is a comparison of the patient's measured BMD to the mean BMD of a healthy, young (20- to 29-year-old), sex-matched white reference population; no adjustments for race or ethnicity. The T-score is the number of standard deviations from the mean of the reference population. The Z-score is similar but compares the patient's BMD to the mean BMD for a healthy sex- and age-matched population. Patient-reported race or ethnicity should be used for the Z-score if available. A Z-score value of ≤ –2.0 is sometimes helpful in determining whether a secondary cause for osteoporosis is present and is used for diagnosis in children, premenopausal women, and men younger than 50 years of age. Followup monitoring for patients identified with normal or low bone density has not been clearly defined, but one study has suggested a recall period of 15 years for those with T-scores > –1.49, 5 years for T-scores between –1.50 and –1.99, and 1 year for T-score between –2.00 and –2.49.[41]

Using the spine DXA image, an assessment of morphometric vertebral fractures, the vertebral fracture assessment (VFA), can be calculated.[1,35] Each vertebra is assessed for compression (wedge, biconcave, and crush) and described as normal or mild (20% to 25%), moderate (25% to 40%), or severe (>40%) compression. This result becomes important for treatment decisions in patients with low bone mass. VFA is recommended in women >70 years old and in men >80 years old.[6,7,35] They further recommend testing in younger postmenopausal women and men with low bone mass (T-score –1.5 or below) or specific risk factors, such as loss of height.

Laboratory Tests

Laboratory testing (see Clinical Presentation) is used to identify secondary causes of bone loss.[1,6,10,20] If a preliminary investigation indicates a possible secondary cause, additional testing related to that specific secondary cause will be conducted.

Serum 25(OH) vitamin D is the best indicator of total body vitamin D status.[1,42,43] The cutpoints for normal, insufficiency, and deficiency are controversial.[43,44] Osteomalacia or severe vitamin D deficiency, which is discussed later in this chapter, can occur at concentrations less than 10 ng/mL (25 nmol/L).

Clinical **Controversy...**

The Institute of Medicine (IOM) defines 20 ng/mL (50 nmol/L; 1 ng/mL = 2.5 nmol/L) as the cutpoint for normal 25(OH) vitamin D,[44,45] below which would be considered a deficiency. However, some experts and guidelines advocate for a goal 25(OH) vitamin D concentration of 30 to 60 ng/mL (75 to 150 nmol/L) or 30 to 100 ng/mL (75 to 250 nmol/L), with concentrations between 20 and 29 ng/mL (50 to 72 nmol/L) considered insufficient and those less than 20 ng/mL (50 nmol/L) considered deficiency.[1,6–8,43] Guideline recommendations are based on data that suggest serum 25(OH) vitamin D concentrations necessary to maximize intestinal calcium absorption are ≥32 ng/mL (80 nmol/L), minimize secondary hyperparathyroidism are 28 to 45 ng/mL (70 to 112 nmol/L), and reduce fracture risk are 28 ng/mL (70 nmol/L) or greater, with some of these studies disputed or interpreted differently by others.[44]

Because vitamin D assays are fairly expensive and large interlaboratory assay variability exists, routine vitamin D screening cannot be recommended at this time. However, a 25(OH) vitamin D concentration should be considered in anyone at higher risk for low vitamin D (e.g., older adults, patients who are obese or who have minimal sun exposure, insufficient vitamin D intake, dark-pigmented skin, or certain medical conditions especially liver and kidney disease, or are on medications known to affect vitamin D metabolism), and patients with low bone density, history of a low-trauma fracture or frequent falls, or history of unexplained muscle weakness and/or bone pain.[42]

Bone Turnover Markers

Increased concentrations of bone resorption markers (≥2 standard deviations above the premenopausal range) have been shown in some studies to predict fracture risk; however, results have been inconsistent.[38] Bone turnover markers are commonly used in clinical trials and have documented responses to therapy and predictive of fracture prevention in some but not all studies.

Clinical utility is less since analytical and patient variability (within patient variability 26% to 43%) limit interpretation and accuracy. Circadian variability, seasonal variations, food intake, and recent exercise can all affect results. Although not diagnostic, these tests might be helpful in identifying accelerated bone turnover and increased fracture risk; however, most of these data are derived from osteoporosis studies in women. Bone turnover markers could be used to monitor therapy effects. Response to therapy can be measured as early as 2 to 3 months, but their utility is less for zoledronic acid and denosumab.[1,6,37]

Urine and serum bone turnover markers are either enzymes or proteins produced during bone formation or breakdown.[1,6,37] Bone-specific alkaline phosphatase, osteocalcin, and procollagen type 1 propeptides (P1NP) are examples of bone formation markers. Hydroxypyridinium crosslinks of collagen pyridinoline and deoxypyridinoline, C-terminal crosslinking telopeptide of type 1 collagen (CTX), and N-terminal crosslinking telopeptide of type 1 collagen (NTX) are examples of bone resorption markers. CTX and P1NP, newer tests that are more accurate, are becoming the preferred tests. For serum markers, fasting morning samples should be obtained with repeat tests done at the same facility with the same assay.

DIAGNOSIS OF OSTEOPOROSIS

The diagnosis of osteoporosis is based on a low-trauma fracture or central hip and/or spine DXA using WHO T-score thresholds. Low bone mass (which is the preferred term) or osteopenia is a T-score between −1 and −2.5, and osteoporosis is a T-score at or below −2.5.[1,6–8,34,35] Although these definitions are based on data from postmenopausal white women, they are also applied to perimenopausal women, men age 50 years and older, and adults from different races and ethnicities. The diagnosis of osteoporosis in children, premenopausal women, and men younger than 50 years of age should be based on a Z-score at or below −2.0 in combination with other risk factors or fracture.[34,35] Children are not given a diagnosis of osteoporosis; "low BMD for chronological age" is the preferred term.[34]

PREVENTION AND TREATMENT
Osteoporosis

The foundation for osteoporosis prevention and treatment is a bone healthy lifestyle beginning at birth and continuing throughout life. Supplements and medications are used when lifestyle habits are suboptimal and/or osteoporosis has developed.

Desired Outcomes

The primary goal of osteoporosis care should be prevention. Optimizing skeletal development and peak bone mass accrual in childhood, adolescence, and early adulthood will ultimately reduce the future incidence of osteoporosis. Once low bone mass or osteoporosis develops, the objective is to stabilize or improve bone mass and strength and prevent fractures. In patients who have already suffered osteoporotic fractures, reducing pain and deformity, improving functional capacity, improving quality of life, and reducing future falls and fractures are the main goals.

General Approach to Prevention and Treatment

4 5 A bone-healthy lifestyle should begin at birth and continue throughout life. Insuring adequate intakes of calcium and vitamin D along with other bone-healthy lifestyle practices are the first steps in prevention and treatment. Recent guidelines and position statements recommend considering prescription therapy in any postmenopausal woman or man age 50 years and older presenting with one of the following scenarios: a hip or vertebral fracture; T-score of −2.5 or lower at the femoral neck, total hip or spine; or low bone mass (T-score between −1.0 and −2.5 at the femoral neck or spine) with a 10-year probability of hip fracture of 3% or more, or a 10-year probability of any major osteoporosis-related fracture of 20% or more.[1,6–8] Figure 73-3 provides an osteoporosis management algorithm for postmenopausal women and men 50 years and older that incorporates both nonpharmacologic and pharmacologic approaches.

Nonpharmacologic Therapy

4 Nonpharmacologic therapy, referred to as a bone-healthy lifestyle, includes proper nutrition, moderation of alcohol intake, smoking cessation, exercise, and fall prevention. A bone healthy lifestyle that is employed early in life will help to optimize peak bone mass and if continued throughout life, it will minimize bone loss over time. Not only does a bone healthy lifestyle target BMD, but it also contributes to decreasing the risk of falls and fragility fractures.

Diet

Overall, a diet well balanced in nutrients and minerals and limited in salt, alcohol, caffeine, and excessive protein is important for bone health.[1,6,46] Certain nutrients are emerging to have direct and indirect effects on bone.[26,46,47] Being thin or having anorexia nervosa are well known to decrease bone mass. In the past, obesity was thought protective because of increased estrogen production and stimulating bone remodeling due to weight bearing; however, emerging literature suggests leptin and adipose have negative impacts on bone health.[26,48]

Calcium 6 Data clearly indicate that adequate calcium intake is necessary for the development of bone mass during growth and for its maintenance throughout life.[2,55] Adequate calcium intake is an essential component of all osteoporosis prevention and treatment strategies. Table 73-4[6–8,45] summarizes the recommended intakes for calcium based on age.[27] This value represents the amount needed for 97.5% of the population; higher amounts might be needed when concomitant diseases and medications negatively affect calcium homeostasis. Using calcium-containing foods, which also contain other essential nutrients, is the preferred method to achieve daily calcium requirements. Milk and other dairy products have the highest amount of calcium per serving and are available in low-fat options.[27] Some food sources are absorbed well but have low elemental calcium content (e.g., broccoli). Carbohydrates, fat, and lactose increase calcium absorption whereas fiber, wheat bran, phytates (e.g., beans), oxylates (e.g., spinach, rhubarb), high-protein diets, caffeine, and smoking decrease absorption. To get the same amount of calcium in one 8-ounce (~240 mL) glass of milk, one would need to eat 2.25 cups (~530 mL) of cooked broccoli or 8 cups (~1900 mL) of cooked spinach.

People should be encouraged to evaluate their food and beverage intake to determine if they are receiving adequate intakes. To calculate the amount of calcium in a serving of food, consumers can add a zero to the percentage of the daily value listed on food labels. For example, a serving of milk (8 oz. [~240 mL]) has 30% of the daily value of calcium. This translates to 300 mg calcium per serving.

Approximately 25% of the U.S. population has some level of lactose intolerance, with the incidence in Asian (80%) and African American (50%) populations being much higher than in whites (10%).[57] Lactose-intolerant patients have several options, including products containing lactase (Lactaid), lactose-reduced milk, lactose-free milk, calcium-fortified soy milk, certain aged cheeses, or yogurt with active cultures along with other nondairy calcium-fortified products (e.g., orange juice, breakfast cereals, and energy bars).

Vitamin D 7 Table 73-4 lists the recommended adequate intakes for Vitamin D.[45] The three main sources of vitamin D are sunlight (cholecalciferol, vitamin D_3), diet, and supplements.[42,43] Vitamin D_3 comes from oily fish, eggs, and fortified dairy products. Vitamin D_2 comes from fungi and eggs. Websites can be used to identify the few foods high in vitamin D.[61] To calculate the amount of vitamin D in a serving of food, multiply the percent daily value of vitamin D listed on the food label by 4 (e.g., 20% vitamin D = 80 units).

Inadequate concentrations of vitamin D are common in all age groups, especially in older adults and individuals who are malnourished or obese, live in an institution (e.g., nursing home), or live in more northern latitudes. Low vitamin D concentrations result from insufficient intake, dietary fat malabsorption, decreased sun exposure, decreased skin production, or decreased liver and renal metabolism. Endogenous synthesis of vitamin D can be decreased by factors that affect exposure to or decrease skin penetration of ultraviolet B light. Sunscreen use, full body coverage with clothing (e.g., women wearing veiled, full-length dresses), and darkly pigmented skin can all cause a decrease in vitamin D production.

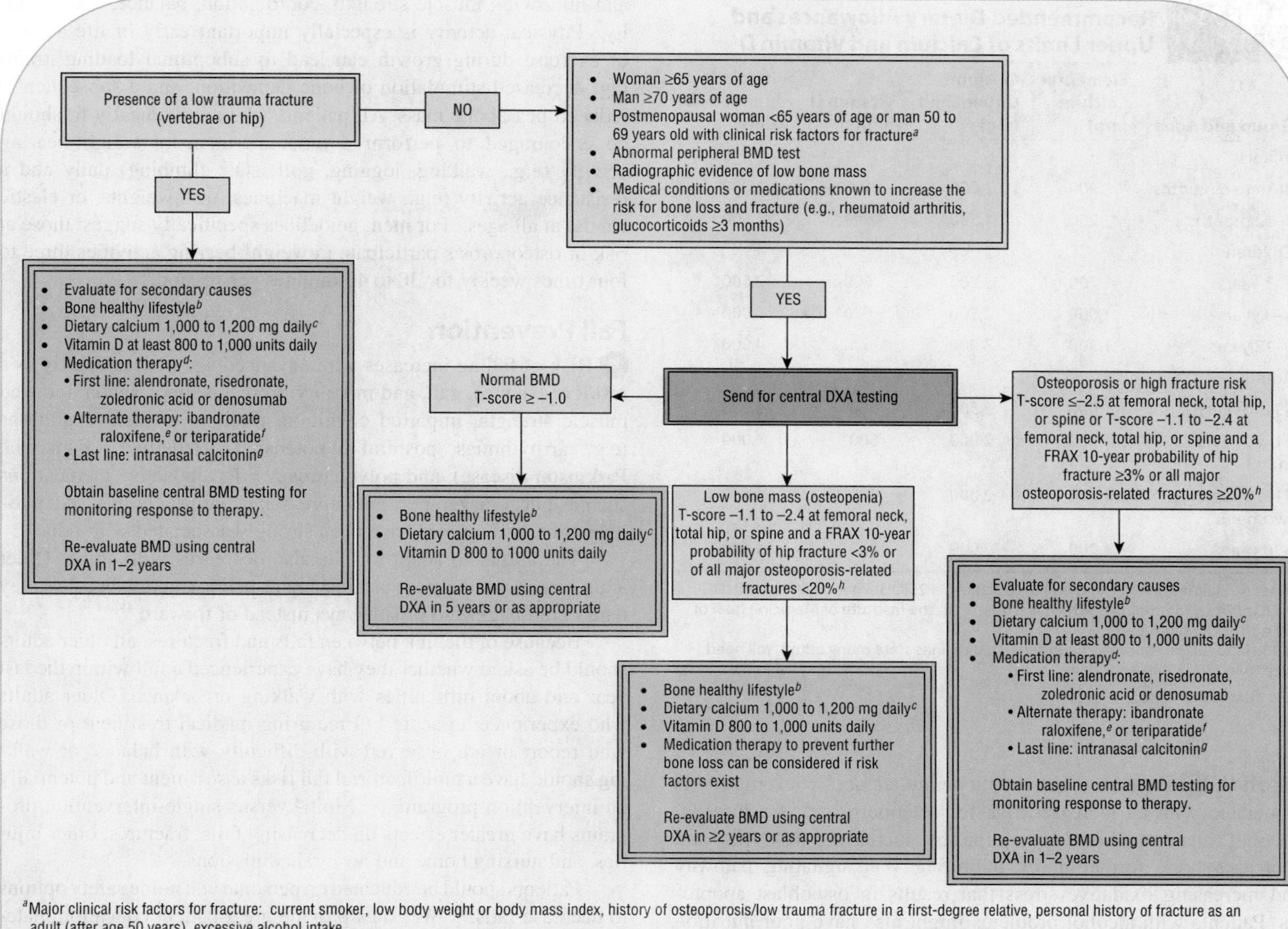

FIGURE 73-3 Algorithm for the management of osteoporosis in postmenopausal women and men aged 50 and older.[1,6–8] (BMD, bone mineral density; DXA, dual-energy x-ray absorptiometry; FRAX, WHO absolute fracture risk assessment tool; WHO, World Health Organization.)

Seasonal variations in vitamin D concentrations are also seen with nadirs in late winter and peaks in late summer. Because few foods are naturally high or fortified with vitamin D, most people, especially older adults, require supplementation.

Other Nutrients and Minerals Vitamin K is a cofactor for carboxylation (activation) of proteins, such as osteocalcin, which are involved in bone formation.[1,13] Vitamin K deficiency can contribute to bone loss and increase fracture risk. Although some vitamin K supplement studies in osteoporosis reported reduced bone loss and fracture risk, data are conflicting and insufficient to recommend routine supplementation. Patients on warfarin should either use calcium products without vitamin K or use supplements with vitamin K consistently after discussion with their healthcare provider. Insufficient to no data exist for routinely using or supplementing other nutrients and minerals such as potassium, boron, magnesium, and vitamins B, C, and E.[1,13] Nutrition research continues to identify more foods that improve bone health, potentially by inhibiting oxidative stress's negative impacts on bone remodeling, increasing BMP and Wnt signaling to increase bone formation, and altering the conversion of mesenchymal cells via PPAR-γ from adipocytes to osteoblasts.[26]

Isoflavones Isoflavone phytoestrogens are plant-derived compounds that possess weak estrogenic agonist and antagonist effects throughout the body.[49] The most common source for isoflavones is dietary soy products. Genistein is the most abundant and biologically active isoflavone in soybeans. Isoflavones are also available as a supplement or part of a calcium combination product. The evidence supporting a positive bone benefit from isoflavone (soy protein or supplements) intake is conflicting[1,49]; however, meta-analyses of randomized placebo-controlled studies have found foods and supplements with at least 75 mg isoflavones increased spine, but not hip, BMD when compared with placebo.[50] Isoflavones from soy foods appear safe, but more information is needed, especially in women with breast cancer and regarding use from supplements.

TABLE 73-4 Recommended Dietary Allowances and Upper Limits of Calcium and Vitamin D

Group and Ages	Elemental Calcium (mg)	Calcium Upper Limit (mg)	Vitamin D (units)[a]	Vitamin D Upper Limit (units)
Infants				
Birth to 6 months	200	1,000	400	1,000
6–12 months	260	1,500	400	1,500
Children				
1–3 years	700	2,500	600	2,500
4–8 years	1,000	2,500	600	3,000
9–18 years	1,300	3,000	600	4,000
Adults				
19–50 years	1,000	2,500	600[b]	4,000
51–70 years (men)	1,000	2,000	600[b]	4,000
51–70 years (women)	1,200	2,000	600[b]	4,000
>70 years	1,200	2,000	800[b]	4,000

[a]Other guidelines recommend intake to achieve a 25(OH) vitamin D concentration of ≥30 ng/mL (75 nmol/L),[6,8] which is higher than the Institute of Medicine goal of ≥20 ng/mL (50 nmol/L).[45]

[b]2013 National Osteoporosis Foundation Guidelines state many adults will need more than 800–1,000 units daily.[7]

Data from reference 45.

Alcohol ❹ Excessive, but not moderate, alcohol consumption is associated with an increased risk for osteoporosis or fractures.[1,26] Alcohol increases bone resorption by increasing RANKL and decreases bone formation by inhibiting Wnt signaling pathway and increasing oxidative stress that results in osteoblast apoptosis. Patients with alcohol problems might also have poor nutrition and have balance impairments resulting in more falls and fractures. Alcohol consumption should not exceed one drink per day for women[1] and two drinks per day for men.[6]

Caffeine ❹ Although results are conflicting, excessive caffeine consumption is associated with increased calcium excretion, increased rates of bone loss, and a modestly increased risk for fracture.[46] Ideally, caffeine consumption should be limited to two servings or less per day. For those with greater intakes, the increased calcium excretion might be compensated by an additional 40 mg calcium intake for each cup of caffeine-containing beverage.

Smoking

❹ Counseling patients of all ages on smoking cessation can help to optimize peak bone mass, minimize bone loss, and ultimately reduce fracture risk.[51] Cigarette smoking is an independent risk factor for osteoporosis and is associated with up to an 80% increased relative risk for hip fracture.[2] The effect is dose and duration dependent. The negative bone effects resulting from poor nutrition and/or lower 25(OH) vitamin D concentrations are associated with reduced intestinal calcium absorption, an increase in bone resorption from a decrease in production and increase in metabolism of estradiol, increase in RANKL and decrease in OPG, decrease in osteoblasts and bone formation secondary to increase in cortisol and dehydroepiandrosterone sulfate (DHEA-S), and impairment of osteoid production and mineralization. The detrimental effects of smoking on neuromuscular function and balance may contribute to an increased risk of falls.

Exercise

❹ Physical activity or exercise is an important nonpharmacologic approach to preventing osteoporotic fractures. Exercise can decrease the risk of falls and fractures by stabilizing bone density and improving muscle strength, coordination, balance, and mobility.[2] Physical activity is especially important early in life as lack of exercise during growth can lead to suboptimal loading/straining, decreased stimulation of bone deposition, and a subsequently reduced peak bone mass. All patients who are medically fit should be encouraged to perform a moderate-intensity weight-bearing activity (e.g., walking, jogging, golf, stair climbing) daily and a resistance activity (e.g., weight machines, free weights, or elastic bands) at all ages.[7] For men, guidelines specifically suggest those at risk of osteoporosis participate in weight-bearing activities three to four times weekly for 30 to 40 minutes per session.[6]

Fall Prevention

❹ Risk of falling increases with advanced age predominantly as a result of balance, gait, and mobility problems, poor vision, reduced muscle strength, impaired cognition, multiple medical conditions (e.g., arrhythmias, postural hypotension, Alzheimer's dementia, Parkinson disease), and polypharmacy.[52] Psychoactive medications such as benzodiazepines, antidepressants, antipsychotics, sedative–hypnotics, and opioids have been strongly associated with falls.

The ability to adapt to falls also decreases with aging. Older adults are more likely to sustain a hip or pelvic fracture because they tend to fall backward or sideways instead of forward.[33]

Because of the link between falls and fractures, all older adults should be asked whether they have experienced a fall within the last year and about difficulties with walking or balance. Older adults who experience an acute fall requiring medical treatment or those who report or are observed with difficulty with balance or walking should have a multifactorial fall risks assessment and potentially an intervention program.[46,52] Multi- versus single-intervention programs have greater effects on decreasing falls, fractures, other injuries, and nursing home and hospital admissions.

Patients should be educated on personal and home safety options to decrease falls.[7,52] Websites provide great patient education materials with solutions for commonly observed safety problems.[32,53,54] Medication profiles should also be reviewed for any unnecessary medications that can affect cognition and balance and potentially increase fall risk. Consideration should be given to replacing high-risk medications with safer alternatives. Vitamin D supplementation has been associated with reduced falls.[42,43,52] Maintenance of a regular individualized exercise program, such as tai chi, should be recommended to improve body strength, balance, and agility.

Other recommendations include resolving vision, low blood pressure, heart rate and rhythm, and foot problems and using proper footwear.

External hip protectors are specialized undergarments designed to pad the area surrounding the hip, decreasing the force of impact from a sideways fall. Conflicting results and poor adherence limit their use.[1,46]

Pharmacologic Therapy

Because nonpharmacologic interventions alone are frequently insufficient to prevent or treat osteoporosis, medication therapy is often necessary. Table 73-5[1,8,55–58] describes fracture and BMD effects, Table 73-6 describes dosing of osteoporosis medications and Table 73-7 outlines adverse effects and monitoring. These medications should always be combined with a bone-healthy lifestyle.

Medication

Drug Treatments of First Choice

❽ Combined with adequate calcium and vitamin D intakes, alendronate, risedronate, zoledronic acid or denosumab are the prescription medication of choice based on evidence of reduced risk of hip and vertebral fractures.[1,7,58,59] Ibandronate, teriparatide, or

TABLE 73-5 Fracture and Bone Mineral Density Effects of Osteoporosis Medications from Pivotal Fracture Trials[a] in Postmenopausal Women

Medication	Vertebral Fracture (%)	Nonvertebral Fracture (%)	Hip Fracture (%)	Change in Spine BMD[b] (%)	Change in Hip BMD[b,c] (%)
Bazedoxifene	42↓	↔	↔	2.2↑	0.5↑
Bazedoxifene with conjugated equine estrogens	ND	ND	ND	0.5–2.3↑	0.2–1.5↑
Bisphosphonates	41–70↓	25–39↓[d]	40–51↓[e]	4.3–6.7↑	2.8–6.0↑
Calcitonin	33↓	↔	↔	0.7↑ (NS)	↔
Denosumab	68↓	20↓	40↓	9.2↑	6.0↑
Estrogen with or without progestogen	33–40↓	13–27↓	34↓	3.5–7↑[f]	1.7–4.1↑[f]
Raloxifene	30–42↓[g]	↔	↔	2.6↑	2.1↑
Teriparatide	65↓	53↓	↔	8.6↑	3.5↑

BMD, bone mineral density; ↓, decrease; ↑, increase; ↔, no significant change; ND, no data.

[a]Fracture reductions are relative risk reductions, no head-to-head fracture studies. Data should only be used for relative between class comparisons, clinical trials with different patient samples and study designs, most pivotal fracture trials 3 years' duration except for teriparatide studies (18 months).

[b]Relative to placebo.

[c]Total hip (alendronate, ibandronate, zoledronic acid, bazedoxifene, denosumab, estrogen, teriparatide) or femoral neck (calcitonin, estrogen, risedronate, raloxifene).

[d]Risedronate and zoledronic acid only; nonvertebral fracture reductions with ibandronate and alendronate were not significant.

[e]Alendronate, risedronate, and zoledronic acid only; hip fracture data not reported with ibandronate.

[f]Data obtained from nonpivotal fracture trials.

[g]In a pivotal bazedoxifene trial with raloxifene as one of the comparators.

Data from references 1, 8, 55–58, and 77.

TABLE 73-6 Dosing of Medications Used in Prevention and Treatment of Osteoporosis

Drug	Brand Name/Formulation	Dose	Comments
Antiresorptive Medications—Nutritional Supplements			
Calcium	Various	*Supplement dose* is the difference between adequate daily intake, which varies by age (200–1,300 mg/day; see Table 73-4), and dietary intake. Might need divided doses.	Available in different salts including carbonate and citrate and different formulations including chewable, liquid. Give calcium carbonate with meals to improve absorption.
Vitamin D D_3 (cholecalciferol)	Over the counter Tablets 400, 1000, and 2000 units Capsules 400, 1,000, 2,000, 5,000, 10,000, and 50,000 units Drops 400, 1,000, and 2,000 units/mL Solution 400 and 5,000 units/mL Spray 1,000 and 5,000 units/spray	*Adequate daily intake:* IOM: 400–800 units/day, varies by age, to achieve adequate intake (see Table 73-4); NOF: 800–1,000 units orally daily. If low 25(OH) vitamin D concentrations, malabsorption or multiple anticonvulsants might require higher doses (>2,000 units daily)	
D_2 (ergocalciferol)	Prescription Capsule 50,000 units Solution 8000 units/mL	*Vitamin D deficiency*: 50,000 units orally once to twice weekly for 8–12 weeks; repeat as needed until therapeutic concentrations	
Antiresorptive Prescription Medications			
Bisphosphonates			
Alendronate	Fosamax Binosto (effervescent tablet)	*Treatment*: 10 mg orally daily or 70 mg orally weekly *Prevention*: 5 mg orally daily or 35 mg orally weekly	70 mg dose is available as a tablet, effervescent tablet, or combination tablet with 2,800 or 5,600 units of vitamin D_3. Administered first thing in the morning on an empty stomach with 6–8 ounces (177–237 mL) of plain water. Do not eat and remain upright for at least 30 minutes following administration. Do not coadminister with any other medication or supplements, including calcium and vitamin D. Avoid if CL_{cr} <35 mL/min (0.58 mL/s)
Ibandronate	Boniva	*Treatment*: 150 mg orally monthly, 3 mg IV quarterly *Prevention*: 150 mg orally monthly	Administration instructions same as for alendronate, except must delay eating and remain upright for at least 60 minutes. Avoid if CL_{cr} <35 mL/min (0.58 mL/s)
Risedronate	Actonel Atelvia (delayed release)	*Treatment and Prevention*: 5 mg orally daily, 35 mg orally weekly, 150 mg orally monthly	Only 35-mg dose also available as a delayed-release product. Administration instructions same as for alendronate, except delayed-release product is taken immediately following breakfast. Avoid if CL_{cr} <30 mL/min (0.5 mL/s)
Zoledronic acid	Reclast	*Treatment*: 5 mg IV infusion yearly; *Prevention*: 5 mg IV infusion every 2 years	May premedicate with acetaminophen or NSAIDs to decrease infusion reaction. Contraindicated if CL_{cr} <35 mL/min (0.58 mL/s) Also marketed under the brand name Zometa with different dosing for prevention of skeletal-related events from bone metastases from solid tumors.

(*continued*)

TABLE 73-6 Dosing of Medications Used in Prevention and Treatment of Osteoporosis (*Continued*)

Drug	Brand Name/Formulation	Dose	Comments
RANK ligand inhibitor			
Denosumab	Prolia	*Treatment*: 60 mcg subcutaneously every 6 months	Administered by a healthcare practitioner. Correct hypocalcemia before administration. Also marketed under the brand name Xgeva with different dosing for prevention of skeletal-related events from bone metastases from solid tumors.
Estrogen agonist antagonist			
Raloxifene	Evista	60 mg daily	
Bazedoxifene	Viviant	20 mg daily	
Bazedoxifene with conjugated equine estrogens	Aprela	20 or 40 mg plus 0.45 or 0.625 mg conjugated equine estrogens daily	
Calcitonin			
Calcitonin (salmon)	Miacalcin Fortical	200 units (1 spray) intranasally daily, alternating nares every other day. 100 units subcutaneously daily	Refrigerate until opened for daily use, then room temperature. Prime with first use.
Formation Medication			
Recombinant human parathyroid hormone (PTH 1–34 units)			
Teriparatide	Forteo	20 mcg subcutaneously daily for up to 2 years	

CL_{cr}, creatinine clearance; IOM, Institute of Medicine; NOF, National Osteoporosis Foundation; NSAID, nonsteroidal antiinflammatory drug; PTH, parathyroid hormone; RANK, receptor activator of nuclear factor κB.

raloxifene are alternatives, and calcitonin is last-line therapy. Duration of bisphosphonate therapy has not been defined, but safety data exist for periods of 10 to 13 years (see below Clinical Controversy). Short-term (18 to 24 months) teriparatide is usually reserved for severe osteoporosis and then followed by bisphosphonate therapy. The algorithm (see Fig. 73-3) helps determine for whom medication therapy should be used. Osteoporosis prescription medications in children, pre- and perimenopausal women, and men younger than 50 years old are controversial and undergoing further investigation.

Published Guidelines and Treatment Protocols

The 2013 National Osteoporosis Foundation's clinician's guide,[7] the 2010 North American Menopause Society's position statement,[1] the American Association of Clinical Endocrinologists' guidelines for women[8] and men,[6] and the Agency for Healthcare Research and Quality[58] provide guidance on osteoporosis prevention and treatment strategies. Applying the National Osteoporosis Foundation's guidelines to a large clinical database, researchers found that approximately 72% of women ≥65 years old and 93% of women ≥75 years old would be eligible for treatment.[60] Even with guidelines and algorithms, many patients are not being evaluated or receiving appropriate osteoporosis therapy, even after a hip fracture.[61]

Drug Class Information

Antiresorptive Therapies

Antiresorptive therapies include calcium, vitamin D, bisphosphonates, estrogen agonists antagonists (known previously as selective estrogen receptor modulators or SERMs), calcitonin, denosumab, estrogen, and testosterone.

Calcium Supplementation ❻ Calcium imbalance can result from inadequate dietary intake, decreased fractional calcium absorption, or enhanced calcium excretion. Adequate calcium intake (see Table 73-4) is considered a foundation for osteoporosis prevention and treatment and should be combined with vitamin D and osteoporosis medications when needed.[45,58] Supplemental calcium intake will be needed in the majority of adults with or at risk for osteoporosis because the average U.S. adult diet contains only 590 to 730 mg calcium per day.[1,62] The amount of the supplement needed is the difference between an individual's dietary consumption and the recommended dietary allowance.

Efficacy Calcium increases BMD, but its BMD effects are less than other antiresorptive and formation osteoporosis medications.[27,58,63] Almost all trials and observational studies showed the children and adults with the higher calcium intakes had greater increases or maintenance of BMD compared to BMD losses with placebo. Calcium's independent role in fracture prevention is less clear. Fracture prevention is only documented with concomitant vitamin D therapy, and some studies were also confounded by poor patient adherence. While there may be insufficient evidence to assess the effect of calcium alone on fractures, it is important to note that clinical trials for the antiosteoporosis medications included adequate calcium intake through supplementation as a part of the study design.

Adverse Events Calcium's most common adverse reaction, constipation, can first be treated with increased water intake, dietary fiber, and exercise. If still unresolved, smaller and more frequent administration or a lower total daily dose can be tried. Calcium carbonate can create gas and cause stomach upset, which might resolve with calcium citrate, a product with fewer GI side effects.

The upper tolerable limit for calcium ranges from 2,000 to 3,000 mg/day depending on age.[45] Calcium supplementation rarely causes kidney stones.[27] Some patients with a history of kidney stones can still ingest adequate amounts of calcium depending on the type of stones and/or will require increased fluid intake and decreased salt intake with their calcium supplementation.[64] Observational data also suggest that calcium supplementation may be linked to a small increased risk of myocardial infarction in women.[65–67] After this chapter was prepared, a similar study demonstrated a similar effect in men and another study provided additional data for women (see Addendum at the end of the text). Because calcium supplements are not without adverse effects and risks, clinicians should encourage dietary calcium and ensure that patients are not getting more than they need.

Drug Interactions Because calcium carbonate requires acid for absorption, drugs such as the proton pump inhibitors may decrease absorption from the carbonate product. Fiber laxatives may decrease

TABLE 73-7 Monitoring of Medications Used in Prevention and Treatment of Osteoporosis

Drug	Adverse Drug Reaction	Monitoring Parameter	Comments
Antiresorptive Medications—Nutritional Supplements			
Calcium	Constipation, gas, upset stomach. *Rare*: kidney stones.	Dietary calcium intake, constipation	Education about a bowel healthy lifestyle (e.g., adequate water, fiber, and exercise).
Vitamin D	Hypercalcemia, (weakness, headache, somnolence, nausea, cardiac rhythm disturbance), hypercalciuria.	Serum 25(OH) vitamin D concentration	Concentrations should be at least 20–30 ng/mL (50–75 nmol/L) and below 50–100 ng/mL (125–250 nmol/L). See text and Table 73-4 for discussion.
Antiresorptive Prescription Medications			
Bisphosphonates			
Bisphosphonates	Transient musculoskeletal pain, nausea, dyspepsia (oral), transient flu-like illness (injectable). *Rare*: GI perforation, ulceration, and/or bleeding (oral); osteonecrosis of the jaw; atypical femoral shaft fracture, severe musculoskeletal pain.	Bone density, fractures, serum calcium for injectable products	Pregnancy category C for alendronate, risedronate, and ibandronate. Pregnancy category D for zoledronic acid. Adherence is suboptimal, thus should be frequently assessed.
RANK ligand inhibitor			
Denosumab	Flatulence, eczema, cellulitis, and infection. *Rare*: osteonecrosis of the jaw.	Serum calcium, bone density, fractures	Pregnancy category X. REMS: Medication guide and monitoring plan due to risks of serious infections, dermatologic adverse reactions, and suppression of bone turnover.
Estrogen agonist antagonist			
Raloxifene	Hot flushes, leg pain, spasms, or cramps, peripheral edema, venous thromboembolism (warm swollen leg, chest pain, shortness of breath, coughing up blood, change in vision).	Bone density, fractures, hot flushes, leg cramps, blood clots	Pregnancy category X. Warning for fatal stroke; rare events predominantly seen in women at high risk for stroke.
Bazedoxifene	Similar to raloxifene.	Bone density, fractures, hot flushes, blood clots	Pregnancy category TBD.
Bazedoxifene with conjugated equine estrogens	Similar to raloxifene and estrogens, plus abdominal pain, yeast infections.	Bone density, fractures, hot flushes, blood clots	Pregnancy category TBD.
Calcitonin			
Calcitonin (salmon)	Nasal: Rhinitis, epistaxis. Injection: nausea, flushing, local inflammation.	Bone density, fractures	Pregnancy category C. Under FDA investigation for slight increase in cancer.
Formation Medication			
Recombinant human parathyroid hormone (PTH 1–34 units)			
Teriparatide	Orthostasis with first few injections, pain at injection site, nausea, headache, dizziness, leg cramps, rare increase in uric acid, slightly increased calcium.	Bone density, fractures, trough serum calcium concentration 1 month after therapy initiation	Pregnancy category C. If serum calcium is high (>10.6 mg/mL [>2.65 mmol/L]), calcium intake should be decreased. Warning about osteosarcoma in rats and therefore contraindicated in patients at high risk for this adverse event. REMS: Medication guide and communication plan due to the increased risk of osteosarcoma and to inform healthcare providers of the 2-year maximum lifetime treatment.

FDA, food and drug administration; GI, gastrointestinal; PTH, parathyroid hormone; REMS, risk evaluation and mitigation strategies; TBD, to be determined.

the absorption of calcium if given concomitantly. Further, calcium may decrease the oral absorption of some drugs including iron, tetracyclines, quinolones, bisphosphonates, and thyroid supplements.

Administration Most children and adults of all race and ethnic backgrounds do not ingest sufficient dietary calcium and therefore require supplements. To ensure adequate calcium absorption, 25(OH) vitamin D concentrations should be maintained in the normal range (30 to 60 ng/mL [75 to 150 nmol/L]).[1,6] Because fractional calcium absorption is dose limited, maximum single doses of 500 to 600 mg or less of elemental calcium are recommended. Because peaks in serum calcium levels after supplementation are hypothesized as a reason for negative cardiovascular effects, limiting doses to 250 mg given more frequently has been proposed.[68] Calcium carbonate is the salt of choice as it contains the highest amount of elemental calcium (40%) and is the least expensive. Calcium carbonate should be taken with meals to enhance absorption in an acidic environment. Calcium citrate absorption (21% calcium) is acid-independent and need not be administered with meals. Although tricalcium phosphate contains 38% calcium, calcium-phosphate complexes could limit overall calcium absorption. This product might be helpful in patients with hypophosphatemia that cannot be resolved with increased dietary intake. Disintegration and dissolution rates vary significantly between products and lots. Products labeled "USP Verified" for "United States Pharmacopeia," which guarantees the identity, strength, purity, and quality of the product, or products from a reputable company should be recommended when possible. Products from unrefined oyster shell or coral calcium should not be recommended because of concerns for high concentrations of lead and other heavy metals. Some calcium products come in alternative dosage forms (e.g., chews, dissolvable tablet, liquid), which can be beneficial for select patients (e.g., swallowing problems). For all products, encourage patients to read the labeling carefully as multiple tablets per day may be needed to obtain adequate calcium intake, especially with noncarbonate salts.

Some commercial calcium supplements contain other nutrients associated with bone physiology such as magnesium, vitamin K and "natural estrogens" or isoflavones. Minimal BMD and no fracture data exist for these combination products.[1,8] These products are also more expensive. Combining too many vitamins and supplements might lead to upper-tolerable nutrient limits being exceeded and a concern for toxicities. Further studies are needed before these combination products can be recommended for osteoporosis.

Vitamin D Supplementation 7 Vitamin D intake is critical for the prevention and treatment of osteoporosis because it maximizes intestinal calcium absorption. Given its safety, low cost, and other benefits of vitamin D, no patient should have an inadequate intake (see Table 73-4).[43,45]

Efficacy Data show that higher dose vitamin D supplementation (≥700 units) is needed for fracture and fall prevention. In one meta-analysis, higher doses of vitamin D (>400 units daily) decreased nonvertebral and hip fractures by approximately 20%.[58,69] A more recent meta-analysis found a fracture benefit only in those patients adherent to at least 800 units daily.[70] Megadose studies (>300,000 units/year) demonstrated an increased fracture rate, and these doses should be avoided.[42] Most studies and a meta-analysis support vitamin D decreasing falls.[42,43,52]

Drug Interactions Some drugs may induce vitamin D metabolism, including rifampin and some anticonvulsants such as phenytoin, barbiturates, valproic acid, and carbamazepine. Vitamin D absorption may be decreased by cholestyramine, colestipol, orlistat, and mineral oil. Vitamin D may enhance the absorption of aluminum; aluminum-containing products should be avoided to prevent aluminum toxicity.

Administration Vitamin D can be taken as a single agent or combination product (see Table 73-4 for daily requirements and guideline recommendations).[6–8,43,45] Several experts believe higher doses (i.e., up to 2,000 units of vitamin D daily) should be recommended to achieve concentrations of at least 30 ng/mL, especially in certain populations.[42,43] This dose is within the safe upper limit of vitamin D (4,000 units per day).[45] The American Association of Clinical Endocrinologists (AACE) guidelines do not recommend a dose, but state supplements should be used to ensure a 25(OH) vitamin D concentration of ≥30 ng/mL.

Although some data support slight differences between vitamin D_3 and D_2 absorption (D_3/D_2 absorption ratio 1.14 (confidence interval [CI] 1.0 to 1.29)),[71] guidelines suggest either agent for prevention and treatment of vitamin D deficiency.[43] Based on a meta-analysis, vitamin D_3 was more efficient than vitamin D_2 at raising 25(OH) vitamin D concentrations, and produced greater BMD changes with bolus dosing but not with lower maintenance doses.[72] The differences could be related to greater metabolism of vitamin D_2 to inactive metabolites. Usual supplementation is with daily nonprescription cholecalciferol products. The relationship between vitamin D_3 dose and the increase in 25(OH) vitamin D concentration varies from 40 units to increase the concentration by 0.8 ng/mL[73] to 100 units[1] to increase the concentration by 0.6 ng/mL[71] to 1 ng/mL,[43] with higher vitamin D doses needed to raise concentrations in obese patients.[73] Higher-dose prescription ergocalciferol regimens administered weekly, monthly, or quarterly can be used for replacement and maintenance therapy. More than one multivitamin or large doses of cod liver oil daily are no longer advocated because of the risk of hypervitaminosis A,[13] which can increase bone loss. Because the half-life of vitamin D is about 1 month, approximately 3 months of therapy are required before a new steady state is achieved, and a repeat 25(OH) vitamin D concentration can be obtained.

Individuals with deficient concentrations of vitamin D are at risk for osteomalacia. Their management is discussed in Other Metabolic Bone Diseases later in the chapter. In patients who are pregnant or obese, have a concomitant disorder (e.g., celiac disease, cystic fibrosis, or Crohn's disease), or take a concomitant medication (e.g., anticonvulsants, glucocorticoids, antifungals, AIDS medications) affecting vitamin D absorption, higher doses and more frequent monitoring are required.[43] In patients with severe hepatic or renal disease, the activated form of vitamin D (calcitriol) might be needed; however, newer research suggests adequate amounts of 25(OH) vitamin D are also important for total body health creating a need for both cholecalciferol and calcitriol coadministration.[74]

Bisphosphonates 8 Alendronate, risedronate, and IV zoledronic acid are FDA indicated for postmenopausal, male, and glucocorticoid-induced osteoporosis. IV and oral ibandronate and some specialized oral formulations of other bisphosphonates are indicated only for postmenopausal osteoporosis.

Pharmacology Bisphosphonates mimic pyrophosphate, an endogenous bone resorption inhibitor. Bisphosphonate antiresorptive activity results from blocking prenylation and inhibiting guanosine triphosphatase-signaling proteins, which lead to decreased osteoclast maturation, number, recruitment, bone adhesion, and life span. Their various R2 side chains produce different bone binding, persistence, and affinities; however, the resulting clinical significances are not known.

Pharmacokinetics Oral bisphosphonates' bioavailability is <1%; and is further decreased by concomitant food and beverages.[75,76] All bisphosphonates become incorporated into bone, giving them long biologic half-lives of up to 10 years. Absorbed bisphosphonates are renally eliminated and elimination decreases linearly with decreasing renal function.

Within 24 hours of an IV administration, approximately 40% of alendronate and zoledronic acid is excreted, whereas approximately 50% to 65% of risedronate and ibandronate is excreted, which coincides with alendronate and zoledronic acid having greater bone absorption, longer bone retention times (less desorption), and more reattachment after bone release.

Efficacy Of the antiresorptive agents, bisphosphonates consistently provide some of the higher fracture risk reductions and BMD increases (see Table 73-5).[1,6,7,58,77,78] Fracture clinical trial data only exist for daily oral bisphosphonate and annual IV therapy, not weekly, monthly, or quarterly regimens. Fracture reductions are demonstrated as early as 6 months, with the greatest fracture reduction seen in patients with lower initial BMD and in those with the greatest BMD changes with therapy. Hip fracture reduction was not seen with daily oral ibandronate. The hip fracture incidence in the placebo group was low, suggesting the study might have been underpowered; the lack of hip fracture reduction data with ibandronate is reflected in evidence-based therapy recommendations (see Fig. 73-3). Although comparative fracture prevention trials do not exist, no differences between oral bisphosphonates and fractures were found based on claims data.[79] Annual IV zoledronic acid has documented both secondary fracture prevention and a decrease in mortality in the treated group.[56] Zoledronic acid has also been documented to decrease bone loss and fractures for patients receiving certain chemotherapy.[1,14] Combination therapy is not recommended.[80]

BMD increases with bisphosphonates are dose dependent and greatest in the first 6 to 12 months of therapy. Small increases continue over time at the lumbar spine, but plateau after 2 to 5 years at the hip. Weekly alendronate, weekly and monthly risedronate, and monthly oral and quarterly IV ibandronate therapy produce equivalent BMD changes to their respective daily regimens. Weekly alendronate therapy increases BMD more than weekly risedronate therapy;[81] however, no evidence indicates that this difference would equate to greater fracture efficacy. Weekly alendronate and monthly ibandronate produced similar BMD effects.[82] After discontinuation, the increased BMD is sustained for a prolonged period of time that varies depending on the bisphosphonate used.[1]

The BMD increases with alendronate, risedronate, zoledronic acid, and oral ibandronate in men are similar to those in postmenopausal women.[6,83] Because of a lack of fracture data from pivotal trials in men, bisphosphonates are only FDA indicated to increase BMD, not to reduce fracture risk in men. Pooled analysis of risedronate studies and one open-label risedronate study document fracture prevention in men, and alendronate has been shown to decrease radiographic but not clinical vertebral fractures in men.[6,29]

Adverse Events If oral bisphosphonates are prescribed correctly and the patient takes them correctly, they are well-tolerated (see Table 73-7).[84] Patients who have serious GI conditions (abnormalities of the esophagus that delay emptying, such as stricture), or who are pregnant should not take bisphosphonates. Although oral bisphosphonates are to be avoided in patients with creatinine clearances less than 30 to 35 mL/min (0.50 to 0.58 mL/s), some experts suggest (not zoledronic acid) can be used in select patients with decreased renal function (see Clinical Controversy and Chap. 29, Chronic Kidney Disease).

Weekly and monthly therapies have similar common but less serious GI effects (perforation, ulceration, GI bleeding) than daily therapy.[8,84] The GI event rates were not increased with concomitant nonsteroidal antiinflammatory medication use. If GI adverse events occur, switching to a different bisphosphonate might resolve the problem. Patients should be encouraged to discuss GI complaints with a healthcare provider. IV ibandronate and zoledronic acid can be used for patients with GI contraindications or intolerances to oral bisphosphonates. Other common bisphosphonate adverse effects include injection reactions and musculoskeletal pain. If severe musculoskeletal pain occurs, the medication can be discontinued temporarily or permanently. Acute phase reactions (e.g., fever, flu-like symptoms, myalgias, arthralgias) are typically associated with IV administration, but rarely have been reported with weekly or monthly oral bisphosphonates. This reaction usually diminishes with subsequent administration.

Rare adverse effects include osteonecrosis of the jaw and subtrochanteric femoral (atypical) fractures.[84] Osteonecrosis of the jaw (ONJ) occurs more commonly in patients with cancer, chemotherapy, radiation, and/or glucocorticoid therapy receiving higher-dose IV bisphosphonate therapy. In osteoporosis treatment, about 1 in 100,000 patients might develop ONJ. When possible, major dental work should be completed before bisphosphonate initiation. For patients already on therapy, some practitioners withhold bisphosphonate therapy during and after major dental procedures, but no data exist to support any beneficial effect of such practice. To date, no causal relationship has been identified between atypical femoral shaft fractures and bisphosphonates. Since some patients with atypical fracture experience prodromal thigh or hip pain, any such pain should be evaluated. For patients with rare and unusual bone fractures while on long-term bisphosphonates, a metabolic bone disease workup should be conducted.

Drug Interactions Because of poor bioavailability, oral bisphosphonates should not be administered at the same time as other medications. The administration instructions described below should be followed.

Dosing and Administration Before bisphosphonates are used, especially before IV administration, the patient's serum calcium concentrations must be normal (see Table 73-6). A dental examination with major dental work completed before initiation is also suggested.[6] Because bioavailability is very poor for bisphosphonates and to minimize GI side effects, each oral tablet should be taken with at least 6 ounces of plain water (not coffee, juice, mineral water, or milk) at least 30 (60 for ibandronate) minutes before consuming any food, supplements (including calcium and vitamin D), or medications. For patients with swallowing difficulties (e.g., after stroke, tube feeding), a buffered, strawberry-flavored effervescent tablet marketed as Binosto, which is dissolved in 4 ounces of room-temperature water, could be used. This formulation has the same food restrictions as traditional oral tablets. Of note, delayed-release risedronate is administered immediately following breakfast with at least 4 ounces of plain water. The patient should also remain upright (i.e., either sitting or standing) for at least 30 minutes after alendronate and risedronate and 1 hour after ibandronate administration. A patient who misses a weekly dose can take it the next day. If more than 1 day has lapsed, that dose is skipped until the next scheduled ingestion. If a patient misses a monthly dose, it can be taken up to 7 days before the next administration.

The IV products need to be administered by a healthcare provider. The quarterly ibandronate injection comes as a prefilled syringe (3 mg/mL) kit with a butterfly needle. The injection is given IV over 15 to 30 seconds. The injection can also be diluted with dextrose 5% in water or normal saline and used with a syringe pump. Once-yearly or every 2-year administration of zoledronic acid should be infused over at least 15 minutes with a pump. Acetaminophen or ibuprofen can be given to decrease acute phase reactions.

9 Although these medications are effective, adherence to daily therapy is poor and results in decreased effectiveness.[85] Once-monthly therapy does not always improve adherence. While dosing frequency is a common barrier to adherence, adverse effects (e.g., GI complaints) and concerns about adverse effects remain important predictors of adherence and persistence. Even after a hip fracture, bisphosphonate persistence is suboptimal.[58,85] To help overcome the barriers associated with dosing frequency, IV ibandronate and zoledronic acid could be used as replacements if cost is not an issue. Weekly alendronate plus vitamin D can potentially help to ensure better adherence with vitamin D intake, but at an increased cost over generic alendronate.

Clinical **Controversy...**

The ideal duration of bisphosphonate therapy is not yet known. Because bisphosphonates are deposited into the bone and continue to suppress bone turnover after discontinuation, some clinicians recommend a "drug holiday."[8,59,86]

Data from studies with a drug holiday after therapy with risedronate for 3 years or alendronate for 5 years show a continued fracture benefit after therapy is discontinued. However, continued treatment with alendronate reduced the risk of new vertebral fracture compared with a drug holiday, and the risk of nonvertebral fracture was reduced in patients with T-scores of −2.5 or below.[59] Based on pharmacology and study results, drug holidays after 5 years of alendronate with reinitiation of therapy in 1 to 2 years, after 5 years of risedronate with reinitiation in 1 year, and after 3 years for zoledronic acid with reinitiation in 2 to 3 years have been proposed.[86]

Another recommendation is based on fracture risk: mild, no need for reinitiation; moderate, reinitiate in 2 to 3 years (depending on bisphosphonate); severe, reinitiate in 1 to 2 years with the same or different medication.[59]

Questions remain regarding which patients a drug holiday might be appropriate, the optimal duration of therapy before a drug holiday, and the length of the drug holiday.

Denosumab 8 Denosumab is FDA approved for treatment of osteoporosis in women and men at high risk for fracture. It is also approved to increase bone mass in men receiving androgen-deprivation therapy for nonmetastatic prostate cancer and in women receiving adjuvant aromatase inhibitor therapy for breast cancer who are at high risk for fracture.

Pharmacology Denosumab is a fully human monoclonal antibody that binds to RANKL, blocking its ability to bind to its RANK receptor on the surface of osteoclast precursor cells and mature osteoclasts. Denosumab inhibits osteoclastogenesis and increases osteoclast apoptosis.

Pharmacokinetics Following subcutaneous injection, the concentration of denosumab peaks in approximately 10 days and slowly declines over a period of 4 to 5 months.[87] The half-life is approximately 25 days. The drug does not accumulate with repeated dosing at 6-month intervals. No dosage adjustment is necessary in renal impairment; however, hypocalcemia is more common in severe renal impairment. There are currently no studies in hepatic impairment.

Efficacy Over 3 years, denosumab significantly decreased vertebral fractures, nonvertebral fractures, and hip fractures in postmenopausal women with low bone density (see Table 73-5).[1,8,58,87] The BMD effects are at least similar to weekly alendronate and can increase BMD in patients with prior alendronate therapy. In men receiving androgen-deprivation therapy, denosumab improved BMD and decreased new vertebral fractures without significant changes in nonvertebral or clinical vertebral fractures. While significant increases in BMD have been demonstrated over 2 years in women with nonmetastatic breast cancer on adjuvant aromatase inhibitor therapy, no fracture data are available.[88] Activity appears to dissipate upon medication discontinuation.[87]

Adverse Events In trials lasting up to 8 years, denosumab was generally well tolerated.[87] Dermatologic reactions not specific to the injection site such as dermatitis, eczema, and rashes were more common than with placebo (see Table 73-7).

Rare, serious adverse effects have included bone turnover suppression and serious infections including skin infections. If any signs of skin infection such as cellulitis appear, patients should be advised to seek medical attention. Because osteonecrosis of the jaw has been reported, major dental work should be completed before use when possible. As with the bisphosphonates, atypical fractures have been reported with this antiresorptive and prodromal pain should be evaluated. Hypocalcemia may occur; adequate calcium and vitamin D supplementation should be ensured and any existing hypocalcemia corrected before therapy initiation. Severe hypocalcemia is more common in patients with underlying kidney dysfunction.

Drug Interactions No drug–drug interactions have been identified with denosumab.

Dosing and Administration Denosumab is administered subcutaneously by a healthcare professional in the upper arm, upper thigh, or abdomen (see Table 73-6). The product is available as a refrigerated prefilled pen or single-use vial that can be stored at room temperature for up to 14 days before administration.

Mixed Estrogen Agonists Antagonists 8 Raloxifene is a second-generation mixed EAA approved for prevention and treatment of postmenopausal osteoporosis and for reducing the risk of invasive breast cancer in postmenopausal women with and without osteoporosis. At the time this chapter was prepared, bazedoxifene was a third-generation EAA under FDA review for prevention of postmenopausal osteoporosis and menopausal symptoms.

Pharmacology EAAs have estrogenic agonist actions in bone and antagonist actions in breast and uterine tissue.[89,90] Bazedoxifene has been combined with conjugated equine estrogens to create a new medication class called the tissue selective estrogen complexes; if approved by FDA, these agents will maximize effects on bone, minimize adverse effects, and eliminate the need for progestogens.[55]

Pharmacokinetics Food has a nonsignificant effect on absorption, which is approximately 2% for raloxifene[91] and 6% for bazedoxifene.[89] Raloxifene is 95% protein bound. Half-life of raloxifene is 28 hours and of bazedoxifene is 30 hours. EAAs are predominantly eliminated via glucuronidation.

Efficacy Raloxifene and bazedoxifene decrease vertebral but not nonvertebral fractures and increase spine and hip BMD, but to a lesser extent than bisphosphonates (see Table 73-5).[1,8,58,89] Raloxifene's vertebral fracture prevention is greater in women without previous fracture. Bazedoxifene's BMD increases are greater, but fracture prevention is similar to raloxifene.[56,89,90] Bazedoxifene with conjugated estrogens produced significantly greater increases in spine and hip BMD than raloxifene and placebo;[55] however, fracture data are not yet available. Raloxifene 7- and 8-year data[8] and bazedoxifene 5-year data[57] support long-term effects and safety in postmenopausal women. After raloxifene discontinuation, the medication effect is lost, with bone loss returning to age- or disease-related rates. Raloxifene's breast cancer prevention benefits might influence its selection for a subset of women at risk for or with osteoporosis and breast cancer.

Raloxifene and bazedoxifene cause some positive lipid effects (decreased total and low-density lipoprotein cholesterol, neutral to increased high-density lipoprotein cholesterol); however, triglycerides can increase slightly.[55] No benefit on cardiovascular disease was demonstrated in the RUTH (Raloxifene Use for the Heart) or MORE-CORE (Multiple Outcomes with Raloxifene study and its continuation) trials; however, when these trials are combined, the raloxifene group had a 10% lower mortality rate due to changes in noncardiovascular and noncancer deaths.[92]

Adverse Events Tolerability is similar with both EAAs (see Table 73-7).[89] Hot flushes are common (<28%).[90] EAAs rarely cause endometrial bleeding; rare but minor vaginal thickenings were seen more frequently with raloxifene than with bazedoxifene.[89] Leg cramps and muscle spasms are common (<17%).[90] Thromboembolic events are uncommon (<1%) but can be fatal. In large trials, no change in overall death, cardiovascular death, or overall stroke incidence was seen; however, a slight increase in fatal stroke (0.7/1,000 women year difference) was documented, resulting in a medication warning for raloxifene.[1,90] Further analysis documented this event in only those with a Framingham stroke risk score ≥13.[1]

Drug Interactions Because of raloxifene's highly protein-bound nature (95%), it can interact with other highly protein-bound medications such as warfarin. Monitoring of both medications is suggested.[91] Cholestyramine can decrease raloxifene absorption. No interactions to date with bazedoxifene.

Dosing and Administration 9 Although once-daily administration is easy (see Table 73-6), adherence and persistence problems exist. Minimal data suggest that dosage adjustments in renal failure are not needed. For severe liver failure, these medications should be used with caution or avoided. EAAs are contraindicated for women with an active or past history of venous thromboembolic disease. Therapy should be stopped if a patient anticipates extended immobility. Women at high risk for a stroke (e.g., Framingham stroke risk score ≥13)[1] or coronary events and those with known coronary artery disease, peripheral vascular disease, atrial fibrillation, or a prior history of cerebrovascular events might not be good candidates for this medication.

Calcitonin ❽ Calcitonin is FDA approved for osteoporosis treatment for women who are at least 5 years past menopause. Because efficacy is less robust than the other antiresorptive therapies, calcitonin is reserved as last-line treatment.

Pharmacology Calcitonin is an endogenous hormone released from the thyroid gland when serum calcium is elevated. The prescription product contains salmon calcitonin, which is more potent and longer lasting than the mammalian form.

Pharmacokinetics Availability is 3% to 5% with nasal administration.[93] Half-life is 18 minutes. Intermittent nasal regimens and an oral product are being explored.

Efficacy Only vertebral fractures have been documented to decrease with intranasal calcitonin therapy (see Table 73-5).[1,8,58] Calcitonin does not consistently affect hip BMD and does not decrease hip fracture risk. Data for use in men have not been published.

Calcitonin might provide some pain relief to some patients with acute vertebral fractures.[1]

Adverse Events Adverse events are listed in Table 73-7.

Drug Interactions Lithium doses might need reduction.[93]

Dosing and Administration ❾ Some patients do not like to administer medications in their nose (see Table 73-6). In clinical trials, a high drop-out rate exists with calcitonin. Subcutaneous administration with 100 units daily is available but rarely used because of more adverse effects and costs.[1] If the nasal product is used for vertebral fracture pain, calcitonin should be prescribed for short-term (4 weeks) treatment and should not be used in place of other more effective and less expensive analgesics nor should it preclude the use of more appropriate osteoporosis therapy.

Estrogen Therapy Estrogens are FDA indicated for prevention of osteoporosis for women at significant risk and for whom other osteoporosis medications cannot be used.[1,8]

Pharmacology Exogenous estrogens provide similar effects as endogenous estrogens. Even though the Women's Health Initiative trials only assessed one dose of conjugated equine estrogens, most clinicians extrapolate the results to all postmenopausal estrogen therapies until data indicate otherwise.

Efficacy Hormone therapy (HT)—estrogen with or without a progestogen—significantly decreases fracture risk (see Table 73-5).[1,8,58] Increases in BMD are less than those with bisphosphonates, denosumab, or teriparatide, but greater than those with raloxifene and calcitonin. Oral and transdermal estrogens at equivalent doses and continuous or cyclic HT regimens have similar BMD effects. Effect on BMD is dose dependent, with some benefit seen with lower estrogen doses; however, fracture risk reduction has not been demonstrated with the lower doses. When HT is discontinued, bone loss accelerates and fracture protection is lost.

Adverse Events and Drug Interactions A complete discussion of adverse events for all estrogen products can be found in Chapter 65, Hormone Therapy in Women.

Dosing and Administration The lowest effective HT dose that prevents and controls menopausal symptoms is used and discontinued as soon as possible. A complete discussion of administration and precautions for all estrogen products can be found in Chapter 65, Hormone Therapy in Women.

Testosterone Decreased testosterone concentrations are seen with certain gonadal diseases, eating disorders, glucocorticoid therapy, oophorectomy, menopause, and andropause. Although it is not FDA indicated for osteoporosis, the male osteoporosis guideline recommends testosterone alone for men with testosterone concentrations <200 ng/dL (6.9 nmol/ L) if low fracture risk and in combination with an osteoporosis medication if fracture risk is high.[6] For men on testosterone maintenance therapy, an anti-osteoporosis medication can be added when risk for osteoporotic fracture is or becomes high. Women with low libido might also be prescribed methyltestosterone.[94] This medication is not solely prescribed for osteoporosis.

Pharmacology Testosterone is converted to estradiol, which decreases bone resorption in men and women.

Efficacy Testosterone has increased BMD in men with low testosterone concentrations, but has no effect if testosterone concentrations are normal.[6] No fracture data are available. Adding alendronate to testosterone therapy in hypogonadal men improved BMD benefits. A few small studies of methyltestosterone in women demonstrated small increases in BMD, but again there are no fracture data.[94]

Adverse Events and Drug Interactions Further discussion of adverse events for testosterone products for men can be found in Chapter 66, Erectile Dysfunction.

Dosing and Administration Testosterone from gels can be transferred to other people from skin and clothing contacts. Patients need to be educated to decrease exposure to partners and children, especially monitoring for virilization adverse effects in children.

Anabolic Therapies

Teriparatide ❽ Teriparatide is FDA indicated for treatment of postmenopausal women who are at high risk for fracture, for increase of BMD in men with idiopathic or hypogonadal osteoporosis who are at high risk for fracture, for men or women intolerant to other osteoporosis medications, and for patients with glucocorticoid-induced osteoporosis. Patients who have a history of osteoporotic fracture, multiple risk factors for fracture, very low bone density (e.g., T-score < –3.5), or who have failed previous bisphosphonate therapy could be candidates for PTH therapy.

Pharmacology Teriparatide is a recombinant product representing the first 34 amino acids in human PTH. Teriparatide increases bone formation, the bone remodeling rate, and osteoblast number and activity. Its actions result from activation of Wnt signaling, induction of runt-related transcription factor (runX2), increased IGF-1 production, and inhibition of osteoblast apoptosis and sclerostin.[24] Both bone mass and architecture are improved. Different PTH analogs (e.g., human PTH 1–31) and parathyroid hormone-related protein are being investigated.[24,25] Full PTH (1–84) is marketed in Europe.[1]

Pharmacokinetics Bioavailability is 95%.[95] The peptide is cleared through hepatic and extrahepatic pathways, with a half-life of 60 minutes. No pharmacokinetic changes are noted with decreasing renal function. No studies have been done in hepatic impairment. Oral, intranasal transdermal, microneedle patch, and implantable microchip PTH formulations, and once-weekly subcutaneous teriparatide are being investigated.[24,25,96,97]

Efficacy Teriparatide reduces vertebral and nonvertebral fracture risk in postmenopausal women (see Table 73-5);[1,8,58] however, no fracture data are available in men or for patients taking glucocorticoids. Lumbar spine BMD increases are greater than other osteoporosis medications. Although wrist BMD is decreased, wrist fractures are not increased. Discontinuation of teriparatide therapy results in a decrease in BMD, which can be alleviated with subsequent antiresorptive therapy.

Because of concern over osteosarcoma, the agent is currently approved for use up to 2 years. Using a second course of teriparatide is controversial.[1] Some advocate no second course.[111] One study found that a second course of teriparatide increased BMD but not to the extent with the first course.[112]

Adverse Events Transient hypercalcemia rarely occurs with teriparatide (see Table 73-7). Because of an increased incidence of osteosarcoma in rats, teriparatide contains a box warning against use in patients at increased baseline risk for osteosarcoma (e.g., Paget's bone disease, unexplained elevations of alkaline phosphatase, pediatric patients, young adults with open epiphyses, or patients with prior radiation therapy involving the skeleton).[95]

Drug Interactions An increased calcium concentration could be a concern if on digoxin therapy.[95]

Dosing and Administration Teriparatide is commercially available as a prefilled "pen" delivery device (see Table 73-6). The pen must be kept refrigerated and can be used immediately after removing from the refrigerator. The daily subcutaneous injection is delivered to the thigh or abdominal area with site rotation. The administration of the first dose should take place with the patient either sitting or lying down in case orthostatic hypotension occurs. The pen must be discarded 28 days after the initial injection. The patient should be reeducated on correct use with each pen refill. Suboptimal adherence decreases efficacy, which might be resolved in the future with newer PTH formulations and less frequent administrations. Besides the conditions listed above, teriparatide should not be used in patients with hypercalcemia, metabolic bone diseases other than osteoporosis, metastatic or skeletal cancers, or premenopausal women of child-bearing potential. Teriparatide should not be used in men with previous radiation therapy.[6]

Teriparatide is the most expensive osteoporosis therapy. Prior authorization may be required. Special arrangements need to be made when patients travel, especially on airplanes.

Combination Therapy

Combinations of different classes of osteoporosis medications have been explored but are not recommended at this time.[8,80,98] Combining two antiresorptive agents (e.g., a bisphosphonate with HT or raloxifene) has demonstrated small additive effects on BMD but with concern that the dual suppression of bone turnover could decrease bone strength. When PTH is combined with raloxifene, zoledronic acid, or HT, greater increases or no additive effects in BMD occurred; however, a blunting of the BMD effect has been seen when PTH was combined with alendronate. Antiresorptive therapy combined with cyclical anabolic therapy has been studied for increased patient convenience and lower cost over daily PTH therapy. Combining alendronate with cyclical PTH (3 months on and 3 months off) has produced similar BMD increases to PTH alone. Recently, the combination denosumab and teriparatide for 12 months was demonstrated to increase BMD at the hip and spine more than monotherapy with either drug.[99] Fracture outcomes from combination therapies are not available. Because no clear benefit with combination therapy exists and such therapy is associated with increased cost and the potential for more adverse effects and nonadherence, combination therapy is not recommended.

Investigational Therapies

❷ Besides the aforementioned investigational products, additional new classes of medications are beginning to show promise in phase II and III studies.[22,24,25] Investigational antiresorptive agents inhibit bone matrix degradation (cathepsin K inhibitors, e.g., odanacatib) or block osteoclast activation (c-src kinase inhibitor, e.g., saracatinib). Anabolic therapies under investigation include subcutaneously administered neutralizing antibodies against sclerostin, (e.g., romosozumab), and DKK-1, which endogenously inhibit osteoblast differentiation and bone formation. Calcilytic drugs stimulate PTH release via antagonism of CaSR by mimicking hypocalcemia. These drugs have the advantage of being given orally while PTH must be administered subcutaneously. However, calcilytic drugs developed to date have a narrow therapeutic index.

Strontium ranelate and tibolone are approved in Europe, and the latter agent is approved in Canada. Most likely, these two medications will not be marketed in the United States.

Vertebroplasty and Kyphoplasty

The use of vertebroplasty and kyphoplasty are controversial in light of randomized controlled trials that suggest at the most short-term but not long-term benefits or cost effectiveness.[46,100] During the procedure, cement is injected into fractured vertebra(e) for patients with debilitating pain 6 to 52 weeks after fracture. In some studies, the procedure stabilized the damaged vertebrae, reduced pain, and decreased opioid intake; the effects are sometimes similar to sham interventions and standard patient care. Long-term adverse outcomes are a concern, including cement leakage into the spinal column (10%), which although frequently asymptomatic can result in nerve damage, and vertebral fracturing around the cement.

SPECIAL POPULATIONS

Osteoporosis is a particular threat in some subgroups because of age, genetic abnormalities, diseases, and medications.

Children

Although rare, osteoporosis in children and adolescents can lead to significant pain, deformity, and chronic disability. Secondary causes are the main contributors to osteoporosis in children (see Tables 73-2 and 73-3),[12,101] but genetic disorders and idiopathic juvenile osteoporosis can be the origin of bone disease.

The diagnosis and treatment of osteoporosis in children and adolescents is challenging.[12,101] No guidelines or consensus recommendations exist. The International Society for Clinical Densitometry's official position is that the diagnosis of osteoporosis in children (<20 years of age) requires the presence of a clinically significant fracture history (long bone fracture of the lower extremity, vertebral compression fracture, or two or more long bone fractures of the upper extremities) in combination with low bone mass.[34] Low bone mass is defined as a Z-score below a −2.0 (adjusted for body size and ethnicity/race) using central DXA of the spine or total body.

After correcting any underlying causes and instituting a bone-healthy lifestyle, pharmacologic treatment should be considered for children with low bone mass and fragility fractures.[12,101] Several small studies, mostly evaluating the IV bisphosphonate pamidronate or oral alendronate, have demonstrated increases in BMD. No studies have demonstrated fracture efficacy in this population. The optimal medication, dose, and duration of therapy are unknown, and more safety data are needed. A major concern with bisphosphonates is their effect on longitudinal bone growth and modeling; however, fracture healing, skeletal growth and maturation, or the appearance of growth plates do not appear to be impaired. Teriparatide cannot be used in children as it has a box warning indicating an increased risk for osteosarcoma.

Premenopausal Women

Clinically significant bone loss and fractures in healthy premenopausal women are rare.[102,103] Approximately 15% of healthy premenopausal women will have low BMD as a normal variation of peak bone mass. Low peak bone mass is a major risk factor for postmenopausal osteoporosis and fractures but thus far is not a predictor of an increased risk for fractures in the premenopausal years. This might be a result of better bone architecture contributing to better bone strength in younger women.

Routine bone density screening and testing are not cost effective and should not be performed in healthy premenopausal women.

No evidence supports that identifying low bone density in healthy premenopausal women results in improved bone-healthy lifestyle practices nor does any evidence exist to support that pharmacologic treatment will reduce future fracture risk.

Most premenopausal women with osteoporosis (Z-score < −2.0) or a history of fragility fracture have an identifiable secondary cause (see Tables 73-2 and 73-3). Therefore, premenopausal women presenting with a history of low-trauma fracture or with a suspected secondary cause for osteoporosis should undergo central DXA testing; if BMD is low, the patient should be considered for pharmacologic therapy. Women with an unidentified cause for osteoporosis and no history of fracture should be treated with a bone-healthy lifestyle and watchful waiting. Therapy may also be considered for premenopausal women experiencing bone loss from cancer chemotherapy or glucocorticoids.

Pharmacologic therapy for osteoporosis should be used with caution in premenopausal women as efficacy and safety have not been adequately demonstrated. Select agents are only FDA-approved for premenopausal women on glucocorticoids. The pregnancy categories are outlined in Table 73-7. Notably, raloxifene and denosumab are in pregnancy category X.

Bisphosphonates are incorporated into the bone matrix and slowly released over time. A theoretical concern is a risk for fetal harm with pregnancies that occur during and after therapy has been stopped. While limited case reports have documented healthy infants after bisphosphonate use, more safety data are needed.

The Older Adult

Osteoporosis and adverse fracture outcomes increase with age.[39] Age is an independent risk factor for osteoporosis and osteoporotic fractures, with the prevalence increasing dramatically with age. The number of older adults with osteoporosis is on the rise, yet the condition is underdiagnosed and undertreated in this population. A challenge is determining the correct screening for nursing home residents; FRAX® slightly overestimated whereas ultrasound underestimated the true osteoporosis incidence in one trial.[104] In another study, 80% of older adults did not receive osteoporosis medication after a fracture.[105] Universal screening of older women with alendronate therapy prescribed only for those with osteoporosis was found to be cost effective, with more cost savings generated with greater age.[106]

Older adults should practice a bone-healthy lifestyle, ingest adequate calcium and vitamin D,[33,45,107] and implement measures to prevent falls.[46,52] Exercise might be difficult in older adults due to osteoarthritis, and or limited by underlying cardiac and respiratory diseases. However, walking and resistance exercise with low weights can stimulate bone remodeling. Lactose intolerance and hypercholesterolemia increases with aging. Dairy products might not be ingested as frequently, increasing the need for calcium supplements. Limited sun exposure due to frailty and institutional residence can increase the need for vitamin D for bone and muscle health.[42,43] Encouraging older adults to do a home safety evaluation for falls can assist with fracture prevention. Multidisciplinary fall prevention programs with multiple interventions generally have greater impact on fall prevention.[52] Many fall prevention materials are available without cost on the Internet.[32,53,54]

Although efficacy and safety data are limited in the oldest older adults,[33,107] evidence consistently shows that those at highest risk for fracture could benefit most from pharmacologic therapy.[108] When deciding whether or not to use prescription medications in older adults, the following factors need to be taken into consideration: remaining life span, ability to take and afford medications, cognitive function, GI disorders, polypharmacy, desire to avoid additional medications, and regimen complexity. Oral bisphosphonate administration is difficult in older adults who are bed bound, have difficulties swallowing, have fluid restrictions for cardiovascular or kidney diseases, or forget to drink adequate amounts of fluid or stay upright for the given time. Osteoporosis medications can put an older adult into the Medicare Part D medication insurance plan "donut hole,"[109] the segment during which the older adult pays most of the medication expenses out of pocket. During this time, older adults might need to make decisions on which medications to continue if finances are an issue. This gap in Part D medication coverage is closing gradually under the Affordable Care Act and is scheduled to be eliminated by 2020.

Chronic Kidney Disease

A bone healthy lifestyle is still required in patients with chronic kidney disease (CKD; glomerular filtration rate [GFR] <60 mL/min/1.73 m^2 [1 mL/s/1.73 m^2]). Vitamin D deficiency exists in 70% of patients with CKD stage 3 (GFR 30 to 59 mL/min [0.5 to 0.99 mL/s]) and 83% of patients with CKD stage 4 (GFR 15 to 29 mL/min [0.25 to 0.49 mL/s]) disease warranting 25(OH) vitamin D monitoring and replacement when needed.[74] Adequate 25(OH) vitamin D concentrations should be achieved in end-stage renal disease (CKD5 – GFR <15 mL/min [<0.25 mL/s] and CKD5D – dialysis) patients as well; however, the data are not yet strong.

Renal osteodystrophy describes a constellation of metabolic bone disorders that develop in patients with stage 4 and 5 CKD as a consequence of intrinsic kidney damage. Bone biopsy might be necessary to differentiate the different types of renal osteodystrophy from osteoporosis in this population. Antiresorptive therapies would be appropriate for the management of osteoporosis; however, they are contraindicated in patients with osteomalacia or adynamic bone and might be ineffective for osteitis fibrosa cystica. In patients with osteoporosis and a creatinine clearance (CL_{cr}) greater than 30 mL/min (0.50 mL/s), routine management can be used (see Fig. 73-3).[110] For patients with osteoporosis and a CL_{cr} less than 30 or 35 mL/min (0.50 or 0.58 mL/s), oral bisphosphonates are not recommended because of potential drug accumulation. Zoledronic acid is contraindicated in patients with CL_{cr} <35 mL/min (0.5 mL/s). Raloxifene has been used in patients with CL_{cr} <45 mL/min (0.75 mL/s). Denosumab is not renally eliminated and might be useful, however, additional research is required for confirmation.

Clinical **Controversy. . .**

Although bisphosphonates are not indicated in stage 4 chronic kidney disease (CKD4), some experts suggest the oral agents or IV ibandronate could be used if the CKD4 is due to aging and not a different pathophysiology.[110] Oral bisphosphonates appear safe and efficacious in the low numbers of patients studied with creatinine clearance (CL_{cr}) as low as 15 mL/min (0.25 mL/s). Some experts recommend decreasing the bisphosphonate dose by 50% or extending the dosing interval, and using the agent for less than 3 years.

DRUG-INDUCED DISEASE

Glucocorticoid-Induced Osteoporosis

10 Current and prior glucocorticoid use is the most common cause of drug-induced osteoporosis.[14,111,112] Approximately 30% to 50% of patients taking chronic oral glucocorticoids will experience a fracture. The relative risk for a vertebral or hip fracture is 5.2 and 2.3 respectively for prednisone doses ≥7.5 mg daily or equivalent.[14] Fracture risk is not increased for patients receiving glucocorticoids for adrenal insufficiency.[113] Although this is a well-documented risk,

many patients receiving glucocorticoids are not evaluated and/or treated for glucocorticoid-induced osteoporosis (GIO).[114]

Bone losses with glucocorticoids are rapid, with the greatest decrease occurring in the first 6 to 12 months of therapy.[111,112] Oral doses as low as 2.5 mg prednisone or equivalent daily have been associated with fractures. GIO has also been associated with inhaled glucocorticoids, although most data suggest no major bone effects.

The pathophysiology of glucocorticoid bone loss is multifactorial. Glucocorticoids decrease bone formation through decreased proliferation and differentiation, and enhanced apoptosis of osteoblasts. They can interfere with the bone's natural repair mechanism through increased apoptosis of osteocytes, the bone's communication cells. Glucocorticoids increase bone resorption by increasing RANKL and decreasing OPG. They can reduce estrogen and testosterone concentrations. A negative calcium balance is created from decreased calcium absorption and increased urinary calcium excretion via alterations in calcium transporters.[27] Risk is greater in patients with a polymorph in the glucocorticoid receptor gene and in older adults partly because of an increase in 11β-hydroxysteroid dehydrogenase 1 that activates the glucocorticoid.[112] The underlying disease requiring this medication sometimes also contributes negatively to bone metabolism.

FRAX® and DXA can be used for BMD evaluation.[111] Based on FRAX® estimates of the 10-year risk of major osteoporotic fracture, patients are risk stratified; low <10%, medium 10% to 20%, high >20%. Because FRAX® does not account for specific dose, duration of therapy, or accumulation of dose, the FRAX® score should be multiplied by various corrections based on patient age to prevent over- and under-estimations.[113] Patients are also classified as high risk if DXA T-score ≤ –2.5 or a history of fragility fracture. A baseline central DXA is recommended before glucocorticoid initiation. Because of the rapid loss of bone that can occur with oral glucocorticoid therapy, central DXA can be repeated yearly thereafter or more often if needed. A vertebral fracture assessment for patients with significant height loss or pain consistent with a vertebral fracture or spine radiography is suggested at baseline and for those already receiving ≥5 mg prednisone or equivalent.

All patients using glucocorticoids should practice a bone-healthy lifestyle (described above) and minimize glucocorticoid exposure when possible.[111] All patients starting or receiving glucocorticoid therapy (any dose or duration) should ingest 1,200 to 1,500 mg elemental calcium and 800 to 1,200 units of vitamin D daily or more to achieve therapeutic 25(OH) vitamin D concentrations. Minimizing fall risk is important. Counseling should occur for all patients using this medication for *more than* 3 months regardless of dose. Glucocorticoids should be used at the lowest dose and for the shortest duration possible.

Current GIO guidelines divide recommendations for prescription medication use by fracture risk, age, menopause and childbearing status, glucocorticoid dose and duration, and fragility fracture (Tables 73-8 and 73-9).[111,112,115] Alendronate and risedronate decrease bone loss and vertebral fractures. IV zoledronic acid and teriparatide produce greater and quicker decreases in bone loss than do oral bisphosphonates. In an observational followup study of patients on glucocorticoids treated with up to 18 months of teriparatide for patients on glucocorticoids, fracture risk was decreased.[116] These agents have FDA indications for prednisone doses ≥7.5 mg daily (bisphosphonates) or at high risk for fracture (teriparatide); this differs from the guideline recommendations. Denosumab is being investigated for GIO and in theory should provide benefit. Recommendations exist for therapy in premenopausal and younger men (<50 years old) if they have already experienced a fragility fracture, but, because of insufficient data, no recommendations provide guidance in those without fracture. Osteoporosis doses and directions for use are the same for postmenopausal and male osteoporosis.

Because glucocorticoids can cause hypogonadism, this condition is frequently evaluated in premenopausal women and men. Although the guidelines no longer include hormone therapy,[111] sometimes this therapy will be prescribed for the symptoms of hypogonadism.[115] While not specifically for osteoporosis treatment, some positive bone effects could occur.

TABLE 73-8 Therapy to Prevent or Treat Glucocorticoid-Induced Osteoporosis in Postmenopausal Women and Men > 50 Years Old

Treatments and Options	Patient Risk Level: Low Risk FRAX® <10%[b]	Medium Risk FRAX® 10–20%[b]	High Risk FRAX® >20%,[b] DXA T-score ≥ –2.5, or Fragility Fracture
Prednisone dose[a]	<7.5 mg daily for ≥3 mo	<7.5 mg daily for ≥3 mo	<5 mg daily for ≤1 month
Medication options	No therapy	Alendronate, risedronate	Alendronate, risedronate, zoledronic acid
Prednisone dose[a]	≥7.5 mg daily for ≥3 mo	≥7.5 mg daily for ≥3 mo	≥5 mg daily for ≤1 month or any dose ≥1 month
Medication options	Alendronate, risedronate, zoledronic acid	Alendronate, risedronate, zoledronic acid	Alendronate, risedronate, zoledronic acid, teriparatide

DXA, dual-energy absorptiometry; FRAX®, World Health Organization fracture risk assessment tool.

[a]Or glucocorticoid equivalent.

[b]Based on the 10-year risk of major osteoporotic fracture estimation.

Data from reference 111.

CANCER TREATMENT–RELATED BONE LOSS

10 Several important risk factors for osteoporosis are found more commonly in patients with cancer.[117] Prostate cancer and breast cancer are the most commonly diagnosed cancers among men and women, respectively. In these patients, antiandrogen and antiestrogen

TABLE 73-9 Therapy to Prevent or Treat Glucocorticoid-Induced Osteoporosis in Premenopausal Women and Men <50 Years Old with a Fragility Fracture

Patient Type	Therapeutic Regimen: Prednisone 5–7.4 mg Daily for 1–3 Months	Prednisone ≥7.5 mg Daily for 1–3 Months	Prednisone <7.5 mg Daily for ≥3 Months	Prednisone ≥7.5 mg Daily for ≥3 Months
Nonchildbearing premenopausal women and men <50 years old	Alendronate, risedronate	Alendronate, risedronate, zoledronic acid	Alendronate, risedronate, zoledronic acid, teriparatide	Alendronate, risedronate, zoledronic acid, teriparatide
Childbearing women	No consensus	No consensus	No consensus	Alendronate, risedronate, teriparatide

Data from reference 111.

therapies increase the risk of osteoporosis. Premature menopause and related ovarian failure induced by chemotherapy may also lead to bone loss. Glucocorticoids used as antiemetic therapy, as a premedication for certain chemotherapies, and in treatment regimens for hematologic malignancies increase bone loss. The need for GIO preventive therapy should be considered if glucocorticoid therapy is planned for 3 months or more.

In addition to the screening recommendations set forth by the National Osteoporosis Foundation (NOF), a baseline DXA is recommended for women taking aromatase inhibitors.[118] Further, the National Comprehensive Cancer Network recommends testing men on androgen-deprivation therapy.[117] When using FRAX® to predict fracture risk, premature menopause and hypogonadism are considered factors contributing to secondary osteoporosis in the risk model. If the fracture risk exceeds the treatment threshold, appropriate therapy should be considered.

For a patient with a history of cancer or active malignancy, individual characteristics will help to guide treatment selection.[117] Some agents have been specifically evaluated for skeletal-related events or for the prevention of cancer therapy–induced bone loss. Data suggest a potential role for bisphosphonates in decreasing recurrence of early stage breast cancer. In women, bisphosphonates have been shown to reduce bone loss associated with chemotherapy-related ovarian failure and ovarian suppression with gonadotropin-releasing hormone and aromatase inhibitors. Raloxifene decreases the risk of invasive breast cancer in high-risk women.

In men with prostate cancer, recommendations include use of denosumab, zoledronic acid, or alendronate.[119] Denosumab is specifically indicated for androgen deprivation-induced bone loss in men with prostate cancer and aromatase inhibitor-induced bone loss in women with breast cancer based on bone mineral density outcomes in these patients.[120]

Because of the risk of osteosarcoma, teriparatide is contraindicated in patients with prior radiation to the skeleton.[117] In all patients with a history of malignancy, clinicians should take a careful history of prior radiation before selecting the most appropriate treatment option.

PERSONALIZED PHARMACOTHERAPY

Bone physiology and pathophysiology are under many genomic and genetic influences. Isolating one or a few genes for correction will unlikely resolve the epidemic of osteoporosis.

Hereditary is important since family history, especially of a hip fracture in a parent, is a strong risk factor for osteoporosis development, and twin studies have suggested that 50% to 85% of variability is due to genetics.[1,121,122] As of early 2013, 62 loci have been identified that influence BMD and 14 loci for fracture risk, ranging from impacts on bone resorption (RANKL, osteoprotegerin) to formation (Wnt, LRP5, sclerostin).

Calcium, vitamin D, and estrogen receptors are also under genetic influence. Genetic modulation is in its infancy for osteoporosis prevention and treatment but might lead to new medications.

EVALUATION OF THERAPEUTIC OUTCOMES

9 Assessment of adherence and tolerability of medication should be performed at each visit. Having a patient repeat back instructions for medication administration will help identify administration problems and enable timely correction. Assessment of fracture, back pain, and height loss can help identify worsening osteoporosis.

To evaluate efficacy, a central DXA BMD measurement can be obtained 1 to 2 years after initiating a medication to monitor response. To minimize test variability, BMD testing should be performed on the same DXA machine. A statistical change must be greater than the least significant change for that specific piece of equipment. Since BMD continues to decrease with aging, no change from baseline can be an acceptable response. Because changes in BMD do not entirely explain changes in fracture risk, many experts believe that decisions on whether or not to continue a particular therapy should not be based solely on BMD response. Central DXAs are then repeated thereafter every 1 to 2 years until BMD is stable, at which time the interval for reassessment could be expanded. In patients with conditions associated with higher rates of bone loss (e.g., glucocorticoid use), more frequent monitoring might be warranted.

Bone turnover markers have been used to determine response as well as use of an osteoporosis prescription medication.[6,8,37,38] The patient either provides a first or second morning voiding urine sample or has blood drawn after an overnight fast to measure the markers 3 to 6 months after therapy initiation. The results are compared with baseline values. To be clinically relevant, changes again need to be greater than the least significant change for that test; beyond that no specific guidelines for interpretation exist. No consensus on result interpretation and high test variability exists, and thus these tests are not yet considered routine.

Osteoporosis Services

9 Currently not all patients are being adequately screened, tested, and treated according to guidelines nor educated about prevention via a bone-healthy lifestyle.[61] All healthcare providers play an important role in screening and monitoring for osteoporosis.[78,123] Community pharmacies and groups can offer health fairs with osteoporosis screenings using ultrasonography and/or FRAX® to identify postmenopausal women and older adult men at risk and then make appropriate referrals for DXA assessment. Healthcare providers can increase bone-healthy lifestyle changes, ensure correct medication use, and resolve medication adverse events. This practice has been financially sustainable in the community pharmacy setting[124] and as part of a patient-centered medical home.[125]

Because adherence is strongly linked to fracture prevention,[58] all healthcare providers should identify and resolve barriers to optimal medication adherence. Some pharmacists are beginning to administer denosumab in community pharmacies to improve adherence and ease of administration. Databases can also be used to ensure that all patients with a low-trauma fracture either have a DXA conducted or osteoporosis medication started. Everyone can work together as interprofessional teams to ensure that health systems and providers meet all quality assurance indicators for optimal patient osteoporosis prevention and treatment.

OTHER METABOLIC BONE DISORDERS

Because of increased interest in bone diseases and newer medications, better therapies are being explored and developed for other bone diseases.

Osteomalacia

Osteomalacia, meaning "soft bones," is a condition seen in adults in which the bone is significantly undermineralized. Rickets is the childhood equivalent of osteomalacia. The most common cause of osteomalacia is severe, prolonged vitamin D deficiency. Disorders that cause hypophosphatemia and, rarely, medications such as long-term anticonvulsant therapy can also cause osteomalacia.[50]

Patients with osteomalacia present with pathologic fractures and/or deep bone pain, proximal muscle weakness, or no obvious symptoms but low BMD. Patients with osteomalacia will have an extremely low 25(OH) vitamin D concentration (<10 ng/mL [<25 nmol/L]) and might have an elevated bone-specific alkaline phosphate, hypophosphatemia and hypocalcemia. The treatment of osteomalacia caused by vitamin D deficiency is high-dose vitamin D replacement therapy. Prescription oral ergocalciferol 50,000 units once to twice weekly for at least 8 weeks is a regimen that is frequently used to raise vitamin D concentrations into the sufficient range. Other high-dose oral and intramuscular vitamin D regimens have also been used. Once 25(OH) vitamin D concentrations are greater than 30 ng/mL (75 nmol/L), chronic maintenance vitamin D therapy can be instituted. Oral ergocalciferol 50,000 units once or twice a month or nonprescription cholecalciferol of 1,000 to 2,000 units once daily are reasonable maintenance options.

CONCLUSION

Osteoporosis prevention begins at birth and continues throughout life by practicing a bone-healthy lifestyle (adequate calcium and vitamin D intake, exercise, no smoking, minimal alcohol use, and fall prevention). Generally osteoporosis occurs in postmenopausal women and older men; however, the disease can occur in all ages as a result of secondary causes such as genetics, diseases, and medications. Central bone densitometry (i.e., DXA) can be used for screening, diagnosis, and monitoring, and the fracture risk assessment tool (i.e., FRAX) can be used for screening and to assist in identifying patients at high risk for fracture requiring treatment.

Alendronate, risedronate, zoledronic acid, and denosumab are first-line therapies since these drugs have been demonstrated to decrease hip, nonvertebral, and vertebral fractures. Teriparatide is the only medication that can build bone; however, cost and subcutaneous administration limit its use. Although medications decrease fracture risk, prescribing of osteoporosis medications and patient adherence to such therapy is suboptimal, leading to less fracture prevention. All healthcare providers need to be actively involved in osteoporosis education, counseling, and prevention across the life span and then attentive to treatment and medication adherence to prevent osteoporotic fractures in patients with osteoporosis. Many diseases and medications can cause secondary osteoporosis. Healthcare providers need to be proactive to achieve better disease control, adjust medications when possible to decrease risk, and prescribe osteoporosis medications when appropriate.

ADDENDUM

As discussed in the adverse effects portion of the Calcium Supplementation section, the link between calcium intake and increased risk of cardiovascular disease and mortality continues to be evaluated.

In a large, prospective, 12-year cohort study following dietary and supplemental calcium intake, the risk of death from heart disease was increased by supplemental calcium (>1,000 mg/d) intake in men but not in women.[126] This effect was not observed from dietary calcium or lower intake of supplements.

Increased overall and cardiovascular mortality was demonstrated in a prospective cohort study of women consuming 1,400 mg or more of calcium daily through diet and/or supplements.[127] There was an increased risk of all-cause mortality, cardiovascular disease mortality, and ischemic heart disease mortality. The risk of all-cause mortality was more pronounced in those who used supplements in addition to a high dietary calcium intake.

While data are conflicting, these studies nonetheless reinforce that clinicians should not promote calcium supplements in patients already consuming adequate dietary amount of this element.

Recent denosumab data documented BMD continues to increase after eight years of therapy with similar side effect profile to the four year data.[128]

ABBREVIATIONS

25(OH) vitamin D	25-hydroxyvitamin D/calcidiol
AACE	American Association of Clinical Endocrinologists
AIDS	acquired immunodeficiency syndrome
ATPase	adenosine triphosphatase
BMD	bone mineral density
BMP	bone morphogenetic protein
CaSR	calcium-sensing receptor
CI	confidence interval
CKD	chronic kidney disease
CL_{cr}	creatinine clearance
CYP	cytochrome P450
CTX	C-terminal crosslinking telopeptide of type 1 collagen
DHEA-S	dehydroepiandrosterone sulfate
DKK-1	Dickkoff-1
DXA	dual-energy x-ray absorptiometry
EAA	estrogen agonist antagonist
FAK	focal adhesion kinase
FDA	Food and Drug Adminstration
FGF	fibroblast growth factor
FRAX®	World Health Organization fracture risk assessment (tool)
FZD	frizzled element
GFR	glomerular filtration rate
GI	gastrointestinal
GIO	glucocorticoid-induced osteoporosis
GSK-3β	glycogen synthase kinase-3β
HT	hormone therapy
IGF	insulin-like growth factor
IL	interleukin
IOM	Institute of Medicine
LRP5/6	lipoprotein receptor-related protein 5 or 6
M-CSF	macrophage colony-stimulating factor
MORE-CORE	Multiple Outcomes with Raloxifene (continuation study)
NCX	sodium/calcium exchanger
NOF	National Osteoporosis Foundation
NTX	N-terminal crosslinking telopeptide of type 1 collagen
ONJ	osteonecrosis of the jaw
OPG	osteoprotegerin
PI3K	phosphatidylinositol 3′-kinase
pDXA	peripheral dual-energy x-ray absorptiometry
PDGF	platelet-derived growth factor
P1NP	procollagen type 1 N-terminal propeptide
PPAR-γ	peroxisome proliferator-activated receptor-γ
PTH	parathyroid hormone
PTHrP	parathyroid hormone-related protein
RANK	receptor activator of nuclear factor-kappa B
RANKL	receptor activator of nuclear factor kappa B ligand
runX2	runt-related transcription factor
RUTH	Raloxifene Use for the Heart (trial)
SERM	selective estrogen receptor modulator
src	tyrosine protein kinase

sFRP	secreted frizzled related protein
TGF	tissue growth factor
TNF	tumor necrosis factor
TRAP	tartrate-resistant acid phosphate
VDR	vitamin D receptor
VFA	vertebral fracture assessment
WHO	World Health Organization
Wnt	wingless tail ligand

REFERENCES

1. The North American Menopause Society. Management of osteoporosis in postmenopausal women; 2010 position statement of the North American Menopause Society. Menopause 2010;17:25–54.
2. National Osteoporosis Foundation. Fast facts on Osteoporosis. February 2, 2013, *nof.org/osteoporosis/diseasefacts.htm.*
3. Orwig DL, Chiles N, Jones M, et al. Osteoporosis in men: Update 2011. Rheum Dis Clin North Am 2011;37:401–414.
4. Burge R, Dawson-Hughes B, Solomon DH, et al. Incidence and economic burden of osteoporosis-related fractures in the United States, 2005–2025. J Bone Miner Res 2007;22: 465–475.
5. Brauer CA, Coca-Perraillon M, Cutler DM, et al. Incidence and mortality of hip fractures in the United States. JAMA 2009;302:1573–1579.
6. Watts NB, Adler RA, Bilezikian JP, et al. Osteoporosis in men: An Endocrine Society clinical practice guideline. J Clin Endocrinol Metab 2012;97:1802–1822.
7. National Osteoporosis Foundation. Clinician's Guide to Prevention and Treatment of Osteoporosis. 2013, *http://www.nof.org/hcp/clinicians-guide.*
8. Watts NB, Bilezikian JP, Camacho PM, et al. American Association of Clinical Endocrinologists medical guidelines for clinical practice for the diagnosis and treatment of postmenopausal osteoporosis. Endocr Pract 2010;16(suppl)3:1–37.
9. International Society for Clinical Densitometry. Official Positions on FRAX. 2010, *www.iscd.org/visitors/pdfs/Official%20Positions%20ISCD-IOF%20FRAX.pdf.*
10. Miller PD. Unrecognized and unappreciated secondary causes of osteoporosis. Endocrinol Metab Clin North Am 2012;41:613–628.
11. Hamdy NA. Osteoporosis: other secondary causes. Premenopausal osteoporosis. Primer on the Metabolic Bone Diseases and Disorders of Mineral Metabolism. Washington, DC: American Society of Bone and Mineral Metabolism, 2008:276–279.
12. Boyce AM, Gafni RI. Approach to the child with fractures. J Clin Endocrinol Metab 2011;96:1943–1952.
13. Ahmadieh H, Arabi A. Vitamins and bone health: Beyond calcium and vitamin D. Nutr Rev 2011;69:584–598.
14. Borgelt LM, Vondracek SF. Osteoporosis and osteomalacia. In: Tisdale JE, Miller DA, eds. Drug-induced Diseases Prevention, Detection, and Management, 2nd ed. Bethesda, MD: American Society of Health-System Pharmacist, 2010:991–1004.
15. Compston J. Skeletal effects of drugs. Primer on the Metabolic Bone Diseases and Disorders of Mineral Metabolism. Washington, DC: American Society of Bone and Mineral Metabolism, 2008:293–297.
16. Seeman E. Bone quality: the material and structural basis of bone strength. J Bone Miner Metab 2008;26:1–8.
17. Healthcare Costs and Utilization Project. Emergency Visits for Injurious Falls among the Elderly, 2006. Statistical brief #80. 2009, *www.hcupus.ahrq.gov/reports/statbriefs/sb80.jsp.*
18. Office of Statistics and Programming National Center for Injury Prevention and Control Centers for Disease Control and Prevention WISQARS Injury Mortality Reports, 1999–2007, United States fall deaths and rates per 100,000. 2007, *webappa.cdc.gov/sasweb/ncipc/mortrate10_sy.html.*
19. Clarke B. Normal bone anatomy and physiology. Clin J Am Soc Nephrol 2008;3(suppl 3):S131–139.
20. The American College of Obstetricians and Gynecologists. Practice Bulletin No. 129: Osteoporosis. Obstet Gynecol 2012;120:718–734.
21. Oury F. A crosstalk between bone and gonads. Ann N Y Acad Sci 2012;1260:1–7.
22. Rachner TD, Khosla S, Hofbauer LC. Osteoporosis: now and the future. Lancet 2011;377:1276–1287.
23. Thompson WR, Rubin CT, Rubin J. Mechanical regulation of signaling pathways in bone. Gene 2012;503:179–193.
24. Toulis KA, Anastasilakis AD, Polyzos SA, et al. Targeting the osteoblast: Approved and experimental anabolic agents for the treatment of osteoporosis. Hormones 2011;10: 174–195.
25. Baron R, Hesse E. Update on bone anabolics in osteoporosis treatment: rationale, current status, and perspectives. J Clin Endocrinol Metab 2012;97:311–325.
26. Ronis MJ, Mercer K, Chen JR. Effects of nutrition and alcohol consumption on bone loss. Curr Osteoporos Rep 2011;9:53–59.
27. Emkey RD, Emkey GR. Calcium metabolism and correcting calcium deficiencies. Endocrinol Metab Clin North Am 2012;41:527–556.
28. Drake MT, Khosla S. Male osteoporosis. Endocrinol Metab Clin North Am 2012;41:629–641.
29. Gielen E, Vanderschueren D, Callewaert F, et al. Osteoporosis in men. Best Pract Res Clin Endocrinol Metab 2011;25:321–335.
30. Syed FA, Ng AC. The pathophysiology of the aging skeleton. Curr Osteoporos Rep 2010;8:235–240.
31. Horstman AM, Dillon EL, Urban RJ, et al. The role of androgens and estrogens on healthy aging and longevity. J Gerontol A Biol Sci Med Sci 2012;67: 1140–1152.
32. Centers for Disease Control and Prevention. Hip fractures among Older Adults. 2010, *www.cdc.gov/HomeandRecreationalSafety/Falls/adulthipfx.html.*
33. Vondracek SF, Linnebur SA. Diagnosis and management of osteoporosis in the older senior. Clin Interv Aging 2009;4:121–136.
34. The International Society for Clinical Densitometry. 2007 Pediatric Official Positions of the International Society for Clinical Densitometry. 2007, *www.iscd.org/wp-content/themes/iscd/pdfs/official-positions/ISCD2007OfficialPositions-Pediatric.pdf.*
35. The International Society for Clinical Densitometry. 2013 ISCD official positions - adult. *www.iscd.org/official-positions/2013-iscd-official-positions-adult/.*
36. Siminoski K. Tools and techniques: Accurate height assessment to detect hidden vertebral fractures. Osteoporosis Update: A Practical Guide for Canadian Physicians 2005;9:4–5.
37. Schousboe JT, Bauer DC. Clinical use of bone turnover markers to monitor pharmacologic fracture prevention therapy. Curr Osteoporos Rep 2012;10:56–63.
38. Szulc P. The role of bone turnover markers in monitoring treatment in postmenopausal osteoporosis. Clin Biochem 2012;45:907–919.

39. Kanis JA, Oden A, Johnell O, et al. The use of clinical risk factors enhances the performance of BMD in the prediction of hip and osteoporotic fractures in men and women. Osteoporos Int 2007;18:1033–1046.
40. United States Preventive Services Task Force. Summaries for patients: Screening for osteoporosis: Recommendations from the U.S. Preventive Services task force. Ann Intern Med 2011;154:356–364.
41. Gourlay ML, Fine JP, Preisser JS, et al. Bone-density testing interval and transition to osteoporosis in older women. N Engl J Med 2012;366:225–233.
42. Haines ST, Park SK. Vitamin D supplementation: What's known, what to do, and what's needed. Pharmacotherapy 2012;32:354–82.
43. Holick MF, Binkley NC, Bischoff-Ferrari HA, et al. Evaluation, treatment, and prevention of vitamin D deficiency: An Endocrine Society clinical practice guideline. J Clin Endocrinol Metab 2011;96:1911–1930.
44. Rosen CJ, Gallagher JC. The 2011 IOM report on vitamin D and calcium requirements for North America: Clinical implications for providers treating patients with low bone mineral density. J Clin Densitom 2011;14:79–84.
45. National Academy of Sciences Institute of Medicine. Dietary reference intakes for calcium and vitamin D: Summary. Washington (DC): National Academies Press, 2011:1–31. *www.nap.edu/catalog.php?record_id=13050*.
46. Body JJ, Bergmann P, Boonen S, et al. Non-pharmacological management of osteoporosis: A consensus of the Belgian Bone Club. Osteoporos Int 2011;22:2769–2788.
47. Banu J, Varela E, Fernandes G. Alternative therapies for the prevention and treatment of osteoporosis. Nutr Rev 2012;70: 22–40.
48. Kawai M, de Paula FJ, Rosen CJ. New insights into osteoporosis: the bone-fat connection. J Intern Med 2012;272:317–329.
49. Pilsakova L, Riecansky I, Jagla F. The physiological actions of isoflavone phytoestrogens. Physiol Res 2010;59:651–664.
50. Taku K, Melby MK, Nishi N, et al. Soy isoflavones for osteoporosis: An evidence-based approach. Maturitas 2011;70:333–338.
51. Yoon V, Maalouf NM, Sakhaee K. The effects of smoking on bone metabolism. Osteoporos Int 2012;23:2081–2092.
52. Panel on Prevention of Falls in Older Persons, American Geriatrics Society and, British Geriatrics Society. Summary of the Updated American Geriatrics Society/British Geriatrics Society clinical practice guideline for prevention of falls in older persons. J Am Geriatr Soc 2011;59: 148–157.
53. Centers for Disease Control and Prevention. Older Adults Fall Publications. 2012, *www.cdc.gov/HomeandRecreationalSafety/Falls/pubs.html*.
54. National Council on Aging. Falls Prevention. 2013, *www.ncoa.org/improve-health/center-for-healthy-aging/falls-prevention/*.
55. Lindsay R, Gallagher JC, Kagan R, et al. Efficacy of tissue-selective estrogen complex of bazedoxifene/conjugated estrogens for osteoporosis prevention in at-risk postmenopausal women. Fertil Steril 2009;92:1045–1052.
56. Silverman SL. New therapies for osteoporosis: Zoledronic acid, bazedoxifene, and denosumab. Curr Osteoporos Rep 2009;7:91–95.
57. Silverman SL, Chines AA, Kendler DL, et al. Sustained efficacy and safety of bazedoxifene in preventing fractures in postmenopausal women with osteoporosis: Results of a 5-year, randomized, placebo-controlled study. Osteoporos Int 2012;23:351–363.
58. Effective Health Care Program Agency for Healthcare Research and Quality. Treatment to prevent osteoporotic fractures: An update. 2012:1–7.
59. Watts NB, Diab DL. Long-term use of bisphosphonates in osteoporosis. J Clin Endocrinol Metab 2010;95:1555–1565.
60. Donaldson MG, Cawthon PM, Lui LY, et al. Estimates of the proportion of older white women who would be recommended for pharmacologic treatment by the new U.S. National Osteoporosis Foundation Guidelines. J Bone Miner Res 2009;24:675–680.
61. Schnatz PF, Marakovits KA, Dubois M, et al. Osteoporosis screening and treatment guidelines: Are they being followed? Menopause 2011;18:1072–1078.
62. Mangano KM, Walsh SJ, Insogna KL, et al. Calcium intake in the United States from dietary and supplemental sources across adult age groups: new estimates from the National Health and Nutrition Examination Survey 2003–2006. J Am Diet Assoc 2011;111:687–695.
63. Spangler M, Phillips BB, Ross MB, et al. Calcium supplementation in postmenopausal women to reduce the risk of osteoporotic fractures. Am J Health Syst Pharm 2011;68:309–318.
64. Bushinsky DA. Calcium nephrolithiasis. Primer on the Metabolic Bone Diseases and Disorders of Mineral Metabolism. American Society of Bone and Mineral Metabolism 2008:460–464.
65. Bolland MJ, Avenell A, Baron JA, et al. Effect of calcium supplements on risk of myocardial infarction and cardiovascular events: Meta-analysis. BMJ 2010;341:c3691.
66. Bolland MJ, Grey A, Avenell A, et al. Calcium supplements with or without vitamin D and risk of cardiovascular events: Reanalysis of the Women's Health Initiative limited access dataset and meta-analysis. BMJ 2011;342:d2040.
67. Chowdhury R, Stevens S, Ward H, et al. Circulating vitamin D, calcium and risk of cerebrovascular disease: A systematic review and meta-analysis. Eur J Epidemiol 2012;27:581–591.
68. Calcium and cardiovascular risk. Pharmacist's Letter 2012;28:280702. *http://pharmacistsletter.therapeuticresearch.com/home.aspx?cs=&s=PL*.
69. Bischoff-Ferrari HA, Willett WC, Wong JB, et al. Prevention of nonvertebral fractures with oral vitamin D and dose dependency: A meta-analysis of randomized controlled trials. Arch Intern Med 2009;169:551–561.
70. Bischoff-Ferrari HA, Willett WC, Orav EJ, et al. A pooled analysis of vitamin D dose requirements for fracture prevention. N Engl J Med 2012;367:40–49.
71. Binkley N, Gemar D, Engelke J, et al. Evaluation of ergocalciferol or cholecalciferol dosing, 1,600 IU daily or 50,000 IU monthly in older adults. J Clin Endocrinol Metab 2011;96:981–988.
72. Tripkovic L, Lambert H, Hart K, et al. Comparison of vitamin D2 and vitamin D3 supplementation in raising serum 25-hydroxyvitamin D status: A systematic review and meta-analysis. Am J Clin Nutr 2012;95:1357–1364.
73. Autier P, Gandini S, Mullie P. A systematic review: influence of vitamin D supplementation on serum 25-hydroxyvitamin D concentration. J Clin Endocrinol Metab 2012;97: 2606–2613.
74. Nigwekar SU, Bhan I, Thadhani R. Ergocalciferol and cholecalciferol in CKD. Am J Kidney Dis 2012;60:139–156.
75. Rizzoli R. Bisphosphonates for post-menopausal osteoporosis: are they all the same? QJM 2011;104:281–300.
76. Cremers S, Papapoulos S. Pharmacology of bisphosphonates. Bone 2011;49:42–49.
77. MacLean C, Newberry S, Maglione M, et al. Systematic review: Comparative effectiveness of treatments to prevent

fractures in men and women with low bone density or osteoporosis. Ann Intern Med 2008;148:197–213.
78. Elias MN, Burden AM, Cadarette SM. The impact of pharmacist interventions on osteoporosis management: A systematic review. Osteoporos Int 2011;22:2587–2596.
79. Harris ST, Reginster JY, Harley C, et al. Risk of fracture in women treated with monthly oral ibandronate or weekly bisphosphonates: The eValuation of IBandronate Efficacy (VIBE) database fracture study. Bone 2009;44:758–765.
80. Compston J. The use of combination therapy in the treatment of postmenopausal osteoporosis. Endocrine 2012;41:11–18.
81. Reid DM, Hosking D, Kendler D, et al. A comparison of the effect of alendronate and risedronate on bone mineral density in postmenopausal women with osteoporosis: 24-month results from FACTS-International. Int J Clin Pract 2008;62:575–584.
82. Emkey R, Delmas PD, Bolognese M, et al. Efficacy and tolerability of once-monthly oral ibandronate (150 mg) and once-weekly oral alendronate (70 mg): Additional results from the Monthly Oral Therapy with Ibandronate for Osteoporosis Intervention (MOTION) study. Clin Ther 2009;31:751–761.
83. Orwoll ES, Binkley NC, Lewiecki EM, et al. Efficacy and safety of monthly ibandronate in men with low bone density. Bone 2010;46:970–976.
84. Lewiecki EM. Safety of long-term bisphosphonate therapy for the management of osteoporosis. Drugs 2011;71:791–814.
85. Imaz I, Zegarra P, Gonzalez-Enriquez J, et al. Poor bisphosphonate adherence for treatment of osteoporosis increases fracture risk: Systematic review and meta-analysis. Osteoporos Int 2010;21:1943–1951.
86. Compston JE, Bilezikian JP. Bisphosphonate therapy for osteoporosis: The long and short of it. J Bone Miner Res Endocrine 2012;27:240–242.
87. Dempster DW, Lambing CL, Kostenuik PJ, et al. Role of RANK ligand and denosumab, a targeted RANK ligand inhibitor, in bone health and osteoporosis: A review of preclinical and clinical data. Clin Ther 2012;34:521–536.
88. Ellis GK, Bone HG, Chlebowski R, et al. Randomized trial of denosumab in patients receiving adjuvant aromatase inhibitors for nonmetastatic breast cancer. J Clin Oncol 2008;26:4875–4882.
89. Duggan ST, McKeage K. Bazedoxifene, a review of its use in the treatment of postmenopausal osteoporosis. Drugs 2011;71:2193–2212.
90. Goldstein SR, Duvernoy CS, Calaf J, et al. Raloxifene use in clinical practice: Efficacy and safety. Menopause 2009;16:413–421.
91. Eli Lilly and Company. Evista prescribing information. 2011:1–18, *pi.lilly.com/us/evista-pi.pdf*.
92. Grady D, Cauley JA, Stock JL, et al. Effect of raloxifene on all-cause mortality. Am J Med 2010;123:469 e1–7.
93. Novartis. Miacalcin nasal spray prescribing information. 2012:1–17, *www.pharma.us.novartis.com/product/pi/pdf/miacalcin_nasal.pdf*.
94. Davey DA. Androgens in women before and after the menopause and post bilateral oophorectomy: Clinical effects and indications for testosterone therapy. Womens Health (Lond Engl) 2012;8:437–446.
95. Eli Lilly and Company. Forteo prescribing information. 2012:1–14, *pi.lilly.com/us/forteo-pi.pdf*.
96. Farra R, Sheppard NF Jr, McCabe L, et al. First-in-human testing of a wirelessly controlled drug delivery microchip. Sci Transl Med 2012;4:122ra21.
97. Nakamura T, Sugimoto T, Nakano T, et al. Randomized teriparatide [human parathyroid hormone (PTH) 1–34] once-weekly efficacy research (TOWER) trial for examining the reduction in new vertebral fractures in subjects with primary osteoporosis and high fracture risk. J Clin Endocrinol Metab 2012;97:3097–3106.
98. Lewiecki EM. Combination therapy: The Holy Grail for the treatment of postmenopausal osteoporosis? Curr Med Res Opin 2011;27:1493–1497.
99. Tsai JN, Uihlein AV, Lee H, et al. Teriparatide and denosumab, alone or combined, in women with postmenopausal osteoporosis: The DATA study randomized trial. 2013;382:50–56.
100. Robinson Y, Olerud C. Vertebroplasty and kyphoplasty-a systematic review of cement augmentation techniques for osteoporotic vertebral compression fractures compared to standard medical therapy. Maturitas 2012;72:42–49.
101. Rauch F, Bishop N. Idiopathic juvenile osteoporosis. In: Primer on the Metabolic Bone Diseases and Disorders of Mineral Metabolism. Washington, DC: American Society of Bone and Mineral Research, 2008:264–266.
102. Vondracek SF, Hansen LB, McDermott MT. Osteoporosis risk in premenopausal women. Pharmacotherapy 2009;29: 305–317.
103. Cohen A, Shane E. Premenopausal osteoporosis. In: Rosen CJ, Compston JE, Lian JB, eds. Primer on the Metabolic Bone Diseases and Disorders of Mineral Metabolism, 7th ed. Hoboken, NJ: Wiley, 2008:289–293.
104. Greenspan SL, Perera S, Nace D, et al. FRAX or fiction: Determining optimal screening strategies for treatment of osteoporosis in residents in long-term care facilities. J Am Geriatr Soc 2012;60:684–690.
105. Greenspan SL, Wyman A, Hooven FH, et al. Predictors of treatment with osteoporosis medications after recent fragility fractures in a multinational cohort of postmenopausal women. J Am Geriatr Soc 2012;60:455–461.
106. Schousboe JT, Ensrud KE, Nyman JA, et al. Universal bone densitometry screening combined with alendronate therapy for those diagnosed with osteoporosis is highly cost-effective for elderly women. J Am Geriatr Soc 2005;53:1697–1704.
107. Gates BJ, Sonnett TE, Duvall CA, et al. Review of osteoporosis pharmacotherapy for geriatric patients. Am J Geriatr Pharmacother 2009;7:293–323.
108. Schousboe JT, Taylor BC, Fink HA, et al. Cost-effectiveness of bone densitometry followed by treatment of osteoporosis in older men. JAMA 2007;298:629–637.
109. Conwell LJ, Esposito D, Garavaglia S, et al. Out-of-pocket drug costs and drug utilization patterns of postmenopausal Medicare beneficiaries with osteoporosis. Am J Geriatr Pharmacother 2011;9:241–249.
110. Jamal SA, West SL, Miller PD. Bone and kidney disease: diagnostic and therapeutic implications. Curr Rheumatol Rep 2012;14:217–223.
111. Grossman JM, Gordon R, Ranganath VK, et al. American College of Rheumatology 2010 recommendations for the prevention and treatment of glucocorticoid-induced osteoporosis. Arthritis Care Res 2010;62:1515–1526.
112. Weinstein RS. Clinical practice. Glucocorticoid-induced bone disease. N Engl J Med 2011;365:62–70.
113. Leib ES, Saag KG, Adachi JD, et al. Official Positions for FRAX® clinical regarding glucocorticoids: The impact of the use of glucocorticoids on the estimate by FRAX® of the 10 year risk of fracture from Joint Official Positions Development Conference of the International Society for Clinical Densitometry and International Osteoporosis Foundation on FRAX®. J Clin Densitom 2011;14:212–219.
114. Majumdar SR, Lix LM, Yogendran M, et al. Population-based trends in osteoporosis management after new

initiations of long-term systemic glucocorticoids (1998–2008). J Clin Endocrinol Metab 2012;97: 1236–1242.

115. Hansen KE, Wilson HA, Zapalowski C, et al. Uncertainties in the prevention and treatment of glucocorticoid-induced osteoporosis. J Bone Miner Res 2011;26:1989–1996.
116. Karras D, Stoykov I, Lems WF, et al. Effectiveness of teriparatide in postmenopausal women with osteoporosis and glucocorticoid use: 3-Year results from the EFOS study. J Rheumatol 2012;39:600–609.
117. Gralow JR, Biermann JS, Farooki A, et al. NCCN Task Force Report: Bone Health in Cancer Care. J Natl Compr Canc Netw 2009;7(suppl 3):S1–32.
118. Hadji P, Body JJ, Aapro MS, et al. Practical guidance for the management of aromatase inhibitor-associated bone loss. Ann Oncol 2008;19:1407–1416.
119. Mohler JL, Armstrong AJ, Bahnson RR, et al. Prostate cancer, Version 3.2012: Featured updates to the NCCN guidelines. J Natl Compr Canc Netw 2012;10:1081–1087.
120. Amgen Manufacturing Limited. Prolia full prescribing information. 2012, *pi.amgen.com/united_states/prolia/prolia_pi.pdf*.
121. Estrada K, Styrkarsdottir U, Evangelou E, et al. Genome-wide meta-analysis identifies 56 bone mineral density loci and reveals 14 loci associated with risk of fracture. Nat Genet 2012;44:491–501.
122. Richards JB, Zheng HF, Spector TD. Genetics of osteoporosis from genome-wide association studies: Advances and challenges. Nat Rev Genet 2012;13:576–588.
123. Solomon DH. Postfracture interventions disseminated through health care and drug insurers: Attempting to integrate fragmented health care delivery. Osteoporos Int 2011;22(suppl 3):465–469.
124. Liu Y, Nevins JC, Carruthers KM, et al. Osteoporosis risk screening for women in a community pharmacy. J Am Pharm Assoc (2003) 2007;47:521–526.
125. Scott MA, Hitch WJ, Wilson CG, et al. Billing for pharmacists' cognitive services in physicians' offices: Multiple methods of reimbursement. J Am Pharm Assoc (2003) 2012;52:175–180.
126. Xiao Q, Murphy RA, Houston DK, Harris TB, Chow WH, Park Y. Dietary and supplemental calcium intake and cardiovascular disease mortality; The National Institutes of Health-AARP diet and health study. JAMA Intern Med 2013;173:639–646.
127. Michaelsson K, Melhus H, Warensjo E, Wolk A, Byberg L. Long term calcium intake and rates of all cause and cardiovascular mortality: community based prospective longitudinal cohort study. BMJ 2013 Feb 12;346:f228.
128. McClung MR, Lewiecki EM, Geller ML, et al. Effect of denosumab on bone mineral density and biochemical markers of bone turnover: 8-year results of a phase 2 clinical trial. Osteoporos Int 2013;24:227–235.

74

Gout and Hyperuricemia

Michelle A. Fravel, Michael E. Ernst, and Elizabeth C. Clark

KEY CONCEPTS

1. In the absence of a history of gout, asymptomatic hyperuricemia may not require treatment.
2. Acute gouty arthritis may be treated effectively with short courses of high-dose nonsteroidal antiinflammatory drugs (NSAIDs), corticosteroids, or colchicine.
3. Low-dose colchicine is highly effective at relieving acute attacks of gout; dose titration leads to more adverse effects but does not improve efficacy.
4. Treatment with urate-lowering drugs to reduce risk of recurrent attacks of gouty arthritis is considered cost-effective for patients having two or more attacks of gout per year.
5. Xanthine oxidase inhibitors are efficacious for the prophylaxis of recurrent gout attacks in both underexcreters and overproducers of uric acid. Either allopurinol or febuxostat should be initiated in patients with one of the following indications for urate-lowering therapy: (a) two or more gout attacks per year, (b) the presence of one or more tophus, (c) chronic kidney disease (stage 2 or worse), or (d) a history of urolithiasis. The dose of the xanthine oxidase inhibitor should be titrated to a goal serum urate concentration of <6 mg/dL (or <5 mg/dL if signs of gout persist at a level of 6 mg/dL).
6. Uricosuric agents should be avoided for patients with renal impairment [a creatinine clearance below 50 mL/min (0.84 mL/s)], a history of renal calculi, or overproduction of uric acid.
7. Low-dose colchicine, NSAID, or corticosteroid therapy should be administered during the first 3 to 6 months of urate-lowering therapy to minimize the risk of acute gout attacks that may occur during this initiation period.
8. Uric acid nephrolithiasis should be treated with adequate hydration (2 to 3 L/day), a daytime urine-alkalinizing agent, and 60 to 80 mEq/day (60 to 80 mmol/L) of potassium bicarbonate or potassium citrate.
9. Patients with hyperuricemia or gout should undergo comprehensive evaluation for signs and symptoms of cardiovascular disease, and aggressive management of cardiovascular risk factors (i.e., weight loss, reduction of alcohol intake, control of blood pressure, glucose, and lipids) should be undertaken as indicated.

The term *gout* describes a heterogeneous clinical spectrum of diseases including elevated serum urate concentration (hyperuricemia), recurrent attacks of acute arthritis associated with monosodium urate crystals in synovial fluid leukocytes, deposits of monosodium urate crystals (tophi) in tissues in and around joints, interstitial renal disease, and uric acid nephrolithiasis.[1]

The underlying metabolic disorder of gout is hyperuricemia, defined physiochemically as serum that is supersaturated with monosodium urate. At 37°C (98.6°F), serum urate concentrations above (or around) 7 mg/dL (416 μmol/L) begin to exceed the limit of solubility for monosodium urate.[1] For determination of the risk of gout, hyperuricemia is defined statistically as serum urate concentrations greater than two standard deviations above the population means for age- and sex-matched healthy populations, usually 7 mg/dL (416 μmol/L) for men and 6 mg/dL (357 μmol/L) for women.[1,2] Although hyperuricemia is fundamental to the development of gout, the mere presence of hyperuricemia itself is often an asymptomatic condition.

EPIDEMIOLOGY

Historically, gout has been referred to as the "disease of kings" since it was often associated with affluent societies and lifestyles of overindulgence, gluttony, and intemperance.[1] Gout continues to occur more commonly in developed countries (e.g., United States, Japan, United Kingdom, and Australia) as compared to developing countries (e.g., China).[3] In the United States, the prevalence of gout is increasing. According to data from the 2007 to 2008 National Health and Nutrition Examination Survey (NHANES), the prevalence of gout in US adults is 3.9%, which corresponds to an estimated 8.3 million people. This represents a 1.2% increase in prevalence compared with NHANES-III survey data from 1988 to 1994.[4]

Elevated serum urate levels are the single most important risk factor for the development of gout, and the relationship between the risk of an attack of acute gouty arthritis and serum urate levels is linearly correlated. The 5-year cumulative risk of gout for patients with serum urate concentrations <7 mg/dL (<416 μmol/L) is 0.6%, compared with a risk of 30.5% for those with urate levels >10 mg/dL (>595 μmol/L).[5] Sustained elevation of serum urate is virtually essential for the development of gout; however, hyperuricemia does not always lead to gout, and many patients with hyperuricemia remain asymptomatic.[2] Although unusual, acute gouty arthritis has been reported to occur in the presence of normal serum uric acid concentrations.[6] The prevalence of hyperuricemia in the United States mirrors the trend seen with gout, affecting 21.4% of adults (43.3 million people) in 2007 to 2008 compared to just 18.2% in 1998 to 1994.[4]

The increased prevalence of gout and hyperuricemia may be partly explained by the aging of the population. Gout and hyperuricemia occur more commonly in the older adult with the highest prevalence, 12.6%, in those 80 years of age and older compared with just 0.4% in those ages 20 to 29 years.[4] Another major contributor to the increased prevalence of gout in the United States is the obesity epidemic. Obese persons are twice as likely to have gout as nonobese counterparts.[7] Dietary and lifestyle factors linked to obesity have also been independently associated with gout. These include consumption of alcohol, sugary beverages, and red meat along with a sedentary lifestyle.[8]

Regarding sex distribution, gout affects men about three times more often than women.[4] The lowest rates of gout are observed in women younger than 45 years, approximately 0.6 cases per 1,000 person-years.[9] Serum uric acid levels in women approach those of men once menopause has occurred; thus, in older age groups the gender gap narrows, and approximately half of newly diagnosed cases of gout are found in women.[10,11] Gout in men younger than 30 years of age or in premenopausal women may indicate an inherited enzyme defect or the presence of renal disease. Although no genetic marker has been isolated for gout, the familial nature of gout strongly suggests an interaction between genetic and environmental factors.

ETIOLOGY AND PATHOPHYSIOLOGY

In humans, the production of uric acid is the terminal step in the degradation of purines. Uric acid serves no known physiologic purpose and is regarded as a waste product. Normal uric acid levels are near the limits of urate solubility, because of the delicate balance that exists between the amount of urate produced and excreted.[2] Humans have higher uric acid levels than other mammals because they do not express the enzyme uricase, which converts uric acid into the more soluble allantoin.[10]

Gout occurs exclusively in humans in whom a miscible pool of uric acid exists. Under normal conditions, the amount of accumulated uric acid is about 1,200 mg in men and about 600 mg in women. The size of the urate pool is increased severalfold in individuals with gout. This excess accumulation may result from either overproduction or underexcretion of uric acid. Several conditions are associated with either decreased renal clearance or an overproduction of uric acid, leading to hyperuricemia. Table 74-1 lists some of these conditions.

Overproduction of Uric Acid

The purines from which uric acid is produced originate from three sources: dietary purine, conversion of tissue nucleic acid into purine nucleotides, and de novo synthesis of purine bases. The purines derived from these three sources enter a common metabolic pathway leading to the production of either nucleic acid or uric acid. Under normal circumstances, uric acid may accumulate excessively if production exceeds excretion. The average human produces about 600 to 800 mg of uric acid each day. Dietary purines play an unimportant role in the generation of hyperuricemia in the absence of some derangement in purine metabolism or elimination. However, diet modifications are important for patients with such problems who develop symptomatic hyperuricemia.

Several enzyme systems regulate purine metabolism. Abnormalities in these regulatory systems can result in overproduction of uric acid. Uric acid may also be overproduced as a consequence of increased breakdown of tissue nucleic acids and excessive rates of cell turnover, as observed with myeloproliferative and lymphoproliferative disorders, polycythemia vera, psoriasis, and some types of anemias. Cytotoxic medications used to treat these disorders can result in overproduction of uric acid secondary to lysis and breakdown of cellular matter.

Two enzyme abnormalities resulting in an overproduction of uric acid have been well described (Fig. 74-1). The first is an increase in the activity of phosphoribosyl pyrophosphate (PRPP) synthetase, which leads to an increased concentration of PRPP. PRPP is a key determinant of purine synthesis and uric acid production. The second is a deficiency of hypoxanthine-guanine phosphoribosyltransferase (HGPRT). HGPRT is responsible for the conversion of guanine to guanylic acid and hypoxanthine to inosinic acid. These two conversions require PRPP as the cosubstrate and are important reactions involved in the synthesis of nucleic acids. A deficiency in the HGPRT enzyme leads to increased metabolism of guanine and hypoxanthine to uric acid and to more PRPP to interact with glutamine in the first step of the purine pathway.[12] Complete absence of HGPRT results in the childhood Lesch–Nyhan syndrome, characterized by choreoathetosis, spasticity, intellectual disability, and markedly excessive production of uric acid. A partial deficiency of the enzyme may be responsible for marked hyperuricemia in otherwise normal, healthy individuals.

TABLE 74-1 Conditions Associated with Hyperuricemia

Primary gout	Obesity
Diabetic ketoacidosis	Sarcoidosis
Myeloproliferative disorders	Congestive heart failure
Lactic acidosis	Renal dysfunction
Lymphoproliferative disorders	Down's syndrome
Starvation	Lead toxicity
Chronic hemolytic anemia	Hyperparathyroidism
Toxemia of pregnancy	Acute alcoholism
Pernicious anemia	Hypoparathyroidism
Glycogen storage disease type 1	Acromegaly
Psoriasis	Hypothyroidism
Hypoxanthine-guanine phosphoribosyltransferase deficiency	Phosphoribosylpyrophosphate synthetase overactivity
Polycythemia vera	Berylliosis
Renal transplantation	

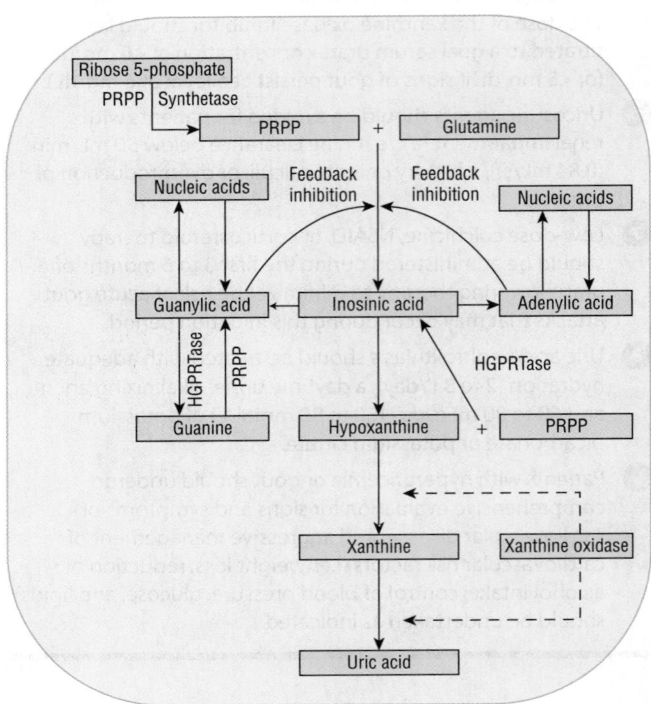

FIGURE 74-1 Purine metabolism. (HGPRT, hypoxanthine-guanine phosphoribosyltransferase; PRPP, phosphoribosyl pyrophosphate.)

CLINICAL PRESENTATION Acute Gouty Arthritis

General

- Gout classically presents as an acute inflammatory monoarthritis. The first metatarsophalangeal joint is often involved ("podagra"), but any joint of the lower extremity can be affected and occasionally gout will present as a monoarthritis of the wrist or finger. The spectrum of gout also includes nephrolithiasis, gouty nephropathy, and aggregated deposits of sodium urate (tophi) in cartilage, tendons, synovial membranes, and elsewhere

Signs and Symptoms

- Fever, intense pain, erythema, warmth, swelling, and inflammation of involved joints

Laboratory Tests

- Elevated serum uric acid levels; leukocytosis

Other Diagnostic Tests

- Observation of monosodium urate crystals in synovial fluid or a tophus
- For patients with long-standing gout, radiographs may show asymmetric swelling within a joint on or subcortical cysts without erosions

Underexcretion of Uric Acid

Normally, uric acid does not accumulate as long as production is balanced with elimination. About two thirds of the daily uric acid production is excreted in the urine and the remainder is eliminated through the GI tract after enzymatic degradation by colonic bacteria. The vast majority of patients (90%) with gout have a relative decrease in the renal excretion of uric acid for an unknown reason (primary idiopathic hyperuricemia).[2]

A decline in the urinary excretion of uric acid to a level below the rate of production leads to hyperuricemia and an increased miscible pool of sodium urate. Almost all the urate in plasma is freely filtered across the glomerulus. The concentration of uric acid appearing in the urine is determined by multiple renal tubular transport processes in addition to the filtered load. Evidence favors a four-component model including glomerular filtration, tubular reabsorption, tubular secretion, and postsecretory reabsorption.

Approximately 90% of filtered uric acid is reabsorbed in the proximal tubule, probably by both active and passive transport mechanisms. There is a close linkage between proximal tubular sodium reabsorption and uric acid reabsorption, so conditions that enhance sodium reabsorption (e.g., dehydration) also lead to increased uric acid reabsorption. The exact site of tubular secretion of uric acid has not been determined; this too appears to involve an active transport process. Postsecretory reabsorption occurs somewhere distal to the secretory site. Table 74-2 lists the drugs that decrease renal clearance of uric acid through modification of filtered load or one of the tubular transport processes. By enhancing renal urate reabsorption, insulin resistance is also associated with gout.

The pathophysiologic approach to the evaluation of hyperuricemia requires determining whether the patient is overproducing or underexcreting uric acid. This can be accomplished by placing the patient on a purine-free diet for 3 to 5 days and then measuring the amount of uric acid excreted in the urine in 24 hours. As it is very difficult to maintain a purine-free diet for several days, this test is done infrequently in clinical practice. Nevertheless, when it is performed, individuals who excrete more than 600 mg on a purine-free diet may be considered overproducers. Hyperuricemic individuals who excrete less than 600 mg of uric acid per 24 hours on a purine-free diet may be classified as underexcreters of uric acid. On a regular diet, excretion of more than 1,000 mg per 24 hours reflects overproduction; less than this is probably normal.

TABLE 74-2 Drugs Capable of Inducing Hyperuricemia and Gout

Diuretics	Ethanol	Ethambutol
Nicotinic acid	Pyrazinamide	Cytotoxic drugs
Salicylates (<2 g/day)	Levodopa	Cyclosporine

CLINICAL PRESENTATION

❶ Gout is diagnosed clinically by symptoms rather than laboratory tests of uric acid. In fact, asymptomatic hyperuricemia discovered incidentally generally requires no therapy because many individuals with hyperuricemia will never experience an attack of gout. These patients should still be encouraged to implement lifestyle measures to reduce serum urate concentrations.

Acute Gouty Arthritis

A classic acute attack of gouty arthritis is characterized by rapid and localized onset of excruciating pain, swelling, and inflammation. The attack is typically monoarticular at first, most often affecting the first metatarsophalangeal joint (great toe) and then, in order of frequency, the insteps, ankles, heels, knees, wrists, fingers, and elbows. In one half of initial attacks, the first metatarsophalangeal joint is affected, a condition commonly referred to as *podagra* (see Fig. 74-2). Up to 90% of patients with gout will experience podagra at some point in the course of their disease.[2]

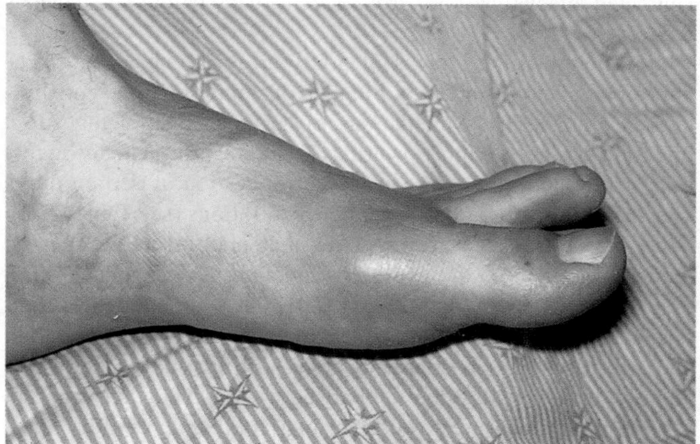

FIGURE 74-2 Acute gout attack of the first metatarsophalangeal joint. *(From Imboden J, Hellmann DB, Stone JH. Current Rheumatology Diagnosis and Treatment, 2nd ed. New York: McGraw-Hill, 2004:316.)*

TABLE 74-3 Clinical Manifestations of Gout

Classic acute gout ("podagra")	Monoarticular arthritis Frequently attacks the first metatarsophalangeal joint, although other joints of the lower extremities are also frequently involved Affected joint is swollen, erythematous, and tender
Interval gout	Asymptomatic period between attacks
Tophaceous gout	Deposits of monosodium urate crystals in soft tissues Complications include soft tissue damage, deformity, joint destruction, and nerve compression syndromes such as carpal tunnel syndrome
Atypical gout	Polyarthritis affecting any joint, upper or lower extremity May be confused with rheumatoid arthritis or osteoarthritis
Gouty nephropathy	Nephrolithiasis Acute and chronic renal impairment

Atypical presentations of gout also occur. For elderly patients, gout can present as a chronic polyarticular arthritis that can be confused with rheumatoid arthritis or osteoarthritis. Additionally, the onset of gout may be less dramatic than the typical acute attack and have fewer clinical findings.[13] Multiple small joints in the hands may be involved, especially in elderly women.[10] Table 74-3 summarizes the different clinical manifestations of gout.

The predilection of acute gout for peripheral joints of the lower extremity is probably related to the low temperature of these joints combined with high intraarticular urate concentration. Synovial effusions are likely to occur transiently in weight-bearing joints during the course of a day with routine activity. At night, water is reabsorbed from the joint space, leaving behind a supersaturated solution of monosodium urate, which can precipitate attacks of acute arthritis. Attacks generally begin at night with the patient awakened from sleep by excruciating pain.

The development of crystal-induced inflammation involves a number of chemical mediators causing vasodilation, increased vascular permeability, complement activation, and chemotactic activity for polymorphonuclear leukocytes.[14] Phagocytosis of urate crystals by the leukocytes results in rapid lysis of cells and a discharge of lysosomal and proteolytic enzymes into the cytoplasm. The ensuing inflammatory reaction is associated with intense joint pain, erythema, warmth, and swelling. Fever is common, as is leukocytosis. Untreated attacks may last from 3 to 14 days before spontaneous recovery.

Although acute attacks of gouty arthritis may occur without apparent provocation, a number of conditions may precipitate an attack. These include stress, trauma, alcohol ingestion, infection, surgery, rapid lowering of serum uric acid by ingestion of uric acid-lowering agents, and ingestion of certain drugs known to elevate serum uric acid concentrations (see Table 74-2). Other crystal-induced arthropathies that may resemble gout on clinical presentation are caused by calcium pyrophosphate dihydrate crystals (pseudogout) and calcium hydroxyapatite crystals, which are associated with calcific periarthritis, tendinitis, and arthritis.[14–17] Acute flares of gouty arthritis may occur infrequently, but over time the interval between attacks may shorten if appropriate measures to correct hyperuricemia are not undertaken. Later in the disease, tophaceous deposits of monosodium urate crystals in the skin or subcutaneous tissues may be found. These tophi can be anywhere but are often found on the hands, wrists, elbows, or knees. It is estimated to take 10 or more years for tophi to develop.

TABLE 74-4 Differential Diagnosis of Acute Monoarthritis

1. Pseudogout (pyrophosphate crystal-related arthritis)
2. Palindromic rheumatism
3. Seronegative inflammatory arthritis
4. Trauma or hemarthrosis
5. Septic arthritis
6. Cellulitis
7. Type II dyslipidemia
8. Unrelated hyperuricemia (as in psoriasis, hypertension) when joint pain is not caused by gout

Diagnostic Evaluation

Table 74-4 lists the differential diagnosis of an acute monoarthritis.[18,19] A definitive diagnosis of gout requires aspiration of synovial fluid from the affected joint and identification of intracellular crystals of monosodium urate monohydrate in synovial fluid leukocytes.[2] Identification of monosodium urate crystals is highly dependent on the experience of the observer. Crystals are needle shaped, and when examined under polarizing light microscopy, they are strongly negatively birefringent (see Fig. 74-3). Crystals can be observed in synovial fluid during asymptomatic periods.[20] If an affected joint is tapped, the resulting synovial fluid may have white cells and appear purulent. Such findings should always raise the question of infection. If any clinical features of infection are present, such as high fever, elevated white blood cell count, multiple joints affected, or an identified source of infection, proper diagnosis and treatment are critical. Patients with gout can have septic arthritis. Diabetes, alcohol abuse, and advanced age increase the likelihood of septic arthritis.

In lieu of obtaining a synovial fluid sample from an affected joint to inspect for urate crystals, the clinical triad of inflammatory monoarthritis, elevated serum uric acid level, and response to colchicine can be used to diagnose gout. However, this approach has limitations, including a failure to recognize atypical gout presentations and the fact that serum uric acid levels can be normal or even low during an acute gout attack.[2,5,21] In addition, use of colchicine

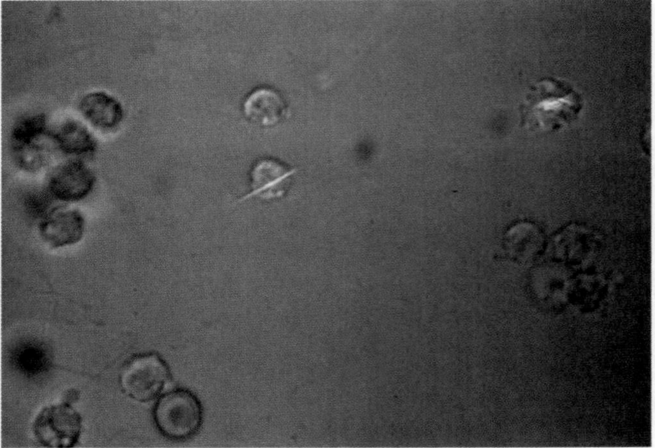

FIGURE 74-3 Urate crystal ingested by a polymorphonuclear leukocyte in synovial fluid. *(From Imboden J, Hellmann DB, Stone JH. Current Rheumatology Diagnosis and Treatment, 2nd ed. New York: McGraw-Hill, 2004:317.)*

TABLE 74-5 EULAR Evidence-Based Recommendations for Gout: Diagnostic Principles

1. In acute attacks the rapid development of severe pain, swelling, and tenderness that reaches its maximum within just 6–12 hours, especially with overlying erythema, is highly suggestive of crystal inflammation though not specific for gout
2. For typical presentations of gout (such as recurrent podagra with hyperuricemia), a clinical diagnosis alone is reasonably accurate but not definitive without crystal confirmation
3. Demonstration of MSU crystals in synovial fluid or tophus aspirates permits a definitive diagnosis of gout
4. A routine search for MSU crystals is recommended in all synovial fluid samples obtained from undiagnosed inflamed joints
5. Identification of MSU crystals from asymptomatic joints may allow definite diagnosis in intercritical periods
6. Gout and sepsis may coexist. When septic arthritis is suspected, gram staining and culture of synovial fluid should still be performed, even if MSU crystals are identified
7. While the most important risk factor for gout, serum uric acid levels do not confirm or exclude gout, as many people with hyperuricemia do not develop gout, and during acute attacks serum levels may be normal
8. Renal uric acid excretion should be determined in selected gout patients, especially those with a family history of young onset gout, onset of gout under age 25, or with renal calculi
9. Although radiographs may be useful for differential diagnosis and may show typical features in chronic gout, they are not useful in confirming the diagnosis of early or acute gout
10. Risk factors for gout and associated comorbidity should be assessed, including features of the metabolic syndrome (obesity, hyperglycemia, hyperlipidemia, hypertension)

EULAR: The European League Against Rheumatism; MSU: monosodium urate.
Data from Reference 22.

as a diagnostic tool for gout is limited by lack of sensitivity and specificity for the disease. Other conditions such as psoriatic arthritis, sarcoidosis, and Mediterranean fever can respond to colchicine therapy. For patients with long-standing gout, radiographs may show punched-out marginal erosions and secondary osteoarthritic changes; however, in an acute first attack radiographs will be unremarkable.[19,22] The presence of chondrocalcinosis on radiographs may indicate pseudogout. Some studies have recently examined the use of magnetic resonance imaging and computed tomography to obtain images for patients with gout; however, this is not currently considered part of normal practice. Table 74-5 shows the European League Against Rheumatism (EULAR) evidence-based diagnostic principles.[22]

Uric Acid Nephrolithiasis

Clinicians should be suspicious of hyperuricemic states for patients who present with kidney stones, as nephrolithiasis occurs in approximately 15% of patients with gout.[23] The frequency of urolithiasis depends on serum uric acid concentrations, acidity of the urine, and urinary uric acid concentration. Typically, patients with uric acid nephrolithiasis have a urinary pH of less than 6. Uric acid has a negative logarithm of the acid ionization constant of 5.5. Therefore, when the urine is acidic, uric acid exists primarily in the unionized, less soluble form. At a urine pH of 5, urine is saturated at a uric acid level of 15 mg/dL (0.89 mmol/L). When the urine pH is 7, the solubility of uric acid in urine is increased to 200 mg/dL (11.9 mmol/L).[1] For patients with uric acid nephrolithiasis, urinary pH typically is less than 6 and frequently less than 5.5. When acidic urine is saturated with uric acid, spontaneous precipitation of stones may occur.

Other factors that predispose individuals to uric acid nephrolithiasis include excessive urinary excretion of uric acid and highly concentrated urine. The risk of renal calculi approaches 50% in individuals whose renal excretion of uric acid exceeds 1,100 mg/day (6.5 mmol/day). In addition to pure uric acid stones, hyperuricosuric individuals are at increased risk for mixed uric acid–calcium oxalate stones and pure calcium oxalate stones. Uric acid stones are usually small, round, and radiolucent. Uric acid stones containing calcium are radiopaque.[24]

Gouty Nephropathy

There are two types of gouty nephropathy: acute uric acid nephropathy and chronic urate nephropathy.[2] In acute uric acid nephropathy, acute renal failure occurs as a result of blockage of urine flow secondary to massive precipitation of uric acid crystals in the collecting ducts and ureters. This syndrome is a well-recognized complication for patients with myeloproliferative or lymphoproliferative disorders and is a result of massive malignant cell turnover, particularly after initiation of chemotherapy.

Chronic urate nephropathy is caused by the long-term deposition of urate crystals in the renal parenchyma. Microtophi may form, with a surrounding giant-cell inflammatory reaction. A decrease in the kidneys' ability to concentrate urine and the presence of proteinuria may be the earliest pathophysiologic disturbances. Hypertension and nephrosclerosis are common associated findings. Although renal failure occurs in a higher percentage of gouty patients than expected, it is not clear if hyperuricemia per se has a harmful effect on the kidneys. The chronic renal impairment seen in individuals with gout may result largely from the coexistence of hypertension, diabetes mellitus, and atherosclerosis.

Tophaceous Gout

Tophi (urate deposits) are uncommon in the general population of gouty subjects and are a late complication of hyperuricemia. The most common sites of tophaceous deposits for patients with recurrent acute gouty arthritis are the base of the fingers, olecranon bursae, ulnar aspect of the forearm, Achilles tendon, knees, wrists, and hands (Fig. 74-4).[2] Eventually, even the hips, shoulders, and spine may be affected. In addition to causing obvious deformities, tophi may damage surrounding soft tissue, cause joint destruction and pain, and even lead to nerve compression syndromes including carpal tunnel syndrome.

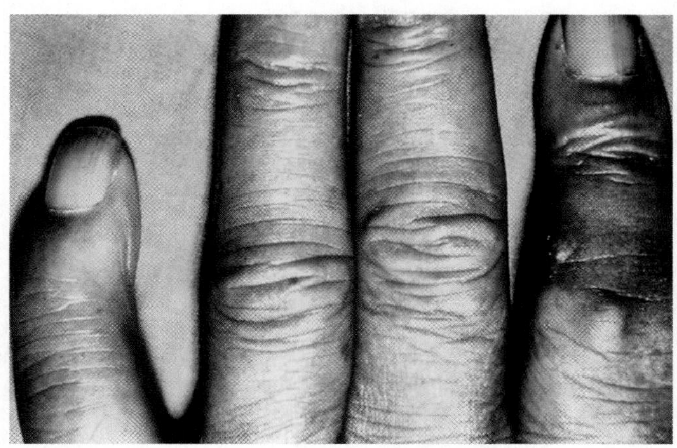

FIGURE 74-4 Tophaceous gout with subcutaneous nodule almost breaking through the skin. *(From South-Paul JE, Matheny SC, Lewis EL. Current Diagnosis and Treatment in Family Medicine. New York: McGraw-Hill, 2004:275.)*

TREATMENT

Desired Outcomes

The goals in the treatment of gout are to terminate the acute attack, prevent recurrent attacks of gouty arthritis, and prevent complications associated with chronic deposition of urate crystals in tissues. These can be accomplished through a combination of pharmacologic and nonpharmacologic methods, including focused patient education efforts. The first-ever American College of Rheumatology (ACR) evidence- and consensus-based guidelines for the management of gout were published in 2012.[25,26] These guidelines provide specific recommendations for treatment of acute gout attacks, management of hyperuricemia in gout, and antiinflammatory prophylaxis of acute gout during initiation of urate-lowering therapy. These guidelines will be discussed throughout the remainder of the treatment section of this chapter. Tables 74-6 and 74-7 summarize dosing and monitoring information for available pharmacotherapy used in management and prevention of gout.

Acute Gouty Arthritis

Nonpharmacologic Therapy

There are limited effective nonpharmacologic therapies for an acute gout attack; therefore, they are recommended strictly as adjunctive treatment.

Local ice application is the most effective.[26] In one small study, adjunctive ice application resulted in significantly greater pain reduction in those receiving the therapy compared with those not treated with ice (difference of 3.33 cm on a 10-cm visual analog pain scale, $P = 0.021$).[27] Complementary and alternative medicines, including flaxseed and celery root, are not recommended in ACR guidelines.[26]

Pharmacologic Therapy

(2) For most patients, acute attacks of gouty arthritis may be treated successfully with nonsteroidal antiinflammatory drugs (NSAIDs), corticosteroids, or colchicine. The ACR guidelines recognize these three modalities as first-line monotherapy for the treatment of acute gout. Treatment should commence within 24 hours of the onset of an attack. In more severe cases, those affecting multiple joints or

TABLE 74-6 Pharmacotherapy of Acute Gout, Antiinflammatory Prophylaxis During Initiation of Urate-Lowering Therapy and Hyperuricemia in Gout[a]

Drug	Brand Name	Initial Dose	Usual Range	Special Population Dose	Other
Acute Gout					
Nonsteroidal antiinflammatory drugs					In general, not recommended in patients with advanced renal disease as NSAID use may decrease renal function; Use with caution in patients with mild to moderate renal impairment
Etodolac	Lodine, various	300 mg twice daily	300–500 mg twice daily		
Fenoprofen	Nalfon, various	400 mg three times daily	400–600 mg three to four times daily		
Ibuprofen	Advil, various	400 mg three times daily	400–800 mg three to four times daily		
Indomethacin	Indocin	50 mg three times daily	50 mg three times daily initially until pain is tolerable then rapidly reduce to complete cessation		
Ketoprofen	Orudis, various	75 mg three times daily or 50 mg four times daily	50–75 mg three to four times daily	Severe renal impairment (GFR < 25 mL/min [0.42 mL/s]): 100 mg maximum daily dose Mildly impaired renal function: 150 mg maximum daily dose Impaired liver function with serum albumin < 3.5 g/dL (<35 g/L): 100 mg maximum daily dose	
Naproxen	Naprosyn, various	750 mg followed by 250 mg every 8 hours until the attack has subsided		Not recommended in severe renal impairment (creatinine clearance <30 mL/min [<0.5 mL/s])	
Piroxicam	Feldene	20 mg once daily or divided twice daily			
Sulindac	Clinoril	200 mg twice a day	150–200 mg twice daily for 7–10 days		
Celecoxib	Celebrex	800 mg followed by 400 mg on day one then 400 mg twice daily for 1 week			Option for patients with GI contraindications to nonselective NSAIDs; unclear risk-to-benefit ratio at this time due to cardiovascular concerns
Oral colchicine	Colcrys	1.2 mg initially, followed by 0.6 mg 1 hour later		See Table 74-8	Dose adjustment recommended when used with selected CYP3A4 and P-glycoprotein inhibitors

(continued)

TABLE 74-6 Pharmacotherapy of Acute Gout, Antiinflammatory Prophylaxis During Initiation of Urate-Lowering Therapy and Hyperuricemia in Gout[a] (*Continued*)

Drug	Brand Name	Initial Dose	Usual Range	Special Population Dose	Other
Corticosteroids					
Oral		0.5 mg/kg prednisone equivalent daily for 5–10 days followed by discontinuation or 0.5 mg/kg daily for 2–5 days followed by tapering for 7–10 days	30–60 mg prednisone equivalent once daily for 3–5 days, then taper in 5-mg decrements spread over 10–14 days until discontinuation		The use of an oral methylprednisolone dose pack may be considered
Intramuscular		Triamcinolone acetonide 60 mg IM once; methylprednisolone 100 mg IM once	Triamcinolone acetonide 60 mg IM once; methylprednisolone 100–150 mg IM daily for 1–2 days		Administration of intramuscular triamcinolone is to be followed by oral prednisone or prednisolone
Intraarticular	Kenalog	Triamcinolone acetonide 10 mg (large joints), 5 mg (small joints)	Triamcinolone acetonide 10–40 mg (large joints), 5–20 mg (small joints)		Intraarticular administration is acceptable when only one to two joints involved and should be used in combination with NSAIDs, colchicine, or oral corticosteroids
Corticotropin	H.P. Acthar Gel	40 units IM or SC every 72 hours	40–80 units IM or SC every 24–72 hours		Contraindicated for IV administration
Interleukin-1 inhibitors					Reserve use for refractory cases
Anakinra	Kineret	100 mg SC daily for 3 days			
Canakinumab	Ilaris	Single dose 150 mg SC			
Antiinflammatory Prophylaxis During Initiation of Urate-Lowering Therapy					
NSAIDs			Lowest effective dosage		
Oral colchicine	Colcrys	0.6 mg daily	0.6 mg once or twice daily	See Table 74-8	
Prednisone or prednisolone		≤10 mg daily			Second-line therapy; recommended only if colchicine and NSAIDs are both contraindicated, ineffective or not tolerated
Interleukin-1 inhibitors					Reserve use for refractory cases
Rilonacept	Arcalyst	320 mg loading dose followed by 160 mg weekly (SC)			Studied for 16-week duration
Canakinumab	Ilaris	Single SC dose (50 mg to 300 mg) or four times weekly SC dosing (50 mg—50 mg—25 mg—25 mg)			
Hyperuricemia in Gout					
Xanthine oxidase inhibitors					
Allopurinol	Lopurin, Zyloprim	100 mg daily	100–800 mg daily to achieve serum urate concentration <6 mg/dL (<357 μmol/L)	Start at dose of 50 mg daily for patients with a glomerular filtration rate <30 mL/min/1.73 m^2	
Febuxostat	Uloric	40 mg daily	40–80 mg/daily	No dosage adjustment necessary for patients with mild-moderate renal dysfunction (creatinine clearance 30–89 mL/min [0.5–1.5 mL/s]) Insufficient data in patients with creatinine clearance <30 mL/min (<0.5 mL/s)	
Uricosurics					
Probenecid	Probalan	250 mg twice daily for one week	500–2000 mg/day [target serum urate concentration <6 mg/dL (<357 mol/L)]	Not recommended if creatinine clearance <50 mL/min (<0.83 mL/s)	
Other					
Pegloticase	Krystexxa	8 mg IV every 2 weeks			Optimal treatment duration has not been established

[a]Agents available in the United States.

TABLE 74-7 Drug Monitoring

Drug	Adverse Drug Reaction	Monitoring Parameter	Comments
NSAIDs	Renal dysfunction, gastritis (worse with concurrent aspirin), fluid retention, blood pressure elevation	Therapeutic Resolution of pain Avoidance of gout attacks when used for prophylaxis Toxic Blood pressure Renal function Edema Dark stools	Avoid for patients with peptic ulcer disease, active bleeding Use caution in congestive heart failure, dehydration, renal impairment Consider coadministration with a proton-pump inhibitor when used long term for patients at risk for GI bleeding
Systemic corticosteroids	GI upset, increased appetite, nervousness/restlessness, transient glucose intolerance, fluid retention, blood pressure elevation	Therapeutic Resolution of pain Avoidance of gout attacks when used for prophylaxis Toxic Glucose levels in patients with diabetes	Limit duration of therapy in patients with diabetes
Intraarticular corticosteroids	Injection pain, rebound arthritis	Therapeutic Resolution of pain Toxic Signs of rebound arthritis (pain relief followed by reemergence of pain)	Avoid if joint sepsis cannot be ruled out
Corticotropin	Increased appetite, nervousness/restlessness, transient glucose intolerance, fluid retention, blood pressure elevation	Therapeutic Resolution of pain	Requires intact pituitary–adrenal axis Less effective for patients receiving long-term oral corticosteroid therapy
Colchicine	Dose-dependent GI adverse effects (diarrhea, nausea, vomiting), rare myelosuppression, and reversible neuromyopathy	Therapeutic Resolution of pain Avoidance of gout attacks when used for prophylaxis Toxic GI symptoms Complete blood count	
Interleukin-1 inhibitors	Injection site reaction, neutropenia, immune hypersensitivity reaction, infectious disease, malignancy	Therapeutic Resolution of pain Avoidance of gout attacks when used for prophylaxis Toxic Neutrophil count (prior to initiation, monthly for the first 3 months of therapy then after 6, 9, and 12 months of therapy) Temperature (periodically to detect infection)	Safety for use in acute gout and gout prophylaxis during initiation of urate-lowering therapy has not yet been established; not FDA approved for use in gout
Allopurinol	Rash, potential for fatal hypersensitivity syndrome	Therapeutic Serum urate level Reduced frequency of gout attacks Toxic Rash Renal function	Can be used in both urate overproduction and urate underexcretion
Febuxostat	Liver enzyme elevation, nausea, arthralgias, and rash	Therapeutic Serum urate level Reduced frequency of gout attacks Toxic Liver function tests Renal function	Can be used in both urate overproduction and urate underexcretion
Probenecid	Urolithiasis	Therapeutic Serum urate level Reduced frequency of gout attacks Toxic Renal function	Useful in urate underexcretion Avoid for patients with history of urolithiasis
Pegloticase	Acute gout attack during treatment initiation, anaphylaxis, GI symptoms (constipation, nausea, vomiting), chest pain, nasopharyngitis	Therapeutic Serum urate levels Reduced frequency of gout attacks Toxic Signs/symptoms of anaphylaxis following infusion	Reserved for patients with gout refractory to conventional therapies Can be used in both urate overproduction and urate underexcretion

causing higher intensity pain, combination or investigational drug therapy may be indicated (Fig. 74-5).[26]

Nonsteroidal Antiinflammatory Drugs

NSAIDs are a mainstay of therapy for acute attacks of gouty arthritis because of their excellent efficacy and minimal toxicity with short-term use. Indomethacin has been historically favored as the NSAID of choice for acute gout flares, but there is little evidence to support one NSAID as being more efficacious than another. Three agents (indomethacin, naproxen, and sulindac) have U.S. Food and Drug Administration (FDA)-approved labeling for the treatment of gout, although several others are likely to be effective.[26] Although

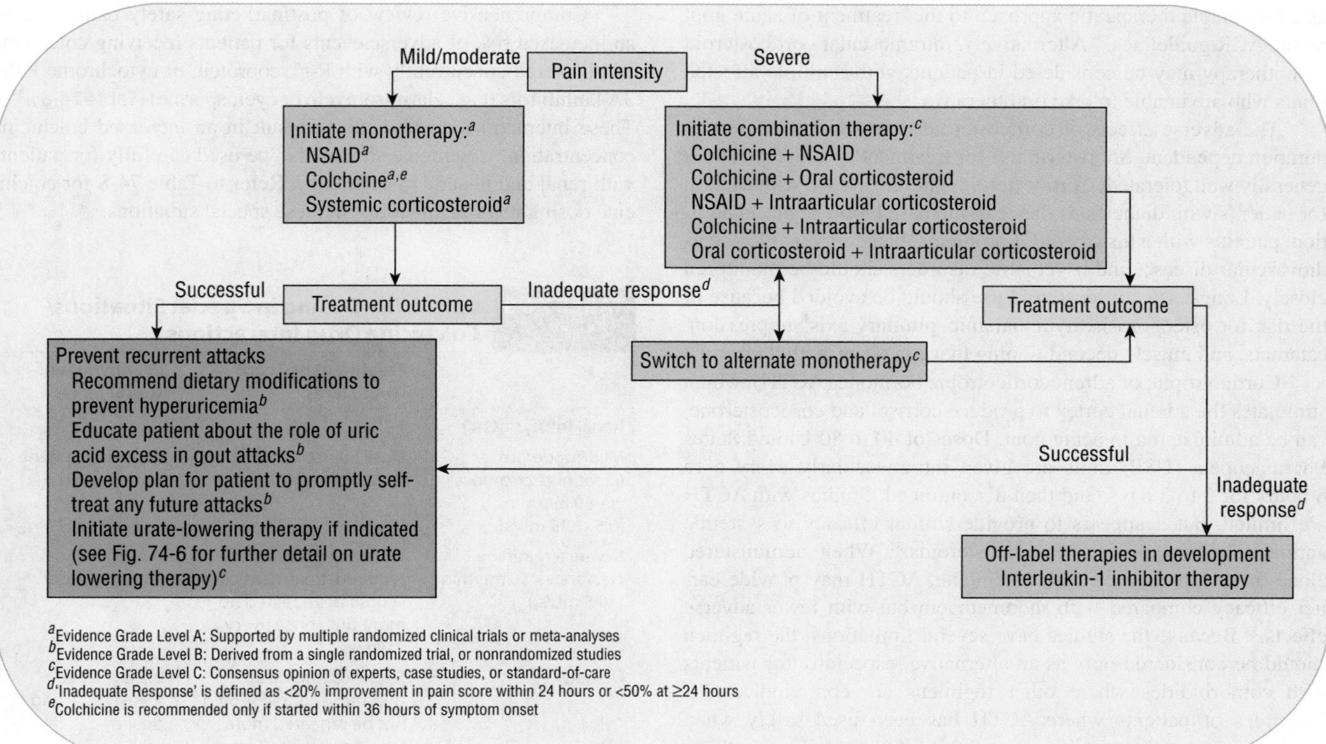

FIGURE 74-5 Algorithm for management of an acute gout attack.

choice of NSAID is not an important determinant of therapeutic success, timing of pharmacotherapy is. It is critical that therapy is initiated within 24 hours of acute gout attack onset and continued until complete resolution.[26] Following resolution of the attack, tapering of NSAID therapy may be considered, especially in patients with comorbidities such as hepatic or renal insufficiency where prolonged therapy would be undesirable.[26] Resolution of an acute attack for most patients generally occurs within 5 to 8 days after initiating therapy.

All NSAIDs have the potential to cause similar adverse effects. The most common areas affected include the GI system (gastritis, bleeding, perforation), kidneys (renal papillary necrosis, reduced creatinine clearance), cardiovascular system (sodium and fluid retention, increased blood pressure), and CNS (impaired cognitive function, headache, dizziness). Caution should be exercised when using NSAIDs for individuals with a history of peptic ulcer disease, congestive heart failure, uncontrolled hypertension, renal insufficiency, coronary artery disease, or who are concurrently receiving anticoagulants or antiplatelets. Patients with active peptic ulcer disease, uncompensated congestive heart failure, severe renal impairment, or a history of hypersensitivity to aspirin or other NSAIDs should not be prescribed an NSAID.

Selective cyclooxygenase-2 (COX-2) inhibitors present a potentially better tolerated alternative to nonselective NSAIDs in patients with GI issues. Specific COX-2 inhibitors, etoricoxib and lumiracoxib, have demonstrated efficacy in the treatment of acute gout in numerous controlled trials; however, these agents are not available in the United States. One study has established effectiveness of high-dose celecoxib (1200 mg on day 1 followed by 400 mg twice daily thereafter) in the treatment of acute gout, but concerns regarding the cardiovascular risk of COX-2 inhibitors must be considered when using these agents (see Chap. 71, Osteoarthritis, for further discussion of COX-2 inhibitors).[28,29] The ACR guidelines recommend celecoxib as an option for patients unable to take NSAIDs but note that the risk-to-benefit ratio of celecoxib use in acute gout is unclear.[26]

Corticosteroids

Corticosteroids have historically been reserved for treatment of acute gout flares when contraindications to other therapies exist, largely due to lack of evidence from controlled clinical trials. However, more recent evidence indicates that corticosteroids are equivalent to NSAIDs in the treatment of acute gout flares.[30] They can be used either systemically or by intraarticular injection. The ACR guidelines recommend that the number of joints involved be considered when choosing the route of corticosteroid administration. If only one or two joints are involved, either intraarticular or oral corticosteroids are recommended. If an attack is polyarticular, systemic therapy is necessary.[26] A hypothetical risk for a rebound attack upon steroid withdrawal exists; therefore, gradual tapering is often employed when discontinuing steroid therapy. The ACR guidelines suggest two different dosing strategies for oral corticosteroid therapy (prednisone or prednisolone) in the treatment of acute gout: (a) 0.5 mg/kg daily for 5 to 10 days followed by abrupt discontinuation or (b) 0.5 mg/kg daily for 2 to 5 days followed by tapering for 7 to 10 days. The guidelines also support the use of a methylprednisolone dose pack for acute treatment of gout, a 6-day regimen that starts with 24 mg on day 1 and decreases by 4 mg each day.[26] Intraarticular administration of triamcinolone acetonide in a dose of 20 to 40 mg may be useful in treating acute gout limited to one or two joints. Injection should be done under an aseptic technique in a joint determined not to be infected. Per ACR guideline recommendations, intraarticular corticosteroid therapy should be used in conjunction with either an NSAID, colchicine, or oral corticosteroid therapy; however, case reports suggest that this therapeutic approach may be as effective as monotherapy.[26,31] A single intramuscular injection of a long-acting corticosteroid, such as methylprednisolone, followed by oral corticosteroid therapy is recognized as a reasonable therapeutic approach to the treatment of acute gout by the ACR guidelines.[26] Alternatively, intramuscular corticosteroid monotherapy may be considered in patients with multiple affected joints who are unable to take oral therapy.

The adverse effects of corticosteroids are generally dose and duration dependent. Short-term use for treatment of acute attacks is generally well tolerated. Corticosteroids should be used with caution for patients with diabetes as they can increase blood sugar. In addition, patients with a history of GI problems, bleeding disorders, cardiovascular disease, and psychiatric disorders should be monitored closely. Long-term corticosteroid use should be avoided because of the risk for osteoporosis, hypothalamic–pituitary axis suppression, cataracts, and muscle deconditioning that can occur with their use.

Corticotropin, or adrenocorticotropic hormone (ACTH), which stimulates the adrenal cortex to produce cortisol and corticosterone, can be administered in acute gout. Doses of 40 to 80 United States Pharmacopeia (USP) units are given intramuscularly every 6 to 8 hours for 2 to 3 days, and then discontinued. Studies with ACTH are limited, but it appears to provide similar efficacy to systemic antiinflammatory doses of corticosteroids.[32] When administered alone or in combination with colchicine, ACTH may provide earlier efficacy compared with indomethacin but with fewer adverse effects.[33] Because the studies have several limitations, the regimen should be considered only as an alternative, especially for patients with comorbidities where other regimens are contraindicated.[34] Examples of patients where ACTH has been used safely when other first-line gout therapies were contraindicated include those with congestive heart failure, chronic renal failure, and history of GI bleeding.[35] The ACR guidelines support the use of ACTH in the treatment of acute gout in patients unable to take oral medications.[26]

Colchicine

(3) Colchicine is an antimitotic drug that is highly effective at relieving acute attacks of gout.[36] When begun within the first 24 hours of an acute attack, colchicine produces a response in two thirds of patients within hours of administration.[37] If the initiation of colchicine is delayed; however, the probability of success with the drug diminishes substantially. For this reason, the ACR guidelines advocate use of colchicine for treatment of acute gout only if started within 36 hours of attack onset.[26]

Although it is a highly effective therapy, oral colchicine can cause dose-dependent GI adverse effects, including nausea, vomiting, and diarrhea. Other important non-GI adverse effects include neutropenia and axonal neuromyopathy, which may be worsened for patients taking other myopathic drugs such as β-hydroxy-β-methylglutaryl-coenzyme A reductase inhibitors (statins) or for those with renal insufficiency.

Colchicine was used for many years as an unapproved drug with no FDA-approved prescribing information, dosage recommendations, or drug interaction warnings. More recently, the FDA approved a 0.6-mg tablet of colchicine (Colcrys®) for oral use. Data submitted in support of the safety and efficacy of colchicine in acute gout flares demonstrated that a substantially lower dose of colchicine (1.2 mg initially, followed by 0.6 mg 1 hour later) was as effective as higher doses traditionally used (continued hourly dosing until symptoms subside or GI symptoms become intolerable).[38] These findings suggest that prior use of high-dose colchicine regimens, may unnecessarily expose patients to increased toxicity with no additional efficacy. In addition to the new low-dose regimen, the ACR guidelines also suggest that colchicine 0.6 mg once or twice daily can be started 12 hours following the initial 1.2 mg dose and continued until the acute attack resolves.[26] This off-label dosing recommendation is based upon pharmacokinetic data that suggests that colchicine levels begin to decline 12 hours after administration.[38]

Comprehensive review of postmarketing safety data revealed an increased risk of adverse events for patients receiving colchicine administered concurrently with P-glycoprotein or cytochrome P450 3A4 inhibitors (e.g., clarithromycin or cyclosporine) (Table 74-8).[39–42] These interactions are thought to result in an increased colchicine concentration. Colchicine should also be used carefully for patients with renal and hepatic insufficiency. Refer to Table 74-8 for colchicine dosing recommendations in these special situations.

TABLE 74-8 Colchicine Dosing in Special Situations/ Colchicine Drug Interactions

	Treatment of Acute Gout Flares	Prophylaxis of Gout Flares
Renal Impairment[a]		
Mild/moderate (creatinine clearance = 30–80 mL/min [0.5–1.25 mL/s])	Dose adjustment not required	Dose adjustment not required
Severe (creatinine clearance <30 mL/min [<0.5 mL/s])	Dose adjustment not required; treatment course should be repeated no more than once every 2 weeks	0.3 mg daily (starting dose)
Dialysis	Single 0.6 mg dose; treatment course should not be repeated more than once every 2 weeks	0.3 mg twice weekly (starting dose)
Hepatic Impairment[b]		
Mild/moderate	Dose adjustment not required	Dose adjustment not required
Severe	Dose adjustment not required; treatment course should be repeated no more than once every 2 weeks	Dose reduction should be considered
Colchicine Drug Interactions		
Strong CYP3A4 inhibitors • Atazanavir • Clarithromycin • Darunavir/ritonavir • Indinavir • Itraconazole • Ketoconazole • Lopinavir/ritonavir • Nefazodone • Nelfinavir • Ritonavir • Saquinavir • Telithromycin • Tipranavir/ritonavir	Single 0.6 mg dose followed by 0.3 mg 1 hour later; dose to be repeated no earlier than 3 days	0.3 mg once every other day to 0.3 mg once daily
Moderate CYP3A4 inhibitors • Amprenavir • Aprepitant • Diltiazem • Erythromycin • Fluconazole • Fosamprenavir • Grapefruit juice and related citrus products • Verapamil	Single 1.2 mg dose; dose to be repeated no earlier than 3 days	0.3 mg to 0.6 mg daily (0.6 mg dose may be given as 0.3 mg twice daily)
P-glycoprotein inhibitors • Cyclosporine • Ranolazine	Single 0.6 mg dose; dose to be repeated no earlier than 3 days	0.3 mg once every other day to 0.3 mg once daily

[a]Treatment of gout flares with colchicine is not recommended in patients with renal impairment who are receiving colchicine for prophylaxis.
[b]Treatment of gout flares with colchicine is not recommended in patients with hepatic impairment who are receiving colchicine for prophylaxis.

IV colchicine has resulted in fatalities and is no longer available.[43]

Interleukin-1 Inhibitors

During acute gout attacks, urate crystals elicit an inflammatory response that triggers the production of interleukin-1 (IL-1).[44] This finding has led to the investigational use of IL-1 inhibitors in the treatment of acute gout.

In small trials, two IL-1 inhibitors, anakinra and canakinumab, have demonstrated efficacy in the treatment of acute gout.[45–48] Neither is approved for treatment of acute gout by the FDA, and their use remains off-label.[44] The ACR guidelines suggest that anakinra 100 mg subcutaneously daily for 3 days or single-dose canakinumab 150 mg subcutaneously can be considered for treatment of severe acute gout attacks refractory to other treatments. However, due to a lack of randomized controlled trials and an uncertain risk-to-benefit ratio, the guidelines note that the role of IL-1 inhibitors in the treatment of acute gout is unclear.[26]

Hyperuricemia in Gout

Nonpharmacologic Therapy

Following treatment and resolution of the intense pain associated with an acute gout attack, the focus shifts to the prevention of future episodes. Recurrent gout attacks can be prevented by maintaining low uric acid levels. Although both nonpharmacologic and pharmacologic efforts to maintain low uric acid levels are critical in the management of gout, trials have shown high rates of nonadherence with urate-lowering therapies.[49] A likely explanation for this lack in patient adherence is the silent nature of intercritical gout (the period of time between two gout attacks). Patient education, therefore, is a critical first step in the management of hyperuricemia.[25,50] Education should address the recurrent nature of the disease and reinforce the objective of each lifestyle/dietary modification and medication therapy recommended.

Weight loss through caloric restriction and exercise should be promoted in all patients with gout and hyperuricemia, as this may enhance renal excretion of urate.[51] Restriction of alcohol intake is of great importance, as this is closely correlated with gout attacks.[52,53] Acute ingestions of alcohol cause lactic acidemia, which reduces renal urate excretion, and long-term alcohol intake promotes production of purines as a by-product of the conversion of acetate to acetyl coenzyme A in the metabolism of alcohol.[54] The ACR guidelines recommend limiting alcohol use in all gout patients and avoidance of any alcohol during periods of frequent gout attacks and in those with advanced gout under poor control.[25] The ACR guidelines also recommend limiting consumption of high-fructose corn syrup and purine-rich foods (organ meats and some seafood), which have been linked to uric acid elevation, and encourage the consumption of vegetables and low-fat dairy products, which have been shown to have urate-lowering effects.[25,55–60]

Another strategy to lower uric acid before initiating urate-lowering pharmacotherapy is to evaluate a patient's medication list for potentially unnecessary drugs that may elevate uric acid levels (Table 74-2). These include thiazide and loop diuretics, calcineurin inhibitors, niacin, and low-dose aspirin. The ACR guidelines consider the potential elimination of uric acid-elevating medications as a baseline recommendation for all gout patients with hyperuricemia; however, the benefit of thiazide diuretics in the treatment of hypertension and of low-dose aspirin in cardiovascular disease prevention is specifically noted.[25]

The presence of gout should not be a contraindication to the use of thiazide diuretics in hypertensive patients, although clinicians should be aware that diuretics are independent risk factors for gout and can increase serum uric acid levels.[9] It may be important to avoid using diuretics if other agents can be used to control blood pressure, particularly if the patient has had frequent gout attacks or continues to have an elevated serum uric acid level despite appropriate therapy for gout. The ACR guidelines specifically recommend against discontinuing low-dose aspirin used for cardiovascular prevention in patients with gout, since aspirin's effect on elevating serum uric acid is negligible.[25]

Pharmacologic Therapy

4 After the first attack of acute gouty arthritis, a decision to institute prophylactic urate-lowering pharmacotherapy must be considered. This decision should carefully balance risk and benefit. Prophylactic pharmacotherapy has been found to be cost-effective if patients have two or more attacks per year, even if the serum uric acid concentration is normal or only minimally elevated.[61,62]

5 Consistent with this finding, the ACR guidelines recognize the occurrence of two or more gout attacks per year as an indication for pharmacologic urate-lowering therapy.[25] Other indications include the presence of one or more tophus, chronic kidney disease (stage 2 or worse), and a history of urolithiasis.[25]

Pharmacologic urate-lowering therapy can be started during an acute gout attack if appropriate antiinflammatory prophylaxis has been initiated[25] (see Antiinflammatory Gout Prophylaxis During Initiation of Pharmacologic Urate-lowering Therapy section and Fig. 74-6 for more detail). The goal of initiating urate-lowering therapies is to achieve and maintain a serum uric acid concentration of less than 6 mg/dL (357 μmol/L), and preferably below 5 mg/dL (297 μmol/L) if signs and symptoms of gout persist.[25,63] Urate lowering should be prescribed for long-term use, as intermittent administration has been less effective in controlling gouty attacks.[25,64] Reduction of serum urate concentrations can be accomplished pharmacologically by decreasing the synthesis of uric acid (xanthine oxidase inhibitors) or by increasing the renal excretion of uric acid (uricosurics).

The ACR guidelines provide a step-wise approach in the treatment of hyperuricemia in gout[25] (Fig. 74-6). Within this strategy, xanthine oxidase inhibitors are recommended as first-line therapy. Probenecid, a potent uricosuric therapy, is recommended as an alternative first-line therapy in patients with a contraindication or intolerance to xanthine oxidase inhibitor therapy. In refractory cases, combination therapy including a xanthine oxidase inhibitor plus an agent with uricosuric properties (probenecid, losartan, or fenofibrate) is suggested. Finally, in severe cases in which the patient cannot tolerate or is not responding to other therapies, pegloticase is recommended.

Xanthine Oxidase Inhibitors

Xanthine oxidase inhibitors reduce uric acid by impairing the ability of xanthine oxidase to convert hypoxanthine to xanthine and xanthine to uric acid. Because they are efficacious for prophylaxis in both underexcreters and overproducers of uric acid, xanthine oxidase inhibitors are the most widely prescribed agents for the long-term prevention of recurrent attacks of gout. For nearly 40 years, allopurinol was the only agent available in the United States; a second xanthine oxidase inhibitor (febuxostat; Uloric) reached the US market in 2009.

Allopurinol is an effective urate-lowering agent, but up to 5% of patients are unable to tolerate it because of adverse effects, and long-term adherence with allopurinol is low.[49,65] Mild adverse effects such as skin rash, leukopenia, GI problems, headache, and urticaria can occur with allopurinol administration. More severe adverse reactions including severe rash (toxic epidermal necrolysis,

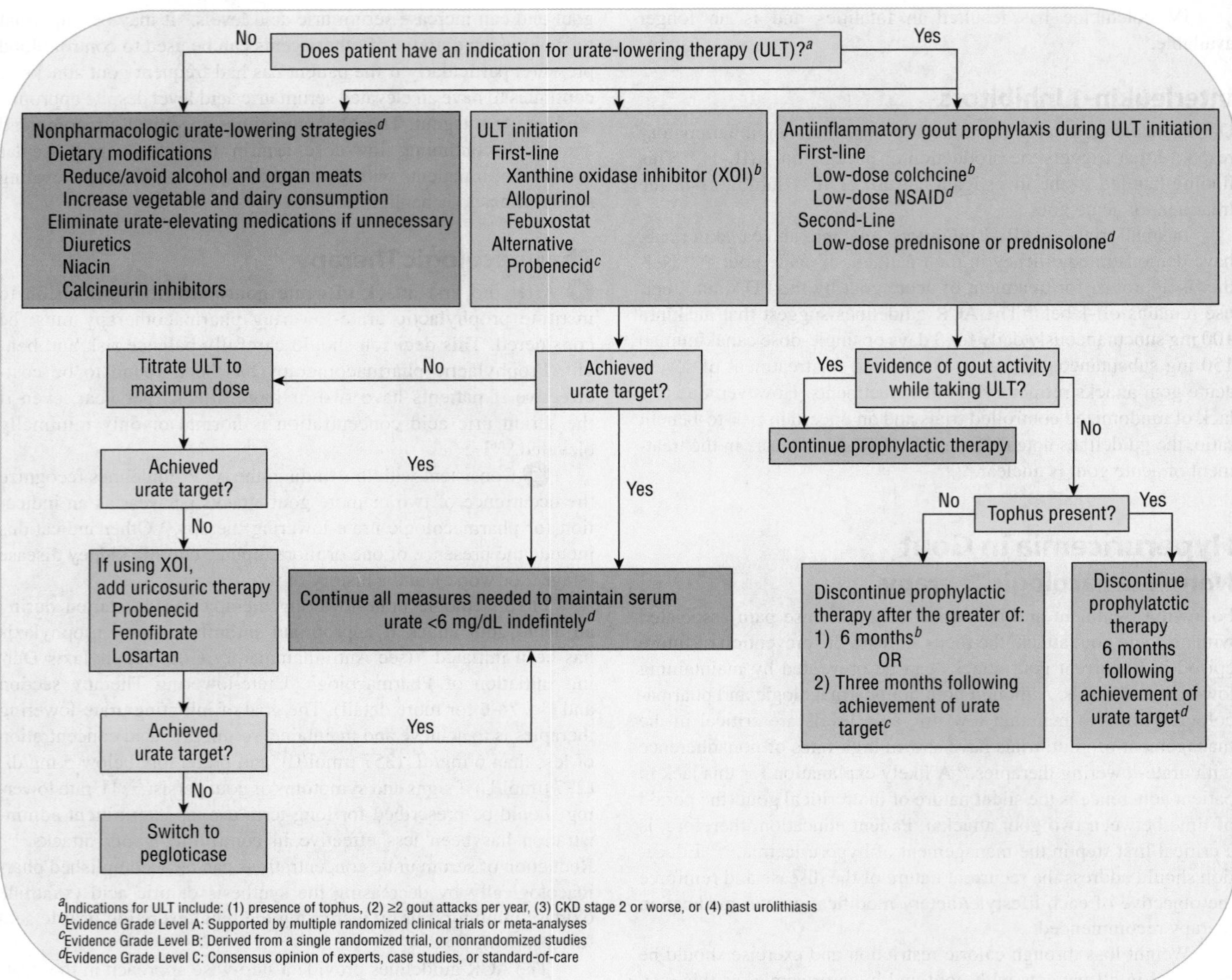

FIGURE 74-6 Algorithm for management of hyperuricemia in gout.

erythema multiforme, or exfoliative dermatitis), hepatitis, interstitial nephritis, and eosinophilia reportedly occur in approximately 1:1,000 patients and are associated with a 20% to 25% mortality.[25] Although direct evidence is lacking, the presence of renal insufficiency and thiazide diuretic use is believed to predispose patients to this "allopurinol hypersensitivity syndrome."[25,66]

Evidence has also linked higher starting doses of allopurinol with an increased incidence of allopurinol hypersensitivity syndrome; therefore, conservative initial dosing is important.[67] ACR guidelines recommended that allopurinol be started at a dose no greater than 100 mg daily and then gradually titrated every 2 to 5 weeks up to a maximum dose of 800 mg/day until the serum urate target is achieved. Patients with chronic kidney disease (stage 4 or worse) should start at a dose no greater than 50 mg per day.[25] This conservative dosing strategy is intended to avoid allopurinol hypersensitivity syndrome and also prevent acute gout attacks common during initiation of urate-lowering therapy.

Traditionally, the maximum daily dose of allopurinol has been reduced for patients with renal insufficiency; however, this recommendation comes from a non-evidence-based algorithm and is therefore not supported by the ACR guidelines.[25,66] It is critical, however, to educate patients with renal impairment taking allopurinol about the signs and symptoms of a serious reaction, including pruritus and rash. These patients should also undergo routine monitoring for elevation of hepatic enzymes and signs of eosinophilia.[25]

Similar to allopurinol, febuxostat lowers serum urate concentrations in a dose-dependent manner.[68,69] In clinical trials, 40 mg/day of febuxostat was noninferior to conventionally dosed allopurinol (300 mg/day) in achieving the primary endpoint of serum urate concentration <6 mg/dL (<357 μmol/L), while 80 mg/day of febuxostat was more effective. The incidence of gout flares occurring during the initial months of administration was similar for both drugs. Febuxostat is well tolerated, with adverse events mostly limited to nausea, arthralgias, and minor liver transaminase elevations.

One criticism of the studies comparing allopurinol and febuxostat is that a fixed dose of allopurinol was used, rather than titrating the dose to achieve the targeted serum urate level. However, the 300 mg/day dosing of allopurinol reflects what has typically been used in the majority of clinical practice.[70] An advantage of febuxostat is that it has been studied in patients with mild-to-moderate hepatic and renal impairment [creatinine clearances of 30 to 89 mL/min (0.50 to 1.49 mL/s)] and does not require dose adjustment in these patients.

Uricosuric Drugs

Uricosuric drugs increase the renal clearance of uric acid by inhibiting postsecretory renal proximal tubular reabsorption of uric acid. The drug used most widely to increase uric acid excretion is probenecid. Several other uricosuric drugs are available in Europe, but not in the United States.

Uricosuric therapies, through their action to increase the elimination of uric acid, cause marked uricosuria and may cause stone formation. Probenecid, specifically, has been associated with a 9% to 11% risk of urolithiasis.[25,71,72] For this reason, patients with a history or urolithiasis should not use potent uricosuric drugs, such as probenecid.[25] The maintenance of adequate urine flow and alkalinization of the urine during the first several days of uricosuric therapy may help to diminish the possibility of uric acid stone formation.[25]

Probenecid is given initially at a dose of 250 mg twice a day for 1 to 2 weeks and then 500 mg twice a day for 2 weeks. Thereafter, the daily dose is increased by 500 mg increments every 1 to 2 weeks until satisfactory control is achieved or a maximum dose of 2 g is reached. In addition to urolithiasis, major adverse effects associated with uricosuric therapy include GI irritation, rash and hypersensitivity, and precipitation of acute gouty arthritis. A disadvantage of uricosurics is that salicylates may interfere with this mechanism and result in treatment failure; however, low doses (325 mg/day or less) of enteric-coated aspirin may be used cautiously. In addition, probenecid can inhibit the tubular secretion of other organic acids; thus, increased plasma concentrations of penicillins, cephalosporins, sulfonamides, and indomethacin can occur.

6 Uricosuric drugs are contraindicated for patients who are allergic to them, for patients with impaired renal function [a creatinine clearance <50 mL/min (<0.84 mL/s)], and for patients who are overproducers of uric acid; for such patients, a xanthine oxidase inhibitor should be used.

Clinical **Controversy...**

Gout and hyperuricemia are highly prevalent in patients with renal impairment. Selection of uric acid-lowering therapy in this population is complicated, given the lack of safety and efficacy data. Renal impairment is a risk factor for allopurinol hypersensitivity syndrome. Reducing the maximum daily dose of allopurinol in patients with renal impairment does not necessarily reduce the risk of allopurinol hypersensitivity syndrome but does compromise efficacy. Normal daily doses of allopurinol may be used in patients with reduced renal function, but slow titration and careful monitoring for symptoms of allopurinol hypersensitivity are necessary.

An alternative uric acid-lowering therapy, febuxostat, is approved for use in patients with creatinine clearance 30 to 60 mL/min (0.5 to 1 mL/s) but has not been studied in those with lower creatinine clearance rates. Uricosuric therapy is not recommended in this population due to lack of evidence for safety and efficacy. It is unclear which uric acid-lowering therapy is the safest, most efficacious, and most cost-effective in patients with renal impairment.

Pegloticase

Pegloticase (Krystexxa) is a pegylated recombinant uricase that works to reduce serum uric acid by converting uric acid to allantoin, a water-soluble and easily excreted substance.

In two 6-month randomized controlled trials, biweekly pegloticase therapy demonstrated efficacy in reducing serum uric acid and resolving tophi in patients with severe gout and hyperuricemia (uric acid ≥8 mg/dL [≥476 μmol/L]) who failed or had a contraindication to allopurinol therapy.[73] Severe gout referred to patients who met at least one of the following criteria: (a) three or more gout flares within the most recent 18 months, (b) one or more tophi, or (c) joint damage due to gout. Far more patients receiving pegloticase therapy compared with placebo achieved the primary outcome, maintenance of uric acid <6 mg/dL (<357 μmol/L) for at least 80% of the time during months 3 and 6 of the trial (42% vs. 0%; $P < 0.001$).

Although clearly efficacious, pegloticase has several drawbacks that limit widespread use. One is the route of administration. The biweekly IV infusions of pegloticase must be given over no less than 2 hours, a potential inconvenience to many patients. Furthermore, given potential infusion-related allergic reactions, patients must be treated with antihistamines and corticosteroids before therapy. Cost is another major consideration. Pegloticase is estimated to cost more than $5,000 per month, not including administration costs associated with an IV infusion.[74] This represents a significantly greater cost burden compared with other urate-lowering therapies.[74]

The ideal duration of pegloticase therapy is currently unknown. Other urate-lowering therapies, xanthine oxidase inhibitors for example, are typically used indefinitely in patients with gout and hyperuricemia. Immunogenicity issues associated with pegloticase therapy may limit the duration with which pegloticase therapy may be used effectively. In the previously cited 6-month pegloticase trials, 134 of 150 patients developed pegloticase antibodies that, for most patients, resulted in a loss of efficacy by month 4.[73]

Given these many limitations and the narrow patient population in which the drug has been studied, pegloticase is an agent of last resort that should be reserved for patients with refractory gout who are unable to take or have failed all other urate-lowering therapies.

Clinical **Controversy...**

Pegloticase is a new recombinant uricase approved for use in chronic refractory gout. Evidence supports its efficacy in maintaining target serum uric acid levels, but little is known about its ability to reduce the frequency of recurrent gout attacks. Also unclear is the optimal duration of pegloticase therapy. Use of pegloticase in special populations at high risk of gout, including those with renal impairment and older patients, has not yet been studied. Given the many unknowns, a clear role for pegloticase in gout therapy is not yet established.

Miscellaneous Agents

Lipid-lowering agents, in particular fenofibrate, can also be prescribed for patients with gout. Although dyslipidemia is common in gout patients, the fibrates are believed to exert their effects as an ancillary benefit by increasing the clearance of hypoxanthine and xanthine, leading to a sustained reduction in serum urate concentrations. Reductions of 20% to 30% in urate levels are observed with fenofibrate use.[75,76] Importantly, fenofibrate does not appear to not cause an acute gout flare when initiated and is well tolerated overall.[77,78]

Losartan, an angiotensin II receptor antagonist, has also demonstrated benefit in reducing serum urate concentrations independent of angiotensin receptor antagonism.[79] Losartan inhibits renal tubular reabsorption of uric acid and increases urinary excretion, and this effect seems to be a unique property of losartan that is not shared with other angiotensin II receptor antagonists.[80] In addition, it alkalinizes the urine, which helps reduce the risk for stone formation.

The ACR guidelines support the use of fenofibrate or losartan in combination with a xanthine oxidase inhibitor in patients with refractory disease.[25]

Antiinflammatory Gout Prophylaxis During Initiation of Pharmacologic Urate-Lowering Therapy

7 Initiation of urate-lowering therapy can prompt an acute attack of gout due to remodeling of urate crystal deposits in joints as a result of rapid lowering of urate concentrations.[26] As such, prophylactic antiinflammatory pharmacotherapy should be employed to prevent gout attacks and, secondarily, to assist in ensuring patient acceptance of and adherence with urate-lowering therapy. The ACR guidelines recommend low-dose oral colchicine (0.6 mg twice daily) and low-dose NSAIDs (e.g., naproxen 250 mg twice/day) as first-line prophylactic therapies, with stronger evidence supporting use of colchicine.[26]

Low-dose corticosteroid therapy (e.g., ≤10 mg/day prednisone) is recommended as an alternative in patients with intolerance, contraindication, or lack of response to first-line therapy.[26] Limited evidence suggests efficacy of IL-1 inhibitors in the prevention of acute gout during the first 16 weeks of urate-lowering therapy initiation [subcutaneous rilonacept 320 mg loading dose followed by 160 mg weekly and subcutaneous canakinumab single dose (50 to 300 mg) or four times weekly dosing (50 mg—50 mg—25 mg—25 mg)].[81,82] Given the limited evidence and lack of FDA approval for this indication, the ACR guidelines do not provide a recommendation for the use of IL-1 inhibitors in this setting.

Pharmacologic prophylaxis should be continued for at least 3 months after achieving target serum uric acid or 6 months total, whichever is longer. For patients with one or more tophi, prophylactic therapy should be continued for 6 months following achievement of serum urate target[26] (Fig. 74-6).

Given the considerable duration of therapy required for acute gout prophylaxis during initiation of urate-lowering therapy, adverse effects of the pharmacologic agents employed must be seriously considered. Although the risk for gastric ulceration and bleeding is relatively small with short-term NASID therapy normally employed when treating acute gout flares, administration of a proton-pump inhibitor or other acid-suppressing therapy is indicated to protect from NSAID-induced gastric problems for patients on long-term prophylactic therapy.[26] Prolonged corticosteroid therapy is clearly linked to many severe adverse effects (i.e., hyperglycemia, Cushing's syndrome, fluid retention, hypertension, osteoporosis, glaucoma, depression/euphoria) and, as suggested above, is not appropriate for first-line therapy for this reason.

Cost is another major consideration when selecting prophylactic pharmacotherapy given the need for an extended duration of therapy (6 months of therapy compared to approximately 1 week for acute gout treatment). While improved dosing recommendations resulted from the recent availability of an FDA-approved colchicine product, the research efforts that provided this additional information have come with a price. Market exclusivity rights were granted to the manufacturer of Colcrys and the resulting lack of competition has caused the price of the medication to increase from approximately \$0.09 per tablet to almost \$5 per tablet.[83] The cost of this brand name colchicine, if not covered by insurance, is a potential challenge to therapy for certain patients. To date there have been no formal pharmacoeconomic studies evaluating colchicine in comparison to other therapies for antiinflammatory prophylaxis during urate-lowering therapy initiation; however, NSAIDs and corticosteroids may present more affordable options for patients.

Nephrolithiasis

8 The medical management of uric acid nephrolithiasis includes hydration sufficient to maintain a urine volume of 2 to 3 L/day, alkalinization of urine, avoidance of purine-rich foods, moderation of protein intake, and reduction of urinary uric acid excretion.

Maintenance of a 24-hour urine volume of 2 to 3 L with an adequate intake of fluids is desirable for all gout patients, but especially for those with excessive uric acid excretion [>1 g/day (>6 mmol/day)]. Alkalinizing agents should be used with the objective of making the urine less acidic. Urine pH should be maintained at 6 to 6.5. In this pH range, up to 85% of uric acid will be in the form of the soluble urate ion.

Reduction of urine acidity is usually accomplished by the administration of potassium bicarbonate or potassium citrate 60 to 80 mEq/day (60 to 80 mmol/day).[84,85] Administration of alkali via sodium salts is a less desirable option for two reasons. First, the sodium-induced volume expansion will increase sodium excretion and can secondarily cause hypercalcemia because calcium passively follows the reabsorption of sodium in the proximal tubule and loop of Henle. In the presence of uric acid, the resultant hypercalcemia can lead to calcium oxalate stone formation. Second, older patients with uric acid kidney stones may also have hypertension, congestive heart failure, or renal insufficiency. Because of these conditions, they should not be overloaded with alkalinizing sodium salts or unlimited fluid intake, as these can worsen these conditions.

Acetazolamide, a carbonic anhydrase inhibitor, produces rapid and effective urinary alkalinization and sometimes is used in conjunction with alkali therapy. When a 250 mg dose of acetazolamide is given at bedtime, the excretion of acidic urine in the early morning hours is avoided. The usual tachyphylaxis (rapid tolerance) to this drug is obviated by a daily repletion dose of bicarbonate.

Since the advent of xanthine oxidase inhibitors, a low-purine, low-protein diet for the patient with uric acid nephrolithiasis is no longer as critical as it once was; however, it is still advisable to instruct the patient to avoid foods rich in purine and to limit protein to no more than 90 g/day. Such a diet is still palatable and reduces appreciably the amount of uric acid in the urine.

The mainstay of drug therapy for recurrent uric acid nephrolithiasis is xanthine oxidase inhibitors. They are effective in reducing both serum and urinary uric acid levels, thus preventing the formation of calculi. Xanthine oxidase inhibitors are recommended as prophylactic treatment for patients who will receive cytotoxic agents for the treatment of lymphoma or leukemia. The marked increase in uric acid production associated with cytolysis of a neoplasm predisposes a patient to the development of uric acid nephrolithiasis.

Asymptomatic Hyperuricemia

Questions are often raised regarding the indication for drug therapy for asymptomatic hyperuricemia. The purported benefits include prevention of acute gouty arthritis, tophi formation, nephrolithiasis, and chronic urate nephropathy. The first three complications are easily controlled should they develop; therefore, antihyperuricemic therapy is not warranted to prevent these conditions. The prevention of urate nephropathy might be a stronger indication because it is irreversible even with proper treatment. Available data indicate, however, that gouty nephropathy is extremely rare in the absence of clinical gout, and evidence that elevation of uric acid by itself may cause renal disease is weak and inconclusive. As discussed previously, renal impairment associated with hyperuricemia is very rare in the absence of concurrent hypertension and atherosclerosis. In addition, it is unclear whether uric acid-lowering therapy protects renal function in such individuals. Thus, the routine treatment of asymptomatic hyperuricemia on the grounds of reducing renal complications is presently not recommended.

The relationship between elevated serum urate concentrations and cardiovascular disease is controversial. In observational studies, hyperuricemia has been shown to be a risk factor for ischemic heart disease.[86–89] However, hyperuricemia is also associated with other known risk factors for cardiovascular disease, such as diabetes mellitus, dyslipidemia, and hypertension, and the individual contribution of hyperuricemia on the risk for cardiovascular disease is difficult to separate from these associated factors. Recently, a 12-year follow-up of the Health Professionals Study revealed a 28% higher risk of death from all causes, 38% higher risk of cardiovascular disease death, 55% higher risk of death from coronary heart disease, and a 59% higher risk of nonfatal myocardial infarction for men with a self-reported history of gout compared with those without this reported history.[90] These associations remained significant even after adjusting for age, body mass index, smoking, family history of myocardial infarction, and comorbidities such as diabetes and hypertension. To date, this study is the only one providing prospective data that implicate gout as an independent risk for coronary heart disease. No studies have examined whether drug treatment of asymptomatic hyperuricemia or gout is protective against coronary artery disease. At this time, it is premature to implement therapy for patients with asymptomatic hyperuricemia in the absence of a history of gout. Instead, efforts should be directed toward aggressive management of cardiovascular risk factors.

Clinical **Controversy. . .**

While asymptomatic hyperuricemia is not generally treated, some clinicians do recommend treatment to reduce the risks of vascular disease, including hypertension, cerebrovascular disease, and kidney disease. Although the link between hyperuricemia and vascular disease has been demonstrated in epidemiologic studies, a direct association has not been established due to the lack of prospective, randomized controlled trials. Furthermore, the impact of normalizing uric acid levels with the use of urate-lowering pharmacotherapy on vascular outcomes is unknown.

Personalized Pharmacotherapy

While the ACR guidelines provide clear recommendations regarding use of pharmacotherapy in the management of gout and hyperuricemia, application of these recommendations requires personalization to fit the needs of a specific patient. When making therapeutic choices for an individual, it is critical to evaluate the adverse effect profile of a particular pharmacotherapeutic agent while considering a patient's baseline risk for those unwanted effects. This involves an analysis of patient demographics and comorbidities.[13]

Allopurinol hypersensitivity syndrome is perhaps the most concerning adverse effect of all potential side effects associated with gout therapies, given the high mortality rate associated with this reaction. As such, it would be ideal if patients at high risk for developing this syndrome could be screened for and, consequently, guided to alternative therapy. Recent research has identified a genetic link in certain populations that increases risk for the development of allopurinol hypersensitivity syndrome. Korean patients with chronic kidney disease (stage 3 or worse), Han Chinese patients, and Thai patients have been identified as being at increased risk for allopurinol hypersensitivity syndrome if found to have a specific genotype (HLA-B*5801 positive).[91–93] The ACR guidelines recommend that HLA-B*5801 testing be considered before allopurinol initiation in these specific subpopulations; for those found to be positive, alternative therapy should be used.[25]

Certain comorbidities may warrant dose adjustment of some gout therapies or, in certain instances, complete avoidance of certain medications. For example, patients with renal impairment should, in general, avoid NSAID therapy and must receive colchicine at reduced doses. Patients with GI disease should also avoid NSAID therapy and may not be able to tolerate colchicine therapy and, therefore, may find most success with corticosteroid therapy. In addition to comorbidities, polypharmacy and cost considerations may affect treatment decisions in an individual patient. Refer to Table 74-9 for an overview of important factors to consider when personalizing pharmacotherapy for an individual patient with gout.

Evaluation of Therapeutic Outcomes

Follow-up of patients with gout depends on the frequency of attacks and on the medications used to treat symptoms. For a patient who is experiencing a first attack of gout, long-term therapy is generally not indicated. As previously mentioned, the ACR guidelines recommend that urate-lowering pharmacotherapy be started only after two or more attacks of gout in one year, because the treatment is long term and relatively expensive, the drugs used are potentially toxic, and adherence for patients without symptoms is generally poor.[25,62,65] Patients having a first attack should be educated about the likelihood of recurrence and what to do if another attack occurs. Approximately 60% of patients have a second attack within the first year, and 78% have a second attack within 2 years. Only 7% of patients do not have a recurrence within a 10-year period.[94]

Baseline blood work for patients receiving hypouricemic medications chronically should include renal function (serum creatinine, blood urea nitrogen), liver enzymes (aspartate aminotransferase, alanine aminotransferase), complete blood count, and electrolytes. There is generally no need to recheck these laboratory parameters for patients undergoing acute therapy with an NSAID or colchicine of limited duration. However, for patients requiring long-term therapy or prophylaxis, they should be rechecked every 6 to 12 months or as clinically indicated. For patients suspected of having an acute attack of gouty arthritis, it is reasonable to check a serum uric acid level, particularly if it is not the first attack and a decision is to be made regarding initiation of prophylactic therapy. However, clinicians should be mindful that acute gouty arthritis can occur in the presence of normal serum uric acid concentrations.[6] During titration of urate-lowering therapy, uric acid should be monitored every 2 to 5 weeks; once the urate target is achieved, uric acid should be monitored every 6 months.[25] This monitoring regimen is recommended not only to ensure appropriate dosing of urate-lowering therapy, but also to serve as an assessment of patient adherence given the known adherence issues with urate-lowering therapies. **9** Because of the high rates of comorbidities associated with gout, including diabetes mellitus, chronic kidney disease, hypertension, obesity, myocardial infarction, heart failure, and stroke, elevated uric acid levels or gout should prompt evaluations for signs of cardiovascular disease and the need for appropriate risk reduction measures.[95] Additionally, clinicians should look for a possible correctable cause of hyperuricemia, such as medications (e.g., thiazide and loop diuretics, niacin, calcineurin inhibitors), obesity, malignancy, and alcohol abuse. Patients should be encouraged to exercise, lose weight, reduce alcohol intake, reduce consumption of syrup-sweetened sodas and increase consumption of low-fat dairy foods and vegetables, and have periodic follow-up to address progress on these goals.

CONCLUSIONS

Hyperuricemia may lead to acute arthritis, chronic gout, or kidney stones or to no sequelae at all. Asymptomatic hyperuricemia may not need to be treated, although lifestyle modifications (e.g., weight loss, reduction of alcohol intake, control of blood pressure) should be encouraged to help reduce serum urate and overall cardiovascular health.

Acute gouty arthritis responds well to short courses of NSAIDs, colchicine, or corticosteroids to treat the underlying inflammatory condition. The management of uric acid nephrolithiasis includes hydration and alkalinization of the urine. Prevention of recurrent

TABLE 74-9 Personalized Pharmacotherapy in Gout

Conditions and Situations	Limitations to Pharmacotherapy	Alternative Therapies
Renal insufficiency	NSAIDs may lead to exacerbation of renal insufficiency	Consider reduced-dose colchicine or corticosteroids for short-term treatment of acute gout Consider reduced-dose colchicine for prophylaxis during initiation of urate-lowering therapy
	Uricosuric therapy is ineffective in patients with renal insufficiency	Consider allopurinol or febuxostat
GI disease	Colchicine may cause GI upset and diarrhea	Consider corticosteroids for treatment of acute gout If monoarticular, consider joint injection
	NSAIDs may cause GI bleeding or ulceration	Consider gastroprotection with coadministration of proton-pump inhibitor when NSAID therapy is used Consider colchicine or corticosteroids for treatment of acute gout Consider low-dose colchicine for prophylaxis during initiation of urate-lowering therapy
Congestive heart failure	NSAIDs may cause a congestive heart failure exacerbation	Consider colchicine for treatment of acute gout Consider colchicine for prophylaxis during initiation of urate-lowering therapy
	Concurrent use of diuretic may increase serum urate	If diuretic remains necessary, consider initiating urate-lowering therapy Consider losartan as a therapy for congestive heart failure given its uricosuric properties
Hypertension	Diuretics may increase uric acid	Consider losartan as alternative or additional antihypertensive therapy given its uricosuric properties Consider addition of urate-lowering therapy if diuretic remains necessary
	NSAIDs may worsen blood pressure control	Consider colchicine or corticosteroids for treatment of acute gout Consider colchicine for prophylaxis during initiation of urate-lowering therapy
Polypharmacy	CYP 3A4 inhibitors and P-glycoprotein inhibitors interact with colchicine leading to elevated colchicine levels	Reduce the dose of colchicine used for the treatment and prophylaxis of acute gout Consider NSAIDs or corticosteroids for treatment of acute gout Consider NSAIDs for prophylaxis during initiation of urate-lowering therapy
	Added pharmacotherapy may be undesirable in a patient with a large medication burden	Consider losartan as urate-lowering therapy in patients with comorbid hypertension Consider fenofibrate as urate-lowering therapy in patients with hypertriglyceridemia
Financial limitations	Febuxostat and colchicine are considerably more costly compared with other gout treatments	Consider allopurinol as urate-lowering therapy Consider NSAIDs or corticosteroids for treatment of acute gout Consider NSAIDs for prophylaxis of gout during initiation of urate-lowering therapy

gouty arthritis or recurrent nephrolithiasis and treatment of chronic gout require hypouricemic therapy with either a uricosuric drug or xanthine oxidase inhibitor. Xanthine oxidase inhibitors are effective in both underexcreters and overproducers of uric acid, making them the hypouricemic drugs of choice for most patients with gout. Finally, antiinflammatory prophylaxis with low-dose colchicine or NSAID therapy is indicated during the initiation of urate-lowering therapy to prevent the development of acute gout due to rapid mobilization or urate.

ABBREVIATIONS

ACR	American College of Rheumatology
ACTH	adrenocorticotropic hormone
HGPRT	hypoxanthine-guanine phosphoribosyltransferase
IL-1	interleukin-1
NSAID	nonsteroidal antiinflammatory drug
PRPP	phosphoribosyl pyrophosphate (synthetase)

REFERENCES

1. Wortmann RL. Chapter 87: Gout and hyperuricemia. In: Firestein GS, Budd RC, Harris ED Jr, et al, eds. Kelley's Textbook of Rheumatology, 8th ed. Philadelphia, PA: WB Saunders, 2008.
2. Edwards NL, Choi HK, Terkeltaub RA. Chapter 12: Gout. In: Klippel JH, Stone, SH, Crofford LJ, et al, eds. Primer on the Rheumatic Diseases, 13th ed. New York, NY: Springer Scientce+Business Media, 2008.
3. Li R, Sun J, Ren L, et al. Epidemiology of eight common rheumatic disease in China: A large-scale cross-sectional survey in Beijing. Rheumatology 2012;51:721–729.
4. Zhu Y, Pandya BJ, Choi HK. Prevalence of gout and hyperuricemia in the US general population: The National Health And Nutrition Examination Survey 2007–2008. Arthritis Rheum 2011;63:3136–3141.
5. Campion EW, Glynn RJ, DeLabry LO. Asymptomatic hyperuricemia. Risks and consequences in the Normative Aging Study. Am J Med 1987;82:421–426.
6. McCarty DJ. Gout without hyperuricemia. JAMA 1994;271:302–303.
7. Juraschek SP, Miller ER, Gelber AC. Body mass index, obesity, and prevalent gout in the United States in 1988–1944 and 2007–2010. Arthritis Care Res 2012;65: 127–132.
8. Choi HK. A prescription for lifestyle change in patients with hyperuricemia and gout. Curr Opin Rheumatol 2010;22: 165–172.
9. Hak AE, Curhan GC, Grodstein F, et al. Menopause, postmenopausal hormone use and risk of incident gout. Ann Rheum Dis 2010;69:1305–1309.
10. Neogi T. Gout. NEJM 2011;364:443–452.
11. Wallace KL, Riedel AA, Joseph-Ridge N, Wortmann R. Increasing prevalence of gout and hyperuricemia over 10 years among older adults in a managed care population. J Rheumatol 2004;31:1582–1587.
12. Wilson JM, Young AB, Kelley WN. Hypoxanthine-guanine phosphoribosyltransferase deficiency. N Engl J Med 1983;309:900–910.

13. Fravel MA, Ernst ME. Management of gout in the older adult. Am J Geriatr Pharmacother 2011;9:271–285.
14. Busso N, Ea HK. The mechanisms of inflammation in gout and pseudogout (CPP-induced arthritis). Reumatismo 2011;63:230–237.
15. McGill NW. Gout and other crystal arthropathies. Med J Aust 1997;166:33–38.
16. Schumacher HR. Crystal-reduced arthritis: An overview. Am J Med 1996;100(Suppl 2A):46S–52S.
17. MacMullan P, McCarthy G. Treatment and management of pseudogout: Insights for the clinician. Ther Adv Musculoskel Dis 2012;4:121–131.
18. Pal B, Foxall M, Dysart T, et al. How is gout managed in primary care? A review of current practice and proposed guidelines. Clin Rheumatol 2000;19:21–25.
19. Eggebeen AT. Gout: an update. Am Fam Physician 2007;76: 801–808.
20. Agudelo CA, Weinberger A, Schumacher HR, et al. Definitive diagnosis of gout by identification of urate crystals in asymptomatic metatarsophalangeal joints. Arthritis Rheum 1979;22:559–560.
21. Logan JA, Morrison E, McGill PE. Serum uric acid in acute gout. Ann Rheum Dis 1997;56:696–697.
22. Zhang W, Doherty M, Pascual E, et al. EULAR evidence based recommendations for gout. Part I. Diagnosis. Report of a task force of the Standing Committee for International Clinical Studies Including Therapeutics (ESCISIT). Ann Rheum Dis 2006;65:1301–1311.
23. Kramer HM, Curhan G. The association between gout and nephrolithiasis: The National Health and Nutrition Examination Survey III, 1988–1994. Am J Kid Dis 2002;40: 37–42.
24. Yu T. Nephrolithiasis in patients with gout. Postgrad Med 1978;63:164–170.
25. Khanna D, Fitzgerald JD, Khanna PP, et al. 2012 American College of Rheumatology guidelines for management of gout. Part 1: Systematic nonpharmacologic and pharmacologic therapeutic approaches to hyperuricemia. Arthritis Care Res 2012;64:1431–1446.
26. Khanna D, Khanna PP, Fitzgerald JD, et al. 2012 American College of Rheumatology guidelines for management of gout. Part 2: Therapy and anti-inflammatory prophylaxis of acute gouty arthritis. Arthritis Care Res 2012;64: 1447–1461.
27. Schlesinger N, Detry MA, Holland BK, et al. Local ice therapy during bouts of acute gouty arthritis. J Rheumatol 2002;29:331–334.
28. Schumacher HR, Berger MF, Li-Yu J, et al. Efficacy and tolerability of celecoxib in the treatment of acute gouty arthritis: A randomized controlled trial. J Rheumatol 2012;39:1859–1866.
29. Mukherjee D, Nissen SE, Topol EJ. Risk of cardiovascular events associated with selective COX-2 inhibitors. JAMA 2001;286:954–959.
30. Janssens HJ, Janssen M, van de Lisdonk EH, et al. Use of oral prednisolone or naproxen for the treatment of gout arthritis: A double-blind, randomised equivalence trial. Lancet 2008;371:1854–1860.
31. Fernandez D, Noguera R, Gonzalez JA, et al. Treatment of acute attacks of gout with a small dose of intraarticular triamcinolone acetonide. J Rheumatol 1999;26: 2285–2286.
32. Siegel LB, Alloway JA, Nashel DJ. Comparison of adrenocorticotropic hormone and triamcinolone acetonide in the treatment of acute gouty arthritis. J Rheumatol 1994;21: 1325–1327.
33. Axelrod D, Preston S. Comparison of parenteral adrenocorticotropic hormone with oral indomethacin in the treatment of acute gout. Arthritis Rheum 1988;31:803–805.
34. Taylor CT, Brooks NC, Kelley KW. Corticotropin for acute management of gout. Ann Pharmacother 2001;35: 365–368.
35. Ritter J, Kerr LD, Valeriano-Marcet J, Spiera H. ACTH revisited: Effective treatment for acute crystal induced synovitis in patients with multiple medical problems. J Rheumatol 1994;21:696–699.
36. Schlesinger N, Schumacher R, Catton M, Maxwell L. Colchicine for acute gout. Cochrane Database Syst Rev 2006;4:CD006190.
37. Ahern MJ, Reid C, Gordon TP, et al. Does colchicine work? The results of the first controlled study in acute gout. Aust NZ J Med 1987;17:301–304.
38. Terkeltaub RA, Furst DE, Bennett K, et al. High versus low dosing of oral colchicine for early acute gout flare: Twenty-four-hour outcome of the first multicenter, randomized, double-blind, placebo-controlled, parallel-group, dose-comparison colchicine study. Arthritis Rheum 2010;62: 1060–1068.
39. Dogukan A, Oymak FS, Taskapan H, et al. Acute fatal colchicine intoxication in a patient on continuous ambulatory peritoneal dialysis (CAPD). Possible role of clarithromycin administration. Clin Nephrol 2001;55:181–182.
40. Rollot F, Pajot O, Chauvelot-Moachon L, et al. Acute colchicine intoxication during clarithromycin administration. Ann Pharmacother 2004;38:2074–2077.
41. Hung IF, Wu AK, Cheng VC, et al. Fatal interaction between clarithromycin and colchicine in patients with renal insufficiency: A retrospective study. Clin Infect Dis 2005;41:291–300.
42. Cheng VC, Ho PL, Yuen KY. Two probable cases of serious drug interaction between clarithromycin and colchicine. South Med J 2005;98:811–813.
43. Bonnel RA, Villalba ML, Karwoski CB, Beitz J. Deaths associated with inappropriate intravenous colchicine administration. J Emerg Med 2002;22:385–387.
44. Kotz J. The gout pipeline crystallizes. Nat Rev Drug Discov 2012;11:425–426.
45. So A, De Meulemeester M, Pikhlak A, et al. Canakinumab for the treatment of acute flares in difficult-to-treat gouty arthritis. Arthritis Rheum 2010;62:3064–3076.
46. So A, De Smedt T, Revaz S, et al. A pilot study of IL-1 inhibition by anakinra in acute gout. Arthritis Res Ther 2007;9:R28.
47. Schlesinger N, De Meulemeester M, Pikhlak A, et al. Canakinumab relieves symptoms of acute flares and improves health-related quality of life in patients with difficult-to-treat gouty arthritis by suppressing inflammation: Results of a randomized, dose-ranging study. Arthritis Res Ther 2011;13:R53.
48. Chen K, Fields T, Mancuso C, et al. Anakinra's efficacy is variable in refractory gout: Report of ten cases. Semin Arthritis Rheum 2010;40:210–214.
49. Harrold LR, Andrade SE, Briesacher BA, et al. Adherence with urate-lowering therapies for the treatment of gout. Arthritis Res Ther 2009;11:R46.
50. Rees F, Jenkins W, Doherty M. Patients with gout adhere to curative treatment if informed appropriately: Proof-of concept observational study. Ann Rheum Dis 2012. E-pub ahead of print.
51. Dessein PH, Shipton EA, Stanwix AE, et al. Beneficial effects of weight loss associated with moderate calorie/carbohydrate restriction, and increased proportional intake of protein and

unsaturated fat on serum urate and lipoprotein levels in gout: A pilot study. Ann Rheum Dis 2000;59:539–543.
52. Choi HK, Atkinson K, Karlson EW, et al. Alcohol intake and risk of incident gout in men: A prospective study. Lancet 2004;363:1277–1281.
53. Zhang Y, Woods R, Chaisson CE, et al. Alcohol consumption as a trigger of recurrent gout attacks. Am J Med 2006;119: 800.e13–18.
54. Schlesinger N. Management of acute and chronic gouty arthritis: Present state-of-the-art. Drugs 2004;64: 2399–2416.
55. Choi HK, Atkinson K, Karlson EW, et al. Purine-rich foods, dairy and protein intake, and the risk of gout in men. N Engl J Med 2004;350:1093–1103.
56. Choi HK, Willett W, Curhan G. Fructose-rich beverages and the risk of gout in women. JAMA 2010;304:2270–2278.
57. Choi HK, Curhan G. Soft drinks, fructose consumption, and ACR Guidelines for Gout Management: Part 1. 1445 the risk of gout in men: Prospective cohort study. BMJ 2008;36: 309–312.
58. Singh JA, Reddy SG, Kundukulam J. Risk factors for gout and prevention: A systematic review of the literature. Curr Opin Rheumatol 2011;23:192–202.
59. Zhang Y, Chen C, Choi H, et al. Purine-rich foods intake and recurrent gout attacks. Ann Rheum Dis 2012;71: 1448–1453.
60. Tsai YT, Liu JP, Tu YK, et al. Relationship between dietary patterns and serum uric acid concentrations among ethnic Chinese adults in Taiwan. Asia Pac J Clin Nutr 2012;21: 263–270.
61. Ferraz MB, O'Brien B. A cost effectiveness analysis of urate lowering drugs in nontophaceous recurrent gouty arthritis. J Rheumatol 1995;22:908–914.
62. Dincer HE, Dincer AP, Levinson DJ. Asymptomatic hyperuricemia: To treat or not to treat. Cleve Clin J Med 2002;69:594–602.
63. Shoji A, Yamanaka H, Kamatani N. A retrospective study of the relationship between serum urate level and recurrent attacks of gouty arthritis: Evidence for reduction of recurrent gouty arthritis with antihyperuricemic therapy. Arthritis Rheum 2004;51:321–325.
64. Bull PW, Scott JT. Intermittent control of hyperuricemia in the treatment of gout. J Rheumatol 1989;16:1246–1248.
65. Riedel AA, Nelson M, Joseph-Ridge N, et al. Compliance with allopurinol therapy among managed care enrollees with gout: A retrospective analysis of administrative claims. J Rheumatol 2004;31:1575–1581.
66. Hande KR, Noone RM, Stone WJ. Severe allopurinol toxicity. Description and guidelines for prevention in patients with renal insufficiency. Am J Med 1984;76: 47–56.
67. Stamp LK, Taylor WJ, Jones PB, et al. Starting dose is a risk factor for allopurinol hypersensitivity syndrome: A proposed safe starting dose of allopurinol. Arthritis Rheum 2012;64:2529–2536.
68. Ernst ME, Fravel MA. Febuxostat: A selective xanthine-oxidase/xanthine-dehydrogenase inhibitor for the management of hyperuricemia in adults with gout. Clin Ther 2009;31:2503–2518.
69. Becker MA, Schumacher HR, Wortmann RL, et al. Febuxostat compared with allopurinol in patients with hyperuricemia and gout. N Engl J Med 2005;353: 2450–2461.
70. Chao J, Terkeltaub R. A critical reappraisal of allopurinol dosing, safety, and efficacy for hyperuricemia in gout. Curr Rheumatol Rep 2009;11:135–140.
71. Perez-Ruiz F, Hernandez-Baldizon S, Herrero-Beites AM, et al. Risk factors associated with renal lithiasis during uricosuric treatment of hyperuricemia in patients with gout. Arthritis Care Res (Hoboken) 2010;62:1299–1305.
72. Thompson GR, Duff IF, Robinson WD, et al. Long term uricosuric therapy in gout. Arthritis Rheum 1962;5: 384–396.
73. Sundy JS, Baraf HS, Yood RA, et al. Efficacy and tolerability of pegloticase for the treatment of chronic gout in patients refractory to conventional treatment: Two randomized controlled trials. JAMA 2011;306:711–720.
74. Shannon JA, Cole SW. Pegloticase: A novel agent for treatment-refractory gout. Ann Pharmacother 2012;46: 368–376.
75. de la Serna G, Cadarso C. Fenofibrate decreases plasma fibrinogen, improves lipid profile, and reduces uricemia. Clin Pharmacol Ther 1999;66:166–172.
76. Feher MD, Hepburn AL, Hogarth MB, et al. Fenofibrate enhances urate reduction in men treated with allopurinol for hyperuricaemia and gout. Rheumatol 2003;42: 321–325.
77. Hepburn AL, Kaye SA, Feher MD. Long-term remission from gout associated with fenofibrate therapy. Clin Rheumatol 2003;22:73–76.
78. Hepburn AL, Kaye SA, Feher MD. Fenofibrate: A new treatment for hyperuricaemia and gout? Ann Rheum Dis 2001;60:984–986.
79. Wurzner G, Gerster JC, Chiolero A, et al. Comparative effects of losartan and irbesartan on serum uric acid in hypertensive patients with hyperuricaemia and gout. J Hypertens 2001;19:1855–1860.
80. Shahinfar S, Simpson RL, Carides AD, et al. Safety of losartan in hypertensive patients with thiazide-induced hyperuricemia. Kidney Int 1999;56:1879–1885.
81. Schumacher HR, Sundy JS, Terkeltaub R, et al. Rilonacept (interleukin-1 trap) in the prevention of acute gout flares during initiation of urate-lowering therapy: Results of a phase II randomized, double-blind, placebo-controlled trial. Arthritis Rheum 2012;64:876–884.
82. Schlesinger N, Mysler E, Lin HY, et al. Canakinumab reduces the risk of acute gouty arthritis flares during initiation of allopurinol treatment: Results of a double-blind, randomised study. Ann Rheum Dis 2011;70:1264–1271.
83. Kesselheim AS, Solomon DH. Incentives for drug development—The curious case of colchicine. NEJM 2010;362:2045–2047.
84. Riese RJ, Sakhaee K. Uric acid nephrolithiasis: Pathogenesis and treatment. J Urol 1992;148:765–771.
85. Pak CY, Sakhaee K, Fuller C. Successful management of uric acid nephrolithiasis with potassium citrate. Kidney Int 1986;30:422–428.
86. Abbott RD, Brand FN, Kannel WB, et al. Gout and coronary heart disease: The Framingham Study. J Clin Epidemiol 1988;41:237–242.
87. Freedman DS, Williamson DF, Gunter EW, et al. Relation of serum uric acid to mortality and ischemic heart disease. The NHANES I Epidemiologic Follow-up Study. Am J Epidemiol 1995;141:637–644.
88. Langford HG, Blaufox MD, Borhani NO, et al. Is thiazide-produced uric acid elevation harmful? Analysis of data from the Hypertension Detection and Follow-up Program. Arch Intern Med 1987;147:645–649.
89. Bengtsson C, Lapidus L, Stendahl C, Waldenstrom J. Hyperuricaemia and risk of cardiovascular disease and overall death. A 12-year follow-up of participants in the

population study of women in Gothenburg, Sweden. Acta Med Scand 1988;224:549–555.
90. Choi HK, Curhan G. Independent impact of gout on mortality and risk for coronary heart disease. Circulation 2007;116:894–900.
91. Jung JW, Song WJ, Kim YS, et al. HLA-B58 can help the clinical decision on starting allopurinol in patients with chronic renal insufficiency. Nephrol Dial Transplant 2011;26:3567–3572.
92. Hung SI, Chung WH, Liou LB, et al. HLA-B*5801 allele as a genetic marker for severe cutaneous adverse reactions caused by allopurinol. Proc Natl Acad Sci USA 2005;102:4134–4139.
93. Tassaneeyakul W, Jantararoungtong T, Chen P, et al. Strong association between HLA-B*5801 and allopurinol-induced Stevens–Johnson syndrome and toxic epidermal necrolysis in a Thai population. Pharmacogenet Genomics 2009;19: 704–709.
94. Gutman AB. The past four decades of progress in the knowledge of gout, with an assessment of the present status. Arthritis Rheum 1973;16:431–445.
95. Zhu Y, Pandya BJ, Choi HK. Comorbidities of gout and hyperuricemia in the US general population: NHANES 2007–2008. Am J Med 2012;125:679–687.

Glaucoma

75

Richard G. Fiscella, Timothy S. Lesar, and Deepak P. Edward

KEY CONCEPTS

1. Primary open-angle glaucoma (POAG) or ocular hypertension is more prevalent outside Asia than closed- or narrow-angle glaucoma.
2. In any form of glaucoma, reduction of intraocular pressure (IOP) is essential.
3. IOP is a very important risk factor for glaucoma, but the most important considerations are progression of glaucomatous changes in the back of the eye (optic disk and nerve fiber layer) and visual field changes when diagnosing and monitoring for POAG or ocular hypertension.
4. Optic nerve changes often occur before visual field changes are exhibited.
5. Recent studies demonstrate that reduction in IOP prevents progression or even onset of glaucoma.
6. Newer medications simplify treatment regimens for patients. Prostaglandin analogs are considered the most potent topical medications for reducing IOP and flattening diurnal variations in IOP.
7. Local adverse events are common with topical glaucoma medications, but patient education and reinforcing adherence are essential to prevent glaucoma progression.

The glaucomas are a group of ocular disorders that lead to an optic neuropathy characterized by changes in the optic nerve head (optic disk) that is associated with loss of visual sensitivity and field. Increased intraocular pressure (IOP), a traditional diagnostic criterion for glaucoma, is thought to play an important role in the pathogenesis of glaucoma, but it is no longer a diagnostic criterion for glaucoma.[1–10] Two major types of glaucoma have been identified: open angle and closed angle. Open-angle glaucoma accounts for the great majority of cases in North America, while closed-angle glaucoma (CAG) is more prevalent in Asia. Either type can be a primary inherited disorder, congenital, or secondary to disease, trauma, or drugs and can lead to serious complications.[1,11–16] Both primary and secondary glaucomas may be caused by a combination of open-angle and closed-angle mechanisms (Table 75-1).

BASIC CONCEPTS

Aqueous Humor Dynamics and Intraocular Pressure

An understanding of IOP and aqueous humor dynamics will assist the reader in understanding the drug therapy of glaucoma.[1,2,17–19]

Aqueous humor is formed in the ciliary body and its epithelium (Figs. 75-1 and 75-2) through both filtration and secretion. Because ultrafiltration depends on pressure gradients, blood pressure and IOP changes influence aqueous humor formation. Osmotic gradients produced by active secretion of sodium and bicarbonate and possibly by other solutes such as ascorbate from the ciliary body epithelial cells into the aqueous humor result in movement of water from the pool of ciliary stromal ultrafiltrate into the posterior chamber, forming aqueous humor. Carbonic anhydrase (primarily isoenzyme type II), α- and β-adrenergic receptors, and sodium- and potassium-activated adenosine triphosphatases are found on the ciliary epithelium and appear to be involved in this secretion of the solutes sodium and bicarbonate.

Receptor systems controlling aqueous inflow have not been elucidated fully. Pharmacologic studies suggest that β-adrenergic agents increase inflow, whereas α_2-adrenergic blocking, β-adrenergic blocking dopamine-blocking, carbonic anhydrase-inhibiting, and adenylate cyclase-stimulating agents decrease aqueous inflow. Aqueous humor produced by the ciliary body is secreted into the posterior chamber at a rate of approximately 2 to 3 μL/min. The pressure in the posterior chamber produced by the constant inflow pushes the aqueous humor between the iris and lens and through the pupil into the anterior chamber of the eye (see Fig. 75-2).[1,2,17–22]

Aqueous humor in the anterior chamber leaves the eye by two routes: (a) filtration through the trabecular meshwork (conventional outflow) to the Schlemm's canal (80% to 85%) and (b) through the ciliary body and the suprachoroidal space (uveoscleral outflow or unconventional outflow). Cholinergic agents such as pilocarpine increase outflow by physically opening the meshwork pores secondary to ciliary muscle contraction. The uveoscleral outflow of aqueous humor is also increased by prostaglandin analogs and β- and α_2-adrenergic agonists. Constant inflow of aqueous humor from the ciliary body and resistance to outflow result in an IOP great enough to produce an outflow rate equal to the inflow rate (see Fig. 75-2).

TABLE 75-1 General Classification of Glaucoma

I. Primary glaucoma
   A. Open angle
   B. Angle closure
      1. With pupillary block
      2. Without pupillary block
II. Secondary glaucoma
   A. Open angle
      1. Pretrabecular
      2. Trabecular
      3. Posttrabecular
   B. Angle closure
      1. Without pupillary block
      2. With pupillary block
III. Congenital glaucoma

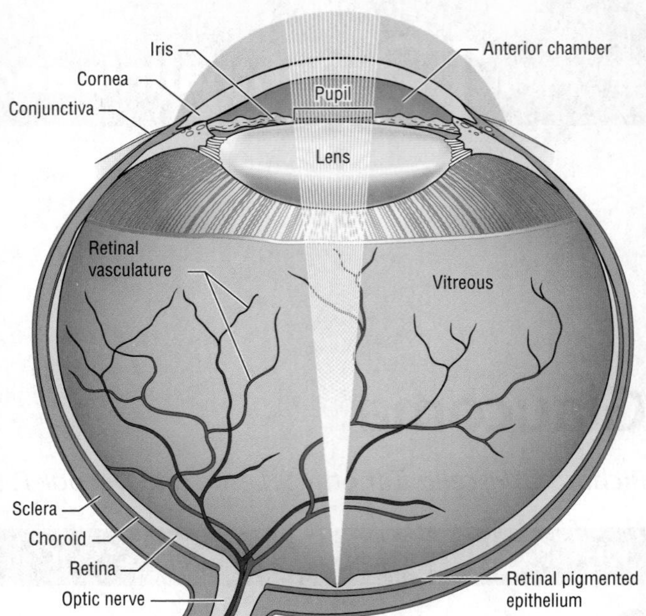

FIGURE 75-1 Anatomy of the eye.

The median IOP measured in large populations is 15.5 ± 2.5 mm Hg (2.1 ± 0.3 kPa); however, the distribution of pressures around the mean is skewed to the right (toward higher readings). IOP is not constant and changes with pulse, blood pressure, forced expiration or coughing, neck compression, and posture. The amount of caffeine in 1 cup of caffeinated coffee (182 mg) increases IOP by about 1 mm Hg after 90 minutes in one study. The authors concluded that the impact of this increase in IOP was not clinically relevant.[9] IOP is measured by tonometry: indentation tonometry, applanation tonometry, or a noncontact method using an air pulse. Newer methods of tonometery include the Pascal tonometer, Icare™ rebound tonometer, and a contact lens-based investigational device that can remotely monitor 24-hour IOP changes from baseline.[10–12] These methods may result in slightly different pressure readings. IOPs consistently greater than 21 mm Hg (2.8 kPa) are found in 5% to 8% of the general population. The incidence increases with age, such that "abnormal" (i.e., >22 mm Hg [>2.9 kPa]) IOP is found in 15% of those 70 to 75 years of age. Intermittently high IOP (>40 mm Hg [>5.3 kPa]) is found in patients with CAG. The increased IOP in all types of glaucoma results from the decreased facility for aqueous humor outflow through the trabecular meshwork. Aqueous humor production in primary open-angle glaucoma (POAG) is normal.[1,2,17–19]

IOP demonstrates considerable circadian variation (often referred to as *diurnal* IOP or the IOP during the daily 24-hour cycle) primarily because of changes in the rate of aqueous humor formation. This circadian variation results in a minimum IOP at approximately 6 PM and a maximum IOP at awakening, although some studies suggest that both healthy and glaucoma patients may have their highest IOP at night after falling asleep.[20] Low systemic blood pressure in conjunction with high IOPs (decreased ocular perfusion pressure) at night can result in optic nerve head damage.[20] Generally, the circadian IOP variation is usually less than 3 to 4 mm Hg (0.4 to 0.5 kPa); however, it may be greater for patients with glaucoma. This circadian variation and the poor relationship of IOP with visual loss make measurement of IOP a poor screening test for glaucoma.

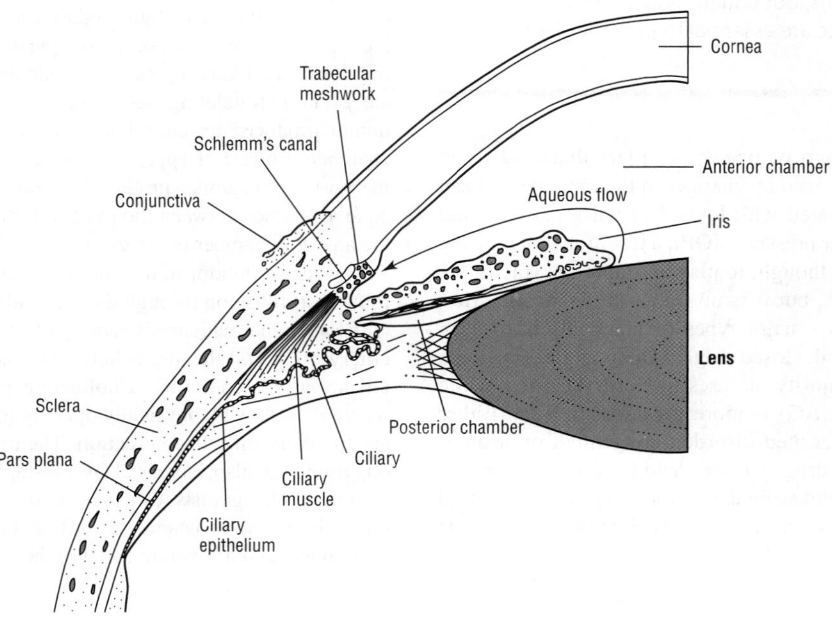

FIGURE 75-2 Anterior chamber of the eye and aqueous humor flow.

Although increased IOP within any range is associated with a higher risk of glaucomatous damage, it is both an insensitive and nonspecific diagnostic and monitoring tool. Of individuals with IOP between 21 and 30 mm Hg (2.8 and 4.0 kPa), only 0.5% to 1% per year will develop optic disk changes and visual field loss (i.e., glaucoma) over 5 to 15 years. However, more subtle retinal damage, such as alteration of color vision or decreased contrast sensitivity, occurs in a higher percentage of patients with IOPs greater than 21 mm Hg (2.8 kPa), and the incidence of visual field defects increases to as high as 28% in individuals with IOPs above 30 mm Hg (4.0 kPa). For a given abnormal IOP, the incidence of glaucoma increases with age. For patients with preexisting optic nerve damage, the worse the existing damage, the more sensitive the eye is to a given IOP. As many as 20% to 30% of patients with glaucomatous visual field loss have an IOP of less than 21 mm Hg (2.8 kPa) (called *normal-tension glaucoma*, referring to the normal IOP). Thus the absolute IOP is a less-precise predictor of optic nerve damage. More direct measurements of therapeutic outcome, such as optic disk examination and visual field evaluation, also must be used as monitors of disease progression.[1–7,17–24] Taking the above factors into consideration, glaucoma medications that provide maximal reduction of IOP over 24 hours and have minimal influence on blood pressure may be advantageous in treating glaucoma patients.

TABLE 75-2 Optic Disk and Visual Field Findings

Optic disk
Cup-to-disk ratio >0.5
Progressive increase in cup size
Cup-to-disk ratio asymmetry >0.2
Vertical elongation of the cup
Excavation of the cup
Increased exposure of lamina cribrosa
Pallor of the cup
Splinter hemorrhages
Cupping to edge of disk
Notching of the cup (usually superior or inferior)
Nerve fiber defects
Visual field findings
General peripheral field constriction
Isolated scotomas (blind spots)
Nasal visual field depression ("nasal step")
Enlargement of blind spot
Large arc-like scotomas
Reduced contrast sensitivity
Reduced peripheral acuity
Altered color vision

Optic Disk and Visual Fields

The optic disk is the portion of the optic nerve ophthalmoscopically visible as it leaves the eye. It consists of approximately 1 million retinal ganglion nerve cell axons, blood vessels, and supporting connective tissue structures (lamina cribrosa). The small depression within the disk is termed the *cup* (Fig. 75-3). A normal physiologic cup does not extend beyond the optic nerve rim and has a varying diameter of less than one third to one half that of the disk (cup-to-disk ratio: 0.33 to 0.5). Table 75-2 lists the common alterations of the optic disk found in glaucoma. These disk changes result from optic nerve axonal degeneration and remodeling of the supporting structures. As the nerve axons die, the cup becomes larger in relation to the whole disk. A loss of retinal nerve fiber layer might be visualized in glaucoma patients with detectable visual field loss. This pattern of changes is consistent with visual field losses and loss of visual sensitivity seen in glaucoma.[1,2,17–24] Damage to the optic nerve can be documented by optic disk photographs, and disease stability or progression may be monitored by examining sequential photographs. Newer methods of assessing damage to the retinal nerve fiber layer and optic disk have been described. These include scanning laser polarimetry (GDX), confocal laser ophthalmoscopy (Heidelberg retinal tomography, or HRT), and optical coherence tomography (OCT). These methods offer the ability to assess the damage to the optic nerve quantitatively.

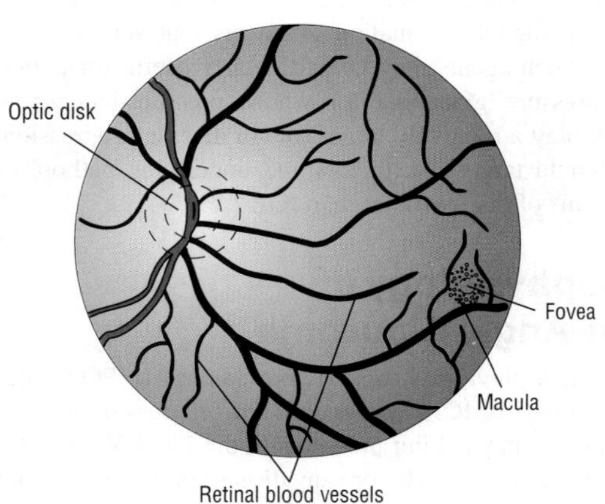

FIGURE 75-3 Normal fundus of the eye and optic disk and cup.

Determination of the visual field allows assessment of optic nerve damage and is an important monitoring parameter in treatment. However, visual field changes lag behind optic disk changes, and a loss of 25% to 35% of retinal ganglion cells is usually required before detectable visual field defects are noted. The peripheral visual field is measured using a visual field instrument called a *perimeter*. Characteristic visual field loss occurs in glaucoma (Fig. 75-4; see also Table 75-2), but loss of central visual acuity usually does not occur until late in the disease. Other indicators, such as color vision changes and contrast sensitivity, may allow earlier and more sensitive detection of glaucomatous changes.[1,2]

Genetics

Glaucoma is often inherited as a complex multifactorial disease, but it can also be inherited as a Mendelian autosomal-dominant or autosomal-recessive trait form. The common age-related adult-onset glaucoma, like POAG, although containing heritability of some significance, is more complex and is influenced by environmental factors. Genetic studies have more clearly defined the underlying molecular events responsible for the Mendelian forms of the disease. However, the chromosome locations identified may play some factor in the more complex forms. A number of major gene loci associated with POAG have been identified. The molecular mechanism of how mutations in any of these genes result in increased IOP with loss of visual field has not been elucidated. The future of genetic studies in glaucoma will include discovery of new glaucoma genes, determination of clinical phenotypes associated with these genes and mutations, understanding how environmental factors interact, and developing a database that can be used for further testing.

Genome-wide association studies have identified new loci that are associated with clinically relevant optic disc parameters, including the optic disc area and vertical cup–disc ratio.[15] Genes associated with chronic angle closure glaucoma have also been identified.[16] Improved understanding of the genetic origins of POAG may lead to

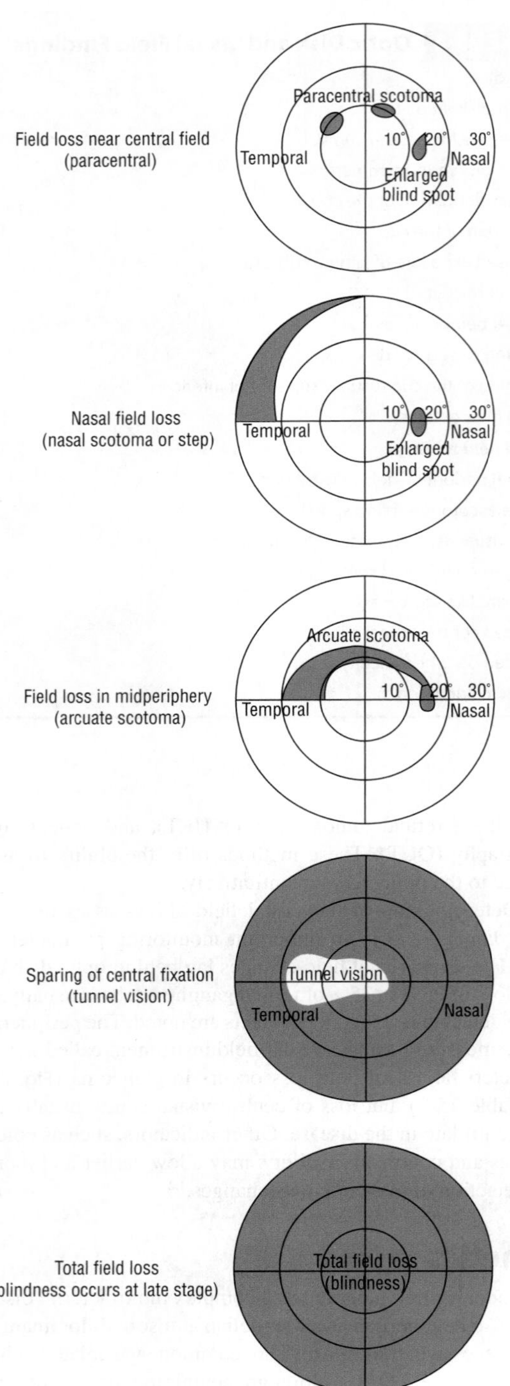

FIGURE 75-4 Schematic of the progression of visual field loss in glaucoma.

new diagnostic tools and therapies that target the underlying causes of the disease.[1,2,15,16,25,26]

Epidemiology of Open-Angle Glaucoma

1 Open-angle glaucoma (OAG) is the second leading cause of blindness, affecting up to 3 million individuals in the United States and up to 60.5 million individuals worldwide. It is estimated that more than 135,000 persons in the United States and about 4.5 million in the world have glaucoma-related bilateral blindness. The prevalence rate varies with age, race, diagnostic criteria, and other factors. In the United States, OAG occurs in 1.5% of the population older than 30 years of age, 1.3% of whites and 3.5% of blacks. Recent study data have also suggested that the prevalence of OAG and ocular hypertension is also high among Latinos of Mexican ancestry, with approximately 4.74% and 3.56% of people affected, respectively.[27] The incidence of OAG increases with increasing age. The incidence of the disease for patients 80 years of age is 3% in whites and 5% to 8% in blacks.

Etiology of Open-Angle Glaucoma

2 The specific cause of glaucomatous optic neuropathy is presently unknown. Previously, increased IOP was considered to be the sole cause of the damage; however, it is now recognized that IOP is only one of many factors associated with the development and progression of glaucoma.[1–10] Increased susceptibility of the optic nerve to ischemia (a reduced or dysregulated blood flow), excitotoxicity, autoimmune reactions, and other abnormal physiologic processes are likely additional contributory factors. The final outcome of these processes is believed to be apoptosis of the retinal ganglion cells, which results in axonal degeneration and finally permanent loss of vision.[11–16] Interestingly enough, there appears to be a fair amount of similarity between neuronal cell death by apoptosis in Alzheimer's disease and glaucoma.[13] Indeed, POAG may represent a number of distinct diseases or conditions that simply manifest the same symptoms. Susceptibility to visual loss at a given IOP varies considerably; some patients do not demonstrate damage at high IOPs, whereas other patients have progressive visual field loss despite an IOP in the normal range (normal-tension glaucoma).

Although IOP poorly predicts which patients will have visual field loss, the risk of visual field loss clearly increases with increasing IOP within any range. In fact, recent studies demonstrate that lowering IOP, no matter what the pretreatment IOP, reduces the risk of glaucomatous progression or may even prevent the onset to early glaucoma in patients with ocular hypertension.[3–7]

The mechanism by which a certain level of IOP increases the susceptibility of a given eye to nerve damage remains controversial. Multiple mechanisms are likely to be operative in a spectrum of combinations to produce the death of retinal ganglion cells and their axons in glaucoma. Pressure-sensitive astrocytes and other cells in the optic disk supportive matrix may produce changes and remodeling of the disk, resulting in axonal death. Vasogenic theories suggest that optic nerve damage results from insufficient blood flow to the retina secondary to the increased perfusion pressure required in the eye, dysregulated perfusion, or vessel wall abnormalities, and results in degeneration of axonal fibers of the retina. Another theory suggests that the IOP may disrupt axoplasmal flow at the optic disk.

Recently, focus on the mechanisms of the retinal ganglion cell apoptosis and the role of excessive glutamate and nitric oxide found in glaucoma patients has broadened the focus of drug therapy research to include evaluation of agents that act as neuroprotectants.[12–15] Such agents may be particularly useful for patients with normal-pressure glaucoma, in whom pressure-independent factors may play a relatively larger role in disease progression. These agents would target risk factors and underlying pathophysiologic mechanisms of disease other than IOP.[11–16]

Pathophysiology of Open-Angle Glaucoma

3 As stated previously, optic nerve damage in POAG can occur at a wide range of IOPs, and the rate of progression is highly variable. Patients may exhibit pressures in the 20 to 30 mm Hg (2.7 to 4.0 kPa) range for years before any disease progression is noticed in the optic disk or visual fields. That is why POAG is often referred to as the "sneak thief of sight."

CLINICAL PRESENTATION Glaucoma

General

- Glaucoma can be detected in otherwise asymptomatic patients, or patients can present with characteristic symptoms, especially vision loss. POAG is a chronic, slowly progressive disease found primarily in patients older than 50 years of age, whereas CAG is more typically associated with symptomatic acute episodes

Symptoms

- POAG: None until substantial visual field loss occurs
- CAG: Nonsymptomatic or prodromal symptoms (blurred or hazy vision with halos around lights that is caused by a hazy, edematous cornea, and occasionally headache) may be present. Acute episodes produce symptoms associated with a cloudy, edematous cornea, ocular pain, or discomfort, nausea, vomiting, abdominal pain, and diaphoresis

Signs

- POAG: Disk changes and visual field loss (see Table 75-2); IOP can be normal or elevated (>21 mm Hg [>2.8 kPa])
- CAG: Acute severe—Hyperemic conjunctiva, cloudy cornea, shallow anterior chamber, and occasionally an edematous and hyperemic optic disk; IOP is generally elevated markedly (40 to 90 mm Hg [5.3 to 12.0 kPa]) when symptoms are present. Chronic—Disk changes and visual field loss (see Table 75-2); IOP can be normal or elevated (>21 mm Hg [>2.8 kPa])

Laboratory Tests

- None

Other Diagnostic Tests

- Emerging tests include optical coherence tomography, retinal nerve fiber analyzers, and confocal scanning laser tomography of the optic nerve

Clinical Presentation of Open-Angle Glaucoma

POAG is a bilateral, often asymmetric, genetically determined disorder constituting 60% to 70% of all glaucomas and 90% to 95% of primary glaucomas (see Clinical Presentation of Glaucoma above). An increased IOP is not required for diagnosis of POAG. Symptoms do not present until substantial visual field constriction occurs. Central visual acuity typically is maintained, even in the late stages of the disease. Even though POAG is a bilateral disease, it may have greater IOP and progression and severity in one eye. As such, each eye is treated individually.

4 Detection and diagnosis involve evaluation of the optic disk and retinal nerve fiber layer, assessment of the visual fields, and measurement of IOP. The presence of characteristic disk changes and visual field loss with or without increased IOP confirms the diagnosis of glaucoma. Typical disk changes and field loss occurring at an IOP of less than 21 mm Hg (2.8 kPa) account for 20% to 30% of patients and are referred to as *normal-tension glaucoma*. Elevated IOP (>21 mm Hg [>2.8 kPa]) without disk changes or visual field loss is observed in 5% to 7% of individuals (known as *glaucoma suspects*) and is referred to as *ocular hypertension*. New technologies such as OCT, retinal nerve fiber analyzers, or confocal scanning laser tomography of the optic nerve head may allow early identification of signs of glaucomatous retinal changes in ocular hypertensives, thus allowing for earlier initiation of therapy.[1–3,17]

Secondary OAG has many causes, including exfoliation syndrome, pigmentary glaucoma, systemic diseases, trauma, surgery, ocular inflammatory diseases, and medications. A system for classifying secondary glaucomas into pretrabecular, trabecular, and posttrabecular forms has been proposed. This classification allows drug therapy to be chosen on the basis of the pathogenic mechanism involved. In pretrabecular forms, a normal meshwork is covered and does not permit aqueous humor outflow. Trabecular forms of secondary glaucoma result from either an alteration of meshwork or an accumulation of material in the intertrabecular spaces. The posttrabecular forms result primarily from disorders causing increased episcleral venous blood pressure.[1,2,15–17]

Prognosis of Open Angle Glaucoma

5 In most cases of POAG, the overall prognosis is excellent when it is discovered early and treated adequately. Even patients with advanced visual field loss can have continued visual field loss reduced if the IOP is maintained at low enough pressures (often <10 to 12 mm Hg [<1.3 to 1.6 kPa]). Progression of visual field loss still occurs in 8% to 20% of patients despite reaching standard therapy IOP goals. However, for untreated patients and for those who fail to achieve target IOP reduction, up to 80% have continued visual field loss. Estimates of progression to bilateral blindness in treated patients range from 4% to 22%. Thus, the keys to medical treatment of POAG are an effective, well-tolerated drug regimen, close monitoring of therapy, and adherence. Medications will control IOP successfully in 60% to 80% of patients over a 5-year period. Availability of newer, highly effective, well-tolerated agents may improve the prognosis further.[1,2,5,17–19,23–28]

Epidemiology of Closed-Angle Glaucoma

The incidence of CAG varies by the ethnic group, with a higher incidence in individuals of Inuit, Chinese, and Asian-Indian descent. Incidence rates of 1% to 4% have been reported in these populations.[1,2] Because of the high frequency of CAG in populous Asia, CAG accounts for approximately one-third of glaucoma worldwide. CAG accounts for a disproportionately high proportion of blindness (estimated at up to 50%) worldwide.[1]

Etiology of Closed-Angle Glaucoma (Angle-Closure Glaucoma)

In North America, primary CAG accounts for a minority of primary glaucomas. When severe acute CAG occurs, it may need to be treated as an emergency to avoid visual loss.

CAG results from mechanical blockage of the (usually normal) trabecular meshwork by the peripheral iris. Partial or complete blockage of the meshwork occurs intermittently, potentially resulting in extreme fluctuations between normal IOP with no symptoms and very high IOP with symptoms of acute CAG. Between attacks of CAG, the IOP is usually normal unless the patient has concomitant POAG or nonreversible blockage of the meshwork with synechiae ("creeping" angle closure) that develops over time in the narrow-angle eye. Primary CAG occurs for patients with inherited shallow anterior chambers (often seen in small eyes), which produce a narrow angle between the cornea and iris or tight contact between the iris and lens (pupillary block). The presence of a narrow angle is determined mainly by visualization of the angle by gonioscopy. Other tests for CAG involve provocation of an angle-closure–induced IOP increase. These tests, which attempt to produce angle closure through mydriasis (darkroom test or mydriasis test) or gravity (prone test), are rarely performed in the clinical setting.

Two major types of classic, reversible primary CAG have been described: CAG with pupillary block and CAG without pupillary block. CAG with pupillary block results when the iris is in firm contact with the lens. This produces a relative block of aqueous flow through the pupil to the anterior chamber (pupillary block), resulting in a bowing forward of the iris, which blocks the trabecular meshwork. CAG with pupillary block occurs most commonly when the pupil is in middilation. In this position, the combination of pupillary block and relaxed iris allows the greatest bowing of the iris; however, angle closure may occur during miosis or mydriasis.

CAG can occur without significant pupillary block for patients with an abnormality called a *plateau iris*. The ciliary processes in these cases are situated anteriorly, which indent the iris forward and cause closure of the trabecular meshwork, especially during mydriasis. The mydriasis produced by anticholinergic drugs or any other drug results in precipitation of both types of CAG glaucoma, whereas drug-induced miosis may produce pupillary block.

Pathophysiology of Closed-Angle Glaucoma

The mechanism of IOP elevation in CAG is clearer than that of POAG. In CAG, a physical blockage of trabecular meshwork is present. In many cases, single or multiple episodes of high IOP that in some patients may exceed 40 mm Hg [>5.3 kPa]) and result in optic nerve damage. Very high IOP (>60 mm Hg [>8.0 kPa]) may result in permanent loss of visual field within a matter of hours to days.

One type of CAG, known as "creeping" angle closure, occurs in patients with narrow angles in which the iris adheres to the trabecular meshwork and may result in continuously increased IOP in ranges more similar to those of POAG, and the clinical behavior is similar to POAG, with individuals differing in the degree and rapidity of visual loss from any given elevated IOP.[1]

Clinical Presentation of Closed-Angle Glaucoma

Most patients with untreated CAG typically experience intermittent nonsymptomatic or prodromal symptoms brought on by precipitating events (see Clinical Presentation of Glaucoma above). Increased IOP during such prodromal episodes is not great enough or long enough to produce the other symptoms of a full-blown attack. Such prodromal attacks last 1 to 2 hours, at which time pupillary block is broken by further mydriasis or miosis, or when miosis or mydriasis occurs in patients with plateau iris. The rate at which IOP increases may be a determinant of when full-blown symptoms occur. Visual fields demonstrate generalized constriction or typical glaucomatous defects as seen in POAG. In approximately 25% of patients, severe attacks may occur and if prolonged, total loss of vision may occur if the IOP is high enough. Tonometry reveals IOPs as high as 40 to 90 mm Hg (5.3 to 12.0 kPa). Patients who have developed adhesions between the iris and meshwork (anterior synechiae) may have chronic IOP elevation with intermittent spikes of high IOP when angle closure occurs.

Drug-Induced Glaucoma

A number of medications are associated with increased IOP or carry labeling that cautions against use of the medication in glaucoma patients. The potential for a medication to produce or worsen glaucoma depends on the type of glaucoma and whether the patient is treated adequately.[25]

Patients with treated, controlled POAG are at minimal risk of induction of an increase in IOP by systemic medications with anticholinergic properties or vasodilators; however, for patients with untreated glaucoma or uncontrolled POAG, the potential of these medications to increase IOP should be considered. Topical anticholinergic agents used to produce mydriasis may result in an increase in IOP. Potent anticholinergic agents such as atropine or homatropine are most likely to increase IOP. Weaker anticholinergics, such as tropicamide, that produce less cycloplegia are less likely to increase IOP and are favored, along with phenylephrine, when mydriasis is desired for POAG patients. Inhaled, nasal, topical, or systemic glucocorticoids may increase IOP for both normal individuals and patients with POAG.

Patients with POAG appear to be particularly susceptible to glucocorticoid-induced increases in IOP. Glucocorticoids reduce the facility of aqueous humor outflow through the trabecular meshwork. The decreased facility of outflow appears to result from the accumulation of extracellular material blocking the trabecular channels. The potential of a glucocorticoid to increase IOP is related to its antiinflammatory potency and intraocular penetration. Thus, patients should be treated with the lowest potency and dose and for the shortest time possible when steroids are indicated.

For patients predisposed to CAG (i.e., narrow anterior chambers), angle closure may be produced by any drug that causes mydriasis (e.g., anticholinergics). A wide range of sulfa compounds causes idiosyncratic reactions that result in anterior choroidal effusions with anterior movement of the iris and lens, resulting in angle closure. The topical use of anticholinergics or sympathomimetic agents most likely will result in angle closure. Systemic and inhaled anticholinergic and sympathomimetic agents also must be used with caution in such patients. As discussed previously, potent miotic agents such as echothiophate may produce angle closure by increasing pupillary block. Table 75-3 lists the drugs associated with potentiation of glaucoma.

TREATMENT

Ocular Hypertension

Treatment of the patient with possible glaucoma (ocular hypertension; i.e., patients with IOP >22 mm Hg [>2.9 kPa]) is less controversial with the recent results of the Ocular Hypertensive Treatment Study (OHTS) than it was in the past.[3] The OHTS helped to identify risk factors for treatment. Patients with IOPs higher than 25 mm Hg (3.3 kPa), vertical cup-to-disk ratio of more than 0.5, and central corneal thickness of less than 555 μm are at greater risk for developing glaucoma. Risk factors such as family history of glaucoma, black ethnicity, severe myopia, and patients with only one eye must

TABLE 75-3 Drugs That May Induce or Potentiate Increased Intraocular Pressure

Open-angle glaucoma
Ophthalmic corticosteroids (high risk)
Systemic corticosteroids
Nasal/inhaled corticosteroids
Fenoldopam
Ophthalmic anticholinergics
Succinylcholine
Vasodilators (low risk)
Cimetidine (low risk)
Closed-angle glaucoma
Topical anticholinergics
Topical sympathomimetics
Systemic anticholinergics
Heterocyclic antidepressants
Low-potency phenothiazines
Antihistamines
Ipratropium
Benzodiazepines (low risk)
Theophylline (low risk)
Vasodilators (low risk)
Systemic sympathomimetics (low risk)
CNS stimulants (low risk)
Serotonin-selective reuptake inhibitors
Imipramine
Venlafaxine
Topiramate
Tetracyclines (low risk)
Carbonic anhydrase inhibitors (low risk)
Monoamine oxidase inhibitors (low risk)
Topical cholinergics (low risk)

also be taken into consideration when deciding which individuals need treatment.

Patients without risk factors typically are not treated and are monitored for the development of glaucomatous changes. Patients with significant risk factors usually are treated with a well-tolerated topical agent such as a prostaglandin analog or β-blocking agent. Other options include an α_2-agonist (brimonidine) or a topical carbonic anhydrase inhibitor (CAI), depending on individual patient characteristics. Optimally, therapy is initiated in one eye to assess efficacy and tolerance. Use of second- or third-line agents (e.g., pilocarpine or dipivefrin) when first-line agents fail to reduce IOP depends on the risk-to-benefit assessment of each patient. The cost, inconvenience, and frequent adverse effects of combination therapies, cholinesterase inhibitors, and oral CAIs result in an unfavorable risk-to-benefit ratio for patients with possible glaucoma.[29]

The goal of therapy is to lower the IOP to a level associated with a decreased risk of optic nerve damage, usually at least a 20%, if not a 25% to 30% decrease from the baseline IOP. Greater decreases may be required in high-risk patients or those with higher initial IOPs. Drug therapy should be monitored by measurement of IOP, examination of the optic disk, assessment of the visual fields, and evaluation of the patient for drug adverse effects and compliance with therapy. Patients who are unresponsive to or intolerant of a drug should be switched to an alternative agent rather than given an additional drug. Many clinicians prefer to discontinue all medications for patients who fail to respond adequately to simple topical therapy, closely monitor for development of disk changes or visual field loss, and treat again when such changes occur.[1,2,17–19,29]

The use of risk calculators has been suggested as a means of determining who are at greatest risk in developing glaucoma. It is hoped that with future improvement in such calculators, one would be able to tailor treatment to those at greatest risk for developing glaucoma.

TREATMENT

Open-Angle Glaucoma

All patients with elevated IOP and characteristic optic disk changes and/or visual field defects not caused by other factors (i.e., glaucoma by definition) should be treated. Recent findings that one in five patients with "normal" IOP and glaucomatous retinal nerve findings (i.e., normal-tension glaucoma) do not have progression of visual field loss if left untreated have prompted recommendations to monitor normal-tension glaucoma patients without immediate threat of loss of central vision and to treat only when progression is documented. Some controversy exists as to whether the initial therapy of glaucoma should be surgical trabeculectomy (filtering procedure), argon or selective laser trabeculectomy, or medical therapy.[1,2,17,18,30–33] Presently, drug therapy remains the most common initial treatment modality. Drug therapy of patients with documented glaucomatous change with either elevated or normal IOP is initiated in a stepwise manner (Fig. 75-5), starting with lower concentrations (when available) of a single, well-tolerated topical agent. The goal of therapy is to prevent further visual loss. A "target" IOP is chosen based on a patient baseline IOP and the amount of existing visual field loss. Typically, an initial target IOP reduction of 30% is desired. Greater reductions may be desired for patients with very high baseline IOPs or advanced visual field loss. Patients with normal baseline IOPs (normal-tension glaucoma) may have target IOPs of less than 10 to 12 mm Hg (1.3 to 1.6 kPa).

Clinical **Controversy...**

How much should the IOP be reduced for patients who may have POAG? Although the major clinical trial (OHTS[3]) required a 20% reduction in IOP for patients with ocular hypertension, many clinicians believe a further lowering of IOP may be more beneficial in preventing the progression of ocular hypertension to glaucoma. The American Academy of Ophthalmology Preferred Practice Guidelines suggest 20% to 30% IOP lowering. It remains to be seen if a more aggressive approach earlier in the treatment of the POAG suspect would be more beneficial.

Pharmacotherapeutic Approach

6 Medications most commonly used to treat glaucoma are the nonselective β-blockers, the prostaglandin analogs, brimonidine (an α_2-agonist), the topical CAIs, and the fixed combination products of timolol/dorzolamide or timolol/brimonidine.[18,21–22]

Before 1996, a β-blocker was used provided no contraindications existed, because this class of drugs has a long history of successful use, providing a combination of clinical efficacy

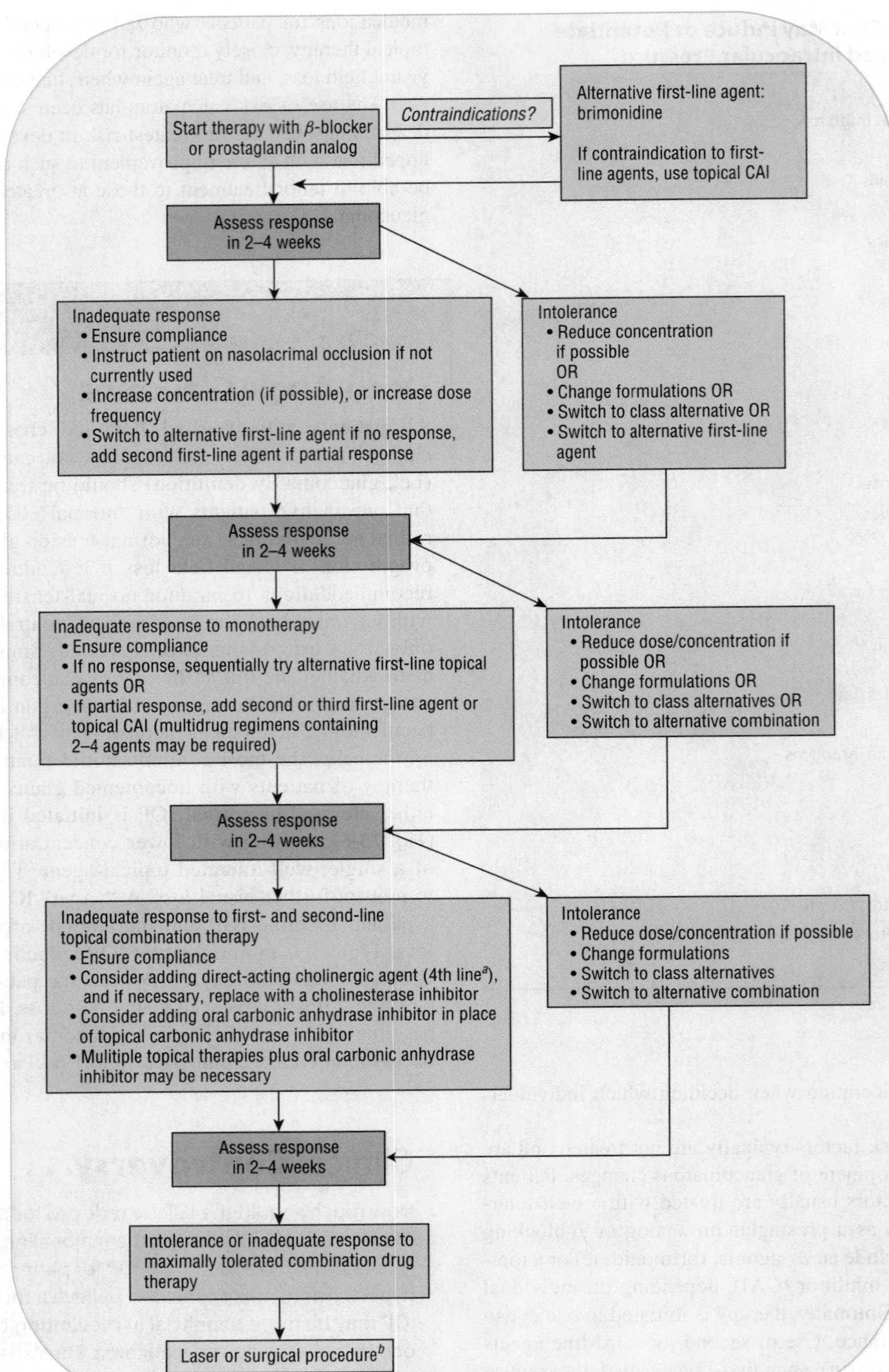

FIGURE 75-5 Algorithm for the pharmacotherapy of open-angle glaucoma. [a]Fourth-line agents not commonly used any longer. [b]Most clinicians believe the laser procedure should be performed earlier (e.g., after three-drug maximum, poorly adherent patient). (CAI, carbonic anhydrase inhibitor.)

and tolerability. The newer agents, in particular the prostaglandin analogs, are often recommended as first-line therapy. They offer once-daily dosing, better IOP reduction, good tolerance and recently, availability of lower-cost generics (see Fig. 75-5). Brimonidine and topical CAIs are also well tolerated and effective agents.[18,34–39] Pilocarpine and dipivefrin are used as third-line therapies because of their increased frequency of adverse effects or reduced efficacy.

Therapy optimally is started as a single agent in one eye (except for patients with very high IOP or advanced visual field loss) to evaluate drug efficacy and tolerance. Monitoring of therapy should be individualized: Initial response to therapy is typically done 4 to 6 weeks after the medication is started. A monocular trial of medication is recommended when possible. Once IOPs reach acceptable levels, the IOP is monitored every 3 to 4 months (more frequently after any change in drug therapy).

Clinical **Controversy. . .**

The American Academy of Ophthalmology has not designated any agent as the drug of choice for initiation of glaucoma treatment. In recent years, many clinicians have used the prostaglandin analogs because they are dosed once daily and achieve the best pressure reduction and are available as less expensive generic products.

Visual fields and disk changes are typically monitored annually or earlier if the glaucoma is unstable or there is suspicion of disease worsening. Patients should always be questioned regarding adherence to and tolerance of prescribed therapy. Initial IOP response does not predict long-term IOP control. Using more than one drop per dose does not improve response, but increases the likelihood of adverse effects and the cost of therapy. When using more than one medication, separation of drop instillation of each agent by at least 5 to 10 minutes is suggested to provide optimal ocular contact for each agent.

The value of an agent with which the patient has shown a drop in IOP following an initial response can be measured by discontinuing the medication completely and determining if an increase in IOP occurs. Patients responding to but intolerant of initial therapy may be switched to another drug or to an alternative dosage form of the same medication. For patients failing to respond to the highest tolerated concentrations of an initial drug, a switch to an alternative agent after 1 day of concurrent therapy should be considered. Alternatively, if only a partial response occurs, addition of another topical drug to be used in combination is a possibility. A number of drugs or drug combinations may need to be tried before an effective and well-tolerated regimen is identified. Because of the frequency of adverse effects, carbachol, topical cholinesterase inhibitors, and oral CAIs are considered last-line agents to be used for patients who fail less-toxic combination topical therapy. IOP responses to ocular hypotensive medication may vary with corneal thickness. The response might be better in those with normal or thin corneas than in those with thicker structures.[22]

Nonpharmacologic Therapy: Laser and Surgical Procedures

When drug therapy fails, is not tolerated, or is excessively complicated, surgical procedures such as laser trabeculoplasty (argon or selective) or a surgical trabeculectomy (filtering procedure) may be performed to improve outflow. Laser trabeculoplasty is usually an intermediate step between drug therapy and trabeculectomy. The newer selective laser trabeculoplasty (SLT) procedure has demonstrated similar IOP reduction as argon laser trabeculoplasty (ALT) and may be repeatable. Recent studies have demonstrated good efficacy for this procedure in comparison with medical treatment options for POAG.[30] Procedures with higher complication rates, such as those involving placement of draining tubes or destruction of the ciliary body (cyclodestruction), may be required when other methods fail (see Fig. 75-2).[1,2,25,31]

Surgical methods for reduction of IOP involve the creation of a channel through which aqueous humor can flow from the anterior chamber to the subconjunctival space (filtering bleb), where it is reabsorbed by the vasculature. A major reason for failure of the procedure is healing and scarring of the site. The use of aqueous shunts or valves to manage glaucoma has been increasing, and the results of a recent study have demonstrated improved safety and efficacy of these devices.[32] Canaloplasty is a minimally invasive surgical treatment that may not be associated with the typical complications of trabeculectomy and drainage implants. It appears to be a well tolerated and an effective, "non-bleb" way to lower IOP and may be useful in mild-to-moderate glaucoma.[32]

Modification of the healing process to maintain patency is possible with the use of antiproliferative agents. The antiproliferative agents 5-fluorouracil and mitomycin C are used for patients undergoing glaucoma-filtering surgery to improve success rates by reducing fibroblast proliferation and consequent scarring. Although used most commonly for patients with increased risk for suboptimal surgical outcome (after cataract surgery and a previous failed filtering procedure), use of these agents also improves success in low-risk patients.[30–33]

TREATMENT

Closed-Angle Glaucoma

The goal of initial therapy for acute CAG with high IOP is rapid reduction of the IOP to preserve vision and to avoid surgical or laser iridectomy on a hypertensive, congested eye. Iridectomy (laser or surgical) is the definitive treatment of CAG; it produces a hole in the iris that permits aqueous humor flow to move directly from the posterior chamber to the anterior chamber, opening up the block at the trabecular meshwork. Drug therapy of an acute attack typically involves administration of pilocarpine, hyperosmotic agents, and a secretory inhibitor (a β-blocker, α_2-agonist, prostaglandin analog, or a topical or systemic CAI). With miosis produced by pilocarpine, the peripheral iris is pulled away from the meshwork. Although traditionally the drug of choice, pilocarpine used as initial therapy is controversial. Miotics may worsen angle closure by increasing pupillary block and producing anterior movement of the lens because of drug-induced accommodation.

At IOPs greater than 60 mm Hg (8.0 kPa), the iris may be ischemic and unresponsive to miotics; as the pressure drops and the iris responds, miosis occurs. During this time, the urge to use excessive amounts of pilocarpine must be resisted. The dose of pilocarpine commonly used is a 1% or 2% solution instilled every 5 minutes for two or three doses and then every 4 to 6 hours. However, many practitioners withhold application of pilocarpine until the IOP has been reduced by other agents, and then apply a single drop of 1% to 2% pilocarpine to produce miosis. In either case, the unaffected contralateral eye should be treated with the miotic every 6 hours to prevent development of angle closure. An osmotic agent also is commonly administered because these drugs produce the most rapid decrease in IOP. Oral glycerin 1 to 2 g/kg can be used if an oral agent is tolerated; if not, IV mannitol 1 to 2 g/kg should be used. Osmotic agents reduce IOP by withdrawing water from the eye secondary to the osmotic gradient between the blood and the eyes. These drugs are among the first-line agents in the short-term treatment of CAG or other forms of acute very high IOP elevations. Topical corticosteroids often are used to reduce the ocular inflammation and reduce the development of synechiae in CAG eyes. In classic CAG, once the IOP is controlled, pilocarpine may be given every 6 hours until iridectomy is performed. Patients failing therapy altogether will require an emergency iridectomy.

Peripheral iridectomy essentially "cures" primary CAG without significant synechiae. Long-term drug therapy is not used unless IOP remains high because of the presence of synechiae blocking the trabecular meshwork or concurrent POAG. In such cases, the pharmacotherapeutic approach is essentially identical to that for the POAG patient, or laser or surgical procedures are performed.[1,2]

PHARMACOLOGIC AGENTS USED IN GLAUCOMA

β-Blocking Drugs

The topical β-blocking agents are one of the most commonly used antiglaucoma medications (Table 75-4). β-Blockers lower IOP by 20% to 30% with a minimum of local ocular adverse effects. These are commonly one of the agents of first choice—along with prostaglandin analogs—in treating POAG if no contraindications exist.[1,2,17–19,34–36]

The β-blocking agents produce ocular hypotensive effects by decreasing the production of aqueous humor by the ciliary body without producing substantial effects on aqueous humor outflow facility. The mechanism by which β-blockers decrease aqueous humor inflow remains controversial, but it is most frequently attributed to β_2-adrenergic receptor blockade in the ciliary body.

Five ophthalmic β-blockers are presently available: timolol, levobunolol, metipranolol, carteolol, and betaxolol. Timolol, levobunolol, and metipranolol are nonspecific β-blocking agents, whereas betaxolol is a relatively β_1-selective agent. Carteolol is a nonspecific blocker with intrinsic sympathomimetic activity. Despite differences in potency, selectivity, lipophilicity, and intrinsic sympathomimetic activity, the five agents reduce IOP to a similar degree, although betaxolol has been reported to produce somewhat less lowering of IOP than timolol and levobunolol. Levobunolol may be more effective than timolol and betaxolol in reducing postcataract surgery IOP increases. Levobunolol solution is more effective in controlling IOP than other agents when given as aqueous solutions on a once-daily schedule (up to 70% of patients). Timolol in the form of a gel-forming solution (Timoptic-XE) provides equivalent IOP control with once-daily administration when compared with the same concentration of the aqueous solution administered twice daily. The choice of a specific β-blocking agent generally is based on differences in adverse effect potential, individual patient response, and cost. Long-term treatment with topical β-blockers results in tachyphylaxis in 20% to 25% of patients. The mean IOP reduction from baseline may be smaller for patients receiving topical β-blockers with concurrent systemic β-blockers.[29]

Local adverse effects with β-blockers usually are tolerable, although stinging on application occurs commonly, particularly with betaxolol solution (less with betaxolol suspension) and metipranolol. Other local effects include dry eyes, corneal anesthesia, blepharitis, blurred vision, and, rarely, conjunctivitis, uveitis, and keratitis. Some local reactions may be a result of preservatives used in the commercially available products. Switching from one agent to another or switching the type of formulation may improve tolerance in patients experiencing local adverse effects.

Systemic effects are the most important adverse effects of β-blockers. Drug absorbed systematically may produce decreased heart rate, reduced blood pressure, negative inotropic effects, conduction defects, bronchospasm, CNS effects, and alteration of serum lipids and may block the symptoms of hypoglycemia. The β_1-specific agents betaxolol and possibly carteolol (as a consequence of intrinsic sympathomimetic activity) are less likely to produce the systemic adverse effects caused by β-adrenergic blockade, such as the cardiac effects and bronchospasm, but a real risk still exists. The use of timolol as a gel-forming liquid or betaxolol as a suspension allows for administration of fewer drugs per day and, therefore, reduces the chance for systemic adverse effects compared with the aqueous solutions.

Because of their systemic adverse effects, all ophthalmic β-blockers should be used with caution for patients with pulmonary diseases, sinus bradycardia, second- or third-degree heart block, congestive heart failure, atherosclerosis, diabetes, and myasthenia gravis, as well as for patients receiving oral β-blocker therapy. Use of the nasolacrimal occlusion (NLO; see Patient Education below for description) technique during administration reduces the risk or severity of systemic adverse effects, as well as optimizes response. Overall, β-adrenergic blocking agents are well tolerated by most patients, and most potential problems can be avoided by appropriate patient evaluation, drug choice, and monitoring of drug therapy. For patients failing or having an inadequate response to single-drug therapy with a β-blocking agent, the addition of a CAI, parasympathomimetic agent, prostaglandin analog, or an α_2-adrenergic receptor agonist usually will result in additional IOP reduction. Dipivefrin added to a β-blocking agent (particularly nonspecific β-blockers) usually results in only minimal additional IOP reduction.[1–3,17–19,29]

α_2-Adrenergic Agonists

Brimonidine and the less lipid-soluble and less receptor-selective apraclonidine are α_2-adrenergic agonists structurally similar to clonidine. Apraclonidine is indicated and brimonidine is effective for prevention or control of postoperative or postlaser treatment increases in IOP. Brimonidine is considered a first-line or adjunctive agent in the therapy of POAG, and apraclonidine is seen as a second-line or adjunctive therapy due to a high incidence of loss of control of IOP (tachyphylaxis) and a more severe and prevalent ocular allergy rate.

α_2-Agonists reduce IOP by decreasing the rate of aqueous humor production (some increase in uveoscleral outflow also occurs with brimonidine). The drugs reduce IOP by 18% to 27% at peak (2 to 5 hours) and by 10% at 8 to 12 hours. Comparative trials demonstrate a reduction in IOP similar to that obtained with 0.5% timolol. Use of brimonidine 0.2% every 8 to 12 hours appears to provide maximum IOP-lowering effects in long-term use. Use of NLO (see Patient Education below) may improve response and allow the longer dosing frequency (i.e., every 12 hours). Combinations of α_2-agonists with β-blockers, prostaglandin analogs, or CAIs produce additional IOP reduction.

An allergic-type reaction characterized by lid edema, eye discomfort, foreign-object sensation, itching, and hyperemia occurs in approximately 30% of patients with apraclonidine. Brimonidine produces this adverse effect in up to 8% of patients. This reaction commonly necessitates drug discontinuation. Systemic adverse effects with brimonidine include dizziness, fatigue, somnolence, dry mouth, and possibly a slight reduction in blood pressure and pulse. α_2-Agonists should be used with caution for patients with cardiovascular diseases, renal compromise, cerebrovascular disease, and diabetes, as well as in those taking antihypertensives and other cardiovascular drugs, monoamine oxidase inhibitors, and tricyclic antidepressants.

Brimonidine is also contraindicated in infants because of apneic spells and hypotensive reactions. In terms of overall efficacy and tolerability, brimonidine approximates that achieved with β-blockers.[1,2,17–19,29]

Brimonidine purite 0.15% or 0.1% is a formulation of brimonidine in a lower concentration than the original product that contains a less-toxic preservative than the most commonly employed benzalkonium chloride. The newer formulations are as effective as the original because the more neutral pH of brimonidine purite (0.15% pH 7.2; 0.1% pH 7.7) allows for higher concentrations of brimonidine in the aqueous humor with a similar reduction in IOP and a reduced incidence of ocular allergy.[29]

A randomized clinical trial of topical brimonidine 0.2% twice daily preserved visual field better than treatment with topical timolol maleate 0.5% in patients with OAG statistically normal IOP.[13] The IOP-lowering efficacy was similar between the two medications, suggesting that this finding was consistent with a non-IOP-related mechanism, possibly a neuroprotective action. However, validation

TABLE 75-4 Topical Drugs Used in the Treatment of Open-Angle Glaucoma

Drug	Pharmacologic Properties	Common Brand Names	Dose Form	Strength (%)	Usual Dose[a]	Mechanism of Action
β-Adrenergic Blocking Agents						
Betaxolol	Relative β_1-selective	Generic	Solution	0.5	One drop twice a day	All reduce aqueous production of ciliary body
		Betoptic-S	Suspension	0.25	One drop twice a day	
Carteolol	Nonselective, intrinsic sympathomimetic activity	Generic	Solution	1	One drop twice a day	
Levobunolol	Nonselective	Betagan	Solution	0.25, 0.5	One drop twice a day	
Metipranolol	Nonselective	OptiPranolol	Solution	0.3	One drop twice a day	
Timolol	Nonselective	Timoptic, Betimol, Istalol	Solution	0.25, 0.5	One drop every day—one to two times a day	
		Timoptic-XE	Gelling solution	0.25, 0.5	One drop every day[a]	
Nonspecific Adrenergic Agonists						
Dipivefrin	Epinephrine prodrug	Propine	Solution	0.1	One drop twice a day	Increased aqueous humor outflow
α_2-Adrenergic Agonists						
Apraclonidine	Specific α_2-agonists	Iopidine	Solution	0.5, 1	One drop two to three times a day	Both reduce aqueous humor production; brimonidine known to also increase uveoscleral outflow; only brimonidine has primary indication
Brimonidine		Alphagan P	Solution	0.15, 0.1	One drop two to three times a day	
Cholinergic Agonists Direct Acting						
Carbachol	Irreversible	Carboptic, Isopto Carbachol	Solution	1.5, 3	One drop two to three times a day	All increase aqueous humor outflow through trabecular meshwork
Pilocarpine	Irreversible	Isopto Carpine, Pilocar	Solution	0.25, 0.5, 1, 2, 4, 6, 8, 10	One drop two to three times a day	
					One drop four times a day	
		Pilopine HS	Gel	4	Every 24 hours at bedtime	
Cholinesterase Inhibitors						
Echothiophate		Phospholine Iodide	Solution	0.125	Once or twice a day	
Carbonic Anhydrase Inhibitors						
Topical						
Brinzolamide	Carbonic anhydrase type II inhibition	Azopt	Suspension	1	Two to three times a day	All reduce aqueous humor production of ciliary body
Dorzolamide		Trusopt Generic	Solution	2	Two to three times a day	
Systemic						
Acetazolamide		Generic	Tablet	125 mg, 250 mg	125–250 mg two to four times a day	
			Injection	500 mg/vial	250–500 mg	
		Diamox Sequels	Capsule	500 mg	500 mg twice a day	
Methazolamide		Generic	Tablet	25 mg, 50 mg	25–50 mg two to three times a day	
Prostaglandin Analogs						
Latanoprost	Prostanoid agonist	Xalatan	Solution	0.005	One drop every night	Increases aqueous uveoscleral outflow and to a lesser extent trabecular outflow
Bimatoprost	Prostamide agonist	Lumigan	Solution	0.01, 0.03	One drop every night	
Travoprost	Prostanoid agonist	Travatan Z	Solution	0.004	One drop every night	
Tafluprost	Prostanoid agonist	Zioptan	Preservative free solution	0.0015%	One drop every night	
Combinations						
Timolol–dorzolamide		Cosopt Generic	Solution	Timolol 0.5% dorzolamide 2%	One drop twice daily	
Timolol–brimonidine		Combigan	Solution	Timolol 0.5% brimonide 0.2%	One drop twice daily	
Brinzolamide–brimonidine		Simrinza		Brinzolamide 1% brimonidine 0.2%	One drop three times daily	

[a]Use of nasolacrimal occlusion will increase the number of patients successfully treated with longer dosage intervals.

of a neuroprotective role for brimonidine requires further research to confirm these results.[13,14]

The combination product timolol 0.5% and brimonidine 0.2% (Combigan) may provide additional IOP lowering than either agent alone.[37]

Clinical **Controversy. . .**

Many animal trials demonstrate that brimonidine has excellent neuroprotective properties.[12–15] Some clinicians believe that one of the major advantages of using brimonidine lies in its potential neuroprotective properties. However, neuroprotection has not been demonstrated in human trials, although a recent article produced the most clinically relevant data to date.[43,44]

Prostaglandin Analogs

The prostaglandin analogs, including latanoprost, travoprost, bimatoprost, and tafluprost, reduce IOP by increasing the uveoscleral and, to a lesser extent, trabecular outflow of aqueous humor. Some differences in receptor sites and mechanisms of action may exist between the two prostaglandins (latanoprost and travoprost), the prostamide (bimatoprost). However both classes appear to produce collagen changes in the ciliary muscle. Bimatoprost may be slightly more effective in lowering IOP, getting a larger percentage of patients to lower IOPs, and for patients unresponsive to latanoprost.[29,38–40] If the patient does not respond to travoprost or latanoprost, a switch to bimatoprost may be beneficial.[39] Generic forms of some prostaglandin analogs are now available, reducing the cost to patients for these agents. Tafluprost is available as a preservative-free solution, which may be useful in patients intolerant of common ophthalmic preservatives or those with corneal surface disorders.

Reduction in IOP with once-daily doses of prostaglandin $F_2\alpha$ analogs (a 25% to 35% reduction) is often greater than that seen with timolol 0.5% twice daily. In addition, nocturnal control of IOP is improved compared with timolol. Interestingly, administration of prostaglandin $F_2\alpha$ analogs twice daily may reduce the IOP similarly to once-daily dosing. The drugs are administered at nighttime, although they are probably as effective if given in the morning.

Prostaglandin analogs are well tolerated and produce fewer systemic adverse effects than timolol. Local ocular tolerance generally is good, but ocular reactions such as punctate corneal erosions and conjunctival hyperemia do occur. Local intolerance occurs in 10% to 25% of patients with these agents.

With prostaglandin analogs, altered iris pigmentation occurs in 15% to 30% of patients, particularly those with mixed-color irises (blue-brown, green-brown, blue-gray-brown, or yellow-brown eyes), which become browner in color over 3 to 12 months. The change in iris pigmentation will often appear within 2 years, and long-term consequences of this pigment change appear to be mostly cosmetic but irreversible upon discontinuation. Hypertrichosis is common and reverses upon discontinuation of the drug. Hyperpigmentation around the lids and lashes has also been reported and appears to reverse upon discontinuation. Topical prostaglandin analogs may produce rates of corneal thinning that are slightly higher than ongoing age-related changes. This effect is unlikely to be clinically relevant.[24]

These agents are associated with uveitis, and caution is recommended for patients with ocular inflammatory conditions. Cystoid macular edema also has been reported. Cases of worsening of herpetic keratitis have been reported.

Prostaglandin analogs can be used in combination with other antiglaucoma agents for additional IOP control because of their unique mechanism of action. Given their excellent efficacy and side-effect profile, prostaglandin analogs provide effective monotherapy or adjunctive therapy for patients who are not responding to or tolerating other agents. The use of prostaglandin analogs as first-line therapy in POAG is approved for latanoprost and bimatoprost. Long-term studies demonstrate these agents are safe, efficacious, and well tolerated in glaucoma therapy.[17–19,29,38,39]

Carbonic Anhydrase Inhibitors

Topical Agents

CAIs reduce IOP by decreasing ciliary body aqueous humor secretion. CAIs appear to inhibit aqueous production by blocking active secretion of sodium and bicarbonate ions from the ciliary body to the aqueous humor.[1,2,29] Topical CAIs such as dorzolamide and brinzolamide are well tolerated and are indicated for monotherapy or adjunctive therapy of POAG and ocular hypertension. Relatively specific inhibitors of carbonic anhydrase enzyme II such as dorzolamide and brinzolamide reduce IOP by 15% to 26%.

Topical CAIs generally are well tolerated. Local adverse effects include transient burning and stinging, ocular discomfort and transient blurred vision, tearing, and, rarely, conjunctivitis, lid reactions, and photophobia. A superficial punctate keratitis occurs in 10% to 15% of patients. Brinzolamide produces more blurry vision but is less stinging than dorzolamide. Systemic adverse effects are unusual despite the accumulation of drug in red blood cells. Because of their favorable adverse-effect profile, topical CAIs provide a useful alternative agent for monotherapy or adjunctive therapy for patients with inadequate response to or who are unable to use other agents. The drugs may add additional IOP reduction for patients using other single or multiple topical agents. The usual dose of a topical CAI is one drop every 8 to 12 hours. Administration every 12 hours produces somewhat less IOP reduction than administration every 8 hours. Use of NLO should optimize response to CAI given at any interval.[1,2,17–19,29,34,36] The combination product timolol 0.5% and dorzolamide 2% (Cosopt) is dosed twice daily and produces equivalent IOP lowering to each product dosed separately. Both dorzolamide and timolol/dorzolamide (Cosopt) are now available as generic formulations.

Systemic Agents

Systemic CAIs are indicated for patients failing to respond to or tolerate maximum topical therapy. Systemic and topical CAIs should not be used in combination because no data exist concerning improved IOP reduction, and the risk for systemic adverse effects is increased. Oral CAIs reduce aqueous humor inflow by 40% to 60% and IOP by 25% to 40%. The available systemic CAIs (see Table 75-4) produce equivalent IOP reduction but differ for potency, adverse effects, dosage forms, and duration of action. Despite their excellent effects on elevated IOP of any etiology, the systemic CAIs frequently produce intolerable adverse effects. As a result, CAIs are considered third-line agents in the treatment of POAG and often used for short-term administration to lower IOP.

On average, only 30% to 60% of patients are able to tolerate oral CAI therapy for prolonged periods. Intolerance to CAI therapy results most commonly from a symptom complex attributable to systemic acidosis and including malaise, fatigue, anorexia, nausea, weight loss, altered taste, depression, and decreased libido. Other adverse effects include renal calculi, increased uric acid, blood dyscrasias, diuresis, and myopia. Elderly patients do not tolerate CAIs as well as younger patients. The available CAIs produce the same spectrum of adverse effects; however, the drugs differ in the frequency and severity of the adverse effects listed.

CAIs should be used with some caution in patients with sulfa allergies (all CAIs, topical or systemic, contain sulfonamide moieties, although cross-sensitivity is thought to be very low), sickle cell disease, respiratory acidosis, pulmonary disorders, renal calculi, electrolyte imbalance, hepatic disease, renal disease, diabetes mellitus, or Addison's disease. Concurrent use of a CAI and a diuretic may rapidly produce hypokalemia. High-dose salicylate therapy may increase the acidosis produced by CAIs, whereas the acidosis produced by CAIs may increase the toxicity of salicylates.[1,2,17–19,21,29,34,35]

Parasympathomimetic Agents

The parasympathomimetic (cholinergic) agents reduce IOP by increasing aqueous humor trabecular outflow. The increase in outflow is a result of physically pulling open the trabecular meshwork secondary to ciliary muscle contraction, thereby reducing resistance to outflow. These agents may reduce uveoscleral outflow. Cholinergic agents work well to decrease IOP, but their use as primary or even adjunctive agents in the treatment of glaucoma has decreased significantly because of local ocular adverse effects and/or frequent dosing requirements.

Pilocarpine, the parasympathomimetic agent of choice in POAG, is available as an ophthalmic solution and a hydrophilic polymer gel (see Table 75-4). Pilocarpine produces similar (20% to 30%) reductions in IOP as those seen with β-blocking agents. Pilocarpine in POAG or "glaucoma suspects" is initiated as 0.5% or 1% solution, one drop three to four times daily. The use of NLO improves response and reduces the need for an every-6-hour dosing frequency. The use of one drop of 2% pilocarpine every 6 to 12 hours and NLO provides optimal response in many patients. Both drug concentration and frequency may be increased if IOP reduction is inadequate. Patients with darkly pigmented eyes frequently require higher concentrations of pilocarpine than do patients with lightly pigmented eyes. Concentrations of pilocarpine above 4% rarely improve IOP control in patients, other than those patients with darkly pigmented eyes.

Pilocarpine 4% gel (Pilopine HS) once daily is equivalent to treatment with pilocarpine solution 4% four times daily or timolol 0.5% twice daily. When using every-24-hour dosing of pilocarpine gel, the adequacy of IOP control late in the dosing interval should be confirmed. Ocular adverse effects of pilocarpine include miosis, which decreases night vision and vision in patients with central cataracts. Visual field constriction may be seen secondary to miosis and should be considered when evaluating visual field changes in a glaucoma patient. Pilocarpine ciliary muscle contraction produces accommodative spasm, particularly in young patients still able to accommodate (prepresbyopic). Pilocarpine may also produce frontal headache, brow ache, periorbital pain, eyelid twitching, and conjunctival irritation or injection early in therapy, which tends to decrease in severity over 3 to 5 weeks of continued therapy.

Cholinergics produce a breakdown of the blood–aqueous humor barrier and may result in a worsening of an ocular inflammatory reaction or condition. Systemic cholinergic adverse effects of pilocarpine—such as diaphoresis, nausea, vomiting, diarrhea, cramping, urinary frequency, bronchospasm, and heart block—are rare but may be seen in patients who are using products with high pilocarpine concentrations (6% to 8%) or in those patients who are using such products overzealously in treatment of acute-angle closure. Other adverse effects associated with direct-acting miotics include retinal tears or detachment, allergic reaction, permanent miosis, cataracts, precipitation of CAG, and, rarely, miotic cysts of the pupillary margin.

Carbachol is a potent direct-acting miotic agent; its duration of action is longer than that of pilocarpine (8 to 10 hours) because of resistance to hydrolysis by cholinesterases. This drug also may act as a weak inhibitor of cholinesterase. Patients with an inadequate response to or intolerance of pilocarpine as a result of ocular irritation or allergy frequently do well on carbachol. The ocular and systemic adverse effects of carbachol are similar to but more frequent, constant, and severe than those of pilocarpine.[1,2,17–19,29,34,35] Clinical use of carbachol is limited and may not be commercially available in the near future.

The cholinesterase inhibitors used most commonly in the treatment of POAG are the long-acting, relatively irreversible agent echothiophate (limited commercial availability; see Table 75-4). This agent is a potent inhibitor of pseudocholinesterase, but also inhibits true cholinesterase. Because of the serious ocular and systemic toxic effects of echothiophate, it is reserved primarily for patients who are either not responding to or are intolerant of other therapy. Because of its cataractogenic properties, most ophthalmologists use this agent only for patients without lenses (aphakia) and for patients with artificial lenses (pseudophakia). The ocular and periocular parasympathomimetic adverse effects are more common and more severe than with pilocarpine or carbachol.

In addition to the parasympathomimetic effects, echothiophate may produce severe fibrinous iritis (particularly with the irreversible inhibitors), synechiae, iris cysts, conjunctival thickening, occlusion of the nasolacrimal ducts, and cataracts. The inhibition of systemic pseudocholinesterase by echothiophate decreases the rate of succinylcholine hydrolysis, resulting in prolonged muscle paralysis. Echothiophate should be discontinued at least 2 weeks before procedures in which succinylcholine is used.

The role of echothiophate in glaucoma is limited by its frequency and potential toxicity. For phakic patients, cholinesterase inhibitors should be administered only if intolerance or failure results with other antiglaucoma medications. Echothiophate has been shown to provide additional IOP-lowering effects when used with β-blockers, CAIs, and sympathomimetic (adrenergic) agents. As with all agents for glaucoma, therapy should be initiated with lower concentrations of these agents. A once-daily administration frequency should be used for most patients unless very high IOP is present.

Use of NLO likely improves response, reduces systemic adverse effects, and should be performed by all patients administering echothiophate. The drug should be used with caution for patients with asthma, retinal detachments, narrow angles, bradycardia, hypotension, heart failure, Down's syndrome, epilepsy, parkinsonism, peptic ulcer, and ocular inflammation, as well as in those receiving cholinesterase inhibitor therapy for myasthenia gravis or exposure to carbamate or organophosphate insecticides and pesticides.[1,2,17–19,29,34,35]

Dipivefrin

The mechanism of action by which dipivefrin (an epinephrine pro-drug) lowers IOP has not been fully elucidated; however, a β_2-receptor–mediated increase in outflow facility through the trabecular meshwork and the uveoscleral route appears to be the primary mechanism. Compared with β-blockers or miotics, dipivefrin is less effective for reducing IOP. With the advent of the better-tolerated and more-efficacious agents to treat glaucoma, the clinical use of epinephrines has decreased dramatically.

A factor limiting the usefulness of dipivefrin is the high frequency of local ocular adverse effects. Tearing, burning, ocular discomfort, brow ache, conjunctival hyperemia, punctate keratopathy, allergic blepharoconjunctivitis, rare loss of eyelashes, stenosis of the nasolacrimal duct, and blurred vision may occur. Prolonged use (>1 year) may result in deposition of pigment (adrenochrome) in the conjunctiva and cornea. Pigment also may deposit in soft contact lenses, turning them black. Dipivefrin may produce mydriasis (particularly when combined with a β-blocker) and may precipitate acute CAG in patients with narrow anterior chambers. A transient increase in IOP may occur with initial therapy, particularly for patients not using other antiglaucoma medications. A relative contraindication to the use of dipivefrin is aphakia (i.e., after cataract removal) or lens dislocation because of the development of swelling of the macular portion of the retina. The edema is dose dependent and disappears with drug discontinuation.

Systemic adverse effects of dipivefrin include headache, faintness, increased blood pressure, tachycardia, arrhythmias, tremor, pallor, anxiety, and increased perspiration. Dipivefrin should be used with caution for patients with cardiovascular diseases, cerebrovascular diseases, aphakia, CAG, hyperthyroidism, and diabetes mellitus, as well as for patients undergoing anesthesia with halogenated hydrocarbon anesthetics. Using NLO with dipivefrin will improve therapeutic response and reduce the risk of systemic adverse effects.[1,2,17–19,29,34,35]

Future Drug Therapies

It is hoped that new agents, improved formulations, and novel approaches to the reduction of IOP and other methods of prevention of glaucomatous visual field loss will provide more effective and better-tolerated therapies. Agents that are neuroprotective and act through mechanisms other than IOP reduction are likely to be part of glaucoma therapy in the future.[13–16,41]

EVALUATION OF THERAPEUTIC OUTCOMES

The ultimate goal of drug therapy for the patient with glaucoma is to preserve visual function through reduction of IOP to a level at which no further optic nerve damage occurs. Because of the poor relationship between IOP and optic nerve damage, no specific target IOP exists. Indeed, drugs used to treat glaucoma may act in part to halt visual field loss through mechanisms separate from or in addition to IOP reduction, such as improvements in retinal or choroidal blood flow. Often a 25% to 30% reduction is desired, but greater reductions (40% to 50%) may be desired for patients with initially high IOPs. For patients with glaucoma, an IOP of less than 21 mm Hg (2.8 kPa) generally is desired, with progressively lower target pressures needed for greater levels of glaucomatous damage. Even lower IOPs (possibly even below 10 mm Hg [1.3 kPa]) are required for patients with very advanced disease, those showing continued damage at higher IOPs, and those with normal-tension glaucoma and pretreatment pressures in the low to middle teens. The IOP considered acceptable for a patient is often a balance of desired IOP and acceptable treatment-related toxicity and of patient quality of life.

PATIENT EDUCATION

❼ An important consideration for patients failing to respond to drug therapy is adherence. Poor adherence or nonadherence occurs in 25% to 60% of glaucoma patients.

A large percentage of patients also fail to use topical ophthalmic drugs correctly. Patients should be taught the following procedure:

1. Wash and dry the hands; shake the bottle if it contains a suspension.
2. With a forefinger, pull down the outer portion of the lower eyelid to form a "pocket" to receive the drop.
3. Grasp the dropper bottle between the thumb and fingers with the hand braced against the cheek or nose and the head held upward.
4. Place the dropper over the eye while looking at the tip of the bottle; then look up and place a single drop in the eye.
5. The lids should be closed (but not squeezed or rubbed) for 1 to 3 minutes after instillation. This increases the ocular availability of the drug.
6. Recap bottle and store as instructed.

Note that many patients are physically unable to administer their own eye drops without assistance. NLO also should be used to improve ocular bioavailability and reduce systemic absorption.[1,2,17–19,29,34,35] The patient induces NLO for 1 to 3 minutes by closing the eyes and placing the index finger over the nasolacrimal drainage system in the inner corner of the eye. This maneuver, as well as eyelid closure itself, decreases nasolacrimal drainage of drug, thereby decreasing the amount of drug available for systemic absorption by the nasopharyngeal mucosa. The use of NLO may improve drug response significantly, reduce adverse effects, and allow less-frequent dosing intervals and the use of lower drug concentrations.

Use of more than one drop per dose increases costs, does not improve response significantly, and may increase adverse effects. When two drugs are to be administered, instillations should be separated by at least 3 to 5 minutes (preferably 10 minutes) to prevent the drug administered first from being washed out. The patient should be taught not to touch the dropper bottle tip with eye, hands, or any surface.

Adherence to glaucoma therapy usually is inadequate, and it always should be considered as a possible cause of drug therapy failure. Assessment of adherence by healthcare providers generally is poor; so all patients should be encouraged continually to administer prescribed therapy diligently as instructed. To improve adherence, the patient, family, and care providers should be fully informed of the expectations of therapy and the need to continue therapy despite a lack of symptoms. Possible adverse effects of the medication and ways to reduce them should be discussed. Adherence will be improved by good communication, simplified and well tolerated dosing regimens, reminder devices, education, close monitoring, and individualized care planning.[1,2,17–19,29,42]

CONCLUSIONS

The glaucomas are a group of primary and secondary diseases whose management presents a considerable challenge to the clinician. Successful therapy requires rational use of antiglaucoma medications and patient adherence to the selected regimen, combined with conscientious monitoring for adverse effects and disease progression. The reward for successful therapy is considerable—the maintenance of vision. The overview of the clinical findings, pathology, and drug therapy presented in this chapter provides the clinician with the fundamentals necessary to understand and treat glaucoma.

ABBREVIATIONS

CAG	closed-angle glaucoma
CAI	carbonic anhydrase inhibitor
IOP	intraocular pressure
NLO	nasolacrimal occlusion
OAG	open-angle glaucoma
OHTS	Ocular Hypertensive Treatment Study
POAG	primary open-angle glaucoma

REFERENCES

1. Quigley HA. Glaucoma. Lancet 2011;377:1367–1377.
2. Kwon YH, Fingert JH, Kuehn MH, Alward WLM. Primary open-angle glaucoma. N Engl J Med 2009;360:1113–1124.
3. Kass MA, Heuer DK, Higginbotham EJ, et al. The ocular hypertension treatment study: A randomized trial determines that topical ocular hypotensive medication delays or prevents the onset of primary open-angle glaucoma. Arch Ophthalmol 2002;120:701–713, discussion 829, 830.

4. Leske MC, Heijl A, Hussein M, et al. Factors for glaucoma progression and the effect of treatment: The early manifest glaucoma trial. Arch Ophthalmol 2003;121:48–56.
5. Van Veldhuisen PC, Schwartz AL, Gaasterland DE, et al. The advanced glaucoma intervention study (AGIS): 7. The relationship between control of intraocular pressure and visual field deterioration. Am J Ophthalmol 2000;130: 429–440.
6. Janz NK, Wren PA, Lichter PR, et al. Quality of life in newly diagnosed glaucoma patients: The collaborative initial glaucoma treatment study. Ophthalmology 2001;108:887–897.
7. Collaborative Normal-Tension Glaucoma Study Group. Comparison of glaucomatous progression between untreated patients with normal-tension glaucoma and patients with therapeutically reduced intraocular pressures. Am J Ophthalmol 1998;126:487–497.
8. Kanner E, Tsai JC. Glaucoma medications use and safety in the elderly population. Drugs Aging 2006;23: 321–332.
9. Jiwani AZ, Rhee DJ, Brauner SC, et al. Effects of caffeinated coffee consumption on intraocular pressure, ocular perfusion pressure, and ocular pulse amplitude: A randomized controlled trial. Eye (Lond) 2012;26(8): 1122–1130.
10. Kotecha A, White E, Schlottmann PG, Garway-Heath DF. Intraocular pressure measurement precision with the Goldmann applanation, dynamic contour, and ocular response analyzer tonometers. Ophthalmology 2010;117:730–737. Epub 2010 Feb 1.
11. Hsiao YC, Dzau JR, Flemmons MS, et al. Home assessment of diurnal intraocular pressure in healthy children using the Icare rebound tonometer. JAAPOS 2012;16(1): 58–60.
12. Mansouri K, Medeiros FA, Tafreshi A, Weinreb RN. Continuous 24-hour monitoring of intraocular pressure patterns with a contact lens sensor: Safety, tolerability, and reproducibility in patients with glaucoma. Arch Ophthalmol 2012;13:1–6. doi: 10.1001/archophthalmol.2012.2280.
13. Krupin T, Liebmann JM, Greenfield DS, et al. A randomized trial of brimonidine versus timolol in preserving visual function: Results from the Low-pressure Glaucoma Treatment Study. Am J Ophthalmol 2011;151:671–681.
14. Quigley HA. Clinical trials for glaucoma neuroprotection are not impossible. Curr Opin Ophthalmol 2012;23: 144–154.
15. Ramdas WD, van Koolwijk LM, Lemij HG, et al. Common genetic variants associated with open-angle glaucoma. Hum Mol Genet 2011;20(12):2464–2471.
16. Vithana EN, Khor CC, Qiao C, et al. Genome-wide association analyses identify three new susceptibility loci for primary angle closure glaucoma. Nat Genet 2012;44: 1142–1146. doi:10.1038/ng.2390.
17. Marquis RE, Whitson JT. Management of glaucoma: Focus on pharmacological therapy. Drugs Aging 2005;22: 1–21.
18. Tanna AP, Rademake AW, Stewart WC, Feldman RM. Meta-analysis of the efficacy and safety of beta-2-adrenergic agonists, adrenergic antagonists, and topical carbonic anhydrase inhibitors with prostaglandin analogs. Arch Ophthalmol 2010;128(7):825–833.
19. Hoyng PF, van Beek LM. Pharmacological therapy for glaucoma: A review. Drugs 2000;59:411–434.
20. Wax MB, Camras CB, Fiscella RG, et al. Emerging perspectives in glaucoma: Optimizing 24-hour control of intraocular pressure. Am J Ophthalmol 2002;133:S1–S10.
21. Law SK. Switching within glaucoma medication class. Curr Opin Ophthalmol 2009;20:100–115.
22. Brandt JD, Beiser JA, Gordon MO, et al. Ocular Hypertension Treatment Study (OHTS) Group. Central corneal thickness and measured IOP response to topical ocular hypotensive medication in the Ocular Hypertension Treatment Study. Am J Ophthalmol 2004;138:717–722.
23. Ocular Hypertension Treatment Study Group; European Glaucoma Prevention Study Group; Gordon MO, Torri V, Miglior S, et al. Validated prediction model for the development of primary open-angle glaucoma in individuals with ocular hypertension. Ophthalmology 2007;114: 10–19.
24. Brandt JD, Gordon MO, Beiser JA, et al. Ocular Hypertension Treatment Study Group. Changes in central corneal thickness over time: The ocular hypertension treatment study. Ophthalmology 2008;115:1550–1556.
25. Triptahi RC, Tripathi BJ, Haggerty C. Drug-induced glaucomas. Drug Saf 2003;26:749–767.
26. Wiggs JL. Genetic etiologies of glaucoma. Arch Ophthalmol 2007;125:30–37.
27. Varma R, Ying-Lai M, Francis BA, et al. Prevalence of open-angle glaucoma and ocular hypertension in Latinos. Ophthalmology 2004;111:1439–1448.
28. Quigley HA, Broman AT. The number of people with glaucoma worldwide in 2010 and 2020. Br J Ophthalmol 2006;90:262–267.
29. Cantor L. Achieving low target pressures with today's glaucoma medications. Surv Ophthalmol 2003;48(Suppl 1):S8–S16.
30. Katz LJ, Steinmann WC, Kabir A, et al. Selective laser trabeculoplasty versus medical therapy as initial treatment of glaucoma: A prospective, randomized trial. J Glaucoma. 2012;21:460–468.
31. Mearza AA, Aslanides IM. Uses and complications of mitomycin C in ophthalmology. Expert Opin Drug Saf 2007;6:27–32.
32. Grover DS, Smith O. Recent clinical pearls from clinical trials in glaucoma. Curr Opin Ophthalmol 2012;23:127–134.
33. Loon SC, Chew PT. A major review of antimetabolites in glaucoma therapy. Ophthalmologica 1999;213:234–245.
34. Schuman JS. Antiglaucoma medications: A review of safety and tolerability issues related to their use. Clin Ther 2000;22:167–208.
35. Kanner E, Tsai JC. Glaucoma medications. Use and safety in the elderly population. Drugs Aging 2006;23:321–332.
36. Han JA, Frishman WH, Sun SW, et al. Cardiovascular and respiratory considerations with pharmacotherapy of glaucoma and ocular hypertension. Cardiol Rev 2008;16:95–108.
37. Sherwood MB, Craven ER, Chou C, et al. Twice-daily 0.2% brimonidine–0.5% timolol fixed-combination therapy vs monotherapy with timolol or brimonidine in patients with glaucoma or ocular hypertension. Arch Ophthalmol 2006;124:1230–1238.
38. Noecker R, Dirks M, Choplin N. A six-month randomized clinical trial comparing the IOP lowering efficacy of bimatoprost and latanoprost in patients with ocular hypertension or glaucoma. Am J Ophthalmol 2003;135:55–63.
39. van der Valk R, Webers CA, Schouten JSAG, et al. Intraocular pressure-lowering effects of all commonly used glaucoma drugs. A meta-analysis of randomized clinical trials. Ophthalmology 2005;112:1177–1185.
40. Drugs for some common eye disorders. Med Lett 2010;8:1–8.

41. Naskar R, Vorwerk CK, Dreyer EB. Saving the nerve from glaucoma: Memantine to caspases. Semin Ophthalmol 1999;14:152–158.
42. Gray TA, Orton LC, Henson D, et al. Interventions for improving adherence to ocular hypotensive therapy. Cochrane Database Syst Rev 2009; 2:CD006132. doi:10.1002/14651858.CD006132.pub2.
43. Krupin T, Liebmann JM, Greenfield DS, et al. A randomized trial of brimonidine versus timolol in preserving visual function: Results from the Low-pressure Glaucoma Treatment Study. Am J Ophthalmol 2011;151:671–681.
44. Quaranta L, Floriani I, Krupin T, et al. The rate of progression and ocular perfusion pressure in the Low-pressure Glaucoma Treatment Study [letters]. Am J Ophthalmol 2011;152:880–881.

76

Allergic Rhinitis

J. Russell May and Philip H. Smith

KEY CONCEPTS

1. Allergic rhinitis is a common disease. Prevention measures and treatment are justified in most cases because of the potential for complications.
2. Because an immune response to allergens results in release of inflammatory mediators that cause allergic rhinitis symptoms, patients must understand the rationale for proper timing and administration of prophylactic regimens.
3. Avoidance of allergens is difficult and it may be impractical to expect full success.
4. Antihistamines offer an effective option for treating both seasonal and persistent allergic rhinitis.
5. Intranasal steroids are highly effective in patients who use them properly.
6. While immunotherapy is the only disease-modifying treatment of allergic rhinitis, expense, potential risks, and the major time commitment required make patient selection critical.

Allergic rhinitis involves inflammation of the nasal mucous membrane. In a sensitized individual, allergic rhinitis occurs when inhaled allergenic particles contact mucous membranes and elicit a specific response mediated by immunoglobulin E (IgE). This acute response involves the release of inflammatory mediators and is characterized by sneezing, nasal itching, and watery rhinorrhea, often associated with nasal congestion. Itching of the throat, eyes, and ears frequently accompanies allergic rhinitis.

Allergic rhinitis may be regarded as seasonal allergic rhinitis, commonly known as *hay fever*, or persistent allergic rhinitis (formerly known as perennial rhinitis). Seasonal rhinitis occurs in response to specific allergens usually present at predictable times of the year, during plants' pollination (typically the spring or fall). Seasonal allergens include pollen from trees, grasses, and weeds. Persistent allergic rhinitis is a year-round disease caused by nonseasonal allergens, such as house dust mites, animal dander, and molds, or multiple allergic sensitivities. It typically results in less variable, chronic symptoms. Many patients have a combination of these two types of allergic rhinitis, with symptoms year-round and seasonal exacerbations.

EPIDEMIOLOGY

1 Allergic rhinitis is one of the most common medical disorders found in humans, affecting 400 million people worldwide.[1] It is the second leading cause of chronic disease in the United States, affecting one person in every four households.[2] In the populations of Europe, United States, Australia, and New Zealand, the prevalence of an IgE sensitization to aeroallergens measured by allergen-specific IgE in serum or skin tests is more than 40% to 50%.[3] Patients may be limited in their ability to carry out normal daily functions; higher levels of general fatigue, mental fatigue, anxiety, depressive disorders, and learning disabilities (secondary to sleep loss and fatigue) are possible.

In addition, the impact of allergic rhinitis goes well beyond these CNS issues. Allergic rhinitis is associated with several other serious medical conditions, including asthma, chronic rhinosinusitis, otitis media, nasal polyposis, respiratory infections, and orthodontic malocclusions.

ETIOLOGY

The development of allergic rhinitis is determined by genetics, allergen exposure, and the presence of other risk factors. A family history of allergic rhinitis, atopic dermatitis, or asthma suggests that rhinitis is allergic. The risk of developing allergic disease appears to increase if one parent is atopic and further increases if two are allergic; however, small sample sizes and the lack of reproducibility prevent generalization.[3]

Allergen exposure is another necessary factor. For allergic rhinitis to occur, an individual must be exposed over time to a protein that elicits the allergic response in that individual. Many potential sufferers never develop symptoms because they do not come into contact with the allergen that would produce symptoms in them.

Evidence suggests microbial exposure in the first years of life could help prevent allergic disease by stimulating a nonatopic immune response.[4] Farm children are exposed to higher concentrations of endotoxin, derived from cell walls of gram-negative bacteria, in barns and dust around the farmhouse. Consumption of nonpasteurized farm milk may cause further exposure. These observations have led to the idea that allergic disease could be prevented by proactively increasing exposure to harmless bacteria early in life (see Alternative Treatment Options below). This could explain why positive skin tests indicating allergen sensitization have been observed more frequently for people in higher socioeconomic classes and for people who live in suburban areas.

Other predisposing factors include an elevated serum IgE (>100 international units/mL [>100 kIU/L]) before the age of 6 years, eczema, and heavy exposure to secondhand cigarette smoke.[5]

Allergens

Allergens that produce seasonal rhinitis include protein components of airborne pollen grains, often enzymes, from a variety of trees, grasses, and weeds. Ragweed and grass pollen are the most common offenders in the United States; however, this varies with the geographic region. In general, tree pollens cause symptoms in the spring, grass pollens cause symptoms in the late spring and summer, and weed pollens are the culprits from late summer through fall. Patients who are hypersensitive to all three may have overlapping problem periods and may be described as having perennial rhinitis when they are actually experiencing prolonged seasonal rhinitis. For this reason and the fact that most patients with seasonal problems are sensitive to at least some of the perennial allergens, there is little practical difference between the two types of allergic rhinitis. To complicate matters further, the antigenic components of many grasses—including fescue, Kentucky bluegrass, orchard, redtop, and timothy—cross-react extensively. By contrast, most tree allergens are antigenically distinct. Trees with allergenic pollen include ash, beech, birch, cedar, hickory, maple, oak, poplar, and sycamore. Flowering plants that depend on insect pollination do not cause allergic rhinitis because their pollen is too heavy and sticky and is not carried in the air.

Smaller mold spores are also important but cause allergy much less frequently. Various spores are present year-round; however, mold growth on decaying vegetation increases seasonally. Just walking through uncut fields or raking leaves can increase exposure. Thus, mold spores can be responsible for both perennial and seasonal allergies.

Indoor allergens are always present. Most important among these are house-dust mite fecal proteins, animal dander, cockroaches, and certain mold species. Dust mite levels are on the rise, possibly because of the construction of energy-efficient homes and offices with reduced ventilation and increased humidity, use of wall-to-wall carpeting, and the popularity of cool-water detergents and cold-water washing.[3]

PATHOPHYSIOLOGY

Knowledge of nasal physiology aids in the understanding of allergic rhinitis. The nose performs three "air conditioning" functions to prepare incoming gases for the lungs. During the fraction of a second that air is in the nose, it is heated, humidified, and cleaned. The cleaning process plays a role in the development of allergic rhinitis. As the air passes through the nose, the turbulence throws particulate matter against a mucous blanket. The rhythmic movements of the nasal cilia cause the mucous blanket to move posteriorly at approximately 9 mm/min, where it is eventually swallowed; thus, trapped foreign particles are removed via the GI tract and do not reach the lungs. It also concentrates foreign protein material into the posterior nasopharynx, where lymph tissues identify them and produce most of the allergic antibody that drives allergic rhinitis.

The vascular tissue in the nose is erectile. Stimulation of sympathetic fibers causes vasoconstriction, reduction in erectile tissue size and the size of the membranes and turbinates, and airway widening. Parasympathetic stimulation causes opposite effects.

Mast cells, in the nasal membranes, participate in the regulation of nasal patency by releasing mediators such as histamine. These are described below.

Immune Response to Allergens

2 Allergic reactions in the nose are mediated by antigen–antibody responses when allergens interact with specific IgE molecules bound to nasal mast cells and basophils. In allergic people, these cells are increased in both number and reactivity. During inhalation, airborne allergens enter the nose and are processed by lymphocytes, which produce antigen-specific IgE, thereby sensitizing genetically predisposed hosts to those agents. Upon nasal reexposure, IgE bound to mast cells interacts with airborne allergen,

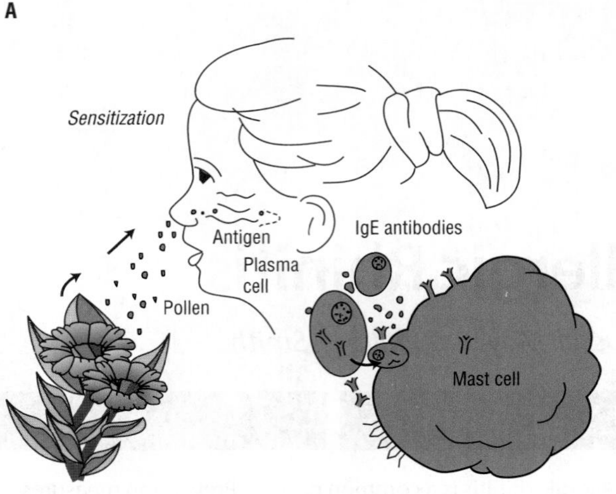

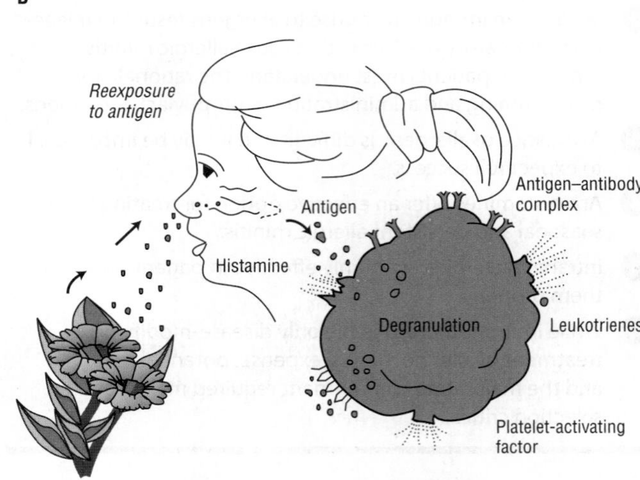

FIGURE 76-1 Allergen sensitization and the allergic response. *A*. Exposure to antigen stimulates IgE production and sensitization of mast cells with antigen-specific IgE antibodies. *B*. Subsequent exposure to the same antigen produces an allergic reaction when mast cell mediators are released.

triggering release of inflammatory mediators in vastly increased quantities (Fig. 76-1).[6]

Both immediate and late-phase reactions are observed after allergen exposure. The immediate reaction occurs within seconds to minutes, resulting in the rapid release of preformed mediators and newly generated mediators from the arachidonic acid cascade as the mast cell membrane is disturbed (Table 76-1). These mediators of immediate hypersensitivity include histamine, some leukotrienes, prostaglandin D_2, tryptase, and kinins.[6] In addition, the mast cell has been found to be a source of several cytokines that probably are relevant to the chronicity of the mucosal inflammation that characterizes allergic rhinitis.[7] Sensory nerve stimulation produces itching, and sneezing occurs via reflex stimulation of efferent vagal pathways. Neuropeptides substance P and calcitonin gene-related peptide from nonadrenergic, noncholinergic nerves affect vascular engorgement directly and via modulation of sympathetic tone. Histamine produces rhinorrhea, itching, sneezing, and obstruction, with the obstruction only partially blocked by H_1- or H_2-blocking agents.[8] Nasal obstruction is also caused by kinins, prostaglandin D_2, and leukotrienes C_4/D_4. Kinins, when directly administered, produce

TABLE 76-1 Mast Cell Mediators

Mediator	Effect
Preformed and rapidly released	
Histamine	Stimulates irritant receptors Pruritus Vascular permeability Mucosal permeability Smooth muscle contraction
Neutrophil chemotactic factor	Influx of inflammatory cells
Eosinophil chemotactic factor	Influx of inflammatory cells
Kinins	Vascular permeability
N-α-tosyl L-arginine methyl esterase	Vascular permeability
Newly generated	
Leukotrienes	Smooth muscle contraction Vascular permeability Mucus secretion Chemotaxis Neutrophil chemotaxis
Thromboxanes	Smooth muscle spasm
Platelet-activating factor	Mucus secretion Airway permeability Chemotaxis Vascular permeability
Granule matrix contents	
Heparin	Antiinflammatory
Tryptase	Protein hydrolysis
Kallikrein	Protein hydrolysis

pain rather than itching.[9] These inflammatory mediators also produce vasodilation, increased vascular permeability, and production of increased nasal secretions.[10]

Four to 8 hours after the initial exposure to an allergen, a late-phase reaction occurs symptomatically in 50% of allergic rhinitis patients.[11] This response, thought to be caused by cytokines released primarily by mast cells and thymus-derived helper lymphocytes, is characterized by profound infiltration and activation of migrating cells. This inflammatory response likely is responsible for the persistent, chronic symptoms of allergic rhinitis, including nasal congestion. The inflamed mucosa becomes hyperresponsive, a state characterized by exacerbation of nasal reactions to nonspecific or irritant triggers. In this state, the patient also reacts to increasingly lower amounts of the same allergen.[12] The process also causes significant increases in nonspecific irritability (as seen in asthma) and the notion among patients that they have become "allergic to everything."

CLINICAL PRESENTATION

The patient with allergic rhinitis typically complains of clear rhinorrhea, paroxysms of sneezing, nasal congestion, postnasal drip, and pruritic eyes, ears, nose, or palate. Symptoms of allergic conjunctivitis are associated more frequently with seasonal than perennial allergic rhinitis, because a majority of the perennial allergens, such as dust mites and molds, are indoors, where air velocity is too low for substantial deposition of allergenic particles on the conjunctivae. However, with heavy exposure from animal or mold allergens, allergic conjunctivitis can be pronounced.

Symptoms secondary to the late-phase reaction, predominantly nasal congestion, begin 3 to 5 hours after antigen exposure and peak at 12 to 24 hours. Subsequent symptoms, both allergic and irritant, are elicited more easily because of the priming effect. For instance, a ragweed-sensitive patient, when exposed to ragweed pollen out of season, responds with modest symptoms and may be very tolerant of irritants such as air pollution or tobacco smoke. During the ragweed season, however, when the nasal mucosa is already inflamed, exposure to small doses of pollen or to irritants to which the patient is usually tolerant elicits a response clinically indistinguishable from the patient's allergy.

Diagnostic Considerations

Allergic rhinitis is distinguished from other causes of rhinitis by a thorough history, physical examination, and certain diagnostic tests. The medical history consists of a careful description of symptoms, environmental factors and exposures, results of previous therapy, use of other medications, previous nasal injuries, previous nasal or sinus surgery, family history, and the presence of other medical problems and medications. Historical identification of specific causative allergens may be difficult. For example, a reaction induced by mowing the lawn may not be caused by grass pollens but may be caused by the disturbance of various weeds, molds, or other plants in the lawn. With perennial allergic rhinitis, the cause–effect and temporal relationships are less clear, making the diagnosis of specific causes more difficult, especially with such covert allergens as house dust mites and molds.

In children, physical examination may reveal allergic shiners—a transverse nasal crease caused by repeated rubbing of the nose—and adenoidal breathing. Pale, bluish, edematous nasal turbinates coated with thin, clear secretions are characteristic of a purely allergic reaction. Tearing, conjunctival injection and edema, and periorbital swelling may be present. Physical findings are generally less clear-cut for adults.

Nasal scrapings will provide a representative sample of cells infiltrating the nasal mucosa and can be helpful in supporting the diagnosis.[13] Microscopic examination of the nasal smear from an allergic individual typically will show numerous eosinophils. The blood eosinophil count may be elevated in allergic rhinitis, but it is nonspecific and has limited usefulness.[14]

Allergy testing can help determine whether a patient's rhinitis is caused by an allergen. Immediate-type hypersensitivity skin tests are used for the diagnosis of allergic rhinitis. These include skin tests performed by the percutaneous route, where the diluted allergen is pricked or scratched into the skin surface, or by the intradermal route, where a small volume (0.01 to 0.05 mL) of diluted allergen is injected between the layers of skin. Percutaneous tests are more commonly performed and are safer and more generally accepted, with intradermal tests reserved for patients requiring confirmation in special circumstances.

In all allergy testing, a positive control (histamine) and a negative control are essential for correct interpretation. After 15 minutes of the application of the allergen, the site is examined for a positive reaction (defined as a wheal-and-flare reaction). Because correct testing is done with extremely minute doses, undetectable by nonsensitized individuals, this reaction is evidence of the presence of mast cell-bound IgE specific to the allergen tested. Many, but not all, common allergens are available as standardized allergenic extracts.

Antihistamines and a few other medications interfere with the wheal-and-flare reaction. First-generation antihistamines should be stopped at least 3 to 5 days before testing, and second-generation, nonsedating antihistamines should be stopped for 10 days before testing.[15] Medications with antihistamine properties (e.g., sympathomimetic agents, phenothiazines, and tricyclic antidepressants) should be discontinued if possible before skin testing.

The radioallergosorbent test (RAST) was the first commonly used method for detecting IgE antibodies in the blood that are specific for a given allergen. Several other quantitative assays that include a reference curve calculated against standardized IgE are available. These tests are highly specific but may be slightly less sensitive than percutaneous tests.

Complications

Not only is allergic rhinitis aggravating, it frequently leads to further complications, particularly if the patient does not receive adequate treatment. Symptoms of untreated rhinitis may lead to disturbed sleep, chronic malaise, fatigue, and poor work or school performance. Patients often are plagued by loss of smell or taste, with sinusitis or polyps underlying many cases of allergy-related hyposmia. Postnasal drip with cough, hoarseness, and even vocal polyps also can be bothersome.

The role of allergic rhinitis in the development of acute otitis media or chronic middle ear effusion is often less clear. Children with allergic rhinitis appear to be at greater risk of these conditions because of nasal obstruction and negative middle ear pressure. Hearing problems in children related to middle ear effusion may lead to delayed development of language in young children or to school problems in older children.

Permanent facial disfigurement can result from chronic allergic rhinitis.[16] The chronic edema and venous stasis may contribute to the development of a high-arched, V-shaped palate. Mouth breathing caused by nasal obstruction can be responsible for dental malocclusion and orthodontic problems. Constant upward rubbing of the nose (allergic salute) can cause a transverse crease across the lower nose; nasal congestion often leads to venous pooling and dark circles under the eyes known as *allergic shiners*.

Allergic rhinitis is clearly associated with asthma. The prevalence of asthma in patients without rhinitis is <2%, while the prevalence of asthma in patients with rhinitis is 10% to 40%.[17] It is not known if allergic rhinitis is an early clinical manifestation of asthma or if the nasal disease itself is causative for asthma.

Recurrent sinusitis and chronic sinusitis are relatively common complications of allergic rhinitis. The structure of the mucus blanket breaks down, with decreased water production by serous glands, leaving hair cells trapped in the thicker mucus layer. This greatly reduces the clearance of trapped bacteria and offers ideal breeding grounds for the bacteria. Nasal polyps are less common but nonetheless bothersome; they require specific therapy but may improve with management of the underlying allergic state. Epistaxis also can be a problem; it is related to mucosal hyperemia and inflammation.

TREATMENT

A number of options exist for the treatment of allergic rhinitis, both nonpharmacologic and pharmacologic. Many of the pharmacologic options are available over-the-counter requiring that patients receive guidance in the selection process by a healthcare professional to obtain the most appropriate therapy. Both over-the-counter and prescription choices must be guided by patient-specific symptomatology and patient characteristics as described in this chapter.

Desired Outcomes

The therapeutic goal for patients with allergic rhinitis is to minimize or prevent symptoms and prevent long-term complications. This goal should be accomplished with no or minimal adverse medication effects and reasonable medication expenses. The patient should be able to maintain a normal lifestyle, including participating in outdoor activities, yard work, and playing with pets as desired.

General Approach to Treatment

Once the causative allergens and the specific symptoms are identified, management consists of three possible approaches: (a) allergen avoidance, (b) pharmacotherapy for prevention or treatment of symptoms, and (c) specific immunotherapy. The pharmacotherapy for symptoms approach includes several options that are based on patient-specific information (Table 76-2). Figure 76-2 depicts an algorithm for treatment options.

Nonpharmacologic Therapy

❸ Avoidance of offending allergens is the most direct method of preventing allergic rhinitis, but it is often the most difficult to accomplish, especially for perennial allergens. Mold growth can be reduced by maintaining household humidity below 50% and removing obvious growth with bleach or disinfectant. Patients sensitive to animals will benefit most by removing pets from the home[18]; however, most animal lovers are reluctant to comply with this approach. Dog and cat allergens may produce symptoms in sensitized individuals.[7] After removing a cat from the home, it may take as long as 20 weeks for the home to reach allergen levels of a

TABLE 76-2 Pharmacotherapeutic Options for Allergic Rhinitis

Medication Class	Symptoms Controlled	Comments
Antihistamines		
Systemic	Sneezing, rhinorrhea, itching, conjunctivitis	For seasonal allergic rhinitis, begin treatment before allergen exposure. Nonsedating agents should be tried first. If ineffective or too expensive for the patient, the older agents may be used. For perennial allergic rhinitis, use an intranasal steroid as an alternative to or in combination with systemic antihistamines
Ophthalmic	Conjunctivitis	Logical addition to nasal steroids if ocular symptoms are present
Intranasal	Sneezing, rhinorrhea, nasal pruritus	Option for seasonal allergic rhinitis. Warn patients of potential drowsiness
Decongestants		
Systemic	Nasal congestion	Only needed when nasal congestion is present
Topical	Nasal congestion	Only needed when nasal congestion is present. Do not exceed 3–5 days
Intranasal corticosteroids	Sneezing, rhinorrhea, itching, nasal congestion	For seasonal allergic rhinitis, an option when congestion is present. Must begin therapy before allergen exposure. Excellent choice for perennial rhinitis
Mast cell stabilizers	See comments	Prevents symptoms; therefore, for seasonal allergic rhinitis, use before offending allergen's season starts. For perennial rhinitis, improvement may not be seen for up to 1 month
Intranasal anticholinergics	Rhinorrhea	Reserve for use when above therapies fail or cannot be tolerated
Leukotriene receptor antagonists	See comments	When combined with antihistamines, more effective than antihistamines alone. May be used as monotherapy in children with asthma and coexisting allergic rhinitis

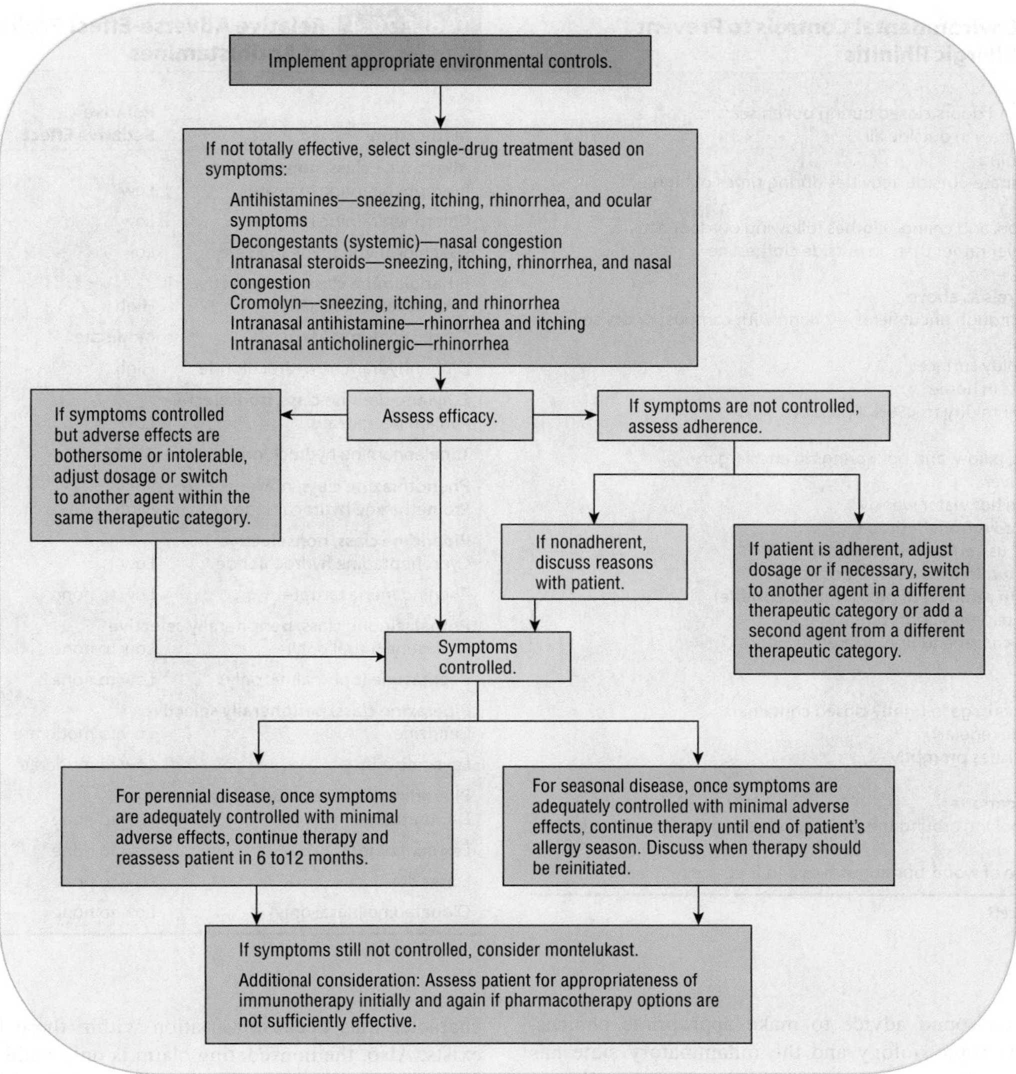

FIGURE 76-2 Treatment algorithm for allergic rhinitis.

pet-free home. Washing cats weekly may reduce allergens but studies are inconclusive.[7] Some dogs display antigens more profusely than do others; clinically, a sensitized person may tolerate one animal better than another.

Evidence to support avoidance measures for house dust mites suggests that accepted notions for reducing exposure have little practical effect.[18] While some evidence shows allergen levels can be reduced by washing bedding on a hot cycle, replacing carpets with hard flooring and using vacuum cleaners with HEPA filters, there is no documented evidence for a clinical benefit. Only encasing bedding in impermeable covers has some clinical benefit in children but not adults. Future studies are needed to determine if environmental control of allergens may be helpful in forestalling further rhinitis and preventing later asthma.

General recommendations have been made to prevent poor air quality in homes.[19] Steps include avoiding wall-to-wall carpeting, using moisture control to prevent the accumulation of molds, and controlling sources of pollution such as cigarette smoke. Patients with seasonal allergic rhinitis should keep windows closed and minimize time spent outdoors during pollen seasons. Immediate hair washing and change of clothes are recommended upon returning indoors. Use of fans that direct outside air into the house should be avoided. Filter masks can be worn while gardening or mowing the lawn. Avoidance of upholstery and stuffed toys in the bedroom are easy steps to accomplish. Table 76-3 summarizes recommendations for environmental control. While these steps are logical, there is little existing evidence that environmental control measures provide clinical benefit. These measures are intended to be a part of a comprehensive treatment strategy that will likely include pharmacotherapy and, in selected cases, immunotherapy.

Other suggested measures for preventing allergic rhinitis include breastfeeding infants and avoidance of exposure to tobacco smoke.[18] Exclusive breastfeeding for the first 3 months of life may help prevent allergies. Avoidance of environmental tobacco smoke (i.e., passive smoking) by children and pregnant woman may also reduce the development of allergies and has been strongly recommended. However, the evidence for both these recommendations is minimal.

Pharmacologic Therapy

First-line therapeutic modalities for treating allergic rhinitis are directed at relief of symptoms (see Table 76-2). Antihistamines and decongestants (both oral and topical) generally are used first in treating allergic rhinitis with medications. Several options in these two categories are available without a prescription, but

TABLE 76-3 Environmental Controls to Prevent Allergic Rhinitis

Pollens
- Keep windows and doors closed during pollen season
- Avoid fans that draw in outside air
- Use air conditioning
- If possible, eliminate outside activities during times of high pollen counts
- Shower, shampoo, and change clothes following outdoor activity
- Use a vented dryer rather than an outside clothesline

Molds
- Use similar controls as above
- Avoid walking through uncut fields, working with compost or dry soil, and raking leaves
- Clean indoor moldy surfaces
- Fix all water leaks in home
- Reduce indoor humidity to <50% if possible

House dust mites
- Encase mattress, pillow, and box springs in an allergen-impermeable cover
- Wash bedding in hot water weekly
- Remove stuffed toys from bedroom
- Minimize carpet use and upholstered furniture
- Reduce indoor humidity to <50% if possible

Animal allergens (if removal of pet is not acceptable)
- Keep pet out of patient's bedroom
- Isolate pet from carpet and upholstered furniture
- Wash pet weekly

Cockroaches
- Keep food and garbage in tightly closed containers
- Take out garbage regularly
- Clean up dirty dishes promptly
- Use roach traps

Other recommendations
- Do not allow smoking around the patient, in the patient's house, or in the family car
- Minimize the use of wood-burning stoves and fireplaces

Adapted from reference 3.

TABLE 76-4 Relative Adverse-Effect Profiles of Antihistamines

Medication	Relative Sedative Effect	Relative Anticholinergic Effect
Alkylamine class, nonselective		
Brompheniramine maleate	Low	Moderate
Chlorpheniramine maleate	Low	Moderate
Dexchlorpheniramine maleate	Low	Moderate
Ethanolamine class, nonselective		
Carbinoxamine maleate	High	High
Clemastinefumarate	Moderate	High
Diphenhydramine hydrochloride	High	High
Ethylenediamine class, nonselective		
Pyrilamine maleate	Low	Low to none
Tripelennamine hydrochloride	Moderate	Low to none
Phenothiazine class, nonselective		
Promethazine hydrochloride	High	High
Piperidine class, nonselective		
Cyproheptadine hydrochloride	Low	Moderate
Phenindamine tartrate	Low to none	Moderate
Phthalazinone class, peripherally selective		
Azelastine (nasal only)	Low to none	Low to none
Bepotastine (ophthalmic only)	Low to none	Low to none
Piperazine class, peripherally selective		
Cetirizine	Low to moderate	Low to none
Levocetirizine	Low to moderate	Low to none
Piperidine class, peripherally selective		
Desloratadine	Low to none	Low to none
Fexofenadine	Low to none	Low to none
Loratadine	Low to none	Low to none
Olopatadine (nasal only)	Low to none	Low to none

patients will need sound advice to make appropriate choices. Knowledge of pathophysiology and the inflammatory state has led to prophylactic therapy for those with more severe disease using agents such as cromolyn and topical steroids. However, in attempting to assess the evidence supporting any particular therapy, clinicians have difficulty interpreting the medical literature for a variety of reasons, including lack of uniformity in the research methodologies, inappropriate drug controls, and failure to identify types of rhinitis in study subjects (perennial vs. seasonal and allergic vs. nonallergic).

Antihistamines

4 Histamine (H_1)-receptor antagonists are competitive antagonists to histamine. They bind to H_1 receptors without activating them, preventing histamine binding and action. Second-generation antihistamines may also affect components of the inflammatory response such as histamine release, generation of adhesion molecules, and influx of inflammatory cells. Although it was once thought that the older antihistamines had no antiinflammatory action, some were shown to have these effects as early as the 1950s.[20] Antihistamines are available in oral, ophthalmic, and intranasal dosage forms.

The oral antihistamines are the most commonly used and can be divided into two major categories: nonselective (first generation) and peripherally selective (second generation). Nonselective agents are commonly referred to as *sedating antihistamines*, and peripherally selective agents are referred to as *nonsedating antihistamines*. These generalizing terms can be misleading. Individual agents should be judged on their specific characteristics because variation within these broad categories exists. Also, the nonsedating claim is only valid when the agents are used at recommended doses.[21] This is of particular concern as some of these antihistamines are available without a prescription. The mechanism for sedation is not well understood, but its central effect depends on the drugs' ability to cross the blood–brain barrier. Most older antihistamines are lipid soluble and cross this barrier easily. The peripherally selective agents have little or no central or autonomic nervous system effects. Table 76-4 lists common antihistamines, their chemical classifications, their relative potential for causing sedation, and their relative anticholinergic effects.

Antihistamines are much more effective in preventing the actions of histamines and essentially do not reverse these actions once they have taken place. Reversal of symptoms is largely caused by the anticholinergic properties of these drugs. This activity is responsible for the drying effect of antihistamines, which reduces the problem of nasal, salivary, and lacrimal gland hypersecretion. Antihistamines antagonize increased capillary permeability, wheal-and-flare formation, and itching.

In general, the antihistamines are well absorbed, have large volumes of distribution, and are metabolized by the liver. Serum half-lives vary considerably between patients. In addition, the therapeutic effects of these agents are more prolonged than might be predicted by their half-lives.

Drowsiness is usually the chief complaint of patients who take antihistamines. It can interfere with a patient's ability to drive a car or operate machinery and may interfere with the patient's ability to function adequately at the workplace. Remember that these problems can also be a reflection of the disease itself. For this reason, many recommend the use of peripherally selective agents as first-line treatment for any patient who is at high risk for the development of adverse events. This includes patients with renal or hepatic impairment, those with small weights (for whom adult doses may provide larger-than-recommended doses on a milligram-per-kilogram basis), patients with preexisting CNS or cardiac disorders, patients who require higher doses, and patients who have shown a tendency to overuse nonprescription or prescription medications.[20]

The sedative effects of antihistamines can be useful for patients who suffer from sleeplessness caused by the symptoms of allergic rhinitis. In these patients, a bedtime dose may prove beneficial. However, they may cause residual daytime sedation, decreased alertness, and performance impairment.

The logic of preferentially using the second-generation agents is not clear-cut. A meta-analysis of performance-impairment trials did not show a clear and consistent distinction between diphenhydramine and the peripherally selective agents.[22] Another study showed that tolerance to sedation secondary to diphenhydramine developed by day 4 of treatment, becoming indistinguishable from placebo,[23] but sedation must be distinguished from impairment since the two are not equivalent. Despite this evidence, recent guidelines recommend the nonsedating agents.[18]

Anticholinergic (drying) effects contribute to the agents' therapeutic efficacy, but they also cause most adverse effects. Dry mouth, difficulty in voiding urine, constipation, and potential cardiovascular effects may be troublesome. Keep in mind that the differences may be small. Patients with a predisposition to urinary retention (e.g., older men and those on concurrent anticholinergic therapy) should use antihistamines with caution. Caution also should be used for patients with increased intraocular pressure, hyperthyroidism, and cardiovascular disease.

Other adverse effects of oral antihistamines include loss of appetite (and paradoxically, weight gain with increased appetite), nausea, vomiting, and epigastric distress.

Antihistamines are only fully effective when taken approximately 1 to 2 hours before anticipated exposure to the offending allergen. This must be discussed with patients who face exposure daily during a pollen season and with those who have indoor perennial allergens where daily scheduled use is necessary. If tolerance develops to the therapeutic effect, a change to an agent in a different chemical class is usually effective.

Patients should be counseled about the proper use of antihistamines. Adverse effects, especially drowsiness, should be emphasized. Patients should be warned against taking other CNS depressants, including the use of alcohol. Patients should be told not to take a double dose when a dose is missed. Taking the antihistamine with meals or at least a full glass of water will help prevent GI adverse effects such as nausea, vomiting, and epigastric distress. Patients should check with their healthcare professional and read labels before taking nonprescription medications. Many cold products and sleep aids contain antihistamines. Patients should be instructed not to use more than one antihistamine at a time. Table 76-5 lists the recommended dosages of the commonly used agents with their prescription status.

Many patients respond to and tolerate the older agents quite well. Because many of the older agents are available generically, they are much less expensive. Patient cost for many of the older nonprescription agents is less than \$5 for a 30-day supply, compared with more than \$20 for some of the nonprescription selective agents and more than \$70 dollars for the selective prescription-only products. Although cost is a concern, patient safety should be the first consideration.

The selective agents have moved ahead of the nonselective choices in a recent survey of pharmacist recommended

TABLE 76-5 Medication Dosing for Allergic Rhinitis

Drug	Brand Name	Dosage	Special Population Dose	Other
Antihistamines				
Oral				
Nonselective:				
Chlorpheniramine maleate	Various	Plain: 4 mg every 6 hours	Pediatrics: 6–12 years: 2 mg every 6 hours 2–5 years: 1 mg every 6 hours	OTC Available as liquid
		Sustained release: 8–12 mg at bedtime or 8–12 mg every 8 hours	6–12 years: 8 mg at bedtime <6 years: not recommended	OTC
Clemastinefumarate	Tavist	1.34 mg every 8 hours	Pediatrics: 6–12 years: 0.67 mg every 12 hours	OTC Available as liquid
Diphenhydramine hydrochloride	Benadryl and others	25–50 mg every 8 hours	Pediatrics: 5 mg/kg per day divided every 8 hours (up to 25 mg per dose)	OTC Available as liquid
Peripherally selective:				
Loratadine	Alavert Claritin	10 mg once daily	Pediatrics: 6–12 years: 10 mg once daily 2–5 years: 5 mg once daily	OTC Available as liquid
Fexofenadine	Allegra	60 mg twice daily or 180 mg once daily	Pediatrics: 2–11 years: 30 mg twice daily	OTC Available as liquid
Ceftirizine	Zyrtec	5–10 mg once daily	Pediatrics: 1–5 years: 2.5 mg daily may increase to twice daily 6–12 months: 2.5 mg once daily	OTC Available as liquid
Levocetirizine	Xyzal	5 mg at bedtime	Pediatrics: 6–11 years: 2.5 mg in the evening 6 months to 5 years: 1.25 mg in the evening	
Nasal				
Azelastine	Astelin Astepro	One to two sprays twice daily	Pediatrics: 5–11 years one spray twice daily (Astelin[R])	
Levocabastine	Livostin	Two sprays twice daily		
Olopantadine	Patanase	Two sprays twice daily	Pediatrics: 6–11 years: one spray twice daily	
Ophthalmic				
Levocabastine	Livostin eye drops	One drop twice daily		
Bepotastine	Bepreve	One drop twice daily		

(continued)

TABLE 76-5 Medication Dosing for Allergic Rhinitis (*Continued*)

Drug	Brand Name	Dosage	Special Population Dose	Other
Decongestants				
Oral				
Pseudoephedrine	Various	60 mg every 4–6 hours Sustained release: 120 mg every 12 hours Controlled release: 240 mg once daily (60 mg immediate release + 180 mg sustained release)	Pediatrics: 6–12 years: 30 mg every 4–6 hours 2–5 years: 15 mg every 4–6 hours	OTC Available as liquid
Phenylephrine	Various	10–20 mg every 4 hours	Pediatrics: 6–12 years: 5 mg every 4 hours 4–6 years: 2.5 mg every 4 hours	OTC Available as liquid
Nasal				
Oxymetazoline	Various	Two to three sprays twice daily		OTC
Phenylephrine	Various	Two to three sprays every 4 hours	Pediatrics: >12 years: use 0.25–0.5% two to three sprays every 4 hours 6–12 years: use 0.25% two to three sprays every 4 hours 2–6 years: use 0.125% one drop every 2–4 hours	OTC
Nasal steroids				
Beclomethasone	Beconase AQ Qnasl	One to two inhalations in each nostril twice daily (Beconase AQ) Two inhalations in each nostril once daily (Qnasl)	Pediatric: (Beconase AQ only) 6–11 years: one inhalation in each nostril twice daily (may increase to two inhalations)	
Budesonide	Rhinocort Aqua	One spray each nostril daily (up to maximum of four sprays each nostril daily)	Pediatrics: <12 years maximum dose two sprays in each nostril daily	
Flunisolide	Various	Two sprays each nostril twice daily	6–14 years: one spray in each nostril three times daily or two sprays in each nostril twice daily	
Fluticasone	Flonase Veramyst	Two sprays in each nostril once daily	Pediatrics: >4 years: one spray in each nostril daily (Flonase) 2–11 years: one spray in each nostril daily (Veramyst)	
Mometasone	Nasonex	Two sprays in each nostril daily	Pediatrics: 2–11 years: one spray in each nostril daily	
Triamcinolone	Nasacort	Two sprays in each nostril daily (reduce to one spray when symptoms controlled)	Pediatrics: 2–11 years: one spray in each nostril once daily	
Other nasal medications				
Cromolyn	Nasalcrom	One spray in each nostril three to four times a day	Pediatrics: >2 years, same as adult dose	OTC
Ipratropium	Atrovent	Two sprays in each nostril two to four times a day	Pediatrics: 5–11 years: two sprays in each nostril three times a day	
Montelukast	Singulair	Oral: 10 mg once daily	Pediatrics: 6–23 months: 4 mg (oral granules) once daily 2–5 years: 4 mg once daily (chewable or granules) 6–14 years: 5 mg once daily (chewable)	

over-the-counter antihistamines.[24] Among the 2 million antihistamine recommendations, the top three were loratadine (41%), cetirizine (33%), and fexofenadine (15%) followed by the nonselective agents diphenhydramine (9%) and chlorpheniramine (2%).

For seasonal and persistent allergic rhinitis, the intranasal antihistamine azelastine is available. The 0.1% product can be used in children for seasonal allergies, while the 0.15% product is labeled for adults only for either type of allergic rhinitis. Despite this labeling, recent guidelines favor the use of the intranasal route for seasonal but not persistent allergic rhinitis.[18] Azelastine has been used successfully for patients who did not respond to loratadine.[25] Using the nasal route offers an alternative to switching to another oral antihistamine. Patient satisfaction has been varied because while the product produces rapid symptom relief, patients complain of drying effects, headache, and diminished effectiveness over time. Patients should be warned of the medication's potential to produce drowsiness, as its systemic availability is approximately 40%.[26,27] Olopatadine, another intranasal antihistamine, may cause less drowsiness as it is a selective H_1-receptor antagonist.

Clinical **Controversy...**

Using intranasal antihistamine for seasonal allergic rhinitis is well accepted, but their role in treating persistent allergic rhinitis is not well defined.

Allergic conjunctivitis, often associated with allergic rhinitis, can be treated with ophthalmic antihistamines such as levocabastine or bepotastine. Because systemic antihistamines usually are also effective for allergic conjunctivitis, one of these ophthalmic agents is a logical addition to nasal steroids when ocular symptoms occur, and it is an acceptable approach for patients whose only symptoms involve the eyes or to add for those whose symptoms persist on oral treatment.

Decongestants

Topical and systemic decongestants are sympathomimetic agents that act on adrenergic receptors in the nasal mucosa, producing

TABLE 76-6 Duration of Action of Topical Decongestants

Medication	Duration (Hour)
Short acting	
Phenylephrine hydrochloride	Up to 4
Intermediate acting	
Naphazoline hydrochloride	4–6
Tetrahydrozoline hydrochloride	
Long acting	
Oxymetazoline hydrochloride	Up to 12
Xylometazoline hydrochloride	

vasoconstriction. Decongestants shrink swollen mucosa and improve ventilation. When nasal congestion occurs with allergic rhinitis, decongestants work well in combination with antihistamines.

Topical Decongestants

Topical decongestants are applied directly to swollen nasal mucosa via drops or sprays. Table 76-6 lists the common topical decongestants and their durations of action. The use of these agents results in little or no systemic absorption.

Because these agents are extremely effective and are available to patients without a prescription, they are widely used. However, prolonged use of these agents (for more than 3 to 5 days) can result in a condition known as *rhinitis medicamentosa*, or *rebound vasodilation*, with even more severe congestion. Patients who develop this condition use increasingly more spray more often with less response. Although the methods used to treat this "addiction" have not been studied formally, several are used commonly. Abrupt cessation works, but it is difficult because of rebound congestion that may leave the patient congested for several days or weeks. Sleeping may become difficult. Nasal steroids have been used successfully, but they take several days to work. Weaning the patient off topical decongestants can be accomplished by decreasing the dosing frequency or the concentration over several weeks. Combining the weaning process with nasal steroids may prove useful. Ultimately, the success of any plan depends on the patient's resolve and clear understanding of the importance of stopping the drug to end the problem.

Other adverse effects of topical decongestants include burning, stinging, sneezing, and dryness of the nasal mucosa.

Patients should be counseled on the use of topical decongestants to prevent rhinitis medicamentosa. Patients should be instructed to use as small a dose as possible as infrequently as possible and only when absolutely necessary (e.g., at bedtime to aid in falling asleep). Duration of therapy always should be limited to 5 days or less.

Systemic Decongestants

Oral decongestants are not as effective on an immediate basis as the topical agents, but their effects sometimes last longer and they cause less local irritation. In addition, rhinitis medicamentosa is not a problem with oral agents. The most commonly used agent is pseudoephedrine. Table 76-5 lists the usual doses for the regular and sustained-release versions. The use of phenylephrine is increasing because of regulations related to pseudoephedrine described below.

Concerns of safety have greatly limited the systemic decongestant options. Legal requirements for the sale of pseudoephedrine were put into place to combat the misuse of the drug as a component in making methamphetamine. Pseudoephedrine must now be sold behind the counter, and the monthly amount a patient can purchase is limited. Until this requirement, pseudoephedrine was the most frequently used systemic decongestant, and it was considered the safest. Doses of 180 mg have been shown to produce no measurable change in blood pressure or heart rate.[28] In higher doses (210 to 240 mg), pseudoephedrine has raised both blood pressure and heart rate.[29] Pseudoephedrine can cause mild CNS stimulation, even at therapeutic doses. Stroke, related to use of oral decongestants such as pseudoephedrine, can occur in patients with hypertension and/or vasospasm.[30] Although stroke complications seem to be associated with higher-than-recommended doses, there is also a stroke risk when these agents are taken properly. Severe hypertensive reactions can occur when pseudoephedrine is given concomitantly with monoamine oxidase inhibitors. Hypertensive patients should, unless necessary, avoid systemic decongestants.

Combination Products

Numerous products combine an antihistamine with a decongestant. While the combination may be rational because of the different mechanisms of action, remember that antihistamines must be taken on a regular schedule, but decongestants should only be used when needed. Both nonselective and peripherally selective antihistamines are available in such combinations. As mentioned previously, patients should read labels to avoid therapeutic duplication. Consideration should be given to how often and how severely the patient is congested before recommending these combinations. Only a short course of a combination product should be used.

Nasal Steroids

5 Nasal steroids are an excellent choice for treating perennial rhinitis, and can be useful in seasonal rhinitis, especially if begun in advance of symptoms. Nasal steroids appear to be effective with minimal adverse effects. Some believe that nasal steroids should be recommended as initial therapy over antihistamines because of their high level of efficacy when used properly and along with avoidance of allergens.[18] Multiple mechanisms are involved with the effects of nasal steroids on the nasal mucosa: reducing inflammation by reducing mediator release, suppressing neutrophil chemotaxis, reducing intracellular edema, causing mild vasoconstriction, and inhibiting mast cell-mediated late-phase reactions. Table 76-5 lists the available nasal steroids and their usual doses.

Topical steroids produce only minor adverse effects, most commonly sneezing, stinging, headache, and epistaxis. Despite concerns about safety of systemic steroids, nasal steroids have been found to have no significant association with hypothalamic–pituitary axis suppression, cataract formation, glaucoma, or bone mineral density changes in the doses used for allergic rhinitis. Growth suppression remains a question with some evidence showing that nasal steroids with higher bioavailability (e.g., beclomethasone) may have a greater growth-suppression effect than less bioavailable agents.[31] These findings require more study. Most likely, all currently available nasal steroids are safe in the majority of patients, and their clinical benefits outweigh any small growth suppressive effect. Other concerns include local infections with *Candida albicans*, which occur rarely.

The therapeutic benefits of topical steroids are not immediate, and they are not decongestants. Patients need to understand this to ensure cooperation and continuation of therapy. Some patients notice improvement in a few days, but peak responses may not be observed for 2 to 3 weeks. Once a response is achieved, the dosage may be reduced. Blocked nasal passages should be cleared with a decongestant or saline irrigation before administration to ensure adequate penetration of the spray. Patients should be advised to avoid sneezing or blowing their noses for at least 10 minutes after administration. Topical steroids should not be used for patients with nasal septum ulcers or recent nasal surgery or trauma.

One additional benefit of nasal steroids in treating allergic rhinitis in individuals with asthma and upper airway conditions is that they may confer some protection against exacerbations of asthma, leading to fewer emergency room visits. The overall relative risk for an emergency visit among asthma patients who received intranasal steroids was 0.7.[32] No effect was seen for patients receiving antihistamines.

Clinical **Controversy. . .**

A recently approved combination of an intranasal steroid with an intranasal antihistamine in fixed doses may provide benefit, but the target patient population has not been well defined.

Other Inhalant Medications

Cromolyn sodium and ipratropium bromide offer two additional approaches for treating allergic rhinitis. Cromolyn sodium is a mast cell stabilizer. Increased interest in this product has resulted from it becoming available without a prescription. Ipratropium bromide is an anticholinergic agent useful in perennial allergic rhinitis.

Cromolyn sodium nasal spray is used for the symptomatic prevention and treatment of allergic rhinitis. It curtails antigen-triggered mast cell degranulation and release of the mediators of allergic reactions, including histamine. Cromolyn sodium has no direct antihistaminic, anticholinergic, or antiinflammatory properties. Similarly to topical steroids, the most common adverse effects—sneezing and nasal stinging—result from local irritation. Dosing information is given in Table 76-5. Cromolyn sodium must cover the entire nasal lining; therefore, patients should be instructed to clear nasal passages before administration. Inhaling gently through the nose during administration aids in this process. Dosing must be repeated at 6-hour intervals to maintain the effect.

For seasonal rhinitis, treatment with cromolyn sodium should be initiated just before the usual start of the offending allergen's season and continued throughout the season. In perennial rhinitis, the effects may not be seen for 2 to 4 weeks; therefore, antihistamines or decongestants may be needed during this initial phase of therapy. As cromolyn sodium begins to work, the need for these medications should decrease.

Ipratropium nasal spray is an anticholinergic agent that exhibits antisecretory properties when applied locally. It provides symptomatic relief of rhinorrhea associated with allergic and other forms of chronic rhinitis. Dosing information is given in Table 76-5. The optimal dose should be determined based on the specific patient's symptoms and response. Adverse effects are mild, with the most common being headache, nosebleeds, and nasal dryness.

Immunotherapy

❻ Experience with immunotherapy has reached the one-century mark, as the first report of the successful use of grass pollen extract injections to treat allergic rhinitis was published in 1911.[33] The therapy was first called *desensitization*; however, this did not seem appropriate because skin reactivity sometimes remained. The name was later changed to *hyposensitization*. Although this term is still used today, *immunotherapy* is used more commonly and is less confusing.

Immunotherapy is the slow, gradual process of injecting increasing doses of antigens responsible for eliciting allergic symptoms into a patient with the hope of inducing tolerance to the allergen when natural exposure occurs. Several mechanisms have been proposed to explain the beneficial effects of immunotherapy, including induction of IgG-blocking antibodies, reduction in specific IgE (long-term), reduced recruitment of effector cells, altered T-cell cytokine balance (a shift from T-helper type 1 to T-helper type 2), T-cell anergy, and alteration of regulatory T-cell actvitiy.[34]

Immunotherapy is moderately expensive, has significant potential risks, and requires a major time commitment from the patient. However, the cost of immunotherapy is usually covered by insurance, including Medicaid. Long-term savings can be realized since decades of treatment with medication can be averted through successful immunotherapy. Candidates for immunotherapy should have significant symptoms unsuccessfully controlled by avoidance and pharmacotherapy or should stand to benefit in other significant ways, such as with asthma. Immunotherapy may postpone the onset of asthma or possibly even prevent it.[35] Patients who are unable to tolerate the adverse effects of properly managed drug therapy also should be considered. Patients must be committed to the necessary regular office visits required to complete this course of therapy over several years.

The effectiveness of immunotherapy for seasonal allergic rhinitis appears to be better than that seen with perennial rhinitis, in part because it is more difficult to determine which allergen is responsible for perennial symptoms, and it is more often due to multiple sensitizations. Effectiveness has been shown in a number of clinical studies using a variety of pollen extracts, even for patients with severe disease resistant to pharmacotherapy.[35] Specific immunotherapy for house dust mites has had good results in appropriately selected patients, but more study is needed. Data indicate that for some patients 3 years of immunotherapy may be sufficient to give lasting benefit[36]; however, many require longer treatment. Sublingual and local nasal specific immunotherapy may offer acceptable alternatives to the traditional subcutaneous route in some patients.[18]

The selection of antigens should be based on patient history and skin test results. Numerous regimens for administration of selected allergens have been suggested. In the beginning, very dilute solutions are given initially one to two times per week. The concentration is increased until the maximum tolerated or highest planned or effective dose is achieved. This maintenance dose is continued in slowly increasing intervals over several years, depending on clinical response. In light of the present understanding of the immunologic results of immunotherapy, it should be given year-round rather than seasonally.

Adverse reactions can occur with immunotherapy and range from mild to life threatening. Among the most common are mild local reactions, consisting of induration and swelling at the site of the injection. These may be immediate or delayed. Other more serious reactions (e.g., generalized urticaria, bronchospasm, laryngospasm, and vascular collapse) occur rarely; deaths can result from anaphylactic reactions. Severe reactions are treated with epinephrine as well as other modalities recommended for anaphylaxis. Because of this potential risk, immunotherapy must not be given without adequate direct observation in a medical facility.

Several patient types are poor candidates for immunotherapy, including patients with any medical condition that would compromise the ability to tolerate an anaphylactic-type reaction, patients with impaired immune systems, and patients with a history of nonadherence to therapy.

Leukotriene Receptor Antagonists

Leukotriene receptor antagonists inhibit the cysteinyl leukotriene receptor. The cysteinyl leukotrienes are one type of inflammatory mediators released from mast cells in allergy. Montelukast is approved for the treatment of perennial allergic rhinitis in children as young as 6 months and for seasonal allergic rhinitis in children as young as 2 years. Montelukast is considered a third choice behind antihistamines and nasal steroids.[18]

Studies published to date show leukotriene receptor antagonists to be no more effective than peripherally selective antihistamines and less effective than intranasal steroids. However, when combined with antihistamines, they are more effective than the antihistamine alone.[37] In children with mild persistent asthma and coexisting allergic rhinitis, montelukast as monotherapy has been recommended.[38] Table 76-5 lists dosage regimens.

Alternative Treatment Options

The development of a monoclonal antibody directed against the binding site of IgE provides an additional way to treat allergic respiratory diseases. Omalizumab, a recombinant humanized anti-IgE monoclonal antibody, was the first to show efficacy in allergic rhinitis.[39] The actual mechanism of how this agent is thought to work is quite complex.[40] Anti-IgE antibodies bind to the site on the IgE molecule that recognizes the IgE receptor, thereby preventing the IgE molecule from binding to mast cells or basophils. The half-life of IgE antibodies on the mast cell surface is about 6 weeks, and as the antibodies are freed, they become available for binding to anti-IgE antibodies. By giving repeated doses of omalizumab, the number of IgE antibodies on the mast cell surface can be reduced significantly over time. The drug-bound IgE molecules are not eliminated but remain in circulation as small immune complexes. IgE receptor numbers on basophils and mast cells are decreased as a result of downregulation. Omalizumab's role should be limited to patients with allergic rhinitis and asthma with a clear IgE-dependent allergic component uncontrolled despite optimal pharmacologic treatment and allergen avoidance.[18]

A few other alternative options have been suggested for treatment of allergic rhinitis. As mentioned earlier in this chapter, microbial exposure in the early years of life could help prevent allergic disease by favoring a nonatopic immune response.[4] However, the use of probiotics may be limited to treatment or prevention of childhood eczema as available evidence shows little benefit in allergic airway diseases.[41] Butterbur, with the active ingredient petasin that exhibits antileukotriene and antihistamine activity, has shown some success but is not recommended for most patients.[18,42] Other treatments that have been tried but are not recommended are homeopathy, acupuncture, and phototherapy.[18]

PERSONALIZED PHARMACOTHERAPY

The two primary pharmacotherapy options for the treatment of allergic rhinitis in adults and children are antihistamines and intranasal steroids. Patient preference should play a role when selecting between these two options. While limited evidence supports intranasal steroids over antihistamines, some patients may prefer simple oral therapy. Either choice requires clear patient counseling to ensure appropriate timing of therapy and expectations of effect.

For patients (both adults and children) who are not immunocompromised, have a high likelihood for adherence, and have adequate insurance and/or financial resources, subcutaneous specific immunotherapy is an excellent choice for treatment of seasonal allergic rhinitis and allergic rhinitis secondary to house dust mites. In some children, immunotherapy may prevent development of asthma.

For patients experiencing an exacerbation of nasal congestion as part of their allergic rhinitis picture, decongestants can be used short term.

Leukotriene receptor antagonists are an appropriate option in adults and children with seasonal allergic rhinitis and in preschool children with persistent allergic rhinitis. Other uses are not indicated due to limited efficacy and high cost.

Cromolyn is another alternative that is effective, but many patients may find its frequent daily dosing (up to six times daily) difficult. As previously mentioned, omalizumab's role should be limited to patients with allergic rhinitis and asthma with a clear IgE-dependent allergic component uncontrolled despite optimal pharmacologic treatment and allergen avoidance.

A drug monitoring summary is shown in Table 76-7. Intranasal and ophthalmic antihistamines may be helpful for specific symptoms

TABLE 76-7 Drug Monitoring

Drug	Adverse Reaction	Monitoring Parameter	Comments
Antihistamines	Drowsiness	Caution patient about the potential for drowsiness, even with nonsedating and intranasal products	Do not mix with alcohol or other CNS depressants
	GI effects	Counsel patient to take with a meal or full glass of water	
	Anticholinergic effects	Watch for dry mouth and difficulty with urination. Caution patient about other medications with anticholinergic effects	Switching to an antihistamine with less anticholinergic effects may be necessary
Decongestants			
Topical	Rebound vasodilation	Watch for decreased response to topical agent	Over prolonged use (>3–5 days)
	Local irritation	Watching for burning, stinging, sneezing, and dryness of mucosa	Self-limiting due to short-term use. May try nasal saline for dryness.
Systemic	Hypertension	If used in a patient with hypertension, monitor blood pressure regularly and discontinue if the pressure increases	Usually not an issue for patients without preexisting hypertension. Use lowest effective dose
	CNS stimulation	Usually mild but discuss with patient	Use lowest effective dose
Nasal steroids	Local effects such as sneezing, stinging, and epistaxis	These effects may vary among products	
Other intranasal agents			
Cromolyn	Local effects such as sneezing, burning, or coughing	Usually mild but tell patient to report bothersome symptoms	If patient cannot tolerate local reactions, choose an alternative agent
Ipratropium	Headache, nosebleeds, and nasal dryness	Usually mild, tell patient to report bothersome symptoms	If patient cannot tolerate local reactions, choose an alternative agent
Montelukast	Behavioral changes	Monitor for mood and behavioral changes including suicidal ideation	Rare but should be monitored
Immunotherapy	Local reactions	Watch for induration or swelling at site of infection	Rare, but should only be given under direct medical supervision with epinephrine available
	Allergic reactions	Monitor for signs of anaphylaxis	

not relieved by first-line choices. An intranasal anticholinergic such as ipratropium is specifically useful for rhinorrhea.

More supportive evidence is needed to determine which patients, if any, would benefit from the other alternative options mentioned earlier.

EVALUATION OF THERAPEUTIC OUTCOMES

With allergic rhinitis, major outcomes include the effect of the disease on a patient's life, the efficacy and tolerability of treatment, and patient satisfaction. Consideration must be given to how the condition is affecting the patient's job or school performance, family and social interactions, and other aspects of quality of life. Drug therapy should prevent or minimize symptoms with few adverse effects. The patient should not have difficulty obtaining needed medication for financial or other reasons. Patients should be questioned about their satisfaction with the management of their allergic rhinitis. The management should result in minimal disruption to their lives.

Methods for assessing patient-reported outcomes and health-related quality of life in clinical trials related to allergy have been recommended.[43] These tools go beyond measuring improvement in symptoms and include such items as sleep quality, nonallergic symptoms (e.g., fatigue, poor concentration, and others), emotions, and participation in a variety of activities. How well each of the current treatment modalities performs and how they compare in improving patient outcomes remain to be determined.

Clinicians caring for allergic rhinitis patients should develop a comprehensive pharmaceutical care plan that addresses several areas. Discuss and agree on therapeutic end points for allergic rhinitis, including the patient's acceptable level of symptom relief, onset of symptom relief expectations, and seasonal starts and stops. Discuss adverse drug reaction self-monitoring and prevention based on treatment selection. Assess patient attitude toward adherence to and persistence with oral, ocular, intranasal, or immunologic therapies. Ensure proper matching of treatment to symptoms and intervene with the prescriber if necessary. Conduct seasonal or annual review with patient.

The therapeutic goal for all patients with allergic rhinitis is to minimize or prevent symptoms. Evaluation of success is accomplished primarily through the discussions with the patient, in whom both relief of symptoms and tolerance of drug therapy must be discussed.

CONCLUSIONS

Allergic rhinitis is a common disease with symptoms ranging from mild to severe. If avoidance measures are unsuccessful, allergic rhinitis should be treated to improve quality of life and prevent long-term complications. Timing of treating is essential. Treatment regimens should be individualized based on patient symptoms and response. Care should be taken to correctly identify allergy as the cause of the patient's rhinitis before committing them to chromic treatment.

ABBREVIATION

IgE immunoglobulin E

REFERENCES

1. Greiner AN, Hellings PW, Rotiroti G, Scadding GK. Allergic rhinitis. Lancet 2011;378:2112–2122.
2. Benninger M, Farrar JR, Blaiss M, et al. Evaluating approved medications to treat allergic rhinitis in the United States: An evidenced-based review of efficacy for nasal symptoms by class. Ann Allergy Asthma Immunol 2010;104:13–29.
3. Bousquet J, Khaltaev N, Cruz AA, et al. Allergic rhinitis and its impact on asthma (ARIA) 2008. Allergy 2008; 63(Suppl 86):8–160.
4. von Mutius E, Radon K. Living on a farm: Impact on asthma induction and clinical course. Immunol Allergy Clin North Am 2008;28:631–647.
5. Wallace DV, Dykewicz MS, Bernstein DI, et al. The diagnosis and management of rhinitis: An updated practice parameter. J Allergy Clin Immunol 2008;122:S1–S83.
6. Wilson SJ, Shute JK, Holgate ST, et al. Localization of interleukin (IL)-4 but not 5 to human mast cell secretory granules by immunoelectron microscopy. Clin Exp Allergy 2000;30:493–500.
7. Riccio AAM, Tosco MA, Cosentino C, et al. Cytokine pattern in allergic and nonallergic chronic rhinosinusitis in asthmatic children. Clin Exp Allergy 2002;32:422–426.
8. Wood-Baker R, Lau L, Howarth PH. Histamine and the nasal vasculature: The influence of H1 and H2-histamine receptor antagonism. Clin Otolaryngol 1996;21:348–352.
9. Howarth PH. Mediators of nasal blockage in allergic rhinitis. Allergy 1997;52(40 Suppl):12–18.
10. Howarth PH. Leukotrienes in rhinitis. Am J Respir Crit Care Med 2000;161:S133–S136.
11. Clark RR, Baroody FM. What drives the symptoms of allergic rhinitis? J Respir Dis 1998;19:S6–S15.
12. Gerth van Wijk R. Perennial allergic rhinitis and nasal hyperreactivity. Am J Rhinol 1998;12:33–35.
13. Klaewsongkram J, Ruxrungtham K, Wannakrairot P, et al. Eosinophil count in nasal mucosa is more suitable than the number of ICAM-1-positive nasal epithelial cells to evaluate the severity of house dust mite-sensitive allergic rhinitis: A clinical correlation study. Int Arch Allergy Immunol 2003;132:68–75.
14. Braunstahl GJ, Fokkens WJ, Overbeek SE, et al. Mucosal and systemic inflammatory changes in allergic rhinitis and asthma: A comparison between upper and lower airways. Clin Exp Allergy 2003;33:579–587.
15. Hill SL, Krouse JH. The effects of montelukast on intradermal wheal and flare. Otolarygol Head Neck Surg 2003;129:199–203.
16. Scadding G. Optimal management of nasal congestion caused my allergic rhinitis in children. Pediatr Drugs 2008;10(3):151–162.
17. Bousquet J, Schunemann HJ, Zuberbier T, et al. Development and implementation of guidelines in allergic rhinitis—An ARIA-GA²LEN paper. Allergy 2012;65: 1212–1221.
18. Brozek JL, Bousquet J, Baena-Cagnani CE, et al. Allergic rhinitis and its impact on asthma (ARIA) guidelines: 2010 revision. J Allergy Clin Immunol 2010;126:466–476.
19. Franchi M, Carrier P, Kotzias D, et al. Working toward healthy air in dwellings in Europe. Allergy 2006;61: 864–868.
20. Casale TB, Blaiss MS, Gelfand E, et al. First do no harm: Managing antihistamine impairment in patients with allergic rhinitis. J Allergy Clin Immunol 2003;111:S835–S842.
21. Sansgiry SS, Shringarpure GS. Springtime confusion: Are consumers getting the right information on how to treat seasonal allergies? J Allergy Clin Immunol 2003;112: 627–628.
22. Bender BG, Berning S, Dudden R, et al. Sedation and performance impairment of diphenhydramine and second-generation antihistamines: A meta-analysis. J Allergy Clin Immunol 2003;111:770–776.

23. Richardson GS, Roehrs TA, Rosenthal L, et al. Tolerance to daytime sedative effects of H1 antihistamines. J Clin Psychopharmacol 2002;22:511–515.
24. Pharmacy Times OTC Guide 2012. *http://www.otcguide.net/conditions/cough-cold-allergy*.
25. Berger WE, White MV. Efficacy of azelastine nasal spray in patients with an unsatisfactory response to loratadine. Ann Allergy Asthma Immunol 2003;91:205–211.
26. Astelin. Product Information. Somerset, NJ: Meda Pharmaceuticals, 2011.
27. Astepro. Product Information. Somerset, NJ: Meda Pharmaceuticals, 2010.
28. Empey DE, Young GA, Letley E, et al. Dose response study of the nasal decongestant and cardiovascular effects of pseudoephedrine. Br J Clin Pharmacol 1980;9:351–358.
29. Drew CDM, Knight GT, Hughes DTD, et al. Comparison of the effects of D-(−)-ephedrine and L-(+)-pseudoephedrine on the cardiovascular and respiratory systems in man. Br J Clin Pharmacol 1978;6:221–225.
30. Cantu C, Arauz A, Murilla-Bonilla LM, et al. Stroke associated with sympathomimetics contained in over-the-counter cough and cold drugs. Stroke 2003;34:1667–1673.
31. Mehle ME. Are nasal steroids safe? Curr Opin Otolaryngol Head Neck Surg 2003;11:201–205.
32. Adams RJ, Fuhlbrigge AL, Finkelstein JA, Weiss ST. Intranasal steroids and the risk of emergency department visits for asthma. J Allergy Clin Immunol 2002;109: 636–642.
33. Noon L. Prophylactic inoculation against hay fever. Lancet 1911;1:1572–1573.
34. Valenta R, Campana R, Marth K, van Hage M. Allergen-specific immunotherapy: From vaccines to prophylactic approaches. J Intern Med 2012;272:144–157.
35. Incorvaia C, Frati F. One century of allergen-specific immunotherapy for respiratory allergy. Immunotherapy 2011;3(5):629–635.
36. Durham SR, Walker SM, Varga EM, et al. Long-term clinical efficacy of grass pollen immunotherapy. N Engl J Med 1999;341:468–475.
37. Rodrigo GT, Yanez A. The role of antileukotriene therapy in seasonal allergic rhinitis: A systematic review randomized trials. Ann Allergy Asthma Immunol 2006;96:779–786.
38. Polos PG. Montelukast is an effective monotherapy for mild asthma and for asthma with co-morbid allergic rhinitis. Prim Care Respir J 2006;15:310–311.
39. Casale TB, Condemi J, LaForce C, et al. Effect of omalizumab on symptoms of seasonal allergic rhinitis. JAMA 2001;286:2956–2967.
40. Frew AJ. Anti-IgE and asthma. Ann Allergy Asthma Immunol 2003;91:117–118.
41. Boyle RJ, Tang ML. The role of probiotics in the management of allergic disease. Clin Exp Allergy 2006;36:568–576.
42. Gray RD, Haggart K, Lee DK, et al. Effects of butterbur treatment in intermittent allergic rhinitis: A placebo-controlled evaluation. Ann Allergy Asthma Immunol 2004;93(1):56–60.
43. Baiardini I, Bousquet PJ, Brzoza Z, et al. Recommendations for assessing patient reported outcomes and health-related quality of life in clinical trials on allergy: A GA^{2}LEN taskforce position paper. Allergy 2010;65:290–295.

Acne Vulgaris

77

Debra Sibbald

KEY CONCEPTS

1. Acne is a highly prevalent disorder affecting many adolescents and adults.
2. It is an extremely complex disease with an etiology originating from multiple causative and contributory factors.
3. Elements of pathogenesis involve defects in epidermal keratinization, androgen secretion, sebaceous function, bacterial growth, inflammation, and immunity.
4. Acne vulgaris cannot be "cured." Goals of treatment of this chronic disorder include control and alleviation of symptoms by reducing the number and severity of lesions, slowing progression, and limiting disease duration and recurrence. Key elements for patient adherence to therapy include prevention of long-term disfigurement associated with scarring and hyperpigmentation and avoidance of psychologic suffering.
5. The most critical target for treatment is the microcomedone, as the entire pathogenic cascade of acne is arrested if follicular occlusion is minimized or reversed. This involves a combination of treatment measures, integrating pharmacologic protocols targeting all four mechanisms involved in acne pathogenesis: increased follicular keratinization, increased sebum production, bacterial lipolysis of sebum triglycerides to free fatty acids, and inflammation.
6. Nondrug measures are aimed at both long-term prevention and treatment. Patients should eliminate aggravating factors, maintain a balanced, low-glycemic load diet, and control stress. They should wash twice daily with a mild soap or soapless cleanser, and restrict cosmetic use to oil-free products. Comedone extraction results in immediate cosmetic improvement in approximately 10% of patients. Shaving should be done as lightly and infrequently as possible, using a sharp blade or electric razor.
7. First-, second-, and third-line therapies should be selected and altered as appropriate for the severity and staging of the clinical presentation.
8. Treatment is directed at controlling the disorder, not curing it. Regimens should be tapered over time, adjusting to response. The smallest number of agents should be used at the lowest possible dosages to ensure efficacy, safety, avoidance of resistance, and patient adherence.
9. Once control is achieved, simplify the regimen but continue with some suppressive therapy. It takes 8 weeks for a microcomedone to mature; thus, any therapy must be continued beyond this duration to assess efficacy in terms of comedonal and inflammatory lesion count, control or progression of severity, and management of associated anxiety or depression. Safety end points include monitoring for adverse effects of treatment.
10. Through empathic and informative counseling, the health professional can motivate the patient to continue long-term therapy.

In this chapter, I review the latest developments in understanding acne vulgaris and its treatment. The contents provide an analysis of the physiology of the pilosebaceous unit; the epidemiology, etiology and pathophysiology of acne; relevant treatment with nondrug measures; and comparisons of pharmacologic agents, including drugs of choice recommended in best-practice guidelines. Options include a variety of alternatives such as retinoids, antimicrobial agents, hormones, and light therapy. Formulation principles are discussed in relation to drug delivery. Patient assessment, general approaches to individualized therapy plans, and monitoring evaluation strategies are presented.

EPIDEMIOLOGY

1 Acne vulgaris is a chronic disease and the most common one treated by dermatologists. The lifetime prevalence of acne approaches 90%, with the highest incidence in adolescents. Prevalence data available from the European Union, United States, Australia, and New Zealand show that acne affects 80% of individuals between puberty and 30 years of age, depending on the method of lesion counting.[1] Other studies have reported acne in 28% to 61% of school children aged 10 to 12 years; 79% to 95% of those 16 to 18 years of age; and even in children aged 4 to 7 years. If mild manifestations were excluded and only moderate or severe manifestations were considered, the frequency in epidemiological studies in Western industrialized countries was still 20% to 35%.[2–4]

The onset of acne vulgaris during puberty occurs at a younger chronologic age in girls than boys. It is triggered in children by the initiation of androgen production by the adrenal glands and gonads, and it usually subsides after the end of growth. However, to some degree, most patients continue to have symptoms into their mid-20s, and there is evidence that the duration of acne may last into middle age for most women, recorded in 54% of women and 40% of men older than 25 years of age.[5] In puberty, acne is often more severe in boys in about 15% of cases, which is tenfold greater than in girls. Women often have more severe forms during adulthood. When untreated, acne usually lasts for several years until it spontaneously remits. After the disease has ended, scars and dyspigmentation are not uncommon permanent negative outcomes.

Genetic factors have been recognized; there is a high concordance among identical twins, and there is also a tendency toward severe acne in patients with a positive family history of acne.

There are believed to be no gender differences in acne prevalence, although such differences are often reported and may represent social biases. In urban clinics, there is a clear preponderance of girls seeking treatment. There is also a perception that acne is less prevalent in rural populations. This is supported by the data from Varanasi where 21.35% of boys (13 to 18 years) from rural areas had acne versus 37.5% of those from the urban areas.[6]

An international group of epidemiologists, community medicine specialists, and anthropologists have questioned whether acne might be predominantly a disease of Western civilization.[7] They assert that since acne vulgaris is nearly universal in westernized societies (afflicting 79% to 95% of the adolescent population), one causative factor might be the Western glycemic diet. While this hypothesis is based on the observation that primitive societies subsisting on traditional (low glycemic) diets have no acne, the theory awaits validation and acceptance by the dermatologic community.

ETIOLOGY

2 Acne is a multifactorial disease. Genetic, racial, hormonal, dietary, and environmental factors have been implicated in its development. Its psychologic impact can be severe.

Four major etiologic factors are involved in the development of acne: increased sebum production, due to hormonal influences; alteration in the keratinization process and hyperproliferation of ductal epidermis; bacterial colonization of the duct with *Propionibacterium acnes*; and production of inflammation with release of inflammatory mediators in acne sites. These are reviewed in the Pathophysiology section later in this chapter.

The role of heredity in acne has not been clearly defined; however, there is a significant tendency toward more serious involvement if one or both parents had severe acne during their youth.

Environmental factors play a major role in determining the severity and extent of acne and may influence the choice of topical treatments. Heat and humidity may induce comedones; pressure or friction caused by protective devices such as helmets, shoulder pads, or pillows, and excessive scrubbing or washing can exacerbate existing acne by causing microcomedones to rupture. Pressure may cause acne lesions to form in patients who do not have acne vulgaris: this variant is called *mechanical acne*. Hair styles that are low on the forehead or neck may cause excessive sweating and occlusion, exacerbating acne. In most cases acne is worse in winter and improves during the summer, suggesting a salutary effect of sunlight. However, in some cases exposure to sunlight worsens the disease.[8]

The importance of psychologic factors in this prolonged and capricious condition has been repeatedly stressed. Emotions such as intense anger and stress can exacerbate acne, causing flares or increasing mechanical manipulation. This is probably the result of increased glucocorticoid secretion by the adrenal glands, which appears to potentiate the effects of androgens.[9]

Dietary influences are the focus of current investigations. In the past, acne was not felt to be influenced by diet, but patients could restrict certain foods they perceived exacerbate acne (chocolate, cola drinks, milk and milk products).[10,11] These recommendations, which still persist in some guidelines, are based on one or two poorly designed studies conducted more than 40 years ago. They have largely been discounted by well-designed current studies. A discussion of the issues surrounding dietary influences is elaborated in the Clinical Controversy on Diet box.

Clinical **Controversy...**

Diet and Acne

The role of dietary influences in acne continues to be disputed in the literature with increasing attention and vigor. Evidentiary studies are currently in progress to elaborate associations between various dietary influences and presentation of acne, following the dismissal of overinterpreted 40-year-old, poorly designed studies that disavowed potential effects of dietary ingestions on acne.[131,132] Researchers are examining nutritional factors both as factors in acne development as well as potential treatment modalities.

Beginning in 2005, a series of studies have linked consumption of dairy products with acne, perhaps due to natural hormonal components and/or other bioactive molecules in milk.[133,134] Acne has been positively associated with the reported quantity of milk ingested, particularly skim milk.[135] Other studies suggest that insulin-like growth factor (IGF), increased by ingestion of high glycemic loads, may play a role in acne.[136,137] Lactoferrin-enriched fermented milk ameliorates acne vulgaris with a selective decrease of tricyloglycerols in skin surface lipids.[138] Lactoferrin is a whey milk protein that has a prominent activity against inflammation. When administered as a dietary supplement on a twice-daily regimen in mild-to-moderate acne vulgaris, it may lead to an overall improvement in acne lesion counts in the majority of affected adolescents and young adults.[139]

The strongest evidence points to a high glycemic load (HGL) diet as a significant factor in acne. In a well-designed randomized controlled trial, a significant reduction in acne was seen in patients who eliminated high glycemic index foods. Patients who consumed a low-glycemic-load diet, compared with a conventional HGL diet, had improvements of facial acne after 12 weeks. Accompanying changes in physical and endocrinologic parameters suggest that decreases in total energy intake, body weight, and indices of androgenicity and insulin resistance may also be associated with observed improvements in acne.[140] Other studies showed correlations between increases in the ratio of saturated to monounsaturated fatty acids and acne lesion counts and increased sebum outflow. This suggests a possible role of desaturase enzymes in sebaceous lipogenesis and the clinical manifestation of acne; these require further investigation.[141] Another study reported an improvement in acne and insulin sensitivity in low-glycemic-load diets compared with controls, suggesting nutrition-related lifestyle factors play a role in the etiology of acne. Independent effects of weight loss versus dietary intervention need to be isolated.[142] In an Australian study, no cases of acne were reported in participants who consumed low glycemic load diets.[135]

A systematic review of dietary influences on acne suggest that a possible role of dietary factors cannot be dismissed, as studies to date have not been sufficiently large or robust. While still controversial, diet is thought to play a role in the development or progression of acne vulgaris and further studies are ongoing. Investigations reviewing antioxidants from nutritional and topical sources and probiotics, as potential acne-fighting agents are now proceeding in early stages.[135]

PATHOPHYSIOLOGY

3 The pathogenesis of acne progresses through the following four major stages:

1. Increased follicular keratinization
2. Increased sebum production
3. Bacterial lipolysis of sebum triglycerides to free fatty acids
4. Inflammation

Improved understanding of acne development on a molecular level suggests that acne is a disease that involves both innate and adaptive immune systems and inflammatory events.

Acne usually begins in the prepubertal period, when the adrenal glands mature, and progresses as androgen production and sebaceous gland activity increase with gonad development.

As shown in Figure 77-1, acne results from the development of an obstructed sebaceous follicle, called a *microcomedone*. Sebaceous glands increase their size and activity in response to circulating androgens. Most patients with acne do not overproduce androgens (with some exceptions); instead, they have sebaceous glands that are hyperresponsive to androgens.[12] Patients with acne have a significantly greater number of lobules per gland compared with unaffected individuals.

Sebaceous lipids are regulated by peroxisome proliferator-activated receptors, which act in concert with retinoid X receptors to regulate epidermal growth and differentiation as well as lipid metabolism. Sterol response element-binding proteins mediate the increase in sebaceous lipids formation induced by insulin-like growth factor-1. Substance P receptors, neuropeptidases, α-melanocyte stimulating hormone, insulin-like growth factor (IGF)-1R and corticotropin-releasing hormone (CRH)-R1 are also involved in regulating sebocyte activity as are ectopeptidases. The sebaceous gland also acts as an endocrine organ in response to changes in androgens and other hormones. Oxidized squalene can stimulate hyperproliferative behavior of keratinocytes, and lipoperoxides produce leukotriene B4, a powerful chemoattractant.[12] The composition of sebum is changed, with a reduction in linoleic acid. The growth of keratinocytes changes. The infrainfundibulum increases its keratinization of cells with hypercornification and development of the microcomedone, the primary lesion of both noninflammatory and inflammatory acne.[13] Cells adhere to each other in an expanding mass, which forms a dense keratinous plug. In particular androgens, hormones could be a stimulus to pilosebaceous duct hypercornification. Sebum, produced in increasing amounts by the active gland, becomes trapped behind the keratin plug and solidifies, contributing to open or closed comedone formation.

Interleukin-1-α upregulation contributes to the development of comedones independently of colonization with *Propionibacterium acnes*. A relative linoleic acid deficiency has also been described.[12]

The pooling of sebum in the follicle provides ideal substrate conditions for proliferation of the anaerobic bacterium *P. acnes*, generating a T cell response, which results in inflammation.[13] *Propionibacterium acnes* produces a lipase that hydrolyzes sebum triglycerides into free fatty acids. These free fatty acids may trigger the changes that lead to an increase in keratinization and microcomedone formation.[14,15] This closed comedone, or whitehead, is the first clinically visible lesion of acne. It takes approximately 5 months to develop. The closed comedone is almost completely obstructed to drainage and has a tendency to rupture.[16–18]

As the plug extends to the upper canal and dilates its opening, an open comedone, or blackhead, is formed. Its dark color is not due to dirt but to either oxidized lipid and melanin or to the impacted mass of horny cells. The cylindrically shaped, open comedone is very stable and may persist for a long time as soluble substances and liquid sebum escape more easily. Acne that is characterized by open and closed comedones is termed *noninflammatory acne*.

Acne produces chemotactic factors and promotes the synthesis of tumor factor-α and interleukin-1β. Cytokine induction by *P. acnes* occurs. Both recruitment of polymorphs into the follicle during the inflammatory process and release of *P. acnes*-generated chemokines lead to pus formation. The pus eventually bursts on the surface with resolution of the inflammation or into the dermis. *Propionibacterium acnes* also produces enzymes that increase the permeability of the follicular wall, causing it to rupture, releasing keratin, hair, and lipids and irritating free fatty acids into the dermis. Several different types of inflammatory lesions may form, including pustules, nodules, and cysts and may lead to scarring.

Hyperpigmentation and scarring are two sequelae of acne. A time delay of up to 3 years between acne onset and adequate treatment correlates to degree of scarring and emphasizes the need for early therapy.[10,11]

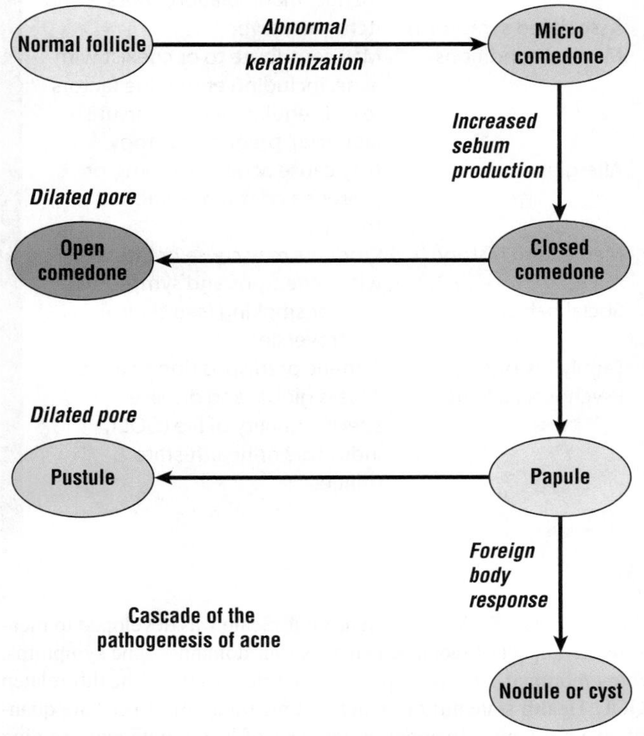

FIGURE 77-1 Cascade of the pathogenesis of acne.

CLINICAL PRESENTATION AND DIAGNOSTIC CONSIDERATIONS

To correctly diagnose acne vulgaris, the clinician considers patient assessment, which includes distinguishing all the presenting signs and symptoms of the clinical presentation, reviewing diagnostic and assessment considerations (see Clinical Presentation box), as well as considering psychosocial issues, differential diagnosis, and the possibility of drug-induced acne.

Psychosocial Issues

Assessment of acne's impact on quality of life is an important consideration in clinical decision making. The negative impact of facial acne is one of the primary motivators for patients to seek and to adhere to treatment.[21] Specific quality of life (QOL) indicators represent patients' perceptions and reactions to their health. Assessing

CLINICAL PRESENTATION

Signs and Symptoms

Lesion Type: Acne Vulgaris Can be Noninflammatory or Inflammatory

- Noninflammatory acne is characterized by open and closed comedones.
  - The closed comedo is visible as a 1–2 mm whitehead most easily seen when the skin is stretched.
    - Is the first clinical sign of acne
    - Has a tendency to rupture
  - The open comedo, or blackhead, is larger, approximately 2–5 mm and is dark-topped with contents extruding.
    - Is relatively stable.
- Inflammatory acne is traditionally characterized as having papulopustular and/or nodular lesions.
  - A pustule is formed from a superficial aggregation of neutrophils.
    - Appears as a raised white lesion filled with pus, usually less than 5 mm in diameter
    - Superficial pustules usually resolve within a few days without scarring
  - A nodule is produced through deeper, dermal, inflammatory infiltration.
    - Is the most severe variant of acne
    - Appears as warm, tender, firm lesions, with a diameter of 5 mm or greater
    - May be suppurative or hemorrhagic within the dermis, may involve adjacent follicles and sometimes extend down to fat
  - Cysts are suppurative nodules named because they resemble inflamed epidermal cysts.
    - Cystic acne may show double comedones, resulting from prior inflammation and fistulous links between neighboring sebaceous units.
  - Progression of inflammatory lesions:
    - Pustules and cysts often rupture spontaneously and drain a purulent or bloody but odorless discharge.[19]
    - Inflammatory lesions may itch as they erupt and can be tender or painful.
    - Often resolution of these lesions leaves erythematous or pigmented macules that can persist for months or longer, especially in dark-skinned individuals.
    - Nodules and deep lesions may result in scarring.

Regions of Involvement

- Acne lesions can occur anywhere on the body apart from the palms and soles.
  - Are usually located on the face, back, neck, shoulders, and chest
  - May extend to buttocks or extremities
  - One or more anatomic areas may be involved in any given patient
  - The pattern of involvement, once present, tends to remain constant.
- Skin, scalp, and hair are frequently oily.

Severity Grading Taxonomies

FDA Investigator Global Assessment 2005[20,22]

Type 1	Almost clear: rare noninflammatory lesions (NIL) with no more than 1 papule
Type 2	Mild, some NIL but no more than a few papules/pustules
Type 3	Moderate: many NIL, some inflammatory lesions (IL), no more than 1 nodule
Type 4	Severe: up to many noninflammatory and inflammatory lesions, but no more than a few nodular lesions

European Union Guidelines Clinical Classification:[12]

I	Comedonal acne
II	Mild-moderate papulopustular acne
III	Severe papulopustular acne, moderate nodular acne *(this level combines FDA types 3 and 4, above)*
IV	Severe nodular acne, conglobate acne *(this is an additional level cf. the FDA types above)*

Diagnostic and Assessment Considerations

Palliating factors	Sunlight
Provoking factors	Premenstrual flares, humid environments, excessive sweating; exposure to chemicals; occlusive clothing; friction; oily cosmetics; manual manipulation; stress
Associated symptoms	Itch, pain, fever
Medical conditions	May contribute to or coexist with acne, including endocrine factors (e.g., irregular menses, hirsutism, alopecia), pregnancy, atopy
Allergies	May cause acne symptoms, or present a contraindication to therapy
Medication history	Products may cause or interact with acne signs and symptoms
Social habits	Diet, or smoking (see clinical controversies)
Family history	Genetic predisposition to acne
Psychosocial issues	Assess global and disease specific quality of life (QOL) indicators or health-state utilities

QOL impairment in patients with acne may aid in management by evaluating psychologic impacts, which may not correlate with clinical severity; aid in detection of depression or need for psychologic care; and improve therapeutic outcomes.

Examples of global scales that have been used to evaluate acne include Skindex[23] and Dermatology QOL Index;[24] examples of acne specific scales include the Acne-specific QOL questionnaire[25] and the Acne QOL Scale.[26] The Acne QOL Scale was developed to measure the impact of facial acne across four domains (acne symptoms, role-emotional, self-perception, and role-social) of health-related QOL. Health-state utilities (such as time trade-off [TTO]) are quantitative measures of patient preferences of health outcomes ranging from 0 (death) to 1 (perfect health) and can be used in clinical trials as outcome measures of treatment effects. TTO utilities for acne in the range of 0.94 to 0.96 can be compared with those of other diseases (e.g., 0.92 for epilepsy, 0.94 for myopia), and help to identify the impact of acne on self-perception and psychologic functioning.[27]

Differential Diagnosis

Acne vulgaris is rarely misdiagnosed. The conditions most commonly mistaken for acne vulgaris include rosacea, perioral dermatitis, gram-negative folliculitis, and drug-induced acne.[28]

Acne rosacea (adult acne) is a chronic relapsing condition, occurring after age 30 years in fair-complexioned persons and involving blood vessels. The first sign is easy flushing followed by development of inflammatory lesions, with edema, papules, and pustules appearing on the nose, cheeks, chin, and forehead, and telangiectasia (spider veins) developing as the condition progresses. The affected area may be sensitive to the touch.

Rosacea (sometimes called adult acne) differs from acne vulgaris in several ways. Its onset is not linked to increased androgens or endocrine changes; comedones are not usually present; aggravating factors are different and include ingestion of alcohol, spicy foods, or hot drinks (especially those containing caffeine); smoking; overexposure to sunlight; and exposure to temperature extremes, friction, irritating cosmetics, and steroids. Rosacea is not curable, progressively worsens, and may ultimately result in rhinophyma (enlarged nose). Refer patients to a physician for treatment, as antibiotics, particularly topical metronidazole, may be required.[29]

Perioral dermatitis occurs primarily in young women and adolescents and is characterized by erythema, scaling, and papulopustular lesions commonly clustered around the nasolabial folds, mouth, and chin. The cause is unknown.[29]

Gram-negative folliculitis *(Proteus, Pseudomonas, Klebsiella)* may complicate acne, with a sudden change to pustules or large inflammatory cysts occurring after long-term treatment of acne with oral antibiotics. Folliculitis may be caused by staphylococci. There is a sudden onset of superficial pustules around the nose, chin, and cheeks. Patients with suspected folliculitis should be referred to a physician.[29]

Several conditions include acne vulgaris as a characteristic component, and understanding the mechanisms involved in these syndromes provides insight into the pathogenesis of acne. These include polycystic ovary syndrome (elevated androgen levels); PAPA syndrome (pyogenic arthritis, pyoderma gangrenosum, acne; early onset arthritis with increased inflammatory activity), and SAPHO syndrome (synovitis, acne, pustulosis, hyperostosis, osteitis syndrome; sterile inflammatory arthro-osteitis, with *P. acnes* as a possible trigger).[13]

Drug-Induced Acne

In addition to the conditions induced by drugs that were presented in eChapter 23, acneiform eruptions can also be caused by medications. Systemic corticosteroids can cause a pustular inflammatory form of acne, especially on the trunk. Onset is abrupt at 2 to 6 weeks after initiation of therapy. Acne has also been associated with most of the potent topical steroids, but not with hydrocortisone, which lacks the ability to inhibit protein synthesis. Discontinuation of the steroid results in an initial worsening of appearance due to removal of the antiinflammatory action of the steroid itself. Caution patients about this reaction, which can be subdued through judicious use of topical hydrocortisone.[30–32]

Antiepileptics and tuberculostatics are the most commonly implicated in drug-induced acne, followed by lithium. Other heavy metals inducing acne include cobalt in vitamin B_{12}.[33] Halogens, especially an excess of iodide in seafood, salt, and health foods, can exacerbate acne. In addition, halogens can provoke de novo acne lesions in individuals who have increased external exposure often due to occupational contact, or pool or hot tub disinfection; this variant is called *chloracne*.

In addition, certain minor ingredients in cosmetics have been implicated in cosmetic acne, including isopropyl myristate, cocoa butter, and fatty acids.

TREATMENT

The first step in determining a safe and efficacious treatment regimen for acne vulgaris is to establish desired outcomes for the patient, regarding both short- and long-term goals.

Desired Outcomes (Goals of Treatment)

4 Acne vulgaris is now approached as a chronic disease for purpose of treatment, as it demonstrates the typical characteristics of chronicity: patterns of recurrence or relapse; a prolonged course; manifests as either acute outbreaks or slow onset; and has psychological and social impact. Two principles should be born in mind: this chronic nature warrants early and aggressive treatment, and maintenance therapy is often needed for optimal outcomes.

Acne requires long-term control, as it cannot be cured. This basic premise needs to be stressed with the patient to establish motivation to adhere to lengthy treatment regimens, which involve both addressing current symptoms and signs and taking preventive measures.

Treatment for acne should aim to reduce both severity (considering objective and subjective grading) and recurrences of skin lesions as well as to improve appearance. A significant percentage change in lesion counts should be noted: most patients empirically validate a margin of 10% to 15% reduction in facial lesion counts as appropriate. Patient global self-assessment of acne improvement is a primary outcome.

Basic goals of treatment include alleviation of symptoms by reducing the number and severity of lesions, slowing the progression of signs and symptoms, limiting the disease duration and recurrence, prevention of long-term disfigurement associated with scarring and hyperpigmentation, and avoidance of psychological suffering.

General Approach to Treatment

5 The most critical target for treatment is the microcomedone, because by eliminating the follicular occlusion the whole cascade of acne is arrested. This will involve a combination of preventive measures to reduce or eliminate risk and aggravating factors and treatment measures. These should integrate nondrug and pharmacologic protocols aimed at cleansing as well as affecting all four mechanisms involved in acne pathogenesis. Combination therapy to target multiple pathogenic steps is often more effective than single therapy, and may offer secondary advantages of decreasing agent-related side effects and minimizing resistance or tolerance to individual treatments.

The approach to acne management is largely determined by:

1. Severity index
2. Lesion type: predominantly noninflammatory or inflammatory
3. Treatment preferences including patient choices
4. Cost implications
5. Skin type and/or ethnic group
6. Patient age
7. Adherence
8. Response to previous therapy

9. Presence of scarring
10. Psychological effects
11. Family history of persistent acne

Topical therapy is the standard of care for mild-to-moderate acne. Those with moderate-to-severe acne will require systemic therapy.

Topical treatments only work where applied. Because topical therapies reduce new lesion development, they require application to the whole affected area rather than individual spots. Most cause initial skin irritation, and some people stop using them because of this. The irritation can be minimized by starting with lower strength preparations and gradually increasing frequency or dose. Where irritation persists, a change in formulation from alcoholic solutions to washes, gels, or more moisturizing creams or lotions might help.

6 7 First-line, second-line, and third-line therapies should be selected and altered as appropriate for the severity and staging of the clinical presentation. Treatment is directed at controlling the disorder, not curing it. Regimens should be tapered over time, adjusting to response. The smallest number of agents should be used at the lowest possible dosages to ensure efficacy, safety, avoidance of resistance, and patient adherence. Once control is achieved, simplify the regimen but continue with some suppressive therapy. It takes 8 weeks for a microcomedone to mature, thus any therapy must be continued beyond this duration in order to assess efficacy.[32] Most topical preparations may be used for years as needed.

Because acne is a chronic disease, lesions typically recur for years. Microcomedones significantly decrease during therapy but rebound almost immediately after therapy is discontinued. Hence, the strategy for treating acne today includes an induction phase followed by a maintenance phase, and is further supported by adjunctive treatments and/or cosmetic routines. A routine part of acne therapy should include maintenance therapy to reduce the potential for recurrence of visible lesions, where maintenance therapy is the regular use of appropriate agents to ensure remission.

For successful long-term treatment, maintenance therapy must be tolerable, appropriate for the patient's lifestyle and convenient, continuing months to years, depending on age. Education about pathophysiology of acne, and the psychosocial benefits of clearer skin are compelling reasons for patient adherence to consistent therapy to sustain remission.

Nonpharmacologic Therapy

8 9 Encourage patients with acne to discontinue or avoid any aggravating factors, maintain a balanced, low-glycemic-load diet and control stress. Evidence shows that by being empathic and informative during counseling, the health professional may motivate the patient to continue long-term therapy.[8,9,28] One of the first approaches to nondrug management of acne is attention to cleansing techniques. Shaving recommendations, comedone extraction, dietary considerations, issues relating to ultraviolet light, and prevention of cosmetic acne should be reviewed with patients.

Cleansing

Cleansers often contain surfactant systems to remove fat from the skin surface. The oil is dispersed from the skin into the surfactant system; however, the active ingredient is sometimes trapped and removed upon rinsing. Also, the balance between cleanliness and drying or irritation should be taken into account. Most patients prefer products with foaming action, and these must contain additional secondary surfactants to enhance the foam and condition the skin.

Soaps are the most widely used cleansing products, but do not lend themselves to efficient delivery of active drug. Two main disadvantages exist. As soaps are rinsed off, the deposit of active agent will be small; and the high pH required in soaps may degrade some active ingredients and be less tolerable on sensitive skin. Soapless cleansers are an alternative to soaps.[34]

Patients should wash no more than twice daily with a mild, nonfragranced opaque or glycerin soap or a soapless cleanser. Acne patients often wash too frequently, attempting to remove surface oils. There is no evidence indicating that this is helpful, as surface lipids do not affect acne. Contributory lipids are deep in the follicle and are not removed through washing. Antiseptic cleansers, while producing a clean, refreshed feeling, remove only surface dirt, oil, and aerobic bacteria. They do not affect *P. acnes*. There is no evidence that any particular washing regimen is superior. Evidence-based studies on the use of cleanser or medicated cleansers are lacking or poorly designed with small numbers of patients.[35] Scrubbing should be minimized to prevent follicular rupture. Soaps produce a drying effect on the skin due to detergent action. As medicated cleansers require increased contact time, this drying action is pronounced, especially with peeling agents. Avoid cream-based cleansers.

Because the acid pH of skin has an antimicrobial effect, it has been proposed that lowering lesional surface pH (with products such as Herpifix, marketed in Europe) may be correlated to the number of acne lesions. Studies are planned.

Polyester cleansing sponges (e.g., Buf-Puf) are synthetics that abrade the skin surface, removing superficial debris. They are unlikely to unseat comedones, considering the structure of these lesions. The sponges are available in soft or coarse textures, with or without soap. Caution patients against using a circular or rubbing motion that will increase irritation, and instruct them to use single, gentle, continuous strokes on each side of the face, from the midline out toward the ears.

Cationic-bond strips that become activated by water are available. The dirt and oil in the pores is anionic. As the strip dries, the cationic-bond binds the anionic dirt and removes it when the strip is peeled off.

Shaving

Males should try both electric and safety razors to determine which is more comfortable for shaving. When using a safety razor, the beard should be softened with soap and warm water or shaving gel. Shaving should be done as lightly and infrequently as possible, using a sharp blade and being careful to avoid nicking lesions. Strokes should be in the direction of hair growth, shaving each area only once.

Comedone Extraction

Comedone extraction is useful and painless and results in immediate cosmetic improvement although it has not been widely tested in clinical trials. Pretreatment with a peeler for 4 to 6 weeks often facilitates the procedure.[32] Following cleansing with hot water, a comedone extractor is placed over the lesion and gentle pressure applied until the contents are expressed. This removes unsightly lesions, preventing progression to inflammation. A correctly sized extractor allows the central keratin plug to extrude through the opening. The small end of a plastic eye dropper, with bulb removed, may also be used. These instruments should be cleaned with alcohol after each use. Some initial reddening may be apparent. If the contents are not expressed with modest pressure, patients should not continue since improper extraction may further irritate the skin. A physician should be consulted if this technique is too difficult for the patient to manage. Since the follicle is difficult to remove completely, comedones may recur between 25 and 50 days following expression. Fewer than 10% of comedone extractions are a complete success, but the process is useful when done properly.[19]

Comedo removal may be helpful in the management of comedones resistant to other therapies, but it has not been well studied despite long-standing clinical use. Also, while the procedure cannot affect the clinical course of the disease, it can improve the patient's appearance, which may positively affect adherence with the treatment program.

Ultraviolet Light

Although ultraviolet light was recommended in the past for desquamation, the practice is no longer advisable because of the well-established carcinogenic and photoaging effects of ultraviolet exposure. Moreover, inflamed skin is more susceptible to the damaging effects of ultraviolet light. Patients taking tretinoin may show heightened sensitivity.[36]

Before exposure to sunlight, patients with acne should apply sunscreens (sun protection factor [SPF] 15) in alcohol or oil-free bases and avoid using the acnegenic benzophenones. Sunscreen should be applied as the first product.

Prevention of Cosmetic Acne

Persistent low-grade acne in women after their mid-20s is frequently caused by heavy cosmetic use. Adolescent acne in younger women may be exacerbated with makeup overuse. The problem is perpetuated when the resultant blemishes are concealed with more cosmetics.

Advise patients to stop using oil-containing cosmetics and avoid cosmetic programs that advocate applying multiple layers of cream-based cleansers and cover-ups. These are advertised through the media and often available through Internet shopping with promotional bonuses. Three-step basic systems usually combine medicated and nonmedicated ingredients, although it may not be apparent by their cosmetic names that therapeutic agents are included. They often start with cleansers, in lotions or creams, which may contain a multitude of unnecessary ingredients, including medicated peelers, oils, fragrances, and preservatives. Often drugs are included in subtherapeutic or low doses, including salicylic acid, sulfur, or benzoyl peroxide. The second step is generally a "toner" or "refresher" which is usually water- or alcohol-based and might contain medicated ingredients such as α-hydroxy acids (e.g., glycolic acid), which are mild comedolytic agents, or even glycerin as a humectant. The final product, often called intensive or repairing solutions, usually contains the lowest strength of peelers such as benzoyl peroxide, sulfur, or salicylic acid; plus potentially sensitizing fragrances and preservatives; or oil-soluble sunscreens that are not identified on the label. Bases may have significant oil content. There may be additional products to supplement as necessary to the base routine of three steps, such as masks or spot treatments. Multiple-step cosmetic programs are often costly, and should be avoided in favor of simple cleansers and more effective single-ingredient peelers at optimal concentrations.

The term *noncomedogenic* may refer to either water-based vehicles or products that are free of substances known to induce comedones. They are not necessarily oil free. Water-based cosmetics may contain significant amounts of oil in the form of undiluted vegetable oils, lanolin, fatty acid esters (butyl stearate, isopropyl myristate), fatty acids (stearic acid), fatty acid alcohols, cocoa butter, coconut oil, red veterinary petrolatum, and sunscreens containing benzophenones. Water-based products are more likely to contribute to pore blockage than oil-free products.

Oil-free makeups are well-tolerated and lipstick, eye shadow, eyeliner, eyebrow pencils, and loose face powders are relatively innocuous. Heavier, oil-based preparations, particularly moisturizers and hairsprays, clog pores and accelerate comedone formation.[37]

The patient should restrict cosmetic use to products labeled oil-free rather than water-based, including makeup, moisturizers, or sunscreens. Coverup cosmetics for acne are available in several skin tones and in lotion and cream forms. They often contain peeling agents, antibacterial agents, or hydroquinone. Most contain sulfur. They may be applied as cosmetics two or three times daily, over the entire face or to individual lesions. However, because the spread time of oil-free makeup is decreased, best results are achieved if applied to one-quarter of the face at a time. Topical medication should be applied after gentle cleansing and a foundation lotion may be used sparingly as a concealer.[38,39,40]

Because the action of most therapeutic acne agents is to dry the skin, the use of moisturizers is counterproductive. Active agents such as α-hydroxy acids (glycolic, lactic, pyruvic, and citric acids) may be present in the cosmetic formulation, since they reduce corneocyte adhesion.[41] Patients with acne should be restricted to oil-free α-hydroxy acid products unless absolutely necessary because of treatment with strong drying agents or isotretinoin.

Vehicles

The formulation of an acne vehicle must consider the technical characteristics of maintaining and delivering the drug in an active state together with the need for an elegant product that the patient will enjoy using, so that it is more likely to be applied as required and deliver the full benefit. Physically and chemically, the vehicle will be used with one or more of the following goals: reduce excess oil, control bacteria associated with acne, reduce the effects of hyperkeratinization, and unclog pores. Performance, safety, and stability should be maximized while addressing technical and commercial factors.

Immiscible liquids might be delivered in oil-in-water or water-in-oil emulsions. In addition to having undesirable oil content, these vehicles also contain humectants, thickeners, preservatives, and fragrance, all of which may be problematic.

Solutions are simpler formulations, and there is a trend to use them as the soaking liquid for wipe products made with fibrous cloths. The viability of these kinds of products must take into consideration whether packages are resealable if they contain multiple wipes, and whether the volatility of the solvent will affect storage and availability of the active agent or cause crystallization. Solutions are used mainly with topical antibiotics, which are often dissolved in specific types of alcohol. Although some antibiotics are only soluble in ethyl alcohol, isopropyl alcohol is generally better able to remove oil from the skin surface and is preferred for nonmedicated vehicles. An 8% glycolic acid solution is available for use alone or for incorporation in topical antibiotic preparations. Solutions and washes can be more easily applied to large areas such as the back.[42]

Nongreasy solutions, gels, lotions, and creams should be selected as bases for topical acne preparations. Gels are very useful as they are totally oil free along with mixtures of water or alcohol. Lotions and creams will contain some oil-phase ingredients. Discourage moisturizers and oil-based products. Lotions are slightly less drying than gels, and creams are more emollient. Many gels contain ethanol or isopropyl alcohol. Propylene glycol is sometimes present in small amounts to add viscosity and lessen the drying effects of strong peeling agents. Gels are drying but may cause a burning irritation in some patients and may prevent certain kinds of cosmetics from adhering to the skin.[37] Propylene glycol gels are easy to apply and dry without a visible or sticky film. Nonalcoholic gels may be as effective and less drying than alcoholic solutions. Alcoholic or acetone gels are usually more drying and provide better penetration of the active ingredient.

The percent contribution of vehicle (placebo) toward reported efficacy of reduction of lesions counts of eight commonly prescribed topical preparations at the end of 10 to 12 weeks of daily administration has been evaluated as a mean value of 55% (range 35% to 82%). This demonstrates the great importance of vehicle effects in topical therapy.[43] Consider the patient's skin type and preferences in the choice of vehicle for topical agents. Patients with oily skin often prefer vehicles with higher proportions of alcohol (solutions and gels), while those with dry or sensitive skin prefer nonirritating lotions and creams. Hydrating and emollient products are often recommended to patients using drying treatment therapies, such as isotretinoin, to control adverse effects and improve adherence to treatment. Lotions can be used with any skin type and can be easily spread over hair-bearing skin, but will cause burning or dryness if they contain propylene glycol. Compatibility of vehicles and agents with cosmetics should also be considered.

How to Use Topical Preparations

Topical preparations should not be applied to individual lesions but to the whole area affected by acne to prevent new lesions from developing, using care around the eyelid, mouth, and neck to avoid chafing. Lotions should be applied with a cotton swab once or twice a day after washing or at bedtime if they leave a visible residue.

Psychologic Approaches, Hypnosis, and Biofeedback

The psychologic effects of acne may be profound and the American Academy of Dermatology expert workgroup unanimously concluded that effective acne treatment can improve the emotional outlook of patients.[44] There is weak evidence of the possible benefit of biofeedback-assisted relaxation and cognitive imagery.[45,46]

Dressings

A pilot double-blind, randomized study of 20 patients has shown some benefit of treatment with a hydrocolloid acne dressing when compared with tape dressings for improving mild to moderate inflammatory acne vulgaris. Results showed greater reduction over 3 to 7 days in the overall severity of acne and inflammation, along with greater improvement in redness, oiliness, dark pigmentation, and sebum casual level. Less ultraviolet B light reaches the skin surface with the hydrocolloid dressing in place.[47,48]

Pharmacologic Therapy

Successful pharmacologic therapy must address one of the four mechanisms involved in the pathogenesis of acne. There are numerous agents available that prove one or more of these actions and are therefore effective (Table 77-2). However, the choice of active pharmacologic therapy depends on severity.

Mechanisms of drug action relating to acne pathogenesis are illustrated in Figure 77-2.

Drug Treatments of First Choice

There is concordance among key opinion leaders in different settings regarding recommendations for drugs of choice for management of acne (the Global Alliance,[49] European Guidelines[12]).

For comedonal, noninflammatory acne, active agents of first choice include those that correct the defect in keratinization by producing exfoliation most efficaciously. Topical retinoids, in particular, adapalene, can be recommended as drugs of choice.[12,49] Benzoyl peroxide or azelaic acid can be considered, as alternatives (lower strength recommendation)[12,49] or a change could be made to an alternate topical retinoid. Limitations can apply that may necessitate the use of a treatment with a lower strength of recommendation as a first-line therapy (e.g., financial resources and reimbursement limitations, legal restrictions, availability, drug licensing). Because the comedone is the initial lesion even in inflammatory acne, these agents are used to correct the defect in keratinization in all cases of acne.

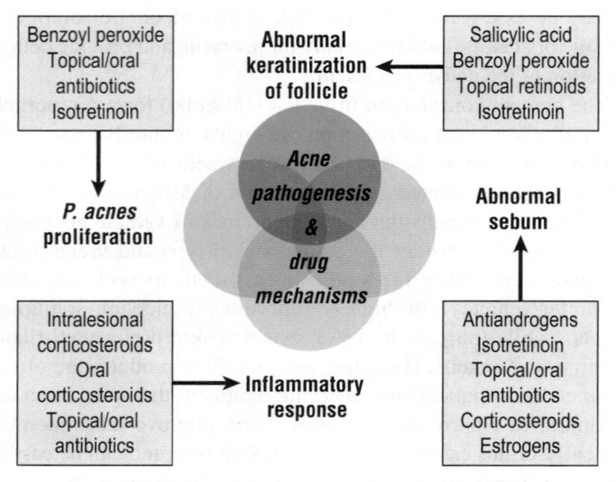

FIGURE 77-2 Acne pathogenesis and drug mechanisms.

For mild-to-moderate papulopustular inflammatory acne, it is important to reduce the population of *P. acnes* in the follicle and the generation of its extracellular products and inflammatory effects. Either the fixed-dose combination adapalene and benzoyl peroxide or the fixed-dose combination of clindamycin and benzoyl peroxide are strongly recommended as first choice therapy (high strength recommendation).[12,49] As alternatives, a different topical retinoid used with a different topical antimicrobial agent could be advised, with or without benzoyl peroxide. Azelaic acid or benzoyl peroxide can also be recommended (medium strength recommendation). In case of more widespread disease, a combination of a systemic antibiotic with adapalene can be recommended for the treatment of moderate papulopustular acne.

Low-strength recommendations are offered as considerations for treatment in the event of limitations that apply in selecting a first-choice agent. The choices would be blue light monotherapy, fixed-dose combination of erythromycin and tretinoin, fixed-dose combination of isotretinoin and erythromycin, or oral zinc. In case of more widespread disease, a combination of a systemic antibiotic with either benzoyl peroxide or with adapalene in fixed combination with benzoyl peroxide can be considered.[12]

For severe papulopustular or moderate nodular acne, oral isotretinoin monotherapy is strongly recommended as the drug of first choice (high strength recommendation). As alternatives, medium strength recommendations can be given for systemic antibiotics in combination with adapalene, with the fixed-dose combination of adapalene and benzoyl peroxide or in combination with azelaic acid.[12,49] In the event of limitations to use of these agents, considerations could be given to oral antiandrogens in combination with oral antibiotics or topical treatments, or systemic antibiotics in combination with benzoyl peroxide (low strength recommendation).

For nodular or conglobate acne, monotherapy with oral isotretinoin is strongly recommended as the drug of first choice (high strength recommendation).[12] As alternative agents, systemic antibiotics in combination with azelaic acid can be recommended (medium strength recommendation). If limitations exist to use of these agents, consideration could be given to oral antiandrogens in combination with oral antibiotics, systemic antibiotics in combination with adapalene, benzoyl peroxide, or the adapalene-benzoyl peroxide fixed-dose combination (low strength recommendation).[12]

For maintenance therapy for acne, the most recommended agents are topical retinoids. The most extensively studied maintenance treatment (four controlled trials) has been adapalene regimens.[12] Other published options include tazarotene or tretinoin. In general, maintenance therapy is begun after a 12-week induction and continues for 3 to 4 months. Continuing improvement using this schema is achieved, with relapse occurring when patients stop treatment, suggesting a longer duration of maintenance therapy is likely to be beneficial. Topical azelaic acid is an alternative to topical retinoids for acne maintenance therapy, with advantageous efficacy and safety profiles for long-term therapy. To minimize antibiotic resistance, long-term therapy with antibiotics is not recommended as an alternative to topical retinoids. If an antimicrobial effect is desired, the addition of benzoyl peroxide to topical retinoid therapy is preferred.

Published Guidelines

In general, recommendations should be based on critical appraisal and interpretation of the literature combined with clinical experience. There is considerable heterogeneity in the acne literature. The large number of products and product combinations, and the scarcity of comparative studies, has led to disparate opinions and few recommendations are evidence-based. Various evidence-based guidelines, available from multiple American, Canadian, European, Scandinavian, and South African sources from 2005 to 2012, do not provide concordance or clarity on all issues.

The 2012 European Guidelines for the Treatment of Acne focus primarily on major treatments, include use of light and laser therapy (see Clinical Controversy on Light Therapy box), but do not review general management issues such as psychological determinants, scarring, diet, and so forth.[12] Where relevant, specific information from multiple sources will be integrated into the therapy section that follows.

Clinical **Controversy...**

Light Therapy

Increasingly, "diverse" light therapies (using various wavelengths) as convenient acne treatments with few[117] or temporary[119] adverse effects are reported. Conclusions based on outcomes with light therapy are contradictory.

Light therapies for acne are believed to work by killing *Propionibacterium acnes* and by damaging and shrinking sebaceous glands, reducing sebum output. Light therapies may be used once or twice weekly as a course of 6 to 10 treatments, with each irradiation lasting 10 to 20 minutes.[119] *P. acnes* produce endogenous porphyrins that absorb light to form highly reactive singlet oxygen, which destroys the bacteria.[119] Since porphyrins have peak absorption at blue light wavelengths, blue light is often used to treat acne. Red light is also absorbed by porphyrins and can penetrate deeper into the skin,[120] where it may directly affect inflammatory mediators. Other light therapies attempt to selectively target and damage sebaceous glands directly, reducing their size and thus sebum output.[121] These include infrared lasers, low-energy pulsed dye lasers, and radiofrequency devices.[119]

Photodynamic therapy (PDT) uses specific light-activating creams, which are absorbed into the skin and amplify the response to light therapy but tend to produce more severe adverse effects. There are concerns that PDT may interfere with the skin's natural immune mechanisms[122] and cause long-term skin damage.

Previously, treatment was not available universally, but accessed privately via dermatologists or clinics, and expensive. Light therapies are increasingly popular among consumers and home-use blue light therapy is now available. Patients find it easier to comply with light treatments because of their short duration.

Medical science continues to debate whether light of different wavelengths is effective.[119] To date, very few trials compare light therapy with conventional acne treatments. The European evidence-based guidelines for the treatment of acne evaluated existing light therapies and concluded published evidence is still very scarce and standardized treatment protocols and widespread experience are still lacking. They were unable to make a recommendation for or against treatment of comedonal; mild to moderate papulopustular (MMPP) or severe papulopustular/nodular acne with monotherapy visible light, visible or infrared wavelengths lasers, or intense pulsed light or PDT because of lack of or conflicting or insufficient evidence. Blue light has a low strength recommendation as a consideration for MMPP.[12]

A Cochrane review protocol is investigating the current state of evidence for use of light therapy in acne.[124]

An expert committee of the American Academy of Dermatology convened in 2007 to define guidelines for acne therapy and identify nine clinical questions to structure the primary issues in diagnosis and management (Table 77-1).[44] These guidelines address the management of adolescent and adult patients presenting with acne but not the consequences of disease, including the scarring, postinflammatory erythema, or postinflammatory hyperpigmentation. The use of light and laser therapy was not addressed in the guidelines. In 2009, The Global Alliance to Improve Outcomes in Acne updated their 2003 recommendations to review new information about pathophysiology and treatment and included current published data on relevant issues. They provided seven summary statements, most of which are based primarily on expert opinion (level V evidence) because of a lack of studies or different designs and methodologies of existing studies (evidence from published studies constitute levels I to IV).[49]

The Alliance consensus statements were as follows:[49]

1. Acne should be approached as a chronic disease.
2. Strategies to limit antibiotic resistance are important in acne management.
3. Combination retinoid-based therapy is first-line therapy for acne.
4. More data are need to define the role of laser and light therapy in acne.
5. Topical retinoids should be first-line agents in acne maintenance therapy.
6. Early, appropriate treatment is best to minimize potential for acne scars.
7. Assess adherence via verbal interview or use of a simple tool.

General Information Regarding Efficacy and Safety

The guidelines and recommendations of the American Academy of Dermatology considered the efficacy and safety of various treatments, such as topical agents, systemic antibacterial agents, hormonal agents, isotretinoin, miscellaneous therapies, complementary and alternative therapies, and dietary restriction, based on levels of evidence and best clinical practice.[44] More specific information about the efficacy and safety of each of these specific modalities is outlined below in sections on each individual agent.

Alternative Drug Treatments

Complementary and Alternative Medications Herbal and alternative therapies have been used to treat acne. Although these products appear to be well tolerated, very limited data exist regarding their safety and efficacy.

A systematic review of complementary and alternative medicine (CAM) treatments for acne in 2006 identified 15 randomized controlled trials covering diverse approaches such as *Aloe vera*, pyridoxine, fruit-derived acids, kampo (Japanese herbal medicine), and ayurvedic herbal treatments.[50] Although mechanisms of potential benefit for some were biologically plausible, the included studies were of poor quality and inconclusive.

Another systematic review of seventeen traditional Chinese medicine randomized controlled trials found some benefit for acupuncture with moxibustion that was better than Western medicines, but the quality of included studies was limited.[50,51]

A review of studies published from 2007 to 2010 showed most studies were level of evidence grade D. Two studies of grade A concluded that topical tea tree oil 5% gel and gluconolactone are efficacious in mild to moderate acne, with the latter agent comparable with benzoyl peroxide 5%. No data supported these claims,

TABLE 77-1 Guidelines for Managing Acne Vulgaris

Clinical Question Issues	Recommendation	Strength of Recommendation[a]	Level of Evidence[a]
I Systems for the grading and classification of acne	Use a grading/classification system	B	II
IIa Role of microbiologic testing	Do microbiologic testing	B	II
IIb Role of endocrinologic testing	Do endocrinologic testing	A	I
III Use of specific agents for topical therapy	Retinoids Benzoyl peroxide Antibiotics Other agents	A A A A	I I I I
IV Efficacy and safety of systemic antibiotics	Tetracyclines Macrolides Trimethoprim-sulfamethoxazole	A A A	I I I
V Efficacy and safety of hormonal agents	Contraceptive agents Spironolactone Antiandrogens Oral corticosteroids	A B B B	I II II II
VI Efficacy and safety of isotretinoin	Isotretinoin	A	I
VII Efficacy and safety of miscellaneous therapy	Intralesional steroids Chemical peels Comedo removal	C C C	III III III
VIII Efficacy and safety of complementary therapy	Herbal agents Psychologic approaches Hypnosis/biofeedback	B C B	I III II
IX Efficacy and safety of dietary restrictions[b]	Effect of diet	B	II

[a]An expert panel of the American Academy of Dermatology developed these clinical recommendations using the best available evidence. The panel rated evidence using the Strength of Recommendation Taxonomy (SORT), which uses this three-point scale:
I. Good quality patient-oriented evidence.
II. Limited quality patient-oriented evidence.
III. Other evidence including consensus guidelines, extrapolations from bench research, opinion, or case studies.

Similarly, recommendations were ranked as follows:
A. Recommendation based on consistent and good quality patient-oriented evidence.
B. Recommendation based on inconsistent or limited quality patient-oriented evidence.
C. Recommendation based on consensus, opinion, or case studies.

[b]See Clinical Controversy: Dietary Influences

Reprinted from reference 44. Copyright © 2007, with permission from Elsevier.

and one study predated the review dimensions (published in 1992). One grade B study compared tea tree oil 5% against benzoyl peroxide 5% without placebo and concluded tea tree oil provided slower relief but less discomfort.[52]

A systematic review of four randomized controlled trials of tea tree oil in 2000 did not find conclusive evidence of benefit.[53]

There is increasing interest in the use of CAM as adjuvant or single therapies: in America, 7% or people report using a complementary medicine, and 2% report seeing a complementary medicine practitioner.[54] Traditional Chinese medicine has been widely used to treat acne for many years, based on a diagnosis from a traditional Chinese medicine perspective according to the different syndromes of acne.

The lack of appropriate data, absence of quality assessment, and inconsistencies in search methodology suggest that CAM cannot be recommended for acne therapy at this time. This is a research gap that needs to be addressed.

The Cochrane collaboration is undertaking a systematic review to assess the effectiveness and safety of any CAM in the management of acne vulgaris.[55]

Glycolic Acid Another agent considered as an alternative therapy for acne vulgaris is glycolic acid. The efficacy and tolerability of a 0.1% retinaldehyde/6% glycolic acid combination (Diacneal) has been evaluated for mild-to-moderate acne vulgaris.[56] Physician and patient ratings of acne symptom severity and tolerance performed at baseline and months 1, 2, and 3 showed mean numbers of papules, pustules, and comedones were significantly reduced from month 1 on, demonstrating that glycolic acid is effective and well tolerated in mild-to-moderate acne vulgaris.

Both glycolic acid–based, salicylic acid or salicylic acid derivative–based, (e.g., lipohydroxyacid) and amino fruit acid-peeling preparations have been used in the treatment of acne. There is very little evidence from clinical trials published in peer-reviewed literature supporting the efficacy of peeling regimens.[44] Further research on the use of peeling in the treatment of acne needs to be conducted to establish best practices for this modality.

Hydroquinone To control pigmentation, hydroquinone, which reversibly damages melanocytes, has been used as a hypopigmenting agent in concentrations of 2% to 4%, in preparations of clear or tinted gels, which are more drying, and as vanishing or opaque, flesh-tinted creams, with or without α-hydroxy acids or sunscreens. Hydroquinone causes fading of epidermal but not dermal pigmentation. Onset of response is usually 3 to 4 weeks, and the depigmentation lasts for 2 to 6 months but is reversible. While effective in the removal of melanin, hydroquinone has been clinically found to be a possible carcinogen and causes a blue-black discoloration known as ochronosis.[57]

After considering new data and information on the safety of hydroquinone, the U.S. Food and Drug Administration (FDA) issued a proposed ruling in 2006 about hydroquinone products. The FDA proposed reversing earlier rules that hydroquinone is generally recognized as safe and effective. As of early 2013, FDA had not yet issued a final ruling on the status of nonprescription hydroquinone, and many physicians consider a ban unnecessary, given the lack of convincing evidence of carcinogenic risk to humans and the rarity of ochronosis occurrence.

Treatment of Scarring Drug and nonmeasures for scar resolution are important in acne vulgaris because many patients are scarred despite adequate treatment. For patients with mild scarring, nonprescription α-hydroxy acids may be used, while severe scarring may be corrected with other treatment modalities that require consultation with a dermatologist. Dermabrasion, local or subcuticular excision, collagen implants, chemical peels (e.g., 70% glycolic acid, trichloroacetic acid) and laser therapy have been used to improve scarring. Atrophic scars can be treated with laser resurfacing. Usually the scar is not completely removed, but a more cosmetically acceptable result is achieved. Keloids and hypertrophic scars can be treated with intralesional triamcinolone, cryotherapy, topical steroids and silicone sheeting. Surgical options for scars include excision, augmentation with collagen or fat, chemical peels, subcision, and injection of autologous fibroblasts.

Special Populations

About 20% of young infants (2 to 3 months of age) develop papules, pustules, and less commonly closed or open comedones, primarily on the cheeks, due to placental transfer of maternal androgens (neonatal acne). The acne subsides within a few months with regular maturation. Boys are affected more often than girls because of a transient increase in testosterone secretion during the third and fourth month of intrauterine life. *Malassezia* spp. may be involved in pathogenesis.[19] Resolution occurs without therapy.[58] Infants with neonatal acne may have more severe teenage acne.[19]

The treatment of acne in children is similar to that in adults. Because topical therapies may be more irritating in children, initiation with low concentrations is preferred. Systemic treatments should be reserved for more extensive cases. Erythromycin is preferred over tetracyclines for children younger than 9 years of age because tetracyclines can affect growing cartilage and teeth.

Although treatment is with isotretinoin has numerous potential minor adverse effects in patients of all ages, an uncommon complication in young patients is premature epiphyseal closure. This generally occurs when isotretinoin is administered in high doses, thus limiting long-term therapy.

Selecting appropriate treatment in pregnant women can be challenging because many acne therapies are teratogenic; all topical and especially oral retinoids should be avoided. Oral therapies such as tetracyclines and antiandrogens are also contraindicated in pregnancy. Topical and oral treatment with erythromycin may be considered.

Acne in skin of color is an increasing problem, presenting unique challenges. Although combination therapy is now the standard of care in acne, concerns exist with the increased potential irritation and dryness in skin of color. Although individual medications can be titrated or applied at different times of day to avoid irritation, this is not always practical or desirable. There is a paucity of clinical studies that evaluate the safety and efficacy of acne medications in skin of color. One study has examined susceptibility to irritation in Fitzpatrick skin types I to III versus types IV to VI and found subjects with darker skin were not more susceptible and tolerability was comparable across the two groups. Hispanic subjects were not more susceptible to irritation compared with total study groups.[59]

Drug Class Information

This section reviews the pharmacology and mechanisms as related to pathophysiology for pharmacologic options recommended in the guidelines for mild, moderate, and severe acne. It will also review evidence of efficacy and safety as well as kinetics, interactions, dosing, and administration when relevant.

Exfoliants (Peeling Agents) Exfoliants induce continuous mild drying and peeling by primary irritation, damaging the superficial layers of the skin, and inciting inflammation. This stimulates mitosis, thickening the epidermis, and increasing horny cells, scaling, and erythema. A decrease in sweating results in a dry, less oily surface and may superficially resolve pustular lesions.

In the past, a rabbit model was used to study the efficacy of topical exfoliants in retarding tar-induced comedone formation and accelerating their loss (comedolysis). In this animal model, retinoic acid (tretinoin) was most active, compared with benzoyl peroxide and salicylic acid, which were respectively less active. Data from peer-reviewed literature regarding the efficacy of sulfur, resorcinol, sodium sulfacetamide, aluminum chloride, and zinc are limited. Traditional nonprescription exfoliants, including phenol, resorcinol, betanaphthol, sulfur, Vleminckx's solution, and sodium thiosulfate, are weak or ineffective. These agents are not comedolytic given that they affect the superficial epidermis rather than the hair canal. They have been supplanted by superior effective agents. A new agent, linoleic acid-rich phosphatidylcholine combined with 4% nicotinamide, is suggested as an emulsion treatment that may be effective in normalization of follicular hyperkeratinization, and also provide antiinflammatory effects.[60,61]

Resorcinol This phenol derivative is less keratolytic than salicylic acid. It is said to be both bactericidal and fungicidal. Products containing resorcinol 1% to 2% have been used for acne, often in combination with other peeling agents, such as sulfur or salicylic acid. The FDA considers resorcinol 2% and resorcinol monoacetate 3%, in combination with sulfur 3% to 8%, to be safe and effective and that the combination may enhance the activity of sulfur. However, the FDA is not convinced that resorcinol and resorcinol acetate are safe and effective when used as single ingredients, and has placed such products in category II (not generally recognized as safe and effective, or misbranded).[61]

Resorcinol is an irritant and sensitizer and should not be applied to large areas of the skin or on broken skin. It produces a reversible, dark brown scale on some dark-skinned individuals.

Protective packaging is important as resorcinol is reactive to light and oxygen. It has good solubility in both water and alcohol and is heat stabile Thus, it is incorporated into a variety of products, including emulsions.[62]

Salicylic Acid Salicylic acid has been used for many years for the treatment of acne, although few well-designed trials of its safety and efficacy exist. It is a natural ingredient in many plants, such as willow tree or willow bark, is a β-hydroxy acid, and penetrates the pilosebaceous unit. It has comedolytic activity, although the concentrations in commercial preparations (less than 2% to 3%) are generally low. While concentrations less than 2% may actually increase keratinization, concentrations between 3% and 6% are keratolytic, softening the horny layer and producing shedding of scales. Its mechanism remains unresolved, attributed to either reduced cohesion of corneocytes or shedding of epidermal cells, rather than breakdown of keratin.

Salicylic acid has no effect on the mitotic activity of normal epidermis and does not influence disordered cornification.[63] It may also provide mild antibacterial value, as it is active against *P. acnes*. It also offers slight antiinflammatory activity at concentrations ranging from 0.5% to 5%. Its efficacy against comedones helps to prevent development of inflamed lesions, thus providing a delayed efficacy.[64]

Salicylic acid is an effective agent. As a peeling agent, its relative strength compared with others in this class varies according to the model used in measurement. It is slightly *less* potent than equal-strength benzoyl peroxide when measured with the rabbit ear animal model, and slightly *more* potent when measured with a biologic microcomedone model.[64] It may have antiinflammatory properties that help dry inflammatory lesions.[62] Its comedolytic properties are considered less potent than topical retinoids. It is often used when patients cannot tolerate a topical retinoid because of skin irritation.[65]

Its keratolytic effect may enhance the absorption of other agents. Salicylic acid may cause some degree of local skin peeling and discomfort (burning or reddening) as it is a mild irritant. It is not a sensitizer. Although the FDA recognizes salicylic acid as safe and effective, the compound offers no advantages over more modern topical agents such as benzoyl peroxide.[61,63,65]

Salicylic acid products are often used as first-line therapy for mild acne because of their widespread availability without a prescription. They are often available in alcohol–detergent impregnated pads as well as washes, bars, and semisolid vehicles. Lower concentrations are sometimes combined with sulfur to produce an additive keratolytic effect. Concentrations of up to 5% to 10% can be used for acne, beginning with a low concentration and increasing as tolerance to the irritation develops. However, the maximum strength allowed in nonprescription acne products is 2%. In high concentrations of 20% to 30% in hydroethanolic vehicles, salicylic acid, either alone or in combination, can be used as a peeling agent for comedonal acne and hyperpigmentation. It has been shown to extrude closed and open comedones several days after peel, but it must be applied under strict control to offer this adjunctive benefit when treating acne vulgaris.[66]

Sulfur Sulfur medications often lessen the severity of acne, presumably because of keratolytic and antibacterial action. Sulfur helps resolve comedones by its exfoliant action. Its popularity is due to its ability to quickly resolve pustules and papules, mask and conceal lesions (similar to a thick foundation lotion), and produce irritation leading to skin peeling and mild antibacterial action. Sulfur is used in the precipitated or colloidal form in concentrations of 2% to 10%, because it is practically insoluble in water and must be well dispersed. Its stability depends on effective maintenance of the dispersion.[62] Sulfur compounds (e.g., sulfides, thioglycolates, sulfites, thiols, cysteines, and thioacetates) are also available and somewhat weaker. Sulfur can cause slight ophthalmic and dermatologic irritation, and patients should be cautioned to avoid eye contact. Use should be discontinued if excessive irritation results. Although it is often combined with salicylic acid or resorcinol to increase its effect, its use is limited by its offensive odor and the availability of more effective agents.[67]

Sulfur has met the criteria of the FDA Advisory Review Panel for nonprescription topical acne products and is considered safe and effective when used alone, although its antibacterial effects were not recognized by this panel. Sodium thiosulfate, zinc sulfate, and zinc sulfide were not considered safe and effective.

Topical Retinoids Normal epithelial cell differentiation is a vitamin A–dependent process, and the most powerful peeling agents identified to date are related retinoid compounds. The effectiveness of topical retinoids in the treatment of acne is well documented. There is no consensus about the relative efficacy of currently available topical retinoids (tretinoin, adapalene, tazarotene) and oral isotretinoin. The rationale for the use of topical retinoids is based on their ability to target key stages in the development of the disease; the agents act by binding to specific nuclear receptors, reducing inflammation, and inhibiting sebocyte proliferation and differentiation, which reduces sebum production.

These agents act to reduce obstruction within the follicle and therefore are useful in the management of both comedonal and inflammatory acne. As a group, the retinoids reverse abnormal keratinocyte desquamation.[68] Thus, the retinoid family are highly active peelers. They improve acne vulgaris by inhibiting microcomedone formation, diminishing the number of mature comedones and subsequently, inflammatory lesions. In addition, they normalize follicular epithelium maturation and desquamation. The third-generation retinoids (i.e., adapalene and tazarotene) are receptor specific. Topical retinoids, unlike isotretinoin, do not decrease production of sebum, but primarily decrease inflammation, normalize keratinocyte differentiation, and increase keratinocyte proliferation and migration.[68]

Retinoids have a secondary effect that facilitates acne clearance. By loosening and decreasing corneocytes, they increase skin permeability, facilitate absorption of other agents, such as antimicrobials or benzoyl peroxide, and increase penetration of oral antibiotics into the follicular canal. This decreases the overall duration of antibiotic treatment and lessens the possibility of resistance. Therefore, combination products with oral or topical antimicrobials are available for increased efficacy, faster onset of effects, decreased total antibiotic use and risk of resistance, and shorter duration of treatment.[68] Retinoids may also improve and prevent postinflammatory hyperpigmentation often seen in people with darker complexions who have acne.

Retinoic acid (vitamin A acid or tretinoin) slows the desquamation process, reducing numbers of both microcomedones and comedones.[14] It is a powerful exfoliant and is not to be used in pregnant women because of risk to the fetus. Gels and creams are less irritating than solutions.

Adapalene is a stable, fast-acting, antiacne treatment that has significant antiinflammatory and comedolytic properties.[68–72] It causes epidermal and follicular epithelium hyperplasia, increased desquamation, keratinocyte differentiation, and loosening of corneocyte connections. Its antiinflammatory effect is due to the inhibition of oxidative metabolism of arachidonic acid and inhibition of chemotactic reponses.[72] It is better at reducing inflammatory lesions and total lesion count[72] and causes less local irritation because of its mechanisms and receptor specificity than tretinoin or tazarotene.[68–75] Release from lotions and hydroalcoholic gels is more effective than from creams and aqueous gels and a microsphere gel formulation may be less irritating.[68,74] It is a good first-line therapy for colder climates or in patients with sensitive skin.[57]

Adapalene is generally regarded as the topical retinoid of first choice for both treatment and maintenance therapy, as it is as effective but less irritating than other topical retinoids.[12,49] It is available in fixed-dose combinations in specialized gel vehicles with benzoyl peroxide to increase the efficacy in comparison with monotherapies. This strategy allows for the synergy of adapalene effects on normalizing desquamation with reduction of inflammation due to benzoyl peroxide action against *P. acnes*.

Tazarotene is also a specific agent with superior efficacy to parent retinoids, reducing both noninflammatory and inflammatory lesions.[68] Its exact mechanism is unknown, but it is thought to activate retinoid receptors and thereby affect keratinocyte differentiation, as well as inhibit proinflammatory transcription factors to decrease cell proliferation and inflammation.[68] It penetrates skin but accumulates in the upper dermis. It is as effective as adapalene in reducing noninflammatory and inflammatory lesion counts when applied half as frequently. Compared with tretinoin, it is as effective for comedonal and more effective for inflammatory lesions when applied once daily.[76–78] Short contact therapy, 1 to 5 minutes every other night, gradually increasing to overnight, is frequently advocated for dosing in patients with sensitive skin, whereas oily complexions may tolerate twice daily short contact time. Tazarotene is not degraded by sunlight.[14]

Retinoids include the systemic agent isotretinoin, which has effects on comedogenesis and sebum control, and is reviewed below under Antisebum Agents.

Retinoids tend to produce remissions that are maintained for extended periods of time, provided the accompanying irritation does not impede patient adherence. However, such adverse effects including erythema, xerosis, burning, and desquamation, are issues for many patients. The concentration and/or vehicle of any particular retinoid may decrease tolerability.[69,70] Most retinoids are unstable and insoluble in water.

Topical retinoids are not teratogenic; however, tretinoin should be used cautiously in pregnancy and tazarotene is contraindicated. Tretinoin and adapalene are in FDA category C, while tazarotene, based on large-surface-area use in psoriasis (see Chap. 78), is in FDA category X.[19]

Skin type and age may influence tolerability in addition to choice of vehicle. Oily skin may be more resistant, and darker skin is more prone to postinflammatory hyperpigmentation due to retinoid dermatitis. To decrease irritation, start with the lowest concentration and increase as tolerated. Application of retinoids should be at night, a half hour after cleansing, starting with every other night for 1 to 2 weeks to adjust to irritation. Short contact time starting with 2 minutes and adding 30 seconds per dose can be advised for patients with sensitive skin or in the winter, discontinuing and resuming after a 3-day rest if undue irritation results. Doses can be increased only after beginning with 4 to 6 weeks of the lowest concentration and least irritating vehicle. Adapalene and tazarotene are photoirritants (not photosensitizers), and sun avoidance and sunscreen use are imperative.[68]

Overall, topical retinoids are the cornerstone of acne treatment and provide safe, effective, and economical means of treating all but the most severe cases of acne vulgaris. They should be the first step in moderate acne, alone or in combination with antibiotics and benzoyl peroxide, reverting to retinoids alone for maintenance once adequate results are achieved. Their lack of effect in inducing bacterial resistance enables long-term maintenance of remission.

A Cochrane systematic evidence-based assessment of all issues regarding acne treatment with topical retinoids is planned to establish optimal treatment regimens, compare efficacy and tolerability of combination therapy, assess effect on *P. acnes* resistance, and evaluate safety.[78]

Antibacterial Agents Choices for antibacterial therapy include benzoyl peroxide, prescription topical and systemic antibiotics, and combination products. These drugs kill *P. acnes* and inhibit the production of proinflammatory mediators by organisms that are not killed.[14]

Benzoyl Peroxide Benzoyl peroxide is a bactericidal agent that has proven effective in the treatment of acne. Because of concerns of resistance, it is often used in the management of patients treated with oral or topical antibiotics. Used alone or in combination, benzoyl peroxide is the standard of care for mild-to-moderate popular-pustular acne.[12,49] It has the ability to prevent or eliminate the development of *P. acnes* resistance.

Benzoyl peroxide is a derivative of coal tar and was first used for acne vulgaris in the mid-1960s, becoming popular once stable formulations aimed at its heat-lability were developed in the mid-1970s.[79] These preparations are the single most useful group of topical nonprescription drugs and agents of first choice for most patients with mild-to-moderate acne vulgaris. Benzoyl peroxide is well absorbed through the stratum corneum and concentrates in the pilosebaceous unit.[80] It has three principle actions useful in both noninflammatory and inflammatory acne. It produces powerful anaerobic antibacterial activity due to slow release of oxygen, thereby acting against gram-positive and gram-negative bacteria, yeasts, and fungi. This nonspecific antibacterial mechanism does not induce resistance with long-term use.[79] It has a rapid (within 2 hours) cidal effect that lasts at least 48 hours. As a result, it may decrease the number of inflamed lesions within 5 days. As an indirect effect, it induces suppression of sebum production; it does not reduce skin surface lipids, but is effective in reducing free fatty acids, which are comedogenic agents and triggers of inflammation.[80] Topical benzoyl peroxide 5% lowers free fatty acids 50% to 60% after daily application for 14 days, and decreases aerobic bacteria by 84% and anaerobic bacteria (primarily *P. acnes*) by 98%. It also produces comedolysis.

While earlier rabbit model studies showed a benzoyl peroxide effect greater than that of salicylic acid, these animal comedones were not physiologic but induced by tar. More recent studies using native microcomedones show an anticomedogenic effect that is only comparatively slight, compared with tretinoin or salicylic acid.[81,82] Finally, a supplementary benefit of benzoyl peroxide is an indirect antiinflammatory action, which is due either to its antibacterial or oxidizing effects. This has been reported in several studies and thus can be used to support treatment of predominantly inflamed lesions.[79] The drug's antiacne effect is augmented by increased blood flow, dermal irritation, local anesthetic properties, and promotion of healing.[83–86] Because the primary effect of benzoyl peroxide is antibacterial, it is most effective for inflammatory acne. Many patients with noninflammatory comedonal acne will respond to its peeling action.

Benzoyl peroxide is available in a variety of preparations including gel, washes, lotions, and creams. There is no clear superiority of different preparations in terms of effectiveness. Newer delivery systems to enhance efficacy and tolerability are also being investigated.

Cleansers containing benzoyl peroxide are available as nonprescription liquid washes and solid bars of various strengths. The desquamative and antibacterial effectiveness in a soap or wash is minimized by limited contact time and removal with proper rinsing. Stable lotions are available in 2.5%, 5%, and 10%. Alcohol and acetone gels facilitate bioavailability and may be more effective, while water-based vehicles are less irritating and better tolerated. A 4% hydrophase gel is available that suspends crystals of benzoyl peroxide in a dimethylisosorbide solvent as the water in the base evaporates. The resulting solution is absorbed by the skin, leaving no film. The manufacturer claims the resulting efficacy is equal to 10% benzoyl peroxide with the minimal irritation of a 2.5% aqueous base gel. This may be an alternative for the patient with easily irritated skin who requires additional potency. This vehicle is easily combined with prepackaged clindamycin or erythromycin powders. Paste vehicles are stiffer and more drying than ointments or creams, which facilitate absorption and allow the active ingredients to stay localized.

Concentrations of 2.5%, 5%, and 10% in a water-based gel have been compared with the vehicle alone. The 2.5% formulation is equivalent to the 5% and 10% formulation in reducing the number of inflammatory lesions. The lower strength may not be as effective a peeler compared to higher strengths, which is due to an irritancy reaction. Thus, irritant side effects with the 2.5% gel are less frequent than with the 10% gel but are equivalent to the 5% gel. The lowest concentration of benzoyl peroxide should be used for treating patients with easily irritated skin and may lessen irritation when used in combination topical therapy with comedolytic agents.

Benzoyl peroxide may bleach hair, bedsheets, and clothing. It produces a mild primary irritant dermatitis that subsides with continued use and is more likely to occur in those with fair complexions, a tendency to irritancy, or propensity to sunburn. This irritation is dependent on the concentration and the vehicle, being higher with alcoholic gels compared with emulsion bases.[80] There are rare reports of contact allergic dermatitis. Cross-reactions with other sensitizers, notably Peruvian balsam and cinnamon, are well established. It may cross-sensitize to other benzoic acid derivatives such as topical anesthetics. Concomitant use of an abrasive cleanser may initiate or enhance sensitization.[87]

Another side effect is body odor from breakdown of the benzoyl peroxide that remains on clothing and bed sheets.

There is no indication that the normal use of benzoyl peroxide in the treatment of acne is associated with an increased risk of facial skin cancer. Although links have been made in experiments with mice, human relevance has not been established. The weak in vitro genotoxic potential is not manifested in vivo based on a lack of initiating or complete carcinogenic activity.[80] Overall, the cutaneous use of benzoyl peroxide is relatively safe, and is recognized by the FDA as category 3, which means that more information is required to make a final determination of safety and efficacy for nonprescription use.[88–91] Safety is also confirmed by the American Academy of Dermatology and the German Best Guideline Acne (BGA) Monograph.[79]

Benzoyl peroxide has been used in combination with other antiacne medications, such as sulfur and chlorhydroxyquinoline, or in formulations with urea to facilitate drug delivery. No significant improvement has been demonstrated.

Benzoyl peroxide has also been combined with prescription agents to improve efficacy, reduce dosing strengths, decrease irritation, and reduce resistance of antibiotics.[92–95]

Benzoyl peroxide is often combined with topical retinoid for an antimicrobial effect or used in conjunction with an antimicrobial. It reduces the likelihood of antibiotic resistance. For long-term maintenance therapy, it is recommended as a highly efficient bactericidal agent to be added to a topical retinoid.[49]

The benefits in efficacy and tolerability of combining topical antibiotics with benzoyl peroxide over using either as monotherapy have been demonstrated in several trials, most in combination with clindamycin. Combination with erythromycin show advantages over oral tetracycline monotherapy.[96]

The adjunctive use of clindamycin/benzoyl peroxide gel with tazarotene cream promotes greater efficacy and may also enhance tolerability. Increased tolerability might be attributed to emollients in the clindamycin/benzoyl peroxide gel formulation.[97] A patented gel formulation of benzoyl peroxide 5%/clindamycin phosphate 1% (clindamycin) containing dimethicone and glycerin was studied both as a monotherapy and in combination with topical retinoid use. Certain additives, such as silicates and specific humectants, reduced irritation by maintaining barrier integrity.[98]

All single-agent preparations of benzoyl peroxide are now available without prescription. Recommend the weakest concentration (2.5%) in a water-based formulation or the 4% hydrophase, for anyone with a history of skin irritation, or who must use combination therapy.[98] There are many suggested routines to initiate therapy. One is to gently cleanse the skin and apply the preparation for 15 minutes the first evening, avoiding the eyes and mucous membranes. A mild stinging and reddening will appear. Each evening the time should be doubled until the product is left on for 4 hours and subsequently all night. Dryness and peeling will appear after a few days. Once tolerance is achieved, the strength may be increased to 5% or the base changed to the acetone or alcohol gels, or to paste. Alternatively, benzoyl peroxide can be applied for 2 hours for four nights, 4 hours for four nights, and then left on all night. It is important to wash the product off in the morning. Other drying agents should be discontinued. Patients with very sensitive skin or demonstrated sensitivity to benzoyl peroxide should not use the product, and it should be discontinued if irritation becomes severe upon use. Contact with eyes, lips, or mouth should be avoided.

A sunscreen is recommended if benzoyl peroxide is used. To avoid interactions, apply the sunscreen during the day and the benzoyl peroxide at night.

Comparison of Salicylic Acid and Benzoyl Peroxide Although both salicylic acid and benzoyl peroxide are used for mild-to-moderate acne, their mechanisms differ and therefore different types of acne respond to each. Benzoyl peroxide is a strong antibacterial agent, while salicylic acid acts primarily through keratolysis.

Studies have shown salicylic acid to be equal or slightly superior to benzoyl peroxide in reducing number of comedones and subsequently number of inflammatory lesions. Any superiority salicylic acid demonstrates is likely because it interferes with an earlier step in pathogenesis—formation of the primary lesion of acne, the microcomedone.[63,65] However, studies of the compound did not use identical formulations. Instead, they compared salicylic acid cleansers to benzoyl peroxide washes and salicylic acid solutions to benzoyl peroxide creams. The effect of different bases is critical in determining differences in efficacy and therefore comparability of action since the base itself has an effect and influences penetration and duration of action.

In summary, the two products have similar efficacy, with salicylic acid noted as stronger in terms of retarding comedone formation. Benzoyl peroxide, as an antibacterial with some peeling effects, is considered the nonprescription and cosmetic gold standard for milder versions of the condition, used alone or in combination to increase efficacy and improve tolerability; however, salicylic acid is included in many of these products because of the perception of efficacy and safety for comedonal acne of type 1 or milder presentation.[64]

Topical Antibacterials The value of topical antibiotics in the treatment of acne has been investigated in many clinical trials. In addition to reduction of *P. acnes* as the primary mechanism for efficacy in acne, certain antibiotic drugs are also potent antiinflammatory agents via other mechanisms.

Macrolides, including topical erythromycin and topical clindamycin, have been demonstrated to be effective and are well-tolerated, well-established acne treatments. However, they have become less effective since the early 1990s because of resistance by *P. acnes*.[99] Decreased sensitivity of *P. acnes* to these antibiotics can limit the use of either drug as a single therapeutic agent. Resistant strains are usually resistant to all of the macrolides. Addition of benzoyl peroxide or topical retinoids to the macrolide antibiotic regimen is more effective than monotherapy and mitigates against survival of resistant *P. acnes* populations.

Clindamycin is the preferred macrolide because of potent action, lack of absorption, and its limited systemic use because it can cause pseudomembranous colitis when given orally or by injection. It is available as a single ingredient topical preparation and can also be combined with benzoyl peroxide. Erythromycin is available alone and in combination with retinoic acid or benzoyl peroxide. Some topical antibiotic–benzoyl peroxide combinations require refrigeration.[44] Other topical antibiotics that are being studied include fluoroquinolones such as 1% nadifloxacin cream but are not available in the American market.

Oral Antibacterials Systemic antibiotics are a standard of care in the management of moderate and severe acne and treatment-resistant forms of inflammatory acne. There is evidence to support the use of tetracycline, doxycycline, minocycline, erythromycin, trimethoprim–sulfamethoxazole, trimethoprim, and azithromycin. Studies do not exist for the use of ampicillin, amoxicillin, or cephalexin. However, any antibiotic that can reduce the *P. acnes* population in vivo and interfere with the organism's ability to generate inflammatory agents should be effective.[44] Although erythromycin is effective, use should be limited to those who cannot use one of the tetracyclines (i.e., pregnant women or children under 8 years of age because of the potential for damage to the skeleton or teeth). Ciprofloxacin, trimethoprim-sulfamethoxazole, and trimethoprim alone are also effective in instances where other antibiotics cannot be used or for patients who do not respond to conventional treatment.[61,100]

The tetracycline antibiotic family has multiple modes of action, well-understood antibacterial effects, and antiinflammatory effects that target an additional aspect of pathogenesis.[99–101] Agents such as tetracycline, minocycline, and doxycycline are used only as systemic agents. Through calcium chelation, they inhibit neutrophil and monocyte chemotaxis. Concentrations below the antibiotic threshold still inhibit inflammation, and improve both acne vulgaris and acne rosacea.

Tetracycline is no longer the drug of choice in this family; its disadvantages include diet-related effects on absorption and the drug's lower antiinflammatory and antibacterial activity.

The incidence of significant adverse effects with oral antibiotic use is low. However, adverse effect profiles may be helpful for each systemic antibiotic used in the treatment of acne. Vaginal candidiasis may complicate the use of all oral antibiotics.[44] Doxycycline is very commonly a photosensitizer especially at higher doses.

Minocycline has been associated with pigment deposition in the skin, mucous membranes, and teeth, particularly among patients receiving long-term therapy and/or higher doses of the medication. In some cases this is irreversible. Pigmentation occurs most often in acne scars, anterior shins, and mucous membranes. Minocycline may cause dose-related dizziness, which resolves with dose titration; urticaria; hypersensitivity syndrome, autoimmune hepatitis, a systemic lupus erythematosus-like syndrome; and serum sickness-like reactions.[44,99]

The Cochrane collaboration has conducted a review into the efficacy and safety of minocycline, examining 39 randomized controlled trials. These studies show that minocycline is an effective treatment for moderate to severe inflammatory acne but present no evidence to support the first-line use of minocycline in acne treatment. The drug is more lipophilic, may act more quickly, and can be taken once daily. However, people treated with minocycline are at a significantly greater risk of developing an autoimmune syndrome than those given tetracycline or no treatment.[102]

Bacterial resistance to antibiotics is an increasing problem particularly because therapy is directed at control over a long period of time.[99] The development of strains with unidentified mutations suggest new mechanisms of resistance are evolving. Combined resistance to clindamycin and erythromycin is much more common than resistance to tetracycline.[12] Use of topical antibiotics can lead to resistance largely confined to the skin of treated sites, whereas oral antibiotics can lead to resistance in commensal flora at all body sites. Resistance is more common in patients with moderate-to-severe acne and in countries with high outpatient antibiotic sales. Resistance is disseminated primarily by person-to-person contact, and thus the spread occurs frequently.

There have been an increasing number of reports of systemic infections caused by resistant *P. acnes* in nonacne patients after surgery. A transmission of factors conferring resistance to bacteria other than *P. acnes* has been described.

The most likely effect of resistance is to reduce the clinical efficacy of antibiotic-based treatment regimens to a level below that in patients with fully susceptible flora. This has been shown as a decreased clinical efficacy of topical erythromycin in clinical trials; there is no evidence to date of this effect in treatments with oral tetracycline or topical clindamycin.

Studies on *P. acnes* resistance have highlighted the need for treatment guidelines to restrict the use of antibiotics to limit the emergence of resistant strains. Patients with less severe forms of acne should not be treated with oral antibiotics, and where possible such therapy should be limited to the shortest feasible duration (e.g., 6 to 8 weeks). Local patterns of resistance should be considered.[96] The use of systemic antibiotics should be limited (both indication and duration) and topical antibiotic monotherapy should be avoided.

There should be early use of combination therapy with retinoids. Often, when oral antibiotics are combined with topical agents, the antibiotic may be discontinued after 6 months of therapy.[103] Nearly 70% of patients with acne require antibiotics for 12 weeks or less if aggressive retinoid therapy is used during that time.[99]

Another potential strategy that had been suggested is to eliminate the use of antibiotics and combine other topical agents. Neither retinoids nor benzoyl peroxide creates selective pressure for resistance and is one combination option. Although this approach has been evaluated for efficacy and safety, there is limited evidence of its effect on microbial resistance. In one open label study of adapalene and benzoyl peroxide, baseline counts of antibiotic resistant strains of *P.* acnes were reduced by week 4.[49,96]

Stricter cross-infection control measures are recommended when assessing acne. Any topical or systemic antibiotic therapy should be combined when possible with broad-spectrum antibacterial agents such as benzoyl peroxide. In addition, isotretinoin use should be initiated earlier in indicated patients, rather than prolonging antibiotic courses.[12]

Azelaic Acid Azelaic acid possesses activity against all four pathogenic factors that produce acne. It has antiinflammatory and antibacterial activities. Azelaic acid also normalizes keratinization, which accounts for its anticomedogenic effect. It is a competitive inhibitor of mitochondrial oxidoreductases and of 5-α-reductase, inhibiting the conversion of testosterone to 5-dehydrotestosterone. It also possesses bacteriostatic activity to both aerobic and anaerobic bacteria including *P. acnes*. Azelaic acid is an antikeratinizing agent, displaying antiproliferative cytostatic effects on keratinocytes and modulating the early and terminal phases of epidermal differentiation.[104] It may produce hypopigmentation. Inhibition of thioredoxin reductase by azelaic acid provides a rationale for its depigmenting property.

Azelaic acid 20% cream is used in the treatment of mild to moderate inflammatory acne, has an excellent safety profile with minimal adverse effects, and is well-tolerated in comparison with other acne treatments. The most common adverse effects, occurring in approximately 1% to 5% of patients, are pruritus, burning, stinging, and tingling. Adverse reactions are generally transient and mild in nature. Other adverse reactions, such as erythema, dryness, rash, peeling, irritation, dermatitis, and contact dermatitis, have been reported in less than 1% of patients.[104]

Azelaic acid has been shown effective in clinical trials studied with topical 2% erythromycin, topical 5% benzoyl peroxide gel, and topical 0.05% tretinoin cream in the treatment of mild to moderate inflammatory acne. However, the agent has limited efficacy, compared with other antiacne therapies.[44] It is an alternative to first choice therapy for comedonal and all types inflammatory acne, particularly in combination.[12] It is an alternative to topical retinoids for maintenance therapy as its efficacy and safety profile are advantageous for long-term therapy.[12]

Azelaic acid should be applied twice a day, in the morning and evening. A majority of patients with inflammatory lesions may experience an improvement in their acne within 4 weeks of beginning treatment. However, treatment may be continued over several months, if necessary.

Azelaic acid is in a pregnancy category B and should only be used in pregnant women if medically necessary. Patients with dark complexions should be monitored for early signs of hypopigmentation.

Dapsone Topical dapsone 5%, a synthetic sulfone, is a recently introduced treatment for acne available as a topical gel. Sulfones have both antiinflammatory and antibacterial properties, and may be used in sulfonamide-allergic patients.

Dapsone's utility is attributable to its antiinflammatory and antimicrobial properties that improve both inflammatory and noninflammatory acne, with more prominent effects occurring in inflammatory lesions. Short- and long-term safety and efficacy have been demonstrated.[105] Topical dapsone is a novel addition to the treatment armamentarium, especially for patients exhibiting sensitivities or intolerance to conventional antiacne agents.[106]

Topical dapsone 5%, alone or in combination, with adapalene 0.1% or benzoyl peroxide 4% has been shown to be safe and efficacious, but may be more irritating than other topical agents.[96,107]

Intralesional Steroids Intralesional corticosteroid injections are effective in the treatment of individual inflammatory acne nodules. The effect of intralesional injection with corticosteroids is a well-established and recognized treatment for large inflammatory lesions. Cystic acne improved in patients receiving intralesional steroids.[44]

Systemic absorption of steroids may occur with intralesional injections. Adrenal suppression was observed in one study. The injection of intralesional steroids may be associated with local atrophy. Lowering the concentration and/or volume of steroid may minimize these complications.

Antisebum Agents No topical agents directly influence the production of sebum. Systemic drugs that influence sebum production include high-dose estrogens, antiandrogens (cyproterone acetate), spironolactone, and the retinoid isotretinoin. Antioxidants, such as sodium l-ascorbyl-2-phosphate 5%, may act to prevent the oxidation of sebum and studies are in preliminary stages.

Oral antiandrogens, such as spironolactone and cyproterone acetate, can also be useful in the treatment of acne. While flutamide can be effective, hepatotoxicity limits its use. There is no evidence to support the use of finasteride. There are limited data to support the effectiveness of oral corticosteroids in the treatment of acne. Oral corticosteroid therapy is of temporary benefit in patients who have severe inflammatory acne. In patients who have well-documented adrenal hyperandrogenism, low-dose oral corticosteroids may be useful in treatment of acne.[44]

Oral Contraceptives Estrogen-containing oral contraceptives can be useful in the treatment of acne in some women. Those currently approved by the FDA for the management of acne contain norgestimate with ethinyl estradiol and norethindrone acetate with ethinyl estradiol. There is good evidence and consensus opinion that other estrogen-containing oral contraceptives are also equally effective.[44]

The Cochrane collaboration conducted a review in 2012 to determine the effectiveness of combination oral contraceptives (COCs) for the treatment of facial acne compared with placebo or other active therapies. Thirty-one trials with a total of 12,579 women were reviewed.[107]

COC use reduced inflammatory and noninflammatory facial lesion counts, severity grades, and self-assessed acne in nine placebo comparison trials, according to the review. Progestins included levonorgestrel, norethindrone acetate, norgestimate, drospirenone, dienogest, and chlormadinone acetate. There were fewer clear differences in trials that compared varying progestin types, showing no superiority, little differences, or conflicting results. No conclusions could be reached regarding the effect of a COC compared with an antibiotic because there was only one underpowered trial.[107]

Most studies assessed women over six treatment cycles, which might not be adequate for a chronic condition like acne. In two trials, patients were more likely to discontinue because of adverse events. Thus even if COCs improve acne, women might not be willing to accept long-term use for acne because of other side effects.

The review concluded that COCs should be considered for women with acne who also want an oral contraceptive. There is a need for more research into comparative effectiveness of COCs in randomized control trials, and into the acceptability and need for long-term use of COCs for acne.[107]

Spironolactone At higher doses, spironolactone is an antiandrogenic compound. Dosages of 50 mg to 200 mg have been shown to be effective in acne. Spironolactone may cause hyperkalemia, particularly when higher doses are prescribed or when there is cardiac or renal compromise. It occasionally causes menstrual irregularity. A 5% spironolactone gel, studied in patients with increased sebum secretion, resulted in a decrease in the total acne lesions with no significant efficacy under the acne severity index.[108]

Cyproterone Acetate Cyproterone combined with ethinyl estradiol (in the form of an oral contraceptive) has been found effective in the treatment of acne in females. Higher doses have been found more effective than lower doses. No cyproterone/estrogen-containing oral contraceptives are approved for use in the United States.[107]

Oral Corticosteroids Oral corticosteroids have two potential modes of activity in the treatment of acne. One study demonstrated that low-dose corticosteroids suppress adrenal activity in patients who have proven adrenal hyperactivity.[109] Expert opinion is that short courses of higher dose oral corticosteroids may be beneficial in patients with highly inflammatory disease.

Oral Isotretinoin Isotretinoin revolutionized the treatment of acne, yet its use and availability are increasingly complex. The risk of potential adverse effects must be weighed against its ability to prevent lifelong and permanent physical and psychological scarring.[110]

A good understanding of this agent's mechanisms and adverse effects is important. Oral isotretinoin is a natural metabolite of vitamin A. Its mechanism is elusive, as it does not bind to retinoid receptors. It has been shown to reduce sebogenesis and may also inhibit sebaceous gland activity, growth of *P. acnes*, inflammation, and improve follicular epithelial differentiation.[111] Systemic isotretinoin exerts a primary effect on comedogenesis, causing a decrease in size and reduction in formation of new comedones.[14] Isotretinoin is the only drug treatment for acne that produces prolonged remission.

Oral isotretinoin is approved for the treatment of severe recalcitrant nodular acne. Oral isotretinoin is also useful for the management of less severe acne that is treatment-resistant (unresponsive to adequate treatment, reasonable courses of antibiotic, or combination peelers and antibiotics administered for 6 weeks to 3 months) or that is producing either physical or psychologic scarring.[44]

The teratogenic effects of oral retinoid therapy are well documented. Because of its teratogenicity and the potential for many other adverse effects, this drug should be prescribed only by those physicians knowledgeable in its appropriate administration and monitoring. Female patients of child-bearing potential must only be treated with oral isotretinoin if they are participating in the approved pregnancy prevention and management program (i.e., iPLEDGE). Two different forms of contraception must be started 1 month before and continue at least 1 month (but normally 4 months) after therapy and pregnancy monitoring undertaken before, during, and after therapy.[110]

The approved dosage of isotretinoin is 0.5 to 2.0 mg/kg/day. The drug is usually given over a 20-week course. Drug absorption is greater when the drug is taken with food. Initial flaring can be minimized with a beginning dose of 0.5 mg/kg/day or less. Alternatively, lower doses can be used for longer time periods, with a total cumulative dose of 120 to 150 mg/kg. In patients with severely inflamed acne, an even greater initial dose reduction may be required. In the most severe cases of acne, consideration of pretreatment with oral corticosteroids may also be appropriate. When used, drying agents must be discontinued, and replaced with moisturizers. Some patients experience a relapse of acne after the first course of treatment with isotretinoin. Relapses are more common in younger adults or when lower doses are used.

Because isotretinoin is a vitamin A derivative, it interacts with many of the biologic systems of the body, and consequently has a significant pattern of adverse effects. The pattern is similar to that seen in hypervitaminosis A. Side effects include those of the mucocutaneous (most common), musculoskeletal, and ophthalmic systems, as well as headaches and central nervous system effects. Most of the adverse effects, such as cheilitis, and dry nose, eyes, and mouth, are temporary and resolve after the drug is discontinued.[110] Laboratory monitoring during therapy should include triglycerides, cholesterol, transaminases, and complete blood counts.

Mood disorders, depression, suicidal ideation, and suicides have been reported sporadically in patients taking this drug. A causal relationship has not been established. These symptoms are quite common in adolescents and young adults, the age range of patients who are likely to receive isotretinoin. This issue and other key unresolved considerations regarding isotretinoin continue to be the subject of investigations and are discussed as a Clinical Controversy in this chapter.

Clinical **Controversy. . .**

Accutane Considerations

After almost three decades of experience with oral isotretinoin, the published data and opinion of experts still differ with respect to its use as first-line or reserve therapy, optimal dosing, and risk of depression. The 2012 European Guidelines for the treatment of acne noted conflicting viewpoints from major opinion leaders.[12] It is important to put into perspective issues surround its responsible and informed use.[110]

Some directives persist in reserving isotretinoin use only for severe acne, nodular or conglobate acne that has not responded to appropriate antibiotics and topical therapy.[125] For many reasons, others recommend that isotretinoin should be considered the first-choice therapy for severe acne, given its clinical effectiveness, prevention of scarring, and quick improvement of a patient's quality of life, including minimizing depression. This position suggesting delaying the use of oral isotretinoin, the most effective choice, poses an ethical problem. Although comparative trials are missing, clinical experience confirms relapse rates after isotretinoin treatment are the lowest among available therapies.[12,126,127]

Evidence on best dosage, including cumulative dosage, is rare and partly conflicting for isotretinoin. In most trials, the higher doses associated with better response rates have less favorable safety/tolerability profiles. Attempts to determine the cumulative dose necessary to obtain an optimal treatment response and low relapse rate have not yet yielded sufficient evidence for a strong recommendation. Current expert opinion recommends for severe cases, a dosage of 0.3 to 0.5 mg, and for conglobate acne, a dose of 0.5 mg/kg or higher. Duration of therapy should be at least 6 months. For insufficient response, prolong treatment. Opinions vary on whether or not to restrict use to patients under 12 years and whether to avoid lasers, peelers or wax epilation for at least 6 months after discontinuation of therapy.[12,128]

The causal relationship between the use of isotretinoin and risk of depression continues to be scrutinized with no consensus. The issue is complex as depression and suicidal ideation occur with severe acne in the absence of isotretinoin.

There are instances in which withdrawal of isotretinoin has resulted in improved mood, and reintroduction of isotretinoin has resulted in the return of mood changes. Treatment of severe acne with isotretinoin is often associated with mood improvement.[44] There is epidemiologic evidence that the incidence of these events is less in patients treated with isotretinoin than in an age-matched general population. There is also evidence that the risk of depressed mood is no greater during isotretinoin therapy than during therapy of an age-matched acne group treated with conservative therapy.[44]

A systematic review published in 2005 did not find any evidence to support worsening of depression after use, and some depressive scores improved with use, but nine of these studies had limitations.[129] A retrospective cohort study in Sweden found attempted suicide increased in users, but an increased risk was present before treatment. An increased risk of attempted suicide was present 6 months after isotretinoin, suggesting patients should be monitored for suicidal behavior after treatment discontinuation.[130]

The current literature is insufficient to support a meaningful causative association, but important study limitations exist. In the absence of definitive evidence, an idiosyncratic effect cannot be excluded. Prescribers of isotretinoin are advised to note prior psychiatric symptoms, monitor patients at each visit for early recognition, and advise patients about a possible risk of depression and suicidal behavior.[12,129,130] This disputed association remains an important area for future research.

Pharmacologic Cleansing Options

Medicated Soaps and Washes Medicated soaps, washes, and foams may contain topical antiseptics such as triclosan; peeling agents such as salicylic acid, sulfur, antimicrobials such as benzoyl peroxide, clindamycin, or azelaic acid, alone or in combination in low concentrations. They may be nonprescription or prescription status.[111] Most washes should remain on the skin from 15 seconds to 5 minutes followed by thorough rinsing. This limits the amount of time the active ingredient is in contact with the skin. Other cleansers are applied after washing and left on the skin without rinsing.

Quaternary ammonium compounds are cationic detergents that are inactivated quickly in the presence of organic material, such as sebum. The duration of action of these products is short.

Bacteriostatic soaps, such as hexachlorophene, carbanilides, and salicylanilides (halogenated hydroxyphenols) may alter normal flora or be acnegenic. Few ordinary soaps induce acne. However, acne patients are particularly susceptible to comedogenic contactants, and if these soaps are applied several times daily for long periods, they may become troublesome.

Soaps containing coal tar, which can induce folliculitis, are not indicated for acne.

In a very small group of patients, a combination cleanser containing triclosan, azelaic acid, and salicylic acid produced a greater histopathologic decrease in inflammatory response compared with a nonmedicated cleanser, but there was no significant difference in noninflammatory lesions in either group.[111] Chlorhexidine inhibits in vitro growth of *P. acnes*.[112] A 4% chlorhexidine gluconate preparation in a detergent base has been shown to be as effective as benzoyl peroxide washes in patients with mild acne, and both preparations reduced the number of inflammatory and noninflammatory lesions after 8 and 12 weeks, compared with vehicle alone.[113]

Alcohol-detergent medicated pads, impregnated with salicylic acid 0.5%, have reduced inflammatory lesions and open comedones in mild to moderate acne. This type of medication is less abrasive, not rinsed off, and convenient.[114]

Alcohol-detergent wipes, swabs, or "pledgets" impregnated with antibiotics, such as clindamycin or lincomycin, are available. The antibiotic is deposited in low concentrations on the surface of the skin, and may not penetrate to the depths of the pilosebaceous duct. Although patients may like the convenience and perception of using an active agent, they should not be recommended over simple cleansing.

Abrasives consist of finely divided particles of fused aluminum or plastic together with cleansing and wetting agents. Abrasives peel and remove surface debris and may assist resorption of papules and pustules. Despite vigorous rubbing, removal of comedones is not accomplished. Particles containing active agents, such as sodium tetraborate decahydrate, dissolve on use, and their abrasiveness is therefore limited.[115] The effectiveness of an abrasive cleanser with and without polyethylene granules showed no difference in results in patients with mild to moderate acne. These products are not indicated in most cases but may be used in a patient who responds empirically.[116]

Personalized Pharmacotherapy

The individualized treatment of certain patient groups, including infants, children, pregnant women, and persons of color is described under Special Populations.

Providers and patients must also weigh costs and drug availability in choosing a treatment regimen. One study showed that the average total cost of treatment per episode across all age groups is US$689.06.[143] Topical retinoids and fixed-dose combination therapies are in general more expensive than benzoyl peroxide preparations. Laser treatments and cosmetic procedures are also very costly. The economics of long-term maintenance therapy should be borne in mind when selecting a regimen. Patients should not spend large amounts on herbals and botanicals, as well as home remedies, given the lack of current good evidence to support their use. As acne is a chronic disease extending over many years, total cost implications are important and affect adherence and response.

Other practical considerations include the need for refrigeration of some products such as antibiotics. Local patterns of resistance should be kept in mind in choosing antibiotics. Extent and area of lesion involvement when large or inaccessible (e.g., the back or trunk) as well as ease of application may determine the choice of route between topical and systemic therapy. The natural skin predilection toward oiliness versus dryness may dictate the choice of vehicle. Dietary interactions should be born in mind with certain drugs such as oral tetracycline. Sunscreens will need to be used with photosensitizers, and applied as the first topical agent.

Regimens that may require more frequency of application may be difficult for students or patients whose occupation limits flexibility. History of poor adherence because of intolerance of topical treatments may be countered by reducing the strength of treatment, using a different preparation of the drug, or switching to an alternative topical agent that causes less irritation.

EVALUATION OF THERAPEUTIC OUTCOMES

10 Provide a monitoring framework for patients with acne. Parameters should be monitored by the patient and recorded in a diary. Therapy should be appropriately tapered in response to improvement or resolution. The healthcare professional should be responsible for ensuring that the treatment plan remains on schedule and is effective with no adverse effects. The patient should be contacted within 2 to 3 weeks to determine progress.

Acne is poorly understood by adolescents. These patients often lack knowledge of the cause of the disorder and aggravating factors, indications for self-care versus prescription treatment, expected onset of effect, sequence of the healing process, duration of treatment, appropriate application of topical agents, maximal achievable effects, expected adverse effects, safety concerns, and the benefit to quality of life. Clinicians should review patient understanding of each of these important factors to ensure patient adherence. There is often a need to supplement counseling sessions with written materials to which the patient can refer at home.

Good adherence is the key to treatment success. Other strategies to increase adherence include use of once-daily regimens, online followup visits, and remote digital imaging for ongoing lesion assessment.[143–145]

Monitoring of the Pharmaceutical Care Plan

Tables 77-2, 77-3, and 77-4 provide a guide for monitoring patients with acne. Table 77-2 outlines individual drugs, their most common adverse effects, parameters to monitor, and issues to note. Table 77-3 outlines general effectiveness and safety end points, monitoring parameters, and degree of change and timeframes for short- and long-term outcomes. Table 77-4 is a guide for monitoring acne patients with consideration to the severity grading of acne types I through IV.

CONCLUSIONS

Considerable gaps remain in the understanding of acne, despite all that is known about the pathogenesis of acne and the mechanisms of effective drugs for controlling its symptoms, progression, and complications at structural, biochemical, and physiologic levels. It is still not possible to precisely define the cause of one of the most common skin diseases, nor is it possible to identify a cure for a condition that affects a very large proportion of the global population.

ABBREVIATIONS

BGA	best guidelines acne
CAM	complementary and alternative medication
COC	combination oral contraceptive
CRH	corticotropin-releasing hormone
FDA	U.S. Food and Drug Administration
HGL	high glycemic load
IGF	insulin-like growth factor
MMPP	mild to moderate papulopustular
P. acnes	*Propionibacterium acnes*
PAPA	pyogenic arthritis, pyoderma gangrenosum, acne
PDT	photodynamic therapy
QOL	quality of life
SAPHO	synovitis, acne, pustulosis, hyperostosis, osteitis syndrome
SPF	sun protection factor
TTO	time trade-off

TABLE 77-2 Monitoring of Medications Used in Acne Treatment and Maintenance Therapy

Drug	Adverse Drug Reaction	Monitoring Parameter	Comments
Exfoliants			
Resorcinol	Irritant and sensitizer	Degree and/or changes in signs or symptoms of irritancy (redness, discomfort, peeling, skin breakdown or dermatitis).	Should not be applied to large areas of the skin or on broken skin.
Sulfur	Avoid eye contact—slight ophthalmic and skin irritation	Degree and/or changes in signs or symptoms of irritancy (redness, discomfort, peeling, skin breakdown or dermatitis). Use should be discontinued if excessive irritation results.	
Salicylic acid	Mild irritant—burning and reddening, local skin peeling	Degree and/or changes in signs or symptoms of irritancy (redness, discomfort, peeling, skin breakdown or dermatitis).	Begin with a low concentration and increase as tolerance develops. Not a sensitizer.
Retinoids			
Isotretinoin	Side effects: mucocutaneous (most common), musculoskeletal, and ophthalmic systems. Common: dryness of mucus membranes (lips, mouth, eyes, nose) dry skin, itching, hair loss, thirst, back pain, myalgia, headaches, and central nervous system effects. Increased cholesterol. Teratogenic. Sun sensitivity. Depression and suicide—controversial.	Test for pregnancy twice before starting. Contraceptive measures must be started 1 month prior, continued during the 2 months of treatment and for at least 1 month after stopping treatment (but normally 4 months). Laboratory monitoring during therapy should include triglycerides, cholesterol, transaminases, and complete blood counts (before, during and after treatment). Degree and/or changes in signs or symptoms of irritancy to skin (redness, discomfort, peeling, skin breakdown or dermatitis). Degree and/or changes in signs or symptoms of irritancy to mucous membranes (mouth, nose, eyes). Instances of headache or central nervous system symptoms. Note prior psychiatric symptoms, monitor patients at each visit for early recognition of changes in mood or psychological well-being (before, during and after treatment).	Drying agents must be discontinued. Sun avoidance strategies and sunscreen use recommended. Vitamin A supplementation. Use moisturizers (lip balm, nasal moisturizers, eye lubricants, temp removal of contacts). Most adverse effects, such as cheilitis, and dry nose, eyes and mouth, are temporary and resolve after the drug is discontinued. Advise patients about a possible risk of depression and suicidal behavior.
Tretinoin/ Retinoic acid	Common: erythema, dryness, burning, photosensitization. Rare: true contact allergy. Use cautiously in pregnancy. (Irritation: tazarotene > retinoic acid > adapalene)	Degree and/or changes in signs or symptoms of irritancy to skin (redness, discomfort, peeling, skin breakdown or dermatitis). Skin changes in areas of sun exposure—dermatitis or hives.	Additive effects with concomitant topical drying medications; products with high concentrations of alcohol, astringents, abrasive soaps, etc. Gels and creams are less irritating than solutions. Sun avoidance strategies and sunscreen use recommended.
Adapalene	Side effects include erythema, xerosis, burning and desquamation. Less irritation than other retinoids. Photoirritation or sensitization.	Degree and/or changes in signs or symptoms of irritancy to skin (redness, discomfort, peeling, skin breakdown or dermatitis). Skin changes in areas of sun exposure—dermatitis or hives.	Less photosensitivity than other agents. Sun avoidance strategies and sunscreen use recommended.
Tazarotene	Side effects include irritation, erythema, xerosis, burning and desquamation.	Skin changes in areas of sun exposure—dermatitis or hives.	Contraindicated in pregnancy due to the large surface area. Short contact therapy, 1–5 minutes every other night, gradually increasing to overnight advocated for dosing in patients with sensitive skin. Oily complexions may tolerate twice daily, short contact time.
Topical Antimicrobial Agents			
Benzoyl peroxide	Dryness and peeling appear after a few days; erythema; burning; pruritus. Rare reports of contact allergic dermatitis. May bleach hair and clothing. Body odor, odor on clothes and bed sheets. Irritation is concentration dependent—most frequent with 10% gel. Irritation from gels used as vehicles—water-based < alcohol = acetone	Once tolerance is achieved, the strength may be increased to 5% or the base changed to the acetone or alcohol gels, or to paste. Degree and/or changes in signs or symptoms of irritancy to skin (redness, discomfort, peeling, skin breakdown or dermatitis). Hives.	Increased skin irritation or drying effect with other medications, soaps, and cosmetics with strong drying effect. Chemically incompatible with retinoic acid. Cross-reactions with other sensitizers, such as Peruvian balsam, cinnamon, and other benzoic acid derivatives (topical anesthetics).
Clindamycin	Erythema, peeling, itching, dryness and burning	Signs or symptoms of irritancy to skin (redness, discomfort, peeling, skin breakdown or dermatitis).	

(*continued*)

TABLE 77-2 Monitoring of Medications Used in Acne Treatment and Maintenance Therapy (*Continued*)

Drug	Adverse Drug Reaction	Monitoring Parameter	Comments
Oral Antibiotics			
Erythromycin	Gastrointestinal upset (nausea, vomiting, diarrhea) Vaginal candidiasis	If gastrointestinal adverse effects occur, monitor hydration Vaginal discharge	Drug interactions: Inhibits CYP1A2 and CYP3A4: carbamazepine, cyclosporine, theophylline, and warfarin. Safe in pregnant women and children.
Tetracyclines	Gastrointestinal intolerance: (tetracycline > erythromycin > doxycycline = minocycline) Vaginal candidiasis Photosensitivity is dose-dependent (doxycycline > tetracycline).	Vaginal discharge. Skin changes in areas of sun exposure—dermatitis or hives.	Contraindicated in pregnant women or in children younger than 9 years of age. Absorption decreased by food, chelated by antacids and milk. To be taken on an empty stomach.
Minocycline	Drug-induced lupus. Pigment changes in skin, mucous membranes, and teeth. Hepatitis. Urticaria. Dose-related dizziness (resolves with dose titration). Autoimmune hepatitis and hypersensitivity syndrome.	Vaginal discharge. Skin changes in areas of sun exposure—dermatitis or hives. Changes or discoloration of skin, teeth, or mucous membranes. Monitor degree of dizziness as dose is titrated. Signs of hypersensitivity syndrome: fever, dermatitis, blistering reactions; systemic symptoms such as malaise, changes in blood pressure or renal function.	Contraindicated in pregnant women or in children younger than 9 years of age. Decreased gastrointestinal absorption with Fe, Ca, Mg, Al. Sun avoidance strategies and sunscreen use recommended.
Doxycycline	Gastrointestinal upset. Photosensitizer (especially at higher doses).	If gastrointestinal side effects occur, monitor hydration. Skin changes in areas of sun exposure—dermatitis or hives.	Contraindicated in pregnant women or in children younger than 9 years of age. Sun avoidance strategies and sunscreen use recommended.
Antisebum			
Combination oral contraceptives	Breakthrough bleeding, headache. Serious: venous thromboembolism, hepatotoxicity.	Spotting or bleeding.	Oral antibiotics may decrease contraceptive efficacy—(significance controversial).
Spironolactone	Common: hyperkalemia, menstrual irregularity, gynecomastia, breast tenderness	Menstrual signs. Breast changes.	
Antiinflammatory			
Azelaic acid	Primary: pruritus, burning, stinging, and tingling Other: erythema, dryness, rash, peeling, irritation, dermatitis, and contact dermatitis - in less than 1% of patients	Skin changes in areas of sun exposure—dermatitis or hives	Adverse reactions are generally transient and mild in nature.
Dapsone	Short- and long-term safety and efficacy demonstrated. Peeling, dryness, and erythema.	Skin changes in areas of sun exposure—dermatitis or hives	Does not induce phototoxicity or photoallergy in human dermal safety studies. Medications such as rifampin, anticonvulsants, trimethoprim/sulfamethoxazole, and St. John's wort may increase formation of dapsone hydroxylamine (toxicity).

Al, aluminum; Ca, calcium; Fe, iron; Mg, magnesium.

TABLE 77-3 Monitoring Therapy for Acne: Parameters and Frequency

Person Responsible and Frequencies for Monitoring:

Patient: daily while on drug therapy; Pharmacist: every 4–8 wk of therapy or next pharmacy visit

Parameter	Time Frame/Degree of Change	Actions
	Short-Term Effectiveness End Points (Acne Resolution/Control)	
Lesion count	Decrease by 10–25% within 4–8 wk, with control, or more than a 50% decrease within 2–4 mo	If end points not achieved, refer to a physician for further therapy.
Comedones	Resolve by 3–4 mo	
Inflammatory lesions	Resolve within a few weeks	
Anxiety, depression	Achieve control or improvement within 2–4 mo	
	Long Term	
Progression of severity	No progression of severity	If end points not achieved, refer to a physician for further therapy.
Recurrent episodes	Lengthening of acne-free periods throughout therapy	
Scarring or pigmentation	No further scarring or pigmentation throughout therapy	
	Safety End Points (Treatment Side Effects)	
Dermatitis, increased dryness, gastrointestinal upset, photosensitivity	No adverse effects	Refer to a physician for alternate therapy, dose reduction, discontinuation or additive palliative treatment or preventative measures for adverse effects.

TABLE 77-4 Monitoring Care Plans for Acne Types I through IV

Acne Type	Description	Suggested Options	Followup Action If Patient Responds	Followup Action If Patient Does Not Respond in 3 Months	Adjustment in Therapy If Patient Does Not Respond Adequately to Previous Action
Type I	Mainly comedones with an occasional small inflamed papule or pustule; no scarring present	Topical retinoid is the drug of choice; can also consider benzoyl peroxide or salicylic acid	Continue until lesions are completely cleared and then stop or taper therapy.	Treat as Type II acne	
Type II	Comedones and more numerous papules and pustules (mainly facial); mild scarring	Topical retinoid plus benzoyl peroxide, topical or antibiotic	Continue until lesions are completely cleared and then stop or taper therapy.	Treat as Type III acne	
Type III	Numerous comedones, papules and pustules, spreading to the back, chest and shoulders, with an occasional cyst or nodule; moderate scarring	Systemic antibiotic plus topical retinoid, or benzoyl peroxide *Or*	Oral antibiotics typically are prescribed for daily use over 4–6 mo, with subsequent tapering and discontinuation as acne improves. Other agents can also be stopped or tapered at this time.	Add oral contraceptive or antiandrogen (women only)	Oral isotretinoin (except in women who are or who may become pregnant); consider safety end points (potential adverse effects) before initiating therapy
Type IV	Numerous large cyst on the face, neck and upper trunk; severe scarring	Systemic antibiotic plus topical retinoid, and benzoyl peroxide ± oral contraceptive or antiandrogen (females only)	Oral antibiotics typically are prescribed for daily use over 4–6 mo, with subsequent tapering and discontinuation as acne improves. Other agents can also be stopped or tapered at this time.	If no response after 3–6 mo, oral isotretinoin (except in women who are or who may become pregnant). Consider safety end points (potential adverse effects) before initiating therapy.	

REFERENCES

1. Cunliffe WJ, Gould DJ. Prevalence of facial acne vulgaris in late adolescence and in adults. Br Med J 1979;1:1109–1110.
2. Rademaker M, Garioch JJ, Simpson NB. Acne in schoolchildren: No longer a concern for dermatologists. BMJ 1989;298:1217–1219.
3. Kilkenny M, Merlin K, Plunkett A, Marks R. The prevalence of common skin conditions in Australian school children, III: Acne vulgaris. Br J Dermatol 1998;139:840–845.
4. Nijsten T, Rombouts S, Lambert J. Acne is prevalent but use of its treatments is infrequent among adolescents from the general population. J Eur Acad Dermatolog Venereol 2007;21:163–168.
5. Smithard A, Glazebrook C, Williams HC. Acne prevalence, knowledge about acne and psychological morbidity in mid-adolescence: A community-based study. Br J Dermatol 2001;41:577–580.
6. Pandey SS. Epidemiology of acne vulgaris. Indian J Dermatol 1983;28:109–110.
7. Kubba R, Bajaj AK, Thappa DM, et al. Acne in India: Guidelines for management—IAA Consensus Document: Epidemiology of acne. Indian J Dermatol Venereol Leprol 2009;75(suppl 1):S3.
8. Shalita AR. Acne vulgaris: Pathogenesis and treatment. Cosmet Toiletries 1983;98:57–60.
9. Malus M, LaChance PA, Lamy L, Macaulay A, Vanasse M. Priorities in adolescent health care: The teenagers' viewpoint. J Fam Pract 1987;25:159–162.
10. Rosenberg EW. Acne diet reconsidered. Arch Dermatol 1981;117(4):193–195.
11. Fulton JE, Plewig G, Kligman AM. Effect of chocolate on acne vulgaris. JAMA 1969;210:2071.
12. Nast A, Dreno B, Bettoli V, et al. Guidelines for the treatment of acne. Journal of the European Academy of Dermatology and Venereology 2012;26(suppl 1):1–29.
13. Chu A. Acne vulgaris. In Lebwohl MG, Heyman WR, Berth-Jones J, Couslon I, eds. Treatment of Skin Diseases, 2nd ed. Philadelphia, PA: Mosby Elsevier, 2006:6–12.
14. Dreno B, Poli F. Epidemiology of acne. Dermatology 2003;206:7–10.
15. Tucker SB, Rogers S, Winkleman RK. Inflammation in acne vulgaris: Leukocyte attraction and cytotoxicity by comedonal material. J Invest Dermatol 1985;74:21–25.
16. Winston MH, Shalita AR. Acne vulgaris. Pediatr Clin North Am 1991;38(4):889–903.
17. Plewig G, Kligman AM. The dynamics of primary comedo formation. In: Plewig G, Kligman AM, eds. Acne: Morphogenesis and Treatment. New York: Springer-Verlag, 1975:58–107.
18. Puissegur-Lupo M. Acne vulgaris, treatments and their rationale. Postgrad Med 1985;78(7):76–88.
19. Batra RS. Acne. In: Arndt KA, Tsu JTS, eds. Manual of Dermatologic Therapeutics, 7th ed. Philadelphia, PA: Lippincott, Williams and Wilkins, 2007:3–18.
20. U.S. Department of Health and Human Services Food and Drug Administration Center for Drug Evaluation and Research (CDER). Guidance for Industry. Acne vulgaris: developing drugs for treatment. 2005, *http://www.fda.gov/dowloads/Drugs/GuidanceComplianceRegulatoryInformation/GuideancesCM071292.pdf.*
21. Harrison-Atlas R, Bernhard JD, O'Connor RC, Weinraub LF. What to do when typical teenage acne strikes. JCOM 1996;3:9.
22. Pochi PE, Shalita AR, Straus JC, et al. Report of the consensus conference on acne classification. J Am Acad Dermatol 1991;24(3):495–500.

23. Chren MM, Lasek RJ, Quinn LM, et al. Skindex, a quality-of-life measure for patients with skin disease. Reliability, validity and responsiveness. J Invest Dermatol 1996;107(5):707–713.
24. Finlay AY, Khan GK. Dermatology Quality of Life Index (DLQI): A simple practical measure for routine clinical use. Clin Exp Dermatol 1994;19(3):210–106.
25. Girman CJ, Hartmaier S, Thiboutot D, et al. Evaluating health-related quality of life in patients with facial acne: Development of a self-administered questionnaire for clinical trials. Qual Life Res 1996;5(5):481–490.
26. Gupta MA, Johnson AM, Gupta AK. The development of an acne quality of life scale: Reliability, validity and relationship to subjective acne severity in mild to moderate acne vulgaris. Acta Derm Venereol 1998;78(6):451–456.
27. Wang KC and Zane LT. Recent advances in acne vulgaris research: Insights and clinical implications. In: James, WD, ed. Advances in Dermatology. Philadelphia, PA: Elsevier, 2008:197–209.
28. Johnson BA, Nunley JR. Topical therapy for acne vulgaris: How do you choose the best drug for each patient? Postgrad Med J 2000;107(3):69–80.
29. Habif TP. Acne, rosacea, and related disorders. In: Klein EA, Menczer BS, eds. Clinical Dermatology. Toronto: Mosby, 1990:756.
30. Kelly AP. Acne and related disorders. In: Sams WM, Lynch PJ, eds. Principles and Practice of Dermatology. New York: Churchill Livingstone, 1990:1014.
31. MacDonald Hull S, Sunliffe WJ. The use of a corticosteroid cream for immediate reduction in the clinical signs of acne vulgaris. Acta Derm Venereol 1989;69(5):452–453.
32. Brodell RT, O'Brien MR. Topical corticosteroid-induced acne: three treatment strategies to break the "addiction cycle." Postgrad Med 1999;106(6):225–229.
33. Hitch JM. Acneform eruption induced by drugs and chemicals. JAMA 1969;200:879.
34. Boothroyd, S. Topical therapy and formulation principles. In: Webster GF, Rawlings AV, eds. Acne and its therapy. New York: Informa Healthcare USA, 2007:253–274.
35. Choi YS, Suh HS, Yoon MY, et al. A study of the efficacy of cleansers for acne vulgaris. J Dermatol Treat 2010;21(3):201–205.
36. Food and Drug Administration. Non-prescription drugs. 2009, *http://www.fda.gov/OHRMS/DOCKETS/98fr/78n-0065-npr0003.pdf.*
37. Russell JJ. Topical therapy for acne. Am Fam Physician 2000;61(2):357–365.
38. Epinette WW, Gresit MC, Osols II. The role of cosmetics in postadolescent acne. Cutis 1982;29(5):500–514.
39. Plewig G, Kligman AM. Acne cosmetica. In: Plewig G, Kligman AM, eds. Acne: Morphogenesis and Treatment. New York: Springer-Verlag, 1975;226–229.
40. Mills OH, Kligman AM. Comedogenicity of sunscreens. experimental observations in rabbits. Arch Dermatol 1982;18(6):417–419.
41. Cappel M Mauger D, Thiboutet D. Correlation between serum levels of insulin-like growth factor 1, dehydroepiandrosterone sulfate, an dihydrotestosterone and acne lesion counts in adult women. Arch Dermatol 2005;141:333.
42. Thiboutot DM. New treatments and therapeutic strategies for acne. Arch Fam Med 2000;9(2):179–187.
43. Chiou WL. Low intrinsic drug activity and dominant vehicle (Placebo) effect in the topical treatment of acne vulgaris. Int J Clin Pharmacol Therapeut 2012;50(6):434–437.
44. Strauss JS, Kowchk DP, Leyden JJ, et al. Guidelines of care for acne vulgaris management. J Am Acad Dermatol 2007;56:651–663.
45. Ellerbroek WC. Hypotheses toward a unified field theory of human behavior with clinical application to acne vulgaris. Perspect Biol Med 1973;16:240–262.
46. Hughes H, Brown BW, Lawlis GF, Fulton JE Jr. Treatment of acne vulgaris by biofeedback relaxation and cognitive imagery. J Psychosom Res 1983;27:185–191.
47. Chao CM, Lai WY, Wu BY, Chang HC, Huang WS, Chen YF. A pilot study on efficacy treatment of acne vulgaris using a new method: Results of a randomized double-blind trial with Acne Dressing. J Cosmet Sci 2006;57(2):95–105.
48. Rhei LD, Zatz JL, Motwani MR. Targeted delivery of actives from topical treatment products to the pilosebaceous unit. In: Webster GF, Rawlings AV, eds. Acne and Its Therapy. New York: Informa Healthcare USA, 2007:223–252.
49. Thiboutot D, Gollnick H, Bettoli V, et al. New Insights into the management of acne: an update from the Global Alliance to Improve Outcomes in Acne Group. J Am Acad Dermatolog 2009;60:S1–S50.
50. Magin PJ, Adams J, Pond CD, et al. Topical and oral CAM in acne: A review of the empirical evidence and a consideration of its context. Complement Ther Med 2006;14:62–76.
51. Li B, Chair H Du YH, et al. Evaluation of therapeutic effect and safety for clinical randomized and controlled trials of treatment of acne with acupuncture and moxibustion. Zhongguo Zhen Jiu 2009;247–251.
52. Reuter J, Merfort I Schempp CM. Botanicals in dermatology: an evidence-based review. Am J Clin Dermatol 2010;11:247–67.
53. Ernst E, Huntley A. Tea-tree oil: A systematic review of randomized clinical trials. Forsch Komplementarmed Klass Natureheilkd 2000;7:17–20.
54. Eisenberg DM, Davis RB, Ettner SL, et al. Trends in alternative medicine use in the United States, 1990–1997: Results of a follow-up national survey. JAMA 1998;280(18):1569–1575.
55. Cae H, Liu JP, Smith CA et a. Complementary therapies for acne vulgaris (Protocol). The Cochrane collaboration, issue 11. New York: Wiley, 2011. *http://www.thecochranelibrary.com.*
56. Poli F, Ribet V, Lauze C, Adhoute H, Morinet P. Efficacy and safety of 0.1% retinaldehyde/6% glycolic acid (Diacneal) for mild to moderate acne vulgaris. A multicentre, double-blind, randomized, vehicle-controlled trial. Dermatol 2005;210(suppl 1):14–21.
57. Food and Drug Administration. Non-prescription drugs. 2009, *http://www.fda.gov/OHRMS/DOCKETS/98fr/78n-0065-npr0003.pdf.*
58. Katsambas AD, Katoulis AC, Stavropoulos P. Acne neonatorum: A study of 22 cases. Int J Dermatol 1999;38(2):128–130.
59. Callender VD. Fitzpatrick skin types and clindamycin phosphate 1.2%/benzoyl peroxide gel: Efficacy and tolerability of treatment in moderate to severe acne. J Drugs Dermatol 2012;11(5):643–648.
60. Brown S. Therapeutic potpourri. Dermatol Clin 1989;7(1):71–74.
61. Sykes NL, Webster GF. Acne: A review of optimum treatment. Drugs 1994;48(1):59–70.
62. Zouboulis CC. Moderne aknetherapie. Akt Dermatol 2003;29:49–57.
63. Zander E, Weisman S. Treatment of acne vulgaris with salicylic acid pads. Clin Ther 1992;14:247–253.
64. Gross, G. Benzoyl peroxide and salicylic acid therapy. In: Webster GF, Rawlings AV, eds. Acne and Its Therapy. New York: Informa Healthcare USA, 2007:117–136.

65. Shalita AR. Treatment of mild and moderate acne vulgaris with salicylic acid in an alcohol-detergent vehicle. Cutis 1981;28:556–561.
66. Kligman D, Kligman AM. Salicylic acid as a peeling agent for the treatment of acne. Cosmetic Dermatol 1997;10:44–47.
67. Lin AN, Reimer RJ, Carter DM. Sulfur revisited. J Am Acad Dermatol 1988;18:553–558.
68. Kroshinsky D, Shalita AR, Topical retinoids. In Webster GF, Rawlings AV, eds. Acne and Its Therapy. New York: Informa Healthcare USA, 2007:103–112.
69. Galvin SA, Gilbert R, Baker M, Guibal F, Tuley MR. Comparative tolerance of adapalene 0.1% gel and six different tretinoin formulations. Br J Dermatol 1998;139(suppl 52):34–40.
70. Mills OH Jr, Berger RS. Irritation potential of a new topical tretinoin formulation and a commercially-available tretinoin formulation as measured by patch testing in human subjects. J Am Acad Dermatol 1998;38:S11–S16.
71. Jeremy AHT, Holland DB, Roberts SG, et al. Inflammatory events are involved in acne lesion initiation. J Invest Dermatol 2003;139:897–900.
72. Shroot B, Michel S. Pharmacology and chemistry of adapalene. J Am Acad Dermatol 1997;36(6):S96–S103.
73. Weiss JS, Shavin JS. Adapalene for the treatment of acne vulgaris. J Am Acad Dermatol 1998;39(2):50–54.
74. Brogden R, Goa K. Adapalene: A review of its pharmacological properties and clinical potential in the management of mild to moderate acne. Drugs 1997;53(3):511–519.
75. Verschoore M, Langner A, Wolska M, Jablonska S, Czernielewski J, Schaefer H. Vehicle controlled study of CD 271 lotion in the topical treatment of acne vulgaris. J Invest Dermatol 1993;100:221.
76. Russell JJ. Topical therapy for acne. Am Fam Physician 2000;61(2):357–365.
77. Kakita L. Tazarotene versus tretinoin or adapalene in the treatment of acne vulgaris. J Am Acad Dermatol 2000; 43(2 pt 3):851–854.
78. Tzellos T, Toulis KA, Dessinioti C, et al. Topical retinoids for the treatment of acne vulgaris (protocol). The Cochrane collaboration, issue 12. New York: Wiley, 2011. *http://www.thecochranelibrary.com.*
79. Gross, G. Benzoyl peroxide and salicylic acid therapy, In: In Webster GF, Rawlings AV, eds. Acne and Its Therapy. New York: Informa Healthcare USA, 2007:117–136.
80. Zander E, Weisman S. Treatment of acne vulgaris with salicylic acid pads. Clin Ther 1992;14:247–253.
81. Zouboulis CC. Moderne aknetherapie. Akt Dermatol 2003; 29:49–57.
82. Gollnick H, Schramm M. Topical drug treatments in acne. Dermatol 1998;196:119–125.
83. Cotterill JA. Benzoyl peroxide. Acta Derm Venereol 1980;89(suppl):57–63.
84. Cunliffe WJ, Holland KT. The effect of benzoyl peroxide on acne. Acta Derm Venereol 1981;61(3):267–269.
85. Lassus A. Local treatment of acne. A clinical study and evaluation of the effect of different concentrations of benzoyl peroxide gel. Curr Med Res Opin 1981;7(6): 370–373.
86. Cunliffe WJ, Dodman B, Eady R. Benzoyl peroxide in acne. Practitioner 1978;220(3):470–482.
87. Maddin S. Benzoyl peroxide. Can J Dermatol 1989;1(4):92.
88. Report of the Expert Advisory Committee on Dermatology. The carcinogenic activity of benzoyl peroxide. Information Letter Ottawa: Health Protection Branch (Canada) 1987;711:1–9.
89. Cunliffe WJ, Burke B. Benzoyl peroxide: Lack of sensitization. Acta Derm Venereol 1982;62(5): 458–459.
90. Tkach JR. Allergic contact urticaria to benzoyl peroxide. Cutis 1982;29(2):187–188.
91. Rietschel RL, Duncan SH. Benzoyl peroxide reactions in an acne study group. Contact Dermatitis 1982;8:323–326.
92. Bowman S, Gold M, Nasir A, Vamvakias G. Comparison of clindamycin/benzoyl peroxide, tretinoin plus clindamycin, and the combination of clindamycin/benzoyl peroxide and tretinoin plus clindamycin in the treatment of acne vulgaris: A randomized, blinded study. J Drug Dermatol 2005;4(5): 611–618.
93. Korkut C, Piskin S. Benzoyl peroxide, adapalene, and their combination in the treatment of acne vulgaris. J Dermatol 2005;2(3):169–173.
94. Bikowski JB. Clinical experience results with clindamycin 1% benzoyl peroxide 5% gel (Duac) as monotherapy and in combination. J Drug Dermatol 2005;4(2):164–171.
95. Burkhart CG, Burkhart CN. Treatment of acne vulgaris without antibiotics: Tertiary amine-benzoyl peroxide combination vs. benzoyl peroxide alone (Proactiv Solution). Int J Dermatol 2007;46(1):89–93.
96. Gamble R, Dunn J, Dawson A, et al. Topical antimicrobial treatment of acne vulgaris: An evidence-based review. Am J Clin Dermatol 2012;13(3):141–152.
97. Tanghetti E, Abramovits W, Solomon B, Loven K, Shalita A. Tazarotene versus tazarotene plus clindamycin/benzoyl peroxide in the treatment of acne vulgaris: A multicenter, double-blind, randomized parallel-group trial. J Drugs Dermatol 2006;5(3):256–261.
98. Del Rosso JQ, Tanghetti E. The clinical impact of vehicle technology using a patented formulation of 5%/clindamycin 1% gel: Comparative assessments of skin tolerability and evaluation of combination use with a topical retinoid. J Drug Dermatol 2006;5(2):160–164.
99. Webster, G. Antimicrobial therapy in acne. In: In Webster GF, Rawlings AV, eds. Acne and Its Therapy. New York: Informa Healthcare USA, 2007:97–102.
100. Bottomly WW, Cunliffe WJ. Oral trimethoprim as a third line antibiotic in the management of acne vulgaris. Dermatol 1993;187:193–196.
101. Dalzeil K, Dykes PJ, Marks R. The effect of tetracycline and erythromycin in a model of acne-type inflammation. Br J Exp Pathol 1987;68:67–70.
102. Garner SE, Eady A, Bennett C, et al. Minocycline for acne vulgaris: efficacy and safety (review). The Cochrane collaboration, issue 9. New York: Wiley, 2012. *http://www.thecochranelibrary.com.*
103. Hughes BR, Murphy CE, Barnett J, Cunliffe WJ. Strategy of acne therapy with long-term antibiotics. Br J Dermatol 1989;121:623–628.
104. Passi S, Picardo M, De Luca C, Nazzaro-Porro M. Mechanism of azelaic acid action in acne. G Ital Dermatol Venereol 1989;10:455–463.
105. Draelos ZD, Carter E, Maloney JM, et al. Two randomized studies demonstrate the efficacy and safety of dapsone gel, 5% for the treatment of acne vulgaris. J Am Acad Dermatol. 2007;56(3):439 p1–10.
106. Fleischer AB, Jr., Shalita A, Eichenfield LF, et al. Dapsone gel 5% in combination with adapalene gel 0.1%, benzoyl peroxide gel 4% or moisturizer for the treatment of acne vulgaris: A 12-week, randomized, double-blind study. J Drugs Dermatol 2010;9(1):33–40.
107. Arowojolu AO, Gall MR, Lopez LM, et al. Combined oral contraceptive pills for treatment of acne. The Cochrane

collaboration, issue 7. New York: Wiley, 2012. *http://www.thecochranelibrary.com.*

108. Afzli BM, Yaghoobi E, Yaghoobi R, et al. Comparison of the efficacy of 5% topical spironolactone gel and placebo in the treatment of mild and moderate acne vulgaris: A randomized controlled trial. J Dermatol Treat 2012;23(1):21–25.
109. Nader S, Rodriguez-Rigau LJ, Smith KD, Steinberger E. Acne and hyperandrogenism: Impact of lowering androgen levels with glucocorticoid treatment. J Am Acad Dermatol 1984;11:256–259.
110. Lowenstein EB, Lowenstein EJ. Isotretinoin systemic therapy and the shadow cast upon dermatology's downtrodden hero. Clin Dermatol 2011;29:652–661.
111. Rawlings, AV. The molecular biology of retinoids and their receptors. In: In Webster GF, Rawlings AV, eds. Acne and Its Therapy. New York: Informa Healthcare USA, 2007:45–53.
112. Choi YS, Suh HS, Yoon MY, et al. A study of the efficacy of cleansers for acne vulgaris. J Dermatol Treat 2010;21(3): 201–205.
113. Stoughton RB, Leyden JJ. Efficacy of 4 percent chlorhexidine gluconate skin cleanser in the treatment of acne vulgaris. Cutis 1987;39(6):551–553.
114. Shalita AR. Treatment of mild and moderate acne vulgaris with salicylic acid in an alcohol-detergent vehicle. Cutis 1982;28(11):556–568.
115. Arndt KA. Acne. In: Arndt KA, ed. Manual of Dermatologic Therapeutics, 4th ed. Toronto: Little Brown, 1989:3–13.
116. Fulgha CC, Caltalano PM, Childers RC, et al. Abrasive cleansing in the management of acne vulgaris. Arch Dermatol 1982;118(9):658–659.
117. Elman M. The effective treatment of acne vulgaris by a high-intensity, narrow band 405–420 nm light source. J Cosmet Laser Ther 2003;5:111.
118. Friedman PM. Treatment of inflammatory facial acne vulgaris with the 1450-nm diode laser: A pilot study. Dermatol Surg 2004;30:147.
119. Mariwalla K. Use of lasers and light-based therapies for treatment of acne vulgaris. Lasers Surg Med 2005;37:33.
120. Ross EV. Optical treatments for acne. Dermatol Ther 2005;18:253.
121. Lloyd JR. Selective photothermolysis of the sebaceous glands for acne treatment. Lasers Surg Med 2002;31:115.
122. Böhm M, Luger TA. The pilosebaceous unit is part of the skin immune system. Dermatol 1998;196(1):75–79.
123. Seaton E. Investigation of the mechanism of action of nonablative pulsed-dye laser therapy in photorejuvenation and inflammatory acne vulgaris. Brit J Dermatol 2006;155:748.
124. Car J, Car M, Hamilton F, et al. Light therapies for acne (protocol). The Cochrane collaboration, issue 4. New York: Wiley, 2009. *http://www.thecochranelibrary.com.*
125. European Directive for systemic isotretinoin prescription. EMEA—Committee for Proprietary Medicinal Products (CPMP). 2012, *http://www.ema.europa.eu/docs/en_GB/document_library/Referrals_document/Isotretinoin_29?WC500010882.pdf.*
126. Ganceviciene R, Zouboulis CC. Isotretinoin: state of the art treatment for acne vulgaris. J Dtsch Dermatol Ges 2010;8(suppl 1):S47–S59.
127. Strauss JS, Krowchuk DP, Leyden JJ, et al. Guidelines for optimal use of isotretinoin in acne. J Am Acad Dermatol 2007;56:651–663.
128. Layton AM, Dreno B, Gollnick HPM, et al. A review of the European Directive for prescribing systemic isotretinoin for acne vulgaris. J Eur Acad Dermatol Venereol 2006; 20: 773–776.
129. Marqueling AL, Zane LT, Depression and suicidal behavior in acne patients treated with isotretinoin: A systematic review. Semin Cutan Med Surg 2005;24:92–102.
130. Sundstrom A, Alfredsson L, Sjolin-Forsberg G, et al. Association of suicide attempts with acne and treatment with isotretinoin: retrospective Swedish cohort study. Br Med J 2010;341:c5812.
131. Anderson, PC. Foods as the cause of acne. Am Fam Physician 1971;3(3):n102–n103.
132. Fulton, JE, Plewig G, Kligman AM. Effect of chocolate on acne vulgaris. JAMA 1969;210(11):2071–2074.
133. Adebamowo CA, Spiegelman D, Danby FW, et al. High school dietary dairy intake and teenage acne. J Am Acad Dermatol 2005;52:360.
134. Danby FW. Acne and milk, the diet myth, and beyond. J Am Acad Dermatol 2005;52:360.
135. Bowers J. Diet and acne. Dermatology World 2011:31–34.
136. Thiboutot D. Acne: hormonal concepts and therapy. Clin Dermatol 2004;22:419.
137. Cappel M, Mauger D, Thiboutet D. Correlation between serum levels of insulin-like growth factor 1, dehydroepiandrosterone sulfate, an dihydrotestosterone and acne lesion counts in adult women. Arch Dermatol 2005;141:333.
138. Kim J, Ko Y, Park YK, et al. Dietary effect of lactoferrin-enriched fermented milk on skin surface lipid and clinical improvement of acne vulgaris. Nutrition 2010;26(9): 902–909.
139. Mueller EA, Trapp S, Frentzel A, et al. Efficacy and tolerability of oral lactoferrin supplementation in mild to moderate acne vulgaris: an exploratory study. Curr Med Res Opin 2011;27(4):793–797.
140. Smith RN, Mann NJ, Braue A, et al. The effect of a high protein, low-glycemic load diet versus a conventional high-glycemic load diet on biochemical parameters associated with acne vulgaris: A randomized, investigator-masked controlled trial. J Am Acad Dermatol 2007;57(2):247–256.
141. Smith RN, Braue A, Varigos GA, Mann NJ. The effect of a low glycemic load diet on acne vulgaris and the fatty acid composition of skin surface triglycerides. J Dermatol Sci 2008;50(1):41–52.
142. Smith RN, Mann NJ, Braue A, Makelainen H, Varigos GA. A low-glycemic-load diet improves symptoms in acne vulgaris patients: a randomized controlled trial. Am J Clin Nutr 2007;86(1):107–115.
143. Yentzer BA, Ade RA, Fountain JM., et al. Simplifying regimens promotes greater adherence and outcomes with topical acne medications: a randomized controlled trial. Cutis 2012; 86(2):103–108.
144. Watson AJ, Bergman H, Williams CM, et al. A randomized trial to evaluate the efficacy of online follow-up visits in the management of acne. Arch Dermatol 2010;146(4): 406–411.
145. Bergman H, Tsai KY, Seo SJ, et al. Remote assessment of acne: the use of acne grading tools to evaluate digital skin images. Telemed J E Health 2009;15(5):426–430.

78

Psoriasis

Rebecca M. Law and Wayne P. Gulliver

KEY CONCEPTS[1]

1. Patients with psoriasis have a lifelong illness that may be very visible and emotionally distressing. There is a strong need for empathy and a caring attitude in interactions with these patients.
2. Psoriasis is a progressive T-lymphocyte–mediated systemic inflammatory disease that results from a complex interplay between multiple genetic factors and environmental influences. Genetic predisposition and precipitating "trigger" factors play a role in the "march of psoriasis." This march of innate and adaptive immune responses result in clinical expressions (e.g., keratinocyte proliferation) and is possibly responsible for psoriatic comorbidities.
3. Diagnosis of psoriasis is usually based on recognition of the characteristic psoriatic lesion and not based on laboratory tests.
4. Treatment goals for patients with psoriasis are to minimize signs such as plaques and scales, alleviate symptoms such as pruritus, reduce the frequency of flare-ups, ensure appropriate treatment of associated comorbid conditions such as psoriatic arthritis or clinical depression, and minimize treatment-related morbidity.
5. Management of patients with psoriasis generally involves both nonpharmacologic and pharmacologic therapies.
6. Nonpharmacologic alternatives such as stress reduction and the liberal use of moisturizers may be very beneficial and should always be considered and initiated when appropriate.
7. Pharmacologic alternatives for psoriasis include topical agents, phototherapy, and systemic agents (both traditional agents and newer biologic response modifiers).
8. Pharmacologic therapy is generally guided by the severity of disease, advancing from topical agents to phototherapy to systemic agents as needed.
9. Rotational therapy (i.e., rotating systemic drug interventions) is a means to minimize drug-associated toxicities. However, continuous treatment has replaced rotational or sequential therapy and is now the standard of care for many dermatologists.
10. Some biologic response modifiers (BRMs) have proven efficacy for psoriasis; however, there are differences among these agents, including mechanism of action, duration of remission, and adverse-effect profile. BRMS are often used for moderate-to-severe psoriasis and may be first-line therapy especially if comorbidities exist.

Psoriasis is a chronic disease that waxes and wanes. It is never cured, and it is now known to be associated with multiple comorbidities including heart disease, diabetes, and the metabolic syndrome. The signs and symptoms of psoriasis may subside totally (go into remission) and then flare up again (exacerbation). Triggers include stress, seasonal changes, and some drugs. Disease severity may vary from mild to disabling. Psoriasis imposes a burden of disease that extends beyond the physical dermatologic manifestations.

(1) Patients with psoriasis have a lifelong illness that may be very visible and emotionally distressing. There is a strong need for empathy and a caring attitude in interactions with these patients. Thus, management of this condition is necessarily long-term and multifaceted, and management modalities may change according to the severity of illness at the time.

EPIDEMIOLOGY

Psoriasis is likely the most common immune-modulated inflammatory disease in North America and Europe, as it is thought to affect 17 million people, or approximately 2% of the population.[2,3] Worldwide prevalences vary between 0.1% and 3%, with reasons for variation ranging from racial to geographic and environmental.[3] Higher prevalences than 3% have been reported occasionally in Canada and the United States. Lower frequencies of between 0.4% and 0.7% are seen for people of African and Asian descent.[4,5] Of interest is the fact that psoriasis is seldom seen in North and South American aboriginal Indians. It affects males and females equally.[3,6] The majority of patients (approximately 75%) have onset before the age of 40 years,[3] but psoriasis has been observed at birth and as late as the ninth decade of life.[3] Many studies report two peak ages of onset: at 20 to 30 and 50 to 60 years of age.[3,5]

ETIOLOGY

(2) Psoriasis is a T-lymphocyte–mediated systemic inflammatory disease that results from a complex interplay between multiple genetic factors and environmental influences. Genetic predisposition coupled with some precipitating factor triggers an abnormal immune response, resulting in the initial psoriatic skin lesions. This has more recently been called the "march of psoraisis"[2] to reflect the innate and adaptive immune responses that are present. This march leads to expressions of psoriasis with keratinocyte proliferation being central to the clinical presentation of psoriasis. Subsequently, this march is possibly responsible for various comorbidities as a consequence of chronic inflammation.[2] For example, there is an association between psoriasis and cardiovascular disease, which appears to be an ongoing, two-way interplay.[2]

Genetics

Dermatologists have recognized the familial tendencies of psoriasis for many years. Monozygotic twins have a concordance rate in the 80% range. Rates of family history in a psoriasis family range between 36% and 91%.[6–9] A study using the founder population of Newfoundland and Labrador noted that more than 80% of the patients had a positive family history.

Genetic studies suggested at least seven loci are involved in psoriasis.[3] In particular, *PSORS1* appears to be a key gene locus determining susceptibility to psoriasis.[2] In 2009, studies of the Newfoundland and Labrador population confirmed that major histocompatibility complex antigen HLA-Cw6 and tumor necrosis factor (TNF)-α as major psoriasis susceptibility genes, along with interleukin (IL)-23 loci that had previously been reported.[3,10] The findings have been confirmed in multiple populations from North America, Europe, and China.[11,12]

Predisposing Factors and Precipitating Factors

Injury to the skin, infection, drugs, smoking, alcohol consumption, obesity, and psychogenic stress have been implicated in development of psoriasis. Examples of these precipitating factors include a horsefly bite causing skin trauma (known as the *Koebner phenomenon*),[13] a viral or streptococcal infection, or the use of β-adrenergic blockers.[14] Factors exacerbating preexisting psoriasis include drugs (e.g., lithium, nonsteroidal antiinflammatory drugs [NSAIDs], antimalarials, β-adrenergic blockers, and withdrawal of corticosteroids), and psoriatic patients commonly have exacerbations during times of stress.[1,14] Stressful situations occur for many patients, and it is thought that patients with a genetic predisposition to psoriasis and a precipitating event or trigger factor play a role.

PATHOPHYSIOLOGY

Psoriasis is a common chronic inflammatory disease that most likely involves both acquired and innate immunity. The interaction between dermal dendritic cells activated T cells of the TH-1, TH-17 lineage in concert with a multitude of cytokines and growth factors are responsible for the epidermal hyperplasia and dermal inflammation that is seen in the skin of patients with psoriasis. These inflammatory cells form lymphoid structures in psoriatic dermis, allowing the unimpeded inflammatory process to continue.[15] When therapeutic intervention is initiated and positive the psoriatic phenotype is completely reversible without residual damage. This is in contrast to significant damage often seen in psoriatic arthritis that, if not treated early, is irreversible.

Comorbidities

It is now well documented that psoriasis patients have significant associated comorbidities.[2] Psoriatic arthritis is one of the most common and well-known extracutaneous manifestations of disease. Other associated comorbidities include metabolic syndrome, other immune-mediated disorders such as Crohn's disease, multiple sclerosis, and some psychological illnesses (anxiety, depression, and alcoholism).[16] Also, malignancies such as cutaneous T-cell lymphoma are associated with psoriasis, and melanoma and nonmelanoma skin cancer are associated with psoriasis treatments.

The National Psoriasis Foundation published a clinical consensus on psoriasis comorbidities with recommendations for screening and addressing issues such as cardiovascular risk, metabolic syndrome, and obesity.[17] The importance of screening for comorbidities in psoriasis patients cannot be overemphasized: Nearly half of the psoriatic patients older than age 65 have at least three comorbidities, (with two-thirds of this patient population having two or more comorbidities).[18] The presence of a specific comorbidity in a patient with psoriasis may influence the choice of pharmacotherapy.

TABLE 78-1 Phenotypic Classifications of Psoriasis

Plaque
Flexural and/or intertriginous
Seborrheic
Scalp
Acrodermatitis of Hallopeau
Palm and/or soles
Erythrodermic
Guttate
Generalized pustular psoriasis

Psoriatic arthritis (PsA) usually develops after the onset of psoriasis,[3] typically 10 years later.[16] However, 10% to 15% of patients report that the PsA appeared first.[3] The prevalence of PsA in psoriatic patients is about 30% but varies by disease severity.[16] In one U.S. study, the prevalences were 14% for patients with mild psoriasis, 18% for those with moderate psoriasis, and 56% for patients with severe psoriasis.[19] TNF-α and HLA-Cw6 are linked to both PsA and psoriasis.[20] Although immunomodulating treatments for psoriasis (such as methotrexate or TNF-α inhibitors) are useful for PsA, NSAIDs effective for joint symptoms of PsA may exacerbate psoriasis.

Metabolic syndrome is a cluster of risk factors including abdominal obesity, atherogenic dyslipidemia, hypertension, insulin resistance or glucose intolerance, prothrombotic state, and proinflammatory state.[17] Patients with psoriasis are at increased risk of developing the metabolic syndrome.[17] The syndrome is a strong predictor of cardiovascular diseases, stroke, and diabetes.[17,21,22] Patients with this syndrome are three times as likely to have a myocardial infarction (MI) or stroke, twice as likely to die from the MI or stroke, and five times as likely to develop type 2 diabetes.[17] A 2010 retrospective analysis of pooled data from three clinical trials (M02-528, CHAMPION, and REVEAL) showed that patients with psoriasis have a 28% and 12% increased 10-year risks of coronary heart disease (CHD) and stroke, respectively.[22]

Patients with psoriasis also have a decreased life expectancy and increased rates of mortality. Psoriasis is an independent risk factor for atherosclerosis, especially for younger patients with severe disease.[17] A 2006 study found that a relative risk (RR) of death for a 30-year-old person with severe psoriasis was 3.10, after controlling for traditional cardiovascular risk factors (e.g., age, gender, hypertension, dyslipidemia, diabetes mellitus, smoking, body mass index [BMI], C-reactive protein [CRP], and family history of cardiovascular disease).[17,23]

Types of Psoriasis

Plaque psoriasis, also known as *psoriasis vulgaris*, is the most common type of psoriasis (Table 78-1) and is seen in about 90% of psoriasis patients. Plaque psoriasis presents as shown in the Clinical Presentation box.

DIAGNOSTIC CONSIDERATIONS

3 The diagnosis of psoriasis is a diagnosis based on recognition of the characteristic psoriatic lesion and not on laboratory tests. Diagnostic testing is rarely performed as a biopsy may be suggested but is not diagnostic of psoriasis.

Psoriasis is traditionally classified into mild, moderate, or severe disease. In 2011, a European consensus (19 countries) formalized the definition of disease severity and treatment goals and defined plaque

CLINICAL PRESENTATION

Signs and Symptoms of Plaque Psoriasis	Description (*from reference 26*)
Lesions (plaques)	Erythematous Red-violet in color At least 0.5 cm in diameter Well demarcated—clearly distinguished from normal skin Typically covered by silver, flaking scales
Skin involvement	Either as single lesions at predisposed areas (e.g., knees, elbows) or Generalized over a wide BSA Mild psoriasis: ≤5% BSA involvement Moderate psoriasis: PASI ≥8 (higher in trials of biologics) Severe psoriasis: The rule of tens: PASI ≥10 or DLQI ≥10 or BSA ≥10% (in some phototherapy trials, BSA ≥20% used as lower limit) Categories in the European consensus: Mild psoriasis: BSA ≤10 and PASI ≤10 and DLQI ≤10. Moderate-to-severe psoriasis: (BSA >10 or PASI >10) and DLQI >10
Pruritus	More than 50% of patients with psoriasis have associated pruritus May be severe in some patients and may require treatment to minimize excoriations from constant scratching
Other associated concerns	Lesions may also be physically debilitating or socially isolating. Potential comorbidities: PsA, depression, hypertension, obesity, diabetes mellitus, Crohn's disease, anxiety, alcoholism

BSA, body surface area; DLQI, Dermatology Life Quality Index; PASI, psoriasis area and severity index; PsA, psoriatic arthritis.

psoriasis severity as two main categories: mild versus moderate-to-severe.[24,25] Both classification systems are in use today. In clinical practice, assessment of the severity of disease includes both an objective evaluation of the extent and symptoms as well as a subjective evaluation of the impact of disease on the patient's quality of life.[26] Assessment typically includes measures of symptom and involvement such as body surface area (BSA), Psoriasis Area and Severity Index (PASI), or Physician's Global Assessment (static PGA), as well as quality-of-life measures such as the Dermatology Life Quality Index (DLQI) or the Short Form (SF-36) Health Survey.[26]

Classification of psoriasis as mild, moderate, or severe disease is generally based on BSA or PASI measurements (see Clinical Presentation box). Practically, to give a rough estimate of BSA involvement, palm size is approximately 1% BSA, head and neck involvement is approximately 10% BSA, both upper limbs approximately 20% BSA, trunk involvement (front and back) approximately 30% BSA, and both lower limbs approximately 40% BSA.

TREATMENT

Treatment of psoriasis is based on managing the underlying pathophysiology. Agents that modulate the abnormal immune response, such as corticosteroids and biologic response modifiers, are important treatment strategies for psoriasis. Topical therapies that affect cell turnover are also effective for psoriasis. In addition, nonpharmacologic therapies are effective adjuncts and should be considered for all patients with psoriasis. A treatment regimen should always be individualized, taking into consideration severity of disease, patient responses, and tolerability to various interventions. Furthermore, if comorbidities exist, they must be taken into treatment considerations and managed early. Optimal psoriasis care needs to maintain a focus on the patient's overall health-related quality of life.

Desired Outcomes

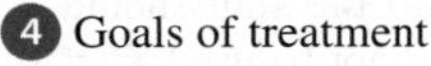

4 Goals of treatment[1]:

- Minimizing or eliminating the signs of psoriasis, such as plaques and scales
- Alleviating pruritus and minimizing excoriations
- Reducing the frequency of flare-ups
- Ensuring appropriate treatment of associated comorbid conditions such as psoriatic arthritis, hypertension, dyslipidemia, diabetes, or clinical depression
- Avoiding or minimizing adverse effects from treatments used (topical, phototherapy, and/or systemic)
- Providing cost-effective therapy
- Providing guidance or counseling as needed (e.g., stress-reduction techniques)
- Maintaining or improving the patient's quality of life

Evaluation of Therapeutic Outcomes

Successful management of psoriasis should include not only clearance of skin lesions, which may take weeks to months depending on the severity of disease, but also control of associated conditions such as itching, and, importantly, comorbidities, including dyslipidemia, hypertension, psoriatic arthritis, and clinical depression. The ultimate goal is to provide enough control of this chronic disease (and its comorbidities, if present) so that the patient's quality of life is minimally affected.

The 2011 European consensus defined induction and maintenance phases and provided separate treatment goals for induction and maintenance.[24,25] The induction phase is defined as the first 16 weeks of treatment for drugs with a rapid induction to remission (such as adalimumab or infliximab), extending the phase to 24 weeks of treatment for less rapidly effective drugs (such as methotrexate or etanercept).[25] To be considered successful therapy, a treatment regimen should result in a reduction of PASI greater than or equal to 75%, or PASI of 50% to 75% coupled with a DLQI less than 5.[25] Otherwise, treatment modifications should be considered. Treatment goals should be assessed at 10 to 16 weeks and then every 8 weeks thereafter.[25]

General Approach to Treatment

5 Management of patients with psoriasis generally involves both nonpharmacologic and pharmacologic therapies. Nonpharmacologic therapies are important and should be used for all patients with psoriasis, regardless of the severity of disease. Pharmacologic therapies are always tailored to the individual patient with psoriasis and different treatment strategies would be used depending on psoriatic disease severity, presence or absence of comorbid illnesses, and any special considerations such as hepatic or renal dysfunction.

Nonpharmacologic Therapy

6 Nonpharmacologic alternatives may be very beneficial and should always be considered and initiated when appropriate.[1] These include stress-reduction strategies, moisturizers, oatmeal baths, and skin protection using sunscreens.[27]

In particular, stress reduction has been shown to improve both the extent and severity of psoriasis and to include methods such as guided imagery and stress-management clinics. Liberal use of nonmedicated moisturizers, applied ad lib, helps to maintain skin moisture, reduces skin shedding, controls associated scaling, and may reduce pruritus. Oatmeal baths further reduce pruritus and with regular use may minimize the need for systemic antipruritic drugs.

Sunscreens, preferably with a sun protection factor (SPF) of 30 or more, should be regularly used because sunburns can trigger an exacerbation of psoriasis. Irritation to the skin should be minimized—harsh soaps or detergents should not be used. Cleansing should be done with tepid water and preferably with lipid-free and fragrance-free cleansers.[1,27]

For patients with comorbidities such as dyslipidemia, obesity, or cardiovascular disease, cessation of nicotine and alcohol consumption, diet control, and increasing physical activity are all important interventions.[2]

Pharmacologic Therapy

7 Pharmacologic alternatives for psoriasis are topical agents, phototherapy, and systemic agents, including biologic response modifiers.

Drug Treatments of First Choice

8 For limited or mild to moderately severe disease, topical treatments are the usual standard of care, with phototherapy and photochemotherapy used in moderate to severe cases. For patients presenting with extensive or moderate-to-severe disease, systemic therapies with or without the use of topical treatments are the usual standard of care. Newer systemic treatments such as biologic response modifiers (BRMs) may be the treatments of choice, especially for patients with comorbidities such as PsA or if traditional systemic treatments (such as methotrexate or cyclosporine) are contraindicated. Once the disease is under control, it would be important to step down to the least potent, least toxic agent(s) that maintain control. 9 Sequential therapy and rotational therapy may minimize drug-associated toxicities; however, continuous treatment is now the standard of care for many dermatologists. Different treatment algorithms are used, depending on the severity of the plaque psoriasis (Figs. 78-1 and 78-2).[1]

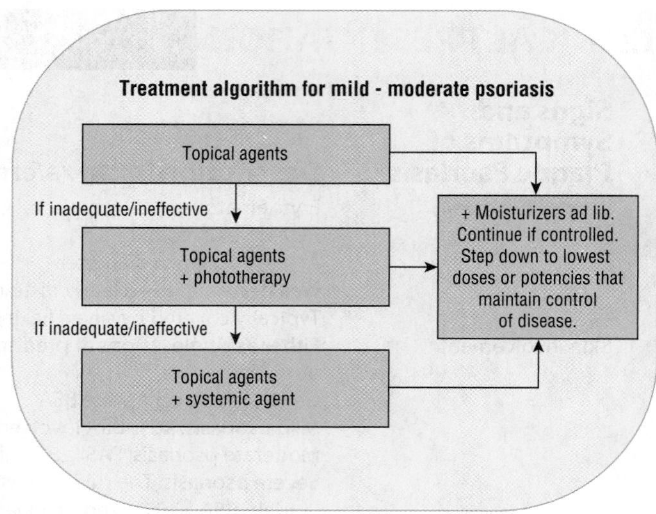

FIGURE 78-1 Treatment algorithm for mild-to-moderate psoriasis. *(Reprinted from reference 1 with permission from the publisher.)*

Published Guidelines or Treatment Protocols Treatment guidelines have recently been updated in both the United States and Canada.[26,28–35] All U.S. guidelines are endorsed by the American Academy of Dermatology or the National Psoriasis Foundation, and Canadian guidelines are endorsed by the Canadian Dermatology Association. In Europe, guidelines from the British Association of Dermatologists[36] and a European 19-country consensus have been published.[24,25] These guidelines represent the current standards of care.

Topical Therapies

Approximately 80% of patients with psoriasis have mild-to-moderate disease,[30] and the majority of these patients can be treated with topical therapies alone.[30] Individualized approaches are essential because of the wide variation in patients' presentations, their psychosocial health, and their personal opinions as to what would be acceptable treatment.[26] Topical therapies include corticosteroids, vitamin D_3 analogs, retinoids, anthralin, and coal tar. These are generally efficacious and safe for this patient population. Topical agents are also used

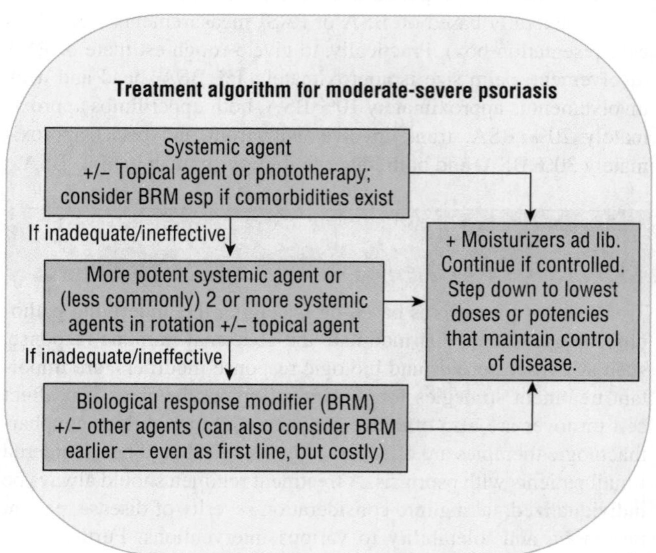

FIGURE 78-2 Treatment algorithm for moderate-to-severe psoriasis. *(Reprinted from reference 1 with permission from the publisher.)*

TABLE 78-2 Topical Corticosteroid Potency Chart

Potency Rating	Corticosteroid—Topical Preparations
Class 1: Superpotent	Betamethasone dipropionate 0.05% ointment (Diprolene and Diprosone ointment) Clobetasone propionate 0.05% lotion/spray/shampoo (Clobex lotion/spray/shampoo, OLUX foam) Clobetasone propionate 0.05% cream and ointment (Cormax, Temovate) Diflorasone diacetate 0.05% ointment (Florone, Psorcon) Halobetasol propionate 0.05% cream and ointment (Ultravate) Flurandrenolide tape 4 mcg/cm² (Cordran)
Class 2: Potent	Amcinonide 0.1% ointment (Cyclocort ointment) Betamethasone dipropionate 0.05% cream/gel (Diprolene cream, gel, and Diprosone cream) Desoximetasone 0.25% cream (Topicort) Fluocinonide 0.05% cream, gel, ointment (Lidex) Halcinonide 0.1% cream (Halog)
Class 3: Upper mid-strength	Amcinonide 0.1% cream (Cyclocort cream) Betamethasone valerate 0.1% ointment (Betnovate/Valisone ointment) Diflorasone diacetate 0.05% cream (Psorcon cream) Fluticasone propionate 0.005% ointment (Cutivate ointment) Mometasone furoate 0.1% ointment (Elocon ointment) Triamcinolone acetonide 0.5% cream and ointment (Aristocort)
Class 4: Mid-strength	Betamethasone valerate 0.12% foam (Luxiq) Clocortolone pivalate 0.1% cream (Cloderm) Desoximetasone 0.05% cream and gel (Topicort LP) Fluocinolone acetonide 0.025% ointment (Synalar ointment) Fluocinolone acetonide 0.2% cream (Synalar-HP) Hydrocortisone valerate 0.2% ointment (Westcort ointment) Mometasone furoate 0.1% cream (Elocon cream) Triamcinolone acetonide 0.1% ointment (Kenalog)
Class 5: Lower mid-strength	Betamethasone dipropionate 0.05% lotion (Diprosone lotion) Betamethasone valerate 0.1% cream and lotion (Betnovate/Valisone cream & lotion) Desonide 0.05% lotion (DesOwen) Fluocinolone acetonide 0.01% shampoo (Capex shampoo) Fluocinolone acetonide 0.01%, 0.025%, 0.03% cream (Synalar cream) Flurandrenolide 0.05% cream and lotion (Cordran) Fluticasone propionate 0.05% cream and lotion (Cutivate cream and lotion) Hydrocortisone butyrate 0.1% cream (Locoid) Hydrocortisone valerate 0.2% cream (Westcort cream) Prednicarbate 0.1% cream (Dermatop) Triamcinolone acetonide 0.1% cream and lotion (Kenalog cream and lotion)
Class 6: Mild	Alclometasone dipropionate 0.05% cream and ointment (Aclovate) Betamethasone valerate 0.05% cream and ointment Desonide 0.05% cream, ointment, gel (DesOwen, Desonate, Tridesilon) Desonide 0.05% foam (Verdeso) Fluocinonide acetonide 0.01% cream and solution (Synalar) Fluocinonide acetonide 0.01% FS oil (Derma-Smoothe)
Class 7: Least Potent	Hydrocortisone 0.5%, 1%, 2%, 2.5% cream, lotion, spray, and ointment (various brands)

Adapted from The National Psoriasis Foundation—Mild Psoriasis: Steroid potency chart, http://www.psoriasis.org/netcommunity/sublearn03_mild_potency. Rosso JD, Friedlander SF. Corticosteroids: Options in the era of steroid-sparing therapy. J Am Acad Dermatol 2005;53:S50–S58; Leung DYM, Nicklas RA, Li JT, et al. Disease management of atopic dermatitis: An updated practice parameter. Ann Allergy Asthma Immunol 2004;93:S1–S17.

as adjunctive therapy for patients with more extensive disease who are being treated concurrently with phototherapy or systemic agents.

To determine the quantity of topical agents required, the fingertip unit[37] can be used. One fingertip unit is approximately 500 mg,[30,37] which is sufficient to cover one hand (front and back) or about 2% BSA.[38] The trunk (front and back) is about 30% BSA; to cover the entire trunk once, about 15 fingertip units, or 7500 mg (7.5 g), would be required.

In a 2012 systematic review of topical and phototherapies for psoriasis by dermatologists in France, nine recommendations based on evidence and expert opinion are offered. However, quality literature was limited, and the recommendations relating to optimal steroid use and optimal first-line treatment for psoriasis did not reach 80% consensus.[37]

Corticosteroids Topical corticosteroids have been the mainstay of therapy for the majority of patients with psoriasis for over half a century. They are generally well tolerated, although adverse effects can occur, including systemic ones on occasion. Table 78-2 provides a summary of topical corticosteroid formulations—including ointments, creams, gels, foams, lotions, sprays, shampoos, tape, and solutions[30]—and potencies.

The choice of vehicle affects corticosteroid potency: Ointments, being the most occlusive, enhance drug penetration and provide the most potent formulations. However, patients may prefer a less greasy formulation, such as a cream or lotion for daytime use, although they may be willing to apply the more effective ointment-based corticosteroid during the night.[30] Providing additional occlusion will increase drug penetration of a topical preparation, resulting in enhanced potency. For example, flurandrenolide cream and lotion are potency class 5, but flurandrenolide tape was found to have higher efficacy than diflorasone diacetate ointment (potency class 1).[30,39,40]

Despite their widespread use, there have been few large-scale, randomized placebo-controlled corticosteroid trials and even fewer head-to-head comparisons with other therapies. The most comprehensive review to date is the analysis of topical psoriasis therapies done in 2002 but recent studies aren't included so this review was already somewhat out of date when published.[26,41] This systematic review found that all topical corticosteroid treatments considered were efficacious and significantly better than placebo; and that the highest potency corticosteroids were the most efficacious, followed by vitamin D_3 analogs.[26] The French group in 2012 found variable efficacy in their systematic review, noting that recommendations about topical steroid use should be mostly based on expert opinion, and that maintenance intermittent treatment may prolong remission.[42]

Corticosteroids have antiinflammatory, antiproliferative, immunosuppressive, and vasoconstrictive effects.[30] These are mediated through a variety of mechanisms. Mechanisms of action include binding to intracellular corticosteroid receptors and regulation of gene transcription (in particular those which code for proinflammatory cytokines).[30]

Appropriate use of topical corticosteroids should include an assessment of disease severity and disease location as well as knowledge of the patient's preference and age. Lower potency corticosteroids should be used for infants and for lesions on the face, intertriginous areas, and areas with thin skin. For other areas of the body in adults, mid- to high-potency agents are generally recommended as initial therapy.[30] The highest potency corticosteroids are generally reserved for patients with very thick plaques or recalcitrant disease, such as plaques on palms and soles. The use of potency class 1 corticosteroids should be limited to a duration of 2 to 4 weeks,[30] recognizing that the risk of cutaneous and systemic side effects increases with continued use.

Cutaneous adverse effects include skin atrophy, acne, contact dermatitis, hypertrichosis, folliculitis, hypopigmentation, perioral dermatitis, striae, telangiectases, and traumatic purpura.[26,30] Systemic adverse effects have been reported not only with superpotent corticosteroids but also with extended or widespread use of mid-potency agents.[30] Systemic adverse effects include hypothalamic–pituitary–adrenal (HPA) axis suppression and less commonly Cushing's syndrome, osteonecrosis of the femoral head, cataracts, and glaucoma.[30]

All topical corticosteroids are pregnancy category C.[30]

Tachyphylaxis can occur with prolonged use, although its clinical significance is difficult to verify.[26] It is recommended that the frequency of use be gradually reduced once clinical response is seen, although there are no established tapering regimens.[30] The French group recommended twice-weekly maintenance therapy.[37] Other approaches include transitioning to weaker potency agents or combination with other nonsteroidal topical therapies.[30] Pulse dosing has also been used to minimize tachyphylaxis and adverse effects.[43]

Vitamin D_3 Analogs Topical vitamin D_3 analogs include calcipotriol (calcipotriene), calcitriol (the active metabolite of vitamin D), and tacalcitol. Only calcipotriol is currently available in the United States[30] and Canada.[26] Other analogs currently under study include maxacalcitol and becocalcidiol.[30] Their mechanisms of action include binding to vitamin D receptors, which results in inhibition of keratinocyte proliferation and enhancement of keratinocyte differentiation.[26,30] They also inhibit T-lymphocyte activity.[26]

The efficacy of calcipotriol for patients with mild psoriasis is well established in randomized double-blind placebo-controlled trials. In head-to-head comparison studies with other topical agents, calcipotriol was found to be more effective than anthralin (dithranol)[44] and comparable or slightly more effective than potency class 3 (upper mid-strength) topical corticosteroid ointments such as betamethasone valerate 0.1% ointment.[26,45,46] In an analysis of topical psoriasis therapies done in 2002,[41] calcipotriol was found to be as effective as all but the most potent topical corticosteroids.[26] Combination therapy with a topical steroid is particularly effective[47] and is discussed later in the chapter.

Vitamin D_3 analogs are generally well tolerated and have a good safety profile in comparison with other topical therapies.[47] Cutaneous adverse effects most commonly include a mild irritant contact dermatitis; others include burning, pruritus, edema, peeling, dryness, and erythema.[26,30] These adverse effects may be mitigated with continued use.[30] Systemic adverse effects, including hypercalcemia and parathyroid hormone suppression, are rare unless patients are using more than the recommended maximum of 5 mg calcipotriol (100 g of calcipotriol 50 mcg/g cream or ointment) per week[26,30] or if there is underlying renal disease or impaired calcium metabolism.[30] When applied sparingly over a BSA <30%, the risk of hypercalcemia is remote.[37]

Calcipotriol is pregnancy category C. It is inactivated by ultraviolet A (UVA) light thus it should be applied after rather than before UVA light exposure.[30]

Retinoids Tazarotene is a topical retinoid that acts through the following mechanisms: normalizing abnormal keratinocyte differentiation, diminishing keratinocyte hyperproliferation, and clearing the inflammatory infiltrate in the psoriatic plaque.[26,30] It is effective in clearing psoriatic plaque lesions and achieving remission.

In a placebo-controlled trial of tazarotene 0.1% and 0.05% gels for patients with plaque psoriasis, tazarotene provided a 50% or greater improvement in 63% (0.1% gel) and 50% (0.05% gel) of patients, respectively, after 12 weeks of use.[48] The therapeutic benefit appears to be maintained for 12 weeks after cessation of therapy.[48] Later clinical trials with tazarotene 0.1% and 0.05% creams versus a placebo vehicle provided similar findings.[49] The 2012 systematic review similarly found that about 50% of patients experienced a 50% or more improvement with no difference in formulations.[37]

Adverse effects of tazarotene include a high incidence of irritation at the site of application, a dose-dependent effect.[26] This results in burning, itching, and erythema, which can occur in lesional and perilesional skin.[30] Irritation may be reduced by using the cream formulation, lower concentration, alternate-day application, or short-contact (30 to 60 minutes) treatment.[30] Ad lib use of moisturizers is also beneficial. Tazarotene is also potentially photosensitizing, due to thinning of the epidermis that can occur with continued use.[30]

Tazarotene is pregnancy category X and should not be used in women of childbearing age unless effective contraception is being used.

Anthralin Anthralin is not as commonly used as other topical therapies currently available for psoriasis; however, there are situations where its use is appropriate and efficacious. It has a direct antiproliferative effect on epidermal keratinocytes,[1,14] normalizing keratinocyte differentiation.[30] Although the exact mechanism of action is unknown, it may have a direct effect on mitochondria[30,50] and reduce the mitotic activity. It also prevents T-lymphocyte activation.[30] Small placebo-controlled studies demonstrated efficacy for anthralin used continuously or as very short contact (1 minute of treatment).[30]

Currently, short-contact anthralin therapy (SCAT) is usually the preferred regimen, where the anthralin ointment is applied only to the thick plaque lesions for 2 hours or less and then wiped off.[1,30] Because lesions are generally well demarcated, zinc oxide ointment or a nonmedicated stiff paste should be applied to the surrounding normal skin to protect it from irritation and burning. Anthralin should be used with caution, if at all, on the face and intertriginous areas because of the risk of severe skin irritation.[30]

Concentrations for SCAT range from 1% to 4% or as tolerated; concentrations for continuous anthralin therapy vary from 0.05% to 0.4%. Aside from significant and often severe skin irritation, other adverse effects include folliculitis and allergic contact dermatitis, but these are uncommon.

Anthralin is pregnancy category C. People who handle the dry anthralin powder should avoid skin contact (e.g., by wearing gloves while compounding).[1]

Coal Tar Coal tar was one of the earliest agents used to treat psoriasis. It is keratolytic and may have antiproliferative and antiinflammatory effects.[1] Coal tar formulations include crude coal tar and tar distillates (liquor carbonis detergens) in ointments, creams, and shampoos. Because of limited efficacy coupled with patient acceptance and compliance issues, coal tar preparations are less commonly used today, especially in North American and European[37] countries.

A 2007 comparative study in Thailand reported that betamethasone valerate was significantly more effective than coal tar.[26,51] Although coal tar may have similar efficacy as calcipotriol, it has a slower onset of action.[26] In addition, coal tar has an unpleasant odor and will stain clothing; thus, it may be cosmetically unappealing to patients.

Adverse effects include folliculitis, acne, local irritation, and phototoxicity.[26] It is carcinogenic in animals, but for humans no convincing data have emerged regarding carcinogenicity with topical use.[30]

Coal tar concentrations as used in psoriasis treatments (0.5% to 5%) are considered safe by the FDA.[33] However, occupational exposure to coal tar, especially in very high concentrations such as coal tar used in industrial paving,[33] was reported to increase the risk of lung cancer, scrotal cancer, and skin cancer.[30,33] The risk of teratogenicity when used in pregnancy is likely to be small, if it exists.[30]

Salicylic Acid Salicylic acid has keratolytic properties and has been used in various formulations including shampoos or bath oils for patients with scalp psoriasis. In combination with topical corticosteroids, it enhances steroid penetration thus increasing efficacy. It should not be used in combination with ultraviolet B (UVB) light phototherapy because of a filtering effect that may reduce efficacy. Systemic absorption and toxicity can occur, especially when applied to more than 20% BSA or when used for patients with renal impairment.

Avoid the use of salicylic acid in children. However, it may be used for limited and localized plaque psoriasis in pregnancy.[30]

Calcineurin Inhibitors Topical calcineurin inhibitors such as pimecrolimus 1% cream (Elidel) are used for the treatment of inflammatory skin diseases such as atopic dermatitis.[52–54] Pimecrolimus was found to be effective for plaque psoriasis when used under occlusion[53] and also effective for patients with moderate to severe inverse psoriasis (intertriginous areas are affected).[54] Because this cream is less irritating than calcipotriol and also avoids steroid adverse effects such as skin atrophy, it may be a useful alternative for patients with lesions in intertriginous areas.

Phototherapies and Photochemotherapy

Phototherapy has been used for treating psoriasis for years and is still an important treatment modality today. It has been known for centuries that some skin diseases improve with sun exposure, and clinical studies with phototherapies have been reported since the late 19th century.[28] Phototherapy consists of using nonionizing electromagnetic radiation, either UVA or UVB, as light therapy to treat psoriatic lesions.[55]

UVB is given alone as either broadband or narrowband UVB (NB-UVB), currently with NB-UVB being the preferred method. Broadband UVB is also given as photochemotherapy with topical agents such as crude coal tar (Goeckerman regimen)[55] or anthralin (Ingram regimen) for enhanced efficacy.[28]

UVA is generally given with a photosensitizer, such as an oral psoralens, to enhance efficacy—this regimen is known as PUVA (photochemotherapy with oral methoxypsoralen and ultraviolet A light).[55]

With respect to comparative efficacy, NB-UVB is more efficacious than broadband UVB, but may be slightly less effective than PUVA.[28,56] PUVA is very effective in the majority of patients, with the potential for long remissions.[28] A meta-analysis showed that more patients are still clear at 6 months with PUVA versus with NB-UVB.[56] However, because of greater availability of UVB treatment centers, more evidence available now of the efficacy of UVB treatments for psoriasis (in particular, NB-UVB), and especially the increasing concerns about PUVA toxicities (including skin cancers), phototherapy for psoriasis currently uses UVB or NB-UVB where available. Failure of NB-UVB may justify PUVA therapy.[55]

UVB interferes with protein and nucleic acid synthesis, leading to decreased proliferation of epidermal keratinocytes.[28] UVA has similar effects on epidermal keratinocytes. However, because of deeper penetration into the dermis, it also has effects on dermal dendritic cells, fibroblasts, endothelial cells, mast cells, and skin-infiltrating inflammatory cells including granulocytes and T lymphocytes.[28]

Adverse effects of phototherapy include erythema, pruritus, xerosis, hyperpigmentation, and blistering, especially with higher dosages. It should be used with caution for patients with photosensitivity concerns, and drug interactions include photosensitizing medications such as tetracyclines. Patients must be provided with eye protection during UVB, NB-UVB, or PUVA treatments, and for 24 hours[55] or the remainder of the day[28] after PUVA treatments. In addition, patients receiving PUVA therapy may experience gastrointestinal symptoms such as nausea or vomiting, which may be minimized by taking the oral psoralens with food or milk.[28] For patients also receiving oral retinoids plus PUVA (RE-PUVA), the UVA dose should be reduced by one-third.[28]

Long-term PUVA use can lead to photoaging and the development of PUVA lentigines. Psoralens bind to proteins in the lens of the eye; thus, there is a potential for increased cataract formation. Furthermore, although UVB has a theoretical risk of photocarcinogenesis, the risk is significantly higher with PUVA and is dose related.[28,55] A meta-analysis reported a 14-fold increase in the incidence of squamous cell carcinoma (SCC) in patients receiving high-dose PUVA when compared with low-dose PUVA, with SCC of the male genitalia particularly elevated.[28,57] PUVA may also increase the risk of basal cell carcinoma and possibly melanoma,[28] which may occur 15 years after the first treatment.[55]

Systemic Therapies

Systemic therapies are the mainstay of treatment for patients with moderate-to-severe psoriasis, with topical therapies remaining as useful adjuncts. However, as discussed below under combination therapies, topical calcipotriol and betamethasone dipropionate ointment may provide sufficient disease control for some patients.[26,58] Conversely, a subset of patients with limited disease may have debilitating symptoms, and the use of systemic therapies would be warranted.[29] Systemic therapies include the following traditional agents acitretin, cyclosporine, methotrexate, mycophenolate mofetil (MMF), and hydroxyurea; as well as the newer BRMs, specifically adalimumab, alefacept, etanercept, infliximab, and ustekinumab.

Acitretin In the 1980s, etretinate became the first oral retinoid, or vitamin A acid derivative, available for the treatment of psoriasis. It has since been replaced by acitretin, its active metabolite.

Retinoids may be less effective than methotrexate or cyclosporine when used as monotherapy. Currently, acitretin is more commonly used in combination with topical calcipotriol or phototherapy.[26,29] Its efficacy appears to be dose dependent,[29] but low-dose acitretin (25 mg/day) is safer and better tolerated than higher-dose (50 mg/day) therapy.[26]

Common adverse effects of acitretin include hypertriglyceridemia and mucocutaneous adverse effects such as dryness of the eyes, nasal and oral mucosa, chapped lips, cheilitis, epistaxis, xerosis, brittle nails, and burning or sticky skin.[26,29] Less commonly, "retinoid dermatitis" may occur. Periungual pyogenic granulomas are sometimes seen after long-term use of acitretin.[29] Rarely, skeletal abnormalities—such as disseminated idiopathic skeletal hyperostosis (DISH) syndrome—may occur.[26]

All retinoids are teratogenic and are pregnancy category X, including topical retinoids. Acitretin should not be used for women of childbearing age unless they are able and willing to use effective birth control not only for the duration of acitretin therapy but also for 3 years after discontinuing the agent.[26,29] Men receiving acitretin should not donate blood for a similar time period.

Ethanol should be avoided during therapy and for 2 months after drug discontinuation because it causes the transesterification of acitretin to etretinate, which has a much longer elimination half-life.

Cyclosporine Cyclosporine is a systemic calcineurin inhibitor. The original formulation, marketed as Sandimmune, was first approved as a posttransplant immunosuppressant to prevent organ rejection. The more bioavailable microemulsion formulation, Neoral, was approved by the FDA in 1997 for the treatment of psoriasis and rheumatoid arthritis.[32]

Cyclosporine is efficacious for both inducing remission and maintenance therapy for patients with moderate to severe plaque psoriasis. It is also effective in treating pustular, erythrodermic, and nail psoriasis.[32]

In comparative randomized controlled trials (RCTs), cyclosporine was significantly more effective than etretinate[59] and similar or slightly better in efficacy than methotrexate.[26,32,60] After inducing remission, maintenance therapy using low doses (1.25 mg/kg/day to 3.0 mg/kg/day) may prevent relapse.[32] The dose should always be titrated to the lowest effective dose for maintenance. In one placebo-controlled study, the relapse rate was 42% for patients on 3.0 mg/kg/day versus 84% for patients on placebo.[61]

For patients discontinuing cyclosporine, a gradual taper of 1 mg/kg/day each week may prolong the time before relapse, as compared with abrupt discontinuation.[29,32] Abrupt discontinuation resulted in a dramatic rebound of psoriasis in a few cases.[26] Because more than half of patients discontinuing cyclosporine will relapse within 4 months, patients should be provided with appropriate alternative treatments shortly before or after discontinuing cyclosporine therapy.[32]

Adverse effects of cyclosporine include cumulative renal toxicity, hypertension, and hypertriglyceridemia. The latter two are particularly significant for patients with prior elevation of diastolic blood pressure or triglycerides.[26] Hypertriglyceridemia can occur in up to 15% of patients with psoriasis who are treated with cyclosporine, although this effect is generally reversible upon cessation of therapy.[29]

The risk of SCC and other nonmelanoma skin cancers increases with duration of treatment[26] and with prior PUVA treatments.[29] Thus, although continuous therapy for up to 2 years may be efficacious,[32] it should be used only in a subset of patients[26] in whom renal function is monitored with annual determinations of glomerular filtration rate (GFR) and monthly measurements of blood pressure and creatinine clearance, with more frequent measurements during the initial 6 weeks of treatment.[26]

Baseline blood pressure, serum creatinine, serum urea nitrogen, triglycerides, complete blood count, uric acid, potassium, and magnesium should be obtained before initiating therapy, every 2 weeks for the first 12 weeks of therapy, and monitored monthly thereafter during therapy.[26,32] Age-appropriate malignancy screens should also be done, and patients should be seen for dental examinations at least yearly because of the risk of gingival hyperplasia.[32]

The 2009 Canadian Guidelines recommended that cyclosporine be normally reserved for intermittent use in periods up to 12 weeks for most patients with psoriasis,[26] although other recommendations are for periods of 1 year or up to 2 years.[32] Risk of toxicity increases with treatment duration.

As a cytochrome P450 isoenzyme 3A4 (CYP3A4) substrate, cyclosporine has significant drug interactions. Serum concentration monitoring is not routinely needed for patients with psoriasis because doses used are lower than in transplant recipients, although monitoring may be advisable for patients taking interacting drugs.

Drugs that can increase cyclosporine concentrations include calcium channel blockers (verapamil, diltiazem, and nicardipine), amiodarone, thiazide diuretics, macrolide antibiotics, allopurinol, oral contraceptives, ezetimibe, selective serotonin reuptake inhibitors (fluoxetine, sertraline), fluoroquinolones (ciprofloxacin, norfloxacin), antifungals (ketoconazole, itraconazole, fluconazole, voriconazole), and cimetidine.[32] Grapefruit juice will also increase cyclosporine concentrations.

Drugs that can reduce cyclosporine concentrations include anticonvulsants (carbamazepine, oxcarbazepine, phenobarbital, phenytoin, valproic acid), efavirenz, and St. John's wort.[32]

Conversely, cyclosporine may also affect the drug levels of some drugs. Concurrent use of potentially interacting drugs should be avoided when possible.

Methotrexate For decades, methotrexate has been the mainstay of systemic therapy for patients with moderate-to-severe psoriasis. It has direct antiinflammatory benefits due to its effects on T-cell gene expression and also has cytostatic effects.[26] It is more efficacious than acitretin and similar or slightly less efficacious than cyclosporine.[26,34]

Although it also has a significant adverse effects profile, methotrexate is generally considered a safer alternative than cyclosporine unless there are preexisting contraindications such as liver disease. In some head-to-head clinical studies more patients dropped out of the cyclosporine treatment arms due to adverse effects.[29,34] While BRMs are undoubtedly more efficacious, they are much more costly, and some insurance companies require an inadequate response or intolerance to methotrexate (the gold standard) as a prerequisite for approving their use.[34] In a recent placebo-controlled comparative study with adalimumab (CHAMPION), the efficacy of methotrexate was 36% versus 80% for adalimumab and 19% for placebo.[62] Adalimumab also provided a more rapid response; however, the duration of remission is unclear. In another recent randomized phase 3 trial (RESTORE), the efficacy of methotrexate was 42% versus 78% for infliximab.[63]

Initial doses of 7.5 to 15 mg/week may be increased to 20 to 25 mg/week if the response is inadequate at 8 to 12 weeks, with appropriate adverse effect monitoring. Methotrexate can be used continuously for years or decades with sustained benefits.[26] Methotrexate inhibits folate biosynthesis; and the use of folate supplementation during prolonged methotrexate therapy as seen in dermatology remains controversial (see Clinical Controversy box).

Clinical **Controversy...**

Folate Supplementation for Methotrexate Therapy

Although some experts recommend folate supplementation for all patients receiving methotrexate for psoriasis, others add folate only when patient issues occur, such as gastrointestinal adverse effects or early bone marrow toxicity (as manifested by an increased mean corpuscular volume) that can be caused by megaloblastic anemia.[29,34] Lack of folate supplementation has also been listed as a risk factor for hepatotoxicity from methotrexate use.[34] One small placebo-controlled study suggested that folate supplementation may result in a slight decrease in efficacy of treatment,[116] but the study methodology has been questioned.[29,34]

The most significant adverse effect is cumulative liver toxicity; and total lifetime dose of methotrexate must be monitored. Traditionally, patients received a pretreatment liver biopsy and subsequent biopsies when a cumulative dose of 1.5 g is reached. Currently, it is recognized that pretreatment liver biopsies may not be practical or appropriate in all cases[26,34] and that baseline liver biopsies only be considered for patients with a history of significant liver disease.[34] It has also been recommended that a baseline liver biopsy be delayed for 2 to 6 months so that medication efficacy and tolerability can first be established[34] (i.e., intention to continue with methotrexate use). Risk factors for hepatotoxicity from methotrexate include the following: a history of or current alcohol consumption, persistent abnormal liver chemistry studies, history of liver disease including chronic hepatitis B or C, family history of inheritable liver disease, history of significant exposure to hepatotoxic drugs or chemicals, diabetes mellitus, obesity, and hyperlipidemia.[29,34] For patients without preexisting risk factors for hepatotoxicity, it is recognized that they would likely have a low risk of fibrosis and would not require a baseline liver biopsy; furthermore, consideration can be made to continue methotrexate treatment for these patients without biopsies at all, to perform a liver biopsy after 3.5 to 4.0 g total cumulative dose, or to switch therapy to an alternate drug at that point.[29,34]

Other adverse effects include significant nausea, pulmonary toxicity, pancytopenia, acute myelosuppression, megaloblastic anemia, and a small but significant increase in lymphoma.[26] Although rare, pancytopenia can occur anytime with the use of low-dose weekly methotrexate and even after single doses of methotrexate.[29] Methotrexate is an abortifacient and is teratogenic (pregnancy category X) and should not be used in pregnancy. After methotrexate therapy is discontinued, it is recommended that men continue an effective birth control for 3 months (since one cycle of spermatogenesis is 74 days), and women should be on effective birth control for at least one ovulatory cycle.[26,29]

Significant drug interactions include serum albumin binding interactions with salicylates, phenytoin, sulfonamides/trimethoprim, ciprofloxacin, and thiazide diuretics, potentially increasing toxicity. Drugs that can reduce methotrexate renal elimination (such as acidic drugs, including salicylates or vitamin C) will also increase serum methotrexate levels and hence increase toxicity. In addition, drugs with hepatotoxic potential may pose an additive risk with methotrexate use.[29]

Systemic Therapy with Biologic Response Modifiers

10 Some BRMs have proven efficacy for psoriasis; however, there are differences among these agents, including mechanism of action, duration of remission, and adverse-effect profile. In general, because of their immunomodulatory effects, there is an increased risk of infection with most of these agents. The use of live or live-attenuated vaccines during therapy is generally contraindicated. Currently, BRMs are often considered for patients with moderate to severe psoriasis when other systemic agents are inadequate or relatively contraindicated. BRMs are sometimes recommended for first-line therapy, alongside conventional systemic agents, for patients with moderate to severe psoriasis; however, in practice, drug access due to cost considerations may be a limiting factor. BRMs may be appropriate as first-line therapy if comorbidities exist. For example, BRMs such as infliximab or adalimumab would be an appropriate treatment option for patients with both plaque psoriasis and active PsA. BRMs currently available for treatment of psoriasis include adalimumab, alefacept, etanercept, infliximab, and ustekinumab.[64,65]

Currently, a number of RCTs describe short-term efficacy of various BRMs for psoriasis but few long-term studies are available. A recent 3-year open-label extension of a 1-year adalimumab phase 3 trial (REVEAL) has demonstrated sustained response with continuous use in initial PASI 75 responders, as discussed below.[66] More clinical evidence has enabled the development of guidelines in an attempt to optimize BRM therapies for psoriasis.[25,65] The current European consensus recommends either adalimumab or infliximab with etanercept as a suggested alternative, but these guidelines are incomplete as other BRMs such as ustekinumab have not been included.[25]

Tumor Necrosis Factor-α Inhibitors Dysregulation of TNF-α production has been associated with various inflammatory conditions, including rheumatoid arthritis, inflammatory bowel disease, ankylosing spondylitis, PsA, and psoriasis.[66–68] Elevated TNF-α levels are seen in both the affected skin and serum of patients with psoriasis; and these elevated levels have a significant correlation with psoriasis severity.[31] The biologic agents etanercept, adalimumab, and infliximab are TNF-α inhibitors. They offer the prospect of more rapid disease control than is commonly seen with the other BRMs.[26] After successful control of psoriasis, TNF-α levels are reduced to normal.[41]

There are safety concerns common to TNF-α inhibitors, mainly from observations made through their use in rheumatoid arthritis and inflammatory bowel disease and more recently psoriasis.[66–68] One concern is an increased risk of infections, most commonly upper respiratory tract infections, and less commonly serious infections including sepsis, new-onset or reactivation tuberculosis, and opportunistic infections such as histoplasmosis, cryptococcosis, aspergillosis, candidiasis, and pneumocystis.[26,31,66–68] There have been reports of serious pulmonary and disseminated histoplasmosis, coccidioidomycosis, and blastomycosis infections,[69,70] sometimes with fatal outcomes when these infections were not consistently recognized and promptly treated in the patients taking TNF-α inhibitors.[69]

A second concern is the development or worsening of autoimmune diseases such as peripheral and central demyelinating disorders including multiple sclerosis and drug-induced lupus-like syndromes.[26,31,70] A third concern is the potential increased risk of malignancies such as lymphoma,[26,31,70] melanoma, and nonmelanoma skin cancer.[31] A fourth concern is the potential for other cutaneous adverse effects including vasculitis, granulomatous reactions, cutaneous infections, psoriasiform eruptions, and infusion or injection site reactions.[67] Flares of pustular psoriasis have been reported primarily for patients undergoing treatment for nondermatologic conditions such as rheumatoid arthritis.[26] There is also a concern about chronic heart failure (CHF), although this has now become controversial because of conflicting studies demonstrating both worsening and improvement.[31]

The current recommendation from the American Academy of Dermatology is that TNF-α inhibitors be avoided in patients with severe CHF (New York Heart Association class III or IV), and those with milder CHF should have their TNF-α inhibitors withdrawn at the onset of new symptoms or worsening of preexisting CHF.[31]

Although the above are safety concerns common to etanercept, adalimumab, and infliximab, their safety profiles are not identical. For example, the risk for tuberculosis (TB) is lowest with etanercept and highest with infliximab.[26] They are pregnancy category B and safe to use in pregnancy.[31]

Adalimumab is a human monoclonal antibody that provides rapid and efficacious control of psoriasis.[31] Clinical trials in patients with moderate-to-severe psoriasis have shown dramatic results. A 2006 12-week RCT with open-label extension to 52 weeks showed significant improvement within 1 week of therapy, with complete or nearly complete clearance in some patients, and clinical benefits were maintained for at least 1 year with continuous therapy for most patients.[26,71]

A 2008 52-week RCT (REVEAL) with an initial 16-week double-blind placebo-controlled (DBPC; period A) phase followed by a 17-week open-label phase (period B) followed by a 19-week DBPC phase (period C) showed a 71% PASI 75 response for adalimumab treated patients versus 7% for placebo-treated patients at week 16. All patients received open-label adalimumab from weeks 17 through 32. At week 33, patients achieving PASI 75 were rerandomized to adalimumab or placebo; patients achieving PASI 50 but <75 were continued on open-label adalimumab; and therapy for patients with PASI <50 was discontinued. At week 52, 5% of patients rerandomized to adalimumab lost adequate response versus 28% of patients rerandomized to placebo. Adalimumab was continued at 40 mg every other week. The study showed that adalimumab can produce rapid and dramatic results which can be sustained on continued use, in patients with moderate-to-severe psoriasis.[72]

Additional 3-year open-label extension study for patients in REVEAL showed that in patients with sustained initial PASI 75 responses, adalimumab efficacy was maintained for more than 3 years of continuous therapy and maintenance was best at PASI 100. Some patients with PASI <75 in REVEAL also achieved long-term PASI 75 responses.[66]

For comparative studies, as discussed in the methotrexate section, a head-to-head study showed that adalimumab was significantly more efficacious than methotrexate.[62]

Adalimumab is given as 80 mg subcutaneously in the first week, then 40 mg the following week, and thereafter 40 mg every other week continuously.[26,31] More frequent dosing has been explored.[26]

Adverse effects in adalimumab clinical trials including the 3-year extension were similar to those already described for this class of BRMs (i.e., tuberculosis and other opportunistic infections such as candidiasis, congestive heart failure, malignancies including nonmelanoma skin cancer that may be related to psoriasis, and allergic reactions).[66,71,72]

Etanercept was one of the earliest BRMs available on the market for use in inflammatory diseases. It has demonstrated efficacy for rheumatoid arthritis. It was approved for use in PsA in the United States in June 2002 and approved in 2004 for use in moderate to severe psoriasis.[70] It is also approved for treatment of juvenile rheumatoid arthritis and ankylosing spondylitis. Thus, as opposed to some of the other BRMs approved for psoriasis, etanercept has been extensively used in rheumatology both for adults and children.

The dosing of etanercept in psoriasis differs from its other indications, reflective of the dosing regimens found to be effective for psoriasis in clinical trials. Etanercept is used continuously, given as 50 mg subcutaneously twice weekly for the first 12 weeks, followed by 25 mg twice weekly[26] or 50 mg once weekly.[31,70] Significant improvement was seen in about 50% of patients in clinical trials by week 12 and more than 50% of participants by week 24; with continuing therapy, weaker responders continued to improve for up to 1 year.[26,29,73] Continuing therapy using 50 mg twice weekly regimens are being explored and may provide greater benefit.[26] Etanercept was efficacious in children and adolescents (aged 4 to 17 years) with plaque psoriasis dosed at 0.8 mg/kg (maximum 50 mg) once weekly.[74]

Infliximab also received approval for rheumatologic diseases before psoriasis and was on the market before adalimumab. Infliximab may be more efficacious than etanercept. A 2011 open-label study showed that psoriatic patients with an inadequate response to etanercept had rapid and sustained improvement when switched to infliximab.[75] Unlike etanercept or adalimumab, infliximab is a chimeric antibody with both murine and human components; thus, antibodies to the drug can develop, resulting in infusion reactions.[31] Regular therapy rather than intermittent dosing on an as-needed basis may minimize this occurrence.[31] The standard dosing regimen is three IV infusions of 5 mg/kg given over a 6-week induction period, followed by regular infusions every 8 weeks.[31]

Clinical response is seen rapidly. In a randomized controlled phase III trial, 80% of patients responded by week 10 (after 3 doses of infliximab); however, the response dropped to about 50% by week 50.[76,77] Rare reports of serious adverse events, including fatal cases of hepatosplenic T-cell lymphomas, have been associated with infliximab use.[28] Other rare instances of cholecystitis and autoimmune hepatitis, which may be a class effect for TNF-α inhibitors, have also been reported.[26]

Alefacept Alefacept was the first BRM to receive approval for the treatment of psoriasis, in January 2003 in the United States and in October 2004 in Canada. Over the years, it has accumulated an extensive and reassuring safety record, with no evidence of increased incidence of infections, cancers, or any other serious adverse events beyond background levels. The exception is that CD4 T lymphocytes can be depleted, and CD4 cell counts must be monitored. CD4 cell counts must be monitored, since those T lymphocytes can be depleted.[26,78]

In comparison with other BRMs, alefacept monotherapy provides only limited control of psoriasis, and as discussed later, it is often explored in combination regimens to enhance response.[26] However, even with monotherapy, long periods of near complete remission can be seen occasionally.[26]

Dosing is intended to be intermittent. Alefacept is given for a 12-week course, then repeated only when the loss of control becomes unacceptable (up to two more courses per year).[26] Maximal response was generally seen by 6 to 8 weeks in responders, and currently there is no measure to predict which patients will respond.[31]

Ustekinumab Ustekinumab is an IL-12/23 monoclonal antibody approved for the treatment of psoriasis in adults 18 years or older with moderate-to-severe plaque psoriasis.[67] It selectively targets IL-12 and IL-23, two cytokines that play a role in the pathogenesis of psoriasis.

Two large randomized placebo-controlled trials (PHOENIX 1 and PHOENIX 2) demonstrated clinical efficacy of ustekinumab, with approximately 70% of patients achieving 75% skin clearance after two doses and maintaining the response for 1 year with continued treatment.[79–81] The improvements were dramatic. The impact of ustekinumab on patients' health-related quality of life (QOL) in PHOENIX 2 was also evaluated.[82] Patients showed a significant improvement not only in skin-related QOL, but also in symptoms of anxiety and depression (as assessed by the Hospital Anxiety and Depression Scale).[82] The subset of patients with PsA in PHOENIX 1 and PHOENIX 2 also showed significant improvement in QOL, anxiety, and depression.[83]

Weight-based dosing rather than fixed-dose was found to be clinically significant for efficacy in PHOENIX 1 and PHOENIX 2—heavier patients required a higher dose.[84] Serum ustekinumab concentrations were also affected by weight.[84] Dosing is 45 mg for patients weighing 100 kg (220 lb) or less, and 90 mg for those of higher weights. Ustekinumab is administered subcutaneously at weeks 0 and 4, then every 12 weeks as maintenance therapy.

Cumulative 3-year safety data from PHOENIX 1 and 2, and a third RCT (ACCEPT) have also been published.[85,86] Common adverse effects include upper respiratory infections, headache, fatigue, pruritus, back pain, injection site reactions, and arthralgia, with the most common events being headache and nasopharyngitis.[85] Ustekinumab does not appear to exacerbate atopic diseases.[85] Serious adverse effects include those seen with other BRMs, including serious tubercular, fungal, viral infections, and cancers. No evidence of a dose-response to infection rates was seen.[86] Serious infections and malignancy rates did not increase with long-term ustekinumab treatment up to 3 years.[85,86] In addition, a reversible posterior leukoencephalopathy syndrome (RPLS) has been reported.[67]

Combination Therapies

Combination therapies may be beneficial in the management of plaque psoriasis: generally to either enhance efficacy or minimize toxicity. As shown in Figures 78-1 and 78-2, combinations can include two topical agents, a topical agents plus phototherapy, a systemic agent plus topical therapy, a systemic agent plus phototherapy, two systemic agents used in rotation, or a systemic agent and a BRM. Rotational therapy is not commonly used in practice, and the use of a BRM added to a systemic agent is still under investigation.

The combination of a topical corticosteroid and a topical vitamin D_3 analog is particularly useful. This was shown in several studies to be efficacious and safe, with less skin irritation than monotherapy with either agent, and the combination product containing calcipotriol and betamethasone dipropionate ointment has demonstrated efficacy in RCTs for patients with relatively severe psoriasis.[26,30] The combination may also be steroid sparing.[30]

The combination of retinoids with phototherapy has also been shown to increase efficacy. Because retinoids may be photosensitizing and increase the risk of burning after ultraviolet (UV) light exposure, doses of phototherapy should be reduced to minimize adverse effects. A RCT with tazarotene and broadband UVB not only showed significant enhancement of UVB efficacy but also reduced the number of UVB treatment sessions needed for response.[28,30,87] The combination of acitretin and broadband UVB reduced the number of needed treatments, compared with UVB alone.[26,88] Acitretin with NB-UVB (RE-UVB) was highly effective for patients with difficult-to-control psoriasis.[30,89] The combination of acitretin and PUVA (RE-PUVA) also showed greater efficacy than monotherapy with either agent.[28,90] RE-PUVA can be used to achieve clearance with up to a twofold reduction in total UV exposure.[26] Phototherapy has also been used with other topical agents, such as UVB with coal tar (Goeckerman regimen)[55] to increase treatment response, because coal tar is also photosensitizing.

BRMs used in combination with other therapies are being explored. Some beneficial combinations have been found. Alefacept and NB-UVB in combination significantly reduced the number of UVB treatments needed with clearance seen in 43% of patients within 12 weeks.[26,91] Infliximab given concurrently with immunosuppressive agents such as methotrexate or azathioprine may result in a lower incidence of infusion reactions to infliximab.[31]

Alternative Drug Treatments

Mycophenolate Mofetil (MMF) is a systemic agent occasionally used for patients with resistant cases of moderate-to-severe psoriasis.[26] This is currently not an approved indication in either Canada or the United States.

A few reports and small studies are available describing the efficacy of MMF when used as monotherapy or adjuvant therapy.[92] In addition, one small study evaluated the switch for eight patients with severe psoriasis from cyclosporine to MMF after a washout period of 2 to 4 weeks. On cyclosporine, seven of these patients had deteriorating renal function and hypertension, and one experienced loss of efficacy.[93] After the switch to MMF, there was significant loss of psoriasis control in five of the eight patients but also significant improvement in renal function for six patients.[92,93]

Conversely, another small study evaluated the sequential use of MMF followed by cyclosporine in eight patients with moderate-to-severe psoriasis.[94] There was significant improvement with MMF in all patients, and all patients further improved when switched to cyclosporine.[94]

MMF has some uncommon but significant adverse effects, including increased incidence of opportunistic infections such as cytomegalovirus, cryptococcosis, candidiasis, and *Pneumocystis jirovecii*.[92] Cases of progressive multifocal leukoencephalopathy have also been reported.[92] There may be an associated risk of malignancy.[95]

Hydroxyurea Hydroxyurea is an antimetabolite usually used for cancer treatments, but it has also been used in the systemic treatment of psoriasis for more than 30 years.[26,29] It is still occasionally tried for patients with recalcitrant severe psoriasis, although BRMs may be a better option for these patients.

Hydroxyurea has been compared with methotrexate for patients with moderate-to-severe psoriasis.[96] Weekly regimens showed greater efficacy for methotrexate with a faster clearance rate, although hydroxyurea was also efficacious. The authors concluded that weekly doses of hydroxyurea may be an alternative to methotrexate for patients experiencing intolerable methotrexate side effects or have reached the recommended cumulative dose.[96]

Adverse effects of hydroxyurea include significant bone marrow suppression, lesional erythema, localized tenderness, and reversible hyperpigmentation.[26,96]

Complementary and Alternative Medicines The use of complementary and alternative medicine (CAM) among patients with psoriasis is common, with a prevalence of 43% to 69% in various studies.[97] Most of these patients use herbs, special diets, or dietary supplements in conjunction with their usual antipsoriatic medications and not as replacements. Most patients do not discuss CAM use with their physicians.[97]

A 2009 systematic review of RCTs found that, although there is a large body of literature on CAM use in psoriasis, the quality of most studies was relatively low.[97] CAM agents and interventions with documented clinical efficacy in psoriasis include *Mahonia aquifolium*, fish oil, climatotherapy (Dead Sea salts), and stress reduction techniques.

Mahonia aquafolium (Oregon grape, Mountain grape, or barberry but *not* European barberry) is an evergreen native to southern British Columbia, western Oregon, and northern Idaho. The rhizome and root contain berberine as the primary active constituent. Berberine is an alkaloid that inhibits keratinocyte growth and reduces keratinocyte proliferation, and it also has antibacterial and antifungal activities. In at least two clinical trials *Mahonia aquifolium* was efficacious in reducing disease severity: In one randomized placebo-controlled study a *Mahonia aquifolium* 10% preparation applied topically twice daily resulted in a significant improvement in the PASI score and the Quality of Life Index (QLI), compared with placebo.[98] Adverse effects in clinical trials included rash, burning sensation, redness, and itching.

Fish oil contains two important long-chain polyunsaturated fatty acids—eicosapentaenoic acid (EPA) and docosahexaenoic acid (DHA). EPA and DHA are omega-3 fatty acids. They act as substrates competing with arachidonic acid for cyclooxygenase and lipoxygenase, thus reducing the production of proinflammatory molecules in psoriatic plaques.[97] Several randomized placebo-controlled and/or comparative trials for patients with psoriasis have demonstrated efficacy of fish oils. One study comparing EPA plus etretinate to etretinate monotherapy found significantly greater efficacy with the combination of EPA plus etretinate.[99]

Climatotherapy refers to the practice of traveling to the Dead Sea and sunbathing and/or bathing in the sea—the beneficial effects are likely from the high salinity of the sea and UV rays.[97] Several studies have demonstrated efficacy, including two studies using saline spa baths. One study used highly concentrated (25% to 27%) saline spa baths plus UVB compared with UVB alone, and the other used low concentrated (4.5% to 12%) saline spa bath plus UVB again compared with UVB alone. In both studies the clinical response was significantly better with the saline spa bath plus UVB combination.[97,100,101]

Stress-reduction techniques have inconsistently shown some benefit. One randomized study demonstrated that both meditation or meditation and imagery were efficacious as adjunctive treatments for patients with scalp psoriasis.[102] A second randomized study for patients with psoriasis receiving either UVB or PUVA therapy showed that the addition of a mindfulness-based stress-reduction audiotape played during light treatments reduced response times for patients receiving UVB but not PUVA therapy.[103] This confirmed the belief that psychological stress plays a role in psoriasis. More recently, in a case-control study of risk factors during the year before the onset of psoriasis, stressful life events were found to be significant.[104,105]

Personalized Pharmacotherapy

Despite the availability of good quality evidence and clinical practice guidelines, patients with psoriasis are still often undertreated or inappropriately managed.[25] A 2007 study in the U.S. involving 1,657 patients from National Psoriasis Foundation surveys found that 40% of patients with psoriasis were receiving no current treatment; of those, 27% had psoriasis involving >10% body surface area.[106] In addition, those receiving care may be undertreated.[106] Early access to care and adherence may also be issues.

Patient-specific therapies that take into consideration comorbid illnesses, adherence, and pharmacoeconomic issues in addition to the patient's psoriatic manifestations and responses to treatments are important, and will ultimately improve the quality of care. Treatment goals need to be defined for both short-term and long-term management time frames.[25] Without optimizing patient care, the concern is that patients with poorly managed psoriasis may follow a "diminished" life course compared with the course they might have taken if they did not have psoriasis, as the disease has significant psychological, social, and economic impacts in addition to its physical manifestations.[107]

To this end, a current focus is defining frameworks[107] and specific treatment goals[25] for implementation of practice guidelines, as described earlier in this chapter. The reader is encouraged to review the noted references for further information.

Special Populations

Psoriasis in Children Pediatric psoriasis is more often attributable to direct precipitating factors such as skin trauma, infections, drugs, or stress.[26,108] Compared with adults, plaque lesions in children are often smaller, thinner, and less scaly, which can make diagnosis more difficult. Face and flexures are more commonly involved than for adults. Psoriatic diaper rash can occur up to age 2. PsA is rare.[26]

Topical treatment is the standard of care for children with psoriasis, with topical corticosteroids often the treatment of first choice.[26] Other useful pharmacologic therapies include calcipotriol and anthralin; calcipotriol with or without topical corticosteroids has also been recommended as treatment of first choice[109] because it produces minimal adverse effects.[26] Since children's skin is thinner and better hydrated than that of adults, they are at higher risk of drug absorption leading to systemic adverse effects. The lowest potency corticosteroid that provides control should be used, and it should be tapered as the lesions improve. If long-term calcipotriol is used, monitoring of ionized calcium is recommended because of the risk of hypercalcemia.[26]

Systemic therapies are reserved for children with severe and recalcitrant psoriasis.[26,109] Methotrexate can provide near to complete clearance[109] and has been safely used to control severe childhood psoriatic episodes and then withdrawn as lesions improve.[26] Regular monitoring for liver and blood toxicity is required.[26] The BRM etanercept was studied in a randomized placebo-controlled trial of 211 children and adolescents (4 to 17 years) with moderate-to-severe plaque psoriasis. It significantly reduced disease severity; however, four serious adverse events occurred (ovarian cyst requiring removal, gastroenteritis, gastroenteritis-associated dehydration, and left basilar pneumonia).[110] Etanercept has been studied in children with polyarticular juvenile rheumatoid arthritis without new safety concerns emerging.[26]

Phototherapy should be used with caution, especially for younger children, because of long-term carcinogenic risks and phototoxicities. For older children and adolescents with severe, extensive, or treatment-resistant disease, UVB may be a treatment option.[26]

Psoriasis in Pregnancy Hormonal changes in pregnancy can improve symptoms for patients with plaque psoriasis. In one study, 55% of patients showed improvements during pregnancy.[26,111] For patients with more than 10% BSA involvement who reported improvement, lesions decreased by more than 80% during pregnancy.[111] This appeared to correlate with high estrogen but not progesterone levels.[111] Thus, some pregnant women may require minimal treatment for their psoriasis.

Some antipsoriatic drugs have significant teratogenic risks, placing them in pregnancy category X. Thus, women of childbearing potential must use effective birth control during therapy, and may need to continue effective contraception after discontinuing therapy for a period of time, as discussed in detail throughout this chapter. In addition, drugs listed as pregnancy category C may carry known teratogenic risks in animal studies or have limited available data for use in pregnancy.

UVB has been considered the safest treatment for extensive psoriasis during pregnancy. It is recommended for patients with widespread disease not controlled by topical agents. One problem with this therapy is an increased potential for reactivation of herpes simplex, which may be transmitted to the infant at delivery.[26]

For more detailed information about antipsoriatic drugs in pregnancy, a systematic, drug-by-drug review of case reports and case-control studies is available.[112] The 2009 Canadian Guidelines for the Management of Plaque Psoriasis provides a drug-by-drug summary of recommendations for topical agents, phototherapy, and systemic agents in pregnancy.[26]

Psoriasis in the Elderly Age-related changes in organ function/drug clearance and greater drug sensitivity increase the risk of adverse drug events for elderly patients with psoriasis.

Methotrexate is hepatotoxic and should be used with caution in the elderly. Cyclosporine has nephrotoxic potential and may also increase blood pressure. Both drugs have significant drug interactions, and polypharmacy, common in older patients, make management of interactions challenging.

In addition, older patients may have preexisting comorbidities, such as hyperlipidemia and metabolic syndrome, and this may further limit drug use. Adalimumab appears equally efficacious in older patients (older than 65) who may have higher incidences of hypertension, hyperlipidemia, depression, obesity, and diabetes.[113] Adverse effects profiles were similar between subgroups (various weights and comorbidities) with no significant differences in serious adverse events.[113] Topical psoriasis treatments are often prescribed for elderly patients as first-line therapy[26]; however, even with topicals, adverse effects—including systemic ones—can occur with greater frequency in these patients.[26]

Psoriasis in Patients with a History of Solid Tumors As discussed throughout this chapter, many antipsoriatic therapies carry significant cancer risks. PUVA, systemic therapies such as cyclosporine, and some BRMs are associated with increased risks of oncologic disorders.

A systematic review of the risk of malignancy associated with therapies for moderate to severe psoriasis confirmed the following[95]: PUVA is associated with an increased risk of cutaneous SCC and malignant melanoma; UVB is a much safer therapeutic modality than PUVA; cyclosporine increases risks of lymphoma, internal malignancies, and skin cancers; methotrexate may be associated with increased melanoma and Epstein–Barr virus–associated lymphomas; MMF may be associated with lymphoproliferative disorders; and the malignancy risk may be increased for biologic agents, especially the TNF-α inhibitors.[95]

The 2009 Canadian guidelines recommend that TNF-α inhibitors be used with caution for patients with a history of malignancy or existing malignancies, and the T-cell modulator alefacept is contraindicated for these patients.[26]

Pharmacoeconomic Considerations

10 The wide gap in costs of agents for psoriasis makes economics and availability of insurance or other coverage important considerations in formulating a therapeutic plan.

Currently, the expensive BRMs are often considered for patients with moderate-to-severe psoriasis when less expensive systemic agents are inadequate or relatively contraindicated. BRMs have also been recommended as first-line therapy, alongside conventional systemic agents, for patients with moderate-to-severe psoriasis; however, in practice, drug access secondary to cost considerations can limit use. These agents may be needed early, though, for some patients with comorbidities.

A recent pharmacoeconomic analysis of BRMs in the treatment of psoriasis suggests that the cost-to-benefit ratio for BRMs may be favorable.[68] There are also cost differences among the BRMs. Of the TNF-α inhibitors, etanercept is the least costly, followed by adalimumab than infliximab.[114] However, etanercept is less efficacious. Adalimumab (at doses of 40 mg every other week) is significantly less costly than ustekinumab, with similar efficacies, in patients with suboptimal response to etanercept.[115]

CONCLUSIONS

Psoriasis is a lifelong illness with no known cure. Significant comorbidities may coexist. Treatment should be patient-specific, with consideration given to disease severity, patient risk factors, age, and comorbidities. Newer treatment modalities, including numerous BRMs, are now parts of the armamentarium available in the management of this disease.

ABBREVIATIONS

BMI	body mass index
BRM	biologic response modifier
BSA	body surface area
CAM	complementary and alternative medicine
CHD	coronary heart disease
CHF	chronic heart failure
CRP	C-reactive protein
CYP3A4	cytochrome P450 isoenzyme 3A4
DBPC	double-blind placebo-controlled
DHA	docosahexaenoic acid
DISH	disseminated (or diffuse) idiopathic skeletal hyperostosis
DLQI	Dermatology Life Quality Index
EPA	eicosapentaenoic acid
FDA	Food and Drug Administration
GFR	glomerular filtration rate
HLA-C	major histocompatibility complex antigen
HPA	hypothalamic–pituitary–adrenal
IL	interleukin
MMF	mycophenolate mofetil
MI	myocardial infarction
NSAIDs	nonsteroidal antiinflammatory drugs
NB-UVB	narrowband ultraviolet B (311 nm ultraviolet B light)
PASI	psoriasis area and severity index
PGA	Physician's Global Assessment
PsA	psoriatic arthritis
PUVA	psoralens with ultraviolet A light
QOL	quality of life
QLI	Quality of Life Index
RCT	randomized controlled trial
RE-PUVA	retinoid plus PUVA (as combination therapy)
RE-UVB	retinoid plus NBUVB (as combination therapy)
RPLS	reversible posterior leukoencephalopathy syndrome
RR	relative risk
SCAT	short-contact anthralin therapy
SCC	squamous cell carcinoma
SF-36	Short Form Health Survey
SPF	sun protection factor
TB	tuberculosis
TNF-α	Tumor necrosis factor-α
UV	ultraviolet
UVA	ultraviolet A (315 to 400 nm ultraviolet A light)
UVB	ultraviolet B, or broadband UVB (28 to 315 nm ultraviolet B light)

REFERENCES

1. Law RM. Chapter 64: Psoriasis. In: Chisholm-Burns M, ed. Pharmacotherapy Principles and Practice, 3rd ed. New York: McGraw-Hill, 2013:1127–1141.
2. Reich K. The concept of psoriasis as a systemic inflammation: Implications for disease management. J Eur Acad Dermatol Venereol 2012;26(suppl 2):3–11.
3. Gulliver WP, Pirzada SM. Psoriasis: More than skin deep. In: Saeland S, ed. Recent Advances in Skin Immunology. Kevala, India: Research Signpost, 2008:167–179.
4. Christopher E. Psoriasis-epidemiology and clinical spectrum. Clin Exp Dermatol 2001;26:314–320.
5. Lowes, MA, Bowcock AM, Krueger JG. Pathogenesis and therapy of psoriasis. Nature 2007;445(7130):866–873.
6. Farber EM, Nall ML. The natural history of psoriasis in 5600 patients. Dermatologica 1974;148:118.
7. Farber E, Bright R, Nall M. Psoriasis: A questionnaire survey of 2144 patients. Arch Dermatol 1974;98:248–259.
8. Lomboldt G. Psoriasis: Prevalence, Spontaneous Course and Genetics: A Census Study on the Prevalence of Skin Disease on the Faroe Islands. Copenhagen: G.E.C. Gad, 1963.
9. Farber EM, Nall ML, Watson W. Natural history of psoriasis in 61 twin pairs. Arch Dermatol 1974;109:207–211.
10. Nall L, Gulliver WP, Charmley P, et al. Search for the psoriasis susceptibility gene: The Newfoundland Study. Cutis 1999;64:323–329.
11. Nair RP, Duffin KC, Helms C, et al. Genome-wide scan reveals association of psoriasis with IL-23 and NF-κB pathways. Nat Genet 2009;41:199–204.
12. Zhang XJ, Huang W, Yang S, et al. Psoriasis genome-wide association study identified susceptibility variants within LCE gene cluster at 1q21. Nat Genet 2009;41:205–210.
13. Raychaudhuri SP, Jiang W-Y, Raychaudhuri SK. Revisiting the Koebner phenomenon. Am J Pathol 2008;172:961–971.
14. Clarke C. Psoriasis—first-line treatments. Pharm J 2005;274:623–626.
15. Nickoloff BJ, Nestle FO. Recent insight into the immunopathogenesis of psoriasis provide new therapeutic opportunities. J Clin Invest 2004;113:1664–1675.
16. Guenther L, Gulliver W. Psoriasis comorbidities. J Cutan Med Surg 2009;13(suppl 2):S77–S87.
17. Kimball AB, Gladman D, Gelfand JM, et al. National Psoriasis Foundation clinical consensus on psoriasis comorbidities and recommendations for screening. J Am Acad Dermatol 2008;58:1031–1042.
18. Gulliver WP. Importance of screening for comorbidities in psoriasis patients. Expert Rev Dermatol 2008;3:133–135.
19. Gelfand JM, Gladman Dd, Mease PJ, et al. Epidemiology of psoriatic arthritis in the population of the United States. J Am Acad Dermatol 2005;53:573–577.
20. Rahman P, O'Reilly DD. Psoriatic arthritis genetic susceptibility and pharmacogenetics. Pharmacogenomics 2008;9:195–205.
21. Wilson PW, D'Agostino RB, Parise H, et al. Metabolic syndrome as a precursor of cardiovascular disease and type 2 diabetes mellitus. Circulation 2005;112:3066–3072.
22. Kimball AB, Guerin A, Latremouille-Viau D, et al. Coronary heart disease and stroke risk in patients with psoriasis: Retrospective analysis. Am J Med 2010;123:350–357.
23. Gelfand JM, Neimann AL, Shin DB, et al. Risk of myocardial infarction in patients with psoriasis. JAMA 2006;296:1735–1741.
24. Mrowietz U, Kragballe K, Reich K, et al. Definition of treatment goals for moderate to severe psoriasis: A European consensus. Arch Dermatol Res 2011;303:1–10.

25. Mrowietz U. Implementing treatment goals for successful long-term management of psoriasis. J Eur Acad Dermatol Venereol 2012;26(suppl 2):12–20.
26. Papp KA, Gulliver W, Lynde CW, Poulin Y (Steering Committee). 2009 Canadian Guidelines for the Management of Plaque Psoriasis—Canadian Guidelines for the Management of Plaque Psoriasis, 1st ed. Endorsed by the Canadian Dermatology Association. 2009, *http://www.dermatology.ca/guidelines/cdnpsoriasisguidelines.pdfwww.der matology.ca/psoriasisguidelines.html.*
27. Law RMT, Gulliver WP. Chapter 110: Psoriasis. In: Schwinghammer TL, Koehler JM, eds. Pharmacotherapy Casebook and Instructor's Guide: A Patient-Focused Approach, 9th ed. New York: McGraw-Hill, 2014, in press.
28. Menter A, Korman NJ, Elmets CA, et al. 2009 guidelines of care for the management of psoriasis and psoriatic arthritis—section 5. Guidelines of care for the treatment of psoriasis with phototherapy and photochemotherapy. J Am Acad Dermatol 2010;62:114–135.
29. Menter A, Korman NJ, Elmets CA, et al. 2009 Guidelines of care for the management of psoriasis and psoriatic arthritis—section 4. Guidelines of care for the management and treatment of psoriasis with traditional systemic agents. J Am Acad Dermatol 2009;61:451–485.
30. Menter A, Korman NJ, Elmets CA, et al. 2009 Guidelines of care for the management of psoriasis and psoriatic arthritis—section 3. Guidelines of care for the management and treatment of psoriasis with topical therapies. J Am Acad Dermatol 2009;60:643–659.
31. Menter A. Gottlieb A, Feldman SR, et al. Guidelines of care for the management of psoriasis and psoriatic arthritis—section 1. Overview of psoriasis and guidelines of care for the treatment of psoriasis with biologics. J Am Acad Dermatol 2008;58:826–850.
32. Rosmarin DM, Lebwohl M, Elewski BE, et al. Cyclosporine and psoriasis: 2008 National psoriasis Foundation Consensus Conference. J Am Acad Dermatol 2010;62:838–853.
33. National Psoriasis Foundation. Topical treatments for psoriasis including steroids. 2009, *http://www.psoriasis.org/NetCommunity/Document.Doc?id=164.*
34. Kalb RE, Strober B, Weinstein G, Lebwohl M. Methotrexate and psoriasis: 2009 National Psoriasis Foundation Consensus Conference. J Am Acad Dermatol 2009;60:824–837.
35. Guenther L, Langley RG, Shear NH, et al. Integrating biologic agents into management of moderate-to-severe psoriasis: a consensus of the Canadian Psoriasis Expert Panel. J Cutan Med Surg 2004;8:321–337.
36. Cohen SN, Baron SE, Archer CB. Guidance on the diagnosis and clinical management of psoriasis. Clin Exp Dermatol 2012;37(suppl 1):13–18.
37. Paul C, Gallini A, Archier E, et al. Evidence-based recommendations on topical treatment and phototherapy of psoriasis: Systematic review and expert opinion of a panel of dermatologists. J Eur Acad Dermatol Venereol 2012;26(suppl 3):1–10.
38. Long CC, Finlay AY. The finger-tip unit—a new practical measure. Clin Exp Dermatol 1991;16:444–447.
39. Menter Kamili. Topical treatment of psoriasis. In: Yawalkar N, ed. Current Problems in Dermatology. Basel, Switzerland: S. Karger AG; 2009.
40. Krueger GG, O'Reilly MA, Weidner M, et al. Comparative efficacy of once-daily flurandrenolide tape versus twice-daily diflorasone diacetate ointment in the treatment of psoriasis. J Am Acad Dermatol 1998;38:186–190.
41. Mason J, Mason AR, Cork MJ. Topical preparations for the treatment of psoriasis: A systemic review. Br J Dermatol 2002;146:351–364.
42. Castela E, Archier E, Devaux S, et al. Topical corticosteroids in plaque psoriasis: A systematic review of efficacy and treatment modalities. J Euro Acad Dermatol Venereol 2012;26(suppl 3):36–46.
43. Katz HI, Prawer SE, Medansky RS, et al. Intermittent corticosteroid maintenance treatment of psoriasis: A double-blind multicenter trial of augmented betamethasone dipropionate ointment in a pulse dose treatment regimen. Dermatol 1991;183:269–274.
44. Wall ARJ, Poyner TF, Menday AP. A comparison of treatment with dithranol and calcipotriol on the clinical severity and quality of life in patients with psoriasis. Br J Dermatol 1998;139:1005–1011.
45. Cunliffe WJ, Berth-Jones J, Claudy A, et al. Comparative study of calcipotriol (MC 903) ointment and betamethasone 17-valerate ointment in patients with psoriasis vulgaris. J Am Acad Dermatol 1992;26:736–743.
46. Kragballe K, Gjertsen BT, De Hoop D, et al. Double-blind, right/left comparison of calcipotriol and betamethasone valerate in treatment of psoriasis vulgaris. Lancet 1991;337:193–196.
47. Devaux S, Castela A, Archier E, et al. Topical vitamin D analogues alone or in association with topical steroids for psoriasis: A systematic review. J Euro Acad Dermatol Venereol 2012;26(suppl 3):52–60.
48. Weinstein GD, Krueger GG, Lowe NJ, et al. Tazarotene gel, a new retinoid, for topical therapy of psoriasis: Vehicle-controlled study of safety, efficacy, and duration of therapeutic effect. J Am Acad Dermatol 1997;37:85–92.
49. Weinstein GD, Koo JY, Krueger GG, et al. Tazarotene cream in the treatment of psoriasis: Two multicenter, double-blind, randomized, vehicle-controlled studies of the safety and efficacy of tazarotene cream 0.05% and 0.1% applied once daily for 12 weeks. J Am Acad Dermatol 2003;48:760–767.
50. McGill A, Frank A, Emmett N, et al. The anti-psoriatic drug anthralin accumulates in keratinocyte mitochondria, dissipates mitochondrial membrane potential, and induces apoptosis through a pathway dependent on respiratory competent mitochondria. FASEB J 2005;19:1012–1014.
51. Thawornchaisit P, Harncharoen K. A comparative study of tar and betamethasone valerate in chronic plaque psoriasis: a study in Thailand. J Med Assoc Thai 2007;90:1997–2002.
52. Stuetz A, Grassberger M, Meingassner JG. Pimecrolimus (Elidel, SDZ ASM 981)—preclinical pharmacologic profile and skin selectivity. Semin Cutan Med Surg 2001;20:233–241.
53. Mrowietz U, Graeber M, Brautigam M, et al. The novel azomycin derivative SDZ ASM 981 is effective for psoriasis when used topically under occlusion. Br J Dermatol 1998;139:992–996.
54. Gribetz C, Ling M, Lebwohl M, et al. Pimecrolimus cream 1% in the treatment of intertriginous psoriasis: A double-blind, randomized study. J Am Acad Dermatol 2004;51:731–738.
55. Matz H. Phototherapy for psoriasis: what to choose and how to use: Facts and controversies. Clin Dermatol 2010;28:73–80.
56. Archier E, Devaux S, Castela E, et al. Efficacy of Psoralen UV-A therapy vs. narrowband UV-B therapy in chronic plaque psoriasis: A systematic literature review. J Euro Acad Dermatol Venereol 2012;26(suppl 3):11–21.
57. Stern RS. Genital tumors among men with psoriasis exposed to psoralens and ultraviolet A radiation (PUVA) and

ultraviolet B radiation: The photochemotherapy follow-up study. N Engl J Med 1990;322:1093–1097.

58. Anstey AV, Kragballe K. Retrospective assessment of PASI 50 and PASI 75 attainment with a calcipotriol/betamethasone dipropionate ointment. Int J Dermatol 2006;45:970–975.
59. Mahrie G, Schulze HJ, Farber L, et al. Low-dose short-term cyclosporine versus etretinate in psoriasis: improvement of skin, nail, and joint involvement. J Am Acad Dermatol 1995;32:78–88.
60. Heydendael VM, Spuls POL, Opmeer BC, et al. Methotrexate versus cyclosporine in moderate-to-severe chronic plaque psoriasis. N Engl J Med 2003;349:658–665.
61. Shupack J, Abel E, Bauer E, et al. Cyclosporine as maintenance therapy in patients with severe psoriasis. J Am Acad Dermatol 1997;36:423–432.
62. Saurat JH, Stingl G, Dubertret L, et al. Efficacy and safety results from the randomized controlled comparative study of adalimumab vs. methotrexate vs. placebo in patients with psoriasis (CHAMPION). Br J Dermatol 2008;158:558–566.
63. Barker J, Hoffmann M, Wozel G, et al. Efficacy and safety of infliximab vs. methotrexate in patients with moderate-to-severe plaque psoriasis: Results of an open-label, active-controlled, randomized trial (RESTORE1). Br J Dermatol 2011;165:1109–1117.
64. Ferrandiz C, Carrascosa JM, Boada A. A new era in the management of psoriasis? The biologics: Facts and controversies. Clin Dermatol 2010;28:81–87.
65. Langley RG. Effective and sustainable biologic treatment of psoriasis: What can we learn from new clinical data? J Euro Acad Dermatol Venereol 2012;26(suppl 2):21–29.
66. Gordon K, Papp K, Poulin Y, et al. Long-term efficacy and safety of adalimumab in patients with moderate to severe psoriasis treated continuously over 3 years: Results from an open-label extension study for patients from REVEAL. J Am Acad Dermatol 2012;66:241–251.
67. Moustou A-E, Matekovits A, Dessinioti C, et al. Cutaneous side effects of anti-tumor necrosis factor biologic therapy: A clinical review. J Am Acad Dermatol 2009;61:486–504.
68. Poulin Y, Langley R, Teiseira HD, et al. Biologics in the treatment of psoriasis: Clinical and economic overview. J Cutan Med Surg 2009;13(suppl 2):S49–S57.
69. Health Canada. Association of Enbrel (etanercept) with Histoplasmosis and Other Invasive Fungal Infections—For Health Professionals. 2009, *http://www.hc-sc.gc.ca/dhp-mps/medeff/advisories-avis/prof/_2009/enbrel_hpc-cps-eng.php*.
70. Bissonnette R. Etanercept for the treatment of psoriasis. Skin Ther Lett 2006;11:1–4, *http://www.skintherapyletter.com/2006/11.1/1.html*.
71. Gordon KB, Langley RG, Leonard C, et al. Clinical response to adalimumab treatment in patients with moderate to severe psoriasis: double-blind, randomized controlled trial and open-label extension study. J Am Acad Dermatol 2006;55:598–606.
72. Menter A, Tyring SK, Gordon K, et al. Adalimumab therapy for moderate to severe psoriasis: A randomized, controlled phase III trial. J Am Acad Dermatol 2008;58:106–15.
73. Leonardi CL, Powers JL, Matheson RT, et al. Etanercept as monotherapy in patients with psoriasis. N Engl J Med 2003;349:2014–2022.
74. Paller AS, Siegfried EC, Langley RG, et al. Etanercept treatment for children and adolescents with plaque psoriasis. N Engl J Med 2008;358:241–251.
75. Gottlieb AB, Kalb RE, Blauvelt A, et al. The efficacy and safety of infliximab in patients with plaque psoriasis who had an inadequate response to etanercept: Results of a prospective, multicenter, open-label study. J Am Acad Dermatol 2011;67:642–650.
76. Reich K, Nestle FO, Papp K, et al. Infliximab induction and maintenance therapy for moderate-to-severe psoriasis: A phase III, multicenter, double-blind trial. Lancet 2005;366:1367–1374.
77. Menter A, Feldman SR, Weinstein GD, et al. A randomized comparison of continuous vs intermittent infliximab maintenance regimens over 1 year in the treatment of moderate-to-severe plaque psoriasis. J Am Acad Dermatol 2007;56:e1–e15.
78. Goffe B, Papp K, Gratton D, et al. An integrated analysis of thirteen trials summarizing the long-term safety of alefacept in psoriasis patients who have received up to nine courses of therapy. Clin Ther 2005;27:1912–1921.
79. Johnson & Johnson. Stelara (ustekinumab) anti IL-12/23—receives FDA approval for treatment of moderate-to-severe plaques psoriasis with four-times-a-year maintenance dosing. 2009, *http://www.jnj.com/connect/news/all/20090925_150000*.
80. Leonardi C, Kimball AB, Papp K, et al. Efficacy and safety of ustekinumab, a human interleukin-12/23 monoclonal antibody, in patients with psoriasis: 76-Week results from a randomized, double-blind, placebo-controlled trial (PHOENIX 1). Lancet 2008;371:1665–1674.
81. Papp KA, Langley RG, Lebwohl M, et al. Efficacy and safety of ustekinumab, a human interleukin-12/23 monoclonal antibody, in patients with psoriasis: 52-Week results from a randomized, double-blind, placebo-controlled trial (PHOENIX 2). Lancet 2008;371:1675–1684.
82. Langley RG, Feldman SR, Han C, et al. Ustekinumab significantly improves symptoms of anxiety, depression, and skin-related quality of life in patients with moderate-to-severe psoriasis: Results from a randomized, double-blind, placebo-controlled phase III trial. J Am Acad Dermatol 2010;63:457–465.
83. Sofen H, Wasel N, Yeilding N, et al. Ustekinumab improves overall skin response and health-related quality of life, in a subset of moderate to severe psoriasis patients with psoriatic arthritis: Analysis of PHOENIX 1 and 2. J Am Acad Dermatol 2011 Feb;64(2 suppl 1):AB156.
84. Lebwohl M, Yeilding N, Szapary P, et al. Impact of weight on the efficacy and safety of ustekinumab in patients with moderate to severe psoriasis: Rationale for dosing recommendations. J Am Acad Dermatol 2010;63:571–579.
85. Lebwohl M, Leonardi C, Griffiths CEM, et al. Long-term safety experience of ustekinumab in patients with moderate-to-severe psoriasis (part I of II): Results from analyses of general safety parameters from pooled phase 2 and 3 clinical trials. J Am Acad Dermatol 2012;66:731–741.
86. Gordon KB, Papp KA, Langley RG, et al. Long-term safety experience of ustekinumab in patients with moderate to severe psoriasis (part II of II): Results from analyses of infections and malignancy from pooled phase II and III clinical trials. J Am Acad Dermatol 2012;66:742–751.
87. Koo JY, Lowe NJ, Lew-Kaya DA, et al. Tazarotene plus UVB phototherapy in the treatment of psoriasis. J Am Acad Dermatol 2000;43:821–828.
88. Lowe NJ, Prystowsky JH, Bourget T, et al. Acitretin plus UVB therapy for psoriasis: comparisons with placebo plus UVB and acitretin alone. J Am Acad Dermatol 1991;24:591–594.
89. Spuls PI, Rozenblit M, Lebwohl M. Retrospective study of the efficacy of narrowband UVB and acitretin. J Dermatol Treat 2003;14(suppl):17–20.
90. Tanew A, Guggenbichler A, Honigsmann H, et al. Photochemotherapy for severe psoriasis without or in

combination with acitretin: A randomized, double-blind comparison study. J Am Acad Dermatol 1991;25:682–684.

91. Legat FJ, Hofer A, Wackernagel A, et al. Narrowband UV-B phototherapy, alefacept, and clearance of psoriasis. Arch Dermatol 2007;143:1016–1022.
92. Orvis AK, Wesson SK, Breza TS, et al. Mycophenolate mofetil in dermatology. J Am Acad Dermatol 2009;60:183–199.
93. Davidson SC, Morris-Jones R, Powles AV, et al. Change of treatment from cyclosporin to mycophenolate mofetil in severe psoriasis. Br J Dermatol 2000;143:405–407.
94. Pedraz J, Dauden E, Delgado-Jimenez Y, et al. Sequential study on the treatment of moderate-to-severe chronic plaque psoriasis with mycophenolate mofetil and cyclosporin. J Eur Acad Dermatol Venereol 2006;20:702–706.
95. Patel RV, Clark LN, Lebwohl M, et al. Treatments for psoriasis and the risk of malignancy. J Am Acad Dermatol 2009;60:1001–1017.
96. Ranjan N, Sharma NL, Shanker V, et al. Methotrexate versus hydroxycarbamide (hydroxyurea) as a weekly dose to treat moderate-to-severe chronic plaque psoriasis: A comparative study. J Dermatol Treat 2007;18:295–300.
97. Smith N, Weymann A, Tausk FA, et al. Complementary and alternative medicine for psoriasis: A qualitative review of the clinical trial literature. J Am Acad Dermatol 2009;61:841–856.
98. Bernstein S, Donsky H, Gulliver W, et al. Treatment of mild to moderate psoriasis with Relieva, a Mahonia aquifolium extract—a double-blind, placebo-controlled study. Am J Ther 2006;13:121–126.
99. Danno K, Sugie N. Combination therapy with low-dose etretinate and eicosapentaenoic acid for psoriasis vulgaris. J Dermatol 1998;25:703–705.
100. Brochow T, Schiener R, Franke A, et al. A pragmatic randomized controlled trial on the effectiveness of highly concentrated saline spa water baths followed by UVB compared to UVB only in moderate to severe psoriasis. J Altern Complement Med 2007;13:725–732.
101. Brochow T, Schiener R, Franke A, et al. A pragmatic randomized controlled trial on the effectiveness of low concentrated saline spa water baths followed by ultraviolet B (UVB) compared to UVB only in moderate to severe psoriasis. J Eur Acad Dermatol Venereol 2007;21:1027–1037.
102. Gaston L, Crombez J, Lassonde M, et al. Psychological stress and psoriasis: Experimental and prospective correlational studies. Acta Derm Venereol 1991;156: 37–43.
103. Kabat-Zinn J, Wheeler E, Light T, et al. Influence of a mindfulness meditation-based stress reduction intervention on rates of skin clearing in patients with moderate to severe psoriasis undergoing phototherapy (UVB) and photochemotherapy (PUVA). Psychosom Med 1998;60:625–632.
104. Treloar V. Integrative dermatology for psoriasis: facts and controversies. Clin Dermatol 2010;28:93–99.
105. Naldi L, Chatenoud L, Linder D, et al. Cigarette smoking, body mass index, and stressful life events as risk factors for psoriasis: results from an Italian case-control study. J Invest Dermatol 2005;125:61–67.
106. Horn EJ, Fox KM, Patel V, et al. Are patients with psoriasis undertreated? Results of National Psoriasis Foundation survey. J Am Acad Dermatol 2007;57:957–962.
107. Augustin M, Alvaro-Gracia JM, Bagot M, et al. A framework for improving the quality of care for people with psoriasis. J Euro Acad Dermatol Venereol 2012;26(suppl 4):1–16.
108. Benoit S, Hamm H. Childhood psoriasis. Clin Dermatol 2007;25:555–562.
109. De Jager MEA, de Jong EMG, van de Kerkhof PCM, et al. Efficacy and safety of treatments for childhood psoriasis: A systemic literature review. J Am Acad Dermatol 2010;62:1013–1030.
110. Paller AS, Siegfried EC, Langley RG, et al. Etanercept treatment for children and adolescents with plaque psoriasis. N Engl J Med 2008;358:241–251.
111. Murase JE, Chan KK, Garite TJ, et al. Hormonal effect on psoriasis in pregnancy and post partum. Arch Dermatol 2005;141:601–606.
112. Lam J, Polifka JE, Dohil MA. Safety of dermatologic drugs used in pregnant patients with psoriasis and other inflammatory skin diseases. J Am Acad Dermatol 2008;59:295–315.
113. Menter A, Gordon KB, Leonardi CL, et al. Efficacy and safety of adalimumab across subgroups of patients with moderate to severe psoriasis. J Am Acad Dermatol 2010;63:448–456.
114. Bonafede M, Watson C, Fox K. Cost of tumor necrosis factor blocker per treated psoriatic arthritis patient using drug utilization data from a US managed care population. J Am Acad Dermatol 2012 Apr: 66(4)suppl 1: AB189 (poster reference no 5165. Poster abstracts. American Academy of Dermatology 70th Annual Meeting, San Diego, California, March 15–20, 2012.).
115. Augustin M, Sundaram M, Mulani PM, et al. Cost per responder with adalimumab versus ustekinumab treatment for moderate to severe psoriasis with suboptimal response to etanercept. J Am Acad Dermatol 2012 Apr: 66(4)suppl 1: AB189 (poster reference no. 5056. Poster abstracts. American Academy of Dermatology 70th Annual Meeting, San Diego, California, March 15–20, 2012.).
116. Salim A, Tan E, Ilchyshyn A, et al. Folic acid supplementation during treatment of psoriasis with methotrexate: a randomized, double-blind, placebo-controlled trial. Br J Dermatol 2006;154:1169–1174.

79

Atopic Dermatitis

Rebecca M. Law and Po Gin Kwa

KEY CONCEPTS

1. Atopic dermatitis is a chronic skin disorder involving inflammation associated with intense pruritus, a hallmark symptom. Management of atopic dermatitis must always include appropriate management of the associated pruritus.
2. Atopic dermatitis is associated with other atopic diseases such as asthma and allergic rhinitis in the same patient or family. The three conditions are known as the *atopic triad*.
3. The prevalence of atopic dermatitis appears to have increased two- to threefold in many developed and developing countries during the last three decades. Recent data indicate age and country or regional differences, with some countries showing no change or even a decrease. Rural areas appear to have lower prevalence rates.
4. There are genetic and environmental factors in the pathogenesis and pathophysiologic manifestations of atopic dermatitis. The inheritance pattern is not straightforward. More than one gene may be involved in the disease, with the filaggrin gene (*FLG*) being a key player.
5. Atopic dermatitis often presents in infants and young children. The clinical presentation differs somewhat depending on the age of the patient.
6. Secondary bacterial skin infections are common in patients with atopic dermatitis and must be promptly treated.
7. Management of atopic dermatitis must always include appropriate nonpharmacologic management of any controllable environmental factors, such as avoidance of identified triggers. These may include aeroallergens (e.g., mold, grass, pollen), foods (e.g., peanuts, eggs, tomatoes), chemicals (e.g., detergents, soaps), clothing material (e.g., wool, polyester), temperature (e.g., excessive heat), and humidity (e.g., low humidity).
8. Nonpharmacologic management of atopic dermatitis entails managing the symptoms associated with pruritus and encouraging appropriate skin care habits such as proper bathing techniques and the copious use of moisturizers, which is a standard of care.
9. Topical corticosteroids are the drugs of first choice for atopic dermatitis.
10. Topical calcineurin inhibitors (tacrolimus and pimecrolimus) are alternate treatment options for adults and children over the age of 2 years.
11. This chronic illness has substantial socioeconomic impact. The cost may be magnified by undertreatment.

❶ Atopic dermatitis (AD) is a common skin disease. It is often referred to as *eczema*, which is a general term for several types of skin inflammation. AD is the most common type of eczema (Table 79-1).[1] It is a chronic skin disorder involving inflammation with pruritus as the hallmark symptom and presentation. This disorder is often the prelude to atopic diathesis, which includes asthma and other allergic diseases.

❷ This form of dermatitis is commonly associated with other atopic disorders, such as allergic rhinitis and asthma. AD, allergic rhinoconjunctivitis, and asthma are known collectively as the *atopic triad*.[2] AD has also been defined as the cutaneous manifestation of atopy.[2]

The disease can have periods of exacerbation, or flareups, followed by periods of remission. These flareups may be disruptive to the patient's quality of life and may affect the entire family. Disease flareups are difficult to manage and may be complicated by secondary infections. About one-half (estimate up to 65%) of cases in children first manifest before age 1 year[1–4]; these cases are termed *early onset atopic dermatitis*.[5] Approximately 85% of patients develop symptoms before age 5 years.[1]

Of the children with AD diagnosed before age 1 year, approximately 40% to 60% will have the same skin condition continuing into their adulthood.[1,3]

Onset after age 30 years is much less common and is often caused by exposure to harsh or wet conditions[1] such as repeated skin trauma or exposure to harsh chemicals. In adults, the prevalence is believed to be 1% to 3%, with an overall lifetime prevalence of approximately 7%.[1]

EPIDEMIOLOGY

❸ The prevalence of AD is generally said to have increased two- to threefold in developed and developing countries during the last three decades.[5] Currently in developed countries, an estimated 15% to 30% of children and 2% to 10% of adults are affected.[5,6] The prevalence appears to be increasing worldwide, as earlier prevalence rates were estimated at 10% to 15% in children.[4]

❸ The largest international study of the prevalence of AD found both age and country differences in prevalence rates.[7] This international study was the International Study of Asthma and Allergies in Childhood (ISAAC), which was conducted in three phases.[8] ISAAC Phase One included 700,000 children from 156 centers in 56 countries between 1992 and 1998. ISAAC Phase Two studied allergic causes from 30 centers in 22 countries. ISAAC Phase Three repeated a multicountry cross-sectional survey (1999 to 2004) and included 187,943 children aged 6 to 7 years from 64 centers in 35 countries and 302,159 adolescents

TABLE 79-1 Types of Eczema (Dermatitis)[1]

- **Allergic contact eczema (allergic contact dermatitis):** A red, itchy, weepy reaction where the skin has come into contact with a substance that the immune system recognizes as foreign, such as poison ivy or certain preservatives in creams and lotions.
- **Atopic dermatitis (or irritant contact dermatitis):** A chronic skin disease characterized by itchy, inflamed skin.
- **Contact eczema:** A localized reaction that includes redness, itching, and burning where the skin has come into contact with an allergen (an allergy-causing substance) or with an irritant such as an acid, cleaning agent, or other chemical.
- **Dyshidrotic eczema:** Irritation of the skin on the palms of hands and soles of the feet characterized by clear, deep blisters that itch and burn.
- **Neurodermatitis:** Scaly patches of the skin on the head, lower legs, wrists, or forearms caused by a localized itch (such as an insect bite) that become intensely irritated when scratched.
- **Nummular eczema:** Coin-shaped patches of irritated skin—most common on the arms, back, buttocks, and lower legs—that may be crusted, scaling, and extremely itchy.
- **Seborrheic eczema:** Yellowish, oily, scaly patches of skin on the scalp, face, and occasionally other parts of the body.
- **Stasis dermatitis:** A skin irritation on the lower legs, generally related to circulatory problems.

aged 13 to 14 years from 105 centers in 55 countries. For children aged 6 to 7 years, most countries showed an increase of 2 standard deviations (SDs) in mean annual prevalence over a 5- to 10-year period. In contrast, for adolescents aged 13 to 14 years, the trends differ from country to country. Large increases in prevalence were seen in developing countries (e.g., Mexico, Chile, Kenya, and Algeria, and seven countries in Southeast Asia). But in other countries with formerly very high prevalences, the mean annual prevalence in eczema symptoms has either leveled off or decreased. Most of the largest decreases (SD ≥2) in prevalence were reported from developed countries in northwest Europe, (e.g., the United Kingdom, Ireland, Sweden, Germany) and New Zealand.[7] The ISAAC study has suggested that a maximum prevalence plateau of approximately 20% has emerged.[7,8]

There were no differences according to the sex of the study participant, or with gross national income at a country level.[7] This is consistent with other reports that AD affects males and females at approximately the same rate.[1] There appears to be a lower prevalence of AD in rural areas when compared with urban areas, suggesting a link to the *hygiene hypothesis*, which postulates that the absence of early childhood exposure to infectious agents increases susceptibility to allergic diseases.[9–11] In contrast, children attending daycare centers before 3 months of age have less atopy and asthma in later childhood,[11,12] and areas with diffuse and chronic helminth infestations have a low prevalence of allergic diseases.[11] In addition, a recent European birth cohort study involving 1,133 newborns showed that children born to farm families had a lower prevalence of sensitization to seasonal inhaled allergens such as grass pollen.[13] Maternal exposure during pregnancy (i.e., prenatal exposure) to animal sheds correlated with the lower prevalence rate in the farm children.[12] However, there were no differences in prevalence related to inhaled perennial allergens.

Reported risk factors associated with higher prevalence include urban environment, higher socioeconomic status, higher level of family education, a family history of AD, female gender (after age 6 years), and smaller family size.[8]

ETIOLOGY

❹ AD is a complex genetic disease that arises from gene–gene and gene–environment interactions. There are two major groups of genes involved. First, there are the genes encoding for epidermal or other epithelial structural proteins. Second, there are genes encoding for the major elements of the immune system.[5]

The inheritance pattern is not straightforward. More than one gene is likely involved in the disease. There is an increased risk for a child to have AD if there is a family history of other atopic diseases, such as hay fever or asthma. The risk is significantly higher if both parents have an atopic disease.[1] Studies of identical twins show that a person whose identical twin has AD is seven times more likely to have AD than someone in the general population.[1] And a person whose fraternal twin has AD is three times more likely to have AD than someone in the general population.[1] Another estimate is 80% concordance in monozygous twins and 20% in heterozygous twins.[10]

Thus, genetic predispositions to developing AD exist. Specifically, there are several possible genes on the chromosomes 3q21, 1q21, 16q, 17q25, 20p, and 3p26. Of these chromosomes, 1q21 has the highest linkage region. This region has a family of epithelium-related genes called the epidermal differentiation complex.[5] One of these genes, the filaggrin gene (*FLG*), on chromosome 1q21.3, was initially identified as the gene involved in ichthyosis vulgaris, and several mutations of this gene were subsequently identified in European and Japanese patients with AD.[14] *FLG* encodes for a key protein in epidermal differentiation. Mutations or deficiency of *FLG* results in an abnormality in permeability barrier function.[15]

Epidermal barrier dysfunction is a prerequisite for the penetration of high-molecular-weight allergens in pollens, house dust mite products, microbes, and food.[5] In mice studies, this barrier abnormality alters thresholds for irritant and acute allergic contact dermatitis, and *FLG* deficiency predisposes to the development of an AD-like dermatosis.[15] In humans, two common *FLG* variants (*R501X* and *2282del4*) with an estimated combined allele frequency of about 6% have been identified in individuals of European descent.[16] Eighteen other less common variants have also been identified in Europeans, with an additional 17 mutations restricted to individuals of Asian descent.[16] Each of these variants leads to nonsense mutations which either prevent or severely diminish the production of filaggrin in the epidermis.[16] Mutations of *FLG* seem to occur mainly in early onset AD patients and may be associated with the development of asthma in patients with AD.[5,16] However, *FLG* mutations are identified in only 30% of European patients with AD; implying that other genetic mutations affecting other epidermal structures may be important (e.g., changes in the cornified envelope proteins involucrin and loricrin, or lipid composition).[5]

There are other genes encoding for the immune system that may be associated with AD, especially those found on chromosome 5q31-33.[5] These genes code for cytokines that regulate IgE synthesis. Cytokines are produced mainly by type 1 and type 2 helper T cells. T-helper type 1 (TH_1) cells produce cytokines, which suppress immunoglobulin E (IgE) production (e.g., interferon-γ and interleukin-12 [IL-12]).[5] T-helper type 2 (TH_2) cells produce cytokines, which increase IgE production (e.g., IL-5 and IL-13).[5,17] In patients with AD, there is an imbalance between TH_1 and TH_2 immune responses. These patients are genetically predisposed to TH_2 predominance, seen as increased TH_2 cell activity.[2,5,17] Increased TH_2 activity causes the release of IL-3, IL-4, IL-5, IL-10, and IL-13, resulting in blood eosinophilia, increased serum IgE, and increased growth and development of mast cells.[2,5,17,18] In addition, these cytokines affect the maturation of B cells and cause a genomic rearrangement in these cells that favors isotype class switching from immunoglobulin M (IgM) to IgE.[5]

In summary, recent data suggest that *FLG* deficiency alone can provoke a barrier abnormality in the epidermis and predispose to the development of dermatitis by enhancing allergen absorption through the skin.[19] Furthermore, there appears to be complex relationships, including genetic and nongenetic risk factors, that modify an individual's susceptibility to allergic disease.[20] Complex genetic factors contribute to the increased susceptibility to AD (*FLG* mutations and gene–gene interactions). These, along with environmental factors (gene–environment interactions), result in the pathophysiologic changes and clinical presentations associated with AD.

PATHOPHYSIOLOGY

The initial mechanisms that trigger inflammatory changes in the skin in patients with AD are unknown. Neuropeptides, irritation, or pruritus-induced scratching may be causing the release of proinflammatory cytokines from keratinocytes. Alternatively, allergens in the epidermal barrier or in food may cause T-cell mediated but IgE-independent reactions. Allergen-specific IgE is not a prerequisite.[5] Characteristic features in pathophysiology are skin barrier dysfunction, and immune deviation toward TH_2 with subsequent increased IgE.[10] The disease is further complicated by microbial colonization with pathologic organisms resulting in increased susceptibility for skin infections.[10]

Skin barrier dysfunction plays a critical role in the development of AD,[10,21,22] and loss of function mutations in the skin structural protein *filaggrin* is a major risk factor.[22] Other factors may include a deficiency of skin barrier proteins, increased peptidase activity, lack of certain protease inhibitors, and lipid abnormalities.[22] There must be epidermal barrier dysfunction for high-molecular-weight allergens in pollens, house dust mite particles, microbes, and foods to penetrate the skin barrier. Atopic skin has reduced antimicrobial peptides (AMPs). AMPs are normally produced by keratinocytes, sebocytes, and mast cells, and they form a chemical shield on the surface of the skin. Reduced AMPs result in a diminished antimicrobial barrier, which correlates with increased susceptibility to infections and superinfections seen in these patients.[23]

On penetration of the epidermal barrier, allergens are met by dendritic cells (DCs). DCs are antigen-presenting cells populating the skin, respiratory tract, and mucosa of the GI tract (i.e., at the front line of pathogen entry).[24] DCs then enhance TH_2 polarization, resulting in increased production of IgE. Keratinocytes in the skin of patients with AD also produce high levels of an IL-7–like protein, which again drives dendritic cells to enhance TH_2 polarization. Epidermal dendritic cells in patients with AD bear IgE and express its high-affinity receptor (FcεRI).[25–27] Serum IgE is often elevated in patients with AD,[1,18] especially during an exacerbation.

However, on initial presentation, patients with early onset AD generally do not have increased IgE levels (i.e., there is no detectable IgE-mediated allergic sensitization). IgE-mediated allergic sensitization may occur several weeks or months after the initial AD lesions appear. Although in some children—mostly girls—this sensitization never occurs.[5]

Predisposing Factors

Several factors can predispose patients to development of AD. These include climate, infection, genetics, environmental aeroallergens, and food.

Hot and extremely cold climates are both poorly tolerated by patients with this condition. Dry weather, common in the winter, causes increased skin dryness. Hot weather causes increased sweating, resulting in pruritus.

Patients with AD are commonly colonized by *Staphylococcus aureus* bacteria. Clinical infections with *S. aureus* frequently cause flareups of AD.

As discussed previously, genetics plays a role in AD. Family history of AD is common.

Exposure to environmental aeroallergens is another risk factor. Dust mites, pollens, molds, cigarette smoke, and dander from animal hair or skin may worsen the symptoms of AD.[1,18]

The role of food as antigens in the pathogenesis of AD is controversial. Small amounts of environmental foods (low-dose exposure from foods on tabletops, hands, dust) may penetrate the skin barrier and be taken up by Langerhans cells, leading to TH_2 responses and IgE production.[28] However, early high-dose oral food consumption induces oral tolerance. The timing and balance of cutaneous and oral exposure determines whether a child will have allergy or tolerance.[28] Increased serum IgE antibodies to a particular food is evidence of sensitization to a food and is consistent with although not proof of a food allergy.[1,29] Eczema may frequently be a manifestation of food allergy,[28] and patients with AD have a higher prevalence of food allergy than those in the general population.[1] Conversely, a current belief is that food allergy may be caused by AD, and in most patients with coexisting AD and food allergy, AD precedes the food allergy. Regardless, the two conditions coexist, and the likelihood of an infant or child with AD also having food allergy or allergies must be kept in mind.[29]

There is a known epidermal barrier dysfunction in AD, allowing for increased low-level skin permeability to allergenic foods. Certain foods may trigger acute reactions, including urticaria and anaphylaxis. The most commonly reported allergenic foods are eggs, milk, peanuts, wheat, soy, tree nuts, shellfish, and fish.[1] Individual food allergies, such as peanut allergy, have increased in prevalence in the last decade;[28,29] new food allergies may also be increasing in prevalence, particularly kiwi allergy[28,30] and sesame seed allergy.[28,31] Consistent with the oral tolerance concept, early results from recent studies using sublingual and oral immunotherapy to specific food allergens (e.g., milk or peanut) appear to indicate that it may be possible to induce oral tolerance, and that it may be possible to desensitize children to some allergenic foods. Currently, these treatment protocols have only been done in highly supervised research settings and with small numbers of patients.[32] For more information about management of food allergies the reader is directed to the 2010 National Institute of Allergy and Infectious Diseases (NIAID)-sponsored expert panel's report, available at *www.niaid.nih.gov*.[29]

CLINICAL PRESENTATION

Diagnosis of AD is generally based on clinical presentation (Table 79-2).[1] There is no objective diagnostic test for the clinical confirmation of AD.[1,33] Filaggrin gene mutations may be associated with persistent and more severe AD as well as early onset cases.[22]

TABLE 79-2 Skin Features Associated with Atopic Dermatitis[1]

- **Atopic pleat (Dennie-Morgan fold):** An extra fold of skin that develops under the eye.
- **Cheilitis:** Inflammation of the skin on and around the lips.
- **Hyperlinear palms:** Increased number of skin creases on the palms.
- **Hyperpigmented eyelids:** Eyelids that have become darker in color from inflammation or hay fever.
- **Ichthyosis:** Dry, rectangular scales on the skin.
- **Keratosis pilaris:** Small, rough bumps, generally on the face, upper arms, and thighs.
- **Lichenification:** Thick, leathery skin resulting from constant scratching and rubbing.
- **Papules:** Small raised bumps that may open when scratched and become crusty and infected.
- **Urticaria:** Hives (red, raised bumps) that may occur after exposure to an allergen, at the beginning of flares, or after exercise or a hot bath.

Clinical Controversy...

Although it has traditionally been thought that food allergies are a predisposing factor for the development of atopic dermatitis, some clinicians are now thinking that atopic dermatitis may be the predisposing factor for the development of food allergies in an individual. Often the signs and symptoms of atopic dermatitis appear before the food allergies.

5 The course of AD varies significantly over time. Studies reviewing the natural course of the disease usually describe the disease pattern as persistent, intermittent, or in remission.[8] A 2004 study found that 43% were in complete remission after age 2 years, with 19% having persistent disease and 38% an intermittent pattern.[8]

The clinical presentation of AD differs depending on the age of the patient. In infancy, the earliest onset of AD usually occurs between 2 and 6 months of age, and especially between the 6th and 12th weeks of life.[1,2] It has been reported that 75% of cases have their onset within the first 6 months.[2] A more conservative estimate is that at least 65% of patients develop symptoms within the first year of life, and at least 85% will have developed symptoms before the age of 5 years.[1] The initial presentation in infancy is an erythematous, papular skin rash that may first appear on the cheeks and chin as a patchy facial rash[1,2] and that can progress to red, scaling, oozing skin.[1] The rash shows a centrifugal distribution affecting the malar region of the cheeks, forehead, scalp, chin, and behind the ears while sparing the central areas (i.e., the nose and paranasal creases).[2] Lesions occur in the flexor surfaces, such as antecubital and popliteal fossae. Over the next few weeks and as the infant becomes more mobile and begins crawling, the lesions spread to the extensors of the lower legs, and eventually the entire body may be involved, with sparing of the diaper area and the nose.[1] These lesions are associated with uncontrollable itchiness, and the infant will become irritable and may try to rub his or her face to relieve the itch. Scratching may occur quite early, and infants with AD may scratch themselves continuously, mainly when they are undressed or during sleep.[2] Excessive rubbing or scratching may result in excoriation and development of secondary infections.

In childhood, the skin often appears dry, flaky, rough, cracked, and may bleed because of scratching. With repeated scratching and rubbing the skin becomes lichenified. Lichenification, usually localized to the flexural folds of the extremities,[33] is characteristic of childhood AD in older children and adults.[33,34] Lichenification signifies repeated rubbing of the skin and is seen mostly over the folds, bony protuberances, and forehead.[34] Excoriations and crusting are also commonly seen, along with secondary infections. Sometimes increased folds are seen underneath the eyes (so-called Dennie–Morgan folds).[34] Lesions are still most commonly seen in the flexor surfaces of the body, particularly the flexural creases of the antecubital and popliteal fossae.[34]

Sleep disturbances also occur. One study reported that there are both brief and longer awakenings associated with scratching episodes that affect sleep efficiency in school-age children with AD.[35]

In adulthood, lesions are more diffuse with underlying erythema. The face is commonly involved and may be dry and scaly. Lichenification may again be seen. A brown macular ring around the neck, representing a localized deposit of amyloid, is typical but not always present.[34]

Although no objective diagnostic test confirms presence of AD,[1] some signs, symptoms, and other factors are commonly used in its diagnosis. These include pruritus, early age of onset, eczematous skin lesions that vary with age, chronic and relapsing courses, dry and flaky skin, IgE reactivity, family or personal history of asthma or hay fever, or other atopic diseases (Table 79-3).[18] In addition, allergy skin testing may be helpful in identifying factors that trigger flares of AD.[1] Negative results may help rule out certain substances as triggers; however, positive results may be unrelated to disease activity, and false positives are common.[1]

TABLE 79-3 Major and Minor Signs and Symptoms of Atopic Dermatitis[1]

Major indicators
- Pruritus (intense itching)
- Characteristic rash in locations typical of the disease
- Chronic or repeatedly occurring symptoms
- Personal or family history of atopic disorders (eczema, hay fever, asthma)

Selected minor indicators
- Early age of onset
- Dry skin that may also have patchy scales or rough bumps
- Increased serum IgE
- Numerous skin creases on the palms
- Hand or foot involvement
- Inflammation around the lips
- Nipple eczema
- Susceptibility to skin infection
- Positive allergy skin tests

1 Pruritus is a quintessential feature of AD, and a diagnosis cannot be made if there is no history of itching.[1–4] AD has been called the itch that, when scratched, erupts.[2] Scratching or rubbing itchy, atopic skin characterizes this type of eczema.[2] Scratching and rubbing further irritates the skin, increases inflammation, and exacerbates itchiness.[3] Atopic skin can itch during sleep. This nighttime itching is a problem for many children with the disease, since there is no conscious control of scratching during sleep.[1,18,35]

Pruritus can be triggered by a variety of factors. The most common triggers of itch have been reported as heat and perspiration (96%), wool (91%), emotional stress (81%), certain foods (49%), alcohol (44%), upper respiratory infections (36%), and house dust mites (>35%).[36]

Once pruritus occurs, the surrounding normally nonpruritic skin area (whether inflamed or noninflamed) may be very sensitive and react to light stimuli and begin itching (allokinesis). Allokinesis is typical of AD.[18,36] As a result of allokinesis, patients with AD may experience pruritic attacks when their skin is touched accidentally by mechanical factors such as clothing,[18] especially wool products.[36]

Elevated serum IgE may be seen, consistent with the genetically predetermined dominance of TH_2 cytokines causing increased IgE. In addition, increased serum IgE antibodies to a particular food, consistent with a food allergy,[3] is common in patients with AD. The radioallergosorbent test (RAST) is an allergen-specific IgE antibody test used to screen for allergy to a specific substance or substances. In some cases the RAST test may be used to monitor immunotherapy or to see if a child has outgrown a specific allergy. Positive (elevated) RAST usually indicates an allergy to a suspected or known allergen. However, the level of IgE may not correlate with the severity of an allergic reaction, and the IgE level may remain elevated for years after an allergy has been outgrown.[18]

A clinically useful set of criteria for the diagnosis of AD is as follows: atopy, pruritus, eczema, and altered vascular reactivity.[18,36]

COMPLICATIONS

6 Patients with AD are prone to skin infections. Atopic skin is drier and the stratum corneum has weakened protective abilities; combined with the abnormal skin barrier function and immune defense, there is an increased risk of secondary bacterial skin infections with staphylococci or streptococci, and viral infections such as herpes simplex or even fungal infections.[1] Constant scratching to relieve

pruritus may cause excoriations, further compromising the integrity of the skin barrier. *S. aureus* is a common cause of secondary bacterial infections in AD.[10] Binding of *S. aureus* is enhanced by skin inflammation as seen in AD.[21] Many patients with AD are colonized with *S. aureus* and may have exacerbations after skin infections of this organism.[10,21] Secondary bacterial infections may present as yellowish crusty lesions and should be promptly treated. Oral (systemic) antibiotics are generally more effective than topical treatment.[1,21]

Patients with AD are also more prone to disseminated infections with herpes simplex or vaccinia virus.[21] Severe viral infections such as eczema herpeticum or eczema vaccinatum might be linked to the severity of atopy.[21] Smallpox vaccination is contraindicated in patients with AD.[21]

TREATMENT

Desired Outcomes

In treating patients with AD, clinicians generally have the following clinical goals in mind:

1. Provide symptomatic relief—control the itching.
2. Control the AD.
3. Identify and, when possible, eliminate triggers and environmental aeroallergens.
4. Identify and minimize predisposing factors for exacerbations including any stressors.
5. Prevent future exacerbations.
6. Provide any social and psychological support needed for the patient, family, and caregivers.
7. Minimize or prevent adverse events from medications and other treatment modalities.
8. Treat to cure any secondary skin infections, if present.

Successful management of AD should include not only clearance of skin lesions, which may take days to weeks depending on the severity of disease, but also control of the itch, minimizing or eliminating triggers, monitoring the patient to minimize or prevent adverse events from medications or other treatment modalities, and providing adequate social and psychological support for the patient, family, and caregivers.

The ultimate goal is to provide enough control of this chronic disease so that future exacerbations are prevented, thus ensuring that the patient's quality of life is minimally affected by AD. Because the course of the disease evolves over time, management strategies may change.

7 Both nonpharmacologic and pharmacologic therapies are important in managing the signs and symptoms of AD. Nonpharmacologic strategies include identifying and minimizing or eliminating preventable risk factors, such as known triggers and allergens, as well as appropriate skin care.

Treatment guidelines and protocols for AD are available. These are listed in Table 79-4.

TABLE 79-4 Useful Sources of Information about Treatment of Atopic Dermatitis

Published Guidelines or Treatment Protocols

- Ring J, Alomar A, Bieber M, et al. Guidelines for treatment of atopic eczema (atopic dermatitis) parts 1 and II. J Eur Acad Dermatol Venereol 2012;26:1045–1060, 1176–1193.
- Rubel D, Thirumoorthy T, Soebaryo W, et al. Consensus guidelines for the management of atopic dermatitis: An Asia-Pacific perspective. J Dermatol 2013;40:160–171.
- Baron SE, Cohen SN, Archer CB. British Association of Dermatologists and Royal College of General Practitioners. Guidance on the diagnosis and clinical management of atopic eczema. Clin Exp Dermatol 2012; 37(suppl 1):7–12.
- Simpson EL. Atopic dermatitis: A review of topical treatment options. Curr Med Res Opin 2010;26(3):633–640.
- Carbone A, Siu A, Patel R. Pediatric atopic dermatitis: A review of the medical management. Ann Pharmacother 2010;44:1448–1458.
- National Institute of Arthritis and Musculoskeletal and Skin Diseases. Handout on Health: Atopic Dermatitis. US Department of Health and Human Services. NIH Publication No. 09-4272. August 2011, *www.niams.nih.gov/Health_Info/Atopic_Dermatitis/default.asp.*
- Lynde C, Barber K, Claveau J, Gratton D, et al. Canadian practical guide for the treatment and management of atopic dermatitis. J Cutan Med Surg 2005;8(suppl 5):1–9. *http://www.springerlink.com/content/r5432000056r2748/fulltext.html.*
- Eichenfield LF, Hanifin JM, Luger TA, et al. Consensus conference on pediatric atopic dermatitis. J Am Acad Dermatol 2003;49:1088–1095.
- Leung DYM, Nicklas RA, Li JT, et al. Disease management of atopic dermatis: An updated practice parameter. Ann Allergy Asthma Immunol 2004;93(9):S1–S21.
- Abramovits W. A clinician's paradigm in the treatment of atopic dermatitis. J Am Acad Dermatol 2005;53:S70–S77.

Useful Websites

- National Institute of Arthritis and Musculoskeletal and Skin Diseases (NIAMS), U.S. National Institutes of Health: *http://www.niams.nih.gov/Health_Info/Atopic_Dermatitis/default.asp*
- American Academy of Allergy Asthma & Immunology (AAAAI): *http://www.aaaai.org/patients/allergic_conditions/atopic_dermatitis.stm*
- American Academy of Dermatology: *http://www.aad.org/public/publications/pamphlets/skin_eczema.html*
- DermNet NZ: *http://dermnetnz.org/dermatitis/atopic.html*
- EczemaNet: *http://www.skincarephysicians.com/eczemanet/phototherapy.html*

Nonpharmacologic Therapy

8 Nonpharmacologic approaches to the treatment of infants and children with AD include the following[1]:

1. Give lukewarm baths.
2. Apply lubricant immediately after bathing (moisturizers are a standard of care).[9,10]
3. Keep child's fingernails filed short.
4. Select clothing made of soft cotton fabrics.
5. Consider using sedating antihistamines to reduce scratching at night.
6. Keep the child cool; avoid situations in which overheating occurs.
7. Learn to recognize skin infections and seek treatment promptly.
8. Attempt to distract the child with activities to keep him or her from scratching.
9. Identify and remove irritants and allergens.

Hydration is crucial, and adequate skin hydration is a fundamental part of managing AD.[3] Transepidermal water loss is greater in atopic skin than in normal skin. Thus, any measures to improve skin moisturization, such as liberal use of moisturizers, would be beneficial. Moisturizers are a standard of care and may be steroid-sparing.[9,10,37–40] They are useful for both prevention and maintenance therapy.[9,10,39,40] They can be categorized based on their specific effects on the skin:

1. *Occlusives:* These agents provide an oily layer on the skin surface to slow transepidermal water loss, increasing the moisture content of the stratum corneum. These are the best moisturizers for patients with AD.[3]
2. *Humectants:* In the stratum corneum, these agents increase the water-holding capacity. However, they are not useful in patients with AD because they have a stinging effect on open skin.[3]

3. *Emollients:* These agents smooth out the surface of the skin by filling the spaces with droplets of oil. These are the least effective moisturizers.[3]

Note that the term "emollients" is sometimes more broadly used to mean all nonmedicated moisturizers, including occlusives.[37,38] Usual active ingredients in moisturizers include mineral oil, petrolatum, ceramide, and urea. Ceramide was shown to improve pruritus and sleep in pediatric patients with AD.[38]

The humidity in the home should be kept at or above 50% and the room temperature kept on the cool side.[18]

Appropriate skin care is crucial in preventing flareups.[1] A daily skin care routine should include the following[18]:

1. Using scent-free moisturizers liberally as needed each day. Large quantities can be used, and currently there are no recommendations regarding the appropriate amount or dosing frequency of moisturizers.[38]
2. Bathing in lukewarm water (never hot) for about 5 minutes[10] once or twice daily.[3,37] Adding a capful of emulsifying oil[10] may help the body retain moisture; baths are better than showers. Bathing daily for 10 to 20 minutes may be desirable as long as a thick moisturizer is applied afterward.[37] Bathing twice daily during disease flares may be a useful method for enhancing skin penetration of topical therapies and for debridement of crusting and staphylococcal colonization.[37] If showering, mild liquid cleansers are preferred over soaps.[3]
3. The skin should be lightly towel dried (pat to dry, avoid rubbing or brisk drying).[1,37,38]
4. Scent-free moisturizer should then be applied while the skin is still moist or slightly damp (within 3 minutes of towel drying).[3,37] Some fragrance-free moisturizers include Aveeno Baby Soothing Relief Moisture Cream, Cetaphil, Neutrogena Hand Cream, and Vanicream products. Lotions may be used on the scalp and other hairy areas and for mild dryness on the face, trunk, and limbs; creams are more occlusive than lotions; ointments are the most occlusive and can be used for drier, thicker, or more scaly areas.[3] Occlusive moisturizers are best.[3]
5. Using nonsoap skin cleansers[1] may cause less skin irritation. Lipid- and fragrance-free skin cleansers may be particularly advantageous (e.g., Cetaphil Gentle Skin Cleanser, Free and Clear Liquid Cleanser, Spectro Derm Cleanser). Aquanil, Dove, Neutrogena, and pHisoderm sensitive skin products have also been recommended as low-irritant products, and some are lipid free.
6. Avoiding alcohol-containing topical products including lotions, swabs, and wipes, as they may be drying.
7. Clothing should be double-rinsed. Mild detergents should be used to wash clothing, with no bleach or fabric softener.[3]

Pharmacologic Therapy

Topical Corticosteroids

9 *Topical corticosteroids* are the standard of care to which other treatments are compared.[9,10,37–40] They remain the drug treatment of choice for AD. However, despite their extensive use, supporting data are limited regarding optimal corticosteroid concentrations, duration and frequency of therapy, and quantity of application.[9,10] The use of long-term intermittent application of topical corticosteroids was beneficial and safe in two randomized controlled trials (RCTs); however, independent studies of other formulations are needed.

To maximize the antiinflammatory benefit and minimize adverse effects, the choice of corticosteroid should be matched with the severity and site of disease.[3] Low-potency corticosteroids, such as hydrocortisone 1%, are suitable for the face, and medium-potency corticosteroids, such as betamethasone valerate 0.1%, may be used for the body.[3] For longer-duration maintenance therapy, low-potency corticosteroids are recommended.[33] Mid-strength and high-potency corticosteroids should be used for short-term management of exacerbations.[33] Ultrahigh- and high-potency corticosteroids, such as betamethasone dipropionate 0.05% or clobetasone propionate 0.05%, are typically reserved for short-term treatment of lichenified areas in adults.[39] Short-term treatments mean brief periods of 1 to 2 weeks.[37,38] After the lesions have cleared or significantly improved, a lower-potency steroid should be used for maintenance when necessary.[39] Potent fluorinated corticosteroids should be avoided not only on the face, but also the genitalia and the intertriginous areas, and in young infants.[33] (For a corticosteroid potency comparison chart, see Table 78-2 in the chapter on psoriasis, or visit the National Psoriasis Foundation website at *http://www.psoriasis.org/netcommunity/sublearn03_mild_potency.*)

It is also important to remember that altering the local environment through hydration and/or occlusion as well as changing the vehicle[41] may alter the absorption and effectiveness of the topical corticosteroid.[10] Some vehicles are better suited for certain body areas,[41] such as a lotion for the scalp and hairy areas. Foams may be more cosmetically pleasing to some patients, as they easily disappear into the skin. The surface area of the skin involved and the skin thickness also play a role.[33] In addition, tachyphylaxis is a clinical concern, but there is no experimental documentation.

Adverse effects of topical corticosteroids may be systemic in nature, and they are directly related to the steroid potency, duration of use, and other factors as discussed above. Local adverse effects include striae and skin atrophy, perioral dermatitis, acne, rosacea, telangiectasias, and allergic contact dermatitis (often related to the vehicle).[33,42] The potential for systemic adverse effects is related to the potency of the topical corticosteroid, the site of application, the occlusiveness of the preparation, the percentage of body surface area covered, and the duration of use.[33] Potential systemic effects include hypothalamic-pituitary-adrenal (HPA) axis suppression, infections, hyperglycemia, cataracts, glaucoma, and growth retardation (in children).[1,3,9,18,37,38,42] However, growth retardation may also be related to the chronicity of the illness rather than to corticosteroid use or dietary factors.[3] Although less likely, systemic adverse effects can occur with low-potency topical corticosteroids. For example, a phase II study of a mild-potency corticosteroid (desonide 0.05% foam) in children and adolescents 3 months to 17 years showed that 4% (3 of 75) of patients experienced mild reversible HPA-axis suppression after a 4-week treatment period.[43]

When topical steroid therapy has failed for efficacy or safety reasons, numerous agents and interventions can be used as alternative or add-on therapy in patients with AD.

Topical Calcineurin Inhibitors

10 Topical immunomodulators such as the calcineurin inhibitors tacrolimus ointment (Protopic) and pimecrolimus cream (Elidel) have been shown to reduce the extent, severity, and symptoms of AD in adults and children.[10,39,40] Tacrolimus has been reported to inhibit the activation of key cells involved in AD, including T cells, dendritic cells, mast cells, and keratinocytes.[33] Pimecrolimus acts similarly to tacrolimus, inhibiting T-cell proliferation, preventing gene transcription of TH_1 and TH_2 cytokines, and reducing mediator release from mast cells and basophils.[33] However, pimecrolimus has more favorable lipophilic characteristics and, in animal studies, appears to preferentially distribute to the skin as opposed to the systemic circulation.[33,44] Both tacrolimus ointment and pimecrolimus cream are approved for AD in adults and children older than age 2 years.[3,10,39,40,44] Although clinical trials conducted in younger

infants (e.g., 2 to 23 months old) also showed significant efficacy without appreciable adverse effects, use in children younger than age 2 years is not FDA approved.[45] Tacrolimus 0.03% ointment is approved for moderate-to-severe AD for ages 2 years and older, with the 0.1% ointment limited to ages 16 years and older; pimecrolimus 1% cream is approved for mild-to-moderate AD for ages 2 years and older.[45] There is limited data comparing topical corticosteroids with tacrolimus or pimecrolimus.

Because of continuing concerns regarding a possible risk of cancer with tacrolimus and pimecrolimus,[45] both drugs are recommended for use as second-line treatments in AD,[9,10,37–40] when the continued use of topical corticosteroids is ineffective or inadvisable.[37] They may be appropriate in patients with corticosteroid-related adverse effects, patients with large body-surface areas of disease, patients unresponsive to corticosteroids, or other reasons where treatment with corticosteroids is inadvisable.[3] Children and adults with a weakened or compromised immune system should not be treated with these agents. Unlike topical corticosteroids, calcineurin inhibitors can be used on all body locations for prolonged periods,[3,10] although episodic use is recommended. Skin atrophy does not occur.[33]

The most common adverse effect of topical calcineurin inhibitors is transient discomfort (burning sensation) at the application site.[3] There is a potential for local skin carcinogenesis as seen in animal studies, or for systemic effects if high blood levels are reached (e.g., increased susceptibility to infections due to immunosuppressive effects).[45] Because there is a possible risk of cutaneous malignancy,[3,37] sun protection is recommended.[3,18,37,45] Patients should be encouraged to apply a high sun protection factor (SPF) broad-spectrum sunblock daily to all exposed skin (e.g., SPF 30 or higher); and this counseling should especially be emphasized for those patients with the highest risk of developing skin cancer, including patients with red hair and/or Fitzpatrick skin types I and II, and patients receiving phototherapy or using tanning beds.[45]

Topical calcineurin inhibitors are very effective in relieving the associated pruritus. Both tacrolimus and pimecrolimus significantly relieve pruritus even after the first few days of treatment in both children and adults (studies report relief after just 3 days).[10]

Clinical **Controversy. . .**

With topical calcineurin inhibitors, there is a potential for local skin carcinogenesis as seen in animal and in vitro studies. In addition, pigmented melanocytic lesions have been seen in treated areas, raising concern about melanoma.[43] The FDA has a black box warning for both tacrolimus ointment and pimecrolimus cream about their potential cancer risk, but no causal relationship has been proven between use of a topical calcineurin inhibitor and the development of lymphoma or nonmelanoma skin cancer.[43]

Phototherapy

Phototherapy is effective for AD and is recommended[10,37–40] especially when the disease is not controlled by tacrolimus or pimecrolimus ointment. Phototherapy may be steroid sparing, allowing for the use of lower-potency topical corticosteroids, or even eliminating the need for maintenance corticosteroids in some cases. Phototherapy may also help prevent secondary bacterial skin infections, commonly seen in patients with AD. However, in a few patients, phototherapy may worsen the AD; it is not recommended in patients whose disease flares up when exposed to sunlight. Relapse following cessation of therapy frequently occurs.[10]

Phototherapy may consist of either ultraviolet light therapy alone, or ultraviolet light therapy alongside drug or topical ointment (commonly called photochemotherapy). Psoralens plus ultraviolet A light (PUVA) is one type of photochemotherapy. The photosensitizer (psoralens) is administered either orally or in a bath immediately prior to ultraviolet A (UVA) light therapy. Topical ointments (such as crude coal tar) may also be used concomitantly with ultraviolet light therapy (e.g., Crude coal tar + ultraviolet B [UVB] light).

Ultraviolet lamps include UVA (315 to 400 nm), UVA1 (340 to 400 nm), broadband UVB (BB-UVB) (280 to 315 nm), and narrowband UVB (NB-UVB) (311 nm). Phototherapies used for AD have included PUVA, high- or medium-dose UVA1, BB-UVB, and NB-UVB.[10,46] There is weaker evidence supporting the use of PUVA in AD[46] and it is not a first-choice therapy.[10] NB-UVB is more effective than BB-UVB therapy and is preferred.[10] BB-UVB may not effectively treat the scalp and skinfold areas. Medium-dose UVA1 is very effective for patients with an acute exacerbation of severe AD; however, the effect may be relatively short-lived and symptoms may recur within 3 months of stopping therapy.[46] An adult study comparing medium-dose UVA1 and NB-UVB found no difference in efficacy; however, the sample size was quite small ($N = 13$), and the follow-up period was confounded by the use of topical corticosteroids.[47] Currently, medium-dose UVA1 is considered similar in efficacy as NB-UVB; and high-dose UVA1 is preferred in severe phases.[10]

Patients need to wear eye protection during ultraviolet (UV) light therapy to prevent damage to the retina. Short-term adverse effects include erythema, skin pain, skin burning or sunburn, pruritus, and pigmentation.[33] Long-term adverse effects include premature aging of the skin (photoaging) and skin cancer.[33,46] For example, PUVA has been associated with squamous cell carcinoma and possibly melanoma, which may occur years after PUVA therapy has ceased.[46]

Coal Tar

Although tar preparations had been widely used for AD and have been recommended as alternative topical therapy, few RCTs support their efficacy.[33] Their antiinflammatory properties are not well characterized, and part of the improvement with the agent may be the result of a placebo effect, which can be significant in AD.[33]

Coal tar products are also staining and malodorous, although newer products may be more cosmetically acceptable. They are not recommended on acutely inflamed skin, since this may result in additional skin irritation.[33]

The use of coal tar in pregnancy has not been studied. Few data are available about tar excretion into breast milk; in addition, safety in children has not been established.[48] Adverse effects include tar folliculitis, acneiform eruptions, irritant dermatitis, burning, stinging, photosensitivity, and a risk of tar intoxication if used extensively in a young child.[48] Although animal studies showed that tar components can be converted to carcinogenic and mutagenic entities, there is inconclusive epidemiologic evidence supporting the claim that human use of topical tar preparations in dermatology leads to skin cancer.[48]

Clinical **Controversy. . .**

Animal studies showed that coal tar components can be converted to carcinogenic/mutagenic entities, and tar keratoses (small nodules that develop from cutaneous tar exposure) have the potential to regress, fall off, or develop into a squamous cell carcinoma. However, there is inconclusive epidemiologic evidence supporting the claim that human use of topical tar preparations in dermatology leads to skin or internal cancers such as bladder cancer or lymphoma.[48]

Systemic Therapies

Systemic therapies for the treatment of AD are generally not well studied or approved by FDA or Health Canada. Small case series or open studies are available for some agents, but few well-conducted RCTs exist. Agents described in published papers have included systemic corticosteroids, cyclosporine, interferon-γ, azathioprine, methotrexate, mycophenolate mofetil, intravenous immunoglobulin (IVIG), and more recently biologic response modifiers.[10]

Systemic corticosteroids, such as oral prednisone, rarely may be required as a short-term treatment[10] for severe, recalcitrant, chronic AD.[33] Although not routinely recommended,[37–40] systemic corticosteroids can provide rapid relief of severe refractory disease during transition to other therapies.[46] The dosage of the drug must be tapered during discontinuance to minimize a rebound flareup.[33,38] Intensified skin care, particularly with topical corticosteroids and moisturizers, is also important during the taper to minimize a rebound flareup.[33]

Cyclosporine is considered effective for severe AD,[10] but its usefulness is limited by significant side effects, including hypertension and nephrotoxicity. There is also the potential for significant drug–drug and drug–food (e.g., grapefruit juice) interactions. It should be reserved for short-term use in adults or children with severe refractory disease.[46] Maximal benefit is usually seen after approximately 2 weeks of use and relapse may occur quickly after cessation of therapy.[10,46] In a meta-analysis of eight RCTs, cyclosporine is more efficacious than placebo, with reduced body surface area, erythema, sleep loss, and glucocorticoid use. However, all scores were back to pretreatment levels 8 weeks after ending cyclosporine therapy.[10]

Recombinant interferon-γ may be effective in a subset of patients with AD.[10] Two randomized placebo-controlled trials in patients with severe AD demonstrated significant improvement in symptoms.[49,50] Short-term adverse effects, such as headache, myalgias, and chills, occurred in substantial proportions of study patients. Transient liver transaminase elevations and granulocytopenia have also occurred.[51] Long-term therapy (up to 24 months) did not appear to be associated with significant adverse events.[33] Some recommend that a higher dose of this agent be used initially followed by a lower dosage during maintenance therapy.[46]

Azathioprine,[33,52] *methotrexate*,[53] *mycophenolate mofetil*,[33] and *IVIG* have shown efficacy in small case series or open-label studies primarily in adults with recalcitrant AD. They are rarely used. Oral methotrexate, with a long history of pediatric use for various inflammatory conditions, appeared to be effective in a case series of children (aged 2 to 16 years) with severe AD.[53]

Biologic response modifiers, unlike for psoriasis, are currently not approved for AD. The safety and efficacy of various biologic response modifiers in patients with AD have been studied,[51] mostly in case reports, small case series, or open-label studies with a limited number of patients. Theoretically, using protein-based therapies is inherently risky in a patient population more prone to developing IgE sensitization to protein antigens than the general population. Type 1 immediate hypersensitivity reactions such as anaphylaxis could result, and patients with severe disease are potentially the patients at greatest risk of anaphylaxis. None has been reported in the published literature, which detail 261 patients with AD treated with various biologics,[51] but these numbers are too small to generalize their findings to larger numbers of people or specific populations.

More specifically, the TNF-α inhibitors infliximab and etanercept appeared effective in a few patients but not others, and adverse events have included infusion reactions with flushing and dyspnea, urticaria, and recurrent skin infections of methicillin-resistant *S. aureus*. Similarly, omalizumab, rituximab, and alefacept have been shown in a few case reports and small case series to be somewhat effective.

Additional research is needed to determine the therapeutic potential and safety of biologics in patients with AD.[51]

Complementary and Alternative Therapies

Traditional Chinese herbal therapy has been studied in placebo-controlled trials and appeared to provide temporary benefit for patients with severe AD. However, the effectiveness may wear off despite continued treatment, and long-term toxicity is unknown.[10,33,54,55]

Mycobacterium vaccae (killed) injected intradermally was found to be effective in reducing the severity of skin disease in a placebo-controlled trial in children with moderate-to-severe AD.[56] This suggests that downregulation of the TH_2 response in AD may potentially be beneficial.[33]

Probiotics of various types have been studied in several RCTs with mixed results. One study group reported that prenatal and postnatal exposure for 6 months to *Lactobacillus rhamnosus GG* halved the frequency of AD at 2, 4, and 7 years but had no effect on atopic sensitization. Other study groups also administered lactobacilli, including *L. rhamnosus GG*, but with mixed results. A recent placebo-controlled study comparing *Bifidobacterium lactis* and *L. rhamnosus HN001* found that *L. rhamnosus HN001* may be effective in preventing the development of AD in high-risk infants, but not Bifidobacterium. However, one study showed that *Lactobacillus acidophilus* supplementation actually increased the sensitization rate (40% vs. 24%) and led to more IgE-associated AD.[57] More research is needed about the role of probiotics in prevention and treatment of AD.[57]

Immunotherapy using allergen-specific desensitization techniques in controlled settings for patients with AD may also be beneficial, and much research is ongoing. Double-blind controlled studies have not shown consistent efficacy.

More research is also needed to adequately assess the role of homeopathy, hypnotherapy, acupuncture, massage therapy, and biofeedback therapy in the treatment of AD.

PERSONALIZED PHARMACOTHERAPY

11 AD may have significant implications not only for the patients themselves, but also their families and caregivers.

In 2006, an international study of 2,002 patients and caregivers from eight countries addressed the effect of AD on the lives of patients and society.[58] This European study found that, on average, patients experienced nine flares per year, with those having severe disease experiencing more flares and taking significantly longer to clear. The flares were associated with disturbed sleep, and 86% of patients avoided at least one type of everyday activity. Schoolwork performance and productivity were negatively affected. Patients missed an average of 2.5 days of school or work per year, and an analysis of adult patient performance at work and occupational absence showed that the social cost of lost productivity could amount to more than 2 billion Euros per year across the European Union. There were also emotional consequences; half of the patients experienced depression or unhappiness about their condition, and one-third reported that AD had eroded their self-confidence. In addition, concern about adverse effects from topical corticosteroid treatments resulted in poor adherence to therapy. On average, patients endured the symptoms of AD without initiating specific treatment 47% of the time they had an exacerbation. Approximately one-half of the respondents were concerned about using topical corticosteroids, and 58% restricted them to particular sites, 39% used them less frequently or for shorter time periods than prescribed, and 66% used them as a last resort. The study concluded that AD is "an undertreated disease that has a significant, yet mostly avoidable, negative effect on patients, their caregivers, and society."[58]

Thus, healthcare professionals play an integral role in providing patient and caregiver education about this disease and specific treatment plans. The importance of adequate and appropriate education for the patient, family, and caregivers about AD and its management cannot be overemphasized. Patients should be involved in their own care.

CONCLUSION

AD is a chronic skin condition that generally presents at an early age. It affects the patient, family, and caregivers. Nonpharmacologic management strategies are important in treatment; these include appropriate skin care, hydration, avoidance of triggers, and psychosocial support. Pharmacologic treatment emphasizes topical corticosteroids as the standard of care. Patient and caregiver education about AD and treatment strategies is critical to minimize nonadherence. Successful outcomes result when patients and caregivers are partners with healthcare professionals in the management of this chronic disease.

ACKNOWLEDGMENT

Portions of this chapter have been adapted with permission from reference 18.

ABBREVIATIONS

AD atopic dermatitis
AMP antimicrobial peptide
BB-UVB broadband ultraviolet B light (280–315 nm)
DC dendritic cell
FDA Food and Drug Administration
FLG filaggrin gene
GI gastrointestinal
HPA hypothalamic-pituitary-adrenal
IgE immunoglobulin E
IgM immunoglobulin M
IL interleukin
ISAAC International Study of Asthma and Allergies in Childhood
IVIG intravenous immunoglobulin
NB-UVB Narrowband ultraviolet B light (311 nm)
NIAID National Institute of Allergy and Infectious Diseases
PUVA psoralens plus ultraviolet A light
RAST radioallergosorbent test
RCT randomized controlled trial
SD standard deviation
SPF sun protection factor
TH_1 T-helper type 1
TH_2 T-helper type 2
UV ultraviolet
UVA ultraviolet A
UVB ultraviolet B

REFERENCES

1. National Institute of Arthritis and Musculoskeletal and Skin Diseases. Handout on Health: Atopic Dermatitis. US Department of Health and Human Services. 2009, *http://www.niams.nih.gov/Health_Info/Atopic_Dermatitis/default.asp*.
2. Gimenez JCM. Atopic dermatitis. Alergol Immunol Clin 2000;15:279–295.
3. Lynde C, Barber K, Claveau J, Gratton D, et al. Canadian practical guide for the treatment and management of atopic dermatitis. J Cutan Med Surg 2005;8(suppl 5):1–9. *http://www.springerlink.com/content/r5432000056r2748/fulltext.html*.
4. Hanifin JM. Epidemiology of atopic dermatitis. Immunol Allergy Clin North Am 2002;22:1–24.
5. Bieber T. Mechanisms of disease: Atopic dermatitis. N Engl J Med 2008;358:1483–494.
6. Williams H, Flohr C. How epidemiology has challenged 3 prevailing concepts about atopic dermatitis. J Allergy Clin Immunol 2006;118:209–213.
7. Williams H, Stewart A, von Mutius E, Cookson W, et al. Is eczema really on the increase worldwide? J Allergy Clin Immunol 2008;121:947–954.
8. DaVeiga SP. Epidemiology of atopic dermatitis: a review. Allergy Asthma Proc 2012;23:227–234.
9. Hanifin JM, Cooper KD, Ho VC, et al. Guidelines of care for atopic dermatitis. J Am Acad Dermatol 2004;50:391–404.
10. Ring J, Alomar A, Bieber M, et al. Guidelines for treatment of atopic eczema (atopic dermatitis) parts 1 and II. J Eur Acad Dermatol Venereol 2012;26:1045–1060, 1176–1193.
11. Akdis CA. New insights into mechanisms of immunoregulation in 2007. J Allergy Clin Immunol 2008;122:700–709.
12. Rothers J, Stern DA, Spangenberg A, Lohman IC, et al. Influence of early day-care exposure on total IgE levels through age 3 years. J Allergy Clin Immunol 2007;120: 1201–1207.
13. Ege MJ, Herzum I, Buchele G, Krauss-Etschmann S, et al. Prenatal exposure to a farm environment modifies atopic sensitization at birth. J Allergy Clin Immunol 2008;122: 407–412.
14. O'Regan GM, Sandilands A, McLean WHI, Irvine AD. Filaggrin in atopic dermatitis. J Allergy Clin Immunol 2008;122:689–693.
15. Scharschmidt TC, Man MQ, Hatano Y, Crumrine D, et al. Filaggrin deficiency confers a paracellular barrier abnormality that reduces inflammatory thresholds to irritants and haptens. J Allergy Clin Immunol 2009;124:496–506.
16. Rodriguez E, Baurecht H, Herberich E, Wagenpfeil S, et al. Meta-analysis of filaggrin polymorphisms in eczema and asthma: robust rick factors in atopic disease. J Allergy Clin Immunol 2009;123:1361–1370.
17. Honey B, Steinhoff M, Ruzicka T, Leung DYM. Cytokines and chemokines orchestrate atopic skin inflammation. J Allergy Clin Immunol 2006;118:178–189.
18. Law RM, Kwa PG. Chapter 111: Atopic dermatitis: The itch that erupts when scratched. In: Schwinghammer TL, Koehler JM, eds. Instructor's Guide: Pharmacotherapy Casebook: A Patient-Focused Approach, 8th ed. New York: McGraw-Hill, 2011:111-1 to 111-5.
19. Leung DYM. Our evolving understanding of the functional role of filaggrin in atopic dermatitis. J Allergy Clin Immunol 2009;124:494–495.
20. Steinke JW, Rich SS, Borish L. Genetics of allergic disease. J Allergy Clin Immunol 2008;121(suppl):S384–S387.
21. Akdis CA, Akdis M, Bieber T, et al. Diagnosis and treatment of atopic dermatitis in children and adults: European Academy of Allergology and Clinical Immunology/ American Academy of Allergy, Asthma and Immunology/ PRACTALL Consensus Report. J Allergy Clin Immunol 2006;118:152–169.
22. Sicherer SC, Leung DYM. Advances in allergic skin disease, anaphylaxis and hypersensitivity reactions to foods, drugs, and insects in 2008. J Allergy Clin Immunol 2009;123:319–327.
23. Schauber J, Gallo RL. Antimicrobial peptides and the skin immune defense system. J Allergy Clin Immunol 2008;122:261–266.

24. Novak N, Bieber T. Dendritic cells as regulators of immunity and tolerance. J Allergy Clin Immunol 2008;121(suppl):S370–S374.
25. Biebe T, de la Salle H, Wollenberg A, et al. Human epidermal Langerhans cells express the high affinity receptor for immunoglobulin E (Fc epsilon RI). J Exp Med 1992;175:1285–1290.
26. Wang B, Rieger A, Kilgus O, et al. Epidermal Langerhans cells from normal human skin bind monomeric IgE via Fc epsilon RI. J Exp Med 1992;175:1353–1365.
27. Novak N, Bieber T. The role of dendritic cell subtypes in the pathophysiology of atopic dermatitis. J Am Acad Dermatol 2005;53(suppl 2):S171–S176.
28. Lack G. Epidemiologic risks for food allergy. J Allergy Clin Immunol 2008;121:1331–1336.
29. Boyce JA, Assa'ad AH, Burks AW, et al. Guidelines for the diagnosis and management of food allergy in the United States. Report of the NIAID-sponsored expert panel. J Allergy Clin Immunol 2010;126(6 suppl):S1–S58. *http://www.niaid.nih.gov/topics/foodAllergy/clinical/Pages/default.aspx.*
30. Lucas JSA, Lewis SA, Jourihane JO'B. Kiwi fruit allergy: A review. Pediatr Allergy Immunol 2003;14:420–428.
31. Cohen A, Goldberg M, Levy B, et al. Sesame food allergy and sensitization in children: The natural history and long-term follow-up. Pediatr Allergy Immunol 2007;18:217–223.
32. Burks AW, Laubach S, Jones SM. Oral tolerance, food allergy, and immunotherapy: Implications for future treatment. J Allergy Clin Immunol 2008;121:1344–1350.
33. Leung DYM, Nicklas RA, Li JT, Bernstein L, et al. Disease management of atopic dermatitis: An updated practice parameter. Ann Allergy Asthma Immunol 2004;93(3):S1–S17.
34. Krafchik BR. Atopic Dermatitis. 2008, *http://emedicine.medscape.com* (eMedicine Specialties > Dermatology > Allergy & Immunology).
35. Stores G, Burrows A, Crawford C. Physiological sleep disturbance in children with atopic dermatitis: A case control study. Pediatr Dermatol 1998;15(4):264–268.
36. Beltrani VS, Boguneiwicz M. Atopic dermatitis. Dermatology Online Journal. 2003, *http://dermatology.cdlib.org/92/reviews/atopy/beltrani.html.*
37. Simpson EL. Atopic dermatitis: A review of topical treatment options. Curr Med Res Opin 2010;26(3):633–640.
38. Carbone A, Siu A, Patel R. Pediatric atopic dermatitis: A review of the medical management. Ann Pharmacother 2010;44:1448–1458.
39. Rubel D, Thirumoorthy T, Soebaryo W, et al. Consensus guidelines for the management of atopic dermatitis: An Asia-Pacific perspective. J Dermatol 2013;40:160–171.
40. Baron SE, Cohen SN, Archer CB. British Association of Dermatologists and Royal College of General Practitioners. Guidance on the diagnosis and clinical management of atopic eczema. Clin Exp Dermatol 2012;37(suppl 1):7–12.
41. Rosso JD, Friedlander SF. Corticosteroids: Options in the era of steroid-sparing therapy. J Am Acad Dermatol 2005;53:S50–S58.
42. Hengge UR, Ruzicka T, Schwartz RA, et al. Adverse effects of topical glucocorticosteroids. J Am Acad Dermatol 2006;54:1–15.
43. Hebert AA; Desonide Foam Phase III Clinical Study Group. Desonide foam 0.05%: Safety in children as young as 3 months. J Am Acad Dermatol 2008;59:334–340.
44. Stuetz A, Grassberger M, Meingassner JG. Pimecrolimus (Elidel, SDZ ASM 981)—Preclinical pharmacologic profile and skin selectivity. Semin Cutan Med Surg 2001;20:233–241.
45. Berger TG, Duvic M, Van Voorhees AS, Frieden IJ. The use of topical calcineurin inhibitors in dermatology: Safety concerns. J Am Acad Dermatol 2006;54:818–823.
46. Abramovits W. A clinician's paradigm in the treatment of atopic dermatitis. J Am Acad Dermatol 2005;53:S70–S77.
47. Majoie IML, Oldhoff JM, van Weelden H, et al. Narrowband ultraviolet B and medium-dose ultraviolet A1 are equally effective in the treatment of moderate to severe atopic dermatitis. J Am Acad Dermatol 2009;60:77–84.
48. Pughdal KV, Schwartz RA. Topical tar: Back to the future. J Am Acad Dermatol 2009;61:294–302.
49. Hanifin JM, Schneider LC, Leung DY, et al. Recombinant interferon gamma therapy for atopic dermatitis. J Am Acad Dermatol 1993;28:189–197.
50. Jang IG, Yang JK, Lee HJ, et al. Clinical improvement and immunohistochemical findings in severe atopic dermatitis treated with interferon gamma. J Am Acad Dermatol 2000;42:1033–1040.
51. Bremmer MS, Bremmer SF, Baig-Lewis S, et al. Are biologics safe in the treatment of atopic dermatitis? A review with a focus on immediate hypersensitivity reactions. J Am Acad Dermatol 2009;61:666–676.
52. Langan S, Rogers S. A retrospective review of the use of azathioprine in the therapy of severe atopic eczema. J Am Acad Dermatol 2005;52(3 suppl 1):P84, abstract P1001.
53. Rouse C, Siegfried E. Methotrexate for atopic dermatitis in children. J Am Acad Dermatol 2008;58(2 suppl 2):AB7, abstract P608.
54. Koo J, Arain S. Traditional Chinese medicine for the treatment of dermatologic disorders. Arch Dermatol 1998;134:1388–1393.
55. Harper J. Traditional Chinese medicine for eczema. BMJ 1994;308:489–490.
56. Arkwright PD, David TJ. Intradermal administration of a killed *Mycobacterium vaccae* suspension (SRL 172) is associated with improvement in atopic dermatitis in children with moderate-to-severe disease. J Allergy Clin Immunol 2001;107:531–534.
57. van der Aa LB, Heymans HAS, van Aalderen WMC, et al. Probiotics and prebiotics in atopic dermatitis: Review of the theoretical background and clinical evidence. Pediatr Allergy Immunol 2010;21:e355–e367.
58. Zuberbier T, Orlow SJ, Paller AS, et al. Patient perspectives on the management of atopic dermatitis. J Allergy Clin Immunol 2006;118:226–232.

80

Anemias

Kristen Cook and William L. Lyons

KEY CONCEPTS

1. Anemia is a group of diseases characterized by a decrease in either hemoglobin (Hb) or the volume of red blood cells (RBCs), which results in decreased oxygen-carrying capacity of the blood. Anemia is defined by the World Health Organization as Hb <13 g/dL (<130 g/L; <8.07 mmol/L) in men and <12 g/dL (<120 g/L; <7.45 mmol/L) in women.
2. Acute-onset anemias are most likely to present with tachycardia, lightheadedness, and dyspnea. Chronic anemia often presents with weakness, fatigue, headache, vertigo, and pallor.
3. Iron-deficiency anemia (IDA) is characterized by decreased levels of ferritin (most sensitive marker) and serum iron, as well as decreased transferrin saturation. Hb and hematocrit decrease later. RBC morphology includes hypochromia and microcytosis. Most patients are adequately treated with oral iron therapy, although parenteral iron therapy is necessary in selected patient populations.
4. Vitamin B_{12} deficiency, a macrocytic anemia, can be due to inadequate intake, malabsorption syndromes, and inadequate utilization. Anemia caused by lack of intrinsic factor, resulting in decreased vitamin B_{12} absorption, is called *pernicious anemia*. Neurologic symptoms can be present and can become irreversible if the vitamin B_{12} deficiency is not treated promptly. Oral or parenteral therapy can be used for replacement.
5. Folic acid deficiency, a macrocytic anemia, results from inadequate intake, decreased absorption, and increased folate requirements. Treatment consists of oral administration of folic acid, even for patients with absorption problems. Adequate folic acid intake is essential in women of childbearing age to decrease the risk of neural tube defects in their children.
6. Anemia of inflammation (AI) is a newer term used to describe both anemia of chronic disease and anemia of critical illness. AI is a diagnosis of exclusion. It results from chronic inflammation, infection, or malignancy and can occur as early as 1 to 2 months after the onset of the disease. The serum iron level usually is decreased, but in contrast to IDA, the serum ferritin concentration is normal or increased. Treatment is aimed at correcting the underlying pathology. Anemia of critical illness occurs within days of acute illness.
7. Anemia is one of the most prevalent clinical problems in the elderly, although not an inevitable complication of aging. Low Hb concentrations are not "normal" among elders. Anemia is associated with an increased risk of hospitalization and mortality, reduced quality of life, and decreased physical functioning in the elderly.
8. IDA is a leading cause of infant morbidity and mortality. Age- and sex-adjusted norms must be used in the interpretation of laboratory results for pediatric patients. Primary prevention of IDA is the goal. A therapeutic trial of oral iron is the standard of care.

Anemia affects a large part of the world's population. According to the World Health Organization, almost 1.6 billion people (25% of the world's population) are anemic. Anemia is defined by the World Health Organization as hemoglobin (Hb) <13 g/dL (<130 g/L; <8.07 mmol/L) in men or <12 g/dL (<120 g/L; <7.45 mmol/L) in women. In the United States, about 3.5 million Americans have anemia based on self-reported data from the National Center for Health Statistics. It is estimated that millions of people are unaware they have anemia, making it one of the most underdiagnosed conditions in the United States. Iron deficiency is the leading cause of anemia worldwide, accounting for as many as 50% of cases.[1] Recent data show that the overall prevalence of anemia has declined in the United States in preschool-aged children and women of childbearing age over the past 20 years, but the prevalence of IDA did not change significantly in these same groups. The reasons for these changes remain unclear.[2] Although nutritional deficiencies occur less often in the United States, obesity surgery, which can cause deficiencies, is becoming increasingly common. Gastric bypass may result in folate, vitamin B_{12}, and iron deficiencies. Prevalence data are confounded by the lack of a standardized definition of anemia and lack of screening guidelines for most populations. The United States Preventive Services Task Force (USPSTF) guidelines for pregnant women recommend routine screening for IDA.

Anemia is not an innocent bystander because it can affect both length and quality of life. Retrospective observational studies of hemodialysis patients and heart failure patients suggest that anemia is an independent risk factor for mortality.[3] In addition, anemia significantly influences morbidity in patients with end-stage renal disease, chronic kidney disease, and heart failure.[4] Anemia is associated with psychomotor and cognitive abnormalities in children. Similarly, anemia is associated with cognitive dysfunction in patients with renal failure or cancer, and among community-dwelling elders.[5] Anemia during pregnancy is associated with increased risk for low birth weights, preterm delivery, and perinatal mortality.[6] Maternal IDA may be associated with postpartum depression in mothers and poor performance by offspring on mental and psychomotor tests. Global goals of treatment in anemic patients are to alleviate signs and symptoms, correct the underlying etiology, and prevent recurrence of anemia.

1 Anemia is a group of diseases characterized by a decrease in either Hb or circulating red blood cells (RBCs), resulting in reduced oxygen-carrying capacity of the blood. Anemia can result from inadequate RBC production, increased RBC destruction, or blood loss. It can be a manifestation of a host of systemic disorders, such as infection, chronic renal disease, or malignancy. Because anemia is a sign of underlying pathology, rapid diagnosis of the cause may be essential.

The functional classification of anemia is shown in Figure 80-1. This chapter focuses on the most common causes of anemia—IDA, anemia associated with vitamin B_{12} or folic acid deficiency, and anemia of inflammation (AI). Some of the other causes of anemia are addressed in other chapters.

Characteristic changes in the size of RBCs seen in erythrocyte indices can be the first step in the morphologic classification and understanding of the anemia. Anemia can be classified by RBC size as macrocytic, normocytic, or microcytic. Vitamin B_{12} deficiency and folic acid deficiency both are macrocytic anemias. An example of a microcytic anemia is iron deficiency, whereas a normocytic anemia may be associated with recent blood loss or chronic disease. More than one etiology of anemia can occur concurrently. Inclusion of the underlying cause of the anemia makes diagnostic terminology easier to understand (e.g., microcytic anemia secondary to iron deficiency).

Microcytic anemias are a result of a quantitative deficiency in Hb synthesis, usually due to iron deficiency or impaired iron utilization. As a result, erythrocytes containing insufficient Hb are formed. Microcytosis and hypochromia are the morphologic abnormalities that provide evidence of impaired Hb synthesis.

Macrocytic anemias can be divided into megaloblastic and nonmegaloblastic anemias. The type of macrocytic anemia can be distinguished microscopically by peripheral blood smear examination. Megaloblasts are distinctive cells that express a biochemical abnormality of retarded DNA synthesis, resulting in unbalanced cell growth. Megaloblastic anemias may affect all hematopoietic cell lines. The most common causes of megaloblastic anemia are vitamin B_{12} and folate deficiency. Nonmegaloblastic macrocytic anemias may arise from liver disease, hypothyroidism, hemolytic processes, and alcoholism. Hemolytic anemias often are macrocytic, reflecting the increased numbers of circulating reticulocytes, which are larger on average than mature red cells.

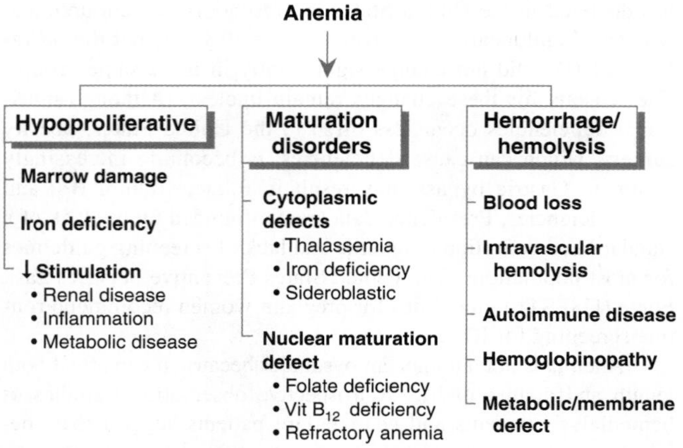

Anemia

Hypoproliferative
- **Marrow damage**
- **Iron deficiency**
- **↓ Stimulation**
  - Renal disease
  - Inflammation
  - Metabolic disease

Maturation disorders
- **Cytoplasmic defects**
  - Thalassemia
  - Iron deficiency
  - Sideroblastic
- **Nuclear maturation defect**
  - Folate deficiency
  - Vit B_{12} deficiency
  - Refractory anemia

Hemorrhage/hemolysis
- **Blood loss**
- **Intravascular hemolysis**
- **Autoimmune disease**
- **Hemoglobinopathy**
- **Metabolic/membrane defect**

FIGURE 80-1 Functional classification of anemia. Each of the major categories of anemia (hypoproliferative, maturation disorders, and hemorrhage/hemolysis) can be further subclassified according to the functional defect in the several components of normal erythropoiesis.

MATURATION AND DEVELOPMENT OF RED BLOOD CELLS

In adults, RBCs are formed in the marrow of the vertebrae, ribs, sternum, clavicle, pelvic (iliac) crest, and proximal epiphyses of the long bones. In children, most bone marrow space is hematopoietically active to meet increased RBC requirements.

In normal RBC formation, a pluripotent stem cell yields an erythroid burst-forming unit. Erythropoietin (EPO) and cytokines such as interleukin-3 and granulocyte–macrophage colony-stimulating factor stimulate this cell to form an erythroid colony-forming unit in the marrow (Fig. 80-2). During this process, the nucleus becomes smaller with each division, finally disappearing in the normal erythrocyte. Hb and iron are incorporated into the gradually maturing RBC, which eventually is released from the marrow into the circulating blood as a reticulocyte. The maturation process usually takes about 1 week. The reticulocyte loses its nucleus and becomes an erythrocyte within several days. The circulating erythrocyte is a nonnucleated, nondividing cell. More than 90% of the protein content of the erythrocyte consists of the oxygen-carrying molecule Hb. Erythrocytes have a normal survival time of 120 days.[7]

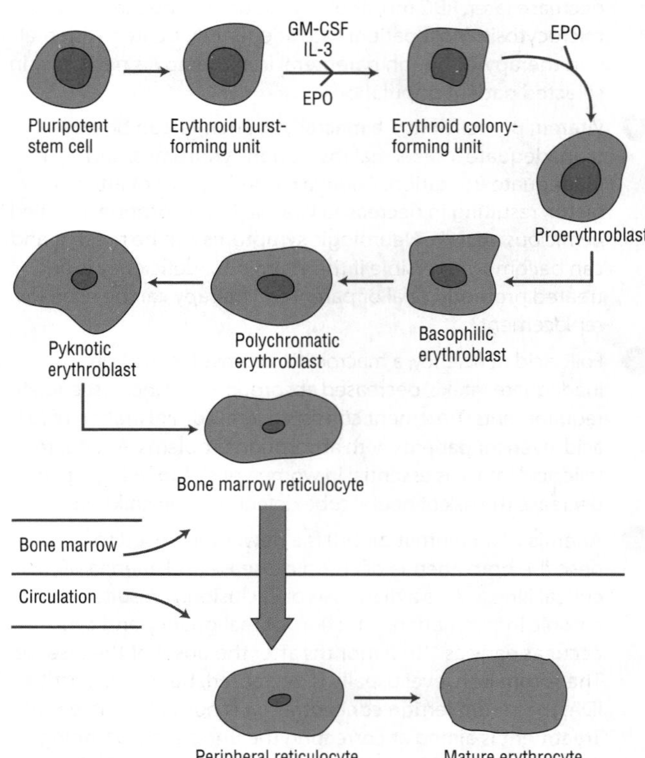

FIGURE 80-2 Erythrocyte maturation sequence (EPO, erythropoietin; GM-CSF, granulocyte-macrophage colony-stimulating factor; IL-3, interleukin-3).

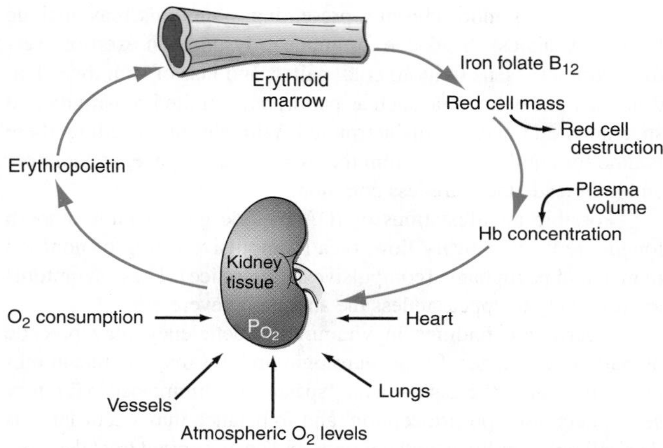

FIGURE 80-3 Physiologic regulation of red cell production by tissue oxygen tension. *(Reproduced with permission from Adamson JW, Longo DL. Anemia and polycythemia. In: Longo DL, Fauci AS, Kasper DL, et al., eds. Harrison's Principles of Internal Medicine. 18th ed. New York: Copyright © McGraw-Hill; 2012: http://www.accessmedicine.com/content.aspx?aID=9113377.)*

Stimulation of Erythropoiesis

The hormone EPO, 90% of which is produced by the kidneys, initiates and stimulates the production of RBCs. Erythropoiesis is regulated by a feedback loop. The main mechanism of action of EPO is to prevent apoptosis, or programmed cell death, of erythroid precursor cells and allow their proliferation and subsequent maturation. A decrease in tissue oxygen concentration signals the kidneys to increase the production and release of EPO into the plasma, which increases production and maturation of RBCs. Under normal circumstances, the RBC mass is kept at an almost constant level by EPO matching new erythrocyte production to the natural rate of loss of RBCs. A summary of erythropoiesis is shown in Figure 80-3. Early appearance of large quantities of reticulocytes in the peripheral circulation (reticulocytosis) is an indication of increased RBC production.[7]

Synthesis of Hemoglobin

Hb contains a protein component with two α-chains and two β-chains. Each chain is linked to a heme group consisting of a porphyrin ring structure with an iron atom chelated at its center, which is capable of binding oxygen. The initial step in the synthesis of heme from the substrate succinyl CoA and glycine requires the presence of pyridoxine phosphate (vitamin B_6) as a catalyst. Following its synthesis in the cytoplasmic mitochondria of the RBC, heme diffuses into the extramitochondrial space, where it combines with the completed α- and β-chains and forms Hb. When hemolytic destruction of RBCs exceeds marrow production capacity and anemia develops, the Hb value decreases to a steady-state level at which production is equal to destruction.

Incorporation of Iron into Heme

Iron is an essential part of Hb. The specific plasma transport protein transferrin delivers iron to the bone marrow for incorporation into the Hb molecule. Transferrin enters cells by binding to transferrin receptors, which circulate and then attach to cells needing iron. Fewer transferrin receptors are present on the surface of cells that do not need iron, thus preventing iron-replete cells from receiving excess iron.[8]

Circulating transferrin normally is about 30% saturated with iron. Transferrin delivers extra iron to other body storage sites, such as the liver, marrow, and spleen, for later use. This iron is stored within macrophages as ferritin or hemosiderin. Ferritin consists of a Fe^{3+} hydroxyphosphate core surrounded by a protein shell called *apoferritin*. Hemosiderin can be described as compacted ferritin molecules with an even greater iron-to-protein shell ratio. Physiologically it is a more stable, but less available, form of storage iron. Since total body iron storage is generally reflected by ferritin levels, low serum levels of ferritin provide strong evidence of IDA.[9]

Normal Destruction of Red Blood Cells

Phagocytic breakdown destroys older blood cells, primarily in the spleen but also in the marrow (Fig. 80-4). Amino acids from the globin chains return to an amino acid pool; heme oxygenase acts on the porphyrin heme structure to form biliverdin and to release its iron. Iron returns to the iron pool to be reused, although biliverdin is further catabolized to bilirubin. The bilirubin is released into the plasma, where it binds to albumin and is transported to the liver for glucuronide conjugation and excretion via bile. If the liver is unable to perform the conjugation, as occurs with intrinsic liver disease or oversaturation of conjugation enzymes by excessive cell hemolysis, the result is an elevated *indirect* (unconjugated) bilirubin. If the biliary excretion pathway for conjugated bilirubin is obstructed, an elevated *direct* bilirubin results. Comparison of direct and indirect bilirubin values helps to determine if the defect in bilirubin clearance occurs before or after bilirubin enters the liver. The Hb in

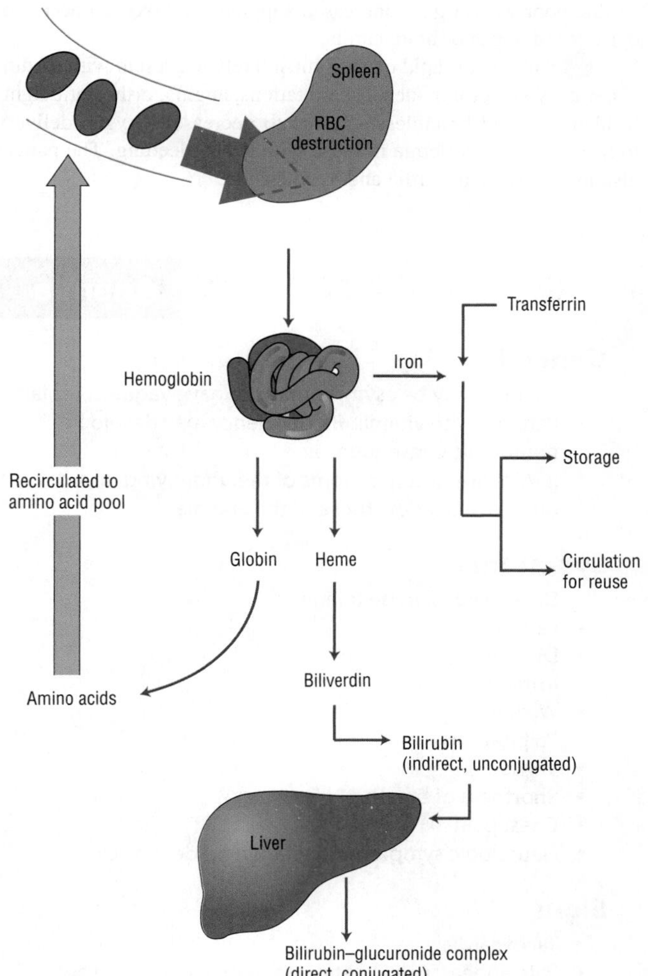

FIGURE 80-4 Destruction of red blood cells (RBCs).

RBCs destroyed by intravascular hemolysis becomes attached to haptoglobin and is carried back to the marrow for processing in the normal manner.[10]

DIAGNOSIS OF ANEMIA

General Presentation

History, physical examination, and laboratory testing are used in the evaluation of the patient with anemia. The workup determines if the patient is bleeding and investigates potential causes of the anemia, such as increased RBC destruction, bone marrow suppression, or iron deficiency. Diet can also be important in identifying causes of anemia. Additionally, information about concurrent nonhematologic disease states and a drug history are essential when evaluating the cause of the anemia (see eChap. 23). History of blood transfusions and exposure to toxic chemicals also should be obtained.

Presenting signs and symptoms of anemia depend on its rate of development and the age and cardiovascular status of the patient. Severity of symptoms does not always correlate with the degree of anemia. Healthy patients may acclimate to very low Hb concentrations if the anemia develops slowly. Mild anemia often is associated with no clinical symptoms and may be found incidentally upon obtaining a complete blood count (CBC) for other reasons. The signs and symptoms in elderly patients with anemia may be attributed to their age or concomitant disease states. The elderly may not tolerate levels of Hb tolerated by younger persons. Similarly, patients with cardiac or pulmonary disease may be less tolerant of mild anemia. Premature infants with anemia may be asymptomatic or have tachycardia, poor weight gain, increased supplemental oxygen needs, or episodes of apnea or bradycardia.

2 Anemia of rapid onset is most likely to present with cardiorespiratory symptoms such as palpitations, angina, orthostatic lightheadedness, and breathlessness due to decreased oxygen delivery to tissues or hypovolemia in those with acute bleeding. The patient also may have tachycardia and hypotension.

If onset is more chronic, presenting symptoms may include fatigue, weakness, headache, orthopnea, dyspnea on exertion, vertigo, faintness, sensitivity to cold, pallor, and loss of skin tone. Traditional signs of anemia, such as pallor, have limited sensitivity and specificity and may be misinterpreted. With chronic bleeding, there is time for equilibration within the extravascular space, so faintness and lightheadedness are less common.

Possible manifestations of IDA include glossal pain, smooth tongue, reduced salivary flow, pica (compulsive eating of nonfood items), and pagophagia (compulsive eating of ice). These symptoms are not likely to appear unless the anemia is severe.

Neurologic findings in vitamin B_{12} deficiency may precede hematologic changes. Early neurologic findings may include numbness and paraesthesias. Ataxia, spasticity, diminished vibratory sense, decreased proprioception, and imbalance may occur later as demyelination of the dorsal columns and corticospinal tract develop. Vision changes may result from optic nerve involvement. Psychiatric findings include irritability, personality changes, memory impairment, depression, and, infrequently, psychosis.

Anemia associated with folate deficiency is typically macrocytic but, unlike B_{12} deficiency, occurs without neurological symptoms. Although the symptoms of anemia will improve with folate replacement and a partial hematologic response will occur, the neurologic manifestations of vitamin B_{12} deficiency will not be reversed with folic acid replacement therapy and consequently may progress or become irreversible if not treated appropriately.

Laboratory Evaluation

The initial evaluation of anemia involves a CBC (including RBC indices), reticulocyte index, and possibly an examination of a stool sample for occult blood. The results of the preliminary evaluation determine the need for other studies, such as examination of a peripheral blood smear. Based on laboratory test results, anemia can be categorized into three functional defects: RBC production failure (hypoproliferative), cell maturation ineffectiveness, or increased RBC destruction or loss (Fig. 80-1).

CLINICAL PRESENTATION Anemia

General

- Patients may be asymptomatic or have vague complaints
- Patients with vitamin B_{12} deficiency may develop neurologic consequences
- In AI, signs and symptoms of the underlying disorder often overshadow those of the anemia

Symptoms

- Decreased exercise tolerance
- Fatigue
- Dizziness
- Irritability
- Weakness
- Palpitations
- Vertigo
- Shortness of breath
- Chest pain
- Neurologic symptoms in vitamin B_{12} deficiency

Signs

- Tachycardia
- Pale appearance (most prominent in conjunctivae)
- Decreased mental acuity
- Increased intensity of some cardiac valvular murmurs
- Diminished vibratory sense or gait abnormality in vitamin B_{12} deficiency

Laboratory Tests

- Hb, hematocrit (Hct), and RBC indices may remain normal early in the disease and then decrease as the anemia progresses
- Serum iron is low in IDA and AI
- Ferritin levels are low in IDA and normal to increased in AI
- TIBC is high in IDA and is low or normal in AI
- Mean cell volume is elevated in vitamin B_{12} deficiency and folate deficiency
- Vitamin B_{12} and folate levels are low in their respective types of anemia
- Homocysteine is elevated in vitamin B_{12} deficiency and folate deficiency
- Methylmalonic acid is elevated in vitamin B_{12} deficiency

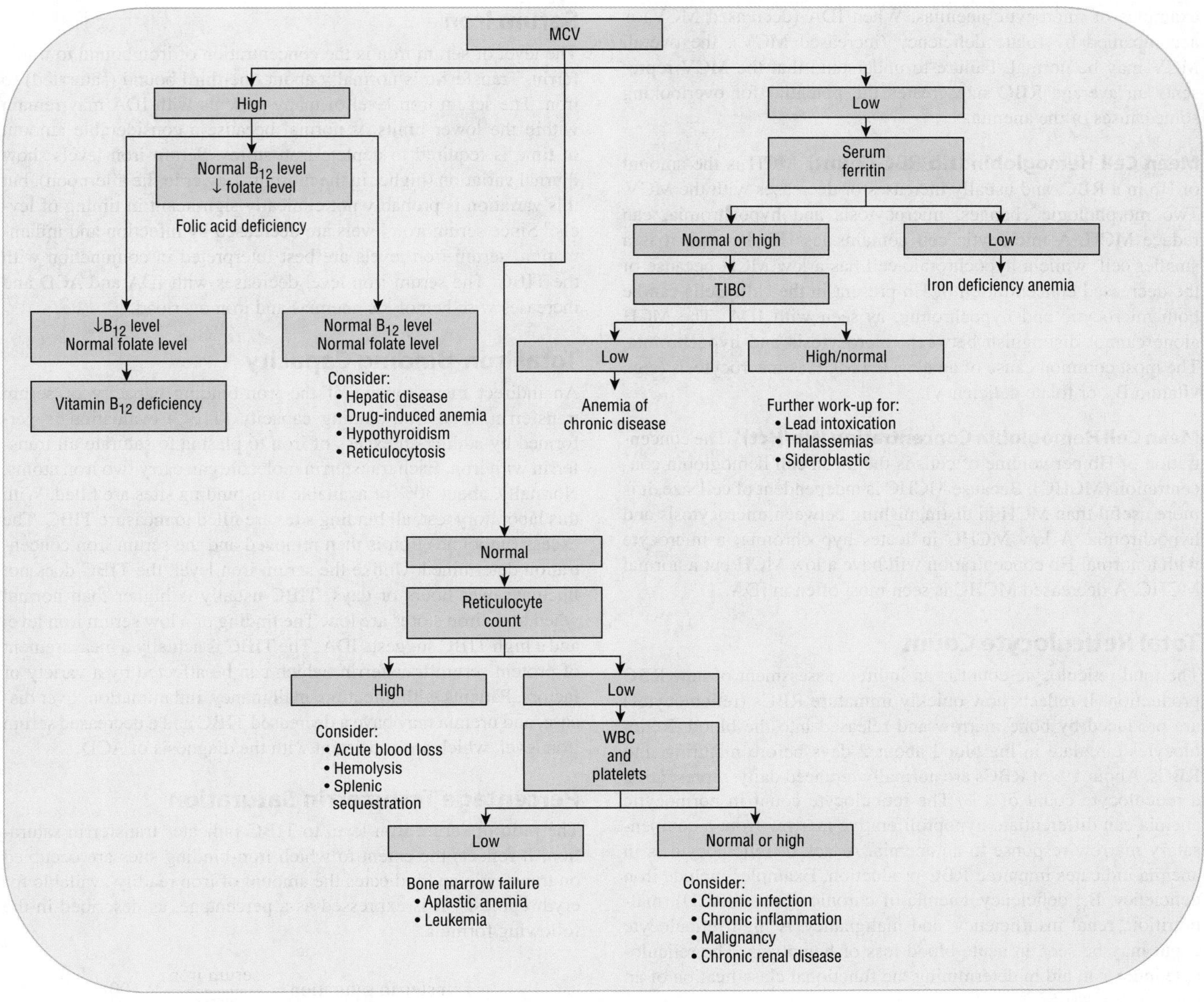

FIGURE 80-5 General algorithm for diagnosis of anemias (↓, decreased; MCV, mean corpuscular volume; TIBC, total iron-binding capacity; WBC, white blood cells).

Figure 80-5 shows a broad, general algorithm for the diagnosis of anemia based on laboratory data. There are many exceptions and additions to this algorithm, but it can serve as a guide to the typical presentation of common types and causes of anemia. The algorithm is less useful in the presence of more than one cause of anemia.

Hemoglobin

Values given for Hb represent the amount of Hb per volume of whole blood. The higher values seen in males are due to stimulation of RBC production by androgenic steroids, whereas the lower values in females reflect the decrease in Hb as a result of blood loss during menstruation. The Hb level can be used as a very rough estimate of the oxygen-carrying capacity of blood. Hb levels may be diminished because of a decreased quantity of Hb per RBC or because of a decrease in the actual number of RBCs.

Hematocrit

Expressed as a percentage, hematocrit (Hct) is the actual volume of RBCs in a unit volume of whole blood. In general, it is about three times the Hb value (when Hb is expressed in g/dL). An alteration in this ratio may occur with abnormal cell size or shape and often indicates pathology. A low Hct indicates a reduction in either the number or the size of RBCs or an increase in plasma volume.

Red Blood Cell Count

The RBC count is an indirect estimate of the Hb content of the blood; it is an actual count of RBCs per unit of blood.

Red Blood Cell Indices

Wintrobe indices describe the size and Hb content of the RBCs and are calculated from the Hb, Hct, and RBC count. RBC indices, such as mean corpuscular volume (MCV) and mean corpuscular hemoglobin (MCH), are single mean values that do not express the variation that can occur in cells.

Mean Cell Volume (Hct/RBC Count) MCV represents the average volume of RBCs. It may reflect changes in MCH. Cells are considered macrocytic if they are larger than normal, microcytic if they are smaller than normal, and normocytic if their size falls within normal limits. Folic acid and vitamin B_{12} deficiency anemias yield macrocytic cells, whereas iron deficiency and thalassemia are examples of microcytic anemias. When IDA (decreased MCV) is accompanied by folate deficiency (increased MCV), the overall MCV may be normal. Failure to understand that the MCV represents an average RBC size creates the potential for overlooking some causes of the anemia.

Mean Cell Hemoglobin (Hb/RBC Count) MCH is the amount of Hb in a RBC, and usually increases or decreases with the MCV. Two morphologic changes, microcytosis and hypochromia, can reduce MCH. A microcytic cell contains less Hb because it is a smaller cell, while a hypochromic cell has a low MCH because of the decreased concentration of Hb present in the cell. Cells can be both microcytic and hypochromic, as seen with IDA. The MCH alone cannot distinguish between microcytosis and hypochromia. The most common cause of an elevated MCH is macrocytosis (e.g., vitamin B_{12} or folate deficiency).

Mean Cell Hemoglobin Concentration (Hb/Hct) The concentration of Hb per volume of cells is the mean cell hemoglobin concentration (MCHC). Because MCHC is independent of cell size, it is more useful than MCH in distinguishing between microcytosis and hypochromia. A low MCHC indicates hypochromia; a microcyte with a normal Hb concentration will have a low MCH but a normal MCHC. A decreased MCHC is seen most often in IDA.

Total Reticulocyte Count

The total reticulocyte count is an indirect assessment of new RBC production. It reflects how quickly immature RBCs (reticulocytes) are produced by bone marrow and released into the blood. Reticulocytes circulate in the blood about 2 days before maturing into RBCs. About 1% of RBCs are normally replaced daily, representing a reticulocyte count of 1%. The reticulocyte count in normocytic anemia can differentiate hypoproliferative marrow from a compensatory marrow response to an anemia. A lack of reticulocytosis in anemia indicates impaired RBC production. Examples include iron deficiency, B_{12} deficiency, anemia of chronic disease (ACD), malnutrition, renal insufficiency, and malignancy. A high reticulocyte count may be seen in acute blood loss or hemolysis. The reticulocyte index can aid in determining the functional classification of an anemia (Fig. 80-5).

Red Blood Cell Distribution Width

The higher the red blood cell distribution width (RDW) is, the more variable is the size of the RBCs. The RDW increases in early IDA because of the release of large, immature, nucleated RBCs to compensate for the anemia, but this change is not specific for IDA. The RDW also can be helpful in the diagnosis of a mixed anemia. A patient can have a normal MCV yet have a wide RDW. This finding indicates the presence of microcytes and macrocytes, which would yield a "normal" average RBC size. Use of RDW to distinguish IDA from ACD is not recommended.

Peripheral Blood Smear

The peripheral blood smear can supplement other clinical data and help establish a diagnosis. Peripheral blood smears provide information on the functional status of the bone marrow and defects in RBC production. Additionally, it provides information on variations in cell size (anisocytosis) and shape (poikilocytosis). Automated blood counters, used for the CBC, can flag specific RBC changes that can be confirmed by a peripheral blood smear. Blood smears are placed on a microscope slide and stained as appropriate. Morphologic examination includes assessment of size, shape, and color. The extent of anisocytosis correlates with increased range of cell sizes. Poikilocytosis can suggest a defect in the maturation of RBC precursors in the bone marrow or the presence of hemolysis.

Serum Iron

The level of serum iron is the concentration of iron bound to transferrin. Transferrin is normally about one-third bound (saturated) to iron. The serum iron level of many patients with IDA may remain within the lower limits of normal because a considerable amount of time is required to deplete iron stores. Serum iron levels show diurnal variation (higher in the morning, lower in the afternoon), but this variation is probably not clinically significant in timing of levels.[9] Since serum iron levels are decreased by infection and inflammation, serum iron levels are best interpreted in conjunction with the TIBC. The serum iron level decreases with IDA and ACD and increases with hemolytic anemias and iron overload.

Total Iron-Binding Capacity

An indirect measurement of the iron-binding capacity of serum transferrin, total iron-binding capacity (TIBC) evaluation is performed by adding an excess of iron to plasma to saturate all transferrin with iron. Each transferrin molecule can carry two iron atoms. Normally, about 30% of available iron-binding sites are filled. With this laboratory test, all binding sites are filled to measure TIBC. The excess (unbound) iron is then removed and the serum iron concentration determined. Unlike the serum iron level, the TIBC does not fluctuate over hours or days. TIBC usually is higher than normal when body iron stores are low. The finding of a low serum iron level and a high TIBC suggests IDA. The TIBC is actually a measurement of protein serum transferrin, which can be affected by a variety of factors. Patients with infection, malignancy, inflammation, liver disease, and uremia may have a decreased TIBC and a decreased serum iron level, which are consistent with the diagnosis of ACD.

Percentage Transferrin Saturation

The ratio of serum iron level to TIBC indicates transferrin saturation. It reflects the extent to which iron-binding sites are occupied on transferrin and indicates the amount of iron readily available for erythropoiesis. It is expressed as a percentage, as described in the following formula:

$$\text{Transferrin saturation} = \frac{\text{serum iron}}{\text{TIBC}} \times 100$$

Transferrin normally is 20% to 50% saturated with iron. In IDA, transferrin saturation of 15% or lower is commonly seen.[10] Transferrin saturation is a less sensitive and specific marker of iron deficiency than are ferritin levels.

Serum Ferritin

The serum concentration of ferritin (storage iron) is proportional to total iron stores and therefore is the best indicator of iron deficiency or iron overload. Ferritin levels indicate the amount of iron stored in the liver, spleen, and bone marrow cells. Low serum ferritin levels are virtually diagnostic of IDA. In contrast, serum iron levels may decrease in both IDA and ACD. Serum ferritin is an acute phase reactant; so chronic infection or inflammation can increase its concentration independent of iron status, masking depleted tissue stores. This limits the utility of the serum ferritin if the level is normal or high for a chronically ill patient. For these patients, iron, even if present in these tissue stores, may not be available for erythropoiesis.

Soluble Transferrin Receptor

The soluble transferrin receptor (sTfR) assay is a laboratory test considered a sensitive, early, highly quantitative marker of iron depletion. The sTfR concentration is inversely correlated with tissue iron stores, and elevated levels are predictive of iron deficiency. Unlike ferritin, the sTfR is not an acute phase reactant; so its level remains normal for patients with chronic disease. It may be a useful test for distinguishing ACD from IDA.[9] The major limitation of this test is that it is not widely available in many laboratories.

Folic Acid

The results of folic acid measurements vary depending on the assay method used. Decreased serum folic acid levels indicate a folate deficiency megaloblastic anemia that may coexist with a vitamin B_{12} deficiency anemia. Erythrocyte folic acid levels are less variable than serum levels because they are slow to decrease in an acute process such as drug-induced folic acid deficiency and slow to increase with oral folic acid replacement. In addition, erythrocyte folic acid levels have the theoretical advantage of less susceptibility to rapid changes in diet and alcohol intake. Limitations with sensitivity and specificity do exist with measurements of erythrocyte folate. It has been proposed that serum folate assay levels be drawn for patients with MCV >110 fL or for patients with a lower MCV and clinical features suggesting a macrocytic anemia. If the serum folate concentration is normal for a patient with suspected folate deficiency, then the erythrocyte folate level should be measured.[11]

Vitamin B_{12}

Low levels of vitamin B_{12} (cyanocobalamin or cobalamin) indicate deficiency. However, a deficiency may exist prior to the recognition of low serum levels. Serum values are maintained at the expense of vitamin B_{12} tissue stores. Vitamin B_{12} and folate deficiency may overlap, thus serum levels of both vitamins should be determined. Vitamin B_{12} levels may be falsely low with folate deficiency, pregnancy, and use of oral contraceptives.[12]

Schilling Test

This test used to be the "gold standard" for assessing vitamin B_{12} absorption. Due to its cost, unavailable test components, and complexity, the test is rarely used today. Tests to replace it are under investigation.[13]

Homocysteine

Vitamin B_{12} and folate both are required for conversion of homocysteine to methionine. Increased serum homocysteine may suggest vitamin B_{12} or folate deficiency. Homocysteine levels also can be elevated in patients with vitamin B_6 deficiency, renal failure, hypothyroidism, or a genetic defect in cystathionine β-synthase.[14]

Methylmalonic Acid

A vitamin B_{12} coenzyme is needed to convert methylmalonyl coenzyme A to succinyl coenzyme A. Patients with vitamin B_{12} deficiency have increased concentrations of serum methylmalonic acid (MMA), which is a more specific marker for vitamin B_{12} deficiency than homocysteine. MMA levels are not elevated in folate deficiency because folate does not participate in MMA metabolism. Levels of both MMA and homocysteine usually are elevated prior to the development of hematologic abnormalities and reductions in serum vitamin B_{12} levels.[12] MMA levels must be interpreted cautiously for patients with renal disease and hypovolemia because the levels may be elevated due to decreased urinary excretion.

IRON-DEFICIENCY ANEMIA

Epidemiology

Iron deficiency is the most common nutritional deficiency in developing and developed countries. Data from the National Health and Nutrition Examination Survey (NHANES) indicate the prevalence of IDA in young children and women of childbearing age is 1.2% and 4.5%, respectively.[2] The normal ranges for Hb and Hct are so wide that a patient may lose up to 15% of RBC mass and still have a Hct within the normal range. Therefore, iron deficiency may precede the appearance of anemia.

Iron Balance

The normal iron content of the body is about 3 to 4 g. Iron is a component of Hb, myoglobin, and cytochromes. About 2 g of the iron exists in the form of Hb, and about 140 mg exists as iron-containing proteins such as myoglobin. About 3 mg of iron is bound to transferrin in plasma, and 1,000 mg of iron exists as storage iron in the form of ferritin or hemosiderin. The rest of the iron is stored in other tissues such as cytochromes.[9] Due to the toxicity of inorganic iron, the body has an intricate system for iron absorption, transport, storage, assimilation, and elimination. Hepcidin is a regulator of intestinal iron absorption, iron recycling, and iron mobilization from hepatic stores. It is a peptide made in the liver, distributed in plasma, and excreted in urine. Hepcidin inhibits efflux of iron through ferroportin. Hepcidin synthesis is increased by iron loading and decreased by anemia and hypoxia. Hepcidin is induced during infections and inflammation, which allows iron to sequester in macrophages, hepatocytes, and enterocytes.[15] As a result, hepcidin is likely an important mediator of AI. Hepicidin is usually suppressed in IDA.[16]

Most people lose about 1 mg of iron daily. Menstruating women can lose up to 0.6% to 2.5% more per day. Pregnancy requires an additional 700 mg of iron and a blood donation can result in as much as 250 mg of iron loss;[17] these patients are at higher risk for deficiency.

Iron is best absorbed in its ferrous (Fe^{2+}) form. The normal daily Western diet contains mainly the ferric (Fe^{3+}) nonabsorbed form. After iron is ionized by stomach acid and then reduced to the Fe^{2+} state, it is absorbed primarily in the duodenum, and to a smaller extent in the jejunum, via intestinal mucosal cell uptake. Subsequently, it is transferred across the cell into the plasma. Iron absorption is not directly proportional to iron intake. Rather as physiologic iron levels decrease, GI absorption of iron increases.

The daily recommended dietary allowance for iron is 8 mg in adult males and postmenopausal females and 18 mg in menstruating females. Children require more iron because of growth-related increases in blood volume, and pregnant women have an increased iron demand brought about by fetal development. In the absence of hemochromatosis, iron overload does not occur, because only the amount of iron lost per day is absorbed. The amount of iron absorbed from food depends on the body stores, the rate of RBC production, the type of iron provided in the diet, and the presence of any substances that may enhance or inhibit iron absorption.

Heme iron, which is found in meat, fish, and poultry, is about three times more absorbable than the nonheme iron found in vegetables, fruits, dried beans, nuts, grain products, and dietary supplements. Gastric acid and other dietary components such as ascorbic acid increase the absorption of nonheme iron. Dietary components that form insoluble complexes with iron (phytates, tannates, and phosphates) decrease absorption. Phytates, a natural component of grains, brans, and some vegetables, can form poorly absorbed complexes and partially explain the increased prevalence of IDA in poorer countries, where grains and vegetables compose a disproportionate amount of the normal diet. Polyphenols bind iron and decrease nonheme iron absorption when large amounts of tea or coffee are consumed with a meal. Although the mechanism is unknown, calcium inhibits absorption of both heme and nonheme iron. Finally, because gastric acid improves iron absorption, patients who have undergone a gastrectomy or have achlorhydria have decreased iron absorption.[18]

Etiology

Iron deficiency results from prolonged negative iron balance, which can occur due to increased iron demand or hematopoiesis, increased loss, or decreased intake/absorption. The onset of iron deficiency depends on an individual's initial iron stores and the imbalance between iron absorption and loss. Multiple etiologic factors usually are involved. Certain groups at higher risk for iron deficiency include children younger than 2 years, adolescent girls, pregnant/lactating females, and those older than 65 years. Patients older than 65 years of age with IDA should be considered for testing for occult GI bleeding.[17] Blood loss must initially be considered a cause of IDA in adults. Blood loss may occur as a result of many disorders, including trauma, hemorrhoids, peptic ulcers, gastritis, GI malignancies, arteriovenous malformations, diverticular disease, copious menstrual flow, nosebleeds, and postpartum bleeding. In less industrialized nations, the risk of IDA is largely related to dietary factors.

The USPSTF recommends routine screening for IDA in all pregnant women.[19] The USPSTF has concluded that evidence is insufficient to recommend for or against routine iron supplementation for nonanemic pregnant women.[17] However, iron deficiency in pregnant women is so common that the Centers for Disease Control and Prevention (CDC) guidelines recommend initiation of low-dose iron supplements or prenatal vitamins with 30 mg/day of iron at each woman's first prenatal visit.

Medication history, specifically regarding recent or past use of iron, alcohol, corticosteroids, warfarin or other anticoagulants, aspirin, and nonsteroidal antiinflammatory drugs (NSAIDs), is a vital part of the history to assess bleeding risk. Other possible causes of hypochromic microcytic anemia include AI, thalassemia, sideroblastic anemia, and heavy metal (mostly lead) poisoning (Fig. 80-4).

Pathophysiology

Iron is vital to the function of all cells. Without iron, cells lose their capacity for electron transport and energy metabolism. Iron deficiency usually is the result of a long period of negative iron balance. Manifestations of iron deficiency occur in three stages. In the initial stage, iron stores are reduced without reduced serum iron levels and can be assessed with serum ferritin measurement. The stores allow iron to be utilized when there is an increased need for Hb synthesis. Once stores are depleted, there still is adequate iron from daily RBC turnover for Hb synthesis. Further iron losses would make the patient vulnerable to anemia development. In the second stage, iron deficiency occurs when iron stores are depleted, and Hb is above the lower limit of normal for the population but may be reduced for a given patient. This can be determined by serial CBC measurements. Findings include reduced transferrin saturation and increased TIBC. The third stage occurs when the Hb falls to less than normal values.

Laboratory Findings

❸ Abnormal laboratory findings for patients with IDA generally include low serum iron and ferritin levels and high TIBC. In the early stages of IDA, RBC size is not changed. Low ferritin concentration is the earliest and most sensitive indicator of iron deficiency. However, ferritin may not correlate with iron stores in the bone marrow because renal or hepatic disease, malignancies, infection, or inflammatory processes may increase ferritin values.[9] Hb, Hct, and RBC indices usually remain normal in early stages.

In the later stages of IDA, Hb and Hct fall below normal values, and a microcytic hypochromic anemia develops. Microcytosis may precede hypochromia, as erythropoiesis is programmed to maintain normal Hb concentration in preference to cell size. As a result, even slightly abnormal Hb and Hct levels may indicate significant depletion of iron stores and should not be ignored. In terms of RBC indices, MCV is reduced earlier in IDA than Hb concentration.

Transferrin saturation (i.e., serum iron level divided by the TIBC) is useful for assessing IDA. Low values may indicate IDA, although low serum transferrin saturation values also may be present in inflammatory disorders. The TIBC may help to differentiate the diagnosis in these patients: TIBC >400 mcg/dL (71.6 mol/L) suggests IDA, while values <200 mcg/dL (35.8 mol/L) usually represent inflammatory disease.

TREATMENT

Iron Deficiency Anemia

Desired Outcomes

The outcomes for all types of anemia in this chapter include: reversal of hematologic parameters to normal, return of normal function and quality of life, and prevention or reversal of long-term complications such as neurologic complications of vitamin B_{12} deficiency.

Dietary Supplementation and Oral Iron Preparations

The severity and cause of IDA determine the approach to treatment. Treatment is focused on replenishing iron stores. Because iron deficiency can be an early sign of other illnesses, treatment of the underlying disease may aid in the correction of iron deficiency.

Treatment of IDA usually consists of dietary supplementation and administration of oral iron preparations. Foods high in iron are listed in Table 80-1. Iron is best absorbed from meat, fish, and poultry. These foods as well as certain iron-fortified cereals can help treat IDA. Orange juice and other ascorbic acid-rich foods can be included with meals to increase absorption. Milk and tea reduce absorption and should be consumed in moderation. In most cases of IDA, oral administration of iron therapy with soluble Fe^{2+} iron salts is appropriate.

Fe^{2+} sulfate, succinate, lactate, fumarate, glutamate, and gluconate are absorbed similarly. The addition of copper, cobalt, molybdenum, or other minerals provides no advantage but increases cost of the product. Iron is best absorbed in the reduced Fe^{2+} form, with maximal absorption occurring in the duodenum, primarily due to the acidic medium of the stomach. Slow-release or sustained-release iron preparations do not undergo sufficient dissolution until they reach the small intestine. In the alkaline environment of the small intestine, iron tends to form insoluble complexes, which significantly reduces absorption. The dose of iron replacement therapy depends on the patient's ability to tolerate the administered iron. Tolerance of iron salts improves with a small initial dose and gradual escalation to the full dose. For patients with IDA, the generally recommended dose is about 150 to 200 mg of elemental iron daily,

TABLE 80-1 Good Sources of Iron

Food	Serving Size	Amount (mg)
Ready to eat cereal, 100% fortified	3/4 cup	18
Instant plain oatmeal, fortified	1 cup	11
Wheat germ	1 oz	2.6
Broccoli	1 medium stalk	2.1
Baked potato	1 medium	2.7
Raw tofu	½ cup	4
Lentils	½ cup	3.3
Beef chuck	3 oz	3.2

TABLE 80-2 Oral Iron Products

Iron Salt	Percent Elemental Iron	Common: Formulations and Elemental Iron Provided
Ferrous sulfate	20	60–65 mg/324–325 mg tablet 60 mg/5 mL syrup 44 mg/ 5 mL elixir 15 mg/1 mL
Ferrous sulfate (exsiccated)	30	65 mg/200 mg tablet 50 mg/160 mg tablet
Ferrous gluconate	12	38 mg/325 mg tablet 28–29 mg/240–246 mg tablet
Ferrous fumarate	33	66 mg/200 mg tablet 106 mg/324–325 mg tablet

TABLE 80-3 Iron Salt–Drug Interactions

Drugs That Decrease Iron Absorption	Object Drugs Affected by Iron
Al-, Mg-, and Ca^{+2}-containing antacids Tetracycline and doxycycline Histamine$_2$ antagonists Proton-pump inhibitors Cholestyramine	Levodopa ↓ (chelates with iron) Methyldopa ↓ (decreases efficacy of methyldopa) Levothyroxine ↓ (decreased efficacy of levothyroxine) Penicillamine ↓ (chelates with iron) Fluoroquinolones ↓ (forms ferric ion quinolone complex) Tetracycline and doxycycline ↓ (when administered within 2 hours of iron salt) Mycophenolate ↓ (decreases absorption)

usually in two or three divided doses to maximize tolerability. If patients cannot tolerate this daily dose of elemental iron, smaller amounts of elemental iron (e.g., single 325 mg tablet of Fe^{2+} sulfate) usually are sufficient to replace iron stores, although at a slower rate. Table 80-2 lists the percentage of elemental iron of commonly available iron salts. The percentage of iron absorbed decreases progressively as the dose increases, although the absolute amount absorbed increases. Iron preferably is administered at least 1 hour before meals because food can interfere with iron absorption. Many patients must take iron with food because they experience GI upset when iron is administered on an empty stomach.

Clinical **Controversy. . .**

Daily ferrous sulfate is not tolerated by all patients and can be difficult to administer in populations of developing countries. Weekly rather than daily supplements have been used, with conflicting efficacy results. The weekly approach follows the natural pattern of mucosal cell turnover.

Adverse reactions to therapeutic doses of iron are primarily GI in nature and consist of dark discoloration of feces, constipation or diarrhea, nausea, and vomiting. GI side effects usually are dose related and are similar among iron salts when equivalent amounts of elemental iron are administered. Administration of smaller amounts of iron with each dose or administration with meals may minimize these adverse effects. Histamine-2 blockers or proton-pump inhibitors reduce gastric acidity and may impair iron absorption. Table 80-3 lists drug interactions with iron.

Failure to respond to appropriate treatment regimens necessitates reevaluation of the patient's condition. A "therapeutic trial of iron" approach will occasionally be used to confirm a presumptive diagnosis of IDA. Common causes of treatment failure include poor patient adherence, inability to absorb iron, incorrect diagnosis, continued bleeding, or a concurrent condition that impairs full reticulocyte response. Even when iron deficiency is present, response may be impaired when a coexisting cause for anemia exists. Rarely a patient has diminished ability to absorb iron, most often due to previous gastrectomy, such as gastric bypass surgery, or celiac disease. Regardless of the form of oral therapy used, treatment should continue for 3 to 6 months after the anemia is resolved to allow for repletion of iron stores and to prevent relapse. Patients should be instructed to store oral iron out of reach of children and pets as small amounts can result in a fatal overdose. Products containing more than 30 mg of elemental iron are required to be packaged as individual dosage units to prevent toxicity. Treatment for acute iron poisoning is discussed in eChapter 10.

Parenteral Iron Therapy

Indications for parenteral iron therapy include intolerance to oral, malabsorption, and long-term nonadherence. Patients with significant blood loss who refuse transfusions and cannot take oral iron therapy also may require parenteral iron therapy. Parenteral iron therapy is also used for patients with chronic kidney disease (see Chap. 29), especially those undergoing hemodialysis, and for some cancer patients receiving chemotherapy on erythropoiesis-stimulating agents (ESAs; see Chap. 104). Four different parenteral iron preparations currently available in the United States are iron dextran, sodium ferric gluconate, iron sucrose, and ferumoxytol (Table 80-4). They differ in their molecular size, pharmacokinetics, bioavailability, and adverse effect profiles. Although toxicity profiles of these agents differ, clinical studies indicate that each is efficacious. Most of the recent research on IV iron has been performed in hemodialysis patients. Iron dextran parenteral preparations have been associated with more anaphylactic reactions. The safety profile of parenteral iron is largely assessed by spontaneous reports to the FDA and observational studies. All parenteral iron preparations carry a risk for anaphylactic reactions but likely to a lesser extent than iron dextran.[20,21] A concern with parenteral iron is that iron may be released too quickly and overload the ability of transferrin to bind it, leading to free iron reactions that can interfere with neutrophil function. In regards to general estimation of total dose of parenteral iron needed to correct anemia, the following formula can be used:

$$\text{Dose of iron (mg)} = \text{whole blood hemoglobin deficit (g/dL)} \times \text{body weight (lb)}$$

An additional quantity of iron to replenish stores should be added (about 600 mg for women and 1,000 mg for men).[9]

Iron dextran, a complex of Fe^{3+} hydroxide and the carbohydrate dextran, contains 50 mg of iron per milliliter and can be given via the intramuscular or IV route. Different brands of iron dextran are available and differ in their molecular weight. They are not interchangeable. Iron dextran must be processed by macrophages for the iron to be biologically available. The absorption and metabolism vary with the route and amount of drug given. The intramuscular route is no longer used routinely.[22] The intramuscular administration of iron dextran requires the Z-tract injection technique to minimize staining of the skin and pain. This technique is used for delivering intramuscular injections of irritating substances to minimize tracking of the medication through surrounding tissues. If intramuscular doses are given, they should not exceed 25 mg for patients weighing less than 5 kg, 50 mg for patients weighing less than 10 kg, and 100 mg for all other patients. Problems with intramuscular administration include patient discomfort, unpredictable delivery, sterile abscesses, tissue necrosis, and atrophy.[23]

TABLE 80-4 Comparison of Parenteral Iron Products

Drug	Brand Name/ Molecular Weight	Amount of Elemental Iron	Usual Adult Dose	Indication	IM Injection	Common Adverse Effects
Ferumoxytol	Feraheme: 750,000 Da	30 mg/mL	Initial 510 mg IV followed by 510 mg IV 3–8 days later (rate 30 mg/s)	Treatment of IDA for adults with chronic kidney disease	No	Hypersensitivity reactions, diarrhea, constipation, nausea, dizziness, hypotension, and peripheral edema
Iron dextran	InFeD: 165,000 Da Dexferrum: 265,000 Da	50 mg/mL	See Table 80-5; Daily dosages should be limited to 100 mg iron (rate not to exceed 50 mg/min) Must administer 0.5 mL test dose and observe 1 hour	Treatment of iron deficiency when oral therapy is infeasible or ineffective	Yes—Z track method	Black box warning: anaphylactic reactions Pain and brown staining at injection site, flushing, hypotension, fever, chills, myalgia, anaphylaxis
Iron sucrose	Venofer: 34,000–60,000 Da	20 mg/mL	Hemodialysis: 100 mg during consecutive dialysis session to 1,000 mg (10 doses) Nondialysis: 200 mg on five different occasions within 14 days (total dose 1000 mg) See the package insert for specific rates Monitor during and at least 30 minutes postdose for anaphylactic reactions	Treatment of IDA for patients with chronic kidney, nondialysis and dialysis dependent	No	Anaphylactic reactions, hypotension, hypertension, nausea, muscle cramps, headaches, upper respiratory infection, edema, dizziness
Sodium ferric gluconate	Ferrlecit: 289,000–444,000 Da	12.5 mg/mL	125 mg elemental iron per dialysis session Most require cumulative dose of 1 g over the eight dialysis session for a favorable response Monitor during and at least 30 minutes postdose for anaphylactic reactions	Treatment of IDA in patients undergoing hemodialysis in conjunction with erythropoietin therapy	No	Hypersensitivity reactions (including anaphylactic reactions), hypotension, hypertension, headache, dizziness, nausea, vomiting, diarrhea, injection site reactions, muscle cramps, dyspnea, chest pain

The iron dextran package insert carries a black-box warning regarding the risk of anaphylaxis. A test dose is required prior to administration of any dose. Fatal reactions have also occurred in patients who tolerated the test dose. The European Medicines Agency is currently considering recommendations to not require a test dose for any parenteral iron preparation. This is based on data that has shown test doses were not necessarily predictive of those that would have anaphylactic reactions. The United States labeling still recommends this with iron dextran at this time. Patients with a history of multiple drug allergies and those who are concomitantly taking angiotensin-converting enzyme inhibitors may be at higher risk. The anaphylactic reactions may be more common with the high molecular weight iron dextrin product.[24] Patients should also be monitored throughout the complete administration of iron dextran and resuscitative equipment should be readily available. Methods of IV administration include multiple slow injections of undiluted iron dextran solution or an infusion of a diluted preparation. This latter method often is referred to as total dose infusion.

Equations for calculating the appropriate doses of parenteral iron dextran for patients with IDA or anemia secondary to blood loss are listed in Table 80-5. Doses given by IV administration should not exceed 50 mg of iron per minute (1 mL/min). It is suggested that all patients considered for an iron dextran injection receive a test dose of 25 mg intramuscularly or IV or a 5- to 10-minute infusion of the diluted solution. Patients should then be observed for more than 1 hour for untoward reactions. An anaphylaxis-like reaction generally responds to IV epinephrine, diphenhydramine, and corticosteroids. If the test dose is tolerated, patients receiving total dose infusions can receive infusion of the remaining solution during the next 2 to 6 hours.[23]

Total replacement doses of IV iron dextran have been given as a single dose. A test dose still is required. The ability to give a total dose infusion is a benefit of iron dextran over the other parenteral iron products.[17] This is not an FDA approved way of administering iron dextran. Iron dextran is best utilized when smaller frequent doses of sodium ferric gluconate or iron sucrose are impractical. Patients who receive total dose infusions are at higher risk for adverse reactions, such as arthralgias, myalgias, flushing, malaise, and fever. Other adverse reactions of iron dextran include staining of the skin, pain at the injection site, allergic reactions, and rarely anaphylaxis. Patients with preexisting immune-mediated diseases, such as active rheumatoid arthritis or systemic lupus erythematosus, are considered at high risk for adverse reactions because of their hyperreactive immune response.

TABLE 80-5 Equations for Calculating Doses of Parenteral Iron Dextran

For patients with iron deficiency anemia:

Adults + children >15 kg

Dose (mL) = 0.0442 (Desired Hb − Observed Hb) × LBW + (0.26 × LBW)

LBW males = 50 kg + 2.3 × (inches over 5 ft)

LBW females = 45.5 kg + 2.3 × (inches over 5 ft)

Children 5–15 kg

Dose (mL) = 0.0442 (Desired Hb − Observed Hb) × W + (0.26 × W)

For patients with anemia secondary to blood loss (hemorrhagic diathesis or long-term dialysis):

mg of iron = blood loss × hematocrit,
where blood loss is in milliliters and hematocrit
is expressed as a decimal fraction

Hb, hemoglobin; LBW, lean body weight; mL, milliliter; W, weight in kg.

Sodium ferric gluconate is a complex of iron bound to one gluconate and four sucrose molecules in a repeating pattern. Its molecular weight is 289 to 440 kDa. Sodium ferric gluconate is available in an aqueous solution. No direct transfer of iron from the Fe^{3+} gluconate to transferrin occurs. The complex is taken up quickly by the mononuclear phagocytic system and has a half-life of about 1 hour in the bloodstream. Sodium ferric gluconate appears to produce fewer anaphylactic reactions than iron dextran does. Side effects of sodium ferric gluconate include cramps, nausea, vomiting, flushing, hypotension, intense upper gastric pain, rash, and pruritus.[25]

Iron sucrose is a polynuclear iron(III) hydroxide in sucrose complex with a molecular weight of 34 to 60 kDa. It is available in 5 mL single-dose vials. Each vial contains 100 mg (20 mg/mL) of iron sucrose. Following IV administration of iron sucrose, the iron is released directly from the circulating iron sucrose to transferrin and is taken up by the mononuclear phagocytic system and metabolized. The half-life is about 6 hours, with a volume of distribution similar to that of iron dextran. Iron sucrose injection should not be administered concomitantly with oral iron preparations because it will reduce the absorption of oral iron.[26] Adverse effects include leg cramps and hypotension.

Ferumoxytol is the newest FDA-approved parenteral product to treat iron deficiency in adults with chronic kidney disease who are on or off dialysis. Ferumoxytol can be administered at a quicker rate than other parenteral iron products with a rate up to 30 mg/s. Typical dosing is 510 mg IV dose followed by a second 510 mg dose 3 to 8 days later. The dose can be readministered after 1 month if anemia persists. No test dose is required but anaphylaxis can occur and patients should be observed for at least 30 minutes after each dose. Compared with oral iron replacement therapy, ferumoxytol has a higher incidence of hypotension and dizziness but less diarrhea, nausea, constipation, and peripheral edema. Clinical experience with this new preparation is still accumulating as it is still relatively new to the market.[27]

MEGALOBLASTIC ANEMIAS

Macrocytic anemias are divided into megaloblastic and nonmegaloblastic anemias. Macrocytosis, as seen in megaloblastic anemias, is caused by abnormal DNA metabolism resulting from vitamin B_{12} or folate deficiency. It also can be caused by administration of various drugs, such as hydroxyurea, zidovudine, cytarabine, methotrexate, azathioprine, 6-mercaptopurine, and cladribine. In vitamin B_{12}- or folate-deficiency anemia, megaloblastosis results from interference with folic acid- and vitamin B_{12}-interdependent nucleic acid synthesis in the immature erythrocyte. The rate of RNA and cytoplasm production exceeds the rate of DNA production. The maturation process is retarded, resulting in immature large RBCs (macrocytosis). RNA and DNA synthesis depend on a series of reactions catalyzed by vitamin B_{12} and folic acid because of their role in the conversion of uridine to thymidine. As shown in Figure 80-6, dietary folates are absorbed in this process and converted to 5-methyl-tetrahydrofolate (A), which then is converted via a B_{12}-dependent reaction (B) to tetrahydrofolate (C). After gaining a carbon, tetrahydrofolate is converted to 5,10-methyl-tetrahydrofolate (D), a folate cofactor used by thymidylate synthetase (E) in the biosynthesis of nucleic acids. The 5,10-methyl-tetrahydrofolate cofactor is converted to dihydrofolate (F) during biosynthesis. Dihydrofolate reductase normally reduces dihydrofolate back to tetrahydrofolate (C), which can again pick up a carbon and be recycled to produce more 5,10-methyl-tetrahydrofolate (D).

Although vitamin B_{12} and folate deficiency are common causes of macrocytosis, other possible causes must be considered if these deficiencies are not found. Other causes of macrocytosis include

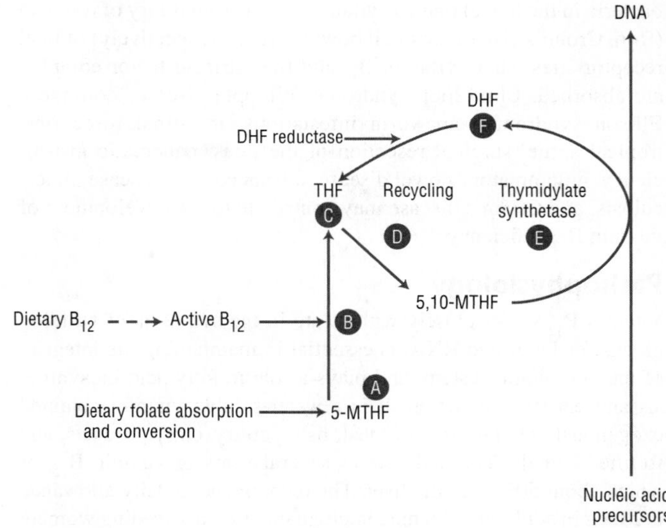

FIGURE 80-6 Drug-induced megaloblastosis (DHF, dihydrofolate; 5-MTHF, 5-methyl-tetrahydrofolate; 5,10-MTHF, 5,10-methyl-tetrahydrofolate; THF, tetrahydrofolate).

(1) a shift to immature or stressed RBCs as seen in reticulocytosis, aplastic anemia, and pure RBC aplasia; (2) a primary bone marrow disorder such as myelodysplastic syndromes, congenital dyserythropoietic anemias, and large granular lymphocyte leukemia; (3) lipid abnormalities as seen with liver disease, hypothyroidism, or hyperlipidemia; and (4) unknown mechanisms resulting from alcohol abuse and multiple myeloma. Macrocytosis is the most typical morphologic abnormality associated with excessive alcohol consumption. Even with adequate folate and vitamin B_{12} levels and the absence of liver disease, patients with high alcohol intake may present with an alcohol-induced macrocytosis. Cessation of alcohol ingestion results in resolution of the macrocytosis within a couple of months.

Vitamin B_{12} Deficiency Anemia

The prevalence of vitamin B_{12} deficiency anemia in the United States is unknown. Risk increases with age.[28] Increased use of gastric acid-suppressing agents, which may inhibit cobalamin release from food, is associated with an increased risk. Older adults in the United States have a high prevalence (up to 15%) of elevated MMA levels and associated low or low-normal vitamin B_{12} levels, likely due to atrophic gastritis and malabsorption of food-bound vitamin B_{12}.[27]

Etiology

4 The three major causes of vitamin B_{12} deficiency are inadequate intake, malabsorption syndromes, and inadequate utilization. Inadequate dietary consumption of vitamin B_{12} is rare. It usually occurs only in patients who are strict vegans and their breast-fed infants, chronic alcoholics, and elderly patients who consume a "tea and toast" diet because of financial limitations or poor dentition. Decreased vitamin B_{12} absorption can occur with loss of intrinsic factor by autoimmune mechanisms (such as pernicious anemia, in which gastric parietal cells are selectively damaged), chronic atrophic gastritis, or stomach surgery. One of the most frequent causes of low serum B_{12} levels is maldigestion, which results from the inability of vitamin B_{12} to be cleaved and released from proteins in food because of inadequate gastric acid production. Treatment of *Helicobacter pylori* may improve vitamin B_{12} status because this bacterial infection is a cause of chronic gastritis.[29] Vitamin B_{12} deficiency may occasionally result from overgrowth of

bacteria in the bowel that use vitamin B_{12} or from injury or removal (from Crohn's disease or small bowel surgery, respectively) of ileal receptor sites where vitamin B_{12} and the intrinsic factor complex are absorbed. Blind loop syndrome, Whipple disease, Zollinger–Ellison syndrome, tapeworm infestations, intestinal resections, tropical sprue, surgical resection of the ileus, pancreatic insufficiency, inflammatory bowel disease, advanced liver disease, tuberculosis, and Crohn's disease may contribute to the development of vitamin B_{12} deficiency.[28]

Pathophysiology

Vitamin B_{12} works closely with folate in the synthesis of building blocks for DNA and RNA, is essential in maintaining the integrity of the neurologic system, and plays a role in fatty acid biosynthesis and energy production. It is a water-soluble vitamin obtained exogenously by ingestion of meat, fish, poultry, dairy products, and fortified cereals. The body stores several years of vitamin B_{12}, of which about 50% is in the liver. The recommended daily allowance is 2 mcg in adults and 2.6 mcg in pregnant or breast-feeding women. The average western diet provides 5 to 15 mcg of vitamin B_{12} daily, of which 1 to 5 mcg is absorbed.[28] Vitamin B_{12} deficiency usually takes several years to develop following vitamin deprivation.

Once dietary cobalamin enters the stomach, pepsin and hydrochloric acid release the cobalamin from animal proteins. The free cobalamin then binds to R-protein, which is released from parietal and salivary cells. In the duodenum, the cobalamin–R-protein complex is degraded, releasing free cobalamin. The cobalamin then binds with intrinsic factor that serves as a cell-directed carrier protein similar to transferrin for iron. This complex attaches to mucosal cell receptors in the distal ileum, the intrinsic factor is discarded, and the cobalamin is bound to transport proteins (transcobalamin I, II, and III). The cobalamin bound to transcobalamin II is secreted into the circulation and is taken up by the liver, bone marrow, and other cells. Most circulating cobalamin is bound to transcobalamin I and transcobalamin III. Passive diffusion is an alternate pathway for vitamin B_{12} absorption independent of intrinsic factor or an intact terminal ileum and accounts for about 1% of vitamin B_{12} absorption.[28]

Vitamin B_{12} deficiency can cause neurologic and hematologic complications. These usually start with bilateral paraesthesia in extremities; deficits in proprioception and vibration can also be present. If not treated, this can progress to ataxia, dementia-like symptoms, psychosis, and vision loss. In children prolonged deficiency can lead to poor brain development.[13,30] Patients with unexplained neuropathies should be evaluated for vitamin B_{12} deficiency.

Laboratory Findings

In macrocytic anemias, MCV is elevated >100 fL, but some patients deficient in vitamin B_{12} may have a normal MCV. If there is a coexisting cause of microcytosis, the MCV may not be elevated.[30] Mild leukopenia and thrombocytopenia are often present because abnormal DNA synthesis can affect all blood cell lines. A peripheral blood smear demonstrates macrocytosis accompanied by hypersegmented polymorphonuclear leukocytes (one of the earliest and most specific indications of this disease), oval macrocytes, anisocytosis, and poikilocytosis. Serum lactate dehydrogenase and indirect bilirubin levels may be elevated as a result of hemolysis or ineffective erythropoiesis.[13] Other laboratory findings include a low reticulocyte count, low serum vitamin B_{12} level (<150 pg/mL [<111 pmol/L]), and low Hct.

In the early stages of vitamin B_{12} deficiency, classic signs and symptoms of megaloblastic anemia may not be evident, and serum levels of vitamin B_{12} may be within normal limits. Therefore, measurement of MMA and homocysteine may be useful because these parameters are typically the first to change. Because MMA and homocysteine are involved in enzymatic reactions that depend on vitamin B_{12}, a deficiency in vitamin B_{12} leads to accumulation of these metabolites. Elevations in MMA are more specific for vitamin B_{12} deficiency. Homocysteine is also elevated in several other situations including: folate deficiency, chronic renal disease, alcoholism, smoking, use of steroid or cyclosporine therapy, and smoking.[30] Low levels of vitamin B_{12} result in hyperhomocysteinemia, which some studies have reported to be an independent risk factor for cerebrovascular, peripheral vascular, coronary, and venous thromboembolic disease.[31]

Blood levels of vitamin B_{12} should be drawn for all patients with suspected vitamin B_{12} deficiency. Vitamin B_{12} values <150 to 200 pg/mL (<111 to 148 pmol/L) are suggestive of B_{12} deficiency. Some patients with clinical B_{12} deficiency manifesting as neurological disease may have normal hematological parameters. Subclinical vitamin B_{12} deficiency is sometimes referred to with vitamin B_{12} levels 200 to 300 pg/mL (148 to 221 pmol/L).[32] A general multivitamin does not typically contain enough vitamin B_{12} to normalize levels in deficient persons. Whether to treat patients in this range is not clear in the absence of neurologic symptoms.

A Schilling test may theoretically be performed to diagnose pernicious anemia, but the usefulness of this test is questionable and rarely alters the clinical management of the vitamin B_{12} deficiency. The Schilling test was once performed to determine whether replacement of vitamin B_{12} should occur via an oral or parenteral route, but evidence now shows that oral replacement is as efficacious as parenteral supplementation because of the vitamin B_{12} absorption pathway independent of intrinsic factor.[28,33]

TREATMENT

Vitamin B_{12} Deficiency Anemia

The goals of treatment for vitamin B_{12} deficiency include reversal of hematologic manifestations, replacement of body stores, and prevention or resolution of neurologic manifestations. Early treatment is of paramount importance because neurologic damage may be irreversible if the deficiency is not detected and corrected within months. In addition to replacement therapy, any underlying etiology that is treatable, such as bacterial overgrowth, should be remedied. Indications for starting oral or parenteral therapy include megaloblastic anemia or other hematologic abnormalities and neurologic disease from deficiency.[30] Those with borderline low levels of B_{12} but no hematologic abnormalities should be followed at yearly intervals.[30] Patients should be counseled on the types of foods high in vitamin B_{12} content such as fortified cereals as seen in Table 80-6. Orally administered vitamin B_{12} can be used effectively to treat pernicious anemia because of the aforementioned alternate pathway of passive absorption, independent of intrinsic factor.[14] Daily oral doses (1,000 to 2,000 mcg) of vitamin B_{12} is as effective as intramuscular administration in achieving hematologic and neurologic responses.[28,33] If vitamin B_{12} levels are marginally low and either MMA or both MMA and homocysteine levels are elevated, administration of 1,000 mcg of oral vitamin B_{12} daily should be strongly considered.[34] Timed-release preparations of oral cobalamin should be avoided.[35] Nonprescription 1,000 mcg cobalamin tablets are available, among several other strengths. A commonly used initial parenteral vitamin B_{12} regimen consists of daily injections of 1,000 mcg of cyanocobalamin for 1 week to saturate vitamin B_{12} stores in the body and resolve clinical manifestations of the deficiency. Thereafter, it can be given weekly for 1 month and monthly thereafter for maintenance. The series of daily parenteral injections may be omitted if administration is difficult or inconvenient. In this case the parenteral injection is then given weekly, sometimes for a longer than 1 month. Parenteral therapy is preferred for patients exhibiting neurologic symptoms until resolution of symptoms and

TABLE 80-6 Good Sources of Vitamin B_{12}

Food	Serving Size	Amount (mcg)
Beef liver, cooked	3 oz	70
Breakfast cereal, fortified (100%)	¾ cup	6
Rainbow trout, cooked	3 oz	3.5
Sockeye salmon, cooked	3 oz	4.9
Beef, cooked	3 oz	2.1
Breakfast cereal, fortified (25%)	¾ cup	1.5
Clams, cooked	3 oz	84.1
Oysters, breaded and fried	6 pieces	1
Tuna, canned in water	3 oz	2.5
Milk	1 cup	1.2
Yogurt	8 oz	1.1

normalization of hematologic indices because the most rapid-acting therapy is necessary.[36] When patients are converted from the parenteral to the oral form of cobalamin, 1,000 mcg of oral cobalamin daily can be initiated on the due date of the next injection. Vitamin B_{12} should be continued for life in pernicious anemia.

In addition to the oral and parenteral forms, vitamin B_{12} is available as a nasal spray for patients in remission following intramuscular vitamin B_{12} therapy who have no nervous system involvement. The nasal spray is administered once weekly. Intranasal administration should be avoided for patients with nasal diseases or those receiving medications intranasally in the same nostril. Patients should not administer the spray 1 hour before or after ingestion of hot foods or beverages, which can impair cobalamin absorption. The efficacy of the nasal spray formulation has not been well studied, and it should be used for maintenance therapy only after hematologic parameters have normalized.

Potential adverse effects with vitamin B_{12} replacement therapy are rare. Uncommon side effects include hyperuricemia and hypokalemia due to marked increase in potassium utilization during production of new hematopoietic cells.

Folic Acid Deficiency Anemia

Epidemiology

Folic acid deficiency is one of the most common vitamin deficiencies occurring in the United States, largely because of its association with excessive alcohol intake and pregnancy.

Etiology

5 Major causes of folic acid deficiency include inadequate intake, decreased absorption, and increased folate requirements. Poor eating habits make this deficiency more common for elderly patients, teenagers whose diets consist of "junk food," alcoholics, food faddists, the impoverished, and those who are chronically ill or demented. Folic acid absorption may decrease for patients who have malabsorption syndromes or those who have received certain drugs. In alcoholics with poor dietary habits, alcohol interferes with folic acid absorption, interferes with folic acid utilization at the cellular level, and decreases hepatic stores of folic acid.

Increased folate requirements may occur when the rate of cellular division is increased, as seen in pregnant women; patients with hemolytic anemia, myelofibrosis, malignancy, chronic inflammatory disorders such as Crohn's disease, rheumatoid arthritis, or psoriasis; patients undergoing long-term dialysis; burn patients; and for adolescents and infants during their growth spurts. This hyperutilization eventually can lead to anemia, particularly when the daily intake of folate is borderline, resulting in inadequate replacement of folate stores.

Several drugs have been reported to cause a folic acid deficiency megaloblastic anemia. Some drugs (e.g., azathioprine, 6-mercaptopurine, 5-fluorouracil, hydroxyurea, and zidovudine) directly inhibit DNA synthesis. Other drugs are folate antagonists; the most toxic is methotrexate (other examples include pentamidine, trimethoprim, and triamterene). A number of drugs (e.g., phenytoin, phenobarbital, and primidone) antagonize folate via poorly understood mechanisms but are thought to reduce vitamin absorption by the intestine (see eChap. 23). Since folic acid doses as low as 1 mg/day may affect serum phenytoin levels, routine folic acid supplementation is not generally recommended. The decline in phenytoin concentration usually occurs within the first 10 days and may decrease phenytoin levels by 15% to 50%.[37]

Pathophysiology

Folic acid is a water-soluble vitamin readily destroyed by cooking or processing. It is necessary for the production of DNA and RNA. It acts as a methyl donor to form methylcobalamin, which is used in the remethylation of homocysteine to methionine. Because humans are unable to synthesize sufficient folate to meet total daily requirements, they depend on dietary sources. Major dietary sources of folate include fresh, green leafy vegetables, citrus fruits, yeast, mushrooms, dairy products, and animal organs such as liver and kidney. Most folate in food is present in the polyglutamate form, which must be broken down into the monoglutamate form prior to absorption in the small intestine. Once absorbed, dietary folate must be converted to the active form tetrahydrofolate through a cobalamin-dependent reaction. In 1997, the United States mandated that grain products be fortified with folic acid in an attempt to increase the dietary intake of folate by 100 mcg of folate daily per person. This amount of supplementation was chosen to decrease the incidence of neural tube defects without masking occult vitamin B_{12} deficiency.

As a result of grain product fortification, neural tube defect frequency has decreased by 25% to 30%.[38] Although body demands for folate are high because of high rates of RBC synthesis and turnover, the minimum daily requirement is 50 to 100 mcg. In the general population, the recommended daily allowance for folate is 400 mcg in nonpregnant females, 600 mcg for pregnant females, and 500 mcg for lactating females.[38] Because the body stores about 5 to 10 mg of folate, primarily in the liver, cessation of dietary folate intake can result in deficiency within 3 to 4 months.

Laboratory Findings

It is of paramount importance to rule out vitamin B_{12} deficiency when folate deficiency is suspected. Laboratory changes associated with folate deficiency are similar to those seen in vitamin B_{12} deficiency, except vitamin B_{12} and MMA levels are normal. Serum folate levels decrease to less than 3 ng/mL (7 nmol/L) within a few days of reduced dietary folate intake. The RBC folate level (<150 ng/mL [<340 nmol/L]) also declines, and levels remain constant throughout the life span of the erythrocyte.[12] If serum or erythrocyte folate levels are borderline, serum homocysteine usually is increased with a folic acid deficiency. If serum MMA levels also are elevated, vitamin B_{12} deficiency must be ruled out given that folate does not participate in MMA metabolism.

TREATMENT

Folic Acid Deficiency Anemia

Therapy for folic acid deficiency consists of administration of exogenous folic acid to induce hematologic remission, replace body stores, and resolve signs and symptoms. In most cases, 1 mg daily is sufficient to replace stores, except in cases of deficiency due to malabsorption, in which case doses of 1 to 5 mg daily may

TABLE 80-7 Good Sources of Folate

Food	Serving	Amount (mcg)
Beef liver	3 oz	215
Cereal, 25% fortified	½ to 1½ cups	100–400
Lentils, cooked	½ cup	180
Chickpeas	½ cup	141
Asparagus	½ cup	132
Spinach, cooked	½ cup	131
Pasta, enriched	½ cup	83
Kidney beans	½ cup	46
White rice, cooked	½ cup	90
Tomato juice	1 cup	48
Brussels sprouts	½ cup	78
Orange	1 medium	47

be necessary. Parenteral folic acid is available but rarely necessary. Synthetic folic acid is almost completely absorbed by the GI tract and is converted to tetrahydrofolate without cobalamin. Therapy should continue for about 4 months if the underlying cause of the deficiency can be identified and corrected to allow for clearance of all folate-deficient RBCs from the circulation. Foods high in folic acid should also be encouraged in the diet as seen in Table 80-7. Long-term folate administration may be necessary in chronic conditions associated with increased folate requirements. Low-dose folate therapy (500 mcg daily) can be administered when anticonvulsant drugs produce a megaloblastic anemia so that discontinuation of anticonvulsant therapy may not be necessary. Adverse effects have not been reported with folic acid doses used for replacement therapy. It is considered nontoxic at high doses and is rapidly excreted in the urine.

Although megaloblastic anemia during pregnancy is rare, the most common cause is folate deficiency. The condition usually manifests as an underweight premature infant and suboptimal health of the mother. Periconceptional folic acid supplementation is recommended to decrease the occurrence and recurrence of neural tube defects, specifically anencephaly and spinal bifida. Folic acid supplementation at a dose of 400 mcg daily is recommended for all women. Women who have previously given birth to offspring with neural tube defects or those with a family history of neural tube defects should ingest 4 mg daily of folic acid.[37–39] Higher levels of folic acid supplementation should not be attained via ingestion of excess multivitamins because of the risk for fat soluble vitamin toxicity.[39] Prenatal vitamins usually have a higher amount of folic acid as compared with general multivitamins to ensure adequate supplementation is attained. It is essential that women in their childbearing years maintain adequate folic acid intake.

ANEMIA OF INFLAMMATION

Epidemiology

6 AI is a newer term used to describe both ACD and anemia of critical illness. This new term was developed to reflect the inflammatory process that underlies both of those types of anemia. The onset of anemia of critical illness is quicker, over days, and typically occurs in a hospital setting. ACD has a similar mechanism, but it develops over months to years from a chronic condition. AI is one of the most common forms of anemia seen clinically, particularly among the elderly. It is especially important in the differential diagnosis of iron deficiency. ACD is associated with common disease states that may mimic the symptoms of anemia, which causes the diagnosis of ACD to sometimes be overlooked in the outpatient setting. Anemia of critical illness is a common complication in critically ill patients and is found almost universally in this patient population.[40] About 95% of patients have less than normal Hb levels by their third day in the intensive care unit.[41]

Etiology

The diagnosis of AI usually is one of exclusion. It is important to exclude IDA as the true or competing etiology. Various conditions associated with ACD may predispose patients to blood loss (malignancy, GI blood loss from treatments with aspirin, NSAIDs, or corticosteroids). ACD is often observed in patients with diseases that last longer than 1 to 2 months, although it can occur in conditions with a more rapid onset of several weeks, such as pneumonia. ACD tends to be a mild (Hb >9.5 g/dL [>95 g/L; >5.90 mmol/L]) or moderate (Hb >8 g/dL [80 g/L; >4.97 mmol/L]) anemia.[42] Anemia associated with human immunodeficiency virus (HIV), autoimmune conditions, cancer, and heart failure are common forms of ACD. The degree of anemia in ACD is generally reflects the severity of underlying disease. Table 80-8 lists common diseases associated with ACD.

Factors that may contribute to anemia in critically ill patients include sepsis, frequent blood sampling, surgical blood loss, immune-mediated functional iron deficiency, decreased production of endogenous EPO, reduced RBC life span, and active bleeding, especially in the GI tract. More commonly, a combination of these factors exists. This combination creates an anemic state over days. Additional comorbid factors include coagulopathies and nutritional deficits such as poor oral intake and altered absorption of vitamins and minerals, including iron, vitamin B_{12}, and folate.[43] Deleterious effects of anemia include an increased risk of cardiac-related morbidity and mortality, especially for patients with known cardiovascular disease. Persistent tissue hypoxia can result in cerebral ischemia, myocardial ischemia, multiple organ deterioration, lactic acidosis, and death. Consequences of anemia in critically ill patients may be enhanced because of the increased metabolic demands of critical illness. Weaning anemic patients from mechanical ventilation may be more difficult.[44]

TABLE 80-8 Diseases Causing Anemia of Inflammation

Common causes

Chronic infections
- Tuberculosis
- Other chronic lung infections (e.g., lung abscess, bronchiectasis)
- Human immunodeficiency virus
- Subacute bacterial endocarditis
- Osteomyelitis
- Chronic urinary tract infections

Chronic inflammation
- Rheumatoid arthritis
- Systemic lupus erythematosus
- Inflammatory bowel disease
- Inflammatory osteoarthritis
- Gout
- Other (collagen vascular) diseases
- Chronic inflammatory liver diseases

Malignancies
- Carcinoma
- Lymphoma
- Leukemia
- Multiple myeloma

Less common causes

Alcoholic liver disease
Congestive heart failure
Thrombophlebitis
Chronic obstructive pulmonary disease
Ischemic heart disease

Pathophysiology

AI is a response to stimulation of the cellular immune system by various underlying disease processes. AI is a hypoproliferative anemia that traditionally has been associated with infectious or inflammatory processes, tissue injury, and conditions associated with release of proinflammatory cytokines. The pathogenesis of AI is multifactorial and is characterized by a blunted EPO response to anemia, an impaired proliferation of erythroid progenitor cells, and a disturbance of iron homeostasis. Increased iron uptake and retention occur within cells. The RBCs have a shortened life span, and the bone marrow's capacity to respond to EPO is inadequate to maintain normal Hb concentration. The cause of this defect is uncertain but appears to involve blocked release of iron from cells in the bone marrow. Iron availability to erythroid progenitor cells then is limited. Various cytokines, such as interleukin-1, interferon-γ, interlukin-6, and tumor necrosis factor released during illness may inhibit the production or action of EPO or the production of RBCs.[42] These cytokines also upregulate hepcidin, which blocks iron release from storage cells.[45] Hepicidin also decreases duodenal absorption of iron.[42]

Laboratory Findings

No definitive test can confirm the diagnosis of AI. The practitioner should maintain a high index of suspicion for any patient with a chronic inflammatory or neoplastic disease. AI may coexist with IDA and folic acid deficiency because many patients with these conditions have poor dietary intake or GI blood loss. Examination of the bone marrow reveals an abundance of iron, suggesting that the release mechanism for iron is the central defect. Patients with AI usually have a decreased serum iron level, but unlike patients with IDA, their serum ferritin level is normal or increased and their TIBC is decreased. Transferrin saturation is typically decreased. AI usually is normocytic and normochromic with mildly depressed Hb. Patients with concurrent AI and IDA usually have microcytes and a more severe anemia. Table 80-9 shows lab values seen in AI and IDA. Erythrocyte survival may be reduced for patients with AI, but a compensatory erythropoietic response does not occur. A low reticulocyte count indicates underproduction of RBCs.[42]

TREATMENT

Anemia of Inflammation

Treatment of AI depends somewhat on the underlying etiology. Guidelines exist for management of anemia for patients with cancer or chronic kidney disease (see Chaps. 29 and 104). Although the goals of therapy should include treating the underlying disorder and correcting reversible causes of anemia, accomplishment of these goals may not totally reverse hematologic and physiologic abnormalities. Iron is effective only if iron deficiency is present. During inflammation, oral or parenteral iron therapy is not as effective. Absorption is impaired because of downregulation of ferroportin and iron diversion mediated by cytokines.[42] Because iron is a required nutrient for proliferating microorganisms, supplementation may theoretically increase the risk of infections. Iron therapy should be reserved for those patients with an established iron deficiency.[42]

TABLE 80-9 Laboratory Value Differences Between Anemia of Inflammation and Iron-Deficiency Anemia

	Anemia of Inflammation	Iron-Deficiency Anemia
Iron	↓	↓
Transferrin	↓ or nl	↑
Transferrin saturation	↓	↓
Ferritin	↑ or nl	↓
Soluble transferrin receptor	nl	↑

nl, normal limits.

Clinical **Controversy...**

The low iron concentrations in critically ill patients may be a defense mechanism, as microbes require iron for sustenance. Therefore, diminished iron levels may inhibit bacterial growth. Further investigation of the net benefit of supplementation with iron is warranted.

RBC transfusions are effective but should be limited to situations in which oxygen transport is inadequate due to concomitant medical problems. Transfusions are typically considered for those with severe anemia (Hb <7 to 8 g/dL [<80 g/L; <4.97 mmol/L]) but can be considered for those between 8 and 10 g/dL (80 to 100 g/L; 4.97 to 6.21 g/L) based on factors such as cost, convenience, and risk of complications. Transfusion risks may include transmission of bloodborne infections, development of autoantibodies, transfusion reactions, and iron overload.

ESAs have been used to stimulate erythropoiesis for patients with AI since a relative EPO deficiency exists for the degree of anemia. Two agents are available: recombinant epoetin alfa and recombinant darbepoetin alfa. Although both agents share the same mechanism of action, darbepoetin alfa has a longer half-life and can be administered less frequently. Although these agents are sometimes used to treat AI, they are not FDA-approved for this indication. Patients with chronic disease may have a relatively impaired response to ESAs. The initial dosage of epoetin alfa and darbepoetin alfa are typically 50 to 100 units per kilogram three times per week and 0.45 mcg per kilogram once weekly, respectively. These doses are typical starting doses for those with chronic kidney disease. Response to ESAs varies depending on dose and cause of the anemia. ESA treatment is effective when the marrow has an adequate supply of iron, cobalamin, and folic acid.

Iron deficiency can occur in patients treated with ESAs; so close monitoring of iron levels is necessary. Some patients develop "functional" iron deficiency, in which the iron stores are normal but the supply of iron to the erythroid marrow is less than necessary to support the demand for RBC production. Therefore, many practitioners routinely supplement ESA therapy with oral iron therapy. Potential toxicities of exogenous ESA administration include increases in blood pressure, nausea, headache, fever, bone pain, and fatigue. Less common adverse effects include seizures, thrombotic events, and allergic reactions such as rashes and local reactions at the injection site. If ESAs are used the practitioner must monitor to ensure the patient's Hb does not exceed 12 g/dL (120 g/L; 7.45 mmol/L) with treatment or that Hb does not rise >1 g/dL (>10 g/L; >0.62 mmol/L) every 2 weeks since both of these events have been associated with increased mortality and cardiovascular events.[46] Tumor progression with these agents can also occur and is discussed in Chapter 104. Further discussion of dosing guidelines and potential adverse outcomes of ESA treatment in populations for which treatment is FDA approved are discussed in Chapters 29 and 104.

Patients who are critically ill require the necessary substrates of iron, folic acid, and vitamin B_{12} for RBC production. Parenteral iron is generally preferred in this population because patients often are undergoing enteral therapy or because of concerns regarding inadequate iron absorption. The disadvantage of parenteral therapy is the theoretical risk of infection.

Pharmacologic doses of ESAs have been used to treat the anemia of critical illness. Few randomized controlled trials have evaluated the role of ESAs in critically ill patients, and the results of these trials have not consistently shown a decrease in transfusion requirements in ESA-treated patients.[47] Further investigation is necessary to determine the effectiveness of ESAs in critically ill patients.[41] These agents are not FDA approved in this setting.

Many critically ill patients receive RBC transfusions despite the inherent risks associated with transfusions. Stored RBCs may not function as well as endogenous blood. Although RBC transfusions may increase oxygen delivery to tissues, cellular oxygen may not increase.[48] Transfusion practices in ICUs vary, and clinicians use different Hb concentrations as thresholds for administering transfusions. The decision to use transfusions must consider the risks, including transmission of infections; volume overload, especially for patients with renal or heart failure; iron overload; and immune-mediated reactions such as febrile reactions, hemolysis, and anaphylaxis. The clinician also must consider administrative, logistic, and economic factors, including the shortage of blood supplies.

ANEMIA IN THE ELDERLY

Epidemiology

7 One of the most common clinical problems observed in the elderly is anemia. Anemia is a prevalent and increasing problem in the elderly, with about 20% of people 85 years and older affected.[49] Elderly patients with the highest incidence of anemia are those who are hospitalized, followed by residents of nursing homes and other institutions, with an estimated rate of 31% to 40%.[50] Although the incidence of anemia is high in the elderly, anemia should not be regarded as an inevitable outcome of aging. The body's set point of Hb does not fall with age. An underlying cause can be identified in about two thirds of older patients. Undiagnosed and untreated anemia has been associated with adverse outcomes, including all-cause hospitalization, hospitalization secondary to cardiovascular disease, and all-cause mortality.[51] Anemia is an independent predictor of death and major clinical adverse events in elderly patients with stable symptomatic coronary artery disease.[52] Anemia can exacerbate neurologic and cognitive conditions and can adversely influence quality of life and physical performance in the elderly.[53] Anemia may be an indication of serious diseases such as GI cancer.

Pathophysiology

Aging is associated with a progressive reduction in hematopoietic reserve, which makes individuals more susceptible to developing anemia in times of hematopoietic stress.[54] Dysregulation of proinflammatory cytokines, most notably interleukin-6, may inhibit EPO production or interact with EPO receptors.[55] Although Hb levels may remain normal, the diminished marrow reserve leaves the elderly patient more susceptible to other causes of anemia. Renal insufficiency, which also is common in elderly patients, may reduce the ability of the kidneys to produce EPO. Older patients often have a normal creatinine level but a diminished glomerular filtration rate. Myelodysplastic syndromes are another common cause of anemia in the elderly, but most anemia cases in the elderly are multifactorial.

Etiology

In the acute care setting, the top three causes of anemia in the elderly are chronic disease (35%), unexplained cause (17%), and iron deficiency (15%), whereas in community-based outpatient clinics, the most common causes are unexplained (36%), infection (23%), and chronic disease (17%).[56]

Another common problem in the elderly is vitamin B_{12} deficiency. The most common causes of clinically overt vitamin B_{12} deficiency are food/cobalamin malabsorption (more than 60% of cases) and pernicious anemia (15% to 20% of cases).[57]

One often-overlooked major factor that may contribute to anemia in the older population is nutritional status. Cognitive and functional impairments in the older population may create barriers for patients to obtain and prepare a nutritious diet. Nutritional deficiencies that are not severe enough to affect the hematopoietic system in the younger population may contribute to anemia in the elderly. Edentulous or infirm elderly who may be too ill to prepare their meals are at risk for nutritional folate deficiency. Risk factors for inadequate folate intake in the elderly include low caloric intake, inadequate consumption of fortified cereals, and failure to take a vitamin/mineral supplement. However, unlike cobalamin levels, folate levels often increase rather than decline with age. High folic acid intake can occur if the elderly patient regularly uses a supplement and consumes fortified cereals.[58,59]

Bleeding with resultant iron deficiency in the elderly may be due to carcinoma, peptic ulcer, atrophic gastritis, drug-induced gastritis, postmenopausal vaginal bleeding, or bleeding hemorrhoids. Elderly women have a much lower incidence of IDA compared with younger, menstruating women. Until proven otherwise, iron deficiency in the elderly should be considered a sign of chronic blood loss. Steps should be taken to rule out bleeding, especially from the GI or female reproductive tract. AI is more common in the elderly, as diseases that contribute to AI such as cancer, infection, and rheumatoid arthritis are more prevalent in this population.

Laboratory Findings

For practical purposes, it is best to use usual adult reference values and WHO criteria for laboratory tests in the elderly. Anemia in elderly persons usually is normocytic and mild, with Hb values ranging between 10 and 12 g/dL (100 to 120 g/L; 6.21 to 7.45 mmol/L) in most anemic patients.[49] Evaluation of an elderly patient should be similar to strategies described previously for younger adults, perhaps with more emphasis on identifying occult blood loss and vitamin B_{12} deficiency. Vitamin B_{12} deficiency may be present even when plasma levels of vitamin B_{12} are within the normal range, but elevated MMA levels will reveal the deficiency. A refractory macrocytic anemia in the elderly should raise suspicion of a myelodysplastic syndrome.

TREATMENT

Anemia in the Elderly

Treatment of anemia in the elderly is the same as that described for each type of anemia discussed in this chapter. With IDA it is essential to treat the underlying cause, if known (i.e., bleeding), and administer iron supplementation. Lower doses of iron supplementation are often recommended in the elderly (e.g., 325 mg of ferrous sulfate once daily) to decrease the incidence of GI adverse effects, which can lead to additional morbidity and poor adherence. The goal of treatment of AI is resolution of the underlying cause, although curing the underlying chronic illness for elderly patients can be difficult. Routine treatment with ESAs is not currently standard of care for AI in the elderly.

ANEMIA IN PEDIATRIC POPULATIONS

Epidemiology

8 IDA is a leading cause of infant morbidity and mortality around the world.[60] Data from NHANES III indicated that 9% of children ages 12 to 36 months in the United States had iron deficiency and 3% had IDA.[61,62] Lack of a normal Hb at birth directly affects nonstorage iron and increases the risk of IDA in the first 3 to 6 months of life. African American or Hispanic-American children have a higher incidence of anemia.[63] Requirements for iron absorption peak during puberty. An anemia of prematurity can occur 3 to 12 weeks after birth in infants younger than 32 weeks' gestation and spontaneously resolves by 3 to 6 months. The prevalence of vitamin B_{12} deficiency has been identified as 1 in 1,255 for levels <100 pg/mL (<74 pmol/L) and 1 in 200 for levels of <200 pg/mL (<148 pmol/L), with the lowest levels in non-Hispanic whites.[64]

Pathophysiology

In contrast to anemias in adults, which tend to be manifestations of a broader underlying pathology, anemias in the pediatric population are more often due to a primary hematologic abnormality. The amount of iron present at birth depends on gestational length and weight. A decrease in EPO production results in a physiologic anemia peaking at 2 months.[65] Iron stores from birth are mostly depleted by 6 months of age.

Etiology

The age of the child can yield some clues regarding the etiology of the anemia. The optimal amount of nutritional iron and folate required varies among individuals based on life-cycle stages. Two peak periods place children at risk of developing IDA. The first peak period occurs during late infancy and early childhood, when children undergo rapid body growth, have low levels of dietary iron, and exhaust stores accumulated during gestation. The second peak period occurs during adolescence, which is associated with rapid growth, poor diets, and onset of menses in girls. Some studies suggest that overweight children are at significantly higher risk for IDA. Proposed factors include genetic influences; physical inactivity, leading to decreased myoglobin breakdown and lower amounts of released iron into the blood; and inadequate diet with limited intake of iron-rich foods.[66]

Conditions in the newborn period that can lead to IDA include prematurity and insufficient dietary intake. Premature infants are at increased risk for IDA because of their smaller total blood volume, increased blood loss through phlebotomy, and poor GI absorption. Factors leading to unbalanced iron metabolism in infants include insufficient iron intake, early introduction of cow's milk, intolerance of cow's milk, medications, and malabsorption. Dietary deficiency of iron in the first 6 to 12 months of life is less common today because of the increased use of iron supplementation during breastfeeding and use of iron-fortified formulas. Iron deficiency becomes more common when children change to regular diets.

When screening for iron deficiency in young children, a careful dietary history can help identify children at risk. High iron needs and the tendency to eat fewer iron-containing foods contribute to the etiology of iron deficiency during adolescence.

Other causes of microcytic anemia include thalassemia, lead poisoning, and sideroblastic anemia. Use of homeopathic or herbal medications and exposure to paint or certain cooking materials may place children at risk for lead exposure. Normocytic anemias in children include infection with human parvovirus B19 and glucose-6-phosphate dehydrogenase (G6PD) deficiency. Macrocytic anemias are caused by deficiencies in vitamin B_{12} and folate, chronic liver disease, hypothyroidism, and myelodysplastic disorders. Folic acid deficiency usually is due to inadequate dietary intake, but human milk and cow's milk provide adequate sources. Folic acid deficiency may be seen in infants and children who primarily consume goat's milk or health food milk alternatives, or in children with insufficient intake of green leafy vegetables. Vitamin B_{12} deficiency due to nutritional reasons is rare but may occur due to a congenital pernicious anemia.

Laboratory Findings

When evaluating laboratory values for pediatric patients, the clinician must use age- and sex-adjusted norms. It is important to know that many blood samples are capillary samples, such as heel or finger sticks, which may have slightly different results than venous samples. The USPSTF has concluded that evidence is insufficient to recommend for or against routine screening for IDA in asymptomatic, low risk, children aged 6 to 12 months. The Hb is a sensitive test for iron deficiency, but it has low specificity in childhood anemias. If an abnormality is found, a CBC should be ordered to evaluate MCV and determine whether the anemia is microcytic, normocytic, or macrocytic. A peripheral blood smear and reticulocyte count also may be helpful. The peripheral blood smear can indicate the etiology based on RBC morphology, and the reticulocyte count helps differentiate between decreased RBC production and increased RBC destruction or loss. Other laboratory tests include serum iron, ferritin, TIBC, and transferrin saturation. Mild hereditary anemias may produce a mild hypochromic microcytic anemia that can be confused with IDAs. The RDW may be high with iron deficiency and is more likely to be normal with thalassemia. Laboratory features of anemia of prematurity include normocytic normochromic cells, low reticulocyte count, low serum EPO concentrations, and decreased RBC precursors in bone marrow. Laboratory diagnosis of vitamin B_{12} and folate deficiency in children is similar to that of adults.

TREATMENT

Anemia in Pediatric Populations

Primary prevention of IDA in infants, children, and adolescents is the most appropriate goal because delays in mental and motor development are potentially irreversible. In 2006, the USPSTF published revised recommendations to screen and supplement iron deficiency in the United States, focusing on children and pregnant women.[17] The USPSTF recommends routine iron supplementation for asymptomatic children aged 6 to 12 months who are at increased risk for IDA. Fair evidence was found that iron supplementation (e.g., iron-fortified formula or iron supplements) might improve neurodevelopmental outcomes in children at risk for IDA. The quality of evidence of benefit for children 6 to 12 months of age not at risk for IDA was poor.

Interventions likely to prevent anemia include diverse foods with bioavailable forms of iron, food fortification for infants and children, and individual supplementation. Routine screening for iron deficiency in nonpregnant adolescents is recommended only for those with risk factors, which include vegetarian diets, malnutrition, low body weight, chronic illness, or history of heavy menstrual blood loss.

Anemia of prematurity is frequently treated with RBC transfusions, with wide variations in transfusion practices among neonatal ICUs. Reasons for transfusions include improved oxygen delivery, increased intravascular volume, reduced fatigue during feeding, and improved growth. ESAs have been used to treat anemia of prematurity, but it is important to note that ESA pharmacokinetics differ depending on the developmental age of the infant. ESA use is controversial because it has not been shown to clearly reduce transfusion requirements. Other questions regarding safety and proper use of ESAs in anemia of prematurity remain unanswered.

For infants aged 9 to 12 months with a mild microcytic anemia, the most cost-effective treatment is a therapeutic trial of iron. Fe^{2+} sulfate at a dose of 3–6 mg/kg/day of elemental iron divided once or twice daily between meals for 4 weeks is recommended. In children who respond, iron should be continued for two more months to replace storage iron pools, along with dietary intervention and patient education.[67] Parenteral iron therapy has a limited role and is rarely necessary.

For the macrocytic anemias in children, folate can be administered in a dose of 1 mg daily. However, vitamin B_{12} deficiency due to congenital pernicious anemia requires lifelong vitamin B_{12} supplementation. Dose and frequency should be titrated according to clinical response and laboratory values. No data regarding the use of oral vitamin B_{12} supplementation in children are available.

PERSONALIZED PHARMACOTHERAPY

In the treatment of the anemias discussed in this chapter, personalized pharmacotherapy is important in a few populations. When treating IDA, the elderly should be treated with lower doses of oral iron therapy. This typically is once daily dosing with ferrous sulfate 325 mg. Patients with immune-mediated disease are at higher risk for having hypersensitivity reactions to parenteral iron therapy. Patients who have neurologic symptoms upon diagnosis of vitamin B_{12} deficiency should strongly be considered for parenteral B_{12} supplementation. If ESAs are used to treat AI, iron status should be closely monitored to ensure efficacy of these agents as functional iron deficiency can develop.

EVALUATION OF THERAPEUTIC OUTCOMES

For IDA, a positive response to a trial of oral iron therapy is characterized by a modest reticulocytosis in days, with an increase in Hb starting after about 2 weeks with continued rapid rise in Hb. As the Hb level approaches normal, the rate of increase slows progressively. Hb should reach a normal level after about 2 months of therapy and often sooner.[9] If the patient does not develop reticulocytosis, reevaluation of the diagnosis or iron replacement therapy is necessary. Iron therapy should continue for a period sufficient for complete restoration of iron stores. Serum ferritin concentrations should return to the normal range prior to discontinuation of iron. The time interval required to accomplish this goal varies, although at least 6 to 12 months of therapy usually is warranted. Patients with negative iron balances caused by bleeding may require iron replacement therapy for only 1 month after correction of the underlying lesion, whereas patients with recurrent negative balances may require long-term treatment with as little as 30 to 60 mg of elemental iron daily.

When large amounts of parenteral iron are administered, by either total dose infusion or multiple intramuscular or IV doses, the patient's iron status should be closely monitored. Patients receiving regular IV iron should be monitored for clinical or laboratory evidence of iron toxicity or overload. Iron overload may be indicated by abnormal hepatic function tests, serum ferritin >800 ng/mL (>800 g/L), or transferrin saturation >50%. Serum ferritin and transferrin saturation should be measured in the first week after larger IV iron doses. Hb and Hct should be measured weekly, and serum iron and ferritin levels should be measured at least monthly.

In the treatment of vitamin B_{12} deficiency anemia, most patients respond rapidly to vitamin B_{12} therapy. The typical patient will experience an improvement in strength and well-being within a few days of treatment initiation. Reticulocytosis is evident in 3 to 5 days. Hb begins to rise after the first week and should normalize in 1 to 2 months. CBC count and serum cobalamin levels usually are drawn 1 to 2 months after initiation of therapy and 3 to 6 months thereafter for surveillance monitoring. Homocysteine and MMA levels can be repeated 2 to 3 months after initiation of replacement therapy to evaluate for normalization of levels, although levels begin to decrease in 1 to 2 weeks. Neuropsychiatric signs and symptoms can be reversible if treated early. If permanent neurologic damage has resulted, progression should cease with replacement therapy. Slow response to therapy or failure to observe normalization of laboratory results may suggest the presence of an additional abnormality such as iron deficiency, thalassemia trait, infection, malignancy, nonadherence, or misdiagnosis.

In folic acid deficiency anemia, symptomatic improvement, as evidenced by increased alertness and appetite, often occurs early during the course of treatment. Reticulocytosis begins in the first week. Hct begins to rise within 2 weeks and should reach normal levels within 2 months. MCV initially increases because of an increase in reticulocytes but gradually decreases to normal.

When using ESAs, one of the earliest responses is an increase in blood reticulocyte count, which usually occurs in the first few days. Baseline iron status should be checked before and during treatment, as many patients receiving ESAs require supplemental iron therapy. The optimal form and schedule of iron supplementation are not known. Hb levels should be monitored twice a week until stabilized. Hb should also be monitored twice weekly for 2 to 6 weeks after a dose adjustment.[46] A fall in Hb during ESA therapy may indicate a need for iron supplementation or signal occult blood loss. Baseline and periodic monitoring of iron, TIBC, transferrin saturation, or ferritin levels may be useful in optimizing iron repletion and limiting the need for ESAs. Patients who do not respond to 8 weeks of optimal dosage should not continue taking ESAs. Target Hb levels should be 11 to 12 g/dL (110 to 120 g/L; 6.83 to 7.45 mmol/L). Cost is an issue with ESA therapy; therefore, drug cost must be weighed against the effects on transfusions and hospitalizations.

Responses and monitoring of treatment are similar in the elderly as described for the general adult population described earlier in the chapter. If the reticulocyte count rises but the anemia does not improve, inadequate absorption of iron or continued blood loss should be suspected. As with any form of anemia, symptomatic improvement should be evident shortly after starting therapy, and Hb/Hct should begin to rise within a few weeks of initiating therapy. A key component of symptom assessment among older adults is the functional domain. Patients should be asked about changes in self-care abilities, mobility, and stamina.

Therapeutic outcomes are assessed in children by monitoring Hb, Hct, and RBC indices 4 to 8 weeks after initiation of iron therapy. For premature infants, Hb or Hct should be monitored weekly.

ABBREVIATIONS

ACD	anemia of chronic disease
AI	anemia of inflammation
AIDS	acquired immunodeficiency syndrome
CBC	complete blood count
CDC	Centers for Disease Control and Prevention
EPO	erythropoietin
ESA	erythropoiesis-stimulating agent
Fe^{2+}	ferrous iron

Fe^{3+}	ferric iron
G6PD	glucose-6-phosphate dehydrogenase
Hb	hemoglobin
Hct	hematocrit
HIV	human immunodeficiency virus
IDA	iron-deficiency anemia
MCH	mean corpuscular hemoglobin
MCHC	mean corpuscular hemoglobin concentration
MCV	mean corpuscular volume
MMA	methylmalonic acid
NHANES	National Health and Nutrition Examination Survey
RBC	red blood cell
RDW	red blood cell distribution width
TIBC	total iron-binding capacity
USPSTF	United States Preventive Services Task Force
WHO	World Health Organization

REFERENCES

1. Benoist B, McLean E, Egli M, et al. Worldwide prevalence of anaemia 1993–2005: WHO global database on anaemia. World Health Organization; 2008.
2. Cusick SE, Mei Z, Freedman DS, et al. Unexplained decline in the prevalence of anemia among US children and women between 1988–1994 and 1999–2002. Am J Clin Nutr 2008; 88:1611–1617.
3. Nissenson A. Anemia not just an innocent bystander. Arch Intern Med 2003;163:1400–1404.
4. Mozaffarian D. Anemia predicts mortality in severe heart failure: The prospective randomized amlodipine survival evaluation (PRAISE). J Am Coll Cardiol 2003;41: 1933–1939.
5. Chaves PHM, Carlson MC, Ferrucci L, et al. Association between mild anemia and executive function impairment in community-dwelling older women: The Women's Health and Aging Study II. J Am Geriatr Soc 2006;54:1429–1435.
6. Anemia in pregnancy. ACOG Practice Bulletin No. 95. American College of Obst and Gynecologists. Obstet Gynecol 2008;112:201–207.
7. Prchal JT. Production of erythrocytes. In: Kaushansky K, Lichtman MA, Beutler E, et al, eds. Williams Hematology, 8th ed. New York: McGraw-Hill; 2010:453–448.
8. Wians FH, Urban JE, Keffer JH, Kroft SH. Discriminating between iron deficiency anemia and anemia of chronic disease using traditional indices of iron status vs. transferrin receptor concentration. Am J Clin Pathol 2001;115:112–118.
9. Beutler E. Disorders of iron metabolism. In: Kaushansky K, Lichtman MA, Beutler E, et al, eds. Williams Hematology, 8th ed. New York: McGraw-Hill; 2010:565–606.
10. Beutler E. Destruction of erythrocytes. In: Kaushansky K, Lichtman MA, Beutler E, et al., eds. Williams Hematology, 8th ed. New York: McGraw-Hill; 2010:449–454.
11. Galloway M, Rushworth L. Red cell or serum folate? Results from the National Pathology Alliance benchmarking review. J Clin Pathol 2003;56:924–926.
12. Snow CF. Laboratory diagnosis of vitamin B_{12} and folate deficiency. Arch Intern Med 1999;159:1289–1298.
13. Green R. Folate, cobalamin, and megaloblastic anemias. In: Kaushansky K, Lichtman MA, Beutler E, et al., eds. Williams Hematology, 8th ed. New York: McGraw-Hill; 2010:533–564.
14. Dharmarajan TS, Norkus EP. Approaches to vitamin B_{12} deficiency. Early treatment may prevent devastating complications. Postgrad Med 2001;110:99–105.
15. Ganz T. Hepcidin—A regulator of intestinal iron absorption and iron recycling by macrophages. Best Pract Res Clin Haematol 2005;18:171–182.
16. Goodnough LT, Nemeth E, Gan T. Detection, evaluation, and management of iron restricted erythropoiesis. Blood 2010;116:4754–4761.
17. Killip S, Bennett J, Chambers M. Iron deficiency anemia. Am Fam Physician 2007;75:671–678.
18. Hershko C, Ianculovich M, Souroujon M. A hematologist's view of unexplained iron deficiency anemia in males: Impact of *Helicobacter pylori* eradication. Blood Cells Mol Dis 2007;38:45–53.
19. U.S. Preventive Services Task Force (USPSTF). Screening for Iron Deficiency Anemia—Including Iron Supplementation for Children and Pregnant Women. Rockville, MD: Agency for Healthcare Research and Quality (AHRQ); 2006.
20. Faich G, Strobos J. Sodium Fe^{3+} gluconate complex in sucrose: Safer IV iron therapy than iron dextrans. Am J Kidney Dis 1999;33:464–470.
21. Chandler G, Harchowal J, Macdougall IC. Intravenous iron sucrose: Establishing a safe dose. Am J Kidney Dis 2001;38:988–991.
22. Silverstein SB, Gilreath JA, Rodgers GM. Intravenous iron therapy: A summary of treatment options and review of guidelines. J Pharm Practice 2008;21:431–443.
23. InFeD [package insert]. Morristown, NJ: Watson Pharma; 2009.
24. Munoz M, Garcia-Erce JA, Remacha AF. Disorders of iron metabolism: Part II: Iron deficiency and iron overload. J Clin Pathol 2011;64:287–296.
25. Ferrlecit [package insert]. Morristown, NJ: Watson Pharma; 2006.
26. Venofer [package insert]. Shirley, NY: American Regent; 2008.
27. Feraheme [package insert]. Lexington, MA: AMAG Pharmaceuticals; 2009.
28. Oh RC, Brown DL. Vitamin B_{12} deficiency. Am Fam Physician 2003;67:979–986, 993–994.
29. Kaptan K, Beyan C, Ural AU, et al. Helicobacter pylori—Is it a novel causative agent in vitamin B_{12} deficiency? Arch Intern Med 2000;160:1349–1353.
30. Hoffbrand AV. Chapter 105. Megaloblastic Anemias. In: Longo DL, Fauci AS, Kasper DL, Hauser SL, Jameson JL, Loscalzo J, eds. Harrison's Principles of Internal Medicine, 18th ed. New York: McGraw-Hill; 2012. *http://www.accessmedicine.com/content.aspx?aID =9117611*.
31. Aronow WS. Homocysteine. The association with atherosclerotic vascular disease in older persons. Geriatrics 2003;58:22–28.
32. Green R. Indicators for assessing folate and vitamin b-12 status and for monitoring the efficacy of intervention strategies. Am J Clin Nutr 2011;94(Suppl):666S–672S.
33. Vidal-Alaball J, Butler CC, Cannings-John R, et al. Oral vitamin B_{12} versus intramuscular vitamin B_{12} for vitamin B_{12} deficiency. Cochrane Database Syst Rev 2005;3:CD004655.
34. Cravens DD, Nashelsky J, Oh RC. How do we evaluate a marginally low B_{12} level? J Fam Pract 2007;56:62–63.
35. Solomon LR. Oral vitamin B_{12} therapy: A cautionary note. Blood 2004;103:2863.
36. Lane LA, Rojas-Fernandez. Treatment of vitamin B_{12}-deficiency anemia: Oral versus parenteral therapy. Ann Pharmacother 2002;36:1268–1272.
37. Yerby MS. Clinical care of pregnant women with epilepsy: Neural tube defects and folic acid supplementation. Epilepsia 2003;44(Suppl 3):33–40.

38. Pitkin RM. Folate and neural tube defects. Am J Clin Nutr 2007;85:285S–288S.
39. American College of Obstetricians and Gynecologists (ACOG). Neural Tube Defects. ACOG Practice Bulletin No. 44. Washington, DC: American College of Obstetricians and Gynecologists, 2003.
40. Corwin HL, Gettinger A, Pearl RG, et al. The CRIT Study: Anemia and blood transfusion in the critically ill—Current clinical practice in the United States. Crit Care Med 2004; 32:39–52.
41. Stubbs JR. Alternatives to blood product transfusion in the critically ill: Erythropoietin. Crit Care Med 2006;34(Suppl): S160–S169.
42. Weiss GW, Goodnough LT. Anemia of chronic disease. N Engl J Med 2005;352:1011–1023.
43. Rodriguez RM, Corwin HL, Gettinger A, et al. Nutritional deficiencies and blunted erythropoietin response as cause of anemia of critical illness. J Crit Care 2001;16:36.
44. Silver MR. Anemia in the long-term ventilator-dependent patient with respiratory failure. Chest 2005;128(Suppl): 568S–575S.
45. Adamson J. The anemia of inflammation/malignancy: Mechanisms and management. Hematology Am Soc Hematol Educ Program 2008;159–165.
46. Procrit [package insert]. Thousand Oaks, CA: Amgen, 2009.
47. Rudis M, Jacobi J, Hassan E, et al. Managing anemia in the critically ill patient. Pharmacotherapy 2004;24: 229–247.
48. Hébert PC, Wells G, Martin C, et al. Do blood transfusions improve outcomes related to mechanical ventilation? Chest 2001;119:1850–1857.
49. Guralnik JM, Eisenstaedt RS, Ferrucci L, et al. Prevalence of anemia in person 65 years and older in the United States: Evidence for a high rate of unexplained anemia. Blood 2004;104:2263–2268.
50. Carmel R. Anemia and aging: An overview of clinical, diagnostic, and biological issues. Blood Rev 2001;15:9–18.
51. Culleton BF, Manns BJ, Zhang J, et al. Impact of anemia on hospitalization and mortality in older adults. Blood 2006;107:3841–3846.
52. Muzzarelli S, Pfisterer M, TIME Investigators. Anemia as independent predictor of major events in elderly patients with chronic angina. Am Heart J 2006;152:991–996.
53. Woodman R, Ferrucci L, Guralnik J. Anemia in older adults. Curr Opin Hematol 2005;12:123–128.
54. Balducci L, Hardy CL, Lyman GH. Hematopoietic growth factors in the older cancer patient. Curr Opin Hematol 2001;8:170–187.
55. Eisenstaedt R, Penninx BW, Woodman RC. Anemia in the elderly: Current understanding and emerging concepts. Blood Rev 2006;20:213–226.
56. Balducci L. Epidemiology of anemia in the elderly: Information on diagnostic evaluation. J Am Geriatr Soc 2003;51(Suppl):S2–S9.
57. Andres E, Loukili N, Noel E, et al. Vitamin B_{12} (cobalamin) deficiency in elderly patients. CMAJ 2004;171:251–259.
58. Mulligan JE, Greene GW, Caldwell M. Sources of folate and serum folate levels in older adults. J Am Diet Assoc 2007;107:495–499.
59. Ford ES, Bowman BA. Serum and red blood cell folate concentrations, race, and education: Findings from the third National Health and Nutrition Examination Survey. Am J Clin Nutr 1999;69:476–481.
60. Milman N. Iron prophylaxis in pregnancy—General or individual and in which dose? Ann Hematol 2006;85: 821–828.
61. Recommendations to prevent and control iron deficiency in the United States. Morb Mortal Wkly Rep 1998;47:1–36.
62. Moy RJ. Prevalence, consequences and prevention of childhood nutritional iron. Clin Lab Haematol 2006;28: 291–298.
63. Coyer S. Anemia: Diagnosis and management. J Pediatr Health Care 2005;19:380–385.
64. Wright JD, Bialostosky K, Gunter EW, et al. Blood folate and vitamin B_{12}: United States, 1988–94. Vital Health Stat 1998;11:1–78.
65. Palis J, Segel GB. Chapter 6. Hematology of the Fetus and Newborn. In: Prchal JT, Kaushansky K, Lichtman MA, Kipps TJ, Seligsohn U, eds. *Williams Hematology*. 8th ed. New York: McGraw-Hill, 2010. *http://www.accessmedicine.com/content.aspx?aID=6107804*.
66. Nead KG, Halterman JS, Kaczorowski JM, et al. Overweight children and adolescents: A risk group for iron deficiency. Pediatrics 2004;114:104–108.
67. Kazal LA. Prevention of iron deficiency in infants and toddlers. Am Fam Physician 2002;66:1217–1224.

Coagulation Disorders

81

Betsy Bickert Poon, Char Witmer, and Jane Pruemer

KEY CONCEPTS

1. Hemophilia is an inherited bleeding disorder resulting from a congenital deficiency in factor VIII or IX.
2. The goal of therapy for hemophilia is to prevent bleeding episodes and their long-term complications and to arrest bleeding if it occurs.
3. Recombinant factor concentrates usually are first-line treatment of hemophilia because they have the lowest risk of infection.
4. Inhibitor formation is the most significant treatment complication in hemophilia. It is associated with significant morbidity and decreased quality of life.
5. The goal of therapy for von Willebrand disease is to increase von Willebrand factor and factor VIII levels to prevent bleeding during surgery or arrest bleeding when it occurs.
6. Factor VIII concentrates that contain von Willebrand factor are the agents of choice for treatment of type 3 von Willebrand disease and some type 2 von Willebrand disease, and for serious bleeding in type 1 von Willebrand disease.
7. Desmopressin acetate often is effective for treatment of type 1 von Willebrand disease. It also may be effective for treatment of some forms of type 2 von Willebrand disease.

The coagulation system is intricately balanced and designed to stop bleeding at the site of vascular injury through complex interactions between the vascular endothelium, platelets, procoagulant proteins, anticoagulant proteins, and fibrinolytic proteins. Hemostasis stops bleeding at the site of vascular injury through the formation of an impermeable platelet and fibrin plug. Three key mechanisms facilitate hemostasis including vascular constriction, primary platelet plug formation (primary hemostasis), and clot propagation through fibrin formation (secondary hemostasis). Derangements in this finely tuned system can lead to either bleeding or thrombosis. Bleeding disorders are the result of either a coagulation factor defect, a quantitative or qualitative platelet defect, or enhanced fibrinolytic activity. The complex system regulating hemostasis is described in the pathophysiology section of Chapter 9.

COAGULATION FACTORS

Secondary hemostasis facilitates propagation and stabilization of the initial platelet plug formed in primary hemostasis through the formation of fibrin on the activated platelet surface. This step is initiated via the tissue factor pathway and is vital for adequate hemostasis. Coagulation factors circulate as inactive precursors (zymogens). Activation of these coagulation proteins entails a cascading series of proteolytic reactions (Fig. 9-2). At each step, a clotting factor undergoes limited proteolysis and becomes an active protease (designated by a lowercase "a," as in Xa).

The coagulation factors can be divided into three groups on the basis of biochemical properties: vitamin K-dependent factors (II, VII, IX, and X), contact activation factors (XI and XII, prekallikrein, and high-molecular-weight kininogen), and thrombin-sensitive factors (V, VIII, XIII, and fibrinogen). Biologic half-life and blood product source varies by coagulation factor (Table 81-1).

CLINICAL MANIFESTATIONS AND DIAGNOSIS

The diagnosis of coagulation disorders can be established from a detailed clinical history, physical examination, and laboratory test results. The clinical history should ascertain if there is a family history of bleeding or known bleeding disorders. Laboratory testing can distinguish bleeding disorders caused by defects in the coagulation pathways (Fig. 9-4), fibrinolytic pathways, or alterations in the number or function of platelets. Table 81-2 describes common coagulation tests.

HEMOPHILIA

1 Hemophilia is a bleeding disorder that results from a congenital deficiency in a plasma coagulation protein. Hemophilia A (classic hemophilia) is caused by a deficiency of factor VIII, whereas hemophilia B (Christmas disease) is caused by a deficiency of factor IX. The incidence of hemophilia is about 1 in 5,000 male births, 80% to 85% hemophilia A and 15% to 20% hemophilia B.[1,2] There are no significant racial differences in the incidence of hemophilia.

About one-third of patients with hemophilia have a negative family history, presumably representing a spontaneous mutation. Both hemophilia A and hemophilia B are recessive X-linked diseases, which mean that the defective gene is located on the X chromosome. The disease primarily affects only males while females are carriers. Affected males have the abnormal allele on their X chromosome and no matching allele on their Y chromosome, their sons would be normal (assuming the mother is not a carrier) and their daughters would be obligatory carriers. Female carriers have one normal allele and therefore do not usually have a bleeding tendency. Although female carriers have lower factor VIII levels than females who are not carriers.[3] Sons of a female carrier and a normal male have a 50% chance of having hemophilia and daughters have a 50% chance of being carriers. Thus, there is a "skipped generation" mode of inheritance in which the female carriers do not express the disease but can pass it on to the next male generation.

TABLE 81-1 Blood Coagulation Factors

Factor[a]	Synonym	Biologic Half-life (h)	Blood Product Source
I	Fibrinogen	100–150	Cryoprecipitate (200–300 mg/bag)
II	Prothrombin	50–80	FFP, PCC
V	Proaccelerin	12–36	FFP
VII	Proconvertin	4–6	Recombinant VIIa, FFP, PCC
VIII	Antihemophilic factor	12–15	FFP, factor concentrates, cryoprecipitate
IX	Christmas factor	18–30	FFP, PCC, factor concentrates
X	Stuart-Power factor	25–60	FFP, PCC
XI	Plasma thromboplastin antecedent	40–80	FFP
XII	Hageman factor	50–70	Not associated with bleeding diathesis
XIII	Fibrin-stabilizing factor	150	FFP, cryoprecipitate, factor concentrate
VWF	von Willebrand factor	8–12	FFP, cryoprecipitate, factor concentrate

FFP, fresh-frozen plasma; PCC, prothrombin complex concentrate.

[a]Coagulation factors are numbered with roman numerals in order of their discovery. The most common synonyms are listed. Factor III (tissue factor) and factor IV (calcium ions) have been omitted. There is no factor VI.

Hemophilia has been observed in a small number of females. It can occur if both factor VIII and IX genes are defective,[4,5] if a female patient has only one X chromosome as in Turner syndrome, or if the normal X chromosome is excessively inactivated through a process called *lyonization* or highly skewed X inactivation.[6–8]

In 1984, researchers isolated and cloned the human factor VIII gene.[9,10] It is a large gene, consisting of 186 kilobases (kb).[11] More than 900 unique mutations in the factor VIII gene, including point mutations, deletions, and insertions, have been reported (*http://hadb.org.uk/*). Deletions and nonsense mutations are often associated with the more severe forms of factor VIII deficiency because no functional factor VIII is produced. In 1993, researchers identified an inversion in the factor VIII gene at intron 22 that accounts for about 45% of severe hemophilia A gene abnormalities.[12] That discovery has greatly simplified carrier detection and prenatal diagnosis in families with this gene mutation. A more recently discovered inversion mutation involving intron 1 of the factor VIII gene accounts for an additional 5% of severe hemophilia mutations.[13]

The factor IX gene, cloned and sequenced in 1982, consists of only 34 kb and thus is significantly smaller than the factor VIII gene.[14] Unlike the factor VIII gene in patients with severe hemophilia A, the factor IX gene in patients with hemophilia B has no predominant mutation. Direct gene mutation analysis is simpler in hemophilia B because of the smaller gene size, and to date more than 900 different mutations have been reported (*http://kcl.ac.uk/ip/petergreen/haemBdatabase.html*). Most of these mutations are single base-pair substitutions. About 3% of factor IX gene mutations are deletions or complex rearrangements, and the presence of these mutations is associated with a severe phenotype.[11]

Hemophilia B Leyden is a rare variant in which factor IX levels initially are low but rise at puberty. The mechanism underlying the pathogenesis of this disorder has been controversial. Some propose that the binding of the androgen receptor and other transcription factors are responsible.[15,16] Other molecular mechanisms for age-related gene regulation has been recently discovered and implicated in factor IX Leyden.[17] Identification of this genotype is clinically important because it confers a better prognosis.

Clinical Presentation

The characteristic bleeding manifestations of hemophilia include palpable ecchymoses, bleeding into joint spaces (hemarthroses), muscle hemorrhages, and excessive bleeding after surgery or trauma. The severity of clinical bleeding generally correlates with the degree of deficiency of either factor VIII or factor IX. Factor VIII and factor IX activity levels are measured in units per milliliter, with 1 unit/mL representing 100% of the factor found in 1 mL of normal plasma.[18] Normal plasma levels range from 0.5 to 1.5 units/mL. Patients with less than 0.01 units/mL (1%) of either factor are classified as having severe hemophilia, those with 0.01 to 0.05 units/mL (1% to 5%) are moderate, and those with greater than 0.05 units/mL (5%) have mild hemophilia (Table 81-3).

Patients with severe disease experience frequent spontaneous hemorrhages, whereas those with moderate disease have excessive bleeding following mild trauma and rarely experience spontaneous hemarthroses. Patients with mild hemophilia may have so few symptoms that their condition can be undiagnosed for many years, and they usually have excessive bleeding only after significant trauma or surgery. Disease severity does not always correlate with disease manifestations. Those with severe disease (less than 1% factor activity) may occasionally not display a severe phenotype, while some with milder forms of the disease may have more severe bleeding.

CLINICAL PRESENTATION Hemophilia

Signs and Symptoms

- Ecchymoses (palpable/raised)
- Hemarthrosis (especially knee, ankle, and elbow)
- Joint pain
- Joint swelling and erythema
- Decreased range of motion
- Muscle hemorrhage
- Swelling at the site of muscle bleeding
- Pain with motion of affected muscle
- Signs of nerve compression
- Significant anemia from an iliopsoas or thigh bleed
- Oral bleeding with dental extractions or trauma
- Hematuria
- Intracranial hemorrhage (spontaneous or following trauma)
- Excessive bleeding with surgery

Laboratory Testing

- Prolonged activated partial thromboplastin time (aPTT)
- Decreased factor VIII or factor IX level
- Normal prothrombin time (PT)
- Normal platelet count
- Normal von Willebrand factor antigen and activity
- Normal bleeding time

TABLE 81-2 Laboratory Procedures

Procedure	Identifies	Coagulation Cause of Abnormal Value	Clinical Manifestations
Prothrombin time (PT)	Factors I, II, V, VII, X	Newborn Vitamin K deficiency Inherited factor deficiencies[a] Warfarin therapy Liver disease Lupus anticoagulant (rare) Afibrinogenemia Dysfibrinogenemia	Bleeding following surgery, trauma, etc Easy bruising
Activated partial thromboplastin time (aPTT)	Factors I, II, V, VIII, IX, X	Inherited factor deficiencies[a] Lupus anticoagulant Heparin therapy Liver disease Afibrinogenemia Dysfibrinogenemia	Joint and muscle bleeding Bleeding after surgery, trauma, etc
	HMWK, prekallikrein		No bleeding manifestations
	Factor XII		Increased incidence of thrombotic disease possible with severe factor XII deficiency
	Factor XI		Variable bleeding tendency Bleeding following surgery, trauma, etc
Thrombin time (TT)	Fibrinogen Inhibitors of fibrin aggregation	Afibrinogenemia Dysfibrinogenemia Heparin therapy	Lifelong hemorrhagic disease Variable clinical symptoms from asymptomatic to either a bleeding diathesis or prothrombotic
Platelet count	Thrombocytopenia	Quantitative platelet disorder, type 2B von Willebrand disease, immune thrombocytopenia, other cause of thrombocytopenia	Mucocutaneous bleeding
Platelet function analyzer	Platelet function	Qualitative platelet defects, von Willebrand disease, antiplatelet therapy Also prolonged in anemia and thrombocytopenia **Insensitive to mild platelet defects and has fallen out of favor as a screening test*	Mucocutaneous bleeding
Platelet aggregation	Gold standard to assess platelet function	Qualitative platelet defects, antiplatelet medications	Mucocutaneous bleeding
Euglobulin clot lysis time (ECLT)	Fibrinolytic defect	A decreased ECLT indicates hyperfibrinolysis, which indicates an abnormality in the fibrinolytic pathway including: plasminogen activator inhibitor 1 deficiency, α_2-plasminogen inhibitor deficiency Hypofibrinogenemia	Bleeding after trauma or surgical procedures especially in oral and urogenital areas

HMWK, high-molecular-weight kininogen.

[a]Bleeding manifestations depend on factor levels.

TABLE 81-3 Laboratory and Clinical Manifestations of Hemophilia

	Severe (<0.01 units/mL)	Moderate (0.01–0.05 units/mL)	Mild (>0.05 units/mL)
Age at diagnosis	≤1 year	1–2 years	2 years to adult
Neonatal symptoms			
PCB	Usually	Usually	Rarely
ICH	Occasionally	Uncommonly	Rarely
Muscle/joint hemorrhage	Spontaneous	Minor trauma	Minor to major trauma
CNS hemorrhage	High risk	Moderate risk	Uncommon
Postsurgical hemorrhage (without prophylaxis)	Frank bleeding, severe	Wound bleeding, common	Wound bleeding
Oral hemorrhage following trauma, tooth extraction	Usually	Common	Common

CNS, central nervous system; ICH, intracranial hemorrhage; PCB, postcircumcisional bleeding.

Normal range of factor VIII/IX activity level is 0.5–1.5 units/mL (50–150%). A value of 1 unit/mL corresponds to 100% of the factor found in 1 mL of normal plasma.

Patients with hemophilia usually present with clinical manifestations after age 1 year, when they begin to walk and increase their risk of bleeding due to falling.

Diagnosis

The diagnosis of hemophilia should be considered in any male with unusual bleeding. A family history of bleeding is helpful in the diagnosis but is absent in up to 50% of patients with about one-third representing spontaneous mutations and the remaining secondary to an unrecognized family history.[11] Brothers of patients with hemophilia should be screened; sisters should undergo carrier testing. Laboratory testing in patients with hemophilia will reveal an isolated prolonged partial thromboplastin time (PTT) and a decreased FVIII or FIX level.

Patients with severe hemophilia A should be tested for the common factor VIII gene inversions. In patients with severe hemophilia A who lack an inversion mutation or patients with moderate or mild hemophilia A, the gene can be sequenced to determine the exact mutation.[19] Techniques for determining the genetic mutation in patients with hemophilia B are similar, but no predominant mutation like the factor VIII inversion has been found. The smaller size of the factor IX gene facilitates direct DNA mutational analysis.[19]

Advances in molecular genetic analysis have greatly improved the accuracy of carrier status evaluation. Thus, female relatives of patients with hemophilia who are at risk of being carriers should be tested. Carrier testing is simplified if the familial mutation has already been identified. Additionally, the appropriate factor level should be measured in female carriers to identify those with levels less than 0.3 units/mL (30%) who themselves might be at risk for bleeding.

Hemophilia can be diagnosed prenatally by chorionic villus sampling in gestational weeks 11 to 14 or by amniocentesis after 15 weeks' gestation.[20] These are invasive procedures with a 0.5% to 1% chance for pregnancy loss.[20] A new noninvasive method uses cell-free fetal DNA that exists in maternal circulation to determine the sex of the fetus helping establish if more invasive testing is required for a male fetus.[20] More recently this method was used to successfully identify hemophilia mutations in 12 subjects.[21] At this time the method of using fetal DNA in maternal circulation to identify hemophilia mutations is still experimental and requires further validation.

TREATMENT
Hemophilia

Desired Outcomes

The comprehensive care of hemophilia requires a multidisciplinary approach. The patient is best managed in specialized centers with trained personnel and appropriate laboratory, radiologic, and pharmaceutical services. The healthcare team includes hematologists, orthopedic surgeons, nurses, physical therapists, dentists, genetic counselors, psychologists, pharmacists, case managers, and social workers. The goal for comprehensive hemophilia care is to preventing bleeding episodes and their long-term sequelae so that patients with hemophilia can live full, active, and productive lives.

2 IV factor replacement therapy for the treatment or prevention of bleeding is the mainstay of treatment for hemophilia. Parents usually learn how to infuse factor concentrate to facilitate home treatment. Older children and adult patients learn self-administration. Home healthcare nursing support may be helpful, particularly for the youngest patients in whom venous access may be difficult. In the setting of poor venous access, central line placement may be indicated. Administration of factor at home is more convenient for families and allows for earlier treatment of acute bleeding episodes. However, serious bleeding episodes always require medical evaluation.

Patients with hemophilia should receive routine immunizations, including immunization against hepatitis B. Hepatitis A vaccine is also recommended for patients with hemophilia because of the risk (albeit small) of transmitting the causative agent through factor concentrates.[22] Use of a small-gauge needle can prevent excessive bleeding. Many healthcare providers advocate subcutaneous rather than intramuscular immunizations to decrease the risk of intramuscular bleeding or hematoma formation, but there is a lack of evidence to support this route of administration.

A few special considerations apply to the perinatal care of male infants of hemophilia carriers. Intracranial or extracranial hemorrhage has been estimated to occur in 1% to 4% of newborns with hemophilia.[23] Vacuum extraction and forceps delivery increase the risk of cranial bleeding. Elective cesarean section has not been shown to prevent intracranial bleeding. There is no clear consensus on the optimal mode of delivery or the use of prophylactic factor replacement in male infants of hemophilia carriers.[23] Circumcision should be postponed until a diagnosis of hemophilia is excluded. Factor levels can be assayed from cord blood samples or from peripheral venipuncture. Arterial puncture should be avoided because of the risk of hematoma formation. If an infant has hemophilia, many clinicians recommend a screening head ultrasound to rule out an intracranial hemorrhage prior to discharge from the nursery.

History of Hemophilia Treatment

Therapy for hemophilia has undergone dramatic advances over the past few decades. Fifty years ago, administration of fresh-frozen plasma was the only available treatment. The introduction of cryoprecipitate in the early 1960s allowed more specific therapy for hemophilia A.[24] Intermediate-purity factor VIII and IX plasma-derived concentrates became available in the 1970s.[24] Plasma-derived factor concentrates are made from the donations of thousands of people. Contamination of plasma pools with hepatitis B, hepatitis C, and the human immunodeficiency virus (HIV) during the late 1970s and early 1980s resulted in transmission to a large portion of patients with hemophilia. Since the mid-1980s, plasma-derived concentrates have been manufactured with a variety of virus-inactivating techniques, including dry heat, pasteurization, and treatment with chemicals (e.g., solvent detergent mixtures).[11] Since 1986, no transmission of HIV through factor concentrates to patients with hemophilia in the United States has been reported.[11] Protein purification techniques, introduced in the 1990s, led to the production of high-purity plasma-derived concentrates with increased amounts of factor VIII or factor IX relative to the product's total protein content. Recombinant factor VIII and then factor IX also became available in the 1990s.[24] Significant improvements have also been made with recombinant products in limiting the risk of infectious transmission from albumin used to stabilize some of the products. Like plasma-derived products, these products use viral inactivation steps. With each subsequent generation of recombinant factor VIII products, the use of human proteins has been reduced.[24]

More recently, there has been significant progress in the development of long-acting factor VIII or IX products. Different methods have been utilized to prolong the half-life of either factor VIII or IX including pegylation, polysialic acid, albumin infusion, and Fc infusion.[25] Clinical trials for factor VIII and FIX products that utilize either pegylation or fusion to an Fc receptor are ongoing.[25]

Hemophilia A

Table 81-4 summarizes the factor VIII products currently available in the United States. Most patients are treated with high-purity products. Products with the lowest risk of transmitting infectious disease should generally be used. Thus, recombinant products, when available, are generally used rather than plasma-derived products.

Recombinant Factor VIII

3 Recombinant factor VIII is produced with recombinant DNA technology and is derived from cultured Chinese hamster ovary cells or baby hamster kidney cells transfected with the human factor VIII gene.[11] Because it is not derived from blood donations, the risk of transmitting infections through administration of recombinant factor VIII is low and recombinant products are generally favored over plasma-derived products. A small risk of viral infection of the cell lines used to produce the clotting factor remains.[26] Furthermore, human and/or animal proteins are utilized in the production process of some recombinant products.[24] Therefore, these products have a theoretical risk of transmitting infection, although hepatitis and HIV infection have never been reported with their use.[11] The presence of parvovirus B19 DNA has been reported in recombinant factor VIII products.[27] First-generation recombinant factor VIII products contain human albumin as a stabilizing protein.[11] Second-generation

TABLE 81-4 Factor Concentrates

Brand Name	Product Type	Viral Inactivation or Exclusion Method	Other Contents
Factor VIII Concentrates			
Alphanate AHF/VWF complex	Plasma	Solvent detergent, dry heat	Albumin, heparin, vWF
Hemofil M AHF	Plasma	Solvent detergent, monoclonal antibody, ion-exchange chromatography	Albumin
Humate-P AHF/VWF complex	Plasma	Pasteurization	Albumin, vWF
Koāte-DVI	Plasma	Solvent detergent, dry heat, gel permeation chromatography	Albumin
Monarc-M	Plasma	Solvent detergent, monoclonal antibody	Albumin
Monoclate P	Plasma	Pasteurization, monoclonal antibody	Albumin
Wilate VWF/FVIII Complex	Plasma	Solvent detergent, dry heat	Sodium citrate, sucrose, vWF
Advate	Recombinant	Solvent detergent, column chromatography, monoclonal antibody	Trehalose
Helixate FS	Recombinant	Solvent detergent, ion-exchange chromatography, monoclonal antibody	Human plasma protein solution (fermentation only); sucrose
Kogenate FS	Recombinant	Solvent detergent, ion-exchange chromatography, monoclonal antibody	Human plasma protein solution (fermentation only); sucrose
Recombinate	Recombinant	Immunoaffinity, chromatography, monoclonal antibody	Albumin
ReFacto B domain deleted	Recombinant	Chromatography	Albumin (fermentation only); sucrose
Xyntha	Recombinant	Chromatography, solvent detergent, nanofiltration	Sucrose
Rixubis	Recombinant	Chromatography, solvent detergent, nanofiltration	Sucrose, mannitol
Factor IX Concentrates			
AlphaNine SD	Plasma	Solvent detergent, nanofiltration	Heparin
Mononine	Plasma	Sodium thiocyanate, dual ultrafiltration	Heparin, mannitol
BeneFix	Recombinant	None	
aPCC			
Feiba VH Immuno	Plasma	Vapor heat	IIa, VIIa, VIIIa, IXa, Xa
PCC			
Bebulin VH	Plasma	Vapor heat	Heparin, II, IX, X
Profilnine S/D	Plasma	Solvent detergent	II, VII, IX, X
Other			
Corifact	Plasma	Heat, precipitation/adsorption, ion exchange chromatography	XIII, albumin
NovoSeven	Recombinant	Solvent detergent	VII

aPCC, activated prothrombin complex concentrate; PCC, prothrombin complex concentrate; vWF, von Willebrand factor.

recombinant factor VIII products add sugar instead of human albumin as a stabilizer, but human albumin is utilized in the culture process. One second-generation product (ReFacto®) has deletion of the B domain of the factor VIII gene, yielding a smaller protein product.[11] This B domain does not appear to be necessary for coagulation function. Third-generation recombinant factor VIII products contain no human protein either in the culture or in the stabilization processes.[24]

Clinical trials have demonstrated that recombinant factor VIII products are comparable in effectiveness to plasma-derived products.[11] The risk of patients with severe hemophilia A developing an inhibitory antibody to factor VIII with use of recombinant factor VIII is 25% to 32%.[28] The risk of inhibitor formation has been reported to be higher in recombinant products as compared with plasma-derived products. In studies of previously untreated patients, the cumulative incidence of inhibitor formation was 10.3% for plasma-derived versus 28.7% for recombinant products.[29] However, it is difficult to compare the cumulative incidence from different studies because of differences in patient population (e.g., heterogeneity in risk factors for inhibitor formation), study methodology, frequency of inhibitor testing, and length of follow-up.[29] Two recent systematic reviews attempted to control for the heterogeneity in studies and were unable to demonstrate a difference in the risk of inhibitor formation.[30,31] In the review by Iorio et al., most of the apparent difference in risk of inhibitor formation was explained by differences in study design, study period, testing frequency, and median follow-up. The source of factor concentrate (recombinant vs. plasma-derived) was not statistically significant.[31] To address this very important clinical question, a prospective international randomized clinical trial (SIPPET—Survey of Inhibitors in Plasma Product Exposed Toddlers) is currently enrolling patients and is comparing inhibitor incidence in previously untreated patients exposed to either plasma or recombinant factor products.[32]

Plasma-Derived Factor VIII Products

Several different plasma-derived factor VIII products are available (Table 81-4). These products are derived from the pooled plasma of thousands of donors and therefore potentially can transmit infection. Donor screening, testing plasma pools for evidence of infection, viral reduction through purification steps, and viral inactivation procedures (e.g., dry heat, pasteurization, and solvent detergent treatment) have resulted in a safer product. No cases of HIV transmission from factor concentrates have been reported since 1986.[11] However, isolated cases of hepatitis C infection with use of plasma-derived products have been reported.[11] Additionally, outbreaks of hepatitis A viral infections associated with plasma-derived products, likely because solvent detergent treatment does not inactivate this nonenveloped virus, have been reported. Parvovirus has been reported to be present in both plasma-derived and recombinant factor VIII products.[26,27] Finally, possible infection with as yet unidentified viruses that currently used methods would not inactivate remains a concern. In addition, Prion disease may be present in plasma-derived factor VIII products.[26,33]

Factor VIII concentrates can be classified according to their level of purity, which refers to the specific activity of factor VIII in the product. Cryoprecipitate is a low-purity product. Cryoprecipitate also contains von Willebrand factor, fibrinogen, and factor XIII. Current American Association of Blood Banks standards call for a minimum of 80 international units of factor VIII per cryoprecipitate pack.[11] This product is no longer considered a primary treatment of factor VIII deficiency in countries where factor VIII concentrates are available because cryoprecipitate does not undergo a viral inactivation process. Intermediate-purity products have a specific factor VIII activity of 5 units/mg of protein and high-purity products have up to 2,000 units/mg of protein.[11] Ultrahigh-purity plasma-derived products are prepared with monoclonal antibody purification steps and have a specific activity of 3,000 units/mg of protein prior to addition of albumin as a stabilizer.

Factor VIII Concentrate Replacement

Appropriate dosing of factor VIII concentrate depends on the half-life of the infused factor, the patient's body weight, and the volume of distribution. The presence or absence of an inhibitory antibody to factor VIII and the titer of this antibody also influence treatment. Recovery studies, which measure the immediate postinfusion factor level, and survival studies, which assess the half-life of the factor, can establish patient-specific pharmacokinetics. The location and magnitude of the bleeding episode determine the percent correction to target as well as the duration of treatment. Serious or life-threatening bleeding requires peak factor levels of greater than 0.75 to 1 units/mL (75% to 100%); less severe bleeding may be treated with a goal of 0.3 to 0.5 units/mL (30% to 50%) peak plasma levels. Table 81-5 provides general guidelines for the management of bleeding in different locations.

Factor VIII is a large molecule that remains in the intravascular space. Therefore, the plasma volume (about 50 mL/kg) can be used to estimate the volume of distribution. In general, each unit of factor VIII concentrate infused per kilogram of actual body weight yields a 2% rise in plasma factor VIII levels. The following equation can be used to calculate an initial dose of factor VIII:

$$\text{Factor VIII (units)} = (\text{Desired level} - \text{Baseline level}) \times 0.5 \times (\text{Weight [in kilograms]})$$

The baseline level usually is omitted from the equation when it is negligible compared to the desired level. The half-life of factor VIII ranges from 8 to 15 hours. It is generally necessary to administer 50% of the initial dose about every 12 hours to sustain the desired level of factor VIII. A single treatment may be adequate for minor bleeding, such as oral bleeding or slight muscle hemorrhages. However, because of the potential for long-term joint damage with hemarthroses, 2 or 3 days of treatment is often recommended for these bleeds. Serious bleeding episodes may require maintenance of 70% to 100% factor activity for 1 week or longer. As previously mentioned, factor VIII dosing depends on several variables, and each case must be considered individually. Individual pharmacokinetics may help guide treatment, particularly for serious bleeding episodes.

Alternatively, factor VIII can be administered as a continuous infusion when prolonged treatment is required (e.g., in the perioperative period or for serious bleeding episodes). Infusion rates ranging from 2 to 4 units/kg per hour usually are given in fixed-dose continuous infusion protocols, with the aim of maintaining a steady-state level of 60% to 100%.[34,35] Administration of factor concentrate via continuous infusion may reduce factor requirements by 20% to 50% because unnecessarily high peaks of factor VIII that occur with bolus injections are avoided.[35] A gradual decrease in factor VIII clearance during the first 5 to 6 days of treatment contributes to the lower factor concentrate requirements.[35] Daily monitoring of factor level can help determine the appropriate rate of infusion.

Administration of factor VIII concentrate via continuous infusion has been shown to be safe and effective, and it may be more convenient than bolus therapy for hospitalized patients.[34,35] The advantages of continuous infusion include maintenance of a steady-state plasma level with avoidance of potentially subtherapeutic trough levels and reduced cost associated with decreased factor requirements. A potential side effect with continuous infusion is thrombophlebitis at the delivery site. Concomitant infusion of saline or the addition of heparin (2 to 5 units/mL) to the infusion bag can minimize this risk.[35] Bacterial contamination of the concentrate is another theoretical concern and preparation of the infusion bag should occur under sterile conditions (i.e., under laminar flow).[35] Finally, concerns about the stability of the formulations appear to

TABLE 81-5 Guidelines for Factor Replacement Therapy for Hemorrhage in Hemophilia A and B

Site of Hemorrhage	Desired Hemostatic Factor Level (% of Normal)	Comments
Joint	50%–70%, 2–3 days	Rest/immobilization/physical therapy rehabilitation following bleed; several doses may be necessary to prevent or treat target joint
Muscle	30%–50% for most sites 70%–100% for thigh, iliopsoas, or nerve compression	Risk of significant blood loss with a thigh or iliopsoas bleed; bed rest for iliopsoas or thigh bleeding
Oral mucosa	30%–50%	May try antifibrinolytic or topical thrombin prior to factor replacement for minor bleeding; higher factor levels are needed for tongue swelling or risk of airway compromise; antifibrinolytic therapy should be used following factor replacement
GI	Initially 100%, then 40%–60%	Endoscopy is highly recommended; antifibrinolytic therapy may be useful. Continue until healing occurs
Hematuria	30%–50% if no trauma 70%–100% if traumatic	If no pain or trauma, consider bed rest and fluids for 24 hours; factor should be given if hematuria persists; evaluate if hematuria persists; if trauma to abdomen or back, perform imaging and give aggressive factor replacement
CNS	Initially 100%, then 50%–100% for 10–21 days	Lumbar puncture requires prophylactic factor coverage
Trauma or surgery	Initially 100%, then 50%–100% until wound healing complete	Perioperative and postoperative management plan must be in place preoperatively; evaluation for inhibitors is crucial prior to elective surgery

aPCC, activated prothrombin complex concentrate; PCC, prothrombin complex concentrate.

be unwarranted, as most high-purity factor VIII concentrates have been shown to remain stable for at least 7 days after reconstitution.[35] Exposure of factor VIII to light for 10 hours after reconstitution can decrease activity by 30%.[35] Therefore, it would be prudent to shield the container with foil wrap or an appropriate bag.

Other Pharmacologic Therapy

Treatment with desmopressin acetate often is adequate for minor bleeding episodes in patients with mild hemophilia A. A synthetic analog of the antidiuretic hormone vasopressin, desmopressin, causes release of von Willebrand factor and factor VIII from endogenous endothelial storage sites. It appears to be most effective in patients with higher baseline factor VIII levels (0.1 to 0.15 units/mL).[36] The recommended dose of desmopressin is 0.3 mcg/kg diluted in 50 mL of normal saline and infused IV over 15 to 30 minutes.[36] Patients with mild or moderate hemophilia A should undergo a desmopressin trial to determine their response to this medication. At least a twofold rise in factor VIII to a minimal level of 0.3 units/mL within 60 minutes is considered an adequate response.[37] In adults with mild hemophilia A, the response rate to desmopressin has been reported to be 80% to 90%.[37] Pediatric studies have reported a lower rate of response ranging from 40% to 47%.[37] Furthermore, the pediatric response rate was related to age; some nonresponding children became responders at an older age.[37]

Infusion of desmopressin can be repeated daily for up to 2 to 3 days. Tachyphylaxis, an attenuated response with repeated dosing, may develop after that time. The factor increase after the second dose of desmopressin is about 30% lower than after the initial dose.[36] Factor concentrate therapy may be necessary if the patient requires additional treatment. Factor levels should be measured to ensure that an adequate response has been achieved. Treatment with desmopressin will not result in hemostasis in patients who have severe hemophilia and those who are only marginally responsive. Desmopressin should not be used as primary therapy for life-threatening bleeding episodes such as intracranial hemorrhage or for major surgical procedures when a minimum and sustained factor VIII concentration of 0.7 to 1 units/mL is required.

Desmopressin can be administered intranasally via a concentrated nasal spray.[36] It elicits a slower and less marked response, with a peak effect in 60 to 90 minutes after administration, which is somewhat longer than with IV administration.[36,37] The dosage is one spray (150 mcg) for patients who weigh less than 50 kg and two sprays (300 mcg) for those who weigh more than 50 kg.[37] The nasal spray may serve as an alternative to the IV formulation, especially in patients with mild bleeding episodes.

Few adverse effects are associated with desmopressin. The most commonly observed side effect is facial flushing.[36] Less frequently reported side effects include mild headaches, increased heart rate, and decreased blood pressure. Thrombosis is a rare complication associated with desmopressin.[37] Because of its antidiuretic effects, desmopressin has the potential to cause water retention, which may lead to severe hyponatremia. This may be a particular problem in children younger than 2 years, in whom hyponatremic seizures have been reported.[36] Therefore, desmopressin should be used with caution in this age group.[37] Patients with congestive heart failure may be at increased risk for developing hyponatremia with use of desmopressin.[37] Fluid restriction for 24 hours after the desmopressin dose and monitoring of urine output are recommended with desmopressin administration.[37]

Antifibrinolytic therapy inhibits clot lysis and therefore is a useful adjunctive therapy for the treatment of hemophilia. Antifibrinolytic agents are particularly beneficial for treatment of oral bleeding because of a high concentration of fibrinolytic enzymes in saliva. Antifibrinolytic therapy can also be helpful as adjuvant therapy in GI bleeding, epistaxis, or menorrhagia. The two currently available antifibrinolytics include aminocaproic acid and tranexamic acid. Aminocaproic acid is given at a dosage of 100 mg/kg (maximum 6 g) every 6 hours and can be administered orally or IV.[11] The dosage of tranexamic acid is 25 mg/kg (maximum 1.5 g) orally every 6 to 8 hours.[11]

Hemophilia B

Therapeutic options for hemophilia B have improved greatly over the past several years, first with the development of monoclonal antibody-purified plasma-derived products and then with the licensure of recombinant factor IX. Products currently available in the United States for treatment of hemophilia B are listed in Table 81-4.

Recombinant Factor IX

Recombinant factor IX was not available until 1998, which is 6 years after the first recombinant factor VIII product.[38] Recombinant factor IX is produced in Chinese hamster ovary cells transfected with the factor IX gene. Blood and plasma products are not used to produce recombinant factor IX or to stabilize the final product; thus, recombinant factor IX has an excellent viral safety profile.[11,38] Clinical trials have shown the product to be safe and efficacious in the treatment of acute bleeding episodes and in the management of bleeding associated with surgical procedures.[11,38] Although the half-life of recombinant factor IX is similar to that of the plasma-derived products, recovery is about 30% lower.[38] As a result, doses of recombinant factor IX concentrate must be higher than those of plasma-derived products to achieve equivalent plasma levels. Because individual pharmacokinetics may vary, recovery and survival studies should be performed to determine optimal treatment.[11] Recombinant factor IX is considered the treatment of choice for hemophilia B.

Plasma-Derived Factor IX Products

High-purity factor IX plasma concentrates have been available in the United States since the early 1990s.[11,38] These products are derived from plasma through biochemical purification and monoclonal immunoaffinity techniques. Other viral inactivation measures, such as solvent detergent or chemical treatment, are also used.

Before the high-purity products were approved for use, hemophilia B patients were treated with factor IX concentrates that also contained other vitamin K-dependent proteins (factors II, VII, and X), known as prothrombin complex concentrates (PCCs). These products contain small amounts of activated factors generated during processing, and their use has been associated with thrombotic complications, including deep-vein thrombosis, pulmonary embolism, myocardial infarction, and disseminated intravascular coagulation.[11,38] The risk of such complications is highest in patients who are receiving high or repeated doses of PCCs, in those who have hepatic disease (the liver removes the activated factors from circulation), in neonates, and in patients who have experienced crush injuries or who are undergoing major surgery.[11,38] Concomitant use of PCCs and antifibrinolytics should be avoided because of the risk for thrombosis.

Because of the lower purity of PCCs and their thrombogenic potential, these products are not first-line treatment of hemophilia B, although they are still used for treatment of patients with hemophilia A or B who have developed inhibitory antibodies against factor VIII or factor IX, respectively. High-purity factor IX concentrates have excellent efficacy in the treatment of bleeding episodes and in the control of bleeding associated with surgical procedures.[38] Their viral safety profile has been reported to be excellent, and the risk of thromboembolic complications is low.[38]

Factor IX Concentrate Replacement

Factor IX is a relatively small protein. Unlike factor VIII, it is not limited to the intravascular space; it also passes into the extravascular compartment.[38] This results in a volume of distribution that is about twice that of factor VIII. For plasma-derived factor IX concentrates, each unit of factor IX infused per kilogram of actual body weight yields about a 1% rise in the plasma level of factor IX (range, 0.67% to 1.28%).[11] The following equation can be used to calculate the initial dose:

Plasma-derived factor IX (units) = (Desired level – Baseline level) × (Weight [in kilograms])

As with the factor VIII dose calculation, the baseline level term can be omitted from the formula if it is negligible compared to the desired level. Because recovery of recombinant factor IX is lower than that of the plasma-derived products, the following adjustment is made:

Pediatric dosing:

Recombinant factor IX (units) = (Desired level – Baseline level) × 1.4 × (Weight [in kilograms]).

Adult dosing:

Recombinant factor IX (units) = (Desired level – Baseline level) × 1.2 × (Weight [in kilograms]).

A recovery study to determine optimal dosing is recommended for patients who receive recombinant factor IX because of the wide interpatient variability in pharmacokinetics.

Because the half-life of factor IX is about 24 hours, dosing can be less frequent than with factor VIII. Table 81-5 provides general guidelines for dosing factor IX based on the site and severity of the bleeding episode.

Prophylactic Replacement Therapy

Traditionally, factor concentrates for hemophilia patients have been given on demand, as the bleeding episode occurs. However, recurrent joint bleeding can damage the joint and lead to the development of severe physical disability. Thus, it would be preferable to prevent bleeding episodes and avoid the resultant damage. Known as *prophylactic factor replacement therapy*, this approach consists of regular infusion of concentrate to maintain the deficient factor at a minimum of 0.01 units/mL (1%). In developed countries, prophylaxis for patients with severe hemophilia is considered standard of care. Patients with moderate hemophilia may sometimes require prophylaxis and it is rarely used in patients with mild hemophilia.

In effect, prophylactic replacement therapy converts severe hemophilia into a milder form of the disease. The rationale for this approach is that patients with moderate hemophilia rarely experience spontaneous hemarthroses, and they have a much lower incidence of chronic arthropathy. Two recent pediatric clinical trials have demonstrated the efficacy of prophylaxis in pediatric patients.[39,40] The first pediatric randomized clinical trial comparing prophylaxis to enhanced episodic treatment to prevent joint disease in boys (age <30 months) with severe hemophilia demonstrated that prophylaxis prevented joint damage and decreased the frequency of joint and other hemorrhages.[41] More recently, a European randomized clinical trial of prophylaxis in pediatric patients with hemophilia A confirmed the efficacy of prophylaxis in preventing bleeds and arthropathy.[39] The efficacy of prophylaxis in adult patients with hemophilia is unclear and is the focus of ongoing clinical trials.

At this time, no consensus exists regarding the timing for the initiation of prophylaxis or the dosing schedule.[25] A common regimen for patients with hemophilia A is 25 to 40 units/kg of factor VIII given every other day or three times per week. For hemophilia B, the usual dosage is 30 to 40 units/kg of factor IX given twice weekly because of the longer half-life of factor IX.[38]

Controversy exists regarding the ideal timing for the initiation of prophylaxis. Primary prophylaxis is regular replacement therapy started at a young age (usually before age 2 years), prior to the onset of joint bleeding.[41] Secondary prophylaxis begins after significant joint bleeding has already occurred.[41] In 2001, the Medical and Scientific Advisory Council of the National Hemophilia Foundation of the United States recommended primary prophylaxis beginning at age 1 to 2 years for children with severe hemophilia. The use of primary prophylaxis has many challenges and has not been widely accepted in the United States. Many institutions continue to use some form of secondary prophylaxis, in which prophylaxis is started after a pattern of bleeding has been established.

Several disadvantages are associated with primary prophylaxis. Perhaps most important is the high cost of prophylactic replacement therapy. Other issues to consider are the inconvenience to families and possible difficulties with compliance. Central venous lines may be necessary for frequent administration of factor concentrates, particularly in children younger than 2 years, who are at the age targeted for initiation of primary prophylaxis regimens. Potential complications of central venous access include surgical risks, infection, and catheter-related deep-vein thrombosis. Catheter-related infections are common in patients with hemophilia and have been reported to occur in up to 0.2 to 2/1,000 catheter days.[42] Catheter-related infections appear to be even more common in hemophilia patients who have developed inhibitory antibodies.[42] Finally, routine use of primary prophylaxis may initially overtreat some patients with severe hemophilia who do not have a severe clinical phenotype.

Clinical **Controversy. . .**

Hemophilia patients may receive prophylactic factor concentrate therapy to prevent or decrease bleeding episodes, or they may receive on-demand factor concentrate therapy in response to a bleeding episode. In addition, prophylaxis may be primary or secondary. Controversy exists over the benefits of prophylaxis in adult patients with hemophilia, appropriate time to initiate prophylaxis in children, and appropriate dosing for prophylaxis.

Treatment of Inhibitors in Hemophilia

Neutralizing antibodies to factor VIII and IX, known as *inhibitors*, develop in a subset of patients with hemophilia. 4 The development of an inhibitor is the most serious complication of factor replacement therapy and is associated with considerable morbidity and a decreased quality of life. The incidence of new factor VIII inhibitors in patients with severe factor VIII deficiency is about 30%.[43] Inhibitors are less common in patients with mild or moderate hemophilia occurring in about 3% to 13% of patients.[44–46] The occurrence of inhibitors in patients with hemophilia B is much lower, occurring in only 1% to 3% of patients.[11]

Most inhibitors develop in childhood, after relatively few exposure days (median 10 to 15 days).[47] Patients with severe hemophilia are much more likely to develop inhibitors than those with milder forms of the disease.[47] It is possible that the low levels of factor produced in patients with mild or moderate hemophilia induce immune tolerance in these individuals. In contrast, factor levels are undetectable in patients with severe hemophilia, so infused factor VIII is regarded as a foreign protein, which may provoke an antibody response. The rate of inhibitor formation varies even among patients with identical mutations, which suggests that host factors modify the risk. The development of an inhibitor is the result of a complex interaction between a patient's immune system and genetic and environmental risk factors.

An inhibitor is a polyclonal high-affinity immunoglobulin G (IgG), directed against the factor VIII or IX protein.[48,49] Inhibitors interfere with infused factor concentrate rendering them ineffective. The presence of an inhibitor is suspected when a decreased clinical response to factor replacement is observed, or it may be discovered incidentally on routine laboratory screening. Inhibitors are measured with the Bethesda assay, and titers are reported in Bethesda units (BUs). One BU is the amount of inhibitor needed to inactivate half of the factor VIII or factor IX in a mixture of inhibitor-containing plasma and pooled normal plasma.[11] Patients with inhibitors to factor VIII or factor IX are divided into two groups: low responders, who have low levels of inhibitors (<5 BU/mL) and generally have little or no rise in antibody titers after exposure to the factor; and high responders (>5 BU/mL), who have higher inhibitor levels and develop an increase in antibody titer after exposure (anamnestic response).[50]

Therapy for patients with inhibitors involves treatment of acute bleeding episodes and treatment directed at eradicating the inhibitor. The inhibitor titer, the site and magnitude of bleeding, and the patient's past response to bypassing therapy determine the approach to the treatment of acute bleeding. For patients with a low inhibitor titer, administration of high doses of the specific factor often can control bleeding episodes. Two to three times the usual replacement dose and more frequent dosing intervals are often necessary to overcome the antibody. Factor-level monitoring and clinical assessments help to evaluate the adequacy of treatment. Additional supportive measures, such as immobilization and administration of antifibrinolytic agents, should be used, where appropriate.

In the presence of a high-titer inhibitor, it is impossible to administer enough factor VIII or factor IX to neutralize the antibody and achieve a hemostatic plasma level. Therefore, the treatment of bleeding episodes consists of using agents that bypass the factor to which the antibody is directed. These bypassing agents include prothrombin complex concentrates (PCCs), activated prothrombin complex concentrates (aPCCs), and recombinant factor VIIa.

PCCs contain the vitamin K-dependent factors II, VII, IX, and X. Small quantities of activated factors are present in these products. Activated aPCCs contain greater quantities of the activated factors primarily factor X and prothrombin.[51] The recommended dosage for aPCCs is 50 to 100 units/kg administered every 8 to 12 hours, depending on the severity of the bleeding episode and the maximum dose should not exceed 200 units/kg/day.[51] Activated PCCs appear to be more effective than PCCs and are preferred in patients with inhibitors. As previously mentioned, there is a risk of serious thrombotic complications, including pulmonary emboli, deep-vein thrombosis, and myocardial infarction associated with use of PCCs and aPCCs.[51] Additionally, because these products contain trace amounts of factor VIII and larger amounts of factor IX, they can stimulate an anamnestic response in patients with hemophilia A and, more commonly, in those with hemophilia B.[51] Other minor side effects include dizziness, nausea, hives, flushing, and headaches. Patients with factor IX inhibitors occasionally develop severe allergic reactions in response to infusion of factor IX-containing products, so these patients should be monitored closely.[38]

Recombinant factor VIIa, a bypassing agent, is thought to be hemostatically active only at the site of tissue injury where the tissue factor is present.[52] Recombinant factor VIIa is not a plasma-derived product, so both viral transmission and anamnestic responses to factor VIII or factor IX are unlikely.[51] The initial recommended dose for bleeding episodes is 90 mcg/kg.[51] However, depending on a patient's response to recombinant factor VIIa, higher doses up to 300 mcg/kg are used. A drawback is the product's short half-life, which necessitates dosing every 2 hours. Continuous infusion of recombinant factor VIIa, which may be more convenient and cost-effective, has been reported, although studies are limited. Patients treated with bypassing agents must be monitored clinically because no laboratory test directly measures the effectiveness of treatment.

Both recombinant factor VIIa and aPCCs have been demonstrated to be effective in the treatment of bleeding for patients with inhibitors.[53–58] A randomized crossover trial of recombinant factor VIIa versus an aPCC (FEIBA) assessed patient-reported efficacy 6 hours after treatment and did not demonstrate statistical equivalence between the two products.[59] However, the confidence interval of the difference only slightly exceeded the 15% boundary (−11.4% to 15.7%, $P = 0.59$).[59] The efficacy between products was rated quite differently by many of the subjects, which shows significant variability in their individual hemostatic response to bypassing agents.

In determining which bypassing product to use in an individual patient, the clinician must consider multiple factors. In a patient with a newly diagnosed inhibitor where the inhibitor titer needs to fall before initiating immune tolerance induction (ITI), it is prudent to use recombinant factor VIIa because aPCCs contain a small amount of factor VIII or IX and have been shown to increase the inhibitor titer. It is also important to consider an individual's response to specific bypassing agents because of the significant variability in response between individuals. In some patients, bleeding can be unresponsive to monotherapy and may require alternating products.[60] Due to the risk of developing thrombosis or disseminated intravascular coagulation from alternating bypassing agents, this therapy should be used with caution and only in an inpatient setting.[61]

In the past, porcine factor VIII was an alternative therapeutic option for patients who have hemophilia A and inhibitors. Porcine factor VIII is not currently available, although a recombinant version is in development.[62] It was removed from the market secondary to contamination with porcine parvovirus.[51] The rationale is that porcine factor VIII is enough like human factor VIII to participate in the coagulation cascade, yet most factor VIII inhibitors have absent or only weak neutralizing activity against nonhuman factor VIII. However cross-reactivity with porcine factor VIII does occur, and a high titer of antibody against porcine factor VIII can develop.

The current hemostatic therapies for patients with an inhibitor have limited effectiveness leading to significant morbidity and a decreased quality of life. The ideal therapy for patients with an inhibitor is total eradication so that optimal hemostatic treatment with either factor VIII or IX is possible. At this time, the only proven method for inhibitor eradication is ITI, which involves the regular infusion of high doses of the factor to induce antigen-specific tolerance.

The majority of ITI data are from patients with hemophilia A. Multiple immune tolerance registries were established to help determine patient- and treatment-related factors associated with immune tolerance outcome.[63–67] Across these registries, a patient's peak historical FVIII inhibitor titer (<200 BU) and the inhibitor titer at the time of ITI induction (<10 BU) were associated with successful immune tolerance. The overall ITI success rate from these registries ranged from 51% to 79%.[63–67] This wide range is likely related to a lack of standardization in study methodologies, treatment protocols, and eradication definitions.

There are conflicting data regarding the ITI factor VIII dose and success of ITI. A variety of different dosing regimens, ranging from 25 units/kg every other day to more than 200 units/kg every day, have been used. The International Immune Tolerance Registry demonstrated improved ITI success with high doses (200 IU/kg), while the North American and Spanish Immune Tolerance Registries demonstrated improved success with lower dosing strategies.[64,65,67] The International Immune Tolerance Study is a multicenter randomized clinical trial that compared high-dose (200 units/kg/day) to low-dose (50 units/kg three times/week) regimens in patients with severe hemophilia A and high titer inhibitors (>5 BU).[68] This study was stopped early due an increased risk of bleeding events in the low-dose arm. At the stopping point, the proportion of ITI success was not significantly different between the two arms, but the time to achieve ITI success was shorter in the high-dose arm. Because the study was stopped early, it lacked statistical power to demonstrate therapeutic equivalence below the 30% boundary of equivalence. It appears that a high-dose strategy achieves tolerance at a faster rate, which explains the lower bleeding rate.

Although not commonly used in ITI protocols, immune modulation has been reported as a method to improve tolerance success. In Sweden, the Malmo protocol uses a combination of immunoabsorption (to acutely decrease the factor VIII inhibitor titer), cyclophosphamide, IV immunoglobulin, and daily high dose factor VIII.[69] The benefit appears to be decreased time to tolerance, but the overall success rate is comparable to other ITI protocols without the risks associated with immune modulation.[70] Rituximab, an anti-CD20 monoclonal antibody that inhibits B-cells and interferes with IgG production, has been used with some success. A phase II single-arm clinical trial used rituximab as a single agent in patients with high titer inhibitors. Only 3 out of 16 subjects (18.8%) had a major response (decline in the inhibitor to <5 BU without an increase in the inhibitor titer after re-challenge to factor VIII).[71] It appears that as a single agent in previously treated patients with inhibitors, rituximab had a small effect but further studies are needed to determine if rituximab could be more effective if used with ITI.

Figure 81-1 summarizes the therapeutic options in the management of hemophilia A patients with inhibitors. The same algorithm can be applied to the management of hemophilia B patients, except that factor IX should be substituted for factor VIII.

Gene Therapy in Hemophilia

Hemophilia is an excellent candidate for gene therapy because tight control of gene expression is not required. Even low levels of factor expression can reduce bleeding episodes in patients with severe hemophilia, which is similar to the rationale of prophylactic factor replacement. Gene therapy for the treatment of hemophilia remains in the early clinical stages. Advances at this time are most apparent in hemophilia B. Recently, a landmark clinical trial reporting the results of a single peripheral venous infusion of an adenovirus associated factor IX transgene vector under the control of a liver-restricted promoter in six patients with severe hemophilia B was published.[72] All of the study subjects demonstrated long-term (over 2 years) expression of the factor IX transgene with therapeutic levels of factor IX (plateau factor IX levels from 1% to 6%).[72,73] At this time, gene therapy for factor VIII deficiency has not progressed to human clinical trials. Potential benefits to gene therapy include patient convenience, viral safety, and decreased cost. Possible drawbacks to gene therapy include a risk of inhibitor formation, tumorigenesis related to possible integration of the viral vector, possible germ-line transmission of the viral vector, and concerns about long-term gene expression.

Pain Management in Hemophilia

Pain, both acute and chronic, can be a common occurrence in patients with hemophilia. The most likely cause of acute pain is bleeding, and treatment should include factor replacement to stop the bleeding, and RICE (Rest, Ice, Compression, Elevation).[74] Acetaminophen can be used for mild pain, although narcotic analgesia may be required for more severe pain. Nonsteroidal anti-inflammatory drugs impair platelet function and may increase bleeding and should not be used during acute bleeding episodes.

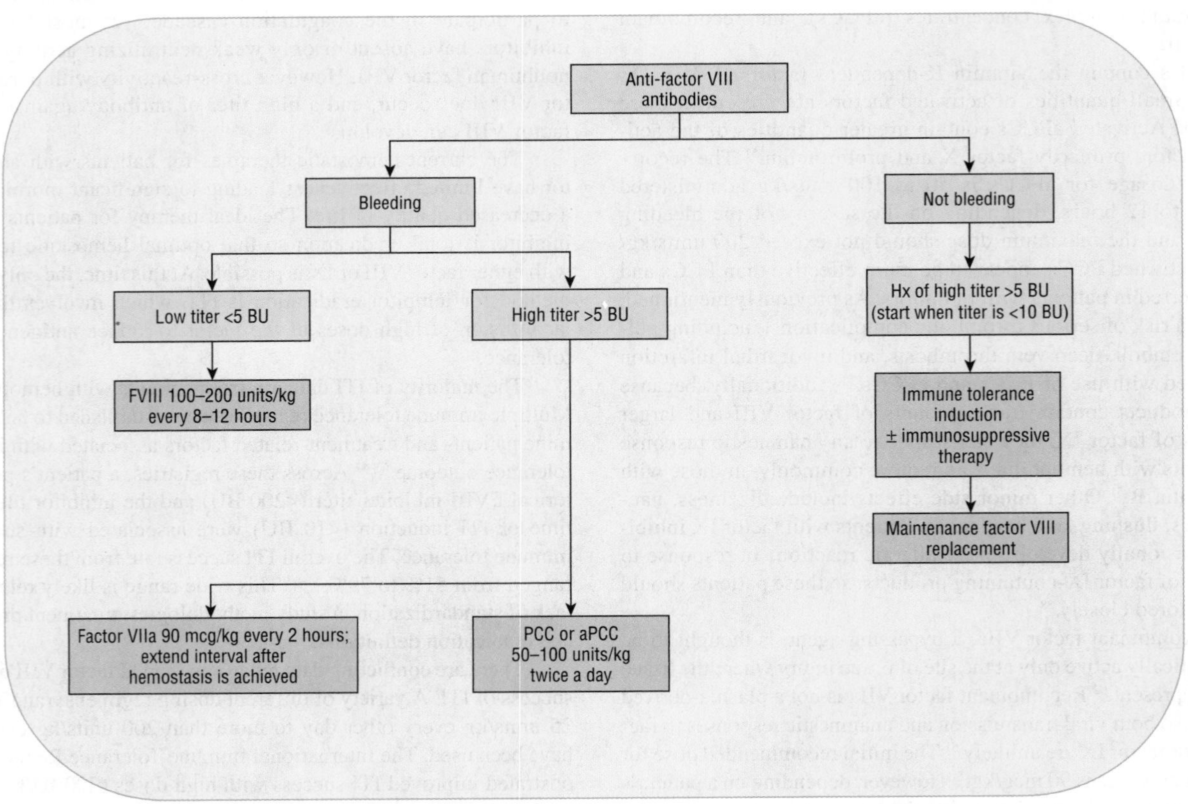

FIGURE 81-1 Treatment algorithm for the management of patients with hemophilia A and factor VIII antibodies. (aPCC, activated prothrombin complex concentrate; BU, Bethesda unit; PCC, prothrombin complex concentrate.)

Cyclooxygenase-2 inhibitors have less antiplatelet activity and are an option for acute pain management.[74]

Chronic pain in patients with hemophilia is typically secondary to hemophilic arthropathy. Hemophilic arthropathy is the direct result of recurrent hemarthrosis. Persistent blood in the joint leads to inflammation, synovial hypertrophy and inflammation, cartilage destruction, and finally bony erosion.[75] Cyclooxygenase-2 inhibitors can also be helpful in managing chronic pain. Surgical interventions may help to alleviate chronic pain. Synovectomy (removal of the hypertrophied synovium) can reduce chronic pain from recurrent bleeding. Patients with more advanced joint disease could benefit from joint replacement.

Surgery in Hemophilia

In the patient with hemophilia undergoing a surgical procedure, the goal of treatment is maintaining factor levels of at least 0.5 to 0.7 units/mL (50% to 70%) during surgery and in the postoperative period in order to prevent excessive bleeding. Intermittent dosing or continuous infusion factor replacement may accomplish this goal. Before surgery, factor concentrate usually is infused to obtain a plasma level of 1 unit/mL (100%). Replacement therapy is continued to maintain plasma levels greater than 0.5 units/mL (50%) for 5 to 7 days or longer, depending on the type of surgery. Preoperative evaluation for elective procedures should include measurement of an inhibitor titer and assessment of the recovery and half-life of infused factor in the patient.

Personalized Pharmacotherapy

The newest approach in hemophilia treatment is "personalized" prophylaxis.[76] Traditionally, standard prophylaxis is prescribed based on a weight-based calculation to increase a patient's trough factor level to greater than 0.01 units/mL (1%). While this approach is successful for many patients, some may still experience breakthrough bleeding. Demonstrating that a single prophylactic regimen is unlikely to be optimal for all patients and that prophylactic dosing and timing may need to be altered to optimally prevent bleeding. Many factors can contribute to breakthrough bleeding including the patient's activity level, individual pharmacokinetics, the presence of a target joint, synovial hypertrophy, and the degree of hemophilic arthropathy present.[76] The prophylaxis regimen should take into account these factors and be adjusted accordingly.

With inhibitor formation as the most significant treatment complication in hemophilia, targeted pharmacotherapy is being evaluated to decrease a patient's risk of inhibitor formation. For example, researchers are working to identify immunodominant epitopes in FVIII that could lead to the creation of new therapeutic FVIII products for high-risk individuals.[77]

Evaluation of Therapeutic Outcomes

The main goal in the treatment of hemophilia is to control and prevent bleeding episodes and their long-term sequelae, such as chronic arthropathies. Pharmacologic and nonpharmacologic interventions should be aimed at achieving this goal. Treatment response can be monitored through clinical parameters, such as cessation of bleeding and resolution of symptoms. Monitoring plasma factor levels also may be helpful, particularly for severe bleeding episodes. Home therapy for administration of factor concentrates is common among patients with hemophilia because this approach can lead to earlier treatment and more independence for the patient. Diaries in which the patient documents symptoms, the dose of factor replacement, adjuvant therapies used, and treatment response can help the caregiver evaluate the success of home therapy. Monitoring the number and type of bleeding episodes and trough plasma factor levels makes it possible to evaluate the adequacy of prophylactic regimens. Physical examination with evaluation of joint range of motion and radiographic imaging of target joints indicates the long-term success of preventing and treating arthropathies.

Clinicians should check for the development of inhibitors, especially in patients with severe disease and exposure to factor concentrates, at least yearly and with any suspicion of poor treatment response. The development of inhibitors challenges the management and control of bleeding episodes. A full understanding of the clinical situation and the titer of the inhibitor are mandatory to address all treatment options for each patient. Because no laboratory test measures the effectiveness of bypassing therapy in patients with inhibitors, close clinical monitoring for worsening or resolution of symptoms is essential for optimizing the outcome.

VON WILLEBRAND DISEASE

The most common congenital bleeding disorder in the United States and in the world, von Willebrand disease, has a prevalence of 1% to 2%.[78,79] von Willebrand disease refers to a family of disorders caused by a quantitative and/or qualitative defect of von Willebrand factor, a glycoprotein that plays a role in both platelet aggregation and coagulation (Table 81-6). von Willebrand factor mediates platelet adhesion to injured blood vessel sites and promotes platelet aggregation. It binds factor VIII and protects it from degradation by plasma proteases, thus prolonging its half-life. Unlike hemophilia, von Willebrand disease has an autosomal inheritance pattern, resulting in an equal frequency of disease in males and females.

The gene for von Willebrand factor is located on chromosome 12 and is 178 kb in length.[80,81] Transcription and translation produce a large primary product that subsequently undergoes complex modifications, resulting in von Willebrand factor multimers of various sizes with molecular weights ranging from 500 to 20,000 kDa.[82] von Willebrand factor is synthesized in endothelial cells, where it is either stored in Weibel–Palade bodies or secreted constitutively.[83] It also is synthesized in megakaryocytes and stored in α-granules, from which it is released following platelet activation.

von Willebrand factor is important for both primary and secondary hemostasis. In response to vascular injury, it promotes platelet adhesion by interacting with the glycoprotein Ib receptor on platelets.[80,83] It can facilitate platelet aggregation by binding to the platelet glycoprotein IIb/IIIa receptor, although fibrinogen is the main ligand for this receptor.[80] The highest-molecular-weight von Willebrand factor multimers appear to be the most important in platelet adhesion because their large surface area contains numerous binding sites for various ligands and receptors. An additional function of von Willebrand factor is that it is the carrier molecule for circulating factor VIII, protecting it from premature degradation and removal.[84] A deficiency of von Willebrand factor reduces

TABLE 81-6 von Willebrand Disease

von Willebrand factor (vWF)
Large multimeric glycoprotein that is necessary for normal platelet adhesion, normal bleeding time, and stabilizing factor VIII

von Willebrand factor antigen (vWF:Ag)
Antigenic determinant(s) on vWF measured by immunoassays; usually low in types 1 and 2; virtually absent in type 3

Ristocetin cofactor activity (RCo)
Functional assay of vWF activity based on platelet aggregation with ristocetin. Reduced by the same degree as vWF:Ag in types 1 and 3, but to a greater extent in type 2 disease (except 2B)

TABLE 81-7 von Willebrand Disease Classification and Laboratory Values *(Modified from Nichols 2009)*

Condition	Description	vWF-RCo (IU/dL)	vWF-Ag (IU/dL)	FVIII	vWF-RCo/vWF-Ag ratio
Definite Type 1	Partial quantitative vWF deficiency	<30	<30	↓ or Normal	>0.5–0.7
"Probable type 1"		30–50	30–50	Normal	>0.5–0.7
Type 2A	↓ vWF-dependent platelet adhesion with selective deficiency of high-MW vWF multimer	<30	<30–200	↓ or Normal	<0.5–0.7
Type 2B	↑ vWF affinity for platelet GP 1b; + ↓ platelet numbers	<30	<30–200	↓ or Normal	Usually <0.5–0.7
Type 2M	↓ vWF-dependent platelet adhesion without selective deficiency of high MW vWF multimers	<30	<30–200	↓ or Normal	<0.5–0.7
Type 2N	Markedly ↓ vWF binding affinity for FVIII	30–200	30–200	↓↓	>0.5–0.7
Type 3	Virtually complete deficiency of vWF	<3	<3	↓↓↓ (<10 IU/DL)	Not applicable
Normal		50–200	50–200	Normal	>0.5–0.7

vWF, von Willebrand factor; RCo, ristocetin cofactor.

the half-life of factor VIII and decreases plasma factor VIII levels. Therefore, von Willebrand factor plays a dual role in hemostasis, affecting both platelet function and coagulation.

Classification of von Willebrand Disease

von Willebrand disease consists of a heterogeneous group of disorders that can be classified into three major subtypes. The National Institutes of Health has developed a classification scheme that characterizes von Willebrand disease according to both the quantity of the von Willebrand clotting factors and their functionality (Table 81-7). Types 1 and 3 are associated with quantitative defects in von Willebrand factor; type 2 mutations refer to functional abnormalities in von Willebrand factor.[85] Determination of the disease subtype is important because it influences treatment.

Type 1 von Willebrand disease is the most common type, accounting for 60% to 70% of cases.[78,86] It is characterized by a mild-to-moderate reduction in the level of von Willebrand factor (although its multimeric structure is normal) and a similar reduction in the level of factor VIII. It usually is inherited in an autosomal-dominant fashion with variable penetrance and expression.[87] Bleeding symptoms often are very mild to moderate.[84] Patients with von Willebrand disease can experience easy bruising, nosebleeds, or other mucosal bleeding such as GI or heavy menstrual bleeding. Subjects may be at risk of bleeding following surgery, traumatic injury, or childbirth.[78]

Type 2 von Willebrand disease, diagnosed in 9% to 30% of affected patients, is characterized by a qualitative abnormality of von Willebrand factor.[84] Bleeding manifestations may be more severe than with type 1 disease. Inheritance most often is autosomal dominant but may be recessive.[87] Type 2 von Willebrand disease can be subdivided into four variants. Type 2A is the most frequent subtype and is characterized by a reduced von Willebrand factor–platelet interaction and an absence of high- and intermediate-molecular-weight factor multimers. Type 2B is a less common variant characterized by an abnormal von Willebrand factor that has an increased affinity for the platelet glycoprotein Ib receptor. This subtype is associated with thrombocytopenia, which usually is mild. In addition, there usually is an absence of high-molecular-weight forms of von Willebrand factor. Type 2M arises from a qualitative defect in von Willebrand factor that impairs its binding to platelets; it is similar to type 2A, except that there is no measurable reduction in the high-molecular-weight multimers.[87] Finally, type 2N von Willebrand disease (Normandy) is a rare form of the disease in which von Willebrand factor has a markedly reduced affinity for factor VIII. This subtype leads to a moderate-to-severe reduction of factor VIII plasma levels with normal von Willebrand factor levels.[87]

Type 3 von Willebrand disease refers to a severe quantitative variant of the disease in which von Willebrand factor is nearly undetectable and factor VIII levels are very low (<20 IU/dL). It often is inherited in an autosomal recessive fashion.[84,86] Type 3 von Willebrand disease is rare, affecting only about 1 person in 1,000,000.[78] The clinical phenotype is severe, reflecting major deficits in primary hemostasis and coagulation.

There is a platelet-type pseudo-von Willebrand disease in which von Willebrand factor is normal but a defect in the platelet glycoprotein Ib receptor causes an increased affinity for normal von Willebrand factor.[84] As a result, platelet-type pseudo-von Willebrand disease is phenotypically similar to type 2B disease but should be distinguished from it because the treatment is different.

Acquired von Willebrand disease is a rare bleeding disorder that is similar to the congenital form of the disease. It has been reported primarily in association with autoimmune disorders, such as systemic lupus erythematosus, lymphoproliferative disorders, myeloproliferative disorders, hypothyroidism, and certain neoplastic diseases such as Wilms' tumor and lymphoma.[84,88] It has been reported in situations of high shear stress, such as aortic stenosis. Certain medications have been associated with acquired von Willebrand disease, including valproic acid, griseofulvin, hydroxyethyl starch, and ciprofloxacin.[88] Bleeding manifestations vary from mild to severe, and the condition often resolves with treatment of the underlying disease. Various mechanisms have been proposed, including autoantibodies to von Willebrand factor resulting in rapid removal from the plasma, adsorption to tumor cells or activated platelets, increased proteolysis, or mechanical destruction.[88]

CLINICAL PRESENTATION von Willebrand Disease

- Clinical manifestations are variable; some patients are asymptomatic
- Mucocutaneous bleeding: epistaxis, gingival bleeding with minor manipulation, menorrhagia
- Easy bruising
- Postoperative bleeding

TABLE 81-8 Replacement Therapy in von Willebrand Disease[a]

Condition	Therapy
Major surgery	Maintain factor VIII level ≥50% for 1 week Prolonged treatment in type 3 patients (>7 days)
Minor surgery	Maintain factor VIII level ≥50% for 1–3 days Maintain factor VIII level >20%–30% for an additional 4–7 days
Dental extraction	Single infusion to achieve factor VIII level >50% Desmopressin prior to procedure for type I
Spontaneous or posttraumatic bleeding	Usually single infusion of 20–40 units/kg

[a]The yield of Factor VIII after first infusion is similar to that observed in hemophilia A (about 2% increment over baseline amount for every 1 unit/kg of factor VIII infused).

Diagnosis

When a patient has a lifelong history of mucocutaneous bleeding and a family history of abnormal bleeding, the clinician should suspect von Willebrand disease. For a review of clinical questions to ask the patient, refer to the National Heart, Lung, and Blood Institute guidelines (Table 81-8).[78] Several different laboratory tests are helpful in the diagnosis of this hemostatic abnormality. Initial screening tests include determinations of PT, activated partial thromboplastin time (aPTT), and platelet count. PT is normal, whereas aPTT may be normal or prolonged in relation to the reduction in plasma factor VIII levels. A normal aPTT does not rule out von Willebrand disease; specific laboratory assessment of the von Willebrand factor is required. The platelet count usually is normal, although thrombocytopenia is common in type 2B and platelet-type pseudo-von Willebrand disease. The bleeding time or PFA-100 may be prolonged but can be normal in patients with milder forms of the disease.

Specific laboratory tests for the diagnosis of von Willebrand disease include measurement of von Willebrand factor antigen (vWF:Ag) level, factor VIII assay, determination of von Willebrand factor (ristocetin cofactor) activity, and von Willebrand factor multimer analysis (Table 81-6). Plasma concentrations of von Willebrand factor increase with age, cigarette smoking, exercise, pregnancy starting in the second trimester, and infection, and with the use of certain medications, such as corticosteroids, high-dose estrogen birth control pills, and desmopressin.[89] Repeated test measurements may be necessary to make the diagnosis because of physiologic variations in plasma levels.

Electroimmunoassay, immunoradiometric assay, or enzyme-linked immunosorbent assay can be used to quantify vWF:Ag.[84] vWF:Ag levels are known to vary with different ABO blood types.[90] The vWF:Ag level is usually low in types 1 and 2 von Willebrand disease and virtually absent in type 3 disease. Factor VIII levels are normal or mildly decreased in patients with type 1 or 2 disease and very low (<10%) in those with type 3 disease.[84] Ristocetin, an antibiotic that causes platelet aggregation in the presence of functional von Willebrand factor, is used to measure von Willebrand factor activity. The assay is performed by mixing platelet-free patient plasma, normal formalin-fixed platelets, and ristocetin and then quantitating the extent of platelet agglutination.[82] Ristocetin cofactor activity usually is reduced in parallel to vWF:Ag levels in types 1 and 3 disease and decreased to a greater extent than vWF:Ag in type 2 disease (except type 2B).[87] Ristocetin-induced platelet agglutination is useful for further distinguishing type 2B disease, as a low concentration of ristocetin induces excessive aggregation in type 2B disease. The reader is referred to Table 81-7 for a summary of the various types of von Willebrand disease.

von Willebrand factor multimers can be analyzed by separating them by size on an agarose gel. All multimer sizes are present in type 1 disease, whereas reduced levels of intermediate- and high-molecular-weight multimers are characteristic of type 2 disease. Type 3 patients lack all types of von Willebrand factor multimers.

The von Willebrand factor gene was cloned in the mid-1980s, and now the role of molecular genetics is coming into play in the diagnosing of von Willebrand disease. Molecular genetic testing for vWD is now a feasible option in some instances.[91] Genetic testing may be used to clarify diagnostic uncertainty that may remain after coagulation testing and clinical evaluation.

TREATMENT
von Willebrand Disease

Desired Outcomes

5 The specific type of von Willebrand disease and the location and severity of bleeding determine the approach to treatment. The comprehensive care of patients with von Willebrand disease requires a team approach. The desired outcome is to prevent bleeding episodes and their short-term and long-term consequences so that patients with von Willebrand disease can live active and productive lives. Local measures, including pressure, ice, and topical thrombin, often can control superficial bleeding. Systemic treatment is used for bleeding that cannot be controlled in this manner and for prevention of bleeding with surgery. The goal of systemic therapy is to correct platelet adhesion and coagulation defects by stimulating the release of endogenous von Willebrand factor or by administering products that contain von Willebrand factor and factor VIII.[83,92] General guidelines for treatment of von Willebrand disease are shown in Figure 81-2. The von Willebrand disease guidelines are available at the National Heart, Lung, and Blood Institute Web site (*http://www.nhlbi.nih.gov/guidelines/vwd/index.htm*). In addition, a consensus guideline for the treatment of von Willebrand disease and other bleeding disorders in women was published in 2009.[93]

Replacement Therapy

6 The treatment of choice for patients with types 2B, 2M, and 3 von Willebrand disease and for patients with type 1 or 2A von Willebrand disease who are unresponsive to desmopressin (which is discussed in the next section) is replacement therapy with plasma-derived von Willebrand factor-containing products.[86,94] Several virus-inactivated, intermediate- or high-purity factor VIII concentrates contain sufficient amounts of functional von Willebrand factor.[94] Four factor-replacement products, all of them plasma-derived, are available in the United States for the treatment of patients with von Willebrand disease (Table 81-4). Two vWF/FVIII complex (human) products that contain high-molecular-weight multimers of vWF are commercially available. Ultrahigh-purity (monoclonal antibody-derived) plasma-derived products and recombinant factor VIII products contain only negligible amounts of von Willebrand factor and are inadequate for treatment of von Willebrand disease. A very high-purity plasma-derived von Willebrand factor concentrate and a recombinant von Willebrand factor product (does not contain blood-based additives) are currently in clinical trials.[95] Data from the Phase I study of the recombinant vWF have been presented at the 2011 International Society on Thrombosis and Haemostasis meeting. Pharmacokinetics of the recombinant factor were found to be similar to that of endogenous vWF. Because these von Willebrand factor concentrates do not contain appreciable factor VIII, concomitant administration of a factor VIII-containing product may be necessary for patients with severe disease and low levels of factor VIII.[96] Cryoprecipitate contains about 80 to 100 units

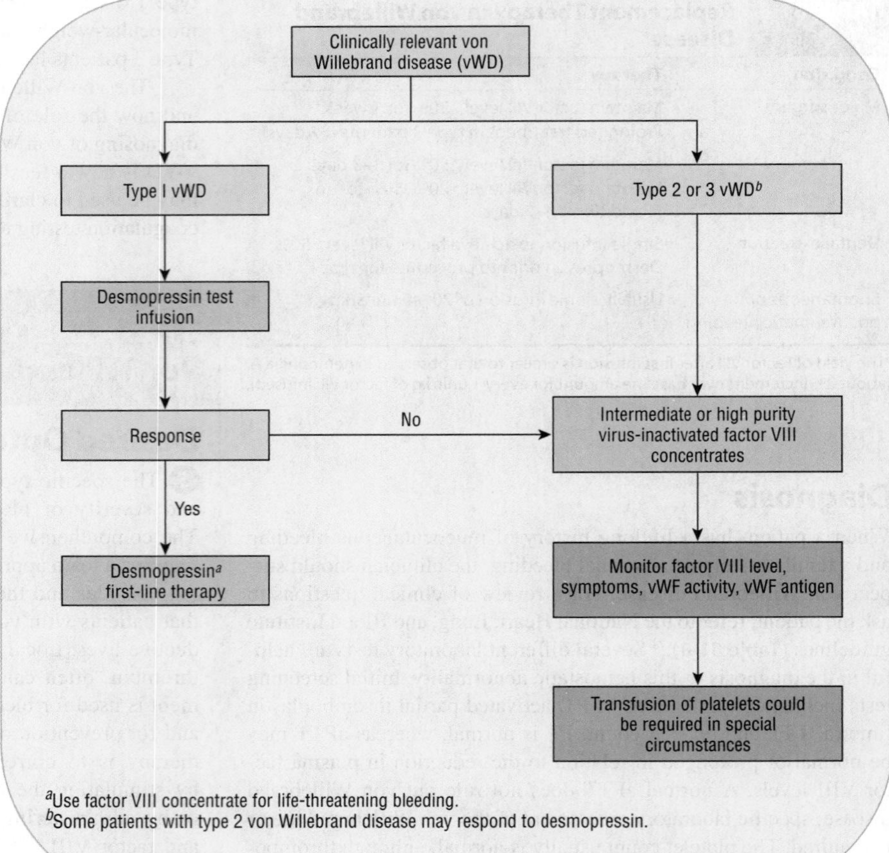

FIGURE 81-2 Guidelines for treatment of von Willebrand disease.

of von Willebrand factor per unit (5 to 10 times more von Willebrand factor and factor VIII than fresh-frozen plasma), and in the past it was the mainstay of therapy for von Willebrand disease.[84] However, because cryoprecipitate is not virally inactivated, it should not be used as first-line treatment. General guidelines for the dosing of replacement therapy in patients with von Willebrand disease unresponsive to desmopressin are provided in Table 81-9.

Other Pharmacologic Therapy

7 Desmopressin stimulates the endothelial cell release of von Willebrand factor and factor VIII. It is effective for patients with von Willebrand disease who have adequate endogenous stores of functional von Willebrand factor. This group includes most patients with type 1 disease and some patients with type 2A disease.

TABLE 81-9 Questions to Ask Patients

1. Have you or a blood relative ever needed medical attention for a bleeding problem or been told you have a bleeding disorder or problem?
   - During or after surgery?
   - With dental procedures or extractions?
   - During childbirth or for heavy menses?
   - Ever had bruises with lungs?
2. Do you have or have you ever had:
   - Liver or kidney disease?
   - A blood or bone marrow disorder?
   - A high or low platelet count?
3. Do you take aspirin, NSAIDs, clopidogrel, warfarin, heparin?

If yes to any of the above questions, ask additional questions:

1. Do you have a blood relative who has a bleeding disorder, such as von Willebrand disease or hemophilia?
2. Have you ever had prolonged bleeding from trivial wounds, lasting more than 15 minutes or recurring spontaneously during the 7 days after the wound?
3. Have you ever had heavy, prolonged, or recurrent bleeding after surgical procedures, such as tonsillectomy?
4. Have you ever had bruising, with minimal or no apparent trauma, especially if you could feel a lump under the bruise?
5. Have you ever had a spontaneous nosebleed that required more than 10 minutes to stop or needed medical attention?
6. Have you ever had heavy, prolonged, or recurrent bleeding after dental extractions that required medical attention?
7. Have you ever had blood in your stool, unexplained by a specific anatomic lesion (such as an ulcer in the stomach or polyp in the colon) that required medical attention?
8. Have you ever had anemia requiring treatment or received a blood transfusion?
9. For women, have you ever had heavy menses, characterized by the presence of clots greater than an inch in diameter and/or changing a pad or tampon more than hourly or resulting in anemia or low iron level?

NSAID, non-steroidal antiinflammatory drug.

Adapted from Nichols WL, Rick ME, Otel TL, et al. Clinical and laboratory diagnosis of von Willebrand disease: a synopsis of the 2008 NHLBI/NIH guidelines. Am J Hematol 2009;84:366–370.

Conversely, desmopressin is not appropriate for patients with type 3 disease, who lack stores of von Willebrand factor.

Desmopressin usually is not recommended for treatment of type 2B disease because the release of additional abnormal von Willebrand factor may exacerbate thrombocytopenia, but it has been reported to be beneficial in some patients with type 2B disease.[84] If desmopressin is used for treatment of type 2B disease, close monitoring is necessary.

Clinical **Controversy. . .**

Some hematologists find desmopressin beneficial in treating patients with type 2B von Willebrand disease, whereas others believe that it may exacerbate thrombocytopenia.

The dose of desmopressin used for treatment of von Willebrand disease is identical to that used for treatment of mild factor VIII deficiency, 0.3 mcg/kg given IV over 15 to 30 minutes. Patients with von Willebrand disease generally have a better response to desmopressin than those with hemophilia, with an average three- to fivefold increase in von Willebrand factor and factor VIII levels.[84] These levels remain elevated for about 6 to 8 hours. The response to desmopressin in a given patient usually is consistent, and a trial of desmopressin should determine if the medication likely will be effective for the individual. Desmopressin is preferable to use of plasma-derived products for patients who have an adequate response because desmopressin does not carry a risk of viral transmission. An added benefit is the substantially lower cost of desmopressin compared to the plasma-derived products. (For a discussion of the side effects of desmopressin, see Treatment of Hemophilia A above.)

Desmopressin can be administered every 12 to 24 hours, but the response diminishes with repeated treatment. After three to four doses, desmopressin often is no longer effective, and alternative replacement therapy may be necessary if prolonged treatment is required. Laboratory monitoring, including vWF:Ag measurements, factor VIII assays, vWF:activity assessments, and clinical examinations, will determine the adequacy of treatment.

Intranasal administration of desmopressin, at the same dosage as that used for mild factor VIII deficiency, can be useful for treatment of mild bleeding episodes. One or two doses administered at the start of menses may be helpful in controlling menorrhagia.[97] Oral contraceptives may also be very effective in controlling this symptom. Antifibrinolytic agents, such as aminocaproic acid and tranexamic acid, may be of special value in tissues rich in plasminogen activators, such as the mouth, especially with tooth extractions.[84] They can also be used in the management of epistaxis, GI bleeding, and menorrhagia. However, these agents should be avoided in urinary tract bleeding because of the risk of thrombosis and obstruction.

In acquired von Willebrand disease, low levels of plasma vWF are the result of accelerated removal of protein from plasma through the action of different pathogenic mechanisms. Acquired von Willebrand disease may be associated with monoclonal gammopathy, lymphoproliferative or myeloproliferative syndromes, or cardiovascular disease. The treatment of the underlying lymphoproliferative disease with rituximab, a monoclonal antibody against CD20 on lymphocytes, has been reported to be relatively ineffective in the management of the acquired von Willebrand disease.[98] IV immune globulin remains an additional therapy in acquired von Willebrand disease, along with vWF concentrate and/or desmopressin.

Gene Therapy

Patients with the most severe bleeding phenotypes of von Willebrand disease (type 3 and some severe cases of types 1 and 2) may be the most likely candidates for gene therapy, which may offer the potential of a long-term, if not lifelong, correction of vWF deficiency. Studies placing vWF cDNA into a lentiviral vector are currently ongoing.[81] Preclinical trials are being conducted to test the feasibility of gene transfer in the management of von Willebrand disease.

Personalized Pharmacotherapy

Current treatment of individual patients with von Willebrand disease is personalized. While the general goal of systemic therapy to correct platelet adhesion and coagulation defects by stimulating the release of vWF or administering products that contain vWF, a single guideline that works for every patient with von Willebrand disease would not be plausible. Each patient's bleeding risk factors must be taken into consideration, and therapy tailored to the individual. The proposed regimen should take into account these risk factors and the most appropriate individualized therapy should be provided.

Evaluation of Therapeutic Outcomes

Since the main goal in the treatment of patients with von Willebrand disease is to prevent or control bleeding and the consequences of such bleeding, assessment of bleeding episodes can be monitored via clinical and laboratory parameters. Monitoring the number and types of bleeding episodes and measurement of plasma concentrations of vWF and Factor VIII make it possible to evaluate the effectiveness of specific prophylactic and treatment regimens. As with hemophilia patients, assessment of patients' activities of daily living gives clinicians a better appreciation of the success of the treatment plan.

OTHER CONGENITAL FACTOR DEFICIENCIES

In addition to deficiencies in factors VIII and IX, congenital deficiencies in fibrinogen, in factors II, V, VII, X, XI, and XIII, and in combinations of factor deficiencies have been reported.[99] Contact factor abnormalities, including deficiencies in factor XII, high-molecular-weight kininogen, and prekallikrein, prolong the aPTT but do not lead to any bleeding diathesis. Identification of these disorders is important so that inappropriate treatment is not given. The only contact factor deficiency associated with bleeding symptoms is factor XI deficiency. Also known as hemophilia C, this deficiency is particularly common in people of Ashkenazi Jewish descent.[99] Bleeding manifestations are variable. Bleeding usually does not occur spontaneously, but excessive bleeding may occur after trauma or surgery. Most other deficiencies are inherited as autosomal recessive disorders and are rare. Some patients with abnormal molecules, such as a dysfibrinogenemia, may have an increased tendency to develop thromboembolic disease. Most of these deficiencies are treated with fresh-frozen plasma. Newer specific concentrates are becoming available. For example, a factor XIII plasma-derived concentrate is available, and recombinant factor VIIa is approved for use in patients with congenital VII deficiency. Cryoprecipitate, which is rich in fibrinogen, can be used to treat patients with fibrinogen deficiency or dysfunctional fibrinogen (dysfibrinogenemia).

COMPLICATIONS OF REPLACEMENT THERAPY

Transmission of bloodborne infectious diseases is always a concern when blood and blood-derived products are used. Most patients with hemophilia who received plasma-derived products were infected with hepatitis viruses and HIV during the 1980s prompting the development of viral inactivation methods for use during the manufacturing of factor concentrates.[26] All currently available plasma-derived factor concentrates come from screened donors and undergo viral inactivation procedures in an effort to reduce the risk of viral transmission. Heat treatment, which includes dry and wet heat, is one method of viral inactivation. Wet heat is applied while the concentrate is in suspension or in solution (pasteurization) and appears to be more effective than dry heat. Other methods of viral inactivation include chemical (solvent detergent) and affinity chromatography with monoclonal antibodies. Solvent detergent treatment inactivates lipid-coated viruses such as HIV and hepatitis B and C, but it is not effective against parvovirus B19, transfusion transmitted virus, hepatitis A, or prions.[26] Parvovirus B19 has been found in both plasma-derived and recombinant factor VIII concentrates (due to the use of albumin as a stabilizer in some recombinant products).[26,27] Parvovirus B19 may be particularly important for patients with hemophilia and HIV infection because it can cause chronic anemia in patients with immune deficiency.[100] Prions are not inactivated by either solvent detergent treatment or by heat, so there is a risk of transmission.[26]

Other complications associated with factor administration include allergic reactions, fever, chills, urticaria, and nausea. PCCs and aPCCs also have the potential to cause thromboembolic complications, including deep-vein thrombosis, pulmonary embolism, myocardial infarction, and DIC, likely related to the presence of activated factors.[101] Antifibrinolytic agents should not be given to patients receiving PCCs or aPCCs to avoid thrombotic complications.

Porcine factor VIII, used in the treatment of patients with inhibitors to factor VIII, is not known to transmit human viruses. However, allergic-type reactions (e.g., fever, chills, skin rashes, nausea, and headaches) have been reported.[102] Patients who experience these reactions can be treated with steroids and/or diphenhydramine. Thrombocytopenia is another potential complication of porcine factor VIII use.[102]

Recombinant factor VIII or IX has a low risk of viral transmission. Adverse effects of these products include metallic taste, mild dizziness, mild rash, burning at the infusion site, and a small drop in blood pressure.

ABBREVIATIONS

aPCC	activated prothrombin complex concentrate
aPTT	activated partial thromboplastin time
BU	Bethesda unit
HIV	human immunodeficiency virus
ITI	immune tolerance induction
PCC	prothrombin complex concentrate
PT	prothrombin time
vWF:Ag	von Willebrand factor antigen

REFERENCES

1. Rosendaal FR, Briet E. The increasing prevalence of haemophilia. Thromb Haemost 1990;63:145.
2. Soucie JM, Evatt B, Jackson D. Occurrence of hemophilia in the United States. The Hemophilia Surveillance System Project Investigators. Am J Hematol 1998;59:288–294.
3. Ay C, Thom K, Abu-Hamdeh F, et al. Determinants of factor VIII plasma levels in carriers of haemophilia A and in control women. Haemophilia 2010;16:111–117.
4. David D, Morais S, Ventura C, Campos M. Female haemophiliac homozygous for the factor VIII intron 22 inversion mutation, with transcriptional inactivation of one of the factor VIII alleles. Haemophilia 2003;9:125–130.
5. Shetty S, Ghosh K, Mohanty D. Hemophilia B in a female. Acta Haematol 2001;106:115–117.
6. Espinos C, Lorenzo JI, Casana P, Martinez F, Aznar JA. Haemophilia B in a female caused by skewed inactivation of the normal X-chromosome. Haematologica 2000;85:1092–1095.
7. Favier R, Lavergne JM, Costa JM, et al. Unbalanced X-chromosome inactivation with a novel FVIII gene mutation resulting in severe hemophilia A in a female. Blood 2000;96:4373–4375.
8. Weinspach S, Siepermann M, Schaper J, et al. Intracranial hemorrhage in a female leading to the diagnosis of severe hemophilia A and Turner syndrome. Klin Padiatr 2009;221:167–171.
9. Gitschier J, Wood WI, Goralka TM, et al. Characterization of the human factor VIII gene. Nature 1984;312:326–330.
10. Toole JJ, Knopf JL, Wozney JM, et al. Molecular cloning of a cDNA encoding human antihaemophilic factor. Nature 1984;312:342–347.
11. Lee C, Berntorp E, Hoots W, eds. Textbook of Hemophilia, 2nd ed. Chichester, West Sussex, UK: Wiley-Blackwell, 2010.
12. Lakich D, Kazazian HH Jr, Antonarakis SE, Gitschier J. Inversions disrupting the factor VIII gene are a common cause of severe haemophilia A. Nat Genet 1993;5:236–241.
13. Bagnall RD, Waseem N, Green PM, Giannelli F. Recurrent inversion breaking intron 1 of the factor VIII gene is a frequent cause of severe hemophilia A. Blood 2002;99:168–174.
14. Kurachi K, Davie EW. Isolation and characterization of a cDNA coding for human factor IX. Proc Natl Acad Sci USA 1982;79:6461–6464.
15. Crossley M, Ludwig M, Stowell KM, De Vos P, Olek K, Brownlee GG. Recovery from hemophilia B Leyden: an androgen-responsive element in the factor IX promoter. Science 1992;257:377–3779.
16. Picketts DJ, Lillicrap DP, Mueller CR. Synergy between transcription factors DBP and C/EBP compensates for a haemophilia B Leyden factor IX mutation. Nat Genet 1993;3:175–179.
17. Kurachi S, Huo JS, Ameri A, et al. An age-related homeostasis mechanism is essential for spontaneous amelioration of hemophilia B Leyden. Proc Natl Acad Sci USA 2009;106:7921–7926.
18. Khorana AA, Streiff MB, Farge D, et al. Venous thromboembolism prophylaxis and treatment in cancer: a consensus statement of major guidelines panels and call to action. J Clin Oncol 2009;27:4919–4926.
19. Peyvandi F, Jayandharan G, Chandy M, et al. Genetic diagnosis of haemophilia and other inherited bleeding disorders. Haemophilia 2006;12(Suppl 3):82–89.
20. Peyvandi F, Garagiola I, Mortarino M. Prenatal diagnosis and preimplantation genetic diagnosis: novel technologies and state of the art of PGD in different regions of the world. Haemophilia 2011;17(Suppl 1):14–17.
21. Tsui NB, Kadir RA, Chan KC, et al. Noninvasive prenatal diagnosis of hemophilia by microfluidics digital PCR analysis of maternal plasma DNA. Blood 2011;117:3684–3691.
22. Steele M, Cochrane A, Wakefield C, et al. Hepatitis A and B immunization for individuals with inherited bleeding disorders. Haemophilia 2009;15:437–447.
23. Ljung RC. Intracranial haemorrhage in haemophilia A and B. Br J Haematol 2008;140:378–384.
24. Franchini M. The modern treatment of haemophilia: a narrative review. Blood Transfus 2012;4:1–6.

25. Berntorp E, Shapiro AD. Modern haemophilia care. Lancet 2012;379:1447–1456.
26. Valentino LA, Oza VM. Blood safety and the choice of anti-hemophilic factor concentrate. Pediatr Blood Cancer 2006;47:245–254.
27. Soucie JM, Siwak EB, Hooper WC, Evatt BL, Hollinger FB. Human parvovirus B19 in young male patients with hemophilia A: associations with treatment product exposure and joint range-of-motion limitation. Transfusion 2004;44:1179–1185.
28. Key NS. Inhibitors in congenital coagulation disorders. Br J Haematol 2004;127:379–391.
29. Mannucci PM, Mancuso ME, Santagostino E. How we choose factor VIII to treat hemophilia. Blood 2012;119:4108–4114.
30. Franchini M, Tagliaferri A, Mengoli C, Cruciani M. Cumulative inhibitor incidence in previously untreated patients with severe hemophilia A treated with plasma-derived versus recombinant factor VIII concentrates: a critical systematic review. Crit Rev Oncol Hematol 2012;81:82–93.
31. Iorio A, Halimeh S, Holzhauer S, et al. Rate of inhibitor development in previously untreated hemophilia A patients treated with plasma-derived or recombinant factor VIII concentrates: a systematic review. J Thromb Haemost 2010;8:1256–1265.
32. Mannucci PM, Gringeri A, Peyvandi F, Santagostino E. Factor VIII products and inhibitor development: the SIPPET study (survey of inhibitors in plasma-product exposed toddlers). Haemophilia 2007;13(Suppl 5):65–68.
33. Jemel A, Siegel R, Ward E, Hao Y, Xu J, Thun MJ. Cancer statistics, 2009. CA Cancer J Clin 2009;59:225–249.
34. Batorova A, Martinowitz U. Continuous infusion of coagulation factors: current opinion. Curr Opin Hematol 2006;13:308–315.
35. Schulman S. Continuous infusion. Haemophilia 2003;9: 368–375.
36. Franchini M, Zaffanello M, Lippi G. The use of desmopressin in mild hemophilia A. Blood Coagul Fibrinolysis 2010;21:615–619.
37. Castaman G. Desmopressin for the treatment of haemophilia. Haemophilia 2008;14(Suppl 1):15–20.
38. Franchini M, Frattini F, Crestani S, Bonfanti C. Haemophilia B: current pharmacotherapy and future directions. Expert Opin Pharmacother 2012;13:2053–2063.
39. Gringeri A, Lundin B, von Mackensen S, Mantovani L, Mannucci PM. A randomized clinical trial of prophylaxis in children with hemophilia A (the ESPRIT Study). J Thromb Haemost 2011;9:700–710.
40. Manco-Johnson MJ, Abshire TC, Shapiro AD, et al. Prophylaxis versus episodic treatment to prevent joint disease in boys with severe hemophilia. N Engl J Med 2007;357:535–544.
41. Blanchette VS. Prophylaxis in the haemophilia population. Haemophilia 2010;16(Suppl 5):181–188.
42. Ljung R. The risk associated with indwelling catheters in children with haemophilia. Br J Haematol 2007;138: 580–586.
43. Lusher JM, Arkin S, Abildgaard CF, Schwartz RS. Recombinant factor VIII for the treatment of previously untreated patients with hemophilia A. Safety, efficacy, and development of inhibitors. Kogenate Previously Untreated Patient Study Group. N Engl J Med 1993;328:453–459.
44. Addiego J, Kasper C, Abildgaard C, et al. Frequency of inhibitor development in haemophiliacs treated with low-purity factor VIII. Lancet 1993;342:462–464.
45. Ehrenforth S, Kreuz W, Scharrer I, et al. Incidence of development of factor VIII and factor IX inhibitors in haemophiliacs. Lancet1992;339:594–598.
46. Sultan Y. Prevalence of inhibitors in a population of 3435 hemophilia patients in France. French Hemophilia Study Group. Thromb Haemost 1992;67:600–602.
47. Gouw SC, van den Berg HM. The multifactorial etiology of inhibitor development in hemophilia: genetics and environment. Semin Thromb Hemost 2009;35:723–734.
48. Fulcher CA, de Graaf Mahoney S, Zimmerman TS. FVIII inhibitor IgG subclass and FVIII polypeptide specificity determined by immunoblotting. Blood 1987;69:1475–1480.
49. Gilles JG, Arnout J, Vermylen J, Saint-Remy JM. Anti-factor VIII antibodies of hemophiliac patients are frequently directed towards nonfunctional determinants and do not exhibit isotypic restriction. Blood 1993;82:2452–2461.
50. White GC, Rosendaal F, Aledort LM, et al. Definitions in hemophilia. Recommendation of the scientific subcommittee on factor VIII and factor IX of the scientific and standardization committee of the International Society on Thrombosis and Haemostasis. Thromb Haemost 2001;85:560.
51. Haya S, Moret A, Cid AR, et al. Inhibitors in haemophilia A: current management and open issues. Haemophilia 2007;13(Suppl 5):52–60.
52. Hedner U. Mechanism of action of factor VIIa in the treatment of coagulopathies. Semin Thromb Hemost 2006;32(Suppl 1):77–85.
53. Buchanan GR, Kevy SV. Use of prothrombin complex concentrates in hemophiliacs with inhibitors: clinical and laboratory studies. Pediatrics 1978;62:767–774.
54. Hilgartner MW, Knatterud GL. The use of factor eight inhibitor by-passing activity (FEIBA immuno) product for treatment of bleeding episodes in hemophiliacs with inhibitors. Blood 1983;61:36–40.
55. Kurczynski EM, Penner JA. Activated prothrombin concentrate for patients with factor VIII inhibitors. N Engl J Med 1974;291:164–167.
56. Lusher JM, Roberts HR, Davignon G, et al. A randomized, double-blind comparison of two dosage levels of recombinant factor VIIa in the treatment of joint, muscle and mucocutaneous haemorrhages in persons with haemophilia A and B, with and without inhibitors. rFVIIa Study Group. Haemophilia 1998;4:790–798.
57. Shapiro AD, Gilchrist GS, Hoots WK, Cooper HA, Gastineau DA. Prospective, randomised trial of two doses of rFVIIa (NovoSeven) in haemophilia patients with inhibitors undergoing surgery. Thromb Haemost 1998;80:773–778.
58. Sjamsoedin LJ, Heijnen L, Mauser-Bunschoten EP, et al. The effect of activated prothrombin-complex concentrate (FEIBA) on joint and muscle bleeding in patients with hemophilia A and antibodies to factor VIII. A double-blind clinical trial. N Engl J Med 1981;305:717–721.
59. Astermark J, Donfield SM, DiMichele DM, et al. A randomized comparison of bypassing agents in hemophilia complicated by an inhibitor: the FEIBA NovoSeven Comparative (FENOC) Study. Blood 2007;109:546–551.
60. Gringeri A, Fischer K, Karafoulidou A, et al. Sequential combined bypassing therapy is safe and effective in the treatment of unresponsive bleeding in adults and children with haemophilia and inhibitors. Haemophilia 2011;17: 630–635.
61. Ingerslev J, Sorensen B. Parallel use of by-passing agents in haemophilia with inhibitors: a critical review. Br J Haematol 2011;155:256–262.

62. Kempton CL, Abshire TC, Deveras RA, et al. Pharmacokinetics and safety of OBI-1, a recombinant B domain-deleted porcine factor VIII, in subjects with haemophilia A. Haemophilia 2012;18:798–804.
63. Coppola A, Margaglione M, Santagostino E, et al. Factor VIII gene (F8) mutations as predictors of outcome in immune tolerance induction of hemophilia A patients with high-responding inhibitors. J Thromb Haemost 2009;7:1809–1815.
64. Dimichele D. The North American Immune Tolerance Registry: contributions to the thirty-year experience with immune tolerance therapy. Haemophilia 2009;15: 320–328.
65. Haya S, Lopez MF, Aznar JA, Batlle J. Immune tolerance treatment in haemophilia patients with inhibitors: the Spanish Registry. Haemophilia 2001;7:154–159.
66. Lenk H. The German Registry of immune tolerance treatment in hemophilia—1999 update. Haematologica 2000;85(10 Suppl):45–47.
67. Mariani G, Scheibel E, Nogao T, et al. Immunetolerance as treatment of alloantibodies to factor VIII in hemophilia. The International Registry of Immunetolerance Protocols. Semin Hematol 1994;31(2 Suppl 4):62–64.
68. Hay CR, DiMichele DM. The principal results of the International Immune Tolerance Study: a randomized dose comparison. Blood 2012;119:1335–1344.
69. Nilsson IM, Berntorp E, Zettervall O. Induction of immune tolerance in patients with hemophilia and antibodies to factor VIII by combined treatment with intravenous IgG, cyclophosphamide, and factor VIII. N Engl J Med 1988;318:947–950.
70. Berntorp E, Astermark J, Carlborg E. Immune tolerance induction and the treatment of hemophilia. Malmo protocol update. Haematologica 2000;85(10 Suppl):48–50; discussion 50-1.
71. Leissinger C, Kruse-Jarres R, Granger S, et al. Phase II trial of rituximab in the treatment of inhibitors in congenital hemophilia A: results of the RICH study. Blood (ASH Annual Meeting Abstracts) 2011;118:27.
72. Nathwani AC, Tuddenham EG, Rangarajan S, et al. Adenovirus-associated virus vector-mediated gene transfer in hemophilia B. N Engl J Med 2011;365:2357–2365.
73. High KA. The gene therapy journey for hemophilia: are we there yet? Hematology Am Soc Hematol Educ Program 2012;2012:375–381.
74. Riley RR, Witkop M, Hellman E, Akins S. Assessment and management of pain in haemophilia patients. Haemophilia 2011;17:839–845.
75. Raffini L, Manno C. Modern management of haemophilicarthropathy. Br J Haematol 2007;136:777–787.
76. Collins PW. Personalized prophylaxis. Haemophilia 2012;18(Suppl 4):131–135.
77. Howard TE, Yanover C, Mahlangu J, et al. Haemophilia management: Time to get personal? Haemophilia 2011;17: 721–728.
78. Nichols WL, Rick ME, Ortel TL. Clinical and laboratory diagnosis of von Willebrand disease: A synopsis of the 2008 NHLBI/NIH guidelines. Am J Hematol 2009;84: 366–370.
79. Blomback M, Eikenboom J, Lane D, Denis C, Lillicrap DP. von Willebrand disease biology. Haemophilia 2012; 18(Suppl 4):141–147.
80. Kreutz W. von Willebrand's disease: From discovery to therapy—Milestones in the last 25 years. Haemophilia 2008;14(Suppl 5):1–2.
81. DeMeyer SF, Deckmyn H, Vanhoorelbeke K. von Willebrand factor to the rescue. Blood 2009;113:5049–5057.
82. Bolton-Maggs PH, Favaloro EJ, Hillarp A, Jennings I, Kohler H. Difficulties and pitfalls in the laboratory diagnosis of bleeding disorders. Haemophilia 2012;18(Suppl 4):66–72.
83. Reininger AJ. Function of von Willebrand factor in haemostasis and thrombosis. Haemophilia 2008; 14(Suppl 5):11–26.
84. Federici AB, Castaman G, Mannucci PM. Guidelines for the diagnosis and management of von Willebrand disease in Italy. Haemophilia 2002;8:607–621.
85. Budde U. Diagnosis of von Willebrand disease subtypes: Implications for treatment. Haemophilia 2008;14(Suppl 5): 27–38.
86. Federici AB, James P. Current management of patients with severe von Willebrand Disease Type 3: A 2012 Update. Acta Haematol 2012;128:88–99.
87. Federici AB, Mannucci PM. Advances in the genetics and treatment of von Willebrand disease. Curr Opin Pediatr 2002;14:23–33.
88. Mohri H. Acquired von Willebrand syndrome: Features and management. Am J Hematol 2006;81:616–623.
89. Kouides PA. Aspects of the laboratory identification of von Willebrand disease in women. Semin Thromb Hemost 2006;32:480–484.
90. Gill JC, Endres-Brooks J, Bauer PJ, Marks WJJ, Montgomery RR. The effect of ABO blood group on the diagnosis of von Willebrand disease. Blood 1987;69:1691–1695.
91. James P, Lillicrap DP. The role of molecular genetics in diagnosing von Willebrand disease. Semin Thromb Hemost 2008;34:502–508.
92. Peyvandi F, Klamroth R, Carcao M. Management of bleeding disorders in adults. Haemophilia 2012;18(Suppl 2):24–36.
93. James AH, Kouides PA, Abdul-Kadir R. Von Willebrand disease and other bleeding disorders in women: Consensus on diagnosis and management from an international expert panel. Am J Obstet Gynecol 2009;201:12e1–12e8.
94. Schramm W. Haemate P von Willebrand factor/factor VIII concentrate: 25 years of clinical experience. Haemophilia 2008;14(Suppl 5):3–10.
95. Berntorp E. Prophylaxis in von Willebrand disease. Haemophilia 2008;14(Suppl 5):47–53.
96. Bolton-Maggs PH, Lillicrap DP, Goudemand J, Berntorp E. von Willebrand disease update: Diagnostic and treatment dilemmas. Haemophilia 2008;14(Suppl 5):56–61.
97. Mannucci PM. Treatment of von Willebrand's disease. N Engl J Med 2004;351:683–694.
98. Mazoyer E, Fain O, Dhote R, Laurian Y. Is rituximab effective in acquired von Willebrand syndrome? (Letter). Br J Haematol 2008;144:967–968.
99. Peyvandi F, Duga S, Akhavan S, Mannucci PM. Rare coagulation deficiencies. Haemophilia 2002;8:308–321.
100. Bolton-Maggs PH, Pasi KJ. Haemophilias A and B. Lancet 2003;361:1801–1809.
101. Lee C, Berntorp E, Hoots W, eds. Textbook of Hemophilia, 1st ed. Malden, MA: Blackwell Publishing Ltd., 2005.
102. Lloyd Jones M, Wight J, Paisley S, Knight C. Control of bleeding in patients with haemophilia A with inhibitors: A systematic review. Haemophilia 2003;9:464–520.

82

Sickle Cell Disease

C. Y. Jennifer Chan and Melissa Frei-Jones

KEY CONCEPTS

1. Sickle cell disease (SCD) is an inherited disorder caused by a defect in the gene for β-globin, a component of hemoglobin, and is called a qualitative hemoglobinopathy. Patients can have one defective gene (sickle cell trait that is not a disease) or two defective genes (SCD).
2. Although SCD usually occurs in persons of African ancestry, other ethnic groups can be affected. Multiple mutation variants result in different clinical manifestations.
3. SCD involves multiple organ systems. Usual clinical signs and symptoms include anemia, pain, splenomegaly, and pulmonary symptoms. SCD can be identified by routine neonatal screening programs. Early diagnosis allows early comprehensive care.
4. Patients with SCD are at risk for infection. Prophylaxis against pneumococcal infection reduces death during childhood in children with sickle cell anemia.
5. Hydroxyurea decreases the incidence of painful episodes, but patients treated with hydroxyurea should be carefully monitored.
6. Neurologic complications caused by vasoocclusion can lead to stroke. Screening with transcranial Doppler ultrasound to identify children at risk accompanied by chronic transfusion therapy programs have been shown to be beneficial in decreasing the occurrence of overt stroke in children with SCD.
7. Patients with fever greater than 38.5°C (101.3°F) should be evaluated, and appropriate antibiotics administered immediately, including coverage for encapsulated organisms, especially pneumococcal organisms.
8. Pain episodes can often be managed at home. Hospitalized patients require parenteral analgesics. Analgesic options include opioids, nonsteroidal antiinflammatory agents, and acetaminophen. The patient characteristics and the severity of the pain should determine the choice of agent and regimen.
9. Patients with SCD should be followed regularly for healthcare maintenance issues and monitored for changes in organ functions.

1 Sickle cell syndromes, which can be divided into sickle cell trait (SCT) and sickle cell disease (SCD), are a group of hereditary conditions characterized by the presence of sickle cell hemoglobin (HbS) in red blood cells (RBCs). SCT is the heterozygous inheritance of one normal β-globin gene producing HbA and one sickle gene producing HbS (HbAS) gene. Individuals with SCT are asymptomatic. SCD can be of homozygous or compounded heterozygous inheritance. Homozygous sickle cell hemoglobin (hemoglobin S) (HbSS) has historically been referred to as sickle cell anemia (SCA). The heterozygous inheritance of HbS with another qualitative or quantitative β-globin mutation results in sickle cell hemoglobin C (HbSC), sickle cell β-thalassemia (HbSβ^+-thal and HbSβ^0-thal), and some other rare phenotypes.[1,2]

Over the years, progress has been made in understanding the relationship between clinical severity and genotype, as well as the natural history of common morbidities associated with SCD. Ongoing research involves investigation of pharmacotherapies used to treat SCD. Recent advances in the care of SCD patients have increased life expectancy.[1–7]

SCD is a chronic illness with significant burden for family and society. Frequent hospitalizations can interrupt schooling and result in employment difficulties.[8–10] Acute complications of the disease can be unpredictable, rapidly progressive, and life threatening. Later in life, chronic organ damage and cognitive or emotional impairments can develop.[1,2] Because of the complexity and gravity of the illness, it is essential that comprehensive care is available to all patients and that all providers involved have a good understanding of the disease and its management.[1,2,8,11]

EPIDEMIOLOGY

2 SCD affects millions of people worldwide and is most common in people with African heritage.[1,12] The most common SCD genotype is HbSS (~60% to 65%), followed by HbSC (~25% to 30%), HbSβ^+-thal and HbSβ^0-thal (~5% to 10%). Other variants account for less than 1% of patients.[1,2] The disease is common among those with ancestors from sub-Saharan Africa, India, Saudi Arabia, and Mediterranean countries.[2,13] In the United States, about 90,000 Americans have SCD with a prevalence of 1 in 2,500 newborns, 1 in 500 African Americans, and 1 in 36,000 Hispanic births.[1,14,15] About 2 million Americans have SCT with a prevalence rate of 1 in 12 African Americans and 1 in 100 Hispanics.[16]

About 275,000 babies are born with SCD every year and 85% occur in Africa.[2,12] The prevalence of SCD in the region is determined by the frequencies of SCT. The distribution of SCT reflects the survival advantage in regions (tropical areas) where malaria is endemic as the gene mutation offers partial protection against serious malarial infection. RBCs carrying the abnormal sickle hemoglobin prevent the normal growth and development of *Plasmodium falciparum* within RBCs. Individuals with SCT are more likely to survive the acute malarial illness whereas individuals with SCD-HbSS often present with more severe disease. The incidence of the sickle gene in a population correlates with the historical incidence of malaria and SCT results in partial resistance to the disease.[1,2,12,17]

The prevalence of SCD is highest in sub-Saharan Africa. Other areas where the sickle mutation can be found include the

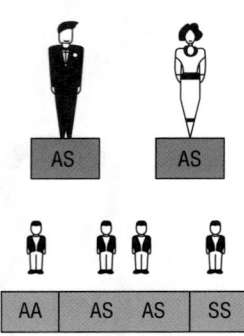

FIGURE 82-1 Sickle cell gene inheritance scheme for both parents with sickle cell trait (SCT). Possibilities with each pregnancy: 25% normal (AA); 50% SCT (AS); and 25% sickle cell anemia (SS). (A, normal hemoglobin; S, sickle cell hemoglobin)

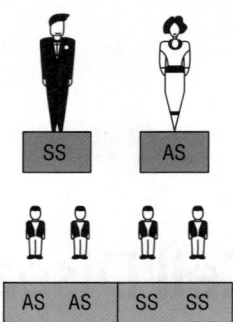

FIGURE 82-3 Sickle cell gene inheritance scheme for one parent with sickle cell trait (SCT) and one parent with sickle cell anemia (SCA). Possibilities with each pregnancy: 50% SCA (SS); 50% SCT (AS). (A, normal hemoglobin; S, sickle cell hemoglobin)

Arabian Peninsula, the Indian subcontinent, and the Mediterranean region. In Africa, the variants are Senegal (Atlantic West Africa), Benin (Central West Africa), Bantu (Central African Republic), and Cameroon. Arab-Indian haplotype is seen in certain areas of Saudi Arabia and India.[2,13] Haplotypes identified through newborn screening programs in the United States showed that the Benin haplotype was the most frequent (63%), followed by Bantu (14%), Senegal (9%), Cameroon (4%), and Saudi Arabian (2%).[13] Genetic analysis shows that the mutation found in Arabic patients is different from the mutation in those of African descent. Sickle gene mutation variants have been associated with different geographic locations and may be responsible for variations in clinical manifestations.[3,5,13]

ETIOLOGY

Normal hemoglobin (hemoglobin A [HbA]) is composed of two α chains and two β chains (α_2 β_2). The biochemical defect that leads to the development of HbS involves the substitution of valine for glutamic acid as the sixth amino acid in the β-polypeptide chain. Another type of abnormal hemoglobin, hemoglobin C (HbC), is produced by the substitution of lysine for glutamic acid as the sixth amino acid in the β-chain. Structurally, the α-chains of HbS, HbA, and HbC are identical. Therefore, it is the chemical differences in the β-chain that account for sickling and its related sequelae.[1–3]

SCA or HbSS is the most common form of SCD and occurs when an individual inherits both maternal and paternal β-globin alleles that code for the HbS. Figures 82-1 to 82-4 show the probability of inheritance with each pregnancy for the offspring of parents with HbA, SCT, and HbSS. If both parents are carriers, the offspring will have a 25% risk of inheriting SCD and a 50% risk of SCT (Fig. 82-1). β-Thalassemia is a quantitative hemoglobinopathy resulting from a genetic defect in β-globin production. β-Thalassemia can be co-inherited with HbS and may vary from no β-globin production (β^0) to some β-globin production (β^+). Individuals with HbSS and HbSβ^0-thal have a more severe course than those with HbSC and HbSβ^+-thal.[2,13] As discussed earlier, several haplotypes characterize the sickle gene, resulting in different clinical and hematologic courses. Included among these types are the three most commonly found in the United States: the Bantu haplotype, characterized by severe disease; the Senegal haplotype, characterized by mild disease; and the Benin haplotype, characterized by a course intermediate to that of the other two haplotypes. Although there are a number of other haplotypes seen around the world, the major types outside of the United States include Saudi Arabian and Cameroon, both with milder courses of illness.[2,3,5]

PATHOPHYSIOLOGY

Normal adult RBCs contain predominantly HbA (96% to 98%). Other forms of hemoglobin are HbA$_2$ (2% to 3%) and fetal hemoglobin (HbF; less than 1%). Normal RBCs are biconcave shape and able to deform to squeeze through capillaries.[1–3,18] HbF is present predominantly in fetal RBCs and is a tetramer of two α globin chains and two γ globin chains ($\alpha_2\gamma_2$). Prior to birth, HbF is the predominant hemoglobin type. Around 32 weeks gestation, a switch from the production of γ chains to β chains occurs and, consequently, an increase in HbA production is seen. Increased HbF production is seen under severe erythroid stress, such as anemia, hematopoietic

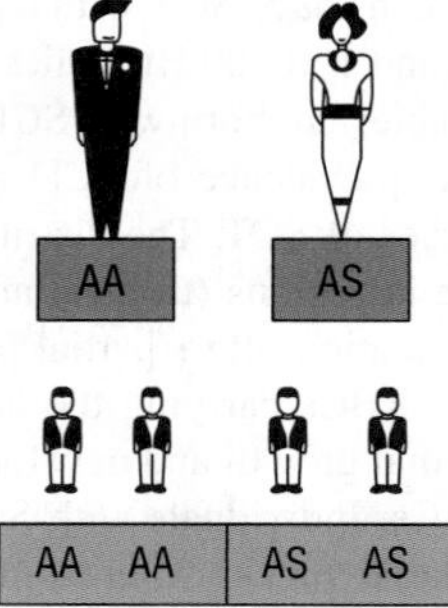

FIGURE 82-2 Sickle cell gene inheritance scheme for one parent with sickle cell trait (SCT) and one parent with no sickle cell gene. Possibilities with each pregnancy: 50% normal (AA); 50% SCT (AS). (A, normal hemoglobin; S, sickle cell hemoglobin)

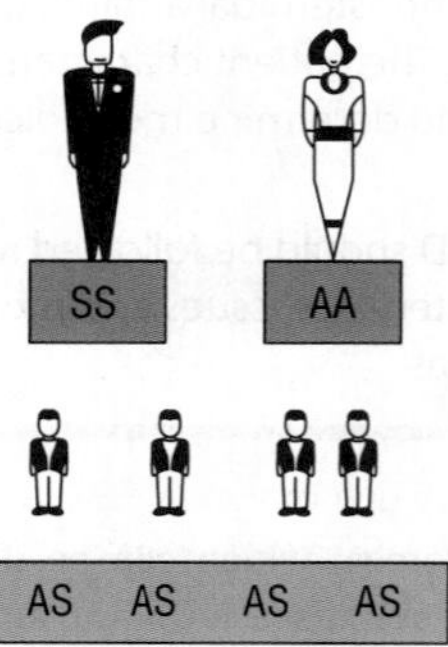

FIGURE 82-4 Sickle cell inheritance scheme for one parent without sickle cell gene and one parent with sickle cell anemia (SCA). Possibilities with each pregnancy: 100% SCT (AS). (A, normal hemoglobin; S, sickle cell hemoglobin)

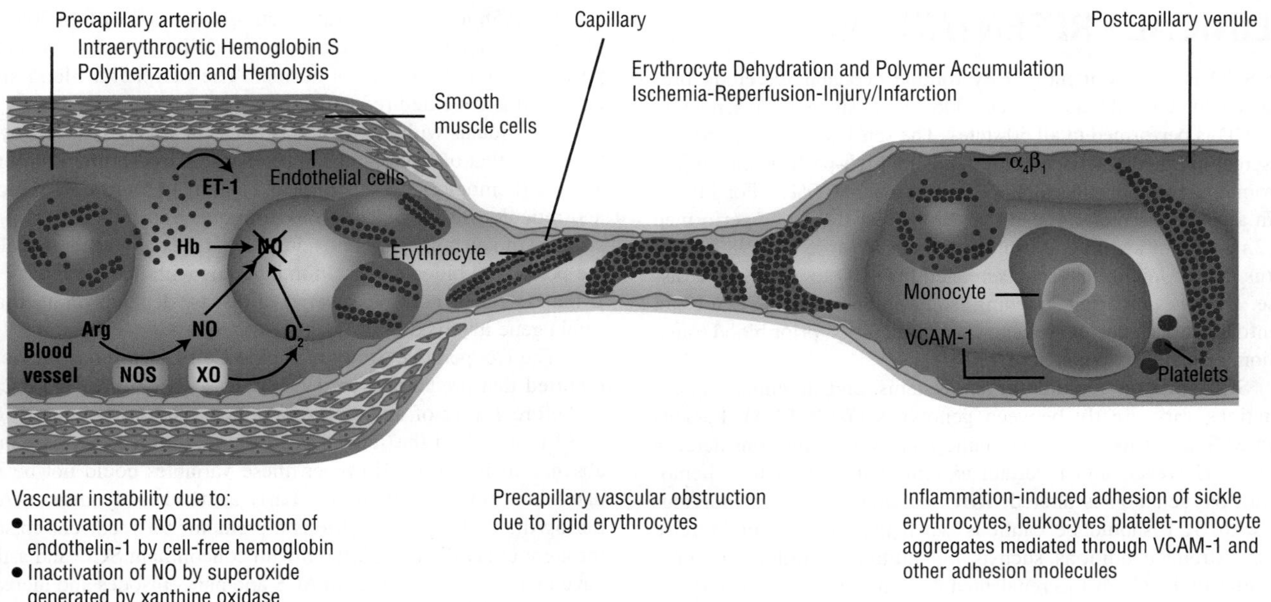

FIGURE 82-5 Pathophysiology of sickle cell disease. (Arg, arginine; ET-1, endothelin-1; Hb, hemoglobin; NO, nitric oxide; NOS, nitrous oxide synthase; VCAM-1, vascular cell adhesion molecule 1; XO, xanthine oxidase.) *(From Kato GJ, Gladwin MT. Sickle cell disease. In: Hall JB, Schmidt GA, Wood LDH, eds. Principles of Critical Care, 3rd ed. New York: McGraw-Hill, 2005:1658.)*

stem cell transplantation (HSCT), or chemotherapy or in the hereditary condition, hereditary persistence of fetal hemoglobin (HPFH) where a mutation in the β-globin gene cluster results in continued HbF production after birth. HPFH is a benign, asymptomatic condition.[3,5,7,19]

In the pathogenesis of SCD, the following are primarily responsible for the various clinical manifestations: impaired circulation, destruction of RBCs, and stasis of blood flow. These changes result directly from two major disturbances involving RBCs: abnormal hemoglobin polymerization and membrane damage (Fig. 82-5).

The solubilities of HbS and HbA are the same under conditions of normal oxygenation. Because of increased hydrophobicity as a result of the valine-substituting glutamic acid substitution, solubility of deoxygenated HbS is reduced. Saturation of deoxy-HbS leads to intermolecular binding and formation of thin bundles of fibers, which initially are unstable. However, the increased binding of deoxy-HbS eventually results in cross-linked fibers and stable polymers. This process is influenced by mean corpuscular hemoglobin concentration (MCHC), temperature, intracellular pH, and the circulating amount of HbS. Polymerization allows deoxygenated hemoglobin molecules to exist as a semisolid gel that protrudes into the cell membrane, leading to distortion of RBCs (sickle shaped) and loss of deformability. The presence of sickled RBCs increases blood viscosity and encourages sludging in the capillaries and postcapillary venules. Such obstructive events lead to local tissue hypoxia, which tends to accentuate the pathologic process.[1,2,6]

When reoxygenated, polymers within the RBCs are lost, the RBCs eventually return to normal shape. This process contributes to the vasoocclusive manifestation in that HbS is able to squeeze into microvasculature when oxygenated, but becomes sickled when deoxygenated. The cycle of sickling and unsickling results in damage to the cell membrane, loss of membrane flexibility, and rearrangement of surface phospholipids. Membrane damage also alters ion transport, resulting in potassium and water loss, which can lead to a dehydrated state that enhancing the formation of sickled forms. After continual repetitions of the process, the RBC membrane develops into rigid irreversibly sickled cell (ISC). Unlike the reversible sickled cells, which have normal morphology when oxygenated, ISCs are elongated cells and remain sickled when oxygenated. More rigid membranes of HbS-containing RBCs retard flow, particularly through the microcirculation. In addition, sickled RBCs tend to adhere to vascular endothelial cells, which further increase polymerization and obstruction.[1,2,6]

Intermolecular binding and polymer formation are reduced by HbF and to a lesser degree by HbA_2. RBCs that contain HbF sickle less readily than cells without. ISCs, not surprisingly, have a low HbF level. Increased levels of HbF, as in the case of the Saudi Arabian genotype, result in more benign forms of SCD. The amount of HbF and HbA_2 in relation to HbS influences the clinical manifestations and accounts for some of the variability in severity among SCD genotypes.[2,5]

Intravascular destruction of sickle cells can occur at an accelerated rate. The stresses of circulation and repetitive sickle–unsickle cycles lead to cell fragmentation. Damage to the cell membrane promotes cell recognition by macrophages. Rigid ISCs are easily trapped, resulting in short circulatory survival and chronic hemolysis. The typical sickled cell survives for about 16 to 20 days, whereas the life span of a normal RBC is 120 days. Anemia triggers the release of immature RBCs (reticuloctyes) from bone marrow prematurely. Surface adhesion proteins that maintain the reticulocytes inside the marrow adhere to the endothelium in postcapillary venules, further blocking the mature HbS-containing RBCs leading to complete occlusion of microvessels.[6,18]

In addition to sickling, other factors are also responsible for the clinical manifestations associated with SCD. Hemolysis releases free hemoglobin resulting in generation of reactive oxygen species, and alternation of nitric oxide (NO) metabolism. Obstruction of blood flow to the spleen by sickle cells can result in functional asplenia, defined as the loss of splenic function with an intact spleen. These patients can also have deficient opsonization. Impaired splenic function increases susceptibility to infection by encapsulated organisms, particularly pneumococcal bacteria. Coagulation abnormalities in SCD can be the result of continuous activation of the hemostatic system or disorganization of the membrane layer.[2,6]

CLINICAL PRESENTATION

❸ SCD is usually identified by routine neonatal screening programs in the United States. Since 2006, universal neonatal screening for SCD is performed in all 50 states. The sensitivity and specificity of screening methods (isoelectric focusing high-performance liquid chromatography, or electrophoresis) approach 100%.[20] For infants with a positive screening result, a second test should be performed by 2 months of age to confirm the diagnosis. More than 98% newborns in the United States are screened for SCD to identify the disease. Despite universal screening, some infants with SCD are not identified at birth because of extreme prematurity, prior blood transfusion, or inability to contact family.[19–21]

SCD involves multiple organ systems, and its clinical manifestations vary greatly between genotypes (Table 82-1). Persons with SCT are usually asymptomatic and SCT is not considered a disease. However, under certain extreme situations where hemoglobin oxygenation is altered, RBC sickling can occur. Individuals with SCT should be cautious when participating in exercise under extreme conditions, such as high altitude or military training. Sickling of RBCs in the renal medulla, an area with low oxygen tension, can result in the inability to concentrate urine. Individuals with such impairment are at risk of dehydration during periods in which the body normally conserves water. Microscopic hematuria has been observed, and gross hematuria can occur after heavy exercise. Other reported complications associated with SCT are venous thromboembolism, renal medullary carcinoma, and chronic kidney disease.[14,17,22] An increased incidence of urinary tract infection in women, especially during pregnancy, was previously reported and specific screening guidelines should be followed.[23]

The cardinal features of SCD are hemolytic anemia and vasoocclusion. In individuals with HbSS, anemia usually develops from 4 to 6 months after birth. The delay in presentation is due to the presence of HbF in the infant's RBCs. However, HbF production is gradually replaced by HbS, which typically leads the clinical manifestations of hemolysis and vasoocclusion, such as pain and swelling of the hands and feet, commonly referred to as *hand-and-foot syndrome* or *dactylitis* in infants.[1,2]

The common clinical signs and symptoms associated with HbSS include chronic anemia and pallor; fever; arthralgia; scleral icterus; abdominal pain; weakness; anorexia; fatigue; enlargement of the liver, spleen, and heart; and hematuria. Laboratory findings include the low hemoglobin level around 6 to 9 g/dL (3.72 to 5.58 mmol/L), elevated reticulocytes of 10% to 20%, and elevated platelet and white blood cell (WBC) counts. Mean corpuscular volume (MCV) is normal. The peripheral blood smear demonstrates sickled red cell forms.[1,14,18]

Individuals with HbSC disease present with less severe symptoms than that of HbSS and can be characterized primarily by mild anemia (hemoglobin levels of 9 to 11 g/dL [5.58 to 6.82 mmol/L] and reticulocytes of 3% to 10%), infrequent episodes of pain, persistence of splenomegaly into adult life, and excessive target cells in the peripheral blood smear. In individuals with heterozygous HbS-β-thalassemia syndrome, severity of disease depends on the thalassemia gene involved.[1,18]

The Cooperative Study of Sickle Cell Disease has previously reported that predictors for severe disease in children are dactylitis before 1 year of age, an average hemoglobin less than 7 g/dL (4.34 mmol/L) in the second year of life, and leukocytosis in the absence of infection. However, these variables could not be validated in a more recent study.[24] Early acute chest syndrome (ACS) during the first 3 years of life is a predictor for recurrent episodes throughout childhood. Children with concomitant SCD and asthma have increased frequencies of ACS and pain episodes and increased mortality. Risk factors for early death in adults with SCD include complications such as sickle cell pain, anemic events, ACS, renal failure, and pulmonary disease.[1,25–27] With longer survival for SCD, chronic manifestations of the disease contribute to the increased prevalence of morbidity later in life.

TABLE 82-1 Clinical Features of Sickle Cell Trait and Common Types of Sickle Cell Disease

Type	Clinical Features
Sickle cell trait (SCT)	Rare painless hematuria; normal Hb level; heavy exercise under extreme conditions can provoke gross hematuria and complications
Sickle cell anemia (SCA-HbSS)	Pain episodes, microvascular disruption of organs (spleen, liver, bone marrow, kidney, brain, and lung), gallstones, priapism, leg ulcers; anemia (Hb 6–9 g/dL)
Sickle cell hemoglobin C (HbSC)	Painless hematuria and rare aseptic necrosis of bone; pain episodes are less common and occur later in life; other complications are ocular disease and pregnancy-related problems; mild anemia (Hb 9–11 g/dL)
Sickle cell β^+-thalassemia (HbSβ^+-thal)	Rare pain; milder severity than HbSS because production of some HbA; Hb 10–12 g/dL with microcytosis
Sickle cell β^0-thalassemia (HbSβ^0-thal)	No HbA production; severity similar to SCA; Hb 6–9 g/dL with microcytosis

Hb, hemoglobin; HbA, hemoglobin A.

COMPLICATIONS

Acute Complications

Fever and Infection

Functional asplenia and failure to make antibodies against encapsulated organisms contribute to the high risk of overwhelming sepsis in individuals with SCD. Penicillin prophylaxis and vaccination have significantly reduced the overall risk of *Streptococcus pneumonia* bacteremia, but an increased incidence of invasive pneumococcal infections with nonvaccine serotypes has been reported.[28–30] Other encapsulated organisms are *Haemophilus influenzae, Neisseria meningitidis*, and *Salmonella*, and the latter has been known to cause osteomyelitis and pneumonia in SCD. *Mycoplasma pneumoniae* and *Chlamydia pneumoniae* should be considered in older children with infiltrates on chest radiograph. Viral infections (e.g., influenza and parvovirus B19) can result in severe morbidity.[1,2,18,28,29,31,32]

All SCD patients with fever greater than 38.3°C (101°F) must be evaluated to determine the risk of infection or sepsis; workup should include physical examination, complete blood count with reticulocyte count, blood culture, chest radiograph, urinalysis, and urine culture. Lumbar puncture may be needed, especially in young and toxic-appearing children. A low threshold for empiric therapy compared to that in the general population is recommended.[1,28,31,33]

Children with SCD may experience a severe complication due to infection that results in impaired bone marrow production of RBCs. An aplastic crisis is characterized by a decrease in the reticulocyte count and the rapid development of severe anemia (Table 82-2). The bone marrow becomes hypoplastic and is most often associated with a viral infection, particularly parvovirus B19.[1,14,31]

Neurologic

Neurologic abnormalities and cognitive deficits are well documented in patients with SCD. Vasoocclusive processes can lead to cerebrovascular occlusion that manifests as signs and symptoms of overt stroke, such as headache, paralysis, aphasia, visual disturbances, facial droop, and convulsions. The risk of stroke is highest for HbSS and lowest for HbSβ^+-thal. The occurrence of cerebral

TABLE 82-2 Acute Sickle Cell Complications

Vasoocclusive pain episodes[a]

Clinical features: Acute painful infarction without changes in Hb; almost all patients with SCA will have episodes of acute pain. Recurrent acute pain results in bone, joint, and organ damage and chronic pain. Vasoocclusive episodes most commonly involve the bones, liver, spleen, brain, lungs, and penis. Acute long bone pains can be accompanied by signs of inflammation, making it difficult to differentiate from osteomyelitis. Abdominal involvement can resemble a surgical abdomen. Precipitating factors include infection, extreme weather conditions, dehydration, and stresses

Signs and symptoms: Deep throbbing pain; local tenderness, erythema, and swelling can be seen. Fever and leukocytosis are common. Dactylitis usually occurs in young infants. Jaundice and increased transaminases present if liver is involved

Evaluation: Frequent physical examination, CBC, reticulocyte count, and urinalysis; based on symptomatology. The following may be needed: needle aspiration to rule out osteomyelitis, abdominal studies (radiograph, computed tomography scan, etc.), liver function tests, bilirubin, culture, and chest radiograph

Aplastic crisis[b]

Clinical features: Acute decrease in Hb with decreased reticulocyte count (usually less than 1%); transient suppression of RBC production in response to bacterial or viral infection, most common being parvovirus B19

Signs and symptoms: Headache, fatigue, dyspnea, pallor, and tachycardia; can also present with fever, upper respiratory or GI infection symptoms

Evaluation: CBC, reticulocyte count, radiograph, cultures (blood, urine, and throat), evaluation of viral infection (e.g., parvovirus titers)

Acute splenic sequestration[c]

Clinical features: Acute exacerbation of anemia due to sequestration of large blood volume by the spleen. More commonly seen in patients with functioning spleens (e.g., infants with HbSS and older children and rarely adults with HbSC disease); onset often is associated with viral or bacterial infections; recurrences are common and can be fatal

Signs and symptoms: Sudden onset of fatigue, dyspnea, and distended abdomen; rapid decrease in Hb and Hct with elevated reticulocyte count, abdominal pain, splenomegaly, vomiting, hypotension, and shock

Evaluation: Close monitoring of vital signs, spleen size, and oxygen saturation, CBC, reticulocyte count, and cultures

CBC, complete blood count; Hb, hemoglobin; HbSC, sickle cell hemoglobin C; Hct, hematocrit; HbSS, homozygous HbS; RBC, red blood cell.

[a]From McCavit,[1] Steinberg,[14] Roseff,[18] and Ballas et al.[44]
[b]From McCavit,[1] Steinberg,[14] and Booth et al.[31]
[c]From McCavit,[1] Steinberg,[14] Roseff,[18] and Brousse et al.[47]

infarct in HbSS is 11% by age 20 years and 24% by age 45 years with a recurrence rate as high as 70% in 3 years. The highest risk occurs during the first decades, in particular ages 2 to 5. The risk is lowest before age 2 secondary to the protective effect of HbF. Ischemic strokes occur in 54% of cerebrovascular accidents with the highest risk before age 10 years and after 30 years of age; whereas hemorrhagic strokes are more common when patients are in their 20s and are associated with poor outcome.[1,2,34]

In addition to neurologic examination, evaluation of acute events include computed tomography (CT) scan and magnetic resonance imaging (MRI), magnetic resonance angiography for asymptomatic infarction, and transcranial Doppler (TCD) ultrasound to detect abnormal velocity and identify individuals at increased risk of stroke. In addition, electroencephalography (EEG) can be used if there is a history of seizure.[1,2]

About 10% to 30% of SCD who have HbSS with no prior history of stroke have been found to have changes on MRI of the brain consistent with infarction or ischemia. These "silent infarcts" can be associated with increased risk of stroke, decreased neurocognitive functions, behavioral changes, and poor academic performances. Finally, lower intelligence, visual-motor impairments, and neuropsychological dysfunctions have been reported in patients not affected by acute or silent strokes and are associated with severity of anemia.[1,34–37]

Acute Chest Syndrome

ACS is the second most common cause of hospitalization and responsible for about 25% of death among individuals with SCD. ACS is defined as a new pulmonary infiltrate associated with one or more of the following: cough, dyspnea, tachypnea, chest pain, fever, wheezing, and new-onset hypoxia. As many as one-half of individuals with SCD experience at least one episode of ACS. Risk factors for ACS and recurrence include young age (peak incidence between age 2 to 4 years), higher Hb, lower HbF, higher leukocytes, history of asthma or bronchial hyper-responsiveness, and smoke exposure. Genotype and haplotype also influence the occurrence. Patients with HbSS and HbSβ^0-thal have higher incidence than those with HbSC and HbSβ^+-thal. The prevalence is higher with African haplotypes than that of Saudi Arabia.[1,25,38,39]

The primary etiology for ACS is pulmonary vascular occlusion. The most common cause of ACS is infectious and may be of bacterial, viral, or mycoplasma in origin. Infections, fat emboli released from bone marrow during pain crisis, or direct adhesion of RBC to the pulmonary vasculature leads to the inflammation and injury of the lung. Predictors for respiratory failure include extensive lobar involvement, platelet count less than 200,000 cells/mm^3 (200×10^9/L), and history of cardiac or neurologic complications. In addition to physical examinations, evaluations should include chest radiographs. In severe cases, CT scan, perfusion scintigraphy, transthoracic echocardiography, and bronchoscopy should also be considered. Pulmonary changes often involve the lower lobes of the lungs and may cause pleural effusions. Bilateral infiltrates or multiple lobe involvements may be an indication of poor prognosis. The mortality rates for ACS are less than 1%, 3%, and 9% for children up to 9 years old, children 10 to 19 years old, and adults, respectively. Pulmonary manifestations must be recognized early and managed aggressively as ACS can rapidly progress to pulmonary failure and death.[25,39,40]

Priapism

Stasis and sickling of erythrocytes within the sinusoids of the corpora cavernosa is the primary mechanism of priapism, a sustained painful erection. In recent years, a better understanding of pathophysiology of priapism has identified other mechanisms at the molecular level, such as NO and adenosine pathways. Stuttering priapism is repeated intermittent attacks up to several hours before remission; whereas ischemic priapism is a persistent painful erection greater than 4 hours and should be considered as an emergency. Thirty to 45% of males with SCD will present with at least one episode of priapism during their lifetime and the first episodes often occur during childhood. Impotence has been reported after repeated episodes and is directly related to the duration prior to treatment. ASPEN (association of sickle cell disease, priapism, exchange transfusion, and neurologic events) syndrome has occurred one to 11 days after partial exchange transfusion in males who presented with priapism. This syndrome can range from headaches and seizures to obtundation requiring ventilation.[41–43]

Sickle Cell Pain

Chronic hemolytic anemia in the SCD patient is periodically interrupted by acute episodes of pain and vasoocclusion, particularly in childhood (Table 82-2). Although fever, infections, dehydration, hypoxia, acidosis, and sudden temperature alterations can precipitate pain, multiple factors often contribute to its development.[44]

Sickle cell pain may be caused by bone or muscle infarction due to vasoocclusion and may affect a single site such as an arm, leg, or back or may involve multiple areas of the body. Acute painful episode is the most common reason of hospitalization. Individuals with HbSS disease experience frequent episodes of pain than those HbSC disease or some other variants.[1,2,14] Biomarker for severity of pain during vasoocclusion episodes include C-reactive protein and lactate dehydrogenase (LDH).[4,45] In addition, higher pain score at presentation and older age are predictors for admission and longer duration of hospitalization.[46] Dactylitis (hand-and-foot syndrome) is a sub-type of sickle cell pain, occurring in infancy and early childhood and is characterized by redness and swelling of the dorsal aspects of the hands, feet, fingers, and toes. The episodes are painful but usually do not result in permanent damage.[1]

Splenic Sequestration

Splenic sequestration is the sudden massive enlargement of the spleen resulting from the sequestration of sickled RBCs in the splenic parenchyma (Table 82-2). Hematocrit and hemoglobin concentrations dramatically fall, with reticulocytosis and no evidence of marrow failure or accelerated hemolysis. Trapping of the sickled RBCs by the spleen also leads to a decrease in circulating blood volume, which can result in hypotension and shock. The condition is most often seen in infants and children because their spleens are intact, and can cause sudden death in young children. Splenic enlargement may also be acutely painful due to rapid capsular expansion. Over time, repeated splenic infarctions lead to autosplenectomy and the spleen can no longer become engorged; the incidence therefore declines as adolescence approaches.[1,47]

Chronic Complications

Pulmonary

Pulmonary hypertension as defined as an elevated tricuspid regurgitation (TR Jet) velocity has been reported to be a risk factor for death in adult patients with SCD.[48] Diagnosis based on screening echocardiogram has been reported in children and adolescents, although its significance has not been established. Since recent studies have reported that screening echocardiogram alone has a high-false positive rate, pulmonary hypertension must be confirmed with right heart catheterization.[48,49]

The prevalence of asthma in children with SCD is similar to that of general population. However, asthma in individuals with SCD is associated with ACS and vasoocclusive pain episodes and increased mortality. Early screening for asthma starting at age 1 and pulmonary function test at least every 5 years starting at age 6 have been recommended. Medications such as inhaled corticosteroids and β-agonists for asthma exacerbation should be utilized for asthma control.[1,27,48]

Skeletal and Skin Diseases

Bone diseases are common in SCD and the vitamin D level has been suggested to be the biomarker.[4] Osteonecrosis, particularly of the femoral or humeral heads, causes permanent damage and disability.[14,50,51] Osteopenia associated with low bone formation has been reported in both males and females with SCD.[52] Children with SCD also have an increased incidence of osteomyelitis; the organism most often responsible is *Salmonella*.[31] In addition to necrosis of joints, chronic leg ulcers most commonly seen in the medial and lateral malleolus (ankles) can become a difficult and painful problem for adult. Ulcers are often seen after trauma or infection and are usually slow to heal.[53]

Ocular Manifestations

Ocular problems seen in patients with SCD include transient monocular blindness, visual field defects from retinal hemorrhage, retinal detachment, vitreous hemorrhage, venous microaneurysms, and neovascularization. The incidence of proliferative retinopathy in SCD patients varies from 5% to 10%. Vasoocclusion in the eye can occur as early as 20 months of age, and clinically detectable retinal diseases usually occur during adolescence and early adulthood. Despite the less systemic manifestations, individuals with HbSC develop serious retinal complications more often and earlier than those with HbSS. Annual examination with retinal evaluation is recommended for patients with SCD to prevent blindness from retinopathy and other complications.[54]

Gastrointestinal Diseases

Cholelithiasis is a common complication of SCD resulting from chronic hemolysis and increased bilirubin production, and leading to biliary sludge and/or stone formation. The risk of gallstones increases with age: 14% by age 10 years and 50% by age 22 years. Cholecystitis, exemplified by pain in the right upper quadrant, can be confused with an acute sickle pain episode in the abdomen. Cirrhosis occurred in 18% of young adults with SCD. Causes for development of chronic hepatic disease include repeated occlusion in the liver, iron overload, and hepatitis.[1,14,55]

Cardiac Diseases

Cardiovascular complications associated with anemia, including cardiac enlargement and various murmurs, can occur in patients with SCD. Patients experience various degrees of exertional dyspnea, tachycardia, and palpitation because of the decreased oxygen-carrying capacity of the blood. Left ventricular diastolic dysfunction has been reported in 18% of adults with SCD and is associated with increased mortality, especially in patients with pulmonary hypertension. Left ventricular stiffness and left ventricular hypertrophy have been reported, and the progression is speculated to lead to diastolic dysfunction later in life. Acute myocardial infarction in adults with SCD may be underrecognized due to the high incidence of sickle cell acute chest pain.[56,57]

Renal

Sickling in the renal medulla, an area with relative hypoxia and low pH, can lead to sickle cell nephropathy. Renal dysfunction in SCD begins during infancy evidenced by glomerular hyperfiltration. Other manifestations include inability to concentrate urine, hematuria, tubular acidosis, papillary necrosis, glomerulonephritis, microalbuminuria, and proteinuria. Enuresis, as a result of increased urine production, is a common complaint. Chronic renal failure has been reported in 30% of adults with SCD, and end-stage renal disease is associated with high mortality.[2,14,58,59]

Growth and Development

Delayed growth and sexual maturation are common in patients with SCD. Despite normal birth weight and length, growth retardation occurs between 6 months and 4 years with height, weight, and bone mass index being affected. The poor growth cannot be explained by nutritional factors alone. Alternations in growth factors as well as increased metabolic rate are factors contributing to the growth failure. Delay in puberty by 1 to 2 years is common in adolescents with SCD and fertility problems tend to occur more often in female SCD patients than in normal women.[60,61]

Psychiatric

Depression and anxiety are more common in children and adults with SCD than in the general population and have a significant impact on quality of life.[62,63] Depression is associated with pain episodes in children with SCD. In addition, the level of depression has been reported to be associated with anxiety between mothers and children.[64] DSM-IV psychiatric diagnosis in adolescents with SCD include attention-deficit-hyperactivity, oppositional defiant, conduct, major depressive, and anxiety disorders.[65]

Pregnancy

Pregnancy introduces an increased risk for the mother with SCD and for the fetus. Some women experience increased pain episodes during pregnancy and the anemia of SCD can lead to intrauterine growth retardation. Preterm labor and premature delivery are common in mothers with SCD, and the risk of spontaneous abortion is increased. The incidence of cesarean delivery and pregnancy-related complications are higher when compared to mothers who do not have SCD.[14,66,67]

TREATMENT
Sickle Cell Disease

Desired Outcomes

The goal of treatment is to reduce hospitalizations, complications, and mortality. Treatment for SCD involves the use of general measures to meet the unique demands for increased erythropoiesis. Additional interventions can be aimed at preventing or treating complications of the disease. When an acute complication occurs, the type and severity of the episode determine the appropriate therapeutic plan.

With availability of public health programs and comprehensive care, most children survive through childhood.[12,26,68] The median survival rate is estimated to be 42 years for males and 48 years for females for HbSS, and 60 years for males and 68 years for females for HbSC.[12] With increased life expectancy, management of SCD should include assessment of health-related quality of care in both adults and children.

Patients with SCD require lifelong multidisciplinary care. All patients with SCD should receive regularly scheduled comprehensive medical evaluations. Because of the complexity of the disease, a multidisciplinary team is needed to provide high-quality medical care, education, counseling, and psychosocial support. Appropriate comprehensive care can have a positive impact on both longevity and quality of life. This care includes the use of evidence-based treatment combining general symptomatic supportive care, preventative medical therapies, and more specific disease-modifying therapies aimed at altering hematologic capacity and function.

Routine Health Maintenance

Immunizations

Administration of routine immunizations is crucial preventive care in managing SCD. Impaired splenic function increases susceptibility to infection by encapsulated organisms, particularly *Pneumococci*. Prior to the routine use of penicillin prophylaxis and the development of pneumococcal vaccines, invasive pneumococcal disease was 20- to 100-fold more common in children with SCD than in healthy children. Reduced mortality has been associated with the introduction of pneumococcal vaccines.[26,68]

Two different pneumococcal vaccines are available. The 13-valent pneumococcal conjugate vaccine (PCV13; Prevnar®) induces good antibody responses in infants and children less than 2 years of age. Immunization with the PCV13 is recommended for all children, regardless of SCD status, younger than 24 months of age. Infants should receive the first dose after 6 weeks of age. Two additional doses should be given at 2-month intervals, followed by a fourth dose at age 12 to 15 months. The 23-valent pneumococcal polysaccharide vaccine (PPSV 23; Pneumovax®23) is recommended for all children with functional or acquired asplenia but must be given after 2 years of age because of poor antibody response. To cover different serotypes, PPSV 23 should be given starting at 2 years of age, and be administered 2 months after the last dose of the 7-valent pneumococcal conjugate vaccine (PCV7)/PCV13. A booster dose of PPSV 23 is recommended 5 years after the first dose. The recommended immunization schedule and catch-up schedule for PCV13 and PPV 23 are presented in Table 82-3. For children ages 2 to 18 years with SCD who did not receive PCV-13 during their routine immunization, a single dose of PCV-13 is recommended.[69]

The risk of meningococcal disease is also higher in SCD and meningococcal vaccination is recommended for individuals with functional or acquired asplenia. Three different meningococcal vaccines are available. Meningococcal groups C and Y and *Haemophilus* b tetanus toxoid conjugate vaccine (Hib-MenCY-TT) are approved for age 6 weeks through 18 months. The quadrivalent (serogroups A, C, Y, and W-135) meningococcal conjugate vaccines, MenACWY-CRM and MenACWY-D, are approved for age 2 through 55 years. In addition, MenACWY-D is available as a two-dose series for age 9 months through 23 months. Infants with functional asplenia should be vaccinated with the four-dose series of Hib-MenCY-TT at age 6 weeks through 18 months. If the first dose of Hib-MenCY-TT is given at or after 12 months of age, two doses should be given at least 8 weeks apart. Infants 9 through 23 months of age should be vaccinated with the two-dose series of MenACWY-D. Children over 2 years and adults with functional or acquired asplenia should receive a primary immunization series with two doses of the quadrivalent vaccine given 8 weeks apart. A booster is recommended every 5 years for individuals with SCD.[70,71] Finally, children 6 months and older and adults with SCD should receive influenza vaccine annually.[27]

Penicillin

4 Penicillin prophylaxis until at least 5 years of age is recommended in children with SCD HbSS or Hb Sβ^0-thal, even if they have received PCV13 or PPSV 23 immunization as prophylaxis against invasive pneumococcal infections. Prophylactic treatment should begin at 2 months of age or earlier. An effective regimen that reduces the risk of pneumococcal infections by 84% is penicillin V potassium at a dosage of 125 mg orally twice daily until the age of 3 years, followed by 250 mg twice daily until the age of 5 years. An alternate regimen is benzathine penicillin, 600,000 units given intramuscularly every 4 weeks for children age 6 months to 6 years, and 1.2 million units every 4 weeks for those over 6 years of age for whom continued therapy is warranted. Individuals who are allergic to penicillin can be given erythromycin 20 mg/kg per day twice daily. Penicillin prophylaxis is not routinely given in older children, based on a study demonstrating no benefit over placebo beyond the age of 5 years. However, continuation of oral pneumococcal prophylaxis should be considered on a case-by-case basis, and is recommended for anyone with a history of invasive pneumococcal infection or surgical splenectomy.[1,27]

Clinical **Controversy...**

The need for routine penicillin prophylaxis in HbSC and HbSβ^+-thal patients is controversial because these patients have less severe disease. The original trial showing decreased morbidity from invasive infection included children with HbSS or SCA.

Fetal Hemoglobin Inducers

HbF reduces polymer formation of HbS due to its high oxygen affinity. Increased HbF levels significantly correlate with decreased RBC sickling and RBC adhesion and observational studies show a relationship between HbF concentration and severity of SCD. Individuals with SCD and low HbF levels experience more frequent pain and higher mortality. HbF levels of 20% or greater reduce the risk of acute sickle cell complications. Based on these observations, HbF induction has become a treatment modality for patients with SCD.

TABLE 82-3 Pneumococcal Immunizations for Children with Sickle Cell Disease

	Recommended Schedule
Previously Unvaccinated	
Age 2–6 months	**PCV13 (Prevnar®)**: Three doses 8 weeks apart; then one dose at 12–15 months
Age 7–11 months	**PCV13 (Prevnar®)**: Two doses 8 weeks apart; then one dose at 12–15 months
Age 12–23 months	**PCV13 (Prevnar®)**: Two doses 8 weeks apart
Age 24–71 months	**PCV13 (Prevnar®)**: Two doses 8 weeks apart **PPSV 23 (Pneumovax®)**: Two doses; first dose at least 8 weeks after the last PCV7/PCV13 dose; second dose 5 years after the first PPSV 23 dose
Age 6 years or older	**PCV13 (Prevnar®)**: One dose **PPSV 23 (Pneumovax®)**: Two doses; first dose at least 8 weeks after the last PCV7/PCV13 dose; second dose 5 years after the first PPSV 23 dose
Previously Vaccinated	
Age 2–6 months	
One dose PCV7/PCV13	**PCV13 (Prevnar®)**: Two doses 8 weeks apart; first dose at least 8 weeks after the last PCV7/PCV13 dose; then one dose at 12–15 months
Two doses PCV7/PCV13	**PCV13 (Prevnar®)**: One dose at least 8 weeks after the last PCV7/PCV13 dose; then one dose at 12–15 months
Age 7–11 months	
One or two doses PCV7/PCV13 before age 7 months	**PCV13 (Prevnar®)**: One dose; then one dose at 12–15 months and at least 8 weeks after the last PCV7/PCV13 dose
Age 12–23 months	
One dose PCV7/PCV13 before age 12 months	**PCV13 (Prevnar®)**: Two doses 8 weeks apart; first dose at least 8 weeks after the last PCV7/PCV13 dose
One dose PCV7/PCV13 at age 12 months or older	**PCV13 (Prevnar®)**: One dose at least 8 weeks after last PCV7/PCV13 dose
Two or three doses PCV7/PCV13 before age 12 months	**PCV13 (Prevnar®)**: One dose at least 8 weeks after last PCV7/PCV13 dose
Received four doses of PCV7	**PCV13 (Prevnar®)**: One dose at least 8 weeks after most recent dose
Age 24–71 months	
Less than three doses PCV7/PCV13 given before age 24 months	**PCV13 (Prevnar®)**: Two doses 8 weeks apart; first dose at least 8 weeks after the last PCV7/PCV13 dose **PPSV 23 (Pneumovax®)**: Two doses; first dose at least 8 weeks after the last PCV7/PCV13 dose; second dose 5 years after the first PPSV 23 dose
Three doses PCV7/PCV13 given before age 24 months of age	**PCV13 (Prevnar®)**: One dose at least 8 weeks after the last PCV7/PCV13 dose **PPSV 23 (Pneumovax®)**: Two doses; first dose at least 8 weeks after last PCV7/PCV13 dose; second dose 5 years after the first PPSV 23 dose
Received four doses of PCV7	**PCV13 (Prevnar®)**: One dose at least 8 weeks after most recent dose **PPSV 23 (Pneumovax®)**: Two doses; first dose at least 8 weeks after the last PCV7/PCV13 dose; second dose 5 years after the first PPSV 23 dose
One dose PPSV 23 given	**PCV13 (Prevnar®)**: Two doses 8 week apart; first dose at least 8 weeks after PPSV 23 dose **PPSV 23 (Pneumovax®)**: Second dose 5 years after first PPSV 23
Age 6 years or older	
Received PPSV 23	**PCV13 (Prevnar®)**: One dose 8 weeks after PPSV 23 **If only received one dose of PPSV 23 (Pneumovax®)**: Second dose 8 weeks after PCV7/PCV13 and 5 years after the first PPSV 23 dose

PCV7, 7-valent pneumococcal conjugated vaccine; PCV13, 13-valent pneumococcal conjugated vaccine; PPSV 23, 23-valent pneumococcal polysaccharide vaccine.
From MMWR.[69]

Hydroxyurea

Hydroxyurea, a chemotherapeutic agent, increases HbF levels by stimulating HbF production. It also increases the number of HbF-containing reticulocytes and intracellular HbF. Its antineoplastic activity is related to inhibition of DNA synthesis by blocking the conversion of ribonucleoside to deoxyribonucleotides. The exact mechanism of HbF production is unknown, but is postulated that the cytotoxic effect in the bone marrow stimulates stress erythropoiesis and triggers rapid erythroid regeneration and shifts erythrocyte hemoglobin production to HbF. In addition, hydroxyurea increases NO levels, reduces neutrophils and monocytes, has antioxidant properties, alters the RBC membrane, increases RBC deformability by increasing intracellular water content, and decreases RBC adhesion to the endothelium.[2,5,7]

Hydroxyurea can prevent acute sickle cell pain and is FDA-approved for adults with SCD based on the result of the Multicenter Study of Hydroxyurea in Sickle Cell Anemia (MSH Trial), a double-blind, placebo-controlled study. In this study, hydroxyurea significantly reduced the frequency of painful episodes, risk of ACS, need for blood transfusions, and number of hospitalizations.[56] The study was terminated early after interim analyses showed significant benefits. The incidence of death, stroke, and hepatic sequestration in the hydroxyurea and placebo groups was not significantly different during the evaluation period. However, a follow-up study showed a 40% reduction in mortality with hydroxyurea over a 9-year period.[2,27,72]

Although hydroxyurea is not FDA approved for use in children and adolescents with SCD, the National Institutes of Health (NIH) has supported several clinical trials investigating its safety and efficacy.[7] Studies in pediatric patients have demonstrated similar results to the MSH Trial with no adverse effects on growth and development. In addition, some patients treated with hydroxyurea therapy had possible recovery or preservation of splenic and brain functions, including cognitive performances. In patients who cannot tolerate chronic transfusion therapy for stroke prevention, hydroxyurea can prevent recurrent strokes and reduce iron overload from transfusion.[2,7,72] The Pediatric Hydroxyurea Phase III Clinical Trial (BABY HUG) evaluated hydroxyurea therapy in young children ages 9 to 18 months.[73] Infants were randomized between hydroxyurea and a placebo; the primary endpoints were splenic and renal function. Investigators found no significant difference in the primary endpoints but did find fewer episodes of pain and dactylitis with no significant toxicities. Hydroxyurea reduced the risk of painful events, ACS, renal enlargement, hospitalizations, and transfusions. In addition, improved urine concentration ability, as demonstrated by higher urine osmolality, was reported. No increased risk of infections or genotoxicity was observed in hydroxyurea-treated children.[74–76]

The most common side effect of hydroxyurea is bone marrow suppression, causing neutropenia, thrombocytopenia, anemia, and/or decreased reticulocyte count. These hematologic side effects usually recover within 2 weeks of therapy discontinuation. Other side effects include dry skin and hyperpigmentation of skin or nails.[1,2,14] Long-term adverse effects of hydroxyurea therapy in patients with SCD are not fully known, although no serious adverse effects were reported in a long-term (17.5 years) follow-up study of the MSH trial.[77] Studies in children have not demonstrated delays in growth or puberty.[72] Myelodysplasia, acute leukemia, and chronic opportunistic infection associated with T-lymphocyte abnormalities have been reported in other patient populations treated with hydroxyurea. Ongoing follow-up is needed to determine the carcinogenic or leukemogenic effects of hydroxyurea in SCD. Reproductive toxicity is also a concern. High-dose hydroxyurea has been shown to be teratogenic in animals, but normal pregnancies have been reported in women with SCD who received hydroxyurea during pregnancy.[78]

Clinical indications for hydroxyurea include frequent painful episodes, severe symptomatic anemia, a history of ACS, or other severe vasoocclusive complications. The starting dose for adult is 15 mg/kg per day as a single daily dose (Fig. 82-6). The Baby HUG study found that children can be safely started at 20 mg/kg.[73] Dosage can be increased by 5 mg/kg up to a maximum of 35 mg/kg after 8 weeks if the patient can tolerate the adverse effects and blood counts are stable. Hydroxyurea dosage should be individualized based on response and toxicity. In general, 3 to 6 months of therapy are required before improvement is observed. Medication adherence can be an issue. Since the MCV generally increases as the level of HbF increases, monitoring MCV is an inexpensive and convenient method to monitor response and adherence.[1,72,79]

5 Patients receiving hydroxyurea should be closely monitored for toxicity. Blood counts should be checked every 4 weeks during dose titration and every 8 weeks thereafter. Treatment should be interrupted if hematologic indices fall below the following values: absolute neutrophil count, 2,000 cells/mm^3 (2×10^9/L); platelet count, 80,000 cells/mm^3 (80×10^9/L); hemoglobin, 5 g/dL (3.1 mmol/L); or reticulocytes, 80,000 cells/mm^3 (80×10^9/L) if the hemoglobin concentration is less than 9 g/dL (5.58 mmol/L). Other laboratory abnormalities warranting temporary discontinuation of therapy are a 50% increase in serum creatinine and a 100% increase in transaminases. After recovery has occurred, treatment should be resumed at a dose that is 2.5 to 5 mg/kg per day lower than the dose associated with toxicity. If no toxicity occurs after 12 weeks with the lower dose, the dose can be increased by 2.5 to 5 mg/kg per day. If the increased dose produces hematologic toxicity, the patient should be maintained at the last tolerated dose with no further escalation except for normal growth or weight gain. If no increase in MCV is observed, possible explanations are that the marrow is unable to respond, the hydroxyurea dose is inadequate, or the patient is nonadherent.[72,79]

5-Aza-2′-Deoxycytidine (Decitabine)

5-Azacytidine and 5-aza-2′-deoxycytidine (decitabine) induce HbF by inhibiting DNA methylation, thus preventing the switch from γ- to β-globin production. Decitabine has been evaluated in a small number of patients with SCD who did not respond to hydroxyurea. In one study of adult patients who were resistant or intolerant to hydroxyurea, an increase in HbF was observed with 5-aza-2′-deoxycytidine at a dose of 0.2 mg/kg one to three times a week subcutaneously. Reduced acute sickle cell pain episodes and improved performance status were reported in four adult patients with severe SCD. The only significant toxicities observed were neutropenia and increased platelet count.[5,7] Long-term clinical effects and adverse effects of decitabine have not been fully evaluated. This agent may have a role in treating patients who fail to respond to hydroxyurea. Currently, two trials investigating the use of decitabine in adults with severe SCD are actively recruiting patients (*http://www.clinicaltrials.gov*; NCT01375608 and NCT01685515).

Chronic Transfusion Therapy

RBC transfusions play an important role in the management of SCD. In acute illness, transfusions can be life saving and the guidelines for acute transfusion are discussed in a later section. Chronic transfusion programs can prevent serious complications of SCD. The primary indication for chronic transfusion is stroke prevention and amelioration of organ damage. Blood transfusion can be administered as a simple transfusion, a manual exchange, or an automated exchange called erythrocytapheresis. Exchange transfusion is associated with higher cost but has the advantage of limiting volume, minimizing hyperviscosity and transfusional iron overload.[1,4,18]

6 In children with an overt stroke, chronic transfusions are used as secondary stroke prevention and reduce stroke recurrence from about 50% to about 10% over 3 years. An initial stroke in SCD can be devastating and transfusions can be given for primary stroke prevention. Prophylactic transfusions significantly reduced the incidence of first stroke over a 2-year period in children 2 to 16 years of age who were at an increased risk for stroke based on TCD ultrasonography. The risk of stroke was reduced from 16% in patients receiving usual care to 2% in those who received prophylactic transfusions.[1,18,34]

Chronic transfusions can also reduce the frequency of vasoocclusive pain and ACS and prevent or delay progression of organ damage. They can also reverse preexisting organ dysfunction and improve quality of life, energy levels, exercise tolerance, growth, and sexual development. Chronic transfusions should be considered in selected children and adults with previous stroke or children with abnormal TCD measurements. Chronic transfusions have also been used in patients with severe or recurrent ACS, debilitating pain, splenic sequestration, recurrent priapism, chronic organ failure, intractable leg ulcers, severe chronic anemia with cardiac failure, and complicated pregnancies, although data supporting the efficacy of chronic transfusion in these situations are limited.[2,14]

The goal of transfusions is to achieve and maintain an HbS concentration of less than 30% of total hemoglobin in the primary and secondary prevention of neurologic complications. Transfusions are usually given every 3 to 4 weeks, but the frequency of transfusion is adjusted to maintain the desired HbS levels. The risk of recurrent stroke decreases after 2 years of transfusion therapy and, in the absence of recurrent stroke, many clinicians will liberalize the HbS goal to less than 50%.[2,14,34] The optimal duration of primary prophylactic transfusion therapy in children with abnormal TCD is not clear, but discontinuation of transfusions has been associated with a 50% stroke recurrence rate within 12 months and abnormal blood flow velocity on TCD in children with SCD. For secondary stroke prevention, transfusions should be continued indefinitely.[14,34] A pilot study suggested that hydroxyurea could be started prior to discontinuation of transfusion for secondary stroke prevention with at least a 6-month overlap with transfusions.[34] However, the phase III trial of switching hydroxyurea for transfusion in secondary stroke

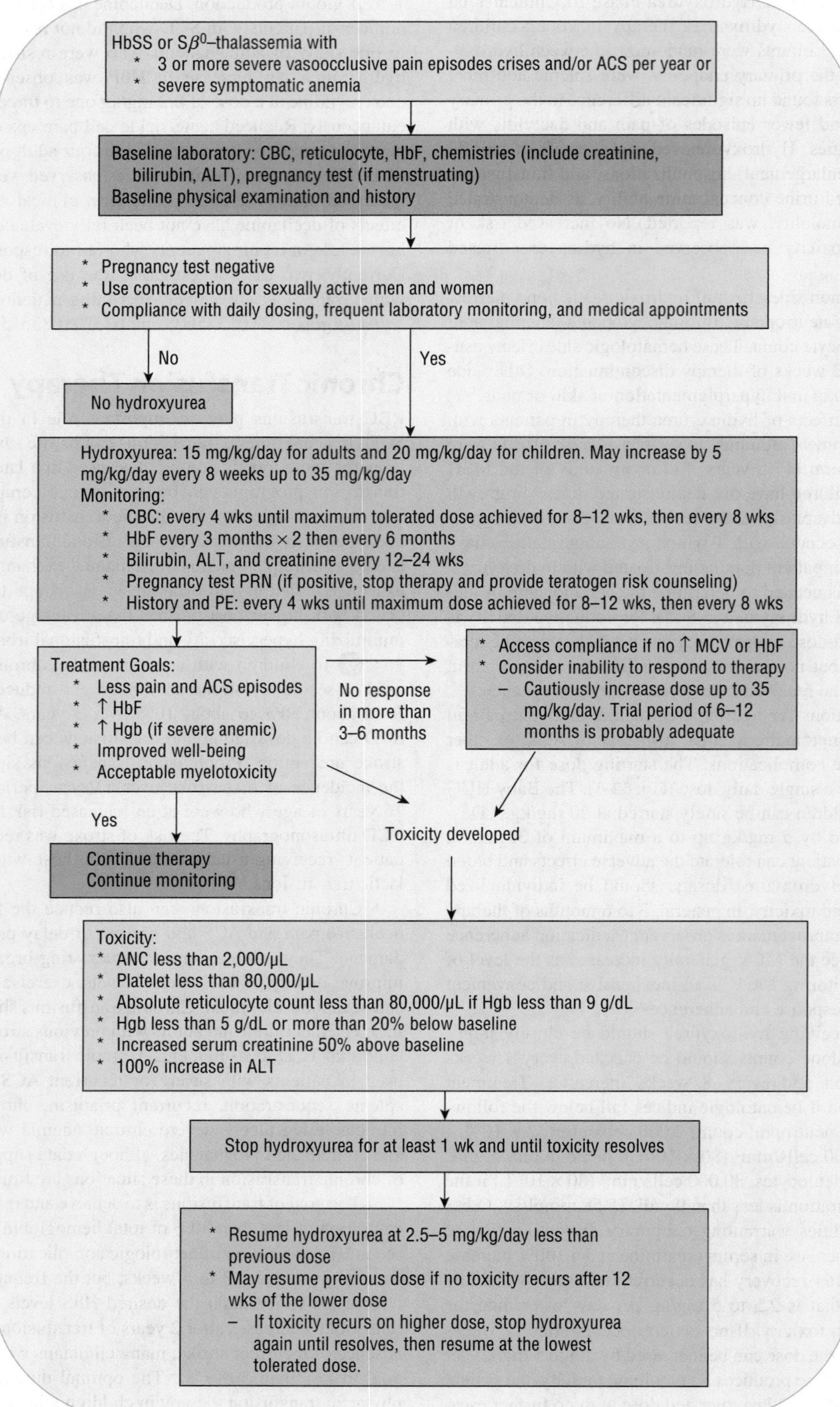

FIGURE 82-6 Hydroxyurea use in sickle cell disease. (ACS, acute chest syndrome; ALT, alanine aminotransferase; ANC, absolute neutrophil count; CBC, complete blood cell count; Hb, hemoglobin; HbF, fetal hemoglobin; HbSS, homozygous sickle cell hemoglobin; HBSSβ^0, sickle cell β^0-thalassemia; MCV, mean corpuscular volume; PE, physical examination; PRN, as needed; RBC, red blood cell.) *(From McCavit,[1] Ware and Aygun,[72] Wang et al.,[73] Ballas et al.,[78] and Heeney and Ware.[79])*

prevention, the SWiTCH trial, was closed early due to an increased risk of recurrent strokes in the hydroxyurea arm when compared to transfusions.[80]

Although the benefits of transfusion therapy are clear in some clinical situations, its role in other situations such as an acute pain episode, priapism, and leg ulcer remains controversial.[2,14,18] The risks of transfusion therapy must be weighed against possible benefits. The risks associated with transfusion therapy include alloimmunization (sensitization to the blood received), hyperviscosity, viral transmission, volume overload, iron overload, and nonhemolytic transfusion reactions. The use of leukocyte-reduced RBC transfusions in chronically transfused patients can reduce the risk of nonhemolytic transfusion reactions and viral transmission.[2,18] Transfusion-related infections also remain a concern. All patients should be immunized with hepatitis A and B vaccines. Other viruses that can be transmitted through blood products are parvovirus B19, hepatitis C, and cytomegalovirus. The risk of contracting human immunodeficiency virus from blood transfusions, although still of concern, has decreased with routine blood screening.[31]

Alloimmunization or alloantibody formation occurs in 19% to 37% of SCD patients who receive RBC transfusions and results from antigen differences on the red cell surface between the primarily Caucasian donor pool and recipients with SCD. Alloimmunization can make it difficult to find cross-matched blood and cause delayed hemolytic transfusion reactions. To prevent alloimmunization, patients receiving chronic transfusions should receive the best cross-matched blood including extended typing of other red cell antigens especially C, E, and Kell or full RBC phenotyping.[2,18,81]

The development of alloimmunization can be life-threatening for individuals with SCD. Delayed hemolytic transfusion reactions (DHTR) usually occur within 7 to 10 days after transfusion but can occur as early as 2 days or as late as 20 days after transfusion. During a DHTR, patients develop symptoms consistent with hemolysis such as worsened pain, especially abdominal pain, severe anemia due to hemolysis of the transfused unit, and reticulocytopenia, further aggravating the anemia. Subsequent transfusions can further worsen the clinical situation because of the presence of multiple antibodies making cross-matching difficult. Life-threatening events can be treated with steroids and IV immunoglobulin. Recombinant erythropoietin has been used in patients with reticulocytopenia. Recovery, as evidenced by reticulocytosis with a gradual increase in the hemoglobin level, may occur only after further transfusions are withheld. Although some patients tolerate further transfusions after recovery, especially if the donor unit is negative for the offending alloantibody, others cannot avoid recurrent transfusions and may experience another hemolytic transfusion reaction. Rituximab has been used in two patients to prevent recurrent DHTR. It is generally preferable to prevent the development of DHTR by performing RBC phenotyping and, at a minimum, transfusing individuals with blood that is C, E, and Kell negative.[2,18,81]

Transfusional iron overload is another complication of RBC transfusions, and patients should be counseled to avoid excess dietary iron. Abnormal liver biopsy results showing mild-to-moderate inflammation or fibrosis have been reported. Chelation therapy should be considered after more than 1 year of chronic transfusions or when serum ferritin is greater than 1,500 to 2,000 ng/mL (1,500 to 2,000 mcg/L). Two chelating agents are available. Deferoxamine has been used as a chelating agent for decades but must be administered by subcutaneous or IV infusion. Deferasirox, an oral chelator given at a dose of 20 to 30 mg/kg once daily, has shown to be equally effective as deferoxamine and has demonstrated acceptable safety profile in a long-term study for up to 5 years. The most common side effects with deferasirox are transient skin rash and GI symptoms such as nausea, vomiting, diarrhea, and abdominal pain.[27,81–83]

Allogeneic Hematopoietic Stem Cell Transplantation

Allogeneic HSCT is currently the only therapy that can cure patients with SCD. The overall survival rate and event-free survival rate for children and young adults with sibling matched donors have been reported at 93% to 97% and 82% to 86%, respectively.[84] The largest series included 87 patients aged 2 to 22 years with severe SCD. Transplant-related deaths occurred in six patients, with graft-versus-host disease (GVHD) being the main cause of death in four patients.[85] The reported incidences of acute and chronic GVHD ranged from 15% to 20% and 12% to 20%, respectively. Other complications included seizures, marrow rejection, and sepsis. Improved growth, stabilization or improvement of CNS abnormalities, and recovery of splenic dysfunction were observed in posttransplant SCD patients, but gonadal failure and delayed sexual development in females requiring hormonal replacements have been reported.[84,86]

The optimal candidates for allogeneic HSCT are SCD patients who are younger than 16 years of age; have a severe form of SCD and complications such as refractory pain, stroke, or recurrent ACS; and have an human leukocyte antigen (HLA)-matched sibling donor. Although allogeneic HSCT in young children before organ damage and alloimmunization occur are associated with an increased success, disease progression is unpredictable, making it difficult to determine the optimal time for transplantation. The risks associated with allogeneic HSCT must be carefully considered, as the transplant-related mortality rate is about 5% to 10%, and graft rejection is about 10%. Other risks associated with allogeneic HSCT include secondary malignancies. Neurologic events, such as intracranial hemorrhage and seizures during transplant, were seen more frequently in patients with a history of stroke.[85,86]

Experience with unrelated HLA-matched or related HLA-mismatched donor transplants is very limited. Unfortunately, many children who are eligible for allogeneic HSCT do not have an HLA-matched sibling donor and unrelated HLA-matched transplants are associated with higher transplant-related mortality. Umbilical cord blood is another potential donor source with specific advantages over marrow donors including a lower incidence of severe GVHD and a larger donor pool from which to select donors, but such advantages are balanced by longer time to engraftment and a higher rate of graft rejection.[85] Finally, a recent study of the use of nonmyeloablative allogeneic HSCT in 10 adult patients reported mixed donor-recipient chimerism and reversal of SCD and several open clinical trials continue to evaluate the role of reduced-intensity conditioning regimens.[87]

Treatment of Acute Complications

General Management

Parents and older children should be educated on the signs and symptoms of complications and conditions that require urgent evaluation. During acute illness, patients should be evaluated promptly, as deterioration can occur rapidly. Fluid balance should be maintained because dehydration and fluid overload can worsen complications associated with SCD. Oxygen saturation by pulse oximetry should be maintained at least 92% or at baseline. New or increasing supplemental oxygen requirements should be investigated.[14,18]

Episodic Transfusions

Indications for RBC transfusions include (a) acute exacerbation of baseline anemia, such as aplastic crisis if the anemia is severe, hepatic or splenic sequestration, or severe hemolysis; (b) ACS, stroke, or acute multiorgan failure; and (c) preparation for procedures that require the use of general anesthesia. Other patients in whom chronic transfusions can be useful include patients with complicated obstetric problems, refractory leg ulcers, or refractory and protracted painful episodes. Acute transfusion is not indicated for priapism, uncomplicated pain, or asymptomatic anemia. Simple transfusion or partial exchange transfusion can be used though red cell exchange has been shown to have superior outcomes when compared to simple transfusion in overt stroke. If simple transfusion is used, volume overload leading to congestive heart failure can occur if anemia is corrected too rapidly in patients with severe anemia. In addition, increases in hemoglobin levels to greater than 10 g/dL (6.2 mmol/L) can cause hyperviscosity and should be avoided.[2,18,81]

Infection and Fever

Patients with SCD should be evaluated as soon as possible for any fever greater than 38.5°C (101.3°F). Criteria for hospitalization include an infant younger than 1 year, history of previous bacteremia or sepsis, temperature greater than 40°C (104°F), WBC greater than 30,000 cells/mm^3 (30 × 10^9/L) or less than 5,000 cells/mm^3 (5 × 10^9/L) and/or platelets less than 100,000 cells/mm^3 (100 × 10^9/L), and evidence of other acute complications or toxic appearance. Outpatient management can be considered in older nontoxic children with reliable family caregivers. Antibiotic choice should provide adequate coverage for encapsulated organisms.[1,31]

7 Ceftriaxone should be used for outpatient management because it provides coverage for 24 hours. If admitted, cefotaxime can also be used. For patients with cephalosporin allergy, clindamycin can be used. Vancomycin should be considered for acutely ill children or if *Staphylococcus* is suspected. A macrolide antibiotic should be added if *M. pneumoniae* is suspected such as in ACS. Penicillin prophylaxis should be discontinued while the patient is receiving broad-spectrum antibiotics. Acetaminophen or ibuprofen can be used for fever control. Increased fluid requirements may be present because of poor oral intake and/or increased insensible losses contributing to dehydration.[1,2,31]

Cerebrovascular Accidents

Patients with acute neurologic events must be hospitalized and monitored closely. Physical and neurologic examination should be performed every 2 hours. Acute treatment for children should include exchange transfusion to maintain hemoglobin at about 10 g/dL (6.2 mmol/L) and HbS less than 30%, anticonvulsants for patients with a seizure history, and therapy for increased intracranial pressure if needed. Chronic transfusion therapy should be initiated for children with ischemic stroke as discussed earlier. In adults presenting with ischemic stroke related to atherosclerotic disease and not occlusion by sickled red cells, thrombolytic therapy should be considered if it is less than 3 hours since the onset of symptoms.[1,14,34]

Acute Chest Syndrome

Patients with ACS should use incentive spirometry frequently (e.g., at least every 2 hours while awake) to reduce atelectasis development. In addition, proper management of pain is important. The goal is to provide relief while avoiding analgesic-induced hypoventilation. Appropriate fluid therapy is important as overhydration can cause pulmonary edema and exacerbate respiratory distress. Early use of broad-spectrum antibiotics, including a macrolide or quinolone in adults, is also recommended. Studies indicate that infection is the most common cause of ACS and can involve gram-positive, gram-negative, or atypical bacteria. Oxygen therapy is indicated for all patients who are hypoxic or in acute distress. In a patient with a history of reactive airway disease, asthma or wheezing on examination, a trial of bronchodilators is appropriate. Transfusions are indicated for severe ACS with worsening hypoxia and increased work of breathing.[1,14,39]

Steroids can decrease inflammation and endothelial cell adhesion. Glucocorticoids can decrease the duration of hospitalization and need for transfusions and other supportive care but can also increase the readmission rate for other SCA-related complications. Another promising therapy is the use of NO, which relaxes and dilates blood vessels. Its hematologic effects include inhibition of platelet aggregation and reduction in the polymerization tendency of HbS. Marked improvement of pulmonary status and cardiac output were reported in a patient with ACS. Inhaled NO and oral L-arginine, the precursor of NO, are being evaluated for management of ACS in both children and adults.[1,27,39,40]

Priapism

Stuttering priapism, episodes that last a few minutes to 2 hours, may resolve spontaneously with exercise, warm bath, and oral analgesics. Prolonged episodes lasting more than 2 to 3 hours require prompt medical attention. The initial goals of treatment are to provide appropriate analgesic therapy, reduce anxiety, produce detumescence, and preserve testicular function and fertility. Treatment given within 4 to 6 hours can usually reduce erection. Aggressive hydration and adequate pain control should be initiated. Use of ice packs is not recommended. Heat (hot water bottles, hot packs, or sitz baths) can provide comfort without precipitating pain crisis. Although transfusions have been given to these patients, the efficacy of this therapeutic intervention has not been established and is associated with severe neurologic sequelae.[42,43]

Clinicians have used both vasoconstrictors and vasodilators in the treatment of priapism. Vasoconstrictors, such as diluted phenylephrine (10 mcg/mL) or epinephrine (1:1,000,000), are thought to work by forcing blood out of the corpus cavernosum into the venous return. In one uncontrolled open-label study, aspiration followed by intrapenile irrigation with epinephrine was effective and well tolerated. In that study, blood was first aspirated from the corpus cavernosum, and then the area was irrigated with a 1:1,000,000 solution of epinephrine. The priapism resolved in 37 of the 39 occasions. A follow-up study reported that 3 out of 20 patients required a repeat procedure within 24 hours. The therapy was well tolerated with no serious immediate or long-term side effects, but on two occasions, a small intrapenile hematoma formed after treatment. Detumescence can be achieved more rapidly using penile irrigation than simple transfusion but the procedure should be performed by an urologist with experience in the treatment of priapism.[43,88–90]

Vasodilators, such as terbutaline and hydralazine, relax the smooth muscle of the vasculature. This relaxation allows oxygenated arterial blood to enter the corpus cavernosum, which displaces or washes out the damaged sickle cells that are stagnant in the corpus cavernosum. Terbutaline has been used to treat priapism, but it has not been formally studied in patients with SCD.[43,90] In one case report, a single oral sildenafil dose at onset of priapism aborted episodes. However, long-term studies of sildenafil have shown an increase in the frequency of pain episodes (*http://www.clinicaltrials.gov* NCT00492531). Surgical interventions used in severe refractory priapism have included a variety of shunt procedures. These surgical procedures have been successful in some cases, but they have a high failure rate and potential serious complications, which include impotence, skin sloughing, cellulitis, and urethral fistulas.[42]

Modalities to prevent priapism are limited and not well studied. Pseudoephedrine (30 or 60 mg/day given orally at bedtime) and leuprolide, a gonadotropin-releasing hormone, have been used to decrease the number of recurrent episodes of priapism. Hydroxyurea therapy can also be useful although the effect of hydroxyurea on the prevalence of priapism has not been formally investigated. Finally, antiandrogens (bicalutamide and finasteride) have been used in SCD for treatment of recurrent or refractory priapism without major side effects. The role of RBC transfusion in preventing priapism remains unclear and transfusion is not recommended for long-term management.[1,43,90]

Clinical **Controversy...**

Some clinicians transfuse patients to maintain an HbS level less than 30% to prevent recurrent priapism. Duration of such regimens should be limited to 6 to 12 months. Clinical practice guidelines do not recommend chronic transfusion to prevent recurrent priapism.

Aplastic Crisis

Treatment of aplastic crisis is primarily supportive, and most patients recover spontaneously in 5 to 10 days. The only treatment may be RBC transfusions if the anemia is severe or symptomatic. The reticulocyte count is used to detect the suppression of red cell production and the need for transfusion. The most common cause, parvovirus B19, is contagious and infected patients should be placed in isolation. In addition, contact with pregnant healthcare providers should be avoided because parvovirus infection during the midtrimester of pregnancy can result in hydrops fetalis and stillbirth.[14,18,31]

Splenic Sequestration

Splenic sequestration crisis is a major cause of mortality in young children with SCD. The sequestration of RBCs in the spleen can result in a rapid drop of hemoglobin, leading to hypovolemia, shock, and death. Immediate treatment with RBC transfusions is indicated to correct hypovolemia. Broad-spectrum antibiotic therapy, which includes coverage for *pneumococci* and *H. influenzae*, can also be beneficial if the patient is febrile as infection can precipitate sequestration.[1]

Recurrent episodes occur in about half of patients and are associated with increased mortality. Options for management of recurrence include observation, chronic transfusion, and splenectomy. Increased risk of invasive infection after splenectomy is a concern in very young children, but most experts agree individuals with HbSS develop splenic dysfunction as early as 6 months of age and have acquired asplenia by 5 years of age and by 10 to 12 years for those with Hb SC. Splenectomy is probably indicated, even after a single sequestration crisis, if that sequestration was life threatening. Splenectomy should be considered after repetitive episodes, even if they are less serious. For children younger than 2 years of age, chronic blood transfusions are recommended by some experts, though not supported by evidence, to prevent sequestration and delay splenectomy until the age of 2 years, when the risk of postsplenectomy septicemia is lower and pneumococcal vaccination has been completed. Finally, splenectomy should also be considered for patients with chronic hypersplenism.[27,91]

Acute Sickle Cell Pain

Hydration and analgesia are the mainstays of treatment for vaso-occlusive (painful) episodes (Table 82-4). Patients with mild pain crisis can be treated as outpatients with rest, increased fluid intake, warm compresses, and oral analgesics. Hospitalization is necessary for moderate to severe pain or when oral analgesics fail to relieve pain. A pain episode may be precipitated by several risk factors including infection. In the setting of pain and fever, an infectious etiology should be evaluated, and appropriate empiric therapy should be initiated in patients who have fever or are critically ill. In patients with severe symptomatic anemia, transfusions may be indicated. Fluid replacement given IV or orally to correct or prevent hydration at 1 to 1.5 times the maintenance requirement is recommended. Close monitoring of fluid status is essential as aggressive hydration, particularly with sodium-containing fluids, can lead to volume overload, ACS, and heart failure.[92,93]

TABLE 82-4 Management of Acute Sickle Cell Pain

Principles
- Treat underlying precipitating factors
- Avoid delays in analgesia administration
- Use pain scale to assess severity
- Choice of initial analgesic should be based on previous pain pattern, history of response, current status, and other medical conditions
- Schedule pain medication; avoid as-needed dosing
- Provide rescue dose for breakthrough pain
- If adequate pain relief can be achieved with one or two doses of morphine, consider outpatient management with a weak opioid; otherwise hospitalization is needed for parenteral analgesics
- Frequently assess to evaluate pain severity and side effects; titrate dose as needed
- Treating adverse effects of opioids is part of pain management
- Consider nonpharmacologic intervention (e.g., relaxation techniques, guided imagery, deep breathing)
- Transition to oral analgesics as the patient improves; choose an oral agent based on previous history, anticipated duration, and ability to swallow tablets; if sustained-release products are used, a product with a rapid onset is also needed for breakthrough pain

Analgesic regimens

Mild-to-moderate pain: nonopioid ± weak opioid
Moderate-to-severe pain: weak opioid or low dose of a strong opioid ± nonopioid
Severe pain: strong opioid + nonopioid

Other adjunct therapy

Hydration, heating pads, relaxation, and distraction
Stool softener and/or stimulants for constipation
Antihistamine for itching
Antiemetics for nausea or vomiting

From Zempsky,[92] Jerrell et al.,[93] and Wright and Ahmedzai.[94]

The frequency and severity of acute pain episodes associated with SCD are variable. Pain should be assessed and analgesic therapy should be tailored for each patient and each individual episode. Several verbal and nonverbal pain assessment tools are available and should be used to measure the intensity of pain. Unfortunately, they have not been validated for sickle cell pain. However, pain scales validated for use in children, such as the Wong-Baker FACES scale, should be used in pediatric patients with SCD pain. The healthcare provider should choose one tool appropriate for age and use it routinely to assess pain. Other useful information to guide choice of analgesics should include previous effective agents and their dosages, response to therapy and previous clinical course, and duration of pain episodes.[14,92,93]

8 Aggressive therapy that relieves pain and enables the patient to attain maximum functional ability should be initiated in patients with acute pain. Mild-to-moderate pain should be treated with nonsteroidal antiinflammatory drugs (NSAIDs) or acetaminophen, unless there are contraindications to their use (Table 82-5). Ketorolac may be useful for patients requiring IV therapy. Because of concerns about GI bleeding, it is recommended to limit the duration of therapy to 5 days or less. Ketorolac has also been associated with acute nonreversible kidney failure in a patient with SCD and should be used with caution and renal function monitored appropriately. When acetaminophen is used, it is important to monitor the total dose of acetaminophen administered in patients who may also be receiving the agent for fever or another acetaminophen-containing product for pain. If mild-to-moderate pain persists, an opioid should be added. Effective combination therapy, such as an NSAID combined with an opioid, can enhance analgesic efficacy while decreasing side effects.[14,92–94]

Severe pain should be treated aggressively until the pain is tolerable. Commonly used opioids include morphine, hydromorphone, fentanyl, and methadone (Table 82-5). The weak opioids, codeine and hydrocodone, are used to manage mild-to-moderate pain usually

TABLE 82-5 Commonly Used Analgesics Dosing Table

Drug	Brand Name	Initial Dose	Comments
Nonopioid			
Ibuprofen	Motrin® Advil®	Children: 10 mg/kg orally every 6–8 hours Adult: 400–800 mg/dose orally every 6–8 hours	• Use with caution in patients with renal failure (dehydration) and bleeding • Individualized dosing based on history and severity of pain
Naproxen	Naprosyn® Aleve®	Children: 5–7 mg/kg orally every 8–12 hours Adult: 250–500 mg/dose every 12 hours	• Use with caution in patients with renal failure (dehydration) and bleeding • Individualized dosing based on history and severity of pain
Ketorolac	Toradol®	Children: 0.5 mg/kg IV up to 30 mg/dose every 6 hours Adults: 30 mg/dose IV every 6 hours	• Maximum 5 days • Use with caution in patients with renal failure (dehydration) and bleeding
Weak Opioid			
Acetaminophen with codeine	Tylenol with codeine	Children: 0.5–1 mg/kg per dose orally every 4–6 hours Adult: 30–60 mg/dose orally every 4–6 hours	• Dose based on codeine • Maximum acetaminophen 3 g/day • Commonly given as needed in combination with weak strong opioid • Individualized dosing based on history and severity of pain
Acetaminophen with hydrocodone	Lortab® Norco® Vicodin®	Children: 0.15–0.2 mg/kg per dose orally every 4–6 hours Adults: 5–10 mg/dose orally every 4–6 hours	• Dose based on hydrocodone • Maximum total acetaminophen 3 g/day • Commonly given as needed in combination with weak strong opioid
Strong Opioid			
Morphine		Children: 0.1–0.2 mg/kg per dose IV every 3–4 hours Adults: 5–10 mg/dose IV every 3–4 hours IV continuous infusion: 0.05–0.2 mg/kg per hour; titrate to effect Patient-controlled analgesics: 0.05 mg/kg per hours basal; demand 0.01–0.03 mg/kg every 20 minutes; 4-hour lock out 0.5–0.6 mg/kg	• For breakthrough, give 1/4 to 1/2 of the scheduled dose as bolus every 1–2 hours; assess amount of rescue dose used in 8–12 hours and readjust scheduled dose or infusion rate as needed • Individualized dosing based on history and severity of pain
Hydromorphone	Dilaudid®	Children: 0.02–0.03 mg/kg per dose IV every 3–4 hours Adults: 1.5–2 mg/dose IV every 3–4 hours Patient-controlled analgesics: 0.003–0.005 mg/kg per hour basal; demand 0.03–0.05 mg/kg every 10 minutes; 4 hour lock out 0.06–0.08 mg/kg	• For breakthrough, give 1/4 to 1/2 of the scheduled dose as bolus every 1–2 hours; assess amount of rescue dose used in 8–12 hours and readjust scheduled dose or infusion rate as needed • Individualized dosing based on history and severity of pain

in the outpatient setting. Meperidine has no advantages as an analgesic and significant negative sequelae. Its duration of action is short compared with the half-life of the metabolite normeperidine, which accumulates and can cause CNS side effects, ranging from dysphoria to seizures. Meperidine is contraindicated for use in children to treat acute pain and should be avoided if possible and used only for a very brief duration in adult patients who are allergic or intolerant to other opioids.[92–94]

Both prior history and current assessment should be considered in the management of acute sickle cell pain. For patients whose typical pain improves in a short time, preparations with a short duration of action are appropriate. For patients whose pain requires many days to resolve, sustained-release preparations combined with a short-acting product for breakthrough pain are more appropriate. If the patient has been on long-term opioid therapy at home, tolerance can develop. In these cases, the acute pain can be treated with an opioid of different potency or a larger dose of the same medication. IV administration provides a rapid onset of action and therefore is preferred for severe pain. Intramuscular injections should be avoided. Children may actually deny pain due to fear of injections. Analgesics should be titrated to pain relief. In patients with continuous pain, the analgesic should be given as a scheduled dose or continuous infusion. Continuous infusion has the advantage of less fluctuation of blood levels between dosing intervals. As needed dosing is only indicated for breakthrough pain. Patient-controlled analgesia (PCA) is commonly prescribed for severe pain episodes. When used properly, PCA allows patients to have control over pain therapy and minimizes the lag time between perception of pain and administration of analgesics. Studies have shown PCA reduced cumulative dosage required for pain control. The transdermal fentanyl patch has also been used successfully, but its role in sickle cell pain crisis is unclear because of its slow onset of onset of pain relief (12 to 16 hours) and fixed dosage form, which makes it difficult to titrate the dose. Other alternative pain management techniques such as physical therapy, massage, biofeedback, and relaxation therapy can be helpful as adjunct therapy.[27,92–94]

Suboptimal pain relief has been reported in both emergency room and hospitalized patients. The most common cause of suboptimal pain control in children and adults with SCD is the suspicion of addiction. This obstacle is especially common in adolescents. In one study, 53% of emergency physicians believed that 20% of SCD patients are psychologically addicted to opioid analgesics. Another barrier to effective pain control is the difference in perception between patients, family, and healthcare providers. Patients with SCD often suffer from chronic pain, and they may cope with the pain by being inactive. Patients who have inadequate pain control can exhibit anxiety and drug-seeking behavior for fear of pain. Tolerance to opioids may also be misinterpreted as drug addiction by healthcare providers and families. Aggressive pain control, frequent monitoring of pain during episodes, and tapering medication according to response are factors that minimize physical dependence. The use of a protocol has been shown to result in optimal management of pain control in SCD.[92–94]

Inhaled NO has been studied as therapy to abort pain at onset of episodes. Significant reduction of pain scores in adult patients received inhaled NO in the emergency room.[95] However, no differences in duration of episodes, hospital stay, or opioid use when given to hospitalized adult and pediatric patients were observed.[96] Systemic corticosteroids, methylprednisolone and dexamethasone, have also been evaluated as an adjunct therapy for pain control. Shorter duration of analgesic therapy and duration of hospitalization were reported but increased risk of readmission was also reported.[97]

PERSONALIZED PHARMACOTHERAPY

The mainstay of treatment in SCD involves medical therapy for supportive care and disease modification. Medical therapy is usually individualized by weight-based dosing. However, newer approaches are being evaluated to personalize therapy based on pharmacokinetics and pharmacodynamics. For example, many adults with SCD have abnormal renal function due to intrarenal sickling. The most important disease modifying medication, hydroxyurea, is renally excreted with urinary recovery of 40% of the administered dose in adults with SCD. A lower initial dose of 7.5 mg/kg per day is recommended for individuals with creatinine clearance of less than 60 mL/min.[7,98] Pharmacokinetic differences between adult and pediatric patients were not reported in the initial study of a small cohort of SCD patients.[7] As a result, investigators designed a prospective clinical trial, the Hydroxyurea Study of Long-Term Effects (HUSTLE, NCT00305175), to evaluate interpatient variability among children taking hydroxyurea. For the first-dose pharmacokinetic studies, 51 of 87 patients showed a "fast" absorption profile with an earlier and higher maximum concentration after a single dose of 20 mg/kg. Pharmacodynamic analysis identified several parameters that were associated with maximum tolerated dose (MTD) and HbF at MTD. However, prediction of response to hydroxyurea based on pharmacokinetic and pharmacodynamic parameters was unsatisfactory and the investigators concluded that standardized dose escalation to myelosuppression remains to be the best option.[99]

Adults and children with SCD require the use of acute and chronic pain medications including opioids to control painful episodes. Some patients have inadequate relief to codeine. Children who failed oral therapy with codeine were found to have a polymorphism in the *CYP2D6* gene which results in a poor metabolizer phenotype. The CYP2D6 enzyme mediates the conversion of codeine to morphine. These results can lead to early discontinuation of codeine analgesics in children with SCD if no response is observed after their first dose and the use of alternative oral analgesics for the treatment of pain at home. In patients with SCD, analgesia is sometimes not obtained even with very high IV opioid doses. Several enzymes that are involved in morphine metabolism may be altered in patients with SCD including UGT2B7, a morphine-metabolizing enzyme; OPRM1, a mu-opioid receptor or ABCB1, a transporter protein at the blood–brain barrier. Further studies are needed to evaluate the importance of genetic variations in these enzymes.[100]

The concept of personalized therapy in SCD is now evolving with the identification of single nucleotide polymorphisms (SNPs) associated with disease severity and HbF responses to hydroxyurea therapy. Genome-wide association studies have identified several loci in HbF expression. BCL11A is a transcription factor that regulates hemoglobin switching and could account for the variability of HbF levels between individuals with high and low HbF. Different biomarkers have been studied in SCD to identify complications and phenotypic variability. The potential use of biomarkers and genome-based modification of phenotype in SCD may allow personalized therapeutic approaches in the future.[2,3,7]

EVALUATION OF THERAPEUTIC OUTCOMES

9 SCD is a complex disorder that requires multidisciplinary comprehensive care. All patients should be medically evaluated regularly to provide preventive care, establish baseline symptoms and laboratory values, monitor changes, and provide education appropriate for age. For infants younger than 1 year old, medical evaluations every 2 to 4 months are needed. Beyond 2 years of age, evaluation can be extended to every 6 to 12 months with modifications depending on severity of the illness.

Routine laboratory evaluation including complete blood cell counts and reticulocyte counts every 3 to 6 months up to 2 years of age, then every 6 to 12 months; the HbF level should be screened annually until 2 years of age, then annually. Evaluation of renal, hepatobiliary, and pulmonary function should be done annually. TCD screening is recommended to start at age 2 years and performed annually for children with HbSS and HbSβ^0. Ophthalmologic examination to screen for retinopathy is recommended at around age 10 to 12 years for those with HbSC and 14 years for HbSS. In patients with recurrent ACS, pulmonary function tests should be done to establish baseline values and identify declines in lung function as well as an evaluation by pulmonology to screen for lower airway hyperresponsiveness.

It is essential that immunizations and prophylactic antibiotics be given. When infections do occur, appropriate antibiotic therapy should be initiated, and the patient should be monitored for laboratory and clinical improvement. The efficacy of hydroxyurea can be measured as a decrease in the number, severity, and duration of sickle cell pain episodes. HbF concentrations or MCV values can also provide some indication of the patient's response to therapy. When painful episodes do occur, the effectiveness of analgesics can be measured by subjective assessments made by the patient, family, and healthcare practitioners. The success of poststroke blood transfusions can be measured by clinical progression or the occurrence of subsequent strokes. Finally, indicators can be used for measurements of quality of care for children with SCD.

ABBREVIATIONS

ASPEN	association of sickle cell disease, priapism, exchange transfusion, and neurologic events
ACS	acute chest syndrome
CT	computed tomography
EEG	electroencephalography
GVHD	graft-versus-host disease
HbA	hemoglobin A
HbAS	one normal (hemoglobin A) and one sickle cell hemoglobin (hemoglobin S) gene
HbC	hemoglobin C
HbF	fetal hemoglobin
HbSβ^+-thal	hemoglobin sickle cell β^+-thalassemia
HbSβ^0-thal	hemoglobin sickle cell β^0-thalassemia
HbSC	sickle cell hemoglobin C
HbSS	homozygous sickle cell hemoglobin (hemoglobin S)
HbS	sickle cell hemoglobin
HLA	human leukocyte antigen
HPFH	hereditary persistence of fetal hemoglobin
HSCT	hematopoietic stem cell transplantation
ISC	irreversibly sickled cell
MCHC	mean corpuscular hemoglobin concentration
MCV	mean corpuscular volume
MRI	magnetic resonance imaging
MSH	Multicenter Study of Hydroxyurea in Sickle Cell Anemia

MTD	maximum tolerated dose
NO	nitric oxide
NSAID	nonsteroidal antiinflammatory drug
PCA	patient-controlled analgesia
PCV7	7-valent pneumococcal conjugate vaccine
PCV13	13-valent pneumococcal conjugate vaccine
PPSV 23	23-valent pneumococcal polysaccharide vaccine
RBC	red blood cell
SCA	sickle cell anemia
SCD	sickle cell disease
SCT	sickle cell trait
SNP	single nucleotide polymorphism
TCD	transcranial Doppler
WBC	white blood cell

REFERENCES

1. McCavit TL. Sickle cell disease. Pediatr Rev 2012;33:195–204; quiz 5–6.
2. Rees DC, Williams TN, Gladwin MT. Sickle-cell disease. Lancet 2010;376:2018–2031.
3. Steinberg MH, Sebastiani P. Genetic modifiers of sickle cell disease. Am J Hematol 2012;87:795–803.
4. Rees DC, Gibson JS. Biomarkers in sickle cell disease. British J Haematol 2012;156:433–445.
5. Eridani S, Mosca A. Fetal hemoglobin reactivation and cell engineering in the treatment of sickle cell anemia. J Blood Med 2011;2:23–30.
6. Odievre MH, Verger E, Silva-Pinto AC, Elion J. Pathophysiological insights in sickle cell disease. Indian J Med Res 2011;134:532–537.
7. Hankins J, Aygun B. Pharmacotherapy in sickle cell disease—State of the art and future prospects. Br J Haematol 2009;145:296–308.
8. Dampier C, LeBeau P, Rhee S, et al. Health-related quality of life in adults with sickle cell disease (SCD): A report from the comprehensive sickle cell centers clinical trial consortium. Am J Hematol 2011;86:203–205.
9. Dale JC, Cochran CJ, Roy L, Jernigan E, Buchanan GR. Health-related quality of life in children and adolescents with sickle cell disease. J Pediatr Health Care 2011;25:208–215.
10. Swanson ME, Grosse SD, Kulkarni R. Disability among individuals with sickle cell disease: Literature review from a public health perspective. Am J Prev Med 2011;41(6 Suppl 4): S390–S397.
11. Wang CJ, Kavanagh PL, Little AA, Holliman JB, Sprinz PG. Quality-of-care indicators for children with sickle cell disease. Pediatrics 2011;128:484–493.
12. Aygun B, Odame I. A global perspective on sickle cell disease. Pediatr Blood Cancer 2012;59:386–390.
13. Creary M, Williamson D, Kulkarni R. Sickle cell disease: Current activities, public health implications, and future directions. J Womens Health 2007;16:575–582.
14. Steinberg MH. In the clinic: sickle cell disease. Ann Intern Med 2011;155:ITC31–15; quiz ITC316.
15. National Institutes of Health, Division of Blood Diseases and Resources, Public Health Service. Who is at risk for sickle cell anemia? September 2012 [cited November 6, 2012]. *http://www.nhlbi.nih.gov/health/health-topics/topics/sca/atrisk.html.*
16. National Human Genome Research Institute N. Learning about sickle cell disease. October 2011 [cited November 2012]. *http://www.genome.gov/10001219.*
17. Key NS, Derebail VK. Sickle-cell trait: Novel clinical significance. Hematology Am Soc Hematol Educ Program 2010;2010:418–422.
18. Roseff SD. Sickle cell disease: A review. Immunohematology 2009;25:67–74.
19. Benson JM, Therrell BL Jr. History and current status of newborn screening for hemoglobinopathies. Semin Perinatol 2010;34:134–144.
20. U. S. Preventive Services Task Force. Screening for Sickle Cell Disease in Newborns: U.S. Preventive Services Task Force Recommendation Statement. AHRQ Publication No 07-05104-EF-2, September 2007 [cited September 17, 2012]. *http://www.uspreventiveservicestaskforce.org/uspstf07/sicklecell/sicklers.htm.*
21. Michlitsch J, Azimi M, Hoppe C, et al. Newborn screening for hemoglobinopathies in California. Pediatr Blood Cancer 2009;52:486–490.
22. Grant AM, Parker CS, Jordan LB, et al. Public health implications of sickle cell trait: A report of the CDC meeting. Am J Prev Med 2011;41(6 Suppl 4):S435–439.
23. Thurman AR, Steed LL, Hulsey T, Soper DE. Bacteriuria in pregnant women with sickle cell trait. Am J Obstet Gynecol 2006;194:1366–1370.
24. Quinn CT, Lee NJ, Shull EP, et al. Prediction of adverse outcomes in children with sickle cell anemia: A study of the Dallas Newborn Cohort Blood 2008;111:544–548.
25. Miller AC, Gladwin MT. Pulmonary complications of sickle cell disease. Am J Resp Crit Care Med 2012;185:1154–1165.
26. Yanni E, Grosse SD, Yang Q, Olney RS. Trends in pediatric sickle cell disease-related mortality in the United States, 1983–2002. J Pediat 2009;154:541–545.
27. Meier ER, Miller JL. Sickle cell disease in children. Drugs 2012;72:895–906.
28. Narang S, Fernandez ID, Chin N, Lerner N, Weinberg GA. Bacteremia in children with sickle hemoglobinopathies. J Pediatr Hematol Oncol 2012;34:13–16.
29. McCavit TL, Xuan L, Zhang S, Flores G, Quinn CT. Hospitalization for invasive pneumococcal disease in a national sample of children with sickle cell disease before and after PCV7 licensure. Pediatr Blood Cancer 2012;58:945–949.
30. McCavit TL, Quinn CT, Techasaensiri C, Rogers ZR. Increase in invasive Streptococcus pneumoniae infections in children with sickle cell disease since pneumococcal conjugate vaccine licensure. J Pediatr 2011;158:505–507.
31. Booth C, Inusa B, Obaro SK. Infection in sickle cell disease: A review. Intern J Infect Dis 2010;14:e2–e12.
32. Richards LH, Howard J, Klein JL. Community-acquired Salmonella bacteraemia in patients with sickle-cell disease 1969–2008: A single centre study. Scand J Infect Dis 2011;43:89–94.
33. Mava Y, Ambe JP, Bello M, Watila I, Nottidge VA. Urinary tract infection in febrile children with sickle cell anaemia. West African J Med 2011;30:268–272.
34. Verduzco LA, Nathan DG. Sickle cell disease and stroke. Blood 2009;114:5117–5125.
35. DeBaun MR, Armstrong FD, McKinstry RC, et al. Silent cerebral infarcts: A review on a prevalent and progressive cause of neurologic injury in sickle cell anemia. Blood 2012;119:4587–4596.
36. Hijmans CT, Grootenhuis MA, Oosterlaan J, et al. Neurocognitive deficits in children with sickle cell disease are associated with the severity of anemia. Pediatr Blood Cancer 2011;57:297–302.
37. Hijmans CT, Fijnvandraat K, Grootenhuis MA, et al. Neurocognitive deficits in children with sickle cell disease: A comprehensive profile. Pediatr Blood Cancer 2011;56:783–788.

38. Poulter EY, Truszkowski P, Thompson AA, Liem RI. Acute chest syndrome is associated with history of asthma in hemoglobin SC disease. Pediatr Blood Cancer 2011;57:289–293.
39. Paul RN, Castro OL, Aggarwal A, Oneal PA. Acute chest syndrome: Sickle cell disease. Eur J Haematol 2011;87:191–207.
40. Gladwin MT, Vichinsky E. Pulmonary complications of sickle cell disease. N Engl J Med 2008;359:2254–2265.
41. Chrouser KL, Ajiboye OB, Oyetunji TA, Chang DC. Priapism in the United States: The changing role of sickle cell disease. Am J Surgery 2011;201:468–474.
42. Broderick GA, Kadioglu A, Bivalacqua TJ, et al. Priapism: Pathogenesis, epidemiology, and management. J Sex Med 2010;7(1 Pt 2):476–500.
43. Crane GM, Bennett NE Jr. Priapism in sickle cell anemia: Emerging mechanistic understanding and better preventative strategies. Anemia 2011;2011:297364.
44. Ballas SK, Gupta K, Adams-Graves P. Sickle cell pain: A critical reappraisal. Blood 2012;120:3647–3656.
45. Najim OA, Hassan MK. Lactate dehydrogenase and severity of pain in children with sickle cell disease. Acta Haematol 2011;126:157–162.
46. Rogovik AL, Li Y, Kirby MA, Friedman JN, Goldman RD. Admission and length of stay due to painful vasoocclusive crisis in children. Am J Emerg Med 2009;27:797–801.
47. Brousse V, Elie C, Benkerrou M, et al. Acute splenic sequestration crisis in sickle cell disease: Cohort study of 190 paediatric patients. Br J Haematol 2012;156:643–648.
48. Caboot JB, Allen JL. Pulmonary complications of sickle cell disease in children. Curr Opin Pediatr 2008;20:279–287.
49. McLaughlin VV, Archer SL, Badesch DB, et al. ACCF/AHA 2009 expert consensus document on pulmonary hypertension: A report of the American College of Cardiology Foundation Task Force on Expert Consensus Documents and the American Heart Association: developed in collaboration with the American College of Chest Physicians, American Thoracic Society, Inc., and the Pulmonary Hypertension Association. Circulation 2009;119:2250–2294.
50. Mahadeo KM, Oyeku S, Taragin B, et al. Increased prevalence of osteonecrosis of the femoral head in children and adolescents with sickle-cell disease. Am J Hematol 2011;86:806–808.
51. Matos MA, dos Santos Silva LL, Brito Fernandes R, Dias Malheiros C, Pinto da Silva BV. Avascular necrosis of the femoral head in sickle cell disease patients. Ortop Traumatol Rehabil 2012;14:155–160.
52. Chapelon E, Garabedian M, Brousse V, et al. Osteopenia and vitamin D deficiency in children with sickle cell disease. Eur J Haematol 2009;83:572–578.
53. Minniti CP, Eckman J, Sebastiani P, Steinberg MH, Ballas SK. Leg ulcers in sickle cell disease. Am J Hematol 2010;85:831–833.
54. Fadugbagbe AO, Gurgel RQ, Mendonca CQ, et al. Ocular manifestations of sickle cell disease. Ann Trop Paediatr 2010;30:19–26.
55. Ebert EC, Nagar M, Hagspiel KD. Gastrointestinal and hepatic complications of sickle cell disease. Clin Gastroenterol Hepatol 2010;8:483–489.
56. Voskaridou E, Christoulas D, Terpos E. Sickle-cell disease and the heart: Review of the current literature. Br J Haematol 2012;157:664–673.
57. Fitzhugh CD, Lauder N, Jonassaint JC, et al. Cardiopulmonary complications leading to premature deaths in adult patients with sickle cell disease. Am J Hematol 2010;85:36–40.
58. Ware RE, Rees RC, Sarnaik SA, et al. Renal function in infants with sickle cell anemia: Baseline data from the BABY HUG trial. J Pediatr 2010;156:66–70.
59. Sharpe CC, Thein SL. Sickle cell nephropathy—A practical approach. Br J Haematol 2011;155:287–297.
60. Bennett EL. Understanding growth failure in children with homozygous sickle-cell disease. J Pediatr Oncol Nursing 2011;28:67–74.
61. Al-Saqladi AW, Cipolotti R, Fijnvandraat K, Brabin BJ. Growth and nutritional status of children with homozygous sickle cell disease. Ann Trop Paediatr 2008;28:165–189.
62. Levenson JL, McClish DK, Dahman BA, et al. Depression and anxiety in adults with sickle cell disease: The PiSCES project. Psychosom Med 2008;70:192–196.
63. Simon K, Barakat LP, Patterson CA, Dampier C. Symptoms of depression and anxiety in adolescents with sickle cell disease: The role of intrapersonal characteristics and stress processing variables. Child Psychiatr Hum Dev 2009;40:317–330.
64. Unal S, Toros F, Kutuk MO, Uyaniker MG. Evaluation of the psychological problems in children with sickle cell anemia and their families. Ped Hematol Oncol 2011;28:321–328.
65. Benton TD, Boyd R, Ifeagwu J, Feldtmose E, Smith-Whitley K. Psychiatric diagnosis in adolescents with sickle cell disease: A preliminary report. Current Psychiatr Rep 2011;13:111–115.
66. Rogers DT, Molokie R. Sickle cell disease in pregnancy. Obstet Gynecol Clin North Am 2010;37:223–237.
67. Barfield WD, Barradas DT, Manning SE, Kotelchuck M, Shapiro-Mendoza CK. Sickle cell disease and pregnancy outcomes: Women of African descent. Am J Prev Med 2010;38(4 Suppl):S542–S549.
68. Quinn CT, Rogers ZR, McCavit TL, Buchanan GR. Improved survival of children and adolescents with sickle cell disease. Blood 2010;115:3447–3452.
69. Nuorti JP, Whitney CG. Prevention of pneumococcal disease among infants and children—Use of 13-valent pneumococcal conjugate vaccine and 23-valent pneumococcal polysaccharide vaccine—Recommendations of the Advisory Committee on Immunization Practices (ACIP). MMWR Recomm Rep 2010;59:1–18.
70. Licensure of a meningococcal conjugate vaccine (Menveo) and guidance for use—Advisory Committee on Immunization Practices (ACIP), 2010. MMWR 2010;59:273.
71. Infant Meningococcal Vaccination: Advisory Committee on Immunization Practices (ACIP) Recommendations and Rationale. MMWR 2013;62:52–54.
72. Ware RE, Aygun B. Advances in the use of hydroxyurea. Hematology Am Soc Hematol Educ Program 2009;2009:62–69.
73. Wang WC, Ware RE, Miller ST, et al. Hydroxycarbamide in very young children with sickle-cell anaemia: A multicentre, randomised, controlled trial (BABY HUG). Lancet 2011;377:1663–1672.
74. Alvarez O, Miller ST, Wang WC, et al. Effect of hydroxyurea treatment on renal function parameters: Results from the multi-center placebo-controlled BABY HUG clinical trial for infants with sickle cell anemia. Pediatr Blood Cancer 2012;59:668–674.
75. Thornburg CD, Files BA, Luo Z, et al. Impact of hydroxyurea on clinical events in the BABY HUG trial. Blood 2012;120:4304–4310.
76. McGann PT, Flanagan JM, Howard TA, et al. Genotoxicity associated with hydroxyurea exposure in infants with sickle cell anemia: Results from the BABY-HUG Phase III Clinical Trial. Pediatr Blood Cancer 2012;59:254–257.

77. Steinberg MH, McCarthy WF, Castro O, et al. The risks and benefits of long-term use of hydroxyurea in sickle cell anemia: A 17.5 year follow-up. Am J Hematol 2010;85:403–408.
78. Ballas SK, McCarthy WF, Guo N, et al. Exposure to hydroxyurea and pregnancy outcomes in patients with sickle cell anemia. J Natl Med Assoc 2009;101:1046–1051.
79. Heeney MM, Ware RE. Hydroxyurea for children with sickle cell disease. Hematol Oncol Clin North Am 2010;24:199–214.
80. Ware RE, Helms RW. Stroke with transfusions changing to hydroxyurea (SWiTCH). Blood 2012;119:3925–3932.
81. Smith-Whitley K, Thompson AA. Indications and complications of transfusions in sickle cell disease. Pediatr Blood Cancer 2012;59:358–364.
82. Vichinsky E, Bernaudin F, Forni GL, et al. Long-term safety and efficacy of deferasirox (Exjade) for up to 5 years in transfusional iron-overloaded patients with sickle cell disease. Br J Haematol 2011;154:387–397.
83. Cancado R, Olivato MC, Bruniera P, et al. Two-year analysis of efficacy and safety of deferasirox treatment for transfusional iron overload in sickle cell anemia patients. Acta Haematol 2012;128:113–118.
84. Khoury R, Abboud MR. Stem-cell transplantation in children and adults with sickle cell disease: An update. Expert Rev Hematol 2011;4:343–351.
85. Thompson LM, Ceja ME, Yang SA. Stem cell transplantation for treatment of sickle cell disease: Bone marrow versus cord blood transplants. Am J Health Syst Pharm 2012;69:1295–1302.
86. Al Jefri AH. Advances in allogeneic stem cell transplantation for hemoglobinopathies. Hemoglobin 2011;35:469–475.
87. Oringanje C, Nemecek E, Oniyangi O. Hematopoietic stem cell transplantation for children with sickle cell disease. Cochrane Database Syst Rev 2009;(1):CD007001.
88. Broderick GA. Priapism and sickle-cell anemia: diagnosis and nonsurgical therapy. The journal of sexual medicine. 2012;9:88–103.
89. Morrison BF, Burnett AL. Stuttering priapism: insights into pathogenesis and management. Current urology reports. 2012;13:268–276.
90. Muneer A, Minhas S, Arya M, Ralph DJ. Stuttering priapism—A review of the therapeutic options. Intern J Clin Pract 2008;62:1265–1270.
91. Lesher AP, Kalpatthi R, Glenn JB, Jackson SM, Hebra A. Outcome of splenectomy in children younger than 4 years with sickle cell disease. J Pediatr Surg 2009;44:1134–1138.
92. Zempsky WT. Evaluation and treatment of sickle cell pain in the emergency department: Paths to a better future. Clin Pediatr Emerg Med 2010;11:265–273.
93. Jerrell JM, Tripathi A, Stallworth JR. Pain management in children and adolescents with sickle cell disease. Am J Hematol 2011;86:82–84.
94. Wright J, Ahmedzai SH. The management of painful crisis in sickle cell disease. Curr Opin Support Palliat Care 2010;4:97–106.
95. Head CA, Swerdlow P, McDade WA, et al. Beneficial effects of nitric oxide breathing in adult patients with sickle cell crisis. Am J Hematol 2010;85:800–802.
96. Gladwin MT, Kato GJ, Weiner D, et al. Nitric oxide for inhalation in the acute treatment of sickle cell pain crisis: A randomized controlled trial. JAMA 2011;305:893–902.
97. Vandy Black L, Smith WR. Evidence-based mini-review: Are systemic corticosteroids an effective treatment for acute pain in sickle cell disease? Hematology Am Soc Hematol Educ Program 2010;2010:416–417.
98. Food and Drug Administration. Package insert for DROXIA (hydroxyurea). 01/2012 [cited Jan 25, 2013]. *http://dailymed.nlm.nih.gov/dailymed/lookup.cfm?setid=740e054b-faac-7c27-f06d-a56efb699355.*
99. Ware RE, Despotovic JM, Mortier NA, et al. Pharmacokinetics, pharmacodynamics, and pharmacogenetics of hydroxyurea treatment for children with sickle cell anemia. Blood 2011;118:4985–4991.
100. Fertrin KY, Costa FF. Genomic polymorphisms in sickle cell disease: Implications for clinical diversity and treatment. Expert Rev Hematol 2010;3:443–458.

Antimicrobial Regimen Selection

83

Grace C. Lee and David S. Burgess

KEY CONCEPTS

1. Every attempt should be made to obtain specimens for culture and sensitivity testing prior to initiating antibiotics.
2. Empirical antibiotic therapy should be based on knowledge of likely pathogens for the site of infection, information from patient history (e.g., recent hospitalizations, work-related exposure, travel, and pets), and local susceptibility.
3. Patients with delayed dermatologic reactions (i.e., rash) to penicillin generally can receive cephalosporins. Patients with type I hypersensitivity reactions (i.e., anaphylaxis) to penicillins should not receive cephalosporins. Alternatives to the cephalosporins include aztreonam, quinolones, sulfonamide antibiotics, or vancomycin based on type of coverage indicated.
4. Creatinine clearance should be estimated for every patient who is to receive antibiotics and the antibiotic dose interval adjusted accordingly. Hepatic function should be considered for drugs eliminated through the hepatobiliary system, such as clindamycin, erythromycin, and metronidazole.
5. All concomitant drugs and nutritional supplements should be reviewed when an antibiotic is added to a patient's therapy to ensure drug–drug interactions will be avoided.
6. Combination antibiotic therapy may be indicated for polymicrobial infections (e.g., intra-abdominal, gynecologic infections), to produce synergistic killing (such as β-lactam plus aminoglycoside vs. *Pseudomonas aeruginosa*), or to prevent the emergence of resistance.
7. All patients receiving antibiotics should be monitored for resolution of infectious signs and symptoms (e.g., decreasing temperature and white blood cell count) and adverse drug events.
8. Antibiotics with the narrowest effective spectrum of activity are preferred. Antibiotic route of administration should be evaluated daily, and conversion from IV to oral therapy should be attempted as signs of infection improve for patients with functioning GI tracts (general exceptions are endocarditis and CNS infections).
9. Patients not responding to an appropriate antibiotic treatment in 2 to 3 days should be reevaluated to ensure (a) the correct diagnosis, (b) that therapeutic drug concentrations are being achieved, (c) that the patient is not immunosuppressed, (d) that the patient does not have an isolated infection (i.e., abscess, foreign body), or (e) that resistance has not developed.

Choosing an antimicrobial agent to treat an infection is far more complicated than matching a drug to a known or suspected pathogen.[1,2] Most clinicians generally follow a systematic approach to select an antimicrobial regimen (Table 83-1). Problems arise when this systematic approach is replaced by prescribing broad-spectrum therapy to cover as many organisms as possible. Consequences of not using the systematic approach include the use of more expensive and potentially more toxic agents, which can, in turn, lead to widespread resistance and difficult-to-treat superinfections. Another abuse of antimicrobial agents is administration when they are not needed such as when they are prescribed for self-limited clinical conditions that are most likely viral in origin (i.e., the common cold).

Initial selection of antimicrobial therapy is nearly always empirical, which is prior to documentation and identification of the offending organism. Infectious diseases generally are acute, and a delay in antimicrobial therapy can result in serious morbidity or even mortality. Thus, empirical antimicrobial therapy selection should be based on information gathered from the patient's history and physical examination and results of Gram stains or of rapidly performed tests on specimens from the infected site. This information, combined with knowledge of the most likely offending organism(s) and an institution's local susceptibility patterns, should result in a rational selection of antibiotics to treat the patient. This chapter introduces a systematic approach to the selection of antimicrobial therapeutic regimens.

CONFIRMING THE PRESENCE OF INFECTION

Fever

The presence of a temperature greater than the expected 37°C (98.6°F) "normal" body temperature is considered a hallmark of infectious diseases. Body temperature is controlled by the hypothalamus. In addition, the circadian rhythm, a built-in temperature

TABLE 83-1 Systematic Approach for Selection of Antimicrobials

Confirm the presence of infection
- Careful history and physical examination
- Signs and symptoms
- Predisposing factors

Identification of the pathogen (see eChap. 24)
- Collection of infected material
- Stains
- Serologies
- Culture and sensitivity

Selection of presumptive therapy considering every infected site
- Host factors
- Drug factors

Monitor therapeutic response
- Clinical assessment
- Laboratory tests
- Assessment of therapeutic failure

cycle, is also operational. The daily temperature rhythm can vary for each individual. In a healthy person, the internal thermostat is set between the morning low temperature and the afternoon peak as controlled by the circadian rhythm. During fever, the hypothalamus is reset at a higher temperature level.

Fever is defined as a controlled elevation of body temperature above the normal range. The average normal body temperature range taken orally is 36.7°C to 37°C (98°F to 98.6°F). Body temperatures obtained rectally generally are 0.6°C (1°F) higher and axillary temperatures are 0.6°C (1°F) lower than oral temperatures, respectively. Skin temperatures are also less than the oral temperature but can vary depending on the specific measurement method.

Fever can be a manifestation of disease states other than infection. Collagen vascular (autoimmune) disorders and several malignancies can have fever as a manifestation. Fever of unknown or undetermined origin is a diagnostic dilemma and is reviewed extensively elsewhere.[3]

Many drugs have been identified as causes of fever.[4] *Drug-induced fever* is defined as persistent fever in the absence of infection or other underlying condition. The fever must coincide temporally with the administration of the offending agent and disappear promptly on its withdrawal, after which the temperature remains normal. Possible mechanisms of drug-induced fever are either a hypersensitivity reaction or development of antigen–antibody complexes that result in the stimulation of macrophages and the release of interleukin 1 (IL-1). Although this is not a common drug effect (accounting for no more than 5% of all drug reactions), it should be suspected when obvious reasons for fever are not present. Almost any medication can produce fever, but *β*-lactam antibiotics, anticonvulsants, allopurinol, hydralazine, nitrofurantoin, sulfonamides, phenothiazines, and methyldopa appear to be responsible more often than others.

Noninfectious etiologies of fever can be referred to as "false-positives." Although these certainly can confuse the clinician, even more troublesome are false-negatives: the absence of fever in a patient with signs and symptoms consistent with an infectious disease. Careful questioning of the patient or family is vital to assess the ingestion of any medication that can mask fever (e.g., aspirin, acetaminophen, nonsteroidal antiinflammatory agents, and corticosteroids). The use of antipyretics should be discouraged during the treatment of infection unless absolutely necessary because they can mask a poor therapeutic response. Moreover, elevated body temperature, unless very high (>40.5°C [105°F]), is not harmful and may be beneficial.

Signs and Symptoms

White Blood Cell Count

Most infections result in elevated white blood cell (WBC) counts (leukocytosis) because of the increased production and mobilization of granulocytes (neutrophils, basophils, and eosinophils), lymphocytes, or both to ingest and destroy invading microbes. The generally accepted range of normal values for WBC counts is between 4,000 and 10,000 cells/mm^3 (4×10^9 and 10×10^9/L). Values above or below this range hold important prognostic and diagnostic value.

Bacterial infections are associated with elevated granulocyte counts, often with immature forms (band neutrophils) seen in peripheral blood smears. Mature neutrophils are also referred to as *segmented neutrophils* or *polymorphonuclear* (PMN) *leukocytes*. The presence of immature forms (left shift) is an indication of an increased bone marrow response to the infection. With infection, peripheral WBC counts can be very high, but they are rarely higher than 30,000 to 40,000 cells/mm^3 (30×10^9 to 40×10^9/L). Because leukocytosis indicates the normal host response to infection, low leukocyte counts after the onset of infection indicate an abnormal response and generally are associated with a poor prognosis.

The most common granulocyte defect is neutropenia, a decrease in absolute numbers of circulating neutrophils. A thorough description of the consequences of neutropenia is given in Chapter 99. Lymphocytosis, even with normal or slightly elevated total WBC counts, generally is associated with tuberculosis and viral or fungal infections. Increases in monocytes can be associated with tuberculosis or lymphoma, and increases in eosinophils can be associated with allergic reactions to drugs or infections caused by metazoa. Many types of infections can be accompanied by a completely normal WBC count and differential.

Local Signs

The classic signs of pain and inflammation can manifest as swelling, erythema, tenderness, and purulent drainage. Unfortunately, these are only visible if the infection is superficial or in a bone or joint. The manifestations of inflammation in deep-seated infections (e.g., meningitis, pneumonia, endocarditis, and urinary tract infection) must be ascertained by examining tissues or fluids. For example, the presence of neutrophils in spinal fluid, lung secretions (sputum), or urine is highly suggestive of a bacterial infection.

Symptoms referable to an organ system must be sought out carefully because not only do they help in establishing the presence of infection, but they also aid in narrowing the list of potential pathogens. For example, a febrile patient with complaints of flank pain and dysuria can well have pyelonephritis. In this situation, enteric gram-negative bacilli, especially *Escherichia coli*, are the predominant pathogens. If a febrile patient has no symptoms suggestive of an organ system but only constitutional complaints, the list of possible infectious diseases is lengthy.[3] A febrile individual with cough and sputum production probably has a pulmonary infection. What is not so evident, however, is the etiologic organism in this situation, because it can be caused by bacteria, mycobacteria, viruses, *Chlamydia*, or mycoplasmas.[5] In this situation, attention to the patient's history and background disease states is important. Even more important is a careful examination of the infected material (in this case sputum) to ascertain the identity of the pathogen.

IDENTIFICATION OF THE PATHOGEN

Microbiology Issues

❶ Infected body materials must be sampled, if at all possible or practical, before institution of any antimicrobial therapy for two reasons. First, a Gram stain of the material might reveal bacteria, or an acid-fast stain might detect mycobacteria or actinomycetes. Second, a delay in obtaining infected fluids or tissues until after antimicrobial therapy is started might result in false-negative culture results or alterations in the cellular and chemical composition of infected fluids. This is particularly true in patients with urinary tract infections, meningitis, and septic arthritis.[6]

Blood cultures usually should be performed in the acutely ill febrile patient. Blood culture collection should coincide with sharp elevations in temperature, suggesting the possibility of microorganisms or microbial antigens in the bloodstream. Ideally, blood should be obtained from peripheral sites as two sets (one set consists of an aerobic bottle and one set an anaerobic bottle) from two different sites approximately 1 hour apart. In selected infections, bacteremia is qualitatively continuous (e.g., endocarditis), so cultures can be obtained at any time.[7]

In addition to the infected materials produced by the patient (e.g., blood, sputum, urine, stool, and wound or sinus drainage), other less accessible fluids or tissues must be obtained if they are suspected to be the infected site (e.g., spinal fluid in meningitis and joint fluid in arthritis). Abscesses and cellulitic areas also should be aspirated.

Interpreting Results

After a positive Gram stain, culture results, or both are obtained, the clinician must be cautious in determining whether the organism recovered is a true pathogen, a contaminant, or a part of the normal flora (see eChap. 24). The latter consideration is especially problematic with cultures obtained from the skin, oropharynx, nose, ears, eyes, throat, and perineum. These surfaces are heavily colonized with a wide variety of bacteria, some of which can be pathogenic in certain settings. For example, coagulase-negative staphylococci are found in cultures of all the aforementioned sites, yet are seldom regarded as pathogens unless recovered from blood, venous access catheters, or prosthetic devices.

Importantly, cultures of specimens from purportedly infected sites that are obtained by sampling from or through one of these contaminated areas might contain significant numbers of the normal flora. For urine cultures, the urinalysis should be used in combination with culture results to assess the presence of WBCs, nitrite, and leukocyte esterase to help confirm infection and rule out colonization.

Particularly problematic are expectorated sputum specimens that must be evaluated carefully by determination of the presence of squamous epithelial cells and leukocytes.[5] A predominance of epithelial cells in sputum specimens reduces the likelihood that recovered bacteria are pathogenic, especially when multiple types of organisms are seen on Gram stain. In contrast, the discovery of leukocytes in large numbers with one predominant type of organism is a more reliable indicator of a valid collection. In general, however, sputum evaluation has poor sensitivity and specificity as a diagnostic test.[5]

Caution also must be used in the evaluation of positive culture results from normally sterile sites (e.g., blood, cerebrospinal fluid [CSF], or joint fluid). The recovery of bacteria normally found on the skin in large quantities (e.g., coagulase-negative staphylococci or diphtheroids) from one of these sites can be a result of contamination of the specimen rather than a true infection. However, these organisms can be pathogenic in certain settings.

Gram-staining techniques, culture methods, and serologic identification, as well as susceptibility testing, are discussed in detail in eChapter 24. Emphasis must be placed on the proper collection and handling of specimens and careful assessment of Gram stain or other test results in guiding the clinician toward appropriate selection of initial antimicrobial therapy.[8]

SELECTION OF PRESUMPTIVE THERAPY

❷ To select rational antimicrobial therapy for a given clinical situation, a variety of factors must be considered. These include the severity and acuity of the disease, host factors, factors related to the drugs used, and the necessity for using multiple agents. In addition, there are generally accepted drugs of choice for the treatment of most pathogens (see Appendix 83-1).

Drugs of choice are compiled from a variety of sources and are intended as guidelines rather than as specific rules for antimicrobial use. These choices are influenced by local antimicrobial susceptibility data rather than information published by other institutions or national compilations. Each institution should publish an annual summary of antibiotic susceptibilities (antibiogram) for organisms cultured from patients. Antibiograms contain both the number of nonduplicate isolates for common species and the percentage susceptible to the antibiotics tested. To further guide empirical antibiotic therapy, some hospitals publish unit-specific antibiograms in unique patient care areas, such as intensive care units or burn units.

Susceptibility of bacteria can differ substantially among hospitals within a community. For example, the prevalence of hospital-acquired methicillin-resistant *Staphylococcus aureus* (HA-MRSA) in some centers is quite high, whereas in other centers the problem might be nonexistent. This particular situation will influence the selection of therapy for possible *S. aureus* infection, where the clinician must choose either a β-lactam or vancomycin. The problem of differing susceptibilities is not limited only to gram-positive bacteria but also is evident in gram-negative organisms, and all drug classes are affected.

Empirical therapy is directed at organisms that are known to cause the infection in question. These organisms are discussed for different sites of infection in Chapters 83 to 102. To define the most likely infecting organisms, a careful history and physical examination must be performed. The place where the infection was acquired should be determined, for example, the home (community acquired), nursing home environment, or hospital acquired (nosocomial). Nursing home patients can be exposed to potentially more resistant organisms because they are often surrounded by ill patients who are receiving antibiotics. Other important questions to ask infected patients regarding the history of present illness include the following:

1. Are any other people sick at home, especially children?
2. Are any unusual pets kept in the home such as pigeons?
3. Where are you employed (i.e., are you exposed to contaminated meat or infectious biohazards)?
4. Has there been any recent travel (i.e., to endemic areas of fungal infections or developing countries)?

Host Factors

Several host factors should be considered when evaluating a patient for antimicrobial therapy. The most important factors are drug allergies, age, pregnancy, genetic or metabolic abnormalities, renal and hepatic function, site of infection, concomitant drug therapy, and underlying disease states.

Allergy

❸ Allergy to an antimicrobial agent generally precludes its use. Careful assessment of allergy histories must be performed because many patients confuse common adverse drug effects (i.e., GI disturbance) with true allergic reactions.[9] Among the most commonly cited antimicrobial allergies are those to penicillin, penicillin-related compounds, or both. In the absence of complete penicillin skin testing capabilities, a rule of thumb for giving cephalosporins to patients allergic to penicillin is to avoid giving them to patients who give a good history for immediate or accelerated reactions (e.g., anaphylaxis, laryngospasm) and to give them under close supervision in patients with a history of delayed reactions, such as a rash.[10] If a gram-negative infection is suspected or documented, therapy with a monobactam may be appropriate because cross-reactivity with other β-lactams is nonexistent.

Age

The patient's age is an important factor both in trying to identify the likely etiologic agent and in assessing the patient's ability to eliminate the drug(s) to be used. The best example of an age determinant of organisms is in bacterial meningitis, where the pathogens differ as the patient grows from the neonatal period through infancy and childhood into adulthood.[6]

For neonates, hepatic and liver functions are not well developed. Therefore, bilirubin excretion is decreased resulting in increased concentration of unconjugated bilirubin that can cause kernicterus. Neonates (especially when premature) can develop kernicterus when given sulfonamides. This results from displacement of bilirubin from serum albumin. In addition, neonates have more body water content that results in a larger volume of distribution leading to adjustments in antibiotic dosing regimens. Additional special drug considerations for pediatric patients include low frequency of adverse effects and compliance-enhancing features (e.g., absorption not affected by food, once- to twice-daily dosing, and good taste).[11]

The major physiologic change in persons older than 65 years of age is a decline in the number of functioning nephrons that, in turn, results in decreased renal function.[12] This is usually manifested by an increased incidence of side effects caused by antimicrobials that are eliminated renally. For example, renal toxicity caused by aminoglycosides may be apparent much sooner during therapy than in younger patients.

Pregnancy

During pregnancy, not only is the fetus at risk for drug teratogenicity, but also the pharmacokinetic disposition of certain drugs can be altered.[13] Penicillins, cephalosporins, and aminoglycosides are cleared from the peripheral circulation more rapidly during pregnancy. This is probably a result of marked increases in intravascular volume, glomerular filtration rate, and hepatic and metabolic activities. The net result is that maternal serum antimicrobial concentrations can be as much as 50% lower during this period than in the nonpregnant state. Increased dosages of certain compounds might be necessary to achieve therapeutic levels during late pregnancy.

Metabolic or Genetic Variation

Inherited or acquired metabolic abnormalities will influence the therapy of infectious diseases in a variety of ways. For example, patients with impaired peripheral vascular flow may not absorb drugs given by intramuscular injection. In addition, certain metabolic states can predispose patients to enhanced drug toxicity. For instance, patients who are phenotypically slow acetylators of isoniazid are at greater risk for peripheral neuropathy.[14] Patients with severe deficiency of glucose-6-phosphate dehydrogenase can develop significant hemolysis when exposed to such drugs as sulfonamides, nitrofurantoin, nalidixic acid, antimalarials, and dapsone. Although mild deficiencies are found in African Americans, the more severe forms of the disease generally are confined to persons of eastern Mediterranean origin. Another example is the antiretroviral drug abacavir, which is associated with a severe hypersensitivity reaction, consisting of fever, rash, abdominal pain, and respiratory distress. This risk has been associated with the presence of a human leukocyte antigen allele HLA-B*5701. Routine screening for the presence of this allele before initiating treatment with abacavir is a recommendation in the current HIV treatment guidelines.

Organ Dysfunction

4 Patients with diminished renal or hepatic function or both will accumulate certain drugs unless the dosage is adjusted.[15,16] Recommendations for dosing antibiotics in patients with liver dysfunction are not as formalized as guidelines for patients with renal dysfunction. Antibiotics that should be adjusted in severe liver disease include clindamycin, erythromycin, metronidazole, and rifampin. Significant accumulation can occur when both liver dysfunction and renal dysfunction are present for the following drugs: cefotaxime, nafcillin, piperacillin, and sulfamethoxazole.

Concomitant Drugs

5 Any concomitant therapy that the patient is receiving can influence the drug selection, dose, and monitoring. For instance, administration of isoniazid to a patient who is also receiving phenytoin can result in phenytoin toxicity secondary to inhibition of phenytoin metabolism by isoniazid. Furthermore, drugs that possess similar adverse effect profiles can increase the risk for effects (i.e., two drugs that cause nephrotoxicity or neutropenia). A detailed review of drug interactions is beyond the scope of this chapter, but an excellent textbook on this subject is available.[17] Lists of potentially severe drug–drug interactions are provided in Table 83-2.

Concomitant Disease States

Concomitant disease states can influence the selection of therapy. Certain diseases will predispose patients to a particular infectious disease or will alter the type of infecting organism. For example, patients with diabetes mellitus and the resulting peripheral vascular disease often develop infections of the lower extremity soft tissue. Moreover, the alterations in peripheral blood flow associated with the disease and perhaps altered immunity make such infections more difficult to treat than in nondiabetics. Patients with chronic lung disease or cystic fibrosis develop frequent pulmonary infections that can be caused by somewhat different microorganisms than are found in otherwise normal hosts.

Patients with immunosuppressive diseases, such as malignancies or acquired immunologic deficiencies, are highly predisposed to infections, and the types of causative or pathogenic organisms can be vastly different from what would be expected (see Chap. 99). For instance, patients undergoing chemotherapy for acute forms of leukemia often are profoundly granulocytopenic and are predisposed to infections caused by bacteria and fungi.[18] Patients with the acquired immunodeficiency syndrome (AIDS) often become infected with an enormous variety of organisms (see Chap. 102).

Many factors predisposing to infection are related to disruption of the host's integumentary barriers. For example, trauma, burns, and iatrogenic wounds induced in surgery can lead to a substantial risk of infection depending on the severity and location of the injury or disruption. For a complete discussion of the various risks involved in surgical procedures, see Chapter 100.

Drug Factors

Pharmacokinetic and Pharmacodynamic Considerations

Integration of both pharmacokinetic and pharmacodynamic properties of an agent is important when choosing antimicrobial therapy to ensure efficacy and to prevent resistance.[19] Early researchers relied

TABLE 83-2 Major Drug Interactions with Antimicrobials

Antimicrobial	Other Agent(s)	Mechanism of Action/Effect	Clinical Management
Aminoglycosides	Neuromuscular blocking agents	Additive adverse effects	Avoid
	Nephrotoxins (N) or ototoxins (O) (e.g., amphotericin B [N], cisplatin [N/O], cyclosporine [N], furosemide [O], NSAIDs [N], radiocontrast [N], vancomycin [N])	Additive adverse effects	Monitor aminoglycoside SDC and renal function
Amphotericin B	Nephrotoxins (e.g., aminoglycosides, cidofovir, cyclosporine, foscarnet, pentamidine)	Additive adverse effects	Monitor renal function
Azoles	See Chapter 98		
Chloramphenicol	Phenytoin, tolbutamide, ethanol	Decreased metabolism of other agents	Monitor phenytoin SDC, blood glucose
Foscarnet	Pentamidine IV	Increased risk of severe nephrotoxicity/ hypocalcemia	Monitor renal function/serum calcium
Isoniazid	Carbamazepine, phenytoin	Decreased metabolism of other agents (nausea, vomiting, nystagmus, ataxia)	Monitor drug SDC
Macrolides/azalides	Digoxin	Decreased digoxin bioavailability and metabolism	Monitor digoxin SDC; avoid if possible
	Theophylline	Decreased metabolism of theophylline	Monitor theophylline SDC
Metronidazole	Ethanol (drugs containing ethanol)	Disulfiram-like reaction	Avoid
Penicillins and cephalosporins	Probenecid, aspirin	Blocked excretion of β-lactams	Use if prolonged high concentration of β-lactam desirable
Ciprofloxacin/norfloxacin	Theophylline	Decreased metabolism of theophylline	Monitor theophylline
Quinolones	Classes Ia and III antiarrhythmics	Increased Q-T interval	Avoid
	Multivalent cations (antacids, iron, sucralfate, zinc, vitamins, dairy, citric acid), didanosine	Decreased absorption of quinolone	Separate by 2 hours
Rifampin	Azoles, cyclosporine, methadone propranolol, PIs, oral contraceptives, tacrolimus, warfarin	Increased metabolism of other agent	Avoid if possible
Sulfonamides	Sulfonylureas, phenytoin, warfarin	Decreased metabolism of other agent	Monitor blood glucose, SDC, PT
Tetracyclines	Antacids, iron, calcium, sucralfate	Decreased absorption of tetracycline	Separate by 2 hours
	Digoxin	Decreased digoxin bioavailability	Monitor digoxin SDC; avoid if possible

PI, protease inhibitor; PT, prothrombin time; SDC, serum drug concentrations.

Azalides: azithromycin; azoles: fluconazole, itraconazole, ketoconazole, and voriconazole; macrolides: erythromycin and clarithromycin; protease inhibitors: amprenavir, indinavir, lopinavir/ritonavir, nelfinavir, ritonavir, and saquinavir; quinolones: ciprofloxacin, gemifloxacin, levofloxacin, and moxifloxacin.

solely on pharmacokinetic properties such as the area under the (drug concentration) curve (AUC), maximum observed concentration (peak), and drug half-life to optimize therapy. Pharmacodynamics is the study of the relationship between drug concentration and the effects on the microorganism. There is an important relationship between both pharmacokinetic and microbiologic parameters that has resulted in measurements such as AUC:minimal inhibitory concentration (MIC) ratio, peak:MIC ratio, and time (T) the concentration is above MIC ($T >$ MIC).[19–23]

Aminoglycosides exhibit concentration-dependent bactericidal effects. An example of the integration of pharmacokinetics and microbiologic activity is the use of high-dose, once-daily aminoglycosides. For these regimens, the drug is given as a single large daily dose to maximize the peak:MIC ratio. Aminoglycosides also possess a postantibiotic effect (persistent suppression of organism growth after concentrations decrease below the MIC) that appears to contribute to the success of high-dose, once-daily administration. Fluoroquinolones exhibit concentration-dependent killing activity, but optimal killing appears to be characterized by the AUC:MIC ratio.

β-Lactams display time-dependent bactericidal effects. Killing activity is enhanced only marginally if drug concentration exceeds the MIC. Therefore, the important pharmacodynamic relationship for these antimicrobials is the duration that drug concentrations exceed the MIC ($T >$ MIC). Effective dosing regimens require serum drug concentrations to exceed the MIC for at least 40% to 50% of the dosing interval. Frequent small doses, continuous infusion, or prolonged infusion of β-lactams appears to be correlated with positive outcomes.

A detailed discussion on antimicrobial pharmacokinetics–pharmacodynamics is beyond the scope of this chapter. However, excellent sources of information on this topic are available.[19–23]

Tissue Penetration

The importance of tissue penetration varies with site of infection. Some of the difficulties in interpreting data include a lack of correlation with clinical outcomes and poor understanding of whether the antimicrobial agents are present in a biologically active form. An example of the former problem is the recognized efficacy of drugs with low biliary fluid concentrations in the treatment of cholecystitis, cholangitis, or both and the absence of the enhanced efficacy of drugs whose primary route of elimination is biliary excretion of active drug. An example of the latter difficulty is with penetration to deep infections, such as abscesses, where various factors such as acid pH, WBC products, and various enzymes can inactivate even high concentrations of certain drugs.

The CNS is one body site where antimicrobial penetration is relatively well defined, and correlations with clinical outcomes are established.[6,24] CSF concentrations of antimicrobial agents necessary to cure bacterial meningitis have been defined, and drugs that do not reach significant concentrations in the CSF should be either avoided or instilled directly, if feasible.

Caution must be exercised when selecting an antimicrobial agent for clinical use on the basis of tissue or fluid penetration.

Body fluids where drug concentration data are clinically relevant include CSF, urine, synovial fluid, and peritoneal fluid. Apart from these areas, more attention should be paid to clinical efficacy, antimicrobial spectrum, toxicity, and cost than to comparative data on penetration into a given body site.

The proper route of administration for an antimicrobial depends on the site of infection. Parenteral therapy is warranted when patients are being treated for febrile neutropenia or deep-seated infections such as meningitis, endocarditis, and osteomyelitis. Severe pneumonia often is treated initially with IV antibiotics and switched to oral therapy as clinical improvement is evident.[5,25] Patients treated in the ambulatory setting for upper respiratory tract infections (e.g., pharyngitis, bronchitis, sinusitis, and otitis media), lower respiratory tract infections, skin and soft-tissue infections, uncomplicated urinary tract infections, and selected sexually transmitted diseases can usually receive oral therapy.

Drug Toxicity

It is incumbent on health professionals to avoid toxic drugs whenever possible. Antibiotics associated with CNS toxicities, usually when not dose-adjusted for renal function, include penicillins, cephalosporins, quinolones, and imipenem. Hematologic toxicities generally are manifested with prolonged use of nafcillin (neutropenia), piperacillin (platelet dysfunction), cefotetan (hypoprothrombinemia), chloramphenicol (bone marrow suppression, both idiosyncratic and dose-related toxicity), and trimethoprim (megaloblastic anemia). Reversible nephrotoxicity classically is associated with aminoglycosides and vancomycin. Irreversible ototoxicity can occur with aminoglycosides. In the outpatient setting, patients must be counseled regarding photosensitivity with azithromycin, quinolones, tetracyclines, pyrazinamide, sulfamethoxazole, and trimethoprim. Lastly, all antibiotics have been implicated in causing diarrhea and colitis secondary to *Clostridium difficile*[26] (see Chap. 91). List of potential antibiotic adverse drug reactions is provided in Table 83-3.

Aside from consideration of drug toxicity, some antimicrobial use requires more intensive risk–benefit analysis. An example of this is the decision to use isoniazid prophylactically to prevent tuberculosis. Because the hepatotoxicity of isoniazid increases in frequency with age, older persons (>45 years of age) who are candidates for isoniazid prophylaxis (positive skin test) must have additional risk factors for tuberculosis to balance the potential toxic effects. These include evidence of recent skin test conversion, immunosuppression, or previous gastrectomy. Older patients without additional risk factors are more likely to suffer toxicity from isoniazid than derive benefit from its use.[27]

Combination Antimicrobial Therapy

6 In selecting a drug regimen for a given patient, consideration must be given to the necessity of using more than one drug.[28] Combinations of antimicrobials generally are used to broaden the spectrum of coverage for empirical therapy, achieve synergistic activity against the infecting organism, and prevent the emergence of resistance.

Broadening the Spectrum of Coverage

Increasing the coverage of antimicrobial therapy generally is necessary in mixed infections where multiple organisms are likely to be present. This is the case in intraabdominal and female pelvic infections, in which a variety of aerobic and anaerobic bacteria can produce disease.[29] Traditionally, a combination of a drug active against aerobic gram-negative bacilli (such as an aminoglycoside) and a drug active against anaerobic bacteria (such as metronidazole or clindamycin) is selected. Newer compounds, which possess good activity against both of these types of organisms, such as the β-lactam/β-lactamase inhibitor combinations, carbapenems, or glycylcyclines, might be adequate to replace the combination and thereby reduce the cost of therapy. The other clinical situation in which an increased spectrum of activity is desirable is with nosocomial infections.[25]

Synergism

The achievement of synergistic antimicrobial activity is advantageous for infections caused by enteric gram-negative bacilli in immunosuppressed patients. Laboratory tests to identify synergy between antibiotic combinations are described in eChapter 24. Traditionally, combinations of aminoglycosides and β-lactams have been used because these drugs together generally act synergistically against a wide variety of bacteria. However, the data supporting superior efficacy of synergistic over nonsynergistic combinations are weak. At best, it would appear that synergistic combinations produce better results in certain infections caused by *Pseudomonas aeruginosa* and *Enterococcus* species.[30–32]

The most obvious example of the use of synergy is the treatment of enterococcal endocarditis. The causative organism is usually only inhibited by penicillins, but it is killed rapidly by the addition of streptomycin or gentamicin to a penicillin.[7] The need for bactericidal activity in the treatment of endocarditis underscores the need for these synergistic combinations.

Preventing Resistance

The use of combinations to prevent the emergence of resistance is applied widely but not often realized. The only circumstance where this has been clearly effective is in the treatment of tuberculosis. The prevalence of resistance to a first-line drug such as isoniazid or rifampin in a population of organisms may be as high as 1 in 10^6 to 10^8. Because the bacterial load in a patient with active tuberculosis often exceeds this, two drugs are given to reduce the likelihood of encountering resistance to less than 1 in 10.[27] There is ample evidence from in vitro data and experimental bacterial infections that combinations of drugs with different mechanisms are effective in the prevention of the emergence of resistance. Data from clinical trials, however, either are conflicting or do not convincingly support this concept.[32]

Clinical **Controversy. . .**

Despite evidence of potential advantages of definitive combination therapy for gram-negative infections from in vitro and animal studies, clinical data have been conflicting, and there is evidence that it may even be harmful. Currently, whether definitive combination antimicrobial therapy is more efficacious than monotherapy for infections with gram-negative bacteria remains a debate.

Disadvantages of Combination Therapy

Although there are potentially beneficial effects from combining drugs, there also are potential disadvantages, including increased cost, greater risk of drug toxicity such as nephrotoxicity with aminoglycosides, amphotericin, and possibly vancomycin, and superinfection with even more resistant bacteria.[30–32]

The combination of two or more antibiotics can result in antagonistic effects. Clinically, the effect of antagonism may be evident when one drug induces β-lactamase production and another drug is β-lactamase unstable. Cefoxitin and imipenem are examples of drugs capable of inducing β-lactamases and may result in more rapid inactivation of penicillins when used together.

TABLE 83-3 Antimicrobial Adverse Drug Reactions

Antimicrobial Class	Adverse Drug Reaction	Monitoring Parameters	Comments
Penicillins	Hypersensitivity reactions and rash, drug fever, diarrhea, emesis, abdominal pain, hepatitis, interstitial nephritis, leukopenia, thrombocytopenia, Coomb's positive-hemolytic anemia, *C. difficile* colitis, electrolyte abnormalities, seizures	Monitor for hypersensitivity reactions (e.g., bronchospasm, anaphylaxis, angioneurotic edema, immediate urticaria). During prolonged therapy and/or high-dose regimens, periodically monitor renal function, hepatic function, and CBC	Most serious reaction is immediate IgE-mediated anaphylaxis. Incidence is 0.05%, but 5–10% can be fatal
Cephalosporins	Hypersensitivity reactions and rash, drug fever, diarrhea, interstitial nephritis, Coomb's positive-hemolytic anemia, leukopenia, thrombocytopenia, coagulopathy, hepatitis, *C. difficile* colitis	Monitor for hypersensitivity reactions (e.g., bronchospasm, anaphylaxis, angioneurotic edema, immediate urticaria) and rash, renal function, hepatic function, and CBC	Patients with a history of IgE-mediated allergic reactions to penicillins should not receive a cephalosporin
Carbapenems	Hypersensitivity reactions and rash, headache, nausea, diarrhea, seizures, drug fever, eosinophilia, thrombocytopenia, hepatitis, *C. difficile* colitis	Monitor for hypersensitivity reactions (e.g., bronchospasm, anaphylaxis, angioneurotic edema, immediate urticaria) and rash, renal function, hepatic function, and CBC	Skin test cross-sensitivity with penicillin reported to be up to 50%, but clinically significant cross-sensitivity reactions in penicillin-allergic patients reported to be as low as 1% Highest incidence of seizures with use of imipenem–cilastatin. More frequent in patients who are elderly, have history of seizure disorders and renal dysfunction
Monobactams	Rash, diarrhea, nausea, hepatitis, thrombocytopenia, *C. difficile* colitis	Monitor renal and hepatic function	May be used in patients with allergy to penicillins/cephalosporins
Aminoglycosides	Tubular necrosis and renal failure, vestibular and cochlear toxicity, neuromuscular blockade, vertigo, anemia, hypersensitivity	Monitor renal function, SDC, serum calcium, magnesium, sodium. Monitor for nausea, vomiting, nystagmus, and vertigo	Nephrotoxicity can be reversible. More frequent in patients with the following risk factors: elderly, history of renal dysfunction, concomitant administration of nephrotoxic drug (i.e., cyclosporine, amphotericin B, radiocontrast, vancomycin), and duration of therapy Ototoxicities can be irreversible
Glycopeptides	Red man syndrome, phlebitis, renal dysfunction, neutropenia, leukopenia, eosinophilia, thrombocytopenia, drug fever	Monitor renal function, CBC, and SDC	Red man syndrome is associated with rapid infusion and nonspecific histamine release. May be prevented by prolonging infusions to over at least 60 minutes and pretreatment with antihistamines
Lipopeptides (daptomycin)	Hepatotoxicity, CPK elevation with or without myopathy, diarrhea, eosinophilic pneumonia, *C. difficile* colitis	Monitor LFTs, development of muscle pain/weakness, or neuropathy Obtain serum CPK levels at baseline and weekly (or more frequently in patients with prior or concomitant statin, renal dysfunction, or patients with elevations in CPK)	CPK elevation is dose-dependent. Obtain baseline and weekly CPK levels. Discontinue daptomycin if CPK exceeds 10 times normal level or if patient develops myopathy and CPK >1,000 international units/L (16.7 μkat/L). Consider stopping statin therapy during treatment with daptomycin
Oxazolidinones	Myelosuppression (thrombocytopenia, leukopenia, and anemia), peripheral neuropathy, optic neuropathy, blindness, lactic acidosis, diarrhea, nausea, serotonin syndrome, interstitial nephritis	Monitor for signs and symptoms of serotonin syndrome particularly in patients with prior or concomitant serotonergic agents, CBC with differential. For prolonged therapy, perform visual function tests, monitor visual acuity and visual field defect	Myelosuppression is reversible and associated with treatment duration >2 weeks
Tetracyclines	GI upset, nausea, vomiting, diarrhea, hepatotoxicity, esophageal ulcerations, photosensitivity, azotemia, visual disturbances, vertigo, hyperpigmentation, deposition on teeth, hemolytic anemia, pseudotumor cerebri, pancreatitis, *C. difficile* colitis	Monitor CBC with differential, LFTs, and renal function	Doxycycline preferred in patients with renal dysfunction Vestibular symptoms more frequent in women than in men Avoid use during pregnancy and in children
Chloramphenicol	Myelosuppression, aplastic anemia, "gray baby syndrome," optic neuritis, peripheral neuropathy, digital paresthesias, GI upset, *C. difficile* colitis, hypersensitivity	Obtain baseline CBC with differential and every 2 days during therapy. Monitor SDC (particularly in children and in patients with hepatic or renal insufficiency), liver and renal function	Bone marrow suppression associated with doses >4 g/day. Serum levels greater than 50 mcg/mL (mg/L; 155 μmol/L) are associated with increased risk for "gray baby syndrome"
Rifamycines	Discoloration of urine, tears, contact lens, sweat, hepatotoxicity, GI upset, flu-like syndrome, hypersensitivity, thrombocytopenia, leukopenia, drug fever, interstitial nephritis, thrombocytopenia	Monitor LFTs, bilirubin, renal function, CBC at baseline; continue to monitor every 2–4 weeks in patients with hepatic impairment or receiving concomitant hepatotoxic drugs	Increased potential for hepatitis with concomitant hepatotoxic drugs (i.e., TB drugs)
Macrolides/azalide	GI intolerance, diarrhea, prolonged QTc, cholestatic hepatitis, reversible ototoxicity, torsade de pointes, rash, hypothermia, exacerbation of myasthenia gravis	Monitor LFTs and ECG in high-risk patients	

(continued)

TABLE 83-3 Antimicrobial Adverse Drug Reactions (*Continued*)

Antimicrobial Class	Adverse Drug Reaction	Monitoring Parameters	Comments
Clindamycin	Diarrhea, *C. difficile* colitis, nausea, vomiting, generalized rash, hypersensitivity	For prolonged therapy, monitor liver and renal function	
Fluoroquinolones	GI intolerance, headache, malaise, insomnia, dizziness, photosensitivity, QTc prolongation, tendon rupture, peripheral neuropathy, crystalluria, seizure, interstitial nephritis, Stevens-Johnson syndrome, allergic pneumonitis, *C. difficile* colitis	Monitor renal function, encephalopathic changes (e.g., confusion, hallucinations, and tremor)	Tendon rupture more frequently seen in the elderly and kidney, heart, and lung transplant recipients, and with concurrent use of corticosteroids
Polymyxins	Nephrotoxicity, neurotoxicity (paresthesia, vertigo, ataxia, blurred vision, slurred speech), neuromuscular blockade, bronchospasm (administered via inhalation)	Obtain baseline renal function tests and regularly during therapy. Monitor for signs of neuromuscular blockade (e.g., respiratory depression, apnea, muscle weakness)	Nephrotoxicity is dose-dependent
Sulfonamides and trimethoprim	GI intolerance, rash, hyperkalemia, bone marrow suppression (anemia with folate deficiency, thrombocytopenia, and leukopenia), serum sickness, hepatitis, photosensitivity, crystalluria with azotemia, urolithiasis, methemoglobinemia, Stevens-Johnson syndrome, toxic epidermal necrolysis, aseptic meningitis, pancreatitis, interstitial nephritis, Sweet's syndrome, neurologic toxicity	Monitor for hypersensitivity reactions and rash, CBC, renal and hepatic function, serum potassium, serum glucose	HIV-infected patients are at increased risk for developing adverse drug reactions Methemoglobinemia due to severe G6PD deficiency
Metronidazole	GI intolerance, headache, metallic taste, dark urine, peripheral neuropathy, disulfiram reactions with alcohol, insomnia, stomatitis, aseptic meningitis, dysarthria	Monitor hepatic function, mental/neurologic status	Peripheral neuropathy is reversible and associated with prolonged treatment

CBC, complete blood count; SDC, serum drug concentrations; LFT, liver function test; CPK, creatine phosphokinase; TB, tuberculosis.

MONITORING THERAPEUTIC RESPONSE

7 After antimicrobial therapy has been instituted, the patient must be monitored carefully for a therapeutic response. Culture and sensitivity reports from specimens sent to the microbiology laboratory must be reviewed and the therapy changed accordingly. Use of agents with the narrowest spectrum of activity against identified pathogens is recommended. If anaerobes are suspected, even if they are not identified, anaerobic therapy should be continued.

Patient monitoring should include many of the same parameters used to diagnose the infection. The WBC count and temperature should start to normalize. Physical complaints from the patient also should diminish (i.e., decreased pain, shortness of breath, cough, or sputum production). Appetite should improve. However, radiologic improvement can lag behind clinical improvement.

Determinations of serum (or other fluid) levels of antimicrobials can be useful in ensuring outcome, preventing toxicity, or both. There are only a few antimicrobials that require serum concentration monitoring and then only in selected situations. These include the aminoglycosides, vancomycin, flucytosine, and chloramphenicol. Achievement of adequate aminoglycoside concentrations within the first few days of therapy of gram-negative infection has been correlated with better therapeutic outcome.[33]

Changes in the volume of distribution can have a significant impact on the efficacy, safety, or both of therapy. An unexpectedly low volume of distribution (such as in the dehydrated patient) will result in higher, potentially toxic drug concentrations, whereas a larger-than-expected volume of distribution (such as in patients with edema or ascites) will result in low, potentially subtherapeutic concentrations. The most effective methods use measured serum concentrations of the drugs rather than estimations from renal function tests to assess true drug clearance from the body.

8 As patients improve clinically, the route of administration should be reevaluated. Streamlining therapy from parenteral to oral (switch therapy) has become an accepted practice for many infections.[5] Criteria that should be present to justify a switch to oral therapy include (a) overall clinical improvement, (b) lack of fever for 8 to 24 hours, (c) decreased WBC count, and (d) a functioning GI tract. Drugs that exhibit excellent oral bioavailability when compared with IV formulations include ciprofloxacin, clindamycin, doxycycline, levofloxacin, metronidazole, moxifloxacin, linezolid, and trimethoprim–sulfamethoxazole.

FAILURE OF ANTIMICROBIAL THERAPY

9 A variety of factors may be responsible for an apparent lack of response to therapy. Patients who fail to respond over 2 to 3 days require a thorough reevaluation. It is possible that the disease is not infectious or is nonbacterial in origin, or there is an undetected pathogen in a polymicrobial infection. Other factors include those directly related to drug selection, the host, or the pathogen. Laboratory error in identification, susceptibility testing, or both (presence of inoculum effect or resistant subpopulations) is a rare cause of antimicrobial failure.

Failures Caused by Drug Selection

Factors related directly to the drug selection include an inappropriate drug selection, dosage, or route of administration. Malabsorption of a drug product because of GI disease (such as a short-bowel syndrome) or a drug interaction (such as complexation of fluoroquinolones with multivalent cations resulting in reduced absorption) can lead to potentially subtherapeutic serum concentrations.

Accelerated drug elimination is also possible. This can occur in patients with cystic fibrosis or during pregnancy, when more rapid clearance or larger volumes of distribution can result in low serum concentrations, particularly for aminoglycosides. A common cause of failure of therapy is poor penetration into the site of infection. This is especially true for sites such as the CNS, eye, and prostate gland. Drug failure also can result from drugs that are highly protein bound or that are chemically inactivated at the site of infection.

Failures Caused by Host Factors

Host defenses must be considered when evaluating a patient who is not responding to antimicrobial therapy. Patients who are immunosuppressed (e.g., granulocytopenia from chemotherapy or AIDS) may respond poorly to therapy because their defenses are inadequate to eradicate the infection despite seemingly adequate drug regimens. A good example is the poor response of infection in granulocytopenic patients that is seen when their WBC counts remain low during therapy. This contrasts with a much better response when granulocyte counts increase during therapy.

Other host factors are related to the need for surgical drainage of abscesses or removal of foreign bodies, necrotic tissue, or both. If these situations are not corrected, they result in persistent infection and, occasionally, bacteremia despite adequate antimicrobial therapy.

Failures Caused by Microorganisms

There are two types of resistance, intrinsic and acquired resistance. Intrinsic resistance is when the antimicrobial agent never had activity against the bacterial species. For example, gram-negative bacteria are naturally resistant to vancomycin because the drug cannot penetrate the outer membrane of gram-negative bacteria. Acquired resistance is when the antimicrobial agent was originally active against the bacterial species but the genetic makeup of the bacteria has changed so the drug can no longer be effective.[34]

The strategies used by bacteria to develop acquired resistance are primarily classified into four general mechanisms of resistance: (a) alteration in the target site, (b) change in membrane permeability, (c) efflux pump, and (d) drug inactivation. Bacteria can use one or more of these mechanisms against a specific antibiotic class. Furthermore, a single mechanism of resistance can result in resistance to multiple related or unrelated classes of antibiotics.

Drug inactivation through either β-lactamases or aminoglycoside-modifying enzymes is the predominant mechanism of resistance. For example, β-lactamases can be either plasmid or chromosomally mediated. In addition, the expression of β-lactamases can be induced or constitutive. There are now multiple types and classes of β-lactamases identified, which is beyond the scope of this chapter. However, there are several outstanding papers discussing all of the different types of β-lactamases.[35–37]

The increase in resistance among bacteria is believed to be a result of continued overuse of antimicrobials in the community, as well as in hospitals, and the increasing prevalence of immunosuppressed patients receiving long-term suppressive antimicrobials for the prevention of infections. These resistance patterns are regionally variable, and susceptibility patterns in the community (or hospital) should be monitored closely to promote rational antimicrobial selection.[34]

Enterococci have been isolated with multiple resistance patterns. They may be resistant to β-lactams (by virtue of β-lactamase production, altered penicillin-binding proteins [PBPs], or both), vancomycin (via alterations in peptidoglycan synthesis), and high levels of aminoglycosides (via enzymatic degradation). Pneumococci resistant to penicillins, certain cephalosporins, and macrolides are increasingly common. These organisms generally are susceptible to vancomycin, the new fluoroquinolones, and cefotaxime or ceftriaxone. However, antimicrobial agents such as linezolid, daptomycin, telavancin, and tigecycline have been targeted at resistant gram-positive bacteria.

Treatment of an infection caused by *Enterobacter*, *Citrobacter*, *Serratia*, or *P. aeruginosa* with a third-generation cephalosporin or aztreonam may produce an initial clinical response by eradicating all the susceptible bacteria in the population. Within a few days, however, the highly resistant subpopulations have a selective advantage and can overgrow the infection site to produce a relapse.[37] These bacteria usually retain susceptibility to aminoglycosides, carbapenems, and fluoroquinolones but are resistant to all other β-lactams. Host defenses are extremely important in this scenario. Debilitated patients with pulmonary infections, abscesses, or osteomyelitis are at high risk for drug failure. In these situations, a combination regimen to prevent the emergence of resistance or the use of carbapenem or a fluoroquinolone may be warranted for empirical therapy.

ANTIMICROBIAL USE MANAGEMENT

Antibiotic Formulary

Institutions must decide which antibiotics to include on their formularies. The decision to have a formulary remains controversial; however, restricting choices does encourage familiarity with a core of antibiotics for residents and attending physicians. Open formularies allow the empirical use of any commercially available antibiotics, with recommended guidelines for changes when culture and sensitivity results are finalized. Many institutions have developed an antibiotic stewardship team.[38,39] The team is generally a multidisciplinary group including representation from microbiology, infection control, administration, information technology, pharmacy including infectious disease-trained clinical pharmacists, and physicians from several disciplines, including infectious disease. The implementation of the guidelines and restrictions recommended by such groups requires the cooperation of the entire medical staff. Education is vital to the success of the antibiotic formulary.[38,39]

Antimicrobial Cycling

An interesting topic in formulary management that gained interest and scientific research is *antimicrobial cycling*. Antimicrobial cycling is a predetermined change in an antimicrobial recommendation for empirical therapy of a specific infection at a predetermined time. It also has been called *rotation of antimicrobials*. This strategy should not be confused with *antimicrobial switch therapy*, which involves changes in the route of administration of antimicrobial therapy (i.e., IV to oral).

Antimicrobial cycling is employed as a mechanism to reduce or prevent antimicrobial resistance. *Proactive cycling* is a planned switch to preempt resistance at a predetermined point or series of points with a predetermined schedule. *Reactive cycling* is a response to high or unacceptable resistance and is often a one-time switch. Most programs incorporate aspects of both types of cycling. Cycling implies returning to the original drug after other choices have been used. Rotation implies several planned changes.

Antimicrobial cycling is based on the assumptions (a) that the resistance problem is caused by the overuse of a particular agent or class of agents and (b) that discontinuation of the particular agent or class of agents will restore susceptibility. These assumptions correlate best with nosocomial gram-negative organisms that can rapidly develop resistance. Theoretically, antimicrobial agents should be sequenced in such an order that mechanisms of resistance do not overlap (i.e., changing drug classes).[39,40] However, data have provided insufficient evidence to clearly demonstrate the usefulness of antibiotic cycling.

Keeping Current

Attention must be paid to the literature on antimicrobials to assist in the selection of therapy. The results from prospective, controlled, randomized clinical trials should be evaluated whenever possible when considering appropriate antimicrobial therapy. Results from prelicensing open trials offer only limited information that can be useful in this regard because patients in these trials generally are not seriously ill and are not infected with multiple resistant bacteria. Other confounding factors found in most clinical situations are excluded by virtue of the study design. Therefore, comparative data in more seriously ill patients are essential for the appropriate application of new agents.

Postmarketing trials are also important because results can demonstrate superiority of one regimen over another, in efficacy, safety, or cost-effectiveness. Appropriate antimicrobial therapy can change as new organisms are discovered, susceptibility patterns change, new drugs become available, and new clinical trial results are published. Classical thinking in the treatment of infectious diseases will continue to change and evolve to maintain antimicrobial efficacy. Optimal use of modern antimicrobials is just beginning to be defined.

ABBREVIATIONS

AIDS	acquired immunodeficiency syndrome
AUC	area under the curve
CSF	cerebrospinal fluid
HA-MRSA	hospital-acquired methicillin-resistant *Staphylococcus aureus*
IL-1	interleukin 1
MIC	minimal inhibitory concentration
PBP	penicillin-binding protein
PMN	polymorphonuclear
WBC	white blood cell

REFERENCES

1. Leekha S, Terrell CL, Edson RS. General principles of antimicrobial therapy. Mayo Clin Proc 2011;86(2):156–167.
2. Slama TG, Amin A, Brunton SA, et al. A clinician's guide to the appropriate and accurate use of antibiotics: The Council for Appropriate and Rational Antibiotic Therapy (CARAT) criteria. Am J Med 2005;118(7A):1S–6S.
3. Mackowiak PA, Durach DT. Fever of unknown origin. In: Mandell GL, Bennett JE, Dolin R, eds. Mandell, Douglas and Bennett's Principles and Practice of Infectious Diseases, 7th ed. New York: Churchill Livingstone, 2010:779–790.
4. Cunha BA. Antibiotic selection in the penicillin-allergic patient. Med Clin North Am 2006;90:1257–1264.
5. Mandell LA, Wunderink RG, Anzueto A, et al. Infectious Diseases Society of America/American Thoracic Society consensus guidelines on the management of community-acquired pneumonia in adults. Clin Infect Dis 2007;44:S27–S72.
6. Tunkel AR, Van de Beek D, Scheld MW. Acute meningitis. In: Mandell GL, Bennett JE, Dolin R, eds. Mandell, Douglas and Bennett's Principles and Practice of Infectious Diseases, 7th ed. New York: Churchill Livingstone, 2010:1189–1230.
7. Baddour LM, Wilson WR, Bayer AS, et al. Infective endocarditis. Diagnosis, antimicrobial therapy, and management of complications: A statement for healthcare professionals from the Committee on Rheumatic Fever, Endocarditis, and Kawasaki Disease, Council on Cardiovascular Disease in the Young, and the Councils on Clinical Cardiology, Stroke, and Cardiovascular Surgery and Anesthesia, American Heart Association. Circulation 2005;111:e394–e434.
8. Croft AC, Woods GL. Specimen collection and handling for diagnosis of infectious diseases. In: McPherson RA, Pincus MR, eds. McPherson: Henry's Clinical Diagnosis and Management by Laboratory Methods, 22nd ed. Pennsylvania: Elsevier Saunders, 2011:1239–1254.
9. Granowitz EV, Brown RB. Antibiotic adverse reactions and drug interactions. Crit Care Clin 2008;24:421–442.
10. Gruchalla RS, Pirmohamed M. Antibiotic allergy. N Engl J Med 2006;354:601–609.
11. Chavez-Bueno S, Stull T. Antibacterial agents in pediatrics. Infect Dis Clin North Am 2009;23(4):265–280.
12. Weber S, Mawdsley E, Kaye D. Antibiotic agents in the elderly. Infect Dis Clin North Am 2009;23(4):881–898.
13. Crider KS, Cleves MA, Reefhuis J, et al. Antibacterial medication use during pregnancy and risk of birth defects: National Birth Defects Prevention Study. Arch Pediatr Adolesc Med 2009;163(11):978–985.
14. Roy PD, Majumder M, Roy B. Pharmacogenomics of anti-TB drugs-related hepatotoxicity. Pharmacogenomics 2008;9:311.
15. Gilbert B, Robbins P, Livornese LL. Use of antibacterial agents in renal failure. Infect Dis Clin North Am 2009;23(4):899–924.
16. Verbeeck RK. Pharmacokinetics and dosage adjustment in patients with hepatic dysfunction. Eur J Clin Pharmacol 2008;64(12):1147–1161.
17. Piscitelli SC, Rodvold KA. Drug Interactions in Infectious Diseases, 2nd ed. Totowa, NJ: Humana Press, 2005.
18. Freifeld AG, Bow EJ, Sepkowitz KA, et al. Clinical practice guideline for the use of antimicrobial agents in neutropenic patients with cancer: 2010 update by the Infectious Diseases Society of America. Clin Infect Dis 2011;52(4):e56–e93.
19. Drusano GL. Pharmacokinetics and pharmacodynamics of antimicrobials. Clin Infect Dis 2007;45:s89–s95.
20. Ambrose PG, Bhavnani SM, Rubino CM, et al. Pharmacokinetics–pharmacodynamics of antimicrobial therapy: It's not just for mice anymore. Clin Infect Dis 2007;44:79–86.
21. Nightingale CH, Ambrose PG, Drusano GL, et al. Antimicrobial Pharmacodynamics in Theory and Clinical Practice, 2nd ed. New York: Marcel Dekker, 2007.
22. DeRyke CA, Lee SY, Kuti JL, et al. Optimising dosing strategies of antibacterials utilizing pharmacodynamic principles. Drugs 2006;66:1–14.
23. George JM, Towne TG, Rodvold KA. Prolonged infusions of β-lactam antibiotics: Implications for antimicrobial stewardship. Pharmacotherapy 2012;32(8):707–721.
24. Sinner SW, Tunkel AR. Antimicrobial agents in the treatment of bacterial meningitis. Infect Dis Clin North Am 2004;18:581–602.
25. American Thoracic Society (ATS), Infectious Diseases Society of America (IDSA). Official ATS and IDSA statement: Guidelines for the management of adults with hospital-acquired, ventilator-associated, and healthcare-associated pneumonia. Am J Respir Crit Care Med 2005;171:388–416.
26. Cohen SH, Gerding DN, Johnson S, et al. Clinical practice guidelines for *Clostridium difficile* infection in adults: 2010 update by the Society of Healthcare Epidemiology

of America (SHEA) and the Infectious Diseases Society of America (IDSA). Infect Control Hosp Epidemiol 2010;31(5):431–455.

27. Taylor Z, Nolan CM, Blumberg HM, American Thoracic Society, Centers for Disease Control and Prevention, Infectious Diseases Society of America. Controlling tuberculosis in the United States. Recommendations from the American Thoracic Society, CDC, and the Infectious Diseases Society of America. MMWR Recomm Rep 2005;54 (RR-12):1–81.
28. Ibrahim EH, Sherman G, Ward S, et al. The influence of inadequate antimicrobial treatment of bloodstream infections on patient outcomes in the ICU setting. Chest 2000;118(1):146–155.
29. Solomkin JS, Mazuski JE, Bradley JS, et al. Diagnosis and management of complicated intra-abdominal infection in adults and children: Guidelines by the Surgical Infection Society and the Infectious Diseases Society of America. Clin Infect Dis 2010;50:133–164.
30. Paul M, Leibovici L. Combination antimicrobial treatment versus monotherapy: The contribution of meta-analyses. Infect Dis Clin North Am 2009;23:277–293.
31. Bliziotis IA, Samonis G, Vardakas KZ, et al. Effect of aminoglycoside and β-lactam combination therapy versus β-lactam monotherapy on the emergence of antimicrobial resistance: A meta-analysis of randomized, controlled trials. Antimicrob Agents Chemother 2005;41:149–158.
32. Tamma PD, Cosgrove SE, Maragakis LL. Combination therapy for treatment of infections with gram-negative bacteria. Clin Microbiol Rev 2012;25(3):450–470.
33. Turnidge J. Pharmacodynamics and dosing of aminoglycosides. Infect Dis Clin North Am 2003;17: 503–528.
34. Chen LF, Chopra T, Kaye KS. Pathogens resistant to antibacterial agents. Med Clin North Am 2011;95:647–676.
35. Queenan AM, Bush K. Carbapenemases: The versatile β-lactamases. Clin Microbiol Rev 2007;20:440–458.
36. Bush K, Jacoby GA. Updated functional classification of β-lactamases. Antimicrob Agents Chemother 2010;54(3):969–976.
37. Jacoby GA. AmpC β-lactamases. Clin Microbiol Rev 2009; 22:161–182.
38. Fishman N, Patterson J, Saiman L, et al. Policy statement on antimicrobial stewardship by the Society for Healthcare Epidemiology of America (SHEA), the Infectious Diseases Society of America (IDSA), and the Pediatric Infectious Diseases Society (PIDS). Infect Control Hosp Epidemiol 2012;33(4):322–327.
39. Dellit TH, Owens RC, McGowan JE, et al. Infectious Diseases Society of America and the Society for Healthcare Epidemiology of America guidelines for developing an institutional program to enhance antimicrobial stewardship. Clin Infect Dis 2007;44:159–177.
40. Brown EM, Nathwani D. Antibiotic cycling or rotation: A systematic review of the evidence of efficacy. J Antimicrob Chemother 2005;55:6–9.

Appendix 83-1

Drugs of Choice, First Choice, *Alternative(s)*

GRAM-POSITIVE COCCI

Enterococcus faecalis (generally not as resistant to antibiotics as *Enterococcus faecium*)

- Serious infection (endocarditis, meningitis, pyelonephritis with bacteremia)
  - Ampicillin (or penicillin G) + (gentamicin or streptomycin)
  - Vancomycin + (gentamicin or streptomycin), daptomycin, linezolid, telavancin, tigecycline[a]
- Urinary tract infection
  - Ampicillin, amoxicillin
  - *Fosfomycin* or *nitrofurantoin*

E. faecium (generally more resistant to antibiotics than *E. faecalis*)

- Recommend consultation with infectious disease specialist.
  - Linezolid, quinupristin/dalfopristin, daptomycin, tigecycline[a]

Staphylococcus aureus/Staphylococcus epidermidis

- Methicillin (oxacillin)-sensitive
  - Nafcillin or oxacillin
  - *FGC,[b,c] trimethoprim–sulfamethoxazole, clindamycin, BL/BLI[d]*
- Hospital-acquired methicillin (oxacillin)–resistant
  - Vancomycin ± (gentamicin or rifampin)
  - *Daptomycin, linezolid, telavancin, tigecycline,[a] trimethoprim–sulfamethoxazole*, or *quinupristin–dalfopristin*
- Community-acquired methicillin (oxacillin)–resistant
  - Clindamycin, trimethoprim–sulfamethoxazole, doxycycline[a]
  - *Daptomycin, linezolid, telavancin, tigecycline,[a]* or *vancomycin*

Streptococcus (groups A, B, C, G, and *Streptococcus bovis*)

- Penicillin G or V or ampicillin
- *FGC,[b,c] erythromycin, azithromycin, clarithromycin*

Streptococcus pneumoniae

- Penicillin-sensitive (minimal inhibitory concentration [MIC] <0.1 mcg/mL [mg/L])
  - Penicillin G or V or ampicillin
  - *FGC,[b,c] doxycycline,[a] azithromycin, clarithromycin, erythromycin*
- Penicillin intermediate (MIC 0.1 to 1 mcg/mL [mg/L])
  - High-dose penicillin (12 million units/day for adults) or ceftriaxone[c] or cefotaxime[c]
  - *Levofloxacin,[a] moxifloxacin,[a] gemifloxacin,[a] or vancomycin*
- Penicillin-resistant (MIC ≥1.0 mcg/mL [mg/L])
  - Recommend consultation with infectious disease specialist.
    - *Vancomycin ± rifampin*
    - *Per sensitivities: cefotaxime, ceftriaxone,[c] levofloxacin,[a] moxifloxacin,[a] or gemifloxacin[a]*

Streptococcus, viridans group

- Penicillin G ± gentamicin[e]
- *Cefotaxime,[c] ceftriaxone,[c] erythromycin, azithromycin, clarithromycin*, or *vancomycin ± gentamicin*

GRAM-NEGATIVE COCCI

Moraxella (Branhamella) catarrhalis

- Amoxicillin–clavulanate, ampicillin–sulbactam
- *Trimethoprim–sulfamethoxazole, erythromycin, azithromycin, clarithromycin, doxycycline,[a] SGC,[c,f] cefotaxime,[c] ceftriaxone,[c]* or *TGCPO[c,g]*

Neisseria gonorrhoeae (also give concomitant treatment for *Chlamydia trachomatis*)

- Disseminated gonococcal infection
  - Ceftriaxone[c] or cefotaxime[c]
  - *Oral followup: cefpodoxime,[c] ciprofloxacin,[a]* or *levofloxacin[a]*
- Uncomplicated infection
  - Ceftriaxone,[c] cefotaxime,[c] or cefpodoxime[c]
  - *Ciprofloxacin[a]* or *levofloxacin[a]*

Neisseria meningitides

- Penicillin G
- *Cefotaxime[c]* or *ceftriaxone[c]*

GRAM-POSITIVE BACILLI

Clostridium perfringens

- Penicillin G ± clindamycin
- *Metronidazole,[a] clindamycin, doxycycline,[a] cefazolin,[c] carbapenem[h,i]*

Clostridium difficile

- Oral metronidazole[a]
- *Oral vancomycin*

GRAM-NEGATIVE BACILLI

Acinetobacter spp.

- Doripenem, imipenem, or meropenem ± aminoglycoside[j] (amikacin usually most effective)
- *Ampicillin–sulbactam, colistin,[i]* or *tigecycline[a]*

Bacteroides fragilis (and others)

- Metronidazole[a]
- *BL/BLI,[d] clindamycin, cefoxitin,[c] cefotetan,[c]* or *carbapenem[h,i]*

Enterobacter spp.

- Carbapenem[h] or cefepime ± aminoglycoside[j]
- *Ciprofloxacin,[a] levofloxacin,[a] piperacillin–tazobactam, ticarcillin–clavulanate*

Escherichia coli

- Meningitis
  - Cefotaxime,[c] ceftriaxone,[c] meropenem
- Systemic infection
  - Cefotaxime[c] or ceftriaxone[c]
  - *BL/BLI,[d] fluoroquinolone,[a,k] carbapenem[h,i]*
- Urinary tract infection
  - Most oral agents: check sensitivities
  - Ampicillin, amoxicillin–clavulanate, doxycycline,[a] or cephalexin[c]
  - *Aminoglycoside,[j] FGC,[b,c] nitrofurantoin, fluoroquinolone[a,k]*

Gardnerella vaginalis

- Metronidazole[a]
- *Clindamycin*

Haemophilus influenzae

- Meningitis
  - Cefotaxime[c] or ceftriaxone[c]
  - *Meropenem[i]*

- Other infections
  - BL/BLI,[d] or if β-lactamase-negative, ampicillin or amoxicillin
  - *Trimethoprim–sulfamethoxazole, cefuroxime,[c] azithromycin, clarithromycin,* or *fluoroquinolone[a,k]*

Klebsiella pneumoniae

- BL/BLI,[d] cefotaxime,[c] ceftriaxone,[c] cefepime[c]
- Carbapenem,[h,i] fluoroquinolone[a,k]

Legionella spp.

- Azithromycin, erythromycin ± rifampin, or fluoroquinolone[a,k]
- Trimethoprim–sulfamethoxazole, clarithromycin, or doxycycline[a]

Pasteurella multocida

- Penicillin G, ampicillin, amoxicillin
- *Doxycycline,[a] BL/BLI,[d] trimethoprim–sulfamethoxazole or ceftriaxone[c]*

Proteus mirabilis

- Ampicillin
- *Trimethoprim–sulfamethoxazole*

Proteus (indole-positive) (including *Providencia rettgeri*, *Morganella morganii*, and *Proteus vulgaris*)

- Cefotaxime,[c] ceftriaxone,[c] or fluoroquinolone[a,k]
- *BL/BLI,[d] aztreonam,[l] aminoglycosides,[j] carbapenem[h,i]*

Providencia stuartii

- Amikacin, cefotaxime,[c] ceftriaxone,[c] fluoroquinolone[a,k]
- *Trimethoprim–sulfamethoxazole, aztreonam,[l] carbapenem[h,i]*

Pseudomonas aeruginosa

- Urinary tract infection only
  - Aminoglycoside[j]
  - *Ciprofloxacin,[a] levofloxacin[a]*
- Systemic infection
  - Cefepime,[c] ceftazidime,[c] doripenem,[i] imipenem,[i] meropenem,[i] piperacillin–tazobactam, or ticarcillin–clavulanate + aminoglycoside[j]
  - *Aztreonam,[l] ciprofloxacin,[a] levofloxacin,[a] colistin[i]*

Salmonella typhi

- Ciprofloxacin,[a] levofloxacin,[c] ceftriaxone,[c] cefotaxime[c]
- *Trimethoprim–sulfamethoxazole*

Serratia marcescens

- Ceftriaxone,[c] cefotaxime,[c] cefepime,[c] ciprofloxacin,[a] levofloxacin[a]
- *Aztreonam,[l] carbapenem,[h,i] piperacillin–tazobactam, ticarcillin–clavulanate*

Stenotrophomonas (Xanthomonas) maltophilia (generally very resistant to all antimicrobials)

- Trimethoprim–sulfamethoxazole.
- *Check sensitivities to ceftazidime,[c] doxycycline,[a] minocycline,[a] and ticarcillin–clavulanate.*

MISCELLANEOUS MICROORGANISMS

Chlamydia pneumoniae

- Doxycycline[a]
- *Azithromycin, clarithromycin, erythromycin, or fluoroquinolone[a,k]*

C. trachomatis

- Azithromycin or doxycycline[a]
- *Levofloxacin,[a] erythromycin*

Mycoplasma pneumoniae

- Azithromycin, clarithromycin, erythromycin, fluoroquinolone[a,k]
- *Doxycycline[a]*

SPIROCHETES

Treponema pallidum

- Neurosyphilis
  - Penicillin G
  - *Ceftriaxone[c]*
- *Primary or secondary*
  - Benzathine, penicillin G
  - *Ceftriaxone[c] or doxycycline[a]*

Borrelia burgdorferi (choice depends on stage of disease)

- Ceftriaxone[c] or cefuroxime axetil,[c] doxycycline,[a] amoxicillin
- *High-dose penicillin, cefotaxime[c]*

---

[a]Not for use in pregnant patients or children.
[b]First-generation cephalosporins—IV: cefazolin; orally: cephalexin, cephradine, or cefadroxil.
[c]Some penicillin-allergic patients may react to cephalosporins.
[d]β-Lactam/β-lactamase inhibitor combination—IV: ampicillin–sulbactam, piperacillin–tazobactam, and ticarcillin–clavulanate; orally: amoxicillin–clavulanate.
[e]Gentamicin should be added if tolerance or moderately susceptible (MIC >0.1 mcg/mL [mg/L]) organisms are encountered; streptomycin is used but can be more toxic.
[f]Second-generation cephalosporins—IV: cefuroxime; orally: cefaclor, cefditoren, cefprozil, cefuroxime axetil, and loracarbef.
[g]Third-generation cephalosporins—orally: cefdinir, cefixime, cefetamet, cefpodoxime proxetil, and ceftibuten.
[h]Carbapenem: doripenem, ertapenem, imipenem/cilastatin, and meropenem.
[i]Reserve for serious infection.
[j]Aminoglycosides: gentamicin, tobramycin, and amikacin; use per sensitivities.
[k]Fluoroquinolones IV/orally: ciprofloxacin, levofloxacin, and moxifloxacin.
[l]Generally reserved for patients with hypersensitivity reactions to penicillin.

Central Nervous System Infections

84

Ramy H. Elshaboury, Elizabeth D. Hermsen, Jessica S. Holt, Isaac F. Mitropoulos, and John C. Rotschafer

KEY CONCEPTS

1. The four most likely pathogens of bacterial meningitis in the United States are *Streptococcus pneumoniae*, group B *Streptococcus*, *Neisseria meningitidis*, and *Haemophilus influenzae* type b, although routine vaccination is having a dramatic effect on the incidence of these pathogens causing infection.
2. In cases of meningitis, initial findings can include (a) presenting signs and symptoms: fever, headache, nuchal rigidity (the classic triad), Brudzinski's or Kernig's sign, and altered mental status; and (b) abnormal cerebrospinal fluid (CSF) chemistries: elevated white blood cell (WBC) count (>1,000 cells/mm^3 [$>1 \times 10^9$/L]), elevated protein (>50 mg/dL [>500 mg/L]), and decreased glucose levels (<45 mg/dL [<2.5 mmol/L).
3. Two main microbiologic tests that should be obtained include a Gram stain and culture of the CSF. Molecular testing such as polymerase chain reaction, latex coagglutination, and enzyme immunoassay (EIA) tests provide for the rapid identification of several causes of meningitis.
4. Three primary goals of treatment in meningitis include (a) eradication of infection, (b) amelioration of signs and symptoms, and (c) prevention of the development of neurologic sequelae, such as seizures, deafness, coma, and death.
5. When selecting antibiotics, the clinician must consider the antibiotic concentration at the site of infection, as well as the spectrum of antibacterial activity. Empirical choices should be based on age, predisposing conditions, and comorbidities. (a) Ceftriaxone or cefotaxime and vancomycin are reasonable initial choices for empirical coverage of community-acquired meningitis in adult patients. (b) *Listeria monocytogenes* is a common pathogen in infants and elderly; therefore, ampicillin with or without gentamicin should be added empirically to antimicrobial coverage.
6. Empirical coverage with an appropriate antibiotic should be started as soon as possible when clinical suspicion of meningitis exists. If there is a delay in doing a lumbar puncture (even 30 to 60 minutes), or if the patient is to undergo neuroimaging, the first dose of an antibiotic should not be withheld. Changes in the CSF after initiation of antibiotics usually take 12 to 24 hours.
7. Antibiotic dosages for the treatment of meningitis should be optimized to ensure adequate CNS penetration.
8. The duration of antibiotic treatment for meningitis has not been standardized; however, the duration generally is based on the causative organism and the individual case and may range from 7 to 21 days.
9. Close contacts and relatives of the index case should be assessed for appropriate prophylaxis, particularly for *N. meningitidis* and *H. influenzae* meningitis.
10. Steroid treatment includes dexamethasone 0.15 mg/kg per dose to be given four times daily for 4 days in infants and children older than 2 months of age with proven or strongly suspected bacterial meningitis. Steroids should be started prior to the first dose of antibiotics.

CNS infections are caused by a variety of pathogens, including bacteria, viruses, fungi, and parasites. Infections are the result of hematogenous spread from a primary infection site, seeding from a parameningeal focus, reactivation from a latent site, trauma, or congenital defects within the CNS. Newer diagnostic techniques have enabled more rapid and definitive diagnoses, thus diminishing the number of unknown "aseptic meningitis" diagnoses and improving targeted therapy. Bacteria resistant to multiple antibiotics present new challenges in the management of meningitis. This chapter presents the etiology, pathophysiology, therapy, and prophylaxis of these infections, concentrating predominantly on bacterial meningitis.

EPIDEMIOLOGY

Approximately 1.2 million cases of acute bacterial meningitis (ABM), excluding epidemics, occur every year around the globe, resulting in ~170,000 deaths.[1,2] Mortality rates for patients with meningitis vary depending on the causative microorganism and age group. About 20% (range 12.3% to 35.3%) of survivors will experience one or more neurologic disabilities.[3] Neurologic sequelae frequently associated with ABM include seizures, sensorineural hearing loss, and hydrocephalus. Risk for the development of neurologic sequelae depends on the infecting organism, with pneumococcal meningitis being associated with the highest risk.[4] Despite the availability of antimicrobial therapy against the most common CNS pathogens, CNS infections continue to have significant morbidity and mortality.

Two findings that have the potential for great epidemiologic impact on bacterial meningitis are the following: (a) passive and active exposures to cigarette smoke are risk factors for bacterial meningitis, especially meningococcal disease,[5] and (b) children with cochlear implants that include a positioner are at increased risk of bacterial meningitis, specifically pneumococcal meningitis. The incidence of meningitis due to *Streptococcus pneumoniae* in children with cochlear implants was more than 30 times the incidence in a similar cohort of the U.S. population without implants.[6] Other risk factors for ABM include respiratory tract infection, otitis media mastoiditis, head trauma, alcoholism, high-dose steroids, splenectomy, sickle cell disease, immunoglobulin (Ig) deficiency, and immunosuppression.

ETIOLOGY

1 CNS infections are caused by a variety of microorganisms. Historically, CNS infections were primarily community acquired; however, an increasing number of cases are now nosocomial.[7] *Haemophilus influenzae* type b was the most commonly identified cause of bacterial meningitis until the introduction of the *H. influenzae* type b (Hib) conjugate vaccine in 1990, when *S. pneumoniae* became the most commonly identified cause in the United States (58%), followed by group B *Streptococcus* (GBS) (18.1%), *Neisseria meningitidis* (13.9%), *H. influenzae* (6.7%), and *Listeria monocytogenes* (3.4%).[8]

Following the release of the heptavalent pneumococcal protein-conjugate vaccine (PCV7) in 2000, the rate of invasive pneumococcal disease steadily dropped from 24.3 cases per 100,000 people in 1999 to 17.3 per 100,000 in 2001 and 13.5 per 100,000 in 2007. The largest impact was in children younger than 2 years of age where a nearly 70% decline in infection rate was reported as a result of implementation in the routine childhood vaccination schedule. Interestingly, the effect carried into the adult population as well with significant reduction in invasive pneumococcal disease across all age groups.[9,10]

As a result of the decline of ABM rates in children, the median age of patients increased from 30.3 years in 1998 to 41.3 years in 2007 in the United States.[8] Both the Hib and pneumococcal vaccines are of limited availability in developing countries where cost is often prohibitive. Thus, rate of invasive disease and case fatalities among children continue to be much higher than in Western countries.

ANATOMY AND PHYSIOLOGY OF THE CENTRAL NERVOUS SYSTEM

Meninges

The skull and vertebrae protect the CNS from blunt or penetrating trauma (Fig. 84-1). The brain is suspended in these structures by cerebrospinal fluid (CSF) and is surrounded by the meninges. The meninges are made up of three separate membranes: dura mater, arachnoid, and pia mater.[11] Dura mater, or pachymeninges, lies directly beneath and is adherent to the skull. The other two membranes are referred to collectively as *leptomeninges*. Pia mater lies directly over brain tissue. Arachnoid, the middle layer, lies between the dura mater and the pia mater. The subarachnoid space, located between the arachnoid and the pia mater, is the conduit for CSF. By definition, meningitis refers to inflammation of the subarachnoid space or spinal fluid, whereas encephalitis is an inflammation of the brain itself. Since infectious microorganisms frequently are an underlying cause of these inflammatory processes, the terms *meningitis* and *encephalitis* frequently are used to denote an infectious process. The decision regarding the diagnosis of meningoencephalitis depends on radiographic, laboratory, and clinical information but would refer to inflammation of both tissue and fluid.

Cerebrospinal Fluid

Approximately 85% of the CSF is produced within the third, fourth, and lateral ventricles by the choroid plexus (Fig. 84-1). CSF volume in the CNS is related to patient age: infants have approximately 40 to 60 mL of CSF, older children have 60 to 100 mL, and adults have 115 to 160 mL. Normally, CSF is produced at the rate of approximately 500 mL/day and flows unidirectionally downward through the spinal cord. The CSF is removed by the arachnoid villi and vertebral venous plexus located in the spinal cord and does not recommunicate with the point of production.[11]

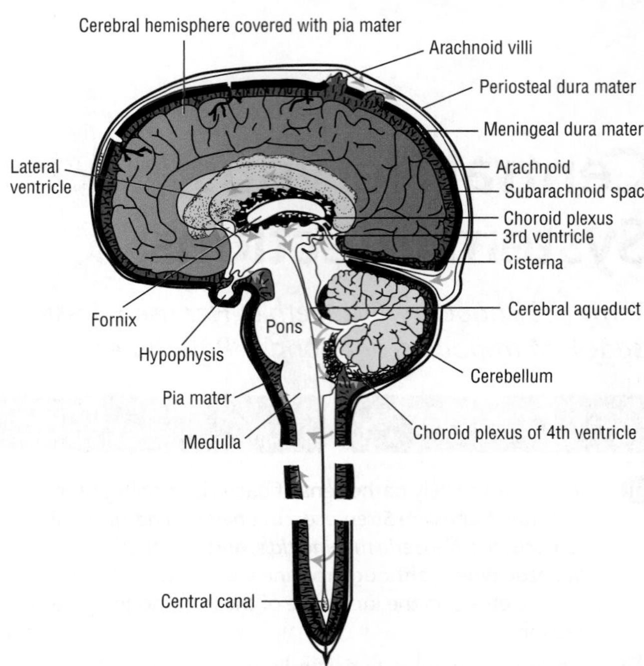

FIGURE 84-1 Diagram of the CNS.

2 The CSF normally is clear, with a protein content of less than 50 mg/dL (500 mg/L), a glucose concentration of approximately 50% to 60% of the simultaneous peripheral serum glucose concentration, and a pH of approximately 7.4. Also, it typically contains fewer than 5 white blood cells (WBCs)/mm^3 (or fewer than 5×10^6/L), all of which should be lymphocytes (Table 84-1). As meninges become inflamed, the constituency of the CSF will change, and these changes can be used diagnostically as markers of infection.

Blood–Brain Barrier/Blood–CSF Barrier

Natural barriers to the exchange of drugs and endogenous compounds among the blood, brain, and CSF are the blood–brain barrier and the blood–CSF barrier (BCSFB) (Fig. 84-2). The blood–brain barrier consists of tightly joined capillary endothelial cells. Drug entry into brain tissue is accomplished by direct passage through the capillary endothelial cells and further penetration of the glial cells that envelop the capillary structure.[11]

Passage of drugs into the CSF is controlled by the BCSFB. This barrier is created by ependymal cells of the choroid plexus, which function as an active transport system similar to the renal tubular epithelial cells. The inflammatory process associated with meningitis inhibits the active transport system of the choroid plexus.[12] As in the active transport system in the kidney, the secretion of substances out of the choroid plexus also can be inhibited by the administration of probenecid.[11]

PATHOPHYSIOLOGY OF THE CNS INFECTION

The development of bacterial meningitis occurs following bacterial invasion of the host and CNS, bacterial multiplication with subsequent inflammation of the CNS, specifically the subarachnoid

TABLE 84-1 Mean Values of the Components of Normal and Abnormal Cerebrospinal Fluid[13,16,19,20,97]

Type	Normal	Bacterial	Viral	Fungal	Tuberculosis
WBC (cells/mm³ or ×10⁶/L)	<5 (<30 in newborns)	1,000–5,000	5–500	100–400	25–500
Differential[a]	Monocytes	Neutrophils	Lymphocytes	Lymphocytes	Variable
Protein (mg/dL)	<50 (<500 mg/L)	Elevated	Mild elevation	Elevated	Elevated
Glucose (mg/dL)	45–80 (2.5–4.4 mmol/L)	Low	Normal	Low	Low
CSF: blood glucose ratio	50–60%	Decreased	Normal	Decreased	Decreased

[a]Initial cerebrospinal fluid (CSF) and while blood cell (WBC) count may reveal a predominance of polymorphonuclear leukocytes (PMNs).

space and the ventricular space, pathophysiologic alterations owing to progressive inflammation, and the resulting neuronal damage.[13] The critical first step in the acquisition of ABM is nasopharyngeal colonization of the host. Igs such as secretory IgA are found in high concentrations within nasopharyngeal secretions and work to inhibit bacterial colonization. However, the mucus barrier is deteriorated by IgA proteases secreted by the bacteria, which then extend pili that allow adherence to the host cell surface receptors. Bacterial pathogens attach themselves to nasopharyngeal epithelial cells and are phagocytized into the host's bloodstream. After accessing the patient's bloodstream, bacteria must overcome the host's defense mechanisms. Commonly, CNS bacterial pathogens will produce an extensive polysaccharide capsule resistant to neutrophil phagocytosis and complement opsonization. *H. influenzae*, *Escherichia coli*, and *N. meningitidis* strains lacking polysaccharide capsules are unable to cause meningitis. Capsular polysaccharides activate the alternate complement pathway, which promotes phagocytosis and clearance of infecting pathogens. Patients unable to activate the alternative complement pathway, such as asplenic and sickle cell patients, are predisposed to bacterial infections caused by encapsulated microorganisms and therefore are at increased risk for meningitis.[13]

Although the exact site and mechanism of bacterial invasion into the CNS is unknown, studies suggest that invasion into the subarachnoid space occurs by continuous exposure of the CNS to large bacterial inocula. Bacteremia with inoculum densities of at least 10^3 colony-forming units (CFU)/mL (10^6 CFU/L) appears to be essential for subarachnoid space invasion.[14] Although several sites of bacterial invasion have been theorized, the most plausible sites are the choroid plexus and/or the cerebral microvasculature. Host defense mechanisms within the subarachnoid space are inadequate to combat bacterial pathogens; therefore, bacteria replicate freely within the CSF until either overgrowth occurs or an effective antibiotic regimen is administered that terminates the process.

The effects of meningitis, namely, inflammation within the subarachnoid space and the ensuing neurologic damage, are not necessarily a direct result of the pathogens themselves. The neurologic sequelae occur due to the activation of the host's inflammatory pathways, which is induced by the pathogens or their products. Bacterial cell lysis and subsequent death can result in the release of cell wall components, such as lipopolysaccharide (LPS), lipid A (endotoxin), lipoteichoic acid, teichoic acid, and peptidoglycan, depending on whether the pathogen is gram-positive or gram-negative (Fig. 84-3).

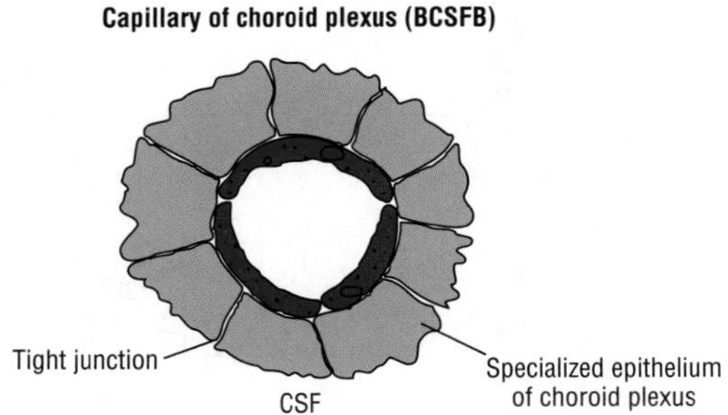

FIGURE 84-2 Schematic representation of a blood–cerebrospinal fluid barrier capillary, brain tissue capillary, and normal tissue capillary (*below*).

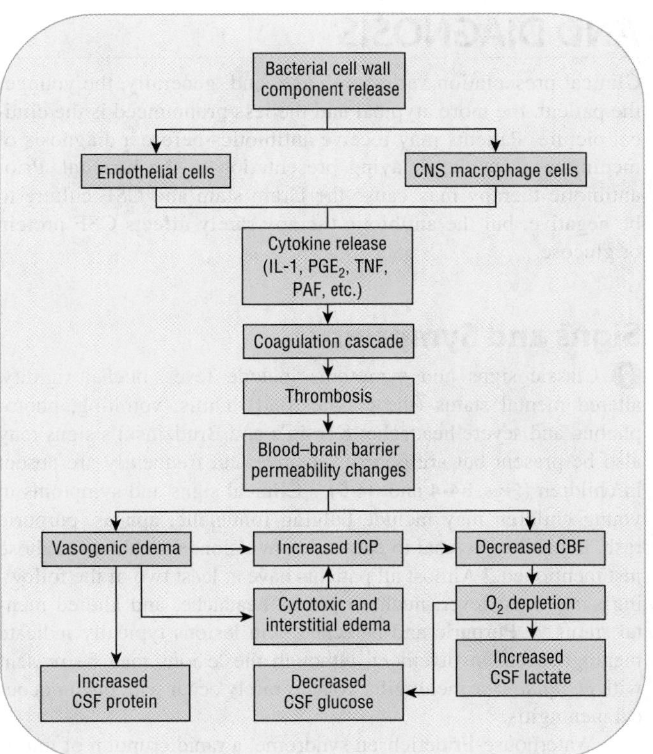

FIGURE 84-3 Hypothetical schema of pathophysiologic events that occur during bacterial meningitis. (IL-1, interleukin 1; TNF, tumor necrosis factor; PAF, platelet-activating factor; CBF, cerebral blood flow; CSF, cerebrospinal fluid; PGE_2, prostaglandin E_2; ICP, intracranial pressure.)

These cell wall components cause capillary endothelial cells and CNS macrophages to release cytokines (interleukin 1 [IL-1] and tumor necrosis factor [TNF]) and other inflammatory mediators (IL-6, IL-8, platelet-activating factor [PAF], nitric oxide, arachidonic acid metabolites [e.g., prostaglandin and prostacycline], and macrophage-derived proteins). Proteolytic products and toxic oxygen radicals are released from the capillary endothelium, causing an alteration in the permeability of the blood–brain barrier. PAF activates the coagulation cascade, and arachidonic acid metabolites stimulate vasodilation. These events propagate other sequential events that lead to cerebral edema, elevated intracranial pressure (ICP), CSF pleocytosis, decreased cerebral blood flow (CBF), cerebral ischemia, and death.[13,14]

Clinical **Controversy. . .**

Procalcitonin (PCT) has emerged as a predictive biomarker for invasive infections, including meningitis, owing to specificity to bacterial infections. Elevation of serum PCT levels was mostly studied in lower respiratory tract and bloodstream infections, but some data support its association with bacterial meningitis. Utility of PCT in predicting bacterial meningitis, differentiating bacterial from viral etiologies, and deciding on starting and stopping antibacterial therapy is controversial. More studies are needed to confirm the impact of serum PCT monitoring on clinical outcomes.

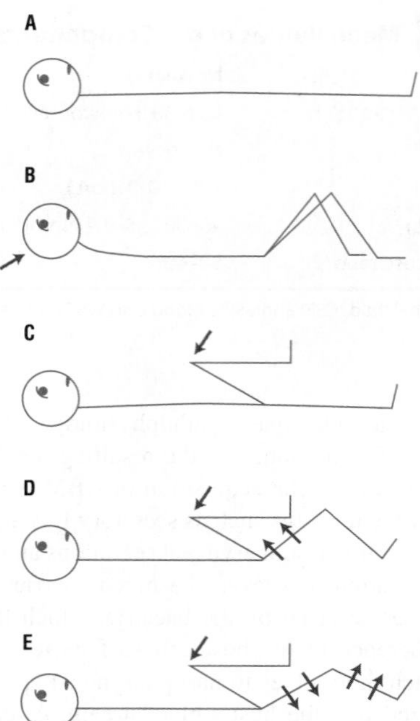

FIGURE 84-4 *A, B.* Brudzinski's neck signs. Hip and knee flexion occurs as a result of flexion of the neck (*B*). *C–E.* Brudzinski's leg signs. *C.* Patient's leg is flexed by examiner (*arrow*). *D.* The contralateral leg begins to flex—identical contralateral sign (*arrows*). *E.* The contralateral leg now begins to extend spontaneously, resembling a little kick (*arrows*).

CLINICAL PRESENTATION AND DIAGNOSIS

Clinical presentation varies with age, and, generally, the younger the patient, the more atypical and the less pronounced is the clinical picture. Patients may receive antibiotics before a diagnosis of meningitis is made, delaying presentation to the hospital. Prior antibiotic therapy may cause the Gram stain and CSF culture to be negative, but the antibiotic therapy rarely affects CSF protein or glucose.

Signs and Symptoms

❷ Classic signs and symptoms include fever, nuchal rigidity, altered mental status (the classic triad), chills, vomiting, photophobia, and severe headache; Kernig's and Brudzinski's signs may also be present but are poorly sensitive and frequently are absent in children (Figs. 84-4 and 84-5).[15] Clinical signs and symptoms in young children may include bulging fontanelle, apneas, purpuric rash, irritability, refusal to eat, and convulsions in addition to those just mentioned.[15] Almost all patients have at least two of the following symptoms: fever, nuchal rigidity, headache, and altered mental status.[4,16] Purpuric and petechial skin lesions typically indicate meningococcal involvement, although the lesions may be present with *H. influenzae* meningitis. Rashes rarely occur with pneumococcal meningitis.[17]

Waterhouse-Friderichsen syndrome, a rapid eruption of multiple hemorrhagic lesions associated with a shock-like state, is associated with meningococcal meningitis. Both *H. influenzae* meningitis and meningococcal meningitis can cause involvement of the joints during the illness. History of head trauma with or without skull fracture or presence of a chronically draining ear is associated with pneumococcal involvement.

Bacterial Meningitis Score

Bacterial Meningitis Score is a validated clinical decision tool aimed to identify children older than 2 months with CSF pleocytosis who are at low risk of ABM. This tool incorporates clinical features such as positive CSF Gram stain, presence of seizure, serum absolute neutrophil count ≥10,000 cells/mm^3 (≥10 × 10^9/L), CSF protein ≥80 mg/dL (≥800 mg/L), and CSF neutrophil count ≥1,000 cells/mm^3 (≥1 × 10^9/L). Treatment is recommended when one or more criteria are present. Certain pediatric patients are excluded including those with purpura, CSF shunt, recent neurosurgery, and Lyme's disease (LD) and those who received oral or IV antibiotics within 72 hours. This scoring tool was validated in several studies showing high accuracy in excluding ABM. One meta-analysis of eight validation studies between 2002 and 2012 (5,312 pediatric patients) showed the tool to be highly accurate, with combined sensitivity of 99.3%, specificity of 62.1%, and negative predictive value of 99.7%.[18]

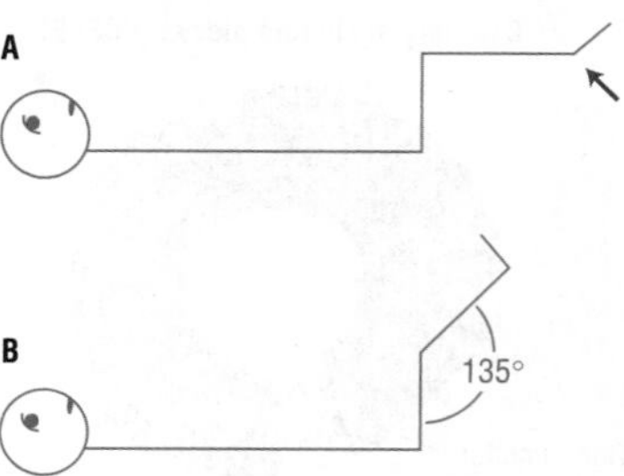

FIGURE 84-5 Kernig's sign. *A.* Knees are raised to form a 90° angle relative to the trunk, and the examiner attempts to extend the knees. *B.* Once the knee angle reaches approximately 135°, contracture or extensor spasm occurs.

Laboratory Tests

Several tubes of CSF are collected via lumbar puncture for chemistry, microbiology, and hematology tests. Theoretically, the first tube has a higher likelihood of being contaminated with both blood and bacteria during the puncture, although the total volume is more important in practice than the tube cultured. CSF should not be refrigerated or stored on ice.

Analysis of CSF chemistries typically includes measurement of glucose and total protein concentrations. An elevated CSF protein of ≥50 mg/dL (≥500 mg/L) and a CSF glucose concentration of less than 50% of the simultaneously obtained peripheral value suggest bacterial meningitis (see Table 84-1).

The values for CSF glucose, protein, and WBC concentrations found with bacterial meningitis overlap significantly with those for viral, tuberculous, and fungal meningitis (see Table 84-1). Therefore, CSF WBC counts and CSF glucose and protein concentrations cannot always distinguish the different etiologies of meningitis.

Other Diagnostic Tests[19–22]

In patients presenting with new-onset seizures, signs of space-occupying lesions or moderate to severe impairment of consciousness, cranial imaging via magnetic resonance imaging (MRI), or cranial computed tomography (CT) should precede a lumbar puncture. MRI is generally preferred as it more clearly identifies areas of cerebral edemas. In these instances, the withdrawal of CSF fluid from a lumbar puncture reduces counterpressure that may result in compression of the brain from above with risk of brain herniation complicating the clinical course. Neuroimaging should not however delay initiation of antibiotic therapy as doing so can result in a poor outcome in this disease.[23,24] MRI is the preferred modality for the diagnosis of encephalitis due to higher specificity and sensitivity (A-I) than CT (B-III) (see Table 84-2 footnotes for rating scale of evidence).

TABLE 84-2 Bacterial Meningitis: Most Likely Etiologies and Empirical Therapy by Age Group[13,19,20]

Age	Most Likely Organisms	Empirical Therapy[a]
<1 month	*S. agalactiae* Gram-negative enterics[b] *L. monocytogenes*	Ampicillin + cefotaxime *or* ampicillin + aminoglycoside
1–23 months	*S. pneumoniae* *N. meningitidis* *H. influenzae* *S. agalactiae*	Vancomycin[c] + third-generation cephalosporin (cefotaxime *or* ceftriaxone)
2–50 years	*N. meningitidis* *S. pneumoniae*	Vancomycin[c] + third-generation cephalosporin (cefotaxime *or* ceftriaxone)
>50 years	*S. pneumoniae* *N. meningitidis* Gram-negative enterics[b] *L. monocytogenes*	Vancomycin[c] + ampicillin + third-generation cephalosporin (cefotaxime *or* ceftriaxone)

Strength of recommendation: (A) Good evidence to support a recommendation for use; should always be offered. (B) Moderate evidence to support a recommendation for use; should generally be offered.
Quality of evidence: (I) Evidence from ≥1 properly randomized, controlled trial. (II) Evidence from ≥1 well-designed clinical trial, without randomization; from cohort or case–control analytic studies (preferably from ≥1 center) or from multiple time series. (III) Evidence from opinions of respected authorities, based on clinical experience, descriptive studies, or reports of expert committees.[19]

[a]All recommendations are A-III.
[b]*E. coli, Klebsiella* spp., and *Enterobacter* spp. common.
[c]Vancomycin use should be based on local incidence of penicillin-resistant *S. pneumoniae* and until cefotaxime or ceftriaxone minimum inhibitory concentration results are available.

Blood and other specimens should be cultured according to clinical judgment because meningitis frequently can arise via hematogenous dissemination or can be associated with infections at other sites. A minimum of 20 mL of blood in each of two to three separate cultures per each 24-hour period is necessary for the detection of most bacteremia.

❸ Gram stain and culture of the CSF are the most important laboratory tests performed for bacterial meningitis. The Gram stain continues to be the most rapid and accurate method of presumptively diagnosing ABM. When performed before antibiotic therapy is initiated, Gram stain is both rapid and sensitive and can confirm the diagnosis of bacterial meningitis in 75% to 90% of cases. The sensitivity of the Gram stain decreases to 40% to 60% in patients who received prior antibiotic therapy. Culture is required to differentiate the various bacterial etiologies.

Polymerase chain reaction (PCR) techniques can be used to diagnose meningitis caused by *N. meningitidis*, *S. pneumoniae*, and Hib. PCR is considered to be highly sensitive and specific, but expense and availability can be limiting. Currently, no U.S. FDA-approved testing is available.

Latex fixation, latex coagglutination, and enzyme immunoassay (EIA) tests provide for the rapid identification of several bacterial causes of meningitis, including *S. pneumoniae*, *N. meningitidis*, and Hib. Rapid-identification latex tests work by bringing potential capsular antigens of the pathogen causing meningitis in contact with a specific antibody, causing an antigen–antibody reaction. This capsular antigen–antibody reaction can be observed visually and quickly without waiting for culture results. The sensitivity and specificity of latex fixation and coagglutination tests can vary with the manufacturer of the antibody, density of the antigen present in the CSF, and pathogen being tested. Latex agglutination is most useful for patients who have been treated with antimicrobials and whose CSF Gram stain and culture are negative (B-III).

Diagnosis of tuberculosis meningitis employs acid-fast staining, culture, and PCR of the CSF. PCR testing of the CSF is the preferred method of diagnosing most viral meningitis infections (A-III). The standard diagnostic tests for fungal meningitis include culture, direct microscopic examination of stained and unstained specimens of CSF, antigen detection of cryptococcal or histoplasmal antigens, and antibody assay of serum and/or CSF.

TREATMENT

Desired Outcome

❹ Goals for the treatment of CNS infections should include eradication of infection, amelioration of signs and symptoms, preventing morbidity and mortality, initiating appropriate antimicrobials, providing supportive care, and preventing disease through timely introduction of vaccination and chemoprophylaxis. Understanding antibiotic selection and the issues surrounding antibiotic penetration will assist in meeting the goals of treatment.

General Approach to Treatment and Nonpharmacologic and Supportive Therapy

This section discusses issues surrounding the approach to treatment, such as antibiotic penetration within the CNS, duration of antibiotic therapy, and supportive treatments. Until a pathogen is identified, prompt empirical antibiotic coverage is often needed. ❺ Based on the patient's profile (i.e., allergies, age, and concurrent medical conditions), extent of antibiotic CNS penetration,[25]

TABLE 84-3 Penetration of Antimicrobial Agents into the CSF[a,25]

Therapeutic Levels in CSF with or Without Inflammation	
Acyclovir	Levofloxacin
Chloramphenicol	Linezolid
Ciprofloxacin	Metronidazole
Fluconazole	Moxifloxacin
Flucytosine	Pyrazinamide
Foscarnet	Rifampin
Fosfomycin	Sulfonamides
Ganciclovir	Trimethoprim
Isoniazid	Voriconazole
Therapeutic Levels in CSF with Inflammation of Meninges	
Ampicillin ± sulbactam	Imipenem
Aztreonam	Meropenem
Cefepime	Nafcillin
Cefotaxime	Ofloxacin
Ceftazidime	Penicillin G
Ceftriaxone	Piperacillin/tazobactam[b]
Cefuroxime	Pyrimethamine
Colistin	Quinupristin/dalfopristin
Daptomycin	Ticarcillin ± clavulanic acid[b]
Ethambutol	Vancomycin
Nontherapeutic Levels in CSF with or Without Inflammation	
Aminoglycosides	Cephalosporins (second generation)[c]
Amphotericin B	Doxycycline[d]
β-Lactamase inhibitors[e]	Itraconazole[f]
Cephalosporins (first generation)	

CSF, cerebrospinal fluid.

[a]Using recommended CNS dosing and compared with MIC of target pathogens.
[b]May not achieve therapeutic levels against organisms with higher MIC, as in *P. aeruginosa*. Tazobactam does not penetrate blood–brain barrier.
[c]Cefuroxime is an exception.
[d]Documented effectiveness for *Borrelia burgdorferi*.
[e]Includes clavulanic acid, sulbactam, and tazobactam.
[f]Achieves therapeutic concentrations for *Cryptococcus neoformans* therapy.

and spectrum of activity, appropriate recommendations can be made, and therapy should last at least 48 to 72 hours or until the diagnosis of bacterial meningitis can be ruled out (Tables 84-2 and 84-3). 6 The first dose of antibiotics should not be withheld, even when lumbar puncture is delayed or neuroimaging is being performed. Changes in the CSF after antibiotic administration usually take 12 to 24 hours. Continued therapy should be based on the assessment of clinical improvement, cultures, and susceptibility testing results. Once a pathogen is identified, antibiotic therapy should be tailored to the specific pathogen (Tables 84-4 and 84-5). Throughout the course of treatment, efficacy parameters, such as signs and symptoms, microbiologic findings, and CSF examination, should be followed to evaluate the success of meeting the desired outcomes.

Supportive care, particularly early in the course of treatment, is critically important. Administration of fluids, electrolytes, antipyretics, and analgesics is indicated for patients presenting with ABM. Additionally, venous thromboembolism prophylaxis and ICP monitoring are often needed. Patients may require the administration of osmotic diuretics such as mannitol 25% or hypertonic 3% saline to maintain an ICP of <15 mm Hg (<2 kPa) and a cerebral perfusion pressure of ≥60 mm Hg (≥8 kPa). Other supportive care measures may include respiratory and circulatory support, GI care, and maintaining normal body temperature. Although supportive care is important initially, appropriate antibiotic therapy (empirical or definitive) should be started as soon as possible.[23,24]

7 Several factors influence the transfer of antibiotic from capillary blood into the CNS, including inflammation of the meninges, which increases antibiotic penetration through damage to tight junctions between capillary endothelial cells and decreases the activity of an energy-dependent efflux pump in the choroid plexus responsible for movement of penicillins and, to a much lesser extent, fluoroquinolones and aminoglycosides (see Table 84-3). Antibiotics having low molecular weights are passed more easily through biologic barriers than compounds of higher molecular weight. Only antibiotics that are nonionized at physiologic or pathologic pH are capable of diffusion. Highly lipid-soluble compounds penetrate more readily than water-soluble compounds. Antibiotics not extensively bound to plasma proteins provide a larger free fraction of drug capable of passing into the CSF. Passage of large, polar antibiotics into the CSF may be assisted, however, by a carrier transport system. Antibiotic dosages in the treatment of CNS infections must be optimized to ensure adequate penetration to the site of infection.

Problems of CSF penetration were traditionally overcome by direct instillation of antibiotics intrathecally, intracisternally, or intraventricularly. Advantages of direct instillation, however, must be weighed against the risks of invasive CNS procedures. Intrathecal administration of antibiotics is unlikely to produce therapeutic concentrations in the ventricles possibly owing to the unidirectional flow of CSF.[26] Although intraventricular administration from a therapeutic standpoint may be preferred over intrathecal administration, the former requires neurosurgical placement of a subcutaneous reservoir. Intraventricular delivery may be necessary in patients who have shunt infections that are difficult to eradicate or who cannot undergo surgical interventions (A-III).[19] The antimicrobial agents often utilized for ABM treatment have adequate CSF penetration, which has limited the need for direct CNS instillation of antibiotics. The European guidelines for meningitis treatment recommend considering the use of intrathecal or intraventricular antibiotics only in patients who fail conventional treatment.[20]

8 Although the length of treatment for bacterial meningitis generally is based on the causative organism, there is no universally accepted standard (Table 84-4). Meningitis caused by *S. pneumoniae* has been treated successfully with 10 to 14 days of antibiotic therapy. Meningitis caused by *N. meningitidis* or *H. influenzae* usually can be treated with a 7-day course of antibiotics. In contrast, a longer duration (≥21 days) has been recommended for patients with *L. monocytogenes*, gram-negative or pseudomonal meningitis (A-III). Therapy should be individualized, and some patients may require enduring courses.[19,20]

Clinical **Controversy...**

Patients with ABM often remain hospitalized for the duration of IV antibiotic treatment. Outpatient treatment may be appropriate in certain patients following the acute phase of infection, typically the first 7 days. Decreasing length of stay and hospital-acquired complications has driven the efforts to complete treatment courses in the outpatient setting. However, only certain patients who are at low risk of developing neurologic complications should be considered for outpatient treatment, and close followup should be arranged.

Causative Organisms

S. pneumoniae (Pneumococcus or Diplococcus)

1 *S. pneumoniae* is the leading cause of meningitis in patients ≥2 months of age in the United States. Overall case-fatality rate is estimated to be 18%. Despite the decline in rates of pneumococcal meningitis since the introduction of PCV7 vaccination in 2000, case-fatality rate did not significantly change from pre-PCV7 era.[8]

TABLE 84-4 Antimicrobial Agents of First Choice and Alternative Choice in the Treatment of Meningitis Caused by Gram-Positive and Gram-Negative Microorganisms[16,19,20]

Organism	Antibiotics of First Choice	Alternative Antibiotics	Recommended Duration of Therapy
Gram-positive Organisms			
Streptococcus pneumoniae[a]			10–14 days
Penicillin susceptible MIC ≤0.06 mcg/mL (mg/L)	Penicillin G or ampicillin (A-III)	Cefotaxime (A-III), ceftriaxone (A-III), cefepime (B-II), or meropenem (B-II)	
Penicillin resistant MIC >0.06 mcg/mL (mg/L)	Vancomycin[b,c] + cefotaxime or ceftriaxone (A-III)	Moxifloxacin (B-II)	
Ceftriaxone resistant MIC >0.5 mcg/mL (mg/L)	Vancomycin[b,c] + cefotaxime or ceftriaxone (A-III)	Moxifloxacin (B-II)	
Staphylococcus aureus			14–21 days
Methicillin susceptible	Nafcillin or oxacillin (A-III)	Vancomycin (A-III) or meropenem (B-III)	
Methicillin resistant	Vancomycin[b,c] (A-III)	Trimethoprim-sulfamethoxazole or linezolid (B-III)	
Group B *Streptococcus*	Penicillin G or ampicillin (A-III) ± gentamicin[b,c]	Ceftriaxone or cefotaxime (B-III)	14–21 days
S. epidermidis	Vancomycin[b,c] (A-III)	Linezolid (B-III)	14–21 days[d]
L. monocytogenes	Penicillin G or ampicillin ± gentamicin[b,c,e] (A-III)	Trimethoprim–sulfamethoxazole (A-III), meropenem (B-III)	≥21 days
Gram-negative Organisms			
Neisseria meningitidis			7–10 days
Penicillin susceptible	Penicillin G or ampicillin (A-III)	Cefotaxime or ceftriaxone (A-III)	
Penicillin resistant	Cefotaxime or ceftriaxone (A-III)	Meropenem or moxifloxacin (A-III)	
Haemophilus influenzae			7–10 days
β-Lactamase negative	Ampicillin (A-III)	Cefotaxime (A-III), ceftriaxone (A-III), cefepime (A-III), or moxifloxacin (A-III)	
β-Lactamase positive	Cefotaxime or ceftriaxone (A-I)	Cefepime (A-I) or moxifloxacin (A-III)	
Enterobacteriaceae[f]	Cefotaxime or ceftriaxone (A-II)	Cefepime (A-III), moxifloxacin (A-III), meropenem (A-III), or aztreonam (A-III)	21 days
Pseudomonas aeruginosa	Cefepime or ceftazidime (A-II) ± tobramycin[b,c] (A-III)	Ciprofloxacin (A-III), meropenem (A-III), piperacillin plus tobramycin[a,b] (A-III), colistin sulfomethate[g] (B-III), aztreonam (A-III)	21 days

[a]European guidelines recommend considering the addition of rifampin to vancomycin therapy.
[b]Direct CNS administration may be considered if failed conventional treatment.
[c]Monitor serum drug levels.
[d]Based on clinical experience; no clear recommendations.
[e]European guidelines recommend adding gentamicin for the first 7 days of treatment.
[f]Includes *E. coli and Klebsiella* spp.
[g]Should be reserved for multidrug-resistant pseudomonal or *Acinetobacter* infections for which all other therapeutic options have been exhausted.

See Table 84-2 footnotes for rating scale of evidence.

Approximately 50% of cases are secondary infections resulting from primary infections of parameningeal foci, such as the ear or paranasal sinuses. Pneumonia, endocarditis, CSF leak secondary to head trauma, splenectomy, alcoholism, sickle cell disease, and bone marrow transplantation may predispose the patient to the development of pneumococcal meningitis.

Neurologic complications, such as coma, hearing impairment, and seizures, are common with pneumococcal meningitis. The prognosis of pneumococcal meningitis depends on a variety of factors, including chronic comorbidities, low Glasgow Coma Scale Score, focal neurologic deficits on admission, low CSF leukocyte count, pneumonia, bacteremia, and intracranial and systemic complications.[27]

Based on resistance patterns and the fact that sufficient CSF concentrations of penicillin are difficult to achieve with standard IV doses, penicillin should not be used as empirical therapy if *S. pneumoniae* is a suspected pathogen. Furthermore, appropriate Clinical Laboratory Standards Institute (CLSI)–approved testing of all CSF isolates for penicillin resistance is recommended. Ceftriaxone and cefotaxime have served as alternatives to penicillin in the treatment of penicillin-resistant pneumococci. Of note, higher cephalosporin minimum inhibitory concentration (MIC) and higher cephalosporin resistance rates were shown in penicillin-resistant isolates.[28] Therapeutic approaches to cephalosporin-resistant pneumococcus include the addition of vancomycin and rifampin. However, only data from animal and experimental trials supporting the use of rifampin are available.[29,30] **6** Therefore, the combination of vancomycin and ceftriaxone has been suggested as empirical treatment until the results of antimicrobial susceptibility testing are available (A-III). Vancomycin should not be used alone even for highly penicillin- and cephalosporin-resistant strains (A-III).[19,20] Some pneumococcal strains exhibit tolerance to vancomycin and were linked to increased meningitis mortality.[31,32]

Based on concern about the limited therapeutic options for penicillin- and cephalosporin-resistant pneumococcal meningitis, newer agents have been evaluated. Meropenem is approved by the U.S. FDA for the treatment of bacterial meningitis in children aged 3 months and older and has shown similar clinical and microbiologic efficacy to cefotaxime or ceftriaxone. It is currently recommended as an alternative to a third-generation cephalosporin in penicillin-nonsusceptible isolates (B-II). Some caution is warranted with the use of imipenem for CNS infections because of the possibility of drug-induced seizures, especially when not properly dose adjusted for declining renal function. Of note, seizures may be caused by meningitis itself or by imipenem, and the cause is difficult to differentiate. The newer fluoroquinolones represent another therapeutic option owing to favorable activity against multidrug-resistant pneumococci and good penetration into the CSF (B-II).[33]

IV linezolid and daptomycin have emerged as therapeutic options for treating multidrug-resistant gram-positive infections. Linezolid in combination with ceftriaxone has been used to treat a

TABLE 84-5 Dosing of Antimicrobial Agents by Age Group[19–22,89,105]

Agent	Infants and Children	Adults	Monitoring/Comments
Antibacterial			
Ampicillin	75 mg/kg every 6 hours	2 g every 4 hours	
Aztreonam	—	2 g every 6–8 hours	Alternative for penicillin allergy
Cefepime	50 mg/kg every 8 hours	2 g every 8 hours	Consider prolonged infusion
Cefotaxime	75 mg/kg every 6–8 hours	2 g every 4–6 hours	Preferred in neonates
Ceftazidime	50 mg/kg every 8 hours	2 g every 8 hours	
Ceftriaxone	100 mg/kg daily	2 g every 12 hours	Avoid in neonates
Ciprofloxacin	10 mg/kg every 8 hours	400 mg every 8–12 hours	Consider higher doses for *P. aeruginosa*
Colistin	5 mg/kg/day	5 mg/kg/day	Consider intraventricular doses Only for MDR organisms Monitor renal function
Gentamicin	2.5 mg/kg every 8 hours	2 mg/kg every 8 hours *or* 5–7 mg/kg daily	TDM is recommended Monitor renal function
Levofloxacin	—	750 mg daily	May prolong QTc
Linezolid	10 mg/kg every 8 hours	600 mg every 12 hours	May cause thrombocytopenia and peripheral neuropathy
Meropenem	40 mg/kg every 8 hours	2 g every 8 hours	Consider prolonged infusion
Moxifloxacin	—	400 mg daily	May prolong QTc
Oxacillin/nafcillin	50 mg/kg every 6 hours	2 g every 4 hours	Nafcillin preferred if renal dysfunction
Penicillin G	0.05 million units/kg every 4 hours	4 million units every 4 hours	
Polymyxin B	—	1.25–1.5 mg/kg every 12 hours	Only for MDR organisms No data in pediatric patients
Tobramycin	2.5 mg/kg every 8 hours	2.5 mg/kg every 8 hours *or* 5–7 mg/kg daily	TDM is recommended Monitor renal function
Trimethoprim–sulfamethoxazole	5 mg/kg every 6–12 hours	5 mg/kg every 6–12 hours	Dose based on trimethoprim
Vancomycin	15 mg/kg every 6 hours	15–20 mg/kg every 8–12 hours	TDM is recommended Monitor renal function
Antimycobacterials			
Isoniazid	10–15 mg/kg daily	5 mg/kg daily	Supplemental vitamin B_6 is recommended
Rifampin	10–20 mg/kg daily (maximum 600 mg daily)	600 mg daily	Many drug–drug interactions
Pyrazinamide	15–30 mg/kg daily	15–30 mg/kg daily	Rarely causes hepatotoxicity
Ethambutol	15–25 mg/kg daily	15–25 mg/kg daily	May cause neutropenia
Antifungals			
Amphotericin B	1 mg/kg daily	0.7–1 mg/kg daily	Monitor renal function Maintain adequate hydration
Lipid amphotericin B	5 mg/kg once daily	3–4 mg/kg daily	Monitor renal function Maintain adequate hydration
Flucytosine	25 mg/kg every 6 hours	25 mg/kg every 6 hours	Consider TDM to avoid bone marrow suppression
Fluconazole	6–12 mg/kg daily	800–1,200 mg daily	Monitor liver function
Itraconazole	—	200 mg every 12 hours	Consider TDM Suspension form is preferred
Posaconazole	—	400 mg every 12 hours	Variable absorption No data in pediatric patients
Voriconazole	7 mg/kg every 12 hours	6 mg/kg every 12 hours × 2 doses, and then 4 mg/kg every 12 hours	Consider TDM Many drug–drug interactions Monitor liver function
Antivirals			
Acyclovir	10–20 mg/kg every 8 hours	10–20 mg/kg every 8 hours	Monitor renal function Maintain adequate hydration
Ganciclovir	—	5 mg/kg every 12 hours	Monitor renal function
Foscarnet	—	60 mg/kg every 8 hours *or* 90 mg/kg every 12 hours	Monitor renal function Maintain adequate hydration

TDM, therapeutic drug monitoring; MDR, multidrug resistant.

limited number of cases of pneumococcal meningitis with outcomes similar to standard treatment.[34] The penetration of daptomycin in the CSF was approximately 6% following a 15 mg/kg bolus achieving maximum concentration approximately 4 hours after the dose in a rabbit meningitis model. The 15 mg/kg dose produces similar serum concentrations in rabbits as the 6 mg/kg dose in humans. In this study, daptomycin was able to clear both the penicillin-resistant and the quinolone-resistant pneumococci from the CSF more rapidly than the standard regimen of vancomycin and ceftriaxone.[35] Additionally, daptomycin may reduce the inflammatory response caused by cell wall components in pneumococcal meningitis compared with ceftriaxone in animal models.[36]

Pneumococcal vaccines help in reducing the risk of invasive pneumococcal disease. Virtually all serotypes of *S. pneumoniae* exhibiting intermediate or complete resistance to penicillin are found in the 23-valent pneumococcal polysaccharide vaccine (PPV23) (Pneumovax 23®). Due to low vaccination rates among people 65 years of age and older, the U.S. Centers for Disease Control and Prevention (CDC) issued stronger recommendations for the use of the pneumococcal polysaccharide vaccine, calling for vaccination of the following high-risk groups: persons over the age of 65 years; persons aged 2 to 64 years who have a chronic illness, who live in high-risk environments (e.g., Alaskan Natives and residents of long-term care facilities), and who lack a functioning spleen (e.g., sickle cell disease and splenectomy); and immunocompromised persons over the age of 2 years, including those with human immunodeficiency virus (HIV) infection. Additionally, the question of whether or not college students living in dormitories, a possible high-risk environment, should be vaccinated remains debatable. Unfortunately, variability in the host's ability to mount an immune response to the vaccine limits its usefulness for penicillin-resistant pneumococci in children younger than 2 years of age and in immunocompromised adults.

In 2000, a heptavalent pneumococcal protein-conjugate vaccine (PCV7) (Prevnar®) was approved for use in children 2 months of age and older. Use of the vaccine has significantly reduced invasive pneumococcal infections, including sepsis and meningitis, as well as possible cost savings.[9,37] Moreover, the vaccine is safe and effective in low-birth-weight and preterm infants.[38] In the decade following the introduction of PCV7, rate of invasive disease caused by non-PCV7 strains increased considerably, especially serotype 19A.[9] This led to the development of a newer vaccine with expanded coverage. Ultimately, the FDA approved a 13-valent pneumococcal conjugate vaccine (PCV13) (Prevnar 13®) in 2010 for childhood vaccination. Current recommendations are for all healthy infants younger than 2 years of age to be immunized with the PCV13 at 2, 4, 6, and 12 to 15 months. The CDC has issued a recommendation that all persons with cochlear implants receive age-appropriate vaccination with the pneumococcal conjugate vaccine, pneumococcal polysaccharide vaccine, or both.[39] In 2011, the FDA approved the use of PCV13 in adults 50 years and older as PCV13 was shown to produce antibody levels that are either comparable to or higher than the levels achieved by PPV23, for the 13 serotypes included in PCV13. Final recommendations from the CDC regarding the routine use of PCV13 in adults will be forthcoming.

N. meningitidis (Meningococcus)

❶ *N. meningitidis* is a leading cause of bacterial meningitis among children and young adults in the United States and around the world.[8,40] The source of infection usually is an asymptomatic carrier. Five of the 13 serogroups of *N. meningitidis* (A, B, C, Y, and W-135) are primarily responsible. Clusters of meningococcal disease, defined as two or more cases of the same serogroup that are closer in time and space than expected for the population or group under observation, generally are associated with crowding as in schools, dormitories, and military barracks.[41] Although some of these clusters have been due to serogroup B, the majority has been due to serogroup C. Serogroup A, although associated with meningococcal outbreaks in Africa and Asia, is a rare cause of disease in the United States. Serogroup Y, although frequently associated with pneumonia, is emerging as an important cause of invasive meningococcal disease in select areas.[42] Overall, *N. meningitidis* accounted for 13.9% of all meningitis cases in the United States during 2003 to 2007, most cases in persons aged 2 to 18 years. According to recent estimates, the case-fatality rate is approximately 10%.[8]

Initially, patients are colonized and, at some point, develop bacteremia, which most likely occurs prior to hospital admission. Meningitis occurs after the bacteria seed into the meninges. After the acute phase of meningitis has resolved, there is a unique immune reaction that distinguishes meningococcal meningitis from other bacterial causes. ❷ The patient develops a characteristic immunologic reaction of fever, arthritis (usually involving large joints), and pericarditis approximately 10 to 14 days after the onset of disease and despite successful treatment. At this time, examination of the synovial fluid reveals a large number of polymorphonuclear cells, elevated protein concentrations, normal glucose concentrations, and sterile cultures. The reaction may last a week or longer, and no additional antibiotic therapy is required; however, patients may benefit from nonsteroidal antiinflammatory agents and supportive care.[17,43]

Seizures and coma are uncommon with meningococcal meningitis. Patients may behave aggressively and often are maniacal. They may develop deafness and transiently impaired ocular movements. Deafness unilaterally or, more commonly, bilaterally may develop early or late in the disease course. Hearing loss secondary to sensory nerve damage (sensorineural hearing) is usually permanent, whereas conductive hearing impairment, such as damage to the tympanic membrane, is often reversible.[17,43]

The presence of petechiae may be the primary clue that the underlying pathogen is *N. meningitidis*. Approximately 60% of adults and up to 90% of pediatric patients with meningococcal meningitis have purpuric lesions, petechiae, or both.[17] Patients may have an obvious or subclinical picture of disseminated intravascular coagulation (DIC), which may progress to infarction of the adrenal glands and renal cortex and cause widespread thrombosis and rapid death.

❻ Third-generation cephalosporins (i.e., cefotaxime and ceftriaxone) are the recommended empirical treatment for meningococcal meningitis (A-III) (see Table 84-4). When final culture results are available, penicillin G or ampicillin is recommended for penicillin-susceptible isolates. Meropenem and fluoroquinolones are also suitable alternatives for the treatment of penicillin-nonsusceptible meningococci (A-III).[19,20]

N. meningitidis is spread by direct person-to-person close contact, including respiratory droplets and pharyngeal secretions. Close contacts of patients contracting *N. meningitidis* meningitis are at an increased risk of developing meningitis. Close contacts include daycare center contacts, members of the household, or anyone who has been exposed to respiratory or oral secretions through activities such as coughing, sneezing, or kissing. Household contacts of people who have sporadic disease are at increased risk for meningococcal meningitis compared with overall population. Secondary cases of meningitis usually develop within the first week following exposure, but may take up to 60 days after contact with the index case.[44] Young children are at the greatest risk of contracting *N. meningitidis*; however, all ages are at risk, especially close contacts exposed via household, daycare, or military contact.

❾ Prophylaxis of close contacts should be started only after consultation with the local health department. In general, rifampin, ceftriaxone, ciprofloxacin, or azithromycin is given for prophylaxis. A systematic review of available data suggests an increased rate of rifampin-resistant isolates.[45] Also, cases of ciprofloxacin-resistant isolates were reported in North America.[46] For regions with reported ciprofloxacin resistance, one dose of azithromycin 500 mg is recommended for prophylaxis. Further discussion of who should receive prophylaxis is beyond the scope of this chapter; interested readers can refer to the recommendations of the CDC and recommendations of the American Academy of Pediatrics.

Two meningococcal vaccines are available for routine immunization. Both vaccines contain antigens to serogroups A, C, Y, and W-135, but lack activity against serogroup B. Meningococcal polysaccharide vaccine (MPSV4) is preferred for adults 56 years and older who have an indication for immunization, while meningococcal conjugate vaccine quadrivalent (MCV4) is preferred for individuals 55 years and younger. Typically, adolescents receive a primary dose of MCV4 at age 11 or 12, and a booster dose at age 16. Please refer to Chapter 102 for Vaccine chapter in this book for further information on meningococcal vaccination and target high-risk groups.

H. influenzae

❶ Historically, Hib was the most common cause of meningitis in children 6 months to 3 years of age. Since the introduction of effective vaccines, the incidence of Hib disease in the United States has declined dramatically. Widespread vaccination of infants and children has effectively decreased the incidence of bacterial meningitis due to *H. influenzae* in children between the ages of 1 month and 5 years, resulting in a significant decline in all cases of bacterial meningitis.[8] In children older than 3 years and adults, meningitis caused by *H. influenzae* may indicate a parameningeal focus of infection such as middle ear infection, paranasal sinus infection, or CSF leakage. Spread of the organism occurs through direct spread from infected sinuses, draining of these areas via the veins, or bacteremia originating from the local focus of infection.[47]

❻ Because approximately 20% of *H. influenzae* strains are ampicillin-resistant, a third-generation cephalosporin is recommended empirically until susceptibilities are available (A-I). If the organism is susceptible to ampicillin, the patient can be switched to ampicillin and the cephalosporin discontinued (A-III). Third-generation cephalosporins (cefotaxime and ceftriaxone) are active against *β*-lactamase–producing and non–*β*-lactamase–producing strains of *H. influenzae*. In addition, they are relatively free of toxicity and do not require serum concentration monitoring. Cefepime (A-I) and fluoroquinolones (A-III) are suitable alternatives regardless of *β*-lactamase activity.[19,20]

❾ Prophylaxis is to protect close contacts from the index case by eliminating nasopharyngeal and oropharyngeal carriage of *H. influenzae*. Invasive disease should be reported to the local public health department and the CDC. Prophylaxis of close contacts should be started only after consultation with the local health department. Widespread vaccination has limited the need for chemoprophylaxis. Further discussion of who should receive prophylaxis is beyond the scope of this chapter; interested readers can refer to the recommendations of the American Academy of Pediatrics.

Vaccination includes a series of doses and usually is begun in children at 2 months of age. In addition to pediatric immunization, the vaccine also should be considered in patients older than 5 years of age with the following underlying conditions: sickle cell disease, asplenia, and immunocompromising diseases. Refer to Chapter 102 for further information on vaccine dosing and administration.

Group B *Streptococcus* (*Streptococcus agalactiae*)

❶ GBS is a leading cause of neonatal meningitis in the United States and around the world.[8,48] The causative organism, *S. agalactiae*, is a gram-positive bacterium with *β*-hemolytic properties that is often implicated in neonatal sepsis, pneumonia, and meningitis. GI and genitourinary colonization in pregnant women is common. Neonates acquire this infection through vertical transmission while passing through the vaginal canal during birth.

Early onset infections are those occurring within the first week of life, while late-onset infections occur after the first week of the child's birth. Universal prenatal screening and intrapartum antimicrobial prophylaxis of colonized pregnant women have significantly decreased rate of early onset invasive disease.[49] While rates of GBS meningitis in the United States did not change significantly during 1998 to 2007, including cases in patients <2 months of age, most cases during 2002 to 2007 were late-onset infections that are not affected by intrapartum prophylaxis.[8]

❻ Ampicillin and penicillin G are the recommended agents for the treatment of presumed GBS (A-III). Addition of an aminoglycoside should also be considered for confirmed GBS meningitis.[19] GBS continues to be susceptible to ampicillin and penicillin; however, reports of isolates with increased MIC have been published.[49,50]

Investigations are undergoing to develop vaccines to reduce maternal colonization and prevent fetal transmission of GBS. Clinical trials have shown promising results; however, to date there are no licensed vaccines available for GBS.

L. monocytogenes

L. monocytogenes is a gram-positive diphtheroid-like organism. This disease primarily affects neonates, alcoholics, immunocompromised adults, and the elderly, while infections in healthy individuals are extremely rare. *L. monocytogenes* is implicated in approximately 10% of meningitis cases in those older than 65 years of age and carries a case-fatality rate of approximately 18% in the United States.[8]

Transmission usually involves colonization of the patient's GI tract with the organisms, which then penetrate the gut lumen. Coleslaw, unpasteurized milk, Mexican-style soft cheese, ready-to-eat foods, and raw beef and poultry all have been identified as sources of this foodborne pathogen.[13] If a sufficient cell-mediated immune response (T lymphocytes, macrophages) is not produced, bacteremia, meningitis, meningoencephalitis, or cerebritis may develop. Infection of the CNS may be diffuse or localized, possibly involving the cerebral hemispheres, thalamus, and brain stem.

Incidence of *L. monocytogenes* meningitis tends to peak in the summer and early fall. As with gram-negative meningitis, presentation may be subtle and insidious, and clinical suspicion should prompt lumbar puncture. ❷ *L. monocytogenes* produces primarily a mononuclear CSF response.[51] One common laboratory error seen with *L. monocytogenes* is a tendency to misidentify the organism on Gram stain as a diphtheroid, *Streptococcus*, or a poorly staining gram-negative rod.

Treatment of *L. monocytogenes* meningitis with penicillin G or ampicillin may result in only a bacteriostatic effect and possible persistence of infection. Usually the combination of penicillin G or ampicillin with an aminoglycoside results in a bactericidal effect. ❽ Patients should be treated for a minimum of 3 weeks (A-III).[19] European guidelines for meningitis treatment recommend considering combination therapy for the first 7 to 10 days of treatment, with the remaining course of therapy completed with penicillin G or ampicillin alone.[20] Despite in vitro activity against *L. monocytogenes*, vancomycin was associated with high failure rates.[52] Third-generation cephalosporins lack in vitro activity against *L. monocytogenes*. Trimethoprim–sulfamethoxazole and meropenem may be effective alternatives because adequate CSF penetration is achieved (A-III).[19,20]

Gram-Negative Meningitis

During the last several years, the incidence of gram-negative bacillary meningitis, excluding *H. influenzae*, has been increasing in both children and adults. *E. coli* is a leading cause of bacterial meningitis in neonates up to 3 months of age.[53] Several factors predispose patients to the development of gram-negative meningitis: congenital defects involving the CNS, accidental cranial trauma, neurosurgery, the use of antimicrobial agents with exclusive gram-positive activity preoperatively in neurosurgery, any form of communication between the skin and subarachnoid space (such as a dermal sinus), diabetes, malignancy, urinary tract infection in neonates, cirrhosis, parameningeal infection, spinal anesthesia, advanced age, immunosuppression, and hospitalization in general.

Elderly debilitated patients are at an increased risk of gram-negative meningitis but typically lack the classic signs and symptoms of the disease. Nuchal rigidity may be difficult to detect secondary to cervical arthritis. Presence of a low-grade fever and changes in mental status without other obvious cause should prompt consideration of meningitis and a lumbar puncture. Neonates are also at risk for gram-negative meningitis with *E. coli* and *Klebsiella pneumoniae*, which are responsible for 40% to 50% of cases.[53]

Treatment of gram-negative meningitis is complex because of the variety of organisms that can infect the CNS. The treatment of meningitis due to *Pseudomonas aeruginosa* remains a unique problem because antibiotics showing good antibacterial activity, such as antipseudomonal penicillins and aminoglycosides, penetrate the CSF poorly. Furthermore, many isolates of *P. aeruginosa* are resistant to multiple, if not all, commonly used agents, and this trend in resistance is increasing. 6 Initially, cases of *P. aeruginosa* meningitis should be treated with an extended-spectrum *β*-lactam such as ceftazidime or cefepime (A-II), or alternatively aztreonam, ciprofloxacin, or meropenem (A-III). The addition of an aminoglycoside—usually tobramycin—to one of the above agents should also be considered (A-III).[19,20] Since aminoglycosides penetrate the CSF poorly, their inclusion is predominantly to aid in the treatment of extracerebral infections. If multidrug-resistant *Pseudomonas* is suspected initially, intraventricular administration of an aminoglycoside should be considered along with IV administration. Preservative-free forms of gentamicin and tobramycin are available and should be used for direct administration into the CSF. Since CSF flows unidirectionally with gravity, intraventricular aminoglycoside administration is more likely to produce therapeutic concentrations throughout the CSF than intrathecal administration. While intraventricular administration of aminoglycosides is considered for treatment of *P. aeruginosa* meningitis, this method produced higher mortality in a sample of infants treated for gram-negative bacillary meningitis.[54] Thus, intraventricular administration of aminoglycosides to infants is not recommended routinely.

Multidrug-resistant *Pseudomonas* and *Acinetobacter* infections are of concern to clinicians because of the limited therapeutic options available. This concern has led to the reemergence of the use of older antibiotics, such as colistin and polymyxin B. Colistin can be used, both IV and intrathecally, in the treatment of multidrug-resistant *Pseudomonas* or *Acinetobacter* CNS infections.[55] Furthermore, synergistic activity with the combination of colistin and ceftazidime against multidrug-resistant *P. aeruginosa* was demonstrated in an in vitro model.[56] The use of colistin should be reserved for only the most severe cases.

Other gram-negative organisms causing meningitis, excluding *P. aeruginosa* and *Acinetobacter* spp., most likely can be treated with a third- or fourth-generation cephalosporin, such as cefotaxime, ceftriaxone, ceftazidime, or cefepime. Ceftazidime, however, may not be the best choice of empirical antibiotic for situations where the offending organism is not known initially because of its lack of reliable gram-positive coverage. Cefotaxime should be used in place of ceftriaxone in the neonatal period because of the potential for the displacement of bilirubin from albumin-binding sites.

Trimethoprim–sulfamethoxazole is useful in the management of the Enterobacteriaceae family and also may be useful in the management of *L. monocytogenes* (A-III). One advantage of trimethoprim–sulfamethoxazole is that its penetration into the CSF does not depend on meningeal inflammation. Trimethoprim–sulfamethoxazole is not bactericidal, which may be a disadvantage. Fluoroquinolones have good penetration into the CSF and are effective in animal models of both gram-negative and gram-positive meningitis; however, there are limited data on their efficacy in clinical practice. Ciprofloxacin is recommended as an alternative agent for the treatment of *E. coli*, other Enterobacteriaceae, and *P. aeruginosa* (A-III). Cefepime, meropenem, and aztreonam represent other therapeutic options for the treatment of gram-negative bacterial meningitis (A-III).[19,20]

8 CSF cultures may remain positive for several days or more with a regimen that eventually will be curative. Therapeutic efficacy can be monitored through bacterial colony counts every 2 or 3 days, which should decrease progressively over the period of therapy. Therapy for gram-negative meningitis should be continued for a minimum of 21 days from the start of treatment with an effective agent.[19,20]

Bacillus anthracis

B. anthracis is a large, endospore-forming, aerobic, gram-positive bacterium capable of producing infection via the cutaneous, pulmonary, or GI routes. Cases of meningitis have been reported following both cutaneous and inhalational infections. Prior to the bioterrorism-related outbreak of 11 inhalational and 12 suspected or confirmed cases of cutaneous anthrax in 2001, only 18 sporadic cases had occurred in the United States in the 20th century, with the last occurrence in 1976.[57]

The major neurologic complication of anthrax infection is fulminant, rapidly fatal hemorrhagic meningoencephalitis. The inhalational form of anthrax seems to be a potent inducer of neurologic symptoms, and death usually occurs within a week for those with neurologic complications.[57] *B. anthracis* typically is susceptible to penicillin, amoxicillin, erythromycin, doxycycline, and ciprofloxacin. The bioterrorism-related strain was susceptible to the fluoroquinolones, rifampin, tetracycline, vancomycin, imipenem, meropenem, chloramphenicol, clindamycin, and the aminoglycoside, but resistant to third-generation cephalosporins and trimethoprim–sulfamethoxazole. Ciprofloxacin or doxycycline plus one of the aforementioned antibiotics, preferably clindamycin to limit toxin production, is the currently recommended regimen for the treatment of inhalational anthrax, but doxycycline is not recommended for the treatment of anthrax meningitis owing to poor CNS penetration, compared with MIC of most bacterial pathogens, and recent in vitro resistance.[57,58]

Dexamethasone as an Adjunctive Treatment for Bacterial Meningitis In addition to antibiotics, dexamethasone is a commonly used therapy in the treatment of meningitis. Corticosteroids inhibit the production of TNF and IL-1, both potent proinflammatory cytokines. In trials that measured inflammatory mediators, lower levels of TNF, PAF, or IL-1 were detected in patients treated with dexamethasone.[59–61] A series of clinical studies assessing the efficacy of corticosteroid therapy for the initial treatment of bacterial meningitis indicate conflicting results.[59–63] A systematic review in 2004 shows treatment with corticosteroids reduces both mortality and neurologic sequelae in adults with community-acquired bacterial meningitis.[64] However, subsequent large randomized clinical trials show conflicting results. A fundamental problem with corticosteroid investigations to date is that the majority of patients in the trials had *H. influenzae* meningitis, which has decreased dramatically following the introduction of polysaccharide conjugate vaccines. Additionally, the majority of studies examining dexamethasone use for pneumococcal meningitis were conducted before widespread penicillin-resistant pneumococcus emerged or in parts of the world where penicillin resistance is minimal.

A systematic review of 24 randomized controlled trials of corticosteroid use in ABM showed that corticosteroids significantly reduced hearing loss and neurologic sequelae, but did not reduce overall mortality, nor were associated with beneficial effects in low-income countries. Subgroup analyses showed reduced mortality in pneumococcal meningitis and reduced severe hearing loss in *H. influenzae* meningitis.[65] Another meta-analysis of five randomized, double-blinded, placebo-controlled trials of dexamethasone for ABM in patients of all ages showed that adjunctive dexamethasone did not seem to significantly reduce death or neurologic disability.[66] Thus, adjunctive corticosteroid use in the management of ABM remains controversial.

Most clinical trials on the use of adjunctive dexamethasone in bacterial meningitis have involved children. A retrospective analysis of pediatric patients with pneumococcal meningitis and one unblinded, noncontrolled trial suggested that adjunctive steroids may decrease the neurologic sequelae and mortality associated with *S. pneumoniae* meningitis.[60,67] A meta-analysis in 1997 suggested benefits in *H. influenzae* meningitis and, if commenced with or before antibiotics, suggested benefit for pneumococcal meningitis in childhood.[68]

(10) Current recommendations call for the use of adjunctive dexamethasone in infants and children with *H. influenzae* meningitis (A-I). The recommended IV dose is 0.15 mg/kg every 6 hours for 2 to 4 days, initiated 10 to 20 minutes prior to or concomitant with, but not after, the first dose of antimicrobials (A-I). Clinical outcome is unlikely to improve if dexamethasone is given after the first dose of antimicrobial and should therefore be avoided (A-I). For infants and children 6 weeks of age and older with pneumococcal meningitis, adjunctive dexamethasone may be considered after weighing the potential benefits and possible risks (C-II).[19,69] If adjunctive dexamethasone is used, careful monitoring of signs and symptoms of GI bleeding and hyperglycemia should be employed. Moreover, the use of dexamethasone may interfere with the interpretation of clinical response to treatment, such as resolution of fever.

If pneumococcal meningitis is suspected or proven, it is recommended that adults receive dexamethasone 0.15 mg/kg (up to 10 mg) every 6 hours for 2 to 4 days with the first dose administered 10 to 20 minutes prior to first dose of antibiotics (A-I). Similar to the pediatric population, clinical outcome is unlikely to improve if dexamethasone is given after the first dose of antibiotics and should therefore be avoided (A-I).[19,20] It is often difficult to ascertain the responsible pathogen on presentation; therefore, some clinicians recommend initiating dexamethasone in all adult patients presenting with meningitis (B-III). Dexamethasone is not routinely recommended for patients with ABM due to other bacterial etiologies.[19,20]

Routine use of dexamethasone in meningitis is not without controversy. A potential concern is that adjunctive dexamethasone therapy may reduce the penetration of antibiotics into the CSF by inhibiting meningeal inflammation. In early experimental models of meningitis, steroids decreased the CSF concentrations of ampicillin, rifampin, vancomycin, and gentamicin.[61,70] Ceftriaxone and vancomycin penetration into CSF was unaffected by concurrent dexamethasone administration in pediatric patients.[71,72] More recent data show that appropriate concentrations of vancomycin in CSF may be obtained even when adjunctive dexamethasone is used, but the small number of subjects studied limits the generalization of these findings. Also, measured serum and CSF levels, with and without dexamethasone, were based on a 15 mg/kg loading dose followed by a continuous infusion of 60 mg/kg/day according to the European guidelines, which is not the standard of care in the United States.[73]

Bacterial Brain Abscess

Approximately 1,500 to 2,500 cases of brain abscess occur annually in the United States, with decreasing incidence due to contiguous spread of infection from the oropharynx, middle ear, and paranasal sinuses and increasing incidence due to contiguous spread from cranial trauma or neurosurgical procedures.[74,75] Other sources of infection include hematogenous spread from distant foci of infection, such as endocarditis or intraabdominal infection.

(2) The clinical presentation varies depending on the number, size, and location of the abscess(es). Headache, mental status changes, focal neurologic deficits, and fever are the most common symptoms of brain abscess, but seizures and nausea and vomiting may also be seen.[75] Diagnosis of brain abscess can be facilitated by CT or MRI, with preference given to MRI due to the ability to better differentiate cerebral tumor, stroke, and abscess.[76] Lumbar puncture is not routinely recommended in patients with brain abscess, while CT-guided aspiration and biopsy can be both diagnostic and therapeutic.

The etiology of brain abscess depends on the initial site of infection. Those arising from spread of infection from oropharynx, middle ear, and paranasal sinuses are commonly caused by streptococci and oral anaerobes (e.g., *Actinomyces* spp., *Bacteroides* spp., *Fusobacterium* spp., *Peptostreptococcus*). Staphylococci and aerobic, gram-negative bacilli are commonly involved in postoperative abscesses or those following head trauma. *P. aeruginosa* and *Nocardia* spp. can also cause brain abscesses but are more commonly seen in immunocompromised patients.[75,76]

(6) Because brain abscesses are commonly polymicrobial, empirical antimicrobial therapy should include antibiotics with activity against gram-positive, gram-negative, and anaerobic organisms. For example, the regimen could include vancomycin plus a third- or fourth-generation cephalosporin plus metronidazole, depending on risk factors. A carbapenem (such as meropenem) could replace the cephalosporin and metronidazole. De-escalation of therapy should occur once a causative organism is identified. While no consensus on treatment duration for brain abscesses exists, duration of therapy should be determined for each individual patient and should include consideration of the causative pathogen, size of abscess, use of surgical treatment, and response to therapy.[75] Because seizure is a common complication of brain abscesses, anticonvulsant therapy is recommended for at least 1 year and may be discontinued when an EEG shows no epileptic activity.[76] (10) The benefit of dexamethasone in the treatment of brain abscess is unclear and is not routinely recommended.

Cryptococcus neoformans

Cryptococcus spp. are encapsulated soil yeasts acquired by inhalation of spores from the environment leading to CNS infection and less commonly pulmonary disease. The two main pathogenic species are *C. neoformans* and *C. gattii*. While cryptococcal infections mainly affect persons with underlying impaired immunity such as HIV-positive (approximately 85% of cases) and HIV-negative immunosuppressed patients, infections in nonimmunosuppressed individuals have been reported in North America.[77] Globally, approximately 958,000 cases of cryptococcal meningitis occur annually, resulting in 3-month case-fatality rate of over 600,000.[78]

The incubation period in acquired immunodeficiency syndrome (AIDS) patients may be very short, as opposed to a relatively normal host, in whom it may be very long. Symptoms of *C. neoformans* meningitis are insidious and may be present for varying periods, depending on the host involved, before the definitive diagnosis is made. (2) Fever and a history of headaches are the most common symptoms, although altered mentation and evidence of focal neurologic deficits may be present. Examination of the CSF usually reveals mildly elevated WBCs, primarily lymphocytes (see Table 84-1). (3) Diagnosis is based on the presence of a positive CSF, blood, sputum, or urine culture for *C. neoformans*. Organisms may be seen by microscope when stained with India ink and are more likely to be seen in AIDS patients compared with other hosts. An additional rapid test helpful in diagnosis is latex agglutination, which detects the presence of cryptococcal antigens. Latex agglutination is associated with overall sensitivities and specificities of 93% to 100% and 93% to 98%, respectively.[77] A cryptococcal antigen detection test needs to be considered in any patient presenting initially with meningitis. Risk factors predictive of a poor outcome include lethargy at presentation, nonimmunosuppressed patients, high CSF cryptococcal antigen titer, low CSF WBC count, low CD4 cell count, fungemia, and elevated CSF pressure.[77,79–81]

Rapid sterilization of CNS through rapid fungicidal activity is the main approach of induction therapy, which ranges from 2 to 6 weeks, followed by consolidation therapy for 8 weeks. Despite poor penetration into the CSF, amphotericin B has long been the drug of choice for the treatment of acute cryptococcal meningitis due to its rapid fungicidal activity.[79] Amphotericin B 0.7 mg/kg/day combined with flucytosine 100 mg/kg/day for 2 weeks (A-I) is more effective than amphotericin alone (B-II) for HIV-positive patients.[82] Additionally, this combination is associated with the most rapidly fungicidal activity, when compared with amphotericin alone, in combination with fluconazole or in combination with fluconazole and flucytosine.[83]

Unfortunately, in the AIDS population, flucytosine is often poorly tolerated, causing bone marrow suppression and GI distress. Careful monitoring of hematologic parameters, therapeutic drug monitoring (TDM), and dose adjustment for patients with renal insufficiency are recommended to avoid flucytosine-associated toxicities. Amphotericin B alone (B-II) or in combination with high-dose fluconazole (B-I) may be a reasonable alternative to standard treatment.[84,85] Lipid formulations of amphotericin B at higher doses (3 to 5 mg/kg/day) can be used for HIV-positive patients with or predisposed to renal dysfunction (B-II) and are recommended for organ transplant recipients (B-III).[86]

Azole therapy is the most studied alternative regimen for the treatment of *C. neoformans* meningitis in HIV-positive patients. Fluconazole and itraconazole have been studied as monotherapy with mixed results. If used alone or in combination with flucytosine, higher fluconazole doses of 800 to 2,000 mg/day are recommended due to higher success rates (B-II).[87] To note, the rate of fluconazole-resistant *C. neoformans* has been increasing in recent years.[88] Itraconazole has limited utility in induction therapy due to limited CSF levels of active drug (C-II). Generally, itraconazole suspension is preferred due to better absorption, and TDM is recommended to ensure optimal drug levels.[89] Voriconazole in combination with amphotericin B shows similar rate of clearance of cryptococcal CFU in CSF samples compared with standard therapy.[85] Posaconazole has demonstrated clinical activity against cryptococcal and other fungal infections of the CNS in patients with refractory disease or otherwise intolerant to standard antifungal agents. Posaconazole appeared well tolerated at oral doses of 800 mg/day and may be an alternative in the treatment of fungal CNS infection due to *C. neoformans*.[90,91] More data are needed to determine what role the new azole antifungal agents will play in future treatment of cryptococcal meningitis.

HIV-positive persons often require extended maintenance or suppressive therapy, minimum of 12 months, because of high relapse rates following primary therapy (induction and consolidation phases) for *C. neoformans*. A large multicenter, controlled trial compared fluconazole 200 mg/day (A-I) and amphotericin B 1 mg/kg/wk (C-I) in the prevention of relapse. Two percent of patients receiving fluconazole versus 18% of patients on amphotericin B relapsed. In addition, the amphotericin B group had significantly more frequent bacterial infections, bacteremia, and drug-related toxicity.[92] Fluconazole (A-I) is superior to itraconazole (C-I) in the prevention of relapse.[93] Current guidelines recommend continuing maintenance therapy until immune reconstitution takes place. Guidelines for the prevention of opportunistic infections in HIV-infected persons are updated frequently and can be found at *www.aidsinfo.nih.gov*. Readers interested in treatment guidelines for cryptococcal meningitis in HIV-negative immunosuppressed, such as transplant recipients, and nonimmunosuppressed individuals are encouraged to review the Infectious Diseases Society of America guidelines for the management of cryptococcal disease.[89]

Viral Encephalitis

Encephalitis is defined by the presence of an inflammatory process of the brain in association with clinical evidence of neurologic dysfunction.[21] Patients with metabolic disturbances, organ dysfunction, and noninfectious encephalitis, including postimmunization encephalitis or encephalomyelitis, can have similar clinical presentation to those with infectious encephalitis. Several infectious organisms have been identified to cause encephalitis, with viral etiologies being the most commonly diagnosed.[94–96] Additionally, meningoencephalitis is a term commonly used to describe meningeal inflammation along with encephalitis.

The epidemiology of viral encephalitis in the United States has changed dramatically since the mid-1960s because of the introduction of large-scale polio, rubella, varicella, and mumps immunization programs. Worldwide, mumps remains a causative agent of viral encephalitis in countries with low vaccination rates. Poliomyelitis, once a significant cause of encephalitis, is now confined to only a few less developed countries. Common causes of viral encephalitis and meningoencephalitis in the United States include herpes simplex virus (HSV), West Nile virus, and the enteroviruses. Additionally, viral encephalitis cases are caused by a variety of other pathogens, such as arboviruses, adenoviruses, influenzae virus A and B, rotavirus, corona virus, cytomegalovirus (CMV), varicella-zoster, Epstein-Barr virus, and lymphocytic choriomeningitis. To note, a confirmed or probable pathogen is not identified in the majority of encephalitis cases.[94–96]

Viral encephalitis is acquired primarily by hematogenous spread or, alternatively, by neuronal spread of the causative pathogen. After entry into the host, viral replication occurs, resulting in dissemination through the reticuloendothelial system or vasculature. Infection of the capillary endothelial cells and choroid plexus may provide a conduit for CNS infections. Viruses such as polio, herpes, and varicella-zoster also may gain access to the CNS by axonal retrograde transmission from peripheral nerve endings. Once a virus gains access to the CNS, the course of infection depends on the virulence of the particular virus and the host immune response. Subsequent neuronal injury is caused by direct cell damage due to viral replication, but inflammatory and immune-mediated responses also contribute to neurologic damage.[16,97]

In contrast with purulent meningitis, host response to viral encephalitis is mediated primarily through cytotoxic T lymphocytes. Increases in concentrations of IL-1, IL-6, and interferon (INF)-α, -β, and -γ may occur. While cytokine assays are available for investigational use, they are not used routinely in the clinical diagnosis of viral encephalitis.[16,97]

2 The clinical syndrome associated with viral encephalitis generally is independent of viral etiology and may vary depending on the patient's age. Common signs in adults include headache, mild fever, nuchal rigidity, malaise, drowsiness, nausea, vomiting, and photophobia. Only fever and irritability may be evident in the infant, and ABM must be ruled out as a cause of fever when no other localized findings are observed in a child. Duration of symptoms generally is 1 to 2 weeks, and specific manifestations outside the meninges also can occur depending on the viral etiology.

Laboratory examination of the CSF usually reveals a pleocytosis with 100 to 1,000 WBCs/mm^3 (100×10^6 to $1{,}000 \times 10^6$/L), which are primarily lymphocytic; however, 20% to 75% of patients with viral encephalitis may have a predominance of polymorphonuclear cells on initial examination of the CSF. On repeat lumbar puncture, 90% of patients presenting initially with a predominance of neutrophils experience a shift to a predominance of mononuclear cells. Other laboratory findings include normal to mildly elevated protein concentrations and normal or mildly reduced glucose concentrations (see Table 84-1).[16,97]

3 As mentioned before, pathogens responsible for viral encephalitis are often not identified.[94–96] Poor laboratory recovery of viral pathogens and limited treatment options for viral encephalitis made the need for specific identification of pathogens of questionable value. Advances in diagnostic laboratory techniques and the potential for decreased costs associated with longer duration of hospitalization for patients with unconfirmed viral encephalitis have led to a reevaluation of the need for confirmatory pathogen diagnosis. When clinical signs warrant pathogen identification, appropriate laboratory diagnostic techniques, including PCR and serologic testing, should be undertaken (A-III). Molecular methods are preferred to conventional laboratory tests, such as viral cultures and brain biopsy, in the diagnosis of viral encephalitis owing to improved sensitivity and specificity, higher yield, and rapid results.[21,22]

Supportive and symptomatic treatments of patients with viral encephalitis are of great importance due to limited treatment options for most viral etiologies. Such treatments may include seizure control, hemodynamic management, venous thromboembolism prevention, ICP management, and secondary bacterial infection prevention. Corticosteroid therapy is generally not recommended in most viral encephalitis cases; however, treatment should be considered for patients with cerebral edema and increased ICP.[21,22]

Although there are numerous pathogenic causes of viral encephalitis, much of the clinical presentation, diagnosis, and treatment are similar. The most commonly isolated viral etiologies are described here.

Both herpes simplex virus type 1 (HSV1) and herpes simplex virus type 2 (HSV2) are considered the most common treatable causes of viral encephalitis. HSV1 is associated with encephalitis in adults, whereas HSV2 is associated predominantly with encephalitis in newborns.[94–96] An HSV infection of the CNS most likely is spread via retrograde movement from the dorsal root ganglion. Sexually active adults acquire herpes simplex meningitis during or after an attack of genital or rectal herpes, whereas neonates acquire the virus during passage through the vaginal canal of mothers with active herpes infection. HSV PCR testing on CSF specimens should be performed for all patients with presumed encephalitis (A-III). Moreover, repeat testing should be considered for patients with an initial negative test after 3 to 7 days (B-III). Establishing the correct diagnosis as early as possible is paramount because of high mortality rate without treatment (approaches 70%), and unlike other viral etiologies, specific and effective therapy is available. As a result, empirical therapy of suspected HSV encephalitis while laboratory results are pending is necessary. Delaying antiviral therapy has been consistently associated with unfavorable outcomes and increased mortality across several studies. In one retrospective study of 184 patients with HSV encephalitis, administration of IV acyclovir within first day of hospital admission was associated with a lower mortality rate (13% vs. 31%).[24] Additionally, a clinical decision to treat may need to be made regardless of test results.

Acyclovir is the drug of choice for herpes simplex encephalitis. In adult patients with normal renal function, acyclovir is usually administered as 10 mg/kg IV every 8 hours for 2 to 3 weeks (A-I).[21,22] Higher doses of acyclovir (20 mg/kg IV every 8 hours) have been used in neonates and are associated with lower mortality rates (A-I).[98] Herpes virus resistance to acyclovir has been reported with increasing incidence, particularly in immunocompromised patients with prior or chronic exposures to acyclovir, ranging from 3.5% to 10% in immunocompromised patients.[99] The alternative treatment for acyclovir-resistant HSV is foscarnet. The dose for patients with normal renal function is 40 to 60 mg/kg infused over 1 hour every 8 to 12 hours for 3 weeks, with the higher dose typically reserved for HIV-infected individuals.[22] Ensuring adequate hydration is imperative to decrease risk of acyclovir- and foscarnet-induced nephrotoxicity. In addition, patients receiving foscarnet should be monitored for seizures related to alterations in plasma electrolyte levels.

Because of the recent epidemic in the United States, a separate discussion of the West Nile virus is warranted. Although West Nile virus is transmitted primarily by mosquitoes, transmission of the virus via blood products, organ transplantation, transplacental transfer, and breast milk has been documented. Similar to the other arboviruses, the incubation period for West Nile virus ranges from 3 days to 2 weeks. Infection with West Nile virus is asymptomatic in most adults or causes a mild flu-like syndrome characterized by fever, malaise, myalgia, and lymphadenopathy. Typically, less than 1% of patients develop neurologic disease, of which approximately two thirds have encephalitis, with the remainder having meningitis without encephalitis. Many patients develop a maculopapular, erythematous rash, which is more common in children than in adults and is uncommon in other forms of viral encephalitis. The other neurologic manifestations include fever, nausea, vomiting, headache, altered mental status, movement disorders, and/or a syndrome much like poliomyelitis.[100] The primary risk factor for this manifestation seems to be advanced age, but alcohol abuse, diabetes, hypertension, immunosuppression, and cardiovascular disease were also identified as potential risk factors for neuroinvasive disease and worse outcomes.[100,101] The poliomyelitis syndrome is characterized by an early prodromic phase of fevers and weakness followed by the sudden onset of flaccid paralysis. Among patients hospitalized with West Nile virus, the mortality rate is approximately 10% to 15%, whereas patients with encephalitis and weakness have a mortality rate of 30%. CSF examination of West Nile virus encephalitis typically shows pleocytosis and a slightly elevated CSF protein concentration. Several diagnostic methods have been developed for West Nile virus, including a PCR assay and enzyme-linked immunosorbent assay (ELISA) tests. However, serologic tests (ELISA) can cross-react with other flaviviruses causing a false-positive result. Moreover, serum IgM antibodies for West Nile virus can persist for up to 1 year, leading to confusion regarding whether the infection is an acute or previous infection. Ribavirin has shown inhibitory effects on the West Nile virus in neural tissue cultures, but this has not been studied in controlled trials. Finally, DNA vaccines were studied in animals and have shown positive results.[100] Treatment is typically supportive, including treatment for seizures and increased ICP, and in the majority of cases, the disease is self-limiting.[21,22]

CMV has emerged as a major cause of morbidity and mortality in immunocompromised patients, including HIV-infected individuals and transplant recipients on immunosuppressants. CNS infections with CMV are often difficult to treat, with higher failure rates and poor outcomes. Combination therapy with ganciclovir and foscarnet (B-III) is recommended for induction treatment due to the higher failure rates and lack of survival benefits when monotherapy with either agent is utilized. Ganciclovir 5 mg/kg every 12 hours and foscarnet 60 mg/kg every 8 hours (or 90 mg/kg every 12 hours) for 3 weeks are recommended during the induction phase, followed by maintenance phase with either agent (B-III).[21,22] Other interventions that may improve survival outcomes include the initiation of HAART in untreated HIV-infected patients and reduction of immunosuppression intensity in transplant recipients.

HIV encephalitis is a common CNS complication associated with AIDS. Frequently, patients may complain of headache, photophobia, or stiff neck at the time of presumed seroconversion. As the disease progresses neurologic symptoms are frequently reported secondary to other opportunistic infections. Diagnosis of viral encephalitis is difficult because mental status and neurologic examinations are not sensitive enough to detect early changes. Direct evidence of HIV encephalitis can be obtained through CSF culture, p24 antigen testing, or qualitative or quantitative PCR for HIV RNA. Diagnostic workup of other potential copathogens, such as HSV, *Toxoplasma gondii*, *Mycobacterium tuberculosis*, *Aspergillus* spp., and *Cryptococcus*, also should be performed. Refer to Chapter 103 for a complete discussion of infectious complications in HIV-positive individuals.

Other Etiologies

M. tuberculosis

M. tuberculosis is the primary cause of tuberculous meningitis and remains the most life-threatening form of extrapulmonary tuberculosis.[102] The incidence of tuberculosis in general has decreased to 3.3 cases per 100,000 individuals in the United States in 2011,[103] with only 138 cases of tuberculous meningitis reported to the CDC in 2010.[104]

The CDC recommends an initial regimen of four drugs for empirical treatment of *M. tuberculosis*. This regimen consists of isoniazid, rifampin, pyrazinamide, and ethambutol 15 to 20 mg/kg/day (maximum 1.6 g/day) for the first 2 months, generally followed by isoniazid plus rifampin for the remaining duration of therapy.[105] The recommended therapy for HIV-positive individuals is the same as for immunocompetent patients, although rifabutin may be considered in place of other rifamycins in an effort to minimize drug interactions with protease inhibitors and non-nucleoside reverse-transcriptase inhibitors. Therapy in HIV-negative and HIV-positive patients should be individualized based on susceptibility patterns and guidelines from the CDC and the American Thoracic Society, which are updated frequently and available on the Internet (*www.cdc.gov/nchstp/tb/pubs/mmwrhtml/maj_guide.htm*). Patients with *M. tuberculosis* meningitis should be treated for 9 months or longer with multiple-drug therapy, and patients with rifampin-resistant strains should receive 18 to 24 months of therapy.

Tuberculous meningitis has a mortality rate of 10% to 50% despite early diagnosis and treatment. The level of patient consciousness at the start of therapy is the most useful prognostic indicator. Patients who are comatose at the beginning of therapy have a mortality rate of approximately 75%. Other negative prognostic factors include old age, poor nutrition, evidence of miliary disease, high initial CSF protein concentrations, presence of hydrocephalus, and evidence of elevated ICP. Between 10% and 30% of patients surviving the disease have physical or mental sequelae, including deafness, vertigo, and short-term memory loss.[106,107]

Treponema pallidum (Neurosyphilis)

Infection of the CNS by *T. pallidum* can occur at any stage of the disease, although it is most commonly seen in tertiary syphilis many years, even decades, after the initial exposure. The incidence of late latent syphilis, which includes neurosyphilis, according to the CDC has remained approximately 6 cases per 100,000 for the last decade. Patients with neurosyphilis may be asymptomatic, or present with signs and symptoms consistent with acute meningitis. Diagnosis is based on CSF findings, neurologic manifestations, and serologic evidence of exposure.[108] Aqueous penicillin G is recommended for treatment as 3 to 4 million units every 4 hours or 18 to 24 million units as a continuous infusion for a duration of 10 to 14 days. CSF examination should be repeated every 6 months until the cell count and protein has returned to normal.[109] For further reading on the manifestations and treatment of syphilis, we refer you to Chapter 95.

Primary Amoebic Meningoencephalitis (PAM)

PAM is a very rare form of CNS infection caused by *Naegleria fowleri*, a unicellular parasite that lives in warm stagnant fresh or brackish waters, and potentially well water. Humans acquire PAM when water is insufflated through the nostrils usually while swimming.[110,111] The pathogen attaches to the olfactory nerve and migrates through the cribriform plate into the brain. Within a few days *N. fowleri* will begin to multiply in numbers as the pathogen consumes the olfactory bulb. The patient may have problems properly identifying odors (parosmia), progressing to an inability to smell (anosmia), and then will lose taste sensation (ageusia). Trophozoites may be seen in the CSF at this time and are often missed visually but can be confirmed using PCR methods.[112] The disease becomes rapidly progressive as the parasite moves further into the brain and meninges causing fever, headache, neck rigidity, nausea, emesis, and possibly seizures. Unfortunately, even if PAM is recognized prospectively, the clinical prognosis is not good. Most cases of PAM are misdiagnosed or the diagnosis is made at autopsy. PAM is almost always a fatal event, which makes defining optimal management practices speculative at best. Most of the available PAM literature consists of case reports or summaries of case reports. Treatment of PAM usually consists of high-dose amphotericin B therapy. In some cases, azithromycin, rifampicin, and fluconazole have been added as adjuvants with some success.[113] Chlorpromazine has been shown to be highly effective in vitro and in animal models against *N. fowleri*; however, the clinical utility of the drug in humans is unknown.

T. gondii

Toxoplasmic encephalitis (TE) is caused by the protozoan *T. gondii*. Approximately 22.5% of the U.S. population 12 years and older has been infected with *T. gondii*. In other parts of the world, up to 95% of populations are infected. The primary routes of transmission are foodborne, animal-to-human (cats serving as the definitive host), mother-to-child (congenital), blood transfusions, and organ transplantation.[114] TE is typically caused by the reactivation of disease in immunocompromised patients, especially those with AIDS, or intrauterine infection in newborns. Clinical manifestations include extrapyramidal signs and symptoms, headache, seizures, confusion, hemiparesis, cranial nerve abnormalities, or fever.[21] In congenital toxoplasmosis, patients may also present with hydrocephalus, intracerebral calcification, microcephaly, convulsions, or chorioretinitis.[21,115] Definitive diagnosis of TE requires a clinical sample via a brain biopsy; therefore, TE is presumptively diagnosed on the basis of clinical symptoms, positive serology for anti-*Toxoplasma* immunoglobulin G (IgG) antibodies, and identification of space-occupying lesions on CT, MRI, or other radiologic imaging. In patients with AIDS, MRI typically shows multiple ring-enhancing lesions. *T. gondii* can also be detected by PCR in CSF; however, the sensitivity is low (50%) and the result is usually negative once treatment has started.[21,115,116] First-line treatment for TE in adults consists of pyrimethamine plus sulfadiazine plus leucovorin (A-I). Leucovorin is typically added to the treatment regimen to reduce the likelihood of hematologic toxicity associated with pyrimethamine. In patients who are unable to tolerate sulfadiazine, clindamycin may be used as an alternative (A-I). Other alternative treatment options include trimethoprim–sulfamethoxazole (B-I), atovaquone plus pyrimethamine plus leucovorin (B-II), atovaquone plus sulfadiazine (B-II), atovaquone monotherapy (B-II), or pyrimethamine plus leucovorin plus azithromycin (B-II). Treatment recommendations are the same in pediatric patients; however, several of the alternative regimens have not been studied in children.[21,115,116]

Borrelia burgdorferi

LD is caused by the spirochete *B. burgdorferi* and is the most common tick-borne infection in North America and Europe.[117] Lyme neuroborreliosis (LNB) is an infectious disorder of the nervous system caused by *B. burgdorferi* and has been reported in up to 10% to 15% of patients with untreated LD. CNS involvement includes meningitis, myelitis, cerebral vasculitis, and encephalitis. Clinical manifestations include fever, headache, fatigue, photosensitivity, phonosensitivity, confusion, hemiparesis, cranial neuropathy (facial neuropathy being the most common), cerebellar ataxia, ocular flutter, apraxia, *opsoclonus-myoclonus syndrome*, or Parkinson's-like symptoms. Poliomyelitis-like syndromes and acute stroke-like symptoms caused by cerebral vasculitis have been documented in single case reports but are considered rare. Unlike the European LD, the North American LD is also characterized by a skin rash called erythema migrans.[117–119] Currently there is no international consensus for the diagnosis of LNB. Diagnosis is primarily based on the presence of neurologic symptoms without other obvious reasons, CSF analysis (lymphocytic pleocytosis, moderately elevated protein, normal glucose), intrathecal *B. burgdorferi* antibody production, blood and CSF serologic testing (ELISA plus Western blot), and MRI demonstrating areas of inflammation.[21,117,118] PCR testing for detection of *B. burgdorferi* in CSF has a sensitivity of less than 10% to 30% and has an unknown specificity; therefore, it is not routinely recommended. Parenteral treatment with ceftriaxone once daily is recommended as first-line treatment of LNB. Patients with cranial neuropathy without clinical signs of meningitis may be treated with oral amoxicillin, doxycycline, or cefuroxime axetil. The European Federation of Neurological Societies (EFNS) guidelines also recommend oral doxycycline as a first-line option for patients with symptoms confined to the meninges, cranial nerves, nerve roots, or peripheral nerves based on its CSF penetration, ability to achieve CSF concentrations above the MIC, and several Class III studies showing similar short- and long-term efficacy to various parenteral regimens.[118] Alternative parenteral options to ceftriaxone include cefotaxime or penicillin G. For patients intolerant to β-lactams, doxycycline oral or IV is suggested.

EVALUATION OF THERAPEUTIC OUTCOMES

Signs and Symptoms

Because of the potential for rapid deterioration associated with meningitis, signs and symptoms of fever, headache, meningismus (e.g., nuchal rigidity, Brudzinski's or Kernig's sign), vital signs, and signs of cerebral dysfunction should be evaluated every 4 hours for the initial 3 days and then daily thereafter. The Glasgow Coma Scale should be used in severely ill patients. Trends in improvement and resolution rather than single evaluations in time are more important in monitoring the signs and symptoms of meningitis.

Microbiologic Findings

CSF and blood samples for Gram stain, cultures, and sensitivity testing should be taken prior to starting antibiotic therapy. If lumbar puncture is delayed, however, antibiotics should be started. Although the CSF cultures may be negative, antibiotic therapy rarely interferes with the protein and/or glucose concentrations in the CSF. Furthermore, if the laboratory is made aware of the antibiotic therapy, steps can be taken to diminish the effects of the antibiotic during the detection process. Gram stain results can be obtained immediately and can guide empirical antibiotic treatment. Identification of the organism can be made within 24 hours, and sensitivities should be available within 48 hours. Repeat cultures should be performed to help determine if sterilization is achieved. A second tube of blood should be taken to allow for latex agglutination tests of antigens to common meningeal pathogens (*H. influenzae*, *S. pneumoniae*, *N. meningitidis*, *E. coli*, and GBS) if the Gram stain has not been helpful.

CSF Examination

In bacterial meningitis, the CSF WBC count usually is greater than 1,000 cells/mm^3 (1,000 × 10^6/L), the CSF protein concentration is elevated, and the CSF glucose concentration (hypoglycorrhachia) is often low (<45 mg/dL [<2.5 mmol/L] or 50% to 60% of a simultaneous blood glucose value). Viral encephalitis, in contrast, results in relatively normal CSF protein and glucose levels and typically does not result in greater than 90% polymorphonuclear leukocytes (PMNs) in the CSF (see Table 84-1).

ABBREVIATIONS

ABM	acute bacterial meningitis
AIDS	acquired immunodeficiency syndrome
BCSFB	blood–cerebrospinal fluid barrier
CBF	cerebral blood flow
CDC	U.S. Centers for Disease Control and Prevention
CFU	colony-forming unit
CLSI	Clinical and Laboratory Standards Institute
CMV	cytomegalovirus
CSF	cerebrospinal fluid
CT	computed tomography
DIC	disseminated intravascular coagulation
EFNS	European Federation of Neurological Societies
EIA	enzyme immunoassay
ELISA	enzyme-linked immunosorbent assay
GBS	group B *Streptococcus*
Hib	*H. influenzae* type b
HIV	human immunodeficiency virus
HSV	herpes simplex virus
HSV1	herpes simplex virus type 1
HSV2	herpes simplex virus type 2
ICP	intracranial pressure
Ig	immunoglobulin
IgG	immunoglobulin G
IL-1	interleukin 1
INF	interferon
LD	Lyme's disease
LNB	Lyme neuroborreliosis
LPS	lipopolysaccharide
MCV4	meningococcal conjugate vaccine quadrivalent
MIC	minimum inhibitory concentration
MPSV4	meningococcal polysaccharide vaccine
MRI	magnetic resonance imaging
PAF	platelet-activating factor
PAM	primary amoebic meningoencephalitis
PCR	polymerase chain reaction
PCT	procalcitonin
PCV7	heptavalent pneumococcal protein-conjugate vaccine
PCV13	13-valent pneumococcal conjugate vaccine
PMN	polymorphonuclear leukocytes
PPV23	23-valent pneumococcal polysaccharide vaccine
TDM	therapeutic drug monitoring
TE	toxoplasmic encephalitis
TNF	tumor necrosis factor
WBC	white blood cell

REFERENCES

1. Scheld WM, Koedel U, Nathan B, Pfister HW. Pathophysiology of bacterial meningitis: Mechanism(s) of neuronal injury. J Infect Dis 2002;186(Suppl 2): S225–S233.
2. World Health Organization. New and Under-Utilized Vaccines Implementation (NUVI): Bacterial Meningitis. February 2012, *http://www.who.int/nuvi/meningitis/en/index.html*.
3. Edmond K, Clark A, Korczak VS, et al. Global and regional risk of disabling sequelae from bacterial meningitis: A systematic review and meta-analysis. Lancet Infect Dis 2010;10(5):317–328.
4. van de Beek D, de Gans J, Spanjaard L, et al. Clinical features and prognostic factors in adults with bacterial meningitis. N Engl J Med 2004;351(18):1849–1859.
5. Gold R. Epidemiology of bacterial meningitis. Infect Dis Clin North Am 1999;13(3):515–525, v.

6. Reefhuis J, Honein MA, Whitney CG, et al. Risk of bacterial meningitis in children with cochlear implants. N Engl J Med 2003;349(5):435–445.
7. van de Beek D, Drake JM, Tunkel AR. Nosocomial bacterial meningitis. N Engl J Med 2010;362(2):146–154.
8. Thigpen MC, Whitney CG, Messonnier NE, et al. Bacterial meningitis in the United States, 1998-2007. N Engl J Med 2011;364(21):2016–2025.
9. Pilishvili T, Lexau C, Farley MM, et al. Sustained reductions in invasive pneumococcal disease in the era of conjugate vaccine. J Infect Dis 2010;201(1):32–41.
10. Whitney CG, Farley MM, Hadler J, et al. Decline in invasive pneumococcal disease after the introduction of protein–polysaccharide conjugate vaccine. N Engl J Med 2003;348(18):1737–1746.
11. Bleck T, Greenlee J. Anatomic considerations in central nervous system infections. In: Mandell GL, Bennett JE, Dolin R, eds. Principles and Practice of Infectious Diseases, 5th ed. New York: Churchill Livingstone, 2000:950–959.
12. Spector R, Lorenzo AV. Inhibition of penicillin transport from the cerebrospinal fluid after intracisternal inoculation of bacteria. J Clin Invest 1974;54(2):316–325.
13. Mace SE. Acute bacterial meningitis. Emerg Med Clin North Am 2008;26(2):281–317, viii.
14. Kim KS. Emerging molecular targets in the treatment of bacterial meningitis. Expert Opin Ther Targets 2003;7(2): 141–152.
15. Curtis S, Stobart K, Vandermeer B, et al. Clinical features suggestive of meningitis in children: A systematic review of prospective data. Pediatrics 2010;126(5):952–960.
16. Ziai WC, Lewin JJ 3rd. Update in the diagnosis and management of central nervous system infections. Neurol Clin 2008;26(2):427–468, viii.
17. Brouwer MC, Tunkel AR, van de Beek D. Epidemiology, diagnosis, and antimicrobial treatment of acute bacterial meningitis. Clin Microbiol Rev 2010;23(3):467–492.
18. Nigrovic LE, Malley R, Kuppermann N. Meta-analysis of Bacterial Meningitis Score validation studies. Arch Dis Child 2012;97(9):799–805.
19. Tunkel AR, Hartman BJ, Kaplan SL, et al. Practice guidelines for the management of bacterial meningitis. Clin Infect Dis 2004;39(9):1267–1284.
20. Chaudhuri A, Martinez-Martin P, Kennedy PG, et al. EFNS guideline on the management of community-acquired bacterial meningitis: Report of an EFNS Task Force on acute bacterial meningitis in older children and adults. Eur J Neurol 2008;15(7):649–659.
21. Tunkel AR, Glaser CA, Bloch KC, et al. The management of encephalitis: Clinical practice guidelines by the Infectious Diseases Society of America. Clin Infect Dis 2008;47(3):303–327.
22. Steiner I, Budka H, Chaudhuri A, et al. Viral meningoencephalitis: A review of diagnostic methods and guidelines for management. Eur J Neurol 2010;17(8): 999–e57.
23. Auburtin M, Wolff M, Charpentier J, et al. Detrimental role of delayed antibiotic administration and penicillin-nonsusceptible strains in adult intensive care unit patients with pneumococcal meningitis: The PNEUMOREA prospective multicenter study. Crit Care Med 2006;34(11): 2758–2765.
24. Poissy J, Wolff M, Dewilde A, et al. Factors associated with delay to acyclovir administration in 184 patients with herpes simplex virus encephalitis. Clin Microbiol Infect 2009;15(6):560–564.
25. Nau R, Sorgel F, Eiffert H. Penetration of drugs through the blood–cerebrospinal fluid/blood–brain barrier for treatment of central nervous system infections. Clin Microbiol Rev 2010;23(4):858–883.
26. Heath PT, Nik Yusoff NK, Baker CJ. Neonatal meningitis. Arch Dis Child Fetal Neonatal Ed 2003;88(3):F173–F178.
27. Kastenbauer S, Pfister H-W. Pneumococcal meningitis in adults: Spectrum of complications and prognostic factors in a series of 87 cases. Brain 2003;126(5):1015–1025.
28. Fenoll A, Gimenez MJ, Robledo O, et al. Influence of penicillin/amoxicillin non-susceptibility on the activity of third-generation cephalosporins against *Streptococcus pneumoniae*. Eur J Clin Microbiol Infect Dis 2008;27(1):75–80.
29. Ribes S, Taberner F, Domenech A, et al. Evaluation of ceftriaxone, vancomycin and rifampicin alone and combined in an experimental model of meningitis caused by highly cephalosporin-resistant *Streptococcus pneumoniae* ATCC 51916. J Antimicrob Chemother 2005;56(5):979–982.
30. Lee H, Song JH, Kim SW, et al. Evaluation of a triple-drug combination for treatment of experimental multidrug-resistant pneumococcal meningitis. Int J Antimicrob Agents 2004;23(3):307–310.
31. Gillis LM, White HD, Whitehurst A, Sullivan DC. Vancomycin-tolerance among clinical isolates of *Streptococcus pneumoniae* in Mississippi during 1999-2001. Am J Med Sci 2005;330(2):65–68.
32. Rodriguez CA, Atkinson R, Bitar W, et al. Tolerance to vancomycin in pneumococci: Detection with a molecular marker and assessment of clinical impact. J Infect Dis 2004;190(8):1481–1487.
33. Rodriguez-Cerrato V, McCoig CC, Saavedra J, et al. Garenoxacin (BMS-284756) and moxifloxacin in experimental meningitis caused by vancomycin-tolerant pneumococci. Antimicrob Agents Chemother 2003;47(1):211–215.
34. Faella F, Pagliano P, Fusco U, et al. Combined treatment with ceftriaxone and linezolid of pneumococcal meningitis: A case series including penicillin-resistant strains. Clin Microbiol Infect 2006;12(4):391–394.
35. Cottagnoud P, Pfister M, Acosta F, et al. Daptomycin is highly efficacious against penicillin-resistant and penicillin- and quinolone-resistant pneumococci in experimental meningitis. Antimicrob Agents Chemother 2004;48(10):3928–3933.
36. Grandgirard D, Oberson K, Buhlmann A, et al. Attenuation of cerebrospinal fluid inflammation by the nonbacteriolytic antibiotic daptomycin versus that by ceftriaxone in experimental pneumococcal meningitis. Antimicrob Agents Chemother 2010;54(3):1323–1326.
37. Isaacman DJ, Fletcher MA, Fritzell B, et al. Indirect effects associated with widespread vaccination of infants with heptavalent pneumococcal conjugate vaccine (PCV7; Prevnar). Vaccine 2007;25(13):2420–2427.
38. Shinefield H, Black S, Ray P, et al. Efficacy, immunogenicity and safety of heptavalent pneumococcal conjugate vaccine in low birth weight and preterm infants. Pediatr Infect Dis J 2002;21(3):182–186.
39. Centers for Disease Control and Prevention. Prevention of pneumococcal disease among infants and children: Recommendations of the Advisory Committee on Immunization Practices (ACIP). MMWR 2010;59(RR-11):1–19.
40. Harrison LH, Trotter CL, Ramsay ME. Global epidemiology of meningococcal disease. Vaccine 2009;27(Suppl 2):B51–B63.
41. Harrison LH. Epidemiological profile of meningococcal disease in the United States. Clin Infect Dis 2010;50(Suppl 2):S37–S44.

42. Harrison LH, Jolley KA, Shutt KA, et al. Antigenic shift and increased incidence of meningococcal disease. J Infect Dis 2006;193(9):1266–1274.
43. Weinstein L. Bacterial meningitis. Specific etiologic diagnosis on the basis of distinctive epidemiologic, pathogenetic, and clinical features. Med Clin North Am 1985;69(2):219–229.
44. Centers for Disease Control and Prevention. Prevention and control of meningococcal disease recommendations of the Advisory Committee on Immunization Practices (ACIP). MMWR 2005;54(RR-7):1–21.
45. Zalmanovici Trestioreanu A, Fraser A, Gafter-Gvili A, Paul M, Leibovici L. Antibiotics for preventing meningococcal infections. Cochrane Database Syst Rev 2011;(8):CD004785.
46. Wu HM, Harcourt BH, Hatcher CP, et al. Emergence of ciprofloxacin-resistant *Neisseria meningitidis* in North America. N Engl J Med 2009;360(9):886–892.
47. Tang LM, Chen ST, Wu YR. *Haemophilus influenzae* meningitis in adults. Diagn Microbiol Infect Dis 1998; 32(1):27–32.
48. Thaver D, Zaidi AK. Burden of neonatal infections in developing countries: A review of evidence from community-based studies. Pediatr Infect Dis J 2009;28(Suppl 1):S3–S9.
49. Verani JR, McGee L, Schrag SJ. Prevention of perinatal group B streptococcal disease—Revised guidelines from CDC, 2010. MMWR Recomm Rep 2010;59(RR-10):1–36.
50. Phares CR, Lynfield R, Farley MM, et al. Epidemiology of invasive group B streptococcal disease in the United States, 1999-2005. JAMA 2008;299(17):2056–2065.
51. Brouwer MC, van de Beek D, Heckenberg SG, et al. Community-acquired *Listeria monocytogenes* meningitis in adults. Clin Infect Dis 2006;43(10):1233–1238.
52. Richards SJ, Lambert CM, Scott AC. Recurrent *Listeria monocytogenes* meningitis treated with intraventricular vancomycin. J Antimicrob Chemother 1992;29(3): 351–353.
53. Zaidi AK, Thaver D, Ali SA, Khan TA. Pathogens associated with sepsis in newborns and young infants in developing countries. Pediatr Infect Dis J 2009;28(Suppl 1): S10–S18.
54. McCracken GH Jr, Mize SG, Threlkeld N. Intraventricular gentamicin therapy in gram-negative bacillary meningitis of infancy. Report of the Second Neonatal Meningitis Cooperative Study Group. Lancet 1980;1(8172): 787–791.
55. Kim BN, Peleg AY, Lodise TP, et al. Management of meningitis due to antibiotic-resistant *Acinetobacter* species. Lancet Infect Dis 2009;9(4):245–255.
56. Gunderson BW, Ibrahim KH, Hovde LB, et al. Synergistic activity of colistin and ceftazidime against multiantibiotic-resistant *Pseudomonas aeruginosa* in an in vitro pharmacodynamic model. Antimicrob Agents Chemother 2003;47(3):905–909.
57. Meyer MA. Neurologic complications of anthrax: A review of the literature. Arch Neurol 2003;60(4):483–488.
58. Inglesby TV, O'Toole T, Henderson DA, et al. Anthrax as a biological weapon, 2002: Updated recommendations for management. JAMA 2002;287(17):2236–2252.
59. Lebel MH, Freij BJ, Syrogiannopoulos GA, et al. Dexamethasone therapy for bacterial meningitis. Results of two double-blind, placebo-controlled trials. N Engl J Med 1988;319(15):964–971.
60. Girgis NI, Farid Z, Mikhail IA, et al. Dexamethasone treatment for bacterial meningitis in children and adults. Pediatr Infect Dis J 1989;8(12):848–851.
61. Schaad UB, Lips U, Gnehm HE, et al. Dexamethasone therapy for bacterial meningitis in children. Swiss Meningitis Study Group. Lancet 1993;342(8869):457–461.
62. Odio CM, Faingezicht I, Paris M, et al. The beneficial effects of early dexamethasone administration in infants and children with bacterial meningitis. N Engl J Med 1991;324(22):1525–1531.
63. Lebel MH, Hoyt MJ, Waagner DC, et al. Magnetic resonance imaging and dexamethasone therapy for bacterial meningitis. Am J Dis Child 1989;143(3):301–306.
64. van de Beek D, de Gans J, McIntyre P, Prasad K. Steroids in adults with acute bacterial meningitis: A systematic review. Lancet Infect Dis 2004;4(3):139–143.
65. Brouwer MC, McIntyre P, de Gans J, et al. Corticosteroids for acute bacterial meningitis. Cochrane Database Syst Rev 2010;(9):CD004405.
66. van de Beek D, Farrar JJ, de Gans J, et al. Adjunctive dexamethasone in bacterial meningitis: A meta-analysis of individual patient data. Lancet Neurol 2010;9(3):254–263.
67. Kennedy WA, Hoyt MJ, McCracken GH Jr. The role of corticosteroid therapy in children with pneumococcal meningitis. Am J Dis Child 1991;145(12):1374–1378.
68. McIntyre PB, Berkey CS, King SM, et al. Dexamethasone as adjunctive therapy in bacterial meningitis. A meta-analysis of randomized clinical trials since 1988. JAMA 1997;278(11):925–931.
69. American Academy of Pediatrics. Pickering LK, ed. Red Book®: 2012 Report of the Committee on Infectious Diseases. 29th ed. Elk Grove Village, IL: American Academy of Pediatrics, 2012.
70. Paris MM, Hickey SM, Uscher MI, et al. Effect of dexamethasone on therapy of experimental penicillin- and cephalosporin-resistant pneumococcal meningitis. Antimicrob Agents Chemother 1994;38(6):1320–1324.
71. Gaillard JL, Abadie V, Cheron G, et al. Concentrations of ceftriaxone in cerebrospinal fluid of children with meningitis receiving dexamethasone therapy. Antimicrob Agents Chemother 1994;38(5):1209–1210.
72. Klugman KP, Friedland IR, Bradley JS. Bactericidal activity against cephalosporin-resistant *Streptococcus pneumoniae* in cerebrospinal fluid of children with acute bacterial meningitis. Antimicrob Agents Chemother 1995;39(9):1988–1992.
73. Ricard JD, Wolff M, Lacherade JC, et al. Levels of vancomycin in cerebrospinal fluid of adult patients receiving adjunctive corticosteroids to treat pneumococcal meningitis: A prospective multicenter observational study. Clin Infect Dis 2007;44(2):250–255.
74. Carpenter J, Stapleton S, Holliman R. Retrospective analysis of 49 cases of brain abscess and review of the literature. Eur J Clin Microbiol Infect Dis 2007;26(1):1–11.
75. Honda H, Warren DK. Central nervous system infections: Meningitis and brain abscess. Infect Dis Clin North Am 2009;23(3):609–623.
76. Muzumdar D, Jhawar S, Goel A. Brain abscess: An overview. Int J Surg 2011;9(2):136–144.
77. Chayakulkeeree M, Perfect JR. Cryptococcosis. Infect Dis Clin North Am 2006;20(3):507–544, v–vi.
78. Park BJ, Wannemuehler KA, Marston BJ, et al. Estimation of the current global burden of cryptococcal meningitis among persons living with HIV/AIDS. AIDS 2009;23(4):525–530.
79. Bicanic T, Meintjes G, Wood R, et al. Fungal burden, early fungicidal activity, and outcome in cryptococcal meningitis in antiretroviral-naive or antiretroviral-experienced patients treated with amphotericin B or fluconazole. Clin Infect Dis 2007;45(1):76–80.

80. Vidal JE, Gerhardt J, Peixoto de Miranda EJ, et al. Role of quantitative CSF microscopy to predict culture status and outcome in HIV-associated cryptococcal meningitis in a Brazilian cohort. Diagn Microbiol Infect Dis 2012;73(1):68–73.
81. Nguyen MH, Husain S, Clancy CJ, et al. Outcomes of central nervous system cryptococcosis vary with host immune function: Results from a multi-center, prospective study. J Infect 2010;61(5):419–426.
82. van der Horst CM, Saag MS, Cloud GA, et al. Treatment of cryptococcal meningitis associated with the acquired immunodeficiency syndrome. National Institute of Allergy and Infectious Diseases Mycoses Study Group and AIDS Clinical Trials Group. N Engl J Med 1997;337(1):15–21.
83. Brouwer AE, Rajanuwong A, Chierakul W, et al. Combination antifungal therapies for HIV-associated cryptococcal meningitis: A randomised trial. Lancet 2004;363(9423):1764–1767.
84. Pappas PG, Chetchotisakd P, Larsen RA, et al. A phase II randomized trial of amphotericin B alone or combined with fluconazole in the treatment of HIV-associated cryptococcal meningitis. Clin Infect Dis 2009;48(12):1775–1783.
85. Loyse A, Wilson D, Meintjes G, et al. Comparison of the early fungicidal activity of high-dose fluconazole, voriconazole, and flucytosine as second-line drugs given in combination with amphotericin B for the treatment of HIV-associated cryptococcal meningitis. Clin Infect Dis 2012;54(1):121–128.
86. Hamill RJ, Sobel JD, El-Sadr W, et al. Comparison of 2 doses of liposomal amphotericin B and conventional amphotericin B deoxycholate for treatment of AIDS-associated acute cryptococcal meningitis: A randomized, double-blind clinical trial of efficacy and safety. Clin Infect Dis 2010;51(2):225–232.
87. Milefchik E, Leal MA, Haubrich R, et al. Fluconazole alone or combined with flucytosine for the treatment of AIDS-associated cryptococcal meningitis. Med Mycol 2008;46(4):393–395.
88. Pfaller MA, Diekema DJ, Gibbs DL, et al. Results from the ARTEMIS DISK Global Antifungal Surveillance Study, 1997 to 2007: 10.5-year analysis of susceptibilities of noncandidal yeast species to fluconazole and voriconazole determined by CLSI standardized disk diffusion testing. J Clin Microbiol 2009;47(1):117–123.
89. Perfect JR, Dismukes WE, Dromer F, et al. Clinical practice guidelines for the management of cryptococcal disease: 2010 update by the Infectious Diseases Society of America. Clin Infect Dis 2010;50(3):291–322.
90. Flores VG, Tovar RM, Zaldivar PG, Martinez EA. Meningitis due to Cryptococcus neoformans: treatment with posaconazole. Curr HIV Res 2012;10(7):620–623.
91. Pitisuttithum P, Negroni R, Graybill JR, et al. Activity of posaconazole in the treatment of central nervous system fungal infections. J Antimicrob Chemother 2005;56(4):745–755.
92. Powderly WG. Therapy for cryptococcal meningitis in patients with AIDS. Clin Infect Dis 1992;14(Suppl 1):S54–S59.
93. Saag MS, Cloud GA, Graybill JR, et al. A comparison of itraconazole versus fluconazole as maintenance therapy for AIDS-associated cryptococcal meningitis. National Institute of Allergy and Infectious Diseases Mycoses Study Group. Clin Infect Dis 1999;28(2):291–296.
94. Glaser CA, Gilliam S, Schnurr D, et al. In search of encephalitis etiologies: Diagnostic challenges in the California Encephalitis Project, 1998-2000. Clin Infect Dis 2003;36(6):731–742.
95. Glaser CA, Honarmand S, Anderson LJ, et al. Beyond viruses: Clinical profiles and etiologies associated with encephalitis. Clin Infect Dis 2006;43(12):1565–1577.
96. Granerod J, Ambrose HE, Davies NW, et al. Causes of encephalitis and differences in their clinical presentations in England: A multicentre, population-based prospective study. Lancet Infect Dis 2010;10(12):835–844.
97. Wright EJ, Brew BJ, Wesselingh SL. Pathogenesis and diagnosis of viral infections of the nervous system. Neurol Clin 2008;26(3):617–633, vii.
98. Whitley R. Neonatal herpes simplex virus infection. Curr Opin Infect Dis 2004;17(3):243–246.
99. Piret J, Boivin G. Resistance of herpes simplex viruses to nucleoside analogues: Mechanisms, prevalence, and management. Antimicrob Agents Chemother 2011;55(2):459–472.
100. Murray KO, Walker C, Gould E. The virology, epidemiology, and clinical impact of West Nile virus: A decade of advancements in research since its introduction into the Western Hemisphere. Epidemiol Infect 2011;139(6): 807–817.
101. Murray KO, Koers E, Baraniuk S, et al. Risk factors for encephalitis from West Nile Virus: A matched case–control study using hospitalized controls. Zoonoses Public Health 2009;56(6–7):370–375.
102. Tung YR, Lai MC, Lui CC, et al. Tuberculous meningitis in infancy. Pediatr Neurol 2002;27(4):262–266.
103. Centers for Disease Control and Prevention. Trends in tuberculosis—United States, 2011. MMWR Morb Mortal Wkly Rep 2012;61(11):181–185.
104. Friedan T. Centers for Disease Control and Prevention. Reported Tuberculosis in the United States, 2010. Atlanta, GA: U.S. Department of Health and Human Services, CDC, October 2011, *http://www.cdc.gov/features/dstb2010data/*.
105. American Thoracic Society, CDC, Infectious Diseases Society of America. Treatment of tuberculosis. MMWR Recomm Rep 2003;52(RR-11):1–77.
106. Leonard JM, Des Prez RM. Tuberculous meningitis. Infect Dis Clin North Am 1990;4(4):769–787.
107. Holdiness MR. Management of tuberculosis meningitis. Drugs 1990;39(2):224–233.
108. Mitsonis CH, Kararizou E, Dimopoulos N, et al. Incidence and clinical presentation of neurosyphilis: A retrospective study of 81 cases. Int J Neurosci 2008;118(9):1251–1257.
109. Workowski KA, Berman S. Sexually transmitted diseases treatment guidelines, 2010. MMWR Recomm Rep 2010;59(RR-12):1–110.
110. Blair B, Sarkar P, Bright KR, et al. *Naegleria fowleri* in well water. Emerg Infect Dis 2008;14(9):1499–1501.
111. Kaushal V, Chhina DK, Ram S, et al. Primary amoebic meningoencephalitis due to *Naegleria fowleri*. J Assoc Physicians India 2008;56:459–462.
112. Schild M, Gianinazzi C, Gottstein B, Muller N. PCR-based diagnosis of *Naegleria* sp. infection in formalin-fixed and paraffin-embedded brain sections. J Clin Microbiol 2007;45(2):564–567.
113. Soltow SM, Brenner GM. Synergistic activities of azithromycin and amphotericin B against *Naegleria fowleri* in vitro and in a mouse model of primary amebic meningoencephalitis. Antimicrob Agents Chemother 2007;51(1):23–27.
114. Centers for Disease Control and Prevention. Parasites—Toxoplasmosis (*Toxoplasma* Infection). Atlanta, GA: U.S. Department of Health and Human Services, CDC, November 2010, *http://www.cdc.gov/parasites/toxoplasmosis/index.html*.

115. Mofenson LM, Brady MT, Danner SP, et al. Guidelines for the prevention and treatment of opportunistic infections among HIV-exposed and HIV-infected children: Recommendations from CDC, the National Institutes of Health, the HIV Medicine Association of the Infectious Diseases Society of America, the Pediatric Infectious Diseases Society, and the American Academy of Pediatrics. MMWR Recomm Rep 2009;58(RR-11):1–166.
116. Kaplan JE, Benson C, Holmes KH, et al. Guidelines for prevention and treatment of opportunistic infections in HIV-infected adults and adolescents: Recommendations from CDC, the National Institutes of Health, and the HIV Medicine Association of the Infectious Diseases Society of America. MMWR Recomm Rep 2009;58(RR-4):1–207 [quiz CE201–CE204].
117. Halperin JJ. Nervous system Lyme disease: Diagnosis and treatment. Rev Neurol Dis 2009;6(1):4–12.
118. Mygland A, Ljostad U, Fingerle V, et al. EFNS guidelines on the diagnosis and management of European Lyme neuroborreliosis. Eur J Neurol 2010;17(1):8–16, e11–e14.
119. Wormser GP, Dattwyler RJ, Shapiro ED, et al. The clinical assessment, treatment, and prevention of Lyme disease, human granulocytic anaplasmosis, and babesiosis: Clinical practice guidelines by the Infectious Diseases Society of America. Clin Infect Dis 2006;43(9):1089–1134.

85 Lower Respiratory Tract Infections

Martha G. Blackford, Mark L. Glover, and Michael D. Reed

KEY CONCEPTS

1. Respiratory infections remain the major cause of morbidity from acute illness in the United States and likely represent the most common reasons why patients seek medical attention.
2. The majority of pulmonary infections follow colonization of the upper respiratory tract with potential pathogens, whereas microbes less commonly gain access to the lungs via the blood from an extrapulmonary source or by inhalation of infected aerosol particles. The competency of a patient's immune status is an important factor influencing the susceptibility to infection, etiologic cause, and disease severity.
3. An appropriate treatment regimen for the patient with uncomplicated lower respiratory tract infection can be established by evaluating the patient history, physical examination, chest radiograph, and properly collected sputum for culture and interpreted in light of current knowledge of the most common lung pathogens and their antibiotic susceptibility patterns within the community.
4. Acute bronchitis is caused most commonly by respiratory viruses and almost always is self-limiting. Therapy targets associated symptoms, such as lethargy, malaise, or fever (ibuprofen or acetaminophen), and fluids for rehydration. Routine use of antibiotics should be avoided and medication to suppress cough is rarely indicated.
5. Chronic bronchitis is caused by several interacting factors, including inhalation of noxious agents (most prominent are cigarette smoke and exposure to occupational dusts, fumes, and environmental pollution) and host factors including genetic factors and bacterial (and possibly viral) infections. The hallmark of this disease is a chronic cough, excessive sputum production, and expectoration with persistent presence of microorganisms in the patient's sputum.
6. Treatment of acute exacerbations of chronic bronchitis includes attempts to mobilize and enhance sputum expectoration (chest physiotherapy, humidification of inspired air), oxygen if needed, aerosolized bronchodilators (albuterol) in select patients with demonstrated benefit, and antibiotics.
7. Respiratory syncytial virus is the most common cause of acute bronchiolitis, an infection that mostly affects infants during their first year of life. In the well infant, bronchiolitis usually is a self-limiting viral illness.
8. The most prominent pathogen causing community-acquired pneumonia in otherwise healthy adults is *S. pneumoniae*, whereas the most common pathogens causing hospital-acquired and healthcare-associated pneumonia are *Staphylococcus aureus* and gram-negative aerobic bacilli. Anaerobic bacteria are the most common etiologic agents in pneumonia that follows aspiration of gastric or oropharyngeal contents.
9. Treatment of community-acquired pneumonia may consist of humidified oxygen for hypoxemia, bronchodilators (albuterol) when bronchospasm is present, rehydration fluids, and chest physiotherapy for marked accumulation of retained respiratory secretions. Antibiotic regimens should be selected based on presumed causative pathogens and pulmonary distribution characteristics and should be adjusted to provide optimal activity against pathogens identified by culture (sputum or blood).
10. Treatment of nosocomial pneumonia requires aggressive therapy with careful consideration of the dominance and susceptibility patterns of the pathogens present within the institution.

❶ Respiratory tract infections remain the major cause of morbidity from acute illness in the United States and most likely represent the single most common reason patients seek medical attention. This chapter focuses on bacterial and viral infections involving the lower respiratory tract, which includes the tracheobronchial tree and lung parenchyma.

❷ The respiratory tract has an elaborate system of host defenses, including humoral immunity, cellular immunity, and anatomic mechanisms.[1] When functioning properly, the host defenses of the respiratory tract are markedly effective in protecting against pathogen invasion and removing potentially infectious agents from the lungs. For the most part, infections in the lower respiratory tract occur only when these defense mechanisms are impaired, as in cases of dysgammaglobulinemia or compromised ciliary function, such as that caused by the chronic inflammation accompanying cigarette smoking. In addition, local defenses may be overwhelmed when a particularly virulent microorganism or excessive inoculum invades lung parenchyma. The majority of pulmonary infections follow colonization of the upper respiratory tract with potential pathogens, which, after achieving sufficiently high concentrations, gain access to the lung via aspiration of oropharyngeal secretions. Less commonly, microbes enter the lung via the blood from an extrapulmonary source or by inhalation of infected aerosolized particles. The specific type of pulmonary infection caused by an invading microorganism is determined by a variety of host factors, including age, anatomic features of the airway, and specific characteristics of the infecting agent.

The most common infections involving the lower respiratory tract are bronchitis, bronchiolitis, and pneumonia. Lower respiratory tract infections in children and adults most commonly result from either viral or bacterial invasion of lung parenchyma. The diagnosis of viral infections rests primarily on the recognition of a characteristic constellation of clinical signs and symptoms. Because treatment is largely supportive, only occasionally does the diagnosis require laboratory confirmation; this is achieved through serologic tests or identification of the organism by culture or antigen detection in respiratory secretions.[2] Laboratory techniques using polymerase chain reaction (PCR), real-time PCR, microarrays, and multiplex ligation-dependent probe amplification, to name a few, have emerged as a means to identify specific pathogens rapidly and accurately.[3]

In contrast, because bacterial pneumonia usually necessitates expedient, effective, and specific antibiotic therapy, its management depends, in large part, on an understanding of the risk factors for acquiring pneumonia, predominant pathogens within the community, and, if necessary, isolation of the etiologic agent by culture from lung tissue or secretions.[4–7] The pharynx is colonized with many organisms that can cause pneumonia; therefore, culture of expectorated sputum can be misleading unless the specimen is examined to ensure that it has originated from the lower respiratory tract. The Gram stain provides the easiest method for distinguishing lower from upper respiratory tract secretions; moreover, through determination of the shape and color of the bacteria, the Gram stain frequently narrows the microbiologic differential diagnosis sufficiently to allow accurate initial therapy. Scanned under low-power microscopy, Gram-stained expectorated upper respiratory tract secretions contain many irregularly shaped epithelial cells with little evidence of inflammation and may not reflect the pathogen. In contrast, a lower-tract specimen from a patient with bacterial pneumonia usually contains multiple neutrophils per high-powered field and a single or predominant bacterial species. Culture of specimens confirmed to originate from the lower tract by Gram stain provides valuable diagnostic information for the majority of patients with bacterial pneumonia. In addition, pneumonia promotes the release of inflammatory mediators and acute-phase proteins such as C-reactive protein, which is significantly elevated in serum in the presence of respiratory tract infections.[8]

(3) An appropriate treatment regimen for the patient with an uncomplicated lower respiratory tract infection usually can be established by history, physical examination, chest radiograph, and properly collected sputum cultures interpreted in light of the most common lung pathogens and their antibiotic susceptibility patterns within the community.[2,4,6,9] More sophisticated or invasive diagnostic methods (e.g., computed tomography, bronchoscopy, and lung biopsy)[2] are reserved for severely ill patients who are unable to expectorate sputum or who are not responding to empirical therapy or for pulmonary infections occurring in immunocompromised patients.

BRONCHITIS

Bronchitis and bronchiolitis are inflammatory conditions of the large and small elements, respectively, of the tracheobronchial tree. The inflammatory process does not extend to the alveoli. Bronchitis frequently is classified as acute or chronic. Acute bronchitis occurs in individuals of all ages, whereas chronic bronchitis primarily affects adults. Bronchiolitis is a disease of infancy.

Acute Bronchitis

Epidemiology and Etiology

Acute bronchitis occurs most commonly during the winter months, following a pattern similar to those of other acute respiratory tract infections. Cold, damp climates and the presence of high concentrations of irritating substances (e.g., air pollution, cigarette smoke) may precipitate attacks.

(4) Respiratory viruses are by far the most common infectious agents associated with acute bronchitis.[10] The common cold viruses (rhinovirus and coronavirus) and lower respiratory tract pathogens (influenza virus and adenovirus) account for the majority of cases. Wider use of reverse transcriptase PCR diagnostic evaluations has identified respiratory viral pathogens not previously described as etiologic agents in acute bronchitis and bronchiolitis including the human metapneumovirus and bocavirus.[11] In children, similar pathogens are observed, with the addition of the parainfluenza viruses. Although the true incidence remains to be defined, *Mycoplasma pneumoniae* appears to be a frequent cause of acute bronchitis. Additionally, *Chlamydophila pneumoniae* (also referred to as *Chlamydophila*)[12] and *B. pertussis*[13] (agent responsible for whooping cough) have been associated with acute respiratory tract infections. Although a variety of bacteria, including *S. pneumoniae*, *Streptococcus* species, *Staphylococcus* species, and *Haemophilus* species, may be isolated from throat or sputum culture, these organisms probably represent contamination by normal flora of the upper respiratory tract rather than true pathogens. Although a primary bacterial etiology for acute bronchitis appears rare, secondary bacterial infection may be involved.

Pathogenesis

(4) Because acute bronchitis is primarily a self-limiting illness and rarely a cause of death, few data describing the pathology are available. In general, infection of the trachea and bronchi yields hyperemic and edematous mucous membranes with an increase in bronchial secretions. Destruction of respiratory epithelium can range from mild to extensive and may affect bronchial mucociliary function. In addition, the increase in desquamated epithelial cells and bronchial secretions, which can become thick and tenacious, further impairs mucociliary activity. The probability of permanent damage to the airways as a result of acute bronchitis remains unclear but appears unlikely. However, epidemiologic evaluations support the belief that recurrent acute respiratory infections may be associated with increased airway hyperreactivity and possibly the pathogenesis of asthma or chronic obstructive pulmonary disease (COPD).

Clinical Presentation

Acute bronchitis usually begins as an upper respiratory infection with nonspecific complaints.[10,14] Cough is the hallmark of acute bronchitis and occurs early. The onset of cough may be insidious or abrupt, and the symptoms persist despite resolution of nasal or nasopharyngeal complaints; cough may persist for up to 3 or more weeks. Frequently, the cough initially is nonproductive but then progresses, yielding mucopurulent sputum. In older children and adults, the sputum is raised and expectorated; in the young child, sputum often is swallowed and can result in gagging and vomiting. Substantial discomfort may result from the coughing. Dyspnea, cyanosis, or signs of airway obstruction are observed rarely unless the patient has underlying pulmonary disease, such as emphysema or COPD. Fever, when present, rarely exceeds 39°C (102.2°F) and appears most commonly with adenovirus, influenza virus, and *M. pneumoniae* infections. The diagnosis typically is made on the basis of a characteristic history and physical examination. Bacterial cultures of expectorated sputum generally are of limited use because of the inability to avoid normal nasopharyngeal flora by the sampling technique. In routine cases, viral cultures are unnecessary and frequently unavailable. Viral antigen detection tests, developed to identify respiratory viral antigens from nasal secretions rapidly, can be obtained in many hospital laboratories and in some practice settings when a specific diagnosis is necessary for clinical or epidemiologic reasons. Cultures, serologic or PCR diagnosis of *M. pneumoniae*, and culture, direct fluorescent antibody detection, or PCR for *B. pertussis* should be obtained in prolonged or severe cases when epidemiologic considerations would suggest their involvement.

TREATMENT

Desired Outcome

In the absence of a complicating bacterial superinfection, acute bronchitis almost always is self-limiting. The goals of therapy are to provide comfort to the patient and, in the unusually severe case, to treat associated dehydration and respiratory compromise.[10]

General Approach to Treatment

4 Treatment of acute bronchitis is symptomatic and supportive in nature. Reassurance and antipyretics frequently are all that are needed. Bedrest for comfort may be instituted as desired. Patients should be encouraged to drink fluids to prevent dehydration and possibly to decrease the viscosity of respiratory secretions. Mist therapy (use of a vaporizer) may promote the thinning and loosening of respiratory secretions.

Pharmacologic Therapy

Mild analgesic–antipyretic therapy often is helpful in relieving the associated lethargy, malaise, and fever. Aspirin or acetaminophen (650 mg in adults or 10 to 15 mg/kg per dose in children; maximum daily adult dose <4 g and pediatric dose 60 mg/kg) or ibuprofen (200 to 800 mg in adults or 10 mg/kg per dose in children; maximum daily adult dose 3.2 g and pediatric dose 40 mg/kg) should be administered every 4 to 6 hours. In children, aspirin should be avoided and acetaminophen used as the preferred agent because of the possible association between aspirin use and the development of Reye's syndrome.[15]

Use of ibuprofen as an antipyretic has increased. The drug's antipyretic efficacy appears identical to that of aspirin or acetaminophen, although its duration of antipyretic effect may be slightly longer (e.g., 3 to 4 hours for aspirin and acetaminophen vs. 5 to 6 hours for ibuprofen). Caution should be exercised in the administration of ibuprofen for patients younger than 6 months, elderly patients, and individuals with poor renal function. Aspirin and ibuprofen inhibit prostaglandin synthesis and may adversely influence renal function in these predisposed patient populations.

Patients may present with mild to moderate wheezing. In otherwise healthy patients, no meaningful benefits have been described with the use of oral or aerosolized β_2-receptor agonists and/or oral or aerosolized corticosteroids. A Cochrane review showed limited benefit of β_2-receptor agonists in both pediatric and adult patients compared with the side effects; however, in adults with airflow obstruction there was a trend toward improvement.[16] Some clinicians, despite no data, may initiate a brief trial (e.g., ~5 to 7 days) of oral or inhaled corticosteroid for patients with persistent (>14 to 20 days), troublesome cough. Despite several studies, none support the use of mucolytic agents.

Patients suffering from acute bronchitis frequently medicate themselves with nonprescription cough and cold remedies containing various combinations of antihistamines, sympathomimetics, and antitussives despite the lack of definitive evidence supporting their effectiveness. In fact, the tendency of these agents to dehydrate bronchial secretions could aggravate and prolong the recovery process. Although not recommended for routine use, persistent, mild cough, which may be bothersome, can be treated with dextromethorphan; more severe coughs may require intermittent codeine or other similar agents.[10,14] In severe cases, the cough may be persistent enough to disrupt sleep, and use of a mild sedative–hypnotic, concomitantly with a cough suppressant (e.g., codeine), may be desirable. However, antitussives should be used cautiously when the cough is productive. The primary or supplemental use of expectorants is questionable because their clinical effectiveness has not been well established.

Routine use of antibiotics for treatment of acute bronchitis should be discouraged due to limited benefit.[10,17] In previously healthy patients who exhibit persistent fever or respiratory symptoms for more than 4 to 6 days or for predisposed patients (e.g., elderly, immunocompromised), the possibility of a concurrent bacterial infection should be suspected. When possible, antibiotic therapy should be directed toward anticipated respiratory pathogen(s) (i.e., *S. pneumoniae*). *M. pneumoniae*, if suspected by history or if confirmed by culture serology or PCR, can be treated with azithromycin. Alternatively and empirically, a fluoroquinolone antibiotic with activity against these suspected pathogens (e.g., levofloxacin) can be used. During known epidemics involving the influenza A virus, amantadine or rimantadine may be effective in minimizing associated symptoms if administered early in the course of the disease, although treatment with adamantanes is no longer recommended by the Centers for Disease Control and Prevention (CDC) due to increasing influenza resistance to these two agents.[18] The neuraminidase inhibitors (e.g., zanamivir and oseltamivir) are active against both influenza A and B viral infections and may reduce the severity and duration of the influenza episode if administered promptly during the onset of the viral infection and are the preferred treatment (see Chap. 87).[19,20] Unfortunately, the incidence of influenza virus resistance to available antiviral drugs is increasing.[18,21]

Chronic Bronchitis

Epidemiology and Etiology

Chronic bronchitis, a component of COPD, is a clinical diagnosis for a nonspecific disease that primarily affects adults. An in-depth presentation of the spectrum and management of COPD is given in Chapter 16. This section will focus solely on chronic bronchitis, a disease that affects most patients with COPD but can develop in patients with normal spirometry.[22] In developed countries the prevalence of chronic bronchitis is slightly higher in men than in women and possibly more common in whites.[22,23]

5 Chronic bronchitis is defined clinically as the presence of a chronic cough productive of sputum lasting more than 3 consecutive months of the year for 2 consecutive years without an underlying etiology of bronchiectasis or tuberculosis. The disease is a result of several contributing factors; the most prominent include cigarette smoking, exposure to occupational dusts, fumes, and environmental pollution, and host factors (e.g., genetic factors and bacterial [and possibly viral] infections). The contribution of each of these factors and of others (either alone or in combination) to chronic bronchitis is unknown. Cigarette smoke is a well-known airway irritant and is believed to be the predominant factor in the etiology of chronic bronchitis. Although previously assumed the most common etiologic cause of chronic bronchitis, more strict prohibition of public smoking and the resultant decrease in chronic tobacco smokers, particularly in developed countries, underscores the importance of other factors as causes of this chronic disease. Additional airway irritants including occupational dust, chemicals, or air pollution, either alone or more probably in combination, are also responsible for the pathogenesis of chronic bronchitis. Furthermore, genome-wide association studies have begun to identify single-nucleotide polymorphisms that may have clinical relevance in COPD; see Chapter 16.[24] Lastly, the influence of recurrent

respiratory tract infections during childhood or young adult life on the later development of chronic bronchitis remains obscure, but recurrent respiratory infections may predispose individuals to the development of chronic bronchitis.[23] Whether these recurrent respiratory tract infections are a result of unrecognized anatomic abnormalities of the airways or impaired pulmonary defense mechanisms is unclear.

Numerous consensus statements and published authoritative guidelines define chronic bronchitis and emphysema as the two main components of COPD/chronic obstructive lung disease (COLD).[22,23,25] The Global Initiative for Chronic Obstruction Lung Disease (GOLD)[22] guidelines document does not distinguish these two diagnoses (e.g., emphysema or chronic bronchitis) in the definition of COPD, but it does define COPD as a disease characterized by airflow obstruction that is not fully reversible and progressive. The GOLD guidelines provide a COPD classification scoring system according to severity that can be helpful in staging patients for intensity of therapy and prognosis.[22] Unfortunately, differences in definitions between authoritative organizations[22,23,25] may cause confusion in the assignment of patients in clinical trials and thus to assessment and applications of study results to clinical care.

Pathogenesis

Chronic inhalation of an irritating noxious substance compromises the normal secretory and mucociliary function of bronchial mucosa.[23] Bronchial biopsy specimens in bronchitic patients underscore the importance of proinflammatory cytokines (e.g., interleukins 1β, 6, and 8, transforming growth factor-β, leukotriene B4, and tumor necrosis factor-α) in the pathogenesis and propagation of the observed inflammatory changes. In chronic bronchitis, the bronchial wall is thickened, and the number of mucus-secreting goblet cells on the surface epithelium of both larger and smaller bronchi is increased markedly. In contrast, goblet cells generally are absent from the smaller bronchi of normal individuals. In addition to the increased number of goblet cells, hypertrophy of the mucous glands and dilation of the mucous gland ducts are observed. As a result of these changes, chronic bronchitics have substantially more mucus in their peripheral airways, further impairing normal lung defenses. This increased quantity of tenacious secretions within the bronchial tree frequently causes mucous plugging of the smaller airways. Accompanying these changes are squamous cell metaplasia of the surface epithelium, edema, and increased vascularity of the basement membrane of larger airways and variable chronic inflammatory cell infiltration. In addition, the amounts of several proteases derived from inflammatory cells are increased and due to COPD-induced defective antiproteases lead to continued destruction of connective tissue. Continued progression of this pathology can result in residual scarring of small bronchi and peribronchial fibrosis augmenting airway obstruction and weakening of bronchial walls.

Clinical Presentation

❺ The hallmark of chronic bronchitis is a cough that may range from a mild to a severe, incessant coughing productive of purulent sputum.[22,23] Coughing may be precipitated by multiple stimuli, including simple, normal conversation. Expectoration of the largest quantity of sputum usually occurs on arising in the morning, although many patients expectorate sputum throughout the day. The expectorated sputum usually is tenacious and can vary in color from white to yellow-green. Patients with chronic bronchitis often expectorate as much as 100 mL/day more than normal. As a result, many patients complain of a frequent bad taste in their mouth and of halitosis.

The diagnosis of chronic bronchitis is based primarily on clinical assessment and history. Any patient who reports coughing sputum on most days for at least 3 consecutive months each year for 2 consecutive years presumptively has chronic bronchitis.[23] The diagnosis of chronic bronchitis is made only when the possibilities of bronchiectasis, cardiac failure, cystic fibrosis, and lung carcinoma have been effectively excluded. In an attempt to be more specific in the diagnosis, some investigators have added the criteria of lost wages for 3 or more weeks. In addition, many clinicians attempt to subdivide their patients based on severity of disease to guide therapeutic interventions. A useful diagnostic/clinical severity-based classification system is often used to categorize patients to assist in defining an acute therapeutic strategy. The classification system used most often utilizes three descriptive categories: (a) *simple chronic bronchitis* best describes patients with no major risk factors and sputum flora reflects the common associated pathogens where the patient usually responds well to first-line oral antibiotic therapy. (b) *Complicated chronic bronchitis* refers to those patients with what would be considered a "simple chronic bronchitis" exacerbation, but the patients have two or more disease-associated risk factors such as forced expiratory volume in the first second of expiration (FEV_1) <50% (<0.50) predicted, age >64 years, >4 exacerbations per year, home oxygen use, underlying cardiac disease, use of immunosuppressants, or use of antibiotics for an exacerbation within the past 3 months. These group II patients may also harbor drug-resistant pathogens. (c) *Severe complicated chronic bronchitis* refers to those patients with group II symptoms but clinically are much worse, for example, FEV_1 <35% (<0.35) predicted, >4 acute exacerbations per year, increased risk for infection with *P. aeruginosa*, and presence of pathogens that are multidrug resistant (MDR). The latter patients often require hospitalization and aggressive parenteral antibiotics including combination therapy. A clinical algorithm for the diagnosis and treatment of chronic bronchitic patients with an acute exacerbation incorporating the principles of the clinical classification system is shown in Figure 85-1. The importance of accurate classification for grouping patients of similar disease involvement cannot be overemphasized with respect to assessing publications outlining treatment strategies for these patients.[26] Although gross, these classifications attempt to capture specific phenotypes of chronic bronchitis patients. It is hoped that within the next 2 to 4 years, pharmacogenomic advances will provide a more sophisticated tool for defining specific phenotypes linked to specific, optimal therapies.[27] The typical clinical presentation of chronic bronchitis is listed in Table 85-1. Comparison of the trends in changes in patient's physical activity, symptoms, and clinical/physical findings from the patient's "routine" is extremely helpful in determining the presence and severity of an acute exacerbation. In general, a good clinical relationship exists between the purulence of the sputum and the bacterial load (>90% of cases) and for sputum color, for example, the greener the color, the greater the amount of leukocyte myeloperoxidase (indicating that more inflammatory cells are present).

In more advanced stages of chronic bronchitis, physical findings associated with cor pulmonale, including cardiac enlargement, hepatomegaly, and edema of the lower extremities, are observed. In general, chronic bronchitics tend to maintain at least normal body weight and commonly are obese. Radiographic studies are of limited value in either the diagnosis or followup of a patient. The microscopic and laboratory assessments of sputum are considered important components in the overall evaluation of patients with chronic bronchitis. A fresh sputum specimen obtained as an early morning sample is preferred. Comparison of the cellular constituents of chronic bronchitic sputum with those of normal sputum can provide insight into the degree of activity of the disease processes. An increased number of polymorphonuclear granulocytes often suggests continual bronchial irritation, whereas an increased number of eosinophils suggests an allergic component that should be further investigated. Gram staining of the sputum often reveals a mixture of both gram-positive and gram-negative bacteria, reflecting

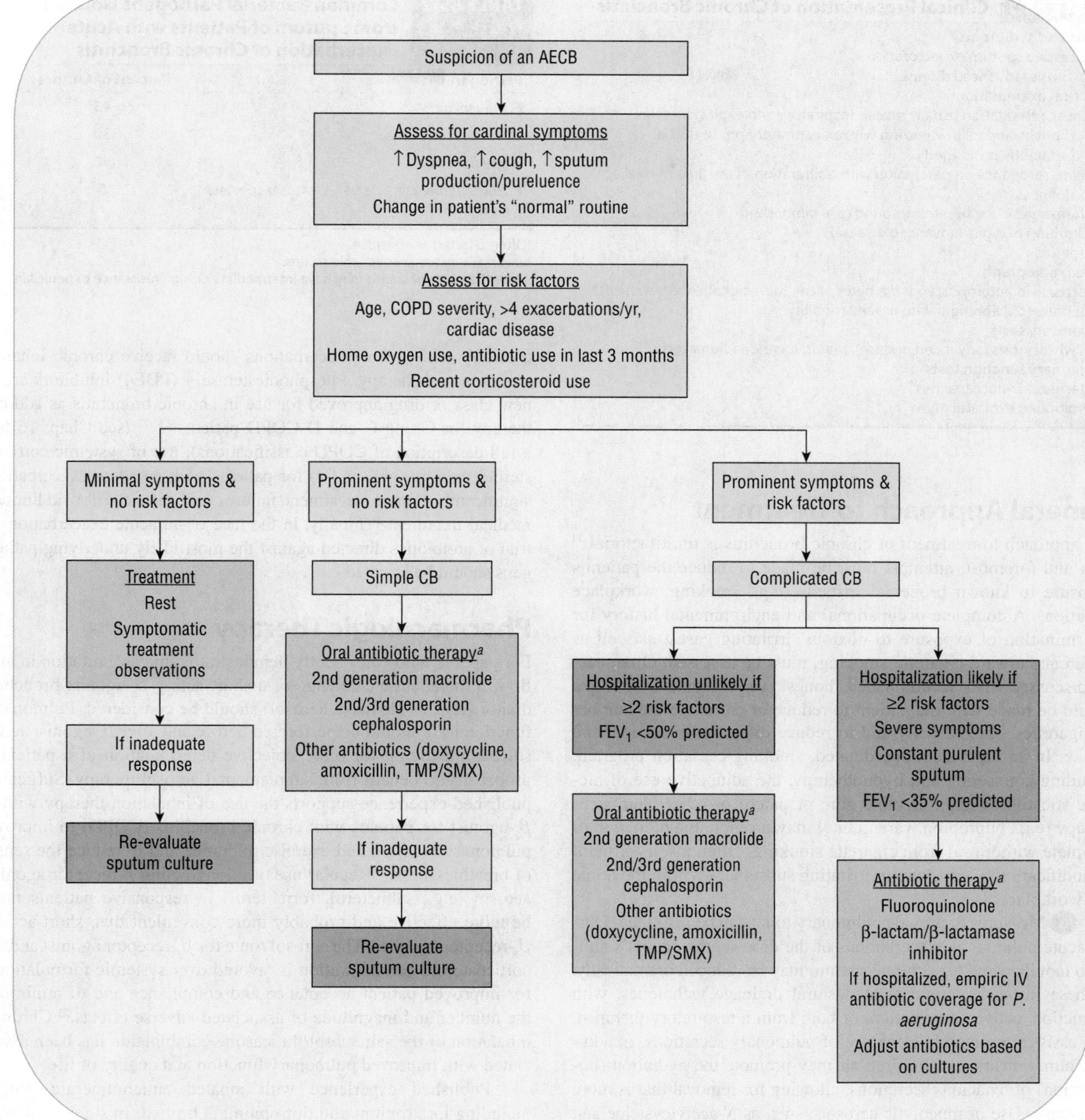

FIGURE 85-1 Clinical algorithm for the diagnosis and treatment of chronic bronchitic patients with an acute exacerbation incorporating the principles of the clinical classification system. (AECB, acute exacerbation of chronic bronchitis; COPD, chronic obstructive pulmonary disease; CB, chronic bronchitis; TMP/SMX, trimethoprim/sulfamethoxazole.) [a]See Table 85-3 for commonly used antibiotics and doses. *(Adapted from reference 34.)*

normal oropharyngeal flora and chronic tracheal colonization (in order of frequency) by nontypeable *H. influenzae*, *S. pneumoniae*, and *M. catarrhalis*. Table 85-2 lists the most common bacterial isolates identified from sputum culture for patients experiencing an acute exacerbation of chronic bronchitis (AECB). For patients with more severe airflow disease (e.g., FEV_1 <40% [<0.40]), enteric gram-negative bacilli, *E. coli*, *Klebsiella* species, *Enterobacter* species, and *P. aeruginosa* may be significant pathogens during acute exacerbations.[28]

TREATMENT

Desired Outcome

The goals of therapy for chronic bronchitis are twofold: to reduce the severity of chronic symptoms and to ameliorate acute exacerbations and achieve prolonged infection-free intervals.

TABLE 85-1 Clinical Presentation of Chronic Bronchitis

Signs and symptoms
- Excessive sputum expectoration
- Cyanosis (advanced disease)

Physical examination
- Chest auscultation usually reveals inspiratory and expiratory rales, rhonchi, and mild wheezing with an expiratory phase that is frequently prolonged
- Hyperresonance on percussion with obliteration of the area of cardiac dullness
- Normal vesicular breathing sounds are diminished
- Clubbing of digits (advanced disease)
- Obesity

Chest radiograph
- Increase in anteroposterior diameter of the thoracic cage (barrel chest)
- Depressed diaphragm with limited mobility

Laboratory tests
- Erythrocytosis (advanced disease), that is, increased hematocrit

Pulmonary function tests
- Decreased vital capacity
- Prolonged expiratory flow

TABLE 85-2 Common Bacterial Pathogens Isolated from Sputum of Patients with Acute Exacerbation of Chronic Bronchitis

Pathogen	Percent of Cultures
H. influenzae[a,b]	45
M. catarrhalis[a]	30
S. pneumoniae[c]	20
E. coli, Enterobacter species, *Klebsiella* species, *P. aeruginosa*	5

[a]Often β-lactamase positive.
[b]Vast majority are nontypeable strains.
[c]More than 25% of strains may have intermediate or high resistance to penicillin.

General Approach to Treatment

The approach to treatment of chronic bronchitis is multifactorial.[23] First and foremost, attempts must be made to reduce the patient's exposure to known bronchial irritants (e.g., smoking, workplace pollution). A complete occupational and environmental history for determination of exposure to noxious, irritating gases, as well as preference toward cigarette smoking, must be assessed. Often easier discussed than accomplished, honest, yet reasonable attempts should be made with the patient to reduce or eliminate the number of cigarettes smoked daily and to reduce exposure to secondhand smoke. In an organized, coordinated, smoking cessation program, including counseling and hypnotherapy, the adjunctive use of nicotine substitutes (e.g., nicotine gum or patch) or other pharmacotherapy (e.g., bupropion, varenicline) may promote the reduction or complete withdrawal from cigarette smoking. Often just as difficult is modification of exposure to irritating substances within the home and workplace.

6 Measures to provide pulmonary toilet can be instituted. During acute pulmonary exacerbations of the disease, the patient's ability to mobilize and expectorate sputum may be reduced dramatically. In these instances, attempts at postural drainage techniques, with instruction, active participation, or both from a respiratory therapist, may assist in promoting clearance of pulmonary secretions. In addition, humidification of inspired air may promote the hydration (liquefaction) of tenacious secretions, allowing for removal that is more productive. Use of mucolytic aerosols, such as *N*-acetylcysteine and DNAse, is of questionable therapeutic value, particularly considering their propensity to induce bronchospasm (*N*-acetylcysteine) and their excessive cost. A Cochrane meta-analysis of mucolytic therapy in subjects with chronic bronchitis or COPD found that treatment with mucolytics was associated with a small reduction in acute exacerbations and did not cause any harm, improve quality of life, or slow the decline of lung function.[29] The clinical benefit may be greater for chronic bronchitics/COPD patients who have frequent or prolonged exacerbations and are unable to utilize inhaled corticosteroids or long-acting β_2-agonists.[29] Although limited data are available, chronic use of oral or aerosolized bronchodilators may be of benefit by increasing mucociliary and cough clearance. For patients with moderate to severe COPD, combination therapy with a long-acting β_2-agonist and inhaled corticosteroid led to decreased exacerbations and rescue medication use while it also improved quality of life, lung function, and symptom scores compared with long-acting β_2-agonist monotherapy.[30] Furthermore, patients may benefit from inhaled corticosteroids; patients with severe disease (FEV_1 <50% [<0.50]) with a history of frequent exacerbations should receive chronic inhaled corticosteroid therapy. Phosphodiesterase 4 (PDE4) inhibitors are a new class of drug approved for use in chronic bronchitis as add-on therapy for Group C and D COPD patients[22,31,32] (see Chap. 16 for a full description of COPD classifications); use of systemic corticosteroid therapy (oral or IV) for patients with an acute exacerbation significantly reduces treatment failures and the need for additional medical treatment.[22] Finally, in the face of an acute exacerbation, a trial of antibiotics directed against the most likely underlying pathogens should be initiated.

Pharmacologic Therapy

For patients who consistently demonstrate clinical limitation in airflow, a therapeutic challenge of a short-acting β_2-agonist bronchodilator (e.g., as albuterol aerosol) should be considered. Pulmonary function tests should be performed before and after β_2-agonist aerosol administration for more objective determination of a patient's propensity to benefit from supplemental aerosol therapy. Sufficient published experience supports the use of inhalation therapy with a β_2-agonist for patients with chronic bronchitis (COPD) to improve pulmonary function and exercise tolerance and to reduce the sense of breathlessness.[23] Regular use of a long-acting β-receptor agonist aerosol (e.g., salmeterol, formoterol) in responsive patients may be more effective and probably more convenient than short-acting β_2-receptor agonists. The aerosol route for β_2-receptor agonist and/or corticosteroid administration is favored over systemic formulations for improved patient acceptance and compliance and to minimize the number and magnitude of associated adverse effects.[22] Chronic inhalation of the salmeterol/fluticasone combination has been associated with improved pulmonary function and quality of life.

Published experience with inhaled anticholinergic drugs, including ipratropium and tiotropium, is limited. In stable patients, long-term inhalation of ipratropium has been associated with a decreased frequency of cough, less severe coughing, and a decrease in the volume of expectorated sputum. Once-daily tiotropium inhalation was associated with significant bronchodilation and dyspnea relief compared with placebo but had no significant effect on the incidence or severity of cough.[22,23] Although chronic theophylline administration has been used extensively in the past, this therapy is used with decreasing frequency in favor of aerosolized β_2-receptor agonists. A salmeterol/fluticasone combination markedly reduced the number of chronic bronchitis–associated emergency room visits and hospitalizations compared with an ipratropium-based regimen.[33]

PDE4 inhibitors, compared with the nonselective phosphodiesterase inhibitor theophylline, only affect phosphodiesterase in the airway smooth muscle, immune (eosinophils, monocytes, and neutrophils), and proinflammatory cells. Roflumilast, the only available PDE4 inhibitor, was approved by the U.S. FDA in 2011 for use in patients with severe COPD with chronic bronchitis and a history of exacerbations. Moderate to severe exacerbations treated with steroids were reduced by 15% to 20% in patients receiving roflumilast and add-on therapy with long-acting β_2-agonists had effects on lung function.[22] GOLD guidelines suggest the use of PDE4 inhibitors as an alternative therapy for COPD Group C patients with chronic bronchitis and as add-on therapy for COPD Group D patients with chronic bronchitis.[22] The side effect profile for PDE4 inhibitor differs from inhaled COPD medications; patients may experience nausea, vomiting, decreased appetite, and sleep disturbances.[22,32] Intolerable nausea and vomiting had occurred with cilomilast, a PDE4 inhibitor primarily targeting isozyme PDE4D located in the CNS compared with isozyme PDE4B, which is located in immune and proinflammatory cells.[31] Roflumilast is nonselective for the PDE4 isozymes and is less likely to cause nausea and vomiting. Unexplained weight loss has also been reported in studies; therefore, a patient's weight should be taken into consideration prior to treatment and monitored during therapy.

Use of antimicrobials for treatment of chronic bronchitis has been controversial but is becoming more accepted. Numerous comparative evaluations, including placebo-controlled studies of antibiotic administration with acute and chronic treatment of chronic bronchitics, have suggested definite clinical benefit, whereas other similar studies have not.[22,25,26,28,34] The antibiotics selected most frequently possess variable in vitro activity against the common sputum isolates *H. influenzae*, *S. pneumoniae*, *M. catarrhalis*, and *M. pneumoniae*. Conflicting published results appear independent of the antibiotic used or the regimen compared. The wide disparity that exists in the results from these studies, combined with the difficulties in recognition and lack of standardized diagnostic criteria for acute exacerbations of chronic bronchitis, serves as the basis for the enormous controversy surrounding the use of antibiotics in this condition.[23] A review of 14 double-blinded, randomized clinical trials compared fluoroquinolones with more standard antibiotic regimens (e.g., macrolides, azalides, oral cephalosporins, and the combination drug amoxicillin/clavulanate).[28] As expected, no significant differences were observed between treatment arms. However, in a small subset of studies ($n = 4$), the sputum culture became negative in a significantly higher number of fluoroquinolone-treated patients. Other studies showed an increase in the interval between acute exacerbations for patients who received fluoroquinolone therapy. An additional advantage of fluoroquinolone therapy is the short course (e.g., 5 days) and once-daily dosing compared with other antibiotic regimens.

A useful paradigm for the assessment and treatment of acute exacerbations of chronic bronchitis and antibiotic decision making is shown in Figure 85-1. Furthermore, many clinicians will use the so-called Anthonisen criteria to determine if antibiotic therapy is indicated.[35] With the Anthonisen criteria if a patient exhibits two of the following three criteria during an AECB, the patient will most likely benefit from antibiotic therapy and, thus, should receive a treatment course: (a) increase in shortness of breath; (b) increase in sputum volume; (c) production of purulent sputum. There are greater healthcare costs for patients who are noncompliant with their antibiotic regimen for their AECB.[36]

The increasing resistance of the common bacterial pathogens to first-line agents further complicates antibiotic selection. As many as 30% to 40% of *H. influenzae* and 95% to 100% of *M. catarrhalis* isolates produce β-lactamases. Moreover, up to 40% of *S. pneumoniae* isolates demonstrate resistance to penicillin (minimum inhibitory concentration [MIC] = 0.1 to 2 mg/L), with approximately 20% of isolates being highly resistant (MIC >2 mg/L). Concern regarding *S. pneumoniae* resistance is increasing, now ≥30% for macrolides. Despite these changes in bacterial susceptibility, the current recommendation is to initiate therapy with first-line agents in less severely affected patients (see Fig. 85-1). Trimethoprim/sulfamethoxazole has been extremely useful for patients with less severe disease.[37] However, the public campaign in the United Kingdom by the Committee of Safety of Medicines to discourage the use of trimethoprim/sulfamethoxazole based on rare but possibly life-threatening cases of Stevens-Johnson syndrome has markedly reduced the use of this agent worldwide. For patients with more moderate to severe disease, many clinicians will begin antibiotic therapy with the second-line agents, amoxicillin/clavulanate, a macrolide (such as azithromycin or clarithromycin, although they are being used less frequently), and more frequently with a fluoroquinolone, such as levofloxacin (see Fig. 85-1).[22,28,34,38]

Regardless of the antibiotic selected, predetermined outcome measures should be monitored closely for each patient to determine the success or failure of the therapeutic intervention. Oral antibiotics with broader antibacterial spectra (e.g., amoxicillin/clavulanate, fluoroquinolones, or azalides) that possess potent in vitro activity against sputum isolates are increasingly becoming first-line antibiotics as initial therapy for treatment of acute exacerbations of chronic bronchitis.[22,28,33,34,37]

An important clinical outcome variable directing drug selection and criteria for beginning antibiotics in individual patients is the infection-free period when chronic bronchitics are off antibiotics. The actual length of the infection-free time period and the change in the number of physician office visits and hospital admissions with a particular antibiotic regimen are extremely important to identify, whenever possible, for each patient. The antibiotic regimen that results in the longest infection-free period defines the "regimen of choice" for specific patients for future acute exacerbations of their disease. Trials of prophylactic antibiotic use may provide a slight benefit in exacerbation rates; however, GOLD guidelines do not currently support this indication.[22]

Antibiotics should be selected that are effective against responsible pathogens, demonstrate the least risk of drug interactions, and can be administered in a manner that promotes compliance. Antibiotics commonly used for treatment of these patients and their respective adult starting doses are listed in Table 85-3. Doses of antibiotics should be adjusted as needed to the desired clinical effect and the lowest incidence of acceptable side effects. A frequently used clinical strategy to enhance the duration of symptom-free periods incorporates higher-dose antibiotic regimens using the upper limit of the

TABLE 85-3 Oral Antibiotics Commonly Used for the Treatment of Acute Respiratory Exacerbations in Chronic Bronchitis

Antibiotic	Brand Name	Usual Adult Dose (mg)	Dose Schedule (Doses/Day)
Preferred Drugs			
Ampicillin	—	250–500	4
Amoxicillin	—	500–875	3–2
Amoxicillin/clavulanate	Augmentin®	500–875	3–2
Ciprofloxacin	Cipro®	500–750	2
Levofloxacin	Levaquin®	500–750	1
Moxifloxacin	Avelox®	400	1
Doxycycline	Monodox®	100	2
Minocycline	Minocin®	100	2
Tetracycline HCl	—	500	4
Trimethoprim/sulfamethoxazole[a]	Bactrim DS™/Septra DS®	1 DS	2
Supplemental Drugs			
Azithromycin	Zithromax®	250–500	1
Erythromycin	Ery-Tab®/Erythrocin®	500	4
Clarithromycin	Biaxin®	250–500	2
Cephalexin	Keflex®	500	4

[a]DS, double-strength tablet (160-mg trimethoprim/800-mg sulfamethoxazole).

recommended daily antibiotic dose for a period of 5 to 7 days. More clinicians are electing to limit their antibiotic treatment regimen to 5 days as compelling data continue to support equal efficacy and possibly less side effects with short-duration antibiotic therapy versus longer treatment regimens (>7 days).[39]

BRONCHIOLITIS

Epidemiology and Etiology

7 Bronchiolitis is an acute viral infection of the lower respiratory tract that affects approximately 50% of children during the first year of life and 100% by age 2 years. The occurrence of bronchiolitis peaks during the winter months and persists through early spring. Bronchiolitis remains the major reason for hospital admission during the first year of life. The incidence of bronchiolitis appears to be more common in males than in females.[40,41]

Respiratory syncytial virus (RSV) is the most common cause of bronchiolitis, accounting for up to 75% of all cases. During epidemic periods, the incidence of RSV-induced bronchiolitis may approach 90% of cases. Other detectable viruses include parainfluenza, adenovirus, and influenza. Bacteria serve as secondary pathogens in a minority of cases.[40,42]

Clinical Presentation

A prodrome suggesting an upper respiratory tract infection, usually lasting from 2 to 8 days, precedes the onset of clinical symptoms (Table 85-4). Due to limited oral intake because of coughing combined with fever, vomiting, and diarrhea, infants frequently are dehydrated. The increased work of breathing and tachypnea most likely further increase fluid loss. In most cases, this clinical picture persists between 3 and 7 days. Although the hospital course of bronchiolitic children often is variable, substantial clinical improvement usually is observed within the first 2 days, with gradual improvement and complete resolution sometimes requiring 4 to 8 weeks.

The diagnosis of bronchiolitis is based primarily on history and clinical findings. It is important for the clinician to attempt to differentiate between bronchiolitis and a host of other clinical entities affecting infants, which may produce a similar picture of dyspnea and wheezing. Asthma, congestive heart failure, anatomic airway abnormalities, cystic fibrosis, foreign bodies, and gastroesophageal reflux are the primary disease entities that may present with wheezing in children. Isolation of a viral pathogen in the respiratory secretions of a wheezing child establishes a presumptive diagnosis of infectious bronchiolitis. However, the ability to identify specific viral pathogens often is hindered by the limited availability of special virology laboratories. In addition, in the elderly and in immunocompromised patients, antigen detection lacks adequate sensitivity, and patients frequently seek medical care after the acute stage of the infection, thus compromising the ability of the available tests to diagnose RSV. However, the proliferation of commercial enzyme-linked immunosorbent assays and fluorescent antibody staining techniques of nasopharyngeal secretions has increased the ability to identify viral antigens within several hours.[40] Identification of RSV by PCR should be available routinely from most clinical laboratories, but its relevance to the clinical management of bronchiolitis remains obscure.

Multiple clinical laboratory determinations have been used to assist in the management of cases of bronchiolitis. Radiographic evaluation of the chest in children with bronchiolitis yields variable findings but may help to distinguish this illness from other entities characterized by wheezing. In children requiring hospitalization, abnormalities in blood gas tensions are frequent and appear to relate to disease severity. Hypoxemia is common and increases the respiratory drive, whereas hypercarbia is seen in only the most severe cases. Despite the presence of moderate degrees of hypoxemia, clinical cyanosis is unusual.

TABLE 85-4 Clinical Presentation of Bronchiolitis

Signs and symptoms
Prodrome with irritability, restlessness, and mild fever
Cough and coryza
Vomiting, diarrhea, noisy breathing, and increased respiratory rate as symptoms progress
Labored breathing with retractions of the chest wall, nasal flaring, and grunting
Physical examination
Tachycardia and respiratory rate of 40–80/min in hospitalized infants
Wheezing and inspiratory rales
Mild conjunctivitis in one third of patients
Otitis media in 5–10% of patients
Laboratory tests
Peripheral white blood cell count normal or slightly elevated
Abnormal arterial blood gases (hypoxemia and, rarely, hypercarbia)

TREATMENT

Desired Outcome

7 In the well infant, bronchiolitis usually is a self-limiting illness, and reassurance, antipyretics, and adequate fluid intake usually are all that are necessary while waiting for resolution of the underlying viral infection. In-hospital support is necessary for the child suffering from respiratory failure or marked dehydration; underlying cardiac and pulmonary diseases potentiate these conditions.

General Approach to Treatment

7 Almost all otherwise healthy babies with bronchiolitis can be followed as outpatients. Such infants are treated for fever, provided generous amounts of oral fluids, and observed closely for evidence of respiratory deterioration.[43] In severely affected children, the mainstays of therapy for bronchiolitis are oxygen therapy and IV fluids. In a subset of patients, aerosolized bronchodilators may have a role. For selected infants, particularly those with underlying pulmonary disease, cardiac disease, or both, therapy with the antiviral agent ribavirin can be considered.[44]

Pharmacologic Therapy

7 Aerosolized β_2-adrenergic therapy appears to offer little benefit for the majority of patients and may even be detrimental.[40,42] However, this therapy may offer some benefit to the child with a predisposition toward bronchospasm. In addition, although clinical trials have demonstrated varied results, nebulized epinephrine seems to be more efficacious than albuterol in hospitalized patients with bronchiolitis.[40,45] For such patients, bronchodilator therapy may be offered initially but should not be pursued in the absence of a clear-cut clinical benefit. Similarly, controlled trials of corticosteroids in bronchiolitic infants have not shown therapeutic effects or significant harmful effects.[42,44] As a result, the routine use of systemically administered corticosteroids is discouraged. Conversely, the combined use of oral dexamethasone with nebulized epinephrine may act synergistically to reduce hospital admissions and shorten the time to discharge and the duration of symptoms; however, more trials are needed to confirm these findings.[45,46] Although placing children with bronchiolitis in mist tents has been common practice, no data have documented the effectiveness of this practice.

Ribavirin may offer benefit to a subset of infants with bronchiolitis. Although ribavirin, a synthetic nucleoside, possesses in vitro antiviral properties against a variety of RNA and DNA viruses, including influenza A, influenza B, parainfluenza, and adenovirus,[41] it is approved only in aerosolized form against RSV. Use of the drug requires special equipment (small-particle aerosol generator) and specially trained personnel for administration via oxygen hood or mist tent. Special care must be taken to avoid drug particle deposition and the resulting clogging of respiratory tubing and valves in mechanical ventilators. Among hospital admissions for RSV infection, ribavirin therapy failed to decrease length of hospital stay, number of days in the intensive care unit, or number of days receiving mechanical ventilation. Consequently, the American Academy of Pediatrics does not recommend the routine use of ribavirin in children with bronchiolitis.[47] In light of this and because of the requirement for special aerosolization equipment and the cost of the drug itself, most experts recommend reserving use of ribavirin for severely ill patients, especially those with chronic lung disease (particularly bronchopulmonary dysplasia), congenital heart disease, prematurity, and immunodeficiency (especially severe combined immunodeficiency and human immunodeficiency virus [HIV] infection).

Clinical **Controversy...**

Because bacteria are not primary pathogens in the etiology of bronchiolitis, antibiotics should not be administered routinely. Despite this, many clinicians frequently administer antibiotics while awaiting culture results because the clinical and radiographic findings in bronchiolitis often are suggestive of possible bacterial pneumonia.

For infants with underlying pulmonary or cardiovascular disease, prophylaxis against RSV may be warranted. When administered monthly during the RSV season, both RSV immune globulin and palivizumab[48] (a monoclonal antibody for RSV) may decrease the number of RSV episodes and the need for hospitalization. Between the two, palivizumab appears to be preferred, given its ease of administration, lack of administration-related adverse effects, and noninterference with select immunizations.

There is no vaccine marketed for RSV. Of note, in the 1960s, a formalin-inactivated vaccine induced a promising IgG response; however, the severity of subsequent infections was increased in immunized patients. In addition, aside from the need to induce immunity to multiple strains of the virus, a series of boosters would be required as natural infection with RSV does not prevent subsequent infections.[44]

PNEUMONIA

Epidemiology

Pneumonia remains the most common cause of severe sepsis and infectious cause of death in children and adults in the United States, with a mortality rate of 30% to 40%.[6,49] Pneumonia occurs throughout the year, with the relative prevalence of disease resulting from different etiologic agents varying with the seasons. It occurs in persons of all ages, although the clinical manifestations are most severe in the very young, the elderly, and the chronically ill.

Pathogenesis

Microorganisms gain access to the lower respiratory tract by three routes. They may be inhaled as aerosolized particles, or they may enter the lung via the bloodstream from an extrapulmonary site of infection; however, aspiration of oropharyngeal contents, a common occurrence in both healthy and ill persons during sleep, is the major mechanism by which pulmonary pathogens gain access to the normally sterile lower airways and alveoli. When pulmonary defense mechanisms are functioning optimally, aspirated microorganisms are cleared from the region before infection can become established; however, aspiration of potential pathogens from the oropharynx can result in pneumonia if lung defenses are impaired.[7] Factors that promote aspiration, such as altered sensorium and neuromuscular disease, may result in an increase in the size of the inoculum delivered to the lower respiratory tract, thereby overwhelming local defense mechanisms. Lung infections with viruses suppress the antibacterial activity of the lung by impairing alveolar macrophage function and mucociliary clearance, thus setting the stage for secondary bacterial pneumonia. Mucociliary transport is also depressed by ethanol and narcotics and by obstruction of a bronchus by mucus, tumor, or extrinsic compression. All these factors can severely impair pulmonary clearance of aspirated bacteria.

8 The most prominent pathogen causing community-acquired pneumonia (CAP) in otherwise healthy adults is *S. pneumoniae* and accounts for up to 75% of all acute cases. Other common pathogens include *M. pneumoniae*, *Legionella species*, *C. pneumoniae*, *H. influenzae*, and a variety of viruses including influenza.[5,50] Healthcare-associated pneumonia (HCAP) is a classification used to distinguish nonhospitalized patients at risk for MDR pathogens (e.g., *P. aeruginosa*, *Acinetobacter species*, and methicillin-resistant *Staphylococcus aureus* [MRSA]) from those with CAP.[5,51] The term *atypical* may be applied to pneumonia to indicate that the pneumonia may be caused by an atypical pathogen (e.g., bilateral lobar pneumonia with a negative sputum Gram stain) such as *M. pneumoniae*, *C. pneumoniae*, or *Legionella* species.[52]

Gram-negative aerobic bacilli, *S. aureus*, and MDR pathogens are the leading causative agents in hospital-acquired pneumonia (HAP).[7] Anaerobic bacteria are the most common etiologic agents in pneumonia that follows the aspiration of gastric or oropharyngeal contents. Ventilator-associated pneumonia (VAP) is also associated with MDR pathogens.

Pneumonia in infants and children is caused by a wider range of microorganisms, and, unlike adults, nonbacterial pathogens predominate. Most pneumonias occurring in the pediatric age group are caused by viruses, especially RSV, parainfluenza, and adenovirus.[6] *M. pneumoniae* is an important pathogen in older children. Beyond the neonatal period, *S. pneumoniae* is the major bacterial pathogen in childhood pneumonia, followed by group A *Streptococcus* and *S. aureus*. *H. influenzae* type b, once a major childhood pathogen, has become an infrequent cause of pneumonia since the introduction of active vaccination against this organism in the late 1980s.

Based on the differences in severity and outcome for patients with CAP, genetic factors likely play a role.[53] Multiple variations in genes affecting inflammation, cough and airway protection, pattern recognition molecules, and organ function along with environmental factors may alter a patient's response to CAP. In the future, as specific genetic polymorphisms are better associated with disease response, therapy should become better targeted.

Clinical Presentation

Bacterial pneumonia is caused most commonly by gram-positive streptococci and staphylococci and by gram-negative organisms that normally inhabit the GI tract (enterics) or soil and water (nonenterics). In addition, *Legionella*, itself a weakly staining gram-negative nonenteric organism, accounts for a small percentage of CAP and HAP, although the true incidence may be underreported.[52] Finally, *M. tuberculosis*, an acid-fast staining bacillus, still remains an important cause of pneumonia in urban centers throughout the United States even though the incidence is much lower compared with that in other countries.[54,55]

TABLE 85-5 Clinical Presentation of Pneumonia

Signs and symptoms
Abrupt onset of fever, chills, dyspnea, and productive cough
Rust-colored sputum or hemoptysis
Pleuritic chest pain
Physical examination
Tachypnea and tachycardia
Dullness to percussion
Increased tactile fremitus, whisper pectoriloquy, and egophony
Chest wall retractions and grunting respirations
Diminished breath sounds over affected area
Inspiratory crackles during lung expansion
Chest radiograph
Dense lobar or segmental infiltrate
Laboratory tests
Leukocytosis with predominance of polymorphonuclear cells
Low oxygen saturation on arterial blood gas or pulse oximetry

A wide array of gram-positive and gram-negative organisms can cause pneumonia, but they usually present a similar clinical appearance (Table 85-5); thus, the epidemiologic and clinical clues will render one more likely than the other. *S. pneumoniae*, *S. aureus*, the enteric gram-negative rods, and occasionally other organisms may produce local irritation or destruction of blood vessels leading to rust-colored sputum or hemoptysis. Pleural effusions, both sterile and empyematous, may be associated with many of these entities, as evidenced by distant breath sounds and a wide area of dulled percussion. The chest radiograph and sputum examination and culture are the most useful diagnostic tests for gram-positive and gram-negative bacterial pneumonia.[5] Typically, the chest radiograph reveals a dense lobar or segmental infiltrate. However, patchy consolidation may be seen occasionally with virtually all these pathogens. Occasionally, pneumonia resulting from hematogenous spread of the organisms results in a diffuse, alveolar pattern on chest radiograph. Gram stain of the expectorated sputum demonstrates many polymorphonuclear cells per high-powered field in the presence of a predominant organism, which is reflected as heavy growth of a single species on culture. Other laboratory tests are less sensitive or specific. Blood cultures may be helpful in identifying the offending organism but are positive in only a minority of patients. The complete blood count usually reflects a leukocytosis with a predominance of polymorphonuclear cells; in some instances, particularly with *S. pneumoniae*, elevation of the white blood cell (WBC) count may be pronounced. Normal or mildly elevated WBC counts, however, do not exclude bacterial pneumonic disease. The patient also may be hypoxic, as reflected by low oxygen saturation on arterial blood gas or pulse oximetry.

Community-Acquired Pneumonia

8 *S. pneumoniae* is the most common community-acquired bacterial pneumonia in adult and pediatric patients.[5,6] It is particularly prevalent and severe for patients with splenic dysfunction, diabetes mellitus, chronic cardiopulmonary or renal disease, or HIV infection. Community-acquired disease with *S. aureus* is identified most frequently in young infants, patients with early cystic fibrosis, and those recovering from an antecedent respiratory viral infection. Group A *Streptococcus* is an uncommon cause of CAP and frequently occurs after a viral respiratory tract infection. Only occasionally is it associated with streptococcal pharyngitis. The organism is pyogenic, and the presentation can be severe. Community-acquired enteric gram-negative pneumonia is identified most frequently among patients with chronic illness, especially alcoholism and diabetes mellitus. In preschool-aged children, viral pathogens more commonly cause CAP compared with bacterial pathogens.[6]

Severity scores (e.g., CURB-65 and PSI), with varying strengths and weaknesses, have been utilized to assist healthcare professionals in predicting intensive care hospitalization and outcomes for patients with CAP.[5,56,57] Definitions of severe CAP may vary depending on the institution; however, patients with severe CAP are more likely to require intensive care or mechanical ventilation, or develop complications with sepsis, bacteremia, or multiorgan failure.[51] Severe CAP may also be difficult to distinguish from HCAP or HAP; however, the pathogens, *S. pneumoniae*, *H. influenzae*, and anaerobic bacteria, are not usually MDR. Patients at greater risk for severe CAP are those with underlying medical conditions or at risk for aspiration, animal exposure, or exposure to other infected patients or seasonal epidemics.[51]

Healthcare-Associated Pneumonia

Over the past several decades, the type of facilities where patients can receive healthcare has changed with infusion therapies, wound care, and dialysis available in an outpatient environment.[58] This, along with patients residing in a nursing home or long-term care facility or patients recently discharged from a hospital, has blurred the distinction between the pneumonia acquired as an inpatient versus an outpatient. See Table 85-6 for HCAP criteria. Patients diagnosed with HCAP are more similar to hospitalized patients based

TABLE 85-6 Pneumonia Classifications and Risk Factors

Type of Pneumonia	Definition	Risk Factors
Community acquired (CAP)	Pneumonia developing in patients with no contact to a medical facility	• Age >65 years • Diabetes mellitus • Asplenia • Chronic cardiovascular, pulmonary, renal and/or liver disease • Smoking and/or alcohol abuse
Healthcare associated (HCAP)	Pneumonia developing in patients not in an acute care medical facility but two or more risk factors for MDR pathogens	• Recent hospitalization ≥2 days within past 90 days • Nursing home or long-term care facility resident • Recent (past 30 days) antibiotic use, chemotherapy, wound care or infusion therapy at either a healthcare facility or home • Hemodialysis patients • Contact with a family member with infection caused by MDR pathogen
Hospital-acquired (HAP)	Pneumonia developing >48 hours after hospital admission	• Witnessed aspiration • COPD, ARDS, or coma • Administration of antacids, H_2-antagonists, or proton pump inhibitor • Supine position • Enteral nutrition, nasogastric tube • Reintubation, tracheostomy, or patient transport • Prior antibiotic exposure • Head trauma, ICP monitoring • Age >60 years • See healthcare associated for MDR risk factors
Ventilator associated (VAP)	Pneumonia developing >48 hours after intubation and mechanical ventilation	• Same as hospital acquired

ARDS, adult respiratory distress syndrome; CAP, community-acquired pneumonia; COPD, chronic obstructive pulmonary disease; HAP, hospital-acquired pneumonia; HCAP, healthcare-associated pneumonia; ICP, intracranial pressure; MDR, multidrug resistant; VAP, ventilator-associated pneumonia.

TABLE 85-7 Pulmonary Complications of Human Immunodeficiency Virus Infection

- Infections
  - Viruses
    - Cytomegalovirus
    - Herpes simplex virus
    - Varicella-zoster virus
    - Respiratory syncytial virus and other common respiratory pathogens (parainfluenza virus, adenovirus)
    - Measles virus
  - Bacteria
    - Pyogenic organisms (especially *S. pneumoniae, H. influenzae*; in late disease, *S. aureus* and gram-negative organisms)
    - *M. tuberculosis*
    - *M. avium* complex and other nontuberculous mycobacteria
  - Fungi
    - *Histoplasma capsulatum*
    - *Coccidioides immitis*
    - *Cryptococcus neoformans*
    - *Candida* species
    - *Aspergillus* species
  - Parasites
    - *Pneumocystis carinii*
    - *Toxoplasma gondii*
    - Cryptosporidia
    - *Strongyloides stercoralis*
- Malignancies
  - Kaposi's sarcoma
  - Non-Hodgkin's lymphoma
  - Smooth muscle tumors
- Lymphocytic interstitial pneumonitis
- Nonspecific interstitial pneumonitis
- Drug-induced pneumonitis

on comorbid conditions (e.g., heart disease, chronic kidney disease, immunocompromised, or dementia) than patients with CAP and are at a greater risk for MDR pathogens.[7,51] The more common pathogens isolated from residents of long-term care facilities/nursing homes have MRSA, enteric gram-negative rods, and *Pseudomonas* species.[7] Compared with patients with CAP, patients with HCAP are more likely to receive inappropriate antibiotics initially and have a higher risk of mortality.[59] Thus, it is important to recognize the difference between HCAP and CAP for appropriate empirical antibiotics.

Pneumonia in the HIV-Infected Patient

A broad range of pathogens can cause pneumonia in HIV infection (Table 85-7) including opportunistic infections such as *P. jiroveci* and *Mycobacterium* species.[60] These patients may be afflicted with pneumonia multiple times in their lifetime, particularly in the advanced stages of the disease, and a given episode may be caused by more than one species. The clinical presentation of pneumonia in HIV-infected persons frequently is not helpful in distinguishing one pathogen from another. The pneumonia usually is subacute in onset and consists of fever, nonproductive cough, and dyspnea. Radiographically, most of these entities produce a multilobular or diffuse pattern. Some practitioners initially treat the HIV-infected patient with pneumonia empirically; however, given the wide array of possible pathogens, more frequently a specific microbiologic diagnosis is aggressively pursued early in the patient's course through sputum induction or bronchoalveolar lavage to allow a rational choice of an antimicrobial regimen. The diagnosis and treatment of HIV-infected patients with pulmonary disease is discussed in detail in Chapter 103.

Pneumonia in the Neutropenic Host

Neutropenia in the cancer patient is a common complication of aggressive chemotherapy but occasionally results from the cancer itself. The risk of infection for the cytopenic patient is increased significantly when the absolute neutrophil count falls below 500 cells mm^3 (500×10^6/L) and the neutropenia persists for more than 7 days. For many patients, the duration of chemotherapy-induced cytopenia can be reduced by judicious application of colony-stimulating factors.[61]

The organisms that cause pneumonia in the cytopenic cancer patient include a broad range of bacteria and fungi. The most prominent among these are gram-positive bacteria (staphylococci and streptococci); others include enteric and nonenteric (particularly *P. aeruginosa*) gram-negative rods as well as the fungi (*Candida, Aspergillus*). The chest radiograph may reveal the lobar pattern typical of bacterial infection in the normal host, or it may exhibit a diffuse pattern. Sometimes the pneumonia remains invisible by chest radiograph until the neutropenia resolves. Noninfectious entities that may cause pulmonary symptoms include toxicity from radiation or chemotherapy or infiltration of the lung parenchyma by the tumor itself.

Hospital-Acquired Pneumonia

After the urinary tract and the bloodstream, the lungs are the most frequent site of infection acquired in the hospital. HAP is seen most commonly in critically ill patients and usually caused by bacteria.[7] Factors predisposing patients to the development of HAP include the severity of illness, duration of hospitalization, supine positioning, witnessed aspiration, coma, acute respiratory distress syndrome, patient transport, and prior antibiotic exposure (see Table 85-6). The strongest predisposing factor, however, is mechanical ventilation (intubation). The length of stay for hospital admissions is increased, on average, by 7 to 9 days for patients who develop HAP.[7]

The organisms most commonly associated with HAP are *S. aureus* and enteric (e.g., *K. pneumoniae* or *E. coli*) and nonenteric (e.g., *P. aeruginosa*) gram-negative bacilli, organisms that colonize the pharynx of the hospitalized, critically ill patient. Patients with longer lengths of hospital admission prior to the development of HAP are more likely to have MDR organisms.[7] The diagnosis of HAP usually is established by the presence of a new infiltrate on chest radiograph, fever, worsening respiratory status, and the appearance of thick, neutrophil-laden respiratory secretions. In actuality, the diagnosis often is difficult to make in the intensively ill patient with underlying lung pathology that itself can be associated with an abnormal changing radiograph, as occurs with congestive heart failure or chronic lung disease. If a patient develops fever, leukocytosis, and purulent sputum, and has positive sputum/tracheal cultures but radiographic imaging does not indicate new infiltrates, he or she may have tracheobronchitis as opposed to HAP.[7] Broad-spectrum antibiotics frequently are started empirically even in equivocal circumstances, with bronchoscopy reserved for poorly responsive patients.[7]

Gram-Positive Bacteria

S. aureus is a prominent cause of HAP and may result from hematogenous spread from a distant source. It is characteristically severe and accompanied by the formation of pneumatoceles (air-containing cavities within the lung). Infections caused by MDR organisms such as MRSA and vancomycin-intermediate and vancomycin-resistant *S. aureus* are increasing among patients with HAP. Group B *Streptococcus*, although rare in adults, is the most common cause of bacterial pneumonia among neonates, in whom it typically causes a clinical and radiographic picture nearly indistinguishable from hyaline membrane disease.[62]

Enteric Gram-Negative Bacteria

The enteric gram-negative bacteria are leading causes of HAP because the upper respiratory tract becomes rapidly colonized with gram-negative organisms after hospitalization, particularly among critically ill patients and those receiving antibiotics.[63] *K. pneumoniae* is the most frequently encountered pathogen among the gram-negative enteric bacteria, although the relative prominence of these organisms varies among hospitals. The gram-negative bacilli are associated with high mortality, sometimes exceeding 50%; their potential to produce significant morbidity and mortality has been enhanced by the emergence of highly MDR organisms in some hospital settings.[7]

Nonenteric Gram-Negative Bacteria

The most prominent nonenteric gram-negative rods associated with pneumonia include *P. aeruginosa*, *H. influenzae*, and *M. catarrhalis*. Like the enteric gram-negative organisms, *P. aeruginosa* is a frequent cause of HAP and is particularly prominent among neutropenic and burn patients.[7] In addition, cystic fibrosis patients suffer from chronic, multilobar infections with *P. aeruginosa*, as well as other *Pseudomonas* species, and *S. maltophilia* is an emerging pathogen[64]; these infections are punctuated with acute exacerbations. *H. influenzae* type b historically has been a prominent pathogen in childhood pneumonia. The incidence of all invasive disease due to this organism in the pediatric age group has dropped dramatically since the introduction of the conjugated *Haemophilus* vaccines in the late 1980s. However, two different clinical presentations of *H. influenzae* pneumonia still are seen in adults. The most common by far is the bronchopneumonia form, which develops most frequently for patients with underlying chronic lung disease and is believed to represent, in most patients, an exacerbation of chronic bronchitis. In the second form of *H. influenzae* pneumonia, segmental or lobar involvement predominates. The course of this illness is more acute, with sudden onset of cough, fever, and pleuritic chest pain. Finally, *M. catarrhalis*, an important cause of otitis media and sinusitis, is an increasingly important cause of lower respiratory tract infections in immunocompromised and hospitalized patients.

Anaerobic Bacteria

8 Anaerobic pneumonitis is most likely to occur in individuals predisposed to aspiration by impaired consciousness or dysphagia as the source for the anaerobic bacteria is generally the oral cavity/gingival crevice.[65] Bronchogenic carcinoma is an associated underlying condition. A variety of gram-positive and gram-negative anaerobic bacteria indigenous to the upper airway may cause pneumonitis when large quantities of oropharyngeal secretions are aspirated into the lower airways. The most common organisms identified are *B. melaninogenicus*, Fusobacteria, and anaerobic streptococci; polymicrobial infections with anaerobes and aerobes, such as *S. aureus*, *S. pneumoniae*, and gram-negative bacilli, are common.[65]

Early in the infection, clinical symptoms are similar to CAP with patients presenting with cough, low-grade fever, pulmonary infiltrates, and leukocytosis. The course of anaerobic pneumonia is typically indolent and patients are unlikely to have rigors. Other characteristic features are lung abscess, necrotizing pneumonia, and empyema. Anaerobic infections should be suspected if patients are predisposed to aspiration or have a chronic course, putrid sputum/breath, pulmonary necrosis, or empyema.[65] Chest radiographs reveal infiltrates typically located in dependent lung segments, and lung abscesses develop in 20% of patients 1 to 2 weeks into the course of the illness.

Ventilator-Associated Pneumonia

VAP is defined as pneumonia occurring >48 hours post–endotracheal intubation. The risk for developing pneumonia in the hospital increases by 6 to 21 times after a patient is intubated[7] because it bypasses the natural airway defenses against the migration of upper respiratory tract organisms into the lower tract. This situation is exacerbated by the wide use of acid-reducing drugs (e.g., H_2-receptor blocking agents, proton pump inhibitors) in the intensive care unit, which increases the pH of gastric secretions and may promote the proliferation of microorganisms in the upper GI tract. Subclinical microaspirations are events that occur routinely in intubated patients and result in the inoculation of bacteria-contaminated gastric contents into the lung and a higher incidence of nosocomial pneumonia.[66] Pneumonia that develops within 4 days of hospitalization is more likely to be caused by an antibiotic sensitive organism such as *S. pneumoniae*, *S. aureus*, or *Haemophilus* species, whereas infections developing later are more likely to be MDR (e.g., *P. aeruginosa*, MRSA, *Acinetobacter* species). Outbreaks of VAP may be caused occasionally by contaminated respiratory therapy equipment.

To date, there is no "gold standard" for diagnosing VAP; thus, an accurate diagnosis is challenging. Most intensivists agree that VAP should be suspected if new or persistent infiltrates are found on chest radiograph along with ≥2 of the following: purulent tracheal secretions, leukocytosis or leucopenia, and body temperature >38.3°C (>100.94°F).[9,66] Invasive (e.g., bronchoalveolar lavage) or noninvasive techniques may be used for obtaining samples of lower respiratory tract secretions for culture and sensitivity testing.[66]

Atypical Pneumonia

Legionella species, *Mycoplasma* species, *Chlamydia* species, viruses, and fungi are recognized causes of pneumonia syndromes in all age groups. The designation *atypical pneumonia*, distinct from the typical bacterial pneumonia course seen most commonly in adults, has been used to describe the illness caused by many of these agents.[52,67]

Legionella pneumophila

Of the several *Legionella* species known to cause pneumonia in humans, *L. pneumophila* is by far the most important, accounting for 4% to 9% of all CAPs in North America and Europe.[52] *Legionella*, a small, gram-negative, non–spore-forming bacilli, is an aquatic organism that is transmitted by inhalation of aerosols containing the organism or by microaspiration of contaminated water. Outbreaks of illness caused by *L. pneumophila* have been linked to excavation sites and to contaminated water from air conditioners and showers. Person-to-person transmission has not been demonstrated. In addition to epidemics, *L. pneumophila* causes sporadic illness that peaks in summer and fall. Individuals who are male, middle aged or older, immunocompromised, chronic bronchitics, or cigarette smokers, or have used tumor necrosis factor-α antagonists are at increased risk.[52]

Infection with *L. pneumophila* is characterized by multisystem involvement and the severity of the infection can range from mild to severe, rapidly progressive pneumonia.[57,67] It has a gradual onset, with prominent constitutional symptoms (e.g., malaise, lethargy, weakness, anorexia) occurring early in the course of the illness. A dry, nonproductive cough is present initially and becomes productive of mucoid or purulent sputum over several days. Fevers exceeding 40°C (104°F) develop in more than half of patients, typically are unremitting, and are associated with a relative bradycardia. Pleuritic chest pain and progressive dyspnea may be seen. Extrapulmonary symptoms, particularly diarrhea, nausea, and vomiting, remain evident throughout the course of the illness. Myalgias and arthralgias also occur. Substantial changes in the patient's mental status, often out of proportion to the degree of fever, are seen in approximately one fourth of patients. Obtundation, hallucinations, grand mal seizures, and focal neurologic findings are also associated with this illness. Chest radiographs initially reveal patchy alveolar infiltrates that may be bilateral and asymmetric. Pulmonary infiltrates may worsen even when the patient is receiving appropriate antibiotics. Progression to lobar or multilobar consolidation is frequent, as are small pleural effusions.

Laboratory findings include leukocytosis with a predominance of mature and immature granulocytes in 50% to 75% of patients. Urinalysis may reveal proteinuria, hematuria, and casts; liver function tests may be abnormal and increases in serum creatine phosphokinase have occurred in patients with *L. pneumophila*.[67] Hyponatremia and hypophosphatemia (typically occurring early in infection) have been reported frequently.[67] Because *L. pneumophila* stains poorly with commonly used stains, routine microscopic examination of sputum is of little diagnostic value. Although it exhibits slow growth and has highly selective growth requirements, *L. pneumophila* has been isolated successfully from tissue using a specialized medium. Direct fluorescent antibody examination of respiratory tract secretions, lung tissue, or pleural fluid is the most rapid means of establishing the diagnosis. The sensitivity of this method approaches 70% for sputum and 90% for lung tissue, and diagnostic specificity is high for both. Commercially available urine antigen tests have been developed for *L. pneumophila*. These tests are 70% sensitive and remain positive for weeks, even after effective antibiotics have been started. Because these diagnostic tests are unavailable in many clinical laboratories, the diagnosis of Legionnaires' disease often is presumptive and based on a suggestive clinical presentation.

M. pneumoniae

The mycoplasmas are included in their own taxonomy labeled *Mollicutes*. Although their small size and filterability are similar to viruses, the structure of their ribosomal RNA indicates that they have evolved from bacteria, and, unlike any virus, they contain cytoplasm and can replicate in an extracellular environment. They are distinguished from eubacteria by their low genetic content and have a parasitic relationship with their hosts.[52] In addition, the mycoplasmas lack a cell wall and are surrounded instead by a lipid membrane. The latter characteristic explains the resistance of these pathogens to cell wall–active antibiotics.

M. pneumoniae causes human disease throughout the year, with a slightly increased incidence in fall and early winter. During the summer months when other causes of pneumonia are less common, *M. pneumoniae* is responsible for a greater proportion of cases. Both infection and disease from *M. pneumoniae* are common, with 10% to 30% of the cases of CAP in children and young adults attributed to this organism.[68] In enclosed populations, such as military recruits and college dormitory residents, it may cause more than 50% of the cases of CAP. Infection is spread by close person-to-person contact, and the incubation period is 2 to 3 weeks. *M. pneumoniae* infections are unusual in children younger than 5 years and show a peak incidence in older children and young adults. Only 3% to 10% of persons infected with *M. pneumoniae* develop pneumonia, with the majority of respiratory tract involvement manifested as pharyngitis and tracheobronchitis. Asymptomatic infection is common.

M. pneumoniae usually presents with a gradual onset of fever, headache, and malaise, with the appearance 3 to 5 days after the onset of illness of a persistent, hacking cough that initially is nonproductive. Sore throat, ear pain, and rhinorrhea often are present. Chills are seen only occasionally, and pleuritic pain is uncommon. Lung findings generally are limited to rales and rhonchi; findings of consolidation are rare. Nonpulmonary manifestations of *M. pneumoniae* are extremely common and include nausea, vomiting, diarrhea, myalgias, arthralgias, polyarticular arthritis, and skin rashes while myocarditis, pericarditis, hemolytic anemia, meningoencephalitis, cranial neuropathies, and Guillain-Barré syndrome have also been reported.[52,69] Systemic symptoms generally clear in 1 to 2 weeks, whereas respiratory symptoms may persist for up to 4 weeks. Although the course of mycoplasma pneumonia usually is benign and self-limited, severe respiratory disease may develop in patients with sickle cell disease, agammaglobulinemia, COPD, and splenectomy.[52,67]

Radiographic findings generally are more impressive than the patient's physical findings and include patchy or interstitial infiltrates, which are seen most commonly in the lower lobes.[67] Small unilateral, transient pleural effusions are common, but large effusions and empyema are rare. Radiographic abnormalities resolve slowly, and 4 to 6 weeks may be required for complete resolution.

Sputum Gram stain may reveal mononuclear or polymorphonuclear leukocytes, with no predominant organism. Although *M. pneumoniae* can be cultured from respiratory secretions using specialized medium, its growth is slow, and 2 to 3 weeks may be necessary for culture identification. Indirect evidence of infection by *M. pneumoniae* is the presence of elevated levels of serum cold hemagglutinins. These immunoglobulin M antibodies develop in approximately half of patients with mycoplasmal pneumonia and can be elevated in other illnesses, especially viral infection. A definitive diagnosis also can be made by demonstrating a fourfold or greater rise in serum antibodies to *M. pneumoniae*. However, because this test also requires 2 to 4 weeks for results, the diagnosis of mycoplasmal pneumonia during the acute phase of the illness must be based on the characteristic history, appropriate clinical setting, and typical physical findings.

C. pneumoniae

C. pneumoniae has received the new taxonomic classification of *Chlamydophila*; however, it may still be referred to as *Chlamydia pneumoniae* in some references.[12] *C. pneumoniae*, formally designated the Taiwan acute respiratory (*TWAR*) agent after the laboratory designations for the first two isolates, is antigenically similar to *C. psittaci*. *C. pneumoniae* infection is ubiquitous worldwide; ~80% of the population has been infected by adulthood,[52] but only a small percentage of infections result in clinically apparent pneumonia. Conversely, approximately 5% to 15% of pneumonia is associated with this pathogen.[12] Primary infection with *Chlamydia* pneumonia typically occurs in young adults and is characterized by mild respiratory symptoms with a gradual onset (e.g., incubation period about 21 days). Constitutional manifestations, particularly fever, headache, and hoarseness, are common.[52] The radiographic findings are nonspecific and usually consist of multilobular interstitial infiltrates with circumscribed lesions.[67] Immunity is incomplete, and reinfection with *C. pneumoniae* is common, particularly among the elderly. Definitive diagnosis of *C. pneumoniae*–associated pneumonia depends on identification of the organism in sputum. Culture of this organism is difficult, and commercially available antigen detection systems are insensitive.

Viral Pneumonia

Viruses are an uncommon cause of pneumonia in adults, except in the immunosuppressed.[7] Influenza virus, usually type A, is the most common viral cause of pneumonia in the adult civilian population[5]; other viruses causing adult CAP include RSV, adenoviruses, parainfluenza, and human metapneumovirus.[5] In contrast, viruses are by far the most common agents producing pneumonia in infants and young children, up to 80% in <2-year-olds, with RSV accounting for most cases; other common viruses in children are parainfluenza, adenovirus, human metapneumovirus, bocavirus, and rhinovirus.[6,40,52]

All viral respiratory tract infections occur more commonly in the winter, and rapid person-to-person spread through susceptible populations is typical. Underlying cardiac or pulmonary disease predisposes to an increased incidence and severity of viral lower respiratory tract infection, especially with influenza virus in adults and RSV in children. Radiographic findings are nonspecific and include bronchial wall thickening and perihilar and diffuse interstitial infiltrates. Pleural effusions may be seen, especially in adenovirus and parainfluenza pneumonia.

The clinical pictures produced by respiratory viruses are sufficiently variable and overlap to such a degree that an etiologic diagnosis cannot be made confidently based on clinical grounds alone. Although virus isolation in tissue culture is still considered the gold standard, it is time consuming and technically demanding; a period of ≥7 days often is required for virus identification[3]; thus, this method usually cannot be used for definitive diagnosis during the acute phase of illness. Serologic tests for virus-specific antibodies are used often in epidemiologic and surveillance studies of viral infections since the diagnostic fourfold rise in titer between acute and convalescent phase sera may require 2 to 3 weeks to develop.[3] Rapid antigen testing for the influenza virus (some tests distinguishing types A and B) and RSV is available; however, cost, high false-positive rates, and 50% to 70% sensitivity are considerations for its utility during nonpeak seasons.[3,5,7] Viral testing with molecular techniques provides increased utility for patient care with high sensitivity, rapid results and the ability to detect new and emerging pathogens. Numerous testing methods are available, not all in the United States, including real-time PCR, solid and liquid microarrays, mass spectrometry, target-enriched multiplexing PCR, and multiplex ligation-dependent probe amplification, to name a few.[3]

Viruses that have emerged in recent decades and caused significant outbreaks include avian influenza H5N1, severe acute respiratory syndrome coronavirus (SARS-CoV), and swine influenza H1N1.[70–72] The first known cases of humans infected with avian H5N1 subtype occurred in Hong Kong in 1997, with 6 deaths among 18 infected patients. Signs and symptoms typical of the H5N1 virus are those common to other subtypes; however, pneumonia, respiratory distress syndrome, lymphopenia, and clotting abnormalities tend to occur rapidly in patients infected with this highly virulent subtype. In April 2009, a novel influenza A virus of swine origin, H1N1, was identified as the causative pathogen in an outbreak of respiratory illness and influenza-like illness in Mexico.[72] Signs and symptoms of the H1N1 virus are similar to other subtypes; however, more serious infections have resulted in hospitalization and death. It has also affected normally healthy young adults as opposed to other flu viruses, which tend to be more severe in the young and the elderly.

SARS-CoV manifested in China in November 2002 and was an extremely contagious atypical pneumonia.[73,74] The virus is transmitted primarily via large-droplet spread; however, surface contamination and airborne and fecal spread are possible. Signs and symptoms associated with SARS include high fever, myalgias, headache, diarrhea, and a dry nonproductive cough. Respiratory symptoms may progress to shortness of breath and hypoxemia, necessitating the need for intubation and mechanical ventilation. Diagnostic tests for patients suspected of contracting SARS should include chest x-ray film, blood cultures, sputum cultures and Gram stain, pulse oximetry, and identification of other potential pathogens, including influenza A and B, *Legionella*, and RSV. For unclear reasons, SARS appears to be less severe for pediatric patients.

Tuberculosis

The acid-fast bacillus *M. tuberculosis* causes tuberculosis and is spread person to person by inhalation of droplets. After years of steady decline, the number of cases of pneumonia caused by *M. tuberculosis* in the United States began to increase in the middle to late 1980s. The new epidemic was a consequence of an increased incidence among prison inmates, IV drug abusers, immigrants, and, most prominently, HIV-infected patients.[75] It is most prominent in urban neighborhoods afflicted with crowded conditions and poor access to healthcare. Unlike previous eras in which tuberculosis was seen most frequently in elderly men, infection currently is identified in increasing numbers of young minority adults. As mentioned, the resurgence of tuberculosis is at least partially related to coinfection with HIV; HIV-infected patients are more likely to develop symptomatic disease with its associated fits of coughing than are their immunocompetent counterparts, and this enables further spread of infection. Other groups prone to tuberculosis include the homeless and patients in chronic care facilities and homes for the elderly. Fortunately, since 1992, the incidence of tuberculosis in the United States has declined, reaching a record low. However, the incidence of tuberculosis worldwide continues to increase. Both the sustained worldwide increase in tuberculosis and the reemergence of tuberculosis in the United States are important reasons for the development of multiple-drug resistance, that is, mycobacteria that are resistant to two or more of the first-line antituberculosis drugs. Infection caused by these organisms is poorly responsive to alternative therapy and is associated with mortality rates exceeding 50% (see Chap. 90 for a detailed discussion on the diagnosis and treatment of tuberculosis).

TREATMENT

Desired Outcome

Eradication of the offending organism through selection of the appropriate antibiotic and complete clinical cure are the goals of therapy for bacterial pneumonia. Therapy should minimize associated morbidity, including one or both of the following: reversible or irreversible disease and drug-induced organ toxicity (e.g., renal, lung, or hepatic dysfunction). Most cases of viral pneumonia are self-limiting, although therapy of influenza pneumonia with specific antiviral agents (oseltamivir and zanamivir) may hasten recovery. All efforts should focus on the design of the most cost-effective approach to therapy. Whenever possible, the oral (vs. parenteral) route for drug administration should be selected, encouraging outpatient management rather than hospitalization.

General Approach to Treatment

9 The first priority in assessing the patient with pneumonia is to evaluate the adequacy of respiratory function and to determine the presence of signs of systemic illness, specifically dehydration or sepsis with resulting circulatory collapse. Oxygen or, in severe cases, mechanical ventilation and fluid resuscitation should be provided as necessary. Further supportive care of the patient with pneumonia includes humidified oxygen for hypoxemia, administration of bronchodilators (albuterol) when bronchospasm is present, and chest physiotherapy with postural drainage if evidence of retained secretions is present. Additional therapeutic adjuncts include adequate hydration (IV if necessary), optimal nutritional support, and control of fever. Appropriate sputum samples may be obtained to determine the microbiologic etiology. Rehydration should be provided to replace losses that may have occurred as a result of fever, poor intake, and/or associated vomiting. Selection of an appropriate antimicrobial must be made based on the patient's probable or documented microbiology, distribution in the respiratory tract, side effects, and cost. Respiratory tract infection diagnosis and treatment guideline reports have been published by authoritative professional organizations that focus on proper treatment regimens and should be consulted for evidence-based treatment recommendations across the spectrum of community- and/or hospital-associated pneumonias.[76,77]

Clinical **Controversy. . .**

Various adjunctive therapy options have been studied for their potential benefits in CAP in recent years. Drugs that have been studied include corticosteroids, prostaglandin inhibitors, statins, immunoglobulin therapy, mediator-specific immunomodulators, angiotensinogen-converting enzyme inhibitors, and oral hypoglycemic agents. Proposed mechanisms for some of the drugs have centered on protective effects (e.g., vasodilation, cough reflex) and antiinflammatory effects. Differences in study design and patient populations have made it difficult to determine if there are any true benefits these therapies may have in CAP.[78]

Pharmacologic Therapy

Antibiotic Concentrations

Antibiotic concentrations in respiratory secretions in excess of the pathogen MIC are necessary for successful treatment of pulmonary infections.[77] The concept of a blood–bronchus barrier, analogous but dissimilar to the blood–brain barrier, has been used to assess the characteristics of drug penetration into pulmonary secretions. The ability of a drug to penetrate respiratory secretions depends on multiple physicochemical factors, including molecular size, lipid solubility, and degree of ionization at serum and biologic fluid pH and extent of protein binding. Studies performed in animals and cystic fibrosis patients suggest that larger molecular size favors the accumulation of drugs in bronchial secretions. This finding contrasts with data on drug penetration of other physiologic compartments, such as the cerebrospinal fluid, and may be a result of the trapping of lower-molecular-weight compounds in mucin pores. Nevertheless, the rate at which a drug may accumulate in certain respiratory secretions appears to remain an important factor relative to the drug's clinical efficacy in treating pulmonary infections. The unionized form of drug and lipid solubility also appears to favor drug penetration. Of note, the pH of the infected bronchi often is more acidic than that of normal tissue and blood. These factors combined underscore the importance of considering the inhaled route of antimicrobial drugs for the treatment of patients with moderate to severe pneumonia, particularly in high-risk patient groups.[79,80]

Clinical **Controversy...**

Prior to the availability of newer β-lactam and fluoroquinolone antibiotics possessing consistently potent activity against multiple gram-negative pathogens, some investigators promoted the administration of antibiotics by direct endotracheal instillation. This method of drug administration attempts to provide increased topical concentrations of antibiotics that do not appear to penetrate respiratory secretions effectively while reducing the likelihood of systemic toxicity. In addition, greater local concentrations of antibiotics, particularly of the polymyxins and aminoglycosides, are believed to overcome partially the substantial decrease in antibiotic bioactivity observed when these agents interact with the purulent material present in infectious foci. Despite these potential theoretical advantages, the role of antibiotic aerosols or direct endotracheal instillation in clinical practice remains controversial and guidelines do not recommend the routine use of aerosolized antibiotics.[7,77,79–81]

Limited data are available for assessing the influence of drug protein binding on the rate and amount of respiratory secretion penetration. Clearly, it is the free antibiotic fraction reaching the infected site capable of binding to the bacterial cell target that is responsible for antibacterial activity. Given that the degree of protein binding influences a drug's ability to traverse membranes, a similar relationship would be expected within the lung. However, focusing on the absolute amount of an antibiotic bound to plasma/tissue proteins without accounting for the drug's overall antibacterial potency is errant. To completely assess an antibiotic's therapeutic potential in the treatment of pneumonia or any infectious process, it is prudent to assess the antibiotic's integrated pharmacokinetic–pharmacodynamic (PK-PD) characteristics (e.g., bacterial killing may be concentration dependent or time dependent) that account for the drug's degree of binding to serum proteins, tissue distribution, and in vitro potency. These concepts relating to antibiotic activity and overall drug penetration of respiratory secretions underscore the importance of applying the advances realized in our knowledge of antimicrobial PK and PD to the design of optimal antibiotic dosing regimens. Integration of an individual antimicrobial drug's PK-PD has afforded the development of just such optimal antibiotic dosing regimens (improved efficacy and safety) based on drug- and patient-specific factors.[76,77] A primary example of antibiotic PK-PD–designed optimal dosing is reflected in the clinical practice of administering certain antibiotics (aminoglycosides) to achieve high peak serum concentrations on the assumption that higher (and possibly more effective) biologic fluid concentrations of the drug will be achieved. The aminoglycosides are large polar molecules that diffuse poorly into tissue and respiratory secretions; however, with increasing concentrations obtained with once-daily dosing, increased target-tissue concentrations would be expected with increasing individual doses. Further, recognizing that the peak drug concentration-to-pathogen MIC ratio (Cmax:MIC) is the primary PK-PD correlate for aminoglycosides and that the target Cmax:MIC ratio for aminoglycosides is ~10, the single daily dose strategy is most likely to achieve the desired PK-PD target at the desired anatomic site. Similar is the case for the so-called respiratory fluoroquinolones (e.g., levofloxacin, moxifloxacin, gemifloxacin) higher individual dose therapy targeting a greater Cmax:MIC ratio or the more commonly targeted area under the concentration–time curve (AUC)-to-pathogen MIC ratio, that is, AUC:MIC, for fluoroquinolones. The target 24-hour AUC:MIC ratio for fluoroquinolones is >35 (possible minimum of 25) for gram-positive and >125 (possible minimum of 100) for gram-negative pathogens. For greatest probability of success, the antibiotic concentrations projected in these PK-PD correlates should include the expected free (not protein-bound) antibiotic concentration. Conversely, concentration-dependent killing characteristics best correlate with successful therapy with the β-lactam/carbapenem and macrolide classes of antimicrobials.[76,77] See eChapter 24 and Chapter 83 for more in-depth discussion of antibiotic concepts.

Sputum is frequently assessed as possibly representing the PD interface for pulmonary infections. It is only one of many pulmonary fluids and secretions, and it may serve as a reservoir for pathogen growth. These beliefs have led many investigators to assess antibiotic concentrations in sputum, frequently describing sputum drug concentrations as a ratio of serum to sputum drug concentration. Although sputum drug concentrations provide some insight into the characteristics of drug penetration of respiratory secretions, caution should be exercised in the interpretation of these data. Data describing sputum drug concentrations often are difficult to interpret because of differences in analytic techniques, method of sputum sampling, and random nature of sampling times relative to drug dose. Moreover, representation of sputum drug concentrations as a ratio of serum drug concentration can be misleading and most probably should be described relative to absolute drug concentration or apparent area under the drug concentration versus time curve in sputum. To more accurately describe the distribution characteristics of antimicrobial agents in sputum, research studies should be designed to allow sequential repeated sputum sampling over a specified dosage interval under both first-dose and steady-state conditions. Thus, until greater sophistication is achieved in our understanding of the relationships between antibiotic concentrations in specific anatomic sites, plasma (blood)-based integrated PK-PD correlates should be used for antibiotic and dose selection.

Selection of Antimicrobial Agents

Treatment of bacterial pneumonia, like the treatment of most infectious diseases, initially involves the empirical use of a relatively broad-spectrum antibiotic that is effective against probable pathogens after appropriate cultures and specimens for laboratory evaluation have been obtained.[5,7,81] Therapy should be narrowed to cover specific pathogens after the results of cultures are known. Multiple factors that help to define the potential pathogens involved include

TABLE 85-8 Evidence-Based Empirical Antimicrobial Therapy for Pneumonia in Adults[a]

Clinical Setting	Usual Pathogens	Empirical Therapy
Outpatient/Community Acquired		
Previously healthy	*S. pneumoniae, M. pneumoniae, H. influenzae, C. pneumoniae, M. catarrhalis*	Macrolide/azalide,[b] or tetracycline[c]
	Viral	Oseltamivir or zanamivir if <48° from onset of symptoms
Comorbidities (diabetes, heart/lung/liver/renal disease, alcoholism)		Fluoroquinolone[d] or β-lactam + macrolide[b]
Elderly	*S. pneumoniae*, gram-negative bacilli	Piperacillin/tazobactam or cephalosporin[e] or carbapenem[f]
Regions with >25% rate of macrolide-resistant *S. pneumoniae*		Fluoroquinolone[d] or β-lactam + macrolide[b]/tetracycline
Inpatient/Community Acquired		
Non-ICU	*S. pneumoniae, H. influenzae, M. pneumoniae, C. pneumoniae, Legionella* sp.	Fluoroquinolone[d] or β-lactam + macrolide[b]/tetracycline
ICU	*S. pneumoniae, S. aureus, Legionella* sp., gram-negative bacilli, *H. influenzae*	β-Lactam + macrolide[b]/fluoroquinolone[d]
	If *P. aeruginosa* suspected	Piperacillin/tazobactam or meropenem or cefepime + fluoroquinolone[d]/AMG/azithromycin; or β-lactam + AMG + azithromycin/respiratory fluoroquinolone[d]
	If MRSA suspected	Above + vancomycin or linezolid
	Viral	Oseltamivir or zanamivir ± antibiotics for 2° infection
Hospital Acquired, Ventilator Associated, or Healthcare Associated		
No risk factors for MDR pathogens	*S. pneumoniae, H. influenzae*, MSSA enteric gram-negative bacilli	Ceftriaxone or fluoroquinolone[d] or ampicillin/sulbactam or ertapenem or doripenem
Risk factors for MDR pathogen	*P. aeruginosa, K. pneumoniae* (ESBL), *Acinetobacter* sp.	Antipseudomonal cephalosporin[e] or antipseudomonal carbapenem or β-lactam/β-lactamase + antipseudomonal fluoroquinolone[d] or AMG[g]
	If MRSA or *Legionella* sp. suspected	Above + vancomycin or linezolid
Aspiration	*S. aereus*, enteric gram-negative bacilli	Penicillin or clindamycin or piperacillin/tazobactam + AMG[g]
	Anaerobes	Clindamycin, β-lactam/β-lactamase, or carbapenem
Atypical Pneumonia[h]		
Legionella pneumophilia		Fluoroquinolone,[d] doxycycline, or azithromycin
Mycoplasma pneumonia		Fluoroquinolone,[d] doxycycline, or azithromycin
Chlamydophila pneumonia		Fluoroquinolone,[d] doxycycline, or azithromycin
SARS		Fluoroquinolone[d] or macrolides[b]
Avian influenza		Oseltamivir
H1N1 influenza		Oseltamivir

MRSA, methicillin-resistant *Staphylococcus aureus*; AMG, aminoglycoside; SARS, severe acute respiratory syndrome; ESBL, extended-spectrum β-lactamases; MDR, multidrug resistant; MSSA, methicillin-sensitive *Staphylococcus aureus*.

[a]See the section Selection of Antimicrobial Agents.
[b]Macrolide/azalide: erythromycin, clarithromycin, and azithromycin.
[c]Tetracycline: tetracycline, HC1, and doxycycline.
[d]Fluoroquinolone: ciprofloxacin, levofloxacin, and moxifloxacin.
[e]Antipseudomonal cephalosporin: cefepime and ceftazidime.
[f]Antipseudomonal carbapenem: imipenem and meropenem.
[g]Aminoglycoside: amikacin, gentamicin, and tobramycin.
[h]For tuberculosis, see Chapter 90.

Data from references 5, 7, and 52.

patient age, previous and current medication history, underlying disease(s), major organ function, and present clinical status. These factors must be evaluated to select an appropriate and effective empirical antibiotic regimen as well as the most appropriate route for drug administration (oral or parenteral). For a more detailed discussion on the principles of antibiotic selection, see Chapter 83.

Numerous antibiotics are available, and many are effective in the treatment of bacterial pneumonia. Superiority of one antibiotic over another when both demonstrate similar dose-normalized in vitro activity and tissue distribution characteristics is difficult to define. Our opinions on appropriate empirical choices for the treatment of bacterial pneumonias relative to a patient's underlying disease are listed in Table 85-8 for adults and Table 85-9 for children. A complete listing of antimicrobial agents for specific pathogens is beyond the scope of this chapter and is presented in Chapter 83.

A patient's medical history of responding/not responding to one of these antibiotics in the recent past will assist greatly in the decision to continue their use. In contrast and for patients with risk factors, regardless of the patient's setting at the time of infection, that is, community, long-term care facility, acute care hospital, etc., the fluoroquinolone antibiotics represent important treatment tools based on their highly favorable PK (tissue and intracellular distribution) and PD (potency, broad spectrum) characteristics combined with ease of administration (IV, oral) and patient tolerability. Furthermore, optimal dosing directed by the projected 24-hour free fluoroquinolone AUC-to-pathogen MIC ratio (see above) has markedly decreased the emergence of pathogen resistance, fostered maximal bacteriologic kill, and enhanced patient safety.

Table 85-10 lists dosages for selected antibiotics used for the treatment of bacterial pneumonia. The large number of expensive drugs mandates critical evaluation for formulary selection and clinical use. Similarities of in vitro activity, resistance to bacterial-inactivating enzymes, and overall effectiveness often make rational therapeutic decisions difficult and even appear random. However, some general principles can be applied to guide rational antibiotic choice, including direct comparison of the antibiotic's likely attainment of the defined PK-PD target correlate for specific bacterial species within the infected site. An understanding and application of

TABLE 85-9 Empirical Antimicrobial Therapy for Pneumonia in Pediatric Patients[a]

Clinical Setting	Usual Pathogen(s)	Empirical Therapy
Outpatient/Community Acquired		
<1 month	Group B *Streptococcus*, *H. influenzae* (nontypeable), *E. coli*, *S. aureus*, *Listeria*	Ampicillin/sulbactam, cephalosporin,[b] carbapenem[c]
	CMV, RSV, adenovirus	Ribavirin for RSV[d]
1–3 months	*C. pneumoniae*, possibly *Ureaplasma*, CMV, *Pneumocystis carinii* (afebrile pneumonia syndrome)	Macrolide/azalide,[e] trimethoprim–sulfamethoxazole
	S. pneumoniae, *S. aureus*	Semisynthetic penicillin[f] or cephalosporin[g]
Preschool-aged children	Viral (rhinovirus, RSV, influenza A and B, parainfluenzae, adenovirus, human metapneumovirus, coronavirus)	Antimicrobial therapy not routinely required
Previously healthy, fully immunized infants and preschool children with suspected mild–moderate bacterial CAP	*S. pneumoniae* *M. pneumoniae*, other atypical	Amoxicillin, cephalosporin[b,g] Macrolide/azalide or fluoroquinolone
Previously healthy, fully immunized school-aged children and adolescents with mild–moderate CAP	*S. pneumoniae* *M. pneumoniae*, other atypical	Amoxicillin, cephalosporin,[b,g] or fluoroquinolone Macrolide/azalide, fluoroquinolone, or tetracycline
Moderate–severe CAP during influenza virus outbreak	Influenza A and B, other viruses	Oseltamivir or zanamivir
Inpatient/Community Acquired		
Fully immunized infants and school-aged children	*S. pneumoniae* CA-MRSA *M. pneumoniae*, *C. pneumoniae*	Ampicillin, penicillin G, cephalosporin[b] *β*-Lactam + vancomycin/clindamycin *β*-Lactam + macrolide/fluoroquinolone/doxycycline
Not fully immunized infants and children; regions with invasive penicillin-resistant pneumococcal strains; patients with life-threatening infections	*S. pneumoniae, PCN resistant* MRSA *M. pneumoniae*, other atypical pathogens	Cephalosporin[b] Add vancomycin/clindamycin Macrolide/azalide[e] + *β*-lactam/doxycycline/fluoroquinolone

CMV, cytomegalovirus; RSV, respiratory syncytial virus; CAP, community-acquired pneumonia; MRSA, methicillin resistant *S. aureus*.

[a]See the section Selection of Antimicrobial Agents.
[b]Third-generation cephalosporin: ceftriaxone and cefotaxime. Note that cephalosporins are not active against *Listeria*.
[c]Carbapenem: imipenem–cilastatin and meropenem.
[d]See text for details regarding possible ribavirin treatment for RSV infection.
[e]Macrolide/azalide: erythromycin and clarithromycin/azithromycin.
[f]Semisynthetic penicillin: nafcillin and oxacillin.
[g]Second-generation cephalosporin: cefuroxime and cefprozil.
Data from reference 6.

inherent drug characteristics appears to be of the utmost importance for the selection of an optimal therapeutic regimen. Thus, whenever possible, identification of the causative pathogen and expected/defined antibiotic activity (e.g., MIC) is of paramount importance to the selection/design of the optimal antibiotic regimen.

Community-Acquired Pneumonia

Tables 85-8 and 85-9 provide evidence-based guidelines for the treatment of CAP in adults[5] and children,[6] respectively. The bacterial causes are relatively constant, even across geographic areas and patient populations. Unfortunately, pathogen resistance to standard antimicrobials is increasing (e.g., penicillin-resistant pneumococci), necessitating careful attention by the clinician to local and regional bacterial susceptibility patterns.[50] Thus, whenever possible, initial therapy should be based on presumed antibacterial susceptibility and consist of older, less-expensive agents, with newer and more expensive antibiotics reserved for unresponsive illness or special circumstances. Indiscriminate use of recently introduced agents increases healthcare costs and, in some instances (e.g., widespread use of fluoroquinolones), induces resistance among a significant percentage of community-acquired organisms.[5] The rapidly evolving epidemiology of bacterial resistance, including the increasing emergence of penicillin-resistant *S. pneumoniae* in many areas of the United States and Europe, forces the clinician to be vigilant and knowledgeable about antibiotic sensitivity patterns in each community. Indiscriminate use of antimicrobials for treatment of pneumonia has contributed to the problem of antimicrobial resistance, underscoring the need for defining the optimal antibiotic regimen for each patient.

9 Evidence-based empirical therapy differs among outpatients, hospitalized patients, and hospitalized patients admitted to an intensive care unit (Tables 85-8 and 85-9).[5,6] Antimicrobial therapy should be initiated for hospitalized patients with acute pneumonia within 8 hours of admission because an increase in mortality has been demonstrated when therapy was delayed beyond 8 hours of admission.

Healthcare-Associated Pneumonia

It is important to identify patients at risk for HCAP and initiate appropriate empirical antibiotic therapy since these patients are at risk for MDR organisms. Delaying treatment of appropriate antibiotics in these patients increases mortality.[51] Antibiotic selection will be similar to those used in HAP and VAP. Broad-spectrum antibiotics should be used empirically for pneumonia developing ≥5 days after hospital admission or if the patient has risk factors for MDR pathogens.[7] See Table 85-8 for recommended empirical antimicrobial therapy.

Hospital-Acquired Pneumonia

10 Antibiotic selection within the hospital environment demands greater care because of constant changes in antibiotic resistance patterns in vitro and in vivo. Ironically, some *β*-lactam antibiotics, which were developed to treat MDR hospital-acquired organisms, can themselves induce broad-spectrum bacterial *β*-lactamases and thereby lead to even greater problems with resistance.[77] These facts underscore the importance of regularly documenting the epidemiology of pathogens and infectious diseases within a specific practice or institution. As a result, an antimicrobial agent for a specific

TABLE 85-10 Antibiotic Doses for Treatment of Bacterial Pneumonia

Antibiotic Class	Antibiotic	Brand Name	Daily Antibiotic Dose[a] Pediatric	Adult (Total Dose/Day)
Penicillin	Ampicillin ± sulbactam	Unasyn®	150–200 mg/kg/day	6–12 g
	Amoxicillin ± clavulanate[b]	Augmentin®	45–100 mg/kg/day	0.75–1 g
	Piperacillin/tazobactam	Zosyn®	200–300 mg/kg/day	12–18 g
	Penicillin		100,000–250,000 units/kg/day	12–18 million units
Extended-spectrum cephalosporins	Ceftriaxone	Rocephin®	50–75 mg/kg/day	1–2 g
	Cefotaxime	Claforan®	150 mg/kg/day	2–12 g
	Ceftazidime	Fortaz®/Tazicef®	90–150 mg/kg/day	4–6 g
	Cefepime	Maxipime®	100–150 mg/kg/day	2–6 g
Macrolide/azalide	Clarithromycin	Biaxin®	15 mg/kg/day	0.5–1 g
	Erythromycin	Ery-Tab®	30–50 mg/kg/day	1–2 g
	Azithromycin	Zithromax®	10 mg/kg × 1 day, and then 5 mg/kg/day× 4 days	500 mg day 1, and then 250 mg/day × 4 days
Fluoroquinolones[c]	Moxifloxacin	Avelox®	—	400 mg
	Gemifloxacin	Factive®	—	320 mg
	Levofloxacin	Levaquin®	8–20 mg/kg/day	750 mg
	Ciprofloxacin	Cipro®	30 mg/kg/day	1.2 g
Tetracycline[d]	Doxycycline	Monodox®/Doxy 100™	2–5 mg/kg/day	100–200 mg
	Tetracycline HCl		25–50 mg/kg/day	1–2 g
Aminoglycosides	Gentamicin		7.5–10 mg/kg/day	7.5 mg/kg
	Tobramycin		7.5–10 mg/kg/day	7.5 mg/kg
Carbapenems	Imipenem	Primaxin®	60–100 mg/kg/day	2–4 g
	Meropenem	Merrem®	30–60 mg/kg/day	1–3 g
Other	Vancomycin		45–60 mg/kg/day	2–3 g
	Linezolid	Zyvox®	20–30 mg/kg/day	1.2 g
	Clindamycin	Cleocin®	30–40 mg/kg/day	1.8 g

[a]Doses can be increased for more severe disease and may require modification for patients with organ dysfunction.
[b]Higher-dose amoxicillin and amoxicillin/clavulanate (e.g., 90 mg/kg/day) are used for penicillin-resistant *S. pneumoniae*.
[c]Fluoroquinolones have been avoided for pediatric patients because of the potential for cartilage damage; however, they have been used for MDR bacterial infection safely and effectively in infants and children (see text).
[d]Tetracyclines are rarely used in pediatric patients, particularly in those younger than 8 years because of tetracycline-induced permanent tooth discoloration.

infectious disease favored in one practice site may not be the most desirable selection in another site despite similarities in size and patient profile. Strict and careful control and, possibly, rotation of empirical antibiotics in the hospital environment may help to limit the emergence of resistant organisms. Newer antibiotics developed for treatment of resistant, hospital-acquired pathogens are costly; therefore, their use must be moderated to some extent in an era where capitated hospital costs and mandated budget cuts will not tolerate careless antibiotic use. Broad-spectrum antibiotics are more appropriate choices for patients with risk factors for MDR pathogens or if HAP develops after at least 5 days of hospitalization.[7] See Table 85-8 for recommended antimicrobial therapy.

Ventilator-Associated Pneumonia

The approach to treating VAP is similar to antibiotic selection in HAP and HCAP (see Table 85-8). Patients should be carefully evaluated to determine whether they are at risk for MDR pathogens as this is essential in selecting appropriate empirical antibiotic therapy.[7] It is also important to identify patients with VAP early since delays in initiating appropriate antibiotic therapy are associated with increased mortality. Aerosolized antibiotic delivery has been considered for more targeted therapy; however, there are limited studies at this time supporting the safety and efficacy in pneumonia.[82]

Atypical Pneumonia

Pneumonia caused by atypical pathogens may be more difficult to treat with antibiotics than "typical" pathogens. It is debatable whether empirical treatment for hospitalized patients with CAP should include antibiotic coverage of atypical pathogens; however, if patients present with extrapulmonary findings, atypical coverage should be given higher consideration.[67] There does not appear to be any benefit in terms of survival or clinical efficacy to providing atypical coverage for all patients.[83] See Table 85-8 for a summary of the evidence-based guidelines on management.

For *Legionella* pneumonia, respiratory fluoroquinolones and doxycycline are superior to macrolides, the previous drug of choice.[84] Double antibiotic coverage is not recommended if one of these agents is used unless the patient is immunocompromised.[67] *Mycoplasma* pneumonia is difficult to treat due to the organism's lack of a cell wall, limiting certain antibiotics, and it is found on epithelial cells in the respiratory tract instead of inside the cells.[52,67] Macrolides and tetracyclines are generally effective against *Mycoplasma*; however, macrolide-resistant strains have been emerging over the past decade.[68] *Chlamydophila* organisms are sensitive to macrolides, doxycycline, and fluoroquinolones. Symptoms such as cough and malaise may be present for months following antibiotic therapy.[52] The management of tuberculosis is further discussed in Chapter 90.

For viral causes of pneumonia, antivirals such as amantadine and oseltamivir can be used, depending on viral susceptibility. Treatment for H5N1 and H1N1 is primarily supportive; patients with H5N1 generally require aggressive oxygen therapy and intensive monitoring[70,71] while the majority of those with H1N1 are treated as outpatients. Both viruses are resistant to amantadine; therefore, the neuraminidase inhibitors oseltamivir and zanamivir are recommended if antivirals are administered. Treatment of SARS involves primarily supportive care and procedures to prevent transmission to others.[73] Owing to the uncertainty associated with the diagnosis of SARS, empirical therapy with broad-spectrum antibiotics should be used including fluoroquinolones or macrolides/azalides. Although its efficacy is unproven, ribavirin also has been used to treat patients and corticosteroids have been used owing to the potential benefit in the presence of progressive pulmonary disease; methylprednisolone has been used in doses ranging from 80 to 500 mg/day.

TABLE 85-11 Evidenced-Based Guidelines for Preventing Healthcare-Associated Pneumonia

Recommendation	Recommendation Grade[a]
For nebulizers, use aerosolized medications in single-dose vials. If multidose medication vials are used, follow manufacturers' instructions for handling, storing, and dispensing the medications	1B
Pneumococcal vaccination is recommended for patients at high risk for severe pneumococcal infections	1A
Unless contraindicated, administer a macrolide to any person who has had close contact with persons having pertussis	1B
In acute care settings, offer vaccine to inpatients and outpatients at high risk for complications from influenza beginning in September and throughout the influenza season	1A
Unless contraindicated, provide prophylactic treatment to all patients without influenza illness in the involved unit with amantadine, rimantadine, or oseltamivir for a minimum of 2 weeks or until approximately 1 week after the end of the outbreak	1A
Unless contraindicated, patients with influenza should receive amantadine, rimantadine, oseltamivir, or zanamivir within 48 hours of the onset of symptoms	1A

[a]Grade 1A, strongly recommended for implementation and strongly supported by well-designed experimental, clinical, or epidemiologic studies; grade 1B, strongly recommended for implementation and supported by certain clinical or epidemiologic studies and by strong theoretical rationale.

Prevention

Prevention of some cases of pneumonia is possible through the use of vaccines and medications against selected infectious agents. Polyvalent polysaccharide vaccines are available for two of the leading causes of bacterial pneumonia, *S. pneumoniae* and *H. influenzae* type b. Children should be vaccinated against *S. pneumoniae*, *H. influenzae* type b, pertussis, and influenza; immune prophylaxis for RSV is recommended for high-risk infants during RSV season. Caregivers for infants <6 months should also be vaccinated against influenza and pertussis. To minimize the risk of developing VAP, healthcare providers should seek to minimize colonization of the aerodigestive tract, prevent aspiration (head raised 45°), and limit the length of mechanical ventilation.[66] In addition, evidence-based guidelines for preventing HCAP have been published (Table 85-11).[85] (See Chap. 87 for a full discussion of prevention of influenza and Chap. 102 for vaccines.)

EVALUATION OF THERAPEUTIC OUTCOMES

After therapy has been instituted, appropriate clinical parameters should be monitored to ensure the efficacy and safety of the therapeutic regimen. For patients with bacterial infections of the upper or lower respiratory tract, the time to resolution of initial presenting symptoms and the lack of appearance of new associated symptomatology are important to determine. For patients with CAP or pneumonia from any source of mild to moderate clinical severity, the time to resolution of cough, decreasing sputum production, and fever, as well as other constitutional symptoms of malaise, nausea, vomiting, and lethargy, should be noted. If the patient requires supplemental oxygen therapy, the amount and need should be assessed regularly. A gradual and persistent improvement in the resolution of these symptoms and therapies should be observed. Initial resolution should be observed within the first 2 days and progression to complete resolution within 5 to 7 days but usually no more than 10 days.

For patients with HAP/HCAP, substantial underlying diseases, or both, additional parameters can be followed, including the magnitude and character of the peripheral blood WBC count, chest radiograph, and blood gas determinations. Similar to patients with less severe disease, some resolution of symptoms should be observed within 2 days of instituting antibiotic therapy. If no resolution of symptoms is observed within 2 days of starting seemingly appropriate antibiotic therapy or if the patient's clinical status is deteriorating, the appropriateness of initial antibiotic therapy should be critically reassessed. The patient should be evaluated carefully for deterioration of underlying concurrent disease(s). Additionally, the caregiver should consider the possibility of changing the initial antibiotic therapy to expand antimicrobial coverage not included in the original regimen (e.g., *Mycoplasma*, *Legionella*, and anaerobes). Furthermore, the need for antifungal therapy (lipid-based amphotericin B) should be considered. Some resolution of symptoms should be observed within 2 days of starting proper antibiotic therapy, with complete resolution expected within 10 to 14 days.

ABBREVIATIONS

AECB	acute exacerbation of chronic bronchitis
AUC	area under the concentration curve
CAP	community-acquired pneumonia
CDC	Centers for Disease Control and Prevention
Cmax	maximum concentration
COLD	chronic obstructive lung disease
COPD	chronic obstructive pulmonary disease
FEV_1	forced expiratory volume in the first second of expiration
GOLD	Global Initiative for Chronic Obstructive Lung Disease
HAP	hospital-acquired pneumonia
HCAP	healthcare-associated pneumonia
HIV	human immunodeficiency virus
MDR	multidrug resistant
MIC	minimum inhibitory concentration
MRSA	methicillin-resistant *Staphylococcus aureus*
PCR	polymerase chain reaction
PDE4	phosphodiesterase 4
PK-PD	pharmacokinetic–pharmacodynamic
RSV	respiratory syncytial virus
SARS	severe acute respiratory syndrome
SARS-CoV	severe acute respiratory syndrome coronavirus
TWAR	Taiwan acute respiratory agent
VAP	ventilator-associated pneumonia
WBC	white blood cell

REFERENCES

1. Eddens T, Kolls JK. Host defenses against bacterial lower respiratory tract infection. Curr Opin Immunol 2012;24(4): 424–430.
2. Jaroszewski DE, Webb BJ, Leslie KO. Diagnosis and management of lung infections. Thorac Surg Clin 2012;22(3): 301–324.
3. Yan Y, Zhang S, Tang YW. Molecular assays for the detection and characterization of respiratory viruses. Semin Respir Crit Care Med 2011;32(4):512–526.
4. Koulenti D, Rello J. Hospital-acquired pneumonia in the 21st century: A review of existing treatment options and their impact on patient care. Expert Opin Pharmacother 2006;7(12):1555–1569.
5. Mandell L, Wunderink R, Anzueto A, et al. Infectious Diseases Society of America/American Thoracic Society

consensus guidelines on the management of community-acquired pneumonia in adults. Clin Infect Dis 2007;44 (Suppl 2):S27–S72.

6. Bradley JS, Byington CL, Shah SS, et al. The management of community-acquired pneumonia in infants and children older than 3 months of age: Clinical practice guidelines by the Pediatric Infectious Diseases Society and the Infectious Diseases Society of America. Clin Infect Dis 2011;53(7): e25–e76.
7. American Thoracic Society, Infectious Diseases Society of America. Guidelines for the management of adults with hospital-acquired, ventilator-associated, and healthcare-associated pneumonia. Am J Respir Crit Care Med 2005; 171(4):388–416.
8. Lippi G, Meschi T, Cervellin G. Inflammatory biomarkers for the diagnosis, monitoring and follow-up of community-acquired pneumonia: Clinical evidence and perspectives. Eur J Intern Med 2011;22(5):460–465.
9. Porzecanski I, Bowton D. Diagnosis and treatment of ventilator-associated pneumonia. Chest 2006;130(2):597–604.
10. Wenzel RP, Fowler AA 3rd. Clinical practice. Acute bronchitis. N Engl J Med 2006;355(20):2125–2130.
11. Brodzinski H, Ruddy R. Review of new and newly discovered respiratory tract viruses in children. Pediatr Emerg Care 2009;25(5):352–360 [quiz 61–63].
12. Blasi F, Tarsia P, Aliberti S. *Chlamydophila pneumoniae*. Clin Microbiol Infect 2009;15(1):29–35.
13. Crowcroft N, Pebody R. Recent developments in pertussis. Lancet 2006;367(9526):1926–1936.
14. Braman S. Chronic cough due to acute bronchitis: ACCP evidence-based clinical practice guidelines. Chest 2006; 129(1 Suppl):95S–103S.
15. Glasgow J. Reye's syndrome: The case for a causal link with aspirin. Drug Saf 2006;29(12):1111–1121.
16. Becker LA, Hom J, Villasis-Keever M, van der Wouden JC. Beta2-agonists for acute bronchitis. Cochrane Database Syst Rev 2011;(7):CD001726.
17. Smucny J, Fahey T, Becker L, Glazier R. Antibiotics for acute bronchitis. Cochrane Database Syst Rev. 2004;(4):CD000245.
18. Hersh A, Maselli J, Cabana M. Changes in prescribing of antiviral medications for influenza associated with new treatment guidelines. Am J Public Health 2009;99(Suppl 2): S362–S364.
19. Jefferson T, Demicheli V, Di Pietrantonj C, Jones M, Rivetti D. Neuraminidase inhibitors for preventing and treating influenza in healthy adults. Cochrane Database Syst Rev 2006;(3):CD001265.
20. Jefferson T, Jones M, Doshi P, Del Mar C. Neuraminidase inhibitors for preventing and treating influenza in healthy adults: Systematic review and meta-analysis. BMJ 2009; 339:b5106.
21. Regoes R, Bonhoeffer S. Emergence of drug-resistant influenza virus: Population dynamical considerations. Science 2006;312(5772):389–391.
22. Rodriguez-Roisin R, Anzueto A, Bourbeau J, et al.; GOLD Executive Committee. Global Strategy for the Diagnosis, Management, and Prevention of Chronic Obstructive Pulmonary Disease (Revised 2011). Global Initiative for Chronic Obstructive Lung Disease (Updated 2011). April 2001.
23. Braman SS. Chronic cough due to chronic bronchitis: ACCP evidence-based clinical practice guidelines. Chest 2006;129(1 Suppl):104S–115S.
24. Qiu W, Cho MH, Riley JH, et al. Genetics of sputum gene expression in chronic obstructive pulmonary disease. PLoS One 2011;6(9):e24395.
25. Pierson D. Clinical practice guidelines for chronic obstructive pulmonary disease: A review and comparison of current resources. Respir Care 2006;51(3):277–288.
26. Wilson R, Jones P, Schaberg T, et al. Antibiotic treatment and factors influencing short and long term outcomes of acute exacerbations of chronic bronchitis. Thorax 2006;61(4): 337–342.
27. Wood A, Tan S, Stockley R. Chronic obstructive pulmonary disease: Towards pharmacogenetics. Genome Med 2009; 1(11):112.
28. Mensa J, Trilla A. Should patients with acute exacerbation of chronic bronchitis be treated with antibiotics? Advantages of the use of fluoroquinolones. Clin Microbiol Infect 2006; 12(Suppl 3):42–54.
29. Poole P, Black PN, Cates CJ. Mucolytic agents for chronic bronchitis or chronic obstructive pulmonary disease. Cochrane Database Syst Rev 2012;8:CD001287.
30. Nannini LJ, Lasserson TJ, Poole P. Combined corticosteroid and long-acting beta(2)-agonist in one inhaler versus long-acting beta(2)-agonists for chronic obstructive pulmonary disease. Cochrane Database Syst Rev 2012;9:CD006829.
31. Field SK. Roflumilast, a novel phosphodiesterase 4 inhibitor, for COPD patients with a history of exacerbations. Clin Med Insights Circ Respir Pulm Med 2011;5:57–70.
32. Pinner NA, Hamilton LA, Hughes A. Roflumilast: A phosphodiesterase-4 inhibitor for the treatment of severe chronic obstructive pulmonary disease. Clin Ther 2012;34(1):56–66.
33. Delea T, Hagiwara M, Dalal A, et al. Healthcare use and costs in patients with chronic bronchitis initiating maintenance therapy with fluticasone/salmeterol vs other inhaled maintenance therapies. Curr Med Res Opin 2009;25(1):1–13.
34. Hayes DJ, Meyer K. Acute exacerbations of chronic bronchitis in elderly patients: Pathogenesis, diagnosis and management. Drugs Aging 2007;24(7):555–572.
35. Anthonisen N, Manfreda J, Warren C, et al. Antibiotic therapy in exacerbations of chronic obstructive pulmonary disease. Ann Intern Med 1987;106(2):196–204.
36. Sorensen S, Baker T, Fleurence R, et al. Cost and clinical consequence of antibiotic non-adherence in acute exacerbations of chronic bronchitis. Int J Tuberc Lung Dis 2009;13(8):945–954.
37. Korbila I, Manta K, Siempos I, et al. Penicillins vs trimethoprim-based regimens for acute bacterial exacerbations of chronic bronchitis: Meta-analysis of randomized controlled trials. Can Fam Physician 2009;55(1):60–67.
38. Dimopoulos G, Siempos I, Korbila I, et al. Comparison of first-line with second-line antibiotics for acute exacerbations of chronic bronchitis: A metaanalysis of randomized controlled trials. Chest 2007;132(2):447–455.
39. Falagas M, Avgeri S, Matthaiou D, et al. Short- versus long-duration antimicrobial treatment for exacerbations of chronic bronchitis: A meta-analysis. J Antimicrob Chemother 2008;62(3):442–450.
40. Stempel H, Martin E, Kuypers J, et al. Multiple viral respiratory pathogens in children with bronchiolitis. Acta Paediatr 2009;98(1):123–126.
41. Wright M, Piedimonte G. Respiratory syncytial virus prevention and therapy: Past, present, and future. Pediatr Pulmonol 2011;46(4):324–347.
42. Smyth RL, Openshaw PJ. Bronchiolitis. Lancet 2006; 368(9532):312–322.
43. Schuh S. Update on management of bronchiolitis. Curr Opin Pediatr 2011;23(1):110–114.
44. Yanney M, Vyas H. The treatment of bronchiolitis. Arch Dis Child 2008;93(9):793–798.

45. Plint AC, Johnson DW, Patel H, et al. Epinephrine and dexamethasone in children with bronchiolitis. N Engl J Med 2009;360(20):2079–2089.
46. Hartling L, Fernandes RM, Bialy L, et al. Steroids and bronchodilators for acute bronchiolitis in the first two years of life: Systematic review and meta-analysis. BMJ 2011;342:d1714.
47. American Academy of Pediatrics Subcommittee on Diagnosis and Management of Bronchiolitis. Diagnosis and management of bronchiolitis. Pediatrics 2006;118(4):1774–1793.
48. Perrin KM, Bégué RE. Use of palivizumab in primary practice. Pediatrics 2012;129(1):55–61.
49. Nseir S, Mathieu D. Antibiotic treatment for severe community-acquired pneumonia: Beyond antimicrobial susceptibility. Crit Care Med 2012;40(8):2500–2502.
50. Feldman C, Anderson R. Antibiotic resistance of pathogens causing community-acquired pneumonia. Semin Respir Crit Care Med 2012;33(3):232–243.
51. Anand N, Kollef M. The alphabet soup of pneumonia: CAP, HAP, HCAP, NHAP, and VAP. Semin Respir Crit Care Med 2009;30(1):3–9.
52. Marrie TJ, Costain N, La Scola B, et al. The role of atypical pathogens in community-acquired pneumonia. Semin Respir Crit Care Med 2012;33(3):244–256.
53. Waterer GW. Community-acquired pneumonia: Genomics, epigenomics, transcriptomics, proteomics, and metabolomics. Semin Respir Crit Care Med 2012;33(3):257–265.
54. Gordin FM, Masur H. Current approaches to tuberculosis in the United States. JAMA 2012;308(3):283–289.
55. Mitruka K, Oeltmann JE, Ijaz K, Haddad MB. Tuberculosis outbreak investigations in the United States, 2002-2008. Emerg Infect Dis 2011;17(3):425–431.
56. Buising K, Thursky K, Black J, et al. A prospective comparison of severity scores for identifying patients with severe community acquired pneumonia: Reconsidering what is meant by severe pneumonia. Thorax 2006;61(5): 419–424.
57. Pereira JM, Paiva JA, Rello J. Assessing severity of patients with community-acquired pneumonia. Semin Respir Crit Care Med 2012;33(3):272–283.
58. Zilberberg M, Shorr A. Epidemiology of healthcare-associated pneumonia (HCAP). Semin Respir Crit Care Med 2009;30(1):10–15.
59. Micek S, Kollef K, Reichley R, et al. Health care-associated pneumonia and community-acquired pneumonia: A single-center experience. Antimicrob Agents Chemother 2007;51(10):3568–3573.
60. Punpanich W, Groome M, Muhe L, et al. Systematic review on the etiology and antibiotic treatment of pneumonia in human immunodeficiency virus-infected children. Pediatr Infect Dis J 2011;30(10):e192–e202.
61. Smith T, Khatcheressian J, Lyman G, et al. 2006 update of recommendations for the use of white blood cell growth factors: An evidence-based clinical practice guideline. J Clin Oncol 2006;24(19):3187–3205.
62. Pettersson K. Perinatal infection with group B streptococci. Semin Fetal Neonatal Med 2007;12(3):193–197.
63. Falcone M, Venditti M, Shindo Y, Kollef MH. Healthcare-associated pneumonia: Diagnostic criteria and distinction from community-acquired pneumonia. Int J Infect Dis 2011;15(8):e545–e550.
64. de Vrankrijker AM, Wolfs TF, van der Ent CK. Challenging and emerging pathogens in cystic fibrosis. Paediatr Respir Rev 2010;11(4):246–254.
65. Bartlett JG. Anaerobic bacterial infection of the lung. Anaerobe 2012;18(2):235–239.
66. Hunter JD. Ventilator associated pneumonia. BMJ 2012; 344:e3325.
67. Cunha B. Atypical pneumonias: Current clinical concepts focusing on Legionnaires' disease. Curr Opin Pulm Med 2008;14(3):183–194.
68. Morozumi M, Takahashi T, Ubukata K. Macrolide-resistant *Mycoplasma pneumoniae*: Characteristics of isolates and clinical aspects of community-acquired pneumonia. J Infect Chemother 2010;16(2):78–86.
69. Narita M. Pathogenesis of extrapulmonary manifestations of *Mycoplasma pneumoniae* infection with special reference to pneumonia. J Infect Chemother 2010;16(3):162–169.
70. Liu J. Avian influenza—A pandemic waiting to happen? J Microbiol Immunol Infect 2006;39(1):4–10.
71. Wong S, Yuen K. Avian influenza virus infections in humans. Chest 2006;129(1):156–168.
72. Centers for Disease Control and Prevention (CDC). Update: Novel influenza A (H1N1) virus infections—Worldwide, May 6, 2009. MMWR Morb Mortal Wkly Rep 2009;58(17):453–458.
73. Sampathkumar P, Temesgen Z, Smith T, Thompson R. SARS: Epidemiology, clinical presentation, management, and infection control measures. Mayo Clin Proc 2003;78(7): 882–890.
74. Coughlin MM, Prabhakar BS. Neutralizing human monoclonal antibodies to severe acute respiratory syndrome coronavirus: Target, mechanism of action, and therapeutic potential. Rev Med Virol 2012;22(1):2–17.
75. Nahid P, Daley C. Prevention of tuberculosis in HIV-infected patients. Curr Opin Infect Dis 2006;19(2):189–193.
76. Sharpe B. Guideline-recommended antibiotics in community-acquired pneumonia: Not perfect, but good. Arch Intern Med 2009;169(16):1462–1464.
77. Owens RJ, Shorr A. Rational dosing of antimicrobial agents: Pharmacokinetic and pharmacodynamic strategies. Am J Health Syst Pharm 2009;66(12 Suppl 4):S23–S30.
78. Wunderink RG, Mandell L. Adjunctive therapy in community-acquired pneumonia. Semin Respir Crit Care Med 2012;33(3):311–318.
79. Safdar A, Shelburne S, Evans S, Dickey B. Inhaled therapeutics for prevention and treatment of pneumonia. Expert Opin Drug Saf 2009;8(4):435–449.
80. Palmer L. Aerosolized antibiotics in critically ill ventilated patients. Curr Opin Crit Care 2009;15(5):413–418.
81. Muscedere J, Dodek P, Keenan S, et al. Comprehensive evidence-based clinical practice guidelines for ventilator-associated pneumonia: Diagnosis and treatment. J Crit Care 2008;23(1):138–147.
82. Luyt C, Combes A, Nieszkowska A, et al. Aerosolized antibiotics to treat ventilator-associated pneumonia. Curr Opin Infect Dis 2009;22(2):154–158.
83. Robenshtok E, Shefet D, Gafter-Gvili A, et al. Empiric antibiotic coverage of atypical pathogens for community acquired pneumonia in hospitalized adults. Cochrane Database Syst Rev 2008;(1):CD004418.
84. Forgie S, Marrie T. Healthcare-associated atypical pneumonia. Semin Respir Crit Care Med 2009;30(1):67–85.
85. Tablan O, Anderson L, Besser R, et al. Guidelines for preventing health-care–associated pneumonia, 2003: Recommendations of CDC and the Healthcare Infection Control Practices Advisory Committee. MMWR Recomm Rep 2004;53(RR-3):1–36.

86

Upper Respiratory Tract Infections

Christopher Frei and Bradi Frei

KEY CONCEPTS

1. Most upper respiratory tract infections have a viral etiology and tend to resolve spontaneously without pharmacologic therapy.
2. The most common bacterial causes are *Streptococcus pneumoniae* (acute otitis media and acute rhinosinusitis) and group A *β*-hemolytic *Streptococcus* (acute pharyngitis).
3. Vaccination against influenza and pneumococcus may decrease the risk of acute otitis media.
4. Because upper respiratory tract infections are so common, antibiotics used to treat them serve as catalysts for the emergence and spread of antibiotic resistance, thereby making prudent antibiotic use critically important.
5. When antibiotics are prescribed, the empirical medications of choice are amoxicillin for acute otitis media, amoxicillin–clavulanate for acute rhinosinusitis, and amoxicillin and penicillin for acute pharyngitis.
6. For otitis media, high-dose amoxicillin (80–90 mg/kg/day) is recommended if the patient is at high risk for a penicillin-resistant pneumococcal infection.

More patients present to physicians' offices and emergency departments for upper respiratory tract infections than any other infectious disease.[1,2] Otitis media, rhinosinusitis, and pharyngitis are the three most common upper respiratory tract infections. Because they are so common, community and emergency health care workers must be familiar with the diagnosis, assessment, and management of patients with these infections. Furthermore, antibiotics used for the treatment of upper respiratory tract infections serve as catalysts for the emergence and spread of antibiotic resistance, thereby making prudent antibiotic use critically important.

ACUTE OTITIS MEDIA

The term *otitis media* comes from the Latin *oto-* for "ear," *itis* for "inflammation," and *medi-* for "middle"; otitis media, then, is an inflammation of the middle ear. There are three subtypes of otitis media: acute otitis media, otitis media with effusion, and chronic otitis media. The three are differentiated by (a) acute signs of infection, (b) evidence of middle ear inflammation, and (c) presence of fluid in the middle ear.[3] Acute otitis media is the subtype with the greatest role for antibiotics and will be discussed in detail.

Epidemiology

Otitis media is one of the leading reasons for physicians' office visits and emergency department visits in the United States, accounting for more than 16 million clinic and emergency department visits annually.[1,2] There are more than 709 million cases of otitis media worldwide each year; half of these cases occur in children under 5 years of age.[4] Many patients with acute otitis media will receive a prescription, and the costs associated with managing otitis media are almost $3 billion annually in the United States.[5]

Etiology

❶ Approximately 40% to 75% of acute otitis media cases are caused by viral pathogens.[6] ❷ Common bacterial pathogens include *Streptococcus pneumoniae* (35% to 40%), nontypeable *Haemophilus influenzae* (30% to 35%), and *Moraxella catarrhalis* (15% to 18%).[7] The microbial etiology has changed as a result of the introduction and widespread use of the seven-valent pneumococcal conjugate vaccine (PCV7). Specifically, the proportion of *S. pneumoniae* cases has declined, and the proportion of *H. influenzae* cases has risen.[3] A new *S. pneumoniae* serotype (19A) has begun to emerge.[8]

S. pneumoniae, *H. influenzae*, and *M. catarrhalis* can all possess resistance to *β*-lactams. *S. pneumoniae* develops resistance through alteration of penicillin-binding proteins, whereas *H. influenzae* and *M. catarrhalis* produce *β*-lactamases. Up to 40% of *S. pneumoniae* isolates in the United States are penicillin nonsusceptible, and up to half of these have high-level penicillin resistance.[9] Approximately 30% to 40% of *H. influenzae* and greater than 90% of *M. catarrhalis* isolates from the upper respiratory tract produce *β*-lactamases.[10–12] Risk factors have been identified for amoxicillin-resistant bacteria. These include attendance at child care centers, recent receipt of antibiotic treatment (within the past 30 days), and age younger than 2 years.[6]

Pathophysiology

Acute otitis media usually follows a viral upper respiratory tract infection that impairs the mucociliary apparatus and causes Eustachian tube dysfunction in the middle ear.[7,13] The middle ear is the space behind the tympanic membrane, or eardrum. A noninfected ear has a thin, clear tympanic membrane. In otitis media, this space becomes blocked with fluid, resulting in a bulging and erythematous tympanic membrane. Bacteria that colonize the nasopharynx enter the middle ear and are not cleared properly by the mucociliary system. The bacteria proliferate and cause infection. Children tend to be more susceptible to otitis media than adults because the anatomy of their Eustachian tube is shorter and more horizontal, facilitating bacterial entry into the middle ear.

Clinical Presentation

Patients or caregivers frequently characterize acute otitis media as having an acute onset of otalgia (ear pain). For parents of young

CLINICAL PRESENTATION Acute Otitis Media

General

- Cases of acute otitis media often follow viral upper respiratory tract infections. A diagnosis of acute otitis media requires the following three criteria: (a) acute signs of infection, (b) evidence of middle ear inflammation, and (c) presence of fluid in the middle ear. The latter two criteria must be determined by otoscopic exam. The signs of infection must be acute and may be nonspecific, including fever (<25% of patients) and otalgia (>75% of patients). Younger children may be irritable, tug on the involved ear, and have difficulty sleeping.

Signs and Symptoms of Middle Ear Inflammation

- Erythema of the tympanic membrane
- Otalgia

Signs and Symptoms of Middle Ear Effusion

- Fullness or bulging of the tympanic membrane (most important sign)
- Limited or absent mobility of the tympanic membrane
- Otorrhea

Compiled from references 6, 7, and 13.

children, irritability and tugging on the ear are often the first clues that a child has acute otitis media.

The diagnoses of acute otitis media and otitis media with effusion are easily confused, and careful attention to history, signs, and symptoms is important. Otitis media with effusion is characterized by fluid in the middle ear without signs and symptoms of acute ear infection, such as pain and a bulging eardrum.[3,7] A diagnosis of acute otitis media requires that three criteria be satisfied: (a) acute signs of infection, (b) evidence of middle ear inflammation, and (c) presence of fluid in the middle ear.[3] Middle ear effusion is indicated by any of the following: bulging of the tympanic membrane, limited or absent mobility of the tympanic membrane, or otorrhea.[6] Signs and symptoms of middle ear inflammation include either distinct erythema of the tympanic membrane or distinct otalgia.[6] A diagnosis is considered to be "uncertain" if the patient does not have all three of these diagnostic criteria.

TREATMENT

Desired Outcome

6 Treatment goals include pain management and prudent antibiotic use. These will be discussed in detail, but, first, it is important to consider primary prevention of acute otitis media through the use of bacterial and viral vaccines.

3 A systematic review demonstrated that the PCV7 reduced the occurrence of acute otitis media episodes by 6% to 7% when the vaccine was administered during infancy.[14] Children with a history of acute otitis media did not benefit when the PCV7 was administered at an older age.[14] In June 2012, a new 13-valent pneumococcal conjugate vaccine was approved for use in adults 19 years of age or older.

The *H. influenzae* type b (Hib) vaccine has been available for two decades and is thought to be responsible for a significant reduction in invasive Hib disease; now it is the nontypeable *H. influenzae* that is of greatest concern in acute otitis media.[15] Other vaccines, including nontypeable *H. influenzae* and *M. catarrhalis* vaccines, are in development.

Finally, because acute otitis media cases often follow influenza cases, influenza vaccination should be considered as a possible means to prevent acute otitis media. Refer to the U.S. Centers for Disease Control and Prevention website (*www.cdc.gov*) and statements from the Advisory Committee on Immunization Practices for the most up-to-date information regarding recommended immunization practices.

General Approach to Treatment

The first step is to differentiate acute otitis media from otitis media with effusion or chronic otitis media, as the latter two types do not benefit substantially from antibiotic therapy. If the patient has acute otitis media, then consider if the disease severity warrants antibiotic therapy. Recognize that amoxicillin is the mainstay of therapy and that penicillin resistance can be overcome, in many cases, with higher doses of amoxicillin. Address the patient's pain as described below. The therapeutic strategy should be changed if complications develop or if symptoms fail to resolve within 3 days.

Nonpharmacologic Therapy

Regardless of the decision to administer antibiotics, acetaminophen or a nonsteroidal antiinflammatory drug, such as ibuprofen, should be offered early to relieve pain in acute otitis media.[6] In addition, eardrops with a local anesthetic, such as amethocaine, benzocaine, or lidocaine, provide pain relief when administered with oral pain medication to children aged 3 to 18 years.[16] Because of minimal benefit and increased side effects, neither decongestants nor antihistamines should be routinely recommended in cases of acute otitis media or otitis media with effusion.[6,17,18]

Pharmacologic Therapy

National clinical practice guidelines for appropriate diagnosis and treatment of acute otitis media were first published in 2004 by the American Academy of Pediatrics (AAP) and the American Academy of Family Physicians (AAFP).[6] These guidelines are focused on children 2 months to 12 years of age with uncomplicated cases. These guidelines do not pertain to children with systemic illness or with underlying conditions that may alter the course of acute otitis media (e.g., anatomic abnormalities, genetic conditions such as Down's syndrome, immunodeficiencies, and cochlear implants).

Systematic reviews and randomized controlled trials have more closely examined the value of antibiotics for acute otitis media.[3,19–22]

Taken together, these studies suggest a moderate benefit of antibiotics for the treatment of acute otitis media, particularly in patients with severe symptoms.

4 Antibiotic therapy for upper respiratory diseases must be balanced with possible increases in adverse drug events and increased antibiotic pressure. One strategy to reduce antibiotic use in this setting is "delayed therapy."[23] Delayed therapy most often means that a healthcare worker provides the patient with a prescription, but encourages the patient to wait to use the medication for 48 to 72 hours to see if the symptoms will resolve on their own. Candidates for delayed therapy include (a) children 6 months to 2 years of age without severe symptoms plus uncertain diagnosis, (b) children 2 years and older without severe symptoms, and (c) children 2 years and older with an uncertain diagnosis.[6] Delayed therapy decreases antibiotic use but also decreases patient satisfaction and may harm patients.[3] A Cochrane review concluded that this strategy is no better than avoiding antibiotics altogether.[23]

5 If antibiotics are to be administered, then amoxicillin should be given to most children (80 to 90 mg/kg/day in two divided doses).[6] *S. pneumoniae* resistance to penicillin can be overcome with this amoxicillin dose. If pathogens that produce β-lactamase are known or suspected, then amoxicillin should be given in combination with a β-lactamase inhibitor: amoxicillin–clavulanate (90 mg/kg/day of amoxicillin with 6.4 mg/kg/day of clavulanate in two divided doses).[6] In patients with moderate to severe illness (temperature greater than 39°C [102°F] and/or severe otalgia), amoxicillin–clavulanate is recommended. Table 86-1 lists antibiotic recommendations for acute otitis media.

Clinical trials have not provided a clear answer as to which antibiotics are most efficacious[3]; therefore, the choice of amoxicillin is largely based on microbiology and pharmacokinetic–pharmacodynamic studies. Amoxicillin has the best pharmacodynamic profile against drug-resistant *S. pneumoniae* of all available oral antibiotics. In addition, amoxicillin has a long record of safety, possesses a narrow spectrum of activity, and is inexpensive. Higher middle ear fluid concentrations of amoxicillin as a result of higher dosing overcome most drug-resistant *S. pneumoniae* even with its increased minimum inhibitory concentration (MIC).[6] Its excellent efficacy against *S. pneumoniae* outweighs the issue of β-lactamase-producing *H. influenzae* and *M. catarrhalis*, against which amoxicillin may not be effective. This is because both *H. influenzae* and *M. catarrhalis* are more likely than *S. pneumoniae* to lead to a spontaneous resolution of the infection.

If treatment failure occurs with amoxicillin, an antibiotic should be chosen with activity against β-lactamase-producing *H. influenzae* and *M. catarrhalis*, as well as drug-resistant *S. pneumoniae*.[6] Amoxicillin–clavulanate is recommended. Other choices are cefuroxime, cefdinir, cefpodoxime, and intramuscular ceftriaxone.[6] Second-generation cephalosporins, though β-lactamase stable, are expensive, have an increased incidence of side effects, and may increase selective pressure for resistant bacteria. Furthermore, most cephalosporins do not achieve adequate middle ear fluid concentrations against drug-resistant *S. pneumoniae* for the desired duration of the dosing interval. Use of trimethoprim–sulfamethoxazole and erythromycin–sulfisoxazole is discouraged because of high rates of resistance.[6] Intramuscular ceftriaxone is the only antibiotic other than amoxicillin that achieves middle ear fluid concentrations above the MIC for greater than 40% of the dosing interval.[6] Although single doses of ceftriaxone have been used, daily doses for 3 days are recommended to optimize clinical outcomes.[6] Ceftriaxone should be reserved for severe and unresponsive infections or for patients for whom oral medication is inappropriate because of vomiting, diarrhea, or possible nonadherence. It is an expensive antibiotic, and the intramuscular injections are painful. The drug can be given IV, but the risk-to-benefit ratio of starting an IV line must also be examined. Tympanocentesis can also be considered for treatment failure or persistent acute otitis media. It has a therapeutic effect of relieving pain and pressure and can be used to collect fluid to identify the causative agent. Clindamycin may also be considered at this point for coverage of documented penicillin-resistant *S. pneumoniae*.[6] Patients with a penicillin allergy can be treated with several alternative antibiotics. If the reaction is not type I hypersensitivity, cefdinir, cefpodoxime, or cefuroxime can be used. If the reaction is type I, a macrolide such as azithromycin or clarithromycin may be used. If *S. pneumoniae* is documented, clindamycin is an alternative. However, the incidence of resistance is much higher with these antibiotics, and of these antibiotics, only clindamycin is recommended by the AAP/AAFP guidelines.[6]

There is ongoing debate regarding the optimal duration of therapy for acute otitis media. Traditional recommendations call for 10 days of antibiotic therapy; however, some experts have speculated that patients can be treated for as little as 3 to 5 days.

TABLE 86-1 Antibiotics and Doses for Acute Otitis Media

Antibiotic	Brand Name	Dose	Comments[a]
Initial Diagnosis			
Amoxicillin	Amoxil®	80–90 mg/kg/day divided twice daily	First-line (nonsevere)
Amoxicillin–clavulanate[b]	Augmentin®	90 mg/kg/day of amoxicillin plus 6.4 mg/kg/day of clavulanate divided twice daily	First-line (severe)
Cefdinir, cefuroxime, cefpodoxime	Omnicef®, Ceftin®, Vantin®		Non–type 1 allergy (nonsevere)
Ceftriaxone (1–3 days)	Rocephin®		Non–type 1 allergy (severe)
Azithromycin, clarithromycin	Zithromax®, Biaxin®		Type 1 allergy (nonsevere)
Failure at 48–72 Hours			
Amoxicillin–clavulanate[b]	Augmentin®	90 mg/kg/day of amoxicillin plus 6.4 mg/kg/day of clavulanate divided twice daily	First-line (nonsevere)
Ceftriaxone (1–3 days)	Rocephin®		First-line (severe) and non–type 1 allergy (nonsevere)
Clindamycin	Cleocin®		Non–type 1 allergy (severe) and type 1 allergy (nonsevere and severe)

[a]Severe: temperature greater than or equal to 39°C (102°F) and/or severe otalgia.
[b]Amoxicillin–clavulanate 90:6.4 or 14:1 ratio is available in the United States; 7:1 ratio is available in Canada (use amoxicillin 45 mg/kg for one dose, amoxicillin 45 mg/kg with clavulanate 6.4 mg/kg for second dose).

From reference 6.

Unfortunately, the data to support this theory are inconclusive, with some studies demonstrating similar outcomes and others demonstrating worse outcomes with short-course therapy.[3] The advantages of short-course therapy are an increased likelihood that the patient will adhere to the full course of treatment, decreased side effects and cost, and decreased bacterial-selective pressure for both the individual and the community. Short-course treatment is not recommended in children younger than 2 years of age. In children at least 6 years old who have mild to moderate acute otitis media, a 5- to 7-day course may be used.

Clinical **Controversy. . .**

The 2004 AAP/AAFP guidelines for acute otitis media recommended a "wait and see" approach prior to administering antibiotics.[6] This is because many cases of acute otitis media will resolve without antibiotics and the guideline authors believed that a "delayed therapy" approach might serve as a mechanism to reduce antibiotic overuse. A systematic review examined studies that have investigated this practice.[3] The review found two studies that reported similar outcomes in patients who received immediate antibiotic therapy as compared with those who received delayed antibiotic therapy; however, two other studies found it detrimental to delay antibiotic therapy. Regardless of the evidence, it appears that prescribers are reluctant to withhold antibiotic therapy and the rate of immediate antibiotic prescribing for acute otitis media has been found to be similar before and after publication of the 2004 AAP/AAFP guidelines (89% vs. 84%, $P = 0.103$).[24]

Recurrent acute otitis media is defined as at least three episodes in 6 months or at least four episodes in 12 months. Recurrent infections are of concern because patients younger than 3 years are at high risk for hearing loss and language and learning disabilities. Clinical studies generally do not favor prophylaxis. Treatment can be delayed until the onset of symptoms of an upper respiratory tract infection or antibiotic prophylaxis can be limited to 6 months' duration during the winter months. Surgical insertion of tympanostomy tubes (T tubes) is an effective method for the prevention of recurrent otitis media. These small tubes are placed through the inferior portion of the tympanic membrane under general anesthesia and aerate the middle ear. Children with recurrent acute otitis media should be considered for T-tube placement.

Personalized Pharmacotherapy

One of the most exciting developments in the world of infectious diseases has to do with clinical biomarkers. Procalcitonin increases in response to bacterial infection and declines as the infection resolves. Clinicians are starting to use procalcitonin blood levels to decide when to initiate and discontinue antibiotics in patients with acute upper respiratory infections (URIs).[25] A Cochrane systematic review of 14 trials with 4,221 participants found that procalcitonin protocols significantly reduced antibiotic consumption without negatively impacting patient survival or treatment failure.[26] The finding was driven by lower prescription rates in primary care and shorter durations of antibiotic therapy in emergency departments and intensive care units.[26] Despite the enthusiasm for this approach, there are still several aspects of procalcitonin monitoring that need to be resolved, including the timing of levels, the procalcitonin cutoff values for different clinical decision points, and the cost-effectiveness of this technology.[27]

Evaluation of Therapeutic Outcomes

Patients with acute otitis media should be reassessed after 3 days. By this time, there should be clinical improvement in the signs and symptoms of infection, including pain, fever, and erythema/bulging of the tympanic membrane. If the patient has not responded and antibiotics were withheld initially, they should be instituted now. If the patient initially received an antibiotic, then the antibiotic should be changed (Table 86-1). Most children will become asymptomatic at 7 days.

Early reevaluation of the eardrum when signs and symptoms are improving can be misleading because effusions persist. Over a period of 1 week, changes in the eardrum normalize, and the pus becomes serous fluid. Air–fluid levels are apparent behind the eardrum, at which point the stage is now referred to as *otitis media with effusion*. This does not represent ongoing infection, nor are additional antibiotics required. Two weeks after an acute otitis media episode, 60% to 70% of children still have a middle ear effusion—40% at 1 month and 10% to 25% at 3 months.[6] Younger children and those with a history of recurrent infections have a further delay in resolution.

Immediate reevaluation is appropriate if hearing loss results from persistent middle ear effusions following infection. Complications of otitis media are infrequent but include mastoiditis, bacteremia, meningitis, and auditory sequelae with the potential for speech and language impairment.[6]

ACUTE BACTERIAL RHINOSINUSITIS

Sinusitis is an inflammation and/or infection of the paranasal sinuses, or membrane-lined air spaces, around the nose.[28] The term *rhinosinusitis* is now preferred because sinusitis typically also involves the nasal mucosa.[28] Even though the majority of rhinosinusitis infections are viral in origin, antibiotics are frequently prescribed. It is thus important to differentiate between viral and bacterial rhinosinusitis to avoid antibiotic overuse.

A new set of clinical practice guidelines for acute bacterial rhinosinusitis was published in 2012.[28] These guidelines provide "a systematic weighting of the strength of recommendation (e.g., 'high, moderate, low, very low') and quality of evidence (e.g., 'strong, weak')" using a well-known rating system.[29] Several of the recommendations in these new guidelines differ substantially from prior guidelines.

Epidemiology

1 Nearly 30 million cases of rhinosinusitis are diagnosed annually in the United States.[30] Acute bacterial rhinosinusitis is overdiagnosed; thus, antibiotics are overprescribed. Most rhinosinusitis infections have a viral etiology; nevertheless, one in five antibiotics prescribed for adults in the United States is for rhinosinusitis.[31,32] Adults with rhinosinusitis miss an average of 6 workdays/y with these infections.[33] Patients with rhinosinusitis are significantly more likely to use the emergency room, spend more than $500/y on medical care, and see a medical specialist.[33]

Etiology

2 Acute bacterial rhinosinusitis is caused, most often, by the same bacteria implicated in acute otitis media: *S. pneumoniae* and *H. influenzae*. These organisms are responsible for ~50% to 70% of bacterial causes of acute bacterial rhinosinusitis in both adults and children.[28] *M. catarrhalis* is also frequently implicated in adults and children (~8% to 16%).[28] *Streptococcus pyogenes*, *Staphylococcus aureus*, gram-negative bacilli, and anaerobes are associated less frequently with acute bacterial rhinosinusitis.[28] Issues of bacterial resistance are similar to those found with acute otitis media.

CLINICAL PRESENTATION AND DIAGNOSIS Acute Bacterial Rhinosinusitis

General

- There are three clinical presentations that are most consistent with acute bacterial versus viral rhinosinusitis:
  - Onset with *persistent* signs or symptoms compatible with acute rhinosinusitis, lasting for ≥10 days without any evidence of clinical improvement (strong, low–moderate)
  - Onset with *severe* signs or symptoms of high fever (≥39°C [102°F]) and purulent nasal discharge or facial pain lasting for at least 3 to 4 consecutive days at the beginning of illness (strong, low–moderate)
  - Onset with *worsening* signs or symptoms characterized by new-onset fever, headache, or increase in nasal discharge following a typical viral URI that lasted 5 to 6 days and were initially improving ("double sickening") (strong, low–moderate)

Signs and Symptoms

- Purulent anterior nasal discharge, purulent or discolored posterior nasal discharge, nasal congestion or obstruction, facial congestion or fullness, facial pain or pressure, fever, headache, ear pain/pressure/fullness, halitosis, dental pain, cough, and fatigue

From reference 28.

Pathophysiology

Similar to acute otitis media, acute bacterial rhinosinusitis is often preceded by a viral respiratory tract infection that causes mucosal inflammation.[34] This can lead to obstruction of the sinus ostia—the pathways that drain the sinuses.[7] Mucosal secretions become trapped, local defenses are impaired, and bacteria from adjacent surfaces begin to proliferate. The maxillary and ethmoid sinuses are the ones most frequently involved.[7] The pathogenesis of chronic rhinosinusitis has not been well studied. Whether it is caused by more persistent pathogens or a subtle defect in the host's immune function, some patients develop chronic symptoms after their acute infection.

Clinical Presentation

The greatest barrier to efficient use of antibiotics in acute bacterial rhinosinusitis is the lack of a simple and accurate diagnostic test. The gold standard for diagnosis is sinus puncture with recovery of bacteria in high density (10^4 colony-forming units/mL [10^7 CFU/L] or greater)[28]; however, sinus puncture is invasive and costly, and can be painful, so it is not routinely done. Sinus radiography can help, but it is not routinely recommended. Because there is no simple and accurate office-based test for acute bacterial rhinosinusitis, clinicians rely on clinical findings to make the diagnosis.

TREATMENT

Desired Outcome

The goals of treatment for acute bacterial rhinosinusitis are to reduce signs and symptoms, achieve and maintain patency of the ostia, limit antibiotic treatment to those who may benefit, eradicate the bacterial infection with appropriate antibiotic therapy, minimize the duration of illness, prevent complications, and prevent progression from acute disease to chronic disease.

General Approach to Treatment

❹ The first step is to delineate viral and bacterial rhinosinusitis. This is based on disease duration, initial severity of illness, and worsening symptomatology. Viral rhinosinusitis typically improves in 7 to 10 days; therefore, a diagnosis of acute bacterial rhinosinusitis requires persistent symptoms (10 days or greater) or a worsening of symptoms after 5 to 6 days. Acute bacterial rhinosinusitis may also be suspected if the patient has severe symptoms at the beginning of his or her illness. Amoxicillin–clavulanate is now recommended as the first-line antibiotic therapy for patients with acute bacterial rhinosinusitis.[28] Adjuvant, non-antibiotic therapies have a limited role.

The next step is to decide if the patient needs to be referred to a specialist. Potential reasons for referral include mental status changes, visual disturbances, immunosuppressive illness, nosocomial infections, anatomic defects causing obstruction and possibly requiring surgery, unusually severe symptoms, multiple recurrent episodes (3 to 4/y), unilateral findings, significant coexisting illnesses, risk factors for unusual or resistant pathogens, and history of antibiotic failure. The specialist may perform computed tomography to assess the severity and extent of disease and identify the underlying causes.

Nonpharmacologic Therapy

Several nonprescription therapies are used in the management of nonbacterial rhinosinusitis for symptomatic relief. These include nasal decongestant sprays that reduce inflammation by vasoconstriction, such as phenylephrine and oxymetazoline. Use should be limited to no more than 3 days to prevent the development of tolerance and/or rebound congestion. Oral decongestants also may aid in nasal/sinus patency. Irrigation of the nasal cavity with saline and steam inhalation may be used to increase mucosal moisture, and mucolytics (e.g., guaifenesin) may be used to decrease the viscosity of nasal secretions.

In contrast, if a patient is suspected of having acute bacterial rhinosinusitis, then decongestants and antihistamines are not recommended (strong, low–moderate).[28] These can dry mucosa and disturb clearance of mucosal secretions. Other therapies are recommended to be used as adjuncts to antibiotics for patients with acute bacterial rhinosinusitis. Intranasal saline irrigation with either physiologic or hypertonic saline is recommended for adults (weak, low–moderate),[28] but the evidence from a Cochrane review is unimpressive.[35] Intranasal corticosteroids are now recommended for patients with a history of allergic rhinitis (weak, moderate) based on good data from a randomized controlled trial and a Cochrane review.[36,37]

Pharmacologic Therapy

Several prestigious groups have published statements and clinical practice guidelines for the management of patients with acute bacterial rhinosinusitis, including the Academy of Pediatrics, the Sinus and Allergy Health Partnership, the American Academy of Otolaryngology–Head and Neck Surgery, the Agency for Healthcare Research and Quality, and the Joint Task Force on Practice Parameters, representing the American Academy of Allergy, Asthma, and Immunology, the American College of Allergy, Asthma, and Immunology, and the Joint Council of Allergy, Asthma, and Immunology. The most recent set of clinical practice guidelines was published by the Infectious Diseases Society of America (IDSA) in 2012[28]; these guidelines are the primary source for many of the statements in this chapter.

5 Amoxicillin–clavulanate is now the first-line treatment for acute bacterial rhinosinusitis in children (strong, moderate) and adults (weak, low) (Tables 86-2 and 86-3).[28] In contrast, prior guidelines, including the ones published by the Canadian government in 2011,[38] list amoxicillin as the first-line treatment option due to its safety, narrow spectrum of activity, good tolerability, and favorable cost. Other randomized controlled trials have even questioned the value of amoxicillin in nonsevere cases of acute bacterial rhinosinusitis.[39–42] Nevertheless, the IDSA guidelines support the choice of amoxicillin–clavulanate based on (a) the emergence of *H. influenzae* as a more common cause of upper respiratory tract infections in children than in the past[3,43] and (b) the high prevalence of *β*-lactam-producing respiratory pathogens in acute bacterial rhinosinusitis (particularly *H. influenzae* and *M. catarrhalis*).[44] Recall that approximately 30% to 40% of *H. influenzae* and greater than 90% of *M. catarrhalis* isolates from the upper respiratory tract produce *β*-lactamases.[10–12] The advantage of amoxicillin–clavulanate, as compared with amoxicillin, is a greater spectrum of coverage. The disadvantage is increased cost, greater risk of adverse effects including diarrhea, and an added risk of hypersensitivity to the clavulanate component.[28] No other antibiotics are recommended as first-line for initial empirical therapy.

High-dose amoxicillin–clavulanate is recommended as second-line for initial empirical therapy in children and adults (weak, moderate); doxycycline is also second-line for adults (weak, low) but should be avoided in children.[28] High-dose amoxicillin–clavulanate is preferred in the following situations: (a) geographic regions with high endemic rates (10% or greater) of invasive penicillin-nonsusceptible *S. pneumoniae*, (b) severe infection, (c) attendance at daycare, (d) age less than 2 or greater than 65 years, (e) recent hospitalization, (f) antibiotic use within the last month, and (g) immunocompromised persons (weak, moderate).[28] Severe infections are those with "evidence of systemic toxicity with fever of 39°C (102°F) or higher, and threat of suppurative complications."[28]

Clinical **Controversy. . .**

The new IDSA guidelines support the use of intranasal corticosteroids for patients with acute bacterial rhinosinusitis, especially those who also have a history of allergic rhinitis; however, the guidelines are silent regarding the use of oral corticosteroids.[28] A Cochrane systematic review addressed this question.[45] The authors of the review identified four randomized controlled trials with a total of 1,008 adult participants with acute bacterial rhinosinusitis. All participants received oral antibiotics and either oral corticosteroids (prednisone 24 to 80 mg daily or betamethasone 1 mg daily) or a control treatment (placebo in three trials, nonsteroidal antiinflammatory drugs in one trial). All four trials observed faster resolution or improvement in symptoms among the patients who received oral corticosteroids. These studies did not report any information regarding the long-term effects of oral corticosteroids, such as relapse and recurrence of acute bacterial rhinosinusitis. This systematic review supports the use of oral corticosteroids as adjuvant therapy to antibiotics for the treatment of acute bacterial rhinosinusitis.

TABLE 86-2 Antibiotics and Doses for Acute Bacterial Rhinosinusitis in Children

Antibiotic	Brand Name	Dose	Comments
Initial Empirical Therapy			
Amoxicillin–clavulanate	Augmentin®	45 mg/kg/day po twice daily	First-line
Amoxicillin–clavulanate	Augmentin®	90 mg/kg/day po twice daily	Second-line
***β*-Lactam Allergy**			
Clindamycin plus cefixime or cefpodoxime	Cleocin®, Suprax®, Vantin®	Clindamycin (30–40 mg/kg/day po three times daily) plus cefixime (8 mg/kg/day po twice daily) or cefpodoxime (10 mg/kg/day po twice daily)	Non–type 1 allergy
Levofloxacin	Levaquin®	10–20 mg/kg/day po every 12–24 hours	Type 1 allergy
Risk for Antibiotic Resistance or Failed Initial Therapy			
Amoxicillin–clavulanate	Augmentin®	90 mg/kg/day po twice daily	
Clindamycin plus cefixime or cefpodoxime	Cleocin®, Suprax®, Vantin®	Clindamycin (30–40 mg/kg/day po three times daily) plus cefixime (8 mg/kg/day po twice daily) or cefpodoxime (10 mg/kg/day po twice daily)	
Levofloxacin	Levaquin®	10–20 mg/kg/day po every 12–24 hours	
Severe Infection Requiring Hospitalization			
Ampicillin–sulbactam	Unasyn®	200–400 mg/kg/day IV every 6 hours	
Ceftriaxone	Rocephin®	50 mg/kg/day IV every 12 hours	
Cefotaxime	Claforan®	100–200 mg/kg/day IV every 6 hours	
Levofloxacin	Levaquin®	10–20 mg/kg/day IV every 12–24 hours	

po, orally.

From reference 28.

TABLE 86-3 Antibiotics and Doses for Acute Bacterial Rhinosinusitis in Adults

Antibiotic	Brand Name	Dose	Comments
Initial Empirical Therapy			
Amoxicillin–clavulanate	Augmentin®	500 mg/125 mg po three times daily, or 875 mg/125 mg po twice daily	First-line
Amoxicillin–clavulanate	Augmentin®	2,000 mg/125 mg po twice daily	Second-line
Doxycycline		100 mg po twice daily or 200 mg po once daily	Second-line
***β*-Lactam Allergy**			
Doxycycline		100 mg po twice daily or 200 mg po once daily	
Levofloxacin	Levaquin®	500 mg po once daily	
Moxifloxacin	Avelox®	400 mg po once daily	
Risk for Antibiotic Resistance or Failed Initial Therapy			
Amoxicillin–clavulanate	Augmentin®	2,000 mg/125 mg po twice daily	
Levofloxacin	Levaquin®	500 mg po once daily	
Moxifloxacin	Avelox®	400 mg po once daily	
Severe Infection Requiring Hospitalization			
Ampicillin–sulbactam	Unasyn®	1.5–3 g IV every 6 hours	
Levofloxacin	Levaquin®	500 mg po once daily	
Moxifloxacin	Avelox®	400 mg po once daily	
Ceftriaxone	Rocephin®	1–2 g IV every 12–24 hours	
Cefotaxime	Claforan®	2 g IV every 4–6 hours	

po, orally.

From reference 28.

If a child has a *β*-lactam allergy, he or she may receive levofloxacin monotherapy (weak, low) or clindamycin plus cefixime or cefpodoxime combination therapy (weak, low).[28] Adults may receive doxycycline, levofloxacin, or moxifloxacin monotherapy (weak, low).[28] The guidelines also provide several options for patients at risk for antibiotic resistance, who failed initial therapy, or who have a severe infection requiring hospitalization (Tables 86-2 and 86-3).[28] Notably, cephalosporins are no longer recommended as monotherapy due to variable rates of resistance against *S. pneumoniae* (weak, moderate).[28] Macrolides are no longer recommended because of high rates of *S. pneumoniae* resistance (strong, moderate).[28] Trimethoprim–sulfamethoxazole has not been recommended for some time due to resistance among *S. pneumoniae* and *H. influenzae* (strong, moderate).[28]

The duration of therapy for the treatment of acute bacterial rhinosinusitis is not well established. Most trials have used 10- to 14-day antibiotic courses for uncomplicated rhinosinusitis,[42] and the guidelines support this treatment duration in children (weak, low–moderate).[28] For adults, the recommended duration is only 5 to 7 days (weak, low–moderate).[28]

Personalized Pharmacotherapy

Scientists are investigating a link between human genetics and the predisposition for chronic rhinosinusitis. There is limited evidence to suggest that people with certain genetic polymorphisms may be at greater risk for chronic rhinosinusitis[46]; however, no such link has been identified for acute bacterial rhinosinusitis. Furthermore, patient genetics are not currently used to guide selection of antibiotic therapy for this condition. It is important to consider patient weight and renal function when selecting antibiotic therapy for acute bacterial rhinosinusitis. Notice that all of the antibiotics recommended for children are dosed according to patient weight. Furthermore, most of the recommended antibiotics are excreted through the kidneys and should be adjusted for renal function as described in the package labeling.

Evaluation of Therapeutic Outcomes

If symptoms persist or worsen after 48 to 72 hours of appropriate antibiotic therapy, then the patient should be reevaluated and alternative antibiotics should be considered (strong, moderate).[28] Patients who do not respond to first- or second-line therapies should be referred to a specialist and worked up more aggressively, potentially with direct sinus aspiration (strong, moderate) or contrast-enhanced computed tomography (weak, low).[28]

ACUTE PHARYNGITIS

❶ ❷ Pharyngitis is an acute infection of the oropharynx or nasopharynx.[47] It is responsible for 1% to 2% of all outpatient visits.[48] Although viral causes are most common, group A *β*-hemolytic streptococci (GABHS; also known as *S. pyogenes*), is the primary bacterial cause[47]; pharyngitis due to GABHS is commonly known as "strep throat."

A new set of clinical practice guidelines for GABHS was published in 2012.[47] These guidelines provide "a systematic weighting of the strength of recommendation (e.g., 'high, moderate, low, very low') and quality of evidence (e.g., 'strong, weak')" using a well-known rating system.[29] Several of the recommendations in these new guidelines differ substantially from prior guidelines.

Epidemiology

Acute pharyngitis accounts for ~2 million emergency department and outpatient department visits per year,[2] at a cost of approximately $1.2 billion total and up to $539 million for children alone.[49] Although viral causes are most common, GABHS is the primary bacterial cause and is associated with rare but severe sequelae if not treated appropriately.[47,50] Nonsuppurative complications include acute rheumatic fever, acute glomerulonephritis, reactive arthritis, peritonsillar abscess, retropharyngeal abscess, cervical lymphadenitis, mastoiditis, otitis media, rhinosinusitis, and necrotizing fasciitis.

Although all age groups are susceptible, epidemiologic data demonstrate certain groups are at higher risk. Children 5 to 15 years of age are most susceptible; parents of school-age children and those who work with children are also at increased risk. Pharyngitis in a child younger than 3 years of age is rarely caused by GABHS.[47]

Seasonal outbreaks occur, and the incidence of GABHS is highest in winter and early spring.[47] The incubation period is 2 to 5 days, and the illness often occurs in clusters.[51] Spread occurs via direct contact (usually from hands) with droplets of saliva or nasal secretions, and transmission is thus worse in institutions, schools, families, and crowded areas.[51] Untreated, patients with streptococcal pharyngitis are infectious during the acute illness and for another week thereafter. Effective antibiotic therapy reduces the infectious period to about 24 hours.

Acute rheumatic fever is rarely seen in developed countries. In the United States, acute rheumatic fever secondary to GABHS infection was a cause of concern in the 1950s and was the major reason for penicillin therapy, but the annual incidence of this disease today is extremely rare (≤1 case per 1 million population); however, some risk does remain. Outbreaks have been reported in the United States as recently as the late 1980s and early 1990s. Furthermore, acute rheumatic fever is widespread in developing countries.

Etiology

❶ Viruses cause the majority of acute pharyngitis cases. Specific etiologies include rhinovirus (20%), coronavirus (5%), adenovirus (5%), herpes simplex virus (4%), influenza virus (2%), parainfluenza virus (2%), and Epstein-Barr virus (1%).[47,52]

❷ A bacterial etiology is far less likely. Of all the bacterial causes, GABHS is the most common (10% to 30% of persons of all ages with pharyngitis) and is the only commonly occurring form of acute pharyngitis for which antibiotic therapy is indicated.[47] In the pediatric population, GABHS causes 15% to 30% of pharyngitis cases. In adults, GABHS is responsible for 5% to 15% of all symptomatic episodes of pharyngitis.[47]

Other, less common causes of acute pharyngitis are groups C and G *Streptococcus*, *Corynebacterium diphtheriae*, *Neisseria gonorrhoeae*, *Mycoplasma pneumoniae*, *Arcanobacterium haemolyticum*, *Yersinia enterocolitica*, and *Chlamydia pneumoniae*.[47] Treatment options for these organisms are not addressed in this chapter.

Pathophysiology

The mechanism by which GABHS causes pharyngitis is not well defined. Asymptomatic pharyngeal carriers of the organism may have an alteration in host immunity (e.g., a breach in the pharyngeal mucosa) and the bacteria of the oropharynx may migrate to cause an infection. Pathogenic factors associated with the organism itself may also play a role. These include pyrogenic toxins, hemolysins, streptokinase, and proteinase.

Clinical Presentation

Sore throat is the most common symptom of pharyngitis. Accurate differentiation of GABHS from pharyngitis caused by other agents is important for treatment decisions; however, this can be difficult even for experienced clinicians. Therefore, microbiologic testing is recommended for symptomatic patients unless they have symptoms suggestive of viral etiology or are younger than 3 years of age (strong, high).[47]

In previous national guidelines, clinical scoring systems such as the Centor criteria or modifications of the Centor criteria have been advocated for clinical diagnosis in adults as a way to overcome the lack of sensitivity and specificity of clinician judgment and to avoid laboratory testing of all patients; however, recent guidelines from Infectious Disease Society of America and the American Heart Association suggest testing be done in all patients with signs and symptoms of streptococcal pharyngitis (strong, high).[47] Only those with a positive test for GABHS require antibiotic treatment.[47,53] Laboratory tests should not be performed unless the patient has symptoms consistent with GABHS pharyngitis. This is because a positive test does not necessarily indicate disease. A positive test may simply indicate that the patient is a carrier for GABHS and is not actively infected.

Approximately 20% of children are carriers; the prevalence is lower among adults.[47] Table 86-4 lists the evidence-based principles for diagnosis of GABHS. There are several options to test

CLINICAL PRESENTATION AND DIAGNOSIS Group A Streptococcal Pharyngitis

General

- A sore throat of sudden onset that is mostly self-limited
- Fever and constitutional symptoms resolving in about 3 to 5 days
- Clinical signs and symptoms are similar for viral causes and nonstreptococcal bacterial causes

Signs and Symptoms of GABHS Pharyngitis

- Sore throat
- Pain on swallowing
- Fever
- Headache, nausea, vomiting, and abdominal pain (especially in children)
- Erythema/inflammation of the tonsils and pharynx with or without patchy exudates
- Enlarged, tender lymph nodes
- Red swollen uvula, petechiae on the soft palate, and a scarlatiniform rash

Signs Suggestive of Viral Origin for Pharyngitis

- Conjunctivitis
- Coryza
- Cough

Laboratory Tests

- Throat swab and culture
- RADT

From reference 47.

TABLE 86-4 Evidence-Based Principles for Diagnosis of Group A *Streptococcus*

Recommendations	Level
Selective use of diagnostic testing only in those with clinical features suggestive of group A *Streptococcus* will increase the proportion of positive tests as well as results of those truly infected, not carriers	A-II
Clinical diagnosis cannot be made with certainty even by the most experienced clinician; bacteriologic confirmation is required	A-II
Throat culture remains the diagnostic standard, with a sensitivity of 90–95% for detection of group A *Streptococcus* if done correctly	A-II
Rapid identification and treatment of patients with disease can reduce transmission, allow patients to return to work or school earlier, and reduce the acute morbidity of the disease	A-II
The majority of rapid antigen-detection tests available have a specificity >95% (minimizes overprescribing to those without disease) and a sensitivity of 80–90% compared with culture	A-II
Early initiation of antibiotic therapy results in faster resolution of signs and symptoms. Delays in therapy (if awaiting cultures) can be made safely for up to 9 days after symptom onset and still prevent major complications such as rheumatic fever	A-I

These guidelines provide a systematic weighting of the strength of the recommendation (A, good; B, moderate; and C, poor) and quality of evidence (I, at least one randomized controlled trial; II, at least one well-designed clinical trial, not randomized, or a cohort or case–control analytical study, or from multiple time series, or from dramatic results of an uncontrolled trial; and III, expert opinion).

From Bisno AL, Gerber MA, Gwaltney JM Jr, et al. Practice guidelines for the diagnosis and management of group A streptococcal pharyngitis: Infectious Diseases Society of America. Clin Infect Dis 2002;35(2):113–125.

for GABHS. A throat swab can be sent for culture or used for the rapid antigen-detection test (RADT). Cultures are the gold standard, but they require 24 to 48 hours for results. The RADT is more practical in that it provides results quickly, it can be performed at the bedside, and it is less expensive than culture. If RADT is positive, it does not require a follow-up throat culture (strong, high).[47] If RADT yields negative test results, it is generally recommended to follow up with a throat culture to confirm the results for children and adolescents but not necessary in adults (strong, moderate).[47] Delaying therapy while awaiting culture results does not affect the risk of complications (although some argue that symptomatic benefit is postponed, and contagion remains), and patients must be educated as to the value of waiting, given the low false-negative rate of RADT.[53]

TREATMENT

Desired Outcome

The goals of treatment for pharyngitis are to improve clinical signs and symptoms, minimize adverse drug reactions, prevent transmission to close contacts, and prevent acute rheumatic fever and suppurative complications, such as peritonsillar abscess, cervical lymphadenitis, and mastoiditis.[47]

General Approach to Treatment

Once the diagnosis of GABHS pharyngitis has been made, the clinician must decide appropriate supportive care, when to initiate antibiotic therapy, the appropriate antibiotic, and the duration of therapy. The selection of appropriate antibiotic therapy will involve careful consideration of cost, safety, efficacy, potential for regimen adherence, and bacterial resistance rates. Clinicians should be aware of the local resistance patterns, which may differ from the national patterns.

4 Antibiotic overuse has been well documented.[47,52] Antibiotics are prescribed for 73% of patients who visit their provider with a complaint of "sore throat."[54] This rate is well above the incidence of GABHS pharyngitis. Antibiotic therapy should be reserved for those patients with clinical and epidemiologic features of GABHS pharyngitis, preferably with a positive laboratory test (strong, high). Empirical therapy is not recommended unless there is a high index of suspicion based on clinical or epidemiologic data and laboratory results are pending. However, it is important to discontinue empirical antibiotics if laboratory results are negative.

Nonpharmacologic Therapy

Supportive care should be offered to all patients with acute pharyngitis. Little evidence is available for nonpharmacologic therapy for pharyngitis. However, pharmacologic supportive care interventions include antipyretic medications, analgesics, and nonprescription lozenges and sprays containing menthol and topical anesthetics for temporary relief of pain (strong, high).[47] There are limited data for use of corticosteroids to reduce the symptoms of GABHS pharyngitis and given the risk of adverse effects its use is not recommended (weak, moderate).[47] Because pain is often the primary reason for visiting a physician, emphasis on analgesics such as acetaminophen and nonsteroidal antiinflammatory drugs to aid in pain relief is strongly recommended.

Pharmacologic Therapy

The most recent set of clinical practice guidelines was published by the IDSA in 2012[47]; these guidelines are the primary source for many of the statements in this chapter. Tables 86-5 and 86-6 outline dosing for acute GABHS pharyngitis and chronic carriers of GABHS.

5 For over 30 years, GABHS isolated in the United States have been susceptible to penicillin, with no reported cases of GABHS resistance to penicillin.[47] Because penicillin and amoxicillin have narrow spectrums of activity and are readily available, safe, and inexpensive, they are considered to be the treatments of choice (strong, high).[47,53] The only controlled studies that have demonstrated that antibiotic therapy prevents rheumatic fever following GABHS pharyngitis were done with procaine penicillin, which was later replaced with benzathine penicillin.[53] Penicillin given by other routes is assumed to be equally efficacious. The ability of other antibiotics to eradicate GABHS has led to extrapolation that these antibiotics will also prevent rheumatic fever.[53]

Amoxicillin may be preferable for children with GABHS pharyngitis because the suspension is more palatable than penicillin.[47] GI adverse effects and rash are more common with amoxicillin. A once-daily, extended-release formulation of amoxicillin has been approved for treatment of GABHS pharyngitis in adults and children aged 12 years and older; however, use of once-daily dosing in GABHS pharyngitis is not recommended by current guidelines.[47]

If patients are unable to take oral medications, intramuscular benzathine penicillin can be given, although it is painful.[47] In penicillin-allergic patients, azithromycin, clarithromycin, clindamycin, or a first-generation cephalosporin such as cephalexin can be used if the reaction is non–IgE-mediated (strong, moderate).[47,53] Newer macrolides such as azithromycin and clarithromycin are equally effective as erythromycin and cause fewer GI adverse effects; therefore, these newer macrolides are preferred to erythromycin. GABHS resistance to macrolides is low (5% to 8%) in the United States, but is higher in some other areas of the world.[47]

TABLE 86-5 Antibiotics and Doses for Group A β-Hemolytic Streptococcal Pharyngitis

Antibiotic	Brand Name	Dose	Duration	Rating
Preferred Antibiotics				
Penicillin V	Pen-V®	Children: 250 mg twice daily or three times daily orally Adult: 250 mg four times daily or 500 mg twice daily orally	10 days	IB
Penicillin G benzathine	Bicillin L-A®	Less than 27 kg: 0.6 million units; 27 kg or greater: 1.2 million units intramuscularly	One dose	IB
Amoxicillin[a]	Amoxil®	50 mg/kg once daily (maximum 1,000 mg); 25 mg/kg (maximum 500 mg) twice daily	10 days	IB
Penicillin Allergy				
Cephalexin	Keflex®	20 mg/kg/dose orally twice daily (maximum 500 mg/dose)	10 days	IB
Cefadroxil	Duricef®	30 mg/kg orally once daily (maximum 1 g)	10 days	IB
Clindamycin	Cleocin®	7 mg/kg/dose orally thrice daily (maximum 300 mg/dose)	10 days	IIaB
Azithromycin[b]	Zithromax®	12 mg/kg orally once daily (maximum 500 mg)	5 days	IIaB
Clarithromycin[b]	Biaxin®	15 mg/kg orally per day divided in two doses (maximum 250 mg twice daily)	10 days	IIaB

These guidelines provide a systematic weighting of the strength of the recommendation (Class I, conditions for which there is evidence and/or general agreement that a given procedure or treatment is beneficial, useful, and effective; Class II, conditions for which there is conflicting evidence and/or a divergence of opinion about the usefulness/efficacy of a procedure or treatment; Class IIa, weight of evidence/opinion is in favor of usefulness/efficacy; Class IIb, usefulness/efficacy is less well established by evidence/opinion; Class III, conditions for which there is evidence and/or general agreement that a procedure/treatment is not useful/effective and in some cases may be harmful) and quality of evidence (A, data derived from multiple randomized clinical trials or meta-analyses; B, data derived from a single randomized trial or nonrandomized studies; C, only consensus opinion of experts, cases studies, or standard of care).

[a]Standard formulation, not extended release.

[b]Resistance of GABHS to these agents may vary and local susceptibilities should be considered with these agents.

From reference 47.

In previous pharyngitis guidelines, clindamycin was only an alternative to erythromycin-resistant strains; however, it is now considered an acceptable alternative for penicillin-allergic patients due to the low GABHS resistance rate of 1%.[47,53] Tonsillectomy is not recommended because a Cochrane review found that its impact on "sore throat" due to pharyngitis is unpredictable (strong, high).[55]

GABHS resistance rates to tetracyclines are high. Sulfonamides and trimethoprim–sulfamethoxazole have poor eradication rates for GABHS; therefore, use of these antibiotics is no longer recommended.[47] Fluoroquinolones are not recommended due to poor activity of the older agents. The newer fluoroquinolones have activity against GABHS but are expensive and have a broad spectrum of activity.[47,53]

The ideal time to start antibiotics has not been established. The immediate start of antibiotics does not affect the risk of developing rheumatic fever, and no evidence suggests it reduces recurrent infection.[53] Clinical guidelines recommend withholding antibiotics unless the patient has a positive laboratory result.[47,53] Nevertheless, a survey of clinicians treating children and adolescents with acute pharyngitis revealed that 42% of clinicians would start antibiotics before diagnostic results were received and many would continue antibiotics despite a negative test result.[56] A retrospective analysis of visits to a primary care clinic for acute pharyngitis demonstrated that 66% of providers did not adhere to any of the recommended pharyngitis guidelines.[54]

The impact of appropriate antibiotic therapy is limited to decreasing the duration of signs and symptoms by 1 or 2 days.[48] It can decrease the severity of pharyngitis symptoms when initiated within 2 or 3 days of onset in patients with proven GABHS. Microbiologic eradication will occur in 48 to 72 hours, which aids in decreasing transmission.[48] The duration of therapy for GABHS pharyngitis is 10 days, except for benzathine penicillin and azithromycin, to maximize bacterial eradication (strong, moderate).[47] Although some clinicians have proposed shorter courses of treatment for pharyngitis, confounding factors from these studies, such as the lack of strict entry criteria or differentiation between new and failed infections, limit the widespread application of short antibiotic courses at this time.[47]

Approximately 25% of household contacts of a person with acute GABHS pharyngitis harbor GABHS in their upper respiratory tracts.[47] Routine testing and/or treating of asymptomatic household contacts of an index patient is not recommended (strong, moderate).[47] GABHS carriers do not need antimicrobial therapy due to very low risk of spreading GABHS pharyngitis or developing suppurative or nonsuppurative complications.[49] If tested, it is not necessary

TABLE 86-6 Antibiotics and Doses for Eradication of Group A β-Hemolytic Streptococcal Pharyngitis in Chronic Carriers

Antibiotic	Brand Name	Dose
Clindamycin	Cleocin®	20–30 mg/kg/day orally in three divided doses (maximum 300 mg/dose)
Amoxicillin–clavulanate	Augmentin®	40 mg/kg/day orally in three divided doses (maximum 2,000 mg/day of amoxicillin)
Penicillin V and rifampin	Pen-V®, Rifadin®	Penicillin V: 50 mg/kg/day in four doses × 10 days (maximum 2,000 mg/day); *and* rifampin: 20 mg/kg/day in one dose × last 4 days of treatment (maximum 600 mg/day)
Penicillin G benzathine and rifampin	Bicillin L-A®, Rifadin®	Penicillin G benzathine: less than 27 kg—0.6 million units; 27 kg or greater—1.2 million units intramuscularly; *and* rifampin: 20 mg/kg/day orally in two doses during last 4 days of treatment with penicillin (maximum 600 mg/day)

From reference 47.

to treat these asymptomatic carriers. It is difficult to ascertain the cause of symptomatic pharyngitis in carriers of GABHS if they do develop symptoms. Providers should pay close attention to the symptoms to help differentiate viral versus bacteriologic cause of pharyngitis because laboratory tests will be positive in these patients (strong, moderate).[47]

Clinical **Controversy...**

A study explored the value of pharmacist-provided care for patients with GABHS pharyngitis. The study measured treatment costs and health outcomes in patients diagnosed and managed by a community pharmacist or usual care.[57] Groups were compared in terms of treatment costs (excluding diagnostic costs) and quality-adjusted life days. The two models scored similarly in terms of quality-adjusted life days; however, the community pharmacist provided care at a lower treatment cost. The feasibility of pharmacist-directed care for patients with GABHS pharyngitis needs to be determined in additional studies involving larger populations.

When acute GABHS pharyngitis occurs in a carrier, a treatment course of appropriate antibiotics is recommended.[47,53] In the treatment of recurring episodes of culture-positive GABHS pharyngitis, there are limited data to support a particular antibiotic regimen. Several alternative antibiotics are preferred over penicillin or amoxicillin with GABHS carriers and recurrent pharyngitis. Amoxicillin–clavulanate, clindamycin, penicillin/rifampin combination, and benzathine penicillin G/rifampin combination may be considered for recurrent episodes of pharyngitis to maximize bacterial eradication in potential carriers and to counter copathogens that produce β-lactamases.[47] Table 86-6 outlines dosing for eradication of GABHS in chronic carriers and those who experience symptomatic episodes.

Patients with documented histories of rheumatic fever (including cases manifested solely by Sydenham's chorea) and those with definite evidence of rheumatic heart disease should receive continuous prophylaxis initiated as soon as the patient is diagnosed and the initial infection has been treated. The duration of secondary prophylaxis is individualized based on patient risk of recurrence of rheumatic fever and/or rheumatic heart disease. Intramuscular benzathine penicillin G every 4 weeks is the recommended regimen for secondary prevention in the United States in most circumstances.[53] Additional options for secondary prophylaxis include oral penicillin V and sulfadiazine. Medication adherence is critical for successful secondary prevention with oral antibiotics. Sulfadiazine is an effective antibiotic for the prevention of infection and is appropriate if the patient is penicillin-allergic. Sulfonamides are not appropriate for treatment of GABHS pharyngitis because they are not effective for eradication of GABHS. If individuals are allergic to penicillin and sulfadiazine, a macrolide or azalide is recommended; however, this recommendation is based on expert opinion rather than clinical trial data.[53]

Personalized Pharmacotherapy

Currently, there are no pharmacogenetic or genomic factors involved in the diagnosis or treatment of GABHS pharyngitis. Factors that should be considered when personalizing therapy for a patient include allergy status, prior antibiotic use, and adherence. Those with a history of antibiotic use for acne may be at higher risk for resistant strains of GABHS. Short-course antibiotics or penicillin G benzathine may be considered in patients with a history of nonadherence.

Evaluation of Therapeutic Outcomes

Most pharyngitis cases are self-limited; however, antibiotics hasten resolution when given early for proven cases of GABHS pharyngitis.[47] Generally, fever and other symptoms resolve within 3 or 4 days of onset without antibiotics; however, symptoms will improve 0.5 to 2.5 days earlier with antibiotic therapy.[47] Follow-up testing is generally not necessary for index cases or in asymptomatic contacts of the index patient[47,50]; however, throat cultures 2 to 7 days after completion of antibiotics are warranted for patients who remain symptomatic or when symptoms recur despite completion of treatment.[53]

ABBREVIATIONS

AAFP	American Academy of Family Physicians
AAP	American Academy of Pediatrics
CFU	colony-forming unit
GABHS	group A β-hemolytic streptococci
Hib	*Haemophilus influenzae* type b
IDSA	Infectious Diseases Society of America
MIC	minimum inhibitory concentration
PCV7	seven-valent pneumococcal conjugate vaccine
RADT	rapid antigen-detection test
T tube	tympanostomy tube
URI	upper respiratory infection

REFERENCES

1. Hsiao CJ, Cherry DK, Beatty PC, Rechtsteiner EA. National Ambulatory Medical Care Survey: 2007 summary. Natl Health Stat Report 2010;(27):1–32.
2. Hing E, Hall MJ, Ashman JJ, Xu J. National Hospital Ambulatory Medical Care Survey: 2007 outpatient department summary. Natl Health Stat Report 2010;(28):1–32.
3. Coker TR, Chan LS, Newberry SJ, et al. Diagnosis, microbial epidemiology, and antibiotic treatment of acute otitis media in children: A systematic review. JAMA 2010;304(19):2161–2169.
4. Monasta L, Ronfani L, Marchetti F, et al. Burden of disease caused by otitis media: Systematic review and global estimates. PLoS One 2012;7(4):e36226.
5. Soni A. Ear Infections (Otitis Media) in Children (0-17): Use and Expenditures, 2006. Statistical Brief #228. Rockville, MD: Agency for Healthcare Research and Quality, 2008, *http://www.meps.ahrq.gov/mepsweb/data_files/publications/st228/stat228.shtml.*
6. American Academy of Pediatrics Subcommittee on Management of Acute Otitis Media. Diagnosis and management of acute otitis media. Pediatrics 2004;113(5):1451–1465.
7. Wald ER. Acute otitis media and acute bacterial sinusitis. Clin Infect Dis 2011;52(Suppl 4):S277–S283.
8. Pichichero ME, Casey JR. Emergence of a multiresistant serotype 19A pneumococcal strain not included in the 7-valent conjugate vaccine as an otopathogen in children. JAMA 2007;298(15):1772–1778.
9. Jones RN, Sader HS, Moet GJ, Farrell DJ. Declining antimicrobial susceptibility of *Streptococcus pneumoniae* in the United States: Report from the SENTRY Antimicrobial Surveillance Program (1998-2009). Diagn Microbiol Infect Dis 2010;68(3):334–336.

10. Harrison CJ, Woods C, Stout G, et al. Susceptibilities of *Haemophilus influenzae*, *Streptococcus pneumoniae*, including serotype 19A, and *Moraxella catarrhalis* paediatric isolates from 2005 to 2007 to commonly used antibiotics. J Antimicrob Chemother 2009;63(3):511–519.
11. Critchley IA, Brown SD, Traczewski MM, et al. National and regional assessment of antimicrobial resistance among community-acquired respiratory tract pathogens identified in a 2005-2006 U.S. Faropenem surveillance study. Antimicrob Agents Chemother 2007;51(12):4382–4389.
12. Sahm DF, Brown NP, Draghi DC, et al. Tracking resistance among bacterial respiratory tract pathogens: Summary of findings of the TRUST Surveillance Initiative, 2001–2005. Postgrad Med 2008;120(3 Suppl 1):8–15.
13. Chonmaitree T, Revai K, Grady JJ, et al. Viral upper respiratory tract infection and otitis media complication in young children. Clin Infect Dis 2008;46(6):815–823.
14. Jansen AG, Hak E, Veenhoven RH, et al. Pneumococcal conjugate vaccines for preventing otitis media. Cochrane Database Syst Rev 2009;(2):CD001480.
15. Agrawal A, Murphy TF. *Haemophilus influenzae* infections in the *H. influenzae* type b conjugate vaccine era. J Clin Microbiol 2011;49(11):3728–3732.
16. Foxlee R, Johansson A, Wejfalk J, et al. Topical analgesia for acute otitis media. Cochrane Database Syst Rev 2006;(3):CD005657.
17. Coleman C, Moore M. Decongestants and antihistamines for acute otitis media in children. Cochrane Database Syst Rev 2008;(3):CD001727.
18. Griffin GH, Flynn C, Bailey RE, Schultz JK. Antihistamines and/or decongestants for otitis media with effusion (OME) in children. Cochrane Database Syst Rev 2006;(4):CD003423.
19. Rovers MM, Glasziou P, Appelman CL, et al. Antibiotics for acute otitis media: A meta-analysis with individual patient data. Lancet 2006;368(9545):1429–1435.
20. Thanaviratananich S, Laopaiboon M, Vatanasapt P. Once or twice daily versus three times daily amoxicillin with or without clavulanate for the treatment of acute otitis media. Cochrane Database Syst Rev 2008;(4):CD004975.
21. Tahtinen PA, Laine MK, Huovinen P, et al. A placebo-controlled trial of antimicrobial treatment for acute otitis media. N Engl J Med 2011;364(2):116–126.
22. Hoberman A, Paradise JL, Rockette HE, et al. Treatment of acute otitis media in children under 2 years of age. N Engl J Med 2011;364(2):105–115.
23. Spurling GK, Del Mar CB, Dooley L, Foxlee R. Delayed antibiotics for respiratory infections. Cochrane Database Syst Rev 2007;(3):CD004417.
24. Coco A, Vernacchio L, Horst M, Anderson A. Management of acute otitis media after publication of the 2004 AAP and AAFP clinical practice guideline. Pediatrics 2010;125(2):214–220.
25. Schuetz P, Briel M, Christ-Crain M, et al. Procalcitonin to guide initiation and duration of antibiotic treatment in acute respiratory infections: An individual patient data meta-analysis. Clin Infect Dis 2012;55(5):651–662.
26. Schuetz P, Muller B, Christ-Crain M, et al. Procalcitonin to initiate or discontinue antibiotics in acute respiratory tract infections. Cochrane Database Syst Rev 2012;9: CD007498.
27. Schuetz P, Amin DN, Greenwald JL. Role of procalcitonin in managing adult patients with respiratory tract infections. Chest 2012;141(4):1063–1073.
28. Chow AW, Benninger MS, Brook I, et al. IDSA clinical practice guideline for acute bacterial rhinosinusitis in children and adults. Clin Infect Dis 2012;54(8):e72–e112.
29. Guyatt GH, Oxman AD, Vist GE, et al. GRADE: An emerging consensus on rating quality of evidence and strength of recommendations. BMJ 2008;336(7650): 924–926.
30. Schiller JS, Lucas JW, Ward BW, Peregoy JA. Summary health statistics for U.S. adults: National Health Interview Survey, 2010. Vital Health Stat 10 2012;(252):1–207.
31. Gill JM, Fleischut P, Haas S, et al. Use of antibiotics for adult upper respiratory infections in outpatient settings: A national ambulatory network study. Fam Med 2006;38(5):349–354.
32. Rosenfeld RM, Andes D, Bhattacharyya N, et al. Clinical practice guideline: Adult sinusitis. Otolaryngol Head Neck Surg 2007;137(3 Suppl):S1–S31.
33. Bhattacharyya N. Contemporary assessment of the disease burden of sinusitis. Am J Rhinol Allergy 2009;23(4): 392–395.
34. Revai K, Dobbs LA, Nair S, et al. Incidence of acute otitis media and sinusitis complicating upper respiratory tract infection: The effect of age. Pediatrics 2007;119(6): e1408–e1412.
35. Kassel JC, King D, Spurling GK. Saline nasal irrigation for acute upper respiratory tract infections. Cochrane Database Syst Rev 2010;(3):CD006821.
36. Williamson IG, Rumsby K, Benge S, et al. Antibiotics and topical nasal steroid for treatment of acute maxillary sinusitis: A randomized controlled trial. JAMA 2007;298(21):2487–2496.
37. Zalmanovici A, Yaphe J. Intranasal steroids for acute sinusitis. Cochrane Database Syst Rev 2009;(4):CD005149.
38. Desrosiers M, Evans GA, Keith PK, et al. Canadian clinical practice guidelines for acute and chronic rhinosinusitis. J Otolaryngol Head Neck Surg 2011;40(Suppl 2): S99–S193.
39. Garbutt JM, Banister C, Spitznagel E, Piccirillo JF. Amoxicillin for acute rhinosinusitis: A randomized controlled trial. JAMA 2012;307(7):685–692.
40. Falagas ME, Giannopoulou KP, Vardakas KZ, et al. Comparison of antibiotics with placebo for treatment of acute sinusitis: A meta-analysis of randomised controlled trials. Lancet Infect Dis 2008;8(9):543–552.
41. Young J, De Sutter A, Merenstein D, et al. Antibiotics for adults with clinically diagnosed acute rhinosinusitis: A meta-analysis of individual patient data. Lancet 2008;371(9616):908–914.
42. Ahovuo-Saloranta A, Borisenko OV, Kovanen N, et al. Antibiotics for acute maxillary sinusitis. Cochrane Database Syst Rev 2008;(2):CD000243.
43. Casey JR, Adlowitz DG, Pichichero ME. New patterns in the otopathogens causing acute otitis media six to eight years after introduction of pneumococcal conjugate vaccine. Pediatr Infect Dis J 2010;29(4):304–309.
44. Tristram S, Jacobs MR, Appelbaum PC. Antimicrobial resistance in *Haemophilus influenzae*. Clin Microbiol Rev 2007;20(2):368–389.
45. Venekamp RP, Thompson MJ, Hayward G, et al. Systemic corticosteroids for acute sinusitis. Cochrane Database Syst Rev 2011;(12):CD008115.
46. Mfuna-Endam L, Zhang Y, Desrosiers MY. Genetics of rhinosinusitis. Curr Allergy Asthma Rep 2011;11(3): 236–246.
47. Shulman ST, Bisno AL, Clegg HW, et al. Clinical practice guideline for the diagnosis and management of group A streptococcal pharyngitis: 2012 update by the Infectious Diseases Society of America. Clin Infect Dis 2012;55: 1279–1282.

48. Snow V, Mottur-Pilson C, Cooper RJ, Hoffman JR. Principles of appropriate antibiotic use for acute pharyngitis in adults. Ann Intern Med 2001;134(6):506–508.
49. Salkind AR, Wright JM. Economic burden of adult pharyngitis: The payer's perspective. Value Health 2008;11(4):621–627.
50. Bisno AL. Acute pharyngitis. N Engl J Med 2001;344(3):205–211.
51. Cooper RJ, Hoffman JR, Bartlett JG, et al. Principles of appropriate antibiotic use for acute pharyngitis in adults: Background. Ann Intern Med 2001;134(6):509–517.
52. Wessels MR. Clinical practice. Streptococcal pharyngitis. N Engl J Med 2011;364(7):648–655.
53. Gerber MA, Baltimore RS, Eaton CB, et al. Prevention of rheumatic fever and diagnosis and treatment of acute streptococcal pharyngitis: A scientific statement from the American Heart Association Rheumatic Fever, Endocarditis, and Kawasaki Disease Committee of the Council on Cardiovascular Disease in the Young, the Interdisciplinary Council on Functional Genomics and Translational Biology, and the Interdisciplinary Council on Quality of Care and Outcomes Research: Endorsed by the American Academy of Pediatrics. Circulation 2009;119(11):1541–1551.
54. Linder JA, Chan JC, Bates DW. Evaluation and treatment of pharyngitis in primary care practice: The difference between guidelines is largely academic. Arch Intern Med 2006;166(13):1374–1379.
55. Burton MJ, Glasziou PP. Tonsillectomy or adeno-tonsillectomy versus non-surgical treatment for chronic/recurrent acute tonsillitis. Cochrane Database Syst Rev 2009;(1):CD001802.
56. Park SY, Gerber MA, Tanz RR, et al. Clinicians' management of children and adolescents with acute pharyngitis. Pediatrics 2006;117(6):1871–1878.
57. Klepser DG, Bisanz SE, Klepser ME. Cost-effectiveness of pharmacist-provided treatment of adult pharyngitis. Am J Manag Care 2012;18(4):e145–e154.

87

Influenza

Jessica C. Njoku and Elizabeth D. Hermsen

KEY CONCEPTS

1. Influenza is a viral illness associated with high mortality and high hospitalization rates among persons older than age 65 years. The aging of the population is contributing to an increased disease burden in the United States.
2. Seasonal influenza epidemics are the result of viral antigenic drift, which is why the influenza vaccine is changed on a yearly basis. Antigenic drift forms the foundation of the recommendation for annual influenza vaccination.
3. The acquisition of a new hemagglutinin and/or neuraminidase by the influenza virus is called *antigenic shift*, which results in a novel influenza virus that has the potential to cause a pandemic.
4. The primary route of influenza transmission is person-to-person via inhalation of respiratory droplets, and transmission can occur for as long as the infected person is shedding virus from the respiratory tract.
5. Clinical diagnosis of influenza is difficult. Classic signs and symptoms include abrupt onset of fever, muscle pain, headache, malaise, nonproductive cough, sore throat, and rhinitis. These signs and symptoms usually resolve within 1 week of presentation.
6. In the United States, the primary mechanism of influenza prevention is annual vaccination. Vaccination not only prevents influenza illness and influenza-related hospitalizations and deaths but also may decrease healthcare resource use and the overall cost to society.
7. The trivalent influenza vaccine (TIV) and the live-attenuated influenza vaccine (LAIV) are the two commercially available vaccines for prevention of seasonal influenza. Both vaccines contain influenza A subtypes H3N2 and H1N1 and influenza B virus, which are initially grown in hens' eggs.
8. Antiviral drugs for prophylaxis of influenza should be considered adjuncts to vaccine and are not replacements for annual vaccination.
9. The sooner the antiviral drugs are started after the onset of illness, the more effective they are.
10. Oseltamivir and zanamivir are neuraminidase inhibitors that have activity against both influenza A and influenza B viruses, while the adamantanes have activity against only some influenza A H1N1 viruses. Antiinfluenza agents are most effective if started within 48 hours of the onset of illness.

Influenza causes significant morbidity and mortality, particularly among young children and the elderly. Seasonal influenza epidemics result in 25 to 50 million influenza cases, approximately 200,000 hospitalizations, and more than 30,000 deaths each year in the United States. Globally, influenza causes nearly 500,000 deaths each year. More people die of influenza than of any other vaccine-preventable illness. Significant societal consequences associated with influenza include visits to physicians' offices and emergency departments and days lost from school and/or work. The societal costs associated with influenza are more than $40 billion in the United States alone.[1]

Vaccination is the primary mechanism of influenza prevention in the United States. The antiviral armamentarium for treatment and prophylaxis of influenza is limited, which further emphasizes the importance of prevention with vaccination and appropriate use of infection control measures during outbreaks. Research toward the development of novel antivirals and vaccines is needed for effective control of seasonal epidemics and for pandemic preparedness.

ETIOLOGY AND EPIDEMIOLOGY

Influenza infection can occur at any time during the year with the highest rates of influenza-associated illness during the winter months. The highest rate of infection occurs in children, but the highest rates of severe illness, hospitalization, and death occur among those older than age 65 years, young children (<2 years old), and those who have underlying medical conditions, including pregnancy and cardiopulmonary disorders, that increase their risk of complications from influenza. (1) The seasonal influenza epidemics from 1993 to 2008 resulted in an average annual influenza-associated hospitalization rate of 63.5 (95% CI, 37.5 to 236.6) per 100,000 person-years. Influenza-associated hospitalization rates were four times higher among infants aged <1 year compared with among those aged 1 to 4 years.[2] Similarly, influenza-associated hospitalization rates were 18 times higher, and 5 times higher, among persons aged ≥65 years compared with among those aged 5 to 49 years, and 50 to 64 years, respectively.[2] In 2006 alone, an estimated 37,000 hospital discharges were attributed to influenza.[1,2] Approximately 90% of seasonal influenza-related deaths occur in those older than age 65 years.[3] Thus, the aging of the population is contributing to an increased disease burden. Deaths associated with influenza often result from secondary bacterial pneumonia, primary viral pneumonia, and/or exacerbation of underlying comorbidities.

Influenza Viruses A, B, and C

Influenza virus types A, B, and C are members of the Orthomyxoviridae family and affect many species, including humans, pigs, horses, and birds. Influenza A and B viruses are the two types that cause disease in humans. Influenza A viruses are responsible for the regular, seasonal epidemics of the flu, whereas influenza B viruses are typically associated with sporadic outbreaks, particularly among residents of long-term care facilities. Influenza A viruses are further categorized into different subtypes based on changes in two surface antigens—hemagglutinin and neuraminidase (NA). Influenza B viruses are not categorized into subtypes.

Hemagglutinin allows the influenza virus to enter host cells by attaching to sialic acid receptors and is the major antigen to which antibodies are directed on exposure.[4] NA allows the release of new viral particles from host cells by catalyzing the cleavage of linkages to sialic acid.[4]

Sixteen hemagglutinin subtypes (H1 to H16) and nine NA subtypes (N1 to N9) of influenza A have been isolated from birds. However, the only influenza A subtypes that have circulated among humans since the 1918 pandemic (see Antigenic Drift and Antigenic Shift below) are H1 to H3 and N1 and N2.[4] The primary subtypes of influenza A that have been circulating among humans for the past 3 decades are H3N2 and H1N1.

Antigenic Drift and Antigenic Shift

❷ Immunity to influenza virus occurs as a result of the development of antibody directed at the surface antigens, particularly hemagglutinin. However, immunity to one influenza subtype does not offer protection against other subtypes or types of influenza. Moreover, immunity to one antigenic variant of a subtype of influenza may not confer protection against other antigenic variants. Antigenic variants are created by point mutations in the surface antigens of a particular subtype, resulting in small changes in the hemagglutinin and/or NA molecules, which is called *antigenic drift*. Antigenic drift is the basis for seasonal epidemics of influenza, the reason for changes in the annual influenza vaccine, and the rationale behind the recommendation for annual vaccination.

Immunity to one subtype of influenza does not confer protection against other subtypes or types. ❸ Antigenic shift occurs when the influenza virus acquires a new hemagglutinin and/or NA via genetic reassortment rather than point mutations.[4] Most likely, the genetic reassortment occurs when an animal that supports the growth of multiple subtypes of influenza, such as a pig, is concurrently infected with two subtypes of the influenza virus. Conversely, antigenic shift may occur directly from avian strains that have gained competency in the human host. Antigenic shift results in the emergence of a novel influenza virus and carries the potential of causing a pandemic. However, novelty alone is insufficient to cause an influenza pandemic; the virus must be able to replicate in humans, spread person-to-person, and affect a susceptible population.[4]

Spanish Influenza of 1918

The influenza pandemic of 1918 was the most significant infectious disease outbreak known to humans, causing approximately 40 to 50 million deaths in a year, with more than 500,000 deaths occurring in the United States.[4–6] Although the reports of the first illnesses associated with this pandemic occurred in Spain, there is no evidence that the virus associated with this pandemic actually originated there, indicating a misnomer. The pandemic occurred almost concurrently in Europe, Asia, and North America.[5]

The 1918 pandemic was caused by a particularly virulent influenza A H1N1 virus, which was entirely of avian origin.[7] In contrast to the other pandemics of the 20th century, the 1918 pandemic resulted in an unusual mortality pattern. The mortality peaked for those younger than age 4 years, those between the ages of 25 and 35 years, and those older than 65 years of age, which resulted in a W-shaped mortality curve, as opposed to the U- or J-shaped curve typically associated with influenza.[6] Over half of the deaths occurred in persons aged 20 to 40 years. The death toll associated with this pandemic culminated in an almost 10-year drop in the life expectancy of the population at the time.[6]

Asian Influenza of 1957

The Asian flu pandemic began when a new H2 subtype of influenza A surfaced in Hunan province in China in 1957.[6] The virus appears to have formed from coinfection with an avian H2N2 virus and a human H1N1 virus in a common host, possibly a pig or a human.[8] The H2N2 virus quickly spread to Japan, South America, the United States, New Zealand, and Europe, resulting in approximately 4 million deaths worldwide, with 70,000 deaths occurring in the United States.[5,6] Unlike the Spanish flu of 1918, the mortality curve for the Asian flu pandemic was U- or J-shaped, with infants and elderly being most affected.[5]

Hong Kong Influenza of 1968

The H2N2 virus of the Asian flu circulated in the human population until 1968, when a new H3 subtype emerged in China and Hong Kong[5] following genetic reassortment with the H2N2 virus.[5,6] The H3N2 virus quickly spread to the United States and later to Europe. This pandemic caused more than 30,000 deaths in the United States and approximately 2 million deaths worldwide.[5,6] The lower morbidity and mortality associated with the Hong Kong flu may be explained by previous exposure of the population to the N2 subtype. Similar to the Asian flu of 1957, the mortality curve for the Hong Kong flu pandemic was U- or J-shaped, primarily affecting infants and elderly.[5]

Avian Influenza

Influenza viruses are in circulation in southern China during all months of the year.[4] Given this fact and the close proximity of dense populations of people, pigs, and wild and domestic birds, this area proves ideal for the development of new influenza viruses via genetic reassortment (antigenic shift), as demonstrated by the pandemics of 1957 and 1968 and, most recently, the emergence of what is known as avian influenza.[4]

The first report of human infection with the avian H5N1 virus occurred in 1997 in Hong Kong in a 3-year-old who had a direct link with chickens and later died.[9] This was followed by 18 confirmed cases and 6 deaths.[10] The virus reemerged in 2003 as an antigenically and genetically different virus that has spread widely through wild and domestic bird populations in Asia, Africa, and Europe as well as infecting humans in 15 countries: Azerbaijan, Bangladesh, Cambodia, China, Djibouti, Egypt, Indonesia, Iraq, Lao People's Democratic Republic, Myanmar, Nigeria, Pakistan, Thailand, Turkey, and Vietnam.[5,11] As of August 10, 2012, a total of 608 cases and 359 deaths caused by H5N1 infection have been reported.[11] The current overall case fatality is 60%.

The spread of avian influenza viruses from person to person has been reported very rarely, and has been limited, inefficient, and unsustained.[12,13] The precise mode of transmission is unknown, but most cases have occurred as a result of close and prolonged person-to-person contact. Cases of transmission via aerosolization have not been reported.[14] Clinical presentation includes high fever and influenza-like illness, and watery diarrhea without blood may occur up to 1 week prior to respiratory symptoms.[16] Almost all patients have clinically apparent pneumonia. Progression to death, most commonly as a consequence of respiratory failure, occurs a mean of 9 to 10 days after the onset of illness.[14] The NA inhibitors, oseltamivir and zanamivir, have activity against the H5N1 virus, although higher doses may be needed. Oseltamivir resistance has been detected in several patients infected with the H5N1 virus who were treated with oseltamivir.[14] Amantadine and rimantadine are ineffective against H5N1. An inactivated monovalent influenza virus vaccine against H5N1 is available for vaccination of persons 18 to 64 years of age at increased risk of exposure to the H5N1 influenza virus. Two 1-mL doses given intramuscularly 28 days apart (range, 21 to 35 days) are recommended. The vaccine is supplied in a 5-mL multidose vial, with ~50 mcg thimerosal per dose added as a preservative.[15] At the present time, the vaccine is being stockpiled for use if H5N1 begins transmitting easily from person to person. Individuals at high risk, for example, those who work with poultry and H5N1 poultry outbreak responders, are encouraged to receive annual seasonal influenza vaccine to minimize the risk of coinfection with human and avian influenza A viruses.

The potential for H5N1 to cause a pandemic is of concern as it could spread more quickly than pandemics of the past because of the mobility of people in today's world. International travel has increased 73% since 1990, with 763 million people crossing international borders in 2004.[16] A severe pandemic, like that of 1918, could cause more than 9 million hospitalizations and more than 1.9 million deaths, whereas a moderate pandemic, like those of 1957 and 1968, could result in more than 800,000 hospitalizations and more than 200,000 deaths in the United States alone.[5]

Swine Influenza of 2009

An outbreak of a novel influenza A H1N1 (formerly swine origin influenza virus [SOIV]) was initially detected in Mexico in March 2009 and subsequently in the United States in April 2009 in California and Texas.[17–19] The virus then spread throughout North America, Europe, Asia, and subsequently worldwide, prompting the World Health Organization (WHO) on June 11, 2009 to declare phase 6, indicating widespread human infection, for the influenza pandemic.[18] Since 1998, triple reassortant swine influenza A (H1) viruses, containing genes from swine, avian, and human lineages, have circulated among swine in the United States.[19] However, the novel influenza A H1N1 virus is unique in that although much of the genome is similar to the triple reassortant swine viruses previously seen in the United States, the genes encoding for NA and matrix (M) proteins are most similar to those circulating in the Eurasian swine population. This particular genetic combination has not been seen before.[19] The virus has since become the predominant influenza A H1N1 in circulation, effectively replacing traditional seasonal influenza A (H1N1).

Several characteristics of the novel influenza A H1N1 outbreak differ from those of a typical seasonal influenza outbreak. Symptomatology associated with the novel influenza include fever (94%), cough (92%), sore throat (66%), diarrhea (25%), and vomiting (25%).[19,20] An estimated 43 to 89 million cases of 2009 H1N1 occurred between April 2009 and April 2010 with a median 274,000 hospitalizations. Globally, 18,500 laboratory-confirmed H1N1-related deaths were reported; however, this may represent an underestimation of true disease burden.[20,21] The majority of the cases occurred in otherwise healthy children and young adults <65 years of age including pregnant women, with the highest incidence reported among those aged 18 to 64 years.[20] Contrary to seasonal influenza where about 60% of hospitalizations and 90% of deaths occur in people ≥65 years, approximately 90% and 87% of 2009 H1N1-related hospitalizations and deaths, respectively, occurred in people <65 years. However, like seasonal influenza, people with underlying health conditions had greater risk of hospitalizations and death. Among those who were deceased due to novel H1N1 infection, the median age was ~40 years and 59% of deaths (respiratory and cardiovascular) occurred in Southeast Asia and Africa.[20,21]

Variant Influenza A (H3N2), 2012

In August 2011, the U.S. Centers for Disease Control and Prevention (CDC) reported the first case of an influenza infection due to influenza A H3N2 variant virus (H3N2v).[22] Since then, 319 cases (12 from 2011, and 307 from 2012) were reported from 12 states in the United States resulting in 13 hospitalizations and 0 deaths.[23] As at the time of this publication, no human infection with H3N2v had been documented outside of the United States. The H3N2v is considered a variant virus because it is different from influenza A viruses circulating among humans. Infections due to variant influenza viruses, for example, A(H1N1)v, A(H3N2)v, and A(H1N2)v of swine origin, have been documented in the past.[22] The H3N2v virus contains genes from avian, swine, and human viruses and the M gene from the 2009 H1N1 pandemic virus (A[H1N1]pdm09).[24] The virus was originally detected in pigs in 2010 but human infection was first documented in July 2011. The virus appears to spread more readily from pigs to people than other variant viruses, but has limited person-to-person transmission. The main risk factor for infection with the virus based on evaluation of available cases is exposure to pigs, mostly in fair settings.[22] Since the virus is related to human flu viruses from the 1990s, most adults have some immunity against it.[25] Hence, most cases to date have occurred in children, who have little immunity against this virus.

The symptoms and severity of H3N2v have mostly been mild and similar to those of seasonal influenza (fever, cough, sore throat, body aches, etc.), but like seasonal influenza, serious illness with H3N2v infection is possible.[22] Vaccination remains key to preventing H3N2v infection. Additionally, the CDC has encouraged people at high risk of influenza complications to stay away from swine barns at the fair.[26] People who are at high risk of serious complications from influenza, including H3N2v virus infection, are: children <5 years old, people ≥65 years old, pregnant women, and people with certain chronic medical conditions (asthma, diabetes, heart disease, immunocompromised, and neurologic or neurodevelopmental conditions). The treatment of H3N2v virus infection is similar to that of seasonal influenza. NA inhibitors are the mainstay of treatment. The adamantanes should not be used due to high resistance.[26]

PATHOGENESIS

4 The route of influenza transmission is person-to-person via inhalation of respiratory droplets, which can occur when an infected person coughs or sneezes.[26] Transmission may also occur if a person touches an object contaminated with respiratory secretions and then touches his or her mucus membranes. The incubation period for influenza ranges between 1 and 7 days, with an average incubation of 2 days.[26] Transmission can occur for as long as the infected person is shedding virus from the respiratory tract. Adults are considered infectious within 1 day before until 7 days after onset of illness. Children, especially younger children, might potentially be infectious for longer periods (>10 days).[22,27] Viral shedding can persist for weeks to months in severely immunocompromised people.

The pathogenesis of influenza in humans is not well understood. The severity of the infection is determined by the balance between viral replication and the host immune response.[4] Severe illness is likely a result of both a lack of ability of host defense mechanisms to inhibit viral replication and an overproduction of cytokines leading to tissue damage in the host.[28]

CLINICAL PRESENTATION Diagnosis of Influenza

General

- The clinical diagnosis of influenza can be difficult because the presentation is similar to a number of other respiratory illnesses. The sensitivity of clinical diagnosis ranges from 38% for children to 77% for adults and largely depends on the relative prevalence of influenza and other respiratory viruses circulating in a community.[29]
- The clinical course and outcome are affected by age, immunocompetence, viral characteristics, smoking, comorbidities, pregnancy, and the degree of preexisting immunity.
- Complications of influenza may include exacerbation of underlying comorbidities, primary viral pneumonia, secondary bacterial pneumonia or other respiratory illnesses (e.g., sinusitis, bronchitis, otitis), encephalopathy, transverse myelitis, myositis, myocarditis, pericarditis, and Reye's syndrome.

Signs and Symptoms

- 5 Classic signs and symptoms of influenza include rapid onset of fever, myalgia, headache, malaise, nonproductive cough, sore throat, and rhinitis.
- Nausea, vomiting, and otitis media are also commonly reported in children.[30]
- Signs and symptoms typically resolve in approximately 3 to 7 days, although cough and malaise may persist for more than 2 weeks.
- Primary viral pneumonia, occurring predominantly in pregnant women and in those with underlying cardiovascular disease, usually begins with fever and dry cough, which changes to a productive cough of bloody sputum. This rapidly progresses to dyspnea, hypoxemia, and cyanosis with radiologic evidence of bilateral interstitial infiltrates.[31]
- Secondary bacterial pneumonia is usually seen in individuals with underlying pulmonary disorders and presents during the early stages of defervescence from the influenza infection. These patients usually present with fever, productive cough, and radiologic evidence of consolidation.[31]

Laboratory Tests

- Complete blood count and chemistry panels should be obtained to assess the overall status of the patient.
- The gold standard for diagnosis of influenza is viral culture, which can provide information on the specific strain and subtype. Viral culture has a high sensitivity but can take as long as a week to develop, limiting the clinical relevance of the results.
- Tests such as the rapid antigen and point-of-care (POC) tests, direct fluorescence antibody (DFA) test, and the reverse-transcription polymerase chain reaction (RT-PCR) assay may be used for rapid detection of virus.

Other Diagnostic Tests

- Cultures of potential sites of infection should be obtained if coinfection, superinfection, or secondary infection is suspected.
- Chest radiograph should be obtained if pneumonia is suspected.

Rapid Tests

- Rapid tests have allowed for prompt diagnosis and initiation of antiviral therapy and decreased inappropriate use of antibiotics. Rapid antigen or POC tests use enzyme immunoassay (EIA) technology to provide results within 1 hour of specimen collection. Appropriate specimens for collection, in decreasing order of sensitivity, are nasopharyngeal aspirates, nasopharyngeal swabs/washes, and oropharyngeal swabs.[29] POC tests allow for differentiation of influenza viruses A and B, with sensitivity and specificity ranging from 57% to 90% and 65% to 99%, respectively.[29] In general, use of POC tests is contraindicated in those who have had symptoms for longer than 3 days, and results may be confounded following recent immunization with live-attenuated influenza vaccine (LAIV).[29]
- DFA testing requires more technical expertise and infrastructure than POC tests. The advantages of DFA are increased sensitivity over POC tests and simultaneous detection of other respiratory viruses, such as respiratory syncytial virus and adenovirus.[30] DFA provides results between 1 and 4 hours after specimen collection and may serve as a confirmatory assay for a POC test.
- RT-PCR assay is a nucleic acid amplification test and is the most sensitive, specific, and versatile diagnostic test for influenza.[29] RT-PCR is replacing viral isolation as the reference standard and can determine the type, subtype, and strain of influenza. Results are provided within 4 to 6 hours of specimen collection.

PREVENTION

The best means to decrease the morbidity and mortality associated with influenza is to prevent infection through vaccination.[26,27] Appropriate infection control measures, such as hand hygiene, basic respiratory etiquette (e.g., cover your cough, throw tissues away), and contact avoidance, are also important in preventing the spread of influenza. Additionally, chemoprophylaxis is useful in certain situations.

Vaccination

6 The primary means of influenza prevention employed in the United States is annual vaccination. Vaccination can help prevent hospitalization and death among those at high risk, decrease influenza-like illness, decrease visits to physicians' offices and emergency rooms, decrease otitis media in children, and prevent school and/or work absenteeism. Annual vaccination is now recommended for all persons aged 6 months or older and caregivers (e.g., parents,

TABLE 87-1 Influenza Vaccination Rates and Goals by Patient Population[26]

Patient Population	Vaccination Coverage (%)	Vaccination Coverage National Goal (2000/2012)
Children aged 6–23 months	41[a]	N/A
Persons aged 18–49 years with high-risk conditions	38[a]	60%/60%
Persons aged 18–49 years without high-risk conditions	29[a]	60%/60%
Persons aged 50–64 years	46[a]	60%/60%
Persons aged 50–64 years with high-risk conditions	55[b]	60%/60%
Persons aged >65 years	69[a]	60%/90%
Nursing home residents	83[c]	80%/90%
Pregnant women without other high-risk conditions	11[b]	N/A
Healthcare workers	35[a]	N/A

N/A, not applicable; no goals established.

[a]2009–2010 data.
[b]2008–2009 data.
[c]1998 data.

teachers, babysitters, nannies) of children <6 months of age. Vaccination is also recommended for those who live with and/or care for people who are at high risk, including household contacts and healthcare workers.

The ideal time for all influenza vaccination is during October or November to allow for the development and maintenance of immunity during the peak of the influenza season.[26,27] Table 87-1 lists the vaccination coverage rates and goals for various patient populations.

7 The two vaccines currently available for prevention of seasonal influenza are the trivalent influenza vaccine (TIV) and the LAIV. Both vaccines contain two influenza A subtypes (H3N2 and H1N1) and influenza B virus; the specific strains included in the vaccine each year change based on antigenic drift. The viruses used for both vaccines are initially grown in embryonated hens' eggs, which explain the precautionary measures for vaccination of persons with a severe allergic reaction to eggs.[26] The Advisory Committee on Immunization Practices (ACIP) has made the following recommendations regarding the vaccinations of persons with reports of egg allergy: (a) vaccination with TIV rather than with LAIV for persons with a history of egg allergy that involves only hives. Vaccination should be done by a healthcare provider who is familiar with possible manifestations of egg allergy and the recipient should be observed for at least 30 minutes after dose. (b) Persons with severe allergic reactions such as angioedema, respiratory distress, light-headedness, or recurrent emesis or required epinephrine after an egg exposure should be referred to a physician with expertise in the management of allergic reactions for the receipt of an influenza vaccination. (c) Severe allergic reaction to influenza vaccine is a contraindication to receiving future vaccinations.[26] The CDC encourages individuals to use the Vaccine Adverse Event Reporting System to aide in collecting and analyzing adverse events following influenza vaccinations.[26]

Trivalent Influenza Vaccine

7 Intramuscular TIV is FDA approved for use in people older than 6 months of age, regardless of their immune status. Of note, several commercial products are available and are approved for different age groups (Table 87-2). The intradermal vaccine, Fluzone Intradermal®, is approved by FDA for use in adults 18 to 64 years of age and is another vaccination option for people in this age group. TIV is made with killed viruses, meaning it cannot cause signs and symptoms of influenza-like illness (Table 87-3). Age and immune status can affect the efficacy of TIV as can the similarity of the vaccine to the viruses in circulation. Afluria® brand of TIV vaccine is contraindicated in patients with hypersensitivity to neomycin or polymyxin. Afluria® is also not recommended first line in children 6 months to 8 years, due to reports of high febrile episodes following administration.[26,32]

In children between 6 and 24 months of age, a 2-year randomized study of intramuscular TIV exhibited 89% seroconversion and

TABLE 87-2 Approved Influenza Vaccines for Different Age Groups—United States, 2012–2013 Season[26]

Vaccine	Trade Name	Manufacturer	Dose/Presentation	Thimerosal Mercury Content (mcg Hg/0.5 mL dose)	Age Group	Number of Doses
TIV	Fluzone	Sanofi Pasteur	0.25-mL prefilled syringe	0	6–35 months	1 or 2[a]
			0.5-mL prefilled syringe	0	≥36 months	1 or 2[a]
			0.5-mL vial	0	≥36 months	1 or 2[a]
			5-mL multidose vial	25	≥6 months	1 or 2[a]
TIV	Agriflu	Novartis Vaccines	0.5-mL prefilled syringe	0	≥18 years	1
TIV	Fluvirin	Novartis Vaccines	0.5-mL prefilled syringe	<1	≥4 years	1 or 2[a]
			5-mL multidose vial	25	≥4 years	1 or 2[a]
TIV	Fluarix	GlaxoSmithKline	0.5-mL prefilled syringe	0	≥3 years	1
TIV	FluLaval	ID Biomedical Corporation	5-mL multidose vial	<25	≥18 years	1
TIV	Afluria	CSL Biotherapies	0.5-mL prefilled syringe	0	≥9 years	1
			5-mL multidose vial	24.5	≥9 years	
TIV High Dose	Fluzone HD	Sanofi Pasteur	0.5-mL prefilled syringe	0	≥65 years	1
TIV intradermal	Fluzone Intradermal	Sanofi Pasteur	0.1-mL prefilled microinjection system	0	18–64 years	1[b]
LAIV	FluMist[c]	MedImmune	0.2-mL sprayer	0	2–49 years	1 or 2[d]

LAIV, live-attenuated influenza vaccine; TIV, trivalent influenza vaccine.

[a]Two doses administered at least 1 month apart are recommended for children aged 6 months to less than 9 years who are receiving influenza vaccine for the first time or received one dose in first year of vaccination during the previous influenza season.
[b]*Given intradermally.* A 0.1-mL dose contains 9 mcg of each vaccine antigen (27 mcg total).
[c]The new quadrivalent formulation of FluMist approved in 2012 will replace currently available seasonal trivalent LAIV formulation beginning 2013–2014 season.
[d]Two doses administered 4 weeks apart are recommended for children aged 2 to less than 9 years who are receiving influenza vaccine for the first time.

TABLE 87-3 Comparison of Trivalent (TIV) and Live-Attenuated Influenza Vaccine (LAIV)

Characteristic	TIV	LAIV
Age groups approved for use	>6 months	2–49 years
Immune status requirements	Immunocompetent or immunocompromised	Immunocompetent
Viral properties	Inactivated (killed) influenza A (H3N2), A (H1N1), and B viruses	Live-attenuated influenza A (H3N2), A (H1N1), and B viruses
Route of administration	Intramuscular/intradermal	Intranasal
Immune system response	High serum IgG antibody response	Lower IgG response and high serum IgA mucosal response

efficacy of 66% in year 1 and 7% in year 2 versus culture-confirmed influenza.[33] In children between 1 and 15 years of age, the efficacy of TIV was 91.4% and 77.3% against culture-confirmed influenza A H1N1 and H3N2, respectively. Two doses of TIV are important for children under the age of 9 years, supporting the rationale for the recommendation of a booster dose of TIV at least 1 month after the initial dose in children between 6 months and less than 9 years of age (see Table 87-2).[26]

TIV is also effective in adult populations under and older than the age of 65 years. A double-blind, randomized controlled trial evaluating intramuscular TIV in healthy adults younger than the age of 65 years demonstrated an efficacy of 50% against serologically confirmed influenza during a season in which the vaccine and the circulating viruses were not well matched and an efficacy of 86% during a season in which the vaccine and the circulating viruses were well matched.[34] These findings were corroborated by a large Cochrane Database System review, which found that TIV had an efficacy of 70% in healthy adults younger than 65 years of age, regardless of virus and vaccine concordance.[35] Vaccination of those younger than 65 years old during seasons when the virus and vaccine are well matched results in decreased work absenteeism and healthcare resource use.[34,35]

Intradermal TIV in adults 18 to 64 years of age provides immune response similar to the intramuscular injection.[36] Both vaccines were similar in their safety profile. In clinical trials Fluzone® intradermal was noninferior to Fluzone® intramuscular in eliciting immune response as measured by hemagglutination inhibition antibody geometric mean titers (GMTs).[36] The rate of seroconversion was similar between the two vaccines against influenza strains A (H1N1 and H3N2), but not for strain B. The most common adverse reactions were injection site related, which were transient (resolving in 3 to 7 days), and include erythema (>75%), swelling (>50%), induration (>50%), pain (>50%), and pruritus (>40%). Compared with the intramuscular vaccine, Fluzone® intradermal contains 40% less antigen (Table 87-2).

Adults older than the age of 65 years benefit from influenza vaccination, including prevention of complications and decreased risk of influenza-related hospitalization and death. However, people in this population may not generate a strong antibody response to the vaccine and may remain susceptible to infection. In patients older than the age of 60 years who do not reside in a long-term care facility, TIV efficacy was 58% against influenza illness.[26] Although the efficacy against influenza illness for those living in long-term care facilities is between 30% and 40%, the vaccine is 50% to 60% effective in preventing influenza-related hospitalization or pneumonia and 80% effective in preventing influenza-related death.[26]

The most frequent adverse effect associated with TIV is soreness at the injection site that lasts for less than 48 hours. TIV may cause fever and malaise in those who have not previously been exposed to the viral antigens in the vaccine.[26] Allergic-type reactions (hives, systemic anaphylaxis) rarely occur after influenza vaccination and are likely a result of a reaction to residual egg protein in the vaccine.

The 1976 swine influenza vaccine was linked to a rise in the incidence of Guillain-Barré syndrome (GBS), and this has propagated the belief that TIV may cause GBS.[26] However, there is insufficient evidence to establish causality. Although several studies have failed to establish a relationship between influenza vaccination and increased frequency of GBS, two studies have demonstrated a small but significant increase in GBS following influenza vaccination.[37,38] Therefore, vaccination should be avoided in persons who are not at high risk for influenza complications and who have experienced GBS within 6 weeks of receiving a previous influenza vaccine.[26] The potential benefits of influenza vaccination in terms of prevention of severe illness, hospitalization, and mortality significantly outweigh the risks of GBS, and vaccination is recommended for all groups previously discussed.

The multidose vials and a few of the single-dose preparations of intramuscular TIV contain trace to small amounts of a preservative, thimerosal, which is a mercury-containing compound (see Table 87-2). Some individuals are concerned about thimerosal exposure, particularly among children, because of the unfounded belief that thimerosal exposure is linked to the development of autism. No scientifically persuasive evidence exists to suggest harm from thimerosal exposure from a vaccine. Conversely, accumulating evidence reports the lack of harm from such exposure.[39–41] Thus, similar to GBS, the potential benefits of influenza vaccination in terms of prevention of severe illness, hospitalization, and mortality significantly outweigh the theoretical risk associated with thimerosal exposure, and vaccination is recommended for all groups previously discussed. However, to maximize the public health benefit and placate concerned individuals, thimerosal-free vaccine is available (see Table 87-2).

Live-Attenuated Influenza Vaccine

7 LAIV is made with live, attenuated viruses and is approved for intranasal administration in healthy people between 2 and 49 years of age (see Table 87-3). Advantages of LAIV include its ease of administration, intranasal rather than intramuscular administration, and the potential induction of broad mucosal and systemic immune response.[26] The mucosal response occurs at the site of viral entry and may prevent infection before viral replication occurs. LAIV is more expensive than TIV and is approved for use in a more limited population.

Controlled studies support the use of LAIV in healthy people between the ages of 2 and 49 years. Although LAIV was previously FDA approved for children who were at least 5 years old, three pivotal trials led the FDA to approve LAIV for children who were at least 2 years old.[42] LAIV recipients aged 2 to 5 years had 52.5% and 54.4% fewer cases of influenza illness against matched and mismatched strains, respectively, as compared with TIV recipients.

Although LAIV is FDA approved for adults younger than the age of 49 years, LAIV is effective in healthy adults between 18 and 64 years old.[43] Vaccination reduced the number of severe febrile illnesses by 18.8% and febrile upper respiratory tract illnesses by 23.6%.[43] Additionally, vaccination led to fewer days of illness, fewer days lost from work, fewer visits to healthcare providers, and decreased use of prescription antibiotics and nonprescription medications.[43]

The adverse effects typically associated with LAIV administration include runny nose, congestion, sore throat, and headache.

Because LAIV contains live, attenuated viruses, viral shedding may occur for several days following vaccination with LAIV, although this should not be equated with person-to-person transmission.[26] Additionally, because LAIV contains live-attenuated viruses, which carry a theoretical infection risk, LAIV should not be given to immunosuppressed patients or given by healthcare workers who are severely immunocompromised. Moreover, for the reasons discussed in Trivalent Influenza Vaccine above, LAIV should not be administered to persons with a history of GBS or hypersensitivity to eggs.

In February 2012, the FDA approved FluMist® Quadrivalent vaccine for influenza prevention in people aged 2 to 49 years.[44] FluMist® Quadrivalent vaccine contains four strains of the influenza viruses, two influenza A strains and two influenza B strains. This is the first influenza vaccine of this modality. The inclusion of a second B strain in the vaccine is thought to increase the likelihood of adequate protection against circulating influenza B strains. Like the already approved FluMist® trivalent, the quadrivalent vaccine is made of attenuated viruses and is administered as a spray into the nose. Studies of FluMist® trivalent, in addition to three new clinical trials with the quadrivalent vaccine in 4,000 children (2 to 17 years) and adults (18 to 49 years) in the United States, provide supporting evidence on the efficacy and safety of FluMist® Quadrivalent.[44] The studies showed that immune responses were similar between FluMist® Quadrivalent and FluMist® trivalent. Also, adverse reactions reported were similar among those receiving FluMist® Quadrivalent and FluMist® trivalent. The most commonly reported adverse reactions were runny or stuffy nose in both children and adults, and headache and sore throat in adults. The quadrivalent vaccine will replace the trivalent LAIV formulation for the 2013 to 2014 influenza season (Table 87-2).

Clinical **Controversy. . .**

LAIV is not recommended in several populations, including people older than 50 years and pregnant women, largely because the vaccine has not been studied extensively in these populations. However, many clinicians believe the use of LAIV in these populations is acceptable.

Postexposure Prophylaxis

8 Antiviral drugs available for prophylaxis of influenza should be considered adjuncts but are not replacements for annual vaccination. Historically, the adamantanes and NA inhibitors are two classes of antiviral drugs available for influenza prophylaxis and treatment. However, the adamantanes are no longer recommended for prophylaxis or treatment in the United States (because of widespread resistance among influenza viruses) until susceptibility is reestablished among influenza A virus.[45–47] Both of the NA inhibitors, oseltamivir and zanamivir, are effective prophylactic agents against influenza in terms of preventing laboratory-confirmed influenza when used for seasonal prophylaxis (67% and 85% effective for zanamivir and oseltamivir, respectively) and preventing influenza illness among persons exposed to a household contact who was diagnosed with influenza (79% to 81% and 68% to 89% effective for zanamivir and oseltamivir, respectively).[38,48,49] Additionally, oseltamivir was 92% effective against influenza and also reduced associated complications when used as seasonal prophylaxis among immunized, institutionalized, elderly patients.[50] Both of these agents remain active against all influenza viruses, including influenza A H3N2v (Tables 87-4 and 87-5). During the time of pandemic H1N1 influenza in 2009, the FDA expanded the use of oseltamivir to children 3 months or older under its emergency use authorization (EUA) guidance. However, the EUA has since expired in June 2010 and oseltamivir is limited to its approved indications in individuals aged 1 year or above. In practice, clinicians continue to apply the expanded dosage recommendations for children 3 to 11 months of age, which are endorsed by the American Academy of Pediatrics and Pediatric Infectious Diseases Society (PIDS).[27,47] Table 87-6 gives dosing recommendations.

TABLE 87-4 Antiviral Susceptibilities of Circulating Viruses

	Oseltamivir	Zanamivir	Adamantanes
Variant influenza A (H3N2), 2012	Susceptible	Susceptible	Resistant
Novel influenza A (H1N1)	Susceptible[a]	Susceptible	Resistant
Seasonal A (H3N2)	Susceptible	Susceptible	Resistant
Influenza B	Susceptible	Susceptible	Resistant
Avian influenza (H5N1)	Susceptible	Susceptible	Variable

[a]Small number of isolates shown to be resistant to oseltamivir.

In those patients who did not receive the influenza vaccination and are receiving an antiviral drug for prevention of disease during the influenza season, the medication should optimally be taken for the entire duration of influenza activity in the community. The use of prophylaxis requires clinical judgment and depends on a variety of factors, but prophylaxis for seasonal influenza should be considered during influenza season for the following groups of patients:

1. Persons at high risk of serious illness and/or complications who cannot be vaccinated
2. Persons at high risk of serious illness and/or complications who are vaccinated after influenza activity has begun in their community since the development of sufficient antibody titers after vaccination takes approximately 2 weeks
3. Unvaccinated persons who have frequent contact with those at high risk
4. Persons who may have an inadequate response to vaccination (e.g., advanced human immunodeficiency virus [HIV] disease)
5. Long-term care facility residents, regardless of vaccination status, when an outbreak has occurred in the institution
6. Unvaccinated household contacts of someone who was diagnosed with influenza

TABLE 87-5 Interim Recommendations for the Selection of Antiviral Treatment Based on Confirmed Influenza Subtypes[45,47]

Laboratory Test	Preferred[a]	Alternative
Not performed or negative, but influenza suspected clinically[a]	Oseltamivir or zanamivir	None
Positive variant H3N2v	Oseltamivir or zanamivir	None
Positive novel H1N1	Oseltamivir or zanamivir	None
Positive A (nonnovel H1N1)	Oseltamivir or zanamivir	None
Positive A (H3N2), or B	Oseltamivir or zanamivir	None
Positive A + B	Oseltamivir or zanamivir	None

[a]Viral surveillance data might help guide antiviral choices if oseltamivir resistance becomes more prevalent.

TABLE 87-6 Recommended Daily Dosage of Influenza Antiviral Medications for Treatment and Prophylaxis—United States[27,45,47]

Drug	Adult Treatment	Adult Prophylaxis[a]	Pediatric Treatment[b]	Pediatric Prophylaxis[c]
Oseltamivir	75-mg capsule twice daily for 5 days	75-mg capsule daily	≤3 months[d]: 12 mg twice daily 3–5 months[d]: 20 mg twice daily 6–11 months[d]: 25 mg twice daily ≥1 year ≤15 kg: 30 mg twice daily 16–23 kg: 45 mg twice daily 23–40 kg: 60 mg twice daily >40 kg: 75 mg twice daily All for 5 days	≤3 months. Not recommended; situation judged critical due to limited data in this group 3–5 months[d]: 20 mg daily 6–11 months[d]: 25 mg daily ≥1 year ≤15 kg: 30 mg daily 16–23 kg: 45 mg daily 23–40 kg: 60 mg daily >40 kg: 75 mg daily
Zanamivir	2 inhalations twice daily × 5 days	2 inhalations daily	2 inhalations twice daily × 5 days for ≥7 years old	2 inhalations daily for ≥5 years old
Rimantadine[e]	200 mg/day in one to two doses × 7 days	200 mg/day in one to two doses	1–9 years old or <40 kg: 6.6 mg/kg/day divided twice daily (maximum 150 mg/day) ≥10 years old: 200 mg/day in one to two doses Treat 5–7 days	1–9 years old: 5 mg/kg daily (maximum 150 mg/day) ≥10 years old: 200 mg/day in one to two doses
Amantadine[e]	200 mg/day in one to two doses until 24–48 hours after symptom resolution	Same as treatment doses	>12 years old: same as adult 1–9 years old: 5 mg/kg/day in one to two doses; maximum 150 mg/day ≥10–12 years old: 100 mg orally twice daily	Same as treatment doses

[a]If influenza vaccine is administered, prophylaxis can generally be stopped 14 days after vaccination for noninstitutionalized persons. When prophylaxis is being administered following an exposure, prophylaxis should be continued for 10 days after the last exposure. In persons at high risk for complications from influenza for whom vaccination is contraindicated or expected to be ineffective, chemoprophylaxis should be continued for the duration that influenza viruses are circulating in the community during influenza season.

[b]Alternate dosing by IDSA/PIDS (2011) is: infants and premature—1 mg/kg/dose q 12 h; 0–8 months—3 mg/kg/dose q 12 h; 9–23 months—3.5 mg/kg/dose q 12 h.[47]

[c]Alternate dosing by IDSA/PIDS (2011) is: 3–8 months—3 mg/kg/dose daily; 9–23 months—3.5 mg/kg/dose daily.[47]

[d]Unlabeled dosing.[27]

[e]*Note:* Although amantadine and rimantadine have been used historically for the treatment and prophylaxis of influenza A viruses, due to high resistance, the CDC no longer recommends the use of these agents for the treatment and/or prophylaxis of influenza.

Prophylaxis for novel H1N1 influenza should be considered in the following groups:

1. Persons at high risk of serious illness and/or complications who have had close contact with persons with laboratory-confirmed or clinically confirmed novel H1N1 infection during those persons' infectious period
2. Healthcare/public health personnel who have had recognized, unprotected close contact with persons with laboratory-confirmed or clinically confirmed novel H1N1 infection during those persons' infectious period

LAIV should not be administered until 48 hours after influenza antiviral therapy has stopped, and influenza antiviral drugs should not be administered for 2 weeks after the administration of LAIV because the antiviral drugs inhibit influenza virus replication.[38] No contraindication exists for concomitant use of TIV and influenza antiviral drugs.

Pregnant Women and Immunocompromised Hosts

Pregnant women and immunocompromised hosts are special populations at increased risk of influenza complications and are also populations in whom careful consideration must be given in regard to prevention strategies.

Pregnant women, regardless of trimester, should receive annual influenza vaccination with TIV but not with LAIV.[26] No studies have demonstrated an increased incidence of adverse effects in mothers or their infants related or potentially related to TIV, but no such data exist for LAIV.[51] TIV is also safe for breast-feeding mothers. No data exist for LAIV and breast-feeding, but caution is warranted because of the potential for viral shedding.[26]

Immunocompromised hosts should receive annual influenza vaccination with TIV but not with LAIV. TIV was 100% effective against laboratory-confirmed influenza in HIV-positive patients with no significant effect on viral load or CD4 cell count.[52] However, antibody titers may not be as high as in immunocompetent individuals and are not improved with a second dose of vaccine.[53] Similarly, antibody titers may not be as high in solid-organ transplant patients as in immunocompetent persons, but, conversely, antibody titers were increased significantly after a second dose of TIV in adult liver transplant patients.[54] Although this suggests a potential benefit from a two-dose regimen, such a regimen is not currently recommended for solid-organ transplant recipients. Data are currently limited in this arena for the intradermal TIV. In a study of intradermal TIV involving immunocompromised patients compared with healthy controls, humoral responses (GMTs and protection rates [PRs]) were significantly better among healthy controls than those among immunocompromised patients.[55] This is not surprising given an already attenuated immune system. But it was also noted that compared with the standard intramuscular TIV, GMTs and PRs were similar within all tested groups. Immune response to vaccine may be less than desired in immunocompromised patients.[26]

Large clinical trials evaluating the use of influenza antivirals for prophylaxis are lacking in immunocompromised hosts. Viral shedding occurs for prolonged periods in this population and may promote the development of antiviral resistance, which has already been documented with oseltamivir in HIV-positive patients.[56,57]

TREATMENT

When prevention efforts fail or are not used, clinicians must turn to the agents available for treatment of influenza. Currently, the antiviral treatment options are limited, particularly in the face of resistance to the adamantanes and oseltamivir.

Goals of Therapy

The four primary goals of therapy of influenza are to control symptoms, prevent complications, decrease work and/or school absenteeism, and prevent the spread of infection.

General Approach to Treatment

In the era of pandemic preparedness and increasing resistance, early and definitive diagnosis of influenza is crucial. 9 The currently available antiviral drugs are most effective if started within 48 hours of the onset of illness. Moreover, the sooner the antiviral drugs are started after the onset of illness, the more effective they are. Antiviral drugs shorten the duration of illness and provide symptom control. Adjunct agents, such as acetaminophen for fever or an antihistamine for rhinitis, may be used concomitantly with the antiviral drugs.

Nonpharmacologic Therapy

Patients suffering from influenza should get adequate sleep and maintain a low level of activity. They should stay home from work and/or school in order to rest and prevent the spread of infection. Appropriate fluid intake should be maintained. Cough/throat lozenges, warm tea, or soup may help with symptom control (cough, sore throat).

Pharmacologic Therapy

The NA inhibitors are the only antiviral drugs available for treatment and prophylaxis of influenza and are oseltamivir and zanamivir. IV peramivir is another NA inhibitor under investigation for treatment of influenza. The adamantanes (amantadine and rimantadine) are no longer recommended due to high resistance among influenza viruses. A limited discussion of adamantanes and peramivir can be found below, but the focus will be on oseltamivir and zanamivir.

Adamantanes

The adamantanes (amantadine and rimantadine) block the M2 ion channel, which is specific to influenza A viruses, and inhibit viral uncoating. Historically, the adamantanes were used for the treatment of seasonal influenza A H1N1, as they do not have activity against influenza A H3N2 or influenza B viruses. The novel influenza A H1N1 that emerged during the 2009 to 2010 influenza season, which has now replaced seasonal influenza A H1N1 as the predominant seasonal virus, was found to be discriminatorily resistant to the adamantanes. Data from the 2009 to 2010 influenza season showed that 81.8% of influenza A (H3N2) and 99.6% of influenza A (2009 H1N1) strains were resistant to adamantanes.[58] As a result, the CDC only recommends the use of NA inhibitors for the treatment and prophylaxis of influenza A, until susceptibility of adamantanes is reestablished among influenza A viruses. Resistance to adamantanes is often conferred by a single point mutation, and this is problematic because it results in cross-resistance to the entire class.[45,46]

Neuraminidase Inhibitors

10 Oseltamivir and zanamivir are NA inhibitors that have activity against both influenza A and influenza B viruses.[45,46] Without NA, release of the virus from infected cells is impaired, and, thus, viral replication is decreased. When administered within 48 hours of the onset of illness, oseltamivir and zanamivir may reduce the duration of illness by approximately 1 day versus placebo.[45] In a pivotal trial, oseltamivir reduced the time to return to normal health in adults by 1.9 days and the time to return to normal activity by 2.8 days.[59] These reductions have a significant effect on not only the quality of life for the patient but also the societal costs associated with influenza. 9 Of note, the benefits of treatment are highly dependent on the timing of the initiation of treatment, with the ideal initiation period being within 12 hours of illness onset.[60]

Oseltamivir treatment in adults and adolescents with documented influenza illness resulted in a 26.7% reduction in overall antibiotic use, a 55% reduction in lower respiratory tract complications (bronchitis, pneumonia), and a 59% reduction in hospitalizations.[61] Zanamivir treatment in adults and adolescents with influenza-like illness resulted in a 28% reduction in antibiotic use and a 40% reduction in lower respiratory tract complications.[62] The data in these studies largely come from healthy individuals rather than those at highest risk for complications associated with influenza. The impact of appropriate treatment in high-risk populations may be even greater than that which has been documented to date.

Oseltamivir is approved for treatment in those older than the age of 1 year, while zanamivir is approved for treatment in those older than the age of 7 years. During the H1N1 pandemic in 2009, the FDA issued an EUA for oseltamivir that expanded its use in children younger than 1 year of age. The EUA has since expired on June 23, 2010[63]; however, the dosages in children 3 to 11 months are still used in clinical practice.[27] The recommended doses vary by agent and age (see Table 87-6), and the recommended duration of treatment for both oseltamivir and zanamivir is 5 days.

During 2009 H1N1 influenza pandemic, FDA allowed the use of investigational peramivir for the treatment of hospitalized adult and pediatric patients under its EUA.[64] However, like oseltamivir, this EUA has expired[63] and individuals in need of peramivir therapy will have to be enrolled in an ongoing study. Preliminary data suggest that peramivir is as effective as oseltamivir, without severe adverse events. Based on an observational study, the 14-day, 28-day, and 56-day survival rates of 31 patients with severe 2009 H1N1 infection treated with peramivir were 77%, 67%, and 59%, respectively.[65] The most common adverse event reported was rash.[66]

Neuropsychiatric complications consisting of delirium, seizures, hallucinations, and self-injury in pediatric patients (mostly from Japan) have been reported following treatment with oseltamivir.[67–69] Since influenza itself can be associated with neuropsychiatric manifestations, a causal relationship between oseltamivir and neuropsychiatric effects has not been delineated.[66,67] However, the label for oseltamivir has been updated to include neuropsychiatric events as a precaution,[67] and their occurrence with use of oseltamivir should not be ignored.

Influenza resistance to the NA inhibitors has been documented but cross-resistance between the NA inhibitors has not been reported.[45] Antiviral resistance remains relatively low. During the 2011 to 2012 influenza season, 98.6% of the tested 2009 H1N1 viruses were susceptible to oseltamivir, and 100% of the 2009 H1N1 viruses tested were susceptible to zanamivir; 100% of influenza A (H3N2) tested were susceptible to both oseltamivir and zanamivir; and 100% of influenza B viruses tested were susceptible to both oseltamivir and zanamivir.[70] Antiviral susceptibility testing of circulating viruses confirmed that seasonal influenza A H3N2 and variant influenza H3N2 maintain susceptibility to oseltamivir and zanamivir.[23,24] The burden of surveillance rests on clinicians to identify local patterns of influenza circulation to guide antiviral therapy.

Clinical **Controversy...**

Some clinicians debate the cost–benefit of the use of diagnostic tests for influenza as well as treatment of influenza in otherwise healthy individuals who are likely to experience resolution without treatment. This controversy is compounded by the fact that the diagnostic tests and the benefits associated with treatment of influenza are highest early in the disease process and many patients present after this time period.

Special Populations

Inadequate data exist regarding the use of antiinfluenza medications in special populations, such as immunocompromised hosts. Furthermore, limited data exist regarding use of influenza antivirals during pregnancy. The adamantanes are embryotoxic and teratogenic in rats, and limited case reports of adverse fetal outcomes following amantadine use in humans have been published. Oseltamivir and zanamivir have been used but lack solid safety clinical data in pregnant women. Pregnancy should not be considered a contraindication to oseltamivir or zanamivir use. Oseltamivir is preferred for treatment of pregnant women because of its systemic activity; however, the drug of choice for chemoprophylaxis is not yet defined. Zanamivir may be preferred because of its limited systemic absorption, but respiratory complications need to be considered, especially in women with underlying respiratory diseases. Both the adamantanes and the NA inhibitors are excreted in breast milk and should be avoided by mothers who are breast-feeding their infants. More studies are needed in these populations who are at high risk for serious disease and complications from influenza.

Clinical **Controversy. . .**

Some debate exists regarding the benefit of antiviral administration >48 hours after onset. While clinicians agree that the most benefit is achieved the earlier the medications are started, some data suggest benefit even beyond 48 hours after onset, albeit more limited.

PANDEMIC PREPAREDNESS

This chapter is not meant to provide an exhaustive review of the biology of influenza or pandemic preparedness. This topic is rapidly changing and interested readers are referred to the following websites: *www.flu.gov*, *www.who.int/influenza/human_animal_interface/en/*, and *www.cdc.gov/h1n1flu*.

A vital component of pandemic preparedness is forethought—plans must be established for how to effectively triage large numbers of ill patients, prioritize and/or ration vaccine and antivirals, and communicate with the public through mass media during a period of severe labor shortage (a result of stress and illness among healthcare workers) and supply shortfall (a result of societal and economic disruption).

EVALUATION OF THERAPEUTIC OUTCOMES

Patients should be monitored daily for resolution of signs and symptoms associated with influenza, such as fever, myalgia, headache, malaise, nonproductive cough, sore throat, and rhinitis. These signs and symptoms will typically resolve within approximately 1 week. If the patient continues to exhibit signs and symptoms of illness beyond 10 days or a worsening of symptoms after 7 days, a physician visit is warranted as this may be an indication of a secondary bacterial infection. Ideally, antiviral therapy should not be started until influenza is confirmed via the laboratory. However, therapy should be initiated within 48 hours of illness onset, emphasizing the need for rapid diagnosis. Repeat diagnostic tests to demonstrate clearance of the virus are not necessary.

ABBREVIATIONS

ACIP	Advisory Committee on Immunization Practices
CDC	U.S. Centers for Disease Control and Prevention
DFA	direct fluorescence antibody
EIA	enzyme immunoassay
EUA	emergency use authorization
GBS	Guillain-Barré syndrome
GMTs	geometric mean titers
HIV	human immunodeficiency virus
LAIV	live-attenuated influenza vaccine
M	matrix
NA	neuraminidase
PIDS	Pediatric Infectious Diseases Society
POC	point of care
PRs	protection rates
RT-PCR	reverse-transcription polymerase chain reaction
SOIV	swine origin influenza virus
TIV	trivalent influenza vaccine
WHO	World Health Organization

REFERENCES

1. American Lung Association. Trends in Pneumonia and Influenza Morbidity and Mortality. American Lung Association. New York: Research and Scientific Affairs Epidemiology and Statistics Unit, 2010.
2. Zhou H, Thompson WW, Viboud CG, et al. Hospitalizations associated with influenza and respiratory syncytial virus in the United States, 1993-2008. Clin Infect Dis 2012;54(10):1427–1436.
3. Centers for Disease Control and Prevention (CDC). Estimates of deaths associated with seasonal influenza—United States, 1976–2007. MMWR Morb Mortal Wkly Rep 2010;59(33):1057–1062.
4. Nicholson KG, Wood JM, Zambon M. Influenza. Lancet 2003;362(9397):1733–1745.
5. Monto AS, Comanor L, Shay DK, Thompson WW. Epidemiology of pandemic influenza: Use of surveillance and modeling for pandemic preparedness. J Infect Dis 2006;194(Suppl 2):S92–S97.
6. Palese P. Influenza: Old and new threats. Nat Med 2004; 10(12 Suppl):S82–S87.
7. Taubenberger JK, Morens DM. 1918 influenza: The mother of all pandemics. Emerg Infect Dis 2006;12(1):15–22.
8. Belshe RB. The origins of pandemic influenza—Lessons from the 1918 virus. N Engl J Med 2005;353(21):2209–2211.
9. Yuen KY, Chan PK, Peiris M, et al. Clinical features and rapid viral diagnosis of human disease associated with avian influenza A H5N1 virus. Lancet 1998;351(9101):467–471.
10. Mounts AW, Kwong H, Izurieta HS, et al. Case–control study of risk factors for avian influenza A (H5N1) disease, Hong Kong, 1997. J Infect Dis 1999;180(2):505–508.
11. Anonymous. Epidemic and Pandemic Alert and Response: Avian Influenza. *http://www.who.int/csr/disease/avian_influenza/en/index.html*.
12. Yang Y, Halloran ME, Sugimoto JD, Longini IM Jr. Detecting human-to-human transmission of avian influenza A (H5N1). Emerg Infect Dis 2007;13:1348–1353.
13. Zaman M, Ashraf S, Dreyer NA, Toovey S. Human infection with avian influenza virus, Pakistan, 2007. Emerg Infect Dis 2011;17(6):1056–1059.
14. Beigel JH, Farrar J, Han AM, et al. Avian influenza A (H5N1) infection in humans. N Engl J Med 2005;353(13):1374–1385.

15. Avian Influenza H5N1 Vaccine. *http://www.fda.gov/downloads/BiologicsBloodVaccines/Vaccines/ApprovedProducts/UCM112836.pdf.*
16. Hill DR. The burden of illness in international travelers. N Engl J Med 2006;354(2):115–117.
17. Centers for Disease Control and Prevention. Update: Novel influenza A (H1N1) virus infections—Worldwide, May 6, 2009. MMWR Morb Mortal Wkly Rep 2009;58:453–458.
18. World Health Organization. Influenza A (H1N1)—Update 14. Geneva: World Health Organization, 2009, *http://www.who.int/csr/don/2009_05_04a/en/index.html.*
19. Dawood FS, Jain S, Finelli L, et al. Novel swine-origin influenza A (H1N1) virus investigation team. Emergence of a novel swine-origin influenza A (H1N1) virus in humans. N Engl J Med 2009;360:2605–2615.
20. Centers for Disease Control and Prevention (CDC). Prevention. Flu Activity & Surveillance [Updated in Weekly CDC Surveillance Reports]. *http://www.cdc.gov/h1n1flu/estimates_2009_h1n1.htm.*
21. Dawood FS, Iuliano AD, Reed C, et al. Estimated global mortality associated with the first 12 months of 2009 pandemic influenza A H1N1 virus circulation: A modeling study. Lancet Infect Dis 2012;12:687–695.
22. Centers for Disease Control and Prevention. Notes from the field: Outbreak of influenza A (H3N2) virus among persons and swine at a county fair—Indiana, July 2012. MMWR Morb Mortal Wkly Rep 2012;61:561.
23. Centers for Disease Control and Prevention. Influenza A (H3N2) Variant Virus Outbreaks. *http://www.cdc.gov/flu/swineflu/h3n2v-case-count.htm.*
24. Lindstrom S, Garten R, Balish A, et al. Human infections with novel reassortant influenza A(H3N2)v viruses, United States, 2011. Emerg Infect Dis 2012;18:834–837.
25. Centers for Disease Control and Prevention. Antibodies cross-reactive to influenza A (H3N2) variant virus and impact of 2010–11 seasonal influenza vaccine on cross-reactive antibodies—United States. MMWR Morb Mortal Wkly Rep 2012;61:237–241.
26. Grohskopf L, Uyeki T, Bresee J, et al. Prevention and control of influenza with vaccines: Recommendations of the Advisory Committee on Immunization Practices (ACIP)—United States, 2012-13 Influenza Season. MMWR Morb Mortal Wkly Rep 2012;61:613–618.
27. American Academy of Pediatrics, Committee on Infectious Diseases. Policy, statement—Recommendations for prevention and control of influenza in children, 2010-2011. Pediatrics 2010;126(4):816–826.
28. Cheung CY, Poon LL, Lau AS, et al. Induction of proinflammatory cytokines in human macrophages by influenza A (H5N1) viruses: A mechanism for the unusual severity of human disease? Lancet 2002;360(9348):1831–1837.
29. Petric M, Comanor L, Petti CA. Role of the laboratory in diagnosis of influenza during seasonal epidemics and potential pandemics. J Infect Dis 2006;194(Suppl 2):S98–S110.
30. Neuzil KM, Zhu Y, Griffin MR, et al. Burden of interpandemic influenza in children younger than 5 years: A 25-year prospective study. J Infect Dis 2002;185(2):147–152.
31. Newton DW, Treanor JJ, Menegus MA. Clinical and laboratory diagnosis of influenza virus infections. Am J Manag Care 2000;6(Suppl 5):S265–S275.
32. Centers for Disease Control and Prevention. Update: Recommendations of the Advisory Committee on Immunization Practices (ACIP) regarding use of CSL seasonal influenza vaccine (Afluria) in the United States during 2010–11. MMWR Morb Mortal Wkly Rep 2010;59:989–992.
33. Hoberman A, Greenberg DP, Paradise JL, et al. Effectiveness of inactivated influenza vaccine in preventing acute otitis media in young children: A randomized controlled trial. JAMA 2003;290(12):1608–1616.
34. Bridges CB, Thompson WW, Meltzer MI, et al. Effectiveness and cost–benefit of influenza vaccination of healthy working adults: A randomized controlled trial. JAMA 2000;284(13):1655–1663.
35. Demicheli V, Rivetti D, Deeks JJ, Jefferson TO. Vaccines for preventing influenza in healthy adults. Cochrane Database Syst Rev 2004;(3):CD001269.
36. Fluzone Intradermal Vaccine [prescribing information]. Swiftwater, PA: Sanofi Pasteur Inc, 2012.
37. Juurlink DN, Stukel TA, Kwong J, et al. Guillain-Barré syndrome after influenza vaccination in adults: A population-based study. Arch Intern Med 2006;166(20):2217–2221.
38. Lasky T, Terracciano GJ, Magder L, et al. The Guillain-Barré syndrome and the 1992–1993 and 1993–1994 influenza vaccines. N Engl J Med 1998;339(25):1797–1802.
39. Centers for Disease Control and Prevention (CDC). Summary of the joint statement on thimerosal in vaccines. American Academy of Family Physicians, American Academy of Pediatrics, Advisory Committee on Immunization Practices, Public Health Service. MMWR Morb Mortal Wkly Rep 2000;49(27):622, 631.
40. Price CS, Thompson WW, Goodson B, et al. Prenatal and infant exposure to thimerosal from vaccines and immunoglobulins and risk of autism. Pediatrics 2010;126:656–664.
41. Institute of Medicine. Adverse Effects of Vaccines: Evidence and Causality. August 25, 2011, *http://www.iom.edu/Reports/2011/Adverse-Effects-of-Vaccines-Evidence-and-Causality.aspx.*
42. Belshe RB, Ambrose CS, Yi T. Safety and efficacy of live attenuated influenza vaccine in children 2-7 years of age. Vaccine 2008;26(Suppl 4):D10–D16.
43. Nichol KL, Mendelman PM, Mallon KP, et al. Effectiveness of live, attenuated intranasal influenza virus vaccine in healthy, working adults: A randomized controlled trial. JAMA 1999;282(2):137–144.
44. FluMist Quadrivalent Vaccine [prescribing information]. Gaithersburg, MD: MedImmune, LLC, 2012.
45. Centers for Disease Control and Prevention (CDC). Influenza Division, National Center for Immunization and Respiratory Diseases. Antiviral agents for the treatment and chemoprophylaxis of influenza—Recommendations of the Advisory Committee on Immunization Practices (ACIP). MMWR Surveill Summ 2011;60(1):1–28.
46. Harper SA, Bradley JS, Englund JA, et al. Expert Panel of the Infectious Diseases Society of America. Seasonal influenza in adults and children—Diagnosis, treatment, chemoprophylaxis, and institutional outbreak management: Clinical practice guidelines of the Infectious Diseases Society of America. Clin Infect Dis 2009;48(8):1003–1032.
47. Bradley JS, Byington CL, Shah SS, et al. The management of community-acquired pneumonia in infants and children older than 3 months of age: Clinical practice guidelines by the Pediatric Infectious Diseases Society and the Infectious Diseases Society of America. Clin Infect Dis 2011;53(7):e25–e76.
48. Hayden FG, Pavia AT. Antiviral management of seasonal and pandemic influenza. J Infect Dis 2006;194(Suppl 2):S119–S126.

49. Monto AS, Pichichero ME, Blanckenberg SJ, et al. Zanamivir prophylaxis: An effective strategy for the prevention of influenza types A and B within households. J Infect Dis 2002;186(11):1582–1588.
50. Peters PH Jr, Gravenstein S, Norwood P, et al. Long-term use of oseltamivir for the prophylaxis of influenza in a vaccinated frail older population. J Am Geriatr Soc 2001; 49(8):1025–1031.
51. Englund JA. Maternal immunization with inactivated influenza vaccine: Rationale and experience. Vaccine 2003;21(24):3460–3464.
52. Tasker SA, Treanor JJ, Paxton WB, Wallace MR. Efficacy of influenza vaccination in HIV-infected persons. A randomized, double-blind, placebo-controlled trial. Ann Intern Med 1999;131(6):430–433.
53. Kroon FP, van Dissel JT, de Jong JC, et al. Antibody response after influenza vaccination in HIV-infected individuals: A consecutive 3-year study. Vaccine 2000;18(26):3040–3049.
54. Soesman NM, Rimmelzwaan GF, Nieuwkoop NJ, et al. Efficacy of influenza vaccination in adult liver transplant recipients. J Med Virol 2000;61(1):85–93.
55. Gelinck LB, van den Bemt BJ, Marijt WA, et al. Intradermal influenza vaccination in immunocompromized patients is immunogenic and feasible. Vaccine 2009;27(18):2469–2474.
56. Ison MG, Gubareva LV, Atmar RL, et al. Recovery of drug-resistant influenza virus from immunocompromised patients: A case series. J Infect Dis 2006;193(6):760–764.
57. Whitley RJ, Monto AS. Prevention and treatment of influenza in high-risk groups: Children, pregnant women, immunocompromised hosts, and nursing home residents. J Infect Dis 2006;194(Suppl 2):S133–S138.
58. Centers for Disease Control and Prevention. Update: Influenza Activity—United States, August 30, 2009–January 1, 2010. MMWR Morb Mortal Wkly Rep 2010;59(2):38–43.
59. Treanor JJ, Hayden FG, Vrooman PS, et al. Efficacy and safety of the oral neuraminidase inhibitor oseltamivir in treating acute influenza: A randomized controlled trial. US Oral Neuraminidase Study Group. JAMA 2000;283(8):1016–1024.
60. Aoki FY, Macleod MD, Paggiaro P, et al. Early administration of oral oseltamivir increases the benefits of influenza treatment. J Antimicrob Chemother 2003;51(1):123–129.
61. Kaiser L, Wat C, Mills T, et al. Impact of oseltamivir treatment on influenza-related lower respiratory tract complications and hospitalizations. Arch Intern Med 2003; 163(14):1667–1672.
62. Kaiser L, Keene ON, Hammond JM, et al. Impact of zanamivir on antibiotic use for respiratory events following acute influenza in adolescents and adults. Arch Intern Med 2000;160(21):3234–3240.
63. US Centers for Disease Control and Prevention. Termination of the Emergency Use Authorization (EUA) of Medical Products and Devices. June 24, 2010, *http://www.cdc.gov/h1n1flu/eua/.*
64. Peramivir Emergency Use Authorization. *http://www.fda.gov/downloads/Drugs/DrugSafety/PostmarketDrugSafetyInformationforPatientsandProviders/UCM187800.pdf.*
65. Hernandez JE, Adiga R, Armstrong R, et al. Clinical experience in adults and children treated with intravenous peramivir for 2009 influenza A (H1N1) under an emergency IND program in the United States. Clin Infect Dis 2011;52:695.
66. Sorbello A, Jones SC, Carter W, et al. Emergency use authorization for intravenous peramivir: Evaluation of safety in the treatment of hospitalized patients infected with 2009 H1N1 influenza A virus. Clin Infect Dis 2012;55:1.
67. Tamiflu [prescribing information]. San Francisco, CA: Genentech USA, Inc/Roche Group, August 2012, *http:/www.rocheusa.com/products/tamiflu/pi.pdf.*
68. Newland JG, Laurich VM, Rosenquist AW, et al. Neurologic complications in children hospitalized with influenza: Characteristics, incidence, and risk factors. J Pediatr 2007; 150:306–310.
69. Chung BH, Tsang AM, Wong VC. Neurologic complications in children hospitalized with influenza: Comparison between USA and Hong Kong. J Pediatr 2007;151:e17–e18.
70. Centers for Disease Prevention and Control. Influenza Antiviral Drug Resistance. *http://www.cdc.gov/flu/about/qa/antiviralresistance.htm.*

88

Skin and Soft-Tissue Infections

Douglas N. Fish and Susan L. Pendland

KEY CONCEPTS

1. Folliculitis, furuncles (boils), and carbuncles begin around hair follicles and are caused most often by *Staphylococcus aureus*. Folliculitis and small furuncles are generally treated with warm, moist heat to promote drainage; large furuncles and carbuncles require incision and drainage. A penicillinase-resistant penicillin such as dicloxacillin is commonly used for extensive or serious infections (e.g., fever). Empiric treatment of purulent infections that have a high suspicion for community-associated methicillin-resistant *S. aureus* (CA-MRSA) should include clindamycin, trimethoprim–sulfamethoxazole, a tetracycline, or linezolid.

2. Erysipelas, a superficial skin infection with extensive lymphatic involvement, is caused by *Streptococcus pyogenes*. The treatment of choice is penicillin, administered orally or parenterally, depending on the severity of the infection.

3. Impetigo is a superficial skin infection that occurs most commonly in children. It is characterized by fluid-filled vesicles that develop rapidly into pus-filled blisters that rupture to form golden-yellow crusts. Effective therapy includes penicillinase-resistant penicillins (dicloxacillin), first-generation cephalosporins (cephalexin), and topical mupirocin. *S. aureus* is the primary cause of impetigo, with infections caused by CA-MRSA emerging in recent years.

4. Lymphangitis, an infection of the subcutaneous lymphatic channels, is generally caused by *S. pyogenes*. Acute lymphangitis is characterized by the rapid development of fine, red, linear streaks extending from the initial infection site toward the regional lymph nodes, which are usually enlarged and tender. Penicillin is the drug of choice.

5. Cellulitis is an infection of the epidermis, dermis, and superficial fascia most commonly caused by *S. pyogenes* and *S. aureus*. Lesions generally are hot, painful, and erythematous, with nonelevated, poorly defined margins. Oral trimethoprim–sulfamethoxazole, doxycycline, minocycline, or clindamycin is used for initial treatment of suspected CA-MRSA in patients with purulent cellulitis (i.e., lesion with purulent drainage or exudate, or nondrainable abscess). Treatment of nonpurulent cellulitis generally consists of a penicillinase-resistant penicillin (dicloxacillin) or first-generation cephalosporin (cephalexin) for 5 to 10 days, with the option of adding coverage for CA-MRSA in certain patients. Severe infections in hospitalized patients should receive empiric therapy with vancomycin.

6. Necrotizing fasciitis is a rare but life-threatening infection of subcutaneous tissue that results in progressive destruction of superficial fascia and subcutaneous fat. Early and aggressive surgical debridement is an essential part of therapy for treatment of necrotizing fasciitis. Mixed infections are treated with broad-spectrum regimens that cover streptococci, gram-negative aerobes, and anaerobes. Infections caused by *S. pyogenes* or *Clostridium* species should be treated with the combination of penicillin and clindamycin.

7. Diabetic foot infections are managed with a comprehensive treatment approach that includes both proper wound care and antimicrobial therapy. Potential pathogens include staphylococci, streptococci, aerobic gram-negative bacilli, and obligate anaerobes. Antimicrobial regimens for diabetic foot infections are based on severity of the infection, expected treatment setting, and risk factors for infection with more resistant pathogens such as methicillin-resistant *S. aureus* (MRSA) and *Pseudomonas aeruginosa*. Outpatient therapy with oral antimicrobials should be used whenever possible for less severe infections, while more severe infections initially require IV therapy.

8. Prevention is the single most important aspect in the management of pressure sores. After a sore develops, successful local care includes a comprehensive approach consisting of relief of pressure, proper cleaning (debridement), disinfection, and appropriate antimicrobial therapy if an infection is present. Good wound care is crucial to successful management.

9. All bite wounds (either animal or human) should be irrigated thoroughly with large volumes of sterile normal saline, and the injured area should be immobilized and elevated. Depending on the severity of the bite wound, amoxicillin–clavulanic acid or ampicillin–sulbactam is often used for treatment of animal bites because of their coverage of *Pasteurella* species, streptococci, *S. aureus*, and anaerobes typically present in the oral flora of dogs and cats.

10. Although antimicrobial prophylaxis of dog bites is not recommended routinely, patients with bite injuries caused by cats or humans should be given prophylactic antimicrobial therapy for 3 to 5 days. Infected bite wounds should be treated for 7 to 14 days with oral or IV antibiotics having activity against *Eikenella corrodens*, streptococci, *S. aureus*, and β-lactamase–producing anaerobes.

Skin and soft-tissue infections (SSTIs) may involve any or all layers of the skin (epidermis, dermis, subcutaneous fat), fascia, and muscle. They also may spread far from the initial site of infection and lead to more severe complications, such as endocarditis, gram-negative sepsis, or streptococcal glomerulonephritis. Sometimes the treatment of SSTIs may necessitate both medical and surgical management. This chapter presents details of the pathogenesis and management of some of the most common infections involving the skin and soft tissues, ranging in severity from superficial to life-threatening.

EPIDEMIOLOGY

Bacterial infections of the skin can be classified as primary or secondary (Table 88-1).[1-3] Primary bacterial infections usually involve areas of previously healthy skin and are caused by a single pathogen. In contrast, secondary infections occur in areas of previously damaged skin and are frequently polymicrobic. SSTIs are also classified as complicated or uncomplicated. Complicated infections are those that involve deeper skin structures (e.g., fascia, muscle layers), require significant surgical intervention, or occur in patients with compromised immune function (e.g., diabetes mellitus, human immunodeficiency virus [HIV] infection).[4] Other categories that are crucial for successful treatment are the differentiation of necrotizing versus nonnecrotizing, as well as purulent versus nonpurulent, SSTIs.[4-7]

SSTIs are among the most common infections seen in community and hospital settings.[8,9] However, most infections are believed to be mild and are treated in an outpatient setting, making it difficult to accurately quantify community-acquired SSTIs. SSTIs were diagnosed in 0.8% of physician office visits between 1993 and 2005; this corresponded to approximately 82 million diagnoses of SSTI, being more common among 70 years of age and older.[3] Emergency room visits for SSTIs have increased dramatically in recent years, attributed primarily to an increase in community-associated methicillin-resistant *Staphylococcus aureus* (CA-MRSA) cellulitis and abscesses.[10,11] A study of emergency department visit rates between 1997 and 2007 found a 3.1-fold increase (11% per year) for abscess SSTIs, with only a minimal increase in nonabscess SSTIs.[11] According to an Agency for Healthcare Research and Quality (AHRQ) report, in 2007 SSTIs were responsible for over 600,000 hospitalizations and represented 2% of all admissions in males and 1.2% in females.[9] Another study examined the rate and occurrence of infectious disease hospitalization using data from the Nationwide Input Sample for 1998 to 2006.[12] A total of 10.1% of hospitalizations during that period were due to cellulitis.

While the exact incidence of SSTIs is unknown, the frequency of infections caused by drug-resistant gram-positive cocci has been increasing.[4-7] While the high incidence of healthcare-associated MRSA (HA-MRSA) has been a major concern for many years,[13] the emergence of CA-MRSA is even more problematic.[5-7,13-19] CA-MRSA are characteristically isolated from patients lacking typical risk factors (e.g., prior hospitalization, long-term care facility) and are often susceptible to non–β-lactam antibiotics such as trimethoprim–sulfamethoxazole, doxycycline, and clindamycin.[1,13,14,16,18,20] They also differ genetically from HA-MRSA with methicillin resistance carried on the type IV staphylococcal chromosomal cassette *mec* (SCC*mec*) element of the *mecA* gene.[1,13] CA-MRSA strains often harbor genes for Panton-Valentine leukocidin (PVL), a cytotoxin responsible for leukocyte destruction and tissue necrosis. In contrast, HA-MRSA strains usually lack genes for PVL and are associated with SCC*mec* alleles I to III.[1,13,16,16,19] While the incidence of HA-MRSA has declined in recent years,[21] the incidence of CA-MRSA has dramatically increased.[4-7,20] Clinicians should suspect CA-MRSA in geographic areas with a high prevalence of these strains, or in recurrent or persistent infections that are not responding to appropriate β-lactam therapy. Concerns for the future are the mixing of community and nosocomial strains, with HA-MRSA strains acquiring virulence genes (PVL) or CA-MRSA strains acquiring antimicrobial resistance via the SCC*mec* element.[13]

In addition to the emergence of CA-MRSA, treatment choices for SSTIs have been further complicated by the increased incidence of macrolide-resistant strains of *S. aureus* and *Streptococcus pyogenes*.[16,20,22] Data from the Minnesota Department of Health found erythromycin susceptibility among CA-MRSA strains decreased from 45% to 13% during the years 2000 to 2005.[20] There is concern about the use of clindamycin for CA-MRSA infections due to the risk of inducible clindamycin resistance in *S. aureus* strains that are erythromycin-resistant, but clindamycin-susceptible.[20] A double-disk test (D-zone test) is recommended to identify erythromycin-resistant strains with inducible clindamycin resistance if treatment with clindamycin is desired.[6,7,13,23] A positive D-zone test, indicating the presence of the *erm* gene, suggests the possibility of the emergence of clindamycin resistance during therapy.[13]

TABLE 88-1 Bacterial Classification of Important Skin and Soft-Tissue Infections[1-3]

Primary Infections	
Erysipelas	Group A streptococci (*Streptococcus pyogenes*)
Impetigo	*Staphylococcus aureus* (including methicillin-resistant strains), group A streptococci
Lymphangitis	Group A streptococci; occasionally *S. aureus*
Cellulitis	Group A streptococci, *S. aureus* (potentially including methicillin-resistant strains); occasionally other gram-positive cocci, gram-negative bacilli, and/or anaerobes
Necrotizing fasciitis	
Type I	Anaerobes (*Bacteroides* spp., *Peptostreptococcus* spp.) and facultative bacteria (streptococci, Enterobacteriaceae)
Type II	Group A streptococci
Type III	*Clostridium perfringens*
Secondary Infections	
Diabetic foot infections	*S. aureus*, streptococci, Enterobacteriaceae, *Bacteroides* spp., *Peptostreptococcus* spp., *Pseudomonas aeruginosa*
Pressure sores	*S. aureus* including methicillin-resistant strains, streptococci, Enterobacteriaceae, *Bacteroides* spp., *Peptostreptococcus* spp., *P. aeruginosa*
Bite wounds	
Animal	*Pasteurella* spp., *S. aureus*, streptococci, *Bacteroides* spp.
Human	*Eikenella corrodens*, *S. aureus*, streptococci, *Corynebacterium* spp., *Bacteroides* spp., *Peptostreptococcus* spp.
Burn wounds	*P. aeruginosa*, Enterobacteriaceae, *S. aureus*, streptococci

ETIOLOGY

The majority of SSTIs are caused by gram-positive organisms present on the skin surface.[7,24] Gram-positive bacteria (coagulase-negative staphylococci, diphtheroids) are the predominant flora of the skin, with gram-negative organisms being relatively uncommon (Table 88-2).[1-3] *S. aureus*, as well as a variety of gram-negative bacteria, including *Acinetobacter* species, can be found in moist

TABLE 88-2 Predominant Microorganisms of Normal Skin[1-3]

Bacteria
Gram-positive
Coagulase-negative staphylococci
Micrococci (*Micrococcus luteus*)
Corynebacterium species (diphtheroids)
Propionibacterium species
Gram-negative
Acinetobacter species
Fungi
Malassezia species
Candida species

CLINICAL PRESENTATION

Folliculitis

- Clustering, pruritic papules localized to hair follicles.
- Generally develop in areas subject to friction and perspiration.
- Papules are generally 5 mm or less in diameter and erythematous.
- Papules evolve into pustules that generally spontaneously rupture in several days.
- Systemic signs (fever, malaise) are uncommon.

Furuncles

- Inflammatory, draining nodule involving a hair follicle.
- Generally develop in areas subject to friction and perspiration.
- Lesions are discrete, whether occurring as singular or multiple nodules.
- Lesion starts as a firm, tender, red nodule that becomes painful and fluctuant.
- Lesions often drain spontaneously.
- Lesions caused by CA-MRSA often have necrotic centers characteristic of "spider bites."
- Systemic signs are uncommon.

Carbuncles

- Formed when adjacent furuncles coalesce to form a single inflamed area.
- Form broad, swollen, erythematous, deep, and painful follicular masses.
- Commonly develop on the back of the neck and are more likely to occur in patients with diabetes.
- Commonly associated with systemic signs (fever, chills, malaise).
- Bacteremia with secondary spread to other tissues is common.

intertriginous areas (e.g., axilla, groin, and toe webs) of the body.[1,2,25] Approximately 30% to 35% of healthy individuals are reported to be colonized with *S. aureus* on the skin or in the anterior nares.[1,3] Colonization, whether transient or permanent, provides a nidus for infection should the integrity of the epidermis be compromised.[1,2,10]

S. aureus and *S. pyogenes* account for the majority of community-acquired SSTIs.[1,10,24] Data from large surveillance studies showed *S. aureus* to be the most common cause (45%) of SSTIs in hospitalized patients.[26] Also of note in these studies was the 36% incidence of methicillin resistance among strains of *S. aureus*. Other common nosocomial pathogens included *Pseudomonas aeruginosa* (11%), enterococci (9%), and *Escherichia coli* (7%).[26]

PATHOPHYSIOLOGY

The skin serves as a barrier between humans and their environment, therefore functioning as a primary defense mechanism against infections. The skin and subcutaneous tissues normally are extremely resistant to infection but may become susceptible under certain conditions. Even when high concentrations of bacteria are applied topically or injected into the soft tissue, resulting infections are rare.[1–3,27,28] Several host factors act together to confer protection against skin infections. Because the surface of the skin is relatively dry and has a pH of approximately 5.6, it is not conducive to bacterial growth.[1,3] Continuous renewal of the epidermal layer results in the shedding of keratocytes, as well as skin bacteria.[2] In addition, sebaceous secretions are hydrolyzed to form free fatty acids that strongly inhibit the growth of many bacteria and fungi. Conditions that may predispose a patient to the development of skin infections include (a) high concentrations of bacteria (>10^5 microorganisms), (b) excessive moisture of the skin, (c) inadequate blood supply, (d) availability of bacterial nutrients, and (e) damage to the corneal layer allowing for bacterial penetration.[2,3,27,28]

The best defense against SSTI is intact skin.[2,27] The majority of SSTIs result from the disruption of normal host defenses by processes such as skin puncture, abrasion, or underlying diseases (e.g., diabetes).[1,2,27,29] The nature and severity of the infection depend on both the type of microorganism present and the site of innoculation.

FOLLICULITIS, FURUNCLES, AND CARBUNCLES

1 Folliculitis is inflammation of the hair follicle and is caused by physical injury, chemical irritation, or infection. Infection occurring at the base of the eyelid is referred to as a stye. While folliculitis is a superficial infection with pus present only in the epidermis,[10,24] furuncles and carbuncles occur when a follicular infection extends from around the hair shaft to involve deeper areas (subcutaneous tissue) of the skin.[29] A furuncle, commonly known as an *abscess* or *boil*, is a walled-off mass of purulent material arising from a hair follicle.[10] The lesions are called *carbuncles* when adjacent furuncles coalesce to form a single inflamed area.[10] This aggregate of infected hair follicles forms deep masses that generally open and drain through multiple sinus tracts.[13,29] *S. aureus* is the most common cause of folliculitis, furuncles, and carbuncles.[13,29] Inadequate chlorine levels in whirlpools, hot tubs, and swimming pools have been responsible for outbreaks of folliculitis caused by *P. aeruginosa*.[1,29] Outbreaks of furunculosis caused by *S. aureus* and CA-MRSA have been reported in settings involving close contact (e.g., families, prisons), especially when skin injury was common (such as with sports).[13,29] In addition, some individuals experience repeated episodes of furunculosis.[24] The major predisposing factor in recurrent infection is the presence of *S. aureus* in the anterior nares.[16,24,29]

TREATMENT
Folliculitis, Furuncles, and Carbuncles

Desired Outcomes

The goals of treatment include relieving discomfort, preventing further spread of the infection, and preventing recurrence. Controlling recurrent furunculosis is key due to the difficulty in treating chronic furunculosis.[24] Treatments should be effective and inexpensive and have minimal adverse effects.

Treatment

Table 88-3 summarizes evidence-based treatment recommendations from clinical guidelines for SSTIs.[5,6,16,30–33] Treatment of folliculitis generally requires only local measures, such as warm moist compresses or topical therapy (e.g., clindamycin, erythromycin, mupirocin, or benzoyl peroxide).[29,31] Topical agents generally are applied two to four times daily for 7 days. Small furuncles generally can be treated with moist heat, which promotes localization and drainage of pus.[29,31] Large and/or multiple furuncles

TABLE 88-3 Evidence-Based Recommendations for Treatment of Skin and Soft-Tissue Infections[5,6,16,30–33]

Recommendations	Recommendation Grade
Folliculitis, Furuncles, Carbuncles	
Folliculitis and small furuncles can be treated with moist heat; large furuncles and carbuncles require incision and drainage. Antimicrobial therapy is unnecessary unless extensive lesions or fever are present	A-II for nondrug management; E-III for recommendation against antibiotics
Erysipelas	
Most infections are caused by *Streptococcus pyogenes*. Penicillin (oral or IV depending on clinical severity) is the drug of choice	A-I
If *Staphylococcus aureus* is suspected, a penicillinase-resistant penicillin or first-generation cephalosporin should be used	A-I
Impetigo	
S. aureus accounts for the majority of infections; consequently, a penicillin-resistant penicillin or first-generation cephalosporin is recommended	A-I
Topical therapy with mupirocin is equivalent to oral therapy	A-I
Cellulitis	
Empiric antibiotics for outpatients with purulent cellulitis should provide activity against community-associated MRSA; coverage of β-hemolytic streptococci is likely not required. Mild–moderate infections can generally be treated with oral agents (dicloxacillin, cephalexin, clindamycin) unless resistance is high in the community	A-II
Empiric antibiotics for outpatients with nonpurulent cellulitis should provide activity against β-hemolytic streptococci; coverage for community-associated MRSA may be considered for patients with systemic toxicity or those who have not responded to β-lactam therapy alone	A-II
Recommended antibiotics for empiric coverage of community-associated MRSA in outpatients include orally administered trimethoprim–sulfamethoxazole, doxycycline, minocycline, clindamycin, and linezolid	A-II for all listed options
If coverage of both β-hemolytic streptococci and community-associated MRSA is desired, empiric antibiotic regimens for outpatient therapy include orally administered clindamycin alone; linezolid alone; or trimethoprim–sulfamethoxazole, doxycycline, or minocycline in combination with amoxicillin	A-II for all listed options
Hospitalized patients with complicated or purulent cellulitis should receive IV antibiotics with activity against MRSA pending culture data. Antibiotic options include vancomycin, linezolid, daptomycin, telavancin, and clindamycin	A-I for all except clindamycin; clindamycin A-III
A β-lactam antibiotic (e.g., cefazolin) may be considered for empiric treatment of nonpurulent cellulitis in hospitalized patients. Antibiotics should be modified to include MRSA coverage if unfavorable clinical response	A-II
In the treatment of *S. aureus* infections, trough serum vancomycin concentrations should always be maintained >10 mg/L (>7 μmol/L) to avoid development of resistance	B-III
Necrotizing Fasciitis	
Early and aggressive surgical debridement of all necrotic tissue is essential	A-III
Necrotizing fasciitis caused by *S. pyogenes* should be treated with the combination of clindamycin and penicillin	A-II
In the treatment of necrotizing fasciitis caused by methicillin-resistant *S. aureus* infections, trough serum vancomycin concentrations of 15–20 mg/L (10–14 μmol/L) are recommended	B-II
Clostridial gas gangrene (myonecrosis) should be treated with clindamycin and penicillin	B-III
Diabetic Foot Infections	
Clinically uninfected wounds should not be treated with antibiotics	A-III
Empiric antibiotic regimens should be selected based on severity of infection and likely pathogens	A-III
Antibiotic therapy should target only aerobic gram-positive cocci in patients with mild to moderate infection who have not received antibiotics within the previous month	C-III
Broad-spectrum empiric antibiotic therapy should be initiated in most patients with severe infections, until culture and susceptibility data are available	A-III
Empiric antibiotics directed against *Pseudomonas aeruginosa* are usually unnecessary except in patients with specific risk factors for infection with this pathogen: patient has been soaking feet, patient has failed previous antibiotic therapy with nonpseudomonal agents, or clinically severe infection	A-III
Empiric antibiotics directed against MRSA should be considered in patients with specific risk factors, including: prior history of infection or colonization with MRSA, high local prevalence of MRSA (e.g., ≥50% for mild infections, ≥30% for severe infection), or clinically severe infection	C-III
Oral agents with high bioavailability may be used in the treatment of most mild, and many moderate, infections	A-II
Parenteral therapy is initially preferred for all severe, and some moderate, infections. After initial response, step-down therapy to oral agents can be considered	C-III
Definitive therapy should be based on results of appropriately collected cultures and sensitivities, as well as clinical response to empiric antimicrobial agents	A-III
Appropriate wound care, in addition to appropriate antimicrobial therapy, is often necessary for healing of infected wounds	A-III
Antibiotic therapy should only be continued until resolution of signs/symptoms of infection, but not necessarily until the wound is fully healed. The duration of therapy should initially be 1–2 weeks for mild infections and 2–3 weeks for moderate to severe infection	C-III

(continued)

TABLE 88-3 Evidence-Based Recommendations for Treatment of Skin and Soft-Tissue Infections[5,6,16,30–33] (*Continued*)

Recommendations	Recommendation Grade
Animal Bites	
Many bite wounds can be treated on an outpatient basis with amoxicillin–clavulanic acid	B-II
Serious infections requiring IV antimicrobial therapy can be treated with a β-lactam/β-lactamase inhibitor combination or second-generation cephalosporin with activity against anaerobes (e.g., cefoxitin)	B-II
Penicillinase-resistant penicillins, first-generation cephalosporins, macrolides, and clindamycin should not be used for treatment of infected wounds because of their poor activity against *Pasteurella multocida*	D-III
Human Bites	
Antimicrobial therapy should provide coverage against *Eikenella corrodens*, *S. aureus*, and β-lactamase–producing anaerobes	B-III

Strength of recommendation: A, good evidence for use; B, moderate evidence for use; C, poor evidence for use, optional; D, moderate evidence to support not using; E, good evidence to support not using. *Quality of evidence*: I, evidence from ≥1 properly randomized controlled trials; II, evidence from ≥1 well-designed clinical trials without randomization, case–control analytic studies, multiple time series, or dramatic results from uncontrolled experiments; III, evidence from expert opinion, clinical experience, descriptive studies, or reports of expert committees.

and carbuncles require incision and drainage.[4,13,16,31,32] Systemic antibiotics are usually not necessary unless accompanied by fever or extensive cellulitis.[4,16] Treatment of more severe infections generally consists of a penicillinase-resistant penicillin (such as dicloxacillin) or a first-generation cephalosporin (such as cephalexin) for 5 to 10 days (refer to Table 88-4 for adult and pediatric doses). An alternative agent for penicillin-allergic patients is clindamycin. Empiric treatment of purulent infections that have a higher suspicion for CA-MRSA should include clindamycin, trimethoprim–sulfamethoxazole, a tetracycline, or linezolid.[4,6,24,32] For individuals with nasal colonization, application of mupirocin ointment twice daily in the anterior nares for the first 5 days of each month decreases recurrent furunculosis by almost half.[16,24] In addition, a single oral daily dose of clindamycin 150 mg for 3 months or 500 mg of azithromycin weekly for 3 months reduced recurrent infections caused by susceptible strains of *S. aureus* by approximately 80%.[24]

Evaluation of Therapeutic Outcomes

Many follicular infections resolve spontaneously without medical or surgical intervention. Lesions should be incised if they do not respond to a few days of moist heat and nonprescription topical agents. Following drainage, most lesions begin to heal within several days without antimicrobial therapy. Any patient who is unresponsive to several days of therapy with a penicillinase-resistant penicillin or first-generation cephalosporin should have a culture and sensitivity performed because of the increasing frequency of CA-MRSA.

ERYSIPELAS

❷ Erysipelas is a distinct form of cellulitis involving the more superficial layers of the skin and cutaneous lymphatics.[5,13,24,34] The intense red color and burning pain associated with this skin infection led to the common name of "St. Anthony's fire." The infection is almost always caused by β-hemolytic streptococci, with the organisms gaining access via small breaks in the skin. Group A streptococci (*S. pyogenes*) are responsible for most infections.[16,24,31] Infections are more common in infants, young children, the elderly, and patients with nephrotic syndrome.[6,31] Erysipelas also commonly occurs in areas of preexisting lymphatic obstruction or edema.[13,31] Diagnosis is made on the basis of the characteristic lesion.

TABLE 88-4 Recommended Oral Drugs or Outpatient Treatment of Mild–Moderate Skin and Soft-Tissue Infections

Infection	Adults	Children
Folliculitis	None; warm saline compresses usually sufficient	
Furuncles and carbuncles	Dicloxacillin Cephalexin Clindamycin[a] Trimethoprim–sulfamethoxazole[b]	Dicloxacillin Cephalexin Clindamycin[a,b] Trimethoprim–sulfamethoxazole[b]
Erysipelas	Procaine penicillin G Penicillin VK Clindamycin[a] Erythromycin[a]	Penicillin VK Clindamycin[a] Erythromycin[a]
Impetigo	Dicloxacillin Cephalexin Cefadroxil Clindamycin[a] Mupirocin ointment[a] Retapamulin ointment[a] Trimethoprim–sulfamethoxazole[b]	Dicloxacillin Cephalexin Cefadroxil Clindamycin[a,b] Mupirocin ointment[a] Retapamulin ointment[a] Trimethoprim–sulfamethoxazole[b]
Lymphangitis	Initial IV therapy, followed by penicillin VK Clindamycin[a]	Initial IV therapy, followed by penicillin VK Clindamycin[a]
Diabetic foot infections	Dicloxacillin Clindamycin Cephalexin Amoxicillin–clavulanate Levofloxacin ± metronidazole or clindamycin[a,c] Ciprofloxacin ± metronidazole or clindamycin[a,c] Moxifloxacin	
Bite wounds (animal or human)	Amoxicillin–clavulanate Doxycycline[a] Moxifloxacin[a] Trimethoprim–sulfamethoxazole + metronidazole or clindamycin[a] Levofloxacin or ciprofloxacin + metronidazole or clindamycin[a] Cefuroxime axetil + metronidazole or clindamycin Dicloxacillin + penicillin VK	Amoxicillin–clavulanate Trimethoprim–sulfamethoxazole + metronidazole or clindamycin[a] Cefuroxime axetil + metronidazole or clindamycin Dicloxacillin + penicillin VK

[a]Recommended for patients with penicillin allergy.
[b]Recommended if CA-MRSA is suspected.
[c]Fluoroquinolone alone may be suitable for mild infections, while addition of drugs with antianaerobic activity may be recommended for more severe infections.

CLINICAL PRESENTATION

General

- Lower extremities are the most common sites.

Symptoms

- Flu-like symptoms (fever, chills, malaise) common prior to the appearance of the lesion
- Infected area described as painful or as a burning pain

Signs

- Lesion is intensely erythematous and edematous, often with lymphatic streaking.
- Lesion has raised border, which is sharply demarcated from uninfected skin.
- Temperature is often mildly elevated.

Laboratory Tests

- Causative organism usually cannot be cultured from the surface skin.
- Needle aspiration or punch biopsies occasionally identify organism.
- Cultures considered for more severe cases (e.g., atypical clinical findings such as fluid-filled blisters).

Other Diagnostic Tests

- A complete blood count is often performed because leukocytosis is common.
- C-reactive protein is also generally elevated.

TREATMENT
Erysipelas

Desired Outcomes

The goal of treatment of erysipelas is rapid eradication of the infection, thereby providing relief of symptoms (pain, tenderness, fever).[34] Preventing recurrent infection is also important, as recurrence is a primary complication, occurring in approximately 20% of patients.[24,34] Treatments should be effective and inexpensive and have minimal adverse effects.

Treatment

Mild to moderate cases of erysipelas are treated with intramuscular procaine penicillin G or penicillin VK for 7 to 10 days (see Table 88-4).[24,31] Recommended doses and monitoring parameters for selected antibiotics are given in Tables 88-5 and 88-6. Penicillin-allergic patients can be treated with clindamycin. For more serious infections, the patient should be hospitalized and aqueous penicillin G administered IV.[24,31] Marked improvement usually is seen within 48 hours, and the patient often may be switched to oral penicillin to complete the course of therapy. Although one study has shown that the median time for cure, IV antibiotics, and hospital stay was reduced in patients receiving prednisolone in addition to antibiotics, further studies are needed before corticosteroids can be recommended for routine use.[16,31,35]

Evaluation of Therapeutic Outcomes

Erysipelas generally responds quickly to appropriate antimicrobial therapy. Temperature and white blood cell count should return to normal within 48 to 72 hours. Erythema, edema, and pain also should resolve gradually.

IMPETIGO

❸ Impetigo is a superficial skin infection that is seen most commonly in children.[6,24,36,37] The infection is generally classified as bullous or nonbullous based on clinical presentation.[10,36,37] Impetigo is most common during hot, humid weather, which facilitates

CLINICAL PRESENTATION

General

- Exposed skin, especially the face, is the most common site.

Symptoms

- Pruritus is common.
- Systemic signs and symptoms of infection are minimal.
- Weakness, fever, and diarrhea occasionally seen with bullous form.

Signs

Nonbullous:

- Lesions start as small, fluid-filled vesicles.
- Vesicles rapidly develop into pustules that rupture readily.
- Purulent discharge dries to form characteristic golden-yellow crusts.

Bullous:

- Lesions start as vesicles that rapidly progress into bullae containing clear yellow fluid.
- Bullae soon rupture, forming thin, light brown crusts.
- Regional lymph nodes may be enlarged.

Laboratory Tests

- Cultures should be collected.
- Crusted tops of lesions should be raised to obtain purulent material at the base for culture.
- Open, draining pustules should not be cultured as they may be colonized with skin flora.

Other Diagnostic Tests

- Complete blood count often performed as leukocytosis is common

TABLE 88-5 Drug Dosing Table[a]

Drug	Brand Name	Initial Dose	Usual Range	Special Population Dose	Other
Oral Agents					
Amoxicillin–clavulanate	Augmentin®	875/125 mg orally two times daily	875/125 mg orally two times daily	Pediatric: 40 mg/kg (of the amoxicillin component) orally in two divided doses	
Cefaclor	Ceclor®	500 mg orally every 8 hours	500 mg orally every 8 hours	Pediatric: 20–40 mg/kg/day (not to exceed 1 g) orally in three divided doses	
Cefadroxil	Duricef®	500 mg orally every 12 hours	250–500 mg orally every 12 hours	Pediatric: 30 mg/kg orally in two divided doses	
Cefuroxime axetil	Ceftin®	500 mg orally every 12 hours	250–500 mg orally every 12 hours	Pediatric: 20–30 mg/kg orally in two divided doses	
Cephalexin	Keflex®	250–500 mg orally every 6 hours	250–500 mg orally every 6 hours	Pediatric: 25–50 mg/kg orally in four divided doses	
Ciprofloxacin	Cipro®	500 mg orally every 12 hours	500–750 mg orally every 12 hours		
Clindamycin	Cleocin®	300–600 mg orally every 6–8 hours	300–600 mg orally every 6–8 hours	Pediatric: 10–30 mg/kg/day orally in three to four divided doses[4]	
Dicloxacillin	Dynapen®	250–500 mg orally every 6 hours	250–500 mg orally every 6 hours	Pediatric: 25–50 mg/kg orally in four divided doses	
Doxycycline	Vibramycin®	100–200 mg orally every 12 hours	100–200 mg orally every 12 hours		May be used for oral treatment of MRSA infection
Erythromycin	E-Mycin® Erythrocin®	250–500 mg orally every 6 hours	250–500 mg orally every 6 hours	Pediatric: 30–50 mg/kg orally in four divided doses[a]	
Levofloxacin	Levaquin®	500–750 mg orally once daily	500–750 mg orally once daily		
Metronidazole	Flagyl®	250–500 mg orally every 8 hours	250–500 mg orally every 8 hours	Pediatric: 30 mg/kg orally in three to four divided doses	
Moxifloxacin	Avelox®	400 mg orally once daily	400 mg orally once daily		
Mupirocin ointment	Bactroban®	Apply to affected areas ointment every 8 hours	Apply to affected areas ointment every 8 hours	Pediatric: apply to affected areas ointment every 8 hours	
Penicillin VK	Veetids® Pen-V®	250–500 mg orally every 6 hours	250–500 mg orally every 6 hours	Pediatric: 25,000–90,000 units/kg orally in four divided doses	
Retapamulin ointment	Altabax®	Apply to affected area every 12 hours	Apply to affected area every 12 hours	Pediatric: apply to affected area every 12 hours	
Trimethoprim–sulfamethoxazole	Bactrim® Septra® Cotrimoxazole®	160/800 mg orally every 12 hours	160 /800 mg orally every 12 hours	Pediatric: 4–6 mg/kg (of the trimethoprim component) orally every 12 hours	Up to double the usual dose may be considered for oral treatment of MRSA infection
Parenteral Agents					
Ampicillin	Omnipen® Polycillin® Principen®	2 g IV every 6 hours	1–2 g IV every 4–6 hours	Pediatric: 200–300 mg/kg/day IV in four to six divided doses	
Aztreonam	Azactam®	1 g IV every 6 hours	1 g IV every 6 hours	Pediatric: 100–150 mg/kg/day IV in four divided doses	
Cefazolin	Ancef® Kefzol®	1 g IV every 8 hours	1 g IV every 6–8 hours	Pediatric: 75 mg/kg/day IV in three divided doses	
Cefepime	Maxipime®	2 g IV every 12 hours	1–2 g IV every 12 hours	Pediatric: 100 mg/kg/day IV in two divided doses	
Cefotaxime	Claforan®	2 g IV every 6 hours	1–2 g IV every 6 hours	150–200 mg/kg/day in three to four divided doses	
Cefoxitin	Mefoxin®	1–2 g IV every 6 hours	1–2 g IV every 6 hours	Pediatric: 30–40 mg/kg/day IV in four divided doses	
Ceftazidime	Fortaz®	2 g IV every 8 hours	1–2 g IV every 8 hours	Pediatric: 150 mg/kg/day IV in three divided doses	
Ceftriaxone	Rocephin®	1 g IV once daily	1 g IV once daily		
Cefuroxime	Zinacef®	1.5 g IV every 8 hours	0.75–1.5 g IV every 8 hours	Pediatric: 150 mg/kg/day IV in three divided doses	
Ciprofloxacin	Cipro®	400 mg IV every 8–12 hours	400 mg IV every 8–12 hours		
Clindamycin	Cleocin®	300–600 mg IV every 6–8 hours	300–600 mg IV every 6–8 hours; 600–900 mg IV every 6–8 hours for necrotizing fasciitis	Pediatric: 30–50 mg/kg/day IV in three to four divided doses	
Daptomycin	Cubicin®	4 mg/kg IV once daily	4 mg/kg IV once daily		For MRSA infection

(continued)

TABLE 88-5 Drug Dosing Table[a] (Continued)

Drug	Brand Name	Initial Dose	Usual Range	Special Population Dose	Other
Doripenem	Doribax®	500 mg IV every 8 hours	500 mg IV every 8 hours		
Ertapenem	Invanz®	1 g IV once daily	1 g IV once daily	Pediatric: 30 mg/kg/day IV in one to two divided doses	
Gentamicin	Garamycin®	Traditional: 2 mg/kg loading dose, followed by 1.5 mg/kg IV every 8 hours. Alternative: 5–7 mg/kg IV once daily	Traditional dosing: guided by measured serum concentrations	Pediatric: 5–7 mg/kg/day IV in three divided doses; doses guided by serum concentrations	
Imipenem–cilastatin	Primaxin®	500 mg IV every 6 hours	250–500 mg IV every 6–8 hours	Pediatric: 40–80 mg/kg/day IV in four divided doses	
Levofloxacin	Levaquin®	750 mg IV once daily	500–750 mg IV once daily		
Linezolid	Zyvox®	600 mg IV or orally every 12 hours	600 mg IV or orally every 12 hours	Pediatric: 20–30 mg/kg/day IV in two to three divided doses	For MRSA infection
Meropenem	Merrem®	1 g IV every 8 hours	1 g IV every 8 hours	Pediatric: 60 mg/kg/day IV in three divided doses	
Metronidazole	Flagyl®	500 mg IV every 8 hours	500 mg IV every 8 hours	Pediatric: 30–50 mg/kg/day IV in three divided doses	
Moxifloxacin	Avelox®	400 mg IV once daily	400 mg IV once daily		
Nafcillin	Nafcil®	2 g IV every 6 hours	1–2 g IV every 4–6 hour	Pediatric: 100–200 mg/kg/day IV in four to six equally divided doses	
Penicillin G	Pfizerpen® Bicillin® Wycillin®	1–2 million units IV every 4–6 hours	1–2 million units IV every 4–6 hours	Pediatric: 100,000–200,000 units/kg/day IV in four divided doses[a]	
Piperacillin–tazobactam	Zosyn®	4.5 g IV every 6 hours	3.375–4.5 g IV every 6 hours	Pediatric: 250–350 mg/kg/day IV in three to four divided doses	
Procaine penicillin G	Bicillin C-R®	600,000 units IM every 12 hours	600,000–1.2 million units IM every 12 hours	Pediatric: 25,000–50,000 units/kg (maximum 1.2 million units) IM once daily	
Tigecycline	Tigacil®	100 mg IV once, and then 50 mg IV every 12 hours	100 mg IV once, and then 50 mg IV every 12 hours		
Tobramycin	Nebcin®	Traditional: 2 mg/kg loading dose, followed by 1.5 mg/kg IV every 8 hours. Alternative: 5–7 mg/kg IV once daily	Traditional dosing: guided by measured serum concentrations	Pediatric: 5–7 mg/kg/day IV in three divided doses; doses guided by serum concentrations	
Vancomycin	Vancocin®	30–40 mg/kg/day IV in two divided doses	Dosing guided by serum concentrations to achieve trough of 15–20 mg/L	Pediatric: 40–60 mg/kg/day IV in three to four divided doses; doses guided by serum concentrations	For MRSA infection

IM, intramuscularly; MRSA, methicillin-resistant *S. aureus*.

[a]Dosing guidelines in patients with normal renal function.

TABLE 88-6 Drug Monitoring

Drug	Adverse Reaction	Monitoring Parameters	Comments
Aminoglycosides (tobramycin, gentamicin)	Nephrotoxicity	Serum creatinine, urine output, serum concentrations	Extended-interval ("once-daily") dosing potentially associated with less renal toxicity, similar efficacy to traditional dosing. Goal trough concentration <1 mcg/mL (mg/L; <2 μmol/L) during extended-interval dosing
Daptomycin	Myopathy	Serum creatine phosphokinase	Most CPK elevations will be asymptomatic; risk of myopathy may be increased with concomitant use of HMG-coA reductase inhibitors
Imipenem–cilastatin	CNS toxicities, seizure	Serum creatinine, mental status, CNS function	Increased incidence with higher dose, failure to adjust dose/interval for reduced renal function. Increased risk compared with meropenem or doripenem
Linezolid	Myelosuppression, thrombocytopenia, optic/peripheral neuropathy, serotonin syndrome	CBC, vision changes, serum lactate, heart rate, blood pressure, temperature, myoclonus	Myelosuppression and neuropathy more common with prolonged use. Weak MAO inhibitor, serotonin syndrome possible with other serotonergic drugs such as SSRIs and SNRIs
Nafcillin	Interstitial nephritis	Serum creatinine, urine output	Reversible, requires switch to alternative β-lactam
Vancomycin	Nephrotoxicity, infusion reactions	Serum creatinine, urine output, blood pressure, heart rate, serum concentrations	Dose adjustment required for renal dysfunction. Pretreatment and slow infusion may decrease incidence of infusion reaction. Goal trough concentration 15–20 mcg/mL (mg/L; 10–14 μmol/L) for serious infections, including necrotizing fasciitis

CBC, complete blood count; MAO, monoamine oxidase; SNRI, serotonin–norepinephrine reuptake inhibitor; SSRI, selective serotonin reuptake inhibitor.

CLINICAL PRESENTATION

General

- Lymphadenitis (acute or chronic inflammation of the lymph nodes) may occur when microorganisms reach the lymph nodes.

Symptoms

- Systemic signs and symptoms (i.e., fever, chills, malaise, and headache) often develop rapidly before any sign of infection is evident at the initial site of inoculation, or after the initial lesion has subsided.
- Systemic signs and symptoms often are more profound than would be expected based on examination of the cutaneous lesion.

Signs

- Peripheral lesion associated with proximal red linear streaks directed toward the regional lymph nodes is diagnostic of acute lymphangitis.
- Lymph nodes usually are enlarged and tender.
- Peripheral edema of the involved extremity often is present.
- Thrombophlebitis and acute lymphangitis in the lower extremities may be confused because both are associated with red linear streaking and tender areas; however, in thrombophlebitis, no portal of entry is identifiable.

Laboratory Tests

- Cultures of the affected lesions often yield negative results.
- Pathogens often identified by Gram stain of the initial lesion if done early in the course of the disease.

Other Diagnostic Tests

- Complete blood count often performed as leukocytosis is common

microbial colonization of the skin.[6,31,36] Minor trauma, such as scratches or insect bites, allows entry of organisms into the superficial layers of skin, and infection ensues.[29,31,37] Impetigo is highly communicable and readily spreads through close contact, especially among siblings and children in daycare centers and schools.[31,36]

Although historically caused by *S. pyogenes*, *S. aureus* has emerged as a principle cause of impetigo (either alone or in combination with *S. pyogenes*).[24,36,37] The bullous form is caused by strains of *S. aureus* capable of producing exfoliative toxins.[24,36] The bullous form most frequently affects neonates,[36] and accounts for approximately 30% of all cases of impetigo.[31,36] Similar to other SSTIs, impetigo has been reported to be increasingly due to CA-MRSA.[24,37]

TREATMENT
Impetigo

Desired Outcomes

The goals of treatment include relieving discomfort, improving the cosmetic appearance of lesions, preventing further spread of the infection, and preventing recurrence. Preventing transmission to others is also important.[36,37] Treatments should be effective and inexpensive and have minimal adverse effects.[36]

Treatment

Although impetigo may resolve spontaneously, antimicrobial treatment is indicated to relieve symptoms, prevent formation of new lesions, and prevent complications such as cellulitis. Penicillinase-resistant penicillins (such as dicloxacillin) are preferred for treatment because of the increased incidence of infections caused by *S. aureus*.[16,24] First-generation cephalosporins (e.g., cephalexin) are also commonly used.[24] Penicillin, administered as a single intramuscular dose of benzathine penicillin G or as oral penicillin VK, is effective for infections known to be caused by *S. pyogenes*. Penicillin-allergic patients can be treated with clindamycin. The duration of therapy is 7 to 10 days. A 7-day course of topical therapy with mupirocin ointment or retapamulin ointment is also effective for mild cases.[16,24] With proper treatment, healing of skin lesions generally is rapid and occurs without residual scarring. Removal of crusts by soaking in soap and warm water also may be helpful in providing symptomatic relief.[24,31]

A review of interventions for impetigo by the Cochrane Collaboration found that topical mupirocin and oral antibiotics (except penicillin and erythromycin) were equally effective for the treatment of impetigo.[38] Conclusions for extensive impetigo could not be made due to lack of data. Adverse effects were more commonly reported with oral antibiotics (GI) than for topical agents. In addition, disinfectant solutions did not show evidence of benefit.

Evaluation of Therapeutic Outcomes

Clinical response should be seen within 7 days of initiating antimicrobial therapy for impetigo. Treatment failures could be a result of noncompliance or antimicrobial resistance. A followup culture of exudates should be collected for culture and sensitivity, with treatment modified accordingly.

LYMPHANGITIS

4 Acute lymphangitis is an inflammation involving the subcutaneous lymphatic channels. Lymphangitis usually occurs secondary to puncture wounds, infected blisters, or other skin lesions. Most infections are caused by *S. pyogenes*.[39]

TREATMENT
Lymphangitis

Desired Outcomes

The goal of treatment of lymphangitis is rapid eradication of the infection, thereby providing relief of symptoms (pain, tenderness, fever). Prevention of systemic complications is also an important goal as thrombophlebitis and abscess formation are possible. Treatments should be effective and inexpensive and have minimal adverse effects.

Treatment

Penicillin is the antibiotic of choice. Because these infections are potentially serious and rapidly progressive, initial treatment should be with IV penicillin G 1 to 2 million units every 4 to 6 hours. Parenteral treatment should be continued for 48 to 72 hours, followed by oral penicillin VK for a total of 10 days.[39] Nondrug therapy includes immobilization and elevation of the affected extremity and warm-water soaks every 2 to 4 hours.[39] For penicillin-allergic patients, clindamycin may be used.

Evaluation of Therapeutic Outcomes

Lymphangitis usually responds rapidly to appropriate therapy; signs and symptoms often are decreased markedly or absent within 24 hours of starting antibiotics.

CELLULITIS

5 Cellulitis is an acute infectious process that represents a serious type of SSTI. It initially affects the epidermis and dermis and may spread subsequently within the superficial fascia.[10] Cellulitis is considered a serious disease because of the propensity of the infection to spread through lymphatic tissue and to the bloodstream. *S. pyogenes* and *S. aureus* are the most frequent bacterial causes.[5,7,13,22,29] However, many bacteria have been implicated in various types of cellulitis (Table 88-1). Approximately 4 million patients were hospitalized for cellulitis between 1998 and 2006, representing 10% of all infection-related admissions.[12,40] The rising incidence of infections caused by methicillin-resistant *S. aureus* (MRSA) is a major concern in both the community and hospital settings.[14–19,26]

Injection drug users are predisposed to several infectious complications, including abscess formation and cellulitis at the site of injection.[16] These SSTIs are often polymicrobic in nature and are believed to originate from the skin and/or oropharynx, as well as from contaminated needles, syringes, and diluents.[16] *S. aureus* is the most common pathogen isolated from injection drug users; the incidence of MRSA is also rising.[14,16,41] Anaerobic bacteria, especially oropharyngeal anaerobes, are also found commonly, particularly in polymicrobic infections.[16] Outbreaks caused by *Clostridium* species have also been reported in injection drug users, particularly in association with contaminated black tar heroin.[16]

Acute cellulitis with mixed aerobic and anaerobic pathogens may occur in diabetics, following traumatic injuries, at sites of surgical incisions to the abdomen or perineum, or where host defenses have been otherwise compromised (vascular insufficiency).[6,10,29] In older patients, cellulitis of the lower extremities also may be complicated by thrombophlebitis. Other complications of cellulitis include local abscess, osteomyelitis, and septic arthritis.[16,42]

TREATMENT
Cellulitis

Desired Outcomes

The goals of therapy of acute bacterial cellulitis are rapid eradication of the infection and prevention of further complications. Effective treatment of cellulitis includes avoidance of unnecessary antimicrobials that contribute to increased resistance, and minimizing toxicities and cost of therapy.

Drug and Nondrug Management of Cellulitis

Local care of cellulitis includes elevation and immobilization of the involved area to decrease swelling.[5,43] Cool sterile saline dressings may decrease pain and can be followed later with moist heat to aid in localization of the cellulitis. Surgical intervention (incision and drainage) as a mode of therapy is rarely indicated in the treatment of uncomplicated cellulitis, but may play an important role in management of more severe or complicated cases. Antimicrobial therapy is directed against the type of bacteria either documented or suspected to be present based on the clinical presentation. Particular attention

CLINICAL PRESENTATION

General

- Usually a history of an antecedent wound from minor trauma, abrasion, ulcer, or surgery

Symptoms

- Patients often experience fever, chills, or malaise and complain that the affected area feels hot and painful.
- Systemic findings such as hypotension, dehydration, and altered mental status are common.

Signs

- Characterized by erythema and edema of the skin.
- Lesions are nonelevated and have poorly defined margins.
- Affected areas generally are warm to touch.
- Inflammation generally is present with little or no necrosis or suppuration of soft tissue.
- Lesions may be associated with purulent drainage, exudates, and/or abscesses.
- Tender lymphadenopathy associated with lymphatic involvement is common.

Laboratory Tests

- Cultures should be collected when possible.
- Gram stain of fluid obtained by injection and aspiration of 0.5 mL of saline (using a small 22-gauge needle) into the advancing edge of the lesion may aid the microbiologic diagnosis but often yields negative results.
- Diagnosis usually is made on clinical grounds rather than by culture.

Other Diagnostic Tests

- Complete blood count often performed as leukocytosis is common
- Blood cultures often useful because bacteremia may be present in up to 30% of cases

must be paid to patients with risk factors for more atypical or resistant bacterial pathogens when selecting antibiotics for treatment of cellulitis. Such organisms include particularly CA-MRSA, but also aerobic gram-negative bacteria and anaerobes.

Because staphylococcal and streptococcal cellulitis are indistinguishable clinically,[22,42] and because of concern regarding appropriate recognition and treatment of MRSA infections, guidelines from the Infectious Diseases Society of America provide detailed recommendations for empiric antibiotic therapy of cellulitis.[32] Infection with CA-MRSA should be considered in patients with skin abscesses, subjective history of insect bites, or more severe infections.[32,42] Appropriate clinical specimens for culture and susceptibility testing should be collected whenever possible in such patients.[5,32,42] Incision and drainage is the primary therapy for infections such as small abscesses and furuncles, and in otherwise uncomplicated patients with mild infections. Systemic antibiotic therapy is often unnecessary in such cases.[32] Antibiotic therapy is recommended along with incision and drainage in patients with more complicated abscesses associated with the following: severe or extensive disease involving multiple sites of infection; rapidly progressive infection in the presence of associated cellulitis; signs and symptoms of systemic illness; complicating factors such as extremes of age, comorbidities, or immunosuppression; abscesses in areas that are difficult to drain, such as hands, face, and genitalia; or lack of response to previous drainage alone.[32,42,44–47]

Antibiotic selection for outpatient treatment of cellulitis is chiefly determined by clinical findings such as appearance of the infected lesion and presence of more severe systemic illness. Purulent cellulitis is defined as infection associated with purulent drainage or exudate in the absence of a drainable abscess.[32] Empiric antibiotics for purulent cellulitis in outpatients should include an orally administered agent with activity against CA-MRSA such as trimethoprim–sulfamethoxazole, a tetracycline, or clindamycin (Table 88-7); infection due to streptococci is less likely in this situation and specific coverage is not required.[32,48–50] Oral linezolid is also recommended in such cases but is significantly more expensive and no more efficacious than other treatment options.[32]

TABLE 88-7 Initial Treatment Regimens for Cellulitis and Necrotizing Fasciitis

Antibiotic	Adult Dose and Route	Pediatric Dose and Route
Cellulitis		
Staphylococcal or unknown gram-positive infection		
Mild to moderate nonpurulent infection	Dicloxacillin or cephalexin orally[a]	Dicloxacillin or cephalexin orally[a]
Mild to moderate purulent infection with suspected CA-MRSA	Trimethoprim–sulfamethoxazole, doxycycline, minocycline, or clindamycin orally	Trimethoprim–sulfamethoxazole or clindamycin orally
Severe nonpurulent infection	IV cefazolin or nafcillin[b]	IV cefazolin or nafcillin[b]
Severe purulent infection	IV vancomycin, linezolid, or daptomycin	IV vancomycin or linezolid
Streptococcal (documented)		
Mild to moderate infection	Penicillin VK orally[a] or IM procaine penicillin G[a]	Penicillin VK orally or IM procaine penicillin G[a]
Severe infection	IV aqueous penicillin G[a]	IV aqueous penicillin G[a]
Gram-negative bacilli		
Mild to moderate infection	Cefaclor or cefuroxime axetil orally[c]	Cefaclor or cefuroxime axetil orally
Severe infection	IV aminoglycoside[d] or IV cephalosporin (first- or second-generation depending on severity of infection or susceptibility pattern)[c]	IV aminoglycoside[d] or IV cephalosporin (first- or second-generation depending on severity of infection or susceptibility pattern)
Polymicrobic infection without anaerobes	IV aminoglycoside[e] + IV penicillin G, nafcillin, or vancomycin depending on isolation of staphylococci or streptococci and risk for MRSA infection	IV aminoglycoside[e] + IV penicillin G, nafcillin, or vancomycin depending on isolation of staphylococci or streptococci and risk for MRSA infection
Polymicrobic infection with anaerobes		
Mild to moderate infection	Amoxicillin/clavulanate orally. *Or* ciprofloxacin or levofloxacin + clindamycin or metronidazole orally. *Or* moxifloxacin orally	Amoxicillin/clavulanate orally
Severe infection	IV aminoglycoside[e] + IV clindamycin or metronidazole. *Or* IV second- or third-generation cephalosporin + IV clindamycin or metronidazole. *Or* IV antianaerobic second-generation cephalosporin. *Or* IV imipenem–cilastatin, meropenem, ertapenem, doripenem, or piperacillin–tazobactam	IV aminoglycoside[e] + IV clindamycin or metronidazole. *Or* IV second- or third-generation cephalosporin + IV clindamycin or metronidazole. *Or* IV antianaerobic second-generation cephalosporin. *Or* IV imipenem–cilastatin, meropenem, ertapenem, or piperacillin–tazobactam
Necrotizing fasciitis		
Type I	IV ampicillin–sulbactam or piperacillin–tazobactam + IV clindamycin + IV ciprofloxacin. *Or* IV cefotaxime + IV clindamycin or metronidazole. *Or* IV imipenem/cilastatin, meropenem, or ertapenem	
Type II	IV penicillin G + IV clindamycin[d]	
Type III	IV penicillin G + IV clindamycin[d]	

CA-MRSA, community-associated methicillin-resistant *Staphylococcus aureus*; IM, intramuscularly.

[a]For penicillin-allergic patients, use clindamycin.
[b]For penicillin-allergic patients, use vancomycin.
[c]For penicillin-allergic adults, use a fluoroquinolone (ciprofloxacin, levofloxacin, or moxifloxacin).
[d]May consider initially adding vancomycin for CA-MRSA coverage if suspicions of staphylococcal involvement (see text).
[e]A fluoroquinolone (adults only) or aztreonam may be used in place of the aminoglycoside in patients with severe renal dysfunction or other relative contraindications to aminoglycoside use.

Clinical **Controversy. . .**

The most appropriate dose of trimethoprim–sulfamethoxazole for the treatment of CA-MRSA is not known. Although higher doses (e.g., two double-strength tablets orally twice daily) have been recommended,[32] a prospective observational study of high dose versus standard dose of trimethoprim–sulfamethoxazole for treatment of SSTIs caused by MRSA found no clinically or statistically significant differences in rates of clinical resolution of infections.[51] Although trimethoprim–sulfamethoxazole is an inexpensive and generally well-tolerated drug, whether higher doses have any true clinical benefit and should be routinely used in most patients remains to be established.

Nonpurulent cellulitis is defined as cellulitis without purulent drainage or exudate and no associated abscess. The role of MRSA in these types of infection is not clear, so empiric therapy of nonpurulent cellulitis is directed primarily against Group A β-hemolytic streptococci. Recommended empiric therapy consists of an orally administered β-lactam such as cephalexin or dicloxacillin, or clindamycin.[32] Oral cephalosporins, such as cefadroxil, cefaclor, cefprozil, cefpodoxime proxetil, and cefdinir, are also effective in the treatment of cellulitis but are more expensive.[16,42] In penicillin-allergic patients, oral or parenteral clindamycin may be used.[32,42] Alternatively, a first-generation cephalosporin may be used cautiously for patients without a history of immediate or anaphylactic reactions to penicillin. In severe cases in which cephalosporins cannot be used because of suspected and/or documented MRSA or severe β-lactam allergies, vancomycin should be administered.[16,32]

Empiric treatment of CA-MRSA should be considered for patients with nonpurulent cellulitis if they have not responded appropriately to β-lactam therapy alone, or if patients exhibit signs of more severe infection with systemic toxicity.[32] Recommended drugs for coverage of CA-MRSA in this setting are the same as those for purulent cellulitis. Clindamycin has reasonably good activity against β-hemolytic streptococci, but the activities of trimethoprim–sulfamethoxazole and the tetracyclines against this organism are not well defined.[32] Therefore, if empiric coverage of both MRSA and β-hemolytic streptococci is desired for patients with nonpurulent cellulitis, it is recommended that they receive clindamycin alone or amoxicillin in combination with trimethoprim–sulfamethoxazole, doxycycline, or minocycline.[32] Although often used for treatment of uncomplicated outpatient cellulitis, fluoroquinolones (e.g., levofloxacin, moxifloxacin) are not recommended for routine use due to their unnecessarily broad spectrum of activity, concerns for resistance, and higher cost compared with other preferred options.

Clinical **Controversy. . .**

Whether antibiotic coverage for both β-hemolytic streptococci and CA-MRSA is required during the initial treatment of nonpurulent cellulitis is controversial. The great majority of nonpurulent cellulitis appears to be caused by β-hemolytic streptococci, and hospitalized patients treated with β-lactam antibiotics alone were reported to have excellent clinical response rates.[52] However, the high prevalence of CA-MRSA has prompted some clinicians to empirically cover this pathogen as part of routine therapy because of benefit-versus-risk considerations.[32,52] Whether the addition of antibiotics having activity against CA-MRSA should be done routinely, or in which specific patients such coverage should be considered, is not known.

Patients in whom specific pathogens have been identified by culture should have empiric antibiotics narrowed according to susceptibility test results. If documented to be a mild cellulitis secondary to streptococci, oral penicillin VK or intramuscular procaine penicillin G may be administered. Since *S. aureus* susceptibilities are more variable, treatment of documented staphylococcal infections will depend on test results for specific isolates. The usual duration of therapy for outpatient therapy of cellulitis, either purulent or nonpurulent, is 5 to 10 days.[16,31,42]

More severe infections should be treated initially with IV antibiotic regimens (Table 88-7). The classification of infections as either purulent or nonpurulent is again useful in the selection of appropriate initial therapy in these patients. Hospitalized patients with more severe or complicated purulent cellulitis should be empirically treated with an antibiotic having activity against MRSA. Vancomycin, linezolid, daptomycin, telavancin, and clindamycin are all acceptable treatment options with comparable efficacy in adults.[31,32,53] In children, vancomycin, linezolid, or clindamycin is the preferred treatment option. Hospitalized patients with nonpurulent cellulitis may be initially treated with IV cefazolin or nafcillin, with change to an agent with activity against MRSA if there is unsatisfactory clinical response.[32] Ceftriaxone 50 to 100 mg/kg as a single daily dose has also been efficacious in the treatment of cellulitis in pediatric patients.[31,43] The recommended duration of therapy for cellulitis in hospitalized patients is 7 to 14 days, but this should be individualized based on patient response.[32]

Linezolid, quinupristin–dalfopristin, daptomycin, ceftaroline, and telavancin all exhibit excellent activity against resistant gram-positive pathogens.[44–47,53] However, significantly higher cost compared with vancomycin, as well as lack of demonstrated advantages in efficacy, makes them most appropriate for treatment of complicated or refractory infections, or those documented as caused by multidrug-resistant pathogens, rather than as initial therapy. The availability of orally administered linezolid may provide a cost-effective "step-down" option as an alternative to prolonged treatment with parenteral agents for many patients with more complicated infections and/or those patients who require initial hospitalization.[48]

Carbapenems (i.e., imipenem, meropenem, ertapenem, and doripenem) and the β-lactam–β-lactamase inhibitor combination antibiotics (ampicillin–sulbactam, ticarcillin–clavulanate, and piperacillin–tazobactam) appear to be equivalent to standard therapies in adults.[5,16,31,42] However, the greater cost of these agents without increased efficacy compared with other reliable regimens, particularly given the increasing problem of MRSA, makes them less desirable for empiric therapy except in serious polymicrobic infections.[5,16,42]

For cellulitis caused by gram-negative bacilli or a mixture of microorganisms, immediate antimicrobial chemotherapy, as determined by Gram stain, is essential (Table 88-7). Surgical debridement of necrotic tissue and drainage also may be appropriate. Gram-negative cellulitis may be treated appropriately with an aminoglycoside (such as gentamicin or tobramycin), or a first- or second-generation cephalosporin (e.g., cephalexin, cefaclor, or cefuroxime). Ceftriaxone, ceftazidime, and the fluoroquinolones are also effective in the treatment of cellulitis caused by both gram-negative and gram-positive bacteria.[5,16,31,42] If gram-positive aerobic bacteria are also present on Gram stain, an additional agent such as penicillin G or a penicillinase-resistant penicillin may need to be added to provide coverage against staphylococci or streptococci as appropriate.[32] Addition of an agent active against MRSA (e.g., vancomycin) may need to be considered for severe, complicated infections in hospitalized patients.[5,16,31,32,42]

Because some polymicrobic infections may also involve anaerobic bacteria, antibiotic therapy may need to be broadened to include agents with good activity against these organisms. Many different treatment regimens are possible depending on the bacteriology of the lesion (Table 88-7). Orally administered antibiotics, as monotherapy or in combination regimens, may be appropriately used in the treatment of mild to moderate infections in outpatients. Monotherapy or combination regimens of IV antibiotics may be necessary for more severe infections in hospitalized patients. Therapy should be 10 to 14 days in duration.[16,31,42]

Because gram-negative and mixed aerobic–anaerobic cellulitis can progress quickly to serious tissue invasion, therapeutic intervention should be immediate.[16,31,42] If treated early, a rapid response can be seen. Unfortunately, because these infections often occur in patients with compromised immune defenses, they may still progress, even with therapeutic intervention. If the infectious process is secondary to a systemic cause (e.g., diabetes), the treatment course often is prolonged and may be associated with high morbidity and mortality.[16,31,42]

Infections in injection drug users generally are treated similarly to those in other types of patients.[16,31,42] It is important that blood cultures be obtained in these cases because 25% to 35% of patients may be bacteremic.[16,31] Also, patients should be assessed for the presence of abscesses; incision, drainage, and culture of these lesions are of extreme importance.[16] Initial antimicrobial therapy while awaiting culture results of abscesses should include broad coverage for gram-negative and anaerobic organisms, in addition to *S. aureus* (including MRSA in areas with high prevalence) and streptococci.[16,31,42]

Evaluation of Therapeutic Outcomes

If treated promptly with appropriate antibiotics, the majority of patients with cellulitis are cured rapidly. Culture and sensitivity results should be evaluated carefully for both the adequacy of culture material and the presence of resistant organisms. Additional high-quality samples for culture may be needed for microbiologic analysis. Failure to respond to therapy also may be indicative of an underlying local or systemic problem or a misdiagnosis.

NECROTIZING SOFT-TISSUE INFECTIONS

Necrotizing soft-tissue infections consist of a group of extremely severe infections, associated with high morbidity and mortality, that require early and aggressive surgical debridement in addition to appropriate antibiotics and intensive supportive care.[4,7,54–57] Different terms have been used to classify necrotizing infections based on factors such as predisposing conditions, onset of symptoms, pain, skin appearance, etiologic agent, gas production, muscle involvement, and systemic toxicity.[5,29,55] However, while many types of necrotizing soft-tissue infections have been designated as unique infectious processes, they all share similar pathophysiologies, clinical features, and treatment approaches.[54–57] The major clinical entities of necrotizing infections are *necrotizing fasciitis* and *clostridial myonecrosis* (gas gangrene).[54–56]

6 Necrotizing fasciitis is a rare but severe infection of the subcutaneous tissue that may be caused by aerobic and/or anaerobic bacteria and results in progressive destruction of the superficial fascia and subcutaneous fat.[5,13,31,55,56] Type I necrotizing fasciitis is the most common type and accounts for approximately 80% of necrotizing soft-tissue infections.[55,56] It generally occurs after trauma or surgery and involves a mixture of anaerobes (*Bacteroides*, *Peptostreptococcus*) and facultative bacteria (streptococci and Enterobacteriaceae) that act synergistically to cause destruction of fat and fascia.[7,55] Type I necrotizing fasciitis is also reported more commonly among injection drug users.[54–57] In type I infections, the skin may be spared, and the speed at which the infection spreads

CLINICAL PRESENTATION

General

- Most frequently involve the abdomen, perineum, and lower extremities.
- Predisposing factors such as diabetes mellitus, local trauma or infection, or recent surgery often present.
- Rapid diagnosis is critical due to the aggressive nature and high associated mortality (20% to 50%).

Symptoms

- Systemic symptoms generally are marked (e.g., fever, chills, and leukocytosis) and may include shock and organ failure, especially in patients with type II infections.
- Pain in the affected area and systemic toxicity are characteristically more pronounced than with cellulitis.

Signs

- May be difficult to differentiate between necrotizing fasciitis and cellulitis early in infection.
- Affected area is initially hot, swollen, and erythematous without sharply demarcated margins.
- Affected area is often shiny, exquisitely tender, and painful.
- Diffuse swelling of the area is followed by the appearance of bullae filled with clear fluid.
- Rapidly progressive infection with the frequent development of a maroon or violaceous color of the skin after several days.
- Infection may rapidly evolve into a frank cutaneous gangrene, sometimes with myonecrosis.

Laboratory Tests

- Tissue samples should be obtained for histologic examination, and culture and susceptibility testing.
- Clostridial myonecrosis shows little inflammation on histologic examination.

Other Diagnostic Tests

- Surgical exploration is the best and most rapid diagnosis of necrotizing infections; computed tomography and magnetic resonance imaging may also be helpful.
- Blood samples should be collected for complete blood count and chemistry profile, as well as for bacterial culture.
- Laboratory tests that may aid in the diagnosis of necrotizing infections (LRINEC score) include C-reactive protein, white blood cell count, hemoglobin, sodium, creatinine, and glucose.

(3 to 5 days) is somewhat slower than that in type II.[29] Necrotizing fasciitis affecting the male genitalia is termed *Fournier's gangrene*.[55] Type II necrotizing fasciitis is caused by virulent strains of *S. pyogenes* and is commonly referred to as *streptococcal gangrene*.[7,55] This type of infection has often been called "flesh-eating bacteria" by the lay press. Unlike previous reports of streptococcal gangrene that affected older individuals with underlying diseases, recent reports have occurred primarily in young, previously healthy adults following some type of minor trauma. It differs from type I infections in its clinical presentation. Type II infections have rapidly extending necrosis (i.e., 24 to 72 hours) of subcutaneous tissues and skin, gangrene, severe local pain, and systemic toxicity.[29,54–57] They are also highly associated with an early onset of shock and organ failure and are present in approximately half the cases of streptococcal toxic shock-like syndrome.[29,54,55] Of note, CA-MRSA is increasingly reported in type II infections, either as a single organism or in combination with streptococci.[9,55,56] Clinicians should consider CA-MRSA in areas that are endemic for CA-MRSA or if patients have risk factors for these organisms.

Clostridial myonecrosis (type III necrotizing fasciitis) is a necrotizing infection that involves the skeletal muscle.[9,55] Type III infections account for less than 5% of necrotizing infections.[55] Gas production and muscle necrosis are prominent features of this infection, which readily explains why this infection is commonly referred to as *gas gangrene*.[54–56] The infection advances rapidly, often over a matter of a few hours.[54–56] Most infections occur after surgery or trauma, with *Clostridium perfringens* identified as the most common etiologic agent.[55]

TREATMENT
Necrotizing Soft-Tissue Infections

Desired Outcomes

The goals of therapy of acute bacterial cellulitis are rapid eradication of the infection, prevention of further complications, and reduction in mortality. Effective treatment of necrotizing soft-tissue infections includes avoidance of unnecessary antimicrobials that contribute to increased resistance, and minimizing toxicities and cost of therapy.

Management of Necrotizing Infections

On diagnosis, immediate and aggressive surgical debridement of all necrotic tissue is essential.[9,54–57] Initial surgical debridement performed greater than 14 hours after the diagnosis of necrotizing infection was independently associated with increased patient mortality, including a 34-fold increased risk of death in patients with septic shock.[58] Patients often require further surgical intervention following initial debridement to ensure that all necrotic tissue has been removed.[16,54–58] Type I necrotizing fasciitis must be empirically treated with broad-spectrum antibiotics that include coverage against streptococci, Enterobacteriaceae, and anaerobes. A number of antibiotic regimens are recommended to successfully treat necrotizing soft-tissue infections (see Table 88-5); these are generally similar to regimens used for polymicrobic cellulitis.[31,54–57] Antibiotic therapy can be modified after Gram stain and culture reports are available.

If a diagnosis of type II necrotizing fasciitis is established, broad-spectrum empiric therapy should be replaced with the combination of penicillin and clindamycin.[55,56] Although *S. pyogenes* remains susceptible to penicillin, clindamycin is more effective.[54,56] Several factors have been postulated to explain the greater efficacy of clindamycin, including the mechanism of action (inhibition of protein synthesis) that may cause decreased production of bacterial exotoxins.[54–57] In addition, clindamycin has immunomodulatory properties that may account for the higher efficacy.[54,56] Clindamycin is also effective against strains of CA-MRSA.[55] The combination of penicillin and clindamycin is also recommended for treatment of clostridial myonecrosis.[16,54,55] Hyperbaric oxygen also may be of some benefit for clostridial myonecrosis.[54–57]

Evaluation of Therapeutic Outcomes

Because of the high mortality associated with necrotizing infections, rapid and complete debridement of all devitalized and necrotic tissue is essential. Surgical debridement, coupled with appropriate antimicrobial therapy and supportive measures for management of shock and organ failure, should stabilize the patient. Vital signs and laboratory tests should be monitored carefully for signs of resolution of the infection. Change in antimicrobial therapy or additional surgical debridement may be needed in patients who do not show signs of improvement.

DIABETIC FOOT INFECTIONS

Three major types of foot infections are seen in diabetic patients: deep abscesses, cellulitis of the dorsum, and mal perforans ulcers.[59,60] Most deep abscesses involve the central plantar space (arch) and are caused by minor penetrating trauma or by an extension of infection of a nail or web space of the toes. Infections of the dorsal area generally arise from infections in the toes that are related to routine care of the nails, nail beds, and calluses of the toes. Mal perforans ulcer is a chronic ulcer of the sole of the foot. The ulcer develops on thickened, hardened calluses over the first or fifth metatarsal. Mal perforans ulcers are associated with neuropathic changes, which are responsible for the misalignment of the weight-bearing bones of the foot.[59,60] Osteomyelitis is one of the most serious complications of diabetic foot infection (DFI) and may occur in 30% to 40% of infections.[30,59]

Epidemiology

DFI is among the most common complications of diabetes, accounting for as many as 20% of all hospitalizations in diabetic patients at an annual cost of $200 to $350 million.[30,59,61] Approximately 15% of diabetic patients experience significant soft-tissue infection during their lifetime.[61] Approximately 71,000 lower-extremity amputations, often sequelae of uncontrolled infection, are performed each year on diabetic patients; this represents up to 70% of all nontraumatic amputations in the United States.[30,59,61] Approximately 20% of diabetics will undergo additional surgery or amputation of a second limb within 12 months of the initial amputation.[30,59]

Etiology

Mild cases of DFI are often monomicrobial. However, more severe infections are typically polymicrobic; up to 60% of hospitalized patients have polymicrobial infections (Table 88-8).[30,59,60,62–67] Wide ranges in the frequency of various bacteria in DFI reflect differences in culture techniques as well as variation among different types and severity of infections. Staphylococci and streptococci are the most common pathogens, although gram-negative bacilli and/or anaerobes occur in up to 50% of cases.[30,62–67] Although *P. aeruginosa* is an important pathogen in DFI, it is usually reported to occur in <10% of wounds and is most commonly associated with more severe infections.[30,63] Obligate anaerobes are also more commonly associated with severe infections in patients with chronic foot ischemia.[30,62,63] MRSA is increasingly important in DFI and has been reported in from 10% to 30% of infected wounds.[30,63,64,67–69] The presence of MRSA in DFI has been associated with increased risk of treatment

TABLE 88-8 Bacterial Isolates from Foot Infections in Diabetic Patients[30,59,60,62–68,71]

Organisms	Percentage of Isolates
Aerobes	63–100
Gram-positive	42–100
Staphylococcus aureus (all)	15–67
S. aureus (MRSA)	7–30
Streptococcus spp.	6–32
Enterococcus spp.	2–25
Coagulase-negative staphylococci	6–10
Other gram-positive aerobes	0–19
Gram-negative	16–55
Proteus spp.	3–7
Enterobacter spp.	1–9
Escherichia coli	3–10
Klebsiella spp.	1–6
Pseudomonas aeruginosa	3–33
Other gram-negative bacilli	3–13
Anaerobes	1–40
Peptostreptococcus spp.	4–28
Bacteroides fragilis group	2–9
Other *Bacteroides* spp.	3–6
Clostridium spp.	0–2
Other anaerobes	7–19

failure and worse patient outcomes, but these findings have not been consistent among studies and the clinical relevance of MRSA in this setting is still unclear.[30,60,68]

Identifying causative pathogens from cultures of diabetic wounds is often difficult. The chronic nature of DFI means that these wounds are often heavily colonized by organisms not playing a role in the infection. Superficial swab cultures are not as reliable as culture specimens obtained from deep tissues via biopsy, tissue scraping (curettage), or needle aspiration of drainage or abscess fluid.[64,67,70] Therefore, cultures and sensitivity tests should be done with specimens obtained from a deep culture of the wound base whenever possible. Before the wound is cultured, it should be scrubbed vigorously with saline-moistened sterile gauze to remove any overlying necrotic debris and further debrided as necessary.[30,64] Bone cultures should also be performed when there is diagnostic uncertainty regarding the presence of osteomyelitis or when therapeutic decisions are dependent on knowing the exact etiology of infection.[30,64]

Pathophysiology

Three key factors are involved in the development of diabetic foot problems: neuropathy, angiopathy and ischemia, and immunologic defects. Any of these disorders can occur in isolation; however, they frequently occur together.[61]

Neuropathic changes to the autonomic nervous system as a consequence of diabetes may affect the motor nerve supply of small intrinsic muscles of the foot, resulting in muscular imbalance, abnormal stresses on tissues and bone, and repetitive injuries.[59,61] Diminished sensory perception causes an absence of pain and unawareness of minor injuries and ulceration. The sympathetic nerve supply may be damaged, resulting in an absence of sweating that may lead to dry cracked skin and secondary infection.[30,59,61]

Atherosclerosis is more common, appears at a younger age, and progresses more rapidly in the diabetic than in the nondiabetic. Diabetics may have problems with both small vessels (microangiopathy) and large vessels (macroangiopathy) that can result in varying degrees of ischemia, ultimately leading to skin breakdown and infection.

Diabetic patients typically have normal humoral immunity, normal levels of immunoglobulins, and normal antibody responses. Patients with diabetes, however, have impaired phagocytosis and intracellular microbicidal function as compared with nondiabetics; this may be related to angiopathy and low tissue levels of oxygen.[30,59,61] These defects in cell-mediated immunity make patients with diabetes more susceptible to certain types of infection and impair the patients' ability to heal wounds adequately.[59,60,61]

TREATMENT
Diabetic Foot Infections

Desired Outcomes

7 The goals of therapy in the management of DFI include the following: (a) successfully treat infected wounds by using effective nondrug and antibiotic therapy; (b) prevent additional infectious

CLINICAL PRESENTATION

General

- Infections are often much more extensive than they appear initially.

Symptoms

- Patients with peripheral neuropathy often do not experience pain; simple complaints of swelling or edema are common.

Signs

- Clinical signs of infection may not be present secondary to angiopathy and neuropathy.
- Lesions vary in size and clinical features (e.g., erythema, edema, warmth, presence of pus, draining sinuses, pain, and tenderness).
- Foul-smelling odor suggests the presence of anaerobic organisms.
- Temperature may be mildly elevated or normal.

Laboratory Tests

- Specimens for culture and sensitivities should be collected.
- Deep-tissue samples obtained during surgical debridement are most useful for culture and susceptibility testing.
- Wounds must be cultured for both aerobic and anaerobic organisms.

Other Diagnostic Tests

- Possible presence of osteomyelitis also must be assessed via radiograph, bone scan, or both, as appropriate.

complications; (c) preserve as much normal limb function as possible; (d) avoid unnecessary use of antimicrobials that contribute to increased resistance; and (e) minimize toxicities and cost while increasing patient quality of life.

Management

Up to 90% of infections can be treated successfully with a comprehensive treatment approach that includes both wound care and antimicrobial therapy.[30,60,64,65] After carefully assessing the extent of the lesion and obtaining necessary cultures, necrotic tissue must be thoroughly debrided, with wound drainage and amputation as required. Wounds must be kept clean and dressings changed frequently (two to three times daily). Because of the relationship between hyperglycemia and immune system defects, glycemic control must be maximized to ensure optimal wound healing. In addition, the patient's activities should be restricted initially to bedrest for leg elevation and control of edema, if present. Adequate pressure relief from a foot wound (i.e., off-loading) is crucial to the healing process.[30,61,64] Finally, appropriate antimicrobials must be initiated.[30,60,61,64,65] However, the optimal antimicrobial therapy for DFI has yet to be defined. Empiric therapy that is totally comprehensive in its coverage of all possible pathogens does not seem to be necessary unless the infection is life- or limb-threatening, assuming that adequate wound care is also being performed.[30,60,64,65] This is particularly true regarding MRSA, *P. aeruginosa*, and anaerobes; the perceived need for empiric coverage of these organisms often leads to use of excessively broad-spectrum drug regimens. Several studies have shown good treatment efficacy despite the fact that treatment regimens did not have consistently good activity against these particular organisms.[30,64,66–68,71]

Proper selection of empiric antibiotics for DFI begins with thorough patient assessment and classification of the severity of the infection. Specific drug regimens, route of administration, and duration of therapy are all then largely dependent on the severity of infection. Although a number of classification systems are available, the most recent DFI treatment guidelines use those summarized in Table 88-9.[30,64] Wounds with no local signs of infection often do not require antibiotic therapy, and the majority of mild, uncomplicated infections can be managed successfully on an outpatient basis with highly bioavailable oral antimicrobials and good wound care (Tables 88-9 and 88-10).[30,60,64,65] Antibiotics for treatment of mild infections should be largely limited to those with activity against skin flora such as streptococci and methicillin-susceptible *S. aureus* (MSSA), except in those patients with risk factors for infection with other types of pathogens (Fig. 88-1).[30,64] Patients with specific risk factors for MRSA (Table 88-10) should empirically receive trimethoprim–sulfamethoxazole or doxycycline orally, while those who have received antibiotics within the past month should also receive empiric antibiotics that provide activity against gram-negative bacilli. Oral antimicrobials should be used cautiously in DFI complicated by osteomyelitis, extensive ulceration, areas of necrosis, or a combination of these. The use of topical antimicrobials, including medical-grade honey, has been advocated for the treatment of DFI in an attempt to minimize the cost of therapy and systemic antibiotic exposure leading to adverse effects and resistance. Although the most recent guidelines allow for consideration of topical therapy in mild infection in selected patients, use of topical agents is quite controversial and not routinely recommended.[30,60,64,72,73]

Appropriate initial therapy for patients with moderate to severe infection is also dependent on the presence of specific risk factors that increase the likelihood of infection with more resistant pathogens such as *P. aeruginosa* and MRSA (Table 88-10).[30,64] Many moderate infections can be successfully treated with orally

TABLE 88-9 Classifications and Treatment Strategies for Diabetic Foot Infections of Varying Severity

Clinical Signs/ Symptoms of Infection	Infection Severity	Treatment Setting
None	Uninfected	Outpatient management; nonantibiotic wound management only
Local infection present (≥2 of the following): local swelling or induration, erythema, local tenderness or pain, local warmth, purulent discharge		
Local infection involving only skin and subcutaneous tissue, without involvement of deeper tissues or SIRS criteria present; if erythema is present, must be >0.5 and ≤2 cm around ulcer	Mild	Outpatient management; topical or oral antibiotics
Local infection with erythema >2 cm around ulcer, or involving structures deeper than skin and subcutaneous tissue (e.g., abscess, osteomyelitis, septic arthritis, fasciitis); no SIRS criteria present	Moderate	Outpatient (or initial inpatient) management; oral (or initial parenteral) antibiotics
Local infection with ≥2 SIRS criteria: • Temperature >38°C or <36°C (>100.4°F or <96.8°F) • HR >90 • RR >20 • WBC >12,000 or <4,000, or ≥10% bands (>12 × 10⁹/L or <4 × 10⁹/L, or ≥0.10 bands)	Severe	Inpatient, followed by outpatient, management; initial parenteral antibiotics, followed by switch to oral when possible

administered antibiotics that provide activity against MSSA, streptococci, and gram-negative aerobic bacilli; coverage of obligate anaerobes may also be considered in patients with chronic or previously treated wounds (Fig. 88-2).[30,64] The addition of orally administered agents with activity against MRSA is recommended in patients with moderate or severe infection and specific risk factors for MRSA; such patients may also be considered for hospitalization and initial treatment with parenteral antibiotics in order to ensure adequate antibiotics for potentially more complex infections.[30,64] Patients with more extensive or chronically unhealed wounds, even though assessed as moderate in severity, may also be more appropriately treated initially with parenteral antibiotics in the hospital setting.[30,64] All patients with severe DFI should be hospitalized initially and treated with broad-spectrum IV antibiotics (Table 88-10 and Fig. 88-2).[30,64] Severe infection is considered a risk factor for *P. aeruginosa*, so most patients with severe DFI will be initially started on antipseudomonal antibiotics.[30,64] Many patients will also be initially started on antibiotics that provide activity against MRSA due to risk-versus-benefit considerations, but assessment of risk factors in individual patients should still be performed in order to minimize the use of excessively broad-spectrum antibiotics when possible.

Current guidelines for management of DFI include options for both monotherapy and combination regimens (Table 88-10).[30] Monotherapy, along with appropriate medical or surgical management, or both, is often effective in treating DFI, including those in which osteomyelitis is present.[30,60,65,66] Monotherapy is particularly attractive because of the potential advantages of convenience, cost, and avoidance of toxicities. Microbiologic and clinical cure rates ranging from 60% to 90% may be expected from any of these agents.[66] Selection of a specific regimen is determined by patient-specific factors including allergies, renal function, history

TABLE 88-10 Suggested Antibiotic Regimens for Empiric Treatment of Diabetic Foot Infections

Severity of Infection	Probable Pathogens	Drug(s)[a]	Duration of Therapy
Mild	*Staphylococcus aureus* (MSSA) *Streptococcus* spp. *S. aureus* (MRSA) • Patients with history of MRSA infection or colonization in past year • Prevalence of MRSA ≥50% in local geographic area • Recent hospitalization	Amoxicillin–clavulanate Cephalexin Dicloxacillin Clindamycin Levofloxacin Moxifloxacin[b]	1–2 weeks; may increase up to 4 weeks if infection slow to resolve
Moderate to severe (initially oral or IV antibiotics for moderately severe infections, IV antibiotics for severe infections)	MSSA *Streptococcus* spp. Enterobacteriaceae Obligate anaerobes	Ampicillin/sulbactam Cefoxitin Ceftriaxone Imipenem/cilastatin Ertapenem Levofloxacin Moxifloxacin Tigecycline Levofloxacin or ciprofloxacin + clindamycin	Moderately severe infection: 1–3 weeks; severe infection: 2–4 weeks
	MRSA • Patients with history of MRSA infection or colonization in past year • Prevalence of MRSA ≥30% in local geographic area • Recent hospitalization • Infection severe enough that not empirically covering MRSA poses unacceptable risk of treatment failure	Add to one of the above regimens: • Vancomycin • Linezolid • Daptomycin	
	Pseudomonas aeruginosa • Patient has been soaking feet • Patient has previously failed therapy with nonpseudomonal antibiotic regimen • Severe infection	Piperacillin/tazobactam	
	Mixed infections potentially including all of the above	Cefepime, ceftazidime, or aztreonam + metronidazole or clindamycin + vancomycin[c] *Or* piperacillin–tazobactam or imipenem–cilastatin or meropenem[b] + vancomycin[c]	

MRSA, methicillin-resistant *S. aureus*; MSSA, methicillin-susceptible *S. aureus*.

[a]Agents not shown in any particular order of preference.
[b]Not specifically recommended in IDSA guidelines but may be appropriate treatment option.
[c]Linezolid or daptomycin may be used in place of vancomycin.

of previous antibiotic use, and cost. In penicillin-allergic patients, metronidazole or clindamycin plus a fluoroquinolone, aztreonam, or possibly a third- or fourth-generation cephalosporin is appropriate.[30,60,65] Vancomycin also is used frequently in severe infections because of its excellent activity against gram-positive pathogens. Linezolid, daptomycin, and tigecycline are specifically recommended alternatives for treatment of this pathogen.[30,60,64,65] Tigecycline may be particularly useful in this setting because of its activity against gram-negative aerobes and anaerobic bacteria, thus allowing it to be used as monotherapy for the treatment of mixed infections in patients where coverage of *P. aeruginosa* is not of great concern. A newer agent, ceftaroline fosamil, has in vitro activity that is suitable for DFI but has not been studied for this indication and its role is not yet defined. Because many patients already have some degree of diabetic nephropathy that may place them at higher risk of nephrotoxicity, strong recommendations have been made against the use of aminoglycoside antibiotics unless no alternative agents are available.[30,60] When an aminoglycoside is used, care must be taken to avoid further compromising renal function. All antibiotic regimens should be adjusted as necessary for renal dysfunction.

Duration of therapy for DFI depends on the severity of the infection, ranging from 1 to 2 weeks for mild infections up to 2 to 4 weeks or more for severe infections.[30,60] In cases of underlying osteomyelitis, treatment should continue for 6 to 12 weeks.[30,60,65] After healing of the infection has occurred, a well-designed program for prevention of further infections should be instituted. The use of adjunctive agents such as colony-stimulating factors, growth factors, and hyperbaric oxygen for either prevention or treatment of DFIs is controversial and not widely recommended.[30]

Evaluation of Therapeutic Outcomes

Therapy should be reevaluated carefully after 48 to 72 hours to assess favorable response. Change in therapy (or route of administration, if oral) should be considered if clinical improvement is not observed at this time. For optimal results, drug therapy should be appropriately modified according to information from deep-tissue culture and the clinical condition of the patient. Infections in diabetic patients often require extended courses of therapy because of impaired host immunity and poor wound healing.

PRESSURE SORES

The terms *decubitus ulcer*, *bed sore*, and *pressure sore* are used interchangeably.[74–76] The decubitus ulcer and the bed sore are types of pressure sores. The term *decubitus ulcer* is derived from the Latin word *decumbere*, meaning "lying down." Pressure sores, however, can develop regardless of a patient's position.

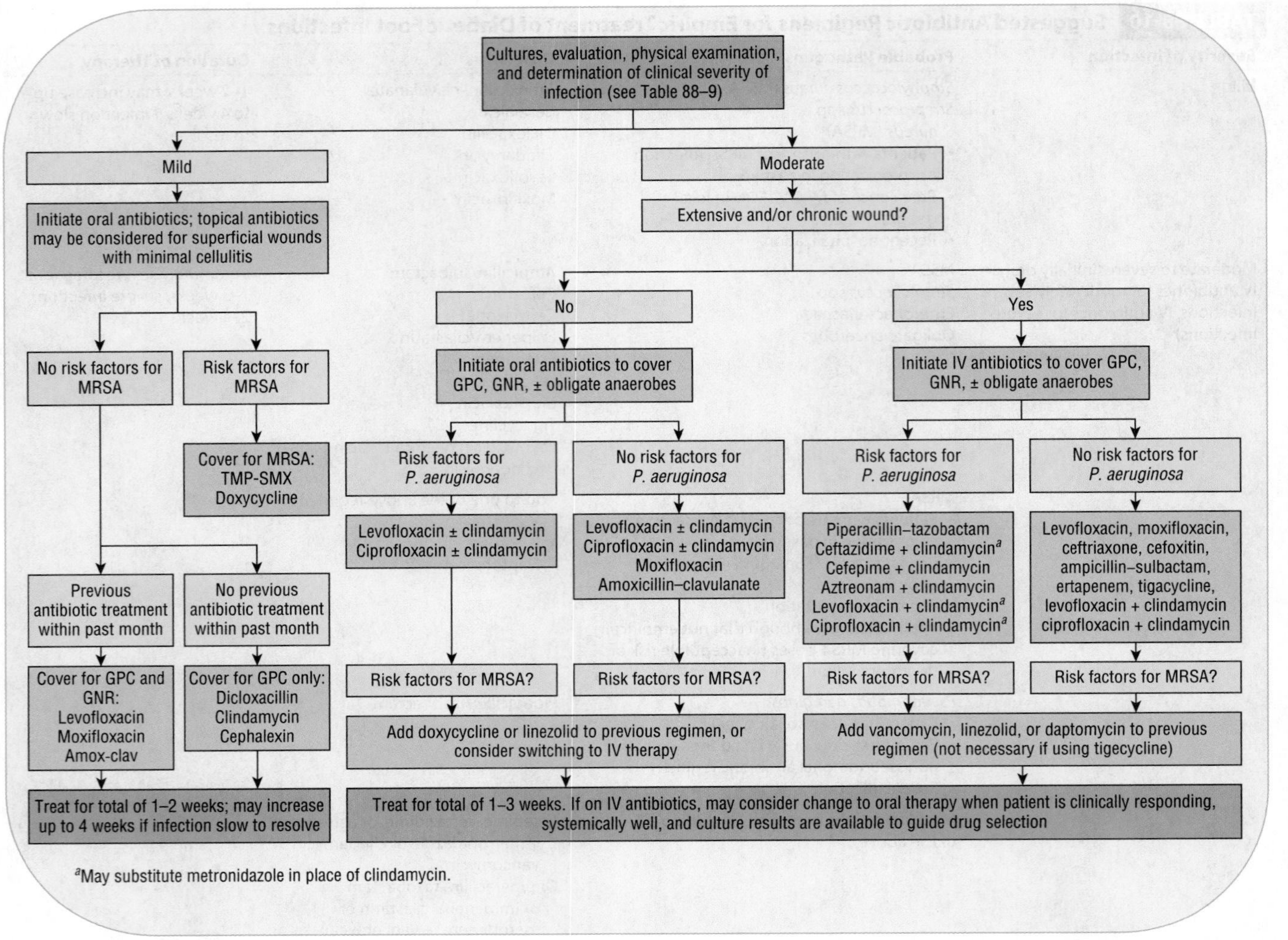

Cultures, evaluation, physical examination, and determination of clinical severity of infection (see Table 88–9)

Mild

Initiate oral antibiotics; topical antibiotics may be considered for superficial wounds with minimal cellulitis

No risk factors for MRSA

Risk factors for MRSA

Cover for MRSA: TMP-SMX Doxycycline

Previous antibiotic treatment within past month

No previous antibiotic treatment within past month

Cover for GPC and GNR: Levofloxacin Moxifloxacin Amox-clav

Cover for GPC only: Dicloxacillin Clindamycin Cephalexin

Treat for total of 1–2 weeks; may increase up to 4 weeks if infection slow to resolve

Moderate

Extensive and/or chronic wound?

No

Initiate oral antibiotics to cover GPC, GNR, ± obligate anaerobes

Risk factors for *P. aeruginosa*

Levofloxacin ± clindamycin
Ciprofloxacin ± clindamycin

No risk factors for *P. aeruginosa*

Levofloxacin ± clindamycin
Ciprofloxacin ± clindamycin
Moxifloxacin
Amoxicillin–clavulanate

Risk factors for MRSA?

Add doxycycline or linezolid to previous regimen, or consider switching to IV therapy

Yes

Initiate IV antibiotics to cover GPC, GNR, ± obligate anaerobes

Risk factors for *P. aeruginosa*

Piperacillin–tazobactam
Ceftazidime + clindamycin[a]
Cefepime + clindamycin
Aztreonam + clindamycin
Levofloxacin + clindamycin[a]
Ciprofloxacin + clindamycin[a]

No risk factors for *P. aeruginosa*

Levofloxacin, moxifloxacin, ceftriaxone, cefoxitin, ampicillin–sulbactam, ertapenem, tigacycline, levofloxacin + clindamycin ciprofloxacin + clindamycin

Risk factors for MRSA?

Add vancomycin, linezolid, or daptomycin to previous regimen (not necessary if using tigecycline)

Treat for total of 1–3 weeks. If on IV antibiotics, may consider change to oral therapy when patient is clinically responding, systemically well, and culture results are available to guide drug selection

[a]May substitute metronidazole in place of clindamycin.

FIGURE 88-1 Recommended treatment algorithm for initial management of mild to moderate diabetic foot infections. (GNR, aerobic gram-negative rods; GPC, aerobic gram-positive cocci; MRSA, methicillin-resistant *Staphylococcus aureus*; TMP-SMX, trimethoprim–sulfamethoxazole.)

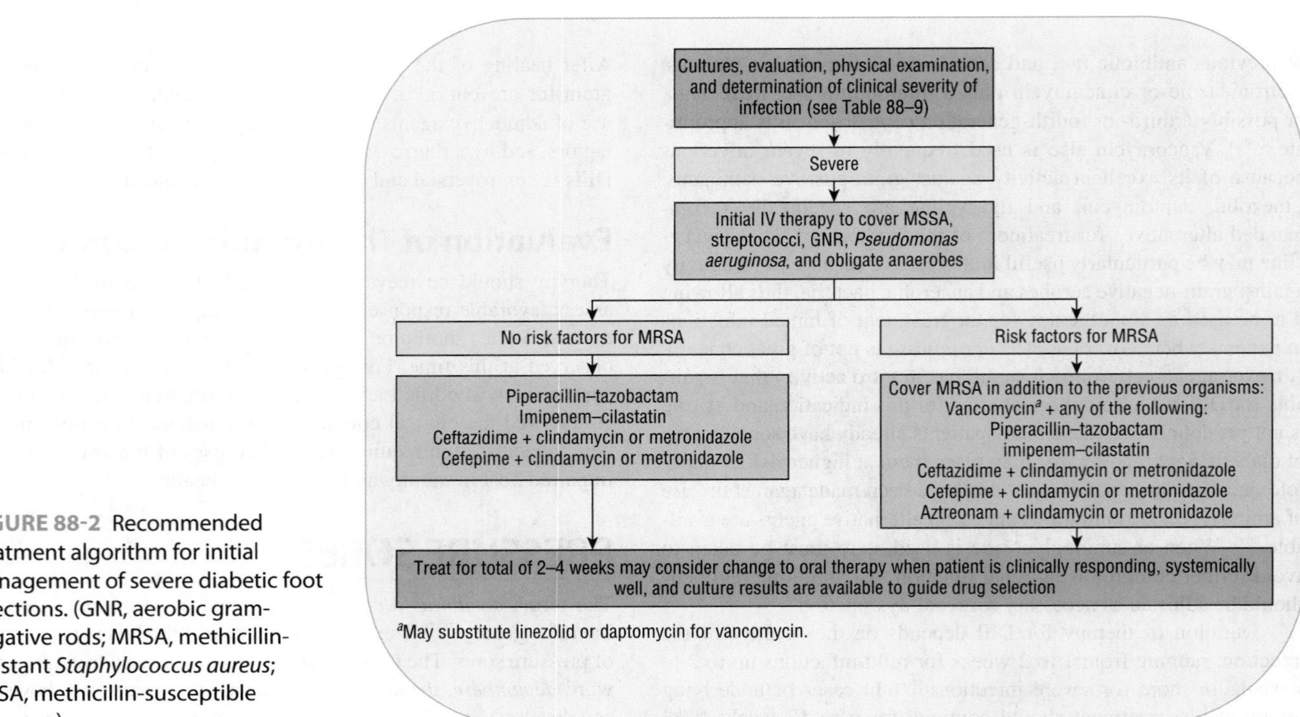

FIGURE 88-2 Recommended treatment algorithm for initial management of severe diabetic foot infections. (GNR, aerobic gram-negative rods; MRSA, methicillin-resistant *Staphylococcus aureus*; MSSA, methicillin-susceptible *S. aureus*.)

TABLE 88-11 Pressure Sore Classification

Suspected deep-tissue injury	Area of discolored intact skin or blood-filled blister due to damage of underlying soft tissue from pressure and/or shear. Area may be preceded by tissue that is painful, firm, mushy, boggy, warmer or cooler as compared with adjacent tissue
Stage 1	Pressure sore is generally reversible, is limited to the epidermis, and resembles an abrasion. Intact skin with nonblanchable redness of a localized area, usually over a bony prominence. The area may be painful, firm, soft, warmer or cooler as compared with adjacent tissue
Stage 2	A stage 2 sore also may be reversible; partial thickness loss of dermis presenting as a shallow open ulcer with a red pink wound bed. May also present as an intact or open/ruptured serum-filled blister, or as a shiny or dry shallow ulcer
Stage 3[a]	Full thickness tissue loss. Subcutaneous fat may be visible, but bone, tendon, or muscles are not exposed. May include undermining and tunneling. Depth of the ulcer varies by anatomical location; may range from shallow to extremely deep over areas of significant adiposity
Stage 4[a]	Full thickness tissue loss with exposed bone, tendon, or muscle; can extend into muscle and/or supporting structures (e.g., fascia, tendon, or joint capsule) making osteomyelitis possible. Often includes undermining and tunneling; depth of the ulcer varies by anatomical location
Unstageable[a]	Full thickness tissue loss in which the base of the ulcer is covered by slough (yellow, tan, gray, green, or brown) and/or eschar (tan, brown, or black) in the wound bed. True depth, and therefore stage, cannot be determined

[a]Stage 3, stage 4, and unstageable lesions are unlikely to resolve on their own and often require surgical intervention.

From reference 77.

Numerous systems for classification of pressure sores have been described. The 2007 recommendations of the National Pressure Ulcer Advisory Panel are shown in Table 88-11 and illustrate the various stages of progression through which a pressure sore may pass.[77]

Complications of pressure sores are not uncommon and may be life-threatening. Infection is one of the most serious and most frequently encountered complications of pressure ulcers.[75,76] Although most pressure sore wounds are heavily colonized, the majority of these eventually heal.[78–80] When true infection is present, however, there is bacterial invasion of previously healthy tissue. Without treatment, an initial small, localized area of ulceration can rapidly progress to large ulcers within days. The visible ulcer is just a small portion of the actual wound[81]; up to 70% of the total wound is below the skin. A pressure-gradient phenomenon is created by which the wound takes on a conical nature; the smallest point is at the skin surface, and the largest portion of the defect is at the base of the ulcer (Fig. 88-3).

Epidemiology

Pressure sores are most common among chronically debilitated persons, the elderly (70% involve persons greater than 70 years of age), and persons with serious spinal cord injury.[28,75,76,81,82] Generally, patients who are at risk for pressure sores are elderly or chronically ill young patients who are immobilized, in either bed or a wheelchair, and who may have altered mental status and/or incontinence.[75,76,81,82]

Etiology

Similar to DFIs, a large variety of aerobic gram-positive and gram-negative organisms, as well as anaerobes, frequently are isolated from wound cultures.[28] Most pressure sores are colonized with microorganisms, making assessment for infection a clinical challenge.[28,78] Curettage of the ulcer base after debridement provides more reliable culture information than does needle aspiration.[78–80] Biopsy specimens give the most reliable data but may not be practical to obtain. Deep-tissue cultures from different sites may give different results. Cultures collected from pressure ulcers reveal polymicrobial growth. A culture collected by swab is likely to identify surface bacteria colonizing the wound rather than to diagnose the infection.[78]

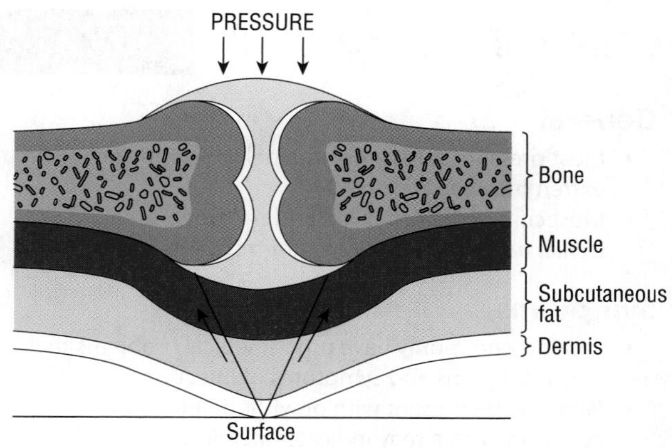

FIGURE 88-3 Distribution of forces involved with sore formation in a conical fashion.

Pathophysiology

Many factors apparently predispose patients to the formation of pressure sores: paralysis, paresis, immobilization, malnutrition, anemia, infection, and advanced age. Factors thought to be most critical to their formation are pressure, shearing forces, friction, and moisture[28,75,83]; however, there is still debate as to the exact pathophysiology of pressure sore formation.[83]

Pressure is the essential element in the formation of pressure sores.[28,76,81,83] The areas of highest pressure are generated most often over the bony prominences.[28,74–76,78,82,83] Both the degree of pressure and the length of time that the pressure is applied are important.[75,76,83]

Shearing occurs when two surfaces move in opposite directions.[28,83] This situation can occur when the head of a bed is raised, causing the upper torso to slide downward, transmitting pressure to the sacrum and other areas. This effect results in occlusion or distortion of vessels, leading to compromise of the dermis. At the same time, sitting and gravity create shearing forces; the posterior sacral skin area can become fixed secondary to friction with the bed. The effects of friction and shearing forces combine, resulting in transmission of force to the deep portion of the superficial fascia and leading to further damage of soft-tissue structures.[28,75,78,83]

Compounding the problems of shearing and friction forces are the macerating effects of excessive moisture in the local environment, resulting from incontinence and perspiration. This factor is of critical importance because when combined with the other forces, it increases the risk of pressure sore formation fivefold.[28,75,79,83]

TREATMENT
Pressure Sores

Desired Outcomes

The primary goal for pressure sores is prevention. Once a pressure sore has developed, the goals of therapy are prevention of complications (i.e., infections), preventing sores from growing larger, and

CLINICAL PRESENTATION

General

- Most pressure sores are in the pelvic region and lower extremities; see Figure 88-4.
- Most common sites: sacral and coccygeal areas, ischial tuberosities, and greater trochanter.

Symptoms

- Patients commonly have other medical problems that may mask signs and symptoms of infection.
- Pain may be present with or without infection; continuous pain may indicate infection.

Signs

- A dark red color on the surface of a pressure sore may indicate local infection.
- Surrounding erythema, swelling, and heat are commonly present with infection.
- Purulent discharge, foul odor, and systemic signs (e.g., fever and leukocytosis) of infection may be present.

Laboratory Tests

- Cultures should be collected from either a biopsy or fluid obtained by needle aspiration.

Other Diagnostic Tests

- Complete blood count often performed for assessment of potential infection.
- Consider magnetic resonance imaging if suspicious of underlying osteomyelitis.

preventing the development of sores in other locations.[81] Eradication of infection should include good wound care and topical therapies, and avoidance of broad-spectrum antimicrobials unless guided by results from appropriately collected cultures or in patients with bacteremia, sepsis, cellulitis, or osteomyelitis.

Drug and Nondrug Management

8 Prevention is the single most important aspect in the management of pressure sores. Skin surveillance and frequent repositioning (i.e., pressure reduction) are key in preventing pressure sores.[76,81] Prevention is far easier and less costly than the intensive care necessary for the healing and eventual closure of pressure sores. Of primary importance, then, is the ability to identify patients who are at high risk so that preventive measures may be instituted. Relief of pressure through proper positioning, and periodic repositioning, is probably the single most important factor in preventing pressure sore formation. Relief for a period of only 5 minutes once every 2 hours is believed to give protection against pressure sore formation.[75,78–81] Repositioning seated patients every 15 to 60 minutes is also recommended.[28,81] Pressure relief devices such as mattresses or overlays filled with air, water, gel, or foam are helpful in preventing pressure sores.[84] Cushions and ankle or heel protectors should also be encouraged.[75,76,78] Skin care and prevention of soilage are also important, with the intent being to keep the surface relatively free of moisture. Patients with problems of incontinence should be cleaned frequently, and efforts should be made to keep the involved areas dry.[75]

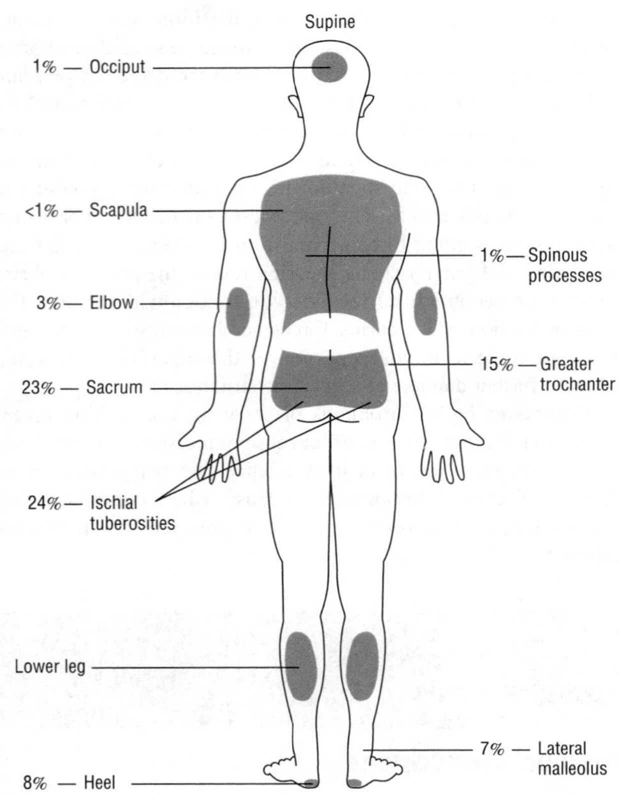

FIGURE 88-4 Supine view of areas where pressure sore formation tends to occur.

The medical approach to the treatment of pressure sores depends on the stage of the disease. Medical management generally is indicated for lesions that are of moderate size and relatively shallow depth (stage 1 or 2 lesions) and are not located over a bony prominence. Depending on their location and severity, from 30% to 80% of these ulcers will heal without an operation. Surgical intervention is almost always necessary for ulcers that extend through superficial layers or into bone (stage 3, stage 4, and unstageable lesions).[77]

The goal of therapy is to clean and decontaminate the ulcer in order to permit formation of healthy granulation tissue that promotes wound healing or prepares the wound for an operative procedure. The main factors to be considered for successful topical therapy (local care) are (a) relief of pressure, (b) debridement of necrotic tissue as needed, (c) wound cleansing, (d) dressing selection, and (e) prevention, diagnosis, and treatment of infection.[28,75,76,78,81,82]

Relief of pressure is important once a pressure sore has developed. The same repositioning methods and pressure-reducing devices used for preventive care also apply to treatment.[28,76]

The goals of debridement and cleansing measures are removal of devitalized tissue and reduction of bacterial contamination, which can slow granulation time and impede healing.[28,75,76] Debridement can be accomplished by surgical, mechanical, or chemical means.[28,75,76] Surgical debridement rapidly removes necrotic material from the wound and is recommended for urgent situations (e.g., cellulitis and sepsis).[78–80] Mechanical debridement generally involves wet-to-dry dressing changes. Saline-soaked gauze is applied to the wound; after drying, the gauze is removed and with it any adherent necrotic tissue. Other effective mechanical therapies include hydrotherapy (use of the whirlpool [Hubbard tank] to remove necrotic tissue and debris), wound irrigation, and dextranomers (beads placed in the wound to absorb exudate and bacteria).[28,76] Chemical debridement includes enzymatic and autolytic agents. Enzymatic debridement involves application of topical debriding agents to remove devitalized tissue. This method is recommended for patients who cannot tolerate surgery or are in a long-term care or home setting.[28,76] Autolytic debridement involves the use of synthetic dressings that allow devitalized tissue to self-digest via enzymes present in wound fluids. Autolytic debridement is contraindicated in the treatment of infected pressure sores.[28]

Pressure sore wounds should be cleaned with normal saline.[76] No cleansing solution or technique has demonstrated greater efficacy on healing.[84] Cleansing agents that are cytotoxic, such as povidone–iodine, iodophor, sodium hypochlorite solution, hydrogen peroxide, and acetic acid, should be avoided.[75,76,79,80] Many of these agents destroy granulation tissue and impair healing. Many different types of dressings are available for pressure sores.[28] Wound dressing materials should keep the wound moist, allow free exchange of air, act as a physical barrier to bacteria, and prevent physical damage.[28,76] Controlled studies of the various types of wound dressings have shown no significant differences in healing outcomes.[70] Occlusive dressings (hydrocolloid, such as DuoDERM™ or Tegaderm™) and transparent dressings (e.g., 3M Tegaderm™) are not recommended for infected wounds.[28,76] If occlusive dressings are used, any infection should be controlled or the dressing frequency increased.

A 2-week trial of topical antibiotics (silver sulfadiazine or triple antibiotic) may be considered for a clean ulcer that is not healing or is producing a moderate amount of exudate despite appropriate care.[79] Systemic treatment of pressure ulcers is generally for infections associated with bacteremia, sepsis, cellulitis, or osteomyelitis.[79,80] Empiric therapy for infected pressure sores or associated infectious complications should cover MRSA, anaerobes, enterococci, and more resistant gram-negative bacteria such as *Pseudomonas* (see Table 88-5).[76] Thereafter, antibiotics should be guided by results from appropriately collected cultures.

Other nonpharmacologic approaches to shortening the healing time have included the use of hyperbaric oxygenation, hydrotherapy, high-frequency/high-intensity sound waves, and electrotherapy.[79,80,84] Electrical stimulation is the only adjunctive therapy that is proven effective.[79,80] Various comorbid conditions (diabetes mellitus, smoking, peripheral vascular disease, malnutrition) may impair wound healing. Eliminating or optimizing these factors is recommended, although studies have not demonstrated benefit.[28,75,76,81–83]

Evaluation of Therapeutic Outcomes

With appropriate wound care and antimicrobial therapy, infected pressure sores can heal. A reduction in erythema, warmth, pain, and other signs and symptoms should be seen in 48 to 72 hours.

ANIMAL AND HUMAN BITE WOUNDS

Approximately half the population in the United States will be bitten by either an animal or another human sometime during their lifetimes.[85,86] Animal bites (typically from dogs or cats) are common causes of injury, particularly to children, and are associated with significant risk of infection without prompt attention to appropriate management. Likewise, human bite wounds are often deceptively severe and frequently require aggressive management to reduce the risk of infectious complications. If left untreated, soft-tissue infection and osteomyelitis may occur, possibly requiring extensive debridement or amputation.

Epidemiology

Dog bites account for approximately 60% of all animal bite wounds requiring medical attention.[85] The Centers for Disease Control and Prevention reports that 386,000 individuals seek emergency room attention for dog bites annually.[86] The rate of dog bite–related injuries is highest in children aged 5 to 9 years. Most dog bites are to the extremities,[85] but the majority of bites to children less than 5 years of age are to the face and neck.[86] Cat bites are the second most common cause of bite wounds in the United States, accounting for up to 20% of all animal bites.[85] Cat bites occur most commonly on the upper extremities and face, with most injuries reported in women and the elderly.[85,87] Human bites are the third most frequent type of bites requiring medical attention.

Infection rates after dog and cat bites are estimated at 20% overall. However, infection may occur in up to 30% to 80% of serious cat bites, a rate more than double those seen with dog bites.[87] Also, bite wounds to the hands become infected in 30% to 40% of cases.[85] Patients at greatest risk of acquiring animal bite–related infection have had a puncture wound (usually to the hand), have not sought medical attention within 8 hours of the injury, and are older than 50 years of age.[85,87]

Infected human bites can occur as bites from the teeth or from blows to the mouth (clenched-fist injuries). Bites by others can occur to any part of the body, but most often involve the hands. Infectious complications occur in 10% to 50% of patients with human bites.[87]

Etiology

Infections in bite wounds are caused predominantly by mouth flora from the animal or human biter, and from the victim's own skin flora (Table 88-12).[85,87–91] Most infections are polymicrobial, with a median of three to nine bacterial isolates per culture.[85,87–91] *Pasteurella* is the most frequent isolate from both dog and cat bites. *Pasteurella multocida* is part of the normal oral flora of up to 90% of cats; dog bites more commonly involve *P. canis* (approximately 26% of infections).[87,89] Tularemia (*Pasteurella tularensis*) and cat scratch disease (*Bartonella henselae*) have also have been transmitted by cat bites, while rabies is associated with dog bites, particularly in developing countries.[89,90,97] Human bite wounds are notable for potential involvement of *Eikenella corrodens* in approximately 30% of infections.

Pathophysiology

The potential for infection from an animal bite is great owing to the pressure that can be exerted during the bite and the vast number of potential pathogens that make up the normal oral flora.[85,87–90] Cats' teeth are slender and extremely sharp. Their teeth easily penetrate into bones and joints, resulting in a higher incidence of septic arthritis and osteomyelitis.[85,87–90] Although a dog's teeth may not be as sharp, they can exert a pressure of 200 to 450 lb/in^2 (~1,400 to 3,100 kPa) and therefore result in a serious crush injury with much devitalized tissue.[85,87–90] In addition, the polymicrobic (aerobic and anaerobic) nature of animal bites provides a synergistic relationship, thus making an infection harder to eradicate.[88]

Human bites generally are more serious and more prone to infection than animal bites, particularly clenched-fist injuries.[88] While the force of a punch may sever a tendon or nerve or break a bone, it most often causes a breach in the capsule of the metacarpophalangeal joint, leading to direct inoculation of bacteria into

TABLE 88-12 Bacterial Isolates from Infections in Animal and Human Bite Wounds[85,87–90]

Organisms	Percentage of Isolates	
	Dog and Cat	Human
Aerobes	74–90	44
Pasteurella spp.	50–75	—
Streptococcus spp.	46–50	52–84
S. anginosus		52
S. mitis	22	12
S. pyogenes	12	14
S. mutans	12	2
Staphylococcus spp.	35–46	54
S. aureus	20	30
S. epidermidis	18	22
Neisseria spp.	32–35	4
Moraxella spp.	10–35	2
Corynebacterium spp.	12–28	12
Enterococcus spp.	10–12	6
Bacillus spp.	8–11	—
Eikenella corrodens	2	30
Enterobacteriaceae	6–12	8–15
Anaerobes	50–70	40–90
Fusobacterium spp.	32–33	32–34
Porphyromonas spp.	28–30	2
Bacteroides spp.	18–28	4
Prevotella spp.	19–28	22–36
Propionibacterium spp.	18–20	4
Peptostreptococcus spp.	8–16	22
Veillonella spp.	2	24
Mixed aerobic and anaerobic	50–75	40–66

the joint or bone.[88,90] When the hand is relaxed, the tendons carry bacteria into deeper spaces of the hand, resulting in more extensive infection.[88,90]

TREATMENT

Desired Outcomes

The goals of therapy of bite wounds, whether caused by animals or humans, are twofold: to provide effective prophylaxis against infection, when appropriate, and to achieve rapid eradication of established infection and prevent further complications. Effective treatment of bite wounds includes avoidance of unnecessary antimicrobials that contribute to increased resistance, and minimizing toxicities and cost of therapy.

Management of Bite Wounds

9 Bite wounds should be irrigated thoroughly with a copious volume of sterile water or saline, and the wound washed vigorously with soap or povidone–iodine in order to reduce the bacterial count in the wound.[87,90] Surgical debridement and immobilization of the affected area is often required in dog and human bites associated with more extensive tissue injury. Clinical failures due to edema have occurred despite appropriate antibiotic therapy.[85] Therefore, it is important to stress to patients that the affected area should be elevated for several days or until edema has resolved. In the case of animal bites, an immunization history of the animal should be obtained. It is also important for the patient's tetanus immune status to be determined. Because transmission of viruses (HIV, herpes, hepatitis B and C) is a possibility with human bites, information about the biter is important. Although the possibility of acquiring HIV through saliva alone is believed to be unlikely, the presence

CLINICAL PRESENTATION

General

Animal bites:

- Only general wound care is required for most patients with dog bites who present early (<12 hours) after injury; infection is more likely in patients presenting late (≥12 hours) after injury.

Human bites:

- Most patients with clenched-fist injuries present for medical care after infection is already established.

Symptoms

- Patients often seek medical care for infection-related complaints (i.e., pain, purulent discharge, and swelling) at the site of the injury.
- Wounds often have a purulent discharge, and decreased range of motion may be present.

Signs

- Erythema, swelling, and clear or purulent discharge at site of infected wound.

Animal bites:

- If *P. multocida* is present, a rapidly progressing cellulitis is observed within 24 to 48 hours of initial injury.
- Fever is uncommon.
- Adenopathy or lymphangitis is uncommon.

Human bites:

- Lymphadenopathy is common.
- In clenched-fist injuries, edema may limit the ability of tendons to glide in their sheaths, thereby limiting a joint's range of motion.

Laboratory Tests

- Samples for bacterial cultures (aerobic and anaerobic) should be obtained from infected wounds.
- Wounds seen less than 8 hours or more than 24 hours after injury that show no signs of infection may not need to be cultured.
- White blood counts should be monitored for resolution of infection if initially elevated.

Other Diagnostic Tests

- Radiographic evaluation should be performed if damage to a bone or joint is suspected.

of virus-containing blood in the saliva makes disease transmission possible.[92,93] Bite victims exposed to blood-tainted saliva may be offered antiretroviral chemoprophylaxis, but each case should be individually assessed based on the potential for significant exposure and potential risks and benefits of antiretroviral therapy.[92,93]

Patients with clenched-fist injuries should be seen by a specialist in hand care to evaluate for penetration into the synovium, joint capsule, and bone.[16,88] Primary closure for human bites generally is not recommended. Tetanus toxoid and antitoxin may be indicated.

⑩ All patients with human bite injuries should receive prophylactic antibiotic therapy for 3 to 5 days due to high infection risk (Table 88-4).[90,91,93] Prophylactic antimicrobial agents should be given as soon as possible to all patients, regardless of the appearance of the wound, unless it can be documented that the wound does not involve hands, feet, or joints and penetrates no deeper than the epidermis.[16,79,90]

The role of prophylactic antimicrobial therapy for early, noninfected animal bite wounds remains controversial.[85,87,88,90] However, prophylactic antibiotics are generally advised unless the wound is very superficial and easily cleaned,[85,87,88] or unless the patient presents 72 hours or more after injury and has no clinical signs of infection.[88] Prophylaxis is more strongly recommended in patients with moderate to severe wounds, or if the wound is considered at high risk for infection. Factors associated with increased risk include the following: age greater than 50 years, immunocompromised patients, chronic comorbidities (e.g., diabetes), cat bites, deep puncture wounds beyond the epidermal layer, and wounds to the face, hands, feet, genitalia, or over joint surfaces.[87,88,90] A 3- to 5-day course of prophylactic antibiotics is recommended.[16,87,88,90]

Clinical **Controversy. . .**

The question whether to provide antibiotic prophylaxis for animal bites, particularly those caused by dogs, remains controversial. Controlled studies have not definitively shown reduction in infection rates through use of prophylactic antibiotics for uninfected bites; however, such studies are few and recommendations are largely based on uncontrolled data. Recommendations in favor of antibiotic prophylaxis are based on the relatively high infection rates and the potential for severe complications such as osteomyelitis and septic arthritis. If used, prophylaxis should be kept to a short duration (i.e., 3 to 5 days) to minimize concerns related to cost, adverse effects, and antibiotic resistance.

Empiric antibiotics for treatment of established infection of bite wounds should be directed at a variety of aerobic and anaerobic flora (Table 88-4). Amoxicillin–clavulanic acid is most commonly recommended for oral outpatient therapy due to excellent activity against all likely pathogens, including *Pasteurella* and *Eikenella*.[16,85,87,88,90] Alternative oral agents include moxifloxacin or doxycycline alone, or trimethoprim–sulfamethoxazole, levofloxacin, ciprofloxacin, or a second- or third-generation cephalosporin in combination with metronidazole or clindamycin to provide activity against oropharyngeal anaerobes. Although the combination of penicillin VK plus dicloxacillin has been recommended traditionally for treatment of bite wounds, its use has become less common in favor of other alternatives. Failure to provide adequate initial treatment of bite wounds results in treatment failures and increased need for hospitalization for parenteral antibiotics.[16,85,87–90]

Hospitalization for minor wounds is unnecessary if surgical repair of vital structures has not been performed. Patients with clenched-fist or other serious bite injuries and severe resultant infection may be considered for IV antibiotics. Treatment options for patients requiring IV therapy include β-lactam–β-lactamase inhibitor combinations (ampicillin–sulbactam, piperacillin–tazobactam), second-generation cephalosporins with antianaerobic activity (e.g., cefoxitin), and ertapenem.[16,90] The combination of doxycycline or a fluoroquinolone with metronidazole or clindamycin may be used in patients with severe β-lactam allergies. The length of antimicrobial therapy depends on the severity of the injury/infection. However, therapy should generally be continued from 7 to 14 days.[16,85,88–90]

Tetanus does not occur commonly after dog bites; however, it is possible. If the immunization history of a patient with anything other than a clean, minor wound is unknown, tetanus–diphtheria (TD) toxoids should be administered.[94,95] Both TD toxoids and tetanus immune globulin should be administered to patients who have never been immunized.[90,96]

Because the rabies virus can be transmitted via saliva, rabies may be a potential complication of a bite. When the symptoms of rabies develop after a bite, the prognosis for survival is poor. Roughly 3% of rabies cases documented in animals were in dogs (the most frequent vectors are skunks, raccoons, and bats).[97,98] In the United States, recommendations for postexposure prophylaxis after a dog bite depend on the health of the dog. If the animal is healthy and able to be observed for a 10-day period, active prophylaxis is only required if the dog develops signs of rabies.[85,87,97] If the dog is known or suspected to be rabid, postexposure procedures should be initiated; current treatment guidelines should be consulted for appropriate management recommendations.[97,98] Outside of the United States, locally applicable guidelines such as those from the World Health Organization should be consulted.[99]

Evaluation of Therapeutic Outcomes

Evaluation of treatment for either animal or human bites should follow the same general guidelines. Bite victims treated on an outpatient basis with oral antimicrobials should be followed up within 24 hours by either phone or office visit.[16] Hospitalization or change to IV therapy should be considered if the infection has progressed. For hospitalized patients with no improvement in signs and symptoms following 24 hours of appropriate therapy, surgical debridement may be needed. Physical therapy may be needed to improve complications such as residual joint stiffness and loss of function, particularly after human bites involving clenched-fist injuries.

PERSONALIZED PHARMACOTHERAPY

Desired treatment outcomes for the various types of SSTIs described in this chapter are achieved through close monitoring and frequent patient assessment, including judicious evaluation of antimicrobial therapies. SSTIs are challenging in that cultures are often not performed due to the unavailability of easily obtained culturable specimens and the low yield of common culturing techniques. Empiric antibiotic selection based on most likely pathogens is an effective strategy in less severe infections such as erysipelas, impetigo, and furuncles. However, treatment of more severe infections such as cellulitis, DFI, and necrotizing fasciitis should be individualized based on properly obtained culture specimens and documented pathogens and susceptibilities whenever possible. Aggressive antimicrobial use must be balanced against unnecessary administration of drugs that may lead to increased antimicrobial resistance, adverse effects, and cost. Proper evaluation of an individual patient's severity of infection and risk of complications allows for selection of appropriate antimicrobials for treatment of infection and selection of appropriate treatment settings (e.g., inpatient vs. outpatient), both of which may allow for the most cost-effective therapy.

ABBREVIATIONS

AHRQ	Agency for Healthcare Research and Quality
CA-MRSA	community-associated methicillin-resistant *S. aureus*
DFI	diabetic foot infection
HA-MRSA	healthcare-associated methicillin-resistant *Staphylococcus aureus*
HIV	human immunodeficiency virus
MRSA	methicillin-resistant *Staphylococcus aureus*
MSSA	methicillin-susceptible *Staphylococcus aureus*
PVL	Panton-Valentine leukocidin
SCC*mec*	staphylococcal chromosomal cassette *mec*
SSTI	skin and soft-tissue infection
TD	tetanus–diphtheria

REFERENCES

1. Cogen AL, Nizet V, Gallo RL. Skin microbiota: A source of disease or defence? Br J Dermatol 2008;158:442–455.
2. Gould D. Skin flora: Implications for nursing. Nurs Stand 2012;26:48–56.
3. Granato PA. Pathogenic and indigenous microorganisms of humans. In: Murray PR, Baron EJ, Jorgensen JH, et al., eds. Manual of Clinical Microbiology, 9th ed. Washington, DC: ASM Press, 2007:46–56.
4. Rajan S. Skin and soft-tissue infections: Classifying and treating a spectrum. Cleveland Clin J Med 2012;79:57–66.
5. Gunderson CG. Cellulitis: Definition, etiology, and clinical features. Am J Med 2011;124:1113–1122.
6. Breen JO. Skin and soft tissue infections in immunocompetent patients. Am Fam Physician 2010;81:893–899.
7. Napolitano LM. Severe soft tissue infections. Infect Dis Clin North Am 2009;23:571–591.
8. Pallin DJ, Espinola JA, Leung DY, et al. Epidemiology of dermatitis and skin infections in United States physicians offices, 1993-2005. Clin Infect Dis 2009;49:901–907.
9. Levit K, Wier L, Stranges E, Ryan K, Elixhauser A. HCUP Facts and Figures: Statistics on Hospital-Based Care in the United States, 2007. Rockville, MD: Agency for Healthcare Research and Quality, 2009, *http://www.hcup-us.ahrq.gov/reports.jsp*.
10. Dawson AL, Dellavalle RP, Elston DM. Infectious skin diseases: A review and needs assessment. Dermatol Clin 2012;30:141–151.
11. Qualls ML, Mooney MM, Camargo CA Jr, Zucconi T, Hooper DC, Pallin DJ. Emergency department visit rates for abscess versus other skin infections during the emergence of community-associated methicillin-resistant *Staphylococcus aureus*, 1997-2007. Clin Infect Dis 2012;55:103–105.
12. Christensen KLY, Holman RC, Steiner CA, Sejvar JJ, Stoll BJ, Schonberger LB. Infectious disease hospitalizations in the United States. Clin Infect Dis 2009;49:1025–1035.
13. Stevens DL. Treatments for skin and soft-tissue and surgical site infections due to MDR gram-positive bacteria. J Infect 2009;59:532–539.
14. Stryjewski ME, Chambers HF. Skin and soft tissue infections caused by community-acquired methicillin-resistant *Staphylococcus aureus*. Clin Infect Dis 2008;46(Suppl 5): S368–S377.
15. Tenover FC, Goering RV. Methicillin-resistant *Staphylococcus aureus* strain USA300: Origin and epidemiology. J Antimicrob Chemother 2009;64:441–446.
16. Stevens DL, Bisno AL, Chambers HF, et al. Practice guidelines for the diagnosis and management of skin and soft-tissue infections. Clin Infect Dis 2005;41:1373–1406.
17. Daum RS. Skin and soft tissue infections caused by methicillin-resistant *Staphylococcus aureus*. N Engl J Med 2007;357:380–390.
18. Moran GJ, Krishnadasan A, Gorwitz RJ, et al. Methicillin-resistant *S. aureus* infections among patients in the emergency department. N Eng J Med 2006;355:666–674.
19. King MD, Humphrey BJ, Wang YF, et al. Emergence of community-acquired methicillin-resistant *Staphylococcus aureus* USA 300 clone as the predominant cause of skin and soft-tissue infections. Ann Intern Med 2006;144: 309–317.
20. Como-Sabetti K, Harriman KH, Buch JM, Giennen A, Boxrud DJ, Lynfield R. Community-associated methicillin-resistant *Staphylococcus aureus*: Trends in case and isolate characteristics from six years of prospective surveillance. Public Health Rep 2009;124:427–435.
21. Centers for Disease Control and Prevention. Active Bacterial Core Surveillance Report, Emerging Infections Program Network, Methicillin-Resistant *Staphylococcus aureus*. 2010, *http://www.cdc.gov/abcs/reports-findings/survreports/mrsa10.html*.
22. Jeng A, Beheshti M, Li J, Nathan R. The role of beta-hemolytic streptococci in causing diffuse, nonculturable cellulitis. Medicine (Baltimore) 2010;89:217–226.
23. Raney PM, Tenover FC, Carey R, McGowan JE Jr, Patel JB. Investigation of inducible clindamycin and telithromycin resistance in isolates of beta-hemolytic streptococci. Diagn Microbiol Infect Dis 2006;55:213–218.
24. Bernard P. Management of common bacterial infections of the skin. Curr Opin Infect Dis 2008;21:122–128.
25. Yu Y, Cheng AS, Wang L, et al. Hot tub folliculitis or hand–foot syndrome caused by *Pseudomonas aeruginosa*. J Am Acad Dermatol 2007;57:596–600.
26. Moet GJ, Jones RN, Biedenbach DJ, Stilwell MG, Fritsche TR. Contemporary causes of skin and soft tissue infections in North America, Latin America, and Europe: Report from the SENTRY Antimicrobial Surveillance Program (1998–2004). Diagn Microbiol Infect Dis 2007; 57:7–13.
27. Reichel M, Heisig P, Kampf G. Identification of variables for aerobic bacterial density at clinically relevant skin sites. J Hosp Infect 2011;78:5–10.
28. Garcia AD, Thomas DR. Assessment and management of chronic pressure ulcers in the elderly. Med Clin North Am 2006;90:925–944.
29. Brook I. Microbiology and management of soft tissue and muscle infections. Int J Surg 2008;6:328–338.
30. Lipsky BA, Berendt AR, Cornia PB, et al. 2012 Infectious Diseases Society of America clinical practice guidelines for the diagnosis and treatment of diabetic foot infections. Clin Infect Dis 2012;54:132–173.
31. Pasternak MS, Swartz MN. Cellulitis, necrotizing fasciitis, and subcutaneous tissue infections. In: Mandell GL, Bennett JE, Dolin R, eds. Mandell, Douglas and Bennett's Principles and Practice of Infectious Diseases, 7th ed. New York: Churchill-Livingstone, 2010:1289–1312.
32. Liu C, Bayer A, Cosgrive SE, et al. Clinical practice guidelines by the Infectious Diseases Society of America for the treatment of methicillin-resistant *Staphylococcus aureus* infections in adults and children. Clin Infect Dis 2011;52:1–38.
33. Rybak MJ, Lomaestro BM, Rotschafer JC, et al. Vancomycin therapeutic guidelines: A summary of consensus recommendations from the Infectious Diseases Society of America, the American Society of Health-System Pharmacists, and the Society of Infectious Diseases Pharmacists. Am J Health Syst Pharm 2009;66:82–98.

34. Krasagakis K, Valachis A, Maniatakis P, Kruger-Krasagakis S, Samonis G, Tosca AD. Analysis of epidemiology, clinical features and management of erysipelas. Int J Dermatol 2010; 49:1012–1017.
35. Kilburn SA, Featherstone P, Higgins B, Brindle R. Interventions for cellulitis and erysipelas. Cochrane Database Syst Rev 2010;(6):CD004299.
36. Cole C, Gazewood J. Diagnosis and treatment of impetigo. Am Fam Physician 2007;75:859–864.
37. Bangert S, Levy M, Hebert AA. Bacterial resistance and impetigo treatment trends: A review. Pediatr Dermatol 2012; 29:243–248.
38. Koning S, Van der Sande R, Verhagen AP, et al. Interventions for impetigo. Cochrane Database Syst Rev 2012;1:CD003261.
39. Pasternak MS, Swartz MN. Lymphadenitis and lymphangitis. In: Mandell GL, Bennett JE, Dolin R, eds. Mandell, Douglas and Bennett's Principles and Practice of Infectious Diseases, 7th ed. New York: Churchill-Livingstone, 2010:1323–1334.
40. Pallin DJ, Egan DJ, Pelletier AJ, et al. Increased US emergency department visits for skin and soft tissue infections, and changes in antibiotic choices, during the emergence of community-associated methicillin-resistant *Staphylococcus aureus*. Ann Emerg Med 2008;51: 291–298.
41. Odell CA. Community-associated methicillin-resistant *Staphylococcus aureus* (CA-MRSA) skin infections. Curr Opin Pediatr 2010;22:273–277.
42. Stevens DL, Eron LL. Cellulitis and soft tissue infections. Ann Intern Med 2009;150:ITC1–ITC11.
43. Bailey E, Kroshinsky D. Cellulitis: Diagnosis and management. Dermatol Ther 2011;24:229–239.
44. Gorwitz RJ, Jernigan DB, Powers JH, et al. Strategies for Clinical Management of MRSA in the Community: Summary of an Experts' Meeting Convened by the Centers for Disease Control and Prevention. 2006, *http://www.cdc.gov/ncidod/dhqp/ar_mrsa_ca.html*.
45. Herman RA, Kee VR, Moores KG, et al. Etiology and treatment of community-acquired methicillin-resistant *Staphylococcus aureus*. Am J Health Syst Pharm 2008;65: 219–225.
46. Moellering RC Jr. Current treatment options for community-acquired methicillin-resistant *Staphylococcus aureus* infection. Clin Infect Dis 2008;46:1032–1037.
47. Nathwani D, Morgan M, Masterton RG, et al. Guidelines for UK practice for the diagnosis and management of methicillin-resistant *Staphylococcus aureus* (MRSA) infections presenting in the community. J Antimicrob Chemother 2008;61:976–994.
48. McKinnon PS, Sorensen SV, Liu LZ, Itani KM. Impact of linezolid on economic outcomes and determinants of cost in a clinical trial evaluating patients with MRSA complicated skin and soft-tissue infections. Ann Pharmacother 2006;40: 1017–1023.
49. Ruhe JJ, Menon A. Tetracyclines as an oral treatment option for patients with community onset skin and soft tissue infections caused by methicillin-resistant *Staphylococcus aureus*. Antimicrob Agents Chemother 2007;51:3298–3303.
50. Cenizal MJ, Skiest D, Luber S, et al. Prospective randomized trial of empiric therapy with trimethoprim–sulfamethoxazole or doxycycline for outpatient skin and soft tissue infections in an area of high prevalence of methicillin-resistant *Staphylococcus aureus*. Antimicrob Agents Chemother 2007;51:2628–2630.
51. Cadena J, Nair S, Henao-Martinez AF, et al. Dose of trimethoprim–sulfamethoxazole to treat skin and skin structure infections caused by methicillin-resistant *Staphylococcus aureus*. Antimicrob Agents Chemother 2011;55:5430–5432.
52. Jeng A, Beheshti M, Li J, et al. The role of beta-hemolytic streptococci in causing diffuse, nonculturable cellulitis: A prospective investigation. Medicine (Baltimore) 2010;89:217–226.
53. Micek ST. Alternatives to vancomycin for the treatment of methicillin-resistant *Staphylococcus aureus* infections. Clin Infect Dis 2007;45(Suppl 3):S184–S190.
54. Cainzos M, Gonzales-Rodriguez FJ. Necrotizing soft tissue infections. Curr Opin Infect Dis 2007;13:433–439.
55. Ustin JS, Malangoni MA. Necrotizing soft-tissue infections. Crit Care Med 2011;39:2156–2162.
56. Morgan MS. Diagnosis and management of necrotizing fasciitis: A multiparametric approach. J Hosp Infect 2010; 75:249–257.
57. Bellapianta JM, Ljungquist K, Tobin E, et al. Necrotizing fasciitis. J Am Acad Orthop Surg 2009;17:174–182.
58. Boyer A, Vargas F, Coste F, et al. Influence of surgical treatment timing on mortality from necrotizing soft tissue infections requiring intensive care management. Intensive Care Med 2009;35:847–853.
59. Lavery LA, Armstrong DG, Wunderlich RP, et al. Risk factors for foot infections in persons with diabetes mellitus. Diabetes Care 2006;29:1288–1293.
60. Rao N, Lipsky BA. Optimising antimicrobial therapy in diabetic foot infections. Drugs 2007;67:195–214.
61. Tecilazich F, Dinh T, Veves A. Treating diabetic ulcers. Expert Opin Pharmacother 2011;12:593–606.
62. Bader MS. Diabetic foot infection. Am Fam Physician 2008; 78:71–79.
63. Lipsky BA, Tabak YP, Johannes RS, et al. Skin and soft tissue infections in hospitalized patients with diabetes: Culture isolates and risk factors associated with mortality, length of stay and cost. Diabetologia 2010;53:914–923.
64. Lipsky BA, Peters EJG, Senneville E, et al. Expert opinion on the management of infections in the diabetic foot. Diabetes Metab Res Rev 2012;28(Suppl 1):163–178.
65. Nelson EA, O'Meara S, Craig D, et al. Systematic review of antimicrobial treatments for diabetic foot ulcers. Diabet Med 2006;23:348–359.
66. Crouzet J, Lavigne JP, Richard JL, et al. Diabetic foot infection: A critical review of recent randomized clinical trials on antibiotic therapy. Int J Infect Dis 2011;15: e601–e610.
67. Ertugrul MB, Baktiroglu S, Salman S, et al. Pathogens isolated from deep soft tissue and bone in patients with diabetic foot infections. J Am Podiatr Med Assoc 2008; 98:290–295.
68. Eleftheriadou I, Tentolouris N, Argiana V, et al. Methicillin-resistant *Staphylococcus aureus* in diabetic foot infections. Drugs 2010;70:1785–1797.
69. Tentolouris N, Petrikkos G, Vallianou N, et al. Prevalence of methicillin-resistant *Staphylococcus aureus* in infected and uninfected diabetic foot ulcers. Clin Microbiol Infect 2006;12:186–189.
70. Kessler L, Piemont Y, Ortega F, et al. Comparison of microbiological results of needle puncture vs. superficial swab in infected diabetic foot ulcer with osteomyelitis. Diabet Med 2006;23:99–102.
71. Lipsky BA, Armstrong DG, Citron DM, et al. Ertapenem versus piperacillin/tazobactam for diabetic foot infections (SIDESTEP): Prospective, randomized, controlled, double-blinded, multicentre trial. Lancet 2005;366:1695–1703.
72. Lipsky BA, Hoey C. Topical antimicrobial therapy for treating chronic wounds. Clin Infect Dis 2009;49:1541–1549.

73. Kwakman PHS, Van den Akker JPC, Guciu A, et al. Medical-grade honey kills antibiotic-resistant bacteria in vitro and eradicates skin colonization. Clin Infect Dis 2008;46: 1677–1682.
74. Reddy M, Gill SS, Kalkar SR, et al. Treatment of pressure ulcers. A systematic review. JAMA 2008;300:2647–2662.
75. Jaul E. Assessment and management of pressure ulcers in the elderly. Drugs Aging 2010;27:311–325.
76. Bluestein D, Javaheri A. Pressure ulcers: Prevention, evaluation, and management. Am Fam Physician 2008;78: 1186–1196.
77. Black J, Baharestani M, Cuddigan J, et al. National Pressure Ulcer Advisory Panel's updated pressure ulcer staging system. Dermatol Nurs 2007;19:343–349.
78. Keast DH, Parslow N, Houghton PE, et al. Best practice recommendations for the prevention and treatment of pressure ulcers: Update 2006. Adv Skin Wound Care 2007;20:447–460.
79. Levi B, Rees R. Diagnosis and management of pressure ulcers. Clin Plast Surg 2007;34:735–748.
80. Ho CH, Bogie K. The prevention and treatment of pressure ulcers. Phys Med Rehab Clin North Am 2007;18:235–253.
81. Tchanque-Fossuo CN, Kuzon WM Jr. An evidence-based approach to pressure sores. Plast Reconstr Surg 2011;127: 932–939.
82. Markova A, Mostow EN. US skin disease assessment: Ulcer and wound care. Dermatol Clin 2012;30:107–111.
83. Dealey C. Skin care and pressure ulcers. Adv Skin Wound Care 2009;22:421–428.
84. Brolmann FE, Ubbink DT, Nelson EA, Munte K, van der Horst CM, Vermeulen H. Evidence-based decisions for local and systemic wound care. Br J Surg 2012;99:1172–1183.
85. Oehler RL, Velez AP, Mizrachi M, et al. Bite-related and septic syndromes caused by cats and dogs. Lancet Infect Dis 2009;9:439–447.
86. Centers for Disease Control and Prevention. Dog Bite: Fact Sheet. 2008, *http://www.cdc.gov/HomeandRecreationalSafety/Dog-Bites/dogbite-factsheet.html.*
87. Thomas N, Brook I. Animal bite-associated infections: Microbiology and treatment. Expert Rev Anti Infect Ther 2011;9:215–226.
88. Brook I. Management of human and animal bite wound infection: An overview. Curr Infect Dis Rep 2009;11:389–395.
89. Abrahamian FM, Goldstein EJC. Microbiology of animal bite wound infection. Clin Microbiol Rev 2011;24:231–246.
90. Goldstein EJC. Bites. In: Mandell GL, Bennett JE, Dolin R, eds. Mandell, Douglas and Bennett's Principles and Practice of Infectious Diseases, 7th ed. New York: Churchill-Livingstone, 2010:3911–3915.
91. Talan DA, Abrahamian FM, Moran PM, et al. Clinical presentation and bacteriologic analysis of infected human bites in patients presenting to emergency departments. Clin Infect Dis 2003;37:1481–1489.
92. Smith DK, Grohskopf LA, Black RJ, et al. Antiretroviral postexposure prophylaxis after sexual, injection-drug use, or other nonoccupational exposure to HIV in the United States. Recommendations from the U.S. Department of Health and Human Services. MMWR Recomm Rep 2005;54(RR-2):1–20.
93. Harrison M. A 4-year review of human bite injuries presenting to emergency medicine and proposed evidence-based guidelines. Injury 2009;40:826–830.
94. Kretsinger K, Broder KR, Cortese MM, et al. Preventing tetanus, diphtheria, and pertussis among adults: Use of tetanus toxoid, reduced diphtheria toxoid and acellular pertussis vaccine. Recommendations of the Advisory Committee on Immunization Practices (ACIP). MMWR Recomm Rep 2006;55(RR-17):1–33.
95. Broder KR, Cortese MM, Iskander JJ, et al. Preventing tetanus, diphtheria, and pertussis among adolescents: Use of tetanus toxoid, reduced diphtheria toxoid and acellular pertussis vaccine. Recommendations of the Advisory Committee on Immunization Practices (ACIP). MMWR Recomm Rep 2006;55(RR-3):1–34.
96. Orenstein WA, Pickering LK, Mawle A, et al. Immunization. In: Mandell GL, Bennett JE, Dolin R, eds. Mandell, Douglas and Bennett's Principles and Practice of Infectious Diseases, 7th ed. New York: Churchill-Livingstone, 2010:3917–3949.
97. Manning SE, Rupprecht CE, Fishbein D, et al. Human rabies prevention—United States, 2008. Recommendations of the Advisory Committee on Immunization Practices (ACIP). MMWR Recomm Rep 2008;57(RR-3):1–28.
98. Nigg AJ, Walker PL. Overview, prevention, and treatment of rabies. Pharmacotherapy 2009;29:1182–1195.
99. World Health Organization. *http://www.who.int/entity/rabies/PEP_prophylaxis_guidelines_June10.pdf.*

89

Infective Endocarditis

Angie Veverka, Michael A. Crouch, and Brian L. Odle

KEY CONCEPTS

1. Infective endocarditis is an uncommon infection usually occurring in persons with preexisting cardiac valvular abnormalities (e.g., prosthetic heart valves) or with other specific risk factors (e.g., IV drug abuse).
2. Three groups of organisms cause a majority of infective endocarditis cases: streptococci, staphylococci, and enterococci.
3. The clinical presentation of infective endocarditis is highly variable and nonspecific, although a fever and murmur are usually present. Classic peripheral manifestations (e.g., Osler's nodes) may or may not occur.
4. The diagnosis of infective endocarditis requires the integration of clinical, laboratory, and echocardiographic findings. The two major diagnostic criteria are bacteremia and echocardiographic changes (e.g., valvular vegetation).
5. Treatment of infective endocarditis involves isolation of the infecting pathogen and determination of antimicrobial susceptibilities, followed by high-dose, parenteral, bactericidal antibiotics for an extended period.
6. Surgical replacement of the infected heart valve is an important adjunct to endocarditis treatment in certain situations (e.g., patients with acute heart failure).
7. β-Lactam antibiotics, such as penicillin G (or ceftriaxone), nafcillin, and ampicillin, remain the drugs of choice for streptococcal, staphylococcal, and enterococcal endocarditis, respectively.
8. Aminoglycoside antibiotics are essential to obtain a synergistic bactericidal effect in the treatment of enterococcal endocarditis. Adjunctive aminoglycosides also may decrease the emergence of resistant organisms (e.g., prosthetic valve endocarditis caused by coagulase-negative staphylococci) and hasten the pace of clinical and microbiologic response (e.g., some streptococcal and staphylococcal infections).
9. Vancomycin is reserved for patients with immediate β-lactam allergies and the treatment of resistant organisms.
10. Antimicrobial prophylaxis is used as an attempt to prevent infective endocarditis for patients who are at the highest risk (such as persons with prosthetic heart valves) before a bacteremia-causing procedure (e.g., dental extraction).

Endocarditis is an inflammation of the endocardium, the membrane lining the chambers of the heart and covering the cusps of the heart valves.[1,2] More commonly, *endocarditis* refers to infection of the heart valves by various microorganisms. Although it typically affects native valves, it also may involve nonvalvular areas or implanted mechanical devices (e.g., mechanical heart valves). Bacteria primarily cause endocarditis, but fungi and other atypical microorganisms can lead to the disease; hence, the more encompassing term *infective endocarditis* is preferred.[2,3]

Endocarditis is often referred to as *acute* or *subacute* depending on the pace and severity of the clinical presentation. The acute, fulminating form is associated with high fevers and systemic toxicity. Virulent bacteria, such as *Staphylococcus aureus*, frequently cause this syndrome, and if untreated, death may occur within days to weeks. On the other hand, subacute infective endocarditis is more indolent, and it is caused by less invasive organisms, such as viridans streptococci, usually occurring in preexisting valvular heart disease. Although infective endocarditis is often referred to as acute or subacute, it is best classified based on the etiologic organism, the anatomic site of infection, and pathogenic risk factors.[1,4,5] Infection also may follow surgical insertion of a prosthetic heart valve, resulting in prosthetic valve endocarditis (PVE), or insertion of a cardiac implantable electronic device, resulting in cardiac device infective endocarditis (CDIE).[6,7]

EPIDEMIOLOGY AND ETIOLOGY

Infective endocarditis is an uncommon, but not rare, infection. Population-based studies have reported incidence rates of 2 to 15 cases per 100,000 person-years.[1,8,9] In the United States, the infection is listed as the primary or secondary diagnosis of 28,000 hospital discharges.[10] The mean male-to-female ratio is approximately 2:1.[11] As the population ages and as valve replacement surgery becomes more common, the mean age of patients with infective endocarditis increases. Overall, most cases occur in individuals older than 50 years of age, and it is uncommon in children.[11–14] PVE and CDIE account for 20% and 6.4% of cases of infective endocarditis, respectively.[11,15] Those with a history of IV drug abuse (IVDA) are also at high risk. Of note, the incidence of healthcare-associated infective endocarditis is rising, especially in the elderly population.[11,12] Other conditions associated with a higher incidence of infective endocarditis include diabetes, long-term hemodialysis, and poor dental hygiene.[5]

(1) Most persons with infective endocarditis have risk factors, such as preexisting cardiac valvular abnormalities. Many types of structural heart disease result in turbulent blood flow that increases the risk for infective endocarditis. A predisposing risk factor, however, may be absent in up to 25% of cases. Some of the more important risk factors include[5,7,11,13,16]:

1. Presence of a prosthetic valve (highest risk)
2. Previous endocarditis (highest risk)
3. Congenital heart disease (CHD)
4. Chronic IV access

5. Diabetes mellitus
6. Healthcare-related exposure
7. Acquired valvular dysfunction (e.g., rheumatic heart disease)
8. Cardiac implantable device
9. Chronic heart failure
10. Mitral valve prolapse with regurgitation
11. IVDA

In the past, rheumatic heart disease was a prevalent risk factor for infective endocarditis, but the incidence of this disease continues to decline. The risk of infective endocarditis in persons with mitral valve prolapse and regurgitation is small; however, because the condition is prevalent, it is an important contributor to the overall number of infective endocarditis cases.[5,11] PVE occurs in 1% to 3% of patients undergoing valve replacement surgery in the first post-operative year.[11,17]

❷ Nearly every organism causing human disease may cause infective endocarditis, but three groups of organisms result in a majority of cases: streptococci, staphylococci, and enterococci (Table 89-1).[1,3,4,11,16] The incidence of staphylococci, particularly *S. aureus*, continues to increase, and case series have documented that staphylococci have surpassed viridans streptococci as the leading cause of infective endocarditis.[11,16] In general, streptococci cause infective endocarditis in patients with community-acquired disease and underlying cardiac abnormalities, such as mitral valve prolapse or rheumatic heart disease. Staphylococci (*S. aureus* and coagulase-negative staphylococci) are the most common cause of PVE within the first year after valve surgery, and *S. aureus* is common in those with a history of IVDA. Although polymicrobial infective endocarditis is uncommon, it is encountered most often in association with IVDA.[1,11,16] Enterococcal endocarditis tends to follow genitourinary manipulations or obstetric procedures.[17] There are many exceptions to the preceding generalizations; thus, isolation of the causative pathogen and determination of its antimicrobial susceptibilities offer the best chance for successful therapy.

The mitral and aortic valves are affected most commonly in cases involving a single valve. Subacute endocarditis tends to involve the mitral valve, whereas acute disease often involves the aortic valve. Up to 35% of cases involve concomitant infections of both the aortic and the mitral valves. Infection of the tricuspid valve is less common, with a majority of these cases occurring in patients with a history of IVDA. It is rare for the pulmonary valve to be infected.[11,16,17]

TABLE 89-1 Etiologic Organisms in Infective Endocarditis[a]

Agent	Percentage of Cases
Staphylococci	30–70
Coagulase positive	20–68
Coagulase negative	3–26
Streptococci	9–38
Viridans streptococci	10–28
Other streptococci	3–14
Enterococci	5–18
Gram-negative aerobic bacilli	1.5–13
Fungi	1–9
Miscellaneous bacteria	<5
Mixed infections	1–2
"Culture negative"	<5–17

[a]Values encompass community-acquired, healthcare-associated, native valve, and prosthetic valve infective endocarditis.

Data from references 3, 11, and 16.

Pathophysiology

The development of infective endocarditis via hematogenous spread, the most common route, requires the sequential occurrence of several factors. These components are complex and not fully elucidated.[18,19]

1. *The endothelial surface of the heart is damaged.* This injury occurs with turbulent blood flow associated with the valvular lesions previously described.
2. *Platelet and fibrin deposition occurs on the abnormal epithelial surface.* These platelet–fibrin deposits are referred to as *nonbacterial thrombotic endocarditis.*
3. *Bacteremia gives organisms access to and results in colonization of the endocardial surface.* Bacteremia is the result of trauma to a mucosal surface with a high concentration of resident bacteria, such as the oral cavity and GI tract. Transient bacteremia commonly follow certain dental, GI, urologic, and gynecologic procedures. Staphylococci, viridans streptococci, and enterococci are most likely to adhere to nonbacterial thrombotic endocarditis, probably because of production of specific adherence factors, such as dextran by some oral streptococci and glycocalyx for staphylococci. Gram-negative bacteria rarely adhere to heart valves and are uncommon causes of infective endocarditis.
4. *After colonization of the endothelial surface, a "vegetation" of fibrin, platelets, and bacteria forms.* The protective cover of fibrin and platelets allows unimpeded bacterial growth to concentrations as high as 10^9 to 10^{10} organisms per gram of tissue.

The pathogenesis of early PVE or CDIE differs from infective endocarditis acquired by the hematogenous route because surgery may directly inoculate prosthetic material with bacteria from the patient's skin or operating room personnel. In the case of early PVE, a recently placed nonendothelialized valve is more susceptible to bacterial colonization than are native valves. Bacteria also may colonize the new valve from contaminated bypass pumps, cannulas, and pacemakers or from a nosocomial bacteremia subsequent to an intravascular catheter.[7,16,17] The mechanism of bacterial colonization and pathogenesis in late PVE is similar to native valve endocarditis (NVE).[17]

The vegetations seen in infective endocarditis may be single or multiple and vary in size from a few millimeters to centimeters. Bacteria within the vegetation grow slowly and are protected from antibiotics and host defenses. The adverse effects of infective endocarditis and the resulting lesions can be far-reaching and include (a) local perivalvular damage, (b) embolization of septic fragments with potential hematogenous seeding of remote sites, and (c) formation of antibody complexes.[17,19]

Formation of vegetations may destroy valvular tissue, and continued destruction can lead to acute heart failure via perforation of the valve leaflet, rupture of the chordae tendineae or papillary muscle, or, for patients with PVE, valve dehiscence. Occasionally, valvular stenosis may occur. Abscesses can develop in the valve ring or in myocardial tissue itself. Even with resolution of the process, fibrosis of tissue with some residual dysfunction is possible.

Vegetations may be friable, and fragments may be released downstream. These infected particles, termed *septic emboli*, can result in organ abscess or infarction. Septic emboli from right-sided endocarditis commonly lodge in the lungs, causing pulmonary abscesses. Emboli from left-sided vegetations commonly affect organs with high blood flow, such as the kidneys, spleen, and brain.[17,19]

Circulating immune complexes consisting of antigen, antibody, and complement may deposit in organs, producing local inflammation and damage (e.g., glomerulonephritis in the kidneys). Other potential pathologic changes that result from immune-complex deposition or septic emboli include the development of "mycotic" aneurysms (although the aneurysm is usually bacterial in origin, not fungal), cerebral infarction, splenic infarction and abscess, and skin manifestations such as petechiae, Osler's nodes, and Janeway's lesions.[5,17,19]

CLINICAL PRESENTATION

3 The clinical presentation of infective endocarditis is highly variable and nonspecific. Fever is the most common finding and is often accompanied by other vague symptoms (Table 89-2). Fever may be relatively low grade, particularly in subacute cases. Heart murmurs are found in a majority of patients, most often preexisting, with some documented as new or changing. Infective endocarditis usually begins insidiously and worsens gradually. Patients may present with nonspecific findings, such as fever, chills, weakness, dyspnea, night sweats, weight loss, or malaise. In contrast, patients with acute disease, such as those with a history of IVDA and *S. aureus* infective endocarditis, may appear with classic signs of sepsis.

Splenomegaly is a frequent finding for patients with prolonged endocarditis. Other important clinical signs especially prevalent in subacute illness may include the following peripheral manifestations ("stigmata") of endocarditis[5,11,12,16]:

1. Osler's nodes: Purplish or erythematous subcutaneous papules or nodules on the pads of the fingers and toes. These lesions are 2 to 15 mm in size and are painful and tender. These nodes are not specific for infective endocarditis and may be the result of embolism, immunologic phenomena, or both.
2. Janeway's lesions: Hemorrhagic, painless plaques on the palms of the hands or soles of the feet. These lesions are believed to be embolic in origin.
3. Splinter hemorrhages: Thin, linear hemorrhages found under the nail beds of the fingers or toes. These lesions are not specific for infective endocarditis and more commonly are the result of traumatic injuries. Distal lesions are more likely the result of trauma, whereas proximal lesions tend to be associated with infective endocarditis.
4. Petechiae: Small (usually 1 to 2 mm in diameter), erythematous, painless, hemorrhagic lesions. These lesions appear anywhere on the skin but more frequently on the anterior trunk, buccal mucosa and palate, and conjunctivae. Petechiae are nonblanching and resolve after a few days.
5. Clubbing of the fingers: Proliferative changes in the soft tissues about the terminal phalanges observed in long-standing endocarditis.
6. Roth's spots: Retinal infarct with central pallor and surrounding hemorrhage.
7. Emboli: Embolic phenomena occur in up to one third of cases and may result in significant complications. Left-sided endocarditis can result in renal artery emboli causing flank pain with hematuria, splenic artery emboli causing abdominal pain, and cerebral emboli, which may result in hemiplegia or alteration in mental status. Right-sided endocarditis may result in pulmonary emboli, causing pleuritic pain with hemoptysis.

Patients with infective endocarditis typically have laboratory abnormalities; however, none of these changes is specific for the disease. Anemia (normocytic, normochromic), leukocytosis, and thrombocytopenia may be present. The white blood cell count is often normal or only slightly elevated, sometimes with a mild left shift. Acute bacterial endocarditis, however, may present with an elevated white blood cell count, consistent with a fulminant infection. The erythrocyte sedimentation rate and C-reactive protein may be elevated in approximately 60% of patients. Often the urinary analysis is abnormal, with proteinuria and microscopic hematuria occurring in approximately 25% of individuals.[5,11]

TABLE 89-2 Clinical Presentation of Infective Endocarditis

General
The clinical presentation of infective endocarditis is highly variable and nonspecific

Symptoms
The patient may complain of fever, chills, weakness, dyspnea, night sweats, weight loss, and/or malaise

Signs
Fever is common, as is a heart murmur (sometimes new or changing).
The patient may have embolic phenomenon, splenomegaly, or skin manifestations (e.g., Osler's nodes, Janeway's lesions)

Laboratory tests
The patient's white blood cell count may be normal or only slightly elevated
Nonspecific findings include anemia (normocytic, normochromic), thrombocytopenia, an elevated erythrocyte sedimentation rate or C-reactive protein, and altered urinary analysis (proteinuria/microscopic hematuria)
The hallmark laboratory finding is continuous bacteremia; three sets of blood cultures should be collected over 24 hours

Other diagnostic tests
An electrocardiogram, chest radiograph, and echocardiogram are commonly performed. Echocardiography to determine the presence of valvular vegetations plays a key role in the diagnosis of infective endocarditis; it should be performed in all suspected cases

The hallmark of infective endocarditis is a continuous bacteremia caused by bacteria shedding from the vegetation into the bloodstream; 90% to 95% of patients with infective endocarditis have positive blood cultures.[1,11,17] Three sets of blood cultures, each from separate venipuncture sites, should be collected over 24 hours, and antibiotics should be withheld until adequate blood cultures are obtained. On the other hand, if a patient has a toxic appearance, several blood cultures should be collected promptly, followed by immediate empirical antimicrobial treatment. The blood cultures for patients who have received previous antibiotics should be monitored more closely because pathogen growth may be suppressed.[1] "Culture-negative" endocarditis describes a patient in whom a clinical diagnosis of infective endocarditis is likely but blood cultures do not yield a pathogen. This condition is often the consequence of previous antibiotic therapy, improperly collected blood cultures, or unusual organisms.[4] When blood cultures from patients suspected of having infective endocarditis show no growth after 48 to 72 hours, the laboratory should be advised and cultures held for up to a month to detect growth of fastidious organisms.[4]

An electrocardiogram, chest radiograph, and echocardiogram are performed for patients suspected of endocarditis. The electrocardiogram rarely shows important diagnostic findings but may reveal heart block, suggesting extension of the infection. The chest radiograph may provide more diagnostic information, especially in a patient with right-sided endocarditis. Septic pulmonary emboli may occur, leading to multiple lung foci. The echocardiogram is the most important test and should be performed for all patients suspected of this infection.

Echocardiography plays an important role in the diagnosis and management of infective endocarditis.[4] The chosen approach, transthoracic echocardiography (TTE) or transesophageal echocardiography (TEE), depends on the clinical setting. The TEE technique is more sensitive for detecting vegetations (90% to 100%) as compared with TTE (58% to 63%), and TEE maintains good specificity (85% to 95%).[1,4] TTE appears reasonable in the evaluation of children or adults in whom the clinical suspicion of infective endocarditis is relatively low.[4,20] TEE is preferred in high-risk patients such as those with prosthetic heart valves, many CHDs, previous endocarditis, new murmur, heart failure, or other stigmata of endocarditis.[4,21,22] The lack of vegetation on echocardiogram does not exclude infection even if the transesophageal approach is used. Conversely, the test may reveal an unsuspected large vegetation, extension of the disease into surrounding tissue, valvular defects, abscess formation, cordial rupture, or an intracardiac fistula. Thus, in addition to helping in the diagnosis of infective endocarditis, the echocardiogram allows the physician to evaluate hemodynamic stability and the need for urgent surgical intervention; it also provides a rough estimate of the likelihood of embolism.[4,22]

DIAGNOSIS

❹ The signs and symptoms of infective endocarditis are not specific, and the diagnosis is often unclear. The identification of infective endocarditis requires the integration of clinical, laboratory, and echocardiographic findings. The Duke diagnostic criteria include major and minor variables (Table 89-3).[23,24] Based on the number of major and minor criteria that are fulfilled, patients suspected of infective endocarditis are categorized into three separate groups: definite infective endocarditis, possible infective endocarditis, or infective endocarditis rejected.[24]

TABLE 89-3 Diagnosis of Infective Endocarditis According to the Modified Duke Criteria

Major Criteria
Blood culture positive for infective endocarditis
Typical microorganisms consistent with infective endocarditis from two separate blood cultures:
Viridans streptococci, *Streptococcus bovis*, HACEK group, *Staphylococcus aureus*; or
Community-acquired enterococci, in the absence of a primary focus; or
Microorganisms consistent with infective endocarditis from persistently positive blood cultures, defined as follows:
At least two positive cultures of blood samples drawn greater than 12 hours apart; or
All of three or a majority of four or more separate cultures of blood (with first and last sample drawn at least 1 hour apart)
Single positive blood culture for *Coxiella burnetii* or antiphase I immunoglobulin G antibody titer >1:800
Evidence of endocardial involvement
Echocardiogram positive for infective endocarditis (transesophageal echocardiography recommended for patients with prosthetic valves, rated at least "possible infective endocarditis" by clinical criteria, or complicated infective endocarditis [paravalvular abscess]; transthoracic echocardiography as first test for other patients), defined as follows:
Oscillating intracardiac mass on valve or supporting structures, in the path of regurgitant jets or on implanted material in the absence of an alternative anatomic explanation; or abscess; or
New partial dehiscence of prosthetic valve
New valvular regurgitation (worsening or changing of preexisting murmur not sufficient)
Minor Criteria
Predisposition, predisposing heart condition, or injection drug use
Fever, temperature >38°C (100.4°F)
Vascular phenomena, major arterial emboli, septic pulmonary infarcts, mycotic aneurysm, intracranial hemorrhage, conjunctival hemorrhages, and Janeway's lesions
Immunologic phenomena: glomerulonephritis, Osler's nodes, Roth's spots, and rheumatoid factor
Microbiologic evidence: positive blood culture but does not meet a major criterion as noted above or serologic evidence of active infection with organism consistent with infective endocarditis
Echocardiographic minor criteria eliminated

HACEK, *Haemophilus* species (*H. parainfluenzae, H. aphrophilus, H. paraphrophilus*), *Actinobacillus actinomycetemcomitans, Cardiobacterium hominis, Eikenella corrodens*, and *Kingella kingae*.

Note: Cases are defined clinically as *definite* if they fulfill two major criteria, one major criterion plus three minor criteria, or five minor criteria; cases are defined as *possible* if they fulfill one major and one minor criterion or three minor criteria. Cases are rejected if there is a firm alternate diagnosis explaining evidence of infective endocarditis; resolution of infective endocarditis syndrome with antibiotic therapy for <4 days; no pathologic evidence of infective endocarditis at surgery or autopsy, with antibiotic therapy for <4 days; or criteria for possible infective endocarditis are not met, as above.

Data from references 23 and 24.

PROGNOSIS

The outcome for endocarditis is improved with rapid diagnosis, appropriate treatment (i.e., antimicrobial therapy, surgery, or both), and prompt recognition of complications should they arise. Factors associated with increased mortality include (a) heart failure, (b) increasing age, (c) endocarditis caused by resistant organisms such as fungi or gram-negative bacteria, (d) left-sided endocarditis caused by *S. aureus*, (e) paravalvular complications, (f) healthcare-acquired infection, and (g) PVE.[4,5,11,16] The presence of heart failure has the greatest negative impact on the short-term prognosis.[4] For left-sided native valve infective endocarditis, mortality rates range from 15% to 45%; lower rates (4% to 16%) occur with community-acquired disease that is most commonly caused by viridans streptococci. Higher rates (25% to 45%) occur with healthcare-associated disease that is more commonly caused by enterococci and staphylococci.[1] Even higher rates of mortality are seen with unusually encountered organisms (e.g., mortality greater than 50% for *Pseudomonas aeruginosa*).[4] The mortality rate for right-sided infective endocarditis associated with IVDA is generally low (e.g., less than 10%).[1,4] For those who relapse after treatment for infective endocarditis, most will do so within the first 2 months after discontinuation of antimicrobials. Relapse rates for viridans streptococcus are generally low (2%), whereas relapse is more likely in those with enterococcal infection (8% to 20%) and PVE (10% to 15%).[5,17] After appropriate treatment and recovery, the risk of morbidity and mortality following infective endocarditis persists for years, although it gradually declines annually. Morbidity remains elevated because of a greater likelihood of recurrent infective endocarditis, heart failure, and embolism or, if a valve is replaced, the risk of anticoagulation, valve thrombosis, or additional valve surgery.[5,21]

TREATMENT

Desired Outcomes

The desired outcomes for treatment and prophylaxis of infective endocarditis are to:

1. Relieve the signs and symptoms of the disease
2. Decrease morbidity and mortality associated with the infection
3. Eradicate the causative organism with minimal drug exposure
4. Provide cost-effective antimicrobial therapy determined by the likely or identified pathogen, drug susceptibilities, hepatic and renal function, drug allergies, and anticipated drug toxicities
5. Prevent infective endocarditis from occurring or recurring in high-risk patients with appropriate prophylactic antimicrobials

General Approach to Treatment

❺ The most important approach in the treatment of infective endocarditis is isolation of the infecting pathogen and determination of antimicrobial susceptibilities, followed by high-dose, parenteral, bactericidal antibiotics for an extended period.[1,5,17] Identification of susceptibilities is crucial given the escalating level of antibiotic resistance to commonly encountered pathogens.

Treatment usually is started in the hospital, but for select patients it is often completed in the outpatient setting so long as defervescence has occurred and followup blood cultures show no growth.[5,25] Large doses of parenteral antimicrobials usually are necessary to achieve bactericidal concentrations within vegetations. An extended duration of therapy is required, even for susceptible pathogens, because microorganisms are enclosed within valvular vegetations and fibrin deposits. These barriers impair host defenses and protect microbes from phagocytic cells. In addition, high bacterial concentrations within vegetations may result in an inoculum effect that further resists killing (see eChap. 24 for additional discussion). Many bacteria are not actively dividing, further limiting the rate of bacterial death. For most patients, a minimum of 4 to 6 weeks of therapy is required.[4]

Nonpharmacologic Therapy

❻ Surgery is an important adjunct in the management of both NVE and PVE. In most surgical cases, valvectomy and valve replacement are performed to remove infected tissue and to restore hemodynamic function. Indications for surgery include heart failure, persistent bacteremia, persistent vegetation, an increase in vegetation size, or recurrent emboli despite prolonged antibiotic treatment, valve dysfunction, paravalvular extension (e.g., abscess), or endocarditis caused by resistant organisms (e.g., fungi or gram-negative bacteria).[4,26,27] More controversial is the appropriate timing of surgery as American and European guidelines have different criteria for emergent or urgent surgical intervention.[26,27] Additionally, studies evaluating postsurgical outcomes and associated mortality are limited such that a specific risk prediction system has not been established.[28–32] Early surgery (e.g., within 48 hours) may be appropriate in patients with severe heart failure and large vegetations, whereas patients with septic shock, advanced age, or neurologic complications of infective endocarditis may have more detrimental outcomes.[28,29,33,34]

Clinical **Controversy...**

The role of surgery in the management of infective endocarditis has expanded; however, criteria to select patients and appropriate timing of surgery have not been well defined. Additionally, more studies are needed to evaluate postsurgical outcomes.

Pharmacologic Therapy

Specific treatment recommendations from the American Heart Association (AHA) provide guidance for the management of infective endocarditis, and these were updated in 2005.[4] Guidelines published in 2009 by the European Society of Cardiology are consistent with the AHA guidelines.[27] Both guidelines use an evidence-based scoring system where recommendations are given a classification as well as level of evidence. Class I recommendations are conditions for which there is evidence, general agreement, or both that a given procedure or treatment is useful and effective. Class II recommendations are conditions for which there is conflicting evidence, a divergence of opinion, or both about the usefulness/efficacy of a procedure or treatment (IIa implies the weight of evidence/opinion is in favor of usefulness/efficacy, whereas IIb implies usefulness/efficacy is less well established by evidence/opinion). Class III recommendations are conditions for which there is evidence, general agreement, or both that the procedure/treatment is not useful/effective and in some cases may be harmful. Level of evidence is listed as A (data derived from multiple randomized clinical trials), B (data derived from a single randomized trial or nonrandomized studies), and C (consensus opinion of experts).

❼ β-Lactam antibiotics, such as penicillin G (or ceftriaxone), nafcillin, and ampicillin, remain the drugs of choice for streptococcal, staphylococcal, and enterococcal endocarditis, respectively. Tables 89-4 to 89-7 summarize these recommendations, which are discussed in more detail in the following sections. Tables 89-8 and 89-9 list drug dosing and monitoring recommendations for adult and pediatric patients. Because these guidelines focus on common causes of endocarditis, readers are referred to other references for more in-depth discussion of unusually encountered organisms.[4,27,35–37]

❽ For some pathogens, such as enterococci, the use of synergistic antimicrobial combinations (including an aminoglycoside) is essential to obtain a bactericidal effect. Combination antibiotics also may decrease the emergence of resistant organisms during treatment (e.g., PVE caused by coagulase-negative staphylococci) and hasten the pace of clinical and microbiologic response (e.g., some streptococcal and staphylococcal infections). Occasionally, combination treatment will result in a shorter treatment course.

Streptococcal Endocarditis

Streptococci are a common cause of infective endocarditis, with most isolates being viridans streptococci. *Viridans streptococci* refer to a large number of different species, such as *Streptococcus sanguinis, Streptococcus oralis, Streptococcus salivarius, Streptococcus mutans*, and *Gemella morbillorum*.[4] These bacteria are common inhabitants of the human mouth and gingiva, and they are especially common causes of endocarditis involving native valves.[1,4,16] During dental surgery, and even when brushing the teeth, these organisms can cause a transient bacteremia. In susceptible individuals, this may result in infective endocarditis. Streptococcal endocarditis is usually subacute, and the response to medical treatment is very good. *Streptococcus bovis* is not a viridans streptococcus, but it is included in this treatment group because it is penicillin sensitive and requires the same treatment as viridans streptococci. *S. bovis* is a nonenterococcal group D *Streptococcus* that resides in the GI tract. Infective endocarditis caused by this organism is often associated with a GI pathology, especially colon carcinoma. Endocarditis caused by *Streptococcus pneumoniae, Streptococcus pyogenes*, and group B, C, and G streptococci are uncommon, and their treatment is not well defined.[4,19]

Antimicrobial regimens for viridans streptococci are well studied, and in uncomplicated cases, response rates as high as 98% can be expected. Viridans streptococci are penicillin susceptible, although some are more susceptible than others. Most are exquisitely sensitive to penicillin G and have minimal inhibitory concentrations (MICs) of less than 0.12 mcg/mL (mg/L).[4,19] Approximately 10% to 20% are moderately susceptible (MIC 0.12 to 0.5 mcg/mL [mg/L]). This difference in in vitro susceptibility led to recommendations that the MIC be determined for all viridans streptococci and that the results be used to guide therapy. Some streptococci are deemed tolerant to the killing effects of penicillin, where the minimal bactericidal concentration (MBC) exceeds the MIC by 32 times. A tolerant organism is inhibited but not killed by an antibiotic normally considered bactericidal.[4] Bactericidal activity is required for successful treatment of infective endocarditis; therefore, infections with a tolerant organism may relapse after treatment. Despite some animal studies of endocarditis suggesting that tolerant strains do not respond as readily to β-lactam therapy as nontolerant ones, this phenomenon is primarily a laboratory finding

TABLE 89-4 Treatment Options for Native Valve Endocarditis by Causative Organism

Agent[a]	Duration	Strength of Recommendation	Comments
Highly Penicillin-Susceptible (MIC ≤0.12 mcg/mL [mg/L]) Viridans Group Streptococci and *Streptococcus Bovis*			
Aqueous crystalline penicillin G sodium	4 weeks	1A	2-Week regimens are not intended for the following patients: • Most patients >65 years of age • Impairment of the eighth cranial nerve function • Renal function with a creatinine clearance <20 mL/min (<0.33 mL/s) • Known cardiac or extracardiac abscess • Infection with *Abiotrophia, Granulicatella*, or *Gemalla* species
Ceftriaxone	4 weeks	1A	
Aqueous crystalline penicillin G sodium plus gentamicin	2 weeks	1B	
Ceftriaxone plus gentamicin	2 weeks	1B	
Vancomycin	4 weeks	1B	Recommended only for patients unable to tolerate penicillin or ceftriaxone
Viridans Group Streptococci and *S. Bovis* Relatively Resistant to Penicillin (MIC >0.12 to ≤0.5 mcg/mL [mg/L])			
Aqueous crystalline penicillin G sodium plus gentamicin	4 weeks 2 weeks	1B	
Ceftriaxone plus gentamicin	4 weeks 2 weeks	1B	
Vancomycin	4 weeks	1B	Recommended only for patients unable to tolerate penicillin or ceftriaxone
Oxacillin-Susceptible Staphylococci[b]			
Nafcillin or oxacillin Optional: gentamicin sulfate[c]	6 weeks 3–5 days	1A	Aqueous crystalline penicillin G sodium may be used as an alternative if the strain is highly penicillin susceptible (MIC ≤0.1 mcg/mL [mg/L]) and does not produce β-lactamase; use similar dosing as streptococci relatively resistant to penicillin
Cefazolin Optional: gentamicin sulfate[c]	6 weeks 3–5 days	1B	For use in patients with nonanaphylactoid-type penicillin allergies; patients with an unclear history of immediate-type hypersensitivity to penicillin should be considered for skin testing
Vancomycin	6 weeks	1B	For use in patients with anaphylactoid-type hypersensitivity to penicillin and/or cephalosporins
Oxacillin-Resistant Staphylococci			
Vancomycin	6 weeks	1B	
Daptomycin	6 weeks	1A	

Please refer to Table 89-6 for treatment of NVE caused by enterococci.

[a]See Tables 89-8 and 89-9 for appropriate dosing, administration, and monitoring information.

[b]Regimens indicate treatment for left-sided endocarditis or complicated right-sided endocarditis; uncomplicated right-sided endocarditis may be treated for shorter durations and is described in the text.

[c]The clinical benefit of synergistic aminoglycoside therapy is discussed briefly in the text.

Data from references 4 and 20.

with little clinical significance.[4,19] Treatment for tolerant strains is identical to that for nontolerant organisms, and measurement of the MBC is not recommended.[4]

An assortment of regimens can be used to treat uncomplicated NVE caused by fully susceptible viridans streptococci (Table 89-4). Two single-drug regimens consist of high-dose parenteral penicillin G or ceftriaxone for 4 weeks. If a shorter course of therapy is desired, the guidelines suggest either high-dose parenteral penicillin G or ceftriaxone in combination with an aminoglycoside.[4] When used in select patients, this combination is as effective as 4 weeks of penicillin alone. Although streptomycin was listed in previous guidelines, gentamicin is the preferred aminoglycoside because serum drug concentrations are obtained easily, clinicians are more familiar with its use, and the few strains of streptococci resistant to the effects of streptomycin–penicillin remain susceptible to gentamicin–penicillin. Other aminoglycosides are not recommended.

The decision of which regimen to use depends on the perceived risk versus benefit. For example, a 2-week course of gentamicin in an elderly patient with renal impairment may be associated with ototoxicity, worsening renal function, or both. Furthermore, the 2-week regimen is not recommended for patients with known extracardiac infection. On the other hand, a 4-week course of penicillin alone generally entails greater expense, especially if the patient remains in the hospital. Monotherapy with once-daily ceftriaxone offers ease of administration, facilitates home healthcare treatment, and may be cost-effective.[1,4,25]

The British Society for Antimicrobial Chemotherapy guidelines suggest that all of the following conditions be present to consider a 2-week treatment regimen for penicillin-sensitive streptococcal endocarditis[35]:

1. Penicillin-sensitive viridans streptococcus or *S. bovis* (penicillin MIC <0.1 mcg/mL [mg/L])
2. No cardiovascular risk factors such as heart failure, aortic insufficiency, or conduction abnormalities
3. No evidence of thromboembolic disease
4. Native valve infection
5. No vegetation of greater than 5 mm diameter on echocardiogram
6. Clinical response within 7 days (the temperature should return to normal, the patient should feel well, and the patient's appetite should return to normal)

9 When a patient has a history of an immediate-type hypersensitivity to penicillin, vancomycin should be chosen for infective endocarditis caused by viridans streptococci. When vancomycin is used, the addition of gentamicin is not recommended.[4] Most patients who report a penicillin allergy have a negative penicillin skin test and consequently are at low risk of anaphylaxis.[38] The published experience with penicillin is more extensive than with alternative regimens; consequently, a thorough allergy history must be obtained before a second-line therapy is administered.

TABLE 89-5 Treatment Options for Prosthetic Valve Endocarditis (PVE) by Causative Organism

Agent[a]	Duration (Weeks)	Strength of Recommendation	Comments
Highly Penicillin-Susceptible (MIC ≤0.12 mcg/mL [mg/L]) Viridans Group Streptococci and *Streptococcus Bovis*			
Aqueous crystalline penicillin G sodium with or without gentamicin	6 2	1B	Combination therapy with gentamicin has not demonstrated superior cure rates compared with monotherapy with a penicillin or cephalosporin and should be avoided in patients with CrCl <30 mL/min (<0.50 mL/s)
Ceftriaxone with or without gentamicin	6 2	1B	
Vancomycin	2	1B	Recommended only for patients unable to tolerate penicillin or ceftriaxone
Relatively Resistant or Fully Resistant (MIC >0.12 mcg/mL [mg/L]) Viridans Group Streptococci and *S. Bovis*			
Aqueous crystalline penicillin G sodium plus gentamicin	6	1B	
Ceftriaxone plus gentamicin	6	1B	
Vancomycin	6	1B	Recommended only for patients unable to tolerate penicillin or ceftriaxone
Oxacillin-Susceptible Staphylococci			
Nafcillin or oxacillin plus rifampin plus gentamicin	≥6 ≥6 2	1B	Aqueous crystalline penicillin G sodium may be used as an alternative if the strain is highly penicillin susceptible (MIC ≤0.1 mcg/mL [mg/L]) and does not produce β-lactamase; use similar dosing as streptococci relatively resistant to penicillin; cefazolin may be substituted for nafcillin or oxacillin in patient with nonimmediate-type hypersensitivity
Vancomycin plus rifampin plus gentamicin	≥6 ≥6 2	1B	Recommended only for patients with anaphylactoid-type hypersensitivity to penicillin and/or cephalosporins
Oxacillin-Resistant Staphylococci			
Vancomycin plus rifampin plus gentamicin	≥6 ≥6 2	1B	

Please refer to Table 89-6 for treatment of PVE caused by enterococci.

[a]See Tables 89-8 and 89-9 for appropriate dosing, administration, and monitoring information.

Data from references 4 and 20.

TABLE 89-6 Treatment Options for Native or Prosthetic Valve Endocarditis Caused by Enterococci

Agent[a]	Duration[b] (Weeks)	Strength of Recommendation	Comments
Ampicillin-, Penicillin-, and Vancomycin-Susceptible Strains			
Ampicillin plus gentamicin	4–6	1A	Symptoms present for <3 months: use 4-week regimen Symptoms present for >3 months: use 6-week regimen
Aqueous crystalline penicillin G sodium plus gentamicin	4–6	1A	
Vancomycin plus gentamicin	6	1B	Recommended only for patients unable to tolerate penicillin or ampicillin
Gentamicin-Resistant Strains			
If susceptible, use streptomycin in place of gentamicin in the regimens listed above			
Penicillin-Resistant Strains			
Ampicillin–sulbactam plus gentamicin (β-lactamase–producing strain)	6	IIaC	Treatment with ampicillin–sulbactam for >6 weeks will be needed if strain is also gentamicin resistant
Vancomycin plus gentamicin (intrinsic penicillin resistance[c])	6	IIaC	May also use in patients with β-lactamase–producing strains who have known intolerance to ampicillin–sulbactam
***Enterococcus Faecium* Strains Resistant to Penicillin, Aminoglycosides, and Vancomycin[c]**			
Linezolid	≥8	IIaC	Antimicrobial cure rates may be <50%; bacteriologic cure may only be achieved with cardiac valve replacement
Quinupristin–dalfopristin	≥8	IIaC	
***Enterococcus Faecalis* Strains Resistant to Penicillin, Aminoglycosides, and Vancomycin[c]**			
Imipenem–cilastatin plus ampicillin	≥8	IIbC	
Ceftriaxone plus ampicillin	≥8	IIbC	

[a]See Tables 89-8 and 89-9 for appropriate dosing, administration, and monitoring information.
[b]All patients with prosthetic valves should be treated for at least 6 weeks.
[c]Infectious disease consult highly recommended.

Data from reference 4.

TABLE 89-7 Treatment Options for Culture-Negative Endocarditis and Endocarditis Caused by Gram-Negative Organisms[a]

Agent[b]	Duration[c] (Weeks)	Strength of Recommendation	Comments
HACEK[d] Microorganisms			
Ceftriaxone	4	1B	Other third- or fourth-generation cephalosporins may be used as an alternative
Ampicillin–sulbactam	4	IIaB	
Ciprofloxacin	4	IIbC	Recommended for patients with known intolerance to cephalosporins or ampicillin; other fluoroquinolones may be used as an alternative
Culture-Negative Endocarditis, Native Valve			
Ampicillin–sulbactam plus gentamicin	4–6	IIbC	
Vancomycin plus gentamicin plus ciprofloxacin	4–6	IIbC	Recommended only for patients unable to tolerate penicillin
Culture-Negative Endocarditis, Early (<1 Year) Prosthetic Valve			
Vancomycin plus cefepime plus rifampin plus gentamicin	6 2	IIbC	
Culture-Negative Endocarditis, Late (>1 Year) Prosthetic Valve			
Ampicillin–sulbactam plus gentamicin plus rifampin	6	IIbC	
Vancomycin plus gentamicin plus ciprofloxacin plus rifampin	6	IIbC	Recommended only for patients unable to tolerate penicillin
Suspected *Bartonella*, Culture-Negative			
Ceftriaxone plus gentamicin with or without doxycycline	6 2 6	IIaB	
Culture-Positive *Bartonella*			
Doxycycline plus gentamicin	6 2	IIaB	Rifampin is recommended as an alternative in patient who cannot be given gentamicin

[a]Infectious disease consult highly recommended.
[b]See Tables 89-8 and 89-9 for appropriate dosing, administration, and monitoring.
[c]All patients with prosthetic valves should be treated for 6 weeks.
[d]Haemophilus parainfluenzae, *Haemophilus aphrophilus, Actinobacillus actinomycetemcomitans, Cardiobacterium hominis, Eikenella corrodens*, and *Kingella kingae*.
Data from reference 4.

For patients with complicated infections (e.g., extracardiac foci) or when the streptococcus has an MIC of 0.12 to less than or equal to 0.5 mcg/mL (mg/L), combination therapy with an aminoglycoside for the first 2 weeks and penicillin (higher dose) or ceftriaxone is recommended, followed by penicillin or ceftriaxone alone for an additional 2 weeks (Table 89-4).[4] Some viridans streptococci have biologic characteristics that complicate diagnosis and treatment, previously referred to as nutritionally variant streptococci. *Abiotrophia defectiva* and *Granulicatella* species have nutritional deficiencies that hinder growth in routine culture media.[4,5,19] These organisms require special broth supplemented with pyridoxal hydrochloride or cysteine. For patients infected with nutritionally variant streptococci or when the *Streptococcus* has an MIC of more than 0.5 mcg/mL (mg/L), treatment should follow the enterococcal endocarditis treatment guidelines.[4]

The rationale for combination therapy of penicillin-susceptible viridans streptococci is that enhanced activity against these organisms usually is observed when cell-wall–active agents are combined with aminoglycosides in vitro.[39] Combined treatment results in quicker sterilization of vegetations in animal models of endocarditis and probably explains the high response rates observed for patients treated for a total of 2 weeks.[4,40] The combined treatment, however, is not superior to penicillin alone. Some authors question the need for combination therapy in relatively resistant streptococci, emphasizing that few human data suggest that patients with endocarditis caused by these organisms respond less well to penicillin alone.[39,41]

For patients with endocarditis of prosthetic valves or other prosthetic material caused by viridans streptococci and *S. bovis*, choices of treatment are similar to those without prosthetic material (e.g., penicillin or ceftriaxone); however, treatment courses are extended to 6 weeks (Table 89-5). In fact, if the organism is relatively resistant, gentamicin is recommended for 6 weeks.

Whether extended-interval aminoglycoside dosing has a role in infective endocarditis continues to be debated. At this time, data support extended-interval dosing for the treatment of streptococcal infective endocarditis, and as compared with three-times-daily dosing this approach may have greater efficacy.[42–45] One study specifically evaluated the combination of ceftriaxone (2 g daily) with gentamicin (3 mg/kg daily) for 2 weeks compared with ceftriaxone (2 g daily) alone for 4 weeks for penicillin-sensitive streptococci. Both regimens were safe and effective with similar clinical cure rates at 3 months following treatment.[40]

Clinical **Controversy...**

In the past, the AHA guidelines recommended traditional aminoglycoside dosing (three times daily) whenever clinicians use these antibiotics. Extended-interval dosing (once-daily administration) is an intriguing dosing strategy, but data only support this approach for the treatment of streptococcal infective endocarditis.

Staphylococcal Endocarditis

Endocarditis caused by staphylococci has become more prevalent, mainly because of increased IVDA, more frequent use of

TABLE 89-8 Drug Dosing Table for Treatment of Infective Endocarditis[a]

Drug	Brand Name	Recommended Dose	Pediatric (Ped) Dose[b]	Additional Information
Ampicillin	NA	2 g IV every 4 hours	50 mg/kg every 4 hours or 75 mg/kg every 6 hours	24-hour total dose may be administered as a continuous infusion: 12 g IV every 24 hours
Ampicillin–sulbactam	Unasyn®	2 g IV every 4 hours	50 mg/kg every 4 hours or 75 mg/kg every 6 hours	
Aqueous crystalline penicillin G sodium	NA			24-hour total dose may be administered as a continuous infusion: 12–18 million units IV every 24 hours (Ped: 200,000 units/kg IV/24 hours)
• MIC <0.12 mcg/mL (mg/L) (native valve only)		3 million units IV every 4 hours or every 6 hours	50,000 units/kg IV every 6 hours	
• All other indications		4 million units IV every 4 hours or 6 million units IV every 6 hours	50,000 units/kg IV every 4 hours or 75,000 units/kg IV every 6 hours	24 million units IV every 24 hours (Ped: 300,000 units/kg IV every 24 hours)
Cefazolin	Ancef®	2 g IV every 8 hours	33 mg/kg IV every 8 hours	
Cefepime	Maxipime®	2 g IV every 8 hours	50 mg/kg IV every 8 hours	
Ceftriaxone sodium	Rocephin®	2 g IV or IM every 24 hours 2 g IV or IM every 12 hours (*E. faecalis only*)	100 mg/kg IV or IM every 24 hours	
Ciprofloxacin	Cipro®	400 mg IV every 12 hours or 500 mg po every 12 hours	20–30 mg/kg IV or po every 12 hours	Avoid use if possible in patients <18 years of age
Daptomycin	Cubicin®	6 mg/kg IV every 24 hours		Doses as high as 8–10 mg/kg IV every 24 hours have been used in adults; doses should be calculated using actual body weight
Doxycline	Vibramycin®	100 mg IV or po every 12 hours	1–2 mg/kg IV or po every 12 hours	
Gentamicin sulfate	NA	1 mg/kg IV or IM every 8 hours	1 mg/kg IV or IM every 8 hours	Doses should be calculated using ideal body weight or adjusted body weight if >120% of ideal body weight; may also be administered as a single dose of 3 mg/kg of actual body weight
Imipenem–cilastatin	Primaxin®	500 mg IV every 6 hours	15–25 mg/kg IV every 6 hours	
Linezolid	Zyvox®	600 mg IV or po every 12 hours	10 mg/kg IV every 8 hours	
Nafcillin or oxacillin	NA	2 g IV every 4 hours	50 mg/kg IV every 6 hours	
Quinupristin–dalfopristin	Synercid®	7.5 mg/kg IV every 8 hours	7.5 mg/kg IV every 8 hours	
Rifampin	Rifadin®	300 mg IV or po every 8 hours	5–7 mg/kg IV or po every 8 hours	
Streptomycin	NA	15 mg/kg IV or IM every 12 hours		
Vancomycin	Vancocin®	15–20 mg/kg IV every 8 hours or every 12 hours	15 mg/kg IV every 6 hours	A loading dose of 25–30 mg/kg may be administered in adults; doses should be calculated using actual body weight; single doses should not exceed 2 g

[a]All doses assume normal renal function.
[b]Should not exceed adult dosage.

peripheral and central venous catheters, and increased frequency of valve replacement surgery.[46,47] *S. aureus* is the most common organism causing infective endocarditis among those with IVDA and persons with venous catheters. Coagulase-negative staphylococci (usually *Staphylococcus epidermidis*) are prominent causes of PVE.

Staphylococcal endocarditis is not a homogeneous disease; appropriate management requires consideration of several questions: Is the organism methicillin resistant? Should combination therapy be used? Is the infection on a native or prosthetic valve? Does the patient have a history of IVDA? Is the infection on the left or right side of the heart? Another consideration in staphylococcal endocarditis is that some organisms may exhibit tolerance to antibiotics. Similar to streptococci, however, the concern for tolerance among staphylococci should not affect antibiotic selection.[4]

Any patient who develops staphylococcal bacteremia is at risk for endocarditis. Many investigators have attempted to develop criteria that identify the bacteremic patient likely to have infective endocarditis.[46] In the past, patients were considered to be at high risk for infective endocarditis if *S. aureus* bacteremia was community acquired versus hospital acquired; however, nosocomial *S. aureus* bacteremia is now considered as a major criterion for development of infective endocarditis.[23,24] The prevalence of infective endocarditis in patients with *S. aureus* bacteremia is approximately 25%, leading some authors to suggest that screening echocardiography be performed in all patients.[48] In hospitalized patients with *S. aureus* bacteremia and an identified focus of infection, such as a vascular catheter, the risk of concomitant infective endocarditis is low, and treatment of the bacteremia can be reduced to 2 weeks. This approach applies only if the patient does not have a prosthetic valve or additional clinical evidence for endocarditis.[49] Additionally, the following parameters predict higher risk of infective endocarditis for patients with *S. aureus* bacteremia: (a) the absence of a primary site of infection, (b) metastatic signs of infection, and (c) valvular vegetations detected by echocardiography.[24,48]

The recommended therapy for patients with left-sided, native valve infective endocarditis caused by methicillin-sensitive

TABLE 89-9 Drug Monitoring of Select Agents

Drug	Major Adverse Drug Reactions	Monitoring Parameters	Comments
Daptomycin	Myopathy, rhabdomyolysis	Creatinine phosphokinase (CPK) at least weekly; monitor for signs and symptoms of muscle pain	More frequent monitoring may be warranted in patients with renal dysfunction or receiving concomitant therapy with HMG-CoA reductase inhibitors; discontinue if symptomatic and CPK >5 times the upper limit of normal (ULN) or if CPK ≥10 times ULN
Gentamicin	Nephrotoxicity, ototoxicity, neuromuscular blockade	When dosed three times daily: • Target peak serum concentrations of 3–4 mcg/mL (mg/L; 6.3–8.4 μmol/L) and trough serum concentrations of <1 mcg/mL (mg/L; <2.1 μmol/L)	Avoid concomitant use of other nephrotoxic agents such as diuretics, nonsteroidal antiinflammatory drugs, and radiocontrast media. Avoid rapid IV administration
Linezolid	Thrombocytopenia, optic, or peripheral neuropathy	Platelet counts at baseline and weekly, visual changes	More common with prolonged therapy (≥2 weeks for thrombocytopenia, >28 days for visual symptoms); avoid concomitant myelosuppressive agents
Quinupristin–dalfopristin	Phlebitis (peripheral administration), myalgias, arthralgias, hyperbilirubinemia	Signs and symptoms of joint or muscle pain	Venous irritation may be alleviated by increasing the infusion volume from 250 to 500 or 750 mL; alternatively administer via a central line
Rifampin	Hepatotoxicity	Baseline liver function tests, and then at least every 2–4 weeks during therapy	Avoid concomitant medications that cause hepatotoxicity; may cause red or orange discoloration of bodily secretions (urine, sweat, tears)
Vancomycin	Nephrotoxicity, red man syndrome	Target trough concentrations of 15–20 mcg/mL[a] (mg/L; 10–14 μmol/L)	Red man syndrome may be managed by prolonging the infusion time from 1 to 2 hours; administration of an antihistamine prior to loading or maintenance doses may also be considered

[a]Measuring peak serum vancomycin concentrations is no longer recommended.

S. aureus (MSSA) is 6 weeks of nafcillin or oxacillin, often combined with a short course of gentamicin (Table 89-4). Four weeks of monotherapy with nafcillin or oxacillin may be sufficient for uncomplicated infections (no perivalvular abscess or septic metastatic complications). From in vitro studies, the combination of an aminoglycoside and penicillinase-resistant penicillin or vancomycin enhances the activity of these drugs for MSSA. In animal models of endocarditis, combinations of penicillin with an aminoglycoside eradicate organisms from vegetations more rapidly than penicillins alone.[39,50] In most human studies, the addition of an aminoglycoside to nafcillin hastens the resolution of fever and bacteremia, but it does not affect survival or relapse rates and can increase renal toxicity.[39,51,52] One small cohort study has demonstrated a decrease in recurrent bacteremia with combination therapy.[53] Traditional twice- or three-times-daily dosing of aminoglycosides is recommended when administered for staphylococcal infective endocarditis; however, there is a report with gentamicin given once a day.[54]

If a patient has a mild, delayed allergy to penicillin, first-generation cephalosporins (such as cefazolin) are effective alternatives, but they should be avoided for patients with a history of immediate-type hypersensitivity reactions to penicillins (see Table 89-4). The potential for a true immediate-type allergy should be assessed carefully. A penicillin skin test should be conducted before giving antibiotic treatment to any patient with infective endocarditis caused by MSSA if there is a questionable penicillin allergy.[55] 9 For a patient with a positive skin test or a history of immediate hypersensitivity to penicillin, vancomycin is chosen. Vancomycin, however, kills *S. aureus* slowly and is regarded as inferior to penicillinase-resistant penicillins for MSSA.[56] Alternatively, patients with immediate-type hypersensitivity reactions to penicillin who fail to respond to vancomycin therapy should be considered for penicillin desensitization.[4] Generally, antibiotic therapy should be continued for 6 weeks. Unfortunately, left-sided infective endocarditis caused by *S. aureus* continues to have a poor prognosis, with a mortality rate between 17% and >50%.[1,47] For reasons discussed in the following section, those with infective endocarditis associated with IVDA have a more favorable response to therapy.

During the past decade, staphylococci more commonly have become resistant to penicillinase-resistant penicillins (e.g., methicillin). 9 Although vancomycin is still the most commonly selected alternative in these cases (see Table 89-4), susceptibility reports with MIC >2 mcg/mL (mg/L) and reports of vancomycin-resistant *S. aureus* strains are increasing.[20] Literature has emerged documenting success with daptomycin or linezolid for these patients.[57–62] Based on available data, daptomycin (at a dose of 6 mg/kg/day) was approved by the FDA in 2006 for the treatment of *S. aureus* bacteremia associated with right-sided NVE and is now a recommended alternative.[20,58] Higher doses of daptomycin (8 to 10 mg/kg/day) have been used in clinical practice and may be preferred by some experts, although prospective, randomized clinical trials are lacking.[20,63–65] To date, linezolid has not been approved by the FDA for use in endocarditis as most available data are based on case reports, and there is concern regarding use of a bacteriostatic agent for this condition.[20,57,66] Furthermore, the FDA issued a warning for linezolid in 2007 following reports from one study that patients with catheter-related bacteremia treated with linezolid had an increased incidence of death due to gram-negative bacillary infections.[67] The presence or lack of a prosthetic heart valve in patients with a methicillin-resistant organism guides therapy and determines whether vancomycin should be used alone or, if a prosthetic valve is present, whether combination therapy is necessary (Table 89-5).[4]

Staphylococcus Endocarditis: IV Drug Abuser

Infective endocarditis in those with IVDA is frequently (60% to 70%) caused by *S. aureus*, although other organisms may be common in certain geographic locations.[1] In this setting, the tricuspid valve is frequently infected, resulting in right-sided infective endocarditis. Most patients have no history of valve abnormalities, are usually otherwise healthy, and have a good response to medical treatment. Nonetheless, surgery may be required.

An uncomplicated, left-sided MSSA endocarditis may be treated sufficiently with 4 weeks of monotherapy with penicillinase-resistant penicillin.[4] For the IV drug abuser, however, the clinical response with right-sided MSSA endocarditis is usually excellent. These patients may be treated effectively (clinical and microbiologic cure exceeding 85%) with a 2-week course of nafcillin or oxacillin plus an aminoglycoside.[68–74] There are limited data on using short-course vancomycin, in place of nafcillin or oxacillin.[69,74] Another trial suggested that a 2-week regimen of a penicillinase-resistant penicillin alone, without the addition of an aminoglycoside, is as effective as combined therapy in MSSA tricuspid valve endocarditis.[75] Although these data suggest that an aminoglycoside is unnecessary for short-course treatment in the IV drug abuser with right-sided infective endocarditis, most clinicians are uncomfortable with monotherapy and choose combination treatment so long as there are no reasons to avoid an aminoglycoside. Short-course therapy should not be used in left-sided endocarditis, and it is inappropriate for patients with underlying acquired immunodeficiency syndrome, renal failure, meningitis, or substantial pulmonary complications, such as lung abscess from right-sided infective endocarditis.[4]

An intriguing therapeutic approach for staphylococcal endocarditis in those with IVDA is oral treatment. One study indicated that short-course IV treatment (primarily nafcillin; mean: 16 days) followed by oral treatment (dicloxacillin or oxacillin; mean: 26 days) might be effective for tricuspid valve MSSA endocarditis.[76] The positive results of this trial can be explained by the duration of IV antibiotics (>2 weeks) being longer than sufficient. Two other studies that predominantly used oral therapy (ciprofloxacin and rifampin) demonstrated efficacy (cure rates exceeding 90%) in addicts with uncomplicated right-sided endocarditis caused by MSSA.[77,78] At this time, concerns with resistance (e.g., ciprofloxacin) and limited published data preclude routine use of oral antibacterial regimens for the treatment of infective endocarditis in the IV drug abuser.[4]

Staphylococcal Endocarditis: Prosthetic Valves

PVE accounts for approximately 15% of all infective endocarditis cases.[8] An episode of PVE occurring within 2 months of surgery strongly suggests that the cause is staphylococci implanted during the procedure. Yet the risk of staphylococcal endocarditis remains elevated for up to 12 months after valve replacement.[79] Because this type of infective endocarditis is typically a nosocomial infection, methicillin-resistant organisms are common, and vancomycin is the cornerstone of therapy. Combination antimicrobials are recommended because of the high morbidity and mortality associated with PVE and its refractoriness to therapy.[4,11,20] Although the addition of rifampin to a penicillinase-resistant penicillin or vancomycin does not result in predictable bacterial synergism, rifampin may have unique activity against staphylococcal infection that involves prosthetic material, where its addition results in a higher microbiologic cure rate.[66] Combination therapy also decreases the emergence of resistance to rifampin, which frequently occurs when it is used alone. For methicillin-resistant staphylococci (both methicillin-resistant *S. aureus* [MRSA] and coagulase-negative staphylococci), vancomycin is recommended with rifampin for 6 weeks or more (see Table 89-5). An aminoglycoside is added for the first 2 weeks if the organism is aminoglycoside susceptible. For MSSA, penicillinase-resistant penicillin is administered in place of vancomycin. PVE responds poorly to medical treatment and has a higher mortality compared with NVE. Valve dehiscence and incompetence can result in acute heart failure, and surgery is often a component of treatment.[4,33]

Twelve months or more after valve replacement, the likely organism for PVE parallels that of NVE. As with NVE, antimicrobial therapy should be based on the identified organism and in vitro susceptibility. If an organism is identified other than staphylococci, the treatment regimen should be guided by susceptibilities and should be at least 6 weeks in duration.[4] Additionally, a concomitant aminoglycoside is recommended if streptococci or enterococci are identified. Once-daily aminoglycoside regimens have not been adequately evaluated in PVE and are not recommended.[4]

The use of anticoagulation is controversial in PVE. In general, those who require anticoagulation for a prosthetic valve should continue the anticoagulant cautiously during endocarditis therapy, unless a contraindication to therapy exists. It is recommended to hold all anticoagulation for at least 2 weeks for patients with *S. aureus* PVE if a recent CNS embolic event has occurred.[4]

Enterococcal Endocarditis

Enterococci are normal inhabitants of the human GI tract and, occasionally, of the anterior urethra. These organisms are usually of low virulence but can become pathogens in predisposed patients following genitourinary manipulations (older men) or obstetric procedures (younger women).[19] Historically, enterococci were considered group D streptococci, but they have been reclassified into the genus *Enterococcus* (*E. faecalis* and *E. faecium*). *E. faecalis* is the most common clinical isolate (approximately 90%) of the two species. Enterococci cause 5% to 18% of endocarditis cases, but they are more resistant to therapy than staphylococci and streptococci. Enterococci are noteworthy for the following reasons: (a) no single antibiotic is bactericidal, (b) MICs to penicillin are relatively high (1 to 25 mcg/mL [mg/L]), (c) intrinsic resistance occurs to all cephalosporins and relative resistance occurs to aminoglycosides (e.g., "low-level" aminoglycoside resistance), (d) combinations of a cell-wall–active agent such as a penicillin or vancomycin and an aminoglycoside are necessary for killing, and (e) resistance to all available drugs is increasing.[4,80,81]

Monotherapy with penicillin for infective endocarditis caused by enterococci results in relapse rates of 50% to 80%. When used alone, penicillins are only bacteriostatic against enterococci, and combination therapy is always recommended for susceptible strains.[4] The relapse rate following penicillin–gentamicin therapy for susceptible strains is less than 15%.[5] The killing of enterococci by the bactericidal combination of an aminoglycoside antibiotic and a penicillin is the best clinical example of antibiotic synergy. Because the aminoglycoside cannot penetrate the bacterial cell in the absence of the penicillin, enterococci usually will appear to be resistant to aminoglycosides by routine susceptibility testing (low-level resistance). However, in the presence of an agent that disrupts the cell wall such as penicillin, the aminoglycoside can gain entry, attach to bacterial ribosomes, and cause rapid cell death. An aminoglycoside–vancomycin combination is also synergistic against enterococci and is appropriate therapy for the penicillin-allergic patient.[4,19]

Enterococcal endocarditis ordinarily requires 4 to 6 weeks of ampicillin or high-dose penicillin G plus an aminoglycoside for cure (Table 89-6). Ampicillin has greater in vitro activity than penicillin G, although there are no clinical data to document differences in efficacy. A 6-week course is recommended for patients with symptoms lasting longer than 3 months and those with PVE. Streptomycin has been the most extensively studied aminoglycoside, but gentamicin is presently favored. Because of resistance, other aminoglycosides, such as tobramycin and amikacin, cannot be substituted routinely. In the treatment of enterococcal endocarditis, relatively low serum concentrations of aminoglycosides appear adequate for successful therapy, such as a gentamicin peak concentration of approximately 3 to 4 mcg/mL (mg/L; 6.3 to 8.4 μmol/L).[4,82] Treatment of enterococcal endocarditis does not have the high success rate seen with infective endocarditis caused by viridans streptococci, presumably because the organism is more resistant to killing.

Although some data support the use of extended-interval aminoglycoside dosing for other types of endocarditis (i.e., streptococci), the data are more vague regarding this strategy in enterococcal infective endocarditis.[83] Even though some studies suggest that extended-interval aminoglycoside dosing and short-interval (traditional) dosing are clinically equivalent,[84–86] discordant studies imply otherwise.[87,88] The paucity of human data precludes routine use of extended-interval aminoglycoside dosing in this setting and the guidelines recommend three-times-daily dosing.[4]

Resistance among enterococci to penicillins and aminoglycosides is increasing.[4] Enterococci that exhibit high-level resistance to streptomycin (MIC >2,000 mcg/mL [mg/L]) are not synergistically killed by penicillin and streptomycin because the aminoglycoside either no longer binds to the ribosome or is inactivated by an aminoglycoside-modifying enzyme, streptomycin adenylase. Because enterococci will appear resistant to aminoglycosides on routine susceptibility testing, the only way to distinguish high-level from low-level resistance is by performing special susceptibility tests using 500 to 2,000 mcg/mL (mg/L) of the aminoglycoside. High-level streptomycin-resistant enterococci occur with a frequency approaching 60%, and high-level resistance to gentamicin is now found in 10% to 50% of isolates. Although most gentamicin-resistant enterococci are resistant to all aminoglycosides (including amikacin), 30% to 50% remain susceptible to streptomycin.[19,80] High-level gentamicin resistance is mediated by a bifunctional aminoglycoside-modifying enzyme, 6-acetyltransferase/2-phosphotransferase, and most strains also possess streptomycin adenylase. These organisms do not commonly cause infective endocarditis; data on appropriate therapy are sparse, and therapeutic options are few.[80,81,89]

In addition to isolates with high-level aminoglycoside resistance, β-lactamase–producing enterococci (especially *E. faecium*) have been reported. If these organisms are discovered, use of vancomycin or ampicillin–sulbactam in combination with gentamicin should be considered. Vancomycin-resistant enterococci are reported increasingly, primarily with *E. faecium*. Vancomycin resistance occurs when the bacterium replaces the normal vancomycin target with a peptidoglycan precursor that does not bind vancomycin.[81]

Treating multidrug-resistant enterococci is difficult, and data on appropriate therapy are sparse. Current guidelines suggest either linezolid or quinupristin–dalfopristin for resistant strains of *E. faecium* and combination β-lactam therapy (ampicillin with either imipenem–cilastatin or ceftriaxone) for *E. faecalis*.[4] Daptomycin has produced conflicting results.[90–94] Surgery and replacement of the infected cardiac valve may be the only cure.

HACEK Group

Fastidious gram-negative bacteria from the group of bacteria including *Haemophilus parainfluenzae, Haemophilus aphrophilus, Actinobacillus actinomycetemcomitans, Cardiobacterium hominis, Eikenella corrodens*, and *Kingella kingae* (HACEK group) account for 5% to 10% of native valve, community-acquired infective endocarditis.[4] Frequently, these types of infective endocarditis present as subacute illnesses with large vegetations and emboli.[19] These oropharyngeal organisms typically are slow growing and should be considered as possible causes of "culture-negative" endocarditis. In the past, high-dose ampicillin with gentamicin for 4 weeks was an acceptable treatment regimen for HACEK endocarditis, but β-lactamase–producing organisms are occurring more often; hence, HACEK organisms should be considered resistant to ampicillin alone. Numerous treatments are reasonable for the treatment of HACEK infective endocarditis, including ceftriaxone and ampicillin–sulbactam; the newest addition to the guidelines is oral ciprofloxacin for select patients (Table 89-7).[4] Treatment is usually for 4 weeks, but it should be extended to 6 weeks in PVE caused by one of these organisms.

Less Common Types of Infective Endocarditis

Atypical Microorganisms

Endocarditis caused by organisms such as *Bartonella*; *Coxiella burnetii*; *Brucella, Candida*, and *Aspergillus* spp.; *Legionella*; and gram-negative bacilli (e.g., *Pseudomonas*) is relatively uncommon. Medical therapy for infective endocarditis caused by these organisms is usually unsuccessful.[4,5] Consultation with an infectious disease expert is warranted when these microorganisms are identified.

In addition to *Pseudomonas* spp., other gram-negative bacilli that have been implicated include *Salmonella* spp., *Escherichia coli, Citrobacter* spp., *Klebsiella–Enterobacter* spp., *Serratia marcescens, Proteus* spp., and *Providencia* spp.[36] Generally, these infections have a poor prognosis, with mortality rates as high as 60% to 80%.[36] Cardiac surgery in concert with extended-course antibacterial therapy is the recommended course (class IIa; level of evidence: B) for most patients with gram-negative bacillary infective endocarditis. Readers are referred to the AHA guidelines for more extensive review of *Pseudomonas* spp. infective endocarditis and unusual gram-negative bacteria treatment regimens.[4]

Fungi cause between 2% and 4% of endocarditis cases; most patients with fungal endocarditis have undergone recent cardiovascular surgery, are IV drug abusers, have received prolonged treatment with IV catheters or antibiotics, or are immunocompromised.[19,95] *Candida* spp. and *Aspergillus* spp. are the most commonly involved, and the mortality rate is high (greater than 80%) for the following reasons: (a) large, bulky vegetations that often form, (b) systemic septic embolization that may occur, (c) the tendency of fungi to invade the myocardium, (d) poor penetration of vegetations by antifungals, (e) the low toxic-to-therapeutic ratio of agents such as amphotericin B, and (f) the lack of consistent fungicidal activity of available antifungal agents.[3,96] When fungal infective endocarditis is identified, the combined medical–surgical approach is recommended. Because these infections occur infrequently, scant clinical data are available to make solid treatment recommendations; however, the use of antifungal agents alone has been globally unsuccessful. Amphotericin B has been the mainstay pharmacologic approach. The availability of newer antifungal agents challenges this historical approach, although clinical trial data are lacking.[4]

C. burnetii (Q fever) may be recovered from blood cultures, but infection is more likely to be identified via serologic tests. It is a common cause of infective endocarditis in certain areas of the world where goat, cattle, and sheep farming are widespread. The most favorable therapy for Q fever is unknown but may include doxycycline with trimethoprim–sulfamethoxazole, rifampin, or fluoroquinolones.[19] *Brucella* are facultative intracellular gram-negative bacilli. Humans are infected by this organism after ingesting infected unpasteurized milk or undercooked meat, inhalation of infectious aerosols, or contact with infected tissues. This type of infective endocarditis is more common in veterinarians and livestock handlers. Cure requires valve replacement and antimicrobial agents including doxycycline with streptomycin or gentamicin or doxycycline with trimethoprim–sulfamethoxazole or rifampin for an extended period (8 weeks to months).[19]

Culture-Negative Endocarditis

Sterile blood cultures are reported in 5% to 20% of patients with infective endocarditis if strict diagnostic criteria are used.[5,11] This type of infective endocarditis may occur as a result of unidentified subacute right-sided infective endocarditis, previous antibiotic therapy, slow-growing fastidious organisms, nonbacterial etiologies (e.g., fungi), and improperly collected blood cultures. When blood cultures from patients suspected of infective endocarditis show no growth after 48 to 72 hours, the laboratory should be advised, and cultures should be held for up to a month to detect growth of fastidious organisms.[4]

The AHA guidelines provide general recommendations for culture-negative infective endocarditis (Table 89-7), although clinicians should individualize therapy, as necessary. Selection of treatment can be difficult, balancing the need to cover all likely organisms against potential toxic drug effects (e.g., aminoglycosides). Antimicrobial selection should be in consultation with an infectious disease specialist. Irrespective of the chosen treatment, extended antimicrobial therapy is required. The empirical approaches for culture-negative infective endocarditis highlight the need for proper collection and monitoring of blood cultures and an extensive medication history.

PERSONALIZED PHARMACOTHERAPY

Infective endocarditis remains an uncommon disease, but the cost of treatment can be substantial. In the past, the long duration of hospitalization required to administer IV antimicrobials was the major expense. In select cases, abbreviated and/or outpatient, oral antimicrobial therapy may appreciably reduce the cost of care.

Shorter-course antimicrobial regimens are advocated when possible. For instance, in exquisitely sensitive streptococcal endocarditis (MICs less than 0.12 mcg/mL [mg/L]), a 2-week regimen of high-dose parenteral penicillin G or ceftriaxone in combination with an aminoglycoside is as effective as 4 weeks of penicillin alone.[4] Uncomplicated right-sided MSSA endocarditis in the IV drug abuser may be treated with a 2-week course. Treatment with nafcillin or oxacillin in combination with an aminoglycoside appears to be cost-effective.

The initiation of outpatient parenteral antibiotics should be considered early in the treatment of infective endocarditis, after the patient is stable clinically and responds favorably to initial antibiotics. Outpatient treatment is safe and cost-effective in select situations.[26,97] Patients considered for home therapy must be hemodynamically stable, compliant with therapy, have careful medical monitoring, understand the potential complications of the disease, and have immediate access to medical care. Advances in technology allow for the outpatient administration of complex antibiotic regimens that significantly reduce the cost of therapy. Simple regimens, such as single daily doses of ceftriaxone for streptococcal infective endocarditis, are particularly attractive. Although endocarditis is common in those with a history of IVDA and home healthcare would substantially reduce the cost of treatment, many clinicians are uncomfortable with outpatient IV therapy because central venous access is required. Sudden cardiac decompensation in an outpatient setting is also of concern.[4,98]

EVALUATION OF THERAPEUTIC OUTCOMES

The evaluation of patients treated for infective endocarditis includes assessment of disease signs and symptoms, blood cultures, microbiologic tests, serum drug concentrations, and other tests that evaluate organ function.

Signs and Symptoms

Fever usually subsides within 1 week of initiating therapy.[5,17,98] Persistence of fever may indicate ineffective antimicrobial therapy, emboli, infections of intravascular catheters, or drug reactions. For some patients, low-grade fever may persist even with appropriate antimicrobial therapy. With defervescence, the patient should begin to feel better, and other symptoms, such as lethargy or weakness, should subside. Echocardiography should be performed when antibiotic therapy has been completed to determine new baseline cardiac function (i.e., ventricular size and function). A TTE is usually sufficient.

Blood Cultures

Blood cultures should be negative within a few days, although microbiologic response to vancomycin may be slower. If bacteria continue to be isolated from blood beyond the first few days of therapy, it may indicate that the antimicrobials are inactive against the pathogen or that the doses are not producing adequate concentrations at the site of infection. After the initiation of therapy, blood cultures should be rechecked until negative. During the remainder of therapy, frequent blood culturing is not necessary. Additional blood cultures should be rechecked after successful treatment (e.g., once or twice within the 8 weeks after treatment) to ensure cure.[4]

Microbiologic Tests

For all isolates from blood cultures, MICs should be determined; MBCs are no longer recommended.[4] The agent currently being used should be tested, as well as alternatives that may be required if intolerance, allergy, or resistance occurs. Occasionally, it is useful to determine whether synergy exists for antimicrobial combinations, although synergistic regimens usually can be predicted from the literature. eChapter 24 summarizes the methods for in vitro determinations of synergy.

Serum bactericidal titers (SBTs; also called *Schlichter's tests*) have been used in the past in association with a number of infectious diseases. The SBT is the greatest dilution of a patient's serum sample that is obtained while receiving antimicrobial treatment that kills greater than 99.9% of an inoculum of the infecting pathogen in vitro over 18 to 24 hours.

Although specific SBTs have been evaluated in endocarditis, at present, SBTs have little value in monitoring treatment of common types of infective endocarditis and should not be recommended routinely.[4,99] This test may be useful when the causative organisms are only moderately susceptible to antimicrobials, when less-well-established regimens are used, or when response to therapy is suboptimal and dosage escalation is being considered.

Serum Drug Concentrations

Of the agents used commonly for infective endocarditis, measurement of serum drug concentrations is routinely available for aminoglycosides (except streptomycin) and vancomycin. Few data, however, support attaining any specific serum concentrations for patients with infective endocarditis. In general, serum concentrations of the antimicrobial should exceed the MBC of the organisms. Aminoglycoside concentrations rarely exceed the MBC for certain organisms, such as streptococci and enterococci, and concentrations of aminoglycosides and vancomycin for staphylococci have not been correlated with response.[99,100]

When aminoglycosides are administered for infective endocarditis caused by gram-positive cocci with a traditional three-times-daily regimen, peak serum concentrations are recommended to be on the low side of the traditional ranges (3 to 4 mcg/mL [mg/L; 6.3 to 8.4 μmol/L] for gentamicin). If extended-interval dosing is used, which is only recommended in streptococcal infective endocarditis, the most appropriate method of monitoring has not been determined. When vancomycin is administered, the most recent treatment guidelines for infective endocarditis recommend serum drug monitoring of peak and trough concentrations.[4] However, it is now generally accepted that peak concentrations of vancomycin have limited clinical applicability and the primary goal of serum vancomycin monitoring is to ensure adequate trough concentrations, in this case 15 to 20 mcg/mL (mg/L; 10 to 14 μmol/L), are achieved.[101]

PREVENTION

10 Antimicrobial prophylaxis is used as an attempt to prevent infective endocarditis for patients who are at the highest risk.[6,18] The use of antimicrobials for this purpose requires consideration of (a) cardiac conditions associated with endocarditis, (b) procedures causing bacteremia, (c) organisms likely to cause endocarditis, and (d) pharmacokinetics, spectrum, cost, adverse effects, and ease of administration of available antimicrobial agents. The objective of prophylaxis is to diminish the likelihood of infective endocarditis in high-risk individuals from procedures that result in bacteremia. Although there are no prospective, controlled human trials demonstrating that prophylaxis in high-risk individuals protects against the development of endocarditis during bacteremia-induced procedures, animal studies suggest possible benefit.[18] Many causes of infective endocarditis, however, appear not to be secondary to an invasive procedure. Bacteremia as a consequence of daily activities may, in fact, be the major culprit, and the value of antibiotic prophylaxis before bacteremia-causing procedures has been questioned.[102] Retrospective human studies, though, support that a reduction of endocarditis occurs for select patients following dental surgery where prophylaxis is employed.[18] The common practice of using antimicrobial therapy in this setting remains controversial. The mechanism of a beneficial effect in humans is unclear, but antibiotics may decrease the number of bacteria at the surgical site, kill bacteria after they are introduced into the blood, and prevent adhesion of bacteria to the valve. Prophylaxis does not reduce the frequency of bacteremia immediately following tooth extraction as compared with a control group, suggesting that a reduction in adhesion or effects after the bacteria adhere to the endocardium are more likely mechanisms.[103,104] Other studies have further questioned the benefit of antibiotic prophylaxis.[105]

Clinical **Controversy...**

The common practice of administering antibiotics to high-risk individuals before a bacteremia-causing procedure is controversial. Despite limited data supporting this approach and the fact that 100% compliance with AHA preventative guidelines would have only a modest benefit, the use of single-dose antibiotics for the prevention of endocarditis remains a standard of care.

Regardless of the controversy about whether prophylactic antibiotics should be used, infective endocarditis prophylaxis is recommended in select situations, specifically dental procedures, in those with underlying high-risk cardiac conditions. The AHA released updated guidelines that better define who should and should not receive infective endocarditis prophylaxis.[18] This update is important as data show overuse of infective endocarditis prophylaxis occurs in low-risk patients and underuse occurs in those at greater risk.[106]

Key points of this report are that (a) only a small number of cases of infective endocarditis might be prevented with antibiotic prophylaxis for dental procedures, even if 100% effective; (b) infective endocarditis prophylaxis for dental procedures should be recommended only for patients with underlying cardiac conditions associated with the highest risk; (c) for those with high-risk underlying cardiac conditions, prophylaxis is recommended for all dental procedures involving manipulation of gingival tissue or the periapical region of teeth or perforation of the oral mucosa; (d) prophylaxis is not recommended based solely on an increased lifetime risk of acquisition of infective endocarditis; and (e) administration of antibiotics solely to prevent endocarditis is not recommended for patients who undergo a genitourinary or GI tract procedure.

TABLE 89-10 Prophylaxis of Infective Endocarditis

Highest Risk Cardiac Conditions	Presence of a prosthetic heart valve Prior diagnosis of infective endocarditis Cardiac transplantation with subsequent valvulopathy Congenital heart disease (CHD)[a]	
Types of procedures	Any that require perforation of the oral mucosa or manipulation of the periapical region of the teeth of gingival tissue	
Antimicrobial Options	**Adult Doses[b]**	**Pediatric Doses[b] (mg/kg)**
Oral amoxicillin	2 g	50
IM or IV ampicillin[c]	2 g	50
IM or IV cefazolin or ceftriaxone[c,d,e]	1 g	50
Oral cephalexin[d,e,f]	2 g	50
Oral clindamycin[e]	600 mg	20
Oral azithromycin or clarithromycin[e]	500 mg	15
IV or IM clindamycin[c,e]	600 mg	20

[a]Includes only the following: unrepaired cyanotic CHD, prophlyaxis within the first 6 months of implanting prosthetic material to repair a congenital heart defect, and repaired CHD with residual defects at or adjacent to prosthetic material.
[b]All one-time doses administered 30–60 minutes prior to initiation of the procedure.
[c]For patients unable to tolerate oral medication.
[d]Should be avoided in patients with immediate-type hypersensitivity reaction to penicillin or ampicillin (e.g., anaphylaxis, urticaria, or angioedema).
[e]Option for patients with nonimmediate hypersensitivity reaction to penicillin or ampicillin.
[f]May substitute with an alternative first- or second-generation cephalosporin at an equivalent dose.

Data from reference 18.

To determine whether a patient should receive prophylactic antibiotics, one needs to assess the patient's risk and whether he or she is undergoing a procedure resulting in bacteremia. When antibiotic prophylaxis is appropriate, a single 2 g dose of amoxicillin is recommended for adult patients at risk, given 30 to 60 minutes before undergoing procedures associated with bacteremia. Because the duration of antimicrobial prophylaxis appears to be relatively short, guidelines do not advocate a second oral dose of amoxicillin, which was recommended previously. Alternative prophylaxis regimens for patients allergic to penicillins or those unable to take oral medications are also provided. A summary of guideline recommendations is available in Table 89-10. Consultation of the full AHA guideline is suggested for more detailed information.[18]

ABBREVIATIONS

AHA	American Heart Association
CDIE	cardiac device infective endocarditis
CHD	congenital heart disease
HACEK	the group of bacteria including *Haemophilus parainfluenzae, Haemophilus aphrophilus, Actinobacillus actinomycetemcomitans, Cardiobacterium hominis, Eikenella corrodens*, and *Kingella kingae*

IVDA	IV drug abuse
MBC	minimal bactericidal concentration
MIC	minimal inhibitory concentration
MRSA	methicillin-resistant *Staphylococcus aureus*
MSSA	methicillin-sensitive *Staphylococcus aureus*
NVE	native valve endocarditis
PVE	prosthetic valve endocarditis
SBT	serum bactericidal titer
TEE	transesophageal echocardiogram
TTE	transthoracic echocardiogram

REFERENCES

1. Qui Y, Moreillon P. Infective endocarditis. Nat Rev Cardiol 2011;8:322–336.
2. Pierce D, Calkins BC, Thornton K. Infectious endocarditis: Diagnosis and treatment. Am Fam Physician 2012;85: 981–986.
3. Fernandez Guerrero ML, Alvarez B, Manzarbeitia F, Renedo G. Infective endocarditis at autopsy: A review of pathologic manifestations and clinical correlates. Medicine 2012;91:152–164.
4. Baddour LM, Wilson WR, Bayer AS, et al. Infective endocarditis: Diagnosis, antimicrobial therapy, and management of complications: A statement for healthcare professionals from the Committee on Rheumatic Fever, Endocarditis, and Kawasaki Disease, Council on Cardiovascular Disease in the Young, and the Councils on Clinical Cardiology, Stroke, and Cardiovascular Surgery and Anesthesia, American Heart Association: Endorsed by the Infectious Diseases Society of America. Circulation 2005;111:e394–e434.
5. Mylonakis E, Calderwood SB. Infective endocarditis in adults. N Engl J Med 2001;345:1318–1330.
6. Nishimura RA, Carabello BA, Faxon DP, et al. ACC/AHA 2008 guideline update on valvular heart disease: Focused update on infective endocarditis: A report of the American College of Cardiology/American Heart Association Task Force on Practice Guidelines: Endorsed by the Society of Cardiovascular Anesthesiologists, Society for Cardiovascular Angiography and Interventions, and Society of Thoracic Surgeons. Circulation 2008;118:887–896.
7. Baddour LM, Epstein AE, Erickson CC, et al.; on behalf of the American Heart Association Rheumatic Fever, Endocarditis, and Kawasaki Disease Committee of the Council on Cardiovascular Disease in the Young; Council on Cardiovascular Surgery and Anesthesia; Council on Cardiovascular Nursing; Council on Clinical Cardiology; and the Interdisciplinary Council on Quality of Care and Outcomes Research. Update on cardiovascular implantable electronic device infections and their management: A scientific statement from the American Heart Association. Circulation 2010;121:458–477.
8. Berlin JA, Abrutyn E, Strom BL, et al. Incidence of infective endocarditis in the Delaware Valley, 1988–1990. Am J Cardiol 1995;76:933–936.
9. Hogevik H, Olaison L, Andersson R, et al. Epidemiologic aspects of infective endocarditis in an urban population. A 5-year prospective study. Medicine (Baltimore) 1995;74:324–339.
10. Roger VL, Go AS, Lloyd-Jones DM, et al.; on behalf of the American Heart Association Statistics Committee and Stroke Statistics Subcommittee. Heart disease and stroke statistics—2012 update: A report from the American Heart Association. Circulation 2012;125:e2–e220.
11. Murdoch DR, Corey GR, Hoen B, et al. Clinical presentation, etiology, and outcome of infective endocarditis in the 21st century: The International Collaboration on Endocarditis-Prospective Cohort Study. Arch Intern Med 2009;169:463–473.
12. Durante-Mangoni E, Bradley S, Selton-Suty C, et al. Current features of infective endocarditis in elderly patients: Results of the International Collaboration on Endocarditis Prospective Cohort Study. Arch Intern Med 2008;168:2095–2103.
13. Hanai M, Hashimoto K, Mashiko K, et al. Active infective endocarditis: Management and risk analysis of hospital death from 24 years' of experience. Circ J 2008;72:2062–2068.
14. Day MD, Gauvreau K, Shulman S, Newburger JW. Characteristics of children hospitalized with infective endocarditis. Circulation 2009;119:865–870.
15. Athan E, Chu VH, Tattevin P, et al. Clinical characteristics and outcome of infective endocarditis involving implantable cardiac devices. JAMA 2012;307:1727–1735.
16. Benito N, Miro JM, de Lazzari E, et al. Health care-associated native valve endocarditis: Importance of non-nosocomial acquisition. Ann Intern Med 2009;150:586–594.
17. Hill EE, Herijgers P, Herregods MC, Peetermans WE. Evolving trends in infective endocarditis. Clin Microbiol Infect 2006;12:5–12.
18. Wilson W, Taubert KA, Gewitz M, et al. Prevention of infective endocarditis: Guidelines from the American Heart Association: A guideline from the American Heart Association Rheumatic Fever, Endocarditis, and Kawasaki Disease Committee, Council on Cardiovascular Disease in the Young, and the Council on Clinical Cardiology, Council on Cardiovascular Surgery and Anesthesia, and the Quality of Care and Outcomes Research Interdisciplinary Working Group. Circulation 2007;116:1736–1754.
19. Bashore TM, Cabell C, Fowler V. Update on infective endocarditis. Curr Probl Cardiol 2006;31:274–352.
20. Liu C, Bayer A, Cosgrove SE, et al. Clinical practice guidelines by the Infectious Diseases Society of America for the treatment of methicillin-resistant *Staphylococcus aureus* infections in adults and children. Clin Infect Dis 2011;52:1–38.
21. Thuny F, Grisoli D, Collart F, et al. Management of infective endocarditis: Challenges and perspectives. Lancet 2012;379:965–975.
22. Sachdev M, Peterson GE, Jollis JG. Imaging techniques for diagnosis of infective endocarditis. Cardiol Clin 2003;21: 185–195.
23. Durack DT, Lukes AS, Bright DK. New criteria for diagnosis of infective endocarditis: Utilization of specific echocardiographic findings. Duke Endocarditis Service. Am J Med 1994;96:200–209.
24. Li JS, Sexton DJ, Mick N, et al. Proposed modifications to the Duke criteria for the diagnosis of infective endocarditis. Clin Infect Dis 2000;30:633–638.
25. Tice AD, Rehm SJ, Dalovisio JR, et al. Practical guidelines for outpatient parenteral antimicrobial therapy. Clin Infect Dis 2004;38:1651–1672.
26. Bonow RO, Carabello BA, Chatterjee K, et al. 2008 focused update incorporated into the ACC/AHA 2006 guidelines for the management of patients with valvular heart disease: A report of the American College of Cardiology/American Heart Association Task Force on Practice Guidelines (Writing Committee to Revise the 1998 Guidelines for the Management of Patients with Valvular Heart Disease): Endorsed by the Society of Cardiovascular Anesthesiologists, Society for Cardiovascular Angiography and Interventions, and Society of Thoracic Surgeons. Circulation 2008;118:e523–e661.

27. Habib G, Hoen B, Tornos P, et al. Guidelines on the prevention, diagnosis, and treatment of infective endocarditis (new version 2009): The Task Force on the Prevention, Diagnosis, and Treatment of Infective Endocarditis of the European Society of Cardiology (ESC). Eur Heart J 2009;30:2369–2413.
28. Gelsomino S, Maessen JG, van der Veen F, et al. Emergency surgery for native mitral valve endocarditis: The impact of septic and cardiogenic shock. Ann Thorac Surg 2012;93:1469–1476.
29. Ramirez-Duque N, Garcia-Cabrera E, Ivanova-Georgieva R, et al. Surgical treatment for infective endocarditis in elderly patients. J Infect 2011;63:131–138.
30. Manne MB, Shrestha NK, Lytle BW, et al. Outcomes after surgical treatment of native and prosthetic valve infective endocarditis. Ann Thorac Surg 2012;93:489–494.
31. Kiefer T, Park L, Tribouilloy C, et al. Association between valvular surgery and mortality among patients with infective endocarditis complicated by heart failure. JAMA 2011;306:2239–2247.
32. De Feo M, Cotrufo M, Carozza A, et al. The need for a specific risk prediction system in native valve infective endocarditis surgery. Sci World J 2012;2012:307571. doi:10.1100/2102/307571.
33. Byrne JG, Rezai K, Sanchez JA, et al. Surgical management of endocarditis: The Society of Thoracic Surgeons clinical practice guideline. Ann Thorac Surg 2011;91:2012–2019.
34. Kang DH, Kim YJ, Kim SH, et al. Early surgery versus conventional treatment for infective endocarditis. N Engl J Med 2012;366:2466–2473.
35. Elliott TS, Foweraker J, Gould FK, et al. Guidelines for the antibiotic treatment of endocarditis in adults: Report of the Working Party of the British Society for Antimicrobial Chemotherapy. J Antimicrob Chemother 2004;54:971–981.
36. Morpeth S, Murdoch D, Cabell CH, et al. Non-HACEK gram-negative bacillus endocarditis. Ann Intern Med 2007;147:829–835.
37. Lefort A, Chartier L, Sendid B, et al. Diagnosis, management and outcome of *Candida* endocarditis. Clin Microbiol Infect 2012;18:E99–E109.
38. Gruchalla RS, Pirmohamed M. Clinical practice. Antibiotic allergy. N Engl J Med 2006;354:601–609.
39. Falagas ME, Matthaiou DK, Bliziotis IA. The role of aminoglycosides in combination with a beta-lactam for the treatment of bacterial endocarditis: A meta-analysis of comparative trials. J Antimicrob Chemother 2006;57: 639–647.
40. Sexton DJ, Tenenbaum MJ, Wilson WR, et al. Ceftriaxone once daily for four weeks compared with ceftriaxone plus gentamicin once daily for two weeks for treatment of endocarditis due to penicillin-susceptible streptococci. Endocarditis Treatment Consortium Group. Clin Infect Dis 1998;27:1470–1474.
41. Paul M, Leibovici L. Combination antimicrobial treatment versus monotherapy: The contribution of meta-analyses. Infect Dis Clin North Am 2009;23:277–293.
42. Blatter M, Fluckiger U, Entenza J, et al. Simulated human serum profiles of one daily dose of ceftriaxone plus netilmicin in treatment of experimental streptococcal endocarditis. Antimicrob Agents Chemother 1993;37: 1971–1976.
43. Francioli P, Ruch W, Stamboulian D. Treatment of streptococcal endocarditis with a single daily dose of ceftriaxone and netilmicin for 14 days: A prospective multicenter study. Clin Infect Dis 1995;21:1406–1410.
44. Francioli PB, Glauser MP. Synergistic activity of ceftriaxone combined with netilmicin administered once daily for treatment of experimental streptococcal endocarditis. Antimicrob Agents Chemother 1993;37:207–212.
45. Gavalda J, Pahissa A, Almirante B, et al. Effect of gentamicin dosing interval on therapy of viridans streptococcal experimental endocarditis with gentamicin plus penicillin. Antimicrob Agents Chemother 1995;39:2098–2103.
46. Fernandez Guerrero ML, Gonzalez Lopez JJ, Goyenechea A, et al. Endocarditis caused by *Staphylococcus aureus*: A reappraisal of the epidemiologic, clinical, and pathologic manifestations with analysis of factors determining outcome. Medicine (Baltimore) 2009;88:1–22.
47. Ferderspiel J, Stearns SC, Peppercorn AF, et al. Increasing US rates of endocarditis with *Staphylococcus aureus*: 1999-2008. Arch Intern Med 2012;172:363–365.
48. Rasmussen RV, Host U, Arpi M, et al. Prevalence of infective endocarditis in patients with *Staphylococcus aureus* bacteremia: The value of screening with echocardiography. Eur J Echocardiogr 2011;12:414–420.
49. Mermel LA, Allon M, Bouza E, et al. Clinical practice guidelines for the diagnosis and management of intravascular catheter-related infection: 2009 update by the Infectious Diseases Society of America. Clin Infect Dis 2009;49:1–45.
50. Graham JC, Gould FK. Role of aminoglycosides in the treatment of bacterial endocarditis. J Antimicrob Chemother 2002;49:437–444.
51. Cosgrove SE, Vigliani GA, Fowler VG Jr, et al. Initial low-dose gentamicin for *Staphylococcus aureus* bacteremia and endocarditis is nephrotoxic. Clin Infect Dis 2009;48: 713–721.
52. Korzeniowski O, Sande MA. Combination antimicrobial therapy for *Staphylococcus aureus* endocarditis in patients addicted to parenteral drugs and in nonaddicts: A prospective study. Ann Intern Med 1982;97:496–503.
53. Lemonovich TL, Haynes K, Lautenbach E, et al. Combination therapy with an aminoglycoside for *Staphylococcus aureus* endocarditis and/or persistent bacteremia is associated with a decreased rate of recurrent bacteremia: A cohort study. Infection 2011;39:549–554.
54. Gavalda J, Lopez P, Martin T, et al. Efficacy of ceftriaxone and gentamicin given once a day by using human-like pharmacokinetics in treatment of experimental staphylococcal endocarditis. Antimicrob Agents Chemother 2002;46: 378–384.
55. Dodek P, Phillips P. Questionable history of immediate-type hypersensitivity to penicillin in staphylococcal endocarditis: Treatment based on skin-test results versus empirical alternative treatment—A decision analysis. Clin Infect Dis 1999;29:1251–1256.
56. Petti CA, Fowler VG Jr. *Staphylococcus aureus* bacteremia and endocarditis. Cardiol Clin 2003;21:219–233.
57. Falagas ME, Manta KG, Ntziora F, Vardakas KZ. Linezolid for the treatment of patients with endocarditis: A systematic review of the published evidence. J Antimicrob Chemother 2006;58:273–280.
58. Fowler VG Jr, Boucher HW, Corey GR, et al. Daptomycin versus standard therapy for bacteremia and endocarditis caused by *Staphylococcus aureus*. N Engl J Med 2006;355: 653–665.
59. Moore CL, Osaki-Kiyan P, Haque N, et al. Daptomycin versus vancomycin for bloodstream infections due to methicillin-resistant *Staphylococcus aureus* with a high vancomycin minimum inhibitory concentration: A case control study. Clin Infect Dis 2012;54:51–58.
60. Levine DP, Lamp KC. Daptomycin in the treatment of patients with infective endocarditis: Experience from a registry. Am J Med 2007;120(10 Suppl 1):S28–S33.

61. Rehm SJ, Boucher H, Levine D, et al. Daptomycin versus vancomycin plus gentamicin for treatment of bacteraemia and endocarditis due to *Staphylococcus aureus*: Subset analysis of patients infected with methicillin-resistant isolates. J Antimicrob Chemother 2008;62:1413–1421.
62. Segreti JA, Crank CW, Finney MS. Daptomycin for the treatment of gram-positive bacteremia and infective endocarditis: A retrospective case series of 31 patients. Pharmacotherapy 2006;26:347–352.
63. Wu G, Abraham T, Rapp J, et al. Daptomycin: Evaluation of a high-dose treatment strategy. Int J Antimicrob Agents 2011;38:192–196.
64. Dutante-Mangoni E, Casillo R, Bernardo M, et al. High-dose daptomycin for cardiac electronic device-related infective endocarditis. Clin Infect Dis 2012;54:347–354.
65. Kullar R, Davis SL, Levine DP, et al. High-dose daptomycin for treatment of complicated gram-positive infections: A large, multicenter, retrospective study. Pharmacotherapy 2011;31:527–536.
66. Gold HS, Pillai SK. Antistaphylococcal agents. Infect Dis Clin North Am 2009;23:99–131.
67. Information for Healthcare Professionals: Linezolid (Marketed as Zyvox). 2012, *http://www.fda.gov/Drugs/DrugSafety/PostmarketDrugSafetyInformationforPatientsandProviders/DrugSafetyInformationforHeathcareProfessionals/ucm085249.htm.*
68. Chambers HF. Short-course combination and oral therapies of *Staphylococcus aureus* endocarditis. Infect Dis Clin North Am 1993;7:69–80.
69. Chambers HF, Miller RT, Newman MD. Right-sided *Staphylococcus aureus* endocarditis in intravenous drug abusers: Two-week combination therapy. Ann Intern Med 1988;109:619–624.
70. DiNubile MJ. Abbreviated therapy for right-sided *Staphylococcus aureus* endocarditis in injecting drug users: The time has come? Eur J Clin Microbiol Infect Dis 1994;13:533–534.
71. DiNubile MJ. Short-course antibiotic therapy for right-sided endocarditis caused by *Staphylococcus aureus* in injection drug users. Ann Intern Med 1994;121:873–876.
72. Espinosa FJ, Valdes M, Martin-Luengo F, et al. Right endocarditis caused by *Staphylococcus aureus* in parenteral drug addicts: Evaluation of a combined therapeutic scheme for 2 weeks versus conventional treatment. Enferm Infecc Microbiol Clin 1993;11:235–240.
73. Torres-Tortosa M, de Cueto M, Vergara A, et al. Prospective evaluation of a two-week course of intravenous antibiotics in intravenous drug addicts with infective endocarditis. Grupo de Estudiode Enfermedades Infecciosas de la Provincia de Cadiz. Eur J Clin Microbiol Infect Dis 1994;13:559–564.
74. Yung D, Kottachchi D, Neupane B, et al. Antimicrobials for right-sided endocarditis in intravenous drug users: A systematic review. J Antimicrob Chemother 2007;60:921–928.
75. Ribera E, Gomez-Jimenez J, Cortes E, et al. Effectiveness of cloxacillin with and without gentamicin in short-term therapy for right-sided *Staphylococcus aureus* endocarditis. A randomized, controlled trial. Ann Intern Med 1996;125:969–974.
76. Parker RH, Fossieck BE Jr. Intravenous followed by oral antimicrobial therapy for staphylococcal endocarditis. Ann Intern Med 1980;93:832–834.
77. Dworkin RJ, Lee BL, Sande MA, et al. Treatment of right-sided *Staphylococcus aureus* endocarditis in intravenous drug users with ciprofloxacin and rifampicin. Lancet 1989;2:1071–1073.
78. Heldman AW, Hartert TV, Ray SC, et al. Oral antibiotic treatment of right-sided staphylococcal endocarditis in injection drug users: Prospective randomized comparison with parenteral therapy. Am J Med 1996;101:68–76.
79. Lopez J, Revilla A, Vilacosta I, et al. Definition, clinical profile, microbiological spectrum, and prognostic factors of early-onset prosthetic valve endocarditis. Eur Heart J 2007;28:760–765.
80. Fernandez Guerrero ML, Goyenechea A, Verdejo C, et al. Enterococcal endocarditis on native and prosthetic valves: A review of clinical and prognostic factors with emphasis on hospital-acquired infections as a major determinant of outcome. Medicine (Baltimore) 2007;86:363–377.
81. Sood S, Malhotra M, Das BK, et al. Enterococcal infections & antimicrobial resistance. Indian J Med Res 2008;128:111–121.
82. Wilson WR, Wilkowske CJ, Wright AJ, et al. Treatment of streptomycin-susceptible and streptomycin-resistant enterococcal endocarditis. Ann Intern Med 1984;100:816–823.
83. Tam VH, Preston SL, Briceland LL. Once-daily aminoglycosides in the treatment of gram-positive endocarditis. Ann Pharmacother 1999;33:600–606.
84. Gavalda J, Cardona PJ, Almirante B, et al. Treatment of experimental endocarditis due to *Enterococcus faecalis* using once-daily dosing regimen of gentamicin plus simulated profiles of ampicillin in human serum. Antimicrob Agents Chemother 1996;40:173–178.
85. Houlihan HH, Stokes DP, Rybak MJ. Pharmacodynamics of vancomycin and ampicillin alone and in combination with gentamicin once daily or thrice daily against *Enterococcus faecalis* in an in vitro infection model. J Antimicrob Chemother 2000;46:79–86.
86. Schwank S, Blaser J. Once-versus thrice-daily netilmicin combined with amoxicillin, penicillin, or vancomycin against *Enterococcus faecalis* in a pharmacodynamic in vitro model. Antimicrob Agents Chemother 1996;40:2258–2261.
87. Fantin B, Carbon C. Importance of the aminoglycoside dosing regimen in the penicillin–netilmicin combination for treatment of *Enterococcus faecalis*-induced experimental endocarditis. Antimicrob Agents Chemother 1990;34:2387–2391.
88. Marangos MN, Nicolau DP, Quintiliani R, et al. Influence of gentamicin dosing interval on the efficacy of penicillin-containing regimens in experimental *Enterococcus faecalis* endocarditis. J Antimicrob Chemother 1997;39:519–522.
89. Lipman ML, Silva J Jr. Endocarditis due to *Streptococcus faecalis* with high-level resistance to gentamicin. Rev Infect Dis 1989;11:325–328.
90. Arias CA, Torres HA, Singh KV, et al. Failure of daptomycin monotherapy for endocarditis caused by an *Enterococcus faecium* strain with vancomycin-resistant and vancomycin-susceptible subpopulations and evidence of in vivo loss of the vanA gene cluster. Clin Infect Dis 2007;45:1343–1346.
91. Cunha BA, Mickail N, Eisenstein L. *E. faecalis* vancomycin-sensitive enterococcal bacteremia unresponsive to a vancomycin tolerant strain successfully treated with high-dose daptomycin. Heart Lung 2007;36:456–461.
92. Hidron AI, Schuetz AN, Nolte FS, et al. Daptomycin resistance in *Enterococcus faecalis* prosthetic valve endocarditis. J Antimicrob Chemother 2008;61:1394–1396.
93. Jenkins I. Linezolid- and vancomycin-resistant *Enterococcus faecium* endocarditis: Successful treatment with tigecycline and daptomycin. J Hosp Med 2007;2:343–344.

94. Forrest GN, Arnold RS, Gammie JS, et al. Single center experience of a vancomycin resistant enterococcal endocarditis cohort. J Infect 2011;63:420–428.
95. Falcone M, Barzaghi N, Carosi G, et al. *Candida* infective endocarditis: Report of 15 cases from a prospective multicenter study. Medicine (Baltimore) 2009;88:160–168.
96. Pierrotti LC, Baddour LM. Fungal endocarditis, 1995–2000. Chest 2002;122:302–310.
97. Rehm S, Campion M, Katz DE, et al. Community-based outpatient parenteral antimicrobial therapy (CoPAT) for *Staphylococcus aureus* bacteraemia with or without infective endocarditis: Analysis of the randomized trial comparing daptomycin with standard therapy. J Antimicrob Chemother 2009;63:1034–1042.
98. Andrews MM, von Reyn CF. Patient selection criteria and management guidelines for outpatient parenteral antibiotic therapy for native valve infective endocarditis. Clin Infect Dis 2001;33:203–209.
99. Weinstein MP, Stratton CW, Ackley A, et al. Multicenter collaborative evaluation of a standardized serum bactericidal test as a prognostic indicator in infective endocarditis. Am J Med 1985;78:262–269.
100. McCormack JP, Jewesson PJ. A critical reevaluation of the "therapeutic range" of aminoglycosides. Clin Infect Dis 1992;14:320–339.
101. Rybak M, Lomaestro B, Rotschafer JC, et al. Therapeutic monitoring of vancomycin in adult patients: A consensus review of the American Society of Health-System Pharmacists, the Infectious Diseases Society of America, and the Society of Infectious Diseases Pharmacists. Am J Health Syst Pharm 2009;66:82–98.
102. Roberts GJ. Dentists are innocent! "Everyday" bacteremia is the real culprit: A review and assessment of the evidence that dental surgical procedures are a principal cause of bacterial endocarditis in children. Pediatr Cardiol 1999; 20:317–325.
103. Hall G, Hedstrom SA, Heimdahl A, et al. Prophylactic administration of penicillins for endocarditis does not reduce the incidence of postextraction bacteremia. Clin Infect Dis 1993;17:188–194.
104. Van der Meer JT, Van Wijk W, Thompson J, et al. Efficacy of antibiotic prophylaxis for prevention of native-valve endocarditis. Lancet 1992;339(8786):135–139.
105. Strom BL, Abrutyn E, Berlin JA, et al. Risk factors for infective endocarditis: Oral hygiene and nondental exposures. Circulation 2000;102:2842–2848.
106. Seto TB, Kwiat D, Taira DA, et al. Physicians' recommendations to patients for use of antibiotic prophylaxis to prevent endocarditis. JAMA 2000;284:68–71.

Tuberculosis

Rocsanna Namdar, Michael Lauzardo, and Charles A. Peloquin

90

KEY CONCEPTS

1. Tuberculosis (TB) is the most prevalent communicable infectious disease on earth. It is the leading cause of death in human immunodeficiency virus (HIV) infection worldwide. It remains out of control in many developing nations. These nations require medical and financial assistance from developed nations in order to control the spread of TB globally.
2. In the United States, TB disproportionately affects ethnic minorities as compared with whites, reflecting greater ongoing transmission in ethnic minority communities. Additional TB surveillance and preventive treatment are required within these communities.
3. Coinfection with HIV and TB accelerates the progression of both diseases, thus requiring rapid diagnosis and treatment of both diseases.
4. Mycobacteria are slow-growing organisms; in the laboratory, they require special stains, special growth media, and long periods of incubation to isolate and identify.
5. TB can produce atypical signs and symptoms in infants, the elderly, and immunocompromised hosts, and it can progress rapidly in these patients.
6. Latent TB infection (LTBI) can lead to reactivation disease years after the primary infection occurred.
7. The patient suspected of having active TB disease must be isolated until the diagnosis is confirmed and the patient is no longer contagious. Often, isolation takes place in specialized "negative-pressure" hospital rooms to prevent the spread of TB.
8. Isoniazid and rifampin are the two most important TB drugs; organisms resistant to both these drugs (multidrug-resistant TB [MDR-TB]) are much more difficult to treat.
9. Directly observed treatment (DOT) is considered the standard of care. DOT should be used whenever possible to reduce treatment failures and the selection of drug-resistant isolates.
10. Never add a single drug to a failing TB treatment regimen!

INTRODUCTION

1 Tuberculosis (TB) remains a leading infectious killer globally. TB is caused by *Mycobacterium tuberculosis*, which can produce either a silent, latent infection or a progressive, active disease.[1] Left untreated or improperly treated, TB causes progressive tissue destruction and, eventually, death. Because of renewed public health efforts, TB rates in the United States continue to decline. In contrast, TB remains out of control in many developing countries—to the point that one third of the world's population currently is infected.[1] Given increasing drug resistance, it is critical that a major effort be made to control TB before the most potent drugs are no longer effective.

TB rates generally have risen with increasing urbanization and overcrowding because it is easier for an airborne disease to spread when people are packed closely together. Hence, TB became a significant pathogen in Europe during the Middle Ages and peaked during the Industrial Revolution, when it caused approximately 25% of all deaths in Europe and in the United States.[1,2] This dire threat led to the rise of public health departments and to procedures such as the isolation of infected patients. Thus, TB was directly responsible for many of the healthcare practices that we take for granted today. Unfortunately, in developing nations, some of these practices are not widely available, and TB continues to rage unabated.

EPIDEMIOLOGY

Globally, roughly 2 billion people are infected by *M. tuberculosis*, and roughly 2 million people die from active TB each year despite the fact that it is curable.[1,2] In the United States, an estimated 9 to 14 million people are latently infected with *M. tuberculosis*, meaning that they are not currently sick but that they could fall ill with TB at any time. In 2011, a total of 10,521 new TB cases were reported in the United States, an incidence of 3.4 cases per 100,000 population, which is 6.4% lower than the rate in 2010. This is the lowest rate recorded since national reporting began in 1953.[3] (For detailed data analysis, visit the Centers for Disease Control and Prevention [CDC] website at *www.cdc.gov/nchstp/tb*.) The annual incidence of TB in the United States declined by approximately 5% per year from 1953 to 1983 (Fig. 90-1).[3] In 1984, this decline slowed, and then the incidence of TB rose from 1988 to 1992, reaching 10.5 cases per 100,000 population. Since 1992, more effective infection control practices and treatment protocols have reduced TB rates significantly as mentioned above. Despite this good news, the eradication of TB from the United States remains very difficult. One reason is that we continue to import new cases from countries where TB remains out of control.[3,4]

Risk Factors for Infection

Location and Place of Birth

Four states (California, Florida, New York, and Texas) continued to report more than 500 cases each in 2011. Combined, these four states accounted for 5,299 TB cases or approximately half (50.4%) of all TB cases reported in 2011.[3] Within these states, TB is most prevalent in large urban areas.[3]

The TB rate among foreign-born persons was 12 times that of U.S.-born persons in 2011.[3] The percentage of foreign-born TB

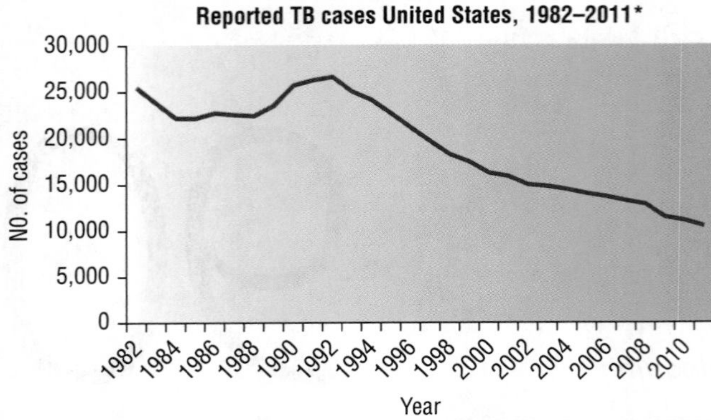

FIGURE 90-1 Reported TB Cases, United States, 1982–2011. *Updated as of June 25, 2012. *(From reference 3.)*

patients in the United States has increased annually since 1986, reaching 62.5% in 2011.[3] The 17.3 per 100,000 population TB rate among foreign-born persons was a 4.8% decrease since 2010 and a 49% decrease since 1993. In 2011, 54.1% of foreign-born persons with TB originated from five countries: Mexico (1,392 cases), the Philippines (750 cases), Vietnam (537 cases), India (498 cases), and China (365 cases).[3] Therefore, healthcare workers must "think TB" when caring for patients from these countries who experience symptoms such as cough, fever, and weight loss.

Close contacts of pulmonary TB patients are most likely to become infected.[2–4] These include family members, coworkers, or coresidents in places such as prisons, shelters, or nursing homes. The more prolonged the contact, the greater is the risk, with infection rates as high as 30%.[3,4] Although many circumstances exist, TB patients frequently have limited access to healthcare, live in crowded conditions, or are homeless.[2–4] Many patients have histories of alcohol abuse or illicit drug use, and many are coinfected with hepatitis B or human immunodeficiency virus (HIV). These concurrent social and health problems make treating some TB patients particularly difficult.

Race, Ethnicity, Age, and Gender

❷ In the United States, TB disproportionately affects ethnic minorities. In 2011, for the first time since the current reporting system began in 1993, non-Hispanic Asians surpassed Hispanics as the largest ethnic group among TB patients. Compared with non-Hispanic whites, the TB rate among non-Hispanic Asians was 25 times greater, and rates among non-Hispanic blacks and Hispanics were 8 and 7 times greater, respectively. Among U.S.-born ethnic groups, the greatest disparity in TB rates occurred among non-Hispanic blacks, whose rate was six times the rate for non-Hispanic whites.[3] TB is most common during early adulthood primarily in the 25- to 44-year age group. In 2010, 6% of cases in the United States were children under 15 years of age, 11% were age 15 to 24, 33% were age 25 to 44, 31% were age 45 to 64, and 20% were at least 65 years old.[4] TB is more common in older whites and Asians compared with younger people from these groups. This reflects reactivation of latent infection acquired many years earlier when TB was very common. Older blacks and Hispanics also have more TB than younger individuals, but the differences by age are not as pronounced.[5] This reflects a greater recent transmission among younger blacks and Hispanics compared with younger whites and Asians. Until the age of 15 years, TB rates are similar for males and females, but after that, the male predominance increases with each decade of life.[5]

Coinfection with Human Immunodeficiency Virus

❸ HIV is the most important risk factor for active TB, especially among people 25 to 44 years of age.[2,4–6] TB and HIV seem to act synergistically within patients and across populations, making each disease worse than it might otherwise be. In 2011, 7.9% of incident cases of TB in the United States were coinfected with HIV.[3] This increase in percentage over previous years was felt to be due largely to improved reporting of HIV status to state TB programs. These numbers are estimates because laws and regulations in some states prohibit sharing HIV status of TB patients with the TB program. HIV coinfection may not increase the risk of acquiring *M. tuberculosis* infection, but it does increase the likelihood of progression to active disease.[1,6] There is evidence for higher mortality rates in HIV coinfected with multidrug-resistant (MDR) and extensively drug-resistant (XDR) TB.[7]

Risk Factors for Disease

Once infected with *M. tuberculosis*, a person's lifetime risk of active TB is approximately 10%.[2,4,6] The greatest risk for active disease occurs during the first 2 years after infection. Children younger than 2 years of age and adults older than 65 years of age have two to five times greater risk for active disease compared with other age groups. Patients with underlying immune suppression (e.g., renal failure, cancer, and immunosuppressive drug treatment) have 4 to 16 times greater risk than other patients. Finally, HIV-infected patients with *M. tuberculosis* infection are 100 times more likely to develop active TB than normal hosts.[4,8] HIV-infected patients have an annual risk of active TB of approximately 10%, rather than a lifetime risk at that rate. Therefore, all patients with HIV infection should be screened for tuberculous infection, and those known to be infected with *M. tuberculosis* should be tested for HIV infection.

ETIOLOGY

M. tuberculosis is a slender bacillus with a waxy outer layer.[2,6] It is 1 to 4 μm in length, and under the microscope, it is either straight or slightly curved in shape.[1,9,10] It does not stain well with Gram stain, so the Ziehl-Neelsen stain or the fluorochrome stain must be used instead.[1,2,6] After Ziehl-Neelsen staining with carbol-fuchsin, mycobacteria retain the red color despite acid–alcohol washes. Hence, they are called *acid-fast bacilli* (AFB).[9] After staining, microscopic examination ("smear") detects about 8,000 to 10,000 organisms per milliliter (8×10^6/L to 10×10^6/L) of specimen, so a patient can be "smear negative" but still grow *M. tuberculosis* on culture. Microscopic examination also cannot determine which of the more than 100 mycobacterial species is present or whether the organisms in the original samples were alive or dead.[1,9,10] On smear, they are all dead. On culture, *M. tuberculosis* grows slowly, doubling about every 20 hours. This is slow compared with gram-positive and gram-negative bacteria, which double about every 30 minutes.

Culture and Susceptibility Testing

❹ Direct susceptibility testing involves inoculating specialized media with organisms taken directly from a concentrated, smear-positive specimen.[1,9,10] This approach produces susceptibility results in 2 to 3 weeks. Indirect susceptibility testing involves inoculating the test media with organisms obtained from a pure culture of the organisms, which can take several more weeks. The most common agar method, known as the *proportion method*, uses the ratio of colony counts on drug-containing agar to that on drug-free agar.[1,10] In the United States, the critical proportion for resistance is 1%. That means that if a drug-containing plate shows only 2% of the growth seen on a drug-free plate, some of the organisms from the specimen were resistant to that drug. Therefore, it is likely that many of the organisms in the patient also are resistant to that drug, and it should not be used to treat that patient.

The proportion method's limitations include many weeks to obtain results, drug degradation during the incubation, and a qualitative result (susceptible or resistant). The newer mycobacterial growth indicator tube (MGIT) (Becton Dickson, Sparks, MD) systems use liquid media and detect live mycobacteria in as few as 9 to 14 days.[11,12]

Rapid-identification tests are now available. Nucleic acid probes such as the AccuProbe (Gen-Probe, San Diego, CA) use DNA probes to identify the presence of complementary ribosomal ribonucleic acid (rRNA) for several mycobacterial species.[6,9,13] DNA fingerprinting using restriction-fragment-length polymorphism analysis has been used to identify clusters of cases.[1,9,13] Amplification of the genetic material can be achieved through polymerase chain reaction (PCR) (Roche Molecular Systems, Branchburg, NJ), the amplified *M. tuberculosis* direct (MTD) test (Gen-Probe), and strand-displacement amplification (SDA; Becton-Dickinson, Sparks, MD).[9,12] Thin-layer chromatography, high-performance liquid chromatography for mycolic acid identification, and gas chromatography for short-chain fatty acids (methyl esters) have been used to speciate mycobacterial isolates.[1,9,13] Other tests are designed to detect common genetic changes associated with drug resistance, such as changes in the *katG* gene associated with isoniazid resistance and the *rpoB* gene associated with rifampin resistance.[6,12,14,15] Two tests, the Gene X-pert (Cepheid, Sunnyvale, CA) and the Hain test (Hain Lifescience, Nehren, Germany), have entered into limited clinical use in the United States. These tests offer clinicians a chance to know rapidly if resistance to rifampin is present (both tests) and what drugs might be good initial choices (Hain Test).

Transmission

M. tuberculosis is transmitted from person to person by coughing or other activities that cause the organism to be aerosolized.[2,6,11] These particles, called *droplet nuclei*, contain one to three bacilli and are small enough (1 to 5 mm) to reach the alveolar surface. This produces "droplet nuclei" that are dispersed in the air. Each droplet nuclei contains one to three organisms. Approximately 30% of individuals who experience prolonged contact with an infectious TB patient will become infected.

A person with cavitary, pulmonary TB and a cough may infect roughly one person per month until that person is treated effectively, although this number can vary significantly. A person with the uncommon laryngeal form of TB can spread organisms even when talking, so the transmission rates can be even higher.

PATHOPHYSIOLOGY

Immune Response

T-lymphocyte responses are essential to controlling *M. tuberculosis* infections.[2,6,16,17] In the mouse model, two different T-cell responses—the T-helper type 1 (TH_1) response and the T-helper type 2 (TH_2) response—have been described. The TH_1 response is the preferred response to TB, and the TH_2 response, including the potentially subversive influence of interleukin (IL) 4, is undesirable.[2,16,17] Some workers have argued that this dichotomy is clearer in the mouse model, and in many humans, the T-cell response may be classified as TH_0 (elements of both TH_1 and TH_2).[16] In either case, T lymphocytes activate macrophages that, in turn, engulf and kill mycobacteria. T lymphocytes also destroy immature macrophages that harbor *M. tuberculosis* but are unable to kill the invaders.[16,17] CD4+ cells are the primary T cells involved, with contributions by $\gamma\delta$ T cells and CD8+ T cells.[20] CD4+ T cells produce interferon-γ (INF-γ) and other cytokines, including IL-2 and IL-10, that coordinate the immune response to TB.[16] Because CD4+ cells are depleted in HIV-infected patients, these patients are unable to mount an adequate defense to TB.[16,17]

Although B-cell responses and antibody production can be demonstrated in TB-infected mammals, these humoral responses do not appear to contribute much to the control of TB within the host.[2,6,16] Tumor necrosis factor-α (TNF-α) and INF-γ are important cytokines involved in coordinating the host's cell-mediated response. Rheumatoid arthritis patients treated with TNF-α inhibitors (such as infliximab) have high rates of reactivation TB.[18] Therefore, patients known to be deficient in the activity of TNF-α or INF-γ should be screened for TB infection and offered appropriate treatment.

M. tuberculosis has several ways of evading or resisting the host immune response.[16,17] In particular, *M. tuberculosis* can inhibit the fusion of lysosomes to phagosomes inside macrophages. This prevents the destructive enzymes found in the lysosomes from getting to the bacilli captured in the phagosomes. This inhibition of destructive mechanisms allows time for *M. tuberculosis* to escape into the cytoplasm. Virulent *M. tuberculosis* is able to multiply in the macrophage cytoplasm, thus perpetuating their spread. Finally, lipoarabinomannan (LAM), the principal structural polysaccharide of the mycobacterial cell wall, inhibits the host immune response.[16,17] LAM induces immunosuppressive cytokines, thus blocking macrophage activation; additionally, LAM scavenges O_2, thus preventing attack by superoxide anions, hydrogen peroxide, singlet oxygen, and hydroxyl radicals.[16,17] These survival mechanisms make *M. tuberculosis* a particularly difficult organism to control. Any defects in the host immune system make it likely that *M. tuberculosis* will not be controlled and that active disease will ensue.

Primary Infection

Primary infection usually results from inhaling airborne particles that contain *M. tuberculosis*.[2,6,17] The progression to clinical disease depends on three factors: (a) the number of *M. tuberculosis* organisms inhaled (infecting dose), (b) the virulence of these organisms, and (c) the host's cell-mediated immune response.[2,3,6,11,17,19] At the alveolar surface, the bacilli that were delivered by the droplet nuclei are ingested by pulmonary macrophages.[22] If these macrophages inhibit or kill the bacilli, infection is aborted.[17] If the macrophages cannot do this, the organisms continue to multiply. The macrophages eventually rupture, releasing many bacilli, and these mycobacteria are then phagocytized by other macrophages. This cycle continues over several weeks until the host is able to mount a more coordinated response.[17] During this early phase of infection, *M. tuberculosis* multiplies logarithmically.[17]

Some of the intracellular organisms are transported by the macrophages to regional lymph nodes in the hilar, mediastinal, and retroperitoneal areas. The cycle of phagocytosis and cell rupture continues. During lymph node involvement, the mycobacteria may be held in check. More frequently, *M. tuberculosis* spreads throughout the body through the bloodstream.[2,6,17] When this intravascular dissemination occurs, *M. tuberculosis* can infect any tissue or organ in the body. Most commonly, *M. tuberculosis* infects the posterior apical region of the lungs. This may be so because of the high oxygen content, and it may be because of a less vigorous immune response in this area.

After about 3 weeks of infection, T lymphocytes are presented with *M. tuberculosis* antigens. These T cells become activated and begin to secrete INF-γ and the other cytokines noted earlier. The processes described in Immune Response above then begin to occur. First, T lymphocytes stimulate macrophages to become bactericidal.[17] Large numbers of activated microbicidal macrophages surround the solid caseous (cheese-like) tuberculous foci (the necrotic area of infection).[17] This process of creating activated microbicidal macrophages is known as *cell-mediated immunity* (CMI).[17]

At the same time that CMI occurs, delayed-type hypersensitivity (DTH) also develops through the activation and multiplication of T lymphocytes. DTH refers to the cytotoxic immune process that kills nonactivated immature macrophages that are permitting intracellular bacillary replication.[17] These immature macrophages are killed when the T lymphocytes initiate Fas-mediated apoptosis (programmed cell death).[17] The bacilli released from the immature macrophages then are killed by the activated macrophages.[17]

By this time (>3 weeks), macrophages have begun to form granulomas to contain the organisms. In a typical tuberculous granuloma, activated macrophages accumulate around a caseous lesion and prevent its further extension.[17] At this point, the infection is largely under control, and bacillary replication falls off dramatically. Depending on the inflammatory response, tissue necrosis and calcification of the infection site plus the regional lymph nodes may occur.

Over 1 to 3 months, activated lymphocytes reach an adequate number, and tissue hypersensitivity results. This is shown by a positive tuberculin skin test. Any remaining mycobacteria are believed to reside primarily within granulomas or within macrophages that have avoided detection and lysis, although some residual bacilli have been found in various types of cells.[2,6,16]

Approximately 90% of infected patients have no further clinical manifestations. Most patients only show a positive skin test (70%), whereas some also have radiographic evidence of stable granulomas. This radiodense area on chest radiograph is called a *Ghon's complex*. Approximately 5% of patients (usually children, the elderly, and the immunocompromised) experience "progressive primary" disease that occurs before skin test conversion, which presents as a progressive pneumonia, usually in the lower lobes.[20] Disease frequently spreads, leading to meningitis and other severe forms of TB.[20] Because of this risk of severe disease, very young, elderly, and immunocompromised patients, including those with HIV, should be evaluated and treated for latent or active TB.

Reactivation Disease

❻ Roughly 10% of infected patients develop reactivation disease at some point in their lives. Nearly half of these cases occur within 2 years of infection.[2,6,11] In the United States, most cases of TB are believed to result from reactivation. Reinfection is uncommon in the United States because of the low rate of exposure and because previously sensitized individuals possess some degree of immunity to reinfection.[2,17] Exceptions include patients coinfected with HIV who live in areas of higher exposure to *M. tuberculosis*.

The apices of the lungs are the most common sites for reactivation (85% of cases).[2] For reasons that are not entirely known (waning cellular immunity, loss of specific T-cell clones, blocking antibody), organisms within granulomas emerge and begin multiplying extracellularly.[17] The inflammatory response produces caseating granulomas, which eventually will liquefy and spread locally, leading to the formation of a hole (cavity) in the lungs.

The immune response contributes to the severity of the lung damage, and DTH allows for intracellular mycobacterial multiplication.[16,17] In addition, there is "innocent bystander" killing of host cells and locally thrombosed blood vessels.[17] The killing of mycobacteria, macrophages, and neutrophils that have entered the battle releases cytokines and lysozymes into the infectious foci. This toxic mixture can be too much for the surrounding alveoli and airway cells, causing regional necrosis and structural collapse.[2,17] These unstable foci liquefy, spreading the infection to neighboring areas of the lung, creating a cavity. Some of this necrotic material is coughed out, producing droplet nuclei. Bacterial counts in the cavities can be as high as 10^8 per milliliter of cavitary fluid. Partial healing may result from fibrosis, but these lesions remain unstable and may continue to expand.[2,17] If left untreated, pulmonary TB continues to destroy the lungs, resulting in hypoxia, respiratory acidosis, and eventually death.

Extrapulmonary and Miliary Tuberculosis

Caseating granulomas at extrapulmonary sites can undergo liquefaction, releasing tubercle bacilli and causing symptomatic disease.[2,6] Extrapulmonary TB without concurrent pulmonary disease is uncommon in normal hosts but more common in HIV-infected patients. Because of these unusual presentations, the diagnosis of TB is difficult and often delayed in immunocompromised hosts.[2,6] Lymphatic and pleural diseases are the most common forms of extrapulmonary TB, followed by bone, joint, genitourinary, meningeal, and other forms.[2,6] Occasionally, a massive inoculum of organisms enters the bloodstream, causing a widely disseminated form of the disease known as *miliary TB*. It is named for the millet seed appearance of the small granulomas seen on chest radiographs, and it can be rapidly fatal.[16] Miliary TB is a medical emergency requiring immediate treatment.

Influence of HIV Infection on Pathogenesis

❸ HIV infection is the strongest single risk factor for active TB.[2,6,16] As CD4+ lymphocytes multiply in response to the mycobacterial infection, HIV multiplies within these cells and selectively destroys them. In turn, the TB-fighting lymphocytes are depleted.[16] This vicious cycle puts HIV-infected patients at 100 times the risk of active TB compared with HIV-negative people.[21] In addition, the combination of HIV infection and certain social behaviors increases the risk of newly acquired TB. In select areas of the United States during the resurgence of TB during the early 1990s, up to 50% of new TB cases were the result of recent infection, particularly among HIV-infected individuals.[21,22]

As mycobacteria spread throughout the body, HIV replication accelerates in lymphocytes and macrophages. This leads to progression of HIV disease.[16,23] HIV-infected patients who are infected with TB deteriorate more rapidly unless they receive antimycobacterial chemotherapy.[24,25] Most clinicians now recommend beginning TB treatment first, and shortly after, beginning HIV treatment. However, this needs to be individualized based on degree of immunosuppression from HIV and the patient's tolerance of the treatment regimen. Some patients will experience paradoxical worsening of the TB.[11,23] This appears to result from a reinvigorated inflammatory response to TB. Because TB can be very dangerous in HIV-positive patients, they should be screened for tuberculous infection or disease soon after they are shown to be HIV-positive.[2,6,16]

CLINICAL PRESENTATION

The classical presentation of TB is shown in Clinical Presentation of Tuberculosis above. The onset of TB may be gradual, and the diagnosis may not be considered until a chest radiograph is performed. Unfortunately, many patients do not seek medical attention until more dramatic symptoms, such as hemoptysis, occur. At this point, patients typically have large cavitary lesions in the lungs. These cavities are loaded with *M. tuberculosis*. Expectoration or swallowing of infected sputum may spread the disease to other areas of the body.[1,2,6,19] Physical examination is nonspecific but suggestive of progressive pulmonary disease. ❺ Patients coinfected with HIV may have atypical presentations.[1,2,6,19] As their CD4+ counts decline, HIV-positive patients are less likely to have positive skin tests, cavitary lesions, or fever. Pulmonary radiographic findings may be minimal or absent. HIV-positive patients have a higher incidence of extrapulmonary TB and are more likely to present with progressive primary disease. Because their symptoms are not specific to TB, a thorough workup for TB is essential.[2,6,16,19]

CLINICAL PRESENTATION Tuberculosis

Signs and Symptoms

- Patients typically present with weight loss, fatigue, a productive cough, fever, and night sweats.[1,2,6,19]
- Frank hemoptysis.

Physical Examination

- Dullness to chest percussion, rales, and increased vocal fremitus are observed frequently on auscultation.

Laboratory Tests

- Moderate elevations in the white blood cell (WBC) count with a lymphocyte predominance

Diagnostic Considerations

- Positive sputum smear
- Fiber-optic bronchoscopy (if sputum tests are inconclusive and suspicion is high)

Chest Radiograph

- Patchy or nodular infiltrates in the apical areas of the upper lobes or the superior segment of the lower lobes[2,6,19]
- Cavitation that may show air–fluid levels as the infection progresses

Extrapulmonary TB typically presents as a slowly progressive decline in organ function.[2,6,19] Patients may have low-grade fever and other constitutional symptoms. Patients with genitourinary TB may present with sterile pyuria and hematuria. Lymphadenitis often involves the cervical and supraclavicular nodes and may appear as a neck mass with spontaneous drainage. Tuberculous arthritis and osteomyelitis occur most commonly in the elderly and usually affect the lower spine and weight-bearing joints. TB of the spine is known as *Pott's disease*.[2] Abnormal behavior, headaches, or convulsions suggest tuberculous meningitis. Involvement of the peritoneum, pericardium, larynx, and adrenal glands also occurs.[2,6,19]

The Elderly

❺ TB in the elderly is easily confused with other respiratory diseases. Many clinical findings are muted or absent altogether. Compared with younger patients, TB in the elderly is far less likely to present with positive skin tests, fevers, night sweats, sputum production, or hemoptysis.[2,19,24] Weight loss may occur but is nonspecific. In contrast, mental status changes are twice as common in the elderly, and mortality is six times higher.[2,19,24] TB is a preventable cause of death in the elderly that should not be overlooked.

Children

❺ TB in children, especially those younger than 12 years of age, may present as a typical bacterial pneumonia and is called *progressive primary TB*.[19,20] Clinical disease often begins 1 to 2 months after exposure and precedes skin-test positivity. Unlike adults, pulmonary TB in children often involves the lower and middle lobes.[19,20] Dissemination to the lymph nodes, GI and genitourinary tracts, bone marrow, and meninges is common. Because of delays in recruitment of cellular immunity, cavitary disease is infrequent, and the number of organisms present typically is smaller than in an adult. Because cavitary lesions are uncommon, children do not spread TB readily. However, TB can be rapidly fatal in a child, and it requires prompt chemotherapy.

DIAGNOSIS

Diagnostic Testing

The key to stopping the spread of TB is early identification of infected individuals.[1,2,6,19] Table 90-1 lists the populations most likely to benefit from testing (column 1 patients are at highest risk for TB,

TABLE 90-1 Criteria for Tuberculin Positivity by Risk Group

Reaction 5 mm of Induration	Reaction ≥10 mm of Induration	Reaction ≥15 mm of Induration
Human immunodeficiency virus (HIV)-positive persons	Recent immigrants (i.e., within the last 5 years) from high-prevalence countries	Persons with no risk factors for TB
Recent contacts of tuberculosis (TB) case patients	Injection-drug users	
Fibrotic changes on chest radiograph consistent with prior TB	Residents and employees[a] of the following high-risk congregate settings: prisons and jails, nursing homes and other long-term care facilities for the elderly, hospitals and other healthcare facilities, residential facilities for patients with acquired immunodeficiency syndrome (AIDS), homeless shelters	
Patients with organ transplants and other immunosuppressed patients (receiving the equivalent of ≥15 mg/day of prednisone for 1 month or more)[b]	Mycobacteriology laboratory personnel Persons with the following clinical conditions that place them at high risk: silicosis, diabetes mellitus, chronic renal failure, some hematologic disorders (e.g., leukemias and lymphomas), other specific malignancies (e.g., carcinoma of the head or neck and lung), weight loss of ≥10% of ideal body weight, gastrectomy, jejunoileal bypass Children younger than 4 years of age or infants, children, and adolescents exposed to adults at high risk	

[a]For persons who are otherwise at low risk and who are tested at the start of employment, a reaction of ≥15 mm induration is considered positive.
[b]Risk of TB for patients treated with corticosteroids increases with higher dose and longer duration.

Adapted from Screening for tuberculosis and tuberculosis infection in high-risk populations: Recommendations of the Advisory Council for the Elimination of Tuberculosis. MMWR Recomm Rep 1995;44(RR-11):19–34.

followed by those in column 2). Members of these high-risk groups should be tested for TB infection and educated about the disease.

The Mantoux test is a TB skin test. It uses tuberculin purified protein derivative (PPD), and unlike the Heaf or tine test, the Mantoux test is quantitative. The standard 5-tuberculin-unit PPD dose is placed intracutaneously on the volar aspect of the forearm with a 26- or 27-gauge needle.[2,19,24] This injection should produce a small, raised, blanched wheal. An experienced professional should read the test in 48 to 72 hours. The area of induration (the "bump") is the important end point, not the area of redness. Table 90-1 lists the criteria for interpretation.[1,2,6,19,24] The CDC does not recommend the routine use of anergy panels.[24,26] Aplisol and Tubersol 5-tuberculin-unit products are available commercially and are similar in sensitivity, specificity, and reactivity. It is important, however, to use one product and notify appropriate users when switching between products.[27,28]

The "booster effect" occurs for patients who do not respond to an initial skin test but show a positive reaction if retested about a week later.[19,26] Patients with past *M. tuberculosis* infection and some patients with past immunization with bacillus Calmette-Guérin (BCG) vaccine or past infection with other mycobacteria may "boost" with a second skin test. Individuals who require periodic skin testing, such as healthcare workers, should receive a two-stage test initially.[19,26,29] Once they are shown to be skin-test negative, any positive skin test later shows recent infection, and this requires treatment.

The PPD skin test is an imperfect diagnostic tool. Up to 20% of patients with active TB are falsely skin-test negative, presumably because their immune systems are overwhelmed.[16,26] False-positive results are more common in low-risk patients and those recently vaccinated with BCG. Despite BCG vaccination, one should not ignore a positive PPD result. These patients require careful evaluation for active disease, and they may be offered preventive treatment because many come from areas where TB infection is common.

Interferon-γ release assays (IGRA) measure the release of INF-γ in blood in response to the TB antigens.[30] They may provide quick and specific results for identifying *M. tuberculosis*. IGRAs do not trigger a booster effect and are more specific for testing *M. tuberculosis* than the PPD. The QuantiFERON-TB Gold test (QFT-G) is an enzyme-linked immunosorbent assay (ELISA) and was approved by the U.S. FDA in 2005.[30] The T-SPOT.TB, an enzyme-linked immunospot assay, was approved by the U.S. FDA in 2008.[31] Both tests can be used for diagnosing latent TB infection (LTBI) and TB disease caused by *M. tuberculosis*. The antigenic proteins are absent from BCG vaccine strains and from most non-TB mycobacteria. Therefore, QFT-G does not trigger a booster effect and is more specific for testing of *M. tuberculosis* than the PPD. Although these tests can provide results to diagnose both latent infection and disease, they cannot differentiate between the two. Results are available within <24 hours, instead of the 2 to 3 days required for the traditional PPD skin test. Therefore, the patient does not have to return to the clinic as required by the PPD skin test, making it more convenient. The CDC has approved the use of these tests in all circumstances in which the PPD is currently used; however, the sensitivity for young children (<5 years) and in immunocompromised patients has not been determined.[32–35]

Additional Tests

When active TB is suspected, attempts should be made to isolate *M. tuberculosis* from the site of infection.[2,6,19,26] Sputum collected in the morning usually has the highest yield.[2,9,19] Daily sputum collection over 3 consecutive days is recommended.

For patients unable to expectorate, sputum induction with aerosolized hypertonic saline may produce a diagnostic sample. Bronchoscopy, or aspiration of gastric fluid via a nasogastric tube, may be attempted for select patients.[19] For patients with suspected extrapulmonary TB, samples of draining fluid, biopsies of the infected site, or both may be attempted. Blood cultures are positive occasionally, especially in AIDS patients.[19,36]

TREATMENT

Desired Outcomes

The desired outcomes during the treatment of TB are:

1. Rapid identification of a new TB case
2. Initiation of specific anti-TB treatment
3. Prompt resolution of the signs and symptoms of disease
4. Achievement of a noninfectious state in the patient, thus ending isolation
5. Adherence to the treatment regimen by the patient
6. Cure of the patient as quickly as possible (generally at least 6 months of treatment)

It is also important that patients with active disease are isolated to prevent spread of the disease and that appropriate samples for smears and cultures are collected. Secondary goals are identification of the index case that infected the patient, identification of all persons infected by both the index case and the new case of TB ("contact investigation"), and completion of appropriate treatments for those individuals.

General Approaches to Treatment

Drug treatment is the cornerstone of TB management.[2,6,11,37] Monotherapy can be used only for infected patients who do not have active TB (latent infection, as shown by a positive skin test). Once active disease is present, a minimum of two drugs, and generally three or four drugs, must be used simultaneously.[2,6,11,37] The duration of treatment depends on the condition of the host, extent of disease, presence of drug resistance, and tolerance of medications. The shortest duration of treatment generally is 6 months, and 2 to 3 years of treatment may be necessary for cases of MDR-TB.[2,6,11,37] Because the duration of treatment is so long and because many patients feel better after a few weeks of treatment, careful followup is required. Directly observed therapy (DOT) by a healthcare worker is a cost-effective way to ensure completion of treatment and is considered the standard of care.[2,6,11,37–39]

Principles for Treating Latent Infection and for Treating Disease

Asymptomatic patients with tuberculous infection have a bacillary load of about 10^3 organisms, compared with 10^{11} organisms in a patient with cavitary pulmonary TB.[2,6] As the number of organisms increases, the likelihood of naturally occurring drug-resistant mutants also increases. Naturally occurring resistant mutants are found at rates of 1 in 10^6 to 1 in 10^8 organisms for the anti-TB drugs.[2,37] When treating asymptomatic latent infection with isoniazid monotherapy, the risk of selecting out isoniazid-resistant organisms is low. The isoniazid mutation rate is about 1 in 10^6, but only about 10^3 organisms are present in the body. In contrast, the risk of selecting out isoniazid-resistant organisms is unacceptably high for patients with cavitary TB. One can prevent selection of these resistant mutants by adding more drugs because the rates for resistance mutations to multiple drugs are additive functions of the individual rates. For example, only 1 in 10^{13} organisms would be naturally resistant to both isoniazid (1 in 10^6) and rifampin (1 in 10^7).[2,37] It is unlikely that such rare organisms are present in a previously untreated patient.

Combination chemotherapy is required for treating active TB disease. The patient should receive at least two drugs to which the isolate is susceptible, and, generally, four drugs are given at the outset of treatment. Rifampin and isoniazid are the best drugs for preventing drug resistance, followed by ethambutol, streptomycin, and pyrazinamide.[2,6,37,40]

Three subpopulations of mycobacteria are proposed to exist within the body, and each appears to respond to certain drugs.[2,37] Most numerous are the extracellular, rapidly dividing bacteria, often found within cavities (about 10^7 to 10^9 organisms). These are killed most readily by isoniazid, followed by rifampin, streptomycin, and the other drugs. A second group resides within caseating granulomas (possibly 10^5 to 10^7 organisms). These organisms appear to be in a semidormant state, with occasional bursts of metabolic activity. Pyrazinamide, through its conversion within *M. tuberculosis* to pyrazinoic acid, appears most active against these organisms. Rifampin and isoniazid also may be active against this subpopulation. The third subset is the intracellular mycobacteria present within macrophages (10^4 to 10^6). Rifampin, isoniazid, and the quinolones appear to be most active against intracellular *M. tuberculosis*. While this appears to explain what happens during the treatment of TB, there is no practical way to quantitate these populations within a given patient.

Nonpharmacologic Therapy

7 Nonpharmacologic interventions aim to (a) prevent the spread of TB, (b) find where TB has already spread using contact investigation, and (c) replenish the weakened (consumptive) patient to a state of normal weight and well-being. The first two items are performed by public health departments. Clinicians involved in the treatment of TB should verify that the local health department has been notified of all new cases of TB.

Workers in hospitals and other institutions must prevent the spread of TB within their facilities.[2,11,24] All such workers should learn and follow each institution's infection control guidelines. This includes using personal protective equipment, including properly fitted respirators, and closing doors to "negative-pressure" rooms. These hospital isolation rooms draw air in from surrounding areas rather than blowing air (and *M. tuberculosis*) into these surrounding areas. The air from the isolation room may be treated with ultraviolet lights and then vented safely outside. However, these isolation rooms work properly only if the door is closed.

Debilitated TB patients may require therapy for other medical problems, including substance abuse and HIV infection, and some may need nutritional support. Therefore, clinicians involved in substance abuse rehabilitation and nutritional support services should be familiar with the needs of TB patients. Surgery may be needed to remove destroyed lung tissue, space-occupying infected lesions (*tuberculomas*), and certain extrapulmonary lesions.[2,11,37] BCG is the only clinically relevant vaccine for TB in use today. Although it is one of the most commonly administered vaccines in history, it is of limited value, and cannot prevent infection by *M. tuberculosis*. BCG (discussed below) may prevent extreme forms of TB in infants.[37,41]

Pharmacologic Therapy

Treating Latent Infection

Isoniazid is the preferred drug for treating LTBI.[2,6,11,37] Generally, isoniazid alone is given for 9 months. The treatment of LTBI reduces a person's lifetime risk of active TB from approximately 10% to approximately 1%. Because TB is spread easily through the air, each case prevented also prevents a second wave of cases that each prevented case would have produced. Historically, the treatment of LTBI has been called *prophylaxis*. Table 90-2 lists the LTBI treatment options.

Because young children, the elderly, and HIV-positive patients are at greater risk of active disease once infected with *M. tuberculosis*, they require careful evaluation. Once active TB is ruled out, they should receive treatment for latent infection.[2,18,19,37]

The keys to successful treatment of LTBI are (a) infection by an isoniazid-susceptible isolate, (b) adherence to the regimen, and (c) no exogenous reinfection.[2] Isoniazid adult doses are usually 300 mg daily (5 to 10 mg/kg of body weight)[37] (see Table 90-2). Lower doses are less effective.[2,42,43] Isoniazid should be given on an empty stomach, and antacids should be avoided within 2 hours of dosing. Rifampin 600 mg daily for 4 months can be used when isoniazid resistance is suspected or when the patient cannot tolerate isoniazid.[2,37] There is a growing body of evidence that 4 months of rifampin may be a safer and more cost-effective alternative to 9 months of isoniazid. Menzies and colleagues showed that 4 months of rifampin was significantly cheaper per patient completing treatment because of better completion and fewer adverse events.[44] The combination of pyrazinamide plus rifampin is no longer recommended because of higher than expected rates of hepatotoxicity. Rifabutin 300 mg daily might be substituted for rifampin for patients at high risk of drug interactions. When resistance to isoniazid and rifampin is suspected in the isolate causing infection, there is no regimen proved to be effective.[2,37] Regimens that *might* be effective include ethambutol plus levofloxacin, but data regarding efficacy are lacking.

TABLE 90-2 Recommended Drug Regimens for Treatment of Latent Tuberculosis (TB) Infection in Adults

Drug	Interval and Duration	Comments	Rating[a] (Evidence)[b] HIV–	HIV+
Isoniazid	Daily for 9 months[b,c]	In human immunodeficiency virus (HIV)-infected patients, isoniazid may be administered concurrently with nucleoside reverse transcriptase inhibitors (NRTIs), protease inhibitors, or non-nucleoside reverse transcriptase inhibitors (NNRTIs)	A (II)	A (II)
	Twice weekly for 9 months[b,c]	Directly observed therapy (DOT) must be used with twice-weekly dosing	B (II)	B (II)
Isoniazid	Daily for 6 months[c]	Not indicated for HIV-infected persons, those with fibrotic lesions on chest radiographs, or children	B (I)	C (I)
	Twice weekly for 6 months[c]	DOT must be used with twice-weekly dosing	B (II)	C (I)
Rifampin	Daily for 4 months	For persons who are contacts of patients with isoniazid-resistant, rifampin-susceptible TB who cannot tolerate pyrazinamide	B (II)	B (III)
Isoniazid and rifapentine	Once weekly for 3 months	DOT must be used with once-weekly dosing. Not recommended for the following: children <2 years old, HIV/AIDS patients taking antiretroviral treatment, isoniazid- or rifampin-resistant strains, pregnant women or women expecting to become pregnant within the 12-week regimen	B (II)	B (II)

[a]Strength of recommendation: A, preferred; B, acceptable alternative; C, offer when A and B cannot be given.
[b]Quality of evidence: I, randomized clinical trial data; II, data from clinical trials that are not randomized or were conducted in other populations; III, expert opinion.
[c]Recommended regimen for children younger than 18 years of age.

Data from Targeted tuberculin testing and treatment of latent tuberculosis infection. American Thoracic Society. MMWR Recomm Rep 2000;49(RR-6):31; reference 46.

In 2011, a randomized controlled trial conducted in Brazil, Spain, Canada, and the United States compared 12 weeks of once-weekly isoniazid and rifapentine by DOT with daily self-administered isoniazid for 9 months.[45] This study, with over 8,000 participants, showed that the 12 weeks of weekly isoniazid and rifapentine given by DOT was not inferior in efficacy to 9 months of self-administered isoniazid, had a significantly higher completion rate (82% vs. 69%), and was associated with fewer grade 3 or 4 adverse reactions (1.6% vs. 3%).[45] It should be noted however that hypersensitivity reactions were more common with the isoniazid/rifapentine regimen and close clinical followup should be undertaken while experience is gained with this new regimen for LTBI therapy. The CDC now recommends the 12-week isoniazid/rifapentine regimen as an equal alternative to 9 months of daily isoniazid for treating LTBI in otherwise healthy patients aged ≥12 years who have a predictive factor for greater likelihood of TB developing, which included recent exposure to contagious TB, conversion from negative to positive on an indirect test for infection (i.e., IGRA or tuberculin skin test), and radiographic findings of healed pulmonary TB.[46] HIV-infected patients who are otherwise healthy and are not taking antiretroviral medications are also included in this category. However, precautions should be taken as HIV-infected patients are more likely to have extrapulmonary TB or pulmonary TB with normal findings on chest radiograph. For recent skin-test converters of all ages, the risk of active TB outweighs the risk for drug toxicity.[24,37] Pregnant women, alcoholics, and patients with poor diets who are treated with isoniazid should receive pyridoxine (vitamin B_6) 10 to 50 mg daily to reduce the incidence of CNS effects or peripheral neuropathies. All patients who receive treatment of LTBI should be monitored monthly for adverse drug reactions and for possible progression to active TB.

Treating Active Disease

8 The CDC, American Thoracic Society (ATS), and the Infectious Diseases Society of America have published an algorithm for the treatment of TB (Fig. 90-2). The treatment of active TB requires the use of multiple drugs. There are two primary anti-TB drugs, isoniazid and rifampin, with the rest of the drugs having specific roles.[37,40] Isoniazid and rifampin should be used together whenever possible. Typically, *M. tuberculosis* is either very susceptible or very resistant to a given drug. Theoretically, minimal inhibitory concentration (MIC) results could be used to guide dosing in the treatment of moderately resistant *M. tuberculosis*, but this remains to be studied prospectively.[2,11,37]

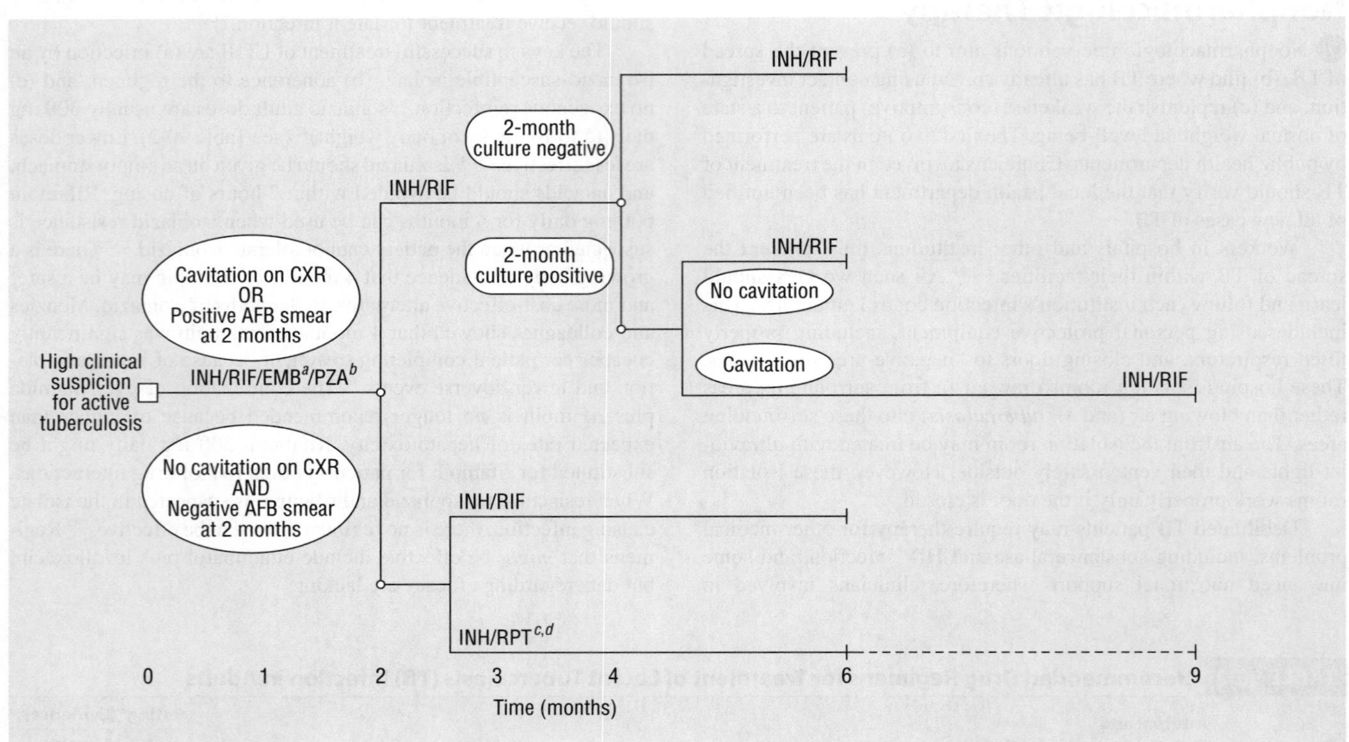

FIGURE 90-2 Treatment algorithm for tuberculosis. Note: Patients in whom tuberculosis is proved or strongly suspected should have treatment initiated with isoniazid, rifampin, pyrazinamide, and ethambutol for the initial 2 months. A repeat smear and culture should be performed when 2 months of treatment has been completed. If cavities were seen on the initial chest radiograph or the acid-fast smear is positive at completion of 2 months of treatment, the continuation phase of treatment should consist of isoniazid and rifampin daily or twice weekly for 4 months to complete a total of 6 months of treatment. If cavitation was present on the initial chest radiograph and the culture at the time of completion of 2 months of therapy is positive, the continuation phase should be lengthened to 7 months (total of 9 months of treatment). If the patient has HIV infection and the CD^+ cell count is <100/μL (<100 × 10^6/L), the continuation phase should consist of daily or three-times-weekly isoniazid and rifampin. In HIV-uninfected patients having no cavitation on chest radiograph and negative acid-fast smears at completion of 2 months of treatment, the continuation phase may consist of either once-weekly isoniazid and rifapentine, or daily or twice-weekly isoniazid and rifampin, to complete a total of 6 months (bottom). Patients receiving isoniazid and rifapentine, and whose 2-month cultures are positive, should have treatment extended by an additional 3 months (total of 9 months). (CXR, chest radiograph; EMB, ethambutol; INH, isoniazid; PZA, pyrazinamide; RIF, rifampin; RPT, rifapentine.) [a]EMB may be discontinued when results of drug susceptibility testing indicate no drug resistance. [b]PZA may be discontinued after it has been taken for 2 months (56 doses). [c]RPT should not be used in HIV-infected patients with tuberculosis or in patients with extrapulmonary tuberculosis. [d]Therapy should be extended to 9 months if the 2-month culture is positive. *(From: American Thoracic Society, Centers for Disease Control and Prevention, Infectious Diseases Society of America. Treatment of tuberculosis. MMWR Recomm Rep 2003;52(RR-11):1-77.)*

Drug susceptibility testing should be done on the initial isolate for all patients with active TB. These data should guide the selection of drugs over the course of treatment.[2,6,11,37] However, some patients are unable to provide a suitable specimen for laboratory testing. If susceptibility data are not available for a given patient, the drug susceptibility data for the suspected source case or regional susceptibility data should be used.[2,37]

Drug resistance should be expected for patients presenting for the retreatment of TB. These patients require retesting of drug susceptibility using freshly collected specimens. It is imperative to learn what drugs the patient received and for how long the patient received them.[2,11,37] A treatment history, often called a "*drug-o-gram*," shows the start and stop dates of all antimycobacterial drugs on a horizontal bar graph.[2,37] A drug-o-gram should be constructed for all retreatment patients.

9 The standard TB treatment regimen is isoniazid, rifampin, pyrazinamide, and ethambutol for 2 months, followed by isoniazid and rifampin for 4 months, a total of 6 months of treatment.[2,11,37] If susceptibility to isoniazid, rifampin, and pyrazinamide is shown, ethambutol can be stopped at any time. Without pyrazinamide, a total of 9 months of isoniazid and rifampin treatment is required. Table 90-3 shows the recommended treatment regimens. When intermittent therapy is used, DOT is essential. Doses missed during an intermittent TB regimen decrease its efficacy and increase the relapse rate. Note that Table 90-3 shows recommendations that differ for HIV-negative and HIV-positive patients. HIV-positive patients should not receive highly intermittent regimens. In general, regimens given daily five times each week or three times weekly can be used for HIV-positive patients. Less frequent dosing is associated with higher failure and relapse rates and the selection of rifampin-resistant organisms.[37]

When a patient's sputum smears convert to a negative, the risk of the patient infecting others is greatly reduced, but it is not zero.[2,17,37] Such patients can be removed from respiratory isolation, but they must be careful not to cough on others and should meet with others only in well-ventilated places. Smear-negative patients still may be culture positive, so they still can transmit TB to others.

Clinical **Controversy...**

Although very effective therapy exists for the treatment of TB, it continues to be a problem in the developing world. Cure rates of 95% to 98% are achievable with appropriate treatment; however, the right social, economic, and political conditions must exist in order for the prolonged, complicated regimen to be administered appropriately. Although individual case management (susceptibility testing, TDM, close followup) is ideal, it is difficult to implement in countries that bear the highest burden of TB. DOT exists in many developing countries, but due to limited resources and other social and political barriers, true DOT is not the standard of care.

TABLE 90-3 Drug Regimens for Culture-Positive Pulmonary Tuberculosis Caused by Drug-Susceptible Organisms

	Initial Phase		Continuation Phase				
Regimen	Drugs	Interval and Dose[c] (Minimal Duration)	Drugs	Interval and Doses[c,d] (Minimal Duration)	Range of Total Doses (Minimal Duration)	Rating[a] (Evidence)[b] HIV–	HIV+
1	Isoniazid, rifampin, pyrazinamide, ethambutol	Seven days per week for 56 doses (8 weeks) or 5 days/wk for 40 doses (8 weeks)[e]	Isoniazid/ rifampin	Seven days per week for 126 doses (18 weeks) or 5 days/wk for 90 doses (18 weeks)[e]	182–130 (26 weeks)	A (I)	A (II)
			Isoniazid/ rifampin	Twice weekly for 36 doses (18 weeks)	92–76 (26 weeks)	A (I)	A (II)[f]
			Isoniazid/ rifapentine[g]	Once weekly for 18 doses (18 weeks)	74–58 (26 weeks)	B (I)	E (I)
2	Isoniazid, rifampin, pyrazinamide, ethambutol	Seven days per week for 14 doses (2 weeks), then twice weekly for 12 doses (6 weeks) or 5 days/ wk for 10 doses (2 weeks),[e] and then twice weekly for 12 doses (6 weeks)	Isoniazid/ rifampin	Twice weekly for 36 doses (18 weeks)	62–58 (26 weeks)	A (II)	B (II)[f]
			Isoniazid/ rifapentine[g]	Once weekly for 18 doses (18 weeks)	44–40 (26 weeks)	B (I)	E (I)
3	Isoniazid, rifampin, pyrazinamide, ethambutol	Three times weekly for 24 doses (8 weeks)	Isoniazid/ rifampin	Three times weekly for 54 doses (18 weeks)	78 (26 weeks)	B (I)	B (II)
4	Isoniazid, rifampin, ethambutol	Seven days per week for 56 doses (8 weeks) or 5 days/wk for 40 doses (8 weeks)[e]	Isoniazid/ rifampin	Seven days per week for 217 doses (31 weeks) or 5 days/wk for 155 doses (31 weeks)[e]	273–195 (39 weeks)	C (I)	C (II)
			Isoniazid/ rifampin	Twice weekly for 62 doses (31 weeks)	118–102 (39 weeks)	C (I)	C (II)

[a]Ratings: A, preferred; B, acceptable alternative; C, offer when A and B cannot be given.
[b]Evidence ratings: I, randomized clinical trial; II, data from clinical trials that were not randomized or were conducted in other populations; III, expert opinion.
[c]When directly observed therapy is used, drugs may be given 5 days/wk, and the necessary number of doses adjusted accordingly. Although there are no studies that compare five with seven daily doses, extensive experience indicates this would be an effective practice.
[d]Patients with cavitation on initial chest radiograph and positive cultures at completion of 2 months of therapy should receive a 7-month (31-week; either 217 doses [daily] or 62 doses [twice weekly]) continuation phase.
[e]Five-day-a-week administration is always given by directly observed therapy. Rating for 5-day-per-week regimens is A (III).
[f]Not recommended for HIV-infected patients with CD4+ cell counts <100 cells/μL (<100 × 10^6/L).
[g]Should be used only in HIV-negative patients who have negative sputum smears at the time of completion of 2 months of therapy and who do not have cavitation on initial chest radiograph (see text). For patients started on this regimen and found to have a positive culture from the 2-month specimen, treatment should be extended an extra 3 months.

Adapted from American Thoracic Society, Centers for Disease Control and Prevention, Infectious Diseases Society of America. Treatment of tuberculosis. MMWR Recomm Rep 2003;52(RR-11):1–77.

Patients who are slow to respond clinically, those who remain culture positive at 2 months of treatment, those with cavitary lesions on chest radiograph, and perhaps HIV-positive patients should be treated for a total of 9 months and for at least 6 months from the time that they convert to smear and culture negativity.[2,6,11,37] Some authors recommend therapeutic drug monitoring (TDM) for such patients.[2,11,40,42] When isoniazid and rifampin cannot be used, treatment durations become 2 years or more regardless of immune status.[2,11,37,40]

Adjustments to the regimen should be made once the susceptibility data are available.[2,11,37] If the organism is drug-resistant, careful consideration of the remaining therapeutic options must be made. Two or more drugs with in vitro activity against the patient's isolate and that the patient has not received previously should be added to the regimen, as needed.[2,11,37] (10) There is no standard regimen for MDR-TB.[2,11,37] Each patient's exposure history, previous treatment history (including toxicity and adherence issues), and current susceptibility data must be considered simultaneously. *It is critical to avoid monotherapy, and it is critical to avoid adding a single drug to a failing regimen.*[2,11,37] Adding one drug at a time leads to the sequential selection of drug resistance until there are no drugs left. TB specialists should be consulted regarding cases of MDR-TB. It may take several months for a patient with MDR-TB to become culture negative because the drugs used lack the potency of isoniazid and rifampin.[2,40] Consequently, prolonged respiratory isolation may be required.

Drug resistance should be considered in the following situations:

1. Patients who have received prior therapy for TB
2. Patients from areas with a high prevalence of resistance (South Africa, Dominican Republic, Peru, Southeast Asia, the Baltic countries, and the former Soviet states)
3. Patients who are homeless, institutionalized, IV drug abusers, or infected with HIV
4. Patients who still have AFB-positive sputum smears after 1 to 2 months of therapy
5. Patients who still have positive cultures after 2 to 4 months of therapy
6. Patients who fail treatment or relapse after treatment
7. Patients known to be exposed to MDR-TB cases

Empirical therapy with four or more drugs may be needed for acutely ill patients.[2,11,37] These regimens may be altered when the susceptibility pattern becomes known. If the index case is known, then the same effective regimen should be employed for the new case. Again, MDR-TB cases should be referred to specialists. A new term in use, *XDR-TB*, refers to "extensively drug-resistant TB." Such organisms are resistant to at least isoniazid, rifampin, a fluoroquinolone, and one second-line injectable drug (amikacin, capreomycin, or kanamycin).[47]

Special Populations

Tuberculous Meningitis and Extrapulmonary Disease Patients with CNS TB usually are treated for longer periods (9 to 12 months instead of 6 months).[2,11,37] In general, isoniazid, pyrazinamide, ethionamide, and cycloserine penetrate the cerebrospinal fluid readily, but rifampin, ethambutol, and streptomycin have variable CNS penetration.[43] Of the quinolones, levofloxacin may be preferred based on current data. Extrapulmonary TB of the soft tissues can be treated with conventional regimens.[2,11,37] TB of the bone typically is treated for 9 months, occasionally with surgical debridement.[2,11,37]

Children TB in children may be treated with regimens similar to those used in adults, although some physicians still prefer to extend treatment to 9 months.[2,11,19,20,37] Pediatric doses of isoniazid and rifampin on a milligram-per-kilogram basis are higher than those used in adults (Table 90-4).[37]

Pregnancy Women with TB should be cautioned against becoming pregnant because the disease poses a risk to the fetus and to the mother. If already pregnant, the usual treatment is isoniazid, rifampin, and ethambutol for 9 months.[47] Isoniazid and ethambutol are relatively safe for use in pregnant women.[2,37,43,48] B vitamins are particularly important during pregnancy and should be provided to women being treated for TB. Rifampin is associated rarely with birth defects, including limb reduction and CNS lesions.[43] In general, rifampin is used in pregnant women with TB. Pyrazinamide has not been studied in large numbers of pregnant women, but anecdotal data suggest that it may be safe.[37]

Streptomycin use during pregnancy may lead to hearing loss in the newborn, including complete deafness. Streptomycin and the other aminoglycosides must be reserved for critical situations where alternatives do not exist.[2,37] Although the polypeptide capreomycin has not been studied, it probably carries the same risks.

Ethionamide may cause premature delivery and congenital deformities when used during pregnancy.[37,43] Down's syndrome also has been reported with ethionamide, so it cannot be recommended in this setting. *p*-Aminosalicylic acid has been used safely in pregnancy, but specific data are lacking.[37,43] Cycloserine is known to cross the placenta, but the effects on the developing fetus are not known. Therefore, cycloserine generally cannot be recommended during pregnancy.[43]

Ciprofloxacin, levofloxacin, moxifloxacin, and the other quinolones are associated with permanent damage to cartilage in the weight-bearing joints of immature animals, especially dogs and rabbits.[37,43] Although these drugs do not frequently cause joint problems in humans, other anti-TB agents should be used during pregnancy.

Pregnant women with LTBI are not at the same level of risk compared with those with active disease. Therapy with isoniazid for LTBI may be delayed until after pregnancy or, if recent skin-test conversion has occurred, started during the second trimester of pregnancy.[37,43,48] Although most anti-TB drugs are excreted in breast milk, the amount of drug received by the infant through nursing is insufficient to cause toxicity. Quinolones should be avoided in nursing mothers, if possible.

HIV Infection Patients with AIDS and other immunocompromised hosts may be managed with chemotherapeutic regimens similar to those used in immunocompetent individuals, although treatment is often extended to 9 months (see Table 90-3).[2,11,37] The precise duration to recommend remains a matter of debate. Highly intermittent regimens (twice or once weekly) are not recommended for HIV-positive TB patients. Prognosis has been particularly poor for HIV-infected patients infected with MDR-TB, so all efforts should be made to reduce the time between clinical presentation, diagnosis of TB, and start of appropriate treatment. Recommendations for management of HIV and TB published by the World Health Organization and others have provided guidance on monitoring of treatment, side effects, and drug interactions of HIV and TB, MDR, XDR-TB.[7,49] Differentiation must be made between infection with *M. tuberculosis* and nontuberculous mycobacteria, such as *Mycobacterium avium* complex (MAC), because the drugs used are different. While awaiting laboratory results, the patient can be treated empirically for TB if there is any doubt about the causative organism. Some patients with AIDS malabsorb their oral medications; this is discussed in Therapeutic Drug Monitoring below.[2,37,40,42] The major issue of drug interactions is discussed in Rifampin below.

TABLE 90-4 Doses[a] of Antituberculosis Drugs for Adults and Children[b,c]

Drug	Preparation	Adults/ Children	Doses			
			Daily	1× Per Week	2× Per Week	3× Per Week
First-line Drugs						
Isoniazid	Tablets (50, 100, 300 mg); elixir (50 mg/5 mL); aqueous solution (100 mg/mL) for IV or intramuscular injection	Adults (maximum)[c]	5 mg/kg (300 mg)	15 mg/kg (900 mg)	15 mg/kg (900 mg)	15 mg/kg (900 mg)
		Children (maximum)[c]	10–15 mg/kg (300 mg)	—	20–30 mg/kg (300 mg)	—
Rifampin	Capsule (150, 300 mg); powder may be suspended for oral administration; aqueous solution for IV injection	Adults[d] (maximum)[c]	10 mg/kg (600 mg)	—	10 mg/kg (600 mg)	10 mg/kg (600 mg)
		Children (maximum)[c]	10–20 mg/kg (600 mg)	—	10–20 mg/kg (600 mg)	—
Rifabutin	Capsule (150 mg)	Adult[d] (maximum)[c]	5 mg/kg (300 mg)	—	5 mg/kg (300 mg)	5 mg/kg (300 mg)
		Children	Appropriate dosing for children is unknown	Appropriate dosing for children is unknown	Appropriate dosing for children is unknown	Appropriate dosing for children is unknown
Rifapentine	Tablet (150 mg, film coated)	Adults[c]	—	10 mg/kg (continuation phase) (600 mg usual adult dose)	—	—
		Children	The drug is not approved for use in children	The drug is not approved for use in children	The drug is not approved for use in children	The drug is not approved for use in children
Pyrazinamide	Tablet (500 mg, scored)	Adults (maximum)[c]	40–55 kg: 1,000 mg (2 g)	—	40–55 kg: 2,000 mg	40–55 kg: 1,500 mg
			56–75 kg: 1,500 mg (2 g)	—	56–75 kg: 3,000 mg	56–75 kg: 2,500 mg
			76–90 kg: 2,000 mg (2 g)	—	76–90 kg: 4,000 mg	76–90 kg: 3,000 mg
		Children (maximum)[c]	15–30 mg/kg (2 g)	—	50 mg/kg (2 g)	—
Ethambutol	Tablet (100, 400 mg)	Adults (maximum)[c]	40–55 kg: 800 mg (1,600 mg)	—	40–55 kg: 2,000 mg	40–55 kg: 1,200 mg
			56–75 kg: 1,200 mg (1,600 mg)	—	56–75 kg: 2,800 mg	56–75 kg: 2,000 mg
			76–90 kg: 1,600 mg (1,600 mg)	—	76–90 kg: 4,000 mg	76–90 kg: 2,400 mg
		Children[d] (maximum)[c]	15–20 mg/kg daily (1 g)	—	50 mg/kg (2.5 g)	—
Second-line Drugs						
Cycloserine	Capsule (250 mg)	Adults (maximum)[c]	10–15 mg/kg/day (1 g in two doses), usually 500–750 mg/day in two doses[e]	There are no data to support intermittent administration	There are no data to support intermittent administration	There are no data to support intermittent administration
		Children (maximum)[c]	10–15 mg/kg/day (1 g/day)	—	—	—
Ethionamide	Tablet (250 mg)	Adults[f] (maximum)[c]	15–20 mg/kg/day (1 g/day), usually 500–750 mg/day in a single daily dose or two divided doses[f]	There are no data to support intermittent administration	There are no data to support intermittent administration	There are no data to support intermittent administration
		Children (maximum)[c]	15–20 mg/kg/day (1 g/day)	There are no data to support intermittent administration	There are no data to support intermittent administration	There are no data to support intermittent administration
Streptomycin	Aqueous solution (1-g vials) for IV or intramuscular administration	Adults (maximum)[c]	15 mg/kg/day[g] (1 g)	[g]	[g]	[g]
		Children (maximum)[c]	20–40 mg/kg/day (1 g)	—	20 mg/kg	—
Amikacin/ kanamycin	Aqueous solution (500-mg and 1-g vials) for IV or intramuscular administration	Adults (maximum)[c]	15 mg/kg/day[g] (1 g)	[g]	[g]	[g]
		Children (maximum)[c]	15–30 mg/kg/day (1 g) IV or intramuscular as a single daily dose	—	15–30 mg/kg	—

(continued)

TABLE 90-4 Doses[a] of Antituberculosis Drugs for Adults and Children[b,c] (Continued)

Drug	Preparation	Adults/ Children	Doses			
			Daily	1× Per Week	2× Per Week	3× Per Week
Capreomycin	Aqueous solution (1-g vials) for IV or intramuscular administration	Adults (maximum)[c]	15 mg/kg/day[g] (1 g)	[g]	15–30 mg/kg	[g]
		Children (maximum)[c]	15–30 mg/kg/day (1 g) as a single daily dose	—		—
p-Aminosalicylic acid (PAS)	Granules (4-g packets) can be mixed with food; tablets (500 mg) are still available in some countries, but not in the United States; a solution for IV administration is available in Europe	Adults[c]	8–12 g/day in two or three doses	There are no data to support intermittent administration	There are no data to support intermittent administration	There are no data to support intermittent administration
		Children (maximum)[c]	200–300 mg/kg/day in two to four divided doses (10 g)	There are no data to support intermittent administration	There are no data to support intermittent administration	There are no data to support intermittent administration
Levofloxacin	Tablets (250, 500, 750 mg); aqueous solution (500-mg vials) for IV injection	Adults[c]	500–1,000 mg daily	There are no data to support intermittent administration	There are no data to support intermittent administration	There are no data to support intermittent administration
		Children[c]	[h]	[h]	[h]	[h]
Moxifloxacin	Tablets (400 mg); aqueous solution (400 mg/250 mL) for IV injection	Adults[c]	400 mg daily	There are no data to support intermittent administration	There are no data to support intermittent administration	There are no data to support intermittent administration
		Children[c]	[i]	[i]	[i]	[i]

Higher doses of rifampin and rifapentine are being studied. Rifabutin dose may need to be adjusted when there is concomitant use of protease inhibitors or non-nucleoside reverse transcriptase inhibitors.

[a]Dose per weight is based on ideal body weight. Children weighing more than 40 kg should be dosed as adults.

[b]For purposes of this document, adult dosing begins at age 15 years.

[c]The authors of this chapter do not agree with the use of maximum doses, since this arbitrarily caps doses for patients who otherwise might need larger doses. These maximum doses were not based on prospective studies in large or overweight individuals, and do not consider patients with documented malabsorption of their medications. Clinical judgment should be used in such circumstances.

[d]The drug can likely be used safely in older children but should be used with caution in children less than 5 years of age, in whom visual acuity cannot be monitored. In younger children, ethambutol at the dose of 15 mg/kg/day can be used if there is suspected or proven resistance to isoniazid or rifampin.

[e]It should be noted that, although this is the dose recommended generally, most clinicians with experience using cycloserine indicate that it is unusual for patients to be able to tolerate this amount. Serum concentration measurements are often useful in determining the optimal dose for a given patient.

[f]The single daily dose can be given at bedtime or with the main meal.

[g]Dose: 15 mg/kg/day (1 g), and 10 mg/kg in persons older than 59 years of age (750 mg). Usual dose: 750–1,000 mg administered intramuscularly or IV, given as a single dose 5–7 days/wk and reduced to two or three times per week after the first 2–4 months or after culture conversion, depending on the efficacy of the other drugs in the regimen.

[h]The long-term (more than several weeks) use of levofloxacin in children and adolescents has not been approved because of concerns about effects on bone and cartilage growth. However, most experts agree that the drug should be considered for children with tuberculosis caused by organisms resistant to both isoniazid and rifampin. The optimal dose is not known.

[i]The long-term (more than several weeks) use of moxifloxacin in children and adolescents has not been approved because of concerns about effects on bone and cartilage growth. The optimal dose is not known.

Data from American Thoracic Society, Centers for Disease Control and Prevention, Infectious Diseases Society of America. Treatment of tuberculosis. MMWR Recomm Rep 2003;52(RR-11):1–77.

Renal Failure For nearly all patients, isoniazid and rifampin do not require dose modification in renal failure. They are eliminated primarily by the liver.[40,43,50] In the unlikely event that peripheral neuropathies develop, the frequency of isoniazid dosing may be reduced. Pyrazinamide and ethambutol typically require a reduction in dosing frequency from daily to three times weekly (Table 90-5).[37,50]

Renally cleared TB drugs include the aminoglycosides (amikacin, kanamycin, and streptomycin), capreomycin, ethambutol, cycloserine, and levofloxacin.[37,43,51] Dosing intervals need to be extended for these drugs (Table 90-5). Ciprofloxacin and moxifloxacin are approximately 50% cleared by the kidneys but may not require a change in dose from once daily, as used for TB. The metabolites of isoniazid, pyrazinamide, and *p*-aminosalicylic acid are cleared primarily by the kidneys. The role of these metabolites in causing toxicity is unknown, so their accumulation in renal failure may carry some risk.

Ethionamide and its sulfoxide metabolite are hepatically cleared, so dosing is unchanged.[37,51] *p*-Aminosalicylic acid is converted largely to metabolites prior to renal elimination; these metabolites may accumulate in renal failure.[51] For patients on hemodialysis, the usual 12-hour dosing interval for *p*-aminosalicylic acid granules seems to be safe. Dialysis will remove the metabolites. Serum concentration monitoring must be performed for cycloserine to avoid dose-related toxicities in renal failure patients.[40,42,51]

Hepatic Failure Anti-TB drugs that rely on hepatic clearance for most of their elimination include isoniazid, rifampin, pyrazinamide, ethionamide, and *p*-aminosalicylic acid.[43] Ciprofloxacin and moxifloxacin are approximately 50% cleared by the liver. Elevations of serum transaminase concentrations generally are not correlated with the residual capacity of the liver to metabolize drugs, so these markers cannot be used as guides for drug dosing. Furthermore, isoniazid, rifampin, pyrazinamide, and, to a lesser degree, ethionamide, *p*-aminosalicylic acid, and, rarely, ethambutol may cause hepatotoxicity.[37,40,43] For some patients with drug-susceptible TB, a "liver-sparing" regimen of streptomycin, levofloxacin, and ethambutol may be used, at least temporarily.[37,40,43] Because this regimen requires 18 or more months of treatment to be successful, patients usually are switched to isoniazid- and rifampin-containing regimens as soon as they are able.

Morbid Obesity Data are not available for dosing the TB drugs for patients with morbid obesity.[43] Relatively hydrophilic drugs (isoniazid, pyrazinamide, the aminoglycosides, capreomycin,

TABLE 90-5 Dosing Recommendations for Adult Patients with Reduced Renal Function and for Adult Patients Receiving Hemodialysis

Drug	Change in Frequency?	Recommended Dose and Frequency for Patients with Creatinine Clearance <30 mL/min (<0.50 mL/s) or for Patients Receiving Hemodialysis[a,b,c,d]
Isoniazid	No change	300 mg once daily, or 900 mg three times per week
Rifampin	No change	600 mg once daily, or 600 mg three times per week
Pyrazinamide	Yes	25–35 mg/kg per dose three times per week (not daily)
Ethambutol	Yes	15–25 mg/kg per dose three times per week (not daily)
Levofloxacin	Yes	750–1,000 mg per dose three times per week (not daily)
Cycloserine	Yes	250 mg once daily, or 500 mg/dose three times per week[e]
Ethionamide	No change	250–500 mg/dose daily
p-Aminosalicylic acid	No change	4 g/dose, twice daily
Streptomycin	Yes	12–15 mg/kg per dose two or three times per week (not daily)
Capreomycin	Yes	12–15 mg/kg per dose two or three times per week (not daily)
Kanamycin	Yes	12–15 mg/kg per dose two or three times per week (not daily)
Amikacin	Yes	12–15 mg/kg per dose two or three times per week (not daily)

[a]Standard doses are given unless there is intolerance.
[b]The medications should be given after hemodialysis on the day of hemodialysis.
[c]Monitoring of serum drug concentrations should be considered to ensure adequate drug absorption, without excessive accumulation, and to assist in avoiding toxicity.
[d]Data currently are not available for patients receiving peritoneal dialysis. Until data become available, begin with doses recommended for patients receiving hemodialysis and verify adequacy of dosing, using serum concentration monitoring.
[e]The appropriateness of 250-mg daily doses has not been established. There should be careful monitoring for evidence of neurotoxicity.

Adapted from American Thoracic Society, Centers for Disease Control and Prevention, Infectious Diseases Society of America. Treatment of tuberculosis. MMWR Recomm Rep 2003;52(RR-11):1–77.

ethambutol, *p*-aminosalicylic acid, and cycloserine) can be dosed initially based on ideal body weight. Very low or very high serum concentrations can be avoided by checking the serum concentrations.

The TB Drugs

The interested reader is referred to several other publications for more detailed information regarding these drugs.[2,10,37,40,42,43] Note that although the ATS/CDC guidelines recommend "maximum" doses (see Table 90-4),[37] in the authors' view, the "maximum" dose for a given patient is the dose that produces the desired response with an acceptable level of toxicity.[40,42] This can only be determined on a case-by-case basis. Artificially capping doses may deprive patients of needed drug.

Primary Antituberculosis Drugs

Isoniazid Isoniazid is one of the two most important TB drugs. It is highly specific for mycobacteria, with a MIC against *M. tuberculosis* of 0.01 to 0.25 mcg/mL (mg/L). It is bactericidal and is thought to inhibit mycolic acid synthesis and disruption of the cell wall in susceptible organisms. Most nontuberculous mycobacteria such as *M. avium* are resistant to isoniazid, although *M. kansasii* and *Mycobacterium xenopi* are susceptible. The most common mechanisms of resistance result from mutations in the *katG* or *inhA* genes.

Isoniazid is readily absorbed from the GI tract and from intramuscular injection sites. It also can be given as a short IV infusion over 5 minutes if diluted in about 20 mL of normal saline.[52] Isoniazid should be given on an empty stomach whenever possible.[53] *N*-Acetyltransferase 2 forms the principal metabolite acetylisoniazid, which lacks antimycobacterial activity. The rate at which humans acetylate isoniazid is determined genetically; slow acetylation is an autosomal recessive trait and reflects a relative lack of *N*-acetyltransferase 2. Fast acetylators have isoniazid half-lives of less than 2 hours. Approximately 50% of whites and blacks and 80% to 90% of Asians and Native Alaskans are rapid acetylators. Slow acetylators have isoniazid half-lives of 3 to 4 hours and may be at an increased risk of neurotoxicity. The association of acetylator status and risk of hepatotoxicity, however, appears to be weak.[54] Poor absorption and rapid clearance of isoniazid for patients receiving highly intermittent therapy are associated with poor clinical outcomes.[55,56]

Transient elevations of the serum transaminases occur in 12% to 15% of patients receiving isoniazid and usually occur within the first 8 to 12 weeks of therapy.[37] Overt hepatotoxicity, however, occurs in only 1% of cases. Risk factors for hepatotoxicity include patient age, preexisting liver disease, excessive alcohol intake, pregnancy, and the postpartum state. Isoniazid also may result in neurotoxicity, most frequently presenting as peripheral neuropathy or, in overdose, as seizures and coma. Patients with pyridoxine deficiency, such as pregnant women, alcoholics, children, and the malnourished, are at increased risk. Isoniazid may inhibit the metabolism of phenytoin, carbamazepine, primidone, and warfarin.[40] Patients who are being treated with these agents should be monitored closely, and appropriate dose adjustments should be made when necessary.

Rifampin The introduction of rifampin into routine use during the 1970s allowed for true short-course treatment of TB (6 to 9 months).[2,11,37] Without rifampin, treatment is generally 18 months or longer. Drug resistance to rifampin is an ominous prognostic factor because it is frequently associated with isoniazid resistance and leaves the patient with few good therapeutic options. Clinicians *must* take care to protect susceptibility to rifampin by carefully treating their patients. Rifampin shows bactericidal activity against *M. tuberculosis* and several other mycobacterial species, including *M. bovis* and *M. kansasii*.[57] It also is active against a broad array of other bacteria. Alteration of the target site on RNA polymerase, primarily through changes in the *rpoB* gene, leads to most forms of rifampin resistance.[37,57]

Rifampin usually is given orally, but it also can be given as a 30-minute IV infusion.[57] Oral doses are best given on an empty stomach.[58] Patients with AIDS, diabetes, and other GI problems appear to have difficulty absorbing rifampin after oral doses, and this has been associated with therapeutic failures in some cases.[40,42,56,59] Rifampin is metabolized to 25-desacetyl rifampin, which retains some of rifampin's activity; most of rifampin and its metabolite are cleared in the bile. Rifampin generally is given at 600 mg daily or intermittently, although this dose does not take full advantage of rifampin's concentration-dependent killing.[40,42] Higher doses should be tested in humans within the context of clinical trials.

Elevations in hepatic enzymes have been attributed to rifampin in 10% to 15% of patients, with overt hepatotoxicity occurring in less than 1%.[37,57] More frequent adverse effects of rifampin include rash, fever, and GI distress. Allergic reactions to rifampin have been reported and occur more frequently with intermittent rifampin doses 900 mg or more twice weekly. These reactions may take the form of a flu-like syndrome with development of fever, chills, headache, arthralgias, and, rarely, hypotension and shock.[37] Alternatively, hemolytic anemia or acute renal failure may occur, requiring permanent discontinuation.

TABLE 90-6 Recommended Regimens for the Concomitant Treatment of Tuberculosis and HIV Infection

Combined Regimen for Treatment of HIV and Tuberculosis	PK Effect of the Rifamycin	Tolerability/Toxicity	Antiviral Activity When Used with Rifampin	Recommendations (Comments)
Efavirenz-based antiretroviral therapy[a] with rifampin-based TB treatment	Well-characterized, modest effect	Low rates of discontinuation	Excellent	Preferred (efavirenz should not be used during the first trimester of pregnancy)
PI-based antiretroviral therapy[a] with rifabutin-based TB treatment	Little effect of rifabutin on PI concentrations, but marked increases in rifabutin concentrations	Low rates of discontinuation (if rifabutin is appropriately dose-reduced)	Favorable, although published clinical experience is not extensive	Preferred for patients unable to take efavirenz[b]
Nevirapine-based antiretroviral therapy with rifampin-based TB treatment	Moderate effect	Concern about hepatotoxicity when used with isoniazid, rifampin, and pyrazinamide	Favorable	Alternative for patients who cannot take efavirenz and if rifabutin not available
Zidovudine/lamivudine/abacavir/tenofovir with rifampin-based TB treatment	50% decrease in zidovudine, possible effect on abacavir not evaluated	Anemia	No published clinical experience	Alternative for patients who cannot take efavirenz and if rifabutin not available
Zidovudine/lamivudine/tenofovir with rifampin-based TB treatment	50% decrease in zidovudine, no other effects predicted	Anemia	Favorable, but not evaluated in a randomized trial	Alternative for patients who cannot take efavirenz and if rifabutin not available
Zidovudine/lamivudine/abacavir with rifampin-based TB treatment	50% decrease in zidovudine, possible effect on abacavir not evaluated	Anemia	Early favorable experience, but this combination is less effective than efavirenz-based regimens in persons not taking rifampin	Alternative for patients who cannot take efavirenz and if rifabutin not available
Superboosted lopinavir-based ART with rifampin-based TB treatment	Little effect	Hepatitis among healthy adults, but favorable experience, among young children (<3 years)	Good, among young children (<3 years)	Alternative if rifabutin not available; preferred for young children when rifabutin not available

ART, antiretroviral therapy.

[a]With two nucleoside analogues.

[b]Includes patients with NNRTI-resistant HIV, those unable to tolerate efavirenz, and women during the first one to two trimesters of pregnancy.

Adapted from Centers for Disease Control and Prevention. Managing Drug Interactions in the Treatment of HIV Related Tuberculosis. 2007.

Rifampin's potent induction of hepatic enzymes, especially cytochrome P450 3A4, may enhance the elimination of many other drugs, most notably the protease inhibitors used to treat HIV (Table 90-6). HIV-positive patients may benefit from the use of rifabutin instead of rifampin.[25,37,49,60] Furthermore, women who use oral contraceptives must use another form of contraception during therapy because increased clearance of the hormones may lead to unexpected pregnancies. Patient records should be reviewed for potential drug interactions before dispensing rifampin. Rifampin may turn urine and other secretions orange-red and may permanently stain some types of contact lenses.

Other Rifamycins Rifabutin is used for disseminated *M. avium* infection in AIDS patients and is quite active against *M. tuberculosis*. Most rifampin-resistant organisms are resistant to rifabutin. Because rifabutin is a less potent enzyme inducer than rifampin, it may be used for patients who are receiving protease inhibitors.[37,49,60,61] For HIV-positive patients, the ATS/CDC recommends regimens with three or more doses of the TB drugs per week (see Table 90-3). Rifapentine is a long-acting rifamycin that can be used once weekly in the continuation phase of treatment (after the first 2 months) in carefully selected HIV-negative patients. It is approximately as potent an enzyme inducer as rifampin, so similar drug interactions are likely.[37,49,60,61]

Pyrazinamide Adding pyrazinamide to the first 2 months of treatment with isoniazid and rifampin shortens the duration to 6 months for most patients.[2,37] Pyrazinamide may be bacteriostatic or bactericidal depending on the concentration and the susceptibility of the organism. It is usually well absorbed and displays a fairly long half-life.[62,63] The most common toxicities of pyrazinamide are GI distress, arthralgias, and elevations in the serum uric acid concentrations.[37] Most patients do not experience true gout. Hepatotoxicity is the major limiting adverse effect and is dose-related when pyrazinamide is given daily.

A fixed-combination product (Rifater, Aventis) of rifampin 120 mg, isoniazid 50 mg, and pyrazinamide 300 mg is designed to prevent drug resistance by keeping the self-medicating patient from using only one drug at a time. If the patient is receiving DOT, there is no particular advantage to this product. The typical dose of Rifater will be five to six tablets daily. When pyrazinamide is discontinued after 2 months of treatment, the combination product Rifamate (isoniazid 150 mg and rifampin 300 mg) can be substituted.

Ethambutol Ethambutol replaced *p*-aminosalicylic acid as a first-line agent in the 1960s because it was better tolerated by patients.[2,37] It is used as a fourth drug for TB while awaiting susceptibility data.[37] If the organism is susceptible to isoniazid, rifampin, and pyrazinamide, ethambutol can be stopped. Ethambutol is active against most mycobacteria, by inhibiting synthesis of metabolites and impairing cell metabolism, and is generally bacteriostatic.

Ethambutol should not be given with antacids.[64] For patients with renal failure, the ethambutol dose should be reduced to three times per week.[50,65] Retrobulbar neuritis is the major adverse effect. Patients may complain of a change in visual acuity, the inability to see the color green, or both. They should be monitored monthly while on the drug using Snellen wall charts for visual acuity and Ishihara red-green color discrimination cards.[31,37]

Second-Line Antituberculosis Drugs

Streptomycin Streptomycin is one of three aminoglycoside antibiotics (along with amikacin and kanamycin) that are active against mycobacteria. It is quite active against MAC and several other mycobacteria, enterococci, *Brucella*, *Yersinia*, and various other bacteria.

Although labeled only for intramuscular dosing, streptomycin can be given safely as IV infusions (100 mL of 5% dextrose in water or normal saline) over 30 minutes, similar to the other aminoglycosides.[66] Streptomycin, like other aminoglycosides, is renally cleared by glomerular filtration and must be given less often to patients with renal dysfunction.[37,40]

Streptomycin occasionally causes nephrotoxicity, although it tends to be mild and reversible. It also is capable of causing ototoxicity (vestibular and cochlear), which may become permanent with continued use.[37] Older patients and those receiving long durations of treatment are most likely to experience hearing loss, whereas vestibular toxicity is highly unpredictable.

Resistance to amikacin and kanamycin is frequently linked but independent of resistance to streptomycin and independent of resistance to capreomycin. Therefore, susceptibility tests should guide the selection of these injectable drugs.

p-Aminosalicylic Acid In the United States, only the enteric-coated, sustained-release granule form (Paser) is available.[67–69] GI disturbances are the most common adverse effects from *p*-aminosalicylic acid. Diarrhea is usually self-limited, with symptoms improving after the first 1 to 2 weeks of therapy. Occasionally, a few doses of an opioid will resolve the problem. It also is important to tell the patient that the empty granules will appear in the stool. Although FDA approved for three daily doses, pharmacokinetic data support twice-daily dosing.[68]

Various types of malabsorption, including steatorrhea, were reported with previous dosage forms of *p*-aminosalicylic acid. Hypersensitivity and, rarely, severe hepatitis may occur. *p*-Aminosalicylic acid is known to produce goiter, with or without myxedema, that seems to occur more frequently with concomitant ethionamide therapy.

Cycloserine Cycloserine is only used to treat MDR-TB. It is well absorbed orally and is best taken on an empty stomach.[70] It is cleared primarily through the kidneys by glomerular filtration and requires dosage reduction in renal failure. Cycloserine can produce dose-related CNS toxicity, including lethargy, confusion, or unusual behavior. Seizures, although reported, are exceedingly rare in U.S. patients.[2,37] Therapy is improved by maintaining 2-hour postdose serum concentrations between 20 and 35 mcg/mL (mg/L; 200 and 349 μmol/L).[40,42] Most patients reach a maximum dose of 750 mg daily, divided unevenly into two doses. This can be achieved by starting with 250 mg daily for 2 days, followed by 250 mg increments over 2-day intervals. This dose of cycloserine can be maintained if the patient complains of only occasional mild CNS effects, such as difficulty concentrating. Serum concentrations can be checked 1 to 2 weeks into therapy. The addition of pyridoxine 50 mg daily may improve patient tolerance of cycloserine.

Ethionamide Ethionamide shares structural features with two other antimycobacterial agents, isoniazid and, more distantly, thiacetazone, a drug not used in the United States. Prothionamide, the *n*-propyl derivative of ethionamide, is used in Europe. Ethionamide is only active against organisms of the genus *Mycobacterium*, and it should be considered primarily bacteriostatic because it is difficult to achieve serum concentrations that would be bactericidal.[37,40,42]

GI toxicity is the dose-limiting adverse effect. The drug should be introduced gradually in 250 mg increments, as described earlier for cycloserine. Rarely will a patient tolerate more than 1,000 mg daily in divided oral doses. Ethionamide may be administered with a light snack or prior to bedtime to minimize GI intolerance. Food does not affect absorption significantly.[71] Little ethionamide is recovered in the urine, so doses remain the same in renal failure. Ethionamide may cause goiter with or without hypothyroidism (especially when given with *p*-aminosalicylic acid), gynecomastia, alopecia, impotence, menorrhagia, photodermatitis, and acne. The management of diabetes also may be more difficult for patients receiving ethionamide. Because of these problems, ethionamide only is used when necessary.

Clofazimine Clofazimine is a drug with good activity against *Mycobacterium leprae* and some activity against *M. tuberculosis* and *M. avium*. It is used in doses of 100 mg daily in advanced cases of MDR-TB or MAC, especially when therapeutic options are limited.[37,40] The drug has a terminal elimination half-life that is weeks long. GI distress and skin discoloration are the most important adverse reactions. Although uncommon, severe GI pain may occur because of deposition of clofazimine crystals within the intestines; this may require surgical correction.

Thiacetazone Thiacetazone is a weak agent used rarely in parts of the developing world because of its low cost. Skin reactions, including rash and Stevens-Johnson syndrome, may occur. Thiacetazone must be discontinued permanently as soon as a rash appears. Similar to trimethoprim–sulfamethoxazole, the incidence of skin reactions is much higher for AIDS patients.[72]

Quinolones Levofloxacin, gatifloxacin (outside of the United States), and moxifloxacin are sometimes used to treat MDR-TB because of their excellent activity against *M. tuberculosis*. Several studies have suggested a potential role for moxifloxacin as a possible replacement for certain first-line agents.[2,11,37,40,73–75] Moxifloxacin has been compared with isoniazid and ethambutol during the first 8 weeks of therapy for pulmonary TB. It did not demonstrate a significant increase in 8-week culture negativity when compared with isoniazid. However, shorter time to culture conversion was seen when compared with ethambutol. Quinolones are useful because most are available in oral and IV dosage forms, so they can be used in critically ill patients. However, resistance of MTB to the fluoroquinolones is a major concern. Resistance is attributed to mutations in the *gyrA* and *gyrB* genes and can develop in a relatively short period of time.[76]

Macrolides/Azalides The macrolide clarithromycin and azalide azithromycin represent substantial advances in the treatment of MAC but demonstrate limited activity against *M. tuberculosis* and are not used frequently for TB.[2,11,37,40]

New Drugs and Delivery Systems Several promising compounds are currently under development for the treatment of MTB. The nitroimidazole derivatives, OPC67683 (delamanid) and PA824, are chemically related to metronidazole and work through inhibiting mycolic acid synthesis. The diarylquinoline TMC207 (bedaquiline) works through targeting the ATP synthase pump, and does not demonstrate cross-resistance with existing TB drugs. All of these agents have potent in vitro and in vivo activity with very low MICs against *M. tuberculosis*.[77–79] Both TMC-207 and OPC67683 have been evaluated in Phase 2b placebo-controlled, double-blind, randomized trials in patients with newly diagnosed MDR-TB and have shown rapid culture conversion and good tolerance.[77,78,80] PA-824 has moved from Phase 1 to Phase 2 trials. Linezolid has been used in some patients with MDR-TB.[81] Long-term use of linezolid requires careful monitoring of hematologic indices for potential anemia and thrombocytopenia. It may be possible to reduce the incidences of these toxicities by giving linezolid 600 mg daily or 300 mg twice daily for the slow-growing *M. tuberculosis* rather than the usual 600 mg twice-daily dose used for gram-positive organisms. Two new compounds in the oxazolidinone class, PNU-100480 and AZD-5847, are currently in Phase 1 studies. Liposomes have been investigated as delivery systems for various agents against mycobacteria, including isoniazid, rifampin, and the aminoglycosides. By changing the pharmacokinetic profile of such agents, their use in the treatment of mycobacterial infections could be enhanced greatly. Currently, no such product is licensed for use against TB.

Corticosteroids Adjunctive therapy with corticosteroids may be of benefit for some patients with tuberculous meningitis or pericarditis to relieve inflammation and pressure.[2,37] They should be avoided in most other circumstances because they detract from the immune response to TB.

Bacille Calmette-Guérin Vaccine The BCG vaccine is an attenuated, hybridized strain of *M. bovis*. It was developed in 1921 and is used as a prophylactic vaccine against TB. Administration of BCG vaccine is compulsory in many developing countries and is officially recommended in many others. Vaccination with BCG produces a subclinical infection resulting in sensitization of T lymphocytes and cross-immunity to *M. tuberculosis*, as well as cutaneous hypersensitivity and, in many cases, a positive tuberculin skin test.

In the published clinical trials, several different BCG preparations were used, and the efficacy of these vaccinations ranged from negative 56% (some patients did worse with the vaccine) to positive 80%.[2,37] Trials within the United States and Puerto Rico have shown efficacy rates of 6% to 29%. The primary benefit of BCG vaccination appears to be the prevention of severe forms of TB in children. Data from the BCG trials show that the incidence of tuberculous meningitis and miliary TB is 52% to 100% lower and that the incidence of pulmonary TB is 2% to 80% lower in vaccinated children younger than 15 years of age than it was in unvaccinated controls.

Unfortunately, BCG does not appear to be very reliable in preventing disease by *M. tuberculosis* in other segments of the population. Side effects occur in 1% to 10% of vaccinated persons and usually include severe or prolonged ulceration at the vaccination site, lymphadenitis, and lupus vulgaris. It is recommended that pregnant women and patients with impaired immune systems, including those with HIV infection, avoid vaccination. The World Health Organization had recommended, however, that in populations where the risk of TB is high, HIV-infected infants who are asymptomatic should receive BCG vaccine at birth or as soon as possible thereafter. Because BCG infection has occurred in AIDS patients given the vaccine, individuals with symptomatic HIV infection should not be vaccinated.[2,37]

In the United States, BCG vaccination is recommended only for uninfected children who are at unavoidable risk of exposure to TB and for whom other methods of prevention and control have failed or are not feasible.[2,37] Its use is very limited.

PERSONALIZED PHARMACOTHERAPY

Health professionals should develop and maintain treatment plans, provide drug information, direct appropriate TDM, and monitor adherence, adverse drug reactions, and interactions to TB therapy through regular assessments. Patients coinfected with HIV will require special attention because of their immunocompromised state and increased risk of drug interactions. TDM may be necessary in certain populations.

Therapeutic Drug Monitoring

TDM, or applied pharmacokinetics, is the use of serum drug concentrations to optimize therapy.[37,40,42,82,83] TDM generally should be used if patients are failing appropriate treatment (no clinical improvement after 2 to 4 weeks or smear positive after 4 to 6 weeks). Patients with AIDS, diabetes, cystic fibrosis, various GI disorders, or MDR-TB may be tested prospectively, before problems arise, to ensure adequate treatment (Table 90-6). Blood samples collected at 2 and 6 hours after a dose have been used with some success, although they may not be the optimal sampling times for all the drugs. Finally, TDM of the TB and HIV drugs is perhaps the most logical way to untangle the complex drug interactions that take place.[84,85]

Clinical **Controversy. . .**

Some TB centers employ TDM for many of their patients at the outset of treatment in order to identify drug-delivery problems early. Other centers wait to see how the patient responds and perform TDM only if problems arise. An argument can be made for either approach. The latter can save money, but delays in effective treatment can affect the patient's outcome adversely.

EVALUATION OF THERAPEUTIC OUTCOMES

Monitoring of the Pharmaceutical Care Plan

The most serious problem with TB therapy is patient nonadherence to the prescribed regimens.[86] Unfortunately, there is no reliable way to identify such patients a priori. Noncompliance rates of up to 89% have been reported with TB therapy.[86] It is critical to the control of TB that such adherence rates be improved dramatically. The most effective way to achieve this end is with DOT.[2,11,37] Despite criticisms that it will cost more money, it is far cheaper in the long run to prevent the further spread of disease with DOT than to track down and treat additional cases of TB continuously.

The homeless and other underprivileged individuals are assumed to constitute the group of patients considered "unreliable," and DOT should be reserved for them; it is also assumed that "responsible" patients cared for by private physicians may be treated with daily, unsupervised therapy. A study conducted in Baltimore, however, compared outcomes (sputum culture conversion to negative at 3 months) for patients with pulmonary TB who were treated by private physicians with outcomes for patients treated via DOT in a city-run clinic. Surprisingly, 3-month culture conversion occurred in only 40% of the private-care patients, compared with 90% in the city clinic-care patients.[82] Clearly, expansion of the use of DOT to nearly all patients with TB may be of benefit.

Patients who are AFB smear positive should have sputum samples sent for AFB stains every 1 to 2 weeks until two consecutive smears are negative. This provides early evidence of a response to treatment.[37] Once on maintenance therapy, sputum cultures can be performed monthly until two consecutive cultures are negative, which generally occurs over 2 to 3 months. If sputum cultures continue to be positive after 2 months, drug susceptibility testing should be repeated, and serum concentrations of the drugs should be checked.

Serum chemistries, including blood urea nitrogen, creatinine, aspartate transaminase, and alanine transaminase, and a complete blood count with platelets should be performed at baseline and periodically thereafter, depending on the presence of other factors that may increase the likelihood of toxicity (e.g., advanced age, alcohol abuse, pregnancy)[2,37] (see Table 90-7). Hepatotoxicity should be suspected for patients whose serum transaminases exceed five times the upper limit of normal or whose total bilirubin concentration exceeds 3 mg/dL (51.3 μmol/L) and for patients with symptoms such as nausea, vomiting, or jaundice. At this point, the offending agent(s) should be discontinued. Sequential reintroduction of the drugs with frequent testing of liver enzymes is often successful in identifying the offending agent; other agents may be continued. Alternative agents should be selected as needed. Audiometric testing should be performed at baseline and monthly for

TABLE 90-7 Antituberculosis Drug Monitoring Table

Drug	Adverse Effects	Monitoring
Isoniazid	Asymptomatic elevation of aminotransferases, clinical hepatitis, fatal hepatitis, peripheral neurotoxicity, CNS effects, lupus-like syndrome, hypersensitivity, monoamine poisoning, diarrhea	LFT monthly in patients who have preexisting liver disease or who develop abnormal liver function that does not require discontinuation of drug; dosage adjustments may be necessary in patients receiving anticonvulsants or warfarin
Rifampin	Cutaneous reactions, GI reactions (nausea, anorexia, abdominal pain), flu-like syndrome, hepatotoxicity, severe immunologic reactions, orange discoloration of bodily fluids (sputum, urine, sweat, tears), drug interactions due to induction of hepatic microsomal enzymes	Liver enzymes and interacting drugs as needed (e.g., warfarin)
Rifabutin	Hematologic toxicity, uveitis, GI symptoms, polyarthralgias, hepatotoxicity, pseudojaundice (skin discoloration with normal bilirubin), rash, flu-like syndrome, orange discoloration of bodily fluids (sputum, urine, sweat, tears)	Drug interactions are less problematic than rifampin
Rifapentine	Similar to those associated with rifampin	Drug interactions are being investigated and are likely similar to rifampin
Pyrazinamide	Hepatotoxicity, GI symptoms (nausea, vomiting), nongouty polyarthralgia, asymptomatic hyperuricemia, acute gouty arthritis, transient morbilliform rash, dermatitis	Serum uric acid can serve as a surrogate marker for adherence; LFTs in patients with underlying liver disease
Ethambutol	Retrobulbar neuritis, peripheral neuritis, cutaneous reactions	Baseline visual acuity testing and testing of color discrimination; monthly testing of visual acuity and color discrimination in patients taking >15–20 mg/kg, having renal insufficiency, or receiving the drug for >2 months
Streptomycin	Ototoxicity, neurotoxicity, nephrotoxicity	Baseline audiogram, vestibular testing, Romberg's testing, and SCr Monthly assessments of renal function and auditory or vestibular symptoms
Amikacin/kanamycin	Ototoxicity, nephrotoxicity	Baseline audiogram, vestibular testing, Romberg's testing, and SCr; monthly assessments of renal function and auditory or vestibular symptoms
Capreomycin	Nephrotoxicity, ototoxicity	Baseline audiogram, vestibular testing, Romberg's testing, and SCr Monthly assessments of renal function and auditory or vestibular symptoms Baseline and monthly serum K^+ and Mg^{2+}
p-Aminosalicylic acid	Hepatotoxicity, GI distress, malabsorption syndrome, hypothyroidism, coagulopathy	Baseline LFTs and TSH TSH every 3 months
Moxifloxacin	GI disturbance, neurologic effects, cutaneous reactions	No specific monitoring recommended

LFT, liver function test; TSH, thyroid-stimulating hormone.

Adapted from American Thoracic Society, Centers for Disease Control and Prevention, Infectious Diseases Society of America. Treatment of tuberculosis. MMWR Recomm Rep 2003;52(RR-11):1–77.

patients who must receive aminoglycosides for more than 1 to 2 months. Vision testing (Snellen visual acuity charts and Ishihara color discrimination plates) should be performed on all patients who receive ethambutol. All patients diagnosed with TB should be tested for HIV infection.

ABBREVIATIONS

AFB acid-fast bacillus
ATS American Thoracic Society
BCG bacillus Calmette-Guérin
CDC Centers for Disease Control and Prevention
CMI cell-mediated immunity
DOT directly observed treatment
DTH delayed-type hypersensitivity
ELISA enzyme-linked immunosorbent assay
HIV human immunodeficiency virus
IGRA interferon-γ release assay
IL interleukin
INF interferon
LAM lipoarabinomannan
LTBI latent tuberculosis infection
MAC *Mycobacterium avium* complex
MDR multidrug resistant
MGIT mycobacterial growth indicator tube
MIC minimal inhibitory concentration
MTD *M. tuberculosis* direct
PCR polymerase chain reaction
PPD purified protein derivative
QFT-G QuantiFERON-TB Gold test
rRNA ribosomal ribonucleic acid
SDA strand-displacement amplification
TB tuberculosis
TDM therapeutic drug monitoring
TH_1 T-helper type 1
TH_2 T-helper type 2
TNF tumor necrosis factor
WBC white blood cell
XDR extensively drug-resistant

REFERENCES

1. WHO. Report on the Global Tuberculosis Epidemic. Geneva: World Health Organization, 2011.
2. Iseman MD. A Clinician's Guide to Tuberculosis. Philadelphia, PA: Lippincott Williams & Wilkins, 2000.
3. Centers for Disease Control and Prevention. Reported Tuberculosis in the United States, 2011. Atlanta, GA: US

Department of Health and Human Services, CDC, 2011, *http://www.cdc.gov/tb/statistics/reports/2011/default.htm.*

4. Centers for Disease Control and Prevention. Tuberculosis in the United States, 2010. Atlanta, GA: Department of Health and Human Services, CDC, 2010, *http://www.cdc.gov/tb/statistics/reports/2010/default.htm.*
5. Hudelson P. Gender differentials in tuberculosis: The role of socio-economic and cultural factors. Tuber Lung Dis 1996;77:391–400.
6. Fitzgerald DW, Sterling TR. *Mycobacterium tuberculosis*. In: Mandell GL, Bennett JE, Dolin R, eds. Principles and Practice of Infectious Diseases, 5th ed. New York: Churchill-Livingstone, 2010:3129–3164.
7. WHO. Guidelines for the Programmatic Management of Drug Resistant Tuberculosis. Geneva: World Health Organization, 2011.
8. Harries AD, Zacharia R, Corbett EL, et al. The HIV associated tuberculosis epidemic—When will we act? Lancet 2010;375:1906–1919.
9. Heifets L. Mycobacteriology laboratory. Clin Chest Med 1997;18:35–53.
10. Heifets LB. Drug susceptibility tests in the management of chemotherapy of tuberculosis. In: Heifets LB, ed. Drug Susceptibility in the Chemotherapy of Mycobacterial Infections. Boca Raton, FL: CRC Press, 1991:89–122.
11. Daley CL, Chambers HF. *Mycobacterium tuberculosis* complex. In: Yu VL, Weber R, Raoult D, eds. Antimicrobial Therapy and Vaccines, Vol I. Microbes, 2nd ed. New York: Apple Trees Productions, 2002:841–865.
12. Issa R, Mohd Hassan NA, Abdul H, et al. Detection and discrimination of *Mycobacterium tuberculosis* complex. Diagn Microbiol Infect Dis 2012;72:62–67.
13. Roberts GD, Böttger EC, Stockman L. Methods for the rapid identification of mycobacterial species. Clin Lab Med 1996;16:603–615.
14. Somoskovi A, Parsons LM, Salfinger M. The molecular basis of resistance to isoniazid, rifampin, and pyrazinamide in *Mycobacterium tuberculosis*. Respir Res 2001;2:164–168.
15. Marin M, Garcia de Viedma D, Ruiz-Serrano MJ, Bouza E. Rapid direct detection of multiple rifampin and isoniazid resistance mutations in *Mycobacterium tuberculosis* in respiratory samples by real-time PCR. Antimicrob Agents Chemother 2004;48:4293–4300.
16. Daniel TM, Boom WH, Ellner JJ. Immunology of tuberculosis. In: Reichman LB, Hershfield ES, eds. Tuberculosis: A Comprehensive International Approach, 2nd ed. New York: Marcel Dekker, 2000:157–185.
17. Piessens WF, Nardell EA. Pathogenesis of tuberculosis. In: Reichman LB, Hershfield ES, eds. Tuberculosis: A Comprehensive International Approach, 2nd ed. New York: Marcel Dekker, 2000:241–260.
18. Long, R, Gardam, M. Tumour necrosis factor-α inhibitors and the reactivation of latent tuberculosis infection. Can Med Assoc J 2003;168:1153–1156.
19. American Thoracic Society/Centers for Disease Control and Prevention. Diagnostic standards and classification of tuberculosis in adults and children. Am J Respir Crit Care Med 2000;161:1376–1395.
20. Cruz AT, Stark JR. Clinical manifestations of tuberculosis in children. Paediatr Respir Rev 2007;8:107–117.
21. Alland D, Kalkut GE, Moss AR, et al. Transmission of tuberculosis in New York City: An analysis of DNA fingerprinting and conventional epidemiologic methods. N Engl J Med 1994;330:1710–1716.
22. Daley CL, Small PM, Schecter GF, et al. An outbreak of tuberculosis with accelerated progression among persons infected with the human immunodeficiency virus: An analysis using restricted-fragment-length polymorphisms. N Engl J Med 1992;326:231–235.
23. Kwan CK, Ernst JD. HIV and tuberculosis: A deadly human syndemic. Clin Microbiol Rev 2011;24:351–376.
24. American Thoracic Society/Centers for Disease Control and Prevention. Targeted tuberculin skin testing and treatment of latent tuberculosis infection. Am J Respir Crit Care Med 2000;161:S221–S247.
25. Akolo C, Adetifa I, Sheppard S, Volmink J. Treatment of latent tuberculosis infection in HIV infected persons. Cochrane Database Syst Rev 2010;(1):CD000171.
26. Anergy skin testing and preventive therapy for HIV-infected persons: Revised recommendations. Centers for Disease Control and Prevention. MMWR Recomm Rep 1997; 46:1–10.
27. Jensen PA, Lambert LA, Iademarco MF, Ridzon R; Centers for Disease Control and Prevention. Guidelines for preventing the transmission of *Mycobacterium tuberculosis* in health care settings. MMWR Recomm Rep 2005; 54(RR-17):1–141.
28. Villarino ME, Burman WJ, Wang Y et al. Comparable specificity of two commercial tuberculin reagents in persons at low risk for tuberculosis infection. JAMA 1999;281: 169–171.
29. Rosenberg T, Manfreda J, Hershfield ES. Two-step tuberculin testing in staff and residents of a nursing home. Am Rev Respir Dis 1993;148:1537–1540.
30. Mazurek GH, Jereb J, Varnon A, et al. Updated guidelines for interferon gamma release assay to detect *Mycobacterium tuberculosis* infection, United States. MMWR Recomm Rep 2010;59(RR-5):1–25.
31. Barnes PF. Weighing gold or counting spots. Am J Respir Crit Care Med 2006;174:731–735.
32. Nicol MP, Davies MA, Wood K, Hatherill M, et al. Comparison of T-SPOT. TB assay and tuberculosis skin test for the evaluation of young children at high risk for tuberculosis in community setting. Pediatrics 2009;123: 38–43.
33. Bergamini BM, Losi M, Vaienti F, et al. Performance of commercial blood tests for the diagnosis of latent tuberculosis infection in children and adolescents. Pediatrics 2009;123:e419–e424.
34. Lighter J, Rigaud M, Eduardo R, Peng CH, et al. Latent tuberculosis diagnosis in children by using the quantiferon-TB gold in tube test. Pediatrics 2009;123:30–37.
35. Richeldi L, Losi M, D'Amico R, et al. Performance of tests for latent tuberculosis in different groups of immunocompromised patients. Chest 2009;136:198–204.
36. Bouza E, Diaz-Lopez MD, Moreno S, et al. *Mycobacterium tuberculosis* bacteremia in patients with and without human immunodeficiency virus infection. Arch Intern Med 1993;153:496–500.
37. American Thoracic Society/Centers for Disease Control/Infectious Disease Society of America. Treatment of tuberculosis. Am J Respir Crit Care Med 2003;167:603–662.
38. Fujiwara PI, Larkin C, Frieden TR. Directly observed therapy in New York City. Clin Chest Med 1997;18:135–148.
39. Weis SE. Universal directly observed therapy. Clin Chest Med 1997;18:155–163.
40. Peloquin CA. Pharmacological issues in the treatment of tuberculosis. Ann N Y Acad Sci 2001;953:157–164.
41. Fourie PB, Ellner JJ, Johnson JL. Whither *Mycobacterium vaccae*—Encore. Lancet 2002;360:1032–1033.
42. Peloquin CA. Therapeutic drug monitoring in the treatment of tuberculosis. Drugs 2002;62:2169–2183.

43. Peloquin CA. Antituberculosis drugs: Pharmacokinetics. In: Heifets LB, ed. Drug Susceptibility in the Chemotherapy of Mycobacterial Infections. Boca Raton, FL: CRC Press, 1991:59–88.
44. Aspler A, Long R, Trajman A, et al. Impact of treatment completion, intolerance and adverse events on health system costs in a randomized trial of 4 months of rifampin or 9 months isoniazid for latent TB. Thorax 2010;65:582–587.
45. Sterling TR, Villarino ME, Borisov AS, et al. Three months of once-weekly rifapentine and isoniazid for *M. tuberculosis* infection. N Engl J Med 2011;365:2155–2166.
46. Centers for Disease Control and Prevention. Recommendations for use of isoniazid–rifapentine regimen with direct observation to treat *Mycobacterium tuberculosis* infection. MMWR Morb Mortal Wkly Rep 2011;60: 1650–1653.
47. Lawn SD, Wilkinson R. Extensively drug resistant tuberculosis. BMJ 2006;333:559–560.
48. Mnyani CN, McIntyre JA. Tuberculosis in pregnancy. Br J Obstet Gynecol 2011;118:226–231.
49. WHO. Antiretroviral Therapy for HIV Infection in Adults and Adolescents: Towards Universal Access. Geneva: World Health Organization, 2006.
50. Malone RS, Fish DN, Spiegel DM, et al. The effect of hemodialysis on isoniazid, rifampin, pyrazinamide, and ethambutol. Am J Respir Crit Care Med 1999;159:1580–1584.
51. Malone RS, Fish DN, Spiegel DM, et al. The effect of hemodialysis on cycloserine, ethionamide, *para*-aminosalicylate, and clofazimine. Chest 1999;116:984–990.
52. Crabbe SJ. Drug InfoSearch—Intravenous isoniazid. P&T 1990;15:1483–1484.
53. Peloquin CA, Namdar R, Dodge AA, Nix DE. Pharmacokinetics of isoniazid under fasting conditions, with food, and with antacids. Int J Tuberc Lung Dis 1999; 3:703–710.
54. Berning SE, Peloquin CA. Antimycobacterial agents: Isoniazid. In: Yu VL, Merigan TC, Barriere S, White NJ, eds. Antimicrobial Chemotherapy and Vaccines. Baltimore: Williams & Wilkins, 2010:654–663.
55. Weiner M, Burman W, Vernon A, et al. Low isoniazid concentration associated with outcome of tuberculosis treatment with once-weekly isoniazid and rifapentine. Am J Respir Crit Care Med 2003;167:1341–1347.
56. Weiner M, Benator D, Burman W, et al. Association between acquired rifamycin resistance and the pharmacokinetics of rifabutin and isoniazid among patients with HIV and tuberculosis. Clin Infect Dis 2005;40:1481–1491.
57. Morris AB, Kanyok TP, Scott J, et al. Rifamycins. In: Yu VL, Merigan TC, Barriere S, White NJ, eds. Antimicrobial Chemotherapy and Vaccines. Baltimore: Williams & Wilkins, 1998:901–963.
58. Peloquin CA, Namdar R, Singleton MD, Nix DE. Pharmacokinetics of rifampin under fasting conditions, with food, and with antacids. Chest 1999;115:12–18.
59. Barroso EC, Pinheiro VG, Facanha MC, et al. Serum concentrations of rifampin, isoniazid, and intestinal absorption, permeability in patients with multidrug resistant tuberculosis. Am J Trop Med Hyg 2009;81:322–329.
60. Mofenson LM, Brady MT, Danner SP, et al. Guidelines for the prevention and treatment of opportunistic infections among HIV-exposed and HIV-infected children: Recommendations from the CDC, the National Institutes of Health, the HIV Medicine Association of Infectious Diseases Society of America, the Pediatric Infectious Disease Society and the American Academy of Pediatrics. MMWR Recomm Rep 2009;58:1–166.
61. Burman WJ, Gallicano K, Peloquin CA. Comparative pharmacokinetics and pharmacodynamics of the rifamycin antibiotics. Clin Pharmacokinet 2001;40:327–341.
62. Peloquin CA, Jaresko GS, Yong CL, et al. Population pharmacokinetic modeling of isoniazid, rifampin, and pyrazinamide. Antimicrob Agents Chemother 1997;41: 2670–2679.
63. Peloquin CA, Bulpitt AE, Jaresko GS, et al. Pharmacokinetics of pyrazinamide under fasting conditions, with food, and with antacids. Pharmacotherapy 1998;18:1205–1211.
64. Peloquin CA, Bulpitt AE, Jaresko GS, et al. Pharmacokinetics of ethambutol under fasting conditions, with food, and with antacids. Antimicrob Agents Chemother 1999;43:568–572.
65. Summers KK, Hardin TC. Treatment of tuberculosis in hemodialysis patients. J Infect Dis Pharmacother 1996;2: 37–55.
66. Peloquin CA, Berning SE. Comment: Intravenous streptomycin. Ann Pharmacother 1993;27:1546–1547.
67. Peloquin CA, Henshaw TL, Huitt GA, et al. Pharmacokinetic evaluation of *p*-aminosalicylic acid granules. Pharmacotherapy 1994;14:40–46 (Correction. Pharmacotherapy 1994;14:2).
68. Peloquin CA, Berning SE, Huitt GA, et al. Once-daily and twice-daily dosing of *p*-aminosalicylic acid (PAS) granules. Am J Respir Crit Care Med 1999;159:932–934.
69. Peloquin CA, Zhu M, Adam RD, et al. Pharmacokinetics of *p*-aminosalicylate under fasting conditions, with orange juice, food, and antacids. Ann Pharmacother 2001;35:1332–1338.
70. Zhu M, Nix DE, Adam RD, et al. Pharmacokinetics of cycloserine under fasting conditions, with orange juice, food, and antacids. Pharmacotherapy 2001;21:891–897.
71. Zhu M, Namdar R, Stambaugh JJ, et al. Population pharmacokinetics of ethionamide in patients with tuberculosis. Tuberculosis 2002;82:91–96.
72. Elliott AM, Foster SD. Thiacetazone: Time to call a halt? Tuber Lung Dis 1996;77:27–29.
73. Burman WJ, Goldberg S, Johnson JL, et al. Moxifloxacin versus ethambutol in the first 2 months of treatment for pulmonary tuberculosis. Am J Respir Crit Care Med 2006;174:331–338.
74. Conde MB, Efron A, Loredo C, et al. Moxifloxacin versus ethambutol in the initial treatment of tuberculosis: A double blind, randomized, controlled phase II trial. Lancet 2009;373:1183–1189.
75. Dorman SE, Johnson JL, Goldberg S, et al. Substitution of moxifloxacin for isoniazid during intensive phase treatment of pulmonary tuberculosis. Am J Respir Crit Care Med 2009;180:273–280.
76. Devasia RA, Blackman A, Gebretsadik T, et al. Fluoroquinolone resistance in *Mycobacterium tuberculosis*: The effect of duration and timing of fluoroquinolone exposure. Am J Respir Crit Care Med 2009;180:365–370.
77. Diacon AH, Pym A, Grobusch M, et al. The diarylquinoline TMC207 for multidrug resistant tuberculosis. N Engl J Med 2009;360:2397–2405.
78. Diacon AH, Dawson R, Hanekom M, et al. Early bactericidal activity of delamanid (OPC-67683) in smear-positive pulmonary tuberculosis patients. Int J Tuberc Lung Dis 2011; 15:949–954.
79. Hu Y, Coates AR, Mitchison DA. Comparison of the sterilizing activities of the nitroimidazopyran PA-824 and moxifloxacin against persisting *Mycobacterium tuberculosis*. Int J Tuberc Lung Dis 2008;12:69–73.
80. Gler MT, Skripconoka V, Sanchez-Garavito E, et al. Delamanid for multidrug resistant pulmonary tuberculosis. N Engl J Med 2012;366:2151–2160.

81. Forun J, Martin-Davila P, Navas E, et al. Linezolid for the treatment of multidrug resistant tuberculosis. J Antimicrob Chemother 2005;56:180–185.
82. Chaulk CP, Friedman M, Dunning R. Modeling the epidemiology and economics of directly observed therapy in Baltimore. Int J Tuberc Lung Dis 2000;4:201–207.
83. Tappero JW, Bradford WZ, Agerton TB, et al. Serum concentrations of antimycobacterial drugs in patients with pulmonary tuberculosis in Botswana. Clin Infect Dis 2005;41:461–469.
84. Perlman DC, Segal Y, Rosenkranz S, et al. The clinical pharmacokinetics of rifampin and ethambutol in HIV-infected persons with tuberculosis. Clin Infect Dis 2005;41:1638–1647.
85. Peloquin CA. Agents for tuberculosis. In: Piscitelli SC, Rodvold KA, eds. Drug Interactions in Infectious Diseases. Totowa, NJ: Humana Press, 2001:109–120.
86. Brudney K, Dobkin J. Resurgent tuberculosis in New York City: Human immunodeficiency virus, homelessness, and the decline of tuberculosis control programs. Am Rev Respir Dis 1991;144:745–749.

91

Gastrointestinal Infections and Enterotoxigenic Poisonings

Steven Martin and Rose Jung

KEY CONCEPTS

1. The etiology of infectious diarrhea includes bacteria, viruses, and protozoans. Viral infections are the leading cause of diarrhea in the world.
2. The common pathogens responsible for watery diarrhea are norovirus and enterotoxigenic *Escherichia coli*. The pathogens that produce dysentery or bloody diarrhea are *Shigella* spp., *Campylobacter jejuni*, nontyphoid *Salmonella*, and enterohemorrhagic *E. coli*.
3. Fluid and electrolyte replacement is the cornerstone of therapy for diarrheal illnesses. Oral rehydration therapy is preferred in most cases of mild and moderate diarrhea.
4. Antibacterial therapy often is not indicated for gastroenteritis because many cases are mild and self-limited or are viral in nature. Antibiotic therapy is recommended in severe cases of diarrhea, moderate-to-severe cases of traveler's diarrhea, most cases of febrile dysenteric diarrhea, and culture-proven bacterial diarrhea.
5. Loperamide offers symptomatic relief in patients with moderate watery diarrhea. However, the use of antimotility agents should be avoided in patients with dysentery diarrhea.
6. Diarrheal illness can be largely prevented by following simple rules of personal hygiene and safe food preparation.
7. Metronidazole is the drug of choice for mild to moderate *Clostridium difficile* infection (CDI). In patients with severe disease, contraindication or intolerance to metronidazole, and inadequate response to metronidazole, oral vancomycin or fidaxomicin, is recommended.
8. The most common pathogens for traveler's diarrhea include enterotoxigenic *E. coli*, *Shigella*, *Campylobacter*, *Salmonella*, and viruses.
9. Patient education in prevention strategies and self-treatment of traveler's diarrhea is recommended. Prophylaxis with antibiotics is not recommended in most situations.
10. Common pathogens responsible for food poisoning include *Staphylococcus*, *Salmonella*, *Shigella*, and *Clostridium*.

GI infections and enterotoxigenic poisonings encompass a wide variety of medical conditions characterized by inflammation of the GI tract. Vomiting and diarrhea are commonly associated with GI inflammation. The resulting dehydration is responsible for much of the morbidity and mortality. Diarrhea is defined as a decrease in consistency of bowel movements (i.e., unformed stool) and an increase in frequency of stools to ≥3 per day.[1] Acute disease is commonly associated with diarrhea lasting ≤14 days in duration while persistent diarrhea lasts >14 days.

This chapter focuses on infectious etiologies of acute GI infections and enterotoxigenic poisonings. A wide variety of viral, bacterial, and parasitic pathogens are responsible for this disease. Chapter 93 discusses the common protozoans that cause gasteroenteritis. Therefore, this chapter focuses on common viral and bacterial etiologies. Because the clinical consequences of bloody or dysenteric diarrhea can be more severe compared with cases of watery or nonbloody diarrhea, the chapter is organized accordingly. Epidemiology, clinical presentation, diagnosis, treatment, and prevention strategies are discussed for all GI infections, and further elaborated in subsequent sections in regards to specific diseases such as *Clostridium difficile*–associated diarrhea, traveler's diarrhea, and foodborne illnesses.

EPIDEMIOLOGY

Dehydration resulting from acute diarrhea is the second leading cause of morbidity and mortality worldwide, and infants and children younger than 5 years of age are at the highest risk. Among the 139 low- to middle-income countries, there were approximately 1.7 billion episodes of childhood diarrhea in 2010. The incidence of diarrhea for all children younger than age 5 years was estimated to be 2.9 episodes per child per year. The incidence of diarrhea was higher in younger children, with 4.5 episodes per child per year among children aged 6 to 11 months, compared with 2.3 episodes per child per year for children 24 to 59 months of age.[2] Younger children also had a higher risk of death from acute dehydrating diarrhea. For children younger than age 1 year and those aged 1 to 4 years, the median mortality rates were 8.5 and 3.8 per 1,000 children per year, respectively.[3] Although incidence of childhood diarrhea has been declining, diarrhea remains a major health problem in children, especially in those younger than 1 year.

In the United States, 179 million episodes of acute gastroenteritis occur each year, resulting in more than 600,000 hospitalizations and more than 5,000 deaths.[4,5] In contrast to the developing world where the risk of death is highest among young children, most of those who die of diarrheal illness in the United States are elderly. During 1979 to 1987, 51% of deaths caused by diarrheal illness were among patients older than age 74 years, and 27% were among the ages of 55 to 74 years; only 11% of deaths were in those younger than age 5 years.[6] Similarly, a study of the McDonnell-Douglas Health Information System database revealed that 25% of all hospitalizations and 85% of all mortality associated with diarrhea involved the elderly (≥age 60 years).[4] In addition to children and elderly, other groups at risk for GI infections include travelers and campers, patients in chronic care facilities, military personnel assigned overseas, and immunocompromised patients such as those with acquired immunodeficiency syndrome (AIDS).

Etiology

1 The etiology of GI infections and enterotoxigenic poisonings includes a wide variety of virus, bacteria, and parasites, but contribution of each is unknown. Etiologic agents are rarely identified due to the infrequency of stool samples collected, or inability of many laboratories to detect the full range of pathogens, especially viruses. In this chapter, discussions of pathogens responsible for watery diarrhea focus on virus (rotavirus and norovirus), enterotoxigenic *Escherichia coli* (ETEC), and cholera. Pathogens commonly associated with dysenteric or bloody diarrhea are *Shigella* spp., *Salmonella* spp., *Campylobacter* spp., enterohemorrhagic *E. coli* (EHEC), *Yersinia enterocolitica*, and *C. difficile*. Characteristics of watery and dysenteric diarrhea and common pathogens responsible for them are outlined in Table 91-1.

Viruses are now recognized as the leading cause of diarrhea in the world. In Asia, Africa, and Latin America, viral gastroenteritis accounts for 3 to 5 billion cases and is associated with 5 to 10 million deaths.[7] Noroviruses, previously known as Norwalk-like viruses, account for greater than 90% of viral gastroenteritis among all age groups and 50% of outbreaks worldwide. In the United States, noroviruses have been estimated to cause 21 million cases of acute gastroenteritis annually including >70,000 hospitalizations and nearly 800 deaths.[5] Outbreaks occur throughout the year and have been documented in families, healthcare systems, cruise ships, and college dormitories.

In infants and children, rotavirus, a double-stranded, wheel-shaped, RNA virus, is the most common cause of diarrhea worldwide, and 1 million people die annually from the infection. In the United States, approximately 3.5 million cases of diarrhea, 500,000 physician visits, 50,000 hospitalizations, and 20 deaths occur each year in children younger than age 5 years.[7] Nearly all children are infected by age 5 years. After the initial infection with rotavirus, 40% of children are protected against subsequent infection, 75% are protected against subsequent gastroenteritis, and up to 88% are protected against severe gastroenteritis. Other viruses, enteric adenovirus, and astrovirus, coronaviruses, enteroviruses, and pestiviruses, are being identified increasingly as causative agents of diarrhea. Characteristics of viral pathogens causing gastroenteritis are outlined in Table 91–2.

2 In the United States, bacterial causes of acute gastroenteritis account for more than 5.2 million cases of diarrhea annually including 46,000 hospitalizations and 1,500 deaths.[4] However, there appears to be substantial underreporting and the cause is identified in less than 3% of cases. In the United States, common pathogens responsible for watery diarrhea are norovirus and ETEC while those associated with dysentery or bloody diarrhea are *Shigella* spp. (15.3%), *Campylobacter* spp. (6.2%), *Salmonella* spp. (5.8%), EHEC (2.6%), and others (0.6%).[8] Other organisms that are responsible for dysentery include *Aeromonas* species, noncholera *Vibrio*, and *Y. enterocolitica*. Characteristics of acute bacterial pathogens causing gastroenteritis are summarized in Table 91-3.

Cholera has been rare in the United States because of advanced water and sanitation systems. However, the disease that causes profuse watery diarrhea is endemic in the Indian subcontinent and sub-Saharan Africa. *Vibrio cholerae* is a gram-negative bacillus sharing similar characteristics with the family Enterobacteriaceae, and the disease is caused by toxigenic *V. cholerae* serogroups O1 or O139. Approximately half of the people infected with *V. cholerae* O1 are symptomatic, whereas only 1% to 5% of those infected with *V. cholerae* O139 manifest symptoms.[9]

E. coli is a gram-negative bacillus commonly found in the human GI tract, and diarrheagenic *E. coli* is differentiated into several distinct categories based on pathogenic features of diarrheal disease: ETEC, enteroinvasive *E. coli* (EIEC), enteropathogenic *E. coli* (EPEC), enteroaggregative *E. coli* (EAEC), and EHEC. ETEC occurs most commonly, and accounts for about half of all cases of *E. coli* diarrhea. There are an estimated 79,000 cases of ETEC in

TABLE 91-1 Acute Infectious Diarrhea Clinical Syndromes: Watery versus Dysentery

	Watery	Dysentery
Percentage of patients	90	5–10
Stools		
Appearance	Watery	Bloody
Volume	Increased: ++/+++	Increased: +/++
Number per day	<10	>10
Reducing substances	0 to +++	0
pH	5–7.5	6–7.5
Occult blood	Negative	Positive
Fecal polymorphonuclear cells	Absent or few	Many
Mechanisms	Toxins Reduced absorption	Toxins Mucosal invasion
Complications		
Dehydration	Could be severe	Mild
Others	Acidosis, shock, electrolyte imbalance	Tenesmus, rectal prolapse, seizures
Etiology	*Vibrio cholerae* Enterotoxigenic *Escherichia coli* (ETEC) Rotaviruses Noroviruses	*Shigella* *Salmonella* *Campylobacter* *Yersinia* Enterohemorrhagic *E. coli* (EHEC) *Clostridium difficile*

TABLE 91-2 Characteristics of Agents Responsible for Acute Viral Gastroenteritis

Virus	Peak Age of Onset	Time of Year	Duration	Mode of Transmission	Common Symptoms
Rotavirus	6 months to 2 years	October to April	3–7 days	Fecal–oral, water, food	Nausea, vomiting, diarrhea, fever, abdominal pain, lactose intolerance
Norovirus	All age groups	Peak in winter	2–3 days	Fecal–oral, food, water, environment	Nausea, vomiting, diarrhea, abdominal cramps, myalgia
Astrovirus	<7 years	Winter	1–4 days	Fecal–oral, water, shellfish	Diarrhea, headache, malaise, nausea
Enteric adenovirus	<2 years	Year-round	7–9 days	Fecal–oral	Diarrhea, respiratory symptoms, vomiting, fever
Pestivirus	<2 years	NR	3 days	NR	Mild
Coronavirus-like particles	<2 years	Fall and early winter	7 days	NR	Respiratory disease
Enterovirus	NR	NR	NR	NR	Mild diarrhea, secondary organ damage

NR, not reported.

TABLE 91-3 Characteristics of Acute Bacterial Gastroenteritis

Bacteria	Incubation Period	Duration	Mode of Transmission	Common Symptoms
Watery Diarrhea				
Vibrio cholerae	2–3 days	1–3 days	Contaminated food or water with human feces usually in areas of inadequate treatment of sewage and drinking water	Profuse watery diarrhea, vomiting, and leg cramps Death can occur within hours without treatment
Enterotoxigenic *E. coli*	1–3 days	3–4 days	Contaminated food or water with animal or human feces	Watery diarrhea and abdominal cramping
Enteropathogenic *E. coli*	9–12 hours	NR	Contaminated food or water with animal or human feces	Acute onset of profuse watery diarrhea, vomiting, and low-grade fever in young children (<2 years of age) in the developing world
Enteroaggregative *E. coli*	NR	NR	Contaminated food or water with animal or human feces	Chronic, watery, mucoid, secretory diarrhea with low-grade fever in immunocompromised persons (HIV infections)
Enteroinvasive *E. coli*	10–18 hours	NR	Contaminated food or water with animal or human feces	Watery diarrhea in young children in the developing world
Dysentery Diarrhea				
Shigella	1–3 days	1–7 days	Fecal–oral Contaminated food or water with infected human feces	Watery or bloody diarrhea (8–10 stools/day), severe abdominal pain, fever, and malaise
Enterohemorrhagic *E. coli*	3–4 days	5–7 days	Contaminated food (particularly cattle) or water with animal or human feces	Severe stomach cramps, diarrhea (often bloody), and vomiting Approximately 5–10% develop hemolytic uremic syndrome
Campylobacter jejuni	2–5 days	5–7 days	Contaminated food (particularly poultry), water, or contact with infected animals	Diarrhea (often bloody), cramping, abdominal pain, and fever
Nontyphoid *Salmonella*	12–36 hours	1–5 days	Contaminated food, water, or contact with infected animals	Diarrhea (sometimes bloody), fever, and abdominal cramps
Yersinia	4–7 days	1–3 weeks	Contaminated food or water	Fever, abdominal pain, and diarrhea (often bloody)

NR, not reported.

the United States each year.[4] ETEC is also the most common cause of traveler's diarrhea and a common cause of food- and water-associated outbreaks. Infections with EIEC and EPEC are primarily a disease of children in developing countries.[10,11] EAEC strains are implicated in persistent diarrhea (≥14 days) in human immunodeficiency virus (HIV)-infected patients.[12] EHEC, also known as Shiga toxin–producing *E. coli* (STEC), causes watery diarrhea that becomes bloody in 1 to 5 days in 80% of patients.[10]

Approximately 165 million cases of shigellosis occur worldwide with 450,000 cases from the United States annually.[13] *Shigella* species are gram-negative bacilli belonging to the family Enterobacteriaceae. Four species most often associated with disease are *Shigella dysenteriae* type 1, *Shigella flexneri*, *Shigella boydii*, and *Shigella sonnei*.[13] In the United States, *S. sonnei* and *S. flexneri* are the most common causes of gastroenteritis. The other two *Shigella* species are commonly acquired during travel to developing countries. Poor sanitation or personal hygiene, inadequate water supply, malnutrition, and increased population density are associated with an increased risk of *Shigella* gastroenteritis epidemics, even in developed countries.

The *Campylobacter* species are flagellated, curved, gram-negative rods. Although there are 14 different species, *Campylobacter jejuni* is the species responsible for more than 99% of *Campylobacter*-associated gastroenteritis. Approximately 2.4 million persons are affected each year in the United States, involving almost 1% of the entire population.[4]

Salmonella enterica are gram-negative bacilli belonging to the family Enterobacteriaceae. The most prevalent *S. enterica* serotypes are Typhi and Paratyphi, which cause enteric fever. Gastroenteritis is caused by *S. enterica* serotypes Typhimurium or Enteritidis. In the United States, the largest burden of *Salmonella* infection is due to nontyphoidal serotypes, causing approximately 1.4 million cases of salmonellosis, 16,000 hospitalizations, and 600 deaths, occurring annually.[14]

Recognized as a common and potentially deadly cause of infectious diarrhea, EHEC is believed to be the major etiologic factor responsible for the development of hemorrhagic colitis and hemolytic uremic syndrome (HUS). The annual disease burden of *E. coli* O157:H7 in the United States is more than 20,000 infections and as many as 250 deaths; however, the failure of many clinical laboratories to screen for this organism greatly complicates any estimates.[15] In the United States, serotype O157:H7 causes 50% to 60% of all EHEC infections, but in the southern hemisphere, including Argentina, Australia, Chile, and South Africa, non-O157:H7 serotypes are often more prevalent. Non-O157 STEC strains in general produce a lower frequency of dysentery than O157 positive strains (62% vs. 85%).

Yersinia species are non–lactose-fermenting gram-negative coccobacilli that are widely distributed in nature. The genus *Yersinia* includes six species known to cause disease in humans. *Y. enterocolitica* and, to a lesser extent, *Yersinia pseudotuberculosis* are most likely associated with intestinal infection, but overall both are a relatively infrequent cause of diarrhea and abdominal pain. More than 50 serotypes of *Y. enterocolitica* exist; of these, serotypes 0:3, 0:8, and 0:9 are associated most frequently with enterocolitis.[16] Children are the most likely to experience illness with *Y. enterocolitica* infection.

PATHOPHYSIOLOGY

Acute gastroenteritis and its resulting diarrhea are caused by altered movement of ions and water resulting in increased colonic secretion. Under normal conditions, the GI tract has the tremendous capacity to absorb fluid and electrolytes allowing only 100 to 200 mL of fluid to be excreted in the stool daily.[17] The classic enteric pathogen that causes secretary diarrhea is *V. cholerae*, but ETEC and rotavirus are also responsible for watery diarrhea.

V. cholerae is an enteric pathogen that causes classical secretory diarrhea due to changes in ion secretion and absorption. Among the toxins produced by *V. cholerae*, the most important is cholera toxin.[9] Cholera toxin consists of two subunits, A and B. The B subunits are responsible for delivery of the A subunit into the cell. The A subunit stimulates adenylate cyclase, which increases intracellular cyclic adenosine monophosphate (cAMP) and results in protein kinase A (PKA)-mediated activation of cystic fibrosis transmembrane conductance regulator (CFTR). This leads to increased chloride secretion and decreased sodium absorption producing the severe watery diarrhea characteristic of the disease.[18] The toxin likely acts along the entire intestinal tract, but most fluid loss occurs in the duodenum. The net effect of the cholera toxin is isotonic fluid secretion (primarily in the small intestine) that exceeds the absorptive capacity of the intestinal tract (primarily the colon).

ETEC also causes watery diarrhea characterized by severe intestinal water secretion by producing plasmid-mediated enterotoxins: heat-labile toxin and heat-stable toxin. The heat-labile toxin has two subunits (A and B) that have similar antigenic properties and action on the gut mucosa as cholera toxin. Heat-labile toxins increase chloride secretion via activation of cAMP. The net effect is luminal accumulation of electrolytes that draws water into the intestine, and production of a cholera-like secretory diarrhea.[19] Heat-stable toxin is thought to be nonantigenic and produces watery diarrhea by acting on the small intestine.

Rotavirus induces changes in transepithelial fluid balance, and causes malabsorption as a consequence of destruction of epithelial lining of intestine, and vascular damage and ischemia of villi. Once rotavirus infects small intestinal villus cells, viroplasms are formed and its toxin, nonstructural protein 4 (NSP4), is released. The viral enterotoxin increases intracellular calcium, and the increase in calcium disrupts microvillus cytoskeleton, as well as barrier function. Changes to the villi include shortening of villus height, crypt hyperplasia, and mononuclear cell infiltration of the lamina propria.[20]

Inflammatory diarrhea is caused by two groups of organisms—enterotoxin-producing, noninvasive bacteria (e.g., EAEC, EHEC) or invasive organisms (e.g., *Salmonella* spp., *Shigella* spp., *Campylobacter* spp.). The enterotoxin-producing organisms adhere to the mucosa, activate cytokines, and stimulate the intestinal mucosa to release inflammatory mediators. Invasive organisms, which can also produce enterotoxin, invade the intestinal mucosa to induce an acute inflammatory reaction, involving the activation of cytokines and inflammatory mediators.

Ingestion of as few as 10 to 200 viable organisms of the *Shigella* species causes disease in healthy adults.[13] *Shigella* multiply and spread within the submucosa of the small bowel, but they rarely extend beyond the mucosa. Inflammatory diarrhea is caused by the pathogens invading the epithelial barrier through M cells where they encounter and eliminate macrophages. The destruction of macrophages after emergence from M cells causes an initial release of interleukin (IL)-1β. This initial inflammatory process is exacerbated by free bacteria binding to toll-like receptor (TLR4) that causes the production of IL-6 and IL-8. Both IL-1β and IL-8 attract polymorphonucleocytes.[21] Release of polymorphonucleocytes activates chloride secretion and subsequent diarrhea. Degranulation and release of toxic substances by neutrophils cause ulceration of the epithelium, distortion of the crypts, death to intestinal epithelium, sloughing of mucosal cells, bloody mucoid exudate into the gut lumen, and submucosal accumulation of inflammatory cells with microabscess formation.[22] Microabscesses eventually may coalesce, forming larger abscesses. Infection frequently involves the entire colon. In addition to the virulence characteristics of invasiveness, *S. dysenteriae* type 1 and, to a lesser degree, *S. flexneri* and *S. sonnei* produce a cytotoxin or Shiga toxin, which can lead to HUS.[10]

The pathogenicity of EHEC is related to the production of Shiga-like toxins, so named because of their resemblance to the Shiga toxin of *S. dysenteriae*.[17] The cytotoxic effect of Shiga-like toxins disrupts the mucosal integrity of the large intestine, causing diarrhea. In addition, the toxin is able to pass through the intestinal epithelium to reach the endothelial cells lining small blood vessels that supply the gut, kidney, and other viscera, causing the myriad metabolic events that eventually lead to HUS.

CLINICAL PRESENTATION AND DIAGNOSIS

Gastroenteritis is an illness characterized by diarrhea, which may be accompanied by nausea, vomiting, fever, and abdominal pain. For the best diagnosis and management, it is important to distinguish secretory diarrhea that produces watery diarrhea from inflammatory diarrhea or dysentery. Most enteric pathogens produce acute diarrhea. Dysentery is defined as passing grossly bloody stools. Not all stools in dysenteric illness may contain visible blood, while most stools contain mucus. Systemic toxicity such as fever is often associated with dysentery of infectious origin. Symptoms of enteric pathogens that cause watery and dysentery diarrhea are listed in Table 91-1.

A physical examination and careful history that includes information about symptoms, the length of time the patient has been sick, the number of individuals affected, and recent history of travel, diet, and medications are important factors in making a diagnosis. Infections with norovirus or ETEC result in mild, self-limiting disease. Cholera produces severe dehydrating diarrhea. Infections with enteric pathogens such as *Shigella* spp., *Salmonella* spp., *Campylobacter* spp., EHEC, and *Y. enterocolitica* can result in dysentery diarrhea and severe complications. The clinical presentation of acute viral and bacterial gastroenteritis is summarized in Tables 91-2 and 91-3, respectively.

❸ Stool culture is an important tool in making an organism-specific diagnosis and determining susceptibility to antimicrobial agents. Due to the low yield, stool cultures are not recommended in most mild to moderate watery diarrhea. Instead, indications for stool cultures include dysenteric diarrhea, persistent diarrhea especially in immunocompromised patients (i.e., persons aged 65 years and older with comorbid diseases, neutropenia, or HIV infection), and diarrhea where an outbreak is suggested.[1] A routine stool culture identifies the presence of *Campylobacter*, *Salmonella*, and *Shigella* species. The yield of stool cultures for other pathogens is increased if the test is ordered specifically based on history and physical examination. For dysenteric diarrhea, the laboratory should be instructed to look for EHEC including *E. coli* O157:H7. In hospitalized patients who develop diarrhea 3 days after hospitalization or in those with recent exposure to antimicrobials or chemotherapy, stool specimen should be sent for *C. difficile* toxins A and B. In addition to stool cultures, microscopic examination for fecal polymorphonuclear cells, or a simple immunoassay for the neutrophil marker lactoferrin, can further provide evidence of an inflammatory process and increase the yield of cultures in patients presenting with dysenteric diarrhea.

Complications

Complications associated with acute watery diarrhea most likely result from dehydration and, therefore, Treatment below focuses on rehydration therapy. Dysenteric diarrhea is more likely to have severe complications, especially in children less than 5 years of age and in elderly. Enteric pathogens responsible for complications include *Shigella* spp., *Salmonella* spp., *Campylobacter* spp., EHEC, and *Y. enterocolitica*.

Bacteremia is the most common complication of gastroenteritis and can be seen after infections with nontyphoid *Salmonella*, *C. jejuni* or *C. fetus*, and *Y. enterocolitica*.[15] Nontyphoid *Salmonella* is most common in children less than 5 years of age, elderly, and patients with hemoglobinopathy, malaria, or immunosuppression. Bacteremia due to *Campylobacter* spp. has been reported in patients with HIV infection, malignancy, transplantation, and hypogammaglobulinemia. Although rare, *Y. enterocolitica* bacteremia has been reported in patients with diabetes mellitus, severe anemia, hemochromatosis, cirrhosis, and malignancy, the elderly, and those who have received frequent red blood cell transfusions (iron overload).[23] The clinical syndrome is characterized by persistent bacteremia and prolonged intermittent fever with chills. Stool cultures frequently are negative. Leukocyte counts are often within the normal range. Vascular complications such as seeding of atherosclerotic plaques or aneurysms in arterial vessels occur in 10% to 25% of adults with bacteremia. Localized infections involving bone, cysts, heart, kidney, liver, lungs, pericardium, and spleen develop in 5% to 10% of patients with bacteremia.

Severe complication in patients infected with EHEC is HUS. HUS is defined by the triad of acute renal failure, thrombocytopenia, and microangiopathic hemolytic anemia.[24] This syndrome is commonly observed in children less than 5 years of age and the elderly. Approximately 2% to 7% of cases infected with O157:H7 strains are complicated by development of HUS. Death may occur rarely, usually as a result of HUS. *S. dysenteriae* type 1 can also cause HUS, although more rarely than observed with EHEC.[13]

Shigella infection may also lead to complications such as generalized seizures, sepsis, toxic megacolon, perforated colon, arthritis, and protein-losing enteropathy. Mortality is rare, but it may be more likely with *S. dysenteriae* type I. Less than 3% of persons who are infected with *S. flexneri* will later develop Reiter's syndrome, characterized by pains in the joints, irritation of the eyes, and painful urination. This can lead to chronic arthritis.[25]

Infection with *C. jejuni* has been associated with Guillain-Barré syndrome (GBS), but the relationship is not well understood.[26] The risk of developing GBS after *C. jejuni* infection appears to be low (approximately 1 case of GBS per 1,000 *C. jejuni* infections). The weakness usually starts in the legs with difficulty in walking and may progress to a complete paralysis of all extremities that lasts several weeks and usually requires intensive care.

Approximately 10% to 30% of adult patients develop a reactive arthritis 1 to 2 weeks after recovery from gastroenteritis secondary to *S. flexneri*, *Salmonella* spp., *C. jejuni*, and *Y. enterocolitica*. This arthritis, involving the knees, ankles, toes, fingers, and wrists, usually resolves in 1 to 4 months but may persist in approximately 10% of patients.[26] This complication is more common in persons with the HLA-B27 antigen.

TREATMENT

Fortunately, diarrheal mortality has declined substantially in the past 2 decades, especially among children younger than 1 year of age. Interventions for diarrheal disease such as improved sanitation, increased use of oral rehydration therapy (ORT), breast-feeding, and better weaning practices are responsible for the decrease in case-fatality rates.

General Approach to Treatment

The cornerstone of management for all GI infections and enterotoxigenic poisonings is to prevent dehydration by correcting fluid and electrolyte imbalances. In mild, self-limiting acute gastroenteritis, a diet of oral fluids and easily digestible foods such as chicken soup and crackers is recommended. In patients with severe dehydrating watery diarrhea and dysenteric diarrhea, IV rehydration therapy, antibiotics, and/or antimotility treatments are needed.

Rehydration Therapy

Initial assessment of fluid loss is essential for successful rehydration therapy and should include acute weight loss, as it is the most reliable means of determining the extent of water loss. However, if accurate baseline weight is not available, clinical signs are helpful in determining approximate deficits (Table 91-4). Physical assessment generally is more reliable in young children and infants than in adults.

TABLE 91-4 Clinical Assessment of Degree of Dehydration in Children Based on Percentage of Body Weight Loss[a]

Variable	Minimal or No Dehydration (<3% Loss of Body Weight)	Mild to Moderate (3–9% Loss of Body Weight)	Severe (≥10% Loss of Body Weight)
Blood pressure	Normal	Normal	Normal to reduced
Quality of pulses	Normal	Normal or slightly decreased	Weak, thready, or not palpable
Heart rate	Normal	Normal to increased	Increased (bradycardia in severe cases)
Breathing	Normal	Normal to fast	Deep
Mental status	Normal	Normal to listless	Apathetic, lethargic, or comatose
Eyes	Normal	Sunken orbits/decreased tears	Deeply sunken orbits/absent tears
Mouth and tongue	Moist	Dry	Parched
Thirst	Normal	Eager to drink	Drinks poorly; too lethargic to drink
Skin fold	Normal	Recoil in <2 seconds	Recoil in >2 seconds
Extremities	Warm, normal capillary refill	Cool, prolonged capillary refill	Cold, mottled, cyanotic, prolonged capillary refill
Urine output	Normal to decreased	Decreased	Minimal
Hydration therapy	None	ORS 50–100 mL/kg over 3–4 hours	Lactated Ringer's solution or normal saline 20 mL/kg in 15–30 minutes IV until mental status or perfusion improves Followed by 5% dextrose 0.5 normal saline IV at twice maintenance rates or ORS 100 mL/kg over 4 hours.
Replacement of ongoing losses	<10 kg body weight: 60–120 mL ORS per >10 kg body weight: 120–240 mL ORS per diarrheal stool or emesis	Same	If unable to tolerate ORS, administer through nasogastric tube or administer 5% dextrose 0.5 normal saline with 20 mEq/L potassium chloride IV

ORS, oral rehydration solution.

[a]Percentages vary among authors for each dehydration category; hemodynamic and perfusion status is most important; when unsure of category, therapy for more severe category is recommended.

3 Fluid replacement is the cornerstone of therapy for dehydration due to diarrhea regardless of etiology. For the treatment of mild to moderate dehydration, ORT is superior to administration of IV fluids. ORT reverses dehydration in nearly all patients with mild to moderate diarrhea with 94% to 97% efficacy.[27] It offers the advantages of being inexpensive and noninvasive, and does not require hospitalization for administration. Moreover, thirst drives use of ORT and provides a safeguard against overhydration. Therefore, treatment of dehydration consists of ORT for rehydration and replacement of ongoing losses as well as continuation of normal feeding.

The necessary components of oral rehydration solutions (ORS) include carbohydrates (typically glucose), sodium, potassium, chloride, and water. In 1979, the World Health Organization (WHO) introduced a glucose-based ORS formulation that is 310 mOsm/L. This original formation known as ORS ≥310 takes advantage of glucose-coupled sodium transport in the small bowel and enhances sodium and subsequently water transport across intestinal walls. Therefore, this glucose-based ORS is effective in replacing the fluid from acute diarrhea but does not reduce stool output or shorten duration of diarrhea. In 2002, the World Health Organization/United Nations Children's Fund (WHO/UNICEF) changed its recommendation to a reduced osmolarity solution (osmolarity = 245 mOsm/L). The use of ORS ≤270 reduced stool volume, shortened duration of diarrhea, and decreased need for unscheduled IV therapy when compared with ORS ≥310.[28] The newer formulation of ORS ≤270 mOsm/L was, however, more likely to cause hyponatremia (blood sodium levels <130 mmol/L).[29]

In restoring fluid and electrolyte balance in cholera infections, polymer-based ORS may be more efficacious than glucose-based ORS. Polymer-based ORS contains rice, wheat, sorghum, or maize. This polymer-based ORS releases glucose more slowly after digestion, and when absorbed in the small bowel, enhances the reabsorption of water and electrolyte secreted into the bowel lumen during diarrhea. In a meta-analysis of 34 trials, polymer-based ORS has been shown to reduce the duration of diarrhea in adults with cholera when compared with glucose-based ORS ≥310 and ≤270.[30]

Guidelines on rehydration therapy based on the degree of dehydration and replacement of ongoing losses are outlined in Table 91-4. ORS should be given in small and frequent volumes (5 mL every 2 to 3 minutes in a teaspoon or oral syringe). Nasogastric administration of ORT is an alternative method of administration in a child with persistent vomiting. For breastfed infants, nursing should be continued. The composition of commercial ORS and commonly consumed beverages is listed in Table 91-5. Clear fluids, such as soft drinks, sweetened fruit drinks, broth, and sports drinks, should be avoided in the treatment of dehydration. Those solutions may cause an osmotic diarrhea and hypernatremia.

In the treatment of severe dehydration, the primary goal of therapy is rapid restoration of fluid losses, correction of metabolic acidosis, and replacement of potassium deficiency. Severely dehydrated patients should be resuscitated initially with lactated Ringer's solution or normal saline IV to restore hemodynamic stability. Lactated Ringer's solution is preferred over normal saline because normal saline does not correct metabolic acidosis. Rapid IV rehydration is preferred over more prolonged replacement regimens for restoring extracellular fluids and electrolytes because it more effectively reestablishes GI and renal perfusion. After rehydration, maintenance fluid is given based on accurate recording of intake and output volumes. ORT should be instituted as soon as it can be tolerated.

Early refeeding with age-appropriate unrestricted diet is recommended in children. Previously, the proponents of late refeeding recommended variable periods of fasting followed by gradual reintroduction of food in order to prevent complications. A meta-analysis of 12 trials showed that early refeeding during or immediately following the start of rehydration did not increase the risk of complications such as unscheduled IV fluids, vomiting, or development of persistent diarrhea compared with late refeeding that ranged from 20 to 48 hours after start of rehydration.[31] Initially, easily digested foods such as bananas, applesauce, and cereal should be introduced. Foods high in fiber, sodium, and sugar should be avoided. Lactase deficiency may be exacerbated among known lactase-deficient patients and may persist up to 10 days.

Antimicrobial Therapy

4 The indiscriminate use of antimicrobial therapy produces increases in antimicrobial resistance, side effects of antimicrobial agents, and the threat of superinfections owing to eradication of normal flora. Increasing fluoroquinolone resistance in *Campylobacter* and multidrug resistance in *Salmonella* species worldwide reinforces the importance of judicious use of antibiotics and prudent infection control measures.[32,33] Antibiotic therapy is recommended in severe cases of diarrhea, moderate-to-severe cases of traveler's diarrhea, most cases of febrile dysenteric diarrhea, and culture-proven bacterial diarrhea. Antimicrobial therapy is not recommended in EHEC diarrhea.

Antibiotic therapy is recommended in severe cases of cholera and ETEC diarrhea. In cases of cholera, antibiotics shorten the duration of diarrhea, decrease fluid loss, and shorten the duration of the carrier state.[9] It is important to take local susceptibility patterns into consideration in the selection of the antimicrobial regimen. In areas of high fluoroquinolone resistance, azithromycin has been effective in patients with cholera. In patients with ETEC diarrhea, empiric antibiotics reduce severity and duration of diarrhea. A short course of therapy with fluoroquinolones (e.g., ciprofloxacin and levofloxacin) is the most commonly recommended therapy due to increased resistance among other drug classes.[34] Rifaximin has been effective

TABLE 91-5 Comparison of Common Solutions Used in Oral Rehydration and Maintenance

Product	Na (mEq/L)	K (mEq/L)	Base (mEq/L)	Carbohydrate (mmol/L)	Osmolarity (mOsm/L)
WHO/UNICEF (2002)	75	20	30	75	245
Naturalyte	45	20	48	140	265
Pedialyte	45	20	30	140	250
Infalyte	50	25	30	70	200
Rehydralyte	75	20	30	140	250
Cola[a]	2	0	13	700	750
Apple juice[a]	5	32	0	690	730
Chicken broth[a]	250	8	0	0	500
Sports beverage[a]	20	3	3	255	330

[a]These solutions should be avoided in dehydration.

TABLE 91-6 Recommendations for Antibiotic Therapy

Pathogen	Children	Adults
Watery Diarrhea		
Vibrio cholerae O1	Erythromycin 30 mg/kg/day divided every 8 hours orally × 3 days; azithromycin 10 mg/kg/day given orally once daily × 3 days	Doxycycline 300 mg orally × 1 day Alternatives: tetracycline 500 mg orally four times daily × 3 days; erythromycin 250 mg orally every 8 hours × 3 days; azithromycin 500 mg orally once daily × 3 days
Enterotoxigenic *Escherichia coli*	Azithromycin 10 mg/kg/day given orally once daily × 3 days; ceftriaxone 50 mg/kg/day given IV once daily × 3 days	Ciprofloxacin 750 mg orally once daily × 1–3 days. Alternatives: rifaximin 200 mg orally three times daily × 3 days; azithromycin 1,000 mg orally × 1 day *or* 500 mg orally daily × 3 days
Dysenteric Diarrhea		
Shigella species[a]	Azithromycin 10 mg/kg/day given orally once daily × 3 days; ceftriaxone 50 mg/kg/day given IV once daily × 3 days	Ciprofloxacin 750 mg orally once daily × 3 days; levofloxacin 500 mg orally once daily × 3 days Alternatives: azithromycin 500 mg orally once daily × 3 days
Salmonella		
Nontyphoidal[a]	Ceftriaxone 100 mg/kg/day divided IV every 12 hours × 7–10 days; azithromycin 20 mg/kg/day orally once daily × 7 days	Ciprofloxacin 750 mg orally once daily × 7–10 days; levofloxacin 500 mg orally once daily × 7–10 days Alternatives: azithromycin 500 mg orally once daily × 7 days For immunocompromised patients, duration should be increased to 14 days for both fluoroquinolones and azithromycin
Campylobacter[a]	Azithromycin 10 mg/kg/day given orally once daily × 3–5 days; erythromycin 30 mg/kg/day divided into two to four doses orally × 3–5 days	Azithromycin 500 mg orally once daily × 3 days; erythromycin 500 mg orally every 6 hours × 3 days
Yersinia species[a]	Treat as shigellosis	Treat as shigellosis
Clostridium difficile	Metronidazole 7.5 mg/kg (maximum: 500 mg) orally or IV every 8 hours × 10–14 days; vancomycin 10 mg/kg (maximum: 125 mg) orally every 6 hours × 10–14 days	Mild to moderate disease: metronidazole 500 mg orally or IV every 8 hours daily × 10–14 days Severe disease: vancomycin 125 mg orally every 6 hours × 10–14 days Alternatives: rifaximin 400 mg orally every 6 hours × 10–14 days; fidaxomicin 200 mg orally every 12 hours × 10–14 days
Traveler's Diarrhea		
Prophylaxis[a]		Norfloxacin 400 mg or ciprofloxacin 750 mg orally daily; rifaximin 200 mg one to three times daily up to 2 weeks
Treatment		Ciprofloxacin 750 mg orally ×1 day or 500 mg orally every 12 hours × 3 days; levofloxacin 1,000 mg orally × 1 day or 500 mg orally daily × 3 days; rifaximin 200 mg three times daily × 3 days; azithromycin 1,000 mg orally × 1 day or 500 mg orally daily × 3 days

[a]For high-risk patients only. See the preceding text for the high-risk patients in each infection.

for ETEC when traveling in Mexico.[35] Further discussions of antibiotic prophylaxis and treatment can be found in Traveler's Diarrhea below. Table 91-6 summarizes antibiotic recommendations. Further details regarding treatment of *C. difficile*–associated diarrhea, traveler's diarrhea, and foodborne illnesses are discussed in respective sections.

Antibiotic therapy is indicated in most febrile dysenteric diarrhea. In shigellosis, antibiotics shorten the period of fecal shedding and attenuate the clinical illness. Antibiotic therapy is reserved for the elderly, those who are immunocompromised, children in day-care centers, malnourished children, and healthcare workers. In the United States, *Shigella* spp. remain susceptible to fluoroquinolones. Fluoroquinolone resistance among *Shigella* spp. is of increasing concern in developing countries, and azithromycin may be a better choice in patients with a recent history of travel to a developing region.[15] Similar antibiotic regimens can be used for high-risk patients who develop *Yersinia* bacteremia (i.e., infants younger than age 3 months and patients with cirrhosis or iron overload) or in patients with bone and joint infections.[36] In Campylobacteriosis, antibiotics are not useful unless started within 4 days of the start of the illness because they do not shorten the duration or severity of diarrhea and only shorten the duration of bacterial excretion. Antibiotics are warranted in patients with high fevers, severe bloody diarrhea, prolonged illnesses (>1 week), pregnancy, and immunocompromised states, including HIV infection. Fluoroquinolone resistance among *Campylobacter* spp. has increased, and is now 10% to 13% in the United States and 41% to 88% in Europe and Asia. Resistance may be the result of the use of fluoroquinolone antibiotics in poultry and other animal feed, and the frequent use of these agents internationally in treating enteric infections. Macrolides such as erythromycin and azithromycin are recommended especially in patients with a recent history of travel to Asia.[34]

Nontyphoid *Salmonella* infection leads to bacteremia in approximately 8% of otherwise healthy adults. Risk of bacteremia is increased in some patient populations and should be treated with antibiotics. High-risk patients include neonates or infants younger than 1 year, persons older than 50 years, and patients with primary or secondary immunodeficiency such as AIDS or chemotherapy-induced inflammatory bowel disease, sickle cell disease, vascular abnormalities (prostatic heart valve or abdominal aneurysm), or prosthetic joints.[15] Susceptibility testing is recommended due to increased resistance.

Outcomes of some bacterial diarrheal illnesses may be worsened by the use of antibiotics, therefore precluding their use. In patients infected with EHEC, use of an antimicrobial agent such as a fluoroquinolone or trimethoprim–sulfamethoxazole may increase the risk of HUS by increasing the production of Shiga-like toxin.[36] Empiric antimicrobial therapy should be withheld when clinical suspicion is high due to the high prevalence of the disease in the region, patient clinical presentation suggestive of EHEC infection, or a known foodborne outbreak of dysentery with an incubation period of longer than 2 days. Antibiotics should not be given to infants or children due to a higher incidence of HUS in this population. Treatment of EHEC infection is primarily limited to supportive care, which may include fluid replacement therapy, hemodialysis, hemofiltration, transfusion of packed erythrocytes, platelet infusions, and other interventions as indicated clinically. Severe disease may cause chronic kidney failure and require renal transplantation.

Antimotility Agents

5 Antimotility drugs such as diphenoxylate and loperamide offer symptomatic relief in patients with watery diarrhea by reducing the number of stools. In dysenteric diarrhea, slowing of fecal transit time with these agents is thought to result in extended toxin-associated damage, worsening diseases such as HUS. Therefore, antimotility drugs are not recommended in patients with many toxin-mediated dysenteric diarrhea (i.e., EHEC, pseudomembranous colitis, shigellosis). However, evidence suggests that in adults with dysenteric diarrhea these agents do not appear to be harmful if given concomitantly with antibacterial therapy.[36]

Clinical **Controversy. . .**

Loperamide should not be used in patients with fever or bloody stool. There is evidence that the use of such agents can increase the risk for development of HUS, possibly by delaying intestinal clearance of the organism and thereby increasing toxin absorption.

Probiotics

Probiotics are preparations of microorganisms and most commercial products have been derived from food sources, particularly cultured milk products. Several systematic reviews and meta-analyses have shown an overall reduction in the duration of diarrhea by approximately 17 to 30 hours with the use of probiotics.[37] No serious adverse effects have been reported in otherwise healthy persons. Probiotics that were effective in at least one controlled trial included *Lactobacillus rhamnosus* GG, *Lactobacillus reuteri*, combination *L. rhamnosus*, *L. reuteri*, and *Bifidobacterium animalis* subsp. *lactis*, and combination *Lactobacillus acidophilus* and *Lactobacillus bifidus*. Unfortunately, the data do not clearly define type, dose, or duration of probiotic treatment that would result in clinical benefit.

Oral Zinc Supplementation

Zinc deficiency is largely due to inadequate dietary intake and is common in many developing countries where morbidity and mortality associated with acute diarrhea in children remain high. In children older than 6 months of age with moderate signs of malnutrition, zinc supplementation may shorten the duration of diarrhea by approximately 27 hours (MD −26.98 hours, 95% CI −14.62 to −39.34).[38] Therefore, oral zinc supplementation of 20 mg/day for 1 to 2 weeks may have an additional benefit over ORS in reducing children mortality in developing countries. Common side effects include metallic taste and vomiting. At high doses, zinc supplementation may cause epigastric pain, lethargy, and fatigue.

PREVENTION OF GASTROINTESTINAL INFECTIONS

6 Public health measures of improved water supply and sanitation facilities and the quality control of commercial products are important for the control of the majority of enteric infections. In addition, many diarrheal diseases can be prevented by following simple rules of personal hygiene and safe food preparation. Hand washing with soap and running water is instrumental in preventing the spread of illness and should be emphasized for caregivers and persons with diarrheal illnesses. Safe food handling and preparation practices can significantly decrease the incidence of certain types of enteric infections.

Reporting suspected outbreaks and cases of notifiable illness to local health authorities is vital to investigation of threats of enteric infection arising from increasingly global and industrialized food supplies. The reporting of specific infectious diseases to the appropriate public health authorities is the cornerstone of public health surveillance, outbreak detection, and prevention and control efforts.

Vaccines are used to boost specific immune processes directed against the bacteria themselves or against adherence appendages, cytotoxins, or enterotoxins. Unfortunately, there are only a few vaccines available for prevention of gastroenteritis. Vaccines for typhoid fever are the parenteral Vi capsular polysaccharide vaccine (ViCPS) and the oral live-attenuated Ty21a vaccine.[39] Efficacy rates for both vaccines range from 50% to 80%. The ViCPS is indicated for children who are ≥2 years of age and a booster dose is administered 2 years later. The Ty21a vaccine is indicated for children ≥6 years of age; one capsule should be swallowed whole every other day for a total of four doses at least 1 week before the potential exposure. A booster should be taken every 5 years if continued protection is needed.

In the United States, routine rotavirus vaccination is recommended for all infants beginning at age 2 months. There are two vaccines, RotaTeq (RV5) and Rotarix (RV1), available for reducing rotaviral gastroenteritis.[40] The RV5 vaccine is a live, oral vaccine that offers 74% efficacy against gastroenteritis of any severity and 98% efficacy against severe disease. This vaccine also decreased office visits by 86%, emergency department visits by 94%, and hospitalizations by 96%. The RV1 vaccine is a live-attenuated human rotavirus vaccine. A trial of this vaccine has shown a clinical efficacy of 79% against gastroenteritis of any severity and 96% efficacy against severe rotavirus disease. Rotarix reduced hospitalizations by 100% and medically attended visits by 92% in the first rotavirus season, and reduced hospitalizations by 96% through two seasons.[40] The RV5 vaccine is administered orally in a three-dose series at ages 2, 4, and 6 months while the RV1 vaccine is administered orally in a two-dose series at ages 2 and 4 months. The first dose may be given between 6 weeks and 14 weeks and 6 days of age and all doses should be given before 8 months of age.

Although not available in the United States, two oral vaccines are available in other countries. Dukoral (Crucell, Stockholm, Sweden) consists of killed *V. cholerae* O1 organisms and the cholera B subunit, and is licensed in over 60 countries. Shanchol (Shantha Biotechnics, Hyderabad, India) consists of killed whole cells from a mix of pathogenic strains of *V. cholerae* (O1 and O139) and is licensed in India.[9] Both vaccines are given in two doses (three doses of Dukoral are required for children 2 to 5 years of age) and administered about 7 to 14 days apart (up to 42 days apart for Dukoral). Dukoral must be administered with a buffer that requires 75 to 150 mL of clean water while Shanchol does not require the buffer. Both vaccines demonstrated protective efficacy of 47% to 87% after two doses but almost none after a single dose. Protection is achieved in approximately 1 week following the last dose and persists for about 2 years. The common side effects were considered mild and included abdominal pain, headache, fever, and nausea. The WHO does not require vaccination for international travel to or from endemic areas because vaccines require two doses and provide incomplete protection for a relatively short period of time.

EVALUATION OF THERAPEUTIC OUTCOMES

Appropriate followup care of patients with acute diarrhea is based on successful restoration of fluid losses. The clinical signs and symptoms that lead to the diagnosis also can assess adequate rehydration, and should be monitored frequently. Since ORT is now preferred, routine laboratory testing often is unnecessary. Electrolytes should be measured in those receiving IV fluids, when oral replacement fails, or when signs of hypernatremia or hypokalemia are present. Followup stool samples to ensure complete evacuation of the infecting pathogen may be necessary only in patients who are at high risk to initiate or contribute to a community outbreak. All patients should be monitored for complications associated with the infecting pathogen, resolution of the diarrhea, and adverse reactions to the pharmacologic agents used. Prompt discharge of hospitalized patients is recommended when rehydration is achieved, IV fluids have not been required, oral intake equals or exceeds losses, or adequate education and medical followup are ensured. For most patients, discharge can occur in 16 to 24 hours.

C. difficile

Epidemiology

C. difficile is the most commonly known cause of infectious diarrhea in hospitalized patients in North America and Europe. *C. difficile* infection (CDI) is associated with use of broad-spectrum antimicrobials, including clindamycin, ampicillin, cephalosporins, and fluoroquinolones. Other agents that have been implicated, albeit at a lower incidence rate, include aminoglycosides, erythromycin, trimethoprim–sulfamethoxazole, vancomycin, and metronidazole. Although in most cases CDI occurs during or shortly after the completion of antimicrobial therapy, disease onset can be delayed for 2 or 3 months.[41] CDI occurs most often in high-risk groups, such as the elderly, debilitated patients, cancer patients, surgical patients, patients receiving antibiotics, patients with nasogastric tubes, and patients who frequently use laxatives. A meta-analysis of 23 studies (~300,000 patients) suggests that proton pump inhibitors increase the incidence of CDI by 65%.[42]

Unfortunately attributable mortality from CDI increased from 5.7 to 23.7 deaths per 1 million persons in the United States from 1999 to 2004.[43] Mortality from the infection has been reported as high as 38%, with many studies indicating a mortality rate of 15% or greater.[44] Increased mortality is assumed to be due to the emergence of a single-strain type (North American pulsed-field type 1 [NAP-1]) in outbreaks.[45] NAP-1 strain is highly resistant to fluoroquinolones and carries deletion mutations in a regulatory gene (tcdC) believed to inhibit toxin production, causing higher levels of toxin production responsible for more serious diseases. The NAP-1 strain is also refractory to standard therapy.

Pathogenesis

C. difficile is a gram-positive spore-forming anaerobic bacillus and causes a toxin-mediated disease. Once antibiotics disrupt normal colonic flora and colonization of *C. difficile* occurs, two toxins (A and B) are released to mediate diarrhea and colitis. This toxin production is essential in disease manifestation. Toxin A is the major pathogenic factor and has been characterized as an enterotoxin that causes intestinal fluid secretion, mucosal injury, and inflammation through actin disaggregation, intracellular calcium release, and damage to neurons. Toxin B is a nonenterotoxic cytotoxin that causes depolymerization of filamentous actin and mediates more potent damage to human colonic mucosa than toxin A. Initially, raised white and yellowish plaques form, and the surrounding mucosa may be inflamed. With progression of disease, these pseudomembranous plaques become enlarged and scatted over the colorectal mucosa.[41]

Clinical Presentation

Clinical diagnosis is based on the onset of diarrhea during or after antimicrobial use and often is associated with abdominal discomfort, fever, and polymorphonuclear leukocytosis. A spectrum of disease ranges from mild diarrhea to life-threatening toxic megacolon and pseudomembranous enterocolitis.[41] In colitis without pseudomembrane formation, patients present with malaise, abdominal pain, nausea, anorexia, watery diarrhea, low-grade fever, and leukocytosis. Fulminant disease is characterized by severe abdominal pain, perfuse diarrhea, high fever, marked leukocytosis, and classic pseudomembrane formation evident with sigmoidoscopic examination.

CDI should be suspected in patients experiencing diarrhea with a recent history of antibiotic use (within the previous 3 months) or in those whose diarrhea began 72 hours after hospitalization. Diagnosis can be established by detection of toxin A or B, stool culture for *C. difficile*, or endoscopy. If the stool sample is negative, a second analysis is recommended because the testing sensitivity may be increased with repeat testing. Endoscopy should be reserved for situations where rapid diagnosis is needed, ileus is present, stool is not available, or other colonic diseases are in the differential diagnosis.

TREATMENT

Initial therapy should include discontinuation of the offending agent.[41] Fluid and electrolyte replacement therapy is necessary. Although diarrhea will resolve in up to 25% of patients within 48 hours of discontinuing the offending agent without therapy, most patients require antibiotics. Metronidazole, vancomycin, and fidaxomicin are all effective agents for treating *C. difficile* diarrhea. Nitazoxanide, rifampin, and bacitracin have also been studied.

In head-to-head comparison studies, vancomycin and metronidazole were similar in duration of diarrhea and toxin or organism clearance, rate of initial cure of infection, rate of recurrence, mortality, and incidence of side effects.[46–48] Vancomycin was superior to metronidazole in a subgroup analysis of 69 patients with severe *C. difficile* diarrhea.[46] When vancomycin has been compared with agents other than metronidazole, including fidaxomicin, the rate of initial cure did not significantly differ between treatment groups. Recurrence was common, ranging from 9% to 37% in clinical trials. Only the comparison between vancomycin and fidaxomicin demonstrated a significant difference in recurrence, 25.4% versus 15.3% ($P = 0.005$).[49]

7 Metronidazole (250 mg four times daily or 500 mg three times daily) is the drug of choice for mild to moderate CDI because its oral formation is less expensive than that of vancomycin or fidaxomicin, and there are concerns for vancomycin-resistant enterococci with oral vancomycin use. In patients with severe disease, contraindication or intolerance to metronidazole, and inadequate response to metronidazole, oral vancomycin or fidaxomicin, is recommended. Vancomycin (125 mg four times daily) must be administered orally because IV vancomycin does not achieve gut lumen concentrations high enough for effective bacterial elimination. Due to cost, many institutions choose to use the injectable form of vancomycin to prepare an oral formulation. In patients with an ileus (where oral vancomycin reaching site of infection is questioned) vancomycin may be delivered by retention enema or adding IV metronidazole. Fidaxomicin is a macrocyclic oral antibiotic (200 mg administered twice daily) that has minimal bioavailability, and is bacteriostatic against *C. difficile*.

Recurrence of CDI occurs in approximately 20% of cases.[50] Patients with one prior episode of relapse have a greater than 40% risk of additional recurrences, whereas those with two or more previous episodes have a greater than 60% risk.[51] Risk factors for recurrent CDI include a history of recurrence, emergency hospital admission, previous GI hospital admission, recent (within 4 to 12 weeks) hospitalization, increasing age, use of additional antimicrobials, and an inadequate protective immune response to *C. difficile* toxins.[50]

Treatment of recurrence has not been well studied. In a subgroup analysis of 128 patients who developed relapse after initial therapy with either vancomycin or fidaxomicin, response to therapy (>90% cure) was similar for both drugs. However, there was significantly less recurrence within 28 days in those treated with fidaxomicin (35.5% vs. 19.7% vancomycin, $P = 0.045$). Management of the first relapse is identical to a primary episode because relapse is rarely due to resistance to the initial agent of treatment. Instead, relapse occurs because treatment fails to eradicate the spore forms of pathogen or treatment makes patients vulnerable to another infection by impairing normal flora. There are some data suggesting that fidaxomicin inhibits spore production in *C. difficile*.[52]

The optimal management of patients with multiple relapses is not clear. A prolonged tapered pulse dosing of oral vancomycin has been suggested for second relapses.[51,53] Alternative regimens that have shown efficacy include drugs in rifamycin class: vancomycin + rifampin[54] or vancomycin followed by rifaximin.[55] Concern with these regimens includes drug interactions with rifampin and development of resistance, especially if either rifampin or rifaximin is used as monotherapy. Nitazoxanide is another alternative agent in patients with relapse following metronidazole therapy.[56] There are two other modalities that have been shown to have efficacy against CDI: IVIG and fecal transplantation. Individuals with low concentration of circulating IgG antitoxin are susceptible to more severe disease and frequent relapses. In those with multiple relapses due to impaired antigenic response to toxins, IVIG 400 mg/kg may be a worthwhile intervention.[56] It is, however, expensive and its efficacy is reported in case series and anecdotal reports. Fecal transplantation uses a small amount of fresh feces from a healthy donor, suspended in saline, filtered, and administered through a nasogastric tube or by retention enema.[57] Although it was efficacious in a case series, it is a difficult option to offer to patients.

Agents that have lost favor due to poor efficacy or resistance include bacitracin, cholestyramine, colestipol, and fusidic acid. Probiotics using *Saccharomyces boulardii* or lactobacilli species to augment colonization resistance and prevent recurrent CDI have been studied in adults and children. A placebo-controlled trial of 204 patients demonstrated no benefit of *S. boulardii* for prevention of CDI in hospitalized adults.[58] However, several trials suggest the probiotic may be effective in prevention of CDI in pediatric patients.[59] Agents that are in clinical trials include ramoplanin (a new lipoglycodepsipeptide), rifamycins (including rifampin, rifaximin, and rifalazil), monoclonal antibodies to *C. difficile* toxins A and B, and CB-315 (a lipopeptide). Tolevamer (a large anionic polymer that binds *C. difficile* toxins A and B) was inferior to metronidazole and vancomycin in the treatment of the first episode of CDI, but the relapse rate was lower.[60] A *C. difficile* toxoid vaccine (Sanofi Pasteur) has received fast-track status through the FDA, and is in phase II testing.

Drugs that inhibit peristalsis, such as diphenoxylate, are contraindicated in CDI.[41] Slowing of fecal transit time is thought to result in extended toxin-associated damage. Strict hand washing and contact precautions are imperative measures in preventing the spread of the organism. *C. difficile* can be cultured in rooms of infected individuals up to 40 days after discharge.

Clinical **Controversy...**

Some investigators have found prophylaxis with competing, nonpathogenic organisms such as *Lactobacillus* spp. or *Saccharomyces* spp. to be helpful in preventing relapses in small numbers of patients with CDI. It is thought that these organisms help to restore the natural flora in the gut and make patients more resistant to colonization by *C. difficile* when used in conjunction with appropriate antibiotics.

TRAVELER'S DIARRHEA

Traveler's diarrhea describes the clinical syndrome manifested by malaise, anorexia, and abdominal cramps followed by the sudden onset of diarrhea that incapacitates many travelers. It interferes with planned activities or work in 30% of those affected. In particular, an increased risk lies with North Americans and Northern Europeans traveling to Latin America, southern Europe, Africa, and Asia. The highest risk is observed with patients with immunocompromised conditions, achlorhydria, inflammatory bowel disease, and people with chronic debilitating medical conditions. Overall, 20% to 50% of people traveling to high-risk areas will develop the illness.[34]

8 The onset of symptoms usually occurs during the first week of travel but can occur anytime during the visit or after returning home. Traveler's diarrhea is caused by contaminated food or water. The most common pathogens are bacterial in nature and include ETEC (20% to 72%), *Shigella* (3% to 25%), *Campylobacter* (3% to 17%), and *Salmonella* (3% to 7%).[8] Viruses (up to 30%) are also potential causes, as are parasites, although they are rare during short-term travels, accounting for less than 5% of cases. Bacterial enteropathogens cause up to 80% of cases. The diarrhea-producing *E. coli* (ETEC) plays more important role in Latin America, Africa, and South Asia. The invasive enteric pathogens (*Campylobacter* spp., *Shigella* spp., and *Salmonella* spp.) are relatively more important causes of traveler's diarrhea in Asia.

The severity of the syndrome is determined by the number of stools per day and the presence or absence of cramping, nausea, and vomiting. Mild diarrhea is defined as one to three loose stools per day that are associated with abdominal cramps lasting less than 14 days. Moderate diarrhea indicates more than four loose stools daily associated with dehydration, and severe diarrhea is defined as the presence of fever or blood in stools. Traveler's diarrhea is rarely life-threatening and in most cases, symptoms resolve in several days without treatment. Travelers to high-risk areas should pack a kit that includes a thermometer, loperamide, 3 days of antibiotics (see Treatment below), ORS salts, and a water purification method.[34]

Prevention

9 Patient education in avoiding high-risk food and beverages should be the best method for minimizing the risk. High-risk foods and beverages include raw or undercooked meat and seafood, moist foods served at room temperature, fruits that cannot be peeled, vegetables, milk from a questionable source, hot sauces on the table, tap water, unsealed bottled water, iced drinks, and food from a street vendor. Slogans such as "Peel it, boil it, cook it, or forget it" remind travelers to avoid contaminated food and to use water purification or reliable bottled beverages. Unfortunately, a meta-analysis concluded that the incidence of diarrhea was similar in travelers who followed the old adage and those who engaged in riskier eating habits.[61] A potential reason for a lack of difference may be due to the fact that cooking foods does not always kill pathogens and food should not be considered safe unless it is cooked until steaming hot. Nonetheless, advisement of avoidance measures regarding safe foods, beverages, and eating establishments is recommended to heighten awareness.

Bismuth subsalicylate 524 mg (two tablets or two tablespoonfuls) orally four times daily for up to 3 weeks is a commonly recommended prophylactic regimen.[34] Bismuth subsalicylate may inhibit enterotoxin activity and prevent diarrhea. Persons taking this regimen should be informed of adverse events, including temporary black discoloration of tongue and stools, and, rarely, tinnitus.

Although the efficacy of prophylactic antibiotics has been documented, their use is not recommended for most travelers due to the potential side effects of antibiotics (e.g., photosensitivity), predisposition to other infections such as CDI or vaginal candidiasis, the increased risk of selection of drug-resistant organisms, cost, lack of data on the safety and efficacy of antibiotics given for more than 2 or 3 weeks, and availability of rapidly effective antibiotics for treatment. Prophylactic antibiotics are recommended only in high-risk individuals or in situations in which short-term illness could ruin the purpose of the trip, such as a military mission. A fluoroquinolone is the drug of choice when traveling to most areas of the world.[34] Due to fluoroquinolone resistance among *Campylobacter* spp., azithromycin can be considered when traveling to South Asia and Southeast Asia.

Rifaximin is a nonabsorbed oral rifamycin that has activity against enteric pathogens and may have a role in the prevention of traveler's diarrhea in select populations. A randomized, double-blind trial of rifaximin 200 mg once, twice, or three times daily with meals for 2 weeks resulted in equal protection of 72% for each of the three dosing regimens compared with placebo.[35] Since rifaximin is effective against traveler's diarrhea due to noninvasive strains of *E. coli*, this agent should be reserved for travel regions where *E. coli* predominates, such as Latin America and Africa. Rifaximin has a tolerability and safety profile comparable to that of placebo. The concern with the class rifamycin is the emergence of resistance when used as monotherapy.

TREATMENT

The goals of treatment are to avoid dehydration, reduce the severity and duration of symptoms, and prevent interruption to planned activities. Fluid and electrolyte replacement should be initiated at the onset of diarrhea. ORT is generally not required in otherwise healthy individuals; flavored mineral water ad libitum offers a good source of sodium and glucose. In infants and young children, elderly, and those with chronic debilitating medical conditions, ORT is recommended. For symptom relief, loperamide (preferred because of its quicker onset and longer duration of relief relative to bismuth) may be taken (4 mg orally initially and then 2 mg with each subsequent loose stool to a maximum of 16 mg/day in patients without bloody diarrhea and fever). Loperamide should be discontinued if symptoms persist for more than 48 hours. Other symptomatic therapy in mild diarrhea includes bismuth subsalicylate 524 mg every 30 minutes for up to eight doses.[34] There is insufficient evidence to warrant the recommendation of probiotics.

Since behavioral modification has limited efficacy and chemoprophylaxis is not recommended in most travelers, the current recommendation relies on self-treatment. Most trials indicate that a single dose of antibiotic and up to 3 days of treatment will improve the condition within 24 to 36 hours, shortening the duration of diarrhea by 1 to 2 days.[34] A single dose of fluoroquinolone is recommended initially and if diarrhea is improved within 12 to 24 hours, antibiotics should be discontinued. Otherwise, it can be continued for up to 3 days. A fluoroquinolone is recommended when traveling to most areas of the world. Where fluoroquinolone-resistant *Campylobacter* is common, such as in South Asia and Southeast Asia, azithromycin can be used.[34] Azithromycin can also be used in pregnant women and children younger than age 16 years. Empiric treatment of young children should be cautioned.

Rifaximin was as effective as a 3-day course of ciprofloxacin in shortening the duration of diarrhea in noninvasive traveler's diarrhea. However, rifaximin was not as effective in patients with fever and bloody diarrhea and in those with invasive pathogens. Therefore, a 3-day course of rifaximin has been approved for the treatment of traveler's diarrhea caused by noninvasive strains of *E. coli* in people ≥12 years of age and can be considered when traveling to areas where *E. coli*–associated traveler's diarrhea is common, such as Mexico and Jamaica.[34]

For rapid improvement in symptoms, antibiotic therapy with adjunctive treatment with loperamide has shown benefit.[62] All clinical trials concluded that the combination therapy was safe, and the worsening of the disease with the use of antimotility treatment has not been encountered.

Clinical **Controversy...**

Most trials have shown that a short course of antibiotic therapy reduces the duration of traveler's diarrhea by 1 to 2 days with mild side effects. Some clinicians advocate a self-treatment with antibiotics for moderate-to-severe traveler's diarrhea, while others urge a more cautious approach. The final decision on self-treatment should rely on discussions with individual travelers, taking into consideration their ability and willingness to adhere to prevention strategies and to tolerate diarrheal illness during the trip.

FOOD POISONING

10 Foodborne illnesses result from the ingestion of food containing pathogenic microorganisms that cause GI infections or preformed toxins that were produced by microorganisms that cause enterotoxigenic poisonings. In the United States, foodborne diseases cause approximately 76 million illnesses, 325,000 hospitalizations, and 5,200 deaths each year.[4] Foodborne transmission may account for up to 80% of acute gastroenteritis. Common enteric pathogens responsible for foodborne diseases have been discussed in the previous sections (norovirus, nontyphoidal *Salmonella*, *Campylobacter* spp., *Shigella*, *E. coli*). Common foodborne pathogens that cause enterotoxigenic poisonings include *Staphylococcus aureus*, *Bacillus cereus*, *Clostridium perfringens*, and *Clostridium botulinum*. Characteristics of pathogens responsible for foodborne illnesses are summarized in Table 91-7.

Because foodborne disease can appear as sporadic cases or outbreaks, the diagnosis should be suspected whenever two or more people present with acute GI or neurologic manifestations after sharing a meal within the previous 72 hours. Important clues about etiologic agents can be gathered from demographic information (age, gender, etc.), the clinical syndrome, incubation period, and medical history, type of foods consumed, seasonality, and geographic location of the outbreak.

Enterotoxigenic poisonings result from ingestion of food contaminated by preformed toxins. Therefore, symptoms are rapid in onset, but most cases of food poisoning are of short duration with recovery occurring within 1 to 2 days. *B. cereus* causes two different types of clinical syndromes. The first one is caused by characterized by a short incubation period and mostly vomiting. The second syndrome has a longer incubation period and is characterized by diarrhea. Foodborne *C. perfringens* infection may present as two distinct syndromes. Type A organisms are seen in Western nations and result in a 24-hour illness characterized by watery diarrhea and epigastric pain. Type C organisms can be found in undercooked pork and occur in underdeveloped tropical regions. They can produce a toxin-related syndrome called *enteritis necroticans*, which is a coagulative transmural necrosis of the intestinal wall. This syndrome can result in intestinal perforation leading to sepsis and mortality in approximately 40% of victims.

Foodborne botulism results from the ingestion of food contaminated with preformed toxins or toxin-producing spores from *C. botulinum*. *C. botulinum* poisoning is relatively rare; only 110 cases are reported per year in the United States.[63] Botulism is almost always associated with improper preparation or storage of food. Seven distinct toxins (A to G) have been described. The

TABLE 91-7 Food Poisonings

Organism	Principal Foods	Peak Incidence (United States)	Time to Symptoms	Duration	Common Symptoms
Enterotoxigenic Poisonings					
Staphylococcus aureus	Salad, pastries, ham, sandwiches, puddings, unpasteurized milk, cheese products	Summer	1–6 hours	1 day	Nausea, vomiting, abdominal cramps, diarrhea
Bacillus cereus	Fried rice, dairy products, spices, bean sprouts, vegetables	None	1–6 hours 6–24 hours	1 day 1 day	Nausea, vomiting Diarrhea
Clostridium botulinum	Home-canned fruits, vegetables, meats, honey	None	18–36 hours		Double vision, blurred vision, drooping eyelids, slurred speech, difficulty swallowing, dry mouth, and muscle weakness
Clostridium perfringens (type A)	Meats, poultry, gravies, dried or precooked foods	Fall, winter, spring	8–12 hours	1 day	Abdominal cramps, diarrhea
GI Infections					
Campylobacter	Poultry, dairy products, clams, water	Spring, summer	2–5 days	7 days	Diarrhea (may be bloody), cramping, abdominal pain, fever
Salmonella spp.	Beef, poultry, water, eggs, dairy products	Summer	12–72 hours	4–7 days	Diarrhea (sometimes bloody), fever, abdominal cramps
Enteropathogenic *E. coli*	Water	None	1–3 days	5–7 days	Severe diarrhea, vomiting, dehydration
Enterotoxigenic *E. coli*	Water, ice, food	None	1–3 days	3–4 days	Profuse watery diarrhea, abdominal cramping
Shigella spp.	Salad, water	Summer	1–2 days	5–7 days	Diarrhea (often bloody), fever, abdominal cramps
Vibrio cholerae	Water	None	2 hours to 5 days	2–3 days	Profuse watery diarrhea, vomiting, leg cramps
Vibrio parahemolyticus	Shellfish (oysters)	Spring, summer, fall	24 hours	3 days	Watery diarrhea, abdominal cramping, nausea, vomiting, fever, chills
Yersinia enterocolitica	Dairy products, raw or undercooked pork products	None	4–7 days	1–3 weeks	Fever, abdominal pain, diarrhea (often bloody)

toxins prevent the release of acetylcholine at the peripheral cholinergic nerve terminal. Toxin activity has prompted the use of minute locally injected doses to treat select spastic disorders, such as blepharospasm, hemifacial spasm, and certain dystonias. Foodborne botulism is suspected when patients present with acute GI symptoms concurrently or just prior to the onset of a symmetric descending paralysis without sensory or central nervous system involvement. Diagnosis is made by culturing *C. botulinum* from the stool. The clinical presentation may resemble GBS associated with *C. jejuni* infection. The difference lies in the onset of neurologic symptoms, which typically occur 1 to 3 weeks after the onset of *C. jejuni* infection, and the condition usually is manifested by an ascending paralysis in *C. jejuni*–associated GBS.

Treatment consists primarily of respiratory support and use of botulinum antitoxin.[64] If evaluation is performed within several hours of ingestion, gastric lavage or induction of vomiting is suggested. Cathartics and enemas also can be used to remove residual toxin from the bowel, but they are contraindicated in cases of ileus. Botulinum antitoxin is a concentrated preparation of equine globulins obtained from horses immunized with toxins A, B, and E. Because trivalent antitoxin is equine in origin, patients should be tested for hypersensitivity before receiving the product IV. Other agents used experimentally as adjunctive therapy are guanidine, which antagonizes the effect of botulinum toxin at the neuromuscular junction, and 4-aminopyridine, which increases acetylcholine release. Newer and more effective methods of treatment and prevention are under development, including a botulinum toxin vaccine consisting of nontoxic botulinum fragments. Prevention always should be stressed. Botulinum toxins are heat labile and readily destroyed by 10 minutes of boiling. All home-canned foods should be processed according to directions and boiled, not just warmed, prior to consumption.

In foodborne illnesses, the cornerstone of therapy remains supportive care. ORT is preferred in replenishing and maintaining fluid and electrolyte balance, and IV fluid therapy should be reserved for those who are severely ill and cannot tolerate oral therapy. Antiemetics and antiperistaltic agents offer symptomatic relief, but the latter should not be given in patients who present with high fever, bloody diarrhea, or fecal leukocytes. Antimicrobial therapy is not effective in the management of *S. aureus*, *C. perfringens*, or *B. cereus* food poisonings. In developed countries, many of the foodborne illnesses can be prevented with proper food selection, preparation, and storage. However, in developing countries, sanitation and clean water supply are larger concerns.

ABBREVIATIONS

AIDS	acquired immunodeficiency syndrome
cAMP	cyclic adenosine monophosphate
CDI	*Clostridium difficile* infection
CFTR	cystic fibrosis transmembrane conductance regulator
EAEC	enteroaggregative *Escherichia coli*
EHEC	enterohemorrhagic *Escherichia coli*
EIEC	enteroinvasive *Escherichia coli*
EPEC	enteropathogenic *Escherichia coli*
ETEC	enterotoxigenic *Escherichia coli*
GBS	Guillain-Barré syndrome
HIV	human immunodeficiency virus
HUS	hemolytic uremic syndrome
IL	interleukin
NAP-1	North American pulsed-field type 1
NSP4	nonstructural protein 4

ORS	oral rehydration solutions
ORT	oral rehydration therapy
PKA	protein kinase A
STEC	Shiga toxin–producing *E. coli*
TLR4	toll-like receptor
UNICEF	United Nations Children's Fund
ViCPS	Vi capsular polysaccharide vaccine
WHO	World Health Organization

REFERENCES

1. Guerrant RL, Van Gilder T, Steiner TS, et al. Practice guidelines for the management of infectious diarrhea. Clin Infect Dis 2001;32(3):331–351.
2. Fischer Walker CL, Perin J, Aryee MJ, Boschi-Pinto C, Black RE. Diarrhea incidence in low- and middle-income countries in 1990 and 2010: A systematic review. BMC Public Health 2012;12:220.
3. Kosek M, Bern C, Guerrant RL. The global burden of diarrhoeal disease, as estimated from studies published between 1992 and 2000. Bull World Health Organ 2003;81(3):197–204.
4. Jones TF, McMillian MB, Scallan E, et al. A population-based estimate of the substantial burden of diarrhoeal disease in the United States; FoodNet, 1996-2003. Epidemiol Infect 2007;135(2):293–301.
5. Scallan E, Griffin PM, Angulo FJ, Tauxe RV, Hoekstra RM. Foodborne illness acquired in the United States—Unspecified agents. Emerg Infect Dis 2011;17(1):16–22.
6. Scallan E, Hoekstra RM, Angulo FJ, et al. Foodborne illness acquired in the United States—Major pathogens. Emerg Infect Dis 2011;17(1):7–15.
7. Charles MD, Holman RC, Curns AT, Parashar UD, Glass RI, Bresee JS. Hospitalizations associated with rotavirus gastroenteritis in the United States, 1993-2002. Pediatr Infect Dis J 2006;25(6):489–493.
8. Talan D, Moran GJ, Newdow M, et al. Etiology of bloody diarrhea among patients presenting to United States emergency departments: Prevalence of *Escherichia coli* O157:H7 and other enteropathogens. Clin Infect Dis 2001;32(4):573–580.
9. Sack DA, Sack RB, Nair GB, Siddique AK. Cholera. Lancet 2004;363(9404):223–233.
10. Holtz LR, Neill MA, Tarr PI. Acute bloody diarrhea: A medical emergency for patients of all ages. Gastroenterology 2009;136(6):1887–1898.
11. Robins-Browne RM, Hartland EL. *Escherichia coli* as a cause of diarrhea. J Gastroenterol Hepatol 2002;17(4):467–475.
12. Flores J, Okhuysen PC. Enteroaggregative *Escherichia coli* infection. Curr Opin Gastroenterol 2009;25(1):8–11.
13. Niyogi SK. Shigellosis. J Microbiol 2005;43(2):133–143.
14. Voetsch AC, Van Gilder TJ, Angulo FJ, et al. FoodNet estimate of the burden of illness caused by nontyphoidal *Salmonella* infections in the United States. Clin Infect Dis 2004;38(Suppl 3):S127–S134.
15. Pfeiffer ML, DuPont HL, Ochoa TJ. The patient presenting with acute dysentery—A systematic review. J Infect 2012;64(4):374–386.
16. Sabina Y, Rahman A, Ray RC, Montet D. *Yersinia enterocolitica*: Mode of transmission, molecular insights of virulence, and pathogenesis of infection. J Pathog 2011;2011:429069.
17. Hodges K, Gill R. Infectious diarrhea: Cellular and molecular mechanisms. Gut Microbes 2010;1(1):4–21.
18. Li C, Dandridge KS, Di A, et al. Lysophosphatidic acid inhibits cholera toxin-induced secretory diarrhea through CFTR-dependent protein interactions. J Exp Med 2005;202(7):975–986.
19. Lucas ML. Enterocyte chloride and water secretion into the small intestine after enterotoxin challenge: Unifying hypothesis or intellectual dead end? J Physiol Biochem 2008;64(1):69–88.
20. Greenberg HB, Estes MK. Rotaviruses: From pathogenesis to vaccination. Gastroenterology 2009;136(6):1939–1951.
21. Rallabhandi P, Awomoyi A, Thomas KE, et al. Differential activation of human TLR4 by *Escherichia coli* and *Shigella flexneri* 2a lipopolysaccharide: Combined effects of lipid A acylation state and TLR4 polymorphisms on signaling. J Immunol 2008;180(2):1139–1147.
22. Fernandez MI, Sansonetti PJ. *Shigella* interaction with intestinal epithelial cells determines the innate immune response in shigellosis. Int J Med Microbiol 2003;293(1):55–67.
23. Haverly RM, Harrison CR, Dougherty TH. *Yersinia enterocolitica* bacteremia associated with red blood cell transfusion. Arch Pathol Lab Med 1996;120(5):499–500.
24. Panos GZ, Betsi GI, Falagas ME. Systematic review: Are antibiotics detrimental or beneficial for the treatment of patients with *Escherichia coli* O157:H7 infection? Aliment Pharmacol Ther 2006;24(5):731–742.
25. Garg AX, Pope JE, Thiessen-Philbrook H, Clark WF, Ouimet J. Arthritis risk after acute bacterial gastroenteritis. Rheumatology (Oxford) 2008;47(2):200–204.
26. Allos BM. *Campylobacter jejuni* infections: Update on emerging issues and trends. Clin Infect Dis 2001;32(8):1201–1206.
27. Organization WH. The Treatment of Diarrhoea: A Manual for Physicians and Other Senior Health Workers. 2005, *http://whqlibdoc.who.int/publications/2005/9241593180.pdf*.
28. Hahn S, Kim S, Garner P. Reduced osmolarity oral rehydration solution for treating dehydration caused by acute diarrhoea in children. Cochrane Database Syst Rev 2002;(1):CD002847.
29. Musekiwa A, Volmink J. Oral rehydration salt solution for treating cholera: </= 270 mOsm/L solutions vs >/= 310 mOsm/L solutions. Cochrane Database Syst Rev 2011;(12):CD003754.
30. Gregorio GV, Gonzales ML, Dans LF, Martinez EG. Polymer-based oral rehydration solution for treating acute watery diarrhoea. Cochrane Database Syst Rev 2009;(2):CD006519.
31. Gregorio GV, Dans LF, Silvestre MA. Early versus delayed refeeding for children with acute diarrhoea. Cochrane Database Syst Rev 2011;(7):CD007296.
32. Payot S, Bolla JM, Corcoran D, Fanning S, Megraud F, Zhang Q. Mechanisms of fluoroquinolone and macrolide resistance in *Campylobacter* spp. Microbes Infect 2006;8(7):1967–1971.
33. Parry CM, Threlfall EJ. Antimicrobial resistance in typhoidal and nontyphoidal salmonellae. Curr Opin Infect Dis 2008;21(5):531–538.
34. Hill DR, Ericsson CD, Pearson RD, et al. The practice of travel medicine: Guidelines by the Infectious Diseases Society of America. Clin Infect Dis 2006;43(12):1499–1539.
35. DuPont HL, Jiang ZD, Okhuysen PC, et al. A randomized, double-blind, placebo-controlled trial of rifaximin to prevent travelers' diarrhea. Ann Intern Med 2005;142(10):805–812.

36. DuPont HL. Clinical practice. Bacterial diarrhea. N Engl J Med 2009;361(16):1560–1569.
37. Allen SJ, Martinez EG, Gregorio GV, Dans LF. Probiotics for treating acute infectious diarrhoea. Cochrane Database Syst Rev 2010;(11):CD003048.
38. Lazzerini M, Ronfani L. Oral zinc for treating diarrhoea in children. Cochrane Database Syst Rev 2012;6:CD005436.
39. Steinberg EB, Bishop R, Haber P, et al. Typhoid fever in travelers: Who should be targeted for prevention? Clin Infect Dis 2004;39(2):186–191.
40. Cortese MM, Parashar UD. Prevention of rotavirus gastroenteritis among infants and children: Recommendations of the Advisory Committee on Immunization Practices (ACIP). MMWR Recomm Rep 2009;58(RR-2):1–25.
41. Leffler DA, Lamont JT. Treatment of *Clostridium difficile*-associated disease. Gastroenterology 2009;136(6):1899–1912.
42. Janarthanan S, Ditah I, Adler DG, Ehrinpreis MN. *Clostridium difficile*-associated diarrhea and proton pump inhibitor therapy: A meta-analysis. Am J Gastroenterol 2012;107(7):1001–1010.
43. Redelings MD, Sorvillo F, Mascola L. Increase in *Clostridium difficile*-related mortality rates, United States, 1999-2004. Emerg Infect Dis 2007;13(9):1417–1419.
44. Mitchell BG, Gardner A. Mortality and *Clostridium difficile* infection: A review. Antimicrob Resist Infect Control 2012;1(1):20.
45. Loo VG, Poirier L, Miller MA, et al. A predominantly clonal multi-institutional outbreak of *Clostridium difficile*-associated diarrhea with high morbidity and mortality. N Engl J Med 2005;353(23):2442–2449.
46. Zar FA, Bakkanagari SR, Moorthi KM, Davis MB. A comparison of vancomycin and metronidazole for the treatment of *Clostridium difficile*-associated diarrhea, stratified by disease severity. Clin Infect Dis 2007;45(3):302–307.
47. Wenisch C, Parschalk B, Hasenhundl M, Hirschl AM, Graninger W. Comparison of vancomycin, teicoplanin, metronidazole, and fusidic acid for the treatment of *Clostridium difficile*-associated diarrhea. Clin Infect Dis 1996;22(5):813–818.
48. Teasley DG, Gerding DN, Olson MM, et al. Prospective randomised trial of metronidazole versus vancomycin for *Clostridium-difficile*-associated diarrhoea and colitis. Lancet 1983;2(8358):1043–1046.
49. Louie TJ, Miller MA, Mullane KM, et al. Fidaxomicin versus vancomycin for *Clostridium difficile* infection. N Engl J Med 2011;364(5):422–431.
50. Eyre DW, Walker AS, Wyllie D, et al. Predictors of first recurrence of *Clostridium difficile* infection: Implications for initial management. Clin Infect Dis 2012;55(Suppl 2):S77–S87.
51. McFarland LV, Elmer GW, Surawicz CM. Breaking the cycle: Treatment strategies for 163 cases of recurrent *Clostridium difficile* disease. Am J Gastroenterol 2002;97(7):1769–1775.
52. Babakhani F, Bouillaut L, Gomez A, Sears P, Nguyen L, Sonenshein AL. Fidaxomicin inhibits spore production in *Clostridium difficile*. Clin Infect Dis 2012;55(Suppl 2):S162–S169.
53. Kelly C. A 76-year-old man with recurrent *Clostridium difficile*-associated diarrhea. JAMA 2009;301(9):954–962.
54. Buggy BP, Fekety R, Silva J Jr. Therapy of relapsing *Clostridium difficile*-associated diarrhea and colitis with the combination of vancomycin and rifampin. J Clin Gastroenterol 1987;9:155–159.
55. Johnson S, Schriever C, Galang M, Kelly CP, Gerding DN. Interruption of recurrent *Clostridium difficile*-associated diarrhea episodes by serial therapy with vancomycin and rifaximin. Clin Infect Dis 2007;44:846–848.
56. Wilcox W. Descriptive study of intravenous immunoglobulin for the treatment of recurrent *Clostridium difficile* diarrhea. J Antimicrob Chemother 2004;53:882–884.
57. Aas J, Gessert C, Bakken JS. Recurrent *Clostridium difficile* colitis: Case series involving 18 patients treated with donor stool administered via a nasogastric tube. Clin Infect Dis 2003;36:580–585.
58. Pozzoni P, Riva A, Bellatorre AG, et al. *Saccharomyces boulardii* for the prevention of antibiotic-associated diarrhea in adult hospitalized patients: A single-center, randomized, double-blind, placebo-controlled trial. Am J Gastroenterol 2012;107(6):922–931.
59. Johnston BC, Supina AL, Ospina M, Vohra S. Probiotics for the prevention of pediatric antibiotic-associated diarrhea. Cochrane Database Syst Rev 2007;(2):CD004827.
60. Louie TJ, Peppe J, Watt CK, et al. Tolevamer, a novel nonantibiotic polymer, compared with vancomycin in the treatment of mild to moderately severe *Clostridium difficile*-associated diarrhea. Clin Infect Dis 2006;43:411–420.
61. Shlim D. Looking for evidence that personal hygiene precautions prevent traveler's diarrhea. Clin Infect Dis 2005;41(Suppl 8):S531–S535.
62. Riddle MS, Arnold S, Tribble DR. Effect of adjunctive loperamide in combination with antibiotics on treatment outcomes in traveler's diarrhea: A systematic review and meta-analysis. Clin Infect Dis 2008;47(8):1007–1014.
63. Sobel J, Tucker N, Sulka A, McLaughlin J, Maslanka S. Foodborne botulism in the United States, 1990-2000. Emerg Infect Dis 2004;10(9):1606–1611.
64. Sobel J. Botulism. Clin Infect Dis 2005;41(8):1167–1173.

Intraabdominal Infections

92

Keith M. Olsen, Alan E. Gross, and Joseph T. DiPiro

KEY CONCEPTS

1. Most intraabdominal infections are "secondary" infections that are polymicrobial and are caused by a defect in the GI tract that must be treated by surgical drainage, resection, and/or repair.
2. Primary peritonitis is generally caused by a single organism (*Staphylococcus aureus* in patients undergoing chronic ambulatory peritoneal dialysis [CAPD] or *Escherichia coli* in patients with cirrhosis).
3. Secondary intraabdominal infections are usually caused by a mixture of bacteria, including enteric Gram-negative bacilli and anaerobes, which enhance the pathogenic potential of the bacteria.
4. For peritonitis, early and aggressive IV fluid resuscitation and electrolyte replacement therapy are essential. A common cause of early death is hypovolemic shock caused by inadequate intravascular volume and tissue perfusion.
5. Treatment is generally initiated on a "presumptive" or empirical basis and should be based on the likely pathogen(s) and local resistance patterns.
6. Antimicrobial regimens for secondary intraabdominal infections should include coverage for enteric Gram-negative bacilli and anaerobes. Antimicrobials that may be used for the treatment of secondary intraabdominal infections depending on severity of illness and microbiology data include (a) third-generation cephalosporin (ceftriaxone or cefuroxime) with metronidazole, (b) ticarcillin–clavulanate or piperacillin–tazobactam, (c) a carbapenem (imipenem, meropenem, doripenem, and ertapenem), and (d) quinolone (levofloxacin or ciprofloxacin) plus metronidazole or moxifloxacin alone.
7. Treatment of patients with peritoneal dialysis-associated peritonitis should include an antistaphylococcal antimicrobial such as a first-generation cephalosporin (cefazolin) or vancomycin (intraperitoneal administration is preferred).
8. The duration of antimicrobial treatment should be for 4 to 7 days for most secondary intraabdominal infections.
9. Patients treated for intraabdominal infections should be assessed for the occurrence of drug-related adverse effects, particularly hypersensitivity reactions (β-lactam antimicrobials), diarrhea (most agents), fungal infections (most agents), and nephrotoxicity (aminoglycosides).

Intraabdominal infections are those contained within the peritoneal cavity or retroperitoneal space. The peritoneal cavity extends from the undersurface of the diaphragm to the floor of the pelvis and contains the stomach, small bowel, large bowel, liver, gallbladder, and spleen. The duodenum, pancreas, kidneys, adrenal glands, great vessels (aorta and vena cava), and most mesenteric vascular structures reside in the retroperitoneum. Intraabdominal infections may be generalized or localized, complicated or uncomplicated, and community or healthcare-associated. Uncomplicated intraabdominal infections are confined within visceral structures, such as the liver, gallbladder, spleen, pancreas, kidney, or female reproductive organs while complicated intraabdominal infections involve anatomical disruption, extend beyond a single organ, and yield peritonitis and/or abscess. *Peritonitis* is defined as the acute inflammatory response of the peritoneal lining to microorganisms, chemicals, irradiation, or foreign-body injury. This chapter deals only with peritonitis of infectious origin.

An *abscess* is a purulent collection of fluid separated from surrounding tissue by a wall consisting of inflammatory cells and adjacent organs. It usually contains necrotic debris, bacteria, and inflammatory cells. These processes differ considerably in presentation and approach to treatment.

EPIDEMIOLOGY

Peritonitis may be classified as primary, secondary, or tertiary.[1–5] Primary peritonitis, also called *spontaneous bacterial peritonitis*, is an infection of the peritoneal cavity without an evident source in the abdomen.[6] Bacteria may be transported from the bloodstream to the peritoneal cavity, where the inflammatory process begins. In secondary peritonitis, a focal disease process is evident within the abdomen. Secondary peritonitis may involve perforation of the GI tract (possibly because of ulceration, ischemia, or obstruction), postoperative peritonitis, or posttraumatic peritonitis (blunt or penetrating trauma). Tertiary peritonitis occurs in critically ill patients and is infection that persists or recurs at least 48 hours after apparently adequate management of primary or secondary peritonitis.

❶ Primary peritonitis occurs in both children and adults, although the rates in children have been declining.[4] Primary peritonitis develops in up to 10% to 30% of patients with alcoholic cirrhosis.[4–7] Patients undergoing chronic ambulatory peritoneal dialysis (CAPD) average one episode of peritonitis every 33 months.[8] Epidemiologic data for secondary and tertiary intraabdominal infections are less understood. Secondary peritonitis may be caused by perforation of a peptic ulcer; traumatic perforation of the stomach, small or large bowel, uterus, or urinary bladder; appendicitis; pancreatitis; diverticulitis; bowel infarction; inflammatory bowel disease; cholecystitis; operative contamination of the peritoneum; or diseases of the female genital tract, such as septic abortion, postoperative uterine infection, endometritis, and salpingitis. Appendicitis is one of the most common causes of intraabdominal infection. In 2006, 353,000 appendectomies were performed in the United States for suspected appendicitis.[9] Most healthcare-associated intraabdominal infections occur as complications following intraabdominal surgeries.

TABLE 92-1 Causes of Bacterial Peritonitis

Primary (spontaneous) bacterial peritonitis
Peritoneal dialysis
Cirrhosis with ascites
Nephrotic syndrome
Secondary bacterial peritonitis
Miscellaneous causes
Diverticulitis
Appendicitis
Inflammatory bowel diseases
Salpingitis
Biliary tract infections
Necrotizing pancreatitis
Neoplasms
Intestinal obstruction
Perforation
Mechanical GI problems
Any cause of small bowel obstruction (adhesions, hernia)
Vascular causes
Mesenteric arterial or venous occlusion (atrial fibrillation)
Mesenteric ischemia without occlusion
Trauma
Blunt abdominal trauma with rupture of intestine
Penetrating abdominal trauma
Iatrogenic intestinal perforation (endoscopy)
Intraoperative events
Solid organ transplant in the abdomen
Peritoneal contamination during abdominal operation
Leakage from GI anastomosis

ETIOLOGY

Primary peritonitis in adults occurs most commonly in association with alcoholic cirrhosis, especially in its end stage, or with ascites caused by postnecrotic cirrhosis, chronic active hepatitis, acute viral hepatitis, congestive heart failure, malignancy, systemic lupus erythematosus, or nephritic syndrome. It may also result from the use of a peritoneal catheter for dialysis or CNS ventriculoperitoneal shunting for hydrocephalus. Rarely, primary peritonitis occurs without apparent underlying disease.

Table 92-1 summarizes many of the potential causes of bacterial peritonitis. Causes include inflammatory processes of the GI tract or abdominal organs, bowel obstruction, vascular occlusions that may lead to gangrene of the intestines, and neoplasia that may cause intestinal perforation or obstruction. Other possible causes include those resulting from traumatic injuries, postoperative infections, or solid organ transplant in the abdomen.

Abscesses are the result of chronic inflammation and may occur without preceding generalized peritonitis. They may be located within one of the spaces of the peritoneal cavity or within one of the visceral organs, and may range from a few milliliters to a liter or more in volume. These collections often have a fibrinous capsule and may take from a few weeks to years to form.

The causes of intraabdominal abscess overlap those of peritonitis and, in fact, may occur sequentially or simultaneously. Appendicitis is the most frequent cause of abscess. Other potential causes of intraabdominal abscess include pancreatitis, diverticulitis, lesions of the biliary tract, genitourinary tract infections, perforation in the abdomen, trauma, and leaking intestinal anastomoses. In addition, pelvic inflammatory disease in women may lead to tuboovarian abscess. For some diseases, such as appendicitis and diverticulitis, abscesses occur more frequently than generalized peritonitis.

Microflora of the Gastrointestinal Tract and Female Genital Tract

A full appreciation of intraabdominal infection requires an understanding of the normal microflora within the GI tract. There are striking differences in bacterial species and concentrations of flora within the various segments of the GI tract (Table 92-2), and this bacterial environment usually determines the severity of infectious processes in the abdomen. Generally, the low gastric pH eradicates bacteria that enter the stomach. With achlorhydria, bacterial counts may rise to 10^5 to 10^7 organisms/mL (10^8 to 10^{10}/L). The normally low bacterial count may also increase by 1,000- or 10,000-fold with gastric outlet obstruction, hemorrhage, gastric cancer, and in patients receiving histamine 2 (H_2)-receptor antagonists, proton pump inhibitors, or antacids.

The biliary tract (gallbladder and bile ducts) is sterile in most healthy individuals, but in people older than 70 years of age, those with acute cholecystitis, jaundice, or common bile duct stones, it is likely to be colonized by aerobic Gram-negative bacilli (particularly *Escherichia coli* and *Klebsiella* spp.) and enterococci.[10] Patients with biliary tract bacterial colonization are at greater risk of intraabdominal infection.

In the distal ileum, bacterial counts of aerobes and anaerobes are quite high. In the colon, there may be 500 to 600 different types of bacteria in stool, with concentrations often reaching 10^{11} organisms/mL (10^{14}/L) and anaerobic bacteria outnumbering aerobic bacteria by more than 1,000 to 1.[2,11] In fact, up to 50% of the dry mass of stool is *Bacteroides* spp. Fortunately, most colonic bacteria are not pathogens because they cannot survive in environments outside the colon. Perforation of the colon results in the release of large numbers of anaerobic and aerobic bacteria into the peritoneum.

The colonic flora are generally consistent unless broad-spectrum antimicrobials have been used. Depending on the type of antibiotic and spectrum, the duration of use, route of administration, and the pharmacokinetic and pharmacodynamic properties, antibiotics can cause shifts in the normal GI microflora including causing increased drug resistance.[12]

The lower female genital tract is generally colonized by a large number of aerobic and anaerobic bacteria. Anaerobes may number 10^9 organisms per milliliter (10^{12}/L) and often include lactobacilli,

TABLE 92-2 Usual Microflora of the GI Tract

		Approximate Concentration (Log No. Organisms/mL [×10³/L])	
Site	**Commonly Found Bacteria**	**Aerobes**	**Anaerobes**
Stomach[a]	*Streptococcus, Lactobacillus*	10–100	Rare
Biliary tract	Normally sterile (*Escherichia coli, Klebsiella*, or enterococci in some patients)	0	0
Proximal small bowel	*Streptococcus* (including enterococci), *E. coli, Klebsiella, Lactobacillus*, diphtheroids	100	Few
Distal ileum	*E. coli, Klebsiella, Enterobacter*, enterococci, *Bacteroides fragilis, Clostridium*, peptostreptococci	10^4–10^6	10^5–10^7
Colon	*Bacteroides* spp., peptostreptococci, *Clostridium, E. coli, Klebsiella*, enterococci, *Enterobacter, Candida*, and many others	10^5–10^8	10^9–10^{11}

[a]With achlorhydria, acid suppressive therapy, gastric cancer, or gastric outlet obstruction, bacterial counts may rise to 10^5/mL.

eubacteria, clostridia, anaerobic streptococci, and, less frequently, *Bacteroides fragilis.* Aerobic bacteria most often are streptococci and *Staphylococcus epidermidis*, and these may number 10^8 organisms per milliliter (10^{11}/L).

PATHOPHYSIOLOGY

Intraabdominal infection results from bacterial entry into the peritoneal or retroperitoneal spaces or from bacterial collections within intraabdominal organs. In primary peritonitis, bacteria may enter the abdomen via the bloodstream or the lymphatic system by transmigration through the bowel wall, through an indwelling peritoneal dialysis catheter, or via the fallopian tubes in females. Hematogenous bacterial spread (through the bloodstream) occurs more frequently with tuberculosis peritonitis or peritonitis associated with cirrhotic ascites. When peritonitis results from peritoneal dialysis, skin surface flora are introduced via the peritoneal catheter. In secondary peritonitis, bacteria most often enter the peritoneum or retroperitoneum as a result of perforation of the GI or female genital tracts caused by diseases or traumatic injuries. In addition, peritonitis or abscess may result from contamination of the peritoneum during a surgical procedure or following anastomotic leak.

The physiologic characteristics of the peritoneal cavity determine the nature of the response to infection or inflammation within it.[1,4] The peritoneum is lined by a highly permeable serous membrane with a surface area approximately that of skin. The peritoneal cavity is lubricated with less than 100 mL of sterile, clear yellow fluid, normally with fewer than 250 cells/mm^3 (250×10^6/L), a specific gravity below 1.016, and protein content below 3 g/dL (30 g/L). These conditions change drastically with peritoneal infection or inflammation, as described below.

After bacteria are introduced into the peritoneal cavity, there is an immediate response to contain the insult. Humoral and cellular defenses respond first; then the omentum adheres to the affected area. A limited bacterial inoculum is handled rapidly by defense mechanisms, including complement activation and a leukocyte response. Under certain conditions, the bacterial insult is not contained, and bacteria disseminate throughout the peritoneal cavity, resulting in peritonitis. This is more likely to occur in the presence of a foreign body, hematoma, dead tissue, a large bacterial inoculum, continuing bacterial contamination, and contamination involving a mixture of synergistic organisms. Protein–calorie malnutrition, antecedent steroid therapy, and diabetes mellitus may also contribute to the formation of an intraabdominal abscess.

When bacteria become dispersed throughout the peritoneum, the inflammatory process involves most of the peritoneal lining. There is an outpouring into the peritoneum of fluid containing leukocytes, fibrin, and other proteins that form exudates on the inflamed peritoneal surfaces and begin to form adhesions between peritoneal structures. This process, combined with a paralysis of the intestines (ileus), may result in confinement of the contamination to one or more locations within the peritoneum. Fluid also begins to collect in the bowel lumen and wall, and distension may result.

The fluid and protein shift into the abdomen (called *third-spacing*) may be so dramatic that circulating blood volume is decreased, which may cause decreased cardiac output and hypovolemic shock. Accompanying fever, vomiting, or diarrhea may worsen the fluid imbalance. A reflex sympathetic response, manifested by sweating, tachycardia, and vasoconstriction, may be evident. With an inflamed peritoneum, bacteria and endotoxins are absorbed easily into the bloodstream (translocation), and this may result in septic shock.[1,4,5] Other foreign substances present in the peritoneal cavity potentiate peritonitis. These adjuvants, notably feces, dead tissues, barium, mucus, bile, and blood, have detrimental effects on host defense mechanisms, particularly on bacterial phagocytosis.

Many of the manifestations of intraabdominal infections, particularly peritonitis, result from cytokine activity. Inflammatory cytokines, such as tumor necrosis factor-α (TNF-α), interleukin (IL) 1, IL-6, IL-8, and interferon γ (INF-γ), are produced by macrophages and neutrophils in response to bacteria and bacterial products or in response to tissue injury resulting from the surgical incision.[1,4] These cytokines produce wide-ranging effects on the vascular endothelium of organs, particularly the liver, lungs, kidneys, and heart. With uncontrolled activation of these mediators, sepsis may result (see Chap. 97, Sepsis and Septic Shock).[13,14]

Peritonitis may result in death because of the effects on major organ systems. Fluid shifts, cytokines and endotoxin may result in hypovolemia, hypoperfusion, and shock. Hypoalbuminemia may result from protein loss into the peritoneum exacerbating intravascular volume loss. Pulmonary function may be compromised by the inflamed peritoneum, producing splinting (muscle rigidity caused by pain) that inhibits adequate diaphragmatic movement leading to atelectasis and pneumonia. Increased lung vascular permeability and resulting shunting of blood may induce onset of the respiratory distress syndrome and associated hypoxemia and hypercarbia. With fluid loss and hypotension, renal and hepatic perfusion may be compromised, and acute renal and hepatic failure are potential threats.

If peritoneal contamination is localized but bacterial elimination is incomplete, an abscess results. This collection of necrotic tissue, bacteria, and white blood cells may be at single or multiple sites and may be within one of the spaces of the peritoneal cavity or in one of the visceral organs. The location of the abscess is often related to the site of primary disease. For example, abscesses resulting from appendicitis tend to appear in the right lower quadrant or the pelvis; those resulting from diverticulitis tend to appear in the left lower quadrant or pelvis.

An abscess begins by the combined action of inflammatory cells (such as neutrophils), bacteria, fibrin, and other inflammatory mediators. Bacteria may release heparinases that cause local thrombosis and tissue necrosis or fibrinolysins, collagenases, or other enzymes that allow extension of the process into surrounding tissues. Neutrophils gathered in the abscess cavity die in 3 to 5 days, releasing lysosomal enzymes that liquefy the core of the abscess. A mature abscess may have a fibrinous capsule that isolates bacteria and the liquid core from antimicrobials and immunologic defenses.

Within the abscess, the oxygen tension is low and anaerobic bacteria thrive; thus, the size of the abscess may increase because it is hypertonic, resulting in an additional influx of fluid. Hypertonicity promotes the formation of bacterial L forms, which are resistant to antimicrobial agents that disrupt cell walls. Abscess formation may continue and mature for long periods of time and may not be readily evident to either patient or physician. In some instances, the abscess may resolve spontaneously, and, infrequently, it may erode into adjacent organs or rupture and cause diffuse peritonitis. If the abscess erodes through the skin, it may result in an enterocutaneous fistula, connecting bowel to skin, or in a draining sinus tract.

The overall outcome from an intraabdominal infection depends on key factors: inoculum size, virulence of the contaminating organisms, the presence of adjuvants within the peritoneal cavity that facilitate infection, the adequacy of host defenses, source control, and the adequacy of initial treatment.[15,16]

Microbiology of Intraabdominal Infection

2 Primary bacterial peritonitis is often caused by a single organism. In children, the pathogen is usually group A *Streptococcus*, *E. coli*, *Streptococcus pneumoniae*, or *Bacteroides* species.[4,17–20] When peritonitis occurs in association with cirrhotic ascites, *E. coli* is isolated most frequently. Other potential pathogens are: *Haemophilus*

TABLE 92-3 Pathogens Isolated from Patients with Intraabdominal Infection

	Secondary Peritonitis[3] (%)	Community-Acquired Infection[25] (%)	Nosocomial Infection[25] (%)
Gram-Negative Bacteria			
Escherichia coli	32–61	29	22.5
Enterobacter	8–26	5.2	8.0
Klebsiella	6–26	2.8	4.5
Proteus	4–23	1.7	2.4
Gram-Positive Bacteria			
Enterococcus	18–24	10.6	18
Streptococcus	6–55	13.7	10
Staphylococcus	6–16	3.1	4.8
Anaerobic Bacteria			
Bacteroides	25–80	13.7	10.3
Clostridium	5–18	3.5	3.4
Fungi	2–5	3	4

influenzae, *Klebsiella* spp., *Pseudomonas* spp., anaerobes, and *S. pneumoniae*.[21] Occasionally, primary peritonitis may be caused by *Mycobacterium tuberculosis*. Peritonitis in patients undergoing peritoneal dialysis is caused most often by common skin organisms, such as coagulase-negative staphylococci, *Staphylococcus aureus*, streptococci, and enterococci. Gram-negative bacteria associated with peritoneal dialysis infections include *E. coli*, *Klebsiella* spp., and *Pseudomonas* spp.[6] Mortality from primary peritonitis caused by Gram-negative bacteria is much greater than that from Gram-positive bacteria.[4,5]

3 Because of the diverse bacteria present in the GI tract, secondary intraabdominal infections are often polymicrobial.[2] The mean number of different bacterial species isolated from infected intraabdominal sites ranged from 2.9 to 3.7, including an average of 1.3 to 1.6 aerobes and 1.7 to 2.1 anaerobes.[21,22] With proper anaerobic specimen collection, anaerobic organisms are isolated in most patients. In one report of patients with gangrenous and perforated appendicitis, an average of 10.2 different organisms was isolated from each patient, including 2.7 aerobes and 7.5 anaerobes.[23] Purely aerobic or anaerobic infections are uncommon, as are infections caused by fungi. Table 92-3 gives the frequencies with which specific bacteria were isolated from patients with peritonitis and other intraabdominal infections.[3,24] Nosocomial infections tend to have a more diverse array of pathogens and higher likelihood of multidrug resistance compared with isolates from community-acquired infections.[25] *E. coli*, *Streptococcus* spp., and *Bacteroides* spp. were isolated most often from the infection site, as well as from blood cultures. In patients diagnosed with severe infections, the pattern of bacterial isolates may change and commonly includes *Candida* spp., enterococci, Enterobacteriaceae, and *S. epidermidis*.

Visceral organ abscesses differ in character from the typical intraabdominal abscess. Hepatic abscesses may be polymicrobial (involving *E. coli*, *Klebsiella* spp., and anaerobes) or occasionally may be caused by amoeba.[11] Pancreatic abscesses are often polymicrobial, involving enteric bacteria that ascend through the biliary system. Splenic abscesses usually result from hematogenous dissemination of bacteria, such as *E. coli, S. aureus*, *Proteus mirabilis*, *Enterococcus* spp., and *K. pneumoniae*, as well as anaerobes.[11] Pelvic inflammatory disease is associated initially with *Neisseria gonorrhoeae* or *Chlamydia trachomatis*. However, tuboovarian abscesses are usually polymicrobial, having a mix of Gram-positive and Gram-negative aerobes and anaerobes.

Bacterial Synergism

The size of the bacterial inoculum and the number and types of bacterial species present in intraabdominal infections influence patient outcome. The combination of aerobic and anaerobic organisms appears to greatly increase the severity of infection. In animal studies, combinations of aerobic and anaerobic bacteria were much more lethal than infections caused by aerobes or anaerobes alone.

Facultative bacteria may provide an environment conducive to the growth of anaerobic bacteria.[2] Although many bacteria isolated in mixed infections are nonpathogenic by themselves, their presence may be essential for the pathogenicity of the bacterial mixture.[7] The role of facultative bacteria in mixed infections can include (a) promotion of an appropriate environment for anaerobic bacterial growth through oxygen consumption, (b) production of nutrients necessary for anaerobes, and (c) production of extracellular enzymes that promote tissue invasion by anaerobes.

Rat models of intraabdominal infection demonstrate that uncontrolled infection with an implanted mix of aerobes and anaerobes leads to a two-stage (biphasic) infectious process. There is an early peritonitis phase with a high mortality rate and isolation of *E. coli* from blood and a late abscess formation phase in all survivors with isolation of anaerobes such as *B. fragilis* and *Fusobacterium varium*. These experiments and others support the concept that aerobic enteric organisms and anaerobes are pathogens in intraabdominal infection. Aerobic bacteria, particularly *E. coli*, appear responsible for the early mortality from peritonitis, whereas anaerobic bacteria are major pathogens in abscesses, with *B. fragilis* predominating.[26]

Enterococcus can be isolated from many intraabdominal infections in humans, but its role as a pathogen is not clear. Enterococcal infection occurs more commonly in postoperative peritonitis, in the presence of specific risk factors indicating failure of the host's defenses (immunocompromised patients), or with the use of broad-spectrum antibiotics.[27,28]

CLINICAL PRESENTATION

Intraabdominal infections have a wide spectrum of clinical features often depending on the specific disease process, the location and magnitude of bacterial contamination, and concurrent host factors. Peritonitis is usually recognized easily, but intraabdominal abscess may often continue for considerable periods of time, either going unrecognized or being attributed to an unrelated disease process. Patients with primary and secondary peritonitis present quite differently (Table 92-4).[1,4,5]

Primary peritonitis can develop over a period of days to weeks and is usually a more indolent process than secondary peritonitis. The first sign of peritonitis may be a cloudy dialysate in patients undergoing peritoneal dialysis or worsening encephalopathy in a cirrhotic patient.

The patient with generalized bacterial peritonitis presents most often in acute distress. The patient lies still, usually on his or her back, possibly with the hips slightly flexed. Any movement of the patient, including rocking the bed or breathing, worsens the generalized abdominal pain.

If peritonitis continues untreated, the patient may experience hypovolemic shock from third-space fluid loss into the peritoneum, bowel wall, and lumen. This may be accompanied by sepsis because the inflamed peritoneum absorbs bacteria and toxins into mesenteric blood vessels and lymph nodes, initiating production of inflammatory cytokines. Hypovolemic shock is the major factor contributing to mortality in the early stage of peritonitis.

Intraabdominal abscess may pose a difficult diagnostic challenge because the symptoms are neither specific nor dramatic. The patient may complain of abdominal pain or discomfort, but these symptoms are not reliable. Fever is usually present; often it is low

TABLE 92-4 Clinical Presentation of Peritonitis

Primary Peritonitis
General
The patient may not be in acute distress, particularly with peritoneal dialysis
Signs and symptoms
The patient may complain of loss of appetite, bloating, nausea, vomiting (sometimes with diarrhea), and abdominal tenderness
Temperature may be only mildly elevated or not elevated in patients undergoing peritoneal dialysis
Bowel sounds are hypoactive
The cirrhotic patient may have worsening encephalopathy
Cloudy dialysate fluid with peritoneal dialysis
Laboratory tests
The patient's white blood cell (WBC) count may be only mildly elevated
Ascitic fluid usually contains greater than 250 leukocytes/mm^3 (250 × 10^6/L), and bacteria may be evident on Gram stain of a centrifuged specimen
In 60–80% of patients with cirrhotic ascites, the Gram stain is negative
Other diagnostic tests
Culture of peritoneal dialysate or ascitic fluid should be positive, particularly if collected prior to initiation of antibiotics
Secondary Peritonitis
Signs and symptoms
Generalized abdominal pain
Tachypnea
Tachycardia
Nausea and vomiting
Temperature is normal initially then increases to 37.8–38.9°C (100–102°F) within the first few hours and may continue to rise for the next several hours
Hypotension, hypoperfusion, and shock if volume is not restored
Decreased urine output due to vascular volume depletion
Physical examination
Voluntary abdominal guarding changing to involuntary guarding and a "board-like abdomen"
Abdominal tenderness and distension
Faint bowel sounds that cease over time
Laboratory tests
Leukocytosis (15,000–20,000 WBC/mm^3 [15 × 10^9 to 20 × 10^9/L]), with neutrophils predominating and an elevated percentage of immature neutrophils (bands)
Elevated hematocrit and blood urea nitrogen because of dehydration
Patient progresses from early alkalosis because of hyperventilation and vomiting to metabolic acidosis
Other diagnostic tests
Abdominal radiographs may be useful because free air in the abdomen (indicating intestinal perforation) or distension of the small or large bowel is often evident

grade, but it may be high, with a spiking pattern. The patient may have a paralytic ileus and abdominal distension. The abdominal examination is unreliable; tenderness and pain may be present, and a mass may be palpated.

Peritonitis may result from an abscess that ruptures, spreading bacteria and toxins throughout the peritoneum. In other patients, the entry of bacterial toxins into the systemic circulation from the abscess may lead to sepsis and progressive multisystem organ failure (e.g., renal, hepatic, pulmonary, or cardiovascular).

Laboratory studies are not generally helpful in the diagnosis of intraabdominal abscess, although most patients will have leukocytosis. Some patients may have positive blood cultures, whereas others, particularly diabetics, may have hyperglycemia. The finding of *Bacteroides* or any two enteric bacteria in the bloodstream is often indicative of an intraabdominal infectious process.

Radiographic methods are used to make the diagnosis of an intraabdominal abscess. Plain radiographs may show air–fluid levels or a shift of normal intraabdominal contents by the abscess mass. GI contrast studies may also demonstrate this displacement of abdominal structures. Both of these modalities provide indirect evidence of abscess presence but are not generally helpful in precisely locating the abscess.

Ultrasound is a frequent first diagnostic method used when an intraabdominal abscess is suspected. The procedure may be done at the bedside, which is particularly helpful when the patient is in the intensive care unit.

Computed tomographic (CT) scanning is the preferred modality used to evaluate the abdomen for the presence of an abscess and is the imaging study of greatest value. If not contraindicated, an oral radiocontrast agent should be given to allow differentiation of the abscess from the bowel. IV radiocontrast material will be taken up preferentially in the wall of the abscess, creating a unique radiographic appearance, so-called rim enhancement. Magnetic resonance imaging offers no significant advantage when compared with CT scanning.

Intraabdominal infection caused by disease processes at specific sites often produces characteristic manifestations that are helpful in diagnosis. For example, a patient with diverticulitis may exhibit stabbing left-lower-quadrant abdominal pain and constipation. Fever and leukocytosis are frequently present, and a tender mass is sometimes palpable. With appendicitis, the findings may be inconsistent, but many patients have a sudden onset of periumbilical or epigastric pain that is usually colicky and later shifts to the right lower quadrant. The location of pain may vary because the appendix can be in many locations (e.g., retrocecal or pelvic) in the abdomen. A mass may be palpable on abdominal, pelvic, or rectal examination. The patient's temperature is generally mildly elevated early and then increases. If perforation and peritonitis occur, findings would include diffuse abdominal pain, rigidity, and sustained fever. More often, however, appendiceal perforation results in a local abscess.

TREATMENT

Desired Outcome

The primary goals of treatment are correction of the intraabdominal disease processes or injuries that have caused infection and the drainage of purulent collections (abscesses). A secondary objective is to achieve a resolution of infection without major organ system complications (pulmonary, hepatic, cardiovascular, or renal failure) or adverse drug effects. Ideally, the patient should be discharged from the hospital after treatment with full function for self-care and routine daily activities.

General Approach to Treatment

The treatment of intraabdominal infection most often requires hospitalization and the coordinated use of three major modalities: (a) prompt drainage of the infected site, (b) hemodynamic resuscitation and support of vital organ functions, and (c) early administration of appropriate antimicrobial therapy to treat infection not eradicated by surgery.[2]

Antimicrobials are an important adjunct to drainage procedures in the treatment of secondary intraabdominal infections; however, the use of antimicrobial agents without surgical intervention is usually inadequate. For most cases of primary peritonitis, drainage procedures may not be required, and antimicrobial agents become the mainstay of therapy.

❹ In the early phase of serious intraabdominal infections, attention should be given to the maintenance of organ system functions. With generalized peritonitis, large volumes of IV fluids are required to restore vascular volume, to improve cardiovascular function, and to maintain adequate tissue perfusion and oxygenation. Adequate urine output should be maintained to ensure adequate resuscitation and proper renal function. Respiratory function can be assisted by a variety of methods, including oxygen therapy, pulmonary physiotherapy, and ventilatory support in severely ill patients. Often the critically ill patient with intraabdominal infection will require intensive care management, particularly if there is cardiovascular or respiratory instability. In addition, isolation procedures may be required if the infectious process poses a threat to other hospitalized patients.

An additional important component of therapy is nutrition. Intraabdominal infections often directly involve the GI tract or disrupt its function (paralytic ileus). The return of GI motility may take days, weeks, and, occasionally, months. In the interim, enteral or parenteral nutrition as indicated facilitates improved immune function and wound healing to ensure recovery.

Nonpharmacologic Treatment

Drainage Procedures

Primary peritonitis is treated with antimicrobials and rarely requires drainage. Secondary peritonitis requires surgical correction of the underlying pathology. The drainage of the purulent material is the critical component of management of an intraabdominal abscess. Without adequate drainage of the abscess, antimicrobial therapy and fluid resuscitation can be expected to fail.

Secondary peritonitis is treated surgically; this is often called *source control*, which refers to all the physical measures undertaken to eradicate the focus of infection.[2,5] At the time of laparotomy (surgical opening and exploration of the abdomen), attempts are made to correct the cause of the peritonitis. This may include patching a perforated ulcer with omentum, removal of a segment of perforated colon, or excision of a portion of gangrenous small intestine. In addition, the surgeon may elect to leave the abdomen open after the laparotomy, plan a re-laparotomy at a later time regardless of the patient's condition, or, perform re-laparotomy if the patient develops reinfection.[5] The goal of all these procedures is to repair or remove the inflamed or gangrenous viscus and to prevent further bacterial contamination. The presence of active inflammation increases the difficulty of the surgical procedure, which results in a higher morbidity and mortality rate than if the same procedures were performed in an elective setting without inflammation.

The presence of active inflammation may make it technically impossible to perform the definitive surgical procedure. In this situation, attempts are made to provide drainage of the infected or gangrenous structures. If an intraabdominal abscess, separate from any intraabdominal organ, is discovered during an exploratory laparotomy, it may be debrided, excised, or drained. If the intraabdominal abscess involves an abdominal structure, then a resection of part or of the entire organ may be required. An example of this situation is an abscess associated with diverticular disease of the colon. Management may include drainage of the abscess and resection of the involved part of the colon. All foreign material, necrotic tissue, feces, blood, or pus should be removed from the operative field, and the peritoneum should be copiously irrigated with 0.9% sodium chloride to decrease the concentrations of bacteria or other noxious substances.

After an abscess is located, it must be drained. This may be performed surgically or with percutaneous, image-guided techniques.[5,29] Typically, image-guided techniques employ ultrasonography or CT scanning. The management of an intraabdominal abscess with percutaneous catheter drainage may be sufficient to resolve the infection. Some patients may require a subsequent procedure to treat the underlying GI conditions; however, a significant advantage is obtained by first draining the abscess percutaneously. This allows the surgical procedure to be performed on a patient who is no longer suffering the systemic manifestations of uncontrolled infection. Drainage techniques may be performed using endoscopy or laparoscopy. These minimal-access techniques may offer advantages when compared with traditional surgery but will probably be used less often than radiologically assisted percutaneous drainage techniques.

The most valuable microbiologic information may be obtained at the time of percutaneous or operative abscess drainage. If pus or fluid is found that is believed to be infected, it is best to aspirate 2 to 3 mL into a syringe, remove any air, and tightly cap the syringe. The specimen should be taken promptly to the microbiology laboratory, where a Gram stain should be performed immediately and cultures prepared for identification of aerobic and anaerobic bacteria. If no fluid is available for collection, culture swab devices may be applied to the infected area; however, anaerobic organisms often are not isolated from swabs.

Fluid Therapy

❹ Patients should be evaluated for signs of hypovolemia, hypoperfusion, and shock. Aggressive fluid repletion and management are required for successful treatment of intraabdominal infections. The Surviving Sepsis Campaign: International Guidelines for Management of Severe Sepsis and Septic Shock recommend treatment goals during the first 6 hours or resuscitation: (a) central venous pressure (CVP) 8 to 12 mm Hg, (b) mean arterial pressure (MAP) ≥65 mm Hg, and (c) maintain urine output ≥0.5 mL/kg/h.[30,31] If the patient is mechanically ventilated a target CVP 12 to 15 mm Hg should be achieved.[30] Fluid therapy is instituted for the purposes of achieving or maintaining proper intravascular volume to ensure adequate cardiac output, tissue perfusion, and correction of acidosis. Loss of fluid through vomiting, diarrhea, or nasogastric suction contributes to dehydration. Intravascular volume can be assessed by blood pressure and heart rate but more accurately by measurement of CVP or urinary output. When a contracted vascular volume is accompanied by hemorrhage, the initial hematocrit may be normal, but if there is no associated hemorrhage, the hematocrit is usually elevated as an indication of hemoconcentration. Urine output should be monitored continuously in severely ill patients by use of a urinary bladder catheter, quantitated hourly, and should equal or exceed 0.5 mL/kg of body weight per hour.

In patients with peritonitis, hypovolemia is often accompanied by metabolic acidosis. IV fluids should consist of a bolus of crystalloids or colloids with additional fluids targeting predefined therapeutic goals.[30,31] In the initial hour of treatment, large volumes of solution may be required to restore intravascular volume. Thereafter, fluids may be required at a rate of 1 L/h or higher. Once targeted therapeutic goals are reached, maintenance fluids should be instituted with 0.9% sodium chloride and potassium chloride (20 mEq/L [20 mmol/L]) or 5% dextrose and 0.45% sodium chloride with potassium chloride (20 mEq/L [20 mmol/L]). The administration rate should be based on estimated daily fluid loss through urine and nasogastric suction, including 0.5 to 1 L for insensible fluid loss. Potassium would not be included routinely if the patient is hyperkalemic or has renal insufficiency. If appropriate fluid management fails to restore target goals of perfusion, vasopressor therapy should be initiated.[30] A more thorough discussion of fluid and vasopressor therapy are presented elsewhere in this text (Chaps. 13, 14, and 96).

In patients with significant blood loss, blood transfusion may be indicated. This is generally in the form of packed red blood cells. The criteria for blood transfusion are controversial, but a hematocrit of 25% is generally accepted. In the individual patient, the decision is often determined by the overall clinical status and the ability of the patient to compensate for the reduction in oxygen-carrying capacity associated with an acute anemia. Additional blood component therapy with fresh-frozen plasma or platelets is also based on the needs of the individual patient. Aggressive fluid therapy must often be continued in the postoperative period because fluid will continue to sequester in the peritoneal cavity, bowel wall, and lumen.

Pharmacologic Treatment

Antimicrobial Therapy

The goals of antimicrobial therapy are (a) to control bacteremia and prevent the establishment of metastatic foci of infection, (b) to reduce suppurative complications after bacterial contamination, and (c) to prevent local spread of existing infection. After suppuration has occurred (e.g., an abscess has formed), a cure by antibiotic therapy alone is very difficult to achieve; antimicrobials may serve to improve the results obtained with surgery.

5 An empirical antimicrobial regimen should be started as soon as the presence of intraabdominal infection is suspected. Therefore, antibiotics are usually initiated after culture specimens are collected but before identification of the infecting organisms is complete. Therapy must be initiated based on the likely pathogens. Increasing resistance to fluoroquinolones, ampicillin–sulbactam, and clindamycin emphasize the importance of utilizing local susceptibility data for empiric therapy and tailoring the antibiotic regimen based on susceptibility results. Predominant pathogens, as discussed in the preceding section, vary depending on the site of intraabdominal infection and the underlying disease process. Table 92-5 lists the likely pathogens against which antimicrobial agents should be directed.

Antimicrobial Experience Many studies have been conducted evaluating or comparing the effectiveness of antimicrobials for the treatment of intraabdominal infections. Substantial differences in patient outcomes from treatment with a variety of agents have not generally been demonstrated.[32]

Important findings from over 20 years of clinical trials regarding selection of antimicrobials for intraabdominal infections are the following:

1. Antimicrobial regimens used for secondary infections should cover a broad spectrum of aerobic and anaerobic bacteria from the GI tract. Empiric treatment should be guided by the local epidemiology of resistant pathogens and patient-specific risk factors for acquisition pathogens of concern.
2. Single-agent regimens (such as antianaerobic cephalosporins, extended-spectrum penicillins with β-lactamase inhibitors, and carbapenems) are as effective but have the benefit of being less nephrotoxic compared to combinations of aminoglycosides with antianaerobic agents. This is also true for antimicrobial treatment of acute bacterial contamination from penetrating abdominal trauma.[33,34]
3. Resistance is now prevalent among *B. fragilis* to clindamycin and cefotetan and *E. coli* to ampicillin–sulbactam and quinolones and therefore these agents should not be routinely used empirically for complicated intraabdominal infections.[35,36]
4. If susceptible, antimicrobial treatment can be completed orally with amoxicillin–clavulanate, metronidazole with either ciprofloxacin or levofloxacin, or moxifloxacin.[37]
5. Four to seven days of antimicrobial treatment is sufficient for most intraabdominal infections with adequate source control.[39]

Intraabdominal infection presents in many different ways and with a wide spectrum of severity. The regimen employed and duration of treatment depends on the specific clinical circumstances (i.e., the nature of the underlying disease process, severity of illness, and risk of resistant pathogens).

Recommendations 6 For most intraabdominal infections, the antimicrobial regimen should be effective against both aerobic and anaerobic bacteria.[38,39] When initial antimicrobial therapy is inactive, morbidity and mortality rates are higher than when initially active therapy is used.[39] Although it is impossible to provide antimicrobial activity against every possible pathogen, agents with activity against enteric Gram-negative bacilli such as *E. coli* and *Klebsiella* spp., and anaerobes such as *B. fragilis* should be administered. If most of the organisms can be eliminated through drainage or antimicrobials, the synergistic effect may be removed, and the patient's defenses may be able to resolve the remaining infection.

Table 92-6 presents the recommended agents for treatment of community-acquired complicated intraabdominal infections from the Infectious Diseases Society of America and the Surgical Infection Society.[39] These recommendations were formulated using an

TABLE 92-5 Likely Intraabdominal Pathogens

Type of Infection	Aerobes	Anaerobes
Primary (Spontaneous) Bacterial Peritonitis		
Children	Group A *Streptococcus*, *E. coli*, pneumococci	—
Cirrhosis	*E. coli*, *Klebsiella*, pneumococci (many others)	—
Peritoneal dialysis	*Staphylococcus*, *Streptococcus*, *E. coli*, *Klebsiella*, *Pseudomonas*	—
Secondary Bacterial Peritonitis		
Gastroduodenal	*Streptococcus*, *E. coli*	—
Biliary tract	*E. coli*, *Klebsiella*, enterococci	*Clostridium* or *Bacteroides* (infrequent)
Small or large bowel	*E. coli*, *Klebsiella*, *Proteus*	*B. fragilis* and other *Bacteroides*, *Clostridium*
Appendicitis	*E. coli*, *Pseudomonas*	*Bacteroides*
Abscesses	*E. coli*, *Klebsiella*, *Streptococcus*, enterococci	*B. fragilis* and other *Bacteroides*, *Clostridium*, anaerobic cocci
Liver	*E. coli*, *Klebsiella*, *Streptococcus*, enterococci, *Staphylococcus*, amoeba	*Bacteroides* (infrequent)
Spleen	*Staphylococcus*, *Streptococcus*, *E. coli*, *Salmonella*	

TABLE 92-6 Recommended Agents for the Treatment of Community-Acquired Complicated Intraabdominal Infections in Adults

Agents Recommended for Mild-to-Moderate Infections	Agents Recommended for High Risk or High Severity Infections
Single Agent	
Cefoxitin[a] Ticarcillin–clavulanate	Piperacillin–tazobactam
Moxifloxacin[b] Ertapenem[c]	Imipenem–cilastatin,[c] Meropenem,[c] doripenem[c]
Combination Regimens	
Cefazolin,[a] cefuroxime,[a] ceftriaxone, cefotaxime each in combination with metronidazole	Cefepime or ceftazidime each in combination with metronidazole
Ciprofloxacin[b] or levofloxacin[b] each in combination with metronidazole	Ciprofloxacin[b] or levofloxacin[b] each in combination with metronidazole

[a]Empiric first- and second-generation cephalosporin use should be avoided unless local antibiograms show >80% to 90% susceptibility of *E. coli* to these agents.

[b]Use of quinolones may be associated with treatment failure due to increasing resistance of enteric pathogens including *E. coli*. Empiric quinolone use should be avoided unless local antibiograms show >80% to 90% susceptibility of *E. coli* to quinolones.

[c]Carbapenems should typically be reserved for settings where there is a high risk of resistance to other agents.

Adapted from Solomkin et al.[39]

evidence-based approach. Table 92-7 lists additional evidence-based recommendations for the treatment of complicated intraabdominal infections. Most community-acquired infections are of mild-to-moderate severity whereas healthcare-associated infections tend to be more severe, more difficult to treat, and more commonly due to resistant pathogens. Table 92-8 presents guidelines for treatment and alternative regimens for specific situations. These are general guidelines; there are many factors that cannot be incorporated into such a table including local resistance patterns to commonly used agents such as quinolones.

Most patients with severe intraabdominal infection, sepsis of intraabdominal source, or healthcare-associated infection should be placed on piperacillin–tazobactam, cefepime with metronidazole, or a carbapenem such as imipenem, doripenem, or meropenem. In

TABLE 92-7 Evidence-Based Recommendations for Treatment of Complicated Intraabdominal Infections

	Grade of Recommendation[a]
Elements of Appropriate Intervention	
An appropriate source control procedure to drain infected foci, control ongoing peritoneal contamination by diversion or resection, and restore anatomic and physiological function to the extent feasible is recommended for nearly all patients with intraabdominal infection	B-2
Community-Acquired Infections of Mild-to-Moderate Severity in Adults	
Antibiotics used for empiric treatment of community-acquired intraabdominal infections should be active against enteric Gram-negative aerobic and facultative bacilli and enteric Gram-positive streptococci	A-1
For patients with mild-to-moderate community-acquired infections, the use of ticarcillin–clavulanate, cefoxitin, ertapenem, moxifloxacin, or tigecycline as single-agent therapy or combinations of metronidazole with cefazolin, cefuroxime, ceftriaxone, cefotaxime, levofloxacin, or ciprofloxacin are preferable to regimens with substantial anti-pseudomonal activity (Table 92-6)	A-1
Empiric coverage of *Enterococcus* is not necessary in patients with mild-to-moderate severity community-acquired intraabdominal infection	A-1
The use of agents listed as appropriate for higher-severity community-acquired infection and healthcare-associated infection is not recommended for patients with mild-to-moderate community-acquired infection, because such regimens may carry a greater risk of toxicity and facilitate acquisition of more resistant organisms	B-2
High-Risk or High-Severity Community-Acquired Infections in Adults[b]	
The empiric use of antimicrobial regimens with broad-spectrum activity against Gram-negative organisms, including meropenem, imipenem–cilastatin, doripenem, piperacillin–tazobactam, ciprofloxacin or levofloxacin in combination with metronidazole, or ceftazidime or cefepime in combination with metronidazole, is recommended for patients with high-severity community-acquired intraabdominal infection	A-1
Aztreonam plus metronidazole is an alternative, but addition of an agent effective against Gram-positive cocci is recommended	B-3
Healthcare-Associated Infections in Adults	
Empiric antibiotic therapy for healthcare-associated intraabdominal infection should be driven by local microbiologic results	A-2
To achieve empiric coverage of likely pathogens, multidrug regimens that include agents with expanded spectra of activity against Gram-negative aerobic and facultative bacilli may be needed. These agents include meropenem, imipenem–cilastatin, doripenem, piperacillin–tazobactam, or ceftazidime or cefepime in combination with metronidazole. Aminoglycosides or colistin may be required	B-3
Antimicrobial Agents Not Recommended	
Ampicillin–sulbactam is not recommended for use because of high rates of resistance to this agent among community-acquired *E. coli*	B-2
Quinolone-resistant *E. coli* have become common in some communities, and quinolones should not be used unless hospital surveys indicate 90% susceptibility of *E. coli* to quinolones	A-2
Cefotetan and clindamycin are not recommended for use because of increasing prevalence of resistance to these agents among the *Bacteroides fragilis* group	B-2
Because of the availability of less toxic agents demonstrated to be at least equally effective, aminoglycosides are not recommended for routine use in adults with community-acquired intraabdominal infection	B-2
Oral Completion Therapy	
For adults recovering from intraabdominal infection, completion of the antimicrobial course with oral forms of moxifloxacin, ciprofloxacin plus metronidazole, levofloxacin plus metronidazole, an oral cephalosporin with metronidazole, or amoxicillin–clavulanic acid is acceptable in patients able to tolerate an oral diet and in patients in whom susceptibility studies do not demonstrate resistance	B-2
Duration of Therapy	
Antimicrobial therapy of established infection should be limited to 4–7 days, unless it is difficult to achieve adequate source control. Longer durations of therapy have not been associated with improved outcome	B-3
For acute stomach and proximal jejunum perforations, in the absence of acid-reducing therapy or malignancy and when source control is achieved within 24 hours, prophylactic antiinfective therapy directed at aerobic Gram-positive cocci for 24 hours is adequate	B-2
Bowel injuries attributable to penetrating, blunt, or iatrogenic trauma that are repaired within 12 hours and any other intraoperative contamination of the operative field by enteric contents should be treated with antibiotics for ≤24 hours	A-1
Acute appendicitis without evidence of perforation, abscess, or local peritonitis requires only prophylactic administration of narrow spectrum regimens active against aerobic and facultative and obligate anaerobes; treatment should be discontinued within 24 hours	A-1
The administration of prophylactic antibiotics to patients with severe necrotizing pancreatitis prior to the diagnosis of infection is not recommended	A-1

(continued)

TABLE 92-7 Evidence-Based Recommendations for Treatment of Complicated Intraabdominal Infections (*Continued*)

	Grade of Recommendation[a]
Anaerobic Coverage	
Coverage for obligate anaerobic bacilli should be provided for distal small bowel, appendiceal, and colon-derived infection and for more proximal GI perforations in the presence of obstruction or paralytic ileus	A-1
Antifungal Therapy	
Antifungal therapy for patients with severe community-acquired or healthcare-associated infection is recommended if *Candida* is grown from intraabdominal cultures	B-2
Anti-MRSA Therapy	
Empiric antimicrobial coverage directed against MRSA should be provided to patients with healthcare-associated intraabdominal infection who are known to be colonized with the organism or who are at risk of having an infection due to this organism because of prior treatment failure and significant antibiotic exposure	B-2
Vancomycin is recommended for treatment of suspected or proven intraabdominal infection due to MRSA	A-3
Antienterococcal Therapy	
Antimicrobial therapy for enterococci should be given when enterococci are recovered from patients with healthcare-associated infection	B-III
Empiric antienterococcal therapy is recommended for patients with high-risk community-acquired infections and healthcare-associated intraabdominal infections, particularly those with postoperative infection, those who have previously received cephalosporins or other antimicrobial agents selecting for *Enterococcus* species, immunocompromised patients, and those with valvular heart disease or prosthetic intravascular materials	B-II
Initial empiric antienterococcal therapy should be directed against *Enterococcus faecalis*. Antibiotics that can potentially be used against this organism, on the basis of susceptibility testing of the individual isolate, include ampicillin, piperacillin/tazobactam, and vancomycin	B-III
Empiric therapy directed against vancomycin-resistant *Enterococcus faecium* is not recommended unless the patient is at very high risk for an infection due to this organism, such as a liver transplant recipient with an intraabdominal infection originating in the hepatobiliary tree or a patient known to be colonized with vancomycin-resistant *E. faecium*	B-III

[a]Strength of recommendations: A, B, C = good, moderate, and poor evidence to support recommendation, respectively. Quality of evidence: 1 = Evidence from ≥1 properly randomized, controlled trial. 2 = Evidence from ≥1 well-designed clinical trial without randomization, from cohort or case-controlled analytic studies; from multiple time series, or from dramatic results from uncontrolled experiments. 3 = Evidence from opinions of respected authorities, based on clinical experience, descriptive studies, or reports of expert communities.

[b]Criteria for high risk or high severity community-acquired infection: APACHE II score ≥15, delay in initial intervention (>24 hours), advanced age, comorbidity and degree of organ dysfunction, low albumin level, poor nutritional status, degree of peritoneal involvement or diffuse peritonitis, inability to achieve adequate debridement or control of drainage, and presence of malignancy.

From Solomkin et al.[39]

patients with IgE-mediated allergic reactions to β-lactams (hives/urticaria, bronchospasm, angioedema, or anaphylaxis), combination therapy with aztreonam–vancomycin and metronidazole may be used. The benefits of systemic empiric antifungal (with fluconazole) have not been established for intraabdominal infection and should not be used routinely.

Aminoglycoside-based treatment regimens are no longer routinely recommended due to their narrow therapeutic index (nephrotoxicity, ototoxicity) relative to the recommended agents such as β-lactams. Aminoglycosides are typically reserved for use in patients with IgE-mediated allergic reactions to alternative agents or as dictated by the susceptibility of the presumed or proven infecting pathogen(s).[32,39]

The initial dosage for aminoglycosides should be determined based on the patient's weight and renal function. Traditionally, gentamicin and tobramycin were administered multiple times daily with specific peak (6 to 10 mcg/mL [mg/L; 13 to 21 μmol/L]) and trough (<1 to 2 mcg/mL [mg/L; <2 to 4 μmol/L]) concentration targets. Because aminoglycosides have concentration-dependent killing and have a relatively long postantibiotic effect for aerobic Gram-negative bacilli, extended-interval dosing of aminoglycosides is possible. For most patients and indications, extended-interval aminoglycoside dosing (i.e., 5 to 7 mg/kg once daily for tobramycin or gentamicin) has replaced traditional dosing given equivalent efficacy and decreased nephrotoxicity.[40–42]

Antimicrobial resistance continues to rise worldwide while at the same time few new agents, particularly for multidrug-resistant Gram-negative pathogens, are being brought to market.[43] These problematic multidrug-resistant bacteria include enteric pathogens producing extended-spectrum β-lactamases (ESBL) which have been increasingly isolated from intraabdominal cultures.[35] For patients with ESBL-producing pathogens, carbapenems (such as imipenem–cilastatin, meropenem, or ertapenem) are typically the drugs of choice. With increased use of carbapenems, pathogens continue to evolve with the development of β-lactamases that hydrolyze carbapenems (e.g., *Klebsiella pneumoniae* carbapenemase [KPC]), multidrug-resistant *Pseudomonas* spp., and carbapenem-resistant *Acinetobacter* spp. Especially in patients with healthcare-associated intraabdominal infections, these multidrug-resistant pathogens have caused clinicians to use more toxic and potentially less effective agents such as the polymyxins/colistin, tigecycline, and aminoglycosides. This increasing resistance highlights the need, from an individual patient and public health standpoint, to ensure that antimicrobials are selected appropriately, at the right dose, and for the right duration.

Clinical **Controversy...**

Due to recent reports of increased risk of mortality associated with tigecycline, some clinicians recommend the drug be reserved for the treatment of infections due to multidrug-resistant pathogens that are sensitive to tigecycline.[44,45] Others cite the lack of clinical trial evidence in seriously ill patients or those with multidrug-resistant pathogens as a reason for hesitation in using tigecycline in these patient populations.[46]

TABLE 92-8 Guidelines for Empiric Antimicrobial Agents for Intraabdominal Infections[39,49]

	Primary Agents	Alternatives
Primary (Spontaneous) Bacterial Peritonitis		
Cirrhosis	Ceftriaxone, cefotaxime	1. Piperacillin–tazobactam, carbapenems 2. Aztreonam combined with an agent active against *Streptococcus* spp. (e.g., vancomycin) or quinolones with significant *Streptococcus* spp. activity (levofloxacin, moxifloxacin)
Peritoneal dialysis	Initial empiric regimens should be active against both Gram-positive (including *S. aureus*) and Gram-negative pathogens: Gram-positive agent (first-generation cephalosporin or vancomycin) plus a Gram-negative agent (third-generation cephalosporin or aminoglycoside)	1. Cefepime or carbapenems may be used alone 2. Aztreonam or an aminoglycoside may be used in place of ceftazidime or cefepime as long as combined with a Gram-positive agent 3. Quinolones may be used in place of Gram-negative agents if local susceptibilities allow
	1. *Staphylococcus* spp.:oxacillin/nafcillin or first-generation cephalosporin	1. Vancomycin should be used if concern for methicillin-resistant *Staphylococcus* spp. 2. Add rifampin for 5–7 days with vancomycin for methicillin-resistant *Staphylococcus aureus*
	2. *Streptococcus* or *Enterococcus*: ampicillin	1. An aminoglycoside may be added for *Enterococcus* spp. 2. Linezolid, daptomycin, or quinupristin/dalfopristin should be used to treat vancomycin-resistant *Enterococcus* spp. not susceptible to ampicillin
	3. Aerobic Gram-negative bacilli: ceftazidime or cefepime	1. The regimen should be based on in vitro sensitivity tests
	4. *Pseudomonas aeruginosa*: two agents with differing mechanisms of action, such as an oral quinolone plus ceftazidime, cefepime, tobramycin, or piperacillin	
Secondary Bacterial Peritonitis		
Perforated peptic ulcer	First-generation cephalosporins	1. Ceftriaxone, cefotaxime, or antianaerobic cephalosporins[a]
Other	Third- or fourth-generation cephalosporin with metronidazole, piperacillin–tazobactam or ticarcillin–clavulanate, carbapenem	1. Ciprofloxacin[b] or levofloxacin[b] each with metronidazole or *moxifloxacin*[b] alone 2. Aztreonam with vancomycin and metronidazole 3. Antianaerobic cephalosporins[a]
Abscess		
General	Third- or fourth-generation cephalosporin with metronidazole, piperacillin–tazobactam, or ticarcillin–clavulanate	1. Imipenem–cilastatin, meropenem, doripenem, or ertapenem 2. Ciprofloxacin[b] or levofloxacin[b] each with metronidazole or moxifloxacin alone
Liver	As above	Use metronidazole if amoebic liver abscess is suspected
Spleen	Ceftriaxone or cefotaxime	Moxifloxacin[b] or levofloxacin[b]
Other Intraabdominal Infections		
Appendicitis	Same management as for community-acquired complicated intraabdominal infections as listed in Table 92-6[39]	
Community-acquired acute cholecystitis	Ceftriaxone or cefotaxime	Severe infection, piperacillin/tazobactam, antipseudomonal carbapenem, aztreonam with metronidazole
Cholangitis	Ceftriaxone or cefotaxime each with or without metronidazole	Vancomycin with aztreonam with or without metronidazole
Acute contamination from abdominal trauma	Antianaerobic cephalosporins[a] or metronidazole with either ceftriaxone or cefotaxime	1. Piperacillin/tazobactam or a carbapenem 2. Ciprofloxacin[b] or levofloxacin[b] each with metronidazole or moxifloxacin alone

[a]Cefoxitin or ceftizoxime; these agents should be avoided empirically unless local antibiograms show >80% to 90% susceptibility of *E. coli* to these agents.
[b]Use of quinolones may be associated with treatment failure due to increasing resistance of enteric pathogens including *E. coli*. Empiric quinolone use should be avoided unless local antibiograms show >80% to 90% susceptibility of *E. coli* to quinolones.

With intraabdominal contamination from the upper GI tract (perforation of a peptic ulcer or biliary tract disease), *B. fragilis* is an uncommon pathogen, and other agents therefore may be substituted for metronidazole. Alternatives include ampicillin, penicillin, or first-generation cephalosporins.

Coverage for enterococci for mild-to-moderate community-acquired intraabdominal infections is not recommended.[39] The failure of host defenses may be a critical factor in the pathogenicity of enterococci. In patients with severe community-acquired intraabdominal infection or patients with healthcare-associated infection, it is recommended to include coverage of enterococcus in the initial regimen.[39] Ampicillin remains the drug of choice for this indication because it is most active in vitro against enterococcus. Vancomycin is active against most enterococci; however, rates of vancomycin-resistant enterococci are increasing, particularly in select patient populations (e.g., liver transplantation, immunocompromised patients).[47] Agents including linezolid or daptomycin are commonly utilized for vancomycin-resistant enterococcus infections. Table 92-7 lists additional evidence-based recommendations for *Enterococcus* spp. coverage.

Clinical Controversy. . .

Enterococci are often isolated from intraabdominal infections, and many antimicrobials are ineffective against enterococci (such as cephalosporins and quinolones). Regimens without activity against enterococci (e.g., cefepime with metronidazole) are generally effective in treating intraabdominal infections; however, there are numerous reports of enterococcal superinfection in immunocompromised patients, particularly after broad-spectrum antimicrobial use. The Infectious Disease Society of America and Surgical Infection Society guidelines[39] recommend empiric coverage of Enterococcus for severe or high-risk community-acquired infection and healthcare-associated infection. The guidelines indicate, "Empiric coverage of Enterococcus is not necessary in patients with (mild-moderate) community-acquired intraabdominal infection."

7 Intraperitoneal administration of antibiotics is preferred over IV therapy in the treatment of peritonitis that occurs in patients undergoing CAPD.[48] The International Society of Peritoneal Dialysis guidelines for the diagnosis and pharmacotherapy of peritoneal dialysis-associated infections provide dosing recommendations for intermittent and continuous therapy based on the modality of dialysis (CAPD or automated peritoneal dialysis) and the extent of the patient's residual renal function.[49] Third-generation cephalosporins, such as ceftriaxone, remain the treatments of choice for primary peritonitis associated with cirrhosis.[50]

Antimicrobial agents effective against both Gram-positive (including *Staphylococcus aureus*) and Gram-negative organisms should be used for initial intraperitoneal empiric therapy for peritonitis in peritoneal dialysis patients. The most important factors to take into consideration for initial antimicrobial selection are the dialysis center's and the patient's history of infecting organisms and their sensitivities. For empiric intraperitoneal therapy, cefazolin (loading dose [LD] 500 mg/L; maintenance dose [MD] 125 mg/L) or vancomycin (LD 1,000 mg/L; MD 25 mg/L) in cases of high prevalence of methicillin-resistant *Staphylococcus aureus* (MRSA) or β-lactam allergy may be utilized for Gram-positive coverage. One of these Gram-positive agents should be combined with a Gram-negative agent such as ceftazidime (LD 500 mg/L; MD 125 mg/L) or cefepime (LD 500 mg/L; MD 125 mg/L) or an aminoglycoside (gentamicin or tobramycin LD 8 mg/L; MD 4 mg/L). Another option is monotherapy with cefepime or imipenem–cilastatin (LD 250 mg/L; MD 50 mg/L). Antimicrobial doses should empirically be increased by 25% in patients with residual renal function (more than 100 mL/day urine output).[49] Antimicrobial therapy should be continued for at least 1 week after the dialysate fluid is clear and for a total of at least 14 days. The reader is referred to these guidelines for additional information.[49]

After acute bacterial contamination, such as with abdominal trauma where GI contents spill into the peritoneum, antibiotics should be administered. If the patient is seen soon after injury (within 2 hours) and surgical measures are instituted promptly, antianaerobic cephalosporins (such as cefoxitin), a third-generation cephalosporin (such as ceftriaxone or cefuroxime) with metronidazole, or piperacillin/tazobactam are effective in preventing most infectious complications. Antimicrobials should be administered as soon as possible after injury.

For appendicitis, the antimicrobial regimen used should depend on the appearance of the appendix at the time of operation, which may be normal, inflamed, gangrenous, or perforated. Because the condition of the appendix is unknown preoperatively, it is advisable to begin antimicrobial agents before the appendectomy is performed. Reasonable regimens would be antianaerobic cephalosporins or, if the patient is seriously ill, piperacillin–tazobactam or a carbapenem (such as imipenem–cilastatin or meropenem). If, at operation, the appendix is normal or inflamed, postoperative antimicrobials are not required. If the appendix is gangrenous or perforated, a treatment course of 4 to 7 days with the agents listed in Table 92-6 is appropriate.

8 The necessary duration of treatment for intraabdominal infections is not clearly defined. Acute intraabdominal contamination, such as after a traumatic injury, may be treated with a very short course (24 hours).[51] For established infections (i.e., peritonitis or intraabdominal abscess), an antimicrobial course limited to 4 to 7 days is justified. This allows eradication of bacteria remaining in the peritoneum after a surgical procedure that may enter the peritoneum through healing suture lines. Under certain conditions, therapy for longer than 7 days would be justified (e.g., if the patient remains febrile or is in poor general condition, or when a focus of infection in the abdomen is still present). For some abscesses, such as pyogenic liver abscess, antimicrobials may be required for a month or longer.

Intraperitoneal irrigation of antimicrobial agents for treatment of intraabdominal infection has been studied, often with conflicting results.[52] Intraoperative antimicrobial irrigation does not improve patient outcomes in comparison with copious intraoperative irrigation with normal saline. Possibly the most important aspect of peritoneal irrigation is the dilutional effect on bacteria and adjuvants that promotes infection (intestinal contents and hemoglobin). Most systemically administered antimicrobials easily cross the peritoneal membrane so that peritoneal fluid concentrations are similar to serum. Confined areas, such as an abscess, can be expected to attain much lower antimicrobial concentrations.

EVALUATION OF THERAPEUTIC OUTCOMES

Whichever antimicrobial regimen is chosen, the patient should be reassessed continually to determine the success or failure of therapies. The clinician should recognize that there are many reasons for poor patient outcome with intraabdominal infection; improper antimicrobial administration is only one. The patient may be immunocompromised, which decreases the likelihood of successful outcome with any regimen. It is impossible for antimicrobials to compensate for a nonfunctioning immune system. There may be surgical reasons for poor patient outcome. Failure to identify all intraabdominal foci of infection or leaks from a GI anastomosis may cause continued intraabdominal infection. Even when intraabdominal infection is controlled, accompanying organ system failure, most often renal or respiratory, may lead to patient demise. Finally, antimicrobial resistance may relate to treatment failure as isolates from intraabdominal infections are increasingly drug resistant.[53]

The outcome from intraabdominal infection is not determined solely by what transpires in the abdomen. Unsatisfactory outcomes in patients with intraabdominal infections may result from complications that arise in other organ systems. Infectious complications commonly associated with mortality after intraabdominal infection are urinary tract infections and pneumonia.[54] A high APACHE (Acute Physiology and Chronic Health Evaluation) II score, low serum albumin concentration, and high New York Heart Association cardiac function status were significantly and independently associated with increased mortality from intraabdominal infection.[55]

9 Once antimicrobials are initiated and the other important therapies described earlier are used, most patients should show

improvement within 2 to 3 days. Usually, temperature will return to near normal, vital signs should stabilize, and the patient should not appear in distress, with the exception of recognized discomfort and pain from incisions, drains, and the nasogastric tube. At 24 to 48 hours, aerobic bacterial culture results should return. If a suspected pathogen is not sensitive to the antimicrobial agents being given, the regimen should be changed if the patient has not shown sufficient improvement. If the isolated pathogen is susceptible to one antimicrobial and the patient is progressing well, antimicrobial therapy may often be deescalated.

With anaerobic culturing techniques and the slow growth of these organisms, anaerobes are often not identified until 4 to 7 days after culture, and sensitivity information is difficult to obtain. For this reason, there are usually few data with which to alter the antianaerobic component of the antimicrobial regimen. A report indicating that anaerobes were not isolated should not be the sole justification for discontinuing antianaerobic drugs because anaerobic bacteria that were present in the infectious process may not have been transported properly to the microbiology laboratory, or other problems may have led to cell death in vitro.

Clinical **Controversy. . .**

Although some investigators suggest that routine culturing of patients with community-acquired intraabdominal infections contributes little to their management,[56] other investigators suggest that antimicrobial therapy should be based on susceptibility of the bacteria collected from the operative site because this correlates with clinical outcome.[57]

Reasons for antimicrobial failure may not always be apparent. Even when antimicrobial susceptibility tests indicate that an organism is susceptible in vitro to the antimicrobial agent, therapeutic failures may occur. Possibly there is poor penetration of the antimicrobial agent into the focus of infection, or bacterial resistance may develop after initiation of antimicrobial therapy. In addition, it is possible that an antimicrobial regimen may encourage the development of infection by organisms not susceptible to the regimen being used. Superinfection in patients being treated for intraabdominal infection can be caused by *Candida*; however, enterococci or opportunistic Gram-negative bacilli such as *Pseudomonas* or *Serratia* may be involved.

Treatment regimens for intraabdominal infection can be judged as successful if the patient recovers from the infection without recurrent peritonitis or intraabdominal abscess and without the need for additional antimicrobials. A regimen can be considered unsuccessful if a significant adverse drug reaction occurs, reoperation or percutaneous drainage is necessary, or patient improvement is delayed beyond 1 or 2 weeks. The costs of treatment can be significantly reduced if parenteral antimicrobials can be switched to oral agents for completion of therapy.[58]

ABBREVIATIONS

APACHE	acute physiology and chronic health evaluation
CAPD	chronic ambulatory peritoneal dialysis
CT	computed tomography
CVP	central venous pressure
ESBL	extended-spectrum β-lactamase
IL	interleukin
INF	interferon
KPC	*Klebsiella pneumoniae* carbapenemase
LD	loading dose
MAP	mean arterial pressure
MD	maintenance dose
MRSA	methicillin-resistant *Staphylococcus aureus*
TNF	tumor necrosis factor

REFERENCES

1. Ordonez CA, Puyana JC. Management of peritonitis in the critically ill patient. Surg Clin North Am 2006;86:1323–1349.
2. Marshall JC. Intra-abdominal infections. Microbes Infect 2004;6:1015–1025.
3. Marshall JC, Innes M. Intensive care unit management of intraabdominal infection. Crit Care Med 2003;31:2228–2237.
4. Levison ME, Bush LM. Peritonitis and intraperitoneal abscesses. In: Mandell GL, Bennett JE, Dolin R, eds. Mandell, Douglas, and Bennett's Principles and Practice of Infectious Diseases, 7th ed. Philadelphia: Saunders, 2010:1011–1034 [chapter 71].
5. Sartelli M, Viale P, Koike K et al. WSES consensus conference: Guidelines for the first-line management of intra-abdominal infections. World J Emerg Surg 2011;6:1–29.
6. Wiest R, Krag A, Gerbes A. Spontaneous bacterial peritonitis: Recent guidelines and beyond. Gut 2012;61:297–310.
7. Mowat C, Stanley AJ. Spontaneous bacterial peritonitis—Diagnosis, treatment, and prevention. Aliment Pharmacol Ther 2001;15:1851–1859.
8. Mujais S. Microbiology and outcomes of peritonitis in North America. Kidney Int 2006;70:555–562.
9. Buie VC, Owings MF, DeFrances CJ, Golosinskiy A. National Hospital Discharge Survey: 2006 summary. National Center for Health Statistics. Vital Health Stat 2010;13(168):22–53.
10. Toloza EM, Wilson SE. Cholecystitis and cholangitis. In: Fry DE, ed. Surgical Infections. Boston: Little, Brown, 1995:254–263.
11. Brook I. Microbiology and management of abdominal infections. Dig Dis Sci 2008;53:2585–2591.
12. Jernberg C, Lofmark S, Edlund C, Jansson JK. Long-term impacts of antibiotic exposure on the human intestinal microbiota. Microbiology 2010;156:3216–3223.
13. Riche FC, Cholley BP, Panis YH, et al. Inflammatory cytokine response in patients with septic shock secondary to generalized peritonitis. Crit Care Med 2000;28:433–437.
14. Solomkin JS, Mazuski J. Intra-abdominal sepsis: Newer interventional and antimicrobial therapies. Infect Dis Clin North Am 2009;23:593–608.
15. Malangoni MA. Contributions to the management of intraabdominal infection. Am J Surg 2005;190:255–259.
16. Herzog T, Chromic, Uhl W. Treatment of complicated intra-abdominal infections in the era of multidrug resistant bacteria. Eur J Med Res 2010;15:525–532.
17. Thompson AE, Marshall JC, Opal SM. Intraabdominal infections in infants and children: Descriptions and definitions. Pediatr Crit Care Med 2005;6:S30–S35.
18. Rice-Townsend SE, Lawrence Moss R, Rangel SJ. Peritonitis. In: Long SS, Pickering LK, Prober CG, eds. Principles and Practice of Pediatric Infectious Diseases, 4th ed. Elsevier Churchill Livingstone; 2012.
19. Guillet-Caruba C, Cheikhelard A, Guillet M, et al. Bacteriologic epidemiology and empirical treatment of pediatric complicated appendicitis. Diagn Microbiol Infect Dis 2011;69:376–381.

20. Lee SL, Islam S, Cassidy LD, et al. Antibiotics and appendicitis in the pediatric population: An American Pediatric Surgical Association Outcomes and Clinical Trials Committee systematic review. J Pediatr Surg 2010;45: 2181–2185.
21. Johnson DH, Cuhna BA. Infections in cirrhosis. Infect Dis Clin North Am 2001;15:363–371.
22. Brook I, Frazier EH. Aerobic and anaerobic microbiology of retroperitoneal abscesses. Clin Infect Dis 1998;26:938–941.
23. Bennion RS, Baron EJ, Thompson JE, et al. The bacteriology of gangrenous and perforated appendicitis—Revisited. Ann Surg 1990;211:165–171.
24. Sawyer RG, Rosenlof LK, Adams RB, et al. Peritonitis into the 1990s: Changing pathogens and changing strategies in the critically ill. Am Surg 1992;58:82–87.
25. Montravers P, Lepape A, Dubreuil L, et al. Clinical and microbiological profiles of community-acquired and nosocomial infections: Results of the French prospective, observational EBIIA study. J Antimicrob Chemother 2009;63:785–794.
26. Onderdonk AB, Bartlett JG, Louie T, et al. Microbial synergy in experimental intraabdominal abscess. Infect Immun 1997;13:22–26.
27. Donskey CJ, Chowdhry TK, Hecker MT, et al. Effect of antibiotic therapy on the density of vancomycin-resistant enterococci in the stool of colonized patients. Ann Surg 2000;343:1925–1932.
28. Sitges-Serra A, Lopez MJ, Girvent M, et al. Postoperative enterococcal infection after treatment of complicated intraabdominal sepsis. Br J Surg 2002;89:361–367.
29. Jaffe TA, Nelson RC, Delong DM, Paulson EK. Practice patterns in percutaneous image-guided intraabdominal abscess drainage: Survey of academic and private practice centers. Radiology 2004;233:750–756.
30. Dellinger RP, Levy MM, Rhodes A, et al. Surviving Sepsis Campaign: International guidelines for management of severe sepsis and septic shock: 2012. Crit Care Med 2013; 41:580–637.
31. Rivers E, Nguyen B, Havstad S, et al. Early goal-directed therapy in the treatment of severe sepsis and septic shock. N Engl J Med 2001;345:1368–1377.
32. Wong PF, Gilliam AD, Kumar S, et al. Antibiotic regimens for secondary peritonitis of gastrointestinal origin in adults. Cochrane Database Syst Rev 2007;2:CD004539.
33. Hooker KD, DiPiro JT, Wynn JJ. Aminoglycoside combinations versus single β-lactams for penetrating abdominal trauma: A meta-analysis. J Trauma 1991;31: 1155–1160.
34. Solomkin JS, Dellinger EP, Christou NV, et al. Results of a multicenter trial comparing imipenem/cilastatin to tobramycin/clindamycin for intraabdominal infections. Ann Surg 1990;212:581–591.
35. Hoban DJ, Bouchillon SK, Hawser SP, Badal RE, Labombardi VJ, DiPersio J. Susceptibility of gram-negative pathogens isolated from patients with complicated intra-abdominal infections in the United States, 2007–2008: Results of the Study for Monitoring Antimicrobial Resistance Trends (SMART). Antimicrob Agents Chemother 2010;54:3031–3034.
36. Snydman DR, Jacobus NV, McDermott LA, et al. Lessons learned from the anaerobe survey: Historical perspective and review of the most recent data (2005–2007). Clin Infect Dis 2010;50(Suppl 1):S26–S33.
37. Hawser SP, Bouchillon SK, Hoban DJ, Badal RE. In vitro susceptibilities of aerobic and facultative anaerobic Gram-negative bacilli from patients with intra-abdominal infections worldwide from 2005–2007: Results from the SMART study. Int J Antimicrob Agents 2009;34: 585–588.
38. Gauzit R, Pean Y, Mistretta F, Lalaude O. Epidemiology, management, and prognosis of secondary non-postoperative peritonitis: A French prospective observational multicenter study. Surg Infect 2009;10:119–127.
39. Solomkin JS, Mazuski JE, Bradley JS, et al. Diagnosis and management of complicated intra-abdominal infection in adults and children: Guidelines by the Surgical Infection Society and the Infectious Diseases society of America. Clin Inf Dis 2010;50:133–164.
40. Nicolau DP, Freeman CD, Belliveau PP, Nightingale CH, Ross JW, Quintiliani R. Experience with a once-daily aminoglycoside program administered to 2184 adult patients. Antimicrob Agents Chemother 1995;39:650–655.
41. Rybak MJ, Abate BJ, Kang SL, Ruffing MJ, Lerner SA, Drusano GL. Prospective evaluation of the effect of an aminoglycoside dosing regimen on rates of observed nephrotoxicity and ototoxicity. Antimicrob Agents Chemother 1999;43:1549–1555.
42. Olsen KM, Rudis MA, Rebuck JA, Gelmont D, Mehdian R, Nelson C, Rupp ME. Effect of single daily dose vs. multiple daily dosing of tobramycin on alanine aminopeptidase and *N*-acetyl-β-D-glucosaminidase excretion. Crit Care Med 2004;32:1678–1682.
43. Boucher HW, Talbot GH, Bradley JS, et al. Bad bugs, no drugs: no ESKAPE! An update from the Infectious Diseases Society of America. Clin Infect Dis 2009;48: 1–12.
44. Mutnick AH, Biedenbach DJ, Jones RN. Geographic variations and trends in antimicrobial resistance among *Enterococcus faecalis* and *Enterococcus faecium* in the SENTRY Antimicrobial Surveillance Program (1997–2000). Diagn Microbiol Infect Dis 2003;46:63–68.
45. Prasad P, Sun J, Danner R, Natanson C. Excess deaths associated with tigecycline after approval based on non-inferiority trials. Clin Infect Dis 2012;54:1699–1709.
46. US Food and Drug Administration. FDA Drug Safety Communication: Increased risk of death with Tygacil (tigecycline) compared to other antibiotics used to treat similar infections. US Food and Drug Administration. 1 September 2010. *http://www.fda.gov/Drugs/DrugSafety/ucm224370.htm.*
47. Powers JH. Asking the right questions: Morbidity, mortality, and measuring what's important in unbiased evaluations of antimicrobials. Clin Infect Dis 2012;54:1710–1713.
48. Wiggins KJ, Craig JC, Johnson DW, Strippoli GF. Treatment for peritoneal dialysis-associated peritonitis. Cochrane Database Syst Rev 2008;(1):CD005284.
49. Li PK, Szeto CC, Piraino B, et al. International Society for Peritoneal Dialysis Peritoneal dialysis-related infections recommendations: 2010 update. Perit Dial Int 2010;30: 393–423.
50. Runyon BA. Management of adult patients with ascites due to cirrhosis: An update. Hepatology 2009;49:2087–2107.
51. Bozorgzadeh A, Pizzi WF, Barie PS, et al. The duration of antibiotic administration in predicting abdominal trauma. Am J Surg 1999;172:125–135.
52. Schein M, Gecelter G, Freinkel W, et al. Peritoneal lavage in abdominal sepsis: A controlled clinical study. Arch Surg 1990;125:1132–1135.
53. Baquero F, Hsueh P, Paterson DL, et al. In vitro susceptibilities of aerobic and facultatively anaerobic gram-negative bacilli isolated from patients with intra-abdominal infections worldwide: 2005 results from study for monitoring

antimicrobial resistance trends. Surg Infect 2009;10: 99–104.

54. Merlino JI, Yowler CJ, Malangoni MA. Nosocomial infections adversely affect the outcomes of patients with serious intraabdominal infections. Surg Infect (Larchmt) 2004;5:21–27.

55. Christou NV, Barie PS, Dellinger EP, et al. Surgical infection society intraabdominal infection study. Arch Surg 1993;128:193–199.

56. Dougherty SH. Antimicrobial culture and susceptibility testing has little value for routine management of secondary bacterial peritonitis. Clin Infect Dis 1997;25(Suppl 2): S258–S261.

57. Montravers P, Gauzit R, Muller C, Marmuse JP, Fichelle A, Desmonts JM. Emergence of antibiotic-resistant bacteria in cases of peritonitis after intraabdominal surgery affects the efficacy of empirical antimicrobial therapy. Clin Infect Dis 1996;23(3):486–494.

58. Paladino JA, Gilliland-Johnson KK, Adelman MH, Coohn SM. Pharmacoeconomics of ciprofloxacin plus metronidazole vs. piperacillin–tazobactam for complicated intra-abdominal infections. Surg Infect 2008;9:325.

93

Parasitic Diseases

JV Anandan

KEY CONCEPTS

1. The drug of choice for giardiasis in a first-term pregnant patient is paromomycin 25 to 35 mg/kg/day in divided doses for 5 to 10 days.
2. Stool samples for amebiasis may not be ideal for differential diagnosis of species and the specific antigen test for *definitive* diagnosis of *Entamoeba histolytica* is the ELISA (*Entamoeba histolytica* II Kit) test.
3. Asymptomatic cyst passers and patients with mild intestinal amebiasis should receive one of the following luminal agents: paromomycin 25 to 35 mg/kg/day three times daily for 7 days, iodoquinol 650 mg three times daily for 20 days, or diloxanide furoate 500 mg three times daily for 10 days.
4. With the unavailability of pyrantel pamoate, either mebendazole (Vermox) or albendazole (Albenza) is the drug of choice for hookworm, ascariasis, enterobiasis, and trichuriasis.
5. Administration of corticosteroids or other immunosuppressive drugs to an infected individual with strongyloidiasis can result in hyperinfections and disseminated strongyloidiasis.
6. The most serious complication of cysticercosis is invasion of the CNS, which results in neurocysticercosis. Neurocysticercosis can cause obstructive hydrocephalus, strokes, and seizures; antihelminthic treatment for these conditions remains controversial.
7. When IV quinidine is not readily available, IV artesunate (available under an investigational new drug (IND) from the CDC at *www.cdc.gov/malaria/features/artesunate_now_available.htm*), a water-soluble artemisinin derivative, administered at 2.4 mg/kg/dose for 3 days at 0, 12, 24, 48, and 72 hours is the recommended drug if severe *Plasmodium falciparum* is suspected.
8. Because *falciparum* malaria is associated with serious complications, including pulmonary edema, hypoglycemia, jaundice, renal failure, confusion, delirium, seizures, coma, and death, careful monitoring of fluid status and hemodynamic parameters is mandatory. Either hemofiltration or hemodiafiltration is indicated in renal failure.
9. The two drugs that are available in the United States (obtained from CDC) to treat *Trypanosoma cruzi* infections are nifurtimox (Lampit) and benznidazole (Rochagan). Benznidazole is used as the drug of choice in South America.
10. Permethrin (1% and 5%) for pediculosis and scabies, respectively, is the preferred agent and remains the safest agent, especially in infants and children. Spinosad crème rinse 0.9% and benzyl alcohol 5% are new agents for head lice.

Parasitic diseases continue to receive increasing attention from clinicians in the United States because of the high frequency of travel, deployment of personnel for humanitarian and military missions (e.g., Peace Corps volunteers), inflow of immigrants from a wider geographic distribution, and the presence of immunosuppressed populations (e.g., acquired immunodeficiency syndrome [AIDS] and transplant patients). Migrant farm workers who work and live in substandard hygienic conditions, the large and growing Central and South American immigrant population, and other inadequately screened immigrants from Asia represent significant sources of parasitic infections in the United States.[1–9] Clinicians need to have a heightened awareness of parasitic diseases and how to treat them. Clinical signs and symptoms, together with the patient's travel history, should be used with other diagnostic aids in the identification of parasitic diseases. Parasitic infections caused by pathogenic protozoa or helminths affect more than 3 billion people worldwide and impose tremendous health and economic burdens on developing countries.[9]

This chapter discusses the major parasitic diseases, including protozoan diseases (giardiasis, amebiasis, malaria, and Chagas disease), helminthic infections (ascariasis, enterobiasis, hookworm, strongyloidiasis, and cestodiasis), and ectoparasitic infestations (head and body lice). Emphasis is placed on diseases seen more frequently in the United States. World distribution of parasites depends on the presence of suitable hosts, habitats, and environmental conditions.[9] A human parasite that does not use an intermediate host is likely to be found in any inhabited region of the world as long as the environmental conditions are suitable. *Ascaris* (roundworm) and *Trichuris* (whipworm) require carelessness of habits for transfer and require time outside the human body, where they are exposed to heat and dryness, to reach the infective stage. The distribution of the hookworm is more limited because the free-living forms are unprotected by resistant shells or cysts. African trypanosomiasis never occurs outside the range of the tsetse fly; malaria normally never occurs beyond the range of the infective *Anopheles* mosquito; and schistosomiasis never occurs in the absence of a specific water snail. The prevalence of clonorchiasis (Chinese liver fluke) is an example of the impact of both environmental and geographic factors. Clonorchiasis requires the simultaneous presence of not only humans, specific snail species, and certain fish, but also unsanitary conditions that make the eggs accessible to the snails, an association of the snail and fish, and the established local habit of eating raw fish. The ability of some parasites to infect hosts other than humans may perpetuate an infection even when human habits preclude the possibility of more than occasional access to the human body. In North America, the broad tapeworm (*Diphyllobothrium latum*) would perish if it were not that dogs and other carnivores, such as the brown bear, serve as reservoir hosts.

HOST–PARASITE RELATIONSHIP

Symbiosis is the association of two species for the purpose of obtaining food for either one or the other. *Parasitism* is a symbiotic relationship in which one species, the host, is injured through the activities of the other. Through evolution, parasites have made specific morphologic adaptations. Adaptation to the host has taken a number of forms: loss of locomotor organelles in the protozoan *Sporozoa*; partial and complete lack of digestive systems in the trematodes and cestodes, respectively; elaboration of proteolytic enzymes to penetrate the host intestinal mucosa by *Entamoeba histolytica*; the cercariae of the blood fluke that penetrate the skin of the host by elaborate enzymes; and, finally, the ability to infect an intermediate host to increase reproductive capacity, as seen among the cestodes and trematodes.[9]

Parasites normally inflict some degree of injury to the host, the extent of which depends on such factors as parasite load, nutritional status, and immunologic competence of the host. *Entamoeba coli* is considered commensal because it subsists on the bacterial flora of the gut and does not cause any harm to the host. Unlike *Entamoeba coli*, *Fasciolopsis buski*, the giant intestinal fluke, can produce severe local damage to the intestinal wall. *Ascaris*, the roundworm, can perforate the bowel wall, cause intestinal obstruction, and invade the appendix and bile duct. Malarial parasites destroy red blood cells by multiplying inside them. *D. latum*, or the broad fish tapeworm, removes vitamin B_{12} from the GI tract, resulting in megaloblastic anemia.[9]

PROTOZOAN DISEASES

Giardiasis

Epidemiology and Etiology

Giardia lamblia (also known as *Giardia intestinalis* or *Giardia duodenalis*), an enteric protozoan, is the most common intestinal parasite responsible for diarrheal syndromes throughout the world.[10–13] *Giardia* is the most frequently identified intestinal parasite in the United States, with a prevalence rate of 15% in some areas. *G. lamblia* is the first enteric pathogen seen in children in developing countries, with prevalence rates between 15% and 30%.[12]

There are two stages in the life cycle of *G. lamblia*: the trophozoite and the cyst. *G. lamblia*, which is found in the small intestine, gallbladder, and biliary drainage, is a pear-shaped trophozoite with four pairs of flagella. Two nuclei lie in the area of the sucking disk, giving the protozoan a characteristic face-like image.

The distribution of giardiasis is worldwide. Children seem to be affected more frequently than adults. Children in day care centers may infect parents and other family members.[12] In less developed countries, fecal contamination of the environment and lack of potable water, education, and housing continue to be risk factors for giardiasis among children.

Pathology

Giardiasis results from ingestion of *G. lamblia* cysts in fecally contaminated water or food. The protozoan excysts under the stimulus of low gastric pH to release the trophozoite.[12] Colonization and multiplication of the trophozoite lead to mucosal invasion, localized edema, and flattening of the villi, resulting in malabsorption states in the host.[10,12]

Lactose intolerance precipitated by giardiasis and iron deficiency can persist even after eradication of the protozoan. Achlorhydria, hypogammaglobulinemia, or deficiency in secretory immunoglobulin A (IgA) are predispositions for giardiasis.[10,12,14] Table 93-1 describes the clinical presentation of giardiasis.

TABLE 93-1 Clinical Presentation of Giardiasis

Acute onset
Diarrhea, cramp-like abdominal pain, bloating, and flatulence[10–12]
Malaise, anorexia, nausea, and belching[12]
Chronic
Diarrhea: foul-smelling, copious, light-colored, fatty stools; weight loss
Periods of diarrhea alternating with constipation
Steatorrhea, lactose intolerance, vitamin B_{12}, and fat-soluble vitamin deficiencies[10,12,14]

Diagnosis of giardiasis is made by examination of fresh stool or a preserved specimen during the acute diarrheal phase. Fresh stool specimens may show the trophozoites, whereas preserved specimens usually yield the cysts. Three stool specimens for ova and parasites (O&P) will yield up to 90% of the parasites.[10] Since detection of the trophozoites or cysts in fecal samples by enzyme-linked immunosorbent assay (ELISA) or immunofluorescence or identification of the *Giardia* antigen by counterimmunoelectrophoresis are readily available in most laboratories, and these tests are frequently utilized to identify *Gardia* before initiating therapy.[10,12,15]

TREATMENT

Desired Outcome

To reduce morbidity and to avoid complications in patients identified with prolonged diarrhea and malabsorption and who have a recent history of travel to an endemic area, rapid identification by the O&P examination or by the antigen detection test should be used to institute appropriate therapy.[10,12]

Pharmacologic Therapy

All symptomatic adults and children older than 8 years of age with giardiasis can be treated with metronidazole 250 mg three times daily for 5 to 10 days, or tinidazole 2 g once, or nitazoxanide 500 mg twice daily for 3 days.[16] The alternative drugs include furazolidone 100 mg four times daily or paromomycin 25 to 35 mg/kg/day in divided doses daily for 1 week.[10,12,16,17] ❶ Paromomycin 25 to 35 mg/kg/day in three doses for 5 to 10 days is a safe agent in pregnancy.[10,12,16] The pediatric dose for metronidazole is 15 mg/kg/day three times daily for 5 to 7 days.[16] The pediatric dose of tinidazole is 50 mg/kg (maximum 2 g) once while nitazoxanide (Alinia) suspension is dosed at 100 mg every 12 hours (1 to 3 years), 200 mg every 12 hours (4 to 11 years), and the adult dose is recommended for children older than 12 years; all are administered for 3 days.[12,16] Quinacrine, which was the drug of choice in giardiasis, has been discontinued by the manufacturer but is obtained in the United States from a specialized pharmacy (see Appendix 93-1). Albendazole 400 mg daily for 5 days has variable cure rates (55% to 95%). Tinidazole (50 mg/kg—single dose) and metronidazole regimen may be considered equivalent in children.[10,13,17]

Evaluation of Therapeutic Outcomes

Patients with symptomatic giardiasis, positive stool samples, or the detection of *Giardia* antigen by counterimmunoelectrophoresis or ELISA should be treated with metronidazole for 5 to 7 days. Metronidazole produces cure rates of between 80% and 90%.[10,17] Diarrhea will stop within a few days, although in some patients it may take 1 to 2 weeks. Cyst excretion will cease within days; however, intestinal dysfunction (manifested as increased transit time) and radiologic changes (irregular thickening of the folds in the upper small intestine) may take a few months to resolve.[10] Patients who fail initial therapy with metronidazole should preferably be treated with a drug from a different class. Nitazoxanide (500 mg twice daily for 3 days) is effective in patients who are not responding to metronidazole.[12] Pregnant patients can receive paromomycin 25 to 35 mg/kg/day in divided doses for 7 days. Metronidazole has been used in the second and third trimesters of pregnancy.[12] Giardiasis can be prevented by good personal hygiene and by caution in food and drink consumption.

Amebiasis

Epidemiology and Etiology

Because of its worldwide distribution and serious GI manifestations, amebiasis is one of the most important parasitic diseases of humans.[9,18–21] The major causative organism in amebiasis is *E. histolytica*, which inhabits the colon and must be differentiated from the *Entamoeba dispar* and a recently identified species, *Entamoeba moshkovskii* that are associated with an asymptomatic carrier state. *E. dispar* is considered nonpathogenic, while the status of *E. moshkovskii* remains to be defined.[19] Although *E. histolytica* and *E. dispar* are indistinguishable morphologically, monoclonal antibodies have been used to separate the two.[20,21] The *E. histolytica* II kit (TechLab, Blacksburg, VA) remains the most specific antigen test for *E. histolytica*.[19] Invasive amebiasis is almost exclusively the result of *E. histolytica* infection. Approximately 50 million cases of invasive disease result each year worldwide, leading to an excess of 100,000 deaths.[21] The incidence of amebiasis is estimated at approximately 1% in the general U.S. population.[21] The highest incidence is found in institutionalized mentally retarded patients, sexually active homosexuals, patients with AIDS, and new immigrants from endemic areas (e.g., Mexico, India, West and South Africa, and portions of Central and South America).[19,21]

Pathology

E. histolytica invades mucosal cells of colonic epithelium, producing necrotizing ulcers in the submucosa.[19–21] The trophozoite has a cytolethal effect on cells through a toxin. If the trophozoite gets into the portal circulation, it will be carried to the liver, where it produces abscess and periportal fibrosis.[19–24] Amebic ulcerations can affect the colon, perineum, and genitalia, and abscesses may occur in the lung and brain.[20–24]

Clinical Presentation

The most frequent clinical manifestations of the disease are GI (Table 93-2).

Amebic liver abscesses can spread to the lungs and pleura.[20,21] Pericardial infections, although rare, may be associated with extension of the amebic abscess from the left lobe of the liver. Erosion of liver abscesses also present as peritonitis.[19–22]

TABLE 93-2 Most Common Manifestations of Amebiasis

Intestinal disease
Vague abdominal discomfort, malaise to severe abdominal cramps, flatulence, bloody diarrhea (heme-positive in 100% of cases) with mucus[19–21]
Eosinophilia is usually absent, although moderate leukocytosis is not unusual[20,21]
Amebic liver abscess
High fever, rigors and profuse sweating, significant leukocytosis with left shift, elevated alkaline phosphatase, and liver tenderness on palpation[21,22,24]
Right-upper-quadrant pain, hepatomegaly, and liver tenderness, with referred pain to the left or right shoulder
Erosion of liver abscesses may also present as peritonitis[19–21]

Review of the patient's history and recent travel should be strongly emphasized. Intestinal amebiasis is diagnosed by demonstrating *E. histolytica* cysts or trophozoites (may contain ingested erythrocytes) in fresh stool or from a specimen obtained by sigmoidoscopy. ❷ Stool samples are insensitive and do not distinguish between *E. histolytica* and the nonpathogenic *E. dispar* or *E. moshkovskii*. Sensitive techniques are available to detect *E. histolytica* in stool (these are rapid tests within 2 hours) including ELISA, antigen detection (*E. histolytica* II kit), and polymerase chain reaction (PCR).[19–21,23] Endoscopy with scraping or biopsy may provide more definitive diagnosis where stool examinations do not provide adequate evidence.[19,21]

When amebic liver abscess is suspected from initial physical examination and history, confirmatory diagnostic procedures will include serology and liver scans (using isotopes by ultrasound or computed tomography) or magnetic resonance imaging.[20,21] Leukocytosis (>10,000/mm^3 [>10 × 10^9/L]) and an elevated alkaline phosphatase concentration (>75%) are common findings. In rare instances, needle aspiration of the hepatic abscess may be attempted using ultrasound guidance.[22,24]

TREATMENT

Desired Outcome

In amebiasis, the goals of therapy are initially to eradicate the parasite by use of specific amebicides and then to render supportive therapy.

Treatment Regimens

A number of different regimens have been suggested depending on the category of amebiasis: asymptomatic cyst passers, intestinal amebiasis, and amebic liver abscess.[16,19–22] Electrolyte replacement, antibiotic therapy, and nutritional support are essential adjunctive treatment modalities. Large hepatic abscess or amebic pericarditis may require needle aspiration, percutaneous catheter drainage, or, rarely, surgery before drug therapy.[20–22] Most regimens require a combination of drugs administered concurrently or sequentially.[19,21,24]

A careful history to exclude concurrent bacterial infection and other tissue complications of *E. histolytica* should be part of consideration when planning therapy for amebiasis.

Pharmacologic Therapy

Metronidazole (Flagyl), dehydroemetine, and chloroquine (Aralen) are tissue-acting agents, whereas iodoquinol (Yodoxin), diloxanide furoate (Furamide), and paromomycin (Humatin) are luminal amebicides. A systemic agent may be so well absorbed that only small amounts of the drug stay in the bowel, which might prove ineffective as a luminal agent.[20–23] A luminal-acting agent, on the other hand, may be too poorly absorbed to be effective in the tissue. In the asymptomatic cyst passer, it is necessary to eradicate the causative agent from the lumen to prevent intestinal amebiasis or the development of amebic liver abscess. Drug effectiveness may be monitored by stool examination, although the ELISA test should be used to verify eradication of *E. histolytica*.[19,21]

❸ Asymptomatic cyst passers and patients with mild intestinal amebiasis should receive one of the following luminal agents: paromomycin 25 to 35 mg/kg/day three times daily for 7 days, iodoquinol 650 mg three times daily for 20 days, or diloxanide furoate 500 mg three times daily for 10 days.[16] Diloxanide furoate is available only from Panorama Compounding Pharmacy (6744 Balboa Blvd., Van Nuys, CA 91406, (800) 247-9767; or Medical Center Pharmacy, New Haven, CT, (203) 688-6816).[16] The pediatric dose for paromomycin is the same as in adults, whereas the dose of iodoquinol is 30 to 40 mg/kg/day (maximum: 2 g) in three doses for 20 days, and the dose of diloxanide furoate is 20 mg/kg/day in three doses for 10 days.[16] Paromomycin is the preferred luminal agent in pregnant patients.[16,21]

Patients with severe intestinal disease or liver abscess should receive metronidazole 750 mg three times daily for 10 days, followed by a course of one of the luminal agents indicated earlier.[16,20–21] Tinidazole 2 g mg once daily for 5 days has been suggested for amebic liver abscess.[16] In the pediatric patient, the dose of oral metronidazole is 50 mg/kg/day in divided doses to be followed by a luminal agent.[16] Patients who are too ill to take oral metronidazole should receive the drug in equivalent doses by the IV route.[21]

Evaluation of Therapeutic Outcomes

Followup in patients with amebiasis should include repeat stool examination, serology, colonoscopy (for colitis), or computed tomography (CT) (for liver abscess) between days 5 and 7, at the end of the course of therapy, and a month after the end of therapy. Most patients with either intestinal amebiasis or colitis will respond in 3 to 5 days with amelioration of symptoms. Patients with liver abscesses may take from 7 to 10 days to respond; patients not responding during this period may require aspiration of abscesses or exploratory laparotomy. Serial liver scans have demonstrated healing of liver abscesses over 4 to 8 months after adequate therapy.[21]

Sanitation and Preventive Measures

Travelers and tourists visiting an epidemic area should avoid local tap water, ice, salads, and unpeeled fruits. Water can be disinfected by the use of iodine (tincture of iodine or commercial sources: Potable Aqua tablet [Wisconsin Pharmacal] or 5% to 10% acetic acid), but boiled water is probably the safest. An alternative or additional measure may be to carry a portable water purifier (such as MSR Mini Works Ex Water Filter. *www.backcountry.com*). Because food handlers in Asia and Latin America may be a source of amebiasis, travelers should avoid eating at food stalls and open markets.

HELMINTHIC DISEASES

Most intestinal helminthic infections may not be associated with clearly defined manifestation of disease, but they can cause significant pathology.[9,25–33] One factor that determines the pathogenicity of helminths is their population density. Light infections may be fairly well tolerated, whereas high populations of intestinal helminths can result in predictable disease presentations. In the United States, these infections are seen most frequently in recent immigrants from Southeast Asia, the Caribbean, Mexico, and Central America.[2,26,27] Other populations that have a high risk of infestation include institutionalized patients (both young and elderly), preschool children in daycare centers, residents of Indian reservations, and homosexual individuals. Certain conditions and drugs (fever, corticosteroids, and anesthesia) can cause atypical localization of worms.[34–38] Immunocompromised hosts can be overwhelmed by some helminthic infections, such as strongyloidiasis.[34]

Nematodes

Hookworm Disease

This is an infection of the small intestine caused by either *Ancylostoma duodenale* or *Necator americanus*. *N. americanus* is found in the southeastern United States, where the temperature and humidity provide the proper environment. *Ancylostoma* is seen rarely in the United States.[25]

TABLE 93-3 Clinical Presentations of Nematode Infections and Cysticercosis

Hookworm[27]
Mild epigastric pain and tenderness, headache, fatigue, anemia, hypoproteinemia, and cutaneous larva migrans
Ascariasis[26]
Abdominal pain, right-upper-quadrant pain, biliary coli, cholangitis, pancreatitis, and abdominal obstruction
Enterobiasis[25]
Mild abdominal discomfort and perianal itch
Strongyloidiasis[35,37]
GI: abdominal pain, bloating, nausea, constipation, and small bowel obstruction
Cardiopulmonary: cough, wheezing, pleural effusion, chest pain, and dyspnea
Dermatologic/hematologic: pruritic linear streaks of lower thighs and buttocks and eosinophilia
CNS: headache, altered mental status, and meningitis
Cysticercosis[42,45]
Abdominal pain, nausea, diarrhea, painless nodules on arms, chest, legs, and myalgia
Neurocysticercosis: headache, intracranial hypertension, hydrocephalus, and seizures

The life cycles of both species of hookworm are similar. The adult worms live in the small intestine attached to the mucosa. The females liberate eggs, which are eliminated in the feces and develop into larvae. Infective larvae enter the host in contaminated food or water or penetrate the skin, where a papular eruption with localized edema and erythema can result.

In the small intestine, where the adult worm lives attached to the mucosa, injury is usually caused by mechanical and lytic destruction of tissue. The loss of blood can lead to anemia and hypoproteinemia (Table 93-3).[26–29]

Stool should be examined for eggs and the rhabditiform larvae. Eosinophilia (30% to 60%) may be present in patients during early infection.

TREATMENT

4 Mebendazole (Vermox), an oral synthetic benzimidazole, is the agent of first choice in hookworm. It is also effective against ascariasis, enterobiasis, and trichuriasis.[16,25] The adult dose for treatment of hookworm infestation is 100 mg twice daily for 3 days. Pediatric patients older than 2 years of age should receive the same dose as adults.[16] Albendazole is an alternative agent.[16]

Ascariasis

Ascariasis is caused by the giant roundworm *Ascaris lumbricoides*. Female worms range from 20 to 35 cm in length. The worm is found worldwide but more commonly in areas where sanitation is poor. In the United States, endemic areas include southeastern parts of the Appalachian range and the Gulf Coast states.

During migration of the larvae through the lungs, patients can present with pneumonitis, fever, cough, eosinophilia, and pulmonary infiltrates.[9,25] Other symptoms of ascariasis include abdominal discomfort, abdominal obstruction, vomiting, and appendicitis (see Table 93-3).[9,25,31,32] Diagnosis is made by demonstrating the characteristic egg in the stool.

TREATMENT

In both adults and pediatric patients older than 2 years of age, the treatment for ascariasis is mebendazole (Vermox) 100 mg twice daily for 3 days.[16] An alternative drug for ascariasis is albendazole 400 mg as a single dose.[16]

Enterobiasis

Enterobiasis, or pinworm infection, is caused by *Enterobius vermicularis*. The pinworm is a small, thread-like, spindle-shaped worm about 1 cm in length. It is the most widely distributed helminthic infection in the world. There are estimated to be 42 million cases in the United States.[25] The majority of those infected are children.

The most common problem with enterobiasis is cutaneous irritation in the perianal region, made by the migrating females or the presence of eggs. However, there are reports of other complications, including appendicitis and intestinal perforation.[25,33] The intense pruritus and scratching can cause dermatitis and secondary bacterial infections. In children, the itching can cause loss of sleep and restlessness (see Table 93-3).

The most effective method of diagnosing pinworm infections is by the use of perianal swab using adhesive Scotch tape. The Scotch tape, which is applied to the perianal region with a tongue depressor, is examined microscopically for eggs.[9,25]

TREATMENT

The common agents for treatment include pyrantel pamoate, mebendazole, or albendazole (Albenza). The dose of pyrantel pamoate is 11 mg/kg (maximum 1 g) as a single dose that can be repeated in 2 weeks. The dose of mebendazole for adults and children older than 2 years of age is 100 mg as a single dose; this may be repeated in 2 weeks.[16,25] The dose of albendazole for adults and children older than 2 years of age is 400 mg, and should be repeated in 2 weeks.[25] Following treatment, all bedding and underclothes should be sterilized by steaming or washing in the hot water cycle of a regular washing machine; this will eradicate the eggs. Bathroom rugs and toilet accessories also should be cleaned in a similar way.

Strongyloidiasis

Strongyloidiasis is caused by *Strongyloides stercoralis*, which has a worldwide distribution and is predominantly prevalent in South America (Brazil and Columbia) and in Southeast Asia. Strongyloidiasis is primarily seen among institutionalized populations (mental homes, mentally disabled children's homes) and immunocompromised individuals (patients with human immunodeficiency virus [HIV], AIDS, and hematologic malignancies).[34–38] The worm is usually found in the upper intestine where the eggs are deposited and hatch to form the rhabditiform larvae. The rhabditiform larvae (male and female) migrate to the bowel where they may be excreted in the feces. If excreted in the feces, the larvae can evolve into either one of two forms after copulation: (a) free-living noninfectious rhabditiform larvae or (b) infectious filariform larvae. The filariform larvae can penetrate host skin, travel to the lungs via the bronchi and glottis, and make their way to the small intestine. At times, the filariform larvae may not pass out in the feces but instead migrate to the lungs and produce progeny, a process called autoinfection. This can result in hyperinfection (i.e., increased number of larvae in intestine, lungs, and other internal organs), especially in immunocompromised hosts.[34–36]

Symptoms with acute infection may appear with localized pruritic rash, but heavy infestations can produce eosinophilia (10% to 15%), diarrhea, abdominal pain, and intestinal obstruction (see Table 93-3).[37–39]

❺ Administration of corticosteroids or other immunosuppressive drugs to an infected individual can result in hyperinfections and disseminated strongyloidiasis.[34,36,38] Diagnosis of strongyloidiasis is made by identification of the rhabditiform larvae in stool, sputum, duodenal fluid, and cerebrospinal fluid, by small bowel biopsy specimens, or by antigen testing (ELISA assay).[37]

TREATMENT

The drug of choice for strongyloidiasis is oral ivermectin 200 mcg/kg/day for 2 days and the alternative is albendazole 400 mg twice daily for 7 days.[16,34,39,40] In a patient with hyperinfection or disseminated strongyloidiasis, immunosuppressive drugs should be discontinued and treatment initiated with ivermectin 200 mcg/kg/day until all symptoms are resolved (duration, 5 to 14 days). Patients should be tested periodically to ensure the elimination of the larvae.[39] Individuals from endemic areas, who are candidates for organ transplantation, must be screened for *S. stercoralis*.

Taenia solium: Cysticercosis and Neurocysticercosis

Tapeworm infection caused by *T. solium* is a result of ingestion of poorly cooked pork that contains the larvae or cysticercus.[41,42] Cysticercus, when released from the contaminated meat by host digestive juices, matures into the adult tapeworm and attaches to the host jejunum. Cysticercosis is a systemic disease caused by the larva of *T. solium* (oncosphere) and is usually acquired by ingestion of eggs in contaminated food or by autoinfection.[41–44] The larvae can penetrate the bowel and migrate through the bloodstream to infect different organs including the CNS (neurocysticercosis).[43,44,46] The larvae matures in about 8 weeks and remain as a semitransparent, oval-shaped, fluid-filled bladder in tissues. In the United States, the highest incidence of cysticercosis has been reported in immigrants from Mexico.[41–43] Cysticercosis in most tissues may not produce major symptoms and usually manifest as subcutaneous nodules, primarily in the arms, legs, and chest. However, penetration of the larval stage (cysticercus) into the CNS can produce hydrocephalus, intracranial hypertension, stroke, and seizure activity.[42] Epileptic seizures (50% to 80%) may be the presenting symptoms in patients with neurocysticercosis (see Table 93-3).[42,45] Clinical presentation, primarily seizure history, together with radiographic demonstration (CT and magnetic resonance imaging) of the cysticercus within the bladder or calcified cysts in the CNS, is diagnostic for neurocysticercosis.[41,42] Serologic diagnosis is made by the use of an enzyme-linked immunoelectrotransfer blot assay, which is considered highly sensitive and specific for cysticercosis.[41,42,45,46]

TREATMENT

Evaluation of Therapeutic Outcome

Morbidity and disease with intestinal nematodes are related to the intensity of infection or worm burden; subjects with transient exposure have less severe disease. The major adverse effects of intestinal nematodes are malnutrition, fatigue, and diminished work capacity. Treatment with antihelminthic agents results in complete eradication and significant change in the well-being of patients. Unlike other nematode infections, strongyloidiasis can perpetuate itself by autoinfection, and in the immunosuppressed host, the filariform larvae can invade various organs (e.g., lungs, CNS, and the like) to produce disseminated infection that can be fatal.[9,43–47]

❻ The most serious complication of cysticercosis is invasion of the CNS, which results in neurocysticercosis. Neurocysticercosis can cause obstructive hydrocephalus, strokes, and seizures; antihelminthic treatment for these conditions remains controversial.[42,45,46]

Clinical Controversy. . .

❻ Cysticercosis (excluding neurocysticercosis) is normally not treated. The management for neurocysticercosis remains controversial but may include surgery, anticonvulsants (neurocysticercosis-induced seizures), and antihelminthic therapy.[42,45,46] Antihelminthic therapy, if one decides this is an option, is albendazole 400 mg twice daily for 8 to 30 days and this regimen can be repeated if necessary.[16] However, the dose and duration of therapy with albendazole is not clearly defined.[42,46]

MALARIA

Malaria represents the most devastating disease in terms of human suffering and economics. It affects the largest number of people (between 300 and 500 million new infections are reported annually) in the world, and between 1 and 2 million deaths worldwide.[5,48–50] In the United States, deaths from malaria are preventable. The primary reasons for deaths are failure to take chemoprophylaxis, inappropriate chemoprophylaxis, delay in seeking medical care, and misdiagnosis.[5,7,50]

Epidemiology

The exact geographic distribution of the various species is not well documented; it is reported that *Plasmodium vivax* is more prevalent in India, Pakistan, Bangladesh, Sri Lanka, and Central America; whereas *P. falciparum* is predominant in Africa, Haiti, Dominican Republic, the Amazon region of South America, and New Guinea. Most of the infections with *Plasmodium ovale* occur in Africa, and the distribution of *Plasmodium malariae* is considered worldwide.[5,49,60]

In the United States, most cases of malaria are reported in immigrants from endemic areas and in American travelers. Blood transfusion also has been cited as a cause of malarial infection.[48,51]

Etiology

Malaria is transmitted by the bite of an infected *Anopheles* mosquito that introduces the sporozoites (tissue parasites) of the plasmodia (*P. falciparum*, *P. vivax*, *P. malariae*, and *P. ovale*) into the bloodstream. The asexual reproduction stage develops in humans, whereas the sexual stage occurs in the mosquito.[9,48,49] The sporozoites invade parenchymal hepatocytes, multiply in stages referred to as *exoerythrocytic stages*, and become hepatic vegetative forms or schizonts. Schizonts rupture to release daughter cells, or merozoites, that then infect erythrocytes.

P. falciparum and *P. malariae* remain in the primary exoerythrocytic stage in the liver for about 4 weeks before invading erythrocytes, whereas *P. vivax* and *P. ovale* can exist in the liver in the latent exoerythrocytic form for extended periods, and, therefore, infected subjects can experience relapses. The merozoites that invade the erythrocytes develop sequentially into ring forms, trophozoites, schizonts, and finally, merozoites, which can invade other erythrocytes or can develop into gametocytes, which undergo the sexual stage in the *Anopheles* vector. Because erythrocytic forms never reinvade the liver without developing into sporozoites in the vector, malaria infections from transfusion never result in the exoerythrocytic, or "liver," form.[9,49] *P. falciparum* can result in high levels of parasitemia because of its ability to invade erythrocytes of all ages, unlike *P. vivax* and *P. ovale*, which only invade young cells.[48,49]

TABLE 93-4 Clinical Presentation of Malaria

Initial presentation
Nonspecific fever, chills, rigors, diaphoresis, malaise, vomiting[48,49,52]
Orthostatic hypotension
Electrolyte abnormalities

Erythrocytic phase
Prodrome: headache, anorexia, malaise, fatigue, and myalgia
Nonspecific complaints such as abdominal pain, diarrhea, chest pain, and arthralgia
Paroxysm: high fever, chills, and rigor[9,49,52,59]
Cold phase: severe pallor and cyanosis of the lips[9,49,52]
Hot phase: fever between 40.5°C (104.9°F) and 41°C (105.8°F)
Sweating phase:
- Follows hot phase by 2–6 hours
- Fever resolves
- Marked fatigue and drowsiness, warm, dry skin, tachycardia, cough, severe headache, nausea, vomiting, abdominal pain, diarrhea, and delirium
- Lactic acidosis and hypoglycemia (with falciparum malaria)[48,49,52,59]

Anemia
Splenomegaly

***P. falciparum* infections**
Hypoglycemia, acute renal failure, pulmonary edema, severe anemia, thrombocytopenia, high-output heart failure, cerebral congestion, seizures and coma, and adult respiratory syndrome[49,52,60]

Pathology

The erythrocytic phase causes extensive hemolysis, which results in anemia and splenomegaly. The most serious complications usually are associated with *P. falciparum* infections.[48–50,52–60] Infants and children younger than 5 years of age and nonimmune pregnant women are at high risk for severe complications from falciparum malaria.[52–56] The complications associated with falciparum malaria are primarily a result of the high parasitemia and the ability of the parasites to sequester in capillaries and postcapillary vessels of organs such as the brain and the kidney. It has been postulated that tissue hypoxia from anemia, together with *P. falciparum*-parasitized red blood cell adherence to endothelial cells in capillaries, contribute to extensive vascular disease and severe metabolic effects.[52,53] *P. malariae* is implicated in immune-mediated glomerulonephritis and nephrotic syndrome (Table 93-4).[49,52]

To ensure a positive diagnosis, blood smears should be obtained every 12 to 24 hours for three consecutive days.[9,49,52] The presence of parasites in the blood 3 to 5 days after initiation of therapy suggests drug resistance. Recent advances for detecting malaria parasite have included DNA or RNA probes by PCR and rapid dipstick tests (ParaSight F, Becton-Dickinson, Cockeysville, MD) and OptiMAL.[48,49,52] The dipstick is reported to have a sensitivity of 88% and a specificity of 97%; however, microscopy is still considered the optimal test.

TREATMENT

Desired Outcome

The primary goal in the management of malaria is the rapid diagnosis of the *Plasmodia* spp. by blood smears (repeated every 12 hours for 3 days) so as to initiate timely antimalarial therapy to eradicate the infection within 48 to 72 hours and to avoid complications such as hypoglycemia, pulmonary edema, and renal failure that are responsible for increased mortality in malaria.[49]

Pharmacologic Therapy

In adults (including pregnant women), the chemoprophylaxis for all species of *Plasmodium* is chloroquine phosphate 300 mg (base) once weekly beginning 1 to 2 weeks prior to departure and continued for 4 weeks after leaving an endemic area.[16,48,49,52,61–63] The pediatric dose of chloroquine phosphate is 5 mg (base) per kilogram of body weight (maximum 300 mg). When departing an area endemic for *P. vivax* or *P. ovale*, primaquine phosphate 30 mg (base) daily for 14 days beginning the last 2 weeks of chloroquine prophylaxis should be added to the regimen. The pediatric dose of primaquine is 0.6 mg (base) per kilogram of body weight per day for 14 days. The pediatric doses of chloroquine can be calculated based on body weight, and the tablets can be pulverized and placed in gelatin capsules. Parents can be instructed to suspend the dose in food, simple syrup, chocolate milk, or in a drink.[61]

In areas where chloroquine-resistant *P. falciparum* (CRPF) strains exist, travelers should receive mefloquine (Lariam) for prophylaxis. The adult dose of mefloquine is 250 mg once weekly beginning 1 week prior to departure and continuing for the full period of exposure, followed by 250 mg for 4 weeks after last exposure.[16,48,49] The pediatric dose of mefloquine for prophylaxis is based on body weight.[16]

Body Weight (kg)	Dose
5 to 10	One-eighth tablet/week
11 to 20	One-quarter tablet/week
21 to 30	One-half tablet/week
31 to 45	Three-quarters tablet/week
>45	One tablet/week

For travelers who are at immediate risk for drug-resistant *falciparum* malaria, a loading dose of mefloquine may be considered (except for travel to Thailand, Myanmar, Vietnam, Laos, and Cambodia, where atovaquone–proguanil combination, one tablet daily 2 days prior to departure and through the stay and 1 week after leaving area, may be an alternative).[49] Mefloquine is administered at 250 mg daily for 3 days before travel, followed by 250 mg once weekly while in the endemic area and continued for 4 weeks after last exposure.[48,49] All patients receiving mefloquine should receive the FDA Medication Guide, and the drug should be avoided in patients with a history of cardiac conduction problems.[48] Patients may experience neuropsychiatric reactions (seizures, psychosis, anxiety, sleep disturbances, insomnia, and dizziness) from mefloquine and may need to be monitored closely.[16,62,63]

An alternative regimen for prophylaxis in chloroquine-resistant areas for those who cannot tolerate mefloquine or Malarone, is to take oral doxycycline 100 mg daily starting 1 to 2 days prior to departure, during the exposure period, and continuing for 4 weeks after leaving the endemic area.[16] Children older than 8 years of age should receive 2 mg/kg/day (up to 100 mg) of doxycycline. Doxycycline is contraindicated in children younger than 8 years of age, in pregnant women, and during breastfeeding.[16,49,63,65]

In an uncomplicated attack of malaria (for all plasmodia except CRPF), the recommended regimen is chloroquine 600 mg (base) initially, followed by 300 mg (base) 6 hours later, and then 300 mg (base) daily for 2 days. In severe illness or when oral therapy is not tolerated or parenteral quinine is not available, quinidine gluconate 10 mg/kg as a loading dose (maximum 600 mg) in 250 mL normal saline should be administered slowly over 1 to 2 hours, followed by continuous infusion of 0.02 mg/kg/minute until oral therapy can be started.[16,48,49] In patients who have received either quinine or mefloquine, the loading dose of quinidine should be omitted. Oral quinine (650 mg every 8 hours) together with doxycycline 100 mg twice daily should follow the IV dose of quinidine to complete a total of 7 days of therapy.[16,48,60] The pediatric dose of IV quinidine gluconate is the same as the dose for adults.[16] The pediatric dose of quinine is 30 mg/kg/day in three divided doses for 7 days. Children younger than age 8 years and pregnant women should get clindamycin 20 mg/kg/day in divided doses for 7 days instead of doxycycline.[16,49,60]

7 When IV quinidine is not readily available, IV artesunate (available under an IND from the CDC at *www.cdc.gov/malaria/features/artesunate_now_available.htm*), a water-soluble artemisinin derivative, administered at 2.4 mg/kg/dose for 3 days at 0, 12, 24, 48, and 72 hours is the recommended drug if severe *P. falciparum* is suspected.[16,58]

In *P. falciparum* (chloroquine-resistant) infections, a dose of 750 mg mefloquine followed by 500 mg 12 hours later is recommended. The pediatric dose of mefloquine is 15 mg/kg (<45 kg body weight) followed by 10 mg/kg 8 to 12 hours later.[16] IV quinidine gluconate (or IV artesunate) followed by oral quinine plus doxycycline to complete a total of 7 days of therapy should follow in a severe illness, as already indicated.[16,49] An alternative oral treatment for CRPF infection in adults, especially in those with a history of seizures, conduction problems, or psychiatric disorders to mefloquine, is the combination of atovaquone 250 mg and proguanil 100 mg (Malarone) (four tablets daily for 3 days).[16,48,49] An alternative to Malarone is the combination product of artemether 20 mg and lumefantrine 120 mg (Coartem) recently approved by the FDA in the United States (for regimen, see *http://www.cdc.gov/malaria/pdf/treatmenttable.pdf*). The IV quinidine regimen requires close monitoring of the electrocardiogram and other vital signs (e.g., hypotension, QT interval prolongation, and hypoglycemia).[16,49,55,60]

8 Because *falciparum* malaria is associated with serious complications, including pulmonary edema, hypoglycemia, jaundice, renal failure, confusion, delirium, seizures, coma, and death, careful monitoring of fluid status and hemodynamic parameters is mandatory.[48,49,55,60] Either hemofiltration or hemodiafiltration is indicated in renal failure.

Malarial infection does not produce immunity in patients, and active research has been initiated to develop a malaria vaccine.[66–68] A vaccine that blocks the entry of sporozoites into the liver cells will prevent malaria at this stage. However, immunity to sporozoites does not protect the host against parasites in the erythrocytic cycle. Infective sporozoites of *P. falciparum* are covered by a polypeptide, circumsporozoite protein. Isolation and identification of the gene encoding for this circumsporozoite protein have led to the development of a monoclonal antibody by recombinant DNA technology; *P. falciparum* sporozoite vaccine is now under investigation.[68]

Evaluation of Therapeutic Outcomes

When advising potential travelers on prophylaxis for malaria, be aware of the incidence of CRPF malaria and the countries where this is prevalent.[16,62,63] Detailed recommendations for prevention of malaria may be obtained by checking the website *www.cdc.gov/travel/* or *www2.cdc.gov/mmwr/*[63,69] or calling the U.S. Centers for Disease Control and Prevention (CDC) (see Appendix 93-1). In view of the increasing incidence of *P. falciparum* resistance to antimalarials, newer drugs are under active study and include the water-soluble artesunate and the oil-soluble artemether and combinations with other agents.[16,49,63,64,70–75]

Acute *P. falciparum* malaria resistant to chloroquine should be treated with IV quinidine or artesunate.[16,58] Patients receiving IV quinidine should have a central venous catheter to follow fluid status, and the electrocardiogram should be monitored closely. Hypoglycemia that is associated with *P. falciparum* should be checked and corrected with dextrose infusions.[48,49,55] Quinidine infusion should be slowed temporarily or stopped if electrocardiogram shows a QT interval of greater than 0.6 seconds, an increase in the QRS complex to greater than 50%, or hypotension unresponsive to fluid challenge results. The suggested quinidine levels should be maintained at 3 to 7 mg/L (9 to 22 μmol/L).[49] Blood smears should be checked every 12 hours until parasitemia is less than 1%. Resolution of fever should take place between 36 and 48 hours after initiation of the IV quinidine therapy and the blood should be clear of parasites in 5 days.[48,49,52] If parenteral therapy is required for more than 48 hours, the dose of quinidine should be lowered by half.[16]

Travelers to endemic areas for malaria should be advised to remain in well-screened areas, to wear clothes that cover most of the body, and to sleep in mosquito nets.[7,49,71] It is prudent to carry the insect repellent DEET (*N,N*-diethyl-metatol) or Picaridin (Cutter Advanced) insect spray for use in mosquito-infested areas. Readers are urged to check publications from the CDC for the list of countries where CRPF exist.[16,69]

Clinical **Controversy...**

Because there remains public concern with mefloquine chemoprophylaxis, primarily about its neuropsychiatric effects and cardiac conduction problems,[16,62] an alternative regimen for chemoprophylaxis may be the combination of atovaquone and proguanil (Malarone): one tablet daily beginning 1 to 2 days prior to travel and continuing for the duration of stay and 1 week after leaving the area.[16,62] Daily primaquine 30 mg (base) also has been suggested for prophylaxis for both *P. vivax* and *P. falciparum* malaria.[16] However, these alternative agents compared to mefloquine, remain less than ideal choice for high CRPF malaria regions.[62]

AMERICAN TRYPANOSOMIASIS

Etiology

Two distinct forms of the genus *Trypanosoma* occur in humans. One is associated with African trypanosomiasis (sleeping sickness) and the other with American trypanosomiasis (Chagas disease).[76–79] *Trypanosoma brucei gambiense*, *T. brucei*, and *T. brucei rhodesiense* are the causative organisms for the African trypanosomiasis. *T. brucei rhodesiense* causes the acute disease and is the more virulent of the three species. African trypanosomiasis is transmitted by various species of tsetse fly belonging to the genus *Glossina*. Further discussion of this subject will focus on American trypanosomiasis.

Trypanosoma cruzi is the agent that causes American trypanosomiasis. American trypanosomiasis is transmitted by a number of species of a reduviid bug (*Triatoma infestans*, *Rhodnius prolixus*) that live in wall cracks of houses in rural areas of North, Central, and South America. The reduviid bug is infected by sucking blood from animals (e.g., opossums, dogs, and cats) or humans infected with circulating trypomastigotes (Table 93-5).

In chronic trypanosomiasis, patients present with cardiomyopathy and heart failure. Electrocardiograms are usually abnormal, demonstrating extrasystoles, first-degree heart block, right bundle-branch block, and other serious conduction disturbances.[77–79] Degeneration of the autonomic ganglia in the smooth muscle of the esophagus and colon leads to uncoordinated peristalsis. The end result has been reported to be "megasyndromes" of affected organs.[78,79] Penetration of the CNS results in meningoencephalitis, strokes, seizures, and focal paralysis.[78–80]

A history to verify the possible exposure to *T. cruzi* should be an important initial diagnostic workup. Recovery of *T. cruzi* is definitive, but this is not always possible, especially in chronic disease.

TABLE 93-5 Clinical Presentation of South American Trypanosomiasis

Acute
Unilateral orbital edema ("Romana's sign")[78,79]
Granuloma or "chagoma"
Fever, hepatosplenomegaly, and lymphadenopathy
Chronic
Cardiac: cardiomyopathy and heart failure
ECG: first-degree heart block, right bundle-branch block, and arrhythmias[76–78]
GI: enlargement of esophagus and colon ("mega" syndrome)[76,78]
CNS: meningoencephalitis, strokes, seizures, and focal paralysis[78–80]

Positive serologic tests using the indirect immunofluorescent antibody test and ELISA (Chagas' EIA, Abbott Laboratories, Abbott Park, IL) may be diagnostic for the disease. The only serologic test available in the United States is Chagas' Kit (Hemagen Diagnostics, Inc., Columbia, MD).[78] A PCR test has also been used for diagnosis of *T. cruzi*[76,81] Specimens may be sent to the CDC for testing. All candidates from an endemic area for Chagas disease who are candidates for transplantation should be tested for *T. cruzi*.[82]

TREATMENT

Desired Outcome

The primary goal of drug therapy in trypanosomiasis is to reduce the duration and severity of the illness and to decrease mortality.

Pharmacologic Therapy

❾ The drugs that have been used to treat *T. cruzi* infections include nifurtimox (Lampit, Bayer 2502) and benznidazole (Rochagan).[16,78,79,83] Both oral nifurtimox and benznidazole are available from the CDC. Oral benznidazole is the drug of choice for *T. cruzi* in South America.[16] Neither of the agents are optimal therapy and there is ongoing search for newer agents.[76,78] The adult oral dose of nifurtimox is 8 to 10 mg/kg/day in divided doses for 30 to 120 days. The pediatric dose (1 to 10 years of age) is 15 to 20 mg/kg/day in four divided doses and children (11 to 16 years) should receive 12.5 to 15 mg/kg/day in four divided doses for 30 to 120 days.[16] Symptomatic treatment for heart failure includes digitalis and diuretics; the GI complications, however, may require surgical revisions and reconstruction.[78,79]

Evaluation of Therapeutic Outcomes

American trypanosomiasis (Chagas disease), which is endemic in all Latin American countries, can be transmitted congenitally, by blood transfusion, and by organ transplantation.[78,79] Treatment with nifurtimox of the acute phase (i.e., fever, malaise, edema of face, generalized lymphadenopathy, and hepatosplenomegaly) produces between 30% and 70% cure rates.[78] Treatment of chronic infection with nifurtimox is not recommended. It is essential to identify *T. cruzi*-infected patients by serology and to monitor the cardiovascular status of these patients by electrocardiogram periodically. The congestive failure of cardiomyopathic Chagas disease is treated the same way as cardiomyopathies from other causes.[76,78]

ECTOPARASITES

A parasite that lives on the outside of the body of the host is called an *ectoparasite*. Millions of people become infested with pediculosis yearly in the United States.[84] Pediculosis usually is associated with poor personal hygiene, and infections are passed from person to person through social and sexual contact. The three types of human lice belong to two genera: *Pediculus*, including the head and body lice, and *Phthirus*, with only one species, the crab louse.[9,84,85] The human louse is detectable to the human naked eye and measures approximately 2 to 3 mm in length.

Lice

The two species that belong to this group include *Pediculus humanus capitis* (head louse) and *Pediculus humanus corporis* (body louse). Female lice deposit eggs on the hair. The eggs (or nits) remain firmly attached to the hair, and in about 10 days, the lice hatch to form nymphs, which mature in 2 weeks. Using both their piercing mouthparts and a pumping device, the larva and adults feed on the blood of the host. The body louse and head louse are essentially identical, although they live on different parts of the body. Unlike the head louse, which lives on the hair, the body louse is more frequently found on clothing of the infected host.

Pubic or crab lice are found on the hairs around the genitals, although they can occur in other areas of the body (e.g., eyelashes, beards, and axillae). Patients usually complain of severe pruritus from papular lesions produced by the bite of the louse. Hypersensitivity to foreign material injected by the lice can produce macular swellings and occasionally can lead to secondary bacterial infections.[84]

TREATMENT

The goal of therapy is to eradicate the causative organisms and provide symptomatic relief to patients. The agent of choice for all three infections (body, head, and crab lice) is 1% permethrin (Nix).[84–88] Permethrin is a derivative of the flowers of the plant *Chrysanthemum cinerariifolium.* The term *pyrethrin* is usually applied to several esters of chrysanthemic acid and pyrethric acid. Permethrin has both pediculicidal and ovicidal activity against *P. humanus* var *capitis.* The cure rate is reported to be in the range of 85% to 95%.[84] Individuals who have a history of ragweed or chrysanthemum allergy should use this compound with caution. The side effects reported with permethrin products include itching, burning, stinging, and tingling. Permethrin 1% is applied to the scalp after the hair has been dried following a shampooing. The scalp should be saturated with permethrin liquid, and a towel should be wrapped around the scalp to allow the application to stay on for 10 minutes. The hair then should be rinsed thoroughly. A cream rinse of permethrin 1% (Nix-Creme Rinse) is also available. To ensure complete eradication, especially of newly hatched lice, it may be necessary to repeat the application. Recently, the FDA approved benzyl alcohol 5% (Ulesfia; Sciele Pharma Inc., Atlanta, GA) as an alternative therapy for head lice.[86]

There is increasing lice resistance to permethrin 1%.[85,88,89] Alternative preparations for lice are 0.5% malathion (Ovide), Spinosad 0.9% crème rinse (which is equally effective as permethrin[89]), and benzyl alcohol 5% (Ulesfia).[16,86,89] To ensure complete eradication of lice infestation, the malathion application should be left on the scalp for about 90 minutes.[87] For the relief of pruritus, a soothing lotion of calamine liniment or lotion with 0.1% menthol may be used. Other members of the family or sexual partners also should be treated. All bedding and clothes should be sterilized by boiling or washing in the hot water cycle of the washing machine to avoid reinfections. Seams of clothes should be examined to verify that all organisms are eradicated. An ocular lubricant (e.g., Lacri-Lube S.O.P.) applied twice daily may be used to remove crab louse infection of the eyelids.

Scabies

Scabies is caused by the itch mite *Sarcoptes scabiei*, which affects both humans and animals. Mange in domestic animals is caused by the same organism. Infection usually affects the interdigital and popliteal folds, axillary folds, the umbilicus, and the scrotum.[90–92]

Patients will complain of severe itching and an inability to sleep and may have excoriations in the interdigital web spaces, wrists, elbows, buttocks, groin, and scalp. Excoriations may lead to secondary bacterial infections. The diagnosis is made by looking for burrows formed by the mite and taking skin scrapings, which will demonstrate the mite on a wet mount.

TREATMENT

Because these infections cause a great deal of discomfort and distress to patients and families, the goals of therapy are to eradicate the infestations rapidly, to institute symptomatic treatment, and to provide counseling and reassurance. The treatment of choice is permethrin 5% (Elimite) cream.[16,90–92] To initiate the treatment, the skin should be scrubbed thoroughly in a warm soapy bath using a soft brush to remove all scabs. The lotion is then applied to the whole body, avoiding the face, mucous membranes, and eyes. The application should be left on for 8 to 14 hours before bathing. A single application eradicates 97% of scabies in subjects.[90] All close contacts should be checked and treated appropriately.

Other agents used to treat scabies include topical crotamiton 10% (Eurax) and oral ivermectin (Stromectol) 200 mcg/kg as a single dose, which may be repeated in 2 weeks.[16,92] Crotamiton and oral ivermectin may be used in patients who have hypersensitivity to permethrin preparations. Topical corticosteroids and antihistamines may be used to decrease pruritus.

10 Permethrin (1% and 5%) for pediculosis and scabies, respectively, is the preferred agent and remains the safest agent, especially in infants and children.[84,92] One application of permethrin is consistently effective in eradicating more than 90% of all infections. However, pruritus may persist for 2 to 4 weeks because of the remnants of mite parts in the skin. Ivermectin is an alternative therapy for scabies. Spinosad 0.9% and benzyl alcohol 5% are new agents approved for head lice.[86,89]

ABBREVIATIONS

AIDS	acquired immunodeficiency syndrome
ELISA	enzyme-linked immunosorbent assay
PCR	polymerase chain reaction

REFERENCES

1. Dawson-Hahn EE, Greenberg SLM, Domachowske JB, Olson BG. Eosinophilia and seroprevalence of Schistosomiasis and Strongyloidiasis in newly arrived pediatric refugees: An examination of Center for Disease Control and Prevention screening guidelines. J Pediat 2010;156:1016–1018.
2. Patel S, Sethi A. Imported tropical diseases. Dermatol Therap 2009;22:538–549.
3. Simmons CP, Farrar JJ, Van Vinh Chau N, Wills B. Dengue. N Engl J Med 2012;366:1423–1432.
4. Munoz P, Valerio M, Puga D, Bouza E. Parasitic infections in solid organ transplant recipients. Infect Dis Clin North Am 2010;24:461–495.

5. Mali S, Kachur SP, Arguin PM. Malaria Surveillance—United States, 2010. MMWR 2012;61(2):1–17.
6. Chen LH, Wilson ME. The role of the traveler in emerging infections and magnitude of travel. Med Clin North Am 2008;92:1409–1432.
7. Whitman TJ, Coyne PE, Magill AJ, et al. An outbreak of *Plasmodium falciparum* malaria in U.S. Marines deployed in Liberia. Am J Trop Med Hyg 2010;83: 258–265.
8. Taylor SM, Molyneux ME, Simel DL, Meshnick SR, Juliano JJ. Does this patient have malaria? JAMA 2010;304: 2048–2056.
9. John DT, Petri WA Jr. Markell and Voge's Medical Parasitology, 9th ed. Philadelphia, PA: WB Saunders, 2006.
10. Hill DR, Nash TE. Intestinal flagellate and ciliate infections: *Giardia lamblia*. In: Guerrant RL, Walker DH, Weller PF, eds. Tropical Infectious Diseases. Principles, Pathogens & Practice, 3rd ed. New York: Saunders/Elsevier, 2011: 623–630.
11. Tejman-Yarden N, Eckmann L. New approaches to the treatment of Giardiasis. Curr Opin Infect Dis 2011;24: 451–456.
12. Hill DR, Nash TE. *Giardia lamblia*. In: Mandell GL, Bennett JE, Dolin R, eds. Principles and Practice of Infectious Diseases, 7th ed. New York: Elsevier/Churchill Livingstone, 2010:3527–3534.
13. Busatti HG, Santos JFG, Gomes MA. The old and new therapeutic approaches to the treatment of giardiasis: Where are we? Biol Targets & Therapy 2009;3:273–287.
14. Fuglestad AJ, Lehmann A, Kroupina MG, et al. Iron deficiency in international adoptees from Eastern Europe. J Pediatr 2008;153:272–277.
15. Youn S, Kabir M, Haque R, Petri Je WA. Evaluation of a screening test for detection of Giardia and Cryptosporidium parasites. J Clin Microbiol 2009;47:451–452.
16. Abramowicz M, ed. Drugs for Parasitic Infections. The Medical Letter on Drugs and Therapeutics, 2nd ed. New Rochelle, NY: The Medical Letter, Inc., 2010:1–81.
17. Escobedo AA, Almirall P, Alfonso M, et al. Treatment of intestinal protozoan infections in children. Arch Dis Child 2009;94:478–482.
18. Stark D, Van Hal SJ, Matthews G, Harkness J, Marriott D. Invasive amebiasis in men who have sex with men, Australia. Emerg Infect Dis 2008;14:1141–1143.
19. Peterson KM, Singh U, Petri WA Jr. Enteric amebiasis. In: Guerrant RL, Walker DH, Weller PF, eds. Tropical Infectious Diseases. Principles, Pathogens & Practice, 3rd ed. New York: Saunders/Elsevier, 2011:614–622.
20. Pritt BS, Clark CG. Amebiasis. Mayo Clin Proc 2008;83:1154–1160.
21. Petri WA Jr, Haque R. *Entamoeba* species, including amebiasis. In: Mandell GL, Bennett JA, Dolin R, eds. Principles and Practice of Infectious Diseases, 7th ed. New York: Elsevier/Churchill Livingstone, 2010: 3411–3425.
22. Zhu MM, Lu H, Wang TR, Zheng Q, Ran ZH. Concurrent amoebic and *Klebsiella pneumoniae* liver abscess in an immunocompetent patient: An unusual case report and review of the literature. J Digest Dis 2010;11:249–253.
23. Solaymani-Mohammadi S, Petri WA Jr. Intestinal invasion by *Entamoeba histolytica.* Subcell Biochem 2008;47: 221–232.
24. Rao S, Solaymani-Mohammadi S, Petri WA Jr, Parker SK. Hepatic amebiasis: A reminder of the complications. Curr Opin Pediatr 2009;21:145–149.
25. Maguire JH. Intestinal nematodes (Roundworms). In: Mandell GL, Bennett JE, Dolin R, eds. Principles and Practice of Infectious Diseases, 7th ed. New York: Elsevier/Churchill-Livingstone; 2010;3577–3586.
26. Mascarini-Serra L. Prevention of soil-transmitted helminth infection. J Glob Infect Dis 2011;3:175–182.
27. Hotez PJ. Hookworm and poverty. Ann NY Acad Sci 2008;1136:38–44.
28. Pasricha S-R, Caruana SR, Phu TQ, et al. Anemia, iron deficiency, meat consumption, and hookworm in women of reproductive age in Northwest Vietnam. Am J Trop Med Hyg 2008;78:375–381.
29. Jarim-Botelho A, Raff S, Gazzinelli MF, et al. Hookworm, *Ascaris lumbricoides* infection and polyparasitism associated with poor cognitive performance in Brazilian schoolchildren. Trop Med Int Health 2008;13:994–1004.
30. Keiser J, Utzinger J. Efficacy of current drugs against soil-transmitted helminth infections: Systematic review and meta-analysis. JAMA 2008;299:1937–1948.
31. Jain MK. Biliary parasites: Diagnostic and therapeutic strategies. Curr Treat Options Gastroenterol 2008;11: 85–95.
32. Ugras SK, Finley DJ, Salem A. *Ascaris lumbricoides* infection causing respiratory distress after coronary artery bypass grafting. Surg Infect 2010;11:177–178.
33. Chang T-K, Liao C-W, Huang Y-C, et al. Prevalence of *Enterobius vermicularis* infection among preschool children in kindergartens of Taipei City, Taiwan in 2008. Korean J Parasitol 2009;47:185–187.
34. Balagopal A, Mills L, Shah A, Subramaniam A. Detection and treatment of *Strongyloides* syndrome following lung transplantation. Transplant Infect Dis 2009;11:149–154.
35. Bush LM, de Almeida KNF, Perez MT. Severe strongyloidiasis associated with subclinical human T-cell leukemia/lymphoma virus-1 infection. An illustrative case and review. Infect Dis Clin Pract 2009;17:84–89.
36. Lichtenberger P, Rosa-Cunha I, Morris M, et al. Hyperinfection strongyloidiasis in a liver transplant recipient treated with parenteral ivermectin. Transplant Infect Dis 2009;11:137–142.
37. Croker C, Reporter R, Redelings M, Mascola L. Strongyloidiasis-related deaths in the United States, 1919–2006. Am J Trop Med Hyg 2010;89:422–426.
38. Marcos LA, terashima A, Canales M, Gotuzzo E. Update on Strongyloidiasis in the immunocompromised host. Curr Infect Dis Rep 2011;13:35–46.
39. Basile A, Simzar S, Bentow J, et al. Disseminated *Strongyloides stercoralis* hyperinfection during medical immunosuppression. J Am Acad Dermal 2010;63:896–902.
40. Fusco DN, Downs JA, Satlin MJ, et al. Case Report: Non-oral treatment with ivermectin for disseminated Strongyloidiasis. Am J Trop Med Hyg 2010;83:979–883.
41. King CH, Farley JK. Cestodes (Tapeworms). In: Mandell GL, Dolin R, Bennett JE, eds. Principles and Practice of Infectious Diseases, 6th ed. New York: Elsevier/Churchill Livingstone, 2010;3607–3616.
42. Garcia HH, Coyle CM, White AC, Jr. Cysticercosis. In: Guerrant RL, Walker DH, Weller PF, eds. Tropical Infectious Diseases. Principles, Pathogens, & Practice, 3rd ed. Philadelphia, PA: Saunders/Elsevier, 2011:815–823.
43. Serpa JA, Graviss EA, Kass JS, White AC, Jr. Neurocysticercosis in Houston, Texas. An update. Medicine 2011;90:81–86.
44. Singhi P. Neurocysticercosis. Ther Adv Neurol Disorder 2011;4:67–81.

45. Garcia HH, Gonzalez AE, Gilman RH. Cysticercosis of central nervous system: How should it be managed? Curr Opin Infect Dis 2011;24:423–427.
46. Solelo H. Clinical manifestations, diagnosis and treatment of neurocysticercosis. Curr Neurol Neurosci Rep 2011;11: 529–535.
47. Singh G, Prabhakar S. The effects of antimicrobial and antiepiletic treatment on the outcome of epilepsy associated with central nervous system (CNS) infections. Epilepsia 2008;49(Suppl 6):42–46.
48. Fairhurst RM, Wellems TE. Plasmodium species (Malaria). In: Mandell GL, Dolin R, Bennett JE, eds. Principles and Practice of Infectious Diseases, 7th ed. New York: Elsevier/ Churchill Livingstone, 2010:3437–3462.
49. White NJ, Breman JG. Malaria. In: Longo DL, Fauci AS, Kasper DL, Hauser SL, et al. eds. Harrison's Principles of Internal Medicine, 18th ed. New York: McGraw-Hill, 2011:1688–1705.
50. O'Donnell FL (Ed.). Armed Forces Health Surveillance Center. Update: Malaria, US Armed Forces, 2011. MSMR 2012;19:1–15.
51. Spencer B, Steele W, Custer B, et al. Risk for malaria in United States donors deferred for travel to malaria-endemic areas. Transfusion 2009;49:2335–2345.
52. Hoffman SL, Campbell CC, White NJ. Malaria. In: Guerrant RL, Walker DH, Weller PF, eds. Tropical Infectious Diseases. Principles, Pathogens and Practice, 3rd ed. New York: Saunders/Elsevier, 2011:646–675.
53. John CC, Bangirana P, Byarugaba J, et al. Cerebral malaria in children is associated with long-term cognitive impairment. Pediatrics 2008;122:e92–e99.
54. Mishra SK, Wiese L. Advances in the management of cerebral malaria in adults. Curr Opin Neurol 2009;22:302–307.
55. John CC, Kutamba E, Mugarura K, Opoka RO. Adjunctive therapy for cerebral malaria and other forms of *Plasmodium falciparum* malaria. Exp Rev Infect Ther 2010;8:997–1008.
56. Phillips A, Bassett P, Zeki S, Newman S, Pasvol G. Risk factors for severe disease in adults with falciparum malaria. Clin Infect Dis 2009;48:871–878.
57. Fernando SD, Rodrigo C, Rajapakse S. The "hidden" burden of malaria: Cognitive impairment following infection. Malar J 2010;9:366.
58. Rosenthal PJ. Artesunate for the treatment of severe Falciparum malaria. N Engl J Med 2008;358:1829–1836.
59. Kopel E, Marhoom E, Sidi Y, Schwartz E. Successful oral treatment for severe falciparum malaria: The World Health Organization Criteria revisited. Am J Trop Med Hyg 2012;86:409–411.
60. Akinosoglou K-A, Pasvol G. The management of malaria in adults. Clin Med 2011;11:497–501.
61. Freedman DO. Malaria prevention in short-term travelers. N Engl J Med 2008;359:603–612.
62. Schlagenhauf P, Adamcova M, Regep L, Schaerer MT, Rhein H-G. The position of mefloquine as a 21st century malaria prophylaxis. Malar J 2010;9:357.
63. Schlagenhauf P, Petersen E. Malaria chemoprophylaxis: Strategies for risk groups. Clin Microb Rev 2008;21:466–472.
64. Makanga M, Bassat Q, Rosenthal PJ, et al. Efficacy and safety of Artemether–Lumefantrine in the treatment of acute, uncomplicated *Plasmodium falciparum* malaria: A pooled analysis. Am J Trop Med Hyg 2011;85:793–804.
65. Poespoprodjo JR, Fobia W, Price RN, et al. Adverse pregnancy outcomes in an area where multiresistant *Plasmodium vivax* and *Plasmodium falciparum* infections are endemic. Clin Infect Dis 2008;46:1374–1381.
66. Greenwood BM, Targett GAT. Malaria vaccines and the new malaria agenda. Clin Microb Infect 2011;17: 1600–1607.
67. The RTS,S Clinical Trials Partnership. First results of Phase 3 trials of RTS,S/AS01 malaria vaccine in African children. N Engl J Med 2011;365:1863–1875.
68. Roestenberg M, McCall M, Hopman J, et al. Protection against a malaria challenge by sporozoite inoculation. N Engl J Med 2009;361:468–477.
69. Keystone JS, Steffen R, Kozarsky P. Health advice for International Travel. In: Guerrant RL, Walker DH, Weller PF, eds. Tropical Infectious Diseases. Principles, Pathogens, & Practice, 3nd ed. Philadelphia, PA: Saunders/ Elsevier;2011:887–901.
70. Campbell CC. Malaria control—Addressing challenges to ambitious goals. N Engl J Med 2009;361:522–523.
71. Stauffer WM, Weinberg M, Newman RD, et al. Pre-departure and post-arrival management of *P. falciparum* malaria in refugees relocating from Sub-Saharan Africa to the United States. Am J Trop Med Hyg 2008;79:141–146.
72. Wongsrichanalai C, Meshnick SR. Declining artesunate–mefloquine efficacy against Falciparum malaria on the Cambodia–Thailand border. Emerg Infect Dis 2008;14: 716–719.
73. Douglas NM, Anstey NM, Angus BJ, Nosten F, Price RN. Artemisinin combination therapy for vivax malaria. Lancet Infect Dis 2010;10:405–416.
74. Dondorp AM, Nosten F, Yi P, et al. Artemisinin resistance in *Plasmodium falciparum* malaria. N Engl J Med 2009;361:455–467.
75. Rosenthal PJ. Antiprotozoal drugs. In: Katzung BG, Masters SB, Trevor AJ, eds. Basic and Clinical Pharmacology, 12th ed. New York: Lange Medical Books/McGraw-Hill, 2012:915–936.
76. Rassi A Jr, Rassi A, Marin-Neto JA. Chagas disease. Lancet 2010;375:1388–1402.
77. Biolo A, Ribeiro AL, Clausell N. Chagas cardiomyopathy—Where do we stand after a hundred years? Prog Cardiovascul Dis 2010;52:300–306.
78. Kirchhoff LV. Trypanosoma species (American trypanosomiasis, Chagas' disease): Biology of trypanosomes. In: Mandell GL, Bennett JE, Dolin R, eds. Principles and Practice of Infectious Diseases, 6th ed. New York: Elsevier/Churchill Livingstone, 2010: 3481–3488.
79. Kirchhoff LV. American trypanosomiasis (Chagas' disease). In: Guerrant RL, Walker DH, Weller PF, eds. Tropical Infectious Diseases. Principles, Pathogens, & Practice, 3rd ed. Philadelphia, PA: Saunders/Elsevier, 2011:689–695.
80. Nunes MCP, Barbosa MM, Ribeiro ALP. Ischemic cerebrovascular events in patients with Chagas cardiomyopathy. A prospective follow-up study. J Neurol Sci 2009;278:96–101.
81. Bern C, Montgomery SP, Katz L, Caglioti S, Stramer SL. Chagas disease and US blood supply. Curr Opin Infect Dis 2008;21:476–482.
82. Kun H, Moore A, Mascola L, et al. Transmission of *Trypanosoma cruzi* by heart transplantation. Clin Infect Dis 2009;48:1534–1540.
83. Bern C. Antitrypanosomal therapy for chronic Chagas' disease. N Engl J Med 2011;364:2527–2534.
84. Diaz JH. Lice (pediculosis). In: Mandell GL, Bennett JR, Dolin R, eds. Principles and Practice of Infectious Diseases, 6th ed. New York: Elsevier/Churchill Livingstone;2010:3629–3632.

85. Diamantis SA, Morrell DS, Burkhart CN. Treatment of head lice. Dermatol Ther 2009;22:273–278.
86. Meinking TL, Villar ME, Vicaria M, et al. The clinical trials supporting benzyl alcohol lotion 5% (Iesfia TM): A safe effective topical treatment for head lice (*Pediculosis humanus capitis*). Pediat Dermatol 2010;27:19–24.
87. Idriss S, Levitt J. Malathion for head lice and scabies: Treatment and safety considerations. J Drugs Dermatol 2009;8:715–720.
88. Burgess IF. Current treatments for *Pediculosis capitis*. Curr Opin Infect Dis 2009;22:131–136.
89. Stough D, Shellabarger S, Quiring J, Gabrielsen AA Jr. Efficacy and safety of Spinosad and Permethrin creme rinses for *Pediculosis capitis* (Head lice). Pediatr 2009;93: e389–e395.
90. Bourresse S, Chosidow O. Scabies in healthcare settings. Curr Opin Infect Dis 2010;23:111–118.
91. Hicks MI, Elston DM. Scabies. Dermatol Ther 2009;22: 279–292.
92. Currie BJ, McCarthy JS. Permethrin and Ivermectin for scabies. N Engl J Med 2010;362:717–725.

Appendix 93-1 Antiparasitic Drugs

Drug	Indications	Side Effects	Comments	References
Albendazole 200 mg tablet (Albenza)	Giardiasis, ascariasis, neurocysticercosis	GI: abdominal pain, nausea, diarrhea, increase in liver function enzymes	Not recommended in children <2 years old	9, 16, 42, 45, 46
Artemether 20 mg/ Lumefantrine 120 mg tablet (Coartem)	Acute uncomplicated Falciparum malaria	Headache, dizziness, asthenia, fatigue, and arthralgia	Approved for patients >5 kg body weight	52, 75
Artesunate[a]	Severe *falciparum* malaria	Rash, dizziness, and pruritus	Obtained by IND from CDC (when IV quinidine is not readily available)	16, 58
Atovaquone 250 mg *plus* proguanil 100 mg (Malarone)[b]	Prevention and treatment of *P. falciparum* malaria	Abdominal pain, nausea, vomiting, and headache		9, 16, 48, 49, 52, 61, 62, 75
Chloroquine phosphate (aralen, nivaquine) 250- and 500-mg tablets; 50 mg/mL (as HCl); 5-mL ampule	Malaria	GI: nausea, vomiting, and diarrhea CNS: dizziness, headache, blurring of vision, confusion, and fatigue Derm: pruritus	Administer oral dose after meals IV route: recommend ECG monitoring *Contraindication*: patients with psoriasis or porphyria	9, 16, 48, 49, 52, 61, 75
Diloxanide furoate[b] (Furamide) 500-mg tablet[c]	Amebiasis	GI: nausea and flatulence Derm: pruritus		9, 16, 19, 20, 21, 75
Furazolidone (Furoxone) 100-mg tablet	Giardiasis	GI: nausea and vomiting	Disulfiram-like reaction with alcohol; avoid in G6PD deficiency; may cause hemolysis; changes color of urine to brown	9, 16
Suspension: 50 mg/5 mL	Alternative to metronidazole	Hypersensitivity: hypotension, fever, arthralgia, and urticaria Other: headache		
Iodoquinol (Yodoxin) 210-mg tablet	Amebiasis	GI: abdominal pain and diarrhea Derm: rash	May interfere with the thyroid function test *Contraindication*: patients with iodine intolerance	9, 16, 19–21, 75
Ivermectin (Stromectol) 6-mg tablet	Strongyloidiasis Pediculosis Scabies	Dizziness, somnolence, tremor, vertigo, pruritus, and abdominal pain	Should be taken with a full glass of water	9, 16, 34, 39, 92
Mebendazole (Vermox) 100-mg chewable tablet	Ascariasis, trichuriasis, hookworm, and pinworm	GI: abdominal pain and diarrhea CNS: headache and dizziness Other: pyrexia and neutropenia	Drug should be taken with meals *Contraindication*: pregnancy *Drug interaction*: can increase serum levels of theophylline	9, 16, 25
Mefloquine (Lariam) 250-mg tablet	*P. falciparum* malaria	Incidence 17% GI: nausea, vomiting, abdominal pain, and diarrhea Card: sinus bradycardia CNS: vertigo, dizziness, confusion, hallucinations, psychosis, and convulsions Derm: itching, skin rash	Patients given doses in excess of 12 mg/kg should be monitored carefully because the side effects are dose related	9, 16, 48–50, 52, 55, 61, 62, 75
Metronidazole (Flagyl)	Amebiasis	GI: nausea, anorexia, vomiting, diarrhea, abdominal cramping, glossitis, and metallic taste	Avoid alcohol; alcohol ingestion will cause the disulfiram reaction: abdominal distress, vomiting, and hypotension	9, 11–13, 16, 19–21
Oral: 250-mg, 500-mg tablets	Giardiasis	CNS: dizziness, vertigo, headache, and paresthesia	*Contraindication*: First trimester of pregnancy	
Nifurtimox[c] (Lampit, Bayer 2502)	South American trypanosomiasis	GI: anorexia and nausea CNS: peripheral neuritis and psychosis Hemat: hemolysis in G6PD deficiency patients	Monitor pulmonary function and hematologic parameters	9, 16, 75, 76, 78, 79
Nitazoxanide (Alinia) 100-mg/5-mL suspension	Cryptosporidiosis Giardiasis	Abdominal pain, diarrhea, vomiting, and headache	Rarely may produce yellow sclerae	12, 16, 17
Primaquine phosphate 26.3-mg tablet	Malaria (*P. vivax*) (*P. ovale*)	GI: nausea and abdominal pain CNS: mental depression	In patients with G6PD deficiency, it can cause hemolysis	9, 16, 48, 49, 52
Pyrimethamine 25 mg *plus* sulfadoxine 500 mg (Fansidar)	*P. falciparum*-resistant malaria	GI: nausea, abdominal pain, stomatitis, headache, and glossitis Hemat: agranulocytosis, aplastic anemia, leukopenia, megaloblastic anemia, hemolytic anemia, and hemolysis in patients with G6PD deficiency	Combination was recently reported to cause the Stevens–Johnson syndrome; patients should be advised to call their physician/pharmacist if a skin rash or other reaction is seen	9, 16, 48, 49, 75

(*continued*)

Appendix 93-1 Antiparasitic Drugs (*Continued*)

Drug	Indications	Side Effects	Comments	References
Quinacrine 100 mg[c]	Giardiasis	GI: nausea, anorexia, and vomiting Headache, toxic psychosis, hepatitis, and aplastic anemia	Avoid in pregnancy, psychosis, and psoriasis	9, 12, 16
Quinidine gluconate 500 mg base/mL; 10 mL	Acute malaria	GI: nausea, vomiting, and diarrhea Card: hypotension, widening of QRS and QT on ECG, and heart block	Administration of IV quinidine requires close monitoring; should normally monitor ECG and all vital signs	9, 16, 48, 49, 52
Quinine sulfate 325-mg and 650-mg tablets	Acute malaria	Cinchonism: flushing, dizziness, nausea, vomiting, and diarrhea (levels over 10 mcg/mL [mg/L; 31 µmol/L]) Card: hypotension and widening of QRS complex Hemat: hemolysis, leukopenia, thrombocytopenia	When drug is administered IV, it should be administered by slow infusion (600 mg over 8 hours); close monitoring of vitals and ECG *Avoid use*: IM administration	9, 16, 48, 49, 52, 75

Card, cardiologic; Derm, dermatologic; ECG, electrocardiogram; G6PD, glucose-6-phosphate dehydrogenase; Hemat, hematologic; IND, investigational new drug.

[a]Investigational new drug from Centers for Disease Control and Prevention, Atlanta, GA 30333 (404-639-3670).

[b]Atovaquone 62.5 mg/proguanil 25 mg (Malarone), pediatric strength.

[c]Investigational drugs obtained from Panorama Compounding Pharmacy, 6744 Balboa Blvd, Van Nuys, CA 91406 (800-247-9767).

Available from CDC drug service, Centers for Disease Control and Prevention, Atlanta, GA 30333 (404-639-3670).

94

Urinary Tract Infections and Prostatitis

Elizabeth A. Coyle and Randall A. Prince

KEY CONCEPTS

1. Urinary tract infections (UTIs) can be classified as uncomplicated and complicated. *Uncomplicated* refers to an infection in an otherwise healthy, premenopausal female who lacks structural or functional abnormalities of the urinary tract. Most often complicated infections are associated with a predisposing lesion of the urinary tract; however, the term may be used to refer to all other infections, except for those in the otherwise healthy, premenopausal adult female.
2. Recurrent UTIs are considered either reinfections or relapses. Reinfection usually happens more than 2 weeks after the last UTI and is treated as a new uncomplicated UTI. Relapse usually happens within 2 weeks of the original infection, and is a relapse of the original infection either because of unsuccessful treatment of the original infection, a resistant organism, or anatomical abnormalities.
3. Seventy-five to ninety-five percent of uncomplicated UTIs are caused by *Escherichia coli* and the remainder are caused primarily by *Staphylococcus saprophyticus*, *Proteus* spp., and *Klebsiella* spp. Complicated infections may be associated with other gram-negative organisms and *Enterococcus faecalis*.
4. Symptoms of lower UTIs include dysuria, urgency, frequency, nocturia, and suprapubic heaviness, whereas upper UTIs involve more systemic symptoms such as fever, nausea, vomiting, and flank pain.
5. Significant bacteriuria traditionally has been defined as bacterial counts of greater than 10^5 organisms (CFU)/mL (10^8/L) of a midstream clean catch urine. Many clinicians, however, have challenged this statement as too general. Indeed, significant bacteriuria in patients with symptoms of a UTI may be defined as greater than 10^2 organisms (CFU)/mL and go ahead and take out the 10^5/L.
6. The goals of treatment of UTIs are to eradicate the invading organism(s), prevent or treat systemic consequences of infections, prevent the recurrence of infection, and prevent antimicrobial resistance.
7. Uncomplicated UTIs can be managed most effectively with short-course (3 days) therapy with either trimethoprim–sulfamethoxazole, one dose of fosfomycin, or 5 days of nitrofurantoin. Due to the possibility of collateral damage, fluoroquinolones should be reserved for suspected pyelonephritis or complicated infections.
8. In choosing appropriate antibiotic therapy, practitioners need to be cognizant of antibiotic resistance patterns, particularly to *E. coli*. Trimethoprim–sulfamethoxazole has diminished activity against *E. coli* in some areas of the country, with reported resistance in some areas greater than 20%.
9. Acute bacterial prostatitis can be managed with many agents that have activity against the causative organism. Chronic prostatitis requires prolonged therapy with an agent that penetrates the prostatic tissue and secretions. Therapy with fluoroquinolone or trimethoprim–sulfamethoxazole is preferred for up to 6 weeks.

Infections of the urinary tract represent a wide variety of syndromes, including urethritis, cystitis, prostatitis, and pyelonephritis. Urinary tract infections (UTIs) are the most commonly occurring bacterial infections and one of the most common reasons for antibiotic exposure, especially in females of childbearing age.[1–3] Approximately 60% of females will develop a UTI during their lifetime with about one fourth having a recurrence within a year.[2] Infections in men occur much less frequently until the age of 65 years at which point the incidence rates in men and women are similar.

A UTI is defined as the presence of microorganisms in the urinary tract that cannot be accounted for by contamination. The organisms present have the potential to invade the tissues of the urinary tract and adjacent structures. Infection may be limited to the growth of bacteria in the urine, which frequently may not produce symptoms. A UTI can present as several syndromes associated with an inflammatory response to microbial invasion and can range from asymptomatic bacteriuria to pyelonephritis with bacteremia or sepsis.

UTIs are classified by lower and upper UTIs. Typically, they have been described by anatomic site of involvement. Lower tract infections correspond to cystitis (bladder), and pyelonephritis (an infection involving the kidneys) represents upper tract infection.

1 Also, UTIs are designated as uncomplicated or complicated. Uncomplicated infections occur in individuals who lack structural or functional abnormalities of the urinary tract that interfere with the normal flow of urine or voiding mechanism. These infections occur in premenopausal females of childbearing age (15 to 45 years) who are otherwise normal, healthy individuals. Infections in males generally are not classified as uncomplicated because these infections are rare and most often represent a structural or neurologic abnormality.

Complicated UTIs are usually the result of a predisposing lesion of the urinary tract, such as a congenital abnormality or distortion of the urinary tract, a stone, indwelling catheter, prostatic hypertrophy, obstruction, or neurologic deficit that interferes with the normal flow of urine and urinary tract defenses. Complicated infections occur in both genders and frequently involve the upper and lower urinary tract.

TABLE 94-1 Diagnostic Criteria for Significant Abacteriuria

≥10^2 CFU coliforms/mL (≥10^5 CFU/L) or ≥10^5 CFU noncoliforms/mL (≥10^8 CFU/L) in a symptomatic female
≥10^3 CFU bacteria/mL (≥10^6 CFU/L) in a symptomatic male
≥10^5 CFU bacteria/mL (≥10^8 CFU/L) in asymptomatic individuals on two consecutive specimens
Any growth of bacteria on suprapubic catheterization in a symptomatic patient
≥10^2 CFU bacteria/mL (≥10^5 CFU/L) in a catheterized patient

CFU, colony-forming unit.

2 Recurrent UTIs in healthy nonpregnant women—two or more UTIs occurring within 6 months or three or more UTIs within 1 year—are a common problem. They are characterized by multiple symptomatic infections with asymptomatic periods occurring between each episode and may be either reinfections or relapses. Reinfections are caused by a different organism than originally isolated and account for the majority of recurrent UTIs. Relapses are the development of repeated infections with the same initial organism and usually indicate a persistent infectious source.[2]

Asymptomatic bacteriuria is a common finding, particularly among those 65 years of age and older when there is significant bacteriuria (>10^5 bacteria/mL [>10^8/L] of urine) in the absence of symptoms. Symptomatic abacteriuria or acute urethral syndrome consists of symptoms of frequency and dysuria in the absence of significant bacteriuria. This syndrome is commonly associated with *Chlamydia* infections.

Significant abacteriuria is a term used to distinguish the presence of microorganisms that represent true infection versus contamination of the urine as it passes through the distal urethra prior to collection. Historically, bacterial counts equal to or greater than 100,000 organisms/mL (10^8/L) of urine in a "clean-catch" specimen were judged to indicate true infection.[4–6] Counts less than 100,000 organisms/mL (10^8/L) of urine, however, may represent true infection in certain situations. For example, with concurrent antibacterial drug administration, rapid urine flow, low urinary pH, or upper tract obstruction.[6] Table 94-1 lists the clinical definitions of significant bacteriuria, which are dependent on the clinical setting and the method of specimen collection.[6] These criteria allow for more appropriate specificity and sensitivity in documenting infection under differing clinical circumstances.

EPIDEMIOLOGY

The prevalence of UTIs varies with age and gender. In newborns and infants up to 6 months of age, the prevalence of abacteriuria is approximately 1% and is more common in boys. Most of these infections are associated with structural or functional abnormalities of the urinary tract and also have been correlated with noncircumcision.[7] Between the ages of 1 and 6 years, UTIs occur more frequently in females. The prevalence of abacteriuria in females and males of this age group is 3% to 7% and 1% to 2%, respectively.[7,8] Infections occurring in preschool boys usually are associated with congenital abnormalities of the urinary tract. These infections are difficult to recognize because of the age of the patient, but they often are symptomatic. In addition, the majority of renal damage associated with UTI develops at this age.[7,8]

Through grade school and before puberty, the prevalence of UTI is approximately 1%, with 5% of females reported to have significant bacteriuria prior to leaving high school. This percentage increases dramatically to 1% to 4% after puberty in nonpregnant females primarily as a result of sexual activity. Approximately 1 in 5 women will suffer a symptomatic UTI at some point in their lives. Many women have recurrent infections with a significant proportion of these women having a history of childhood infections. In contrast, the prevalence of bacteriuria in adult men is very low (<0.1%).[9]

In the elderly, the ratio of bacteriuria in women and men is dramatically altered and is approximately equal in persons older than age 65 years.[10] The overall incidence of UTI increases substantially in this population with the majority of infections being asymptomatic. The rate of infection increases further for elderly persons who are residing in nursing homes, particularly those who are hospitalized frequently. The increase is probably the result of factors such as obstruction from prostatic hypertrophy in males, poor bladder emptying as a result of prolapse in females, fecal incontinence in demented patients, and neuromuscular disease including strokes and increased urinary instrumentation (catheterization).

ETIOLOGY

3 The bacteria causing UTIs usually originate from bowel flora of the host. Although virtually every organism is associated with UTIs, certain organisms predominate as a result of specific virulence factors. The most common cause of uncomplicated UTIs is *Escherichia coli*, which accounts for 80% to 90% of community-acquired infections. Additional causative organisms in uncomplicated infections include *Staphylococcus saprophyticus*, *Klebsiella pneumoniae*, *Proteus* spp., *Pseudomonas aeruginosa*, and *Enterococcus* spp.[11] Because *Staphylococcus epidermidis* is frequently isolated from the urinary tract, it should be considered initially a contaminant. Repeat cultures should be performed to help confirm the organism as a real pathogen.

Organisms isolated from individuals with complicated infections are more varied and generally are more resistant than those found in uncomplicated infections. *E. coli* is a frequently isolated pathogen, but it accounts for less than 50% of infections. Other frequently isolated organisms include *Proteus* spp., *K. pneumoniae*, *Enterobacter* spp., *P. aeruginosa*, staphylococci, and enterococci. Enterococci represent the second most frequently isolated organisms in hospitalized patients.[11–13] In part, this finding may be related to the extensive use of third-generation cephalosporin antibiotics, which are not active against the enterococci. Vancomycin-resistant *Enterococcus faecalis* and *Enterococcus faecium* (vancomycin-resistant enterococci) have become more widespread, especially in patients with long-term hospitalizations or underlying malignancies. Vancomycin-resistant enterococci are major therapeutic and infection control issues because these organisms are susceptible to few antimicrobials.[12,13]

Staphylococcus aureus infections may arise from the urinary tract, but they are more commonly a result of bacteremia producing metastatic abscesses in the kidney. *Candida* spp. are common causes of UTI in the critically ill and chronically catheterized patient.

Most UTIs are caused by a single organism; however, in patients with stones, indwelling urinary catheters, or chronic renal abscesses, multiple organisms may be isolated. Depending on the clinical situation, the recovery of multiple organisms may represent contamination and a repeat evaluation should be done.

PATHOPHYSIOLOGY

Route of Infection

Organisms typically gain entry into the urinary tract via three routes: the ascending, hematogenous (descending), and lymphatic pathways. The female urethra usually is colonized by bacteria believed to originate from the fecal flora. The short length of the female urethra and its proximity to the perirectal area make colonization of the urethra likely. Other factors that promote urethral colonization include the use of spermicides and diaphragms as methods of contraception.[2,3] Although there is evidence in females that bladder infections follow colonization of the urethra, the mode of ascent of the microorganisms is incompletely understood. Massage of the female urethra and sexual intercourse allow bacteria to reach the bladder.[14] Once bacteria have reached the bladder, the organisms quickly multiply and can ascend the ureters to the kidneys. This sequence of events is more likely to occur if vesicoureteral reflux (reflux of urine into the ureters and kidneys while voiding) is present. UTIs are more common in females than in males because the anatomic differences in location and length of the urethra tend to support the ascending route of infections as the primary acquisition route.

Infection of the kidney by hematogenous spread of microorganisms usually occurs as the result of dissemination of organisms from a distant primary infection in the body. Infections via the descending route are uncommon and involve a relatively small number of invasive pathogens. Bacteremia caused by *S. aureus* may produce renal abscesses. Additional organisms include *Candida* spp., *Mycobacterium tuberculosis*, *Salmonella* spp., and enterococci. Of particular interest, it is difficult to produce experimental pyelonephritis by IV administering common gram-negative organisms such as *E. coli* and *P. aeruginosa*. Overall, less than 5% of documented UTIs result from hematogenous spread of microorganisms.

There appears to be little evidence supporting a significant role for renal lymphatics in the pathogenesis of UTIs. There are lymphatic communications between the bowel and kidney, as well as between the bladder and kidney. There is no evidence, however, that microorganisms are transferred to the kidney via this route.

After bacteria reach the urinary tract, three factors determine the development of infection: the size of the inoculum, the virulence of the microorganism, and the competency of the natural host defense mechanisms. Most UTIs reflect a failure in host defense mechanisms.

Host Defense Mechanisms

The normal urinary tract generally is resistant to invasion by bacteria and is efficient in rapidly eliminating microorganisms that reach the bladder. The urine under normal circumstances is capable of inhibiting and killing microorganisms. The factors thought to be responsible include a low pH, extremes in osmolality, high urea concentration, and high organic acid concentration. Bacterial growth is further inhibited in males by the addition of prostatic secretions.[14,15]

The introduction of bacteria into the bladder stimulates micturition with increased diuresis and efficient emptying of the bladder. These factors are critical in preventing the initiation and maintenance of bladder infections. Patients who are unable to void urine completely are at greater risk of developing UTIs and frequently have recurrent infections. Also, patients with even small residual amounts of urine in their bladder respond less favorably to treatment than patients who are able to empty their bladders completely.[16]

An important virulence factor of bacteria is their ability to adhere to urinary epithelial cells resulting in colonization of the urinary tract, bladder infections, and pyelonephritis. Various factors that act as antiadherence mechanisms are present in the bladder preventing bacterial colonization and infection. The epithelial cells of the bladder are coated with a urinary mucus or slime called *glycosaminoglycan*. This thin layer of surface mucopolysaccharide is hydrophilic and strongly negatively charged. When bound to the uroepithelium, it attracts water molecules and forms a layer between the bladder and urine. The antiadherence characteristics of the glycosaminoglycan layer are nonspecific and when the layer is removed by dilute acid solutions, rapid bacterial adherence results.[17]

In addition, the Tamm–Horsfall protein is a glycoprotein produced by the ascending limb of Henle and distal tubule that is secreted into the urine and contains mannose residues. These mannose residues bind *E. coli* that contain small surface-projecting organellae on their surfaces called *pili* or *fimbriae*. Type 1 fimbriae are mannose-sensitive and this interaction prevents the bacteria from binding to similar receptors present on the mucosal surface of the bladder. Other factors that possibly prevent adherence of bacteria include immunoglobulins (Ig) G and A. Investigators have documented both systemic and local kidney immunoglobulin synthesis in upper tract infections. The role of immunoglobulins in preventing bladder infection is less clear. Patients with reduced urinary levels of secretory IgA are, however, at increased risk of infections of the urinary tract.

After bacteria have invaded the bladder mucosa, an inflammatory response is stimulated with the mobilization of polymorphonuclear leukocytes (PMNs) and resulting phagocytosis. PMNs are primarily responsible for limiting the tissue invasion and controlling the spread of infection in the bladder and kidney. They do not play a role in preventing bladder colonization or infections and actually contribute to renal tissue damage.

Other host factors that may play a role in the prevention of UTIs are the presence of *Lactobacillus* in the vaginal flora and circulating estrogen levels. In premenopausal women, circulating estrogen supports the vaginal tract growth of lactobacilli, which produce lactic acid to help maintain a low vaginal pH, thereby preventing *E. coli* vaginal colonization.[18] Topical estrogens are used for the prevention of UTI in postmenopausal women who have more than 3 recurrent UTI episodes per year and are not on oral estrogens.[19]

Bacterial Virulence Factors

Pathogenic organisms have differing degrees of pathogenicity (virulence), which play a role in the development and severity of infection. Bacteria that adhere to the epithelium of the urinary tract are associated with colonization and infection. The mechanism of adhesion of gram-negative bacteria, particularly *E. coli*, is related to bacterial fimbriae that are rigid, hair-like appendages of the cell wall.[9] These fimbriae adhere to specific glycolipid components on epithelial cells. The most common type of fimbriae is type 1, which binds to mannose residues present in glycoproteins. Glycosaminoglycan and Tamm–Horsfall protein are rich in mannose residues that readily trap those organisms that contain type 1 fimbriae, which are then washed out of the bladder.[20] Other fimbriae are mannose resistant and are associated more frequently with pyelonephritis, such as P fimbriae, which bind avidly to specific glycolipid receptors on uroepithelial cells. These bacteria are resistant to washout or removal by glycosaminoglycan and are able to multiply and invade tissue, especially the kidney. In addition, PMNs, as well as secretory IgA antibodies, contain receptors for type 1 fimbriae, which facilitate phagocytosis, but are lacking receptors for P fimbriae.

Other virulence factors include the production of hemolysin and aerobactin.[21] Hemolysin is a cytotoxic protein produced by bacteria that lyses a wide range of cells, including erythrocytes, PMNs, and monocytes. *E. coli* and other gram-negative bacteria require iron for aerobic metabolism and multiplication. Aerobactin facilitates the binding and uptake of iron by *E. coli*; however, the significance of this property in the pathogenesis of UTIs remains unknown.

PREDISPOSING FACTORS TO INFECTION

The normal urinary tract typically is resistant to infection and colonization by pathogenic bacteria. In patients with underlying structural abnormalities of the urinary tract, the typical host defenses previously discussed usually are lacking or compromised. There are several known abnormalities of the urinary tract system that interfere with its natural defense mechanisms, the most important of which is obstruction. Obstruction can inhibit the normal flow of urine disrupting the natural flushing and voiding effect in removing bacteria from the bladder and resulting in incomplete emptying. Common conditions that result in residual urine volumes include prostatic hypertrophy, urethral strictures, calculi, tumors, bladder diverticula, and drugs such as anticholinergic agents. Additional causes of incomplete bladder emptying include neurologic malfunctions associated with stroke, diabetes, spinal cord injuries, tabes dorsalis, and other neuropathies. Vesicoureteral reflux represents a condition in which urine is forced up the ureters to the kidneys. Urinary reflux is associated not only with an increased incidence of UTIs and pyelonephritis, but also with renal damage.[8,16] Reflux may be the result of a congenital abnormality or, more commonly, bladder overdistension from obstruction.

Other risk factors include urinary catheterization, mechanical instrumentation, pregnancy, and the use of spermicides and diaphragms.

CLINICAL PRESENTATION

❹ The presenting signs and symptoms of UTIs in adults are recognized easily (Table 94-2). Women frequently will report gross hematuria. Systemic symptoms, including fever, typically are absent in this setting. Unfortunately, large numbers of patients with significant bacteriuria are asymptomatic. These patients may be normal, healthy patients, elderly patients, children, pregnant patients, and patients with indwelling catheters. It is important to note that attempts at differentiating upper tract from lower tract infections on the basis of symptoms alone are not reliable.

Elderly patients frequently do not experience specific urinary symptoms, but they will present with altered mental status, change in eating habits, or GI symptoms. In addition, patients with indwelling catheters or neurologic disorders commonly will not have lower tract symptoms. Instead, they may present with flank pain and fever. Many of the aforementioned patients, however, frequently will develop upper tract infections with bacteremia and no or minimal urinary tract symptoms.

Symptoms alone are unreliable for the diagnosis of bacterial UTIs. The key to the diagnosis of UTI is the ability to demonstrate significant numbers of microorganisms in an appropriate urine specimen to distinguish contamination from infection. The type and extent of laboratory examination required depends on the clinical situation.

TABLE 94-2 Clinical Presentation of Urinary Tract Infections in Adults

Signs and symptoms
- Lower UTI: dysuria, urgency, frequency, nocturia, and suprapubic heaviness
- Gross hematuria
- Upper UTI: flank pain, fever, nausea, vomiting, and malaise

Physical examination
- Upper UTI: costovertebral tenderness

Laboratory tests
- Bacteriuria
- Pyuria (white blood cell count $>10/mm^3$ [$\geq 10 \times 10^6/L$])
- Nitrite-positive urine (with nitrite reducers)
- Leukocyte esterase-positive urine
- Antibody-coated bacteria (upper UTI)

UTI, urinary tract infection.

Urine Collection

Examination of the urine is the cornerstone of laboratory evaluation for UTIs. There are three acceptable methods of urine collection. The first is the *midstream clean-catch method*. After cleaning the urethral opening area in both men and women, 20 to 30 mL of urine is voided and discarded. The next part of the urine flow is collected and should be processed immediately (refrigerated as soon as possible). Specimens that are allowed to sit at room temperature for several hours may result in falsely elevated bacterial counts. The midstream clean-catch is the preferred method for the routine collection of urine for culture. When a routine urine specimen cannot be collected or contamination occurs, alternative collection techniques must be used.

The two acceptable alternative methods include catheterization and suprapubic bladder aspiration. Catheterization may be necessary for patients who are uncooperative or who are unable to void urine. If catheterization is performed carefully with aseptic technique, the method yields reliable results. Note, however, that introduction of bacteria into the bladder may result and the procedure is associated with infection in 1% to 2% of patients. Suprapubic bladder aspiration involves inserting a needle directly into the bladder and aspirating the urine. This procedure bypasses the contaminating organisms present in the urethra and any bacteria found using this technique generally are considered to represent significant bacteriuria.[22–25] Suprapubic aspiration is a safe and painless procedure that is most useful in newborns, infants, paraplegics, seriously ill patients, and others in whom infection is suspected and routine procedures have provided confusing or equivocal results.

Bacterial Count

❺ The diagnosis of UTI is based on the isolation of significant numbers of bacteria from a urine specimen. Microscopic examination of a urine sample is an easy-to-perform and reliable method for the presumptive diagnosis of bacteriuria. The examination may be performed by preparing a Gram stain of unspun or centrifuged urine. The presence of at least one organism per oil-immersion field in a properly collected uncentrifuged specimen correlates well with more than 100,000 colony-forming units (CFU)/mL (10^5 CFU/mL or 10^8 CFU/L) of urine. For detecting smaller numbers of organisms, a centrifuged specimen is more sensitive. Such examinations detect more than 10^5 bacteria/mL (10^8 CFU/L) with a sensitivity of greater than 90% and a specificity of greater than 70%.[22,23] A quantitative count of greater than or equal to 10^5 CFU/mL (10^8 CFU/L) is considered indicative of a UTI; however, up to 50% of women will present with clinical symptoms of a UTI with lower counts (10^3 CFU/mL [10^6 CFU/L]).[4]

Pyuria, Hematuria, and Proteinuria

Microscopic examination of the urine for leukocytes is used to determine the presence of pyuria. The presence of pyuria in a symptomatic patient correlates with significant bacteriuria.[24] Pyuria is defined as a white blood cell (WBC) count of greater than 10 WBC/mm^3 (10×10^6/L) of urine. A count of 5 to 10 WBC/mm^3 (5×10^6 to 10×10^6/L) is accepted as the upper limit of normal. It should be emphasized that pyuria is nonspecific and signifies only the presence of inflammation and not necessarily infection. Thus patients with pyuria may or may not have infection. Sterile pyuria has long been associated with urinary tuberculosis, as well as chlamydial and fungal urinary infections.

Hematuria, microscopic or gross, is frequently present in patients with UTI, but is nonspecific. Hematuria may indicate the presence of other disorders, such as renal calculi, tumors, or glomerulonephritis. Proteinuria is found commonly in the presence of infection.

Chemistry

Several biochemical tests have been developed for screening urine for the presence of bacteria. A common dipstick test detects the presence of nitrite in the urine, which is formed by bacteria that reduce nitrate normally present in the urine. False-positive tests are uncommon. False-negative tests are more common and frequently are caused by the presence of gram-positive organisms or *P. aeruginosa* that do not reduce nitrate.[25] Other causes of false tests include low urinary pH, frequent voiding, and dilute urine.

The leukocyte esterase dipstick test is a rapid screening test for detecting the presence of pyuria. Leukocytes esterase is found in primary neutrophil granules and indicates the presence of WBCs. The leukocyte esterase test is a sensitive and highly specific test for detecting more than 10 WBC/mm^3 (10×10^6/L) of urine. When the leukocyte esterase test is used with the nitrite test, the reported positive predictive value and specificity is 79% and 82%, respectively, for the detection of bacteriuria.[26,27] These tests can be useful in the outpatient evaluation of uncomplicated UTIs. However, urine culture is still the "gold standard" test in determining the presence of UTIs.

Culture

The most reliable method of diagnosing UTI is by quantitative urine culture. Urine in the bladder is normally sterile making it statistically possible to differentiate contamination of the urine from infection by quantifying the number of bacteria present in a urine sample. This criterion is based on a properly collected midstream clean-catch urine specimen. Patients with infection usually have greater than 10^5 bacteria/mL (10^8/L) of urine. It should be emphasized that as many as one third of women with symptomatic infection have less than 10^5 bacteria/mL (10^8/L). Also, a significant portion of patients with UTIs, either symptomatic or asymptomatic, have less than 10^5 bacteria/mL (10^8/L) of urine.

Several laboratory methods are used to quantify bacteria present in the urine. The most accurate method is the pour-plate technique. This method is unsuitable for a high-volume laboratory because it is expensive and time-consuming. The streak-plate method is an alternative that involves using a calibrated-loop technique to streak a fixed amount of urine on an agar plate. This method is used most commonly in diagnostic laboratories because it is simple to perform and less costly.

After identification and quantification are complete, the next step is to determine the susceptibility of the organism. There are several methods by which bacterial susceptibility testing may be performed. Knowledge of bacterial susceptibility and achievable urine concentration of the antibiotics puts the clinician in a better position to select an appropriate agent for treatment.

Infection Site

Several methods have been evaluated to determine the location of infection within the urinary system and differentiate upper tract from lower tract involvement. The most direct method is a ureteral catheterization procedure as described by Stamey and colleagues.[28] The method involves the passage of a catheter into the bladder and then into each ureter, where quantitative cultures are obtained. History and physical examination were of little value in predicting the site of infection. Although this method provides direct quantitative evidence for UTI, it is invasive, technically difficult, and expensive. The Fairley bladder washout technique is a modification of the Stamey procedure that involves Foley catheterization only.[29] After the catheter is passed into the bladder, bladder samples are obtained and the bladder is washed out with culture samples taken at 10, 20, and 30 minutes. The procedure shows that up to 50% of patients have renal involvement, regardless of signs and symptoms. Other investigators found 10% to 20% of tests to be equivocal.[29]

Noninvasive methods of localization may be more acceptable for routine use; however, they have limited clinical value. Patients with pyelonephritis can have abnormalities in urinary concentrating ability. The use of concentrating ability for localization of UTIs, however, is associated with high false-positive and false-negative responses and is not useful clinically.[25] The antibody-coated bacteria test is an immunofluorescent method that detects bacteria coated with Ig in freshly voided urine indicating upper UTI. The sensitivity and specificity of this test to localize the site of infection are reported to average 88% and 76%, respectively.[30] Because of the high incidence of false-positive and false-negative results, antibody-coated bacteria testing is not used routinely in the management of UTIs.

Virtually all patients with uncomplicated lower tract infections can be cured with a short course of antibiotic therapy and this assumption sometimes can be used to distinguish between patients with lower and upper tract infections. Patients who do not respond or who relapse may do so because of upper tract involvement. It is rarely necessary to localize the site of infection to direct the clinical management of such patients.

TREATMENT

Desired Outcomes

6 The goals of UTI treatments are (a) to eradicate the invading organism(s), (b) to prevent or to treat systemic consequences of infection, (c) to prevent the recurrence of infection, and (d) to decrease the potential for collateral damage with too broad of antimicrobial therapy.

Management

The management of a patient with a UTI includes initial evaluation, selection of an antibacterial agent, and duration of therapy and follow-up evaluation. The initial selection of an antimicrobial agent for the treatment of UTI is based primarily on the severity of the presenting signs and symptoms, the site of infection and whether the infection is determined to be uncomplicated or complicated. Other considerations include antibiotic susceptibility, side-effect potential, cost, current antimicrobial exposure, and the comparative inconvenience of different therapies.[1]

Various pharmacologic factors may affect the action of antibacterial agents. Certainly, the ability of the agent to achieve appropriate concentrations in the urine is of utmost importance. Factors that affect the rate and extent of excretion through the kidney include the patient's glomerular filtration rate and whether or not the agent is actively secreted. Filtration depends on the molecular size and degree of protein binding of the agent. Agents such as sulfonamides, tetracyclines, and aminoglycosides enter the urine via filtration. As the glomerular filtration rate is reduced, the amount of drug that enters the urine is reduced. Most β-lactam agents and quinolones are filtered and are actively secreted into the urine. For this reason, most of these agents achieve high urinary concentrations despite unfavorable protein-binding characteristics or the presence of renal dysfunction.

The ability to eradicate bacteria from the urine is related directly to the sensitivity of the microorganism and the achievable concentrations of the antimicrobial agent in the urine. Unfortunately, most susceptibility testing is directed at achievable concentrations in the blood. There is a poor correlation between achievable blood concentrations of antimicrobial agents and the eradication of bacteria from the urine.[31] In the treatment of lower tract infections, plasma concentrations of antibacterial agents may not be important, but achieving appropriate plasma concentrations appears critical in patients with bacteremia and renal abscesses.

Nonspecific therapies have been advocated in the treatment and prevention of UTIs. Fluid hydration has been used to produce rapid dilution of bacteria and removal of infected urine by increased voiding. A critical factor appears to be the amount of residual volume remaining after voiding. As little as 10 mL of residual urine can alter the eradication of infection significantly.[16] Paradoxically, increased diuresis also may promote susceptibility to infection by diluting the normal antibacterial properties of the urine. Often in clinical practice the concentrations of antimicrobial agents in the urine are so high that dilution has little effect on efficacy.

The antibacterial activity of the urine is related to the low pH, which is the result of high concentrations of various organic acids. Large volumes of cranberry juice increase the antibacterial activity of the urine and prevent the development of UTIs.[3,32,33] Apparently, the fructose and other unknown substances (condensed tannins, proanthocyanidin) in cranberry juice act to interfere with adherence mechanisms of some pathogens, thereby preventing infection or reinfection. Acidification of the urine by cranberry juice does not appear to play a significant role. The use of other agents (ascorbic acid) to acidify the urine to hinder bacterial growth does not achieve significant acidification. Consequently, attempts to acidify urine with systemic agents are not recommended. *Lactobacillus* probiotics also may aid in the prevention of female UTIs by decreasing the vaginal pH, thereby decreasing *E. coli* colonization.[19,33] In postmenopausal women, estrogen replacement may be of help in the prevention of recurrent UTIs. After 1 month of topical estrogen replacement, decreases in vaginal *Lactobacillus*, as well as decreases in vaginal pH and *E. coli* colonization, have been found.[18,33]

Clinical **Controversy. . .**

The use of cranberry juice or lactobacilli in the prevention of UTIs has long been discussed. *Lactobacillus* potentially helps keep the vaginal pH in the normal range (pH 4 to 4.5), regulating genitourinary bacteria therefore aiding in the prevention of UTIs.[32] Possible clinical benefits with cranberry juice in sexually active adult women with recurrent UTI by decreasing the adherence of bacteria to the bladder epithelial cells. However, a placebo controlled trial with cranberry juice in the prevention of recurrent UTIs in college age females showed no benefit with cranberry juice.[32] Unfortunately, the consistency of study results has varied, as have the types of cranberry products tested, leading to overall inconclusive evidence.[32,33] More reliable and thorough studies on the overall effectiveness of cranberry juice or lactobacilli need to be performed before a uniform opinion on the role of these agents in UTIs can be stated.

Urinary analgesics such as phenazopyridine hydrochloride are used frequently by many clinicians.[3] If the pain or dysuria present in a UTI is a consequence of infection, then urinary analgesics have little clinical role because most patients' symptoms respond quite rapidly to appropriate antibacterial therapy. Also, urinary analgesics may mask signs and symptoms of UTIs not responding to antimicrobial therapy.[34,35,36]

Clinical **Controversy. . .**

Phenazopyridine hydrochloride is an over the counter urinary anesthetic/analgesic that can be used for symptom relief in UTIs. Common brand names are Pyridium®, Azo-Standard®, and Uristat®. It is utilized frequently by patients as self-medication to alleviate the dysuria associated with UTIs. The use of phenazopyridine in the treatment of UTIs is controversial. It has no antimicrobial properties and has a number of adverse effects such as red-orange discoloration of body fluids, rash, anaphylaxis, and rare effects such as hemolytic anemia, methemoglobinemia, and acute renal failure. In addition, its use can mask the symptoms of an untreated or inappropriately treated UTI. Unfortunately, there are not any guidelines for its role in the treatment of UTIs; however, experts agree that if phenazopyridine is utilized, only use the recommended dose (maximum 200 mg three times a day) and it should be limited to 1 to 2 days for symptomatic relief of the dysuria with UTIs.[34,35] In addition, it should be used with the combination of appropriate antibiotic therapy.

Pharmacologic Therapy

Ideally, the antimicrobial agent chosen should be well tolerated, well absorbed, achieve high urinary concentrations, and have a spectrum of activity limited to the known or suspected pathogen(s). Table 94-3 lists the most common agents used in the treatment of UTIs along with comments concerning their general use. Table 94-4 presents an overview of various therapeutic options for outpatient therapy of UTI. Table 94-5 describes empirical treatment regimens for selected clinical situations.

8 The therapeutic management of UTIs is best accomplished by first categorizing the type of infection: acute uncomplicated cystitis, symptomatic abacteriuria, asymptomatic bacteriuria, complicated UTIs, recurrent infections, or prostatitis. In choosing the appropriate antibiotic therapy, it is important to be aware of the increasing resistance of *E. coli* and other pathogens to many frequently prescribed antimicrobials. Resistance to *E. coli* is as high as 37% for amoxicillin and ampicillin.[1,37] Overall, most *E. coli* remain susceptible to trimethoprim–sulfamethoxazole, although resistance is continuing to increase and has been reported as high as 27%.[38] Although resistance to the fluoroquinolones remains low, these agents are being utilized more frequently and the incidence of fluoroquinolone-resistant *E. coli* is increasingly being reported and is of great concern.[37–43] Current or recent antibiotic exposure is the most significant risk factor associated with *E. coli* resistance and with the extensive use of the fluoroquinolones and trimethoprim–sulfamethoxazole for various infections, including UTIs, resistance will continue to increase.[37–42] In addition, broad-spectrum antimicrobials such as fluoroquinolones and broad-spectrum cephalosporins have a high impact on GI flora, increasing the risk of collateral damage or the selection of resistant *E. coli* pathogens.[37–40,43,44] In light of rising resistance and in order to decrease the overuse of broad-spectrum antimicrobials, agents such as nitrofurantoin and fosfomycin are now considered first-line treatments along with trimethoprim–sulfamethoxazole in acute uncomplicated cystitis. Both nitrofurantoin and fosfomycin have little effects on the gut flora and *E. coli* susceptibility still remains high.[3,44–48] Antibiotic therapy should be determined based on the geographic resistance patterns, as well as the patient's recent history of antibiotic exposure.

TABLE 94-3 Commonly Used Antimicrobial Agents in the Treatment of Urinary Tract Infections

Drug	Brand Name	Adverse Drug Reactions	Monitoring Parameters	Comments
Oral Therapy				
Trimethoprim–sulfamethoxazole	Bactrim®, Septra®	Rash, Stevens–Johnson Syndrome, renal failure, photosensitivity, hematologic (neutropenia, anemia, etc.)	Serum creatinine, BUN, electrolytes, signs of rash, and CBC	This combination is highly effective against most aerobic enteric bacteria except *P. aeruginosa*. High urinary tract tissue concentrations and urine concentrations are achieved, which may be important in complicated infection treatment. Also effective as prophylaxis for recurrent infections
Nitrofurantoin	Macrobid®	GI intolerance, neuropathies, and pulmonary reactions	Baseline serum creatinine and BUN	This agent is effective as both a therapeutic and prophylactic agent in patients with recurrent UTIs. Main advantage is the lack of resistance even after long courses of therapy
Fosfomycin	Monurol®	Diarrhea, headache, and angioedema	No routine tests recommended	Single-dose therapy for uncomplicated infections, low levels of resistance, use with caution in patients with hepatic dysfunction
Fluoroquinolones Ciprofloxacin Levofloxacin	 Cipro® Levaquin®	Hypersensitivity, photosensitivity, GI symptoms, dizziness, confusion, and tendonitis (black box warning)	CBC, baseline serum creatinine, and BUN	The fluoroquinolones have a greater spectrum of activity, including *P. aeruginosa*. These agents are effective for pyelonephritis and prostatitis. Avoid in pregnancy and children. Moxifloxacin should not be used owing to inadequate urinary concentrations
Penicillins Amoxicillin–clavulanate	 Augmentin®	Hypersensitivity (rash, anaphylaxis), diarrhea, superinfections, and seizures	CBC, signs of rash, or hypersensitivity	Due to increasing *E. coli* resistance, amoxicillin–clavulanate is the preferred penicillin for uncomplicated cystitis
Cephalosporins Cefdnir Cefpodoxime-proxetil	 Omnicef® Vantin®	Hypersensitivity (rash, anaphylaxis), diarrhea, superinfections, and seizures	CBC, signs of rash, or hypersensitivity	There are no major advantages of these agents over other agents in the treatment of UTIs, and they are more expensive. These agents are not active against enterococci
Parenteral Therapy				
Aminoglycosides Gentamicin Tobramycin Amikacin	 Garamycin® Nebcin® Amikin®	Ototoxicity, nephrotoxicity	Serum creatinine and BUN, serum drug concentrations, and individual pharmacokinetic monitoring	These agents are renally excreted and achieve good concentrations in the urine. Amikacin generally is reserved for multidrug-resistant bacteria
Penicillins Ampicillin–sulbactam Piperacillin–tazobactam	 Unasyn® Zosyn®	Hypersensitivity (rash, anaphylaxis), diarrhea, superinfections, and seizures	CBC, signs of rash, or hypersensitivity	These agents generally are equally effective for susceptible bacteria. The extended-spectrum penicillins are more active against *P. aeruginosa* and enterococci and often are preferred over cephalosporins. They are very useful in renally impaired patients or when an aminoglycoside is to be avoided
Cephalosporins Ceftriaxone Ceftazidime Cefepime	 Rocephin® Fortaz® Maxipime®	Hypersensitivity (rash, anaphylaxis), diarrhea, superinfections, and seizures	CBC, signs of rash, or hypersensitivity	Second- and third-generation cephalosporins have a broad spectrum of activity against gram-negative bacteria, but are not active against enterococci and have limited activity against *P. aeruginosa*. Ceftazidime and cefepime are active against *P. aeruginosa*. They are useful for nosocomial infections and urosepsis due to susceptible pathogens
Carbapenems/Monobactams Imipenem–cilistatin Meropenem Doripenem Ertapenem Aztreonam	 Primaxin® Merrem® Doribax® Invanz® Azactam®	Hypersensitivity (rash, anaphylaxis), diarrhea, superinfections, and seizures	CBC, signs of rash, or hypersensitivity	Carbapenems have a broad spectrum of activity, including gram-positive, gram-negative, and anaerobic bacteria. Imipenem, meropenem, and doripenem are active against *P. aeruginosa* and enterococci, but ertapenem is not. Aztreonam is a monobactam that is only active against gram-negative bacteria, including some strains of *P. aeruginosa*. Generally useful for nosocomial infections when aminoglycosides are to be avoided and in penicillin-sensitive patients
Fluoroquinolones Ciprofloxacin Levofloxacin	 Cipro® Levaquin®	Hypersensitivity, photosensitivity, GI symptoms, dizziness, confusion, and tendonitis (black box warning)	CBC, baseline serum creatinine, and BUN	These agents have broad-spectrum activity against both gram-negative and gram-positive bacteria. They provide urine and high-tissue concentrations and are actively secreted in reduced renal function

TABLE 94-4 Overview of Outpatient Antimicrobial Therapy for Lower Tract Infections in Adults

Indications	Antibiotic	Dose[a]	Interval	Duration
Lower tract infections				
Uncomplicated	Trimethoprim–sulfamethoxazole	1 DS tablet	Twice a day	3 days
	Nitrofurantoin monohydrate	100 mg	Twice a day	5 days
	Fosfomycin	3 g	Single dose	1 day
	Ciprofloxacin	250 mg	Twice a day	3 days
	Levofloxacin	250 mg	Once a day	3 days
	Amoxicillin–clavulanate	500 mg	Every 8 hours	5–7 days
Complicated	Trimethoprim–sulfamethoxazole	1 DS tablet	Twice a day	7–10 days
	Ciprofloxacin	250–500 mg	Twice a day	7–10 days
	Levofloxacin	250 mg	Once a day	10 days
		750 mg	Once a day	5 days
	Amoxicillin–clavulanate	500 mg	Every 8 hours	7–10 days
Recurrent infections	Nitrofurantoin	50 mg	Once a day	6 months
	Trimethoprim–sulfamethoxazole	1/2 SS tablet	Once a day	6 months
Acute pyelonephritis	Trimethoprim–sulfamethoxazole	1 DS tablet	Twice a day	14 days
	Ciprofloxacin	500 mg	Twice a day	14 days
		1000 mg ER	Once a day	7 days
	Levofloxacin	250 mg	Once a day	10 days
		750 mg	Once a day	5 days
	Amoxicillin–clavulanate	500 mg	Every 8 hours	14 days

DS, double strength; SS, single strength.

[a]Dosing intervals for normal renal function.

Acute Uncomplicated Cystitis

Acute uncomplicated cystitis is the most common form of UTI. These infections typically occur in women of childbearing age and often are related to sexual activity. Although the presence of dysuria, frequency, urgency, and suprapubic discomfort frequently is associated with lower tract infection, a significant number of patients have upper tract involvement as well.[3] Because these infections are predominantly caused by *E. coli*, antimicrobial therapy initially should be directed against this organism. Other common causes include *S. saprophyticus* and occasionally *K. pneumoniae* and *Proteus mirabilis*. Because the causative organisms and their susceptibility generally are known, many clinicians advocate a cost-effective approach to management. This approach includes a urinalysis and initiation of empirical therapy without a urine culture (Fig. 94-1).[1] Therefore, the susceptibility patterns of the geographic area drive the choice of empiric therapy.

TABLE 94-5 Evidence-Based Empirical Treatment of Urinary Tract Infections and Prostatitis

Diagnosis	Pathogens	Treatment Recommendation	Comments
Acute uncomplicated cystitis	*Escherichia coli*, *Staphylococcus saprophyticus*	1. Nitrofurantoin × 5 days (A, I)[a] 2. Trimethoprim–sulfamethoxazole × 3 days (A, I)[a] 3. Fosfomycin × 1 dose (A, I)[a] 4. Fluoroquinolone × 3 days (A, I)[a] 5. β-Lactams × 3–7 days (B,I)[a]	Short-course therapy more effective than single dose Reserve fluoroquinolones as alternatives to development of resistance (A-III)[a] β-Lactams as a group are not as effective in acute cystitis then trimethoprim–sulfamethoxazole or the fluoroquinolones, do not use amoxicillin or ampicillin[a]
Pregnancy	As above	1. Amoxicillin–clavulanate × 7 days 2. Cephalosporin × 7 days 3. Trimethoprim–sulfamethoxazole × 7 days	Avoid trimethoprim–sulfamethoxazole during the third trimester
Acute pyelonephritis			
Uncomplicated	*E. coli*	1. Quinolone × 7 days (A, I)[a] 2. Trimethoprim–sulfamethoxazole (if susceptible) × 14 days (A,I)[a]	Can be managed as outpatient
	Gram-positive bacteria	1. Amoxicillin or amoxicillin–clavulanic acid × 14 days	
Complicated	*E. coli* *P. mirabilis* *K. pneumoniae* *P. aeruginosa* *Enterococcus faecalis*	1. Quinolone × 14 days 2. Extended-spectrum penicillin plus aminoglycoside	Severity of illness will determine duration of IV therapy; culture results should direct therapy Oral therapy may complete 14 days of therapy
Prostatitis	*E. coli* *K. pneumoniae* *Proteus* spp. *P. aeruginosa*	1. Trimethoprim–sulfamethoxazole × 4–6 weeks 2. Quinolone × 4–6 weeks	Acute prostatitis may require IV therapy initially Chronic prostatitis may require longer treatment periods or surgery

[a]Strength of recommendations: A, good evidence for; B, moderate evidence for; C, poor evidence for and against; D, moderate against; E, good evidence against. Quality of evidence: I, at least one proper randomized, controlled study; II, one well-designed clinical trial; III, evidence from opinions, clinical experience, and expert committees.

Data from reference 1.

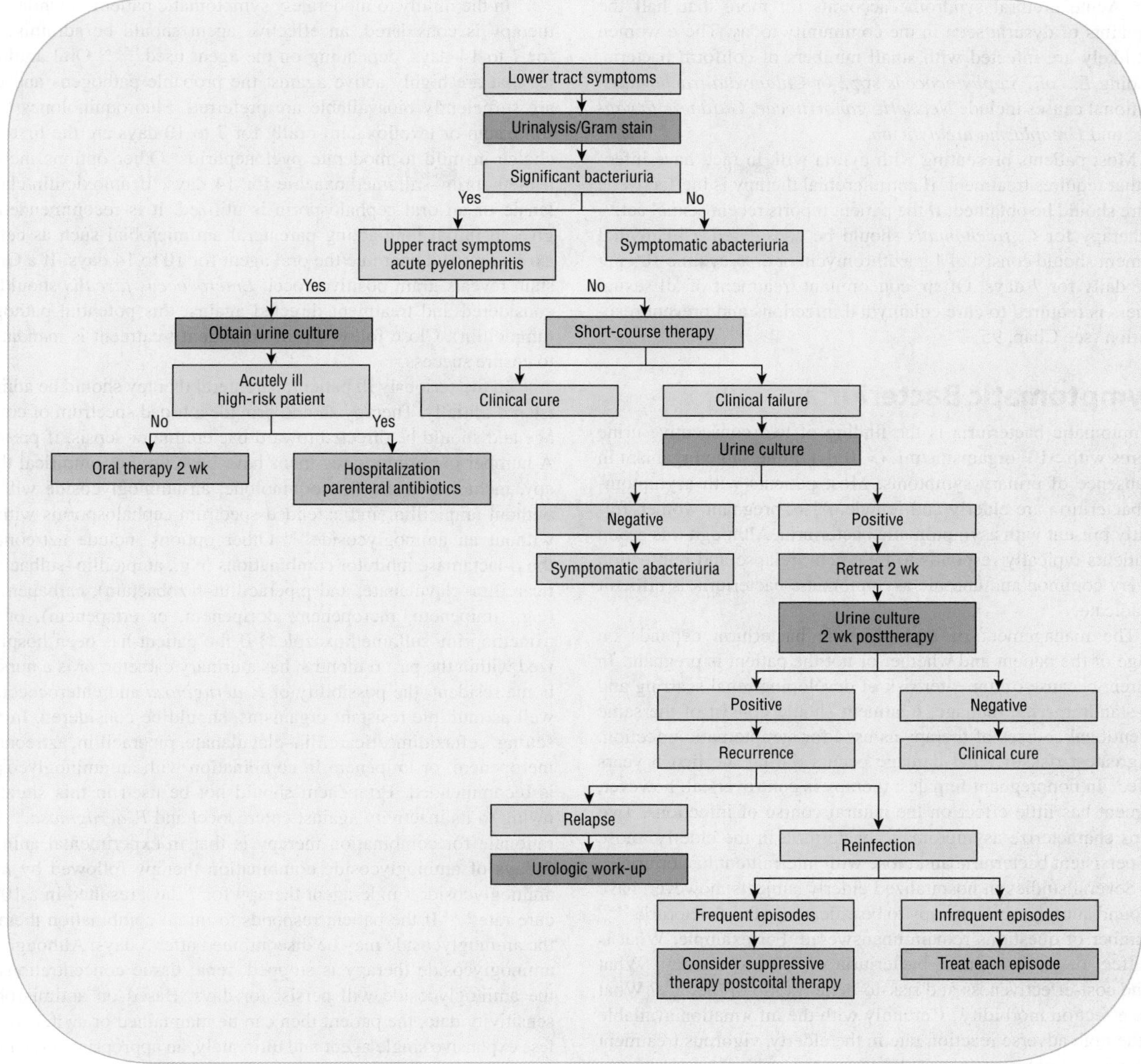

FIGURE 94-1 Management of UTIs in females.

The goal of treatment for uncomplicated cystitis is to eradicate the causative organism and to reduce the incidence of recurrence caused by relapse or reinfection. The ability to reduce the chance of recurrence depends on the agent's efficacy in eradicating the uropathogenic bacteria from the vaginal and GI reservoir. In the past, conventional therapy consisted of an effective oral antibiotic administered for 7 to 14 days. However, acute cystitis is a superficial mucosal infection that can be eradicated with much shorter courses of therapy (3 days). Advantages of short-course therapy include increased adherence, fewer side effects, decreased cost, and less potential for the development of resistance.

7 Three-day courses of trimethoprim–sulfamethoxazole or a fluoroquinolone (e.g., ciprofloxacin or levofloxacin, not moxifloxacin) are superior to single-dose therapies.[47,49–51] Although the fluoroquinolones have shown excellent efficacy in acute cystitis, the newest guidelines recommend reserving these agents for patients with suspected or possible pyelonephritis due to the collateral damage risk. Instead, a 3-day course of trimethoprim–sulfamethoxazole, a 5-day course of nitrofurantoin, or a one-time dose of fosfomycin should be considered as first-line therapy.[1,45,46,50,52] In areas where there is >20% resistance of *E. coli* to trimethoprim–sulfamethoxazole, nitrofurantoin or fosfomycin should be utilized. Amoxicillin or ampicillin should not be utilized due to the high incidence of resistant *E. coli*. Instead, if a *β*-lactam must be utilized, amoxicillin/clavulanate, cefdinir, cefaclor, or cefpodoxime proxetil for 3 to 7 days are the preferred choices. For most adult females, short-course therapy is the treatment of choice for uncomplicated lower UTIs. Short-course therapy is inappropriate for patients who have had previous infections caused by resistant bacteria, for male patients, and for patients with complicated UTIs. If symptoms recur or do not respond to therapy, a urine culture should be obtained and conventional therapy with a suitable agent instituted.[1]

Symptomatic Abacteriuria

Symptomatic abacteriuria or acute urethral syndrome represents a clinical syndrome in which females present with dysuria and pyuria, but the urine culture reveals less than 10^5 bacteria/mL (10^8/L) of urine. Acute urethral syndrome accounts for more than half the complaints of dysuria seen in the community today. These women most likely are infected with small numbers of coliform bacteria, including *E. coli*, *Staphylococcus* spp., or *Chlamydia trachomatis*. Additional causes include *Neisseria gonorrhoeae*, *Gardnerella vaginalis*, and *Ureaplasma urealyticum.*

Most patients presenting with pyuria will, in fact, have infection that requires treatment. If antimicrobial therapy is ineffective, a culture should be obtained. If the patient reports recent sexual activity, therapy for *C. trachomatis* should be considered. Chlamydial treatment should consist of 1 g azithromycin or doxycycline 100 mg twice daily for 7 days. Often, concomitant treatment of all sexual partners is required to cure chlamydial infections and prevent reacquisition (see Chap. 95).

Asymptomatic Bacteriuria

Asymptomatic bacteriuria is the finding of two consecutive urine cultures with $>10^5$ organisms/mL ($>10^8$/L) of the same organism in the absence of urinary symptoms. Most patients with asymptomatic bacteriuria are elderly and female. Also, pregnant women frequently present with asymptomatic bacteriuria. Although this group of patients typically responds to treatment, relapse and reinfection are very common and chronic asymptomatic bacteriuria is difficult to eradicate.

The management of asymptomatic bacteriuria depends on the age of the patient and whether or not the patient is pregnant. In children, because of a greater risk of developing renal scarring and long-standing renal damage, treatment should consist of the same conventional courses of therapy as used for symptomatic infection. The greatest risk of renal damage occurs during the first 5 years of life.[53] In nonpregnant females, therapy is controversial; however, treatment has little effect on the natural course of infections. Two groups characterize asymptomatic bacteriuria in the elderly: those with persistent bacteriuria and those with intermittent bacteriuria.

Several studies in hospitalized elderly subjects, however, have not found antimicrobial therapy to be efficacious for abacteruria.[54–57] A number of questions remain unanswered. For example: What is the effect of eradication of bacteriuria on life expectancy? What are the cost-effectiveness and risk-to-benefit ratio of therapy? What is the effect on morbidity? Certainly with the information available and the high adverse reaction rate in the elderly, vigorous treatment and screening programs cannot be advocated.

Complicated Urinary Tract Infections

Acute Pyelonephritis

The presentation of high-grade fever (>38.3°C [100.9°F]) and severe flank pain should be treated as acute pyelonephritis and warrants aggressive management. Severely ill patients with pyelonephritis should be hospitalized and IV antimicrobials administered initially (see Table 94-5). However, milder cases may be managed with orally administered antibiotics in an outpatient setting. Signs and symptoms of nausea, vomiting, and dehydration may require hospitalization.

At the time of presentation, a Gram stain of the urine should be performed along with a urinalysis, culture, and sensitivity tests. The Gram stain should indicate the morphology of the infecting organism(s) and help to direct the selection of an appropriate antibiotic. However, the precise identity and susceptibility of the infecting organism(s) will be unknown initially, warranting empirical therapy. The goals of treatment include the achievement of therapeutic concentrations of an antimicrobial agent in the bloodstream and urinary tract to which the invading organism is susceptible and sufficient therapy to eradicate residual infection in the tissues of the urinary tract.

In the mildly to moderately symptomatic patient in whom oral therapy is considered, an effective agent should be administered for 7 to 14 days, depending on the agent used.[1,58–63] Oral antibiotics that are highly active against the probable pathogens and that are sufficiently bioavailable are preferred. Fluoroquinolones (ciprofloxacin or levofloxacin) orally for 7 to 10 days are the first-line choice in mild to moderate pyelonephritis. Other options include trimethoprim–sulfamethoxazole for 14 days. If amoxicillin/clavulanate or an oral cephalosporin is utilized, it is recommended to give an initial long-acting parenteral antimicrobial such as ceftriaxone first and continue the oral agent for 10 to 14 days. If a Gram stain reveals gram-positive cocci, *Enterococcus faecalis* should be considered and treatment directed against this potential pathogen (ampicillin). Close follow-up of outpatient treatment is mandatory to ensure success.

In the seriously ill patient, parenteral therapy should be administered initially. Therapy should provide a broad spectrum of coverage and should be directed toward bacteremia or sepsis, if present. A number of antibiotic regimens have been used as empirical therapy, including an IV fluoroquinolone, an aminoglycoside with or without ampicillin, and extended-spectrum cephalosporins with or without an aminoglycoside.[1,64] Other options include aztreonam, the β-lactamase inhibitor combinations (e.g., ampicillin–sulbactam, ticarcillin–clavulanate, and piperacillin–tazobactam), carbapenems (e.g., imipenem, meropenem, doripenem, or ertapenem), or IV trimethoprim–sulfamethoxazole.[65] If the patient has been hospitalized within the past 6 months, has a urinary catheter, or is a nursing home resident, the possibility of *P. aeruginosa* and enterococci, as well as multiple resistant organisms, should be considered. In this setting, ceftazidime, ticarcillin–clavulanate, piperacillin, aztreonam, meropenem, or imipenem in combination with an aminoglycoside is recommended. Ertapenem should not be used in this situation owing to its inactivity against enterococci and *P. aeruginosa*.[64] The rationale for combination therapy is that in experimental animals 3 days of aminoglycoside combination therapy followed by non-aminoglycoside single-agent therapy for 7 days resulted in a 100% cure rate.[58,63] If the patient responds to initial combination therapy, the aminoglycoside may be discontinued after 3 days. Although the aminoglycoside therapy is stopped, renal tissue concentrations of the aminoglycoside will persist for days. Based on antimicrobial sensitivity data, the patient then can be maintained or switched to a less expensive single agent and ultimately, an appropriate oral agent may be used.

Effective therapy should stabilize the patient within 12 to 24 hours. A significant reduction in urine bacterial concentrations should occur in 48 hours. If bacteriologic response has not occurred, an alternative agent should be considered based on susceptibility testing. If the patient fails to respond clinically within 3 to 4 days or has persistently positive blood or urine cultures, further investigation is needed to exclude bacterial resistance, possible obstruction, papillary necrosis, intrarenal or perinephric abscess, or some other disease process. Usually by the third day of therapy, the patient is afebrile and significantly less symptomatic. In general, after the patient has been afebrile for 24 hours, parenteral therapy may be discontinued and oral therapy instituted to complete a 2-week course. Follow-up urine cultures should be obtained 2 weeks after completion of therapy to ensure a satisfactory response and detect possible relapse.

Urinary Tract Infections in Males

The management of UTIs in males is distinctly different and often more difficult than in females. Infections in male patients are considered to be complicated because endogenous bacteria in the presence of functional and/or structural abnormalities that disrupt the normal defense mechanisms of the urinary tract cause them. The incidence of infections in males younger than 60 years of age is much less than

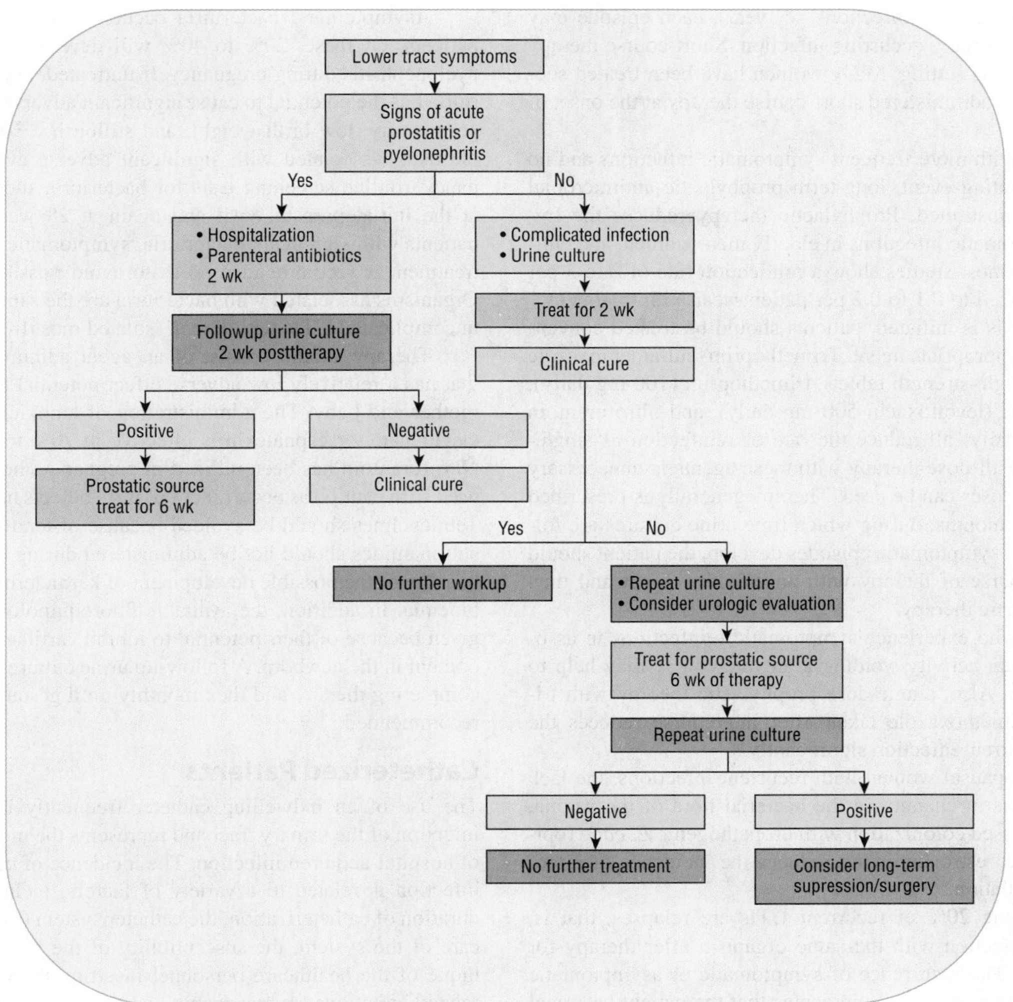

FIGURE 94-2 Management of UTIs in males.

the incidence in females. During the adult years, the occurrence of infection can be related directly to some manipulation of the urinary tract. The most common causes are instrumentation of the urinary tract, catheterization, and renal and urinary stones. Uncomplicated infections are rare, but they may occur in young males as a result of homosexual activity, noncircumcision, and having sex with partners who are colonized with uropathogenic bacteria. As the patient ages, the most common cause of infection is related to bladder outlet obstruction because of prostatic hypertrophy. In addition, the prostate gland may become infected and provide a nidus for recurrent infection in males.

The conventional view is that therapy in males requires prolonged treatment (Fig. 94-2). A urine culture should be obtained before treatment because the cause of infection in men is not as predictable as in women. Single-dose or short-course therapy is not recommended in males. Considerably fewer data are available comparing various antimicrobial agents in males as compared with females. If gram-negative bacteria are presumed, trimethoprim–sulfamethoxazole or the quinolone antimicrobials should be considered because these agents achieve high renal tissue, urine, and prostatic concentrations.[66]

Initial therapy should be for 10 to 14 days. Factors associated with treatment success are isolation of a single organism, the absence of significant obstruction or anatomic abnormalities, a normally functioning urinary tract, and the absence of prostatic involvement. Parenteral therapy may be required in certain situations, such as in severely ill patients, in the presence of acute prostatitis or epididymitis and in patients who cannot tolerate oral medications. A comparison of 2-week versus 6-week therapy in males with recurrent infections who were given trimethoprim–sulfamethoxazole had cure rates of 29% and 62%, respectively.[67] Other investigators advocate longer treatment periods in males, as well.[68] Follow-up cultures at 4 to 6 weeks after treatment are important in males to ensure bacteriologic cure. Many patients require longer periods of treatment and possible alterations in antibiotics, depending on culture and sensitivity results and clinical response.

Recurrent Infections

Recurrent episodes of UTI account for a significant portion of all UTIs. Of the patients suffering from recurrent infections, 80% can be considered reinfections, that is, the recurrence of infection by an organism different from the organism isolated from the preceding infection. These patients most commonly are female and recurrence develops in approximately 20% of females with cystitis. Reinfections can be divided into two groups: those with less than three episodes per year and those who develop more frequent infections.

Management strategies depend on predisposing factors, number of episodes per year, and the patient's preference. Factors commonly associated with recurrent infections include sexual intercourse and diaphragm or spermicide use for birth control. Therapeutic options include self-administered therapy, postcoital therapy, and continuous low-dose prophylaxis. In patients with infrequent infections (less than three infections per year), each episode may be treated as a separately occurring infection. Short-course therapy is appropriate in this setting. Many women have been treated successfully with self-administered short-course therapy at the onset of symptoms.[36,69]

In patients with more frequent symptomatic infections and no apparent precipitating event, long-term prophylactic antimicrobial therapy may be instituted. Prophylactic therapy reduces the frequency of symptomatic infections in elderly men, women, and children. In women, most studies show a reinfection rate of 2 to 3 per patient-year reduced to 0.1 to 0.2 per patient-year with treatment.[69] Before prophylaxis is initiated, patients should be treated conventionally with an appropriate agent. Trimethoprim–sulfamethoxazole (one-half of a single-strength tablet), trimethoprim (100 mg daily), a fluoroquinolone (levofloxacin 500 mg daily), and nitrofurantoin (50 or 100 mg daily) all reduce the rate of reinfection as single-agent therapy.[69] Full-dose therapy with these agents is unnecessary and single daily doses can be used. Therapy generally is prescribed for a period of 6 months, during which time urine cultures are followed monthly. If symptomatic episodes develop, the patient should receive a full course of therapy with an effective agent and then resume prophylactic therapy.

In women who experience symptomatic reinfections in association with sexual activity, voiding after intercourse may help to prevent infection. Also, single-dose prophylactic therapy with trimethoprim–sulfamethoxazole taken after intercourse reduces the incidence of recurrent infection significantly.[69]

In postmenopausal women with recurrent infections, the lack of estrogen results in changes in the bacterial flora of the vagina, resulting in increased colonization with uropathogenic *E. coli*. Topically administered estrogen cream reduces the incidence of infections in this population.[18,19]

The remaining 20% of recurrent UTIs are relapses, that is, persistence of infection with the same organism after therapy for an isolated UTI. The recurrence of symptomatic or asymptomatic bacteriuria after therapy usually indicates that the patient has renal involvement, a structural abnormality of the urinary tract or chronic bacterial prostatitis. In the absence of structural abnormalities, relapse often is related to renal infection and requires a long duration of treatment. Women who relapse after short-course therapy should receive a 2-week course of therapy. In patients who relapse after 2 weeks of therapy, therapy should be continued for another 2 to 4 weeks. If relapse occurs after 6 weeks of therapy, urologic evaluation should be performed and any obstructive lesion should be corrected. If this is not possible, therapy for 6 months or longer may be considered. Asymptomatic adults who have no evidence of urinary obstruction should not receive long-term therapy.

In males, relapse usually indicates bacterial prostatitis, the most common cause of persistent bacteriuria. Although many agents have been used for long-term therapy of relapses, trimethoprim–sulfamethoxazole and the fluoroquinolones appear to be highly effective.

Special Conditions

UTIs in Pregnancy

During pregnancy, significant physiologic changes occur to the entire urinary tract that dramatically alter the prevalence of UTIs and pyelonephritis. Severe dilation of the renal pelvis and ureters, decreased ureteral peristalsis, and reduced bladder tone occur during pregnancy.[70] These changes result in urinary stasis and reduced defenses against reflux of bacteria to the kidneys. In addition, increased urine content of amino acids, vitamins, and nutrients encourages bacterial growth. All of these factors increase the incidence of bacteriuria resulting in symptomatic infections, especially during the third trimester.

Asymptomatic bacteriuria occurs in 4% to 7% of pregnant patients. Of these, 20% to 40% will develop acute symptomatic pyelonephritis during pregnancy. If untreated, asymptomatic bacteriuria has the potential to cause significant adverse effects, including prematurity, low birth weight, and stillbirth.[71,72] Because pyelonephritis is associated with significant adverse events during pregnancy, routine screening tests for bacteriuria should be performed at the initial prenatal visit and again at 28 weeks' gestation. In patients with significant bacteriuria, symptomatic or asymptomatic, treatment is recommended so as to avoid possible complications. Organisms associated with bacteriuria are the same as those seen in uncomplicated UTIs with *E. coli* isolated most frequently.

Therapy should consist of an agent administered for 7 days that has a relatively low adverse effect potential and is safe for the mother and baby. The administration of amoxicillin, amoxicillin–clavulanate, or cephalexin is effective in 70% to 80% of patients. Nitrofurantoin has been utilized in pregnancy; however, it must be used with caution as occurrences of birth defects have been reported. Tetracyclines should be avoided because of teratogenic effects and sulfonamides should not be administered during the third trimester because of the possible development of kernicterus and hyperbilirubinemia. In addition, the available fluoroquinolones should not be given because of their potential to inhibit cartilage and bone development in the newborn. A follow-up urine culture 1 to 2 weeks after completing therapy and then monthly until gestation is complete is recommended.

Catheterized Patients

The use of an indwelling catheter frequently is associated with infection of the urinary tract and represents the most common cause of hospital-acquired infection. The incidence of catheter-associated infection is related to a variety of factors, including method and duration of catheterization, the catheter system (open or closed), the care of the system, the susceptibility of the patient, and the technique of the healthcare personnel inserting the catheter. Catheter-related infections are reasonably preventable infections and are now considered one of the hospital-acquired complications chosen by the Centers for Medicare and Medicaid Services (CMS) in which hospitals will no longer receive reimbursement for treatment.[73,74]

Bacteria may enter the bladder in a number of ways. During the catheterization, bacteria may be introduced directly into the bladder from the urethra. Once the catheter is in place, bacteria may pass up the lumen of the catheter via the movement of air bubbles, by motility of the bacteria, or by capillary action. In addition, bacteria may reach the bladder from around the exudative sheath that surrounds the catheter in the urethra. Cleaning the periurethral area thoroughly and applying an antiseptic (povidone-iodine) can minimize infection occurring during insertion of the catheter. The use of closed drainage systems has reduced significantly the ability of bacteria to pass up the lumen of the catheter and cause infection. Presently, a bacterium passing around the catheter sheath in the urethra is probably the most important pathway for infection. Avoiding manipulation of the catheter and trauma to the urethra and urethral meatus can minimize this path of acquisition.

Patients with indwelling catheters acquire UTIs at a rate of 5% per day.[73–75] The closed systems are capable of preventing bacteriuria in most patients for up to 10 days with appropriate care. After 30 days of catheterization, however, there is a 78% to 95% incidence of bacteriuria, despite use of a closed system.[74,76] Unfortunately, UTI symptoms in catheterized patient are not clearly defined. Fever, peripheral leukocytosis, and urinary signs and symptoms may be of little predictive value.[73,74] When bacteriuria occurs in the asymptomatic, short-term catheterized patient (<30 days), the use of systemic antibiotics should be withheld and the catheter removed as soon as possible. If the patient becomes symptomatic, the catheter should be removed and treatment as described for complicated infections started. The optimal duration of therapy is unknown. In the long-term catheterized patient (>30 days), bacteriuria is inevitable.[73,74] The administration of systemic antibiotics active against the infecting organism will sterilize the urine; however, reinfection occurs rapidly in more than 50% of patients. In addition, resistant organisms recolonize the urine. Symptomatic patients must be treated because they are at risk of developing pyelonephritis and bacteremia. Bacteria adhere to the catheter and produce a biofilm consisting of bacterial glycocalyces, Tamm–Horsfall protein, as well as apatite and struvite salts, that act to protect the bacteria from antibiotics.[75] Recatheterization with a new sterile unit should be performed in those symptomatic patients, if the existing catheter has been in place for more than 2 weeks.

Various methods have been proposed to prevent the development of bacteriuria and infection in the patient with an indwelling catheter (see Table 94-5). The success of these methods depends on the type of catheter and the length of time it is in place. The use of constant bladder irrigation with antiseptic or antibacterial solutions reduces the incidence of infection in those with open drainage systems, but this approach has no advantage in those with closed systems. The use of prophylactic systemic antibiotics in patients with short-term catheterization reduces the incidence of infection over the first 4 to 7 days.[74,76] In long-term catheterized patients, however, antibiotics only postpone the development of bacteriuria and lead to the emergence of resistant organisms. Therefore, antibiotic prophylaxis should not be utilized in short-term or long-term catheterized patients.

PROSTATITIS

Bacterial prostatitis is an inflammation of the prostate gland and surrounding tissue as a result of infection. It is classified as either acute or chronic. By definition, pathogenic bacteria and significant inflammatory cells must be present in prostatic secretions and urine to make the diagnosis of bacterial prostatitis. Prostatitis occurs rarely in young males, but it is commonly associated with recurrent infections in persons older than 30 years of age. As many as 50% of all males develop some form of prostatitis at some period in their life.[77–79] The acute form typically is an acute infectious disease characterized by a sudden onset of fever, tenderness, and urinary and constitutional symptoms. Chronic prostatitis presents with few symptoms related to the prostate but rather symptoms of urinating difficulty, low back pain, perineal pressure, or a combination of these. It represents a recurring infection with the same organism that results from incomplete eradication of bacteria from the prostate gland.

Pathogenesis and Etiology

The exact mechanism of bacterial infection of the prostate is not well understood. The possible routes of infection are the same as those for UTIs. Reflux of infected urine into the prostate gland is thought to play an important role in causing infection. Intraprostatic reflux of urine occurs commonly and results in direct inoculation of infected urine into the prostate.[77–79] In addition, intraprostatic reflux of sterile urine can result in a chemical prostatitis and may be the cause of nonbacterial prostatitis. Sexual intercourse may contribute to infection of the prostate gland because prostatic secretions from men with chronic prostatitis and vaginal cultures from their sexual partners grow identical organisms. Other known causes of bacterial prostatitis include indwelling urethral and condom catheterization, urethral instrumentation, and transurethral prostatectomy in patients with infected urine.

Physiologic factors are believed to contribute to the development of prostatitis. Functional abnormalities found in bacterial prostatitis include altered prostate secretory functions. Prostatic fluid obtained from normal males contains prostatic antibacterial factor. This heat-stable, low-molecular-weight cation is a zinc-complexed polypeptide that is bactericidal to most urinary tract pathogens.[80] The antibacterial activity of prostatic antibacterial factor is related directly to the zinc content of prostatic fluid. Prostate fluid zinc levels and prostatic antibacterial factor activity also appear diminished in patients with prostatitis, as well as in the elderly.[80] Whether these changes are a cause or effect of prostatitis remains to be determined.

The pH of prostatic secretions in patients with prostatitis is altered.[81] Normal prostatic secretions have a pH in the range of 6.6 to 7.6. With increasing age, the pH tends to become more alkaline. In patients with inflammation of the prostate, prostatic secretions may have an alkaline pH in the range of 7 to 9. These changes suggest a generalized secretory dysfunction of the prostate that not only can affect the pathogenesis of prostatitis but also can influence the mode of therapy.

Gram-negative enteric organisms are the most frequent pathogens in acute bacterial prostatitis.[77–79] *E. coli* is the predominant organism, occurring in 75% of cases. Other gram-negative organisms frequently isolated include *K. pneumoniae*, *P. mirabilis*, and less frequently, *P. aeruginosa*, *Enterobacter* spp., and *Serratia* spp. Infrequently, cases of gonococcal and staphylococcal prostatitis occur.

E. coli most commonly causes chronic bacterial prostatitis with other gram-negative organisms isolated less frequently. The importance of gram-positive organisms in chronic bacterial prostatitis remains controversial. *S. epidermidis*, *S. aureus*, and diphtheroids have been isolated in some studies.

Clinical Presentation

Acute bacterial prostatitis presents as other acute infections (Table 94-6). Massage of the prostate will express a purulent discharge that will readily grow the pathogenic organism. Prostatic massage is contraindicated in acute bacterial prostatitis, however, because of the risk of inducing bacteremia and the associated local pain. The diagnosis of acute bacterial prostatitis can be made from the patient's clinical presentation and the presence of significant bacteriuria. As with other UTIs, the infecting organism can be isolated from a midstream specimen.

In contrast, chronic bacterial prostatitis is more difficult to diagnose and treat. Chronic bacterial prostatitis typically is characterized by recurrent UTIs with the same pathogen and is the most common cause of recurrent UTI in males. The patient's clinical presentation can vary widely (see Table 94-6). Many adults, however, are asymptomatic.

Because physical examination of the prostate is often normal, urinary tract localization studies are critical to the diagnosis

TABLE 94-6 Clinical Presentation of Bacterial Prostatitis

Signs and symptoms
Acute bacterial prostatitis: high fever, chills, malaise, myalgia, localized pain (perineal, rectal, sacrococcygeal), frequency, urgency, dysuria, nocturia, and retention
Chronic bacterial prostatitis: voiding difficulties (frequency, urgency, dysuria), low back pain, and perineal and suprapubic discomfort

Physical examination
Acute bacterial prostatitis: swollen, tender, tense, or indurated gland
Chronic bacterial prostatitis: boggy, indurated (enlarged) prostate in most patients

Laboratory tests
Bacteriuria
Bacteria in expressed prostatic secretions

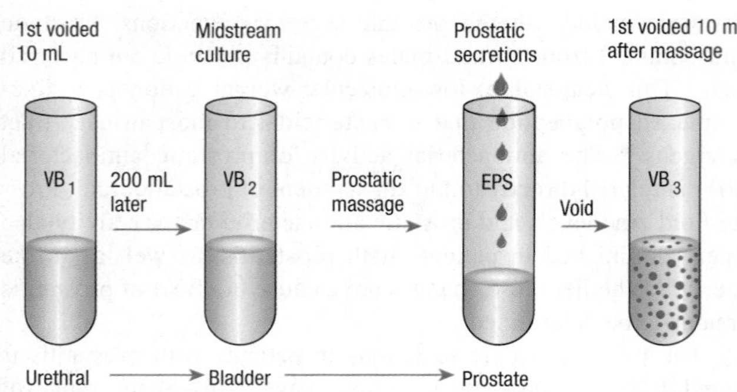

FIGURE 94-3 Segmented cultures of the lower tract in men. (EPS, expressed prostatic secretions; VB_1, voiding bladder 1; VB_2, voiding bladder 2; VB_3, voiding bladder 3.)

of chronic bacterial prostatitis. The method of quantitative localization culture, as described by Meares and Stamey,[15,82] remains the diagnostic standard (Fig. 94-3). The method compares the bacterial growth in sequential urine and prostatic fluid cultures obtained during micturition. The first 10 mL of voided urine is collected (voiding bladder 1, or VB_1) and constitutes urethral urine. After approximately 200 mL of urine has been voided, a 10-mL midstream sample is collected (VB_2). This specimen represents bladder urine. After the patient voids, the prostate is massaged and expressed prostatic secretions (EPS) are collected. After prostatic massage, the patient voids again and 10 mL of urine is collected (VB_3).

The diagnosis of bacterial prostatitis is made when the number of bacteria in EPS is 10 times that of the urethral sample (VB_1) and midstream sample (VB_2). If no EPS is available, the urine sample following massage (VB_3) should contain a bacterial count 10-fold greater than that of VB_1 or VB_2. If significant bacteriuria is present, ampicillin, cephalexin, or nitrofurantoin should be given for 2 to 3 days to sterilize the urine prior to performing the localization study.

Treatment

9 In general, the goals in the management of bacterial prostatitis are the same as those for UTIs. Acute bacterial prostatitis responds well to appropriate antimicrobial therapy that is directed at the most commonly isolated organisms. Prostatic penetration of antimicrobials occurs because the acute inflammatory reaction alters the cellular membrane barrier between the bloodstream and the prostate. Most patients can be managed with oral antimicrobial agents, such as trimethoprim–sulfamethoxazole and the fluoroquinolones (e.g., ciprofloxacin, levofloxacin) (see Table 94-5). Other effective agents in this setting include cephalosporins and β-lactam–β-lactamase combinations. Although IV therapy is rarely necessary for total treatment, IV to oral sequential therapy with trimethoprim–sulfamethoxazole or the fluoroquinolones is appropriate. The conversion to an oral antibiotic can be considered after the patient is afebrile for 48 hours or after 3 to 5 days of IV therapy. The total course of antibiotic therapy should be 4 weeks in order to reduce the risk of development of chronic prostatitis, although in some cases 2 weeks may be sufficient. Therapy may be prolonged with chronic prostatitis (6 to 12 weeks). Long-term suppressive therapy also may be initiated for recurrent infections, such as three times weekly ciprofloxacin, trimethoprim–sulfamethoxazole regular-strength tablet daily, or nitrofurantoin 100 mg daily.[82]

Chronic bacterial prostatitis often presents a more vexing situation because cures are obtained rarely. Despite high serum concentrations of antibacterial drugs in excess of the minimal inhibitory concentrations of the infecting organisms, bacteria persist in prostatic fluid. Most likely the failure to eradicate sensitive bacteria is caused by the inability of antibiotics to reach sufficient concentrations in the prostatic fluid and cross the prostatic epithelium.

Several factors that determine antibiotic diffusion into prostatic secretions were delineated from the canine model. Lipid solubility is a major determinant in the ability of drugs to diffuse from plasma across epithelial membranes. The degree of ionization in plasma also affects the diffusion of drugs. Only unionized molecules can cross the lipid barrier of prostatic cells, and the drug's pK_a (negative logarithm of acid ionization constant) directly determines the fraction of unchanged drug.

The pH gradient across the membrane has an influence on tissue penetration, as well. A pH gradient of at least one pH unit between separate compartments allows for ion trapping. As the unionized drug crosses the epithelial barrier into prostatic fluid, it becomes ionized allowing less drug to diffuse back across the lipid barrier. In early studies with the canine model, the prostatic pH was reported to be acidic (6.4).[81] In humans, however, the pH of prostatic secretions from an inflamed prostate is actually basic (8.1 to 8.3).[81]

The choice of antibiotics in chronic bacterial prostatitis should include agents that are capable of reaching therapeutic concentrations in the prostatic fluid and which possess the spectrum of activity to be effective. Agents that achieve therapeutic prostatic concentrations include trimethoprim and the fluoroquinolones. Sulfamethoxazole penetrates poorly and probably contributes very little to trimethoprim activity when used in combination. The fluoroquinolones appear to provide the best therapeutic options in the management of chronic bacterial prostatitis. Therapy should be continued for 4 to 6 weeks initially. Longer treatment periods may be necessary in some cases. If therapy fails with these regimens, chronic suppressive therapy may be used or surgery considered.

PERSONALIZED PHARMACOTHERAPY

Patient-centered pharmacotherapy and management of UTIs require knowledge of the pathogenesis and causative organisms associated with the various clinical syndromes described in this chapter. Individualizing the antimicrobial therapy will depend on many factors, first and foremost being the susceptibility of the offending pathogen. As was discussed in the chapter, *E. coli* resistance is continuing to increase, therefore it is imperative for the healthcare professional to be familiar with the resistance trends in their geographical area when prescribing therapy. In addition, the prevention of increasing resistance and collateral damage should be considered when selecting antimicrobial therapy.[1] Other factors to consider in selecting therapy would be a patient's allergies and recent antimicrobial exposure. Lastly, cost may factor into compliance enhancing the effectiveness of therapy. The costs include both direct and indirect costs associated with treatment.

Direct costs are those associated with diagnosis, treatment, and follow-up. The cost of pharmaceuticals varies according to the agents used and the duration of therapy. Trimethoprim–sulfamethoxazole and amoxicillin–clavulanate are rather inexpensive. However, when considering rates of resistance leading to therapeutic failure, overall costs increase dramatically. The fluoroquinolones also are highly effective agents, but generally are more expensive and a rise in their utilization is now being associated with increasing resistance.[64,83] In general, the outcome and total cost depend on whether therapy is empirical or definitive (based on a culture diagnosis for acute infection) and if the individual patient is adherent with the regimen. As a healthcare professional, working with and counseling the individual patient in order to select an appropriate therapy is essential in achieving positive therapeutic outcomes.

ABBREVIATIONS

CFU colony-forming unit
EPS expressed prostatic secretions
PMN polymorphonuclear leukocyte
UTI urinary tract infection
WBC white blood cell

REFERENCES

1. Gupta K, Hooton TM, Naber KG, et al. International clinical practice guidelines for the treatment of acute uncomplicated cystitis and pyelonephritis in women: A 2010 update by the Infectious Diseases Society of America and the European Society for Microbiology and Infectious Diseases. Clin Infect Dis 2011;52(5):e103–e120.
2. Naber KG, Cho YH, Matsumoto T, et al. Immunoactive prophylaxis of recurrent urinary tract infections: A meta-analysis. Int J Antimicrob Agents 2009;33:111–119.
3. Kallen AJ, Welch HG, Sirovich BE. Current antibiotic therapy for isolated urinary tract infections in women. Arch Intern Med 2006;166:635–639.
4. Nicolle LE. Uncomplicated urinary tract infection in adults including uncomplicated pyelonephritis. Urol Clin North Am 2008;35:1–12.
5. Little P, Turner S, Rumsby K, et al. Developing clinical rules to predict urinary tract infection in primary care settings: Sensitivity and specificity of near patient tests (dipsticks) and clinical scores. Br J Gen Pract 2006;56:606–612.
6. Platt R. Quantitative definition of bacteriuria. Am J Med 1983;75:44–52.
7. Alper BS, Curry SH. Urinary tract infection in children. Am Fam Physician 2005;72(12):2483–2488.
8. Habib S. Highlights for management of a child with a urinary tract infection. Int J Pediatr 2012; Epub Jul 19.
9. Sobel JD, Kaye D. Urinary tract infections. In: Mandell GL, Bennett JE, Dolin R, eds. Principles and Practice of Infectious Diseases, 7th ed. New York: Churchill-Livingstone, 2009:957–985.
10. Shortliffe LM, McCue JD. Urinary tract infections at the age extremes: Pediatrics and geriatrics. Am J Med 2002;113(Suppl 1A):55S–66S.
11. Nicolle L, Anderson PAM, Conly J, et al. Uncomplicated urinary tract infection in women, current practice and the effect of antibiotic resistance on empiric treatment. Can Fam Phys 2006;52:612–618.
12. Shigemura K, Arakawa S, Tanaka K, et al. Clinical investigation of isolated bacteria from urinary tracts of hospitalized patients and their susceptibilities to antibiotics. J Infect Chemother 2009;15:18–22.
13. Heintz BH, Haliloric J, Christensen CL. Vancomycin resistant enterococcal urinary tract infections. Clin Infect Dis 2010;30(11):1136–1149.
14. Stamatiou C, Bovis C, Panagopoulos P, Petrakos G, Economou A, Lycoudt A. Sex-induced cystitis—Patient burden and other epidemiological features. Clin Exp Obstet Gynecol 2005;32(13):180–182.
15. Stamey TA, Fair WR, Timothy MM, et al. Antibacterial nature of prostatic fluid. Nature 1968;218:444–447.
16. Shand DG, Nimmon CC, O'Grady F, et al. Relation between residual urine volume and response to treatment of urinary infection. Lancet 1970;1:1305–1306.
17. Parsons CL, Schrom SH, Hanno P, et al. Bladder surface mucin: Examination of possible mechanisms for its antibacterial effect. Invest Urol 1978;6:196–200.
18. Raz R, Stamm WE. A controlled trial of intravaginal estriol in post-menopausal women with recurrent urinary tract infections. N Engl J Med 1993;329:753–756.
19. Stamm WE. Estrogens and urinary tract infection. J Infect Dis 2007;195:623–624.
20. Orskov I, Ferencz A, Orskov F. Tamm–Horsfall protein or uromucoid is the normal urinary slime that traps type-1 fimbriated *Escherichia coli*. Lancet 1980;1:887.
21. Measley RE, Levison ME. Host defense mechanisms in the pathogenesis of urinary tract infection. Med Clin North Am 1991;75:275–286.
22. Jenkins RD, Fenn JP, Matsen JM. Review of urine microscopy for bacteriuria. JAMA 1986;255:3397–3403.
23. Pezzlo M. Detection of urinary tract infections by rapid methods. Clin Microbiol Rev 1988;2:268–280.
24. Stamm WE. Measurement of pyuria and its relation to bacteriuria. Am J Med 1983;75(Suppl 1):53–58.
25. Pappas PG. Laboratory in the diagnosis and management of urinary tract infections. Med Clin North Am 1991;75:313–325.
26. St John A, Boyd JC, Lowes AJ, Price CP. The use of urinary dipstick tests to exclude urinary tract infection: A systematic review of the literature. Am J Clin Pathol 2006;126(3):428–436.
27. Nys S, van Merode T, Bartelds AIM, et al. Urinary tract infections in general practice patients: Diagnostic tests versus bacteriological culture. J Antimicrob Chemother 2006;57:955–958.
28. Stamey TA, Govan DE, Palmer JM. The localization and treatment of urinary tract infections: The role of bactericidal urine levels as opposed to serum levels. Medicine (Baltimore) 1965;44:1–36.
29. Fairley KF, Bond AG, Brown RB, et al. Simple test to determine the site of urinary tract infection. Lancet 1967;2:427–428.
30. Thomas VC, Forland M. Antibody-coated bacteria in urinary tract infection. Kidney Int 1982;21:1–7.
31. Stamey TA, Fair WR, Timothy MM, et al. Serum versus urinary antimicrobial concentrations in cure of urinary tract infections. N Engl J Med 1974;291:1159–1163.
32. Barbosa-Cesnik C, Brown MB, Buxton M, et al. Cranberry juice fails to prevent recurrent urinary tract infection: Results from a randomized placebo-controlled trial. Clin Infect Dis 2011;52(1):23–30.
33. Barrons R, Tassone D. Use of *Lactobacillus* probiotics for bacterial genitourinary infections in women: A review. Clin Ther 2008;30(3):453–468.
34. Gaines KK. Phenazopyridine hydrochloride: The use and abuse of an old Standby for UTI. Urol Nurs 2004;24(3):207–209.
35. Zelenitsky S, Zhanel G. Phenazopyridine in urinary tract infections. Ann Pharmacother 1996;30:866–868.
36. Masson P, Matheson S, Webster AC. Meta-analyses in prevention and treatment of urinary tract infections. Infect Dis Clin North Am 2009;23:355–385.
37. Olson RP, Harrell LJ, Kaye KS. Antibiotic resistance in urinary isolates of *Escherichia coli* from college women with urinary tract infections. Antimicrob Agents Chemother 2009;53(3):1285–1286.
38. Colgan R, Johnson JR, Kuskowski M, Gupta K. Risk factors for trimethoprim–sulfamethoxazole resistance in patients with acute uncomplicated cystitis. Antimicrob Agents Chemother 2008;52:846–851.
39. Bergman M, Nyberg ST, Huovinen P, et al. Association between antimicrobial consumption and resistance

in *Escherichia coli*. Antimicrob Agents Chemother 2009;53(3):912–917.
40. Talan DA, Krishnadasan A, Abrahamian FM, et al. Prevalence and risk factor analysis of trimethoprim–sulfamethoxazole and fluoroquinolone-resistant *Escherichia coli* infection among emergency department patients with pyelonephritis. Clin Infect Dis 2008;47:1150–1158.
41. Paterson DL. "Collateral damage" from cephalosporin or quinolone antibiotic therapy. Clin Infect Dis 2004;38 (Suppl 4):S341–S345.
42. Karlowsky JA, Hoban DJ, DeCarby MR, Laing NM, Zhanel GG. Fluoroquinolone-resistant urinary isolates of *Escherichia coli* from outpatients are frequently multi-drug resistant: Results from the North American urinary tract infection collaborative. Antimicrob Agents Chemother 2006;50:2251–2254.
43. Johnson L, Sabel A, Burman WJ, et al. Emergence of fluoroquinolone resistance in outpatient urinary *Escherichia coli* isolates. Am J Med 2008;121(10):876–884.
44. Wagenlehner FME, Weidner W, Naber KG. An update on uncomplicated urinary tract infections in women. Curr Opin Urol 2009;19:368–374.
45. Kashanian J, Hakimian P, Blute M, et al. Nitrofurantoin: The return of an old friend in the wake of growing resistance. BJU Int 2008;102:1634–1637.
46. Knottnerus BJ, Nys S, ter Riet G, et al. Fosfomycin tromethamine as a second agent for the treatment of acute, uncomplicated urinary tract infections in adult female patients in the Netherlands? J Antimicrob Chemother 2008;62:356–359.
47. Tice AD. Short course therapy of acute cystitis: A brief review of therapeutic strategies. J Antimicrob Chemother 1999;43(Suppl A):85–93.
48. Stein GE. Comparison of single-dose fosfomycin and a 7-day course of nitrofurantoin in female patients with uncomplicated urinary tract infections. Clin Ther 1999;21:1864–1872.
49. Cox CE, Marbury TC, Pittman WG, et al. A randomized, double-blind, multicenter comparison of gatifloxacin versus ciprofloxacin in the treatment of complicated urinary tract infection and pyelonephritis. Clin Ther 2002;24:223–236.
50. Irvani A, Klimberg I, Briefer C, et al. A trial comparing low-dose, short-course ciprofloxacin and standard 7-day therapy with cotrimoxazole or nitrofurantoin in the treatment of uncomplicated urinary tract infections. J Antimicrob Chemother 1999;43(Suppl A):67–75.
51. Stass H, Kubitza D. Pharmacokinetics and elimination of moxifloxacin after oral and intravenous administration in man. J Antimicrob Chemother 1999;43(Suppl B):83–90.
52. Gupta K, Hooton TM, Roberts PL, et al. Short-course nitrofurantoin for the treatment of acute uncomplicated cystitis in women. Arch Intern Med 2007;167(20):2207–2212.
53. Chang SL, Shortliffe LD. Pediatric urinary tract infections. Pediatr Clin North Am 2006;53(3):379–400.
54. Nicolle LE, Bradley S, Colgan R, et al. Infectious disease society of America guidelines for diagnosis and treatment of asymptomatic bacteriuria in adults. Clin Infect Dis 2005;40:643–654.
55. U.S. Preventive Services Task Force. Screening for asymptomatic bacteriuria in adults: U.S. Preventive Services Task Force Reaffirmation Recommendation Statement. Ann Intern Med 2008;149:43–47.
56. Juthani-Mehta M, Quagliarello V, Perrelli E, et al. Clinical features to identify urinary tract infection in nursing home residents: A cohort study. J Am Geriatr Soc 2009;57:963–970.
57. Nicolle LE, Bjornson J, Harding GKM, et al. Bacteriuria in elderly institutionalized men. N Engl J Med 1983;309:1420–1425.
58. Neal DE. Complicated urinary tract infections. Urol Clin North Am 2008;35:13–22.
59. Talan DA, Stamm WE, Hooton TM, et al. Comparison of ciprofloxacin (7 days) and trimethoprim–sulfamethoxazole (14 days) for acute uncomplicated pyelonephritis in women: A randomized trial. JAMA 2000;283(12):1583–1590.
60. van Nieuwkoop C, van't Wout JW, Assendelft WJJ, et al. Treatment duration of febrile urinary tract infection (FUTIRST trial): A randomized placebo-controlled multicenter trial comparing short (7 days) antibiotic treatment with conventional treatment (14 days). BMC Infect Dis 2009;9:131–140.
61. Katchman EA, Milo G, Paul M, Christiaens T, Baerheim A, Leibovici L. Three days vs. longer duration of antibiotic treatment for cystitis in women: A systemic review and meta-analysis. Am J Med 2005;118(11):1196–1207.
62. Peterson J, Kaul S, Khashab M, et al. A double-blind, randomized comparison of levofloxacin 750 mg once-daily for five days with ciprofloxacin 400/500 mg twice-daily for 10 days for the treatment of complicated urinary tract infections and acute pyelonephritis. Urology 2008;71(1):17–22.
63. Brown P, Moran K, Foxman B. Acute pyelonephritis among adults, cost of illness and considerations for the economic evaluation of therapy. Pharmacoeconomics 2005;23(11):1123–1142.
64. Curran MP, Simpson D, Perry CM. Ertapenem, a review of its use in the management of bacterial infections. Drugs 2003;63:1855–1878.
65. Wagenlehner FME, Wagenlehner C, Redman R, et al. Urinary bactericidal activity of doripenem versus that of levofloxacin in patients with complicated urinary tract infections or pyelonephritis. Antimicrob Agents Chemother 2009;53(4):1567–1573.
66. Naber KG. Management of bacterial prostatitis: What's new? BJU Int 2008;101(Suppl 3):7–10.
67. Gleckman R, Crowley M, Natsios GA. Therapy of recurrent invasive urinary tract infection in men. N Engl J Med 1979;301:878–880.
68. Lipsky GA. Urinary tract infections in men: Epidemiology, pathophysiology, diagnosis, and treatment. Ann Intern Med 1989;110:138–150.
69. Lichtenberger P, Hooton TM. Antimicrobial prophylaxis in women with recurrent urinary tract infections. Int J Antimicrob Agents 2011;385:36–41.
70. Macejko AM, Shaeffer AJ. Asymptomatic bacteriuria and symptomatic urinary tract infections during pregnancy. Urol Clin North Am 2007;34(1):35–42.
71. Christensen B. Which antibiotics are appropriate for treating bacteriuria in pregnancy? J Antimicrob Chemother 2000;46(Suppl S1):29–34.
72. McDermott S, Daguise V, Mann H, Szwejbka L, Callaghan W. Perinatal risk for mortality and mental retardation associated with maternal urinary tract infections. J Fam Pract 2001;50:433–437.
73. Saint S, Meddings JA, Calfee D, et al. Catheter-associated urinary tract infection and the medicare rule changes. Ann Intern Med 2009;150(12):877–884.

74. Hooten TM, Bradley SF, Cardenas DD, et al. Diagnosis, prevention, and treatment of catheter-associated urinary tract infections in adults: 2009 International Clinical Practice Guidelines from the Infectious Diseases Society of America. Clin Infect Dis 2010;50:625–663.
75. Ohkawa M, Sugata T, Sawaki M, et al. Bacterial and crystal adherence to the surfaces of indwelling urethral catheters. J Urol 1990;143:717–721.
76. Johnson JR, Duskowski MA, Wilt TJ. Systemic review: Antimicrobial urinary catheters prevent catheter-associated urinary tract infections in hospital patients. Arch Intern Med 2006;144(2):116–126.
77. Murphy AB, Macejko A, Taylor A, et al. Chronic prostatitis management strategies. Drugs 2009;69(1):71–84.
78. Sharp VJ, Takacs EB. Prostatitis: Diagnosis and treatment. Am Fam Physician 2010;82(4):397–406.
79. Lipsky BA, Byren I, Hoey CT. Treatment of bacterial prostatitis. Clin Infect Dis 2010;50(12):1641–1652.
80. Fair WR, Couch J, Wehner M. Prostatic antibacterial factor: Identity and significance. Urology 1976;7:169–177.
81. Pfau A, Perlberg S, Shapiro A. The pH of prostatic fluid in health and disease: Implications of treatment in chronic bacterial prostatitis. J Urol 1978;119:384–387.
82. Wagenlehner FM, Naber KG. Current challenges in the treatment of complicated urinary tract infections and prostatitis. Clin Microbiol Infect 2006;12(Suppl 3):67–80.
83. Alam MF, Cohen D, Butler C, et al. The additional costs of antibiotics and re-consultations for antibiotic-resistant *Escherichia coli* urinary tract infections managed in general practice. Int J Antimicrob Agents 2009;33:255–257.

95

Sexually Transmitted Diseases

Leroy C. Knodel

KEY CONCEPTS

1. All recommended treatment regimens for gonorrhea include antibiotic therapy directed against *Chlamydia* species because of the high prevalence of coexisting infections, unless chlamydia has been ruled out.
2. Parenteral penicillin is the treatment of choice for all syphilis infections. For patients who are penicillin allergic, few well-studied alternative agents are available, and all are oral medications that require 2 to 4 weeks of therapy to be effective. Patient compliance and thus efficacy are a concern when alternative regimens must be used.
3. Chlamydia genital tract infections represent the most frequently reported communicable disease in the United States. In females, these infections are frequently asymptomatic or minimally symptomatic and, if left untreated, are associated with the development of pelvic inflammatory disease and attendant complications such as ectopic pregnancy and infertility. As a result, all sexually active females aged 20 to 25 years and sexually active women with multiple sexual partners should be screened annually for this infection.
4. Oral acyclovir, famciclovir, and valacyclovir are effective in reducing viral shedding, duration of symptoms, and time to healing of first-episode genital herpes infections, with maximal benefits seen when therapy is initiated at the earliest stages of infection. The benefit of these agents for recurrent infections has not been demonstrated. Patient-initiated, single-day antiviral therapy started within 6 to 12 hours of prodromal symptom onset offers an alternative to continuous suppressive therapy of recurrent infection in some individuals.
5. Metronidazole and tinidazole are the only agents currently approved in the United States to treat trichomoniasis. Although a single 2-g dose of either agent is widely used for compliance and other reasons, the alternative 7-day metronidazole regimen may be a better choice if sexual partners of treated individuals cannot be treated concurrently.

The spectrum of sexually transmitted diseases (STDs) has broadened from the classic venereal diseases—gonorrhea, syphilis, chancroid, lymphogranuloma venereum, and granuloma inguinale—to include a variety of pathogens known to be spread by sexual contact (Table 95-1). Because of the large number of infected individuals, the diversity of clinical manifestations, the changing drug-susceptibility patterns of some pathogens, and the high frequency of multiple STDs occurring simultaneously in infected individuals, the diagnosis and management of patients with STDs are much more complex today than they were even a decade ago.[1–4]

Despite a higher reported incidence of most major STDs in men, the complications of STDs generally are more frequent and severe in women. In particular, serious effects on maternal and infant health during pregnancy are well documented.[1,4] Damage to reproductive organs, increased risk of cancer, complications associated with pregnancy, and transmission of disease to the fetus or newborn are associated with several STDs. As a result of the physiologic, psychosocial, and economic consequences of STDs, and because of the increasing prevalence of some viral STDs, such as human immunodeficiency virus (HIV) and genital herpes, for which curative therapy is not available, there is continuing research into STDs and the primary prevention of these diseases.[2–5]

With the exception of HIV infection, which is reviewed in detail in Chapter 103, the most frequently occurring STDs in the United States are discussed in this chapter. For other less common STDs, only recommended treatment regimens are presented. The most current information on the epidemiology, diagnosis, and treatment of STDs provided by the U.S. Centers for Disease Control and Prevention (CDC) can be obtained at the CDC Website (*www.cdc.gov*).

Numerous interrelated factors contribute to the epidemic nature of STDs. Sociocultural, demographic, and economic factors, together with patterns of sexual behavior, host susceptibility to infection, changing properties of the causative pathogens, disease transmission by asymptomatic individuals, and environmental factors, are important determinants of the frequency and distribution of STDs in the United States and worldwide.

Age is one of the most important demographic determinants of STD incidence. Two thirds of STD cases each year occur in persons in their teens and twenties, the peak years of sexual activity. With increasing age, the incidence of most STDs decreases exponentially. In sexually active teenagers, STD rates are highest in the youngest, suggesting that physiologic differences may contribute to increased susceptibility.[2–5]

Age-specific rates of STDs are higher in men than in women; however, reported rates may not represent true gender differences but rather may reflect greater ease of detection in men. In recent years, the ratio of male-to-female cases for most STDs has declined, possibly reflecting improvements in the diagnosis of STDs in asymptomatic women or changes in female sexual behavior following the availability of improved methods of contraception. Although some racial disparity exists for rates of STD infection, it is possible that this is a reflection of socioeconomic differences.[1–5]

The single greatest risk factor for contracting STDs is the number of sexual partners. As the number of sexual partners increases, the risk of being exposed to someone infected with an STD increases. Sexual preference also plays a major role in the

TABLE 95-1 Sexually Transmitted Diseases

Disease	Associated Pathogens
Bacterial	
Gonorrhea	*Neisseria gonorrhoeae*
Syphilis	*Treponema pallidum*
Chancroid	*Haemophilus ducreyi*
Granuloma inguinale	*Calymmatobacterium granulomatis*
Enteric disease	*Salmonella* spp., *Shigella* spp., *Campylobacter* fetus
Campylobacter infection	*Campylobacter jejuni*
Bacterial vaginosis	*Gardnerella vaginalis, Mycoplasma hominis, Bacteroides* spp., *Mobiluncus* spp.
Group B streptococcal infections	Group B *Streptococcus*
Chlamydial	
Nongonococcal urethritis	*Chlamydia trachomatis*
Lymphogranuloma venereum	*Chlamydia trachomatis*, type L
Viral	
Acquired immunodeficiency syndrome	Human immunodeficiency virus
Herpes genitalis	Herpes simplex virus, types I and II
Viral hepatitis	Hepatitis A, B, C, and D viruses
Condylomata acuminata	Human papillomavirus
Molluscum contagiosum	Poxvirus
Cytomegalovirus infection	Cytomegalovirus
Mycoplasmal	
Nongonococcal urethritis	*Ureaplasma urealyticum*
Protozoal	
Trichomoniasis	*Trichomonas vaginalis*
Amebiasis	*Entamoeba histolytica*
Giardiasis	*Giardia lamblia*
Fungal	
Vaginal candidiasis	*Candida albicans*
Parasitic	
Scabies	*Sarcoptes scabiei*
Pediculosis pubis	*Phthirus pubis*
Enterobiasis	*Enterobius vermicularis*

transmission of STDs. For all major STDs, rates are disproportionately greater in men who have sex with men (MSM) than in heterosexuals. In addition, a number of less common STDs, including several caused by enteric protozoans and bacterial pathogens, occur primarily in MSM. The major risk factors for MSM appear to be related to the greater number of sexual partners and the practice of unprotected anal–genital, oral–genital, and oral–anal intercourse. In addition, prostitution and illicit drug use are associated with a higher incidence of most STDs.[1–5]

Some of the most serious sequelae of STDs are associated with congenital or perinatal infections. Most neonatal infections are acquired at birth, after infant passage through an infected cervix or vagina. Neonatal *Chlamydia trachomatis*, *Neisseria gonorrhoeae*, and herpes simplex virus (HSV) infections are associated with this type of spread. For pregnant women with syphilis, infection is usually transmitted transplacentally, producing a congenital infection. Depending on the organism, neonatal infections can manifest in a variety of ways, produce significant morbidity, and in some cases result in infant death.[1–4]

Other than complete abstinence, the most effective way to prevent STD transmission is by maintaining a mutually monogamous sexual relationship between uninfected partners. Short of this, use of barrier contraceptive methods, such as the male and female condoms, diaphragm, cervical cap, vaginal sponges, and vaginal spermicides alone or in combination, provides varying degrees of protection from a number of STDs. When used correctly and consistently, male latex condoms with or without spermicide are more effective than natural skin condoms in protecting against STD transmission, including HIV, gonorrhea, chlamydia, trichomoniasis, HSV, and human papillomavirus (HPV). When lubrication is desired with latex condoms, water-based products, such as K-Y jelly, are recommended because oil-based agents (e.g., petroleum jelly) can weaken latex condoms and reduce their effectiveness. For latex-allergic individuals, other synthetic condoms (e.g., polyurethane) appear to possess efficacy against STD transmission similar to latex condoms. The female condom is a lubricated polyurethane sheath with a diaphragm-like ring on each end that can be used as a protective device for women with male sexual partners who do not desire to use a condom. Limited data suggest that the female condom blocks penetration of viruses, including HIV; for nonviral STDs, the female condom provides STD protection similar to the male condom.[1,3,5,6] At one time, use of nonoxynol-9, a vaginal spermicide with cytolytic activity, was advocated to reduce the transmissibility of several STDs. This was based in large part on in vitro and animal data. However, nonoxynol-9 does not reduce the risk of transmission of common STDs and actually can increase the risk of HIV transmission. Frequent use of nonoxynol-9 damages vaginal, cervical, and rectal epithelium, leading to increased transmissibility of HIV and possibly other STDs. Diaphragms may protect against cervical gonorrheal, chlamydial, and trichomonal infections.[1,5–8]

The varied spectrum of clinical syndromes produced by common STDs is determined not only by the etiologic pathogen(s) but also by differences in male and female anatomy and reproductive physiology. For a number of STDs, the signs and symptoms overlap sufficiently to prevent accurate diagnosis without microbiologic confirmation. Frequently, symptoms are minimal or absent despite the presence of infection. Table 95-2 lists common clinical syndromes associated with STDs.[1–4]

GONORRHEA

Epidemiology and Etiology

The gram-negative diplococcus *N. gonorrhoeae* is the causative organism of gonorrhea. Although the rate of reported cases in the United States has remained relatively stable over the past decade, over 300,000 cases were reported in 2010. However, because of the increasing incidence of resistance to available antibiotics, there is concern that this number may dramatically increase in the future.[1,9] Of concern also are the substantial number of infections that remain undiagnosed and unreported.[1,9] Humans are the only known natural host of this intracellular parasite. Because of its rapid incubation period and the large number of infected individuals with asymptomatic disease, gonorrhea is difficult to control.[1,10–15]

Although the risk of a female acquiring a cervical infection after a single episode of vaginal intercourse with an infected male partner is high and increases with multiple exposures, the risk of transmission from an infected female to an uninfected male is not as great following a single act of coitus. No data are available on the risk of transmission after other types of sexual contact.[10–14]

Pathophysiology

On contact with a mucosal surface lined by columnar, cuboidal, or noncornified squamous epithelial cells, the gonococci attach to cell membranes by means of surface pili and are then pinocytosed. The virulence of the organism is mediated primarily by the presence of pili and other outer membrane proteins. After mucosal damage is established, polymorphonuclear (PMN) leukocytes invade the tissue, submucosal abscesses form, and purulent exudates are secreted.[10–15]

TABLE 95-2 Selected Syndromes Associated with Common Sexually Transmitted Pathogens

Syndrome	Commonly Implicated Pathogens	Common Clinical Manifestations[a]
Urethritis	*Chlamydia trachomatis*, herpes simplex virus, *Neisseria gonorrhoeae*, *Trichomonas vaginalis*, *Ureaplasma urealyticum*	Urethral discharge, dysuria
Epididymitis	*C. trachomatis*, *N. gonorrhoeae*	Scrotal pain, inguinal pain, flank pain, urethral discharge
Cervicitis/vulvovaginitis	*C. trachomatis*, *Gardnerella vaginalis*, herpes simplex virus, human papillomavirus, *N. gonorrhoeae*, *T. vaginalis*	Abnormal vaginal discharge, vulvar itching/irritation, dysuria, dyspareunia
Genital ulcers (painful)	*Haemophilus ducreyi*, herpes simplex virus	Usually multiple vesicular/pustular (herpes) or papular/pustular (*H. ducreyi*) lesions that can coalesce; painful, tender lymphadenopathy[b]
Genital ulcers (painless)	*Treponema pallidum*	Usually single papular lesion
Genital/anal warts	Human papillomavirus	Multiple lesions ranging in size from small papular warts to large exophytic condylomas
Pharyngitis	*C. trachomatis* (?), herpes simplex virus, *N. gonorrhoeae*	Symptoms of acute pharyngitis, cervical lymphadenopathy, fever[c]
Proctitis	*C. trachomatis*, herpes simplex virus, *N. gonorrhoeae*, *T. pallidum*	Constipation, anorectal discomfort, tenesmus, mucopurulent rectal discharge
Salpingitis	*C. trachomatis*, *N. gonorrhoeae*	Lower abdominal pain, purulent cervical or vaginal discharge, adnexal swelling, fever[d]

[a]For some syndromes, clinical manifestations can be minimal or absent.
[b]Recurrent herpes infection can manifest as a single lesion.
[c]Most cases of pharyngeal gonococcal infection are asymptomatic.
[d]Salpingitis increases the risk of subsequent ectopic pregnancy and infertility.

Clinical Presentation

Individuals infected with gonorrhea can be symptomatic or asymptomatic, have complicated or uncomplicated infections, and have infections involving several anatomic sites. Interestingly, most of the symptomatic patients who are not treated become asymptomatic within 6 months, with only a few becoming asymptomatic carriers of the disease.[10–13] The most common clinical features of gonococcal infections are presented in Table 95-3.

Complications associated with untreated gonorrhea appear more pronounced in women, likely a result of a high percentage who experience signs and symptoms that are nonspecific and minimally symptomatic. As a result, many women do not seek treatment until after the development of serious complications, such as pelvic inflammatory disease (PID). Approximately 15% of women with gonorrhea develop PID. Left untreated, PID can be an indirect cause of infertility and ectopic pregnancies. In 0.5% to 3% of patients with gonorrhea, the gonococci invade the bloodstream and produce disseminated disease. Disseminated gonococcal infection (DGI) is three times more common in women than in men. The usual clinical manifestations of DGI are tender necrotic skin lesions, tenosynovitis, and monoarticular arthritis.[1,10–14]

Diagnosis

Diagnosis of gonococcal infections can be made by gram-stained smears, culture, or methods based on the detection of cellular components of the gonococcus (e.g., enzymes, antigens, DNA, or lipopolysaccharide [LPS]) in clinical specimens. Various stains have been used to identify gonococci microscopically, with the Gram stain the most widely used in clinical practice. Gram-stained smears are positive for gonococci when gram-negative diplococci of typical kidney bean morphology are identified within PMN leukocytes.[1,10–14] In the presence of equivocal smears (extracellular gonococcal forms that can be nonpathogenic, commensal *Neisseria*, or gram-negative diplococci of atypical morphology), culture is mandatory. In urethral smears from men with symptomatic urethritis, the smear is highly sensitive and specific, and is considered diagnostic for infection. Because of their low sensitivity, gram-stained smears are not recommended in the diagnosis of endocervical, rectal, cutaneous, and asymptomatic male urethral infections. Because of the presence of nonpathogenic *Neisseria* in the pharynx, the Gram stain is not useful in the diagnosis of pharyngeal infection.[1,10,12–14]

Although no longer considered the most sensitive of diagnostic tests for gonorrhea, culture is considered the test of choice because

TABLE 95-3 Presentation of Gonorrhea Infections

	Males	Females
General	Incubation period 1–14 days Symptom onset in 2–8 days	Incubation period 1–14 days Symptom onset in 10 days
Site of infection	Most common: urethra Others: rectum (usually caused by rectal intercourse in MSM), oropharynx, eye	Most common: endocervical canal Others: urethra, rectum (usually caused by perineal contamination), oropharynx, eye
Symptoms	Can be asymptomatic or minimally symptomatic Urethral infection: dysuria and urinary frequency Anorectal infection: asymptomatic to severe rectal pain Pharyngeal infection: asymptomatic to mild pharyngitis	Can be asymptomatic or minimally symptomatic Endocervical infection: usually asymptomatic or mildly symptomatic Urethral infection: dysuria, urinary frequency Anorectal and pharyngeal infection; symptoms same as for men
Signs	Purulent urethral or rectal discharge can be scant to profuse Anorectal: pruritus, mucopurulent discharge, bleeding	Abnormal vaginal discharge or uterine bleeding; purulent urethral or rectal discharge can be scant to profuse
Complications	Rare (epididymitis, prostatitis, inguinal lymphadenopathy, urethral stricture) Disseminated gonorrhea	Pelvic inflammatory disease and associated complications (i.e., ectopic pregnancy, infertility) Disseminated gonorrhea (three times more common than in men)

MSM, men who have sex with men.

of its high specificity in medicolegal situations (e.g., suspected abuse, rape); in diagnosing anorectal, pharyngeal, and conjunctival infections; and in screening populations with a low prevalence. Anatomic sites to be cultured depend on the individual's sexual preferences and body areas exposed. In women, because the urethra and other sites are rarely the sole locus of infection, cervical cultures produce the highest yield and frequently are performed in conjunction with rectal cultures. Urethral cultures are recommended in women who have had hysterectomies and heterosexual men.[1,10–14]

Because technical constraints and cost preclude the use of culture techniques in many office settings and clinics, alternative methods of diagnosis have been developed, including enzyme immunoassay (EIA), DNA probe techniques, and nucleic acid amplification techniques (NAATs). With the exception of Gram stain for symptomatic gonococcal urethritis, these tests offer increased sensitivity and/or specificity over both Gram stain and culture.[10,13,14,16] Additionally, many of these tests can provide a more rapid means of diagnosis than culture. Of particular clinical importance is the high sensitivity of NAATs for detecting *N. gonorrhoeae* using noninvasive specimens (e.g., self-collected urine specimens, vaginal swabs). As a result, NAAT is considered the standard of care for the diagnosis of gonorrhea. This technology is also being used to concurrently test for *C. trachomatis* using a single specimen. However, a major drawback of NAATs is their inability to provide resistance data on isolated gonococcal strains. In cases of documented treatment failure, antimicrobial susceptibility testing is recommended.[1,14–16]

TREATMENT

1 In 2010 the CDC issued an update to their recommended treatment regimens for gonorrhea. This update eliminated oral cephalosporins from the recommended treatment regimens for gonorrhea, leaving parenteral ceftriaxone as the only recommended agent for treating gonorrhea[14] (Table 95-4). The ceftriaxone-based regimens are the only regimens that have well-documented efficacy in the treatment of urethral, cervical, rectal, and pharyngeal infections. Coexisting chlamydial infection, which is documented in up to 50% of women and 20% of men with gonorrhea, constitutes the major cause of postgonococcal urethritis, cervicitis, and salpingitis in patients treated for gonorrhea for whom concurrent chlamydial infection has not been ruled out.[1,14] As a result, concomitant treatment with azithromycin or doxycycline is recommended in all patients treated for gonorrhea. If a cefixime-based regimen is used to treat gonorrhea, it is recommended that patients return in 1 week for a test of cure. While azithromycin (2 g) as a single dose appears highly effective in eradicating both gonorrhea and chlamydia, it is not recommended as a preferred alternative to ceftriaxone because of concerns regarding the development of resistance. In cephalosporin-allergic individuals, azithromycin (2 g) is currently the only alternative available to treat gonorrhea.[1,14,17,18]

Although oral therapy with cefixime may offer a more patient acceptable alternative to intramuscular ceftriaxone, the declining susceptibility of gonorrheal isolates in the United States to cefixime has resulted in its move from a recommended regimen of choice to an alternative regimen. Additionally, only ceftriaxone is effective in treating pharyngeal gonorrhea and eradicating both gonorrhea and incubating syphilis in a patient coinfected with both organisms. The latter is particularly beneficial in areas with a high rate of syphilis.[1,10,12–15]

Pregnant women infected with *N. gonorrhoeae* should be treated with ceftriaxone. For presumed or diagnosed concurrent *C. trachomatis* infection, azithromycin or amoxicillin is the preferred treatment.[1,10,11]

Ceftriaxone is the recommended therapy for DGI, gonococcal meningitis, endocarditis, and any type of gonococcal infection in children. In cases of DGI, patients should be hospitalized and treated with ceftriaxone or one of the alternative parenteral cephalosporin antibiotics (see Table 95-4). Although marked improvement is usually noted within 48 hours of initiating therapy, treatment should be continued for at least 7 days.[1,13,14] Gonococcal ophthalmia

TABLE 95-4 Treatment of Gonorrhea

Type of Infection	Recommended Regimens[a]	Alternative Regimens[a]
Uncomplicated infections of the cervix, urethra, and rectum in adults	Ceftriaxone 250 mg IM once *plus* Azithromycin 1 g PO once, or doxycycline 100 mg PO twice daily for 7 days[b]	Cefixime 400 mg PO once *plus* Azithromycin 1 g PO once, or doxycycline 100 mg PO twice daily for 7 days (plus test of cure in 1 week)[c,d,e]
Uncomplicated infections of the pharynx	Ceftriaxone 250 mg IM once *plus* Azithromycin 1 g PO once, or doxycycline 100 mg PO twice daily for 7 days	Consult with infectious disease expert
Disseminated gonococcal infection in adults (>45 kg)	Ceftriaxone 1 g IM or IV every 24 hours[f]	Cefotaxime 1 g IV every 8 hours[f] or ceftizoxime 1 g IV every 8 hours[f]
Uncomplicated infections of the cervix, urethra, and rectum in children (≤45 kg)	Ceftriaxone 125 mg IM once	
Gonococcal conjunctivitis in adults	Ceftriaxone 1 g IM once[g]	
Ophthalmia neonatorum	Ceftriaxone 25–50 mg/kg IV or IM once (not to exceed 125 mg)	
Infants born to mothers with gonococcal infection (prophylaxis)	Erythromycin (0.5%) ophthalmic ointment in a single application[h]	Ceftriaxone 25–50 mg/kg IM or IV once (not to exceed 125 mg)

CDC, Centers for Disease Control and Prevention; *C. trachomatis*, *Chlamydia trachomatis*; NAAT, Nucleic Acid Amplification Test; PO, orally.

[a]Recommendations are those of the CDC.

[b]Tetracyclines are contraindicated during pregnancy. Pregnant women should be treated with recommended cephalosporin-based combination therapy. Women who cannot tolerate a cephalosporin should receive azithromycin 2 g PO once and have a test of cure 1 week later.

[c]Ideally performed using culture; if culture is not available, use a NAAT for *N. gonorrhoeae*.

[d]Patients who are treatment failures with alternative regimens should be treated with ceftriaxone 250 mg IM once plus azithromycin 2 g PO once in consultation with an infectious disease expert.

[e]For patients with severe cephalosporin allergy, azithromycin 2 g PO once is recommended plus a test of cure in a week.

[f]Parenteral treatment regimens should be continued for 24–48 hours after improvement begins; at this time therapy can be switched to cefixime 400 mg PO twice daily (tablet or suspension) to complete a 7-day course of treatment.

[g]A single lavage of the infected eye with normal saline should be considered; empiric therapy for *C. trachomatis* is recommended.

[h]Efficacy in preventing chlamydial ophthalmia is unclear.

is highly contagious in adults and neonates and requires ceftriaxone therapy. Single-dose therapy is adequate for gonococcal conjunctivitis, although some physicians recommend continuing therapy until cultures are negative at 48 to 72 hours. Topical antibiotics are not sufficiently effective when used alone for ocular infections and are not necessary with appropriate systemic therapy. Infants with any evidence of ocular infection should be evaluated for signs of DGI.[1,10,13–14,19]

Clinical **Controversy...**

Some clinicians advocate that a single 2-g dose of azithromycin should be the treatment of choice for gonorrhea because it is also effective in eradicating concomitant chlamydial infection. However, because of concerns regarding the development of resistance and the relatively high incidence of GI side effects, azithromycin monotherapy is not recommended as a first-line therapy.

Treatment of gonorrhea during pregnancy is essential to prevent ophthalmia neonatorum. Gonococcal infection in newborns results primarily from passage through an infected birth canal, but it also can be transmitted in utero. Ophthalmia neonatorum is the most common ophthalmic infection in newborns (1.6% to 12%), although membranes of the vagina, pharynx, or rectum also can become colonized. Conjunctival involvement usually develops within 7 days of delivery and is characterized by intense, bilateral conjunctival inflammation with chemosis. If not treated promptly, corneal ulceration and blindness can develop. Because the law in most states requires neonatal prophylaxis with topical ocular antimicrobials, gonococcal ophthalmia neonatorum is rare in the United States. The CDC recommends that erythromycin (0.5%) ophthalmic ointment be instilled in each conjunctival sac immediately postpartum.[1,10–14,19]

Evaluation of Therapeutic Outcomes

In the past, persistence of gonorrhea symptoms a short time following treatment with a recommended regimen against gonorrhea usually indicated reinfection rather than treatment failure and, as such, reflected the need for improved patient education and sex partner referral. However, with antimicrobial resistance increasingly being reported in recent years, reinfection can no longer be assumed as the cause. As a result, the CDC recommends that all apparent treatment failures be assessed using culture and sensitivity testing. Persistence of symptoms also can be due to other infectious causes, such as *C. trachomatis*.[1,10–15] While the CDC does not recommend routine follow-up of patients treated with a recommended regimen, it is recommend that any patient treated with an alternative regimen be tested for cure 1 week following treatment.

SYPHILIS

Epidemiology and Etiology

During the 2000s, the number of reported cases of primary and secondary syphilis in the United States has remained relatively constant at around 14,000.[9] Of these newly diagnosed cases, two-thirds are reported in MSM. In addition to being highly contagious, syphilis is of major concern because, if left untreated, it can progress to a chronic systemic disease that can be fatal or seriously disabling.[20–29] Syphilis usually is acquired by sexual contact with infected mucous membranes or cutaneous lesions, although on rare occasions it can be acquired by nonsexual personal contact, accidental inoculation, or blood transfusion. The causative organism of syphilis is *Treponema pallidum*, a spirochete. The risk of acquiring syphilis from an infected individual after a single sexual encounter is approximately 50% to 60%. After sexual contact, the organism penetrates the intact mucous membrane or a break in the cornified epithelium, and spirochetemia occurs.[21,24,25–29]

There is strong evidence of an association between syphilis and HIV infection. Syphilis, similar to other sexually transmitted genital ulcer diseases, can increase the risk of acquiring HIV in exposed individuals. In addition, immunologic defects in HIV-infected individuals can produce an atypical serologic response to syphilis. In particular, the possibility of delayed seroreactivity, markedly elevated serologic titers, and increased false-positive results could complicate the diagnosis, as well as assessment of treatment efficacy, in HIV-positive individuals infected with syphilis. Furthermore, anecdotal evidence suggests that compromised immune function can result in an accelerated progression of syphilis, particularly to neurosyphilis, requiring more aggressive antibiotic therapy in comparison with an immunocompetent host. As a result of this association, the CDC recommends that all patients diagnosed with syphilis be tested for HIV infection.[1,20,22–24,26,27]

Clinical Presentation

The clinical presentation of syphilis is varied with progression through multiple stages possible in untreated or inadequately treated patients (Table 95-5).

Primary Syphilis

The primary stage, characterized by the appearance of a chancre on cutaneous or mucocutaneous tissue exposed to the organism, is highly infectious. Even without treatment, chancres persist only for 1 to 8 weeks before healing spontaneously. Because syphilitic chancres can be confused with other infectious etiologies, appropriate diagnostic testing is important.[20–24,26,28]

TABLE 95-5 Presentation of Syphilis Infections

General	
Primary	Incubation period 10–90 days (mean, 21 days)
Secondary	Develops 2–8 weeks after initial infection in untreated or inadequately treated individuals
Latent	Develops 4–10 weeks after secondary stage in untreated or inadequately treated individuals
Tertiary	Develops in approximately 30% of untreated or inadequately treated individuals 10–30 years after initial infection
Site of Infection	
Primary	External genitalia, perianal region, mouth, and throat
Secondary	Multisystem involvement secondary to hematogenous and lymphatic spread
Latent tertiary	Potentially multisystem involvement (dormant) CNS, heart, eyes, bones, and joints
Signs and Symptoms	
Primary	Single, painless, indurated lesion (chancre) that erodes, ulcerates, and eventually heals (typical); regional lymphadenopathy is common; multiple, painful, purulent lesions possible but uncommon
Secondary	Pruritic or nonpruritic rash, mucocutaneous lesions, flulike symptoms, lymphadenopathy
Latent	Asymptomatic
Tertiary	Cardiovascular syphilis (aortitis or aortic insufficiency), neurosyphilis (meningitis, general paresis, dementia, tabes dorsalis, eighth cranial nerve deafness, blindness), gummatous lesions involving any organ or tissue

Secondary Syphilis

The secondary stage of syphilis is characterized by a variety of mucocutaneous eruptions resulting from widespread hematogenous and lymphatic spread of *T. pallidum*. Skin lesions can be either generalized or localized to a small portion of the body and, with the exception of follicular lesions, are nonpruritic. Generalized lymphadenopathy also is seen in the majority of patients, as are nonspecific symptoms such as mild and transitory malaise, fever, pharyngitis, headache, anorexia, and arthralgia. If untreated, secondary syphilis disappears in 4 to 10 weeks; however, lesions can recur at any time within 4 years.[20–28]

Latent Syphilis

By definition, persons with a positive serologic test for syphilis but with no other evidence of disease have latent syphilis. Latent syphilis is further divided into early and late latency. During early latency, the patient is considered potentially infectious because of the 25% risk of spontaneous mucocutaneous relapse. The U.S. Public Health Service defines early latency as 1 year from the onset of infection, although other investigators propose a longer interval, such as 2 to 4 years. With the exception of pregnancy in which the mother can pass the disease to the fetus, late latency is considered noninfectious, although the patient remains a host.[1,20–28]

Most untreated patients with late latent syphilis have no further sequelae; however, approximately 25% to 30% progress either to neurosyphilis or to late syphilis with clinical manifestations other than neurosyphilis. Treatment of all patients with latent syphilis is essential because there is no way to predict which patients will have progression of their disease.[20–28]

Tertiary Syphilis and Neurosyphilis

If left untreated, syphilis can slowly produce an inflammatory reaction in virtually any organ in the body. Manifestations of this disease progression were referred to previously as *tertiary syphilis*. These clinical manifestations now are differentiated into two subgroups based on the presence or absence of CNS involvement: neurosyphilis or tertiary syphilis (i.e., gumma and cardiovascular syphilis).[1,20–28]

Currently, the term *neurosyphilis* encompasses any patient with cerebrospinal fluid (CSF) abnormalities consistent with CNS infection. Approximately 40% of patients with primary or secondary syphilis exhibit such abnormalities, although most remain asymptomatic. Persistence of CSF abnormalities into late latency is associated with a greater risk of progression to symptomatic neurosyphilis. Although data are conflicting, some investigators suggest that HIV-infected patients are at greater risk of developing symptomatic neurosyphilis than patients with intact immune systems.[1,20–28]

Rarely seen, the most common manifestations of disease progression from late latency are benign gumma formation and cardiovascular syphilis. The gumma, a nonspecific granulomatous lesion, is the classic lesion of late syphilis and develops in 50% of patients with disease progression. These chronic, destructive lesions characteristically infiltrate the skin, bone, soft tissue, and liver but can be found in any organ or tissue. Gummas of critical organs, such as the heart or brain, can be fatal.[1,20–24,27]

Congenital Syphilis

In pregnant women with syphilis, *T. pallidum* can cross the placenta at any time during pregnancy. The risk of fetal infection is greatest in pregnant women with primary and secondary syphilis and declines in pregnant women with late disease. Transmission of syphilis during pregnancy occurs primarily transplacentally and can result in fetal death, prematurity, or congenital syphilis. Symptoms can be seen during the first months of life (early congenital syphilis) or later in childhood or adolescence (late congenital syphilis). Manifestations of early congenital syphilis resemble those of secondary syphilis, whereas those of late congenital syphilis correspond to the tertiary stage in adults.[20,22–24]

Diagnosis

Because *T. pallidum* is difficult to culture in vitro, diagnosis is based primarily on microscopic examination of serous material from a suspected syphilitic lesion or on results from serologic testing. In primary syphilis, diagnosis is established by the presence of *T. pallidum* on dark-field microscopic examination of material from cutaneous lesions and enlarged lymph nodes in patients with secondary syphilis. In incubating syphilis, confirmation frequently is by dark-field microscopic examination because serologic tests can be unreactive early in the disease. Another method of direct microscopic examination, the direct fluorescent-antibody (test) for *T. pallidum* (DFA-TP), which uses monoclonal or polyclonal antibodies specific for *T. pallidum*, has greater specificity and sensitivity than dark-field examination, and does not require the immediate examination of fresh specimens.[24–29]

Serologic tests are the mainstay in the diagnosis of syphilis and traditionally are categorized as nontreponemal or treponemal. Common nontreponemal tests include the Venereal Disease Research Laboratory (VDRL) slide test, rapid plasma reagin (RPR) card test, unheated serum reagin (USR) test, and the toluidine red unheated serum test (TRUST). Nontreponemal tests, which are inexpensive and easily performed, rely on the detection of treponemal antibodies directed against an alcoholic solution of cardiolipin, lecithin, and cholesterol contained in these tests. A positive nontreponemal test can indicate the presence of any stage of syphilis or congenital syphilis, although incubating syphilis and very early primary syphilis produce a negative reaction; however, because they are nonspecific tests, false-positive reactions occur, making them inappropriate to confirm the diagnosis alone. Transiently false-positive results can be seen in patients with acute febrile illnesses, after immunizations, and during pregnancy. Chronic false-positive results are commonly associated with heroin addiction, aging, chronic infections, autoimmune diseases, and malignant disease. In some cases, false-positive reactions are familial and are related to abnormal serum globulin levels.[23–29]

Nontreponemal tests are used primarily as screening tests; however, because *T. pallidum* antibody titers also can be quantitated by testing serial dilutions of the patient's serum for reactivity, they are useful in following the progression of the disease, recovery after therapy, and possible reinfection. Because antibody titers vary to some extent between tests, it is important that sequential serologic testing be performed using the same method each time. In patients treated successfully for primary and secondary syphilis, nontreponemal tests almost always will return to seronegativity. If these tests are going to return to negative in patients with early latent syphilis, they will do so within the first 4 years after adequate therapy; patients with disease of longer duration usually remain seropositive for life. In addition to their use in serologic testing, nontreponemal tests often are used on CSF to diagnose neurosyphilis.[23–29]

In some patients with secondary syphilis, a prozone phenomenon occurs that produces a negative VDRL test despite the presence of high reaginic antibody titers. This is corrected by diluting the patient's serum prior to testing.[26,27] For HIV-positive individuals with syphilis, the reactivity of nontreponemal tests can vary depending on the stage of the HIV infection. In the early stages, reaginic titers higher than in non–HIV-infected patients have been seen, resulting in the prozone phenomenon. During the later stages of HIV infection, however, when immune function deteriorates to a greater extent, serologic responses can be reduced or delayed. As a result, the diagnosis of syphilis in HIV-infected individuals can be more difficult.[1,24–29]

In diagnosing all stages of syphilis, treponemal tests are more sensitive than nontreponemal tests. Because these tests are technically more demanding and are more expensive, they are used primarily as confirmatory rather than as screening tests. For many years, the fluorescent treponemal antibody absorption (FTA-ABS) test was the most frequently used treponemal test. The FTA-ABS test uses the *T. pallidum* antigen to detect specific antibodies to treponemal organisms. However, the FTA-ABS test has largely been replaced by card assays such as the *T. pallidum* hemagglutination assay (TPHA), the microhemagglutination assay for antibodies to *T. pallidum* (MHA-TP), and the *T. pallidum* particle agglutination assay (TPPA) which can be automated and are less expensive to perform. Despite adequate antibiotic therapy for any stage of syphilis, the antibody tests usually remain reactive for life and therefore are not useful in assessing serologic response to therapy, relapse, or reinfection.[1,24–29]

Several EIAs for *T. pallidum* have become available and are gaining wide use as confirmatory tests. Polymerase chain reaction (PCR)-based tests also are being investigated, particularly in situations in which serologic testing has poor sensitivity and specificity (e.g., congenital syphilis, early primary syphilis, and neurosyphilis). Additionally, multiplex PCR tests that can identify the presence of *T. pallidum*, herpes simplex virus type 1 (HSV-1) and herpes simplex virus type 2 (HSV-2), and *Haemophilus ducreyi* from genital ulcer specimens are under study. The CDC recommends that all patients diagnosed with syphilis be tested for HIV infection.[1,22–24,29]

TREATMENT

Table 95-6 presents the CDC's treatment recommendations.[1] Parenteral penicillin G is the treatment of choice for all stages of syphilis. Because *T. pallidum* multiplies slowly, single doses of short- or intermediate-acting penicillins do not provide the prolonged, low-level exposure to penicillin required for eradication of the treponeme. As a result, benzathine penicillin G is the only penicillin effective for single-dose therapy.[1,22–28]

The recommended treatment for syphilis of less than 1 year's duration is benzathine penicillin G 2.4 million units as a single dose. Although the relapse rate for this regimen is less than 3%, some investigators advocate that 2.4 million units be administered once a week for two consecutive weeks. In patients with syphilis of longer than 1 year's duration and normal CSF examination, benzathine penicillin G is administered weekly for three successive doses. Although not specifically recommended by the CDC, this three-dose regimen is used by some experts to treat HIV-infected patients with syphilis of less than 1 year's duration based on data suggesting a greater risk of treatment failure with single-dose therapy.[1,24–28]

Patients with abnormal CSF findings should be treated as having neurosyphilis. Preferred regimens for neurosyphilis provide

TABLE 95-6 Drug Therapy and Follow-up of Syphilis

Stage/Type of Syphilis	Recommended Regimens[a,b]	Follow-up Serology
Primary, secondary, or early latent syphilis (<1 year's duration)	Benzathine penicillin G 2.4 million units IM in a single dose	Quantitative nontreponemal tests at 6 and 12 months for primary and secondary syphilis; at 6, 12, and 24 months for early latent syphilis[c]
Late latent syphilis (>1 year's duration) or latent syphilis of unknown duration or tertiary syphilis	Benzathine penicillin G 2.4 million units IM once a week for 3 successive weeks (7.2 million units total)	Quantitative nontreponemal tests at 6, 12, and 24 months[d,e]
Neurosyphilis	Aqueous crystalline penicillin G 18–24 million units IV (3–4 million units every 4 hours or by continuous infusion) for 10–14 days[f] *or* Aqueous procaine penicillin G 2.4 million units IM daily plus probenecid 500 mg PO four times daily, both for 10–14 days[f]	CSF examination every 6 months until the cell count is normal; if it has not decreased at 6 months or is not normal by 2 years, retreatment should be considered
Congenital syphilis (infants with proven or highly probable disease)	Aqueous crystalline penicillin G 50,000 units/kg IV every 12 hours during the first 7 days of life and every 8 hours thereafter for a total of 10 days *or* Procaine penicillin G 50,000 units/kg IM daily for 10 days	Serologic follow-up only recommended if antimicrobials other than penicillin are used
Penicillin-Allergic Patients[g]		
Primary, secondary, or early latent syphilis	Doxycycline 100 mg PO two times daily for 14 days[g,h] *or* Tetracycline 500 mg PO four times daily for 14 days[h] *or* Ceftriaxone 1 g IM or IV daily for 8–10 days	Same as for non–penicillin-allergic patients
Late latent syphilis (>1 year's duration) or syphilis of unknown duration	Doxycycline 100 mg PO twice a day for 28 days[h,i] *or* Tetracycline 500 mg PO four times daily for 28 days[h,i]	Same as for non–penicillin-allergic patients

CDC, Centers for Disease Control and Prevention; CSF, cerebrospinal fluid; PO, orally.

[a]Recommendations are those of the CDC.
[b]The CDC recommends that all patients diagnosed with syphilis be tested for HIV infection.
[c]More frequent follow-up (i.e., 3, 6, 9, 12, and 24 months) recommended for HIV-infected patients.
[d]More frequent follow-up (i.e., 6, 12, 18, and 24 months) recommended for HIV-infected patients.
[e]No specific recommendations exist for tertiary syphilis because of the lack of available data.
[f]Some experts administer benzathine penicillin G 2.4 million units IM once per week for up to 3 weeks after completion of the neurosyphilis regimens to provide a total duration of therapy comparable to that used for late syphilis in the absence of neurosyphilis.
[g]For nonpregnant patients; pregnant patients should be treated with penicillin after desensitization.
[h]Pregnant patients allergic to penicillin should be desensitized and treated with penicillin.
[i]Limited data suggest that ceftriaxone may be effective, although the optimal dosage and treatment duration are unclear.

treatment over 10 to 14 days with parenteral penicillin G administered every 4 hours. Benzathine penicillin G alone in standard weekly doses and procaine penicillin G in doses under 2.4 million units do not consistently provide treponemicidal levels in the CSF and have resulted in treatment failures. Because *T. pallidum* resistance to penicillin has not emerged, the primary need for alternative drugs in treating syphilis is for penicillin-allergic patients.[1,24–28]

❷ Alternative regimens recommended for penicillin-allergic patients are doxycycline 100 mg orally twice daily or tetracycline 500 mg orally four times daily for 2 to 4 weeks depending on the duration of syphilis infection. These regimens should be used only in cases of documented penicillin allergy, and given concerns regarding patient compliance with these regimens, follow-up serologic testing is of particular importance.[1,24–28]

Other antibiotics used successfully in treating syphilis include various β-lactam antibiotics; however, none offers significant advantages over benzathine penicillin G. Even though ceftriaxone is considered effective in eradicating incubating syphilis when given as a single 125-mg dose, higher doses and more frequent administration (e.g., 1,000 mg daily for 8 to 10 days) appear necessary for more advanced syphilis, and treatment failures are reported in HIV-infected patients. Although azithromycin 2 g as a single dose produces good results in patients with early syphilis, treatment failures and resistance to azithromycin are reported.[1,21,24–28]

Clinical **Controversy. . .**

Some experts even prefer to treat all patients with syphilis of less than 1 year's duration with the three-dose regimen because single-dose therapy is not consistently effective in eradicating treponemes from the CSF; this is of primary concern in patients with undiagnosed CSF involvement, such as in HIV-infected individuals.

For pregnant patients, penicillin is the treatment of choice at the dosage recommended for that particular stage of syphilis. To ensure treatment success and prevent transmission to the fetus, some experts advocate an additional IM dose of benzathine penicillin G 2.4 million units 1 week after completion of the recommended regimen. In women allergic to penicillin, safe and effective alternatives are not available; therefore, skin testing should be performed to confirm a penicillin allergy. It is recommended that women with positive skin tests undergo penicillin desensitization and receive the appropriate treatment regimen for their stage of disease.[1,22–24]

Most patients treated for primary and secondary syphilis experience the Jarisch-Herxheimer reaction after treatment. This benign, self-limiting reaction is characterized by flulike symptoms, such as transient headache, fever, chills, malaise, arthralgia, myalgia, tachypnea, peripheral vasodilation, and aggravation of syphilitic lesions. The exact mechanism of the reaction is unknown, although proposed etiologies, including immunologic mechanisms and release of endotoxin or other toxic treponemal products, are not substantiated. The Jarisch-Herxheimer reaction is independent of the drug and dose used and should not be confused with penicillin allergy. It usually begins within 2 to 4 hours of initiating therapy, peaks at 8 hours, and is complete within 12 to 24 hours. Most reactions can be managed symptomatically with analgesics, antipyretics, and rest. Steroids and antihistamines have been administered prior to initiation of syphilitic therapy but are of limited value.[1,22–24]

Evaluation of Therapeutic Outcomes

Table 95-6 lists the CDC recommendations for serologic follow-up of patients treated for syphilis.[1] Quantitative nontreponemal tests should be performed at 6 and 12 months in all patients treated for primary and secondary syphilis and at 6, 12, and 24 months for early and late latent disease. The CDC recommends more frequent monitoring of HIV-infected individuals (i.e., 3, 6, 9, 12, and 24 months after therapy). In general, the time to reach seronegativity is proportional to the duration of the disease. Table 95-6 also includes specific testing recommendations for other stages of syphilis. Despite adequate therapy, some patients can remain seropositive based on nontreponemal test results. In these cases, stabilization of low antibody titers is indicative of adequate therapy. For women treated during pregnancy, monthly quantitative nontreponemal tests are recommended in those at high risk of reinfection.[22–24]

CHLAMYDIA TRACHOMATIS

Epidemiology and Etiology

Based on CDC data for 2010, over 1.3 million cases of chlamydia infection were reported, making it the most frequently reported infectious disease in the United States.[1,9] Because of the silent nature of many infections, the presumptive treatment of many cases, and the underreporting of many cases, it is estimated that more than double this number of cases actually occur annually. Chlamydial infections also are the primary causes of nongonococcal urethritis (NGU), accounting for as much as 50% of such infections.[1,30–34]

Pathophysiology

C. trachomatis is an obligate intracellular parasite that shares properties of both viruses and bacteria. Like viruses, chlamydiae require cellular material from host cells for replication; however, unlike viruses, chlamydiae maintain their cellular identity throughout development. Although *C. trachomatis* lacks a cell-wall peptidoglycan, its major outer membrane is similar to gram-negative bacteria. At least 18 serovars (subspecies) of *C. trachomatis* exist, of which only the lymphogranuloma venereum strains produce potentially invasive infections. The remaining serovars are involved primarily with superficial infection of epithelial cells.[30–34]

The risk of transmissibility of chlamydia after exposure is unknown but is believed to be less than that following exposure to *N. gonorrhoeae*. Coinfection with chlamydia occurs in a substantial number of individuals with gonorrhea and all individuals diagnosed with *N. gonorrhoeae* should be assumed also to have *C. trachomatis* present, if chlamydial infection has not been ruled out.[1] Of major concern is that chlamydial infections are associated with a significantly increased risk of acquiring HIV infection. In addition to genital infections, ocular infections in adults owing to autoinoculation and infants owing to vaginal delivery through an infected birth canal are reported. Pharyngeal and rectal infections can develop secondary to orogenital or receptive anal intercourse, respectively, with an infected individual.[1,30–37]

Clinical Presentation

In comparison with gonorrhea, chlamydial genital tract infections are more frequently asymptomatic, and when present, symptoms tend to be less noticeable. Urethral discharge usually is less profuse and more mucoid or watery than the urethral discharge associated with gonorrhea.[31–34] Table 95-7 summarizes the usual clinical presentation of chlamydial infections.

Similar to gonorrhea, chlamydia can be transmitted to an infant during contact with infected cervicovaginal secretions. Nearly two-thirds of infants acquire chlamydial infection after endocervical exposure, with the primary morbidity associated with seeding of the infant's eyes, nasopharynx, rectum, or vagina. In exposed infants,

TABLE 95-7 Presentation of *Chlamydia* Infections

	Males	Females
General	Incubation period: 35 days Symptom onset: 7–21 days	Incubation period: 7–35 days Usual symptom onset: 7–21 days
Site of infection	Most common: urethra Others: rectum (receptive anal intercourse), oropharynx, eye	Most common: endocervical canal Others: urethra, rectum (usually caused by perineal contamination), oropharynx, eye
Symptoms	More than 50% of urethral and rectal infections are asymptomatic Urethral infection: mild dysuria, discharge Pharyngeal infection: asymptomatic to mild pharyngitis	More than 66% of cervical infections are asymptomatic Urethral infection: usually subclinical; dysuria and frequency uncommon Rectal and pharyngeal infection: symptoms same as for men
Signs	Scant to profuse, mucoid to purulent urethral or rectal discharge Rectal infection: pain, discharge, bleeding	Abnormal vaginal discharge or uterine bleeding, purulent urethral or rectal discharge can be scant to profuse
Complications	Epididymitis, Reiter's syndrome (rare)	Pelvic inflammatory disease and associated complications (i.e., ectopic pregnancy, infertility) Reiter's syndrome (rare)

neonatal conjunctivitis develops in as many as 50%, and pneumonia develops in up to 16%. Inclusion conjunctivitis in newborns is usually self-limited, but it can result in scarring and micropannus of the cornea. Interstitial pneumonitis occurring secondary to carriage in the nasopharynx typically is mild, but it can be severe and require hospitalization.[1,31–34,36]

Diagnosis

3 Because of the high rate of asymptomatic disease and the high prevalence of chlamydial infection in sexually active females 25 years of age or younger and sexually active women with new sex partners or multiple sex partners, the CDC recommends routine annual screening in these individuals. Laboratory confirmation of chlamydial infection is important because of the relative lack of specificity of symptoms when present.[1]

Cell culture is the reference standard against which all other diagnostic tests are measured. Because chlamydiae are obligate intracellular parasites, specimens for culture must be obtained from endocervical (women) or urethral (men) epithelial cell scrapings rather than from urine or urethral discharges. Although tissue culture techniques have close to 100% specificity, the sensitivity is reported to be as low as 70% in part because of problems of improper specimen collection, transport, or processing. Because of the technical demands, expense, and length of time until results are available (3 to 7 days), culture is not used widely for diagnostic purposes today. However, culture remains the diagnostic standard in medicolegal cases such as sexual assault and child abuse because of its high specificity and ability to detect only viable organisms.[31–34,37–40]

Tests that detect chlamydial antigens and nucleic acid provide more rapid results, are technically less demanding to perform, are less costly, and in some situations have greater sensitivity than culture. Commonly used nonculture tests for detection of *C. trachomatis* are the enzyme immunosorbent assay (EIA), DNA hybridization probe, and NAATs.[32,34,37,39]

Although still widely used both as rapid office tests and as laboratory-based tests, EIA methods for diagnosis of *C. trachomatis* are no longer recommended because of their poor sensitivity in comparison to NAATs. NAATs, which can detect small amounts of chlamydial DNA, are highly sensitive and specific for detecting infection in urogenital and anal specimens, as well as in urine. Use of self-collected vaginal or anal specimens or first-void urine samples offers greater patient acceptability, particularly when used to screen asymptomatic individuals. A further advantage of tests that can screen urine for the presence of infection is that up to 30% of women are reported to have urethral infection only, which would be missed using a test on endocervical samples. Because of their ability to detect as little as a single gene copy in a specimen, nucleic acid residues that persist following successful antibiotic therapy of a chlamydial infection can result in a false-positive test for several weeks following eradication of the organism.[33,34]

TREATMENT

A number of antimicrobials, including tetracyclines, macrolides, azithromycin, and some fluoroquinolones, display good in vitro and in vivo activity against *C. trachomatis*. In most clinical trials, cure rates exceeding 90% are reported for these agents. All these antimicrobials also appear to have good efficacy against *Ureaplasma urealyticum*, the second most common cause of NGU.[31–34]

Azithromycin 1 g orally as a single dose and doxycycline 100 mg orally twice daily for 7 days are the regimens of choice for the treatment of uncomplicated chlamydial infections[1] (Table 95-8). Because of its prolonged serum and tissue half-life, azithromycin is the only single-dose therapy that is effective in treating *C. trachomatis*. Of the fluoroquinolones, ofloxacin and levofloxacin are included in the CDC recommendations, but neither appears to offer an advantage over other first-line nor alternative therapies. Although ciprofloxacin and some other fluoroquinolones have

TABLE 95-8 Treatment of *Chlamydial* Infections

Infection	Recommended Regimens[a]	Alternative Regimen
Uncomplicated urethral, endocervical, or rectal infection in adults	Azithromycin 1 g PO once, or doxycycline 100 mg PO twice daily for 7 days	Ofloxacin 300 mg PO twice daily for 7 days, or levofloxacin 500 mg PO once daily for 7 days, or erythromycin base 500 mg PO four times daily for 7 days, or erythromycin ethylsuccinate 800 mg PO four times daily for 7 days
Urogenital infections during pregnancy	Azithromycin 1 g PO as a single dose or amoxicillin 500 mg PO three times daily for 7 days	Erythromycin base 500 mg PO four times daily for 7 days, or erythromycin base 250 mg PO four times daily for 14 days, or erythromycin ethylsuccinate 800 mg PO four times daily for 7 days (or 400 mg PO four times daily for 14 days)
Conjunctivitis of the newborn or pneumonia in infants	Erythromycin base 50 mg/kg/day PO in four divided doses for 14 days[b]	

CDC, Centers for Disease Control and Prevention; PO, orally.

[a]Recommendations are those of the CDC.

[b]Topical therapy alone is inadequate for ophthalmia neonatorum and is unnecessary when systemic therapy is administered.

activity against *C. trachomatis* and *U. urealyticum*, high dosages have not consistently eradicated chlamydial infections.[1,31–37]

For pregnant women with chlamydial urogenital infections, treatment can reduce the risk of pregnancy complications and transmission to the newborn significantly. Because the use of tetracyclines and fluoroquinolones is contraindicated during pregnancy, azithromycin and amoxicillin are the recommended drug treatments (see Table 95-8). When compliance with a multiday regimen is a concern, azithromycin is the preferred treatment in women, regardless of pregnancy status. It is recommended that posttreatment cultures be obtained for pregnant patients treated for chlamydial infections to ensure eradication of the infection. Persons treated for chlamydia should abstain from sexual intercourse for 7 days following the initiation of treatment.[1,34–37,41,42]

C. trachomatis transmission during perinatal exposure can result in infections of the eye, oropharynx, lungs, urogenital tract, and rectum of the neonate or infant. Despite its efficacy in preventing gonococcal ophthalmia, topical erythromycin ointment (0.5%) appears less effective in preventing chlamydial ophthalmia. Additionally, topical therapy has no effect on nasal carriage or colonization of other parts of the infant's body, so the potential for other infections, including pneumonia, remains. Because of the high percentage of treatment failures, topical therapy is not recommended to treat ophthalmia caused by *C. trachomatis*. Instead, an oral erythromycin regimen is recommended.[1,31–34]

Evaluation of Therapeutic Outcomes

Treatment of chlamydial infections with the recommended regimens is highly effective; therefore, posttreatment laboratory testing is not recommended routinely unless symptoms persist or there are other specific concerns (e.g., pregnancy). Posttreatment tests should not be performed for at least 3 weeks following completion of therapy.[1] When posttreatment tests are positive, they usually represent noncompliance, failure to treat sexual partners, or laboratory error rather than inadequate therapy or resistance to therapy. Infants with pneumonitis should receive follow-up testing because erythromycin is only 80% effective, and a second course of therapy can be necessary.[1,31–34]

GENITAL HERPES

Epidemiology and Etiology

Genital herpes infections represent the most common cause of genital ulceration seen in the United States. More than 50 million Americans have genital herpes, and this number is increasing by at least 500,000 each year.[1,43–48] Because of its morbidity, recurrent nature, and potential for complications, as well as its ability to be transmitted asymptomatically, genital herpes is of major public health importance.[45–54] Similar to syphilis and other STDs, the presence of genital herpes lesions is associated with an increased risk of acquiring HIV following exposure.[1,43–49]

Pathophysiology

Herpes comes from the Greek word meaning "to creep" and is used to describe two distinct but antigenically related serotypes of HSV. HSV-1 is associated most commonly with oropharyngeal disease, and HSV-2 is associated most closely with genital disease; however, each virus is capable of causing clinically indistinguishable infections in both anatomic areas.[43–45,48]

Humans are the sole known reservoir for HSV. Infection is transmitted via inoculation of virus from infected secretions onto mucosal surfaces (e.g., urethra, oropharynx, cervix, and conjunctivae) or through abraded skin. Evidence that the virus survives for a limited time on environmental surfaces suggests the possibility of fomitic transfer as a nonvenereal route of transmission.[43–45,48]

The cycle of HSV infection occurs in five stages: primary mucocutaneous infection, infection of the ganglia, establishment of latency, reactivation, and recurrent infection. After viral inoculation, HSV infection is associated with cytoplasmic granulation, ballooning degeneration of cells, and production of mononucleated giant cells. Initially, the cellular response is predominantly PMN, followed by a lymphocytic response. Replication occurs with viral spread to contiguous cells and peripheral sensory nerves. Latency then is established in sensory or autonomic nerve root ganglia. Latency appears to be lifelong, interrupted only by reactivation of the viral infection. It is unclear what factors are important in maintaining latency, but immune responses and emotional and physical stresses appear important in reactivating latent virus.[43–45,48]

Clinical Presentation

The signs and symptoms of genital herpes infection are influenced by many factors, including previous exposure to HSV, viral type, and host factors such as age and site of infection. Because a high percentage of initial and recurrent infections are asymptomatic, and because viral shedding can occur in the absence of apparent lesions or symptoms, identification and education of individuals with genital herpes are essential in controlling its transmission.[43–52] A summary of the clinical presentation of genital herpes is provided in Table 95-9.

Complications

Complications from genital herpes infections result from both genital spread and autoinoculation of the virus and occur most commonly with primary first episodes. Lesions at extragenital sites, such as the eye, rectum, pharynx, and fingers, are not uncommon. CNS involvement is seen occasionally and can take several forms, including an aseptic meningitis, transverse myelitis, or sacral radiculopathy syndrome.[43–52]

A major concern is the effect of genital herpes on neonates exposed during pregnancy. Neonatal herpes is associated with a high mortality and significant morbidity. It is transmitted to the newborn primarily through exposure to HSV in the birth canal but, in rare cases, also is transmitted transplacentally. The risk of transmission during birth appears much greater for first-episode primary infections than for recurrent infections. Neonatal herpes infection has a case-fatality rate of approximately 50%, with a large proportion of surviving infants experiencing significant morbidity, including permanent neurologic damage.[43,44,48]

Diagnosis

Confirmation of a genital herpes infection can be made only with laboratory testing. Tissue culture is the most specific (100%) and sensitive method (80% to 90%) of confirming the diagnosis of first-episode genital herpes; however, culture is relatively insensitive in detecting HSV in ulcers in the latter stages of healing and in recurrent infections, as a result, in part, of reduced viral load. Viral culture is expensive and time-consuming, and improper collection or transport of specimens can result in false-negative results. In most situations, HSV isolation on tissue culture takes 48 to 96 hours. Following isolation, it is recommended that typing of the virus be performed because of prognostic implications (HSV-1 is associated with a lower rate of asymptomatic and symptomatic recurrence). In instances in which rapid detection is necessary, such as an impending birth, other detection methods can be more useful. Amplified culture techniques that combine cell culture for 24 hours and subsequent staining for HSV antigen have sensitivities and specificities only slightly less than those of culture.[43–48,53–55]

Several serologic tests capable of distinguishing HSV-1 and HSV-2 antibodies are available. These tests detect antibodies to type-specific HSV-1 and HSV-2 proteins gG-1 and gG-2, respectively. Although antibody formation begins immediately following a primary herpes infection, complete seroconversion (i.e., complete

TABLE 95-9 Presentation of Genital Herpes Infections

General	Incubation period 2–14 days (mean, 4 days) Can be caused by either HSV-1 or HSV-2
Classification of infection	
First-episode primary	Initial genital infection in individuals lacking antibody to either HSV-1 or HSV-2
First-episode nonprimary	Initial genital infection in individuals with clinical or serologic evidence of prior HSV (usually HSV-1) infection
Recurrent	Appearance of genital lesions at some time following healing of first-episode infection
Signs and symptoms	
First-episode infections	Most primary infections are asymptomatic or minimally symptomatic Multiple painful pustular or ulcerative lesions on external genitalia developing over a period of 7–10 days; lesions heal in 2–4 weeks (mean, 21 days) Flulike symptoms (e.g., fever, headache, malaise) during first few days after appearance of lesions Others—local itching, pain, or discomfort; vaginal or urethral discharge, tender inguinal adenopathy, paresthesias, urinary retention Severity of symptoms greater in females than in males Symptoms are less severe (e.g., fewer lesions, more rapid lesion healing, fewer or milder systemic symptoms) with nonprimary infections Symptoms more severe and prolonged in the immunocompromised On average viral shedding lasts approximately 11–12 days for primary infections and 7 days for nonprimary infections
Recurrent	Prodrome seen in approximately 50% of patients prior to appearance of recurrent lesions; mild burning, itching, or tingling are typical prodromal symptoms Compared to primary infections, recurrent infections associated with (1) fewer lesions that are more localized, (2) shorter duration of active infection (lesions heal within 7 days), and (3) milder symptoms Severity of symptoms greater in females than in males Symptoms more severe and prolonged in the immunocompromised On average viral shedding lasts approximately 4 days Asymptomatic viral shedding is more frequent during the first year after infection with HSV
Therapeutic implications of HSV-1 versus HSV-2 genital infection	Primary infections caused by HSV-1 and HSV-2 virtually indistinguishable Recurrent infections and subclinical viral shedding are less frequent with HSV-1 Recurrent infections with HSV-2 tend to be more severe
Complications	Secondary infection of lesions; extragenital infection because of autoinoculation; disseminated infection (primarily in immunocompromised patients); meningitis or encephalitis; neonatal transmission

HSV-1, herpes simplex virus type 1; HSV-2, herpes simplex virus type 2.

antibody development) can take several months. Until the full expression of all antigenic determinants of HSV-1 and HSV-2 occurs, these tests are not useful in differentiating HSV-1 and HSV-2 infection. Older antibody detection tests, some of which are still marketed, are unable to distinguish between HSV-1 and HSV-2 owing to the considerable cross-reactivity between the two serotypes. Given the high prevalence of HSV-1 antibody in the adult population, accurate interpretation of positive results is not possible.[43–48,53–55]

PCR assays that detect HSV DNA and differentiate HSV-1 and HSV-2 infections are more sensitive than culture and are considered the diagnostic test of choice for suspected CNS infections (i.e., HSV encephalitis and HSV meningitis). PCR assays are highly sensitive in detecting asymptomatic viral shedding.[43–48,53–55]

Although the diagnosis of genital herpes can be confirmed only by laboratory tests, less stringent diagnostic criteria (e.g., characteristic physical findings or clinical history) frequently are used in clinical practice. A presumptive diagnosis of genital herpes commonly is made based on the presence of dark-field-negative, vesicular, or ulcerative genital lesions. A prior history of similar lesions or recent sexual contact with an individual with similar lesions also is useful in making the diagnosis. Other STDs, including chancroid, lymphogranuloma venereum, and granuloma inguinale, and causes such as trauma, allergic reactions, and bacterial or fungal infections are considered in the differential diagnosis.[43–48,53–55]

TREATMENT

The most achievable goals in the management of genital herpes are to relieve symptoms and to shorten the clinical course, to prevent complications and recurrences, and to decrease disease transmission. Although research has focused primarily on the treatment of active infection and suppression of recurrences, increasing emphasis is being placed on various approaches, including immunotherapy that might provide protection from disease transmission or possibly eliminate established latency.[47–48]

Palliative and supportive measures are the cornerstone of therapy for patients with genital herpes. Pain and discomfort usually respond to warm saline baths or the use of analgesics, antipyretics, or antipruritics; good genital hygiene can prevent the development of bacterial superinfection.

4 Specific chemotherapeutic approaches to treating genital herpes include antiviral compounds, topical surfactants, photodynamic dyes, immune modulators, vaccines, and interferons. Few of these have undergone extensive evaluation, however, and only the antiviral agents have demonstrated any consistent clinical efficacy. The most recent CDC recommendations for the treatment of genital herpes include the antiviral agents acyclovir, valacyclovir, and famciclovir[1] (Table 95-10). The overall efficacy of these agents in treating genital HSV infection appears comparable, although patient compliance can be improved with regimens requiring less frequent dosing.[1,43,44]

First-Episode Infections

Oral formulations of acyclovir, famciclovir, and valacyclovir have demonstrated efficacy in reducing viral shedding, duration of symptoms, and time to healing of first-episode genital herpes infections, with maximal benefits seen when therapy is initiated at the earliest stages of infection. Table 95-10 lists the recommended acyclovir, famciclovir, and valacyclovir oral regimens for first-episode infections. In immunocompromised patients or those with severe symptoms or complications necessitating hospitalization, parenteral acyclovir can be beneficial; however, the IV regimen has been associated with renal, GI, bone marrow, and CNS toxicity, particularly

TABLE 95-10 Treatment of Genital Herpes

Type of Infection	Recommended Regimens[a,b]	Alternative Regimen
First clinical episode of genital herpes[c]	Acyclovir 400 mg PO three times daily for 7–10 days,[d] *or* Acyclovir 200 mg PO five times daily for 7–10 days,[d] *or* Famciclovir 250 mg PO three times daily for 7–10 days,[d] *or* Valacyclovir 1 g PO twice daily for 7–10 days[d]	Acyclovir 5–10 mg/kg IV every 8 hours for 2–7 days or until clinical improvement occurs, followed by oral therapy to complete at least 10 days of total therapy[e]
Recurrent infection		
Episodic therapy	Acyclovir 400 mg PO three times daily for 5 days,[f] *or* Acyclovir 800 mg PO twice daily for 5 days,[f] *or* Acyclovir 800 mg PO three times daily for 2 days,[f] *or* Famciclovir 125 mg PO twice daily for 5 days,[f] *or* Famciclovir 1 g PO twice daily for 1 day,[f] *or* Famciclovir 500 mg PO once, followed by 250 mg PO twice daily for 2 days,[f] *or* Valacyclovir 500 mg PO twice daily for 3 days,[f] *or* Valacyclovir 1 g PO once daily for 5 days[f]	
Suppressive therapy	Acyclovir 400 mg PO twice daily, *or* Famciclovir 250 mg PO twice daily, *or* Valacyclovir 500 mg or 1,000 mg PO once daily[g]	

CDC, Centers for Disease Control and Prevention; HIV, human immunodeficiency virus; PO, orally.

[a]Recommendations are those of the CDC.
[b]HIV-infected patients can require more aggressive therapy.
[c]Primary or nonprimary first episode.
[d]Treatment duration can be extended if healing is incomplete after 10 days.
[e]Only for patients with severe symptoms or complications that necessitate hospitalization.
[f]Requires initiation of therapy within 24 hours of lesion onset or during the prodrome that precedes some outbreaks.
[g]Valacyclovir 500 mg appears less effective than other valacyclovir and acyclovir regimens in patients with 10 or more recurrences per year.

in patients with renal dysfunction receiving high doses. No antiviral regimen is known to prevent latency or alter the subsequent frequency and severity of recurrences in humans.[1,43–48,51,52,56–59]

Recurrent Infections

There are two approaches to management of recurrent episodes: episodic or chronic suppressive therapy. Episodic therapy is initiated early during the course of the recurrence, preferably within 6 to 12 hours of the onset of prodromal symptoms but no more than 24 hours after the appearance of lesions. In most patients, appreciable effects on symptomatology are not seen. Patients with prolonged episodes of recurrent infection or severe symptomatology are most likely to benefit from episodic therapy. Table 95-10 lists the recommended acyclovir, famciclovir, and valacyclovir suppressive regimens. One concern with episodic therapy is that some patients continue to shed virus despite the absence of lesions or presence of prodromal symptoms. Because of the relative mildness and brevity of recurrent infections, parenteral administration of acyclovir usually is not justifiable.[1,43–48,51,52,56–59]

Suppressive therapy with recommended antivirals reduces the frequency and severity of recurrences in 70% to 80% of patients experiencing frequent recurrences. Asymptomatic viral shedding is markedly reduced in patients receiving suppressive therapy; however, the extent to which this decreases disease transmission to sexual partners remains to be determined. Despite antiviral suppressive therapy, low-level virus shedding still occurs. However, this virus shedding may be less than that seen in patients treated episodically for recurrences, and thus may be associated with a lower risk of disease transmission. Because the frequency of recurrences tends to diminish over time, periodic "drug holidays" are advocated to assess changes in the underlying recurrence rate and determine if continued suppressive therapy is warranted.[1,43–48,51,52,56–59]

Clinical **Controversy...**

The role of antiviral agents in the treatment of most recurrent genital herpes episodes is controversial. Because signs and symptoms of recurrent infections generally are milder and of shorter duration than those of first-episode infections in immunocompetent hosts, demonstration of clinically important therapeutic benefits is difficult. However, as episodic, asymptomatic viral shedding is common in HSV-2 infection, suppressive therapy in combination with use of condoms provides some protection to uninfected sexual partners.

Resistant HSV isolates have been identified in some patients experiencing breakthrough recurrences while taking acyclovir. Although there is concern about the development of resistant strains with suppressive therapy, clinical trials have found no evidence of cumulative toxicity or significant resistance in patients treated continuously with the recommended antivirals.[43–48]

Selected Populations

Immunocompromised patients are at greatest risk for severe and recurrent HSV infections. Acyclovir, valacyclovir, and famciclovir have been used to prevent reactivation of infection in patients seropositive for HSV who undergo transplantation procedures or induction chemotherapy for acute leukemia. Immunocompromised individuals, such as patients with acquired immunodeficiency syndrome (AIDS), who fail treatment or prophylaxis with recommended antiviral doses frequently demonstrate improved response with higher doses. If resistance is suspected or confirmed with recommended first-line antivirals, foscarnet is usually effective. However, its use is associated with a greater risk of serious adverse effects. Lesional application of an extemporaneous compounded cidofovir (1%) gel or trifluridine ophthalmic solution appears to offer some benefits also.[1,43–48]

The safety of acyclovir, famciclovir, and valacyclovir during pregnancy is not established, although considerable experience with acyclovir in pregnant patients has produced no evidence of teratogenic effects. Because of the high maternal and infant morbidity associated with first-episode primary genital infections or severe recurrent infections at or near term, many clinicians advocate the use of systemic acyclovir as the standard of care in such cases; however, the effectiveness of such therapy is unknown. The use of acyclovir to suppress recurrent episodes near term is more controversial primarily because of the lack of data demonstrating significant benefits in this situation.[1,43–48,60–63]

With the increasing prevalence of genital herpes worldwide, the potential exists for widespread use and misuse of acyclovir, valacyclovir, and famciclovir, resulting in development of resistant HSV isolates. In vitro resistance to these three agents usually is mediated by alterations in viral thymidine kinase; most resistant isolates are either thymidine kinase-deficient or have altered thymidine kinase. The incidence and clinical implications of HSV resistance require further study particularly with respect to immunocompromised hosts, in whom resistance can develop with greater frequency and be of greater clinical importance. Unlike acyclovir, valacyclovir, and famciclovir, foscarnet does not require the presence of thymidine kinase to be effective.[43–48]

Numerous agents for the prophylaxis and treatment of genital herpes infections are being studied. Neither topical nor systemic interferons have demonstrated consistent beneficial effects in genital HSV infections; however, a reduction in pain and time of healing of lesions has been reported with an interferon preparation incorporated into a gel containing nonoxynol-9. Other treatments under investigation include cidofovir and immune modulators such as imiquimod and resiquimod.[43–48] Agents that can eliminate ganglionic latency and prevent recurrent HSV infections are not expected to be available in the near future. Development of vaccines capable of protecting against HSV infection has proved challenging given the relative lack of protection offered by humoral and cell-mediated immunity in preventing naturally occurring recurrent infections. Safety concerns with live attenuated virus vaccines resulted in research focused primarily on recombinant protein vaccines that have exhibited relatively poor immunogenicity. Use of heterologous vaccines (bacillus Calmette–Guérin and influenza vaccines) to stimulate the immune system in patients with recurrent genital herpes has proved of no significant benefit.[43–48,64]

Evaluation of Therapeutic Outcomes

Available antiviral compounds are of greatest benefit in patients experiencing first-episode primary infections, immunocompromised patients, and patients with frequent or severe recurrent infections. Antivirals, however, are palliative and not curative, and patients receiving these agents should be monitored closely for adverse drug effects. CDC guidelines suggest that discontinuation of suppressive therapy after 1 year should be considered to assess for possible changes in the patient's intrinsic pattern of recurrence. In many patients, decreases in recurrence rates and the severity of symptoms occur over time. However, some clinicians prefer to continue suppressive therapy indefinitely because it significantly reduces asymptomatic viral shedding, a potential benefit in reducing the risk of disease transmission to uninfected sexual partners.[1,43–48]

TRICHOMONIASIS

Epidemiology and Etiology

Trichomonas vaginalis, a flagellated, motile protozoan is responsible for 3 to 5 million cases of trichomoniasis annually in the United States. Humans are host to two other *Trichomonas* species, *Trichomonas tenax* and *Trichomonas hominis*, but *T. vaginalis* is the only species thought to be pathogenic. Although infection by nonsexual contact is reported, it is rare. Contamination of inanimate objects and spread of infection via communal bathing or contact with infected bath or toilet articles is possible because *T. vaginalis* can survive for up to 45 minutes on moist surfaces. Neonatal infections also represent another possible nonvenereal route of disease transmission.[65–69]

Coinfection with other STDs is not unusual in patients diagnosed with trichomoniasis. Women infected with *T. vaginalis* are three times more likely to have gonorrhea than those who do not have trichomoniasis; approximately 20% of men with gonococcal urethritis also have trichomoniasis.[65–69] In patients treated appropriately for genital *C. trachomatis* or *U. urealyticum* infection, persistent urethritis can result from coexisting trichomonal infection. Although not well documented, the inflammatory response produced by trichomoniasis may increase the risk of acquiring HIV.[1,65–70]

Pathophysiology

Trichomonads typically can be isolated from the vagina, urethra, and paraurethral ducts and glands in the majority of infected women. Infrequently, they are recovered from the endocervix. Extragenital sites are epidemiologically important because infection can persist and result in reinfection of the vagina if local therapy alone is used. This may account for the higher relapse rates reported for local versus systemic therapy. After attachment to the vaginal or urethral mucosa, trichomonads usually elicit an inflammatory response that manifests as a discharge containing large numbers of PMN leukocytes.[65–74]

Clinical Presentation

Trichomonal infections are reported more commonly in women than in men. In part this might be because of the smaller number of organisms found in the male urethra making detection more difficult, greater disease transmission rates from males to females, and the nature of male infections, which have a high spontaneous cure rate even in the absence of treatment.[66,67,70–72,75] The typical clinical presentation of trichomoniasis in males and females is presented in Table 95-11.

TABLE 95-11 Presentation of *Trichomonas* Infections

	Males	Females
General	Incubation period 3–28 days Organism can be detectable within 48 hours after exposure to infected partner	Incubation period 3–28 days
Site of infection	Most common: urethra Others: rectum (usually caused by rectal intercourse in MSM), oropharynx, eye	Most common: endocervical canal Others: urethra, rectum (usually caused by perineal contamination), oropharynx, eye
Symptoms	Can be asymptomatic (more common in males than females) or minimally symptomatic Urethral discharge (clear to mucopurulent) Dysuria, pruritus	Can be asymptomatic or minimally symptomatic Scant to copious, typically malodorous vaginal discharge (50–75%) and pruritus (worse during menses) Dysuria, dyspareunia
Signs	Urethral discharge	Vaginal discharge Vaginal pH 4.5–6 Inflammation/erythema of vulva, vagina, and/or cervix Urethritis
Complications	Epididymitis and chronic prostatitis (uncommon) Male infertility (decreased sperm motility and viability)	Pelvic inflammatory disease and associated complications (i.e., ectopic pregnancy, infertility) Premature labor, premature rupture of membranes, and low-birth-weight infants (risk of neonatal infections is low) Cervical neoplasia

MSM, men who have sex with men.

Diagnosis

T. vaginalis produces nonspecific symptoms also consistent with bacterial vaginosis; as a result, laboratory diagnosis is required. Because *T. vaginalis* requires a pH range of 4.9 to 7.5 for survival, a vaginal discharge pH of greater than 5 usually indicates the presence of either *T. vaginalis* or *Gardnerella vaginalis*, a common cause of bacterial vaginosis. The simplest and most reliable means of diagnosis is a wet-mount examination of the vaginal discharge.[67,70–72,75] Trichomoniasis is confirmed if characteristic pear-shaped, flagellating organisms are observed. The wet mount is only about 60% to 80% sensitive in detecting the presence of trichomonads, with lower sensitivities reported in men and in women with low-grade, subacute, or chronic infections.[68–70,72,74]

Although the presence of trichomonads may be reported on a Papanicolaou smear (Pap), the sensitivity of this cytologic technique is less than for wet mount and also is associated with a high number of false-positive and false-negative results. Stained smears of cervical specimens have been used in diagnosis, but they are less sensitive and more time-consuming than the wet mount and therefore are not recommended. Culture techniques for trichomonads are highly specific and more sensitive than the wet mount, but they are not useful in rapid diagnosis because up to 48 hours or longer is necessary for growth. Cultures can be necessary, however, to confirm the diagnosis in the absence of a positive wet mount or to determine antimicrobial susceptibility in intractable cases.[1,65–72,74,75]

Newer diagnostic tests such as monoclonal antibody or DNA probe techniques, as well as PCR tests that can detect small amounts of trichomonal DNA, have been developed. These office-based tests are highly sensitive and specific for detecting infection in both vaginal specimens and urine. However, these tests are still not widely used.[65–69]

In males, demonstration of trichomonads in urethral specimens or urine sediment by wet mount is difficult, and diagnosis depends largely on culture. Specimens from males should be taken prior to first voiding because the small number of trichomonads in males may be reduced by micturition.[65–71]

TREATMENT

Recommended and alternative treatment regimens for *T. vaginalis* include either metronidazole or tinidazole, both of which produce high cure rates in these infections. In only a few cases have *T. vaginalis* isolates been resistant to standard metronidazole or tinidazole doses. In these instances, longer courses of therapy or doses higher than those recommended routinely as initial therapy usually produce a cure.[1,65–69,72,75,76]

Table 95-12 provides treatment recommendations for trichomonas infections.[1] The standard therapy for trichomoniasis is either metronidazole or tinidazole 2 g orally as a single dose; cure rates are comparable with the recommended alternative regimen of metronidazole 500 mg twice daily for 7 days. When sexual partners are treated simultaneously, cure rates greater than 95% are reported. If sexual partners are not treated concurrently, cure rates are somewhat lower. In limited clinical testing, single metronidazole doses of less than 1.5 g are associated with high failure rates.[1,65–69,72,75,76]

Advantages of single-dose therapy over the multidose alternative regimen include better patient compliance, lower total dose, lower cost, and shorter exposure of the patient's GI and urogenital anaerobic bacterial flora to the drug. As a result of the latter, the likelihood of developing pseudomembranous colitis or symptomatic candidal vulvovaginitis is decreased.[65–69,72] Because high doses of metronidazole have mutagenic effects in bacteria and oncogenic effects in mice, a reduced time of exposure in humans can be beneficial. There is no conclusive evidence for either of these effects in humans after short-term therapy with recommended doses. GI complaints (e.g., anorexia, nausea, vomiting, and diarrhea) are more common with the single 2-g dose of either metronidazole or tinidazole, occurring in 5% to 10% of treated patients. Some patients also complain of a bitter metallic taste in the mouth with metronidazole. Patients intolerant of the single 2-g dose because of GI adverse effects usually tolerate the alternative metronidazole multidose regimen.[65–69,72,75,76]

TABLE 95-12 Treatment of Trichomoniasis

Type	Recommended Regimen[a]	Alternative Regimen
Symptomatic and asymptomatic infections	Metronidazole 2 g PO in a single dose[b] *or* Tinidazole 2 g PO in a single dose	Metronidazole 500 mg PO two times daily for 7 days[c] *or* Tinidazole 2 g PO for 5 days[d]
Treatment in pregnancy	Metronidazole 2 g PO in a single dose[e]	

CDC, Centers for Disease Control and Prevention; PO, orally.

[a]Recommendations are those of the CDC.

[b]Treatment failures to single dose metronidazole should be treated with metronidazole 500 mg PO twice daily for 7 days. Persistent failures should be managed in consultation with an expert. Metronidazole or tinidazole 2 g PO daily for 5 days has been effective in patients infected with *Trichomonas vaginalis* strains mildly resistant to metronidazole, but experience is limited; higher doses also have been used.

[c]Metronidazole labeling approved by the FDA does not include this regimen. Dosage regimens for treatment of trichomoniasis included in the product labeling are the single 2 g dose; 250 mg three times daily for 7 days; and 375 mg twice daily for 7 days. The 250 mg and 375 mg dosage regimens are currently not included in the CDC recommendations.

[d]For treatment failures with metronidazole 2 g as a single dose and metronidazole 500 mg PO two times daily for 7 days.

[e]Metronidazole is pregnancy category B and tinidazole is pregnancy category C; both drugs are contraindicated in the first trimester of pregnancy. Some clinicians recommend deferring metronidazole treatment in asymptomatic pregnant women until after 37 weeks gestation.

5 To achieve maximal cure rates and prevent relapse with either metronidazole or tinidazole as a single 2-g dose, simultaneous treatment of infected sexual partners is necessary. In women treated with the alternative 7-day course, however, relapse rates are not appreciably different regardless of whether or not sexual partners are treated. It is speculated that in men, spontaneous resolution of trichomonal infection or a reduction in the number of trichomonads below the inoculum necessary to transmit disease may occur during the 7 days of a female's therapy. In patients who fail to respond to an initial course of metronidazole therapy, a second course of therapy with metronidazole 500 mg twice daily for 7 days or a single 2-g dose of tinidazole is recommended. Patients refractory to a second course of treatment usually respond to a regimen using higher dosages of either agent (i.e., 2 to 4 g daily for 5 to 14 days). Good response rates also are reported for metronidazole 2 to 3 g orally plus either a single 500-mg tablet administered intravaginally or intravaginal metronidazole gel (0.75%) for 7 to 14 days.[61,65–69,71,76,77] Topical vaginal therapy alone is associated with low cure rates because infections involving the urethra or periurethral glands are unaffected and can serve as the source of reinfection.[67] Use of IV metronidazole can be warranted for rare cases of intolerance to oral medication or infections resistant to high-dose oral metronidazole. Sexual partners of all patients who require retreatment also should be treated or retreated because the majority of apparent treatment failures appear to be caused by reinfection or noncompliance.[65–69]

Concerns regarding the use of metronidazole in women who are pregnant or breast-feeding have been raised. Because metronidazole is secreted in breast milk, it is recommended that breast-feeding be interrupted for 12 to 24 hours after maternal ingestion of a single 2-g dose. Metronidazole (pregnancy category B) and tinidazole (pregnancy category C) are contraindicated during the first trimester of pregnancy based on FDA-approved labeling. Although some experts recommend avoiding use of either agent throughout pregnancy, others advocate the use of metronidazole during any stage of pregnancy because of the potential adverse pregnancy outcomes associated with trichomoniasis. Currently no consensus exists on whether or how to treat trichomonas infections in pregnant women.[1,65–69]

Various local therapies for trichomoniasis have been proposed, particularly for pregnant patients. Clotrimazole vaginal suppositories, 100 mg at bedtime for 1 to 2 weeks, relieve symptoms in many women and produce cure rates of 50% or greater. An alternative therapy is gentle douching with either a diluted solution of vinegar or a 1% zinc sulfate solution until symptoms improve and then less frequently thereafter. This therapy generally provides some symptomatic improvement but few cures. Although once recommended, povidone-iodine douches should be avoided during pregnancy because of the risk of fetal thyroid suppression.[65–69]

Several other nitroimidazole antibiotics related to metronidazole and tinidazole (e.g., nimorazole, ornidazole, and carnidazole) are being investigated worldwide for the treatment of trichomoniasis. Unfortunately, none of these agents differs significantly from metronidazole or tinidazole in terms of efficacy (i.e., cross-resistance is high) or toxicity against metronidazole-susceptible strains of *T. vaginalis*.[65–69]

EVALUATION OF THERAPEUTIC OUTCOMES

Follow-up is considered unnecessary in patients who become asymptomatic after treatment with recommended therapy. When patients remain symptomatic, it is important to determine if reinfection has occurred. In these cases, a repeat course of therapy, as well as identification and treatment or retreatment of infected sexual partners, is recommended. In situations in which reinfection can be excluded, a relative resistance to metronidazole or tinidazole should be assumed, and an alternative regimen should be prescribed. Culture and sensitivity are warranted for infections unresponsive to alternative regimens.

HUMAN PAPILLOMAVIRUS AND OTHER STDS

Several STDs other than those just discussed occur with varying frequency in the United States and throughout the world. Although an in-depth discussion of these diseases is beyond the scope of this chapter, Table 95-13 lists recommended treatment regimens.[1] Of notable

TABLE 95-13 Treatment Regimens for Miscellaneous Sexually Transmitted Diseases

Infection	Recommended Regimen[a]	Alternative Regimen
Chancroid (*Haemophilus ducreyi*)	Azithromycin 1 g PO in a single dose, *or* Ceftriaxone 250 mg IM in a single dose, *or* Ciprofloxacin 500 mg PO twice daily for 3 days,[b] *or* Erythromycin base 500 mg PO four times daily for 7 days	
Lymphogranuloma venereum	Doxycycline 100 mg PO twice daily for 21 days[c]	Erythromycin base 500 mg PO four times daily for 21 days[d]
Human papillomavirus (HPV) infection		
External genital/perianal warts	*Provider-Administered Therapies:* Cryotherapy (e.g., liquid nitrogen or cryoprobe); repeat weekly as necessary, *or* Podophyllin resin 10–25% in compound tincture of benzoin applied to lesions; repeat weekly as necessary,[e,f] *or* Trichloroacetic acid (TCA) 80–90% *or* bichloracetic acid (BCA) 80–90% applied to warts; repeat weekly as necessary, *or* Surgical removal (tangential scissor excision, tangential shave excision, curettage, or electrosurgery) *Patient-Applied Therapies:* Podofilox 0.5% solution or gel applied twice daily for 3 days, followed by 4 days of no therapy; cycle is repeated as necessary for up to four cycles,[f] *or* Imiquimod 5% cream applied at bedtime three times weekly for up to 16 weeks,[f] *or* Sinecatechins 15% ointment applied three times daily for up to 16 weeks	Intralesional interferon *or* Photodynamic therapy *or* Topical cidofovir
Vaginal and anal warts	Cryotherapy with liquid nitrogen, or TCA or BCA 80–90% as for external HPV warts; repeat weekly as necessary[g] Surgical removal (not for vaginal or urethral meatus warts)	
Urethral meatus warts	Cryotherapy with liquid nitrogen, or podophyllin resin 10–25% in compound tincture of benzoin applied at weekly intervals[f,h]	
Prevention	Gardasil® (human papillomavirus quadrivalent [types 6, 11, 16, and 18]) recombinant vaccine 0.5 mL IM on day 1; a second and third dose are administered 2 and 6 months following the first dose[i,j,k] Cervarix® (human papillomavirus bivalent [types 16 and 18]) recombinant vaccine 0.5 mL IM on day 1; a second and third dose are administered 1 and 6 months following the first dose[i,l]	

[a]Recommendations are those of the Centers for Disease Control and Prevention (CDC).
[b]Ciprofloxacin is contraindicated for pregnant and lactating women and for persons aged <18 years.
[c]Azithromycin 1 g PO once weekly for 3 weeks can be effective.
[d]Pregnant patients should be treated with erythromycin.
[e]Some experts recommended washing podophyllin off after 1–4 hours to minimize local irritation.
[f]Safety during pregnancy is not established.
[g]Surgical removal of anal warts is also a recommended treatment.
[h]Some specialists recommend the use of podofilox and imiquimod for treating distal meatal warts.
[i]CDC recommendations: vaccination is recommended in girls 11–12 years of age, and in females aged 13–26 years who either were not previously vaccinated, or who did not complete the vaccination series.
[j]FDA approved labeling for Gardasil®: indicated in girls and women 9 through 26 years of age for the prevention of cervical, vulvar, vaginal, and anal cancer caused by HPV types 16 and 18, genital warts (condyloma acuminata) caused by HPV types 6 and 11, and precancerous or dysplastic lesions caused by HPV types 6, 11, 16, and 18.
[k]Vaccination is recommended in males aged 9–26 years to prevent genital warts and anal cancer.
[l]FDA approved labeling for Cervarix®: indicated in females 9 through 25 years of age for the prevention of cervical cancer, cervical intraepithelial neoplasia grade 2 or worse, adenocarcinoma in situ, and cervical intraepithelial neoplasia grade 1 caused by HPV types 16 and 18.

importance among these other STDs, however, is genital HPV infection, the most common viral STD in the United States. More than 100 HPV types have been characterized by genomic makeup, with approximately 30 types associated with genital tract lesions.[79–81] Of these, types 6 and 11 are associated most commonly with the development of low-grade dysplasia manifested as exophytic genital warts. In most individuals, genital infection with HPV is subclinical, and patients with visible acuminate warts represent less than 1% of all infected individuals. When present, genital warts can be large and multifocal, producing variable degrees of discomfort. Based on HPV DNA detection methods, most warts will regress spontaneously within 1 to 2 years of their initial appearance. However, reinfection is common in young, sexually active populations.[1,78,79]

Infection with several HPV types, particularly HPV-16 and HPV-18, is considered the major risk factor for the development of cervical neoplasia, the second most common cancer in women worldwide. Although epidemiologic, virologic, and clinical data strongly support this association, HPV infection alone is insufficient to cause cervical cancer development because only a small percentage of infected women develop the disease. It appears that the interplay of host immune defenses, genetic factors, and infection with HPV types containing a more aggressive variant all contribute to the risk of developing cervical neoplasia.[78,79]

The Pap smear is the most frequently used and cost-effective diagnostic test for detecting clinical and subclinical (i.e., no visible signs of condylomata) HPV in women. However, Pap smears are neither specific for HPV nor useful in detecting latent infections. Frequently, visual inspection of genital surfaces under magnification can assist in making the diagnosis. Various tests for detecting HPV DNA, RNA, or capsid protein also are available, and unlike the Pap smear do not require subjective interpretation of the results. The HPV-specific tests are only approved in women with abnormal Pap smears or women older than 30 years of age. However, use of HPV DNA testing as a routine screening test in lieu of Pap smears is expected in the near future. In women identified to have high-risk HPV infections by these tests, follow-up cytology would be performed.[78,79]

No consensus exists on the best approach to treating patients with genital HPV infection, particularly because most cases appear to be transient with spontaneous regression of lesions. A number of treatments are recommended (see Table 95-13), but none is clearly superior to the others. Treatment generally is directed toward patients with manifestations of genital warts, with the goal of removing or destroying these lesions and grossly infected surrounding tissue. Because such treatment neither stops viral expression in surrounding tissue nor eliminates viral latency, recurrence of lesions is not uncommon.[78,79]

Two HPV vaccines are marketed in the United States. Cervarix, a bivalent vaccine for HPV-16 and -18, and Gardasil, a quadrivalent vaccine for HPV-6, -11, -16, and -18. Both vaccines are indicated for preventing cervical precancers and cervical cancer in females 9 to 26 years of age. In addition, Gardasil is indicated in males between the ages of 9 and 26 years for the prevention of genital warts caused by HPV-6 and -11, and for the prevention of anal cancer caused by HPV-16 and -18. Clinically important differences in the magnitude and duration of the immune response, as well as prevention of HPV infections and cervical cancer remain to be determined.[80–83]

ABBREVIATIONS

AIDS	acquired immunodeficiency syndrome
CDC	Centers for Disease Control and Prevention
CSF	cerebrospinal fluid
DFA-TP	direct fluorescent-antibody (test) for *T. pallidum*
DGI	disseminated gonococcal infection
EIA	enzyme immunoassay
FTA-ABS	fluorescent treponemal antibody absorption
HIV	human immunodeficiency virus
HPV	human papillomavirus
HSV	herpes simplex virus
HSV-1	herpes simplex virus type 1
LPS	lipopolysaccharide
MHA-TP	microhemagglutination assay for antibodies to *T. pallidum*
MSM	men who have sex with men
NAATs	nucleic acid amplification tests
NGU	nongonococcal urethritis
Pap	Papanicolaou smear
PCR	polymerase chain reaction
PID	pelvic inflammatory disease
PMN	polymorphonuclear
RPR	rapid plasma reagin
STD	sexually transmitted disease
TPHA	*T. pallidum* hemagglutination assay
TPPA	*T. pallidum* particle agglutination assay
TRUST	toluidine red unheated serum test
USR	unheated serum reagin
VDRL	Venereal Disease Research Laboratory

REFERENCES

1. Workowski KA, Berman SM, Centers for Disease Control and Prevention. Sexually transmitted diseases treatment guidelines 2010. MMWR Recomm Rep 2010;21;59(RR 12):1–111.
2. Marrazzo JM, Holmes KK. Sexually transmitted diseases: Overview and clinical approach. In: Longo DL, Fauci AS, Kasper DL, Hauser SL, Jameson JL, Loscalzo J, eds. Harrison's Principles of Internal Medicine, 18th ed. [electronic version]; New York: McGraw-Hill, 2012. *http://www.accessmedicine.com.libproxy.uthscsa.edu/content.aspx?aID=9119937.*
3. Aral SO, Holmes KK. The epidemiology of STIs and their social and behavioral determinants: Industrialized and developing countries. In: Holmes KK, Sparling PF, Stamm WE, et al., eds. Sexually Transmitted Diseases, 4th ed. New York: McGraw-Hill, 2008:53–92.
4. Sulak PJ. Sexually transmitted diseases. Semin Reprod Med 2003;21:399–413.
5. Cohen MS. Approach to the patient with a sexually transmitted disease. In: Goldman L, Schafer AI, eds. Goldman's Cecil Medicine, 24th ed. [electronic version]; 2011. *http://www.mdconsult.com.libproxy.uthscsa.edu/books/page.do?eid=4-u1.0-B978-1-4377-1604-7..00293-1&isbn=978-1-4377-1604-7&uniqId=368839637-2#4-u1.0-B978-1-4377-1604-7..00293-1--c00293.*
6. Steiner MJ, Warner L, Stone KM, Cates W Jr. Condoms and other barrier methods for prevention of STD/HIV infection and pregnancy. In: Holmes KK, Sparling PF, Stamm WE, et al., eds. Sexually Transmitted Diseases, 4th ed. New York: McGraw-Hill, 2008:1821–1829.
7. Obiero J, Mwethera PG, Wiysonge CS. Topical microbicides for prevention of sexually transmitted infections. Cochrane Database Syst Rev 2012;6:CD007961.
8. Food and Drug Administration, HHS. Over-the-counter vaginal contraceptive and spermicide drug products containing nonoxynol 9; required labeling. Final rule. Fed Regist 2007;72:71769–71785.
9. Centers for Disease Control and Prevention. Sexually Transmitted Disease Surveillance, 2010. Atlanta, GA: U.S. Department of Health and Human Services, 2011. *http://www.cdc.gov/std/stats10/surv2010.pdf.*

10. Ram S, Rice PA. Gonococcal infections. In: Longo DL, Fauci AS, Kasper DL, Hauser SL, Jameson JL, Loscalzo J, eds. Harrison's Principles of Internal Medicine, 18th ed. [electronic version]. 2012. *http://www.accessmedicine.com.libproxy.uthscsa.edu/content.aspx?aID=9121197.*
11. Marrazzo JM, Handsfield HH, Sparling PF. *Neisseria gonorrhoeae.* In: Mandell GL, Bennett JE, Dolin R, eds. Mandell, Douglas, and Bennett's Principles and Practice of Infectious Diseases, 7th ed. [electronic version]; MD Consult, 2010. *http://www.mdconsult.com.libproxy.uthscsa.edu/book/player/book.do?method=display&type=about Page&decorator=header&eid=4-u1.0-B978-0-443-06839-3..X0001-X-TOP&isbn=978-0-443-06839-3&uniq=177288689.*
12. Newman LM, Moran JS, Workowski KA. Update on the management of gonorrhea in adults in the United States. Clin Infect Dis 2007;44:S84–S101.
13. Marrazzo JM, Hofmann J. Infections due to *Neisseria.* In: Nabel EG (editor in chief), Federman DD (founding editor). ACP Medicine [electronic version]; 2009. *http://online.statref.com.libproxy.uthscsa.edu/Document/Document.aspx?docAddress=SaoWxNG8S1byvtPckclkVw%3d%3d&offset=7&SessionId=11469E6MHHSOSKLN.*
14. Centers for Disease Control and Prevention. Cephalosporin-resistant *Neisseria gonorrhoeae* public health response plan. Atlanta, GA: U.S. Department of Health and Human Services, 2012. *http://www.cdc.gov/std/treatment/Ceph-R-ResponsePlanJuly30-2012.pdf.*
15. Centers for Disease Control and Prevention. Update to CDC's sexually transmitted diseases treatment guidelines, 2010: Oral cephalosporins no longer a recommended treatment for gonococcal infections. MMWR Morb Mortal Wkly Rep 2012;61(31):590–594. *http://www.cdc.gov/mmwr/preview/mmwrhtml/mm6131a3.htm?s_cid=mm6131a3_w*
16. Gaydos CA. Nucleic acid amplification tests for gonorrhea and chlamydia: Practice and applications. Infect Dis Clin North Am 2005;19:367–386.
17. Lyss SB, Kamb ML, Peterman TA, et al. *Chlamydia trachomatis* among patients infected with and treated for *Neisseria gonorrhoeae* in sexually transmitted disease clinics in the United States. Ann Intern Med 2003;139:178–185.
18. Ison CA. Antimicrobial resistance in sexually transmitted infections in the developed world: Implications for rational treatment. Curr Opin Infect Dis 2012;25:73–78.
19. Woods CR. Gonococcal infections in neonates and young children. Semin Pediatr Infect Dis 2005;16:258–270.
20. LaFond RE, Lukehart SA. Biological basis for syphilis. Clin Microbiol Rev 2006;19:29–49.
21. Carlson JA, Dabiri G, Cribier B, Sell S. The immunopathobiology of syphilis: The manifestations and course of syphilis are determined by the level of delayed-type hypersensitivity. Am J Dermatopathol 2011;33:433–460.
22. Lukehart SA. Syphilis. In: Longo DL, Fauci AS, Kasper DL, Hauser SL, Jameson JL, Loscalzo J, eds. Harrison's Principles of Internal Medicine, 18th ed. [electronic version]; 2012. *http://www.accessmedicine.com.libproxy.uthscsa.edu/content.aspx?aid=9102029.*
23. Augenbraun M. Syphilis. In: Klausner JD, Hook EW III, eds. Current Diagnosis & Treatment of Sexually Transmitted Diseases [electronic version]; AccessMedicine, 2007. *http://www.accessmedicine.com.libproxy.uthscsa.edu/content.aspx?aID=3025480.*
24. Sparling PF, Swartz MN, Musher DM, Healy BP. Clinical manifestations of syphilis. In: Holmes KK, Sparling PF, Stamm WE, et al., eds. Sexually Transmitted Diseases, 4th ed. New York: McGraw-Hill, 2008:661–688.
25. Lee V, Kinghorn G. Syphilis: An update. Clin Med 2008;8:330–333.
26. Goh BT. Syphilis in adults. Sex Transm Infect 2005;81:448–452.
27. Kent ME, Romanelli F. Reexamining syphilis: An update on epidemiology, clinical manifestations, and management. Ann Pharmacother 2008;42:226–236.
28. Eccleston K, Collins L, Higgins SP. Primary syphilis. Int J STD AIDS 2008;19:145–151.
29. Sena AC, White BL, Sparling PF. Novel *Treponema pallidum* serologic tests: A paradigm shift in syphilis screening for the 21st century. Clin Infect Dis 2010;51:700–708.
30. Hafner L, Beagley K, Timms P. *Chlamydia trachomatis* infection: Host immune responses and potential vaccines. Mucosal Immunol 2008;1:116–130.
31. Stamm WE, Batteiger BE. *Chlamydia trachomatis* (trachoma, perinatal infections, lymphogranuloma venereum, and other genital infections). In: Mandell GL, Bennett JE, Dolin R, eds. Mandell, Douglas, and Bennett's Principles and Practice of Infectious Diseases, 7th ed [electronic version]; MD Consult, 2010. *http://www.mdconsult.com.libproxy.uthscsa.edu/book/player/book.do?method=display&type=aboutPage&decorator=header&eid=4-u1.0-B978-0-443-06839-3..X0001-X-TOP&isbn=978-0-443-06839-3&uniq=177288689.*
32. Gaydos CA, Quinn TC. Chlamydial infections. In: Longo DL, Fauci AS, Kasper DL, Hauser SL, Jameson JL, Loscalzo J, eds. Harrison's Principles of Internal Medicine, 18th ed. [electronic version]; 2012. *http://www.accessmedicine.com.libproxy.uthscsa.edu/content.aspx?aid=9102676.*
33. Stamm WE. *Chlamydia trachomatis* infections of the adult. In: Holmes KK, Sparling PF, Stamm WE, et al., eds. Sexually Transmitted Diseases, 4th ed. New York: McGraw-Hill, 2008:575–593.
34. Geisler WM, Stamm WE. Genital chlamydial infections. In: Klausner JD, Hook EW III, eds. Current Diagnosis & Treatment of Sexually Transmitted Diseases [electronic version]; AccessMedicine, 2007. *http://www.accessmedicine.com.libproxy.uthscsa.edu/content.aspx?aID=3025480.*
35. Mylonas I Female genital *Chlamydia trachomatis* infection: Where are we heading? Arch Gynecol Obstet 2012;285:1271–1285.
36. Zar HJ. Neonatal chlamydial infections: Prevention and treatment. Paediatr Drugs 2005;7:103–110.
37. Paavonen J. *Chlamydia trachomatis* infections of the female genital tract: State of the art. Ann Med 2012;44:18–28.
38. Kalwij S, Macintosh M, Baraitser P. Screening and treatment of *Chlamydia trachomatis* infections. BMJ 2010;340:912–917.
39. Bebear C, de Barbeyrac B. Genital *Chlamydia trachomatis* infections. Clin Microbiol Infect 2009;5:4–10.
40. Hammerschlag MR, Kohlhoff SA. Treatment of chlamydial infections. Expert Opin Pharmacother 2012;13:545–552.
41. Geisler WM. Diagnosis and management of uncomplicated *Chlamydia trachomatis* infections in adolescents and adults: Summary of evidence reviewed for the 2010 Centers for Disease Control and Prevention Sexually Transmitted Diseases Treatment Guidelines. Clin Infect Dis 2011;53(Suppl 3):S92–S98.
42. Anonymous. Drugs for sexually transmitted infections. Treat Guidel Med Lett 2010;8:53–50. [Erratum appears in Treat Guidel Med Lett 2010;8:82]
43. Leone P. Genital Herpes. In: Klausner JD, Hook EW III, eds. Current Diagnosis & Treatment of Sexually Transmitted Diseases [electronic version]; AccessMedicine, 2007. *http://www.accessmedicine.com.libproxy.uthscsa.edu/content.aspx?aID=3025480.*

44. Schiffer, JT, Corey L. Herpes simplex virus. In: Mandell GL, Bennett JE, Dolin R, eds. Mandell, Douglas, and Bennett's Principles and Practice of Infectious Diseases, 7th ed. [electronic version]; MD Consult, 2010. *http://www.mdconsult.com.libproxy.uthscsa.edu/book/player/book.do?method=display&type=aboutPage&decorator=header&eid=4-u1.0-B978-0-443-06839-3..X0001-X-TOP&isbn=978-0-443-06839-3&uniq=177288689.*
45. Gupta R, Warren T, Wald A. Genital herpes. Lancet 2007;370:2127–2137.
46. Kimberlin DW, Rouse DJ. Genital herpes. N Engl J Med 2004;350:1970–1977.
47. Corey L, Wald A. Genital herpes. In: Holmes KK, Sparling PF, Stamm WE, et al., eds. Sexually Transmitted Diseases, 4th ed. New York: McGraw-Hill, 2008:399–437.
48. Corey L. Herpes simplex viruses. In: Fauci AS, Kasper DL, Longo DL, et al., eds. Harrison's Principles of Internal Medicine, 17th ed. [electronic version]; 2008. *http://online.statref.com.libproxy.uthscsa.edu/Document/Document.aspx?docAddress=41ATb9F8ccLkXnJpdO9gbw%3d%3d&offset=71&SessionId=11465DDAHROTSXMQ.*
49. Dwyer DE, Cunningham AL. Herpes simplex and varicella-zoster virus infections. Med J Aust 2002;177:267–273.
50. Chayavichitslip P, Buckwalter JV, Krakowski AC, Friedlander SF. Herpes simplex. Pediatr Rev 2009;30:119–130.
51. Simmons A. Clinical manifestations and treatment considerations of herpes simplex virus infection. J Infect Dis 2002;186(Suppl 1):S71–S77.
52. Beauman JG. Genital herpes: A review. Am Fam Physician 2005;72:1527–1534.
53. Wald A, Ashley-Morrow R. Serological testing for herpes simplex virus (HSV)-1 and HSV-2 infection. Clin Infect Dis 2002;35(Suppl 2): S173–S182.
54. Wald A. Testing for genital herpes: How, who, and why. Curr Clin Top Infect Dis 2002;22:166–180.
55. Scoular A. Using the evidence base on genital herpes: Optimising the use of diagnostic tests and information provision. Sex Transm Infect 2002;78:160–165.
56. Cernik C, Gallina K, Brodell RT. The treatment of herpes simplex infections: An evidence-based review. Arch Intern Med 2008;168:1137–1144.
57. Martinez V, Caumes E, Chosidow O. Treatment to prevent recurrent genital herpes. Curr Opin Infect Dis 2008;21:42–48.
58. Mell HK. Management of oral and genital herpes in the emergency department. Emerg Med Clin North Am 2008;26:457–473.
59. Patel R, Stanberry L, Whitley RJ. Review of recent HSV recurrent-infection treatment studies. Herpes 2007;14:23–26.
60. Hill J, Roberts S. Herpes simplex virus in pregnancy: New concepts in prevention and management. Clin Perinatol 2005;32:657–670.
61. Mills J, Mindel A. Genital herpes simplex infections: Some therapeutic dilemmas. Sex Transm Dis 2003;30:232–233.
62. Jones CA. Vertical transmission of genital herpes: Prevention and treatment options. Drugs 2009;69:421–434.
63. Hollier LM, Wendell GD. Third trimester antiviral prophylaxis for preventing maternal genital herpes simplex virus (HSV) recurrences and neonatal infection. Cochrane Database Syst Rev 2008;1:CD004946.
64. Stanberry LR. Clinical trials of prophylactic and therapeutic herpes simplex virus vaccines. Herpes 2004;11(Suppl 3): 161A–169A.
65. Weller PF. Protozoal intestinal infections and trichomoniasis. In: Fauci AS, Kasper DL, Longo DL, et al., eds. Harrison's Principles of Internal Medicine, 17th ed. [electronic version]; 2008. *http://online.statref.com.libproxy.uthscsa.edu/Document/Document.aspx?docAddress=41ATb9F8ccLkXnJpdO9gbw%3d%3d&offset=71&SessionId=11465DDAHROTSXMQ.*
66. Soper D. Trichomoniasis: Under control or undercontrolled? Am J Obstet Gynecol 2004;190:281–290.
67. Hobbs MM, Sena AC, Swygard H, Schwebke JR. *Trichomonas vaginalis* and trichomoniasis. In: Holmes KK, Sparling PF, Stamm WE, et al., eds. Sexually Transmitted Diseases, 4th ed. New York: McGraw-Hill; 2008:771–793.
68. Schwebke J. Trichomoniasis. In: Klausner JD, Hook EW III, eds. Current Diagnosis & Treatment of Sexually Transmitted Diseases [electronic version]; AccessMedicine, 2007. *http://www.accessmedicine.com.libproxy.uthscsa.edu/content.aspx?aID=3025480.*
69. Schwebke JR. *Trichomonas vaginalis.* In: Mandell GL, Bennett JE, Dolin R, eds. Mandell, Douglas, and Bennett's Principles and Practice of Infectious Diseases, 7th ed. [electronic version]; MD Consult, 2010. *http://www.mdconsult.com.libproxy.uthscsa.edu/book/player/book.do?method=display&type=aboutPage&decorator=header&eid=4-u1.0-B978-0-443-06839-3..X0001-X-TOP&isbn=978-0-443-06839-3&uniq=177288689.*
70. Schwebke JR, Burgess D. Trichomoniasis. Clin Microbiol Rev 2004;17:794–803.
71. Wendel KA, Workowski KA. Trichomoniasis: Challenges to appropriate management. Clin Infect Dis 207;44(Suppl 3): S123–S129.
72. Say PJ, Jacyntho C. Difficult-to-manage vaginitis. Clin Obstet Gynecol 2005;48:753–768.
73. Faro S. Vaginitis: Differential Diagnosis and Management. Boca Raton, FL: Parthenon Publishing, 2004:67–92.
74. Eckert LO. Acute vulvovaginitis. N Engl J Med 2006;355:1244–1252.
75. Sobel JD. What's new in bacterial vaginosis and trichomoniasis. Infect Dis Clin North Am 2005;19:387–406.
76. Forna F, Gülmezoglu AM. Interventions for treating trichomoniasis in women. Cochrane Database Syst Rev 2003;2:CD000218.
77. Cudmore SL, Delgaty KL, Hayward-McClelland SF, et al. Treatment of infections caused by metronidazole-resistant *Trichomonas vaginalis*. Clin Microbiol Rev 2004;17: 783–793.
78. Huh WK. Human papillomavirus infection: A concise review of natural history. Obstet Gynecol 2009;114:139–143.
79. Winer RL, Koutsky LA. Genital human papillomavirus infection. In: Holmes KK, Sparling PF, Stamm WE, et al., eds. Sexually Transmitted Diseases, 4th ed. New York: McGraw-Hill, 2008:489–508.
80. Hutchinson DJ, Klein KC. Human papillomavirus disease and vaccines. Am J Health Syst Pharm 2008;65:2105–2112.
81. Hershey JH, Velez LF. Public health issues related to HPV vaccination. J Public Health Manag Pract 2009;15:384–392.
82. Hager WD. Human papilloma virus infection and prevention in the adolescent population. J Pediatr Adolesc Gynecol 2009;22:197–204.
83. Medeiros LR, Rosa DD, da Rosa MI, et al. Efficacy of human papillomavirus vaccines: A systematic quantitative review. Int J Gynecol Cancer 2009;19:1166–1176.

96

Bone and Joint Infections

Edward P. Armstrong and Ziad Shehab

KEY CONCEPTS

1. The most common cause of osteomyelitis (particularly that acquired by hematogenous spread) and infectious arthritis is *Staphylococcus aureus*.
2. Culture and susceptibility information are essential as a guide for antimicrobial treatment of osteomyelitis and infectious arthritis.
3. Joint aspiration and examination of synovial fluid are extremely important to evaluate the possibility of infectious arthritis.
4. The most important treatment modality of acute osteomyelitis is the administration of appropriate antibiotics in adequate doses for a sufficient length of time.
5. Antibiotics generally are given in high doses so that adequate antimicrobial concentrations are reached within infected bone and joints.
6. The standard duration of antimicrobial treatment for acute osteomyelitis is 4 to 6 weeks.
7. Oral antimicrobial therapies can be used for osteomyelitis to complete a parenteral regimen in children who have had a good clinical response to IV antibiotics and in adults without diabetes mellitus or peripheral vascular disease when the organism is susceptible to the oral antimicrobial, a suitable oral agent is available, and compliance is ensured.
8. The three most important therapeutic approaches to the management of infectious arthritis are appropriate antibiotics, joint drainage, and joint rest.
9. Monitoring of antibiotic therapy is important and typically involves noting clinical signs of inflammation, periodic white blood cell (WBC) counts, C-reactive protein, erythrocyte sedimentation rate (ESR) determinations, and radiographic findings.

Bone and joint infections are comprised of two disease processes known, respectively, as *osteomyelitis* and *septic* or *infectious arthritis*. They are unique and separate infectious entities with different signs and symptoms and infecting organisms. Despite advances in therapy, these infections continue to cause significant morbidity from residual damage and chronic or recurring infections. Emphasis on initiating antibiotic therapy as soon as possible is important in reducing long-term complications.

EPIDEMIOLOGY

Osteomyelitis generally is an uncommon disease. One classic publication reported that 247 patients had osteomyelitis in a prominent American teaching hospital during a 4-year period.[1] Acute osteomyelitis has an estimated annual incidence of 0.4 per 1,000 children.[2] In adults, osteomyelitis caused by contiguous spread, including postoperative, direct puncture, and that associated with adjacent soft tissue infections, comprises 47% of infections. Hematogenous osteomyelitis comprises 19% of infections, and osteomyelitis occurring in patients with significant peripheral vascular disease comprises 34% of infections. A review of osteomyelitis cases based on duration of disease shows that acute disease constitutes 56% of patients and that chronic osteomyelitis, defined as having a previous hospitalization for the same infection, constitutes 44% of patients. Another classification system has defined acute osteomyelitis as <2 weeks duration, subacute as 2 to 4 weeks duration, and chronic as >4 weeks duration.

Infectious or septic arthritis is an inflammatory reaction within the joint space. Distinct from osteomyelitis, septic arthritis is one of the most common causes of new cases of arthritis. The incidence of proven or likely septic arthritis is 4 to 10 cases per 100,000 patient-years per year.[3] The incidence of septic arthritis increases to 70 cases per 100,000 patient-years among patients that have rheumatoid arthritis.[4]

ETIOLOGY

Osteomyelitis

The most common method of classifying osteomyelitis is based on the mode of acquisition of the bone infection. Disease that results from spread through the bloodstream is termed *hematogenous osteomyelitis*, while that reaching the bone from an adjoining soft tissue infection is termed *contiguous osteomyelitis*. Patients with peripheral vascular disease are at risk for the development of contiguous osteomyelitis, and they present unique management features. Osteomyelitis that results from direct inoculation, such as from trauma, puncture wounds, or surgery, generally is also classified as inoculation osteomyelitis.

Osteomyelitis also can be classified based on the duration of the disease. Acute osteomyelitis describes infections of recent onset, usually several days to 1 week, whereas chronic infections are those of a longer duration. Some authors describe chronic infections as those with symptoms for more than 1 month before therapy, whereas other authors define chronic infections as relapse of an initial infection. Hematogenous osteomyelitis almost always involves one bone whereas contiguous osteomyelitis can present in multiple bones, especially when vascular insufficiency is an underlying risk factor.

Infectious Arthritis

Infectious arthritis can occur from many different types of microorganisms.[5] Most infecting organisms produce an infection in a single joint, termed *monoarticular infections*; however, infections also can involve two or more joints.[6] As with osteomyelitis, joint infections also can be classified according to the mechanisms by which the infecting organism reaches the joint. Infectious arthritis can result by spread from an adjacent bone infection, direct contamination of the joint space, or hematogenous dissemination. Hematogenous spread of the disease comprises the majority of infections; spread from osteomyelitis and direct inoculation is much less frequent. Septic arthritis is most prevalent in children and the elderly. Approximately, one-third of people with septic arthritis are children younger than 2 years of age.[7]

PATHOPHYSIOLOGY

Hematogenous Osteomyelitis

Hematogenous osteomyelitis is typically a disease of the growing bone in children and most cases occur in patients younger than 16 years of age. Table 96-1 summarizes the primary characteristics of osteomyelitis. Less commonly, these infections occur in adults. Osteomyelitis of the vertebrae is also acquired hematogenously and occurs most frequently in patients older than 50 years of age.[8]

Unique features of the anatomy and physiology of long bones appear to predispose them to become infected.[9] Their vascular structure appears to predispose them for hematogenous infections that begin within the metaphyses (Fig. 96-1). The nutrient arteries of the long bones divide within the medullary canal of the bone into small arterioles. These end in hairpin turns near the growth plate and flow into veins, of much wider diameter, that drain the medullary cavity.[1] An infection in hematogenous disease is initiated within the bend of the arterioles where there is considerable slowing of blood flow passing through the hairpin capillary loops. This sludging of blood flow allows bacteria present within the bloodstream to settle and initiate an inflammatory response. They have access to the bone by gaps in the endothelial layer and the absence of a basement membrane. In addition to these structural features, there also appears to be less active phagocytosis within the metaphysis. After the bacteria settle in the bone, avascular necrosis can occur from occlusion of the nutrient vessels and release of bacterial enzymes.

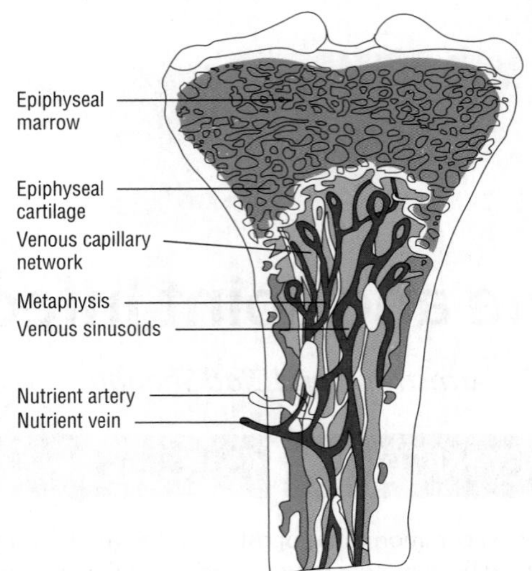

FIGURE 96-1 Cross section of normal bone.

TABLE 96-1 Types of Osteomyelitis, Age Distribution, Common Sites, and Risk Factors

Type of Osteomyelitis	Typical Age (years)	Site(s) Involved	Risk Factors
Hematogenous	Less than 1	Long bones and joints	Prematurity, umbilical or other central venous catheter or venous cutdown, respiratory distress syndrome, and perinatal asphyxia
	1–20	Long bones (femur, tibia, and humerus)	Infection (pharyngitis, cellulitis, and respiratory infections), trauma, and sickle cell disease
	Older than 50	Vertebrae	Diabetes mellitus, blunt trauma to spine, and urinary tract infection
Contiguous	Older than 50	Femur, tibia, and mandible	Hip fractures and open fractures
Puncture	Less than 18	Foot	Puncture injury to foot
Vascular insufficiency	Older than 50	Feet and toes	Diabetes mellitus, peripheral vascular disease, and pressure sores

In addition to these anatomic and functional features, there is some evidence that trauma is associated with developing an infection in specific bones. Children who develop hematogenous osteomyelitis may report some type of trauma before the onset of their symptoms and animal data indicate that traumatized bone is more likely to become infected than normal bone.

Once the infection is initiated, exudate begins to form within the bone marrow and the fluid accumulates under increased pressure. The age of the patient largely determines the next stage in the pathophysiology. In children older than 12 to 18 months, the infection that started in the metaphysis of a long bone is prevented from spreading into the epiphysis and the adjacent joint space because of the epiphyseal growth plate that acts as a physical barrier; however, the exudate often dissects from the medulla through the soft cortex to the subperiosteal space as the periosteum in these children is loosely attached to the underlying cortex. The periosteum is thick and not easily ruptured thus containing the pus in the subperiosteal space, sometimes forming a subperiosteal abscess. If there is significant damage to the periosteum, the pus can decompress into a soft-tissue abscess. The cortex obtains most of its blood supply from the periosteum and a subperiosteal abscess can impair the blood flow to the outer portion of the cortical bone resulting in a devitalized piece of dead bone termed a *sequestrum*. The elevated periosteum remains viable because its blood supply, derived from the overlying muscle, is unaffected. The raised periosteum will continue to produce bone; however, this new bone is now separated from the cortex because the periosteum has been raised from the infection. This new bone that is deposited under the periosteum is termed *involucrum*.

In adults, the periosteum is tightly bound to the cortex that is thick. These anatomic features generally cause the infections to remain intramedullary. As expected, subperiosteal abscess formations are less common in adults. The infection can spread to subperiosteal structures through the Haversian and Volkmann's canals.

The vascular supply of long bones in neonates also has unique anatomic characteristics that affect their presentation. Bridging blood vessels go across the epiphyseal plate from the metaphysis into the epiphysis thus enabling an infection that started within the metaphyseal area to spread easily to involve the epiphyses and then into the joint.[10] Therefore, in infants, not only can the infection spread to involve the periosteum and the shaft as in older children, but the infection also can spread directly to involve the joint.[11]

In children, hematogenous osteomyelitis typically involves a single bone and has a predilection for involvement of the long bones, such as the femur, tibia, humerus, and fibula.[11] In contrast, neonatal infections commonly involve multiple bones. Vertebral infections are common in patients older than 50 years of age.[12] Vertebral disease in young children usually involves the disk space and the two vertebral facets adjoining it because of the nature of the vascular supply of the vertebrae at that age. This entity is known as diskitis. Vertebral osteomyelitis involving the body of the vertebra can be seen in children older than 8 years of age.

Chronic osteomyelitis is more likely to occur if large segments of bone become avascular and necrotic. This results in a piece of devitalized bone to which antimicrobial delivery is impaired. As a result, this infection is prone to exacerbations and may lead to weakening of that bone or to the formation of draining sinuses to the skin.

1 The bacteriology of hematogenous osteomyelitis is unique in that one pathogen, *Staphylococcus aureus*, is responsible for more than 80% of these infections, with group A Streptococci and *Streptococcus pneumoniae* accounting for a few cases. *Kingella kingae*, an organism that is part of the oral flora is emerging as a pathogen in children less than 3 years of age. *Haemophilus influenzae* type b (Hib), which used to be an important pathogen, has been almost completely eliminated with the use of the conjugate vaccine and is now a rare pathogen in bone and joint infections.[9] Similarly, pneumococcal disease is anticipated to decrease in prevalence as invasive pneumococcal disease is prevented by the use of the conjugate pneumococcal vaccine in infants. While *S. aureus* is also the major pathogen in neonatal osteomyelitis, disease in this age group can also result from infections with group B streptococcus, and *Escherichia coli*. They are multifocal in half the cases.

Vertebral osteomyelitis has several unique features and occurs most commonly in adults 50 to 60 years of age. The lumbar and thoracic regions are the locations of most infections. Hematogenous infections are most likely to develop in the vascular areas near the subchondral plate region of the vertebral body. Staphylococci cause approximately 60% of these infections; however, gram-negative organisms now play a significant role.[13] These gram-negative organisms, particularly *E. coli*, most likely originate within the urinary tract. *E. coli* vertebral infections have been associated with urinary tract infections, positive urine cultures, and bacteremias. *Mycobacterium tuberculosis* and *Coccidioides immitis/posadasii* also are known to cause infections in the spine. Skin and respiratory tract infections are other sources of infection known to lead to vertebral infections.

While infections of the spine can involve the vertebrae in 1% to 2% of older children with osteomyelitis, they more commonly involve the disk space of the lumbar vertebrae in children less than 5 years of age.

Osteomyelitis in the IV drug user has unique features.[14] More than 50% of such infections involve the vertebral column and less than 20% of infections are located in either the sternoarticular or pelvic girdle. Infections are much less frequent within the extremities. They also have an unusual spectrum of organisms with gram-negative organisms being responsible for 88% of infections. *Pseudomonas aeruginosa*, either singly or in combination with other organisms, is cultured in 78% of all infections. *Klebsiella*, *Enterobacter*, and *Serratia* species also can be found but less commonly. In addition, staphylococcal and streptococcal organisms are sometimes cultured.

Patients with sickle cell anemia and related hemoglobinopathies also represent a unique population in that two thirds of bone infections in these patients are caused by *Salmonella* species, while the rest are usually caused by staphylococci and other gram-negative organisms.[15] Bowel infarctions from the sickle cell disease can facilitate the entry of salmonellae from the colon into the bloodstream with resultant hematogenous spread to the bone. Osteomyelitis in patients with sickle cell disease may occur in any bone, but it most commonly involves the medullary cavity of long or tubular bones. Because of the difficulty in separating bone pain during a sickle cell crisis from that of an infection, osteomyelitis can be relatively advanced in these patients by the time the diagnosis is made.

Direct Inoculation Osteomyelitis

This category of osteomyelitis includes infections caused by direct entrance of organisms from a source outside the body. Penetrating wounds (e.g., trauma), open fractures, and various invasive orthopedic procedures can result in direct inoculation of organisms into the bone. More than 80% of cases of postoperative osteomyelitis are known to occur following open reductions of fractures. Specifically, these infections occur most commonly after internal fixation of a hip fracture or femoral or tibial shaft fracture. Osteomyelitis resulting from puncture injuries to the feet are associated with gram-negative infection or the bone and cartilage (sometimes classified as *osteochondritis*), especially infections caused by *P. aeruginosa*. *S. aureus* is also a significant pathogen in these patients.

Contiguous-Spread Osteomyelitis

Osteomyelitis secondary to spread from an adjacent soft tissue infection is called contiguous osteomyelitis. It can result from pressure ulcers or from adjacent soft tissue infections and most often involves the distal extremities. Less commonly, infections can spread from infected teeth to involve the mandible or occur secondary to sinus infections by spreading through the mucosal lining of the sinuses into the vascular system surrounding the bone.[16,17]

In contrast to hematogenous osteomyelitis, which occurs most commonly in children, contiguous-spread osteomyelitis occurs most commonly in patients older than age 50, most likely because of predisposing factors, such as hip fractures or vascular disease, are more common in this age group.

Contiguous-spread disease has several important differences compared with hematogenous osteomyelitis. Although *S. aureus* is still the most common organism isolated, infections with multiple organisms, including gram-negative bacilli, occur frequently. *P. aeruginosa*, streptococcus, *E. coli*, *Staphylococcus epidermidis*, and anaerobes can be isolated.

Patients with osteomyelitis in association with severe vascular insufficiency are extremely difficult to manage.[18] As anticipated, most of these patients have diabetes mellitus or severe atherosclerosis, and they develop their infections by contiguous spread. Generally, these patients are between the ages of 50 and 70 years. Frequently, patients with vascular disease develop osteomyelitis in their toes and fingers, and there is usually an adjacent area of infection, such as cellulitis or dermal ulcers. Importantly, infections in these patients are almost always polymicrobial and often include staphylococcus and streptococcus or the combination of staphylococcus, streptococcus, and Enterobacteriaceae. Enterococci and anaerobic organisms also can be involved.

Anaerobic organisms also play a role in osteomyelitis. When anaerobes are grown from cultures, they usually are found in association with other organisms, including aerobic bacteria. Predisposing factors in patients who have anaerobic osteomyelitis include vascular disease, bites, contiguous infections, peripheral neuropathy, hematogenous spread, and trauma.[19] The anaerobic infections in association with diabetes mellitus almost always occur within the feet. *Bacteroides fragilis* and *Bacteroides melaninogenicus* comprise the majority of anaerobic isolates.

Infectious Arthritis

Infectious arthritis usually is acquired by hematogenous spread.[6] The synovial tissue is highly vascular and does not have a basement membrane, so organisms in the blood can easily reach the synovial fluid. Table 96-2 summarizes the characteristics of acute infectious arthritis.

TABLE 96-2 Characteristics of Acute Infectious Arthritis

Feature	Finding
Peak incidence	Children younger than 16 years Adults older than 50 years
Clinical findings	Fever of 38–40°C (100.4–104°F) in children; painful swollen joint in the absence of trauma Physical examination: Effusion, restriction of joint motion, tenderness, redness, and warmth of joint
Most commonly affected joints	Knee, hip, ankle, elbow, wrist, and shoulder
Laboratory findings	
Erythrocyte sedimentation rate	Elevated in 90% of cases
White blood cell count	Elevated in 30–60% of cases
Left shift	Seen in two thirds of patients
Blood culture	Positive in 40% of cases
Needle aspiration of joint	Gram-stain diagnostic in 30–50% of cases. Synovial fluid cultures are positive in 60–80% of cases. Synovial fluid differential reveals 90% polymorphonuclear leukocytes. Synovial fluid glucose decreased relative to serum glucose. Lactic acid levels elevated in nongonococcal infectious arthritis, but not in gonococcal infectious arthritis

Some organisms, such as *Neisseria gonorrhoeae*, are especially likely to infect a joint during bacteremia. Risk factors associated with adult infectious arthritis (more than one factor may be present) are systemic corticosteroid use, preexisting arthritis, arthrocentesis, distant infection, diabetes mellitus, trauma, and other diseases.[20]

Organisms also can gain access to the joint from a deep-penetrating wound injury, intraarticular steroid injections, arthroscopy, prosthetic joint surgery, and spread to the joint from a contiguous focus of osteomyelitis. Trauma also appears to be a risk factor in facilitating microbial entry into the synovial space. Unlike children, adults often have significant systemic diseases that predispose them to infectious arthritis, such as diabetes mellitus, immunosuppressive states (e.g., cancer or liver disease), or preexisting arthritis. IV drug abusers and individuals with intravascular infections such as endocarditis also are prone to develop septic arthritis.

Preexisting abnormal joint architecture, joint trauma, and surgery are other important risk factors because chronic inflammation or trauma makes the joint more susceptible to infection. In addition, individuals with rheumatoid arthritis can be prone to bacterial infection because of an inherent phagocytic defect, as well as concomitant corticosteroid therapy. Women are more prone to develop disseminated gonococcal infections than men. The second and third trimesters of pregnancy and the time of menses appear to be the times of greatest risk for developing gonococcal bacteremia.

After bacteria gain access to the joint, the organisms begin to multiply and produce a purulent exudate within the joint. If this joint effusion is present beyond 7 days, chronic, and sometimes irreversible, damage can occur to the bone and joint as a result of proteolytic enzymes and pressure necrosis. Purulent effusions can promote cartilage destruction by increasing leukocyte enzyme activity. In conjunction with the development of the effusion, almost all patients will develop a hot, swollen, painful joint.

2 *S. aureus*, the single most common infecting organism, is found in 37% to 65% of cases of nongonococcal bacterial arthritis.[7] Streptococcal infections are the second most common and gram-negative organisms are less common. Among the latter, *E. coli* is the most common; however, *P. aeruginosa* is the most frequent organism in IV drug abusers. Neonates may have infectious arthritis because of a broad range of organisms, with *S. aureus*, group B Streptococcus, and gram-negative organisms being most common. *S. aureus* and streptococcus are the most common pathogens in children younger than 5 years of age. Hib, which used to be the most common pathogen in these children, has essentially been eliminated by immunization with the conjugate Hib vaccine. Pneumococcal arthritis is also decreasing in incidence as a result of conjugate pneumococcal vaccine administration to infants. If a child has not been fully vaccinated or is immunocompromised, Hib may be a cause. Within the adult population, *S. aureus* is responsible for the vast majority of nongonococcal infections. Gonococcal arthritis is a common manifestation of disseminated gonococcal infection occurring in 42% to 85% of such patients.[7] Gonococcal arthritis is now uncommon in North America and Europe although it remains an important concern in developing countries. Although rare, osteomyelitis and infectious arthritis can be caused by fungi and in the case of arthritis by viruses such as varicella-zoster, rubella, or parvovirus.[21] Arthritis is rarely caused by Salmonella, Corynebacteria, Brucella, *Neisseria meningitides*, *Mycoplasma pneumoniae*, or *Ureaplasma urealyticum*. Penetrating injury of the joint can result in an infection due to Pasteurella in dog bites, Capnocytophaga in human bites, and Pantoea when the injury is induced by a thorn.

CLINICAL PRESENTATION

The clinical presentation of acute hematogenous osteomyelitis is summarized in Table 96-3. Although neonatal hematogenous osteomyelitis can spread rapidly to involve the joint, often there are few associated systemic symptoms.[22] A joint effusion is present in 60% to 70% of neonatal infections. Decreased limb motion or edema over the affected area may be the only signs from which to suspect the diagnosis. Vertebral osteomyelitis produces nonspecific symptoms, such as constant back pain, fever or night sweats, and weight loss.[23] The pain typically is present at rest and increases in severity with movement. Serious neurologic complications can occur if the infection extends and compresses the spinal cord. With contiguous-spread osteomyelitis there is often an area of localized tenderness, warmth, edema, and erythema over the infected site. Patients with significant vascular insufficiency usually have local symptoms, such as pain, swelling, and redness. Less commonly, they also can have fever and elevated white blood cell (WBC) count. The presentation of osteomyelitis after surgery or trauma depends on the precipitating cause. If the infection follows surgery or bone trauma, the symptoms usually are noted within 1 month. The most frequent symptom is pain in the area of infection. Less commonly, patients also can develop a fever and elevated WBC count.

Patients with nongonococcal bacterial arthritis almost always present with a fever, and 50% of patients have an elevated WBC

TABLE 96-3 Clinical Presentation of Hematogenous Osteomyelitis

Signs and symptoms
Significant tenderness of the affected area, pain, swelling, fever, chills, decreased motion, and malaise

Laboratory tests
Elevated erythrocyte sedimentation rate, C-reactive protein, and white blood cell count
50% of patients will have positive blood cultures

Diagnostic studies
Bone changes observed on radiographs 10–14 days after the onset of infection. Magnetic resonance imaging and technetium scans positive as early as 1 day after the onset of infection

count (see Table 96-2). The average initial synovial WBC count is $10 \times 10^3/\text{mm}^3$ (10×10^9/L) or greater in nongonococcal bacterial disease. The most frequent initial sign of disseminated gonococcal infections is the triad of dermatitis, tenosynovitis, and migratory polyarthralgia or polyarthritis.

Nongonococcal bacterial arthritis is almost always monoarticular. The knee is the most commonly involved joint, but infections also can occur in the shoulder, wrist, hip, ankle, interphalangeal joints, and elbow joints. Usually, the initial focus of infection that acted as the source for bacterial or microbial entrance can be identified. Common routes for bacterial entrance include infections of the respiratory tract, skin, and urinary tract; often no specific source can be identified. Blood cultures are important in these patients because they can be positive in 50% of patients.

Another type of infectious arthritis occurs following prosthetic joint surgery. The most common symptom is pain. Local signs of inflammation and fever are common in acute infections while chronic infections present in a more subtle fashion, typically with pain alone and often loosening of the prosthesis. With these infections, the C-reactive protein usually is elevated, although a leukocytosis often is absent. Infections that result from postoperative contamination usually become apparent within 1 year of surgery.

Radiologic and Laboratory Tests

The evaluation of a patient who may have osteomyelitis has several unusual aspects. Radiographs of the involved area should be obtained to rule out other processes such as a fracture; bone changes characteristic of osteomyelitis appear late and are not typically seen until at least 10 to 14 days after the onset of the infection as more than 50% of the bone matrix must be removed before the lesions can be detected radiologically. Magnetic resonance imaging is the most sensitive and commonly used diagnostic imaging modality and offers the advantage of better anatomic definition, especially of abscesses or joint effusions. Radionuclide bone scanning is useful in identifying the focus of osteomyelitis.[24,25]

Despite the seriousness of osteomyelitis, often there are few laboratory abnormalities. The erythrocyte sedimentation rate (ESR), C-reactive protein, and WBC count may be the only laboratory abnormalities.[11] The degree of abnormality of these laboratory findings does not correlate with the disease outcome; however, they are useful for monitoring therapy. C-reactive protein can be elevated because of the presence of inflammation, and it can be substituted for the ESR. C-reactive protein is generally the more sensitive marker of response to therapy and often increases and decreases before the ESR.

When a clinical assessment of osteomyelitis is suspected, it is important to establish a bacteriologic diagnosis by culture of the infected bone. Accurate culture information is especially important as a guide for treatment of osteomyelitis in this era of increasing antimicrobial resistance. Bone aspiration and bone biopsy are valuable in determining an accurate bacteriologic diagnosis. In addition, they help determine whether or not there is an abscess present. If an abscess is identified, it must be drained and the pus is cultured, and a Gram stain is performed. Aspirates of subperiosteal pus or metaphyseal fluid yield a pathogen in 70% of cases. Cultures should be done for both aerobic and anaerobic bacteria. A Gram stain of the aspirate can be useful in initiating appropriate empirical antibiotic therapy.

If a specimen is obtained from a previously undrained or unopened wound abscess, the pathogen usually can be identified. In chronic osteomyelitis, however, identification can be more difficult.[26] Open wounds and draining sinuses frequently are contaminated with other organisms and thus provide inaccurate culture information.[27] They cannot be relied on to reflect the pathogen unless consecutive deep sinus tract cultures reveal the same pathogens.[28] Cultures of loculated pus aspirates in the area of orthopedic devices removed from infected bone can be trusted, however, to identify the infecting organism. In diabetic patients that may have osteomyelitis, bone infections are most common in patients with foot ulcers greater than 3 mm and in patients with C-reactive protein levels greater than 3.2 mg/dL (32 mg/L).[29] The preferable time to obtain culture material in a patient with a chronic draining sinus is at the time of open surgical debridement.

In addition to performing cultures from the involved bone, it also is important to obtain cultures from any site believed to be the source of a bacteremia. Blood cultures should be obtained. Approximately 50% of patients with hematogenous osteomyelitis will have positive blood cultures and may obviate the need for bone aspiration in these patients.

3 When evaluating the possibility of a patient having infectious arthritis, immediate joint aspiration with subsequent analysis of the synovial fluid is extremely important. The presence of purulent fluid usually indicates the presence of a septic joint. The synovial fluid WBC count is usually 50 to $200 \times 10^3/\text{mm}^3$ (50×10^9 to 200×10^9/L) when an infection is present. However, serum WBC, ESR, and C-reactive protein may not be useful acutely in septic arthritis.[30] Approximately half the patients with an infected joint have a low synovial glucose level, usually less than 40 mg/dL (2.2 mmol/L). Gram stains of joint fluid demonstrate bacteria in 50% of patients with septic arthritis; however, such stains are positive in only 25% of patients with gonococcal arthritis. Synovial fluid cultures usually are positive in patients with nongonococcal infections. Both blood and joint fluid should be cultured aerobically and anaerobically in a patient suspected of having an infected joint. Blood cultures are positive in one half of patients with nongonococcal infections but in only 20% of those with gonococcal infections. Pharyngeal, rectal, cervical, or urethral smears and cultures, as well as cultures of cutaneous lesions, should be performed if a disseminated gonococcal infection is considered. As with osteomyelitis, most patients will have an elevated C-reactive protein concentration and ESR. Radiographs of infected joints often reveal distension of the joint capsule with soft tissue swelling in the adjacent space. Magnetic resonance imaging can be helpful in identifying an infected joint, especially the hip. In patients who have developed an infected prosthetic joint, loosening of the prosthesis can be seen radiographically.

TREATMENT

Desired Outcome

The goals of treatment are resolution of the infection and prevention of long-term sequelae. The ultimate outcome of osteomyelitis depends on the acute or chronic nature of the disease and how rapidly appropriate therapy is initiated. Patients with acute osteomyelitis have the best prognosis. Cure rates exceeding 80% can be expected for patients with acute osteomyelitis who have surgery when indicated and receive appropriate antibiotics for 4 to 6 weeks. When the growth plate is involved in children, discrepancies in the growth of bones or angular bone deformities can result.

In contrast, patients with chronic osteomyelitis have a much poorer prognosis. Dead bone and other necrotic material from the infection act as a bacterial reservoir and make the infection very difficult to eliminate. Adequate surgical debridement to remove all the dead bone and necrotic material, combined with prolonged administration of antibiotics, provides the best chance to obtain a cure.[31] The inability to remove all the dead bone can allow residual infection and require suppressive antibiotics to control the infection.

While many patients who develop infectious arthritis recover with no long-term sequelae, 50% are left with decreased joint function or mobility. Gonococcal arthritis usually resolves rapidly with antibiotics and has a lower rate of sequelae. Individuals at greatest risk for long-term sequelae are those who have symptoms present for more than 7 days before starting therapy and those with infections occurring within the hip joint and infections caused by gram-negative organisms. Common long-term residual effects following infectious arthritis are limited joint motion and persistent pain.

General Approach to Treatment

4 Following completion of the steps needed to determine the infecting organism, the most important treatment modality of acute osteomyelitis is the administration of appropriate antibiotics in adequate doses for a sufficient length of time. It is important to stress that early antibiotic therapy can mitigate the need for surgery, subsequent sepsis, chronic infection, disruption of longitudinal bone growth, and angular deformity of the bone.[32] A delay in treatment can allow bone necrosis to occur and make eradication of the infection much more difficult. In these patients with chronic osteomyelitis, exacerbations of the infection can result if all necrotic tissue is not removed surgically and all microorganisms eliminated. Chronic suppressive antimicrobial therapy and adjunctive treatment with hyperbaric oxygen or antibiotic-impregnated implants during surgery also has been used.[33,34]

If a patient with hematogenous osteomyelitis does not respond by having a decrease in fever, local swelling, redness, and pain following the initiation of adequate antibiotic therapy, the patient should undergo surgical debridement of the infected area. It is important to emphasize the priority of starting antibiotics immediately after the cultures have been obtained.

Pharmacologic Therapy

Antibiotic Bone Concentration

5 Antibiotics used in the management of acute osteomyelitis generally are given in high doses (adjusted for weight, renal function, hepatic function, or both) so that adequate antimicrobial concentrations are reached within the infected bone and joint.[35] Between 8 and 12 g/day of a penicillinase-resistant penicillin (nafcillin or oxacillin), ampicillin, or cephalosporin or a similar large dose of another parenteral antibiotic is used in the initial management of adults with osteomyelitis.[36] These dosing recommendations, however, are empirical; the relationship between a specific dose of a given antibiotic and its resulting concentration within the infected bone is largely unknown. Semisynthetic penicillins, cephalosporins, clindamycin, and the aminoglycosides can be detected in bone homogenates soon after their administration.

Daptomycin may also be an effective empiric therapy for the treatment of osteomyelitis in adults caused by most methicillin-susceptible and methicillin-resistant *S. aureus* (MRSA), but the data are limited.[37] Further prospective studies are needed to define the situations in which daptomycin might be best utilized and its optimal dosing.

Clinical **Controversy. . .**

The impact of resistant organisms has created some controversy regarding whether empiric therapy should be adjusted. Some clinicians recommend empirical coverage for MRSA when staphylococcal infection is suspected. However, others believe that culture results and susceptibility testing or lack of response to routine staphylococcal antibiotics should instead trigger use of antibiotics directed against MRSA. The frequency of MRSA in a community may help guide which approach is used.

Duration of Antibiotic Therapy

6 The specific duration of antibiotic therapy needed in the management of osteomyelitis is usually 4 to 6 weeks.[38,39] Failure rates approaching 20% have been observed in children treated with parenteral antibiotics for 3 weeks or less. One analysis in children with hematogenous osteomyelitis recommended 20 days of antibiotic therapy after initial parenteral therapy as long as the C-reactive protein level normalized within 7 to 10 days.[40] Although these data were largely evaluated in children, this duration of therapy recommendation is also used in adults.[41] Treatment failures may be due to the presence of infected necrotic bone or infected hardware (wires, plates, screws, and rods) that could not be removed.[42]

A modification of this recommendation has been used in some patients. Children receiving an appropriate oral antibiotic regimen and adults receiving an oral fluoroquinolone antibiotic, such as ciprofloxacin, have been treated successfully with a 6-week course. Improvement in the patient's clinical signs and symptoms and normalization of the C-reactive protein level or ESR are important parameters to assess therapy.[43] If signs or symptoms are still present at 6 weeks, therapy should be extended. Short course therapy for children who have had a puncture wound of the foot resulting in *P. aeruginosa* osteochondritis, and who have had surgical debridement of infected material, can be used with parenteral antibiotics for as little as 10 days.

Oral Antibiotic Therapy

7 One of the most significant changes in the management of osteomyelitis is the use of oral antibiotics to complete therapy.[44] Criteria for the use of oral outpatient antibiotic therapy for osteomyelitis include all of the following:

1. Confirmed osteomyelitis
2. Initial clinical response to parenteral antibiotics
3. Suitable oral agent available
4. Compliance ensured

Suitable candidates are children with good clinical response to IV therapy and adults without diabetes mellitus or peripheral vascular disease. There have been two primary populations that have benefited from oral treatment. Children responding to initial parenteral therapy may be excellent candidates to receive follow-up oral therapy with an agent such as dicloxacillin, cephalexin, clindamycin, or amoxicillin depending on their culture and susceptibility results.[45] Although more controversial, the other population to benefit from oral therapy is adults with an infecting organism susceptible to a fluoroquinolone.[46] These two populations now no longer routinely require expensive and complicated courses of long-term parenteral antibiotics.

The use of oral antibiotics is well studied in children.[47] Typically, injectable antibiotics are used initially and then switched to oral antibiotics when there was a decrease in the signs of inflammation and the C-reactive protein or when the patient was afebrile for 3 days. If pus was obtained on the initial needle aspirate, or if a reduction in fever, local swelling, and tenderness did not occur despite adequate rest, immobilization, and intensive antibiotic therapy, the patients underwent surgical drainage. The patients enrolled in oral antibiotic trials generally had disease of recent onset, identification of a specific infecting organism, enforced compliance, and surgery as indicated. In patients who meet these criteria, oral antibiotics appear to offer a great advantage in the treatment of osteomyelitis.[48] Patients not meeting these criteria may have a higher risk of developing chronic osteomyelitis if oral therapy is inappropriate or not strictly adhered to. Limited retrospective data in adults indicated that parenteral therapy for less than 4 weeks followed by oral therapy may be effective.[49]

Ciprofloxacin is effective in the treatment of osteomyelitis caused by gram-negative bacteria, such as *Enterobacter cloacae* and *Serratia marcescens*; however, many strains of streptococci are relatively resistant. Activity of ciprofloxacin against gram-negative bacilli allows patients to be treated orally and avoids the potential toxic complications of 4 to 6 weeks of aminoglycoside therapy.[50] Ciprofloxacin and other fluoroquinolones also have demonstrated effectiveness in the treatment of chronic osteomyelitis along with adequate surgical debridement. Another benefit with this agent is that it can be administered on an every-12-hour schedule. An important limitation of this antibiotic class, however, is that fluoroquinolones should not be used in children younger than 16 to 18 years of age or in pregnant women because of the potential to cause cartilage damage. Ciprofloxacin also has poor coverage against anaerobic organisms and staphylococci and emergence of resistant *P. aeruginosa* can be a problem. Newer fluoroquinolones have additional gram-positive activity; however, additional well-controlled clinical trials are needed to determine most appropriately their role in the treatment of osteomyelitis.[50]

Concern has been raised about staphylococcal resistance to fluoroquinolones. MRSA infections do not respond well to ciprofloxacin; however, resistance also can be troublesome for methicillin-susceptible strains. It is recommended that when ciprofloxacin is used to treat osteomyelitis with mixed etiologies that include *S. aureus*, it should be combined with an antistaphylococcal drug such as dicloxacillin, cephalexin, or clindamycin.

Clinical **Controversy. . .**

The role of fluoroquinolones may be debated. Some clinicians believe that oral fluoroquinolones should be preferred treatments for osteomyelitis; however, others believe that there have been inadequate studies to date to determine their comparative clinical effectiveness.

Antibiotic Selection

A critical component in the management of osteomyelitis is the selection of appropriate antibiotics. Empirical therapy must be selected on the basis of the most likely infecting organism while the results of culture and susceptibility data are pending. Table 96-4 summarizes empirical therapy recommendations. It is difficult to make evidence-based recommendations on the treatment of these infections as little high-quality clinical evidence exists. Experimental evidence, case series, and published expert opinion are used to suggest preferred treatment options. Dosages expressed in terms of milligrams per kilogram per day generally are given in divided doses every 6 to 8 hours (three to four times a day).

Because *S. aureus*, group B streptococci, and *E. coli* are the most common infecting organisms in newborns, an IV dosage of 150 mg/kg per day (given in four divided doses) of oxacillin or nafcillin plus cefotaxime 150 mg/kg per day (given in three to four divided doses) is appropriate. For children 5 years of age or younger, *S. aureus* and group A streptococci are the most common infecting organisms. Appropriate therapy in this age group is nafcillin or oxacillin 150 to 200 mg/kg per day IV or cefazolin 100 mg/kg per day. If the patient is immunocompromised or has not been fully vaccinated, empirical therapy is needed to also cover Hib. In this setting, IV cefuroxime 150 mg/kg per day is appropriate empirical therapy. For children older than 5 years, *S. aureus* is the most likely infecting organism, and either nafcillin or oxacillin 150 to 200 mg/kg per day IV or cefazolin 100 mg/kg per day IV is recommended. If patients are allergic to penicillins or cephalosporins or are infected with MRSA, vancomycin, clindamycin, or linezolid can be used.[51–53] Children with culture-negative osteomyelitis can be managed as presumed staphylococcal disease with excellent long-term results. Empiric therapy may need to be modified if community-acquired MRSA is prevalent.[54] The antimicrobial therapy should then be adjusted based on susceptibility testing results. Children with osteomyelitis usually can be treated successfully with 4 weeks of parenteral therapy or parenteral followed by oral therapy.

TABLE 96-4 Empirical Treatment of Osteomyelitis

Patient Subtype	Likely Infecting Organism	Antibiotic[a]	Recommendation Grades[b]
Newborn	*Staphylococcus aureus*, group B *streptococci*, *Escherichia coli*	Nafcillin or oxacillin 50–150 mg/kg/day IV plus cefotaxime 100–200 mg/kg/day IV	B-3
Children 5 years of age or younger	1. If vaccinated for *Haemophilus influenzae* type b: *S. aureus* or streptococci	1. Nafcillin or oxacillin 150–200 mg/kg/day IV or cefazolin 100 mg/kg/day IV	B-3
	2. If not vaccinated against *H. influenzae* type b	2. Cefuroxime 150 mg/kg/day IV	B-3
Children older than 5 years of age	*S. aureus*	Nafcillin or oxacillin 150–200 mg/kg/day IV or cefazolin 100 mg/kg/day IV	A-3
Adults	*S. aureus*	Nafcillin or oxacillin 2 g IV every 4 hours or cefazolin 2 g IV every 8 hours	A-3
IV drug abusers	*Pseudomonas*	Ciprofloxacin 750 mg PO twice daily or ceftazidime or cefepime 2 g IV every 8 hours	B-3
Postoperative or posttrauma patients	Gram-positive and gram-negative organisms	Nafcillin or oxacillin 2 g IV every 4 hours plus ceftazidime or cefepime 2 g IV every 8 hours or ticarcillin–clavulanate 3.1 g IV every 4 hours	B-3
Patients with vascular insufficiency	Gram-positive and gram-negative organisms	Nafcillin or oxacillin 2 g IV every 4 hours or cefazolin 2 g IV every 8 hours plus ceftazidime or cefepime 2 g IV every 8 hours	B-3
	If anaerobes suspected	Cefotetan 2 g IV every 12 hours or clindamycin 900 mg IV every 8 hours plus ceftazidime or cefepime 2 g IV every 8 hours	C-3

PO, orally.

[a]Dosage should be adjusted for some agents in patients with renal and/or hepatic dysfunction.

[b]Strength of recommendations: A, B, C = good, moderate, and poor evidence to support recommendation, respectively. Quality of evidence: 1 = Evidence from more than one properly randomized, controlled studies or multiple time series; or dramatic results from uncontrolled experiments. 2 = Evidence from more than one well-designed clinical trial with randomization, from cohort or case-controlled analytic studies. 3 = Evidence from opinions of respected authorities, based on clinical experience, descriptive studies, or reports of expert communities.

An oral regimen can be an alternative to the previous recommendation in many cases of osteomyelitis in children. Children who have undergone surgery, if needed, and have had a good clinical response to IV therapy may be candidates for the alternate oral antibiotic regimen.[55] Parenteral antibiotic therapy should be initiated and continued until there has been a resolution in the erythema, swelling, and tenderness and until the patient is afebrile. Dicloxacillin, cloxacillin, and cephalexin (100 mg/kg per day) are effective oral agents. Patients should be monitored with periodic WBC counts, C-reactive protein, and ESR determinations. When oral antibiotics are used, the total duration of oral and injectable therapy is usually at least 4 weeks. As stated previously, because of the risk of cartilage damage, fluoroquinolones should not be used in children. Hematogenous osteomyelitis in adults is caused most frequently by *S. aureus* and thus is treated appropriately with 8 to 12 g/day of a penicillinase-resistant penicillin such as nafcillin or a first-generation cephalosporin (e.g., cefazolin). Clindamycin 2.4 g/day, or vancomycin 2 g/day (with normal renal function) can be used in adults allergic to penicillin; however, if the infection is located within the vertebrae, *E. coli* must be considered, and thus, depending on the culture and susceptibility data, a switch to a cephalosporin may be needed. After institution of appropriate antibiotic therapy, the antimicrobial agent should be continued for at least 4 to 6 weeks total (parenteral plus oral).

Clinical **Controversy...**

H. influenzae vaccination has decreased the frequency of *H. influenzae* infections. Some clinicians believe that empirical therapy of osteomyelitis and septic arthritis in a child younger than 5 years of age no longer requires Hib coverage; however, others are concerned about children not being fully vaccinated and desire to use an antibiotic with activity against this organism.

Special Populations Osteomyelitis in patients with sickle cell hemoglobinopathies is commonly caused by either *Salmonella* or *S. aureus*.[15] Thus, empirical antibiotics of first choice include ceftriaxone or cefotaxime. Alternatives are chloramphenicol and ciprofloxacin (in adults).

Bone infections in adults with a history of IV drug abuse require coverage for gram-negative organisms; therefore, empirical treatment with ceftazidime or defepime 2 g IV every 8 hours. If compliance can be ensured, these patients are excellent candidates to receive oral ciprofloxacin 750 mg twice daily. Antibiotic therapy in these patients should be continued for at least 4 to 6 weeks.

As discussed previously, several microorganisms can cause bone infections that occur after surgery or from contiguous spread of an adjacent soft tissue infection. *S. aureus* is the single most common organism, but multiple organisms can be involved. To provide the required broad-spectrum coverage, nafcillin 2 g IV every 4 hours plus ceftazidime or cefepime 2 g IV every 8 hours should be used as initial therapy. Alternative single agents are ticarcillin–clavulanate potassium 3.1 g IV every 4 hours or piperacillin–tazobactam in adults; however, there is less experience with these agents. Other broad-spectrum alternatives can be cefepime and imipenem. The antibiotic regimen requires reevaluation after culture and susceptibility information is available. Ciprofloxacin can be an appropriate oral alternative for these patients if the susceptibility data are favorable. Frequently, the antibiotics must be continued for 6 weeks to obtain a cure, and surgery often is required to remove any infected or devitalized tissue.

Patients with established vascular insufficiency who subsequently develop osteomyelitis are extremely difficult to manage.[56] Impaired blood flow to the extremities impedes the healing process, possibly requiring vascular bypass surgery. Infections in these patients involve a wide range of organisms, including *S. aureus*, *Streptococcus*, anaerobes, and gram-negative organisms. Bone culture-guided antibiotic therapy has been associated with cure in diabetics with osteomyelitis of the foot.[57] Broad-spectrum therapy with a penicillinase-resistant penicillin in combination with ceftazidime is the preferred initial therapy.[58] If anaerobes are suspected, an antianaerobic cephalosporin (e.g., cefoxitin) or clindamycin plus ceftazidime can be substituted. Ampicillin may need to be added to the regimen to provide coverage against enterococci. Despite aggressive antibiotic therapy along with surgical debridement, these patients continue to have low cure rates.[59,60] Amputation of the involved area may be required to obtain a cure of the infection.[61]

Home Antibiotic Therapy Because the management of bone and joint infections frequently requires prolonged parenteral antibiotics, newer antibiotic regimens have been used. Administration of antibiotics in the home environment and the use of antibiotics with extended elimination half-lives are commonly used. Although acute osteomyelitis is one of the more common infectious diseases that can be treated with home IV antibiotics, not all patients are acceptable candidates for home administration. Patients must be screened to include only those who are receiving a stable treatment program, those who are interested and are motivated in participating, and those who have good venous access, as well as those who have support from family members or neighbors and have home facilities for storage and refrigeration. Patients with adequate vascular access may be able to use a peripheral IV catheter; however, a central IV catheter may be required if venous access difficulties occur. Certain exclusion criteria also must be considered. Complications of other preexisting diseases such as diabetic retinopathy, intention tremor, disabling inflammation or degenerative joint disease, coagulopathies, or various neurologic disorders can prevent individuals from receiving home antibiotics. A history of alcoholism or of IV drug abuse also is important exclusion criteria. Patients who are fluent in only a foreign language and patients who are illiterate or hard of hearing may have to be excluded if a qualified guardian is unavailable. In addition to meeting these initial screening criteria, patients must successfully complete a thorough training program before hospital discharge. Aseptic technique, proper catheter care, and correct administration techniques must be documented. Once a patient is receiving therapy in the home environment, continued monitoring of their antimicrobial therapy and drug levels when indicated is important. It is vital to ensure compliance with the antimicrobial regimen. Catheter-related complications are common in patients receiving prolonged courses of parenteral antibiotics.[62]

In addition, the specific antibiotic regimen characteristics must be considered when evaluating a patient for home antibiotics. Some important features are microbiologic culture and susceptibility data, the number of required daily antimicrobial doses, antibiotic stability data, and requirements for unique monitoring for the specific antimicrobial regimen, such as serum creatinine and drug level monitoring with aminoglycosides or vancomycin. Although an organism can be susceptible to several antimicrobial agents, one antibiotic can provide practical benefits over other agents.

Infectious Arthritis 8 The three most important therapeutic maneuvers in the management of infectious arthritis are appropriate antibiotics, joint drainage, and joint rest. Smears of the synovial fluid can be useful to select appropriate antibiotic therapy initially.[7] If bacteria are not observed on the Gram stain in a patient who has a purulent joint effusion, antibiotics still should be initiated because of the low sensitivity of the Gram stain. A delay in initiating antibiotics significantly increases the likelihood for long-term complications.[63,64]

The specific antibiotic selected depends on the most likely infecting organism.[65] In infants younger than 1 month of age, the infecting organisms vary widely, and empirical therapy thus must provide broad-spectrum coverage. A penicillinase-resistant penicillin such as nafcillin or oxacillin plus a third-generation cephalosporin is appropriate. Children younger than 5 years of age who have been immunized for Hib should receive nafcillin, oxacillin, or cefazolin.[66]

In children older than 5 years of age and in adults, initial therapy with a penicillinase-resistant penicillin or first-generation cephalosporin is appropriate to provide the necessary coverage against *S. aureus*. Therapy should be changed to clindamycin, vancomycin, or linezolid if the *S. aureus* is resistant to methicillin.[67,68] They can be converted to oral therapy after initial IV therapy.[40] As with osteomyelitis, IV drug abusers require coverage for *P. aeruginosa*, and therefore, combination therapy with an aminoglycoside, fluoroquinolone, or anti-pseudomonal cephalosporin is needed. The antibiotics usually are administered parenterally and achieve sufficient concentrations within the synovial fluid, and thus intraarticular antibiotic injections are unnecessary. Although studies to define clearly the appropriate length of therapy have not been conducted, 2 to 3 weeks of antibiotic therapy generally is adequate in nongonococcal infections.[69] Less than 2 weeks of therapy combined with one joint aspiration was effective in closely monitored children with infectious arthritis.[70] Joint fluid cultures usually are no longer positive after 7 days of antibiotics.

Disseminated gonococcal infections often respond quickly to antibiotics. Ceftriaxone 1 g/day for 7 to 10 days is the treatment of choice for adults. After culture and susceptibility results are available and the organism is determined to be susceptible, therapy can be switched on the fourth day to cefixime, oral amoxicillin or to doxycycline or tetracycline to complete the 7- to 10-day course. Clinical resolution of signs and symptoms usually is rapid.

Closed-needle aspiration is recommended for all infected joints except the hip.[71] Joint drainage can be repeated daily for 5 to 7 days until effusions no longer reaccumulate. Open drainage is required in hip infections because closed-needle aspiration is difficult and inadequate. During the initial phase of the infection, weight bearing, such as walking, on the joint should be avoided. Passive range-of-motion exercises should be initiated when the pain begins to subside to maintain joint mobility.[72] Approximately one third of patients with bacterial arthritis have a poor joint outcome, such as severe functional deterioration. Poor joint outcomes are associated with older patients, those with preexisting joint disease, and patients with an infected joint containing synthetic material. Treatment guidelines for septic arthritis of the hip may be helpful in managing these patients.[73]

PERSONALIZED PHARMACOTHERAPY

Individualized therapy is important in the treatment of osteomyelitis and infectious arthritis. Patient's quality of life can be significantly diminished if long-term sequelae develop, such as impaired joint motion or draining sinus tracts, or if amputation is required. Patient demographics, infection characteristics (e.g., infecting organism and its susceptibility patterns), treatment cost, and quality-of-life issues all play a major role in evaluating individualized treatment alternatives (oral therapy or home antibiotic treatment) rather than requiring patients to remain hospitalized to receive 4 to 6 weeks of parenteral antibiotics. In addition, adverse events commonly occur with prolonged outpatient parenteral antibiotic therapy. One study in 45 children noted that 85.7% of patients receiving vancomycin had adverse drug events and 42.9% of patients required the drug be discontinued.[74] This analysis also noted that cefazolin had the lowest rate of adverse drug events in this population. Monitoring is important to ensure that personalized therapy is effective to both cure the infection as well as minimize the risk for complications.

TABLE 96-5 Monitoring Protocol

Parameter	Frequency	Notes
Culture and susceptibility	At initiation of treatment	
White blood cell count	One time per week until within normal range	
C-reactive protein or erythrocyte sedimentation rate	Weekly	May not decrease to normal range until several weeks of therapy
Clinical signs of inflammation (redness, pain, swelling, tenderness, and fever)	Daily during initiation of therapy	
Compliance of outpatient therapy	Reinforce before starting oral therapy and with each healthcare visit	Compliance is critical if treatment is to be successful

EVALUATION OF THERAPEUTIC OUTCOMES

9 Patients with bone and joint infections must be monitored closely. Table 96-5 summarizes a pharmaceutical care monitoring protocol. An assessment of a therapy's success or failure is based on the patient's clinical findings and laboratory values. The clinical signs of inflammation, such as swelling, tenderness, pain, redness, and fever, should resolve with appropriate therapy. Initially, the clinical signs are assessed daily until improvement and then periodically thereafter. Elevations in WBC count also should decline gradually. The ESR usually is determined weekly. Elevations in the C-reactive protein or ESR may not return to normal until after several weeks of therapy. The WBC count usually is obtained once or twice per week until it returns to the normal range. If by the end of the 4- to 6-week antibiotic course the clinical findings of osteomyelitis are no longer present and the C-reactive protein and ESR are within normal limits, the patient can be considered a clinical cure. Patients can relapse, however, after initially appearing to be cured. No relapse for 1 year generally is considered a complete cure.

If a patient fails to resolve the clinical signs and symptoms of inflammation after appropriate empirical antibiotics, surgical debridement may be needed. In addition, the patient might have a resistant or an atypical infecting organism that may require a modification of the antibiotic therapy. It is especially important to identify the infecting organism and its susceptibility pattern. Follow-up cultures at subsequent debridements can be useful to assess the antibiotic therapy.

Despite apparently adequate surgery and antibiotics, some patients can fail therapy and have recurrent relapses in their infection.[75] This scenario is more common in the population with chronic osteomyelitis. These patients can require long-term oral suppressive antimicrobial therapy to keep the infection under control.

ABBREVIATIONS

ESR erythrocyte sedimentation rate
MRSA methicillin-resistant *Staphylococcus aureus*
WBC white blood cell

REFERENCES

1. Waldvogel FA, Medoff G, Swartz MN. Osteomyelitis: A review of clinical features, therapeutic considerations and unusual aspects. N Engl J Med 1970;282:198–206, 260–266, 316–322.
2. Van den Bruel A, Bartholomeeusen S, Aertgeerts B, Truyers C, Buntinx F. Serious infections in children: An incidence study in family practice. BMC Fam Pract 2006;7–23.
3. Mathews CJ, Weston VC, Jones A, Field M, Coakley G. Bacterial septic arthritis in adults. Lancet 2010;375:846–855.
4. Garcia-De La Torre I, Nava-Zavala A. Gonococcal and nongonococcal arthritis. Rheum Dis Clin North Am. 2009;35:63–73.
5. Lavy CBD, Thyoka M. For how long should antibiotics be given in acute paediatric septic arthritis? A prospective audit of 96 cases. Trop Doct 2007;37:195–197.
6. Smith JW, Chalupa P, Shabaz HM. Infectious arthritis: Clinical features, laboratory findings and treatment. Clin Microbial Infect 2006;12:309–314.
7. Garcia-Arias M, Balsa A, Mola EM. Septic arthritis. Best Pract Res Clin Rheumatol 2011;25:407–421.
8. Zimmerli W. Vertebral osteomyelitis. N Engl J Med 2010;362:1022–1029.
9. Harik NS, Smeltzer MS. Management of acute hematogenous osteomyelitis in children. Expert Anti Infect Ther 2010;8:175–181.
10. Dessi A, Crisafulli M, Accossu S, et al. Osteoarticular infections in newborns: Diagnosis and treatment. J Chemother 2008;20:542–550.
11. Offiah AC. Acute osteomyelitis, septic arthritis and discitis: Differences between neonates and older children. Eur J Radiol 2006;60(2):221–232.
12. Livorsi DJ, Daver NG, Atmar RL, et al. Outcomes of treatment for hematogenous *Staphylococcus aureus* vertebral osteomyelitis in the MRSA Era. J Infect 2008;57:128–131.
13. Dartnell J, Ramachandran M, Katchburian M. Haematogenous acute and subacute paediatric osteomyelitis. J Bone Joint Surg Br 2012;94:584–595.
14. Chihara S, Segreti J. Osteomyelitis. Dis Mon 2010;56:6–31.
15. Marti-Carvajal AJ, Agreda-Perez LH, Cortes-Jofre M. Antibiotics for treating osteomyelitis in people with sickle cell disease. Cochrane Database Syst Rev 2009;2:CD007175.
16. Prasad KC, Prasad SC, Mouli N, Agarwal S. Osteomyelitis in the head and neck. Acta Oto-Laryngol 2007;127:194–205.
17. Ducic Y. Osteomyelitis of the mandible. South Med J 2008;101:465.
18. Howell WR, Goulston C. Osteomyelitis: An update for hospitalists. Hosp Pract (Minneap) 2011;39:153–160.
19. Brook I. Microbiology and management of joint and bone infections due to anaerobic bacteria. J Orthop Sci 2008;13:160–169.
20. Smith JW, Chalupa P, Hasan MS. Infectious arthritis: Clinical features, laboratory findings and treatment. Clin Microbiol Infect 2006;12:309–314.
21. Horowitz DL, Katzap E, Horowitz S, Barilla-LaBarca ML. Approach to septic arthritis. Am Fam Physician 2011;84:653–660.
22. Copley LAB. Pediatric musculoskeletal infection: Trends and antibiotic recommendations. J Am Acad Orthop Surg 2009;17:618–626.
23. Conrad DA. Acute hematogenous osteomyelitis. Pediatr Rev 2010;31:464–471.
24. Jaramillo D. Infection: Musculoskeletal. Pediatr Radiol 2011;41(Suppl 1):S127–S134.
25. Kan JH, Hilmes MA, Martus JE, et al. Value of MRI after recent diagnostic or surgical intervention in children with suspected osteomyelitis. Am J Roentgenol 2008;191: 1595–1600.
26. Coviello V, Stevens MR. Contemporary concepts in the treatment of chronic osteomyelitis. Oral Maxillofac Surg Clin North Am 2007;19:523–534.
27. Elamurugan TP, Jagdish S, Kate V, Parija SC. Role of bone biopsy specimen culture in the management of diabetic foot osteomyelitis. Int J Surg 2011;9:214–216.
28. Bernard L, Uckay I, Vuagnat A, et al. Two consecutive deep sinus tract cultures predict the pathogen of osteomyelitis. Int J Infect Dis 2010;14:e390–e393.
29. Fleischer AE, Didyk AA, Woods JB, Burns SE, Wrobel JS, Armstrong DG. Combined clinical and laboratory testing improves diagnostic accuracy for osteomyelitis in the diabetic foot. J Foot Ankle Surg 2009;48:39–46.
30. Carpenter CR, Schuur JD, Everett WW, Pines JM. Evidence-based diagnostics: Adult septic arthritis. Acad Emerg Med 2011;18:781–786.
31. Garcia-Lechuz J, Bouza E. Treatment recommendations and strategies for the management of bone and joint infections. Expert Opin Pharmacother 2009;10:35–55.
32. Rao N, Ziran BH, Lipsky BA. Treating osteomyelitis: Antibiotics and surgery. Plast Reconstr Surg 2011;127 (Suppl 1):177S–187S.
33. Sancineto CF, Barla JD. Treatment of long bone osteomyelitis with a mechanically stable intramedullar antibiotic dispenser: Nineteen consecutive cases with a minimum of 12 months follow-up. J Trauma 2008;65: 1416–1420.
34. Wright BA, Roberts CS, Seligson CS, et al. Cost of antibiotic beads is justified: A study of open fracture wounds and chronic osteomyelitis. J Long Term Eff Med Implants 2007;17:181–185.
35. Pea F. Penetration of antibacterials into bone: What do we really need to know for optimal prophylaxis and treatment of bone and joint infections. Clin Pharmacokinet 2009;48: 125–127.
36. Mouzopoulos G, Kanakaris NK, Kontakis G, Obakponovwe O, Townsend R, Giannoudis PV. Management of bone infections in adults: The surgeon's and microbiologist's perspectives. Injury 2011;42(Suppl 5):S18–S23.
37. Lamp KC, Friedrich LV, Mendez-Vigo L, et al. Clinical experience with daptomycin for the treatment of patients with ostomyelitis. Am J Med 2007;120:S13–S20.
38. Howard-Jones AR, Isaacs D. Systematic review of systemic antibiotic treatment for children with chronic and sub-acute pyogenic osteomyelitis. J Paediatr Child Health 2010;46:736–741.
39. Weichert S, Sharland M, Clarke NMP, Faust SN. Acute haematogenous osteomyelitis in children: Is there any evidence for how long we should treat? Curr Opin Infect Dis 2008;21:258–262.
40. Peltola H, Paakkonen M, Kallio P, Kallio MJT. Prospective, randomized trial of 10 days versus 30 days of antimicrobial treatment, including a short-term course of parenteral therapy, for childhood septic arthritis. Clin Infect Dis 2009;48:1201–1210.
41. Roblot F, Besnier JM, Juhel L, et al. Optimal duration of antibiotic therapy in vertebral osteomyelitis. Semin Arthritis Rheum 2007;36:269–277.
42. Haidar R, Boghossian AD, Atiyeh B. Duration of post-surgical antibiotics in chronic osteomyelitis: Empiric or evidence-based? Int J Infect Dis 2010;14:e752–e758.

43. Paakkonen M, Peltola H. Simplifying the treatment of acute bacterial bone and joint infections in children. Expert Rev Anti Infect Ther 2011;9:1125–1131.
44. Hatzenbuehler J, Pulling TJ. Diagnosis and management of osteomyelitis. Am Fam Physician 2011;84:1027–1033.
45. Paakkonen M, Peltola H. Antibiotic treatment for acute haematogenous osteomyelitis of childhood: Moving towards shorter courses and oral administration. Int J Antimicrob Agents 2011;38:273–280.
46. Karamanis EM, Matthaiou DK, Moraitis LI, Falagas ME. Fluoroquinolones versus β-lactam based regimens for the treatment of osteomyelitis. A meta-analysis of randomized controlled trials. Spine 2008;33:E297–E304.
47. Zaoutis T, Localio AR, Leckerman K, et al. Prolonged intravenous therapy versus early transition to oral antimicrobial therapy for acute osteomyelitis in children. Pediatrics 2009;123:636–642.
48. Bachur R, Pagon Z. Success of short-course parenteral antibiotic therapy for acute osteomyelitis of childhood. Clin Pediatr 2007;46:30–35.
49. Daver NG, Shelburne SA, Atmar RL, et al. Oral step-down therapy is comparable to intravenous therapy for *Staphylococcus aureus* osteomyelitis. J Infect 2007;54: 539–544.
50. Spellberg B, Lipsky BA. Systemic antibiotic therapy for chronic osteomyelitis in adults. Clin Infect Dis 2012;54: 393–407.
51. Chen CJ, Chiu CH, Lin TY, et al. Experience with linezolid therapy in children with osteoarticular infections. Pediatr Infect Dis J 2007;26:985–988.
52. Joshi AY, Huskins WC, Henry NK, Boyce TG. Empiric antibiotic therapy for acute osteoarticular infections with suspected methicillin-resistant *Staphylococcus aureus* or *Kingella*. Pediatr Infect Dis J 2008;27:765–767.
53. Kaplan SL. Challenges in the evaluation and management of bone and joint infections and the role of new antibiotics for gram positive infections. Adv Exp Med Biol 2009;634: 111–120.
54. Afghani B, Kong V, Wu FL. What would pediatric infectious disease consultants recommend for management of culture-negative acute hematogenous osteomyelitis? J Pediatr Orthop 2007;27:805–809.
55. Paakkonen M, Kallio PE, Kallio MJT, Peltola H. Management of osteoarticular infections caused by *Staphylococcus aureus* is similar to that of other etiologies. Analysis of 199 Staphylococcal bone and joint infections. Pediatr Infect Dis J 2012;31:436–438.
56. Game F. Management of osteomyelitis of the foot in diabetes mellitus. Nat Rev Endocrinol 2010;6:43–47.
57. Senneville E, Lombart A, Beltrand E, et al. Outcome of diabetic foot osteomyelitis treated nonsurgically. Diabetes Care 2008;31:637–642.
58. Byren I, Peters EJG, Hoey C, Berendt A, Lipsky BA. Pharmacotherapy of diabetic foot osteomyelitis. Expert Opin Pharmacother 2009;10:3033–3047.
59. Berendt AR, Peters EJG, Bakker K, et al. Specific guidelines for treatment of diabetic foot osteomyelitis. Diabetes Metab Res Rev 2008;24(Suppl 1):S190–S191.
60. Berendt AR, Peters EJG, Bakker K, et al. Diabetic foot osteomyelitis: A progress report on diagnosis and a systematic review of treatment. Diabetes Metab Res Rev 2008;24(Suppl 1):S145–S161.
61. Game FL, Jeffcoate WJ. Primarily non-surgical management of osteomyelitis of the foot in diabetes. Diabetologia 2008;51:962–967.
62. Pulcini C, Couadau T, Bernard E, et al. Adverse effects of parenteral antimicrobial therapy for chronic bone infections. Eur J Clin Microbiol Infect Dis 2008;27:1227–1232.
63. Balabaud L, Gaudias J, Boeri C, et al. Results of treatment of septic knee arthritis: A retrospective series of 40 cases. Knee Surg Sports Traumatol Arthrosc 2007;15:387–392.
64. Nunn TR, Cheung WY, Rollinson PD. A prospective study of pyogenic sepsis of the hip in childhood. J Bone Joint Surg Br 2007;89:100–106.
65. Mathews CJ, Kingsley G, Field M, et al. Management of septic arthritis: A systematic review. Postgrad Med J 2008;84:265–270.
66. Kang SN, Sanghera T, Mangwani J, Paterson JMH, Ramachandran M. The management of septic arthritis in children. J Bone Joint Surg Br 2009;91:1127–1133.
67. Rao N, Hamilton CW. Efficacy and safety of linezolid for gram-positive orthopedic infections: A prospective case series. Diagn Microbiol Infect Dis 2007;59:173–179.
68. Falagas ME, Siempos II, Papagelopoulos PJ, Vardakas KZ. Linezolid for the treatment of adults with bone and joint infections. Int J Antimicrob Agents 2007;29:233–239.
69. Paakkonen M, Peltola H. Management of a child with suspected acute septic arthritis. Arch Dis Child 2012;97: 287–292.
70. Bradley JS. What is the appropriate treatment course for bacterial arthritis in children? Clin Infect Dis 2009;48: 1211–1212.
71. Mathews CJ, Coakley G. Septic arthritis: Current diagnostic and therapeutic algorithm. Curr Opin Rheumatol 2008;20:457–462.
72. Mathews CJ, Coakley G. Acute hot joint. Br J Hosp Med 2006;67:232–234.
73. Ravindran V, Logan I, Bourke BE. Septic arthritis: Clinical audits would help optimize the management. Clin Rheumatol 2008;27:1565–1567.
74. Faden D, Faden HS. The high rate of adverse drug events in children receiving prolonged outpatient parenteral antibiotic therapy for osteomyelitis. Pediatr Infect Dis J 2009;28: 539–541.
75. Peltola H, Paakkonen M, Kallio P, Kallio MJ. Short- versus long-term antimicrobial treatment for acute hematogenous osteomyelitis of childhood. Prospective, randomized trial on 131 culture-positive cases. Pediatr Infect Dis J 2010;29:1123–1128.

Severe Sepsis and Septic Shock

S. Lena Kang-Birken

97

KEY CONCEPTS

1. The spectrum of microorganisms associated with sepsis has changed from predominantly gram-negative bacteria in the late 1970s and 1980s to gram-positive bacteria as the major pathogens since the late 1980s.
2. Candidemia is a major cause of morbidity and mortality. *Candida albicans* remains the most common pathogen (45.6%); however, non–*albicans Candida* species collectively is more frequently isolated (54.4%).
3. Sepsis presents a complex pathophysiology, characterized by the activation of multiple overlapping and interacting cascades leading to systemic inflammation, a procoagulant state, and decreased fibrinolysis.
4. Mortality rates with sepsis are higher for older patients with preexisting disease, intensive care unit care, and multiple organ failure.
5. Prompt initiation of broad-spectrum, parenteral antibiotic therapy is required due to the high incidence of complications and mortality with sepsis.
6. A significant volume of fluid leaks from the vasculature occurs with sepsis, and initial fluid resuscitation with large volumes of fluid is required. There is no difference in clinical outcomes between colloid and crystalloid fluid resuscitation.
7. Norepinephrine is generally preferred over dopamine as the vasopressor to correct hypotension in septic shock.
8. Early goal-directed therapy during the first 6 hours, consisting of hemodynamic monitoring with a central venous catheter, volume resuscitation, inotropic therapy, and red blood cell transfusions, demonstrated a significant clinical outcome benefit with a 16% absolute reduction in 28-day mortality.
9. A blood glucose level less than 150 mg/dL (8.3 mmol/L) is recommended for the majority of critically ill patients to reduce morbidity and mortality without the detrimental effects associated with hypoglycemia.
10. IV hydrocortisone is recommended for adult patients with septic shock whose blood pressure is unresponsive to fluids and vasopressors.

Sepsis and severe sepsis continue to pose major healthcare burden. The incidence of sepsis in the United States increased from 82.7 cases per 100,000 population in 1979 to 240.4 cases per 100,000 population in 2000, for an annualized increase of 8.7 percent.[1] Severe sepsis increased from 200 cases per 100,000 in 2003 to 300 cases per 100,000 in 2007, a 50% increase.[2] Despite aggressive medical care and advances, overall in-hospital deaths increased from 75 per 100,000 in 2003 to 87 per 100,000 in 2007, a 16% increase.[2] With increasing total hospital costs to $24.3 billion, there is a vital need for clinicians to comprehend the pathophysiology and to appreciate the management options for acutely ill patients with severe sepsis or septic shock.[2]

DEFINITIONS

In 1992, a joint committee of the American College of Chest Physicians and the Society of Critical Care Medicine standardized the terminology related to sepsis for several reasons: (a) widespread confusion with the use of these terms, (b) the need to provide a flexible classification scheme for patient identification, (c) identification of an earlier therapeutic intervention, and (d) standardization of research protocols.[3]

The criteria for the new terms provide specific physiologic variables that can be used to categorize a patient as having bacteremia, systemic inflammatory response syndrome (SIRS), sepsis, severe sepsis, septic shock, or multiple-organ dysfunction syndrome (MODS), suggesting an important continuum of progressive physiologic decline (Table 97-1). The classification of sepsis was modified to include severe sepsis, septic shock, and refractory septic shock (Fig. 97-1).[4] *Severe sepsis* refers to patients with an acute organ dysfunction, such as acute renal failure or respiratory failure. *Septic shock* refers to sepsis patients with arterial hypotension that is refractory to adequate fluid resuscitation, thus requiring vasopressor administration. It is important to note that progression from sepsis to MODS can occur in the absence of an intervening period of septic shock. Finally, *refractory septic shock* exists if dopamine IV infusion greater than 15 mcg/kg/min or norepinephrine greater than 0.25 mcg/kg/min is required to maintain a mean blood pressure greater than 60 mm Hg.

INFECTION SITES AND PATHOGENS

Predisposing factors of septic shock include age, male gender, nonwhite ethnic origin in North Americans, comorbid diseases, malignancy, immunodeficiency or immunocompromised state, chronic organ failure, alcohol dependence, genetic factors, and seasonal variation.[1,5–8]

The leading primary sites of microbiologically documented infections that lead to sepsis are the respiratory tract (39% to 50%), intraabdominal space (8% to 16%), and urinary tract (5% to 37%).[2,9] Although almost any microorganism can be associated with sepsis and septic shock, the most common etiologic pathogens are gram-positive bacteria (52% of patients), followed by gram-negative bacteria (37.6%), polymicrobial infections (4.7%), anaerobes (1.0%), and fungi (4.6%).[1,10]

TABLE 97-1 Definitions Related to Sepsis

Condition	Definition
Bacteremia (fungemia)	Presence of viable bacteria (fungi) in the bloodstream
Infection	Inflammatory response to invasion of normally sterile host tissue by the microorganisms
Systemic inflammatory response syndrome (SIRS)	Systemic inflammatory response to a variety of clinical insults, which can be infectious or noninfectious. The response is manifested by two or more of the following conditions: temperature >38°C (104°F) or <36°C (98.8°F); HR >90 beats/min; RR >20 breaths/min or $PaCO_2$<32 mm Hg (<4.3 kPa); WBC >12,000 cells/mm^3 (>12 × 10^9/L), <4,000 cells/mm^3 (4 × 10^9/L), or >10% (>0.10) immature (band) forms; positive fluid balance (>20 mL/kg over 24 hours); hyperglycemia; plasma C-reactive protein/procalcitonin >2 SD above normal value; arterial hypotension; CI >3.5 L/min (>0.058 L/s); arterial hypoxemia; acute oliguria; creatinine increase >0.5 mg/dL (>0.44 μmol/L); coagulation abnormalities; ileus, platelets <100,000 /mm^3 (>100 × 10^9/L); bilirubin >4 mg/dL (>68 μmol/L); hyperlactatemia; decreased capillary refill
Sepsis	SIRS secondary to infection
Severe sepsis	Sepsis associated with one or more organ dysfunctions, hypoperfusion, or hypotension. Hypoperfusion and perfusion abnormalities may include, but are not limited to, lactic acidosis, oliguria, and acute alteration in mental status
Septic shock	Sepsis with persistent hypotension despite fluid resuscitation, along with the presence of perfusion abnormalities. Patients who are on inotropic or vasopressor agents may not be hypotensive at the time perfusion abnormalities are measured
Refractory septic shock	Persistent septic shock, requiring dopamine >15 mcg/kg/min or norepinephrine >0.25 mcg/kg/min to maintain mean arterial blood pressure
Multiple organ dysfunction syndrome (MODS)	Presence of altered organ function requiring intervention to maintain homeostasis

CI, cardiac index; HR, heart rate; RR, respiratory rate; SD, standard deviation; T, temperature; WBC, white blood cell (count).

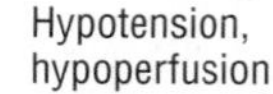

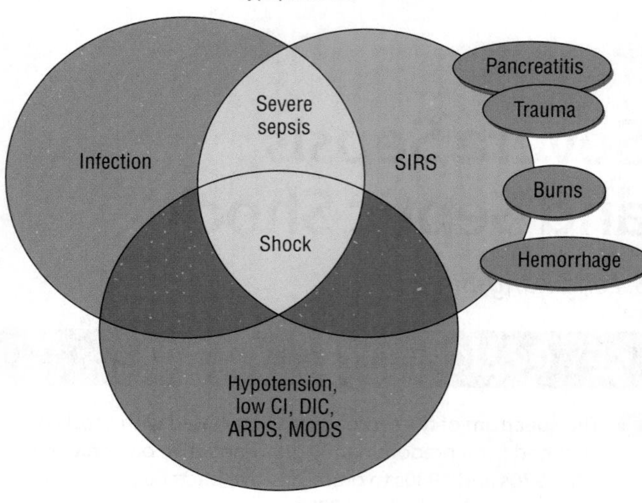

FIGURE 97-1 Relationship of infection, systemic inflammatory response syndrome (SIRS), sepsis, severe sepsis, and septic shock. (ARDS, acute respiratory distress syndrome; CI, cardiac index; DIC, disseminated intravascular coagulation; MODS, multiple-organ dysfunction syndrome.)

Gram-Positive Bacterial Sepsis

❶ Since 1987, gram-positive organisms have been the predominant pathogens in sepsis and septic shock, accounting for 52.1% of all cases.[1] They are commonly caused by *Staphylococcus aureus*, *Streptococcus pneumoniae*, coagulase-negative staphylococci, and *Enterococcus* species.[9–12]

S. aureus bacteremia is associated with an overall mortality rate ranging between 10% and 30%.[13] Factors related to a higher mortality include older age, shock, preexisting renal failure, and the presence of a rapidly fatal underlying disease. *Staphylococcus epidermidis* is most often related to infected intravascular devices, such artificial heart valves and stents, and the use of IV and intra-arterial catheters. Enterococci are isolated most commonly in blood cultures following a prolonged hospitalization and treatment with broad-spectrum cephalosporins.

Gram-Negative Bacterial Sepsis

While the overall percentage of gram-negative sepsis has decreased, the number of cases remains substantial.[1,10] *Escherichia coli* (8% to 30%), *Klebsiella* species (8% to 23%), and *Pseudomonas aeruginosa* (7% to 18%) are the most commonly isolated gram-negative microorganisms in sepsis.[9–12,14] Other common gram-negative pathogens include *Serratia* species, *Enterobacter* species, and *Proteus* species. *P. aeruginosa* and *Acinetobacter* species are more likely to be associated with prior antibiotic exposure.[14]

A greater proportion of patients with gram-negative bacteremia develop clinical sepsis, and also more likely to produce septic shock in comparison to gram-positive organisms, 50% versus 25%, respectively.[9,10,12] Specifically, *P. aeruginosa* sepsis has been associated in a higher mortality rate.[10,14] The major factor associated with the outcome of gram-negative sepsis appears to be the severity of any underlying conditions. Patients with rapidly fatal conditions, such as acute leukemia, aplastic anemia, and burn injury to >70% of the body's surface, have a significantly worse prognosis than those patients with nonfatal underlying conditions such as diabetes mellitus and chronic renal insufficiency.[1,2]

Anaerobic and Miscellaneous Bacterial Sepsis

Anaerobic bacteria such as *Bacteroides fragilis* and *Clostridium* species are usually considered low-risk organisms for the development of sepsis. If present, anaerobes are often found together with other pathogenic bacteria that are commonly found in sepsis. Polymicrobial infections accounted for 5% to 39% of sepsis.[1,10–12,14] Mortality rates associated with polymicrobial infections are similar to sepsis caused by a single organism. Although some clinicians believe the particular combination of organisms present in polymicrobial sepsis can provide clues to the source of infection, no clear source for the infection can be identified in up to 25% of cases.

Fungal Sepsis

❷ Candidemia is among the most common fungal etiologic agents of bloodstream infections. Although *Candida albicans* was the most commonly isolated fungus from blood cultures (45.6%), collectively, non-*albicans Candida* species were more frequently isolated (54.4%).[10–12,15,16] Non-*albicans Candida* species include *C. glabrata*

(26%), *C. parapsilosis* (15.7%), *C. tropicalis* (8.1%), and *C. krusei* (2.5%). Other fungi identified as causes of sepsis are *Cryptococcus*, *Coccidioides*, *Fusarium*, and *Aspergillus*.[11] Risk factors for fungal infection include abdominal surgery, poorly controlled diabetes mellitus, prolonged granulocytopenia, broad-spectrum antibiotic treatment, corticosteroid treatment, prolonged hospitalization, central venous catheter, total parenteral nutrition, hematologic malignancy, and chronic indwelling bladder (Foley) catheter. Recent exposure to azoles is an important risk factor for infection with fluconazole-resistant *Candida* spp.[17] Furthermore, a prospective nationwide surveillance study of candidemia suggested a close correlation between antibacterial drug exposure and bloodstream infection with *C. glabrata* and fluconazole-resistant *Candida* isolates.[17]

In a prospective analysis of the Antifungal Therapy Alliance database, the overall crude 12-week mortality rate for sepsis due to candidemia was 35.2%.[15] A higher in-hospital mortality was reported (61%) among healthcare-associated candidemia.[16] The highest mortality rate of 52.9% was observed in patients with *C. krusei* candidemia; *C. parapsilosis* candidemia was associated with the lowest 12-week mortality rate (23.7%). Hematologic diseases, neutropenia, and a higher number of positive blood cultures were associated with poor outcome irrespective of the patient's gender, age, or days of antifungal drug treatment.

PATHOPHYSIOLOGY

Sepsis is the result of complex interactions among the invading pathogen, the host immune system, and the inflammatory responses. The inflammatory response leads to damage to host tissue, and the antiinflammatory response causes leukocytes to activate. Once the balance to control the local inflammatory process to eradicate the invading pathogens is lost, systemic inflammatory response occurs, converting the infection to sepsis, severe sepsis, or septic shock.

Cellular Components for Initiating the Inflammatory Process

The pathophysiologic focus of gram-negative sepsis has been on the lipopolysaccharide component of the gram-negative bacterial cell wall. Commonly referred to as endotoxin, this substance is unique to the outer membrane of the gram-negative cell wall and is generally released with bacterial lysis. Lipid A, the innermost region of the lipopolysaccharide, is highly immunoreactive and is considered responsible for most of the toxic effects. Although lipid A can affect tissues directly, its predominant effect is to activate macrophages and trigger inflammatory cascades critical in the progression to sepsis and septic shock.[18] Endotoxin forms a complex with an endogenous protein called a lipopolysaccharide-binding protein, which then engages the CD14 receptor on the surface of a macrophage. Subsequently, cytokine mediators are activated and released by the macrophages.

In gram-positive sepsis, the exotoxin peptidoglycan on the cell wall surface appears to exhibit proinflammatory activity. Although it competes with lipid A for similar binding sites on CD14, the potency of peptidoglycan is less than that of endotoxin.[18] However, an important feature of gram-positive bacteria such as *S. aureus* and *S. pyogenes* is the production of potent exotoxins, some of which have been associated with septic shock.

Pro- and Antiinflammatory Mediators

Sepsis involves activation of inflammatory pathways, and a complex interaction between proinflammatory and antiinflammatory mediators plays a major role in the pathogenesis of sepsis. The key proinflammatory mediators are tumor necrosis factor-α (TNF-α), interleukin-1 (IL-1), and interleukin-6 (IL-6), which are released by activated macrophages.[18–20] Other mediators that may be important for the pathogenesis of sepsis are interleukin-8 (IL-8), platelet-activating factor (PAF), leukotrienes, and thromboxane A_2.

The TNF-α levels in plasma can be increased in patients with a variety of diseases and in many healthy people. However, there is a correlation of plasma TNF-α levels with the severity of sepsis. It is highly elevated early in the inflammatory response in most patients with sepsis.[19–21] The TNF-α release leads to activation of other cytokines (IL-1 and IL-6) associated with cellular damage. In addition, TNF-α stimulates the release of cyclooxygenase-derived arachidonic acid metabolites (thromboxane A_2 and prostaglandins) that contribute to vascular endothelial damage. Higher levels of IL-6 and IL-8 have been reported in patients with septic shock than those with SIRS.[8]

The significant antiinflammatory mediators include interleukin-1 receptor antagonist (IL-1RA), interleukin-4 (IL-4), and interleukin-10 (IL-10).[18,19] These antiinflammatory cytokines inhibit the production of the proinflammatory cytokines and down regulate some inflammatory cells. Levels of IL-10 and IL-1RA are higher in septic shock than in sepsis, and higher levels are found among nonsurviving patients than in survivors.[19,20]

The activation and secretion of pro- and antiinflammatory mediators in septic shock occur as a simultaneous immune response as early as the first 24 hours of diagnosis.[14] As Fig. 97-2 illustrates, the balance between pro- and antiinflammatory mechanisms determines the degree of inflammation, ranging from local antibacterial activity to systemic tissue toxicity, organ failure, or death.[19–21]

Cascade of Sepsis

3 The cascade leading to development of sepsis is complex and multifactorial, involving various mediators and cell lines.

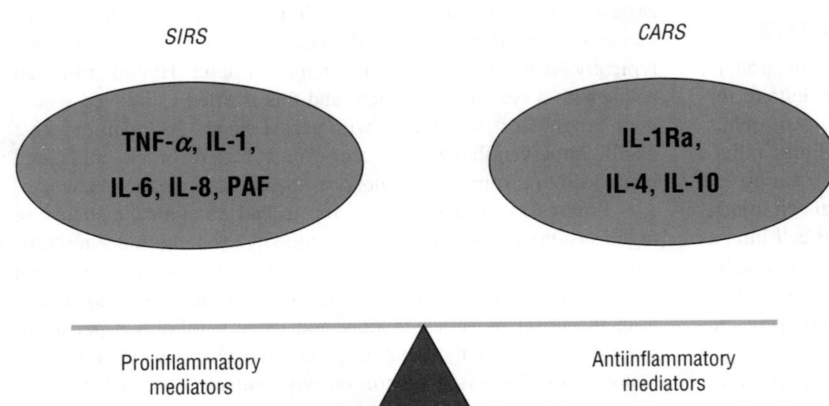

FIGURE 97-2 The balance between pro- and antiinflammatory mediators. (CARS, compensatory antiinflammatory response syndrome; IL, interleukin; IL-1RA, interleukin-1 receptor antagonist; SIRS, systemic inflammatory response syndrome; TNF, tumor necrosis factor.)

Endothelial cells produce a variety of cytokines that mediate a primary mechanism of injury in sepsis. When injured, endothelial cells allow circulating cells such as granulocytes and plasma constituents to enter inflamed tissues, which can result in organ damage.

The microcirculation is affected by sepsis-induced inflammation. The arterioles become less responsive to either vasoconstrictors or vasodilators. The capillaries are less perfused even at the early phases of septic shock, and there is neutrophil infiltration and protein leakage into the venules.[22]

The inflammatory process in sepsis is also directly linked to the coagulation system. Proinflammatory mechanisms that promote sepsis are also procoagulant and antifibrinolytic, whereas fibrinolytic mechanisms can be antiinflammatory.[23] A key endogenous substance involved in inflammation of sepsis is activated protein C, which enhances fibrinolysis and inhibits inflammation. Levels of protein C are reduced in patients with sepsis.[23]

COMPLICATIONS

Septic shock is the most ominous complication associated with sepsis, and it may lead to several complications including disseminated intravascular coagulation (DIC), acute respiratory distress syndrome (ARDS), and multiple organ failure. The organs that failed most frequently are lungs (18%) and kidneys (15%).[1] The less frequent are cardiovascular failure (7%), hematologic failure (6%), metabolic failure (4%), and neurologic failure (2%).[1] Mortality occurs in approximately half of the patients with septic shock.

Disseminated Intravascular Coagulation

DIC is the inappropriate activation of the clotting cascade that causes formation of microthrombi, resulting in consumption of coagulation factors, organ dysfunction, and bleeding. Sepsis remains the most common cause of DIC, and the incidence of DIC increases as the severity of sepsis increases. In sepsis alone, the incidence was 16% in comparison to 38% in septic shock.[24,25] DIC occurs in up to 50% of patients with gram-negative sepsis, but it is also common in patients with gram-positive sepsis.

DIC begins with the activation and production of the proinflammatory cytokines, such as TNF, IL-1, and IL-6, which appear to be the principal mediators, along with endotoxin. The combination of excessive fibrin formation, inhibited fibrin removal from a depressed fibrinolytic system, and endothelial injury result in microvascular thrombosis and DIC.

Complications of DIC vary and depend on the target organ affected and the severity of the coagulopathy. DIC can produce acute renal failure, hemorrhagic necrosis of the GI mucosa, liver failure, acute pancreatitis, ARDS, and pulmonary failure. Furthermore, as the procoagulant state appears to be the key in the pathogenesis of MODS, coagulation dysfunction and MODS often coexist in sepsis.

Acute Respiratory Distress Syndrome

Pulmonary dysfunction, the most common organ dysfunction in sepsis, usually precedes other organs, and it can even initiate the development of SIRS with resultant MODS. Activated neutrophils and platelets adhere to the pulmonary capillary endothelium, initiating multiple inflammatory cascades with a release of a variety of toxic substances. There is diffuse pulmonary endothelial cell injury, increased capillary permeability, and alveolar epithelial cell injury. Consequently, interstitial pulmonary edema occurs that gradually progresses to alveolar flooding and collapse. The end result is loss of functional alveolar volume, impaired pulmonary compliance, and profound hypoxemia.

Coagulation is locally upregulated in the injured lung, whereas fibrinolytic activity is depressed. These abnormalities occur concurrently and favor alveolar fibrin deposition. Anticoagulant interventions that block the extrinsic coagulation pathway can protect against the development of pulmonary fibrin deposition as well as lung dysfunction and acute inflammation.[25] Overall, fibrin deposition in the injured lung and abnormalities of coagulation and fibrinolysis are integral to the pathogenesis of ARDS.

Hemodynamic Effects

The hallmark of the hemodynamic effect of sepsis is the hyperdynamic state characterized by high cardiac output and an abnormally low systemic vascular resistance (SVR).[22,26] TNF-α and endotoxin directly depress cardiovascular function. Endotoxin depresses left ventricular (LV) function independent of changes in LV volume or vascular resistance. Myocardial dysfunction is common in severe sepsis and septic shock, affecting 64% of patients, and involves LV in more than half of the patients.[26]

Persistent hypotension raises concern for the balance of oxygen delivery (DO_2) to the tissues and oxygen consumption (VO_2) by the tissues. Sepsis results in a distributive shock characterized by inappropriately increased blood flow to particular tissues at the expense of other tissues, which is independent of specific tissue oxygen needs. This perfusion defect is accentuated by an increased precapillary atrioventricular shunt. If perfusion decreases, oxygen extraction increases, and the arteriovenous oxygen gradient widens. Cellular DO_2 is decreased, but VO_2 remains unaffected. When increased oxygen demand occurs without increased blood flow, the increased VO_2 is compensated by increased oxygen extraction. If perfusion decreases sufficiently in the face of high metabolic demands, then the reserve DO_2 can be exceeded, and tissue ischemia results. Significant tissue ischemia leads to organ dysfunction and failure. Therefore, systemic DO_2 relative to VO_2 should be optimized by increasing oxygen delivery or decreasing oxygen consumption in a hypermetabolic patient.

Acute Renal Failure

Early acute kidney injury occurs in 42% to 64% of adult patients with sepsis and septic shock.[27,28] Without normal urine output, fluid overload in extravascular space including the lungs develops, leading to impairment of pulmonary gas exchange and severe hypoxemia. Consequently, compromised oxygen delivery exacerbates peripheral ischemia and organ damage. Adequate renal perfusion and a trial of loop diuretics should be initiated promptly in oliguric or anuric patients with MODS along with dialysis to facilitate volume and electrolytes.

CLINICAL PRESENTATION

Table 97-2 lists some of the common clinical features of sepsis, although several of these findings are not limited to infectious processes. The initial clinical presentation can be referred to as signs and symptoms of early sepsis, defined as the first 6 hours. They are typically fever, chills, and change in mental status. Hypothermia can occur with a systemic infection, and this is often associated with a poor prognosis.[29] In patients with sepsis caused by gram-negative bacilli, hyperventilation can occur even before fever and chills, and it can lead to respiratory alkalosis as the earliest metabolic change.

Progression of uncontrolled sepsis leads to clinical evidence of organ system dysfunction as represented by the signs and symptoms attributed to late sepsis. With the exception of rapidly progressing cases as in meningococcemia, *P. aeruginosa*, or *Aeromonas* infection, the onset of shock is slow and usually follows a period of several hours of hemodynamic instability. Oliguria often follows hypotension. Increased glycolysis with impaired clearance of the resulting lactate by the liver and kidneys and tissue hypoxia because

TABLE 97-2 Signs and Symptoms Associated with Sepsis

Early Sepsis	Late Sepsis
Fever or hypothermia	Lactic acidosis
Rigors, chills	Oliguria
Tachycardia	Leukopenia
Tachypnea	DIC
Nausea, vomiting	Myocardial depression
Hyperglycemia	Pulmonary edema
Myalgias	Hypotension (shock)
Lethargy, malaise	Hypoglycemia
Proteinuria	Azotemia
Hypoxia	Thrombocytopenia
Leukocytosis	ARDS
Hyperbilirubinemia	GI hemorrhage
	Coma

ARDS, acute respiratory distress syndrome; DIC, disseminated intravascular coagulation.

of hypoperfusion result in elevated lactate levels, contributing to metabolic acidosis. Altered glucose metabolism, including impaired gluconeogenesis and excessive insulin release, is evidenced by either hyperglycemia or hypoglycemia.

PROGNOSIS

❹ As the patient progresses from SIRS to sepsis to severe sepsis to septic shock, mortality increases in a stepwise fashion. Mortality rates are higher for patients with advanced age, preexisting disease, including chronic obstructive pulmonary disease, neoplasm, and human immunodeficiency virus disease, intensive care unit (ICU) care, more failed organs, positive blood cultures, and *Pseudomonas* species infection.[10,13] In one analysis of cases, mortality increased with age from 10% in children to 38.4% in those 85 years or older.[1] ICU admission was required in 51.1% of patients with severe sepsis; of those patients, mortality was reported in 34.1%.[1] Mortality from severe sepsis and MODS is most closely related to the number of dysfunctioning organs. As the number of failing organs increased from two to five, mortality increased from 54% to 100% (Fig. 97-3).[30] Duration of organ dysfunction can also affect the overall mortality rate.

An elevated lactate concentration of >4 mmol/L in the presence of SIRS significantly increases ICU admission rates, and persistent elevations in lactate for more than 24 hours are associated with a mortality rate as high as 89%.[31] Inversely, patients with higher lactate clearance after 6 hours of emergency department intervention have improved outcome compared with those with lower lactate clearance. There was an ~11% decrease in the likelihood of mortality for each 10% increase in lactate clearance.[31]

Diagnosis and Identification of Pathogen

The presence of clinical features suggesting sepsis should prompt further evaluation of the patient. In addition to obtaining a careful history of any underlying conditions and recent travel, injury, animal exposure, infection, or use of antibiotics, a complete physical examination should be performed to determine the source of the infection.

A collection of specimens should be sent for culture prior to initiating any antimicrobial therapy. In critically ill septic patients, two or three sets of blood cultures should be collected without temporal separation between the sets.[32,33] With suspected catheter-related infection, a pair of blood cultures should be drawn through every lumen of each vascular access device.[33] In severe community-acquired pneumonia, blood cultures and respiratory secretions must be obtained. Urinary antigen detection of *Legionella* sero group 1 is recommended during outbreaks. To document a soft tissue infection, a Gram stain and bacterial culture of any obvious wound exudates should be performed. A needle aspiration of a closed infection such as cellulitis or abscess may be needed for stain and bacterial culture. In abdominal infections, fluid collections identified by imaging studies should be aspirated for Gram stains and aerobic and anaerobic cultures. Recent development of accurate and rapid identification tests has demonstrated positive impact on prescribing appropriate therapy in bloodstream infections such as methicillin-resistant *Staphylococcus aureus* (MRSA) and *Candida* spp.[34,35]

A lumbar puncture is indicated in the case of mental alteration, severe headache, or a seizure, assuming that there are no focal cranial lesions identified by computed tomography scan. Further tests may be indicated to assess any systemic organ dysfunction caused by severe sepsis. The laboratory tests should include hemoglobin, white blood cell (WBC) count with differential, platelet count, complete chemistry profile, coagulation parameters, serum lactate, procalcitonin (PCT), and arterial blood gases.

TREATMENT

In 2008, a "surviving sepsis" campaign guideline for management of severe sepsis and septic shock was published as an international effort to increase awareness and improve outcome in severe sepsis.[32] The primary goals of therapy for patients with sepsis are (a) timely diagnosis and identification of the pathogen, (b) rapid elimination

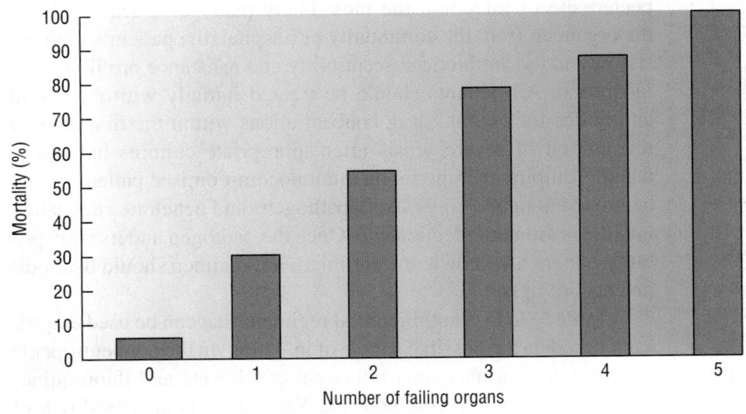

FIGURE 97-3 Mortality related to the number of failing organs.

of the source of infection medically and/or surgically, (c) early initiation of aggressive antimicrobial therapy, (d) interruption of pathogenic sequence leading to septic shock, and (e) avoidance of organ failure. Supportive care such as stress ulcer prophylaxis and nutritional support is important to prevent complications during the stay in the ICU. Table 97-3 describes the summary of the surviving sepsis campaign treatment recommendations.

Elimination of the Source of Infection

After the source of infection is identified, prompt efforts to eradicate that source should be made.[32] With an infected intravascular catheter, the catheter should be removed and cultured. Urinary tract catheters should be removed if association with sepsis is suspected. Suspicion of soft tissue (cellulitis or wound infection) or bone involvement should lead to aggressive debridement of the affected area. Evidence of an abscess or sepsis associated with any intraabdominal pathology should prompt surgical intervention.

TABLE 97-3 Evidence-based Treatment Recommendations for Sepsis and Septic Shock

Recommendations	Recommendation Grades[a]
Initial Resuscitation (First 6 Hours)	
Early goal-directed goals, including CVP 8–12 mm Hg, MAP ≥65 mm Hg, central venous oxygen saturation ≥70% (≥0.70)	1C
Antibiotic Therapy	
IV broad-spectrum antibiotic within 1 hour of diagnosis of septic shock and severe sepsis against likely bacterial/fungal pathogens	1B
Reassess antibiotic therapy daily with microbiology and clinical data to narrow coverage	1C
Fluid Therapy	
No clinical outcome difference between colloids and crystalloids	1B
Fluid challenges of 1000 mL of crystalloids or 300–500 mL of colloids over 30 minutes	1D
Vasopressors	
Norepinephrine and dopamine are the initial choices	1C
Maintain MAP ≥65 mm Hg	1C
Inotropic Therapy	
Use dobutamine when cardiac output remains low despite fluid resuscitation and combined inotropic/vasopressor therapy	1C
Glucose Control	
Use IV insulin to keep blood glucose ≤150 mg/dL (≤8.3 mmol/L)	2C
Steroids	
IV hydrocortisone for septic shock when hypotension remains poorly responsive to adequate fluid resuscitation and vasopressors	2C
Hydrocortisone dose should be <300 mg/day	1A
Deep Vein Thrombosis Prophylaxis	
Use either low-molecular-weight heparin or low-dose unfractionated heparin in preventing deep vein thrombosis	1A
Stress Ulcer Prophylaxis	
H2 receptor blocker or proton pump inhibitor is effective	1A, 1B

CVP, central venous pressure; MAP, mean arterial pressure.

[a]Grades of Recommendation, Assessment, Development, and Evaluation (GRADE) system: a structured system for rating quality of evidence and grading strength of recommendation in clinical practice. Quality of evidence: high (grade A), moderate (grade B), low (grade C), or very low (grade D). Strength of recommendation: strong (grade 1) or weak (grade 2).

Adapted from Dellinger RP, Levy MM, Carlet JM, et al. Surviving sepsis campaign: International guidelines for management of severe sepsis and septic shock: 2008. Crit Care Med 2008;36:296–327.

Antimicrobial Therapy

5 The most recent guidelines from the Surviving Sepsis Campaign recommended starting IV antibiotic therapy as early as possible because early administration of broad-spectrum antibiotics is critical in decreasing the risk of mortality.[32] Early administration (within 1 hour vs. 6 hours of diagnosis) of broad-spectrum antibiotics was independently associated with lower hospital mortality in patients with severe sepsis.[36,37]

Delays in the initiation of effective antimicrobial therapy after the onset of hypotension were significant predictors of mortality.[38] In a large retrospective study, inappropriate initial antimicrobial therapy occurred in about 20% of patients with septic shock, and was associated with a fivefold reduction in survival in comparison to those who received appropriate therapy (52.0% vs. 10.3%, respectively).[12] Therefore, early administration of appropriate antimicrobial therapy is critical in the treatment of severe sepsis and septic shock.

Pharmacokinetics of Antimicrobial Agents in Critically Ill Patients

Pathophysiologic changes have been reported in sepsis that can affect drug distribution, and adjusted dosing regimens are required in critically ill patients with sepsis.[39] Initially high creatinine clearance can be seen in patients with normal serum creatinine because of increased renal preload. Volume of distribution can increase because of fluid accumulation from leaky capillaries and/or altered protein binding. Consequently, some antimicrobial agents, especially for hydrophilic antimicrobials including aminoglycosides, β-lactams, carbapenems, and vancomycin can result in lower peak serum concentrations with usual doses.[40] However, as sepsis progresses, organ perfusion decreases because of significant myocardial depression and leads to multiple organ dysfunction. Consequently, clearance of antimicrobial agents is decreased, prolonging the elimination half-life and accumulation of metabolites. Hence, in addition to selecting the most appropriate antimicrobial agents, a clinician must ensure effective antibiotic usage, such as proper dosing, interval of administration, optimal duration of treatment, monitoring of drug levels when appropriate, and avoidance of unwanted drug interactions. The lack of adherence to these requirements can lead to suboptimal or excessive tissue concentrations that can promote antibiotic resistance, toxicity, and inadequate efficacy despite appropriate antibiotic selection.

Selection of Antimicrobial Agents

The selection of an empiric regimen should be based on the suspected site of infection, the most likely pathogens, acquisition of the organism from the community or hospital, the patient's immune status, and the antibiotic susceptibility and resistance profile for the institution. All patients should be treated initially with parenteral antibiotics for optimal drug concentrations within the first hour of recognition of severe sepsis after appropriate cultures have been taken.[32] Empiric therapy for an immunocompromised patient should be broad enough to cover likely pathogens and penetrate adequately into the presumed infection site. Once the pathogen and its susceptibility pattern are known, the antimicrobial regimen should be modified accordingly.

Table 97-4 lists antimicrobial regimens that can be used empirically based on the possible source of infection. In the nonneutropenic patient with a urinary tract infection, ceftriaxone and fluoroquinolones are generally recommended. When there is increased risk of

TABLE 97-4 Empiric Antimicrobial Regimens in Sepsis

Infection (Site or Type)	Antimicrobial Regimen: Community-acquired	Antimicrobial Regimen: Hospital-acquired
Urinary tract	Ceftriaxone or ciprofloxacin/levofloxacin	Ciprofloxacin/levofloxacin or ceftriaxone or ceftazidime
Respiratory tract	Levofloxacin[a]/moxifloxacin or ceftriaxone + clarithromycin/azithromycin	Piperacillin/tazobactam or ceftazidime or cefipime + levofloxacin/ciprofloxacin or aminoglycoside
Intraabdominal	Ertapenem or tigecycline orciprofloxacin/levofloxacin + metronidazole	Piperacillin/tazobactam or carbapenem[b]
Skin/soft tissue	Vancomycin or linezolid or daptomycin	Vancomycin + piperacillin/tazobactam
Catheter-related		Vancomycin
Unknown		Piperacillin/tazobactam or ceftazidime/cefipime or imipenem/meropenem } ±vancomycin not gentamicin

[a]750 mg orally once daily.
[b]Imipenem, meropenem, and doripenem.

P. aeruginosa in sepsis or hospital-acquired infections, an antipseudomonal antibiotic, such as ceftazidime, is recommended.[41]

S. pneumoniae is the most common cause of community-acquired pneumonia, and it accounts for ~60% of all deaths. The rising incidence of penicillin-resistant *S. pneumoniae* requires empiric use of newer "respiratory" fluoroquinolones. Levofloxacin or moxifloxacin can be used as monotherapy, as they offer excellent coverage against penicillin-resistant pneumococci and aerobic gram-negative bacteria, as well as atypical pathogens, including *Legionella pneumophila, Mycoplasma pneumoniae,* and *Chlamydophila pneumoniae.*[42] Addition of a macrolide to a β-lactam empirical therapy improves outcome in severe pneumonia, and clarithromycin and azithromycin are effective against atypical pathogens and better tolerated than erythromycin.[43]

In nosocomial pneumonia, enteric gram-negative bacteria such as *Enterobacter* and *Klebsiella* species and *P. aeruginosa* are the major pathogens in addition to *S. aureus.* If *P. aeruginosa* infection is suspected, β-lactam antipseudomonal agents (ceftazidime or cefepime), antipseudomonal fluoroquinolone (ciprofloxacin or levofloxacin), or an aminoglycoside should be included in the regimen.[44] When *S. aureus* is likely to be methicillin-resistant, linezolid may be preferred to vancomycin because of the poor penetration of vancomycin into the lungs, as well as the worldwide emergence of glycopeptide intermediately resistant *S. aureus.*[45,46]

Secondary peritonitis as a consequence of perforation of the GI tract is usually polymicrobial involving enteric aerobes and anaerobes, and as many as five organisms are isolated per patient. In general, if resistance for a given antibiotic is greater than 10% to 20% for a common intraabdominal pathogen in the community, that agent should be avoided. Because of widespread resistance of *Escherichia coli* to ampicillin/sulbactam, it is no longer recommended.[47,48] Emerging fluoroquinolone-resistant *E. coli* and the local prevalence of extended-spectrum β-lactamase-producing strains of *Klebsiella* species and *E. coli* should be considered in choosing empiric therapy.[47] *Bacteroides fragilis*, the major pathogen, has shown uniform susceptibility to metronidazole, carbapenems, and β-lactam/β-lactamase inhibitors.[49] High resistance rates were observed for clindamycin and moxifloxacin (as high as 60% for clindamycin and >80% for moxifloxacin), with relatively stable low resistance (5.4%) for tigecycline.

In addition to surgical intervention, broad-spectrum antibiotics, such as β-lactamase inhibitor combination agent (piperacillin/tazobactam) and tigecycline are appropriate in treating intraabdominal infections.[48] Carbapenems such as imipenem, meropenem, and doripenem are indicated in the treatment of resistant pathogens, including Enterobacteriaceae and *P. aeruginosa*, in critically ill patients.[48]

Skin and soft tissue infections (SSTIs) range from cellulitis to rapidly progressive necrotizing fasciitis, which may be associated with septic shock and toxic shock syndrome. Staphylococci and streptococci long have been the leading causes of SSTIs, but severe SSTIs can be caused also by indigenous aerobes and anaerobes such as *Clostridium* species.[50] Early initiation of appropriate empiric broad-spectrum antimicrobial therapy is essential and should include coverage against MRSA due to the high prevalence of community-associated MRSA strains.[45,50] Vancomycin, daptomycin, and linezolid have comparable clinical efficacy and safety data for complicated skin and skin-structure infections caused by MRSA.[45,51,52] A multicenter study of MRSA, vancomycin-resistant *Enterococcus* (VRE) *faecium* and coagulase-negative staphylococci bacteremic patients with sepsis suggested 70% success rate with daptomycin.[53]

Combination therapy does not appear to be more effective than monotherapy in reducing organ failure or mortality.[11] However, the greatest benefit of combination therapy appeared to be in patients with *Pseudomonas* or multidrug-resistant gram-negative bacteremia and in neutropenic patients with severe sepsis or septic shock.[32,54,55]

The antimicrobial regimen should be reassessed after 48 to 72 hours based on the microbiological and clinical data. Once the culture results and antimicrobial susceptibility data return, therapy should be directed toward the isolated pathogen as part of good antibiotic stewardship to prevent drug toxicities and the development of nosocomial superinfections with *Candida* species, *Clostridium difficile*, or VRE.[56] Furthermore, improved patient care outcomes have been demonstrated with such de-escalation of antibiotic therapy.[57]

Antifungal Therapy

Candida species are most frequently associated with fungal infections, and the resulting candidemia is frequently associated with sepsis syndrome and a high mortality rate.[15,58] Septic shock caused by *C. albicans* demonstrated 24.6% survival with initial appropriate therapy but only 4.6% survival without (ninefold decrease).[12] Of the patients with candidemia, delayed appropriate antifungal treatment and failure to achieve timely source control were independently associated with a greater risk of hospital mortality.[59,60] Accurate and rapid identification of candida would prompt timely initiation of appropriate therapy.[35]

Treatment of invasive candidiasis involves amphotericin B-based preparations, azole antifungal agents, and echinocandin antifungal agents, or combinations. The choice depends on the clinical status of the patient, the fungal species and its susceptibility, relative drug toxicity, presence of organ dysfunction that would affect drug clearance, and the patient's prior exposure to antifungal agents.

Empirical fluconazole therapy for suspected nosocomial bloodstream infections can be appropriate for hospitalized patients at high risk for fungal infections, including those receiving total parenteral nutrition, with bowel perforation, *Candida* colonization, malignancy, emergency surgery, or with persistent or new signs and symptoms of infections despite receiving broad-spectrum antibacterial therapy.[61,62] However, recent exposure to antibiotics and fluconazole have been associated with fluconazole-resistant *Candida* species.[17,63] A global survey evaluating the Candida bloodstream infections reported a low overall fluconazole resistance (5% of ICU isolates and 4.4% of non-ICU isolates).[64] Only *C. glabrata* was the only species to exhibit resistance to both azoles and echinocandins. Further investigation of in vitro susceptibilities of 1,669 bloodstream infection isolates of *C. glabrata* reported 9.7% resistance to fluconazole, of which 8% to 9.3% were resistant to enchinocandins.[65]

Caspofungin, the first echinocandin antifungal agent, appears to be potent against all *Candida* species, including *C. glabrata, C. krusei*, and *Candida lusitaniae*, as well as *Aspergillus* species. IV caspofungin was equally effective but better tolerated than amphotericin B deoxycholate for invasive candidiasis.[66] In an international, randomized, double-blind trial, the micafungin 100-mg group was noninferior to caspofungin for the treatment of candidemia and other forms of invasive candidiasis demonstrated (76.4% vs. 72.3%).[67] Anidulafungin, the latest echinocandin to be approved, achieved a success rate of 73.2% against invasive candidiasis in comparison to the 61.1% treatment success rate of fluconazole.[68] The difference was not statistically significant.

In general, suspected systemic mycotic infection leading to sepsis in nonneutropenic patients should be treated empirically with parenteral fluconazole, caspofungin, anidulafungin, or micafungin.[62] An echinocandin is preferred for a patient with recent azole exposure or if the patient is clinically unstable because of its greater activity against fluconazole-resistant *Candida* species and non-*albicans* species, including *C. glabrata* and *C. krusei*.[62] In neutropenic patients, a lipid formulation of amphotericin, caspofungin, or voriconazole is recommended. Azoles should be avoided for empiric therapy in patients who have received an azole for prophylaxis.[62]

Duration of Therapy

The average duration of antimicrobial therapy in the normal host with sepsis is 7 to 10 days, and fungal infections can require 10 to 14 days.[32,44,62] However, the duration can be longer in patients with a slow clinical response, undrainable focus of infection, or neutropenia. In a neutropenic patient, therapy is usually continued until the patient is no longer neutropenic and has been afebrile for at least 72 hours. After the patient is hemodynamically stable, afebrile for 48 to 72 hours, has a normalizing WBC count, and is able to take oral medications, then a "step-down" from parenteral to oral antibiotics can be considered for the remaining duration of therapy.

PCT is a biomarker that increases in response to endotoxins and inflammatory cytokines that are released during systemic bacterial infections. Hence, the PCT level may also be used to guide the length of antibiotic therapy. PCT has been studied as a marker to initiate and discontinue antibiotics in patients with severe sepsis or septic shock and surgical intensive care patients.[69] However, the survival benefit has not been clearly defined.

Clinical **Controversy...**

The biomarker PCT rises early in severe sepsis by pneumonia and bloodstream infections, and a growing body of evidence supports the use of PCT to differentiate bacterial from vial respiratory diagnoses, to help risk stratify patients, and to guide antibiotic therapy decisions in terms of initiating and optimizing duration of therapy.[69,70,71] Randomized controlled trials further suggested that clinical algorithms based on PCT levels resulted in reduced antibiotic use.[70] However, a systematic review of randomized controlled trials investigating PCT algorithms for antibiotic decisions in adult patients with respiratory tract infections and sepsis found no significant difference in mortality between PCT-treated and control patients overall (odds ratio (OR), 0.91; 95% confidence interval (CI), 0.73 to 1.14).[72] There was a consistent reduction in antibiotic prescriptions and duration of therapy. The Procalcitonin and Survival Study Group in Demark compared the standard of care arm and the PCT arm using a strategy of escalation of broad-spectrum antimicrobials and intensified diagnostics based on daily PCT measurements in the multidisciplinary ICU.[73] No significant difference in mortality between the PCT arm and the standard of care arm (31.5% vs. 32.0%; absolute risk reduction 0.6%) was reported. PCT-guided antimicrobial escalation leads to increased use of broad-spectrum antimicrobials, organ-related harm, and prolonged admission to the ICU. Further trials are needed to determine the safety and efficacy of antibiotic sparing PCT strategies in critically ill patients.

Hemodynamic Support

A high cardiac output and a low SVR characterize septic shock. Patients can have hypotension as a result of low SVR and abnormal distribution of blood flow in the microcirculation, resulting in compromised tissue perfusion. Because approximately half of patients with septic shock die of multiple organ system failure, they should be monitored carefully, and aggressive hemodynamic support should be initiated.

Hemodynamics change rapidly in sepsis, and noninvasive evaluation can give inaccurate assessment of filling pressures and cardiac output, requiring a right-sided heart catheter in the ICU setting.[32] Hemodynamic support can be divided into three main categories: fluid therapy, vasopressor therapy, and inotropic therapy.

Fluid Therapy

❻ Septic patients have enormous fluid requirements as a result of peripheral vasodilation and capillary leakage. In ~50% of septic patients who initially present with hypotension, fluids alone will reverse hypotension and restore hemodynamic stability. Rapid fluid resuscitation improves the 28-day survival rate in patients with sepsis-induced hypoperfusion.[32] The goal of fluid therapy is to maximize cardiac output by increasing the LV preload, which will ultimately restore tissue perfusion. Fluid administration should be titrated to clinical end points such as heart rate, urine output, blood pressure, and mental status. Increased serum lactate, a by-product of cellular anaerobic metabolism, should normalize as tissue perfusion improves.

Isotonic crystalloids, such as 0.9% sodium chloride (normal saline) and lactated Ringer solution, are commonly used for fluid resuscitation. A patient in septic shock typically requires up to 10 L of crystalloid solution during the first 24-hour period. These solutions distribute into the extracellular compartment. Approximately 25% of the infused volume of crystalloid remains in the intravascular space, whereas the balance distributes to extravascular spaces. Although this could impair diffusion of oxygen to tissues, clinical impact is unproven.

The most commonly used colloids are 5% albumin, a naturally occurring plasma protein, and 6% hetastarch, a synthetic colloid formulation. These solutions offer more rapid restoration of intravascular volume because they produce greater intravascular volume expansion per quantity of volume infused. Colloids produce less peripheral edema than crystalloid, but there is no significant clinical impact. However, synthetic colloids cause dose-related renal impairment and increased bleeding.[74] The use of colloid solutions and blood products can be particularly important if there is significant blood loss associated with sepsis or if the patient had severe preexisting anemia.

The Saline versus Albumin Fluid Evaluation (SAFE) trial found no difference in the 28-day mortality rate in critically ill patients (21.1% with saline vs. 20.9% with albumin).[75] Although crystalloid solutions require two to four times more volume than colloids, they are generally recommended for fluid resuscitation because of the lower cost. However, colloids can be preferred, especially when the serum albumin is less than 2 g/dL (20 g/L).

Central venous pressure (CVP) is used to monitor fluid status in patients with septic shock. Initial fluid resuscitation should target a CVP between 8 and 12 mm Hg within the first 6 hours of presentation.[32] Fluid challenges should continue until hemodynamic stability is reached as long as CVP is at goal. The rate of fluid administration should be reduced if hemodynamic measures do not improve despite adequate or increasing cardiac filling pressures. Resuscitation typically includes IV normal saline 500 mL every 15 minutes until the target CVP is reached.

Patients receiving fluid challenges require close monitoring of volume status to avoid pulmonary and systemic edema. Aggressive volume expansion can cause an increase in pulmonary capillary pressure, leading to an increase in lung water and associated hypoxemia.[76] There is no significant difference in the incidence of pulmonary edema between the crystalloid and colloid solutions.

Vasopressor and Inotropic Therapy

When fluid resuscitation alone provides inadequate arterial pressure and organ perfusion, vasopressors and inotropic agents should be initiated. Inotropic agents such as dopamine and dobutamine have been effective in improving cardiac output by increasing cardiac contractility. Vasopressors such as norepinephrine should be considered when a systolic blood pressure is less than 90 mm Hg or mean arterial pressure (MAP) is <65 mm Hg after adequate LV preload and inotrope therapy. Although inotropes and vasopressors are effective in life-threatening hypotension and in improving cardiac index (CI), there are significant complications such as tachycardia and myocardial ischemia and infarction as a result of the change in myocardial oxygen consumption in patients with coexisting coronary disease. Thus, a catecholamine infusion should be titrated gradually to restore MAP without impairing stroke volume.

7 Agents commonly considered for vasopressor or inotropic support include dopamine, dobutamine, norepinephrine, phenylephrine, and epinephrine (Table 97-5).[77] Norepinephrine should generally be considered to be the first-choice vasopressor in septic shock after failure to restore adequate blood pressure and organ perfusion with appropriate fluid resuscitation. Norepinephrine is a potent α-adrenergic agent with less pronounced β-adrenergic activity. It increases MAP and SVR because of its vasoconstrictive effects on peripheral vascular beds. Doses of 0.01 to 3 mcg/kg/min can reliably increase blood pressure with little changes in heart rate or CI. Despite the earlier concern of decreased renal blood flow associated with norepinephrine, data in humans and animals demonstrate a norepinephrine-induced renal blood flow as well as urine and cardiac output.[77] Norepinephrine is a more potent agent than dopamine in refractory septic shock. Norepinephrine resulted in greater increases in arterial blood pressure in comparison to patients with septic shock who were treated with dopamine (93% with norepinephrine vs. 31% with dopamine).[77] In a meta-analysis evaluation the randomized trials comparing norepinephrine and dopamine, dopamine was associated with a higher risk of death and more frequently associated with arrythmias.[78]

Dopamine is a natural precursor of norepinephrine and epinephrine, and it exhibits dose-dependent pharmacologic effects. It is an α- and β-adrenergic agent with dopaminergic activity. Doses >5 mcg/kg/min increase MAP and cardiac output, primarily because of the increase in heart rate and cardiac contractility through stimulation of β-adrenergic receptors. At higher doses, α-adrenergic effects predominate, resulting in arterial vasoconstriction. Because of combined vasopressor and inotropic effects, dopamine is more useful in patients with hypotension and compromised systolic function. However, it is also more arrhythmogenic and can cause more tachycardia.[32,77,79] It should be used with caution in patients who have underlying heart disease.

Phenylephrine, a selective α_1-agonist, has rapid onset, short duration, and primary vascular effects, and it is least likely to produce tachycardia. Limited data suggest it can increase blood pressure modestly in fluid-resuscitated patients, and it does not appear to impair cardiac or renal function. Phenylephrine appears useful when tachycardia limits the usage of other vasopressors.[77]

Epinephrine is a nonspecific α- and β-adrenergic agonist. Ranging from 0.1 to 0.5 mcg/kg/min, cardiac output is increased at lower doses, and vasoconstriction occurs predominantly at higher doses. Epinephrine should be reserved for patients who fail to respond to traditional therapies for increasing or maintaining blood pressure, as it impairs blood flow to the splanchnic system, increases the lactate level, and causes dysrhythmia more frequently than other vasoactive agents.[77]

During hypotension, endogenous vasopressin levels increase and maintain arterial blood pressure, as vasopressin is a direct vasoconstrictor without inotropic or chronotropic effects. However, there is a vasopressin deficiency in septic shock most likely caused by inadequate production. Low doses of vasopressin (0.01 to 0.04 units/min) produce a significant increase in MAP in septic shock, and it may be beneficial to add vasopressin in severe sepsis and septic shock that is refractory to other vasopressors.[77] Vasopressin should not be used as a single agent for refractory hypotension. Although it can be used to reduce norepinephrine requirements, this has not been shown to improve mortality rates.[80]

Dobutamine is a β-adrenergic inotropic agent that many clinicians consider to be the preferred drug for improvement of cardiac output and oxygen delivery, particularly in early sepsis

TABLE 97-5 Receptor Activity of Cardiovascular Agents Commonly Used in Septic Shock

Agent	α_1	α_2	β_1	β_2	Dopaminergic
Dopamine	++/+++	?	++++	++	++++
Dobutamine	+	+	++++	++	0
Norepinephrine	+++	+++	+++	+/++	0
Phenylephrine	++/+++	+	?	0	0
Epinephrine	++++	++++	++++	+++	0

α_1, α_1-adrenergic receptor; α_2, α_2-adrenergic receptor; β_1, β_1-adrenergic receptor; β_2, β_2-adrenergic receptor; 0, no activity; ++++, maximal activity; ?, unknown activity.

before significant peripheral vasodilation has occurred. Doses of 2 to 20 mcg/kg/min increase the CI, ranging from 20% to 66%. However, heart rate often increases significantly.[77] Dobutamine should be considered in severely septic patients with low CI but adequate filling pressures and blood pressure. A vasopressor such as norepinephrine and an inotrope such as dobutamine can be used to maintain both MAP and cardiac output.

In summary, for the septic patient with clinical signs of shock and significant hypotension unresponsive to aggressive fluid therapy, norepinephrine is the preferred agent for increasing MAP. Epinephrine should be considered for refractory hypotension. Dopamine and epinephrine are more likely to induce or exacerbate tachycardia than norepinephrine and phenylephrine. In a septic patient with low CI after adequate fluid therapy and adequate MAP, dobutamine is the first-line agent. Alternatively, dopamine in moderate doses (5 to 10 mcg/kg/min) can also be used as an initial agent because of its selective effect on increasing cardiac output with its minimal effect on SVR.

Early Goal-Directed Therapy

8 Initial resuscitation of a patient in severe sepsis or sepsis-induced tissue hypoperfusion should begin as soon as the syndrome is recognized. A randomized, controlled trial evaluated the timing of the goal-directed therapy involving adjustments of cardiac preload, afterload, and contractility to balance oxygen delivery with demand prior to admission to the ICU.[81] The goals during the first 6 hours included CVP of 8 to 12 mm Hg, MAP ≥65 mm Hg, urine output ≥0.5 mL/kg/h, and a central venous or mixed venous oxygen saturation ≥70% (≥0.70). During the first 6 hours of resuscitation, the early goal-directed therapy group had a central venous catheter placed and received more fluid than with traditional therapy (5 vs. 3.5 L), dobutamine therapy to a maximum of 20 mcg/kg/min, and red blood cell transfusions. The 28-day mortality rate was 30% in the early goal-directed therapy group, in comparison to 46.5% in the traditional therapy group consisting of fluid resuscitation, followed by vasopressor therapy if required. Increased oxygen delivery from the red blood cell transfusions to achieve a hematocrit of ≥30% (≥0.30) in the early goal-directed therapy group appeared to be the primary difference between the two groups.

Compliance with the goals of early goal-directed group was closely correlated with the overall mortality rate. At 18 hours after diagnosis of severe sepsis and septic shock patients meeting goals had a greater reduction in mortality than those who did not (26.8% vs. 9.4%, $P < 0.01$).[82] A decade later, over 50 publications involving 18,000 adult patients have shown early goal-directed therapy to decrease in progression of organ failure, reduction in mortality, and decrease in overall healthcare cost by 20%, primarily due to shorter length of hospital stay.[83,84]

Adjunctive Therapies

ARDS and hypoxia are common in septic patients, even in those without pulmonary infection. Oxygen therapy is indicated to maintain oxygen saturation greater than 90% (0.90), and with progressive pulmonary insufficiency, the patient can require assisted ventilation.

9 Hyperglycemia and insulin resistance are frequently associated with sepsis regardless of the presence of diabetes prior to sepsis, and more severe hyperglycemia is associated with higher morbidity and mortality.[32] However, intensive insulin therapy is no longer the standard of care in critically ill patients. Results from a randomized control trial showed that more patients receiving intensive insulin therapy (target serum glucose of 81 to 108 mg/dL [4.5 to 6 mmol/L]) had a higher incidence of severe hypoglycemia and increased mortality at 90 days compared with patients receiving conventional insulin therapy (target ≤180 mg/dL [≤10.0 mmol/L]).[85] Further analysis of patients with moderate (41 to 70 mg/dL [2.3 to 3.9 mmol/L]) and severe hypoglycemia (≤40 mg/dL [≤2.2 mmol/L]) reported death rate of 23.5% with moderate hypoglycemia and 35.4% with severe hypoglycemia.[86] Severe hypoglycemia in the absence of insulin therapy was also associated with a higher risk of death. A glucose range of less than 150 mg/dL (8.3 mmol/L) is recommended for the majority of critically ill patients to improve the outcome while reducing the risk of hypoglycemia.[32]

10 Cortisol levels vary widely in patients with septic shock, and some studies have suggested increased mortality associated with both low and high serum cortisol levels. An adrenocorticotropic hormone (ACTH) stimulation test has been used to identify those patients who have a relative adrenal insufficiency who should then receive supplemental steroid.[32] Corticosteroids have been studied as adjunctive therapy in patients with severe sepsis and septic shock to decrease the duration of shock and to decrease mortality.

A multicenter, randomized, controlled trial demonstrated significant shock reversal and decrease in mortality (absolute reduction 10%) in patients with severe septic shock who were given low-dose corticosteroids within 8 hours after the onset of shock.[87] Fludrocortisone 50 mcg orally and hydrocortisone 200 to 300 mg/day for 7 days in three or four divided doses or by continuous infusion were used in patients with adrenal insufficiency, requiring high-dose or increasing vasopressor therapy within the first 8 hours of septic shock.[87] A subsequent meta-analysis of 12 randomized trials reported decreased mortality compared to placebo (38% vs. 44%; relative risk 0.84).[88] There was no benefit for those patients without adrenal insufficiency. However, in the large multicenter trial, the Corticosteroid Therapy of Septic Shock (CORTICUS), no significant benefit was noted in patients regardless of ACTH stimulation test outcome.[89]

Clinical **Controversy...**

A systematic review reported a significant reduction in 28-day all-cause mortality and hospital mortality in patients receiving prolonged courses (>5 days) of low-dose corticosteroid therapy (≤300 mg hydrocortisone or equivalent/day).[88] The CORTICUS trial found no survival benefit among patients who received prolonged courses of hydrocortisone, but reported a trend in shock reversal for patients who received hydrocortisone.[89] Based on the current Surviving Sepsis guidelines, corticosteroids should be reserved for patients who continue to be hypotensive despite adequate fluids and vasopressor therapy, are maintained on an outpatient corticosteroid regimen, or may be initiated at physician discretion.

Corticosteroids should be weaned once the patient is off vasopressors, although comparative clinical trials comparing whether steroids should be abruptly discontinued or tapered are lacking.

Deep vein thrombosis prophylaxis with either low-dose unfractionated heparin or low-molecular-weight heparin should be initiated in general ICU patients, including those with severe sepsis and septic shock.[32] Similarly, stress ulcer prophylaxis should be initiated in all patients with severe sepsis and septic shock.[32] Proton pump inhibitors and H_2 receptor antagonists are equivalent in their ability to increase gastric pH.

HMG-CoA reductase inhibitors (statins) have diverse pharmacologic effects ranging from decreasing low-density lipoproteins to antiinflammatory and antithrombotic properties. As severe sepsis is characterized by a dysregulation of inflammation and coagulation, statins have been evaluated for their role in the treatment or prevention of severe sepsis. Most studies suggested a clinical benefit for stains, and yet, others have shown no benefit but possible harm.

Clinical **Controversy...**

A variety of observational studies reported mixed results in the role of statins in treatment of sepsis.[90–94] Meta-analysis for various infection-related outcomes revealed ORs in favor of statin use versus no statin (0.61; 95% CI 0.48 to 0.73) for 30 day mortality and 0.40 (95% CI, 0.23-0.57) for sepsis-related mortality.[90] A multicenter cohort study evaluated 1,895 patients hospitalized with pneumonia and sepsis for benefits of prior use of statin and continuation of statin in hospital.[92] No protective effect for statin on clinical outcomes was observed. After adjusting for patient characteristics, there was no mortality benefit for prior use (OR, 0.90 (0.63 to 1.29); $P = 0.57$) or continued statin use (OR, 0.73 (0.47 to 1.13); $P = 0.15$). More prospective trials are needed to clearly define the role of prior statins in severe sepsis and septic shock as well as to develop strategies to continue or discontinue statin once admitted in the ICU for sepsis.

Immunotherapy

Despite the initial enthusiasm for immunotherapeutic interventions for sepsis, overall results have been generally disappointing including drotrecogin alfa (recombinant human activated protein C, rhAPC), an endogenous anticoagulant with antiinflammatory properties. During severe sepsis, the activation of protein C is inhibited by inflammatory cytokines.

Drotrecogin, the first antiinflammatory agent to be approved for sepsis, promotes fibrinolysis and the inhibition of coagulation and inflammation. The Recombinant Human Activated Protein C Worldwide Evaluation in Severe Sepsis (PROWESS) trial showed all-cause mortality at 28 days reduced significantly from 30.8% with placebo to 24.7% in those receiving drotrecogin.[95] However, serious bleeding, including intracranial hemorrhage and a life-threatening bleeding episode, occurred in 3.5% of patients who received drotrecogin in comparison to 2% of patients in the placebo group. Since the approval, ongoing debate on the study's methodology and outcomes has questioned the effectiveness, safety, and place in therapy of drotrecogin alfa. Consequently, the PROWESS-SHOCK study, a randomized, multinational, placebo-controlled, double-blind clinical trial, was initiated in March 2008 to help refine appropriate patient identification for treatment with drotrecogin alfa and to confirm the benefit-risk profile.[96] Planned enrollment was 1,700 patients with severe sepsis and persistent shock, and data collection ended in September 2011. Study design details and the outcomes have not been reported. However, a preliminary analysis submitted to the FDA suggested that the PROWESS-SHOCK study did not meet the primary endpoint of a significant reduction in 28-day all-cause mortality in patients with septic shock treated with drotrecogin alfa compared with placebo. Among 1,680 patients who completed the study, the all-cause mortality rates were 26.4% (223 of 846) in patients treated with drotrecogin alfa and 24.2% (202 of 834) in the placebo group, for a relative risk of 1.09 (95% CI, 0.92 to 1.28; $P = 0.31$). Severe bleeding events occurred in 1.2% and 1% of the drotrecogin alfa and place groups, respectively, suggesting no increased harm. The study failed to demonstrate overall improvement in survival, and without clear demonstration of benefits outweighing the risks, the product was withdrawn from the market worldwide.[96]

PERSONALIZED PHARMACOTHERAPY

Patients presenting with severe sepsis and septic shock are critically ill and their management in an intensive care setting can be overwhelming. While it is critical to manage the complications involving multiple organ systems to ultimately sustain life during the initial hours, infection source identification is imperative as severe sepsis and subsequent multiorgan dysfunction arise from an uncontrolled infection. Clinical presentation of each patient should be considered carefully and should prompt further evaluation of any underlying conditions, recent travel, injury, animal exposure, infection or use of antibiotics along with a complete physical examination to determine the possible source of infection. Based on the individual patients' findings and the most likely source of infection, the empiric regimen may be completely different from one patient to another. A patient presenting with sepsis secondary to a community-acquired pneumonia may receive ceftriaxone and azithromycin where another patient presenting with secondary peritonitis as a consequence of perforation of the GI tract may require a broad-spectrum regimen such as ertapenem or piperacillin/tazobactam.[42,43,48] Catheter-related sepsis may require a removal of the line as well as initiating vancomycin. There is abundant evidence in the literature demonstrating a correlation between the prompt and appropriate antibiotics and the overall survival rate.[36,37] Severe sepsis and complications such as shock, ARDS, and DIC result from an acute infection. As such, prompt identification of the source of infection in an individual patient and customizing the empiric antibiotic regimen may be the key to controlling the multiorgan dysfunctions and overall mortality rate.

ABBREVIATIONS

ACTH	adrenocorticotropic hormone
ARDS	acute respiratory distress syndrome
CI	cardiac index
CORTICUS	Corticosteroid Therapy of Septic Shock (trial)
CVP	central venous pressure
DIC	disseminated intravascular coagulation
DO_2	oxygen delivery to tissues
ICU	intensive care unit
IL	interleukin
IL-1RA	interleukin-1 receptor antagonist
LV	left ventricular
MAP	mean arterial pressure
MODS	multiple-organ dysfunction syndrome
MRSA	methicillin-resistant *Staphylococcus aureus*
PAF	platelet activating factor
PCT	procalcitonin
PROWESS	Recombinant Human Activated Protein C Worldwide Evaluation in Severe Sepsis (trial)
SIRS	systemic inflammatory response syndrome
SSTIs	skin and soft tissue infections
SVR	systemic vascular resistance
TNF	tumor necrosis factor
VO_2	oxygen consumption
VRE	vancomycin-resistant enterococci
WBC	white blood cell

REFERENCES

1. Martin GS, Mannino DM, Eaton S, et al. The epidemiology of sepsis in the United States from 1979 through 2000. N Engl J Med 2003;348:1546–1554.
2. Lagu T, Rothberg MB, Shieh MS, et al. Hospitalizations, costs, and outcomes of severe sepsis in the United States 2003 to 2007. Crit Care Med 2012;40:754–761.
3. American College of Chest Physicians/Society of Critical Care Medicine Consensus Conference. Definitions for sepsis and organ failure and guidelines for the use of innovative therapies in sepsis. Crit Care Med 1992;20:864–874.
4. Levy MM, Fink MP, Marshall JC, et al. 2001 SCCM/ESICM/ACCP/ATS/SIS International Sepsis Definitions Conference. Crit Care Med 2003;31:1250–1256.
5. Tiruvoipati R, Ong K, Gangopadhyay H, et al. Hypothermia predicts mortality in critically ill elderly patients with sepsis. MCB Geriatr 2010;10:70–78.
6. Danai PA, Moss M, Mannino DM, et al. The epidemiology of sepsis in patients with malignancy. Chest 2006;129:1432–1440.
7. Netea MG, van der Meer JWM. Immunodeficiency and genetic defects of pattern-recognition receptors. N Engl J Med 2011;364:60–70.
8. Danai PA, Sinha S, Moss M, et al. Seasonal variation in the epidemiology of sepsis. Crit Care Med 2007;35:410–415.
9. Zahar JR, Timsit JF, Garrouste-Orgeas M, et al. Outcomes in severe sepsis and patients with septic shock: Pathogen species and infection sites are not associated with mortality. Crit Care Med 2011;39:1886–1895.
10. Vincent JL, Sakr Y, Sprung CL, et al. Sepsis in European intensive care units: Results of the SOAP study. Crit Care Med 2006;34:344–353.
11. Brunkhorst FM, Oppert M, Marx G, et al. Effect of empirical treatment with moxifloxacin and meropenem vs meropenem on sepsis-related organ dysfunction in patients with severe sepsis. JAMA 2012;307:2390–2399.
12. Kumar A, Ellis P, Arabi Y, et al. Initiation of inappropriate antimicrobial therapy results in a fivefold reduction of survival in human septic shock. Chest 2009;136:1237–1248.
13. van Hal SJ, Jensen SO, Vaska VL, et al. Predictors of mortality in *Staphylococcus aureus* bacteremia. Clin Microbiol Rev 2012;25:362–386.
14. Johnson MT, Reichley R, Hoppe-Bauer J, et al. Impact of previous antibiotic therapy on outcome of gram-negative severe sepsis. Crit Care Med 2011;39:1859–1865.
15. Horn DL, Neofytos D, Anaissie EJ, et al. Epidemiology and outcomes of candidemia in 2019 patients: Data from the prospective antifungal therapy alliance registry. Clin Infect Dis 2009;48:1695–1703.
16. Diekema D, Arbefeville S, Boyken L, et al. The changing epidemiology of healthcare-associated candidemia over three decades. Diagn Microb Infect Dis 2012;73:45–48.
17. Ben-Ami R, Olshtain-Pops K, Krieger M, et al. Antibiotic exposure as a risk factor for fluconazole-resistant *Candida* bloodstream infection. Antimicrob Agents Chemother 2012;56:2518–2523.
18. Tamayo E, Fernandez A, Almansa R, et al. Pro- and anti-inflammatory responses are regulated simultaneously from the first moments of septic shock. Eur Cytokine Network 2011;22:82–87.
19. Andaluz-Ojeda D, Bobillo E, Iglesias V, et al. A combined score of pro- and anti-inflammatory interleukins improves mortality prediction in severe sepsis. Cytokine 2012;57:332–336.
20. De Pablo R, Monserrat J, Reyes E, et al. Mortality in patients with septic shock correlates with anti-inflammatory but not proinflammatory immunomodulatory molecules. J Intensive Care Med 2011;26:125–132.
21. Heper Y, Akalin EH, Mistik R, et al. Evaluation of serum C-reactive protein, procalcitonin, tumor necrosis factor alpha, and interleukin-10 levels as diagnostic and prognostic parameters in patients with community-acquired sepsis, severe sepsis, and septic shock. Eur J Clin Microbiol Infect Dis 2006;25:481–491.
22. Kanoore Edul VS, Enrico C, Laviolle B, et al. Quantitative assessment of the microcirculation in healthy volunteers and in patients with septic shock. Crit Care Med 2012;40:1443–1448.
23. Fourrier F. Severe sepsis, coagulation, and fibrinolysis: Dead end or one way? Crit Care Med 2012;40:2704–2708.
24. Semeraro N, Ammollo CT, Semeraro F, et al. Sepsis-associated disseminated intravascular coagulation and thromboembolic disease. Mediter J Hematol Infect Dis 2010;2:e2010024.
25. Levi M, Toh CH, Thachil J, et al. Guidelines for the diagnosis and management of disseminated intravascular coagulation. Br J Haematol 2009;145:24–33.
26. Pulido JN, Afessa B, Masaki M, et al. Clinical spectrum, frequency, and significance of myocardial dysfunction in severe sepsis and septic shock. Mayo Clin Proc 2010;87:620–628.
27. Bagshaw SM, George C, Bellomo R. Early acute kidney injury and sepsis: A multicentre evaluation. Crit Care 2008;12:R47.
28. Bagshaw SM, Lapinsky S, Dial S, et al. Acute kidney injury in septic shock: Clinical outcomes and impact of duration of hypotension prior to initiation of antimicrobial therapy. Intensive Care Med 2009;35:871–881.
29. Cunha BA. With sepsis: If fever is good, then hypothermia is bad! Crit Care Med 2012;40:2926–2927.
30. Awad SS. State-of-the-art therapy for severe sepsis and multisystem organ failure. Am J Surg 2003;186:23S–30S.
31. Nguyen HB, Rivers EP, Knoblich BP, et al. Early lactate clearance is associated with improved outcome in severe sepsis and septic shock. Crit Care Med 2004;32:1637–1642.
32. Dellinger RP, Levy MM, Carlet JM, et al. Surviving sepsis campaign: International guidelines for management of severe sepsis and septic shock: 2008. Crit Care Med 2008;36:296–327.
33. Coelho FR, Martins JO. Diagnostic methods in sepsis: The need of speed. Rev Assoc Med Bras 2012;58:498–504.
34. Davies J, Gordon CL, Tong SY, et al. Impact of results of a rapid *Staphylococcus aureus* diagnostic test on prescribing of antibiotics for patients with clustered gram-positive cocci in blood cultures. J Clin Microbiol 2012;50:2056–2058.
35. Aittakorpi A, Kuusela P, Koukila-Kahkola P, et al. Accurate and rapid identification of *Candida* spp. frequently associated with fungemia by using PCR and the microarray-based Prove-it sepsis assay. J Clin Microbiol 2012:50:3635–3640.
36. Ferrer R, Artigas A, Suarez D, et al. Effectiveness of treatments for severe sepsis: A prospective, multicenter, observational study. Am J Respir Crit Care Med 2009;180:861–866.
37. Gaieski DF, Mikkelsen ME, Band RA, et al. Impact of time to antibiotics on survival in patients with severe sepsis or septic shock in whom early goal-directed therapy was initiated in the emergency department. Crit Care Med 2010;38:1045–1053.

38. Kumar A, Roberts D, Wood KE, et al. Duration of hypotension before initiation of effective antimicrobial therapy is the critical determinant of survival in human septic shock. Crit Care Med 2006;34:1589–1596.
39. Pea F. Plasma pharmacokinetics of antimicrobial agents in critically ill patients. Curr Clin Pharmacol 2013;8:5–12 [Epub ahead of print].
40. Baptista JP, Sousa E, Martins PJ, et al. Augmented renal clearance in septic patients and implications for vancomycin optimisation. Int J Antimicrob Agents 2012;39:420–423.
41. Hooton TM, Bradley SF, Cardenas DD, et al. Diagnosis, prevention, and treatment of catheter-associated urinary tract infection in adults: 2009 International clinical practice guidelines from the Infectious Diseases Society of America. Clin Infect Dis 2010;50:625–663.
42. Mandell LA, Wunderinnk RG, Anzueto A, et al. Infectious Disease Society of America/American Thoracic Society consensus guidelines on management of community-acquired pneumonia in adults. Clin Infect Dis 2007;44: S27–S72.
43. Pereira JM, Paiva JA, Rello J. Severe sepsis in community-acquired pneumonia—Early recognition and treatment. Eur J Intern Med 2012;23:412–419.
44. American Thoracic Society Documents. Guidelines for the management of adults with hospital-acquired, ventilator-associated, and healthcare-associated pneumonia. Am J Respir Crit Care Med 2005;171:388–416.
45. Liu C, Bayer A, Cosgrove SE, et al. Clinical practice guidelines by the Infectious Diseases Society of America for the treatment of methicillin-resistant *Staphylococcus aureus* infections in adults and children. Clin Infect Dis 2011;52: 1–38.
46. Mullins CD, Kuznik A, Shaya FT, et al. Cost-effectiveness analysis of linezolid compared with vancomycin for the treatment of nosocomial pneumonia caused by methicillin-resistant *Staphylococcus aureus.* Clin Ther 2006;28: 1184–1198.
47. Baquero F, Hsueh PR, Paterson DL, et al. In vitro susceptibilities of aerobic and facultatively anaerobic gram-negative bacilli isolated from patients with intra-abdominal infections worldwide: 2005 results from Study for Monitoring Antimicrobial Resistance Trends (SMART). Surg Infect 2009;10:99–104.
48. Solomkin JS, Mazuski JE, Bradley JS, et al. Diagnosis and management of complicated intra-abdominal infection in adults and children: Guidelines by the Surgical Infection Society and the Infectious Diseases Society of America. Clin Infect Dis 2010;50:133–164.
49. Snydman DR, Jacobus NV, McDermott LA, et al. Update on resistance of *Bacteroides fragilis* group and related species with special attention to carbapenems 2006–2009. Anaerobe 2011;17:147–151.
50. Lipsky BA, Moran GJ, Napolitano LM, et al. A prospective, multicenter, observational study of complicated skin and soft tissue infections in hospitalized patients: Clinical characteristics, medical treatment, and outcomes. BMC Infect Dis 2012;12:227.
51. Bliziotis IA, Plessa E, Peppas G, et al. Daptomycin versus other antimicrobial agents for the treatment of skin and soft tissue infections: A meta-analysis. Ann Pharmacother 2010;44:97–106.
52. Bounthavong M, Hsu DI. Efficacy and safety of linezolid in methicillin-resistant *Staphylococcus aureus* (MRSA) complicated skin and soft tissue infection (cSSTI): A meta-analysis. Curr Med Res Opin 2010;26: 407–421.
53. Brown JE, Fominaya C, Christensen KJ, et al. Daptomycin experience in critical care patients: Results from a registry. Ann Pharmacother 2012;46:495–502.
54. Tamma PD, Cosgrove SE, Maragakis LL. Combination therapy for treatment of infections with gram-negative bacteria. Clin Microbiol Rev 2012;25:450–470.
55. Qureshi ZA, Paterson DL, Potoski BA, et al. Treatment outcome of bacteremia due to KPC-producing *Klebsiella pneumoniae*: Superiority of combination antimicrobial regimens. Antimicrob Agents Chemother 2012;56: 2108–2113.
56. Dellit TH, Owens RC, McGowan JE Jr, et al. Infectious Disease Society of America and the Society for Healthcare Epidemiology of America guidelines for developing an institutional program to enhance antimicrobial stewardship. Clin Infect Dis 2007;44:159–177.
57. Heenen S, Jacobs F, Vincent JL. Antibiotic strategies in severe nosocomial sepsis: Why do we not de-escalate more often? Crit Care Med 2012;40:1404–1409.
58. Shorr AF, Gupta V, Sun X, et al. Burden of early-onset candidemia: Analysis of culture-positive bloodstream infections from a large U.S. database. Crit Care Med 2009;37:2519–2526.
59. Grim SA, Berger K, Teng C, et al. Timing of susceptibility-based antifungal drug administration in patients with *Candida* bloodstream infection: Correlation with outcomes. J Antimicrob Chemother 2012;67:707–714.
60. Kollef M, Micek S, Hampton N, et al. Septic shock attributed to *Candida* infection: Importance of empiric therapy and source control. Clin Infect Dis 2012;54:1739–1746.
61. Azoulay E, Dupont H, Tabah A, et al. Systemic antifungal therapy in critically ill patients without invasive fungal infection. Crit Care Med 2012;40:813–822.
62. Pappas PG, Kauffman CA, Andes D, et al. Clinical practice guidelines for management of candidiasis: 2009 update by the Infectious Diseases Society of America. Clin Infect Dis 2009;48:503–535.
63. Shah DN, Yau R, Lasco TM, et al. Impact of prior inappropriate fluconazole dosing on isolation of fluconazole-nonsusceptible *Candida* species in hospitalized patients with candidemia. Antimicrob Agents Chemother 2012;56: 3239–3243.
64. Pfaller MA, Messer SA, Moet GJ, et al. Candida bloodstream infections: Comparison of species distribution and resistance to echinocandin and azole antifungal agents in Intensive Care Unit (ICU) and non-ICU settings in the SENTRY Antimicrobial Surveillance Program (2008–2009). Int J Antimicrob Agents 2011;38:65–69.
65. Pfaller MA, Castanheira M, Lockhart SR, et al. Frequency of decreased susceptibility and resistance to echinocandins among fluconazole-resistant bloodstream isolates of *Candida glabrata*. J Clin Microbiol 2012;50:1199–1203.
66. Mora-Duarte J, Betts R, Rotstein R, et al. Comparison of caspofungin and amphotericin B for invasive candidiasis. N Engl J Med 2002;347:2020–2029.
67. Pappas PG, Rotstein CMF, Betts RF, et al. Micafungin versus caspofungin for treatment of candidemia and other forms of invasive candidiasis. Clin Infect Dis 2007;45:883–893.
68. Reboli AC, Rotstein C, Pappas PG, et al. Anidulafungin versus fluconazole for invasive candidiasis. N Engl J Med 2007;356:2472–2482.
69. Schroeder S, Hochreiter M, Koehler T, et al. Procalcitonin-guided algorithm reduces length of antibiotic treatment in surgical intensive care patients with severe sepsis: Results of a prospective randomized study. Langenbecks Arch Surg 2009;394:221–226.

70. Schuetz P, Amin DN, Greenwald JL. Role of procalcitonin in managing adult patients with respiratory tract infections. Chest 2012;141:1063–1073.
71. Layios N, Lambermont B, Canivet JL, et al. Procalcitonin usefulness for the initiation of antibiotic treatment in intensive care unit patients. Crit Care Med 2012;40:2304–2309.
72. Schuetz P, Chiappa V, Briel M, et al. Procalcitonin algorithms for antibiotic therapy decisions. Arch Intern Med 2011;171:1322–1331.
73. Jensen JU, Hein L, Lundgren B, et al. Procalcitonin-guided interventions against infections to increase early appropriate antibiotics and improve survival in the intensive care unit: A randomized trial. Crit Care Med 2011;39:2048–2058.
74. Bayer O, Reinhart K, Kohl M, et al. Effects of fluid resuscitation with synthetic colloids or crystalloids alone on shock reversal, fluid balance, and patient outcomes in patients with severe sepsis: A prospective sequential analysis. Crit Care Med 2012;40:2543–2551.
75. Finfer S, Bellomo R, Boyce N, et al. A comparison of albumin and saline for fluid resuscitation in the intensive care unit. N Engl J Med 2004;350:2247–2256.
76. Durairaj L, Schmidt GA. Fluid therapy in resuscitated sepsis: Less is more. Chest 2008;133:252–263.
77. Hollenberg SM. Inotrope and vasopressor therapy of septic shock. Crit Care Nurs Clin North Am 2011;23: 127–148.
78. Backer DD, Aldecoa C, Njimi H, et al. Dopamine versus norepinephrine in the treatment of septic shock: A meta-analysis. Crit Care Med 2012;40:725–730.
79. Sakr Y, Reinhart K, Vincent JL, et al. Dose dopamine administration in shock influence outcome? Results of the sepsis occurrence in acutely ill patients (SOAP) study. Crit Care Med 2006;34:589–597.
80. Russell JA, Walley KR, Singer J, et al. Vasopressin versus norepinephrine infusion in patients with septic shock. N Engl J Med 2008;358:877–887.
81. Rivers E, Nguyen B, Havstad S, et al. Early goal–directed therapy in the treatment of severe sepsis and septic shock. N Engl J Med 2001;345:1368–1377.
82. Coba V, Whitmill M, Mooney R, et al. Resuscitation bundle compliance in severe sepsis and septic shock: Improves survival, is better late than never. J Intensive Care Med 2011;26:304–313.
83. Rivers EP, Katranji M, Jaehne KA, et al. Early interventions in severe sepsis and septic shock: A review of the evidence one decade later. Minerva Anestesiol 2012;78: 712–724.
84. Shorr AF, Micek ST, Jackson WL, et al. Economic implications of an evidence-based sepsis protocol: Can we improve outcomes and lower costs? Crit Care Med 2007;35:1257–1262.
85. The NICE-SUGAR Investigators. Intensive versus conventional glucose control in critically ill patients. N Engl J Med 2009;360:1283–1297.
86. The NICE-SUGAR Investigators. Hypoglycemia and risk of death in critically ill patients. N Engl J Med 2012;367: 1108–1118.
87. Annane D, Sebille V, Charpentier C, et al. Effects of treatment with low-dose hydrocortisone and fludrocortisone on mortality in patients with septic shock. JAMA 2002;288:862–871.
88. Annane D, Bellissant E, Bollaert PE, et al. Corticosteroids in the treatment of severe sepsis and septic shock in adults: A systematic review. JAMA 2009;301:2362–2375.
89. Sprung CL, Annane D, Keh D, et al. Hydrocortisone therapy for patients with septic shock. N Engl J Med 2008;358: 111–124.
90. Janda S, Young A, Fitzgerald JM, et al. The effect of statins on mortality from severe infections and sepsis: A systematic review and meta-analysis. J Crit Care 2010;25:656.e7–22.
91. Al Harbi SA, Tamim HA, Arabi YM. Association between statin therapy and outcomes in critically ill patients: A nested cohort study. BMC Clin Pharmacol 2011;11:12.
92. Yende S, Milbrandt EB, Kellum JA, et al. Understanding the potential role of statins in pneumonia and sepsis. Crit Care Med 2011;39:1871–1878.
93. Kruger PS, Harward ML, Jones MA, et al. Continuation of statin therapy in patients with presumed infection: A randomized controlled trial. Am J Respir Crit Care Med 2011;183:774–781.
94. Goodin J, Manrique C, Dulohery M, et al. Effect of statins on the clinical outcomes of patients with sepsis. Anaesth Intensive Care 2011;39:1051–1055.
95. Bernard GR, Vincert JL, Laterre PF, et al. Efficacy and safety of recombinant human activated protein C for severe sepsis. N Engl J Med 2001;344:699–709.
96. FDA Drug Safety Communication: Voluntary market withdrawal of Xigris (drotrecogin alfa, activated) due to failure to show a survival benefit. *http://www.fda.gov/Drugs/DrugSafety/ucm277114.htm.*

98

Superficial Fungal Infections

Thomas E. R. Brown and Linda D. Dresser

KEY CONCEPTS

1. Vulvovaginal candidiasis (VVC) is a fungal infection of the vagina that can be classified as uncomplicated or complicated. This classification is useful in determining appropriate pharmacotherapy.
2. *Candida albicans* is the major pathogen responsible for VVC. The number of cases of non–*C. albicans* species appears to be increasing.
3. Signs and symptoms of VVC are not pathognomonic, and reliable diagnosis must be made with laboratory tests including vaginal pH, saline microscopy, and 10% potassium hydroxide (KOH) microscopy.
4. *C. albicans* is the predominant species causing all forms of mucosal candidiasis. Important host and exogenous risk factors have been identified that predispose an individual to the development of mucosal candidiasis. In oropharyngeal and esophageal candidiasis, the key risk factor is impaired host immune system.
5. A topical antimycotic agent is the first choice for treating oropharyngeal candidiasis. Systemic therapy can be used in patients who are not responding to an adequate trial of topical treatment or are unable to tolerate topical agents and in those at high risk for systemic candidiasis. Fluconazole and itraconazole are the most effective azole antimycotic agents.
6. For esophageal candidiasis, topical agents are not of proven benefit; fluconazole or itraconazole solution is the first choice.
7. Optimal antiretroviral therapy is important for the prevention of recurrent and refractory candidiasis in patients with human immunodeficiency virus (HIV) infection.
8. Primary or secondary prophylaxis of fungal infection is not recommended routinely for HIV-infected patients; use of secondary prophylaxis should be individualized for each patient.
9. Topical antimycotic agents are first-line treatment for fungal skin infections. Oral therapy is preferred for the treatment of extensive or severe infection and those with tinea capitis or onychomycosis.
10. Oral antimycotic agents such as terbinafine and itraconazole are first-line treatment for toenail and fingernail onychomycosis.

Superficial mycoses are among the most common infections in the world and the second most common vaginal infections in North America. Mucocutaneous candidiasis can occur in three forms—oropharyngeal, esophageal, and vulvovaginal disease—with oropharyngeal and vulvovaginal disease being the most common. These infections were reported in humans as far back as 1839. Over the past 15 to 20 years, the occurrence rates of some fungal infections have increased dramatically. The prevalence of fungal skin infections varies throughout different parts of the world, from the most common causes of skin infections in the tropics to relatively rare disorders in the United States. This chapter reviews the pharmacotherapy of vulvovaginal candidiasis, oropharyngeal and esophageal candidiasis, and common dermatophyte infections.

VULVOVAGINAL CANDIDIASIS

1 *Vulvovaginal candidiasis* (VVC) refers to infections in individuals with or without symptoms who have positive vaginal cultures for *Candida* species. Depending on episodic frequency, VVC can be classified as either sporadic or recurrent.[1] This classification is essential to understanding the pathophysiology, as well as the pharmacotherapy, of VVC. Furthermore, VVC may be defined as uncomplicated, which refers to sporadic infections that are susceptible to all forms of antifungal therapy regardless of the duration of treatment, or complicated, in which consideration of factors affecting the host, microorganism, and pharmacotherapy all have an essential role in successful treatment.[1] Complicated VVC includes recurrent VVC, severe disease, non–*Candida albicans* candidiasis, and host factors, including diabetes mellitus, immunosuppression, and pregnancy.[1]

Epidemiology

Minimal information on the incidence and prevalence of VVC exists. Healthcare workers are not required to report cases of VVC; therefore, estimates are derived from self-reported histories. Epidemiologic data are limited because VVC usually is diagnosed without microscopy and/or cultures, and antifungal nonprescription preparations are available for self-treatment.[1] By 25 years of age, approximately 50% of college women will have had at least one episode of VVC.[1] It is rare before menarche and increases dramatically at about 20 years of age, with the peak incidence between age 30 and 40 years. It is associated with the initial act of sexual intercourse. As many as 75% of women experience one bout of symptomatic VVC in their lifetime. Between 40% and 50% of women who experience one episode of VVC experience a second episode, and 5% experience recurrent VVC.[2,3] Black women appear to be at higher risk than white women of developing VVC (62.8% vs. 55%, respectively).[4] The incidence after menopause remains unknown. However, one study of 149 healthy postmenopausal women with vulvar conditions reported significantly more women taking hormone replacement therapy (HRT) were prone to developing VVC than those who were not taking HRT (culture-positive, clinical VVC in 49% on HRT versus 1% on those not on HRT).[5]

Costs from VVC can be direct (medical visits and self-treatment) and indirect (nonmedical expenses, e.g., time losses from work, costs of travel, and time required in obtaining treatment). There are an estimated 6 million visits to healthcare providers each year, resulting in more than $1 billion spent annually on these medical visits and self-treatment.[6]

Pathophysiology

❷ *Candida albicans* is the major pathogen responsible for VVC, accounting for 80% to 92% of symptomatic episodes. The remainder are caused by non–*C. albicans* species, with *Candida glabrata* dominating.[7] The number of cases of non–*C. albicans* candidiasis appears to be increasing, possibly related to the use of nonprescription vaginal antifungal preparations and short-course therapy and/or the increased use of long-term maintenance therapy in preventing recurrent infections.[1]

Candida species can act as commensal members of the vaginal flora. Asymptomatic colonization with *Candida* species has been found in 10% to 20% of women of reproductive age.[7,8] *Candida* organisms are dimorphic; blastospores are believed to be responsible for colonization (transmission and spread), whereas germinated *Candida* forms are associated with tissue invasion and symptomatic infections.[9] To colonize the vagina, *Candida* species must be able to attach to the mucosa. The attachment process is complex. Not only are candidal surface structures important for attachment, but appropriate receptors for attachment must be present in the epithelial tissue. Not all women have the same range of receptors, which may explain variation in colonization.[8] Changes in the host's vaginal environment or response are necessary to induce a symptomatic infection. Unfortunately, in most cases of symptomatic VVC, no precipitating factor can be identified.[9]

Risk Factors

Several factors predispose a woman to VVC. VVC is not considered to be a sexually transmitted disease, although sexual factors can be important. There is a dramatic increase in the frequency of VVC when women become sexually active. In addition, oral-genital contact can increase the risk.[1] However, current guidelines do not recommend the treatment of asymptomatic partners.[7] Contraceptive agents, including the diaphragm with spermicide, the contraceptive sponge, and the intrauterine device, increase the risk of VVC. An in vitro adherence demonstrated that four different isolates of *Candida* species were capable of adhering to the contraceptive vaginal ring.[10] Oral contraceptive users demonstrated increased risk of candidiasis; however, these reports were with the higher-dose oral contraceptive pills, and the risk may not be as great with the lower-estrogen-dose oral contraceptives.[11]

Antibiotic use can increase the risk of VVC, but it is significant in only a small number of women. The mechanism by which antibiotics can increase the risk of VVC is unknown; colonization, however, is a prerequisite.[1] A small pilot study of short course antibiotic use of 3 days of antibiotics increased the prevalence of asymptomatic vaginal colonization of *Candida* and the incidence of symptomatic VVC.[12] Diet (excess refined carbohydrates), douching, and tight-fitting clothing often are listed as important risk factors; however, no association has been established between these factors and increased risk of VVC.[1]

Clinical Presentation

❸ The clinical presentation of VVC is given in Table 98-1.[1,7] These signs and symptoms are not pathognomonic, and a reliable diagnosis cannot be made without laboratory tests. Self-diagnosis has a sensitivity of 35%, a specificity of 89%, and a positive predictive value of 62%.[4] More than 50% of women who had self-diagnosed VVC did not have yeast as the causative agent.[13] This limits the value of self-diagnosis and the success of self-treatment. The American College of Obstetricians and Gynecologists (ACOG) recommends that whenever possible women requesting treatment for VVC should be examined and evaluated. They only recommend self-diagnosis in compliant women with multiple confirmed prior cases of VVC who report the same symptoms. They further recommend that if these individuals fail to improve on a short course of therapy, they be evaluated for a further diagnosis.[14] Therefore, in most instances the diagnosis should be based on both clinical presentation and investigations, including vaginal pH, saline microscopy, and 10% potassium hydroxide (KOH) microscopy. The vaginal pH remains normal in VVC, and microscopic investigations should detect blastospores or pseudohyphae. *Candida* cultures usually are not required in the diagnosis of uncomplicated VVC; however, they are recommended when an individual presents with classic signs and symptoms of VVC, has a normal vaginal pH, but microscopy is inconclusive or recurrence is suspected.[7]

TABLE 98-1 Clinical Presentation of Vulvovaginal Candidiasis

General	Often involves both the vulva and the vagina
Symptoms	Intense vulvar itching, soreness, irritation, burning on urination, and dyspareunia
Signs	Erythema, fissuring, curdy "cheese"-like discharge, satellite lesions, edema
Laboratory tests	Vaginal pH—normal, saline and 10% KOH microscopy—blastospores or pseudohyphae
Other diagnostic tests	*Candida* cultures not recommended unless classic signs and symptoms with normal vaginal pH and microscopy are inconclusive or recurrence is suspected

KOH, potassium hydroxide.

TREATMENT

Goals of Therapy

The goal of therapy is complete resolution of symptoms in patients who have symptomatic VVC. A test of the cure is not necessary if symptoms resolve.[7] Antimycotic agents used in the treatment of VVC do not meet the definition of being fungicidal agents because of their slower killing rate. At the end of therapy, the number of viable organisms drops below the detectable range. However, by 6 weeks after a course of therapy, 25% to 40% of women will have positive yeast cultures and remain asymptomatic.[1] Asymptomatic colonization with *Candida* species does not require therapy.

General Approaches to Treatment

The approach to therapy is to remove or improve any predisposing factors if they can be identified. A pharmacologic antimycotic agent should have limited local and systemic side effects, a high cure rate, and easy administration. Additionally, it would be advantageous to use a therapy that is able to resolve symptoms within 24 hours, that has broad antimycotic activity (to cover increasing rates on non–*C. albicans* species), that prevents recurrence, and that can be used over a shortened period of time, such as 1 to 3 days. Many topical azoles medications (such clotrimazole, miconazole, etc) are available without a prescription, and although this may increase public access to these medications, there is concern that having them available without a prescription may lead to inappropriate use. A study conducted using 10 actors as simulated patients who visited 60 pharmacies found that vaginal antimycotics were more likely to be supplied to appropriate individuals as more information was exchanged, if interactions involved a pharmacist, and if questions regarding specific symptoms were used.[15]

Patients should be advised to avoid harsh soaps and perfumes that can cause or worsen vulvar irritation. The genital area must be kept clean and dry by avoiding constrictive clothing and frequent or prolonged exposure to hot tub use.[3] Douching is not recommended for either prevention or treatment.[13] Cool baths can soothe the skin.[3] The oral use of lactobacillus remains unclear. A small trial of 55 women being treated for VVC showed that the addition of oral lactobacillus to single dose oral fluconazole augmented the cure rate compared to the use of fluconazole alone.[16] A trial of a mixture of oral consumption of bee-honey and yogurt showed some efficacy with mycotic cure rates of 76.9% compared to cure rates with antifungal agents of 91.5%.[17] Daily ingestion of 240 mL yogurt containing *Lactobacillus acidophilus* decreased colonization and symptomatic infections of VVC in women with recurrent infections.[18] However, a subsequent study showed that the addition of oral lactobacillus to itraconazole therapy in the treatment of recurrent VVC did not confer any additional benefit. This same trial showed that treatment using classic homeopathy was less effective than the use of itraconazole in recurrent VVC.[19]

Treatment of VVC will be considered to have positive outcomes if the symptoms of VVC are resolved within 24 to 48 hours and no adverse medication events are experienced. Self-assessment of symptom relief is appropriate for most cases of VVC. If symptoms remain unresolved or recur, then further testing and treatment can be required.

Pharmacologic Treatments

Uncomplicated Vulvovaginal Candidiasis

Cure rates for uncomplicated VVC are between 80% and 95% with topical or oral azoles and between 70% and 90% with nystatin preparations. Table 98-2 lists available topical and oral preparations for the treatment of uncomplicated VVC. There are many topical nonprescription preparations for the treatment of VVC. No significant differences in in vitro activity or clinical efficacy exist between the topical azole agents.[1,3,7,14] The selection of a topical azole antimycotic agent should be based primarily on an individual patient's preference as to product formulation. Some topical products can cause vaginal burning, stinging, or irritation; conversely, the vehicle used in topical creams or gels can provide initial symptomatic relief.[1] Of note, most topical preparations can decrease the efficacy of latex condoms and diaphragms.

Oral azoles (such as fluconazole or itraconazole) have been used in the treatment of VVC. Patients may prefer oral therapy because of its convenience.[20] Oral and topical therapies are therapeutically equivalent.[1] A Cochrane review of 19 trials analyzing 22 oral versus topical antifungal comparisons concluded that there were no differences between the routes in short-term mycologic cure rates. There was a significant difference between long-term cure rates in favor of long-term followup; however, the authors stated that the clinical significance of this finding is uncertain.[21]

In the treatment of uncomplicated VVC, the duration of therapy is not critical. Cure rates with different lengths of treatment have not demonstrated that one duration of therapy is significantly better.[20,21,22] Shorter-duration therapies (e.g., clotrimazole 1-day therapy) consist of higher concentrations of azoles that maintain the local therapeutic effect for up to 72 hours and allow for resolution of signs and symptoms.[23] A review of 14 trials that examined 1-day treatments showed less than 7% difference in short-term cure rates or improvement between any two treatments in any two studies and no significant differences in short- or long-term clinical cure rates among 1-day regimens.[22] Table 98–2 lists the therapeutic options for the treatment of uncomplicated VVC.

TABLE 98-2 Treatment for Uncomplicated Vulvovaginal Candidiasis

Active Ingredient	Preparation	Regimen
Nonprescription/Topical Vaginal Products		
Butoconazole	2% cream	One applicator × 3 days
Clotrimazole	1% cream	One applicator × 1 day
	100 mg tablet	One 100 mg tablet × 7 days
	2% cream	One applicator × 1 day
	200 mg tablet	One 200 mg tablet × 3 days
	10% cream	One applicator × 1 day
	500 mg tablet	One 500 mg tablet × 1 day
Miconazole[a]	2% cream	One applicator × 1 day
	100 mg suppository	One 100 mg suppository × 7 days
	200 mg suppository	One 200 mg suppository × 3 days
	1,200 mg ovule	One ovule × 1 day
Ticonazole	2% cream	One applicator × 3 days
	6.5% cream	One applicator × 1 day
Prescription/Topical		
Nystatin	100,000 unit tablet	One tablet × 14 days
Terconazole	0.4% cream	One applicator × 7 days
	0.8% cream	One applicator × 3 days
Oral Products		
Fluconazole	150 mg	One tablet × 1 day

[a]The FDA warns of the possible increase in the anticoagulant effects of warfarin with concomitant use.

Clinical Controversy...

Self-diagnosis of vulvovaginal candidiasis (VVC) is unreliable; however, the availability of nonprescription antifungal agents encourages self-diagnosis and self-treatment for the majority of women. Therefore, women who self-treat should be monitored to ensure that the infection clears within a few days, or they need to see a physician for an accurate diagnosis.

Complicated Vulvovaginal Candidiasis

Complicated VVC occurs in patients who are immunocompromised or have uncontrolled diabetes mellitus.[1] These individuals need a more aggressive treatment plan.[14] Current recommendations are to lengthen therapy to 10 to 14 days regardless of the route of administration.[14] Therapeutic options include those listed in Table 98-2; however, regimens should be continued for 10 to 14 days. A study of oral fluconazole therapy in women with complicated VVC demonstrated that cure rates increased from 67% with single-dose therapy to 80% when the 150 mg dose of fluconazole was repeated 72 hours after the initial dose.[24]

VVC during pregnancy can be considered complicated because consideration of host factors such as hormonal changes that can affect normal flora are essential in selecting therapeutic regimens. Topical agents are considered to be safe throughout pregnancy. A systematic review of 10 trials demonstrated that imidazole topical agents (such as fluconazole) were more effective than nystatin. Two of the trials showed that treatment for 7 days was more effective than treatments of 4 days or less.[25] Oral agents are contraindicated in pregnancy because of the concern for fetal complications. A prospective assessment of pregnancy outcomes in 226 women exposed to fluconazole in the first trimester did not indicate increased risk of congenital abnormalities or other adverse outcomes.[26] The median dose of fluconazole was 200 mg, with 46.5% of the cohort receiving a single dose of fluconazole 150 mg.[27] However, the ACOG recommends avoiding oral therapy, as larger doses of fluconazole have been linked to birth defects.[27] Instead, the ACOG recommends a topical imidazole therapy for 7 days.[14]

Recurrent Vulvovaginal Candidiasis

Recurrent vulvovaginal candidiasis (RVVC) is defined as having more than four episodes of VVC within a 12-month period.[1,7] Fewer than 5% of women develop RVVC, and its pathogenesis is poorly understood. A proper diagnosis should be obtained to rule out other infections or nonmycotic contact dermatitis. RVVC is best treated in two stages: an initial intensive stage followed by prolonged antifungal therapy to achieve mycologic remission. This was demonstrated in a randomized controlled trial in which women were assigned to receive 150 mg fluconazole daily for 10 days followed by 6 months of either fluconazole 150 mg weekly or placebo. Ninety percent of women receiving both active treatments were symptom free for the 6 months following initial treatment (during the weekly fluconazole therapy), and there were 50% fewer symptomatic episodes in the 6 months following weekly suppressive therapy.[28] The Infectious Diseases Society of America stated that there is good evidence from more than one properly randomized controlled trial to recommend 10 to 14 days of induction therapy with a topical or oral azole, followed by 150 mg of fluconazole once weekly for 6 months for recurring *Candida* VVC.[29]

Antifungal-Resistant Vulvovaginal Candidiasis

Resistance to azole antimycotics should be considered in individuals who have persistently positive yeast cultures and fail to respond to therapy despite adherence to prescribed regimens.[1] These infections can be treated with boric acid or 5-flucytosine.[30,31] Boric acid is administered as a 600 mg intravaginal capsule daily for 14 days of induction therapy, followed by a maintenance regimen of one capsule intravaginally twice weekly. Boric acid should not be administered orally, as it is toxic. 5-Flucytosine cream is administered vaginally, 1,000 mg inserted nightly for 7 days. The prevalence of *C. glabrata* is higher in those with diabetes. In a study of 111 consecutive diabetic patients with VVC, 68% had isolates for *C. glabrata* compared with 28.8% for *C. albicans.* Those with *C. glabrata* had significantly higher mycological cure rates with 600 mg of boric acid suppositories for 14 days compared with a single dose of fluconazole 150 mg.[32]

OROPHARYNGEAL AND ESOPHAGEAL CANDIDIASIS

Oropharyngeal candidiasis (OPC), or *thrush,* is a common and localized infection of the oral mucosa caused by the yeast *Candida. Candida albicans,* a common oral commensal organism, is the most frequent infecting species. OPC is also referred to as *candidiasis* (or the more correct but less commonly used term *candidosis*). The infection may extend into the esophagus, causing esophageal candidiasis.

Microbiology and Epidemiology

Candida is a commensal fungus found in the oral cavity in up to 65% of healthy individuals with higher prevalence in healthy children and young adults.[33,34] *Candida* carriage increases under immunocompromised conditions and also among hospitalized patients.[34] Even in the era of highly active antiretroviral therapy (HAART) up to 80% of human immunodeficiency virus (HIV)-infected persons may demonstrate oral yeast colonization.[35] The organism is capable of transition to a pathogen causing symptomatic mucosal infections in association with predisposing host factors.[34] *Candida albicans* is the predominant colonizing *Candida* species (70% to 80%), but any of the non–*C. albicans* species can be colonizers. Colonization rates are influenced by the severity and nature of the underlying medical illness and the duration of hospitalization, as well as age (highest in infants younger than 18 months of age and in adults older than 60 years of age). A variety of host and exogenous factors (Table 98-3) can lead to the transformation of asymptomatic colonization to symptomatic disease, such as oropharyngeal and esophageal candidiasis. *C. albicans* is the most common species causing all forms of mucosal candidiasis in humans. Less frequently, non–*C. albicans* species can be pathogenic and cause disease. These include *C. glabrata, Candida tropicalis, Candida krusei,* and *Candida parapsilosis.*[35,36] *Candida krusei,* although relatively uncommon, generally is recovered from mucosal surfaces of neutropenic patients with hematologic malignancies.[36] Another species, *Candida dubliniensis,* has been identified in both HIV-infected and noninfected patients, and may cause ~15% of infections previously ascribed to *C. albicans.*[36] In patients with cancer, non–*C. albicans* species account for almost half of all *Candida* infections.

Oropharyngeal candidiasis is the most common opportunistic infection in patients with HIV disease, and it may be the first clinical manifestation of the HIV infection in the majority of untreated patients. OPC occurs in 50% to 90% of HIV-infected patients at some point during the progressive course of the disease to acquired immunodeficiency syndrome (AIDS),[33,35,36] although significant reductions in the incidence have been observed after the introduction of highly active antiretroviral therapy. The absolute CD4 T-cell count has been suggested to be the primary risk factor for development of OPC with the greatest risk at CD4 T-cell levels <200 cells/mm^3 (<0.2 × 10^9/L). Also, the HIV viral load has been identified as a predictor of OPC development; OPC is thought to increase with HIV viral loads >10,000 copies/mL (>10 × 10^6/L). This finding correlates with the observation that initiation of antiretroviral therapy and subsequent increase in CD4 T-cell counts does not fully account for the decrease in OPC incidence.[35] Regardless of the CD4 T-cell count, or HIV viral load OPC is predictive for the development of AIDS-related illnesses if left untreated.[33,36]

In non-HIV diseases, such as cancer, the incidence of OPC varies depending on the type of malignant neoplastic disease, level of immune suppression, and type and duration of treatment, but it is less common than in HIV-infected patients. OPC was initially reported in ~25% of patients with solid tumors and up to 60% in those with hematologic malignancies or bone marrow transplant recipients.[37] Current rates of OPC have decreased significantly in these patients because of widespread use of antifungal prophylaxis. Incidence in other patient populations predisposed to OPC such as the hospitalized patient administered broad-spectrum antibiotics or denture and other oral appliance users is not well quantified, however, do represent at-risk individuals where the clinical pharmacist has an important patient-care role.[34,37]

OPC can predispose patients to develop more invasive disease, including esophageal candidiasis.[37] The esophagus is the second most common site of GI candidiasis. The prevalence of esophageal candidiasis has increased mainly because of the number of individuals with AIDS, as well as the increased numbers of other severely immunocompromised patients, especially those with hematologic malignancies.[36] Esophageal candidiasis is the first opportunistic infection in 3% to 10% of HIV-infected patients and is the second most common AIDS-defining disease after *Pneumocystis jiroveci* pneumonia.[36] The mean incidence of esophageal candidiasis among HIV-infected patients is less than OPC and ranges from 15% to 20%.[36] The risk of esophageal candidiasis is increased in HIV-infected patients when the CD4 T-cell count has dropped below 100 to 200 cells/mm^3 (0.1 × 10^9 to 0.2 × 10^9/L), as well as in those with

TABLE 98-3 Risk Factors for the Development of Oropharyngeal and/or Esophageal Candidiasis

Local Factors	Potential Mechanisms
Use of steroids and antibiotics	Suppression of cellular immunity and inhibition of phagocytosis by steroids, including chronic use of inhaled and topical steroids
	Alteration of endogenous oral flora by broad-spectrum antibiotics, especially when used with steroids, creates a milieu for proliferation of *Candida* species because of reduced environmental and nutritional competition
Dentures	Enhanced adherence of *Candida* species to the acrylic material of dentures, reduced saliva flow under surfaces of denture fittings, improperly fitted dentures, and poor oral hygiene provide a milieu conducive to the survival of microorganisms
Xerostomia caused by drugs (e.g., tricyclic antidepressants and phenothiazine), chemotherapy, radiotherapy to the head/neck, and various diseases (e.g., Sjögren's syndrome, HIV, and cancer of the head/neck), as well as bone marrow transplant recipients	Reduced dilutional and cleansing effect caused by low secretion rate and low pH in saliva: Saliva and mucosa secretions have defense factors, such as lactoferrin, sialoperoxidase, isozyme, histidine-rich polypeptide, secretory IgA antibodies, specific anti-*Candida* antibodies that help prevent adhesion and overgrowth of *Candida* species
Smoking	
Disruption of oral mucosa caused by chemotherapy and radiotherapy, ulcers, endotracheal intubation trauma, and burns	Oral mucositis induced by radiation and breaks in the physical barrier of the oral epithelium, which is protective against invasion by microorganisms; altered rate of mucosa regeneration by cancer chemotherapy, which increases vulnerability to infection
Systemic Factors	**Potential Mechanisms**
Drugs (e.g., cytotoxic agents, corticosteroids, and immunosuppressants after organ transplant), omeprazole, and environmental chemicals (e.g., benzene and pesticides)	Reduced immunity because of drug-induced neutropenia or cell-mediated immunity; potent inhibition of gastric acid by PPIs can facilitate the growth of *Candida* species; PPIs also can inhibit the cytotoxic effect of lymphocytes and reduce salivary secretion
Neonates or the elderly	Immature immune system of neonates who usually acquire infection during birth to a mother with vaginal candidiasis or from exposure to infected bottle nipples or to skin of adult caregiver
	Elderly—unclear if this is the direct effect of age per se or contribution from dentures or underlying comorbidity
HIV infection/AIDS	Depletion of CD4 T lymphocytes especially below 200–300 cells/mm^3 ($0.2 \times 10^9 - 0.3 \times 10^9$/L); anti-*Candida* protective mechanism of T lymphocytes at a mucosal level is unclear but can be caused by altered cytokines, especially interferon-γ, that inhibit transformation of *Candida* blastoconidia to the more invasive hyphal phase
Diabetes	Higher than normal numbers of *Candida albicans* cultured from saliva of diabetic patients; can be related to the elevated glucose levels and reduced chemotactic factor in saliva, altered neutrophil function, and reduced saliva volume and flow
Malignancies (e.g., leukemia and head/neck cancer)	Use of intensive radiotherapy and chemotherapy can disrupt oral mucosa and cause xerostomia; prolonged use of broad-spectrum antibiotics in neutropenic patients can alter the normal oral flora; because of the prolonged neutropenia, the principal immune defect, seen especially in leukemic patients, the initial oropharyngeal candidiasis can become systemic or invasive
Nutritional deficiencies (e.g., iron, folate, and vitamins B1, B2, B6, B12, and C)	Can be related to dietary restriction or GI absorption problems; deficiencies can serve to enhance the pathogenic potential of the *Candida* inhabitants, alter host defense mechanisms, or change epithelial barrier integrity

AIDS, acquired immunodeficiency syndrome; GI, gastrointestinal; HIV, human immunodeficiency virus; IgA, immunoglobulin A; PPI, proton pump inhibitor.

OPC.[37,38] However, the absence of OPC does not necessarily exclude the possibility of esophageal disease. Like OPC, the presence of esophageal candidiasis can help predict HIV disease progression and prognosis.[37] The incidence of esophageal candidiasis in non-HIV-infected immunocompromised patients is not well established. *Candida albicans* is the most common cause of esophageal candidiasis, accounting for ~80% of cases, with the rest being caused by non–*C. albicans* species.[35]

The introduction of HAART appears to have resulted in a significant decline in the incidence of OPC and esophageal candidiasis.[35,36] In addition, the widespread use of the azole agents for treatment and prophylaxis has led to a decline in the prevalence of mucosal candidiasis while leading to the emergence of refractory infections that are more challenging to treat.

Pathogenesis and Host Defenses

The pathogenesis of OPC is most clearly elucidated in the setting of HIV infection. There appear to be several levels of immune defense against the development of OPC in HIV-infected persons, and they involve both systemic and local immunity. The primary line of host defense against *C. albicans* is cell-mediated immunity (CMI) at the mucosal surfaces, which is mediated by CD4 T cells.[33] The efficacy of the CD4 T cells is reduced when the number of cells drops below a protective threshold, and protection against infection becomes dependent on secondary or local immune mechanisms.[33,35] When the number of CD4 T cells drops too low, recruitment of these cells to the oral cavity is impaired. The CD4 T-cell count has been considered as the hallmark predictor for development of OPC. However, HIV viral load may have a stronger association with OPC than CD4 cell number.[35,39] The possibility that HIV plays a strong role in susceptibility to infection is supported clinically by the observation that OPC is more common in HIV-infected persons than in those with similar immunosuppression, such as lymphoma and bone marrow transplant. When the primary line of defense fails, the secondary host defenses become crucial. These include the CD8 T cells, salivary cytokines, and other innate immune cells, such as the neutrophils, macrophages, and epithelial cells (with anti-*Candida* activity). Deficiencies or dysfunction in any of these can result in increased susceptibility to OPC. The problem with the CD8 T cells is caused more by a dysfunction of the microenvironment, specifically, reduction in the E-cadherin adhesion molecule that promotes migration of the cells through mucosal tissues.[36] The role of humoral immunity by antibodies as a protective mechanism is

TABLE 98-4 Clinical Classification of Oropharyngeal Candidiasis

Types	Population at Risk	Clinical Signs and Appearance
Pseudomembranous (thrush)	Neonates, patients with HIV or cancer, the debilitated elderly, patients on broad-spectrum antibiotics or steroid inhalers, patients with dry mouth from various causes, and smokers	Classic "cottage cheese" appearance, yellowish white, soft plaques (or milk curds) overlying areas of erythema on the buccal mucosa, tongue, gums, and throat; plaques are easily removed by vigorous rubbing but can leave red or bleeding sites when removed; lesions on the tongue dorsum give it a bald, depapillated appearance
Erythematous (acute atrophic)	Patients with HIV, patients on broad-spectrum antibiotics or steroid inhalers	Sensitive and painful erythematous mucosa with few, if any, white plaques; lesions are generally on the dorsal surface of the tongue or the hard palate, occasionally on the soft palate, but any part of the mucosa can be involved; appear as flat red patches on the palate or atrophic patches on the tongue dorsum with loss of papillae
Hyperplastic (candidal leukoplakia)	Smokers; uncommon in patients with HIV	Thick white and adherent keratotic plaques commonly seen on the buccal mucosa and lateral border of the tongue; can also be seen on the lips and the bottom of the mouth; plaques cannot be easily scraped off or only partially removed; this condition is distinct from oral hairy leukoplakia, and it can progress to severe dysplasia or malignancy
Angular cheilitis	Patients with HIV, denture wearers	Painful red, ulcerative, cracking, or fissuring lesion at one or both comers of the mouth because of an inflammatory reaction; usually lesions are small and rather punctate, but occasionally they can extend in a linear fashion from the angles onto the facial skin
Denture stomatitis (chronic atrophic)	Denture wearers who tend to be elderly and have poor oral hygiene	Red, flat lesions on the mucosa beneath the denture and extend right up to the denture border; more commonly located beneath a maxillary denture, although they can be encountered beneath a mandibular denture

HIV, human immunodeficiency virus.

unclear and controversial. The changeover of the role of *Candida* species from commensal to pathogenic in the human host usually occurs when breakdown in these host defenses occurs. The pathogenesis of OPC is still not completely understood. It is important to develop a better understanding of the pathogenesis and role of host defenses, including the mechanism of CD8 T-cell activity, reduced adhesion molecules, and whether other cofactors, such as HIV viral load, HAART, and injection drug use, play a role. Immunotherapeutic modalities can then be developed to eliminate the susceptibility factors and significantly reduce OPC in the at-risk populations.

Significant differences exist in the virulence among *Candida* species in mucosal candidiasis. One virulence factor is the ability of the organism to adapt and survive in response to changes in the host environment.[35] The genes required for virulence are regulated in response to the environmental signals indigenous to the host environment (e.g., temperature, pH, osmotic pressure, iron and calcium ion concentrations, oxygenation, and carbon and nitrogen availability). The ability of *C. albicans* to undergo reversible morphologic transition between the budding pseudohyphal and the more invasive hyphal growth forms is also a determinant of virulence, and genes are recognized to play a role.[33] Other virulence factors are the adhesive ability of *C. albicans* to epithelial cells and proteins and its ability to invade host cells by means of phospholipase and proteinase enzymes. This may be one of the factors leading to OPC in non–HIV-infected individuals. Other components of the pathogenesis in the absence of HIV that have been postulated are the ability of the *Candida* species to adhere to buccal epithelial cells. A close correlation between adhesion of *Candida* species and their ability to cause infection has been demonstrated in animal model studies.[40] This is hypothesized to be a key element in the development of OPC in patients with altered microflora, including those receiving broad-spectrum antimicrobial therapy.

Risk Factors

4 Several host and exogenous factors contribute to the ability of *Candida* species to cause infection (see Table 98-3). Local and systemic factors, as well as characteristics of the organism itself, can increase the susceptibility of an individual to *Candida* infections.[33] Endocrine disorders besides diabetes mellitus, such as hypothyroidism, hypoparathyroidism, and hypoadrenalism, also can predispose patients to *Candida* species overgrowth. Patients with primary immune deficiencies such as lymphocytic abnormalities, phagocytic dysfunction, immunoglobulin A (IgA) deficiency, viral-induced immune paralysis, and severe congenital immunodeficiencies are also at risk for oropharyngeal candidiasis as well as disseminated candidiasis. Oral mucosal disease, such as lichen planus, can be preexistent causes of candidiasis. Smoking has been suggested as a predisposing risk factor. In many cases, multiple concurrent predisposing factors to candidiasis can exist, for example, xerostomia with mucositis and a break in the epithelial surface or immunosuppression, such as might occur in a leukemic patient receiving radiation and chemotherapy. The severity and extent of *Candida* infections increase with the number and severity of predisposing risk factors.[34]

Clinical Presentation and Diagnosis

Oropharyngeal candidiasis can manifest in several major forms (Table 98-4).[33,34] The clinical signs and symptoms of OPC and the locations of the lesions can be quite diverse (Table 98-5). A presumptive diagnosis of OPC usually is made by the characteristic appearance on the oral mucosa, with resolution of signs and symptoms after antifungal therapy. Pseudomembranous candidiasis, commonly known as *oral thrush,* is the classic and most common form seen in immunosuppressed and immunocompetent hosts. Erythematous and hyperplastic candidiasis and angular cheilitis occur less commonly in the HIV-infected population. Dysphagia, odynophagia, and retrosternal chest pain are common complaints of esophageal candidiasis, which is usually, but not always, accompanied by the presence of OPC. Clinical symptomatology, along with a therapeutic trial of antifungal, can provide a reliable presumptive diagnosis of esophageal candidiasis. If antifungal therapy does not lead to resolution, more invasive tests such as upper GI endoscopy can be undertaken.

TABLE 98-5 Clinical Presentation of Oropharyngeal and Esophageal Candidiasis

Oropharyngeal Candidiasis	Esophageal Candidiasis
General The clinical features can be quite diverse (see Table 98-4)	**General** This usually occurs as an extension of OPC; however, the esophagus can be the only site involved; the distal two-thirds, rather than the proximal one-third, is the most common site
Symptoms Symptoms are diverse and range from none to sore, painful mouth, burning tongue, metallic taste, and dysphagia and odynophagia with involvement of the hypopharynx	**Symptoms** Typically, the symptoms are dysphagia, odynophagia, and retrosternal chest pain but can be asymptomatic in some patients; although rare, epigastric pain can be the dominant symptom
Signs Signs are variable and can include diffuse erythema and white patches on the surfaces of the buccal mucosa, throat, tongue, or gums; constitutional signs are absent	**Signs** Constitutional signs, including fever, occasionally occur; physical findings can range from a few to numerous white or beige plaques of variable size Plaques can be hyperemic or edematous, with ulceration in more severe cases Most advanced cases can occur with increased mucosal friability and narrowing of lumen Uncommon complications include perforation and aortic–esophageal fistula formation
Laboratory tests Scraping of an active lesion for microscopic examination can help confirm the diagnosis (presence of pseudohyphae and budding yeast) but is usually not necessary Cultures are not necessary because isolation of *Candida* species does not distinguish between colonization and true infection; cultures can be taken in patients responding poorly to therapy to determine the infecting species and to predict likely drug resistance	**Laboratory tests** The best test is upper GI endoscopy (more useful than barium swallow); helps exclude other causes of esophagitis (e.g., viral, aphthous ulcers); diagnosis is confirmed by the histologic presence of *Candida* species in biopsy lesions taken during endoscopy Cultures to look for drug-resistant *Candida* species are warranted in patients who require endoscopy

GI, gastrointestinal; OPC, oropharyngeal candidiasis.

TREATMENT

Desired Outcomes

The primary desired outcome in the management of OPC is a clinical cure, that is, elimination of clinical signs and symptoms. Even when the patient is relatively asymptomatic, it is important to treat the initial episode of OPC to avoid progression to more extensive disease. In the most severe cases, the patient's quality of life can be impaired; this can result in decreased fluid and nutritional intake. Lack of appropriate treatment of OPC can lead to more extensive oral disease, especially in patients who are immunocompromised. The most serious complication of untreated OPC is extension of the infection to esophageal candidiasis. Because esophageal candidiasis is more debilitating, the patient's quality of life is more affected. It is important to initiate appropriate antifungal therapy for both OPC and esophageal candidiasis. Preventing or minimizing the number of future recurrences of both types of candidiasis is an equally important outcome. The approach depends largely on the underlying predisposing conditions. Mycologic cure is not a necessary treatment outcome because it may not be feasible or realistic, given that *Candida* species exist commonly as part of the normal mouth flora.

Minimizing toxicities and drug–drug interactions of systemic antifungal agents, as well as maximizing adherence by ensuring that the patient understands the importance of therapy and the directions to take the medication appropriately, are important secondary outcomes of therapy.

General Approach to Treatment

The management of OPC should be individualized for each patient, taking into consideration the underlying immune status, other concurrent mucosal and medical diseases, concomitant medications, and exogenous infectious sources. In HIV-infected patients with inadequately controlled disease, antifungal treatment produces only a transient clinical response, and the relapse rates are higher than in other patient populations. These patients usually require frequent courses of antifungal treatment. Therefore, in patients with HIV disease, treatment with effective HAART is paramount because this would provide the best prophylaxis against recolonization and recurrence of symptoms.[34,35,41]

Whenever feasible, it is desirable to minimize all predisposing factors, such as administration of corticosteroids, chemotherapeutic agents, and antimicrobials, as well as institute proper oral hygiene and resolve concurrent conditions, such as denture stomatitis. Selection of an appropriate antifungal agent for treatment of candidiasis requires consideration of several factors, including the patient's drug adherence, adequate saliva for dissolution of solid topical medications, risk of caries from sucrose- or dextrose-containing preparations, potential drug interactions, coexisting medical conditions (e.g., liver disease), location and severity of the infection, and the need for long-term maintenance therapy. Another factor that could affect drug selection is overuse of fluconazole, leading to the emergence of fluconazole-resistant species of *C. albicans*, and in some cases to all azoles, and other intrinsically more resistant species, such as *C. krusei*, *C. glabrata*, and *C. tropicalis*.

❺ Topical antimycotic therapies should be the first choice for milder forms of infections.[41] The efficacy of antimycotic agents for OPC varies in different patient populations. Until the polyene antimycotic agents became available in the 1950s, gentian violet, an aniline dye, was used to treat OPC. Problems with gentian violet include fungal resistance, skin irritation, and especially the unaesthetic staining of the oral mucosa. In resource limited areas gentian violet remains a therapeutic option. A study of different concentrations of gentian violet demonstrated that a 0.00165% solution does not stain the oral mucosa and has potent antifungal activity.[42] Topical agents, such as nystatin and clotrimazole, have been the standard of treatment for uncomplicated OPC and generally are effective for treatment in otherwise healthy adults and infants with no underlying immunodeficiencies. Topical agents are available in an assortment of formulations, including oral rinses (suspension), troches, powder, vaginal tablets, creams and most recently as a mucoadhesive tablet[37,41,43] (Table 98-6).

Topical agents require frequent applications because of the short contact time with the oral mucosa; the ideal contact time is 20 to 30 minutes. Sufficient saliva is needed to dissolve clotrimazole troches, and this can be problematic for patients with xerostomia. Also, the rough surface of the tablet can become irritating to the oral soft tissue. Troches also contain dextrose, which has cariogenic potential. Nystatin suspension might be a better choice for patients with xerostomia, but it is difficult to maintain adequate contact time with the oral mucosa. Some patients complain of the unpleasant taste of nystatin, which can cause nausea and vomiting; this is especially

TABLE 98-6 Therapeutic Options for Mucosal Candidiasis

Initial Episodes of OPC:[a] Treat for 7–14 Days	Common/Significant Side Effects
Clotrimazole 10 mg troche: hold 1 troche in mouth for 15–20 minutes for slow dissolution 5 times daily (B-2)	Altered taste, mild nausea, vomiting
Nystatin 100,000 units/mL suspension: 5 mL swish and swallow 4 times daily (B-2)	Mild nausea, vomiting, diarrhea
Miconazole 50 mg mucoadhesive buccal tablets 50 mg daily (A-1)	Diarrhea, headache, nausea, dysgeusia, upper abdominal pain, and vomiting
Fluconazole 100 mg tablets:[b] 100–200 mg daily (A-1)	GI upset, hepatitis not common
Itraconazole 10 mg/mL solution:[c] 200 mg daily (A-2)	GI upset, not common: hepatotoxicity, CHF, pulmonary edema with long-term use[e]
Posaconazole 40 mg/mL suspension: 400 mg daily with a full meal (A-2)	GI upset, fever, headache, increased hepatic transaminases not common
Fluconazole-Refractory OPC: Treat for ≥14 Days	
Itraconazole 10 mg/mL solution: 200 mg daily (A-3)	See above
Voriconazole 200 mg tablets: 200 mg twice daily (>40 kg), taken on empty stomach (A-3)	GI upset, rash, reversible visual disturbance (altered light perception, photopsia, chromatopsia, photophobia), increased hepatic transaminases, hallucinations, or confusion
Posaconazole 40 mg/mL suspension: 400 mg twice daily × 3 days, then 400 mg daily × 28 days (A-2)	See above
Amphotericin B 100 mg/mL suspension:[d] 1–5 mL swish and swallow 4 times daily (B-2)	Oral: nausea, vomiting, diarrhea with higher dose
Amphotericin B deoxycholate 50 mg injection: 0.3–0.7 mg/kg/day IV daily (B-2)	IV: fever, chills, sweats, nephrotoxicity, electrolyte disturbances, bone marrow suppression
Caspofungin 50 mg IV daily (B-2)	Fever, headache, infusion-related reactions (<5%) (e.g., rash, facial swelling, pruritus, vasodilation), hypokalemia, increased hepatic transaminases, anemia, neutropenia
Micafungin 150 mg IV daily (B-2)	Similar to caspofungin
Anidulafungin 200 mg IV daily (B-2)	Similar to caspofungin
Esophageal Candidiasis:[a] Treat for 14–21 Days	
Fluconazole 100 mg tablets: 200–400 mg (3–6 mg/kg) daily (A-1)	See above
Echinocandin: see above (B-2)	See above
Amphotericin B deoxycholate 50 mg injection: 0.3–0.7 mg/kg/day IV daily (B-2)	See above
Posaconazole 40 mg/mL suspension: 400 mg twice daily (A-3)	See above
Itraconazole 10 mg/mL solution:[c] 200 mg daily (A-3)	See above
Voriconazole 200 mg tablets: 200 mg twice daily (>40 kg) (A-3)	See above
Voriconazole and echinocandins (A-1): generally reserved for refractory cases	See above
Fluconazole-Refractory EC: Treat for 21–28 Days	
Itraconazole 10 mg/mL solution: 200 mg daily (A-2)	See above
Posaconazole 40 mg/mL suspension: 400 mg twice daily (A-3)	See above
Voriconazole 200 mg tablets: 200 mg twice daily (>40 kg), taken on empty stomach (A-3)	See above
Caspofungin 50 mg IV daily (B-2)	See above
Micafungin 150 mg IV daily (B-2)	Similar to caspofungin
Anidulafungin 100 mg IV on day 1, then 50 mg IV daily (B-2)	Similar to caspofungin
Amphotericin B deoxycholate: 0.3–0.7 mg/kg/day IV, or lipid-based amphotericin 3–5 mg/kg/day IV (B-2)	See above

CHF, congestive heart failure; GI, gastrointestinal; OPC, oropharyngeal candidiasis.

[a]Initial episodes of OPC can be adequately treated first with topical agents before resorting to systemic therapy (B-2), but systemic therapy is required for effective treatment of esophageal candidiasis. (A-2) Suppressive therapy is recommended for patients with frequent or severe recurrences (A-1).
[b]Fluconazole is more effective than ketoconazole (A-1).
[c]Solution is more effective than capsule (A-1); solution is better taken on an empty stomach.
[d]Suspension is not marketed; can be prepared extemporaneously by pharmacy.[50]
[e]See discussion under onychomycosis.

Recommendation grades:

Strength of recommendation: **A**—Both strong evidence for efficacy and substantial clinical benefit to support recommendation for use. *Should always be offered.* **B**—Moderate evidence for efficacy but only limited clinical benefit, to support recommendation for use. *Should generally be* offered. **C**—Evidence for efficacy is insufficient to support recommendation for or against use; or evidence for efficacy might not outweigh adverse consequences or cost of the treatment under consideration. *Optional.* **D**—Moderate evidence for lack of efficacy or adverse outcome supports a recommendation against use. *Should generally not be offered.*

Quality of evidence: **1**—Evidence from at least one properly designed randomized, controlled trial. **2**—Evidence from at least one well-designed trial without randomization, from cohort or case-controlled analytic studies (preferably from more than one center), or from multiple time-series studies, or dramatic results from uncontrolled experiments. **3**—Evidence from opinions of respected authorities based on clinical experience, descriptive studies, or reports of expert committees. (UR) Evidence currently unrated.

problematic in cancer patients experiencing chemotherapy-induced nausea. The high sucrose content of nystatin suspension is cariogenic in dentate patients, and it should be used with caution in diabetic patients.[34,37] Miconazole 50 mg mucoadhesive tablets are the first buccal adherent miconazole product approved for the local treatment of OPC in adults and adolescents older than age 16 years.[44] This product offers the advantage of a once-daily formulation that is tasteless, odorless, and sugar free.[43] Topical creams, such as clotrimazole, ketoconazole, miconazole, and nystatin (usually mixed with a steroid), are more appropriate for application three times daily to the corners of the mouth in treating angular cheilitis, the inflammation, drying, and cracking of the corners of the mouth.[41]

Systemic therapy is necessary in patients with OPC that is refractory to topical treatment, those who cannot tolerate topical agents, moderate-to-severe disease, and those at high risk for disseminated systemic or invasive candidiasis. Effective treatment of esophageal candidiasis generally requires the use of systemic antifungal agents. However, these agents have the disadvantage of producing more side effects (see Table 98-6) and drug–drug interactions (see Chap. 99). Fluconazole is inexpensive and generally well tolerated, and its absorption is unaffected by food or gastric acidity. Ketoconazole requires gastric acidity for absorption, which can be problematic in AIDS patients with achlorhydria; hence, it is best given with an acidic beverage. Ketoconazole is not recommended today with the availability of more effective triazoles. Itraconazole capsules also have the same absorption problem and are no longer recommended. In contrast, itraconazole solution has enhanced absorption and is best taken in a fasting state; in addition, the solution provides the benefit of both topical effects to the oral mucosa and systemic effects and is beneficial to patients with mucositis or swallowing problems. Whenever possible, it is generally beneficial to limit the use of systemic azole agents to prevent unnecessary drug exposure and to minimize the potential for occurrence of drug-resistant candidiasis, particularly from fluconazole resistance.

When patients become unresponsive to topical agents or fluconazole and itraconazole, alternative agents are available.[37,38,41,45,46] These include amphotericin B and newer triazoles (voriconazole and posaconazole) and echinocandins (caspofungin, micafungin, and anidulafungin) (see discussion below).

Clinical **Controversy...**

The optimal strategy for the management of recurrent oral mucosal candidiasis is unclear. Specific criteria for use of secondary prophylaxis are not well defined, and a wide range of approaches can be seen in clinical practice.

Oropharyngeal Candidiasis: Human Immuodeficiency Virus–Infected Patients

It is appropriate to start therapy with topical agents for initial or recurrent episodes of OPC, provided that clinical symptoms are not severe and that there is minimal risk of esophageal involvement.[36,41] Clinical responses with the resolution of signs and symptoms generally occur within 5 to 7 days of initiating treatment. Clotrimazole appears to be the most effective topical agent and demonstrates comparable clinical response rates with both fluconazole and itraconazole.[36,41] However, topical therapy is associated with more frequent relapses than with fluconazole.[38,41] This may be of limited clinical significance in patients receiving effective HAART because of their decreased susceptibility to opportunistic infection. In practice, nystatin suspension is still used frequently in initial episodes of OPC, although it is the least effective agent and is associated with frequent treatment failures and early relapses, especially in patients with advanced HIV disease or neutropenia.[34,37] The safety and efficacy of miconazole mucoadhesive tablets (MMT) for the treatment of OPC in HIV infected patients were studied in a randomized, double-blind, multicenter trial. Clotrimazole troches 10 mg five times daily was the comparator arm in this noninferiority study. The authors concluded that the clinical cure rate of MMT 50 mg once daily was noninferior to clotrimazole treated patients in both the intention to treat (61% vs. 65% respectively) and per protocol (68% vs. 74% respectively) populations at the test of cure visit. Safety and tolerability was also similar between treatment groups.[44]

Systemic oral azoles should be reserved for use in the more severe episodes of OPC unresponsive to topical agents or in patients with concurrent esophageal involvement.[37,41] In clinical practice, fluconazole usually is the systemic azole agent of choice because of its proven efficacy, favorable absorption, safety, and drug-interaction profiles, and it is relatively inexpensive. Fluconazole is superior to ketoconazole and itraconazole capsules.[37,41] Current guidelines suggest a fluconazole regimen of 100 to 200 mg/day for 7 to 14 days.[41] There is evidence from one study showing a single dose of fluconazole 750 mg orally is as effective as fluconazole 150 mg orally for 14 days, which warrants further evaluation, given the potential advantages of adherence and cost-effectiveness.[45] Itraconazole oral solution with an improved absorption profile compared with the capsule formulation is as effective as fluconazole, with comparable clinical and mycologic response and relapse rates.[37,41] However, it carries a higher risk of drug interactions because it is a potent inhibitor of the cytochrome P450 enzymes, and it is associated with more nausea than fluconazole. Posaconazole is an extended-spectrum triazole with potent in vitro activity against both *C. albicans* and non–*C. albicans* species. It is equivalent to fluconazole in terms of efficacy, safety, and tolerability.[46] Posaconazole has joined itraconazole solution and voriconazole as the azole alternatives to fluconazole in the management of moderate-to-severe OPC.[40] Other agents that are effective are amphotericin B and the echinocandins (caspofungin, micafungin, and anidulafungin). They are better reserved for refractory OPC, however, because of their greater toxicity. They are also more expensive and are less convenient to use.

Oropharyngeal Candidiasis: Non-Human Immunodeficiency Virus–Infected Patients

This patient population includes patients with hematologic malignancy (e.g., leukemias) or blood and bone marrow transplantation (BMT) with a long duration of neutropenia and chronic graft-versus-host disease, patients with solid tumors, patients with solid-organ transplants who are receiving immunosuppressive therapy, and patients with diabetes mellitus, as well as patients on prolonged courses of antibiotics or corticosteroids and the debilitated elderly. Factors to consider in deciding whether to use topical or systemic antifungal therapy include the severity and extent of mucosal involvement (oropharyngeal vs. esophageal), predisposing risk factors, and risk for dissemination. Patients who develop neutropenia (e.g., leukemic and BMT patients) are usually at high risk for disseminated and invasive fungal disease, and treatment of oral candidiasis is more aggressive. Patients with cell-mediated immune deficits but normal or near-normal granulocyte function and number (e.g., solid tumors, solid-organ transplants, or diabetic patients) are at low risk for dissemination of infection.

Specific antifungal therapy can be unnecessary for asymptomatic patients at relatively low risk for disseminated candidiasis, such as those who are not granulocytopenic or who are expected to have a short duration of granulocytopenia.[41] Many of these infections will clear spontaneously after recovery of the granulocytes or discontinuation of antibiotic and/or immunosuppressive therapy. However, antifungal therapy usually is required for patients who have persistent infection or significant symptoms, usually pain, or who are granulocytopenic with a relatively high risk of fungal dissemination. Topical agents first can be given a therapeutic trial depending on the severity of infection and the degree of immunosuppression. Although both nystatin and clotrimazole can be effective in treating OPC, nystatin suspension does not effectively reduce the incidence of either oropharyngeal or systemic *Candida* infections in immunocompromised patients receiving chemotherapy or radiation; its use often is associated with treatment failures and early relapses.[41] Clotrimazole appears to be more effective in reducing colonization and treating acute episodes in cancer patients who are immunocompromised. Miconazole mucoadhesive tablets were evaluated in patients with head and neck cancer and found to be superior in terms of achieving a complete response to therapy when compared to miconazole oral gel.[47] MMT has not been studied against clotrimazole in this patient population specifically but is approved for use in adults with OPC.

Systemic azole agents are used for treating OPC in patients who have failed or who are unable to take topical therapy.[37,41,46] The preceding discussion on the relative efficacy of fluconazole, itraconazole, and ketoconazole in HIV-infected patients can be extrapolated to the non-HIV-infected population. Oral fluconazole 100 to 200 mg daily is used more commonly because of more extensive experience with its use, and it is more effective and has a more favorable absorption and side-effect profile compared with other available azoles.[41] If the oral route is not feasible for reasons such as severe chemotherapy-induced mucositis, fluconazole can be administered IV. In patients unresponsive to azoles, IV amphotericin B in relatively low doses of 0.1 to 0.3 mg/kg/day can be tried.[41] Because of the higher risk for dissemination in patients who are severely neutropenic ($<0.1 \times 10^9$ neutrophils/L) or clinically unstable (hypotensive or febrile), some clinicians prefer to initiate therapy with IV amphotericin B at 0.6 mg/kg/day, with therapy continued until the neutropenia has resolved.[41] The echinocandins caspofungin, micafungin, and anidulafungin have all been studied for the treatment of OPC and found to be effective, thus offering another option in the patient with refractory disease.[41]

Topical therapy with clotrimazole or nystatin for 7 days is usually adequate for treating mucocutaneous candidiasis in most solid-organ transplant patients.[37] Use of topical therapy will reduce the number of systemic drugs that these patients receive and hence minimize the risk of drug–drug interactions. Failure to respond to topical agents warrants the use of fluconazole. Low-dose amphotericin B solution as "swish and swallow" (100 mg/mL, 1 mL four times daily) for 7 to 10 days is reserved for the unusual cases of treatment failure.

Patients who develop OPC because of prolonged antibiotic use or aerosolized corticosteroids use can be managed successfully by discontinuation of the offending agent, and the infection usually will resolve. If there is a strong desire to treat because of discomfort or need to hasten symptom resolution or an inability to stop the offending agent, therapy with a topical agent, either miconazole MT, clotrimazole or nystatin, is effective in most cases. The advantage of systemic azoles is the convenience of less frequent dosing. Symptoms usually improve in 3 or 4 days. Infants should be given smaller amounts more frequently (e.g., nystatin 100,000 units every 2 to 3 hours) to ensure better contact time. For denture-related OPC, or candidal stomatitis, effective therapy requires treatment of both the mouth and the dentures to avoid relapse. The dentures must be brushed vigorously and disinfected every night by soaking in antiseptic solution, such as chlorhexidine gluconate 0.25% or a product such as Polident or Efferdent.[37,41] Topical antifungal therapy of the oral cavity is required. Consistent proper oral hygiene and care of the dentures can help prevent relapse.

Esophageal Candidiasis: Human Immunodifiency Virus–Infected Patients

6 Treatment of esophageal candidiasis has not been as well studied as OPC. Because of the significant morbidity of esophageal candidiasis and the absence of evidence supporting the efficacy of topical antifungals, treatment requires systemic antifungal agents.[32,35] Fluconazole is superior to ketoconazole and itraconazole capsules with respect to endoscopic cure and clinical response and usually produces a more rapid onset of action and resolution of symptoms. Fluconazole is as effective as itraconazole solution, with reported response rates of >80% to 90%.[38,41] However, itraconazole solution causes more nausea and drug interactions because of inhibition of the cytochrome P450 enzymes. Amphotericin B, voriconazole, posaconazole, and the echinocandins are also effective in esophageal candidiasis, but they are generally reserved for patients with advanced or inadequately controlled HIV disease where the candidiasis tends to recur or becomes refractory to azole therapy.[48–51]

Esophageal Candidiasis: Non–Human Immunodifiency Virus–Infected Patients

As in the case of HIV-infected patients, treatment of esophageal candidiasis requires systemic therapy. Patients can be started on fluconazole 200 to 400 mg/day for 14 to 21 days.[41] Higher fluconazole doses (up to 400 mg/day) have been suggested for patients with severe symptoms or those who are neutropenic.[52] Other agents currently recommended if fluconazole is not an option are an echinocandin or amphotericin B at 0.3 to 0.7 mg/kg. Itraconazole solution, posaconazole, and voriconazole are effective alternatives that may be considered for those not responding adequately to fluconazole. An echinocandin or IV amphotericin B may be selected over fluconazole for initial therapy in neutropenic patients who present with severe symptoms or who are at high risk for dissemination of *Candida* species, such as those receiving other aggressive immunosuppressive therapy (e.g., corticosteroids, total-body irradiation, or antithymocyte globulin) and who have documented evidence of esophageal candidiasis or who have failed an initial empirical trial of oral nonabsorbable agents or systemic azoles.[41] Therapy should be continued at least until the neutropenia resolves. For patients whose symptoms have resolved and who are afebrile and clinically stable, therapy should be discontinued, and the patients should be monitored closely for infection recurrence. In high-risk patients, particularly those with persistent fever and neutropenia, the potential presence of clinically occult, diffuse GI or disseminated candidiasis should be considered. The echinocandins and newer azole agents (voriconazole and posaconazole) offer less toxic alternatives or oral agents and are preferred in patients who are intolerant of amphotericin B deoxycholate or who have preexisting renal impairment.[37,52,53] There are limited data on the clinical efficacy of anidulafungin compared with fluconazole, 95% versus 89% cure rates, respectively, in the non-HIV-infected patients.[53]

Antifungal-Refractory Oral Mucosal Candidiasis

Treatment failure is generally defined as persistence of signs and symptoms of OPC or esophageal candidiasis after an appropriate trial of antifungal therapy.[36] Treatment of refractory oral mucosal candidiasis is frequently unsatisfactory, and clinical response is usually short-lived, with rapid and periodic recurrences. The key risk factors for occurrence of refractory candidiasis are advanced stage of AIDS with low CD4 cell counts (<50 cells/mm^3 [$<0.05 \times 10^9$/L]) and repeated or prolonged courses of various systemic antifungal agents, in particular systemic azoles.[37,41] Frequent or prolonged use of fluconazole can be associated with fluconazole-refractory candidiasis because of selection of more resistant non–*C. albicans* species. An important initial management strategy is to assess and optimize the antiretroviral therapy of the patient with refractory OPC to help improve the immune function. With the widespread use of HAART, fluconazole-refractory OPC is now less commonly encountered. It is also important to identify and rectify potentially correctable causes of clinical failures of mucosal candidiasis, such as poor drug adherence, adequate dosing, reduced drug absorption associated with hypochlorhydria, and drug–drug interactions.

There have been few controlled studies that assess the effectiveness of antifungal agents. Doubling of the fluconazole dosage to 400 or 800 mg/day can be effective in some patients with infection caused by *Candida* species of intermediate resistance, although the response may be only transient.[38] Fluconazole oral suspension can be beneficial in some patients because of increased salivary concentrations obtained when the suspension is taken with the swish and swallow technique.[41] Patients with fluconazole-refractory mucosal candidiasis can be treated with itraconazole oral suspension because it can be effective in 64% to 80% of patients; however, the benefit is short-lived if chronic suppressive therapy is not maintained.[36,41] Posaconazole suspension has been reported to be successful in ~74% of patients with refractory oral or esophageal candidiasis; voriconazole may also be efficacious in these patients. Amphotericin B oral suspension is another alternative for azole-refractory patients.[38,41] It has broad-spectrum activity against many fungal species and low likelihood of *Candida* species resistance. There are limited data and experience on its use in immunosuppressed patients, and results from small studies have yielded mixed results.[54] Amphotericin B suspension is no longer available commercially in the United States, but it can be prepared extemporaneously by the pharmacy.[54]

Clinical **Controversy...**

Several antifungal agents, in both the triazole and echinocandin class, are available for the treatment of oral mucosal candidiasis. Although they have demonstrated efficacy, their place in therapy remains to be defined. It is not established which specific agent should be used next after failing fluconazole or itraconazole, and current guidelines suggest an echinocandin or amphotericin. Factors to consider in the selection can include the underlying clinical condition, the risk for drug, and side effect profiles.

Until recently, IV amphotericin B deoxycholate has been the alternative for patients with endoscopically proven disease who have failed fluconazole or itraconazole therapy. Patients with severe disease unresponsive to other agents require IV amphotericin B 0.3 to 0.7 mg/kg/day for 7 to 10 days to achieve clinical response; higher dose or longer treatment duration can be needed in more severe disease.[38,41] After response, suppressive therapy with amphotericin B is required to increase disease-free intervals. Patients who fail to respond to amphotericin B and require >1 mg/kg/day might be candidates for liposomal amphotericin B preparations because of renal and/or bone marrow toxicities, although at a markedly higher cost. Flucytosine usually is not used as monotherapy because of rapid development of resistance but can be used in combination with an azole or amphotericin B.[38] Less toxic agents that are also effective are voriconazole and the echinocandins.[52,53] Voriconazole, a triazole antifungal available in both oral and IV preparations, appears to be as effective as fluconazole for esophageal candidiasis, and it has shown success in treatment of fluconazole-refractory disease.[51] However, voriconazole has more side effects and multiple pharmacokinetic drug interactions compared to fluconazole.[51] Caspofungin is the first of the echinocandins to be approved for esophageal candidiasis; more recently, micafungin and anidulafungin have been approved for this indication. All three echinocandins have similar efficacy and tolerability profile as fluconazole, although higher relapse has been reported with caspofungin and anidulafungin compared with fluconazole.[41,53] Because the echinocandins require IV administration and are expensive, they are primarily used in patients who are refractory to the triazoles or have serious triazole-related adverse effects. As a class, the echinocandins have a favorable adverse effect profile. They are less toxic than amphotericin B (see Table 98-6) and have less impact on the cytochrome P450 enzymes than either itraconazole or voriconazole. Immunomodulation with adjunctive granulocyte-macrophage colony-stimulating factor and interferon have been used for refractory oral candidiasis in very limited numbers of patients.[41]

Antifungal Prophylaxis

7 Ensuring that the HIV-infected patient is receiving appropriate antiretroviral therapy to enhance the immune system is perhaps the most important measure in preventing future episodes of mucosal candidiasis (oropharyngeal, esophageal, and vulvovaginal).[41] Initial success of treatment often is followed by symptomatic recurrences, especially in patients with advanced or poorly controlled HIV disease. Long-term suppressive therapy with fluconazole is effective in preventing recurrences or new infections of OPC in AIDS and in patients with cancer.[41] However, the indications for antifungal prophylaxis and the best long-term management strategy still have not been well established. Fluconazole does not provide complete protection, and breakthrough infections can occur.[38] The reduced risk of recurrence of OPC also has not been demonstrated to improve survival. In addition, chronic exposure to azole therapy is a concern in that it might lead to the development of refractory disease or emergence of azole resistance.[41] However, in a randomized trial of continuous versus episodic fluconazole therapy, continuous therapy did not result in a higher rate of refractory OPC or esophageal disease.[53] Currently, HIV specialists do not recommend primary or secondary prophylaxis for OPC.[38] The rationale includes effectiveness of therapy for acute episodes of OPC, low incidence of serious invasive fungal disease, low mortality associated with mucosal candidiasis, potential for drug interactions, potential for emergence of drug resistance, and the prohibitive long-term cost of prophylaxis.

8 The decision to use secondary prophylaxis should be individualized for each patient. Secondary prophylaxis can be considered in patients with multiple recurrent episodes of symptomatic OPC or when the disease is sufficiently severe and affecting the quality of life.[38] Patients with a history of one or more episodes of documented esophageal candidiasis and a CD4 T-cell count still <200 cells/mm^3 (<0.2 × 10^9/L) despite being on HAART are candidates for secondary prophylaxis. Oral fluconazole 100 mg daily is the usual regimen recommended for OPC and esophageal candidiasis,[38,41] although 200 mg three times weekly also appears to be effective.[55] Once-weekly oral fluconazole (200 mg) is also effective for preventing OPC recurrences in those with less-advanced AIDS.[38] Itraconazole solution 200 mg daily orally is an alternative as suppressive therapy for OPC.[41]

Patients with malignant neoplastic diseases who are receiving irradiation, cytotoxic, and/or immunosuppressive therapy are at high risk for fungal infections in addition to bacterial and viral infections. Prophylaxis of *Candida* infection is controversial, and the results of studies have been conflicting and difficult to evaluate. In the hematopoietic stem cell transplant (HSCT) population, fluconazole prophylaxis is recommended prior to engraftment. Cross-resistance to other azoles may occur among *Candida* species; this should be a treatment consideration in a patient who develops a breakthrough fungal infection. Micafungin is an alternative to fluconazole prophylaxis of candidiasis.[56] The value of antifungal prophylaxis in these patients needs to be considered in the broader context of not only reducing colonization and the risk of superficial candidiasis but also, more importantly, reducing the risk for invasive candidiasis and improving survival. Management of these infections in this patient population is discussed further in Chapter 100.

Evaluation of Therapeutic Outcomes

Efficacy end points for oropharyngeal and esophageal candidiasis include rapid relief of symptoms and prevention of complications

TABLE 98-7 Patient Counseling Tips for Managing Oropharyngeal Candidiasis

1. Clean the oral cavity prior to administering the topical antifungal agent. Daily fluoride rinses can help reduce the risk of caries when using an agent containing sucrose or dextrose.
2. Use the topical antifungal agent after meals, as saliva flow and mouth movements can reduce the contact time.
3. Troches should be slowly dissolved in the mouth, not chewed or swallowed whole, over 15 to 30 minutes, and the saliva swallowed.
4. Suspension should be swished around the mouth in the oral cavity to cover all areas for as long as possible, ideally at least 1 minute, then gargled and swallowed.
5. Remove dentures while medication is being applied to the oral tissues.
6. Use a suspension or buccal mucoadhesive tablet instead of a troche if xerostomia is present; if a troche is preferred, the patient should rinse or drink water prior to dosing. For xerostomia, suggest nonpharmacologic measures for symptomatic relief (e.g., ice chips, sugarless gum or hard candy, citrus beverages).
7. Dentures should be removed and disinfected overnight using an antiseptic solution (e.g., chlorhexidine 0.12–0.2%). Disinfect oral tissues in addition to dental prosthesis.
8. Complete treatment course even though symptomatic improvement can occur in 48–72 hours.
9. Maintain good oral hygiene. Brush teeth daily (twice daily) and floss, rinse mouth, or brush teeth after eating sweets.
10. Stop smoking; avoid alcohol.

From reference 52.

without early relapse after completion of the course of therapy.[38,41] Sterilization of the oral cavity is not a feasible end point because mycologic eradication is rarely achievable, especially in HIV-positive patients. Symptomatic relief of presenting signs and symptoms (see Table 98-5) generally occurs within 48 to 72 hours of starting therapy, with complete resolution by 7 to 10 days. Patients should be advised about the time course and told to return for reassessment when signs and symptoms recur. It is usually unnecessary for the patient to be reassessed soon after finishing the treatment course. However, HIV patients should be questioned and examined for the occurrence of mucosal candidiasis as part of their regular followup. The frequency of monitoring can be more often in neutropenic patients because of concern for dissemination of candidiasis. During the period of neutropenia, temperature should be monitored daily, as well as signs of dissemination.

Efficacy of the antifungal agent is partly influenced by patient adherence to the medication regimen. Patients must be counseled on proper administration and dosing, in particular for topical agents (Table 98-7).[52] Safety end points include monitoring for occurrence of the relevant drug side effects and drug interactions (see Table 98-6). Mild GI intolerance can occur with topical therapy, but serious adverse effects are rare. It is still prudent to monitor for hypersensitivity reactions, especially rash and pruritus, that might occur with any medication. GI intolerance is more associated with the oral azoles. Hepatotoxicity can occur when azole therapy is prolonged beyond 7 to 10 days or high doses are used. Periodic monitoring of liver enzymes (alanine transaminase and aspartate amino-transferase) should be considered, especially if prolonged therapy (longer than 21 days) is anticipated. Patients who are receiving IV amphotericin B require daily monitoring by a pharmacist.

MYCOTIC INFECTIONS OF THE SKIN, HAIR, AND NAILS

Superficial mycotic infections of the skin are referred to as *dermatophytoses.* They are common infections that usually are caused by dermatophytes classified by genera: *Trichophyton*, *Epidermophyton*, and *Microsporum.*[57,58] Dermatophytes have the ability to penetrate keratinous structures of the body. These infections affect both male and female genders and all races. Reservoirs of mycotic infections include humans, animals, and soil.[58,59] Individuals can develop an infection if they come in contact with a reservoir in addition to having a conducive environment for mycotic growth (i.e., moist conditions).[60] Risk factors for the development of an infection include prolonged exposure to sweat, maceration, intertriginous folds, sharing personal belongings such as combs, close living quarters (dormitories, barracks).[59,60]

Mycotic infections of the skin have a classic appearance that consists of a central clearing surrounded by an advancing red, scaly, elevated border.[60] Infections of the nail can appear chalky and dull yellow or white and become brittle and crumbly.

Diagnosis usually is based on patient history, as well as the physical examination.[61] Diagnostic tests include direct microscopic examination of a specimen after the addition of KOH or fungal cultures. The KOH test is quick, inexpensive, and easy to perform, whereas cultures are more expensive and take longer to obtain results. Diagnostic tests are recommended when systemic therapy is likely to be prescribed.[61]

9 A general approach to treatment of superficial mycotic infections includes keeping the infected area dry and clean and limiting exposure to the infected reservoir. Topical agents generally are considered to be first-line therapy for infections of the skin. Oral therapy is preferred when the infection is extensive or severe or when treating tinea capitis or onychomycosis.[62–64] Table 98-8 lists specific treatments for each mycotic infection. Superficial mycotic infections are categorized by the pattern and site of infection.[59] The most commonly occurring infections in North America are detailed in the following sections.

Tinea Pedis

Tinea pedis is the most common dermatophytoses (affecting ~70% of adults). It is better known as "athlete's foot" and occurs in hot weather, with exposure to surface reservoirs (locker room floors), and with use of occlusive footwear.[60] Treatment with topical therapy for 2 to 4 weeks often is adequate for mild infections; however, severe infections or involvement of the nails require oral therapy[60] (see Table 98-8). Recurrence of infection occurs in up to 70% of individuals. Prolonged treatment with either topical or systemic therapy may be required.[59,62]

Tinea Manuum

Tinea manuum usually involves the palmar surface of the hands, is unilateral, and can involve the feet. Treatment of this infection is similar to tinea pedis (see Table 98-8). Emollients that contain lactic acid also can be useful.[60]

Tinea Cruris

Tinea cruris is an infection of the proximal thighs and buttocks.[63] It is referred to as "jock itch" and is more common in males. The scrotum and penis often are spared from infection. Treatment with topical therapy is recommended and should continue for 1 to 2 weeks after symptom resolution. Severe infections can require oral therapy (see Table 98-8). Relief of pruritus and burning can be facilitated by the use of short-term (2 or 3 days) topical steroids (2.5% hydrocortisone).[60]

Tinea Corporis

Tinea corporis is an infection of the glabrous skin of the trunk and extremities.[63] Therapy is similar to that for tinea pedis, tinea manuum, and tinea cruris (see Table 98-8).

Tinea Capitis

Tinea capitis is a mycotic infection involving the scalp, hair follicles, and adjacent skin that primarily affects children.[64,65] Treatment

TABLE 98-8 Treatment of Mycoses of the Skin, Hair, and Nails

	Topical[a,b]	Oral[c]
Tinea pedis	Butenafine, daily Sertaconazole, twice daily	Fluconazole 150 mg 1 per week × 1–4 weeks
Tinea manuum	Ciclopirox, twice daily	Ketoconazole 200 mg daily × 4 weeks
Tinea cruris	Clotrimazole, twice daily	Itraconazole 200–400 mg/day × 1 week
Tinea corporis	Econazole, daily Haloprogin, twice daily Ketoconazole cream, daily Miconazole, twice daily Naftifine cream, daily; gel, twice daily Oxiconazole, twice daily Sulconazole, twice daily Terbinafine, twice daily Tolnaftate, twice daily Triacetin cream, solution, 3 times daily Undecylenic acid, various preparations: apply as directed	Terbinafine 250 mg/day × 2 weeks
Tinea capitis	Shampoo only in conjunction with oral therapy or for treatment of asymptomatic carriers	Terbinafine 250 mg/day × 4–8 weeks
Tinea barbae	Ketoconazole twice weekly × 4 weeks Selenium sulfide daily × 2 weeks	Ketoconazole 200 mg daily × 4 weeks Itraconazole 100–200 mg/day × 4–6 weeks Griseofulvin 500 mg/day × 4–6 weeks
Pityriasis versicolor	Clotrimazole, twice daily Econazole, daily Haloprogin, twice daily Ketoconazole, daily Miconazole, twice daily Oxiconazole cream only, twice daily Sulconazole, twice daily Tolnaftate, three times daily	Ketoconazole Fluconazole Itraconazole 200 mg daily × 3–7 days
Onychomycosis	Ciclopirox 8% nail lacquer: apply solution at night for up to 48 weeks	Terbinafine 250 mg/day × 6 weeks (finger), 12 weeks (toe)
Fingernail		Itraconazole 200 mg twice daily × 1 week per month; repeat for total of two pulses (finger) or three pulses (toe)
Toenail		Itraconazole 200 mg daily for 6 weeks (finger) or 12 weeks (toe) Fluconazole 50 mg daily or 300 mg once weekly for ≥6 months (finger) or 12 months (toe)

[a]Other products are available, including combination products.
[b]Length of therapy depends on mycotic sensitivity and severity of infection.
[c]Only capsule formulation studied; give with food for increased absorption.

should consist of oral therapy, as well as the cleaning of combs and brushes, which can be contaminated (see Table 98-8). Daily shampooing is recommended for removal of scales. Some children and adults can be asymptomatic carriers, thereby facilitating spread of the infection.[64] Family members who culture positive for Trichophyton tonsurans should be treated with an antifungal shampoo (e.g., ketoconazole, selenium sulfide, or povidone-iodine).[64]

Tinea Barbae

Tinea barbae affects the hairs and follicles of beards and mustaches.[64] Treatment is similar to that for tinea capitis (see Table 98-8). Removal of the beard or mustache is recommended.[60]

Pityriasis Versicolor

Hyper- and hypopigmented scaly patches characterize pityriasis versicolor, which is also known as *tinea versicolor*. It is caused by yeasts of the *Malassezia* genus which with the exception of *Malassezia pachydermatis*, are all lipophilic. The seborrheic areas (scalp, face, back and front of the trunk) of the human body are always colonized by one or more *Malassezia* spp., such as *M. globosa*, *M. sympodialis*, *M. sloffiae*, and *M. restricta* are the most common colonizers; *M. globosa* and *M. furfur* are most frequent clinical infection isolates. The lesions are found on the trunk, face and extremities.[59] It is more common in adults and in areas with tropical ambient temperatures. Topical treatment usually is adequate unless there is extensive involvement, recurrent infections, or failure of topical therapy.[66] A study of 100 subjects treated with either ketoconazole 2% shampoo or selenium sulfide 2.5% shampoo showed that ketoconazole was significantly more effective that selenium sulfide (89% vs. 35% cure rate).[66] Recurrence of infection after cessation of treatment may be as high as 60% in the first year and 80% the second year. Suppressive maintenance therapy either orally or topically may be used in these cases.[58]

Onychomycosis (Tinea Unguium)

Onychomycosis is a fungal infection of the nail apparatus and is the most common single cause of nail dystrophy, affecting up to 8% of the general population and accounting for up to 50% of all nail problems.[66–69] Onychomycosis more commonly affects the toenails (2% to 14% of adults), ~4 to 19 times more frequently than fingernails, with prevalence increasing with age.[69] This can be because of the slower growth of toenails (three times slower than fingernails), making it easier for fungi to establish infection. Onychomycosis has a significant impact on quality of life, both functional and psychosocial. In addition, the affected nails can disrupt the integrity of the surrounding skin, potentially increasing the risk of secondary bacterial infections.[69]

Onychomycosis is due to infection by dermatophytes (tinea unguium), yeasts and nondermatophyte fungi.[70] Dermatophytes are the most frequent causes of onychomycosis (~90% in toenail and ~50% in fingernail infections).[71] The dermatophytes responsible for causing >90% of cases of onychomycosis are *Trichophyton rubrum* (71%) and *Trichophyton mentagrophytes* (20%).[64,65] Less common fungi causing onychomycosis are the nondermatophytic molds (2.3% to 11%) and yeasts (5.6%). *Candida albicans* is the most commonly isolated yeast and typically affects fingernails rather than toenails.[66,72] Risk factors for dermatophytic onychomycosis are increasing age (especially older than 40 years), family history and genetic factors, immunodeficiency (e.g., HIV, renal transplant, immunosuppressive therapy, and defective polymorphonuclear chemotaxis), diabetes mellitus, psoriasis, peripheral vascular disease, smoking, prevalence of tinea pedis, frequent nail trauma, and sporting activities such as swimming.[72,73] These risk factors also appear to apply to recurrence of onychomycosis. Mold onychomycosis does not seem to be associated with systemic or local predisposing factors, but there is a risk of systemic dissemination in immunosuppressed patients.[72] *Candida* onychomycosis seems to always occur in immunosuppressed patients.[72]

Onychomycosis can present in four or five different major clinical forms, of which lateral distal subungual onychomycosis (DSO) is the most common type.[66,72,74] In DSO, the nail plate, the nail bed, and, in advanced cases, the matrix are all affected, and *T. rubrum* is the most common etiologic cause. The worst case of onychomycosis is progression of the infection to total dystrophic onychomycosis, characterized by almost complete destruction of the nail plate. White superficial onychomycosis (WSO) is usually caused by *T. mentagrophytes*, where the infection is localized to the surface of the nail plate. In proximal subungual onychomycosis (PSO), the fungi (usually *T. rubrum*) invade the nail through the proximal nail fold and spread to the nail plate and matrix. Although PSO is relatively uncommon in the general population, it occurs most frequently in severely immunocompromised patients and is often considered a marker for AIDS.[72,74] Because of the multifactorial etiology of onychomycosis, it is important to differentiate onychomycosis from other causes of nail dystrophies so that the patient receives appropriate therapy and is not subjected to prolonged treatment with unnecessary drugs. Besides clinical history and physical examination, proper diagnosis of onychomycosis can include the combination of direct microscopy of scrapings from the appropriate nail area to look for fungal hyphae and fungal cultures, and, if necessary, histologic examination.[68,75,76] Table 98-9 provides a differential diagnosis for fungal nail diseases.[77]

TABLE 98-9 Differential Diagnosis of Fungal Nail Infections

Diagnosis	Features Consistent with Diagnosis
Psoriasis	Nail pitting, rash elsewhere on body, family history of psoriasis
Lichen planus	Nail atrophy, scarring at proximal aspect of the nail
Periungual squamous cell carcinoma	Single nail affected, pain, warty nail fold change, or ooze from the edge of nail
Yellow nail syndrome	Multiple nails turn yellow, grow slowly, increased longitudinal and transverse curvature, intermittent pain and shedding, associated with chronic sinusitis, bronchiectasis, lymphedema
Trauma	Single nail affected, homogeneous alteration of nail color and altered shape of nail

From reference 77.

TREATMENT

General Approach

Onychomycosis merits proper assessment and treatment consideration because it is a debilitating disease and can exert a negative impact on quality of life (e.g., cosmetic and psychosocial effects, pain, discomfort, and decreased ambulation).[68,70,72,78] It is reasonable to not treat persons with minimal toenail involvement and no associated symptoms.[77] Although definitive data are lacking regarding the risk of progression of untreated disease, it can lead to complications such as cellulitis or reduced mobility, which can further compromise peripheral circulation in those with diabetes or peripheral vascular disease; additionally, infected nails can serve as a source of transmission of fungi to other areas of the body, as well as to other people, such as close household contacts, or in communal bathing places.[69,70,72,78,79] Treatment decisions should be made on an individual basis. The primary end point of treatment is eradication of the organism, with secondary end points being clinical cure and improvement.[69] Assessment of clinical success (cure or improvement) requires followup for several months after the end of treatment because of the slow growth rate of nails, especially toenails (1 mm/month).[68,72] Successful eradication of the fungus does not always result in normalization of the nails because they can have been dystrophic prior to infection. This can cause patient dissatisfaction, especially if this is not explained before starting treatment.[74] There are several factors that must be taken into account on a patient-by-patient basis to ensure appropriate treatment decisions (Table 98-10). The impact of patient adherence on the success of treatment cannot be overemphasized. Patients need to be educated about their disease, expectations of treatment, and prevention of recurrence, and various strategies have been suggested to improve treatment success.[76]

In general, onychomycosis of the toenail is more difficult to treat than fingernails, requires longer treatment duration, and is associated with a higher recurrence. The treatment options for onychomycosis include oral and topical therapies, mechanical or chemical nail avulsion, or a combination of these. Mechanical or chemical nail avulsion is used primarily as adjunct to oral therapy in patients with total dystrophic onychomycosis, in whom there is severe onycholysis and extensive nail thickening or longitudinal spikes. This is to enhance penetration of the antifungal agent to the entire nail plate and unit.[68,70,76,79]

Topical Therapy

(10) Conventional topical antifungal products are available as creams, ointments, powders, and solutions. Because these formulations do not penetrate through the nail plate to the nail bed, they are

TABLE 98-10 Factors That May Impact Treatment Decisions and Outcomes

- Type and severity of onychomycosis
- Causative organism—dermatophyte versus molds or yeast
- Infection of the finger versus toenail
- Extent of disease—involvement of matrix, one or two lateral edges, number of nails
- Thickness of nail plate
- Other sites of mycotic infection (palms, soles, toe webs)
- Other nail alterations affecting outcome (onycholysis, paronychia, dermatophytoma, etc.)
- Other nail diseases and symptoms
- Age and underlying medical conditions (diabetes, poor perfusion, immunocompromised)
- Drug interactions and adverse effects
- Cost of therapy

Data from references 67, 76, 78, and 79.

most appropriately used when the nail plate has been removed.[70,79] Even then cure rates are still low and variable and are influenced by patient adherence.[70,72,79] Nail lacquer represents the latest advance in topical formulation. The volatile vehicle, used to deliver the drug, evaporates and leaves an occlusive film with a high drug concentration on the nail surface.[72,79] There are only two marketed nail lacquers, amorolfine 5% and ciclopirox 8% solution (Penlac), the latter being the only one approved in the United States for the treatment of mild-to-moderate onychomycosis caused by *T. rubrum* without lunula involvement.[72,78,79] Ciclopirox, a hydroxypyridine, has a broad spectrum of antifungal activity (dermatophytes, *Candida* species, and some molds) and requires treatment for 1 year. Although ciclopirox was significantly better than vehicle alone, the mycologic cure rate was only 32% with ciclopirox versus 10% for vehicle alone after 48 weeks of treatment; the overall treatment cure (mycologic cure with 0% to 10% involvement of the target nail) was 9% versus 0.9% for drug and vehicle, respectively.[72,79] However, higher mycologic cure rates of 45% to 65% have been reported in a variety of open-label trials involving 6 to 12 months of treatment.[72] Amorolfine appears to produce higher mycologic and treatment cure rates than ciclopirox.[70,78] Most experts consider topical therapy a feasible option when the infection is superficial involving the nail plate without matrix involvement, such as WSO, involves a partial area of the nail plate not exceeding 50% (owing to difficulty of applying treatment to the margin of the nail), is limited to a few (three or four) nails, is in the very early stages of DSO when infection is still confined to the distal edge of the nail, or when systemic therapy is contraindicated.[68,72,78] Combining topical therapy with debridement of the affected nail (thus diminishing the amount of nail requiring treatment) may increase the likelihood of successful treatment, although there is no strong supporting evidence.[77] Topical therapy is not associated with systemic adverse effects or drug interactions. Any adverse effect will be localized to the application site, such as mild erythema in the adjacent skin area.

Clinical **Controversy. . .**

Treatment of onychomycosis is associated with a high failure rate of 20% to 50%. There appears to be a sound pharmacologic rationale behind the use of combination therapy, which has been used to improve overall efficacy. However, the best combination of agents for use in treating onychomycosis is unclear, and there is no consensus on when to use such agents.

Systemic Therapy

Oral antifungal therapy is considered to be more effective than topical for treating onychomycosis. Terbinafine and itraconazole (capsule), the current first-line agents for treatment, have yielded higher efficacy rates using shorter treatment periods (generally 3 months or shorter) for toenail and fingernail onychomycosis compared with the traditional agents, such as griseofulvin and ketoconazole, which are rarely used nowadays. Terbinafine, an allylamine, exerts fungicidal activity and demonstrates the greatest in vitro activity against dermatophytes compared with the other oral antifungals; it has good activity against nondermatophyte molds and only marginal activity against *Candida* species.[68,79] Like other azoles, itraconazole is fungistatic, has a broad antifungal spectrum, and is very active against dermatophytes, nondermatophytes, and *Candida* species.[68,79] Both agents have lipophilic and keratinophilic properties, which explains their excellent penetration (appearing in the nail plate within days of treatment initiation) and accumulation in the nails, achieving concentrations far exceeding the minimal inhibitory concentration (MIC) of most dermatophytes. Nail terbinafine concentrations are detected within 1 week of starting therapy, whereas itraconazole can be detected 1 (fingernails) to 2 weeks (toenails) after starting therapy.[72] Both drugs are slowly eliminated from the nail, with effective drug concentrations persisting in nails for 30 to 36 weeks after completion of treatment with terbinafine and for 27 weeks with itraconazole.[74] The persistence of drug in the nails explains in part the long-term protection against relapses after the end of treatment and also permits use of intermittent (pulse) dosing.

The treatment of toenail onychomycosis requires a 12-week course, whereas a 6-week course is adequate for fingernail onychomycosis with either drug.[69,74] In general, cure rates of 80% to 90% for fingernail infection and 70% to 80% for toenail infection can be expected.[68] Terbinafine is licensed for daily dosing (see Table 98-8).[69,74,80] Various terbinafine pulse regimens have been evaluated;[73] in some trials, pulse dosing was less effective than continuous dosing, and it did not provide clear safety advantages.[75,76] One trial demonstrated similar efficacy of pulse terbinafine compared with continuous therapy and better outcomes compared with pulse itraconazole treatment.[81] Itraconazole pulse therapy is the preferred method over continuous dosing for fingernail infections, and it is licensed as twice-daily dosing for a 1-week cycle per month for 2 consecutive months (i.e., two pulses), or as daily therapy for 6 weeks (see Table 98-8).[74,80] Although itraconazole pulse therapy is not approved by the U.S. Food and Drug Administration (FDA), three or four pulses are effective for toenail infections; otherwise, half the dose is taken daily for 3 months (see Table 98-8).[74,80] In addition to lower drug cost, the potential advantages of itraconazole pulse therapy compared with continuous therapy are a lower risk of adverse drug effects and improved patient adherence.

Terbinafine is generally considered by most experts as the first-line agent for onychomycosis; itraconazole is the alternative. Direct comparative trials generally have shown that terbinafine is more effective than itraconazole either by continuous or pulse dosing.[68,78,79] Mycologic cure rates for terbinafine range from 77% to 100% depending on the study.[72,82,83] In a cumulative meta-analysis of randomized, controlled trials, mycologic cure rates for terbinafine, itraconazole pulse, itraconazole continuous, fluconazole, and griseofulvin were 76% ± 3%, 63% ± 7%, 59% ± 5%, 60% ± 6%, and 48% ± 5%, respectively.[84] An earlier meta-analysis and systematic review also reported that continuous terbinafine was the most effective therapy for toenail onychomycosis.[84,85,86] In addition, terbinafine was reported to achieve high cure rates in high-risk immunosuppressed patients, such as diabetics and organ transplant recipients, comparable to the immunocompetent population, with no significant adverse effects or drug interactions. It also appears to be effective in HIV patients and nondermatophyte infections.[80,87] A pharmacoeconomic analysis of oral and topical (ciclopirox) therapies showed that from a managed-care perspective, terbinafine was the most cost-effective therapy in terms of highest success rate, lowest relapse rate, and highest number of disease-free days for both fingernail and toenail infections.[88] An analysis that looked only at oral therapy estimated that the cost per cure with the use of terbinafine (based on cure rates from clinical trials) ranged from $2,439 to $7,944, depending on disease severity.[89] Compared with the amount of money a patient would consider reasonable to spend on treatment, the current charges for a course of systemic therapy are considerably higher.[89,90]

Both terbinafine and itraconazole generally are well tolerated. The more common adverse effects reported with terbinafine are GI (e.g., diarrhea, dyspepsia, nausea, and abdominal pain), dermatologic (e.g., rash, urticaria, and pruritus), and headache; less common adverse effects are taste disturbances, fatigue, inability to concentrate, and asymptomatic liver enzyme abnormalities.[74,78,80] Terbinafine can cause transient decrease in absolute lymphocyte counts; hence, monitoring of complete blood counts can be useful, especially in immunocompromised patients.[80] Although uncommon, severe adverse effects have been reported with terbinafine, including erythema multiforme, Stevens-Johnson's syndrome, toxic epidermal necrolysis, pancytopenia, lupus erythematosus, psoriasis, hair loss, and hepatotoxicity. Although the incidence of severe hepatotoxicity is considered rare, the FDA issued a public health advisory in 2001 regarding the association of terbinafine tablets with 16 possible cases of liver failure, including 2 liver transplants and 11 deaths.[91] Terbinafine thus is not recommended for patients with chronic or active liver disease, although hepatotoxicity can occur in patients with no preexisting liver disease or serious underlying medical condition. Prior to initiating terbinafine treatment, it is recommended to obtain appropriate nail specimens for laboratory testing to confirm the diagnosis of onychomycosis. Liver function parameters (serum transaminases) should be assessed at baseline and periodically during treatment with terbinafine.[80,91]

The common adverse effects of itraconazole are similar to those of terbinafine, such as GI disturbance, dermatologic disorders, and headache; less common adverse effects include dizziness, fatigue, fever, decreased libido, and asymptomatic liver enzyme abnormalities (1% to 5% with continuous dosing and ~2% with pulse dosing).[74,78,92] Although still considered rare, 24 serious cases of liver failure, including transplantation and death, have been reported with the use of itraconazole, resulting in an FDA public health advisory warning.[91] Some of these patients did not have preexisting liver disease or serious underlying medical conditions, and some developed within the first week of treatment. Itraconazole should be avoided in patients with elevated liver enzymes or active liver disease or in those who have experienced other drug-induced liver toxicity. Liver function parameters (serum transaminases) should be assessed prior to and periodically during treatment. However, some experts have suggested that frequent monitoring is not as necessary if pulse therapy is used because symptomatic hepatotoxicity has not been reported with pulse therapy.[92] In addition, there is an FDA warning on the risk of developing congestive heart failure (CHF) associated with the use of itraconazole, possibly related to its potential negative inotropic effect.[69,82] Therefore, itraconazole should not be used in patients with evidence of ventricular dysfunction, such as CHF. Symptomatic assessment for the development of CHF also should be included as part of therapy monitoring. Before a patient is subjected to several months of itraconazole treatment, it is important to confirm the diagnosis of onychomycosis.

In contrast to the azoles, terbinafine does not inhibit the cytochrome P450 (CYP)3A4 isoenzymes, but it is a potent inhibitor of the CYP2D6 isoenzymes, which are responsible for metabolism of tricyclic antidepressants and other psychotropic drugs.[69,74,80] The most significant drug interactions with terbinafine are decreased clearance of 33% by cimetidine and increased clearance of 100% by rifampin. Other drug interactions of variable clinical significance are tricyclic antidepressants, cyclosporine, caffeine, theophylline, and terfenadine. Itraconazole and its major metabolite can inhibit the CYP3A4 isoenzymes and result in numerous clinically significant drug interactions where coadministration with several drugs are contraindicated (e.g., alprazolam, midazolam, triazolam, pimozide, lovastatin, simvastatin, cisapride, and terfenadine).[68,74,80]

Fluconazole is also active against dermatophytes, *Candida* species, and some nondermatophytes;[74,78] however, it does not have current FDA-approved indication for treatment of onychomycosis. The overall mycologic cure rate of fluconazole is 48%, which is lowest compared with all other oral agents.[84] The most effective dose and treatment duration have not been clearly established, with a variety of dosing regimens used, ranging from 50 mg daily to 300 mg once weekly for 6 to 12 months (see Table 98-8).[74,80] The advantages of fluconazole include a relatively good safety profile and fewer drug interactions compared with itraconazole.[74,80]

These three oral antifungal agents have superseded the use of griseofulvin and ketoconazole as treatments of choice for onychomycosis.[68,78,79] Griseofulvin has a narrow antifungal spectrum, low clinical efficacy, especially for toenail infections, high relapse rates, and the need for prolonged treatment duration (up to 12 to 18 months for toenails). Use of ketoconazole is also associated with high relapse rates, and the prolonged treatment duration carries an increased risk of hepatotoxicity.

Treatment Response and Recurrence

Treatment failures and recurrence rates of infection following initial cure are high, ranging from 20% to 50%.[69,77] Recurrence could be either a relapse (original infection not completely cured) or reinfection (new infection after achieving a cure of the original). Factors associated with poor response to systemic therapy include a compromised immune system (AIDS), reduced blood flow (diabetes, peripheral vascular disease, vasculitis, connective tissue disease, and CHF), coexisting nail disease (psoriasis), nail factors (slow growth, thick nails, and severe disease), drug-resistant organisms because of extensive prior drug exposure, and reduced bioavailability (absorption problems, poor compliance, and drug interactions).[74,77] To improve treatment outcomes and reduce recurrence, patients should be counseled on the importance of proper foot hygiene, for example, wearing breathable footwear and 100% cotton socks with frequent changes, keeping the nails short and clean, keeping the feet dry, protecting the feet in shared bathing areas, treating tinea pedis, and controlling other predisposing medical conditions.[77]

The use of combination therapy (topical–oral or oral–oral agents) can improve cure rates and shorten treatment duration, as this approach provides complementary mechanisms of attack.[77,78] Studies in Europe have reported favorable results achieved with itraconazole or terbinafine combined with amorolfine.[77,78] To date, no specific combination has been approved or endorsed for use. Other novel approaches include giving supplemental therapy and use of boosted therapy.[77,78] The efficacy and role of either approach remain to be defined.

Clinical **Controversy...**

There is controversy regarding the cost–benefit ratio of treating onychomycosis. People commonly receive treatment without a proper diagnosis of onychomycosis. These patients are not accounted for in any pharmacoeconomic analysis as such this inappropriate treatment will markedly increase the cost per cure. Also relevant to decision making are the risks of treatment and the effects of treatment on quality of life. A study translating these considerations into an amount of money a patient would consider reasonable to spend on treatment found the current costs of a course of therapy are much greater than this sum.[84]

ABBREVIATIONS

ACOG	American College of Obstetricians and Gynecologists
AIDS	acquired immune deficiency syndrome
BMT	bone marrow transplantation
CHF	congestive heart failure
CMI	cell-mediated immunity
CYP	cytochrome P450
DSO	distal subungual onychomycosis
FDA	Food and Drug Administration
GI	gastrointestinal
HAART	highly active antiretroviral therapy
HIV	human immunodeficiency virus
HRT	hormone replacement therapy

HSCT	hematopoietic stem cell transplant
IgA	immunoglobulin A
KOH	potassium hydroxide
MIC	minimum inhibitory concentration
MMT	miconazole mucoadhesive tablet
OPC	oropharyngeal candidiasis
PSO	proximal subungual onychomycosis
RVVC	recurrent vulvovaginal candidiasis
VVC	vulvovaginal candidiasis
WSO	white superficial onychomycosis

REFERENCES

1. Sobel JD, Faro S, Force R, et al. Vulvovaginal candidiasis: Epidemiologic, diagnostic and therapeutic considerations. Am J Obstet Gynecol 1998;178:203–211.
2. Center for Disease Control and Prevention. Vaginal Discharge-STD Treatment Guidelines. 2006, *www.cdc.gov/std/treatment/2006/vaginaldischarge.htm.*
3. Haefner HK. Current evaluation and management of vulvovaginitis. Clin Obstet Gynecol 1999;42:184–195.
4. Foxman B, Barlow R, D'arcy H, et al. *Candida* vaginitis self-reported incidence and associated costs. Sex Transm Dis 2000;27:230–235.
5. Fischer G, Bradford J. Vulvovaginal candidiasis in postmenopausal women: The role of hormone replacement therapy. J Low Genit Tract Dis 2011;15:263–237.
6. Lipsky MS, Waters T, Sharp LK. Impact of vaginal antifungal products on utilization of health care services: Evidence from physician visits. J Am Board Fam Pract 2000;13:178182.
7. Clinical Effectiveness Group. National guideline for the management of vulvovaginal candidiasis. Sex Transm Infect 1999;75(suppl 1):S19–S20.
8. Larsen B. Vaginal flora in health and disease. Clin Obstet Gynecol 1993;36:107–121.
9. Sobel JD. Clinical vulvovaginitis. Clin Obstet Gynecol 1993;36:153–165.
10. Camacho DP, Consolaro ME, Patussi EV, Donatti L, Gasparetto A, Svidzinski TL. Vaginal yeast adherence to the combined contraceptive vaginal ring (CCVR). Contraception 2007;76:439–443.
11. Barbone F, Austin H, Louv WC, Alexander WJ. A follow-up study of the methods of contraception, sexual activity, and rates of trichomoniasis, candidiasis, and bacterial vaginosis. Am J Obstet Gynecol 1990;163:510–514.
12. Xu J, Schwartz K, Bartoces M, Monsur J, Severson RK, Sobel JD. J Am Board Fam Med 2008;21:261–268.
13. Ferris DG, Dekle C, Litaker MS. Women's use of over-the-counter antifungal pharmaceutical products for gynecologic symptoms. J Fam Pract 1996;42:595–600.
14. ACOG practice bulletin: Clinical management guidelines for obstetrician-gynecologists. Obstet Gynecol 2006;107: 1195–1206.
15. Watson MC, Bond CM, Grimshaw J, Johnston M. Factors predicting the guideline compliant supply (or non-supply) of non-prescription medicines in the community pharmacy setting. Qual Saf Health Care 2006;15:53–57.
16. Martinez RC, Franceschini Sa, Patta MC, et al. Improved treatment of vulvaovaginal candidiasis with fluconazole plus probiotic Lactobacillus rhamnosus GR-1 and Lactobacillus reuteri RC-14. Lett Appl Microbiol 2009;48:269–274.
17. Abdelmonem AW, Rasheed SM, Mohamed AS. Bee-honey and yogurt: a novel mixture for treating patients with vulvovaginal candidiasis during pregnancy. Arch Gynecol Obstet 2012;8: Epub ahead of print.
18. Hilton E, Isenberg HD, Alperstein P, et al. Ingestion of yogurt containing *Lactobacillus acidophilus* as prophylaxis for candidal vaginitis. Ann Intern Med 1992;116:353–357.
19. Witt A, Kaufmann U, Bitschnau M, et al. Monthly itraconazole versus classic homeopathy for the treatment of recurrent vulvovaginal candidiasis: a randomized trial. Br J Obstet Gynecol 2009;116:1499–1505.
20. Tooley PJ. Patient and doctor preferences in the treatment of vaginal candidiasis. Practitioner 1985;229:655–662.
21. Nurbhai M, Grimshaw J, Watson M, Bond CM, Mollison JA, Ludbrook A. Oral versus intravaginal imidazole and triazole antifungal treatment of uncomplicated vulvovaginal candidiasis (thrush). Cochrane Database Syst Rev 2007;4:CD002845, DOI:10.1002/14651858.CD002845.pub2.
22. Edelman DA, Grant S. One-day therapy for vaginal candidiasis a review. J Reprod Med 1999;44:543–547.
23. Mendling W, Plempel M. Vaginal secretion levels after 6 days, 3 days and 1 day of treatment with 100-, 200-, 500-mg vaginal tablets of clotrimazole and their therapeutic efficacy. Chemotherapy 1982;28(suppl 1):43–47.
24. Sobel JD, Kapernick PS, Zervos M, et al. Treatment of complicated candida vaginitis: Comparison of single and sequential doses of fluconazole. Am J Obstet Gynecol 2001;185:363–369.
25. Young G, Jewell D. Topical treatment for vaginal candidiasis (thrush) in pregnancy. Cochrane Database Syst Rev 2001;4:CD000225, DOI:10.1002/14651858.CD000225.
26. Mastroiacovo P, Mazzone T, Botto L, et al. Prospective assessment of pregnancy outcomes after first-trimester exposure to fluconazole. Am J Obstet Gynecol 1996;175:1645–1650.
27. Pursley TJ, Blomquist IK, Abraham J, Andersen HF, Bartley JA. Fluconazole-induced congenital anomalies in three infants. Clin Infect Dis 1996;22:336–340.
28. Sobel JD, Wiesenfeld HC, Martens M, et al. Maintenance fluconazole therapy for recurrent vulvovaginal candidiasis. N Engl J Med 2004;351:363–369.
29. Pappas PG, Kauffman CA, Andes DA, et al. Clinical practice guidelines for the management of candidiasis: 2009 update by the infectious diseases society of America. Clin Infect Dis 2009;48:503–535.
30. Sobel JD, Chiam W, Nagappan V, Leaman D. Treatment of vaginitis caused by *Candida glabrata*: Use of topical boric acid and flucytosine. Am J Obstet Gynecol 2003;189:1297–1300.
31. Sobel JD, Chaim W. Treatment of *Torulopsis glabrata* vaginitis: Retrospective review of boric acid therapy. Clin Infect Dis 1996;22:336–340.
32. Ray D, Goswami R, Banerjee U, Dadhawl V, et al. Prevalence of *Candida glabrata* and its response to boric acid vaginal suppositories in comparison with oral fluconazole in patients with diabetes and vulvovaginal candidiasis. Diabetes Care 2007;30:312–317.
33. Leigh JE, Shetty K, Fidel Jr PL. Oral opportunistic infections in HIV-positive individuals: Review and role of mucosal immunity. AIDS Patient Care STDS 2004;18:443–456.
34. Farah CS, Lynch N, McCullough MJ. Oral fungal infections: An update for the general practitioner. Aust Dent J 2010;55(1 suppl):48–54.
35. Thompson III GR, Patel PK, Kirkpatrick WR, et al. Oropharyngeal candidiasis in the era of antiretroviral therapy. Oral Surg Oral Med Oral Pathol Oral Radiol Endod 2010;109:488–495.
36. Delgado ACD, de Jesus PR, Aoki FH, et al. Clinical and microbiological assessment of patients with long-term

diagnosis of human immunodeficiency virus infection and *Candida* oral colonization. Clin Microbiol Infect 2009;15:364–371.

37. Laudenbach JM, Epstein JB. Treatment strategies for oropharyngeal candidiasis. Expert Opin Pharmaocother 2009;10(9):1413–1421.
38. Benson CA, Kaplan JE, Masur H, et al. Treating opportunistic infections among HIV-infected adults and adolescents: Recommendations from CDC, the National Institutes of Health, and the HIV Medicine Association/ Infectious Diseases Society of America. Clin Infect Dis 2004;40:S131–S235.
39. Mercante DE, Leigh JE, Lilly EA, et al. Assessment of the association between HIV viral load and CD4 cell count on the occurrence of oropharyngeal candidiasis in HIV-infected patients. J Acquir Immune Defic Syndr 2006;42:578–583.
40. Soysa NS, Samaranayake LP, Ellepola ANB. Antimicrobials as a contributory factor in oral candidosis: A brief overview. Oral Dis 2008;14:138–143.
41. Pappas PG, Kauffman CA, Andes D, et al. Guidelines for management of candidiasis: 2009 update by the Infectious Diseases Society of America. Clin Infect Dis 2009;48: 503–535.
42. Jurevic RJ, Traboulsi RS, Mukherjee PK, et al. Identification of gentian violet concentration that does not stain oral mucosa, possesses anti-candidal activity and is well tolerated. Eur J Clin Microbiol Infect Dis 2011;30(5):629–633.
43. Lalla RV, Bensadoun RJ. Miconazole mucoadhesive tablet for oropharyngeal candidiasis. Expert Rev Anti Infect Ther 2011;9(1):13.
44. Vazquez JA, Patton LL, Epstein JB et al. Randomized, comparative, double-blind, double-dummy, multicenter trial of miconazole buccal tablet and clotrimazole troches for the treatment of oropharyngeal candidiasis: Study of Miconazole Lauriad® Efficacy and Safety (SMiLES). HIV Clin Trials 2010;11(4):186–196.
45. Hamza OJM, Matee MIN, Bruggemann RJM, et al. Single-dose fluconazole versus standard 2-week therapy for oropharyngeal candidiasis in HIV-infected patients: A randomized, double-blind, double-dummy trial. Clin Infect Dis 2008;47:1270–1276.
46. Vasquez JA, Skiest DJ, Nieto L, et al. A multicenter randomized trial evaluating posaconazole versus fluconazole for the treatment of oropharyngeal candidiasis in subjects with HIV/AIDS. Clin Infect Dis 2006;42: 1179–1186.
47. Bensadoun RJ, Daoud J, El Gueddari B et al. Comparison of the efficacy and safety of miconazole 50 mg mucoadhesive buccal tablets with miconazole 500 mg gel in the treatment of oropharyngeal candidiasis: a prospective, randomized, single-blind, multicenter, comparative, phase III trial in patients treated with radiotherapy for head and neck cancer. Cancer 2008;112(1):204–211.
48. Villanueva A, Arathoon EG, Gotuzzo E, et al. A randomized double-blind study of caspofungin versus amphotericin for the treatment of candidal esophagitis. Clin Infect Dis 2001;33:1529–1535.
49. Arathoon EG, Gotuzzo E, Noriega LM, et al. Randomized, double-blind, multicenter study of caspofungin versus amphotericin B for treatment of oropharyngeal and esophageal candidiasis. Antimicrob Agents Chemother 2002;46:451–457.
50. Villanueva A, Gotuzzo E, Arathoon EG, et al. A randomized, double-blind study of caspofungin versus fluconazole for the treatment of esophageal candidiasis. Am J Med 2002;113:294–299.
51. Deresinski SC, Stevens DA. Caspofungin. Clin Infect Dis 2003;36:1445–1457.
52. Akpan A, Morgan R. Oral candidiasis. Postgrad Med J 2002;78:455–459.
53. Morris MI, Villmann. Echinocandins in the management of invasive fungal infections, part 1. Am J Health Syst Pharm 2006;63:1693–1703.
54. Grim SA, Smith KM, Romanelli F, Ofotokun I. Treatment of azole-resistant oropharyngeal candidiasis with topical amphotericin B. Ann Pharmacother 2002;36:1383–1386.
55. Goldman M, Cloud GA, Wade KD, et al. A randomized study of the use of fluconazole in continuous versus episodic therapy in patients with advanced HIV infection and a history of oropharyngeal candidiasis: AIDS clinical trials group study 323/mycoses study group 40. Clin Infect Dis 2005;41:1473–1480.
56. Marr KA, Bow E, Chiller T, et al. Fungal infection prevention after hematopoietic cell transplantation. Bone Marrow Transplant 2009;44:483–487.
57. Nowak MA, Brodell RT. Rapid diagnosis of superficial fungal infections. Postgrad Med 1999;2:179–180.
58. Schwartz RA. Superficial fungal infections. Lancet 2004;364:1173–1182.
59. Mendez-Tovar LJ. Pathogenesis of dermatophytosis and tinea versicolor. Clin Dermatol 2010;28:185–189.
60. Goldstein AO, Smith KM, Ives TJ, Goldstein B. Mycotic infections. Effective management of conditions involving the skin, hair, and nails. Geriatrics 2000;55:40–52.
61. Drake LA, Dinehart SM, Farmer ER, et al. Guidelines of care for superficial mycotic infections of the skin: Tinea corporis, tinea cruris, tinea faciei, tinea manuum, and tinea pedis. J Am Acad Dermatol 1996;34:282–286.
62. Gupta AK, Chow M, Daniel CR, Aly R. Treatments of tinea pedis. Dermatol Clin 2003;21:431–462.
63. Gupta AK, Chaudhry M Elewski B. Tinea corporis, tinea cruris, tinea nigra, and piedra. Dermatol Clin 2003;21: 395–400.
64. Drake LA, Dinehart SM, Farmer ER, et al. Guidelines of care for superficial mycotic infections of the skin: Tinea capitis and tinea barbae. J Am Acad Dermatol 1996;34:290–294.
65. Higgins EM, Fuller LC, Smith CH. Guidelines for the management of tinea capitis. Br J Dermatol 2000;143:53–58.
66. Ansarun H, Ghaffarpour G. Comparison of effectiveness between ketoconazole 2% and selenium sulfide 2% shampoos in the treatment of tinea versicolor. Iranian J Derm 2005;8:21–25.
67. Effendy I, Lecha M, Feuilhade de Chauvin M, et al. Epidemiology and clinical classification of onychomycosis. J Eur Acad Dermatol Venereol 2005;19(suppl 1):8–12.
68. Roberts DT, Taylor WD, Boyle J. Guidelines for treatment of onychomycosis. Br J Dermatol 2003;148:402–410.
69. Nunley KS, Cornelius L. Current management of onychomycosis. J Hand Surg 2008;33A:1211–1214.
70. Welsh O, Vera-Cabrera L, Welsh E. Onychomycosis. Clin Dermatol 2010;28:151–159.
71. Kaur R, Kashyap B, Bhalla P. Onychomycosis—Epidemiology, diagnosis and management. Indian J Med Microbiol 2008;26(2):108–116.
72. Baran R, Kaoukhov A. Topical antifungal drugs for the treatment of onychomycosis: An overview of current strategies for monotherapy and combination therapy. J Eur Acad Dermatol Venereol 2005;19:21–29.
73. Tosti A, Hay R, Arenas-Guzman R. Patients at risk of onychomycosis—Risk factor identification and active prevention. J Eur Acad Dermatol Venereol 2005;19(suppl 1): 13–16.

74. Iorizzo M, Piraccini BM, Rech G, Tosti A. Treatment of onychomycosis with oral antifungal agents. Expert Opin Drug Deliv 2005;2:435–440.
75. Feuilhade de Chauvin M. New diagnostic techniques. J Eur Acad Dermatol Venereol 2005;19(suppl 1):20–24.
76. Gupta AK, Tu LQ. Onychomycosis therapies: Strategies to improve efficacy. Dermatol Clin 2006;24:381–386.
77. de Berker D. Fungal nail disease. N Engl J Med 2009;360: 2108–2116.
78. Lecha M, Effendy I, Feuilhade de Chauvin M, et al. Treatment options—Development of consensus guidelines. J Eur Acad Dermatol Venereol 2005;19(suppl 1):25–33.
79. Gupta AK, Tu LQ. Therapies for onychomycosis: A review. Dermatol Clin 2006;24:375–379.
80. Gupta AK, Ryder JE, Skinner AR. Treatment of onychomycosis: Pros and cons of antifungal agents. J Cutan Med Surg 2004;8:25–30.
81. Gupta AK, Lynch LE, Kogan N, et al. The use of intermittent terbinafine for the treatment of dermatophyte toenail onychomycosis. J Eur Acad Dermatol Venereol 2009;23:256–262.
82. Sigurgeirsson B, Elewski EE, Rich PA, et al. Intermittent versus continuous terbinafine in the treatment of toenail onychomycosis: A randomized, double-blind, comparison. J Dermatol Treat 2006;17:38–44.
83. Warshaw EM, Fett DD, Bloomfield HE, et al. Pulse verus continuous terbinafine for onychomycosis: A randomized, double-blind, controlled trial. J Am Acad Dermatol 2005;53: 578–584.
84. Gupta AK, Ryder JE, Johnson AM. Cumulative meta-analysis of systemic antifungal agents for the treatment of onychomycosis. Br J Dermatol 2004;150:537–544.
85. Haugh M, Helou S, Boissel JP, Cribier BJ. Terbinafine in fungal infections of the nails: A meta-analysis of randomized clinical trials. Br J Dermatol 2002;147:118–121.
86. Crawford F, Young P, Godfrey C, et al. Oral treatments for toenail onychomycosis: A systematic review. Arch Dermatol 2002;138:811–816.
87. Cribier BJ, Bakshi R. Terbinafine in the treatment of onychomycosis: A review of its efficacy in high-risk populations and in patients with nondermatophyte infections. Br J Dermatol 2004;150:414–420.
88. Casciano J, Amaya K, Doyle J, et al. Economic analysis of oral and topical therapies for onychomycosis of the toenails and fingernails. Manag Care 2003;12:47–54.
89. Schram SE, Warshaw EM. Costs of pulse versus continuous terbinafine for onychomycosis. J Am Acad Dermatol 2007;56:525–527.
90. Cham PM, Chen SC, Grill JP, et al. Reliability of self-reported willingness-to-pay and annual income in patients treated for toenail onychomycosis. Br J Dermatol 2007;156:922–928.
91. Food and Drug Administration. FDA issues health advisory regarding the safety of Sporanox products and Lamisil tablets to treat finger nail infections. 2001, *www.fda.gov/cder/drug/advisory/sporanox-lamisil/advisory.htm.*
92. Gupta AK, Chwetzoff, Del Rosso J, Baran R. Hepatic safety of itraconazole. J Cutan Med Surg 2002;6:210–213.

99

Invasive Fungal Infections

Peggy L. Carver

KEY CONCEPTS

1. Systemic mycoses can be caused by pathogenic fungi and include histoplasmosis, coccidioidomycosis, cryptococcosis, blastomycosis, paracoccidioidomycosis, and sporotrichosis, or infections by opportunistic fungi such as *Candida albicans*, *Aspergillus* species, *Trichosporon*, *Candida glabrata*, *Fusarium*, *Alternaria*, and *Mucor*.
2. The diagnosis of fungal infection generally is accomplished by careful evaluation of clinical symptoms, results of serologic tests, and histopathologic examination and culture of clinical specimens.
3. Histoplasmosis is caused by *Histoplasma capsulatum* and is endemic in parts of the central United States along the Ohio and Mississippi River valleys. Although most patients experience asymptomatic infection, some can experience chronic, disseminated disease.
4. Asymptomatic patients with histoplasmosis are not treated, although patients who do not have acquired immune deficiency syndrome (AIDS) patients with evident disease are treated with either oral ketoconazole or IV amphotericin B; AIDS patients are treated with amphotericin B and then receive lifelong suppression.
5. Blastomycosis is caused by *Blastomyces dermatitidis*. In the immunocompetent host, acute pulmonary blastomycosis can be mild and self-limited and may not require treatment. However, consideration should be given to treating all infected individuals to prevent extrapulmonary dissemination. All persons with moderate to severe pneumonia, disseminated infection, or those who are immunocompromised require antifungal therapy.
6. Coccidioidomycosis is caused by *Coccidioides immitis* and is endemic in some parts of the southwestern United States. It can cause nonspecific symptoms, acute pneumonia, or chronic pulmonary or disseminated disease. Primary pulmonary disease (unless severe) frequently is not treated, whereas extrapulmonary disease is treated with amphotericin B, and meningitis is treated with fluconazole.
7. Cryptococcosis is caused by *Cryptococcus neoformans*, which occurs primarily in immunocompromised patients, and *Cryptococcus gattii*, which occurs primarily in nonimmunocompromised patients. Patients with acute meningitis are treated with amphotericin B with flucytosine. Patients infected with human immunodeficiency virus (HIV) often require long-term suppressive therapy with fluconazole or itraconazole.
8. A variety of *Candida* species (including *C. albicans*, *C. glabrata*, *Candida tropicalis*, *Candida parapsilosis*, and *Candida krusei*) can cause diseases such as mucocutaneous, oral, esophageal, vaginal, and hematogenous candidiasis, as well as candiduria. Candidemia can be treated with a variety of antifungal agents; the optimal choice depends on previous patient exposure to antifungal agents, potential drug interactions and toxicities of each agent, and local epidemiology of intensive care unit (ICU) or hematology–oncology centers.
9. Aspergillosis can be caused by a variety of *Aspergillus* species that can cause superficial infections, pneumonia, allergic bronchopulmonary aspergillosis (BPA), or invasive infection. Voriconazole has emerged as the drug of choice of most clinicians for primary therapy of most patients with invasive aspergillosis (IA). Combination therapy, while widely used, lacks clinical trial data to support its use.

For many years, fungal infections were classified as either superficial "nuisance diseases," such as athlete's foot or vulvovaginal candidiasis, or as relatively rare infections confined primarily to endemic areas of the country. When invasive fungal infections were encountered, amphotericin B was the only consistently effective, systemically active agent available for the treatment of systemic mycoses. (1) Advances in medical technology including organ and bone marrow transplantation, cytotoxic chemotherapy, the widespread use of indwelling IV catheters, and the increased use of potent broad-spectrum antimicrobial agents all have contributed to the dramatic increase in the incidence of fungal infections worldwide.

Fungal infections have emerged as a major cause of death among cancer patients and transplant recipients.[1–3] In addition, patients with acquired immune deficiency syndrome (AIDS) experience substantially more frequent and severe forms of cryptococcosis, histoplasmosis, coccidioidomycosis, and mucocutaneous (esophageal, oral, and vulvovaginal) candidiasis.

Problems remain in the diagnosis, prevention, and treatment of fungal infections. Unlike the available diagnostic techniques for most bacterial pathogens, there remains a host of unresolved issues regarding standardization of susceptibility testing methods, in vitro and in vivo models of infection, the usefulness of monitoring antifungal plasma concentrations, and the development and identification of resistant pathogens.[1,4–6] The Infectious Diseases Society of America (IDSA) publishes guidelines for the treatment of many commonly encountered fungal infections.[7–12] These guidelines provide summaries of the literature and a consensus of expert opinions regarding the treatment of these difficult infections.

MYCOLOGY

Fungi are eukaryotic organisms with a defined nucleus enclosed by a nuclear membrane; a cytoplasmic membrane containing lipids, glycoproteins, and sterols, mitochondria, Golgi apparatus, and ribosomes bound to endoplasmic reticulum; and a cytoskeleton with microtubules, microfilaments, and intermediate filaments. Fungi have rigid cell walls composed of chitin, cellulose, or both that stain with Gomori methenamine silver or periodic acid–Schiff reagent. Most fungi, except *Candida* species, are too weakly gram-positive to be seen well on Gram stain. *Cryptococcus neoformans* has a polysaccharide capsule surrounding the cell wall.[1]

Morphologically, pathogenic fungi can be grouped as either filamentous molds or unicellular yeasts (Fig. 99-1). *Molds* grow as multicellular branching, threadlike filaments (hyphae) that are either septate (divided by transverse walls) or coenocytic (multinucleate without cross walls). On agar media, molds grow outward from the point of inoculation by extension of the tips of filaments and then branch repeatedly, interweaving to form fuzzy, matted growths called *mycelia*. Yeasts are oval or spherically shaped unicellular forms that generally produce pasty or mucoid colonies on agar medium similar to those observed with bacterial cultures. Yeasts have rigid cell walls and reproduce by budding, a process in which daughter cells arise from pinching off a portion of the parent cell.

Many pathogenic fungi, termed *dimorphic fungi*, exist as either a yeast or a mold, depending on pathogen, site of growth (in the host or in the laboratory setting), and temperature. Usually yeasts are the parasitic form that invades human or animal host tissue, whereas molds are the free-living form found in the environment. For example, *Histoplasma capsulatum* exists as a yeast in humans and as a mold in the laboratory.[1]

Susceptibility Testing of Antifungal Agents

Most laboratories do not routinely perform susceptibility tests on fungal isolates, but standardized methods for performing these tests are being developed and are now available for testing selected yeasts.

The Clinical and Laboratory Standards Institute (CLSI) defined clinical breakpoints (CBPs) for fluconazole, itraconazole, voriconazole, and flucytosine for all *Candida* species. Breakpoints are antimicrobial concentrations (MICs) obtained from susceptibility testing, which are used to define isolates as susceptible, intermediate, or resistant. No CBPs have been established for posaconazole or amphotericin B versus *Candida*.[6] (Tables 99-1 and 99-2). Reliable and convincing interpretive breakpoints are not yet available for amphotericin B since available methodology does not reliably identify amphotericin B-resistant isolates.[5–7] The breakpoints should be used following testing with the standardized, reproducible laboratory methodology used to develop the test and they should be interpreted in the context of the delivered dose of the antifungal agent.

Host factors contribute greatly to clinical outcome. A patient may respond clinically to treatment with an antifungal agent despite resistance to that agent in vitro because the patient's own immune system may eradicate the infection, or the agent may reach the site of infection in high concentrations.[13] Thus, in vitro susceptibility does *not* necessarily equate with in vivo clinical success, and in vitro resistance might *not* always correlate with treatment failure.

CBPs are based primarily on pharmacokinetic–pharmacodynamic relationships but do take into account other factors, such as differences in dosing regimens, toxicology, resistance mechanisms, intended or approved indications for use, clinical outcome data, and wild type (WT; i.e., the typical strain as it occurs in nature) MIC distributions. CBPs can be used to differentiate strains for which there is a high likelihood of treatment success (organisms which are clinically susceptible, or [S]), from those for which treatment is more likely to fail (clinically resistant [R]). A clinically intermediate (I) or susceptible dose-dependent (SDD) category can be assigned to pathogens for which the level of antimicrobial agent activity is associated with uncertain therapeutic effect, implying that infections due to the isolate may be appropriately treated in body sites where the drugs are physically concentrated or when a high dosage of drug can be used. Although CBPs are designed to guide therapy, they do not distinguish between fungal isolates with or without resistance mechanisms, nor do they always allow for early detection of resistant isolates.

Susceptibility testing occasionally is indicated, for example, in a patient with prolonged fungemia with a presumed susceptible isolate. Because of wide interlaboratory variability in test results, isolates should be tested at specialty laboratories that routinely perform these specialized tests. Susceptibility testing is most helpful in dealing with infections caused by non-*albicans* species of *Candida*.[5–7]

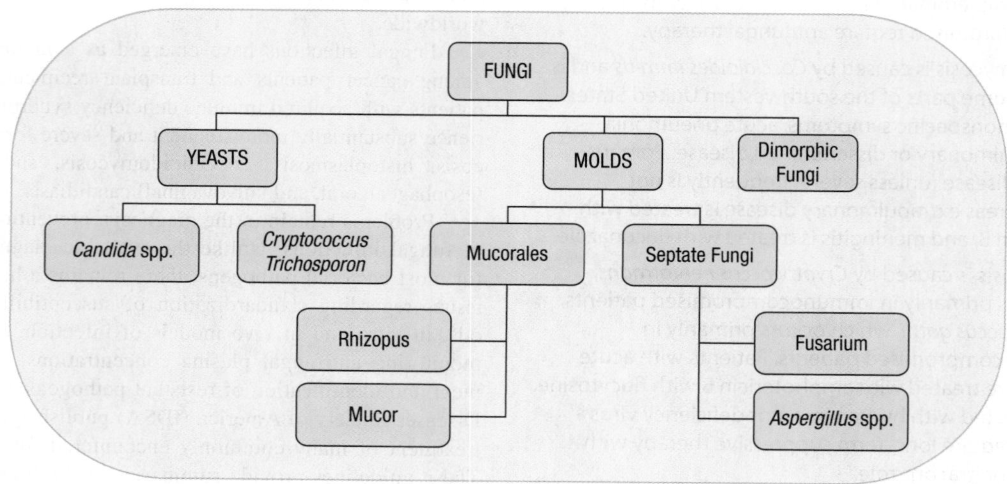

FIGURE 99-1 Morphologically, pathogenic fungi can be grouped as either filamentous molds or unicellular yeasts. *Molds* grow as multicellular branching, thread-like filaments (hyphae) that are either septate (divided by transverse walls) or coenocytic (multinucleate without cross walls).

TABLE 99-1 General Patterns of Susceptibility and Interpretive Breakpoints of *Candida* Species[a]

Candida Species	Patterns of Susceptibility							
	Azoles			*Echinocandins*			*Amphotericin*	
	Fluconazole	**Itraconazole**	**Voriconazole**	**Posaconazole**	**Caspofungin**	**Micafungin**	**Anidulafungin**	**Amphotericin B**
C. albicans	+++ S	+++ S	+++ S	S	+++	+++	+++	+++
C. tropicalis	+++ S	+++ S	+++ S	+++ S	+++ S	+++ S	+++ S	+++ S
C. parapsilosis	S	S	S	S	S[d]	S[d]	S[d]	S
C. glabrata	++ S-DD to R[b]	++ S-DD to R[c]	++	S	S	S	S	S-I[e]
C. krusei	R	S-DD to R[c]	S	S	S	S	S	S-I[e]
C. lusitaniae	S	S	S	S	S	S	S	S to R[f]

Current Interpretive Clinical Breakpoints[5,6]			
	Susceptible	**Susceptible-Dose Dependent**	**Resistant**
Fluconazole	≤8	16–32	≥64
Voriconazole	≤1	2	≥4
Itraconazole	≤0.125	0.25–0.5	≥1
	Susceptible	**Intermediate**	**Resistant**
Flucytosine	≤4	8–16	≥32
Echinocandins	≤2	NA	NA

Proposed Interpretive Clinical Breakpoints[5,6]			
	Susceptible	**Susceptible-Dose Dependent**	**Resistant**
Fluconazole	*C. albicans, C. tropicalis,* and *C. parapsilosis* ≤2	4	≥8
	C. glabrata —	≤32	≥64
	Susceptible	**Intermediate**	**Resistant**
Voriconazole	*C. albicans, C. tropicalis* and *parapsilosis* ≤0.125	0.25–0.5	≥1
	C krusei ≤0.5	1	≥2
Caspofungin Micafungin Anidulafungin	*C. albicans, C. tropicalis* and *C. krusei* ≤0.25	0.5	≥1
	C. parapsilosis ≤2	4	≥8
Caspofungin	*C. glabrata*		
Anidulafungin	≤0.12	0.25	≥0.5
Micafungin	≤0.06	0.12	≥0.25
Posaconazole		Interpretive criteria have not been established	
Amphotericin B		Interpretive criteria have not been established	

For antifungal drugs and pathogens for which susceptibility breakpoints have been established (fluconazole, itraconazole, voriconazole): S, susceptible; S-DD, susceptible-dose dependent (see the text); I, intermediate; R, resistant; NA, not applicable (has not been established for this antifungal against this pathogen). For antifungal drugs and pathogens for which susceptibility breakpoints have not been established, an estimate of relative activity: +++, reliable activity with occasional resistance; ++, moderate activity but resistance is noted; +, occasional activity; 0, no meaningful activity.

[a]Except for amphotericin B, interpretations are based on the use of a broth sensitivity test.
[b]Approximately 15% of *C. glabrata* isolates are resistant to fluconazole.
[c]Approximately 46% of *C. glabrata* isolates and 31% of *C. krusei* isolates are resistant to itraconazole.
[d]Most isolates of *C. parapsilosis* have reduced susceptibility to echinocandins.
[e]A significant proportion of *C. glabrata* and *C. krusei* isolates has reduced susceptibility to amphotericin B.
[f]Although frank resistance to amphotericin B is not observed in all isolates, it is well described for isolates of *C. lusitaniae*.

Data from Pfaller et al.[5] and Eschenauer et al.[6]

Resistance to Antifungal Agents

It is important to distinguish between clinical resistance and microbial resistance. *Clinical resistance* refers to failure of an antifungal agent in the treatment of a fungal infection that arises from factors other than microbial resistance, such as failure of the antifungal agent to reach the site of infection or inability of a patient's immune system to eradicate a fungus whose growth is retarded by an antifungal agent.[13]

Microbial resistance can refer to *primary* or *secondary* resistance, as determined by in vitro susceptibility testing using standardized methodology. *Primary* or *intrinsic resistance* refers to resistance recorded prior to drug exposure in vitro or in vivo. *Secondary* or *acquired resistance* develops on exposure to an antifungal agent and can be either reversible, owing to transient adaptation, or acquired as a result of one or more genetic alterations. The clinical consequences of antifungal resistance can be observed in treatment failures and in changes in the prevalences of *Candida* species causing disease.[13]

The most exhaustive and definitive accounts of antifungal resistance have been described in *Candida* species, in particular *Candida*

TABLE 99-2 General Patterns of In Vitro Susceptibility of Non-Candida Fungal Pathogens[a]

	Patterns of Susceptibility							
	Azoles			*Echinocandins*			*Amphotericin B*	
Pathogen	**Fluconazole**	**Itraconazole**	**Voriconazole**	**Posaconazole**	**Caspofungin**	**Micafungin**	**Anidulafungin**	**Amphotericin B**
Aspergillus								
A. fumigatus	No	Yes	Yes	Yes	Yes	Yes	Yes	Yes
A. flavus	No	Yes	Yes	Yes	Yes	Yes	Yes	Yes
A. terreus	No	Yes	Yes		Yes			No
Fusarium	No	No	Yes (but break-through infections are seen)	Conflicting data (species dependent)	No	No	No	Yes but occasional resistance
Scedosporium	No	No	Yes	Yes (apiospermum)	No	No	No	No
Zygomycetes[b]	No	No	No	Yes	No	No	No	Yes
Trichosporon	No	No	Yes	Yes	No	No	No	No
Cryptococcus	Yes	Yes	Yes	Yes	No	No	No	
Histoplasma	Yes	Yes	Yes	Yes	No[c]	No[c]	No[c]	Yes
Coccidioides	Yes	Yes	Yes	Yes	No[c]	No[c]	No[c]	Yes

[a]No = has minimal or no in vitro activity versus the pathogen; Yes = possesses adequate in vitro activity versus the pathogen.
[b]Includes *Rhizopus*, *Mucor*, and *Absidia* species.
[c]While the echinocandins display activity against the mycelial forms of endemic fungi such as *Histoplasma* spp., *Blastomyces* spp., and *Coccidioides* spp., they display significantly higher MIC values against the yeast forms of these organisms, and should not be used to treat these infections.
Data from Eschenauer et al.[52] and Dodds Ashley et al.[78]

albicans and, to a lesser extent, *Candida glabrata*, *Candida tropicalis*, and *Candida krusei*, as well as in a few *C. neoformans* isolates.[14] There are four different mechanisms that result in azole resistance: (a) mutations or upregulation of *ERG11* (an enzyme involved in the ergosterol biosynthesis pathway), (b) expression of multidrug efflux transport pumps that decrease antifungal drug accumulation within the fungal cell, (c) alteration of the structure or concentration of antifungal drug target proteins, and (d) alteration of membrane sterol proteins (Fig. 99-2). It is beyond the scope of this chapter to provide a complete discussion of the biochemical mechanisms of fungal resistance. Interested readers are referred to several excellent reviews concerning this topic.[13,14]

Among hospitalized patients, there is increasing evidence for a shift toward isolation of other resistant species, such as *C. glabrata*

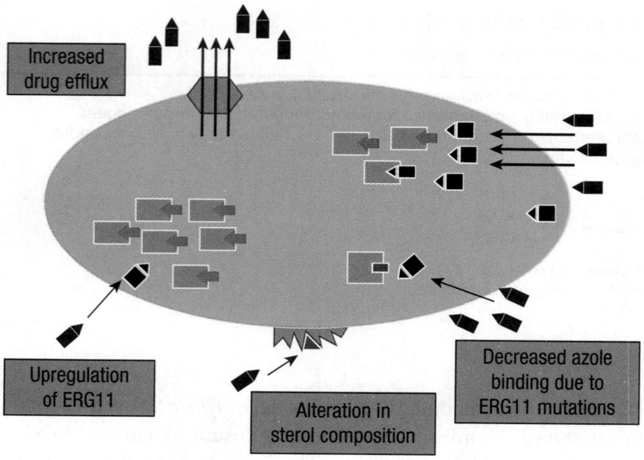

FIGURE 99-2 Mechanisms of azole resistance. Four different mechanisms result in azole resistance: (a) mutations or upregulation of *ERG11*, the target enzyme of azoles, (b) expression of multidrug efflux transport pumps that decrease antifungal drug accumulation within the fungal cell, (c) alteration of the structure or concentration of antifungal drug target proteins, and (d) alteration of membrane sterol proteins.

and *C. krusei*, that have moderate or high-level resistance to fluconazole. This phenomenon has been especially common among patients in whom fluconazole has been used extensively.[3]

The most commonly reported mechanisms of azole resistance among *C. albicans* isolates include reduced permeability of the fungal cell membrane to azoles, alteration in the target fungal enzymes (cytochrome P450, CYP) resulting in decreased binding of the azole to the target site, and overproduction of the fungal CYP enzymes. Studies also suggest the presence of efflux pumps capable of actively pumping azoles from the target pathogen, thereby conferring multidrug resistance to azole antifungals.[13,14] *C. glabrata* isolates are increasingly resistant to both azole and echinocandin antifungal agents.

Although rare, in vitro intrinsic resistance to amphotericin B is described, primarily in *Candida lusitaniae*, *Candida guilliermondii*, and some molds (*Fusarium* spp. and *Pseudallescheria boydii*).[6] Although the rate of apparent resistance to amphotericin B appears to be quite low, breakthrough bacteremias in patients treated with amphotericin B have been observed. *C. glabrata*, *C. guilliermondii*, *C. krusei*, and *C. lusitaniae* appear to have a higher propensity than other *Candida* species to develop resistance to amphotericin B; this point should be kept in mind when treating patients with infections caused by one of these pathogens.[6,13] Acquired resistance of *Aspergillus* species to azoles or echinocandins is relatively uncommon.

Resistant isolates of *C. neoformans* have been reported to have a mutation in the C8 isomerization step of ergosterol synthesis.[6] Current guidelines for the management of cryptococcal infections recommend susceptibility testing only for patients in whom primary treatment has failed, patients with relapse, and for those with recent exposure to antifungals.[6] Acquired resistance of *Candida* species to echinocandins is typically mediated via one of several mechanisms: acquisition of, or intrinsic possession of point mutations in the FKS genes encoding the major subunit of its target enzyme.[6]

PATHOGENESIS AND EPIDEMIOLOGY

Systemic mycoses caused by primary or pathogenic fungi include histoplasmosis, coccidioidomycosis, cryptococcosis, blastomycosis, paracoccidioidomycosis, and sporotrichosis. Primary pathogens can cause disease in both healthy and immunocompromised individuals, although disease generally is more severe or disseminated in the immunocompromised host. In contrast, mycoses caused by opportunistic fungi such as *C. albicans*, *Aspergillus* species, *Trichosporon*, *Torulopsis (Candida) glabrata*, *Fusarium*, *Alternaria*, and *Mucor* generally are found only in the immunocompromised host.[1]

Most fungal infections are acquired as a result of accidental inhalation of airborne conidia. For example, *H. capsulatum* is found in soil contaminated by bat, chicken, or starling excreta, and *C. neoformans* is associated with pigeon droppings. Although some fungi, including *C. albicans*, *C. neoformans*, and *Aspergillus* species, are ubiquitous pathogens with worldwide distribution, other fungi have regional distributions associated with specific geographic environments.[1]

Systemic fungal infections are a major cause of morbidity and mortality in the immunocompromised patient. Fungal infections account for 20% to 30% of fatal infections in patients with acute leukemia, 10% to 15% of fatal infections in patients with lymphoma, and 5% of fatal infections in patients with solid tumors. The frequency of fungal infections among transplant recipients ranges from 0% to 20% for kidney and bone marrow transplant recipients, to 10% to 35% for heart transplant recipients, and 30% to 40% for liver transplant recipients.[15,16]

Approximately 2% to 4% of all hospitalized patients develop a nosocomial infection. Of these, bacteria comprise the most common etiologic agent.[1] Fungi, however, are becoming increasingly significant nosocomial pathogens. Fungi account for 10% of all bloodstream isolates. *Candida* species (primarily *C. albicans*) are the fourth most commonly isolated bloodstream isolate and account for 78% of all nosocomial fungal infections.[17]

Nosocomially acquired fungal infections can arise from either exogenous or endogenous flora. Endogenous flora can include normal commensal organisms of the skin, GI, genitourinary, or respiratory tract. *C. albicans* is found as a normal commensal of the GI tract in 20% to 30% of humans.

A complex interplay of host and pathogen factors influences the acquisition and development of fungal infections. Intact skin or mucosal surfaces serve as primary barriers to infection. Desiccation, epithelial cell turnover, fatty acid content, and low pH of the skin are believed to be important factors in host resistance. Bacterial flora of the skin and mucous membranes compete with fungi for growth. Alterations in the balance of normal flora caused by the use of antibiotics or alterations in nutritional status can allow the proliferation of fungi such as *Candida*, increasing the likelihood of systemic invasion and infection.[1]

Tissue reaction in the presence of fungi varies with fungal species, site of proliferation, and duration of infection. Phagocytosis by neutrophils and macrophages is the earliest mechanism that prevents the establishment of fungi. Consequently, patients with decreased neutrophil counts or decreased neutrophil function are at higher risk of infections, particularly infections caused by *Candida* and *Aspergillus* species. Some mycoses are characterized by a low-grade inflammatory response that does not eliminate the fungi. Fungal cells sometimes can persist within macrophages without being killed, perhaps because of resistance to the effects of lysosomal enzymes.[1]

DIAGNOSIS

2 The diagnosis of invasive fungal infections generally is accomplished by careful evaluation of clinical symptoms, results of serologic tests, and histopathologic examination and culture of clinical specimens. Skin tests generally are not useful diagnostically because they do not distinguish between active and past infection. They remain useful as screening tools and in epidemiologic studies to determine endemic areas. It is beyond the scope of this chapter to discuss the relative merits of each of the immunologic tests used in the diagnosis of invasive fungal infections. Interested readers, however, are referred to several excellent reviews concerning this topic.[18,19]

TREATMENT
Invasive Mycoses

Strategies for the prevention or treatment of invasive mycoses can be classified broadly as prophylaxis, early empirical therapy, empirical therapy, and secondary prophylaxis or suppression.[1] In patients undergoing cytotoxic chemotherapy, antifungal therapy is directed primarily at the prevention or treatment of infections caused by *Candida* and *Aspergillus* species. Prophylactic therapy with topical, oral, or IV antifungal agents is administered prior to and throughout periods of granulocytopenia (absolute neutrophil count <1,000 cells/L). The potential benefits of prophylactic therapy must be weighed against the potential risks inherent in each regimen, including safety, efficacy, cost, the prevalence of infection, and the potential consequences (e.g., resistance) of widespread use.

Early empirical therapy is the administration of systemic antifungal agents at the onset of fever and neutropenia. Empirical therapy with systemic antifungal agents is administered to granulocytopenic patients with persistent or recurrent fever despite the administration of appropriate antimicrobial therapy.

Secondary prophylaxis (or suppressive therapy) is the administration of systemic antifungal agents (generally prior to and throughout the period of granulocytopenia) to prevent relapse of a documented invasive fungal infection that was treated during a previous episode of granulocytopenia.

Although these treatment classifications also have been applied to the treatment of fungal infections in AIDS, patients with AIDS rarely acquire systemic infections caused by *Candida* or *Aspergillus* species, unless they become granulocytopenic because of disease or drugs. The use of antifungal prophylaxis is much less widely studied in this population, although studies suggest that early antifungal prophylaxis with fluconazole or itraconazole decreases the incidence of invasive cryptococcal disease among adult patients who have advanced human immunodeficiency virus (HIV) disease and severe immune suppression (CD4 count <50 cells/mm^3 [<50 × 10^6/L]). However, neither of these interventions showed a clear effect on mortality.[9] Suppressive therapy generally is necessary following acute therapy for histoplasmosis, coccidioidomycosis, and cryptococcosis because of the high rates of relapse when antifungal therapy is discontinued.

HISTOPLASMOSIS

In humans, histoplasmosis is caused by inhalation of dust-borne microconidia of the dimorphic fungus *H. capsulatum*. Although there exist two dimorphic varieties of *H. capsulatum*, the small-celled (2 to 5 microns) form (var. *capsulatum*) occurs globally, whereas the large-celled (8 to 15 microns) form (var. *duboisii*) is confined to the African continent and Madagascar. In tissues stained by conventional techniques, *H. capsulatum* appears as an oval or round, narrow-pore, budding, unencapsulated yeast.[20]

Epidemiology

3 Although histoplasmosis is found worldwide, certain areas of North and Central America are recognized as endemic areas. In the United States, most disease is localized along the Ohio and Mississippi River valleys, where more than 90% of residents may be

affected. Precise reasons for this endemic distribution pattern are unknown but are thought to include moderate climate, humidity, and soil characteristics. *H. capsulatum* is found in nitrogen-enriched soils, particularly those heavily contaminated by avian or bat guano, which accelerates sporulation. Blackbird or pigeon roosts, chicken coops, and sites frequented by bats, such as caves, attics, or old buildings, serve as "microfoci" of infections; once contaminated, soils yield *Histoplasma* for many years. Although birds are not infected because of their high body temperature, bats (mammals) may be infected and can pass yeast forms in their feces, allowing the spread of *H. capsulatum* to new habitats. Air currents carry the spores for great distances, exposing individuals who were unaware of contact with the contaminated site.[20]

Pathophysiology

At ambient temperatures, *H. capsulatum* grows as a mold. The mycelial phase consists of septate branching hyphae with terminal micro- and macroconidia that range in size from 2 to 14 microns in diameter. When soil is disturbed, these conidia become aerosolized and reach the bronchioles or alveoli.[20]

Animal studies demonstrate that within 2 to 3 days after reaching lung tissue, the conidia germinate, releasing yeast forms that begin multiplying by binary fission. During the next 9 to 15 days, organisms are ingested but not destroyed by large numbers of macrophages that are recruited to the infected site, resulting in small infiltrates. Infected macrophages migrate to the mediastinal lymph nodes and other sites within the mononuclear phagocyte system, particularly the spleen and liver. At this time, the onset of specific T-cell immunity in the nonimmune host activates the macrophages, rendering them capable of fungicidal activity. Tissue granulomas form, many of which develop central caseation and necrosis over the next 2 to 4 months. Over a period of several years, these foci become encapsulated and calcified, often with viable yeast trapped within the necrotic tissue.[20,21]

Cellular immunity, as measured by histoplasmin skin-test reactivity, wanes in the absence of occasional reexposure. Although exposure to heavy inocula can overcome these immune mechanisms, resulting in severe disease, reinfection occurs frequently in endemic areas. In the immune individual, the reactions of acquired immunity begin 24 to 48 hours after the appearance of yeast forms, resulting in milder forms of illness and little proliferation of organisms. Although viable organisms can be found within granulomas years after initial infection, the organisms appear to have little ability to proliferate within the fibrous capsules, except in immunocompromised patients.[20,21]

Clinical Presentation

The outcome of infection with *H. capsulatum* depends on a complex interplay of host, pathogen, and environmental factors.[10,20,21] Host factors include the degree of immunosuppression and the presence of immunity (from prior infection). Environmental factors include inoculum size, exposure within an enclosed area, and duration of exposure. Hematogenous dissemination from the lungs to other tissues probably occurs in all infected individuals during the first 2 weeks of infection before specific immunity has developed but is nonprogressive in most cases, which leads to the development of calcified granulomas of the liver and/or spleen. Progressive pulmonary infection is common in patients with underlying centrilobular emphysema.

Acute and chronic manifestations of histoplasmosis appear to result from unusual inflammatory or fibrotic responses to the pathogen, including pericarditis and rheumatologic syndromes during the first year after exposure, with chronic mediastinal inflammation or fibrosis, broncholithiasis, and enlarging parenchymal granulomas later in the course of disease.

Acute Pulmonary Histoplasmosis

In the vast majority of patients, low-inoculum exposure to *H. capsulatum* results in mild or asymptomatic pulmonary histoplasmosis. The course of disease generally is benign, and symptoms usually abate within a few weeks of onset. Patients exposed to a higher inoculum during an acute primary infection or reinfection can experience an acute, self-limited illness with flu-like pulmonary symptoms, including fever, chills, headache, myalgia, and a nonproductive cough. Patients with diffuse pulmonary histoplasmosis can have diffuse radiographic involvement, become hypoxic, and require ventilatory support. A low percentage of patients present with arthritis, erythema nodosum, pericarditis, or mediastinal granuloma.

Chronic Pulmonary Histoplasmosis

Chronic pulmonary histoplasmosis generally presents as an opportunistic infection imposed on a preexisting structural abnormality, such as lesions resulting from emphysema. Patients demonstrate chronic pulmonary symptoms and apical lung lesions that progress with inflammation, calcified granulomas, and fibrosis. Patients with early, noncavitary disease often recover without treatment. Progression of disease over a period of years, seen in 25% to 30% of patients, is associated with cavitation, bronchopleural fistulas, extension to the other lung, pulmonary insufficiency, and often death.

Disseminated Histoplasmosis

In patients exposed to a large inoculum and in immunocompromised hosts, successful containment of the organism within macrophages may not occur, resulting in a progressive illness characterized by yeast-filled phagocytic cells and an inability to produce granulomas. This disease, termed *disseminated histoplasmosis*, is characterized by persistent parasitization of macrophages. The clinical severity of the diverse forms of disseminated histoplasmosis (Table 99-3) generally parallels the degree of macrophage parasitization observed.

Acute (infantile) disseminated histoplasmosis is characterized by massive involvement of the mononuclear phagocyte system by yeast-engorged macrophages. Classically, this severe type of infection is seen in infants and young children and (rarely) in adults with Hodgkin's disease or other lymphoproliferative disorders. In infants or children, acute disseminated histoplasmosis is characterized by unrelenting fever, anemia, leukopenia or thrombocytopenia, enlargement of the liver, spleen, and visceral lymph nodes, and GI symptoms, particularly nausea, vomiting, and diarrhea. The chest roentgenogram often demonstrates remnants of the initiating acute pulmonary lesion. Untreated disease is uniformly fatal in 1 to 2 months. A less severe "subacute" form of the disease, which occurs in both infants and immunocompetent adults, is characterized by focal destructive lesions in various organs, weight loss, weakness, fever, and malaise. Untreated disease generally is fatal in approximately 10 months.

Most adults with disseminated histoplasmosis demonstrate a mild, chronic form of the disease. Untreated patients often are ill for 10 to 20 years, demonstrating long asymptomatic periods interrupted by relapses of clinical illness characterized primarily by weight loss, weakness, and fatigue. Chronic disseminated histoplasmosis can be seen in patients with lymphoreticular neoplasms (Hodgkin's disease) and patients undergoing immunosuppressant chemotherapy for organ transplantation or for rheumatic diseases. Although CNS involvement occurs in 10% to 20% of patients with severe underlying immunosuppressive conditions, focal organ involvement is uncommon. The disease is characterized by the development of focal granulomatous lesions, often with bone marrow involvement resulting in thrombocytopenia, anemia, and leukemia. Fever, hepatosplenomegaly, and GI ulceration are common.

TABLE 99-3 Clinical Manifestations and Therapy of Histoplasmosis

Type of Disease and Common Clinical Manifestations	Approximate Frequency (%)[a]	Therapy/Comments
Nonimmunosuppressed Host		
Acute pulmonary histoplasmosis		
Asymptomatic or mild to moderate disease	50–99	*Asymptomatic, mild, or symptoms <4 weeks:* No therapy generally required. Itraconazole (200 mg three times daily for 3 days and then 200 mg once or twice daily for 6–12 weeks) is recommended for patients who continue to have symptoms for 11 months *Symptoms >4 weeks:* Itraconazole 200 mg once daily × 6–12 weeks[b]
Self-limited disease	1–50	*Self-limited disease:* Amphotericin B[c] 0.3–0.5 mg/kg/day × 2–4 weeks (total dose 500 mg) or ketoconazole 400 mg orally daily × 3–6 months can be beneficial in patients with severe hypoxia following inhalation of large inocula; antifungal therapy generally not useful for arthritis or pericarditis; NSAIDs or corticosteroids can be useful in some cases
Mediastinal granulomas	1–50	Most lesions resolve spontaneously; surgery or antifungal therapy with amphotericin B 40–50 mg/day × 2–3 weeks or itraconazole 400 mg/day orally × 6–12 months can be beneficial in some severe cases; mild to moderate disease can be treated with itraconazole for 6–12 months
Moderately severe to severe diffuse pulmonary disease		Lipid amphotericin B 3–5 mg/kg/day followed by itraconazole 200 mg twice daily for 3 days then twice daily for a total of 12 weeks of therapy; alternatively, in patients at low risk for nephrotoxicity, amphotericin B deoxycholate 0.7–1 mg/kg/day can be utilized; methylprednisolone (0.5–1 mg/kg daily IV) during the first 1–2 weeks of antifungal therapy is recommended for patients who develop respiratory complications, including hypoxemia or significant respiratory distress
Inflammatory/fibrotic disease	0.02	*Fibrosing mediastinitis:* The benefit of antifungal therapy (itraconazole 200 mg twice daily × 3 months) is controversial but should be considered, especially in patients with elevated ESR or CF titers ≤1:32; surgery can be of benefit if disease is detected early; late disease cannot respond to therapy *Sarcoid-like:* NSAIDs or corticosteroids[d] can be of benefit for some patients *Pericarditis:* Severe disease: corticosteroids 1 mg/kg/day or pericardial drainage procedure
Chronic cavitary pulmonary histoplasmosis	0.05	Antifungal therapy generally recommended for all patients to halt further lung destruction and reduce mortality *Mild–moderate disease:* Itraconazole (200 mg three times daily for 3 days and then one or two times daily for at least 1 year; some clinicians recommend therapy for 18–24 months due to the high rate of relapse; itraconazole plasma concentrations should be obtained after the patient has been receiving this agent for at least 2 weeks *Severe disease:* Amphotericin B 0.7 mg/kg/day for a minimum total dose of 25–35 mg/kg is effective in 59–100% of cases and should be used in patients who require hospitalization or are unable to take itraconazole because of drug interactions, allergies, failure to absorb drug, or failure to improve clinically after a minimum of 12 weeks of itraconazole therapy
Histoplasma endocarditis		Amphotericin B (lipid formulations may be preferred, due to their lower rate of renal toxicity) plus a valve replacement is recommended; if the valve cannot be replaced, lifelong suppression with itraconazole is recommended
CNS histoplasmosis		Amphotericin B should be used as initial therapy (lipid formulations at 5 mg/kg/day, for a total dosage of 175 mg/kg may be preferred, due to their lower rate of renal toxicity) for 4–6 weeks, followed by an oral azole (fluconazole or itraconazole 200 mg two or three times daily) for at least a year; some patients may require lifelong therapy; response to therapy should be monitored by repeat lumbar punctures to assess *Histoplasma* antigen levels, WBC, and CF antibody titers; blood levels of itraconazole should be obtained to ensure adequate drug exposure
Immunosuppressed Host		
Disseminated histoplasmosis	0.02–0.05	*Disseminated histoplasmosis:* Untreated mortality 83–93%; relapse 5–23% in non-AIDS patients; therapy is recommended for all patients
Acute (Infantile)		*Nonimmunosuppressed patients:* Ketoconazole 400 mg/day orally × 6–12 months or amphotericin B 35 mg/kg IV
Subacute		*Immunosuppressed patients (non-AIDS) or endocarditis or CNS disease:* Amphotericin B >35 mg/kg × 3 months followed by fluconazole or itraconazole 200 mg orally twice daily × 12 months
Progressive histoplasmosis (immunocompetent patients and immunosuppressed patients without AIDS)		*Moderately severe to severe:* Liposomal amphotericin B (3 mg/kg daily), amphotericin B lipid complex (ABLC, 5 mg/kg daily), or deoxycholate amphotericin B (0.7–1 mg/kg daily) for 1–2 weeks, followed by itraconazole (200 mg twice daily for at least 12 months) *Mild to moderate:* Itraconazole (200 mg twice daily for at least 12 months)
Progressive disease of AIDS	25–50[e]	Amphotericin B 15–30 mg/kg (1–2 g over 4–10 weeks)[f] or itraconazole 200 mg three times daily for 3 days then twice daily for 12 weeks, followed by lifelong suppressive therapy with itraconazole 200–400 mg orally daily; although patients receiving secondary prophylaxis (chronic maintenance therapy) might be at low risk for recurrence of systemic mycosis when their CD4+ T-lymphocyte counts increase to >100 cells/μL (>100 × 10^6/L) in response to HAART, the number of patients who have been evaluated is insufficient to warrant a recommendation to discontinue prophylaxis

AIDS, acquired immunodeficiency syndrome; CF, complement fixation; ESR, erythrocyte sedimentation rate; HAART, highly active antiretroviral therapy; NSAIDs, nonsteroidal antiinflammatory drugs; PO, orally.

[a]As a percentage of all patients presenting with histoplasmosis.

[b]Itraconazole plasma concentrations should be measured during the second week of therapy to ensure that detectable concentrations have been achieved. If the concentration is below 1 mcg/mL (mg/L; 1.4 μmol/L), the dose may be insufficient or drug interactions can be impairing absorption or accelerating metabolism, requiring a change in dosage. If plasma concentrations are greater than 10 mcg/mL (mg/L; 14 μmol/L), the dosage can be reduced.

[c]Deoxycholate amphotericin B.

[d]Effectiveness of corticosteroids is controversial.

[e]As a percentage of AIDS patients presenting with histoplasmosis as the initial manifestation of their disease.

[f]Liposomal amphotericin B (AmBisome) may be more appropriate for disseminated disease.

Data from Wheat et al.,[10] Deepe,[20] and Kauffman.[21]

Histoplasmosis in HIV-Infected Patients

Adult patients with AIDS demonstrate an acute form of disseminated disease that resembles the syndrome seen in infants and children. Progressive disseminated histoplasmosis (PDH), which is defined as a clinical illness that does not improve after at least 3 weeks of observation and that is associated with physical or radiographic findings and/or laboratory evidence of involvement of extrapulmonary tissues, can occur as the direct result of initial infection or because of the reactivation of dormant foci. In endemic areas, 50% of AIDS patients demonstrate PDH as the first manifestation of their disease. PDH is characterized by fever (75% of patients), weight loss, chills, night sweats, enlargement of the spleen, liver, or lymph nodes, and anemia. Pulmonary symptoms occur in only one third of patients and do not always correlate with the presence of infiltrates on chest roentgenogram. A clinical syndrome resembling septicemia is seen in approximately 25% to 50% of patients.[21]

Diagnosis

Detection of single, yeastlike cells 2 to 5 microns in diameter with narrow-based budding by direct examination or by histologic study of blood smears or tissues should raise strong suspicion of infection with *H. capsulatum* because colonization does not occur as with *Aspergillus* or *Candida* infection. Identification of mycelial isolates from clinical cultures can be made by conversion of the mycelium to the yeast form (requires 3 to 6 weeks) or through a rapid (2 hours) and 100% sensitive chemiluminescent DNA probe that recognizes ribosomal DNA. In patients with suspected disseminated or chronic cavitary histoplasmosis, 2 to 3 blood, sputum, and bone marrow cultures and stains should be obtained using the lysis centrifugation (Isolator tube) technique, and the cultures should be held for 14 to 21 days for optimal yield of *H. capsulatum*. In patients with acute self-limited histoplasmosis, extensive testing to verify the diagnosis may not be necessary.

In most patients, serologic evidence remains the primary method in the diagnosis of histoplasmosis. Results obtained from commercially available complement fixation (CF), immunodiffusion (ID), and latex agglutination (LA) antibody tests are used alone or in combination. In general, the use of histoplasmin skin tests is of little value except in epidemiologic studies because histoplasmin reactivity waxes in the absence of occasional reexposure. In addition, histoplasmin skin testing can result in a false increase in the CF titer for mycelial antigen (CF-M) to *H. capsulatum*. A fourfold rise in the CF titer is usually indicative of recent infection, although some patients with severe disease or profound immunosuppression can demonstrate a weaker antibody response. CF titers remain positive for many years, since CF antibodies persist after infection. Because the ID test is more specific but less sensitive than CF, it should be used to assess the importance of weakly reactive results obtained by CF rather than as a screening procedure.

In the AIDS patient with PDH, the diagnosis is best established by bone marrow biopsy and culture, which yield positive cultures in more than 90% of patients, although blood cultures and histopathologic examination and culture of pulmonary tissue, sputum, skin, and lymph nodes also can be helpful. Detection of *H. capsulatum* polysaccharide antigen (HPA) in urine, blood, or cerebrospinal fluid (CSF) by enzyme-linked immunosorbent assay (ELISA) or by modified radioimmunoassay (RIA) offer promising new techniques for the rapid diagnosis of histoplasmosis. The HPA (by RIA) levels also have been used successfully to monitor the course of therapy and to detect relapses in patients with AIDS, and the clearance of antigen from serum and urine correlates with clinical efficacy during maintenance therapy with itraconazole.[21]

TREATMENT

Non–HIV-Infected Patient

❹ Table 99-3 summarizes the recommended therapy for the treatment of histoplasmosis. In general, asymptomatic or mildly ill patients and patients with sarcoid-like disease do not benefit from antifungal therapy. In the vast majority of patients, low-inoculum exposure to *H. capsulatum* results in *mild* or *asymptomatic* pulmonary histoplasmosis. The course of disease generally is benign, and symptoms usually abate within a few weeks of onset. Therapy can be helpful in symptomatic patients whose conditions have not improved during the first month of infection. Fever persisting more than 3 weeks can indicate that the patient is developing progressive disseminated disease, which can be aborted by antifungal therapy. Whether antifungal therapy hastens recovery or prevents complications is unknown because it has never been studied in prospective trials.

Fluconazole remains a second-line agent for the treatment of histoplasmosis. Clinical data regarding the use of newer azoles such as voriconazole and posaconazole are limited. While both have activity against *Histoplasma*, posaconazole appears to be more active than itraconazole in the immune compromised and nonimmune compromised mouse model of infection, while voriconazole has not been tested in animal models. Both agents have been used successfully in a few patients. Of note, the echinocandins have no activity against *Histoplasma*.

Patients with mild, self-limited disease, chronic disseminated disease, or chronic pulmonary histoplasmosis who have no underlying immunosuppression usually can be treated with either oral itraconazole or IV amphotericin B. The goals of therapy are resolution of clinical abnormalities, prevention of relapse, and eradication of infection whenever possible, although chronic suppression of infection can be adequate in immunosuppressed patients, including those with HIV disease.[10,21]

HIV-Infected Patient

In AIDS patients, intensive 12-week primary antifungal therapy (induction and consolidation therapy) is followed by lifelong suppressive (maintenance) therapy with itraconazole. Amphotericin B dosages of 50 mg/day (up to 1 mg/kg per day) should be administered IV to a cumulative dose of 15 to 35 mg/kg (1 to 2 g) in patients who require hospitalization. Amphotericin B can be replaced with itraconazole 200 mg orally twice daily when the patient no longer requires hospitalization or IV therapy to complete a 12-week total course of induction therapy. In patients who do not require hospitalization, itraconazole therapy for 12 weeks can be used.

Fluconazole 800 mg/day orally as induction, followed by 400 mg/day, was effective in 88% of patients, but relapses occurred in approximately one third of patients, and in vitro resistance developed in approximately 50% of patients who relapsed.

In regions experiencing high rates of histoplasmosis (>5 cases/100 patient-years), itraconazole 200 mg/day is recommended as prophylactic therapy in HIV-infected patients. Fluconazole is not an acceptable alternative because of its inferior activity against *H. capsulatum* and its lower efficacy for the treatment of histoplasmosis.[10]

Although patients receiving secondary prophylaxis (chronic maintenance therapy) might be at low risk for recurrence of systemic mycosis when their CD4+ T lymphocyte counts increase to >100 cells/μL ($>100 \times 10^6$/L) in response to highly active antiretroviral therapy (HAART), the number of patients who have been evaluated is insufficient to warrant a recommendation to discontinue prophylaxis.

Evaluation of Therapeutic Outcomes

Response to therapy should be measured by resolution of radiologic, serologic, and microbiologic parameters and by improvement in signs and symptoms of infection. Although investigators are limited by the lack of standardized criteria to quantify the extent of infection, degree of immunosuppression, or treatment response, response rates (based on resolution or improvement in presenting signs and symptoms) of greater than 80% have been reported in case series in AIDS patients receiving varied dosages of amphotericin B. Rapid responses are reported, with the resolution of symptoms in 25% and 75% of patients by days 3 and 7 of therapy, respectively.

After the initial course of therapy for histoplasmosis is complete, lifelong suppressive therapy with oral azoles or amphotericin B (1 to 1.5 mg/kg weekly or biweekly) is recommended because of the frequent recurrence of infection. Relapse rates in AIDS patients not receiving maintenance therapy range from 50% to 90%.[10]

Antigen testing can be useful for monitoring therapy in patients with disseminated histoplasmosis. Antigen concentrations decrease with therapy and increase with relapse.

BLASTOMYCOSIS

North American blastomycosis is a systemic fungal infection caused by *Blastomyces dermatitidis*, a dimorphic fungus that infects primarily the lungs. Patients, however, can present with a variety of pulmonary and extrapulmonary clinical manifestations. Pulmonary disease can be acute or chronic and can mimic infection with tuberculosis, pyogenic bacteria, other fungi, or malignancy. Blastomycosis can disseminate to virtually every other body organ, and approximately 40% of patients with blastomycosis present with skin, bone and joint, or genitourinary tract involvement without any evidence of pulmonary disease.[8,22]

Pulmonary infection probably occurs by inhalation of conidia, which convert to the yeast form in the lung. A vigorous inflammatory response ensues, with neutrophilic recruitment to the lungs followed by the development of cell-mediated immunity and the formation of noncaseating granulomas.

Epidemiology

Blastomycosis was renamed *North American blastomycosis* in 1942, when Conant and Howell named a similar fungus endemic to South America, *Blastomyces braziliensis*, and the disease it caused *South American blastomycosis*. Although the disease is now recognized to be endemic to the southeastern and south central states of the United States (especially those bordering on the Mississippi and Ohio River basins) and the midwestern states and Canadian provinces bordering the Great Lakes, numerous cases of North American blastomycosis have been diagnosed in Africa, northern parts of South America, India, and Europe. Endemic areas have been defined primarily by analysis of sporadic cases and epidemics or clusters of disease because the lack of a dependable skin or laboratory test makes wide-scale epidemiologic testing to determine the incidence of infection unfeasible at present.[8,19,22] Although initial review of sporadic cases suggested that males with outdoor occupations that exposed them to soil were at greatest risk for blastomycosis, there is no sex, age, or occupational predilection for blastomycosis.[8,19,22]

Although *B. dermatitidis* generally is considered to be a soil inhabitant, attempts to isolate the organism in nature frequently have been unsuccessful. *B. dermatitidis* has been isolated from soil containing decayed vegetation, decomposed wood, and pigeon manure, frequently in association with warm, moist soil of wooded areas that is rich in organic debris.[8,19,22]

Pathophysiology and Clinical Presentation

Colonization does not occur with *Blastomyces*.[8,19,22] *Acute pulmonary blastomycosis* generally is an asymptomatic or self-limited disease characterized by fever, shaking chills, and productive, purulent cough, with or without hemoptysis, in immunocompetent individuals. The clinical presentation can be difficult to differentiate from other respiratory infections, including bacterial pneumonia, on the basis of clinical symptoms alone.

Sporadic (nonepidemic) pulmonary blastomycosis can present as a more chronic or subacute disease, with low-grade fever, night sweats, weight loss, and productive cough that resembles tuberculosis rather than bacterial pneumonia. *Chronic pulmonary blastomycosis* is characterized by fever, malaise, weight loss, night sweats, chest pain, and productive cough. Patients often are thought to have tuberculosis and frequently have evidence of disseminated disease that can appear 1 to 3 years after the primary pneumonia has resolved. Reactivation of disease can occur in the lungs or as the focus of new infection in other organs.

In approximately 40% of patients, dissemination is not accompanied by reactivation of pulmonary disease. The most common sites for disseminated disease include the skin and bony skeleton, although less commonly the prostate, oropharyngeal mucosa, and abdominal viscera are involved. CNS disease, while exceedingly uncommon, is associated with the highest mortality rate.

Laboratory and Diagnostic Tests

The simplest and most successful method of diagnosing blastomycosis is by direct microscopic visualization of the large, multinucleated yeast with single, broad-based buds in sputum or other respiratory specimens following digestion of cells and debris with 10% potassium hydroxide.[8,19] Histopathologic examination of tissue biopsies and culture of secretions also should be used to identify *B. dermatitidis*, although it can require up to 30 days to isolate and identify a small inoculum.

No reliable skin test exists to determine the incidence and prevalence of disease in endemic populations, and reliable serologic diagnosis of blastomycosis has long been hampered by the lack of specific and standardized reagents. Serologic response does not always correlate with clinical improvement, although some investigators have noted that a decline in the number of precipitins or CF titers can offer evidence of a favorable prognosis in patients with established disease.

Acute pulmonary blastomycosis generally is an asymptomatic or self-limited disease characterized by fever, shaking chills, and productive, purulent cough, with or without hemoptysis, in immunocompetent individuals. The clinical presentation can be difficult to differentiate from other respiratory infections, including bacterial pneumonia, on the basis of clinical symptoms alone. Sporadic (nonepidemic) cases of pulmonary blastomycosis can present as a more chronic or subacute disease with low-grade fever, night sweats, weight loss, and productive cough that resembles tuberculosis rather than bacterial pneumonia.

TREATMENT

Non–HIV-Infected Patient

5 In the immunocompetent host, acute pulmonary blastomycosis can be mild and self-limited and may not require treatment. However, consideration should be given to treating all infected individuals to prevent extrapulmonary dissemination. All individuals with moderate to severe pneumonia, disseminated infection, or those who are immunocompromised require antifungal therapy.

In patients with mild to moderate pulmonary blastomycosis, itraconazole is effective; however, in patients with moderately severe to severe pulmonary disease, the clinical presentation of the patient, the immune competence of the patient, and the toxicity of the antifungal agents are the main determinants of the choice of antifungal therapy. All immunocompromised patients and patients with progressive pulmonary disease or with extrapulmonary disease should be treated (Table 99-4). In the case of disease limited to the lungs, cure might have occurred without treatment before the diagnosis is made. Regardless of whether or not the patient receives treatment, however, he or she must be followed carefully for many years for evidence of reactivation or progressive disease.[8,19,22]

Some authors recommend azole therapy for the treatment of self-limited pulmonary disease, with the hope of preventing late extrapulmonary disease; however, data supporting the efficacy of these regimens are lacking.[8,22] Itraconazole 200 to 400 mg/day demonstrated 90% efficacy as a first-line agent in the treatment of non–life-threatening non-CNS blastomycosis, and for compliant patients who completed at least 2 months of therapy, a success rate of 95% was noted. No therapeutic advantage was noted with the higher (400 mg) dosage as compared with patients treated with 200 mg.

All patients with disseminated blastomycosis, as well as those with extrapulmonary disease, require therapy. Due to its adverse effects, variable oral absorption, and lack of CNS penetration, ketoconazole is now reserved as an alternative therapy for mild to moderate pulmonary and non-CNS disease. However, older studies demonstrate that ketoconazole 400 mg/day orally for 6 months cures more than 80% of patients with chronic pulmonary and non-meningeal disseminated blastomycosis. Amphotericin B is more efficacious but more toxic and therefore is reserved for noncompliant patients and patients with overwhelming or life-threatening disease, CNS infection, and treatment failures.[8,22] Lipid preparations of amphotericin B have largely replaced conventional amphotericin B for treatment of blastomycosis, despite their higher cost, due to their decreased renal toxicity. Surgery has only a limited role in the treatment of blastomycosis.

HIV-Infected Patient

For unclear reasons, blastomycosis is an uncommon opportunistic disease among immunocompromised individuals, including AIDS patients; however, blastomycosis can occur as a late (CD4 lymphocytes <200 cells/mm^3 [<200 × 10^6/L]) and frequently fatal complication of HIV infection. In this population, overwhelming disseminated disease with frequent involvement of the CNS is common.[8,22] Following induction therapy with amphotericin B (total cumulative dose of 1 g), HIV-infected patients should receive chronic suppressive therapy with an oral azole antifungal.[8,22]

TABLE 99-4 Therapy of Blastomycosis

Type of Disease	Preferred Treatment
Pulmonary[a]	
Moderately severe to severe disease	Lipid formulation of amphotericin B 3–5 mg/kg IV daily or amphotericin B[b] 0.7–1 mg/kg IV daily (total dose 1.5–2.5 g) × 1–2 weeks or until improvement is noted, followed by itraconazole[c,d] 200 mg orally three times daily for 3 days, then 200 mg twice daily, × total of 6–12 months
Mild to moderate disease	Itraconazole[c,d] 200 mg orally three times daily for 3 days, then 200 mg twice daily, for a total of 6 months[c]
CNS disease	*Induction*: Lipid formulation of amphotericin B 5 mg/kg IV daily × 4–6 weeks, followed by an oral azole as consolidation therapy *Consolidation*: Fluconazole[d] 800 mg orally daily, or itraconazole[d] 200 mg two or three times orally daily, or voriconazole[d] 200–400 mg orally twice daily, for ≥12 months and until resolution of CSF abnormalities
Disseminated or Extrapulmonary Disease	
Moderately severe to severe disease	Lipid formulation of amphotericin B 3–5 mg/kg IV daily or amphotericin B[b] 0.7–1 mg/kg IV daily × 1–2 weeks or until improvement is noted, followed by itraconazole[c,d] 200 mg orally three times daily for 3 days, then 200 mg twice daily × 6–12 months. Treat osteoarticular disease with 12 months of antifungal therapy Most clinicians prefer to step-down to itraconazole[d] therapy once the patient's condition improves
Mild to moderate	Itraconazole[c,d] 200 mg orally three times daily for 3 days, then 200 mg once or twice daily × ≥12 months. Treat osteoarticular disease with 12 months of antifungal therapy
Immunocompromised Host (Including Patients with AIDS, Transplants, or Receiving Chronic Glucocorticoid Therapy)	
Acute disease	Lipid formulation of amphotericin B 3–5 mg/kg IV daily or amphotericin B[b] 0.7–1 mg/kg IV daily × 1–2 weeks or until improvement is noted, then give suppressive therapy for a total of at least 12 months of therapy
Suppressive therapy	Itraconazole[c,d] 200 mg orally three times daily for 3 days, then 200 mg twice daily for a total of at least 12 months of therapy; lifelong suppressive therapy with oral itraconazole[d] 200 mg daily may be required for immunosuppressed patients in whom immunosuppression cannot be reversed, and in patients who experience relapse despite appropriate therapy

AIDS, acquired immunodeficiency syndrome.

[a]In the immunocompetent host, acute pulmonary blastomycosis can be mild and self-limited and may not require treatment.

[b]Desoxycholate amphotericin B.

[c]Serum levels of itraconazole should be determined after the patient has received itraconazole for ≥2 weeks, to ensure adequate drug exposure

[d]Azoles should not be used during pregnancy

Data from Chapman and Sullivan[22] and Kauffman.[21]

COCCIDIOIDOMYCOSIS

Epidemiology

Coccidioidomycosis is caused by infection with *Coccidioides immitis*, a dimorphic fungus found in the southwestern and western United States, as well as in parts of Mexico and South America. In North America, the endemic regions encompass the semiarid areas of the southwestern United States from California to Texas known as the Lower Sonoran Zone, where there is scant annual rainfall, hot summers, and sandy, alkaline soil. *C. immitis* grows in the soil as a mold, and mycelia proliferate during the rainy season. During the dry season, resistant arthroconidia form and become airborne when the soil is disturbed.

Although generally considered to be a regional disease, coccidioidomycosis has increased in importance in recent years because of the increased tourism and population in endemic areas, the increased use of immunosuppressive therapy in transplantation and oncology, and the AIDS epidemic. Although there is no racial, hormonal, or immunologic predisposition for acquiring primary disease, these factors affect the risk of subsequent dissemination of disease (Table 99-5).[11]

Pathophysiology

When individuals come in contact with contaminated soil during ranching, dust storms, or proximity to construction sites or

TABLE 99-5 Factors for Severe, Disseminated Infection with Coccidioidomycosis

Race (Filipinos > African Americans > Native Americans > Hispanics > Asians)
Pregnancy (especially when infection is acquired or reactivated in the second or third trimester)
Compromised cellular immune system, including
- AIDS patients
- Patients receiving
  - Corticosteroids
  - Immunosuppressive agents
  - Chemotherapy

Male gender
Neonates
Patients with B or AB blood types

AIDS, acquired immune deficiency syndrome.
Data from Galgiani et al.[11]

archaeologic excavations, arthroconidia are inhaled into the respiratory tree, where they transform into spherules, which reproduce by cleavage of the cytoplasm to produce endospores. The endospores are released when the spherules reach maturity. Similar to histoplasmosis, an acute inflammatory response in the tissue leads to infiltration of mononuclear cells, ultimately resulting in granuloma formation.[11]

Clinical Presentation of Coccidioidomycosis

Coccidioidomycosis encompasses a spectrum of illnesses ranging from primary uncomplicated respiratory tract infection that resolves spontaneously to progressive pulmonary or disseminated infection.[11,19,23] Initial or primary infection with *C. immitis* almost always involves the lungs. Although approximately one third of the population in endemic areas is infected, the average incidence of symptomatic disease is only approximately 0.43%.

Signs and Symptoms

Primary Coccidioidomycosis ("*Valley Fever*") Approximately 60% of infected patients have an asymptomatic, self-limited infection without clinical or radiological manifestations. The remaining 40% of patients exhibit nonspecific symptoms that are often indistinguishable from ordinary upper respiratory infections, including fever, cough, headache, sore throat, myalgias, and fatigue that occur 1 to 3 weeks after exposure to the pathogen. More commonly, a diffuse, mild erythroderma or maculopapular rash is observed. Patients can have pleuritic chest pain and peripheral eosinophilia.

A fine, diffuse rash can appear during the first few days of the illness. Primary pneumonia can be the first manifestation of disease, characterized by a productive cough that can be blood-streaked, as well as single or multiple soft or dense homogeneous hilar or basal infiltrates on chest roentgenogram. *Chronic, persistent pneumonia or persistent pulmonary coccidioidomycosis* (primary disease lasting more than 6 weeks) is complicated by hemoptysis, pulmonary scarring, and the formation of cavities or bronchopleural fistulas.

Necrosis of pulmonary tissue with drainage and cavity formation occurs commonly. Most parenchymal cavities close spontaneously or form dense nodular scar tissue that can become superinfected with bacteria or spherules of *C. immitis*. These patients often have persistent cough, fevers, and weight loss.

Disseminated disease occurs in less than 1% of infected patients. The most common sites for dissemination are the skin, lymph nodes, bone, and meninges, although the spleen, liver, kidney, and adrenal gland also can be involved. Occasionally, miliary coccidioidomycosis occurs, with rapid, widespread dissemination, often in concert with positive blood cultures for *C. immitis*. Patients with AIDS frequently present with miliary disease. Coccidioidomycosis in AIDS patients appears to be caused by reactivation of disease in most patients. Dissemination also is more likely if infection occurs during pregnancy, especially during the third trimester or in the immediate postpartum period.[23]

CNS infection occurs in approximately 16% of patients with disseminated coccidioidomycosis. Patients can present with meningeal disease without previous symptoms of primary pulmonary infection, although disease usually occurs within 6 months of the primary infection. The signs and symptoms are often subtle and nonspecific, including headache, weakness, changes in mental status (lethargy and confusion), neck stiffness, low-grade fever, weight loss, and occasionally, hydrocephalus. Space-occupying lesions are rare, and the main areas of involvement are the basilar meninges.

Diagnosis

The diagnoses of coccidioidomycosis generally utilizes identification or recovery of *Coccidioides* spp. from clinical specimens and detection of specific anticoccidioidal antibodies in serum or other body fluids.[19]

TREATMENT

General Guidelines

6 Therapy for coccidioidomycosis is difficult, and the results are unpredictable. Guidelines[11] are available for treatment of this disease; however, optimal treatment for many forms of this disease still generates debate. The efficacy of antifungal therapy for coccidioidomycosis often is less certain than that for other fungal etiologies, such as blastomycosis, histoplasmosis, or cryptococcus, even when in vitro susceptibilities and the sites of infections are similar. The refractoriness of coccidioidomycosis can relate to the ability of *C. immitis* spherules to release hundreds of endospores, maximally challenging host defenses.[11,23] Fortunately, only approximately 5% of infected patients require therapy.[23]

Goals of Therapy

Desired outcomes of treatment are resolution of signs and symptoms of infection, reduction of serum concentrations of anticoccidioidal antibodies, and return of function of involved organs. It would also be desirable to prevent relapse of illness on discontinuation of therapy, although current therapy is often unable to achieve this goal.

Specific Agents Used for the Treatment of Coccidioidomycosis

Azole antifungals, primarily fluconazole and itraconazole, have replaced amphotericin B as initial therapy for most chronic pulmonary or disseminated infections. Amphotericin B is now usually reserved for patients with respiratory failure because of infection with *Coccidioides* species, those with rapidly progressive coccidioidal infections, or women during pregnancy. Therapy often ranges from many months to years in duration, and in some patients, lifelong suppressive therapy is needed to prevent relapses. Specific antifungals (and their usual dosages) for the treatment of coccidioidomycosis include IV amphotericin B (0.5 to 1.5 mg/kg per day), ketoconazole (400 mg/day orally), IV or oral fluconazole (usually 400 to 800 mg/day, although dosages as high as 1,200 mg/day have been used without complications), and itraconazole (200 to 300 mg orally twice daily or three times daily, as either capsules or solution).[11,23] If itraconazole is used, measurement of serum concentrations can be helpful to ascertain whether oral bioavailability is adequate.

Amphotericin B generally is preferred as initial therapy in patients with rapidly progressive disease, whereas azoles generally are preferred in patients with subacute or chronic presentations. The lipid formulations of amphotericin B have not been studied extensively in coccidioidal infection but can offer a means of giving more drug with less toxicity. Fluconazole probably is the most frequently used medicine given its tolerability, although high relapse rates have been reported in some studies. Relapse rates with itraconazole therapy can be lower than those with fluconazole.[11,23]

The usefulness of newly available antifungal agents of possible benefit for the treatment of refractory coccidioidal infections has not been adequately assessed and they are not yet FDA approved for use in this population. Case reports have suggested that voriconazole can be effective in selected patients. Caspofungin has been effective in treating experimental murine coccidioidomycosis, but in vitro susceptibility of isolates varies widely, and there is only one report regarding its value. Posaconazole was shown to be an effective treatment in a small clinical trial and in patients with refractory infections. Its efficacy relative to other triazole antifungals is unknown.

Clinical **Controversy. . .**

Because of the lack of prospective, controlled trials, there is continued disagreement among experts in endemic areas whether patients with coccidioidomycosis should be treated, and if so, which ones and for how long. The excellent tolerability of oral azoles has lowered the threshold for deciding to treat primary infection, and some clinicians treat all primary infections. Rationales for treating a primary self-limiting infection include the ability to lessen the morbidity associated with the acute infection and the possible ability to reduce the development of more serious complications. However, there is currently no evidence that treatment of the primary infection accomplishes either of these goals.[25]

Combination therapy with members of different classes of antifungal agents has not been evaluated in patients, and there is a hypothetical risk of antagonism. However, some clinicians feel that outcome in severe cases is improved when amphotericin B is combined with an azole antifungal. If the patient improves, the dosage of amphotericin B can be slowly decreased while the dosage of azole is maintained.[11,23]

Primary Respiratory Infection

Although most patients with symptomatic primary pulmonary disease recover without therapy, management should include followup visits for 1 to 2 years to document resolution of disease or to identify as early as possible evidence of pulmonary or extrapulmonary complications.

Patients with a large inoculum, severe infection, or concurrent risk factors (e.g., HIV infection, organ transplant, pregnancy, or high doses of corticosteroids) probably should be treated, particularly those with high CF titers, in whom incipient or occult dissemination is likely. Because some racial or ethnic populations have a higher risk of dissemination, some clinicians advocate their inclusion in the high-risk group. Common indicators used to judge the severity of infection include weight loss (>10%), intense night sweats persisting more than 3 weeks, infiltrates involving more than one half of one lung or portions of both lungs, prominent or persistent hilar adenopathy, CF antibody titers of greater than 1:16, failure to develop dermal sensitivity to coccidial antigens, inability to work, or symptoms that persist for more than 2 months.[11,23]

Commonly prescribed therapies include currently available oral azole antifungals at their recommended doses for courses of therapy ranging from 3 to 6 months.[11,23] In patients with diffuse pneumonia with bilateral reticulonodular or miliary infiltrates, therapy usually is initiated with amphotericin B; several weeks of therapy generally are required to produce clear evidence of improvement. Consolidation therapy with oral azoles can be considered at that time. The total duration of therapy should be at least 1 year, and in patients with underlying immunodeficiency, oral azole therapy should be continued as secondary prophylaxis. Although HIV-infected patients receiving secondary prophylaxis might be at low risk for recurrence of systemic mycosis when their CD4+ T-lymphocyte counts increase to >100 cells/μL (>100 × 10^6/L) in response to HAART, the number of patients who have been evaluated is insufficient to warrant a recommendation to discontinue prophylaxis.

Infections of the Pulmonary Cavity

Many pulmonary infections that are caused by *C. immitis* are benign in their course and do not require intervention. In the absence of controlled clinical trials, evidence of the benefit of antifungal therapy is lacking, and asymptomatic infections generally are left untreated. Symptomatic patients can benefit from oral azole therapy, although recurrence of symptoms can be seen in some patients once therapy is discontinued. Surgical resection of localized cavities provides resolution of the problem in patients in whom the risks of surgery are not too high.[11,23]

Extrapulmonary (Disseminated) Disease

Nonmeningeal Disease

Almost all patients with disease located outside the lungs should receive antifungal therapy; therapy usually is initiated with 400 mg/day of an oral azole. Amphotericin B is an alternative therapy and can be necessary in patients with worsening lesions or with disease in particularly critical locations such as the vertebral column. Approximately 50% to 75% of patients treated with amphotericin B for nonmeningeal disease achieve a sustained remission, and therapy usually is curative in patients with infections localized strictly to skin and soft tissues without extensive abscess formation or tissue damage. The efficacy of local injection into joints or the peritoneum, as well as intraarticular or intradermal administration, remains poorly studied. Amphotericin B appears to be most efficacious when cell-mediated immunity is intact (as evidenced by a positive coccidioidin or spherulin skin test or low CF antibody titer). Controlled trials that document these clinical impressions are lacking, however.[11,23]

Meningeal Disease

Fluconazole has become the drug of choice for the treatment of coccidioidal meningitis. A minimum dose of 400 mg/day orally leads to a clinical response in most patients and obviates the need for intrathecal amphotericin B. Some clinicians will initiate therapy with 800 or 1,000 mg/day, and itraconazole dosages of 400 to 600 mg/day are comparably effective. It is also clear, however, that fluconazole only leads to remission rather than cure of the infections; thus suppressive therapy must be continued for life. Ketoconazole cannot be recommended routinely for the treatment of coccidioidal meningitis because of its poor CNS penetration following oral administration. Patients who do not respond to fluconazole or itraconazole therapy are candidates for intrathecal amphotericin B therapy with or without continuation of azole therapy. The intrathecal dose of amphotericin B ranges from 0.01 to 1.5 mg given at intervals ranging from daily to weekly. Therapy is initiated with a low dosage and is titrated upward as patient tolerance develops.[11,23]

CRYPTOCOCCOSIS

Epidemiology

Cryptococcosis is a noncontagious, systemic mycotic infection caused by the ubiquitous encapsulated soil yeast *Cryptococcus*, which is found in soil, particularly in pigeon droppings, although disease occurs throughout the world, even in areas where pigeons are absent. Infections caused by *C. neoformans* var. *grubii* (serotype A) are seen worldwide among immunocompromised hosts, followed by *C. neoformans* var. *neoformans* (serotype D). On the other hand, *Cryptococcus gattii* (serotypes B and C) is geographically more restricted and in contrast to *C. neoformans*, rarely infects immunosuppressed patients, is not associated with HIV infection, and the infections are more difficult to treat. *C. gattii* is not associated with birds; its main reservoir was thought to be limited to certain species of eucalyptus tree. Until recently, it was most common in tropical and subtropical areas, such as Australia, South America, Southeast Asia, and central Africa, with the highest incidence in Papua New Guinea and Northern Australia, although infections occur in nontropical areas such as North America and Europe. *C. gattii* emerged on Vancouver Island, British Columbia, Canada, in 1999, and subsequently spread to the Vancouver lower mainland, Washington state, and Oregon.[24]

Infection is acquired by inhalation of the organism. The incidence of cryptococcosis has risen dramatically in recent years, reflecting the increased numbers of immunocompromised patients, including those with malignancies, diabetes mellitus, chronic renal failure, and organ transplants and those receiving immunosuppressive agents. The AIDS epidemic also has contributed to the increased numbers of patients; cryptococcosis is the fourth most common infectious complication of AIDS and the second most common fungal pathogen. In most developed countries, widespread use of HAART has significantly decreased the incidence of cryptococcosis; however, the incidence and mortality of this infection are still extremely high in areas with limited access to HAART and a high incidence of HIV.[25]

Cell-mediated immunity appears to play a major role in host defense against infection with *C. neoformans*; 29% to 55% of patients with cryptococcal meningitis have a predisposing condition. Many patients with disseminated cryptococcosis demonstrate defects in cell-mediated immunity. The predilection of *C. neoformans* for the CNS appears to be caused by the lack of immunoglobulins and complement and the excellent growth medium afforded by CSF.[25]

Disease can remain localized in the lungs or can disseminate to other tissues, particularly the CNS, although the skin also can be affected. Hematogenous spread generally occurs in the immunocompromised host, although it also has been seen in individuals with intact immune systems.

Clinical Presentation of Cryptococcosis

Primary cryptococcosis in humans almost always occurs in the lungs, although the pulmonary focus usually produces a subclinical infection.[23–28] Symptomatic infections usually are manifested by cough, rales, and shortness of breath that generally resolve spontaneously. Cryptococcus can present as part of an immune reconstitution inflammatory syndrome (IRIS), a paradoxical worsening of preexisting infectious processes following the initiation of HAART in HIV-infected individuals. In non-AIDS patients, the symptoms of cryptococcal meningitis are nonspecific. Headache, fever, nausea, vomiting, mental status changes, and neck stiffness generally are observed. Less common symptoms include visual disturbances (photophobia and blurred vision), papilledema, seizures, and aphasia. In AIDS patients, fever and headache are common, but meningismus and photophobia are much less common than in non-AIDS patients. Approximately 10% to 12% of AIDS patients have asymptomatic disease, similar to the rate observed in non-AIDS patients.[25,27,28] Intracerebral mass lesions (cryptococcomas) are more common in *C. gattii* than in *C. neoformans*, presumably due to their different host immune responses.[24]

Laboratory Tests

With cryptococcal meningitis, the CSF opening pressure generally is elevated. There is a CSF pleocytosis (usually lymphocytes), leukocytosis, a decreased glucose concentration, and an elevated CSF protein concentration. There is also a positive cryptococcal antigen (detected by LA). The test is rapid, specific, and extremely sensitive, but false-negative results can occur. False-positive tests can result from cross-reactivity with rheumatoid factor and *Trichosporon beigelii*. *C. neoformans* can be detected in approximately 60% of patients by India ink smear of CSF, and it can be cultured in more than 96% of patients. Occasionally, large volumes of CSF are required to confirm the diagnosis.

The CSF parameters in patients with AIDS are similar to those seen in non-AIDS patients, with the exception of a decreased inflammatory response to the pathogen, resulting in a strikingly low number of leukocytes in CSF and extraordinarily high cryptococcal antigen titers.

TREATMENT

The choice of treatment for disease caused by *C. neoformans* depends on both the anatomic sites of involvement and the host's immune status, and thus, treatment recommendations are divided into three specific risk groups: (a) HIV-infected individuals, (b) transplant recipients, and (c) non–HIV-infected and nontransplant hosts (Table 99-6).[9] The management of cryptococcosis includes systemic antifungal therapy, control of elevated ICP, and supportive care. When possible, immune defects should be addressed. Despite the lack of randomized clinical trials, outcomes of treatment for CNS cryptococcosis (without mass lesions or hydrocephalus) appear to be similar for disease due to either *C. neoformans* or *C. gattii*, although no randomized clinical trials have been performed to address this.[24]

Nonimmunocompromised Patients

7 Prior to the introduction of amphotericin B, cryptococcal meningitis was an almost uniformly fatal disease; approximately 86% of patients died within 1 year. The use of large (1 to 1.5 mg/kg) daily doses of amphotericin B resulted in cure rates of approximately 64%. When amphotericin B is combined with flucytosine, a smaller dose of amphotericin B can be employed because of the in vitro and in vivo synergy between the two antifungal agents. Resistance develops to flucytosine in up to 30% of patients treated with flucytosine alone, limiting its usefulness as monotherapy.[26,27] Combination therapy with amphotericin B and flucytosine will sterilize the CSF within 2 weeks of treatment in 60% to 90% of patients, and most immunocompetent patients will be treated successfully with 6 weeks of combination therapy.[25] However, because of the need for prolonged IV therapy and the potential for renal and hematologic toxicity with this regimen, alternative regimens utilizing lipid formulations of amphotericin B and the use of shorter (2 weeks) courses of amphotericin B followed by consolidation therapy with fluconazole for 8 weeks, then maintenance therapy with a lower dosage of fluconazole for 6 to 12 months has been advocated.[9,27–29]

For asymptomatic, immunocompetent hosts with isolated mild to moderate pulmonary disease and no evidence of CNS disease,

TABLE 99-6 Therapy of Cryptococcosis[a,b]

Type of Disease and Common Clinical Manifestations	Therapy/Comments
Nonimmunocompromised Patients (Non–HIV-Infected, Nontransplant)	
Meningoencephalitis *without* neurological complications, in patients in whom CSF yeast cultures are negative after 2 weeks of therapy	*Induction*: Amphotericin B[c] IV 0.7–1 mg/kg/day *plus* flucytosine 100 mg/kg/day orally in four divided doses × ≥4 weeks A lipid formulation of amphotericin B may be substituted for amphotericin B in the second 2 weeks
Follow all regimens with suppressive therapy	*Consolidation*: Fluconazole 400–800 mg orally daily × 8 weeks *Maintenance*: Fluconazole 200 mg orally daily × 6–12 months
Meningoencephalitis *with* neurological complications	*Induction*: Same as for patients without neurologic complications, but consider extending the induction therapy for a total of 6 weeks. A lipid formulation of amphotericin B may be given for the last 4 weeks of the prolonged induction period *Consolidation*: Fluconazole 400 mg orally daily × 8 weeks
Mild-to-moderate pulmonary disease (Nonmeningeal disease)	Fluconazole 400 mg orally daily × 6–12 months
Severe pulmonary cryptococcosis	*Same as CNS disease × 12 months*
Cryptococcemia (nonmeningeal, nonpulmonary disease)	*Same as CNS disease × 12 months*
Immunocompromised Patients	
Severe pulmonary cryptococcosis	*Same as CNS disease × 12 months*
HIV-infected Patients	
Primary therapy; induction and consolidation[g]	*Preferred regimen*: *Induction*: Amphotericin B[d] IV 0.7–1 mg/kg IV daily *plus* flucytosine 100 mg/kg/day orally in four divided doses for ≥ 2 weeks
Follow all regimens with suppressive therapy	*Consolidation*: Fluconazole 400 mg [6 mg/kg] orally daily × ≥8 weeks Liposomal amphotericin B 3–4 mg/kg IV daily, or amphotericin B lipid complex (ABLC) 5 mg/kg IV daily, for ≥2 weeks can be substituted for amphotericin B[d] in patients with or at risk for renal dysfunction *Alternative regimens, in order of preference:* Amphotericin B[d] IV 0.7–1 mg/kg IV daily × 4–6 weeks *or* liposomal amphotericin B 3–4 mg/kg IV daily[f] × 4–6 weeks *or* ABLC 5 mg/kg IV daily × 4–6 weeks *or* Amphotericin B[d] IV 0.7 mg/kg IV daily, *plus* fluconazole 800 mg (12 mg/kg) orally daily × 2 weeks, followed by fluconazole 800 mg [12 mg/kg] orally daily × ≥8weeks *or* Fluconazole ≥ 800 mg (1,200 mg/day is preferred) orally daily *plus* flucytosine 100 mg/kg/day orally in four divided doses × 6 weeks *or* Fluconazole 800–1,200 mg/day orally daily × 10–12 weeks (a dosage ≥1,200 mg/day is preferred when fluconazole is used alone)[e] *or* Itraconazole 200 mg orally twice daily × 10–12 weeks (use of itraconazole, which produces minimal concentrations of active drug in the CSF is discouraged)[i]
Suppressive/maintenance therapy[h]	Preferred: Fluconazole 200 mg orally daily × ≥1 year *or* Itraconazole[i] 200 mg orally twice daily × ≥1 year *or* Amphotericin B[j] IV 1 mg/kg weekly × ≥1 year
Organ Transplant Recipients	
Mild-moderate non-CNS disease or mild-to-moderate symptoms without diffuse pulmonary infiltrates	Fluconazole 400 mg (6 mg/kg) orally daily × 6–12 months
CNS disease, moderately severe or severe CNS disease or disseminated disease without CNS disease, or severe pulmonary disease without evidence of extrapulmonary or disseminated disease	*Induction*: Liposomal amphotericin B 3–4 mg/kg IV daily,[f] or ABLC 5 mg/kg IV daily *plus* flucytosine 100 mg/kg/day orally in four divided doses × ≥2 weeks If induction therapy does not include flucytosine, consider a lipid formulation of amphotericin B for ≥4–6 weeks of induction therapy. Consider the use of a lipid formulation of amphotericin B lipid formulation (6 mg/kg IV daily) in patients with a high-fungal burden disease or relapse of disease. *Consolidation*: Fluconazole 400–800 mg (6–12 mg/kg) per day orally for 8 weeks *Maintenance*: Fluconazole 200–400 mg per day orally for 6–12 months

HIV, human immunodeficiency virus; IT, intrathecal.

[a]When more than one therapy is listed, they are listed in order of preference.
[b]See the text for definitions of induction, consolidation, suppressive/maintenance therapy, and prophylactic therapy.
[c]Deoxycholate amphotericin B.
[d]In patients with significant renal disease, lipid formulations of amphotericin B can be substituted for deoxycholate amphotericin B during the induction.
[e]Or until cerebrospinal fluid (CSF) cultures are negative.
[f]Liposomal amphotericin B has been given safely up to 6 mg/kg daily; could be considered in treatment failure or in patients with a high fungal burden.
[g]Initiate HAART therapy 2–10 weeks after commencement of initial antifungal treatment.
[h]Consider discontinuing suppressive therapy during HAART in patients with a CD4 cell count ≥100 cells/μL (≥100 × 10^6/L) and an undetectable or very low HIV RNA level sustained for ≥ 3months (with a minimum of 12 months of antifungal therapy). Consider reinstitution of maintenance therapy if the CD4 cell count decreases to <100 cells/μL (<100 × 10^6/L).
[i]Drug level monitoring is strongly advised.
[j]Use is discouraged except in azole intolerant patients, since it is less effective than azole therapy, and is associated with a risk of IV catheter-related infections.

Data from Perfect et al.[9]

careful observation can be warranted; in the case of symptomatic infection, fluconazole for 6 to 12 months is warranted. In individuals with non-CNS cryptococcemia, a positive serum cryptococcal antigen titer (>1:8), cutaneous infection, a positive urine culture, or prostatic disease, the clinician must decide whether to follow the regimen for isolated pulmonary disease or the more aggressive regimen for patients with CNS (disseminated) disease.[9]

Pilot studies evaluating combination therapy with fluconazole plus flucytosine as initial therapy yielded unsatisfactory results, and this approach is discouraged even in "low-risk" patients. Ketoconazole has been used successfully in the treatment of cutaneous cryptococcosis, but it is not useful in the treatment of CNS disease, probably because of its poor penetration into the CNS.[9]

Despite low CSF concentrations of amphotericin B (2% to 3% of those observed in plasma), the use of intrathecal amphotericin B is not recommended for the treatment of cryptococcal meningitis except in very ill patients or in patients with recurrent or progressive disease despite aggressive therapy with IV amphotericin B. The dosage of amphotericin B employed is usually 0.5 mg administered through the lumbar, cisternal, or intraventricular (through an Ommaya reservoir) route two or three times weekly. Side effects of intrathecal amphotericin B include arachnoiditis and paresthesias. Intrathecal amphotericin B therapy should be administered in combination with IV amphotericin B.[29]

The recommended management of raised intracranial pressure (ICP) in cryptococcal meningitis (without hydrocephalus, a mass lesion, or a shift on computed tomography [CT] scan) has been repeated CSF removal by spinal tap. Those who do not respond and have ongoing raised ICP should have ophthalmologic monitoring for possible vision loss, and should be considered for ventriculoperitoneal shunt surgery. Neither corticosteroids (in the absence of IRIS) nor acetazolamide is recommended for management of raised ICP. Symptomatic, medically refractory mass lesions that may be compressing vital structures should be considered for surgical therapy.[24]

Immunocompromised Patients

Immunocompromised hosts with isolated severe pulmonary and extrapulmonary disease (including cryptococcemia) without CNS disease should be treated similarly to nonimmunocompromised patients with CNS disease. Immunocompromised patients with CNS infection require more prolonged therapy; treatment regimens are based on those used in the HIV-infected population and follow induction therapy with amphotericin B and consolidation therapy with 6 to 12 months of suppressive therapy with fluconazole.[9]

Organ Transplant Recipients

Cryptococcosis has been documented in an average of 2.8% of solid-organ transplant recipients, with ~25% to 54% having pulmonary infection (of whom 6% to 33% have disease that is limited to the lungs), ~25% of patients having fungemia, and 52% to 61% having CNS involvement and disseminated (involvement of ≥2 sites) infections.[9] The median time to disease onset is 21 months after transplantation; 68.5% of the cases occur >1 year after transplantation.

Fluconazole maintenance therapy should be continued for at least 6 to 12 months. Immunosuppressive management should include sequential or stepwise reduction of immunosuppressants, with consideration of lowering the corticosteroid dose first.[20] Amphotericin B should be used with caution in transplant recipients and is not recommended as first-line therapy in this patient population due to the risk of nephrotoxicity in this population that frequently has reduced renal function. If used, the tolerated dosage of amphotericin B is uncertain, but 0.7 mg/kg daily is suggested with frequent renal function monitoring. Regardless of the agent utilized, all antifungal dosages need to be carefully monitored.[11]

HIV-Infected Patients

Primary antifungal prophylaxis for cryptococcosis is not routinely recommended in HIV-infected patients in the United States and Europe. However, in areas with limited HAART availability, high levels of antiretroviral drug resistance, and a high burden of disease, clinicians may wish to consider the use of either prophylactic therapy or a preemptive strategy with serum cryptococcal antigen testing for asymptomatic antigenemia.[9]

Fluconazole is beneficial for both acute and chronic maintenance therapy for cryptococcal meningitis. Amphotericin B 0.4 to 0.5 mg/kg IV daily was compared with oral fluconazole 200 mg/day. Although the overall 10-week mortality was the same in both groups, the time until the CSF culture became negative was longer, and there were more deaths in the first 2 weeks of therapy in the fluconazole group.[28] In later trials,[29] amphotericin B 0.7 mg/kg IV daily for 2 weeks (with or without oral flucytosine 100 mg/kg per day), followed by consolidation therapy with either itraconazole 400 mg/day orally or fluconazole 400 mg/day orally, led to markedly improved outcomes in comparison with earlier regimens. This study confirmed the benefit of early high-dose (0.7 mg/kg per day) amphotericin B use, the usefulness of flucytosine added to amphotericin B for induction therapy, and the slight superiority of fluconazole over itraconazole for consolidation therapy.

Amphotericin B combined with flucytosine is the initial treatment of choice.[9] In patients who cannot tolerate flucytosine, amphotericin B alone is an acceptable alternative. After the initially successful 2-week induction period, consolidation therapy with fluconazole can be administered for 8 weeks or until CSF cultures are negative. In patients in whom fluconazole cannot be given, itraconazole is an acceptable, albeit less effective, alternative. Combination therapy with fluconazole plus flucytosine is effective; however, it is recommended as an alternative to the preceding therapies because of its potential for toxicity. Lipid formulations of amphotericin B are effective, but the optimal dosage is unknown.[9]

In HIV-infected patients, mortality is highly associated with elevated ICP (CSF opening pressure >250 mm H_2O [>2.5 kPa]). At the initiation of antifungal therapy, lumbar drainage should remove enough CSF to reduce the opening pressure by 50%. Patients initially should undergo daily lumbar punctures to maintain CSF opening pressure in the normal range. When the CSF pressure is normal for several days, the procedure can be suspended. Adjunctive steroid treatment is not recommended because therapy has resulted in mixed results and its impact on outcome is unclear. Similarly, neither mannitol nor acetazolamide therapy provides any clear benefit in the management of elevated ICP.[9]

Suppressive (Maintenance) Therapy for Cryptococcal Meningitis in the HIV-Infected Patient

Relapse of *C. neoformans* meningitis occurs in approximately 50% of AIDS patients after completion of primary therapy. Persistence of asymptomatic urinary *C. neoformans* has been documented in a high percentage of AIDS patients despite seemingly adequate courses of therapy for primary meningeal disease. The prostate appears to act as a sequestered reservoir of infection in these patients, resulting in systemic relapse.

Patients appear to be at low risk for recurrence of cryptococcosis when they have successfully completed a course of initial therapy for cryptococcosis, remain asymptomatic with regard to signs and symptoms of cryptococcosis, have received antifungal therapy for >3 of the previous 6 months, have a serum cryptococcal antigen titer <1:512, or have a sustained increase (e.g., >6 months) in their CD4+ T-lymphocyte counts to >100 to 200 cells/μL ($>100 \times 10^6$ to 200×10^6/L) and an HIV viral load of fewer than 50 copies/mL (50×10^3/L).[9,27–29]

In HIV-infected patients requiring chronic suppressive therapy of cryptococcal meningitis, oral fluconazole 200 mg/day is superior to IV administration of amphotericin B 1 mg/kg weekly in preventing relapse, results in a lower incidence of adverse drug reactions and bacterial infections, and is superior to itraconazole as maintenance therapy.[29]

Until recently, lifelong maintenance therapy to prevent disease relapse was recommended for all patients with AIDS after successful completion of primary induction therapy for cryptococcal meningoencephalitis. However, several studies indicate that the risk of relapse is low and that discontinuation of maintenance therapy is reasonable, provided patients have successfully completed primary therapy, are free of symptoms and signs of active cryptococcosis, and have been receiving HAART with a sustained CD4 cell count >100 cells/mL (>100 × 10^3/L) and an undetectable viral load.[9]

Evaluation of Therapeutic Outcomes

Once the CNS is involved, the usual course is weeks to months of progressive deterioration, with 80% of untreated patients dying within the first year. The prognosis of cryptococcal meningitis depends largely on the underlying predisposing factors of the host. Although cryptococcal antigen is positive in 90% of patients with cryptococcal meningitis, fewer than one half of the patients with cryptococcal meningitis develop antibody to capsular polysaccharide. Those who produce antibody have a slightly improved prognosis. In contrast, the presence of headache is a favorable symptom, presumably because it leads to an earlier diagnosis. A favorable outcome is also associated with a normal mental status on diagnosis and a CSF white blood cell (WBC) count of less than 20 cells/mm^3 (20 × 10^6/L). A poor outcome is predicted, however, by the presence of one or more underlying diseases (including hematopoietic disorders and AIDS), corticosteroid or immunosuppressive therapy, pretreatment serum cryptococcal antigen titers of 1:32, and posttherapy serum antigen titers of 1:8. In non-AIDS patients, the cryptococcal antigen titer can be followed during therapy to assess response to antifungal therapy. In AIDS patients, decreasing titers are not necessarily predictive of success, and titers rarely become negative at the completion of therapy.

CANDIDA INFECTIONS

Candida species are yeasts that exist primarily as small (4 to 6 microns), unicellular, thin-walled, ovoid cells that reproduce by budding. On agar medium, they form smooth, white, creamy colonies resembling staphylococci. Although there are more than 150 species of *Candida*, eight species—*C. albicans, C. tropicalis, Candida parapsilosis, C. krusei, Candida stellatoidea, C. guilliermondii, C. lusitaniae*, and *C. glabrata*—are regarded as clinically important pathogens in human disease.[17] Yeast forms, hyphae, and pseudohyphae can be found in clinical specimens.

Pathophysiology

8 *C. albicans* is a normal commensal of the skin, female genital tract, and entire GI tract of humans. Therefore, the mere presence of hyphae or pseudohyphae in a clinical specimen is insufficient for the diagnosis of invasive disease. The majority of infections with *C. albicans* are acquired endogenously, although human-to-human transmission also can occur. Oral candidiasis in the newborn probably is acquired during passage through the birth canal, and balanitis in the uncircumcised male can be acquired through contact with a female with vaginal candidiasis. Although the term *fungemia* refers to the presence of fungi in the blood, the most commonly isolated organism is *C. albicans*. Candidiasis can cause mucocutaneous or systemic infection, including endocarditis, peritonitis, arthritis, and infection of the CNS. (Mucocutaneous infections caused by *Candida* are discussed in further detail in Chap. 98.)

The role of an intact integument is crucial in the prevention of mucocutaneous or hematogenous candidiasis. After *Candida* invades the dermis or enters the bloodstream, polymorphonuclear (PMN) leukocytes play a major role in the defense of the patient because PMN leukocytes are capable of damaging pseudohyphae and can phagocytize and kill blastoconidia. In addition to neutrophils, lymphocytes, monocytes, macrophages, complement, and eosinophils play a role in the prevention of infection. Adherence of *C. albicans* is important in the pathogenesis of oral candidiasis and subsequent colonization of the GI tract. Because evidence suggests that the GI tract is often the portal of entry for *Candida* in disseminated disease, factors that alter the adherence of *Candida* are crucial in the development of local and systemic infection. *C. tropicalis* adheres to intravascular catheters at a higher rate than *C. albicans*, a factor that may help to account for the increased incidence of systemic infections caused by this pathogen.

HEMATOGENOUS CANDIDIASIS

Epidemiology

The incidence of fungal infections caused by *Candida* species has increased substantially in the past three decades, and *Candida* infections currently constitute a significant cause of morbidity and mortality among severely ill patients. *Candida* species now constitute the fourth most common cause of bloodstream infections (BSIs) for patients hospitalized in ICUs in the United States, following coagulase-negative staphylococci, *Staphylococcus aureus*, and enterococci. The Centers for Disease Control and Prevention's (CDC) National Nosocomial Infection Survey implicated fungi as the cause of 8% of nosocomial infections. Although *C. albicans* accounted for approximately 50% of *Candida* species, non-*albicans* species of *Candida*, including *C. glabrata, C. tropicalis, C. krusei*, and *C. parapsilosis*, are increasingly frequent causes of invasive candidal infections.[30,31] *C. lusitaniae* infections are a cause of breakthrough fungemia in cancer patients; *C. parapsilosis* has emerged as the second most common pathogen, following *C. albicans*, in neonatal ICU patients, where it is often associated with central lines and parenteral nutrition (PN), and fungemias in patients outside the United States, in particular in South America. Fungemia caused by *C. glabrata* is observed more commonly in adults older than 65 years of age.[32] The change in species is of concern clinically because certain pathogens such as *C. krusei* and *C. glabrata* are intrinsically more resistant to commonly used triazole drugs (see Table 99-1).

Pathophysiology

Candida generally is acquired via the GI tract, although organisms also can enter the bloodstream via indwelling IV catheters. Immunosuppressed patients, including those with lymphoreticular or hematologic malignancies, diabetes, and immunodeficiency diseases and those receiving immunosuppressive therapy with high-dose corticosteroids, immunosuppressants, antineoplastic agents, or broad-spectrum antimicrobial agents, are at high risk for invasive fungal infections. However, a number of prospective, randomized, controlled trials have validated the efficacy of antifungal prophylaxis and the use of antifungal agents for the treatment of persistently febrile patients with neutropenia who do not respond to antibiotics, and in the prophylaxis of patients undergoing hematopoietic stem cell transplantation (HSCT), in particular in HSCT patients with graft-versus-host disease (GVHD).[33] These efforts have resulted in a reduction in the frequency of BSIs caused by *Candida* species and systemic candidiasis in patients with neutropenia. Retrospective studies have identified a number of risk factors for candidal BSIs in ICU patients, most of which have been verified in multiple studies, although some remain controversial[34] (Table 99-7). Major risk factors include the use of central venous catheters (CVCs), total PN, receipt of multiple antibiotics, extensive surgery and burns, renal failure and hemodialysis, mechanical ventilation, and prior fungal colonization. Patients who have undergone surgery (particularly surgery of the GI tract) are increasingly susceptible to disseminated candidal infections.[15,34]

Clinical Presentation of Hematogenous Candidiasis

Dissemination of *C. albicans* can result in infection in single or multiple organs, particularly the kidney, brain, myocardium, skin, eye, bone, and joints.[17] In most patients, multiple micro- and macroabscesses are formed. Infection of the liver and spleen is becoming recognized as a particularly common and difficult-to-treat site of infection that characteristically occurs in patients undergoing chemotherapy for acute leukemia or lymphoma.

TABLE 99-7 Risk Factors for Invasive Candidiasis

Colonization
Corrected colonization index (CCI) ≥ 0.4[a]
Colonization index (CI) ≥ 0.8[a]
Candida spp. cultured from sites other than blood
Candiduria
Antibiotic use
Number of antibiotics prior to infection (per additional antibiotics)
Use of two or more antibiotics
Use of broad-spectrum antibiotics in previous 10 days
Surgery
Surgery on ICU admission
Gastro-abdominal surgery
Abdominal drainage
Elective surgery
Cardiopulmonary bypass time > 120 minutes
Hickman catheter
Foreign devices
Central venous catheter
Triple lumen catheter in patients who have undergone surgery
Bladder catheter
Renal failure and dialysis
Prior hemodialysis
Hemofiltration procedures
Increased serum creatinine[b]
New-onset hemodialysis within 3 days of admission to ICU
Acute renal failure
Underlying disease/baseline characteristics
Total PN
Diabetes mellitus
Apache II (per point)
Signs of severe sepsis
Diarrhea at any time
Mechanical ventilation ≥10 days
Hospital-acquired bacterial infection
Bacterial peritonitis by ICU day 11
GI disease
ICU length of stay
Transferred from other hospital
Use of corticosteroids
Profound neutropenia (ANC < 100/mm^3 [<100 × 10^6/L])

[a]CI = the ratio of number of nonblood distinct body sites (dbs) heavily colonized with identical strains to the total number of dbs; CCI = the product of the CI and the ratio of the number of dbs showing heavy growth (≥10^5 CFU/mL [≥10^8 CFU/L]) to the total of dbs growing *Candida* spp.

[b]Serum creatinine >1.2 mg/dL (>106 μmol/L) in females, >1.6 mg/dL (>141 μmol/L) in males.

Data from Lam et al.[34]

Laboratory Tests

Although a variety of serologic tests have been proposed for the detection of *Candida* protein antigens, serum antibodies to *Candida*, and antibodies to cell wall components such as mannan, no test has demonstrated reliable accuracy in the clinical setting for the diagnosis of disseminated infection with *Candida*. Only 25% to 45% of neutropenic patients with disseminated candidiasis at autopsy had a positive blood culture with *C. albicans* prior to death. The interpretation of positive surveillance cultures of the skin, mouth, sputum, feces, or urine is hampered by their occurrence as commensal pathogens and in distinguishing colonization from invasive disease.

Until recently, a rapid presumptive identification of *C. albicans* could be made by incubation of the organism in serum; formation of a germ tube (the beginning of hyphae, which arise as perpendicular extensions from the yeast cell, with no constriction at their point of origin) within 1 to 2 hours offered a positive identification of *C. albicans*. Unfortunately, *C. dubliniensis*, a new species of *Candida* that was identified recently as an important cause of mucosal colonization and infection in HIV-infected individuals, also can produce a germ tube. A negative germ tube test does not rule out the possibility of *C. albicans*, but further biochemical tests must be performed to differentiate between other non-*albicans* species.[35]

In patients with hepatosplenic candidiasis, as the WBC count increases to >1,000 cells/mm^3 (>1 × 10^9/L), imaging studies can detect the presence of abscess or microabscesses in the liver and spleen, often found with acute suppurative and granulomatous reactions.

The peptide nucleic acid (PNA) fluorescence in situ hybridization (FISH) method uses fluorescein-labeled PNA probes that target *C. albicans* 26S rRNA for the identification of *C. albicans*. The test has excellent sensitivity (99% to 100%) and specificity (100%) in the direct identification of *C. albicans* from blood cultures.[18]

Matrix-assisted laser desorption/ionization time-of-flight intact cell mass spectrometry (MALDI-TOF-ICMS) is a promising tool for the rapid detection and identification of pathogenic *Candida* species.

TREATMENT

The list of risk factors for invasive candidiasis in critically ill patients is extensive, and trying to decipher which patients may benefit from antifungal prophylaxis or empirical therapy based on risk factors in an ICU is exceedingly difficult. In addition, the number of risk factors present in ICU patients changes over time, and the majority of ICU patients will have more than one risk factor. Thus, recent studies have focused on combining risk factors to devise clinically useful, practical predictive algorithms and "scoring systems" that can identify high-risk patients early during their ICU admission. To maximize its clinical utility as a decision-making tool, the ideal algorithm would identify high-risk populations (ones with a rate of invasive candidiasis of 10% to 15%), providing clinicians with a means of administering prophylaxis to a minimal number of patients, while preventing the maximal number of invasive candidiasis cases. However, a scoring system is not yet available for use in clinical practice.[34]

Hematogenous Candidiasis

There is a high rate of mortality in nonneutropenic patients with fungal blood cultures.[36] Mortality was highest in patients with sustained positive blood cultures, those who did not receive antifungal therapy, and those infected with non-*albicans* strains of *Candida*.

This study clearly documented the importance of early recognition and treatment of positive fungal blood cultures. Prompt initiation of therapy is important. Delays in empiric antifungal treatment greater than 12 hours after obtaining a positive blood sample are associated with greater hospital mortality.[37–39] Despite increased awareness of the importance of treating patients with positive blood cultures, mortality associated with candidemia remains high.[40]

Current guidelines recommend that the treatment of candidiasis should be guided by knowledge of the infecting species; the clinical status of the patient; when available, the antifungal susceptibility of the infecting isolate; and whether the patient has received antifungal therapy previously (Table 99-8). Therapy should be continued for 2 weeks after the last positive blood culture and resolution of signs and symptoms of infection. All patients should undergo an ophthalmologic examination to exclude the possibility of candidal endophthalmitis.[7] Amphotericin B can be switched to fluconazole (IV or oral) for the completion of therapy. Susceptibility testing of the infecting isolate is a useful adjunct to species identification during selection of a therapeutic approach because it can be used to identify isolates that are unlikely to respond to fluconazole or amphotericin B. However, this is not currently available at many institutions.[6]

Clinical **Controversy. . .**

A meta-analysis of individual patient-level data of 1,915 patients, compiled from seven randomized clinical trials, compared a variety of antifungal therapies for the treatment of candidemia and reported improved survival and greater clinical success with the use of an echinocandin and removal of CVCs.[41,42] Overall, 30-day all-cause mortality was 31.4%; however, mortality was 27% for echinocandins versus 36% for other regimens ($P < 0.0001$). By comparison, mortality was 36% for triazoles versus 30% for other drugs ($P < 0.006$), and 35% for polyenes versus 30% for other drugs ($P = 0.04$). In addition, they reported that mortality for CVC removal 28% versus 41% for patients in whom CVCs were retained ($P < 0.0001$). Based on their findings, echinocandins should be considered as initial therapy not only for critically ill patients, those with prior triazole exposure, and those infected with less susceptible *Candida* spp. such as *C. glabrata* or *C. krusei*, but for most patients with candidemia, and that CVC removal should be performed. Limitations of this study include the exclusion of patients who fall into extremes, and that these studies undertaken during a 15-year period, during which time treatment practices have changed. There was a lack of information regarding the timing of CVC removal, and that only three of the seven randomized clinical trials compared the use of an echinocandin with other antifungals, and in those studies, the mortality rate of patients receiving an echinocandin was similar to that of patients receiving other antifungal therapy.

Nonimmunocompromised Patient

Prophylaxis

In ICUs, the use of fluconazole for prophylaxis or empirical therapy has increased exponentially in the past decade. However, studies that demonstrated benefit in the prevention of invasive candidal BSIs did so either by using highly selective criteria or by studying patients in an unusually high-risk ICU setting, and the role of antifungal prophylaxis in the surgical ICU remains extremely controversial. For a study to demonstrate efficacy in clinical trials, the baseline rate of invasive candidiasis must be >10%, and that prophylaxis must result in > fourfold reduction of disease.[7] Although ICU-specific, a >10% rate of invasive candidiasis is generally found only in the setting of high-risk transplant patients (e.g., patients undergoing liver transplantation), or in patients with one or more of the following risk factors by day 3 of their ICU stay: new-onset dialysis, receipt of broad-spectrum antibiotics, the presence of diabetes, and in patients receiving PN.[42,43] Prophylactic antifungals are indicated in patients with recurrent intestinal perforations and/or anastomotic leak as these patients are at extremely high risk for invasive candidiasis (35%) and the use of empiric fluconazole has been shown to significantly decrease the incidence of infection to 4%.[34]

"Empirical" Therapy (Also Known as Preemptive Therapy)

The term "preemptive" antifungal therapy is often used to describe early antifungal therapy given to high-risk patients with persistent signs and symptoms and clinical, laboratory, or radiologic surrogate markers of infection but without mycological evidence of infection, or those heavily colonized with *Candida*. Few data are available for assessing the role of antifungals as empirical therapy for *suspected* fungemia in patients who do not yet exhibit a positive blood culture, or for isolates other than *C. albicans*.

In a double-blind randomized placebo controlled trial, the empiric use of fluconazole 800 mg daily in 270 high-risk patients with a baseline rate of IC of 9% decreased the incidence of invasive candidiasis only to 5% ($P = 0.24$). The authors concluded that the use of empiric fluconazole cannot be recommended for ICU populations with similar risk factors as those included in the trial.

Initial Antifungal Therapy in Patients with Documented Candidemia

Several large randomized studies in nonneutropenic patients have demonstrated that azoles (fluconazole or voriconazole) and deoxycholate amphotericin B are similarly effective for the therapy of documented candidemia; however, fewer adverse effects are observed with azole therapy (Tables 99-8 and 99-9). Similarly, echinocandins are at least as effective as amphotericin B or fluconazole in (primarily nonneutropenic) adult patients with candidemia with fewer drug-related adverse events. Although the use of combination therapy (high-dose fluconazole plus amphotericin B) was demonstrated recently to be superior to treatment with fluconazole alone, it was associated with a higher rate of nephrotoxicity, and the routine use of combination therapy in this patient population is not yet recommended. Alternatives to fluconazole should be considered when patients have a history of recent exposure to fluconazole or other azoles, when a broader spectrum is desirable (e.g., persistently neutropenic patient), when non-*albicans* species are isolated during or immediately following azole therapy, and in unstable or severely immunocompromised patients.[44–51]

Neonates with disseminated candidiasis usually are treated with amphotericin B because of its low toxicity in this patient population and because of the lack of experience with other agents in this population; however, micafungin or caspofungin may offer safe, effective alternatives.[7,40,52] Treatment should continue until 2 weeks following the last positive blood culture and resolution of signs and symptoms of infection.

Among the lipid-associated formulations of amphotericin B, only liposomal amphotericin B (AmBisome) and amphotericin B lipid complex (ABLC; Abelcet) have been approved for use in proven cases of candidiasis; however, patients with invasive candidiasis also have been treated successfully with amphotericin B colloid dispersion (ABCD, Amphotec or Amphocil). The lipid-associated formulations are less toxic but as effective as amphotericin B deoxycholate.

TABLE 99-8 Antifungal Therapy of Invasive Candidiasis[7,34]

Type of Disease and Common Clinical Manifestations	Therapy/Comments
Prophylaxis of Candidemia	
Nonneutropenic patients[a]	Not recommended except for severely ill/high-risk patients in whom fluconazole IV/PO 400 mg daily should be used (see the text)
Neutropenic patients[a]	The optimal duration of therapy is unclear but at a minimum should include the period at risk for neutropenia: Fluconazole IV/PO 400 mg daily *or* itraconazole solution 2.5 mg/kg every 12 hours PO *or* micafungin 50 mg (1 mg/kg in patients under 50 kg) IV daily
Solid-organ transplantation, liver transplantation	*Patients with two or more key risk factors[b]:* Amphotericin B IV 10–20 mg daily *or* liposomal amphotericin B (AmBisome) 1 mg/kg/day *or* fluconazole 400 mg orally daily
Empirical (Preemptive) Antifungal Therapy	
Suspected disseminated candidiasis in febrile nonneutropenic patients	None recommended; data are lacking defining subsets of patients who are appropriate for therapy (see the text)
Initial Antifungal Therapy (Documented Candidemia with Unknown Candida Species)	
Febrile neutropenic patients with prolonged fever despite 4–6 days of empirical antibacterial therapy	*Treatment duration:* Until resolution of neutropenia An echinocandin[d] is a reasonable alternative; voriconazole can be used in selected situations (see the text)
Less critically ill patients with no recent azole exposure	An echinocandin[d] or fluconazole (loading dose of 800 mg [12 mg/kg], then 400 mg [6 mg/kg] daily)
Additional mold coverage is desired	Voriconazole
Antifungal Therapy of Documented Candidemia and Acute Hematogenously Disseminated Candidiasis, Unknown Species	
Nonimmunocompromised host[c]	*Treatment duration:* 2 weeks after the last positive blood culture and resolution of signs and symptoms of infection *Remove existing central venous catheters when feasible plus fluconazole (loading dose of 800 mg [12 mg/kg], then 400 mg [6 mg/kg] daily) or an echinocandin[d]*
Patients with recent azole exposure, moderately severe or severe illness, or who are at high risk of infection due to *C. glabrata* or *C. krusei*	An echinocandin[d] Transition from an echinocandin to fluconazole is recommended for patients who are clinically stable and have isolates (e.g., *C. albicans*) likely to be susceptible to fluconazole
Patients who are less critically ill and who have had no recent azole exposure	Fluconazole
Antifungal Therapy of Specific Pathogens	
C. albicans, C. tropicalis, and *C. parapsilosis*	Fluconazole IV/PO 6 mg/kg/day *or* an echinocandin[d] or amphotericin B IV 0.7 mg/kg/day *plus* fluconazole IV/PO 800 mg/day; amphotericin B deoxycholate 0.5–1 mg/kg daily or a lipid formulation of amphotericin B (3–5 mg/kg daily) are alternatives in patients who are intolerant to other antifungals; transition from amphotericin B deoxycholate or a lipid formulation of amphotericin B to fluconazole is recommended in patients who are clinically stable and whose isolates are likely to be susceptible to fluconazole (e.g., *C. albicans*); voriconazole (400 mg [6 mg/kg] twice daily × two doses then 200 mg [3 mg/kg] twice daily thereafter) is efficacious, but offers little advantage over fluconazole; it may be utilized as step-down oral therapy for selected cases of candidiasis due to *C. krusei* or voriconazole-susceptible *C. glabrata* *Patients intolerant or refractory to other therapy[e]:* Amphotericin B lipid complex IV 5 mg/kg/day Liposomal amphotericin B IV 3–5 mg/kg/day Amphotericin B colloid dispersion IV 2–6 mg/kg/day
C. krusei	Amphotericin B IV ≤1 mg/kg/day *or* an echinocandin[d]
C. lusitaniae	Fluconazole IV/PO 6 mg/kg/day
C. glabrata	An echinocandin[d] (transition to fluconazole or voriconazole therapy is not recommended without confirmation of isolate susceptibility)
Neutropenic host[f]	*Treatment duration:* Until resolution of neutropenia *Remove existing central venous catheters when feasible, plus:* Amphotericin B IV 0.7–1 mg/kg/day (total dosages 0.5–1 g) *or patients failing therapy with traditional amphotericin B:* Lipid formulation of amphotericin B IV 3–5 mg/kg/day
Chronic disseminated candidiasis (hepatosplenic candidiasis)	*Treatment duration:* Until calcification or resolution of lesions *Stable patients:* Fluconazole IV/PO 6 mg/kg/day *Acutely ill or refractory patients:* Amphotericin B IV 0.6–0.7 mg/kg/day
Urinary candidiasis	*Asymptomatic disease:* Generally no therapy is required *Symptomatic or high-risk patients[g]:* Removal of urinary tract instruments, stents, and Foley catheters, +7–14 days therapy with fluconazole 200 mg orally daily *or* amphotericin B IV 0.3–1 mg/kg/day

PO, orally.

[a]Patients at significant risk for invasive candidiasis include those receiving standard chemotherapy for acute myelogenous leukemia, allogeneic bone marrow transplants, or high-risk autologous bone marrow transplants. However, among these populations, chemotherapy or bone marrow transplant protocols do not all produce equivalent risk, and local experience should be used to determine the relevance of prophylaxis.

[b]Risk factors include retransplantation, creatinine of more than 2 mg/dL (177 μmol/L), choledochojejunostomy, intraoperative use of 40 units or more of blood products, and fungal colonization detected within the first 3 days after transplantation.

[c]Therapy is generally the same for acquired immunodeficiency syndrome (AIDS)/non-AIDS patients except where indicated and should continued for 2 weeks after the last positive blood culture and resolution of signs and symptoms of infection. All patients should receive an ophthalmologic examination. Amphotericin B can be switched to fluconazole (IV or oral) for the completion of therapy. Susceptibility testing of the infecting isolate is a useful adjunct to species identification during selection of a therapeutic approach because it can be used to identify isolates that are unlikely to respond to fluconazole or amphotericin B. However, this is not currently available at most institutions.

[d]Echinocandin = caspofungin 70 mg loading dose, then 50 mg IV daily maintenance dose, or micafungin 100 mg daily, or anidulafungin 200 mg loading dose, then 100 mg daily maintenance dose.

[e]Often defined as failure of ≥500 mg amphotericin B, initial renal insufficiency (creatinine ≥2.5 mg/dL [≥221 μmol/L] or creatinine clearance <25 mL/min [< 0.42 mL/s]), a significant increase in creatinine (to 2.5 mg/dL [221 μmol/L] for adults or 1.5 mg/dL [133 μmol/L] for children), or severe acute administration-related toxicity.

[f]Patients who are neutropenic at the time of developing candidemia should receive a recombinant cytokine (granulocyte colony-stimulating factor or granulocyte–monocyte colony-stimulating factor) that accelerates recovery from neutropenia.

[g]Patients at high risk for dissemination include neutropenic patients, low-birth-weight infants, patients with renal allografts, and patients who will undergo urologic manipulation.

Data from Pappas et al.[7]

TABLE 99-9 Initial Antifungal Therapy of Candidemia in the Nonneutropenic Host

Year Published	Study Drugs and Dosages	Study Design	Results and Comments
1994	Fluconazole versus amphotericin B	Randomized, nonblinded, multicenter	Similar outcomes but higher rate of nephrotoxicity in the amphotericin B group
2002	Caspofungin (70 mg IV × 1 loading dose; then 50 mg IV daily) versus amphotericin B (0.6–0.7 mg/kg/day IV) each antifungal agent was changed to fluconazole after ≥10 days to complete therapy	Randomized, multicenter	Successful outcome was achieved in 73.9% and 61.7% of patients receiving caspofungin and amphotericin B, respectively, but there was a higher rate of nephrotoxicity in the amphotericin B group
2003	Fluconazole 800 mg/day + placebo versus fluconazole 800 mg/day + amphotericin B 0.7 mg/kg/day	Randomized, blinded, multicenter	The study was confounded by differences in the severity of illness of the two study populations (the fluconazole group had more severe illness). The regimens were comparable and noted a trend toward better response (based principally on more effective bloodstream clearance) in the group receiving combination therapy
2005	Voriconazole (6 mg/kg IV every 12 hours on day 1; 3 mg/kg every 12 hours IV on days 2 and 3; then 200 mg PO every 12 hours) versus amphotericin B (≤0.7 mg/kg/day) followed by fluconazole (≥400 mg PO/IV daily)	Randomized, nonblinded, multicenter	Voriconazole was as effective as the regimen of amphotericin B followed by fluconazole in the clearing of blood cultures; treatment discontinuations cased by all-cause adverse events were more frequent in the voriconazole group, although most discontinuations were caused by non–drug-related events, and there were significantly fewer serious adverse events and cases of renal toxicity than in the amphotericin B/fluconazole group
2005	Anidulafungin (200 mg loading dose × 1, then 100 mg/day) versus IV fluconazole (800 mg loading dose × 1, then 400 mg/day)	Randomized, double-blind	A statistically significantly greater response was observed with anidulafungin in the microbiologic intent-to-treat arm at the end of IV therapy, and at the 2- and 6-week followups in patients with APACHE II scores of >20; survival was improved with anidulafungin
2005	Micafungin (100 mg/day IV) versus liposomal amphotericin B (3 mg/kg/day) × 2–4 weeks	Randomized, double-blind	Micafungin treatment was considered effective (clinical plus mycological response) in 89.6% of patients (181:202), compared to 89.5% (170:190) in the amphotericin B group. The amphotericin B group had a significantly higher incidence of side effects, including infusion-related reactions and increases in serum creatinine
2006	Caspofungin (70 mg IV × one loading dose; then 50 mg IV daily) versus micafungin 100 mg/day versus micafungin 150 mg/day	Randomized, double-blind	Micafungin was found noninferior to caspofungin; higher dosages of micafungin (150 mg/day vs. 100 mg/day) were not more efficacious; the safety profiles for the three treatments were similar

APACHE, Acute Physiology and Chronic Health Evaluation; PO, orally.

Data from Rex et al.,[45,48] Reboli et al.,[46] Mora-Duarte et al.,[47] Kullberg et al.,[49] Kuse et al.,[50] and Pappas et al.[51]

Antifungal Therapy for Specific *Candida* Species

C. krusei infections should be treated with large doses of amphotericin B (≥1 mg/kg per day) or with caspofungin (70-mg IV loading dose, followed by 50 mg/day IV) (Table 99-8).[7] *C. tropicalis*, and *C. parapsilosis* can be treated with either amphotericin B at 0.6 mg/kg per day or fluconazole at 6 mg/kg per day. Amphotericin B resistance remains relatively rare despite more than 45 years of clinical use, although it has been reported in *C. lusitaniae* (now *Clavispora lusitaniae*) and *C. guilliermondii*. *Candida rugosa* often is considered to be "polyene tolerant," and these isolates are believed to be selected owing to the wide use of amphotericin B.

Immunocompromised Patients

In immunocompromised patients, the presence of candidemia is associated with evidence of disseminated disease in more than 70% of patients and with a 70% to 80% fatality rate. Therapy should include removal of the catheter and administration of systemic antifungal therapy.[7] The optimal agent, dose, and duration of therapy are unclear, and patients must be monitored carefully with serial blood cultures and careful physical examinations, particularly of the retina. Patients who are neutropenic at the time of developing candidemia should receive a recombinant cytokine (granulocyte colony-stimulating factor or granulocyte-monocyte colony-stimulating factor) that accelerates recovery from neutropenia.[7]

Prophylaxis

Recognition of the role of the GI tract in invasive *Candida* infections has led to efforts to decrease infections by prophylactic administration of topical or systemically absorbed antifungal agents in immunocompromised patients. The use of systemically absorbable agents such as azole antifungal agents appears to decrease the risk of invasive fungal infections.[7,53,54]

Fluconazole (400 mg/day), posaconazole (200 mg three times daily), or micafungin (50 mg daily) from the start of the conditioning regimen until day 75 can reduce the frequency of invasive *Candida* infections and decrease mortality at day 110 in patients undergoing allogeneic bone marrow transplantation.[7,16,54,55] IV caspofungin (50 mg daily) was compared with IV itraconazole (200 mg twice daily for 2 days, then 200 mg once daily). Mortality was similar in both groups. Micafungin 50 mg daily was compared to IV fluconazole 400 mg daily in patients undergoing HSCT. Significantly fewer patients in the micafungin arm versus the fluconazole arm required empiric antifungal therapy, and mortality was decreased, although not significantly, in the micafungin arm. Based on this limited data, micafungin and caspofungin may provide options for prophylaxis in patients undergoing HSCT. However, more compelling data have been demonstrated with posaconazole. In a double-blinded, multi-center clinical trial of the prophylaxis of invasive fungal infections in patients who had undergone HSCT with GVHD, posaconazole (200 mg every 8 hours) was superior to fluconazole (400 mg daily) in preventing aspergillosis and comparable to fluconazole in preventing other breakthrough invasive fungal infections.[16,56]

In less risk-selected patients with hematologic malignancies who are undergoing remission-induction chemotherapy, fluconazole (400 mg/day), posaconazole (200 mg three times daily), or caspofungin (50 mg daily), during induction chemotherapy for the duration of neutropenia, are effective in preventing systemic infection and death caused by *Candida* species.[7,57,58] Itraconazole cyclodextrin (2.5 mg/kg orally twice daily) is an option for less risk-selected patients, but it offers little advantage over other agents and is less well tolerated.[16]

For solid-organ transplant recipients, fluconazole (200 to 400 mg [3 to 6 mg/kg] daily) or liposomal amphotericin B (1 to 2 mg/kg daily for 7 to 14 days) is recommended as postoperative antifungal prophylaxis for liver, pancreas, and small bowel transplant recipients at high risk of candidiasis.[7,15]

The use of prophylactic fluconazole (400 mg [6 mg/kg] daily) can decrease the incidence of fungal infections in select high-risk groups of patients. However, despite decreases in the rate of invasive candidiasis, to date, no mortality benefit has been demonstrated in any clinical trial. Widespread use of prophylactic fluconazole in all ICU patients is not warranted and may lead to an increase in resistance and adverse events. If utilized, prophylactic fluconazole should target high-risk patients with a presumed risk of invasive candidiasis of 10% to 15%.[7,34]

Empirical Therapy for Febrile Neutropenic Patients

Many clinicians advocate early institution of empirical IV amphotericin B in patients with neutropenia and persistent (>5 to 7 days) fever.[16] However, the potential toxicities (particularly nephrotoxicity) of this agent preclude its routine use in all patients. Suggested criteria for the empirical use of amphotericin B include: (a) fever of 5 to 7 days' duration that is unresponsive to antibacterial agents, (b) neutropenia of more than 7 days' duration, (c) no other obvious cause for fever, (d) progressive debilitation, (e) chronic adrenal corticosteroid therapy, and (f) indwelling intravascular catheters. In patients who fail therapy with amphotericin B, lipid formulations of amphotericin B can be used (3 to 5 mg/kg per day). Comparative trials have indicated that lipid formulations of amphotericin B can be used as alternatives to amphotericin B deoxycholate for empirical therapy. Although they do not appear to be substantially more effective, there is less drug-related toxicity (Table 99-10).[16]

Itraconazole and fluconazole have demonstrated efficacy equivalent to that of deoxycholate amphotericin B in patients with hematologic malignancy (not treated with allogeneic HSCT).[59,60] However, as fluconazole is not active against filamentous fungi, its use in patients at high risk for these pathogens should be avoided. If itraconazole is used, the IV formulation should be used because the bioavailability of the oral formulations (including the solution) is unreliable; however, it is no longer available. Voriconazole and caspofungin were compared with liposomal amphotericin B in large randomized, multicenter trials of empirical antifungal therapy in febrile neutropenic patients. Voriconazole did not fulfill the protocol-defined criteria for noninferiority (a difference in success rates between voriconazole and amphotericin B of no more than 10 percentage points) to liposomal amphotericin; however, it was superior in reducing documented breakthrough infections, infusion-related toxicity, and nephrotoxicity. Patients who received voriconazole had more frequent episodes of transient visual disturbances and hallucinations. Caspofungin demonstrated equivalent efficacy but was superior in the successful treatment of baseline invasive fungal infections.[52,61]

Specific Therapy

Amphotericin B, the azoles, and the echinocandins have roles in the treatment of hematogenous candidiasis, and the choice of therapy is guided by weighing the greater activity of amphotericin B for some non-*albicans* species (e.g., *C. krusei*) against the lower toxicity and ease of administration of fluconazole and the echinocandins.[7]

Most clinicians recommend amphotericin B in total dosages of 0.5 to 1 g administered over approximately 1 to 2 weeks in patients with *Candida* endophthalmitis and in all neutropenic patients with candidemia. Longer courses of therapy can be needed in some patients.[17] Fluconazole and amphotericin B appear similarly effective for the treatment of *C. albicans* BSIs in the neutropenic patient; controlled data, however, are lacking. In patients with uncomplicated *C. albicans* fungemia who have not received systemic prophylaxis with antifungal azoles, therapy with fluconazole 400 to 800 mg/day IV can be considered.[62] However, in patients

TABLE 99-10 Comparative Trials for Initial Antifungal Therapy in the Febrile Neutropenic Host

Year Published	Study Drugs	Study Design	Results and Comments
1982	Placebo versus amphotericin B	Randomized	Favored amphotericin B
1989	Placebo versus amphotericin B	Randomized	Favored amphotericin B
1996	Fluconazole versus amphotericin B	Randomized	Defervescence: equivalence; safety analysis favored fluconazole
1998	Fluconazole versus amphotericin B	Randomized	Composite: equivalence; secondary analysis favored fluconazole
2000	Fluconazole versus amphotericin B	Randomized	Composite: equivalence; safety analysis favored fluconazole
1999	Liposomal amphotericin B versus amphotericin B	Randomized, double blind	Composite: equivalence; secondary analysis favors liposomal amphotericin B
2000	Liposomal amphotericin B versus amphotericin B lipid complex	Randomized, double blind	Liposomal amphotericin B had superior safety versus amphotericin B lipid complex and a similar therapeutic success rate
2001	Itraconazole versus amphotericin B	Randomized, open label	Composite: equivalence; secondary analysis favors itraconazole
2002	Voriconazole versus liposomal amphotericin B	Randomized, open label	Composite: equivalence; secondary analysis variable (voriconazole failed to meet criteria for noninferiority); fewer breakthrough infections with voriconazole
2004	Caspofungin versus liposomal amphotericin B	Randomized, double blind	Composite: equivalence; secondary analysis favored caspofungin for treatment of baseline infections
2005	Liposomal amphotericin B loading regimen (10 mg/kg/day × 14 day) versus standard dosing (3 mg/kg/day)	Randomized, prospective, double blind	Loading regimen did not demonstrate any benefit in overall response or survival and was associated with higher rates of nephrotoxicity and hypokalemia

Data from Boogaerts et al.,[59] Winston et al.,[60] Walsh et al.,[61] and Cornely et al.[81]

who have undergone allogeneic HSCT, the role of fluconazole is becoming more limited because of its widespread use for antifungal prophylaxis. In this setting, particularly if the patient has been treated previously with an azole antifungal agent, the possibility of microbiologic resistance must be considered.[7] Infections with fluconazole-resistant *Candida* species, including *C. glabrata*, *C. krusei*, and fluconazole-resistant *C. albicans*, or with *Aspergillus* species are more likely.

Clinical **Controversy. . .**

Because *C. glabrata* demonstrates reduced susceptibility in vitro to both fluconazole and amphotericin B, optimal therapy is unclear. Larger doses of fluconazole (800 mg/day in a 70-kg patient) have been used in less critically ill patients or amphotericin B (≥0.7 mg/kg per day). However, observational studies demonstrated no difference in mortality in nonneutropenic patients administered fluconazole versus amphotericin B for BSIs caused by *C. glabrata*.[40] In vitro, echinocandin antifungal agents appear very active against *C. glabrata*. Current guidelines recommend the use of echinocandins, instead of fluconazole, for the treatment of fungemia caused by *C. glabrata*; however, their usefulness in vivo has not been adequately assessed in controlled trials.[7,40]

In patients intolerant to amphotericin B or fluconazole, one of the lipid formulations can be used. In a randomized trial, ABLC was found to be equivalent to 0.6 to 1 mg/kg per day of amphotericin B, and open-label therapy with ABCD has been successful.

CANDIDURIA

Within the urinary tract, most common lesions are either *Candida* cystitis or hematogenously disseminated renal abscesses. *Candida* cystitis often follows catheterization or therapy with broad-spectrum antimicrobial agents. The diagnosis of *Candida* cystitis can be problematic because of the frequent presence of *Candida* pseudohyphae and yeast cells in urine specimens secondary to urethral colonization. The usefulness of urine colony counts or antibody coating techniques is questionable. The recovery of 10,000 organisms or visualization of both yeast and pseudohyphae from fresh midstream urine or from bladder urine obtained by single catheterization (not indwelling) is suggestive of genitourinary candidiasis. In most patients, the infection is asymptomatic and clears spontaneously without specific antifungal therapy.

Initial therapy of candidal cystitis should focus on removal of urinary catheters whenever possible. Changing the catheter will eliminate candiduria in only 20% of patients, whereas discontinuation will eradicate *Candida* in 40% of patients. Asymptomatic candiduria rarely requires therapy. Therapy should be used in symptomatic patients and in neutropenic patients, as well as in patients with renal allografts and those who will undergo urologic manipulation, because of the risk of dissemination.[63,64]

Fluconazole 200 mg/day for 14 days hastens the time to a negative urine culture as compared with placebo treatment, but 2 weeks after the end of therapy, the frequency of a negative urine culture remains the same with both treatments.[64] Short courses of therapy are not recommended; treatment should include removal of catheters and stents whenever possible plus 7 to 14 days of therapy. Bladder irrigation with amphotericin B (50 mg in 500 mL sterile water instilled twice daily into the bladder via a three-way catheter) is only transiently effective. Minimal quantities (<3%) of amphotericin B are absorbed systemically from the bladder.[64,65]

Role of Catheter Removal

Although it is common practice in today's standard of care to place indwelling catheters in patients for the administration of medications and PN, catheter-related infections are a common complication. These foreign bodies (especially triple-lumen catheters) double as entry ports for normal skin flora or other nosocomial pathogens, and they provide a readily available site for the binding of pathogens through microbiotic biofilms. Their subsequent role as a source of BSIs is facilitated by frequent use, PN, and the potential for contamination of catheters by medical staff who are colonized with *Candida* species.

Most consensus recommendations urge that, if feasible, initial nonmedical management should include removal of all existing tunneled CVCs and implantable devices, particularly in patients with fungemia caused by *C. parapsilosis*, which is very frequently associated with catheters.[7] Arguments against the removal of all catheters in patients with candidemia include the prominent role of the gut as a source for disseminated candidiasis, the significant cost and potential for complications, and the problems that can be encountered in patients with difficult vascular access.[66] However, in an individual patient it is often difficult to determine the relative contribution of gut versus catheter as the primary source of fungemia. The evidence for this recommendation is weakest in cancer patients with severe neutropenia and mucositis (e.g., acute leukemia, stem cell transplant), in whom candidemia is almost always primarily of gut origin, and removal of the catheter is least likely to have an impact on mortality. Nucci and Anaissie[62,66] have proposed that CVCs be removed in nonneutropenic patients without a short life expectancy who have one of the following criteria: (a) otherwise unexplained hemodynamic instability, (b) lack of clinical improvement or resolution of candidemia after more than 72 hours of an optimal dose of an appropriate antifungal agent, (c) established or at high risk for endocarditis or septic thrombophlebitis, or (d) a pocket infection or cellulitis. In patients with more than one CVC, they recommend removal if one tunneled or implanted catheter is the likely source of infection and the patient meets the preceding criteria.[62]

ASPERGILLOSIS

Epidemiology

Aspergillus is a ubiquitous mold that grows well on a variety of substrates, including soil, water, decaying vegetation, moldy hay or straw, and organic debris. Although more than 300 species of *Aspergillus* have been characterized, three species are most commonly pathogenic: *Aspergillus fumigatus*, *Aspergillus flavus*, and *Aspergillus niger*. The varying degrees of pathogenicity of each species depend on their relative geographic prevalence, conidial size and shape, thermotolerance, and production of mycotoxins. For example, transport of *A. fumigatus* conidia into the lungs is facilitated by their smaller diameter in comparison with *A. flavus* and *A. niger*.

9 The term *aspergillosis* may be broadly defined as a spectrum of diseases attributed to allergy, colonization, or tissue invasion caused by members of the fungal genus *Aspergillus*. A single satisfactory classification system for these disease entities is difficult because different populations of patients can develop the same type of infection. For example, osteomyelitis can result from local trauma or hematogenous dissemination in an immunocompromised host. Colonization in normal hosts can lead to allergic diseases ranging from asthma to allergic BPA or, rarely, invasive disease.[67]

Pathophysiology

Aspergillosis generally is acquired by inhalation of airborne conidia that are small enough (2.5 to 3 microns) to reach alveoli or the paranasal sinuses. Each conidiophore releases 10^4 conidia that remain suspended for long periods and are viable for months in dry locations. Although some authors advocate monitoring of hospital air for *Aspergillus* conidia, guidelines for interpreting results do not exist. The use of high-efficiency particulate air (HEPA) filters in operating rooms and laminar flow rooms and removal of immunocompromised patients from hospital renovation sites can be helpful in preventing infection in this population. Although the fate of *Aspergillus* conidia in the GI tract has not been closely studied, limited evidence suggests that this route may provide an important portal of entry for disseminated infections in humans.[68]

Superficial Infection

Superficial or locally invasive infections of the ear, skin, or appendages often can be managed with topical antifungal therapy. Skin infections in patients with burn wounds, although uncommon, can progress to deep-tissue invasion despite the use of topical or parenteral antifungal agents. Risk factors for deep infection include extensive thermal injuries, malnutrition, cirrhosis, and previous infection with *Pseudomonas aeruginosa*.[68]

Allergic Bronchopulmonary Aspergillosis

Allergic manifestations of *Aspergillus* range in severity from mild asthma to allergic BPA. BPA, which is almost always caused by *A. fumigatus*, is characterized by severe asthma with wheezing, fever, malaise, weight loss, chest pain, and a cough productive of blood-streaked sputum. Following recurrent episodes of severe asthma, the disease usually progresses to fibrosis and bronchiectasis with granuloma formation. When *Aspergillus* conidia become trapped in the viscous mucus of asthmatic patients, BPA develops. The fungus grows, releasing toxins and antigens. The resulting host sensitization results in a variety of immune reactions. Early in the course of disease, an immunoglobulin E (IgE)-mediated (type I) immune reaction results in bronchospasm, eosinophilia, and immediate skin reactivity. The ensuing fibrosis and pulmonary infiltrates appear to be mediated by circulating or precipitating antibody complexes of IgG antibody, followed by granuloma formation and mononuclear infiltration because of a type IV delayed hypersensitivity reaction. Therapy is aimed at minimizing the quantity of antigenic material released in the tracheobronchial tree. Management of acute asthma attacks minimizes trapping of *Aspergillus* by bronchial secretions, and administration of parenteral corticosteroids clears lung infiltrates.[68] Antifungal therapy generally is not indicated in the management of allergic manifestations of aspergillosis, although some patients have demonstrated a decrease in their corticosteroid dose following therapy with itraconazole. A double-blind, randomized, placebo-controlled trial showed that itraconazole 200 mg orally twice daily for 16 weeks resulted in significant differences in the amelioration of disease, as measured by the reduction in corticosteroid dose and improvement in exercise tolerance and pulmonary function.[67]

Aspergilloma

In the nonimmunocompromised host, *Aspergillus* infections of the sinuses most commonly occur as saprophytic colonization (aspergillomas or "fungus balls") of previously abnormal sinus tissue. An aspergilloma is composed of intertwined *Aspergillus* hyphae matted together with fibrin, mucus, and cellular debris. Infection usually is localized in the maxillary sinus and rarely is associated with local invasion of adjacent bone or brain tissue. Sinus aspergillosis also can present as allergic sinusitis with nasal drainage of brownish mucous plugs. Therapy with corticosteroids and surgery generally is successful. In the immunocompromised host, subacute, chronic, or fulminant invasive disease can be seen, and a combination of antifungal and surgical therapy generally is required.[12,68]

Pulmonary aspergillomas are fungus balls arising in preexisting cavities because of tuberculosis, histoplasmosis, lung tumors, or radiation fibrosis, although occasionally no previous pulmonary disease is present. The diagnosis of aspergilloma generally is made on the basis of chest radiographs, on which aspergillomas appear as a solid rounded mass, sometimes mobile, of water density within a spherical or ovoid cavity and separated from the wall of the cavity by an airspace of variable size and shape. Patients generally experience chest pain, dyspnea, and sputum production. Hemoptysis is observed in 50% to 80% of patients, probably because of ulceration of the epithelial lining of the cavity with formation of granulation tissue, and hemoptysis is the cause of death in up to 26% of patients with aspergilloma. A poor prognosis is associated with increasing size or number of aspergillomas, immunosuppression (including corticosteroids), increasing *Aspergillus*-specific titers, underlying sarcoidosis, and HIV infection. Although *Aspergillus* can be cultured in only 50% to 60% of patients, precipitating antibodies are positive in virtually 100% of patients.

Invasive disease occurs rarely, and therapy therefore is controversial. There are no controlled clinical trials with which to guide therapy, and recommendations for treatment have been generated from uncontrolled trials and case reports.[12] Concern regarding the risk of severe hemorrhage has led some clinicians to use aggressive surgical excision of aspergillomas or pulmonary resection in patients with hemoptysis. Complications, including bronchopulmonary fistulas, hemorrhage, empyema, and persistent airspace problems, have led to the recommendation that surgical intervention be reserved for patients with severe (>500 mL/24 h) hemoptysis, however. Bronchial artery embolization has been used to occlude the vessel that supplies the bleeding site in patients experiencing hemoptysis. Unfortunately, bronchial artery embolization generally is unsuccessful or only temporarily effective. Collateral circulation eventually develops, supplying blood flow to the affected area, and hemoptysis often recurs; consequently, reembolization is often unsuccessful. Bronchial artery embolization should be used as a temporizing procedure in a patient with life-threatening disease who might respond to more definitive therapy if hemoptysis is stabilized. Mild to moderate hemoptysis should be managed conservatively. Although IV amphotericin B generally is not useful in eradicating aspergillomas, inhaled or intracavitary instillation of amphotericin B has been employed successfully in a limited number of patients. Itraconazole has been efficacious in uncontrolled studies; however, the dose and duration of therapy have not been standardized. Hemoptysis generally ceases when the aspergilloma is eradicated.[12,68]

Invasive Aspergillosis

Although exposure to *Aspergillus* conidia is nearly universal, impaired host defenses are required for the development of invasive disease. Phagocytes (neutrophils, monocytes, and macrophages) rather than antibodies or lymphocytes constitute the primary host defense system against invasive disease with aspergillosis. Macrophages prevent germination of conidia and also eradicate conidia, providing the first line of defense against invasive disease. Administration of corticosteroids appears to impair the killing of conidia by macrophages and to impair mobilization of neutrophils. Neutrophils halt hyphal growth and dissemination and kill mycelia, constituting a second line of defense. Prolonged neutropenia appears to be the most important predisposing factor to the development of IA, accounting for the high frequency of disease in patients with acute leukemia. Complement provides a source of chemotactic factor and facilitates neutrophil damage to hyphae and monocyte killing of conidia. Complement is not necessary for the attachment or ingestion of conidia by human alveolar macrophages.[68,69]

Aspergillosis is an uncommon fungal infection in patients with AIDS. AIDS patients may be at less risk for aspergillosis than other fungal infections because the primary cellular defect in AIDS patients is in the T-lymphocytes, whereas neutrophils and macrophages constitute the primary lines of defense to infection with aspergillosis. Aspergillosis was reported as a late complication of disease in AIDS patients with additional risk factors for aspergillosis, such as corticosteroid use, neutropenia, previous *Pneumocystis carinii* or cytomegalovirus pneumonia, marijuana smoking, or the use of broad-spectrum antibiotics. However, approximately 50% of patients with aspergillosis have no classic risk factors. The majority of these patients had CD4 counts <50 cells/mm^3 (<50 × 10^6/L). Although some patients diagnosed early in their infection responded to treatment, most patients do not respond to therapy with amphotericin B 0.5 mg/kg per day or itraconazole 200 to 600 mg/day.[70]

Invasive disease with *Aspergillus* can arise de novo or from any of the allergic or colonizing forms of aspergillosis. Predisposing factors to the development of IA include glucocorticoid therapy, particularly following chronic administration or with higher dosages (30 to 200 mg/day of prednisone), cytotoxic agents, and recent or concurrent therapy with broad-spectrum antimicrobial agents. Patients with chronic hepatitis, alcoholism, diabetes mellitus, chronic granulomatous disease, leukopenia (<1,000 cells/mm^3 [<1 × 10^9/L]), leukemia (particularly acute lymphocytic or myelogenous leukemia), lymphoma, and acute rejection of an organ transplant are also at a higher risk of invasive disease. Although rare, IA has been reported in apparently normal hosts.[68]

Clinical Presentation

The lung is the most common site of invasive disease.[12,68] In the immunocompromised host, aspergillosis is characterized by vascular invasion leading to thrombosis, infarction, necrosis of tissue, and dissemination to other tissues and organs in the body. Survival beyond 2 or 3 weeks is uncommon. If bone marrow function returns, cavitation of the pulmonary lesion generally occurs, and the spread of infection can be halted. The progressive nature of the disease and its refractoriness to therapy are, in part, caused by the organism's rapid growth and its tendency to invade blood vessels.

Signs and Symptoms

Patients often present with classic signs and symptoms of acute pulmonary embolus: pleuritic chest pain, fever, hemoptysis, and friction rubs. The CNS, liver, spleen, heart, GI tract, pericardium, and other body sites are involved in a substantial minority of cases. In neutropenic patients with *Aspergillus* pneumonia, hyphae invade the walls of bronchi and surrounding parenchyma, resulting in an acute necrotizing, pyogenic pneumonitis. As a result, patients often present with classic signs and symptoms of acute pulmonary embolus: pleuritic chest pain, fever, hemoptysis, and friction rubs.

Diagnosis

The diagnosis of aspergillosis is complicated by the presence of *Aspergillus* as a normal commensal in the human GI tract and respiratory secretions, and establishment of a definitive diagnosis of disease is difficult. Although suggestive of infection, the presence of hyphae in a smear or biopsy specimen is not diagnostic. Demonstration of *Aspergillus* by repeated culture and microscopic examination of tissue provides the most firm diagnosis. The appearance of *Aspergillus* in tissues varies with increasing host resistance from the normal vegetative hyphae found with necrotic tissue and exudate in the alveoli of immunocompromised hosts to the compact, tangled filaments (*granules*) observed in fungal balls. Identification of *Aspergillus* generally is based on the appearance of 2- to 4-micron-wide septate hyphae that are dichotomously branched at 45° angles. Sporulation is observed rarely in tissue. Although growth on Sabouraud dextrose or brain-heart infusion agar can be used for primary culture, bronchoscopy or bronchoalveolar lavage cultures are positive in only 40% of histopathologically identified specimens. Blood, CSF, and bone marrow cultures are rarely positive for *Aspergillus*.

Many clinicians treat positive respiratory cultures of *Aspergillus* as a common contaminant and argue that a minimum of two to three positive cultures is necessary before antifungal therapy is indicated. Any positive culture, however, can be indicative of true infection in the immunocompromised host, and the positive predictive value can be as high as 80% to 90% in patients with leukemia or bone marrow transplants.

Diagnostic Tests Galactomannan is a cell-wall polysaccharide specific to *Aspergillus* species that is detectable in serum and other body fluids during IA. Galactomannan levels, reported as optical density values, can be measured in body fluids by means of a double-sandwich enzyme immunosorbent assay (EIA).

The Platelia *Aspergillus* EIA test (Bio-Rad Laboratories) is FDA-approved for use in the diagnosis of IA in HSCT recipients and in patients with leukemia; its usefulness in solid-organ transplant and pediatric populations needs to be established. The use of mold-active antifungals can decrease the sensitivity of the test. In most patients, circulating antigen can be detected at a mean of 8 days before diagnosis by other means. However, false-positive galactomannan assay results have been reported for patients receiving piperacillin–tazobactam and amoxicillin–clavulanate, those with bifidobacteria infections, and in neonates.[18,19,57]

The BG test (Fungitell; Associates of Cape Cod) detects (1,3)-β-D-glucan (BG) in the serum of patients with symptoms of or medical conditions predisposing to invasive fungal infections and aids in the diagnosis of deep-seated mycoses and fungemia. BG is a cell-wall constituent of many pathogenic fungi, including *Aspergillus* and *Candida* species, and is detectable in patients' serum during invasive disease due to these organisms. In addition to patients with IA and candidiasis, BG is also detectable in patients with infections caused by species of *Fusarium*, *Trichosporon*, *Saccharomyces*, and *Acremonium*, which are less common but very important fungal pathogens, especially in immunocompromised hosts. Detection of BG in serum uses a chromogenic variant of the limulus amoebocyte lysate assay. Although a positive test result for the presence of BG does not identify the infecting fungus, the practical application of this test includes its use as a screening assay (presumptive marker) for invasive fungal infection to allow the earlier initiation of antifungal therapy. Other tests are necessary for the confirmation and identification of the fungal pathogen.[18]

Late findings on radiographic studies include wedge-shaped pleural-based infiltrates or cavities on chest radiographs. Findings on CT scans include the halo sign (an area of low attenuation surrounding a nodular lung lesion) initially (caused by edema or bleeding surrounding an ischemic area) and, later, the crescent sign (an air crescent near the periphery of a lung nodule caused by contraction of infarcted tissue). CT abnormalities are best documented in neutropenic marrow transplant recipients and commonly precede plain chest radiograph abnormalities.[57]

TREATMENT
Invasive Aspergillosis

Therapy for IA is far from optimal at this time in part because of the difficulties in establishing a diagnosis and in part because of a lack of truly effective antifungal agents. Administration of amphotericin B appears to decrease mortality from more than 90% to approximately 45%. These data, however, are difficult to interpret because many patients were diagnosed postmortem, or amphotericin B therapy was not administered until the patient had very advanced disease. Mortality from pulmonary aspergillosis in bone marrow transplant recipients exceeds 94% regardless of therapy.[68] Although early diagnosis and administration of antifungal therapy can result in higher response rates, correction of underlying immune deficits (in particular, return of neutrophil counts) is of paramount importance in eradication of infection.[12]

Until the diagnosis of aspergillosis can be determined more rapidly and definitively, empirical therapy must be instituted when invasive disease is suspected. In patients at highest risk for invasive disease (acute leukemia and bone marrow transplant recipients), the most important predisposing factors include prolonged severe neutropenia (<100 cell/μL [$<100 \times 10^6$/L] for more than 1 week), graft rejection, chronic administration of corticosteroids, and tissue damage from preexisting infection. In these patients, antifungal therapy should be instituted in any of these conditions: (a) persistent fever or progressive sinusitis unresponsive to antimicrobial therapy, (b) an eschar over the nose, sinuses, or palate, (c) the presence of characteristic radiographic findings, including wedge-shaped infarcts, nodular densities, and new cavitary lesions, or (d) any clinical manifestation suggestive of orbital or cavernous sinus disease or an acute vascular event associated with fever. Isolation of *Aspergillus* species from nasal or respiratory tract secretions should be considered confirmatory evidence in any of the previously mentioned clinical settings.[68]

Non–HIV-Infected Patient

Prophylaxis

Unfortunately, effective chemoprophylaxis against infections by *Aspergillus* species has not been demonstrated thus far.[7] As noted above in the discussion of prophylaxis for *Candida* infections in immunocompromised hosts, prophylaxis with azoles or echinocandins can reduce the incidence of fungal infections in select high-risk populations.

Specific Therapy

Even though older azole antifungal agents (miconazole and ketoconazole) possess poor in vitro activity against *Aspergillus* species, newer triazoles demonstrate improved activity both in vitro and in animal models of infection.[71] Voriconazole has emerged as the drug of choice of most clinicians for primary therapy of most patients with IA.[72] A randomized trial, which compared voriconazole with amphotericin B (followed by other licensed antifungal therapy) for primary therapy of aspergillosis, noted better responses, improved survival, and fewer severe side effects with voriconazole.[73]

In patients who are unable to tolerate voriconazole, amphotericin B can be used. Because *Aspergillus* is only moderately susceptible to amphotericin B, full doses (1 to 1.5 mg/kg/day) are generally recommended, with response measured by defervescence and radiographic clearing. To treat microfoci, therapy should be continued after resolution of clinical and radiographic abnormalities until cultures (if they can be obtained) are negative, and reversible underlying predispositions have abated. Clinical response rather than any arbitrary total dose should guide duration of therapy. The optimal dosage or duration of amphotericin B therapy for the treatment of invasive disease is unknown and dependent on the extent of disease, the response to therapy, and the patient's underlying disease(s) and immune status. Unfortunately, the response rate averages only 37% (range, 14% to 83%), and the response to therapy is largely related to the extent of aspergillosis at the time of diagnosis, and host factors, such as resolution of neutropenia and the return of neutrophil function, lessening immunosuppression, and the return of graft function from a bone marrow or organ transplant.

Lipid formulations of amphotericin B can be indicated in patients with impaired renal function, and in those patients who develop nephrotoxicity while receiving deoxycholate amphotericin B. The lipid-based formulations may be preferred as initial therapy in patients with marginal renal function or in patients receiving other nephrotoxic drugs. Although these preparations appear less toxic than standard preparations, only limited data regarding their relative efficacy for IA are available at this time, as the studies with the lipid preparations have been open-label or with historical conventional amphotericin B controls.[70,74]

Caspofungin was approved by the FDA for use as salvage therapy in patients who are intolerant or who fail therapy with one of the amphotericin B formulations.[52] Caspofungin has in vitro activity against *Aspergillus* species and is indicated for the treatment of IA in patients who are refractory to or intolerant of other therapies such as conventional amphotericin B, lipid formulations of amphotericin B, and/or itraconazole. Caspofungin has not yet been studied as first-line therapy for patients with aspergillosis. Because of the high risk of mortality from IA even following treatment with standard therapy such as amphotericin B or itraconazole, caspofungin can offer a new mechanism for salvage therapy for patients with this disease.

The use of adjuvant therapies, such as granulocyte transfusions or recombinant colony-stimulating factors, remains controversial, and controlled trials are lacking at this time. Although some authors advocate combination therapy with azoles, flucytosine, or rifampin plus amphotericin B, controlled clinical studies verifying the efficacy of these combination therapies are lacking.

Secondary Prophylaxis

The use of prophylactic antifungal therapy to prevent primary infection or reactivation of aspergillosis during subsequent courses of chemotherapy is controversial.[12] Studies assessing the utility of IV administration of amphotericin B in low doses (0.1 mg/kg per day) as prophylactic therapy or with higher dosages (0.5 to 0.6 mg/kg per day) as empirical therapy for invasive fungal infections in patients with granulocytopenia have not included sufficient numbers of patients to enable detection of differences in the number of *Aspergillus* infections.

In granulocytopenic patients who recover from an episode of IA, the risk of relapse of aspergillosis during subsequent courses of chemotherapy is greater than 50%. Secondary prophylaxis of aspergillosis with empirical administration of high-dose amphotericin B decreases the risk of relapse. Amphotericin B 1 mg/kg per day is started 24 to 48 hours prior to the start of chemotherapy and continued throughout the period of granulocytopenia.

EMERGING PATHOGENS

The increased frequency of fungal pathogens that were once rare is gaining attention from the medical community. Mucormycosis, previously known Zygomycosis, is a term describing infections caused by fungi belonging to the order Mucorales. Permissive environmental conditions, selective antifungal pressure, and increased numbers of immunosuppressed patients have led to increased numbers of infections caused by the Mucorales (e.g., *Mucor*, *Rhizopus* spp., or *Absidia*) or filamentous fungi such as *Scedosporium* or *Fusarium* species. Posaconazole appears promising for the treatment of Mucorales infections. Breakthrough mucormycosis has been increasingly observed in patients with leukemia and recipients of HSCT receiving *Aspergillus*-active drugs, such as voriconazole or an echinocandin, as neither agent has activity against Mucorales. Of currently available systemic antifungals, only amphotericin B (including the lipid formulations) and posaconazole exhibit good in vitro activity against Mucorales. Echinocandins, which demonstrate modest in vivo activity against some Mucorales, demonstrate enhanced activity when coadministered with lipid amphotericin B formulations. Prompt initiation of antifungal therapy is crucial, as treatment delays are associated with increased mortality.[75]

Unfortunately, the early presentation of *Fusarium* and *Scedosporium* infections often mimics that of aspergillosis. On histopathology, *Scedosporium* species resembles *Aspergillus* species with dichotomously branching, septate hyphae and has a tendency for invasion of vascular structures.[76] These pathogens often demonstrate intrinsic resistance to amphotericin B and are associated with high mortality rates.[73] For example, mortality caused by *Scedosporium prolificans*, previously known as *Scedosporium inflatum*, exceeds 85%; *Scedosporium apiospermum* (the asexual state of *P. boydii)* was uniformly fatal in 23 solid-organ transplant recipients with disseminated disease.[76] However, in vitro data suggest that *S. prolificans* is more sensitive to voriconazole than to amphotericin B or itraconazole.[76,77] Voriconazole recently received FDA approval for the treatment of serious fungal infections caused by *S. apiospermum* and *Fusarium* species, including *Fusarium solani*, in patients intolerant of or refractory to other therapy.[78]

ANTIFUNGAL THERAPY

The antifungal armamentarium for the treatment of invasive fungal infections includes: (a) inhibitors of the fungal cell membrane such as polyenes (e.g., amphotericin B) and azole antifungals, (b) inhibitors of DNA (5-flucytosine), and more recently, (c) inhibitors of cell wall biosynthesis (echinocandins).[78]

Antifungal therapy generally uses one or more of these agents, depending on the severity of infection and the patients' immune status. Rarely are the agents used in combination. Often therapy is initiated with an IV agent such as amphotericin B, and therapy is changed to an oral (azole) regimen as the patient's clinical status improves and oral therapy is tolerated. The most widely used combination therapy consists of flucytosine plus amphotericin B. The role of combination therapy is unclear at this time; controlled trials are lacking and the possibility of therapeutic antagonism when using azoles in combination with amphotericin B remains debated. Controlled trials are needed to define the role of azoles plus amphotericin B and azoles or amphotericin B plus an echinocandin.[79]

Amphotericin B

Amphotericin B remains the therapy of choice for many systemic fungal infections despite a lack of controlled clinical trials documenting the optimal dosage, duration of therapy, or relative efficacy of this agent in comparison with newer azole antifungal agents. During pregnancy, amphotericin B remains the treatment of choice for most fungal infections because azole antifungals are teratogenic.[65,80]

The side effects of amphotericin B generally are categorized as acute (infusion-related) or long term. Gallis et al.[65] recently reviewed the side effects and clinical uses of amphotericin B.

Lipid Formulations of Amphotericin B

The use of deoxycholate amphotericin B frequently is associated with the development of induced nephrotoxicity. In an attempt to decrease the incidence of nephrotoxicity, three lipid formulations of amphotericin B have been developed and approved for use in humans: ABLC (Abelcet; Enzon Pharmaceuticals), ABCD (Amphotec; Intermune Pharmaceuticals), and liposomal amphotericin B (AmBisome; Gilead Pharmaceuticals). In these preparations, amphotericin B is incorporated into the phospholipid bilayer membrane rather than in the enclosed aqueous phase.

The various lipid formulations of amphotericin B exhibit markedly different pharmacokinetics; however, the clinical implications of these differences remain unclear. Although larger doses of these preparations are required to achieve similar pharmacologic effects as the deoxycholate form of amphotericin B, the toxicity appears to be much lower.[80] Although the FDA-approved dosages of these agents are 5 mg/kg per day (ABLC), 3 to 6 mg/kg per day (ABCD), and 3 to 5 mg/kg per day (liposomal amphotericin B), the agents appear generally equipotent. The optimal dose of these compounds for serious *Candida* infections is unknown; however, dosages of 3 to 5 mg/kg per day appear reasonable. Liposomal amphotericin B administered at 3 mg/kg per day was equally as effective but less toxic than a dosage of 10 mg/kg per day as initial therapy for invasive mold infections.[81] The relative efficacy of these agents is unknown; whether differences in pharmacokinetic features result in different outcomes in the treatment of specific types of infections (e.g., CNS infections) is unclear.[7]

Lipid formulations of amphotericin B are indicated for patients intolerant of, refractory to, or at high risk of being intolerant to conventional antifungal therapy.[7,82] Intolerance generally is defined as initial renal insufficiency (creatinine >2.5 mg/dL [>221 μmol/L] or creatinine clearance <25 mL/min [<0.42 mL/s]), a significant increase in creatinine (to 2.5 mg/dL [221 μmol/L] for adults or 1.5 mg/dL [133 μmol/L] for children), or severe acute administration-related toxicity, whereas refractory infections are defined as therapeutic failure of more than 500 mg amphotericin B.

Clinical **Controversy. . .**

Owing to the higher cost and paucity of randomized trials showing the efficacy of lipid-associated formulations of amphotericin B against proven invasive candidiasis, many clinicians limit their first-line use for the treatment of these infections to individuals who are intolerant to, at high risk of intolerance to, or refractory to amphotericin B deoxycholate. However, the data demonstrating up to a 6.6-fold increase in mortality in patients with amphotericin B-induced nephrotoxicity have convinced other clinicians that high-risk patients (e.g., residence in an ICU care or intermediate care unit at the time of initiation of amphotericin B therapy) warrant first-line therapy with these agents.

Only ABLC and liposomal amphotericin B have been approved for use in proven candidiasis. Both in vivo and clinical studies indicate that these compounds are less toxic but as effective as amphotericin B when used in appropriate dosages. Nevertheless, their higher cost and the paucity of randomized trials in proven invasive candidiasis limit their front-line use in these infections.[82]

Flucytosine

Flucytosine (also known as 5-flucytosine) is a fluorinated pyrimidine analog that is highly water-soluble. Patients with creatinine clearances of less than 40 mL/min (0.67 mL/s) should receive 100 to 150 mg/kg daily in four divided doses. The dosage should be reduced by 50% in patients with a creatinine clearance of 25 to 50 mL/min (0.42 to 0.83 mL/s) and by 75% in patients with a clearance of 13 to 25 mL/min (0.21 to 0.42 mL/s). Peak serum concentrations (2 hours after an oral dose) should be monitored in all patients (particularly those with a creatinine clearance of less than 10 mL/min [0.17 mL/s]) to maintain peak serum concentrations of more than 100 mg/L (775 μmol/L).[26]

Flucytosine generally is associated with few side effects in patients with normal renal, GI, and hematologic function, although rash, GI discomfort, diarrhea (5% to 10%), and reversible elevations in hepatic enzymes are observed occasionally. In patients with renal dysfunction or concomitant amphotericin B therapy, leukopenia, thrombocytopenia, and (rarely) enterocolitis can occur. Although studies have suggested that little or no conversion of flucytosine to fluorouracil occurs in vitro, serum concentrations of greater than 1,000 ng/mL (~7.7 μmol/L) (therapeutic for the treatment of malignancies) have been documented in some patients. Investigators have theorized that flucytosine may be secreted into the GI tract, deaminated by intestinal bacteria, and reabsorbed as 5-fluorouracil.[26]

Flucytosine is used in combination with amphotericin B or fluconazole in the treatment of cryptococcosis or (less commonly) candidiasis. The rapid development of resistance to flucytosine, however, precludes its use as single-agent therapy. Mechanisms for drug resistance can include loss of deaminase and decreased permeability to the drug.[26]

Echinocandins

The echinocandins (caspofungin, micafungin, and anidulafungin) are a new class of antifungal agents that act as concentration-dependent, noncompetitive inhibitors of BG synthase, an essential component of the cell wall of susceptible filamentous fungi that is absent in mammalian cells.[52]

All echinocandins display linear pharmacokinetics following administration of IV dosages, and are degraded primarily by the liver (also in the adrenals and spleen) by hydrolysis and *N*-acetylation. Following initial distribution, echinocandins are taken up by red blood cells (micafungin) and the liver (caspofungin and micafungin) where they undergo slow degradation to mainly inactive metabolites, although two uncommon metabolites of micafungin possess antifungal activity. Degradation products are excreted slowly over many days, primarily through the bile. Among the echinocandins, anidulafungin is unique in being eliminated almost exclusively by slow chemical degradation rather than undergoing hepatic metabolism.[52]

Echinocandins are available only as parenteral formulations, are not dialyzable, and do not require dosage adjustment in patients with renal insufficiency. They have minimal CSF penetration, largely because of their high protein binding and large molecular weights, although the clinical relevance of these findings can be disputed, given that several other antifungal agents (amphotericin B and itraconazole) are effective for the treatment of fungal meningitis despite low CSF concentrations.

Adverse effects of echinocandins include histamine release resulting in rash, facial swelling, and itchiness. Limited experience suggests that caspofungin and micafungin are safe to use in pediatric patients; the safety and effectiveness of anidulafungin in pediatric patients has not been established. At the time of FDA approval, there were concerns regarding the safety of caspofungin when combined with cyclosporine. However, three retrospective analyses of the use of caspofungin and cyclosporine in patients do not support a risk of clinically relevant hepatotoxicity.[52]

Azole Antifungal Agents

The introduction of the azole antifungal agents has rapidly expanded the armamentarium of agents useful in the treatment of systemic fungal infections.[9] Adverse effects of azoles include GI disturbances (primarily nausea, vomiting, epigastric pain, and diarrhea), which appear to be more common in patients receiving ketoconazole and the solution formulation of itraconazole. Although cyclodextrin is not absorbed following oral administration, use of the IV formulations of itraconazole and voriconazole is limited to 2 weeks because of concerns for potential nephrotoxicity secondary to accumulation of the cyclodextrin vehicle.[83] Fluconazole is well tolerated; intestinal complaints are the most frequently reported, followed by headaches and rash. Unlike ketoconazole, fluconazole does not inhibit testicular or adrenal steroidogenesis in healthy volunteers or hospitalized patients. Reversible alopecia occurs not infrequently and usually appears after several months of treatment with higher doses of fluconazole. Azoles are potentially teratogenic and should be avoided in pregnant women.[78,80]

Itraconazole

Itraconazole is triazole antifungal with a broad spectrum of antifungal activity. Despite its marked structural similarity to ketoconazole, itraconazole differs in several important respects. Itraconazole appears to have greater specificity against fungal versus mammalian CYP, resulting in greater potency and a decrease in CYP-mediated side effects. In addition, itraconazole possesses excellent in vitro activity against *Aspergillus* and *Sporothrix* species.[4]

Like ketoconazole, the capsule formulation of itraconazole depends on the availability of low gastric pH for dissolution and absorption. Administration with food appears to enhance significantly the bioavailability of itraconazole capsules, whereas it decreases the bioavailability of the oral solution. Because itraconazole exhibits pH-dependent dissolution and absorption, absorption of the capsule formulation is impaired in patients receiving antacids or H_2-receptor antagonists and in patients with achlorhydria.[83] Plasma concentrations of itraconazole following a single oral dose (capsules) in HIV-infected patients are approximately 50% lower than concentrations observed in healthy volunteers. The capsule formulation of itraconazole exhibits unpredictable oral bioavailability, particularly in subjects with hypochlorhydria and in patients with enteropathy caused by mucositis or graft-versus-host gut disease. An oral suspension formulation of itraconazole is available; that uses cyclodextrin as a solubilizing vehicle to increase the solubility of the drug. The oral bioavailability of the solution is unaffected by alterations in gastric pH or in patients with enteropathy.[7,83]

Fluconazole

Fluconazole is a triazole antifungal agent with markedly different pharmacologic features than other marketed azole antifungals. The small molecular weight, low protein binding, and increased water solubility of fluconazole result in rapid, essentially complete absorption of drug following oral administration. Because fluconazole is excreted primarily (>80%) as unchanged drug in the urine, dosage adjustments are necessary in patients with renal dysfunction.[71]

Voriconazole

The hepatic biotransformation of voriconazole is fairly complex and involves CYP2C19, CYP3A4, and CYP2C9, with most metabolism mediated through CYP2C19. Two of the CYPs involved in voriconazole metabolism (CYP2C19 and CYP2C9) exhibit genetic polymorphism; variability in the CYP2C19 genotype accounts for approximately 30% of the overall between-subject variability in voriconazole pharmacokinetics. About 3% to 5% of white and African human populations are poor metabolizers, while 15% to 20% of Asian populations are poor metabolizers. Drug levels can be as much as fourfold greater in poor metabolizers than in individuals who are homozygous extensive metabolizers. Coadministration of voriconazole with drugs that are potent CYP450 enzyme inducers can significantly reduce voriconazole levels. Voriconazole drug interactions are dose-dependent, as they exhibit unpredictable nonlinear pharmacokinetics; thus, drug interactions are more difficult to predict and manage.

The most common side effect of voriconazole is a reversible disturbance of vision (photopsia), which occurs in approximately 30% of patients but rarely leads to discontinuation of the drug. Symptoms tend to occur during the first week of therapy and decrease or disappear despite continued therapy. Patients experience altered color discrimination, blurred vision, the appearance of bright spots and wavy lines, and photophobia. Patients should be cautioned that driving can be hazardous because of the risk of visual disturbances. The visual effects are associated with changes in electroretinogram tracings, which revert to normal when treatment with the drug is stopped; no permanent damage to the retina has been demonstrated.[71]

Clinical **Controversy. . .**

Controversy has arisen about whether single-drug therapy or combination therapy (e.g., voriconazole plus an echinocandin or voriconazole plus a lipid formulation of amphotericin B) is optimum therapy. At present, the highest interest concerns combination therapy in the treatment of aspergillosis, given the continued high mortality of these infections.[83] However, in vitro and animal data have produced conflicting results. Several retrospective studies have suggested an improvement in mortality with combination therapy with two or three antifungal agents; however, prospective, controlled human studies are lacking. Thus, there are as yet no firm recommendations regarding the use of such combinations in humans.[12]

Posaconazole

Posaconazole has a broad spectrum of antifungal activity, including *Aspergillus* and *Candida* species and zygomycetes. In vitro studies demonstrate that posaconazole is an inhibitor but not a substrate of hepatic (but not total) CYP3A4, and both a substrate and an inhibitor of P-glycoprotein (Pgp), suggesting that it may exhibit a drug interaction profile similar to other azoles. In addition, posaconazole undergoes glucuronidation by uridine diphosphate (UDP)-glucuronosyltransferase enzymes.[71]

Drug Interactions with Antifungal Agents

Drug interactions with azole antifungals generally can be placed into three broad categories: (a) decreases in azole bioavailability because of chelation or secondary to increases in gastric pH, (b) interactions with other CYP-metabolized drugs, and (c) interactions caused by inhibition of Pgp. Drug interactions in the latter two categories can result in increases or decreases in the azole antifungal, in the interacting drug, or in both drugs.

The interaction of azole antifungal agents with other CYP-metabolized drugs is well recognized. The azoles appear to be metabolized almost entirely via the CYP3A4 subfamily. As expected, they interact with other drugs metabolized partly or wholly through this enzyme pathway. In addition, fluconazole and voriconazole use the CYP2C19 pathway. Numerous clinically significant interactions have been documented with azole antifungals and a variety of other drugs. In most cases, the azole interferes with the metabolism of the other CYP-metabolized drug.[71]

The interaction between ketoconazole and cyclosporine has been exploited to reduce drug costs associated with administration of cyclosporine following organ transplantation. Relative to ketoconazole and itraconazole, fluconazole appears to be intermediate in its ability to inhibit human cytochromes P450. The magnitude of fluconazole-induced inhibition of cyclosporine metabolism appears, however, to depend on the dosage of fluconazole.

Predictably, drugs such as rifampin, rifabutin, isoniazid, phenytoin, and carbamazepine, which are known to induce the activity of cytochromes P450, result in increased metabolism of the azole antifungals and can result in therapeutic failures. Increased dosages of azole antifungals can be required in patients receiving these combinations of drugs.

Itraconazole is an inhibitor of intestinal Pgp. Significant increases in digoxin (a Pgp substrate) have been observed in patients receiving both agents concurrently. Interactions with other substrates of Pgp would be expected to occur.

Echinocandins are not inducers of CYP enzymes, nor do they interact with Pgp, and are considered poor substrates of CYP3A4. Nevertheless, cyclosporine increases the area under the plasma-concentration versus time curve (AUC) of caspofungin by ~35%, and tacrolimus AUC, peak, and 12-hour concentrations are decreased by approximately 20% during concomitant administration with caspofungin. Additionally, when caspofungin was administered concurrently with tacrolimus, tacrolimus levels were reduced by 20% compared to administration with tacrolimus alone. The mechanism for these interactions is not yet known. Rifampin both inhibits (acutely) and induces (after chronic administration) caspofungin metabolism. A dosage increase is recommended in patients receiving other enzyme inducers, such as efavirenz, nevirapine, phenytoin, dexamethasone, and carbamazepine. Although micafungin does not significantly affect the clearance (or AUC) of tacrolimus, it increases the AUC of sirolimus by 21%, and of nifedipine by 18%, and decreases the clearance of cyclosporine by 16%. Monitoring of cyclosporine levels during combination therapy with micafungin is recommended.[52]

Plasma Concentration Monitoring of Antifungal Agents

Routine therapeutic plasma drug concentration monitoring (TDM) of plasma concentrations of antifungal agents to assess efficacy or toxicity of these agents generally is not available. Correlations between plasma concentrations of antifungal agents and therapeutic outcomes have been poorly studied. However, the available, good-quality, prospectively obtained data in the prophylactic or therapeutic setting are insufficient to justify the routine use of therapeutic drug monitoring. In addition, logistics, cost, and incorporation of therapeutic drug monitoring have yet to be worked out in modern prophylactic algorithms.[84,85]

Under certain circumstances, serum or plasma concentration monitoring is warranted. Given the tremendous interpatient and intrapatient variability in voriconazole metabolism, and poor oral bioavailability of posaconazole, monitoring is often warranted, particularly in patients with GVHD of the gut, mucositis, or diarrhea, or poor oral intake or those receiving concomitant therapy with proton-pump inhibitors. Additional settings include patients susceptible to flucytosine toxicity, to document adequate oral absorption of poorly bioavailable azoles in cases of suspected treatment failure or concern about compliance or absorption, solubility and finally, when drug interactions that might reduce or accelerate the metabolism of azoles is suspected (Table 99-11).[17,84,85]

Combination Antifungal Therapy for Invasive Fungal Infections

Based on extensive experience in the management of bacterial, and more recently, retroviral infections, the use of combination agents for synergistic or additive effects is now common practice, particularly for the treatment of IA.[79] High-dose fluconazole, alone or in combination with amphotericin B, in nonimmunocompromised patients with candidemia demonstrated no antagonism and a trend toward improved success and more rapid clearance of *Candida* from the bloodstream.[48]

TABLE 99-11 Plasma Concentration Monitoring of Antifungal Agents[78,84,85]

	Serum Concentration Monitoring Necessary?	Target Concentration Range	Timing of Sample
Echinocandins	No	NA	NA
Amphotericin B (including lipids)	No	NA	NA
Fluconazole	No	NA	NA
Itraconazole	Yes, to ensure absorption and efficacy	*Efficacy*: Prophylaxis: >0.5 mcg/mL (mg/L; >0.7 μmol/L) Treatment: >1 mcg/mL (mg/L; >1.4 μmol/L) *Toxicity*: <5 mcg/mL (mg/L; <7 μmol/L)	Trough 7 days after initiation of therapy
Voriconazole	Yes—in all patients treated for IFI, altered liver function, potential drug–drug interactions, lack of response *Low* concentrations are associated with poor outcome; *high* concentrations are associated with adverse effects Variable metabolism due to nonlinear PK and genetic variability in CYP2C19 → unpredictable dose–exposure relationship	*Efficacy*: Prophylaxis: trough >0.5–2 mcg/mL (mg/L; >1.4–5.7 μmol/L) Treatment: trough >1–2 mcg/mL (mg/L; >2.9–5.7 μmol/L) Concentrations >2.05 mcg/mL (mg/L; >5.7 μmol/L) are associated with improved outcome; 2–5.5 mcg/mL (mg/L; 5.7–15.7 μmol/L) is probably the best target *Toxicity*: concentrations >5.5 mcg/mL (mg/L; >15.7 μmol/L) are associated with ↑ risk of visual and hepatic adverse events	Trough after 5–7 days therapy if no loading dose administered; 48 hours after administration of loading dose in critically ill patient (time to steady state is unpredictable due to nonlinear metabolism)
Posaconazole	"Probably"—in all patients treated for IFI to ensure absorption, in patients receiving PPIs or with altered GI function, lack of response Outcomes (but not adverse events) correlate with higher plasma concentrations in prophylaxis and possibly treatment	*Efficacy*: Prophylaxis: >0.7 mcg/mL (mg/L; >1 μmol/L) Treatment: Not well studied; concentrations >1.25 mg/L (1.78 μmol/L) needed ? *Toxicity*: Correlation with toxicity poorly defined	Random level at SS (>7 days therapy). The long $t_{1/2}$ ensures little fluctuation in peaks and troughs at SS
Flucytosine	Yes—High concentrations are associated with toxicity	*Toxicity*: "Peak" <80–100 mcg/mL (mg/L; <620–775 μmol/L) *Efficacy*: Trough >30 mcg/mL (mg/L; >232 μmol/L)	2 hours postdose "peak", 3 to 5 days after initiation of therapy

NA, not applicable.

ABBREVIATIONS

AIDS	acquired immunodeficiency syndrome
ABCD	amphotericin B colloid dispersion
ABLC	amphotericin B lipid complex
AUC	area under the plasma-concentration versus time curve
BG	(1,3)-β-D-Glucan
BPA	bronchopulmonary aspergillosis
BSI	bloodstream infection
CBP	clinical breakpoint
CDC	Centers for Disease Control and Prevention
CT	computed tomography
CVC	central venous catheter
CSF	cerebrospinal fluid
CF-M	CF titer for mycelial antigen
CF	complement fixation
CYP	cytochrome P450
ELISA	enzyme-linked immunosorbent assay
FISH	fluorescence in situ hybridization
GVHD	graft-versus-host disease
HEPA	high-efficiency particulate air
HAART	highly active antiretroviral therapy
HPA	*H. capsulatum* polysaccharide antigen
HSCT	hematopoietic stem cell transplantation
ID	immunodiffusion
ICP	intracranial pressure
ICUs	intensive care units
IDSA	Infectious Diseases Society of America
IRIS	immune reconstitution inflammatory syndrome
LA	latex agglutination
PMN	polymorphonuclear
PDH	progressive disseminated histoplasmosis
PNA	peptide nucleic acid
RIA	radioimmunoassay
SDD	susceptible dose-dependent
TDM	therapeutic plasma drug concentration monitoring
PN	parenteral nutrition
WBC	white blood cell
WT	wild type

REFERENCES

1. Bennett JE. Introduction to mycoses. In: Mandell, Douglas, and Bennett's Principles and Practice of Infectious Diseases, 7th ed. Philadelphia, PA: Churchill Livingstone, 2010:3221–3224.
2. Pfaller MA, Jones RN, Messer SA, Edmond MB, Wenzel RP. National surveillance of nosocomial blood stream infection due to *Candida albicans*: Frequency of occurrence and antifungal susceptibility in the SCOPE program. Diagn Microbiol Infect Dis 1998;31:327–332.
3. Pfaller MA, Jones RN, Doern GV, et al. International surveillance of blood stream infections due to *Candida* species in the European SENTRY Program: Species distribution and antifungal susceptibility including the investigational triazole and echinocandin agents. SENTRY Participant Group (Europe). Diagn Microbiol Infect Dis 1999;35:19–25.
4. Pfaller MA, Diekema DJ. Progress in antifungal susceptibility testing of *Candida* spp. by use of Clinical and Laboratory Standards Institute Broth Microdilution Methods, 2010 to 2012. J Clin Microbiol 2012;50(9):2846–2856.
5. Pfaller MA, Andes D, Diekema DJ, Espinel-Ingroff A, Sheehan D. Wild-type MIC distributions, epidemiological

cutoff values and species-specific clinical breakpoints for fluconazole and Candida: Time for harmonization of CLSI and EUCAST broth microdilution methods. Drug Resist Updat 2010;13:180–195.
6. Eschenauer GA, Carver PL. The evolving role of antifungal susceptibility testing. Pharmacotherapy, 2013 Apr 1. doi: 10.1002/phar.1233. [Epub ahead of print]
7. Pappas PG, Kauffman CA, Andes D, et al. Clinical practice guidelines for the management of candidiasis: 2009 update by the Infectious Diseases Society of America. Clin Infect Dis 2009;48(5):503–535.
8. Chapman SW, Dismukes WE, Proia LA, et al. Clinical practice guidelines for the management of blastomycosis: 2008 update by the Infectious Diseases Society of America. Clin Infect Dis 2008;46(12):1801–1812.
9. Perfect JR, Dismukes WE, Dromer F, et al. Clinical practice guidelines for the management of cryptococcal disease: 2010 update by the Infectious Diseases Society of America. Clin Infect Dis 2010;50(3):291–322.
10. Wheat LJ, Freifeld AG, Kleiman MB, et al. Clinical practice guidelines for the management of patients with histoplasmosis: 2007 update by the Infectious Diseases Society of America. Clin Infect Dis 2007;45(7):807–825.
11. Galgiani JN, Ampel NM, Blair JE, et al. Practice guidelines for the treatment of coccidioidomycoses. Clin Infect Dis 2005;41:1217–1223.
12. Walsh TJ, Anaissie EJ, Denning DW, et al. Treatment of aspergillosis: Clinical practice guidelines of the Infectious Diseases Society of America. Clin Infect Dis 2008;46(3):327–360.
13. Sanglard D, Odds FC. Resistance of *Candida* species to antifungal agents: Molecular mechanisms and clinical consequences. Lancet Infect Dis 2002;2:73–85.
14. White TC, Marr KA, Bowden RA. Clinical, cellular, and molecular factors that contribute to antifungal drug resistance. Clin Microbiol Rev 1998;11:382–402.
15. Eschenauer GA, Lam SW, Carver PL. Antifungal prophylaxis in liver transplant recipients. Liver Transpl 2009;15(8):842–858.
16. McCoy D, DePestel DD, Carver PL. Primary antifungal prophylaxis in adult hematopoietic stem cell transplant recipients: Current therapeutic concepts. Pharmacotherapy 2009;29(11)1306–1325.
17. Edwards JE. *Candida* species. In: Mandell, Douglas, and Bennett's Principles and Practice of Infectious Diseases, 7th ed. Philadelphia, PA: Churchill Livingstone, 2010:3225–3240.
18. Alexander BD, Pfaller MA. Contemporary tools for the diagnosis and management of invasive mycoses. Clin Infect Dis 2006; 43:S15–S27.
19. O'Shaughnessy EM, Shea YM, Witebsky FG. Laboratory diagnosis of invasive mycoses. Infect Dis Clin North Am 2003;17(1):135–158.
20. Deepe GS. *Histoplasma capsulatum*. In: Mandell, Douglas, and Bennett's Principles and Practice of Infectious Diseases, 7th ed. Philadelphia, PA: Churchill Livingstone, 2010:3305–3318.
21. Kauffman CA. Histoplasmosis: A clinical and laboratory update. Clin Microbiol Rev 2007;20(1):115–132.
22. Chapman SW, Sullivan DC. *Blastomyces dermatitidis*. In: Mandell, Douglas, and Bennett's Principles and Practice of Infectious Diseases, 7th ed. Philadelphia, PA: Churchill Livingstone, 2010:3319–3332.
23. Parish JM, Blair JE. Coccidioidomycosis. Mayo Clin Proc 2008;83(3):343–348.
24. Hoang LMN, Philips P, Galanis E. *Cryptococcus gattii*: A review of the epidemiology, clinical presentation, diagnosis, and management of this endemic yeast in the Pacific Northwest. Clin Microbiol Newslett 2011;33(24):187–195.
25. Bennett JE, Dismukes WE, Duma RJ, et al. A comparison of amphotericin B alone and combined with flucytosine in the treatment of cryptococcal meningitis. N Engl J Med 1979;301:126–131.
26. Francis P, Walsh TJ. Evolving role of flucytosine in immunocompromised patients: New insights into safety, pharmacokinetics, and anti-fungal therapy. Clin Infect Dis 1992;15:1003–1018.
27. Powderly WG, Saag MS, Cloud GA, et al. A controlled trial of fluconazole or amphotericin B to prevent relapse of cryptococcal meningitis in patients with the acquired immunodeficiency syndrome. N Engl J Med 1992;326: 793–798.
28. Saag MS, Powderly WG, Cloud GA, et al. Comparison of amphotericin B with fluconazole in the treatment of acute AIDS-associated cryptococcal meningitis: The NIAID Mycoses Study Group and the AIDS Clinical Trials Group. N Engl J Med 1992;326:83–89.
29. van der Horst CM, Saag MS, Cloud GA, et al. Treatment of cryptococcal meningitis associated with the acquired immunodeficiency syndrome. N Engl J Med 1997;37:15–21.
30. Pfaller MA, Jones RN, Doern GV, et al. International surveillance of bloodstream infections due to *Candida* species: Frequency of occurrence and antifungal susceptibilities of isolates collected in 1997 in the United States, Canada, and South America for the SENTRY program. J Clin Microbiol 1998;36:1886–1889.
31. Winston DJ, Chandrasekar PH, Lazarus HM, et al. Fluconazole prophylaxis of fungal infections in patients with acute leukemia: Results of a randomized placebo-controlled, double-blind, multicenter trial. Ann Intern Med 1993;118:495–503.
32. Rangel-Frausto MS, Wiblin T, Blumberg HM, et al. National Epidemiology of Mycoses Survey (NEMIS): Variations in rates of blood stream infections due to *Candida* species in seven surgical intensive care units and six neonatal intensive care units. Clin Infect Dis 1999;29:253–258.
33. Edmond MB, Wallace SE, McClish DK, et al. Nosocomial bloodstream infections in United States hospitals: A three-year analysis. Clin Infect Dis 1999;29:239–244.
34. Lam SW, Eschenauer GA, Carver PL. Evolving role of early antifungals in the adult intensive care unit. Crit Care Med 2009;37(5):1580–1593.
35. Sullivan DJ, Moran GP, Coleman DC. Candida dubliniensis: Ten years on. FEMS Microbiol Lett 2005;253(1):9–17.
36. Fraser VJ, Jones M, Dunkel J, et al. Candidemia in a tertiary care hospital: Epidemiology, risk factors, and predictors of mortality. Clin Infect Dis 1992;15(3):414–21.
37. Morrell M, Fraser VJ, Kollef MH. Delaying the empiric treatment of candida bloodstream infection until positive blood culture results are obtained: A potential risk factor for hospital mortality. Antimicrob Agents Chemother 2005;49:3640–3645.
38. Gudlaugsson O, Gillespie S, Lee K, et al. Attributable mortality of nosocomial candidemia, revisited. Clin Infect Dis 2003;37:1172–1177.
39. Garey KW, Rege M, Pai MP, et al. Time to initiation of fluconazole therapy impacts mortality in patients with candidemia: A multi-institutional study. Clin Infect Dis 2006;43(1):25–31.
40. Pappas PG, Rex JH, Lee J, et al. A prospective observational study of candidemia: Epidemiology, therapy, and influences on mortality in hospitalized adult and pediatric patients. Clin Infect Dis 2003;37:634–643.

41. Andes DR, Safdar N, Baddley JW, et al. Impact of treatment strategy on outcomes in patients with candidemia and other forms of invasive candidiasis: A patient-level quantitative review of randomized trials. Clin Infect Dis 2012;54(8):1110–1122.
42. Eggimann P, Francioli P, Bille J, et al. Fluconazole prophylaxis prevents intraabdominal candidiasis in high-risk surgical patients. Crit Care Med 1999;27:1066–1072.
43. Rocco TR, Reinert SE, Simms H. Effect of fluconazole administration in critically ill patients. Arch Surg 2000; 135:160–165.
44. Winston DJ, Hathorn JW, Schuster MG, et al. A multicenter, randomized trial of fluconazole versus amphotericin B for empiric antifungal therapy of febrile neutropenic patients with cancer. Am J Med 2000;108(4):282–289.
45. Rex JH, Bennett JE, Sugar AM, et al. A randomized trial comparing fluconazole with amphotericin B for the treatment of candidemia in patients without neutropenia. N Engl J Med 1994;331:1325–1330.
46. Reboli AC, Rotstein C, Pappas PG, et al. Anidulafungin versus fluconazole for invasive candidiasis. N Engl J Med 2007;356(24):2472–2482.
47. Mora-Duarte J, Betts R, Rotstein C, et al. Comparison of caspofungin and amphotericin B for invasive candidiasis. N Engl J Med 2002;347:2020–2029.
48. Rex JH, Pappas PG, Karchmer AW, et al. A randomized and blinded multicenter trial of high-dose fluconazole plus placebo versus fluconazole plus amphotericin B as therapy for candidemia and its consequences in nonneutropenic subjects. Clin Infect Dis 2003;36:1221–1228.
49. Kullberg BJ, Sobel JD, Ruhnke M, et al. Voriconazole versus a regimen of amphotericin B followed by fluconazole for candidemia in nonneutropenic patients: A randomised non-inferiority trial. Lancet 2005;366(9495):1435–1442.
50. Kuse ER, Chetchotisakd P, da Cunha CA, et al. Micafungin versus liposomal amphotericin B for candidaemia and invasive candidosis: A phase III randomised double-blind trial. Lancet 2007;369(9572):1519–1527.
51. Pappas PG, Rotstein CM, Betts RF, et al. Micafungin versus caspofungin for treatment of candidemia and other forms of invasive candidiasis. Clin Infect Dis 2007;45(7): 883–893.
52. Eschenauer G, DePestel DD, Carver PL. Comparison of echinocandin antifungals. Ther Clin Risk Manag 2007; 3(1):71–97.
53. Goodman JL, Winston DJ, Greenfield RA, et al. A controlled trial of fluconazole to prevent fungal infections in patients undergoing bone marrow transplantation. N Engl J Med 1992;326:845–851.
54. Slavin MA, Osborne B, Adams R, et al. Efficacy and safety of fluconazole prophylaxis for fungal infections after marrow transplantation: A prospective, randomized, double-blind study. J Infect Dis 1995;171:1545–1552.
55. Marr KA, Seidel K, Slavin MA, et al. Prolonged fluconazole prophylaxis is associated with persistent protection against candidiasis-related death in allogeneic marrow transplant recipients: Long-term follow-up of a randomized, placebo-controlled trial. Blood 2000;96:2055–2061.
56. Ullmann AJ, Lipton JH, Vesole DH, et al. A multicenter trial of oral posaconazole vs. fluconazole for the prophylaxis of invasive fungal infections in recipients of allogeneic hematopoietic stem cell transplantation with graft-vs.-host disease. Mycoses 2005;48(Suppl 2):26a–27a.
57. Menichetti F, Del Favero A, Martino P, et al. Itraconazole oral solution as prophylaxis for fungal infections in neutropenic patients with hematologic malignancies: A randomized, placebo-controlled, double-blind, multicenter trial. GIMEMA Infection Program. Gruppo Italiano Malattie Ematologiche dell'Adulto. Clin Infect Dis 1999;28:250–255.
58. Rotstein C, Bow EJ, Laverdiere M, et al. Randomized placebo-controlled trial of fluconazole prophylaxis for neutropenic cancer patients: Benefit based on purpose and intensity of cytotoxic therapy. Clin Infect Dis 1999;28: 331–340.
59. Boogaerts M, Winston DJ, Bow EJ, et al. Intravenous and oral itraconazole versus intravenous amphotericin B as empirical antifungal therapy for persistent fever in neutropenic patients with cancer who are receiving broad-spectrum antibacterial therapy. Ann Intern Med 2001;135:412–422.
60. Winston DJ, Hathorn JW, Schuster MG, et al. A multicenter, randomized trial of fluconazole versus amphotericin B for empiric antifungal therapy of febrile neutropenic patients with cancer. Am J Med 2000;108:282–289.
61. Walsh TJ, Pappas P, Winston DJ, et al. Voriconazole compared with liposomal amphotericin B for empirical antifungal therapy in patients with neutropenia and persistent fever. N Engl J Med 2002;346:225–234.
62. Anaissie EJ, Darouiche RO, Abi-Said D, et al. Management of invasive candidal infections: Results of a prospective, randomized, multicenter study of fluconazole versus amphotericin B and review of the literature. Clin Infect Dis 1996;23:964–972.
63. Kauffman CA, Vazquez JA, Sobel JD, et al. Prospective multicenter surveillance study of funguria in hospitalized patients. Clin Infect Dis 2000;30:14–18.
64. Sobel JD, Kauffman CA, McKinsey D, et al. Candiduria: A randomized, double-blind study of treatment with fluconazole and placebo. Clin Infect Dis 2000;30:19–24.
65. Gallis HA, Drew RH, Pickard WW. Amphotericin B: 30 years of clinical experience. Rev Infect Dis 1990;12:308–329.
66. Nucci M, Anaissie E. Should vascular catheters be removed from all patients with candidemia? An evidence-based review. Clin Infect Dis 2002;34:591–599.
67. Stevens DA, Schwartz HJ, Lee JT, et al. A randomized trial of itraconazole in allergic bronchopulmonary aspergillosis. N Engl J Med 2000;342:756–762.
68. Steinbach WJ, Stevens DA. Review of newer antifungal and immunomodulatory strategies for invasive aspergillosis. Clin Infect Dis 2003;37(Suppl 3):S157–187.
69. Lin SJ, Schranz J, Teutsch SM. Aspergillus case fatality rate: Systematic review of the literature. Clin Infect Dis 2001;32:358–366.
70. Holding KJ, Dworkin MS, Wan PCT, et al. Aspergillosis among people infected with human immunodeficiency virus: Incidence and survival. Clin Infect Dis 2000;31:1253–1257.
71. Saad A, DePestel DD, Carver PL. Factors influencing the magnitude and clinical significance of drug interactions between azole antifungals and select immunosuppressants. Pharmacotherapy 2006;26:1730–1744.
72. Dismukes, WE. Antifungal therapy: Lessons learned over the past 27 years. Clin Infect Dis 2006;42:1289–1296.
73. Herbrecht R, Denning DW, Patterson TF, et al. Voriconazole versus amphotericin B for primary therapy of invasive aspergillosis. N Engl J Med 2002;347:408–415.
74. Ellis M, Spence D, de Pauw B, et al. An EORTC international multicenter randomized trial (EORTC no. 19923) comparing two dosages of liposomal amphotericin B for treatment of invasive aspergillosis. Clin Infect Dis 1998;27:1406–1412.
75. Kontoyiannis DP, Lewis RE. How I treat mucormycosis. Blood 2011;118(5):1216–1224.

76. Castiglioni B, Sutton DA, Rinaldi MG, et al. *Pseudallescheria boydii* (anamorph *Scedosporium apiospermum*) infection in solid organ transplant recipients in a tertiary medical center and review of the literature. Medicine 2002;81:333–348.
77. Lamaris, GA, Chamilos G, Lewis, RE, et al. Scedosporium infection in a tertiary care cancer center: A review of 25 cases from 1989–2006. Clin Infect Dis 2000;43:1580–1584.
78. Dodds Ashley ES, Lewis R, Lewis JS, Martin C, Andes D. Pharmacology of systemic antifungal agents. Clin Infect Dis 2006;43:S28–S39.
79. Marr KA, Boeckh M, Carter RA, et al. Combination antifungal therapy for invasive aspergillosis. Clin Infect Dis 2004;39:797–802.
80. King CT, Rogers PD, Cleary JD, et al. Antifungal therapy during pregnancy. Clin Infect Dis 1998;27: 1151–1160.
81. Cornely OA, Maertens J, Bresnik M, et al. Liposomal amphotericin B as initial therapy for invasive mould infection: A randomized trial comparing a high-loading dose regimen with standard dosing (AmBiLoad trial). Clin Infect Dis 2007;44(10):1289–1297.
82. Ostrosky-Zeichner L, Marr KA, Rex JH, Cohen SH. Amphotericin B. Time for a new "gold standard." Clin Infect Dis 2003;37:415–425.
83. Stevens DA. Itraconazole in cyclodextrin solution. Pharmacotherapy 1999;19:603–611.
84. Smith J, Andes D. Therapeutic drug monitoring of antifungals: Pharmacokinetic and pharmacodynamic considerations. Ther Drug Monit 2008;30(2): 167–172.
85. Goodwin ML, Drew RH. Antifungal serum concentration monitoring: An update. J Antimicrob Chemother 2008;61(1):17–25.

Infections in Immunocompromised Patients

100

Douglas N. Fish and Scott W. Mueller

KEY CONCEPTS

1. An *immunocompromised host* is a patient with defects in host defenses that predispose to infection. Risk factors include neutropenia, immune system defects (from disease or immunosuppressive drug therapy), compromise of natural host defenses, environmental contamination, and changes in normal flora of the host.
2. Immunocompromised patients are at high risk for a variety of bacterial, fungal, viral, and protozoal infections. Bacterial infections caused by gram-positive cocci (staphylococci and streptococci) occur most frequently, followed by gram-negative bacterial infections caused by Enterobacteriaceae and *Pseudomonas aeruginosa*. Fungal infections caused by *Candida* and *Aspergillus*, as well as certain viral infections (herpes simplex virus, cytomegalovirus [CMV]), are also important causes of morbidity and mortality.
3. Risk of infection in neutropenic patients is associated with both the severity and duration of neutropenia. Patients with severe neutropenia (absolute neutrophil count < 500 cells/mm^3 [$<0.5 \times 10^9$/L]) for greater than 7 to 10 days are considered to be at high risk of infection.
4. Fever (single oral temperature of ≥38.3°C [101°F], or a temperature of ≥38°C [100.4°F] for ≥1 hour) is the most important clinical finding in neutropenic patients and is usually the stimulus for further diagnostic workup and initiation of antimicrobial treatment. Infection should be considered as the cause of fever until proven otherwise. Usual signs and symptoms of infection may be altered or absent in neutropenic patients. Appropriate empiric broad-spectrum antimicrobial therapy must be rapidly instituted to prevent excessive morbidity and mortality.
5. Empiric antimicrobial regimens for neutropenic infections should take into account patients' individual risk factors, as well as institutional infection and susceptibility patterns. The significant morbidity and mortality associated with gram-negative infections require that initial empiric regimens for treatment of febrile neutropenia have good activity against *P. aeruginosa* and Enterobacteriaceae. Inpatient parenteral regimens most commonly recommended for initial treatment include monotherapy with an antipseudomonal *β*-lactam, or a combination regimen consisting of an antipseudomonal *β*-lactam, plus an aminoglycoside. Low-risk patients may be successfully treated with oral antibiotics (ciprofloxacin plus amoxicillin/clavulanate), with the treatment setting determined by the patient's clinical status.
6. Neutropenic patients who remain febrile after 3 to 5 days of initial antimicrobial therapy should be reevaluated to determine whether treatment modifications are necessary. Common regimen modifications include addition of vancomycin (if not already administered) and antifungal therapy (amphotericin B or fluconazole). Therapy should be directed at causative organisms, if identified, but broad-spectrum regimens should be maintained during neutropenia.
7. The optimal duration of therapy for febrile neutropenia is controversial. The decision to discontinue antimicrobials is based on resolution of neutropenia, defervescence, culture results, and clinical stability of the patient.
8. Prophylactic antimicrobials are administered to cancer patients expected to experience prolonged neutropenia, as well as to both hematopoietic stem cell and solid-organ transplant recipients. Prophylactic regimens may include antibacterial, antifungal, antiviral, or antiprotozoal agents, or a combination of these, selected according to risk of infection with specific pathogens. Optimal prophylactic regimens should take into account individual patient risk for infection and institutional infection and susceptibility patterns.
9. Patients undergoing hematopoietic stem cell transplantation are at an extremely high risk of infection because of prolonged neutropenia following intensive chemotherapy ± irradiation, while solid-organ transplant recipients are at high risk because of prolonged administration of immunosuppressive drugs. Fungal (*Aspergillus*) and viral (CMV) infections are particularly troublesome in these populations, and prophylactic regimens directed against these pathogens are commonly used. When documented, these infections must be treated aggressively in order to optimize patient outcomes. Nevertheless, mortality rates are often high despite appropriate and aggressive antimicrobial therapy.
10. Immunocompromised patients must be continuously assessed for evidence of infection and response to antimicrobial therapy. Because a large number of antimicrobials may potentially be used, the occurrence of drug-related adverse effects must also be carefully assessed. Efforts should be directed at designing cost-effective treatment strategies that promote optimal patient outcomes.

An immunocompromised host is a patient with intrinsic or acquired defects in host immune defenses that predispose to infection. Advances in modern medicine have created more immunocompromised hosts than ever before. Historically, many of these patients died of their underlying diseases. Dramatic improvements in survival have been achieved by more aggressive therapy of underlying diseases and improved supportive care. However, because such aggressive therapy often renders patients profoundly immunosuppressed for long periods, opportunistic infections remain important causes of morbidity and mortality. This chapter focuses on risk factors for infection, common pathogens and infection sites, and prevention and management of suspected or documented infections in cancer patients (including hematopoietic stem cell transplantation [HSCT] patients) and solid-organ transplant (SOT) recipients. Chapter 103 discusses infectious complications associated with human immunodeficiency virus (HIV) infection.

RISK FACTORS FOR INFECTION/EPIDEMIOLOGY

Many factors influence the degree of immunosuppression and also influence the epidemiology of the associated infections.

Neutropenia

❶❷❸ Neutropenia is defined as an abnormally reduced number of neutrophils circulating in peripheral blood. Although exact definitions of neutropenia can vary, an absolute neutrophil count (ANC) of less than 1,000 cells/mm^3 (1.0×10^9/L) indicates a reduction sufficient to predispose patients to infection.[1] ANC is the sum of the absolute numbers of both mature neutrophils (polymorphonuclear cells [PMNs], also called *polys* or *segs*) and immature neutrophils (*bands*). The absolute number of PMNs and bands is determined by dividing the total percentage of these cells (obtained from the white blood cell [WBC] differential) by 100 and then multiplying the quotient obtained by the total number of WBCs (expressed in cells/mm^3).

The degree or severity of neutropenia, rate of neutrophil decline, and duration of neutropenia are important risk factors for infection.[1–5] All neutropenic patients are considered to be at risk for infection, but those with ANC less than 500 cells/mm^3 (0.5×10^9/L) are at greater risk than those with ANCs of 500 to 1,000 cells/mm^3 (0.5×10^9 to 1.0×10^9/L). Most treatment guidelines use ANC less than 500 cells/mm^3 (0.5×10^9/L) as the critical value in making therapeutic decisions regarding the management of suspected or documented infections.[1–5] Risk of infection and death are greatest among patients with less than 100 neutrophils/mm^3 (0.1×10^9/L) ("profound neutropenia").[1,2,5] In patients with chemotherapy-induced neutropenia, the risk of infection is also increased according to both the rapidity of ANC decline and duration of neutropenia. Patients with severe neutropenia of more than 7 to 10 days' duration are considered to be at especially high risk for serious infections.[3,5] The duration of chemotherapy-induced neutropenia varies considerably among subsets of cancer patients according to the specific chemotherapeutic agents used and the intensity of treatment. Patients undergoing HSCT may have no detectable granulocytes in peripheral blood for up to 3 to 4 weeks and are at particular risk for severe infections with a variety of pathogens.[6]

Bacteria and fungi commonly cause infections in neutropenic patients. Gram-positive cocci (*Staphylococcus aureus*, *Staphylococcus epidermidis*, and other coagulase-negative staphylococci, streptococci, and enterococci) have emerged as the most common cause of acute bacterial infections among neutropenic patients. Gram-negative bacilli (*Escherichia coli*, *Klebsiella pneumoniae*, *Pseudomonas aeruginosa*) traditionally were the most common causes of bacterial infection and remain frequent pathogens.[4,7–9] Although now not as common as gram-positive bacteria, the incidence of gram-negative infections may again be increasing.[3,8] Gram-negative infections are associated with significant morbidity and mortality, in large part due to increasing antibiotic resistance.[7–9] Patients who are neutropenic for extended periods and who receive broad-spectrum antibiotics are at high risk for fungal infections, usually due to *Candida* or *Aspergillus* spp.[2,3,10,11] Viral infections, although not as common as bacterial and fungal infections, also may cause severe infection in neutropenic patients.[2,3,5,6] Successful treatment of infections in neutropenic patients depends on resolution of neutropenia.[1–3,5]

Although not readily quantifiable, abnormalities may exist in granulocyte function as well as in cell numbers. Defects in phagocyte function may be caused by underlying disease (e.g., leukemia) or its treatment (e.g., corticosteroids, antineoplastic agents, and radiation).[3,12]

Immune System Defects

In addition to neutropenia, defects in T-lymphocyte and macrophage function (cell-mediated immunity), B-cell function (humoral immunity), or both predispose patients to infection. Cellular immune dysfunction is the result of underlying disease or immunosuppressive drug therapy; these defects result in a reduced ability of the host to defend against intracellular pathogens. Patients with Hodgkin's disease and transplant patients receiving a wide variety of immunosuppressive drugs, such as cyclosporine, tacrolimus, sirolimus, mycophenolate, corticosteroids, azathioprine, and antineoplastic agents, are at risk for a variety of bacterial, fungal, viral, and protozoal infections (Table 100-1). Although some of these pathogens are associated with asymptomatic or mild disease in normal hosts, they may cause disseminated, life-threatening infections in immunocompromised hosts.

Underlying disease also frequently causes defects in humoral immune function. Patients with multiple myeloma and chronic lymphocytic leukemia have progressive hypogammaglobulinemia that results in defective humoral immunity. Splenectomy performed as a part of the staging process for Hodgkin's disease places patients at risk for infectious complications. Disease states with humoral immune dysfunction predispose the patient to serious, life-threatening infection with encapsulated organisms such as *Streptococcus pneumoniae*, *Haemophilus influenzae*, and *Neisseria meningitidis*.

Destruction of Protective Barriers

Loss of protective barriers is a major factor predisposing immunocompromised patients to infection. Damage to skin and mucous membranes by surgery, venipuncture, IV and urinary catheters, radiation, and chemotherapy disrupts natural host defense systems, leaving patients at high risk for infection. Chemotherapy-induced mucositis may erode mucous membranes of the oropharynx and GI tract and establish a portal for subsequent infection by bacteria, herpes simplex virus (HSV), and *Candida*.[3,5,6] Medical and surgical procedures, such as transplant surgery, indwelling IV catheter placement, bone marrow aspiration, biopsies, and endoscopy, further damage the integument and predispose patients to infection. Infections resulting from disruption of protective barriers usually are a result of skin flora, such as *S. aureus*, *S. epidermidis*, and various streptococci.[1,3,5,12]

Environmental Contamination/Alteration of Microbial Flora

Infections in immunocompromised patients are caused by organisms either colonizing the host or acquired from the environment. Microorganisms may be transferred easily from patient to patient on the hands of hospital personnel unless strict infection control guidelines are followed. Contaminated equipment, such as nebulizers or

TABLE 100-1 Risk Factors and Common Pathogens in Immunocompromised Patients

Risk Factor	Patient Conditions	Common Pathogens
Neutropenia	Acute leukemia Chemotherapy	Bacteria: *Staphylococcus aureus*, *Staphylococcus epidermidis*, *Escherichia coli*, *Klebsiella pneumoniae*, *Pseudomonas aeruginosa*, streptococci, enterococci Fungi: *Candida*, *Aspergillus*, *Zygomycetes* Viruses: Herpes simplex
Impaired cell-mediated immunity	Lymphoma Immunosuppressive therapy (steroids, cyclosporine, chemotherapy)	Bacteria: *Listeria*, *Nocardia*, *Legionella*, Mycobacteria Fungi: *Cryptococcus neoformans*, *Candida*, *Aspergillus*, *Histoplasma capsulatum* Viruses: Cytomegalovirus, varicella-zoster, herpes simplex Protozoal: *Pneumocystis jiroveci*
Impaired humoral immunity	Multiple myeloma Chronic lymphocytic leukemia Splenectomy Immunosuppressive therapy (steroids, chemotherapy)	Bacteria: *S. pneumoniae*, *H. influenzae*, *N. meningitidis*
Loss of protective skin barriers	Venipuncture, bone marrow aspiration, urinary catheterization, vascular access devices, radiation, biopsies	Bacteria: *S. aureus*, *S. epidermidis*, *Bacillus* spp., *Corynebacterium jeikeium* Fungi: *Candida*
Mucous membranes	Respiratory support equipment, endoscopy, chemotherapy, radiation	Bacteria: *S. aureus*, *S. epidermidis*, streptococci, Enterobacteriaceae, *P. aeruginosa*, *Bacteroides* spp. Fungi: *Candida* Viruses: Herpes simplex
Surgery	Solid-organ transplantation	Bacteria: *S. aureus*, *S. epidermidis*, Enterobacteriaceae, *P. aeruginosa*, *Bacteroides* spp. Fungi: *Candida* Viruses: Herpes simplex
Alteration of normal microbial flora	Antimicrobial therapy Chemotherapy Hospital environment	Bacteria: Enterobacteriaceae, *P. aeruginosa*, *Legionella*, *S. aureus*, *S. epidermidis* Fungi: *Candida*, *Aspergillus*
Blood products, donor organs	Bone marrow transplantation Solid-organ transplantation	Fungi: *Candida* Viruses: Cytomegalovirus, Epstein–Barr virus, hepatitis B, hepatitis C Protozoal: *Toxoplasma gondii*

ventilators, and contaminated water supplies have been responsible for outbreaks of *P. aeruginosa* and *Legionella pneumophila* infections, respectively. Foods, such as fruits and green leafy vegetables, which often are colonized with gram-negative bacteria and fungi, are sources of microbial contamination in immunocompromised hosts.[3,6,13]

Most infections in cancer patients are caused by organisms colonizing body sites, such as the skin, oropharynx, and GI tract.[1,3,5,6,13] Approximately 80% of infecting bacterial pathogens are from the patient's own endogenous flora.[1,3] The GI tract is the most common site from which infections in immunocompromised hosts originate. Periodontitis, pharyngitis, esophagitis, colitis, perirectal cellulitis, and bacteremias are caused predominantly by normal flora of the gut; bloodstream infections are thought to arise from microbial translocation across injured GI mucosa.[1,5,6,13] Normal flora may be significantly disrupted and altered; oropharyngeal flora rapidly change to primarily gram-negative bacilli in hospitalized patients. Many cancer patients may already be colonized with gram-negative bacilli on admission as a result of frequent prior hospitalizations and clinic visits. In hospitalized cancer patients, however, up to 50% of infections are caused by colonizing organisms acquired after admission.[1,3]

Although hospitalization and severity of illness are important risk factors for colonization by gram-negative bacilli, administration of broad-spectrum antimicrobial agents has the greatest impact on flora of immunocompromised hosts. Use of these agents disrupts GI tract flora and predisposes patients to infection with more virulent pathogens. Antineoplastic drugs (e.g., cyclophosphamide, doxorubicin, and fluorouracil) and acid-suppressive therapy (e.g., H_2-receptor antagonists, proton-pump inhibitors, and antacids) also may result in changes in GI flora and possibly predispose patients to infection.[1,3,13]

Numerous factors, such as underlying disease, immunosuppressive drug therapy, and antimicrobial administration, determine the immunocompromised host's risk of developing infection. Several risk factors are present concomitantly in many patients (see Table 100-1).

ETIOLOGY OF INFECTIONS IN NEUTROPENIC CANCER PATIENTS

2 Infection remains a significant cause of morbidity and mortality in neutropenic cancer patients. More than 50% of febrile neutropenic patients have an established or occult infection.[1,5] Patients with profound neutropenia are at greatest risk for systemic infection, with at least 20% of these individuals developing bacteremia.[1,5] Areas of impaired or damaged host defenses, such as the oropharynx, lungs, skin, sinuses, and GI tract, are common sites of infection. These local infections may progress to cause systemic infection and bacteremia.[5] Febrile episodes in neutropenic cancer patients can be attributed to microbiologically documented infection in approximately 30% to 40% of cases, about half of which are due to bacteremia. Further, infections can be documented clinically (but not microbiologically) in another 30% to 40% of patients, with the remaining 20% to 40% of patients manifesting infection only by fever.[3,4,8,12]

Table 100-1 lists organisms commonly infecting immunocompromised patients. Approximately 45% to 70% of bacteremic episodes in cancer patients are the result of gram-positive organisms compared with less than 30% of episodes documented during the 1970s and 1980s.[1,4,7,12,14,15] This shift is attributed to the frequent use of indwelling central and peripheral IV catheters, frequent use of broad-spectrum antibiotics with excellent gram-negative activity but relatively poor gram-positive coverage, higher rates of mucositis caused by aggressive cancer treatments, and prophylaxis with trimethoprim–sulfamethoxazole or quinolones.[1,4,7,12] Staphylococci (especially *S. epidermidis*) account for most infections, but *Bacillus* spp. and *Corynebacterium jeikeium* are also important pathogens.[1,5,12,15] Rates of infection due to methicillin-resistant *Staphylococcus aureus* (MRSA) have increased in the hospital and community setting.[16,17] Viridans streptococci, which may be resistant to β-lactams, also have emerged as important pathogens, particularly in patients with chemotherapy-induced mucositis of the oropharynx.[4,12,18,19] Enterococci, including vancomycin-resistant strains, also may be problematic in many institutions.[2,19] Bacteremia caused by vancomycin-resistant enterococci (VRE) in neutropenic patients is associated with a mortality rate exceeding 70%.[4,20]

Gram-positive infections do not always cause immediately life-threatening infections and are associated with somewhat lower mortality rates (approximately 5% to 10%) compared with gram-negative infections.[1,12,15] However, increasing rates of antibiotic resistance have made treatment of gram-positive infections in immunocompromised patients more challenging.[7,12] MRSA infections are associated with increased morbidity, mortality, and hospital costs compared with susceptible organisms.[21] Methicillin resistance among coagulase-negative staphylococci, which may cause 40% to 80% of infections in certain populations, is common (70% to 90% of isolates).[6,7,16] Organisms that are resistant to vancomycin are increasing in importance.[1,5,7,19] Thus, prevention and timely diagnosis and treatment of gram-positive infections are clearly of great importance in the management of neutropenic cancer patients.

Gram-negative infections remain important causes of morbidity and mortality (approximately 20%) in immunocompromised cancer patients.[12,15] However, the relative frequency of infection owing to specific pathogens has been shifting among gram-negative infections. *E. coli* and *Klebsiella* remain the most common isolates at many centers.[15] Strains of *Klebsiella* producing plasmid-mediated extended-spectrum β-lactamases that hydrolyze extended-spectrum cephalosporins have emerged and are cause for concern.[1,5,7,19] The frequency of infections resulting from other gram-negative organisms, such as *Enterobacter*, *Serratia*, and *Citrobacter*, has been increasing.[1,5] Infections with these particular organisms may be difficult to treat because of the ease of β-lactamase induction and the more frequent development of resistance to multiple antibiotics.[1,3,5,12,19]

P. aeruginosa has long been an important pathogen in cancer patients. *P. aeruginosa* infection rates are decreasing in patients with solid tumors but not in patients with hematologic malignancies.[4,7] Infections caused by *P. aeruginosa* are associated with significant morbidity and mortality in neutropenic patients, with mortality rates of 31% to 75% reported.[12,15] The frequency of infection caused by difficult-to-treat organisms such as *Stenotrophomonas maltophilia* and *Burkholderia cepacia* appears to be increasing at many centers, probably because of selective pressures of broad-spectrum antimicrobial use.[4,12] As with gram-positive organisms, antibiotic resistance among gram-negative organisms has continued to increase at alarming rates and has made appropriate antibiotic selection for treatment of febrile neutropenia more difficult.[1,16] Although the GI tract is a common site of bacterial infection, severe infections caused by anaerobic organisms are relatively infrequent. Anaerobes are found most frequently in mixed infections, such as perirectal cellulitis and mucositis-associated oropharyngeal infections.[12]

In addition to bacterial infections, neutropenic cancer patients are at risk for invasive fungal infections. Patients with extended periods of profound neutropenia who have been receiving broad-spectrum antibiotics, corticosteroids, or both are at the highest risk for invasive fungal infection. Up to one third of febrile neutropenic patients who do not respond to 1 week of broad-spectrum antibiotic therapy will have a systemic fungal infection.[1,5,12] Large autopsy studies have documented that up to 40% of patients with hematologic malignancies had deep fungal infections, fully 75% of which were undiagnosed prior to death. Causative pathogens were usually either *Candida* spp. (35%) or *Aspergillus* spp. (55%).[22]

Candida albicans is the most common fungal pathogen in neutropenic cancer patients.[4,12,23] However, non-*albicans* species of *Candida* including *C. glabrata*, *C. tropicalis*, *C. parapsilosis*, and *C. krusei* are being isolated with increasing frequency and are more common than *C. albicans* infections in some studies.[11,23] Increased infections caused by pathogens such as *Trichosporon* spp., *Fusarium* spp., and *Curvularia* have also been reported.[23–25] The shift toward more frequent infection with non-*albicans Candida* is important because of significantly decreased rates of susceptibility among many of these strains.[26] Because *Candida* spp. are normal flora, alteration of body host defenses is an important risk factor for the development of these infections. Oral thrush is the most common clinical manifestation of fungal infection. Mucous membranes damaged from chemotherapy and radiation serve as areas of *Candida* surface colonization and subsequent entry into the bloodstream; disease then may disseminate throughout the body. Organs such as the liver, spleen, kidney, and lungs are commonly involved in disseminated disease.[22,24] Hepatosplenic candidiasis is a particularly important infection in patients with hematologic malignancies.[3,22,24] Diagnosis of *Candida* infections is difficult and often requires invasive tissue sampling.[6] In patients with invasive candidiasis, overall attributable mortality is as high as 35% to 50%.[4,11,23]

Invasive infections caused by *Aspergillus* are a serious complication of neutropenia, with mortality approaching 80% in patients with prolonged neutropenia and/or patients undergoing allogeneic HSCT.[4,12] These infections are particularly prevalent in patients with hematologic malignancies and in patients undergoing HSCT.[4,24,25,27] Infections resulting from *Aspergillus* species (including *A. fumigatus*, *A. terreus*, *A. flavus*, and *A. niger*) usually are acquired via inhalation of airborne spores. After colonizing the lungs, *Aspergillus* invades the lung parenchyma and pulmonary vessels, resulting in hemorrhage, pulmonary infarcts, and a high mortality rate. Invasive pulmonary disease is the dominant manifestation of infection in patients with neutropenia. However, *Aspergillus* also may cause other infections, including sinusitis, cutaneous infection, and disseminated disease involving multiple organs, including the CNS.[27] Prolonged neutropenia is the primary risk factor for invasive pulmonary aspergillosis in patients with acute leukemia; use of corticosteroids also may predispose patients to disease.[27] Invasive aspergillosis should be suspected in neutropenic cancer patients colonized with *Aspergillus* (in sputum and/or nasal cultures) who remain persistently febrile despite at least 1 week of broad-spectrum antibiotic therapy.[1,5,27]

Chemotherapy-induced mucous membrane damage may predispose neutropenic cancer patients to reactivation of HSV, manifesting as gingivostomatitis or recurrent genital infections. Untreated oropharyngeal HSV infections may spread to involve the esophagus and often coexist with *Candida* infections. Clinical disease resulting from HSV occurs most often in patients with serologic evidence (e.g., serum antibodies to HSV) of prior infection. Both HSV-seropositive HSCT patients and HSV-seropositive leukemics receiving intensive chemotherapy are at high risk for recurrent HSV disease during periods of immunosuppression.[3,4,5,6,12]

Pneumocystis jiroveci and *Toxoplasma gondii* are the most common parasitic pathogens found in immunocompromised cancer patients. Patients with hematologic malignancies (i.e., acute lymphocytic leukemia, lymphoma, and Hodgkin's disease) and those receiving high-dose corticosteroids as part of chemotherapy regimens are at the greatest risk of infection.[3,4,6,12] Routine use of trimethoprim–sulfamethoxazole prophylaxis has reduced substantially the incidence of these infections.[1,5,6]

Because the majority of infecting organisms in cancer patients are from the host's own flora, some centers have used routine surveillance cultures in an attempt to prospectively identify causes of fever and suspected infection. In a typical surveillance culture program, cultures of the nose, mouth, axillae, and perirectal area are performed twice weekly, and culture results are correlated with the clinical status of the patient. Because these cultures are costly and have low diagnostic yield, the utility of surveillance culture programs is believed to be limited.[1,5] However, surveillance cultures are useful as research tools and in patients with prolonged profound neutropenia and in institutions that have high rates of antimicrobial resistance or have problems with virulent pathogens such as *P. aeruginosa* or *Aspergillus* spp. Surveillance cultures should be limited to the anterior nares for detecting colonization with MRSA, *Aspergillus*, and penicillin-resistant pneumococci and to the rectum for detecting *P. aeruginosa*, multiple-antibiotic-resistant gram-negative rods, and VRE.[1,12]

Knowledge of infection rates and local susceptibility patterns is essential for guiding optimal management of febrile neutropenia. These parameters must be monitored closely because the spectrum of infectious complications is related to multiple factors, including cancer chemotherapy regimens and antimicrobial therapy used for treatment and prophylaxis.

CLINICAL PRESENTATION

❹ The most important clinical finding in the neutropenic cancer patient is fever. Because of the potential for significant morbidity and mortality associated with infection in these patients, fever should be considered to be the result of infection until proved otherwise.[1–3,8,12] At the appearance of fever, the patient should be evaluated carefully for other signs and symptoms of infection.

TREATMENT

Management of patients with febrile neutropenia, including both treatment and prophylaxis of infectious complications, can be extremely challenging. Although published guidelines are available, the most optimal clinical management of these patients remains unclear in many aspects.

Febrile Episodes in Neutropenic Cancer Patients

Desired outcomes

❹ ❺ The goals of therapy in neutropenic cancer patients with fever are the following: (a) protect the neutropenic patient from early death caused by undiagnosed infection; (b) prevent breakthrough bacterial, fungal, viral, and protozoal infections during periods of neutropenia; (c) effectively treat established infections; (d) reduce morbidity and allow for administration of optimal antineoplastic therapy; (e) avoid unnecessary use of antimicrobials that contribute to increased resistance; and (f) minimize toxicities and cost of antimicrobial therapy while increasing patient quality of life. Empirical broad-spectrum antibiotic therapy is effective at reducing early mortality.[13]

CLINICAL PRESENTATION Febrile Neutropenia[1,3,4,6]

General

- Due to high risk for serious infections, frequent (at least daily) careful clinical assessments must be performed to search for possible evidence of infection
- Physical assessment should include examination of all common sites of infection, including mouth/pharynx, nose and sinuses, respiratory tract, GI tract, urinary tract, skin, soft tissues, perineum, and intravascular catheter insertion sites

Symptoms

- Usual signs and symptoms of infection may be absent or altered in neutropenic patients owing to low numbers of leukocytes and an inability to mount an inflammatory response (e.g., no infiltrate on chest x-ray film, urinary tract infection without pyuria)
- Pain may be present at the infection site(s)

Signs

- Fever in this setting is defined as a single oral temperature ≥38.3°C (≥101°F) in the absence of other causes or temperature ≥38°C (≥100.4°F) for 1 hour or more. Other causes of fever unrelated to infection in this patient population include reactions to blood products, chemotherapeutic agents (and other drugs, including biologics), cell lysis, and underlying malignancy
- Usual signs of infection may be absent or altered; patients with bacteremia commonly exhibit no signs of infection other than fever

Laboratory Tests

- Neutropenia (ANC ≤1,000 cells/mm^3 [≤1.0 × 10^9/L])
- Blood cultures (two or more sets, including vascular access devices) for bacteria and fungi; cultures of other suspected infection sites (infection can be documented microbiologically in only about 30% of cases, about half of which are due to bacteremia)
- Other cultures should be obtained as indicated clinically according to the presence of signs or symptoms
- Recent surveillance cultures (nasal, rectal) should be reviewed, if available
- Complete blood count and blood chemistries should be obtained frequently to monitor neutropenia, plan supportive care, guide drug dosing, and assess patient's overall status

Other Diagnostic Tests

- Chest x-ray film
- Aspiration, biopsy of skin lesions
- Other diagnostic tests as indicated clinically on the basis of physical examination and other assessments

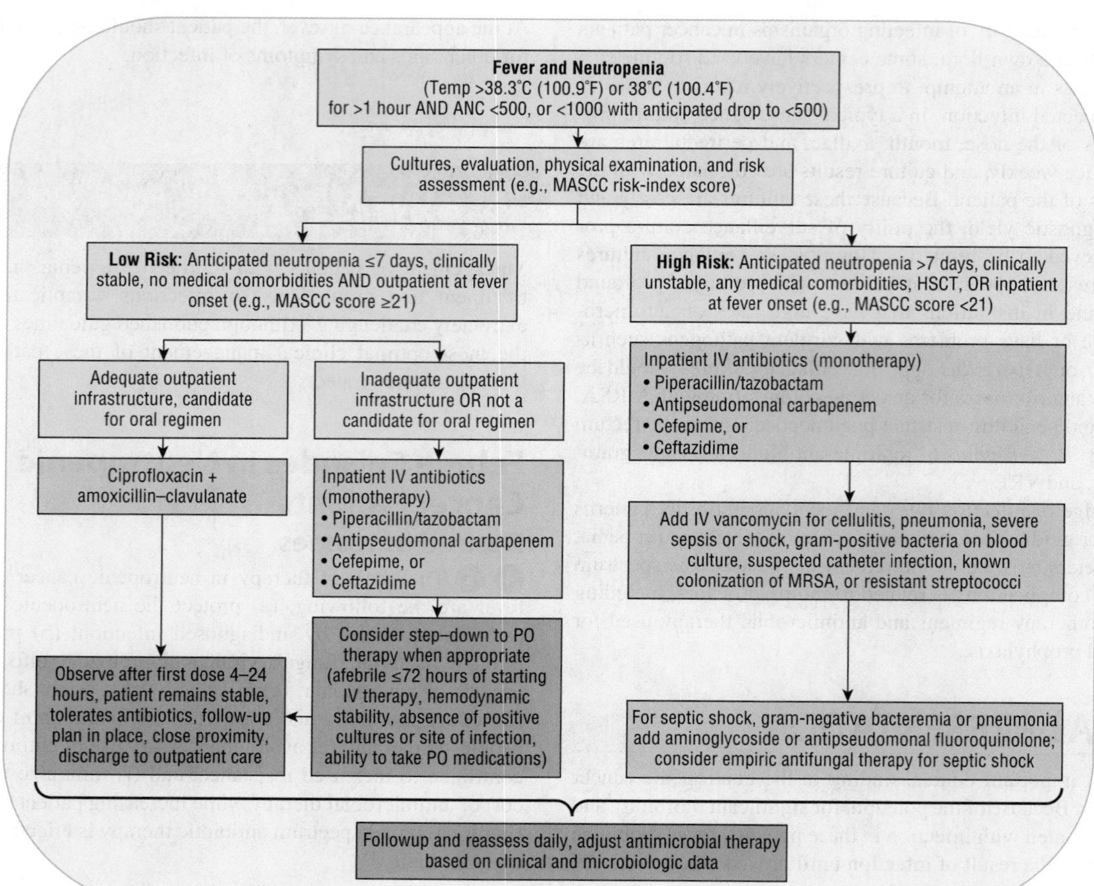

FIGURE 100-1 Initial management of febrile episodes in neutropenic patients. (ANC, absolute neutrophil count; HSCT, hematopoietic stem cell transplantation; MASCC, Multinational Association for Supportive Care in Cancer; PO, oral.)

Approach to Treatment

General guidelines for management of febrile episodes and documented infections in neutropenic patients are shown in Figures 100-1 and 100-2.[1] Although many controversies remain regarding optimal management of these patients, updated evidence-based guidelines from the Infectious Diseases Society of America (IDSA) for the management of febrile neutropenia were published in 2010.[1] Similarly, the National Comprehensive Cancer Network (NCCN) published updated clinical practice guidelines for the prevention and treatment of cancer-related infections in 2012.[5] Selected specific recommendations are discussed in the following sections of this chapter, and their associated evidence-based rankings are summarized in Table 100-2.

Fever in the neutropenic cancer patient is considered to be caused by infection until proved otherwise. High-dose broad-spectrum bactericidal, usually parenteral, empirical antibiotic therapy should be initiated at the onset of fever or at the first signs or symptoms of infection. Withholding antibiotic therapy until an organism is isolated results in unacceptably high mortality rates. Undiagnosed infection in immunocompromised patients can rapidly disseminate and result in death if left untreated or if treated improperly. Failure to initiate appropriate antibiotic therapy for *P. aeruginosa* bacteremia at the onset of fever in neutropenic cancer patients resulted in mortality rates of 15% and 70% within 12 and 48 hours, respectively.[1,5] Empirical antibiotic therapy is 70% to 90% effective at reducing early morbidity and mortality.[1,5,7,12] Therapy must be appropriate and initiated promptly. Antimicrobial therapy must also be initiated promptly in afebrile cancer patients with clinical signs and symptoms of infection.

When designing optimal empirical antibiotic regimens, clinicians must consider infection patterns and antimicrobial susceptibility trends in their respective institutions. Patient factors such as risk for infection, drug allergies, concomitant nephrotoxins, and previous antimicrobial exposure (including prophylaxis) must be considered.[1,4,5] Assessment of the patient's risk of infection will help determine the appropriate route and setting for antibiotic administration (Fig. 100-1). Neutropenic patients with fever can be divided into low- and high-risk groups for complications of severe infection. Risk stratification drives both type and setting of antimicrobial therapy. The Multinational Association for Supportive Care in Cancer (MASCC) risk-index score is recommended by many clinical guidelines to assess a patient's risk of complications.[1,5] Most experts agree that, in general, low-risk patients have an anticipated duration of neutropenia ≤7 days, are clinically stable, and have no or few comorbidities and no bacterial focus or systemic signs of infection other than fever. In contrast, high-risk patients are those with an anticipated duration of neutropenia >7 days or profound neutropenia, are clinically unstable or have comorbid medical problems (e.g., focal or systemic signs of infection, GI symptoms, nausea, vomiting, diarrhea, hypoxemia, and chronic lung disease), or have a high-risk cancer (e.g., acute leukemia) and/or have undergone high intensity chemotherapy. High-risk patients (MASCC <21) should be hospitalized for parenteral antibiotics whereas low-risk patients may be candidates for oral or outpatient antibiotics. Even with such classifications, careful selection of low-risk patients for oral outpatient management is important (discussed in "Oral Antibiotic Therapy for Management of Febrile Neutropenia" section below).[1,5,28–30]

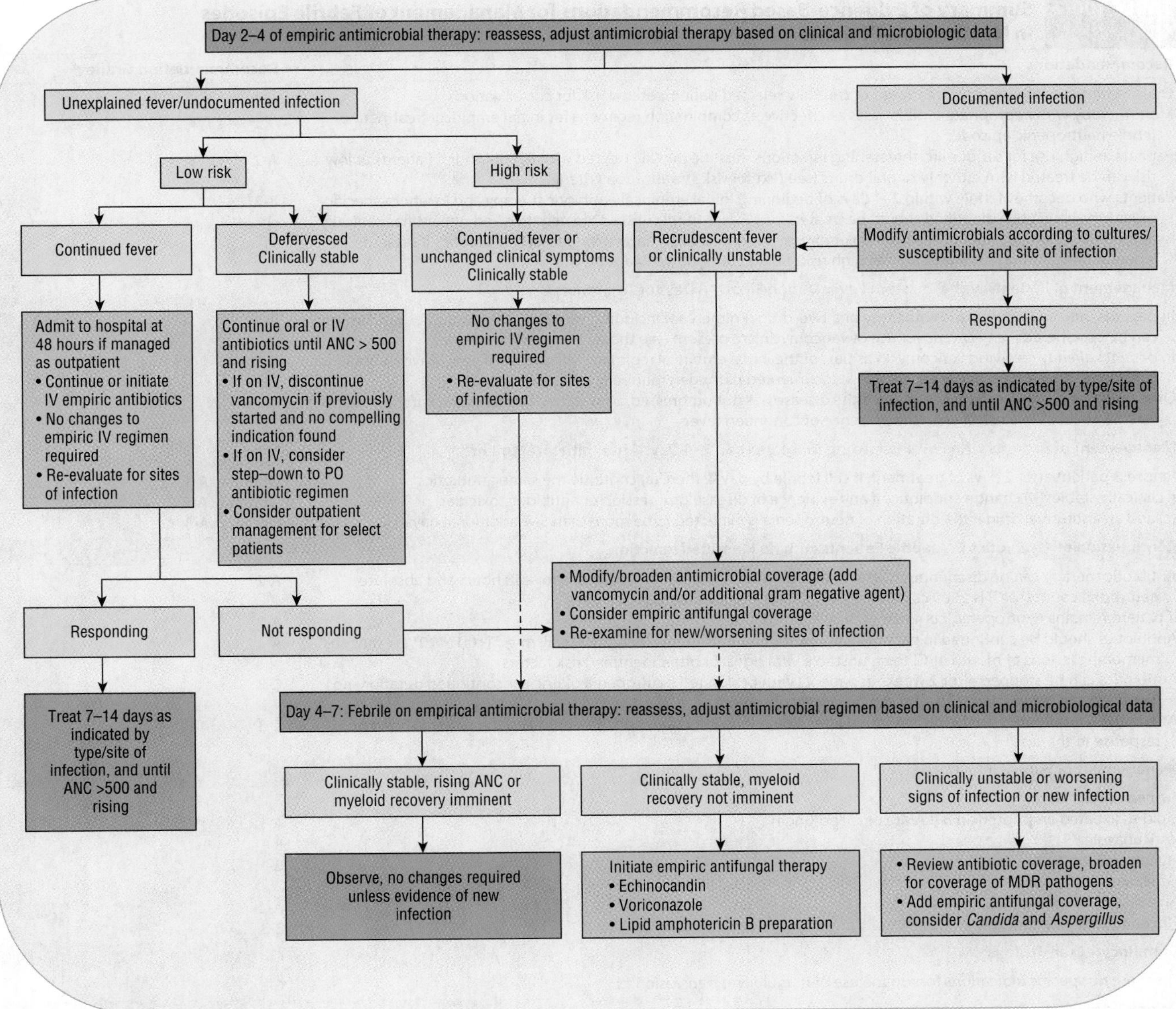

FIGURE 100-2 Subsequent management of febrile episodes in neutropenic patients who have already received empirical antimicrobial therapy for 2–4 days. (ANC, absolute neutrophil count; MDR, multidrug-resistant; PO, oral.)

The optimal antibiotic regimen for empirical therapy in febrile neutropenic cancer patients remains controversial, but it is clear that no single regimen can be recommended for all patients. Because of their frequency and relative pathogenicity, *P. aeruginosa* and other gram-negative bacilli and staphylococci remain the primary targets of empirical antimicrobial therapy.[1,12] Although *P. aeruginosa* is documented in fewer than 5% of bloodstream infections in the population of hospitalized patients, adequate antipseudomonal antibiotic coverage still must be included in empirical regimens because of the significant morbidity and mortality associated with this pathogen.[1,4,12,16] All empirical regimens must be carefully monitored and appropriately revised on the basis of documented infections, susceptibilities of bacterial isolates, development of more defined clinical signs and symptoms of infection, or a combination of these factors.

Although there are some differences among them, consensus guidelines generally recognize three different types of empirical parenteral antibiotic regimens: (a) monotherapy with an antipseudomonal β-lactam such as a cephalosporin (cefepime or ceftazidime), a carbapenem (imipenem–cilastatin, meropenem, or doripenem), or piperacillin–tazobactam; (b) two-drug combination therapy with an antipseudomonal β-lactam plus either an aminoglycoside or an antipseudomonal fluoroquinolone (ciprofloxacin or levofloxacin); and (c) monotherapy or two-drug combination therapy as above, plus the addition of vancomycin (Fig. 100-1).[1,5] Each of these regimens has advantages and disadvantages, which are summarized in Table 100-3. There is no overwhelming evidence that any one of these regimens is superior to the others. The overall response to empirical antibiotic regimens in febrile neutropenic cancer patients is approximately 70% to 90% regardless of whether a pathogen is isolated or which antimicrobial regimen is used.[1,4,5,7,12] Additionally, other alternative regimens may also appropriate based on specific patient characteristics or susceptibilities of suspected pathogens.

β-Lactam Monotherapy

Monotherapy with an antipseudomonal β-lactam is recommended by IDSA 2010 and NCCN 2012 guidelines as initial parenteral therapy for management of febrile neutropenia without suspected or proven resistant organisms or complications (e.g., pneumonia, hypotension,

TABLE 100-2 Summary of Evidence-Based Recommendations for Management of Febrile Episodes in Neutropenic Patients

Recommendations	Recommendation Grades[a]
Oral antibiotics are feasible for treatment of carefully selected patients at low risk for complications	A-1
Monotherapy with appropriate antibiotics is as effective as combination regimens for initial empirical treatment of febrile neutropenic episodes	A-1
Patients at high risk for serious life-threatening infections must be initially treated with IV antibiotics. Patients at low risk can be treated with either IV or oral drugs (see text for risk stratification criteria)	A-2
Patients who become afebrile within 2–4 days of beginning initial empirical antibiotic therapy and in whom specific organisms have been identified should be treated for ≥7 days (until cultures are negative and patient has clinically recovered). Low-risk patients in whom no organism is identified can be switched to oral antibiotics if desired, whereas patients originally classified as high risk should continue on IV antibiotics	B-2
Management of Patients with Persistent Fever During First 2–4 Days of Treatment	
In patients initially receiving monotherapy or a two-drug regimen *not* including vancomycin, addition of vancomycin can be considered if any criteria for use of vancomycin are present (see the text for specific criteria)	B-3
In patients *already* receiving vancomycin as part of the initial empirical regimen, withdrawal of vancomycin should be considered after 2 days in the absence of a documented pathogen requiring continued therapy	A-2
Other initial antibiotics can be continued if the disease has not progressed, or switched to oral therapy if the patient was classified as low risk even in the presence of continued fever	A-1
Management of Patients with Fever Persisting for More Than 2–4 Days After Initial Treatment	
Reassess patient after 2 days of treatment. If still febrile by day 4, then: (a) continue the same antibiotics if clinically stable; (b) change antibiotics if any evidence of disease progression or antibiotic toxicities; or (c) add an antifungal drug if the duration of neutropenia is expected to be more than 5–7 additional days	Option a: A-1 Option b: A-3 Option c: A-3
Continuation of Antibiotics in Afebrile Patients with no Identified Infection	
Antibiotic therapy can be discontinued after 3 days of treatment if patient is afebrile for ≥48 hours and absolute neutrophil count (ANC) is ≥500 cells/mm³ (≥0.5 × 10^9/L) for two consecutive days	A-2
If patient remains neutropenic, continue IV or oral antibiotics	A-2
Antibiotics should be continued in patients with profound neutropenia (ANC <100 cells/mm³ [<0.1 × 10^9/L]), mucous membrane lesions of mouth or GI tract, unstable vital signs, or other identified risk factors	A-2
Antibiotics can be stopped after 2 weeks in patients with prolonged neutropenia of unclear continued duration, no identified site of infection, and who can be closely observed	C-3
Alternatively, antibiotics can be discontinued after 4 days if no infection is documented and the patient shows no response to therapy	C-3
Management of Fungal Infections	
Suspected candidiasis:	
Lipid-associated amphotericin B (LAMB) or caspofungin	A-1
Voriconazole	B-1
Fluconazole or itraconazole	B-1
Candidemia:	
An echinocandin or LAMB	A-2
Fluconazole or voriconazole	B-3
Granulocyte Transfusions	
There are no specific indications for routine use of granulocyte transfusions	C-2
Colony-Stimulating Factors	
Colony-stimulating factors are not indicated for routine treatment of neutropenia in either febrile or afebrile patients	B-2
Prophylactic use of colony-stimulating factors should be considered for patients in whom the anticipated risk of fever and neutropenia is ≥20%	A-2
Antimicrobial Prophylaxis in Neutropenic Patients	
Fluoroquinolone prophylaxis should be considered for high-risk patients with profound neutropenia (ANC ≥500 cells/mm³ [≥0.5 × 10^9/L]) expected to last >7–10 days	B-1
Antibacterial prophylaxis is not required in routinely recommended in low-risk patients who are expected to be neutropenic <7 days	A-3
Prophylaxis with trimethoprim–sulfamethoxazole should be administered to all patients at risk for *Pneumocystis jiroveci* pneumonia, regardless of whether they are neutropenic	A-1
Prophylaxis with fluconazole, posaconazole, voriconazole, or caspofungin is recommended in high-risk patients, starting with induction chemotherapy and continued for duration of neutropenia; itraconzole is an effective alternative agent	A-1 for all agents except voriconazole and caspofungin (both B-2)
In HSCT, prophylaxis with fluconazole, micafungin, posaconazole, itraconzole, voriconazole, or LAMB is recommended during the period of risk of neutropenia	A-1 for fluconazole and micafungin, all others B-2
In HSCT patients with graft-versus-host disease, or neutropenic patients with hematologic malignancies, prophylaxis with posaconazole is recommended for prevention of invasive fungal infections	A-1
HSV-seropositive patients undergoing HSCT or leukemia induction therapy should receive acyclovir prophylaxis during neutropenia, and for at least 30 days after HSCT	A-1 for prophylaxis, A-2 for duration
In HSCT, prophylaxis with acyclovir should be administered during neutropenia and for at least 1 year afterward to prevent VZV infection or reactivation	A-2

[a]Strength of recommendations: A, B, C = good, moderate, and poor evidence to support recommendation for use, respectively; D = moderate evidence to support a recommendation against use.
Quality of evidence: 1 = evidence from ≥1 properly randomized, controlled trial; 2 = evidence from ≥1 well-designed clinical trial without randomization, from cohort or case–control analytic studies, from multiple time series, or from dramatic results from uncontrolled experiments; 3 = evidence from opinions of respected authorities, based on clinical experience, descriptive studies, or reports of expert committees.

Data from references 1, 5, 23, and 27.

TABLE 100-3 Comparative Advantages and Disadvantages of Various Antibiotic Regimens for Empiric Therapy of Febrile Neutropenic Cancer Patients

Regimen	Potential Advantages	Potential Disadvantages
β-Lactam monotherapy (ceftazidime, cefepime, piperacillin–tazobactam, imipenem–cilastatin, or meropenem)	Efficacy comparable to combination regimens; decreased drug toxicities; ease of administration; possibly less expensive	Possibly less efficacy in profound neutropenia or prolonged neutropenia; limited gram-positive activity; no potential for additive/synergistic effects; increased selection of resistant organisms; increased colonization and superinfection rates
Antipseudomonal β-lactam plus aminoglycoside (e.g., gentamicin or tobramycin + cefepime, ceftazidime, or piperacillin–tazobactam)	Traditional regimen, broad-spectrum coverage; optimal therapy of *Pseudomonas aeruginosa*; rapidly bactericidal; synergistic activity; decreased bacterial resistance; reduction of superinfections	Limited gram-positive activity; potential for nephrotoxicity; need for therapeutic monitoring of aminoglycoside concentrations
Antipseudomonal β-lactam plus fluoroquinolone (ciprofloxacin or higher-dose levofloxacin + ceftazidime, cefepime, or piperacillin–tazobactam)	Efficacy similar to other regimens when used in combination therapy; no cross-resistance with β-lactams; possibility for oral administration; may be useful in patients with renal impairment in whom aminoglycosides are undesirable	Marginal gram-positive activity; fluoroquinolones not recommended as monotherapy; resistance may develop rapidly
Empirical regimens containing vancomycin (added to antipseudomonal β-lactam ± aminoglycoside or fluoroquinolone)	Early effective therapy of gram-positive infections	No demonstrated benefit of vancomycin empirical therapy versus addition of vancomycin if needed later; increased risk of selection for vancomycin-resistant enterococci; risk of toxicities; excessive cost; need for therapeutic monitoring of vancomycin concentrations
Oral antibiotic regimens (e.g., ciprofloxacin or levofloxacin + amoxicillin–clavulanate or clindamycin)	Efficacy comparable with parenteral therapy in low-risk patients; less expensive; reduced exposure of patients to nosocomial pathogens	Least studied treatment approach; less potent than parenteral antibiotics; requires compliant patient with 24-hour access to medical care should clinical instability develop

Data from references 1–5, and 12.

vascular access infection, etc.)[1,5] Several β-lactam antibiotics in current use have been evaluated as monotherapy for management of febrile episodes in neutropenic cancer patients, including antipseudomonal cephalosporins (ceftazidime and cefepime), piperacillin–tazobactam, and antipseudomonal carbapenems (imipenem–cilastatin and meropenem).[1,3,5,12,14] Three different meta-analyses assessing as many as 46 clinical trials involving more than 7,600 patients found no significant differences overall between monotherapy and combination therapy (β-lactam/aminoglycoside) in rates of survival, treatment response, and bacterial/fungal superinfections.[31–33] One study also found a higher rate of adverse effects in aminoglycoside-containing combination regimens.[32] In addition, one analysis found that cefepime monotherapy was associated with a significantly higher risk of mortality compared with the other β-lactams evaluated.[1,5,33] A follow-up analysis conducted by the FDA using additional studies and patient-level data failed to confirm an increased risk of mortality with cefepime, concluding that it is as efficacious as other β-lactams.[1,5,34] Significantly lower response rates for ceftazidime (but not cefepime) monotherapy have been reported in another review of the clinical literature.[1,5] However, until the results of these studies can be validated, ceftazidime is still are among the monotherapy regimens routinely recommended as appropriate initial therapy of febrile neutropenic patients, although with a lower strength of evidence in 2012 NCCN guidelines.[1,5,12,33,34] Institutional susceptibility patterns and patient characteristics should drive drug selection.

Doripenem has an appropriate overall spectrum of antibacterial activity with good activity against *P. aeruginosa* and other gram-negative organisms as well as many gram-positive pathogens. Neither the 2012 NCCN nor the 2010 IDSA consensus guidelines specifically recommend doripenem as appropriate for monotherapy due to a lack of supportive clinical evidence at the time the guidelines were written.[1,5] Doripenem is, however, considered by many clinicians to be appropriate for this use.

Use of monotherapy has several potential advantages and disadvantages (see Table 100-3). Perhaps the most common concerns are those regarding the selection of resistant strains of organisms, such as *P. aeruginosa*, *Enterobacter* spp., and *Serratia* spp., through extended-spectrum β-lactamases and type 1 β-lactamases, especially with ceftazidime.[1,5,7,12,19] Activity against gram-positive organisms such as coagulase-negative staphylococci, MRSA, enterococci (including VRE), penicillin-resistant *S. pneumoniae*, and some strains of viridans streptococci is poor with some single β-lactams, but cefepime and antipseudomonal carbapenems have good activity against viridans streptococci and pneumococci.[1,5] Although ceftazidime has been studied widely and used for treatment of febrile neutropenia, newer agents may be more effective owing to ceftazidime's susceptibility to β-lactamase induction and lower activity against gram-positive organisms.[1,7,19,33] Ertapenem, a carbapenem, and tigecycline, a glycylcycline antibiotic, have excellent activity against many gram-negative organisms but should not be used in the empirical treatment of febrile neutropenia due to their weaker activity against *P. aeruginosa*.

As with all empirical antibiotic regimens, patients receiving monotherapy should be monitored closely for treatment failure, secondary infections, and development of resistance. Use of monotherapy may not be appropriate in institutions with high rates of gram-positive infections or infections caused by relatively resistant gram-negative pathogens such as *P. aeruginosa* and *Enterobacter*. The carbapenems are less susceptible to inducible β-lactamases and often may be used effectively in these institutions. Overall, similar efficacy has been observed with monotherapy with antipseudomonal β-lactams compared to aminoglycoside combination therapy for treatment of *P. aeruginosa* infections.[1,5,12,32,33]

Aminoglycoside Plus Antipseudomonal β-Lactam

Regimens consisting of an aminoglycoside plus an antipseudomonal β-lactam traditionally have been the most commonly used for empirical treatment of febrile neutropenia, although many such regimens may lack adequate gram-positive activity (see Table 100-3).[1,5] This relative lack of activity remains a concern because of the increasing frequency of gram-positive infections. The choice of aminoglycoside and β-lactam for inclusion in empirical regimens should be based on institutional epidemiology and antimicrobial susceptibility patterns. Similar efficacy is observed with an antipseudomonal β-lactam in combination with an aminoglycoside.[1,5]

Combinations of broad-spectrum β-lactams and aminoglycosides often provide synergistic activity against bacteria commonly infecting neutropenic patients. The exact role of synergy in the outcome of febrile neutropenic patients treated with empirical antibiotic therapy is somewhat controversial, particularly in light of the efficacy of single-drug regimens. Nevertheless, synergistic combinations of antibiotics appear to be beneficial in patients with persistent profound neutropenia. Moreover, administration of antipseudomonal β-lactams in combination with an aminoglycoside may result in a lower rate of drug resistance.[4]

Aminoglycoside toxicity may be a concern in patients receiving these regimens who are already receiving other nephrotoxic drugs, such as cisplatin and cyclosporine. Administration of aminoglycosides in large single daily doses (once-daily dosing) may be as effective, less costly, and no more toxic than conventional dosing methods.[41] Although once-daily aminoglycoside dosing regimens appear to be safe and effective in these patients, standard dosing regimens are recommended for infections where data are not sufficient to recommend once-daily dosing (e.g., endocarditis).[1,5,12]

Fluoroquinolones as a Component of Empirical Regimens

Because the fluoroquinolone antibiotics have broad-spectrum activity (particularly against gram-negative pathogens), rapid bactericidal activity, and favorable pharmacokinetic and toxicity profiles, these agents have been investigated as empirical therapy for febrile neutropenic patients. Ciprofloxacin is the preferred agent for use in this clinical setting because of its relatively better activity against *P. aeruginosa* and more extensive evidence-based support for its use.[1,12] Response rates to quinolone-containing combination regimens are comparable to those obtained with the other regimens described previously.[1,4,5] Ciprofloxacin is not recommended for monotherapy, however, because of its relatively poor activity against gram-positive pathogens, particularly streptococci, and variable response rates in clinical studies.[1,5] Fluoroquinolones should also not be used as empirical therapy in patients who have received quinolones as infection prophylaxis because of the risk of drug resistance.[1,5,12] Rates of fluoroquinolone resistance are increasing, and streptococcal treatment failures are a concern.[16,19] Although fluoroquinolones are not generally considered first-line empirical therapy, they may be useful as one component of combination regimens in patients with allergies or other contraindications to first-line agents.[1,5]

Empirical Regimens Containing Vancomycin

The inclusion of vancomycin in initial empirical therapy of febrile neutropenic cancer patients is not currently recommended by IDSA 2010 or NCCN 2012 guidelines unless the patient has specific risk factors; however, this remains an ongoing debate. This controversy continues because of the increasing incidence of gram-positive infections in this population, particularly MRSA. One approach is to include vancomycin in the initial empirical antibiotic regimen, thereby providing early effective treatment of possible gram-positive infections. Inclusion of vancomycin in initial empirical regimens may be more appropriate today because of higher rates of MRSA infections as well as aggressive chemotherapy regimens causing significant mucosal damage that increases the risk for streptococcal infections. Decreased mortality from penicillin-resistant viridans streptococcal infections has been observed when vancomycin was included in initial therapy.[1,5,12] A second approach is to withhold vancomycin from initial empirical regimens, later adding the drug if gram-positive organisms are isolated from cultures or if there is no response to initial therapy. Support for both these approaches can be found in the medical literature.[1,5,12,35,36] Prospective studies and at least two meta-analyses have failed to document increased response rates or decreased mortality with the routine addition of vancomycin to initial empirical regimens, provided that vancomycin can be added later as needed.[1,5,12,35,36] In addition to increased costs of therapy, vancomycin was also associated with increased adverse effects, including nephrotoxicity.[35,36] Finally, concerns remain regarding selection of resistant gram-positive bacteria such as VRE with excessive vancomycin use.[1,5,12]

Vancomycin is currently recommended for inclusion in initial empirical regimens only in patients at high risk for gram-positive infection, particularly due to MRSA and coagulase-negative staphylococci (including patients with evidence of infection of central venous catheters and other indwelling lines), high risk for viridans streptococcal infection due to severe mucositis, or pneumonitis or soft tissue infection in hospitals with high rates of MRSA infections.[1,3,5,7,12,35,36] Rates of β-lactam resistance among viridans streptococci range from 18% to 29%.[5] Empirical vancomycin use may be justified in institutions using empirical or prophylactic antibiotic regimens without good activity against streptococci (e.g., ciprofloxacin) and in patients known to be colonized with MRSA or β-lactam–resistant pneumococci. In patients with preliminary culture results indicating gram-positive infection, empirical vancomycin is appropriate while the susceptibility results are pending. Lastly, empirical use of vancomycin may be recommended in patients with hypotension or other evidence of cardiovascular impairment or sepsis without an identified pathogen.[1,5,35,36] If empirical vancomycin therapy is initiated and no evidence of gram-positive infection is found after 48 to 72 hours, the drug should be discontinued.[1,4,5] Continuing vancomycin when not warranted results in higher costs, more toxicities, and greater risk of development of VRE.[1,5]

Other antimicrobial agents, such as quinupristin–dalfopristin, linezolid, daptomycin, telavancin, and ceftaroline, should be reserved for documented infections caused by multiresistant gram-positive pathogens that are not susceptible to, or are unresponsive to, vancomycin. The role of these drugs in the routine treatment of fever in neutropenic patients is undetermined, and linezolid is associated with myelosuppression.[1,5]

Oral Antibiotic Therapy for Management of Febrile Neutropenia

An individual patient's risk for complications of severe infection determines appropriate antibiotic therapy and the proper setting for administration (see Table 100-3).[1,4,5] Risk stratification is based on several parameters (e.g., MASCC score as mentioned above) as well as response to empirical antimicrobial therapy if IV therapy is initially given.[1] Because of the excellent spectrum of activity and favorable pharmacokinetics of currently available oral antibiotics, particularly the fluoroquinolones, oral antibiotics have an important role in the management of selected patients. In patients at low risk for severe or complicated bacterial infection, empirical therapy with broad-spectrum oral antibiotic agents achieves similar patient outcomes as parenteral antibiotics, with response rates of 77% to 95%.[1,4,12,28–30] This has made possible the treatment of febrile neutropenia in low-risk patients in the outpatient setting. Patients judged to be low risk with reliable follow-up may be appropriate candidates for oral antibiotic therapy administered on an outpatient basis.[1,4,12,28–30] Ciprofloxacin in combination with amoxicillin–clavulanate (or clindamycin for penicillin-allergic patients) for enhanced gram-positive coverage has been most commonly studied for outpatient therapy in low-risk patients and is recommended by IDSA and NCCN guidelines.[1,5] In general, monotherapy with ciprofloxacin should be avoided due to relatively poor gram-positive activity. Levofloxacin has been used as monotherapy for outpatient treatment of low-risk patients, due to enhanced gram-positive activity; however, this regimen has not been well studied and is not formally recommended by IDSA or NCCN guidelines. If used, only the higher-dose levofloxacin 750 mg regimen should be administered in order to provide adequate activity against organisms such as *P. aeruginosa*.[1,5] Careful patient selection obviously is required for such management strategies. Important criteria include patient and provider comfort, a history of medication compliance, good caregiver support, a follow-up plan, and close proximity, prompt access and transportation to appropriate medical care around the clock in the event of failure to respond to outpatient antibiotic therapy. If a patient qualifies for oral therapy based on social and clinical status, the first dose of oral regimen should be given and the patient observed for 4 to 24 hours to ensure tolerance and the patient remains clinically stable. Benefits of oral therapy on an outpatient basis include increased convenience and quality of life for patients and caregivers and reduced exposure to multidrug-resistant institutional pathogens.[1,5] Outpatient therapy of low-risk patients now is common practice in most institutions.

In patients at low risk for severe bacterial infection who were initiated on IV antibiotics, oral antibiotics may play a role in step-down therapy. Carefully selected neutropenic patients may be safely switched from broad-spectrum parenteral therapy to oral antibiotic regimens (e.g., ciprofloxacin plus amoxicillin–clavulanate) with response rates comparable to patients remaining on IV therapy.[12,28–30] Patient selection criteria generally include defervescence within 72 hours of initiation of parenteral therapy, hemodynamic stability, absence of positive cultures or a discernible site of infection, and ability to take oral medications. Many of these patients are able to complete their course of therapy at home.[1,5,12,28–30] Changing parenteral antimicrobials to oral regimens in carefully selected patients is now relatively common practice and allows for less expensive hospitalizations and earlier patient discharges.

Antimicrobial Therapy After Initiation of Empirical Therapy

6 After initiation of empirical antimicrobial therapy (Table 100-4), judicious assessment of febrile neutropenic cancer patients is mandatory to evaluate response, clinical status, laboratory data, and potential need for therapy adjustments. After 2 to 4 days of empirical antimicrobial therapy, the clinical status and culture results of febrile neutropenic patients should be reevaluated to determine whether therapeutic modifications are necessary (Fig. 100-2). Modifications of antimicrobial therapy should be based on clinical and laboratory data; antibiotic therapy should be optimized based on culture results. However, during periods of neutropenia, patients generally should continue to receive broad-spectrum therapy because of risk of secondary infections or breakthrough bacteremias when antimicrobial coverage is too narrow.[1,5,12] The treatment duration for a documented infection should be appropriate for the particular organism and site, and should continue for at least the duration of neutropenia (until ANC ≥500 cells/mm^3 [≥0.5 × 10^9/L]) or longer if clinically necessary.

In patients who become afebrile after 2 to 4 days of therapy with no infection identified, it is generally optimal to continue antibiotic therapy until neutropenia has resolved (ANC ≥500 cells/mm^3 [≥0.5 × 10^9/L]). Some clinicians switch therapy to an oral regimen (e.g., ciprofloxacin plus amoxicillin–clavulanate) after 2 days of IV therapy in low-risk patients who become afebrile and have no evidence of infection. In high-risk patients, parenteral antibiotic regimens should be continued until resolution of neutropenia.[1,5] However, in afebrile patients with prolonged neutropenia but no signs or symptoms of infection, consideration can be given to discontinuing antibiotic therapy or switching to fluoroquinolone prophylaxis (discussed in "Prophylaxis of Infections in Neutropenic Cancer Patients" below), provided that patients can be observed carefully and have ready access to medical care.

The optimal management of patients who remain febrile in the absence of microbiologic or clinical documentation of infection remains highly controversial. Persistently febrile patients should be evaluated carefully, but modifications generally are not made to initial antimicrobial regimens within the first 2 to 4 days of therapy unless there is evidence of clinical deterioration (see Fig. 100-1).[1,4,5] It is important to note that the persistence of fever does not necessarily mean failure of a given antimicrobial regimen; up to 25% of neutropenic patients have fever due to noninfectious causes.[8] This is particularly true if patients are otherwise clinically stable. Fever after 2 or more days of antibiotic therapy can be due to a number of causes, including nonbacterial infection, resistant bacterial infection or infection slow to respond to therapy, emergence of a secondary infection, inadequate drug concentrations, drug fever, fever at an avascular site (e.g., catheter infection or abscess), or noninfectious causes such as tumor or administration of blood products.[1,4,5,12] Patients with documented infection who are receiving appropriate antimicrobial therapy (based on in vitro susceptibility tests) often remain febrile until resolution of neutropenia occurs. Therefore, the same antibiotic regimen can be continued in patients who remain febrile despite 2 to 4 days of antibiotic therapy but are otherwise clinically stable, especially if neutropenia is expected to resolve within 1 week. However, antibiotic regimens may require modification in patients experiencing toxicities (Table 100-5) as well as in patients with evidence of progressive disease, clinical instability, or documentation of an organism not covered by the initial regimen.[1,3,4,5,12] If not already part of the regimen, vancomycin should be considered as warranted by clinical and laboratory findings. However, if vancomycin was included in the initial empirical regimen and the patient is still febrile after 2 to 3 days of therapy without isolating a gram-positive pathogen, discontinuation of vancomycin should be considered to reduce the risk of toxicities or resistance.[1,5]

Initiation of Antifungal Therapy

Neutropenic patients who remain febrile despite more than 4 to 7 days of broad-spectrum antibiotic therapy are candidates for antifungal therapy. A high percentage of febrile patients who die during prolonged neutropenia have evidence of invasive fungal infection on autopsy, even though many had no evidence of fungal disease before death.[26] Persistence of fever or development of a new fever during broad-spectrum antibiotic therapy may indicate the presence of a fungal infection, most commonly due to *Candida* or *Aspergillus* spp.[12,22] Blood cultures are positive in fewer than 50% of neutropenic patients with invasive fungal infections.[12,25] Sensitivity and specificity of fungal galactomannan assay may vary and should only be used when *Aspergillus* is suspected. Rapid, sensitive diagnostic tests for fungi such as serum β-D-glucan or fungal DNA assay are not yet in common usage, and waiting for isolation of fungal organisms is associated with high morbidity and mortality. The empirical addition of antifungal therapy is thus justified in this clinical setting.[1,12,25] Therefore, empirical antifungal therapy should be initiated after 4 to 7 days of broad-spectrum antibiotic therapy in persistently febrile patients if the duration of neutropenia is expected to be >1 week. Administered doses must be adequate to treat undiagnosed fungal infection and prevent fungal superinfection in high-risk febrile neutropenic patients.[1,5,23]

Evidence-based recommendations from published guidelines for management of suspected or documented fungal infections in neutropenic patients are summarized in Table 100-2.[23,27] Empirical coverage for both *Candida* spp. and *Aspergillus* should be considered because these organisms are responsible for more than 90% of fungal infections in neutropenic cancer patients.[6,22] *Aspergillus* is particularly common in patients with hematologic malignancies and in patients with hematologic malignancies undergoing HSCT; therefore, amphotericin B traditionally has been preferred for these patients.[1,5,12,37] In the setting of febrile neutropenia, lipid-associated amphotericin B (LAMB) products are similar in efficacy to conventional amphotericin B while causing fewer toxicities. LAMB products are thus almost exclusively recommended over conventional amphotericin B despite the significantly higher cost without clear improvement in efficacy.[1,5,23,27,37,38] Although the use of higher doses of LAMB has been advocated in an effort to improve efficacy, one

TABLE 100-4 Drug Dosing Table[a]

Drug	Brand Name	Initial Dose	Usual Range	Special Population Dose	Other
Antibacterial Agents					
Amoxicillin–clavulanate	Augmentin®	875 mg orally two times daily	875 mg orally two times daily		In combination with ciprofloxacin for outpatient treatment
Ceftazidime	Fortaz®	2 g IV every 8 hours	1–2 g IV every 8 hours		
Cefepime	Maxipime®	2 g IV every 12 hours	1–2 g IV every 12 hours		
Piperacillin–tazobactam	Zosyn®	4.5 g IV every 6 hours	3.375–4.5 g IV every 6 hours		
Imipenem–cilastatin	Primaxin®	500 mg IV every 6 hours	250–500 mg IV every 6 hours		
Meropenem	Merrem®	1 g IV every 8 hours	1 g IV every 8 hours		
Doripenem	Doribax®	500 mg IV every 8 hours	500 mg IV every 8 hours		
Tobramycin	Nebcin®	Traditional: 2 mg/kg loading dose, followed by 1.5 mg/kg IV every 8 hours. Alternative: 5–7 mg/kg IV once daily	Traditional dosing: Guided by measured serum concentrations		
Gentamicin	Garamycin®	Traditional: 2 mg/kg loading dose, followed by 1.5 mg/kg IV every 8 hours. Alternative: 5–7 mg/kg IV once daily	Traditional dosing: Guided by measured serum concentrations		
Ciprofloxacin	Cipro®	400 mg IV every 8 hours	400 mg IV every 8–12 hours	Outpatient treatment: 500 mg orally every 8 hours	May be given orally in low-risk patients
Levofloxacin	Levaquin®	750 mg IV once daily	500–750 mg IV once daily		May be given orally in low-risk patients
Vancomycin	Vancocin®	30–40 mg/kg/day IV in two divided doses	Dosing guided by serum concentrations to achieve trough of 15–20 mg/L		For methicillin-resistant *S. aureus* infection
Nafcillin	Nafcil®	2 g IV every 6 hours	1–2 g IV every 4–6 hours		For methicillin-susceptible *S. aureus* infection
Linezolid	Zyvox®	600 mg IV or orally every 12 hours	600 mg IV or orally every 12 hours		For infection due to vancomycin-resistant enterococci
Ampicillin	Omnipen®, Polycillin®, Principen®	2 g IV every 6 hours	1–2 g IV every 4–6 hours		In combination with gentamicin for *Listeria* infection
Erythromycin	E-mycin®, Erythrocin®	1 g IV every 6 hours	1–2 g IV every 4–6 hours		For *Legionella* infection
Antifungal Agents					
Clotrimazole	Mycelex Troche®	10 mg orally five times daily	10 mg orally five times daily		Administered as oral troche; dissolve in mouth
Nystatin	Nystatin Oral®	100,000 units orally every 6 hours	100,000 units orally every 4–6 hours		Administered as suspension; swish and swallow
Fluconazole	Diflucan®	800 mg IV or orally once, then 400 mg IV or orally once daily	100–800 mg IV or orally once daily	Prophylaxis of *Candida* infection: 400 mg IV or orally once daily	
Itraconazole	Sporanox®	200 mg orally twice daily	200–400 mg/day orally divided twice daily	Prophylaxis of *Candida* infection: 200 mg orally twice daily	
Voriconazole	Vfend®	6 mg/kg IV every 12 hours for two doses, then 4 mg/kg IV every 12 hours	4 mg/kg IV or 200 mg orally every 12 hours	Prophylaxis in high-risk patients: 200 mg orally twice daily	
Posaconazole	Noxafil®	400 mg orally two times daily	400 mg orally two times daily	Prophylaxis in high-risk patients: 200 mg orally three times daily	Administer with full meal or enteral nutritional supplements
Lipid-associated amphotericin B (LAMB)	AmBisome®, Abelcet®	3–5 mg/kg IV once daily	3–5 mg/kg IV once daily	Prophylaxis in high-risk patients: 1 mg/kg IV once daily	
5-Flucytosine	Ancobon®	25 mg/kg/day orally four times daily	25 mg/kg/day orally four times daily		In combination with LAMB for cryptococcal meningitis
Caspofungin	Cancidas®	70 mg IV once, then 50 mg IV once daily	50 mg IV once daily		

(continued)

TABLE 100-4 Drug Dosing Table[a] (*Continued*)

Drug	Brand Name	Initial Dose	Usual Range	Special Population Dose	Other
Micafungin	Mycamine®	100 mg IV once daily	100 mg IV once daily	Prophylaxis in high-risk patients: 50 mg IV once daily	
Anidulafungin	Eraxis®	200 mg IV once, then 100 mg IV once daily	100 mg IV once daily		
Antiviral Agents					
Acyclovir	Zovirax®	5 mg/kg IV every 8 hours, or 800 mg orally five times daily	5–10 mg/kg IV every 8 hours, or 800 mg orally two to five times daily	Prophylaxis of HSV or VZV: 800–1600 mg orally twice daily; CMV prophylaxis in allogeneic HSCT: 800 mg orally four times daily	
Valacyclovir	Valtrex®	1 g orally three times daily	1 g orally three times daily	Prophylaxis of HSV or VZV: 500 mg orally two or three times daily; CMV prophylaxis in allogeneic HSCT: 2 g orally four times daily	
Ganciclovir	Cytovene®	CMV treatment or preemptive therapy: 5 mg/kg IV daily for 2 weeks	CMV treatment or preemptive therapy: After first 2 weeks, 5–6 mg/kg IV daily 5 days/wk	CMV prophylaxis: 5–6 mg/kg IV daily 5 days/wk	
Valganciclovir	Valcyte®	CMV preemptive therapy: 900 mg orally twice daily for 2 weeks	CMV preemptive therapy: After first 2 weeks, 900 mg orally daily	CMV prophylaxis: 900 mg orally daily	
Foscarnet	Foscavir®	CMV treatment: 90 mg/kg IV every 12 hours for 2 weeks; CMV preemptive therapy: 60 mg/kg IV every 12 hours for 2 weeks	CMV treatment: after first 2 weeks, 120 mg/kg IV daily; CMV preemptive therapy: after first 2 weeks, 90 mg/kg IV daily 5 days/wk	CMV prophylaxis: 60 mg/kg IV two or three times daily for 7 days, then 90–120 mg/kg IV daily	
CMV hyperimmune globulin	Cytogam®	400 mg/kg IV every other day for three to five doses	400 mg/kg IV every other day for three to five doses		Recommended in combination with ganciclovir or foscarnet for treatment of CMV pneumonia
Antiprotozoal/Antiparasitic Agents					
Trimethoprim–sulfamethoxazole	Bactrim®, Cotrimoxazole®	15–20 mg/kg/day IV divided every 6 hours[b]	15–20 mg/kg/day IV divided every 6 hours[b]	Prophylaxis of *P. jirovecii*: 160 mg/800 mg orally three times weekly	
Atovaquone	Mepron®	750 mg orally every 12 hours	750 mg orally every 12 hours		
Pentamidine	Pentam®	4 mg/kg IV once daily	4 mg/kg IV once daily		
Clindamycin	Cleocin®	450–600 mg orally every 6 hours	450–600 mg orally every 6 hours		In combination with primaquine for *P. jerovicii*, or with pyrimethamine for toxoplasmosis
Primaquine	Aralen® Primaquine®	15 mg orally once daily	15 mg orally once daily		In combination with clindamycin for *P. jerovicii*
Dapsone	Dapsone®	100 mg orally once daily	100 mg orally once daily		In combination with trimethoprim for *P. jerovicii*
Trimethoprim	Triprim®	15–20 mg/kg/day orally divided every 6 hours	15–20 mg/kg/day orally divided every 6 hours		In combination with dapsone for *P. jerovicii*
Pyrimethamine	Daraprim®	50 mg orally once daily[c]	50–100 mg orally once daily[c]		In combination with sulfadiazine for toxoplasmosis
Sulfadiazine	Sulfadiazine®	1 g orally every 6 hours	1 g orally every 4–6 hours		In combination with pyrimethamine for toxoplasmosis
Thiabendazole	Mintezol®	25 mg/kg orally every 12 hours	25 mg/kg orally every 12 hours (maximum 3 g/day)		For *Strongyloides* and other intestinal worm infections

CMV, cytomegalovirus; HSV, herpes simplex virus; VZV, varicella zoster virus.

[a]Dosing guidelines in patients with normal renal and hepatic function.
[b]Based on the trimethoprim component of the combination.
[c]Folinic acid (5–10 mg/day) often recommended in conjunction with pyrimethamine-containing regimens for prevention of bone marrow toxicity.

TABLE 100-5 Drug Monitoring of Selected Antimicrobials for Febrile Neutropenia, HSCT, and SOT

Drug	Adverse Reaction	Monitoring Parameters	Comments
Antibaterial Agents			
Aminoglycosides (Tobramycin, Gentamicin)	Nephrotoxicity	Serum creatinine, urine output, serum concentrations	Extended-interval ("once daily") dosing potentially associated with less renal toxicity, similar efficacy to traditional dosing. Goal trough concentration <1 mcg/mL (mg/L) during extended-interval dosing
Imipenem–cilastatin	CNS toxicities, seizure	Serum creatinine, mental status, CNS function	Increased incidence with higher dose, failure to adjust dose/interval for reduced renal function. Increased risk compared to meropenem or doripenem
Linezolid	Myelosuppression, thrombocytopenia, optic/peripheral neuropathy, serotonin syndrome	CBC, vision changes, serum lactate, heart rate, blood pressure, temperature, myoclonus	Myelosuppression and neuropathy more common with prolonged use. Short course unlikely to affect marrow recovery in HSCT. Weak MAO inhibitor, serotonin syndrome possible with other serotonergic drugs such as SSRIs and SNRIs
Nafcillin	Interstitial nephritis	Serum creatinine, urine output	Reversible, requires switch to alternative β-lactam
Vancomycin	Nephrotoxicity, infusion reactions	Serum creatinine, urine output, blood pressure, heart rate, serum concentrations	Dose adjustment required for renal dysfunction. Pretreatment and slow infusion may decrease incidence of infusion reaction. Goal trough concentration 15–20 mcg/mL (mg/L; 10–14 μmol/L) for serious infections
Antifungal Agents			
Amphotericin B (lipid-associated)	Nephrotoxicity, hepatotoxicity, electrolyte disturbances, infusion reactions	Serum creatinine, electrolytes, LFTs, blood pressure, heart rate	Liposomal preparations associated with less renal toxicity, similar efficacy to standard preparation. Electrolyte disturbances occur before creatinine alterations. Pretreatment and slow infusion may decrease incidence of infusion reaction
5-Flucytosine	Myelosuppression, GI toxicities	CBC, GI symptoms, serum creatinine, 5-flucytosine serum concentrations	Dose adjustment required for renal dysfunction. Goal serum concentrations are peak <100 mcg/mL (mg/L; <775 μmol/L) and trough 10–50 mcg/mL (mg/L; 77–387 μmol/L)
Posaconazole	Hepatotoxicity, rash; interactions with CYP450 3A4	LTs, skin	Multiple interactions with drugs metabolized by CYP 3A4, including immunosuppressants; close monitoring needed. Poor absorption may warrant serum concentration monitoring if available, goals of >0.7 mcg/mL (mg/L; >1.0 μmol/L) for treatment and >0.5 mcg/mL for (mg/L; >0.7 μmol/L) prophylaxis
Voriconazole	Mental status changes, headache, hallucinations, visual disturbances, hepatotoxicity, QTc prolongation; interactions with CYP450 2C9, 2C19, and 3A4	Mental status, visual function, LFTs, ECG, voriconazole serum concentrations	Mental status/visual changes associated with elevated troughs >5.5 mcg/mL (mg/L; >16 μmol/L); goal trough >1 mcg/mL (mg/L; >3 μmol/L) for treatment and >0.5 mcg/mL (mg/L; >1.4 μmol/L) for prophylaxis. Parenteral formulation contains SBECD, not recommended for patients with CrCL<50 mL/min (<0.83 mL/s). Multiple interactions with drugs metabolized by CYP enzymes, including immunosuppressants; close monitoring needed
Antiviral Agents			
Foscarnet	Nephrotoxicity, hypocalcemia	Serum creatinine, electrolytes	IV hydration prior to administration. Dose adjustment required for renal dysfunction
Ganciclovir, valganciclovir	Myelosuppression, thrombocytopenia	CBC, serum creatinine	Dose adjustment required for renal dysfunction
Antiprotozoal/Antiparasitic Agents			
Dapsone	Hemolytic anemia, hypersensitivity (fever, jaundice, eosinophilia), peripheral neuropathy	CBC, bilirubin, LFTs, muscle strength, G6PD testing before use	Higher incidence of hemolytic anemia in G6PD-deficient patients
Pentamidine (IV)	Nephrotoxicity, leukopenia, hypotension, QTc prolongation, pancreatitis, hypo/hyperglycemia	Serum creatinine, serum blood glucose, blood urea nitrogen, CBC, blood pressure, heart rate; ECG	Adequate hydration recommended
Primaquine	Hemolytic anemia	CBC, bilirubin, G6PD testing before use	Avoid use in G6PD-deficient patients (hemolytic anemia)
Pyrimethamine	Bone marrow suppression	CBC	Folinic acid 5–10 mg/day often used for prevention of bone marrow toxicity
Trimethoprim–sulfamethoxazole	Myelosuppression, hyperkalemia, rash	Serum creatinine, electrolytes, CBC, skin	Dose adjustment required for renal dysfunction

CBC, complete blood count; ECG, electrocardiogram; G6PD, glucose-6-phosphate dehydrogenase; HSCT; hematopoietic stem cell transplantation; LFT, liver function test; MAO, monoamine oxidase; PFT, pulmonary function test; QTc, corrected Q-T interval; SBECD, sulfobutylether-β-cyclodextrin; SOT, solid-organ transplantation; SSNRI, selective serotonin–norepinephrine reuptake inhibitor; SSRI, selective serotonin reuptake inhibitor.

study demonstrated that lower doses (3 mg/kg) of liposomal amphotericin B were as efficacious as higher doses (10 mg/kg) with lower cost and fewer toxicities.[39]

The azole compounds fluconazole, itraconazole, and voriconazole are also used in the management of febrile neutropenia.[23,27,40] Despite the increased cost and toxicities of LAMB, concerns regarding the emergence of *Candida* strains with decreased azole susceptibility and unclear efficacy advantages relative to other agents have prevented these agents from replacing amphotericin B as the gold standard in persistently febrile neutropenic patients.[25,27,37] Fluconazole has good efficacy against *C. albicans* but lacks activity against molds such as *Aspergillus*. The use of fluconazole as an alternative to amphotericin B for empirical antifungal therapy is thus perhaps most appropriate in hospitals in which infections due to *Aspergillus* or non-*albicans* strains of *Candida* are not common.[1,5,37] If fluconazole is used as antifungal prophylaxis in cancer patients, it should not be included in empirical antifungal regimens. Voriconazole is effective in the treatment of documented invasive fungal infections and is recommended as a reliable option for febrile neutropenia despite failing to meet noninferiority criteria when compared against LAMB for empiric therapy in febrile neutropenic patients.[1,5,25,37,40–42] Itraconazole has similar efficacy as amphotericin B, with fewer toxicities. However, current lack of a parenteral dosage form, sometimes erratic oral absorption that often necessitates the use of serum concentration monitoring, numerous potential drug–drug interactions, and availability of many other antifungal options limit the use of itraconazole for empiric therapy.[40–42]

The echinocandin antifungals (caspofungin, micafungin, and anidulafungin) are attractive agents for treatment of febrile neutropenia because of their broad spectrum of antifungal activity and favorable adverse effect profiles. Caspofungin is as effective as, and also generally better tolerated than, liposomal amphotericin B for empirical treatment of neutropenic patients with persistent fever.[40–42] Therefore, caspofungin is considered an appropriate alternative to LAMB and voriconazole.[1,5,23,25,27,37,41] Micafungin and anidulafungin have not been as well studied specifically in this capacity; however, some experts consider them likely as effective.[1,5,23,27]

Clinical **Controversy...**

As with antibiotic therapy, the optimal duration of antifungal therapy remains controversial. Most clinicians agree that antifungal therapy can be discontinued when neutropenia has resolved in clinically stable patients with no evidence of fungal infection. In neutropenic patients, antifungal therapy generally should be continued for at least 2 weeks in the absence of signs and symptoms of active fungal disease, but many experts advocate continuing therapy until resolution of the neutropenia.[4,12,23,37] In neutropenic patients with documented fungal disease, antifungal therapy should be directed at the causative organism, and therapy should be continued for at least 2 weeks after clinical and culture data indicate resolution of the infection.[23] In addition to fungal infections, other causes of persistent fever of unknown origin include resistant bacterial infection, tissue necrosis as a result of underlying tumor, nonbacterial and nonfungal infection (e.g., viral, mycobacterial, or parasitic), and drug or blood product administration. The persistence of fever should not be considered the sole indication for modification of antifungal regimens, assuming that an agent active against *Aspergillus* was initially selected.[25,37] Treatment recommendations for specific fungal infections are given in Table 100-6.

Initiation of Antiviral Therapy

Febrile neutropenic patients with vesicular or ulcerative skin or mucosal lesions should be evaluated carefully for infection due to HSV or varicella-zoster virus (VZV). Mucosal lesions from viral infections provide a portal of entry for bacteria and fungi during periods of immunosuppression. If viral infection is presumed or documented, neutropenic patients should receive aggressive antiviral therapy to aid healing of primary lesions and prevent disseminated disease. Acyclovir traditionally has been used in this population. However, the newer antivirals valacyclovir and famciclovir have better oral absorption and more convenient dosing schedules. Routine use of antiviral agents in the management of patients without mucosal lesions or other evidence of viral infection generally is not recommended.[1,5] Treatment recommendations for viral infections are given in Table 100-6.

Duration of Antimicrobial Therapy

7 The optimal duration of antimicrobial therapy in the neutropenic cancer patient remains controversial. Decisions regarding discontinuation of empirical antimicrobial therapy often are more difficult and complex than those regarding initiation of therapy (see Fig. 100-1). One point on which experts agree, however, is that the most important determinant of the total duration of antibiotic therapy is the patient's ANC.[1,3,5,12] If ANC is ≥500 cells/mm^3 (≥0.5 × 10^9/L) for two consecutive days, if the patient is afebrile and clinically stable for 48 hours or more, and if no pathogen has been isolated, then antibiotics can be discontinued. Some clinicians advocate that patients with ANC less than 500 cells/mm^3 (0.5 × 10^9/L) be maintained on antibiotic therapy until resolution of neutropenia, even if they are afebrile. However, prolonged antibiotic use has been associated with superinfections resulting from resistant bacteria and fungi and increases the risk of antibiotic-related toxicities.[1,5,12] If low-risk patients are stable clinically with negative cultures but the ANC still is less than 500 cells/mm^3 (0.5 × 10^9/L) antibiotics may be discontinued after a total of 5 to 7 afebrile days. However, patients with profound neutropenia (ANC <100 cells/mm^3 [<0.1 × 10^9/L]), mucosal lesions, or unstable vital signs or other risk factors should continue to receive antibiotics until ANC has increased ≥500 cells/mm^3 (≥0.5 × 10^9/L) and the patient is stable clinically.[1,5,12]

Patients who are persistently neutropenic and febrile, but who are stable clinically with no active site of infection, often can be successfully discontinued from antimicrobials after at least 2 weeks of therapy. However, these patients must be monitored carefully because reinstitution of antibiotics may be necessary.[1,5,12] An alternative approach is to place these patients on antimicrobial prophylaxis (discussed in "Prophylaxis of Infections in Neutropenic Cancer Patients" below). Patients with documented infections should receive antimicrobial therapy until the infecting organism is eradicated and signs and symptoms of infection have resolved (at least 10 to 14 days of therapy).

Consensus guidelines provide useful information regarding the management of febrile episodes in cancer patients with neutropenia.[1,5] However, therapy (including initial empirical regimens, modifications, and duration of treatment) must be individualized based on individual patient parameters and response to therapy.

Colony-Stimulating Factors

Because resolution of neutropenia is arguably the most important determinant of patient outcome from both febrile episodes and documented infections, numerous studies have evaluated hematopoietic colony-stimulating factors (CSFs) (sargramostim [granulocyte-macrophage colony-stimulating factor] and filgrastim [granulocyte colony-stimulating factor]) as adjunct therapy to antimicrobial treatment of febrile neutropenic cancer patients.[43] These studies consistently found that use of CSFs reduces the total duration and

TABLE 100-6 Infectious Complications During Neutropenia, and After Hematopoietic Stem Cell and Solid-Organ Transplantation: Syndromes of Disease and Treatment Guidelines

Pathogen	Syndromes of Disease	Recommended Treatment
Bacterial		
Gram-negative aerobic bacilli (Enterobacteriaceae, *Pseudomonas aeruginosa, Haemophilus influenzae*)	Blood, urinary tract, pulmonary, abdomen	*Empiric:* Ceftazidime + aminoglycoside,[a,b] cefepime + aminoglycoside[a,b]; piperacillin–tazobactam; imipenem-cilastatin ± aminoglycoside[a,b] *Definitive:* According to culture and sensitivity results
Gram-positive cocci (*Staphylococcus aureus, Staphylococcus epidermidis, Streptococcus pneumoniae, Enterococcus faecalis*)	Skin, blood, urinary tract, pulmonary, abdomen	*Empiric:* Nafcillin; vancomycin *Definitive:* According to culture and sensitivity results
Legionella spp.	Pulmonary	Erythromycin; ciprofloxacin; levofloxacin
Listeria monocytogenes	CNS	Ampicillin with gentamicin[a]; trimethoprim–sulfamethoxazole
Nocardia spp.	Skin, pulmonary, CNS	Sulfadiazine; trimethoprim–sulfamethoxazole
Fungal		
Candida spp.[c]	Blood, urinary tract, mucous membranes, skin, disseminated disease	Clotrimazole; nystatin; fluconazole; itraconazole; amphotericin B ± 5-flucytosine; lipid-associated amphotericin B (LAMB); caspofungin; micafungin; anidulafungin
Aspergillus spp.[d]	Skin, pulmonary, CNS	Voriconazole; LAMB; caspofungin; micafungin; posaconazole; itraconazole
Cryptococcus neoformans	Skin, pulmonary, CNS	LAMB + 5-flucytosine; fluconazole
Zygomycetes (*Mucor*)	Rhinocerebral disease	LAMB; posaconazole
Viral		
Herpes simplex virus	Skin, CNS, mucous membranes, pulmonary	Acyclovir; foscarnet
Human herpesvirus-6	CNS, hepatic, bone marrow	Ganciclovir; foscarnet
Cytomegalovirus	Pulmonary, blood, urinary tract, GI tract	Ganciclovir; foscarnet; hyperimmune globulins
Varicella-zoster virus	Skin, disseminated disease	Acyclovir; foscarnet
Epstein–Barr virus	Lymphoproliferative disease	No effective treatment
Papovaviruses (BK, JC)	Skin, CNS	No effective treatment
Protozoal/Parasitic		
Pneumocystis jiroveci	Pulmonary	Trimethoprim–sulfamethoxazole; atovaquone; pentamidine; dapsone + trimethoprim; clindamycin + primaquine
Toxoplasma gondii	CNS	Pyrimethamine + sulfadiazine; pyrimethamine + clindamycin
Strongyloides stercoralis	Pulmonary, CNS	Thiabendazole

[a]Choice of specific agent determined according to institutional susceptibilities to individual drugs.
[b]For penicillin-allergic adults, use aztreonam or ciprofloxacin + an aminoglycoside.
[c]Refer to the Clinical Practice Guidelines of the Infectious Diseases Society of America (*reference 23*) for selection and dosing of antifungal agents for specific infections.
[d]Refer to the Clinical Practice Guidelines by the Infectious Diseases Society of America (*reference 27*) for selection and dosing of antifungal agents for specific infections.

severity of chemotherapy-related neutropenia; some studies have also shown fewer hospitalizations and decreased hospital length of stay.[1,5,43,44] However, these studies have failed to demonstrate consistent benefits of CSFs compared with placebo in relation to important outcomes such as decreased overall mortality or infection-related mortality.[5,44] Evidence-based guidelines from the IDSA, American Society of Clinical Oncology (ASCO), and the NCCN recommend that CSFs should not be routinely initiated in patients with uncomplicated fever and neutropenia.[1,5,43,44] However, CSFs should be considered in patients who are at high risk for infection-associated complications, or who have factors that are predictive of poor clinical outcomes.[5,43,44] These factors are summarized in Table 100-7. Patients with prolonged neutropenia and documented severe infections who are not responding to appropriate antimicrobial therapy may also benefit from treatment with CSFs.[43,44] Clinical judgment must be exercised in determining which patients may benefit from judicious use of these expensive agents.

Direct transfusion of neutrophils has also been studied for treatment of febrile neutropenia or documented infections.[45,46] Routine use of neutrophil transfusions is not generally supported by data demonstrating improved clinical outcomes. However, use may be considered in patients with profound prolonged neutropenia with severe documented infections and in whom causative organisms have not been eradicated with appropriate antimicrobial therapy in combination with CSFs.[1,5,45] At present, the use of neutrophil transfusions is considered investigational and is not recommended for routine management of febrile neutropenic patients.[45]

Prophylaxis of Infections in Neutropenic Cancer Patients

8 Owing to the potential morbidity and mortality of infections in neutropenic cancer patients, environmental modifications and prophylactic antimicrobial regimens have been implemented to prevent these complications. The overall goal of antimicrobial prophylaxis in cancer patients is to decrease the number and severity of systemic infections during prolonged periods of neutropenia. As with febrile neutropenia, patient risk factors for development of infection and complications should be assessed prior to initiation of prophylaxis (Table 100-8).

General Measures

Because approximately 50% of pathogens infecting neutropenic cancer patients are acquired in the hospital, reducing acquisition of infectious organisms from the environment is a basic component in controlling nosocomial infections.[1,2,5,6,12] Neutropenic patients

TABLE 100-7 Recommendations for Use of Colony-Stimulating Factors in the Management of Neutropenic Cancer Patients and Those Undergoing Hematopoietic Stem Cell Transplantation

A. Primary prophylaxis of febrile neutropenia
1. Colony-stimulating factors (CSFs) (filgrastim, pegfilgrastim, or sargramostim) may be considered in patients who have a high risk of FN (>20% incidence) based on myelotoxicity of the planned chemotherapy regimen
2. When risk of febrile neutropenia is 10–20%, CSFs may be considered in the presence of certain patient and clinical factors predisposing to increased complications from prolonged neutropenia, including: patient age >65 years; poor performance status; extensive prior treatment including large radiation ports; administration of combined chemoradiotherapy; cytopenias due to bone marrow involvement by tumor; poor nutritional status; presence of open wounds or active infections; previous surgery; poor renal function; liver dysfunction, particularly when evidenced by increased bilirubin; and lack of antibiotic prophylaxis

B. Secondary prophylaxis of febrile neutropenia
1. CSFs (filgrastim, pegfilgrastim, or sargramostim) recommended for patients who experienced neutropenic complications from prior cycles of chemotherapy, and in which a reduced dose may compromise disease-free or overall survival or treatment outcome

C. Therapeutic use in febrile neutropenia
1. CSFs should not be routinely used for patients with neutropenia who are afebrile
2. CSFs (filgrastim or sargramostim only) may be considered in patients with febrile neutropenia who are at high risk for infection-associated complications, or who have prognostic factors that are predictive of poor clinical outcomes, including: profound neutropenia (absolute neutrophil count <100 cells/mm^3 [<0.1 × 10^9/L]); expected prolonged period of neutropenia (>10 days); patient age >65 years; uncontrolled primary disease; sepsis syndrome, or severe infection manifest by hypotension and multiorgan dysfunction; pneumonia; invasive fungal infection; other clinically documented infection; hospitalized at the time of the development of fever; or severe complications during previous episode of febrile neutropenia

D. Reduction in duration of neutropenia in HSCT
1. CSFs are recommended to mobilize peripheral-blood progenitor cells (PBPC) prior to chemotherapy and to reduce the duration of neutropenia after autologous PBPC transplantation

Data from references 43, 44, and 49.

should be placed in reverse isolation (isolation to protect patients from contracting infections after exposure to others) with standard barrier precautions, and strict adherence to infection control guidelines by hospital personnel.[1,5,6,12] Plants and fresh or dried flowers are usually prohibited as part of standard neutropenic precautions in order to minimize risk of exposure to pathogenic bacteria. Proper meticulous handwashing by hospital personnel is a simple yet very effective infection control measure. Most neutropenic patients do not require specific room ventilation; however, HSCT recipients should be placed in a private positive-pressure room with >12 air exchanges per hour and HEPA filtration.[1,5,6,12]

TABLE 100-8 Risk-Based Prophylactic Strategies for Patients with Neutropenia

Risk Group	Patient Characteristics	Prophylactic Strategies
High risk	*Neutropenia:* Severe (absolute neutrophil count <100/mm^3 [<0.1 × 10^9/L]) and/or prolonged (≥10 days) *Malignancy/treatment:* Hematologic malignancy (acute leukemia), allogeneic HSCT, GVHD with high dose steroids, or use of alemtuzumab	Consider bacterial prophylaxis with fluoroquinolone for duration of neutropenia. Give fungal prophylaxis with product and duration based on patient-specific factors. Consider viral prophylaxis with product and duration based on patient-specific factors
Moderate risk	*Neutropenia:* Moderate duration (7–10 days) *Malignancy/treatment:* Autologous HSCT, multiple myeloma, lymphoma, chronic lymphocytic leukemia, purine analog therapy	Consider bacterial prophylaxis with fluoroquinolone for duration of neutropenia. Consider fungal prophylaxis with product and duration based on patient-specific factors. Give/consider viral prophylaxis with product and duration based on patient-specific factors
Low risk	*Neutropenia:* Short duration (≤7 days) *Malignancy/treatment:* Solid tumor treated with conventional chemotherapy	Antibacterial and antifungal prophylaxis not indicated. Viral prophylaxis considered during neutropenia if patient has prior HSV episode

GVHD, graft versus host disease; HSCT, hematopoietic stem cell transplant; HSV, herpes simplex virus.

Data from references 1, 4, 5, 12, and 28–30.

Bacterial Infections

Combinations of oral nonabsorbable antibiotics, such as gentamicin, nystatin, vancomycin, polymyxin B, and colistin, have been widely studied as a means of reducing colonization of the GI tract with virulent pathogens. Although clinical trials have demonstrated that selective intestinal decontamination with oral nonabsorbable antibiotics successfully reduces infections, these regimens are not routinely recommended for prophylaxis because of problems that include unpalatability, high cost, frequent adverse effects (e.g., nausea, vomiting, and diarrhea), and development of resistance.[1,2,4–6,12]

Many prospective clinical trials have shown that prophylaxis with orally administered, systemically available antibiotics such as trimethoprim–sulfamethoxazole and fluoroquinolones is more effective and better tolerated than nonabsorbable antibiotics.[1,5] Although trimethoprim–sulfamethoxazole is effective as prophylaxis against *P. jiroveci*, its lack of activity against *P. aeruginosa* is worrisome when used as prophylaxis against bacterial infection, particularly in institutions where pseudomonal infections are frequent.[1] Other concerns with trimethoprim–sulfamethoxazole prophylaxis include selection of resistant organisms, predisposition to development of oral fungal infections, and delay in bone marrow recovery resulting in prolonged neutropenic episodes.[1,5,6]

Numerous studies have shown that oral fluoroquinolones are more effective than placebo, nonabsorbable antibiotics, or trimethoprim–sulfamethoxazole in preventing gram-negative infections in neutropenic cancer patients.[47,48] Fluoroquinolone prophylaxis during periods of neutropenia decreases the incidence of fever and microbiologically documented gram-negative infections and may decrease the risk of death in these patients.[47,48] However, there are several potential limitations to their use. In particular, ciprofloxacin may lack adequate gram-positive activity and may not be the preferred fluoroquinolone for this reason. Although fluoroquinolone prophylaxis has been associated with the development of resistant gram-negative organisms, two meta-analysis reports suggest that the risk of infection with resistant pathogens is not significantly increased.[47,48] Also the risk of colonization or infection with strains resistant to the prophylactic agent is lower with fluoroquinolones than with trimethoprim–sulfamethoxazole. However, patients experiencing breakthrough infection during fluoroquinolone prophylaxis should not be subsequently placed on a fluoroquinolone-containing empirical antibiotic regimen.[1,5]

Although studies have concluded that the benefits of prophylaxis with fluoroquinolones outweigh the potential risks in neutropenic patients with intermediate to high risk for infection (Table 100-8), antibacterial prophylaxis in general remains somewhat controversial due to continued concerns regarding the potential for development of resistant bacteria, high cost, and lack of impact on patient survival.[1,2,5] Therefore, antibacterial prophylaxis is not recommended routinely for all neutropenic patients. Prophylaxis with ciprofloxacin or levofloxacin generally is indicated for intermediate- to high-risk patients expected to be profoundly neutropenic for more than 1 week, such as HSCT patients.[1,5,6] High dose levofloxacin may be preferred by some clinicians due to enhanced gram-positive activity, but many other clinicians consider them similar in efficacy. If fluoroquinolone prophylaxis is used, strategic monitoring of gram-negative resistance to the drugs should be employed. Neutrophil recovery eliminates the need for continued prophylaxis, and recovery may be facilitated by use of CSFs.[43] CSFs have also been formally recommended by the ASCO and the European Organisation for Research and Treatment of Cancer (EORTC) for primary prevention of febrile neutropenia in high-risk patients (see Table 100-7).[43,49]

Fungal Infections

Because neutropenic patients are at risk for mucocutaneous and invasive fungal infections that are difficult to diagnose and treat in this population, antifungal prophylaxis can be considered in intermediate- to high-risk patients at institutions where fungal infections in cancer patients occur frequently.[1,5] The goal of antifungal prophylaxis is to prevent development of invasive fungal infections during periods of risk, thereby reducing morbidity and mortality. A meta-analysis of antifungal prophylaxis in 38 trials involving more than 7,000 cancer patients reported a decrease in the use of parenteral antifungal therapy, superficial and invasive systemic fungal infections, and fungal infection-related mortality rate.[50] Antifungal prophylaxis in these studies resulted in decreased mortality in patients with prolonged neutropenia and HSCT but no effect on rates of invasive *Aspergillus* infections.

Although the choice of antifungal prophylaxis agents remains controversial, fluconazole prophylaxis has been particularly well studied and reduces the incidence of both superficial and systemic fungal infections; it also significantly decreases mortality from fungal infections in patients with leukemia and HSCT recipients.[5,50] However, use of fluconazole prophylaxis has contributed to the emergence of infections caused by *C. krusei* and *C. glabrata*, pathogens that frequently are resistant to fluconazole and other azole-type antifungal agents.[5,26] Therefore, antifungal prophylaxis with oral fluconazole, itraconazole, posaconazole, caspofungin, or micafungin is now recommended starting with induction chemotherapy.[23] The choice of a specific agent should be determined by the types of fungal isolates at individual institutions.[1,5,23] Patients in whom prophylaxis should be considered include those at intermediate to high infection risk as shown in Table 100-8. After initiation, antifungal prophylaxis should be continued until resolution of neutropenia or the need for institution of antifungal therapy for suspected/documented infection.[23]

Itraconazole, low to moderate doses of amphotericin B, intranasal and aerosolized amphotericin B, LAMB products, voriconazole, and the echinocandin agents have been investigated for *Aspergillus* prophylaxis in neutropenic patients.[6,27,51] Posaconazole was more effective than either fluconazole or itraconazole in the prevention of *Aspergillus* and other invasive fungal infections in patients with hematologic malignancies and prolonged neutropenia.[5,27,51] However, outside of the HSCT setting, posaconazole is currently only recommended for routine prevention of *Aspergillus* infections in neutropenic patients with hematologic malignancies.[27]

Other Infections

Use of trimethoprim–sulfamethoxazole in cancer patients at risk for *P. jiroveci* pneumonia has substantially reduced the incidence of this protozoal infection.[1,5] Antiviral prophylaxis with acyclovir, valacyclovir, or famciclovir is used in most centers to reduce the risk of HSV reactivation in patients with acute leukemia undergoing intensive chemotherapy. Varicella vaccine provides good protection (90%) in leukemic children and may be useful in seronegative adults, although the vaccine has been less well studied in this population.

When considering use of antimicrobial (antibacterial, antifungal, antiprotozoal, and antiviral) prophylaxis in neutropenic patients with cancer, the risks and benefits of prophylaxis must be weighed against issues with development of resistance, toxicities, and other concerns.

Evaluation of Therapeutic Outcomes

10 Close monitoring of febrile neutropenic patients, including both clinical and laboratory parameters, is essential for early detection and treatment of infectious complications. Three general therapeutic outcomes have been defined in the setting of febrile neutropenia: (a) success (survival during the febrile episode until resolution of neutropenia by judicious selection of empirical antimicrobial therapy), (b) success with modification (same as [a] but with additions/modifications to empirical therapy), and (c) failure (death during febrile neutropenia).[13] Because many of the drugs that can be used in this setting (e.g., aminoglycosides and amphotericin B) have significant toxicity potential, careful attention must be paid to prevention and management of drug-related adverse effects. Evaluations of the parameters given in the Clinical Presentation are appropriate to help monitor and guide therapy. In addition, the NCCN guidelines for febrile neutropenia provide comprehensive recommendations on clinical/laboratory monitoring parameters, including schedules.[5] The reader is referred to individual chapters within this book for more detailed discussions of monitoring parameters related to specific types of infections (e.g., pneumonia and urinary tract infections).

INFECTIONS IN PATIENTS UNDERGOING HSCT

1 Infection remains a major barrier to successful HSCT.[52,53] Recipients of HSCT are at enhanced risk for infection because of prolonged periods of neutropenia. In addition, patients receiving allogeneic or matched unrelated donor transplants receive prolonged immunosuppressive drug therapy for prevention and treatment of graft-versus-host disease (GVHD). Intensive pretransplant conditioning regimens (high-dose chemotherapy and total-body irradiation), as well as GVHD itself, often disrupt protective barriers, such as mucous membranes, skin, and the GI tract, placing patients at further risk of infection. Although infectious complications are still associated with considerable morbidity and mortality, studies have documented significant reduction in mortality after HSCT in association with reductions in disease caused by bacterial, fungal, and viral infections.[53]

Etiology and Clinical Presentation of Infections

2 10 The timing with which specific types of infections typically occur following HSCT is shown in Figure 100-3, but the relative

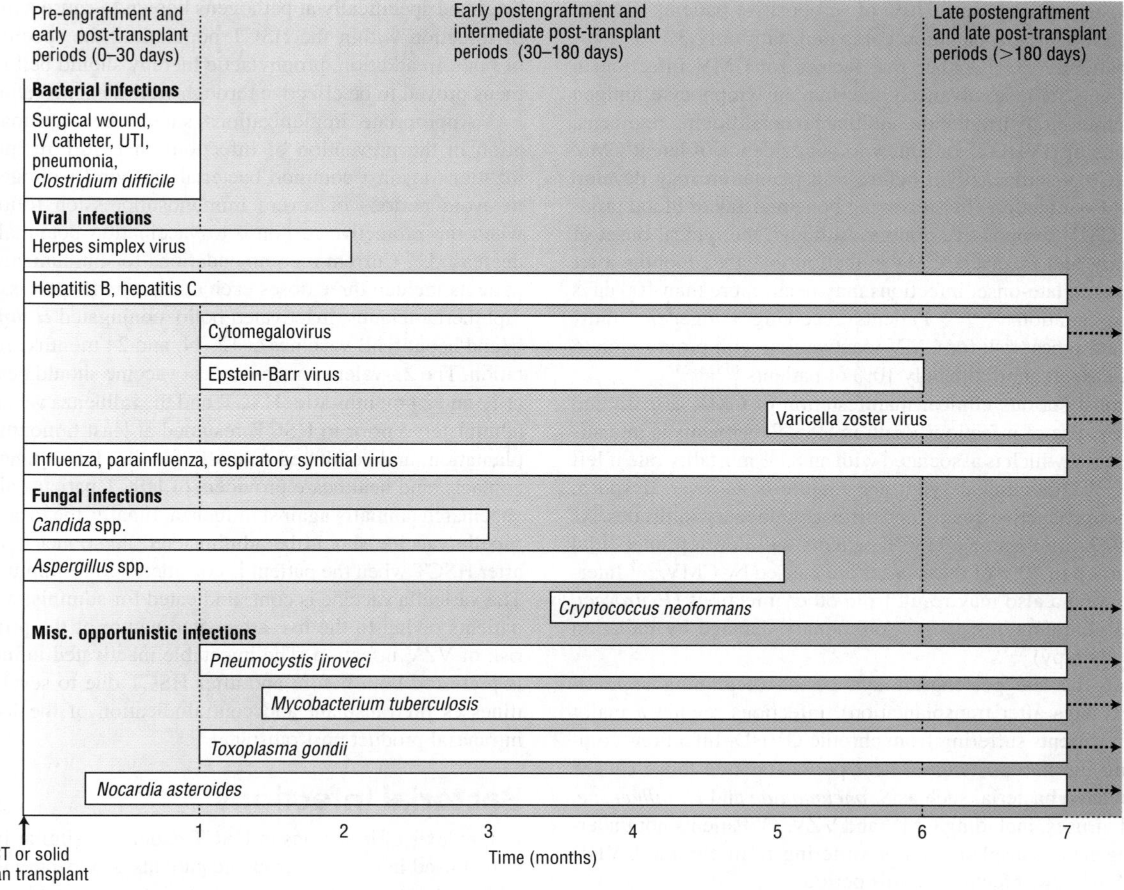

FIGURE 100-3 Timetable for the occurrence of infections in hematopoietic stem cell transplantation (HSCT) and solid-organ transplant patients. (UTI, urinary tract infection.)

incidence and importance of specific pathogens vary greatly according to the specific type of HSCT performed. Patients receiving allogeneic transplants are at greatest risk for infection after HSCT and are predisposed to earlier and more severe infections with opportunistic pathogens such as *Aspergillus*. The presence of GVHD also has an impact on the incidence and timing of various infections, including invasive fungal infections.

After administration of intensive conditioning regimens to eliminate malignant cells and prevent rejection of donor cells, patients may remain profoundly neutropenic for 3 to 4 weeks. During this preengraftment period, patients are at risk for the same types of infectious complications that occur in other granulocytopenic cancer patients (e.g., bacterial and fungal infections) and should be managed accordingly (see Table 100-1). Table 100-6 lists regimens for treatment of specific infections.

HSCT recipients remain at high risk for infection after bone marrow engraftment has occurred.[5,52,53] Significant defects in neutrophil function and cell-mediated and humoral immunity, persisting for several months after transplantation, predispose patients to infectious complications. Acute and chronic GVHD also result in prolonged periods of immunosuppression and increased infection rates.

Patients undergoing HSCT are at significant risk for serious bacterial infections.[52–54] The risk of bacterial infection is particularly increased in patients undergoing allogeneic transplantation and those with GVHD. Gram-negative bacteremia occur in approximately 20% of patients, and mortality rates may reach 25%.[54]

Fungal infections, especially those caused by *Candida* and *Aspergillus* spp., are serious and often result in fatal complications. Fungi remain a serious cause of infection, particularly in allogeneic HSCT recipients, for up to 1 to 2 years following transplantation and may occur in as many as 20% of patients.[52,53,55] Mortality rates associated with invasive aspergillosis infections may be as high as 90%.[52,53,55,56]

HSCT recipients are also at risk for serious viral infections, particularly HSV and cytomegalovirus (CMV). HSV infections may include gingivostomatitis, esophagitis, genital lesions, and, rarely, pneumonia during the first month after transplant.[52,57] Clinical disease is more common in patients with serologic evidence of prior exposure and latent HSV infection pretransplant. Therefore, reactivation of latent disease during periods of immunosuppression is the most common etiology of HSV infection. Without prophylaxis, as many as 80% of HSV-seropositive patients experience mucocutaneous disease after intensive chemotherapy compared with less than 25% of seronegative patients.[10,52,57] HSV infections often coexist with *Candida* infection and mucositis secondary to chemotherapy, radiation, or both.[10,57] Painful swallowing associated with these conditions often makes it difficult for patients to take oral medications and maintain adequate nutritional intake. Because of the considerable morbidity associated with HSV reactivation after transplantation, the HSV serologic status of patients should be determined prior to transplant.

HSCT recipients are at high risk for CMV infections during the early postengraftment period. Infections range in severity from asymptomatic infection with viral shedding (urine, throat, and lungs), to life-threatening disseminated disease and interstitial pneumonia.[10,52,57]

As with HSV, patients seropositive for CMV before transplantation are at high risk for reactivation of infection during periods of immunosuppression; up to 70% of seropositive patients develop reactivation after transplantation compared with only 3% of seronegative patients.[10,52,53,57] Other risk factors for CMV infection in HSCT patients include advanced age, human lymphocyte antigen mismatch, total-body irradiation, multiagent conditioning regimens, and presence of GVHD.[57] Patients without evidence of latent CMV infection (CMV-seronegative) before transplantation may develop primary CMV infection after receiving bone marrow or blood products from CMV-seropositive donors. Although the typical onset of both primary and recurrent CMV infection is 1 to 2 months after transplantation, late-onset infections may occur more than 100 days after transplantation.[10,52,53,57] Patients receiving allogeneic transplants are at highest risk for CMV reactivation, with progression to clinical disease in approximately 10% of patients.[10,52,53,57]

The most serious clinical manifestation of CMV disease and the leading cause of infectious death in HSCT recipients is interstitial pneumonia, which is associated with an 85% mortality rate if left untreated.[52,57] This clinical syndrome manifests as fever, dyspnea, hypoxia, nonproductive cough, and diffuse pulmonary infiltrates. As many as 40% of allogeneic HSCT patients will develop interstitial pneumonia; up to 40% of these cases are caused by CMV.[52,57] Interstitial pneumonia also may result from other infectious (*P. jiroveci*, VZV) and noninfectious causes (pulmonary damage by radiation and chemotherapy).[52,57]

During the late postengraftment period (beginning approximately 180 days after transplantation), infections remain a major problem in patients suffering from chronic GVHD. Infections common during the late postengraftment period include those caused by encapsulated bacteria, such as *S. pneumoniae* and *H. influenzae*, fungi, and viruses, including CMV and VZV.[52,57] Patients not undergoing allogeneic transplantation or suffering from chronic GVHD generally have few infections in this period.

Up to 50% of all patients surviving up to 10 months after transplantation develop an infection caused by VZV.[52,57] Infection with VZV is most common in allogeneic HSCT recipients with acute or chronic GVHD.[10,57] Both primary (varicella) or recurrent disease (herpes zoster) usually present as skin lesions, most of which remain contained to local areas; however, 30% to 45% of these infections may disseminate to other cutaneous areas or body organs, causing mortality as high as 50%.[10,57]

TREATMENT

Desired Outcomes

The goals of therapy in managing HSCT recipients include the following, from the neutropenic period through the late postengraftment period: (a) protect the patient from early death caused by undiagnosed infection; (b) employ effective prophylactic therapy to prevent common bacterial, fungal, viral, and protozoal/parasitic infections; (c) effectively and aggressively treat established infections; (d) avoid unnecessary use of antimicrobials that contribute to increased resistance; and (e) minimize toxicities and cost while increasing patient quality of life.

Prophylaxis and Management of Infections in Recipients of HSCT

8 9 The overall goal of prophylaxis and treatment of infection in HSCT patients is prevention of infectious morbidity and mortality. Specific goals of antimicrobial drug use in HSCT patients include (a) prevention of bacterial, fungal, viral, and protozoal infections during preengraftment and postengraftment periods and (b) effective treatment of established infections. These goals must be achieved at the lowest possible toxicity and cost. Prophylactic therapy should be aimed specifically at pathogens known to cause a high incidence of infection within the HSCT population, the specific institution, or both. In addition, prophylactic therapy should be limited to regimens proved to be effective through well-designed clinical trials.

Appropriate immunizations should be a primary consideration in the prevention of infections in HSCT recipients. Immunizations against common bacterial and viral pathogens are timed to avoid periods of severe immunosuppression following HSCT when the protective response to vaccination potentially would be decreased.[5,6] Current recommendations for immunization of HSCT patients include three doses each of diphtheria–pertussis–tetanus or diphtheria–tetanus, inactivated polio, conjugated *H. influenzae* type b, and hepatitis B vaccines at 12, 14, and 24 months after transplantation. The 23-valent pneumococcal vaccine should be administered at 12 and 24 months after HSCT, and the influenza vaccine should be administered prior to HSCT, resumed at least 6 months after transplantation, and continued annually for life. Family members, close contacts, and healthcare providers of HSCT patients also should be vaccinated annually against influenza. Finally, the measles–mumps–rubella vaccine should be administered no sooner than 24 months after HSCT when the patient is considered to be immunocompetent. The varicella vaccine is contraindicated for administration to HSCT patients owing to the live-attenuated nature of the product and the risk of VZV infection. The injectable inactivated influenza vaccine is preferred both before and after HSCT due to severe underlying illnesses pretransplant and contraindication of the live-attenuated intranasal product posttransplant.[1,5,6]

Bacterial Infections

Prophylaxis of infections in HSCT patients is similar in many ways to that used in other neutropenic patients. Antibacterial prophylaxis with oral antimicrobials is used commonly; considerations are the same as those discussed previously in the "Prophylaxis of Infections in Neutropenic Cancer Patients" section. Although many studies have shown decreased rates of bacteremia and other bacterial infections after HSCT, overall mortality rates have not been consistently reduced.[1,5,6,57] Therefore, routine use of prophylactic antibiotics in HSCT is still controversial but should be considered in patients at moderate to high risk of infection (Table 100-8). Fluoroquinolones are the most frequently used agents, with levofloxacin preferred over ciprofloxacin due to enhanced gram-positive activity.[1,5,6,57] These regimens usually are started either within 72 hours of beginning the chemotherapy conditioning regimens or on the day of hematopoietic stem cell infusion and continued throughout the neutropenic period. Patients who become febrile while receiving prophylaxis should be managed according to general guidelines for febrile neutropenic patients.

Clinical **Controversy...**

Prophylaxis of infection in HSCT patients with parenteral vancomycin has been studied because of the high incidence of gram-positive infections following transplantation. Vancomycin prophylaxis appears to decrease the overall incidence of gram-positive bacterial infections, number of days of empirical antimicrobial therapy, and cost of therapy.[5,6] However, important mortality benefits have not been demonstrated consistently, and there are significant concerns regarding the selection of vancomycin-intermediate *S. aureus* and VRE. Thus, prophylactic vancomycin use is not recommended except in institutions with high rates of MRSA infection among HSCT recipients.[1,5,6] There currently is no defined role in prophylaxis for other agents with anti-MRSA activity (e.g., linezolid).

Antibiotic prophylaxis against bacterial infection is also recommended in the late postengraftment period (>100 days after transplantation) in certain high-risk patients, specifically allogeneic transplant recipients with chronic GVHD.[5,6] Antibiotics should be targeted against encapsulated bacteria, particularly *S. pneumonia*, and should be selected based on local susceptibility patterns for these organisms; penicillin is preferred in areas with low rates of penicillin-resistant pneumococci.[5] Patients receiving trimethoprim–sulfamethoxazole for prophylaxis of other opportunistic infections may be protected adequately and do not necessarily require an additional antibiotic.[5,6] Prophylaxis should be continued as long as the chronic GVHD is being actively treated.

Viral Infections

Prophylaxis of recurrent HSV infection is recommended for all HSV-seropositive patients undergoing HSCT.[1,5,6,57] Approximately 0% to 10% of HSV-seropositive patients receiving acyclovir experienced viral shedding, clinical symptoms of viral reactivation, or both compared with 60% to 80% of patients receiving placebo.[6,57] IV acyclovir therapy eventually is necessary in many patients because of the development of severe mucositis from conditioning regimens. However, oral acyclovir, valacyclovir, or famciclovir is effective and considerably less expensive in patients who can take oral medications. Valacyclovir has replaced acyclovir as first-line therapy in many institutions.[5,6,57,58] The antiviral agent usually is started at the time of the conditioning regimen and continued until bone marrow engraftment or resolution of mucositis (approximately 30 days after HSCT), although longer durations of prophylaxis may be considered in allogeneic HSCT recipients with GVHD or frequent HSV reactivations before transplantation.[5,6,57,58] In addition to preventing recurrence of HSV disease, acyclovir prophylaxis may reduce the incidence of CMV reactivation.[5,6] Patients receiving ganciclovir or foscarnet for prophylaxis or treatment of CMV infection do not need additional antiviral therapy for prevention of HSV or VZV.[5] Patients developing active HSV or VZV infection should be treated with high-dose acyclovir.[57]

Oral acyclovir or valacyclovir given for up to 12 months after transplantation also significantly reduces reactivation of VZV infections and prevents the occurrence of severe VZV disease.[1,5] Patients receiving either allogeneic or autologous HSCT may therefore be considered for long-term (up to 1 year after transplantation) prophylaxis against VZV.[5] Patients who received HSCT within the previous 24 months, or those more than 24 months after HSCT who have chronic GVHD or are undergoing immunosuppressive therapy, should receive varicella-zoster immunoglobulin 625 units intramuscularly within 48 to 96 hours after close contact with persons with chickenpox or shingles for prevention of VZV-related disease.[6]

Acyclovir-resistant HSV has been reported occasionally in HSCT patients receiving acyclovir prophylaxis. Foscarnet is a drug of choice for treatment of documented infection with acyclovir-resistant HSV and should be reserved for this use.[5,6,57]

Prevention of CMV disease has been studied extensively in HSCT patients and is a well-accepted indication for prophylaxis because of the high associated infectious morbidity and mortality. If possible, CMV-seronegative patients should receive donor cells and supportive blood products from seronegative donors only; however, CMV-seropositive patients are not at significant additional risk by receiving blood or donor cells from seropositive donors.[57] Although acyclovir has relatively poor in vitro activity against CMV, a decrease in CMV infection and an improvement in overall survival were reported in HSV- and CMV-seropositive allogeneic HSCT recipients receiving IV acyclovir.[5,6]

Ganciclovir has been well studied for prophylaxis because of its superior activity against CMV compared with acyclovir.[5,6] Oral valganciclovir has also been well studied in the setting of HSCT.[5,58] Valganciclovir has excellent pharmacokinetics and produces serum levels of ganciclovir, which are at least similar to those achieved after IV administration.[59] Valganciclovir is routinely used in many centers based on the favorable pharmacokinetic properties and convenience of oral dosing in certain patients.[5,58,59] Although administration of prophylactic ganciclovir to CMV-seropositive patients may significantly decrease the occurrence of CMV disease, studies have found no clear survival benefit, and ganciclovir-related bone marrow suppression frequently was problematic. Therefore, ganciclovir prophylaxis is somewhat controversial and is not universally recommended for routine use.[5,6,57] It may, however, be considered for allogeneic HSCT recipients for the first 100 days after transplantation.[5,6,57]

Perhaps a more appropriate role for ganciclovir and valganciclovir is preemptive therapy, in which ganciclovir is administered at first isolation of CMV from the blood or bronchoalveolar lavage fluid. Detection of CMV can be accomplished by use of either a monoclonal antibody-based test for viral antigens or by detection of viral DNA through polymerase chain reaction (PCR)-based tests. Preemptive therapy significantly reduced the occurrence of CMV disease (including CMV pneumonia) and improved survival significantly up to 180 days after transplantation.[5,57] Because CMV viremia and bronchoalveolar lavage cultures are highly predictive of subsequent CMV disease, preemptive ganciclovir or valganciclovir therapy should be considered for autologous HSCT recipients within the first 100 days after transplantation or in allogeneic HSCT recipients at any time after transplantation.[5,6,57] The doses of ganciclovir or valganciclovir for preemptive therapy are the same as those used for prophylaxis. Foscarnet can also be used for either prophylaxis or preemptive therapy of CMV disease in patients intolerant of ganciclovir. CSFs are beneficial in this setting (Table 100-6), providing benefits similar to those noted in neutropenic patients with acquired immunodeficiency syndrome receiving ganciclovir therapy for CMV retinitis.[43,44]

Prophylaxis of CMV disease with either IV immunoglobulin (IVIG) or cytomegalovirus hyperimmune globulin (CMVIG) produced variable and inconclusive results, and their use is not currently recommended.[60,61]

Ganciclovir or valganciclovir are the drugs of choice for treatment of active CMV infection in HSCT patients (see Table 100-5). Foscarnet also may be of benefit for treatment or prevention of infections in HSCT patients and may be used as an alternative to ganciclovir/valganciclovir because of its relative lack of bone marrow toxicity. Foscarnet-related nephrotoxicity may be problematic, however, especially in the posttransplant period when patients may be receiving other nephrotoxic agents. Cidofovir has not been well studied in HSCT patients and is also associated with nephrotoxicity, but this agent may also be considered for preemptive therapy or treatment of active disease.[5]

Numerous single-agent treatments, such as vidarabine, interferon, and ganciclovir, have been used unsuccessfully as treatment for CMV pneumonitis. However, the combination of high-dose IVIG and ganciclovir may decrease the mortality of the syndrome from 85% to only 30% to 50%.[57,60,62] Ganciclovir plus hyperimmune CMVIG also is considered effective for treatment of CMV disease, although this regimen has not been studied as extensively in the HSCT population in a controlled fashion. The potential for ganciclovir-associated bone marrow suppression prior to marrow engraftment and in patients who are just recovering from granulocytopenia remains a concern, especially in patients with unstable renal function. Ganciclovir plus CMVIG is used widely as the treatment regimen of choice for severe or life-threatening CMV disease, this use being based on benefit-versus-risk considerations more than definitive clinical data.[5] Ganciclovir plus IVIG may also be used, although CMVIG has replaced IVIG in many institutions.[5,60,62]

Fungal Infections

Prophylaxis with antifungal agents is efficacious and generally recommended for prevention of mucocutaneous and disseminated fungal infections in high-risk HSCT patients (Tables 100-2 and 100-8).[5,6,23,25,51,57,63–66] Patients specifically recommended for prophylaxis include all allogeneic recipients and autologous transplant recipients who are expected to have prolonged neutropenia, have received intensive conditioning regimens associated with extensive mucositis, or have recently received fludarabine.[5,6,23,25,51,57,63,64] Fluconazole is the most commonly used agent; it is started on the day of transplantation and continued until resolution of neutropenia or, in allogeneic HSCT, for at least 75 days after transplantation.[5,6,23,57,64] The variable activity of fluconazole against non-*albicans* species of *Candida* may be problematic in this population, as is lack of activity against *Aspergillus*.[25,26,51,64] Prophylaxis with fluconazole (as well as itraconazole), although effectively reducing colonization and infection with yeasts, has not been consistently demonstrated to reduce overall mortality or invasive infections such as aspergillosis in HSCT recipients.[5,25,51,57,63–66] Micafungin was more efficacious than fluconazole in the prevention of early-onset *Candida* infections in patients with neutropenia prior to engraftment, and also showed a trend to fewer episodes of invasive aspergillosis.[5] Posaconazole was also more effective than fluconazole in the late prevention of invasive *Aspergillus* and other fungal infections in HSCT patients with GVHD. In a meta-analysis, prophylaxis with agents active against *Aspergillus* were also associated with a 33% reduction in mortality related to invasive fungal infections compared to fluconazole.[66] Fluconazole, posaconazole, and micafungin, along with itraconazole, voriconazole, and LAMB products, are all recommended for prophylaxis of fungal infections in HSCT. Posaconazole is the preferred agent in high-risk HSCT patients with GVHD (Table 100-2).[5,25,27,51,63–65]

Protozoal Infections

Pulmonary infection with *P. jiroveci* is a relatively infrequent complication of HSCT. However, mortality rates in this population are approximately 60% and are especially high in patients with GVHD.[5,6,52] Prophylactic trimethoprim–sulfamethoxazole is recommended for a period of 3 to 6 months after autologous HSCT, and for at least 6 months and while receiving immunosuppressive therapy after allogeneic HSCT. Toxoplasmosis is not a common infection in HSCT patients but is associated with mortality rates of approximately 70%.[67] Toxoplasmosis should also be prevented by trimethoprim–sulfamethoxazole prophylaxis.[5,6]

Use of Colony-Stimulating Factors

Filgrastim, pegfilgrastim, and sargramostim have been studied in HSCT patients in an effort to speed bone marrow recovery, reduce the period of neutropenia, and decrease infectious complications. CSFs appear effective as well as safe following autologous transplantation, although increased rates of GVHD and mortality have been reported with use of CSFs following allogeneic transplantation.[43] The use of CSFs is now routinely recommended to mobilize blood progenitor cells and reduce the period of neutropenia in autologous transplants (Table 100-6).[5,43,44]

Evaluation of Therapeutic Outcomes

10 Close monitoring of HSCT patients, including clinical and laboratory data, is essential for early detection and treatment of infectious complications. In addition, because many of the drugs commonly used in this setting (e.g., ganciclovir, amphotericin B, and trimethoprim–sulfamethoxazole) have significant toxicity potential in HSCT patients, careful attention must be paid to prevention and management of drug-related adverse effects. Monitoring parameters related to specific types of infections (e.g., pneumonia and urinary tract infections) should be applied as appropriate. The reader is referred to other chapters within this book for more specific information.

INFECTIONS IN SOLID-ORGAN TRANSPLANT RECIPIENTS

Solid-organ transplantation (SOT) has become an established mode of treatment for end-stage diseases of the heart, lungs, kidney, liver, pancreas, and small bowel. Patient and allograft survival rates have greatly improved due to improvements in immunosuppressive drug therapy, candidate selection, and transplant surgery techniques and more experience in the management of complications (including infection) in these patients. Despite advances in diagnostic techniques and antimicrobial therapy, infectious complications remain important causes of morbidity and mortality after SOT.

Risk Factors

1 Many risk factors for infection are present in SOT patients (see Table 100-1). The most important risk factor in this population is immunosuppressive drug therapy for prevention and treatment of allograft rejection. Risk of infection depends on specific immunosuppressive drug regimens as well as the intensity (dose) and duration of immunosuppression. Most opportunistic infections in transplant patients occur during the first 6 months after transplantation, when the intensity and total cumulative doses of immunosuppressive therapy are very high.[68,69]

Immunosuppressive drugs, often in escalated doses, are used to treat episodes of graft rejection include immunoglobulins directed against T cells (e.g., antithymocyte globulin), murine monoclonal antibodies (muromonab), antibodies against interleukin 2 receptors (daclizumab and basiliximab), T-cell–depleting antibodies (alemtuzumab), and high-dose corticosteroids. Rejection episodes often occur during the period 2 to 4 months posttransplant when the overall cumulative dose or net state of immunosuppression is highest.[68,70] Therefore, patients already at risk for infection are placed at even higher risk if additional immunosuppressive therapy is needed to treat one or more episodes of graft rejection. Immunosuppressive drug therapy must be evaluated carefully when infections occur because, in many cases, immunosuppression may have to be reduced to allow patients to survive the infectious episode, at the expense of increased risk of graft rejection. Risk of increased infectious complications from immunosuppressive therapy used to treat rejection episodes is determined, at least in part, by the specific therapy used.[68–70]

Etiology

2 As with cancer patients, microorganisms infecting SOT patients are present before transplantation or are acquired from exogenous sources. All transplant recipients are at risk for mucocutaneous candidiasis from species colonizing body sites. Invasive fungal infection is less common following kidney and pancreas transplantation (5% to 15%) but may occur in 30% to 60% of heart, lung, liver, and small bowel transplant recipients. Rates are highest following lung, liver, and small bowel transplantation and are associated with mortality rates up to 60% to 80%.[68,71–73] Approximately 50% to 90% of all systemic fungal infections in transplant recipients are caused by *Candida* spp.[68,71,72] Abdominal surgery, especially the more complex procedures required for liver and small bowel transplantation, predispose patients to serious fungal disease, most likely as a consequence of entering an area already colonized with *Candida* spp.[71]

Lung and heart transplant recipients are particularly at risk for invasive aspergillosis; these infections may occur in up to 10% of patients.[71–73] Liver and lung transplant recipients are at high risk for serious gram-negative bacterial infections as a result of the technically difficult surgical procedures.[68] Although opportunistic viral, fungal, and protozoal infections may occur commonly, bacterial infections remain the most frequent infectious complications after transplantation in all allograft recipients.

Organisms present as latent tissue infections may reactivate and cause clinical disease with administration of immunosuppressive drug therapy. Disease resulting from infection reactivation has been noted with viruses (HSV, human herpesvirus-6, CMV, VZV, Epstein–Barr virus), protozoa (*T. gondii*, *P. jiroveci*), and mycobacteria (*Mycobacterium tuberculosis*).[74,75] Serologic or immunologic tests are performed prior to transplantation to assess the risk for reactivation infection and identify other subclinical infections (e.g., hepatitis B, hepatitis C, *Legionella*). Many patients with reactivated infection have no clinical symptoms; often the only evidence of active infection is a rise in antibody titer from the pretransplant baseline, positive culture, or histologic evidence. Reactivation of latent infection may result in severe life-threatening disease in immunosuppressed hosts.[75]

Exogenous sources of infection in transplant patients include environmental contamination and transmission of microorganisms via transplanted organs and blood products. Environmental sources of infection are similar to those noted in other immunocompromised hosts, such as cancer patients. Airborne pathogens, especially fungi such as *Aspergillus* and *Cryptococcus neoformans*, may cause infections in transplant patients; this is thought to be a direct cause of increased *Aspergillus* infections among lung transplant patients.[68,71] Transplant patients are at high risk for nosocomial infections (*P. aeruginosa*, *Acinetobacter*). Optimal prevention and management of nosocomial infections in transplant patients require knowledge of the current epidemiology of infections and susceptibility patterns in the institution.

Infections transmitted via donor organs or blood products are major causes of morbidity and mortality in transplant patients and may include HSV, *T. gondii*, and hepatitis B and C. The most important infections transmitted from the donor, however, are caused by CMV. These infections may cause serious disease, and predispose patients to other opportunistic infections, and contribute to acute and chronic allograft dysfunction or rejection, posttransplant lymphoproliferative disorders, and cardiac complications and atherosclerosis in heart transplant recipients.[68,76] In contrast to reactivation disease, transplant patients contracting primary CMV disease are at increased risk for serious life-threatening infections.[68,77–79] The most important source of primary CMV infection in transplant patients is the donor organ. Efforts are made to avoid transplanting organs from CMV-seropositive donors into CMV-seronegative recipients because of the potentially severe consequences. With the relative scarcity of suitable organs and the rapidity with which transplant decisions often must be made, however, this is not always possible. The consequences of transplanting an organ from a CMV-seropositive donor into an already CMV-seropositive recipient are less clear. CMV reinfection (as well as reactivation) syndromes may occur in these patients.[68,69,79] In addition to transmission from donor organs, primary CMV disease may be transmitted from seropositive blood products, although this is a much less common mode of transmission.

Organs from donors seropositive for *T. gondii* or HSV generally are not withheld from seronegative patients. Organs from known HIV-infected donors, however, are not used for transplantation. Asymptomatic HIV-seropositive individuals with $CD4^+$ lymphocyte count greater than 400 cells/mm^3 (0.4×10^9/L) may be considered for SOT (as well as HSCT) without prohibitively high risk for acceleration of HIV disease.[80] However, this practice is not widespread because of the shortage of donor organs. The impact of protease inhibitors and highly active antiretroviral therapy on long-term outcome of HIV-infected patients following transplantation is not precisely known but is believed to have improved the overall feasibility of transplanting these individuals.[80]

Timing of Infections After Transplantation

As with HSCT, the overall time course for infections can be divided into three general periods after transplantation (see Fig. 100-3). Although risk of infection with specific pathogens varies with the type of transplant, the time course of infections is similar in all transplant recipients. During the early posttransplant period (within the first month after transplantation), patients are at risk for infections already present and brought forward from the pretransplant period (e.g., hepatitis B); postoperative infections, such as surgical wound and catheter infections; infection resulting from colonized donor organs (pneumonia following lung transplant); and reactivation of HSV.[68,69,75] In the intermediate posttransplant period (2 to 6 months after transplant), risk is highest for viral infections, including CMV, Epstein–Barr virus, and hepatitis B and C. The combination of these "immunomodulating" viruses plus sustained immunosuppressive therapy leads to a high risk for opportunistic infections with pathogens such as *P. jiroveci*, *Aspergillus*, and *Nocardia asteroides*.[68,69,71,75] In the late post-transplant period (>6 months after transplant), patients are at risk for persistent infections (particularly viral) from earlier posttransplant periods, reactivation of VZV and *C. neoformans*, and routine infections affecting the general population.[68] In addition, patients who required additional immunosuppression therapy for acute or chronic rejection are at continued high risk for opportunistic infections (*Aspergillus* and *P. jiroveci*).[68,69,71] Although Figure 100-3 illustrates infection patterns common to all solid-organ transplants, the relative incidence and importance of a particular pathogen vary according to the type of transplant.

Types of Infections and Clinical Presentation

10 Transplant patients are at risk for infections occurring at a variety of sites, including skin, surgical wound, urinary tract, lungs, blood, abdomen, and CNS. However, most infections occur at or near the site of the transplanted organ. For example, heart transplant and heart and lung transplant recipients most often are infected within the lungs or thoracic cavity. Urinary tract infections remain an important cause of morbidity in renal transplant patients, especially in the early posttransplant period. Administration of prophylactic antibiotics (e.g., trimethoprim–sulfamethoxazole) to these patients has reduced the incidence and severity of urinary tract infections.[68,69] Serious bacterial and fungal infections originating from the abdomen and GI tract are most common after liver transplantation and are related to variables such as length of surgery and surgical procedures performed. Risk of bacteremia, usually originating from the gut, is highest in liver transplant patients. Renal transplant recipients are at the lowest risk for infections and infectious deaths, whereas patients receiving heart, lung, and liver transplants are at the highest risk for infection-related morbidity and mortality.[68,69,71]

In contrast to febrile neutropenic patients, the threshold for initiating empirical antimicrobial therapy is higher in febrile transplant patients. Appropriate therapy for the large numbers of pathogens that may cause infections in transplant patients varies greatly from organism to organism (Table 100-5). Therefore, careful attempts at definitive diagnosis of suspected infections must be made. If comprehensive workup reveals no source of infection, careful observation of the febrile transplant patient (rather than empirical therapy)

CLINICAL PRESENTATION Infections in Solid-Organ Transplant Patients

General

- Because transplant patients are at high risk for serious infections, frequent (at least daily), careful clinical assessments must be performed to search for evidence of infection
- Clinical presentation of infection is variable and depends on the type and site of infection, type of transplant, time after transplantation, immune status of the host, and dose and duration of immunosuppressive therapy
- Primary viral disease usually is more symptomatic and severe than disease caused by reactivation
- Physical assessment should include examination of all common sites of infection, including mouth/pharynx, nose and sinuses, respiratory tract, GI tract, urinary tract, skin, soft tissues, perineum, and intravascular catheter insertion sites

Symptoms

- Usual signs and symptoms of infection may be absent or altered in patients receiving intensive immunosuppressive regimens owing to an inability to mount a typical inflammatory response (e.g., no infiltrate on chest x-ray film, urinary tract infection without pyuria)
- Pain may be present at infection site(s)

Signs

- Fever is the single most important clinical sign indicating the presence of infection. Other causes of fever unrelated to infection in this patient population include reactions to blood products, drugs, embolic events, and ischemic injury
- Usual signs of infection may be absent or altered
- Signs of allograft dysfunction may be related to infection. Distinguishing fever caused by allograft rejection from that caused by infection often is difficult and frequently requires allograft biopsy

Laboratory Tests

- Blood cultures (at least two sets, including vascular access devices) for bacteria and fungi; cultures of other suspected or potential infection sites (urine, lungs, surgical wounds, and soft tissue infections)
- Other cultures should be obtained as clinically indicated according to the presence of signs or symptoms
- Complete blood count and chemistries should be obtained frequently to monitor allograft function, plan supportive care, guide drug dosing, and assess patient's overall status
- Surveillance cultures for CMV and HSV may be useful during first 3 months after transplantation for early detection of infection

Other Diagnostic Tests

- Chest x-ray film
- Aspiration, biopsy of skin lesions
- Other diagnostic tests as indicated clinically on the basis of physical examination and other assessments

is common practice. Surveillance cultures may be useful during the first 3 months for detecting CMV and HSV infections.[68,71,77,78,81] Management and monitoring of documented infections are similar to that in other types of patients.

TREATMENT

Desired Outcomes

The goals of therapy in managing SOT recipients are similar to those in HSCT and include the following: (a) protect the patient from early death caused by undiagnosed infection, from the surgical procedure through the late postengraftment period; (b) employ effective prophylactic therapy to prevent common bacterial, fungal, viral, and protozoal/parasitic infections; (c) effectively and aggressively treat established infections; (d) avoid unnecessary use of antimicrobials; and (e) minimize toxicities and cost while increasing patient quality of life and avoiding harm to the engrafted organ(s).

Prevention of Infection in Solid-Organ Transplantation

8 The goals of antimicrobial drug use in solid-organ transplant recipients are (a) prevention of infectious complications in the immediate postoperative period, (b) prevention of late infectious complications associated with prolonged periods of immunosuppression, and (c) effective treatment of established infections in order to prevent graft dysfunction and rejection and decrease patient morbidity and mortality. All of these goals must be achieved at the lowest possible toxicity and cost.

Prevention of infection in the transplant patient can be accomplished in a number of ways. First, risk of environmental contamination should be minimized.[82] Patients should be protected from institutional infectious outbreaks. Transplant patients should receive the pneumococcal vaccine once and the influenza vaccine yearly; however, their immunologic responses to these vaccines may be blunted by immunosuppressive therapy.[68]

Because the most important source of primary CMV infection is an infected donor organ, CMV-seronegative patients should not receive organs or blood products from seropositive donors if possible. A number of pharmacologic strategies have been studied in an attempt to prevent CMV infection. Prophylaxis with IV ganciclovir or oral valganciclovir is effective in reducing the incidence of both primary and reactivated CMV infection in SOT.[58,62,68,69,76–79] Ganciclovir prophylaxis also may significantly reduce reactivation of CMV infection in seropositive patients receiving antithymocyte globulin or muromonab for treatment of acute rejection.[69,78,79] High-dose oral acyclovir effectively reduces the incidence of CMV infection and disease following renal transplantation. However, acyclovir is less efficacious in high-risk renal transplant patients (donor positive, recipient negative for CMV serum antibodies) and other nonrenal transplant types.[68,69,76–79,83] Preemptive ganciclovir or valganciclovir (initiated after actual isolation of CMV from blood, urine, bronchoalveolar lavage fluid, or other site) is more effective than acyclovir in preventing CMV disease in liver transplant recipients. Preemptive ganciclovir effectively prevents CMV disease in other types of solid-organ transplants as well.[77,78,81] Ganciclovir-related bone marrow suppression is not as problematic in solid-organ transplant recipients as in HSCT patients; most studies report that the drug is reasonably well tolerated.[62,68,77,78,81,83]

Whether prophylaxis or preemptive therapy is the best approach to preventing CMV disease is controversial.[62,68,73,77–79,81,84–86] Prophylaxis is effective and easy to administer without the need for careful discrimination among suitable patients. However, universal prophylaxis results in unnecessary exposure of low-risk individuals to adverse effects of drugs, and there are concerns that prolonged exposure may increase the risk of viral resistance to drugs.[77,78,83–85] Preemptive therapy is effective and results in exposure of fewer patients to drugs. Prophylactic therapy is recommended primarily in patients at highest risk of disease (i.e., seronegative patients receiving organs from seropositive donors), whereas other lower-risk patients are often recommended to receive only preemptive therapy.[68,73,77,78,81,83–86] However, the risk of CMV infection and disease in lung transplant recipients is so high and is associated with such severe consequences (i.e., chronic graft dysfunction, decreased survival) that prophylaxis is routinely recommended for all lung transplant recipients.[73,86] The duration of prophylactic therapy in SOT recipients is typically 100 days, although data suggest that the duration may be extended to 6 months in high-risk kidney transplant recipients and to 12 months in high-risk lung transplant patients.[73,85,86]

Clinical **Controversy. . .**

CMVIG may be valuable in decreasing the incidence and severity of CMV disease following kidney, heart, lung, and liver transplantation.[62,68,76–79,82] Although prophylaxis with CMVIG has been strongly recommended for CMV-seronegative transplant recipients receiving organs from seropositive donors, the benefits of CMVIG relative to other therapies (e.g., prophylactic or preemptive ganciclovir) are not well known, and available studies have conflicting results. Whether the combination of CMVIG plus ganciclovir offers advantages over the use of either agent alone, either for primary prophylaxis or for treatment of established CMV disease, in SOT is unclear.[62,68,77] However, some authorities recommend use of CMVIG in combination with ganciclovir for treatment of severe, life-threatening CMV pneumonitis in solid-organ transplant recipients.[5,60,62]

Although use of prophylactic acyclovir in HSV-seropositive patients undergoing HSCT is well accepted, prophylaxis in solid-organ transplant recipients remains controversial. Reactivation disease caused by HSV occurs in approximately 25% of HSV-seropositive patients who are not receiving prophylaxis.[68] Oral or genital mucocutaneous disease is the most common presentation, but HSV pneumonitis also is seen occasionally and is associated with a mortality rate of approximately 75%.[68] Acyclovir is therefore used at some centers because of the high incidence of clinical HSV infection after transplantation. Acyclovir for prophylaxis of HSV infection may be considered in patients following a preemptive strategy for management of CMV infection, but would not be necessary in patients receiving ganciclovir or valganciclovir for CMV prophylaxis.

Prophylactic antimicrobial agents are also of benefit to SOT patients in certain other clinical situations. Antibiotic prophylaxis, with agents such as cefazolin started perioperatively and continued for less than 24 hours, is considered to reduce wound infection rates effectively following renal transplantation.[68,82] Although the benefits of perioperative prophylaxis have not been well demonstrated in other types of transplantation procedures, surgical prophylaxis usually is considered mandatory for liver, heart, lung, or small bowel transplant patients because of the high risk of perioperative bacterial infections.[68,82] Pulmonary infections are particularly common in lung and heart-lung transplant recipients. They often are caused by bacteria colonizing the airways of the diseased organs prior to transplantation. Therefore, perioperative antibiotics for lung and heart and lung procedures often are selected based on pretransplant sputum cultures and/or known colonizations.[68,82] In addition, posttransplant antibiotic prophylaxis is effective in decreasing the number of bacterial infections in renal transplant patients. Prophylactic trimethoprim–sulfamethoxazole traditionally has been used because it is inexpensive and well tolerated; other antibiotics, such as the fluoroquinolones, also have been evaluated.[68] Administration of oral low-dose trimethoprim–sulfamethoxazole (one double-strength tablet daily) for 6 to 12 months for prevention of *P. jiroveci* infection following heart and lung transplantation is common, although the efficacy and optimal duration are somewhat controversial.[68,85] Selective bowel decontamination with nonabsorbable antibiotics in combination with a low-bacterial diet (no fresh fruits and vegetables) effectively reduces oropharyngeal and GI colonization with gram-negative aerobes and *Candida* in liver transplant patients. However, selective bowel contamination is less efficacious when administered for a period of less than 1 week prior to transplantation.[82] Because liver transplantation usually is performed without advance notice as organs become emergently available, the practice of selective bowel decontamination remains controversial and is not recommended routinely.[68,82]

Because immunosuppressed transplant recipients are at risk for mucocutaneous fungal infections, prophylactic oral or topical antifungal agents may be indicated in these patients. Liver, pancreas, and small bowel transplant recipients are clearly at high risk for invasive fungal infections and should receive prophylaxis with fluconazole.[23,68,71,85] Prophylaxis has also been suggested for lung and heart–lung transplant recipients due to the high incidence of invasive fungal infections in these patients. Prophylaxis with inhaled LAMB, high-dose fluconazole, itraconazole, voriconazole, and echinocandins have all been reported; however, data supporting either the general recommendation for prophylaxis or choice of specific agent are largely lacking and center-to-center variability is great.[23,71,73,85] Concentrations of immunosuppressant drugs should be monitored closely in transplant patients receiving azole-type antifungal agents (fluconazole, itraconazole, and voriconazole).

Transplant patients, especially heart and heart and lung recipients, without serologic evidence of prior exposure to *T. gondii* who receive organs from seropositive donors are at high risk for toxoplasmosis.[68,85] Many of these patients will be receiving trimethoprim–sulfamethoxazole for prophylaxis of *P. jiroveci* infection; this agent will also provide effective prophylaxis against *T. gondii* as well as *N. asteroides*. Although prophylaxis is not given routinely at all centers, this therapy may be justified in high-risk patients because of the delays in diagnosis and serious infections associated with toxoplasmosis.[68,85]

PERSONALIZED PHARMACOTHERAPY

Desired treatment outcomes in febrile neutropenia and in HSCT and SOT recipients are achieved through close monitoring and frequent patient assessment, including judicious evaluation of antimicrobial therapies based on suspected or documented infections. Treatment of known infections must be individualized based on documented pathogens and antimicrobial susceptibilities; effective treatment may require durations of therapy well beyond recovery of ANC in febrile neutropenic patients. High intensity of immunosuppression regimens in HSCT and SOT, as well as the presence of GVHD in HSCT, also dictate aggressive antimicrobial use with potentially long durations of therapy. However, such aggressive antimicrobial use must be balanced against unnecessary administration of drugs, which may lead to increased antimicrobial resistance, adverse effects, and cost. Proper evaluation of an individual patient's risk of complications during febrile neutropenia or after transplantation allows for determination of proper prophylaxis regimens, selection of appropriate antimicrobials for treatment of infection, and selection of appropriate treatment settings (e.g., inpatient versus outpatient), all of which may allow for the most cost-effective therapy and contribute to an increased quality of life for the patient.

ABBREVIATIONS

ANC	absolute neutrophil count
ASCO	American Society of Clinical Oncology
CMV	Cytomegalovirus
CMVIG	Cytomegalovirus hyperimmune globulin
CSF	colony-stimulating factor
EORTC	European Organisation for Research and Treatment of Cancer
GVHD	graft-versus-host disease
HSCT	hematopoietic stem cell transplantation
HSV	herpes simplex virus
IDSA	Infectious Diseases Society of America
LAMB	lipid-associated amphotericin B
MASCC	Multinational Association for Supportive Care in Cancer
MRSA	methicillin-resistant *Staphylococcus aureus*
NCCN	National Comprehensive Cancer Network
PCR	polymerase chain reaction
PMN	polymorphonuclear leukocyte
SOT	solid-organ transplantation
VRE	vancomycin-resistant enterococci
VZV	varicella-zoster virus
WBC	white blood cell

REFERENCES

1. Freifeld AG, Bow EJ, Sepiowitz KA, et al. Clinical practice guideline for the use of antimicrobial agents in neutropenic patients with cancer: 2010 update by the infectious disease society of America. Clin Infect Dis 2011;52(4): e56–e93.
2. Bow EJ. Management of the febrile neutropenic cancer patient: Lessons from 40 years of study. Clin Microbiol Infect 2005;11(Suppl 5):24–29.
3. Viscoli C, Varnier O, Machetti M. Infections in patients with febrile neutropenia: Epidemiology, microbiology, and risk stratification. Clin Infect Dis 2005;40(Suppl 4): S240–S245.
4. Ellis M. Febrile neutropenia. Evolving strategies. Ann NY Acad Sci 2008;1138:329–350.
5. National Comprehensive Cancer Network. Prevention and treatment of cancer-related infections. Clinical Practice Guidelines in Oncology (NCCN Guidelines®), v.1.2012. September 18, 2012. *http://www.nccn.org/professionals/physician_gls/pdf/infections.pdf.*
6. Tomblyn M, Chiller T, Einsele H, et al. Guidelines for preventing infectious complications among hematopoietic cell transplantation recipient: A global perspective. Biol Blood Marrow Transplant 2009;15:1143–1238.
7. Klastersky J, Awada A, Paesmans MM, Aoun M. Febrile neutropenia: A critical review of the initial management. Crit Rev Oncol Hematol 2011;78:185–194.
8. Toussaint E, Bahel-Ball E, Vekemans M, et al. Causes of fever in cancer patients (prospective study over 477 episodes). Support Care Cancer 2006;14:763–769.
9. Feld R. Bloodstream infections in cancer patients with febrile neutropenia. Int J Antimicrob Agents 2008; 32(Suppl):S30–S33.
10. Neuburger S, Maschmeyer G. Update on management of infections in cancer and stem cell transplant patients. Ann Hematol 2006;85:345–356.
11. Horn DL, Neofytos D, Anaissie EJ, et al. Epidemiology and outcomes of candidemia in 2019 patients: Data from the prospective antifungal therapy alliance registry. Clin Infect Dis 2009;48:1695–1703.
12. Antoniadou A, Giamarellou H. Fever of unknown origin in febrile leukopenia. Infect Dis Clin N Am 2007;21: 1055–1090.
13. Pascoe J, Cullen M. The prevention of febrile neutropenia. Curr Opin Hematol 2006;18:325–329.
14. Viscoli C, Cometta A, Kern WV, et al. Piperacillin–tazobactam monotherapy in high-risk febrile neutropenic cancer patients. Clin Microbiol Infect 2006;12:212–216.
15. Klastersky J, Ameye L, Maertens J, et al. Bacteraemia in febrile neutropenic cancer patients. Int J Antimicrob Agents 2007;30(Suppl 1):S51–S59.
16. Hidron A, Edwards JR, Patel J, et al. Antimicrobial-resistant pathogens associated with healthcare-associated infections: Annual summary of data reported to the National Healthcare Safety Network at the Centers for Disease Control and Prevention, 2006–2007. Infect Control Hosp Epidemiol 2008;29(11):996–1011.
17. King MD, Humphrey BJ, Wang YF, et al. Emergence of community-acquired methicillin-resistant *Staphylococcus aureus* USA 300 clone as the predominant cause of skin and soft-tissue infections. Ann Intern Med 2006;144: 309–317.
18. Reilly AF, Lange BJ. Infections with viridans group streptococci in children with cancer. Pediatr Blood Cancer 2007;49:774–780.
19. Bow EJ. Fluoroquinolones, antimicrobial resistance and neutropenic cancer patients. Curr Opin Infect Dis 2011;24:545–553.
20. Avery R, Kalaycio M, Pohlman B, et al. Early vancomycin-resistant enterococcus (VRE) bacteremia after allogeneic bone marrow transplantation is associated with a rapidly deteriorating clinical course. Bone Marrow Transplant 2005;35:497–499.
21. Lodise TP, McKinnon PS. Burden of methicillin-resistant *Staphylococcus aureus*: Focus on clinical and economic outcomes. Pharmacotherapy 2007;27(7):1001–1012.
22. Chamilos G, Luna M, Lewis RE, et al. Invasive fungal infections in patients with hematologic malignancies in a tertiary care cancer center: An autopsy study over a 15-year period (1989–2003). Haematologica 2006;91:986–989.
23. Pappas PG, Kauffman CA, Andes D, et al. Clinical practice guidelines for the management of candidiasis: 2009 update by the Infectious Diseases Society of America. Clin Infect Dis 2009;48:503–535.
24. Pagano L, Caira M, Candoni A, et al. The epidemiology of fungal infections in patients with hematologic malignancies: The SEIFEM-2004 study. Haematologica 2006;91: 1068–1075.
25. Segal BH, Almyroudis NG, Battiwalla M, et al. Prevention and early treatment of invasive fungal infection in patients

with cancer and neutropenia and in stem cell transplant recipients in the era of newer broad-spectrum antifungal agents and diagnostic adjuncts. Clin Infect Dis 2007;44: 402–409.

26. Ruan S-Y, Chu C-C, Hsueh P-R. In vitro susceptibilities of invasive isolates of *Candida* species: Rapid increase in rates of fluconazole susceptible-dose dependent *Candida glabrata* isolates. Antimicrob Agents Chemother 2008;52:2919–2922.
27. Walsh TJ, Anaissie EJ, Denning DW, et al. Treatment of aspergillosis: Clinical practice guidelines of the Infectious Diseases Society of America. Clin Infect Dis 2008;46: 327–360.
28. Kern WV. Risk assessment and treatment of low-risk patients with febrile neutropenia. Clin Infect Dis 2006;42:533–540.
29. Moores KG. Safe and effective outpatient management of adults with chemotherapy-induced neutropenic fever. Am J Health Syst Pharm 2007;64:717–722.
30. Carstensen M, Sorensen JB. Outpatient management of febrile neutropenia: Time to revise the present treatment strategy. J Support Oncol 2008;6:199–208.
31. Furno P, Bucaneve G, Del Favero A. Monotherapy or aminoglycoside-containing combinations for empirical antibiotic treatment of febrile neutropenic patients: A meta-analysis. Lancet Infect Dis 2002;2:231–242.
32. Paul M, Soares-Weiser K, Grozinsky S, Leibovici L. β-Lactam versus β-lactam-aminoglycoside combination therapy in cancer patients with neutropaenia. Cochrane Database Syst Rev 2003;3:CD003038.
33. Paul M, Yahav D, Bivas A, Fraser A, Leibovici L. Anti-pseudomonal beta-lactams for the initial, empirical, treatment of febrile neutropenia: Comparison of beta-lactams. Cochrane Database Syst Rev 2010; 10(11):CD005197.
34. U.S. Food and Drug Administration. Information for Healthcare Professionals: Cefepime (marketed as Maxipime), 2009. Retrieved September 26, 2012, from *http://www.fda.gov/Drugs/DrugSafety/PostmarketDrugSafetyInformationforPatientsandProviders/DrugSafetyInformationforHeathcareProfessionals/ucm167254.htm*.
35. Paul M, Borok S, Fraser A, et al. Additional anti-Gram-positive antibiotic treatment for febrile neutropenic cancer patients. Cochrane Database Syst Rev 2005;(3):CD003914.
36. Paul M, Borok S, Fraser A, et al. Empirical antibiotics against Gram-positive infections for febrile neutropenia: Systematic review and meta-analysis of randomized controlled trials. J Antimicrob Chemother 2005;55: 436–444.
37. Goldberg E, Gafter-Gvili A, Robenshtok E, et al. Empirical antifungal therapy for patients with neutropenia and persistent fever: Systematic review and meta-analysis. Eur J Cancer 2008;44:2192–2203.
38. Moen MD, Lyseng-Williamson KA, Scott LJ. Liposomal amphotericin B: A review of its use as empirical therapy in febrile neutropenia and in the treatment of invasive fungal infections. Drugs 2009;69:361–392.
39. Cornely OA, Maertens J, Bresnik M, et al. Liposomal amphotericin B as initial therapy for invasive mold infection: A randomized trial comparing a high-loading dose regimen with standard dosing (AmBiLoad trial). Clin Infect Dis 2007;44:1289–1297.
40. Zonios DI, Bennett JE. Update on azole antifungals. Sem Resp Crit Care Med 2008;29:198–210.
41. Rogers TR, Frost S. Newer antifungal agents for invasive fungal infections in patients with haematological malignancy. Br J Haematol 2009;144:629–641.
42. Naeger-Murphy N, Pile JC. Clinical indications for newer antifungal agents. J Hosp Med 2009;4:102–111.
43. Smith TJ, Khatcheressian J, Lyman GH, et al. 2006 update of recommendations for the use of white blood cell growth factors: An evidence-based clinical practice guideline. J Clin Oncol 2006;24:3187–3205.
44. National Comprehensive Cancer Network. Myeloid growth factors. National Comprehensive Cancer Network. Clinical Practice Guidelines in Oncology (NCCN Guidelines®), v.1.2012; February 22, 2012. *http://www.nccn.org/professionals/physician_gls/pdf/myeloid_growth.pdf.*
45. Atallah E, Schiffer CA. Granulocyte transfusion. Curr Opin Hematol 2006;13:45–49.
46. Seidel MG, Peters C, Wacker A, et al. Randomized phase III study of granulocyte transfusions in neutropenic patients. Bone Marrow Transplant 2008;42:679–684.
47. Gafter-Gvili A, Paul M, Fraser A, Leibovici L. Effect of quinolone prophylaxis in afebrile neutropenic patients on microbial resistance: Systematic review and meta-analysis. J Antimicrob Chemother 2007;59:5–22.
48. Leibovici L, Paul M, Cullen M, et al. Antibiotic prophylaxis in neutropenic patients: New evidence, practical decisions. Cancer 2006;107:1743–1751.
49. Aaproa MS, Cameron DA, Pettengell R, et al. EORTC guidelines for the use of granulocyte-colony stimulating factor to reduce the incidence of chemotherapy-induced febrile neutropenia in adult patients with lymphomas and solid tumours. Eur J Cancer 2006;42:2433–2453.
50. Bow EJ, Laverdiere M, Lussier N, et al. Antifungal prophylaxis for severely neutropenic chemotherapy recipients: A meta-analysis of randomized-controlled clinical trials. Cancer 2002;94:3230–3246.
51. Ullmann AJ, Cornely OA. Antifungal prophylaxis for invasive mycoses in high risk patients. Curr Opin Infect Dis 2006;19:571–576.
52. Afessa B, Peters SG. Major complications following hematopoietic stem cell transplantation. Semin Respir Crit Care Med 2006;27:297–309.
53. Gooley TA, Chien JW, Pergam SA, et al. Reduced mortality after allogeneic hematopoietic-cell transplantation. N Engl J Med 2010;363:2091–2101.
54. Mikulska M, Del Bono V, Raiola AM, et al. Blood stream infections in allogeneic hematopoietic stem cell transplant recipients: Reemergence of gram-negative rod and increasing antibiotic resistance. Biol Blood Marrow Transplant 2009;15:47–53.
55. Camps IR. Risk factors for invasive fungal infections in haematopoietic stem cell transplantation. Int J Antimicrob Agents 2008;32(Suppl 2):S119–S123.
56. Bhatti Z, Shaukat A, Almyroudis NG, Segal BH. Review of epidemiology, diagnosis, and treatment of invasive mould infections in allogeneic hematopoietic stem cell transplant recipients. Mycopathologia 2006;162:1–15.
57. Angarone M, Ison MG. Prevention and early treatment of opportunistic viral infections in patients with leukemia and allogeneic stem cell transplantation recipients. J Natl Compr Canc Netw 2008;6:191–201.
58. Busca A, de Fabritiis P, Ghisetti V, et al. Oral valganciclovir as preemptive therapy for cytomegalovirus infection post allogeneic stem cell transplantation. Transpl Infect Dis 2007;9:102–107.
59. Einsele H, Reusser P, Bornhaeuser M, et al. Oral valganciclovir leads to higher exposure to ganciclovir than intravenous ganciclovir in patients following allogeneic stem cell transplantation. Blood 2006;107: 3002–3008.

60. Ichihara H, Nakamae H, Hirose A, et al. Immunoglobulin prophylaxis against cytomegalovirus infection in patients at high risk of infection following allogeneic hematopoietic cell transplantation. Transplant Proc 2011;43:3927–3932.
61. Raanani P, Gafter-Gvili A, Paul M, et al. Immunoglobulin prophylaxis in hematopoietic stem cell transplantation: Systematic review and meta-analysis. J Clin Oncol 2008;27:770–781.
62. Crumpacker CS, Zhang J-L. Cytomegalovirus. In: Mandell GL, Bennett JE, Dolin R, eds. Principles and Practice of Infectious Diseases, 7th ed. New York: Churchill Livingstone, 2010:1971–1987.
63. Ziakas PD, Kourbeti IS, Voulgarelis MV, Mylonakis E. Effectiveness of systemic antifungal prophylaxis in patients with neutropenia after chemotherapy: A meta-analysis of randomized controlled trials. Clin Ther 2010;32:2316–2336.
64. Michallet M, Ito JI. Approaches to the management of invasive fungal infections in hematological malignancy and hematopoietic cell transplantation. J Clin Oncol 2009;27:3398–3409.
65. Nucci M, Anaissie E. Fungal infections in hematopoietic stem cell transplantation and solid-organ transplantation—Focus on aspergillosis. Clin Chest Med 2009;30:295–306.
66. Ethier MC, Science M, Beyenne J, et al. Mould-active compared with fluconazole prophylaxis to prevent invasive fungal diseases in cancer patients receiving chemotherapy or haematopoietic stem-cell transplantation: A systematic review and meta-analysis of randomized controlled trials. Br J Cancer 2012;106:1626–1637.
67. Cavattoni I, Ayuk F, Zander AR, et al. Diagnosis of *Toxoplasma gondii* infection after allogeneic stem cell transplant can be difficult and requires intensive scrutiny. Leuk Lymphoma 2010;51:1530–1535.
68. Fishman JA, Issa NC. Infection in organ transplantation: Risk factors and evolving patterns of infection. Infect Dis Clin N Am 2010;24:273–283.
69. Grim SA, Clark NM. Management of infectious complications in solid-organ transplant recipients. Clin Pharmacol Ther 2011;90:333–342.
70. Issa NC, Fishman JA. Infectious complications of antilymphocyte therapies in solid organ transplantation. Clin Infect Dis 2009;48:772–786.
71. Person AK, Kontoyiannis DP, Alexander BD. Fungal infections in transplant and oncology patients. Infect Dis Clin N Am 2010;24:439–459.
72. San Juan R, Aguado JM, Lumbreras C, et al. Incidence, clinical characteristics and risk factors of late infection in solid organ transplant recipients: Data from the RESITRA study group. Am J Transplant 2007;7:964–971.
73. Kotton CN. Zoonoses in solid-organ and hematopoietic stem cell transplant recipients. Clin Infect Dis 2007;44:857–866.
74. Weikert BC, Blumberg EA. Viral infection after renal transplantation: Surveillance and management. Clin J Am Soc Nephrol 2008;3:S76–S86.
75. Pescovitz MD. Benefits of cytomegalovirus prophylaxis in solid organ transplantation. Transplantation 2006;82: S4–S8.
76. Jancel T, Penzak SR. Antiviral therapy in patients with hematologic malignancies, transplantation, and aplastic anemia. Semin Hematol 2009;46:230–247.
77. Zhang L-F, Wang Y-T, Tian J-H, et al. Preemptive versus prophylactic protocol to prevent cytomegalovirus infection after renal transplantation: A meta-analysis and systematic review of randomized controlled trials. Transpl Infect Dis 2011;13:622–632.
78. Torres-Madriz G, Boucher HW. Immunocompromised hosts: Perspectives in the treatment and prophylaxis of cytomegalovirus disease in solid-organ transplant recipients. Clin Infect Dis 2008;47:702–711.
79. Trullas JC, Cofan F, Tuset M, et al. Renal transplantation in HIV-infected patients: 2010 update. Kidney Int 2011;79:825–842.
80. Strippoli GFM, Hodson EM, Jones C, Craig JC. Preemptive treatment for cytomegalovirus viremia to prevent cytomegalovirus disease in solid organ transplant recipients. Transplantation 2006;81:139–145.
81. Hanson K, Alexander B. Strategies for the prevention of infection after solid organ transplantation. Expert Rev Anti Infect Ther 2006;4:837–852.
82. Razonable RR. Management of viral infections in solid organ transplant recipients. Exp Rev Antiinfect Ther 2011;9:685–700.
83. Hantz S, Garnier-Geoffroy F, Mazeron M-C, et al. Drug-resistant cytomegalovirus in transplant recipients: A French cohort study. J Antimicrob Chemother 2010;65: 2628–2640.
84. Subramanian AK. Antimicrobial prophylaxis regimens following transplantation. Curr Opin Infect Dis 2011;24:344–349.
85. Patel N, Snyder LD, Finlen Copeland CA, Palmer SM. Is prevention the best treatment? CMV after lung transplantation. Am J Transplant 2012;12:539–544.
86. Sims KD, Blumberg EA. Common infections in the lung transplant recipient. Clin Chest Med 2011;32:327–341.

Antimicrobial Prophylaxis in Surgery

101

Salmaan Kanji

KEY CONCEPTS

1. Prophylactic antibiotic therapy differs from presumptive and therapeutic antibiotic therapy in that the latter two involve treatment regimens for documented or presumed infections, whereas the goal of prophylactic therapy is to prevent infections in high-risk patients or procedures.
2. The risk of a surgical site infection (SSI) is determined from both the type of surgery and the patient-specific risk factors; however, most commonly used classification systems account for only procedure-related risk factors.
3. The timing of antimicrobial prophylaxis is of paramount importance. Antibiotics should be administered within 1 hour before surgery to ensure adequate drug levels at the surgical site prior to the initial incision.
4. Antimicrobial agents with short half-lives (e.g., cefazolin) may require intraoperative redosing during long (>3 hours) procedures.
5. The type of surgery, intrinsic patient risk factors, most commonly identified pathogenic organisms, institutional antimicrobial resistance patterns, and cost must be considered when choosing an antimicrobial agent for prophylaxis.
6. Single-dose prophylaxis is appropriate for many types of surgery. First-generation cephalosporins (e.g., cefazolin) are the mainstay for prophylaxis in most surgical procedures because of their spectrum of activity, safety, and cost.
7. Vancomycin as a prophylactic agent should be limited to patients with a documented history of life-threatening β-lactam hypersensitivity or those in whom the incidence of infections with organisms resistant to cefazolin (e.g., methicillin-resistant *Staphylococcus aureus*) is documented or high enough to justify use.

According to the National Center for Health Statistics, some 46 million surgical procedures are performed annually in the United States, the majority of which are done in an outpatient setting.[1] Infection is the most common complication of surgery.[2] Surgical site infections (SSIs) occur in ~3% to 6% of patients and prolong hospitalization by an average of 7 days at a direct annual cost of $5 billion to $10 billion.[3,4] SSIs are the third (14% to 16%) most frequent cause of nosocomial infections among hospitalized patients and the primary (40%) cause of nosocomial infection in surgical patients.[3] Prophylactic administration of antibiotics decreases the risk of infection after many surgical procedures and represents an important component of care for this population.

Antibiotics administered prior to the contamination of previously sterile tissues or fluids are called prophylactic antibiotics. The goal of therapy is to prevent an infection from developing. Although eradication of distal (preexisting, unrelated to surgery) infections lowers the risk for subsequent postoperative infections, it does not per se constitute a prophylactic regimen. In fact, surgical prophylaxis often is prescribed concurrently under these circumstances because of important antimicrobial spectrum- and timing-related concerns. Both SSIs and infections not directly related to the surgical site (e.g., urinary tract infections and pneumonia) are termed *nosocomial.* Prevention of hospital-acquired infections is a major goal of antibiotic prophylaxis.

1 Presumptive antibiotic therapy is administered when an infection is suspected but not yet proven. Clinical scenarios where presumptive therapy is used commonly include acute cholecystitis, open compound fractures, and acute appendicitis of less than 24 hours' duration. In these situations, if signs of perforation or infection are absent during surgery, then routine prophylactic treatment rather than presumptive therapy is warranted. An operative finding of a gangrenous gallbladder or a perforated appendix, however, is suggestive of an established infectious process, and a therapeutic antibiotic regimen is required.[3]

According to the Centers for Disease Control and Prevention's (CDC) National Nosocomial Infections Surveillance System (NNIS),[3] SSIs can be categorized as either incisional (e.g., cellulitis of the incision site) or organ/space (e.g., meningitis; Fig. 101-1). Incisional SSIs are subcategorized into superficial (involving only the skin or subcutaneous tissue) and deep (fascial and muscle layers) infections. Organ/space SSIs can involve any anatomic area other than the incision site. For example, a patient who develops bacterial peritonitis after bowel surgery has an organ/space SSI. By definition, SSIs must occur within 30 days of surgery. If a prosthetic implant is involved, a deep incisional or organ/space SSI can be reported up to 1 year from the date of surgery. Although microbiologic testing of surgical drainage material or sites may help to guide care, the specificity of a negative culture is poor and generally does not rule out an SSI.[3]

RISK FACTORS FOR SURGICAL SITE INFECTIONS

2 SSI incidence depends on both procedure- and patient-related factors. Traditionally, the risk for SSIs has been stratified by surgical procedure in a classification system developed by the National Research Council (NRC; Table 101-1).[5] The NRC classification system proposes that the risk of an SSI depends on the microbiology of the surgical site, the presence of a preexisting infection, the likelihood of contaminating previously sterile tissue during surgery, and the events during and after surgery.[5,6] A patient's NRC procedure classification is the primary determinant of whether antibiotic

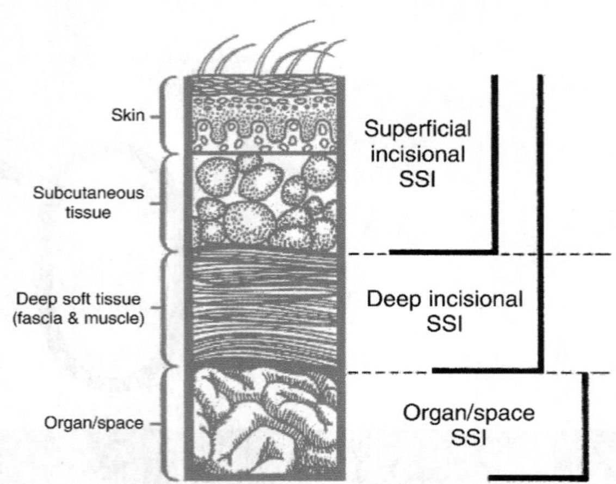

FIGURE 101-1 Cross section of abdominal wall depicting Centers for Disease Control and Prevention classifications of surgical site infections (SSI). *(Reprinted from reference 3 with permission from Elsevier and the Association for Professionals in Infection Control and Epidemiology.)*

prophylaxis is warranted. However, because a patient's NRC wound classification is influenced by surgical findings (e.g., gangrenous gallbladder) and perioperative events (e.g., major technique breaks), categorization generally occurs intraoperatively.[7]

Inherent Patient Risk

The NRC classification system does not account for the influence of underlying patient risk factors for SSI development, instead categorizing the risks for SSIs simply based on a specific surgical procedure. Disease states and conditions known to increase SSI risk are listed in Table 101-2. Preexisting distal infections increase SSI rates and should be resolved prior to surgery whenever possible. Diabetic patients have an increased risk for SSIs, especially those with uncontrolled perioperative blood sugars. Preoperative smoking has been identified as an independent risk factor for SSI because of the deleterious effects of nicotine on wound healing. Preoperative immunosuppression, including corticosteroid use, may increase infection risk. Patients coinfected with human immunodeficiency virus (HIV) and hepatitis C are at approximately double the risk of SSI as the general population.[8] Malnutrition is a well-described risk factor for postoperative complications, including SSI, impaired wound and colonic anastomosis healing, and prolonged hospital stay. Although enteral feeding during the perioperative period can reduce bacterial translocation by maintaining the integrity of the intestinal mucosa, nutritional supplementation does not decrease the incidence of infection.[9]

Colonization of the nares with *Staphylococcus aureus* is a well-described SSI risk factor.[3] Although intranasal application of mupirocin ointment reduces the rate of nasal carriage of *S. aureus*, one large, randomized, double-blind study of 4,030 surgical patients found that prophylactic intranasal mupirocin did not reduce the rate of *S. aureus* SSI, although it did reduce the rate of nosocomial *S. aureus* infections among patients who were *S. aureus* carriers.[10] Other factors shown to increase the risk of SSI are age, length of preoperative hospital stay, and obesity.[3]

Identifying SSI Risk

Two large epidemiologic studies have objectively quantified SSI risk based on specific patient- and procedure-related factors. The Study on the Efficacy of Nosocomial Infection Control (SENIC) analyzed more than 100,000 surgery cases to identify and validate risk factors for SSI.[11] Abdominal operations, operations lasting longer than 2 hours, contaminated or "dirty" procedures (as per NRC classification), and more than three underlying medical diagnoses each was associated with an increased incidence of SSI. When NRC classification was stratified by number of SENIC risk factors present, SSI incidence varied by as much as a factor of 15 within the same NRC operative category (Table 101-3).[12]

In a subsequent analysis of more than 84,000 surgical cases, the NNIS attempted to simplify and refine the SENIC system by quantifying intrinsic patient risk using the American Society of Anesthesiologists' (ASA) preoperative assessment score (Table 101-4).[14,15] An ASA score ≥3 was a strong predictor for the development of an SSI. Other factors associated with increased SSI incidence are contaminated or "dirty" operations (NRC criteria) and surgical procedures lasting longer than average. As in the SENIC study, the SSI rate was linked to the number of risk factors present and varied considerably within NRC class. The NNIS basic SSI risk index is composed of the following criteria: ASA score = 3, 4, or 5; wound class; and duration of surgery. Overall, for 34 of the 44 NNIS procedure categories, SSI rates increased proportionally with the number of risk factors present.[13] The SSI rate was generally lower when the procedure was done laparoscopically.

TABLE 101-1 National Research Council Wound Classification, Risk of Surgical Site Infection, and Indication for Antibiotics

	SSI Rate (%)			
Classification	Preoperative Antibiotics	No Preoperative Antibiotics	Criteria	Antibiotics
Clean	5.1	0.8	No acute inflammation or transection of GI, oropharyngeal, genitourinary, biliary, or respiratory tracts; elective case, no technique break	Not indicated unless high-risk procedure[a]
Clean–contaminated	10.1	1.3	Controlled opening of aforementioned tracts with minimal spillage/minor technique break; clean procedures performed emergently or with major technique breaks	Prophylactic antibiotics indicated
Contaminated	21.9	10.2	Acute, nonpurulent inflammation present; major spillage/technique break during clean–contaminated procedure	Prophylactic antibiotics indicated
Dirty	N/A	N/A	Obvious preexisting infection present (abscess, pus, or necrotic tissue present)	Therapeutic antibiotics required

N/A, not applicable; SSI, surgical site infection.

[a]High-risk procedures include implantation of prosthetic materials and other procedures where surgical site infection is associated with high morbidity (see the text).

Adapted from references 5 and 11.

TABLE 101-2 Patient and Operation Characteristics That May Influence the Risk of Surgical Site Infection

Patient	Operation
Age	Duration of surgical scrub
Nutritional status	Preoperative skin preparation
Diabetes	Preoperative shaving
Smoking	Duration of operation
Obesity	Antimicrobial prophylaxis
Coexisting infections at distal body sites	Operating room ventilation
Colonization with resistant microorganisms	Sterilization of instruments
Altered immune response	Implantation of prosthetic materials
Length of preoperative stay	Surgical drains Surgical technique

Reprinted from reference 3 with permission from Elsevier and the Association for Professionals in Infection Control and Epidemiology.

Although evidence-based recommendations for antimicrobial prophylaxis during surgery are best established using the results of randomized clinical trials, many studies have small sample sizes and do not stratify patients according to overall SSI risk. Future studies, particularly those involving clean procedures, should be stratified by SSI risk so that the subset of high-risk patients who might benefit the most from prophylaxis is clearly established.

BACTERIOLOGY

The most important consideration when choosing antibiotic prophylaxis is the bacteriology of the surgical site. Organisms involved in an SSI are acquired by one of two ways: endogenously (from the patient's own normal flora) or exogenously (from contamination during the surgical procedure). Based on the type and anatomic location of the procedure and the NRC classification (see Table 101-1), resident flora can be predicted and appropriate antibiotic choices made. According to NNIS data, *S. aureus,* coagulase-negative staphylococci, enterococci, *Escherichia coli*, and *Pseudomonas aeruginosa* are the pathogens most commonly isolated (Table 101-5).[14] With the widespread use of broad-spectrum antibiotics, however, *Candida* species and methicillin-resistant *Staphylococcus aureus* (MRSA) are becoming more prevalent.[14]

TABLE 101-3 Surgical Site Infection Incidence (%) Stratified by NRC Wound Classification and SENIC Risk Factors[a]

Number of SENIC Risk Factors	Clean	Clean–Contaminated	Contaminated	Dirty
0	1.1	0.6	N/A	N/A
1	3.9	2.8	4.5	6.7
2	8.4	8.4	8.3	10.9
3	15.8	17.7	11.0	18.8
4	N/A	N/A	23.9	27.4

N/A, not applicable.

[a]Study on the Efficacy of Nosocomial Infection Control (SENIC) risk factors include abdominal operation, operations lasting >2 hours, contaminated or dirty procedures by National Research Council (NRC) classification, and more than three underlying medical diagnoses.

Reprinted from reference 13 with permission.

TABLE 101-4 American Society of Anesthesiologists' Physical Status Classification

Class	Description
1	Normal healthy patient
2	Mild systemic disease
3	Severe systemic disease that is not incapacitating
4	Incapacitating systemic disease that is a constant threat to life
5	Not expected to survive 24 hours with or without operation

Data from reference 15.

Factors affecting the ability of an organism to induce an SSI depend on organism count, organism virulence, and host immunocompetency. Organisms in the commensal flora generally are not pathogenic. These organisms often serve the host as a form of protection against invasive organisms that otherwise would colonize the surgical site. Opportunistic organisms usually are kept in check by normal flora and rarely are problematic unless they are present in large numbers. The loss of normal flora through the use of broad-spectrum antibiotics can destabilize homeostasis, allowing pathogenic bacteria to proliferate and infection to occur.[4]

Normal flora translocated to a normally sterile tissue site or fluid during a surgical procedure can become pathogenic. For example, *S. aureus* or *Staphylococcus epidermidis* may be translocated from the surface of the skin to deeper tissues or *E. coli* from the colon to the peritoneal cavity, bloodstream, or urinary tract. Studies in animals and healthy volunteers have shown bacterial virulence to be an important determinant in the development of secondary infections.[16,17] Whereas more than one million *S. aureus* per square centimeter or gram of tissue are required to produce infection in animals, less than 100,000 *Streptococcus pyogenes* per square centimeter or gram of tissue are required at the same site.[17,18]

Impaired host defense reduces the number of bacteria required to establish an infection. A breach of normal host defenses through surgical intervention (e.g., insertion of a prosthetic device) may enable organisms to cause infection. In addition,

TABLE 101-5 Major Pathogens in Surgical Wound Infections

Pathogen	Percent of Infections[a]
Staphylococcus aureus	20
Coagulase-negative staphylococci	14
Enterococci	12
Escherichia coli	8
Pseudomonas aeruginosa	8
Enterobacter species	7
Proteus mirabilis	3
Klebsiella pneumoniae	3
Other *Streptococcus* species	3
Candida albicans	3
Group D streptococci	2
Other gram-positive aerobes	2
Bacteroides fragilis	2

[a]Data reported by the National Nosocomial Infections Surveillance System from January 1992 through June 2004.

Adapted from reference 5.

the loss of specific immune factors, such as complement activation, tissue-derived inhibitors (e.g., proinflammatory cytokines), cell-mediated response (e.g., T-cell function), and granulocytic or phagocytic function (e.g., neutrophils or macrophages) can greatly increase the risk for SSI development.[19] Vascular occlusive states related to the surgical procedure or those occurring from hypovolemic shock can greatly affect blood flow to the surgical site, thus diminishing host defense mechanisms against microbial invasion. Traumatized tissue, hematomas, and the presence of foreign material also lead to more infections. When a foreign body is introduced during a surgical procedure, fewer than 100 bacterial colony-forming units are required to cause an SSI.[20] Studies examining *S. aureus*-contaminated wound infections on the skin of healthy volunteers demonstrate a 10,000-fold reduction in the number of organisms required to establish a wound infection if sutures are not present.[16]

ANTIMICROBIAL RESISTANCE

Colonization of the host with antibiotic-resistant hospital flora prior to or during surgery may lead to an SSI that is unresponsive to routine antibiotic therapy. The most common cause of nosocomially acquired multiresistant organisms is transmission from hospital personnel.[21] Patients treated with broad-spectrum antibiotic therapy are at increased risk for colonization with hospital flora.

With cephalosporins established as first-line agents for prophylaxis, organisms resistant to cephalosporins represent the majority of pathogens causing SSIs. MRSA and coagulase-negative staphylococci have emerged as the most common pathogens in patients who develop SSIs despite prophylaxis with cephalosporins particularly in cardiothoracic, vascular, orthopedic, and neurologic surgery. Methicillin resistance not only limits the treatment/prophylaxis options available, but it also is associated with increased mortality, longer hospital lengths of stay, and increased costs.[22,23] Although the use of vancomycin for prophylaxis may be appropriate for some operations performed in hospitals with a high rate of infection due to MRSA, there is little guidance on what constitutes a "high rate" of MRSA infection and whether providing prophylaxis with vancomycin alone will result in fewer SSIs.[24] A more effective strategy would be to screen elective surgical candidates for MRSA colonization preoperatively. MRSA colonization is predictive of MRSA SSI and thus effective prophylaxis with vancomycin is then reserved for carriers only. Some single center studies evaluating the decolonization of MRSA carriers preoperatively (i.e., with intranasal mupirocin, chlorhexidine showers) yield mixed results and may not be cost-effective.[25,26]

Although cefazolin remains a mainstay in cardiovascular SSI prophylaxis, its failure has been reported in cases involving methicillin-sensitive *Staphylococcus aureus* (MSSA). In a comparison trial between cefamandole and cefazolin, significantly more failures were attributed to cefazolin, even though the primary pathogen was MSSA.[27] However, a similar trial comparing cefazolin and cefuroxime did not show any difference in SSI incidence between the two regimens.[27] The β-lactamase expressed by some MSSA may be capable of hydrolyzing cefazolin more readily than cefuroxime or cefamandole. Although this trend is disturbing, the overall incidence of cefazolin failure remains low, and cefazolin remains the drug of choice for SSI prophylaxis in cardiovascular surgery.[27]

The increase in frequency of fungal infections in surgical patients has drawn concern. In hospitalized patients, the incidence of nosocomial *Candida* infections nearly doubled from 1992 to 2004.[14,28] Overzealous use of broad-spectrum antibiotics is the most likely cause for this increase. A study of patients undergoing cardiovascular surgery identified sex (female), length of stay in the ICU, and duration of central venous catheterization as risk factors for postoperative *Candida* infections.[29] Although presurgical *Candida* colonization is associated with a higher risk of fungal SSIs, routine preoperative use of prophylactic antifungal agents is not being advocated at this time.[28,30]

SCHEDULING ANTIBIOTIC ADMINISTRATION

❸ ❹ The following principles must be considered when providing antimicrobial surgical prophylaxis: (a) the agents should be delivered to the surgical site prior to the initial incision, and (b) bactericidal antibiotic concentrations should be maintained at the surgical site throughout the surgical procedure. Although animal and human models have demonstrated the efficacy of a single dose of an antibiotic administered just prior to bacterial contamination, long operations often require intraoperative doses of antibiotics to maintain adequate concentrations at the surgical site for the duration of surgery.[31] Antibiotics should be administered with anesthesia just prior to the initial incision. Administration of antibiotics too early may result in concentrations below the MIC toward the end of the operation, and administration too late leaves the patient unprotected at the time of initial incision. In a study examining the timing of antibiotic administration to 2,847 patients receiving prophylaxis, Classen et al.[31] evaluated patients who received prophylaxis early (2 to 24 hours before surgery), preoperative prophylaxis (0 to 2 hours prior to surgery), perioperative prophylaxis (up to 3 hours after first incision), and postoperative prophylaxis (>3 hours after the first incision). The risk of infection was lowest (0.6%) for patients who received preoperative prophylaxis, moderate (1.4%) for those who received perioperative antibiotics, and greatest for those who received postoperative antibiotics (3.3%) or preoperative antibiotics too early (3.8%). The risk for an SSI increases dramatically with each hour from the time of initial incision to the time when antibiotics are eventually administered. For these reasons, prophylactic antibiotics should not be prescribed to be given "on call to the operating room (OR)," which can occur two or more hours prior to the initial incision, nor should concurrent therapeutic antibiotics be relied on to provide adequate protection. In both situations, the chance for improperly timed doses is high. Although the landmark study by Classen et al.[31] confirmed that antimicrobial prophylaxis should be administered within 2 hours prior to the initial incision, administration immediately prior to the incision may not allow enough time for the drug to distribute throughout the tissues involved in the surgery.

In a large prospective observational study of 3,836 visceral, trauma, and vascular surgeries where antimicrobial prophylaxis with cefuroxime and metronidazole was employed, the incidence of SSIs was analyzed according to the timing of antimicrobial administration. When antimicrobial prophylaxis was administered within 30 minutes or between 1 and 2 hours before the initial incision, the risk of SSI was greater when compared to antimicrobial prophylaxis administered 30 to 59 minutes prior to the initial incision. The authors conclude that the optimal window for antimicrobial (cefuroxime and metronidazole) is between 30 and 59 minutes prior to the initial incision.[32] This effect may be a function of the pharmacodynamics and pharmacokinetics of the antimicrobial chosen for the prophylactic regimen. A larger study of 4,472 patients undergoing cardiac, orthopedic, and gynecologic surgery with a variety of antimicrobial prophylactic regimens also evaluated the temporal relationship between SSI occurrence and the timing of antibiotics.

After excluding patients who received drugs with prolonged infusion times (i.e., fluoroquinolones and vancomycin), there was a statistically nonsignificant trend toward fewer SSIs in patients who received their prophylactic regimen within the 30 minutes prior to incision as compared with those who received the regimen 31 to 60 minutes prior to incision (odds ratio, OR: 1.74; 95% confidence interval: 0.98 to 3.04).[33]

Despite the importance of appropriately timed prophylactic antibiotic therapy, few patients receive antibiotics at the optimal time in relation to surgery. Potential barriers include antibiotics ordered after the patient has arrived in the OR, delayed antibiotic preparation or delivery, and use of antibiotics that require long infusion times. One study assessed the timing of prophylactic antibiotics in 100 patients and found that only 26% of patients received an antibiotic dose within 2 hours of the initial surgical incision.[34]

Although most studies comparing single versus multiple doses of prophylactic antibiotics have failed to show a benefit of multidose regimens, the duration of operations in these studies may not be as long as that frequently observed in clinical practice. Proponents of administering a second antibiotic dose during lengthy operations suggest that the risk for SSI is just as great at the end of surgery (during wound closing) as it is during the initial incision. One study of patients undergoing clean–contaminated operations suggests that procedures longer than 3 hours require a second intraoperative dose of cefazolin or substitution of cefazolin with a longer-acting antimicrobial agent.[4] A second study of patients undergoing elective colorectal surgery suggests that low serum antimicrobial concentrations at the time of surgical closure is the strongest predictor of postoperative SSI.[35] Studies of patients undergoing cardiac surgery also have demonstrated a higher infection rate among patients with undetectable antibiotic serum concentrations at the conclusion of the procedure.[36]

One strategy to ensure appropriate redosing of prophylactic antibiotics during long operations is use of a visual or auditory reminder system. One hospital reported its experience with such a system, finding that an automated reminder improved compliance and reduced SSIs. However, even with the reminder system, intraoperative redosing was done in only 68% of eligible patients.[37] Another strategy currently being evaluated is the role of continuous infusions of cefazolin, which one pilot study has found to be a feasible way to ensure adequate serum concentrations of antibiotic during prolonged surgeries.[38] Further trials are required before such an intervention can be recommended.

ANTIMICROBIAL CHOICE

5 The choice of prophylactic antibiotic depends on the type of surgical procedure, the most frequent pathogens seen with this procedure, safety and efficacy profiles of the antimicrobial agent, current literature evidence supporting its use, and cost. Although most SSIs involve the patient's normal flora, antimicrobial selection also must take into account the susceptibility patterns of nosocomial pathogens within each institution. Typically, gram-positive coverage should be included in the choice of surgical prophylaxis because organisms such as *S. aureus* and *S. epidermidis* are encountered commonly as skin flora. The decision to broaden antibiotic prophylaxis to agents with gram-negative and anaerobic spectra of activity depends on both the surgical site (e.g., upper respiratory, GI, or genitourinary tract) and whether the operation will transect a hollow viscous or mucous membrane that may contain resident flora.[3]

Although antimicrobial prophylaxis can be administered through a variety of routes (e.g., oral, topical, or intramuscular), the parenteral route is favored because of the reliability by which adequate tissue concentrations may be acheived.[39] Cephalosporins are the most commonly prescribed agents for surgical prophylaxis because of their broad antimicrobial spectrum, favorable pharmacokinetic profile, low incidence of adverse side effects, and low cost. First-generation cephalosporins, such as cefazolin, are the preferred choice for surgical prophylaxis, particularly for clean surgical procedures.[3,4,7] In cases where broader gram-negative and anaerobic coverage is desired, antianaerobic cephalosporins, such as cefoxitin and cefotetan, are appropriate choices. Although third-generation cephalosporins (e.g., ceftriaxone) have been advocated for prophylaxis because of their increased gram-negative coverage and prolonged half-lives, their inferior gram-positive and anaerobic activity and high cost have discouraged the widespread use of these agents.[3,4,7]

Allergic reactions are the most common side effects associated with cephalosporin use. Reactions can range from minor skin manifestations at the site of infusion to rash, pruritus, and rarely anaphylaxis (<0.02%). The structural similarity between penicillins and cephalosporins (each contains a β-lactam ring) has led to considerable confusion about the cross-allergenicity between these two classes of drugs. Twenty percent of the general population is labeled "penicillin allergic," yet of these patients, only 10% to 20% have positive results of a penicillin skin test.[40] The rate of cross-reactivity is ~2%, but as only 20% of all "penicillin-allergic" patients truly are penicillin allergic, the true incidence of cross-reactivity likely is less than 1%. Routine penicillin skin testing is not cost-effective.[40] In summary, the administration of cephalosporins is both safe and cost-effective for many patients who are labeled "penicillin allergic," and they can be used by patients who have not experienced an immediate or type I penicillin allergy.

Vancomycin can be considered for prophylactic therapy in surgical procedures involving implantation of a prosthetic device in which the rate of MRSA is high.[23,41] If the risk of MRSA is low, and a β-lactam hypersensitivity exists, clindamycin can be used for many procedures instead of cefazolin to limit vancomycin use. Infusion-related side effects, such as thrombophlebitis and hypotension, particularly with vancomycin, usually can be controlled by adequate dilution and slower administration rates.[42]

Pseudomembranous colitis secondary to cephalosporins is uncommon and generally easily treated with a short course of oral metronidazole. Although infrequent, bleeding abnormalities related to cephalosporin use have been reported.[43] The primary hematologic effect appears to be inhibition of vitamin K-dependent clotting factors that results in prolongation of the prothrombin time. The mechanism for this effect, most commonly seen with cefotetan, is related to the methylthiotetrazole side chain of the β-lactam molecule. Patients at greatest risk for this hypoprothrombinemic effect have received a prolonged course of these agents and have underlying risk factors for vitamin K deficiency, such as malnutrition.[44]

Because inappropriate prophylactic antibiotic use not only can induce antibiotic resistance but also can negatively affect an institution's antibiotic budget, initiatives to curtail inappropriate antibiotic use have become the focus of many drug use evaluation efforts. Potential sources of inappropriate antibiotic prophylaxis include the use of broad-spectrum antimicrobials when a narrow-spectrum agent is warranted, extending prophylaxis for durations beyond that recommended in published guidelines, and using expensive antibiotics when equivalent, less expensive agents are available. The most effective tools for ensuring appropriate prophylactic antibiotic prescribing are knowledge of the institutional postoperative infection rate for each type of surgical procedure and familiarity with the bacterial epidemiology patterns for each surgical population.

Individualized institutional guidelines that take into account the best literature evidence, institution-based antibiotic susceptibility data, and surgeon preference are important tools for rationalizing antibiotic prophylaxis use.[45]

RECOMMENDATIONS FOR SPECIFIC TYPES OF SURGERY

Guidelines for surgical prophylaxis usually are structured according to the tissues affected during an operation. Although many different surgical procedures may be performed at any one anatomic site, this method of categorization still is optimal because the factors related to the success of a prophylactic regimen, such as the endogenous flora that are expected and the pharmacokinetics, pharmacodynamics, and spectrum of selected antimicrobials, generally are constant for a particular surgical site (see the discussion above). The choice of antimicrobial prophylaxis is always best evaluated using the results of properly conducted clinical trials. In the absence of studies specific to the procedure in question, extrapolation from data on regimens for different procedures in the same anatomic site in question usually can be made. Subsequent modifications to each prophylactic regimen should be based on intraoperative findings or events.

6 A comprehensive review of the surgical prophylaxis literature is beyond the scope of this chapter, but important factors are reviewed here for each type/site of surgery. Specific recommendations are summarized in Table 101-6. The reader is referred to published guidelines and review articles.[2,3,4,7,39,46,47]

Gastrointestinal Surgery

GI surgery can be categorized according to surgical site and infectious risk. Gastroduodenal surgery and hepatobiliary surgery generally are considered to be clean or clean–contaminated surgeries, with SSI rates generally less than 5%. Colorectal surgery, including appendectomies, is considered contaminated because of the large quantities and polymicrobial nature of bacterial flora within the colon. SSI rates for these types of surgeries generally range from 15% to 30%. Emergent abdominal surgery involving bowel perforation or peritonitis is considered a dirty surgical procedure, associated with a greater than 30% risk of SSI, and should be treated with therapeutic rather than prophylactic antibiotics.[3]

Gastroduodenal Surgery

Insignificant numbers of bacteria usually are found in the stomach and duodenum because of their acidity. The rate of SSIs in gastroduodenal surgery generally is low, so procedures in this region can be classified as clean. The risk for an SSI in this population increases with any condition that can lead to bacterial overgrowth, such as obstruction, hemorrhage, or malignancy, or increasing the pH of gastroduodenal secretions with concomitant acid suppression therapy. Antimicrobial prophylaxis is of clinical benefit only in this high-risk population. In most cases, a single dose of IV cefazolin will provide adequate prophylaxis.[48] For patients with a β-lactam allergy, oral ciprofloxacin is as efficacious as parenteral cefuroxime as prophylactic therapy for gastroduodenal surgery.[48] Antimicrobial prophylaxis is indicated in esophageal surgery only in the presence of obstruction. Postoperative therapeutic antibiotics may be indicated if perforation is detected during surgery, depending on whether an established infection is present.

Use of antibiotic prophylaxis for percutaneous endoscopic gastrostomy placement is controversial.[49] Although postoperative peristomal infection can occur in up to 30% of patients, clinical trials with cefazolin given 30 minutes preoperatively in this population are conflicting.[49] A pharmacoeconomic study that incorporated a meta-analysis of available studies to determine efficacy suggested that antibiotic prophylaxis was cost-effective for patients undergoing percutaneous endoscopic gastrostomy placements.[50]

Hepatobiliary Surgery

Although bile normally is sterile, and the SSI rate after biliary surgery is low, antibiotic prophylaxis is of benefit in this population. Bile contamination (bactobilia) can increase the frequency of SSIs and is present in many patients (e.g., those with acute cholecystitis or biliary obstruction and those of advanced age).[46] In general, however, the correlation between bactobilia in surgical specimens and the subsequent pathogens implicated in an SSI is poor. The most frequently encountered organisms are *E. coli*, *Klebsiella* species, and enterococci. *Pseudomonas* is an uncommon finding in the absence of cholangitis. Trials comparing first-, second-, and third-generation cephalosporins have not demonstrated benefit over single-dose cefazolin prophylaxis even in high-risk patients (e.g., age >60 years, previous biliary surgery, acute cholecystitis, jaundice, obesity, diabetes, and common bile duct stones).[51] Ciprofloxacin and levofloxacin are effective alternatives for β-lactam-allergic patients undergoing open cholecystectomy.[52,53] In fact, orally administered levofloxacin appears to provide similar intraoperative gallbladder tissue concentrations.[53] For low-risk patients undergoing elective laparoscopic cholecystectomy, antibiotic prophylaxis is not of benefit and is not recommended.[54] The risk for SSIs in cirrhotic patients undergoing transjugular intrahepatic portosystemic shunt surgery may be reduced with a single prophylactic dose of ceftriaxone,[55] but not with single doses of shorter-acting cephalosporins.[56]

Although surgeons may use presumptive antibiotic therapy for patients with acute cholecystitis or cholangitis and defer surgery until the patient is afebrile in an effort to decrease the risk of subsequent infections, this practice is controversial. Detection of an active infection during surgery (e.g., gangrenous gallbladder and suppurative cholangitis) is an indication for a course of postoperative therapeutic antibiotics. In either case, antibiotics with additional antianaerobic activity (e.g., cefoxitin or cefotetan) are indicated.[57]

Appendectomy

Suspected appendicitis is a frequent cause of abdominal surgery. Numerous antibiotic regimens, all with activity against gram-positive and gram-negative aerobes and anaerobic pathogens, are effective in reducing SSI incidence.[46] A cephalosporin with antianaerobic activity, such as cefoxitin or cefotetan, is recommended as first-line therapy; however, a comparative trial of cefoxitin and cefotetan suggests that cefotetan may be superior, possibly because of its longer duration of action.[58] In patients with β-lactam allergy, metronidazole in combination with gentamicin is an effective regimen. Broad-spectrum antibiotics covering nosocomial pathogens (e.g., *Pseudomonas*) do not further reduce SSI risk and instead may increase the cost of therapy and promote bacterial resistance.[59] Although single-dose therapy with cefotetan is adequate, prophylaxis with cefoxitin may require intraoperative dosing if the procedure extends beyond 3 hours. Established intraabdominal infections (e.g., gangrenous or perforated appendix) require an appropriate course of postoperative therapeutic antibiotics. Laparoscopic appendectomy produces lower postoperative infection rates than open appendectomy; however, antimicrobial prophylaxis was used for all patients in these studies; thus, the role for prophylaxis in this population remains poorly studied.[60]

Colorectal Surgery

In the absence of adequate prophylactic therapy, the risk for SSI after colorectal surgery is high because of the significant bacterial counts in fecal material present in the colon (frequently $>10^9$ per gram).

TABLE 101-6 Most Likely Pathogens and Specific Recommendations for Surgical Prophylaxis

Type of Operation	Likely Pathogens	Recommended Prophylaxis Regimen[a]	Comments	Grade of Recommendation[b]
GI Surgery				
Gastroduodenal	Enteric gram-negative bacilli, gram-positive cocci, oral anaerobes	Cefazolin 1 g × 1 (see the text for recommendations for percutaneous endoscopic gastrostomy)	High-risk patients only (obstruction, hemorrhage, malignancy, acid suppression therapy, morbid obesity)	IA
Cholecystectomy	Enteric gram-negative bacilli, anaerobes	Cefazolin 1 g × 1 for high-risk patients Laparoscopic: none	High-risk patients only (acute cholecystitis, common duct stones, previous biliary surgery, jaundice, age >60 years, obesity, diabetes mellitus)	IA
Transjugular intrahepatic portosystemic shunt (TIPS)	Enteric gram-negative bacilli, anaerobes	Ceftriaxone 1 g × 1	Longer-acting cephalosporins preferred	IA
Appendectomy	Enteric gram-negative bacilli, anaerobes	Cefoxitin or cefotetan 1 g × 1	Second intraoperative dose of cefoxitin may be required if procedure lasts longer than 3 hours	IA
Colorectal	Enteric gram-negative bacilli, anaerobes	Orally: neomycin 1 g + erythromycin base 1 g at 1, 2, and 11 PM 1 day preoperatively plus mechanical bowel preparation IV: cefoxitin or cefotetan 1 g × 1	Benefits of oral plus IV is controversial except for colostomy reversal and rectal resection	IA
GI endoscopy	Variable, depending on procedure, but typically enteric gram-negative bacilli, gram-positive cocci, oral anaerobes	Orally: amoxicillin 2 g × 1 IV: ampicillin 2 g × 1 or cefazolin 1 g × 1	Recommended only for high-risk patients undergoing high-risk procedures (see the text)	IA
Urologic Surgery				
Prostate resection, shock-wave lithotripsy, ureteroscopy	*Escherichia coli*	Ciprofloxacin 500 mg orally or Trimethoprim–sulfamethoxazole 1 DS tablet	All patients with positive preoperative urine cultures should receive a course of antibiotic treatment	IA–IB
Removal of external urinary catheters, cystography, urodynamic studies, simple cystourethroscopy	*E. coli*	Ciprofloxacin 500 mg orally or Trimethoprim–sulfamethoxazole 1 DS tablet	Should be considered only in patients with risk factors (see the text)	IB
Gynecological Surgery				
Cesarean section	Enteric gram-negative bacilli, anaerobes, group B streptococci, enterococci	Cefazolin 2 g × 1	Can be given before initial incision or after cord is clamped	IA
Hysterectomy	Enteric gram-negative bacilli, anaerobes, group B streptococci, enterococci	Vaginal: cefazolin 1 g × 1 Abdominal: cefotetan 1 g × 1 or cefazolin 1 g × 1	Metronidazole 1 g IV × 1 is recommended alternative for penicillin allergy	IA
Head and Neck Surgery				
Maxillofacial surgery	*Staphylococcus aureus*, streptococci oral anaerobes	Cefazolin 2 g or clindamycin 600 mg	Repeat intraoperative dose for operations longer than 4 hours	IA
Head and neck cancer resection	*S. aureus*, streptococci oral anaerobes	Clindamycin 600 mg at induction and every 8 hours × 2 more doses	Add gentamicin for clean–contaminated procedures	IA
Cardiothoracic Surgery				
Cardiac surgery	*S. aureus*, *Staphylococcus epidermidis*, *Corynebacterium*	Cefazolin 1 g every 8 hours × 48 hours	Patients >80 kg (176 lb) should receive 2 g of cefazolin instead; in areas with high prevalence of *S. aureus* resistance, vancomycin should be considered	IA
Thoracic surgery	*S. aureus*, *S. epidermidis*, *Corynebacterium*, enteric gram-negative bacilli	Cefuroxime 750 mg IV every 8 hours × 48 hours	First-generation cephalosporins are deemed inadequate, and shorter durations of prophylaxis have not been adequately studied	IA
Vascular Surgery				
Abdominal aorta and lower extremity vascular surgery	*S. aureus*, *S. epidermidis*, enteric gram-negative bacilli	Cefazolin 1 g at induction and every 8 hours × 2 more doses	Although complications from infections may be infrequent, graft infections are associated with significant morbidity	IB

(continued)

TABLE 101-6 Most Likely Pathogens and Specific Recommendations for Surgical Prophylaxis (*Continued*)

Type of Operation	Likely Pathogens	Recommended Prophylaxis Regimen[a]	Comments	Grade of Recommendation[b]
Orthopedic Surgery				
Joint replacement	*S. aureus*, *S. epidermidis*	Cefazolin 1 g × 1 preoperatively, then every 8 hours × 2 more doses	Vancomycin reserved for penicillin-allergic patients or where institutional prevalence of methicillin-resistant *S. aureus* warrants use	IA
Hip fracture repair	*S. aureus*, *S. epidermidis*	Cefazolin 1 g × 1 preoperatively, then every 8 hours for 48 hours	Compound fractures are treated as if infection is presumed	IA
Open/compound fractures	*S. aureus*, *S. epidermidis*, gram-negativebacilli, polymicrobial	Cefazolin 1 g × 1 preoperatively, then every 8 hours for a course of presumed infection	Gram-negative coverage (i.e., gentamicin) often indicated for severe open fractures	IA
Neurosurgery				
CSF shunt procedures	*S. aureus*, *S. epidermidis*	Cefazolin 1 g every 8 h × 3 doses or ceftriaxone 2 g × 1	No agents have been shown to be better than cefazolin in randomized comparative trials	IA
Spinal surgery	*S. aureus*, *S. epidermidis*	Cefazolin 1 g × 1	Limited number of clinical trials comparing different treatment regimens	IB
CSF shunt procedures	*S. aureus*, *S. epidermidis*	Cefazolin 1 g every 8 h × 3 doses or ceftriaxone 2 g × 1	No agents have been shown to be better than cefazolin in randomized comparative trials	IA
Craniotomy	*S. aureus*, *S. epidermidis*	Cefazolin 1 g × 1 or cefotaxime 1 g × 1	IV × 1 can be substituted for patients with penicillin allergy Trimethoprim–sulfamethoxazole (160/800 mg)	IA

CSF, cerebrospinal fluid; DS, double strength.

[a]One-time doses are optimally infused at induction of anesthesia except as noted. Repeat doses may be required for long procedures. See the text for references.
[b]Strength of recommendations:
Category IA: Strongly recommended and supported by well-designed experimental, clinical, or epidemiologic studies.
Category IB: Strongly recommended and supported by some experimental, clinical, or epidemiologic studies and strong theoretical rationale.
Category II: Suggested and supported by suggestive clinical or epidemiologic studies or theoretical rationale.

Anaerobes and gram-negative aerobes predominate, but gram-positive aerobes also may play an important role. Reducing this bacterial load with a thorough bowel preparation regimen (4 L of polyethylene glycol solution or 90 mL of sodium phosphate solution administered orally the day before surgery) is controversial; however, 99% of surgeons in a survey routinely use mechanical preparation.[61] Risk factors for SSIs include age over 60 years, hypoalbuminemia, poor preoperative bowel preparation, corticosteroid therapy, malignancy, and operations lasting longer than 3.5 hours.[7]

Antimicrobial prophylaxis reduced mortality from 11.2% to 4.5% in a pooled analysis of trials comparing antimicrobial prophylaxis with no prophylaxis for colon surgery.[62] Effective antibiotic prophylaxis reduces even further the risk for an SSI. Several oral regimens designed to reduce bacterial counts in the colon have been studied.[46] The combination of 1 g neomycin and 1 g erythromycin base given orally 19, 18, and 9 hours preoperatively is the regimen most commonly used in the United States.[63] Neomycin is poorly absorbed, but provides intraluminal concentrations that are high enough to effectively kill most gram-negative aerobes. Oral erythromycin is only partially absorbed but still produces concentrations in the colon that are sufficient to suppress common anaerobes. If surgery is postponed, the antibiotics must be readministered to maintain efficacy. Optimally, the bowel preparation regimen should be completed prior to starting the oral antibiotic regimen. This is of particular concern because most procedures now are performed electively on a "same-day surgery" basis. In this case, the bowel preparation regimen is self-administered by the patient at home on the day prior to hospital admission, and compliance cannot be monitored carefully.

Patients who cannot take oral medications should receive parenteral antibiotics. Cefoxitin or cefotetan is used most commonly, but other second- and some third-generation cephalosporins also are effective.[64] The role of metronidazole in combination with cephalosporin therapy is unclear. Only retrospective evidence suggests that the addition of metronidazole to a cephalosporin or extended-spectrum penicillin provides additional benefit.[65] Until this finding is confirmed in prospective studies, metronidazole should be reserved for combination therapy with cephalosporins with poor anaerobic coverage (e.g., cefazolin). At this time, the evidence recommending the addition of metronidazole to cephalosporins with anaerobic activity (e.g., cefotaxime, cefoxitin, and ceftriaxone) is insufficient.[66] For β-lactam-allergic patients, perioperative doses of gentamicin and metronidazole have been used. Combination therapy (i.e., oral and IV therapy) is controversial. A Cochrane review suggests that combination therapy is superior to either oral or IV antibiotics alone.[66] However, the largest study (491 patients) comparing combination therapy with only IV therapy, which showed no benefit with combination therapy, was not included in the meta-analysis.[67] Postoperative antibiotics generally are unnecessary in the absence of any untoward events or findings during surgery. IV antibiotics are required for colostomy reversal and rectal resection because enterally administered antibiotics will not reach the distal segment that is to be reanastomosed or resected.[68]

Clinical **Controversy...**

A randomized trial of 380 patients undergoing elective colorectal surgery suggests that SSIs are not reduced by preoperative mechanical bowel preparation.[69] This finding was confirmed in a meta-analysis showing that mechanical bowel preparation does not reduce the risk of anastomotic leakage or other complications, including postoperative infection.[70] Despite this new evidence, mechanical bowel preparations continue to be a standard of practice prior to elective bowel surgery.

Gastrointestinal Endoscopy

Despite the large number of endoscopic procedures performed each year, the rate of postprocedural infection is relatively low. The highest bacteremia rates have been reported in patients undergoing esophageal dilation for stricture or sclerotherapy for management of esophageal varices. Although postprocedural bacteremia can occur in as many as 22% of patients, the bacteremia usually is transient (<30 minutes) and rarely results in clinically significant infection. Therefore, antimicrobial prophylaxis is routinely recommended only for high-risk patients (e.g., patients with prosthetic heart valves, a history of endocarditis, systemic-pulmonary shunt, synthetic vascular graft <1 year old, complex cyanotic congenital heart disease, obstructed bile duct, or liver cirrhosis, as well as immunocompromised patients) undergoing high-risk procedures (e.g., stricture dilation, variceal sclerotherapy, and endoscopic retrograde cholangiopancreatography, ERCP).[71] Single-dose preprocedural regimens similar to those for endocarditis prophylaxis are most common (amoxicillin for patients who can tolerate oral premedication or either IV ampicillin or cefazolin). A meta-analysis of antimicrobial prophylaxis for endoscopic placement of percutaneous feeding tubes also suggests that a single preoperative dose of antibiotics reduces the risk of postoperative infection compared with no antibiotic (6.4% vs. 24%).[72] Consensus guidelines have adopted this recommendation and suggest a single dose of cefazolin within 30 minutes prior to the procedure.[71]

Urologic Surgery

Preoperative bacteriuria is the most important risk factor for development of an SSI after urologic surgery. All patients should have a preoperative urinalysis and should receive therapeutic antibiotics if bacteriuria is detected. Patients with sterile urine preoperatively are at low risk for developing an SSI, and the benefit of prophylactic antibiotics in this setting is controversial. Antibiotic prophylaxis is recommended for all patients undergoing transurethral resection of the prostate or bladders tumors, shock-wave lithotripsy, percutaneous renal surgery, or ureteroscopy.[73] The exact incidence of SSIs in this population is obscured by the frequent use of postoperative urinary catheters and the subsequent risk of bacteriuria. *E. coli* is the most frequently encountered organism. Routine use of broad-spectrum antibiotics, such as third-generation cephalosporins and fluoroquinolones, does not decrease SSI rates more than cefazolin, but the ability to administer fluoroquinolones orally rather than IV makes antimicrobial prophylaxis with ciprofloxacin easier and less expensive.[74] First- or second-generation cephalosporins are considered the antimicrobial agents of choice for patients undergoing open or laparoscopic procedures involving entry into the urinary tract and any urologic surgical procedures involving the intestine, rectum, vagina, or implanted prosthesis.[73] The evidence for antimicrobial prophylaxis for the removal of external urinary catheters, cystography, urodynamic studies, simple cystourethroscopy, and open or laparoscopic urologic procedures that do not involve entry into the urinary tract is not as evident. Only patients considered to have risk factors (patients of advanced age; those with anatomic anomalies, poor nutritional history, externalized catheters, colonized endogenous/exogenous material, or distant coexistent infection; smokers; immunocompromised patients; and those who are hospitalized for a prolonged stay) should receive antimicrobial prophylaxis.[73]

Obstetric and Gynecologic Surgeries

Cesarean Section

Cesarean section is the most frequently performed surgical procedure in the United States.[7] Prophylactic antibiotics are given to prevent endometritis, the most commonly occurring SSI. In the past, antibiotics were recommended for only high-risk patients, including those with premature membrane rupture or those not receiving prenatal care. Several large trials, as well as a meta-analysis of 81 trials, have shown benefit in administering prophylactic antibiotics to all women undergoing emergent or elective cesarean section regardless of their underlying risk factors.[75] Cefazolin remains the drug of choice despite the wide spectrum of potential pathogens, and a single 2 g dose appears to be superior to single or multiple 1 g doses.[76] Providing a broader spectrum of coverage with cefoxitin (for anaerobes) or piperacillin (for *Pseudomonas* or enterococci) does not further reduce postoperative infection rates. For patients with a β-lactam allergy, preoperative metronidazole is an acceptable alternative.[75]

Clinical **Controversy. . .**

During a cesarean section, unlike other surgical procedures, the most appropriate timing of antibiotic administration is controversial. Traditionally, antimicrobials were administered after the initial incision and when the umbilical cord was clamped in an attempt to minimize infant drug exposure, which theoretically could mask the signs of neonatal sepsis and select resistant organisms in infants who develop infections. Recent studies and systematic reviews, however, suggest that preincision antibiotics are more effective at preventing postoperative endometritis and other SSIs.[77–79]

Hysterectomy

The most important factor affecting the incidence of SSI after hysterectomy is the type of procedure performed. Vaginal hysterectomies are associated with a high rate of postoperative infection when performed without the benefit of prophylactic antibiotics because of the polymicrobial flora normally present at the operative site.[80] As with cesarean sections, cefazolin is the drug of choice for vaginal hysterectomies despite the wide spectrum of possible pathogens.[80] The American College of Obstetricians and Gynecologists (ACOG) recommends a single dose of either cefazolin or cefoxitin.[81] For patients with a β-lactam allergy, a single preoperative dose of either metronidazole or doxycycline also is effective.[81]

Prophylactic antibiotics are recommended for abdominal hysterectomy despite the lack of bacterial contamination from the vaginal flora. Both cefazolin and antianaerobic cephalosporins (e.g., cefoxitin and cefotetan) have been studied extensively. Single-dose cefotetan is superior to single-dose cefazolin,[82] and the investigators suggest that cefotetan should be the drug of choice for abdominal hysterectomies. However, other investigators suggest that either agent is appropriate, provided 24 hours of antimicrobial coverage is not exceeded.[7] The ACOG guidelines suggest that first-, second-, or third-generation cephalosporins can be used for prophylaxis.[81] Metronidazole also is effective and can be used if patients are allergic to β-lactam antibiotics.[80] Antibiotic prophylaxis may not be required in laparoscopic gynecologic surgery or tubal microsurgery.[83] As with other surgical procedures, perioperative events and findings may require the use of therapeutic antibiotics after surgery.

Head and Neck Surgery

The use of prophylactic antibiotics during head and neck surgery depends on the procedure type. Clean procedures (per NRC definition), such as parotidectomy and simple tooth extraction, are associated with a low incidence of SSI. Head and neck procedures involving an incision through a mucosal layer are associated with a higher risk for SSI. The normal flora of the mouth is polymicrobial; both anaerobes and gram-positive aerobes predominate. Although typical doses of cefazolin usually are ineffective for anaerobic infections, a 2 g dose produces concentrations high enough to inhibit these organisms. A pharmacokinetic study suggested that a single dose of clindamycin is adequate for prophylaxis in maxillofacial surgery unless the procedure lasts longer than 4 hours, when a second dose should be administered intraoperatively.[84] For most head and neck cancer resection surgeries, including free-flap reconstruction, 24 hours of clindamycin is appropriate, and no additional benefit of extending therapy beyond 24 hours is seen. A combination of clindamycin and gentamicin to cover aerobic, anaerobic, and gram-negative bacteria in clean-contaminated oncologic surgery is recommended.[85] Topical therapy with clindamycin, amoxicillin–clavulanate, and ticarcillin–clavulanate has been described in small trials, but the exact role of topical antibiotics is not defined.[86] Antimicrobial prophylaxis is not indicated for endoscopic sinus surgery without nasal packing.[39]

Cardiothoracic Surgery

Although cardiac surgery generally is considered a clean procedure, antibiotic prophylaxis lowers SSI incidence.[46] The substantial morbidity related to an SSI in this population, coupled with the routine implementation of prosthetic devices, further justifies the routine use of prophylaxis.[87] Patients who develop SSIs after coronary artery bypass graft surgery have a mortality rate of 22% at 1 year compared with 0.6% for those who do not develop an SSI.[88] Risk factors for developing an SSI after cardiac surgery include obesity, renal insufficiency, connective tissue disease, reexploration for bleeding, and poorly timed administration of antibiotics.[87] Skin flora pathogens predominate; gram-negative organisms are rare.

Cefazolin has been studied extensively and is considered the drug of choice. Although several studies and a meta-analysis advocate the use of second-generation cephalosporins (e.g., cefuroxime) rather than cefazolin, various methodologic flaws in these studies have limited the extrapolation of these results to practice. Cefazolin was as effective as cefuroxime in a large randomized trial of 702 patients undergoing open heart surgery and thus remains the standard of care.[89] Both patient weight and timing of cefazolin administration relative to surgery must be considered when developing a dosing strategy. Patients weighing >80 kg (176 lb) should receive 2 g cefazolin rather than 1 g. Doses should be administered no earlier than 60 minutes before the first incision and no later than the beginning of induction.[85] Extending therapy beyond 48 hours does not further reduce SSI rates. Single-dose cefazolin therapy may be sufficient but is not recommended by the Society of Thoracic Surgeons at this time pending further study.[90]

7 Routine vancomycin administration may be justified in hospitals having a high incidence of MRSA or when sternal wounds are to be explored surgically for possible mediastinitis. However, a large comparative trial enrolling almost 900 patients in a single center with a high prevalence of MRSA infections found that both cefazolin and vancomycin had similar efficacy in preventing SSI in patients undergoing cardiac surgery that required sternotomy.[91] Mediastinitis constitutes a failure of a prior prophylactic regimen. Continued postoperative vancomycin should be guided by culture and sensitivity data.[40] Subsequent antibiotic therapy is guided by intraoperative findings.

Pulmonary resection is associated with significant SSI risk, and prophylactic antibiotics have an established role in preventing postoperative infectious morbidity. Pleuropulmonary infections are much more common than wound infections, and pathogenic organisms likely migrate from the oral cavity or pharynx.[92] First-generation cephalosporins are inadequate; 48 hours of cefuroxime is preferred. A regimen of ampicillin–sulbactam is superior to first-generation cephalosporins, but further studies are required before this agent can be recommended as first-line prophylactic therapy.[93]

Vascular Surgery

Vascular surgery, like cardiac surgery, generally is considered clean by NRC criteria. Although vascular graft infections occur infrequently (3% to 5%), the associated morbidity and mortality are extensive because treatment often requires surgical graft removal along with therapeutic antibiotic therapy.[94] Prophylactic antibiotics are of benefit, particularly for procedures involving the abdominal aorta and the lower extremities. Cefazolin is regarded as the drug of choice.[95] Twenty-four hours of prophylaxis with cefazolin is adequate; longer courses may lead to bacterial resistance.[96] For patients with β-lactam allergy, 24 hours of oral ciprofloxacin has been shown to be effective.[94]

Orthopedic Surgery

Most orthopedic surgery is clean by definition; thus, prophylactic antibiotics generally are indicated only when prosthetic materials (e.g., pins, plates, and artificial joints) are implanted.[20] A late-occurring infectious complication in this surgical population can result in substantial morbidity and may lead to prosthesis failure and subsequent removal. Staphylococci are the most frequently encountered pathogens; gram-negative aerobes are infrequent. The use of cefazolin is supported by substantial evidence in the literature and therefore is the prophylactic agent of choice. Vancomycin, although effective, is not recommended for routine use unless a patient has a documented history of a serious allergy to β-lactams, or the propensity for MRSA infections at a particular institution necessitates its use. The current recommended duration of prophylaxis for joint replacement and hip fracture surgery is 24 hours.[7] Antibiotic-impregnated cement and beads have been used to lower SSI rates, but conclusive data regarding their efficacy are lacking.[20]

Duration of prophylaxis for the surgical repair of long bone fractures depends on the nature of the fracture. Multiple doses of prophylactic antibiotics offer no advantage over a single preoperative dose for repair of closed bone fractures and is more cost effective.[97,98] Patients suffering open (compound) fractures are particularly susceptible to infection because bacterial contamination almost always has occurred already. Under these circumstances, the use of antibiotics is presumptive. In this setting, cefazolin often is combined with an aminoglycoside, but controlled trials are lacking.[99] A clinical trial comparing clindamycin and cloxacillin suggests that clindamycin is superior and may be appropriate as monotherapy for Gustilo type I and II open fractures but not for type III fractures, for which added gram-negative activity is recommended.[100] Duration of antibiotic therapy is highly variable and depends on surgical findings during debridement, results of intraoperative cultures, and clinical status. A prospective trial comparing short (<24 hours) and long (>24 hours) courses of antimicrobial prophylaxis for severe trauma suggests that longer courses of antibiotics do not offer additional benefit and may be associated with the development of resistant infections.[101] However, established joint infections and osteomyelitis require an extended course of therapeutic antibiotics.

Neurosurgery

Definitive recommendations on the role of antibiotic prophylaxis in neurosurgery cannot be made at this time.[102] Although the rates of SSI after these generally clean operations are low, the morbidity and mortality of SSI, should they occur, are high. Procedures involving cerebrospinal fluid (CSF) shunt placement should be considered separately because this procedure involves placement of a foreign body and is associated with higher infection rates. When choosing an antibiotic, considerations include not only the spectrum of activity but also the penetration of the agent into the site of action (CSF). A meta-analysis suggested that single doses of cefazolin or, where required, vancomycin appear to lower SSI risk after craniotomy.[103] The largest prospective randomized trial to date of 826 patients undergoing clean neurosurgical procedures suggested that a single dose of ceftizoxime was as effective as a combination regimen of single-dose vancomycin and gentamicin. The authors also reported that ceftizoxime was better tolerated and more consistently achieved adequate CSF levels to inhibit the most common organisms.[104] A study of 780 patients undergoing neurosurgical procedures that included shunt surgery reported that single doses of cefotaxime and trimethoprim–sulfamethoxazole were equally effective in preventing SSIs.[105] Most studies of procedures involving a shunt have been small in size and do not consistently show lower infection rates with antibiotic prophylaxis, although the results of a systematic review and meta-analysis suggest that a significant improvement in the incidence of shunt infection with 24 hours of systemic antibiotics (i.e., cefazolin) and the use of antibiotic-impregnated catheters independently.[106]

SSIs associated with spinal surgery are rare but devastating when they occur. The use of antimicrobial prophylaxis in this setting is warranted and recommended by a meta-analysis.[107] Large randomized, controlled trials are lacking, but cefazolin is the antibiotic recommended most commonly. Cephalosporin penetration into the vertebral disk has been questioned. Some small studies suggest that the addition of gentamicin, which has better penetration, might be warranted; however, there is a paucity of clinical trials comparing these two regimens.[108]

Minimally Invasive and Laparoscopic Surgery

Laparoscopic surgeries are being performed frequently for a variety of different operations, including gynecologic, orthopedic, and colorectal surgeries. This minimally invasive technique is associated with smaller wounds, fewer infectious complications, smaller inflammatory response, and therefore a better-preserved immune response to infection compared with the open surgical approach.[109] In colorectal surgery the laparoscopic approach is associated with a 40% reduction in SSI when compared to the open surgical approach.[110,111] The role of antimicrobial prophylaxis in this setting depends on the type of surgery performed and preexisting risk factors for infection. Unfortunately, few large prospective, placebo-controlled trials have determined in which patients and surgeries antimicrobial prophylaxis is warranted.

In addition to the recommendations for previously mentioned laparoscopic procedures, there is a variety of levels of evidence for prophylaxis in other laparoscopic and endoscopic procedures. Patients undergoing ERCP do not need antimicrobial prophylaxis unless biliary obstruction is evident. In these situations, a single 1 g dose of cefazolin will suffice.[112] The role of antimicrobial prophylaxis for transurethral resection of the prostate is better established. A third-generation cephalosporin such as ceftriaxone (or cotrimoxazole for severely β-lactam-allergic patients) can be recommended as single-dose prophylaxis, especially for patients with nonsterile urine preoperatively or indwelling catheters.[112] Insertion of peritoneal dialysis catheters by the laparoscopic technique is associated with significantly lower rates of postoperative infection. With SSI rates less than 5%, prophylactic antimicrobial therapy may not be warranted, but this has not been studied in a sufficiently large placebo-controlled trial. If the decision to provide antimicrobial prophylaxis is made, a single dose of cefazolin will suffice.[112]

NONPHARMACOLOGIC INTERVENTIONS

Strategies other than antimicrobial and aseptic technique for reducing postoperative infections have been investigated in different types of surgeries. The most commonly cited and practiced interventions include intraoperative maintenance of normothermia, provision of supplemental oxygen in the perioperative period, and aggressive perioperative glucose control.

Clinical **Controversy...**

Although interventions to maintain normothermia intraoperatively, provide supplemental oxygen in the perioperative period, and aggressively control perioperative glucose show a significant reduction in SSI, they cannot be generalized to all types of surgeries. However, given the simplicity and low cost of these interventions, many clinicians consider applying these measures outside of the studied population(s). At this time, pending further research, these interventions can be recommended for routine use only in the type of patient or surgery for which they were studied.

Core body temperature can fall by 1 to 1.5°C (33.8 to 34.7°F) intraoperatively in patients under general anesthesia. Intraoperative hypothermia has been associated with impaired immune function, decreased blood flow to the surgical site, decreased tissue oxygen tension, and an increased risk of SSI. Efforts to maintain intraoperative normothermia should be exercised and may include the use of warming blankets and IV fluid warmers to maintain core body temperature above 36.1°C (97°F). One prospective trial of 200 patients undergoing colorectal surgery found that maintenance of normothermia reduced postoperative infection rates along with other morbidity parameters, including length of stay.[113]

Clinical **Controversy...**

Several studies have investigated the role of specialized enteral formulas fortified with a variety of immunomodulating micronutrients thought to enhance the immune response and gut function after trauma or surgery. Although many clinicians are exploring the role of supplements such as glutamine, arginine, omega fatty acids, and nucleotides, no study to date has shown a significant reduction in postoperative infection rates using these formulations.

Low oxygen tension in the tissues that make up the surgical site increases the risk of bacterial colonization and subsequent SSI by decreasing the efficiency of neutrophil activity. Administration of high concentrations of oxygen (80% via ventilator or 12 L/min via a nonrebreather mask) reduced postoperative infection rates significantly in a multicenter randomized trial of 500 patients undergoing colorectal surgery.[114]

Diabetes and poor glucose control are well-known risk factors for SSI. The increased risk of infection is thought to be due to both macrovascular (vasculopathy and venoocclusive disease) and microvascular (subtle immunologic deficiencies, including neutrophil dysfunction and reduced complement and antibody activity)

TABLE 101-7 Strategies for Implementing an Institutional Program to Ensure Appropriate Use of Antimicrobial Prophylaxis in Surgery

1. Educate
Develop an educational program that enforces the importance and rationale of timely antimicrobial prophylaxis
Make this educational program available to all healthcare practitioners involved in the patient's care
2. Standardize the ordering process
Establish a protocol (e.g., a preprinted order sheet) that standardizes antibiotic choice according to current published evidence, formulary availability, institutional resistance patterns, and cost
3. Standardize the delivery and administration process
Use system that ensures antibiotics are prepared and delivered to the holding area in a timely fashion
Standardize the administration time to less than 1 hour preoperatively
Designate responsibility and accountability for antibiotic administration
Provide visible reminders to prescribe/administer prophylactic antibiotics (e.g., checklists)
Develop a system to remind surgeons/nurses to readminister antibiotics intraoperatively during long procedures
4. Provide feedback
Follow up with regular reports of compliance and infection rates

complications. Aggressive control of perioperative blood glucose level decreases the incidence of SSI in diabetics undergoing cardiac surgery and is being evaluated in other types of surgery and in nondiabetic patients.[115]

PERSONALIZED PHARMACOTHERAPY

Prophylactic antibiotics are only effective when therapeutic concentrations in the surgical field are maintained for the entire duration of the surgery. While consideration of drug half-life in the context of the duration of surgery has been discussed earlier in this chapter, other patient-related factors may influence the effectiveness of antibiotic prophylaxis and warrant consideration when choosing a prophylactic regimen (Table 101-7).

Obese patients require larger doses of prophylactic antibiotics to maintain therapeutic drug levels when compared to nonobese patients. Pharmacokinetic studies suggest that patients with a body mass index greater than 40 are more likely to have subtherapeutic concentrations at the end of surgery with cefazolin 1 g preoperatively (and intraoperative for surgeries >3 hours) and thus should receive 2 g doses.[116,117] Underlying disease states that may affect antibiotic metabolism and/or elimination should be considered when developing a prophylactic regimen. For example, patients with thermal burn and spinal cord injuries eliminate certain classes of antibiotics, primarily the aminoglycosides and β-lactams, at unusually high rates compared with controls and will need more frequent intraoperative dosing. Conversely, individuals with renal failure may need less frequent dosing of renally cleared antibiotics. For example, while intraoperative dosing for cefazolin should be every 3 to 4 hours in patients with normal renal function, this interval should be extended to 8 hours for patients with creatinine clearances of less than 50 mL/min (83 mL/s). Individuals who are aggressively fluid resuscitated pre- or intraoperatively or those undergoing cardiac bypass may have altered antibiotic disposition related to increased volume of distribution and reduced total body clearance and may need larger doses (i.e., 2 g cefazolin).

EVALUATION OF THERAPEUTIC OUTCOMES

When evaluating the outcome of surgical antibiotic prophylaxis, it is important to differentiate any potential SSI from other postoperative infection or complication. Although fever and leukocytosis are common in the immediate postoperative period, they typically resolve with prompt ambulation, timely removal of invasive devices, prevention and/or resolution of atelectasis through optimal respiratory care, and effective analgesia. It is important to remember that the emergence of distal infections, such as pneumonia, does not constitute a failure of surgical prophylaxis. Prophylaxis should be as short as possible because prolonged prophylactic regimens may contribute to the selection of resistant organisms and may make any infection more difficult to treat.

Surgical site appearance is the most important determinant of the presence of an infection. Drainage of pus from the incision accompanied by redness, warmth, and pain or tenderness is highly suggestive of an SSI. By definition, any surgical site that requires incision and drainage by the surgeon is considered infected regardless of appearance. Failure to heal and wound dehiscence also are seen with SSIs, although the surgical technique and nutritional status may be important contributing factors.

The presentation of signs and symptoms consistent with an SSI in relation to previous surgery is an important consideration when evaluating therapeutic outcomes after surgical prophylaxis. Many SSIs will not be evident during acute hospitalization. In fact, SSIs may not become evident until up to 30 days later or, in the case of prosthesis implantation, up to 1 year later. Thus, the true incidence of SSI can be determined only by completing comprehensive postdischarge surveillance. All studies investigating the efficacy of surgical prophylaxis must include adequate postdischarge follow-up to be able to thoroughly assess the success of any prophylactic regimen.

ABBREVIATIONS

ACOG	American College of Obstetricians and Gynecologists
ASA	American Society of Anesthesiologists
CDC	Centers for Disease Control and Prevention
CSF	cerebrospinal fluid
MRSA	methicillin-resistant *Staphylococcus aureus*
MSSA	methicillin-sensitive *Staphylococcus aureus*
NNIS	National Nosocomial Infections Surveillance System
NRC	National Research Council
SENIC	Study on the Efficacy of Nosocomial Infection Control
SSI	surgical site infection

REFERENCES

1. Mitka M. Preventing surgical infection is more important than ever. JAMA 2000;283:44–45.
2. Alexander JW, Solomkin JS, Edwards MJ. Updated recommendations for control of surgical site infections. Ann Surg 2011;253:1082–1093.
3. Mangram AJ, Horan TC, Pearson ML, et al. Guideline for prevention of surgical site infection, 1999. Centers for Disease Control and Prevention (CDC) Hospital Infection Control Practices Advisory Committee. Am J Infect Control 1999;27:97–132.
4. Hendrick TL, Anastacio MM, Sawyer RG. Prevention of surgical site infection. Expert Rev Anti Infect Ther 2006; 4:223–233.

5. National Academy of Sciences, National Research Council. Postoperative wound infections: The influence of ultraviolet irradiation of the operating room and of various other factors. Ann Surg 1964;160:32–135.
6. Cruse PJE, Foord R. A five-year prospective study of 23,649 surgical wounds. Arch Surg 1973;107:206–210.
7. ASHP Commission on Therapeutics. ASHP therapeutic guidelines on antimicrobial prophylaxis in surgery. In: Deffenbaugh J, ed. Best Practices for Health System Pharmacy. Bethesda, MD: ASHP, 1999:349–396.
8. Drapeau CMJ, Pan A, Bellacosa C, et al. Surgical site infections in HIV-infected patients: Results from an Italian prospective multicenter observational study. Infection 2009;37:455–460.
9. Dionigi R, Rovera F, Dionigi G, et al. Risk factors in surgery. J Chemother 2001;13:6–11.
10. Perl TM, Cullen JJ, Wenzel RP, et al. Intranasal mupirocin to prevent postoperative *Staphylococcus aureus* infections. N Engl J Med 2002;346:1871–1877.
11. Haley RW, Culver DH, Morgan WM, et al. Identifying patients at high risk of surgical wound infection: A simple multivariate index of patient susceptibility and wound contamination. Am J Epidemiol 1985;127:206–215.
12. Wilson AP, Hodgson B, Liu M, et al. Reduction in wound infection rates by wound surveillance with postdischarge follow-up and feedback. Br J Surg 2006;93:630–638.
13. Gaynes RP, Culver DH, Horan TC, et al. Surgical site infection (SSI) rates in the United States, 1992–1998: The National Nosocomial Infections Surveillance System basic SSI risk index. Clin Infect Dis 2001;33(Suppl 2):S69–S77.
14. National Nosocomial Infections Surveillance (NNIS) System Report, data summary from January 1992 through June 2004 issued October 2004. Am J Infect Control 2004;32:470–485.
15. Owens WD, Felts JA, Spitznagel EL. ASA physical status classifications: A study of consistency of ratings. Anesthesiology 1978;49:239–243.
16. Elek SD, Conen PE. The virulence of *Staphylococcus pyogenes* for man: A study of the problems of wound infection. Br J Exp Pathol 1958;38:573–586.
17. Burke JF. Identification of the sources of staphylococci contaminating the surgical wound during operation. Ann Surg 1963;158:898–904.
18. Kaiser AB, Kernodle DS, Parker RA. Low-inoculum model of surgical wound infection. J Infect Dis 1992;166:393–399.
19. Esposito S. Immune system and surgical site infection. J Chemother 2001;13:12–16.
20. De Lalla F. Antibiotic prophylaxis in orthopedic prosthetic surgery. J Chemother 2001;13:48–53.
21. Halwani M, Solaymani-Dodaran M, Grundman H, et al. Cross transmission of nosocomial pathogens in an adult intensive care unit: Incidence and risk factors. J Hosp Infect 2006;63:39–46.
22. Crawford T, Rodvold KA, Solomkin JS. Vancomycin for surgical prophylaxis? Clin Infect Dis 2012;54:1474–1479.
23. Weigelt JA, Lipsky BA, Tabak YP et al. Surgical site infection: Causative pathogens and associated outcomes. Am J Infect Control 2010;38:112–120.
24. Chambers D, Worthy G, Myers L, et al. Glycopeptide vs. non-glycopeptide antibiotics for prophylaxis of surgical site infections: A systematic review. Surg Infect (Larchmt) 2010;11:455–462.
25. Ramirez MC, Marchessault M, Govednik-Horny C, et al. The impact of MRSA colonization on surgical site infection following major gastrointestinal surgery. J Gastrointest Surg 2013;17:144–152; DOI 10.1007/s11605-012-1995-2.
26. Kim DH, Spencer M, Davidson SM, et al. Institutional prescreening for detection and eradication of methicillin-resistant *Staphylococcus aureus* in patients undergoing elective orthopaedic surgery. J Bone Joint Surg Am 2010; 92:1820–1826.
27. Lowy FD, Waldhausen JA, Miller M, et al. Report of the National Heart, Lung and Blood Institute–National Institute of Allergy and Infectious Diseases working group on antimicrobial strategies and cardiothoracic surgery. Am Heart J 2004:147:575–581.
28. Munoz P, Burrillo A, Bouza E. Criteria used when initiating antifungal therapy against *Candida* spp. in the intensive care unit. Int J Antimicrob Agents 2000;15:83–90.
29. Lipsett PA. Surgical critical care: Fungal infections in surgical patients. Crit Care Med 2006;34:S25–S24.
30. McKinnon PS. Goff DA, Kern JW, et al. Temporal assessment of *Candida* risk factors in the surgical intensive care unit. Arch Surg 2001;136:1401–1408.
31. Classen DC, Evans RS, Pestotnik SL, et al. The timing of prophylactic administration of antibiotics and the risk of surgical wound infection. N Engl J Med 1992;326:281–286.
32. Weber WP, Marti WR, Zwahlen M, et al. The timing of surgical antimicrobial prophylaxis. Ann Surg 2008;247: 918–926.
33. Steinberg JP, Braun BI, Hellinger WC, et al. Timing of antimicrobial prophylaxis and the risk of surgical site infections: Results from the trial to reduce antimicrobial prophylaxis errors. Ann Surg 2009;250:10–16.
34. Bratzler DW, Houck PM, Richards C, et al. Use of antimicrobial prophylaxis for major surgery: Baseline results from the National Surgical Infection Prevention Project. Arch Surg 2005;140:174–182.
35. Zelenitzky SA, Ariano RE, Harding GKM, et al. Antibiotic pharmacodynamics in surgical prophylaxis: An association between intraoperative antibiotic concentrations and efficacy. Antimicrob Agents Chemother 2002;46:3026–3030.
36. Goldman DA, Hopkins CC, Karchmer AW. Cephalothin prophylaxis in cardiac valve surgery: A prospective, double-blind comparison of two-day and six-day regimen. J Thorac Cardiovasc Surg 1977;73:470–479.
37. Zanetti G, Flanagan HL Jr, Cohn LH, et al. Improvement of intraoperative antibiotic prophylaxis in prolonged cardiac surgery by automated alerts in the operating room. Infect Control Hosp Epidemiol 2003;24:7–9.
38. Waltrip T, Lewis R, Young V, et al. A pilot study to determine the feasibility of continuous cefazolininfusion. Surg Infect 2002;3:5–9.
39. Weed HG. Antimicrobial prophylaxis in the surgical patient. Med Clin North Am 2003;27:59–75.
40. Salkind AR, Cuddy PG, Foxworth JW. The rational clinical examination: Is this patient allergic to penicillin? An evidence-based analysis of the likelihood of penicillin allergy. JAMA 2001;285:2498–2505.
41. Gemmel CG, Edwards DI, Fraise AP, et al. Guidelines for the prophylaxis and treatment of methicillin *Staphylococcus aureus* (MRSA) infections in the UK. J Antimicrob Chemother 2006;57:589–608.
42. Hadaway L, Chamallas SN. Vancomycin: New perspectives on an old drug. J Infus Nurs 2003;26:278–284.
43. Wong RS, Cheng G, Chang NP, et al. Use of cefoperazone still needs a caution for bleeding from induced vitamin K deficiency. Am J Hematol 2006;81:76.
44. Williams KJ, Bax RP, Brown H, Machin SJ. Antibiotic treatment and associated prolonged prothrombin time. J Clin Pathol 1991;44:738–741.

45. Frighetto L, Marra CA, Stiver HG, et al. Economic impact of standardized orders for antimicrobial prophylaxis program. Ann Pharmacother 2000;34:154–160.
46. Bratzler DW, Houck PM. Antimicrobial prophylaxis for surgery: An advisory statement from the National Surgical Infection Prevention Project. Clin Infect Dis 2004;38: 1706–1715.
47. Anderson DJ. Surgical site infections. Infect Dis Clin North Am 2011;25:135–153.
48. McArdle CS, Morran CG, Anderson JR, et al. Oral ciprofloxacin as prophylaxis in gastroduodenal surgery. J Hosp Infect 1995;30:211–216.
49. Sharma VK, Howden CW. Meta-analysis of randomized, controlled trials of antibiotic prophylaxis before percutaneous endoscopic gastrostomy. Am J Gastroenterol 2000;95: 3133–3136.
50. Kulling D, Sonnenberg A, Fried M, Bauerfeind P. Cost analysis of antibiotic prophylaxis for PEG. Gastrointest Endosc 2000;51:152–156.
51. Jewesson PJ, Stiver G, Wai A, et al. Double-blind comparison of cefazolin and ceftizoxime for prophylaxis against infections following elective biliary tract surgery. Antimicrob Agents Chemother 1996;40:70–74.
52. Agrawal CS, Sehgal R, Singh RK, Gupta AK. Antibiotic prophylaxis in elective cholecystectomy: A randomized, double-blinded study comparing ciprofloxacin and cefuroxime. Ind J Physiol Pharmacol 1999;43:501–504.
53. Swoboda S, Oberdorfer K, Klee F, et al. Tissue and serum concentrations of levofloxacin 500 mg administered intravenously or orally for antibiotic prophylaxis in biliary surgery. J Antimicrob Chemother 2003;51:459–462.
54. Koc M, Zulfikaroglu B, Kece C, et al. A prospective, randomized study of prophylactic antibiotics in elective laparoscopic cholecystectomy. Surg Endosc 2003;17: 1716–1718.
55. Gulberg V, Deibert P, Ochs A, et al. Prevention of infectious complications after transjugular intrahepatic portosystemic shunt in cirrhotic patients with a single dose of ceftriaxone. Hepatogastroenterology 1999;46:1126–1130.
56. Deibert P, Schwartz S, Olschewski M, et al. Risk factors and prevention of early infection after implantation or revision of transjugular intrahepatic portosystemic shunts: Results of a randomized study. Dig Dis Sci 1998;43:1708–1713.
57. Sheen-Chen SM, Chen WJ, Eng HL, et al. Bacteriology and antimicrobial choice in hepatolithiasis. Am J Infect Control 2000;28:298–301.
58. Liberman MA, Greason KL, Frame S, Ragland JJ. Single-dose cefotetan or cefoxitin versus multiple-dose cefoxitin as prophylaxis in patients undergoing appendectomy for acute nonperforated appendicitis. J Am Coll Surg 1995;180:77–80.
59. Colliza S, Rossi S. Antibiotic prophylaxis and treatment of surgical abdominal sepsis. J Chemother 2001;13:193–201.
60. Chung RS, Rowland DY, Li P, Diaz J. A meta-analysis of randomized, controlled trials of laparoscopic versus conventional appendectomy. Am J Surg 1999;177:250–256.
61. Zmora O, Wexner SD, Hajjar L, et al. Trend in preparation for colorectal surgery: Survey of the members of the American Society of Colon and Rectal Surgeons. Am Surg 2003;69:150–154.
62. Baum ML, Anish DS, Chalmers TC, et al. A survey of clinical trials of antibiotic prophylaxis in colon surgery: Evidence against further use of no-treatment controls. N Engl J Med 1981;305:795–799.
63. Solla JA, Rothenberger DA. Preoperative bowel preparation: A survey of colon and rectal surgeons. Dis Colon Rectum 1990;33:154–159.
64. Fujita S, Saito N, Yamada T, et al. Randomized, multicenter trial of antibiotic prophylaxis in elective colorectal surgery: Single dose vs 3 doses of a second-generation cephalosporin without metronidazole and oral antibiotics. Arch Surg 2007;142:657–661.
65. Mittelkotter U. Antimicrobial prophylaxis for abdominal surgery: Is there a need for metronidazole? J Chemother 2001;13:27–34.
66. Kobayashi M, Mohri Y, Tonouchi H, et al. Randomized clinical trial comparing intravenous antimicrobial prophylaxis alone with oral and intravenous antimicrobial prophylaxis for the prevention of a surgical site infection in colorectal cancer surgery. Surg Today 2007;37:383–388.
67. Nelson RL, Glenny AM, Song F. Antimicrobial prophylaxis for colorectal surgery. Cochrane Database Syst Rev 2009;1:CD001181.
68. Ghorra SG, Rzeczycki TP, Natarajan R, Pricolo VE. Colostomy closure: Impact of preoperative risk factors on morbidity. Am Surg 1999;65:266–269.
69. Zmora O, Mahajna A, Bar-Zakai B, et al. Colon and rectal surgery without mechanical bowel preparation: A randomized, prospective trial. Ann Surg 2003;237:363–367.
70. Cao F, Li J, Li F. Mechanical bowel preparation for elective colorectal surgery: Updated systematic review and meta-analysis. Int J Colorectal Dis 2012;27:803–810.
71. Hirota WK, Petersen K, Baron TH, et al. Guidelines for antibiotic prophylaxis for GI endoscopy. Gastrointest Endosc 2003;58:475–482.
72. Sharma VK, Howden CW. Meta-analysis of randomized, controlled trials of antibiotic prophylaxis before percutaneous endoscopic gastrostomy. Am J Gastroenterol 2001;96:1951–1952.
73. Wolf Jr JS, Bennett CJ, Dmochowski RR, Hollenbeck BK, Pearles MS, Schaeffer AJ. Best practice policy statement on urologic surgery antimicrobial prophylaxis. J Urol 2008;179:1379–1390.
74. Christiano AP, Hollowell CM, Kim H, et al. Double-blind, randomized comparison of single-dose ciprofloxacin versus intravenous cefazolin in patients undergoing outpatient endourologic surgery. Urology 2000;55:182–185.
75. Smaill F, Hofmeyr GJ. Antibiotic prophylaxis for cesarean section. Cochrane Database Syst Rev 2002;2:CD000933.
76. Rouzi AA, Khalifa F, Ba'aqeel H, et al. The routine use of cefazolin in cesarean section. Int J Gynaecol Obstet 2000;69:107–112.
77. Tita ATN, Rouse DJ, Blackwell S, Saade GR, Spong CY, Andrews WW. Emerging concepts in antibiotic prophylaxis for cesarean delivery: A systematic review. Obstet Gynecol 2009;113:675–682.
78. Witt A, Donner M, Petricevic L, et al. Antibiotic prophylaxis before surgery vs after cord clamping in elective cesarean delivery: A double-blind, prospective, randomized, placebo-controlled trial. Arch Surg 2011;146:1404–1409.
79. Macones GA, Cleary KL, Parry S, et al. The timing of antibiotics at cesarean: A randomized controlled trial. Am J Perinatol 2012;29:273–276.
80. Guaschino S, De Santo D, De Seta F. New perspectives in antibiotic prophylaxis for obstetric and gynaecological surgery. J Hosp Infect 2002;50(Suppl A):S13–S16.
81. American College of Obstetricians and Gynecologists. Antibiotic prophylaxis for gynecologic procedures. Obstet Gynecol 2006;108:225–234.
82. Hemsell DL, Johnson ER, Hemsell PG, et al. Cefazolin is inferior to cefotetan as single dose prophylaxis for women undergoing elective total abdominal hysterectomy. Clin Infect Dis 1995;20:677–684.

83. Sturlese E, Retto G, Pulia A, et al. Benefits of antibiotic prophylaxis in laparoscopic gynaecological surgery. Clin Exp Obstet Gynecol 1999;26:217–218.
84. Meuller SC, Henkel KO, Neumann J, et al. Perioperative antibiotic prophylaxis in maxillofacial surgery: Penetration of clindamycin into various tissues. J Craniomaxillofac Surg 1999;27:172–176.
85. Simo R, French G. The use of prophylactic antibiotics in head and neck oncological surgery. Curr Opin Otolaryngol Head Neck Surg 2006;14:55–61.
86. Grandis JR, Vickers RM, Rihs JD, et al. Efficacy of topical amoxicillin plus clavulanate–ticarcillin plus clavulanate and clindamycin in contaminated head and neck surgery: Effect of antibiotic spectra and duration of therapy. J Infect Dis 1994;170:729–732.
87. Roy MC. Surgical-site infections after coronary artery bypass graft surgery: Discriminating site-specific risk factors to improve prevention efforts. Infect Control Hosp Epidemiol 1998;19:229–233.
88. Hollenbeak CS, Murphy DM, Koenig S, et al. The clinical and economic impact of deep chest surgical site infections following coronary artery bypass graft surgery. Chest 2000; 118:397–402.
89. Curtis JJ, Boley TM, Walls JT, et al. Randomized, prospective comparison of first- and second-generation cephalosporins as infection prophylaxis for cardiac surgery. Am J Surg 1993;166:734–737.
90. Edwards FH, Egleman RM, Houck P, et al. The Society of Thoracic Surgeons Practice Guidelines Series: Antibiotic prophylaxis in cardiac surgery, part 1: duration. Ann Thorac Surg 2006;81:397–404.
91. Finkelstein R, Rabino G, Masiah T, et al. Vancomycin versus cefazolin prophylaxis for cardiac surgery in the setting of a high prevalence of methicillin-resistant staphylococcal infections. J Thorac Cardiovasc Surg 2002;123:326–332.
92. Sok M, Dragas AZ, Erzen J, et al. Sources of pathogens causing pleuropulmonary infections after lung cancer resection. Eur J Cardiothorac Surg 2002;22:23–27.
93. Boldt J, Piper S, Uphus D, et al. Preoperative microbiologic screening and antibiotic prophylaxis in pulmonary resection operations. Ann Thorac Surg 1999;68:208–211.
94. Pratesi C, Russo D, Dorigo W, et al. Antibiotic prophylaxis in clean surgery: Vascular surgery. J Chemother 2001;13: 123–128.
95. Douglas A, Udy AA, Wallis S, et al. Plasma and tissue pharmacokinetics of cefazolin in patients undergoing elective and semielective abdominal aortic aneurysm open repair surgery. Antimicrob Agents Chemother 2011;55: 5238–5242.
96. Terpstra S, Noorkhoek GT, Voesten HG, et al. Rapid emergence of resistant coagulase-negative staphylococci on the skin after antibiotic prophylaxis. J Hosp Infect 1999;43:195–202.
97. Slobogean GP, Kennedy SA, Davidson, et al. Single- versus multiple-dose antibiotic prophylaxis in the surgical treatment of closed fractures: A meta-analysis. J Orthop Trauma 2008;22:264–269.
98. Slobogean PG, O'Brien PJ, Brauer CA. Single-dose versus multiple-dose antibiotic prophylaxis for the surgical treatment of closed fractures: A cost-effective analysis. Acta Orthop 2010;81:256–262.
99. Gillespie WJ, Walenkamp G. Antibiotic prophylaxis for surgery for proximal femoral and other closed long bone fractures. Cochrane Database Syst Rev 2001;1:CD000244.
100. Vasenius J, Tulikoura I, Vainionpaa S, Rokkanen P. Clindamycin versus cloxacillin in the treatment of 240 open fractures: A randomized, prospective study. Ann Chir Gynaecol 1998;87:224–228.
101. Velmahos GC, Toutouzas KG, Sarkisyan G, et al. Severe trauma is not an excuse for prolonged antibiotic prophylaxis. Arch Surg 2002;137:537–541.
102. Hosein IK, Hill DW, Hatfield RH. Controversies in the prevention of neurosurgical infection. J Hosp Infect 1999; 43:5–11.
103. Barker FG. Efficacy of prophylactic antibiotics for craniotomy: A meta-analysis. Neurosurgery 1994;35:484–492.
104. Pons VG, Denlinger SL, Guglielmo BJ, et al. Ceftizoxime versus vancomycin and gentamicin in neurosurgical prophylaxis: A randomized, prospective, blinded clinical trial. Neurosurgery 1993;33:416–422.
105. Whitby M, Johnson BC, Atkinson RL, et al. The comparative efficacy of intravenous cefotaxime and trimethoprim/ sulfamethoxazole in preventing infection after neurosurgery: A prospective, randomized study. Brisbane Neurosurgical Infection Group. Br J Neurosurg 2000;14:13–18.
106. Ratilal B, Costa J, Sampaio C. Antibiotic prophylaxis for surgical introduction of intracranial ventricular shunts: A systematic review. J Neurosurg Pediatr 2008;1:48–56.
107. Barker FG. Efficacy of prophylactic antibiotic therapy in spinal surgery: A meta-analysis. Neurosurgery 2002;51: 391–400.
108. Riley LH 3rd. Prophylactic antibiotics for spine surgery: Description of a regimen and its rationale. J South Orthop Assoc 1998;7:212–217.
109. Balague Ponz C, Trias M. Laparoscopic surgery and surgical infection. J Chemother 2001;13:17–22.
110. Aimaq R, Akopian G, Kaufman HS. Surgical site infection rates in laparoscopic versus open colorectal surgery. Am Surg 2011;77:1290–1294.
111. Kiran RP, El-Gazzaz GH, Vogel JD, et al. Laparoscopic approach significantly reduces surgical site infections after colorectal surgery: Data from national surgical quality improvement program. J Am Coll Surg 2010;211:232–238.
112. Wilson APR. Antibiotic prophylaxis in endoscopic and minimally invasive surgery. J Chemother 2001;13:102–107.
113. Kurz A, Sessler DI, Lenhardt R. Perioperative normothermia to reduce the incidence of surgical-wound infection and shorten hospitalization. Study of Wound Infection and Temperature Group. N Engl J Med 1996;334:1209–1215.
114. Greif R, Akca O, Horn EP, et al. Supplemental perioperative oxygen to reduce the incidence of surgical-wound infection. Outcomes Research Group. N Engl J Med 2000;342:161–167.
115. Kao LS, Meeks D, Moyer VA, Lally KP. Peri-operative glycaemic control regimens for preventing surgical site infections in adults. Cochrane Database Syst Rev 2009;3: CD006806.
116. Edmiston CE, Krepel C, Kelly H, et al. Perioperative antibiotic prophylaxis in the gastric bypass patient: Do we achieve therapeutic levels? Surgery 2004;136:738–747.
117. Ho VP, Nicolau DP, Dakin GF, et al. Cefazolin dosing for surgical prophylaxis in morbidly obese patients. Surg Infect (Larchmt) 2012;13:33–37.

Vaccines, Toxoids, and Other Immunobiologics

Mary S. Hayney

102

KEY CONCEPTS

1. Live vaccines may confer life-long immunity but cannot be administered to the immunosuppressed.
2. Inactivated and subunit vaccines and toxoids often require multiple doses to protect from infection and generally booster doses are needed following the primary series.
3. Children less than 2 years of age are unable to mount T-cell–independent immune responses that are elicited by polysaccharide vaccines.
4. Severely immunocompromised individuals should not receive live vaccines, and their responses to inactivated, polysaccharide, toxoid, and recombinant vaccines may be poor.
5. The childhood, adolescent, and adult immunization schedules are updated frequently and published annually. These documents can be used to develop an immunization plan for children.
6. Immunoglobulin (Ig) provides rapid postexposure protection from measles, hepatitis A, varicella, and other infections that wanes over time.
7. Ig adverse effects are often secondary to infusion rate. Slowing the IV infusion rate ameliorate chills, nausea, and fever that may develop during administration.
8. Rh_o(D) Ig prevents Rh-negative mothers from mounting an immune response against hemolytic disease of the newborn. Hemolytic disease of the newborn results when Rh-negative mothers are sensitized to the Rh(D) antigen on the red blood cells of their fetuses.

Immunization is defined as rendering a person protected from an infectious agent. Immunity to an infectious agent can be acquired by exposure to the disease, by transfer of antibodies from mother to fetus, through administration of immunoglobulin (Ig), and from vaccination. Immunization is the process of introducing an antigen into the body to induce protection against the infectious agent without causing disease. An *antigen* is a substance that induces an immune response. An *antibody* produced by the humoral arm of the immune system usually is the response that is measured as evidence of successful vaccination. However, the cellular immune response, which is more difficult to measure, is also an important aspect of vaccine response.

This chapter introduces three groups of agents: vaccines, toxoids, and immune sera (together known as *immunobiologics*). Agents with a limited scope of use, such as agents for bioterrorism or travel, are beyond the scope of this chapter.

PRODUCTS USED TO IMMUNIZE

Vaccines and toxoids are separate and distinct products. However, both types of products induce active immunity—that is, immunity generated by a natural immunologic response to an antigen. Vaccines can be live attenuated or inactivated. Inactivated vaccines may consist of whole or split particles derived from the pathogen. Bacterial vaccines generally are killed whole bacteria or specific bacterial antigens or conjugates. Live-attenuated vaccines induce an immunologic response more consistent with that occurring with natural infection. (1) Because the organisms in live-attenuated vaccines undergo limited replication in the vaccinated individual after administration, they may confer lifelong immunity with one dose (as does a natural infection). (2) Multiple doses of killed vaccines usually are needed to induce long-lasting, effective immunity. Additional doses at varying time intervals (booster doses) often are required to maintain immunity. Booster doses of such vaccines elicit memory responses from the B cells that produce immunoglobulin G (IgG). The immune system already has developed an array of antibodies to the antigen. Upon restimulation with a booster dose, the B cells, which produce the most specific antibodies against the antigen, are activated. Restimulation allows the most active antibodies against the antigen to be selected and maintained in the "immunologic memory." Thus, the booster dose results in a rapid, intense antibody response that is long lasting. Inactivated vaccines also can differ in immunity potential, depending on their composition. For example, polysaccharide vaccines tend to be poorly immunogenic in infants, whereas protein–polysaccharide conjugated vaccines of the same antigen tend to be highly immunogenic (e.g., pneumococcal polysaccharide vaccine vs. pneumococcal conjugated vaccine). (3) T-cell–independent immune response is made to polysaccharide antigens that stimulate B cells directly.[1] There is no maturation or booster response with a T-cell–independent immune response, and children younger than 2 years cannot make this type of response. Protein–polysaccharide conjugate vaccines stimulate T cells and promote interactions between T cells and B cells when producing the protective immune responses consisting of immunologic memory and high-affinity IgG.

Toxoids are inactivated bacterial toxins that generally are combined with aluminum salts to enhance their antigenicity by prolonging antigen absorption and exposure. These adjuvants also increase local tissue irritation when injected. Toxoids stimulate the production of antibodies against the bacterial toxins rather than the infecting bacterial pathogens.

Immune sera are sterile solutions containing antibody derived from human (Ig) sources. Igs are derived from donor pools of blood plasma and are processed using cold ethanol fractionation in order to inactivate known potential pathogens. These sera are indicated for induction of passive immunity (temporary immunity to infection as a result of administration of antibodies not produced by the host; see Other Immunobiologics below).

In addition to the active component in an immunobiologic, other active and inert ingredients are often present. Suspending agents, such as water, saline, or complex fluids containing proteins (e.g., albumin), are used as the vehicle for the immunobiologic agent. Preservatives, stabilizers, and antibiotics may be added to help maintain the integrity of the product. Immunized individuals may respond with allergic reactions not to the immunobiologic agent itself but to the other components of the pharmaceutical preparation. Different manufacturers of the same immunobiologic may have different active and inert ingredients or different quantities of these ingredients in their products.

Certain vaccines manufactured by various companies are considered interchangeable. Hepatitis A, hepatitis B, and *Haemophilus influenzae* type b (Hib) conjugate vaccines from different manufacturers used for the primary series of three doses are considered interchangeable. It is preferable to use diphtheria, tetanus toxoids, and acellular pertussis (DTaP) vaccine from the same manufacturer to complete the entire primary series. However, immunization should not be delayed if the particular type of vaccine administered for the initial doses cannot be ascertained easily.[1]

In general, vaccines and toxoids must be kept refrigerated because breaking the "cold chain" may result in loss of potency. Varicella vaccine and zoster vaccines must be stored frozen. Immune sera generally should be kept refrigerated and not frozen except for lyophilized human IV immunoglobulin (IVIG), which can be stored at room temperature. Careful attention to appropriate storage of all vaccines and immunobiologics is absolutely imperative. Directions for appropriate storage can be found in the package inserts.

FACTORS AFFECTING RESPONSE TO IMMUNIZATION

Various factors are known to affect response to vaccines and toxoids. Viability of the antigen is an important factor (live attenuated vs. inactivated), as discussed previously. Total dose also is important because there seems to exist a threshold dose above which no further increase in antibody titer is seen. The interval between immunization doses, number of doses given, or both may change immune response to an agent. Among hepatitis B vaccine nonresponders, a significant proportion of individuals mount a vaccine response when given additional doses of vaccine.[2] In contrast, additional doses of influenza vaccine are minimally effective in individuals with chronic illness.[3] Generally, intervals longer than those recommended between vaccine doses do not reduce immune response.[1]

The route and site of administration of the immunobiologic are important. This is best illustrated by the hepatitis B vaccine, which elicits a satisfactory antibody response when given in the deltoid muscle but not a consistent response when administered in the gluteal area. Injections should be administered at a site with little likelihood of site damage. Immunobiologics containing adjuvants should be given into a muscle mass because they can cause irritation when given subcutaneously or intradermally.[1]

Host factors influence vaccine response. Immunocompromise, increasing age, underlying disease, and genetic background have been associated with poor response rates.[1,4–6]

VACCINE ADMINISTRATION

Subcutaneous injections should be administered into the thigh of infants and in the upper arm area over the triceps of older children and adults. A ⅝-inch, 25-gauge needle (0.508 mm × 1.6 cm) should be used, taking care not to administer the dose intradermally or intramuscularly (IM). For IM injection, the anterolateral aspect of the upper thigh (infants and toddlers) or the deltoid muscle of the upper arm (children and adults) should be used. When giving an IM injection to an adult weighing less than 60 kg, a ⅝-inch or 1-inch needle (1.6 cm or 2.5 cm) can be used. If a ⅝-inch needle (1.6 cm) is used, the skin over the injection site must be stretched tight and the needle must enter the skin at a 90° to assure that the needle reaches the muscle. A 1-inch needle (2.5 cm) should be used for adults who weigh 60 to 70 kg. Immunizers can choose either a 1-inch or 1½-inch needle (2.5 cm or 3.8 cm) for women who weigh 70 to 90 kg and for men who weigh 70 to 118 kg. For women weighing more than 90 kg and men who weigh more than 118 kg a 1½-inch needle (3.8 cm) must be used.[1] The buttock should not be used because of the potential for inadequate immunologic response and the potential risk of injury to the sciatic nerve. When the buttock must be used (as for large doses of Ig), only the upper outer quadrant should be used with the needle inserted anteriorly. An influenza vaccine for intradermal administration is supplied in an injection device that reliably delivers the vaccine to the intradermal space. The intradermal injection is administered over the deltoid.[7]

The rotavirus vaccines are administered orally. The tube of vaccine should be squeezed inside the infant's mouth toward the inner cheek until the dosing tube is empty. If the infant regurgitates or spits out the vaccine, readministration is not recommended.[8]

Live-attenuated influenza vaccine is administered intranasally.[3] A specially designed sprayer is inserted just inside the nostril, and the dose is sprayed by depressing the plunger of the sprayer. The clip is removed from the plunger so that the second half of the dose can be administered into the other nostril. The vaccinated individual should breathe normally. The dose does not need to be repeated if the individual sneezes during or shortly after administration.

Questions often arise concerning the simultaneous administration of vaccines. In general, inactivated and live-attenuated vaccines can be administered simultaneously at separate sites. If two or more inactivated vaccines cannot be administered simultaneously, they can be administered without regard to spacing between doses. Inactivated and live vaccines can be administered simultaneously or, if they cannot be administered simultaneously, at any interval between doses, except for cholera (killed) and yellow fever (live) vaccines, which should be given at least 3 weeks apart. If live vaccines are not administered simultaneously, their administration should be separated by at least 4 weeks. Live viral vaccines may interfere with purified protein derivative response; thus, tuberculin testing should be postponed 4 to 6 weeks after administration of live-virus vaccine.[1]

Simultaneous administration of Ig and live-attenuated vaccines may inhibit host antibody response because of impairment of viral replication. A dose relationship exists between administration of Ig and inhibition of immune response to a vaccine (Table 102-1). Whole blood and other blood products containing antibodies may interfere with the response to the measles, mumps, and rubella (MMR) and varicella vaccines. In any patient, if vaccination with MMR or varicella is followed by emergency Ig administration, the vaccine can be repeated or seroconversion to viral antigens can be confirmed after sufficient time has elapsed (see Table 102-1). Ig does not interfere with the response to oral vaccines, zoster vaccine, or yellow fever vaccine.[1]

Inactivated vaccines and Igs may be administered simultaneously. However, different sites are recommended for killed vaccine and Ig administration.

VACCINE STORAGE

Appropriate storage is critical to maintaining the integrity of vaccines because improperly stored vaccines can fail to protect the individuals to whom they are administered. Refrigerator temperature is defined

TABLE 102-1 Recommended Intervals Between Administration of Immunoglobulin and Measles- or Varicella-Containing Vaccine[1]

Product/Indication	Dose, Including mg Immunoglobulin G (IgG)/kg Body Weight	Recommended Interval Before Measles or Varicella-Containing[a] Vaccine Administration
RSV monoclonal antibody (Synagis®)[b]	15 mg/kg intramuscularly (IM)	None
TIG	250 units (10 mg IgG/kg) IM	3 months
HAIG		
Contact prophylaxis	0.02 mL/kg (3.3 mg IgG/kg) IM	3 months
International travel	0.06 mL/kg (10 mg IgG/kg) IM	3 months
HBIG	0.06 mL/kg (10 mg IgG/kg) IM	3 months
RIG	20 IU/kg (22 mg IgG/kg) IM	4 months
Measles prophylaxis IG		
Standard (i.e., nonimmunocompromised) contact	0.25 mL/kg (40 mg IgG/kg) IM	5 months
Immunocompromised contact	0.5 mL/kg (80 mg IgG/kg) IM	6 months
Blood tranfusion		
RBCs, washed	10 mL/kg negligible IgG/kg IV	None
RBCs, adenine-saline added	10 mL/kg (10 mg IgG/kg) IV	3 months
Packed RBCs (Hct 65%) [0.650][c]	10 mL/kg (60 mg IgG/kg) IV	6 months
Whole blood (Hct 35%–50%)[0.35–0.50][c]	10 mL/kg (80–100 mg IgG/kg) IV	6 months
Plasma/platelet products	10 mL/kg (160 mg IgG/kg) IV	7 months
Cytomegalovirus IV immunoglobulin (IGIV)	150 mg/kg maximum	6 months
IVIG		
Replacement therapy for immune deficiencies[d]	300–400 mg/kg IV[c]	8 months
Immune thrombocytopenic purpura	400 mg/kg IV	8 months
Immune thrombocytopenic purpura	1 g/kg IV	10 months
Postexposure varicella prophylaxis[e]	400 mg/kg IV	8 months
Kawasaki's disease	2 g/kg IV	11 months

HAIG, Hepatitis A IG; HBIG, Hepatitis B IG; RBCs, Red blood cells; RIG, Rabies IG; TIG, Tetanus IG.

[1]This table is not intended for determining the correct indications and dosages for using antibody-containing products. Unvaccinated persons might not be fully protected against measles during the entire recommended interval, and additional doses of Ig or measles vaccine might be indicated after measles exposure. Concentrations of measles antibody in an Ig preparation can vary by manufacturer's lot. Rates of antibody clearance after receipt of an Ig preparation also might vary. Recommended intervals are extrapolated from an estimated half-life of 30 days for passively acquired antibody and an observed interference with the immune response to measles vaccine for 5 months after a dose of 80 mg IgG/kg.

[a]Varicella-containing vaccine, as used here, does not include zoster vaccine. Zoster vaccine may be given without regard to antibody-containing blood products.
[b]Contains antibody only to respiratory syncytial virus (RSV).
[c]Assumes a serum IgG concentration of 16 mg/mL (g/L).
[d]Measles and varicella vaccinations are recommended for children with asymptomatic or mildly symptomatic human immunodeficiency virus (HIV) infection but are contraindicated for persons with severe immunosuppression from HIV or any other immunosuppressive disorder.
[e]The investigational product VariZIG, similar to licensed VZIG, is a purified human Ig preparation made from plasma containing high levels of anti-varicella antibodies (immunoglobulin class G [IgG]). The interval between VariZIG and varicella vaccine is 5 months.

as between 2.2°C and 7.8°C (36°F to 46°F) and freezer temperature as −15°C (5°F) or colder. Inactivated vaccines are stored refrigerated. Varicella and zoster vaccines must be stored frozen. MMR vaccine can be stored in either the freezer or refrigerator. Live-attenuated influenza vaccine is stored in the refrigerator. Specific storage conditions for individual vaccines can be found in the package insert.

IMMUNIZATION OF SPECIAL POPULATIONS

Groups of individuals may have precautions to vaccines. Many precautions are temporary, and vaccines can be administered later.

Infants

The age of the recipient is an important determining factor in vaccine and toxoid response. In the first few months of life, maternal antibodies acquired via transplacental transfer during the third trimester of gestation protect an infant. However, the maternal antibodies also inhibit the immune response to live vaccines because the circulating antibodies neutralize the vaccine before the infant has the opportunity to mount an immune response. For this reason, live vaccines are not administered until maternal antibodies have waned, generally by infant age 12 months.[1]

Premature infants should be vaccinated at the same chronologic age using the same schedule and precautions for full-term infants. The full recommended doses of vaccines should be used, regardless of age or birth weight. Breastfed infants should be vaccinated according to standard pediatric schedules.

Pregnant Women and Postpartum Immunization

Most vaccines are pregnancy category C. As with most drugs, the vaccines are given this category assignment not because of a known risk to the fetus but because of lack of information. No birth defect has ever been attributed to vaccine exposure.[1] For example, no cases of congenital rubella syndrome from inadvertent administration of rubella vaccine to a pregnant woman have ever been reported. Universal influenza immunization is recommended for women who will be or are pregnant during influenza season. Pregnant women should receive Tdap during the late second trimester or third trimester of pregnancy.[9] Although live vaccines generally are avoided because of the theoretical risk of transmission of the vaccine organism to the fetus, inactivated vaccines may be administered to pregnant women when the benefits outweigh the risks.[1] Hepatitis B, hepatitis A, meningococcal, inactivated polio, and pneumococcal polysaccharide vaccines should be administered to pregnant women who are at risk for contracting these infections.[10]

Administration of live vaccines, such as rubella or varicella, are deferred until postpartum and are routinely recommended for new mothers who do not have evidence of immunity prior to hospital discharge. These live vaccines can be administered without regard to administration of Rh_o(D) Ig in the postpartum period. Additionally, Tdap is recommended for all new mothers who have not received a Tdap before because household contacts are frequently implicated as the source of pertussis infection in a young infant.[12]

Immunocompromised Hosts

4 Vaccination in compromised hosts (e.g., those with chronic disease, such as diabetes or connective tissue disease, alcoholics, or those with cancer or HIV disease) must be individualized based on the disease state and its treatment. In general, severely immunocompromised individuals should not receive live vaccines. Administration of other vaccines may be indicated, but responses may be lower than those mounted by healthy individuals, but may still confer protection.[6]

Patients with chronic pulmonary, renal, hepatic, or metabolic disease who are not receiving immunosuppressants can receive both live-attenuated and killed vaccines and toxoids to induce active immunity. These patients often need higher doses of vaccines or more frequent dosing to induce immunity. Generally, immunization should be considered early in the course of the disease in an attempt to induce immunity at a point when the disease is less severe.

Patients with active malignant disease can receive killed vaccines or toxoids but should not be given live vaccines. The MMR vaccine is not contraindicated for close contacts, however. Live-virus vaccines can be administered to persons with leukemia who have not received chemotherapy for at least 3 months. Vaccines should be timed so that they do not coincide with the start of chemotherapy or radiation therapy.[1] Zoster vaccine should be administered at least 2 weeks prior to the start of immunosuppressing therapy.[11] Annual influenza vaccine should be administered 2 weeks prior to chemotherapy or between cycles.[12] If vaccines cannot be given at least 2 weeks before the start of these therapies, immunization should be postponed until 3 months after the therapy has been completed. Passive immunization with Ig can be used in place of active immunization regardless of the history of immunization.

Glucocorticoids may cause suppressed responses to vaccines. For the purposes of immunization, the immunosuppressing dose of corticosteroids is prednisone 20 mg or more daily or 2 mg/kg daily, or an equivalent dose of another steroid, for at least 2 weeks. Patients receiving long-term, alternate-day steroid therapy with short-acting agents, administration of maintenance physiologic doses of steroids (e.g., 5 to 10 mg/day of prednisone) topical, aerosol, intraarticular, bursal, or tendon steroid injections require no special consideration for immunization. If patients have been receiving high-dose corticosteroids or have had a course lasting longer than 2 weeks, then at least 1 month should pass before immunization with live-virus vaccines.[1]

Patients with HIV infection require special consideration. Responses to live and inactivated vaccines generally are suboptimal and decrease as the disease progresses because HIV produces defects in cell-mediated immunity and humoral immunity. The routinely recommended vaccines should be administered to children. Two doses of MMR vaccine should be administered at least 1 month apart as soon as possible after the first birthday. MMR and varicella virus should be administered only to children who have no or only moderate evidence of immunosuppression.[1] Two doses of varicella vaccine separated by 3 months are recommended only for children with no evidence of immunosuppression. Adults should receive routinely recommended vaccines. Zoster vaccine may be administered to individuals with HIV infection who do not have clinical manifestations of AIDS and have CD4 counts >200/mm^3 (>200 × 10^6/L).[11]

Solid Organ Transplant Patients

Organ transplantation has become routine treatment of end-stage organ disease of many causes. Although the number of organ transplants performed is severely limited by the availability of donor organs, survival of transplant recipients is increasing. Solid-organ transplant patients remain on immunosuppressive regimens for the rest of their lives. These immunosuppressive regimens result in a higher risk of infection and decrease the protection conferred by immunization.[13]

Whenever possible, transplant patients should be immunized prior to transplantation. Live vaccines generally are not given after transplantation. Posttransplantation diphtheria, tetanus, pneumococcal, and influenza vaccine responses are unpredictable. Decreased immune response has been documented following hepatitis B vaccine.

Hematopoietic Stem Cell Transplant Patients

Reimmunization of patients with hematopoietic stem cell transplantation is necessary because antibody concentrations wane rapidly. Annual influenza immunization may begin as soon as 6 months after successful engraftment. Reimmunization with inactivated vaccines should begin approximately 6 months after hematopoietic stem cell transplantation. Hematopoietic stem cell transplant recipients are at increased risk for fulminant infection with encapsulated bacteria, so 13-valent pneumococcal vaccine (PCV13), the 23-valent pneumococcal polysaccharide vaccine (PPSV23), meningococcal vaccine (MCV4), and Hib vaccines are recommended. MMR vaccine (MMR) can be administered at 24 months. Varicella vaccine is not routinely recommended but can be considered on a case-by-case basis. Immunization of household contacts and healthcare workers also is necessary.[1]

CONTRAINDICATIONS AND PRECAUTIONS

There are few contraindications to the use of vaccines except those outlined earlier. The contraindications include a history of anaphylactic reactions to the vaccine or a component of the vaccine. Unexplained encephalopathy occurring within 7 days of a dose of pertussis vaccine is a contraindication to future doses of pertussis vaccines. Immunosuppression and pregnancy are temporary contraindications to live vaccines. An interval of time must elapse based on the dose of Ig before a live vaccine can be administered (see Table 102-1). Precautions for DTaP administration include hypotonic hyporesponsive episode, fever of 40.5°C (104.9°F) or greater, crying lasting more than 3 hours within 48 hours of a previous dose, and seizures with or without fever within 3 days after a dose. A personal or family history of seizures is a precaution for receiving the combination MMR–varicella vaccine. Immunizers may choose to use MMR and varicella vaccines separately.[1] Generally, mild-to-moderate local reactions, mild acute illnesses, concurrent antibiotic use, prematurity, family history of adverse events, diarrhea, and lactation or breastfeeding are not contraindications to immunization.

OBTAINING AN IMMUNIZATION HISTORY

An immunization history should be obtained from every patient, regardless of the reason for the healthcare visit. Ideally, any history provided by the patient from memory should be verified by reviewing the patient's personal written immunization record or a database that contains the complete immunization history. State-based or other public health jurisdiction-based immunization information systems (IIS), also called immunization registries, have been developed to improve immunization coverage by allowing healthcare providers access to records at any contact with the healthcare system. Registries are aimed primarily at facilitation of childhood immunization records.[14] If an official written record is not available, patient characteristics (e.g., military service, travel history, and occupation) may provide clues to the immunization history. Serologic testing for immunity against certain diseases can provide specific information but is used routinely for only a few selected diseases (e.g., measles, rubella, hepatitis A and B, and varicella) and selected circumstances (e.g., employment in a healthcare facility). If a written record does not exist, one should be generated at the time of initiation of immunization. Patients without a written record should be considered susceptible, and an immunization program started and completed unless a serious adverse reaction occurs. As a general rule, the risks associated with overimmunization are minimal relative to the risks associated with contracting vaccine-preventable diseases.[1]

Every healthcare visit, regardless of its purpose, should be viewed as an opportunity to review a patient's immunization status and to administer needed vaccines. Immunization is perhaps the most cost-effective health intervention available. Each visit should include assessment of individuals' vaccine needs, administration of indicated vaccines, and documentation of immunization histories. The outcome measurement of what percentage of patients in a particular practice site is completely immunized is extremely important because the benefits of optimal vaccine use extend beyond the individual patient to the public as a whole.

NATIONAL VACCINE INJURY COMPENSATION PROGRAM

The National Childhood Vaccine Injury Act of 1986 was passed by the U.S. Congress in response to reports of vaccine side effects and liability concerns of vaccine manufacturers and healthcare providers. With vaccine safety being questioned and manufacturers ceasing the development and marketing of vaccines, the National Vaccine Injury Compensation Program was implemented to offer a no-fault alternative means to compensate individuals for injury following vaccination. The program offers liability protection to manufacturers and an efficient means of recovering damages for individuals potentially injured by vaccines. Compensation for vaccine-related injuries is outlined in the Health Resources and Services Administration's Vaccine Injury Table (*http://www.hrsa.gov/vaccinecompensation/vaccinetable.html*). Healthcare providers must report all events requiring medical attention within 30 days of vaccination to the Vaccine Adverse Event Reporting System (VAERS), which serves as a central depot for vaccine-related adverse effects. Only a temporal association between the adverse event and vaccine administration needs to be made. No adverse event rates can be determined because only the number of adverse events reported is known; the number of vaccines administered is not known. This database can be used to survey for changes in the frequencies of adverse events, to evaluate risk factors for adverse events, and to find rare adverse events.[15] VAERS report forms can be obtained by calling 1-800-822-7967, or reports can be made online at *https://vaers.hhs.gov/esub/index*.

USE OF VACCINES AND TOXOIDS

The Advisory Committee on Immunization Practices (ACIP) makes recommendations for use of vaccines for the United States. Other professional organizations, for example, the American Academy of Pediatrics, the American Academy of Family Physicians, or the American College of Obstetrics and Gynecology, publish guidelines. Usually, these guidelines are the same as those issued by the ACIP or the groups try to reconcile their recommendations.

❺ The appendices show the recommended schedules for routine immunization of children and adults. The latest vaccine schedules can be found at *http://www.cdc.gov/vaccines/schedules/hcp/index.html*. All states require children to be fully immunized prior to entering elementary school; however, optimal protection is achieved by immunizing at the recommended ages, which requires special attention to children younger than 2 years. Adults and adolescents also require vaccination and often are unaware of this need. An early adolescent preventive health visit is recommended. This visit is an opportunity to catch up on missed immunizations and to administer meningococcal conjugate, Tdap, and human papillomavirus (HPV) vaccines. All individuals older than 6 months of age should receive an annual seasonal influenza vaccine. Adults should receive routine tetanus–diphtheria (Td) or Tdap boosters and be immune to measles, mumps, rubella, and varicella by either immunization or history of infection. Older adults need zoster vaccine after age 60 years, and pneumococcal polysaccharide vaccine after age 65 years. Certain individuals with conditions or lifestyles that put them at high risk for vaccine-preventable diseases also should be immunized as described in the following text and outlined in the immunization schedules in the appendices.

TOXOIDS

Diphtheria Toxoid Adsorbed

Diphtheria is an acute illness caused by the toxin released by a *Corynebacterium diphtheriae* infection. The toxin inhibits cellular protein synthesis, and membranes form on mucosal surfaces. Systemic toxemia can result in myocarditis, neuritis, and thrombocytopenia. Membrane formation can cause respiratory obstruction, and significant toxin absorption can lead to severe illness and death.

Diphtheria toxoid adsorbed is a sterile suspension of modified toxins of *C. diphtheriae* that induces immunity against the exotoxin of this organism. Two strengths of diphtheria toxoid are available in the United States: pediatric strength (D) and adult strength (d), which contains less antigen. The widespread use of diphtheria toxoid essentially has eliminated diphtheria from the United States.

Primary immunization with diphtheria toxoid (D) is indicated for children older than 6 weeks. The toxoid is given in combination with tetanus toxoid and acellular pertussis vaccine (as DTaP or in combination with additional childhood vaccines that have been licensed to decrease the number of injections required to complete the childhood immunization recommendations) at age 2, 4, and 6 months. Additional doses are given at age 15 to 18 months and again at age 4 to 6 years.[16] Completing the primary diphtheria toxoid immunization series usually induces immunity of at least 10 years' duration in 90% of persons. Booster doses should be given every 10 years.

For unimmunized adults, a complete three-dose series of diphtheria toxoid should be administered, with the first two doses given at least 4 weeks apart and the third dose given 6 to 12 months after the second. The combined Td preparation is recommended for adults because it contains less diphtheria toxoid than the pediatric dose and is associated with fewer reactions to the diphtheria component. One of the vaccine doses in this series should be Tdap. All adults should receive booster doses of Td every 10 years.[17] Adverse effects of diphtheria toxoid include mild-to-moderate tenderness, erythema, and induration at the injection site. Systemic reactions occur very rarely.

Tetanus Toxoid Adsorbed and Tetanus Immunoglobulin

Tetanus is a severe acute illness caused by the exotoxin of *Clostridium tetani*. Tetanus is the only vaccine-preventable disease that is not contagious. It is acquired from the environment. Sustained muscle contractions are characteristic of tetanus. Tetanus toxin interferes with neurotransmitters that promote muscle relaxation, leading to continuous muscle spasms. Death can be due to the tetanus toxin itself or secondary to a complication such as aspiration

TABLE 102-2 Tetanus Prophylaxis[19]

Vaccination History	Clean, Minor		All Other	
	Td[a]	TIG	Td[a]	TIG
Unknown or fewer than three doses	Yes	No	Yes	Yes
Three or more doses	No[a,b]	No	No[a,c]	No

[a]A single dose of Tdap should be used for the next dose of tetanus–diphtheria toxoid for individuals aged ≥10 years.
[b]Yes, if more than 10 years since last dose.
[c]Yes, if more than 5 years since last dose.

pneumonia, dysregulation of the autonomic nervous system, or pulmonary embolism.

Tetanus toxoid adsorbed (adsorbed onto aluminum hydroxide, phosphate, or potassium sulfate to increase antigenicity) is a sterile suspension of the toxoid derived from *C. tetani.* A series of three 0.5-mL doses of tetanus toxoid elicits protection in virtually all individuals. Primary vaccination provides protection for at least 10 years.[17,18] Additional doses of tetanus toxoid (combined with diphtheria toxoid, i.e., Td) are recommended as part of wound management if a patient has not received a dose of tetanus toxoid within the preceding 5 years.[19] For minor or clean wounds, no dose is given. Table 102-2 summarizes these recommendations. Tetanus Ig should be given to individuals who have received fewer than three doses of tetanus toxoid and have more serious wounds. It can be administered with tetanus toxoid, provided that separate syringes and separate injection sites are used.

In children, primary immunization against tetanus usually is offered in conjunction with diphtheria and pertussis vaccination (using DTaP or a combination vaccine that includes other antigens used to decrease the number of injections to complete the childhood immunization schedule). A 0.5-mL dose is recommended at age 2, 4, 6, and 15 to 18 months, but the first dose can be administered as early as age 6 weeks.[16] In children 7 years and older and in adults who have not been immunized previously, a series of three 0.5-mL doses of a tetanus toxoid-containing vaccine is administered IM initially. The first two doses are given 1 to 2 months apart, and the third dose is recommended at 6 to 12 months after the second dose. Boosters are recommended every 10 years, and unless there is contraindication to diphtheria toxoid, Td should be used.[16,20] Tetanus toxoid can be given simultaneously with other killed and live vaccines, and, if indicated, it can be given to immunosuppressed patients.

Adverse reactions to tetanus toxoid include mild-to-moderate local reactions at the injection site, such as warmth, erythema, and induration. Occasionally, a nodule at the injection site develops and remains for a few weeks. Very rare major local reactions occur within 2 to 8 hours of administration to patients with high serum tetanus antitoxin levels. This type of reaction is indicative of high preexisting antibody concentrations, and additional doses of toxoid should not be given any sooner than 10 years. Local reactions do not limit the use of the toxoid for further dosing.[21]

Tetanus Ig is a sterile, concentrated, nonpyrogenic solution of Igs prepared from hyperimmunized humans. It is used to provide passive immunity to tetanus after the occurrence of traumatic wounds in nonimmunized or suboptimally immunized persons (see Table 102-2).[22] A dose of 250 to 500 units IM should be administered. When administered with tetanus toxoid, separate sites for administration should be used. Tetanus Ig also is used for treatment of tetanus. In this setting, a single dose of 3,000 to 6,000 units IM is administered.

Adverse effects of tetanus Ig include pain, tenderness, erythema, and muscle stiffness at the injection site, which may persist for several hours. Systemic reactions occur rarely. IV administration has been associated with severe adverse reactions and is not recommended.

VACCINES

Haemophilus Influenzae Type B Vaccines

Before 1995, Hib was responsible for thousands of cases of serious illnesses (e.g., meningitis, epiglottitis, pneumonia, sepsis, and septic arthritis). The incidence of Hib disease has declined more than 99% since introduction of the conjugate vaccines based on the organism's capsular substance, polyribosylribitol phosphate (PRP).[23]

The Hib vaccines used are conjugate products consisting of either a polysaccharide or an oligosaccharide of PRP covalently linked to a protein carrier. The protein carrier is important because it provides for T-lymphocyte–dependent immunologic response, whereas earlier Hib vaccines that consisted of only unconjugated PRP elicited a response that was T-cell independent. T-cell involvement in the response provides for (a) a greater antibody response regardless of the age of the patient receiving the vaccine, (b) immunologic response at an earlier age (including infants), and (c) a booster effect on subsequent exposure to the Hib capsule, whether through revaccination or natural exposure. The protein carrier is not considered a vaccine and should not be substituted for immunization against tetanus, diphtheria, or *Neisseria meningitidis.*

Hib conjugate vaccines are indicated for routine use in all infants and children younger than 5 years. Multiple products in various combinations are available for use in infants and children of different ages. The primary series of Hib vaccination consists of a 0.5-mL IM dose at ages 2, 4, and 6 months. If Hib PRP-OMP (outer membrane protein of *Neisseria meningitides* as the protein conjugate) is being used, the primary series consists of doses given at ages 2 and 4 months. The series should not be initiated in an infant younger than 6 weeks. Although use of one product for the entire primary series is desirable, adequate protection is achieved even when different products are used during the initial doses. Following the primary series, a booster dose is recommended at age 12 to 15 months. Any of the Hib conjugate vaccines are suitable for the booster dose regardless of which conjugate was used for the primary series of doses.[23]

Schedules are more complex for infants who do not begin Hib immunization at the recommended age or who have fallen behind in the immunization schedule. For infants 7 to 11 months of age who have not been vaccinated, three doses of Hib vaccine should be given: two doses spaced 4 weeks apart and then a booster dose at age 12 to 15 months (but at least 8 weeks since the second dose). For unvaccinated children ages 12 to 14 months, two doses should be given, with an interval of 2 months between doses. In a child older than 15 months, a single dose of any of the vaccine preparations is indicated.[16]

Vaccines for Hib are recommended for routine use only for patients up to age 59 months; beyond this age, most individuals will have natural immunity to Hib infection. Patients with certain underlying conditions (e.g., HIV infection, IgG_2 subclass deficiency, sickle cell disease, splenectomy, and hematopoietic stem cell transplants and those receiving chemotherapy for malignancies) are at higher than normal risk for Hib infection, and use of at least one dose of vaccine in these patients should be considered, although efficacy data in most of these situations are lacking.[1,16,20]

Adverse reactions to the Hib vaccine are uncommon. Erythema and induration at the injection site occur in approximately 5% to 30% of children and resolve within 12 to 24 hours. Fever, diarrhea, and vomiting are reported occasionally.[23]

Hepatitis Vaccines

Information on vaccination for viral hepatitis is given in Chapter 26.

Human Papillomavirus Vaccine

HPV infections are the most common sexually transmitted infections, with the highest prevalence of infection in sexually active young adults.[24] Although more than 120 different HPV types have been identified, at least 40 different types of HPV infect the anogenital tract. These 40 different viruses are grouped into low-risk and high-risk types. Low-risk types can cause genital warts and mild abnormalities on Papanicolaou (Pap) tests. Ninety percent of all cases of genital warts are caused by types 6 and 11. As many as 18 types are considered high risk as they have the ability to penetrate the nucleus of an epithelial cell to transform it to a precancerous cell. They cause abnormal Pap test results and may lead to cancer of the cervix, vulva, vagina, anus, or penis. Types 16 and 18 cause about 70% of all cervical cancers. High-risk HPV infections are necessary but not sufficient for the development of cervical cancer and for the majority of other anogenital and oral squamous cell cancers.

A bivalent HPV (Cervarix, GSK) containing virus-like particles for types 16 and 18 was licensed in late 2009. The quadrivalent vaccine (Gardasil, Merck Vaccines) is directed against cervical cancer-causing types 16 and 18 and types 6 and 11. ACIP recommends either of these HPV vaccine preparations for the prevention of cervical cancer and precancerous lesions. No head-to-head comparison of these vaccines is available, but both vaccines are very efficacious for the prevention of precancerous lesions caused by types 16 and 18.[25] Both vaccines offer some protection against oncogenic nonvaccine strains too.[26–28] Both vaccines are administered as a three-dose series using a harmonized schedule of 0, 1 to 2, and 6 months. The vaccines are recommended for females aged 11 to 12 years and for all females aged 13 to 26 years. Although administration of these vaccines before sexual debut is preferable, the vaccines can be administered without regard to history of sexual activity.[25]

The quadrivalent HPV vaccine is licensed for the prevention of genital warts, anal cancer, and precancerous lesions in males aged 9 to 26 years. Types 6 and 11 cause approximately 90% of genital warts—about 250,000 cases in males each year. Approximately, 7,000 cancers in males are associated with HPV types 16 or 18 infection annually. Additional clinical information showing HPV4 to be effective in the prevention of anal intraepithelial neoplasia (a precursor to anal cancer) among men who have sex with men (MSM) was published.[29] MSM are at a higher risk for infection with HPV, genital warts, and anal cancer.[30] The incidence of cancers associated with HPV is higher among MSM, and the rate of anal cancer among MSM continues to rise.[29,30] The ACIP recommends routine HPV4 vaccine series for males at age 11 to 12 years. Vaccination of males aged 13 to 21 years who have not been vaccinated or who have not completed all three doses of the HPV4 series is also recommended. In addition, males aged 21 to 26 years may receive HPV4. Routine vaccination with HPV4 for MSM through age 26 years is also recommended.[30]

The vaccines are well tolerated, with injection-site reactions and systemic reactions (e.g., headache and fatigue) occurring as commonly in immunized individuals as in the groups receiving placebo. Although syncope is possible with any immunization, the target population of adolescents and young adults has a higher incidence of syncope, including with administration of the HPV vaccine.[25]

These effective vaccines is an important advance, but the need for a Pap test for cervical cancer screening remains. Surveillance for duration of protection conferred by the vaccine series is ongoing; the need for future booster doses is not yet known.

Influenza Virus Vaccine

Information on vaccination for influenza is given in Chapter 87.

Measles Vaccine

Measles (rubeola) is a highly contagious viral illness characterized by rash and high fever. Complications of measles infections include severe diarrhea, otitis media, pneumonia, and encephalitis. Measles results in one to two deaths per 1,000 cases, with a much higher death rate in developing countries. With widespread vaccination, measles is on the verge of elimination from the Western Hemisphere.

The measles vaccine is a live-attenuated viral vaccine that produces a subclinical, noncommunicable infection. Approximately 95% of vaccine recipients mount a protective immune response after a single dose, and most individuals are protected for life.[25] Most persons who do not respond to the first dose of measles vaccine will respond after receiving a second dose, and this forms the basis for the two-dose vaccine strategy that was implemented in the United States in 1989.

The measles vaccine is administered subcutaneously as a 0.5-mL dose in the arm (or in the thigh if the patient is younger than 15 months). The vaccine is administered routinely for primary immunization to persons 12 to 15 months of age. Two combinations of measles containing vaccines are available—measles–mumps–rubella (MMR) or measles–mumps–rubella–varicella (MMRV). The measles vaccine is not administered earlier than 12 months (except in certain outbreak circumstances) because persisting maternal antibody that was acquired transplacentally late in gestation can neutralize the vaccine virus before the vaccinated person can mount an immune response. A second dose of measles-containing vaccine is recommended when children are 4 to 6 years old.[16] The second dose of vaccine results in seroconversion in 95% of individuals who were first-dose nonresponders.

Measles-containing vaccine should not be given to pregnant women or immunosuppressed patients. The one exception is HIV-infected patients, who are at very high risk for severe complications if they develop measles. Persons with HIV infection who have never had measles or have never been vaccinated against it should be given measles-containing vaccine unless there is evidence of severe immunosuppression. The second dose should be given 1 month later rather than waiting for entry to school.[31,32]

Recent administration of Ig interferes with measles vaccine response, so the recommended interval between the Ig and vaccine is determined by the dose of Ig (see Table 102-1).[1] Live vaccines not administered during the same visit must be delayed for at least 30 days following measles or MMR vaccine. Live measles vaccine may suppress a positive tuberculin skin test for up to 6 weeks postadministration.[1] Mild febrile illness and upper respiratory tract infections are not contraindications to vaccination.

Measles vaccination is indicated in all persons born after 1956 or in those who lack documentation of wild virus infection by either history or antibody titers. Two doses of a measles-containing vaccine are required for college students and healthcare workers who were born in 1957 or later. If two doses are needed (the person has never been vaccinated), the doses should be given at least 1 month apart.[16,20]

The measles vaccine has an excellent safety record. The most common side effect following vaccination is fever, which occurs in 5% to 15% of vaccinees. Transient generalized rash may occur in approximately 5% of vaccine recipients. These reactions generally appear 5 to 12 days postvaccination and last 2 to 5 days. Other adverse effects, such as headache, cough, sore throat, eye pain, malaise, and transient thrombocytopenia, occur less frequently.

Meningococcal Polysaccharide and Conjugate Vaccines

N. meningitidis is a leading cause of meningitis and sepsis in children and young adults in the United States. The infection is transmitted by respiratory droplets from infected individuals and asymptomatic carriers. Symptoms include severe headache, sensitivity to light, stiff neck, nausea and vomiting, and high fever. Mortality occurs in 24 to 48 hours following onset of symptoms in 10% to 13% of infected individuals.[33]

Two meningococcal conjugate vaccines combining the same serotypes are licensed for use in individuals aged 9 months to 55 years old (Menactra®, Sanofi-Pasteur) or 2 to 55 years old (Menveo®, Novartis). A quadrivalent vaccine containing capsular polysaccharides for serotypes A, C, Y, and W-135 (Menimmune®, Sanofi-Pasteur) has been available since the early 1970s. Although infections with serogroup B occur at rates that vary with age, it has not been incorporated into the vaccine because group B polysaccharide is not immunogenic. The meningococcal conjugate vaccine is indicated in adolescents at ages 11 to 12 years with a second dose at age 16 years. The vaccine is also recommended for high-risk populations, such as those exposed to the disease, those in the midst of uncontrolled outbreaks, travelers to areas with epidemic or hyperendemic meningococcal disease, and individuals who have terminal complement component deficiencies or asplenia. Reimmunization at 5-year intervals is recommended for individuals who are at high risk.[34] The polysaccharide vaccine should be reserved for those older than 55 years of age who require immunization.

Injection-site reactions are the most common adverse effects following administration of either the meningococcal conjugate or polysaccharide vaccine.

Mumps Vaccine

Mumps is a viral illness that classically causes bilateral parotitis 16 to 18 days after exposure. Fever, headache, malaise, myalgia, and anorexia may precede the parotitis. Serious complications are rare but more common in adults.

The mumps vaccine is a lyophilized live-attenuated vaccine prepared from chick embryo cultures. Each 0.5-mL dose of the vaccine also contains neomycin 25 mcg. The vaccine is available in combinations with measles, rubella (as MMR), and varicella (MMRV) vaccines.

The vaccine is administered as a 0.5-mL subcutaneous injection in the upper arm. Dosing recommendations coincide with those for measles vaccine, with the first dose administered at age 12 to 15 months and the second dose prior to the child's entry into elementary school. Two doses of mumps-containing vaccine are recommended for school-aged children, international travelers, students in post-high school educational institutions, and healthcare workers born after 1956.[31] A single dose of vaccine is acceptable documentation of immunity to mumps for other adults considered at lower risk of mumps infection, including adults born after 1956 and those with an uncertain history of wild virus infection.

Mumps vaccine should not be given to pregnant women or immunosuppressed patients.[1] The effect of Ig preparations on mumps vaccine response is unknown, but the response to measles, rubella, and varicella is compromised if the vaccine is administered after Igs. The recommended interval between the Ig and vaccine is determined by the dose of Ig (see Table 102-1).[1] The vaccine should not be given to individuals with anaphylactic reactions to neomycin.

Serious adverse reactions to the vaccine are reported rarely. Parotitis, rash, pruritus, and purpura occur rarely. Local reactions, including soreness, burning, and stinging, may occur at the injection site.

Pertussis Vaccine

Pertussis is caused by a bacterial infection with *Bordetella pertussis*. The infection starts with signs and symptoms of an acute respiratory infection, called the catarrhal stage. The coughing spells manifest about a week later. Typically, young children will have the characteristic whoop as they struggle to inhale while coughing. Adolescents and adults are more likely to have prolonged periods of coughing. Pertussis can affect any age group, but young infants are at much higher risk for pneumonia, seizures, brain damage, and death. Their rate of hospitalization is much higher than for other age groups. The individual is contagious during the catarrhal stage and the first two weeks of the cough.[17,18]

Acellular pertussis vaccines contain components of the *B. pertussis* organism. All acellular vaccines contain pertussis toxin, and some contain one or more additional bacterial components (e.g., filamentous hemagglutinin, pertactin [a 69-kDa outer membrane protein], and fimbriae types 2 and 3). Acellular pertussis vaccine is recommended for all doses of the pertussis schedule at 2, 4, 6, and 15 to 18 months of age. A fifth dose of pertussis vaccine is given to children 4 to 6 years of age.[16] Pertussis vaccine is administered in combination with diphtheria and tetanus (DTaP). Administration of an acellular pertussis-containing vaccine is also recommended for adolescents once between ages 11 and 18 years. In addition, they should receive a pertussis-containing vaccine with their next dose of Td toxoids.[17,18] Special attention is warranted for the immunization of individuals who have close contact with young infants. Tdap should be administered to women in their late second or third trimester of pregnancy. Tdap should also be administered to all close contacts, including household contacts and out of home care providers.[9]

Local administration site reactions are relatively common. Systemic reactions, such as moderate fever, occur in 3% to 5% of vaccinees. Very rarely, high fever, febrile seizures, persistent crying spells, and hypotonic hyporesponsive episodes occur following vaccination. Allergy to a vaccine component and encephalopathy without known cause within 7 days of a pertussis vaccine are contraindications to future doses of vaccine.

Pneumococcal Vaccines

Streptococcus pneumoniae is a common pathogen with a range of manifestations, including asymptomatic upper respiratory tract colonization, sinusitis, acute otitis media, pharyngitis, pneumonia, meningitis, and bacteremia. Rates of invasive infections are highest in children younger than 2 years and in the elderly.[35,36] Invasive pneumococcal infections cause approximately 40,000 deaths annually. Most of the deaths occur in the elderly or in those with underlying medical conditions. Approximately half the deaths could be preventable by vaccine. Two pneumococcal vaccine preparations, PCV13 and 23-valent pneumococcal polysaccharide vaccine (PPV23) are available. The vaccines have different indications and are not interchangeable.

Pneumococcal Polysaccharide Vaccine

Pneumococcal polysaccharide vaccine (Pneumovax 23) is a mixture of highly purified capsular polysaccharides from 23 of the most prevalent or invasive types of *S. pneumoniae* seen in the United States. Serotypes included are 1, 2, 3, 4, 5, 6B, 7F, 8, 9N, 9V, 10A, 11A, 12F, 14, 15B, 17F, 18C, 19A, 19F, 20, 22F, 23F, and 33F. These 23 types represent 85% to 90% of all blood isolates and 85% of pneumococcal isolates from other generally sterile sites seen in the United States. The vaccine is administered IM or subcutaneously as a single 0.5-mL dose. Each 0.5-mL dose of vaccine contains 25 mcg of each polysaccharide type dissolved in isotonic saline solution (for a total of 575 mcg polysaccharide) and 0.25% phenol as preservative.

PPSV23 is recommended for the following individuals:[37]

1. Persons 65 years and older (if an individual received vaccine more than 5 years earlier and was younger than 65 years at the time of administration, revaccination should be given).
2. Persons aged 2 to 64 years with a chronic illness (congestive heart failure, cardiomyopathy, chronic pulmonary disease, diabetes, alcoholism, and liver disease).
3. Persons aged 2 to 64 years with functional or anatomic asplenia (when splenectomy is planned, PPSV23 should be

given at least 2 weeks before surgery; a single revaccination is recommended at 5 years in subjects older than 10 years and at 3 years in subjects younger than 10 years).

4. Persons aged 19 to 64 years who smoke cigarettes or have asthma.
5. Persons with cochlear implants.

PPSV23 is recommended for immunocompromised persons 2 years and older with (a) HIV infection, (b) leukemia, (c) lymphoma, (d) Hodgkin's disease, (e) multiple myeloma, (f) generalized malignancy, (g) chronic renal failure or nephrotic syndrome, (h) patients receiving immunosuppressive therapy including corticosteroids, and (i) organ and bone marrow transplant recipients. A single revaccination should be given if 5 years or more have passed since the first dose in subjects older than 10 years. In subjects 10 years of age and younger, revaccination should be given 3 years after the previous dose.

PPSV23 induces type-specific antibodies (T-cell–independent mechanisms) with a twofold rise within 2 to 3 weeks in 80% of young healthy adults. No correlation of antibody levels and protection has been determined. Antibody levels to these strains remain elevated for at least 5 years. In certain individuals, these levels decline within 10 years. Children may be protected for only 3 to 5 years. Elderly individuals and patients with chronic disease may have lower antibody levels produced with the vaccine. Children younger than 2 years do not respond adequately to the vaccine.

A number of other groups, including immunocompromised patients (e.g., leukemia, lymphoma, and multiple myeloma), dialysis patients, and patients with acquired immune deficiency syndrome, have reduced antibody production with the vaccine. Asymptomatic HIV-infected patients respond sufficiently to the vaccine. Patients with Hodgkin's disease respond to the vaccine better before splenectomy, chemotherapy, or radiation therapy.

PPSV23 vaccine efficacy has been debated in the literature. Study results generally point to a reduction in invasive pneumococcal disease in the general population and in the elderly. In immunosuppressed populations, the reduction in invasive disease is estimated at 50% to 80% with immunization.[37] Adults hospitalized with community-acquired pneumonia are significantly less likely to die if they have been immunized. In addition, immunized patients were less likely to have respiratory failure and had hospitalization stays that were shorter by 2 days.[38]

PPSV23 safety is well documented. Local reactions occur frequently within the first 48 hours and generally are mild. Local erythema and induration (30%), local discomfort (40%), and local swelling (3%) are the side effects observed most commonly. Revaccination has been associated with self-limited injection-site reactions more commonly than after the first dose. Severe systemic reactions occur rarely and consist of weakness, myalgia, headache, photophobia, chills, and fever.

Pneumococcal Conjugate Vaccine

Invasive pneumococcal disease occurs even more frequently in children younger than 2 years than in those older than 65 years. The infection ranges goes from nasopharyngeal carriage to bacteremia and meningitis. Because of the lack of immune responsiveness in children younger than 2 years when exposed to polysaccharide vaccines, a conjugate vaccine was developed to protect young children from certain strains of *S. pneumoniae.* However, the 13-valent vaccine is also licensed for individuals aged 50 years and older. The 13 valent vaccine (Prevnar-13) contains the conjugated capsular polysaccharides of serotypes 1, 3, 4, 5, 6A, 6B, 7F, 9V, 14, 18C, 19A, 19F, and 23F. In clinical use, the vaccine is associated with a dramatic decline in invasive disease not only in immunized young children but also in individuals in all age groups.[39]

TABLE 102-3 ACIP Recommendations for Use of PCV13 and PPSV23[40]

Vaccine naïve adults
- PCV13 first with PPSV23 administered at least 8 weeks later
- Second dose of PPSV23 at 5-year interval and PPSV23 at age 65 years and at least 5 years after last dose

PPSV23-immunized adults
- PCV13 at least 1 year after last dose of PPSV23
- Second dose of PPSV23 at 5 year interval and PPSV23 at age 65 years and at least 5 years after last dose

Indications for PCV13 for adults 19 years and older
- Functional or anatomic asplenia
- Immunocompromising conditions
  - Congenital or acquired immunodeficiencies
  - HIV infection
  - Chronic renal failure or nephrotic syndrome
  - Leukemias, lymphomas, Hodgkin's lymphoma
  - Generalized malignancy
  - Diseases requiring treatment with immunosuppressive drugs, including long-term systemic corticosteroids or radiation therapy
  - Solid organ transplantation
  - Multiple myeloma
- Cerebral spinal fluid leaks or cochlear implants

PCV13, 13-valent pneumococcal conjugate vaccine. PPSV23, 23-valent pneumococcal polysaccharide vaccine.

Immunization of Children PCV13 is administered as a 0.5-mL IM injection at 2, 4, and 6 months of age and between 12 and 15 months of age. A single dose of PCV13 should be administered to children aged 6 to 18 years with sickle cell disease or splenic dysfunction, HIV infection, immunocompromising conditions, cochlear implant, or cerebral spinal fluid leak should be immunized. PPSV23 can be used in conjunction with PCV13. PPSV23 should be administered after age 2 years and at least 2 months after the last dose of PCV13.[16]

Immunization of Adults The 13-valent pneumococcal conjugate vaccine (PCV13) offers some additional protection over pneumococcal polysaccharide vaccine (PPSV23) alone in this adult high-risk population. Several studies have shown protection that is at least as good as PPSV23. PCV13 is safe in these populations.[40] Based on this information, the ACIP recommended PCV13 for adults with immunocompromising conditions[40] (Table 102-3). PCV13 should be administered prior to PPSV23 in adults who have not been immunized previously. PCV13 should be administered with at least a year interval in those immunocompromised adults for whom it has been recommended and have already received one or more doses of PPSV23. No recommendations have been made for the use of PCV13 in other adult populations.

Poliovirus Vaccines

Poliomyelitis is a contagious viral infection that usually causes asymptomatic infection; however, in its serious form it causes acute flaccid paralysis. Poliovirus is spread via the fecal–oral route. The virus replicates in the upper respiratory tract, GI tract, and local lymphatics. The vast majority of polio infections are subclinical and asymptomatic. Indigenous polio has been absent from the United States since 1979, and the last case in Western Hemisphere was reported in 1991. Global eradication efforts are entering the final stages, and the eradication of polio should be accomplished in the next few years.

An inactivated trivalent vaccine developed by Jonas Salk was licensed for use in 1955. In 1987, an enhanced-potency inactivated polio vaccine (IPV) was introduced and has replaced the original inactivated vaccine. A live-attenuated oral polio vaccine (OPV) was developed by Albert Sabin in 1962. OPV was the primary immunizing agent for poliovirus infection. Widespread OPV use is responsible for eradication of wild-type polio in most of the world. However, with no poliovirus circulation in the United States for years, IPV is the recommended vaccine for the primary series and booster dose for children.[41] OPV will continue to be used in areas of the world that have circulating poliovirus. The CDC maintains a stockpile of OPV to be used only in case of an outbreak.

The IPV series is administered routinely to children at ages 2, 4, and 6 to 18 months, and 4 to 6 years. Protective antibodies to all three serotypes develop in 90% to 100% of children after two doses of vaccine. After three doses, 99% to 100% develop protective immunity, and the fourth dose results in long-term immunity.[41]

Primary poliomyelitis immunization is recommended for all children up to age 18 years. Primary immunization of adults over age 18 years is not recommended routinely because a high level of immunity already exists in this age group and the risk of exposure in developed countries is exceedingly small. However, unimmunized adults who are at increased risk for exposure because of travel, residence, or occupation should receive IPV series. Incompletely immunized adults or children should complete the series of IPV regardless of the interval since initiation of primary immunization. Adults do not need a booster dose routinely unless they are at increased risk of exposure (travel), in which case a single dose of IPV can be given.[42]

Allergies to any component of IPV, including streptomycin, polymyxin B, and neomycin, are contraindications to vaccine use. No serious side effects are attributable to IPV. Pregnant women should be given IPV only if there is a clear need, such as women who will be traveling or living in an area with endemic or epidemic poliovirus.

The routine use of OPV in the United States has been discontinued because OPV is rarely associated with vaccine-associated paralytic poliomyelitis in vaccinees (1 in 6.2 million doses) or contacts (1 in 7.6 million doses). Because individuals with primary immune deficiency are at increased risk for this adverse reaction, OPV is not recommended for persons who are immunodeficient or for normal individuals who reside in a household with an immunocompromised person. The use of OPV is reserved for polio outbreak control.[42]

Rabies Vaccine and Immunoglobulin

Rabies is a virtually universally fatal infection in humans. Although all mammals are susceptible to rabies, carnivorous mammals are reservoirs of the virus and responsible for persistence of the virus in nature.[43] In the United States, most human cases of rabies are from exposure to rabid bats, but raccoons, foxes, skunks, and coyotes are also associated with possible exposure. Worldwide, canines are the primary vectors. Transmission of rabies can occur via percutaneous, permucosal, or airborne exposure to the rabies virus. Circumstances favoring such transmission include animal bites and attacks and contamination of scratches, cuts, abrasions, and mucous membranes with saliva or other infectious material (brain tissue). Unprovoked attacks and daytime attacks by nocturnal animals are considered highly suspect. A few cases of person-to-person transmission have been reported.

Symptoms of rabies are nonspecific during the prodomal stage—fever, headache, malaise, irritability, nausea, and vomiting. The acute neurologic phase is characterized by hyperexcitability, hyperactivity, hallucinations, salivation, a fear of water, and air. A minority of patients present with limp paralysis. Patients die within 5 days of presentation with these neurologic symptoms.

Human diploid cell vaccine (HDCV), and purified chick embryo cell (PCECV) rabies vaccine are killed vaccines used for preexposure and postexposure rabies virus prophylaxis. Preexposure indications for using HDCV, rabies vaccine, adsorbed (RVA), or PCECV rabies vaccine include persons whose vocation or avocation place them at high risk for rabies exposure, such as veterinarians, animal handlers, laboratory workers in rabies research or diagnostic laboratories, cavers, wildlife officers where animal rabies is common, and anyone who handles bats. Travelers who will be in a country or area of a country where there is a constant threat of rabies, whose stay is likely to extend beyond 1 month, and who may not have readily available medical services (e.g., Peace Corps workers and missionaries) should be considered for preexposure prophylaxis. Rabies immunization of immunocompromised individuals should be postponed until the immunosuppression has resolved, or activities should be modified to minimize the potential exposure to rabies. If the vaccine is used in immunocompromised persons, antibody titers should be checked postimmunization. Pregnancy is not a contraindication if the risk of rabies is great. Both vaccine preparations can be administered for preexposure prophylaxis as a three-dose series of 1 mL IM on days 0 and 7 and once between days 21 and 28.[43] Individuals with ongoing risk of exposure—either continuous risk (e.g., research laboratory staff or those involved in rabies biologics production) or individuals with frequent exposures (e.g., those involved with rabies diagnosis, spelunkers, veterinarians, animal control workers, and wildlife workers in rabies-enzootic areas)—should undergo serologic testing every 6 months and 2 years, respectively, to monitor rabies antibody concentrations. A booster dose is recommended if the complete virus neutralization is <1:5 serum dilution by the rapid fluorescent focus inhibition test.

Preexposure prophylaxis does not eliminate the need for postexposure therapy. Persons previously immunized with HDCV or PCECV rabies vaccine or those who previously received postexposure prophylaxis should receive two 1-mL IM doses of HDCV or PCECV rabies vaccine on postexposure days 0 and 3. Rabies Ig should not be given to this group.

Postexposure prophylaxis should be given after percutaneous or permucosal exposure to saliva or other infectious material from a high-risk source. Each case must be considered individually. Consideration needs to be given to the geographic area, species of animal, circumstances of the incident, and type of exposure. Local or state health departments should be contacted for assistance. Thorough cleansing of the wound with soap and water followed by irrigation with a virucidal agent such as povidone–iodine solution is an extremely important part of the management of rabies-prone wounds. Individuals who have not been immunized previously should receive the recommended regimen of rabies Ig (see Rabies Immunoglobulin below) and four doses of HDCV or PCECV rabies vaccine 1 mL IM on days 0, 3, 7, and 14 after exposure. However, a fifth dose in a series should be considered if the exposed individual is immunocompromised. Vaccine response for these individuals should be checked.[44] Rabies vaccine must be administered in the deltoid muscle in adults and in the anterolateral thigh in children. The gluteal region should not be used.[1,44]

Adverse reactions to rabies biologicals are less common and less serious with the currently available vaccines compared with previously used preparations. Local or mild systemic symptoms can typically be managed with antiinflammatory medications or antihistamines. Systemic allergic reactions ranging from hives to anaphylaxis occur in a very small number of subjects. Given the lack of alternative therapy and the fact that rabies infection is almost always fatal, persons exposed to rabies who do have adverse reactions should continue the vaccine series in a setting with medical support services.[43]

Human rabies Ig is used in conjunction with rabies vaccine as part of postexposure rabies management for previously unvaccinated individuals. The product is derived from plasma obtained from donors who have been hyperimmunized with rabies vaccine and have high titers of circulating antibody.

In persons who previously have not been immunized against rabies, rabies Ig is given simultaneously with HDCV or PCECV rabies vaccine to provide optimal coverage in the interval before immune response to the vaccine occurs. The efficacy of this regimen has been clearly demonstrated. In situations where a vaccine has been used alone, mortality rates of 50% to 60% have been observed. Mortality after the combination vaccine and rabies Ig regimens is exceedingly rare; however, deaths have been reported when the wound was not infiltrated with rabies Ig.[44]

Rabies Ig does not interfere with vaccine-induced antibody formation. Its use is not recommended beyond 8 days after initiation of the vaccine series nor in persons previously immunized to rabies.

Human rabies Ig is administered in a dose of 20 international units/kg (0.133 mL/kg). If anatomically feasible, the entire dose should be infiltrated around the wound(s). Any remaining volume should be administered IM at a site distant from the rabies vaccination site. This product should never be administered by the IV route. Because other antibodies in the rabies Ig may interfere with the response to live-virus vaccines (MMR and varicella), it is recommended that these immunizations be delayed for 3 months.[1]

Side effects are rare but may include local soreness at the wound or IM injection site and mild temperature elevations. Caution is advised when administering the product to persons with known systemic allergies to Ig or thimerosal. Pregnancy is not a contraindication to its use.

Rubella Vaccine

Rubella (German measles) is characterized by an erythematous rash, lymphadenopathy, arthralgia, and low-grade fever. The most important consequence of rubella infection occurs during pregnancy, particularly during the first trimester. Congenital rubella syndrome is associated with auditory, ophthalmic, cardiac, and neurologic defects. Rubella infection during pregnancy also can result in miscarriage or stillbirth. The primary goal of rubella immunization is to prevent congenital rubella syndrome. Rubella is no longer endemic in the United States, but high immunization rates are necessary to prevent rubella outbreaks from imported cases.[45]

Rubella vaccine contains lyophilized live-attenuated rubella virus grown in human diploid cell culture. The vaccine is available in combination with measles vaccine, mumps vaccine, and varicella vaccine. Each 0.5-mL dose also contains 25 mcg neomycin and is administered subcutaneously.

Rubella vaccine induces antibodies that are protective against wild-virus infection. The duration of immunity has not been established. A second dose is recommended, however, at the same time measles vaccine is administered (as a second dose of MMR). The vaccine is indicated for children older than 1 year of age. Individuals born before 1957 are assumed to be immune to rubella except for women who could become pregnant. Therefore, all women of childbearing potential should have documentation of receiving at least one dose of a rubella-containing vaccine or laboratory evidence of immunity.[45] Recent administration of Ig interferes with rubella vaccine response for at least 3 months and depends on the dose of Ig that is administered.[1,45] Table 102-1 can be used as a guide for the recommended interval. The vaccine should not be given to immunosuppressed individuals, although MMR vaccine should be administered to young children with HIV infection without severe immunosuppression as soon as possible after their first birthday.[45,46] The vaccine should not be given to individuals who have experienced anaphylactic reactions to neomycin.

Adverse effects of the rubella virus vaccine tend to increase with the age of the recipient. Mild symptoms are similar to wild-virus infection and include lymphadenopathy, rash, urticaria, fever, malaise, sore throat, headache, myalgias, and paresthesias of the extremities. These symptoms occur 7 to 12 days after vaccination and last 1 to 5 days. Joint symptoms occur more often in susceptible postpubertal females. Arthralgia occurs in 25% of vaccinees, and 10% have arthritis-like symptoms. These symptoms usually begin 1 to 3 weeks after vaccination and persist for 1 day to 3 weeks. A very small excess risk of chronic arthropathy exists.[45] The vaccine may cause suppression of tuberculin skin tests for up to 6 weeks after vaccination. The vaccine virus may be excreted in nose and throat secretions, but it is not contagious.

The rubella vaccine has never been associated with congenital rubella syndrome, but its use during pregnancy is contraindicated. However, routine pregnancy testing prior to vaccination is not recommended. Women should be counseled not to become pregnant for 4 weeks following vaccination.[47] Termination of pregnancy is not indicated in women who are accidentally given the vaccine or who become pregnant during the month after vaccination.

Varicella and Zoster Vaccines

Varicella is a highly contagious disease caused by varicella-zoster virus. The clinical illness is characterized by the appearance of successive waves of pruritic vesicles that rapidly crust over. Malaise and fever are common and last for 2 to 3 days. The virus remains dormant in the dorsal ganglia and reactivates as herpes zoster, also known as *shingles.* Although the exact stimulus for reactivation is unknown, a decrease in varicella-specific cell-mediated immunity associated with age or immunosuppression appears to be necessary but not sufficient for reactivation.

Varicella Vaccine

Live-attenuated varicella vaccine contains the Oka/Merck strain of varicella virus, which was attenuated by propagation through several different cell culture lines. Varicella vaccine is a lyophilized product that must be kept frozen and protected from light. Once reconstituted, it must be administered subcutaneously within 30 minutes. Each 0.5-mL dose contains a minimum of 1,350 plaque-forming units of virus as well as 12.5 mg of hydrolyzed gelatin and trace amounts of neomycin, fetal bovine serum, and residual components from cell culture.[48]

The varicella vaccine is safe and immunogenic in healthy children and adults. In clinical studies, varicella vaccine has been 70% to more than 95% effective in preventing chickenpox. Vaccinated individuals who develop chickenpox typically experience milder disease, often with low or no fever and fewer skin lesions, many of which do not vesiculate.[48]

The varicella vaccine is recommended for all children at 12 to 18 months of age, with a second dose prior to entering school between ages 4 and 6 years.[16] A second dose is also recommended for individuals older than this age if they have not already had chickenpox. Varicella vaccine can be used for postexposure prophylaxis. The vaccine is effective in the prevention or modification of varicella infection when given within 3 days and possibly 5 days of exposure. Because the varicella vaccine is a live vaccine, it is contraindicated in pregnant women and in immunocompromised individuals. An exception is children with asymptomatic or mildly symptomatic HIV infection, who should receive two doses of varicella vaccine 3 months apart. In addition, children with humoral immune deficiencies may be immunized. Varicella vaccination is contraindicated in individuals with a history of anaphylactic reaction to any component of the vaccine. Persons who have received blood, plasma, or Ig products in the recent past should not receive varicella vaccine because of concern that passively acquired antibody will interfere with response to the vaccine. The recommended time interval between antibody-containing products and varicella vaccine depends on the dose of Ig (see Table 102-1). Although no adverse events associated with salicylate use after vaccination have been reported, salicylates should be avoided for 6 weeks after vaccination because of the association of salicylate use and Reye's syndrome following varicella infection.[48]

The varicella vaccine has an excellent safety record. Pain, local swelling, and erythema at the injection site occur in up to 32% of patients and fever in 10% to 15%. A varicella-like rash occurs in approximately 4% of vaccinees, accompanied by few, if any, systemic symptoms. The rash may be localized at the injection site or generalized. Lesions usually are few in number (2 to 10) and often papular rather than vesicular. Transmission of vaccine virus to susceptible close contacts has occurred but is rare and believed to occur only when the vaccinee develops a rash. Because the risk of vaccine virus transmission is very low and primary infection can be very severe, vaccination of household contacts of immunocompromised patients is recommended to prevent introduction of varicella into the household.[48]

Zoster Vaccine

After the primary infection with varicella-zoster virus manifested as chicken pox, the virus remains latent in the dorsal ganglia. Herpes zoster, more commonly known as *shingles*, occurs upon reactivation of varicella-zoster virus replication. Herpes zoster can occur at any age, but the incidence dramatically increases with increasing age. The rate of disease increases sharply after age 50 years. The disease rate in individuals older than 80 years of age is 11 cases per 1,000 person-years.[49] Patients with HIV, cancer, or other conditions associated with immunosuppression are at increased risk for disease.[50] The development of the disease is associated with declining cellular immunity to varicella-zoster virus.

The clinical presentation of herpes zoster usually is a vesicular eruption limited to one dermatome. The most common complication is postherpetic neuralgia, which is pain that persists after the skin lesions have healed. Postherpetic neuralgia can persist for weeks to years. The risk of postherpetic neuralgia increases dramatically with age. Virtually no risk of developing postherpetic neuralgia with herpes zoster exists prior to age 50 years, but the risk increases to 50% to 75% after ages 60 and 75 years, respectively. The pain can be so severe as to limit activities of daily living and quality of life.[11]

The zoster vaccine contains 19,000 plaque-forming units of Oka/Merck strain live varicella-zoster virus. Although the same strain of vaccine virus is contained in the childhood varicella vaccines, the doses of vaccine virus are dramatically different, and the vaccines are *not* interchangeable. Zoster vaccine reduces the burden of disease by 60%. The burden of disease is a composite measure considering incidence, severity, and duration of herpes zoster. The incidence of zoster is cut in half and the development of postherpetic neuralgia can be decreased by 67%.[51]

The zoster vaccine is licensed for individuals 50 years of age and older. However, the ACIP recommends the zoster vaccine for routine use in individuals aged 60 years and older. This live vaccine should not be used in immunocompromised individuals, including those on high-dose corticosteroids or with HIV (CD4 cell count $<200/\text{mm}^3$) [$<200 \times 10^6$/L] or malignancies.[11] Immunization of some special populations can be done (see Table 102-4). The duration of protection conferred by immunization is unknown.

TABLE 102-4 Zoster Vaccine Use in Special Populations[11]

- Immunize patients with a history of shingles
- Screening patients for a history of chickenpox is not necessary. Assume anyone born before 1980 is immune to varicella[47]
- Zoster vaccine may be administered to individuals on inhaled, topical, or intraarticular steroids or low-dose oral steroids
- Zoster vaccine may be administered to individuals treated with low-dose methotrexate (<0.4 mg/kg/wk) or 6-mercaptopurine (<1.5 mg/kg/day). These therapies are often used for autoimmune diseases
- The vaccine may be administered to individuals anticipating immunosuppressive therapy. The minimum duration between immunization and initiation of immunosuppressive therapy is 14 days, and some clinicians recommend 1 month
- Stop antiviral therapy at least 24 hours before immunization and restart it at least 14 days after immunization
- Zoster vaccine can be administered without regard to blood product or Ig administration
- Do not administer zoster vaccine to
  - Individuals with AIDS or clinical manifestations of HIV, such as a $CD4^+$ count less than 200 per mm^3 (200×10^6/L)
  - Patients on high doses of steroids (prednisone or its equivalent of 20 mg daily or more for more than 2 weeks)
- Risks and benefits of administering zoster vaccine to individuals on immune modulators, such as tumor necrosis factor agents, must be determined on a case-by-case basis. Immunize prior to initiating therapy if possible

Varicella-Zoster Immunoglobulin

Varicella-zoster Ig is used after exposure to varicella for passive immunization of susceptible immunodeficient patients or other susceptible individuals at particularly high risk for complications of varicella infection. Postexposure prophylaxis with varicella-zoster Ig is indicated for the following susceptible individuals: (a) immunocompromised patients, (b) neonates whose mothers develop varicella within 5 days before or 2 days after delivery, (c) preterm infants (<28 weeks' gestation or weight <1,000 g) who are exposed to varicella while hospitalized, and (d) susceptible pregnant women (e) immunocompromised individuals without evidence of immunity.[52] If varicella is prevented, vaccination should be offered at a later date. Exposure to varicella is defined as direct indoor contact for more than 1 hour with an infectious person. A negative history of clinical disease is not a reliable indicator of varicella susceptibility. Most people with a negative clinical history will have detectable antibody on laboratory testing. Caution is warranted when interpreting a low-positive result in an immunosuppressed patient who has received blood products or Ig because the circulating antibody may be acquired passively.

For maximum effectiveness, varicella-zoster Ig must be given as soon as possible and not more than 10 days following exposure.[52] Because this agent may only attenuate infection, patients who receive varicella-zoster Ig still may have a period of communicability, and varicella-zoster Ig may prolong the incubation period to 28 days. Antiviral therapy can be initiated if signs and symptoms of varicella infection become apparent.

Administration of varicella-zoster Ig is by the IM route at doses of 125 plaque-forming units per 10 kg of body weight up to 625 units (five vials) for patients weighing more than 40 kg. The dose for newborn infants is 125 units.[48]

OTHER IMMUNOBIOLOGICS

Immunoglobulin

Ig is available as both an intramuscular immunoglobulin (IMIG) and an IV immunoglobulin (IVIG) preparation. The IMIG preparation, or the Cohn fraction II, is prepared from pooled plasma of several thousand donors by cold ethanol fractionation. It typically contains greater than 95% IgG and trace amounts of IgM, IgA, and other plasma proteins. Because Ig is harvested from a large donor pool, it contains a wide spectrum of IgG antibodies to the pathogens prevalent in the area from which the donors were obtained. In the fractionation process, high-molecular-weight IgG aggregates are formed, which can activate complement in the absence of antigen and precipitate anaphylactoid reactions. For this reason, IMIG is unsuitable for IV administration. IMIG typically contains 15% to 18% protein and not less than 90% IgG. A number of IVIG preparations are available commercially in the United States. Generally, these preparations contain greater than 90% IgG monomers and trace to small amounts of IgA. These products are available as lyophilized powders or solutions.

When administered either IV or IM, Ig distributes in approximately 5% of the body weight of the recipient. The plasma half-life of Ig ranges from 18 to 32 days. This range of half-life probably is attributable to the variation in the half-life of IgG subclasses. Peak

TABLE 102-5 Indications and Dosage of Intramuscular Immunoglobulin in Infectious Diseases

Primary immunodeficiency states	1.2 mL/kg IM then 0.6 mL/kg every 2–4 weeks
Hepatitis A exposure	0.02 mL/kg IM within 2 weeks if <1 year or >39 years of age
Hepatitis A prophylaxis	0.02 mL/kg IM for exposure <3 months' duration 0.06 mL/kg IM for exposure up to 5 months' duration
Hepatitis B exposure	0.06 mL/kg (HBIG preferred in known exposures)
Measles exposure	0.5 mL/kg (maximum dose 15 mL) as soon as possible 0.5 mL/kg (maximum dose 15 mL) as soon as possible for immunocompromised individuals
Varicella exposure	0.6–1.2 mL/kg as soon as possible when VZIG not available

serum concentrations occur immediately with IVIG but within 2 days with IMIG. After the initial period of equilibration, circulating IgG levels are superimposable between IV and IM equivalent dosages. No dosage adjustment is necessary in patients with renal insufficiency, hepatic insufficiency, or both, dialysis patients, or geriatric patients.

6 Ig is indicated in a wide variety of circumstances to provide passive immunity to individuals. The indications for IMIG differ from those for IVIG. IMIG is indicated for providing passive immunity in patients with hepatitis A infections in those <1 year and older than 39 years, hepatitis B exposures (however, hepatitis B Ig is significantly more effective), measles, varicella, and primary immunodeficiency diseases. Although IMIG is indicated for treatment of primary immunodeficiency, IVIG is better tolerated and is more effective. IMIG is not indicated for prevention of rubella, mumps, or poliomyelitis. Table 102-5 lists the suggested dosages of IMIG for prevention or attenuation of various infectious diseases.

There are many licensed indications, as well as off-label uses, for IVIG.[53] The therapeutic dose of IVIG is set empirically at 2 g/kg, often given as five daily doses of 400 mg/kg each.[54] Mechanisms of IVIG action for treatment of these conditions have been hypothesized.[55]

1. *Primary Immunodeficiency States.*[56] In primary immunodeficiency states, monthly doses of between 100 and 800 mg/kg are administered; the average dose is 200 to 400 mg/kg. The immunodeficiency states for which IVIG is indicated include both antibody deficiencies and combined immune deficiencies. Significant reactions can occur in patients with low intrinsic levels of IgA given IVIG with greater amounts of IgA. An IVIG product with very low amounts of IgA should be used for these patients.
2. *Idiopathic (Immune) Thrombocytopenic Purpura.*[57] For treatment of hemorrhage associated with idiopathic (immune) thrombocytopenic purpura (ITP), doses of 1 g/kg daily for 2 to 3 days plus high-dose methylprednisolone are indicated. Adults tend to respond less well to IVIG than do children. IVIG is acceptable for treatment of both chronic and acute ITP, and IVIG has been used for ITP associated with pregnancy without adverse effects on the fetus. Corticosteroids remain the drugs of choice for adult ITP. In thrombotic thrombocytopenia purpura, IVIG is reported to be effective in patients who do not respond to plasmapheresis. Other platelet disorders in which IVIG may be useful include neonatal immune thrombocytopenia, perinatal autoimmune thrombocytopenia, drug-induced thrombocytopenia, thrombocytopenia secondary to infection, and transfusion-refractory thrombocytopenia; however, the data supporting these uses are minimal.
3. *Chronic Lymphocytic Leukemia.* IVIG is used as a prophylactic measure in patients with chronic lymphocytic leukemia who have had a serious bacterial infection. Doses of 400 mg/kg every 3 to 4 weeks are used.
4. *Kawasaki's Disease (Mucocutaneous Lymph Node Syndrome).* This disease, which generally occurs in children, carries the hallmark of development of coronary artery abnormalities. Generally, the American Academy of Pediatrics recommends that if the strict criteria for Kawasaki's disease are met, an IVIG dose of 400 mg/kg/day for 4 consecutive days be used or, preferably, 2 g/kg as a single dose. The dose should be administered within 10 days of disease onset. Aspirin therapy also should be initiated.[58]
5. *Varicella-Zoster.* Another licensed indication for IVIG is for prophylaxis of varicella-zoster if varicella-zoster Ig is not available.

A number of other proposed uses of IVIG have been identified. It is important to note that these uses are off-label but may be generally accepted in the medical community for routine treatment.[53,54,59] Off-label uses include the following:

1. *Neonatal Sepsis.* Neonatal sepsis can cause significant morbidity within 24 hours of birth. Group B *Streptococcus* and *Escherichia coli* are the primary infecting organisms, but other bacteria and fungi may be associated with sepsis. IVIG appears to be effective in neonates older than 34 weeks' gestational age or who weigh less than 1,500 g. Routine use is not recommended; however, IVIG may be useful in neonates with recurrent infections.[54]
2. *Guillain–Barré Syndrome.* IVIG is effective and is considered an alternative to plasmapheresis.[59]
3. *Autoimmune Diseases.* IVIG may be effective in self-limited immunoregulatory diseases but less effective in chronic diseases such as systemic lupus erythematosus. Overall, little evidence indicates that IVIG is useful for management of autoimmune diseases, except for patients with severe active disease who have not responded to or tolerated other interventions.[53]
4. *Intractable Epilepsy.* IVIG may be useful for patients with confirmed IgG deficiency. IVIG may be considered for certain syndromes, such as West or Lennox–Gastaut syndrome.[60]
5. *Chronic Inflammatory Demyelinating Polyneuropathy.* Although steroids are the first-line therapy, IVIG may be used in patients who do not respond to or do not tolerate steroids.[56]

7 Adverse effects of Ig vary with the route of administration. Following IMIG, pain, tenderness, and muscle stiffness persisting for hours or days are common. Repeat courses may cause sensitization with resulting allergic reactions. With IVIG, adverse effects occur in fewer than 1% of immunocompetent patients and in fewer than 10% of other patients. Chills, fever, nausea, and vomiting often are related to the rate of the infusion. Infusion should be given at a rate of 0.01 to 0.02 mL/kg/min for 30 minutes. If no reactions occur, then the rate can be increased to 0.02 to 0.04 mL/kg/min. If reactions do occur, the infusion should be stopped for 30 minutes and restarted at a lower rate. Although recommendations for infusion rate vary slightly depending on the preparation, the guidelines presented can be followed for the various IV preparations.[61]

Most adverse reactions are mild and transient. Arthralgia, myalgia, fever, pruritus, nausea, vomiting, chest tightness, palpitations, diaphoresis, dizziness, pallor, and respiratory distress have been reported. Rarely, aseptic meningitis has occurred from a few hours to 2 days after high-dose infusion. The syndrome resolves within days without sequelae. Acute renal failure has been reported, primarily in individuals with underlying renal dysfunction, diabetes, sepsis, volume depletion, or other nephrotoxic drugs or in patients older than 65 years. To minimize the risk, ensure adequate hydration prior to infusion and choose an IVIG product that does not contain high sucrose concentrations for individuals at high risk.[62]

Ig products are derived from human blood. Precautions such as donor screening and fractionation procedures and solvent–detergent treatment during the manufacturing process render the IVIG products free of HIV and hepatitis B and C viruses. Although no manufacturing process can guarantee no viral contamination, the potential infection risk from Ig preparations is very small.[62]

Rh_o(D) Immunoglobulin

Second only to the ABO blood group system, Rhesus antigen D [Rh_o(D)] is an important antigen in human blood. The Rh_o(D) locus encodes this antigen, but this locus is absent in approximately 15% of the population. **8** Individuals lacking the Rh_o(D) locus are Rh_o(D) negative and have the potential to mount an antibody response to erythrocytes with the Rh_o(D) present. Rh_o(D) incompatibility during pregnancy can lead to sensitization of the mother. The maternal antibodies developed following normal fetal leakage of erythrocytes to the mother can cause hemolytic disease of the newborn during subsequent pregnancies.

Rh_o(D) Ig is a sterile solution of Igs prepared from human sera with high titers of Rh_o(D) antibody. Rh_o(D) Ig suppresses the antibody response and formation of anti-Rh_o(D) in Rh_o(D)-negative women exposed to Rh_o(D)-positive blood. Administration of Rh_o(D) Ig prevents hemolytic disease of the newborn in subsequent pregnancies with a Rh_o(D)-positive fetus. When administered within 72 hours of delivery of a full-term infant, Rh_o(D) Ig reduces active antibody formation from 12% to 1% to 2%. The reduction in antibody formation is lower when Rh_o(D) Ig is given beyond 72 hours postpartum. Smaller doses of Rh_o(D) Ig are used after abortion, miscarriage, amniocentesis, or abdominal trauma. In addition, Rh_o(D) Ig is used in the case of a premenopausal woman who is Rh_o(D) negative and has inadvertently received Rh_o(D)-positive blood or blood products.

The dosage of Rh_o(D) Ig varies with the indication. A standard dose of 300 mcg is given within 72 hours of a term delivery. Occasionally, when the fetus is known to be Rh_o(D) positive, a 300-mcg dose is given at 28 weeks' gestation and within 72 hours after delivery. For postpregnancy termination occurring up to 13 weeks' gestation, one microdose (50 mcg) vial is given within 72 hours. For pregnancy termination after 13 weeks, one standard dose (300 mcg) is given within 72 hours. In other circumstances, such as in abdominal trauma, amniocentesis, or transfusion accidents, the dosage (number of standard dose vials) is based on the estimated packed red blood cell volume of fetal/maternal hemorrhage divided by 15. Rh_o(D) Ig is administered IM only.

When considering use of Rh_o(D) Ig use, the mother's Rh_o(D) antigen status must be known with certainty. Rh_o(D) Ig should not be given to individuals positive for this antigen or to those with anti-Rh_o(D) antibodies. Occasionally, a large fetal bleed of Rh_o(D)-positive blood may make cross-matching of the mother difficult. In these cases, Rh_o(D) Ig should be given only if previous tests have shown that the mother is Rh_o(D) negative with no anti-Rh_o(D) antibody.

Adverse reactions to Rh_o(D) Ig include injection-site tenderness and fever. Rh_o(D) does not interfere with response to rubella vaccine. Rubella-seronegative women should be immunized at hospital discharge even if they received Rh_o(D) Ig postpartum.

Cytomegalovirus Immunoglobulin

Cytomegalovirus (CMV) causes a generally mild infection in immunocompetent individuals. However, immunocompromised individuals are at risk for serious complications, including pneumonia, retinitis, GI manifestations, and hepatitis. CMV causes a latent infection that can be transmitted from a previously infected solid organ donor to a seronegative recipient. Cytomegalovirus IV immunoglobulin (CMV-IVIG) contains IgG antibodies obtained from healthy persons with high titers of antibodies to CMV.

Attenuation of primary CMV disease associated with solid-organ transplantation in seronegative recipients of seropositive organs is the indication for CMV-IVIG. It is dosed using a tapering schedule that varies depending on the type of transplant. CMV-IVIG is administered IV every 2 weeks, with the final dose administered 16 weeks posttransplantation. Use of CMV-IVIG has resulted in a significant decrease in CMV-related syndromes.

Adverse effects of CMV-IVIG are seen in fewer than 5% of recipients and include flushing, chills, muscle cramps, back pain, chest tightness, fever, nausea, vomiting, hypotension, and tachycardia. These adverse events may be related to the infusion rate and can be managed by temporarily discontinuing the infusion. The infusion can be restarted at a decreased rate. Anaphylaxis occurs rarely and should be considered if hypotension develops during the infusion. Because CMV-IVIG contains other antibodies, live-virus vaccines should be withheld until 3 months after CMV-IVIG administration.

VACCINE INFORMATION RESOURCES

The field of vaccinology is developing ever more rapidly, with numerous changes in recommendations for vaccine use made each year. Keeping up to date with the current recommendations can be a challenge. The childhood, adolescent, and adult immunization schedules are updated frequently and published annually. Recommendations for the use of influenza vaccine are issued annually. Healthcare providers involved in primary care and immunization delivery must keep themselves abreast of these changes in a systematic way. Reading electronic newsletters and browsing reliable Websites are efficient methods for obtaining information (Table 102-6). Although several excellent, reliable, and timely Websites exist, hundreds of sites with misleading and incorrect information also exist. Many of these sites are targeted at parents.

Although the medical community has moved past the controversy, the public still has questions regarding the possible connection between vaccine exposure and autism. The only study to demonstrate a link between vaccines and autism was a series of case reports published in 1998 that has since been withdrawn, and its lead author has been accused of fraud. [63] None of nine studies that have

TABLE 102-6 Web Resources for Vaccine Information

Recommended Internet Sites for Vaccine Information	
http://www.cdc.gov/vaccines/	Vaccines & Immunizations Centers for Disease Control and Prevention
www.immunize.org	Immunization Action Coalition
www.nfid.org/	National Foundation for Infectious Diseases
www.cdc.gov/mmwr/	Morbidity and Mortality Weekly Report
www.iom.edu/	Institute of Medicine of the National Academies
http://www.hrsa.gov/vaccinecompensation/	Vaccine Injury Compensation Program
http://www.chop.edu/service/vaccine-education-center/	Vaccine Education Center Children's Hospital of Philadelphia
http://vaers.hhs.gov/index	Vaccine Adverse Event Reporting System
Recommended Electronic Newsletters	
www.immunize.org/express	The Immunization Action Coalition's newsletter
www.cdc.gov/mmwr/	Morbidity and Mortality Weekly Report

been conducted have found a connection between vaccine exposure and the development of autism.[64] The Vaccine Education Center at the Children's Hospital of Philadelphia has several documents for parents who have questions about vaccines and neurodevelopmental disorders. *http://www.chop.edu/service/vaccine-education-center/hot-topics/*. The CDC is another source of information for parents. *http://www.cdc.gov/vaccinesafety/Concerns/Autism/Index.html.*

PERSONALIZED PHARMACOTHERAPY

Immunization programs are an important part of public health for all people. Therefore, immunization schedules are used across the population with little consideration of individual variability. Recommendations for some vaccines are based on risks, occupation, lifestyle, or age.

However, pharmacogenomics can be used to predict which individuals may be likely to have a vigorous or poor response to a vaccine. Some apparently healthy individuals fail to mount an immune response to a particular vaccine.[65] The consequence of these research findings are not yet ready to be used in clinical care of patients. As the field matures, these polymorphisms may be considered for vaccine design or immunization scheduling.

Vaccines are the only class of medications to which nearly every patient is exposed. Knowledge of these agents is critical to providing pharmaceutical care. Dramatic progress in public health has been made through the appropriate use of immunization. Additional improvements in quality of life and mortality can be made through continued increases in vaccination coverage with careful attention to this aspect of care by all healthcare providers.

ABBREVIATIONS

ACIP	Advisory Committee on Immunization Practices
CDC	U.S. Centers for Disease Control and Prevention
CMV-IVIG	Cytomegalovirus IV immunoglobulin
DTaP	diphtheria, tetanus toxoids, and acellular pertussis
HDCV	human diploid cell rabies vaccine
Hib	*Haemophilus influenzae* type b
HPV	human papillomavirus
Ig	immunoglobulin
IIS	immunization information systems
IMIG	intramuscular immunoglobulin
IPV	inactivated polio vaccine
ITP	idiopathic (immune) thrombocytopenic purpura
IVIG	IV immunoglobulin
MMRV	measles–mumps–rubella vaccine
MSM	men who have sex with men
OPV	oral polio vaccine
PCECV	purified chick embryo cell rabies vaccine
PCV	pneumococcal conjugate vaccine
PPSV23	23-valent pneumococcal polysaccharide vaccine
PRP	polyribosylribitol phosphate
Td	tetanus–diphtheria
Tdap	tetanus–diphtheria–acellular pertussis
VAERS	Vaccine Adverse Event Reporting System

REFERENCES

1. Centers for Disease Control and Prevention. General recommendations on immunization. Recommendations of the Advisory Committee on Immunization Practices (ACIP). MMWR Morb Mortal Wkly Rep 2011;60:1–64.
2. Centers for Disease Control and Prevention. A comprehensive immunization strategy to eliminate transmission of hepatitis B virus infection in the United States. Recommendations of the Advisory Committee on Immunization Practices (ACIP). Part II: Immunization of adults. MMWR Morb Mortal Wkly Rep 2006;55:1–33.
3. Centers for Disease Control and Prevention. Prevention and control of influenza with vaccines. Recommendations of the Advisory Committee on Immunization Practices (ACIP), 2010. MMWR Morb Mortal Wkly Rep 2010;59:1–61.
4. Song JY, Cheong HJ, Hwang IS, et al. Long-term immunogenicity of influenza vaccine among the elderly: Risk factors for poor immune response and persistence. Vaccine 2010;28:3929–35.
5. Poland GA, Ovsyannikov I, Jacobson RM. Application of pharmacogenomics to vaccines. Pharmacogenomics 2009;10:837–52.
6. Löbermann M, Boršo D, Hilgendorf I, Fritzsche C, Zettl UK, Reisinger EC. Immunization in the adult immunocompromised host. Autoimmun Rev 2012;11:212–218.
7. Sanofi pasteur Inc. Influenza Vaccine Virus, Fluzone Product Information. Package Insert 2012:1–8.
8. Centers for Disease Control and Prevention. Prevention of rotavirus gastroenteritis among infants and children. Recommendations of the Advisory Committee on Immunization Practices (ACIP). MMWR Morb Mortal Wkly Rep 2009;58:1–24.
9. Centers for Disease Control and Prevention. Updated recommendations for use of tetanus toxoid, reduced diphtheria toxoid and acellular pertussis (Tdap) vaccine in pregnant women and persons who have or anticipate having close contact with an infant aged <12 months—Advisory Committee on Immunization Practices (ACIP), 2011. MMWR Morb Mortal Wkly Rep 2011;60:1424–1426.
10. Centers for Disease Control and Prevention. Guidelines for vaccinating pregnant women. In; July 2012:1–12.
11. Centers for Disease Control and Prevention. Prevention of herpes zoster. Recommendations of the Advisory Committee on Immunization Practices (ACIP). MMWR Morb Mortal Wkly Rep 2008;57:1–30.
12. Boehmer LM, Waqar SN, Govindan R. Influenza vaccination in patients with cancer: An overview. Oncology 2010;24:1–7.
13. Danzinger-Isakov L, Kumar D, the ASTIDCoP. Guidelines for vaccination of solid organ transplant candidates and recipients. Am J Transplant 2009;9:S258–S62.
14. Centers for Disease Control and Prevention. Immunization information systems progress—United States, 2010. MMWR Morb Mortal Wkly Rep 2012;61:464–467.
15. Varricchio F, Iskander J, DeStefano F, et al. Understanding vaccine safety information from the Vaccine Adverse Event Reporting System. Pediatr Infect Dis J 2004;23:287–294.
16. Centers for Disease Control and Prevention. Recommended immunization schedule for persons aged 0 through 18 years—United States, 2012. MMWR Morb Mortal Wkly Rep 2012; QuickGuide 61:1–4.
17. Centers for Disease Control and Prevention. Updated recommendations for use of tetanus toxoid, reduced diphtheria toxoid, and acellular pertussis (Tdap) vaccine in adults aged 65 years and older—Advisory Committee on Immunization Practices (ACIP), 2012. MMWR Morb Mortal Wkly Rep 2012;61:468–470.
18. Centers for Disease Control and Prevention. Updated recommendations for use of tetanus toxoid, reduced diphtheria toxoid and acellular pertussis (Tdap) vaccine from the Advisory Committee on Immunization Practices, 2010. MMWR Morb Mortal Wkly Rep 2011;60:13–15.

19. Centers for Disease Control and Prevention. Prevention of pertussis, tetanus, and diphtheria among pregnant and postpartum women and their infants. MMWR Morb Mortal Wkly Rep 2008;57:1–51.
20. Centers for Disease Control and Prevention. Recommended adult immunization schedule by vaccine and age group—United States, 2012. MMWR Morb Mortal Wkly Rep 2012; QuickGuide 61:1–7.
21. Centers for Disease Control and Prevention. Tetanus. In: Atkinson W, Wolfe CS, Hanborsky J, eds. Epidemiology and Prevention of Vaccine-Preventable Diseases. 12th ed. Washington, DC: Public Health Foundation; 2012:291–300.
22. Centers for Disease Control and Prevention. Preventing tetanus, diphtheria, and pertussis among adolescents: Use of tetanus toxoid, reduced diphtheria toxoid and acellular pertussis vaccines. Recommendations fo the Advisory Committee on Immunization Practices (ACIP). MMWR Morb Mortal Wkly Rep 2006;55:1–42.
23. Centers for Disease Control and Prevention. *Haemophilus influenzae* type b. In: Atkinson W, Wolfe CS, Hanborsky J, eds. Epidemiology and Prevention of Vaccine-Preventable Diseases. Washington, DC: Public Health Foundation, 2012:87–100.
24. Dunne EF, Unger ER, Sternberg M, et al. Prevalence of HPV infection among females in the United States. JAMA 2007;297:813–819.
25. Centers for Disease Control and Prevention. FDA licensure of bivalent human papillomavirus vaccine (HPV2, Cervarix) for use in females and updated HPV vaccination recommendations from the Advisory Committee on Immunization Practices (ACIP). MMWR Morb Mortal Wkly Rep 2010;59:626–629.
26. Brown DR, Kjaer Susanne K, Sigurdsson K, et al. The impact of quadrivalent human papillomavirus (HPV; Types 6, 11, 16, and 18) L1 virus-like particle vaccine on infection and disease due to oncogenic nonvaccine HPV types in generally HPV-naive women aged 16–26 years. J Infect Dis 2009;199:926–935.
27. Paavonen J, Naud P, Salmerón J, et al. Efficacy of human papillomavirus (HPV)-16/18 AS04-adjuvanted vaccine against cervical infection and precancer caused by oncogenic HPV types (PATRICIA): Final analysis of a double-blind, randomised study in young women. Lancet 2009;374:301–314.
28. Wheeler Cosette M, Kjaer Susanne K, Sigurdsson K, et al. The impact of quadrivalent human papillomavirus (HPV; Types 6, 11, 16, and 18) L1 virus-like particle vaccine on infection and disease due to oncogenic nonvaccine HPV types in sexually active women aged 16–26 years. J Infect Dis 2009;199:936–944.
29. Palefsky JM, Giuliano AR, Goldstone S, et al. HPV vaccine against anal HPV infection and anal intraepithelial neoplasia. N Engl J Med 2011;365:1576–1585.
30. Centers for Disease Control and Prevention. Recommendations on the use of quadrivalent human papillomavirus vaccine in males—Advisory Committee on Immunization Practices (ACIP), 2011. MMWR Morb Mortal Wkly Rep 2011;60:1705–1708.
31. Stermole BM, Grandits GA, Roediger MP, et al. Long-term safety and serologic response to measles, mumps, and rubella vaccination in HIV-1 infected adults. Vaccine 2011;29:2874–2880.
32. Scott P, Moss WJ, Gilani Z, Low N. Measles vaccination in HIV-infected children: Systematic review and meta-analysis of safety and immunogenicity. J Infect Dis 2011;204: S164–S178.
33. Centers for Disease Control and Prevention. Meningococcal disease. In: Atkinson W, Wolfe CS, Hanborsky J, eds. Epidemiology and Prevention of Vaccine-Preventable Diseases. Washington, DC: Public Health Foundation, 2012:193–204.
34. Centers for Disease Control and Prevention. Updated recommendations for the use of meningococcal conjugate vaccines—Advisory Committee on Immunization Practices (ACIP), 2010. MMWR Morb Mortal Wkly Rep 2011;60: 72–76.
35. Weycker D, Strutton D, Edelsberg J, Sato R, Jackson LA. Clinical and economic burden of pneumococcal disease in older US adults. Vaccine 2010;28:4955–4960.
36. Centers for Disease Control and Prevention. Prevention of pneumococcal disease among infants and children—Use of 13-valent pneumococcal conjugate vaccine and 23-valent pneumococcal polysaccharide vaccine. Recommendations of the Advisory Committee on Immunization Practices (ACIP). MMWR Morb Mortal Wkly Rep 2010;59:1–18.
37. Centers for Disease Control and Prevention. Updated recommendations for the prevention of invasive pneumococcal disease among adults using the 23-valent pneumococcal polysaccharide vaccine (PPSV23). MMWR Morb Mortal Wkly Rep 2010;59:1102–1106.
38. Fisman DN, Abrutyn E, Spaude KA, Kim A, Kirchner C, Daley J. Prior pneumococcal vaccination is associated with reduced death, complications, and length of stay among hospitalized adults with community-acquired pneumonia. Clin Infect Dis 2006;42:1093–1101.
39. Pilishvili T, Lexau C, Farley MM, et al. Sustained reductions in invasive pneumococcal disease in the era of conjugate vaccine. J Infect Dis 2010;201:32–41.
40. Centers for Disease Control and Prevention. Use of 13-valent pneumococcal conjugate vaccine and 23-valent pneumococcal polysaccharide vaccine for adults with immunocompromising conditions: Recommendations of the Advisory Committee on Immunization Practices (ACIP). MMWR Morb Mortal Wkly Rep. 2012;61(40):816–819.
41. Centers for Disease Control and Prevention. Updated recommendations of the Advisory Committee on Immunization Practices (ACIP) regarding routine poliovirus vaccination. MMWR Morb Mortal Wkly Rep 2009;58: 829–830.
42. Centers for Disease Control and Prevention. Poliomyelitis prevention in the United States: Updated recommendations of the Advisory Committee on Immunization Practices (ACIP). MMWR Morb Mortal Wkly Rep 2000;49:1–22.
43. Centers for Disease Control and Prevention. Human rabies prevention—United States, 2008. Recommendations of the Advisory Committee on Immunization Practices. MMWR Morb Mortal Wkly Rep 2008;57:1–28.
44. Centers for Disease Control and Prevention. Use of a reduced (4-dose) vaccine schedule for postexposure prophylaxis to prevent human rabies. Recommendations of the Advisory Committee on Immunization Practices. MMWR Morb Mortal Wkly Rep 2010;59:1–9.
45. Centers for Disease Control and Prevention. Measles, mumps, and rubella—Vaccine use and strategies for elimination of measles, rubella, and congenital rubella syndrome and control of mumps: Recommendations of the Advisory Committee on Immunization Practices (ACIP). MMWR Morb Mortal Wkly Rep 1998;47:1–57.
46. Mofenson L, Brady M, Danner S, et al. Guidelines for the Prevention and Treatment of Opportunistic Infections among HIV-exposed and HIV-infected children: Recommendations from CDC, the National Institutes of Health, the HIV Medicine Association of the Infectious Diseases Society of America, the Pediatric Infectious Diseases Society, and the

American Academy of Pediatrics. MMWR Morb Mortal Wkly Rep 2009;58:1–166.
47. Centers for Disease Control and Prevention. Revised ACIP recommendation for avoiding pregnancy after receiving a rubella-containing vaccine. MMWR Morb Mortal Wkly Rep 2001;50:1117.
48. Centers for Disease Control and Prevention. Prevention of varicella. Recommendations of the Advisory Committee on Immunization Practices (ACIP). MMWR Morb Mortal Wkly Rep 2007;56:1–39.
49. Yawn BP, Saddier P, Wollan PC, St Sauver JL, Kurland MJ, Sy LS. A population-based study of the incidence and complication rates of herpes zoster before zoster vaccine introduction. Mayo Clin Proc 2007;82:1341–1349.
50. Zhang J, Xie F, Delzell E, et al. Association between vaccination for herpes zoster and risk of herpes zoster infection among older patients with selected immune-mediated diseases. JAMA 2012;308:43–49.
51. Oxman MN, Levin MJ, Johnson GR, et al. A vaccine to prevent herpes zoster and postherpetic neuralgia in older adults. N Engl J Med 2005;352:2271–2284.
52. Centers for Disease Control and Prevention. FDA approval of an extended period for administering VariZIG for postexposure prophylaxis of varicella. MMWR Morb Mortal Wkly Rep 2012;61:212.
53. Leong H, Stachnik J, Bonk ME, Matuszewski KA. Unlabeled uses of intravenous immune globulin. Am J Health Syst Pharm 2008;65:1815–1824.
54. Stiehm ER, Orange JS, Ballow M, Lehman H. Therapeutic use of immunoglobulins. Advances in Pediatrics 2010;57:185–218.
55. Jolles S, Kaveri SV, Orange J. Current understanding and future directions. Clin Exp Immunol 2009;158:68–70.
56. Berger M. Choices in IgG replacement therapy for primary immune deficiency diseases: Subcutaneous IgG vs. intravenous IgG and selecting an optimal dose. Curr Opin Allergy Clin Immunol 2011;11:532–538.
57. Stasi R, Evangelista M, Stipa E, Buccisano F, Venditti A, Amadori S. Idiopathic thrombocytopenic purpura: Current concepts in pathophysiology and management. Thromb Haemost 2008;99:4–13.
58. Scuccimarri R. Kawasaki disease. Pediatr Clin North Am 2012;59:425–445.
59. Hughes R, Swan A, Doorn P. Intravenous immunoglobulin for Guillain–Barre syndrome. Cochrane Database Syst Rev 2012;(7):1–63.
60. Özkara Ç, Vigevano F. Immuno- and antiinflammatory therapies in epileptic disorders. Epilepsia 2011;52:45–51.
61. Murphy E, Martin S, Patterson JV. Developing practice guidelines for the administration of intravenous immunoglobulin. J Infusion Nurs 2005;28:265–272.
62. Carbone J. Adverse reactions and pathogen safety of intravenous immunoglobulin. Curr Drug Saf 2007;2:9–18.
63. Hawkes N. College investigates whether Wakefield was guilty of scientific fraud. BMJ 2011;342.
64. Centers for Disease Control and Prevention. CDC: Immunization safety and autism—thimerosal and autism research chart. *http://www.cdc.gov/vaccinesafety/00_pdf/CDCStudiesonVaccinesandAutism.pdf.*
65. Poland G, Ovsyannikova I, Jacobson R. Application of pharmacogenomics to vaccines. Pharmacogenomics 2009;10:837–852.

Appendix 102-1

2012 Childhood and Adolescent Immunization Schedules

Figure 1. Recommended immunization schedule for persons aged 0 through 18 years—2013.
(FOR THOSE WHO FALL BEHIND OR START LATE, SEE THE CATCH-UP SCHEDULE [FIGURE 2]).

These recommendations must be read with the footnotes that follow. For those who fall behind or start late, provide catch-up vaccination at the earliest opportunity as indicated by the green bars in Figure 1. To determine minimum intervals between doses, see the catch-up schedule (Figure 2). School entry and adolescent vaccine age groups are in bold.

Vaccines	Birth	1 mo	2 mos	4 mos	6 mos	9 mos	12 mos	15 mos	18 mos	19–23 mos	2-3 yrs	**4-6 yrs**	7-10 yrs	**11-12 yrs**	13–15 yrs	16–18 yrs
Hepatitis B[1] (HepB)	←1st dose→	←2nd dose→			←3rd dose→											
Rotavirus[2] (RV) RV-1 (2-dose series); RV-5 (3-dose series)			←1st dose→	←2nd dose→	See footnote 2											
Diphtheria, tetanus, & acellular pertussis[3] (DTaP: <7 yrs)			←1st dose→	←2nd dose→	←3rd dose→			←4th dose→				←5th dose→				
Tetanus, diphtheria, & acellular pertussis[4] (Tdap: ≥7 yrs)														(Tdap)		
Haemophilus influenzae type b[5] (Hib)			←1st dose→	←2nd dose→	See footnote 5		←3rd or 4th dose, see footnote 5→									
Pneumococcal conjugate[6a,c] (PCV13)			←1st dose→	←2nd dose→	←3rd dose→		←4th dose→									
Pneumococcal polysaccharide[6b,c] (PPSV23)																
Inactivated Poliovirus[7] (IPV) (<18years)			←1st dose→	←2nd dose→	←3rd dose→							←4th dose→				
Influenza[8] (IIV; LAIV) 2 doses for some : see footnote 8					Annual vaccination (IIV only)						Annual vaccination (IIV or LAIV)					
Measles, mumps, rubella[9] (MMR)							←1st dose→					←2nd dose→				
Varicella[10] (VAR)							←1st dose→					←2nd dose→				
Hepatitis A[11] (HepA)							←2 dose series, see footnote 11→									
Human papillomavirus[12] (HPV2: females only; HPV4: males and females)														(3-dose series)		
Meningococcal[13] (Hib-MenCY ≥ 6 weeks; MCV4-D≥9 mos; MCV4-CRM ≥ 2 yrs.)			see footnote 13											←1st dose→		booster

Range of recommended ages for all children | Range of recommended ages for catch-up immunization | Range of recommended ages for certain high-risk groups | Range of recommended ages during which catch-up is encouraged and for certain high-risk groups | Not routinely recommended

This schedule includes recommendations in effect as of January 1, 2013. Any dose not administered at the recommended age should be administered at a subsequent visit, when indicated and feasible. The use of a combination vaccine generally is preferred over separate injections of its equivalent component vaccines. Vaccination providers should consult the relevant Advisory Committee on Immunization Practices (ACIP) statement for detailed recommendations, available online at http://www.cdc.gov/vaccines/pubs/acip-list.htm. Clinically significant adverse events that follow vaccination should be reported to the Vaccine Adverse Event Reporting System (VAERS) online (http://www.vaers.hhs.gov) or by telephone (800-822-7967).Suspected cases of vaccine-preventable diseases should be reported to the state or local health department. Additional information, including precautions and contraindications for vaccination, is available from CDC online (http://www.cdc.gov/vaccines) or by telephone (800-CDC-INFO [800-232-4636]).

This schedule is approved by the Advisory Committee on Immunization Practices (http://www.cdc.gov/vaccines/acip/index.html), the American Academy of Pediatrics (http://www.aap.org), the American Academy of Family Physicians (http://www.aafp.org), and the American College of Obstetricians and Gynecologists (http://www.acog.org).

NOTE: The above recommendations must be read along with the footnotes of this schedule.

Footnotes — Recommended immunization schedule for persons aged 0 through 18 years—United States, 2013

For further guidance on the use of the vaccines mentioned below, see: http://www.cdc.gov/vaccines/pubs/acip-list.htm.

1. **Hepatitis B (HepB) vaccine. (Minimum age: birth)**
   Routine vaccination:
   At birth
   - Administer monovalent HepB vaccine to all newborns before hospital discharge.
   - For infants born to hepatitis B surface antigen (HBsAg)–positive mothers, administer HepB vaccine and 0.5 mL of hepatitis B immune globulin (HBIG) within 12 hours of birth. These infants should be tested for HBsAg and antibody to HBsAg (anti-HBs) 1 to 2 months after completion of the HepB series, at age 9 through 18 months (preferably at the next well-child visit).
   - If mother's HBsAg status is unknown, within 12 hours of birth administer HepB vaccine to all infants regardless of birth weight. For infants weighing <2,000 grams, administer HBIG in addition to HepB within 12 hours of birth. Determine mother's HBsAg status as soon as possible and, if she is HBsAg-positive, also administer HBIG for infants weighing ≥2,000 grams (no later than age 1 week).

   Doses following the birth dose
   - The second dose should be administered at age 1 or 2 months. Monovalent HepB vaccine should be used for doses administered before age 6 weeks.
   - Infants who did not receive a birth dose should receive 3 doses of a HepB-containing vaccine on a schedule of 0, 1 to 2 months, and 6 months starting as soon as feasible. See Figure 2.
   - The minimum interval between dose 1 and dose 2 is 4 weeks and between dose 2 and 3 is 8 weeks. The final (third or fourth) dose in the HepB vaccine series should be administered no earlier than age 24 weeks, and at least 16 weeks after the first dose.
   - Administration of a total of 4 doses of HepB vaccine is recommended when a combination vaccine containing HepB is administered after the birth dose.

   Catch-up vaccination:
   - Unvaccinated persons should complete a 3-dose series.
   - A 2-dose series (doses separated by at least 4 months) of adult formulation Recombivax HB is licensed for use in children aged 11 through 15 years.
   - For other catch-up issues, see Figure 2.
2. **Rotavirus (RV) vaccines. (Minimum age: 6 weeks for both RV-1 [Rotarix] and RV-5 [RotaTeq]).**
   Routine vaccination:
   - Administer a series of RV vaccine to all infants as follows:
     1. If RV-1 is used, administer a 2-dose series at 2 and 4 months of age.
     2. If RV-5 is used, administer a 3-dose series at ages 2, 4, and 6 months.
     3. If any dose in series was RV-5 or vaccine product is unknown for any dose in the series, a total of 3 doses of RV vaccine should be administered.

   Catch-up vaccination:
   - The maximum age for the first dose in the series is 14 weeks, 6 days.
   - Vaccination should not be initiated for infants aged 15 weeks 0 days or older.
   - The maximum age for the final dose in the series is 8 months, 0 days.
   - If RV-1(Rotarix) is administered for the first and second doses, a third dose is not indicated.
   - For other catch-up issues, see Figure 2.
3. **Diphtheria and tetanus toxoids and acellular pertussis (DTaP) vaccine. (Minimum age: 6 weeks)**
   Routine vaccination:
   - Administer a 5-dose series of DTaP vaccine at ages 2, 4, 6, 15–18 months, and 4 through 6 years. The fourth dose may be administered as early as age 12 months, provided at least 6 months have elapsed since the third dose.

   Catch-up vaccination:
   - The fifth (booster) dose of DTaP vaccine is not necessary if the fourth dose was administered at age 4 years or older.
   - For other catch-up issues, see Figure 2.
4. **Tetanus and diphtheria toxoids and acellular pertussis (Tdap) vaccine. (Minimum age: 10 years for Boostrix, 11 years for Adacel).**
   Routine vaccination:
   - Administer 1 dose of Tdap vaccine to all adolescents aged 11 through 12 years.
   - Tdap can be administered regardless of the interval since the last tetanus and diphtheria toxoid-containing vaccine.
   - Administer one dose of Tdap vaccine to pregnant adolescents during each pregnancy (preferred during 27 through 36 weeks gestation) regardless of number of years from prior Td or Tdap vaccination.

   Catch-up vaccination:
   - Persons aged 7 through 10 years who are not fully immunized with the childhood DTaP vaccine series, should receive Tdap vaccine as the first dose in the catch-up series; if additional doses are needed, use Td vaccine. For these children, an adolescent Tdap vaccine should not be given.
   - Persons aged 11 through 18 years who have not received Tdap vaccine should receive a dose followed by tetanus and diphtheria toxoids (Td) booster doses every 10 years thereafter.
   - An inadvertent dose of DTaP vaccine administered to children aged 7 through 10 years can count as part of the catch-up series. This dose can count as the adolescent Tdap dose, or the child can later receive a Tdap booster dose at age 11–12 years.
   - For other catch-up issues, see Figure 2.
5. ***Haemophilus influenzae* type b (Hib) conjugate vaccine. (Minimum age: 6 weeks)**
   Routine vaccination:
   - Administer a Hib vaccine primary series and a booster dose to all infants. The primary series doses should be administered at 2, 4, and 6 months of age; however, if PRP-OMP (PedvaxHib or Comvax) is administered at 2 and 4 months of age, a dose at age 6 months is not indicated. One booster dose should be administered at age 12 through15 months.
   - Hiberix (PRP-T) should only be used for the booster (final) dose in children aged 12 months through 4 years, who have received at least 1 dose of Hib.

   Catch-up vaccination:
   - If dose 1 was administered at ages 12-14 months, administer booster (as final dose) at least 8 weeks after dose 1.
   - If the first 2 doses were PRP-OMP (PedvaxHIB or Comvax), and were administered at age 11 months or younger, the third (and final) dose should be administered at age 12 through 15 months and at least 8 weeks after the second dose.
   - If the first dose was administered at age 7 through 11 months, administer the second dose at least 4 weeks later and a final dose at age 12 through 15 months, regardless of Hib vaccine (PRP-T or PRP-OMP) used for first dose.
   - For unvaccinated children aged 15 months or older, administer only 1 dose.

For further guidance on the use of the vaccines mentioned below, see: http://www.cdc.gov/vaccines/pubs/acip-list.htm.

- For other catch-up issues, see Figure 2.

Vaccination of persons with high-risk conditions:

- Hib vaccine is not routinely recommended for patients older than 5 years of age. However one dose of Hib vaccine should be administered to unvaccinated or partially vaccinated persons aged 5 years or older who have leukemia, malignant neoplasms, anatomic or functional asplenia (including sickle cell disease), human immunodeficiency virus (HIV) infection, or other immunocompromising conditions.

6a. Pneumococcal conjugate vaccine (PCV). (Minimum age: 6 weeks)

Routine vaccination:

- Administer a series of PCV13 vaccine at ages 2, 4, 6 months with a booster at age 12 through 15 months.
- For children aged 14 through 59 months who have received an age-appropriate series of 7-valent PCV (PCV7), administer a single supplemental dose of 13-valent PCV (PCV13).

Catch-up vaccination:

- Administer 1 dose of PCV13 to all healthy children aged 24 through 59 months who are not completely vaccinated for their age.
- For other catch-up issues, see Figure 2.

Vaccination of persons with high-risk conditions:

- For children aged 24 through 71 months with certain underlying medical conditions (see footnote 6c), administer 1 dose of PCV13 if 3 doses of PCV were received previously, or administer 2 doses of PCV13 at least 8 weeks apart if fewer than 3 doses of PCV were received previously.
- A single dose of PCV13 may be administered to previously unvaccinated children aged 6 through 18 years who have anatomic or functional asplenia (including sickle cell disease), HIV infection or an immunocompromising condition, cochlear implant or cerebrospinal fluid leak. See MMWR 2010;59 (No. RR-11), available at http://www.cdc.gov/mmwr/pdf/rr/rr5911.pdf.
- Administer PPSV23 at least 8 weeks after the last dose of PCV to children aged 2 years or older with certain underlying medical conditions (see footnotes 6b and 6c).

6b. Pneumococcal polysaccharide vaccine (PPSV23). (Minimum age: 2 years)

Vaccination of persons with high-risk conditions:

- Administer PPSV23 at least 8 weeks after the last dose of PCV to children aged 2 years or older with certain underlying medical conditions (see footnote 6c). A single revaccination with PPSV should be administered after 5 years to children with anatomic or functional asplenia (including sickle cell disease) or an immunocompromising condition.

6c. Medical conditions for which PPSV23 is indicated in children aged 2 years and older and for which use of PCV13 is indicated in children aged 24 through 71 months:

- Immunocompetent children with chronic heart disease (particularly cyanotic congenital heart disease and cardiac failure); chronic lung disease (including asthma if treated with high-dose oral corticosteroid therapy), diabetes mellitus; cerebrospinal fluid leaks; or cochlear implant.
- Children with anatomic or functional asplenia (including sickle cell disease and other hemoglobinopathies, congenital or acquired asplenia, or splenic dysfunction);
- Children with immunocompromising conditions: HIV infection, chronic renal failure and nephrotic syndrome, diseases associated with treatment with immunosuppressive drugs or radiation therapy, including malignant neoplasms, leukemias, lymphomas and Hodgkin disease; or solid organ transplantation, congenital immunodeficiency.

7. Inactivated poliovirus vaccine (IPV). (Minimum age: 6 weeks)

Routine vaccination:

- Administer a series of IPV at ages 2, 4, 6–18 months, with a booster at age 4–6 years. The final dose in the series should be administered on or after the fourth birthday and at least 6 months after the previous dose.

Catch-up vaccination:

- In the first 6 months of life, minimum age and minimum intervals are only recommended if the person is at risk for imminent exposure to circulating poliovirus (i.e., travel to a polio-endemic region or during an outbreak).
- If 4 or more doses are administered before age 4 years, an additional dose should be administered at age 4 through 6 years.
- A fourth dose is not necessary if the third dose was administered at age 4 years or older and at least 6 months after the previous dose.
- If both OPV and IPV were administered as part of a series, a total of 4 doses should be administered, regardless of the child's current age.
- IPV is not routinely recommended for U.S. residents aged 18 years or older.
- For other catch-up issues, see Figure 2.

8. Influenza vaccines. (Minimum age: 6 months for inactivated influenza vaccine [IIV]; 2 years for live, attenuated influenza vaccine [LAIV])

Routine vaccination:

- Administer influenza vaccine annually to all children beginning at age 6 months. For most healthy, nonpregnant persons aged 2 through 49 years, either LAIV or IIV may be used. However, LAIV should NOT be administered to some persons, including 1) those with asthma, 2) children 2 through 4 years who had wheezing in the past 12 months, or 3) those who have any other underlying medical conditions that predispose them to influenza complications. For all other contraindications to use of LAIV see MMWR 2010; 59 (No. RR-8), available at http://www.cdc.gov/mmwr/pdf/rr/rr5908.pdf.
- Administer 1 dose to persons aged 9 years and older.

For children aged 6 months through 8 years:

- For the 2012–13 season, administer 2 doses (separated by at least 4 weeks) to children who are receiving influenza vaccine for the first time. For additional guidance, follow dosing guidelines in the 2012 ACIP influenza vaccine recommendations, MMWR 2012; 61: 613–618, available at http://www.cdc.gov/mmwr/pdf/wk/mm6132.pdf.
- For the 2013–14 season, follow dosing guidelines in the 2013 ACIP influenza vaccine recommendations.

9. Measles, mumps, and rubella (MMR) vaccine. (Minimum age: 12 months for routine vaccination)

Routine vaccination:

- Administer the first dose of MMR vaccine at age 12 through 15 months, and the second dose at age 4 through 6 years. The second dose may be administered before age 4 years, provided at least 4 weeks have elapsed since the first dose.
- Administer 1 dose of MMR vaccine to infants aged 6 through 11 months before departure from the United States for international travel. These children should be revaccinated with 2 doses of MMR vaccine, the first at age 12 through 15 months (12 months if the child remains in an area where disease risk is high), and the second dose at least 4 weeks later.
- Administer 2 doses of MMR vaccine to children aged 12 months and older, before departure from the United States for international travel. The first dose should be administered on or after age 12 months and the second dose at least 4 weeks later.

Catch-up vaccination:

- Ensure that all school-aged children and adolescents have had 2 doses of MMR vaccine; the minimum interval between the 2 doses is 4 weeks.

10. Varicella (VAR) vaccine. (Minimum age: 12 months)

Routine vaccination:

- Administer the first dose of VAR vaccine at age 12 through 15 months, and the second dose at age 4 through 6 years. The second dose may be administered before age 4 years, provided at least 3 months have elapsed since the first dose. If the second dose was administered at least 4 weeks after the first dose, it can be accepted as valid.

Catch-up vaccination:

- Ensure that all persons aged 7 through 18 years without evidence of immunity (see MMWR 2007;56 [No. RR-4], available at http://www.cdc.gov/mmwr/pdf/rr/rr5604.pdf) have 2 doses of varicella vaccine. For children aged 7 through 12 years the recommended minimum interval between doses is 3 months (if the second dose was administered at least 4 weeks after the first dose, it can be accepted as valid); for persons aged 13 years and older, the minimum interval between doses is 4 weeks.

11. Hepatitis A vaccine (HepA). (Minimum age: 12 months)

Routine vaccination:

- Initiate the 2-dose HepA vaccine series for children aged 12 through 23 months; separate the 2 doses by 6 to 18 months.
- Children who have received 1 dose of HepA vaccine before age 24 months, should receive a second dose 6 to 18 months after the first dose.
- For any person aged 2 years and older who has not already received the HepA vaccine series, 2 doses of HepA vaccine separated by 6 to 18 months may be administered if immunity against hepatitis A virus infection is desired.

Catch-up vaccination:

- The minimum interval between the two doses is 6 months.

Special populations:

- Administer 2 doses of Hep A vaccine at least 6 months apart to previously unvaccinated persons who live in areas where vaccination programs target older children, or who are at increased risk for infection.

12. Human papillomavirus (HPV) vaccines. (HPV4 [Gardasil] and HPV2 [Cervarix]). (Minimum age: 9 years)

Routine vaccination:

- Administer a 3-dose series of HPV vaccine on a schedule of 0, 1-2, and 6 months to all adolescents aged 11-12 years. Either HPV4 or HPV2 may be used for females, and only HPV4 may be used for males.
- The vaccine series can be started beginning at age 9 years.
- Administer the second dose 1 to 2 months after the **first** dose and the third dose 6 months after the **first** dose (at least 24 weeks after the first dose).

Catch-up vaccination:

- Administer the vaccine series to females (either HPV2 or HPV4) and males (HPV4) at age 13 through 18 years if not previously vaccinated.
- Use recommended routine dosing intervals (see above) for vaccine series catch-up.

13. Meningococcal conjugate vaccines (MCV). (Minimum age: 6 weeks for Hib-MenCY, 9 months for Menactra [MCV4-D], 2 years for Menveo [MCV4-CRM]).

Routine vaccination:

- Administer MCV4 vaccine at age 11–12 years, with a booster dose at age 16 years.
- Adolescents aged 11 through 18 years with human immunodeficiency virus (HIV) infection should receive a 2-dose primary series of MCV4, with at least 8 weeks between doses. See MMWR 2011; 60:1018–1019 available at: http://www.cdc.gov/mmwr/pdf/wk/mm6030.pdf.
- For children aged 9 months through 10 years with high-risk conditions, see below.

Catch-up vaccination:

- Administer MCV4 vaccine at age 13 through 18 years if not previously vaccinated.
- If the first dose is administered at age 13 through 15 years, a booster dose should be administered at age 16 through 18 years with a minimum interval of at least 8 weeks between doses.
- If the first dose is administered at age 16 years or older, a booster dose is not needed.
- For other catch-up issues, see Figure 2.

Vaccination of persons with high-risk conditions:

- For children younger than 19 months of age with anatomic or functional asplenia (including sickle cell disease), administer an infant series of Hib-MenCY at 2, 4, 6, and 12-15 months.
- For children aged 2 through 18 months with persistent complement component deficiency, administer either an infant series of Hib-MenCY at 2, 4, 6, and 12 through 15 months or a 2-dose primary series of MCV4-D starting at 9 months, with at least 8 weeks between doses. For children aged 19 through 23 months with persistent complement component deficiency who have not received a complete series of Hib-MenCY or MCV4-D, administer 2 primary doses of MCV4-D at least 8 weeks apart.
- For children aged 24 months and older with persistent complement component deficiency or anatomic or functional asplenia (including sickle cell disease), who have not received a complete series of Hib-MenCY or MCV4-D, administer 2 primary doses of either MCV4-D or MCV4-CRM. If MCV4-D (Menactra) is administered to a child with asplenia (including sickle cell disease), do not administer MCV4-D until 2 years of age and at least 4 weeks after the completion of all PCV13 doses. See MMWR 2011;60:1391–2, available at http://www.cdc.gov/mmwr/pdf/wk/mm6040.pdf.
- For children aged 9 months and older who are residents of or travelers to countries in the African meningitis belt or to the Hajj, administer an age-appropriate formulation and series of MCV4 for protection against serogroups A and W-135. Prior receipt of Hib-MenCY is not sufficient for children traveling to the meningitis belt or the Hajj. See MMWR 2011;60:1391–2, available at http://www.cdc.gov/mmwr/pdf/wk/mm6040.pdf.
- For children who are present during outbreaks caused by a vaccine serogroup, administer or complete an age-and formulation-appropriate series of Hib-MenCY or MCV4.
- For booster doses among persons with high-risk conditions refer to http://www.cdc.gov/vaccines/pubs/acip-list.htm#mening.

Additional information

- For contraindications and precautions to use of a vaccine and for additional information regarding that vaccine, vaccination providers should consult the relevant ACIP statement available online at http://www.cdc.gov/vaccines/pubs/acip-list.htm.
- For the purposes of calculating intervals between doses, 4 weeks = 28 days. Intervals of 4 months or greater are determined by calendar months.
- Information on travel vaccine requirements and recommendations is available at http://wwwnc.cdc.gov/travel/page/vaccinations.htm.
- For vaccination of persons with primary and secondary immunodeficiencies, see Table 13, "Vaccination of persons with primary and secondary immunodeficiencies," in General Recommendations on Immunization (ACIP), available at http://www.cdc.gov/mmwr/preview/mmwrhtml/rr6002a1.htm; and American Academy of Pediatrics. Passive immunization. In: Pickering LK, Baker CJ, Kimberlin DW, Long SS eds. Red book: 2012 report of the Committee on Infectious Diseases. 29th ed. Elk Grove Village, IL: American Academy of Pediatrics.

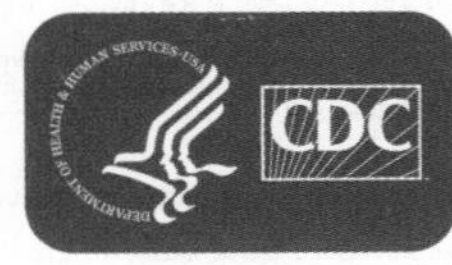

U.S. Department of Health and Human Services
Centers for Disease Control and Prevention

Appendix 102-2

Catch-up Schedule for Person Age 4 Months to 18 years

FIGURE 2. Catch-up immunization schedule for persons aged 4 months through 18 years who start late or who are more than 1 month behind —United States, 2013

The figure below provides catch-up schedules and minimum intervals between doses for children whose vaccinations have been delayed. A vaccine series does not need to be restarted, regardless of the time that has elapsed between doses. Use the section appropriate for the child's age. Always use this table in conjunction with Figure 1 and the footnotes that follow.

Vaccine	Minimum Age for Dose 1	Minimum Interval Between Doses			
		Dose 1 to dose 2	Dose 2 to dose 3	Dose 3 to dose 4	Dose 4 to dose 5
Persons aged 4 months through 6 years					
Hepatitis B[1]	Birth	4 weeks	8 weeks and at least 16 weeks after first dose; minimum age for the final dose is 24 weeks		
Rotavirus[2]	6 weeks	4 weeks	4 weeks[2]		
Diphtheria, tetanus, pertussis[3]	6 weeks	4 weeks	4 weeks	6 months	6 months[3]
Haemophilus influenzae type b[5]	6 weeks	4 weeks if first dose administered at younger than age 12 months 8 weeks (as final dose) if first dose administered at age 12–14 months No further doses needed if first dose administered at age 15 months or older	4 weeks[5] if current age is younger than 12 months 8 weeks (as final dose)[5] if current age is 12 months or older and first dose administered at younger than age 12 months and second dose administered at younger than 15 months No further doses needed if previous dose administered at age 15 months or older	8 weeks (as final dose) This dose only necessary for children aged 12 through 59 months who received 3 doses before age 12 months	
Pneumococcal[6]	6 weeks	4 weeks if first dose administered at younger than age 12 months 8 weeks (as final dose for healthy children) if first dose administered at age 12 months or older or current age 24 through 59 months No further doses needed for healthy children if first dose administered at age 24 months or older	4 weeks if current age is younger than 12 months 8 weeks (as final dose for healthy children) if current age is 12 months or older No further doses needed for healthy children if previous dose administered at age 24 months or older	8 weeks (as final dose) This dose only necessary for children aged 12 through 59 months who received 3 doses before age 12 months or for children at high risk who received 3 doses at any age	
Inactivated poliovirus[7]	6 weeks	4 weeks	4 weeks	6 months[7] minimum age 4 years for final dose	
Meningococcal[13]	6 weeks	8 weeks[13]	see footnote 13	see footnote 13	
Measles, mumps, rubella[9]	12 months	4 weeks			
Varicella[10]	12 months	3 months			
Hepatitis A[11]	12 months	6 months			
Persons aged 7 through 18 years					
Tetanus, diphtheria; tetanus, diphtheria, pertussis[4]	7 years[4]	4 weeks	4 weeks if first dose administered at younger than age 12 months 6 months if first dose administered at 12 months or older	6 months if first dose administered at younger than age 12 months	
Human papillomavirus[12]	9 years	Routine dosing intervals are recommended[12]			
Hepatitis A[11]	12 months	6 months			
Hepatitis B[1]	Birth	4 weeks	8 weeks (and at least 16 weeks after first dose)		
Inactivated poliovirus[7]	6 weeks	4 weeks	4 weeks[7]	6 months[7]	
Meningococcal[13]	6 weeks	8 weeks[13]			
Measles, mumps, rubella[9]	12 months	4 weeks			
Varicella[10]	12 months	3 months if person is younger than age 13 years 4 weeks if person is aged 13 years or older			

NOTE: The above recommendations must be read along with the footnotes of this schedule.

Footnotes — Recommended immunization schedule for persons aged 0 through 18 years—United States, 2013

For further guidance on the use of the vaccines mentioned below, see: http://www.cdc.gov/vaccines/pubs/acip-list.htm.

1. **Hepatitis B (HepB) vaccine. (Minimum age: birth)**
   Routine vaccination:
   At birth
   - Administer monovalent HepB vaccine to all newborns before hospital discharge.
   - For infants born to hepatitis B surface antigen (HBsAg)–positive mothers, administer HepB vaccine and 0.5 mL of hepatitis B immune globulin (HBIG) within 12 hours of birth. These infants should be tested for HBsAg and antibody to HBsAg (anti-HBs) 1 to 2 months after completion of the HepB series, at age 9 through 18 months (preferably at the next well-child visit).
   - If mother's HBsAg status is unknown, within 12 hours of birth administer HepB vaccine to all infants regardless of birth weight. For infants weighing <2,000 grams, administer HBIG in addition to HepB within 12 hours of birth. Determine mother's HBsAg status as soon as possible and, if she is HBsAg-positive, also administer HBIG for infants weighing ≥2,000 grams (no later than age 1 week).

   Doses following the birth dose
   - The second dose should be administered at age 1 or 2 months. Monovalent HepB vaccine should be used for doses administered before age 6 weeks.
   - Infants who did not receive a birth dose should receive 3 doses of a HepB-containing vaccine on a schedule of 0, 1 to 2 months, and 6 months starting as soon as feasible. See Figure 2.
   - The minimum interval between dose 1 and dose 2 is 4 weeks and between dose 2 and 3 is 8 weeks. The final (third or fourth) dose in the HepB vaccine series should be administered no earlier than age 24 weeks, and at least 16 weeks after the first dose.
   - Administration of a total of 4 doses of HepB vaccine is recommended when a combination vaccine containing HepB is administered after the birth dose.

   Catch-up vaccination:
   - Unvaccinated persons should complete a 3-dose series.
   - A 2-dose series (doses separated by at least 4 months) of adult formulation Recombivax HB is licensed for use in children aged 11 through 15 years.
   - For other catch-up issues, see Figure 2.
2. **Rotavirus (RV) vaccines. (Minimum age: 6 weeks for both RV-1 [Rotarix] and RV-5 [RotaTeq]).**
   Routine vaccination:
   - Administer a series of RV vaccine to all infants as follows:
     1. If RV-1 is used, administer a 2-dose series at 2 and 4 months of age.
     2. If RV-5 is used, administer a 3-dose series at ages 2, 4, and 6 months.
     3. If any dose in series was RV-5 or vaccine product is unknown for any dose in the series, a total of 3 doses of RV vaccine should be administered.

   Catch-up vaccination:
   - The maximum age for the first dose in the series is 14 weeks, 6 days.
   - Vaccination should not be initiated for infants aged 15 weeks 0 days or older.
   - The maximum age for the final dose in the series is 8 months, 0 days.
   - If RV-1 (Rotarix) is administered for the first and second doses, a third dose is not indicated.
   - For other catch-up issues, see Figure 2.
3. **Diphtheria and tetanus toxoids and acellular pertussis (DTaP) vaccine. (Minimum age: 6 weeks)**
   Routine vaccination:
   - Administer a 5-dose series of DTaP vaccine at ages 2, 4, 6, 15–18 months, and 4 through 6 years. The fourth dose may be administered as early as age 12 months, provided at least 6 months have elapsed since the third dose.

   Catch-up vaccination:
   - The fifth (booster) dose of DTaP vaccine is not necessary if the fourth dose was administered at age 4 years or older.
   - For other catch-up issues, see Figure 2.
4. **Tetanus and diphtheria toxoids and acellular pertussis (Tdap) vaccine. (Minimum age: 10 years for Boostrix, 11 years for Adacel).**
   Routine vaccination:
   - Administer 1 dose of Tdap vaccine to all adolescents aged 11 through 12 years.
   - Tdap can be administered regardless of the interval since the last tetanus and diphtheria toxoid-containing vaccine.

For further guidance on the use of the vaccines mentioned below, see: http://www.cdc.gov/vaccines/pubs/acip-list.htm.

- Administer one dose of Tdap vaccine to pregnant adolescents during each pregnancy (preferred during 27 through 36 weeks gestation) regardless of number of years from prior Td or Tdap vaccination.

Catch-up vaccination:
- Persons aged 7 through 10 years who are not fully immunized with the childhood DTaP vaccine series should receive Tdap vaccine as the first dose in the catch-up series; if additional doses are needed, use Td vaccine. For these children, an adolescent Tdap vaccine should not be given.
- Persons aged 11 through 18 years who have not received Tdap vaccine should receive a dose followed by tetanus and diphtheria toxoids (Td) booster doses every 10 years thereafter.
- An inadvertent dose of DTaP vaccine administered to children aged 7 through 10 years can count as part of the catch-up series. This dose can count as the adolescent Tdap dose, or the child can later receive a Tdap booster dose at age 11–12 years.
- For other catch-up issues, see Figure 2.

5. ***Haemophilus influenzae* type b (Hib) conjugate vaccine. (Minimum age: 6 weeks)**

Routine vaccination:
- Administer a Hib vaccine primary series and a booster dose to all infants. The primary series doses should be administered at 2, 4, and 6 months of age; however, if PRP-OMP (PedvaxHib or Comvax) is administered at 2 and 4 months of age, a dose at age 6 months is not indicated. One booster dose should be administered at age 12 through15 months.
- Hiberix (PRP-T) should only be used for the booster (final) dose in children aged 12 months through 4 years, who have received at least 1 dose of Hib.

Catch-up vaccination:
- If dose 1 was administered at ages 12-14 months, administer booster (as final dose) at least 8 weeks after dose 1.
- If the first 2 doses were PRP-OMP (PedvaxHIB or Comvax), and were administered at age 11 months or younger, the third (and final) dose should be administered at age 12 through 15 months and at least 8 weeks after the second dose.
- If the first dose was administered at age 7 through 11 months, administer the second dose at least 4 weeks later and a final dose at age 12 through 15 months, regardless of Hib vaccine (PRP-T or PRP-OMP) used for first dose.
- For unvaccinated children aged 15 months or older, administer only 1 dose.
- For other catch-up issues, see Figure 2.

Vaccination of persons with high-risk conditions:
- Hib vaccine is not routinely recommended for patients older than 5 years of age. However one dose of Hib vaccine should be administered to unvaccinated or partially vaccinated persons aged 5 years or older who have leukemia, malignant neoplasms, anatomic or functional asplenia (including sickle cell disease), human immunodeficiency virus (HIV) infection, or other immunocompromising conditions.

6a. **Pneumococcal conjugate vaccine (PCV). (Minimum age: 6 weeks)**

Routine vaccination:
- Administer a series of PCV13 vaccine at ages 2, 4, and 6 months with a booster at age 12 through 15 months.
- For children aged 14 through 59 months who have received an age-appropriate series of 7-valent PCV (PCV7), administer a single supplemental dose of 13-valent PCV (PCV13).

Catch-up vaccination:
- Administer 1 dose of PCV13 to all healthy children aged 24 through 59 months who are not completely vaccinated for their age.
- For other catch-up issues, see Figure 2.

Vaccination of persons with high-risk conditions:
- For children aged 24 through 71 months with certain underlying medical conditions (see footnote 6c), administer 1 dose of PCV13 if 3 doses of PCV were received previously, or administer 2 doses of PCV13 at least 8 weeks apart if fewer than 3 doses of PCV were received previously.
- A single dose of PCV13 may be administered to previously unvaccinated children aged 6 through 18 years who have anatomic or functional asplenia (including sickle cell disease), HIV infection or an immunocompromising condition, cochlear implant or cerebrospinal fluid leak. See MMWR 2010;59 (No. RR-11), available at http://www.cdc.gov/mmwr/pdf/rr/rr5911.pdf.
- Administer PPSV23 at least 8 weeks after the last dose of PCV to children aged 2 years or older with certain underlying medical conditions (see footnotes 6b and 6c).

6b. **Pneumococcal polysaccharide vaccine (PPSV23). (Minimum age: 2 years)**

Vaccination of persons with high-risk conditions:
- Administer PPSV23 at least 8 weeks after the last dose of PCV to children aged 2 years or older with certain underlying medical conditions (see footnote 6c). A single revaccination with PPSV should be administered after 5 years to children with anatomic or functional asplenia (including sickle cell disease) or an immunocompromising condition.

6c. **Medical conditions for which PPSV23 is indicated in children aged 2 years and older and for which use of PCV13 is indicated in children aged 24 through 71 months:**
- Immunocompetent children with chronic heart disease (particularly cyanotic congenital heart disease and cardiac failure); chronic lung disease (including asthma if treated with high-dose oral corticosteroid therapy), diabetes mellitus; cerebrospinal fluid leaks; or cochlear implant.
- Children with anatomic or functional asplenia (including sickle cell disease and other hemoglobinopathies, congenital or acquired asplenia, or splenic dysfunction);
- Children with immunocompromising conditions: HIV infection, chronic renal failure and nephrotic syndrome, diseases associated with treatment with immunosuppressive drugs or radiation therapy, including malignant neoplasms, leukemias, lymphomas and Hodgkin disease; or solid organ transplantation, congenital immunodeficiency.

7. **Inactivated poliovirus vaccine (IPV). (Minimum age: 6 weeks)**

Routine vaccination:
- Administer a series of IPV at ages 2, 4, 6–18 months, with a booster at age 4–6 years. The final dose in the series should be administered on or after the fourth birthday and at least 6 months after the previous dose.

Catch-up vaccination:
- In the first 6 months of life, minimum age and minimum intervals are only recommended if the person is at risk for imminent exposure to circulating poliovirus (i.e., travel to a polio-endemic region or during an outbreak).
- If 4 or more doses are administered before age 4 years, an additional dose should be administered at age 4 through 6 years.
- A fourth dose is not necessary if the third dose was administered at age 4 years or older and at least 6 months after the previous dose.
- If both OPV and IPV were administered as part of a series, a total of 4 doses should be administered, regardless of the child's current age.
- IPV is not routinely recommended for U.S. residents aged 18 years or older.
- For other catch-up issues, see Figure 2.

8. **Influenza vaccines. (Minimum age: 6 months for inactivated influenza vaccine [IIV]; 2 years for live, attenuated influenza vaccine [LAIV])**

Routine vaccination:
- Administer influenza vaccine annually to all children beginning at age 6 months. For most healthy, nonpregnant persons aged 2 through 49 years, either LAIV or IIV may be used. However, LAIV should NOT be administered to some persons, including 1) those with asthma, 2) children 2 through 4 years who had wheezing in the past 12 months, or 3) those who have any other underlying medical conditions that predispose them to influenza complications. For all other contraindications to use of LAIV see MMWR 2010; 59 (No. RR-8), available at http://www.cdc.gov/mmwr/pdf/rr/rr5908.pdf.
- Administer 1 dose to persons aged 9 years and older.

For children aged 6 months through 8 years:
- For the 2012–13 season, administer 2 doses (separated by at least 4 weeks) to children who are receiving influenza vaccine for the first time. For additional guidance, follow dosing guidelines in the 2012 ACIP influenza vaccine recommendations, MMWR 2012; 61: 613–618, available at http://www.cdc.gov/mmwr/pdf/wk/mm6132.pdf.
- For the 2013–14 season, follow dosing guidelines in the 2013 ACIP influenza vaccine recommendations.

9. **Measles, mumps, and rubella (MMR) vaccine. (Minimum age: 12 months for routine vaccination)**

Routine vaccination:
- Administer the first dose of MMR vaccine at age 12 through 15 months, and the second dose at age 4 through 6 years. The second dose may be administered before age 4 years, provided at least 4 weeks have elapsed since the first dose.
- Administer 1 dose of MMR vaccine to infants aged 6 through 11 months before departure from the United States for international travel. These children should be revaccinated with 2 doses of MMR vaccine, the first at age 12 through 15 months (12 months if the child remains in an area where disease risk is high), and the second dose at least 4 weeks later.
- Administer 2 doses of MMR vaccine to children aged 12 months and older, before departure from the United States for international travel. The first dose should be administered on or after age 12 months and the second dose at least 4 weeks later.

Catch-up vaccination:
- Ensure that all school-aged children and adolescents have had 2 doses of MMR vaccine; the minimum interval between the 2 doses is 4 weeks.

10. **Varicella (VAR) vaccine. (Minimum age: 12 months)**

Routine vaccination:
- Administer the first dose of VAR vaccine at age 12 through 15 months, and the second dose at age 4 through 6 years. The second dose may be administered before age 4 years, provided at least 3 months have elapsed since the first dose. If the second dose was administered at least 4 weeks after the first dose, it can be accepted as valid.

Catch-up vaccination:
- Ensure that all persons aged 7 through 18 years without evidence of immunity (see MMWR 2007;56 [No. RR-4], available at http://www.cdc.gov/mmwr/pdf/rr/rr5604.pdf) have 2 doses of varicella vaccine. For children aged 7 through 12 years the recommended minimum interval between doses is 3 months (if the second dose was administered at least 4 weeks after the first dose, it can be accepted as valid); for persons aged 13 years and older, the minimum interval between doses is 4 weeks.

11. **Hepatitis A vaccine (HepA). (Minimum age: 12 months)**

Routine vaccination:
- Initiate the 2-dose HepA vaccine series for children aged 12 through 23 months; separate the 2 doses by 6 to 18 months.
- Children who have received 1 dose of HepA vaccine before age 24 months should receive a second dose 6 to 18 months after the first dose.
- For any person aged 2 years and older who has not already received the HepA vaccine series, 2 doses of HepA vaccine separated by 6 to 18 months may be administered if immunity against hepatitis A virus infection is desired.

Catch-up vaccination:
- The minimum interval between the two doses is 6 months.

Special populations:
- Administer 2 doses of Hep A vaccine at least 6 months apart to previously unvaccinated persons who live in areas where vaccination programs target older children, or who are at increased risk for infection.

12. **Human papillomavirus (HPV) vaccines. (HPV4 [Gardasil] and HPV2 [Cervarix]). (Minimum age: 9 years)**

Routine vaccination:
- Administer a 3-dose series of HPV vaccine on a schedule of 0, 1-2, and 6 months to all adolescents aged 11-12 years. Either HPV4 or HPV2 may be used for females, and only HPV4 may be used for males.
- The vaccine series can be started beginning at age 9 years.
- Administer the second dose 1 to 2 months after the **first** dose and the third dose 6 months after the **first** dose (at least 24 weeks after the first dose).

Catch-up vaccination:
- Administer the vaccine series to females (either HPV2 or HPV4) and males (HPV4) at age 13 through 18 years if not previously vaccinated.
- Use recommended routine dosing intervals (see above) for vaccine series catch-up.

13. **Meningococcal conjugate vaccines (MCV). (Minimum age: 6 weeks for Hib-MenCY, 9 months for Menactra [MCV4-D], 2 years for Menveo [MCV4-CRM]).**

Routine vaccination:
- Administer MCV4 vaccine at age 11–12 years, with a booster dose at age 16 years.
- Adolescents aged 11 through 18 years with human immunodeficiency virus (HIV) infection should receive a 2-dose primary series of MCV4, with at least 8 weeks between doses. See MMWR 2011; 60:1018–1019 available at: http://www.cdc.gov/mmwr/pdf/wk/mm6030.pdf.
- For children aged 9 months through 10 years with high-risk conditions, see below.

Catch-up vaccination:
- Administer MCV4 vaccine at age 13 through 18 years if not previously vaccinated.
- If the first dose is administered at age 13 through 15 years, a booster dose should be administered at age 16 through 18 years with a minimum interval of at least 8 weeks between doses.
- If the first dose is administered at age 16 years or older, a booster dose is not needed.
- For other catch-up issues, see Figure 2.

Vaccination of persons with high-risk conditions:
- For children younger than 19 months of age with anatomic or functional asplenia (including sickle cell disease), administer an infant series of Hib-MenCY at 2, 4, 6, and 12-15 months.
- For children aged 2 through 18 months with persistent complement component deficiency, administer either an infant series of Hib-MenCY at 2, 4, 6, and 12 through 15 months or a 2-dose primary series of MCV4-D starting at 9 months, with at least 8 weeks between doses. For children aged 19 through 23 months with persistent complement component deficiency who have not received a complete series of Hib-MenCY or MCV4-D, administer 2 primary doses of MCV4-D at least 8 weeks apart.
- For children aged 24 months and older with persistent complement component deficiency or anatomic or functional asplenia (including sickle cell disease), who have not received a complete series of Hib-MenCY or MCV4-D, administer 2 primary doses of either MCV4-D or MCV4-CRM. If MCV4-D (Menactra) is administered to a child with asplenia (including sickle cell disease), do not administer MCV4-D until 2 years of age and at least 4 weeks after the completion of all PCV13 doses. See MMWR 2011;60:1391–2, available at http://www.cdc.gov/mmwr/pdf/wk/mm6040.pdf.
- For children aged 9 months and older who are residents of or travelers to countries in the African meningitis belt or to the Hajj, administer an age-appropriate formulation and series of MCV4 for protection against serogroups A and W-135. Prior receipt of Hib-MenCY is not sufficient for children traveling to the meningitis belt or the Hajj. See MMWR 2011;60:1391–2, available at http://www.cdc.gov/mmwr/pdf/wk/mm6040.pdf.
- For children who are present during outbreaks caused by a vaccine serogroup, administer or complete an age and formulation-appropriate series of Hib-MenCY or MCV4.
- For booster doses among persons with high-risk conditions refer to http://www.cdc.gov/vaccines/pubs/acip-list.htm#mening.

Additional information
- For contraindications and precautions to use of a vaccine and for additional information regarding that vaccine, vaccination providers should consult the relevant ACIP statement available online at http://www.cdc.gov/vaccines/pubs/acip-list.htm.
- For the purposes of calculating intervals between doses, 4 weeks = 28 days. Intervals of 4 months or greater are determined by calendar months.
- Information on travel vaccine requirements and recommendations is available at http://wwwnc.cdc.gov/travel/page/vaccinations.htm.
- For vaccination of persons with primary and secondary immunodeficiencies, see Table 13, "Vaccination of persons with primary and secondary immunodeficiencies," in General Recommendations on Immunization (ACIP), available at http://www.cdc.gov/mmwr/preview/mmwrhtml/rr6002a1.htm; and American Academy of Pediatrics. Passive immunization. In: Pickering LK, Baker CJ, Kimberlin DW, Long SS eds. Red book: 2012 report of the Committee on Infectious Diseases. 29th ed. Elk Grove Village, IL: American Academy of Pediatrics.

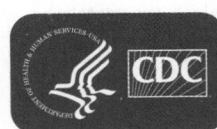

U.S. Department of Health and Human Services
Centers for Disease Control and Prevention

Appendix 102-3

2012 Adult Immunization Schedule

Recommended Adult Immunization Schedule—United States - 2013

Note: These recommendations must be read with the footnotes that follow containing number of doses, intervals between doses, and other important information.

VACCINE ▼ / AGE GROUP ►	19-21 years	22-26 years	27-49 years	50-59 years	60-64 years	≥ 65 years
Influenza [2,*]	1 dose annually					
Tetanus, diphtheria, pertussis (Td/Tdap) [3,*]	Substitute 1-time dose of Tdap for Td booster; then boost with Td every 10 yrs					
Varicella [4,*]	2 doses					
Human papillomavirus (HPV) Female [5,*]	3 doses					
Human papillomavirus (HPV) Male [5,*]	3 doses					
Zoster [6]					1 dose	
Measles, mumps, rubella (MMR) [7,*]	1 or 2 doses					
Pneumococcal polysaccharide (PPSV23) [8,9]	1 or 2 doses					1 dose
Pneumococcal 13-valent conjugate (PCV13) [10]	1 dose					
Meningococcal [11,*]	1 or more doses					
Hepatitis A [12,*]	2 doses					
Hepatitis B [13,*]	3 doses					

*Covered by the Vaccine Injury Compensation Program

- [light shading] For all persons in this category who meet the age requirements and who lack documentation of vaccination or have no evidence of previous infection; zoster vaccine recommended regardless of prior episode of zoster
- [dark shading] Recommended if some other risk factor is present (e.g., on the basis of medical, occupational, lifestyle, or other indication)
- [no shading] No recommendation

Report all clinically significant postvaccination reactions to the Vaccine Adverse Event Reporting System (VAERS). Reporting forms and instructions on filing a VAERS report are available at www.vaers.hhs.gov or by telephone, 800-822-7967.

Information on how to file a Vaccine Injury Compensation Program claim is available at www.hrsa.gov/vaccinecompensation or by telephone, 800-338-2382. To file a claim for vaccine injury, contact the U.S. Court of Federal Claims, 717 Madison Place, N.W., Washington, D.C. 20005; telephone, 202-357-6400.

Additional information about the vaccines in this schedule, extent of available data, and contraindications for vaccination is also available at www.cdc.gov/vaccines or from the CDC-INFO Contact Center at 800-CDC-INFO (800-232-4636) in English and Spanish, 8:00 a.m. - 8:00 p.m. Eastern Time, Monday - Friday, excluding holidays.

Use of trade names and commercial sources is for identification only and does not imply endorsement by the U.S. Department of Health and Human Services.

The recommendations in this schedule were approved by the Centers for Disease Control and Prevention's (CDC) Advisory Committee on Immunization Practices (ACIP), the American Academy of Family Physicians (AAFP), the American College of Physicians (ACP), American College of Obstetricians and Gynecologists (ACOG) and American College of Nurse-Midwives (ACNM).

VACCINE ▼ / INDICATION ►	Pregnancy	Immuno-compromising conditions (excluding human immunodeficiency virus [HIV])[4,6,7,10,15]	HIV infection CD4+ T lymphocyte count[4,6,7,10,14,15] < 200 cells/μL	HIV infection CD4+ T lymphocyte count ≥ 200 cells/μL	Men who have sex with men (MSM)	Heart disease, chronic lung disease, chronic alcoholism	Asplenia (including elective splenectomy and persistent complement component deficiencies)[10,14]	Chronic liver disease	Kidney failure, end-stage renal disease, receipt of hemodialysis	Diabetes	Healthcare personnel
Influenza [2,*]	1 dose IIV annually				1 dose IIV or LAIV annually	1 dose IIV annually					1 dose IIV or LAIV annually
Tetanus, diphtheria, pertussis (Td/Tdap) [3,*]	1 dose Tdap each pregnancy	Substitute 1-time dose of Tdap for Td booster; then boost with Td every 10 yrs									
Varicella [4,*]	Contraindicated			2 doses							
Human papillomavirus (HPV) Female [5,*]		3 doses through age 26 yrs				3 doses through age 26 yrs					
Human papillomavirus (HPV) Male [5,*]		3 doses through age 26 yrs				3 doses through age 21 yrs					
Zoster [6]	Contraindicated				1 dose						
Measles, mumps, rubella (MMR) [7,*]	Contraindicated			1 or 2 doses							
Pneumococcal polysaccharide (PPSV23) [8,9]	1 or 2 doses										
Pneumococcal 13-valent conjugate (PCV13) [10]		1 dose									
Meningococcal [11,*]	1 or more doses										
Hepatitis A [12,*]	2 doses										
Hepatitis B [13,*]	3 doses										

*Covered by the Vaccine Injury Compensation Program

- [light shading] For all persons in this category who meet the age requirements and who lack documentation of vaccination or have no evidence of previous infection; zoster vaccine recommended regardless of prior episode of zoster
- [dark shading] Recommended if some other risk factor is present (e.g., on the basis of medical, occupational, lifestyle, or other indications)
- [no shading] No recommendation

These schedules indicate the recommended age groups and medical indications for which administration of currently licensed vaccines is commonly indicated for adults ages 19 years and older, as of January 1, 2013. For all vaccines being recommended on the Adult Immunization Schedule: a vaccine series does not need to be restarted, regardless of the time that has elapsed between doses. Licensed combination vaccines may be used whenever any components of the combination are indicated and when the vaccine's other components are not contraindicated. For detailed recommendations on all vaccines, including those used primarily for travelers or that are issued during the year, consult the manufacturers' package inserts and the complete statements from the Advisory Committee on Immunization Practices (www.cdc.gov/vaccines/pubs/acip-list.htm). Use of trade names and commercial sources is for identification only and does not imply endorsement by the U.S. Department of Health and Human Services.

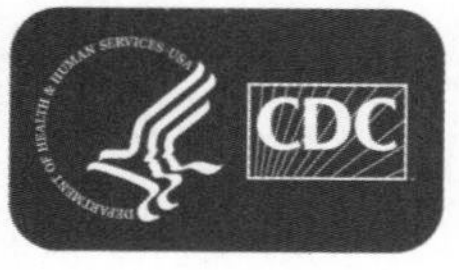

U.S. Department of Health and Human Services
Centers for Disease Control and Prevention

Footnotes — Recommended Immunization Schedule for Adults Aged 19 Years and Older—United States, 2013

1. Additional information

- Additional guidance for the use of the vaccines described in this supplement is available at http://www.cdc.gov/vaccines/pubs/acip-list.htm.
- Information on vaccination recommendations when vaccination status is unknown and other general immunization information can be found in the General Recommendations on Immunization at http://www.cdc.gov/mmwr/preview/mmwrhtml/rr6002a1.htm.
- Information on travel vaccine requirements and recommendations (e.g., for hepatitis A and B, meningococcal, and other vaccines) are available at http://wwwnc.cdc.gov/travel/page/vaccinations.htm.

2. Influenza vaccination

- Annual vaccination against influenza is recommended for all persons aged 6 months and older.
- Persons aged 6 months and older, including pregnant women, can receive the inactivated influenza vaccine (IIV).
- Healthy, nonpregnant persons aged 2–49 years without high-risk medical conditions can receive either intranasally administered live, attenuated influenza vaccine (LAIV) (FluMist), or IIV. Health-care personnel who care for severely immunocompromised persons (i.e., those who require care in a protected environment) should receive IIV rather than LAIV.
- The intramuscularly or intradermally administered IIV are options for adults aged 18–64 years.
- Adults aged 65 years and older can receive the standard dose IIV or the high-dose IIV (Fluzone High-Dose).

3. Tetanus, diphtheria, and acellular pertussis (Td/Tdap) vaccination

- Administer one dose of Tdap vaccine to pregnant women during each pregnancy (preferred during 27–36 weeks' gestation), regardless of number of years since prior Td or Tdap vaccination.
- Administer Tdap to all other adults who have not previously received Tdap or for whom vaccine status is unknown. Tdap can be administered regardless of interval since the most recent tetanus or diphtheria-toxoid containing vaccine.
- Adults with an unknown or incomplete history of completing a 3-dose primary vaccination series with Td-containing vaccines should begin or complete a primary vaccination series including a Tdap dose.
- For unvaccinated adults, administer the first 2 doses at least 4 weeks apart and the third dose 6–12 months after the second.
- For incompletely vaccinated (i.e., less than 3 doses) adults, administer remaining doses.
- Refer to the Advisory Committee on Immunization Practices (ACIP) statement for recommendations for administering Td/Tdap as prophylaxis in wound management (see footnote #1).

4. Varicella vaccination

- All adults without evidence of immunity to varicella (as defined below) should receive 2 doses of single-antigen varicella vaccine or a second dose if they have received only 1 dose.
- Special consideration for vaccination should be given to those who have close contact with persons at high risk for severe disease (e.g., health-care personnel and family contacts of persons with immunocompromising conditions) or are at high risk for exposure or transmission (e.g., teachers; child care employees; residents and staff members of institutional settings, including correctional institutions; college students; military personnel; adolescents and adults living in households with children; nonpregnant women of childbearing age; and international travelers).
- Pregnant women should be assessed for evidence of varicella immunity. Women who do not have evidence of immunity should receive the first dose of varicella vaccine upon completion or termination of pregnancy and before discharge from the health-care facility. The second dose should be administered 4–8 weeks after the first dose.
- Evidence of immunity to varicella in adults includes any of the following:
  - — documentation of 2 doses of varicella vaccine at least 4 weeks apart;
  - — U.S.-born before 1980 except health-care personnel and pregnant women;
  - — history of varicella based on diagnosis or verification of varicella disease by a health-care provider;
  - — history of herpes zoster based on diagnosis or verification of herpes zoster disease by a health-care provider; or
  - — laboratory evidence of immunity or laboratory confirmation of disease.

5. Human papillomavirus (HPV) vaccination

- Two vaccines are licensed for use in females, bivalent HPV vaccine (HPV2) and quadrivalent HPV vaccine (HPV4), and one HPV vaccine for use in males (HPV4).
- For females, either HPV4 or HPV2 is recommended in a 3-dose series for routine vaccination at age 11 or 12 years, and for those aged 13 through 26 years, if not previously vaccinated.
- For males, HPV4 is recommended in a 3-dose series for routine vaccination at age 11 or 12 years, and for those aged 13 through 21 years, if not previously vaccinated. Males aged 22 through 26 years may be vaccinated.
- HPV4 is recommended for men who have sex with men (MSM) through age 26 years for those who did not get any or all doses when they were younger.
- Vaccination is recommended for immunocompromised persons (including those with HIV infection) through age 26 years for those who did not get any or all doses when they were younger.
- A complete series for either HPV4 or HPV2 consists of 3 doses. The second dose should be administered 1–2 months after the first dose; the third dose should be administered 6 months after the first dose (at least 24 weeks after the first dose).
- HPV vaccines are not recommended for use in pregnant women. However, pregnancy testing is not needed before vaccination. If a woman is found to be pregnant after initiating the vaccination series, no intervention is needed; the remainder of the 3-dose series should be delayed until completion of pregnancy.
- Although HPV vaccination is not specifically recommended for health-care personnel (HCP) based on their occupation, HCP should receive the HPV vaccine as recommended (see above).

6. Zoster vaccination

- A single dose of zoster vaccine is recommended for adults aged 60 years and older regardless of whether they report a prior episode of herpes zoster. Although the vaccine is licensed by the Food and Drug Administration (FDA) for use among and can be administered to persons aged 50 years and older, ACIP recommends that vaccination begins at age 60 years.
- Persons aged 60 years and older with chronic medical conditions may be vaccinated unless their condition constitutes a contraindication, such as pregnancy or severe immunodeficiency.
- Although zoster vaccination is not specifically recommended for HCP, they should receive the vaccine if they are in the recommended age group.

7. Measles, mumps, rubella (MMR) vaccination

- Adults born before 1957 generally are considered immune to measles and mumps. All adults born in 1957 or later should have documentation of 1 or more doses of MMR vaccine unless they have a medical contraindication to the vaccine, or laboratory evidence of immunity to each of the three diseases. Documentation of provider-diagnosed disease is not considered acceptable evidence of immunity for measles, mumps, or rubella.

Measles component:

- A routine second dose of MMR vaccine, administered a minimum of 28 days after the first dose, is recommended for adults who
  - — are students in postsecondary educational institutions;
  - — work in a health-care facility; or
  - — plan to travel internationally.
- Persons who received inactivated (killed) measles vaccine or measles vaccine of unknown type during 1963–1967 should be revaccinated with 2 doses of MMR vaccine.

Mumps component:

- A routine second dose of MMR vaccine, administered a minimum of 28 days after the first dose, is recommended for adults who
  - — are students in a postsecondary educational institution;
  - — work in a health-care facility; or
  - — plan to travel internationally.
- Persons vaccinated before 1979 with either killed mumps vaccine or mumps vaccine of unknown type who are at high risk for mumps infection (e.g., persons who are working in a health-care facility) should be considered for revaccination with 2 doses of MMR vaccine.

Rubella component:

- For women of childbearing age, regardless of birth year, rubella immunity should be determined. If there is no evidence of immunity, women who are not pregnant should be vaccinated. Pregnant women who do not have evidence of immunity should receive MMR vaccine upon completion or termination of pregnancy and before discharge from the health-care facility.

HCP born before 1957:

- For unvaccinated health-care personnel born before 1957 who lack laboratory evidence of measles, mumps, and/or rubella immunity or laboratory confirmation of disease, health-care facilities should consider vaccinating personnel with 2 doses of MMR vaccine at the appropriate interval for measles and mumps or 1 dose of MMR vaccine for rubella.

8. Pneumococcal polysaccharide (PPSV23) vaccination

- Vaccinate all persons with the following indications:
  - — all adults aged 65 years and older;
  - — adults younger than age 65 years with chronic lung disease (including chronic obstructive pulmonary disease, emphysema, and asthma); chronic cardiovascular diseases; diabetes mellitus; chronic renal failure; nephrotic syndrome; chronic liver disease (including cirrhosis); alcoholism; cochlear implants; cerebrospinal fluid leaks; immunocompromising conditions; and functional or anatomic asplenia (e.g., sickle cell disease and other hemoglobinopathies, congenital or acquired asplenia, splenic dysfunction, or splenectomy [if elective splenectomy is planned, vaccinate at least 2 weeks before surgery]);
  - — residents of nursing homes or long-term care facilities; and
  - — adults who smoke cigarettes.
- Persons with immunocompromising conditions and other selected conditions are recommended to receive PCV13 and PPSV23 vaccines. See footnote #10 for information on timing of PCV13 and PPSV23 vaccinations.
- Persons with asymptomatic or symptomatic HIV infection should be vaccinated as soon as possible after their diagnosis.
- When cancer chemotherapy or other immunosuppressive therapy is being considered, the interval between vaccination and initiation of immunosuppressive therapy should be at least 2 weeks. Vaccination during chemotherapy or radiation therapy should be avoided.
- Routine use of PPSV23 is not recommended for American Indians/Alaska Natives or other persons younger than age 65 years unless they have underlying medical conditions that are PPSV23 indications. However, public health authorities may consider recommending PPSV23 for American Indians/Alaska Natives who are living in areas where the risk for invasive pneumococcal disease is increased.
- When indicated, PPSV23 should be administered to patients who are uncertain of their vaccination status and there is no record of previous vaccination. When PCV13 is also indicated, a dose of PCV13 should be given first (see footnote #10).

9. Revaccination with PPSV23

- One-time revaccination 5 years after the first dose is recommended for persons aged 19 through 64 years with chronic renal failure or nephrotic syndrome; functional or anatomic asplenia (e.g., sickle cell disease or splenectomy); and for persons with immunocompromising conditions.
- Persons who received 1 or 2 doses of PPSV23 before age 65 years for any indication should receive another dose of the vaccine at age 65 years or later if at least 5 years have passed since their previous dose.
- No further doses are needed for persons vaccinated with PPSV23 at or after age 65 years.

10. Pneumococcal conjugate 13-valent vaccination (PCV13)

- Adults aged 19 years or older with immunocompromising conditions (including chronic renal failure and nephrotic syndrome), functional or anatomic asplenia, CSF leaks or cochlear implants, and who have not previously received PCV13 or PPSV23 should receive a single dose of PCV13 followed by a dose of PPSV23 at least 8 weeks later.
- Adults aged 19 years or older with the aforementioned conditions who have previously received one or more doses of PPSV23 should receive a dose of PCV13 one or more years after the last PPSV23 dose was received. For those that require additional doses of PPSV23, the first such dose should be given no sooner than 8 weeks after PCV13 and at least 5 years since the most recent dose of PPSV23.
- When indicated, PCV13 should be administered to patients who are uncertain of their vaccination status history and there is no record of previous vaccination.
- Although PCV13 is licensed by the Food and Drug Administration (FDA) for use among and can be administered to persons aged 50 years and older, ACIP recommends PCV13 for adults aged 19 years and older with the specific medical conditions noted above.

11. Meningococcal vaccination

- Administer 2 doses of meningococcal conjugate vaccine quadrivalent (MCV4) at least 2 months apart to adults with functional asplenia or persistent complement component deficiencies.
- HIV-infected persons who are vaccinated also should receive 2 doses.
- Administer a single dose of meningococcal vaccine to microbiologists routinely exposed to isolates of Neisseria meningitidis, military recruits, and persons who travel to or live in countries in which meningococcal disease is hyperendemic or epidemic.
- First-year college students up through age 21 years who are living in residence halls should be vaccinated if they have not received a dose on or after their 16th birthday.
- MCV4 is preferred for adults with any of the preceding indications who are aged 55 years and younger; meningococcal polysaccharide vaccine (MPSV4) is preferred for adults aged 56 years and older.
- Revaccination with MCV4 every 5 years is recommended for adults previously vaccinated with MCV4 or MPSV4 who remain at increased risk for infection (e.g., adults with anatomic or functional asplenia or persistent complement component deficiencies).

12. Hepatitis A vaccination

- Vaccinate any person seeking protection from hepatitis A virus (HAV) infection and persons with any of the following indications:
  - — men who have sex with men and persons who use injection or noninjection illicit drugs;
  - — persons working with HAV-infected primates or with HAV in a research laboratory setting;
  - — persons with chronic liver disease and persons who receive clotting factor concentrates;
  - — persons traveling to or working in countries that have high or intermediate endemicity of hepatitis A; and
  - — unvaccinated persons who anticipate close personal contact (e.g., household or regular babysitting) with an international adoptee during the first 60 days after arrival in the United States from a country with high or intermediate endemicity. (See footnote #1 for more information on travel recommendations). The first dose of the 2-dose hepatitis A vaccine series should be administered as soon as adoption is planned, ideally 2 or more weeks before the arrival of the adoptee.
- Single-antigen vaccine formulations should be administered in a 2-dose schedule at either age 0 and 6–12 months (Havrix), or age 0 and 6–18 months (Vaqta). If the combined hepatitis A and hepatitis B vaccine (Twinrix) is used, administer 3 doses at 0, 1, and 6 months; alternatively, a 4-dose schedule may be used, administered on days 0, 7, and 21–30, followed by a booster dose at month 12.

13. Hepatitis B vaccination

- Vaccinate persons with any of the following indications and any person seeking protection from hepatitis B virus (HBV) infection:
  - — sexually active persons who are not in a long-term, mutually monogamous relationship (e.g., persons with more than one sex partner during the previous 6 months); persons seeking evaluation or treatment for a sexually transmitted disease (STD); current or recent injection-drug users; and men who have sex with men;
  - — health-care personnel and public-safety workers who are potentially exposed to blood or other infectious body fluids;
  - — persons with diabetes younger than age 60 years as soon as feasible after diagnosis; persons with diabetes who are age 60 years or older at the discretion of the treating clinician based on increased need for assisted blood glucose monitoring in long-term care facilities, likelihood of acquiring hepatitis B infection, its complications or chronic sequelae, and likelihood of immune response to vaccination;
  - — persons with end-stage renal disease, including patients receiving hemodialysis; persons with HIV infection; and persons with chronic liver disease;
  - — household contacts and sex partners of hepatitis B surface antigen-positive persons; clients and staff members of institutions for persons with developmental disabilities; and international travelers to countries with high or intermediate prevalence of chronic HBV infection; and
  - — all adults in the following settings: STD treatment facilities; HIV testing and treatment facilities; facilities providing drug-abuse treatment and prevention services; health-care settings targeting services to injection-drug users or men who have sex with men; correctional facilities; end-stage renal disease programs and facilities for chronic hemodialysis patients; and institutions and nonresidential daycare facilities for persons with developmental disabilities.
- Administer missing doses to complete a 3-dose series of hepatitis B vaccine to those persons not vaccinated or not completely vaccinated. The second dose should be administered 1 month after the first dose; the third dose should be given at least 2 months after the second dose (and at least 4 months after the first dose). If the combined hepatitis A and hepatitis B vaccine (Twinrix) is used, give 3 doses at 0, 1, and 6 months; alternatively, a 4-dose Twinrix schedule, administered on days 0, 7, and 21–30 followed by a booster dose at month 12 may be used.
- Adult patients receiving hemodialysis or with other immunocompromising conditions should receive 1 dose of 40 µg/mL (Recombivax HB) administered on a 3-dose schedule at 0, 1, and 6 months or 2 doses of 20 µg/mL (Engerix-B) administered simultaneously on a 4-dose schedule at 0, 1, 2, and 6 months.

14. Selected conditions for which Haemophilus influenzae type b (Hib) vaccine may be used

- 1 dose of Hib vaccine should be considered for persons who have sickle cell disease, leukemia, or HIV infection, or who have anatomic or functional asplenia if they have not previously received Hib vaccine.

15. Immunocompromising conditions

- Inactivated vaccines generally are acceptable (e.g., pneumococcal, meningococcal, and influenza [inactivated influenza vaccine]), and live vaccines generally are avoided in persons with immune deficiencies or immunocompromising conditions. Information on specific conditions is available at http://www.cdc.gov/vaccines/pubs/acip-list.htm.

Human Immunodeficiency Virus Infection

103

Peter L. Anderson, Thomas N. Kakuda, and Courtney V. Fletcher

KEY CONCEPTS

1. Infection with human immunodeficiency virus (HIV) occurs through three primary modes: sexual, parenteral, and perinatal. Sexual intercourse, primarily receptive anal and vaginal intercourse, is the most common method for transmission.
2. HIV infects cells expressing cluster of differentiation 4 (CD4) receptors, such as T-helper lymphocytes, monocytes, macrophages, dendritic cells, and brain microglia. Infection occurs via an interaction between glycoprotein 160 (gp160) on HIV with CD4 (primary interaction) and chemokine coreceptors (secondary interactions) present on the surfaces of these cells.
3. The hallmark of untreated HIV infection is profound CD4 T-lymphocyte depletion and severe immunosuppression that puts patients at significant risk for infectious diseases caused by opportunistic pathogens. Opportunistic infections (OIs) in settings without access to antiretroviral drugs are the chief cause of morbidity and mortality associated with HIV infection.
4. The current goal of ART is to achieve maximal and durable suppression of HIV replication, taken to be a level of HIV-RNA in plasma (viral load) less than the lower limit of quantitation. Another equally important outcome is an increase in CD4 lymphocytes because this closely correlates with the risk for developing OIs.
5. General principles for the management of OIs include preventing or reversing immunosuppression with antiretroviral therapy (ART), preventing exposure to pathogens, vaccination, prospective immunologic monitoring, primary chemoprophylaxis, treatment of acute episodes, secondary chemoprophylaxis, and discontinuation of such prophylaxes following ART and subsequent immune recovery.
6. Clinical use of antiretroviral agents is complicated by drug–drug interactions. Some interactions are beneficial and used purposely; others may be harmful, leading to dangerously elevated or inadequate drug concentrations. For these reasons, clinicians involved in the pharmacotherapy of HIV infection must exercise constant vigilance and maintain a current knowledge of drug interactions.
7. Current recommendations for the initial treatment of HIV advocate a minimum of three active antiretroviral agents from at least two drug classes. The typical regimen consists of two nucleoside/nucleotide analogs with either a protease inhibitor (PI; pharmacokinetically enhanced by coadministration with a CYP3A inhibitor), a nonnucleoside reverse transcriptase inhibitor, or an integrase strand transfer inhibitor (InSTI).
8. Inadequate suppression of viral replication allows HIV to select for antiretroviral-resistant HIV variants, a major factor limiting the ability of antiretroviral drugs to inhibit virus replication. Current recommendations for treating drug-resistant HIV include choosing at least two drugs (preferably three) to which the patient's virus is susceptible. Susceptibility can be assessed using either (virtual) genotypic or phenotypic resistance testing.
9. The reduction of viral load with ART lowers the risk of transmission to others. Additionally, prophylaxis with antiretroviral agents in at-risk persons lowers HIV acquisition risk.
10. The longer life span conferred by antiretroviral treatment has given rise to other medical issues. First, a wide spectrum of complications associated with older age have become common, some of which are adverse effects from antiretroviral drugs. Second, hepatitis C virus (HCV) coinfection is an important cause of morbidity and mortality. Medical management of these contemporary HIV complications is constantly evolving.

Acquired immunodeficiency syndrome (AIDS) was first recognized in a cohort of young, previously healthy homosexual men with new-onset profound immunologic deficits, *Pneumocystis carinii* (now *P. jirovecii*) pneumonia (PCP), and/or Kaposi's sarcoma. A retrovirus, human immunodeficiency virus type 1 (HIV-1), is the major cause of AIDS. A second retrovirus, HIV-2, also is recognized to cause AIDS, although it is less virulent, transmissible, and prevalent than HIV-1. These retroviruses are transmitted primarily by sexual contact and by contact with infected blood or blood products. Several risk behaviors for the acquisition of HIV infection have been identified in the United States, most notably the practice of anorectal intercourse and the sharing of blood-contaminated needles by injection-drug users. In many resource-limited countries, the majority of HIV transmission occurs via heterosexual intercourse and from childbearing women to their offspring. Initially, the medical management of HIV consisted of repeated treatments for opportunistic infections (OIs) and eventual palliative care. In the mid-1990s, a new era in the pharmacotherapy for HIV, known as *combination antiretroviral therapy* (ART), was born. ART consists of combinations of antiretroviral agents with different mechanisms of action that potently and durably suppress HIV replication, delay the onset of AIDS, reverse HIV-associated immunologic deficits, reduce HIV transmissions, and significantly prolong survival. Modern antiretroviral drugs and ART regimens have improved upon tolerability and efficacy. Unfortunately, therapeutic challenges remain in the ART era and include the need for continuous adherence to medication and care, drug–drug interactions, drug-resistant HIV, acute and long-term drug toxicities, and other complications associated with a prolonged life span. Progress has been made in the treatment access for this disease, but large numbers of HIV-infected persons remain outside of care. Antiretroviral drugs can prevent HIV acquisition in persons exposed to HIV, but they cannot cure established HIV infection, and no viable vaccine is available.

EPIDEMIOLOGY

The epidemiologic characteristics of HIV infection differ according to geographic region and depend upon the mode of transmission, governmental prevention efforts and resources, and cultural factors.[1,2]

1 Infection with HIV occurs through three primary modes: sexual, parenteral, and perinatal. Sexual intercourse, primarily anal and vaginal intercourse, is the most common method for transmission. The probability of HIV transmission depends upon the type of sexual exposure. The highest risk appears to be from receptive anorectal intercourse at about 0.5% to 3% per sexual act.[3] Transmission risk is lower for receptive vaginal or oral intercourse and each is lower for insertive versus receptive sex acts.[4] Condom use reduces risk of transmission by approximately 20-fold.[4] Other factors that affect the probability of infection include the stage of HIV disease and viral load in the index partner. For example, transmission is higher when the index partner has early or late HIV compared with asymptomatic HIV, as these disease stages are associated with higher viral loads.[5] Individuals with genital ulcers or sexually transmitted diseases are at greater risk for contracting HIV. HIV incidence and prevalence are lower in cultures that advocate male circumcision, which is estimated to reduce risk of male acquisition of HIV during heterosexual intercourse by 60%.[2,5] However, male circumcision may not have the same protective effects for receptive anal intercourse or for an uninfected partner.[6] Casual contact with patients with AIDS or HIV infection is not a significant risk factor for HIV transmission.[2]

Prevention of sexual transmission has focused primarily on education that encourages abstinence (especially for adolescents), use of condoms, and reduction of high-risk behavior (anal intercourse or promiscuity with partners of unknown HIV status).[1] Combination ART dramatically lowers viral replication and infectiousness, significantly reducing the risk of transmission to others.[7] Chemoprophylaxis with antiretroviral drugs is also effective at preventing HIV acquisition.[8–10] A combined approach has been advocated for optimal prevention. Prevention strategies under investigation include HIV vaccines and topical vaginal/rectal microbicides.[11,12]

Parenteral transmission of HIV broadly encompasses infections due to infected blood exposure from needle sticks, IV injection with used needles, receipt of blood products, and organ transplants. Use of contaminated needles or other injection-related paraphernalia by drug abusers has been the main cause of parenteral transmissions. The risk of HIV transmission from sharing needles is approximately 0.67% per episode.[3] Prevention strategies include stopping drug abuse, obtaining needles from credible sources (e.g., pharmacies), never reusing any paraphernalia, using sterile procedures in all injecting activities, and safely disposing of used paraphernalia.[4]

Before widespread screening, HIV was readily transmitted in blood products.[3] However, blood and tissue products in the healthcare system are now rigorously screened for HIV. The estimated risk for receiving tainted blood or blood products in the United States is approximately 1:2,000,000 and that for receiving a tainted tissue transplant is 1:55,000.[13,14] Healthcare workers have a small but definite occupational risk of contracting HIV through accidental injury. Most cases of occupationally acquired HIV have been the result of a percutaneous needle stick injury, which carries an estimated 0.3% risk of transmitting HIV.[15] Mucocutaneous exposures (e.g., tainted blood splash in eyes, mouth, nose) carries a transmission risk of approximately 0.09%.[15] Significant risk factors for seroconversion with a needle stick include deep injury, injury with a device visibly contaminated with blood, and advanced HIV disease in the index patient (high viral load). The risk of transmission from an HIV-infected healthcare worker to a patient is extremely remote. Comprehensive medical guidelines, including antiretroviral drug prophylaxis, have been developed to minimize the hazard of HIV transmission for healthcare workers and for persons exposed by rape or other means.[3,15]

Perinatal infection, or vertical transmission, is the most common cause of pediatric HIV infection.[16] Most infections occur during or near to the time of birth, although a fraction can occur in utero. The risk of mother-to-child transmission is approximately 25% in the absence of ART. Factors that increase the likelihood of vertical transmission include prolonged rupture of membranes, chorioamnionitis, genital infection during pregnancy, preterm delivery, vaginal delivery, birth weight less than 2.5 kg, illicit drug use during pregnancy, and high maternal viral load. Breast-feeding also can transmit HIV. The estimated frequency of breast milk transmission is approximately 4% to 16%, with the majority of infections developing within the first 6 months.[17] High levels of virus in breast milk and in the mother are associated with higher risk of transmission.[17] Formula feeding prevents breast milk transmission of HIV but may not improve mortality from other causes early in life in some settings.[18] Whenever formula feeding is acceptable, feasible, affordable, sustainable, and safe, HIV-infected mothers are recommended not to breast-feed. A separate and comprehensive set of medical guidelines including antiretroviral drug prophylaxis have been developed to minimize the hazard of mother-to-child HIV transmission.[16]

Persons with HIV infection are broadly categorized as those living with HIV and those with an AIDS diagnosis. An AIDS diagnosis is made when the presence of HIV is laboratory-confirmed and the cluster of differentiation 4 (CD4; T-helper cell) count drops below 200 cells/mm^3 (200×10^6/L) or after an AIDS indicator condition is diagnosed.[19] Further distinctions regarding the stage of HIV and AIDS are given in the Revised Centers for Disease Control and Prevention (CDC) surveillance case definition (Table 103-1).[19] In the United States, new HIV/AIDS cases are reported by healthcare providers to a public health department.[20] The cumulative number of reported HIV/AIDS diagnoses in the United States is approximately 1.7 million; more than 550,000 persons have already died.[21] The estimated prevalence of HIV infections including AIDS cases in the United States is about 1.2 million individuals. Each year the CDC estimates that 55,000 new cases of HIV infection occur in the United States.[21,22] Approximately 20% of persons with HIV are unaware of their infection and approximately 50% of those who are aware of their infection are retained in care.[22,23] Therefore, the majority of HIV-infected persons (~60%) are not receiving ART regularly, which contributes to the ongoing transmission of HIV infection.[23]

The epidemic in the United States initially was established in white men who have sex with men (MSM), and the prevalence of HIV in this population still is high.[22] New trends in transmission include more cases in women (currently ~25%) and African Americans and Hispanics, a proportion of whom are not well linked to appropriate prevention, care, and treatment services.[21] Approximately half of new cases occur in African Americans (who make up only 12% of the general population), about one third in Caucasians, and less than one fourth in Hispanics.[20] The main risk factor for transmission in women is heterosexual intercourse (~80% of cases) and injection-drug use (~20% of cases). For men the main risks are MSM (~65%), heterosexual sex (~15%), and injection-drug use (~15%).[24]

The estimated number of individuals living with HIV/AIDS worldwide has stabilized at approximately 34 million persons. The new infection rate is declining.[25] Approximately 2.7 million were infected in 2010, including 390,000 children, down from

TABLE 103-1 Surveillance Case Definition for HIV Infection among Adults and Adolescents (≥13 years)—United States, 2008

Stage	Laboratory Evidence (Laboratory-Confirmed HIV Infection *plus*)	Clinical Evidence
Stage 1	CD4+ cell count ≥500 cells/mm³ (500 × 10⁶/L) or CD4+ percentage ≥29	None required (but no AIDS-defining condition)
Stage 2	CD4+ cell count 200–499 cells/mm³ (200 × 10⁶–499 × 10⁶/L) or CD4+ percentage 14–28	None required (but no AIDS-defining condition)
Stage 3 (AIDS)	CD4+ cell count <200 cells/mm³ (200 × 10⁶/L) or CD4+ percentage <14	or documentation of an AIDS-defining condition (with laboratory-confirmed HIV infection)
Stage unknown	No information on CD4+ counts	and no information on presence of AIDS-defining conditions

AIDS Indicator Conditions	
Candidiasis of bronchi, trachea, or lungs	Lymphoma, Burkitt
Candidiasis, esophageal	Lymphoma, immunoblastic
Cervical cancer, invasive	Lymphoma, primary, or brain
Coccidioidomycosis, disseminated or extrapulmonary	*Mycobacterium avium* complex or *Mycobacterium kansasii*, disseminated or extrapulmonary
Cryptococcosis, extrapulmonary	*Mycobacterium tuberculosis*, any site (pulmonary or extrapulmonary)
Cryptosporidiosis, chronic intestinal (duration >1 month)	*Mycobacterium*, other species or unidentified species, disseminated or extrapulmonary
Cytomegalovirus disease (other than liver, spleen, or nodes)	*Pneumocystis jirovecii* pneumonia (PCP)
Cytomegalovirus retinitis (with loss of vision)	Pneumonia, recurrent
Encephalopathy, HIV-related	Progressive multifocal leukoencephalopathy
Herpes simplex: chronic ulcer(s) (duration >1 month); or bronchitis, pneumonitis, or esophagitis	*Salmonella* septicemia, recurrent
	Toxoplasmosis of brain
Histoplasmosis, disseminated or extrapulmonary	Wasting syndrome due to HIV
Isosporiasis, chronic intestinal (duration >1 month)	
Kaposi's sarcoma	

From reference 19.

approximately 3.3 million new infections in 1998.[25] About 1.8 million people succumbed to AIDS in 2010. Globally, the highest concentration of HIV/ AIDS cases is in sub-Saharan Africa, where approximately 23 million people are infected. However, new infections rates in many sub-Saharan African countries have declined by approximately 25% since 1997.[25] Heterosexual transmission is the most common mode of transmission in sub-Saharan Africa and worldwide (85% of cases). Women in sub-Saharan Africa and resource-limited countries are at disproportionately high risk for acquiring HIV because of biological and cultural factors that foster HIV transmission, such as limited ability to refuse sex.[1,25] Other important epidemiologic features of the HIV epidemic include growing prevalence in eastern Europe and central Asia (e.g., Russian Federation and Ukraine).[25] Injection-drug use is fueling these epidemics.

ETIOLOGY

HIV is an enveloped single-stranded RNA virus and a member of the Lentivirinae (*lenti*, meaning "slow") subfamily of retroviruses. Lentiviruses are characterized by their indolent infectious cycle. There are two related but distinct types of HIV: HIV-1 and HIV-2. HIV-2, found mostly in western Africa, consists of seven phylogenetic lineages designated as subtypes (clades) A through G. HIV-1 also can be categorized based on phylogeny.[26] Three groups of HIV-1 are recognized: M (main or major), N (non-M, non-O), and O (outlier). A new HIV-1 virus was classified as group P (pending the identification of further cases).[27] The nine subtypes of HIV-1 group M are identified as A through D, F through H, and J and K. Mixtures of subtypes are referred to as *circulating recombinant forms* (CRFs). Group M, subtype B, is primarily responsible for the epidemic in North America and western Europe.[26]

The accumulated evidence suggests that HIV in humans was the result of a cross-species transmission (zoonosis) from primates infected with simian immunodeficiency virus (SIV). Phylogenetic and geographic relationships suggest that HIV-2 arose from SIV that infects sooty mangabeys and HIV-1 group M and N arose from SIVcpz, a virus that infects chimpanzees (*Pan troglodytes troglodytes*). Groups O and P may have arisen from a SIV variant that infects wild gorillas. Cultural practices, such as preparation and eating of bush meat or keeping animals as pets, may have allowed the virus to jump from primates to humans. The earliest known human infection with HIV has been traced to central Africa in 1959, but cross-species transmissions probably date back to the early 1900s.[28] Modern transportation, promiscuity, and drug abuse have caused the rapid spread of the virus within the United States and throughout the world.[1,28] This chapter focuses on HIV-1 group M, which is the predominant strain likely to be encountered in the western world.

DETECTION OF HIV AND SURROGATE MARKERS OF DISEASE PROGRESSION

The preferred method for diagnosing HIV-1 infection is an enzyme-linked immunosorbent assay (ELISA), which detects antibodies against HIV-1.[24] ELISA is both highly sensitive (>99%) and highly specific (>99%), but rare false-positive results can occur in multiparous women; recent recipients of hepatitis B, HIV, influenza, or rabies vaccine; patients with multiple blood transfusions, liver disease, and renal failure; or those undergoing chronic hemodialysis. False-negative results may occur and most commonly are attributed to new infection where antibody production is not yet adequate. An HIV-RNA test can detect viremia approximately 2 weeks prior to antibody production.[29] The minimum time to develop antibodies is 3 to 4 weeks from initial exposure, with greater than 95% of individuals developing antibodies after 6 months. Convenient methods for obtaining an ELISA sample from blood or saliva have been developed, including a rapid (20 to 40 minutes) turnaround oral test marketed as a home kit.

Positive ELISA results are repeated in duplicate, and if one or both tests are reactive, a confirmatory test is performed for final diagnosis. Western blot is the most commonly used confirmatory test, although an indirect immunofluorescence assay is available. A reactive ELISA test and a positive confirmatory test indicate an established HIV infection. If the confirmatory test is indeterminate, the individual should be retested 4 weeks later.[24]

HIV testing is recommended when HIV infection is suspected because of symptoms and/or high-risk behavior. Additionally, the CDC now recommends routine HIV screening in all healthcare settings in persons 13 to 64 years, a new policy called "opt-out" testing.[24] The policy states that consent for medical care will imply consent for HIV testing; however, the person must be informed of the test and can opt out of taking it. Because states may have different HIV consent laws, the local requirements for HIV testing should be consulted. The rationale for the opt-out strategy is to diagnose those who unknowingly carry HIV so as to improve their prognosis and reduce further transmission.

Once diagnosed, HIV disease is monitored primarily by two surrogate biomarkers, viral load and CD4 cell count.[30] The viral load test quantifies the degree of viremia by measuring the number of copies of viral RNA (HIV RNA) in the plasma. Methods for determining HIV RNA include reverse-transcription polymerase chain reaction (RT-PCR), branched-chain DNA, transcription-mediated amplification, and nucleic acid sequence-based assay. RT-PCR is used more widely than the other techniques. Irrespective of the method used, viral load is reported as the number of viral RNA copies per milliliter of plasma. Each assay has its own lower limit of sensitivity to viral subtypes, and results can vary from one assay method to the other; therefore, it is recommended that the same assay method be used consistently within patients. Reductions in viral load often are reported in base 10 logarithm. For example, if a patient presents initially with a viral load of 100,000 copies/mL (10^5 copies/mL or 10^8 copies/L) and subsequently has a viral load of 10,000 copies/mL (10^4 copies/mL or 10^7 copies/L), the decrease in viral load is 1 $\log_{10}$. Given that HIV RNA varies within patients, a clinical response is generally considered when the decline in viral load is more than 0.5 $\log_{10}$.[30] Viral load is a major prognostic factor for monitoring disease progression and the effects of treatment.

Because HIV attacks and leads to the destruction of cells bearing the CD4 receptor, the number of CD4 lymphocytes (T-helper cells) in the blood is a critical surrogate marker of disease progression. The normal adult CD4 lymphocyte count ranges from 500 to 1,600 cells/mm^3, or 40% to 70% of total lymphocytes. CD4 counts in children are age dependent, with younger children having higher CD4 counts. The hallmark of HIV disease is depletion of CD4 cells and the associated development of OIs and malignancies.

PATHOGENESIS

2 Understanding the life cycle of HIV (Fig. 103-1) is necessary because the current strategies used for treatment of HIV target various points in this cycle. Once HIV enters the human body, the outer glycoprotein (gp160) on its surface, which is composed of two subunits (gp120 and gp41), has affinity for CD4 receptors, proteins present on the surface of T-helper lymphocytes, monocytes, macrophages, dendritic cells, and brain microglia.[31] The gp120 subunit is responsible for CD4 binding. Once initial binding occurs, the intimate association of HIV with the cell is enhanced by further binding to chemokine coreceptors. The two major chemokine receptors used by HIV are Chemokine (C–C motif) receptor 5 (CCR5) and chemokine (C-X-C motif) receptor 4 (CXCR4). HIV isolates may contain a mixture of viruses that target one or the other of these coreceptors, and some viral strains may be dual-tropic (i.e., can use both coreceptors). The HIV strain that preferentially uses CCR5, R5 viruses, is macrophage-tropic and typically implicated in most cases

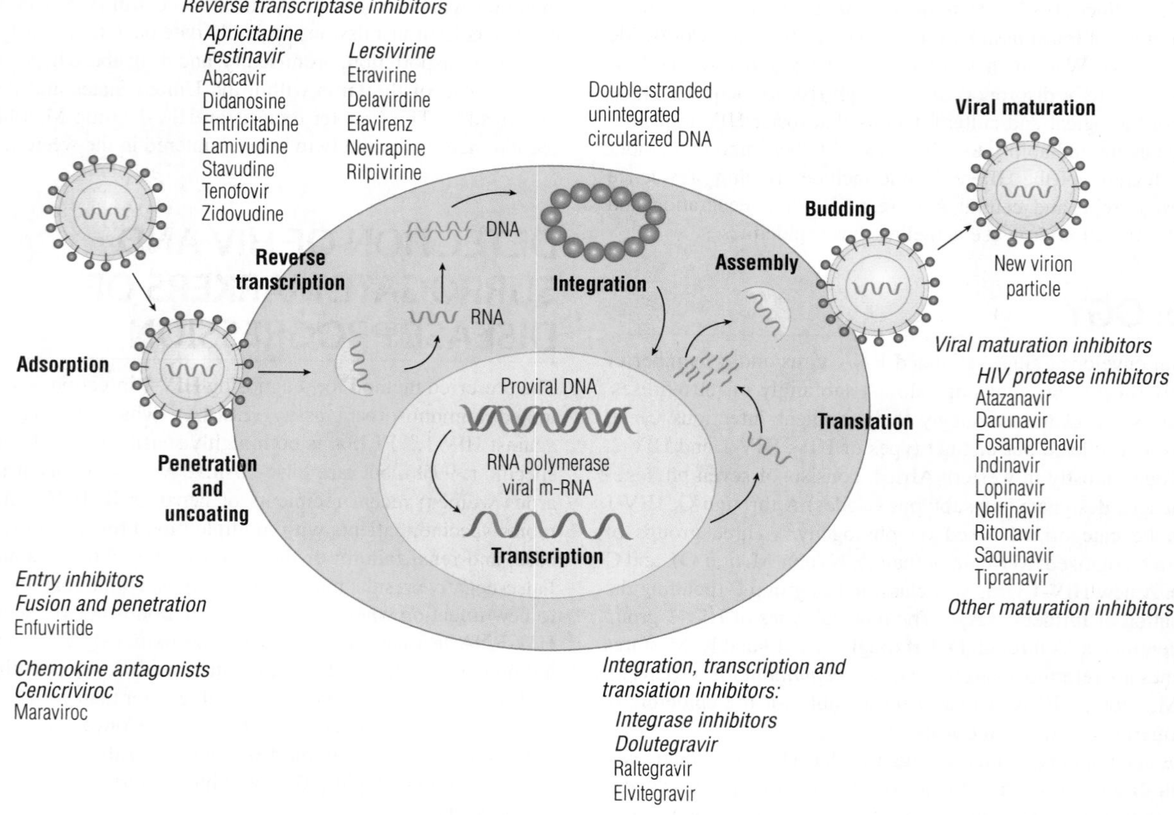

FIGURE 103-1 Life cycle of human immunodeficiency virus with potential targets where replication may be interrupted. Italicized compounds were in development at the time of this writing. *(Reprinted with permission, Courtney V. Fletcher, 2012.)*

of sexually transmitted HIV. Individuals with a common 32-base-pair deletion in the CCR5 gene are protected from progression of HIV disease, and those who are homozygous for the 32-base-pair deletion have a degree of resistance to acquisition of HIV-1.[32,33] The HIV strain that targets CXCR4, designated X4 virus, is T-cell–tropic and often is predominant in the later stage of disease. Other chemokine coreceptors and galactosyl ceramide may also serve as a binding site for HIV. CD4 and coreceptor attachment of HIV to the cell promotes membrane fusion, which is mediated by gp41, and finally internalization of the viral genetic material and enzymes necessary for replication.

After internalization, the viral protein shell surrounding the nucleic acid (capsid) is uncoated in preparation for replication.[31] The genetic material of HIV is positive-sense single-stranded RNA; the virus must transcribe this RNA into DNA (transcription normally occurs from DNA to RNA; HIV works backward, hence the name *retrovirus*). To do so, HIV is equipped with the unique enzyme RNA-dependent DNA polymerase (reverse transcriptase). HIV reverse transcriptase first synthesizes a complementary strand of DNA using the viral RNA as a template. The RNA portion of this DNA–RNA hybrid is then partially removed by ribonuclease H (RNase H), allowing HIV reverse transcriptase to complete the synthesis of a double-stranded DNA molecule. The fidelity of HIV reverse transcriptase is poor, and many mistakes are made during the process. These errors in the final DNA product contribute to the rapid mutation of the virus, which enables the virus to evade the immune response (thus complicating vaccine development), and promotes the evolution of drug resistance during partially suppressive therapy. Following reverse transcription, the final double-stranded DNA product migrates into the nucleus and is integrated into the host cell chromosome by integrase, another enzyme unique to HIV.

The integration of HIV into the host chromosome is troublesome. Most notably, HIV can establish a persistent, latent infection, particularly in long-lived cells of the immune system such as memory T lymphocytes. The virus is effectively hidden in these cells, and this characteristic has greatly inhibited the ability to cure HIV infection. Second, random integration of HIV may cause cellular abnormalities and induce apoptosis.

After integration, HIV preferentially replicates in activated cells. Activation by antigens, cytokines, or other factors stimulates the cell to produce nuclear factor kappa B (NF-κB), an enhancer-binding protein. NF-κB normally regulates the expression of T-lymphocyte genes involved in growth but also can inadvertently activate replication of HIV. HIV encodes six regulatory and accessory proteins: Tat, Nef, Rev, Vpu, Vif, and Vpr, which enhance replication and inhibit innate immunity. For example, the Tat protein is a potent amplifier of HIV gene expression; it binds to a specific RNA sequence of HIV that initiates and stabilizes transcription elongation. Vif is a viral protein that binds human ABOBEC 3G, a cytidine deaminase that converts viral RNA cytosine to uracil and thereby provides innate cellular immunity.[34] Vpu inhibits tetherin, a human cellular membrane protein that prevents diffusion of virus particles after budding from infected cells, thereby allowing HIV to detach from the infected cell.[35] Assembly of new virion particles occurs in a stepwise manner beginning with the coalescence of HIV proteins beneath the host cell lipid bilayer. The nucleocapsid subsequently is formed with viral single-stranded RNA and other components packaged inside. Once packaged, the virion then buds through the plasma membrane, acquiring the characteristics of the host lipid bilayer. After the virus buds, the maturation process begins. Within the virion, protease, another enzyme unique to HIV, begins cleaving a large precursor polypeptide (gag-pol) into functional proteins that are necessary to produce a complete virus. Without this enzyme, the virion is immature and unable to infect other cells.

The characteristics of viral replication and pathogenesis exhibit three general phases: acute, chronic, and terminal (AIDS).[36,37] Initial rounds of HIV replication during acute infection take place largely in the mucosal CD4+ CCR5+ T cell pools in the gut resulting in a massive CD4 T-cell depletion in these tissues.[36,37] Cells are destroyed by various mechanisms, including cell lysis from newly budding virions, cytotoxic T-lymphocyte–induced cell killing, and induction of apoptosis. Following this destruction of the mucosal CD4 T cell pool, which lasts for 2 to 3 weeks, a state of heightened immune activation ensues during the chronic infection phase, which can last for several years. The activated state is characterized by high levels of activation markers on circulating T cells and proinflammatory cytokines and may result from HIV antigen as well as translocation of microbial antigens from the T-cell depleted gut mucosa. Heightened activation enables further HIV replication and ultimately leads to continued depletion of CD4+ CCR5+ T cells. HIV-1 exhibits a very high turnover rate during this chronic phase, with an estimated 10 billion new viruses produced each day. More than 99% of these viruses are produced in newly infected activated cells. Nevertheless, the immune system is able to operate well enough during the chronic phase to prevent overt OIs that herald AIDS. Eventually, the depletion of CD4 cells and the continuous cellular activation leads to a final collapse of the immune system, or AIDS. HIV may use CXCR4 coreceptor during this last phase of infection and these viruses infect a broader range of CD4 cells (naïve and central-memory) speeding the disease progression. It is this unrelenting destruction of CD4 cells that causes the profoundly compromised immune system and AIDS.[36,37]

CLINICAL PRESENTATION

❸ Clinical presentation of primary HIV infection varies, but most patients (40% to 90%) have an acute retroviral syndrome or mononucleosis-like illness (Table 103-2).[38] Symptoms often last 2 weeks, and hospitalization may be required for 15% of patients. Primary infection is associated with a high viral load (>10^6 copies/mL [>10^9/L]) and a precipitous drop in CD4 cells. After several weeks an immune response is mounted, the amount of HIV RNA in plasma falls substantially, CD4 cells rebound slightly, and symptoms resolve gradually. However, as described above, this clinically latent period is not virologically latent because HIV replication is continuous (~10 billion viruses per day) and immune system destruction is ongoing. A steady decrease in CD4 cells is the most measurable aspect of this immune system deterioration. Plasma viral load, on the other hand, will appear to have stabilized at a particular level or "set point." The set point that is established correlates directly with the time to AIDS and morbidity. The Multicenter AIDS Cohort Study measured viral load in 181 HIV-positive men and followed them for as long as 11 years. The mortality rates within 5 years for those with a viral load below 4530 copies/mL (4.53×10^6/L) was 5% compared with 49% for those with a viral load above 36,270 copies/mL (36.27×10^6/L).[39] Thus, a higher viral set point is associated with

TABLE 103-2 Clinical Presentation of Primary Human Immunodeficiency Virus Infection in Adults

Symptoms
Fever, sore throat, fatigue, weight loss, myalgia
40%–80% of patients exhibit a morbilliform or maculopapular rash usually involving the trunk
Diarrhea, nausea, vomiting
Lymphadenopathy, night sweats
Aseptic meningitis (fever, headache, photophobia, stiff neck) may be present in 25% of presenting cases
Other
High viral load (may exceed 1,000,000 copies per milliliter or 10^9/L)
Persistent decrease in CD4 lymphocytes

From reference 38.

TABLE 103-3 Centers for Disease Control and Prevention 2008 Revised Classification System for Human Immunodeficiency Virus Infection in Children Younger Than 13 Years

Immunologic Categories	12 Month CD4 Cells/μL or 10^6/L (%[a])	1–5 Years CD4 Cells/μL or 10^6/L (%[a])	6–12 Years CD4 Cells/μL or 10^6/L (%[a])	
1. No evidence of suppression	≥1,500 (≥25%)	≥1,000 (≥25%)	≥500 (≥25%)	
2. Evidence of moderate suppression	750–1,499 (15%–24%)	500–999 (15–24%)	200–499 (15–24%)	
3. Severe suppression	<750 (<15%)	<500 (<15%)	<200 (<15%)	
Immunologic Categories	**N: No Signs/Symptoms**	**A: Mild Signs/Symptoms**	**B: Moderate Signs/Symptoms**	**C: Severe Signs/ Symptoms**
1. No evidence of suppression	N1	A1	B1	C1
2. Evidence of moderate suppression	N2	A2	B2	C2
3. Severe suppression	N3	A3	B3	C3

[a]Percentage of total lymphocytes.

From reference 19.

poorer prognosis. Not all individuals infected with HIV progress to AIDS—these so-called "long-term nonprogressors" may be infected with a defective virus (e.g., nef-deficient HIV) or may have an intrinsic ability to resist infection (e.g., CCR5 mutation).[33]

Most children born with HIV are asymptomatic. On physical examination, children often present with nonspecific signs, such as lymphadenopathy, hepatomegaly, splenomegaly, failure to thrive, weight loss or unexplained low birth weight (in prenatally exposed infants), and fever of unknown origin.[40] Laboratory findings include anemia, hypergammaglobulinemia (primarily immunoglobulin [Ig] A and IgM), altered mononuclear cell function, and altered T-cell subset ratios. Of note, the normal range for CD4 cell counts in young children is much different from the range in adults (Table 103-3). Children have different susceptibility and/or exposures to OIs compared with adults.[40] Bacterial infections, including *Streptococcus pneumoniae*, *Salmonella* spp., and *Mycobacterium tuberculosis*, may be more prevalent in children with AIDS than in adults with the disease. Kaposi's sarcoma is rare in children. Children with HIV infection may develop lymphocytic interstitial pneumonitis without evidence of *P. jirovecii* or other pathogens on lung biopsy. Some children (~25%) will progress to AIDS rapidly within the first year of life. A presentation of serious OIs such as *P. jirovecii* pneumonia, encephalopathy, failure to thrive, and a precipitous drop in CD4 cells are common in these infants.[40] The current CDC pediatric AIDS surveillance definition (see Table 103-3) excludes children with congenital or perinatally acquired cytomegalovirus or other identified causes of congenital immunodeficiency; laboratory-confirmed HIV-infection is required.[19] General management of the HIV-infected child involves principles similar to those used for the adult: ART, treatment and prophylaxis of OIs, and supportive care.[41,42]

TREATMENT

Desired Outcome

❹ The central goals of ART are to decrease morbidity and mortality, improve quality of life, restore and preserve immune function, and prevent further transmission. The most important and effective way to achieve these goals is maximal suppression of HIV replication, which is interpreted as plasma HIV RNA less than the lower limit of quantitation (i.e., undetectable; usually <50 copies/mL [<50 × 10^3/L]).[30] Such a profound reduction in HIV RNA is associated with reduced transmissions and long-term response to therapy (i.e., durability), as well as increases in CD4 lymphocytes that closely correlates with a reduced risk for developing OIs. While undetectable HIV RNA almost always corresponds with a rise in CD4 lymphocytes, some patients respond virologically or immunologically without the other.[30]

General Approach to Treatment

❺ Prior to 1996, HIV infection was treated with one or two nucleoside analog reverse transcriptase inhibitors (NRTI), which were generally not effective at controlling viremia. Thus, the mainstay of treatment was pharmacologic management of OIs and palliative care. At that time, the prognosis for HIV infection was dire and most patients were disabled and eventually died. In 1995, HIV protease inhibitors (PIs) were introduced followed by NNRTIs, and a new paradigm in HIV treatment was born. Combinations of three active antiretroviral agents from two pharmacologic classes were shown to profoundly inhibit HIV replication to undetectable levels, prevent and reverse immune deficiency, and substantially decrease morbidity and mortality—constituting the ART era.[43] At the same time, multiple other major medical advances were introduced, such as the discovery that HIV establishes a long-lived reservoir in chronically infected cells, and the viral load test (plasma HIV-RNA). With this backdrop of dramatic changes, in 1997 the National Institutes of Health Office of AIDS Research convened a panel to define the scientific principles that might serve as a guide for the clinical use of antiretroviral agents.[44] The 11 principles presented here are an amalgamation of knowledge of the life cycle of HIV, the consequences of HIV replication, clinical trials of antiretroviral agents, and scientific opinion. These foundational principles are still relevant today.

1. Ongoing HIV replication leads to immune system damage and progression to AIDS. HIV infection is always harmful, and true long-term survival free of clinically significant immune dysfunction is unusual.
2. Plasma HIV RNA levels indicate the magnitude of HIV replication and its associated rate of CD4 cell destruction, whereas CD4 cell counts indicate the extent of HIV-induced immune damage already suffered. Regular periodic measurement of plasma HIV RNA levels and CD4 cell counts is necessary to determine the risk of disease progression in an HIV-infected individual and to determine when to initiate or modify antiretroviral treatment regimens.
3. Because rates of disease progression differ among individuals, treatment decisions should be individualized by level of risk indicated by plasma HIV RNA levels and CD4 cell counts.
4. Use of potent combination ART to suppress HIV replication to below the levels of detection of sensitive plasma HIV RNA assays limits the potential for selection of antiretroviral-resistant HIV variants, the major factor limiting the ability of antiretroviral drugs to inhibit virus replication and delay disease progression. Therefore, maximum

achievable suppression of HIV replication should be the goal of therapy.

5. The most effective means for accomplishing durable suppression of HIV replication is simultaneous initiation of combinations of effective anti-HIV drugs with which the patient has not been treated previously and that are not cross-resistant with antiretroviral agents with which the patient has been treated previously.
6. Each of the antiretroviral drugs used in combination therapy regimens always should be used according to optimal schedules and dosages.
7. The available effective antiretroviral drugs are limited in number and mechanism of action, and cross-resistance between specific drugs has been documented. Therefore, any change in ART increases future therapeutic constraints.
8. Women should receive optimal ART regardless of pregnancy status.
9. The same principles of ART apply to both HIV-infected children and adults, although treatment of HIV-infected children involves unique pharmacologic, virologic, and immunologic considerations.
10. Persons with acute primary HIV infections should be treated with combination ART to suppress virus replication to levels below the limit of detection of sensitive plasma HIV RNA assays.
11. HIV-infected persons, even those with viral loads below detectable limits, should be considered infectious and should be counseled to avoid sexual and drug-use behaviors that are associated with transmission or acquisition of HIV and other infectious pathogens.

The extent to which these 11 principles will continue to stand the test of time is unknown; new information on the pathogenesis and treatment of HIV accrues constantly. One continuing source of controversy is whether to treat patients with acute HIV infection. As of October 2012, 27 distinct antiretroviral compounds have been approved by the FDA; two (amprenavir and zalcitabine) have since been removed from the market. Table 103-4 presents the state of the art for treatment of HIV-infected individuals as of October 2012.[30] Treatment is recommended for all HIV-infected persons with a CD4 lymphocyte count below 500 cells/mm^3 (500 × 10^6/L). Many clinicians would also favor starting therapy in asymptomatic patients with CD4 counts above 500 cells/mm^3 (500 × 10^6/L). Other indications for therapy at any CD4 count include pregnancy, history of AIDS-defining illness, HIV-associated nephropathy, or HIV/hepatitis B virus coinfection.

Clinical **Controversy. . .**

Treatment of persons with acute primary HIV infection with combination ART to suppress virus replication to levels below the limit of detection of sensitive plasma HIV RNA assays is controversial. Well-designed trials with clinical end points that define the long-term safety and efficacy of initiating combination ART during acute HIV infection are lacking. Theoretical benefits are decreasing the severity of acute disease; perhaps lowering the initial viral load set point, which affects progression rates; preserving immune function; and reducing the risk for viral transmission. However, these potential benefits must be weighed against the issues imposed by early intervention of chronic therapy, which may be many years ahead of normal initiation of therapy (discussed below).

The optimal time to initiate therapy in chronic HIV infection has been a matter of debate over the last 15 years. The challenges of life-long ART must be balanced against the higher relative risk of ongoing HIV transmissions and disease progression in asymptomatic HIV-infected individuals when ART is delayed. Randomized trials demonstrate that deaths and disease progression are higher if therapy is delayed until CD4 cells fall below 350 cells/mm^3 (350 × 10^6/L).[7,30,45] Epidemiological studies show significantly higher mortality if treatment is delayed in those with a CD4 count of 351 to 500 cells/mm^3 (351 × 10^6 to 500 × 10^6/L) or CD4 counts >500 cells/mm^3 (>500 × 10^6/L) compared with deferring therapy until CD4 counts drop to lower levels.[46] Other epidemiological studies show similar benefits in terms of the composite endpoint of disease progression and death for earlier initiation of therapy.[47,48] Together, these studies support early initiation of ART in patients who are ready and willing to commit to life-long treatment including an understanding of its risks and benefits and the need to maintain a high level of adherence. Healthcare professionals involved in the care of HIV-infected persons must consult the most current literature on the principles and strategies for therapy. Better patient outcomes are demonstrated when clinicians have significant HIV expertise. An excellent source for information on treatment guidelines, which is regularly updated, is available at *www.AIDSinfo.NIH.gov*. Additional guidelines and electronic resources for HIV clinicians are provided in reference 24.

Clinical **Controversy. . .**

The precise time to start therapy is controversial. Early in the ART era, the mantra was "hit early and hit hard," with hopes that the drugs would be well tolerated and the virus could be eradicated. When it became clear that treatment was long term and that these earlier drugs had potential long-term side effects, the mantra changed to a drug-sparing paradigm where therapy was initiated as late as possible. Newer agents have improved upon tolerability, but lack long-term safety data. The benefits of early therapy include preventing the known detriments of unchecked viral replication, including irreversible immune damage and increased likelihood of viral transmission. The potential risks of initiating combination ART include the lifestyle demands of continuous therapy, drug toxicities, and development of antiretroviral drug resistance.

Pharmacologic Therapy

Conceptually the four primary methods of therapeutic intervention against HIV are direct inhibition of chronic viral replication or prevention of HIV acquisition including as virucidal topical formulations (chemicals that destroy intact viruses) to prevent HIV infection, vaccination to stimulate a more effective immune response, and restoration of the immune system with immunomodulators; the latter three approaches are mostly investigational. Several approaches for an HIV vaccine are in development, including whole killed virus, subunit and peptide vaccination, recombinant live vector, and naked DNA delivery. A randomized placebo-controlled trial demonstrated a modest 30% reduction in HIV transmission in a modified-intention to treat analysis of ALVAC-HIV plus AIDSVAX vaccine in 16,402 volunteers.[49] The modified analysis excluded subjects who were found to be HIV-infected prior to randomization. However, the efficacy difference was not significant in the per-protocol analysis. Therefore, the findings must be considered tentative until more definitive data become available. Overall,

TABLE 103-4 Treatment of Human Immunodeficiency Virus Infection: Antiretroviral Regimens Recommended in Antiretroviral-Naïve Persons

	Preferred Regimens	Limitation
NNRTI-based	Efavirenz + tenofovir+ emtricitabine (AI)	Not recommended in the first trimester of pregnancy or in women without adequate contraception
HIV PI-based	Darunavir + ritonavir + tenofovir + emtricitabine (AI)	Rash (darunavir has sulfonamide moiety)
	Atazanavir + ritonavir + tenofovir + emtricitabine (AI)	Not with high doses of proton-pump inhibitors, unconjugated hyperbilirubinemia
InSTI-based	Raltegravir + tenofovir + emtricitabine (AI)	Twice daily (not once daily)
Alternative Regimens (Some Potential Disadvantages vs. Preferred Regimens)		
NNRTI-based	Efavirenz + abacavir + lamivudine (BI)	Possible reduced efficacy for high viral loads (abacavir)
	Rilpivirine + tenofovir + emtricitabine (BI)	Possible reduced efficacy for high viral loads; no proton-pump inhibitors (rilpivirine)
	Rilpivirine + abacavir + lamivudine (BIII)	See above
HIV PI-based	Atazanavir + ritonavir + abacavir + lamivudine (BI)	See above
	Darunavir + ritonavir + abacavir + lamivudine (BII)	See above
	Lopinavir–ritonavir (once or twice daily) either with abacavir + lamivudine or tenofovir + emtricitabine (BI)	GI intolerance, lipids
	Fosamprenavir/ritonavir (once or twice daily) either with abacavir + lamivudine or tenofovir + emtricitabine) (BI)	Rash
InSTI-based	Raltegravir + abacavir + lamivudine (BIII)	See above
	Elvitegravir + cobicistat + tenofovir + emtricitabine (BI)	Should not be used when creatinine clearance <70 mL/min (<1.17 mL/s)
Acceptable Regimens (Potential Additional Disadvantages or Pending Additional Data)		
NNRTI-based	Efavirenz + zidovudine + lamivudine (CI)	Nausea, anemia, lipoatrophy (zidovudine)
	Nevirapine + zidovudine + lamivudine or tenofovir + emtricitabine (CI)	Not in moderate/severe hepatic impairment; not in women with pre-ART CD4 count >250 cells/mm^3 (> 250 × 10^6/L) and men with pre-ART CD4 count >400 cells/mm^3 (> 400 × 10^6/L)
	Nevirapine + abacavir + lamivudine (CIII)	See above
	Rilpivirine + zidovudine + lamivudine (CIII)	See above
HIV PI-based	Atazanavir + (abacavir or zidovudine) + lamivudine (CI)	Lower atazanavir concentrations compared with atazanavir–ritonavir
	(Fosamprenavir + ritonavir or atazanavir + ritonavir) + zidovudine + lamivudine (CI)	See above
	(Darunavir + ritonavir or lopinavir + ritonavir) + zidovudine + lamivudine (CIII)	See above
CCR5-inhibitor-based	Maraviroc + zidovudine + lamivudine (CI)	Lower virologic activity versus efavirenz, need tropism test
	Maraviroc + (tenofovir + emtricitabine or abacavir + lamivudine) (CIII)	See above
InSTI-based	Raltegravir + zidovudine + lamivudine (CIII)	See above
Regimens or Components that should not be used as Initial Therapy		
Regimen or component		**Comment**
Any all NRTI regimen (DI)		Inferior virologic efficacy
Lamivudine (or emtricitabine) + didanosine (DIII)		Inferior virologic efficacy
Didanosine + tenofovir (DII)		Inferior virologic efficacy, CD4 declines
Stavudine (DI)		Toxicity including subcutaneous fat loss, peripheral neuropathy, and lactic acidosis
Darunavir, fosamprenavir, saquinavir, or tipranavir without ritonavir (DI-DIII)		Insufficient plasma concentrations and efficacy or not studied
Delavirdine (DIII)		Inferior virologic efficacy and inconvenient dosing
Enfuvirtide (DIII)		Not studied in naïve patients, inconvenient injections
Etravirine (DIII)		Insufficient data in naïve patients
Indinavir with or without ritonavir (DIII)		Nephrolithiasis, fluid requirements and inconvenient
Nelfinavir (without ritonavir) (DI)		Inferior virologic efficacy
Ritonavir at virologic doses (DIII)		GI intolerance
Tipranavir–ritonavir (DI)		Inferior virologic efficacy

Tenofovir, tenofovir disoproxil fumarate.
Evidence-based rating definition.
Rating strength of recommendation:
A: Both strong evidence for efficacy and substantial clinical benefit support recommendation for use; should always be offered.
B: Moderate evidence for efficacy or strong evidence for efficacy but only limited clinical benefit, supports recommendation for use; should usually be offered.
C: Evidence for efficacy is insufficient to support a recommendation for or against use, or evidence for efficacy might not outweigh adverse consequences (e.g., drug toxicity, drug interactions) or cost of treatment under consideration; use is optional.
D: Moderate evidence for lack of efficacy or for adverse outcome supports recommendation against use; should usually not be offered.
E: Good evidence for lack of efficacy or for adverse outcome supports a recommendation against use; should never be offered.
Rating Quality of Evidence Supporting the Recommendation:
I: Evidence from at least one correctly randomized, controlled trial with clinical outcomes and/or validated laboratory endpoints.
II: Evidence from at least one well-designed clinical trial without randomization or observational cohorts with long-term clinical outcomes.
III: Evidence from opinions of respected authorities based on clinical experience, descriptive studies, or reports of consulting committees.
Lamivudine and emtricitabine are considered interchangeable.

Adapted from Department of Health and Human Services (DHHS) Panel on Antiretroviral Guidelines for Adults and Adolescents. Guidelines for the use of antiretroviral agents in HIV-1-infected adults and adolescents. Updated March 27, 2012. http://AIDSinfo.NIH.gov. From reference 30.

progress has been slow for the vaccine field. Genetic variability in HIV and a nascent understanding of the role of the immune system in suppressing viral replication are significant barriers to the development of an effective HIV vaccine with long-lasting and protective immunity. Immunomodulators, such as aldesleukin (interleukin-2), provide mild benefits in terms of increased CD4 cells; however, aldesleukin is also associated with significant toxicities and no apparent clinical benefit.[50] Additional immunotherapies are in earlier phases of study. Topical virucidal or antiretroviral drug formulations for use vaginally or rectally to prevent sexual transmission of HIV are in various phases of development. Vaginal application of tenofovir 1% gel before and after intercourse reduced HIV infection by 39% in women.[12] However, another study showed that daily tenofovir 1% gel vaginally did not reduce HIV acquisition, indicating that additional trials will be needed before licensing decisions are made.

Antiretroviral Agents

Direct inhibition of viral replication with combinations of potent antiretroviral agents has been the most clinically successful strategy. Four general classes of drugs are used today: entry inhibitors, reverse transcriptase inhibitors, InSTIs, and HIV PIs (Table 103-5).[30] Reverse transcriptase inhibitors consist of two classes: those that are chemical derivatives of purine- and pyrimidine-based nucleosides and nucleotides (nucleoside/nucleotide reverse transcriptase inhibitors [NRTIs]) and those that are not (nonnucleoside reverse transcriptase inhibitors [NNRTIs]). NRTIs include the thymidine analogs stavudine (d4T) and zidovudine (AZT or ZDV); the deoxycytidine analogs emtricitabine (FTC) and lamivudine (3TC); the deoxyguanosine analog abacavir sulfate (ABC); and the deoxyadenosine analogs of which didanosine (ddI) is an inosine derivative and tenofovir disoproxil fumarate (TDF) is a deoxyadenosine-monophosphate nucleotide analog (a nucleotide is a nucleoside with one or more phosphates). **Note that drug abbreviations are provided here and below for reference, but their use is discouraged because they may lead to prescribing or administration errors.** As a class, the NRTIs require phosphorylation to the 5′-triphosphate moiety to become pharmacologically active. Intracellular phosphorylation occurs by cytoplasmic or mitochondrial kinases and phosphotransferases (not viral kinases). The 5′-triphosphate moiety acts in two ways: (a) it competes with endogenous deoxyribonucleotides for the catalytic site of reverse transcriptase, and (b) it prematurely terminates DNA elongation, if taken up and incorporated, as it lacks the requisite 3′-hydroxyl for sugar-phosphate linking.[42] Although NRTI triphosphates (or diphosphate for tenofovir) are specific for HIV reverse transcriptase, their adverse effects may be caused in part by inhibition of mitochondrial DNA or RNA synthesis.[51] Toxicities include peripheral neuropathy, pancreatitis, lipoatrophy (subcutaneous fat loss), myopathy, anemia, and rarely life-threatening lactic acidosis with fatty liver.[52] Use of stavudine and didanosine has declined in favor of more tolerable NRTIs (e.g., emtricitabine, lamivudine, and tenofovir).[30] Emtricitabine, lamivudine, and tenofovir are active against hepatitis B virus, and a combination of these agents should be used in HIV–hepatitis B coinfected patients. With some exceptions (e.g., abacavir), NRTIs are mainly eliminated by the kidney and dose adjustments are required for renal insufficiency (and abacavir should not be used in advanced hepatic impairment). Resistance has been reported for all NRTIs, including cross-resistance within the class as multiple and/or specific mutations accrue.[53]

NNRTIs are a chemically heterogeneous group of agents that bind noncompetitively to reverse transcriptase adjacent to the catalytic site. Unlike NRTIs, NNRTIs do not require intracellular activation, do not compete against endogenous deoxyribonucleotides, and do not have potent antiviral activity against HIV-2. Given the different site of binding to reverse transcriptase, NNRTIs can be used with NRTIs effectively. Available NNRTIs include delavirdine (DLV), efavirenz (EFV), etravirine (ETR), nevirapine (NVP), and rilpivirine (RPV).[30] As a class, the NNRTIs are generally associated with rash and elevated liver function tests, including life-threatening cases rarely, particularly for nevirapine.[51] NNRTIs tend to have long plasma half-lives and are mainly cleared by liver and/or gut-mediated metabolism through the cytochrome P450 (CYP) enzyme system, and caution should be used for those with advanced hepatic insufficiency (nevirapine should not be used in moderate or advanced hepatic insufficiency). NNRTI can be perpetrators of drug–drug interactions associated with CYP metabolism. The NNRTIs are unique in that a single mutation is needed to confer high-level cross-resistance for the class (except etravirine), which has been termed a *low-genetic barrier* to resistance.[53]

The HIV PIs include atazanavir (ATV), darunavir (DRV), fosamprenavir (FPV), indinavir (IDV), lopinavir (LPV), nelfinavir (NFV), ritonavir (RTV), saquinavir (SQV), and tipranavir (TPV). HIV PIs competitively inhibit the cleavage of the gag-pol polyprotein, which is a crucial step in the viral maturation process, thereby resulting in the production of immature, noninfectious virions. HIV PIs are generally associated with GI distress and metabolic changes, such as increased lipids, insulin insensitivity, and changes in body fat distribution.[52] HIV PIs are cleared by liver- and gut-mediated metabolism (mainly CYP3A), and dose adjustments may be required in hepatic insufficiency (tipranavir/ritonavir should not be used in moderate to severe hepatic insufficiency). HIV PIs are almost always used with low doses of ritonavir (or potentially cobicistat in the future), i.e., CYP3A inhibitors, to increase the plasma concentrations of the HIV PI of interest. CYP3A-mediated drug interactions with concomitant medications are important considerations for PIs. Resistance to the HIV PIs generally requires the buildup of multiple mutations, termed a *high-genetic barrier*. Multiple mutations can lead to cross-resistance.[53]

There are currently two types of entry inhibitors: fusion inhibitors and CCR5 antagonists. Enfuvirtide (ENF) is the only fusion inhibitor available at this time. Enfuvirtide is a synthetic 36-amino-acid peptide that binds gp41, which inhibits envelope fusion of HIV-1 with the target cell, but does not have activity against HIV-2. Because of the peptide nature of enfuvirtide, oral delivery is impossible, and subcutaneous injection is the preferred route of administration. Injection-site reactions (pain, erythema, nodules) are the most common adverse effect, nearing 100% incidence. Enfuvirtide is cleared via protein catabolism and amino acid recycling. Enfuvirtide appears to have a low genetic barrier to resistance.[53] Maraviroc is a CCR5 antagonist. Unlike the other available antiretrovirals that interact with a viral target, CCR5 antagonists block a human receptor. The long-term consequences of blocking CCR5 are unknown but may include increased susceptibility to infection by flaviviruses (e.g., West Nile virus and tickborne encephalitis virus).[54] One advantage of targeting a human receptor is that resistance to CCR5 antagonists may be more difficult to develop. Because CCR5 antagonists are only effective against R5 virus and not X4 virus, a viral tropism assay must be performed prior to using a CCR5 antagonist. Maraviroc is a CYP3A and P-glycoprotein substrate and is therefore susceptible to drug-drug interactions and caution should be used in those with advanced hepatic insufficiency. Resistance mutations have been identified for enfuvirtide, but assays for maraviroc resistance have not been developed other than the R5 versus X4 tropism test.

Raltegravir (RAL) and elvitegravir (EVG) are approved InSTI, and dolutegravir is in late development. InSTI bind to HIV integrase while it is in a specific complex with viral DNA. As a result, viral DNA cannot become incorporated into the human genome and cellular enzymes degrade unincorporated viral DNA.

TABLE 103-5 Selected Pharmacologic Characteristics of Antiretroviral Compounds

Drug	F (%)	$t_{1/2}$ (h)[a]	Adult Dose[b] (doses/day)	Plasma C_{max}/C_{min} (μM)	Distinguishing Adverse Effect
Integrase Inhibitors (InSTI)					
Elvitegravir (coformulated with cobicistat)	?	13	150 mg (1)	3.8/1	Diarrhea, nausea, headache
Raltegravir	?	9	400 mg (2)	1.74/0.22	Increased creatine phosphokinase
Nucleoside (Nucleotide) Reverse Transcriptase Inhibitors (NtRTIs)					
Abacavir	83	1.5/20	300 mg (2) *or* 600 mg (1)	5.2/0.03 7.4[c]	Hypersensitivity
Didanosine	42	1.4/24	200 mg (2) *or* 400 mg (1)	2.8/0.03 5.6[c]	Peripheral neuropathy, pancreatitis
Emtricitabine	93	10/39	200 mg (1)	7.3/0.04	Pigmentation on soles and palms in non-whites
Lamivudine	86	5/22	150 mg (2) *or* 300 mg (1)	6.3/1.6 10.5/0.5	Headache, pancreatitis (children)
Stavudine	86	1.4/7	40 mg (2)	2.4/0.04	Lipoatrophy, peripheral neuropathy
Tenofovir disoproxil fumarate	40	17/150	300 mg (1)	1.04/0.4	Renal toxicity (proximal tubulopathy)
Zidovudine	85	2/7	200 mg (3) *or* 300 mg (2)	0.2 3[c]	Anemia, neutropenia, myopathy
Nonnucleoside Reverse Transcriptase Inhibitors (NNRTIs)					
Delavirdine	85	5.8	400 mg (3) *or* 600 mg (2)	35/14	Rash, elevated liver function tests
Efavirenz	43	48	600 mg (1)	12.9/5.6	CNS disturbances and potential teratogenicity
Etravirine	?	41	200 mg (2)	1.69/0.86	Rash, nausea
Nevirapine	93	25	200 mg (2)[d]	22/14	Potentially serious rash and hepatotoxicity
Rilpivirine	?	50	25 mg (1)	0.7/0.3	Possibly depression
Protease Inhibitors (PIs)					
Fosamprenavir[e]			1400 mg (1)[e,f]	14.3/2.9	Rash
Atazanavir	68	7	400 mg (1) *or* 300 mg (1)[f]	3.3/0.23 6.2/0.9	Unconjugated hyperbilirubinemia
Darunavir	82	15	800 mg (1)[f] *or* 600 mg (2)[f]	11.9/6.5	Hepatitis, rash
Indinavir	60	1.5	800 mg (3) *or* 400–800 mg (2)[f]	13/0.25	Nephrolithiasis
Lopinavir[g]	?	5.5	800 mg (1) *or* 400 mg (2)	13.6/7.5	Hyperlipidemia/GI intolerance
Nelfinavir	?	2.6	750 mg (3) *or* 1250 mg (2)	5.3/1.76 7/1.2	Diarrhea
Ritonavir	60	3–5	600 mg (2)[d] *or* "Boosting doses"	16/5	GI intolerance
Saquinavir	4	3	1,000 mg (2)[f]	3.9/0.55	QT prolongation
Tipranavir	?	6	500 mg (2)[f]	77.6/35.6	Hepatotoxicity, intracranial hemorrhage
Entry Inhibitors—Fusion Inhibitor					
Enfuvirtide	84	3.8	90 mg (2)	1.1/0.73	Injection-site reactions
Coreceptor Inhibitor					
Maraviroc	33	15	300 mg (2)	1.2/0.066	Hepatitis, allergic reaction

C_{max}, maximum plasma concentration; C_{min}, minimum plasma concentration; *F*, bioavailability; $t_{1/2}$, elimination half-life.

[a]NtRTIs: Plasma NtRTI $t_{1/2}$/intracellular (peripheral blood mononuclear cells) NtRTI-triphosphate $t_{1/2}$; plasma $t_{1/2}$ only for other classes.

[b]Dose adjustment may be required for weight, renal or hepatic disease, and drug interactions.

[c]C_{min} concentration typically below the limit of quantification.

[d]Initial dose escalation recommended to minimize side effects.

[e]Fosamprenavir is a tablet phosphate prodrug of amprenavir. Amprenavir is no longer available.

[f]Must be boosted with low doses of ritonavir (100 to 200 mg).

[g]Available as coformulation 4:1 lopinavir to ritonavir.

Adapted from Department of Health and Human Services (DHHS) Panel on Antiretroviral Guidelines for Adults and Adolescents. Guidelines for the use of antiretroviral agents in HIV-1-infected adults and adolescents. Updated March 27, 2012. http://AIDSinfo.NIH.gov and product information for agents.

Alternatively, recombination and repair mechanisms may form long-terminal repeat (LTR) circular DNA from the unincorporated viral DNA. Raltegravir and dolutegravir are primarily glucuronidated by UGT1A1 and are not susceptible to CYP-mediated drug interactions. Elvitegravir is extensively metabolized by CYP3A and is co-formulated with cobicistat, a potent CYP3A inhibitor, to optimize drug exposure and enable once daily dosing. Cobicistat, which is devoid of antiretroviral activity, is also being studied as a pharmacokinetic enhancer of HIV PIs. InSTI should be used with caution in advanced hepatic insufficiency. Updated dosing recommendations for hepatic and renal insufficiency for all antiretroviral drugs are included in the Department of Health and Human Services Guidelines.[30] Multiple mutations have been identified conferring resistance to InSTI including cross-resistance as mutations accrue. Dolutegravir was designed to be active against raltegravir and elvitegravir resistant strains.

Novel antiviral agents in the classes listed above and novel agents in new drug classes that exploit other steps in the HIV life cycle (see Fig. 103-1) are in development, with a focus on long-lasting activity and/or high activity against drug-resistant virus.[55]

The anti-herpes and anti-hepatitis B antivirals acyclovir, foscarnet, entecavir, and adefovir exhibit modest anti-HIV activity.[56,57] If these antivirals are used in HIV-infected patients, it should be with suppressive ART therapy.

Drug Interactions

6 Medical use of antiretroviral agents is complicated by clinically significant drug–drug interactions that can occur with many of these agents.[30,58] Some interactions are beneficial and used purposely (e.g., ritonavir and cobicistat); others may be harmful, leading to dangerously elevated or inadequate drug concentrations. Clinicians involved in the pharmacotherapy of HIV must understand the mechanistic basis for these interactions and maintain a current knowledge of drug interactions for these reasons.

Many clinically significant antiretroviral-associated drug interactions involve CYP3A-mediated metabolism and clearance. The HIV PIs, except nelfinavir, the NNRTIs delavirdine, etravirine, and rilpivirine, the CCR5 antagonist maraviroc, and the InSTI elvitegravir are metabolized by CYP3A. In general, efavirenz, etravirine and nevirapine are inducers of CYP3A, whereas delavirdine and the PIs inhibit CYP3A. Ritonavir is a potent inhibitor of CYP3A-mediated metabolism and is now used almost exclusively at lower doses as a pharmacokinetic enhancer of other HIV PIs. Darunavir, lopinavir, saquinavir, and tipranavir must be taken with ritonavir to achieve optimal plasma concentrations. Atazanavir, fosamprenavir, and indinavir are also primarily used with ritonavir for the same reason. Nelfinavir is not effectively boosted by ritonavir given its CYP2C19-mediated metabolism. Cobicistat, which is an analog of ritonavir without antiretroviral activity, is also a potent inhibitor of CYP3A activity and is under study as a booster of HIV-PIs. Many potential concomitant drugs on the market are also metabolized by CYP3A and therefore susceptible to clinically relevant drug interactions with HIV PIs, NNRTIs, and cobicistat.[30,58] Agents with narrow therapeutic indices and/or that exhibit major changes in pharmacokinetics with CYP3A inhibition are most important in this regard. Examples include, but are not limited to, simvastatin, lovastatin, corticosteroids (including inhaled and intranasal), ergot derivatives, oral hormonal contraceptives, hepatitis C PIs (boceprevir/telaprevir), and some antiarrhythmics. The drug interaction potential of antimycobacterium agents, specifically the rifamycins, are particularly relevant given the high potential for such infections in HIV-infected patients.[58] Rifampin, a potent inducer of CYP3A metabolism and conjugation enzymes, is contraindicated with use of most HIV PIs, etravirine, rilpivirine, and maraviroc because concentrations are reduced substantially even with ritonavir enhancement. Raltegravir dose should be doubled in the presence of rifampin; efavirenz is an alternative agent. Ritonavir enhancement generally allows coadministration of HIV PIs with rifabutin.[58] In such cases, the rifabutin dose will require adjustment given its CYP3A-mediated clearance.

The herbal product St. John's wort (*Hypericum perforatum*) is a potent inducer of metabolism and is contraindicated with PIs, NNRTIs, and maraviroc.[30] It must be stressed that the pharmacology of CYP3A interactions may be complicated by simultaneous induction/inhibition of drug transporter-mediated (e.g., P-glycoprotein) clearance and/or other phase I or phase II enzymes. Furthermore, some antiretroviral drugs require acidic environments for optimal absorption creating interactions with antacids, particularly proton-pump inhibitors (e.g., atazanavir, rilpivirine). Clinicians who treat HIV must stay abreast of antiretroviral drug interaction data. Websites are available that catalog and regularly update HIV drug-interaction information (*http://www.hiv-druginteractions.org/*), and the Department of Health and Human Services guidelines for antiretroviral use provide, and regularly update, excellent summaries of known clinically relevant drug interactions.[30,58]

NRTIs are not metabolized by CYP3A, but other drug interaction considerations are important. Generally, NRTIs of the same nucleobase should not be coadministered. For example, zidovudine and stavudine are both thymidine analogs and phosphorylated by the same cellular enzymes. Antagonism occurs between these two drugs both in vitro and in vivo; thus, the two should never be given together. Similarly, deoxycytidine analogs should not be coadministered. The deoxyadenosine analogs didanosine and tenofovir exhibit a plasma drug interaction whereby didanosine concentrations are significantly increased.[30] Furthermore, the two adenosine analogs are less effective together compared with other recommended NRTI regimens and there is concern for CD4 lymphotoxicity, a troubling effect that appears unique to this NRTI combination. Coadministration of didanosine and tenofovir is not recommended.[30]

Landmarks in the Evolution of Antiretroviral Therapy

7 ART has undergone major changes over the past decades. Illustrating these changes is important for a thorough understanding of current treatment strategies. The fundamental landmarks in the use of antiretroviral agents are as follows:

1. An early study demonstrated that zidovudine monotherapy confers a survival benefit in persons who have AIDS.[59] This study showed that a single drug provided moderate clinical benefit.
2. Further investigation showed that combination regimens of two NRTIs (e.g., zidovudine and didanosine or zalcitabine) were superior to zidovudine monotherapy in immunologic and virologic parameters, particularly in patients with no previous ART, and conferred a superior survival benefit.[60] This established that NRTI monotherapy was inferior to dual NRTI therapy.
3. A pivotal study showed that dual NRTI therapy was inferior to triple therapy consisting of 2 NRTIs and the HIV PI indinavir.[61] Use of triple therapy with combinations of two NRTIs with NNRTIs or HIV PIs was associated with a durable response as well as significantly reduced incidence of OIs and improved survival, thus establishing the current paradigm of ART.[62]
4. Evolution of triple-therapy regimens utilizing boosted HIV PIs, co-formulations, new drug classes, and better tolerated agents showed improvements in convenience, tolerability, safety, and virologic efficacy, all helping usher in the current era of ART.[63,64]

7 Taken together, the pivotal studies described above established that HIV should not be treated with single or dual NRTIs. Current recommendations for initial treatment of HIV infection advocate a minimum of three active antiretroviral agents: tenofovir disoproxil fumarate (TDF) plus emtricitabine with either a ritonavir-enhanced PI (darunavir or atazanavir), the NNRTI efavirenz, or the InSTI, raltegravir.[30] Multiple alternative regimens are also safe and effective, but have one or two disadvantages compared with the preferred regimens such as lack of long-term follow-up, weaker virologic responses with high viral loads, lower tolerability, or greater risk of long-term toxicities such as subcutaneous fat loss. Preferred and alternative antiretroviral regimens are listed in Table 103-4.[30] The World Health Organization (WHO) also updated its treatment recommendations for resource-limited settings. The main updates to the WHO guidelines are the recommendation to treat at higher CD4 count thresholds (350 cell/mm^3 [350 × 10^6/L]) and not to include stavudine as initial therapy, due to elevated risk of mitochondrial toxicity.[65]

Adherence

The simplest definition of adherence is the patient's ability to take medication as directed. Variable adherence to ART is common, and a leading cause of therapeutic failure.[66] Factors associated with poor adherence include major psychiatric illnesses, active substance abuse, unstable social circumstances, adverse events, and poor adherence with clinic visits.[30] Studies consistently show that average adherence rates range from 60% to 80% for both HIV PI and NNRTI-based regimens including 30% of subjects who miss >7 consecutive days of dosing.[67–69] The odds of persistent or breakthrough viremia are several-fold higher in patients with adherence below 60% to 80%, and the risk mounts with longer dosing "holidays".[67–69] As clinicians, it is critical to establish a relationship of trust with the patient and to communicate to the patient the importance of proper medication taking. Education should be aimed at understanding the disease process, monitoring, and goals of therapy. An individual's "readiness" to take medications should be clearly established before any treatment is initiated.[30] Help from caregivers, friends, and/or family members should be leveraged by the patient because social and psychological support are among the most important factors that influence adherence in this patient population.

Efficacy

Based on clinical trial data, approximately 70% to 90% of patients will achieve undetectable viral loads with modern ART regimens. The preferred NRTI combination, TDF plus emtricitabine, has demonstrated virologic and tolerability advantages compared with zidovudine/lamivudine and abacavir/lamivudine.[70] An open-labeled trial of 517 antiretroviral naive patients randomized to TDF-emtricitabine versus zidovudine–lamivudine both with efavirenz demonstrated that significantly more patients in the TDF-emtricitabine arm achieved less than 400 copies/mL (400 × 10^3/L) at 48 weeks (84%) compared with patients randomized to zidovudine–lamivudine (73%).[70] Part of this difference was attributed to more patients discontinuing zidovudine–lamivudine due to adverse events compared with TDF–emtricitabine. Subcutaneous fat loss and lipid elevations were also higher in the zidovudine–lamivudine group through 48 weeks. Another randomized study compared abacavir–lamivudine to TDF–emtricitabine in a blinded manner in combination with either efavirenz or atazanavir/ritonavir (open labeled) in 1858 antiretroviral naïve adults. Among subjects with >100,000 copies/mL (>100 × 10^6/L) of plasma HIV-RNA at screening, those randomized to abacavir–lamivudine experienced twice the virologic failure rate and significantly more adverse events compared with those randomized to TDF-emtricitabine.[71] However, other studies have also evaluated virologic efficacy and safety of abacavir–lamivudine in subjects with >100,000 copies/mL (>100 × 10^6/L) at baseline and have found high rates of efficacy and safety regardless of baseline viral load.[72]

Large, randomized, controlled trials have compared TDF–emtricitabine based regimens and demonstrated comparable potency for raltegravir versus efavirenz,[73] and atazanavir/ritonavir versus lopinavir/ritonavir,[74] and increased potency for darunavir/ritonavir over lopinavir/ritonavir.[75] Lopinavir/ritonavir was less tolerable than atazanavir/ritonavir and darunavir/ritonavir in terms of GI distress.[74,75] These studies established the preferred initial regimens for HIV infection listed above. Trials of new combinations such as coformulated elivitegravir–cobicistat–tenofovir disproxil fumarate–emtricitabine versus preferred regimens demonstrate comparable safety and efficacy over 48 weeks, but lack longer-term follow-up compared with the preferred regimens above.[76] Recommended preferred regimens are continuously updated as longer-term follow-up data accrue. Patients with sustained undetectable HIV-RNA taking out-of-date drug regimens may be candidates to simplify to one of the preferred regimens or a more desirable alternative regimen based on past treatment history and other variables. Simplified regimens should continue to include three active drugs. If abacavir is to be used in any regimen, a test for the presence of human leukocyte antigen (HLA)-B*5701 should be done as its presence has been strongly correlated with the development of abacavir hypersensitivity. Should this test be positive, an abacavir allergy should be added to the patient's chart and abacavir should not be used in the patient. Similarly, a tropism test is required prior to using maraviroc to establish that the patient's virus uses the CCR5 coreceptor.[30]

Resistance

8 Regimen failure is commonly associated with antiretroviral resistance, and testing for such resistance is a useful clinical tool.[53] The two types of resistance tests available are phenotype and genotype. A phenotype test determines the concentration of antiretroviral agent necessary to inhibit 50% (IC_{50}) replication of the patient's viral isolate (inhibitory concentration of 50% [IC_{50}]) in a recombinant in vitro viral assay. Results usually are expressed as a fold change in susceptibility (IC_{50}) compared with a wild-type laboratory strain virus. Generally, the fold-change in IC_{50} increases as HIV accumulates additional mutations that confer resistance to a particular drug. However, a single mutation may confer a very high fold-change in IC_{50} for some drugs (e.g., lamivudine, emtricitabine, efavirenz, nevirapine) rendering them ineffective after a single mutation. Although small-to-moderate increases in the fold change suggests reduced susceptibility to that antiretroviral agent, resistance may not be absolute, and partial susceptibility may remain. Theoretically, drug concentrations may be increased to overcome reduced susceptibility. The strengths of phenotypic testing is to provide resistance information for complex mutation patterns, but it is also associated with higher cost, limited number of commercial providers, and slower turnaround time for results. Genotyping assesses genetic mutations and associated codon changes in gp41, reverse transcriptase, integrase or protease in the patient's virus and compares it with the wild-type sequence. Mutations, when present, are listed by the wild-type amino acid followed by the position in the protein or enzyme and end with the mutation found in the patient's virus. For example, a common mutation caused by lamivudine and emtricitabine is the M184V mutation: a substitution of valine (V) for methionine (M) at the 184 position of reverse transcriptase. Mutations can confer varying degrees of antiretroviral drug resistance and in some cases, weighting algorithms have been developed to predict the relative impact of mutation combinations on antiretroviral activity. Algorithms have also been developed to predict a phenotype from a genotype test (i.e., virtual phenotype). Not all mutations, however, are only detrimental—for example, while M184V confers significant resistance to lamivudine and emtricitabine, it is also associated with

a less fit virus.[77] New genetic mutations are discovered occasionally and are catalogued and maintained on websites (e.g., *www.iasusa.org/resistance_mutations*). Interpretation of genotypes resistance tests is complex; therefore, the reader is encouraged to obtain expert advice and consult the most recent guidelines on HIV resistance testing.[53]

Treatment of Special Populations

Pregnancy

Several considerations are relevant to the treatment of pregnant women, including the health of the mother, prevention of HIV transmission to the fetus, potential for teratogenicity, and dosing issues based on pharmacokinetic changes during pregnancy. Treatment recommendations should be consulted to address the specific requirements for HIV-infected pregnant women and the prevention of vertical transmission.[16] Generally, pregnant women should be treated as would nonpregnant women, with some exceptions. In general, efavirenz should be avoided when possible in pregnant women during the first trimester or in women trying to conceive because of potential teratogenicity. Drugs that cross the placental barrier should be included such as, abacavir, emtricitabine, lamivudine, tenofovir, or zidovudine. IV zidovudine is recommended intrapartum depending on the mother's viral load, based on early studies demonstrating clear prophylactic effectiveness as well as extensive familiarity with the side effect profile.[16] Infants also receive zidovudine (± several doses of nevirapine) prophylaxis for 6 weeks after birth. Lopinavir–ritonavir has also been studied extensively in pregnant women, and is recommended in this population. Currently, HIV transmission rates have been reduced to <0.5% for women who are treated with ART and when zidovudine prophylaxis is used.[16]

In resource-limited settings or when HIV infection is detected very close to delivery, an abbreviated course of zidovudine with a single dose of nevirapine also can reduce transmission substantially. In these cases, a 7-day course of zidovudine–lamivudine is given to the mother intrapartum and postpartum to reduce the substantial risk of nevirapine resistance due to its low genetic barrier to resistance and the long decay half-life leading to prolonged suboptimal concentrations.[78] Zidovudine (± nevirapine) is also recommended in the infant. If breast-feeding is necessary because alternatives are not safe or feasible, extended nevirapine prophylaxis in the infant significantly lowers the risk of HIV transmission from the mother.[79]

Chemoprophylaxis

9 In addition to fetal and infant chemoprophylaxis, protection of healthcare workers from accidental exposure to HIV and in cases of rape or high-risk postcoital and postinjection drug-use episodes are important concerns. The CDC has issued guidelines governing antiretroviral treatment of occupational and other high-risk HIV exposures.[3,15] These guidelines should be consulted for updates as the knowledge in this field evolves. The principles of the guidelines are to grade the exposure risk and treat as soon as possible after high-risk exposures to prevent HIV infection. The makeup of the treatment depends upon the risk. Postexposure prophylaxis (PEP) with a triple-drug regimen consisting of two NRTIs and a boosted-PI is recommended for percutaneous blood exposure involving significant risk (e.g., large-bore needle, visible blood from patients with advanced AIDS). Two NRTIs may be offered to the healthcare worker with lower risk of exposure, such as cases involving superficial exposures to the mucous membrane or broken skin. Urine, saliva, nasal secretions, stool, and sputum are not considered infectious unless visibly contaminated with blood. The optimal duration of treatment is unknown, but at least 4 weeks of therapy is advocated. Treatment ideally should be initiated within 1 to 2 hours of exposure, but treatment is recommended up to 72 hours postexposure. Expert consultation is needed when exposure to drug-resistant virus is suspected or confirmed, but this should not delay initiation of PEP.[3,15]

Preexposure prophylaxis (PrEP) using the antiretroviral drugs emtricitabine and TDF was recently approved for preventing sexual HIV acquisition. The approach involves adding tenofovir disoproxil fumarate–emtricitabine to traditional prevention strategies (e.g., condoms) in HIV-negative persons at high risk of HIV acquisition to prevent infection if HIV-exposed PrEP is effective in MSM, serodiscordant couples, and at-risk heterosexual men and women.[8,10,80] The key considerations to maximize PrEP effectiveness are to document an HIV-negative test prior to initiating PrEP, to monitor for HIV infection and renal function regularly, and to promote adherence and the continued use of safe sex practices.

EVALUATION OF THERAPEUTIC OUTCOMES

Two laboratory tests are used to evaluate response to ART: the plasma HIV RNA and the CD4 count.[30] These tests should be established at baseline, along with hematology, chemistries, and serologies for coinfections. A HIV resistance test is recommended upon entry into care. After therapy is initiated, patients are generally monitored at 3-month intervals until HIV-RNA reaches undetectable levels. An assessment at 2 to 8 weeks is warranted to document early response. Monitoring may be increased to every 6 months in stabilized patients. The two main indications for a change in therapy are significant toxicity and treatment failure. Should a single agent be responsible for an intolerable side effect, that agent often can be singly changed out of the regimen, for example, the patient who experiences intolerable CNS disturbances during initiation of efavirenz can switch to a boosted PI without changing the dual NRTI backbone. Caution must be exercised when drugs in the regimen have overlapping toxicities, which makes changing a single agent problematic. Serious and life-threatening toxicities warrant cessation of the whole regimen before deciding upon a subsequent therapy.

As a general guide, the following events indicate treatment failure and should prompt consideration for changing therapy:

1. Less than 1 $\log_{10}$ reduction in HIV RNA 1 to 4 weeks after initiation of therapy or a failure to achieve less than 200 copies/mL (200×10^3/L) by 24 weeks or less than 50 copies/mL (50×10^3/L) by 48 weeks.
2. After HIV RNA suppression, repeated detection of HIV-RNA.
3. Clinical disease progression, usually the development of a new OI.

Therapeutic Failure

8 The most important measure of therapeutic failure is suboptimal suppression of viral replication. Many reasons may underlie suboptimal suppression of viral replication such as nonadherence to medication, development of drug resistance, intolerance to one or more medications, adverse drug–drug or drug–food interactions, or pharmacokinetic–pharmacodynamic variability.[30] In cases of suboptimal suppression of viral replication, these potential causes should be investigated and addressed, if possible. As a general rule, drug resistance develops for regimens that do not maximally suppress HIV replication. Drug resistance testing is recommended while the patient is undergoing the failing regimen or within 4 weeks after stopping the regimen as long as the HIV RNA count is greater than 500 copies/mL (500×10^3/L), which is the threshold for resistance assays (~500 to 1000 copies/mL [~500×10^3

to 1000 × 10^3/L]).[53] Virus may revert to wild-type if more than 4 to 6 weeks has elapsed between regimen discontinuation and the resistance test. Most clinicians use the genotype assay because it is less expensive and results typically are available sooner compared with the phenotype assay. Resistance results usually require expert interpretation. Treating patients with drug-resistant HIV utilizes the same general treatment approaches described for initial therapy above. Patients should be treated with at least two (preferably three) fully active antiretroviral drugs based on medication history, resistance tests, and new mechanistic drug classes (e.g., maraviroc and raltegravir). The goal of therapy is to suppress HIV-RNA to <50 copies/mL (<50 × 10^3/L). In cases when <50 copies/mL (<50 × 10^3/L) cannot be attained, maintenance on the regimen is preferred over drug discontinuation so as to prevent rapid immunological and clinical decline.

The two newest PIs darunavir and tipranavir and the NNRTI, etravirine, have demonstrated activity in persons with multidrug-resistant HIV in controlled clinical trials.[30] The drugs in the newer drug classes, raltegravir, maraviroc, and enfuvirtide, are also active against NRTI-, NNRTI-, and PI-resistant viruses in highly treatment experienced patients in controlled trials.

Previous strategies for therapeutic failure have proven largely ineffective, including drug holidays, structured or strategic treatment interruptions, and structured intermittent therapy. The overall premise of these strategies was similar: stop all antiretrovirals and allow the patient time off medication. Reinitiation of therapy was intended to reestablish control of viral replication, as wild-type virus would be expected to predominate, although the resistant virus is likely archived in long-lived cells. A landmark clinical trial tested the hypothesis that episodic ART guided by the CD4 count would lower morbidity and mortality, including that associated with drug toxicity compared with continuous therapy.[81] However, the patients randomized to episodic therapy (drug-sparing) experienced significantly increased risk of opportunistic disease or death from any cause, including non-AIDS causes.[82] Most morbidity and mortality were consequences of lowering the CD4 count and increasing the viral load, but increased drug-related toxicity was also observed. This and other studies have established that viral replication is damaging to the immune system and end organs and drug-sparing approaches are generally not advocated. Finally, it is important to consider the implications of stopping all drugs simultaneously for regimens containing drugs with short half-lives (e.g., zidovudine) as well as drugs with long half-lives (e.g., efavirenz and nevirapine). The result may be functional monotherapy for the drug with the longest half-life once the shorter half-life drugs are cleared, which can lead to resistance mutations especially for drugs with low genetic barriers (e.g., NNRTIs).[83] At this time, the optimal time sequence for staggered component discontinuation has not been determined.

Clinical **Controversy. . .**

There is a compelling theoretical rationale for therapeutic drug monitoring in the experienced patient, but this approach is currently controversial. Drug susceptibility is founded on the premise that increasing drug concentration corresponds with stronger inhibition of replication up to a maximal effectiveness. This principle holds for drug-resistant variants, except higher drug concentrations are needed for the same levels of inhibition. Therefore, drug concentration monitoring could guide dose adjustments needed to attain the higher target drug concentrations required for optimal viral inhibition. Currently, therapeutic drug monitoring is suggested as a consideration for patients with multidrug-resistant HIV as well as in other select clinical situations. However, limitations to therapeutic drug monitoring include the lack of established target concentrations, intrapatient pharmacokinetic variability, lack of randomized clinical trials proving benefit or cost effectiveness, and few analytical laboratories and experts available for interpretation. Most antiretrovirals are not suitably formulated for minor dose adjustments.

COMPLICATIONS OF HIV INFECTION AND AIDS

3 In the pre-ART era, the major therapeutic focus was prevention and treatment of OIs associated with uncontrolled HIV replication and a steady decline in CD4 cells.[43] Uncontrolled HIV is an insidious disease; persons infected often present with OIs, a consequence of the weakened immune system rather than HIV per se. Most OIs are caused by organisms that are common in the environment and often represent the reactivation of quiescent, hidden infections common in the population. The probability of developing specific OIs is closely related to CD4 count thresholds (Fig. 103-2). These CD4 thresholds serve as a basis for initiating primary OI chemoprevention.

5 In the ART era, the main principle in the management of OIs is treating HIV infection to enable CD4 cell recovery and maintenance above safe levels.[58] Additional important principles regarding management of OIs are as follows:

1. Prevent exposure to opportunistic pathogens
2. Vaccinations to prevent first-episode disease (consult HIV-specific guidelines)
3. Primary chemoprophylaxis at certain CD4 thresholds to prevent first-episode disease
4. Treat emergent OI
5. Secondary chemoprophylaxis to prevent disease recurrence
6. Discontinuation of certain prophylaxes with sustained ART-associated immune recovery

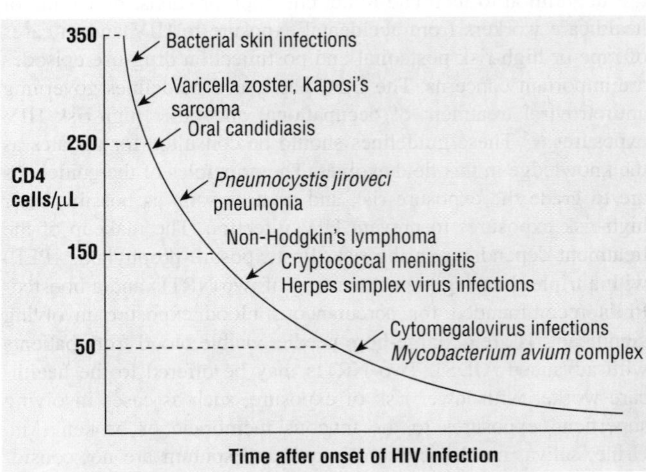

FIGURE 103-2 Natural history of opportunistic infections associated with human immunodeficiency virus infection. *(Reprinted with permission, © Courtney V. Fletcher, 2009.)*

Several considerations are required for the patient who presents with an OI and is simultaneously diagnosed with HIV and who thus needs both OI and ART treatment.[58] Immediate initiation of ART is indicated for OIs that respond to CD4 recovery, such as cryptosporidiosis, progressive multifocal leukoencephalopathy, and Kaposi's sarcoma. However, for other OIs such as cryptococcal meningitis, tuberculosis, *Mycobacterium avium* complex (MAC), and PCP, several potential problems complicate the timing of when to initiate ART relative to OI therapy. First, drug–drug interactions and the complexity of adhering to concomitant regimens can be daunting. Second, potentially overlapping drug toxicities can limit the options for clinicians trying to stop specific drugs thought to be eliciting the toxicity event. Third, an immune reconstitution syndrome (IRIS) has been associated with initiation of ART in the presence of underlying OIs. IRIS is generally characterized by fever and worsening of OI manifestations in the first few months after ART, and the reaction may take weeks to months to resolve.[58,84] Risk factors for IRIS are a low CD4 count, a rapid virologic response to ART, and a high antigenic burden.[85] An ART-associated rapid-onset immune reconstitution against the smoldering OI infection is thought to be the mechanism of IRIS. Treatment of IRIS is supportive, but may also include interruption of ART or antiinflammatory drugs.[84,85]

The AIDS Clinical Trials A5164 study compared immediate versus deferred ART in subjects treated for an acute OI (63% PCP, 12% *Cryptococcal meningitis*, and 12% bacterial infections). Subjects had advanced HIV infection with an average CD4 count of 29 cells/mm^3 (29 × 10^6/L) and viral load >100,000 copies/mL (>100 × 10^6/L). Subjects with tuberculosis were excluded. The immediate ART arm (N = 141) initiated ART within 12 days after OI treatment was started versus within 45 days for the deferred ART arm (N = 141). The rate of AIDS progression or death was significantly greater in the deferred ART arm compared with early ART arm (14% vs. 24%).[86] Other studies have demonstrated similar mortality improvements when initiating ART within 2 weeks of tuberculosis therapy compared with delaying ART by 8 to 12 weeks, particularly in those with low CD4 cell counts.[87–89] However, early ART in patients with cryptococcal meningitis may increase mortality risk compared with beginning ART after the completion of antifungal therapy.[90,91] Expert consultation should be used in the management of ART initiation in patients with OIs.

The three major OIs (PCP, MAC, and cytomegalovirus retinitis) all have decreased substantially in incidence with the advent of ART.[43,58] Furthermore, primary and secondary chemoprophylaxes for OIs have contributed to the same decreases. Nevertheless, opportunistic diseases continue to be complications of HIV disease and occur at low CD4 lymphocyte counts in patients who are unaware of their HIV infection, or who have not responded to ART therapy or OI prophylaxis because of adherence issues or inadequate engagement with the healthcare system.[58]

The spectrum of OIs observed in HIV-infected individuals and recommended first-line regimens for treatment are given in Table 103-6. Recommended therapies for primary prophylaxis are given in Table 103-7.[58] These lists of recommendations are not as extensive as in the published guidelines, which include multiple additional alternatives and cover other less common OIs.[58] The following brief discussion of PCP provides an overview of the epidemiology, diagnosis, clinical manifestations, and results of treatment and serves as an illustration for the principles discussed earlier.

Pneumocystis Jirovecii Pneumonia

5 *Pneumocystis jirovecii* (*carinii*) pneumonia (PCP) has been and continues to be the most common life-threatening OI in patients with AIDS.[92] *P. jirovecii* was formerly named *P. carinii*; the name change was made to distinguish the organism that infects humans (*P. jirovecii*) from the strain that infects rodents (*P. carinii*). The acronym PCP is still used today. Early in the AIDS epidemic 80% of patients experienced PCP at some point during their lifetime.[58,93] Although the incidence of PCP has fallen substantially since the advent of ART and effective prophylaxis for PCP, it still occurs in persons unaware of their HIV infection, and breakthrough PCP can occur in those with variable adherence to ART and/or prophylaxis.[58]

P. jirovecii is a fungus that has protozoan characteristics as well.[92,93] Exposure to *P. jirovecii* is widespread; two thirds of the population have developed serum antibodies by age 2 to 4 years.[58] The organism appears to reside without consequence in humans unless the host becomes immunologically impaired.[94] Disease associated with immunosuppression probably occurs from both new acquisition and reactivation. Ninety percent of PCP cases in AIDS patients occurred in those with CD4 counts less than 200 cells/mm^3 (200 × 10^6/L).[58] Other risk factors include oral thrush, recurrent bacterial pneumonia, unintentional weight loss, and high plasma HIV RNA. Past episodes of PCP increase risk for future episodes, which provides the basis for secondary chemoprophylaxis, as described below.[58]

The presentation of PCP in AIDS often is insidious.[58,92] Characteristic symptoms include fever and dyspnea. Clinical signs are tachypnea with or without rales or rhonchi and a nonproductive or mildly productive cough occurring over a period of weeks, although more fulminant presentations can occur. Chest radiographs may show florid or subtle infiltrates but occasionally are normal. Infiltrates usually are interstitial and bilateral, however. Arterial blood gases may show minimal hypoxia (PaO_2 80 to 95 mm Hg [10.6 to 12.6 kPa]) but in more advanced disease may be markedly abnormal. The diagnosis of PCP usually is made by identification of the organism in induced sputum or in specimens obtained from bronchoalveolar lavage. Less commonly, transbronchial or open lung biopsy is used to locate the organism. Diagnostic PCR tests are available in some institutions.[92]

Untreated PCP has a mortality rate of nearly 100%. Several potential treatments are available for PCP, but the treatment of choice is trimethoprim–sulfamethoxazole (or cotrimoxazole), which is associated with a response rate of 60% to 100%.[58] Parenteral pentamidine is equally efficacious but significantly more toxic. Trimethoprim–sulfamethoxazole is also the regimen of choice for primary and secondary prophylaxis of PCP in patients with and without HIV.[58,92]

When used for treatment of PCP, the dose of trimethoprim–sulfamethoxazole is 15 to 20 mg/kg/day (based on the trimethoprim component) as three to four divided doses.[58,92] Treatment duration typically is 21 days but also must be based on clinical response. Trimethoprim–sulfamethoxazole usually is initiated by the IV route, although oral therapy may suffice in mildly ill and reliable outpatients or for completion of a course of therapy after a response has been achieved with IV administration. Patients with moderate-to-severe PCP should be treated with corticosteroids as soon as possible after starting PCP therapy and certainly within 72 hours, in order to blunt the deterioration seen just after initiation of PCP therapy. Alternative regimens include pentamidine for moderate-to-severe disease and dapsone with trimethoprim, primaquine with clindamycin, and atovaquone for mild-to-moderate PCP.[58] Early initiation of ART is also generally recommended as long as there are no contraindications.[86]

Adverse reactions to trimethoprim–sulfamethoxazole and pentamidine are common, occurring in 20% to 85% of patients in this setting.[58] The more common adverse reactions seen with trimethoprim–sulfamethoxazole are rash (rarely including Stevens–Johnson syndrome), fever, leukopenia, elevated serum transaminase levels, and thrombocytopenia. The incidence of these adverse reactions is higher in HIV-infected individuals than in those not infected with HIV. Mild rashes should be watched closely for progression to more severe reactions but are not an absolute

TABLE 103-6 Therapies for Common Opportunistic Pathogens in HIV-Infected Individuals

Clinical Disease	Preferred Initial Therapies for Acute Infection in Adults (Strength of Recommendation in Parentheses)	Common Drug- or Dose-Limiting Adverse Reactions
Fungi		
Candidiasis, oral	Fluconazole 100 mg orally for 7–14 days (AI)	Elevated liver function tests, hepatotoxicity, nausea, and vomiting
	or Nystatin 500,000 units oral swish (~5 mL) four times daily for 7–14 days (BII)	Taste, patient acceptance
Candidiasis, esophageal	Fluconazole 100–400 mg orally or IV daily for 14–21 days (AI)	Same as above
	or Itraconazole 200 mg/day orally for 14–21 days (AI)	Elevated liver function tests, hepatotoxicity, nausea, and vomiting
Pneumocystis jirovecii pneumonia	Trimethoprim–sulfamethoxazole IV or orally 15–20 mg/kg/day as trimethoprim component in three to four divided doses for 21 days[a] (AI) moderate or severe therapy should be started IV	Skin rash, fever, leucopenia Thrombocytopenia
	or Pentamidine IV 4 mg/kg/day for 21 days[a] (AI)	Azotemia, hypoglycemia, hyperglycemia, arrhythmias
	Mild episodes Atovaquone suspension 750 mg (5 mL) orally twice daily with meals for 21 days[a] (BI)	Rash, elevated liver enzymes, diarrhea
Cryptococcal meningitis	Amphotericin B 0.7 mg/kg/day IV for a minimum of 2 weeks with flucytosine 100 mg/kg/day orally in four divided doses (AI) *followed by*	Nephrotoxicity, hypokalemia, anemia, fever, chills Bone marrow suppression Elevated liver enzymes
	Fluconazole 400 mg/day, orally for 8 weeks or until CSF cultures are negative (AI)[a]	Same as above
Histoplasmosis	Liposomal amphotericin B 3 mg/kg/day IV for 2 weeks (AI) *followed by* Itraconazole 200 mg orally thrice daily for 3 days then twice daily, for 12 months (AII)[a]	Same as above
Coccidioidomycosis	Amphotericin B 0.7–1 mg/kg/day IV until clinical improvement (usually after 500–1,000 mg) then switch to azole (AII)[a]	Same as above
	or Fluconazole 400–800 mg once daily (meningeal disease) (AII)[a]	Same as above
Protozoa		
Toxoplasmic encephalitis	Pyrimethamine 200 mg orally once, then 50–75 mg/day	Bone marrow suppression
	plus Sulfadiazine 1–1.5 g orally four times daily	Allergy, rash, drug fever
	and Leucovorin 10–25 mg orally daily for 6 weeks (AI)[a]	
Isosporiasis	Trimethoprim and sulfamethoxazole: 160 mg trimethoprim and 800 mg sulfamethoxazole orally or IV four times daily for 10 days (AII)[a]	Same as above
Bacteria		
Mycobacterium avium complex	Clarithromycin 500 mg orally twice daily, *plus* ethambutol 15 mg/kg/day orally (AI), *and*	GI intolerance, optic neuritis, peripheral neuritis
	For advanced disease, rifabutin 300 mg/day (dose may need adjustment with ART) (AI)[a]	Rash, GI intolerance Neutropenia, discolored urine, uveitis
Salmonella enterocolitis or bacteremia	Ciprofloxacin 500–750 mg orally (or 400 mg IV) twice daily for 14 days (longer duration for bacteremia or advanced HIV) (AIII)	GI intolerance
Campylobacter enterocolitis	Ciprofloxacin 500 mg orally twice daily *or* Azithromycin 500 mg orally daily for 7 days (or 14 days with bacteremia) (BIII)	Same as above
Shigella enterocolitis	Ciprofloxacin 500 mg orally twice daily for 5 days (or 14 days for bacteremia) (AIII)	Same as above
Viruses		
Mucocutaneous herpes simplex	Acyclovir 5 mg/kg IV every 8 hours until lesions regress, then acyclovir 400 mg orally three times daily until complete healing (famciclovir or valacyclovir is alternative) (AII)	GI intolerance, crystalluria
Primary varicella-zoster	Acyclovir 10–15 mg/kg every 8 hours IV for 7–10 days, then switch to oral acyclovir 800 mg five times daily after defervescence (famciclovir or valacyclovir is alternative) (AIII)	Obstructive nephropathy, CNS symptoms
Cytomegalovirus (retinitis)	Ganciclovir intraocular implant *plus* valganciclovir 900 mg twice daily for 14–21 days then once daily until immune recovery from ART (AI)[a]	Neutropenia, thrombocytopenia
Cytomegalovirus esophagitis or colitis	Ganciclovir 5 mg/kg IV every 12 hours for 21 to 28 days (BII)	Same as above

ART, antiretroviral therapy; CSF, cerebrospinal fluid; HIV, human immunodeficiency virus.

[a]Maintenance therapy is recommended.
See Table 103-4 for levels of evidence-based recommendations.

From reference 58.

TABLE 103-7 Therapies for Prophylaxis of Select First-Episode Opportunistic Diseases in Adults and Adolescents

Pathogen	Indication	First Choice (Strength of Recommendation in Parentheses)
I. Standard of care		
Pneumocystis jirovecii	CD4+ count <200/mm³ (<200 × 10⁶/L) *or* oropharyngeal candidiasis	Trimethoprim–sulfamethoxazole, one double-strength tablet orally once daily (AI) or one single-strength tablet orally once daily (AI)
Mycobacterium tuberculosis		
Isoniazid-sensitive	(Active TB should be ruled out): + test for latent TB infection with no prior TB treatment history *or* – test for latent TB infection, but close contact with case of active tuberculosis *or* history of untreated or inadequately treated healed TB regardless of latent TB infection test results	Isoniazid 300 mg orally plus pyridoxine, 50 mg orally once daily for 9 months (AII) *or* Isoniazid 900 mg orally twice weekly (BII) plus pyridoxine 50 mg orally daily for 9 months (BIII)
For exposure to drug-resistant TB	Consult public health authorities	
Toxoplasma gondii	Immunoglobulin G antibody to *Toxoplasma* and CD4+ count <100/mm³(<100 × 10⁶/L)	Trimethoprim–sulfamethoxazole one double-strength tablet orally once daily (AII)
Mycobacterium avium complex	CD4+ count <50/mm³ (<50 × 10⁶/L)	Azithromycin 1,200 mg orally once weekly (AI) or 600 mg orally twice weekly (BIII) or clarithromycin 500 mg orally twice daily (AI)
Varicella zoster virus (VZV)	Preexposure: CD4 ≥200/mm³ (≥200 × 10⁶/L), no history of varicella infection, or, if available, negative antibody to VZV Postexposure: Significant exposure to chicken pox or shingles for patients who have no history of either condition or, if available, negative antibody to VZV	Varicella vaccination; two doses, 3 months apart (CIII) Varicella-zoster immune globulin, 125 IU per 10 kg (maximum of 625 IU) IM, within 96 hours after exposure to a person with active varicella or herpes zoster (AIII)
Streptococcus pneumoniae	CD4 count ≥200 cells/mm³ (≥200 × 10⁶/L) or no receipt of vaccination in past 5 years. Consider for those with CD4<200/mm³ (<200 × 10⁶/L) and those with an CD4 increase to > 200/mm³ (>200 × 10⁶/L) on ART (CIII)	23-valent polysaccharide vaccine, 0.5 mL intramuscularly (BII) revaccination every 5 years may be considered (CIII)
Hepatitis B virus	All susceptible patients	Hepatitis B vaccine, three doses (AII) Anti-HBs should be obtained 1 month after the vaccine series completion (BIII)
Influenza virus	All patients (annually, before influenza season)	Inactivated trivalent influenza virus vaccine (annual): 0.5 mL intramuscularly (AIII)
Hepatitis A virus	All susceptible (anti-hepatitis A virus–negative) patients at increased risk for hepatitis A infection (e.g., chronic liver disease, illegal drug users, men who have sex with men)	Hepatitis A vaccine: two doses (AII) antibody response should be assessed 1 month after vaccination; with revaccination as needed (BIII)
Human papillomavirus (HPV) infection	15–26 year old women	HPV quadravalent vaccine months 0, 2, and 6 (CIII)
Histoplasma capsulatum	CD4+ count <150/mm³, (<150 × 10⁶/L) endemic geographic area and high risk for exposures	Fluconazole 100–200 mg orally once daily (CI)

See Table 103-4 for levels of evidence-based recommendations.
From reference 58.

contraindication to continuing therapy.[58] This highlights the need for thoughtful consideration of ART components because of overlapping toxicities with some antiretrovirals such as abacavir and nevirapine, which also are associated with rash and hypersensitivity, including life-threatening cases. For pentamidine, side effects are pronounced and include hypotension, tachycardia, nausea, vomiting, severe hypoglycemia or hyperglycemia, pancreatitis, irreversible diabetes mellitus, elevated serum transaminase levels, nephrotoxicity, leukopenia, and cardiac arrhythmias. Some of these reactions appear to be related to the infusion rate (e.g., hypotension and tachycardia) and can be minimized by infusing pentamidine over 1 hour or more.[93] Dosage modification or pharmacokinetic monitoring can reduce the toxicity of both pentamidine and trimethoprim–sulfamethoxazole.[95] Dose reduction of pentamidine from 4 to 3 mg/kg/day appears to be successful in minimizing further rises in serum creatinine levels.[93] Maintenance of serum trimethoprim concentrations between 5 and 8 mcg/mL (mg/L; 17 to 28 μmol/L) may help to prevent severe myelosuppression.[95] Early addition of adjunctive corticosteroid therapy to anti-PCP regimens decreases the risk of respiratory failure and improves survival in patients with AIDS and moderate-to-severe PCP (PaO_2 ≤70 mm Hg [≤ 9.3 kPa] or alveolar–arterial gradient ≥35 mm Hg [≥ 4.7 kPa]).[58,92] The adverse effects associated with corticosteroid therapy in these patients were minimal, primarily an increased incidence of herpetic lesions, although some concerns exist about the potential for reactivation of tuberculosis or cytomegalovirus and/or long-term effects on bones.[93,96]

Prevention of PCP is clearly a preferable treatment strategy. Primary prophylaxis is recommended for any HIV-infected person who has a CD4 lymphocyte count less than 200 cells/mm³ (200 × 10⁶/L) (or CD4 percentage of total lymphocytes <14%) or a history of oropharyngeal candidiasis.[58,92] Secondary PCP prophylaxis is recommended for all HIV-infected individuals who have had a previous episode of PCP.

Trimethoprim–sulfamethoxazole is the most effective and least expensive agent and is the preferred therapy for both primary and secondary prophylaxis of PCP in adults and adolescents.[58,92] It also appears to confer cross-protection against toxoplasmosis and many bacterial infections. The recommended dose in adults and adolescents is one double-strength tablet daily, although other regimens, such as one double-strength tablet thrice weekly or one single-strength tablet daily and gradual dose escalation using liquid trimethoprim–sulfamethoxazole, have been used in an attempt to reduce the incidence of adverse reactions and improve compliance.

Alternative prophylactic regimens are available if trimethoprim–sulfamethoxazole cannot be tolerated.

In the ART era, the profound reduction in HIV replication and restoration in CD4 cell count to levels rarely associated with the development of OIs provides a basis for the discontinuation of primary and secondary prophylaxis.[58] For PCP, primary prophylaxis should be discontinued in patients receiving and responding to ART who have a CD4 cell count greater than 200 cells/mm^3 (200×10^6/L) sustained for at least 3 months, but should be reinstated if the CD4 count drops to less than 200 cells/mm^3 (200×10^6/L). The same criteria apply for both discontinuation and reinitiation of secondary prophylaxis of PCP. However, continued secondary prophylaxis should be considered when the original PCP episode occurred at a CD4 count greater than 200 cells/mm^3 (200×10^6/L).[58]

In summary, comprehensive recommendations are available for management of PCP and other OIs in the context of HIV infection including prevention and treatment.[58] Readers are advised that data continue to emerge on new OI therapies, the safety of stopping primary and secondary prophylaxis, as well as criteria for when to restart secondary prophylaxes. The most current guidelines always should be consulted. Similar OI guidelines have been developed and are updated regularly that are specific to children.[41]

Complications in the ART Era

(10) As with any medication, adverse reactions occur with antiretroviral agents that can range from life-threatening to minor intolerances. Characteristic side effects for each antiretroviral agent are listed in Table 103-5. A comprehensive discussion of all the adverse effects during ART is beyond the scope of this chapter, but can be found in various other sources.[30,51,52] The purpose of this section is to highlight certain medical issues that have emerged in the ART era as HIV-infected patients live longer and are exposed to antiretroviral drugs for many years.

A broad spectrum of complications usually associated with aging appear to occur earlier in HIV-infected patients in the ART era.[82,97] These complications include osteoporosis and osteopenia, renal insufficiency, metabolic syndrome, neurocognitive decline, atherosclerotic disease, frailty, and malignancy. The cause of the early manifestation of these complications is not entirely clear, but evidence suggests that immune-damage or dysregulation (e.g., a state of persistent heightened cellular activation) and ongoing viral replication play a role, as well as adverse events from antiretroviral medications.[82,96]

While contemporary ART has reduced the incidence of some HIV-related cancers such as Kaposi's sarcoma and non-Hodgkin's lymphoma, other non-AIDS-related malignancies plague HIV-infected individuals at significantly elevated rates such as Hodgkin's lymphoma and anal, lung, skin, and hepato-carcinoma.[98] Part, but not all, of this increased risk in HIV-infected patients may be attributed to elevated exposures to human papillomavirus (anal cancer), smoking (lung carcinoma), and chronic hepatitis B and/or C coinfection (liver cancer). Some concern has been raised that antiretroviral drugs may contribute directly to these increased cancer rates, as some agents have caused cancers in laboratory animals as well as genotoxicity in vitro.[16] However, studies have shown similar cancer rates in organ transplant recipients with medication-induced immunosuppression, which suggests that it is the impairment to the immune system associated with HIV-infection that is driving much of these higher cancer rates.[99] While the approach to treatment of AIDS-related malignancies in HIV-infected patients is similar to that in non-HIV-infected patients, treatment is complicated by drug–drug interactions that may exist between the antiretrovirals and the oncolytics.[98]

Antiretroviral drugs may contribute to several complications. Tenofovir has been associated with renal proximal tubulopathy (including rare cases of Fanconi's syndrome and renal failure) as well as osteopenia.[100] PIs and zidovudine–lamivudine have also been associated with osteopenia, although the precise mechanism for these effects is not clear.[101,102] Relationships exist between PIs, efavirenz, and the thymidine analog NRTIs and dyslipidemia (increased triglycerides and low-density lipoproteins [LDL] and decreased high-density lipoproteins [HDL]), abnormal glucose homeostasis (insulin resistance and impaired glucose tolerance), body fat abnormalities (lipoatrophy of the face and extremities and central lipoaccumulation), and lactic acidosis with hepatosteatosis (all the NRTIs).[103,104] These metabolic abnormalities may occur in combination. Notably, some of the same abnormalities are also associated with the HIV infection itself, such as hypertriglyceridemia and insulin resistance.[103] Distinguishing the contribution of disease versus drug and ascertaining whether one abnormality precipitates the development of other abnormalities is difficult.[97,104,105] Various mechanistic hypotheses have been put forward, including NRTI-induced mitochondrial toxicity, and PI/NNRTI interactions with various cellular processes, such as glucose uptake, altered apolipoprotein degradation or synthesis, adipocyte differentiation, and lipolysis.[103,105] Some agents within these classes are less associated with these complications including atazanavir for the PIs, nevirapine for NNRTIs, and lamivudine, emtricitabine, tenofovir, and abacavir for the NRTIs.[103] Early evidence also suggests that raltegravir and maraviroc are less associated with metabolic complications as well.[73,106]

Metabolic complications create several challenges and concerns. First, the metabolic abnormalities may increase the risk of adverse cardiovascular events, and some evidence gives credence to this concern.[107] A large observational prospective cohort study of 23,468 HIV-infected patients applied the Framingham cardiovascular risk algorithm and compared the estimated cardiovascular event rate with the actual event rate.[108] The algorithm takes into account known risk factors, many of which are associated with ART, such as diabetes and dyslipidemia as well as sex, age, smoking, and blood pressure. The estimated event rate paralleled the actual event rate, and both increased with years on ART. This finding suggests that increased cardiovascular risk can be explained by conventional risk factors, which are aggravated by ART. Therefore, the metabolic abnormalities precipitated by ART and HIV should be treated as cardiovascular disease risk factors and may warrant medical intervention. Finally, some observational studies have found an association between myocardial infarction and abacavir and didanosine use.[107,109] However, these associations for abacavir have not been duplicated when evaluating data from randomized controlled trials, indicating the need for additional study.[110]

A second concern and challenge is how to manage the changes in body fat distribution.[111] Preferred agents such as tenofovir, emtricitabine, efavirenz, darunavir, atazanavir, and raltegravir are less associated with lipoatrophy compared with older agents such as stavudine, zidovudine, and indinavir. However, all therapies appear to be associated with visceral abdominal adiposity.[111] Controlled trials of antiretroviral substitution have demonstrated that patients randomized to switch away from stavudine to either abacavir or tenofovir have had small gains in subcutaneous fat.[112] Small controlled studies have demonstrated modest but inconsistent gains in subcutaneous fat with thiazolidinedione therapy.[113] Central fat accumulation is difficult to treat. Lifestyle changes, such as reducing calorie intake and increasing aerobic exercise, should be the first-line approach. Metformin reduces central fat accumulation, but lean body mass and subcutaneous fat may exhibit unwanted declines.[113] Tesamorelin, a growth hormone releasing analog was approved to safely reduce central adiposity, although a drawback is that visceral fat returns within months of discontinuation.[111] Unfortunately, both lipoatrophy and fat accumulation eventually may lead to reconstructive surgery strategies in severe or refractory cases. The best management of body fat changes is prevention through initiation of preferred regimens less likely to cause such changes (see current recommendations for initial therapy).[30]

ART-associated hyperlipidemia can create several therapeutic challenges. Antiretroviral substitution studies have shown lipid improvements after switching away from older PIs to either NNRTIs or atazanavir, but direct pharmacologic intervention may be required.[113] Elevated LDL may respond to β-hydroxy-β-methylglutaryl-coenzyme A (HMG-CoA) reductase inhibitor (statin) therapy. However, serious concerns exist regarding drug–drug interactions between PIs and statins, especially for lovastatin and simvastatin.[30,113] The plasma area under the concentration–time curve of these statins can be increased >10-fold and may increase the risk for rhabdomyolysis. Generally, fluvastatin, pitavistatin, and pravastatin are recommended as alternatives. Atorvastatin or rosuvastatin should be used with caution[30] including initiation with low doses with careful monitoring. Other HIV-specific recommendations exist for lifestyle modifications, and the use of fibrates, niacin, and/or fish oil for isolated hypertriglyceridemia.[111] Current guidelines should always be consulted, as new information regarding the special concerns and challenges associated with HIV lipodystrophy continue to accrue.

Many HIV-infected patients are coinfected with hepatitis C (HCV), which poses another challenge in the ART-era. HIV–HCV coinfection is common because of the shared blood–borne route of transmission.[114,115] Approximately 30% of HIV-infected patients in the United States have HIV–HCV (approximately 300,000 individuals). Up to 90% of injection–drug users and 90% of hemophiliacs with HIV are coinfected with HCV.[114] HIV worsens the prognosis of HCV by reducing the chance of HCV clearance and accelerating HCV progression. After acute HCV infection, approximately 20% of patients without HIV will clear HCV compared with only 5% to 10% of those who also have HIV. With chronic HCV infection, progression to fibrosis, cirrhosis, and liver failure is several-fold faster in HIV–HCV patients versus HCV-monoinfected patients.[115] For these reasons, ART is recommended for HIV–HCV coinfected patients.

A challenge in HIV–HCV patients is the potential for liver toxicity to ART. Coinfected patients have several-fold higher risk of ART-associated transaminase elevations versus patients infected with HIV but not HCV.[114,115] Nevirapine and full-dose ritonavir appear to carry the highest risk of transaminase elevations, whereas stavudine has been linked with steatosis. Ritonavir-boosted PIs generally do not carry the same elevated risk as full-dose ritonavir with the exception of tipranavir–ritonavir, which is associated with risk of clinical hepatitis and hepatic decompensation in those with HCV or hepatitis B infections. Stavudine and didanosine are generally not recommended in combination with HCV therapy owing to risk of mitochondrial toxicity including noncirrhotic portal hypertension for didanosine.[114,115] Other than these examples, the general threat of major liver toxicity is low overall, and this concern should not dissuade the use of ART in HIV–HCV-coinfected persons given the known benefits of therapy.[30,114,115]

HCV therapy should be offered to HIV–HCV coinfected patients according to HCV guidelines, although beginning when CD4 cell counts are above 200 cells/mm^3 (200×10^6/L) is preferable. A significant consideration is potential drug–drug interactions between ART and HCV therapies. In addition to the considerations listed above, severe anemia is possible when zidovudine is used with ribavirin and interferon.[114,115] This appears to be a pharmacodynamic interaction, as zidovudine reduces red blood cell output and ribavirin causes hemolysis. Zidovudine should be avoided when possible.[114,115] Concomitant HCV PIs, boceprevir or telaprevir, with HIV PIs results in a bi-way interaction resulting in reduced concentrations of both drug classes. These interactions were not predicted based on the known pharmacology of these drugs, underscoring the need to study drug–drug interactions prospectively. Drug interactions were not observed between boceprevir or telaprevir with raltegravir, suggesting that raltegravir-based therapy may be a good choice for concomitant therapy. It is likely that the list of drug–drug interactions among HIV and HCV medications will grow as more HCV therapies become available underscoring the importance for consulting the most current literature when managing HIV–HCV coinfection.

PERSONALIZED PHARMACOTHERAPY

A great number of considerations go into choosing the optimal drug regimen for a given patient. A resistance test is generally recommended when the patient enters HIV care, as resistant virus is transmitted in 6% to 16% of new infections. Resistance results should help guide therapy. Other considerations include avoidance of PIs in patients taking contraindicated concomitant medications such as rifampin (efavirenz would be an alternative), avoidance of tenofovir in patients with preexisting renal dysfunction (abacavir would be an alternative), and avoidance of efavirenz in women of childbearing age trying to conceive or not using stable and reliable contraception (PIs would be an alternative). Several once-daily fixed-dose combination formulations are available, which enhances convenience by minimizing the number of tablets or capsules required per dose. Many antiretroviral regimens have important requirements for dosing relative to a meal to optimize absorption.[30] Several factors contribute to whether the patient will mount a durable response to initial therapy, including adherence, pharmacologic effectiveness, and convenience/tolerability.

ACKNOWLEDGMENTS

This work was supported by Grants UO1 AI84735 and AI68636, R01AI093319, and PO1 AI074340 from the National Institute of Allergy and Infectious Disease.

DISCLOSURES

Thomas Kakuda is an employee of Janssen Pharmaceuticals, LLC, a Johnson & Johnson company and a stock holder of Johnson & Johnson.

ABBREVIATIONS

AIDS	acquired immunodeficiency syndrome
ART	antiretroviral therapy
CD	cluster of differentiation
CCR5	Chemokine (C–C motif) receptor 5
CDC	Centers for Disease Control and Prevention
CRFS	circulating recombinant forms
CXCR4	Chemokine (C-X-C motif) Receptor 4
CYP	cytochrome P450
ELISA	enzyme-linked immunosorbent assay
gp	glycoprotein
HCV	hepatitis C virus
HIV	human immunodeficiency virus
IC_{50}	concentration of antiretroviral agent necessary to inhibit 50% of viral replication
InSTI	integrase strand transfer inhibitor
IRIS	immune reconstitution syndrome
LDL	low-density lipoprotein
LTR	long-terminal repeat

MAC	*Mycobacterium avium* complex
MSM	men who have sex with men
NNRTI	nonnucleoside reverse transcriptase inhibitor
NRTI	nucleoside/nucleotide reverse transcriptase inhibitor
OI	opportunistic infection
PCP	*Pneumocystis jirovecii* (*carinii*) pneumonia
PCR	polymerase chain reaction
PI	protease inhibitor
PEP	postexposure prophylaxis
PrEP	preexposure prophylaxis
RT-PCR	reverse-transcription polymerase chain reaction
SIV	simian immunodeficiency virus
TDF	tenofovir disoproxil fumarate
WHO	World Health Organization

REFERENCES

1. Simon V, Ho DD, Abdool Karim Q. HIV/AIDS epidemiology, pathogenesis, prevention, and treatment. Lancet 2006;368(9534):489–504.
2. De Cock KM, Jaffe HW, Curran JW. The evolving epidemiology of HIV/AIDS. AIDS 2012;26(10):1205–1213.
3. Smith DK, Grohskopf LA, Black RJ, et al. Antiretroviral postexposure prophylaxis after sexual, injection-drug use, or other nonoccupational exposure to HIV in the United States: Recommendations from the U.S. Department of Health and Human Services. MMWR Recomm Rep 2005;54(RR-2):1–20.
4. Incorporating HIV prevention into the medical care of persons living with HIV. Recommendations of CDC, the Health Resources and Services Administration, the National Institutes of Health, and the HIV Medicine Association of the Infectious Diseases Society of America. MMWR Recomm Rep 2003;52(RR-12):1–24.
5. Boily MC, Baggaley RF, Wang L, et al. Heterosexual risk of HIV-1 infection per sexual act: Systematic review and meta-analysis of observational studies. Lancet Infect Dis 2009;9(2):118–129.
6. Wiysonge CS, Kongnyuy EJ, Shey M, et al. Male circumcision for prevention of homosexual acquisition of HIV in men. Cochrane Database Syst Rev 2011(6): CD007496.
7. Cohen MS, Chen YQ, McCauley M, et al. Prevention of HIV-1 infection with early antiretroviral therapy. N Engl J Med 2011;365(6):493–505.
8. Baeten JM, Donnell D, Ndase P, et al. Antiretroviral prophylaxis for HIV prevention in heterosexual men and women. N Engl J Med 2012;367(5):399–410.
9. Chasela CS, Hudgens MG, Jamieson DJ, et al. Maternal or infant antiretroviral drugs to reduce HIV-1 transmission. N Engl J Med 2010;362(24):2271–2281.
10. Grant RM, Lama JR, Anderson PL, et al. Preexposure chemoprophylaxis for HIV prevention in men who have sex with men. N Engl J Med 2010;363(27):2587–2599.
11. Rotheram-Borus MJ, Swendeman D, Chovnick G. The past, present, and future of HIV prevention: Integrating behavioral, biomedical, and structural intervention strategies for the next generation of HIV prevention. Annu Rev Clin Psychol 2009;5:143–167.
12. Abdool Karim Q, Abdool Karim SS, Frohlich JA, et al. Effectiveness and safety of tenofovir gel, an antiretroviral microbicide, for the prevention of HIV infection in women. Science. 2010;329(5996):1168–1174.
13. Stramer SL, Glynn SA, Kleinman SH, et al. Detection of HIV-1 and HCV infections among antibody-negative blood donors by nucleic acid-amplification testing. N Engl J Med 2004;351(8):760–768.
14. Zou S, Dodd RY, Stramer SL, Strong DM. Probability of viremia with HBV, HCV, HIV, and HTLV among tissue donors in the United States. N Engl J Med 2004;351(8):751–759.
15. Panlilio AL, Cardo DM, Grohskopf LA, Heneine W, Ross CS. Updated U.S. Public Health Service guidelines for the management of occupational exposures to HIV and recommendations for postexposure prophylaxis. MMWR Recomm Rep 2005;54(RR-9):1–17.
16. Public Health Services Task Force. Recommendations for Use of Antiretroviral Drugs in Pregnant HIV-1-Infected Women for Maternal Health and Interventions to Reduce Perinatal HIV-1 Transmission in the United States—Living document last updated, July 31, 2012; Available at http://www.AIDSinfo.NIH.gov.
17. Shapiro RL, Smeaton L, Lockman S, et al. Risk factors for early and late transmission of HIV via breast-feeding among infants born to HIV-infected women in a randomized clinical trial in Botswana. J Infect Dis 2009;199(3):414–418.
18. Thior I, Lockman S, Smeaton LM, et al. Breastfeeding plus infant zidovudine prophylaxis for 6 months vs formula feeding plus infant zidovudine for 1 month to reduce mother-to-child HIV transmission in Botswana: a randomized trial: The Mashi Study. JAMA 2006;296(7):794–805.
19. Schneider E, Whitmore S, Glynn KM, Dominguez K, Mitsch A, McKenna MT. Revised surveillance case definitions for HIV infection among adults, adolescents, and children aged <18 months and for HIV infection and AIDS among children aged 18 months to <13 years—United States, 2008. MMWR Recomm Rep 2008;57(RR-10):1–12.
20. Hall HI, Song R, Rhodes P, et al. Estimation of HIV incidence in the United States. JAMA 2008;300(5):520–529.
21. Lubinski C, Aberg J, Bardeguez AD, et al. HIV policy: The path forward—A joint position paper of the HIV Medicine Association of the Infectious Diseases Society of America and the American College of Physicians. Clin Infect Dis 2009;48(10):1335–1344.
22. Centers for Disease Control and Prevention. HIV surveillance—United States, 1981–2008. MMWR 2011;60(21):689–693.
23. Gardner EM, McLees MP, Steiner JF, Del Rio C, Burman WJ. The spectrum of engagement in HIV care and its relevance to test-and-treat strategies for prevention of HIV infection. Clin Infect Dis 2011;52(6):793–800.
24. Aberg JA, Kaplan JE, Libman H, et al. Primary care guidelines for the management of persons infected with human immunodeficiency virus: 2009 update by the HIV medicine association of the infectious diseases society of America. Clin Infect Dis 2009;49(5):651–681.
25. UNAIDS World AIDS Day Report 2011. Joint United Nations Programme on HIV/AIDS (UNAIDS). Available at: http://www.unaids.org/en/media/unaids/contentassets/documents/unaidspublication/2011/JC2216_WorldAIDSday_report_2011_en.pdf.
26. Robertson DL, Anderson JP, Bradac JA, et al. HIV-1 nomenclature proposal. Science 2000;288(5463):55–56.
27. Plantier JC, Leoz M, Dickerson JE, et al. A new human immunodeficiency virus derived from gorillas. Nat Med 2009;15(8):871–872.
28. Kallings LO. The first postmodern pandemic: 25 years of HIV/ AIDS. J Intern Med 2008;263(3):218–243.
29. Branson BM. The future of HIV testing. J Acquir Immune Defic Syndr 2010;55:S102–S105.
30. Panel on Antiretroviral Guidelines for Adults and Adolescents. Guidelines for the use of antiretroviral agents in

HIV-1-infected adults and adolescents. Department of Health and Human Services. Living document last updated March 27, 2012. Available at http://www.aidsinfo.nih.gov.
31. Tang H, Kuhen KL, Wong-Staal F. Lentivirus replication and regulation. Annu Rev Genet 1999;33:133–170.
32. Huang Y, Paxton WA, Wolinsky SM, et al. The role of a mutant CCR5 allele in HIV-1 transmission and disease progression. Nat Med 1996;2(11):1240–1243.
33. Stewart GJ, Ashton LJ, Biti RA, et al. Increased frequency of CCR-5 delta 32 heterozygotes among long-term non-progressors with HIV-1 infection. The Australian Long-Term Non-Progressor Study Group. AIDS 1997;11(15):1833–1838.
34. Cullen BR. Role and mechanism of action of the APOBEC3 family of antiretroviral resistance factors. J Virol 2006;80(3):1067–1076.
35. Neil SJ, Zang T, Bieniasz PD. Tetherin inhibits retrovirus release and is antagonized by HIV-1 Vpu. Nature 2008;451(7177):425–430.
36. Siewe B, Landay A. Key concepts in the early immunology of HIV-1 infection. Curr Infect Dis Rep 2012;14(1):102–109.
37. Grossman Z, Meier-Schellersheim M, Paul WE, Picker LJ. Pathogenesis of HIV infection: What the virus spares is as important as what it destroys. Nat Med 2006;12(3): 289–295.
38. Kahn JO, Walker BD. Acute human immunodeficiency virus type 1 infection. N Engl J Med 1998;339:33–39.
39. Mellors JW, Rinaldo CR Jr, Gupta P, White RM, Todd JA, Kingsley LA. Prognosis in HIV-1 infection predicted by the quantity of virus in plasma. Science 1996;272:1167–1170.
40. Khoury M, Kovacs A. Pediatric HIV infection. Clin Obstet Gynecol 2001;44(2):243–275.
41. Mofenson LM, Brady MT, Danner SP, et al. Guidelines for the Prevention and Treatment of Opportunistic Infections among HIV-exposed and HIV-infected children: Recommendations from CDC, the National Institutes of Health, the HIV Medicine Association of the Infectious Diseases Society of America, the Pediatric Infectious Diseases Society, and the American Academy of Pediatrics. MMWR Recomm Rep 2009;58(RR-11):1–166.
42. Panel on Antiretroviral Therapy and Medical Management of HIV-Infected Children. Guidelines for the Use of Antiretroviral Agents in Pediatric HIV Infection. Living document last updated, Nov 5, 2012; Available at http://www.AIDSinfo.NIH.gov.
43. Walensky RP, Paltiel AD, Losina E, et al. The survival benefits of AIDS treatment in the United States. J Infect Dis 2006;194(1):11–19.
44. NIH Panel to Define Principles of Therapy of HIV Infection. Report of the NIH panel to define principles of therapy of HIV infection. MMWR 1998;47(RR-5):1–41.
45. Severe P, Jean Juste MA, Ambroise A, et al. Early versus standard antiretroviral therapy for HIV-infected adults in Haiti. N Engl J Med 2010;363(3):257–265.
46. Kitahata MM, Gange SJ, Abraham AG, et al. Effect of early versus deferred antiretroviral therapy for HIV on survival. N Engl J Med 2009;360(18):1815–1826.
47. When To Start C, Sterne JA, May M, et al. Timing of initiation of antiretroviral therapy in AIDS-free HIV-1-infected patients: A collaborative analysis of 18 HIV cohort studies. Lancet 2009;373(9672):1352–1363.
48. Cascade Collaboration. Timing of HAART initiation and clinical outcomes in human immunodeficiency virus type 1 seroconverters. Arch Intern Med 2011;171(17):1560–1569.
49. Rerks-Ngarm S, Pitisuttithum P, Nitayaphan S, et al. Vaccination with ALVAC and AIDSVAX to prevent HIV-1 infection in Thailand. N Engl J Med 2009.
50. Abrams D, Levy Y, Losso MH, et al. Interleukin-2 therapy in patients with HIV infection. N Engl J Med 2009;361(16):1548–1559.
51. Calmy A, Hirschel B, Cooper DA, Carr A. A new era of antiretroviral drug toxicity. Antivir Ther 2009;14(2):165–179.
52. Carr A. Toxicity of antiretroviral therapy and implications for drug development. Nat Rev Drug Discov 2003;2:624–634.
53. Hirsch MS, Gunthard HF, Schapiro JM, et al. Antiretroviral drug resistance testing in adult HIV-1 infection: 2008 recommendations of an International AIDS Society-USA panel. Clinl Infect Dis 2008;47(2):266–285.
54. Telenti A. Safety concerns about CCR5 as an antiviral target. Curr Opin HIV AIDS 2009;4(2):131–135.
55. Stellbrink HJ. Novel compounds for the treatment of HIV type-1 infection. Antivir Chem Chemother 2009;19(5): 189–200.
56. McMahon MA, Siliciano JD, Lai J, et al. The antiherpetic drug acyclovir inhibits HIV replication and selects the V75I reverse transcriptase multidrug resistance mutation. J Biol Chem 2008;283(46):31289–31293.
57. Canestri A, Ghosn J, Wirden M, et al. Foscarnet salvage therapy for patients with late-stage HIV disease and multiple drug resistance. Antivir Ther 2006;11(5):561–566.
58. Kaplan JE, Benson C, Holmes KH, Brooks JT, Pau A, Masur H. Guidelines for prevention and treatment of opportunistic infections in HIV-infected adults and adolescents: Recommendations from CDC, the National Institutes of Health, and the HIV Medicine Association of the Infectious Diseases Society of America. MMWR Recomm Rep 2009;58(RR-4):1–207; quiz CE201–204.
59. Fischl MA, Richman DD, Grieco MH, et al. The efficacy of azidothymidine (AZT) in the treatment of patients with AIDS and AIDS-related complex. N Engl J Med 1987;317:185–191.
60. Hammer SM, Katzenstein DA, Hughes MD, et al. A trial comparing nucleoside monotherapy with combination therapy in HIV-infected adults with CD4 cell counts from 200 to 500 per cubic millimeter. N Engl J Med 1996;335: 1081–1090.
61. Hammer S, Squires K, Hughes M, et al. A controlled trial of two nucleoside analogues plus indinavir in persons with human immunodeficiency virus infection and CD4 cell counts of 200 per cubic millimeter or less. AIDS Clinical Trials Group 320 Study Team. N Engl J Med 1997;337:725–733.
62. Palella FJ Jr, Delaney KM, Moorman AC, et al. Declining morbidity and mortality among patients with advanced human immunodeficiency virus infection. N Engl J Med 1998;338:853–860.
63. Walmsley S, Bernstein B, King M, et al. Lopinavir–ritonavir versus nelfinavir for the initial treatment of HIV infection. N Eng J Med 2002;346:2039–2046.
64. Gulick RM, Ribaudo HJ, Shikuma CM, et al. Triple-nucleoside regimens versus efavirenz-containing regimens for the initial treatment of HIV-1 infection. N Engl J Med 2004;350(18):1850–1861.
65. World Health Organization. Antiretroviral therapy for HIV infection in adults and adolescents recommendations for a public health approach: 2010 revision. Available at: http://whqlibdoc.who.int/publications/2010/9789241599764_eng.pdf.
66. Lima VD, Harrigan R, Bangsberg DR, et al. The combined effect of modern highly active antiretroviral therapy regimens and adherence on mortality over time. J Acquir Immune Defic Syndr 2009;50(5):529–536.
67. Genberg BL, Wilson IB, Bangsberg D, et al. Patterns of ART adherence and impact on HIV RNA among patients in North America. AIDS 2012;26(11):1415–1423.

68. Ortego C, Huedo-Medina TB, Llorca J, et al. Adherence to highly active antiretroviral therapy (HAART): A meta-analysis. AIDSBehav 2011;15(7):1381–1396.
69. Parienti J-J, Das-Douglas M, Massari V, et al. Not all missed doses are the same: Sustained NNRTI treatment interruptions predict HIV rebound at low-to-moderate adherence levels. PloS One 2008;3(7):e2783.
70. Gallant JE, DeJesus E, Arribas JR, et al. Tenofovir DF, emtricitabine, and efavirenz vs. zidovudine, lamivudine, and efavirenz for HIV. N Engl J Med 2006;354(3):251–260.
71. Sax PE, Tierney C, Collier AC, et al. Abacavir/lamivudine versus tenofovir DF/emtricitabine as part of combination regimens for initial treatment of HIV: Final results. J Infect Dis 2011;204(8):1191–1201.
72. Ha B, Liao QM, Dix LP, Pappa KA. Virologic response and safety of the abacavir/lamivudine fixed-dose formulation as part of highly active antiretroviral therapy: Analyses of six clinical studies. HIV Clin Trials 2009;10(2):65–75.
73. Lennox JL, DeJesus E, Lazzarin A, et al. Safety and efficacy of raltegravir-based versus efavirenz-based combination therapy in treatment-naive patients with HIV-1 infection: A multicentre, double-blind randomised controlled trial. Lancet 2009;374(9692):796–806.
74. Molina JM, Andrade-Villanueva J, Echevarria J, et al. Once-daily atazanavir/ritonavir versus twice-daily lopinavir/ritonavir, each in combination with tenofovir and emtricitabine, for management of antiretroviral-naive HIV-1-infected patients: 48 week efficacy and safety results of the CASTLE study. Lancet 2008;372(9639):646–655.
75. Ortiz R, Dejesus E, Khanlou H, et al. Efficacy and safety of once-daily darunavir/ritonavir versus lopinavir/ritonavir in treatment-naive HIV-1-infected patients at week 48. AIDS 2008;22(12):1389–1397.
76. Sax PE, DeJesus E, Mills A, et al. Co-formulated elvitegravir, cobicistat, emtricitabine, and tenofovir versus co-formulated efavirenz, emtricitabine, and tenofovir for initial treatment of HIV-1 infection: A randomised, double-blind, phase 3 trial, analysis of results after 48 weeks. Lancet 2012;379(9835):2439–2448.
77. Turner D, Brenner BG, Routy JP, Petrella M, Wainberg MA. Rationale for maintenance of the M184v resistance mutation in human immunodeficiency virus type 1 reverse transcriptase in treatment experienced patients. New Microbiol 2004;27(2 Suppl 1):31–39.
78. McIntyre JA, Hopley M, Moodley D, et al. Efficacy of short-course AZT plus 3TC to reduce nevirapine resistance in the prevention of mother-to-child HIV transmission: A randomized clinical trial. PLoS Med 2009;6(10):e1000172.
79. World Health Organization. Antiretroviral drugs for treating pregnant women and preventing HIV infection in infants: Recommendations for a public health approach. 2010 version. Available at: *http://whqlibdoc.who.int/publications/2010/9789241599818_eng.pdf*.
80. Thigpen MC, Kebaabetswe PM, Paxton LA, et al. Antiretroviral preexposure prophylaxis for heterosexual HIV transmission in Botswana. N Engl J Med 2012;367(5):423–434.
81. El-Sadr WM, Lundgren JD, Neaton JD, et al. CD4+ count-guided interruption of antiretroviral treatment. N Engl J Med 2006;355(22):2283–2296.
82. Phillips AN, Neaton J, Lundgren JD. The role of HIV in serious diseases other than AIDS. AIDS 2008;22(18):2409–2418.
83. Taylor S, Boffito M, Khoo S, Smit E, Back D. Stopping antiretroviral therapy. AIDS 2007;21(13):1673–1682.
84. Meintjes G, Scriven J, Marais S. Management of the immune reconstitution inflammatory syndrome. Curr HIV/AIDS Rep 2012;9(3):238–250.
85. Beishuizen SJ, Geerlings SE. Immune reconstitution inflammatory syndrome: Immunopathogenesis, risk factors, diagnosis, treatment and prevention. Neth J Med 2009;67(10):327–331.
86. Zolopa A, Andersen J, Powderly W, et al. Early antiretroviral therapy reduces AIDS progression/death in individuals with acute opportunistic infections: A multicenter randomized strategy trial. PloS One 2009;4(5):e5575.
87. Abdool Karim SS, Naidoo K, Grobler A, et al. Integration of antiretroviral therapy with tuberculosis treatment. N Engl J Med 2011;365(16):1492–1501.
88. Havlir DV, Kendall MA, Ive P, et al. Timing of antiretroviral therapy for HIV-1 infection and tuberculosis. N Engl J Med 2011;365(16):1482–1491.
89. Blanc F-X, Sok T, Laureillard D, et al. Earlier versus later start of antiretroviral therapy in HIV-infected adults with tuberculosis. N Engl J Med 2011;365(16):1471–1481.
90. Thompson M, Aberg J, Hoy J et al. Antiretroviral treatment of adult HIV infection: 2012 recommendations of the international antiviral society—USA panel. JAMA 2012;308(4):387–402.
91. Makadzange AT, Ndhlovu CE, Takarinda K, et al. Early versus delayed initiation of antiretroviral therapy for concurrent HIV infection and Cryptococcal meningitis in Sub-Saharan Africa. Clin Infect Dis 2010;50(11):1532–1538.
92. Krajicek BJ, Thomas CF Jr, Limper AH. Pneumocystis pneumonia: Current concepts in pathogenesis, diagnosis, and treatment. Clin Chest Med 2009;30(2):265–278, vi.
93. Santamauro J, Stover D. *Pneumocystis carinii* pneumonia. Med Clin North Am 1997;81:299–318.
94. Kovacs JA, Masur H. Evolving health effects of pneumocystis: One hundred years of progress in diagnosis and treatment. JAMA 2009;301(24):2578–2585.
95. Wharton J, Coleman D, Wofsy C, et al. Trimethorprim–sulfamethoxazole or pentamidine for *Pneumocystis carinii* pneumonia in the acquired immunodeficiency syndrome. Ann Intern Med 1986;105:37–44.
96. Morse CG, Kovacs JA. Metabolic and skeletal complications of HIV infection: The price of success. JAMA 2006;296(7):844–854.
97. Deeks SG. HIV infection, inflammation, immunosenescence, and aging. Annu Rev Med 2011;62(1):141–155.
98. Spano JP, Costagliola D, Katlama C, Mounier N, Oksenhendler E, Khayat D. AIDS-related malignancies: State of the art and therapeutic challenges. J Clin Oncol 2008;26(29):4834–4842.
99. Grulich AE, van Leeuwen MT, Falster MO, Vajdic CM. Incidence of cancers in people with HIV/AIDS compared with immunosuppressed transplant recipients: A meta-analysis. Lancet 2007;370(9581):59–67.
100. Izzedine H, Harris M, Perazella MA. The nephrotoxic effects of HAART. Nat Rev Nephrol 2009;5(10):563–573.
101. van Vonderen MG, Lips P, van Agtmael MA, et al. First line zidovudine/lamivudine/lopinavir/ritonavir leads to greater bone loss compared to nevirapine/lopinavir/ritonavir. AIDS 2009;23(11):1367–1376.
102. Brown TT, Qaqish RB. Antiretroviral therapy and the prevalence of osteopenia and osteoporosis: A meta-analytic review. AIDS 2006;20(17):2165–2174.
103. Kotler DP. HIV and antiretroviral therapy: Lipid abnormalities and associated cardiovascular risk in HIV-infected patients. JAcquir Immune Defic Syndr 2008;49(Suppl 2):S79–S85.

104. Koutkia P, Grinspoon S. HIV-associated lipodystrophy: Pathogenesis, prognosis, treatment, and controversies. Annu Rev Med 2004;55:303–317.
105. Grinspoon S, Carr A. Cardiovascular risk and body-fat abnormalities in HIV-infected adults. N Engl J Med 2005;352(1):48–62.
106. Vandekerckhove L, Verhofstede C, Vogelaers D. Maraviroc: Perspectives for use in antiretroviral-naive HIV-1-infected patients. J Antimicrob Chemother 2009;63(6):1087–1096.
107. Worm SW, Sabin C, Weber R, et al. Risk of myocardial infarction in patients with HIV infection exposed to specific individual antiretroviral drugs from the 3 major drug classes: The data collection on adverse events of anti-HIV drugs (D:A:D) study. J Infect Dis 2010;201(3): 318–330.
108. Law MG, Friis-Moller N, El-Sadr WM, et al. The use of the Framingham equation to predict myocardial infarctions in HIV-infected patients: Comparison with observed events in the D:A:D Study. HIV Med 2006;7(4):218–230.
109. Sabin CA, Worm SW, Weber R, et al. Use of nucleoside reverse transcriptase inhibitors and risk of myocardial infarction in HIV-infected patients enrolled in the D:A:D study: A multi-cohort collaboration. Lancet 2008;371(9622):1417–1426.
110. Ding X, Andraca-Carrera E, Cooper C, et al. No association of abacavir use with myocardial infarction: Findings of an FDA meta-analysis. J Acquir Immune Defic Syndr 2012 Dec 1;61(4):441–447..
111. Stanley TL, Grinspoon SK. Body Composition and Metabolic Changes in HIV-Infected Patients. J Infect Dis 2012;205(Suppl 3):S383–S390.
112. Moyle GJ, Sabin CA, Cartledge J, et al. A randomized comparative trial of tenofovir DF or abacavir as replacement for a thymidine analogue in persons with lipoatrophy. AIDS 2006;20(16):2043–2050.
113. Wohl DA, McComsey G, Tebas P, et al. Current concepts in the diagnosis and management of metabolic complications of HIV infection and its therapy. Clin Infect Dis 2006;43(5): 645–653.
114. Lo Re V 3rd, Kostman JR, Amorosa VK. Management complexities of HIV/hepatitis C virus coinfection in the twenty-first century. Clin Liver Dis 2008;12(3):587–609, ix.
115. Matthews GV, Dore GJ. HIV and hepatitis C coinfection. J Gastroenterol Hepatol 2008;23(7 Pt 1):1000–1008.

104 Cancer Treatment and Chemotherapy

Stacy S. Shord and Patrick J. Medina

KEY CONCEPTS

1. Carcinogenesis is a multistep process that includes initiation, promotion, conversion, and progression. The growth of normal and cancerous cells is genetically controlled by the balance or imbalance of oncogene and tumor suppressor gene protein products. Multiple genetic mutations are required to convert normal cells to cancerous cells. Apoptosis and cellular senescence (aging) are normal mechanisms for cell death.
2. Several signaling pathways are dysregulated in many common cancers. Several agents have been developed to prevent signal transduction through these pathways. Monoclonal antibodies, which competitively bind to extracellular receptors or their natural ligands, and targeted drugs, which target a component of the intracellular signal transduction pathway, are available for several cancers.
3. Tumors must develop new blood vessels through the process of angiogenesis in order to grow. This process, regulated by proangiogenic and antiangiogenic factors, becomes dysregulated in several cancers and can lead to tumor growth, invasion, and metastasis. New anticancer agents can target this process and decrease tumor growth.
4. Because patients with clinically evident metastatic cancer can rarely be cured, early detection is critical. Screening programs are designed to detect cancers in asymptomatic people who are at risk of a specific cancer. Knowing the early warning signs of cancer is also important in early detection, when cancers are most likely to be localized.
5. Treatment for cancer should not begin until the presence of cancer is confirmed by a tissue (e.g., histologic) diagnosis. Clinical cancer staging provides prognostic information, and in conjunction with the patient's treatment goals, guides the selection of anticancer treatment. The goals include cure, prolongation of life, and palliation. Surgery and radiation provide the best chance of cure for patients with localized cancers, but systemic treatment methods are required for disseminated cancers.
6. Adjuvant therapy is systemic therapy that is administered to treat any existing micrometastases remaining after surgical excision of localized disease. Because adjuvant therapy is given to patients with no remaining clinical evidence of cancer, the benefit of the treatment cannot be proven for an individual patient but only for patient populations. Treatment decisions are based largely on an assessment of the presence of risk factors in an individual patient and their estimated risk for cancer recurrence. The effectiveness of adjuvant therapy is measured by the relative and absolute reduction in the risk of recurrence.
7. Traditional chemotherapy affects rapidly proliferating cells. Chemotherapy can be either "cell-cycle phase specific," targeting one specific phase of the cell cycle, or "cell-cycle phase nonspecific," targeting all proliferating cells regardless of their place in the cell cycle. Whereas cell-cycle phase-specific chemotherapies are generally given more frequently or as continuous infusions, cell-cycle phase-nonspecific chemotherapies are usually given as a single dose.
8. Monoclonal antibodies recognize an antigen that is expressed preferentially on cancer cells or target growth factors responsible for cancer growth. These therapies can vary in the amount of foreign component that can be used to predict tolerability. Monoclonal antibodies that target cellular antigens induce cell death by a variety of mechanisms that involve the host immune system. These antibodies can also be used to deliver drugs, radioisotopes, or toxins to the antigen-expressing cells.
9. Understanding the mechanism of toxicities can lead to more effective prevention and treatment of these toxicities. Prospective dose modification of some chemotherapy and targeted therapies are essential in patients with impaired organ function to reduce the risk of severe adverse events. Identification of genetic variations that affect activation and metabolism may permit the development of individualized therapy that optimize effectiveness and minimize toxicity.
10. Myelosuppression is the acute dose-limiting toxicity for most nonspecific chemotherapy. Whereas anemia can cause fatigue in patients with cancer, the risk of infection in patients is related to the depth and duration of neutropenia. Unexplained fever in neutropenic patients requires prompt initiation of empiric antibiotic therapy. Colony-stimulating factors are available to improve fatigue in patients with anemia and reduce the risk of febrile neutropenia. Evidence-based clinical guidelines should direct the use of these supportive care measures.

INTRODUCTION

Cancer is a group of more than 100 different diseases that are characterized by uncontrolled cellular growth, local tissue invasion, and distant metastases.[1] It is now the leading cause of death in Americans younger than age 85 years. Nearly 1.7 million cases of cancer were projected for 2013 with an estimated 580,350 lives claimed in the United States.[2] Figure 104-1 illustrates the estimated incidence of common cancers and cancer-related deaths. The four most common cancers are prostate, breast, lung, and colorectal cancer. The most common cause of cancer-related deaths in the United States is lung cancer, which accounts for about 160,000 deaths each year. These cancers are discussed in further detail in the chapters that follow.

The roles of healthcare providers in the management of patients with cancer can be very diverse. Thorough knowledge of the pharmacology and the pharmacokinetics of anticancer agents is essential to prevent and manage toxicities. Supportive care issues, such as nutritional support, pain management, infection, and nausea and vomiting, require application of clinical, pharmacologic, and economic principles. Provision of drug information to other healthcare providers and to patients and their families is another critical role. Experienced healthcare providers are able to fulfill these roles and make valuable contributions to patient care in the oncology setting.

This chapter introduces the basic concepts of carcinogenesis, tumor growth, and anticancer treatment; provides general information on the pharmacology and clinical use of anticancer agents; and presents an overview of supportive care issues.

ETIOLOGY OF CANCER

Carcinogenesis

1 The mechanisms by which cancers occur are incompletely understood. A cancer is thought to develop from a cell in which the normal mechanisms for control of growth and proliferation are altered. Current evidence supports the concept of carcinogenesis as a multistage process that is genetically regulated.[3–6] The first step in this process is *initiation*, which requires exposure of normal cells to carcinogenic substances. These carcinogens produce genetic damage that, if not repaired, results in irreversible cellular mutations. This mutated cell has an altered response to its environment and a selective growth advantage, giving it the potential to develop into a clonal population

Estimated new cases*

Males			Females		
Prostate	238,590	28%	Breast	232,340	29%
Lung and bronchus	118,080	14%	Lung and bronchus	110,110	14%
Colorectum	73,680	9%	Colorectum	69,140	9%
Urinary bladder	54,610	6%	Uterine corpus	49,560	6%
Melanoma of the skin	45,060	5%	Thyroid	45,310	6%
Kidney and renal pelvis	40,430	5%	Non-Hodgkin lymphoma	32,140	4%
Non-Hodgkin lymphoma	37,600	4%	Melanoma of the skin	31,630	4%
Oral cavity and pharynx	29,620	3%	Kidney and renal pelvis	24,720	3%
Leukemia	27,880	3%	Pancreas	22,480	3%
Pancreas	22,740	3%	Ovary	22,240	3%
All sites	**854,790**	**100%**	**All sites**	**805,500**	**100%**

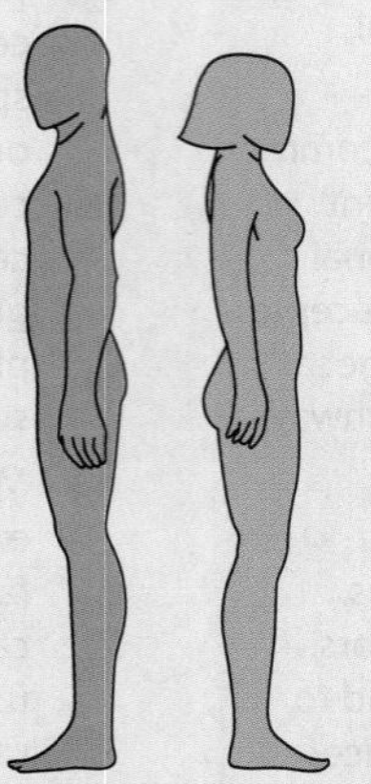

Estimated deaths

Males			Females		
Lung and bronchus	87,260	28%	Lung and bronchus	72,220	26%
Prostate	29,720	10%	Breast	39,620	14%
Colorectum	26,300	9%	Colorectum	24,530	9%
Pancreas	19,480	6%	Pancreas	18,980	7%
Liver and intrahepatic bile duct	14,890	5%	Ovary	14,030	5%
Leukemia	13,660	4%	Leukemia	10,060	4%
Esophagus	12,220	4%	Non-Hodgkin lymphoma	8,430	3%
Urinary bladder	10,820	4%	Uterine corpus	8,190	3%
Non-Hodgkin lymphoma	10,590	3%	Liver and intrahepatic bile duct	6,780	2%
Kidney and renal pelvis	8,780	3%	Brain and other nervous system	6,150	2%
All sites	**306,920**	**100%**	**All sites**	**273,430**	**100%**

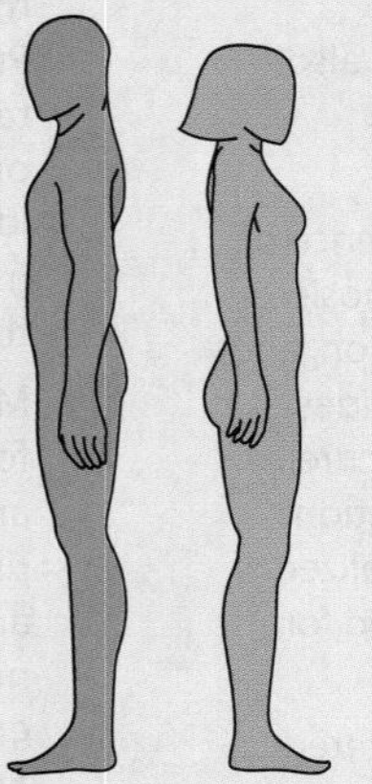

FIGURE 104-1 Estimated 2013 cancer incidences (*top*) and deaths (*bottom*) in the United States for males and females. *Estimates are rounded to the nearest 10 and exclude basal cell and squamous cell skin cancers and in situ carcinoma except urinary bladder. *(Reproduced with permission from Siegel et al.[2])*

of neoplastic cells. During the second phase, known as *promotion*, carcinogens or other factors alter the environment to favor growth of the mutated cell population over normal cells. The primary difference between initiation and promotion is that promotion is a reversible process. Because it is reversible, the promotion phase may be the target of future chemoprevention strategies, including changes in lifestyle and diet. At some point, however, the mutated cell becomes cancerous (*conversion* or *transformation*). Depending on the cancer, 5 to 20 years may elapse between the initiation and promotion and the development of a clinically detectable cancer. The final stage of neoplastic growth, called *progression*, involves further genetic changes leading to increased cell proliferation. The critical elements of this phase include tumor invasion into local tissues and the development of metastases.

Substances that may act as carcinogens or initiators include chemical, physical, and biologic agents.[5] Exposure to chemicals may occur by virtue of occupational and environmental means, as well as lifestyle habits. The association of aniline dye exposure and bladder cancer is one such example. Benzene is known to cause leukemia. Some drugs and hormones used for therapeutic purposes are also classified as carcinogenic chemicals (Table 104-1). Physical agents that act as carcinogens include ionizing radiation and ultraviolet light; radiation induces mutations by forming free radicals that damage DNA (deoxyribonucleic acid) and other cellular components. Viruses are biologic agents that are associated with certain cancers. The Epstein-Barr virus (EBV) is believed to be an important factor in the initiation of Burkitt lymphoma. Likewise, infection with human papilloma virus (HPV) is known to be a major cause of cervical cancer and head and neck cancers. All of the previously mentioned carcinogens, as well as age, gender, diet, growth factors, and chronic irritation, are among the factors considered to be promoters of carcinogenesis.

TABLE 104-1 Selected Drugs and Hormones Known to Cause Cancer in Humans

Drug or Hormone	Type of Cancer Caused
Alkylating agents (e.g., chlorambucil, mechlorethamine, melphalan, nitrosoureas)	Leukemia
Anabolic steroids	Liver
Analgesics containing phenacetin	Renal, urinary bladder
Anthracyclines (e.g., doxorubicin)	Leukemia
Antiestrogens (tamoxifen)	Endometrium
Coal tars (topical)	Skin
Estrogens	
Nonsteroidal (diethylstilbestrol)	Vagina or cervix, endometrium, breast, testes
Steroidal (estrogen replacement therapy, oral contraceptives)	Endometrium, breast, liver
Epipodophyllotoxins (etoposide, teniposide)	Leukemia
Immunosuppressive drugs (cyclosporine, azathioprine)	Lymphoma, skin
Oxazaphosphorines (cyclophosphamide, ifosfamide)	Urinary bladder, leukemia

Adapted from Compagni and Christofori[4] and Stricker and Kumar.[6]

Genetic and Molecular Basis of Cancer

1 In recent years, there has been marked progress in our understanding of the genetic changes that lead to the development of cancer, largely because of improvements in research techniques and new genomic information.[3,5–7] Two major classes of genes are involved in carcinogenesis: oncogenes and tumor suppressor genes. Figure 104-2 illustrates the acquired capabilities of cancer cells that differ from normal cellular function.[8] Oncogenes develop from normal genes, called protooncogenes, and may have important roles in all phases of carcinogenesis. Protooncogenes are present in all cells and are essential regulators of normal cellular functions, including the cell cycle. Genetic alteration of the protooncogene through point mutation, chromosomal rearrangement, or gene amplification activates the oncogene. These genetic alterations may be caused by carcinogenic agents such as radiation, chemicals, or viruses (somatic mutations), or they may be inherited (germ-line mutations). After activation, the oncogene produces either excessive amounts of the normal gene product or an abnormal gene product. The result is dysregulation of normal cell growth and proliferation, which imparts a distinct growth advantage to the cell and increases the probability of neoplastic transformation. An example is the human epidermal growth factor receptor (*HER*) family of oncogenes. This family of receptor tyrosine kinases contains four members: epidermal growth factor receptor (EGFR), HER2, HER3, and HER4. When activated, these receptors mediate cell proliferation and differentiation of cells through activation of intracellular tyrosine kinase receptors and downstream signaling pathways. As an oncogene, the gene product is overexpressed

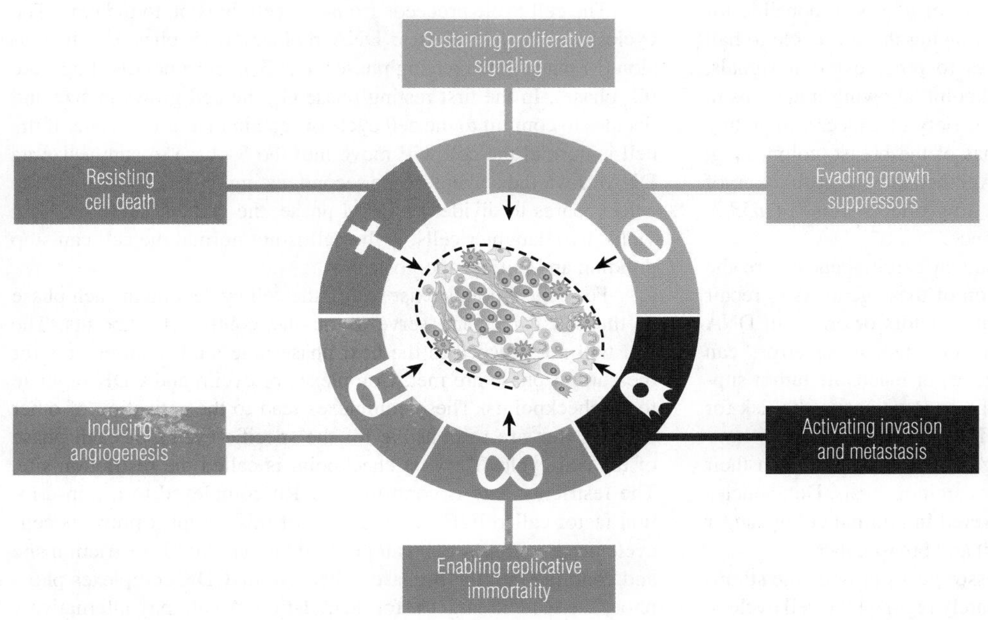

FIGURE 104-2 Functional capabilities acquired by cancer cells, including angiogenesis, self-proliferation, insensitivity to antigrowth signals and limitless growth potential, metastasis, and antiapoptotic effects. It is thought that most, if not all, cancer cells acquire these functions through a variety of mechanisms, including activation of oncogenes and mutations in tumor suppressor genes. *(Reprinted from Cell, Vol 144(5), Hanahan D, Weinberg RA, The Hallmarks of Cancer: The Next Generation, Copyright © 2011, with permission from Elsevier.)*

TABLE 104-2 Examples of Oncogenes and Tumor Suppressor Genes

Gene	Function	Associated Human Cancer
Oncogenes		
Genes for growth factors or their receptors		
EGFR	Codes for epidermal growth factor (EGFR) receptor	Glioblastoma, breast, head and neck, and colon cancers
HER2	Codes for a growth factor receptor	Breast, salivary gland, prostate, bladder, and ovarian cancers
RET	Codes for a growth factor receptor	Thyroid cancer
Genes for cytoplasmic relays in stimulatory signaling pathways		
K-RAS and N-RAS	Code for guanine nucleotide-proteins with GTPase activity	Lung, ovarian, colon, pancreatic binding cancers Neuroblastoma, acute leukemia
Genes for transcription factors that activate growth-promoting genes		
c-MYC		Leukemia and breast, colon, gastric, and lung cancers
N-MYC		Neuroblastoma, small cell lung cancer, and glioblastoma
Genes for cytoplasmic kinases		
BCR-ABL	Codes for a nonreceptor tyrosine kinase	Chronic myeloid leukemia
Genes for other molecules		
BCL-2	Codes for a protein that blocks apoptosis	Indolent B-cell lymphomas
Tumor-Suppressor Genes		
Genes for proteins in the cytoplasm		
APC	Step in a signaling pathway	Colon and gastric cancer
NF-1	Codes for a protein that inhibits the stimulatory Ras protein	Neurofibroma, leukemia, and pheochromocytoma
NF-2	Codes for a protein that inhibits the stimulatory Ras protein	Meningioma, ependymoma, and schwannoma
Genes for proteins in the nucleus		
RB1	Codes for the pRB protein, a master brake of the cell cycle	Retinoblastoma, osteosarcoma, and bladder, small cell lung, prostate, and breast cancers
p53	Codes for the p53 protein, which can halt cell division and induce apoptosis	Involved in a wide range of cancers
Genes for protein whose cellular location is unclear		
BRCA1	DNA repair, transcriptional regulation	Breast and ovarian cancers
BRCA2	DNA repair	Breast cancer
VHL	Regulator of protein stability	Renal cell cancer
MSH2, MLH1, PMS1, PMS2, MSH6	DNA mismatch repair enzymes	Hereditary nonpolyposis colorectal cancer

Data from Liotta et al,[3] Stricker and Kumar,[6] and Weinberg.[7]

or amplified, resulting in excessive cellular proliferation, metastasis, angiogenesis, and cell survival in several cancers. Table 104-2 lists examples of oncogenes by their cellular function.[9]

In contrast, tumor suppressor genes regulate and inhibit inappropriate cellular growth and proliferation.[3,6,7] Gene loss or mutation results in loss of control over normal cell growth. Two common examples of tumor suppressor genes are the retinoblastoma (Rb) and *p53* genes. Mutation of *p53* is one of the most common genetic changes associated with cancer, and it is estimated to occur in half of all cancers.[7] The normal gene product of *p53* is responsible for negative regulation of the cell cycle, allowing the cell cycle to halt for repairs, corrections, and responses to other external signals. Inactivation of *p53* removes this checkpoint, allowing mutations to occur. Mutation of *p53* is linked to a variety of cancers, including brain tumors (astrocytoma); carcinomas of the breast, colon, lung, cervix, and anus; and osteosarcoma. Another important function of *p53* may be modulation of cytotoxic drug effects. Loss of *p53* is associated with anticancer drug resistance.

Another group of genes important in carcinogenesis are the DNA repair genes. The normal function of these genes is to repair DNA that is damaged by environmental factors or errors in DNA that occur during replication.[6] If not corrected, these errors can result in mutations that activate oncogenes or inactivate tumor suppressor genes. As more mutations in the genome occur, the risk for malignant transformation increases. The DNA repair genes have been classified as tumor suppressor genes, because a loss in their function results in an increased risk for carcinogenesis. Deficiencies in DNA repair genes have been discovered in familial colon cancer (hereditary nonpolyposis colon cancer) and breast cancer.

1 Oncogenes and tumor suppressor genes provide the stimulatory and inhibitory signals that ultimately regulate the cell cycle.[3,7] These signals converge on a molecular system in the nucleus known as the cell-cycle clock. The function of the clock in normal tissue is to integrate the signal input and to determine if the cell cycle should proceed. The clock is composed of a series of interacting proteins, the most important of which are cyclins and cyclin-dependent kinases (CDKs). Cyclins (especially cyclin D_1) and CDKs promote entry into the cell cycle and are overexpressed in several cancers, including breast cancer. CDK inhibitors have been identified as important negative regulators of the cell cycle.

The cell cycle proceeds from one cell division to the next. The cycle involves five phases: DNA replication (S phase), cell division (M phase), two resting phases (G_1, G_2), and a nondividing state (G_0 phase). In the first resting phase G_1, the cell grows in size and decides to commit to the cell cycle or remain in a resting state. If the cell is normal the cell will move into the S phase to synthesize its DNA. Next, the cell enters the second resting phase G_2, in which the cell prepares to divide. In the M phase, the cell enters mitosis and yields two daughter cells. If the cell is not normal the cell can stop dividing and initiate apoptosis.

Four checkpoints exist within the cell cycle, one in each phase of the cell cycle, and serve as quality control checkpoints. The cell will not proceed to the next phase unless all requirements for the current phase are met. Complexes of cyclin and CDK regulate these checkpoints. These complexes lead to the activation of other proteins that are responsible for the specific events of each phase of the cell cycle. The first checkpoint is called the restriction site. The restriction site is controlled by Rb complexed to a transcription factor called E2F. The presence of this complex prevents cell-cycle progression. A cell can proceed beyond the G_1 restriction site and continue into the S phase, when cyclin–CDK complexes phosphorylate Rb and target it for degradation. A cell may alternatively withdraw into the G_0 phase in the presence of antimitogenic or the absence of mitogenic factors.[10]

1 When the normal regulatory mechanisms for cellular growth fail, backup defense systems may be activated. The secondary defenses include apoptosis (programmed cell death or suicide) and cellular senescence (aging). Apoptosis is a normal mechanism of cell death required for tissue homeostasis.[3,7,11] This process is regulated by oncogenes and tumor suppressor genes and is also a mechanism of cellular death after exposure to cytotoxins. Overexpression of oncogenes responsible for apoptosis may produce an "immortal" cell, which has increased potential for malignancy. The *bcl-2* oncogene is an example. The most common chromosomal abnormality found in lymphoid malignancies is the t(14;18) translocation. The *bcl-2* protooncogene is normally located on chromosome 18. Translocation of this protooncogene to chromosome 14 in proximity to the immunoglobulin heavy chain gene leads to overexpression of *bcl-2*, which decreases apoptosis and confers a survival advantage to the cell. Studies show that *p53* is also a regulator of apoptosis. Loss of *p53* disrupts normal apoptotic pathways, imparting a survival advantage to the cell. Apoptosis may also play an important role as a mechanism of inherent resistance to chemotherapy.[11]

Cellular senescence is another important defense mechanism.[6,7] Laboratory studies demonstrate that after a cell population has undergone a preset number of doublings, growth stops, and cells die. This is known as senescence, a process that is regulated by telomeres. Telomeres are the DNA segments or caps at the ends of chromosomes. They are responsible for protecting the end of the DNA from damage. With each replication, the length of the telomeres is shortened. After the telomeres are shortened to a critical length, senescence is triggered. In this way, telomeres tally and limit the number of cell doublings. In cancer cells, the function of telomeres is overcome by overexpression of an enzyme known as telomerase. Telomerase replaces the portion of the telomeres that is lost with each cell division, thereby avoiding senescence and permitting an infinite number of cell doublings. Telomerase is a target for anticancer agent development.

1 As information regarding the role of oncogenes and tumor suppressor genes accumulated, it became evident that a single mutation is probably insufficient to initiate cancer.[4–7] Scientists postulate that combinations of mutations are required for carcinogenesis and that each mutation is inherited by the next generation of cells. Thus, several detectable genetic mutations may be present in an established tumor. Whereas early mutations are found in both premalignant lesions and established tumors, later mutations are found only in the established tumor. This theory of sequential genetic mutations resulting in cancer has been demonstrated in colon cancer. In colon cancer, the initial genetic mutation is believed to be loss of the *adenomatous polyposis coli* gene, which results in formation of a small benign polyp. Oncogenic mutation of the *ras* gene is often the next step, leading to enlargement of the polyp. Loss of function of DNA mismatch repair enzymes may occur at many points in the progression of malignant transformation. Loss of the *p53* gene and another gene, believed to be the *deleted in colorectal cancer* (*DCC*) gene, completes the transformation into a malignant lesion. Loss of *p53* is thought to be a late event in the development and progression of the malignancy.

Identification of genes and other proteins involved in carcinogenesis has several important clinical implications. They may be used in cancer screening to identify individuals at increased risk for cancer and are being used to design new anticancer agents and gene therapies, several of which have recently been approved for use. Specific genetic abnormalities are so commonly associated with some cancers that the presence of that abnormality may aid in the diagnosis of that cancer. If the presence of these genes (i.e., gene expression profile) can reliably predict the clinical course of a cancer or response to certain cancer therapies, then genetic analysis may also become an important prognostic and treatment decision tool. An example of this is overexpression of HER2 predicting response to trastuzumab.[9]

Oncogenes and Tumor Suppressor Genes

Recent advances in molecular biology have identified many oncogenes and tumor suppressor genes that contribute to the functional capabilities that are acquired by cancer cells. These activated oncogenes and mutated tumor suppressor genes can be segregated into families and identified by their interactions with specific intracellular signaling pathways. Monoclonal antibodies (MoABs) have been developed to target the extracellular receptors or their natural ligands and prevent ligand binding to the receptor. In addition, small molecular inhibitors that target intracellular tyrosine kinases receptors or signal transduction pathways are available. The net effect of both strategies is to prevent downstream activation of the signal transduction resulting in a decrease in cell proliferation (Fig. 104-3). Some common receptors and pathways targeted by available targeted drugs and MoABs include HER, vascular endothelial growth factor (VEGF), mitogen-activated protein kinase pathway (MAPK) and phosphatidylinositide 3-kinase (PI3K) pathway.

Human Epidermal Growth Factor Receptors

2 Targeting the HER pathway is currently used to treat a variety of solid tumors. The HER family of receptors contains four known members, which upon binding to growth factor ligands result in intracellular phosphorylation of transcription factors and cell proliferation (Fig. 104-4).[9,12,13] EGFR and HER2 are known to be overexpressed in several cancers, including breast, lung, gastric, and colon cancers. Activation of these receptors leads to uncontrolled cellular growth and proliferation, tumor metastasis, and the prevention of apoptosis in cancer cells.[12] The roles of HER3 and HER4 in cancer growth and proliferation are still under investigation. All members of this family contain a transmembrane glycoprotein extracellular ligand binding site, a transmembrane domain, and a cytosolic tyrosine kinase tail. Members of the HER family are inactive by themselves and must form a dimer (a molecule composed of two subunits) either with a member of the same family (homodimer) or with a member of a different HER family (heterodimer).[22] Dimerization of the receptor leads to tyrosine kinase phosphorylation and subsequent activation of downstream pathways required to activate signal transduction and cell growth.

Vascular Endothelial Growth Factor

3 Vascular endothelial growth factor (VEGF) is a protein that stimulates angiogenesis, which is the development of new blood vessels. Angiogenesis is a process important for normal physiologic processes, but becomes unregulated in several malignancies and can lead to tumor growth, invasion, and metastasis. This process is regulated by pro- and antiangiogenic growth factors, which are released in response to hypoxia and other stresses to the cell.[14] Proangiogenic growth factors include VEGF, fibroblast growth factors, platelet-derived growth factor (PDGF), tumor necrosis factor-α (TNF-α), and keratinocyte growth factor. Antiangiogenic growth factors include interleukin-12 (IL-12), interferons (IFNs), platelet factor 4, and tissue inhibitors of metalloproteinase.[15]

The best studied proangiogenic factor is VEGF, whose elevated levels have been associated with a poor prognosis and an increased risk of metastases in a variety of malignancies, including acute myelogenous leukemia (AML), breast cancer, hepatocellular carcinoma, non–small cell lung cancer (NSCLC), ovarian cancer, and colon cancer.[15] Similar to other growth factors, VEGF binds to

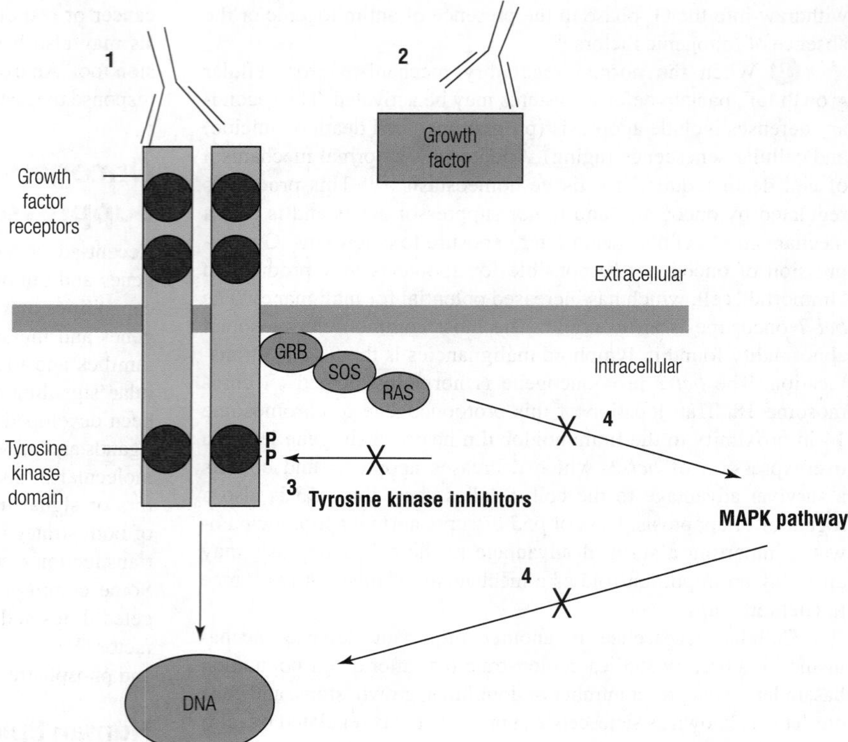

FIGURE 104-3 Common elements of intracellular signaling pathways and targeted strategies that inhibit these pathways, such as (1) monoclonal antibodies (MoABs) against the growth factor receptor, (2) MoABs against the growth factor itself, (3) molecules that target intracellular tyrosine kinases and prevent phosphorylation of tyrosine residues and subsequent activation of downstream signals, and (4) targeting downstream signals. All targeted therapies have the same goal of decreasing cell proliferation and increasing cell death of cancer cells. (MAPK, mitogen-activated protein kinase.)

specific receptors located on the extracellular domain of growth factor receptors. Three known receptors of VEGF have been identified: VEGFR-1, -2, and -3.[15] The VEGFR-1 and VEGFR-2 receptors are expressed primarily in endothelial cells and in some cancer cells and mediate the biologic effects of VEGF. Each of the receptors induces a different signal transduction pathway. These pathways eventually result in the generation of proteases that are necessary for the breakdown of the extracellular matrix, the first step of angiogenesis. Interference with their ability to develop new blood vessels by means of antiangiogenic agents can limit or prevent tumor growth.[15]

Intracellular Signaling Pathways

Well-described intracellular signaling pathways include PI3K, JAK-STAT (Janus kinase–signal transducers and activators of transcription), and MAPK pathways; when activated, they promote cell proliferation and survival. These pathways consist of a chain of proteins that ultimately communicate a signal to the DNA found in the nucleus from a cell surface receptor (e.g., EGFR). A protein within a signaling pathway communicates by adding a phosphate group to its neighboring protein; the phosphate groups act as "on" or "off" switch for the pathway. In cancer, a mutated protein permits

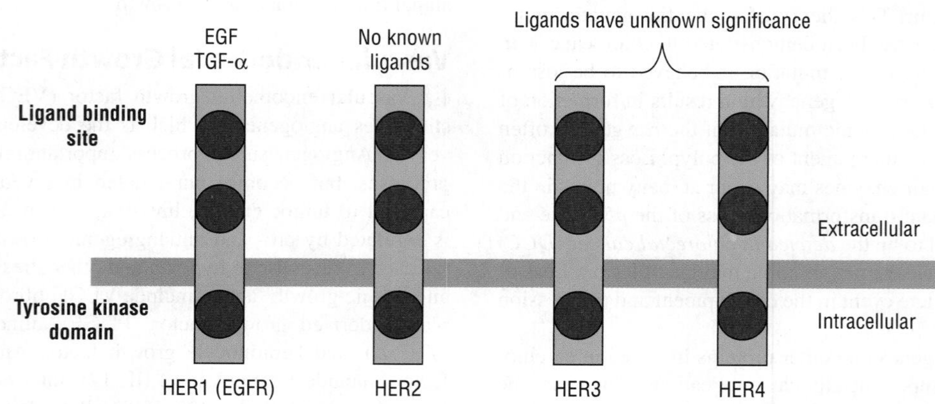

FIGURE 104-4 The human epidermal growth factor receptor (HER) family of growth factor receptors. All members of the HER family contain a transmembrane glycoprotein, an extracellular ligand binding site, and a hydrophobic intracellular portion with a tyrosine kinase domain. HER1 (or more commonly called EGFR [epidermal growth factor receptor]) has several known ligands, and HER2 has no known ligands, but the significance of ligands for HER3 and HER4 is unknown at this time. After the molecule binds to another member of the HER family, the tyrosine kinase domain is phosphorylated, and genes regulating proliferation, antiapoptosis, and cell transformation are turned on. (TGF, transforming growth factor.)

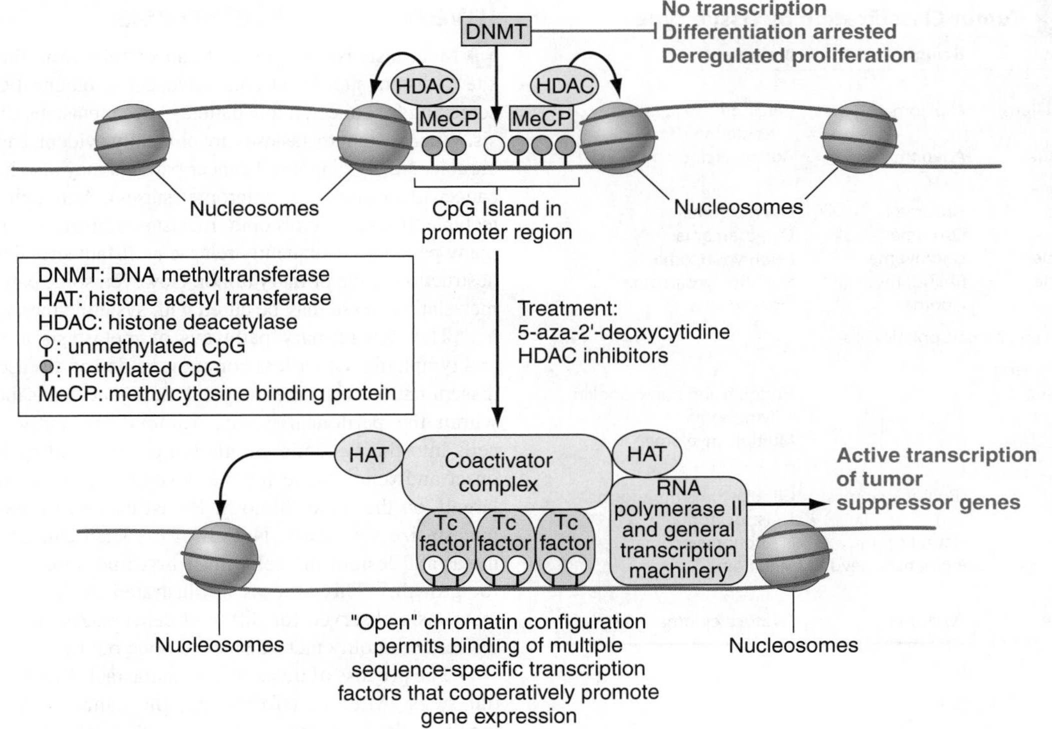

FIGURE 104-5 Epigenetic regulation of gene expression in cancer cells. CpG islands within the promoter and enhancer regions of the gene are methylated, resulting in the complexes with histone deacetylase (HDAC) activity. Chromatin is in a condensed conformation that inhibits transcription *(upper figure)*. Inhibitors of DNMT in combination with inhibitors of HDAC confer a chromatin structure that allows transcription *(lower figure)*. *(From Longo DL. Cancer Cell Biology and Angiogenesis. In: Longo DL, Fauci AS, Kasper DL, et al. eds. Harrison's Principles of Internal Medicine, 18th ed. New York, NY: McGraw-Hill, 2012.)*

the pathway to remain in the "on" or "off" position. The downstream effectors of these pathways also initiate cell cycle progression by promoting the expression of cyclins and repressing the expression of CDK inhibitors.

The MAPK signaling pathways regulates many fundamental cellular processes, including cell differentiation, proliferation, and senescence. These pathways relay the intracellular signals through a series of Ras, Raf, MEK (MAPK/ERK) and ERK (extracellular signaling receptor kinase) proteins that subsequently phosphorylate and regulate nuclear and cytoplasmic structures. Some of these proteins are commonly mutated in pancreatic, melanoma, colorectal, hepatocellular, and other solid tumors.[16]

The PI3K signaling pathway also regulates cell proliferation, growth, survival, and mobility. PI3K becomes activated in response to growth hormones, and it ultimately activates AKT, a serine–threonine kinase that serves as a master switch for the cell cycle progression. Fully activated AKT translocates to the nucleus, where it can inhibit proapoptotic signals and activate antiapoptotic substrates. It can also phosphorylate mammalian target of rapamycin (mTOR). After being activated, mTOR stimulates protein synthesis by phosphorylating translation regulators. mTOR also contributes to protein degradation and angiogenesis.[17] Phosphatase and tensin homolog (PTEN) is a tumor suppressor gene that blocks intracellular signaling through this pathway and is frequently inactivated in several solid tumors.[18,19]

The JAK-STAT signaling pathway helps regulate the immune system. This pathway contains three main components: extracellular receptors, JAKs, and STAT. The pathway is initiated when cytokines or growth factors bind to the receptor, activate JAK, and subsequently recruit STAT. The STAT proteins then translocate to the nucleus and modify gene expression. Altered JAK signaling has been associated with JAK mutations in patients with myelofibrosis.[20]

Epigenetics

Epigenetics refers to changes in gene expression that occur without altering the DNA sequence.[21] The two most common mechanisms of epigenetic regulation include methylation and histone modification. DNA methylation commonly occurs at CpG dinucleotides (or islands) and is catalyzed by DNA methyltransferases (DNMT). Histones are basic proteins associated with DNA in the nucleosome. These proteins may be modified by acetylation, methylation, or phosphorylation on their N-terminal tail. These modifications play a role in transcriptional regulation. For example, whereas histone deacetylases (HDACs) repress transcription, histone acetylases activate transcription. Epigenetic changes may be involved in the development of cancer by either priming the cell and making it susceptible to genetic changes associated with the development of cancer or initiating malignant transformation. As an example, hypermethylation at CpG dinucleotides found near tumor suppressor genes can switch these genes off and promote the development of cancer. Anticancer agents, identified as inhibitors of DNMT or HDAC, target these modifications. Figure 104-5 shows the effects of these inhibitors on methylation, chromatin formation, and transcription.

PATHOLOGY OF CANCER

Tumor Origin

Tumors may arise from any of four basic tissue types: epithelial tissue, connective tissue (i.e., muscle, bone, and cartilage), lymphoid tissue, and nerve tissue. Most cancer cells retain enough traits to identify their basic tissue type; therefore, tumors are typically

TABLE 104-3 Tumor Classification by Tissue Type

Tissue of Origin	Benign	Malignant
Epithelial		
Surface epithelium	Papilloma	Carcinoma (squamous, epidermoid)
Glandular tissue	Adenoma	Adenocarcinoma
Connective tissue		
Fibrous tissue	Fibroma	Fibrosarcoma
Bone	Osteoma	Osteosarcoma
Smooth muscle	Leiomyoma	Leiomyosarcoma
Striated muscle	Rhabdomyoma	Rhabdomyosarcoma
Fat	Lipoma	Liposarcoma
Lymphoid tissue and hematopoietic cells		
Bone marrow elements		
Lymphoid tissue		Hodgkin and non-Hodgkin lymphoma
Plasma cell		Multiple myeloma
Neural tissue		
Glial tissue	"Benign" gliomas	Glioblastoma multiforme, astrocytoma
Nerve sheath	Neurofibroma	Neurofibrosarcoma
Melanocytes	Pigmented nevus	Melanoma
Mixed tumors		
Gonadal tissue	Teratoma	Teratocarcinoma

Adapted from Cotran et al.[6]

named based on the tissue of origin. For example, benign tumors are named for their cell or tissue of origin followed the suffix *-oma*. Table 104-3 lists common tumor nomenclature by tissue type.[6]

Some cancers are preceded by cellular changes that are abnormal but not yet malignant. Correcting these early changes could potentially prevent the occurrence of a cancer. These precancerous lesions may be described as consisting of either hyperplastic or dysplastic cells. Hyperplasia is an increase in the number of cells in a particular tissue or organ, which results in an increased size of the organ. It should not be confused with hypertrophy, which is an increase in the size of the individual cells. Hyperplasia occurs in response to a stimulus and reverses when the stimulus is removed. Dysplasia is defined as an abnormal change in the size, shape, or organization of cells or tissues. Hyperplasia and dysplasia may precede the appearance of a cancer by several months or years.

Cancer cells are divided into those of epithelial origin or the other tissue types. Carcinomas are malignant growths arising from epithelial cells and sarcomas are malignant growths of muscle or connective tissue. *Carcinoma in situ* is a preinvasive stage of malignancy in which the cancer is limited to the epithelial cells or origin. Malignancies of hematologic origin, such as leukemias and lymphomas, are classified separately. Leukemias and lymphomas are discussed in later chapters.

Tumor Characteristics

Tumors may be either benign or malignant. Benign tumors are noncancerous growths that are often encapsulated, localized, and indolent. The cells of benign tumors resemble the cells from which they developed. These masses seldom metastasize, and after being removed, they rarely recur. In contrast, malignant tumors invade and destroy the surrounding tissue. The cells of malignant tumors are genetically unstable, and loss of normal cell architecture results in cells that are atypical of their tissue or cell of origin. These cells lose the ability to perform their usual functions. This loss of structure and function is called anaplasia. Malignant tumors tend to metastasize, and consequently, recurrences are common after removal or destruction of the primary tumor.

Invasion and Metastasis

❹ Metastasis is the spread of cancer cells from the primary tumor site to distant sites.[5,22] Despite advances in diagnostic techniques and screening for cancer, many patients have metastatic disease at diagnosis. When distant metastases are clinically evident, cancers are seldom curable. Newly diagnosed cancer patients may also have microscopic cancer metastases (i.e., micrometastases). Although clinically undetectable, these microscopic metastases must be present because many patients subsequently relapse at distant sites despite removal or destruction of the primary tumor. However, some patients with micrometastatic disease may be cured with systemic therapy.

The two primary pathways of metastasis are hematogenous and lymphatic. Other less common modes of disease spread include dissemination via cerebrospinal fluid and transabdominal spread within the peritoneal cavity. Tumors constantly shed neoplastic cells into the systemic circulation or surrounding lymphatics. The onset and time course for the development of metastasis depends largely on the tumor biology. Breast cancer, for example, tends to metastasize very early. Not all of the shed cancer cells result in a metastatic lesion; the cells must first find an environment suitable for growth.[22] This process is illustrated in the diverse patterns of metastasis observed for different cancers. As an example, prostate cancer commonly metastasizes to bone but rarely to the brain.

The process of invasion and metastasis involves several essential steps. After transformation, the cancer cells and surrounding host tissue secrete substances that stimulate angiogenesis.[23] Cancer cells must then detach from the primary mass and invade surrounding blood and lymph vessels. The cancer cells or cell aggregates detach and embolize through these vessels, but most do not survive circulation. The disseminated cells must then attach to the vascular endothelium. The cells may proliferate within the lumen of the vessel but most commonly extravasate into the surrounding tissue. The local microenvironment may provide growth factors that can serve as "fertilizer" to potentiate the proliferation of the metastasis. At every step, the potential metastatic cell must fight the host immune system. Finally, the metastasis must again initiate angiogenesis to ensure continued growth and proliferation. Because angiogenesis has been recognized as a critical element in primary tumor growth as well as metastasis, it has become a target for development of new anticancer agents, which are described later in the chapter.

DIAGNOSIS AND STAGING

Screening

Because cancers are most curable before they have metastasized, early detection and treatment have obvious potential benefits. Cancer screening programs are designed to detect signs of cancer in people who have not yet developed symptoms from cancer. Lack of effective screening methods and inaccessible anatomic sites limit the availability of screening methods for some cancers. Other limitations of screening methods include false-negative test results (related to the sensitivity of the test), false-positive test result (related to the specificity), and overdiagnosis (true positives that will not become clinically significant). For example, most abnormal test results identified by a screening mammography are false-positive results, although the specificity of this screening method exceeds 90%. Public education on the early warning signs of common cancers is extremely important for facilitating early detection. Effective screening procedures exist for some cancers. The Papanicolaou (Pap) smear test, for example, is an effective tool to detect cervical cancer in its early stages. The American Cancer Society publishes yearly guidelines for routine screening examinations (Table 104-4).[24]

TABLE 104-4 Screening Guidelines for Early Detection of Cancer in Average-Risk, Asymptomatic People

Disease	Test or Procedure	Sex	Age (y)	Frequency
Breast cancer	Breast self-examination	F	≥20	Monthly[a]
	Clinical breast examination	F	20–39	Every 3 years
			≥40	Every year
	Mammography	F	≥40	Every year[b]
Colorectal cancer	One of the following examination schedules should be followed:			
	Fecal occult blood test (FOBT) or fecal immunochemical test (FIT)	M and F	≥50	Every year
	Stool DNA test	M and F	≥50	Uncertain
	Flexible sigmoidoscopy	M and F	≥50	Every 5 years
	Annual FOBT or FIT and flexible sigmoidoscopy[c]	M and F	≥50	Every 5 years
	Colonoscopy	M and F	≥50	Every 10 years
	Computed tomography colonography	M and F	≥50	Every 5 years
	Double-contrast barium enema	M and F	≥50	Every 5 years
Prostate cancer	Digital rectal examination and prostate-specific antigen (PSA) blood test	M	≥50	Not specified[d]
Cervical cancer	Conventional pap test or liquid-based pap test	F	3 years after beginning vaginal intercourse	Every year[e]
Endometrial cancer	Information on risks and symptoms	F	Menopause	Once
Cancer-related check-up	Health counseling and physical examination[f]	M and F	20–40	Every 3 years
			≥40	Every year

[a]Beginning in their early 20s, women should be told about the benefits and limitations of breast self-examination (BSE). The importance of prompt reporting of any new breast symptoms to a healthcare professional should be emphasized. It is acceptable for women to choose not to do BSE or to do BSE irregularly.

[b]Women at increased risk (e.g., family history, genetic tendency, or past breast cancer) should talk with their physician about benefits and limitations of starting earlier, having additional tests, or more frequent examinations.

[c]Flexible sigmoidoscopy together with FOBT or FIT is preferable to either test alone, although annual FOBT or FIT alone and flexible sigmoidoscopy every 5 years without FOBT or FIT has some benefit. People at moderate to high risk for colorectal cancer should discuss a different testing schedule with their physician.

[d]Men who have at least a 10-year life expectancy should have an opportunity to make an informed decision with their healthcare provider about whether to be screened for prostate cancer, after receiving information about the potential benefits, risks, and uncertainties associated with prostate cancer screening. Prostate cancer screening should not occur without an informed decision-making process.

[e]Cervical cancer screening should begin about 3 years after a woman begins having vaginal intercourse but no later than age 21 years. Screening should be performed every year with conventional Pap tests or every 2 years using liquid-based Pap tests. At or after age 30 years, women who have had three normal test results in a row may get screened every 2 to 3 years with cervical cytology (either conventional or liquid-based Pap test) alone or every 3 years with a human papillomavirus DNA test plus cervical cytology. Women age 70 years and older who have had three or more normal Pap test results and no abnormal Pap tests within the last 10 years and women who have undergone a total hysterectomy may choose to stop cervical cancer screening.

[f]To include examination for cancers of the mouth, thyroid, testicles, skin, lymph nodes, and ovaries, as well as health counseling about tobacco, sun exposure, diet and nutrition, risk factors, sexual practices, and environmental and occupational exposures.

From Smith RA, Cokkinides V, Brawley OW. Cancer screening in the United States, 2012: A review of current American Cancer Society guidelines and issues in cancer screening. CA Cancer J Clin 2012;62:129–42.

Diagnosis

The presenting signs and symptoms of cancer vary widely and depend on the cancer. The presentation in adults may include any of cancer's seven warning signs (Table 104-5), pain, or loss of appetite.[25] The warning signs of cancer in pediatrics are different and reflect the tumors more common in this population (Table 104-6).[25] Even with increased public awareness, the fear of a cancer diagnosis can deter people from seeking medical attention. The definitive diagnosis of cancer relies on the procurement of a sample of the tissue or cells suspected of malignancy and pathologic assessment of this sample. This sample can be obtained by numerous methods, including biopsy, exfoliative cytology, or fine-needle aspiration. A tissue diagnosis is essential, because many benign conditions can masquerade as cancer. Definitive treatment should not begin without a pathologic diagnosis.

Staging and Workup

5 In addition to tissue diagnosis, tumors should be staged to determine the extent of disease before any definitive treatment is initiated. The process is dictated by knowledge of the biology of the tumor and by the signs and symptoms elicited in the history and physical examination. Staging provides information on prognosis

TABLE 104-5 Cancer's Seven Warning Signs

Change in bowel or bladder habits
A sore that does not heal
Unusual bleeding or discharge
Thickening or lump in the breast or elsewhere
Indigestion or difficulty in swallowing
Obvious change in wart or mole
Nagging cough or hoarseness
If YOU have a warning signal, see your doctor!

American Cancer Society Study Communicating Cancer Information Through Mass Distribution Leaflets—an American Cancer Society Study. CA Cancer J Clin 1967;17:291–293.

TABLE 104-6 Cancer's Warning Signs in Children

Continued, unexplained weight loss
Headaches with vomiting in the morning
Increased swelling or persistent pain in bones or joints
Lump or mass in abdomen, neck, or elsewhere
Development of a whitish appearance in the pupil of the eye
Recurrent fevers not caused by infections
Excessive bruising or bleeding
Noticeable paleness or prolonged tiredness

Data from American Cancer Society. http://www.cancer.org/docroot/CRI/content/CRI_2_2_3x_Can_Childhood_Cancers_Be_Detected_Early.asp?sitearea=CRI.

and guides treatment selection. A staging workup may involve radiographs, computed tomography scans, magnetic resonance imaging, positron emission tomography scans, ultrasonograms, bone marrow biopsies, bone scans, lumbar puncture, and a variety of laboratory tests (including appropriate tumor markers). After treatment is implemented, the staging workup is usually repeated to evaluate the effectiveness of the treatment. Some cancers produce antigens or other substances; these tumor markers are often nonspecific and may be elevated in many different cancers or in patients with nonmalignant diseases. As a result, tumor markers are generally more useful for monitoring response and detecting recurrence than as diagnostic tools. Examples are human chorionic gonadotropin and alfa-fetoprotein in patients with testicular cancer or prostate-specific antigen in prostate cancer.[6]

The most commonly applied staging system for solid tumors is the TNM classification, where T = tumor, N = node, and M = metastases. A numerical value is assigned to each letter to indicate the size or extent of disease. The designated rating for a tumor describes the size of the primary mass and ranges from T_1 to T_4. Carcinoma in situ is designated as T_{is}. Nodes are described in terms of the extent of the spread of regional lymph nodal involvement (N_0 to N_3). Metastases are generally scored depending on their presence or absence (M_0 or M_1). To simplify the staging process, most cancers are classified according to the extent of disease by a numerical system involving stages I through IV. Stage I usually indicates localized tumor, stages II and III represent local and regional spread of disease, and stage IV denotes the presence of distant metastases. The assigned TNM rating translates into a particular stage classification. For example, T_3 N_1 M_0 describes a moderate- to large-sized primary mass, with regional lymph node involvement and no distant metastases and for most cancers is stage III. The criteria for classifying disease extent are quite specific for each different cancer.[26] For some tumors, such as prostate cancer, alternative alphabetical systems (stage A, B, C, or D) are used in clinical practice. Leukemias and lymphomas follow alternate staging systems that are discussed in subsequent chapters.

TREATMENT
Modalities of Cancer

Five primary modalities are used to treat cancer: surgery, radiation, traditional chemotherapy, targeted drug therapy, and biologic therapy. The oldest treatment modality is surgery, which plays a major role in the diagnosis and treatment of cancer. Surgery remains the treatment of choice for most solid tumors diagnosed in the early stages. Radiation therapy was first used for cancer treatment in the late 1800s and remains a mainstay in the management of cancer. Although very effective for treating many cancers, surgery and radiation are local treatments. These modalities are likely to produce a cure in patients with truly localized disease. Because most patients with cancer have micrometastatic or metastatic disease at diagnosis, localized anticancer treatment often fail to completely eliminate the cancer. In addition, systemic diseases such as leukemia cannot be treated with a localized modality. Chemotherapy, targeted drug therapies, and biologic therapies all access the systemic circulation and can theoretically treat the primary tumor or metastatic disease. Biologic therapies are made from a living organism or its products and include antibodies, vaccines, growth factors, and cytokines.

❻ Many solid tumors or lymphomas appear to be eliminated by surgery or radiation. However, the high incidence of disease recurrence implies that the primary tumor metastasized before it was removed. Adjuvant therapy is the use of systemic therapy to eradicate micrometastatic disease after localized modalities, such as surgery or radiation. The goal of adjuvant therapy is to reduce recurrence rates and prolong long-term survival. Thus, adjuvant therapy is given to patients with potentially curable malignancies who have no clinically detectable disease after surgery or radiation. Because adjuvant therapy is given at a time when the cancer is undetectable (i.e., no measurable disease), its effectiveness is evaluated by recurrence rates and survival. The value of adjuvant therapy is best established in colorectal and breast cancers. Systemic therapy may also be given in the neoadjuvant or preoperative setting. The goals in these instances are to make other treatment modalities more effective by reducing tumor burden and destroying micrometastases. For example, in breast cancer, it is often used to reduce the size of the primary tumor and allow for a less invasive surgical procedure.

These modalities may be used alone, but are typically used in combination. Early-stage breast cancer is a good example of the use of a combined-modality approach. The primary tumor is removed surgically, and radiation therapy is delivered to the remaining breast (after lumpectomy) or to the axilla (if there is marked lymph node involvement). Adjuvant therapy, including chemotherapy and biologic therapy, is then administered to eradicate any micrometastatic disease. Neoadjuvant therapy may sometimes be administered before definitive surgery to increase the likelihood of a tumor resection compared with a mastectomy.

The management of hematologic malignancies also involves the use of combined modalities, but the terminology is different. Chemotherapy that is administered to eradicate the cancer cells is called induction therapy. When a complete remission (the disappearance of all signs of the cancer) is documented, postremission or consolidation therapy is administered. These therapies are designed to eradicate any remaining disease, similar to adjuvant therapy for solid tumors, and can include systemic therapy, a hematopoietic stem cell transplant, or radiation therapy. Maintenance therapy is sometimes administered after consolidation therapy. This therapy is given to prevent the cancer from recurring and may include combination chemotherapy.

When an anticancer agent is administered to patients with local or regional disease, the treatment is often administered to cure the patient and may be labeled curative therapy. However, when the cancer has metastasized to distant sites, cure is usually not possible. Anticancer agents can be administered to patients with metastatic disease to slow the progression of cancer and prolong survival by months to years. Anticancer agents administered to patients with terminal cancer with the goal of reducing symptoms is called palliative therapy.

The era of modern cancer chemotherapy was born in 1941 when Goodman and Gilman first administered nitrogen mustard to patients with lymphoma.[27] Since then, numerous anticancer agents have been developed, and a variety of treatment regimens have been investigated in every cancer. Table 104-7 lists tumors and their responsiveness to chemotherapy.[6,28] Chemotherapy may be indicated as a curative or palliative. Treatment with chemotherapy is the primary curative modality for a few diseases, including leukemias, lymphomas, choriocarcinomas, and testicular cancer. Most solid tumors are not curable with chemotherapy alone, either because of the biology of the tumor or because of advanced disease at presentation. Chemotherapy in this setting is often initiated for palliative purposes. It is often possible to decrease tumor size or to retard growth enough to reduce untoward symptoms caused by the tumor.

MOLECULAR AND CELLULAR BASIS

Principles of Tumor Growth

The study of tumor growth forms the foundation for many of the basic principles of modern cancer chemotherapy. The growth of most tumors is illustrated by the gompertzian tumor growth

TABLE 104-7 The Role of Chemotherapy in the Treatment of Cancer

Chemotherapy Used Alone with Curative Intent	
Acute lymphoblastic leukemia	Acute myelogenous leukemia
Burkitt lymphoma	Diffuse large B-cell lymphoma
Hodgkin lymphoma	Testicular cancer
Choriocarcinoma (gestational trophoblastic neoplasm)	
Chemotherapy Used as Adjuvant Therapy with Curative Intent	
Breast cancer	Colorectal cancer
Ewing sarcoma	Osteosarcoma
Wilms tumor	Ovarian cancer
Chemotherapy Used as Neoadjuvant Therapy	
Anal carcinoma[a]	Bladder cancer
Breast cancer (locally advanced)[a]	Cervical cancer
Esophageal cancer	Head and neck cancers[a]
Osteosarcoma[a]	Rectal cancer
Soft tissue sarcoma[a]	
Chemotherapy Used to Palliate Symptoms in Advanced Disease	
Bladder cancer[a]	Brain tumors
Breast cancer[a]	Carcinoid tumors
Cervical cancer	Chronic lymphocytic leukemia
Chronic myeloid leukemia[a]	Colorectal cancer[a]
Endometrial cancer	Esophageal cancer
Gastric cancer	Head and neck cancers
Hairy cell leukemia[a]	Kaposi sarcoma
Indolent non-Hodgkin lymphomas	Metastatic melanoma
Multiple myeloma[a]	Mycosis fungoides
Neuroblastoma[a]	Non–small cell lung cancer
Osteosarcoma	Ovarian cancer[a]
Pancreatic cancer	Prostate cancer
Small cell lung cancer[a]	Soft tissue sarcoma
Chemotherapy Has Little or No Effect on Palliation	
Hepatocellular cancer	Renal cell carcinoma
Thyroid cancer	

[a]Significant increase in survival is achieved.

Data from Stricker and Kumar[6] and Buick.[28]

curve (Fig. 104-5).[6,28,29] Gompertz was an insurance actuary who described the relationship between age and expected death. This mathematical model also approximates tumor cell proliferation. In the early stages, tumor growth is exponential, which means that the tumor takes a constant amount of time to double its size. During this early phase, most cancer cells are actively dividing. This population of cells is called the *growth fraction*. The doubling time, or time required for the tumor to double in size, is very short. Because most anticancer agents have greater effect on rapidly dividing cells, tumors are most sensitive to their effects when the tumor is small and the growth fraction is high. However, as the tumor grows, the doubling time is slowed.[28,29] The growth fraction is decreased, probably owing to the tumor's outgrowing its blood and nutrient supply or the inability of blood and nutrients to diffuse throughout the tumor mass. Wide variability exists in measured doubling times for different cancers. The doubling time of most solid tumors is about 2 to 3 months. However, some tumors have doubling times of only days (e.g., aggressive non-Hodgkin lymphomas [NHLs]), and others have even longer doubling times (e.g., some salivary gland tumors).[6]

Figure 104-6 also illustrates the impact of tumor burden. It takes about 10^9 cancer cells (1-g mass, 1 cm in diameter) for a tumor to be clinically detectable by palpation or radiography. Such a tumor has undergone about 30 doublings in cell number. It only takes 10 additional doublings for this 1-g mass to reach 1 kg in size. A tumor possessing 10^{12} cells (1-kg mass) is considered lethal. Thus, a tumor is clinically undetectable for most of its life span. Tumor burden also impacts response to treatment. The cell kill hypothesis states that a certain percentage of cells (not a certain number of cells) will be killed with each treatment course. For example, if a tumor consists of 1,000 cells and the treatment kills 90% of the cells, then 10% or 100 cells remain. The second treatment course kills another 90% of cells, and again only 10% or 10 cells remain. According to this hypothesis, the tumor burden will never reach zero. Tumors consisting of less than 10^4 cells are believed to be small enough for elimination by host factors, including immunologic mechanisms, and these factors must be in place for a cure to be possible. The limitations of this theory are that it assumes all cancers are equally responsive and that resistance to anticancer agents and metastases do not occur.[1,6,28,29]

Tumor Proliferation

Both cancer cells and normal cells reproduce in a series of steps known as the cell cycle as described earlier in the chapter. Figure 104-7 depicts the cell cycle and the phases of activity for some traditional chemotherapies.[28,29]

7 All cancer cells do not proliferate faster than normal cells; some cancer cells reproduce more rapidly, but others are more indolent. Many chemotherapies target rapidly proliferating cells (both normal and cancerous cells), and these therapies might act at selective or multiple sites of the cell cycle. Chemotherapy that demonstrates major activity in a particular phase of the cell cycle are known as cell-cycle phase-specific chemotherapies. For example, antimetabolites exert their major effect during the S phase. Cell-cycle phase-specific therapies may also be active to a lesser extent in other phases of the cycle. Cell-cycle phase-nonspecific chemotherapy are those with significant activity in multiple phases. Alkylating agents, such as nitrogen mustards, are examples of a cell-cycle nonspecific agent. In many cases, the cytotoxic effects of an agent may result from interactions with other intracellular activities and are not related to specific cell-cycle events. Endocrine therapies and targeted drugs are examples of these anticancer agents.

Knowledge of cell-cycle specificity has been use to optimize the scheduling of chemotherapy. By definition, cell-cycle phase-specific chemotherapies exert their major activity when cells are in a particular phase of the cell cycle. At any given time, the heterogeneous cell populations within a tumor are at various phases in the cell cycle. By giving cell-cycle phase-specific chemotherapies as a continuous infusion or in multiple repeated fractions, health-care providers can theoretically target more cells as they progress into the sensitive phase. Thus, cell-cycle phase-specific chemotherapies are also termed *schedule dependent*. In contrast, cell-cycle phase-nonspecific chemotherapies are active in many phases and consequently are not schedule dependent. The activity of these chemotherapies depends on the dose and these chemotherapies are termed *dose dependent*.

Biologic therapies and targeted drugs interfere with cancer cell proliferation in a different manner compared with traditional chemotherapy. These therapies stop cancer progression by blocking aberrant intracellular signaling pathways that govern cell responses, movement, and division. Some of these agents can cause cancer cell death by inducing apoptosis or stimulating the immune system to destroy the cancer cells. Some targeted drug therapies and biologic therapies are used in combination with traditional chemotherapy.

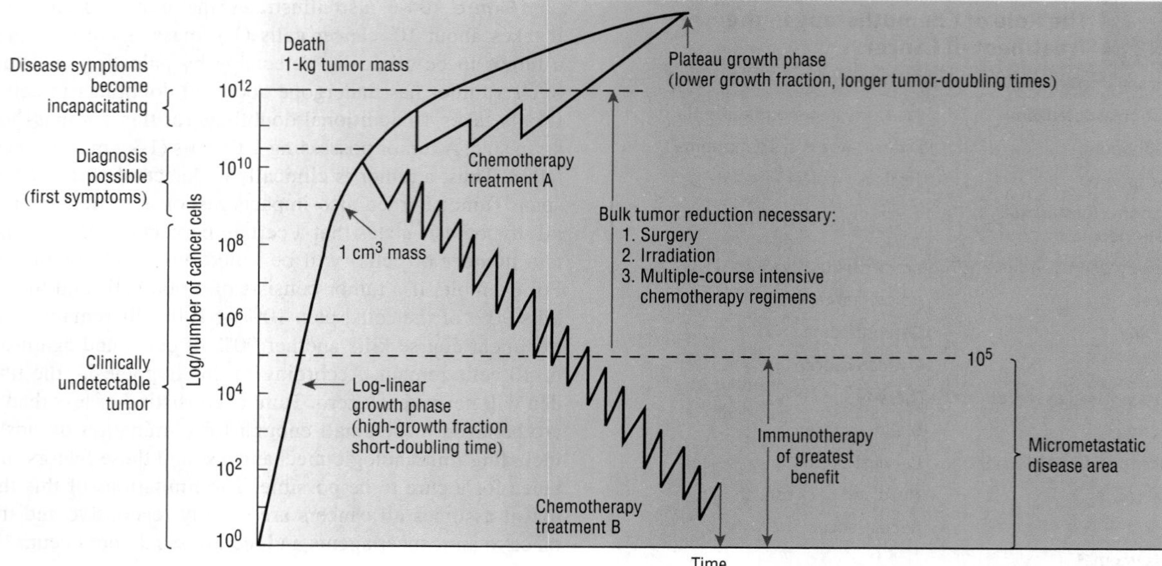

FIGURE 104-6 Gompertzian kinetics tumor-growth curve: relationship to symptoms, diagnosis, and various treatment regimens. *(Reproduced with permission from Buick RN. Cellular basis of chemotherapy. In: Dorr RT, Von Hoff DD, eds. Cancer Chemotherapy Handbook, 2nd ed. New York: Appleton & Lange/McGraw-Hill, 1994:3–14.)*

Molecular Biology

Because many anticancer agents interfere with the cellular synthesis of DNA, RNA, and proteins, it is important to review the basic principles of molecular biology.[3] Each normal human cell contains 46 chromosomes, which are composed of DNA. DNA carries hereditary information in units called genes. A single chromosome can contain 20,000 or more genes. Genes code for specific proteins that regulate cellular activity and inherited traits (some of which affect carcinogenesis and cancer growth, as well as the efficacy and metabolism of anticancer agents). The genetic information is encoded in DNA by precise sequencing of subunits known as nucleotides. Each nucleotide consists of a sugar (deoxyribose), phosphoric acid, and a base. Four bases exist in DNA: adenine, thymine, guanine, and cytosine. Adenine and guanine are purines, and thymine and cytosine are pyrimidines (Fig. 104-8). These nucleotides are connected linearly to form a chain. Each DNA molecule is made up of two chains of nucleotides, which wind around each other to form a double helix. The two strands are held together by chemical bonding between the bases. The bonding process is very specific—adenine binds only with thymine, and guanine binds only with cytosine. This is known as complementary base pairing. RNA is important in the

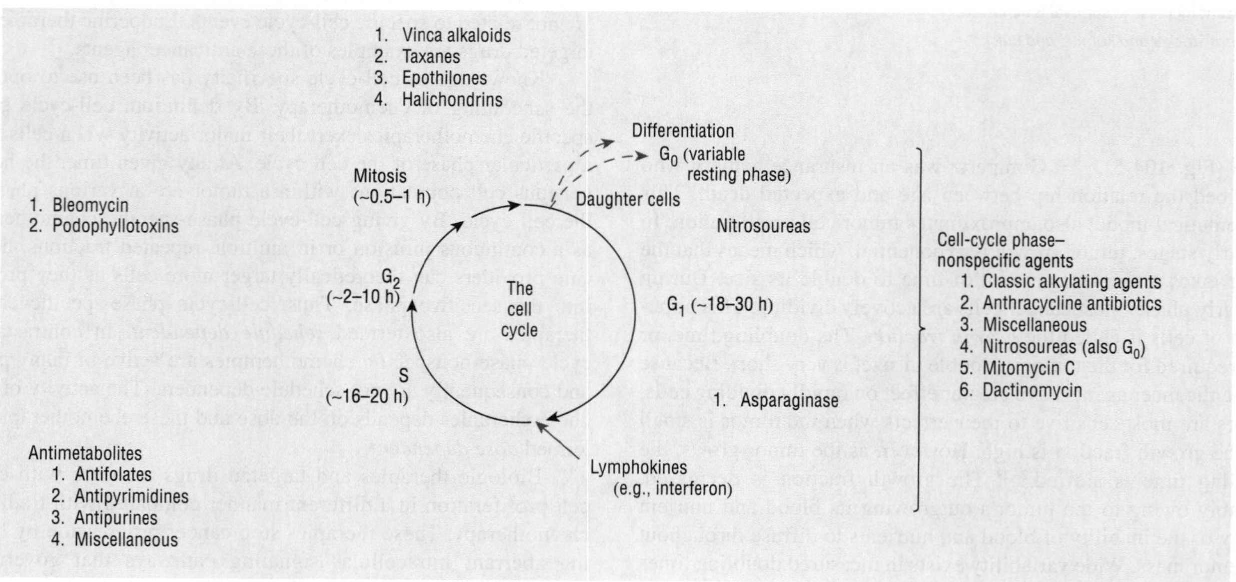

FIGURE 104-7 Cell-cycle activity for anticancer drugs. Cell-cycle phase-specific chemotherapies appear to be most active during a particular phase but may also be active in another phase. Cell-cycle phase-nonspecific chemotherapies may have greater activity in one phase than another but not to the degree of cell-cycle phase-specific chemotherapies. In many cases, it is likely that chemotherapy cytotoxicity involves multiple intracellular sites of action and may not be linked to specific cell-cycle events.

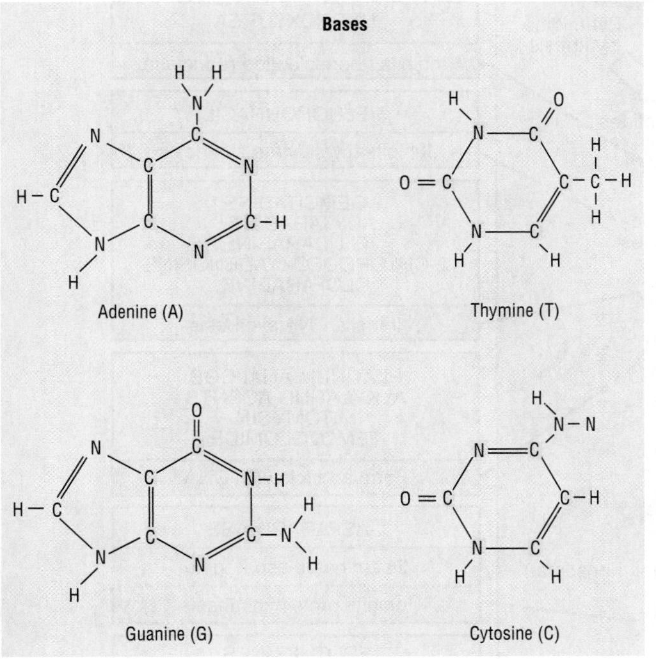

FIGURE 104-8 Structures of DNA bases.

DNA-directed synthesis of proteins or enzymes. RNA differs from DNA in that it is composed of a single strand of nucleotides, the sugar is ribose, and the base uracil is substituted for thymine. There are three known types of RNA: messenger RNA (mRNA), transfer RNA (tRNA), and ribosomal RNA (rRNA).

DNA Synthesis

During the DNA synthesis phase (S phase cell cycle), which takes place in the cell nucleus, the DNA unwinds and exposes its nucleotides. When DNA unwinds for replication or protein synthesis, only the portion of the molecule containing the needed nucleotides needs to be exposed. Rather than unwinding the entire strand, topoisomerase I and II enzymes cleave the DNA strands to facilitate unwinding of the section that is needed. The enzyme DNA polymerase matches free complementary nucleotides from the environment to the exposed nucleotides of the DNA. The newly created strands rewind, resulting in two complete double helices. The topoisomerase enzymes are also responsible for resealing the cleaved DNA strands. Most traditional chemotherapies interfere with DNA synthesis.

Protein Synthesis

The synthesis of proteins is a more complex process. Proteins consist of chains of amino acids in very specific sequences. As in DNA synthesis, the double helix must unwind. However, in protein synthesis, only the portion of the DNA molecule that codes for the desired protein is exposed. The enzyme RNA polymerase matches free complementary RNA nucleotides to the exposed DNA nucleotides, and the resultant chain of nucleotides is called mRNA. This process is called transcription. The mRNA travels to ribosomes in the cytoplasm, where protein synthesis occurs. Each three nucleotides of the mRNA chain compose a codon, whose sequence is specific for a particular amino acid. The codon is recognized by tRNA, which then carries the amino acid to the ribosome, where it is added to the growing peptide chain. This process is known as translation. The completed protein is then ready for its intended use as an enzyme or as a structural component. Targeted therapies, such as targeted drugs and MoABs, typically affect protein synthesis, including aberrant growth factor receptors, dysregulated intracellular signaling pathways, and defective apoptosis and angiogenesis. Whereas MoABs affect cell surface receptors, targeted drugs tend to inhibit intracellular signaling. Other anticancer agents that affect proteins include asparaginase and chemotherapy that interfere with microtubules.

CLINICAL PHARMACOLOGY OF ANTICANCER AGENTS

Anticancer agents are commonly categorized by their mechanism of action or by their origin. Akylators exert their effects on DNA and protein synthesis by binding to DNA and preventing the unwinding of the DNA molecule. Antimetabolites resemble naturally occurring nuclear structural components ("metabolites"), such as the nucleotide bases, or inhibit enzymes involved in the synthesis of DNA and proteins. Antitumor antibiotics derive their name from their source; they are fermentation products of *Streptomyces* species. Figure 104-9 shows the sites of action of common categories of anticancer agents, including traditional chemotherapy, biologic therapies, and targeted drugs. The following sections address these classes of chemotherapies used in the treatment of cancer. The clinical uses, mechanisms, adverse events, and practical patient management for commonly used chemotherapies in each class are detailed. Table 104-8 summarizes dose modifications of individual chemotherapies.

Antimetabolites

Antimetabolites are similar to the nucleotides that make up DNA and RNA. The body mistakes these anticancer agents for the naturally occurring nucleotide bases and metabolizes these agents as the natural nucleotides. These anticancer agents ultimately disrupt replication and cell division by interfering with the production of nucleic acids, DNA, and RNA. Unfortunately, these compounds are not selective for cancer cells, and rapidly dividing normal cells may be poisoned. The most common adverse events associated with the antimetabolites are secondary to a direct cytotoxic effect on rapidly dividing normal cells, such as the bone marrow cells. The three major classes of antimetabolites include pyrimidines, purines, and folate antagonists.

Fluorinated Pyrimidines

5-Fluorouracil 5-Fluorouracil (5-FU) is a fluorinated analog of uracil that was originally synthesized in the late 1950s. It is a prodrug and undergoes sequential phosphorylation to a mono-, di-, and triphsophate similar to natural nucleotide bases to become an active anticancer agent. In the presence of folates, the monophosphate binds tightly to and interferes with the function of thymidylate synthase. This enzyme is required for synthesis of thymidine. The triphosphate metabolite is incorporated into RNA as a false base and interferes with its function. Interference with both thymidine formation and RNA function is important in producing the cytotoxic effects of 5-FU. Although 5-FU nucleotides can also be incorporated directly into DNA and affect its stability, the contribution to cell damage remains unclear. The method of administration influences the mechanism of action, with thymidylate synthesis inhibition playing a greater role in continuous-infusion regimens and incorporation into RNA being more important for intermittent bolus schedules.[30]

Several pharmacologic strategies have been attempted to increase the cytotoxicity of 5-FU against cancer cells and decrease its toxicity to normal cells. The most common strategy combines 5-FU with the reduced folate leucovorin. Folates increase the stability of the monophosphate–thymidylate synthase complex, thereby

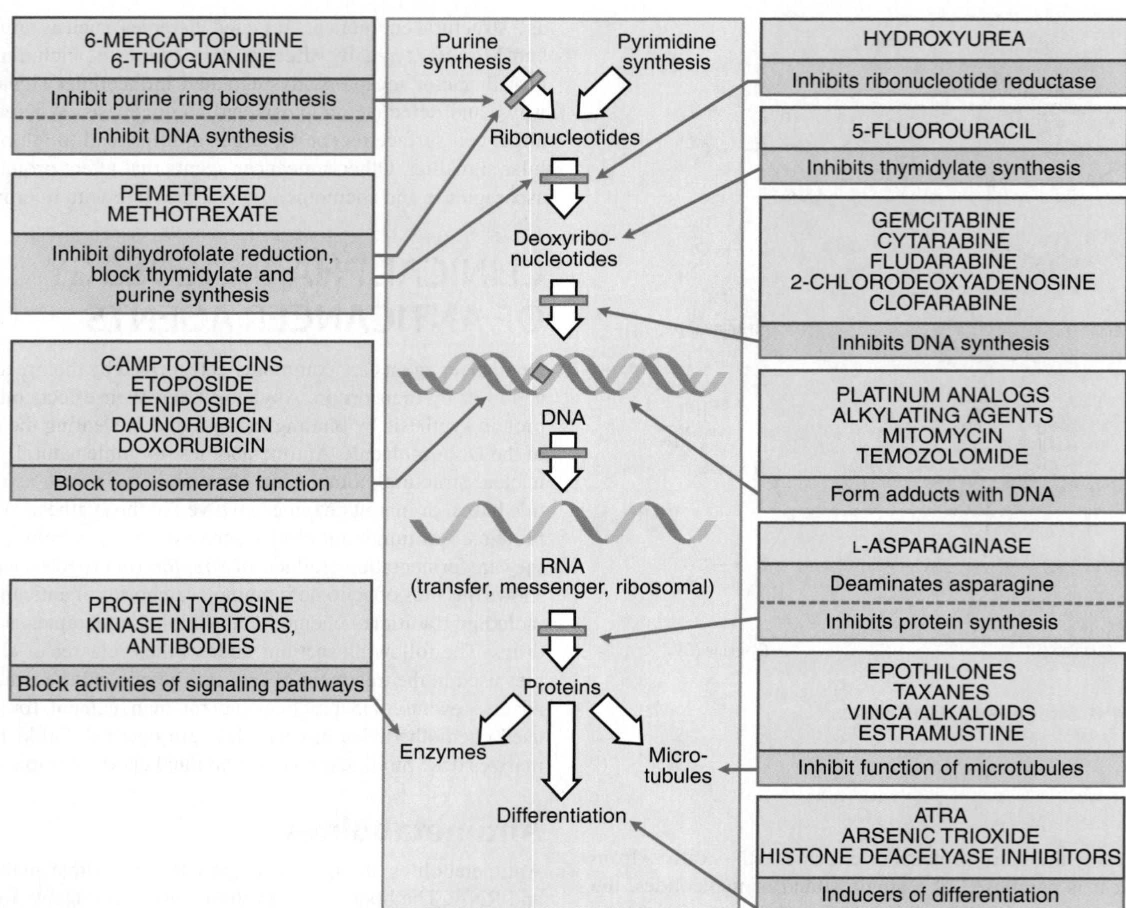

FIGURE 104-9 Mechanisms of action of commonly used anticancer agents. (ATRA, all-*trans*-retinoic acid.) *(From Chabner BA. General Principles of Chemotherapy. In: Brunton LL, Chabner BA, Knollman BC (eds). Goodman & Gilman's The Pharmacologic Basis of Therapeutics, 12th ed. New York: McGraw-Hill, 2010.)*

increasing the cytotoxicity and clinical activity of 5-FU.[30] Dihydropyrimidine dehydrogenase (DPD) catabolize 5-FU and reduced expression of this enzyme has been associated with severe adverse events.[31]

Capecitabine Capecitabine is an oral pyrimidine uracil analog and is a prodrug of 5-FU. Because capecitabine is enzymatically converted to 5-FU, it shares the same mechanisms of action. It generates higher levels of 5-FU selectively within some tumors as compared with normal tissues. Because chronic twice-daily oral dosing of capecitabine produces sustained 5-FU levels similar to continuous IV infusions of 5-FU, the toxicity pattern is similar to that of a continuous infusion of 5-FU.[30,32]

The most common toxicities of fluoropyrimidines include neutropenia, thrombocytopenia, and anemia when administered as an IV bolus administration and hand–foot syndrome and diarrhea when administered as a continuous IV infusion.[30,32]

Cytidine Analogs

Cytarabine Cytarabine (ara-C) is an arabinose analog of cytosine. It is phosphorylated to its active triphosphate within cancer cells and inhibits DNA polymerase, an enzyme responsible for strand elongation. It is also incorporated directly into DNA, where it inhibits the replication of DNA and acts as a chain terminator to prevent DNA elongation. Deaminase enzymes, particularly cytidine deaminase, degrades ara-C.[30,33]

Cytidine deaminase levels are very low in the central nervous system (CNS). Therefore, cytotoxic concentrations of ara-C are maintained in the CNS for several hours after intrathecal administration of traditional cytarabine formulations and for more than 2 weeks after administration of a depot formulation.

The toxicity of cytarabine is dose dependent. The most characteristic toxicity associated with high-dose ara-C (>1 g/m^2 per dose) is a cerebellar syndrome that manifests as dysarthria, nystagmus, and ataxia. The risk of CNS toxicity is strongly correlated with advanced age and renal dysfunction. Renal dysfunction permits accumulation of high levels of the triphosphate, which is believed to be neurotoxic. Hepatic dysfunction, high cumulative doses, and bolus dosing may also increase the risks of neurotoxicity.[30,33]

Gemcitabine Gemcitabine is a fluorine-substituted deoxycytidine analog that is related structurally to cytarabine. Its activation and mechanism of action are similar to those of cytarabine. Gemcitabine is incorporated into DNA, where it inhibits DNA polymerase activity. It also inhibits ribonucleotide reductase, which is the enzyme required to convert ribonucleotides into the deoxyribonucleotides that are needed for both DNA synthesis and repair. Compared with cytarabine, gemcitabine achieves intracellular concentrations about 20 times higher, secondary to increased penetration of cell membranes and greater affinity for the activating enzyme deoxycytidine kinase. Gemcitabine that is incorporated into DNA has a prolonged intracellular half-life. Its stereoconfiguration causes another normal base pair to be added next to the fraudulent gemcitabine base pair in the DNA strand. This "masked chain termination" protects the gemcitabine from excision and elimination.[30,33]

TABLE 104-8 Monitoring of Anticancer Drugs[a]

Agent	Major Adverse Effects	Monitoring Parameters	Comments
Antimetabolites			
Capecitabine	Diarrhea; hand–foot syndrome (palmar–plantar erythema); mild nausea and vomiting	Stool count; hands and feet for early signs of skin breakdown	Dose should be adjusted for patients with decreased renal function Oral prodrug of 5-FU Drug interactions: warfarin results in increased anticoagulant effects; may require phenytoin dose reduction
Cladribine	Myelosuppression; fever (onset by day 6, persisting for about 3 days); immunosuppressive; severe opportunistic infections occur	CBC; signs of infection	Prophylaxis against PJP and other infectious complications required
Clofarabine	Myelosuppression; elevated LFT results; nausea and vomiting; TLS	CBC; LFTs; uric acid	
Cytarabine and liposomal cytarabine for intrathecal use	Myelosuppression; nausea and vomiting; diarrhea; mucositis; TLS; flulike syndrome; rash HDAC toxicities: worsening of above and cerebellar toxicity; conjunctivitis	CBC; signs of infection; renal function; neurologic examinations (signs of confusion)	HDAC infusions should be administered over 2–3 hours to decrease risk of CNS toxicity; use steroid eye drops during treatment and for 48 hours posttreatment to prevent conjunctivitis with HDAC Increased HDAC neurotoxicity in patients with impaired renal function
Fludarabine	Myelosuppression, including decreased T cells; diarrhea; rare CNS toxicity: somnolence, peripheral neuropathies, hearing and visual changes, altered mental status, seizures; pulmonary toxicity; TLS	CBC; signs of infection; renal function; neurologic examinations	Dose should be adjusted for patients with decreased renal function Risk of opportunistic infections necessitate prophylactic antibiotics for PJP and HSV
5-Fluorouracil	Mucositis; diarrhea; hand–foot syndrome; myelosuppression; nausea and vomiting; hyperpigmentation; photosensitivity; ocular toxicity; myocardial ischemic symptoms	CBC; stool count; hands and feet for early signs of skin breakdown	Deficiency of DPD correlates with increased toxicity Drug interaction with warfarin: increased anticoagulant effect
Gemcitabine	Myelosuppression; flulike syndrome; rash; elevations in liver transaminases; nausea and vomiting	CBC; LFTs	Generally very well tolerated; rash may respond to topical steroids; fevers may respond to acetaminophen
6-Mercaptopurine	Myelosuppression; dry skin; rash; photosensitivity; hepatotoxicity: jaundice and hyperbilirubinemia; nausea and vomiting	CBC; LFTs	Allopurinol increases the toxicity of 6-MP by interfering with metabolism 6-MP reduces anticoagulant effects of warfarin
Methotrexate	Myelosuppression; mucositis; renal dysfunction at high doses; nausea and vomiting; CNS toxicity (more severe with IT administration); hepatotoxicity	CBC; LFTs; renal function; urine pH and methotrexate drug levels with high-dose therapy	Dose should be adjusted or avoid use in patients with decreased renal function; avoid drugs that decrease renal excretion of methotrexate (e.g., NSAIDs, PPIs, sulfas and penicillins) Methotrexate distributes readily into third-space fluids (ascites, pleural effusions), prolonging exposure and increasing toxicity; may be contraindication for use Monitor methotrexate levels with high-dose administration; these must include leucovorin rescue to prevent excessive myelosuppression; sodium bicarbonate also given for high-dose therapy to prevent nephrotoxicity (maintain urine pH >7) Use preservative-free preparations for IT and high-dose administration
Pemetrexed	Myelosuppression; stomatitis; pharyngitis; rash; desquamation	CBC; renal function; skin examinations	Avoid in patients with decreased renal function Avoid NSAIDs during administration Supplementation with folic acid (400 mcg daily starting 1 week before first dose; continued days after last dose) and vitamin B_{12} (1000 mcg IM during week before first dose and even cycles thereafter) to decrease myelosuppression Premedication with dexamethasone (day before, the day of, and day after) to decrease incidence of rash

(continued)

TABLE 104-8 Monitoring of Anticancer Drugs[a] (Continued)

Agent	Major Adverse Effects	Monitoring Parameters	Comments
Microtubule-Targeting Drugs			
Cabazitaxel	Myelosuppression; infection; hypersensitivity reactions; diarrhea; asthenia; renal failure; nausea and vomiting	CBC; signs of infection; stool count; renal function; signs of hypersensitivity reactions; LFTs	Avoid in patients with hepatic impairment Premedicate with H_1 and H_2 antagonist plus dexamethasone to decrease risk of hypersensitivity
Docetaxel	Myelosuppression; fluid retention and edema; pleural effusions; ascites; alopecia; rash; peripheral neuropathy; hypersensitivity reactions	CBC; fluid status; LFTs	Contraindicated in patients with hepatic impairment (hyperbilirubinemia, elevated transaminases, or elevated alkaline phosphatase) Dexamethasone 8 mg orally twice daily for 3 days (starting 1 day before docetaxel) is recommended to lower risk of fluid retention
Paclitaxel and nab-paclitaxel	Myelosuppression; infection; hypersensitivity reactions; peripheral neuropathy; myalgias or arthralgias; mucositis; cardiac arrhythmias; alopecia	CBC; signs of infection; signs of hypersensitivity reactions; signs of peripheral neuropathies; LFTs	Avoid or dose should be adjusted in patients with hepatic impairment Premedicate patients to prevent hypersensitivity reactions (dexamethasone, diphenhydramine, and ranitidine) 30 minutes before paclitaxel; nab-paclitaxel associated with decreased hypersensitivity reactions because it does not contain Cremophor and does not require premedication Neurotoxicity may be severe enough to require discontinuation Products are not interchangeable
Vinblastine and vinorelbine	Myelosuppression; mucositis; neurotoxicity: less common than with vincristine; myalgias; SIADH (rarely); vesicant	CBC; LFTs	Dose should be adjusted in patients with elevated bilirubin Treat extravasation injury with warm soaks and injection of hyaluronidase
Vincristine	Peripheral neuropathy (highest of vinca alkaloids); motor, sensory, autonomic, and cranial nerves may all be affected (paresthesias, ileus, urinary retention, facial palsies) and can be irreversible; SIADH; vesicant; myelosuppression (rare; much less than vinblastine or vinorelbine)	Signs of neurotoxicity (tingling in extremities; constipation, CNS toxicity); LFTs	Dose should be adjusted in patients with elevated bilirubin Prevent ileus: treat constipation aggressively Doses are commonly capped at 2 mg to minimize neurotoxicity LETHAL if administered intrathecally Treat extravasation similar to vinblastine
Eribulin	Myelosuppression; peripheral neuropathies; asthenia; alopecia; nausea; constipation	CBC; LFTs; renal function (CrCL); potassium and magnesium levels	Dose reduce for Child-Pugh class A or B hepatic impairment and moderate renal impairment May cause QT prolongation in patients with electrolyte or congenital abnormalities (avoid other drugs that may prolong QT interval)
Ixabepilone	Myelosuppression; peripheral neuropathies; hypersensitivity reactions; asthenia; arthralgias; alopecia	CBC; signs of infection; signs of hypersensitivity reactions; signs of peripheral neuropathies; LFTs	Avoid or dose should be adjusted in patients with elevated hepatic transaminases or bilirubin CYP3A4 substrate, levels may be effected by inducers or inhibitors, avoid use or dose adjustment to ixabepilone may be necessary Premedicate or H_1 and H_2 antagonist
Topoisomerase Inhibitors			
Irinotecan	Diarrhea: acute (within 1 hour of completion; related to cholinergic effects) and delayed (>12 hours after administration; usually after the second or third dose); nausea and vomiting; myelosuppression (neutropenia); alopecia; fatigue; increased LFT results; pulmonary toxicity: diffuse infiltrates, fever, dyspnea	CBC; GI symptoms (bowel movements); fluid and electrolytes	Acute diarrhea is best treated or prevented with atropine; delayed diarrhea is managed with antimotility agents Dose should be adjusted (or not given) in patients with elevated total bilirubin or uridine diphosphate-glucuronosyltransferase (UGT) 1A1 deficiency
Topotecan	Myelosuppression (neutropenia and thrombocytopenia); mucositis; reversible elevations in transaminases; less nausea and diarrhea than irinotecan	CBC; LFTs; renal function	Dose should be adjusted for patients with decreased renal function
Daunorubicin and liposomal daunorubicin	Myelosuppression (dose related); mucositis; nausea and vomiting; alopecia; vesicant: severe extravasation injury; cardiac toxicities: acute—not related to cumulative dose; arrhythmias, pericarditis; chronic—cumulative injury to myocardium (total dose >550 mg/m^2	CBC; LVEF; LFTs	Dose should be adjusted in patients with elevated bilirubin LVEF should be >50% to administer safely Liposomal form: decreased risk of cardiac and vesicant toxicity
Doxorubicin and liposomal doxorubicin	Similar to daunorubicin; cardiac toxicity associated with cumulative doses >450–550 mg/m^2; radiation recall reactions	CBC; LVEF; LFTs	Dose should be adjusted in patients with elevated bilirubin LVEF should be >50% to administer safely May discolor urine (red-orange) Liposomal form: decreased risk of cardiac and vesicant toxicities

Epirubicin	Similar to daunorubicin; cardiac toxicity associated with cumulative doses >900 mg/m^2	CBC; LVEF; LFTs	Dose should be adjusted in patients with elevated bilirubin LVEF should be >50% to administer safely
Etoposide	Myelosuppression; nausea and vomiting: may be worse with oral and high-dose regimens; alopecia; mucositis; hypotension: infusion rate–related; hypersensitivity reactions	CBC; blood pressure	Dose should be adjusted for patients with decreased renal function Requires large volumes of fluid for IV administration because of limited solubility (maximum concentration, 0.4 mg/mL) Available orally in liquid-filled gelatin capsules; ~50% bioavailability, but absorption is variable and greater at lower oral doses
Idarubicin	Similar to daunorubicin Total cumulative dose not well established; >150 mg/m^2 reported to be associated with decreased LVEF	CBC; LVEF; LFTs	Dose should be adjusted in patients with elevated bilirubin LVEF should be >50% to administer safely
Mitoxantrone	Myelosuppression; nausea and vomiting; mucositis; alopecia; less cardiotoxic than the anthracyclines	CBC; LVEF; LFTs	Not a vesicant (may cause vein irritation but not associated with severe tissue injury such as anthracyclines) May discolor urine blue-green
Alkylating Agents			
Bendamustine	Myelosuppression; infection; dermatologic reactions, including Stevens-Johnson's syndrome; TLS; infusion reactions	CBC; signs of infection; signs of dermatologic toxicity; uric acid	Not studied in patients with decreased renal function Allopurinol may increase risk for Stevens-Johnson's syndrome
Busulfan	Myelosuppression; skin hyperpigmentation; pulmonary fibrosis; gynecomastia; adrenal insufficiency High (HSCT) dose toxicities: seizures; hepatic venoocclusive disease; severe nausea and vomiting	CBC; pulmonary status; LFTs; signs of edema (weight gain, fluid status)	Bone marrow recovery may be delayed (3–6 weeks); pulmonary fibrosis associated with >3 years exposure, prior chest radiation Seizure prophylaxis with HSCT doses Pharmacokinetic monitoring is required with IV busulfan IV and oral preparations are not interchangeable; put tablets in gelatin capsules for easier administration with high-dose administration
Carboplatin	Myelosuppression (thrombocytopenia); nausea and vomiting (acute and delayed); risk of hypersensitivity reactions at higher cumulative doses (frequently results in cross-hypersensitivity to cisplatin)	CBC; renal function	Calvert formula used to dose carboplatin Lower incidence of nephrotoxicity, neurotoxicity, and nausea and vomiting than cisplatin
Chlorambucil	Myelosuppression; increased LFT results; skin rash; menstrual irregularities; pulmonary toxicity; risk of secondary malignancies; causes infertility and sterility; teratogenic	CBC; LFTs; pulmonary function	Oral agent that should be taken on an empty stomach; food decreases absorption May be dosed in low daily-dosing regimens or in higher dose, "pulse," or intermittent dosing schedules administered biweekly or monthly; pulse dosing may require patients to take several tablets (e.g., 10–20 tablets) per dose
Cisplatin	Nephrotoxicity; potassium and magnesium wasting; severe nausea and vomiting (acute or delayed onset); neurotoxicity (peripheral neuropathy that is cumulative and dose related and ototoxicity); generally not myelosuppressive (anemia seen with chronic dosing)	Renal function (CrCL and urine output); potassium and magnesium levels; GI symptoms (nausea and vomiting)	Dose should be adjusted or avoid in patients with decreased renal function Hydration required (1–2 L of 0.9% sodium chloride minimum before and after administration; ensure good urine output (>100 mL/h); potassium chloride and magnesium sulfate in IV fluid to replace losses; dose reduce or consider carboplatin for patients with impaired renal function Aggressive antiemetics required pretreatment and for 3–5 days after to prevent delayed nausea and vomiting Amifostine chemoprotective agent may reduce cisplatin renal toxicity Doses should not exceed 100 mg/m^2 (maximum single dose and per-cycle dose)
Cyclophosphamide	Hemorrhagic cystitis; nausea and vomiting (acute and delayed); myelosuppression; alopecia; SIADH, typically with high doses (>2 g/m^2); secondary malignancies (bladder cancers, acute leukemia); infertility; sterility	CBC; renal function; urine output; urinalysis	Dose should be adjusted for patients with decreased renal function Hydration needed to prevent hemorrhagic cystitis (oral or IV ~3 L/day × 72 h); mesna may be required with high-dose regimens (see ifosfamide) Instruct patients to take oral tablets in the morning to allow for elimination of toxic metabolite; absorbed through skin: avoid spills Drug interactions: CYP450 inducers (e.g., barbiturates) may increase formation of toxic metabolites; CYP450 inhibitors (e.g., cimetidine) may increase myelosuppression

(*continued*)

TABLE 104-8 Monitoring of Anticancer Drugs[a] (*Continued*)

Agent	Major Adverse Effects	Monitoring Parameters	Comments
Ifosfamide	Hemorrhagic cystitis; nephrotoxicity; myelosuppression; CNS effects: somnolence, confusion, disorientation, cerebellar symptoms that are dose-related; nausea and vomiting (acute and delayed); alopecia	CBC; daily urinalysis for blood; renal function	Dose should be adjusted for patients with decreased renal function 3–4 L/day fluid for hydration; potassium, magnesium, and phosphate may be required to replace losses Mesna is always given (typically 60%–100% of ifosfamide dose), may be delivered in same IV bag CNS toxicity and nausea and vomiting may be more severe with rapid infusion; case reports suggest methylene blue may be effective treatment for CNS toxicity
Mechlorethamine	Myelosuppression; severe nausea and vomiting; vesicant; secondary malignancies; sterility and infertility	CBC; GI symptoms (nausea and vomiting)	Antidote for extravasation is sodium thiosulfate
Nitrosoureas (carmustine and lomustine)	Myelosuppression; severe nausea and vomiting; cumulative nephrotoxicity; pulmonary fibrosis; facial flushing during infusion	CBC; renal function; pulmonary function	Bone marrow recovery may require 6–8 weeks Carmustine is a vein irritation, and facial flushing may be related to alcohol vehicle; also available in wafer form for implantation into brain tumor cavities after resection Lomustine is administered orally
Oxaliplatin	Peripheral neuropathy >50% patients: acute form: <14 days, rapid onset, reversible, exacerbated by cold; chronic form: onset >14 days and may be permanent; pharyngolaryngeal dysesthesias; nausea and vomiting; anaphylaxis risk	CBC; renal function; acute and chronic neuropathies	Dose should be adjusted for patients with decreased renal function 1 g of magnesium and calcium before and after may be used to prevent neuropathies Avoid exposure to cold
Procarbazine	Myelosuppression; diarrhea; neurotoxicity; neuropathy; flulike syndrome; infertility and sterility; secondary malignancies	CBC	Administered as a single daily dose on an empty stomach MAOIs that interactions with tyramine-rich foods and may precipitate hypertensive crisis; drug interactions: TCAs and SSRIs, sympathomimetics; disulfiram-like reaction with alcohol
Thiotepa	Myelosuppression; nausea and vomiting; mucositis; pruritus and dermatitis	CBC; dermatologic toxicities	Most commonly used in HSCT preparative regimens
Triazenes (dacarbazine and temozolamide)	Myelosuppression; severe nausea and vomiting; increased liver enzymes; flulike syndrome (may last for several days after dacarbazine administration); facial flushing; photosensitivity	CBC; LFTs	Dacarbazine is an IV agent that is light sensitive; dispense in a lightproof bags Temozolamide is an oral prodrug that crossed the blood–brain barrier; may cause lymphosuppression when given with radiation therapy and requires PJP prophylaxis
Miscellaneous Agents			
Arsenic trioxide	Differentiation syndrome (pulmonary infiltrates, respiratory distress, fever, and hypotension); QT prolongation; electrolyte abnormalities (hypokalemia or hyperkalemia and hypomagnesemia); hyperglycemia; rash; lightheadedness; fatigue; musculoskeletal pain	ECG and serum electrolytes (calcium, magnesium, potassium) before each course; renal function	Differentiation syndrome must be treated promptly with corticosteroids Do not give if QTc >500 msec Replace electrolytes before therapy
Bleomycin	Anaphylaxis and hypersensitivity reactions; fever and flulike symptoms; mucositis; pulmonary fibrosis	Obtain PFTs before use and if signs of pulmonary toxicity develop; monitor for anaphylactic reactions	Dose should be adjusted for patients with decreased renal function Test dose (1 unit) is recommended but controversial; premedicate for subsequent doses with acetaminophen Pulmonary toxicity associated with cumulative dose >400 units and preexisting pulmonary disease
Hydroxyurea	Myelosuppression; rash; skin hyperpigmentation; TLS; secondary leukemias	CBC; uric acid	Dose may need to be adjusted for patients with decreased renal function (use with caution) Used to decrease white blood cell counts rapidly to prevent adverse effects of leukocytosis
Mitomycin C	Myelosuppression (delayed and prolonged); mucositis; nausea and vomiting; vesicant; pulmonary fibrosis; hemolytic anemia and uremic syndrome	CBC; renal function; pulmonary function	Apply ice or cold packs to site for extravasation
Omacetaxine	Thrombocytopenia, increased risk of hemorrhage; anemia; neutropenia; diarrhea; nausea; fatigue; asthenia; injection site reaction; pyrexia; infection; lymphopenia; hyperglycemia	CBC; blood glucose	Active in T315I-resistant CML

Retinoids			
Bexarotene	Peripheral edema; insomnia; headache; fever; increased triglycerides and cholesterol; hypothyroidism; leukopenia and anemia; dry skin; increased LTFs; pancreatitis; photosensitivity	CBC; LFTs; cholesterol and triglyceride levels; Thyroid-stimulating levels (TSH)	CYP3A4 substrate Avoid gemfibrozil to treat elevated triglycerides Limit vitamin A supplements May cause hypoglycemia in patients receiving insulin, sulfonylureas, or metformin Teratogenic; contraindicated in pregnancy; female patients should be educated about proper contraceptive measures
Tretinoin (ATRA)	Headache; differentiation syndrome; "ATRA syndrome" consisting of pulmonary symptoms, fever, hypotension, and pleural effusions); dry skin and mucous membranes; mucositis; elevations in transaminases and bilirubin	CBC; LFTs; signs of differentiation syndrome	Differentiation syndrome must be treated promptly with corticosteroids Teratogenic; contraindicated in pregnancy; female patients should be educated about proper contraceptive measures
BCR-ABL Inhibitors			
Bosutinib	Nausea and vomiting; edema; pleural effusions and ascites; myelosuppression; CHF; arthralgias; rash; diarrhea; increased LFT results; hypophosphatemia	CBC; LFTs; phosphate levels; Philadelphia chromosome levels; signs of edema	Dose should be adjusted in patients with Child-Pugh class A, B, or C hepatic impairment CYP3A4 substrate; inhibitor of Pgp Avoid antacids and PPIs Maintenance dose based on CBC
Dasatinib	Nausea and vomiting; edema; pleural effusions and ascites; myelosuppression; CHF; arthralgias; fatigue; rash; diarrhea; increased LFT results; QT prolongation; hypophosphatemia and hypocalcemia	CBC; LFTs; calcium, magnesium, phosphate, and potassium levels; signs of edema; Philadelphia chromosome levels	CYP3A4 substrate and inhibitor Avoid antacids and drugs that decrease gastric pH Maintenance dose based on CBC
Imatinib	Nausea and vomiting; edema; pleural effusions and ascites; myelosuppression; CHF; arthralgias; rash; diarrhea; increased LFT results; hypophosphatemia	CBC; LFTs; phosphate levels; Philadelphia chromosome levels; signs of edema	Dose adjustments should be considered in patients with severe liver and moderate renal impairment CYP3A4 substrate and inhibitor; also inhibits CYP2C19 and CYP2D6; may increase warfarin effects Maintenance dose based on CBC Take with meals and a full glass of water
Nilotinib	Nausea and vomiting; edema; myelosuppression; increased lipase; hyperglycemia; arthralgias; rash; diarrhea; increased LFTs; QT prolongation	CBC; LFTs; serum lipase; glucose levels; magnesium and potassium levels; Philadelphia chromosome levels	Dose should be adjusted in patients with Child-Pugh class A, B, or C hepatic impairment Take on an empty stomach CYP3A4 substrate, avoid inhibitors; inhibitor of CYP3A4, CYP2C8, CYP2C9, and CYP2D6; also induces CYP2B6, CYP2C8, and CYP2C9; drug concentrations of these substrates may be altered Maintenance dose based on CBC
Ponatinib	Myelosuppression; hypertension; rash; abdominal pain; fatigue; headache; dry skin; constipation; arthralgia; nausea; pyrexia; arterial thrombosis, cardiovascular, cerebrovascular, and peripheral vascular thrombosis have occurred; hepatotoxicity; congestive heart failure; pancreatitis; hemorrhage, mostly in occurring in patients with grade 4 thrombocytopenia; fluid retention	Signs and symptoms of congestive heart failure; blood pressure; serum lipase; fluid retention; symptoms of arrhythmias; CBC; LFTs	May need to decrease or hold therapy if hepatotoxicity develops Substrate of CYP3A4; inhibits P-glycoprotein Avoid antacids and drugs that decrease gastric pH
Histone Deacetylase Inhibitors			
Romidepsin	Neutropenia; lymphopenia; thrombocytopenia; infection; nausea; fatigue; vomiting; anorexia; anemia; ECG T-wave changes	CBC; cardiovascular monitoring in patients with congenital long QT syndrome, a history of significant cardiovascular disease, and patients taking other medications that may prolong the QT interval; monitor potassium and magnesium	Substrate of CYP3A4, monitor INR if patient on warfarin
Vorinostat	Diarrhea; fatigue; nausea; thrombocytopenia; anorexia; dysgeusia; PE and DVT have been reported; hyperglycemia has been observed	CBC; signs and symptoms of PE or DVT; electrolytes; chemistry tests, including glucose and Scr	Dose should be adjusted or avoided in patients with hepatic impairment Increase in INR has been observed with concomitant warfarin Severe thrombocytopenia and GI bleeding have been reported with concomitant use with vorinostat and other HDAC inhibitors (e.g., valproic acid)

(continued)

TABLE 104-8 Monitoring of Anticancer Drugs[a] (*Continued*)

Agent	Major Adverse Effects	Monitoring Parameters	Comments
DNA Methyltransferase Inhibitors			
Azacitidine and decitabine	Myelosuppression and infection; constitutional symptoms; musculoskeletal symptoms (arthralgias); cough; dyspnea	CBC; signs of infection	
mTOR Pathway Inhibitors			
Everolimus	Rash; asthenia; stomatitis; nausea; edema; anorexia; anemia; pneumonitis; hyperglycemia; hyperlipidemia; hypertriglyceridemia; hypophosphatemia; elevated liver enzymes; elevated Scr; lymphopenia; thrombocytopenia; leukopenia; infection	Blood glucose; cholesterol and triglyceride levels; CBC, Scr; LFTs; phosphorous levels	Dose should be adjusted in patients with Child-Pugh class A, B, or C hepatic impairment Initiation or increase in cholesterol or diabetic medications often needed Substrate of CYP3A4 and Pgp, may required dose adjustment based on concurrent medication administered
Temsirolimus	Similar to everolimus with addition of infusion-related reactions	Similar to everolimus; monitor for infusion and allergic reactions	Dose should be adjusted in patients with mild hepatic impairment In addition to everolimus, requires diphenhydramine premedication
EGFR Pathway Inhibitors			
Erlotinib	Rash; diarrhea; rare but potentially fatal pulmonary toxicity (ILD); hepatic and renal failure reported	LFTs; monitor renal function and electrolytes in patients at risk of dehydration; monitor for pulmonary symptoms; inflammatory or infectious sequelae of the skin	Dose reductions or delays may be required for rash, but supportive care should be attempted first Therapy should be interrupted (or discontinued) if patients develop symptoms of ILD CYP3A4 substrate; also has a major interaction with warfarin, leading to increased bleeding risk Drugs that alter gastric pH may decrease drug levels Take on an empty stomach and without as food increases absorption and possibly toxicity
Gefitinib	Similar to erlotinib	LFTs; monitor for pulmonary symptoms	Similar precautions and drug interactions as with erlotinib Limited access to patients demonstrating benefit from gefitinib
Lapatinib	Diarrhea; rash; nausea; vomiting; fatigue; decreases in LVEF have been reported; hepatotoxicity; QT prolongation; ILD	LFTs; ECG and electrolyte monitoring; signs and symptoms of ILD; MUGA or ECG before initiating and periodically throughout therapy	Dose should be adjusted in patients with Child-Pugh class C hepatic impairment Take on empty stomach Substrate of CYP3A4; Inhibits CYP3A4 and Pgp Avoid strong CYP3A4 inhibitors, (if unavoidable, consider dose reduction); avoid strong CYP3A4 inducers (if unavoidable, consider gradual dose increases)
Multikinase Inhibitors			
Axitinib	Diarrhea; rash; hand–foot syndrome; bleeding; thrombotic events; hypertension; hepatotoxicity; hypothyroidism; proteinuria; GI perforation; fatigue; rare reports of progressive multifocal leukoencephalopathy	CBC; LFTs; blood pressure; TSH levels; urine protein; signs of bleeding or thrombotic events; neurologic symptoms	Dose should be adjusted in patients with Child-Pugh class B hepatic impairment Substrate of CYP3A4; may require dose adjustment based on concurrent medication administered
Cabozantinib	Diarrhea; stomatitis; hand–foot syndrome; decreased weight; decreased appetite; nausea; fatigue; oral pain; hair color changes; dysgeusia; hypertension; abdominal pain; constipation; increased LFTs; proteinuria; lymphopenia; neutropenia; thrombocytopenia; hypocalcemia; hypophosphatemia; GI perforations and fistulas and hemorrhage have been reported	Signs and symptoms of bleeding; blood pressure; urine protein; CBC; LFTs	Take on an empty stomach Substrate of CYP3A4, monitor for drug interactions
Pazopanib	Diarrhea; hypertension; hair color changes; nausea; anorexia; vomiting; decreased weight; fatigue; musculoskeletal pain; dysguesia; dyspnea; skin hypopigmentation; hypothyroidism; proteinuria; fatal hepatotoxicity has been observed; PE and DVT have occurred	LFTs; ECG in patients at high risk for QT prolongation; blood pressure; signs and symptoms of PE and DVT; TSH; urine protein	Dose should be adjusted in patients with moderate hepatic impairment Take on empty stomach Substrate of CYP1A2, CYP2C8, and CYP3A4; inhibits CYP2C8, CYP2D6, CYP3A4 Reduce dose of pazopanib when administered with strong CYP3A4 inhibitors; avoid CYP3A4 inducers; concomitant use with simvastatin increases liver transaminases
Regorafenib	Asthenia; fatigue; decreased appetite; hand–foot syndrome; diarrhea; mucositis; weight loss; infection; hypertension; dysphonia; reports of hepatotoxicity have been reported; hemorrhage	LFTs; blood pressure	Take with food, low-fat breakfast that contains <30% fat Substrate of CYP3A4; inhibits Pgp Because of an increase risk of hemorrhage with regorafenib, monitor INR closely if on concomitant warfarin

Sorafenib	Diarrhea; rash; hand–foot syndrome; fatigue; hypertension; prolonged QT interval; cardiac events (including MI); drug-induced hepatitis	Blood pressure; LFTs; monitor for prolonged QT intervals and electrolyte abnormalities	Administer on an empty stomach Inhibits CYP2B6, CYP2C8, and CYP2C9; substrate of CYP3A4 May increase the anticoagulation effects of warfarin
Sunitinib	Diarrhea; rash; bleeding; CHF and cardiac effects; QT prolongation; fatigue; hypertension; hepatotoxicity; thyroid dysfunction	CBC; LFTs; signs and symptoms of CHF; blood pressure; signs and symptoms of hypo- or hyperthyroidism; monitor for prolonged QT intervals and electrolyte abnormalities	Substrate of CYP3A4; may required dose adjustment based on concurrent medication administered
Vandetanib	Diarrhea; rash; acne; nausea; hypertension; headache; fatigue; upper respiratory tract infections; decreased appetite; abdominal pain; prolonged QT interval, torsades de pointes, and sudden death have been reported; ILD; rare cases of hemorrhage have been reported	Calcium, potassium, and magnesium; ECG monitoring if on other medications known to prolong the QT interval; pulmonary status, bleeding	Dose should be adjusted in patients with moderate to severe renal impairment Substrate of CYP3A4; inhibits Pgp Avoid other medications that prolong the QT interval Advise patients to wear sunscreen and protective clothing when exposed to sun
Proteasome Inhibitors			
Carfilzomib	Fatigue; anemia; thrombocytopenia; nausea; diarrhea; dyspnea; pyrexia; infusion-related reactions; rare reports of cardiac arrest, CHF, and MI have occurred	Symptoms of dyspnea; CBC; LFTs; cardiac complications	Premedicate with dexamethasone before all cycle 1 doses, during the first cycle of dose escalation, and if infusion reaction symptoms develop
Bortezomib	Fatigue or malaise; nausea; diarrhea; anorexia; constipation; vomiting; myelosuppression, especially thrombocytopenia; hyponatremia; hypokalemia; peripheral neuropathy, cumulative and dose-related; fever	CBC; LFTs; symptoms of neuropathy	Dose should be adjusted in patients with moderate to severe hepatic impairment Can be administered IV or SC (SC administration has been shown to decrease neuropathies) Increased risk of severe neuropathy in patients with preexisting neuropathy Co-administration with strong CYP3A4 inhibitors can increase bortezomib concentrations
Miscellaneous Small Molecule Inhibitors			
Crizotinib	Pneumonitis; hepatotoxicity; QT prolongation; nausea; vomiting; diarrhea; vision changes	LFTs; pulmonary function; monitor for prolonged QT intervals and electrolyte abnormalities	May need to decrease or hold therapy if hepatotoxicity develops Substrate and inhibitor of CYP3A4
Thalidomide, lenalidomide, and pomalidomide	Thalidomide: somnolence; constipation; dizziness or orthostatic; hypotension; rash; peripheral neuropathies; thromboembolic clots Lenalidomide: fatigue; peripheral neuropathy; neutropenia and thrombocytopenia; thromboembolic clots	CBC; signs of thrombosis; signs of peripheral neuropathies	For lenalidomide, dose should be adjusted in patients with moderate to severe renal impairment Prophylactic anticoagulant therapy may be required
Vemurafenib	Arthralgia; rash; alopecia, fatigue; photosensitivity reaction; nausea; pruritus; skin papilloma; cutaneous squamous cell carcinomas; QT prolongation; serious ophthalmologic reactions, including uveitis, iritis, and retinal vein occlusion, have been reported	Dermatologic evaluations; ECG and electrolytes; LFTs; monitor for ophthalmologic reactions	Substrate of CYP3A4; inhibits CYP1A2, CYP2D6, and Pgp; Induces CYP3A4; if patient on warfarin, monitor INR closely Advise patients to avoid sun exposure
Vismodegib	Muscle spasms; alopecia; dysgeusia; ageusia; weight loss; fatigue; nausea; vomiting; diarrhea; decreased appetite; constipation; arthralgias; black box warning for embryo or fetal death and severe birth defects	Female patients should receive a pregnancy test within 1 week before treatment initiation	Patients should not donate blood or blood products while receiving vismodegib and for at least 7 months after the last dose Drugs that affect gastric pH (H_2 antagonists, antacids, and PPIs) may decrease the concentration of vismodegib
Monoclonal Antibodies that Target Cell Surface Glycoproteins			
Alemtuzumab	Myelosuppression and immunosuppression; infection; infusion-related reactions; nausea and vomiting; fever; hypotension; rash; headache; fatigue	CBC; infusion-related reactions; CMV; $CD4^+$ counts	Patients should be started on antiviral and PJP prophylaxis during and 6 months posttreatment
Brentuximab vedotin	Neutropenia; peripheral sensory neuropathy; fatigue; nausea or vomiting; anemia; diarrhea; rash; thrombocytopenia; infusion-related reactions; TLS; rare reports of progressive multifocal leukoencephalopathy	CBC; symptoms of neuropathy; infusion-related reactions; uric acid	Antibody-drug conjugate

(continued)

TABLE 104-8 Monitoring of Anticancer Drugs[a] (*Continued*)

Agent	Major Adverse Effects	Monitoring Parameters	Comments
Ibritumomab tiuxetan	Must consider toxicities of rituximab also because always given in combination; delayed hematologic toxicity; infusion-related reactions; asthenia; nausea; chills; fever; tumor pain	Infusion-related reactions; CBC	Radiopharmaceutical; to be prepared and administered only by personnel trained in radiopharmaceuticals; patients must be trained in precautions to decrease radiation exposure
Ofatumumab	Neutropenia; pneumonia; pyrexia; cough; diarrhea; anemia; fatigue; dyspnea; rash; nausea; bronchitis; upper respiratory infection	Infusion-related reactions; CBC	Patients at high risk of hepatitis B should be screened for before therapy Premedicate with acetaminophen, H_1 antagonist, and corticosteroid For dose 1 initiate infusion at a rate of 3.6 mg/h, dose 2 initiate rate at 24 mg/h, and for doses 3–12 initiate infusion at a rate of 50 mg/h; in the absence of infusional toxicity, the rate of infusion may be increased every 30 minutes
Rituximab	Hypersensitivity reactions; infusion-related side effects (flushing, chills, fever, rigors, hypotension, bronchospasm, dyspnea, and angioedema); TLS (especially with large tumor burden); myelosuppression and infection; rare reports of progressive multifocal leukoencephalopathy; severe skin reactions; myalgias; tachycardia	Infusion-related reactions; CBC; neurologic examination	Patients at high risk of hepatitis B should be screened for before therapy because reactivation of the virus may occur Infusion-related reactions may be severe; increase rate of infusion gradually and premedicate with acetaminophen and diphenhydramine; use meperidine IV as needed for rigors
Tositumomab	Myelosuppression (especially thrombocytopenia and neutropenia) that is severe and prolonged; abdominal pain; diarrhea; infusion reactions; anaphylaxis may occur; hypothyroidism; asthenia; myalgias; cough; rash	Infusion-related reactions; CBC; thyroid function tests	Similar radiation safety procedures as ibritumomab Premedicate with acetaminophen and diphenhydramine Thyroprotective regimen required
Monoclonal Antibodies that Target Growth Factor Receptors and Ligands			
Cetuximab	Rash; paronychial cracking in fingers or toes; asthenia; abdominal pain; nausea; constipation; diarrhea; infusion and hypersensitivity reactions; electrolyte wasting; cardiopulmonary arrest	Electrolytes (magnesium, potassium, and calcium); infusion-related reactions; inflammatory or infectious sequelae of the skin	Dose reductions or delays may be required for rash but supportive care should be attempted first Premedicate with diphenhydramine to decrease infusion-related reactions
Panitumumab	Similar to cetuximab	Similar to cetuximab	Decreased infusion-related reactions to panitumumab and does not appear to be cross reactive; therefore, a patient can receive panitumumab if they react to cetuximab See cetuximab
Pertuzumab	Diarrhea; nausea; alopecia; rash; neutropenia; fatigue; peripheral neuropathy; embryo and fetal toxicity; left ventricular dysfunction; infusion-related reactions	LVEF; signs and symptoms of infusion-related reactions	Given in combination with trastuzumab
Trastuzumab	Cardiac toxicity: congestive cardiomyopathy, usually reversible with medical management; infusion-related reactions	Signs and symptoms of infusion-related reactions; LVEF	Do not administer with anthracyclines because of increased cardiotoxicity
Bevacizumab	GI bleeding or perforation, sometimes with intraabdominal abscess formation; impaired wound healing; hypertension; proteinuria; thrombotic events; rare severe pulmonary hemorrhage; rare reports of progressive multifocal leukoencephalopathy	Blood pressure; urine protein; neurologic examination; signs of GI perforation	GI bleeding or perforation risk not correlated with duration of therapy; evaluate with each dose
Miscellaneous Monoclonal Antibodies			
Ipilimumab	Fatigue; diarrhea; pruritus; rash; colitis; can cause severe and fatal immune-mediated reactions caused by T-cell activation and proliferation (enterocolitis, dermatitis, neuropathy, endocrinopathy, hepatitis)	Thyroid function tests; serum chemistries; signs and symptoms of enterocolitis; bowel perforation; LFTs; dermatitis; symptoms of sensory neuropathy; signs and symptoms of hypophysitis; adrenal insufficiency; and hyper- or hypothyroidism	The immune-mediated reactions can occur weeks to months after treatment with ipilimumab; the treatment of immune-related reactions is corticosteroids, ipilimumab may need to be held or permanently discontinued

Enzymes			
Escherichia coli–derived asparaginase, pegaspargase, and asparaginase *Erwinia chrysanthemi*	Hypersensitivity reactions (fever, hypotension, rash, dyspnea in 25%), much lower risk with polyethylene glycol form and asparaginase *E. chrysanthemi;* pancreatitis; decreased synthesis of proteins, clotting factors; CNS: lethargy	Amylase; LFTs; coagulation parameters (fibrinogen, PT, PTT); hypersensitivity reactions; signs and symptoms of pancreatitis; blood glucose; CBC	Skin test before administration of *E. coli*–derived asparaginase; anaphylaxis precautions Pegaspargase complexes with polyethylene glycol to decrease immunogenicity and prolong duration of action Asparaginase *E. chrysanthemi* was developed for patients who have developed hypersensitivity to *E. coli*–derived asparaginase To substitute a dose of Asparaginase *E. chrysanthemi* for pegasparagase: 25,000 IU/m^2 IM 3 times weekly for 6 doses each planned dose of pegasparagase; to substitute for native *E. coli* asparagase: 25,000 IU/m^2 IM for each scheduled dose
Cytokines			
Interferon-alfa	Flulike symptoms; fatigue; serious or fatal neuropsychiatric (e.g., depression, suicide), autoimmune, ischemic, and infectious complications; pulmonary symptoms; thyroid disorders; hyperglycemia	Signs of mental status changes; infectious complications; pulmonary and cardiac function; blood glucose	Fatigue and flu symptoms tend to decrease with duration of therapy Exists in a pegylated form that has a prolonged half-life
Interleukin-2	Flulike syndrome: fevers, chills, malaise; vascular or capillary leak syndrome: hypotension, pulmonary and peripheral edema; GI: nausea and vomiting, diarrhea; nephrotoxicity; myelosuppression (thrombocytopenia and leukopenia); bacterial infections; CNS: somnolence, confusion; arrhythmias; rash; itching	Intense monitoring required; serum chemistries; LFTs, Scr; electrolytes; CBC; thallium stress test; pulmonary function tests; cardiac monitoring during IL-2 administration	Vasopressor support and fluid resuscitation may be necessary during treatment because of hypotension Pulmonary edema can be managed with cautious use of diuretics; short courses of albumin may also be beneficial Itching may respond to treatment with H_1 antagonists; emollient skin creams or occlusive agents are effective for dry, peeling skin Avoid corticosteroids because they may counteract the antitumor effects of IL-2 Patients on beta-blockers will need to be tapered off before initiation of aldesleukin
Fusion Proteins			
Denileukin difitox	Pyrexia; nausea; fatigue; rigors; vomiting; diarrhea; headache; peripheral edema; cough; dyspnea; pruritus; infusion reactions; capillary leak syndrome; loss of visual acuity	Signs and symptoms of infusion reactions; weight gain; blood pressure; serum albumin, level should be at least 3 g/dL before initiating; visual acuity and color vision	Premedicate with an antihistamine and acetaminophen
Ziv-aflibercept	Neutropenia; diarrhea; proteinuria; elevated transaminases; stomatitis; fatigue; thrombocytopenia; hypertension; weight decreased; decreased appetite; epistaxis; abdominal pain; dysphonia; serum creatinine increased; headache; hemorrhage; GI perforation; compromised wound healing; arterial thromboembolic events; fistula formation	Blood pressure; urine protein; signs and symptoms of GI bleeding and other serious bleeding; signs and symptoms of GI perforation; CBC; LFTs	Should be held at least 4 weeks before elective surgery and restarted at least 4 weeks after major surgery and until the surgical wound is fully healed

ATRA, all-*trans*-retinoic acid; CBC, complete blood count; CHF, congestive heart failure; CML, CML, chronic myeloid leukemia; CMV, cytomegalovirus; CNS, central nervous system; CrCL, creatinine clearance; CYP450, cytochrome P450 isoenzyme; DPD, dihydropyrimidine dehydrogenase; DVT, deep vein thrombosis; ECG, electrocardiogram; GI, gastrointestinal; G6PD, glucose-6-phosphate dehydrogenase; HDAC, high-dose ara-c (cytarabine); HSV, herpes simplex virus; H_1 and H_2, histamine 1 and 2; HDAC, histone deacetylase; HSCT, hematopoietic stem cell transplantation; ILD, interstitial lung disease; INR, international normalized ration; IT, intrathecal; IM, intramuscular; LFT, liver function test; LVEF, left ventricular ejection fraction; MAOI, monoamine oxidase inhibitor; MI, myocardial infarction; mTOR, mammalian target of rapamycin; MUGA, multigated acquisition scan; NSAID, nonsteroidal antiinflammatory drug; PE, pulmonary embolism; PFT, pulmonary function tests; Pgp, P-glycoprotein; PJP, *Pneumocystis jiroveci* pneumonia; PPI, proton pump inhibitor; PT, prothrombin time; PTT, partial thromboplastin time; SC, subcutaneous; Scr, serum creatinine; SIADH, syndrome of inappropriate secretion of antidiuretic hormone; SSRI, selective serotonin reuptake inhibitor; TCA, tricyclic antidepressant; TLS, tumor lysis syndrome; TSH, thyroid-stimulating hormone; UGT1A1, ????????.

[a]Only approximate guidelines can be given. Consult current references before dispensing as not all dose adjustments and monitoring parameters are provided in the table.

Adapted from Chabner BA, Longo DL, ed. Cancer Chemotherapy and Biotherapy: Principles and Practice, 5th ed. Philadelphia: Lippincott Williams & Wilkins, 2010 and prescribing information package inserts.

Purines and Purine Antimetabolites

Mercaptopurine and Thioguanine 6-Mercaptopurine (6-MP) and its analog thioguanine are rapidly converted to ribonucleotides that inhibit purine biosynthesis. They also undergo purine interconversion reactions needed to supply purine precursors for synthesis of nucleic acids. Clinical cross-resistance is generally observed.[30] Both anticancer agents are metabolized by thiopurine methyltransferase (TPMT) and hypoxanthine phosphoribosyl transferase to produce multiple metabolites responsible for the efficacy, hepatic toxicity, and myelosuppression. Genetic polymorphisms of TPMT are associated with reduced enzyme activity and decreased tolerance of standard doses of 6-MP.

6-MP depends on xanthine oxidase for an initial oxidation step. Its metabolism is markedly decreased by concomitant administration of the xanthine oxidase inhibitor allopurinol, and serious toxicity may result. Oral 6-MP doses must be reduced when allopurinol is administered together with 6-MP.[30]

Fludarabine Monophosphate Fludarabine monophosphate is an analog of the purine adenine. Similar to cytarabine, fludarabine interferes with DNA polymerase, causing chain termination. Fludarabine also incorporates into RNA, resulting in inhibited transcription. The usual dose-limiting toxicity is myelosuppression. Fludarabine is also immunosuppressive, with associated opportunistic infections resulting from its effect on T cells and a subsequent decrease in CD4 counts; prophylactic antibiotics and antiviral medications are recommended and should continue until CD4 counts normalize.[30,34]

Cladribine and Pentostatin Cladribine and pentostatin are purine nucleoside analogs with slightly different mechanisms of action. Cladribine is resistant to inactivation by adenosine deaminase and triphosphorylated to an active form that is incorporated into DNA, resulting in inhibition of DNA synthesis and early chain termination. Its antitumor activity is unusual for an antimetabolite in that it affects both actively dividing and resting cancer cells. Pentostatin is a potent inhibitor of adenosine deaminase. Adenosine deaminase is an enzyme critical in purine base metabolism and is found in high concentrations in lymphatic tissue. Similar to fludarabine, these chemotherapies have immunosuppressive effects that place patients at risk for serious opportunistic infections.[30,33]

Antifolates

Folate vitamins are essential cofactors in DNA synthesis. These vitamins carry one-carbon groups in transfer reactions that are required for purine and thymidylic acid synthesis. Natural folates circulating in the blood have a single glutamic acid group, but natural folates within cells are converted to polyglutamates, which are more efficient cofactors and preferentially retained inside cells.[35]

Dietary folates must be chemically reduced to their tetrahydrofolate forms to be active. The enzyme responsible for this reduction is dihydrofolate reductase (DHFR). Antifolates are associated with neutropenia and thrombocytopenia, mucositis, and nausea and vomiting.

Methotrexate Methotrexate (MTX) inhibits DHFR, which results in the depletion of intracellular pools of reduced folates (tetrahydrofolates) essential for thymidylate and purine synthesis. Lack of either thymidine or purines prevents synthesis of DNA. The DHFR-mediated effects of antifolates on normal and tumor cells may be neutralized by supplying reduced folates exogenously. The reduced folate used clinically for "rescue" is leucovorin (folinic acid), which bypasses the metabolic block induced by DHFR inhibitors.[35]

Amplification of DHFR can lead to tumor cell resistance. Other potential causes of resistance are slow rates of thymidylate synthesis, decreased affinity for DHFR, lack of polyglutamation within cancer cells and saturated transport. In high doses, passive diffusion may overcome tumor cell resistance caused by saturated active transport systems. Malignant cells may achieve greater MTX polyglutamate levels than normal cells, which may, in part, explain the selective effects of MTX on malignant versus normal cells.[35]

Accurate and readily available assays for serum MTX levels have made therapeutic drug monitoring of MTX a valuable clinical tool. The threshold for cytotoxic effects of MTX is about 0.02 mg/L (50 nmol/L). Toxicity and efficacy relates not only to peak concentrations, but more importantly to time that concentrations remain above this threshold level. For MTX doses requiring leucovorin rescue (generally doses greater than 1,000 mg/m^2), leucovorin must be administered until levels fall below 0.02 mg/L (50 nmol/L). Therapeutic drug monitoring is also an effective means of increasing the likelihood of therapeutic success by individualizing doses based on target levels.[35] Renal tubular necrosis is seen with high-doses of MTX and vigorous hydration with or without alkalinization of the urine necessary to decrease risk of renal failure.

Glucarpidase has been approved for the treatment of toxic plasma MTX concentrations in patients with delayed MTX clearance because of impaired renal function. It is important to note that MTX concentrations within 48 hours after glucarpidase administration can only be reliably measured by chromatographic methods. Immunoassays can overestimate MTX concentration because of interference from metabolites.[36]

Pralatrexate Pralatrexate is an antifolate drug approved for patients with relapsed or refractory peripheral T-cell leukemias. It competitively inhibits DHFR. It is also a competitive inhibitor for polyglutamylation by the enzyme folylpolyglutamyl synthetase. This inhibition results in the depletion of thymidine and other synthesis of biological molecules that depends on single carbon transfer.[37]

Pemetrexed Pemetrexed is a multitargeted antifolate that inhibits at least three biosynthetic pathways in thymidine and purine synthesis. In addition to inhibiting DHFR, it also inhibits thymidine synthase and glycinamide ribonucleotide formyltransferase, decreasing the risk of the development of drug resistance. Severe hematologic toxicity and deaths associated with neutropenic sepsis have been reported in clinical trials. Elevated baseline cystathionine or homocysteine concentrations correlated with this unexpected toxicity. Routine supplementation of folic acid and vitamin B_{12} lowers levels of these substances and lowers the risk of mortality related to neutropenic sepsis. The approved labeling of pemetrexed requires administration of folic acid and vitamin B_{12} throughout the duration of treatment.[27]

Microtubule-Targeting Drugs

Vinca Alkaloids

Vincristine, vinblastine, and vinorelbine are natural alkaloids derived from the periwinkle (vinca) plant. They act as mitotic inhibitors, or "spindle poisons." Although the alkaloids are very similar structurally, they have different activities and patterns of toxicity. Whereas vinorelbine and vinblastine are associated with dose-limiting myelosuppression, vincristine causes mild myelosuppressive effects but is more neurotoxic.

Vinca alkaloids bind to tubulin, the structural protein that polymerizes to form microtubules. These hollow tubes make up the mitotic spindle and are important in nerve conduction and neurotransmission. Vinca alkaloids disrupt the normal balance between polymerization and depolymerization of microtubules, inhibiting assembly of microtubules and disrupting microtubule dynamics. This interferes with formation of the mitotic spindle and causes cells to accumulate in mitosis. They also disturb a variety of microtubule-related processes in cells and induce apoptosis. Resistance to the vinca alkaloids develops primarily from P-glycoprotein (Pgp)–mediated multidrug resistance, which decreases drug accumulation and retention within cancer cells.[38]

Taxanes

Paclitaxel and docetaxel are taxane plant alkaloids with antimitotic activity. Paclitaxel was isolated from the bark of the Pacific yew tree, *Taxus brevifolia*, but is now produced semisynthetically from the needles of the European yew, *Taxus baccata*. Docetaxel is a semisynthetic taxoid extracted from 10-deacetyl baccatin III, a noncytotoxic precursor found in the renewable needle biomass of yew plants.[38]

Paclitaxel and docetaxel both act by binding to tubulin, but unlike the vinca alkaloids, they do not interfere with tubulin assembly. Instead, the taxanes promote microtubule assembly and therefore interfere with microtubule disassembly. They induce tubulin polymerization, resulting in formation of inappropriately stable, nonfunctional microtubules. The stability of the microtubules damages cells by disrupting the dynamics of microtubule-dependent structures required for mitosis and other cellular functions. Taxanes also have some nonmitotic actions that can promote cancer cell death, such as inhibition of angiogenesis. Resistance to the antitumor effects of the taxanes is attributable to alterations in tubulin or tubulin binding sites or to Pgp multidrug resistance. Although paclitaxel and docetaxel have very similar mechanisms of action, cross-resistance between the two chemotherapies is incomplete.[38] Myelosuppression is common with both taxanes, but other adverse events can differ. While increased fluid retention is seen with docetaxel, increased neurotoxicity and hypersensitivity reactions are seen with paclitaxel.[27,38] Both require premedications with corticosteroids; paclitaxel also requires antihistamines to decrease the likelihood of hypersensitivity reactions.

To circumvent the hypersensitivity reactions with paclitaxel and to possibly increase its efficacy, paclitaxel was formulated to be bound to albumin (nab-paclitaxel). This new dosage form is devoid of the Cremophor excipient that is believed to mediate the hypersensitivity reactions and exacerbate myelosuppression with the conventional formulation. This formulation appears to be selectively activated by cancer cells to the active paclitaxel compound.[39] In clinical trials, nab-paclitaxel has shown comparable activity to the conventional formulation of paclitaxel with a lower incidence of hypersensitivity reactions. Peripheral neuropathies remain a common adverse event with this formulation.

Cabazitaxel is a new semisynthetic derivative of docetaxel that has been demonstrated to elicit an antitumor response in tumors resistant to paclitaxel and docetaxel despite having the same mechanism of action. This is partially because of its lack of affinity for Pgp mentioned earlier that allows cabazitaxel to remain inside the cancer cells. Adverse events and premedications are similar to traditional taxanes.[40]

Epothilones

Similar to the taxanes, the epothilones work in the M phase of the cell cycle. Epothilone binding to microtubules is distinct from taxanes with activity demonstrated in paclitaxel-resistant cell lines.[41] Epothilones appear to be poor substrates for Pgp and their cytotoxicity is not affected by its overexpression. Natural epothilones are macrolide derivatives that have stability and pharmacokinetic problems. Synthetic anticancer agents have been developed with the epothilone, ixabepilone, approved for the treatment of metastatic breast cancer. Toxicities are similar to those of the taxanes; premedication with antihistamines are required, although no corticosteroid is administered unless the patient experiences a hypersensitivity reaction to a previous dose.

Halichondrins

Eribulin is a nontaxane antimicrotuble analogue of the macrolide halichondrin B. It was originally isolated from the marine sponge *Halichondria okadai* but is now fully synthetic. Similar to the vinca alkaloids, eribulin inhibits tubulin polymerization by inhibiting microtubule growth; however, in contrast, it does not shorten or promote depolymerization of microtubules.[42] Additionally, eribulin only binds to the β-tubulin subunit and has demonstrated the ability to overcome taxane resistance conferred by β-tubulin mutations.[42] Adverse events are similar to those of vinblastine (e.g., neutropenia), with a decreased incidence of neuropathy compared with vincristine and taxanes.

Estramustine

Estramustine is an unusual drug, because it structurally combines the alkylating agent *nor*-nitrogen mustard with estradiol.[27] It was designed with the intent that the estradiol portion of the molecule would facilitate uptake of the alkylating agent into hormone-sensitive prostate cancer cells. Despite the inclusion of an alkylator, estramustine does not function in vivo as an alkylating agent. The estradiol is released after its administration and is responsible for most of the toxicity associated with estramustine, but it is not believed to contribute to its cytotoxic effect. In the mid 1980s, estramustine was redefined as an antimicrotubule agent. It binds covalently to microtubule-associated proteins that are part of the structural support for microtubules. The binding causes the separation of microtubule-associated proteins from the microtubules, inhibiting microtubule assembly and eventually causing their disassembly.[27]

Topoisomerase Inhibitors

Topoisomerases are essential enzymes involved in maintaining DNA topologic structure during replication and transcription. DNA topoisomerase enzymes relieve torsional strain during DNA unwinding by producing strand breaks. They cleave DNA strands and form intermediates with the strands, producing a gap through which DNA strands can pass, and then reseal the strand breaks. Topoisomerase I produces single-strand breaks; topoisomerase II produces double-strand breaks.[43] Several important anticancer agents interact with topoisomerase enzymes: camptothecins, anthracyclines, and the epipodophyllotoxins.

Camptothecin Derivatives

The camptothecin analogs irinotecan and topotecan were synthesized to reduce toxicity and improve therapeutic effects of camptothecin, a plant alkaloid derived from *Camptotheca acuminata*. Topotecan and irinotecan, through its active metabolite SN-38, inhibit topoisomerase I enzyme activity. Topoisomerase I enzymes stabilize DNA single-strand breaks and inhibit strand resealing.[43,44] Irinotecan undergoes metabolism to SN-38 by the polymorphic enzyme uridine diphosphate glucosyltransferase, and variant tandem repeats in the promoter of this gene are associated with a higher risk of diarrhea and neutropenia.

Etoposide and Teniposide

Etoposide and teniposide are semisynthetic podophyllotoxin derivatives that bind to tubulin and interfere with microtubule formation. Etoposide and teniposide also damage cancer cells by causing strand breakage through inhibition of topoisomerase II.[43] Resistance may be caused by differences in topoisomerase II levels, increased cell ability to repair strand breaks, or increased levels of Pgp. Etoposide and teniposide are usually clinically cross-resistant. They are cell-cycle phase specific and arrest cells in the S or early G_2 phase. As a result, activity is much greater when they are administered in divided doses over several days rather than in large single doses.

Anthracene Derivatives

The most widely used and best understood anthracene derivative is doxorubicin (Adriamycin or "Adria"). Other members of the anthracene group include daunorubicin (daunomycin), idarubicin, epirubicin, and mitoxantrone. All of these derivatives, except mitoxantrone, are anthracyclines and share a common, four-membered anthracene ring complex with an attached aglycone or sugar portion. The ring complex is a chromophore and accounts for the intense colors of these derivatives.[43,45]

Doxorubicin, Daunorubicin, Idarubicin, and Epirubicin Anthracyclines are classified as antitumor antibiotics, but they have multiple mechanisms of action. Although anthracyclines can intercalate into DNA and cause structural changes that interfere with DNA and RNA synthesis, this is not their primary mechanism of cytotoxicity. Intercalating anticancer agents insert or stack between base pairs of DNA. However, anthracyclines primarily inhibit topoisomerase II, producing double-strand DNA breaks.[27,43,45]

The anthracyclines also undergo electron reductions to reactive compounds that can damage DNA and cell membranes. Free radicals formed from reduction of the anthracyclines first donate electrons to oxygen to make superoxide, which can react with itself to make hydrogen peroxide. Cleavage of hydrogen peroxide produces the highly reactive and destructive hydroxyl radical. This last step requires iron, and anthracyclines are potent iron binders. Iron–anthracycline complexes can then bind to DNA and react rapidly with hydrogen peroxide to produce the hydroxyl radicals that actually cleave DNA. Human cells have natural defenses against oxygen radical damage, in the form of enzymes that can convert the radicals to less reactive compounds, or that can repair DNA damage. Differences in distribution of these defensive enzymes may account for the cumulative dose limiting cardiotoxicity associated with anthracyclines. For example, cardiac muscle has low levels of defensive enzymes and high levels of enzymes that activate anthracyclines. Oxygen free-radical formation is firmly established as a cause of cardiac damage and extravasation injury but is not a major mechanism of tumor-cell killing. Resistance to anthracyclines is usually secondary to Pgp-dependent multidrug resistance. Altered topoisomerase II activity may contribute to the development of resistance.[27,45]

Mitoxantrone Mitoxantrone was synthesized in an attempt to develop a chemotherapy with comparable antitumor activity to doxorubicin but with an improved safety profile. Similar to the anthracyclines, mitoxantrone is an intercalating topoisomerase II inhibitor, but its potential for free-radical formation is much less than that of the anthracyclines. This decreased tendency for free-radical formation may explain the reduced risks of cardiac toxicity and ulceration after extravasation.[27,45]

Alkylating Agents

The alkylating agents are among the oldest and most useful classes of anticancer agents. Their clinical use evolved from the observation of bone marrow suppression and lymph node shrinkage in soldiers exposed to sulfur mustard gas warfare during World War I.[27] In an effort to develop similar agents that might be useful in treating cancerous overgrowths of lymphoid tissues, less reactive derivatives were synthesized. Their effectiveness as anticancer agents was confirmed by clinical trials in the mid-1940s.

All alkylating agents work by covalently bonding to highly reactive alkyl groups or substituted alkyl groups with nucleophilic groups of proteins and nucleic acids. Some agents react directly with biologic molecules, but others form an intermediate compound that reacts with these molecules. The most common binding site for alkylating agents is the seven-nitrogen group of the DNA base guanine. These covalent interactions result in cross-linking between two DNA strands or between two bases in the same strand of DNA. Reactions between DNA and RNA and between drug and proteins may also occur, but the main insult that results in cell death is inhibition of DNA replication because the interlinked strands do not separate as required. Because the alkylating agents can damage DNA during any phase of the cell cycle, they are not cell-cycle phase specific. However, their greatest effect is seen in rapidly dividing cells.

As a class, alkylators are cytotoxic, mutagenic, teratogenic, carcinogenic, and myelosuppressive. Resistance to these chemotherapies can occur from increased DNA repair capabilities, decreased entry into or accelerated exit from cells, increased inactivation inside cells, or lack of cellular mechanisms to result in cell death after DNA damage. They react with water and are inactivated by hydrolysis, making spontaneous degradation an important component of their elimination.[46]

Nitrogen Mustards

Cyclophosphamide and Ifosfamide Cyclophosphamide and ifosfamide are nitrogen mustard derivatives and are widely used in the treatment of solid tumors and hematologic malignancies. These mustards are closely related in structure, clinical use, and toxicity. Neither agent is active in its parent form and must be activated by cytochrome P450 (CYP) enzymes. One of the active metabolites of cyclophosphamide is phosphoramide mustard and of ifosfamide is ifosfamide mustard. The CYP-mediated metabolites 4-hydroxycyclophosphamide and 4-hydroxyifosfamide are also cytotoxic compounds. Acrolein, a metabolite of both cyclophosphamide and ifosfamide, has little antitumor activity, but is responsible for the hemorrhagic cystitis associated with ifosfamide and sometimes high-dose cyclophosphamide.[46] Encephalopathy after ifosfamide can occur within 48 to 72 hours after the infusion and is reversible. The increased production of dechloroethylated metabolites after administration of ifosfamide compared with cyclophosphamide may explain the increased risk of CNS toxicity associated with ifosfamide.[47]

Bendamustine Bendamustine is an alkylating agent (nitrogen mustard derivative) with a benzimidazole ring (purine analog) that demonstrates only partial cross-resistance (in vitro) with other alkylating agents.[48] It leads to cell death via single- and double-strand DNA cross-linking, and it is active against quiescent and dividing cells. The primary cytotoxic activity is due to bendamustine rather than its metabolites. It is used primarily to treat lymphoid malignancies, such as chronic lymphocytic leukemia (CLL) and NHL.

Nitrosoureas

The nitrosoureas are alkylating agents characterized by lipophilicity and ability to cross the blood–brain barrier. Carmustine or bischloroethylnitrosourea (BCNU) and lomustine (CCNU) are commercially available. BCNU is available as an IV preparation and as a drug-impregnated biodegradable wafer (Gliadel) for direct application to residual tumor tissue after surgical resection of brain tumors. The nitrosoureas decompose to reactive alkylating metabolites and to isocyanate compounds that have several effects on reproducing cells.[46]

Nonclassic Alkylating Agents

Several other cytotoxic chemotherapies appear to act as alkylators, although their structures do not include the classic alkylating groups. They are capable of binding covalently to cellular components and include procarbazine, dacarbazine, temozolomide, and the heavy metal compounds.[46]

Dacarbazine and Temozolomide Dacarbazine and temozolomide are nonclassic alkylating agents. Both compounds undergo demethylation to the same active intermediate (monomethyl triazeno-imidazole-carboxamide [MTIC]) that interrupts DNA replication by causing methylation of guanine. Unlike dacarbazine, temozolomide does not require the liver for activation and is chemically degraded to MTIC at physiologic pH. Both agents inhibit DNA, RNA, and protein synthesis.[27,46]

Important pharmacokinetic differences exist between these two agents. Dacarbazine is poorly absorbed and must be administered by IV infusion. Temozolomide is rapidly absorbed after oral administration and is nearly 100% bioavailable when given on a completely empty stomach. Dacarbazine penetrates the CNS poorly, but temozolomide readily crosses the blood–brain barrier, achieving therapeutically active concentrations in cerebrospinal fluid and brain tumor tissues.[27,46]

Cisplatin, Carboplatin, and Oxaliplatin The platinum derivatives—cisplatin, carboplatin, and oxaliplatin—are anticancer agents with remarkable usefulness in cancer treatment. Recognition of cisplatin's cytotoxic activity was the result of a serendipitous observation that bacterial growth in culture was altered when an electric current was delivered to the media through platinum electrodes. The growth change was noted to be similar to that produced by alkylating agents and radiation. It was found that a platinum–chloride complex, now known as cisplatin, generated by the current was responsible for the changes. Carboplatin is a structural analog of cisplatin in which the chloride groups of the parent compound are replaced by a carboxycyclobutane moiety. It shares a similar spectrum of clinical activity with cisplatin, and cross-resistance is common. Oxaliplatin is an organoplatinum compound in which the platinum is complexed with an oxalate ligand as the leaving group and to diaminocyclohexane. Its spectrum of activity differs substantially from the other platinum compounds and includes notable activity against colorectal cancers.[27,46]

The cytotoxicity of the platinum derivatives depends on platinum binding to DNA and the formation of intrastrand cross-links or adducts between neighboring guanines. These intrastrand links cause a major bending of the DNA. They may cause cellular damage by distorting the normal DNA conformation and preventing bases that are normally paired from lining up with each other. Interstrand cross-links also occur.[27,46]

The cytotoxic form of cisplatin is the aquated species in which hydroxyl groups or water molecules replace the two chloride groups. This reaction occurs readily in low concentrations of chloride, such as the concentrations present within cells, and produces a positively charged compound that can react with DNA. The aquated species is responsible for both the efficacy and toxicity of cisplatin. Carboplatin also undergoes aquation but at a slower rate. Oxaliplatin becomes active when the oxalate ligand is displaced in physiologic solutions.[27,46]

Resistance to the therapeutic effects of platinum compounds may occur through several mechanisms. The ability to repair platinum-induced DNA damage may be increased, or the compounds may be inactivated by increased levels of intracellular glutathione, metallothioneins, or other thiol-containing proteins. Altered uptake into cells may also affect sensitivity to platinum compounds.[27,46]

Cisplatin is a highly toxic anticancer agent that can cause serious nephrotoxicity, ototoxicity, peripheral neuropathy, emesis, and anemia. The significant efficacy of cisplatin against many tumors makes it a valuable agent despite these toxicities, most of which can be prevented or managed with aggressive supportive care measures.[27] In contrast, carboplatin administration is limited by hematologic toxicity. Patients with compromised renal function require dose reductions to limit myelosuppressive toxicity.[27,46] The most widely used dosage schema, the Calvert formula (Table 104-9), uses a target area under the curve and renal function parameters to estimate the carboplatin dose. Carboplatin's potential to cause renal damage, peripheral neuropathy, ototoxicity, and nausea and vomiting is much less than that of comparable cisplatin doses.[46] Oxaliplatin is not nephrotoxic or ototoxic and is moderately emetogenic, but it can cause peripheral neuropathies and unique cold-induced neuropathies.[49] All of the platinum derivatives have potential to cause hypersensitivity reactions, including anaphylaxis, after a threshold exposure is reached.

TABLE 104-9 Dosing Formulas for Chemotherapy

DuBois and DuBois
BSA (m^2) = Wt (kg)$^{0.425}$ × Ht (cm)$^{0.725}$ × 0.007184
Mosteller
BSA (m^2) = $\sqrt{(\text{Ht (cm)} \times \text{Wt (kg)}/3600)}$
Calvert (for carboplatin)
Dose (mg)^a = AUC^b × (CrCl^c + 25)

[a]Note that the dose is in total milligrams to be administered, not mg/m^2.
[b]AUC needs to be stated in the dosing protocol.
[c]Cockcroft and Gault equation often clinically used.
AUC, area-under-the-curve; BSA, body surface area; CrCl, creatinine clearance in mL/min; Ht, height; Wt, weight.

Data from Haskell CM. Principles of cancer chemotherapy. In: Haskell CM, ed. Cancer Treatment, 5th ed. Philadelphia, PA: WB Saunders, 2001:62–86.

Endocrine Therapies

Perhaps the earliest successful approach to target the growth processes of cancer cells was the use of endocrine therapies. Endocrine manipulation is an option for management of cancers from tissues whose growth is under gonadal hormonal control, especially breast, prostate, and endometrial cancers. These cancers may regress if the "feeding" hormone is eliminated or antagonized. Major organ system toxicity is uncommon from endocrine therapies, making it the least toxic of systemic anticancer agents. Specific anticancer agents such as the selective estrogen receptor modulators (SERMs) and aromatase inhibitors (AIs) have increased the utility of hormonal therapies in the treatment of cancer.[50–52] These therapies are discussed in detail in Chapters 105 and 108 (Table 104-8).

Corticosteroids are also useful anticancer agents because of their lymphotoxic effects. Their primary use is in management of hematologic malignancies, especially lymphoid malignancies such as lymphomas, lymphocytic leukemias, and multiple myeloma. In addition to their cytotoxic effects, corticosteroids have many other applications as supportive care. Corticosteroids have diverse toxicities in chronic or high-dose use, but are generally well tolerated in the short-term therapies usually used in cancer patient care.[53]

Miscellaneous Agents

Bleomycin

Bleomycin is an antitumor antibiotic. It is a mixture of peptides from fungal *Streptomyces* species and its strength is expressed in units of drug activity.[27] One unit is roughly equal to 1 mg of polypeptide protein. The predominant peptide is bleomycin A2, which makes up about 70% of the commercial drug product. Its cytotoxicity is secondary to DNA strand breakage, or scission, which it produces via free-radical formation. Cytotoxicity depends on binding of the bleomycin–iron complex to DNA. The bleomycin–iron complex then reduces molecular oxygen to free oxygen radicals that cause primarily single-strand breaks in DNA. Bleomycin has greatest effect on cells in the G_2 and M phases of the cell cycle.[27]

Bleomycin is inactivated within cells by the enzyme aminohydrolase. This enzyme is widely distributed but is present in only low concentrations in the skin and the lungs, explaining the predominant toxicities of bleomycin to those sites. Baseline pulmonary function tests and monitoring for pulmonary toxicity are necessary during bleomycin therapy. The presence of hydrolase enzymes in cancer cells is the primary mechanism of resistance to bleomycin. Cells can also become resistant by repairing the DNA breaks produced by bleomycin.[27]

Hydroxyurea

Hydroxyurea is a unique drug that inhibits ribonucleotide reductase. Cells accumulate in the S phase, because DNA synthesis is inhibited and only abnormally short DNA strands are produced.[30] This drug is often used to cause a rapid decline in a patient's white blood cells (WBCs) before more potent chemotherapy is initiated.

Arsenic Trioxide

Arsenic is an organic element and a well-known poison that is an effective treatment for acute promyelocytic leukemia.[54] As an anticancer agent, arsenic trioxide acts as a differentiating agent, inducing the growth progression of cancerous cells into mature, more normal cells. It also induces programmed cell death or apoptosis. This chemotherapy is discussed in more detail in Chapter 111.

Retinoids

Vitamin A and its metabolites, collectively referred to as the retinoids, play important roles in numerous biologic processes, including normal cellular differentiation. Because cancerous growth is characterized by abnormal cellular differentiation, retinoids may play important therapeutic roles in the treatment and perhaps in the prevention of cancers. Tretinoin (all-*trans*-retinoic acid) is a naturally occurring derivative of vitamin A (retinol). Other retinoids indicated for treatment of cancers include alitretinoin (9-*cis*-retinoic acid), available in gel form for topical management of Kaposi's sarcoma lesions, and bexarotene (Targretin®) gel or capsules for treatment of cutaneous T-cell lymphoma.[27,55]

Retinoids are classed as morphogens, small molecules released from one type of cell that can affect the growth and differentiation of neighboring cells. Their normal roles in the human body are to induce differentiation of some cells, stop the differentiation of others, and both suppress and induce apoptosis in different cell types. Their diverse actions come from the diversity of their receptors. The two classes of retinoid receptors are retinoid X receptors (RXRs) and retinoic acid receptors (RARs), each with α, β, and γ subclasses. RXRs are versatile; they bind to RARs and to other nuclear receptors, such as thyroid hormone receptors. After being activated, the receptors act as transcription factors that in turn regulate the expression of genes that control cellular growth and differentiation.[27,55]

Tretinoin binds primarily to the RAR-α receptors. Alitretinoin is considered a panagonist, which means that it binds to all known retinoid receptors, producing diverse regulatory effects. Bexarotene is synthetic and is classed as a rexinoid. It is the first RXR-selective retinoid agonist. The exact mechanism of action of alitretinoin and bexarotene as anticancer agents is unknown.[27,55]

Mitomycin C

Mitomycin C is a natural product that is sometimes classified as an antitumor antibiotic.[46,56] It has similarities to nitrogen mustard compounds and may function as an alkylating agent, although its toxicity pattern differs from conventional alkylating agents.

Omacetaxine Mepesuccinate

Omacetaxine mepesuccinate (previously referred to as homoharringtonine) is a plant alkaloid that inhibits protein translation, thus preventing the initial elongation step of protein synthesis. It appears to decreases cancer stem cells; proliferation proteins; and cell survival proteins, such as c-MYC, in chronic myeloid leukemia (CML) cells *in vitro*. Omacetaxine was approved for the treatment of patients with CML who have failed two or more approved targeted drugs for this disease. Additionally, synergy with these inhibitors has been demonstrated in a few clinical studies. and additional combination trials are ongoing.[57]

CLINICAL PHARMACOLOGY OF TARGETED DRUGS

BCR-ABL Inhibitors

Imatinib

Imatinib is a selective inhibitor of the tyrosine kinase activity of *BCR-ABL* fusion gene, the product of the Philadelphia chromosome.[58] The Philadelphia chromosome is the hallmark finding of CML and is a translocation of genetic material between chromosomes 9 and 22. Imatinib binds to the kinase binding site of the *BCR-ABL* gene, competitively blocking access to adenosine triphosphate (ATP). This prevents tyrosine-kinase phosphorylation of the gene and downstream activation of cellular proliferation.[59] Imatinib also causes apoptosis or arrest of growth in cells expressing *BCR-ABL*. An additional effect of imatinib is its ability in blocking the tyrosine kinase activity of c-KIT (stem-cell factor receptor) and platelet-derived growth factor receptor (PDGFR).[58,60]

Imatinib is a standard treatment option for newly diagnosed Philadelphia chromosome–positive (Ph^+) CML and for c-KIT–positive gastrointestinal stromal tumors (GIST). A major advantage of imatinib is that it can eliminate the Philadelphia chromosome, resulting in cytogenetic responses (elimination of the genetic defect). Imatinib and the other *BCR-ABL* inhibitors are further discussed in Chapter 112. Imatinib is also approved for the treatment of (Ph^+) acute lymphoblastic leukemia (ALL) and other rare diseases.

Adverse events observed with imatinib are usually mild to moderate in severity. Severe fluid retention (pleural effusion, pericardial effusion, and ascites) occurs in fewer than 10% of patients taking imatinib. Patients should be monitored regularly for early signs and symptoms of fluid retention (leg swelling, shoes no longer fitting, and shortness of breath) and instructed to call their healthcare providers when symptoms first develop. Additional adverse events include mild or moderate superficial edema, elevation of liver enzymes, nausea, muscle cramps, headache, and rash.[61] A rash may require early intervention because rare cases of Stevens-Johnson's syndrome have been reported with imatinib and may require permanent discontinuation of imatinib.[61]

Dasatinib, Nilotinib, and Bosutinib

These targeted drugs are next-generation tyrosine kinase inhibitors (TKIs) that share the same binding site on the BCR-ABL tyrosine kinase ATP-binding domain with imatinib.[62,63] These inhibitors maintain clinical activity in patients with CML with some mutations in the BCR-ABL binding site that confer imatinib resistance with the exception of one polymorphism (T351I) in which all four inhibitors appear resistant. Nilotinib and dasatinib are approved for the treatment of patients with CML resistant or intolerant to imatinib in addition to approval for first-line treatment of newly diagnosed CML. These two inhibitors are also approved for the treatment of (Ph^+) ALL. Bosutinib is approved for the treatment of patients resistant or intolerant to the other inhibitors. Both bosutinib and dasatinb also inhibit a family of tyrosine kinases called SRC kinases that are believed to mediate cellular differentiation, proliferation, and survival; SRC kinases have been implicated in modulating multiple oncogenic signal transduction pathways.[59,63]

Overall, these targeted drugs have a toxicity profile similar to that of imatinib with myelosuppression, nausea and vomiting, headache, and fluid retention being commonly reported, although bosutinib does not inhibit the c-KIT or PDGFR, which may account for its reported decrease in myelosuppression.[63] Similar to other TKIs, these anticancer agents could interact with substrates, inducers, or inhibitors of multiple CYP enzymes.

Ponatinib

As mentioned earlier, the T351I mutation, often referred to as the gatekeeper mutation, confers resistance to the above TKIs of BCR-ABL. Ponatinib was developed using a computational chemistry–based approach to inhibit this mutated conformation of BCR-ABL as well as nonmutated forms providing an effective treatment for this traditional resistant tumor.[64] Ponatinib is also approved for patients with (Ph^+) ALL that is resistant or intolerant to prior therapy. The more common adverse events reported are similar to other TKIs, such as hypertension, rash, headache, constipation, fever, and nausea. Arterial thrombosis and hepatic toxicity have been observed.

Histone Deacteylase Inhibitors

Vorinostat and romidepsin both inhibit HDAC; these inhibitors likely inhibit class I and II HDAC enzymes. As described in the section on epigenetics, HDAC catalyzes the removal of acetyl groups from the lysine residues of proteins, including histones and transcription factors.[21,65] By inhibiting HDAC activity, these inhibitors cause the accumulation of acetylated histones and induce cell-cycle arrest and apoptosis of tumor cells. Romidepsin is approved for the treatment of patients with cutaneous T-cell lymphoma who have received at least one prior therapy, and vorinostat is approved for the treatment of patients with cutaneous T-cell lymphoma who have received at least two prior therapies. Adverse events observed with romidepsin include nausea, vomiting, arrhythmias, and infection. Adverse events reported with vorinostat include pulmonary embolism and deep vein thrombosis along with dose-related thrombocytopenia and anemia; other adverse events that have been reported are nausea, diarrhea, hypertriglyceridemia, and hyperuricemia, hypoglycemia, hypokalemia, hyponatremia, hyperkalemia, hypercholesterolemia, hypophosphatemia, and proteinuria.

DNA Methyltransferase Inhibitors

Azacytidine and decitabine are approved for the treatment of patients with myelodysplastic syndrome, a disorder of hematopoietic cell maturation that can progress to AML (see Chap. 114). These agents are nucleoside analogs that demonstrate dose-dependent effects. At lower doses, these analogs exert their effects by directly incorporating into DNA and inhibiting DNMT, which leads to cellular differentiation and apoptosis.[24] At higher doses, these agents might cause the formation of covalent adducts between DNMT and active drug being incorporated into DNA, particularly in cells actively dividing. Hypomethylation also appears to normalize the function of genes that control cell differentiation and proliferation, promoting normal cell maturation.[66]

These inhibitors have demonstrated efficacy in slowing the progression of myelodysplastic syndrome to AML, reducing transfusion requirements, and allowing for the improvement of normal hematopoiesis over time. The primary toxicity is myelosuppression, particularly during early phases of treatment as the malignant clone driving the myelodysplastic syndrome is cleared from the bone marrow and normal hematopoiesis is slowly restored. As a result, infectious complications occur frequently.

mTOR Pathway Inhibitors

Temsirolimus

Temsirolimus binds to the intracellular protein FKBP-12, and this protein–drug complex inhibits mTOR by blocking its kinase activity.[26] mTOR inhibition suppresses the production of proteins that regulate progression through the cell cycle and angiogenesis as described earlier in this chapter. Temsirolimus is approved for metastatic renal cell carcinoma.

The most common adverse reactions with temsirolimus are rash, fatigue, mucositis, nausea, edema, and loss of appetite. The most common laboratory abnormalities are increases in serum creatinine and liver function test results, thrombocytopenia, and neutropenia. Additionally, hyperglycemia and hyperlipidemia that require monitoring of glucose and lipid profiles should be expected.[26] Rare but potentially serious adverse events include interstitial lung disease, immunosuppression (and infection), and renal failure. Temsirolimus is metabolized by CYP3A4, and possible drug interactions requiring dosage adjustments may be necessary.

Everolimus

Everolimus is an oral mTOR inhibitor that is approved for the treatment of patients with advanced renal cell carcinoma after failure of treatment with sunitinib or sorafenib, postmenopausal women with breast cancer in combination with exemestane after failure of treatment with letrozole or anastrozole, adult and pediatric patients with subependymal giant cell astrocytoma with tubular sclerosis complex (TSC), patients with renal angiomyolipoma and TSC, and patients with pancreatic neuroendocrine tumors.[26] It is available as traditional oral tablets and tablets for oral suspension. Adverse reactions and potential drug interactions are similar to those of temsirolimus. Drug interactions with inducers or inhibitors of CYP3A4 and inhibitors of Pgp might warrant discontinuation of the concomitant drug or a reduced dose of everolimus.

Epidermal Growth Factor Receptor Pathway Inhibitors

Erlotinib

Erlotinib is an oral selective EGFR TKI. By competing with ATP for its binding site on the EGFR tyrosine kinase cytosolic domain, it blocks the intracellular downstream signaling and ultimately interferes with the proliferation and growth of cancer cells.[67,68]

Erlotinib is indicated for the treatment of patients with locally advanced or metastatic NSCLC as a second-line agent.[68] It appears effective in patients with or without EGFR-activating mutations, but it appears to be more effective in patients with EGFR-activating mutations.[69] Erlotinib is also approved for use in pancreatic cancer in combination with gemcitabine. Erlotinib has also demonstrated activity in a variety of other tumors, such as head and neck and brain tumors.

Rash and diarrhea are the most common adverse events reported with erlotinib. Some studies suggest that the development of a rash may be predictive of a response to therapy and correlates with clinical benefit.[70] Interstitial lung disease is a rare adverse event reported in patients taking erlotinib. Possible drug interactions include warfarin and CYP3A4 inhibitors or inducers.

Lapatinib

Lapatinib is a 4-anilinoquinazoline kinase inhibitor that inhibits the intracellular kinase domains of both EGFR and HER2.[71] It has demonstrated clinical activity in combination with capecitabine in patients with breast cancer who overexpress HER2 and who have previously received therapy with trastuzumab, an anthracycline, and a taxane.[71] Toxicity for lapatinib was notable for an increased incidence of diarrhea, hepatotoxicity, rash, and QT interval prolongation. Lapatinib has significant CYP-mediated interactions. A specific mutation observed in the HLA-DQA gene has been associated with an increased risk of hepatotoxicity.[72]

Multikinase Inhibitors

Sunitinib, Sorafenib, Pazopanib, and Axitinib

Sunitinib and sorafenib inhibit multiple growth factor receptors (VEGFR-2 and PDGFR), cell surface proteins (c-KIT), and cytokine receptors (FLT3) and thus disrupt multiple aberrant intracellular signaling pathways. In addition, sorafenib inhibits Raf, which is part of the MAPK signaling pathway as described earlier.[73] Sunitinib is approved for GIST and pancreatic neuroendocrine tumors and, sorafenib is approved for metastatic hepatocellular cancers.

Pazopanib and axitinib are second-generation inhibitors. Pazopanib inhibits VEGFR-1, -2, and -3 with additional activity against c-KIT and PDGFR, and axitinib has enhanced potency and selectivity to all VEGFR tyrosine kinases (VEGFR-1, -2, and -3) with minor activity against PDGFR and c-KIT.[74,75] These drugs are approved for the treatment of advanced renal cell cancers. Ponatinib is also approved from sarcomas.

Gastrointestinal adverse events such as diarrhea are common with these drugs, as are rash, fatigue, and hypertension (Table 104-8).

Regorafenib

Regorafenib is an oral multikinase inhibitor that blocks the activity of several protein kinases, including those involved in the regulation of tumor angiogenesis (VEGFR-1, -2, and -3), oncogenes and downstream targets (c-KIT, RET, RAF1, and BRAF), as well as PDGFR and fibroblast growth factor receptor (FGFR).[76] Because many of these targets are important in colon cancer, regorafenib has demonstrated activity and is approved for the treatment of patients with metastatic colorectal cancer. Serious adverse events reported with regorafenib include hepatotoxicity, hemorrhage, and gastrointestinal perforation.

Vandetanib

Vandetanib is a small molecule inhibitor of RET, VEGFR-2 and -3, and EGFR.[77] Because most medullary thyroid cancers express mutated RET, vandetanib has demonstrated activity in this tumor. It is approved for the treatment of metastatic medullary thyroid cancer. Observed adverse events include diarrhea, hypertension, rash, and QT interval prolongation.

Cabozantinib

Cabozantinib is a small molecule inhibitor of numerous receptor kinases, most importantly the RET, VEGFR-2, and the MET membrane receptor.[78] MET is required for several important processes during embryogenesis (e.g., angiogenesis) but leads to abnormal growth and proliferation of several tumors. Because medullary thyroid cancers express mutated RET as well as VEGFR-2 and MET, cabozanitinib has demonstrated activity in this tumor. Cabozantinib is approved for the treatment of patients with metastatic medullary thyroid cancers. Its clinical activity in prostate cancer and other tumors is currently being evaluated. Adverse events reported in clinical trials included diarrhea, hand–foot syndrome, lymphopenia, hypocalcemia, hypertension, transaminitis, and stomatitis.

Proteasome Inhibitors

The proteasome is an enzyme complex that is responsible for degrading proteins that control the cell cycle. Some of the proteins degraded by proteosomes regulate critical functions for cancer growth, such as regulation of the cell cycle, transcription factors, apoptosis, angiogenesis, and cell adhesion.[14]

Bortezomib

Bortezomib has very specific affinity for the catalytic portion of the 26S proteasome. It is a specific inhibitor of this proteasome, which results in accumulation of IκB, an inhibitor of the major transcription factor nuclear factor κB (NF-κB). NF-κB induces transcription of genes that block cell death pathways and promote cell proliferation. Its activity depends on its release from its inhibitory partner protein, IκB, in the cytoplasm and its move to the nucleus. When IκB fails to degrade, through the actions of bortezomib, NF-κB remains in the cytoplasm, preventing it from transcribing the genes that promote cancer growth. Bortezomib is approved for the treatment of multiple myeloma and mantle cell lymphoma.[14]

The most commonly reported adverse events are asthenia (fatigue, malaise, and weakness), nausea, and diarrhea, occurring in more than 50% of patients. Additional adverse events include decreased appetite, nausea, constipation, myelosuppression, peripheral neuropathies, and fever.[14] Most of these adverse events are mild to moderate and managed with supportive care measures. Of these common adverse events, severe adverse events were limited to thrombocytopenia, neutropenia, asthenia, and peripheral neuropathies. Bortezomib is administered every 72 hours to minimize cumulative toxicity by permitting the restoration of proteasome function between doses.

Carfilzomib

Carfilzomib is a second-generation proteasome inhibitor approved for relapsed or refractory multiple myeloma. Whereas it irreversibly and rapidly binds to the proteolytic core particle within the 26S proteasome, bortezomib exhibits reversible inhibition of multiple proteasome targets.[79] This decreases the systemic exposure to the drug while maintaining efficacy. Carfilzomib has been demonstrated to overcome bortezomib resistance in cell lines.

Miscellaneous

Thalidomide, Lenalidomide, and Pomalidomide

Thalidomide, the infamous drug that caused severe limb deformities (phocomelia or "seal limbs") when used by pregnant women as a nonprescription sedative in the 1960s, is approved for treatment of leprosy and multiple myeloma. Thalidomide is a glutamic acid derivative and is broadly classified as an immunomodulatory drug. Lenalidomide and pomalidomide are analogs of thalidomide with similar therapeutic activity but different adverse event profiles.[80] Lenalidomide has been approved for multiple myeloma in patients who have received prior therapy and in patients with transfusion-dependent anemia caused by myelodysplastic syndrome with a specific mutation. Pomalidomide has been approved for the treatment of patients with multiple myeloma with disease progression after prior therapy. These drugs have many potential mechanisms of action, with the main hypothesis thought to be through angiogenesis inhibition, an action also linked to its teratogenic effects. Other possible mechanisms include direct inhibition of cancer cells, free radical oxidative damage to DNA, interfering with adhesion of cancer cells, inhibiting TNF-α production, or altering secretion of cytokines that affect the growth of cancer cells.[80]

The most common adverse events for thalidomide include somnolence, constipation, dizziness, orthostatic hypotension, rash, and peripheral neuropathies. Neutropenia is extremely rare. In contrast, lenalidomide is associated with much less somnolence and neuropathies compared with thalidomide.[80] Neutropenia, thrombocytopenia, and thrombotic issues are prevalent with both lenalidomide and pomalidomide. Because these drugs are teratogenic, these drugs are only available under a special restricted distribution programs.

Crizotinib

Crizotinib binds to the ATP intracellular domain of activated anaplastic lymphoma kinase (ALK), thereby inhibiting phosphorylation and subsequent downstream signaling, similar to other targeted drugs. ALK rearrangements were first identified in large cell lymphomas and later in NSCLC (and a variety of other tumors). In NSCLC, the most common rearrangement involves inversion of chromosome 2p that is primarily fused to the echinoderm microtubule-like protein 4 (EML4), which forms the ALK-EML4 oncogene fusion protein. This rearrangement leads to the activation of downstream signaling pathways (through the Ras pathway) and inhibition of apoptosis.[81] Crizotinib also inhibits the c-MET tyrosine kinase. Crizotinib is approved for the treatment of patients with locally advanced or metastatic NSCLC that is ALK positive as detected by an approved test.

Vemurafenib

Vemurafenib is approved for the treatment of patients with previously untreated metastatic or unresectable melanoma with the BRAF V600E mutation as detected by an approved test, and it is in various stages of clinical trials in additional solid tumors (e.g., colon and thyroid cancers). The BRAF gene is mutated in a variety of solid tumors with most mutations occurring at codon 600. This codon is in the activation loop of BRAF and increases kinase activity and downstream proliferation of cancer cells. The V600E mutation (replacing valine with glutamic acid) is the most common V600 mutation and is seen in about 50% of all melanomas. Vemurafenib inhibits BRAF V600E and blocks downstream phosphorylation in BRAF-mutated cells. Cutaneous squamous cell carcinomas have been reported in patients treated with vemurafenib.[82]

Vismodegib

Vismodegib is an oral small molecule inhibitor of the Hedgehog signaling pathway that it is abnormally activated in a variety of solid tumors, including basal cell carcinoma, medulloblastoma, and ovarian cancers. This pathway is essential for early embryogenesis; therefore, both men and women must use highly effective contraception for up to at least 2 months after their last dose. Vismodegib binds to smoothened receptor (SMO), which prevents downstream signaling and activation of the Hedgehog pathway and inhibits tumor growth.[83] It is currently approved for metastatic basal cell cancer but is actively being investigated in a variety of solid tumors.

Ruxolitinib

Ruxolitinib is an oral inhibitor of JAK1 and JAK2 of the JAK-STAT signaling pathway; these kinases are involved in the regulation of blood and immunologic functioning. It is approved for the treatment of myelofibrosis. The most common adverse events include thrombocytopenia, anemia, dyspnea, headache, diarrhea, and nausea.[84]

CLINICAL PHARMACOLOGY OF BIOLOGIC THERAPIES

Biologic therapies include cytokines, MoABs, growth factors, and vaccines. MoABs are designed to target pathways critical for the survival and growth of cancer cells. These therapies are designed to improve outcomes while minimizing adverse events. MoABs can bind to either the extracellular receptor or to its natural ligand and prevent the activation of the downstream intracellular signaling. Several biologic therapies are available to treat both solid and hematologic malignancies.

8 MoABs consist of immunoglobulin sequences that are known to recognize a specific antigen or protein on the surface of cells. There are five classes of immunoglobulins (IgA, IgD, IgE, IgG, and IgM), with IgG the most commonly used therapeutically. The fundamental structure of all antibodies is identical and consists of two heavy and two light chains joined to form a molecule that resembles the letter Y. The variable region (Fab fragment) of antibodies differs greatly and is composed of three complementary determining regions. The Fab portion is composed of heavy (V_H) and light chains (V_L) that are responsible for binding to antigens. The constant region (Fc fragment) determines the effector function of the antibody.[85]

Two main classes of MoABs are used in the treatment of cancer, the most common of which are unconjugated or naked MoABs. The other class is immunoconjugates, in which MoABs are conjugated to a toxin (immunotoxin), chemotherapy (antibody drug conjugate), or radioactive particle (radioimmunoconjugate). MoABs may also be divided into agents that target cell surface antigens and those that target growth factor receptors or ligands.[85]

Standardized nomenclature exists for naming MoABs.[86] The suffix -mab is used for all MoABs and fragments and is always preceded by the identification of the animal source of the product. The letters *o*, *u*, *xi*, and *zu* before the -mab suffix indicate a murine, human, chimeric, and humanized, respectively. The general disease state the MoABs is treating precedes the source and is identified using a code. Currently, most approved MoABs used in cancer have the code syllabus *-tu(m)* that designates it for use against miscellaneous tumors. If the product is conjugated, a separate word is added for to identify the toxin, chemotherapy, or radioactive particle.

6 The first MoABs used in humans were murine, but most of the MoABs used today are chimeric, humanized or human. These agents differ in the amount of foreign component. Hypersensitivity and infusion-related reactions, with or without the development of antiproduct antibodies (APAs), are generally greatest with murine antibodies and least with humanized antibodies.[85,60] The severity of these reactions can range from mild (e.g., fever, chills, nausea, and rash) to severe, life-threatening anaphylaxis with cardiopulmonary collapse. Patients with a hypersensitivity or infusion-related reaction may also experience chest or back pain during the infusion. Patients with circulating cancer cells in the bloodstream are at highest risk for more severe reactions. Patients must be monitored closely during infusion. The reactions tend to be more severe with the initial infusion, and subside with subsequent treatments. Some MoABs require premedication with antihistamines and acetaminophen to minimize hypersensitivity reactions. Recommended infusion rates are usually lower for the initial dose, with incremental increases as tolerated by the patient. For patients experiencing signs or symptoms of infusion-related reactions, the infusion should be interrupted and prompt treatment with antihistamines, corticosteroids, and other supportive measures should be initiated. Pulmonary toxicity may occur as part of the infusion-related reaction or may occur as a distinct entity.[60,85,87]

The development of APAs can also increase the clearance of the MoAB from the body and subsequently decrease the half-life of the MoAB. These antibodies could also decrease the ability of the MoAB to bind to its target antigen and potentially decrease its efficacy over time.

Additionally, the toxicities of the MoABs will be determined by the selectivity of the target antigen. Antibodies against antigens found on normal and cancer cells will have increased toxicity compared with tumor-specific antigens found only on tumor tissues.

Unconjugated MoABs that target antigens on the cell surface of cancer cells may induce death of cancer cells by several mechanisms. These MoABs could directly mediate cell killing through complement activation (complement-dependent cytotoxicity [CDC]), antibody-dependent cellular toxicity (ADCC), or inhibiting intracellular signaling.[60,85,88] CDC occurs when the Fc portion of the MoAB activates the complement system, leading to tumor cell lysis, and ADCC occurs when effector cells that contain Fc receptors bind to the Fc portion of the MoAB and either lyses or phagocytosizes the antibody-containing cell. Natural killer cells, monocytes, and macrophages are all capable of mediating ADCC. Finally, antibody binding may result in the transmission of signals that induce apoptosis, or programmed cell death in the targeted cell.

Antibody conjugates deliver chemotherapy, toxins, or radioactive particles to a cell targeted by the antibody. After being bound to target antigens, the conjugated drug, toxin, or radioparticle is internalized by the target cell and kills cancer cells through traditional mechanisms of action.[89] In addition to killing the target cell, these conjugates are capable of killing antigen-negative cancer cells sometimes termed the "bystander" effect. Theoretically, immunoconjugates deliver therapy to specific sites of disease while limiting systemic exposure to the chemotherapy or radiation or toxin. The antibody might also contribute to the observed anticancer effects.

Monoclonal Antibodies and Immunoconjugates that Target Cell Surface Glycoproteins

Monoclonal Antibodies and Immunoconjugates that Target CD20

Rituximab Rituximab is a chimeric MoAB directed against the CD20 antigen found on the surface of normal and cancerous B cells.[52] The Fab domain of rituximab binds to the CD20 antigen on B lymphocytes and the Fc domain recruits immune effector functions to mediate B-cell lysis.[90] Possible explanations for its anticancer effect include CDC- and ADCC-mediated killing of malignant B cells along with a direct apoptotic effect.[90]

Rituximab is approved for the treatment of relapsed or refractory, low-grade or follicular, CD20-positive, B-cell NHL and as first-line therapy for patients with aggressive and indolent NHL in combination with chemotherapy. It is also approved for use in patients with other malignancies with CD20-antigen expression (e.g., CLL) in combination with standard chemotherapy.[90,91] Rituximab is also approved for the treatment of refractory rheumatoid arthritis and has an evolving role in a variety of immune-mediated diseases, such as Waldenström macroglobulinemia and aplastic anemia.

Most of the adverse events of rituximab occur during the first infusion and are components of an infusion-related complex secondary to the amount of circulating B cells. After the first infusion, the incidence and the severity of these reactions decrease dramatically.[90,91] The most common events in the infusion-related complex are transient fever, chills, nausea, asthenia, and headache.

Ofatumumab Ofatumumab is a human antibody that also targets the CD20 antigen. Its mechanism of action is similar to that of rituximab; however, ofatumumab targets a different epitope then rituximab, has greater affinity for the antigen, and dissociates from the epitope slower than rituximab.[92] In particular, ofatumumab binds to two regions of the CD20 antigen, the small extracellular loop and the *N*-terminal region of the large extracellular loop. This allows it to demonstrate anticancer activity in patients who have progressed on rituximab in a variety of B-cell cancers.[92] Adverse reactions are similar to rituximab with fewer infusion-related reactions and a higher rate of infectious complications (Table 104-8).

Ibritumomab Tiuxetan Ibritumomab tiuxetan is an radioimmunoconjugate that consists of the murine anti-CD20 MoAB ibritumomab and tiuxetan, a linker chelator, that allows the attachment of indium-111 (used for imaging and dosimetry) and yttrium-90 (active radiotherapy).[93] The therapeutic regimen consists of two steps.[93,94] Y-90–ibritumomab is the therapeutic radiation isotope and selectively delivers radiation to B cells that express the CD20 antigen.

The radiation-induced cytotoxicity delivered by Y-90–ibritumomab not only affects the cancer cells it binds but also other cells that are within the path length of the radioisotope's emissions (bystander effect).[88,93,94] Consequently, Y-90–ibritumomab can induce cell death in CD-20–positive and –negative tumors and eradicate a large number of cancer cells. Ibritumomab tiuxetan also induces ADCC, CDC, and apoptosis.[89,93,94]

Ibritumomab tiuxetan is indicated for the treatment of relapsed or refractory, low-grade or follicular, or transformed B-cell NHL, including rituximab-refractory NHL. Because ibritumomab is derived from murine sources, only one course of therapy is recommended to prevent the development of human antimouse antibody (HAMA) reactions.

Adverse reactions include severe infusion-related reactions, such as anaphylaxis.[89,93,94] Myelosuppression is common with ibritumomab as a consequence of the radioisotope.[89,93] Ibritumomab tiuxetan results in prolonged thrombocytopenia and neutropenia, and dose modifications are necessary based on baseline neutrophil and platelet blood counts.[93] The median durations of thrombocytopenia and neutropenia were 24 and 22 days, respectively, and monitoring and management of cytopenias, along with their complications (e.g., febrile neutropenia, bleeding) is necessary for up to 3 months after the completion of treatment.[93,94]

Tositumomab Tositumomab is another murine anti-CD20 radioimmunoconjugate similar to ibritumomab. One important difference is that tositumomab is combined with the radioisotope iodine I-131, which has therapeutic and safety implications. The tositumomab regimen also consists of two steps.[89] The mechanisms of cell death are similar to ibritumomab as is the indication for refractory NHL.

Most adverse events are similar to ibritumomab with infusion-related reactions requiring appropriate premedications along with prolonged myelosuppression, primarily neutropenia and thrombocytopenia. Complete blood counts should be obtained weekly for 10 to 12 weeks to assess recovery of normal blood counts. To prevent iodine uptake by the thyroid gland, and subsequent delivery of ionizing radiation to the thyroid gland, thyroid protective agents, such as saturated solution of potassium iodide, should be initiated before the start of the tositumomab regimen and continued for 14 days after the therapeutic dose.[89,95]

Monoclonal Antibodies and Immunoconjugates that Target Other Cell Surface Receptors

Alemtuzumab Alemtuzumab is a recombinant humanized MoAB that is directed against CD52. CD52 is expressed on the surface of B and T lymphocytes, natural killer cells, monocytes, and macrophages.[96] Its anticancer activity comes from binding to the CD52 antigen present on leukemic lymphocytes and inducing cell lysis and death.[96]

Alemtuzumab is indicated for the treatment of B-cell CLL in patients who have been treated with alkylating agents and who have failed fludarabine. It is also being investigated as part of conditioning regimens for hematopoietic stem cell transplants, treatment of autoimmune hematologic disorders, indolent NHL, and treatment of graft-versus-host disease.[94,96]

Alemtuzumab is associated with severe infusion-related reactions, hematologic toxicity, and opportunistic infections that are severe enough to warrant a box warning in the product labeling.[85,96]

Hematologic toxicity consisting of severe prolonged neutropenia and thrombocytopenia occur in most patients. Healthcare providers should monitor blood counts prior to alemtuzumab administration to determine if the dose needs to be delayed or reduced.[84,93,95]

Because CD52 is expressed on lymphocytes, alemtuzumab can induce profound lymphopenia including a decrease in CD4 and CD8 counts.[85,94,96] Patients should receive prophylaxis for *Pneumocystis jiroveci* pneumonia and herpes virus, which should be continued for up to 6 months after alemtuzumab therapy or until recovery of CD4 counts to prevent complications.[85,96]

Brentuximab Vedotin Brentuximab vedotin is the first new agent approved for Hodgkin lymphoma in more than 30 years. Brentuximab vedotin is an antibody–drug conjugate that targets the CD30 antigen found on cancer cells. Upon binding to the CD30 antigen, brentuximab vedotin is internalized by endocytosis, and the dipeptide bond that links the naked MoAB to the chemotherapy monomethylauristatin E (MMAE) is cleaved.[97] MMAE then binds to microtubules and acts as an inhibitor of microtubule polymerization. It may also induce apoptosis by inhibiting NF-κB. Brentuximab vedotin is indicated for Hodgkin lymphoma after failure of autologous hematopoietic stem cell transplant (or in patients who are not transplant candidates) and relapsed anaplastic large cell lymphoma.

Monoclonal Antibodies that Target Growth Factor Receptors and Ligands

Epidermal Growth Factor Receptor Signaling Pathway Inhibitors

Cetuximab and Panitumumab Cetuximab is a chimeric MoAB that binds specifically to the extracellular domain of EGFR[60,85,98] on both normal and cancer cells and competitively inhibits the binding of epidermal growth factor and other ligands, such as transforming growth factor-α.[60,98] Binding of cetuximab to the EGFR inhibits cell growth, induces apoptosis, and inhibits VEGF production. Cetuximab is given as monotherapy or in combination with other anticancer agents in the treatment of metastatic colorectal cancer.[98,99] Cetuximab is also approved for use in head and neck cancer either alone or in combination with radiation.[100] The most serious adverse events associated with cetuximab are infusion-related reactions and development of an acne-like rash.[85,99,101] Skin reactions occur in most patients receiving cetuximab and can be severe. This reaction is similar between all EGFR inhibitors and appears to be related to the function of EGFR in skin follicles.[70] These reactions are characterized by multiple follicular or pustular appearing lesions that generally appear within the first 2 weeks of therapy. Although the reactions usually resolve after cessation of treatment, resolution can be slow, continuing beyond 28 days in nearly half of cases. In patients who develop a severe rash, dose modifications may be necessary. Interestingly, a trend for improved responses with increasing severity of skin reactions has been reported and requires further follow-up to assess the clinical importance of these reactions.[70,99] Other common adverse events with cetuximab include fatigue, gastrointestinal complaints (nausea, vomiting, diarrhea, and constipation), and abdominal pain.[99]

Panitumumab is a MoAB that also binds to the cell surface EGFR. It is an IgG2 antibody and the first fully human MoAB approved to treat cancer.[102] Panitumumab is approved as a single agent in refractory metastatic colon cancer. Adverse reactions are similar to cetuximab, although severe reactions appear to be rare because it does not have a murine component.[102]

Both antibodies appear to be more effective in patients with tumors that are KRAS wild type, then patients with tumors that are KRAS mutation positive; therefore, patients with metastatic colorectal cancer should not receive anti-EGFR antibody therapy if a KRAS mutation is detected.[103] Genetic testing in patients with colorectal cancer is discussed in further detail in the Chapter 107.

Trastuzumab Trastuzumab is a humanized MoAB that selectively binds to HER2.[91,95] HER2 is overexpressed in about 33% of breast cancers, in about 22% of gastroesophageal junction and gastric cancers, and to varying degrees in other malignancies (e.g., ovarian, lung, prostate).[9,91,104] Trastuzumab inhibits cell cycle progression by decreasing cells entering the S phase of the cell cycle, which leads to downregulation of HER2 receptors on cancer cells and decreased cell proliferation.[103] Trastuzumab also leads to ADCC and CDC and directly induces apoptosis in cells overexpressing HER2.[105] In addition, synergy between trastuzumab and traditional chemotherapy has been demonstrated, resulting in trastuzumab often being used in combination with chemotherapy.

Trastuzumab is approved for the treatment of metastatic breast cancer as a single agent or in combination with paclitaxel. It is also approved for adjuvant treatment as part of a combination chemotherapy regimen or as a single agent after multimodality anthracycline-based chemotherapy. It is not recommended to administer trastuzumab concomitantly with an anthracycline because of concerns of additive cardiotoxicity. Trastuzumab is also approved in combination with chemotherapy for the treatment of patients with HER2 overexpressing metastatic gastric or gastroesophageal junction adenocarcinoma. The tumors should overexpress HER2 as measured by diagnostic tests that can qualify gene amplification or protein expression.

Trastuzumab is administered as a loading dose followed by weekly infusions.[105] Trastuzumab has been administered every 3 weeks in combination with chemotherapy to simplify the treatment regimen.[106]

The most serious adverse reactions caused by trastuzumab include cardiomyopathy, infusion-related reactions, hypersensitivity reactions (including anaphylaxis), and increased myelosuppression. An evaluation of cardiac function should be performed before administration and extreme caution should be exercised in patients with preexisting cardiac dysfunction and in those who have received prior anthracyclines. In patients who develop a clinically significant decrease in left ventricular function (ejection fraction <50% or greater than 10% decrease), discontinuation of therapy should be considered. Similar to most MoABs, the symptoms associated with a hypersensitivity reaction are most common with the initial infusions of trastuzumab and occur infrequently thereafter. Myelosuppression is infrequent after the administration of trastuzumab as a single agent, but the incidence of neutropenia and febrile neutropenia is higher when trastuzumab is given with myelosuppressive chemotherapy as compared with giving the chemotherapy alone.[105]

Pertuzumab Pertuzumab is a humanized MoAB that targets the HER2 receptor. It is synergistic with trastuzumab and is effective in tumors that have developed resistance to trastuzumab. Pertuzumab binds to extracellular domain II of HER2, a site distinct from trastuzumab, and inhibits ligand-dependent HER2–HER3 dimerization, which subsequently decreases tumor proliferation and resistance pathways.[107] Dual targeting of the HER2 receptor allows for increased efficacy against variant forms of the HER2 receptor, including truncated HER2 receptors. Similar to trastuzumab it appears to induce ADCC in cancer cells. Pertuzumab is currently approved in combination with trastuzumab and docetaxel for the treatment of HER2 overexpressed refractory metastatic breast cancer.

Ado-Trastuzumab Ematansine Ado-trastuzumab ematansine is indicated for the treatment of patients with HER2-positive, metastatic breast cancer who previously received trastuzumab and a taxane. It is an antibody–drug conjugate that consists of the humanized anti-HER2 monoclonal antibody trastuzumab covalently linked to the microtubule-targeting inhibitor DM1.[108]

Vascular Endothelial Growth Factor Signaling Pathway Inhibitors

Bevacizumab Bevacizumab is a humanized MoAB directed against circulating VEGF.[24] It binds to all biologically active circulating isoforms of VEGF and prevents the activation and promotion of angiogenesis.[24]

Bevacizumab is approved, in combination with chemotherapy, for the initial treatment of metastatic colorectal cancer[109] and in combination with chemotherapy, for first-line treatment of patients with advanced nonsquamous NSCLC. Additional uses approved by the Food and Drug Administration (FDA) include metastatic renal cell carcinoma and progressive glioblastoma with off-label use in other cancers.

Several serious adverse events have been associated with bevacizumab, including hypertension, bleeding, and thrombotic events.[109,110] Hypertension is more common in patients with a history of hypertension and responds to oral antihypertensive medications. Although the most common bleeding episodes are transient nosebleeds, fatal CNS and gastrointestinal hemorrhages have been reported. The product labeling includes a box warning regarding the risk of gastrointestinal perforation, wound dehiscence, and fatal hemoptysis.[110] Bevacizumab is not recommended for use within 28 days of major surgery and patients should be instructed to report abdominal pain (an initial sign of gastrointestinal hemorrhage) to their healthcare providers immediately. Paradoxically, bevacizumab also has been associated with thrombotic events, including deep vein thrombosis, pulmonary embolism, and myocardial infarction, especially in elderly patients with a history of cardiac events. Another potentially serious adverse event associated with bevacizumab is proteinuria, and patients should be monitored for the development or worsening of proteinuria with serial urine dipsticks. Patients with a 2+ or greater urine dipstick should undergo further assessment.

Miscellaneous Monoclonal Antibodies

Ipilimumab

Ipilimumab is a human MoAB that blocks cytotoxic T-lymphocyte antigen (CTLA-4) that is approved for the treatment of metastatic melanoma. CTLA-4 acts a negative regulator of T-cell function, decreasing the ability of the immune system to mount an antitumor response. By binding to CTLA-4, ipilimumab allows for enhanced T-cell stimulation, proliferation, and antitumor activity.[111] It can take 3 months or longer to demonstrate a response in patients with melanoma. Based on its enhanced immune response, several severe and fatal immune-mediated adverse reactions have been observed, including enterocolitis, hepatitis, dermatitis, neuropathy, and endocrinopathy (Table 104-8).

Enzymes

L-Asparaginase

L-Asparaginase is unique among anticancer agents in its unusual mechanism of action, patterns of toxicity, and source. It is an enzyme produced by *Escherichia coli* or *Erwinia chrysanthemi*. L-Asparagine is a nonessential amino acid that can be synthesized by most mammalian cells except for those of certain lymphoid human malignancies, which lack or have very low levels of the synthetase enzyme required for L-asparagine formation.[27] L-Asparagine is degraded by the enzyme L-asparaginase, which depletes existing supplies and inhibits protein synthesis. Increased L-asparagine synthetase activity within cancer cells causes resistance to L-asparaginase treatment.[27] L-Asparaginase is a component of multiagent chemotherapy regimen used for the treatment of ALL and multiple products are available as listed in Table 104-8.

Cytokines

Interferons

Interferons are a family of proteins produced by nucleated cells or recombinant DNA technology with antiviral, antiproliferative, and immunoregulatory activities. These proteins are classified as α, β, or γ IFNs based on antigenic, biologic, and pharmacologic properties. IFN alfa has been approved for hairy cell leukemia, melanoma, Kaposi's sarcoma, and CML. A pegylated INF-alfa has been approved for adjuvant treatment of metastatic melanoma.

The mechanisms by which IFNs exert their anticancer effects is unknown, but IFNs likely exert their effect by binding to specific membrane receptors and initiating various intracellular signaling pathways. IFNs can prolong the cell cycle, inhibit angiogenesis, and cause cytostasis and apoptosis. They can increase the expression of antigens on tumor cell surfaces, making the cancerous cells more easily recognized by immune effector cells. IFNs also inhibit certain oncogenes that can direct the unregulated cell growth that is characteristic of cancerous cells. Alterations in gene expression may change the levels of receptors for other cytokines or the concentration of regulatory proteins on immune cells or may activate enzymes that alter cellular growth and function.[59]

The most frequent adverse events are flu-like symptoms and elevated transaminases. Potentially serious adverse events include neuropsychiatric, autoimmune, ischemic, and infectious disorders.

Interleukin-2 (Aldesleukin)

Interleukin-2 is a cytokine produced by recombinant DNA technology that promotes B- and T-cell proliferation and differentiation and initiates a cytokine cascade with multiple interacting immunologic effects. The IL-2 receptor is expressed in increased amounts on activated T cells and mediates most of the effects of aldesleukin. Anticancer activity depends on proliferation of cytotoxic immune cells that can recognize and destroy cancer cells without damaging normal cells. Some of these cytotoxic cells are natural killer cells, lymphokine-activated killer (LAK) cells, and tumor-infiltrating lymphocytes.[112] Aldesleukin has been approved for the treatment of metastatic renal cell carcinoma and melanoma.

The toxicity of aldesleukin is related to dose, route, and duration of therapy, but aldesleukin is toxic therapy that requires vigorous supportive care. The most common dose-limiting toxicities are hypotension, fluid retention, and renal dysfunction. Aldesleukin decreases peripheral vascular resistance, producing peripheral vasodilation, tachycardia, and hypotension. A characteristic vascular or capillary leak syndrome produces fluid retention, which in turn can cause respiratory compromise. These toxicities require administration of vasopressors in most patients, judicious use of fluid support and diuretics, and supplemental oxygen. Patients with underlying cardiovascular or renal abnormalities are more susceptible to these adverse events, making careful patient selection important.[112] Most patients treated with aldesleukin experience thrombocytopenia, anemia, eosinophilia, reversible cholestasis, and skin erythema with burning and pruritus, and some have neuropsychiatric changes, hypothyroidism, and bacterial infections.[112] In general, the toxicities from aldesleukin reverse quickly after therapy is stopped and can be managed or prevented by careful prospective monitoring and supportive care.

Fusion Proteins

Denileukin Diftitox

Denileukin diftitox is a recombinant fusion protein that combines the active sections of both IL-2 and diphtheria toxin. Unconjugated diphtheria toxin is much too toxic to administer to humans. As the "payload" of the fusion protein, however, its cytotoxic effects are directed toward cells that express the high-affinity form of the IL-2 receptor, such as cancer cells of some patients with cutaneous T-cell lymphoma. When denileukin diftitox interacts with IL-2 receptors, the toxin inhibits protein synthesis in the cancer cells and causes cell death.[113] It has been approved for the treatment of cutaneous T-cell lymphomas.

Although denileukin diftitox is directed therapy, its targeting of cells that express high-affinity IL-2 receptors is not specific because these receptors are expressed on cells other than cancer cells. Denileukin diftitox produces acute hypersensitivity reactions, flu-like symptoms, diarrhea, visual impairment, and vascular leak syndrome. It differs from the vascular leak syndrome produced by high-dose aldesleukin in that it occurs in fewer patients, is delayed in onset, is usually self-limited, and does not consistently recur on retreatment.[112,113] Patients with an albumin concentration less than 3 g/dL (30 g/L) are at increased risk for vascular leak syndrome, and use in these patients is not recommended.

Ziv-Aflibercept

Ziv-aflibercept is a soluble recombinant fusion protein that was designed to block multiple signals that stimulate the angiogenic process. It was developed by fusing sections of the VEGFR-1 and VEGFR-2 immunoglobulin domains to the F_c portion of human IgG1. Ziv-aflibercept blocks VEGF-A, VEGF-B, and PIGF by "trapping" the ligands before they get to the native transmembrane receptors and thus decreasing proangiogenic signaling and tumor growth. It is approved in combination with chemotherapy in patients with resistant or progressive metastatic colorectal cancer and has adverse events similar to other anti-VEGF therapies.[114]

RESPONSE CRITERIA

The response to anticancer agents and other treatment modalities could be described as a cure, complete response (CR), partial response (PR), stable disease, or progression.[115] A cure implies that the patient is entirely free of disease and has the same life expectancy as a cancer-free individual. Because of our inability to detect small numbers of cancer cells we can never be absolutely certain that an individual patient is cured. Cancers that are curable with treatment are characterized by a stable plateau in the survival curve where the risk of relapse is very low. For most curable cancers, the survival curve has plateaued by about 5 years. Therefore, patients with a curable cancer who are alive 5 years from the time of diagnosis without disease recurrence are often considered "cured." However, patients with some malignancies, such as breast cancer and melanoma, are still at significant risk for relapse after 5 years.

In an attempt to simply and unify response definitions in both clinical practice and published reports, the RECIST (Response Evaluation Criteria in Solid Tumors) criteria were developed in 2000 and revised in 2009.[115] A *complete response* means complete disappearance of all cancer without evidence of new disease for at least 1 month after treatment. The terms *cure* and *CR* are not synonymous. Although an individual must have a CR to be cured, many individuals who achieve a CR will eventually relapse. A *partial response* is defined as a 30% or greater decrease in the tumor size or other objective disease markers and no evidence of any new disease for at least 1 month. Overall objective response rates for a given treatment are calculated by adding the CR and PR rates. *Progressive disease* is defined as a 20% increase in the tumor size or the development of any new lesions while receiving treatment. A patient whose tumor size neither grows nor shrinks by the above criteria is termed to have *stable disease*. Some patients may experience subjective improvement in the symptoms caused by their cancer without a defined response. Although clinically important, this does not indicate an objective response. The term *clinical benefit response* was recently developed to document these subjective responses; it refers to patients who have clinical benefit as measured by decreases in pain or analgesic consumption or improved quality of life or performance status.

These response definitions are applicable to solid tumors because leukemias and multiple myeloma are not characterized by discrete, measurable masses. Responses in these cancers are measured by elimination of abnormal cells (e.g., return to normal hematology parameters and normal bone marrow in leukemia), return of tumor markers to normal levels (e.g., normal serum protein electrophoresis in multiple myeloma), or improved function of affected organs (e.g., improved renal function after obstructive uropathy). Cytogenetic markers and molecular techniques have an increasingly important role in determining whether all cancer has been truly eliminated. For example, in CML, the Philadelphia chromosome can be detected by polymerase chain reaction (PCR) techniques even when no leukemia is evident in the bone marrow or bloodstream. Patients without evidence of the Philadelphia chromosome are classified as having a *complete cytogenetic response*. Measuring cytogenetic responses is increasingly common in patients with known cytogenetic abnormalities, and the absence of complete cytogenetic responses may predict disease relapse.

The FDA publishes guidance for industry to facilitate the drug development process.[116] New therapies must demonstrate a favorable risk-to-benefit ratio in adequate and well-controlled clinical trials. Overall survival and symptom improvement is considered an appropriate measure of effectiveness. Accelerated approval promulgated in 1992 supported the approval of therapies intended to treat life-threatening or serious illnesses in which the new therapy demonstrated improvement compared to current therapies or provided therapy in the absence of current therapy based on surrogate end points that are likely to predict clinical benefit. Possible surrogate end points include disease-free survival, progression-free survival, objective response rates, and CR rates; overall response rate is the most common surrogate end point used to support accelerated approval. A clinical trial after accelerated approval must be conducted with due diligence and demonstrate clinical benefit, or the product may be removed from the market. In the period from 1990 to 2003, 75% of the new therapies for cancer were approved based on end points other than survival.[116]

Factors Affecting Response to Therapy

Factors affecting response include tumor burden, cancer cell heterogeneity, drug resistance, dose intensity, and patient-specific factors. The significance of tumor burden was discussed earlier in the Principles of Tumor Growth section. Tumors consist of a heterogeneous population of cells. Because of the genetic instability of cancer cells compared with normal cells, mutations commonly occur during cell division; thus, large tumors have undergone many cell divisions and express multiple mutations, resulting in genetically varied populations.[6,28] In 1979, Goldie and Coldman proposed that these cytogenetic changes were not completely random and were highly associated with the development of the ability of tumors to develop drug resistance.[1,6,28] The probability of developing resistant cell populations increases as tumor size increases. It is believed that a small percentage of resistant cancer cells may survive initial therapy. Resistant populations later proliferate and eventually become the dominant population, which could explain the common pattern of an initial response to therapy followed by progressive tumor regrowth despite continuing the same treatment.

Drug resistance may be either an acquired or inherited. Mechanisms of drug resistance include altered drug transport systems, metabolism, and target enzymes; inability to repair drug-induced damage; and insensitivity to drug-induced apoptosis.[6,11,28] For example, multidrug resistance has been observed with natural chemotherapies (i.e., anthracyclines, vinca alkaloids, epipodophyllotoxins, and taxanes), and it occurs when some cancer cells are exposed to increasing concentrations of a specific chemotherapy.[28,117] Surprisingly, these same cells also become resistant to other structurally unrelated chemotherapies and are therefore considered multidrug resistant. The resistant cancer cells possess the transporter Pgp, which enhances the export of these chemotherapies. Other potential mechanisms of drug resistance include inactivation of chemotherapy by glutathione metabolism, upregulation of drug targets, alternative intracellular signaling pathways, and decreased apoptosis. The last mechanism can be mediated by *bcl-2* oncogene overexpression or loss of the *p53* gene, as discussed in the oncogene section.

The relationship between dose and response has been extensively explored for traditional chemotherapies[1] because dose is believed to be a critical factor in determining response for many cancers. *Dose intensity* is defined as the dose delivered to the patient over a specified period of time. The three main variables that determine delivered dose intensity are the dose per course, the interval between doses, and the total cumulative dose. *Dose density* refers to shortening of the usual interval between doses (e.g., every 2 weeks instead of every 3 weeks) and is designed to maximize the effects of therapy on tumor growth kinetics. This strategy has been most extensively studied in breast cancer, with positive results from adjuvant therapy given to patients with high-risk node-positive disease. The delivery of optimal dose intensity is often compromised by the toxicities of the anticancer agent. Treatment cycles are commonly delayed because of inadequate recovery from toxicity, especially myelosuppression. Subsequent doses of the anticancer agents are often reduced to prevent or reduce the severity of these toxicities. The impact on patient outcome has been proven in studies showing reduced rates of response and survival in individuals receiving less-than-optimal doses.[1] Understanding the pathophysiology of toxicities has led to the development of more effective agents to prevent and manage these toxicities. The development of agent- and toxicity-specific chemoprotective agents has facilitated application of dose-intensity principles.[1] For example, the colony-stimulating factors avert neutropenia and permit delivery of dose-intensive or dose-dense regimens that are myelosuppressive. The issue of dose intensity is particularly important in the setting of high-dose chemotherapy with autologous hematopoietic stem cell support. Although lethal myelosuppression is avoided by administering hematopoietic stem cells, other severe end-organ toxicities emerge as doses of the anticancer agents are increased.

Patient-specific factors create unpredictable variability in response to anticancer therapy. For example, interindividual variations in absorption, distribution, elimination, or metabolism could lead to sub- or supratherapeutic levels of anticancer agents and their metabolites. The genetic mutations that resulted in the cancer can also affect response. For example, breast cancers that overexpress HER2 are often sensitive to anthracycline-based regimens.[105] As a result, both efficacy and tolerability can be affected. Until recently, healthcare providers in oncology have modified dose based on variations in body size, blood counts, and organ function. Prospective dose modifications based on these parameters are still very important to optimize the effectiveness of therapy and minimize toxicity. But more specific tools are becoming available as we learn how to identify and apply differences in the genetic makeup of the patient and cancer to their anticancer therapy. *Pharmacogenomics* is the study of the role of inheritance in individual variation in drug response.[118] In oncology, several clinically relevant genetic polymorphisms or variations have been identified that can affect pharmacokinetics and pharmacodynamics. Examples include polymorphisms in genes responsible for the activity of the enzymes DPD (responsible for 5-FU metabolism), TPMT (responsible for thiopurine metabolism), and UGT1A1 (responsible for irinotecan metabolism).[118] Patients with deficiencies in these enzymes can experience significant, and possibly life-threatening, toxicity. Identifying these genetic variants could permit individualization of regimens containing these agents to avoid toxicity. Monitoring of anticancer agents concentrations could also improve the therapeutic index. For example, pharmacokinetic and pharmacodynamic modeling is associated with improved responses and decreased toxicity in children with ALL.

The presence of other disease states (e.g., comorbidities) may also affect response to treatment by limiting treatment options. The overall functional status of a patient may be assessed using performance status scales, such as the Karnofsky and Eastern Cooperative Oncology Group scales (Table 104-10).[119] These scales can be used to predict patient tolerance of anticancer therapy and to assess the effects of therapy on the patient's level of activity and quality of life. For many cancers, performance status at diagnosis is the most important prognostic indicator.

Today's oncology health professionals have a wealth of information to consider when designing a personalized treatment approach. Patient-specific factors (e.g., performance status, comorbidities, organ function, and pharmacogenomics), tumor-specific factors (e.g., pathology, stage and molecular profile), and treatment goals (e.g., palliation and cure) are all considered when determining the best treatment option. Treatment cost can also be an important consideration.

COMBINATION THERAPY

Although single agents are sometimes used, the more common approach to anticancer therapy involves administration of multiple agents to overcome factors for decreased patient response noted previously.[1,27,119] Initially, this approach was based on the Goldie-Coldman hypothesis, which addresses the issue of tumor cell heterogeneity and the inevitable development of drug resistance. Combination therapy is given to inhibit the many different cancer cells. The individual agents selected for combination therapy considers drug-specific factors, such as mechanism of action, cancer activity, and toxicity. Drugs that possess minimally overlapping mechanisms of action and toxicities are combined when possible. For example, myelosuppressive agents are typically combined with nonmyelosuppressive agents to minimize bone marrow suppression while gaining additive anticancer effects. The selected agents should each have significant activity against the cancer. If a synergistic reaction is known to exist for two agents, they may be combined in various treatment regimens.

With the availability of new targeted therapies, one area of research is to determine the optimal ways to combine these therapies, both with traditional chemotherapy and other targeted therapies. In theory, these therapies make ideal combination agents because they target the underlying cancer biology while usually avoiding the common adverse events associated with traditional chemotherapy. Healthcare providers must be careful when combining agents based on clinical data that demonstrate additive or synergistic benefit. Combinations of chemotherapy and targeted therapies have proven successful in breast and colon cancer. Predictive markers might be available to identify which patients may benefit from combinations of chemotherapy and targeted therapies for patients with breast and colon cancers.

ADMINISTRATION

Dosing and Administration

Healthcare providers should monitor several clinical and laboratory values before the administration of myelosuppressive agents. In general, a WBC count of 3,000 cells/mm^3 (3×10^9/L) or above or an

TABLE 104-10 Performance Status Scales

Description: Karnofsky Scale	Karnofsky Scale (%)	Zubrod Scale (ECOG)	Description: ECOG Scale
No complaints; no evidence of disease	100	0	Fully active, able to carry on all predisease activity
Able to carry on normal activity; minor signs or symptoms of disease	90		
Normal activity with effort; some signs or symptoms of disease	80	1	Restricted in strenuous activity but ambulatory and able to carry out work of a light or sedentary nature
Cares for self; unable to carry on normal activity or to do active work	70		
Requires occasional assistance but able to care for most personal needs	60	2	Out of bed more than 50% of time; ambulatory and capable of self-care, but unable to carry out any work activities
Requires considerable assistance and frequent medical care	50		
Disabled; requires special care and assistance	40	3	In bed more than 50% of time; capable of only limited self-care
Severely disabled; hospitalization indicated, although death not imminent	30		
Very sick; hospitalization necessary; requires active supportive treatment	20	4	Bedridden; cannot carry out any self-care; completely disabled
Moribund; fatal processes progressing rapidly	10		
Dead	0		

ECOG, Eastern Cooperative Oncology Group.
Adapted from Cersosimo.[91]

absolute neutrophil count (ANC) of 1,500 cells/mm^3 ($\geq 1.5 \times 10^9$/L) or above and a platelet count of 100,000 cells/mm^3 ($\geq 100 \times 10^9$/L) or above are usually required before administering myelosuppressive agents. In addition, a chemistry panel is drawn to assess organ function, especially for agents eliminated via those routes. Table 104-8 lists agents that require dosing adjustments and require specific laboratory tests before administration; failure to do so may result in overdosing and excessive toxicity.

Anticancer agents might be dosed based on body weight or body surface area (BSA) or as a fixed dose. Chemotherapy is generally dosed based on BSA.[120] BSA is commonly used as an estimate of cardiac output and subsequent distribution to the liver and kidneys, the primary determinants of drug elimination. The most common methods used to determine BSA are the Mosteller and DuBois formulas, which are listed in Table 104-9. Body-sized dosing is also commonly used for MoABs and other therapeutic proteins, but the effect of body size on interpatient variability should be explored to determine optimal dosing approach. In contrast, most oral targeted agents are dosed as a fixed dose based on available tablet or capsule strengths.

Clinical **Controversy. . .**

The use of actual versus ideal body weight for calculating BSA is a source of debate in oncology. Although actual body weight is most often used, some healthcare providers prefer to use an adjusted body weight in obese patients. Healthcare providers need to clearly state the weight used in the BSA calculation. New methods of dosing using individual patient- and tumor-specific factors are an area of active research.

New dosing methods are being developed to improve the accuracy of chemotherapy dosing and prevent both over- and underdosing. For example, carboplatin is now commonly dosed based on the patient's estimated glomerular filtration rate. This method, listed in Table 104-9, is known as the Calvert formula and has been demonstrated to achieve adequate levels of carboplatin without excessive toxicity.[121] Therapy might also be dosed based on drug levels (i.e., MTX), and healthcare providers should be proficient in these calculations before dosing and administering any chemotherapy. The health care provider should also be aware of diagnostic tests warranted before administering targeted agents, such as tamoxifen, AIs, trastuzumab, vemurafenib, and crizotinib. Additional methods using pharmacogenomic testing are being studied to individualize doses.

Safety and Handling Issues

All anticancer agents regardless of the route of administrations should be handled with care to avoid inadvertent exposure of healthcare providers.[122] Consequently, all healthcare facilities should have written procedures for handling these drugs safely, and all personnel should be oriented to these procedures. Additionally, pharmacists should provide information about safe handling and disposal to patients and their families when a patient is prescribed oral anticancer agents. Safe handling includes avoiding skin contact and inhalation, but guidelines regarding safe handling of oral anticancer agents have not been developed.[123]

The United States Pharmacopeia Chapter 797 regulates the preparation of extemporaneously compounded sterile preparations and should be used by providers that prepare IV chemotherapy.[122] The most common avenue of exposure is via inhalation of aerosolized drug. Individuals preparing IV chemotherapy should work in a class II biologic safety cabinet and wear gowns and powder-free disposable latex gloves. The gowns should be made of lint-free, low-permeability fabric with a solid front, long sleeves, and tight-fitting elastic cuffs. Negative-pressure techniques should be used in drug preparation to minimize aerosolization. Healthcare providers administering chemotherapy should take similar precautions to avoid exposure. Kits for cleaning up chemotherapy spills should be located in all areas where chemotherapy is handled. Cytotoxic waste should be disposed of properly, and patients should be informed of proper methods of disposing of potentially contaminated body excreta and cytotoxic waste.

GENERAL SUPPORTIVE CARE ISSUES

9 The treatment of cancer with most anticancer agents is complicated by the risk of multiple serious adverse events, many of which are life threatening. Adverse events are commonly graded on a scale from no toxicity to death; a common scale used in clinical trials is the common terminology criteria for adverse events developed by the National Cancer Institute, and the standard adverse event reporting classification system used in the United States for all drugs is the Medical Dictionary for Regulatory Activities. Specific adverse events, such as doxorubicin-induced cardiotoxicity and bleomycin-related pulmonary toxicity, were summarized earlier. Several adverse events are common to many anticancer agents. For example, nausea and vomiting, myelosuppression, mucositis, alopecia, infertility, and carcinogenesis have been observed with traditional chemotherapy. With the addition of targeted therapies, new adverse events now need to be addressed by healthcare providers. The events observed with targeted therapies appear to depend on the intracellular signaling pathways that are inhibited. For example, rash has been observed with agents that affect the EGFR signaling pathway, and hemorrhage and thrombosis have been observed with agents that affect the VEGFR signaling pathway. Nutritional support and pain management are also important supportive care issues. The management of chemotherapy-induced nausea and vomiting and the basic principles of nutritional support and pain management are discussed in detail in other chapters.

Because many traditional chemotherapies affect DNA synthesis, all rapidly proliferating cells are more sensitive to the toxic effects. Normal tissues, such as the bone marrow, intestinal mucosa, and hair follicles, are tissues in which chemotherapy's effects are manifested.

Myelosuppression

10 Although not seen with all anticancer agents, myelosuppression is the most common dose-limiting adverse event observed with chemotherapy. Myelosuppression is increased when chemotherapy is administered concurrently with radiation to the chest or pelvic region. Bone marrow suppression does not usually occur immediately after chemotherapy administration because blood components that have already been produced must be consumed before the effect is evident. WBCs, especially neutrophil precursors, are most significantly affected because of their rapid proliferation and short life span (6–12 hours). Platelets (5- to 10-day life span) are also affected but to a much less degree than neutrophils. Erythrocytes, with a 120-day life span, are affected the least. Usual nadirs, or lowest blood cell counts, occur at 10 to 14 days after chemotherapy administration, with recovery by 3 to 4 weeks. There are some exceptions to this general rule. The nitrosoureas, mitomycin C, and radiolabeled antibodies exhibit a delayed nadir (4–6 weeks) and recovery (6–8 weeks). Chemotherapy should be delayed until the suggested blood counts for a patient to safely receive myelosuppressive chemotherapy as listed in the previous section are achieved. Patients with leukemia or receiving a hematopoietic stem cell transplant may have a more rapid nadir of about 5 to 7 days.

Neutropenia, particularly with fever, is an undesirable adverse event during chemotherapy for most cancers. If significant neutropenia has occurred with prior courses, the doses of the offending chemotherapy in subsequent courses may be reduced. The magnitude of dose reduction is dictated by the degree of myelosuppression incurred and the incidence and severity of infection or bleeding. Empiric dose reductions may be made for the first chemotherapy treatment if the patient has a low baseline WBC or platelet count, has diminished bone marrow reserve, has impaired drug elimination, or is to receive a combination of several myelosuppressive agents. Patients who have received multiple prior courses of other myelosuppressive chemotherapy or extensive radiation therapy, especially to the pelvis or chest, may have a decreased bone marrow reserve. Therefore, these patients are more sensitive to the myelosuppressive effects of chemotherapy, and normal doses may produce profound bone marrow toxicity. Patients with impaired organ function may have compromised elimination of the chemotherapy and are at increased risk for severe bone marrow suppression if the dose is not appropriately adjusted (Table 104-8).

However, in some tumors (e.g., breast cancer, lymphoma), dosage reduction may compromise response, leading to worse patient outcomes.[1] In patients who are responding well to treatment, some degree of myelosuppression is accepted by most healthcare providers if it is not compromising the patient's quality of life and the cancer is responding to therapy. In these patients, empiric use of hematopoietic growth factors provides an alternative to dose reduction.

Anemia

Although usually not life threatening, anemia is the most common hematologic complication of chemotherapy.[124] The incidence of anemia depends on several factors, including the type and duration of therapy and the type and stage of the underlying malignancy. For example, carboplatin is more commonly associated with anemia than other chemotherapies. Multiple conditions are known to cause anemia in cancer patients, including chronic gastrointestinal blood loss, nutrient deficiency (e.g., iron and folate), chemotherapy and radiation therapy, bone marrow invasion, hemolysis, renal dysfunction, and anemia of chronic disease. Of all the signs and symptoms of anemia, fatigue is most common in patients with cancer.[124] In fact, fatigue is the most commonly reported symptom overall in patients undergoing chemotherapy. The presence of fatigue is correlated with the severity of anemia; treatment of anemia may result in improvement in fatigue and quality of life. Anemia is only one of many possible causes of fatigue in patients with cancer. Other common causes of fatigue include insomnia, depression, unrelieved pain, and the underlying malignancy.

The treatments for chemotherapy-related anemia include red blood cell transfusions and human erythropoietic products (epoetin alfa and darbepoetin alfa).[124] Both epoetin alfa and darbepoetin alfa can increase hemoglobin and hematocrit and decrease transfusion requirements. One difference between the products is that darbepoetin has longer half-life, which allows for less frequent administration of darbepoetin.[125]

Clinical practice guidelines for the treatment of cancer- and chemotherapy-related anemia are available.[124] The first step is to evaluate the underlying cause of the anemia and initiate specific therapy as indicated. Red blood cell transfusions are the mainstay of treatment, but erythropoiesis-stimulating agents could be considered for patients with underlying kidney disease and for patients receiving palliative treatment. These agents must be prescribed and used under a risk management program. The presence of functional iron deficiency should be determined before administering these products.

Serious adverse events related to erythropoiesis-stimulating agents include thrombosis and pure red cell aplasia, which may result in an increased mortality rate from use. These events have generally occurred when the target hemoglobin of 12 g/dL (120 g/L; 7.45 mmol/L) is exceeded or the hemoglobin rises too quickly.[124] Other rare and generally mild adverse events include pain at injection site, rash, flulike symptoms, seizures, and hypertension.

Neutropenia

When the ANC falls below 500 cells/mm^3 (0.5×10^9/L), the risk of infection increases.[126] The ANC may be calculated by multiplying the percentage of neutrophils (segmented plus banded neutrophils) by the total WBC count. The risk of infection is also directly proportional to the duration of neutropenia. Other risk factors for infection include alteration in the integrity of physical defense barriers and the functional integrity of the WBCs. The underlying cancer, chemotherapy, and radiation can affect neutrophil function. The diagnosis of infection in the neutropenic patient is complicated by the lack of WBCs. Usual signs and symptoms of infection, such as pus, abscesses, and infiltrates on chest radiography, are often absent as a result of the lack of WBCs. Subsequently, healthcare providers must rely on fever as an indication of infection in these patients. Definitive culture results may take days, and a septic neutropenic cancer patient can die within hours if not treated. Therefore, empiric antibiotics are promptly initiated based on reliable coverage of the most likely organisms, antibiotic sensitivities at the institution, the patient's signs and symptoms (if present), side effect profiles, and cost.[126] The most common source of infection in these patients is self-infection with body flora, which includes both gram-positive and gram-negative bacteria. Specific treatment of infections in immunocompromised hosts is discussed in Chapter 100.

Numerous methods have been explored to prevent infections in patients with cancer. Colony-stimulating factors (CSFs) are commonly used for this purpose.[126] These factors are naturally occurring proteins that are essential for the normal growth and maturation of blood cell components (Fig. 104-10). CSFs have the ability to enhance the production and the function of their target cells. Two recombinant products, G-CSF (granulocyte colony-stimulating factor) and GM-CSF (granulocyte-macrophage colony-stimulating factor), are commercially available in the United States. G-CSF (filgrastim) specifically stimulates the production of neutrophilic granulocytes, and GM-CSF (sargramostim) promotes the proliferation of granulocytes (neutrophils and eosinophils) and monocytes and macrophages.[127] Although GM-CSF stimulates megakaryocytes, no consistent effect on platelet production has been observed in clinical trials. Both factors initially enhance demargination and mobilization of mature cells from the marrow and then provide constant stimulation of stem cell progenitors. Pegfilgrastim is a long-acting CSF created by adding a polyethylene glycol molecule to G-CSF.[128] Clinical trials have demonstrated that a single dose of pegfilgrastim provides equivalent effects to 10 to 11 days of daily G-CSF, with similar adverse events.

These growth factors may be used as primary or secondary prophylaxis of neutropenia. Primary prophylaxis refers to the use of CSFs to prevent neutropenia with the first cycle of chemotherapy.

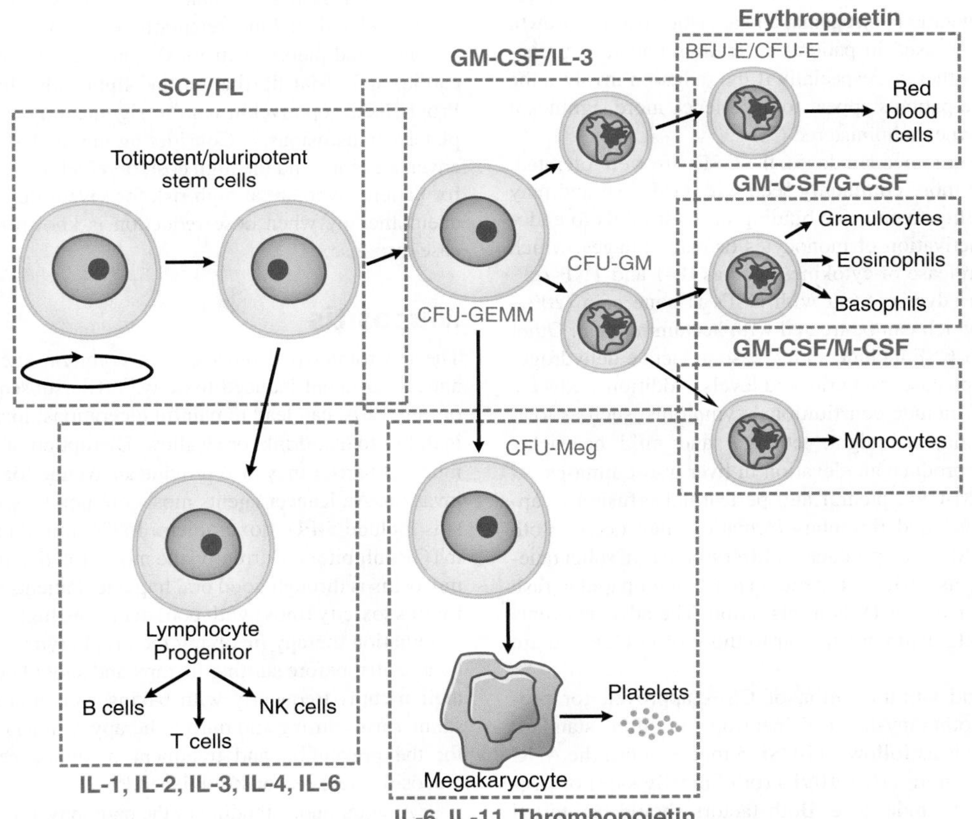

FIGURE 104-10 Sites of action of hematopoietic growth factors in the differentiation and maturation of marrow cell lines. A self-sustaining pool of marrow stem cells differentiates under the influence of specific hematopoietic growth factors to form a variety of hematopoietic and lymphopoietic cells. Stem cell factor (SCF), FTL-3 ligand (FL), interleukin-3 (IL-3), and granulocyte-macrophage colony-stimulating factor (GM-CSF), together with cell–cell interactions in the bone marrow, stimulate stem cells to form a series of burst-forming units (BFU) and colony-forming units (CFUs): CFU-GEMM, CFU-GM, CFU-Meg, BFU-E, and CFU-E (GEMM, granulocyte, erythrocyte, monocyte, and megakaryocytes; GM, granulocyte and macrophage; Meg, megakaryocyte; E, erythrocyte). After considerable proliferation, further differentiation is stimulated by synergistic interactions with growth factors for each of the major cell lines—granulocyte colony-stimulating factor (G-CSF), monocyte/macrophage-stimulating factor (M-CSF), thrombopoietin, and erythropoietin. Each of these factors also influences the proliferation; maturation; and, in some cases, the function of the derivative cell line. (NK, natural killer.) *(From Kaushansky K, Kipps TJ. Hematopoietic agents: Growth factors, minerals and vitamins. In: Brunton LL, Chabner BA, Knollman BC (eds). Goodman & Gilman's The Pharmacologic Basis of Therapeutics, 12th ed. New York: McGraw-Hill, 2010.)*

Recently, the American Society of Clinical Oncology stated that this strategy is clinically and economically appropriate for patients who are receiving a chemotherapy regimen with a 20% or higher risk of febrile neutropenia.[129] Secondary prophylaxis refers to the use of growth factors to prevent recurrent neutropenia in patients who had experienced neutropenia with the prior cycle of chemotherapy. It is recommended that secondary prophylaxis be reserved for patients with chemosensitive cancers when dose reduction may affect disease-free or overall survival.[130]

The role of these factors in the treatment of established neutropenia is less well defined. Most studies suggest no or only minimal clinical benefit from use of CSFs in treating neutropenia; therefore, CSFs should not be routinely used in patients with established neutropenia regardless of the presence of fever. However, certain high-risk patients with fever and neutropenia may benefit from CSFs, including those with neutropenia for more than 10 days, ANC below 100 cells/mm^3 (>0.1 × 10^9/L), age younger than 65 years, and infectious complications (pneumonia, sepsis, or invasive fungal infections) as well as those who are hospitalized at the time of the development of neutropenic fever.[126,130]

Both G-CSF and GM-CSF have also proven effective in accelerating hematopoietic engraftment and in treating graft failure after hematopoietic stem cell transplantation. Other uses for the CSFs include peripheral blood stem cell mobilization, neutropenia in patients with acquired immune deficiency syndrome, myelodysplastic syndromes, congenital neutropenia, and aplastic anemia. Growth factors should not be used in patients receiving concomitant chemotherapy and radiotherapy, especially if the radiation involves the mediastinum. These patients appear to experience more significant thrombocytopenia when administered CSFs.

At currently recommended doses, the CSFs are well tolerated. Adverse events are more commonly seen with GM-CSF and may be related to its ability to enhance binding of neutrophils to endothelial cells or to activation of monocytes or macrophages, which may stimulate the release of cytokines such as IL-1 and TNF-α.[127] The most common adverse event with CSFs is bone pain (20%–25% of patients), which can be treated with acetaminophen. Other adverse events of G-CSF include an increase in lactate dehydrogenase, alkaline phosphatase, and uric acid levels. Additional adverse events of GM-CSF include constitutional symptoms, such as low-grade fever, myalgia, arthralgia, lethargy, and mild headache. GM-CSF may also produce an elevation in liver transaminases. At higher doses of GM-CSF, pleural and pericardial effusions, capillary leak syndrome, and thrombus formation may occur. Both G-CSF and GM-CSF may produce mild erythema at subcutaneous injection sites, as well as a generalized maculopapular rash with either subcutaneous or IV administration. The adverse events observed with pegfilgrastim are similar to those of G-CSF and are treated the same.[128]

The dosing and administration of CSFs approved for prophylaxis of chemotherapy-induced neutropenia after standard dose chemotherapy is as follows: G-CSF 5 mcg/kg until the ANC reaches 10,000 cells/mm^3 (10 × 10^9/L) (or clinically safe) or pegfilgrastim 6 mg as a single dose. Both factors should be started between 24 and 72 hours after chemotherapy; G-CSF can be stopped the day before chemotherapy, but pegfilgrastim needs to be stopped within 14 days of the next dose because of its long half-life. The dose for other uses varies, such as the dose of 10 mcg/kg per day usually used in the setting of peripheral blood stem cell mobilization. The recommended dose of GM-CSF is 250 mcg/m^2 per day. Pharmacokinetic data favor subcutaneous injection as the most effective route. However, in patients in whom subcutaneous injections are not feasible (e.g., anasarca), G-CSF and GM-CSF may be given IV. Pegfilgrastim should not be given IV. Because of the high cost associated with CSF use, alternative dosing regimens have been explored. These regimens attempt to decrease the total amount of CSF used by delaying the start, decreasing the dose, or decreasing the duration of therapy. Standardized doses of 300 mcg or 480 mcg of G-CSF and 500 mcg of GM-CSF, based on product vial sizes, are often used to minimize waste. Specifically, the posttreatment target ANC of 10,000 cells/mm^3 (10 × 10^9/L) recommended by product information is often reduced in clinical practice to 5,000 cells/mm^3 (5 × 10^9/L) or lower. For patients receiving pegfilgrastim, it is important that additional CSFs not be administered for the 10 days after administration because additional benefit is not realized.[128]

Thrombocytopenia

Chemotherapy-induced thrombocytopenia puts the patient at risk for significant bleeding. To date, platelet transfusions remain the mainstay of management. At most centers, platelet transfusions are reserved for patients with a platelet count of less than 10,000 cells/mm^3 (<10 × 10^9/L) unless they are actively bleeding, must undergo a surgical procedure, or have documented infections or fever. For patients with nonmyeloid malignancies who experience significant thrombocytopenia with chemotherapy, oprelvekin (IL-11) may be considered as secondary prophylaxis in subsequent cycles.[131] When used after chemotherapy associated with a high risk of thrombocytopenia, oprelvekin decreased the need for platelet transfusions, as well as the numbers of platelets required for transfusion. Unfortunately, oprelvekin is associated with some significant adverse events, mostly related to fluid retention (e.g., edema, dilutional anemia, dyspnea, and pleural effusions). Cardiac toxicity, especially tachycardia, and atrial fibrillation and flutter also have been observed. Prophylactic oprelvekin also is significantly more expensive than platelet transfusions.[132] Considering the modest clinical benefit, the adverse events, and the high cost, oprelvekin use should be reserved for patients who are at high risk for severe thrombocytopenia from chemotherapy when dose reduction is known to compromise disease response.

Mucositis

The gastrointestinal mucosa is a common site of chemotherapy-anticancer agent induced toxicity.[133] The subsequent inflammation, or mucositis, can lead to painful ulcerations; local infection; and an inability to eat, drink, or swallow. Disruption of the gastrointestinal mucosal barrier may also provide an avenue for systemic microbial invasion. Anticancer agents most commonly associated with mucositis include 5-FU, doxorubicin, MTX, multikinase inhibitors, and mTOR inhibitors. Currently, the most effective means of preventing mucositis is through good oral hygiene. Patients who are at high risk for this toxicity (those with poor dentition, high-dose chemotherapy, or radiation therapy involving the oropharynx) should be evaluated by a dentist before starting therapy and should be instructed to rinse their mouths frequently with baking soda and salt water or plain saline rinses during and during therapy. Clinical practice guidelines for the prevention and treatment of anticancer therapy–induced mucositis were recently published.[133]

A better understanding of the pathophysiology of mucositis has resulted in identification of promising new agents to better prevent mucositis. The keratinocyte growth factor palifermin is approved for use in patients receiving high-dose chemoradiotherapy before hematopoietic stem cell transplantation. Palifermin is given IV at a dose of 60 mcg/kg/day for 3 consecutive days immediately before the initiation of conditioning therapy and then again for 3 days after hematopoietic stem cell transplantation.[134] The effect of palifermin on solid tumor growth is unknown, and its use in nonhematologic cancers is not recommended.

After mucositis has developed, treatment is mainly supportive, including use of topical or systemic analgesics and oral hygiene (including the rinses described).[133] Viscous lidocaine, diphenhydramine liquid, and dyclonine are commonly used topical anesthetics. Severe cases of mucositis may lead to dehydration and require IV hydration and pain medications, including patient-controlled analgesia pumps. Local infections caused by *Candida* species and reactivation of herpes simplex viruses are common in these patients. Suspicious lesions should be cultured, and appropriate antifungal, or antiviral treatment should then be instituted. Antifungal therapy may be delivered topically for mild infections (thrush) with clotrimazole troches or nystatin oral suspension. For more severe oral or esophageal fungal infections, systemic treatment with oral fluconazole or IV antifungals is indicated.

Mucosal damage can occur at any point along the entire length of the gastrointestinal tract. In the lower portion of the gastrointestinal tract, this damage is usually manifested as diarrhea (mild to life threatening in nature) and abdominal pain. Support with IV fluids and electrolyte supplementation should be initiated promptly in severe cases. After infectious causes have been ruled out, diarrhea can safely be treated with antispasmodics, such as Lomotil or loperamide. The somatostatin analog octreotide has also been used successfully to treat severe cases of chemotherapy-induced diarrhea; guidelines exist to assist healthcare providers in treating diarrhea.[133,135]

Cutaneous Reactions

Chemotherapy-induced cutaneous reactions are generally reversible and self-limiting upon dose reductions or delays. Common reactions include localized rash, photosensitivity, skin hyperpigmentation, nail changes, and hand–foot syndrome. Hand–foot syndrome reactions can be uncomfortable and interfere with daily activities. Emollients, cooling procedures, and over-the-counter pain relievers can minimize discomfort. Common chemotherapies associated with cutaneous reactions include cytarabine, 5-FU, capecitabine, doxorubicin, and bleomycin.

Cutaneous reactions, such as rash and hand–foot syndrome, have also been observed with some targeted therapies; for example, rash is often the most common adverse event associated with therapy that inhibits EGFR signaling pathways and requires prompt recognition by healthcare providers to prevent drug discontinuation. Some studies suggest that the rash may be a surrogate marker of response to these agents, perhaps indicating a genetic predisposition to response with EGFR-targeted agents. Rash occurs in up to two-thirds of patients taking EGFR inhibitors, most commonly in the first month of treatment with the typical site of presentation being the face and upper torso. Although no clear guidelines exist for the treatment of this rash, patients should be supported based on their presentation.[70] Anecdotal reports indicate that emollients help if patients complain of dry skin, topical and systemic antibiotics may help if the rash becomes infected, and steroids may help prevent itching and inflammation.[70] Hand–foot syndrome has been reported with several multikinase inhibitors, including sorafenib and sunitinib. The management is the same as for the development of hand–foot syndrome with chemotherapy.

Alopecia

Many patients find alopecia the most distressing adverse event. Alopecia from chemotherapy is usually temporary, and the degree of hair loss varies widely.[136] Hair loss is not limited to the scalp; any area of the body may be affected. Patients receiving a taxane as part of their chemotherapy regimen are especially prone to total body alopecia. Hair loss usually begins 1 to 2 weeks after chemotherapy, and regrowth may begin before the chemotherapy courses are completed. Cryotherapy (local application of ice) and scalp tourniquets have both been investigated as methods of preventing alopecia. Both techniques produce vasoconstriction, resulting in decreased exposure of hair follicles to the chemotherapy. These techniques are not uniformly effective and are contraindicated in patients with cancers that may metastasize to the scalp, such as leukemia and lymphoma.

Extravasation

Vesicants are agents that may cause severe tissue damage if they escape from the vasculature.[129] These agents include the anthracyclines, actinomycin D, the vinca alkaloids, mitomycin C, nitrogen mustard, and the taxanes. The anthracyclines are the most notorious agents and the most extensively investigated. The tissue damage may result in prolonged pain, tissue sloughing, infection, and loss of mobility. Prompt initiation of the appropriate interventions is important to minimize morbidity. Unfortunately, most information on extravasation management is anecdotal; few controlled clinical trials have been conducted to determine optimal intervention strategies. Consequently, prevention is the focus of extravasation management. The most important method of prevention is good administration technique, but extravasations may occur despite good administration technique.[129] The vein selected for administration should be on the distal portion of the arm. The large veins of the forearm are desirable because if a drug does extravasate, there is adequate soft tissue coverage to protect crucial structures such as nerves and tendons, and joint function is not put at risk. Peripherally administered vesicants should be given slowly via IV injection (IV push) through the side arm of a running IV line. The person administering the vesicant should verify needle stability and adequate blood return after each 1 to 2 mL of drug is injected. Vesicants should not be administered by IV infusion unless the patient has a central venous catheter. For extravasation of vesicants, one of the most important interventions is the application of ice packs to the affected area. One exception to this rule is the vinca alkaloids, which are better managed with application of heat. Only a few antidotes to vesicant agents are used clinically. Sodium thiosulfate is used to neutralize nitrogen mustard extravasations, and hyaluronidase (if available) can improve the outcome after extravasation of vinca alkaloids, etoposide, and taxanes. Topical application of dimethyl sulfoxide (DMSO) may be an effective method for managing anthracycline and mitomycin C extravasations.[129] Dexrazoxane, marketed as Totect, has been approved to treat anthracycline extravasation and is given as an IV infusion.[137]

Infertility

Advances in the treatment of some cancers, such as Hodgkin lymphoma and testicular cancer, have produced long-term survivors and the opportunity to examine the late consequences of chemotherapy. Infertility and secondary cancers have emerged as important late effects. The gonadal toxicities of chemotherapy have not received much attention in the past because they are not life threatening. High rates of fertility deficits and sexual dysfunction have been noted for both men and women.[138] In men, chemotherapy can produce severe oligospermia or azoospermia, as well as infertility. Serum testosterone levels are rarely altered. The recovery of spermatogenesis after completing therapy is unpredictable. Men receiving combination chemotherapy appear to sustain more long-lasting adverse events on fertility than do men receiving single-agent chemotherapy. Age, total dose, duration of therapy, and the chemotherapy mechanism are other important variables. In women, toxic effects on the ovaries result clinically in amenorrhea, vaginal epithelial atrophy, and menopausal symptoms. These effects are related to dose and age. Younger patients are more resistant to the effects on the ovaries. As with men, the recovery of fertility is unpredictable, but women younger than 25 years of age appear to have the best outcomes. The effects of the alkylating agents on fertility have been extensively studied. These agents exert profound and consistently detrimental effects on reproductive function.[138] The impact of this drug-induced amenorrhea on patient survival has been less clear with some trials demonstrating a benefit to patients who achieve chemotherapy-induced amenorrhea. Trial results have been mixed, though, and conclusive statements cannot be made at this time. Less is known about commonly used agents such as doxorubicin, taxanes, and platinum compounds. The risk of infertility should be discussed with all patients before they receive anticancer agents, and they should be informed about options for fertility preservation.

Secondary Malignancies

Secondary cancers induced by chemotherapy and radiation are serious long-term complications.[139] Although many solid tumors have been reported as chemotherapy-induced malignancies, AML and myelodysplastic syndromes are the most common secondary cancers. AML and myelodysplastic syndrome have been reported after successful treatment of Hodgkin lymphoma and NHL, acute leukemias, multiple myeloma, breast cancer, and advanced ovarian cancer. For curable cancers, the relatively small risk for occurrence of secondary malignancies is far outweighed by the benefits of survival in large numbers of patients. However, for cancers such as ovarian cancer, the risk of leukemia is not offset by improved survival in patients treated with chemotherapy. The issue of secondary malignancies is of particular concern in patients receiving adjuvant chemotherapy. As with the late complication of infertility, the anticancer agents primarily associated with secondary cancers are the alkylating agents. Etoposide, teniposide, radionucleotides, and the anthracyclines also are linked to secondary leukemias. Solid tumors as secondary malignancies occur more commonly after treatment with radiation than with chemotherapy.

ABBREVIATIONS

ADCC	antibody-dependent cellular cytotoxicity
AI	aromatase inhibitor
ALL	acute lymphoblastic leukemia
ALK	anaplastic lymphoma kinase
AML	acute myelogenous leukemia
ANC	absolute neutrophil count
APA	antiproduct antibodies
ara-C	cytarabine
ATP	adenosine triphosphate
BCNU	carmustine
BSA	body surface area
CCNU	lomustine
CDC	complement-dependent cytotoxicity
CDK	cyclin-dependent kinases
CLL	chronic lymphocytic leukemia
CML	chronic myeloid leukemia
CNS	central nervous system
CR	complete response
CSF	colony-stimulating factor
CTLA-4	cytotoxic T-lymphocyte antigen
CYP	cytochrome P450
DCC	deleted in colorectal cancer
DHFR	dihydrofolate reductase
DMSO	dimethyl sulfoxide
DNA	deoxyribonucleic acid
DNMT	DNA methyltransferase
DPD	dihydropyrimidine dehydrogenase
EGFR	epidermal growth factor receptor
EML	echinoderm microtubule-like protein
ERK	extracellular signal-regulated kinases
FGFR	fibroblast growth factor receptor
5-FU	fluorouracil
G_0	dormant phase of the cell cycle
G_1	first gap phase of the cell cycle
G_2	second gap or premitotic phase of the cell cycle
G-CSF	granulocyte colony-stimulating factor
GIST	gastrointestinal stromal tumor
GM-CSF	granulocyte-macrophage colony-stimulating factor
HAMA	human antimouse antibodies
HER	human epidermal growth factor receptor
HDAC	histone deacetylases
IL	interleukin
IFN	interferon
JK	Janus kinase
LAK	lymphokine-activated killer
M	mitosis
MAPK	mitogen-activated protein kinase
MEK	mitogen-activated protein kinase- extracellular signal-regulated kinases
MMAE	monomethylauristatin E
MoAB	monoclonal antibody
mRNA	messenger RNA
MTIC	monomethyl triazeno-imidazole-carboxamide
mTOR	mammalian target of rapamycin
MTX	methotrexate
NSCLC	non–small cell lung cancer
NF-κB	nuclear factor-κB
NHL	non-Hodgkin lymphoma
Ph^+	Philadelphia chromosome–positive
Pap	Papanicolaou
Pgp	p-glycoprotein
PIGF	phosphatidylinositol-glycan biosynthesis class F
PDGFR	platelet-derived growth factor receptor
PI3K	phosphatidylinositide 3-kinases
PR	partial response
PTEN	phosphatase and tensin homolog
RAR	retinoic acid receptor
Rb	retinoblastoma
RECIST	Response Evaluation Criteria in Solid Tumors
RET	rearranged during transfection receptor
RNA	ribonucleic acid
rRNA	ribosomal RNA
RXR	retinoid X receptor
S	DNA synthesis phase of the cell cycle
SERM	selective estrogen receptor modulator
6-MP	6-mercaptopurine
STAT	signal transducers and activators of transcription
TKI	tyrosine kinase inhibitor
TPMT	thiopurine methyltransferase
tRNA	transfer RNA
VEGF	vascular endothelial growth factor
WBC	white blood cell

REFERENCES

1. Chabner BA. Clinical strategies for cancer treatment: The role of drugs. In: Chabner BA, Longo DL, eds. Cancer Chemotherapy and Biotherapy: Principles and Practice, 5th ed. Philadelphia: Lippincott Williams & Wilkins, 2010.
2. Siegel R, Naishadham D, Jemal A. Cancer statistics, 2013. CA Cancer J Clin 2013;63:11–30.
3. Liotta LA, Liotta LA, Petricoin EF. Genomics and proteomics. In: DeVita VT, Hellman S, Rosenberg SA, eds. Cancer: Principles and Practice of Oncology, 8th ed.

Philadelphia, PA: Lippincott Williams & Wilkins, 2008: 13–34.
4. Compagni A, Christofori G. Recent advances in research on multistage tumorigenesis. Br J Cancer 2000;83:1–5.
5. Weston A, Harris CC. Chemical carcinogenesis. In: Waun KH, Bast RC, Hait WN, et al., eds. Cancer Medicine, 8th ed. Shelton, CT: People's Medical Publishing House-USA, 2010:225–236.
6. Stricker TP, Kumar V. Neoplasia. In: Kumar V, Abbas AK, Aster JC, Fausto N, eds. Robbins and Cotran Pathologic Basis of Disease, 8th ed. Philadelphia, PA: Saunders, 2010:259–330.
7. Weinberg RA. How cancer arises. Sci Am 1996;275:62–71.
8. Hanahan D, Weinberg RA. Hallmarks of cancer: The next generation. Cell 2011;144:646–674.
9. Gross ME, Shazer RL, Agus DB. Targeting the HER-kinase axis in cancer. Semin Oncol 2004;31(Suppl 3):9–20.
10. Schwartz GK, Shah MA. Targeting the cell cycle: a new approach to cancer therapy. J Clin Oncol. 2005;23: 9408–9421.
11. Ghobrial IM, Witzig TE, Adjei AA. Targeting apoptosis pathways in cancer therapy. CA Cancer J Clin. 2005;55: 178–194.
12. Syed S, Rowinsky E. The new generation of targeted therapies for breast cancer. Oncology (Williston Park) 2003;17:1339–1351.
13. Rowinsky EK. Signal events: Cell signal transduction and its inhibition in cancer. Oncologist 2003;8(Suppl 3):5–17.
14. Curran MP, McKeage K. Bortezomib: A review of its use in patients with multiple myeloma. Drugs 2009;69: 859–888.
15. Zondor SD, Medina PJ. Bevacizumab: An angiogenesis inhibitor with efficacy in colorectal and other malignancies. Ann Pharmacother 2004;38:1258–1264.
16. Santarpia L, Lippman SM, El-Naggar AK. Targeting the MAPK-RAS-RAF signaling pathway in cancer therapy. Expert Opin Ther Targets. 2012;16:103–119.
17. Kapoor A, Figlin RA. Targeted inhibition of mammalian target of rapamycin for the treatment of advanced renal cell carcinoma. Cancer 2009;115:3618–3630.
18. Morgensztern D, McLeod HL. PI3K/Akt/mTOR pathway as a target for cancer therapy. Anticancer Drugs 2005;16: 797–803.
19. Georgescu M-M. PTEN tumor suppressor network in PI3K-Akt pathway control. Genes Cancer 2010;1: 1170–1177.
20. Murray PJ. The JAK-STAT signaling pathway: input and output integration. J Immunol 2007;178:2623–2629.
21. Esteller M, Garcia-Foncillas J, Andion E, et al. Inactivation of the DNA-repair gene MGMT and the clinical response of gliomas to alkylating agents. N Engl J Med 2008;358: 1148–1159.
22. Minn AJ, Massave J. Invasion and metastases. In: DeVita VT, Hellman S, Rosenberg SA, eds. Cancer: Principles and Practice of Oncology, 9th ed. Philadelphia, PA: Lippincott Williams & Wilkins, 2011.
23. Heymach JV, Sledge GW, Jain RK. Tumor angiogenesis. In: Waun KH, Bast RC, Hait WN, et al., eds. Cancer Medicine, 8th ed. Shelton, CT: People's Medical Publishing House-USA, 2010:149–169.
24. Smith RA, Cokkinides V, Brawley OW. Cancer screening in the United States, 2012: A review of current American Cancer Society guidelines and issues in cancer screening. CA Cancer J Clin 2012;62:129–142.
25. American Cancer Society. Warning Signs of Cancer. Atlanta, GA: American Cancer Society, 2007.
26. Edge SB, Byrd DR, Compton CC, Fritz AG, Greene FL, Trotti A, eds. AJCC Cancer Staging Manual, 7th ed. New York: Springer-Verlag, 2010.
27. Chabner BA, Amrein PC, Druker BJ, et al. Antineoplastic agents. In: Brunton LL, Lazo JS, Parker KL, eds. Goodman & Gilman's The Pharmacological Basis of Therapeutics, 11th ed. New York: McGraw-Hill, 2006: 1315–1403.
28. Buick RN. Cellular basis of chemotherapy. In: Dorr RT, Von Hoff DD, eds. Cancer Chemotherapy Handbook, 2nd ed. New York: McGraw-Hill, 1994:3–14.
29. Norton L, Gilewski TA. Cytokinetics. In: Waun KH, Bast RC, Hait WN, et al., eds. Cancer Medicine, 8th ed. Shelton, CT: People's Medical Publishing House-USA, 2010: 550–557.
30. Pizzorno G, Sharma S, Cheng Y-C. Pyrimidines and purine antimetabolites. In: Waun KH, Bast RC, Hait WN, et al., eds. Cancer Medicine, 8th ed. Shelton, CT: People's Medical Publishing House-USA, 2010:621–632.
31. Amstutz U, Froehlich TK, Largiadèr CR. Dihydropyrimidine dehydrogenase gene as a major predictor of severe 5-fluorouracil toxicity. Pharmacogenomics 2011;12: 1321–1336.
32. Wagstaff AJ, Ibbotson T, Goa KL. Capecitabine: A review of its pharmacology and therapeutic efficacy in the management of advanced breast cancer. Drugs 2003;63: 217–236.
33. Johnson SA. Clinical pharmacokinetics of nucleoside analogues: Focus on haematological malignancies. Clin Pharmacokinet 2000;39:5–26.
34. Plosker GL, Figgitt DP. Oral fludarabine [see comment]. Drugs 2003;63:2317–2323.
35. Cole PD, Kamen BA, Bertino JR. Folate antagonists. In: Waun KH, Bast RC, Hait WN, et al., eds. Cancer Medicine, 8th ed. Shelton, CT: People's Medical Publishing House-USA, 2010:611–620.
36. Schwartz S, Borner K, Müller K, et al. Glucarpidase (carboxypeptidase g2) intervention in adult and elderly cancer patients with renal dysfunction and delayed methotrexate elimination after high-dose methotrexate therapy. Oncologist 2007;12: 1299–1308.
37. Hui J, Przespo E, Elefante A. Pralatrexate: A novel synthetic antifolate for relapsed or refractory peripheral T-cell lymphoma and other potential uses. J Oncol Pharm Pract 2012;18:275–283.
38. Rowinsky E. Microtubule-targeting natural products. In: Waun KH, Bast RC, Hait WN, et al., eds. Cancer Medicine, 8th ed. Shelton, CT: People's Medical Publishing House-USA, 2010:655–678.
39. Gradishar WJ, Tjulandin S, Davidson N, et al. Phase III trial of nanoparticle albumin-bound paclitaxel compared with polyethylated castor oil-based paclitaxel in women with breast cancer. J Clin Oncol 2005;23:7794–7803.
40. Mita AC, Figlin R, Mita MM. Cabazitaxel: More than a new taxane for metastatic castrate-resistant prostate cancer? Clin Cancer Res 2012;18:6574–6579.
41. Goodin S. Ixabepilone: A novel microtubule-stabilizing agent for the treatment of metastatic breast cancer. Am J Health Syst Pharm 2008;65:2017–2026.
42. Jain S, Vahdat LT. Eribulin mesylate. Clin Cancer Res 2011;17:6615–6622.
43. Rubin EH, Hait WN. Drugs that target DNA topoisomerase. In: Waun KH, Bast RC, Hait WN, et al., eds. Cancer Medicine, 8th ed. Shelton, CT: People's Medical Publishing House-USA, 2010:645–654.

44. Ulukan H, Swaan PW. Camptothecins: A review of their chemotherapeutic potential. Drugs 2002;62: 2039–2057.
45. Danesi R, Fogli S, Gennari A, et al. Pharmacokinetic-pharmacodynamic relationships of the anthracycline anticancer drugs. Clin Pharmacokinet 2002;41: 431–444.
46. Colvin M. Alkylating agents and platinum antitumor compounds. In: Waun KH, Bast RC, Hait WN, et al., eds. Cancer Medicine, 8th ed. Shelton, CT: People's Medical Publishing House-USA, 2010:633–644.
47. Ajlthkumar T, Parkinson C, Shamshad F, et al. Ifosfamide encephalopathy. Clin Oncol 2007;19:108–114.
48. Cheson BD, Rummel MJ. Bendamustine: Rebirth of an old drug. J Clin Oncol 2009;27:1492–1501.
49. Grothey A, Goldberg RM. A review of oxaliplatin and its clinical use in colorectal cancer. Expert Opin Pharmacother 2004;5:2159–2170.
50. Buzdar AU, Dawood S, Harvey HA, Jordan VC. Antiestrogens, progestins and aromatase inhibitors. In: Waun KH, Bast RC, Hait WN, et al., eds. Cancer Medicine, 8th ed. Shelton, CT: People's Medical Publishing House-USA, 2010:737–749.
51. Swaby RF, Sharma CGN, Jordan VC. SERMs for the treatment and prevention of breast cancer. Rev Endocr Metab Disord 2007;8:229–239.
52. Denmeade SR. Androgen deprivation strategies in the treatment of advanced prostate cancer. In: Waun KH, Bast RC, Hait WN, et al., eds. Cancer Medicine, 8th ed. Shelton, CT: People's Medical Publishing House-USA, 2010: 750–758.
53. McKay LI, Cidlowski JA. Corticosteroids. In: Kufe DW, Bast RC, Hait WN, et al., eds. Cancer Medicine, 7th ed. Hamilton, Ontario: BC Decker, 2006:817–827.
54. Powell BL, Moser B, Stock W, et al. Arsenic trioxide improves event-free and overall survival for adults with acute promyelocytic leukemia: North American Leukemia Intergroup Study C9710. Blood. 2010;116:3751–3757.
55. Altucci L, Leibowitz MD, Oglivie KM, et al. RAR and RXR modulation in cancer and metabolic disease. Nat Rev Drug Discov 2007;6:793–810.
56. Bradner WT. Mitomycin C. A clinical update. Cancer Treat Rev 2001;27:35–50.
57. Wetzler M, Segal D. Omacetaxine as an anticancer therapeutic: What is old is new again. Curr Pharm Res 2011;17:59–64.
58. Deininger M, Buchdunger E, Druker BJ. The development of imatinib as a therapeutic agent for chronic myeloid leukemia. Blood 2005;105:2640–2653.
59. Borden EC. Interferons. In: Waun KH, Bast RC, Hait WN, et al., eds. Cancer Medicine, 8th ed. Shelton, CT: People's Medical Publishing House-USA, 2010:679–685.
60. Rotea W Jr, Saad ED. Targeted drugs in oncology: New names, new mechanisms, new paradigm. Am J Health Syst Pharm 2003;60:1233–1243.
61. Gleevec (imatinib mesylate). East Hanover, NJ: Novartis Pharmaceutical Corporation; February 2013.
62. McFarland KL, Wetzstein GA. Chronic myeloid leukemia therapy: Focus of second-generation tyrosine-kinase inhibitors. Cancer Control 2009;16:132–140.
63. Keller-V Amsberg G, Brummendorf TH. Novel aspects of therapy with the dual Src and Abl kinase inhibitor bosutinib in chronic myeloid leukemia. Expert Rev Anticancer Ther 2012;12:1121–1127.
64. Gibbons DL, Pricl S, Kantarjian H, Cortes J, Quintas-Cardama A. The rise and fall of gatekeeper mutations? The BCR-ABL1 T315I paradigm. Cancer 2012;118: 293–299.
65. Bolden JE, Peart MJ, Johnstone RW. Anticancer activities of histone deacetylase inhibitors. Nat Rev Drug Discov 2006;5:769–784.
66. Fandy TE. Development of DNA methyltransferase inhibitors for the treatment of neoplastidiseases. Curr Med Chem 2009;16:2075–2085.
67. Cersosimo RJ. Gefitinib: A new antineoplastic for advanced non-small-cell lung cancer [see comment]. Am J Health Syst Pharm 2004;61:889–898.
68. Tang PA, Tsao M-S, Moore MJ. A review of erlotinib and its clinical use. Expert Opin Pharmacother 2006;7: 177–193.
69. Pallis AG, Syrigos KN. Epidermal growth factor receptor tyrosine kinase inhibitors in the treatment of NSCLC. Lung Cancer 2013; Feb 2.
70. Li T, Perez-Soler R, Saltz L. Skin toxicities associated with epidermal growth factor inhibitors. Target Oncol 2009;4:107–119.
71. Medina PJ, Goodin S. Lapatinib: A dual inhibitor of human epidermal growth factor receptor tyrosine kinases. Clin Ther 2008;30:1426–1447.
72. Spraggs CF, Budde LR, Briley LP, et al. HLA-DQA1*02:01 is a major risk factor for lapatinib-induced hepatotoxicity in women with advanced breast cancer. J Clin Oncol 2011;29:667–673.
73. Rini BI, Campbell SC, Escdier B. Renal cell carcinoma. Lancet 2009;373:1119–1132.
74. Ward JE, Stadler WM. Pazopanib in renal cell carcinoma. Clin Cancer Res 2010;16:5923–5927.
75. Hu-Lowe DD, Zou HY, Grazzini ML, et al. Nonclinical antiangiogenesis and antitumor activities of axitinib (AG-013736), an oral, potent, and selective inhibitor of vascular endothelial growth factor receptor tyrosine kinases 1, 2, 3. Clin Cancer Res 2008;14:7272–7283.
76. Wilhelm SM, Dumas J, Adnane L, et al. Regorafenib (BAY 73-4506): A new oral multikinase inhibitor of angiogenic, stromal and oncogenic receptor tyrosine kinases with potent preclinical antitumor activity. Int J Cancer. 2011;129:245–255.
77. Chau NG, Haddad RI. Vandetanib for the treatment of medullary thyroid cancer. Clin Cancer Res 2013;19: 524–529.
78. Yakes FM, Chen J, Tan J, et al. Cabozantinib (XL184), a novel MET and VEGFR2 inhibitor, simultaneously suppresses metastasis, angiogenesis, and tumor growth. Mol Cancer Ther 2011;10:2298–2308.
79. Kuhn DJ, Orlowski RZ. The immunoproteasome as a target in hematologic malignancies. Semin Hematol 2012;49: 258–262.
80. Rajkumar SV, Kyle RA. Multiple myeloma: Diagnosis and treatment. Mayo Clin Proc 2005;80:1371–1382.
81. Camidge DR, Bang YJ, Kwak EL, et al. Activity and safety of crizotinib in patients with ALK-positive non-small-cell lung cancer: Updated results from a phase 1 study. Lancet Oncol 2012;13:1011–1019.
82. Bollag G, Tsai J, Zhang J, et al. Vemurafenib: The first drug approved for BRAF-mutant cancer. Nat Rev Drug Discov 2012;11:873–886.
83. Rudin CM. Vismodegib. Clin Cancer Res 2012;18:3218–3222.
84. Mesa RA. Ruxolitinib, a selective JAK1 and JAK2 inhibitor for the treatment of myeloproliferative neoplasms and psoriasis. Drugs 2010;13:394–403.
85. Toma MB, Medina PJ. Update on targeted therapy-focus on monoclonal antibodies. J Pharm Pract 2008;21:4–16.

86. American Medical Association. Monoclonal Antibodies. http://www.ama-assn.org/ama/pub/physician-resources/medical-science/united-states-adopted-names-council/naming-guidelines/naming-biologics/monoclonal-antibodies.page.
87. Harris M. Monoclonal antibodies as therapeutic agents for cancer. Lancet Oncol 2004;5:292–302.
88. Villamor N, Montserrat E, Colomer D. Mechanism of action and resistance to monoclonal antibody therapy. Semin Oncol 2003;30:424–433.
89. Cheson BD. Radioimmunotherapy of non-Hodgkin's lymphomas. Blood 2003;101:391–398.
90. Plosker GL, Figgitt DP. Rituximab: A review of its use in non-Hodgkin's lymphoma and chronic lymphocytic leukaemia. Drugs 2003;63:803–843.
91. Cersosimo RJ. Monoclonal antibodies in the treatment of cancer, part 1. Am J Health Syst Pharm 2003;60:1531–1548.
92. Cheson BD. Ofatumumab, a novel anti-CD20 monoclonal antibody for the treatment of B-cell malignancies. J Clin Oncol 2010;28:3525–3530.
93. Hernandez MC, Knox SJ. Radiobiology of radioimmunotherapy with 90Y ibritumomab tiuxetan (Zevalin). Semin Oncol 2003;30(Suppl 17):6–10.
94. Cersosimo RJ. Monoclonal antibodies in the treatment of cancer, Part 2. Am J Health Syst Pharm 2003;60:1631–1641.
95. Kaminski MS, Zelenetz AD, Press OW, et al. Pivotal study of iodine I 131 tositumomab for chemotherapy-refractory low-grade or transformed low-grade B-cell non-Hodgkin's lymphomas [see comment]. J Clin Oncol 2001;19:3918–3928.
96. Gribben JG, Hallek M. Rediscovering alemtuzumab: Current and emerging therapeutic roles. Br J Haematol 2009;144:818–831.
97. Katz J, Janik JE, Younes A. Brentuximab vedotin (SGN-35). Clin Cancer Res 2011;17:6428–6436.
98. Finley RS. Overview of targeted therapies for cancer. Am J Health Syst Pharm 2003;60(Suppl 9):S4–S10.
99. Cunningham D, Humblet Y, Siena S, et al. Cetuximab monotherapy and cetuximab plus irinotecan in irinotecan-refractory metastatic colorectal cancer [see comment]. N Engl J Med 2004;351:337–345.
100. Bonner JA, Harari PM, Giralt J, et al. Radiotherapy plus cetuximab for squamous-cell carcinoma of the head and neck [see comment]. N Engl J Med 2006;354:567–578.
101. Chung CH, Mirakhur B, Chan E, et al. Cetuximab-induced anaphylaxis and IgE specific for galactose–1,3-galactose. N Engl J Med 2008;358:1109–1117.
102. Hoy SM, Wagstaff AJ. Panitumumab in the treatment of metastatic colorectal cancer. Drugs 2006;66:2005–2014.
103. Allegra CJ, Jessup JM, Somerfield MR, et al. American Society of Clinical Oncology provisional clinical opinion: Testing for KRAS gene mutations in patients with metastatic colorectal carcinoma to predict response to anti-epidermal growth factor receptor monoclonal antibody therapy. J Clin Oncol 2009;27:2091–2096.
104. Okines AF, Cunningham D. Trastuzumab in gastric cancer. Eur J Cancer 2010;46:1949–1959.
105. Hudis CA. Trastuzumab—Mechanism of action and use in clinical practice. N Engl J Med 2007;357:39–51.
106. Leyland-Jones B, Gelmon K, Ayoub JP, et al. Pharmacokinetics, safety, and efficacy of trastuzumab administered every three weeks in combination with paclitaxel. J Clin Oncol 2003;21:3965–3971.
107. Capelan M, Pugliano L, De Azambuja E, et al. Pertuzumab: new hope for patients with HER2-positive breast cancer. Ann Oncol 2013;24:273–282.
108. Verma S, Miles D, Gianni L, et al. Trastuzumab emtansine for HER2-positive advanced breast cancer. N Engl J Med 2012;367:1783–1791.
109. Hurwitz H, Fehrenbacher L, Novotny W, et al. Bevacizumab plus irinotecan, fluorouracil, and leucovorin for metastatic colorectal cancer [see comment]. N Engl J Med 2004;350:2335–2342.
110. Avastin (bevacizumab). Prescribing information. San Francisco, CA: Genentech, 2009.
111. Mellman I, Coukos G, Dranoff G. Cancer immunotherapy comes of age. Nature 2011;480:480–489.
112. Ekmekcioglu S, Grimm EA, Kurzrock R. Cytokines and hematopoietic growth factors. In: Waun KH, Bast RC, Hait WN, et al., eds. Cancer Medicine, 8th ed. Shelton, CT: People's Medical Publishing House-USA, 2010: 686–709.
113. Foss F. Clinical experience with denileukin diftitox (ONTAK). Semin Oncol 2006;33(Suppl 3):S11–S16.
114. Zaltrap (ziv-afibercept). Prescribing information. Chattanooga, TN: Sanofi U.S., Inc., 2012.
115. Therasse P, Arbuck SG, Eisenhauer EA, et al. New guidelines to evaluate the response to treatment in solid tumors. J Natl Cancer Inst 2000;92:205–216.
116. Johnson JR, Williams G, Pazdur R. End points and United States Food and Drug Administration approval of oncology drugs. J Clin Oncol 2003;21:1404–1411.
117. Kellen JA. The reversal of multidrug resistance: An update. J Exp Ther Oncol 2003;3:5–13.
118. Lee W, Lockhart AC, Kim RB, Rothenberg ML. Cancer Pharmacogenomics: Powerful tools in cancer chemotherapy and drug development. Oncologist 2005;10:104–111.
119. Haskell CM. Principles of cancer chemotherapy. In: Haskell CM, ed. Cancer Treatment, 5th ed. Philadelphia, PA: WB Saunders, 2001:62–86.
120. Mathijssen RH, de Jong FA, Loos WJ, et al. Flat-fixed dosing versus body surface area based dosing of anticancer drugs in adults: does it make a difference? Oncologist 2007;12:913–923.
121. Calvert AH, Newell DR, Gumbrell LA, et al. Carboplatin dosage: Prospective evaluation of a simple formula based on renal function. J Clin Oncol 1989;7:1748–1756.
122. American Society of Hospital Pharmacists. ASHP guidelines on handling hazardous drugs. Am J Health Syst Pharm 2006;63:1172–1193.
123. Goodin S, Griffith N, Chen B, et al. Safe Handling of oral chemotherapeutic agents in clinical practice: Recommendations from an international pharmacy panel. J Oncol Pract 2011;7:7–12.
124. The NCCN Cancer- and Chemotherapy-Induced Anemia Clinical Practice Guidelines in Oncology (version 1.2013). National Comprehensive Cancer Network, Inc. 2013, *http://www.nccn.org/professionals/physician_gls/pdf/anemia.pdf.*
125. Siddiqui MAA, Keating GM. Darbepoetin alfa: A review of its use in the treatment of anaemia in patients with cancer receiving chemotherapy. Drugs 2006;66:997–1012.
126. Freifeld AG, Bow EJ, Sepkowitz KA, et al. Clinical practice guideline for the use of antimicrobial agents in neutropenic patients with cancer: 2010 Update by the Infectious Diseases Society of America. Clin Infect Dis 2011;52:427–431.
127. Metcalf D. The colony-stimulating factors and cancer. Nat Rev Cancer 2010;10:425–434.
128. Wolf T, Densmore JJ. Pegfilgrastim use during chemotherapy: Current and future applications. Curr Hematol Rep 2004;3:419–423.
129. McCurdy MT, Shanholtz CB. Oncologic emergencies. Crit Care Med 2012;40:2212–2222.

130. Smith TJ, Khatcheressian J, Lyman GH, et al. 2006 Update of recommendations for the use of white blood cell growth factors: An evidence-based clinical practice guideline. J Clin Oncol 2006;24:3187–3205.
131. Vadhan-Raj S. Management of chemotherapy-induced thrombocytopenia: Current status of thrombopoietic agents. Semin Hematol 2009;46(1 Suppl 2):S26–S32.
132. Cantor SB, Elting LS, Hudson DV Jr, Rubenstein EB. Pharmacoeconomic analysis of oprelvekin (recombinant human interleukin-11) for secondary prophylaxis of thrombocytopenia in solid tumor patients receiving chemotherapy. Cancer 2003;97:3099–3106.
133. Keefe DM, Schubert MM, Elting LS, et al. Updated clinical practice guidelines for the prevention and treatment of mucositis. Cancer 2007;109:820–831.
134. Spielberger R, Stiff P, Bensinger W, et al. Palifermin for oral mucositis after intensive therapy for hematologic cancers. N Engl J Med 2004;351:2590–2598.
135. Benson AB, III, Ajani JA, Catalano RB, et al. Recommended guidelines for the treatment of cancer treatment-induced diarrhea. J Clin Oncol 2004;22:2918–2926.
136. Karakunnell J, Berger AM. Hair loss. In: DeVita V, Hellman S, Rosenberg SA, eds. Cancer Principles and Practice of Oncology, 9th ed. Philadelphia, PA: Lippincott Williams & Wilkins, 2011.
137. Reeves D. Management of anthracycline extravasation injuries. Ann Pharmacother 2007;41:1238–1242.
138. Lee SJ, Schover LR, Partridge AH, et al. American Society of Clinical Oncology recommendations on fertility preservation in cancer patients. J Clin Oncol 2006;24:2917–2931.
139. Travis LB, Bhatia S, Allan JM, Oeffinger KC, Ng A. Second primary cancers. In: DeVita VT, Hellman S, Rosenberg SA, eds. Cancer Principles and Practice of Oncology, 9th ed. Philadelphia, PA: Lippincott Williams & Wilkins, 2011.

105

Breast Cancer

Chad M. Barnett, Laura Boehnke Michaud, and Francisco J. Esteva

KEY CONCEPTS

1. Breast cancer is usually diagnosed in the early stages when it is a highly curable malignancy.
2. Local therapy of early-stage breast cancer consists of modified radical mastectomy or lumpectomy plus external-beam radiation therapy. The surgical approach to the ipsilateral axilla may consist of a lymph node mapping procedure with sentinel lymph node biopsy or a full level I/II axillary lymph node dissection.
3. Adjuvant endocrine therapy reduces the rates of relapse and death in patients with hormone receptor–positive early breast cancer. Adjuvant chemotherapy reduces the rates of relapse and death in all patients with early-stage breast cancer.
4. The choice of the most appropriate chemotherapy, endocrine therapy, and anti-*HER2* regimen is complex and rapidly changing as results from ongoing randomized clinical trials are reported.
5. Neoadjuvant chemotherapy and biotherapy are appropriate for selected patients with early breast cancer and most patients with locally advanced breast cancer and inflammatory breast cancer followed by local therapy and further adjuvant systemic therapy as indicated.
6. Whereas the goal of adjuvant and neoadjuvant chemotherapy is curative, the goal of chemotherapy in the metastatic setting is palliative.
7. Initial therapy of metastatic breast cancer in most women with hormone receptor–positive tumors should include endocrine therapy.
8. About 60% of women with metastatic breast cancer will respond to chemotherapy regimens; anthracycline- and taxane-containing regimens are the most active.
9. Anti-*HER2* therapies and other biologic or targeted agents (e.g., everolimus) in combination with chemotherapy or endocrine therapy have significantly improved outcomes for selected patients with metastatic breast cancer.
10. Although controversial, regular screening mammography in women younger than 50 years of age is beneficial, and many national and international studies demonstrate a reduction in the breast cancer mortality rate from annual or biennial screening mammography in women ages 50 to 74 years.

INTRODUCTION

Breast cancer is the most common site of cancer and is second only to lung cancer as a cause of cancer death in American women. It was estimated that 234,580 new cases of breast cancer will be diagnosed and that 40,030 people will die of breast cancer in 2013.[1] In addition to invasive breast cancers, it is estimated that 64,640 cases of noninvasive, or in situ, cancer will be diagnosed among women in the United States in 2013.

Female breast cancer incidence rates vary considerably across racial and ethnic groups. The average annual age-adjusted incidence rate from 2004 to 2008 was 122.3 cases per 100,000 among whites, 116.1 cases among African Americans, 92.3 cases in Hispanics, 89.2 cases in American Indians and Alaska Natives, and 84.9 cases among Asian Americans and Pacific Islanders.[2] Reasons for the higher incidence rates in whites than in other racial and ethnic groups may include differences in reproductive and lifestyle factors and access to and use of screening.

Female breast cancer incidence rates have increased for all women combined since 1980, although the rate of increase slowed in the 1990s and has decreased starting in 2000 after peaking in 1999. The decrease in breast cancer incidence of about 7% from 2002 to 2003 is thought to be related to decreased use of postmenopausal hormone replacement therapy (HRT).[2] Incidence rates were stable from 2004 to 2008. The incidence of ductal carcinoma in situ (DCIS) also increased rapidly between the early and late 1980s and continues to increase. The increase in DCIS is largely attributed to an increased use of screening mammography because most cases of DCIS manifest solely as clustered microcalcifications seen on mammography.[1]

(1) For all racial and ethnic groups, most breast cancers are diagnosed at an early stage when tumors are small and localized. However, a higher proportion of disease is diagnosed at more advanced stages in African American and other minority women than in white women. The death rate is also higher among African American women than white women despite the lower incidence. From 2004 to 2008, the breast cancer death rate was highest in African Americans (32.0 cases per 100,000 women) followed by whites (22.8), American Indians and Alaska Natives (17.2), Hispanics (15.1), and Asian Americans and Pacific Islanders (12.2).[2] The cause of this disparity between white and African American women is widely debated and multifactorial, with possible explanations including access to care, socioeconomic status, cultural differences, higher stage at diagnosis, and more aggressive biologic features. Despite these differences, overall mortality rates from breast cancer in the United States have declined since 1990. These declines

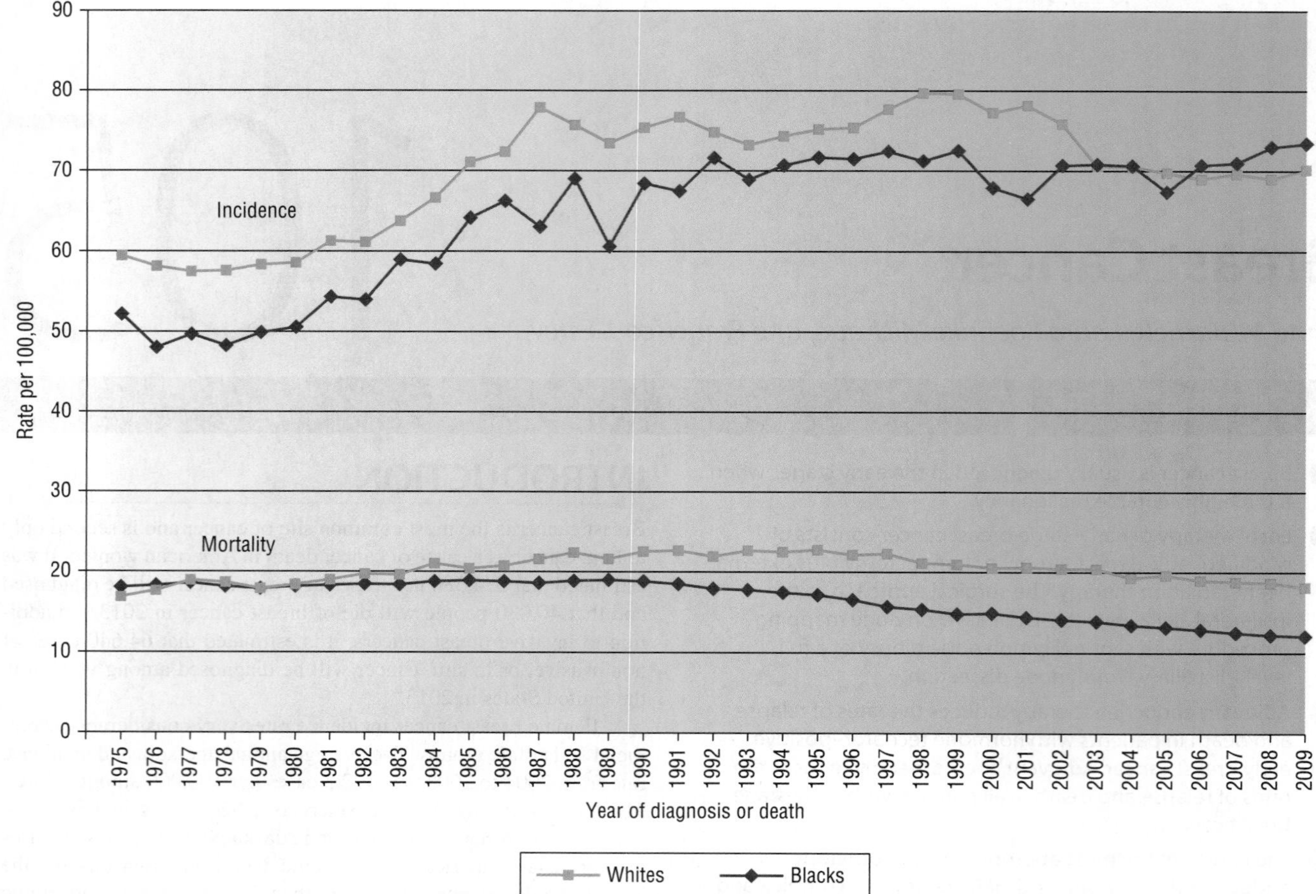

FIGURE 105-1 Breast cancer incidence and mortality rates by race, 1975 to 2009. *(Data from Howlader N, Noone AM, Krapcho M, et al. SEER Cancer Statistics Review, 1975–2009 [Vintage 2009 Populations]. Bethesda, MD: National Cancer Institute. 2009, http://seer.cancer.gov/csr/1975_2009_pops09.)*

have been attributed to increased use of screening and effectiveness of adjuvant treatment.[3–5] Figure 105-1 shows the temporal trends in incidence and mortality by race.

The median age at diagnosis for breast cancer is between the ages of 60 and 65 years.[2] Although lung cancer is the leading cause of cancer deaths for women regardless of age, breast cancer is the leading cause of cancer deaths for females between the ages of 20 and 59 years.[1]

EPIDEMIOLOGY AND ETIOLOGY

The two variables most strongly associated with the occurrence of breast cancer are gender and age. Although one commonly thinks of breast cancer as a disease confined to women, about 2,240 cases of male breast cancer were estimated to be diagnosed in the United States in 2013.[1] Male gender had been considered a poor prognostic factor in some investigations, but it is now believed that higher mortality rates in men are attributable to more advanced disease at the time of diagnosis. When stage and other known prognostic factors are controlled for, the clinical outcome for men with breast cancer is comparable to that of women.[6] Treatment of breast cancer in men is similar to treatment of breast cancer in women.

The incidence of breast cancer increases with advancing age. A frequently quoted breast cancer statistic is that one in eight women will develop breast cancer during her lifetime. It should be emphasized that this is a cumulative lifetime risk of developing the disease from birth to death. The one-in-eight women figure is often misinterpreted by women who assume that it translates into one in eight women being diagnosed with breast cancer each year. A more useful method of presenting the risk data is based on age intervals.[7] Table 105-1 shows that the risk of a woman developing breast cancer before the age of 40 years is about one in 203, and more than half the risk occurs after age 60 years.

An understanding of the relationship between age and the incidence of breast cancer is particularly relevant when one discusses "risk factors" or factors other than age that increase a woman's probability of developing breast cancer. The relative risk (RR) of developing breast cancer for an individual woman in a defined risk group is usually multiplied by the probability of a woman developing breast cancer during her lifetime, and this figure is taken as the cumulative lifetime risk of that individual developing breast cancer. However, the risk of developing breast cancer depends on age.

TABLE 105-1 Risk of Developing Breast Cancer, Women, All Races, 2006 to 2008

Age Interval	Probability (%) of Developing Invasive Breast Cancer During the Interval
Birth–39 y	0.49 or 1 in 203
40–59 y	3.76 or 1 in 27
60–69 y	3.53 or 1 in 28
70 y and older	6.58 or 1 in 15
From birth to death	12.29 or 1 in 8

Data from Cancer Facts & Figures 2012.[2]

Therefore, a more meaningful way to counsel patients regarding their risk of developing breast cancer based on the presence of a known risk factor incorporates an age-specific incidence rate, not cumulative lifetime risk. For example, if a 40-year-old woman with a strong family history of breast cancer has a RR ratio of 2.0, her risk of developing breast cancer by the age of 50 years is only 7.6% (2 × 3.8), not 24.6% (2 × 12.3) (Table 105-1). It is also important to note that recognized risk factors are not additive in a simple mathematical sense. Finally, most women with breast cancer have no identifiable major risk factor, indicating that the search for the etiology of this disease is largely incomplete.

A number of calculators are available to estimate a patient's risk of developing breast cancer. The National Cancer Institute has an online version of the Breast Cancer Risk Assessment Tool (*www.cancer.gov/bcrisktool/Default.aspx*). This tool is based on a statistical model known as the Gail model, derived from data from the Breast Cancer Detection and Demonstration Project, a mammography screening project conducted in the 1970s. The Breast Cancer Risk Assessment Tool was designed for healthcare professionals to project a woman's individualized risk for invasive breast cancer over a 5-year period and over her lifetime. This model has been shown to provide accurate estimates in white women, but it has not been validated for other racial and ethnic groups and other subgroups, including those with genetic risk factors. Other risk assessment models also exist, each taking into account different risk factors. Gail and colleagues have developed a similar model for assessing the risk of developing breast cancer in African American women.[8] These empiric models may not be as useful for women with a history suggestive of hereditary breast cancer. Thus, no one model is appropriate for every patient.

Endocrine Factors

A number of endocrine factors have been linked to the incidence of breast cancer.[9,10] Many of these relate to the total duration of menstrual life. Early menarche, generally defined as menstruation beginning before age 12 years, increases the cumulative lifetime risk of breast cancer development. Similarly, a late age of natural menopause (age 55 years or later) increases the risk of breast cancer development, although to a lesser degree than early menarche.[9] Conversely, bilateral oophorectomy before age 40 years reduces the risk of developing breast cancer.

Nulliparity and a late age at first birth (≥30 years) are reported to increase the lifetime risk of developing breast cancer. It is suggested that the period between the onset of menses and the age of first pregnancy provides a "window of initiation" for the development of breast cancer. This is a time when an unbalanced hormonal environment reacts with the abundant and highly responsive breast tissue. Investigators postulate that international differences in age of menarche, age at menopause, and childbearing may account for a substantial part of the international differences in the incidence of breast cancer.

Many studies have evaluated the relationship between exogenous hormones and the development of breast cancer. Postmenopausal estrogen replacement therapy has been the subject of several epidemiologic studies and meta-analyses, with conflicting results. The National Cancer Institute (NCI)–funded Women's Health Initiative (WHI) is a series of clinical trials designed to investigate the risks and benefits of treatment strategies that could affect women's health issues, such as breast cancer. The estrogen plus progestin trial randomized more than 16,000 postmenopausal women to take conjugated equine estrogen combined with medroxyprogesterone or a placebo.[11] This study reported an increased risk of breast cancer (38 vs. 30 cases per 10,000 person-years; RR ratio = 1.26; 95%; confidence interval [CI], 1.00–1.59) in women taking combined estrogen and progestin for an average of 5.2 years compared with those receiving placebo. Analysis of the National Cancer Institute's Surveillance, Epidemiology, and End Results (SEER) registries showed that the age-adjusted incidence rate of breast cancer in women in the United States in 2003 fell by 6.7% compared with 2002.[12] This decrease in breast cancer incidence seems to be temporally associated with the first report of the WHI study and subsequent decrease in estrogen and progestin HRT use among postmenopausal women. Additional follow-up of patients in this trial confirms a decrease in breast cancer incidence after cessation of estrogen and progestin.[13] In the estrogen alone trial, more than 10,000 women who had a hysterectomy and therefore did not require progestin therapy because of a decreased risk of endometrial carcinoma were randomized to estrogen alone or placebo.[14] The risk of breast cancer was not increased in women who received estrogen alone compared with those who received placebo. With additional follow-up, the incidence of breast cancer in women in this study was actually lower in patients who received estrogen compared with those who received placebo.[15] However, the authors concluded that estrogen alone may not reduce the incidence of breast cancer in patients at increased risk and therefore should not be used specifically for breast cancer risk reduction. Unresolved issues remain as to whether lower doses or short-term use of estrogen or estrogen–progestin for menopausal symptoms can be safe and effective. A longer duration of HRT and concurrent use of progestins appear to contribute to breast cancer risk. The use of postmenopausal HRT in women with a history of breast cancer is generally contraindicated. Women who are considering HRT should carefully consider the risks versus benefits (see Chap. 65) for a detailed discussion of HRT).

Epidemiologic studies of oral contraceptives do not show a consistent relationship between use of birth control pills and breast cancer risk. Results are conflicting, and assessment of the studies should consider the particular oral contraceptive products involved, daily and cumulative doses of the hormones administered, and latency period for development of breast cancer. A meta-analysis of 13 prospective cohort studies conducted between the years of 1989 and 2010 reported a nonsignificant increase in breast cancer incidence for patients who used oral contraceptives compared with those who had never used oral contraceptives.[16] Newer formulations of oral contraceptives contain lower hormone concentrations, and the authors of this meta-analysis were not able to differentiate breast cancer risk based on the formulations of oral contraceptives. It is also important to note that oral contraceptives are known to reduce the risk of ovarian and endometrial cancers. Most experts believe that the safety and benefits of low-dose oral contraceptives currently outweigh the potential risks.

Genetic Factors

Both personal and family histories influence a woman's risk of developing breast cancer. A personal history of breast cancer is associated with an increased risk of developing contralateral breast cancer. Cancers of the uterus and ovary are also associated with an increased risk of developing breast cancer. A number of cancer family syndromes include breast cancer in association with other types of cancers.

Many women have "lumpy breasts" or have a clinical diagnosis of fibrocystic breast disease or benign breast disease. Nonproliferative lesions, such as cysts or simple fibroadenomas, do not increase the risk of breast cancer. Proliferative lesions without atypia, such as intraductal papillomatosis, are associated with a mildly elevated breast cancer risk of about 1.5 to 2.0 times that of the general population. Atypical hyperplasias are classified as either ductal or lobular units, and these lesions may increase a woman's risk for breast cancer to about 4.5 to 5.0 times that of the general population.[17]

Dense breast tissue reduces the sensitivity of mammography in detecting breast cancer and is associated with an increased risk of breast cancer. The risk of breast cancer in women with dense breasts (defined by mammography) has been estimated to be between two and six times that of women of the same age with little density.[18] Many variables, including age, weight, menopausal status, HRT, and parity, can influence mammographic breast density. Genetic factors may also play a role in this finding because mammographic breast density has been shown to have high heritability and is also strongly associated with a positive family history of breast cancer.

The percentage of all breast cancers in the U.S. population that can be attributed to family history is about 10%. Empirical estimates of the risks associated with particular patterns of family history of breast cancer indicate the following[19]:

1. Having any first-degree relative with breast cancer increases a woman's risk of breast cancer about 1.5- to 3-fold. Risk increases with increasing numbers of affected first-degree relatives.
2. The risk is affected by both a woman's own age and the age of the relative when diagnosed. A higher risk is seen when a woman and her relative at diagnosis are younger than 50 years.
3. The risk associated with having any second-degree relative with breast cancer is complex and depends on other family history patterns. However, the risk is generally lower than that of first-degree relatives.
4. Affected family members on both the maternal and the paternal sides are important to consider in evaluation of risk.

Although women with a family history of breast cancer are at increased risk for the disease, the diagnosis of breast cancer is still uncommon in young women even with a positive family history.

Germ-line mutations in either *BRCA1 or BRCA2* are associated with an increased risk for breast and ovarian cancer. These genes function as tumor suppressor genes, maintaining genomic integrity and DNA repair. Compared with an average woman's 13% lifetime risk of developing breast cancer, the probability of developing breast or ovarian cancer by the age of 70 years in women with a *BRCA1* or *BRCA2* mutation is estimated to be 57% and 49% for breast cancer and 40% and 18% for ovarian cancer, respectively.[20]

The probability of being a *BRCA* gene mutation carrier is related to ethnicity and family history. Jewish people of Eastern European decent (Ashkenazi Jews) have an unusually high (2.5%) carrier rate of germ-line mutations in *BRCA1* and *BRCA2* compared with the rest of the U.S. population. Conversely, it is estimated that clinically significant *BRCA* mutations occur at a frequency of about one in 500 persons in the general, non-Jewish U.S. population.[21] Testing for *BRCA1* and *BRCA2* mutations is now widely available, but testing is generally recommended only when there is personal or family history suggestive of hereditary cancer, when the test results can be adequately interpreted, and when results will assist with diagnosis and management. The decision to test an individual for a genetic mutation related to breast cancer risk is complex, and several organizations have published recommendations on genetic susceptibility testing for individuals who meet the criteria for increased risk.[22–25]

Although most genetic causes of breast cancer are attributed to *BRCA1* and *BRCA2,* other genes that have been identified as being associated with hereditary breast cancer include *TP53*, *CHK2*, *PTEN*, *ATM*, and others.[26]

Environmental and Lifestyle Factors

Breast cancer incidence rates vary considerably among countries, which suggests that environmental and lifestyle factors play an important role in the etiology. Compelling evidence is derived from studies of Asian women who migrated to the United States. Although the incidence of breast cancer in Asian women is quite low, the incidence of breast cancer in Asian women who were born in the United States or who migrated from Asia to the United States gradually increases over the individual's lifetime to equal that of the white population in the same geographic area.[27]

Diet is an important and modifiable environmental risk factor. Possible relationships between fat intake and steroid hormone metabolism have led to an emphasis on dietary fat as a possible etiologic agent for breast cancer. Epidemiologic data show a positive correlation between higher dietary fat intake and breast cancer risk, which is stronger in postmenopausal than in premenopausal women. In a meta-analysis of 31 case-control and 14 cohort studies on dietary fat and breast cancer, Boyd et al. reported a small but significant RR ratio of 1.13 (95% CI, 1.03–1.25) when comparing the highest and lowest fat intake categories.[28] To confirm this association prospectively, the hypothesis that low dietary fat intake reduces breast cancer risk was further tested in the WHI Randomized Controlled Dietary Modification Trial.[29] More than 48,000 postmenopausal women were randomized to a dietary intervention that consisted of reducing total fat intake to 20% of energy and consuming at least five servings of fruits and vegetables daily and six servings of grains daily versus a comparison group without any dietary interventions. Over an 8-year mean follow-up period, the incidence of invasive breast cancer was not significantly different between the two groups (annualized incidence rate, 0.42% vs. 0.45%; hazard ratio [HR], 0.91; 95% CI, 0.83–1.01). Although there is still much to be learned about the effects of diet on the risk of developing breast cancer, a low-fat diet seems to be a reasonable approach to potentially reduce the risk of breast cancer.

An additional dietary factor to be explored in the breast cancer population includes food-derived heterocyclic amines, which are known carcinogens found commonly in cooked red meat or processed meat. Studies of red or processed meat ingestion and breast cancer incidence are inconsistent, and no association was reported in one meta-analysis.[30]

Many studies have also examined the association between breast cancer and intake of dietary fiber and micronutrients, including β-carotene, and vitamins A, C, and E. The relationship between vitamins and breast cancer is unclear. No consistent benefit of fruits or vegetable consumption and the risk of breast cancer has been demonstrated.[30]

Another dietary factor that deserves mention is the possible effect of phytoestrogens on breast cancer risk. Phytoestrogens are natural plant estrogens found in soybean products, seeds, berries, and nuts. The two most studied classes of dietary phytoestrogens are isoflavones and lignans; isoflavones are richer in Asian diets, and lignans are the main source of phytoestrogens in the Western diet.[31,32] Because these compounds exhibit weak estrogenic properties, some experts believe that they may function as relative antiestrogens by displacing natural estradiol. However, studies have also reported a potential stimulatory effect on breast tissue. A meta-analysis of observational studies that evaluated phytoestrogen use and the risk of breast cancer suggests that any potential associated risk reduction is modest and may be limited to postmenopausal patients.[31] Nonetheless, the effect of phytoestrogens on breast cancer is very controversial, and further research is needed.

Both body weight and height are associated with the incidence of breast cancer. Most studies of premenopausal women show either no relationship with body weight or slightly declining breast cancer risks with increasing body weight. Most studies in postmenopausal women show increasing breast cancer risks with increasing body weight. Accordingly, a meta-analysis by Renehan et al. found that an increase in body mass index was associated with an increase in the risk of breast cancer for postmenopausal women (RR, 1.12; 95% CI, 1.08–1.16; P <0.0001) but had the opposite effect in premenopausal women (RR, 0.92; 95% CI, 0.88–0.97; P <0.001).[33] An increase in circulating estrogen is postulated to be the most likely explanation for these results. Although height is not a modifiable risk factor, weight and body composition are modifiable and should be studied further. Maintaining a healthy weight and body composition appear to be beneficial and promote many different health benefits but requires further study in association with the incidence of breast cancer.

Many studies report an inverse association between physical activity and breast cancer risk.[34] A review of 19 cohort and 29 case-control studies suggests that the association is stronger for postmenopausal breast cancer than for premenopausal breast cancer. Exercise may provide modest protection against breast cancer, but the relationship is complex. Possible explanations include the effects of physical activity on menstrual characteristics (in premenopausal women), body size, weight, and serum hormone levels. Estrogen-related pathways or other metabolic hormones such as insulin and insulin-like growth factors may influence this relationship. Making healthy choices appears to be the best health advice for women.

Many epidemiologic studies have evaluated the relationship between alcohol and breast cancer. Studies indicate both a modest positive association between alcohol and breast cancer and a dose–response relationship.[35] The risk increases with consumption of alcohol in general regardless of the beverage type or woman's menopausal status. Although the exact mechanism is unknown, the most plausible biologic hypothesis relates to increased levels of estrogen or other reproductive steroid hormones caused by impaired liver function. Although a causal relationship between alcohol consumption and breast cancer has not been proven in a prospective trial, the weight of the available evidence suggests that a relationship (direct or indirect) may exist. Because alcohol consumption is a modifiable risk factor, use in moderation appears to be a sensible approach.

Radiation to the breast tissue is associated with an increased risk of breast cancer, particularly with exposure at a young age (<20 years), again suggesting that a "window of initiation" for breast cancer occurs at a relatively early age. Much of the knowledge about radiation-related breast cancer comes from epidemiologic studies of patients exposed to diagnostic or therapeutic radiation and of Japanese survivors of the atomic bombs.[36] Women treated with chest irradiation for Hodgkin lymphoma in childhood or adolescence and survivors of other childhood cancers (in which radiation is used as a mainstay of therapy) are among the populations at greater risk for secondary breast cancers. The risk increases linearly with radiation dose. Exposure to diagnostic x-rays, including annual screening mammography, does not impart a sufficient dose of radiation for clinical concern in the general population. However, the risk of breast cancer after radiation exposure even in low levels in those with genetic risk factors is unclear and is an ongoing area of research.

In conclusion, numerous studies have been performed to investigate potential causative factors in the etiology of breast cancer. Several endocrine, genetic, environmental, and lifestyle factors are associated with the development of breast cancer to varying degrees. Some factors are modifiable, but others are not. Additionally, the impact of individual risk factors may vary depending on other confounding variables such as age, family history, estrogen use, and menopausal status. Although epidemiologic studies provide a large body of the current evidence, they have their limitations, and results are varied. Meta-analyses summarize numerous study results, but heterogeneity of studies may limit the applicability of the evidence. Additional prospective, randomized controlled trials are needed to confirm the importance of factors that are associated with the risk of developing breast cancer.

CLINICAL PRESENTATION

A painless lump is the initial sign of breast cancer in most women. The typical malignant mass is solitary, unilateral, solid, hard, irregular, and nonmobile. In small numbers of cases, stabbing or aching pain is the first symptom. Less commonly, nipple discharge, retraction, or dimpling may herald the onset of the disease. In more advanced cases, prominent skin edema, redness, warmth, and induration of the underlying tissue may be observed.

The breast is a complex organ composed of skin, subcutaneous tissue, fatty tissue, and branching ductal and glandular structures (Fig. 105-2). Various diseases that affect these structures can produce a palpable mass. In addition, the physiologic changes associated with the menstrual cycle can cause normal breast changes. Common causes of breast masses in young women are fibroadenoma, fibrocystic disease, carcinoma, and fat necrosis.

Many women detect some breast abnormality themselves, but in the United States, it is increasingly common for breast cancer to be detected during routine screening mammography in asymptomatic women. It is widely accepted that the smaller the mass, the higher the likelihood of cure. Thus, as the number of breast cancer cases found by screening mammography increases, overall survival

CLINICAL PRESENTATION

General

- The patient may not have any symptoms because breast cancer may be detected in asymptomatic patients through routine screening mammography.

Local Signs and Symptoms

- A painless, palpable lump is most common.
- Less common: pain; nipple discharge, retraction, or dimpling; skin edema, redness, or warmth
- Palpable local–regional lymph nodes may also be present.

Signs and Symptoms of Systemic Metastases

- Depend on the site of metastases, but may include bone pain, difficulty breathing, abdominal pain or enlargement, jaundice, or mental status changes

Laboratory Tests

- Tumor markers such as cancer antigen (CA 27.29) or carcinoembryonic antigen (CEA) may be elevated.
- Alkaline phosphatase or liver function test results may be elevated in patients with metastatic disease.

Other Diagnostic Tests

- Mammography (with or without ultrasonography, breast MRI, or both).
- Biopsy for pathology review and determination of tumor ER or PR status and *HER2* status.
- Systemic staging tests may include chest radiography, chest computed tomography (CT), bone scan, abdominal CT or ultrasonography, or MRI

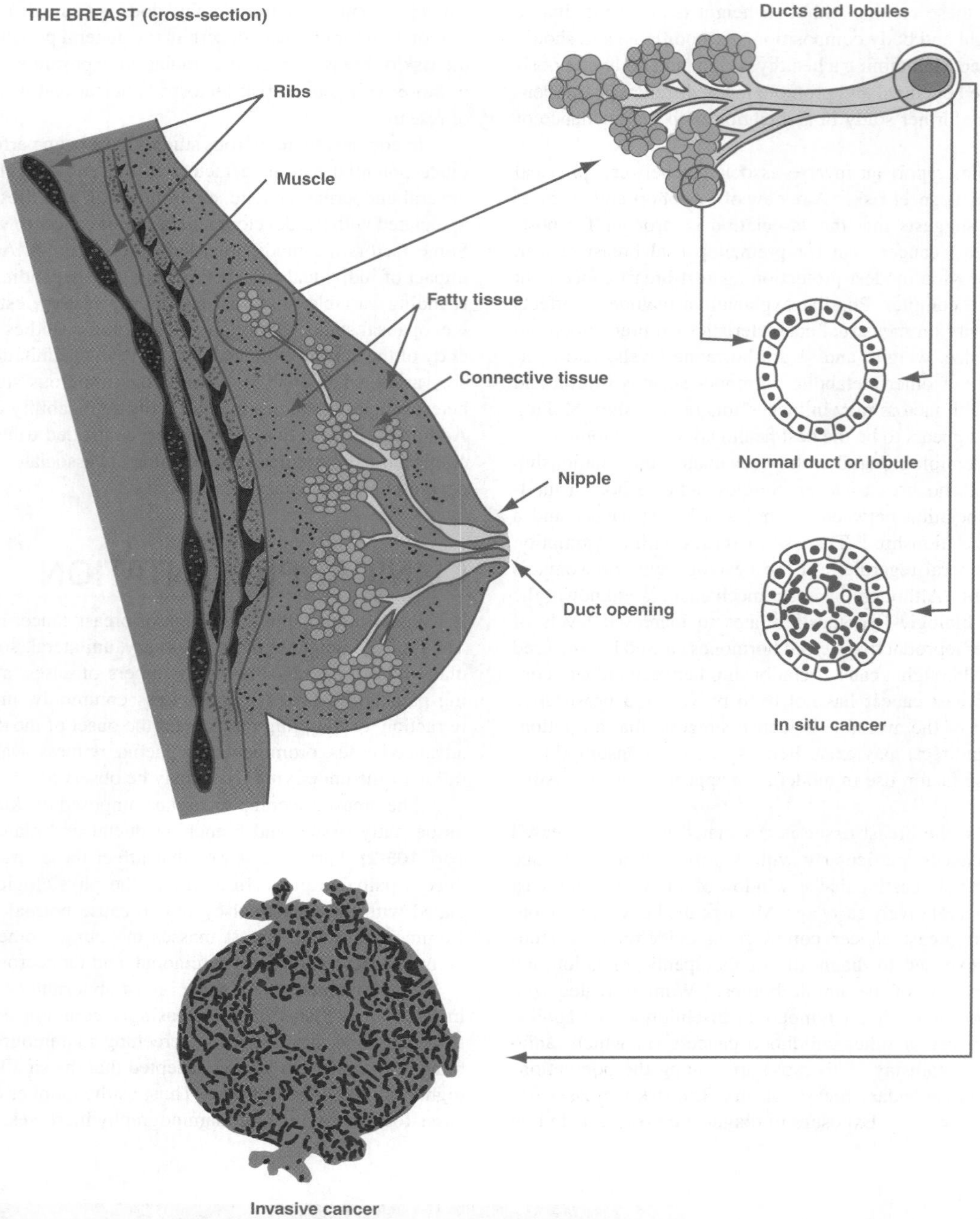

FIGURE 105-2 Breast anatomy.

(OS) of breast cancer patients has improved; however, this decreasing mortality rate is also related to improved systemic therapy.

Breast cancer that is confined to a localized breast lesion is often referred to as *early*, *primary*, *localized*, or *curable*. Breast cancer that has spread to local–regional lymph nodes is still considered early stage (Fig. 105-3). Unfortunately, breast cancer cells often spread by contiguity, through lymph channels, and through the blood to distant sites. This often occurs early in breast cancer growth, and deposits of tumor cells form in distant sites that are undetected with current diagnostic methods and equipment (micrometastases). When breast cancer cells can be detected clinically or radiologically in sites distant from the breast, the disease is referred to as *advanced* or *metastatic* breast cancer. Tissues most commonly involved with distant metastases are lymph nodes (other than local–regional lymph nodes), skin, bone, liver, lungs, and brain. Symptoms of bone pain, difficulty breathing, abdominal enlargement, jaundice, and mental status changes may herald the clinical presentation of metastatic breast cancer. A small percentage of women have signs and symptoms of distant metastases when they first seek treatment. In virtually all of them, a neglected breast mass has been present for several months to years. In addition, about half of all patients who initially are treated for localized disease eventually develop signs and symptoms of metastatic breast cancer.

DIAGNOSIS

The initial workup for a woman presenting with a breast mass or symptoms suggestive of breast cancer should include a careful history, physical examination of the breast, three-dimensional

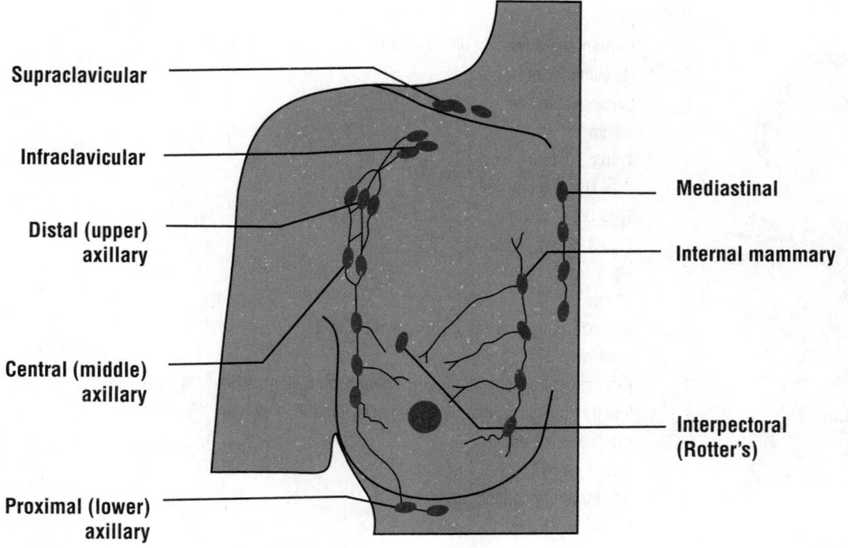

FIGURE 105-3 Lymph node anatomy.

mammography, and possibly other breast imaging techniques such as ultrasonography or magnetic resonance imaging (MRI). Most breast cancers can be visualized on a mammogram as a mass, a cluster of calcifications, or a combination of these findings. Specific mammographic features associated with the highest risk of malignancy include masses with spiculated margins or an irregular shape and calcifications with a linear or segmental distribution.[37] One major factor that affects the ability of mammography to detect cancer includes breast density (the fat-to-glandular tissue ratio of the breast), which may be affected by age, menopausal status, and HRT use. Ultrasonography, MRI, and digital mammography are alternate breast imaging methods that are being investigated for women with dense breasts or other specific subsets of patients with breast cancer (e.g., MRI in patients with inflammatory breast cancer).[38] The technical quality of the examination and the expertise of the radiologist are also important factors.

The Breast Imaging Reporting and Data System (BI-RADS) was developed by the American College of Radiology to standardize mammographic reporting.[39] There are seven assessment categories (0–6) with four possible recommendations: (a) additional imaging evaluation, (b) routine interval screening, (c) short-term follow-up, and (d) biopsy. The probability of a biopsy positive for malignancy increases from less than 2% for BI-RADS category 3 mammograms to 20% to 30% for category 4 mammograms, to greater than 95% for category 5 mammograms. Similar categories for reporting have also been developed for breast MRI and ultrasonography.

Breast biopsy is indicated for a mammographic abnormality that suggests malignancy or for a palpable mass on physical examination. Three techniques are available: fine-needle aspiration, core-needle biopsy, and excisional biopsy.[40] Excisional biopsy completely removes the abnormal tissue. Needle biopsies are performed percutaneously and include both core-needle biopsy (which removes a core of tissue) and fine-needle aspiration (which removes cells from the suspicious site). Core-needle biopsy is the preferred biopsy method for mammographically detected, nonpalpable abnormalities.[38] Core-needle biopsy offers a more definitive histologic diagnosis, avoids inadequate samples, and can distinguish invasive from in situ breast cancer (which fine needle biopsy cannot). After confirmation of malignancy via core-needle biopsy, subsequent surgical procedures are performed (either before or after systemic therapy) to assure complete removal of the abnormal tissue.

STAGING AND PROGNOSIS

Breast cancer stage is defined on the basis of the primary tumor extent and size (T_{1-4}), presence and extent of lymph node involvement (N_{1-3}), and presence or absence of distant metastases (M_{0-1}) (Table 105-2 and Fig. 105-4). Although many possible combinations of T and N are possible within a given stage, simplistically, stage 0 represents carcinoma in situ (T_{is}) or disease that has not invaded

TABLE 105-2 Tumor, Node, Metastasis Stage Grouping for Breast Cancer

Stage Grouping			
0	T_{is}	N_0	M_0
IA	T_1^a	N_0	M_0
IB	T_0	N_1mi	M_0
	T_1^a	N_1mi	M_0
IIA	T_0	N_1^b	M_0
	T_1^a	N_1^b	M_0
	T_2	N_0	M_0
IIB	T_2	N_1	M_0
	T_3	N_0	M_0
IIIA	T_0	N_2	M_0
	T_1^a	N_2	M_0
	T_2	N_2	M_0
	T_3	N_1	M_0
	T_3	N_2	M_0
IIIB	T_4	N_0	M_0
	T_4	N_1	M_0
	T_4	N_2	M_0
IIIC	Any T	N_3	M_0
IV	Any T	Any N	M_1

TNM, tumor, node, metastasis.

[a] T_1 includes T_1mi.

[b] T_0 and T_1 tumors with nodal micrometastasis only are excluded from stage IIa and are classified as stage IB.

Used with the permission of the American Joint Committee on Cancer (AJCC), Chicago. The original source for this material is the AJCC Cancer Staging Manual, 7th ed. (2010) published by Springer Science and Business Media LLC, www.springer.com.

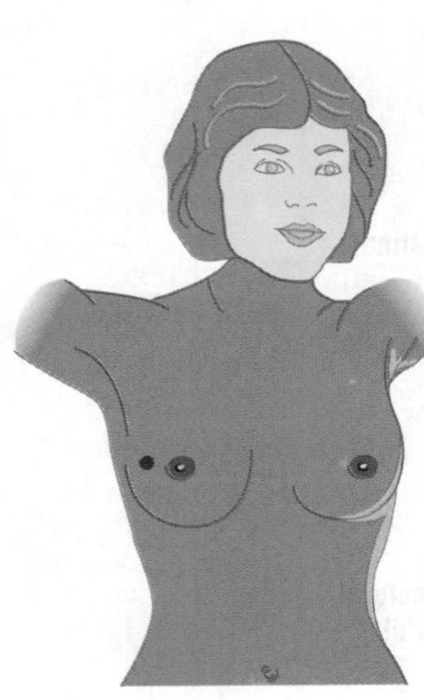

Tumor (T)

T_x	Primary tumor cannot be assessed
T_0	No evidence of tumor
T_{is}	Carcinoma in situ
T_1	≤2 cm
	T_1 mic ≤0.1 cm
	T_{1a} > 0.1–0.5 cm
	T_{1b} > 0.5–1 cm
	T_{1c} > 1–2 cm
T_2	>2–5 cm
T_3	>5 cm
T_4	Any size; with direct extension to chest wall or skin
T_{4a}	Extension to chest wall (not including pectoralis muscle)
T_{4b}	Edema (including peau d'orange) or ulceration of skin or satellite skin nodules
T_{4c}	Both T_{4a} and T_{4b}
T_{4d}	Inflammatory carcinoma

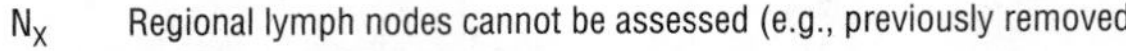

Clinical Nodes (N)

N_X	Regional lymph nodes cannot be assessed (e.g., previously removed)
N_0	No regional lymph node metastasis
N_1	Metastasis in movable ipsilateral axillary lymph node(s)
N_2	Metastases in ipsilateral axillary lymph nodes fixed or matted or in clinically detected ipsilateral internal mammary nodes in the absence of clinically evident axillary lymph node metastasis
	N_{2a} Metastasis in ipsilateral axillary lymph nodes fixed to one another (matted) or to other structures
	N_{2b} Metastasis only in clinically detected ipsilateral internal mammary nodes and in the absence of clinically evident axillary lymph node metastasis
N_3	Metastasis in ipsilateral infraclavicular lymph node(s) or in clinically detected ipsilateral internal mammary lymph node(s) and in the presence of clinically evident axillary lymph node metastasis or metastasis in ipsilateral supraclavicular lymph node(s) with or without axillary or internal mammary lymph node involvement
	N_{3a} Metastasis in ipsilateral infraclavicular lymph node(s) and axillary lymph node(s)
	N_{3b} Metastasis in ipsilateral internal mammary lymph node(s) and axillary lymph node(s)
	N_{3c} Metastasis in ipsilateral supraclavicular lymph node(s)

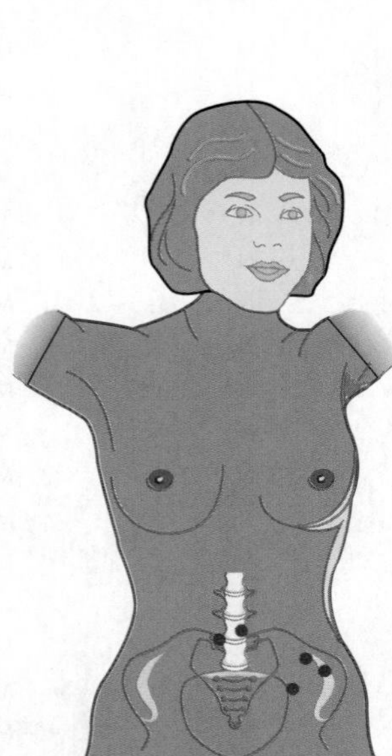

Pathologic Nodes (pN)*

pN0	No regional lymph node metastasis histologically
pN1mi	Micrometastasis (>0.2 mm but none >2.0 mm)
pN1	Metastasis in one to three axillary lymph nodes and/or internal mammary nodes with microscopic disease detected by sentinel lymph node dissection but not clinically detected
pN2	Metastasis in four to nine axillary lymph nodes or in clinically detected internal mammary lymph nodes in the absence of axillary lymph node metastasis
pN3	Metastasis in 10 or more axillary lymph nodes, in infraclavicular lymph nodes, or in clinically detected ipsilateral internal mammary lymph nodes in the presence of one or more positive axillary lymph nodes; in more than three axillary lymph nodes with clinically negative microscopic metastasis in internal mammary lymph nodes; or in ipsilateral supraclavicular lymph nodes

*Based on axillary lymph node dissection with or without sentinel lymph node dissection

Metastasis (M)

M_X	Distant metastasis cannot be assessed
M_0	No distant metastases
M_1	Distant metastasis

FIGURE 105-4 TNM (tumor, node, metastasis) staging system for breast cancer. *(Used with the permission of the American Joint Committee on Cancer [AJCC], Chicago, Illinois. The original source for this material is the AJCC Cancer Staging Manual, 7th ed. [2010] published by Springer Science and Business Media LLC, www.springer.com.)*

the basement membrane of the breast tissue. Stage I represents a small primary invasive tumor without lymph node involvement or with micrometastatic nodal involvement, and stage II disease usually involves regional lymph nodes. Stages I and II are often referred to as *early breast cancer*. It is in these early stages that the disease is highly curable (99% 5-year survival in patients with disease confined to the breast, node negative). Stage III, also referred to as *locally advanced disease*, usually represents a large tumor with extensive nodal involvement in which either node or tumor is fixed to the chest wall. Stage IV disease is characterized by the presence of metastases to organs distant from the primary tumor and is often referred to as *advanced or metastatic disease* as described earlier (23% 5-year survival rate in patients with distant metastases). Most breast cancer today presents in early stages where the prognosis is favorable (93% of newly diagnosed patients have disease confined to the breast or local lymph nodes).[2]

Staging for breast cancer is separated into two groups, clinical and pathologic. Clinical staging is assigned before surgery and is based on physical examination (assessment of tumor size and presence of axillary lymph nodes), imaging (mammography, ultrasonography, and so on), and pathologic examination of tissues (e.g., biopsy results). Pathologic staging occurs after surgery and uses information from clinical staging but adds data from surgical exploration and resection, such as tumor size at surgery and the involvement of micro- or macro-invasive tumor in the lymph nodes or other metastatic sites. Because of the advent of sentinel lymph node biopsy (SLNB; see the Treatment of Early Breast Cancer section), the assessment of lymph node status has become more complex. The American Joint Committee for Cancer (AJCC) publishes staging criteria for cancers, and the breast cancer criteria were most recently updated in January 2010.[41] This staging system is widely accepted and used in all breast cancer patients to determine prognosis and assist with treatment decisions. It is also used to report and track breast cancer diagnoses in tumor registries and databases.

PATHOLOGY

The pathologic evaluation of breast tissue serves to establish the histologic diagnosis and to confirm the presence or absence of other factors believed to influence prognosis.

Invasive Carcinoma

Invasive breast cancers are a histologically heterogeneous group of lesions. Most breast cancers are adenocarcinomas and are classified on the basis of their microscopic appearance as ductal or lobular, corresponding to the ducts and lobules of the normal breast (Fig. 105-2). The various histologic types of breast cancer have different prognoses, but it is unknown whether their response to therapy differs because patients in therapeutic trials are not typically stratified according to histologic type. The five most common types of invasive breast cancer are briefly described.[42]

Invasive or *infiltrating ductal carcinoma* is the most common histology, accounting for about 75% of all invasive breast cancers. These tumors commonly spread to the axillary lymph nodes, and their prognosis is poorer than for other histologic types (specifically tubular, medullary, and mucinous). *Invasive or infiltrating lobular carcinoma* accounts for 5% to 10% of breast tumors. Both clinical and radiologic findings for these tumors may be quite subtle. The typical presentation is an area of ill-defined thickening in the breast in contrast to a prominent lump characteristic of infiltrating ductal carcinoma. *Infiltrating lobular carcinoma* can also be more difficult to detect by mammography. Overall, *infiltrating lobular carcinoma* and *infiltrating ductal carcinoma* have similar likelihoods of axillary node involvement and disease recurrence and death, yet the sites of metastases may differ. Whereas *Infiltrating ductal carcinoma* more frequently metastasizes to the bone or to the liver, lung, or brain, *infiltrating lobular carcinoma* tends to metastasize to the leptomeninges, peritoneal surfaces, retroperitoneum, gastrointestinal tract, reproductive organs, and other unusual sites.

The three most common special types of invasive cancer are *medullary*, *mucinous*, and *tubular*. The prognosis may be more favorable with these unusual histologies. *Medullary carcinoma* accounts for fewer than 7% of all breast carcinomas, *mucinous (or colloid) carcinoma* constitutes about 3%, *and tubular carcinoma* accounts for about 2% of all breast cancers. Histologies rarely reported include adenocystic carcinoma, carcinosarcomas, metaplastic, cribriform, and papillary carcinoma.

Special situations seen clinically and histologically include Paget's disease of the breast, phyllodes tumors, and inflammatory breast cancer. Paget's disease of the breast occurs in 1% to 4% of all patients with breast cancer and is characterized by neoplastic cells in the nipple areolar complex. The patient presents clinically with eczematous changes in the nipple with itching, burning, oozing, bleeding, or some combination of these. In most cases, the nipple changes are associated with an underlying carcinoma in the breast that is usually palpable.

Phyllodes tumors of the breast (also known as cystosarcoma phyllodes) are rare tumors with subtypes that range from benign to malignant. These tumors often enlarge rapidly, are painless, and can appear as fibroadenomas.[43]

Inflammatory breast cancer is characterized clinically by prominent skin edema, redness and warmth, and induration of the underlying tissue. Biopsies of the involved skin reveal cancer cells in the dermal lymphatics. Inflammatory breast cancer typically has a very rapid onset and is often mistaken for an infectious cellulitis or mastitis. Although it may look somewhat similar to a neglected mass, its presentation with rapid onset and progression of local symptoms distinguishes it from other cases of locally advanced breast cancer. The prognosis of patients with inflammatory breast cancer is poor even if the disease is apparently localized.[44]

Noninvasive Carcinoma

As with invasive carcinoma, the noninvasive lesions may be divided broadly into ductal and lobular categories. Evidence supports that the development of malignancy is a multistep process and that invasive breast cancer has a preinvasive, in situ phase. During the carcinoma in situ phase, normal epithelial cells undergo genetic alterations that result in malignant transformation. Transformed epithelial cells proliferate and pile up within lobules or ducts but lack the required genetic alterations that enable the cells to penetrate the basement membrane. Therefore, carcinoma in situ is diagnosed when malignant transformation of cells has occurred but the basement membrane is intact.

The widespread use of screening mammography with subsequent biopsy and greater recognition of noninvasive breast carcinoma by pathologists has resulted in a significant increase in the diagnosis of in situ breast cancer over the past decade. Assuming a consistent incidence and survival rates, researchers estimate that the prevalence of noninvasive (in situ) breast will exceed 1 million cases by 2016.[45] The natural history of these disorders is not well described, and thus the debate continues regarding carcinoma in situ: Is carcinoma in situ preinvasive cancer or simply a marker of unstable epithelium that represents an increased risk for the development of subsequent aggressive cancer?[46,47] Answering this question may change the way noninvasive breast cancers are treated.

Ductal carcinoma in situ is more frequently diagnosed than lobular carcinoma in situ (LCIS). Most cases of DCIS today are found by biopsies performed for clustered microcalcifications seen on screening mammography, a hallmark of this disorder.

The ultimate goal of treatment for noninvasive carcinomas is to prevent the development of invasive disease. If left untreated, it is estimated that 14% to 50% of DCIS lesions will progress to invasive breast cancer.[46] Therefore, up to 50% of these tumors do not progress to invasive disease, but identifying this group of patients is not yet feasible, and all diagnoses should be treated. Locoregional treatment of DCIS depends on its location, size, and pathology.[48] Treatment options include (a) local excision alone with negative margins, (b) local excision (with negative margins) followed by breast irradiation, and (c) traditional total mastectomy with or without reconstruction. Whole-breast irradiation is recommended after excision to significantly decrease the risk of local recurrence, although there is no evidence that survival differs between the previously mentioned options.[48] Excision with negative margins alone without radiation may be considered in patients with small and low-grade DCIS. Mastectomy had been the standard treatment of DCIS for several decades, but long-term survival appears to be equivalent with mastectomy versus local excision and irradiation, and the latter option allows for breast conservation. If more than one area of the breast is involved with DCIS, a mastectomy is the preferred option. Axillary lymph node dissection (ALND) is generally not indicated, although sentinel lymph node biopsy (see the Early Breast Cancer section) may be considered in selected patients.[48] Cytotoxic chemotherapy has no role in the treatment of patients with pure DCIS. It is important to determine hormone receptor status on the cancer cells. Tamoxifen treatment for 5 years may be considered in some women with hormone receptor–positive DCIS. The National Surgical Adjuvant Breast and Bowel Project (NSABP) B-24 trial, which randomized women with DCIS to lumpectomy with radiation plus either tamoxifen or placebo, showed a benefit with tamoxifen in reducing ipsilateral breast cancer recurrence (44% reduction; $P = 0.03$).[49] Further subgroup analyses of this trial suggest a benefit for patients with estrogen receptor (ER)–positive DCIS. Ongoing clinical trials are evaluating the role of aromatase inhibitors (AIs) in the treatment of postmenopausal hormone receptor–positive DCIS. These treatment decisions are often difficult to discuss with patients because these treatments have toxicities that are worrisome to most patients. Nonetheless, an open and honest conversation regarding the risks and benefits is warranted.

Lobular carcinoma in situ is a microscopic diagnosis. In these cases, there is generally no palpable mass, and no specific clinical abnormality is noted. Unlike DCIS, LCIS does not generally demonstrate calcifications on mammography and in fact is usually undetectable by mammography. Consequently, the diagnosis of LCIS is usually an incidental finding in biopsy specimens obtained because of symptoms or mammography findings consistent with benign lesions. It is unclear whether LCIS is a precursor lesion to invasive carcinoma or serves as a marker of risk for invasive carcinoma developing somewhere in the breast. The risk for developing invasive carcinoma is about 0.5% to 1% per year, and both invasive ductal carcinoma and invasive lobular carcinoma can occur. In about 30% to 50% of patients, there are multiple foci of LCIS in the ipsilateral breast, and the contralateral breast is also affected. Thus, the risk for the development of breast cancer is equally high in either breast, which makes the management of LCIS very controversial.[47] Some experts favor a program of observation, with semiannual physical examination and annual mammography.[48] In selected patients with high-risk genetic mutations or strong family history and in women who are particularly anxious about the development of cancer, bilateral mastectomies with or without reconstruction may be considered.[50] Radiation and systemic chemotherapy have no role in the management of LCIS. The use of chemoprevention with tamoxifen in premenopausal women or tamoxifen, raloxifene, or exemestane in postmenopausal women may also be considered for risk reduction in these patients.[50] See Prevention and Early Detection later for details.[51–53]

PROGNOSTIC FACTORS

The natural history of breast cancer varies among patients, with some having extremely aggressive disease that progresses rapidly and others following a more indolent course. The ability to predict prognosis is extremely important in designing treatment recommendations to maximize quantity and quality of life. A number of pathologic prognostic and predictive factors have been identified. Prognostic factors are characteristics or measurements available at diagnosis or time of surgery that in the absence of adjuvant systemic therapy are associated with recurrence rate, death rate, or other clinical outcomes. Predictive factors are measurements available at diagnosis that are associated with response to a specific therapy. Prognostic and predictive factors fall into three general categories: (a) patient characteristics that are independent of the disease such as age; (b) cancer characteristics such as tumor size or histologic type; and (c) other biomarkers that are measurable parameters in tissues, cells, or fluids, such as hormone receptor status. Ideally, the use of prognostic and predictive factors can limit a specific treatment to patients who are most likely to derive benefit, thus sparing unwanted toxicities in those who are unlikely to benefit.

Age at diagnosis and ethnicity are patient characteristics that may affect prognosis. Some younger patients, particularly those younger than 35 years of age, have more aggressive forms of breast cancer and a worse prognosis. Younger patients are more likely to present with poor prognostic features, such as affected lymph nodes, large tumor size, and tumors negative for hormone receptors. Race and ethnicity may also play a role in breast cancer prognosis. African American women have decreased survival periods compared with white women. The cause of this racial disparity is widely debated, with possible explanations including access to care, socioeconomic status, cultural differences, higher stage at diagnosis, and more aggressive biologic features.

Potentially modifiable prognostic factors include alcohol use, dietary factors, weight, and exercise. The association between breast cancer prognosis and alcohol consumption is not as strong as with alcohol and breast cancer risk. A review of seven observational studies showed that postdiagnosis alcohol consumption was not associated with breast cancer outcomes.[54] Two randomized controlled studies examined the effects of diet on the risk of breast cancer with conflicting results, primarily focusing on lowering dietary fat.[55,56] One study found an improvement in disease-free survival (DFS) with incorporation of a low-fat diet (less than 15% dietary fat per day versus no intervention),[56] but another study found no difference in recurrence rates between two dietary intervention approaches (both incorporating a low-fat, high-fiber approach).[55] Although these studies asked different questions and had many confounding variables that potentially affected the results, most clinicians recommend that breast cancer survivors eat a low-fat, high-fiber diet and maintain a healthy weight. Obesity at the time of a breast cancer diagnosis has been shown to increase the risk of breast cancer–specific and overall mortality compared with nonobese breast cancer patients, although the impact of weight loss in this population is unclear.[54] Observational studies have reported that exercise in women after a diagnosis of breast cancer may also decrease the likelihood of breast cancer recurrence and breast cancer–related death.[54] Based on these data, agencies such as the American Cancer Society (ACS) have recognized that physical activity, weight control, and diet are potentially modifiable risk factors for reducing the risk of recurrent breast cancer and other comorbidities (e.g., heart disease, diabetes).[57]

Disease characteristics that have been shown to provide important prognostic information include lymph node status, tumor size, histologic subtype, nuclear or histologic grade, lymphatic and vascular invasion, and proliferation indices.

Tumor size and the presence and number of involved lymph nodes are established primary factors in assessing the risk for breast

TABLE 105-3 Five-Year Survival Rates (%) According to Tumor Size and Axillary Lymph Node Status

	Tumor Size		
Lymph Node Status	**<2 cm**	**2–5 cm**	**>5 cm**
Negative	96	89	82
1–3 positive	87	80	73
≥4 positive	66	59	46

Data from Dillon DA, Guidi AJ, Schnitt SJ. Pathology of invasive breast cancer. In: Harris JR, Lippman ME, Morrow M, Osborne CK, eds. Diseases of the Breast, 4th ed. Philadelphia, PA: Lippincott Williams & Wilkins, 2010:374–407.

cancer recurrence and subsequent metastatic disease. Table 105-3 shows 5-year survival rates according to size of the primary tumor and axillary node involvement. The major factor that influences the likelihood of recurrence is the presence of positive lymph nodes. However, regardless of lymph node status, the size of the primary tumor remains an independent prognostic factor for disease recurrence.

The number of affected lymph nodes is directly related to the risk of disease recurrence. The revised staging system for breast cancer recognizes the absolute number of positive nodes as a prognostic factor: N_1 represents one to three positive nodes, N_2 represents four to nine positive nodes, and N_3 represents 10 or more positive nodes in its pathologic staging system.[41] The relationship between tumor size and lymph node status is complex and not a simple grouping (see discussion below).

Certain histologic subtypes and clinical presentation of breast cancer have prognostic importance. As mentioned earlier, because women with pure *tubular* or *mucinous* tumors have more favorable outcomes than those with *invasive ductal carcinomas*, treatment recommendations may differ.[48] Inflammatory breast cancer, although a clinical designation and not a distinct histologic subtype, is associated with a poor prognosis.[44]

Nuclear grade and tumor (histologic) differentiation are known independent prognostic indicators. Several histologic grading systems have been developed, most of which grade tumors with a score from 1 to 3: grade 1, well differentiated; grade 2, moderately differentiated; and grade 3, poorly differentiated. Higher grade tumors are associated with higher rates of distant metastasis and poorer survival. This factor aids in making treatment decisions, particularly for patients with small tumors and negative lymph nodes.

Lymphatic and vascular invasion (LVI), defined as evidence of tumor emboli in lymphatic or vascular spaces, is a poor prognostic factor likely representing ability of the cancer to spread via hematogenous routes. However, the utility of this as a prognostic factor is largely unknown and is not currently included in either staging or treatment guidelines.[41,48]

The rate of tumor cell proliferation also is associated with risk of breast cancer recurrence. Rate of cell proliferation can be evaluated with various techniques, including (1) mitotic index, which counts the number of mitotic bodies; (2) thymidine-labeling index or S-phase fraction with DNA flow cytometry, which determines the percentage of tumor cells actively dividing; or (3) the use of monoclonal antibodies (MoABs) to antigens present on proliferating cells, such as Ki-67. In a meta-analysis of 85 studies and nearly 33,000 patients, proliferation markers (including Ki-67, mitotic index, proliferating cell nuclear antigen, and thymidine or bromodeoxyuridine labeling index) were associated with significantly shorter disease-free and OS periods.[58] These proliferation indices are additional factors that may be useful in decision making and may predict for responsiveness to chemotherapy, although this is still controversial.

Hormone receptors are not strong prognostic markers but are used clinically to predict response to endocrine therapy. Hormone receptors are nuclear transcription factors that, upon ligand binding, activate a variety of signal transduction pathways that result in cell growth and proliferation. Determination of both ER and progesterone receptor (PR) status is an established procedure that is important in the management of breast cancer. Immunohistochemistry is used to determine the level (i.e., quantity) of hormone receptors, which is important for predictive ability. Other methods of determining ER and PR status, such as mRNA expression, are under investigation but have not been validated as predictive markers. Hormone receptors are most valuable in predicting response to endocrine therapy. About 60% to 70% of patients with ER-positive and PR-positive tumors will respond to hormonal manipulation. More recently, the importance of PR has come under question because response to tamoxifen has been shown to be related to ER status independent of PR status.[4] Guidelines for testing of ER and PR status are available and recommend standards for what tumors to test and methodologic guidelines for pathologists.[59] About 50% to 70% of patients with primary or metastatic breast cancer have hormone receptor–positive tumors. Hormone receptor positivity, more common in postmenopausal women, is associated with a higher response to endocrine therapy and a longer DFS.

The *HER2/neu (HER2)* gene is located on chromosome 17q21 and encodes a 185-kilodaton transmembrane tyrosine kinase growth factor receptor. The *HER2* protein is normally expressed at low levels in the epithelial cells of normal breast tissue. *HER2* is a member of the HER growth factor receptor family, and its overexpression is associated with transmission of growth signals that control aspects of normal cell growth and division. *HER2* overexpression occurs in about 20% to 30% of breast cancers and is associated with increased tumor aggressiveness, increased rates of recurrence, and increased mortality rates. In some studies, *HER2* gene amplification and protein overexpression, measured by fluorescence in situ hybridization (FISH) and immunohistochemistry (IHC), respectively, correlates with factors associated with a poor prognosis. *HER2*-positive status clearly predicts response to trastuzumab, which is a MoAB directed against the extracellular domain of the *HER2* receptor. Tumors that are either IHC 3+ or FISH positive for gene amplification are considered to be positive for *HER2*.[60] For equivocal results of IHC (2+) or FISH, confirmatory testing with the alternate test is recommended. *HER2* gene amplification or protein overexpression has traditionally been considered a poor prognostic factor. However, more recent data suggest that patients with *HER2*-positive metastatic breast cancer treated with trastuzumab have improved survival rates compared with patients with *HER2*-negative metastatic breast cancer or patients with *HER2*-positive metastatic breast cancer who do not receive trastuzumab.[61] These results demonstrate the powerful impact trastuzumab therapy has made on improving patient outcomes.

Although there is a growing understanding of the prognostic significance of individual factors, it is not clear how each factor contributes to the overall prognosis for an individual patient. Computer-aided models, including Adjuvant! (*www.adjuvantonline.com*), are available that combine patient- and tumor-related variables to estimate overall prognosis for individual patients with early stage breast cancer and aid in decisions regarding adjuvant systemic therapy.[62] Such programs have limitations and should be used by healthcare professionals and not directly by patients because of the importance of accurate data entry, selection of different treatment options, and appropriate interpretation of results (see Systemic Adjuvant Therapy later).

Genetic profiling is also being used to provide prognostic and predictive information on clinical outcomes of breast cancer.[62] The Oncotype DX assay uses a reverse-transcription polymerase chain reaction (RT-PCR) assay of 21 genes to predict the likelihood of distant recurrence in lymph node–negative and ER-positive breast cancer patients treated with tamoxifen. MammaPrint is another molecular prognostic test that uses DNA microarray analysis to measure the activity of a set of 70 genes to determine the likelihood of breast cancer recurrence in women with stage I or II breast cancer, tumor size 5 cm or smaller, and no lymph node involvement. Further details on these assays are available in the Systemic Adjuvant Therapy section later.

Novel molecular markers that have shown prognostic and predictive significance include urokinase-type plasminogen activator and its inhibitor, plasminogen activator inhibitor type 1, cyclin E, and the presence of tumor cells in bone marrow or circulating blood.[63] Prospective validation studies will determine whether these tests can be used to assist decision making in individual patients.

In summary, lymph node status and tumor size are two significant prognostic factors that assist clinicians in estimating prognosis and making treatment recommendations for most breast cancer patients (see also Systemic Adjuvant Therapy later). Although the risk of recurrence is clearly high in patients with large primary tumors or lymph node–positive disease, many patients with small primary tumors and lymph node–negative disease will still develop metastases, yet our ability to accurately identify these individual patients is limited. Evaluation of additional prognostic factors can help identify which patients will have a good outcome with local therapy alone and which patients with aggressive features who would benefit from more aggressive, multimodality treatment. Despite these markers, a large proportion of patients will likely be treated unnecessarily with systemic adjuvant therapy (see later discussion), and better prognostic and predictive tools are needed to better select patients to undergo these toxic and costly treatments and procedures.

TREATMENT

Early Breast Cancer (Stage I and II)

Desired Outcomes

The desired therapeutic outcome of adjuvant therapy of breast cancer differs significantly from that of metastatic disease. Adjuvant therapy—chemotherapy, biologic therapy, and hormonal therapy—is administered with curative intent. The rationale for adjuvant therapy is that breast cancer, even when diagnosed in early stages when clinical evidence of distant spread is not apparent, is a systemic disease that spreads early to distant sites. Adjuvant therapy is intended to eradicate micrometastases and thus cure the patient of breast cancer. A predetermined number of cycles of adjuvant therapy or years of biologic or hormonal therapy (or both) are administered. The goals of neoadjuvant therapy are to eradicate micrometastatic disease, determine prognosis, and potentially conserve the breast tissue for a better cosmetic result. Adjuvant and neoadjuvant chemotherapy is often associated with significant toxicity. Clinicians and patients must weigh the short- and long-term risks of chemotherapy, biological therapy, and endocrine therapy with the benefits of lowering the risk of breast cancer recurrence.

Locoregional Therapy

❷ Most patients presenting with breast cancer today have an in situ tumor, a small invasive tumor with negative lymph nodes (stage I), or a small invasive tumor with axillary lymph node involvement (stage II). Surgery alone can cure most, if not all, patients with in situ cancers; 70% to 80% of patients with stage I; and about half of all patients with stage II cancers. The choice of surgical procedures has changed drastically over the past 50 years. This is partly a result of changes in our understanding of the biology of breast cancer and is partly a result of a series of well-conducted clinical trials performed over this time period.

Over the years, many trials have investigated reducing the amount of surgery required to maintain acceptable cosmetic results and rates of local and distant recurrence and mortality. Breast-conserving therapy (BCT) includes removal of part of the breast, surgical evaluation of the axillary lymph node basin, and radiation therapy to the breast. The amount of breast tissue removed as a part of BCT varies from just removing the cancerous "lump" (a lumpectomy) with a small margin of adjacent normal-appearing tissue to removing the "lump" with a wider excision of adjacent normal-appearing tissue (a wide local excision) to removing the entire quadrant of the breast that includes the cancerous "lump" (a quadrantectomy). All of these techniques are referred to as a *segmental or partial mastectomy*. A meta-analysis of 18 clinical trials in almost 10,000 women found no difference in OS for patients who received BCT compared with mastectomy.[64] However, this and other meta-analyses have suggested the potential for a small increase in the risk of locoregional recurrence with BCT.[64,65]

Most patients diagnosed today with breast cancer can be treated with BCT. Several factors should be considered in selecting patients for BCT, including any additional risk the remaining breast tissue poses despite the local effects of radiation therapy. The National Comprehensive Cancer Network (NCCN) recommends that women who carry a known *BRCA1* or *BRCA2* mutation undergo mastectomy and consider additional risk reduction strategies (e.g., bilateral mastectomies).[48] Bilateral total mastectomy and oophorectomy reduce the risk of breast cancer occurrence in patients with *BRCA1* or *BRCA2* mutations, but both breast and ovarian cancers have been reported in patients who have had prophylactic removal of these organs. Multiple sites of cancer within the breast and the inability to attain negative pathologic margins on the excised breast specimen are predictive for an increased risk of recurrence with BCT and are indications for mastectomy. Some preexisting collagen vascular diseases (e.g., scleroderma, systemic lupus erythematosus) are relative contraindications for the use of BCT because of an increased risk of radiation-related adverse effects. Although local recurrence after BCT has not been consistently associated with an increased mortality rate, it is distressing to the patient and requires surgical removal of the breast. In addition, reconstructive therapy is often not feasible in a breast that has previously received irradiation. Another major consideration in selecting patients for BCT is the expected cosmetic result. For some patients, preservation of a limited amount of breast tissue may not justify the inconvenience of radiation therapy. Another approach to therapy for these patients is primary (neoadjuvant) systemic therapy to potentially shrink the tumor and minimize surgery (see the Systemic Adjuvant Therapy and Locally Advanced Breast Cancer sections for further details). Aside from the probability of local recurrence and the ability to achieve a satisfactory cosmetic result, consideration must be given to the availability of an external-beam radiation facility and the patient's willingness to comply with the prescribed course of radiotherapy. In most instances, external-beam radiation therapy used in conjunction with BCT involves 4 to 6 weeks of radiation therapy directed to the entire breast tissue (typically a total of 50 Gy [5000 Rad] administered in 25 daily doses Mondays through Fridays with an optional boost of radiation to the tumor bed) to eradicate residual disease. Complications associated with radiation therapy to the breast are generally minor and include reddening and erythema of the breast tissue and subsequent shrinkage of the total breast mass beyond that predicted on the basis of breast tissue removal. Clinical trials are investigating the use of accelerated partial breast irradiation, intraoperative radiotherapy, or no radiation after segmental mastectomy for certain patient populations with a very low risk of recurrence.[66] Until the results of these studies are available, the standard approach to BCT includes full-breast radiation therapy.

Postmastectomy radiation therapy to the chest wall may also be required in certain situations when tumors are large or the number of positive axillary lymph nodes is high (see the Locally Advanced Breast Cancer section). However, these criteria are also widely debated and are the subject of several meta-analyses. Despite the controversy, it is clear that some women may benefit from local radiation therapy even after removal of the entire breast (i.e., total mastectomy). The NCCN Guidelines state that women with four or more positive axillary lymph nodes should undergo postmastectomy radiation therapy. Patients with one to three positive ipsilateral axillary lymph nodes should strongly consider postmastectomy radiation, although conflicting data exist in this patient population.[48] Patients with (a) positive surgical margins, (b) a tumor larger than 5 cm, or (c) tumors less than 5 cm with close margins (<1 mm of normal adjacent tissue) should consider postmastectomy chest wall radiation therapy. Finally, patients with surgical margins of at least 1 mm, tumor size of 5 cm or less, and negative axillary lymph nodes do not require postmastectomy chest wall radiation therapy. The optimal sequence of radiation therapy and chemotherapy is somewhat controversial. Concurrent administration of chemotherapy and radiation therapy is usually avoided because of an increase in local adverse effects. Most clinicians administer systemic chemotherapy immediately after surgery (if chemotherapy was not administered before surgery) given the hypothetical presence of systemic micrometastases that cannot be eradicated by local radiation therapy. Radiation therapy is then administered after chemotherapy, leaving hormone therapy (which is given for many years) for the end (see the Adjuvant Biologic Therapy section for a discussion of sequencing trastuzumab).

Accurate assessment of the spread of breast cancer cells to the axillary lymph nodes is critical for prognosis and the determination of the utility of both local and systemic treatments. ALND with histopathologic study of the full axillary specimen, including level I and II lymph nodes, was the gold standard for detecting axillary nodal involvement and determining the number of lymph nodes containing tumor. The number of positive axillary lymph nodes remains the most powerful predictor of breast cancer recurrence and survival, but other benefits may include a therapeutic effect of removing the lymph nodes and obtaining information to guide treatment selection. However, axillary dissection is associated with significant morbidity, with an acute complication rate as high as 20% to 30% and rates of chronic lymphedema as high as 20% to 30%.[67,68] Recent studies indicate that about 60% of patients with early stage breast cancer present with lymph node–negative disease, which indicates that many women would derive no therapeutic benefit but would be exposed to the complications from the procedure.

For these reasons, a procedure involving lymphatic mapping and SLNB is recommended at many centers across the United States, and guidelines regarding recommendations for this procedure are now available.[69] The sentinel lymph node(s) is the first lymph node(s) that receives lymph drainage from the primary tumor. Injection of a vital blue dye, a radiocolloid, or both around the primary breast tumor identifies the sentinel lymph node(s) in most patients, and the status of this lymph node(s) may predict the status of the remaining nodes in the nodal basin. Patients with lymph nodes that are suspicious for cancer involvement either by physical examination or imaging should have a biopsy performed to exclude lymph node involvement. SLNB has become the standard of care for patients with clinically negative axillary lymph nodes.[48] Patients with a positive sentinel node or in whom the sentinel node is not identified should proceed to a level I and II ALND, although ALND after a positive lymph node found with SLNB is also controversial in certain patient populations. Data from a single randomized trial suggest that ALND after SLNB in women with clinically node negative tumors smaller than 5 cm, fewer than three involved sentinel lymph nodes, and undergoing BCT with subsequent breast irradiation resulted in higher morbidity, no improvement in local recurrence, and no difference in DFS or OS with SLNB alone.[70]

Despite differences in the mapping technique, the experience of the surgeon, or the patient populations studied, recent studies show that this approach identified the sentinel lymph node(s) in more than 90% of patients.[71] In studies that incorporated completion axillary dissections for comparison, the SLNB procedure accurately predicted the status of the remaining axillary nodes in more than 90% of patients. Considerable controversy exists over the use of this procedure in women with large tumors (>5 cm) or locally advanced disease, palpable axillary lymph nodes, a multifocal or multicentric breast tumor, prior neoadjuvant (preoperative) chemotherapy, or prior surgery involving the breast or axilla. Patients who are pregnant or lactating are generally not considered candidates for this procedure because of concerns regarding the effects of the blue dye or the radiocolloid on the fetus. The decision of whether to use the sentinel lymph node procedure or a full axillary dissection is complex, and readers are referred to an excellent review for further information.[72]

Simple or *total mastectomy* involves removal of the entire breast without dissection of the underlying muscle or axillary nodes. The major disadvantage of this procedure is that axillary nodal status is not determined, and therefore important prognostic information may be lost. This procedure is used in patients with carcinoma in situ, in whom there is a 1% incidence of axillary node involvement, or in cases of in-breast recurrences after BCT.

The early trials investigating less extensive surgical approaches to breast cancer are widely credited with the finding that BCT is an appropriate primary therapy for most women with stages I and II disease and is preferable because it arguably provides survival rates equivalent to those of modified radical mastectomy. These historical trials provided valuable information regarding the natural history of the disease and identified pathologic prognostic factors associated with early cancer spread. The preponderance of information available regarding selection of women most likely to benefit from systemic adjuvant therapy was derived from pathologic evaluation of tissues archived from these early trials. It is hoped that further investigation into less extensive local therapy (now focused on the surgical approach to the axilla and radiation therapy) will continue to provide valuable information for the future.

Systemic Adjuvant Therapy

3 *Systemic adjuvant therapy* is defined as the administration of systemic therapy after definitive local therapy (surgery, radiation, or a combination of these) when there is no evidence of metastatic disease but a high likelihood of disease recurrence. By the time breast cancers become clinically detectable, they have likely been present for a number of years and have had ample opportunity to establish distant micrometastases. Micrometastatic disease can travel from the primary breast tumor and spread to distant organs through several different routes (e.g., hematogenous spread through blood vessels, lymphangitic spread through lymph channels, local extension to surrounding structures). Because local therapies such as breast surgery and irradiation do not address distant micrometastases, systemic therapy may be required to target these tumor cells that have escaped the local area of the breast. The likelihood of micrometastatic disease presence is used to attempt to identify patients with a high risk of recurrence who would require systemic adjuvant therapy. Many collaborative research groups have conducted stepwise series of studies designed to identify appropriate candidates for systemic adjuvant therapy and the optimal regimens and duration of therapy. Several hundred randomized clinical trials evaluating various systemic adjuvant modalities have been reported. Most published results confirm that administration of chemotherapy, endocrine therapy, or both, results in improved DFS or OS for all treated patients or more commonly for patients in specific prognostic subgroups (e.g., nodal involvement, menopausal status, hormone receptor status, or *HER2* status). The huge amounts of data generated by these trials have resulted in a great deal of controversy, with different conclusions being reached by various experts.

4 Interpretation of results of systemic adjuvant therapy is difficult because of differences in the patient populations studied, the variation in natural history of breast cancer, the absence of

information regarding pathologic prognostic factors in many studies, and differences in treatment approach and methods of analysis. Several groups around the world have conducted meta-analyses of similar breast cancer trials in hopes of gaining more insight regarding adjuvant systemic therapy than a single study can provide. One such effort, organized by the Early Breast Cancer Trialists' Collaborative Group (EBCTCG), is based on a worldwide collaboration involving multiple randomized trials and is continually updated with results from new clinical trials. The EBCTCG's overview analyses are updated periodically as new data become available. The most recent updates, published in 2011 and 2012, reflect the long-term effects on breast cancer recurrence and survival for adjuvant tamoxifen and chemotherapy, respectively.[4,5] Many important questions regarding the optimal way to administer adjuvant chemotherapy and endocrine therapy and the magnitude of benefit as measured by DFS or OS in clinically relevant subsets of patients have been answered by these overview analyses. Simply stated, the results of these analyses support the use of adjuvant endocrine therapy in all patients with positive hormone receptor status regardless of age, menopausal status, involvement of axillary lymph nodes, or tumor size.[4] The results of these overview analyses also support the use of adjuvant chemotherapy in most women with lymph node metastases or with primary breast cancers larger than 1 cm in diameter (both node negative and node positive).[5] It is important to note that data from clinical trials incorporating modern AIs or trastuzumab into adjuvant regimens are not included in these analyses because sufficient long-term follow-up has not been reached. Results from these more recent clinical trials are discussed later (see the Adjuvant Biologic Therapy and Adjuvant Endocrine Therapy sections).

Clinicians need to understand the relative and absolute magnitude of benefit associated with adjuvant systemic therapy in breast cancer if they are to help patients understand their treatment options and make informed decisions regarding their care. A proportional reduction of 25% might equivalently be described as an odds ratio (OR), RR ratio, or HR of 0.75; a RR or odds reduction of 25%; or a 25% reduction in the risk of death or death rate. For a given proportional reduction in death rate, the absolute improvement in 15-year survival will depend on the baseline risk of death with no treatment, which varies based on prognostic factors that include patient characteristics, disease characteristics, and biomarkers identified earlier in this chapter. Table 105-4 shows the number of deaths avoided per 100 patients treated in several hypothetical subsets of patients with different estimated 15-year survivals without adjuvant therapy as a function of different estimates of treatment benefit shown as the proportional reductions in mortality if they did receive adjuvant therapy. About 15 of every 100 patients benefited at 15 years from adjuvant therapy when a 30% proportional reduction in mortality is observed in the highest risk subgroups (50% death rate with no adjuvant therapy). In contrast, the same 30% proportional reduction in mortality translated into a benefit for only three of 100 patients in the lowest risk subset (10% death rate with no adjuvant therapy). Thus, the absolute benefit of adjuvant therapy depends on both the proportional reduction in mortality and the risk of disease recurrence, with the greatest benefit observed in the highest risk treatment groups.

TABLE 105-4 Absolute Reduction in Mortality at 10 Years per 100 Patients Treated

Estimated 10-year Death Rate with No Therapy	Hypothetical Proportional Reduction in Mortality as a Result of Treatment				
	50%	40%	30%	20%	10%
50% (5-cm tumor, one positive node)	25	20	15	10	5
30% (4-cm tumor, negative nodes)	15	12	9	6	3
10% (1.5-cm tumor, negative nodes)	5	4	3	2	1

TABLE 105-5 Absolute Benefits of Adjuvant Chemotherapy by Age and Nodal Status

	With Polychemotherapy (%)	With No Polychemotherapy (%)	Absolute Benefit (%)
Disease-Free Survival			
Age <50 years			
Node negative	82.5	72.6	9.9
Node positive	59.4	44.8	14.6
Age 50–69 years			
Node negative	85.7	80.4	5.3
Node positive	63.3	57.4	5.9
Survival[a]			
Age <50 years	67.6	57.6	10
Age 50–69 years	52.6	49.6	3

[a]Younger women, 35% node positive; older women, 70% node positive.

Data from Early Breast Cancer Trialists' Collaborative Group.[109]

Table 105-5 uses data from the overview analyses to show the absolute benefits of adjuvant chemotherapy in terms of age and nodal status. In the highest risk group, node-positive women younger than 50 years of age, only 44.8% were alive and disease free at 5 years with no polychemotherapy compared with 59.4% with polychemotherapy, which translates into an absolute DFS benefit of 14.6%. However, in the node-negative group, patients younger than 50 years old in whom DFS with no polychemotherapy was highest (i.e., 72.6%), the addition of polychemotherapy produced an absolute benefit of only 9.9%. It should be pointed out that all of these differences in DFS are clearly statistically significant and form the basis for national and international guidelines that recommend offering cytotoxic chemotherapy to most women with early stage breast cancer.[48,73] However, the absolute survival benefit in node-positive women 50 to 69 years old is quite small (3%), and depending on other disease characteristics and comorbid conditions, patients may elect not to pursue treatment. Although a 3% absolute reduction in death attributable to polychemotherapy may appear small, at least two investigators report that most patients with breast cancer would accept severe toxicity from treatment to achieve as little as a 1% to 5% absolute improvement in survival.[74,75]

Several international and national groups have developed guidelines for treatment of early stage breast cancer based on specific patient and disease characteristics and the results of the overview analyses. The two most commonly referenced guidelines are the St. Gallen International Expert Consensus Conference and the NCCN guidelines.[48,73] The St. Gallen guidelines are updated every 2 years by an international group of researchers that meets in St. Gallen, Switzerland to review available evidence and create consensus recommendations for selection of adjuvant systemic therapies in specific patient populations outside of the framework of clinical trials. The NCCN has also developed practice guidelines for the treatment of breast cancer that are updated annually or more often based on the available evidence. Recommendations from the NCCN for patients with tumors 1 cm or larger or positive lymph nodes are summarized in Figure 105-5. For patients with tumors smaller than 1 cm, micrometastatic lymph node involvement, or negative lymph nodes, treatment is highly individualized and based on multiple patient- and tumor-related factors, including hormone receptor status, *HER2* status, comorbidities, and patient preferences. Specific treatment recommendations are complex, and readers are referred to the guidelines for further details.

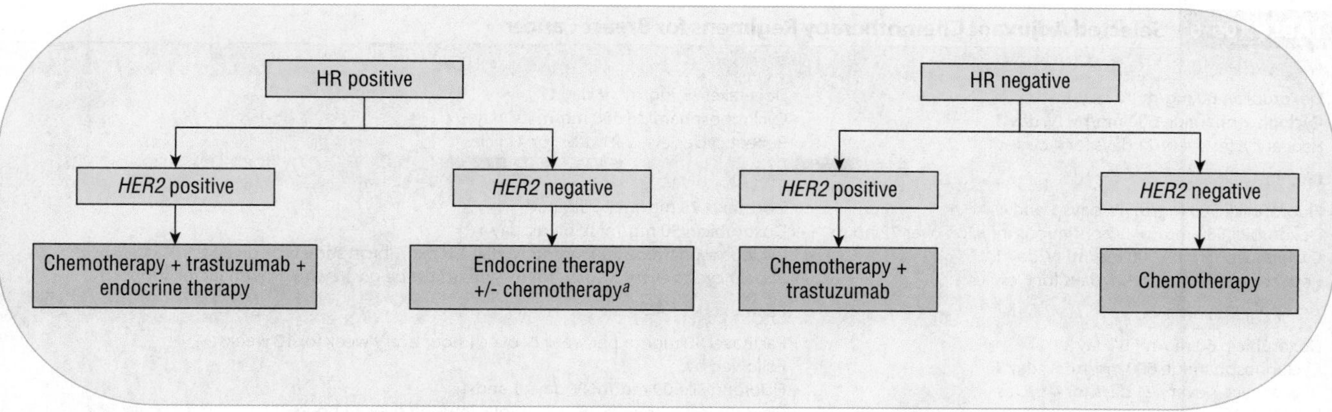

FIGURE 105-5 Treatment of patients with breast cancers larger than 1 cm or with positive lymph nodes. Refer to the text for definitions of HR and *HER2* positivity. Refer to the text for management of patients with tumors smaller than 1 cm, micrometastatic lymph node involvement, or negative lymph nodes. [a]Oncotype DX may identify patients who derive little benefit from chemotherapy (lymph node–negative patients only) (see Systemic Adjuvant Therapy section for details). (HR, hormone receptor; *HER2*, human epidermal growth factor receptor-2.)

5 The use of preoperative systemic therapy is gaining favor in both early stage and locally advanced breast cancers. This approach to therapy, referred to as *neoadjuvant* or *primary systemic therapy*, usually consists of chemotherapy but in special circumstances may also include endocrine therapy (e.g., in inoperable patients with significant comorbidities or in patients with high sensitivity to endocrine therapy). Advantages of preoperative systemic therapy include (a) a decrease in the size of the tumor to minimize surgery, (b) determination of the response to chemotherapy or hormone therapy in vivo (an important prognostic indicator), and (c) other theoretical advantages (e.g., delivery of chemotherapy through an intact vascular system). In a pivotal study conducted by the NSABP (Trial B18), preoperative chemotherapy was compared with traditional chemotherapy given after surgery (the same chemotherapy and the same number of cycles).[76,77] Although no difference was found in DFS or OS, rates of BCT were higher in the group receiving preoperative chemotherapy (67.8% vs. 59.8%).[77] This study also identified a small subset of patients (13%) who had a pathologic complete response (pCR; no tumor left at surgery) after chemotherapy. These patients went on to have a significantly longer DFS compared with patients who did not achieve a pCR ($P < 0.0001$).[77] Importantly, even after 16 years of follow-up, patients who achieved a pCR continued to have superior DFS and OS compared with patients who did not achieve a pCR.[78] Although this approach to therapy was historically reserved for patients with inoperable tumors (locally advanced), the use of preoperative systemic therapy in patients with early stage breast cancer is increasing in popularity because of the ability to assess the response to therapy in vivo as well as the potential to decrease the size of the tumor, allowing for less radical surgery and better cosmetic results.

Intensive research efforts are directed toward identifying characteristics of the primary tumor (e.g., pathologic or molecular prognostic factors) that may predict for a higher or lower likelihood of distant metastases and death in node-negative patients. Although many prognostic factors are being investigated, no single factor or combination of factors sufficiently identifies those at risk of metastases or is sufficiently standardized to be reproducibly applicable to all patients. Currently, two commercially available genetic tests are being prospectively validated as decision-support tools for adjuvant chemotherapy. Oncotype DX® is one of these tests that screens for expression of 21 genes using RT-PCR and results in a recurrence score that can be used to determine the risk of distant recurrence or death from breast cancer in women with ER-positive, node-negative, invasive breast cancer.[62] The tumor tissue used for this test is paraffin-embedded tumor from archived samples. A low recurrence score (<18) indicates a low risk of recurrence with endocrine therapy alone indicating that perhaps adjuvant chemotherapy could be avoided. A high recurrence score (≥31) indicates a high risk of recurrence despite endocrine therapy, suggesting a need for adjuvant chemotherapy followed by endocrine therapy. The utility of chemotherapy in patients with an intermediate score (18–30) is unclear, and ongoing clinical trials hope to further elucidate the role of Oncotype DX in this patient population and in patients with one to three positive lymph nodes after surgery. A second test, MammaPrint, was approved to estimate prognosis in breast cancer patients with early-stage disease, regardless of hormone receptor status. MammaPrint screens the tumor for 70 genes using microarray technology. The assay requires fresh-frozen tissue and reports the predicted rates of recurrence as high or low. This information has been shown to accurately predict for recurrence in a subset of patients not receiving systemic adjuvant therapy. The MINDACT (Microarray In Node-negative Disease may Avoid ChemoTherapy) trial, ongoing in Europe, will compare the predictive capabilities of MammaPrint against the standard prognostic factors to assess which patients with node-negative, ER-positive breast cancer will benefit from adjuvant chemotherapy. Although many clinicians use these tools for individual patients, we await further information to guide the appropriate use of these novel pharmacogenomic tools.

A clinical tool that has been widely adopted for clinical use is an Internet-based tool called Adjuvant! (*www.adjuvantonline.com*), which helps clinicians and patients make informed decisions regarding adjuvant therapy for breast, colon, and lung cancers. The tool allows healthcare professionals to estimate the risks of negative outcomes (e.g., cancer recurrence, death), and the potential benefits of therapy (e.g., reductions in risks of recurrence and death). This is a validated, evidence-based tool that incorporates multiple prognostic and predictive factors into a mathematical model in which each factor is weighted based on established evidence from clinical trials and is placed in the background of the SEER database for patients living in the United States.[62] By entering the patient's age, comorbidities, ER status, tumor grade, tumor size, and nodal status, the clinician can use the tool to estimate the breast cancer mortality and recurrence risk at 10 years and determine the impact of chemotherapy, hormone therapy, or both on these risks. The results are then projected in a graphic format that is easy to understand and

TABLE 105-6 Selected Adjuvant Chemotherapy Regimens for Breast Cancer

AC[b]	TC[a,c]
Doxorubicin 60 mg/m² IV, day 1 Cyclophosphamide 600 mg/m² IV, day 1 Repeat cycles every 21 days for 4 cycles	Docetaxel 75 mg/m² IV, day 1 Cyclophosphamide 600 mg/m² IV, day 1 Repeat cycles every 21 days for 4 cycles
FAC[d,m]	**TAC[a,e]**
Fluorouracil 500 mg/m² IV, days 1 and 4 Doxorubicin 50 mg/m² IV continuous infusion over 72 hours Cyclophosphamide 500 mg/m² IV, day 1 Repeat cycles every 21–28 days for 6 cycles	Docetaxel 75 mg/m² IV, day 1 Doxorubicin 50 mg/m² IV bolus, day 1 Cyclophosphamide 500 mg/m² IV, day 1 (doxorubicin should be given first) Repeat cycles every 21 days for 6 cycles (must be given with growth factor support)
AC → Paclitaxel[a,f]	**Paclitaxel → FAC[g,m]**
Doxorubicin 60 mg/m² IV, day 1 Cyclophosphamide 600 mg/m² IV, day 1 Repeat cycles every 21 days for 4 cycles Followed by: Paclitaxel 80 mg/m² IV weekly Repeat cycles every 7 days for 12 cycles	Paclitaxel 80 mg/m² per week IV over 1 hour every week for 12 weeks Followed by: Fluorouracil 500 mg/m² IV, days 1 and 4 Doxorubicin 50 mg/m² IV continuous infusion over 72 hours Cyclophosphamide 500 mg/m² IV, day 1 Repeat cycles every 21–28 days for 4 cycles[g]
FEC[h]	**CEF[i]**
Fluorouracil 500 mg/m² IV, day 1 Epirubicin 100 mg/m² IV bolus, day 1 Cyclophosphamide 500 mg/m² IV, day 1 Repeat cycle every 21 days for 6 cycles	Cyclophosphamide 75 mg/m² per day orally on days 1–14 Epirubicin 60 mg/m² IV, days 1 and 8 Fluorouracil 600 mg/m² IV, days 1 and 8 Repeat cycles every 21 days for 6 cycles (requires prophylactic antibiotics or growth factor support)
CMF[j,k]	**Dose-Dense AC → Paclitaxel[a,l,n]**
Cyclophosphamide 100 mg/m² per day orally, days 1–14 Methotrexate 40 mg/m² IV, days 1 and 8 Fluorouracil 600 mg/m² IV, days 1 and 8 Repeat cycles every 28 days for 6 cycles *Or* Cyclophosphamide 600 mg/m² IV, day 1 Methotrexate 40 mg/m² IV, day 1 Fluorouracil 600 mg/m² IV, days 1 and 8 Repeat cycles every 21 days for 6 cycles	Doxorubicin 60 mg/m² IV bolus, day 1 Cyclophosphamide 600 mg/m² IV, day 1 Repeat cycles every 14 days for 4 cycles (must be given with growth factor support) Followed by: Paclitaxel 175 mg/m 2 IV over 3 hours Repeat cycles every 14 days for 4 cycles (must be given with growth factor support)

AC, Adriamycin (doxorubicin), Cytoxan (cyclophosphamide); CAF, Cytoxan (cyclophosphamide), Adriamycin (doxorubicin), 5-fluorouracil; CEF, cyclophosphamide, epirubicin, 5-fluorouracil; CMF, cyclophosphamide, methotrexate, 5-flourouracil; FAC, 5-fluorouracil, Adriamycin (doxorubicin), cyclophosphamide; FEC, 5-fluorouracil, epirubicin, cyclophosphamide; TAC, Taxotere (docetaxel), Adriamycin (doxorubicin), cyclophosphamide; TC, Taxotere (docetaxel), cyclophosphamide.

[a]Designated as a preferred regimen in the NCCN Breast Cancer Guidelines.
[b]From Fisher B, Brown AM, Dimitrov NV, et al. Two months of doxorubicin-cyclophosphamide with and without interval reinduction therapy compared with 6 months of cyclophosphamide, methotrexate, and fluorouracil in positive-node breast cancer patients with tamoxifen-nonresponsive tumors: results from the National Surgical Adjuvant Breast and Bowel Project B-15. J Clin Oncol 1990;8:1483.
[c]From Jones SE, Savin MA, Holmes FA, et al. Phase III trial comparing doxorubicin plus cyclophosphamide with docetaxel plus cyclophosphamide as adjuvant therapy for operable breast cancer. J Clin Oncol 2006;24:5381.
[d]From Buzdar AU, Hortobagyi GN, Singletary SE, et al. In: Salmon S, ed. Adjuvant Therapy of Cancer, VIII. Philadelphia, PA: Lippincott-Raven, 1997:93–100.
[e]From Martin M, Dienkowski T, Mackey J, et al. Adjuvant docetaxel for node-positive breast cancer. N Engl J Med 2005;352:2302.
[f]From Sparano JA, Wang M, Martino S, et al. Weekly paclitaxel in the adjuvant treatment of breast cancer. N Engl J Med 2008;358:1663–1671.
[g]From Green MC, Buzdar AU, Smith T, et al. Weekly paclitaxel improves pathologic complete remission in operable breast cancer when compared with paclitaxel once every 3 weeks. J Clin Oncol 2005;23:5983.
[h]From French Adjuvant Study Group. Benefit of a high-dose epirubicin regimen in adjuvant chemotherapy for node-positive breast cancer patients with poor prognostic factors: 5-year follow-up results of French Adjuvant Study Group 05 randomized trial. J Clin Oncol 2001;19:602.
[i]From Levine MN, Bramwell VH, Pritchard KI, et al. Randomized trial of intensive cyclophosphamide, epirubicin, and fluorouracil chemotherapy compared with cyclophosphamide, methotrexate, and fluorouracil in premenopausal women with node-positive breast cancer. National Cancer Institute of Canada Clinical Trials Group. J Clin Oncol 1998;16:2651.
[j]From Bonadonna G, Brusamolino E, Valagussa P, et al. Combination chemotherapy as an adjuvant treatment in operable breast cancer. N Engl J Med 1976;294:405.
[k]From Fisher B, Redmond C, Dimitrov NV, et al. A randomized clinical trial evaluating sequential methotrexate and fluorouracil in the treatment of patients with node-negative breast cancer who have estrogen-receptor-negative tumors. N Engl J Med 1989;320:473.
[l]From Citron ML, Berry DA, Cirrincione C, et al. Randomized trial of dose-dense versus conventionally scheduled and sequential versus concurrent combination chemotherapy as postoperative adjuvant treatment of node-positive primary breast cancer: first report of Intergroup Trial C9741/Cancer and Leukemia Group B Trial 9741. J Clin Oncol 2003;21:1431–1439.
[m]FAC may also be given with bolus doxorubicin administration, and the fluorouracil dose is then given on days 1 and 8.
[n]Another way to give these agents in a dose-dense manner is A → P → C as sequential single agents, in the same doses indicated above, every 14 days for 4 cycles each with growth factor support.

explain to patients. Some of the limitations of Adjuvant! include the limited information regarding outcome in patients with tumors that are smaller than 1 cm and no axillary lymph node involvement; it does not incorporate proliferation markers or *HER2* status of the primary tumor; and it does not consider potential adverse effects of therapy for individual patients. Estimates of outcome with the Adjuvant! program may also vary in specific subgroups of patients, such as women who are diagnosed with breast cancer at a younger age.

Adjuvant Chemotherapy Cytotoxic drugs that have been used alone and in combination as adjuvant therapy for breast cancer include doxorubicin, epirubicin, cyclophosphamide, methotrexate, fluorouracil, paclitaxel, docetaxel, melphalan, prednisone, vinorelbine, and vincristine. Table 105-6 lists some of the most common combination chemotherapy regimens used in the adjuvant setting.

The basic principle of adjuvant therapy for any cancer type is that the regimen with the highest response rate in advanced disease should be the optimal regimen for use in the adjuvant setting.

However, results from individual clinical trials investigating specific regimens in the adjuvant setting are required to identify the benefits and risks in a specific patient population. Early administration of effective combination chemotherapy at a time when the tumor burden is low should increase the likelihood of cure and minimize the emergence of drug-resistant tumor cell clones. Historically, combination chemotherapy regimens (polychemotherapy) have been more effective than single-agent chemotherapy. Anthracyclines (doxorubicin and epirubicin) and more recently taxanes (paclitaxel and docetaxel) have become the cornerstones of modern chemotherapy for the adjuvant treatment of breast cancer. The overview analysis of adjuvant chemotherapy (discussed previously) analyzed the use of CMF- (cyclophosphamide, methotrexate, fluorouracil) or anthracycline-based chemotherapy regimens (polychemotherapy) compared with no chemotherapy. Patients who received polychemotherapy had a 23% ± 2% reduction in annual odds of recurrence and a 14% ± 2% reduction in annual odds of death compared with patients who did not receive chemotherapy, establishing adjuvant chemotherapy as a powerful option for reducing breast cancer recurrence. The authors also analyzed results from 20 trials that directly compared an anthracycline-containing regimen with a CMF-type regimen and demonstrated a significant advantage with the anthracycline regimens.[5] In that meta-analysis, anthracycline-containing regimens were modestly superior in reducing recurrence and death compared with regimens without anthracyclines. A 7% ± 3% reduction in annual odds of recurrence and a 9% ± 3% reduction in annual odds of death were reported in the 2012 update with the anthracycline-containing regimens. It should be noted that regimens with higher cumulative doses of anthracycline (at least 240 mg/m^2 of doxorubicin and at least 360 mg/m^2 of epirubicin) were associated with improvements in the relative risk of recurrence (11% ± 4%) and overall survival (16% ± 4%) compared with standard CMF regimens. Until the 2012 update, adjuvant chemotherapy regimens with taxanes did not have sufficient follow-up to be included in the EBCTCG analyses. This meta-analysis reported data from 33 clinical trials and discovered that incorporation of a taxane reduced the risk of distant recurrence (13% ± 3%), any recurrence (14% ± 2%), and overall mortality (11% ± 3%) compared with a nontaxane regimen.[5] These trials included both sequential and concurrent taxane therapy (paclitaxel or docetaxel) in conjunction with anthracyclines (with or without cyclophosphamide, fluorouracil, or methotrexate). Proportional reductions in recurrence and breast cancer mortality were largely independent of age, nodal status, tumor size, tumor differentiation, or ER status. Most of these trials enrolled node-positive patients only, but some high-risk node-negative patients were also included. There is no apparent biologic reason why patients with node-negative disease should respond differently to the taxanes than those with node-positive disease. However, the absolute benefits for this population may not be large enough to require that all patients with node-negative disease receive an anthracycline- and taxane-based chemotherapy regimen. Because the addition of a taxane may predispose patients to peripheral neuropathy, myelosuppression, and alopecia, adverse events should also be considered. Taxane-containing, non-anthracycline regimens were not included in the meta-analysis but may be appropriate for some patients with a low risk of disease recurrence based on the results from a single randomized clinical trial.[79] However, this subject remains widely debated, and no single adjuvant chemotherapy regimen is preferred.

Cytotoxic chemotherapy is a particularly important treatment modality for patients with tumors that do not express ER or PR and do not overexpress *HER2* (so called triple-negative breast cancers [TNBCs]).[80] Patients with TNBC treated with anthracycline- and taxane-based chemotherapy have significantly decreased survival compared with patients with other breast cancer subtypes. Ironically, this subgroup of patients is more likely to respond to neoadjuvant chemotherapy. Therefore, patients with TNBC who achieve a pCR have an excellent long-term survival, but those who have residual disease at the time of surgery have a worse prognosis than non-TNBC patients. The optimal type and duration of chemotherapy for patients with TNBC is unknown. Because none of the previously identified molecular targets are present in TNBC, incorporation of nontraditional chemotherapy (e.g., platinum agents) into these regimens is under investigation. Identification of meaningful molecular targets is much needed and is where most research is ongoing. Molecular targets of interest include epidermal growth factor receptor (EGFR), vascular endothelial growth factor (VEGF), and poly-ADP ribose polymerase (PARP).

Although the optimal duration of adjuvant chemotherapy administration is unknown, it appears to be on the order of 12 to 24 weeks and depends on the regimen being used. Optimally, chemotherapy should be initiated within 12 weeks of surgical removal of the primary tumor.[81] "Dose intensity" and "dose density" appear to be critical factors in achieving optimal outcomes in adjuvant breast cancer therapy. *Dose intensity* is defined as the amount of drug administered per unit of time and is typically reported in milligrams per square meter of body surface area per week (mg/m^2/wk). Increasing dose, decreasing time between doses, or both can increase dose intensity. *Dose density* is one way of achieving dose intensity but not by increasing the amount of drug given, as occurs with dose escalation, but instead by decreasing the time between treatment cycles. The importance of dose intensity first received wide attention in 1981 when the Milan group reported in a retrospective analysis of their original CMF adjuvant study that only patients who received at least 85% of their planned CMF dose benefited significantly from adjuvant therapy, and those receiving less than 65% of the planned dose had the same DFS and OS as the group of control patients treated with surgery alone.[82] Therefore, dose reductions for standard treatment regimens should be avoided unless necessitated by severe toxicity. But increasing doses beyond those contained in standard treatment regimens does not appear to be beneficial and may be harmful.

Several studies investigating the impact of *dose density* have now been reported. Interest in this approach to adjuvant therapy was stimulated when the Cancer and Leukemia Group B (CALGB) reported results from their trial 9741, which tested not only dose density but also the question of using sequential versus combination chemotherapy regimens. Using a 2 × 2 factorial design, investigators randomized node-positive breast cancer patients after surgery to compare sequential versus concurrent chemotherapy and standard dose versus dose density.[83] The arms of the study were group 1, sequential doxorubicin (A) for 4 cycles followed by paclitaxel (P) for 4 cycles followed by cyclophosphamide (C) for 4 cycles, with all cycles given every 3 weeks; group 2, sequential A for 4 cycles followed by P for 4 cycles followed by C for cycles with all cycles given every 2 weeks with filgrastim; group 3, concurrent AC for 4 cycles followed by P for 4 cycles with all cycles given every 3 weeks; and group 4, concurrent AC for 4 cycles followed by P for 4 cycles with all cycles given every 2 weeks with filgrastim. After a median follow-up period of 36 months, the patients receiving chemotherapy every 2 weeks had a significantly prolonged DFS (at 3 years: 85% vs. 81%; RR, 0.74; $P = 0.01$) and OS (92% vs. 90%; RR, 0.69; $P = 0.013$) compared with chemotherapy every 3 weeks.[83] The use of sequential versus concurrent chemotherapy did not show a benefit for one over the other in terms of DFS or OS, but sequential therapy did appear to be less toxic. Patients in the concurrent every 2 week group (group 4) had significantly more regimen-related toxicity, including a very high rate of red blood cell transfusions for anemia (13% of cycles).[83] Red blood cell transfusions are rarely required with most other standard adjuvant chemotherapy regimens used for breast cancer.

Dose intensity appears to be important for some drugs but not for others. Many studies with anthracyclines (without taxanes) appear to indicate no benefit from a dose-dense approach to drug administration. These data seem to contradict the CALGB 9741 data. However, data with the taxanes, especially paclitaxel, appear to support a dose-dense (not intense) approach, with weekly therapy producing optimal outcomes.[84] Data with paclitaxel given weekly versus every 3 weeks indicate that this drug is more effective when given weekly in the adjuvant, neoadjuvant, and metastatic settings.[84–86] Thus, some speculate that the different paclitaxel schedule is the primary reason for the success with this approach to therapy. A direct comparison between taxane dosing intervals was evaluated in the North American Breast Cancer Intergroup Trial E1199, which randomized patients to receive doxorubicin and cyclophosphamide for 4 cycles every 3 weeks followed by either weekly or every 3 week paclitaxel or docetaxel.[84] Although this study does not directly address the question of dose density because of the lower doses given in the weekly arms, it appears to support the pharmacologic advantage of a taxane given more frequently as the essential factor driving the beneficial outcomes seen with "dose density" in the CALGB 9741 trial. Although no differences in DFS or OS were observed between the weekly or every 3 week schedule or the different taxanes in the E1199 trial, a subgroup analysis indicated that the weekly paclitaxel arm resulted in improved DFS (OR, 1.27; 95% CI, 1.03–1.57; P = 0.006) and OS (OR, 1.32; 95% CI, 1.02–1.72; P = 0.01) compared with paclitaxel administered every 3 weeks. Docetaxel, when administered every 3 weeks, resulted in improved DFS (OR, 1.23; 95% CI, 1.00–1.52; P = 0.02) but not OS (OR, 1.13; 95% CI, 0.88–1.46; P = 0.25) compared with paclitaxel administered every 3 weeks. DFS and OS with weekly docetaxel were not significantly different from paclitaxel administered every 3 weeks. Although other trials have attempted to investigate dose-dense regimens, they also have other variables that were altered that could potentially impact the outcomes. A meta-analysis by Bonilla et al. evaluated four trials of chemotherapy given in a dose-dense fashion compared with conventional administration.[87] In these studies, patients who received dose-dense chemotherapy had statistically improved DFS and OS compared with patients who received conventionally administered chemotherapy. Unfortunately, none of the trials, with the exception of the CALGB 9741 study, adequately evaluated the true impact of dose density.[88] This remains an area of continued research.

A major focus of clinical investigations in the past was the use of high-dose chemotherapy regimens as adjuvant therapy. Because bone marrow suppression is the dose-limiting toxicity for most chemotherapeutic agents, high-dose chemotherapy regimens followed by colony-stimulating factors or reinfusion of autologous hematopoietic stem cells were developed. Several cooperative groups have conducted trials of high-dose chemotherapy with stem cell support versus conventional adjuvant therapy. In an evaluation of 15 clinical trials, the use of high-dose chemotherapy significantly reduced the risk of disease recurrence compared with standard chemotherapy, but no difference in OS was observed.[89] Based on the available evidence, this approach to therapy is currently not recommended outside the context of a clinical trial.

The short-term toxic effects of chemotherapy used in the adjuvant setting are generally well tolerated. Although a number of investigators have demonstrated a reduction in quality of life, most patients are able to maintain a reasonable level of function and emotional and social well-being during treatment.[90,91] Supportive therapy of patients receiving systemic adjuvant chemotherapy has improved over the past decades. Increased attention to the impact of symptoms on quality of life may account for some of this improvement. In addition, more effective antiemetics have become available to assist in managing chemotherapy-induced nausea and vomiting, and myeloid growth factors are often helpful in preventing febrile neutropenia, particularly in elderly patients and patients receiving dose-dense chemotherapy regimens. Despite the use of newer antiemetics for prevention of nausea and vomiting, many women still have difficulty with this side effect, and delayed nausea and vomiting remains problematic in some patients. Aprepitant, a novel neurokinin-1 antagonist, may be considered in addition to serotonin receptor antagonists and dexamethasone to improve outcomes for some patients receiving anthracycline-based chemotherapy, but clinicians should be aware of the potential for clinically significant drug–drug interactions between aprepitant and other drugs, including some chemotherapy. The use of myeloid growth factors to support some adjuvant chemotherapy regimens may be required (e.g., with dose-dense regimens), but these are not routinely used for all adjuvant chemotherapy regimens. Because erythropoiesis-stimulating agents have potential effects on cancer cells and the cellular environment that may negatively impact the antitumor effects of chemotherapy or enhance adverse effects related to the chemotherapy, they should be avoided in patients receiving chemotherapy with a curative intent.[92]

Many other side effects are common with the chemotherapy regimens used for the treatment of early stage breast cancer, and patients should be appropriately counseled regarding the likelihood of alopecia, weight gain, and fatigue. Patients who are menstruating often experience a cessation of menses that may not return; cessation of menses may be accompanied by signs and symptoms of menopause. Deep-vein thrombosis (DVT) has been reported in women receiving combination chemotherapy regimens.[93] Leukemia and other hematologic disorders have long been associated with the alkylating agents (e.g., cyclophosphamide) and the topoisomerase II inhibitors (e.g., doxorubicin and epirubicin). Several studies have estimated a 0% to 1.5% cumulative incidence of leukemia or myelodysplasia after adjuvant chemotherapy with median follow-up period of 3 to 11 years.[94] To date, the dose-dense regimens have not been associated with an excess rate of leukemias, but the follow-up period for these trials is relatively short.

Cardiomyopathy induced by doxorubicin occurs in fewer than 1% of women whose total dose of doxorubicin is less than 320 mg/m^2.[95] This risk may be further decreased by use of continuous infusion or weekly doxorubicin. It should be noted that epirubicin in the adjuvant setting is usually given at a dose of 100 to 120 mg/m^2.[48] At this dose, epirubicin has an equal chance of causing cardiomyopathy as standard doxorubicin doses when both agents are given as bolus or short infusions. Taxanes are often associated with hypersensitivity reactions, peripheral neuropathy, or myalgias and arthralgias for a few days after the infusion.

It is important to note that the magnitude of survival benefit for adjuvant chemotherapy in stages I and II breast cancer is modest, with an absolute reduction in mortality rate of only 5% at 10 years for patients with negative axillary lymph nodes and 10% for patients with positive axillary lymph nodes. In addition, it is currently not possible to accurately predict who will attain this survival benefit. The advent of genetic prognostic tools, such as Oncotype DX, can help to identify patients who may derive little or no benefit from chemotherapy. However, these tests are only appropriate in specific subsets of patients. Studies have reported that most breast cancer patients would accept severe toxicity from treatment to achieve as little as a 1% to 5% improvement in survival.[74,75] Thus, in the absence of the ability to predict who will benefit, it is likely that most patients with stage I and stage II breast cancer would choose adjuvant chemotherapy.

The optimal chemotherapy regimen for use in the adjuvant setting has yet to be identified, and the choice of chemotherapy regimen for a specific patient is complex. Many adjuvant chemotherapy regimens are available, and most of these regimens have not been directly compared in randomized clinical trials. In some cases, the choice of chemotherapy regimen may be geographic, particularly if a regimen has been developed and studied by a particular institution.

Based on data from clinical trials and the previously mentioned pooled analysis, the concomitant or sequential addition of a taxane to an anthracycline-based chemotherapy regimen has become the standard of care for women with node-positive breast cancer. The use of taxanes in combination with anthracyclines is more controversial in patients with node-negative disease, although data from meta-analyses and a single trial specifically in patients with high-risk node negative disease support the use of anthracycline- and taxane-based chemotherapy regimens in this patient population.[5,96] Results from a single trial that evaluated a taxane-containing (non-anthracycline) regimen are available, and this regimen may be an appropriate treatment in a subset of patients at low risk of disease recurrence. NCCN recommendations are purposefully vague, and they do not differentiate between patients with node-positive or -negative breast cancer. The NCCN has designated preferred chemotherapy regimens, as listed in Table 105-6, although detailed information is not provided regarding the rationale behind these designations.

Adjuvant Biologic Therapy As biologic agents continue to demonstrate significant activity against metastatic breast cancer, they are subsequently tested in the adjuvant or neoadjuvant setting. Trastuzumab is a MoAB targeted against the *HER2*-receptor protein. It has demonstrated significant survival benefits when administered with chemotherapy in women with metastatic, *HER2*-positive breast cancer. Several published trials support the use of trastuzumab in combination with or sequentially after adjuvant chemotherapy for patients with early stage, *HER2*-positive breast cancer (Table 105-7).[97] Results from these trials report up to a 50%

TABLE 105-7 Selected Trastuzumab-Based Regimens for Early-Stage Breast Cancer

Regimen	Drugs	Doses	Frequency	Cycles
		Adjuvant		
AC ⇒ PH ⇒ H[a]	Doxorubicin	60 mg/m² IV	Every 21 days	4
	Cyclophosphamide	600 mg/m² IV	Every 21 days	4
	followed by			
	Paclitaxel	175 mg/m² IV over 3 h	Every 21 days	4
	or			
	Paclitaxel	80 mg/m² IV over 1 h	Every 7 days	12 wk
	with Trastuzumab	4 mg/kg IV → 2 mg/kg IV	Every 7 days	12 wk
	followed by			
	Trastuzumab	2 mg/kg IV or 6 mg/kg IV	Every 7 days or every 21 days	Complete 1 year
TCH[b]	Docetaxel	75 mg/m² IV	Every 21 days	6
	Carboplatin	AUC 6 IV	Every 21 days	6
	Trastuzumab	4 mg/kg IV → 2 mg/kg IV	Every 7 days	18 wk
	followed by			
	Trastuzumab	6 mg/kg IV	Every 21 days	Complete 1 year
Chemo ⇒ H[c]	Chemotherapy	See reference for details		At least 4
	followed by			
	Trastuzumab	8 mg/kg IV→ 6 mg/kg IV	Every 21 days	1 year
AC ⇒ TH[b]	Doxorubicin	60 mg/m² IV	Every 21 days	4
	Cyclophosphamide	600 mg/m² IV	Every 21 days	4
	followed by			
	Docetaxel	100 mg/m² IV	Every 21 days	4
	Trastuzumab	4 mg/kg IV → 2 mg/kg IV	Every 7 days	12 wk
	followed by			
	Trastuzumab	6 mg/kg IV	Every 21 days	Complete 1 year
		Neoadjuvant		
PH ⇒ FEC/H[d]	Paclitaxel	225 mg/m² IV over 24 h	Every 21 days	4
	or			
	Paclitaxel	80 mg/m² IV over 1 h	Every 7 days	12 wk
	with trastuzumab	4 mg/kg IV → 2 mg/kg IV	Every 7 days	12 wk
	followed by			
	Fluorouracil	500 mg/m² IV (days 1 and 4)	q 21 days	4
	Epirubicin	75 mg/m² IV	q 21 days	4
	Cyclophosphamide	500 mg/m² IV	q 21 days	4
	with Trastuzumab	2 mg/kg IV	q 7 days	12 wk

AC, Adriamycin (doxorubicin), Cytoxan (cyclophosphamide); FEC, fluorouracil, epirubicin, cyclophosphamide; H, Herceptin (trastuzumab); PH, paclitaxel, Herceptin (trastuzumab); TH, Taxotere (docetaxel), Herceptin (trastuzumab); TCH, Taxotere (docetaxel), carboplatin, Herceptin (trastuzumab).

[a]From Romond EH, Perez EA, Bryant J, et al. Trastuzumab plus adjuvant chemotherapy for operable HER2-positive breast cancer. N Engl J Med 2005;353:1673–1684.
[b]From Slamon D, Eiermann W, Robert N, et al. Adjuvant trastuzumab in HER2-positive breast cancer. N Engl J Med 2011;365:1273–1283.
[c]From Smith I, Procter M, Gelber RD, et al. 2-year follow-up of trastuzumab after adjuvant chemotherapy in HER2-positive breast cancer: a randomised controlled trial. Lancet 2007;369:29–36.
[d]From Buzdar AU, Ibrahim NK, Francis D, et al. Significantly higher pathologic complete remission rate after neoadjuvant therapy with trastuzumab, paclitaxel, and epirubicin chemotherapy: results of a randomized trial in human epidermal growth factor receptor 2-positive operable breast cancer. J Clin Oncol 2005;23:3676.

reduction in the risk of recurrence with the addition of trastuzumab to an adjuvant chemotherapy regimen. A meta-analysis of the six available clinical trials investigating the addition of trastuzumab to chemotherapy involving almost 14,000 women revealed superior DFS (OR, 0.69; 95% CI, 0.59–0.80; P <0.001) and OS (OR, 0.78; 95% CI, 0.69–0.88; P <0.001) in patients with *HER2*-positive breast cancer who received trastuzumab with chemotherapy compared with those that received chemotherapy alone.[98] This difference in DFS translated into a 31% overall lower relative risk for disease progression or death from any cause for patients who received trastuzumab. Although clearly the benefit of adding trastuzumab to these regimens is obvious, the type of chemotherapy, sequence of administration, and duration of trastuzumab differed among the trials, making the optimal trastuzumab-based regimen less obvious.

Most of the regimens investigated in these adjuvant trials included an anthracycline and a taxane given concurrently with trastuzumab or sequentially before trastuzumab. From the available evidence, it appears that administration of a taxane with trastuzumab may be more effective than trastuzumab administered after chemotherapy. In the previously mentioned meta-analysis, sequential and concomitant use of trastuzumab with chemotherapy both prolonged DFS compared with chemotherapy alone; whereas concomitant trastuzumab also improved OS, sequential trastuzumab did not.[98] The adjuvant use of trastuzumab without an anthracycline has been reported in one trial (Breast Cancer International Research Group 006) and appears to provide similar benefit with diminished cardiac adverse effects as compared with traditional anthracycline-containing adjuvant trastuzumab regimens.[99] The duration of trastuzumab therapy in these adjuvant trials ranges from 9 to 104 weeks in the published studies. The optimal duration of trastuzumab therapy is unknown, although the most current data support the use of trastuzumab for a total of 52 weeks. The most commonly used trastuzumab-based adjuvant chemotherapy regimens are listed in Table 105-7.

The incidence of adverse cardiac effects associated with the addition of trastuzumab appears to increase when an anthracycline is included in the regimen before administration of trastuzumab. The incidence of symptomatic heart failure with adjuvant trastuzumab ranges from 0.5% to 4% in highly selected patients who participated in the clinical trials.[99,100] The higher risk of cardiac complications may be acceptable in many patients given the significant reductions in breast cancer recurrence and death rates. Sequential administration of trastuzumab after chemotherapy (as in the HERA trial) appears to produce a lower incidence of cardiac toxicity (symptomatic congestive heart failure = 2% with trastuzumab). Also, the use of a non–anthracycline-based regimen in the BCIRG 006 trial (Table 105-7) was associated with a low incidence (0.4%) of symptomatic heart failure compared with other regimens.[99] However, cross-trial comparisons are challenging because the definition of cardiac events in each trial was different. Therefore, application of these results to individual patients is fraught with difficulties, and many different regimens may be appropriate for a given patient. Concurrent administration of trastuzumab with an anthracycline is very controversial because of potentially higher rates of cardiac dysfunction (see the Anti-*HER2* Agents of Metastatic Breast Cancer section). Concurrent administration of an anthracycline and trastuzumab in the neoadjuvant setting has been reported with extremely promising rates of pCR and limited cardiac complications.[101] This combination should be administered with caution, and patients should be carefully monitored for signs and symptoms of cardiac dysfunction. Similar to many MoABs, trastuzumab is associated with infusion-related reactions such as fever, chills, and rigors temporally associated with trastuzumab infusions. Postmarketing surveillance data have identified "pulmonary toxicity" and "anaphylaxis" as rare but potentially life-threatening reactions associated with trastuzumab. Chemotherapy-related adverse effects, including neutropenia, infection, and diarrhea, are slightly more frequent with the addition of concurrent trastuzumab therapy, but these toxicities are easily managed and do not preclude the use of trastuzumab in patients with early stage breast cancer.

All of these adjuvant trials continued trastuzumab administration during adjuvant radiation therapy and endocrine therapy. The administration of trastuzumab during radiation therapy was evaluated in patients that participated in the N9831 clinical trial. Patients that received concurrent radiation therapy with adjuvant trastuzumab did not experience a significant increase in cardiac events or acute radiation-related adverse events with the exception of transient leukopenia.[102] Therefore, if radiation therapy is clinically indicated, trastuzumab is typically administered concomitantly with radiation.

Many questions remain regarding the optimal use of trastuzumab in the adjuvant or neoadjuvant therapy of early stage breast cancer. The use of trastuzumab with chemotherapy in the adjuvant or neoadjuvant setting is now considered to be the standard of care for patients with node-positive and high-risk node-negative *HER2*-positive breast cancer.[48] Several retrospective analyses of patients with *HER2*-positive tumors smaller than 1 cm who did not receive trastuzumab appear to indicate a poor prognosis, suggesting that these patients may also benefit from trastuzumab-based adjuvant chemotherapy.[103] Although controversial, treatment with trastuzumab in patients with small, *HER2*-positive, node-negative tumors may be considered. A similar approach has been used in the neoadjuvant treatment of *HER2*-positive breast cancer as well (see the Locally Advanced Breast Cancer section). Clinical trials involving other novel anti-*HER2* therapies, such as lapatinib and pertuzumab, in the adjuvant and neoadjuvant settings are ongoing.

Clinical **Controversy. . .**

Trastuzumab clearly has improved the outcomes for women with lymph node–positive and high-risk lymph node–negative early-stage, *HER2*-positive breast cancer. However, patients with small (<1 cm) tumors with negative lymph nodes were not included in prospective clinical trials with trastuzumab. Retrospective data suggest that patients with small *HER2*-positive tumors who did not receive trastuzumab-based chemotherapy have a poor prognosis. Questions remain regarding optimal use of trastuzumab in this patient population, and each patient must weigh the risks versus benefits for his or her individual circumstance.

Adjuvant Endocrine Therapy Endocrine therapies that have been studied in the treatment of primary or early-stage breast cancer include tamoxifen, toremifene, oophorectomy, ovarian irradiation, luteinizing hormone–releasing hormone (LHRH) agonists, and AIs. The choice of agent(s) depends on menopausal status and is based on a multitude of clinical trials completed in this setting that establish different roles for different therapies.

Tamoxifen was traditionally the gold standard adjuvant endocrine therapy and has been used in the adjuvant setting for more than 3 decades. Tamoxifen is antiestrogenic in breast cancer cells, but it appears to have estrogenic properties in other tissues and organs.[104,105] More recent studies show that tamoxifen and other similar drugs have many estrogenic and antiestrogenic effects that depend on the tissue and the gene in question, and they are more appropriately called selective estrogen receptor modulators (SERMs). Women receiving adjuvant tamoxifen therapy have reduced risk of recurrence and mortality compared with women not receiving adjuvant tamoxifen therapy.[4] This observation, coupled with evidence supporting tolerability of tamoxifen, including beneficial estrogenic effects on the lipid profile and bone density, led to tamoxifen's being the endocrine agent of choice for both pre- and postmenopausal women compared with older, more toxic therapies (e.g., megestrol acetate). In the United States, tamoxifen is generally considered the adjuvant endocrine therapy of choice for premenopausal women. However, many ongoing clinical trials are investigating the use of the LHRH agonists or oophorectomy instead of tamoxifen or in addition to tamoxifen or AIs in this group of women.

The optimal dose of tamoxifen is widely debated. The EBCTCG overview showed that the reduction in recurrence was greater in studies that used higher tamoxifen doses ($P = 0.02$ for the trend between 20, 30, or 40 mg/day).[4] However, a dose effect did not exist for tamoxifen and breast cancer mortality. Therefore the current recommended dose for tamoxifen in the adjuvant, metastatic, and risk reduction settings is 20 mg/day. If chemotherapy and radiation therapy are not required, adjuvant tamoxifen therapy is generally initiated shortly after surgery or as soon as pathology results are known and the decision to administer tamoxifen as adjuvant therapy is made.

When adjuvant chemotherapy is also required, tamoxifen should be administered after chemotherapy is completed. This recommendation is based on laboratory and clinical evidence from a phase III trial suggesting tamoxifen administered concurrently with chemotherapy may antagonize the beneficial effect of chemotherapy.[106] In the phase III clinical trial, administration of sequential tamoxifen resulted in a marginally superior DFS compared with concurrent use of tamoxifen with chemotherapy (HR, 0.84; 95% CI, 0.70–1.01; $P = 0.061$).[106] Some clinicians also advocate the initiation of tamoxifen after completion of radiation therapy, but this subject is very controversial, and few trials have addressed the issue of concurrent versus sequential endocrine therapy and radiation therapy.

The optimal duration of tamoxifen therapy in the adjuvant setting is currently 5 years. Studies of prolonged administration (e.g., 10 years) have produced mixed results. In the ATLAS trial, patients with ER-positive breast cancer who had 10 years of tamoxifen had improved DFS and OS compared with those with 5 years of treatment.[107] Previous randomized trials comparing 5 years of tamoxifen treatment with longer than 5 years of tamoxifen treatment have shown opposite results and, in fact, were stopped early because of these detrimental outcomes.[108] Also, patients in the ATLAS trial who received 10 years of tamoxifen had increased risk of developing endometrial cancer and pulmonary embolism compared with those receiving tamoxifen for 5 years (a consistent finding in other randomized trials as well).[107] With these conflicting data regarding efficacy and the possibility of increased toxicity related to a longer duration of tamoxifen therapy, the optimal dose appears to remain 5 years until data from other clinical trials investigating this question become available and either confirm or refute the benefits of the 5-year duration.

Clinical **Controversy. . .**

For premenopausal women with early-stage or locally advanced hormone-receptor-positive breast cancer, the optimal duration of tamoxifen therapy is currently under scrutiny. Clinical trials investigating 5 versus 10 years of tamoxifen therapy have reported conflicting results, with one demonstrating benefit and the other a detriment to prolonged use. Clinical trials further investigating this question are ongoing. Providers should discuss the risks and benefits of extended tamoxifen therapy individually with each patient.

The most reliable information regarding the side effects of tamoxifen comes from the NSABP Breast Cancer Prevention Trial (P1).[51] This trial randomized 13,388 women 35 years of age or older who were at increased risk for breast cancer to placebo ($n = 6,707$) or to 20 mg/day of tamoxifen ($n = 6,681$) for 5 years. Although the primary finding of this study is that tamoxifen reduces the risk of invasive breast cancer by 49%, this study also provides an excellent opportunity to determine the risk of side effects associated with tamoxifen. Information was prospectively collected with regard to the occurrence of hot flashes, vaginal discharge, irregular menses, fluid retention, nausea, skin changes, diarrhea, and weight gain or loss. The self-administered depression scale and a global quality-of-life and a sexual function scale were administered at each follow-up visit. The only symptomatic differences noted between the placebo and tamoxifen group were related to hot flashes and vaginal discharge, both of which occurred more often in the tamoxifen group. No important differences between the two groups were observed in the various self-reporting instruments. Tamoxifen did not increase the risk of ischemic heart disease but did reduce the risk of hip radius and spine fractures. Of note, the rates of stroke, pulmonary embolism, and DVT were elevated in the tamoxifen group (stroke: RR, 1.59; pulmonary embolism: RR, 3.01; and DVT: RR, 1.60), particularly in women age 50 years or older. The rate of endometrial cancer was increased in the tamoxifen group (RR, 2.53), and this increased risk occurred predominantly in women age 50 years or older. The increased risk of endometrial carcinoma is similar in magnitude to that associated with postmenopausal estrogen replacement therapy and is likely a consequence of an estrogenic effect of tamoxifen on the endometrium. Some experts argue that this risk is acceptable because the endometrial cancer induced by tamoxifen is low stage, low grade, and easily treated with surgery or other means and does not pose a life-threatening risk to women. Tamoxifen was also associated with an increased risk of uterine sarcomas (a more aggressive form of endometrial cancer), but this risk appears to be lower than the more common endometrial cancers identified in the NSABP P-1 study. Routine endometrial biopsy is not currently recommended for women receiving tamoxifen therapy. However, women receiving tamoxifen therapy should be counseled to have regular gynecologic examinations and immediately report unusual vaginal bleeding to their primary clinicians for further evaluation.

In premenopausal women, the use of LHRH agonists (ovarian suppression) or ovarian ablation provides benefit in the adjuvant setting. In the EBCTCG overview analysis published in 2005, the overall benefit of ovarian ablation or suppression was significant compared with no treatment but was smaller than previously reported in 1996 (reduction in annual odds of recurrence = 25% ± 12% in women younger than 40 years old and 29% ± 6% in women 40–49 years old).[109] Many of the ongoing trials with the LHRH agonists were not yet included in this analysis, and most of the clinical trials analyzed included patients with hormone receptor–positive, –negative, and unknown tumor status. In an update of this analysis, study inclusion was restricted to patients treated with ovarian suppression with LHRH agonists (not ovarian oblation or oophorectomy) and patients with tumors known to be hormone receptor positive.[110] The addition of a LHRH agonist reduced the rates of recurrence by 25%, deaths after recurrence by 28%, and all deaths by 27% in women younger than 40 years; no significant reductions in recurrence or death were noted in patients older than 40 years. Also, a similar benefit was observed with goserelin as compared with CMF chemotherapy in hormone-sensitive premenopausal breast cancer patients but not in patients with hormone receptor–negative tumors.[110] It is not clear whether the benefit of chemotherapy in this population is a result of the actual effects of chemotherapy or a result of the endocrine effects of chemotherapy-induced amenorrhea. Consequently, some studies have investigated the benefits of adding ovarian ablation or suppression to chemotherapy either with or without tamoxifen. Results from these studies clearly indicate a benefit from ceasing menses regardless of whether this is caused by chemotherapy or ovarian ablation or suppression.[110] It is not clear whether the addition of an LHRH agonist to tamoxifen is advantageous in women with hormone receptor–positive tumors who continue to menstruate after chemotherapy. The optimal duration of adjuvant LHRH agonist use is unknown, with trials ranging from 18 months to 5 years of treatment. Multiple ongoing trials are evaluating whether an LHRH agonist alone with tamoxifen or with an AI is the most effective therapy for premenopausal women. Currently, the only trial with available results is a study by the Austrian Breast and Colorectal Cancer Study Group (ABCSG-12), which randomized premenopausal patients with hormone receptor–positive early-stage breast cancer to 3 years of tamoxifen or anastrozole, both concomitantly with goserelin for ovarian suppression.[111] After a median follow-up period of 62 months, there was no significant difference in DFS between the two groups (HR, 1.08; $P = 0.591$). However, in a retrospective analysis of patients with disease recurrence, the relative risk of death was significantly higher in patients who received anastrozole than in patients who received tamoxifen (HR, 2.0; 95% CI, 1.23–3.24; $P = 0.005$). Until additional data are available, ovarian suppression in combination with an AI should not be considered as an appropriate adjuvant therapy for premenopausal women outside of a clinical trial. It should also be noted that a tamoxifen-only arm was not included in this trial, which makes comparison to the current standard of care for premenopausal women (tamoxifen alone) impossible.

In postmenopausal women, incorporation of AIs is the standard of care in the adjuvant setting. Four different approaches to therapy have been undertaken with these agents: (a) direct comparison with tamoxifen for adjuvant endocrine therapy; (b) sequential use after 5 years of adjuvant tamoxifen therapy; (c) sequential use after 2 to 3 years of adjuvant tamoxifen; and (d) 2 years of treatment with an AI followed by 3 years of adjuvant tamoxifen. Anastrozole and letrozole have been individually, directly compared with tamoxifen as initial therapy in postmenopausal women with hormone receptor–positive, early-stage breast cancer (ATAC [Arimidex, Tamoxifen, Alone or in Combination] Trial and BIG [Breast International Group] 1–98 Trial).[112] These comparisons show an advantage with the AIs over tamoxifen in terms of DFS. Other approaches to adjuvant endocrine therapy with AIs include sequential use of newer agents after either 5 years or 2 to 3 years of tamoxifen. In the MA-17 study, 5 additional years of letrozole was compared with placebo in postmenopausal breast cancer patients who had completed 5 years of tamoxifen therapy.[113] After a median follow-up period of 2.4 years, letrozole was associated with superior estimated 4-year DFS compared with placebo (93% vs. 87%; $P < 0.001$). In a pooled analysis of trials investigating a switch to an AI, 9,015 patients who had completed 2 to 3 years of adjuvant tamoxifen therapy were randomized to continue tamoxifen or crossover to anastrozole or exemestane for the remainder of 5 years.[112] The results of this analysis show a decreased risk of recurrence at 6 years after randomization in patients who switched to an AI compared with those who continued with tamoxifen alone (12.6% vs. 16.0%; $P < 0.00001$). The BIG 1–98 trial, which compared letrozole with tamoxifen, also included two separate arms that investigated the value of switching from tamoxifen to an AI or vice versa. With 71 months of follow-up period, the sequential arms did not improve estimated 5-year DFS compared with letrozole alone in either comparison.[114] Clinical trials are also investigating longer durations of AI use to assess the benefits and harms of continued estrogen deprivation, the results of which are greatly anticipated.

Most national and international guidelines currently recommend incorporation of an AI into the adjuvant endocrine therapy regimen for all postmenopausal, hormone-sensitive breast cancers.[48] The current NCCN guidelines for breast cancer management state that any of the following are acceptable endocrine therapy regimens for these women: (a) an AI for 5 years (or longer based on expert opinion); (b) tamoxifen for 2 to 3 years followed by an AI for a total of 5 years of endocrine therapy, or (c) tamoxifen for 5 years followed by an AI for another 5 years (total of 10 years of endocrine therapy).[48] The NCCN panel believes that the three available AIs (anastrozole, letrozole, and exemestane) have similar antitumor efficacy and toxicity profiles, and many other clinicians agree. Therefore, the optimal endocrine therapy regimen in the adjuvant setting has yet to be determined, and incorporation of biologic therapies into these regimens is also being examined. Results from ongoing trials are eagerly awaited to more clearly define a treatment strategy for women facing this clinical dilemma.

Aromatase inhibitors are generally well tolerated. Adverse effects include bone loss or osteoporosis, hot flashes, myalgia or arthralgia, vaginal dryness or atrophy, mild headaches, and diarrhea. Although concerns surrounding loss of bone density and an increased risk of osteoporosis are evident in these adjuvant trials, the overall impact on quality of life and long-term survival are still being evaluated. Bisphosphonates are coadministered with the AI in many patients in the metastatic setting and may also be beneficial in the adjuvant setting. Other adverse events that are worrisome include questionable effects on the cardiovascular system (e.g., hypercholesterolemia), cognitive functioning, and joint health. Longer follow-up from these trials will continue to provide valuable information to guide treatment decisions and management of adverse effects.

In summary, tamoxifen has been used in the adjuvant setting for nearly 30 years and has a very well-defined safety and efficacy profile in this setting. The roles of other agents such as AIs in postmenopausal women and LHRH agonists in premenopausal women have changed the landscape of adjuvant endocrine therapy, and incorporation of other biologic therapies may further impact outcomes.

The pharmacologic disposition of tamoxifen in humans is very complex and has only recently been elucidated (Fig. 105-6). Tamoxifen is now considered to be a prodrug. Although the parent compound has significant clinical activity, tamoxifen is metabolized through multiple enzymes, including CYP3A4, CYP2C19, CYP2D6, and others, to metabolites that appear to be more active than the parent compound.[115] The active metabolites 4-hydroxytamoxifen (4OH-TAM) and 4-hydroxy-*N*-desmethyltamoxifen (endoxifen) have nearly a 100-fold higher affinity for the ER compared with tamoxifen. Endoxifen is present in the serum at a six- to 12-fold higher concentrations compared with 4OH-TAM; hence, endoxifen is thought to be the most important metabolite for the clinical activity of tamoxifen. The formation of endoxifen is highly dependent on the enzymatic activity of CYP2D6. However, multiple other pathways may also be important for determining activity, including deactivation pathways (e.g., SULT-1-A1, UGT). Polymorphisms in CYP2D6 can lead to increased or decreased formation of endoxifen and may be related to improved or diminished clinical outcomes, respectively. Although clinical data suggest that certain polymorphisms in CYP2D6 may result in poorer DFS or relapse-free survival in patients receiving tamoxifen, other studies show either no relationship or the opposite effect between clinical outcomes and CYP2D6 polymorphisms. Multiple commercially available assays for CYP2D6 are available, but widespread testing for patients receiving tamoxifen is not currently recommended based on available evidence.[48,73] Excellent reviews on this subject are available).[115] Potent inhibitors of CYP2D6, such as paroxetine and fluoxetine, may decrease levels of endoxifen in patients receiving tamoxifen.[116] The clinical outcomes related to such drug–drug interactions in an individual patient are largely unknown and may depend on their underlying CYP2D6 genetic status (e.g., poor metabolizer, extensive metabolizer). In one population-based cohort study, concomitant use of tamoxifen and paroxetine (but not other antidepressants) resulted in increased risk of breast cancer death.[117] Even though high-quality data on strong CYP2D6 inhibitors and

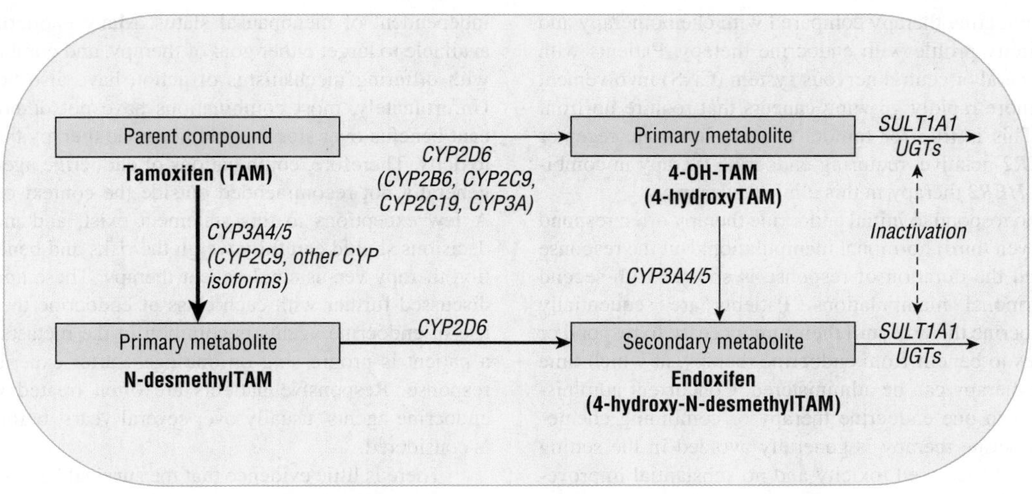

FIGURE 105-6 Tamoxifen metabolism. Widths of the arrows approximate allocation of parent compound to various metabolites. See text for further explanation.

breast cancer outcomes in patients receiving tamoxifen are limited, common sense would dictate avoiding known strong inhibitors of CYP2D6, if possible, in patients receiving tamoxifen.

Locally Advanced Breast Cancer (Stage III)

5 *Locally advanced breast cancer* generally refers to breast carcinomas with significant primary tumor and nodal disease but in which distant metastases cannot be documented. A wide variety of clinical scenarios can be seen within this group of patients, including neglected tumors that have spread locally, to inflammatory breast cancers that are a unique clinical entity. Inflammatory breast cancer is associated with similar clinical findings compared with neglected, locally advanced breast tumors (e.g., erythema representing skin involvement). The distinction between the two diagnoses lies in the rapidity of onset of symptoms. Many locally advanced breast cancers are diagnosed in patients who have had symptoms for months to years and have neglected to seek medical attention. Although these women have a poor prognosis because of the delay in diagnosis, they are not classified as inflammatory breast cancer. The hallmark of inflammatory breast cancers is the rapid onset of symptoms within weeks to months, including erythema of the skin with or without a detectable underlying breast mass. These patients are often inappropriately treated for cellulitis with antibiotics for several weeks to months. Because of the aggressive nature of this disease, a delay in diagnosis can be fatal for some of these women.

The natural history of locally advanced breast cancer shows that even when local–regional control is accomplished, systemic relapse and death from breast cancer eventually occur in most patients if systemic therapy is not used.[118] That observation led to interest in the use of neoadjuvant or primary chemotherapy in locally advanced breast cancer, which renders inoperable tumors resectable and can increase rates of BCT. Other potential benefits related to early initiation of systemic therapy include delivery of drugs through an intact vasculature, in vivo assessment of response to therapy, and the opportunity to study the biologic effects of the systemic treatment. For patients with inoperable breast cancer, including inflammatory breast cancer, the initial approach to therapy should be chemotherapy with the goal of achieving resectability. The NCCN guidelines addressing the management of locally advanced disease recommend primary chemotherapy with an anthracycline- and taxane-containing regimen.[48]

After neoadjuvant chemotherapy, most tumors respond with more than a 50% decrease in tumor size; about 70% of patients experience a reduction in their stage of disease. The chemotherapy regimens used in this setting are similar to those used in the adjuvant setting, but the regimens usually include an anthracycline, incorporate a taxane in some manner, and may have a higher dose density or dose intensity. For patients with *HER2*-positive tumors, the incorporation of trastuzumab with chemotherapy is appropriate.[119] For more detailed information regarding the specific regimen-related information, readers are referred to the referenced review.[120] Neoadjuvant endocrine therapy may be an option for patients who have unresectable hormone receptor–positive tumors who are unable to receive chemotherapy (e.g., multiple comorbid conditions).[121] However, this approach to therapy is not common.

Local therapy usually follows chemotherapy, and the extent of surgery is determined by response to chemotherapy, the wishes of the patient, and the cosmetic results likely to be achieved. However, many patients may be able to have BCT if an acceptable response to chemotherapy is accomplished. Adjuvant radiation therapy should be administered to all locally advanced breast cancer patients to minimize local recurrences regardless of the type of surgery used for that individual patient (e.g., mastectomy or segmental mastectomy). Inoperable tumors that are unresponsive to systemic chemotherapy may require radiation therapy for local management and may not be eligible for surgical resection after radiation. These patients are not commonly encountered but have a very poor prognosis. For most patients with locally advanced breast cancer, cure is still the primary goal of therapy and can be achieved in a large number of patients when all treatment modalities are used.

Metastatic Breast Cancer (Stage IV)

6 Treatment of metastatic breast cancer (MBC) with cytotoxic, biologic, or endocrine therapy often results in regression of disease and improvements in quality of life. The choice of therapy for metastatic disease is based on the presence or absence or certain tumor characteristics and site of disease involvement. The most important factors predicting response to therapy are the presence of estrogen, progesterone, and *HER2* receptors in the primary tumor tissue. Tumors expressing high levels of ER, PR, or both are more likely to respond to endocrine therapy. Tumors overexpressing *HER2* receptor protein are more likely to benefit from anti-*HER2* therapy. The site of disease is also an important factor to consider. Endocrine therapy is the treatment of choice for patients with hormone receptor–positive tumors who exhibit the first sign of metastatic disease in soft tissue, bone, or pleura because of the equal probability

of response to endocrine therapy compared with chemotherapy and a preferable toxicity profile with endocrine therapy. Patients with symptomatic visceral or central nervous system (CNS) involvement generally have more rapidly growing cancers that require up-front chemotherapy. This is true for tumors that are hormone receptor positive and *HER2*-positive, requiring endocrine therapy in combination with anti-*HER2* therapy in this clinical scenario.

Patients who respond to initial endocrine therapy often respond to a second (or even third) hormonal manipulation. But the response rate is lower, and the duration of response is shorter with second (and third) hormonal manipulations. Patients are sequentially treated with endocrine therapy until their tumors cease to respond or the patient ceases to benefit from endocrine therapy, at which time cytotoxic chemotherapy can be administered. Concurrent administration of more than one endocrine therapy or combining chemotherapy plus endocrine therapy is generally avoided in the setting of MBC because of increased toxicity and no substantial improvement in efficacy. Women with hormone receptor–negative tumors; with rapidly progressive or symptomatic lung, liver, or bone marrow involvement (a visceral crisis); and with progressive disease while on initial endocrine therapy are usually treated initially with cytotoxic chemotherapy. All breast cancer patients with metastases to the bone should be considered for treatment with a bone-modifying agent (e.g., pamidronate, zoledronic acid, or denosumab) because these agents have been shown to decrease the rates of skeletal-related events, such as fractures, spinal cord compression, and pain, and the need for radiation to the bones or surgery.[122] These agents do not act as anticancer agents and should be coadministered with chemotherapy, endocrine therapy, or anti-*HER2* therapy.

Desired Outcomes

After breast cancer has advanced beyond local–regional disease, breast cancer is currently incurable. However, some patients live for many years with metastatic disease, making this a chronic disease requiring long-term management strategies that incorporate improvements or maintenance of quality of life. Palliation is the desired therapeutic outcome in the treatment of MBC. Optimizing benefits and minimizing toxicity are general therapeutic goals of any therapy administered in this setting. Therefore, sequential single-agent chemotherapy is often chosen over combination regimens, but individual circumstances may call for more rapid responses in which combination therapy may be indicated. Endocrine therapy is generally less toxic than chemotherapy and may be a more appropriate option for patients with hormone receptor–positive breast cancer. Tumor response to a particular treatment regimen may be measured by changes in laboratory tests, diagnostic imaging, and physical signs and symptoms. If a patient is tolerating therapy well, clear evidence of disease progression on imaging or physical examination is required to warrant changing therapy. Unless the patient clearly cannot tolerate the regimen or the cancer is clearly progressing at a rate that will quickly cause symptoms (or is causing symptoms already), there is not a sound reason to change therapy. Optimizing quality of life is an important therapeutic end point in the treatment of patients with MBC and eventually requires discontinuation of active cancer therapy and a shift to supportive care with hospice services. Balancing between quantity and quality of life is a frequent battle waged by many oncology clinicians with their patients, and difficult decisions are faced during this time.

Endocrine Therapy

7 The pharmacologic goal of endocrine therapy for breast cancer is to either (a) decrease circulating levels of estrogen or (b) prevent the effects of estrogen at the breast cancer cell (targeted therapy) by blocking the hormone receptors or downregulating the presence of these receptors. Achievement of the first goal depends on the menopausal status of the patient, but achievement of the second goal is independent of menopausal status. Many endocrine therapies are available to target either goal of therapy, and combinations of drugs with differing mechanisms of action have also been investigated. Unfortunately, most combinations have not demonstrated significant benefits over single-agent hormone therapy but have increased toxicity. Therefore, combinations of endocrine agents for MBC are generally not recommended outside the context of a clinical trial. A few exceptions to this statement exist, and individual clinical decisions should carefully weigh the risks and benefits of combination therapy versus single-agent therapy. These approaches will be discussed further with each class of endocrine therapy. Sequential use of endocrine agents is common in the metastatic setting when a patient is progressing on one agent after experiencing an initial response. Responsive patients are often treated with a series of endocrine agents, usually over several years, before chemotherapy is considered.

There is little evidence that the survival benefit from one endocrine therapy is clearly superior to that achieved with other therapies in women with MBC. Randomized controlled trials have shown that antiestrogens, AIs, progestins, estrogens, and androgens as well as surgical procedures, including oophorectomy, adrenalectomy, and hypophysectomy, are associated with similar OS in patients with MBC. Consequently, the choice of a particular endocrine therapy is based primarily on the mechanism of action, toxicity, and patient preference (Tables 105-8 and 105-9). Based on these criteria, tamoxifen is the preferred initial agent when metastases are present in a premenopausal woman except when the patient's cancer recurs at the same time or within 1 year of occurrence of adjuvant tamoxifen therapy. In these cases, other agents are generally used. For postmenopausal women, the AIs are generally used first followed by other endocrine therapies upon progression.[48,123]

In postmenopausal and castrated women, the main source of estrogen is derived from the peripheral conversion of androstenedione, produced by the adrenal gland, into estrone and estradiol. This conversion requires the enzyme aromatase. Aromatase also catalyzes the conversion of androgens to estrogens in the ovary in premenopausal women and in extraglandular tissue, including the breast and breast cancer cells, in postmenopausal women. Therefore, AIs effectively reduce the levels of circulating estrogens and estrogens in the target organ. Aminoglutethimide was the prototype AI but was a nonspecific, weak enzyme inhibitor associated with much toxicity and is no longer available in the United States. Several analogs and derivatives of aminoglutethimide, as well as novel endocrine compounds, have been tested over the years to try and improve on the therapeutic ratio of this agent. Third-generation AIs available in the United States include anastrozole, letrozole, and exemestane. These agents have far greater selectivity and higher potency for the aromatase enzyme than aminoglutethimide. A major advantage of these specific compounds is their preferable toxicity profile, which consists mainly of bone loss or osteoporosis, mild nausea, hot flashes, arthralgias or myalgias, and mild fatigue. Anastrozole and letrozole are nonsteroidal compounds that exhibit reversible, competitive inhibition of aromatase. These are triazole compounds and have no intrinsic hormonal activity. Exemestane is a steroidal compound that binds irreversibly to aromatase, forming a covalent bond. Although this mechanism may have theoretical advantages to the reversible binding seen with the nonsteroidal agents, there is no clinical evidence that this drug is superior to other agents in this class. Exemestane does possess some androgenic properties at doses that are much higher than those used clinically and may have unique toxicities in some patients.[123]

Third-generation AIs have been compared with several other endocrine therapies since their approval. Although results are somewhat mixed, there appears to be at least equivalent activity seen with all three of the AIs compared with tamoxifen as first-line therapy and megestrol acetate as second-line therapy after progression on

TABLE 105-8 Endocrine Therapies Used for Metastatic Breast Cancer

Drug	Brand Name	Initial Dose	Usual Range	Special Population Dose	Comments
Aromatase Inhibitors: Nonsteroidal					
Anastrozole	Arimidex, generic	1 mg orally daily			
Letrozole	Femara, generic	2.5 mg orally daily		Caution in severe liver impairment[a]	
Aromatase Inhibitor: Steroidal					
Exemestane	Aromasin	25 mg orally daily			Take after meals
Antiestrogens: SERMs					
Tamoxifen	Nolvadex, generic	20 mg orally daily		See text regarding CYP2D6	See text regarding CYP2D6
Toremifene	Fareston	60 mg orally daily			
Antiestrogen: SERD					
Fulvestrant	Faslodex	500 mg IM every 28 days (after loading days 1, 15, 29)	250–500 mg (see text for details)	Moderate liver impairment[a] administer 250 mg IM every 28 days (after loading days 1, 15, 29)	
LHRH Agonists					
Goserelin	Zoladex	3.6 mg SC every 28 days		Premenopausal women only	
Leuprolide	Lupron (IM), generic	3.75 mg IM (SC) every 28 days	Other formulations and doses are not used for breast cancer	Premenopausal women only	Not FDA approved for breast cancer; other formulations are administered differently
Triptorelin	Trelstar	3.75 mg IM every 28 days		Premenopausal women only	Not FDA-approved for breast cancer
Progestins					
Megestrol acetate	Megace, generic	40 mg orally 4 times a day	80 mg twice daily also appropriate		Absorption maybe increased when taken with food
Medroxyprogesterone	DepoProvera, generic	400 mg IM every week	400–1000 mg IM every week	May need to decrease dose in severe liver impairment[a]	
Androgens					
Fluoxymesterone	Androxy, generic	10 mg orally twice a day	10–20/day in divided doses	Avoid in severe renal or liver impairment[a]	
Estrogens					
Ethinyl estradiol	Multiple generics	1 mg orally 3 times a day	Lower doses not effective	Avoid in jaundice or "marked" liver disease	Take with food
Conjugated estrogens	Premarin	2.5 mg orally 3 times a day	Lower doses not effective	Avoid in jaundice or "marked" liver disease	Take with food

IM, intramuscular; LHRH, luteinizing hormone-releasing hormone; SC, subcutaneous; SERD, selective estrogen receptor downregulator SERM, selective estrogen receptor modulator.

[a]Severe liver impairment: Child-Pugh class C; moderate liver impairment: Child-Pugh class B.

tamoxifen in postmenopausal women with positive or unknown hormone receptor status.[123] Compared with tamoxifen, there appears to be a lower incidence of thromboembolic events and vaginal bleeding in patients who received selective AIs. As second-line therapy after tamoxifen, more nausea, vomiting, and hot flashes are seen with the AIs and more weight gain, fluid retention, and thromboembolism with megestrol acetate. Although generally considered therapeutically equivalent, the use of a steroidal AI (exemestane) after a patient progresses on a nonsteroidal inhibitor (anastrozole or letrozole) may provide some benefit and is a common practice based on limited data. The opposite sequence also has shown some benefit; thus, patients may receive two AIs (first-line and second-line) sequentially, especially patients who progress while on adjuvant tamoxifen therapy.[48]

The AIs should only be used in postmenopausal women. Based on the available evidence, pre- or perimenopausal women, whose ovaries are functioning, are inappropriate candidates for these therapies. Use of the AIs in addition to ovarian ablation (e.g., oophorectomy or LHRH agonists) is under investigation. Interestingly, the use of AIs in men with advanced breast cancer is controversial due to concerns that the pituitary feedback loop may be activated, increasing the levels of follicle-stimulating hormone, luteinizing hormone (LH), and possibly testosterone. Therefore, although objective responses are seen with single-agent AI therapy in men with breast cancer, consensus has yet to be reached regarding the clinical utility of these agents in men, and some clinicians are investigating the combination of an LHRH agonist with an AI in this population.[124] Until further clinical trials are completed, the efficacy and safety of this treatment approach are unknown.

Antiestrogens bind to ERs, which inhibit receptor-mediated gene transcription and therefore block the effect of estrogen on the end target. This class of agents is now subdivided into two pharmacologic categories, SERMs and pure antiestrogens. SERMs include tamoxifen and toremifene (and raloxifene for breast cancer risk reduction in high-risk women) and demonstrate tissue-specific activity, both estrogenic and antiestrogenic, as described previously. The agonistic activity is thought to be responsible for many of the adverse reactions seen with these agents, including the increased

TABLE 105-9 Drug Monitoring for Endocrine Therapies

Drug	Adverse Drug Reaction	Monitoring Parameters	Comments
Aromatase inhibitors	Hot flashes Arthralgia or myalgias Osteoporosis Hypercholesterolemia	Patient assessment BMD Lipid panel	Interval of monitoring controversial
Antiestrogens: SERMs[a]	Hot flashes Endometrial hyperplasia or cancer Venous thromboembolism Osteopenia (premenopausal women only)	Patient assessment Annual gynecologic assessment Consider BMD for premenopausal women	Routine transvaginal ultrasonography and endometrial biopsies are not recommended in the absence of symptoms
Antiestrogens: SERDs[a]	Hot flashes Injection-site reactions	Patient assessment	
LHRH agonists	Hot flashes Injection-site reactions Osteoporosis	Patient assessment BMD	
Progestins[a]	Weight gain Vaginal bleeding or spotting Nausea Venous thromboembolism	Patient assessment Periodic weights	
Androgens[a]	Hirsutism Acne Masculinization Increased hemoglobin Nausea Venous thromboembolism	Patient assessment Complete blood counts	
Estrogens[a]	Nausea or vomiting Venous and arterial thromboembolism Fluid retention Breast tenderness Endometrial hyperplasia or cancer	Patient assessment Annual gynecologic assessment	Routine transvaginal ultrasonography and endometrial biopsies are not recommended in the absence of symptoms

BMD, bone mineral density; LHRH, luteinizing hormone-releasing hormone; SERD, selective estrogen receptor downregulator; SERM, selective estrogen receptor modulator.
[a]Liver function tests obtained periodically to screen for changes in hepatic elimination, hepatotoxicity, and the presence of hepatic metastases.

risk of endometrial cancer, and has led to the development of pure ER antagonists that lack estrogen agonist activity. Pure antiestrogens are also referred to as selective estrogen receptor downregulators (SERDs). These molecules bind to the ER, inhibit estrogen binding, and degrade the drug–ER complex, thus decreasing the amount of ER on the tumor cell surface. Fulvestrant is currently the only pure antiestrogen commercially available in the United States.

Tamoxifen is generally considered to be the antiestrogen of choice in premenopausal women with MBC who have hormone receptor–positive tumors. The toxicities of tamoxifen are described in the Adjuvant Endocrine Therapy section earlier. The only additional toxicity that may be observed in the setting of MBC (specifically bone metastases) is a tumor flare or hypercalcemia, which occurs in about 5% of patients after the initiation of any SERM therapy and is not an indication to discontinue SERM therapy. It is generally accepted that this reaction is associated with response to endocrine therapy, but patients who do not experience such a reaction may still respond. This reaction is seen less frequently with the concurrent use of bisphosphonates as a result of their inhibition of osteoclasts, subsequently preventing the release of calcium from the bone.

Toremifene is another commercially available SERM for the treatment of breast cancer. It exhibits similar efficacy and tolerability compared with tamoxifen in the metastatic setting. Cross-resistance to toremifene has been demonstrated in patients with tamoxifen-refractory disease.[125] Thus, at the current time, toremifene appears to be an alternative to tamoxifen in postmenopausal patients with positive or unknown hormone receptor status with MBC. Raloxifene, another SERM, was originally approval for prevention of osteoporosis in postmenopausal women. Available data with raloxifene as a treatment for breast cancer show very low response rates and no significant clinical benefit. Consequently, use of this agent for breast cancer treatment should be discouraged. The use of raloxifene for breast cancer risk reduction in high-risk women has been reported (see Prevention and Early Detection).

Fulvestrant is approved for the second-line therapy of postmenopausal MBC patients with hormone receptor–positive tumors. It is unique in that it is given as an intramuscular injection. The dosing of fulvestrant has been controversial, and many comparative studies used what is now thought to be an insufficient dose; therefore, its place in therapy is also not clearly defined. Studies have compared this agent with anastrozole, exemestane, and tamoxifen in the treatment of postmenopausal women with MBC. Biologically, fulvestrant should produce similar outcomes in premenopausal women, but no data exist to confirm the safety or efficacy in premenopausal women. In the comparative trials with fulvestrant and an AI (anastrozole or exemestane), similar efficacy and safety were demonstrated with both agents when given after patients progressed on tamoxifen therapy.[123] When compared directly with tamoxifen, time to progression was slightly shorter in the fulvestrant arm, but the difference did not reach statistical significance. That trial failed to confirm statistical noninferiority, which indicates that the trial could not show that fulvestrant was equivalent to tamoxifen.[123] Subsequent pharmacokinetic data confirming a dose–response relationship with fulvestrant led investigators to design a dose comparison study of fulvestrant 250 mg versus 500 mg.[126] Results from this trial confirm that the appropriate dose of fulvestrant for MBC should be 500 mg intramuscularly administered every 2 weeks for 3 doses (days 1, 15, and 29) followed by administration every 28 days. This loading approach to dosing facilitates reaching steady-state plasma levels more rapidly, allowing for a response to be seen within a clinically relevant time frame. To accomplish this dosing, two injections of 5 mL each are administered simultaneously. Although cumbersome and slightly more uncomfortable, patients appear to tolerate this higher dose relatively well, exhibiting similar toxicity profiles regardless of the dose administered.

A subsequent randomized, phase II study comparing this dosing strategy with anastrozole in postmenopausal women with hormone receptor–positive MBC demonstrated superior time to progression with fulvestrant with similar objective responses seen with subsequent hormone therapy administered to both groups.[127] Although the power of this phase II study is limited and survival data are not yet available, it is encouraging to better understand how dosing may impact response with this novel endocrine agent. Combining therapy with anastrozole and fulvestrant has been investigated in two randomized phase III trials with conflicting results.[128,129] Although the combination does appear to be well tolerated, the overall benefits (if any) appear to be modest, and sequential single agents are most commonly administered in the palliative setting of metastatic disease. Adverse events related to fulvestrant include injection-site reactions, hot flashes, asthenia, and headaches. Based on the results of the comparative trial, the dose of fulvestrant approved by the Food and Drug Administration (FDA) was changed to 500 mg given intramuscularly every 28 days with an extra dose administered on day 14. This choice of therapy is covered by Medicare Part B and is a good option for patients who are unable to take an oral medication.

Another goal of endocrine therapy in premenopausal women is to reduce estrogen production with surgery, irradiation, or medication. Ovarian ablation (surgically or chemically) is still commonly used in some parts of the United States and is considered by many specialists to be the endocrine therapy of choice in premenopausal women. The mortality rate with surgical oophorectomy is low, usually less than 3% in appropriately selected patients. Irradiation of the ovaries was a means of castration many years ago but was associated with multiple complications and is no longer performed for these purposes. Chemical castration with LHRH analogs is increasingly used instead of oophorectomy in premenopausal women.

Medical castration with LHRH analogs induces responses in about one third of unselected premenopausal MBC cases. This is accomplished through downregulation of LHRH receptors in the pituitary, decreasing levels of LH, which subsequently lead to a decrease in circulating estrogen to castrated levels. Thus, the effect of LHRH analogs on circulating estrogen levels in premenopausal breast cancer simulates oophorectomy. The three agents available and used in the United States are leuprolide, goserelin, and triptorelin, but only goserelin is FDA approved for the treatment of MBC. These agents are administered as an injection every 4 weeks (all products have extended formulations, lasting 3 months to 1 year, but they are not recommended for the treatment of breast cancer) and are associated with minimal side effects, including amenorrhea, bone loss or osteoporosis, hot flashes, and occasional nausea (Table 105-9). LHRH agonists may also produce a flare response because of an initial surge in LH and estrogen production lasting 2 to 4 weeks. This flare response is similar to that seen with tamoxifen, and patients with high-volume, bulky disease should be monitored for increasing pain and hypercalcemia during the initiation period. A meta-analysis was conducted of several trials that combined tamoxifen and LHRH agonists versus LHRH agonists alone in premenopausal patients with MBC.[130] With a median follow-up period of 6.8 years, there was a significant survival benefit and progression-free survival (PFS) benefit in favor of the combined treatment. The overall response rate was significantly higher with combined endocrine treatment. However, this analysis did not compare tamoxifen alone with the combination of an LHRH agonist with tamoxifen. Therefore, if an LHRH agonist is used as first-line therapy for MBC, it should be used in combination with tamoxifen. But if tamoxifen is used as first-line therapy for MBC, the addition of a LHRH agonist is controversial because of the lack of clinical data to support any additional benefit.[48]

Progestins such as megestrol acetate and medroxyprogesterone acetate have been compared with tamoxifen in randomized trials and have been found to yield equivalent response rates. Whereas medroxyprogesterone acetate is more frequently used in Europe, megestrol acetate is more frequently used in the United States. Based on efficacy and tolerability, these agents are generally reserved as third-line therapy after patients have failed an AI and an antiestrogen (tamoxifen, toremifene, or fulvestrant). The most common side effect of megestrol acetate is weight gain, occurring in 20% to 50% of patients. Patients experiencing weight gain may also have fluid retention, but fluid retention is not totally responsible for the weight gain. In cachectic cancer patients, the weight gain may be desirable, but this is not uniformly true of all patients with MBC. Other side effects associated with progestins include vaginal bleeding in 5% to 10% of patients, either while taking the progestational agent or when it is discontinued, and less than a 10% incidence of hot flashes. Thromboembolic complications are also associated with these agents.[131]

High-dose estrogens and androgens are rarely used today because of their side effect profile and the availability of better tolerated alternatives (e.g., AIs). About one-third of patients placed on high-dose estrogens will discontinue them because of side effects, the most important of which are thromboembolic events, vomiting, and fluid retention. Less common side effects include areolar hyperpigmentation, breast tenderness and engorgement, vaginal discharge, incontinence, hot flashes, and phlebitis. All of the effective androgens cause masculinizing effects, including hirsutism and acne, in more than 50% of patients. The mechanism by which these agents exert a therapeutic effect in breast cancer is unknown. However, these agents may inhibit aromatase, among other pharmacologic effects that antagonize estrogen.

Other agents recently approved for the treatment of metastatic prostate cancer are under investigation for the treatment of MBC. Abiraterone is an analog of ketoconazole that is administered with prednisone for metastatic prostate cancer and affects androgen biosynthesis. Because androgens are converted to estrogens in the presence of aromatase, the impact of abiraterone on estrogen synthesis is also being investigated. Ongoing clinical trials in women and men with MBC may yield positive results, but use of this agent for management of MBC is not currently recommended. Investigation into mechanisms of endocrine resistance have met with some success, leading to the FDA approval of everolimus, an inhibitor of mammalian target of rapamycin (mTOR), in combination with exemestane for patients with MBC progressing on a nonsteroidal AI. This combination is discussed further in the Biologic or Targeted Therapy section.

Cytotoxic Therapy

8 Cytotoxic chemotherapy is eventually required in most patients with MBC. Patients with hormone receptor–negative tumors require chemotherapy as initial therapy of metastases. Hormone-sensitive tumors that fail to respond to endocrine therapy or that initially respond to endocrine therapy, eventually ceasing to respond, require chemotherapy when endocrine options have been exhausted. Combination chemotherapy results in an objective response in about 60% of patients previously unexposed to chemotherapy. Combination chemotherapy regimens are associated with higher response rates than are single-agent therapies in the treatment of MBC, but the higher response rates have not usually translated into clinically significant differences in time to progression and OS in individual clinical trials.[132] Combination regimens are associated with greater toxicity. In the palliative metastatic setting, the least toxic approach is preferred when efficacy is considered equal. In clinical practice, patients who require a rapid response to chemotherapy (e.g., those with symptomatic bulky metastases) often receive combination therapy despite the added toxicity. This decision is complex and should be made on an individual patient basis.

Most patients experience partial responses, but complete disappearance of disease occurs in fewer than 10% of patients treated. The median duration of response is 5 to 12 months, but some patients have an excellent response to an initial course of chemotherapy and may live 5 to 10 years or longer without evidence of disease. The median survival period of patients after treatment with commonly used drug combinations for MBC ranges between 14 and 33 months. The median time to response ranges from 2 to 3 months in most studies, but this period depends on the site of measurable disease and can range from 3 weeks (skin and lymph node metastases) to 18 weeks (bone metastases). After a chemotherapy regimen has been initiated, it is usually continued until there is unequivocal evidence of progressive disease or intolerable side effects. Table 105-10 lists some selected chemotherapy agents used in the metastatic setting.[132]

Factors associated with an increased likelihood of response to chemotherapy include a good performance status, a limited number (one to two) of disease sites (or involved organ systems), and a prolonged previous response to chemotherapy or hormonal therapy (i.e., long disease-free interval). Patients who have progressive disease during chemotherapy have a lower likelihood of response to a subsequent chemotherapy. However, this is not necessarily true for patients who are given chemotherapy after a treatment-free interval of substantial duration (e.g., more than 1 year). Treatments may be repeated if some time has passed between therapies, but this is rarely done because of the large number of agents now available to treat breast cancer. Hormone receptor–positive tumors that are resistant to endocrine therapy are as likely to respond to chemotherapy as patients who receive upfront chemotherapy. Age, menopausal status, and receptor status do not appear to be directly associated with response to chemotherapy. However, there continues to be much debate surrounding the potential association between hormone receptor status and response to chemotherapy (e.g., ER status and anthracyclines). Most clinical decisions regarding chemotherapy are not currently influenced by hormone-receptor status.

TABLE 105-10 Selected Chemotherapy Regimens for Metastatic Breast Cancer

Single-Agent Chemotherapy	
Paclitaxel[a,b] Paclitaxel 175 mg/m² IV over 3 hours Repeat cycles every 21 days *or* Paclitaxel 80 mg/m²/week IV over 1 hour Repeat dose every 7 days	**Vinorelbine**[c] Vinorelbine 30 mg/m² IV, days 1 and 8 Repeat cycles every 21 days *or* Vinorelbine 25–30 mg/m²/week IV Repeat cycles every 7 days (adjust dose based on absolute neutrophil count; see product information)
Docetaxel[d,e] Docetaxel 60–100 mg/m² IV over 1 hour Repeat cycles every 21 days *or* Docetaxel 30–35 mg/m²/week IV over 30 minutes Repeat dose every 7 days	**Gemcitabine**[f] Gemcitabine 600–1,000 mg/m²/week IV, days 1, 8, and 15 Repeat cycles every 28 days (may need to hold day 15 dose based on blood counts)[q]
Protein-Bound Paclitaxel[g,h] Protein-bound Paclitaxel 260 mg/m² IV over 30 minutes Repeat cycles every 21 days *or* Protein-bound paclitaxel 100–150 mg/m² IV over 30 minutes on days 1, 8, and 15 Repeat cycle every 28 days	**Ixabepilone**[i] Ixabepilone 40 mg/m² IV over 3 hours Repeat cycles every 21 days **Eribulin**[k] Eribulin 1.4 mg/m²/dose IV over 2–5 minutes on days 1 and 8 Repeat dose every 21 days
Capecitabine[j] Capecitabine 2,000–2,500 mg/m² per day orally, divided twice daily for 14 days Repeat cycles every 21 days	**Liposomal Doxorubicin**[l] Liposomal doxorubicin 30–50 mg/m² IV over variable duration Repeat cycles every 28 days
Combination Chemotherapy Regimens	
Docetaxel + Capecitabine[m] Docetaxel 75 mg/m² IV over 1 hour, day 1 Capecitabine 2,000–2,500 mg/m² per day orally divided twice daily for 14 days Repeat cycles every 21 days	**Paclitaxel + Gemcitabine**[n] Paclitaxel 175 mg/m² IV over 3 hours, day 1 Gemcitabine 1250 mg/m² IV days 1 and 8 Repeat cycles every 21 days
Ixabepilone + Capecitabine[i] Ixabepilone 40 mg/m² IV over 3 hours, day 1 Capecitabine 1,750–2,000 mg/m²/day orally divided twice daily for 14 days Repeat cycles every 21 days	**Paclitaxel + Bevacizumab**[o] Paclitaxel 90 mg/m² IV over 1 hour, days 1, 8, and 15 Bevacizumab 10 mg/kg IV over 30–90 minutes, days 1 and 15 Repeat cycles every 28 days

[a]From Taxol (paclitaxel) product information. Princeton, NJ: Bristol-Myers Squibb, July 2007.
[b]From Perez EA, Vogelci, Irwin DH, et al. Multicenter phase II trial of weekly paclitaxel in women with metastatic breast cancer. Clin Oncol 2001;19:4216.
[c]From Zelek L, Bartheir S, Riofrio M, et al. Weekly vinorelbine is an effective palliative regimen after failure with anthracyclines and taxanes in metastatic breast carcinoma. Cancer 2001;92:2267.
[d]From Taxotere (docetaxel) product information. Bridgewater, NJ: Sanofi-Aventis, 2008.
[e]From Hainsworth JD, Burris HA 3rd, Erlaud JB, et al. Phase I trial of docetaxel administered by weekly infusion in patients with advanced refractory cancer. J Clin Oncol 1998;16:2164.
[f]From Carmichael J, Possinger K, Philip P, et al. Advanced breast cancer: a phase II trial with gemcitabine. J Clin Oncol 1995;13:2731.
[g]From Abraxane (paclitaxel protein-bound particles for injectable suspension) product information. Bridgewater, NJ: Abraxis Bioscience, September 2009.
[h]From Gradishar WJ, Krasnojon D, Cheporov S, et al. Significantly longer progression-free survival with nab-paclitaxel compared with docetaxel as first-line therapy for metastatic breast cancer. J Clin Oncol 2009;27:3611–3619.
[i]From Boehnke Michaud L. The optimal therapeutic use of ixabepilone in patients with locally advanced or metastatic breast cancer. J Oncol Pharm Pract 2009;15(2):95–106.
[j]From Gralow, JR. Optimizing the treatment of metastatic breast cancer. Breast Cancer Res Treat 2005;89(Suppl 1):S9–S15.
[k]From Halaven (eribulin) product information. Woodcliff Lake, NJ: Eisai Inc., February 2012.
[l]From O'Brien ME, Wigler N, Inbar M, et al. Reduced cardiotoxicity and comparable efficacy in a phase III trial of pegylated liposomal doxorubicin HCl (CAELYX/Doxil) versus conventional doxorubicin for first-line treatment of metastatic breast cancer. Ann Oncol 2004;15(3):440–449.
[m]From O'Shaughnessy J, Miles D, Vukelja S, et al. Superior survival with capecitabine plus docetaxel combination therapy in anthracycline-pretreated patients with advanced breast cancer: phase III trial results. J Clin Oncol 2002;20(12):2812–2823.
[n]From Gemzar (gemcitabine) product information. Indianapolis, IN: Eli Lilly and Co, May 2007.
[o]From Miller K, Wang M, Gralow J, et al. Paclitaxel plus bevacizumab versus paclitaxel alone for metastatic breast cancer. N Engl J Med 2007;357(26):2666–2676.

A number of chemotherapeutic agents have demonstrated activity in the treatment of breast cancer, including doxorubicin, epirubicin, paclitaxel (conventional and protein bound), docetaxel, capecitabine, fluorouracil, cyclophosphamide, methotrexate, vinblastine, vinorelbine, gemcitabine, ixabepilone, eribulin, mitoxantrone, mitomycin C, thiotepa, and melphalan. The most active classes of chemotherapy in MBC are the anthracyclines and the taxanes, producing response rates as high as 50% to 60% in patients who have not received prior chemotherapy for metastatic disease.[132] Doxorubicin (conventional and liposomal) and epirubicin have demonstrated significant efficacy in the metastatic setting and are generally considered therapeutically equivalent when dosed appropriately. Administration of these agents is limited by their cumulative cardiotoxicity. Paclitaxel, docetaxel, and protein-bound paclitaxel are also FDA approved for the treatment of MBC and are generally considered therapeutically equivalent. Taxane administration is limited by cumulative peripheral neuropathy.[132] Most patients will receive each of these agents at some point in the course of their MBC because cross-resistance is incomplete.

An increasing number of patients diagnosed with MBC have been exposed to adjuvant chemotherapy consisting of an anthracycline and a taxane. If metastases are found within 6 to 12 months of completing treatment with these agents, many clinicians will choose treatment from a different chemotherapy class. If it has been longer since their adjuvant therapy, then retreating with the same agents may be considered. However, given the cardiotoxicity associated with the anthracyclines, the use of these agents in the metastatic setting has been generally avoided until the availability of liposomal anthracycline. Pegylated liposomal doxorubicin is associated with less cardiotoxicity and similar efficacy compared with conventional doxorubicin and is a viable option for women who recur more than 1 year after their adjuvant anthracycline regimen.

Weekly administration of paclitaxel and protein-bound paclitaxel results in higher response rates, time to progression, and survival in addition to a more favorable side effect profile compared with administration every 3 weeks.[132] The most useful weekly dose of conventional paclitaxel in the metastatic setting appears to be 80 mg/m^2/week with no breaks in therapy. With this approach, the toxicity profile of paclitaxel changes with less myelosuppression and delayed onset of peripheral neuropathy but slightly more fluid retention and skin and nail changes. Although the incidence of hypersensitivity reactions is also slightly less at these lower doses (requiring fewer premedications), it remains at about 3% despite incorporation of all available preventive measures. There is currently debate regarding the most appropriate weekly dose of protein-bound paclitaxel in the metastatic setting. Doses of 100 to 150 mg/m^2/week administered on days 1, 8, and 15 of a 28-day cycle have been investigated, demonstrating some evidence of a dose–response relationship. In the metastatic palliative setting, a lower dose is generally chosen, minimizing toxicity while not significantly compromising efficacy.[132] Docetaxel is most appropriately dosed on an every-3-week schedule for MBC. Weekly dosing did not produce improvements in disease response and was associated with significantly more toxicities than the every-3-week dosing strategy.[132]

After patients have been treated with an anthracycline and a taxane, single-agent capecitabine, vinorelbine, or gemcitabine have resulted in response rates of 20% to 25%.[132] Of these agents, only capecitabine is FDA approved as a single agent for MBC. Gemcitabine is only FDA approved in combination with paclitaxel for MBC. However, all of these are included in most national and international guidelines as appropriate therapy for MBC. Decisions regarding which agent to choose are based on patient characteristics, expected toxicities, and previous exposure to chemotherapy.

Other antimicrotubule agents have also been approved for the management of MBC, demonstrating significant benefits in patients who have had prior exposure to multiple other chemotherapy agents. Ixabepilone is an epothilone compound with a similar but distinct mechanism of action from the taxanes, binding to β-microtubulin in a unique manner but ultimately leading to microtubule stabilization and cell death in a similar manner compared with the taxanes. It is approved for use in combination with capecitabine and as a single agent for the management of MBC.[132] Eribulin is another antimicrotubule agent with a unique mechanism of action. The first synthetic analogue of halochondrin B, eribulin effectively inhibits polymerization of tubulin into microtubules and suppresses the microtubule growth phase similar to the vinca alkaloids. The mechanism of eribulin's antitumor efficacy differs from the vinca alkaloids in that eribulin does not appear to have any effect on the microtubule shortening phase. These subtle differences are thought to be important for eribulin's efficacy in patients who have been exposed to multiple therapies, including other antimicrotubule agents. It is approved for use as a single agent for the management of MBC patients who have received at least two prior chemotherapies for their metastatic disease.[132]

Both of these agents are associated with similar toxicities compared with the taxanes and vinca alkaloids, respectively (e.g., myelosuppression, neuropathy, myalgias or arthralgias, alopecia, and skin and nail changes with ixabepilone and myelosuppression and neuropathy with eribulin). Hypersensitivity is occasionally seen with ixabepilone because it is also solubilized in Cremophor-EL, the likely causative agent in paclitaxel-associated hypersensitivity. However, eribulin has not been associated with hypersensitivity reactions and is not formulated in a complex solvent system that may predispose patients to allergic-type reactions. Neuropathy may become problematic in patients who have received numerous sequential neurotoxic chemotherapy agents; therefore, careful monitoring of the impact on quality of life is imperative because these therapies are administered in a palliative setting. Ongoing clinical trials are investigating these agents in other combinations and in earlier stages of the disease, and these results are eagerly awaited.[132]

Biologic or Targeted Therapy

Therapies that focus on molecular targets through novel mechanisms are often referred to as biologic or targeted therapy. These agents, while using the biologic knowledge gained from decades of research, are designed to specifically target cancer cells while generally sparing normal tissues. For breast cancer, several agents are available that focus on a myriad of targets that are differentially expressed in breast cancer cells and play a critical role in their proliferation and survival.

9 Anti-*HER2* Agents *HER2*, in selected breast cancers, is a very important protein for maintenance of breast cancer cell proliferation and survival. Currently, three anti-*HER2* agents are available in the United States (trastuzumab, lapatinib, and pertuzumab), and a fourth is nearing approval (trastuzumab emtansine).

As mentioned previously, trastuzumab is a MoAB targeted against the *HER2*-receptor protein. Pertuzumab is also a MoAB but binds to a different epitope on *HER2* and prevents protein dimerization and subsequent cell signaling. Lapatinib is a small-molecule tyrosine kinase inhibitor (TKI) targeted against the *HER2* protein and the *HER1* (EGFR) protein, leading to dual signaling blockade.

Evidence supporting the use of these agents differs greatly, with the majority of data focusing on trastuzumab administered in different combination regimens with chemotherapy, endocrine therapy, or other biologic therapies. Trastuzumab also has significant clinical activity as a single agent, albeit less than trastuzumab-combination regimens. Lapatinib has a fair amount of evidence to support its use in MBC in combination with chemotherapy, endocrine therapy, and other biologics. To date, single-agent lapatinib therapy has a limited role in the management of breast cancer. Pertuzumab was recently approved in the United States for first-line therapy of *HER2*-positive

MBC in combination with trastuzumab and docetaxel. This limited role is likely to expand rapidly as many ongoing clinical trial results mature.

Single-agent treatment with trastuzumab yields a response rate of 15% to 20% and a clinical benefit rate of nearly 40% in patients with *HER2*-overexpressing MBCs.[133] Moreover, the results of a large randomized trial demonstrated that trastuzumab has at least additive, and perhaps synergistic, activity with other chemotherapeutic agents.[134] In this pivotal trial comparing chemotherapy in combination with trastuzumab versus chemotherapy alone, the addition of trastuzumab increased response rates, time to progression, and OS compared with chemotherapy alone. Patients who were anthracycline naive were treated with an anthracycline (mostly doxorubicin; some epirubicin) plus cyclophosphamide and patients who had received an adjuvant anthracycline regimen were treated with paclitaxel. During this trial, patients who received the anthracycline–trastuzumab combination had a very high incidence of cardiotoxicity (27%), leading to discontinuation of this arm of the study and a black box warning regarding this contraindication in the product information for trastuzumab. Many investigators are attempting to circumvent this toxicity while giving these two classes of agents together (e.g., liposomal doxorubicin, continuous-infusion doxorubicin, lower dose epirubicin). However, until further information regarding the safety of these approaches becomes available, anthracyclines administered concurrently with trastuzumab should not be given outside the context of a clinical trial in patients with MBC.[134]

Many other chemotherapy agents have successfully been administered with trastuzumab, including docetaxel, protein-bound paclitaxel, vinorelbine, gemcitabine, capecitabine, and the platinum agents (carboplatin and cisplatin). In phase III trials, single-agent docetaxel or capecitabine was found to be inferior to the same chemotherapy plus trastuzumab in terms of response rates, time to progression and OS (survival benefit only demonstrated with docetaxel–trastuzumab). In phase II trials, vinorelbine in combination with trastuzumab has shown very high response rates even in heavily pretreated patients.[134] In another phase III trial, the triplet combination of paclitaxel, carboplatin, and trastuzumab was compared with paclitaxel and trastuzumab as dual therapy. This study demonstrated superior response rates and time to progression with the triplet regimen versus the doublet regimen.[134] A similar trial designed to confirm this data using docetaxel instead of paclitaxel failed to demonstrate any advantage with the addition of carboplatin to a taxane–trastuzumab regimen. These conflicting results indicate that the benefit of adding a platinum compound to these regimens remains questionable. Toxicities with the addition of carboplatin are significantly greater in terms of myelosuppression and nausea, which should be considered when making treatment decisions in the setting of MBC in which quality of life is paramount.[134]

Significant cross-talk exists between the growth factor pathways (e.g., *HER2*) and hormone receptor pathways (e.g., ER). This has generated a hypothesis that combining endocrine therapies with anti-*HER2* therapies may be synergistic or at least additive in their anticancer effects. The TAnDEM trial randomized patients with *HER2*-positive MBC to anastrozole with or without trastuzumab. The addition of trastuzumab improved PFS from 2.4 months to 4.8 months (P = 0.0016), and overall response rate and clinical benefit rate were also significantly improved.[134] Many other trials are seeking to confirm this information. Although confirming information is awaited, these combinations are frequently used in current clinical practice for patients with hormone receptor–positive, *HER2*-positive MBC.

Upon disease progression, trastuzumab is generally continued while the chemotherapy agent is switched. This clinical practice of continuing trastuzumab beyond progression is well accepted and supported by clinical evidence. von Minckwitz et al. randomized patients who were progressing on front-line trastuzumab-containing regimens to receive either capecitabine alone or capecitabine with continued trastuzumab therapy.[134] Median time to progression was 5.6 months with capecitabine alone and 8.2 months with capecitabine plus trastuzumab (HR, 0.69; 95% CI, 0.48–0.97; P = 0.034). Although there were methodological problems with this trial (e.g., slow accrual led to early closure, open-label design), results support the decade-long clinical practice of continuing trastuzumab beyond progression but raise other questions as to the comparative benefit with this approach versus a lapatinib-based regimen (see later discussion).

Lapatinib is a TKI that dually targets *HER2* and the epidermal growth factor receptor (EGFR or *HER1*). This small molecule works intracellularly to actively shut down the signaling pathway from these two receptors and thus inhibit cell growth and division. Lapatinib is an oral agent with modest activity against breast cancer as a single agent. In combination with capecitabine in women with *HER2*-positive MBC who were previously treated with an anthracycline, a taxane, and trastuzumab, lapatinib improved response rates and time to progression as compared to capecitabine alone.[135] Based on this evidence, the FDA approved lapatinib in this setting. In combination with paclitaxel as first-line therapy for MBC (*HER2*-positive and -negative), the addition of lapatinib did not appear to improve outcomes for patients with *HER2*-negative disease. However, for patients with *HER2*-positive MBC, the addition of lapatinib significantly improved time to progression, event-free survival, objective response rates, and clinical benefit rate, although the *HER2*-positive patients on the paclitaxel–placebo arm did not receive any *HER2*-directed therapy.[136]

Lapatinib has also been combined with endocrine therapy in hopes of taking advantage of the cross-talk between the growth factor receptor and the hormone receptor pathways as mentioned previously. In a large randomized phase III study, letrozole was administered with either lapatinib or placebo in hormone receptor–positive patients with MBC (*HER2* negative and positive).[137] The addition of lapatinib in *HER2*-positive patients improved PFS from 3 months to 8.2 months (HR, 0.71; 95% CI, 0.53–0.96; P = 0.019). In *HER2*-negative patients, no significant benefit was observed with the addition of lapatinib. Another interesting approach to *HER2*-positive MBC has been to combine *HER2*-targeted agents with differing mechanisms of action. Blackwell and colleagues compared lapatinib alone with lapatinib plus trastuzumab in patients with MBC progressing on trastuzumab therapy. PFS was significantly improved with the combination (12 vs. 8.4 weeks; P = 0.029).[138] However, the clinical significance of this small difference (less than 1 month) is debatable, and the expense of this regimen is obvious. Nonetheless, this regimen is well tolerated and commonly used. Treatment beyond progression with lapatinib is not generally considered.

Because lapatinib is a small molecule and can readily cross the blood–brain barrier, investigation has ensued to ascertain its effects on brain metastases. Trastuzumab does not cross the blood–brain barrier, and the CNS is often a sanctuary site for progressive metastases, representing the first site of recurrence in a relatively large number of patients. Phase II trials investigating the efficacy of lapatinib in patients with treated brain metastases failed to demonstrate any significant response. However, in the large randomized trial with capecitabine ± lapatinib, the addition of lapatinib was associated with a lower rate of the CNS as a site of first progression (2% with lapatinib vs. 6% with capecitabine alone; P = 0.045).[135] Ongoing adjuvant trials with lapatinib will continue to evaluate this relationship and determine the value of lapatinib for prevention of CNS metastases.

Resistance to trastuzumab and lapatinib naturally develops, and patients eventually progress on trastuzumab- or lapatinib-based regimens. Pertuzumab, another MoAB targeted against *HER2*, binds to a different epitope of the *HER2* receptor extracellular domain compared with trastuzumab. Similar to trastuzumab, pertuzumab receptor binding stimulates antibody-dependent cellular-mediated cytotoxicity, but pertuzumab also prevents *HER2* from dimerizing with other *HER* receptors (most notably *HER3*), leading to more comprehensive signal blockade. Therefore, the mechanisms of trastuzumab and pertuzumab are thought to be complementary, and regimens that combine these MoABs have shown activity in *HER2*-positive MBC. Phase II trials combining the MoABs alone (without chemotherapy) have shown significant clinical benefit rates of 50% after progression on previous trastuzumab-based therapy.[139] Single-agent therapy with pertuzumab alone in a similar cohort of patients resulted in a clinical benefit rate of only 10%, with an increased clinical benefit rate (up to 40%) when trastuzumab was introduced upon progression on pertuzumab.[139] Although it is confusing as to why pertuzumab is largely ineffective as a single agent, it is interesting that reintroduction of *HER2* blockade is effective in some patients. Therefore, it is likely that single agent pertuzumab will not be used. However, further clinical evidence will be forthcoming guiding the use of this and other new biologic therapies targeting *HER2* and other molecular pathways.

Clinical **Controversy. . .**

Many options now exist for treatment of *HER2*-positive MBC, with multiple new agents approved with potential to significantly impact this disease. Determining the optimal treatment and sequence of therapies for trastuzumab-treated patients is extremely difficult. Many ongoing trials are attempting to better define the role of (a) continuing trastuzumab with different chemotherapies; (b) switching or adding pertuzumab, lapatinib, or TDM1; (c) multiple targeted therapies with or without chemotherapy/endocrine therapy; or (d) some combination of all of these approaches.

In the pivotal, registration trial for pertuzumab, combination therapy with trastuzumab and chemotherapy (docetaxel) demonstrated significant improvements in PFS compared with trastuzumab and chemotherapy alone with manageable increases in the rates of clinically significant toxicity (e.g., febrile neutropenia and grade 3 diarrhea greater with pertuzumab; cardiotoxicity similar).[140] Similar data were reported in abstract form with dual *HER2* therapy plus weekly paclitaxel, leading to addition of this agent (in combination with trastuzumab plus a taxane) to the NCCN guidelines for management of breast cancer.[48] Developments of other anti-*HER2* therapies are well underway, with a fourth agent expected to reach the market in the United States within the next few months. Trastuzumab emtansine is an antibody–drug conjugate consisting of trastuzumab with a potent cytotoxic agent (mertansine) being investigated alone and in combination with other anti-*HER2* agents and chemotherapy. Promising results from early clinical trials with this agent will hopefully lead to FDA approval. The rapidity of available information and new drugs makes treatment decisions difficult in patients with *HER2*-positive MBC. Incorporation of new agents into treatment algorithms will likely become increasingly clear as more data become available to guide clinicians in the optimal use of these combinations and single agents. Until that time, individual treatment approaches become increasingly complex, but the hope these new agents bring to patients progressing on existing therapy is immense. Investigations into the use of these agents in early-stage breast cancer are also underway and may change the landscape for management of *HER2*-positive breast cancer in all stages of the disease. Adverse effects of the anti-*HER2* therapies have been identified and are primarily related to the heart. Therefore, all therapies in this class, regardless of their exact mechanism of receptor blockade, have some degree of cardiotoxicity that should be acknowledge and monitored for. The type of cardiotoxicity differs depending on the agent in question. Trastuzumab and likely pertuzumab are associated with myocardial damage leading to heart failure clinically similar to anthracycline-associated cardiomyopathy. As mentioned earlier, the incidence of heart failure is approximately 5% with single-agent trastuzumab, and the risk is unacceptably high when trastuzumab is given concurrently with an anthracycline.[141] Fortunately, heart failure seen with trastuzumab is somewhat reversible with pharmacologic management, and some patients have continued therapy with trastuzumab after their left ventricular ejection fraction has returned to normal with medical management. Although there are no guidelines for cardiac monitoring with trastuzumab, close monitoring for clinical signs and symptoms of heart failure is recommended in order to intervene with appropriate cardiac treatments. The incidence of cardiotoxicity with pertuzumab administered in combination with trastuzumab is largely unknown. One early study with pertuzumab was stopped early because of cardiotoxicity that surpassed 50% at the time of study discontinuation. Subsequent studies have not demonstrated an increased rate of cardiotoxicity beyond that seen with trastuzumab alone.[139] This discrepancy is likely to be better characterized as further clinical evidence and experience is gained with this new agent. Nonetheless, careful clinical monitoring is required.

Because of concerns regarding the role of *HER2* in normal cardiac functioning, lapatinib may also increase the risk for cardiac dysfunction. However, in a review of more than 3,689 patients who received lapatinib in phase I to III trials, cardiotoxicity occurred in only 1.6% of patients.[142] Although these data are reassuring, it does not rule out the possibility of expanded toxicity when this agent is used in patients not included in the clinical trials such as those with underlying cardiac risks. Rare QT prolongation has also been reported with lapatinib, but the exact clinical significance of this effect is widely debated. Drug interactions that increase systemic exposure to lapatinib may predispose patients to this rare complication (see below).

Adverse events associated with MoABs are seen with trastuzumab and pertuzumab and include infusion-related reactions (primarily fever and chills). These occur in about 40% of patients receiving trastuzumab during the initial infusion and generally go unrecognized by patients. Other infusion-related reactions with trastuzumab include mild nausea, pain at tumor sites, rigors, headaches, dizziness, hypotension, rash, and asthenia, which are much less common.[141] A rare but more severe reaction consisting of severe hypersensitivity or pulmonary reactions has been reported in postmarketing surveillance with trastuzumab. It is important to educate patients regarding the pulmonary reactions because these may occur up to 24 hours after the infusion and can be fatal if not promptly treated. Trastuzumab may increase the incidence of infection, diarrhea, and other adverse events slightly when given with chemotherapy, but most of these increases are not clinically significant for an individual patient. The adverse effects of pertuzumab appear to be similar, with increases in febrile neutropenia and grade 3 diarrhea evident in the phase III trial with docetaxel.[139] As clinicians gain more experience with this agent outside the context of clinical trials, the true incidence and severity of these adverse events will become more evident.

Other adverse events associated with lapatinib include primarily rash and diarrhea. These adverse effects appear to be more significant when combined with chemotherapy (e.g., capecitabine, paclitaxel) but are generally manageable with aggressive antidiarrheal therapy or dose reductions. Other rare effects have been reported (QT prolongation, hepatotoxicity, and interstitial lung disease), and patients should be counseled regarding these effects. Drug–drug and drug–food interactions are particularly important with lapatinib because of its metabolism through the cytochrome P450 system (3A4) and other pharmacokinetic and pharmacodynamic issues.[143] Many of the adverse effects listed previously may be exacerbated caused by drug or food interactions, and careful review of patients' medication lists and education regarding these issues are extremely important.

It should be noted that only 20% to 30% of patients with MBC overexpress *HER2*, and commercially available IHC tests that are reported as 2+ for *HER2* are often negative by the more sensitive and specific FISH technique. To date, there is no benefit associated with the administration of trastuzumab to patients with *HER2*-negative tumors (IHC score of 0 to 1+, or FISH negative) and a very questionable benefit associated with administration of trastuzumab to women with tumors that are 2+ for *HER2* by IHC staining alone. The patients who benefit most from trastuzumab therapy include those whose tumors express *HER2* protein at the 3+ level or who clearly demonstrate gene amplification by FISH testing. Further analyses investigating what other predictive markers may be clinically useful are currently ongoing.[144]

Other Targeted Agents As previously mentioned, treatments for MBC rarely eliminate all cancer cells, and cures are rarely seen after the cancer has spread beyond the local area of the breast and axilla. Acquired drug resistance develops in nearly all patients. Alterations in cell signaling, cell cycle control, and apoptotic signaling are among the common mechanisms of resistance with chemotherapy, endocrine therapy, and anti-*HER2* therapy. The phosphatidylinositol 3-kinase (PI3K)/protein kinase-B (also called Akt) pathway includes many different proteins, one of the most important being the mTOR tyrosine kinase. mTOR is an important mediator for cell proliferation and regulation of apoptosis, angiogenesis, and cellular metabolism. Use of mTOR inhibitors to treat MBC has resulted in conflicting results. Temsirolimus, an IV mTOR inhibitor, was administered with letrozole as first-line therapy for MBC in a large randomized phase III trial, resulting in no improvement in PFS.[145] Everolimus, an oral mTOR inhibitor, was administered with exemestane as second-line therapy for MBC after an AI and produced significant improvements in PFS.[146] In combination with tamoxifen, everolimus demonstrated superior clinical benefit rate and time to progression in a randomized phase II trial. Preliminary results from this trial also appear to indicate a survival advantage.[147] Further investigation of this combination is eagerly awaited.

Targeting mTOR also appears to be important for *HER2*-positive MBC patients progressing on trastuzumab, limited data have explored the use of everolimus with trastuzumab–taxane combinations that appear to be promising, but added toxicities and cost are important factors to consider when adding an mTOR inhibitor to a patient's regimen.[147] The most common adverse events experienced in the everolimus–exemestane trial were mucositis, fatigue or asthenia, cough, pyrexia, and hyperglycemia.[146] As more patients receive this combination outside the context of a clinical trial, adverse effects related to metabolic effects (hypercholesterolemia, hypertriglyceridemia, hyperglycemia) and pneumonitis may become more prevalent because these are evident in patients receiving everolimus for other cancer types (e.g., renal cell carcinoma).

Targeting tumor blood vessels is another strategy to fight breast cancer and potentially reverse drug resistance. One of the most important growth factors that regulates the development of new blood vessels (angiogenesis) is VEGF. Bevacizumab is a MoAB targeted against VEGF and is FDA approved for use with chemotherapy for the management of a variety of malignancies. Bevacizumab has also been tested in clinical trials with capecitabine and paclitaxel in patients with MBC. Conflicting results have been reported with the use of bevacizumab in combination with chemotherapy in patients with MBC, and in 2012, the FDA withdrew the approval for bevacizumab in combination with paclitaxel for management of newly diagnosed MBC. Nonetheless, NCCN guidelines for management of breast cancer continue to list bevacizumab–paclitaxel as one option for the management of *HER2*-negative MBC. Continuing controversy exists regarding this agent in the management of MBC.[148,149] Many other biologic or targeted agents are being investigated and may end up changing the overall management of breast cancer for both early and metastatic disease.

Radiation Therapy

Radiation is an important modality in the treatment of symptomatic metastatic disease. The most common indication for treatment with radiation therapy is painful bone metastases or other localized sites of disease refractory to systemic therapy. Radiation therapy provides significant pain relief to about 90% of patients who are treated for painful bone metastases. Radiation is also an important modality in the palliative treatment of metastatic brain lesions and spinal cord lesions, which respond poorly to systemic therapy, as well as eye or orbit lesions and other sites where significant accumulation of tumor cells occurs. Skin and lymph node metastases confined to the chest wall area may also be treated with radiation therapy for palliation (e.g., open wounds or painful lesions). Chemotherapy may also be added to radiation for sensitization purposes.

PREVENTION AND EARLY DETECTION

Current efforts at breast cancer prevention are directed toward the identification and removal of risk factors often referred to as risk reduction strategies. Unfortunately, a number of risk factors associated with development of breast cancer, such as family history of breast cancer or personal history of breast or other gynecologic malignancies, cannot be modified. Isolation and cloning of breast cancer susceptibility genes now allow screening of women with histories suggestive of "breast cancer families" and identification of appropriate candidates for prophylactic bilateral mastectomies or bilateral salpingo-oophorectomy. These surgeries are considered for women who are at very high risk for the development of breast or ovarian cancer, particularly if the women's breasts are difficult to evaluate by both physical examination and mammography and if the women have persistent disabling fears that they will be diagnosed with cancer. Guidelines for the incorporation of surgical risk reduction strategies are largely based on genetics and other known risk factors for the development of breast (or ovarian) cancer.

In the last 20 years, there has been increasing interest in pharmacologic risk reduction for breast cancer. Two important classes of agents being studied in this setting are the SERMs and AIs.

The drugs with the most clinical information as risk reduction agents for breast cancer are the SERMs, tamoxifen and raloxifene. As previously described, tamoxifen is useful as an adjunct after treatment of primary breast cancer. In randomized trials of tamoxifen as an adjuvant treatment for breast cancer, women who received tamoxifen were also found to have a reduced incidence of contralateral primary breast carcinomas.[109] In a large, randomized, placebo-controlled study, the NSABP demonstrated significant reductions in risk of invasive and noninvasive breast cancers with 5 years of tamoxifen therapy (20 mg/day) in women at high risk for developing the disease.[51] Although this study is controversial, other studies from around the world also have been reported that investigated the role of tamoxifen as a risk reduction strategy. A meta-analysis of these trials indicates a consistent benefit with tamoxifen in reducing the incidence of ER-positive breast cancers (48% reduction; 95% CI, 36%–58%; P <0.0001).[150] Tamoxifen has been repeatedly shown to be a relatively safe drug with an acceptable toxicity profile when used to treat patients with breast cancer. However, its estrogenic effects on the uterus and the coagulation system increase the risk of serious adverse effects that may be critical for patients taking this agent as a risk reduction strategy. Toxicities associated with tamoxifen were previously described in the Adjuvant Endocrine Therapy section. Any decision to use tamoxifen for risk reduction should be made after a thorough discussion of the woman's risk of breast cancer, the potential benefits of tamoxifen, and the potential serious adverse events associated with tamoxifen.

A second trial has been reported that compared tamoxifen with raloxifene in a similar population of high-risk women. The Study of Tamoxifen and Raloxifene (STAR or P2) was published in 2006 and demonstrated a similar rate of invasive breast cancers with the two drugs.[52] However, the rates of noninvasive breast cancer were numerically higher in the raloxifene arm of the trial, although this difference did not reach statistical significance. In 2010, an updated analysis was published, reporting that raloxifene retained 76% of tamoxifen's effectiveness in preventing invasive breast cancer.[151] Rates of endometrial cancer and DVT were more frequent in the tamoxifen arm, but overall quality of life was similar between the two agents.[52] Based on these results, the FDA maintains raloxifene's approval for breast cancer risk reduction in women at high risk of the disease.

A similar reduction in the incidence of contralateral primary breast cancers was demonstrated in the adjuvant clinical trials with the AIs, leading to the premise that AIs may also play a role in risk reduction of breast cancer.[152] Goss and colleagues published the first results of a randomized, placebo-controlled, phase III trial comparing exemestane with placebo for 5 years in high-risk women.[153] Eligibility criteria were similar to the P-1 and STAR trials, and this report represented a median follow-up period of only 34 months. Nonetheless, significant reductions were seen in the rates of invasive breast cancers with exemestane (HR, 0.35; 95% CI, 0.18–0.70; $P = 0.002$) with tolerable adverse events. The authors suggest that adherence was poor, which is common in studies of drugs taken for a long duration in relatively well women. Despite this nonadherence, the benefits appear to be quite large. Ongoing clinical trials with the available AIs are underway, and results from these trials should further elucidate the role of these agents in breast cancer risk reduction strategies.[152]

The NCCN has established guidelines for risk reduction strategies, including mastectomy, oophorectomy, and pharmacologic agents.[50] These guidelines are based on risk assessment tools such as the Gail, BRCAPRO, or Claus models as well as other established risk factors. Much of the guideline depends on a woman's wishes for intervention. The American Society of Clinical Oncology also has published recommendations guiding the use of the pharmacologic agents for breast cancer risk reduction.[154] These guidelines are similar to the NCCN's guidelines in that they recommend the use of tamoxifen or raloxifene for postmenopausal women at high risk (as defined by the Gail or other models) and tamoxifen for premenopausal women at high risk based on the woman's wishes.

The rationale for early detection of breast cancer is based on the relationship between stage of breast cancer at diagnosis and the probability for cure. If all breast cancer cases could be detected at a very early stage of the disease (i.e., small primary tumor and negative lymph nodes), then more patients theoretically could be cured of their disease. Screening guidelines for early detection of breast cancer in women at average risk have been developed by several organizations, including but not limited to the ACS, the United States Preventive Services Task Force (USPSTF), and the NCCN.[38,155,156] The ACS guidelines are most commonly cited. However, it is important to note that the expert panels developing these guidelines often differ in their approach and analysis of the available data, as is evident in the controversies that currently exist.

The ACS currently recommends that all women 20 years and older be informed of the benefits and limitations of breast self-examinations (BSEs).[155] Several studies have investigated the benefits of BSE. These trials were primarily conducted before the routine use of mammographic screening and demonstrated an inferential benefit in diagnosis of earlier stages of breast cancer. One trial, the Shanghai trial, appeared to indicate no benefit, but there was a higher rate of biopsies in women who were taught BSE than in women who were not taught BSE.[157] The investigators from this trial caution that this was a study of BSE instruction and not BSE performance. Compliance and competency with the BSE were neither guaranteed nor evaluated in this trial. Because of the lack of direct evidence to support or refute a benefit with BSE and the apparent associated increase in biopsy rates, the ACS has taken the position that it is optional, but women of all ages should be encouraged to be aware of their breasts in order to recognize any changes and promptly report them to a health professional.[155] Other organizations have taken a similar approach to their recommendations regarding BSE or simply state that there are insufficient evidence to recommend this practice.[38,156]

Recommendations for breast examination by a healthcare professional (clinical breast examination) vary among the screening guidelines most often cited. The rate of breast cancer detection using clinical breast examination (CBE) alone is low, with even lower rates in younger women and women with higher body weight.[155] Randomized clinical trials have reported inconsistent results and often evaluated CBE in conjunction with mammograms. The ACS recommends CBE in conjunction with mammography for women ages 40 years and older.[155] For younger patients (in their 20s and 30s), it is recommended as part of a periodic health examination every 3 years, but this recommendation is based on weak evidence. The USPSTF concluded that there is insufficient evidence to assess the benefits and risks of CBE beyond screening mammography in women older than the age of 40 years.[156]

10 The most controversial screening recommendation for breast cancer is related to annual mammography. It is clear that screening mammography decreases mortality from breast cancer. The controversies surround the balance of benefits and harms associated with a less than perfect screening test in women at average risk of developing breast cancer but of differing ages. Multiple clinical trials have been completed over the years, and multiple meta-analyses of these trials have been conducted as well. Most of the trials included women 50 to 74 years of age, and the interval between testing ranged from 12 to 33 months. The most recent meta-analysis of these data estimated a "number needed to invite for screening to extend one woman's life" (NNI) as 1,339 for women aged 50 to 59 years.[158] Some trials also included women aged 40 to 49 years, albeit significantly fewer women in this age group were included in the meta-analyses. The estimated NNI for women aged 40 to 49 years was reported as 1,904. The largest benefit was found in women ages 60 to 69 years with an estimated NNI of 377. None of the trials included women 75 years of age or older; therefore, there are no data to support or refute the benefit of screening mammography in this population.[158]

Incorporation of this new information into national guidelines differs with each organization. The ACS continues to recommend annual screening mammography for women ages 40 years and older (as long as they are in good health).[155] This recommendation allows for individualized decisions to be made based on the overall health of the woman but does not limit access to younger or older women who may benefit from screening. The USPSTF took a different approach, stating that "the decision to start regular, biennial screening mammography before the age of 50 years should be an individualized one and take patient context into account, including the patient's values regarding specific benefits and harms."[159] For women 50 to 74 years of age, the USPSTF recommends biennial screening mammography. This interval recommendation was based on assumptions of risks and benefits based on the available studies. Although the upper limit for screening varies among guidelines, most experts agree that mammograms in women older than the age of 74 are not supported by the current body of evidence, but some women may benefit if they are otherwise in good health and have a life expectancy of 10 years or more. There are also many other

TABLE 105-11 Breast Cancer Screening Guidelines

Risk Category	ACS[155]	USPTF[156,159]	NCCN[38]
Average Risk			
BSE	Age ≥20 y: optional (discuss benefits and limitations)	Not recommended	Age ≥20 y: breast awareness
CBE	Age ≥20–39 y: every 3 years Age ≥40 y: annually	Insufficient evidence	Age ≥20–39 y: every 1–3 years Age ≥40 y: annually
Mammography	Age ≥40 y: annually (as long as in good health)	Age 50–74 y: biennial Age <50 y: individualized decision	Age ≥40 y: annually
High Risk[a,b]			
BSE	NA	NA	All ages: breast awareness
CBE	NA	NA	All ages: every 6–12 months
Mammography	Age ≥30 y: Annually with MRI	NA	Prior RT or strong family history or genetic predisposition, age ≥25 y: annually (+ CBE) All other categories: annually (+ CBE)
Breast MRI	Age ≥30 y: Annually with mammogram Consider in moderate risk women as well	NA	Consider annually with mammogram + CBE for (a) prior RT, age ≥25 y; (b) lifetime risk >20%; (c) strong family history or genetic predisposition, age ≥25 y; (d) history of LCIS

ACS, American Cancer Society; USPTF, United States Preventive Task Force; NCCN, National Comprehensive Cancer Network; BSE, breast self-examination; CBE, clinical breast examination by a healthcare professional; LCIS, lobular carcinoma in situ; MRI, magnetic resonance imaging; NA, not addressed; RT, thoracic radiation therapy.

[a]High risk is defined by the ACS as women with (a) a known *BRCA1/2* gene mutation; (b) untested woman with first-degree relative with a known *BRCA1/2* gene mutation; (c) lifetime risk of breast cancer of 20%–25% or greater using a risk assessment tool based largely on family history; (d) radiation therapy to the chest between the ages of 10 and 30 years; (e) LiFraumeni's syndrome, Cowden's syndrome, or Bannayan-Riley-Ruvalcaba's syndrome or have first-degree relatives with one of these syndromes. Moderately increased risk is defined as a woman with (a) a lifetime risk of breast cancer of 15%–20% using a risk assessment tool based largely on family history; (b) personal history of breast cancer, DCIS, LCIS, or ADH; or (c) extremely dense breasts or unevenly dense breasts when viewed by mammograms.

[b]High risk is defined by the NCCN as women with (a) prior thoracic radiation therapy before age 30 y, (c) 5-year risk of ≥1.7% of invasive breast cancer in women ≥35 years old, (c) lifetime risk of >20% as defined by models that are largely based on family history, (d) strong family history or genetic predisposition, (e) LCIS, (f) prior history of breast cancer.

debates within this controversial area, and readers are referred to these references for further details.[38,155,156,158,159]

Other radiologic methods of breast imaging are also being investigated (e.g., digital mammography, ultrasonography, and MRI), and minimal data exist to support these methods in some high-risk populations. Recommendations for women with a high risk of breast cancer are not fully established, and definitions of "high risk" vary among different guidelines. The ACS include breast screening MRI as an adjunct to mammography for the following groups of high-risk women: (a) known *BRCA* mutation carriers; (b) untested individuals with a first-degree relative with a *BRCA* mutation; (c) women with a 20% or greater lifetime risk of breast cancer based on models that largely depend on family history; (d) women who had radiation to the chest between the ages of 10 and 30 years of age; (f) women with LiFraumeni's syndrome, Cowden's syndrome, or Bannayan-Riley-Ruvalcaba's syndrome or who have a first-degree relative with one of these syndromes.[155,160] The NCCN also has adopted consensus guidelines for women at high risk of breast cancer, incorporating breast MRI with other established screening tools for women as young as 25 years old (Table 105-11).[25]

It should also be noted that there are risks associated with any screening procedure, and they should be discussed with all patients so they are able to make an informed decision regarding these procedures. The risks involved with screening mammograms include false-negative results, false-positive results, overdiagnosis (true positives that will not become clinically significant), and radiation risk. The rate of false-negative results with the current technology is about 20%, which explains why CBE is an important adjunct to screening for many women. Although the specificity of mammography is quite high (90%), most abnormal examinations are false–positive results, leading to additional biopsies and psychological distress. The issue of overdiagnosis refers primarily to the growth in detection of DCIS from screening mammography. The biologic significance of these tumors is unknown because only some of them would become invasive if left in place. So the question remains: Are we treating women who do not require treatment? Experts in the field continue to debate this issue. Radiation exposure also has been discussed in the context of screening mammography, but the small doses of radiation exposure with mammograms (2–4 mGy [0.2–0.4 Rad] per standard two-view examination) appears to be overshadowed by other benefits in terms of reduction in mortality as a consequence of early cancer detection.[156]

Significant advances in the safety and efficacy of screening mammography have occurred during the last 2 decades. These advances have enabled superior visualization of breast and breast tissue with a lower dose of radiation being delivered. Despite these advances, about 10% of all palpable masses are not detected by mammography. This is most commonly observed in premenopausal women and may be directly related to the increased density of breast tissue in this estrogen-rich environment.

Although the safety and efficacy of screening mammography in terms of image quality and dosimetry are very acceptable, the need for greater quality control in mammography was recognized for some time. The Mammography Quality Standards Act (MQSA) of 1992 ensures that all mammographic facilities achieve a common high standard of quality assurance. Responsibility for operation of the act was given to the FDA, and all facilities that offer mammography must be FDA certified to remain open. The MQSA has now been updated to include full-field digital mammography as well, although the use of this new technology has not yet been incorporated into national screening guidelines. Passage of this landmark legislation, as well as provision of appropriate levels of funding to conduct this program, represents an important contribution to the health of women. Similar quality assurance measures will need to be implemented for breast MRIs and ultrasonography, given the recommendations to use these imaging methods for early detection and diagnosis, respectively, in high-risk women and those with suspicious masses. All women should be aware that breast MRIs and ultrasonography are not currently regulated and should choose to have these tests performed at a reputable facility to ensure quality. The American College of Radiology has developed reporting guidelines to standardize the way these images are interpreted. These are referred to as the BI-RADS and are available for mammography, breast ultrasonography, and breast MRIs.[39] This reporting method allows for uniformity among facilities and better comparisons over time. Nonetheless, differences remain between breast imaging quality and interpretation, and it is best to have imaging conducted at the same facility over time if possible.

PERSONALIZED PHARMACOTHERAPY

Personalized pharmacotherapy is a very broad term that includes many old and new scientific approaches to predict which patients should be treated, how they should be treated, and their likelihood of response or toxicity to treatment. These approaches may be focused on the tumor(s) itself or on patient or host factors. Breast cancer clinicians have been using these approaches to therapeutic decisions for decades and continue to search for novel characteristics to further individualize the choice of therapies.

Most scientific studies in breast cancer focus on tumor-specific markers either individually or as a panel of markers. Since the mid 1970s, clinicians have been using biomarkers to individualize therapy for patients with breast cancer. Initially, the tumor's ER or PR status was used to determine whether endocrine therapy (starting with tamoxifen) would benefit patients with MBC. Although these data have been widely available for many years, ER and PR testing in all breast cancers worldwide has been a relatively new phenomenon. Other biomarkers have been developed over the decades, with *HER2* being the most widely accepted alternate marker for breast cancer. *HER2* was initially studied as a prognostic biomarker in an attempt to ascertain an individual patient's risk of breast cancer recurrence and chemotherapy sensitivity or resistance. Although these applications of *HER2* testing remain controversial, the use of *HER2* testing to establish the likelihood of response or benefit to anti-*HER2* therapies is well established and required for all breast tumors at diagnosis. (See the Adjuvant Systemic Therapy section.)

It is clear from these individual biomarker studies that breast cancers are very heterogeneous, and interaction among markers is also important. Incorporation of multiple markers into biomathematical formulas that predict the likelihood of recurrence of cancer have been developed and are used across the United States to assist clinicians and patients in making informed decisions regarding adjuvant systemic therapy (e.g., Adjuvant! Online). These predictive formulas are useful but do not incorporate several markers that have since been validated individually (e.g., *HER2*, Ki-67, LVI). Genetic panels such as Oncotype DX were developed to screen for and quantify multiple genetic markers in tumor cells and are used as prognostic biomarkers to determine the risk of recurrence in early-stage breast cancer patients. The exact role these genetic panels will play in treatment decisions in the future is uncertain, but scientists and clinicians have embraced the technology, and the copious amounts of data collected from these analyses are being analyzed and incorporated into clinical trials and new standards every day.

Although these are all examples of tools that are used to individualize or personalize pharmacotherapy, very few markers are currently used clinically to represent host or patient differences. One promising area of research is in pharmacogenomics related to drug pharmacokinetics or pharmacodynamics. Results from studies with tamoxifen and CYP2D6 genotyping have been mixed, which is probably related to the complex metabolism of tamoxifen and large number of other prognostic factors (see the Adjuvant Endocrine Therapy section). Throughout this chapter are examples of characteristics that are used to individualize therapy. As more research is done in this field, the amount of tools available to clinicians to assist with treatment decisions will expand greatly.

EVALUATION OF THERAPEUTIC OUTCOMES

The desired therapeutic outcome of adjuvant therapy of breast cancer differs significantly from that of metastatic disease. Adjuvant therapy—chemotherapy, biologic therapy, and hormonal therapy—is administered with curative intent. The rationale for adjuvant therapy is that breast cancer, even when diagnosed in early stages when clinical evidence of distant spread is not apparent, is a systemic disease that spreads early to distant sites. Adjuvant therapy is intended to eradicate micrometastases and thus cure the patient of breast cancer. Therefore, the overall goal of adjuvant therapy is to cure the disease, which is something that cannot be fully evaluated for years after initial diagnosis and treatment. In addition, because disease cannot be detected at the time adjuvant therapy is started, assessment of disease response is not possible. Instead, a predetermined number of cycles of adjuvant therapy or years of biologic or hormonal therapy are administered. Adjuvant chemotherapy is often associated with significant toxicity. Maintaining dose intensity has been demonstrated to be important in the cure of disease, and therefore optimizing supportive care measures such as antiemetics and growth factors is highly recommended. The concept of dose density, using growth factors to maintain blood counts while decreasing the interval between chemotherapy administrations, is very controversial in the management of early-stage breast cancer. Multiple studies investigating this approach to adjuvant chemotherapy have been conducted with conflicting results and many more trials continue to be analyzed in hopes of determining the long-term outcomes related to this approach to therapy. The goals of therapy with neoadjuvant chemotherapy are slightly different. These goals focus on earlier end points of tumor response so as to minimize surgery, determine prognosis, and potentially conserve the breast tissue for a better cosmetic result. The other outcomes discussed with adjuvant therapy also apply to this scenario in terms of improving survival and decreasing recurrences compared with no systemic therapy.

Palliation is the therapeutic outcome in treatment of MBC. Optimizing benefits and minimizing toxicity are general therapeutic goals of any therapy administered in this setting. Therefore, sequential single agents are often chosen over combination regimens, but individual circumstances may call for more rapid responses in which combination therapy may be indicated. Tumor response to a particular treatment regimen may be measured by changes in laboratory tests, diagnostic imaging, or physical signs or symptoms. Periodic testing is clinical useful in some circumstances, but careful interpretation of results is required. If a patient is tolerating therapy well, clear evidence of disease progression on imaging or physical examination is required to warrant changing therapy. Unless the patient clearly cannot tolerate the regimen or the cancer is clearly progressing at a rate that will quickly cause symptoms (or is causing symptoms already), there is not a sound reason to change therapy. Optimizing quality of life is an important therapeutic end point in the treatment of patients with MBC. A number of valid and reliable tools are available for objective assessment of quality of life in patients with breast cancer.

ABBREVIATIONS

ABCSG	Austrian Breast and Colorectal Cancer Study Group
ACS	American Cancer Society
AI	aromatase inhibitor
AJCC	American Joint Committee for Cancer
ALND	axillary lymph node dissection
ATAC	Arimidex, Tamoxifen, Alone or in Combination
BCT	breast-conserving therapy

BIG	Breast International Group
BI-RADS	Breast Imaging Reporting and Data System
BSE	breast self-examination
CALGB	Cancer and Leukemia Group B
CBE	clinical breast examination
CI	confidence interval
CMF	cyclophosphamide, methotrexate, fluorouracil (regimen)
CNS	central nervous system
CYP	cytochrome P450 enzyme
DCIS	ductal carcinoma in situ
DFS	disease-free survival
DVT	deep-vein thrombosis
EBCTCG	Early Breast Cancer Trialists' Collaborative Group
EGFR	epidermal growth factor receptor; also known as HER1
ER	estrogen receptor
FDA	Food and Drug Administration
FISH	fluorescence in situ hybridization
HER2	human epidermal growth factor receptor-2
HR	hazard ratio
HRT	hormone replacement therapy
IHC	immunohistochemistry
LCIS	lobular carcinoma in situ
LH	luteinizing hormone
LHRH	luteinizing hormone–releasing hormone
LVI	lymphatic and vascular invasion
MBC	metastatic breast cancer
MINDACT	Microarray In Node-negative Disease may Avoid ChemoTherapy
MoAB	Monoclonal antibody
MQSA	Mammography Quality Standards Act
MRI	magnetic resonance imaging
mTOR	mammalian target of rapamycin
NCCN	National Comprehensive Cancer Network
NCI	National Cancer Institute
NNI	number needed to invite for screening to extend one woman's life
NSABP	National Surgical Adjuvant Breast and Bowel Project
OR	odds ratio
OS	overall survival
PARP	poly-ADP ribose polymerase
pCR	pathologic complete response
PFS	progression-free survival
PI3K	phosphatidylinositol 3-kinase
PR	progesterone receptor
RR	relative risk
RTPCR	reverse-transcription polymerase chain reaction
SEER	Surveillance, Epidemiology, and End Results
SERD	selective estrogen receptor downregulator
SERM	selective estrogen receptor modulators
SLNB	sentinel lymph node biopsy
STAR	Study of Tamoxifen and Raloxifene
TKI	tyrosine kinase inhibitor
TNBC	triple negative breast cancer
USPSTF	United States Preventive Services Task Force
VEGF	vascular endothelial growth factor
WHI	Women's Health Initiative

REFERENCES

1. Siegel R, Naishadham D, Jemal A. Cancer statistics, 2013. CA Cancer J Clin 2013;63:11–30.
2. Cancer Facts & Figures 2012: American Cancer Society. 2012, *http://www.cancer.org/downloads/STT/500809web.pdf.*
3. Berry DA, Cronin KA, Plevritis SK, et al. Effect of screening and adjuvant therapy on mortality from breast cancer. N Engl J Med 2005;353:784–792.
4. Davies C, Godwin J, Gray R, et al. Relevance of breast cancer hormone receptors and other factors to the efficacy of adjuvant tamoxifen: Patient-level meta-analysis of randomised trials. Lancet 2011;378:771–784.
5. Peto R, Davies C, Godwin J, et al. Comparisons between different polychemotherapy regimens for early breast cancer: Meta-analyses of long-term outcome among 100,000 women in 123 randomised trials. Lancet 2012;379:432–444.
6. Korde LA, Zujewski JA, Kamin L, et al. Multidisciplinary meeting on male breast cancer: summary and research recommendations. J Clin Oncol 2010;28:2114–2122.
7. Fay MP, Pfeiffer R, Cronin KA, et al. Age-conditional probabilities of developing cancer. Stat Med 2003;22: 1837–1848.
8. Gail MH, Costantino JP, Pee D, et al. Projecting individualized absolute invasive breast cancer risk in African American women. J Natl Cancer Inst 2007;99:1782–1792.
9. Collaborative Group on Hormonal Factors in Breast C. Menarche, menopause, and breast cancer risk: Individual participant meta-analysis, including 118 964 women with breast cancer from 117 epidemiological studies. Lancet Oncol 2012;13:1141–1151.
10. Clemons M, Goss P. Estrogen and the risk of breast cancer. N Engl J Med 2001;344:276–285.
11. Rossouw JE, Anderson GL, Prentice RL, et al. Risks and benefits of estrogen plus progestin in healthy postmenopausal women: Principal results from the Women's Health Initiative randomized controlled trial. J Am Med Assoc 2002;288:321–333.
12. Ravdin PM, Cronin KA, Howlader N, et al. The decrease in breast-cancer incidence in 2003 in the United States. N Engl J Med 2007;356:1670–1674.
13. Chlebowski RT, Kuller LH, Prentice RL, et al. Breast cancer after use of estrogen plus progestin in postmenopausal women. N Engl J Med 2009;360:573–587.
14. Anderson GL, Limacher M, Assaf AR, et al. Effects of conjugated equine estrogen in postmenopausal women with hysterectomy: The Women's Health Initiative randomized controlled trial. J Am Med Assoc 2004;291:1701–1712.
15. Anderson GL, Chlebowski RT, Aragaki AK, et al. Conjugated equine oestrogen and breast cancer incidence and mortality in postmenopausal women with hysterectomy: Extended follow-up of the Women's Health Initiative randomised placebo-controlled trial. Lancet Oncol 2012;13:476–486.
16. Zhu H, Lei X, Feng J, Wang Y. Oral contraceptive use and risk of breast cancer: A meta-analysis of prospective cohort studies. Eur J Contraception and Reproductive Hlt Care 2012;17:402–414.
17. Meisner AL, Fekrazad MH, Royce ME. Breast disease: benign and malignant. Med Clin North Am 2008;92: 1115–1141.
18. McCormack VA, dos Santos Silva I. Breast density and parenchymal patterns as markers of breast cancer risk: A meta-analysis. Cancer Epidemiol Biomarkers Prev 2006;15:1159–1169.
19. Collaborative Group on Hormonal Factors in Breast C. Familial breast cancer: Collaborative reanalysis of individual data from 52 epidemiological studies including 58,209 women with breast cancer and 101,986 women without the disease. Lancet 2001;358:1389–1399.
20. Chen S, Parmigiani G. Meta-analysis of BRCA1 and BRCA2 penetrance. J Clin Oncol 2007;25:1329–1333.

21. Nelson HD, Huffman LH, Fu R, Harris EL. Genetic risk assessment and BRCA mutation testing for breast and ovarian cancer susceptibility: Systematic evidence review for the U.S. Preventive Services Task Force. Ann Intern Med 2005;143:362–379.
22. United States Preventive Services Task Force. Genetic risk assessment and BRCA mutation testing for breast and ovarian cancer susceptibility: Recommendation statement. Ann Intern Med 2005;143:355–361.
23. Susceptibility AWGoGTfC. American Society of Clinical Oncology policy statement update: Genetic testing for cancer susceptibility. J Clin Oncol 2003;21:2397–2406.
24. Robson ME, Storm CD, Weitzel J, et al. American Society of Clinical Oncology policy statement update: Genetic and genomic testing for cancer susceptibility. J Clin Oncol 2010;28:893–901.
25. National Comprehensive Care Network. NCCN Clinical Practice Guidelines in Oncology: Genetic/Familial High-Risk Assessment: Breast and Ovarian v.1. 2012, *http://www.nccn.org/professionals/physician_gls/PDF/genetics_screening.pdf.*
26. Zhang B, Beeghly-Fadiel A, Long J, Zheng W. Genetic variants associated with breast-cancer risk: Comprehensive research synopsis, meta-analysis, and epidemiological evidence. Lancet Oncol 2011;12:477–488.
27. Velie EM, Nechuta S, Osuch JR. Lifetime reproductive and anthropometric risk factors for breast cancer in postmenopausal women. Breast Dis 2005;24:17–35.
28. Boyd NF, Stone J, Vogt KN, et al. Dietary fat and breast cancer risk revisited: A meta-analysis of the published literature. Br J Cancer 2003;89:1672–1685.
29. Prentice RL, Caan B, Chlebowski RT, et al. Low-fat dietary pattern and risk of invasive breast cancer: The Women's Health Initiative Randomized Controlled Dietary Modification Trial. J Am Med Assoc 2006;295:629–642.
30. Thomson CA. Diet and breast cancer: Understanding risks and benefits. Nutr Clin Pract 2012;27:636–650.
31. Velentzis LS, Cantwell MM, Cardwell C, et al. Lignans and breast cancer risk in pre- and post-menopausal women: Meta-analyses of observational studies. Br J Cancer 2009;100:1492–1498.
32. Velentzis LS, Woodside JV, Cantwell MM, et al. Do phytoestrogens reduce the risk of breast cancer and breast cancer recurrence? What clinicians need to know. Eur J Cancer 2008;44:1799–1806.
33. Renehan AG, Tyson M, Egger M, et al. Body-mass index and incidence of cancer: A systematic review and meta-analysis of prospective observational studies. Lancet 2008;371:569–578.
34. Monninkhof EM, Elias SG, Vlems FA, et al. Physical activity and breast cancer: A systematic review. Epidemiology 2007;18:137–157.
35. Pelucchi C, Tramacere I, Boffetta P, et al. Alcohol consumption and cancer risk. Nutr Cancer 2011;63:983–990.
36. Ronckers CM, Erdmann CA, Land CE. Radiation and breast cancer: A review of current evidence. Breast Cancer Res 2005;7:21–32.
37. Helvie MA. Imaging Analysis: Mammograpy. In: Harris JR, Lippman ME, Morrow M, et al., eds. Diseases of the Breast, 4th ed. Philadelphia: Lippincott Williams & Wilkins, 2010:116–130.
38. National Comprehensive Care Network. NCCN Clinical Practice Guidelines in Oncology: Breast Cancer Screening and Diagnosis Guidelines v.1. 2012, *http://www.nccn.org/professionals/physician_gls/PDF/breast-screening.pdf.*
39. D'Orsi CJ, Bassett LW, Berg WA, et al. BI-RADS: Mammography, 4th edition. In: D'Orsi CJ, Mendelson EB, Ikeda DM, et al., eds. Breast Imaging Reporting and Data System: ACR BI-RADS—Breast Imaging Atlas. Reston, VA: American College of Radiology, 2003.
40. Bleicher RJ. Management of the palpable breast mass. In: Harris JR, Lippman ME, Osborne CK, Morrow M, eds. Diseases of the Breast, 4th ed. Philadelphia: Lippincott Williams & Wilkins, 2010:32–41.
41. American Joint Commission on Cancer. Edge SB, Byrd DR, Compton, CC, et al., eds. AJCC Cancer Staging Manual, 7th ed. American Joint Committee on Cancer (AJCC), 2010.
42. Dillon DA, Guidi AJ, Schnitt SJ. Pathology of invasive breast cancer. In: Harris JR, Lippman ME, Osborne CK, Morrow M, eds. Diseases of the Breast, 4th ed. Philadelphia: Lippincott Williams & Wilkins, 2010:374–407.
43. Telli ML, Horst KC, Guardino AE, et al. Phyllodes tumors of the breast: natural history, diagnosis, and treatment. J Natl Compr Canc Netw 2007;5:324–330.
44. Dawood S, Merajver SD, Viens P, et al. International expert panel on inflammatory breast cancer: consensus statement for standardized diagnosis and treatment. Ann Oncol 2011;22:515–523.
45. Sprague BL, Trentham-Dietz A. Prevalence of breast carcinoma in situ in the United States. J Am Med Assoc 2009;302:846–848.
46. Kuerer HM, Albarracin CT, Yang WT, et al. Ductal carcinoma in situ: State of the science and roadmap to advance the field. J Clin Oncol 2009;27:279–288.
47. Venkitaraman R. Lobular neoplasia of the breast. Breast J 2010;16:519–528.
48. National Comprehensive Care Network. NCCN Clinical Practice Guidelines in Oncology: Breast Cancer v.3. 2012, *http://www.nccn.org/professionals/physician_gls/PDF/breast.pdf.*
49. Fisher B, Dignam J, Wolmark N, et al. Tamoxifen in treatment of intraductal breast cancer: National Surgical Adjuvant Breast and Bowel Project B-24 randomised controlled trial. Lancet 1999;353:1993–2000.
50. National Comprehensive Care Network. NCCN Clinical Practice Guidelines in Oncology: Breast Cancer Risk Reduction v.1. 2012, *http://www.nccn.org/professionals/physician_gls/PDF/breast_risk.pdf.*
51. Fisher B, Costantino JP, Wickerham DL, et al. Tamoxifen for prevention of breast cancer: report of the National Surgical Adjuvant Breast and Bowel Project P-1 Study. J Natl Cancer Inst 1998;90:1371–1388.
52. Vogel VG, Costantino JP, Wickerham DL, et al. Effects of tamoxifen vs raloxifene on the risk of developing invasive breast cancer and other disease outcomes: The NSABP Study of Tamoxifen and Raloxifene (STAR) P-2 trial. J Am Med Assoc 2006;295:2727–2741.
53. Goss PE, Ingle JN, Ales-Martinez JE, et al. Exemestane for breast-cancer prevention in postmenopausal women. N Engl J Med 2011;364:2381–2391.
54. Ligibel J. Lifestyle factors in cancer survivorship. J Clin Oncol 2012;30:3697–3704.
55. Pierce JP, Natarajan L, Caan BJ, et al. Influence of a diet very high in vegetables, fruit, and fiber and low in fat on prognosis following treatment for breast cancer: The Women's Healthy Eating and Living (WHEL) randomized trial. J Am Med Assoc 2007;298:289–298.
56. Chlebowski RT, Blackburn GL, Thomson CA, et al. Dietary fat reduction and breast cancer outcome: Interim efficacy results from the Women's Intervention Nutrition Study. J Natl Cancer Inst 2006;98:1767–1776.
57. Doyle C, Kushi LH, Byers T, et al. Nutrition and physical activity during and after cancer treatment: An American

Cancer Society guide for informed choices. CA Cancer J Clin 2006;56:323–353.
58. Stuart-Harris R, Caldas C, Pinder SE, Pharoah P. Proliferation markers and survival in early breast cancer: A systematic review and meta-analysis of 85 studies in 32,825 patients. Breast 2008;17:323–334.
59. Hammond ME, Hayes DF, Dowsett M, et al. American Society of Clinical Oncology/College of American Pathologists guideline recommendations for immunohistochemical testing of estrogen and progesterone receptors in breast cancer. J Clin Oncol 2010;28:2784–2795.
60. Wolff AC, Hammond ME, Schwartz JN, et al. American Society of Clinical Oncology/College of American Pathologists guideline recommendations for human epidermal growth factor receptor 2 testing in breast cancer. J Clin Oncol 2007;25:118–145.
61. Dawood S, Broglio K, Buzdar AU, et al. Prognosis of women with metastatic breast cancer by HER2 status and trastuzumab treatment: an institutional-based review. J Clin Oncol 2009;28:92–98.
62. Hornberger J, Alvarado MD, Rebecca C, et al. Clinical validity/utility, change in practice patterns, and economic implications of risk stratifiers to predict outcomes for early-stage breast cancer: A systematic review. J Natl Cancer Inst 2012;104:1068–1079.
63. Harris L, Fritsche H, Mennel R, et al. American Society of Clinical Oncology 2007 update of recommendations for the use of tumor markers in breast cancer. J Clin Oncol 2007;25:5287–5312.
64. Yang SH, Yang KH, Li YP, et al. Breast conservation therapy for stage I or stage II breast cancer: A meta-analysis of randomized controlled trials. Ann Oncol 2008;19:1039–1044.
65. Jatoi I, Proschan MA. Randomized trials of breast-conserving therapy versus mastectomy for primary breast cancer: A pooled analysis of updated results. Am J Clin Oncol 2005;28:289–294.
66. Buchholz TA. Radiation therapy for early-stage breast cancer after breast-conserving surgery. N Engl J Med. 2009;360:63–70.
67. Ivens D, Hoe AL, Podd TJ, et al. Assessment of morbidity from complete axillary dissection. Br J Cancer 1992;66:136–138.
68. Keramopoulos A, Tsionou C, Minaretzis D, et al. Arm morbidity following treatment of breast cancer with total axillary dissection: A multivariated approach. Oncology 1993;50:445–449.
69. Lyman GH, Giuliano AE, Somerfield MR, et al. American Society of Clinical Oncology guideline recommendations for sentinel lymph node biopsy in early-stage breast cancer. J Clin Oncol 2005;23:7703–7720.
70. Giuliano AE, Hunt KK, Ballman KV, et al. Axillary dissection vs no axillary dissection in women with invasive breast cancer and sentinel node metastasis: A randomized clinical trial. J Am Med Assoc 2011;305: 569–575.
71. Kim T, Giuliano AE, Lyman GH. Lymphatic mapping and sentinel lymph node biopsy in early-stage breast carcinoma: A metaanalysis. Cancer 2006;106:4–16.
72. D'Angelo-Donovan DD, Dickson-Witmer D, Petrelli NJ. Sentinel lymph node biopsy in breast cancer: A history and current clinical recommendations. Surg Oncol 2012;21:196–200.
73. Goldhirsch A, Wood WC, Coates AS, et al. Strategies for subtypes—Dealing with the diversity of breast cancer: Highlights of the St. Gallen International Expert Consensus on the Primary Therapy of Early Breast Cancer 2011. Ann Oncol 2011;22:1736–1747.
74. Ravdin PM, Siminoff IA, Harvey JA. Survey of breast cancer patients concerning their knowledge and expectations of adjuvant therapy. J Clin Oncol 1998;16:515–521.
75. Lindley C, Vasa S, Sawyer WT, Winer EP. Quality of life and preferences for treatment following systemic adjuvant therapy for early-stage breast cancer. J Clin Oncol 1998;16:1380–1387.
76. Fisher B, Brown A, Mamounas E, et al. Effect of preoperative chemotherapy on local-regional disease in women with operable breast cancer: Findings from National Surgical Adjuvant Breast and Bowel Project B-18. J Clin Oncol 1997;15:2483–2493.
77. Fisher B, Bryant J, Wolmark N, et al. Effect of preoperative chemotherapy on the outcome of women with operable breast cancer. J Clin Oncol 1998;16:2672–2685.
78. Rastogi P, Anderson SJ, Bear HD, et al. Preoperative chemotherapy: Updates of National Surgical Adjuvant Breast and Bowel Project Protocols B-18 and B-27. J Clin Oncol 2008;26:778–785.
79. Jones S, Holmes FA, O'Shaughnessy J, et al. Docetaxel with cyclophosphamide is associated with an overall survival benefit compared with doxorubicin and cyclophosphamide: 7-year follow-up of US Oncology Research Trial 9735. J Clin Oncol 2009;27:1177–1183.
80. Foulkes WD, Smith IE, Reis-Filho JS. Triple-negative breast cancer. N Engl J Med 2010;363:1938–1948.
81. Lohrisch C, Paltiel C, Gelmon K, et al. Impact on survival of time from definitive surgery to initiation of adjuvant chemotherapy for early-stage breast cancer. J Clin Oncol 2006;24:4888–4894.
82. Bonadonna G, Valagussa P, Moliterni A, et al. Adjuvant cyclophosphamide, methotrexate, and fluorouracil in node-positive breast cancer: The results of 20 years of follow-up. N Engl J Med 1995;332:901–906.
83. Citron ML, Berry DA, Cirrincione C, et al. Randomized trial of dose-dense versus conventionally scheduled and sequential versus concurrent combination chemotherapy as postoperative adjuvant treatment of node-positive primary breast cancer: First report of Intergroup Trial C9741/ Cancer and Leukemia Group B Trial 9741. J Clin Oncol 2003;21:1431–1439.
84. Sparano JA, Wang M, Martino S, et al. Weekly paclitaxel in the adjuvant treatment of breast cancer. N Engl J Med 2008;358:1663–1671.
85. Seidman AD, Berry D, Cirrincione C, et al. Randomized phase III trial of weekly compared with every-3-weeks paclitaxel for metastatic breast cancer, with trastuzumab for all HER-2 overexpressors and random assignment to trastuzumab or not in HER-2 nonoverexpressors: final results of Cancer and Leukemia Group B protocol 9840. J Clin Oncol 2008;26:1642–1649.
86. Green MC, Buzdar AU, Smith T, et al. Weekly paclitaxel improves pathologic complete remission in operable breast cancer when compared with paclitaxel once every 3 weeks. J Clin Oncol 2005;23:5983–5992.
87. Bonilla L, Ben-Aharon I, Vidal L, et al. Dose-dense chemotherapy in nonmetastatic breast cancer: A systematic review and meta-analysis of randomized controlled trials. J Natl Cancer Ins. 2010;102:1845–1854.
88. Herbolsheimer P, Swain SM. Meta-analysis: Should it be more than the sum of its parts? J Natl Cancer Inst 2010;102:1817–1819.
89. Berry DA, Ueno NT, Johnson MM, et al. High-dose chemotherapy with autologous stem-cell support as adjuvant therapy in breast cancer: Overview of 15 randomized trials. J Clin Oncol 2011;29:3214–3223.

90. Moore HC. Impact on quality of life of adjuvant therapy for breast cancer. Curr Oncol Rep 2007;9:42–46.
91. Groenvold M, Fayers PM, Petersen MA, et al. Breast cancer patients on adjuvant chemotherapy report a wide range of problems not identified by health-care staff. Breast Cancer Res Treat 2007;103:185–195.
92. Rizzo JD, Brouwers M, Hurley P, et al. American Society of Clinical Oncology/American Society of Hematology clinical practice guideline update on the use of epoetin and darbepoetin in adult patients with cancer. J Clin Oncol 2010;28:4996–5010.
93. Levine MN, Gent M, Hirsh J, et al. The thrombogenic effect of anticancer drug therapy in women with stage II breast cancer. N Engl J Med 1988;318:404–407.
94. Matesich SM, Shapiro CL. Second cancers after breast cancer treatment. Semin Oncol. 2003;30:740–748.
95. Henderson IC, Sloss LJ, Jaffe N, et al. Serial studies of cardiac function in patients receiving adriamycin. Cancer Treat Rep 1978;62:923–929.
96. Martin M, Segui MA, Anton A, et al. Adjuvant docetaxel for high-risk, node-negative breast cancer. N Engl J Med 2010;363:2200–2210.
97. Costa RB, Kurra G, Greenberg L, Geyer CE. Efficacy and cardiac safety of adjuvant trastuzumab-based chemotherapy regimens for HER2-positive early breast cancer. Ann Oncol 2010;21:2153–2160.
98. Yin W, Jiang Y, Shen Z, et al. Trastuzumab in the adjuvant treatment of HER2-positive early breast cancer patients: A meta-analysis of published randomized controlled trials. PloS One 2011;6:e21030.
99. Slamon D, Eiermann W, Robert N, et al. Adjuvant trastuzumab in HER2-positive breast cancer. N Engl J Med 2011;365:1273–1283.
100. Telli ML, Witteles RM. Trastuzumab-related cardiac dysfunction. J Natl Compr Canc Netw 2011;9:243–249.
101. Buzdar AU, Ibrahim NK, Francis D, et al. Significantly higher pathologic complete remission rate after neoadjuvant therapy with trastuzumab, paclitaxel, and epirubicin chemotherapy: Results of a randomized trial in human epidermal growth factor receptor 2-positive operable breast cancer. J Clin Oncol 2005;23:3676–3685.
102. Halyard MY, Pisansky TM, Dueck AC, et al. Radiotherapy and adjuvant trastuzumab in operable breast cancer: Tolerability and adverse event data from the NCCTG Phase III Trial N9831. J Clin Oncol 2009;27:2638–2644.
103. Banerjee S, Smith IE. Management of small HER2-positive breast cancers. Lancet Oncol 2010;11:1193–1199.
104. Love RR, Wiebe DA, Newcomb PA, et al. Effects of tamoxifen on cardiovascular risk factors in postmenopausal women. Ann Intern Med 1991;115:860–864.
105. Love RR, Mazess RB, Barden HS, et al. Effects of tamoxifen on bone mineral density in postmenopausal women with breast cancer. N Engl J Med 1992;326:852–856.
106. Albain KS, Barlow WE, Ravdin PM, et al. Adjuvant chemotherapy and timing of tamoxifen in postmenopausal patients with endocrine-responsive, node-positive breast cancer: A phase 3, open-label, randomised controlled trial. Lancet 2009;374:2005–2063.
107. Davies C, Pan H, Godwin J, et al. Long-term effects of continuing adjuvant tamoxifen to 10 years versus stopping at 5 years after diagnosis of oestrogen receptor-positive breast cancer: ATLAS, a randomised trial. Lancet 2013;381(9869):805–816.
108. Fisher B, Dignam J, Bryant J, Wolmark N. Five versus more than five years of tamoxifen for lymph node-negative breast cancer: Updated findings from the National Surgical Adjuvant Breast and Bowel Project B-14 randomized trial. J Natl Cancer Inst 2001;93:684–690.
109. Early Breast Cancer Trialists' Collaborative Group. Effects of chemotherapy and hormonal therapy for early breast cancer on recurrence and 15-year survival: An overview of the randomised trials. Lancet 2005;365:1687–1717.
110. Cuzick J, Ambroisine L, Davidson N, et al. Use of luteinising-hormone-releasing hormone agonists as adjuvant treatment in premenopausal patients with hormone-receptor-positive breast cancer: A meta-analysis of individual patient data from randomised adjuvant trials. Lancet 2007;369:1711–1723.
111. Gnant M, Mlineritsch B, Stoeger H, et al. Adjuvant endocrine therapy plus zoledronic acid in premenopausal women with early-stage breast cancer: 62-month follow-up from the ABCSG-12 randomised trial. Lancet Oncol 2011;12:631–641.
112. Dowsett M, Cuzick J, Ingle J, et al. Meta-analysis of breast cancer outcomes in adjuvant trials of aromatase inhibitors versus tamoxifen. J Clin Oncol 2010;28:509–518.
113. Goss PE, Ingle JN, Martino S, et al. A randomized trial of letrozole in postmenopausal women after five years of tamoxifen therapy for early-stage breast cancer. N Engl J Med 2003;349:1793–1802.
114. Mouridsen H, Giobbie-Hurder A, Goldhirsch A, et al. Letrozole therapy alone or in sequence with tamoxifen in women with breast cancer. N Engl J Med 2009;361:766–776.
115. Hertz DL, McLeod HL, Irvin WJ Jr. Tamoxifen and CYP2D6: A contradiction of data. Oncologist 2012;17:620–630.
116. Sideras K, Ingle JN, Ames MM, et al. Coprescription of tamoxifen and medications that inhibit CYP2D6. J Clin Oncol 2010;28:2768–2776.
117. Kelly CM, Juurlink DN, Gomes T, et al. Selective serotonin reuptake inhibitors and breast cancer mortality in women receiving tamoxifen: A population based cohort study. BMJ 2010;340:c693.
118. Giordano SH. Update on locally advanced breast cancer. Oncologist 2003;8:521–530.
119. Khasraw M, Bell R. Primary systemic therapy in HER2-amplified breast cancer: A clinical review. Expert Rev Anticancer Ther 2012;12:1005–1013.
120. Hanrahan EO, Hennessy BT, Valero V. Neoadjuvant systemic therapy for breast cancer: An overview and review of recent clinical trials. Expert Opin Pharmacother 2005;6:1477–1491.
121. Chia YH, Ellis MJ, Ma CX. Neoadjuvant endocrine therapy in primary breast cancer: Indications and use as a research tool. Br J Cancer 2010;103:759–764.
122. Van Poznak CH, Temin S, Yee GC, et al. American Society of Clinical Oncology executive summary of the clinical practice guideline update on the role of bone-modifying agents in metastatic breast cancer. J Clin Oncol 2011;29:1221–1227.
123. Sainsbury R. The development of endocrine therapy for women with breast cancer. Cancer Treat Rev Forthcoming 2012.
124. Doyen J, Italiano A, Largillier R, et al. Aromatase inhibition in male breast cancer patients: Biological and clinical implications. Ann Oncol 2010;21:1243–1245.
125. Stenbygaard LE, Herrstedt J, Thomsen JF, et al. Toremifene and tamoxifen in advanced breast cancer—A double-blind cross-over trial. Breast Cancer Res Treat 1993;25:57–63.
126. Di Leo A, Jerusalem G, Petruzelka L, et al. Results of the CONFIRM phase III trial comparing fulvestrant 250 mg with fulvestrant 500 mg in postmenopausal women with estrogen receptor-positive advanced breast cancer. J Clin Oncol 2010;28:4594–4600.

127. Robertson JF, Lindemann JP, Llombart-Cussac A, et al. Fulvestrant 500 mg versus anastrozole 1 mg for the first-line treatment of advanced breast cancer: Follow-up analysis from the randomized 'FIRST' study. Breast Cancer Res Treat 2012;136:503–511.
128. Mehta RS, Barlow WE, Albain KS, et al. Combination anastrozole and fulvestrant in metastatic breast cancer. N Engl J Med 2012;367:435–444.
129. Bergh J, Jonsson PE, Lidbrink EK, et al. FACT: An open-label randomized phase III study of fulvestrant and anastrozole in combination compared with anastrozole alone as first-line therapy for patients with receptor-positive postmenopausal breast cancer. J Clin Oncol 2012;30:1919–1925.
130. Klijn JG, Blamey RW, Boccardo F, et al. Combined tamoxifen and luteinizing hormone-releasing hormone (LHRH) agonist versus LHRH agonist alone in premenopausal advanced breast cancer: A meta-analysis of four randomized trials. J Clin Oncol 2001;19:343–353.
131. Cardoso F, Bischoff J, Brain E, et al. A review of the treatment of endocrine responsive metastatic breast cancer in postmenopausal women. Cancer Treat Rev 2013;39(5):457–465.
132. Gogineni K, DeMichele A. Current approaches to the management of Her2-negative metastatic breast cancer. Breast Cancer Res 2012;14:205.
133. Cobleigh MA, Vogel CL, Tripathy D, et al. Multinational study of the efficacy and safety of humanized anti-HER2 monoclonal antibody in women who have HER2-overexpressing metastatic breast cancer that has progressed after chemotherapy for metastatic disease. J Clin Oncol 1999;17:2639–2648.
134. Amar S, Roy V, Perez EA. Treatment of metastatic breast cancer: Looking towards the future. Breast Cancer Res Treat 2009;114:413–422.
135. Geyer CE, Forster J, Lindquist D, et al. Lapatinib plus capecitabine for HER2-positive advanced breast cancer. N Engl J Med 2006;355:2733–2743.
136. Di Leo A, Gomez HL, Aziz Z, et al. Phase III, double-blind, randomized study comparing lapatinib plus paclitaxel with placebo plus paclitaxel as first-line treatment for metastatic breast cancer. J Clin Oncol 2008;26:5544–5552.
137. Johnston S, Pippen J, Jr., Pivot X, et al. Lapatinib combined with letrozole versus letrozole and placebo as first-line therapy for postmenopausal hormone receptor-positive metastatic breast cancer. J Clin Oncol 2009;27:5538–5546.
138. Blackwell KL, Burstein HJ, Storniolo AM, et al. Overall survival benefit with lapatinib in combination with trastuzumab for patients with human epidermal growth factor receptor 2-positive metastatic breast cancer: Final results from the EGF104900 study. J Clin Oncl 2012;30:2585–2592.
139. Capelan M, Pugliano L, De Azambuja,et al. Pertuzumab: New hope for patients with HER2-positive breast cancer. Ann Oncol 2013;24;273–282.
140. Baselga J, Cortes J, Kim SB, et al. Pertuzumab plus trastuzumab plus docetaxel for metastatic breast cancer. N Engl J Med 2012;366:109–119.
141. Genetech, Inc. Herceptin (trastuzumab) product information. 2010, *http://www.gene.com/download/pdf/herceptin_prescribing.pdf.*
142. Perez EA, Koehler M, Byrne J, et al. Cardiac safety of lapatinib: pooled analysis of 3689 patients enrolled in clinical trials. Mayo Clin Proc 2008;83:679–686.
143. Paul B, Trovato JA, Thompson J. Lapatinib: A dual tyrosine kinase inhibitor for metastatic breast cancer. Am J Health System Phar 2008;65:1703–1710.
144. Ross JS, Slodkowska EA, Symmans WF, et al. The HER-2 receptor and breast cancer: ten years of targeted anti-HER-2 therapy and personalized medicine. Oncologist 2009;14:320–368.
145. Wolff AC, Lazar AA, Bondarenko I, et al. Randomized phase III placebo-controlled trial of letrozole plus oral temsirolimus as first-line endocrine therapy in postmenopausal women with locally advanced or metastatic breast cancer. J Clin Oncol 2013;31:195–202.
146. Baselga J, Campone M, Piccart M, et al. Everolimus in postmenopausal hormone-receptor-positive advanced breast cancer. N Engl J Med 2012;366:52.
147. Keck S, Glencer AC, Rugo HS. Everolimus and its role in hormone-resistant and trastuzumab-resistant metastatic breast cancer. Future Oncol 2012;8:1383–1396.
148. Cortes J, Calvo E, Gonzalez-Martin A, et al. Progress against solid tumors in danger: The metastatic breast cancer example. J Clin Oncol 2012;30:3444–3447.
149. Lyman GH, Burstein HJ, Buzdar AU, et al. Making genuine progress against metastatic breast cancer. J Clin Oncol 2012;30:3448–3451.
150. Cuzick J, Powles T, Veronesi U, et al. Overview of the main outcomes in breast-cancer prevention trials. Lancet 2003;361:296–300.
151. Vogel VG, Costantino JP, Wickerham DL, et al. Update of the National Surgical Adjuvant Breast and Bowel Project Study of Tamoxifen and Raloxifene (STAR) P-2 Trial: Preventing breast cancer. Cancer Prev Res 2010;3:696–706.
152. Litton JK, Arun BK, Brown PH, Hortobagyi GN. Aromatase inhibitors and breast cancer prevention. Expert Opin Pharmacother 2012;13:325–331.
153. Goss PE, Ingle JN, Ales-Martinez JE, et al. Exemestane for breast-cancer prevention in postmenopausal women. N Engl J Med 2011;364:2381–2391.
154. Visvanathan K, Chlebowski RT, Hurley P, et al. American Society of Clinical Oncology clinical practice guideline update on the use of pharmacologic interventions including tamoxifen, raloxifene, and aromatase inhibition for breast cancer risk reduction. J Clin Oncol 2009;27:3235–3258.
155. Smith RA, Cokkinides V, Brawley OW. Cancer screening in the United States, 2009: A review of current American Cancer Society guidelines and issues in cancer screening. CA Cancer J Clin 2009;59:27–41.
156. Screening for breast cancer: U.S. Preventive Services Task Force recommendation statement. Ann Intern Med 2009;151:716–726.
157. Thomas DB, Gao DL, Self SG, et al. Randomized trial of breast self-examination in Shanghai: Methodology and preliminary results. J Natl Cancer Inst 1997;89:355–365.
158. Nelson HD, Tyne K, Naik A, et al. Screening for breast cancer: An update for the U.S. Preventive Services Task Force. Ann Intern Med 2009;151:727–737.
159. United States Preventive Services Task Force. Screening for Breast Cancer. 2009, *http://www.uspreventiveservicestaskforce.org/uspstf/uspsbrca.htm.*
160. Saslow D, Boetes C, Burke W, et al. American cancer society guidelines for breast screening with MRI as an adjunct to mammography. CA Cancer J Clin 2007;57:75–89.

106

Lung Cancer

Val R. Adams and Susanne M. Arnold

KEY CONCEPTS

1. Lung cancer is the leading cause of cancer deaths in both men and women in the United States. The overall 5-year survival rate for all types of lung cancer is about 15%.
2. Cigarette smoking is responsible for most lung cancers. Smoking cessation should be encouraged, particularly in those receiving curative treatment (i.e., stages I to IIIA non–small cell lung cancer [NSCLC] and limited-stage small cell lung cancer [SCLC]).
3. NSCLC is diagnosed in most (~80%) lung cancer patients. NSCLC typically has a slower growth rate and doubling time than SCLC.
4. Screening test is currently recommended to identify lung cancer in high-risk individuals. However, several studies are evaluating the optimal frequency and duration, as well as the impact of false-positive tests.
5. Treatment decisions are guided by the stage of disease, which is characterized by tumor size and spread. Patient-specific factors (i.e., performance status, comorbid conditions, etc.) must also be considered when developing a treatment plan.
6. The treatment goals in lung cancer are cure (early stage disease), prolongation of survival, and maintenance or improvement of quality of life through alleviation of symptoms.
7. Early stage lung cancer has the highest cure rates when surgical resection of the tumor is used with or without chemotherapy for NSCLC and chemoradiotherapy for SCLC.
8. Advanced-stage lung cancer is primarily treated with systemic therapy. Doublet chemotherapy regimens are superior in response to single-agent regimens and should be used when the patient can tolerate the associated toxicity. Platinum-containing doublets are first-line treatment in most cases of NSCLC and SCLC.
9. Optimal patient care needs to include prevention and treatment of adverse events from chemotherapy. Adverse events may cause delays in chemotherapy administration, increase morbidity, and contribute to treatment failure.

Lung cancer is a major cause of morbidity and mortality. It has reached epidemic proportions in many industrialized countries and is the most frequently fatal malignancy in the world. It is estimated that 228,190 new cases of lung cancer were diagnosed in the United States in 2013.[1] Despite major advances in the understanding and management of lung cancer, the overall 5-year survival rate for all types of lung cancer remains a dismal 16%. In the United States, lung cancer accounts for about 14% of all newly diagnosed cancer in adults.[1] (1) It remains the leading cause of cancer death in both adult men and women, with about 159,480 deaths in 2013.[1] The incidence and death rate caused by lung cancer are declining, which has been attributed to decreased tobacco use over the last 50 years. In comparison to whites, the incidence and mortality of lung cancer is greater in African American men and slightly lower in African American women.[1]

The incidence of lung cancer increases with age, with about two thirds of cases diagnosed between 60 and 79 years.[1] Early lung cancer screening studies failed to demonstrate a survival advantage, but in November 2010, the largest trial of its kind, the National Lung Screening Trial, demonstrated a 20% reduction in the relative risk of death from lung cancer in moderate- to high-risk individuals (95% confidence interval [CI], 6.8 to 26.7; $P = 0.004$). Among subjects enrolled in lung cancer screening trials, the rate of malignancy in the pulmonary nodule detected on low-dose chest computed tomography (CT) scan is low, and surgical procedures are not without risk. Consequently, patients who receive scans as part of lung cancer screening or for another purpose should have other criteria or tests done before considering a biopsy to evaluate for malignant pathology.[2]

Patients with lung cancer may undergo surgery, chemotherapy, radiation, or multimodality therapy, depending on the histologic type of the tumor, its size and location, and the presence of metastases at diagnosis.[3] Two leading oncology groups representing leading clinicians in the United States have published clinical practice guidelines for the treatment of lung cancer. The National Comprehensive Cancer Network (NCCN) has developed consensus-based guidelines that provide recommendations regarding the screening, staging, and treatment of both small cell lung cancer (SCLC) and non–small cell lung cancer (NSCLC).[4,5] The American Society of Clinical Oncology (ASCO) first published evidence-based guidelines regarding the staging and treatment of NSCLC in 1997, which were subsequently updated in 2003; the stage IV NSCLC guideline was updated in 2011.[6]

ETIOLOGY

Lung carcinomas arise from normal bronchial epithelial cells that have acquired multiple genetic lesions and are capable of expressing a variety of phenotypes.[2] Significant advances have been made recently in understanding the molecular genetic changes involved in lung cancer pathogenesis.[3] A large variety of molecular lesions result in abrogation of key cellular regulatory and growth control pathways. Activation of a proto-oncogene, inhibition or mutation of tumor suppressor genes, and production of autocrine (self-stimulatory) growth factors contribute to cellular proliferation and malignant transformation.[3] Many of these molecular alterations are common to both SCLC and NSCLC, but certain mutations are found more frequently in specific subtypes of lung cancer and offer more targeted interventions to prevent or treat lung cancer. In autocrine loop abnormalities, SCLC frequently overexpresses C-KIT (a protein tyrosine kinase receptor that is specific for stem cell factor [aka, CD117]), whereas NSCLC frequently overexpresses epidermal growth factor receptor (EGFR).[7] EGFR inhibitors, such as erlotinib, are used clinically to treat NSCLC and offer a potential method of lung cancer chemoprevention. Crizotinib, a drug that targets the EML4-ALK gene rearrangement protein, demonstrates the importance of this pathway in a subset of adenocarcinoma lung cancer patients.[8]

2 Smoking is a major cause of lung cancer, with about 80% of lung cancer deaths in the United States directly attributed to tobacco use. Tobacco smoke contains many substances, including tumor promoters, carcinogens, and cocarcinogens,[1,7] which are proven carcinogens. The association between environmental tobacco smoke (ETS; also referred to as passive smoking) and lung cancer risk in nonsmokers is not as clear. Most studies have consistently found that spouses of smokers have higher rates of lung cancer than spouses of nonsmokers (about 25% higher risk). In addition, workplace exposure to environmental smoke increases the risk of lung cancer by about 17%. It is currently estimated that ETS contributes to about 3,000 lung cancers annually. Although many of these studies have methodologic flaws, the data seem consistent and seem to indicate a dose–risk relationship, with no safe level of exposure.[9] Smoking cessation is associated with a gradual decrease in the risk, but more than 5 years is necessary before an appreciable decline in risk occurs,[1,7] and the risk never returns to that of a nonsmoker. Because of the public health implications, the United States has several, mainly state-led, tobacco control efforts, including antismoking campaigns, increased tobacco taxes, and smoke-free areas in many public areas. Although the prevalence of cigarette smoking has slowly decreased, it remains at about 19% in 2010 and 2011.[10]

Although most cases of lung cancer are attributable to cigarette smoking, less than 20% of smokers develop lung cancer, which suggests that other risk factors are relevant. An increased risk of lung cancer has been associated with exposure to other environmental respiratory carcinogens (e.g., asbestos, benzene, and arsenic). Genetic risk factors are also important, with an increased risk of lung cancer observed in those with first-degree relatives diagnosed with the disease. Lung cancer risk is associated with polymorphisms that affect the expression and/or function of enzymes regulating metabolism of tobacco carcinogens, DNA repair, or inflammation. Patients with a history of chronic obstructive airway disease and adults with asthma are at an increased risk for lung cancer.[1,7,9] Further studies to better identify which patients are at highest risk of developing lung cancer will be key for new lung cancer screening trials and in chemoprevention trials.

HISTOLOGIC CLASSIFICATION

Before treatment begins, it is critical that an experienced lung cancer pathologist reviews the pathologic material because of the different treatment regimens for NSCLC and SCLC. 3 NSCLC is diagnosed in most (80%) lung cancer patients. NSCLC typically has a slower growth rate and doubling time than SCLC. The histologic classification of NSCLC is well defined and widely accepted (Table 106-1).[11] In the most recent classification, the histologic types, subtypes, and identifiable variants convey information about tumors' natural behavior and in some cases influence therapeutic decisions.[4,5,7,11]

Four major cell types of carcinomas (squamous cell, adenocarcinoma, large cell, and small cell) account for more than 90% of all lung tumors. Early studies with localized disease demonstrated that radiation could cure small cell histology, while surgery did not. Studies with the other histologic types demonstrated better outcomes with surgery than with radiation; hence, the general classification of SCLC and NSCLC was created. Historically, systemic treatment for metastatic squamous cell, adenocarcinoma, and large cell carcinomas was the same and resulted in a similar overall prognosis, which again supported a general classification of SCLC and NSCLC. Trials over the last decade with newer agents have shown differences in efficacy and toxicity with regard to NSCLC histologic types and, consequently, knowledge concerning the histology is essential to optimize drug therapy.[4,5,7]

TABLE 106-1 Histologic Classification of Non-Small Cell Lung Carcinomas

1. Squamous cell carcinoma
   - Papillary
   - Clear cell
   - Small cell (probably should be discontinued)
   - Basaloid
2. Adenocarcinoma
   - Minimally invasive adenocarcinoma (MIA)
   - Invasive adenocarcinoma
   - Lepidic predominant (previously classified as bronchioalveolar carcinoma [BAC])
   - Acinar predominant
   - Papillary predominant
   - Micropapillary predominant
   - Solid predominant with mucin
   - Variants of invasive adenocarcinoma
   - Invasive mucinous adenocarcinoma (previously classified as BAC)
   - Colloid
   - Fetal (low and high grade)
   - Enteric
3. Large cell carcinoma
   - Variants
   - Large cell neuroendocrine carcinoma
   - Combined large cell neuroendocrine carcinoma
   - Basaloid carcinoma
   - Lymphoepithelioma-like carcinoma
   - Clear cell carcinoma
   - Large cell carcinoma with rhabdoid phenotype
4. Adenosquamous carcinoma
5. Sarcomatoid carcinomas
   - Pleomorphic carcinoma
   - Spindle cell carcinoma
   - Giant cell carcinoma
   - Carcinosarcoma
   - Pulmonary blastoma
   - Other
6. Carcinoid tumor
   - Typical carcinoid (TC)
   - Atypical carcinoid (AC)
7. Carcinomas of salivary gland type
   - Mucoepidermoid carcinoma
   - Adenoid cystic carcinoma
   - Epimyoepithelial carcinoma

Adapted from 2004 WHO classification and the 2011 IASCL/ATS/ERS classification as described in reference 11.

Squamous cell carcinoma was once the most common histology, but it now represents less than 30% of all lung cancers. Squamous cell carcinomas have a much higher incidence in smokers and among males and appear to have a strong dose–response relationship to tobacco exposure. Most of these tumors occur centrally, but the incidence of peripheral presentation is increasing. Studies describing the natural history of lung cancer in the era of screening with low-dose CT (LDCT) scans have revealed a relatively constant tumor volume doubling time (104 to 122 days), while the other histologies indicate that smaller tumors found with a CT scan are more indolent (e.g., doubling times three to four times longer with CT-discovered tumors).[12] Squamous cell tumors are slower to metastasize, but they eventually spread to the hilar and mediastinal lymph nodes, liver, adrenal glands, kidneys, bone, and GI tract. [3,11]

Adenocarcinoma accounts for about one-half of lung cancers and is increasing in frequency. It is the most common histology in nonsmoking lung cancer patients. The natural history of adenocarcinoma in the lung shows that small tumors discovered with CT screening are relatively slow growing and the tumor doubling time increases as they get larger; volume doubling time of tumors discovered with CT screening is about 576 days, while those found with routine care double every 169 days.[12] This information is most important when considering screening and the potential for lead time bias. Patients with adenocarcinoma can present with a single nodule, multifocal nodules, or rapidly progressing, bilateral, diffuse processes. This histology is likely to metastasize from a relatively small tumor (often before the diagnosis of the primary tumor) and spread widely to distant sites, including the contralateral lung, liver, bone, adrenal glands, kidneys, and CNS. As a result, adenocarcinoma has a worse prognosis than squamous cell carcinoma, but the prognosis is similar when controlled for stage.[3,4]

Table 106-1 shows several subclassifications and variants of adenocarcinoma. The importance of these subtypes to treatment is currently limited, but newer targeted therapies may work best in certain subtypes, thus allowing more individualized treatment selection. For example, erlotinib was approved because it was effective in NSCLC, but it appears more effective in adenocarcinoma, particularly those with a mutation in the EGFR. The 3% to 13% of NSCLC tumors that have an EML4-ALK rearrangement is almost exclusively adenocarcinoma, which is important to know for testing and if positive will impact therapy.[4,13]

Large cell carcinomas are undifferentiated epithelial tumors, which are often a diagnosis of exclusion. These tumors tend to be large and bulky tumors arising in the periphery of the lung, have a propensity to metastasize in a pattern quite similar to adenocarcinomas, and are associated with a similar poor prognosis.[3,4]

SCLCs account for about 15% of all lung tumors. Nearly all SCLCs are immunoreactive for keratin, epithelial membrane antigen, and thyroid transcription factor 1, and many stain positively for markers of neuroendocrine differentiation. They are distinguished by a proliferation of neoplastic cells with round to oval nuclei. These tumors occur in both the major bronchi and the periphery of the lung. SCLC is a very aggressive and rapidly growing tumor, with about 60% to 70% of patients initially presenting with disseminated disease outside of the hemithorax. These tumors commonly express neuroendocrine differentiation, which may account for some of the paraneoplastic syndromes frequently associated with this disease. SCLC secretes gastrin-releasing peptide that acts as an autocrine growth factor. Secretion of other peptide hormones, cytogenetic abnormalities, and amplification and increased expression of oncogenes are also common. This disease has a propensity to metastasize to the lymph nodes, opposite lung, liver, adrenal glands and other endocrine organs, bone, bone marrow, and CNS.[3,5]

Lung can exhibit more than one histologic cell type (e.g., adenosquamous), which may impact therapy. Patients can also occasionally have multiple lung nodules arising in different lobes or the contralateral lung. They can be the same or different histology. This is referred to as synchronous tumors, and the nodules may be of similar or different cell types. This usually worsens the patient's overall prognosis.[3]

CLINICAL PRESENTATION

At the time of diagnosis, 15% of lung cancers are localized, 22% have regional spread, and 56% have distant metastases (the remaining were not staged).[1] Location and extent of the tumor determine the presenting signs and symptoms. A lesion in the central portion of the bronchial tree is more likely to cause symptoms at an earlier stage as compared with a lesion in the periphery of the lung, which may remain asymptomatic until the lesion is large or has spread to other areas. The most common initial signs and symptoms include cough, dyspnea, and chest pain or discomfort, with or without hemoptysis.[3] Unfortunately, many patients with lung cancer also have chronic pulmonary and/or cardiovascular diseases (usually related to smoking), and such symptoms may go unnoticed or be attributed to the concomitant disease. Many patients also exhibit systemic symptoms of malignancy such as anorexia, weight loss, and fatigue. Disseminated disease can cause extrapulmonary signs and symptoms such as neurologic deficits resulting from CNS metastases, bone pain or pathological fractures secondary to bone metastases, or liver dysfunction resulting from tumor involvement in the liver.[3]

CLINICAL PRESENTATION Lung Cancer

Local Signs and Symptoms Associated with Primary Tumor or Regional Spread within the Thorax

- Cough
- Hemoptysis
- Dyspnea
- Rust-streaked or purulent sputum
- Chest, shoulder, or arm pain
- Wheeze and stridor
- Superior vena cava obstruction
- Pleural effusion or pneumonitis
- Dysphagia (secondary to esophageal compression)
- Hoarseness (secondary to laryngeal nerve paralysis)
- Horner's syndrome
- Phrenic nerve paralysis
- Pericardial effusion/tamponade
- Tracheal obstruction

Extrapulmonary Signs and Symptoms Associated with Metastatic Involvement

- Bone pain and/or pathologic fractures
- Liver dysfunction
- Neurologic deficits
- Spinal cord compression

Paraneoplastic Syndromes

- Weight loss
- Cushing's syndrome
- Hypercalcemia (most commonly in squamous cell lung cancer)
- Syndrome of inappropriate secretion of antidiuretic hormone (most commonly in SCLC)
- Pulmonary hypertrophic osteoarthropathy
- Clubbing
- Anemia
- Eaton-Lambert's myasthenic syndrome
- Hypercoagulable state

Paraneoplastic syndromes are signs and symptoms that occur at sites away from the primary tumor or its metastases and are not associated with direct tumor involvement. They may be caused by the production of biologically active substances (e.g., peptide hormones) or antibodies, or by other undefined mechanisms. Paraneoplastic syndromes occur more frequently with lung cancer than with any other tumor, and more frequently with SCLC than with NSCLC. These syndromes may be the first signs of a tumor and may prompt the search for an underlying malignancy.[3]

SCREENING AND PREVENTION

4 Most lung cancer patients are diagnosed with advanced disease, which is a key factor in the poor prognosis associated with this disease. Surgery (NSCLC) and radiation (SCLC) are the most effective treatment modalities, which generally limit curative intent to patients diagnosed at an early clinical stage.[3–5] Therefore, it is important to diagnose lung cancer earlier, which implies a potential improvement with screening. Several screening techniques, including chest x-ray, CT, and positron emission tomography (PET), scanning have been investigated to detect lung cancer at an earlier stage. The mortality results from screening with a chest x-ray have been negative, but positive results for LDCT scans to screen for lung cancer have been reported. A recent systematic review of the potential benefit and harm from LDCT screening was reported with accompanying recommendations.[14] The largest and only positive study was known as the National Lung Cancer Screening trial that enrolled more than 54,000 high-risk smokers. The study reported a decrease in overall (7% vs. 7.5%) and lung cancer–specific (1.3% vs. 1.7%) mortality with LDCT versus control, respectively. The resulting recommendation is to offer annual LDCT screening to individuals aged 55 to 74 years with a 30-pack-year history who are still smoking or have quit for less than 15 years. These recommendations come with a few caveats, including the fact that the most important step is for current smokers to quit. The optimal frequency and duration of screening is unknown and the harm from screening, including frequent false-positive findings, is unknown.[14] Consequently, patients interested in screening should be enrolled in a clinical trial so answers to these important questions can be answered.

The term *chemoprevention* refers to the use of prophylactic medications to prevent the development of cancer. Many studies of potential chemopreventive agents, including nonsteroidal anti-inflammatory drugs (NSAIDs), retinoids, inhaled glucocorticoids, vitamin E, selenium, and green tea extracts, have been conducted, but none have been successful.[15] Large randomized clinical trials have evaluated β-carotene as a lung cancer chemopreventive agent in high-risk patients (older smokers). Rather than prevent lung cancer, the trials clearly show that older people who smoke have a higher risk of developing and dying of lung cancer if they take a β-carotene supplement. Nonsmokers do not appear to have an altered risk of lung cancer with β-carotene consumption.[16] The impact of selenium and/or vitamin E supplementation was evaluated in older men as part of a large prostate cancer prevention study (Selenium and Vitamin E Cancer Prevention Trial [SELECT]). Unfortunately, no benefit was seen with selenium or vitamin E supplementation.[15,16]

Because the net benefit of screening is still being defined and chemoprevention trials have not proven to provide a survival benefit, the current recommendation is to avoid smoking and maintain a healthy diet with high amounts of fruits and vegetables.[17]

DIAGNOSIS

A patient suspected of having lung cancer should undergo a diagnostic evaluation. Diagnosis of lung cancer requires both visualization of the cancerous lesion and tissue sampling for pathologic assessment. All patients must have a thorough history and physical examination with emphasis on detecting signs and symptoms of the primary tumor, regional spread of the tumor, distant metastases, and paraneoplastic syndromes. The patient's performance status should be assessed to determine whether or not a patient may be able to tolerate surgery and/or chemotherapy.[3–5]

Visualization of the suspected tumor provides the clinician with the information necessary to choose the most appropriate sampling technique. Chest radiographs, endobronchial ultrasound, CT scans, and PET scans are among the most valuable diagnostic tests.[18] Chest radiography is the primary method of lung cancer detection and may also be used to measure tumor size, establish gross lymph node enlargement, and detect other tumor-related findings, such as pleural effusion, lobar collapse, and metastatic bone involvement of ribs, spine, and shoulders. In addition, CT scans may be helpful in the evaluation of parenchymal lung abnormalities, detection of masses only suspected on the chest radiography, and assessment of mediastinal and hilar lymph nodes. PET scans are more accurate than CT scans in distinguishing malignant from benign lesions, detecting mediastinal lymph node metastases, and identifying metastatic spread. Most recently, the use of integrated CT-PET technology has been reported to improve the diagnostic accuracy in the staging of NSCLC over either CT or PET technology alone.[19]

Once the tumor has been located, pathologic examination of tumor tissue is necessary to establish the diagnosis of lung cancer. Tissue is typically obtained through the least invasive method likely to result in an adequate sample; methods include sputum cytology, tumor biopsy by bronchoscopy, mediastinoscopy, percutaneous needle biopsy, or open-lung biopsy. The tissue sample not only confirms malignancy but is also necessary to determine the histology (i.e., squamous cell, adenocarcinoma, large cell, or small cell) and to provide adequate tissue for molecular analysis. Once the diagnosis is established, additional radiologic tests may be required to evaluate lymph nodes and potential metastatic sites for accurate staging. Surgical candidates will have additional sampling of their mediastinal nodes to determine those with stage IIIB (N_3) disease (Table 106-2).[3–5,19]

STAGING

5 Once the diagnosis of lung cancer is confirmed, the extent of disease must be determined to estimate prognosis and guide therapy. For NSCLC, tumor growth and spread are staged with the American Joint Committee on Cancer (AJCC) tumor, node, and metastasis (TNM) staging system. SCLC is typically staged with the Veterans Administration Lung Cancer Study Group method.[3–5,19]

Non–Small Cell Lung Cancer

Clinical staging of NSCLC with the TNM system evaluates the size of the tumor, extent of nodal involvement, and presence of metastatic sites. The TNM criteria have recently been updated,[20] and went into effect in January 2010.[4] The combination of these three evaluations determines the stage. Clinical stages and associated survival rates are described in Table 106-2. For comparison of various therapeutic modalities, a simpler stage grouping system is used in which stage I refers to tumors confined to the lung without lymphatic spread, stage II refers to large tumors with ipsilateral peribronchial or hilar lymph node involvement, stage III includes other lymph node and regional involvement, and stage IV includes tumor with distant metastases. Local disease is associated with the highest cure and survival rates, whereas those with advanced disease have less than a 10% 5-year survival rate.

TABLE 106-2 Tumor (T), Node (N), Metastasis (M) Staging for Non–Small Cell Lung Cancer

Primary Tumor	Description
T_1	Tumor ≤3 cm in diameter, surrounded by lung or visceral pleura, without invasion more proximal than lobar bronchus
T_{1a}	Tumor ≤2 cm in diameter
T_{1b}	Tumor >2 cm but ≤3 cm in diameter
T_2	Tumor >3 cm but ≤7 cm, or tumor with any of the following features: – Involves main bronchus, ≥2 cm distal to carina – Invades visceral pleura – Associated with atelectasis or obstructive pneumonitis that extends to the hilar region but does not involve the entire lung
T_{2a}	Tumor >3 cm but ≤5 cm
T_{2b}	Tumor >5 cm but ≤7 cm
T_3	Tumor >7 cm or any of the following: – Directly invades any of the following: chest wall, diaphragm, phrenic nerve, mediastinal pleura, parietal pericardium, main bronchus <2 cm from carina (without involvement of carina) – Atelectasis or obstructive pneumonitis of the entire lung – Separate tumor nodules in the same lobe
T_4	Tumor of any size that invades the mediastinum, heart, great vessels, trachea, recurrent laryngeal nerve, esophagus, vertebral body, carina, or with separate tumor nodules in a different ipsilateral lobe
Regional Lymph Nodes (N)	
N_0	No regional lymph node metastases
N_1	Metastasis in ipsilateral peribronchial and/or ipsilateral hilar lymph nodes and intrapulmonary nodes, including involvement by direct extension
N_2	Metastasis in ipsilateral mediastinal and/or subcarinal lymph node(s)
N_3	Metastasis in contralateral mediastinal, contralateral hilar, ipsilateral or contralateral scalene, or supraclavicular lymph node(s)
Distant Metastasis (M)	
M_0	No distant metastasis
M_1	Distant metastasis
M_{1a}	Separate tumor nodule(s) in a contralateral lobe; tumor with pleural nodules or malignant pleural or pericardial effusion
M_{1b}	Distant metastasis

Stage	T	N	M	5-Year Survival
Stage IA	T_{1a}–T_{1b}	N_0	M_0	73%
Stage IB	T_{2a}	N_0	M_0	58%
Stage IIA	T_{1a}, T_{1b}, T_{2a}	N_1	M_0	46%
	T_{2b}	N_0	M_0	
Stage IIB	T_{2b}	N_1	M_0	36%
	T_3	N_0	M_0	
Stage IIIA	T_{1a}, T_{1b}, T_{2a}, T_{2b}	N_2	M_0	
	T_3	N_1, N_2	M_0	24%
	T_4	N_0, N_1	M_0	
Stage IIIB	T_4	N_2	M_0	9%
	Any T	N_3	M_0	
Stage IV	Any T	Any N	M_{1a} or M_{1b}	13%

From references 4 and 19.

Small Cell Lung Cancer

The most commonly used system of staging SCLC was developed originally by the Veterans Administration Lung Cancer Study Group. This system categorizes SCLC into two stages: limited and extensive disease. When evidence of the tumor is confined to a single hemithorax and can be encompassed by a single radiation port, the disease is considered limited. Any progression beyond this point is extensive disease. About 60% to 70% of patients initially present with extensive-stage disease. The initial pretreatment evaluation of an SCLC patient should include a medical history, a clinical examination, and laboratory survey, as well as a CT scan of the chest, abdomen, and head. Typically the approach is to identify tumor spread that would demonstrate extensive stage, at which time the workup can stop. For patients without extrathoracic disease identified by these tests, a bone scan and bone marrow biopsy should be performed to confirm limited-stage disease.[3,5]

TREATMENT

Desired Outcomes

6 The desired outcomes of lung cancer treatment depend on tumor histology, stage of disease, and patient characteristics such as age, history, and performance status.[3] These aspects must be assessed before appropriate treatment can be recommended. In the development of a patient care plan, keep in mind the ultimate goals of therapy. In patients with early stage disease that can tolerate aggressive treatment, a definitive cure is the desired outcome of treatment, although this end point is not always met. With advanced stage disease the desired outcomes of treating lung cancer patients who can tolerate aggressive therapy include prolongation of survival. Regardless of treatment based on survival, all therapies should ultimately improve quality of life through alleviation of symptoms. The goals of treatment must be considered when selecting a therapeutic plan. Delivering aggressive treatment that may prolong survival by a few months but includes a high potential for toxicity that could significantly decrease patient quality of life needs to be considered. Treatment decisions must include both the healthcare team and an informed and well-counseled patient.

Non–Small Cell Lung Cancer

If left untreated, patients with advanced NSCLC will die within 3 to 5 months and those with early stage disease found with routine care will die within 10 to 11 months.[12] Surgery, radiation therapy, and systemic therapy with cytotoxic chemotherapy and/or targeted therapies are all used in the management of NSCLC patients. The applications of these treatment modalities are determined by stage and other patient-specific factors (e.g., age, performance status).[3,4] Table 106-3 lists commonly used chemotherapy regimens including doses and schedules.[4,6]

Local Disease

7 Local disease is associated with a favorable prognosis, and the goal of therapy is cure. Surgery is the mainstay of treatment and may be used alone or in some situations with radiation and/or chemotherapy. Patients who have comorbid conditions preventing them from being surgical candidates can be treated with radiation in place of surgery with curative intent, although the cure rates are lower. Stage IA and IB tumors are treated with surgery alone; when complete resection is achieved, adjuvant therapy is not routinely recommended.[21] If surgical margins are positive, re-resection is recommended. Alternatively, patients may receive radiotherapy

TABLE 106-3 Common Chemotherapy Regimens Used to Treat Lung Cancer

Non–small cell lung cancer[4]	
Carboplatin/paclitaxel/bevacizumab	Carboplatin AUC 6 IV mg/mL/min on day 1 Paclitaxel 200 mg/m² IV on day 1 Bevacizumab 15 mg/kg IV on day 1 Repeat cycle every 3 weeks—continue bevacizumab until progression
Carboplatin/pemetrexed	Carboplatin AUC 5 mg/mL/min IV on day 1 Pemetrexed 500 mg/m² IV on day 1 Repeat cycle every 3 weeks
Cetuximab/cisplatin/vinorelbine	Cetuximab 400 mg/m² IV first dose on day 1, and then 250 mg/m² IV weekly Cisplatin 80 mg/m² IV on day 1 Vinorelbine 25 mg/m² IV on days 1 and 8 Repeat cycle every 3 weeks
Cisplatin/paclitaxel (CP)	Cisplatin 75 mg/m² IV on day 1 Paclitaxel 175 mg/m² over 24 hours IV on day 1; repeat cycle every 21 days *Or* Cisplatin 80 mg/m² IV on day 1 Paclitaxel 175 mg/m² IV over 3 hours on day 1; repeat cycle every 21 days[87]
Gemcitabine/cisplatin (GC)	Gemcitabine 1,000 mg/m² IV on days 1, 8, 15 Cisplatin 100 mg/m² IV on day 1; repeat cycle every 28 days[42]
Gemcitabine/cisplatin (GCq21)	Gemcitabine 1,200 mg/m² on days 1 and 8 Cisplatin 80 mg/m² IV on day 1; repeat cycle every 21 days[88] *Or* Gemcitabine 1,250 mg/m² on days 1 and 8 Cisplatin 80 mg/m² IV on day 1; repeat cycle every 21 days[87]
Docetaxel/cisplatin (DC)	Docetaxel 75 mg/m² IV on day 1 Cisplatin 75 mg/m² IV on day 1; repeat cycle every 21 days[42]
Paclitaxel/carboplatin (PCb)	Paclitaxel 225 mg/m² IV over 3 hours on day 1 Carboplatin AUC 6 mcg h/mL IV on day 1; repeat cycle every 21 days *Or* Paclitaxel 175 mg/m² IV over 3 hours on day 1 Carboplatin AUC 6 mcg h/mL IV on day 1; repeat cycle every 21 days for 6 cycles
Vinorelbine/cisplatin (VC)	Vinorelbine 25 mg/m² IV weekly Cisplatin 100 mg/m² IV on day 1; repeat cycle every 28 days[43] *Or* Vinorelbine 30 mg/m² IV on days 1 and 8 Cisplatin 80 mg/m² IV on day 1; repeat cycle every 21 days
Etoposide/cisplatin (EP)	Etoposide 100 mg/m² IV on days 1–3 Cisplatin 100 mg/m² IV on day 1; repeat cycle every 28 days
Vinorelbine/gemcitabine (VG)	Vinorelbine 25 mg/m² IV on days 1 and 8 Gemcitabine 1,000 mg/m² on days 1 and 8 Repeat cycle every 21 days
Paclitaxel/gemcitabine (PG)	Paclitaxel 175 mg/m² IV over 3 hours on day 1 Gemcitabine 1,250 mg/m² on days 1 and 8; repeat cycle every 21 days
Gemcitabine/docetaxel (GD)	Gemcitabine 1,000 mg/m² IV on days 1 and 8 Docetaxel 100 mg/m² IV on day 8; repeat cycle every 21 days
Paclitaxel/vinorelbine (PV)	Paclitaxel 135 mg/m² IV on day 1 Vinorelbine 25 mg/m² IV on day 1; repeat cycle every 14 days for 9 cycles[89]
Small cell lung cancer[5]	
Etoposide/cisplatin (EP)	Cisplatin 80 mg/m² IV on day 1 Etoposide 100 mg/m² IV on days 1–3; repeat cycle every 3 weeks[83,92] *or* Cisplatin 60 mg/m² IV on day 1 Etoposide 120 mg/m² IV on days 1–3; repeat cycle every 3 weeks
Cisplatin/irinotecan (IP)	Cisplatin 60 mg/m² IV on day 1 Irinotecan 60 mg/m² IV on days 1, 8, and 15; repeat cycle every 4 weeks *Or* Cisplatin 30 mg/m² IV on day 1 Irinotecan 65 mg/m² IV on days 1 and 8; repeat cycle every 3 weeks

AUC, area under the curve.

with or without chemotherapy. Although controversial, patients with IB tumors and high-risk features (poorly differentiated tumors, vascular invasion, wedge resection, minimal margins, tumors >4 cm, or visceral pleural involvement) may also receive adjuvant chemotherapy.[3,4,21] Postoperative radiation therapy with older techniques may be detrimental and is not recommended.[4,21]

Stage IIA and IIB disease is primarily treated with surgery, which should be followed by adjuvant chemotherapy. The adjuvant treatment regimen of choice is not clear, but the positive clinical trials used platinum-based regimens, with arguably the best data coming from cisplatin–vinorelbine (Table 106-4).[4,21,22] The absolute benefit in terms of 5-year overall survival in large randomized trials ranges from no benefit to 15%, with a recent systematic review reporting an absolute difference of 5%.[4,21] Adjuvant radiation should be avoided in patients who have complete resection and clean margins because it has not demonstrated to be beneficial and can be detrimental. In those with resected lung cancer and N_2 nodal disease, radiation is recommended followed by adjuvant chemotherapy. Radiation, or more commonly chemoradiotherapy, is the treatment of choice for stage II patients who are medically inoperable. Concurrent rather than sequential administration of chemotherapy and radiation therapy is preferred. The chemotherapy portion of concurrent chemoradiotherapy is platinum-based, with the preferred regimen being cisplatin and etoposide.[4]

Locally Advanced Disease (Stage III)

7 Patients with more advanced local disease have large tumors, multiple tumors, and/or nodal involvement—particularly mediastinal nodal involvement (N_2). Collectively this group of patients is heterogeneous and few well-defined large trials are available to guide treatment. Consequently, treatment is best planned by a multimodality team where individual features and patient input are considered. Optimal outcomes are achieved with multimodality therapy that typically includes systemic chemotherapy. Patients with operable disease should be considered for surgery preceded or followed by systemic chemotherapy. Adjuvant chemotherapy after surgery in selected patients improves overall survival (Table 106-4).[4,21–31] The primary adjuvant trials included patients with stage IIIA disease as well as early stage disease; 5-year survival in these studies improved by about 5%. Chemotherapy administration prior to surgery (i.e., neoadjuvant) should also be considered. Hypothetically, it will treat micrometastatic disease prior to surgery and reduce the tumor size making surgery easier and better tolerated. However, it is possible that the tumor will grow and become inoperable during therapy. Two meta-analyses have reported that neoadjuvant chemotherapy improves 5-year survival by about 5% compared with surgery alone.[32,33] Although a randomized trial comparing neoadjuvant and adjuvant therapy has not been reported, it appears that both approaches are roughly equivalent and better than surgery alone.

TABLE 106-4 Adjuvant Chemotherapy for Early Stage Lung Cancer

Trial	Stage	Number of Participants	Treatment Arms	Number of Cycles	Postoperative Radiotherapy	5-Year Survival	*P*-Value
BLT	I–IV	381	Observation		Per individual institutional policy	60% (2-year)	0.90
			Cisplatin plus vindesine; mitomycin/ifosfamide; mitomycin/vinblastine; or vinorelbine	3		74% (2-year)	
IALT	I–III	1,867	Observation		Per individual institutional policy	40.4%	0.03
			Cisplatin-based doublet (etoposide, vindesine, vinorelbine, vinblastine)			44.5%	
ALPI	I–IIIA	1,209	Observation		Per individual institutional policy	No difference in overall survival	0.585
			Cisplatin, mitomycin, and vindesine	3			
ANITA	I–IIIA	840	Observation	4	Per individual institutional policy	43%	0.017
			Vinorelbine/cisplatin			51%	
JBR.10	IB–II	482	Observation	4	None	54%	0.002
			Vinorelbine/cisplatin			69%	
CALGB 9633	IB	344	Observation	4	None	57%	0.32
			Paclitaxel/carboplatin			60%	

ALPI, Adjuvant Lung Cancer Project Italy; ANITA, Adjuvant Navelbine International Trialist Association; BLT, Big Lung Trial; CALGB, Cancer and Leukemia Group B; IALT, International Adjuvant Lung Cancer Trial; JBR.10, National Cancer Institute of Canada JBR10.10.

From references 21–31.

Radiation may be given in place of surgery as the local treatment modality combined with chemotherapy. Although a large definitive trial has not been performed, this research question has been evaluated in small randomized trials. The largest trial randomized 333 stage IIIA (N_2) patients who responded to three cycles of induction chemotherapy to radiation or surgery. No significant difference in median overall survival (17.5 months vs. 16.3 months for radiation and surgery, respectively) or overall 5-year survival was observed.[34] This study suggests that surgery could be avoided by administering chemoradiotherapy, although it does not improve survival. Based on the knowledge that dual-modality therapy was better than a single modality, researchers tested trimodal therapy in small studies. None of the studies to date have demonstrated a survival benefit with chemotherapy, radiation, and surgery so it is considered investigational. The results of a randomized trial (SAKK-16/00) addressing this question are scheduled to be reported in the fall of 2013. It is currently recommended that patients with resectable stage IIIA NSCLC be treated with chemotherapy plus either radiation or surgery, depending on individual patient and tumor features.[35]

Patients with stage IIIA disease who are not surgical candidates or have a tumor that cannot reasonably be resected and nearly all stage IIIB patients are usually treated with both an active platinum-containing regimen and concurrent radiotherapy. Patients with tumors that cannot fit safely in a radiation port may receive induction chemotherapy followed by chemoradiotherapy. Responding patients may then become surgical candidates. Patients who are not surgical candidates should continue treatment with concurrent chemotherapy and radiation. Patients who are not candidates for radiation are treated like stage IV disease as discussed below.[4]

Clinical **Controversy. . .**

Multimodality therapy improves outcomes for patients with stage III disease, but the sequence and use of surgery or radiation remains to be defined for the stage as a whole.

Advanced-Stage Disease (Stage IIIB and IV)

8 About two-thirds of NSCLC patients present with advanced disease (unresectable stage IIIB or IV) at the time of diagnosis.[1,3] Most of these advanced tumors are not surgically resectable and have disseminated metastatic disease. A few patients with single metastatic sites may undergo surgical resection of both the primary tumor and the metastatic site.[4] For patients who have a tumor that will fit in a tolerable radiation port, chemoradiotherapy should be considered, but systemic therapy is the primary treatment modality for most of these patients.

The intent of first-line chemotherapy is to palliate symptoms, improve quality of life, and increase the duration of survival. Interestingly, the benefits of cytotoxic chemotherapy—as measured by overall survival and quality of life—were not clearly established until the 1990s. The Non–Small Cell Lung Cancer Collaborative Group reported the pivotal results of a large meta-analysis of 52 clinical trials of chemotherapy in the management of NSCLC.[36] The results of this meta-analysis showed that chemotherapy, either alone or combined with surgery or radiotherapy, improves median survival for patients with advanced-stage NSCLC by 2 to 4 months and increases the 1-year absolute survival rate from 10% to 20%.[36,37] Since chemotherapy became the standard treatment, new agents and targeted therapies have extended these modest gains in survival, while in some cases decreasing toxicity profiles. Current guidelines and experts agree that most patients with advanced-stage disease should receive at least one chemotherapy regimen.[3,4,6]

Patient selection for treatment of advanced-stage NSCLC depends on patient-specific factors that include age, performance status, and comorbid conditions. The patient's current performance status (Eastern Cooperative Oncology Group [ECOG] performance status of 0 to 2) appears to be the most consistent predictor of a better response and improved survival after chemotherapy. All patients with a good performance status without significant comorbidities, including elderly patients, should receive first-line therapy. Patients with an ECOG performance status 2 or significant comorbidities should be considered for less intensive therapy (e.g., single-agent chemotherapy). Patients with poor ECOG performance status (≥3) do not respond well to chemotherapy. Patients with an unfavorable prognosis (poor performance status or significant concomitant diseases) should receive best supportive care and palliative radiation when necessary.[3,4,6,37]

Until the mid-1990s, first-line chemotherapy with etoposide and cisplatin (EP) was regarded as the most active regimen in the treatment of advanced NSCLC. Subsequently, a platinum-based doublet with a newer cytotoxic chemotherapy agent became the standard due to superior response rates or median survival rates.[3,38] Each of these newer chemotherapeutic agents had single-agent activity of greater than 20% in NSCLC and included plant alkaloids (i.e., vinorelbine), taxanes (i.e., paclitaxel and docetaxel), antimetabolites (i.e., gemcitabine), antifolates (i.e., pemetrexed), and topoisomerase I inhibitors (i.e., topotecan and irinotecan).[39] Results from many published trials combining these new chemotherapy agents with platinum-based regimens suggest improved 1-year survival rates in advanced NSCLC of 30% to 40% versus 15% to 25% with older cisplatin-based combination regimens.[38,40,41] A pivotal intergroup study[38] compared four of these newer doublet regimens: cisplatin and paclitaxel, gemcitabine and cisplatin, docetaxel and cisplatin, and carboplatin and paclitaxel. Although all of the regimens had overall survival, gemcitabine and cisplatin had the longest time-to-disease progression. When considering all grade 4 and 5 toxic effects, the carboplatin and paclitaxel doublet was lowest at 57%. The investigators concluded that all four regimens are acceptable, but ECOG chose the carboplatin and paclitaxel regimen for future studies due to the lower risk of grade 4 and 5 toxicity.[38] Table 106-5 shows the outcomes of this study and other selected phase III trials of chemotherapy in patients with advanced NSCLC.[30,38,40,42–45] Patients with a contraindication to a platinum agent achieve similar survival results with gemcitabine in combination with paclitaxel or docetaxel.[6] Survival with this doublet cytotoxic therapy approach reached a survival plateau that prevailed for about a decade. Then in 2006, bevacizumab was proven to increase the efficacy of first-line carboplatin and paclitaxel.[46] Not only did this demonstrate the value of adding a targeted therapy to first-line chemotherapy, it also started a new era where we divide NSCLC in two histologic groups: squamous cell and nonsquamous cell. Although there continues to be multiple acceptable regimens, decision making in the current guidelines depends on classifying advanced-stage NSCLC tumors by their histology (squamous and nonsquamous) as well as genetic mutations or rearrangements.[4] Not all targeted agents are associated with additional benefit when added to a platinum doublet. The clinical benefit of adding erlotinib to doublet platinum-based chemotherapy has been studied in two large, randomized controlled trials, with each enrolling more than 1,000 patients.[47,48] These studies and others suggest that small molecule tyrosine kinase inhibitors are not synergistic with chemotherapy, while monoclonal antibodies can be synergistic with chemotherapy in lung cancer.

Squamous Cell Histology Little has changed for patients diagnosed with advanced-stage squamous cell lung cancer since the mid-1990s. The standard of care continues to be a platinum doublet as described above.[4] The lack of progress represents the failure or minor improvement of targeted therapies to be safe and effective in this histology. The only regimen with a targeted agent consists of cetuximab, cisplatin, and vinorelbine. Support of this combination as first-line treatment of advanced NSCLC came from the First-Line ErbituX (FLEX) trial. The primary study end point involving 1,125 patients showed that cetuximab prolonged median overall survival by 1.2 months (11.3 months vs. 10.1 months [hazard ratio for death 0.87, 95% CI 0.762 to 0.996; $P = 0.044$).[49] Although the study met the primary end point, some have questioned whether the survival advantage is large enough to justify an expensive drug that has toxicity, especially since the goal of treatment is to improve quality and duration of life.[50] Because the available data from this trial and others are generally outdated and enrollment was not restricted to patients with only squamous histology, we rely on overall outcomes and subset analysis to evaluate different regimens. Combination chemotherapy regimens that have consistently reported response rates exceeding 30% have used various combinations of

TABLE 106-5 First-Line Combination Regimens in Stage IIIB or IV Non–Small Cell Lung Cancer

Reference	Number Evaluable/ Performance Status	Regimen	Overall Response Rate (%)	Median Survival Duration	Median 1-Year Survival (%)	Time-to-Disease Progression
Scagliotti et al.[51]	1,725	GC	28.2%	10.3 months	41.9%	5.1 months
	All PS 0-1	Pem/C	30.6%	10.3 months	43.5%	4.8 months
Schiller et al.	1,155	CP	21%	7.8 months	31%	3.4 months
(ECOG 1594)[38]	1,083 PS-0-1, 63 PS-2	GC	22%	8.1 months	36%	4.2 months[a]
		DC	17%	7.4 months	31%	3.7 months
		PCb	17%	8.1 months	34%	3.1 months
Kelly et al. (SWOG)[40]	408	PCb	PR 27%	8 months	36%	NR
	All PS-0-1	VC	PR 27%	8 months	33%	NR
		EP	22%	7.2 months	NR	7.2 months
Gridelli et al.[43]	503	VG	25%	8 months	31%	4.3 months
	PS-0-2	GCq21	30%	9.5 months	38%	5.8 months
		VCq21				
Smit et al. (EORTC)[44]	458	CP	32%	8.1 months	36%	4.2 months
	PS-0-2	GCq21	37%	8.9 months	33%	5.1 months
		PG	28%	6.7 months	27%	3.5 months[b]
Georgoulias et al.[42]	389	GD	30%	9 months	34%	4 months
	PS-0-2	VC	39%	9.7 months	41%	5 months
Stathopoulos et al.[45]	360	PV	43%	10 months	38%	6 months
	PS-0-2	PCb	46%	11 months	43%	7 months

CP, cisplatin and paclitaxel; DC, docetaxel and cisplatin; ECOG, Eastern Cooperative Oncology Group; EORTC, European Organization for Research and Treatment of Cancer; EP, etoposide and cisplatin; GC, gemcitabine and cisplatin; GCq21, gemcitabine and cisplatin repeated every 21 days; GD, gemcitabine and docetaxel; NR, not reported; PCb, paclitaxel and carboplatin; Pem/C, pemetrexed and cisplatin; PG, paclitaxel and gemcitabine; PR, partial response; PS, performance status; PV, paclitaxel and vinorelbine; SWOG, Southwest Oncology Group; VC, vinorelbine and cisplatin; VG, vinorelbine and gemcitabine.

[a]Statistically significant difference.

[b]Statistically significant difference between CP and PG, but not CP and GCq21.

cisplatin, carboplatin, and gemcitabine, paclitaxel, docetaxel, and vinorelbine (see Tables 106-3 and 106-5). Analysis of a trial comparing cisplatin and gemcitabine versus cisplatin and pemetrexed showed that the results depended on histology. Patients with squamous histology had a significant improvement in survival with cisplatin and gemcitabine versus cisplatin and pemetrexed ($n = 473$; 10.8 months vs. 9.4 months, respectively). Therefore, some clinicians have extrapolated these data and other subset analyses to support cisplatin and gemcitabine as the platinum doublet of choice for squamous histology.[51] However, cisplatin and vinorelbine with or without cetuximab, or carboplatin and paclitaxel are also reasonable options.[4]

A number of trials and meta-analyses have been performed to determine if carboplatin and cisplatin are equally effective or if one is more effective in NSCLC.[52–55] Individual clinical trials have produced equivocal data; even meta-analyses evaluating both agents disagree.[52,54,55] One meta-analysis of doublet regimens reported that cisplatin was slightly superior when combined with a "newer" agent; cisplatin improved survival by 11% ($P = 0.039$).[53] Clinical trials comparing the two agents have also demonstrated a different toxicity profile. Cisplatin is associated with more GI (severe nausea and vomiting) and renal toxicity than carboplatin. However, carboplatin is associated with more hematologic toxicity (thrombocytopenia) than cisplatin.[54] Although neither is clearly superior to the other, many clinicians have historically used carboplatin because of its more tolerable GI toxicity, but over the past few years the trend has reversed toward increased use of cisplatin, which could be attributed to improved antiemetics (i.e., the neurokinin-1 receptor antagonist aprepitant).

Nonplatinum doublets (e.g., gemcitabine plus paclitaxel or docetaxel) have been evaluated in the setting of first-line therapy of advanced NSCLC. The results of a meta-analysis comparing platinum-based regimens with either the same regimen without the platinum or the platinum replaced by another agent demonstrated that platinum provides a modest benefit.[56,57] One meta-analysis evaluated 17 trials with a total of 4,792 patients and found a small but significant 1-year survival benefit with a platinum-based combination regimen compared with nonplatinum combination regimens (relative risk = 1.08, 95% CI 1.01 to 1.16).[57] Further analysis of carboplatin regimens and cisplatin regimens demonstrated that benefit was only seen with cisplatin-based regimens. Although platinum-based combination regimens remain the preferred treatment, nonplatinum-based combinations are acceptable and recommended in patients with a contraindication to a platinum agent.

Addition of a third drug to a platinum doublet has been extensively studied. Although combinations of three cytotoxic agents usually increase response rates, they do not consistently prolong overall survival and increase toxicity.[58] Because the goal of treatment for advanced-stage disease is to prolong life and improve quality of life, the use of three cytotoxic agents has not become a standard of care.

The duration of first-line therapy has also been studied. The optimal number of cycles remains controversial.[59] Response rates and quality of life were not improved with administration of six as compared with three cycles of mitomycin, cisplatin, and vinblastine.[60] For those receiving paclitaxel–carboplatin, administration of chemotherapy until disease progression had no clinically significant benefit in survival, response rate, or quality of life, but increased toxicity as compared with administration of four cycles.[61] Many large randomized trials have used six cycles as a standard. Current guidelines recommend a total of four to six cycles of first-line platinum-based doublet chemotherapy for advanced squamous cell lung cancer that is stable or responding to chemotherapy.[4] The one exception to this recommendation is when cetuximab is added to cisplatin plus vinorelbine, where the chemotherapy portion stops after six cycles, but the cetuximab continues until progress (continuation maintenance).[49]

Nonsquamous Histology Patients with advanced nonsquamous histology have new treatment options that have improved outcomes. Selecting therapy begins at the time of diagnosis where tumor tissue samples should undergo genetic testing. More specifically, tumor tissue needs to be tested for mutations in the kinase domain of EGFR, exon 19 and mutation of exon 21 (del746-750 and L858R), as well as for the EML4-ALK rearrangement. Tumors that harbor one of these genetic mutations (positive findings) will have a different treatment plan.[4]

Patients who have a tumor that harbors a mutation in the EGFR receptor should receive first-line erlotinib. A recent trial that compared first-line erlotinib, a relatively nontoxic EGFR tyrosine kinase inhibitor to standard platinum-doublet therapy (EUTRAC trial), found erlotinib to be superior.[62] The study was stopped at the interim analysis because of the difference in progression-free survival (9.7 months vs. 5.2 months). As expected the patients receiving erlotinib had less severe adverse events than the patients who received the platinum doublet (6% vs. 20%, respectively). The different toxicities were consistent with prior studies with these regimens; grade 3 to 4 rash occurred in 13% of erlotinib patients and none of the chemotherapy patients, while grade 3 to 4 neutropenia occurred in 22% of platinum doublet patients and none of the erlotinib patients.[62] It is also noteworthy that the erlotinib is continued until disease progression or intolerable toxicity.

The NCCN guidelines recommend that patients whose tumors have an ALK rearrangement should be treated with crizotinib, an ALK tyrosine kinase inhibitor.[4] FDA approval was based on a single-arm phase II trial because of the very impressive results seen in pretreated patients. The original study reported that more than one half had received two or more prior treatments, and 41% had received three or more prior treatments. The response rate in this heavily pretreated patient population was 57%, and one patient achieved a complete response.[63] After its approval, crizotinib has been evaluated in a randomized phase III trial where it was compared with standard second-line chemotherapy (pemetrexed or docetaxel). Patients treated with crizotinib had a higher response rate (65% vs. 20%; P <0.0001) and longer progression-free survival (7.7 months vs. 3 months, P <0.0001). Although first-line crizotinib is currently being evaluated in a phase III trial, the impressive activity in the relapsed setting led the panel to recommend crizotinib as first-line therapy.[64] Toxicity was comparable in patients treated with second-line crizotinib and single-agent chemotherapy (59% all grades in both groups), but clearly differed by type of toxicity. Crizotinib toxicity was GI in nature (diarrhea 53%, nausea 52%, vomiting 44%, and elevated liver enzymes 36%), while the chemotherapy had comparable nausea (35%), but more myelosuppression (neutropenia 22%) and alopecia (20%). An additional measure of toxicity is the proportion of patients who discontinued treatment because of toxicity; 6% of crizotinib patients and 10% of chemotherapy patients discontinued treatment because of drug toxicity, which was consistent with crizotinib's improved quality of life.

For advanced-stage patients whose tumor does not have one of these mutations, better options than the historical four to six cycles of a platinum doublet are available. Bevacizumab was the first targeted agent that improved outcomes compared with a platinum doublet and also started the movement toward individualized therapy based on histology (based on toxicity). A phase II trial randomized 99 chemotherapy-naïve patients with advanced or recurrent NSCLC to carboplatin and paclitaxel, either alone or combined with bevacizumab 7.5 or 15 mg/kg.[65] Patients with CNS metastases, nonhealing wounds, significant cardiovascular disease, significant peripheral vascular disease, active secondary malignancy, pregnancy, or major surgery within 4 weeks of starting therapy, and those requiring anticoagulation were excluded from the trial because of concern over excessive toxicity to the angiogenesis inhibitor. An independent review faculty evaluated the data and found a response rate of 40%, 22%, and 31% and a median survival of 17.7, 11.6, and 14.9 months for the high-dose bevacizumab arm, the low-dose bevacizumab arm, and the control arm, respectively. Nineteen patients in the control arm crossed over to bevacizumab monotherapy on disease progression. Five patients had disease stabilization, and 1-year survival was 47% following crossover. Adverse effects of chemotherapy were not statistically different with the addition of bevacizumab. However, leucopenia, diarrhea, fever, headache, rash, and chills were slightly more common in the bevacizumab-containing arms. In addition, several patients in the bevacizumab arms developed hypertension, proteinuria, and bleeding. Bleeding events included minor mucocutaneous hemorrhage (most commonly grade 1 or 2 epistaxis) and major hemoptysis. Four patients died as a result of hemoptysis or hematemesis; two others experienced life-threatening bleeding complications. All six patients had centrally located tumors, five had necrosis of tumors, and four of the patients had squamous cell carcinoma.[65] This trial led to a prospective, randomized trial evaluating the addition of bevacizumab 15 mg/kg every 3 weeks until progression to carboplatin and paclitaxel for six cycles compared with carboplatin and paclitaxel alone.[46] The bevacizumab was continued until progression or unacceptable toxicity. As a result of bleeding complications seen in the phase II trial, patients with squamous cell carcinoma or brain metastases were excluded. The addition of bevacizumab led to longer progression-free survival from 4.5 to 6.2 months (P <0.001), median survival from 10.3 to 12.3 months ($P = 0.003$), and 1-year survival from 44% to 51%. The risk of bleeding events was significantly higher in the bevacizumab-containing arm (4.4% vs. 0.7%, P <0.001). Seventeen treatment-related deaths occurred during the study: 2 in the carboplatin and paclitaxel group and 15 in the carboplatin, paclitaxel, and bevacizumab group. Other adverse events seen more frequently in the carboplatin, paclitaxel, and bevacizumab group include hypertension, neutropenia, febrile neutropenia, thrombocytopenia, hyponatremia, rash, and headache (P <0.05).[46] NCCN guidelines recommend the addition of bevacizumab to chemotherapy for patients with advanced NSCLC of nonsquamous cell histology, no history of recent significant hemoptysis, no CNS metastasis, and not receiving therapeutic anticoagulation.[4] Interestingly, a recently published study that randomized patients to cisplatin and gemcitabine with or without bevacizumab did not find any survival benefit with the addition of bevacizumab.[66] This trial indicates that bevacizumab is not synergistic with all chemotherapy regimens and consequently should only be used in combination with carboplatin and paclitaxel for lung cancer at this time.

Another study that reported differentiated response by histology was a phase III trial comparing six cycles of cisplatin and either gemcitabine or pemetrexed. Overall survival with cisplatin and pemetrexed was noninferior to cisplatin and gemcitabine in all patients (10.3 months vs. 10.3 months, respectively) and in those with nonsquamous histology (11.8 months vs. 10.4 months, hazard ratio 1.23; 95% CI 1 to 1.51; $P = 0.05$). The cisplatin and pemetrexed had less neutropenia, anemia, and thrombocytopenia but more nausea than cisplatin and gemcitabine.[51] This study supports the concept that pemetrexed has limited activity in squamous cell histology, but is as good as other new agents when combined with a platinum agent.

Several studies demonstrate that continuation or switch maintenance therapy improves survival of NSCLC patients with nonsquamous histology. Continuation maintenance therapy is continuing at least one of the agents used in a combination for four to six cycles until progression. Alternatively, switch maintenance therapy is starting a new agent in responding patients after four to six cycles. Pemetrexed and erlotinib are the agents that have proven survival benefit as maintenance (switch or continuation).[4]

Two large trials have evaluated pemetrexed as maintenance therapy.[67,68] In the largest phase III trial, 663 patients who responded to platinum-doublet therapy were randomized (2:1) to pemetrexed maintenance (switch maintenance) or no further therapy until relapse. The results show that pemetrexed maintenance therapy prolonged median overall survival (13.4 months vs. 10.6 months, $P = 0.012$).[33] Interestingly, the benefit was only seen in patients with nonsquamous histology, and the best results occurred in patients with adenocarcinoma (median survival 16.8 months vs. 11.5 months for placebo, hazard ratio 0.73, 95% CI 0.56 to 0.96). This histology specificity is consistent with pemetrexed as first-line therapy in combination with cisplatin and also as second-line monotherapy.[67] The second large study enrolled 939 nonsquamous histology patients and treated them with four cycles of cisplatin and pemetrexed. The 539 patients who showed benefit from treatment (responders and stable disease) were randomized to continuation maintenance with pemetrexed or placebo. Continuation maintenance with pemetrexed resulted in a longer median overall survival (13.9 months vs. 11 months) and 1-year survival (58% vs. 45%).[68] These two studies clearly established maintenance therapy as standard therapy, but for patients who start a doublet with bevacizumab, it is unclear if both bevacizumab and pemetrexed should be used as continuation maintenance. Initial results from the Alimta/Avastin vs. Avastin Alone (AVAPERL) study show that bevacizumab and pemetrexed are superior than bevacizumab alone based on progression-free survival.[69] However, a larger study that compared carboplatin, paclitaxel, and bevacizumab with bevacizumab continued maintenance to carboplatin, pemetrexed, and bevacizumab with bevacizumab and pemetrexed continuation maintenance found no difference in overall survival.[70] Results of large ongoing studies will address this important research question.

Clinical **Controversy. . .**

The benefit of maintenance pemetrexed and bevacizumab for patients with nonsquamous cell stage IV NSCLC is proven. However, the benefit of bevacizumab and pemetrexed versus pemetrexed alone as maintenance is unknown. Additional clinical trial results to clarify optimal maintenance therapy for patients with nonsquamous stage IV NSCLC are needed.

Another recently reported randomized phase III trial shows that maintenance therapy with erlotinib prolongs disease-free survival versus placebo (Sequential Tarceva in Unresectable NSCLC [SATURN] study).[71] A total of 1,949 patients received four cycles of a platinum doublet; the 889 patients without progressive disease were then randomized to erlotinib or placebo. Erlotinib maintenance prolonged survival by 1 month (11 months vs. 12 months), which included all patients (11% with EGFR mutation and 89% EGFR wild type). Interestingly, erlotinib maintenance appeared to be most effective in patients with adenocarcinoma histology and in those with an EGFR mutation. Although this study is compelling, pemetrexed is more commonly used because those with an EGFR mutation should receive first-line erlotinib and continue it until progression.[4]

Studies evaluating gemcitabine[72] and docetaxel[73] maintenance therapy have been reported with some compelling data. Both studies demonstrate that maintenance therapy improved progression-free survival, with a nonsignificant trend for improved overall survival. These agents should be considered in patients with a contraindication to pemetrexed and erlotinib.

In summary, patients with advanced-stage nonsquamous histology NSCLC should have their tumor tested for an EGFR mutation or ALK rearrangement. Patients with a positive mutation should receive erlotinib (positive EGFR mutation) or crizotinib (ALK rearrangement). Those patients without a mutation should receive four to six cycles of a platinum doublet with bevacizumab or alternatively cetuximab. For those with a contraindication to bevacizumab, treatment with just a doublet is recommended. For patients who have stable disease after or respond to four to six cycles of doublet therapy with or without bevacizumab, maintenance therapy should be initiated.[4]

Second-Line Chemotherapy Second-line chemotherapy is usually offered to those patients with an ECOG performance status of 0 to 2 who experience disease progression to or after first-line chemotherapy. Third-line therapy can be offered if disease progression continues in a patient with adequate performance status. Best supportive care is recommended by the NCCN guidelines for those patients with disease progression and ECOG performance status worse than 2.[4]

Monotherapy with docetaxel, pemetrexed, or erlotinib is an options for second-line therapy in patients with a good performance status who progress during or after first-line chemotherapy.[4,6] Docetaxel was the first to receive FDA approval for the treatment of advanced NSCLC after failure of a platinum-based chemotherapy regimen. The initial docetaxel dose of 100 mg/m^2 IV over 1 hour every 21 days was decreased to 75 mg/m^2 after an interim analysis showed a greater risk of severe neutropenia with the higher dose. Docetaxel, at the 75 mg/m^2 dose, was superior to best supportive care in terms of time-to-disease progression (10.6 weeks vs. 6.7 weeks, $P = 0.001$), median survival (7.5 months vs. 4.6 months; $P = 0.047$), and 1-year survival (37% vs. 11%; $P = 0.003$).[74] Both doses had a statistically significant improvement in 1-year survival when compared with a control regimen of vinorelbine or ifosfamide (32%, 21%, and 19%, respectively).[75]

Subsequently, pemetrexed (Alimta) was FDA approved for second-line treatment of advanced NSCLC based on results of a phase III trial.[76] In that trial, 571 patients were randomized to receive either pemetrexed 500 mg/m^2 with folate and cyanocobalamin supplementation or docetaxel 75 mg/m^2. No significant differences in overall response rate, stable disease, or median survival between the pemetrexed and docetaxel arms were observed. Docetaxel had significantly more hematologic toxicities as compared with pemetrexed, leading to more hospitalizations and use of hematopoietic growth factors and erythropoiesis-stimulating agents. Patients receiving docetaxel had a significantly higher incidence of alopecia, while patients receiving pemetrexed had a significantly higher elevation of alanine aminotransferase.[76]

Erlotinib, a relatively nontoxic agent that targets the EGFR, was approved in November 2004 as a single agent for patients with advanced NSCLC whose disease progressed after at least one prior chemotherapy regimen. Its approval was based on an international, multicenter, randomized, double-blind phase III trial (BR.21)[77] in 731 patients with locally advanced or metastatic NSCLC who had failed at least one prior chemotherapy regimen. Patients were randomized to receive either erlotinib 150 mg or placebo orally once daily. Patients in the erlotinib group had a significantly higher objective response rate (9% vs. 1%, $P < 0.001$) and longer median progression-free and overall survival (9.9 weeks vs. 7.9 weeks, $P < 0.001$ and 6.7 months vs. 4.7 months [hazard ratio = 0.73], $P < 0.001$, respectively) than those in the placebo group. Patients in the erlotinib group also had significantly improved symptom control, specifically time-to-deterioration of cough, dyspnea, and pain.[77] Although these benefits are relatively modest, some individual patients show a profound response. This has led researchers to search for patient and tumor-specific factors (i.e., biomarkers) that can be used to select patients who are likely to respond to an EGFR inhibitor. Patients who have the following characteristics are most likely to respond to EGFR inhibitors: never smokers, women,

Asians, and those with adenocarcinoma histology, particularly the bronchial alveolar carcinoma subset of adenocarcinoma. Analysis of predictive biomarkers led to EGFR mutational testing and to the recommendation that patients who have EGFR mutation-positive tumors should receive first-line erlotinib.[4,62]

In summary, patients with a good performance status should receive second-line therapy, which is determined by histology and first-line treatment. In general, drugs are not repeated, and patients with squamous histology do not receive pemetrexed or erlotinib. Other active agents can be used as monotherapy.

Elderly and Poor-Performance Status Patients Single-agent chemotherapy is an alternative in elderly patients or those with an ECOG performance status of 2.[4,6] First-line, single-agent chemotherapy has objective response rates of 5% to 25% with no significant effect on overall survival. Complete responses are rare and responses that do occur are of brief duration (i.e., 2 to 4 months).[3,78] Among the most active cytotoxic chemotherapy agents in NSCLC are cisplatin, carboplatin, docetaxel, paclitaxel, etoposide, gemcitabine, ifosfamide, irinotecan, topotecan, mitomycin, vinblastine, vinorelbine, and pemetrexed.[4] Erlotinib and crizotinib are also active as a single agent and should be considered in patients with a mutation-positive tumor.

Historically, patients with a ECOG performance status 2 were excluded from NSCLC trials because of excessive toxicity with minimal benefit from combination cytotoxic therapy. A recent randomized phase III trial[79] comparing single-agent weekly docetaxel (n = 171) with docetaxel and gemcitabine (n = 174) in elderly or poor performance status (35% of patients) had disappointing results. No survival differences were observed with docetaxel and gemcitabine versus weekly docetaxel in the 122 poor-performance status patients (3.8 months vs. 2.9 months, respectively), and the median survival is short compared with patients with good performance status.[79] Another randomized phase III trial[80] compared single-agent gemcitabine (n = 85) with gemcitabine/carboplatin (n = 85) in PS-2 patients. The median overall survival was not different between gemcitabine and gemcitabine/carboplatin (5.1 months vs. 6.7 months, respectively). The authors concluded that single-agent therapy is still the standard in this setting.[80] The updated ASCO guidelines state that available data support the use of single-agent chemotherapy and data are insufficient to recommend combination therapy.[6] A recent meta-analysis shows that patients with performance status 2 benefit from treatment.[81]

Personalized Pharmacotherapy

The translation of basic science to the clinic has resulted in personalized pharmacotherapy plans. Treatment decisions are influenced by tumor biology and patient characteristics (e.g., comorbidities and performance status). The primary tumor biology issues evolve around new targeted therapies where histology (squamous vs. nonsquamous histology) and genetic mutations determine the most effective therapy (EGFR mutation, EML4-ALK rearrangement) and duration of therapy. The histology can also correlate with risk of toxicity, such as major bleeding with bevacizumab-treated squamous cell histology patients.

Treatment guidelines generally apply to patients who are fit and desire aggressive therapy. Patient-specific factors that can alter these recommendations include age and comorbid conditions that serve as a relative or absolute contraindication to aggressive platinum-based doublet therapy and even some targeted therapies such that the risk of toxicity outweighs the benefit. For example, elderly patients or those with an ECOG performance status of 2 have a modest benefit to aggressive platinum-doublet therapy; patients with an ECOG performance status of 3 have little to no benefit and a high risk of toxicity. Other considerations include renal dysfunction and the use of a platinum agent, and history of hemoptysis and the use of bevacizumab. Although these examples appear to provide clear guidance, risk is often a continuum and it is sometimes not clear how to treat individual patients (e.g., a fully functioning 50-year-old with angina and a serum creatinine of 1.7 mg/dL and stage IIIB squamous cell lung cancer).

Evaluation of Therapeutic Outcomes

For patients who have undergone surgical resection with or without chemotherapy, radiation, or both, a physical examination and chest radiography are recommended every 3 to 4 months for the first 2 years, then every 6 months for 3 years, and then annually. In addition, a low-dose spiral chest CT scan is recommended annually to monitor for evidence of local recurrence. Suspicious symptoms or physical findings (e.g., bone pain, visual abnormalities, headache, or elevated liver function tests) should prompt an evaluation to rule out distant metastases.[3–5]

Tumor response to chemotherapy is generally evaluated at the end of the second or third cycle and at the end of every second cycle thereafter. Patients with stable disease, with objective response, or with measurable decrease in tumor size (complete or partial response) should continue until four to six cycles have been administered. Patients with nonsquamous histology tumors who respond (i.e., nonprogressive disease) should be considered for maintenance therapy with pemetrexed. Following initial therapy for NSCLC, patients must be monitored for evidence of disease progression.[3–5]

Small Cell Lung Cancer

SCLC is a rapidly dividing malignancy that spreads early in the disease course. Consequently, most patients present with extensive-stage disease (about 60% to 70% of new cases). When patients with SCLC are not treated, the disease quickly becomes fatal. Fortunately, small cell carcinomas are very responsive to chemotherapy and radiation. Chemotherapy with or without radiotherapy is the treatment of choice for most patients. Even after a complete response to therapy, the cancer usually recurs within 6 to 8 months, and survival time following recurrence is typically short (about 4 months). With treatment, median survival rates for patients with limited and extensive disease are 14 to 20 and 9 to 11 months, respectively. Treatment planning starts with stage of disease (i.e., limited vs. extensive stage), but must also take into account other factors, including performance status (treatment usually restricted to performance status 0 or 1), patient age, comorbid conditions (e.g., renal failure), and patient desire to receive treatment.[3,5]

Limited Disease

(7) When a single SCLC mass is found, local therapy with radiation or surgery is considered, although the use of surgery in SCLC is limited to solitary nodules, without evidence of metastasis to lymph nodes. One of the factors differentiating SCLC and NSCLC is the fact that radiation is favored for treatment of local disease over surgery. Radiation is always combined with chemotherapy in limited-stage SCLC, and the regimen of choice is EP. Carboplatin may be substituted for cisplatin to reduce nausea and vomiting, nephrotoxicity, or neurotoxicity,[82] although increased myelosuppression in the form of thrombocytopenia may result. In European countries, a three-drug combination containing an anthracycline has been the mainstay of therapy, but mounting clinical evidence shows that these regimens are inferior to EP plus concurrent radiation and have more toxicity.[83] Consequently, the guidelines recommend that the EP regimen be used with concurrent radiotherapy.[5] Because patients with SCLC commonly have a recurrence in the CNS, trials have been performed to evaluate the benefit of prophylactic cranial irradiation (PCI). A pivotal study showed that PCI reduces the incidence of brain metastasis and increases 3-year survival from 15% to 21%.[84,85] Therefore, patients who achieve a complete response with treatment should be offered PCI.

Extensive Disease

8 Platinum regimens are also the treatment of choice in extensive disease, and many studies have failed to show superiority to the EP regimen as first-line treatment. A combination of irinotecan and cisplatin in one Japanese study demonstrated an increased median survival time by about 3 months over the EP regimen. This regimen showed a lower incidence of severe neutropenic side effects but exhibited higher rates of moderate- to high-grade diarrhea in an Asian population.[86] However, irinotecan and cisplatin failed to improve survival as compared with EP in a study conducted in the United States.[87] Therefore, EP remains the regimen of choice for treating extensive-stage SCLC in the United States, with irinotecan and cisplatin reserved as an acceptable alternative. Concurrent radiotherapy is not used routinely in extensive disease. However, a recent study that randomized extensive-stage patients responding to chemotherapy to observation or PCI reported that PCI decreased the 1-year risk of brain metastasis (14.6% vs. 40.4%), and prolonged survival (27.1% vs. 13.3% at 1 year).[88] This study led to guideline revisions recommending PCI for patients with extensive disease responding to chemotherapy.[5]

Recurrent Disease

SCLC patients who relapse or progress after first-line chemotherapy have a median survival of 4 to 5 months. Unfortunately, when disease recurs, it is usually less sensitive to chemotherapy. The decision of whether or not to use second-line chemotherapy is often based on the length of time between completion of the induction chemotherapy regimen and relapse. If this interval is less than 3 months, the patient has refractory SCLC and is unlikely to respond to second-line therapy; hence, they should receive best supportive care or be enrolled in a clinical trial. For those with greater than a 3-month time interval between first-line chemotherapy and relapse, the expected response rate to treatment is approximately 25%, and second-line therapy should be considered.[3,5] Topotecan (IV and oral) is the only FDA-approved second-line therapy for SCLC. The pivotal trial[89] leading to the approval randomized patients to IV topotecan or the cyclophosphamide, doxorubicin, and vincristine (CAV) regimen. The response rates (24% vs. 18%), time-to-disease progression (13 weeks vs. 12 weeks), and overall survival (25 weeks vs. 25 weeks) were not different between groups. Interestingly, the proportion of patients experiencing symptom improvement was higher in the topotecan arm. The hematologic toxicity was similar between arms; there was slightly more neutropenia in the CAV arm and more anemia and thrombocytopenia in the topotecan arm. Nonhematologic toxicity appears to be higher in the CAV arm; 11% of patients required a dose reduction compared with 1% in the topotecan arm.[89] Oral topotecan appears to be equally effective and similar in terms of dosing, toxicity, and effectiveness as IV topotecan.[90] Based on these studies, topotecan should be considered as the second-line treatment of choice, but because of the modest efficacy other agents warrant consideration. Agents that are recommended in national guidelines[5] include single-agent topotecan, irinotecan, gemcitabine, paclitaxel, docetaxel, and vinorelbine; CAV regimen; and participation in a clinical trial.

Personalized Pharmacotherapy

Personalized pharmacotherapy based on tumor biology has not become a standard for SCLC. However, there is a significant push in research to identify targeted drug therapy that will improve the outcomes of all or subpopulations of patients with SCLC. Current trials are looking at drugs that inhibit specific targets including insulin growth factor receptor 1R, PI3K, AKT, mTOR, Hedgehog, and apoptosis. In order to increase the likelihood of success with these agents, trials are enrolling patients where the relevant pathway appears to be active. If a drug inhibiting a specific pathway proves to be beneficial, then optimal treatment may be individualized based on the tumor biology. Until then, we will continue to choose treatment primarily based on stage, comorbid conditions, and performance status. Similar to NSCLC, patients without comorbid conditions and good performance status will typically receive a platinum doublet (cisplatin and etoposide), but elderly patients, those with significant comorbid conditions, or those with an ECOG performance status of 2 may receive less aggressive treatment (a single agent), and those with extensive-stage disease who are bedridden will not be given cytotoxic therapy because of a lack of benefit.

Evaluation of Therapeutic Outcomes

The effectiveness of first-line therapy is evaluated after two to three cycles of treatment. At this point, therapy is continued for four to six cycles of therapy in patients with a complete or partial response or stable disease, and discontinued or changed to a non–cross-resistant regimen in patients demonstrating evidence of progressive disease. In the case of SCLC, those with response benefit from the addition of PCI following initial therapy. After recovery from first-line therapy, followup visits should occur every 3 months for years 1, 2, and 3, then every 4 to 6 months for years 4 and 5, and then annually for patients with either a partial or complete response.[5]

Complications and Supportive Care

Patients with lung cancer frequently have numerous concurrent medical problems. Such problems may be related to invasion of the primary tumor and its metastases, paraneoplastic syndromes (see Clinical Presentation earlier), chemotherapy and radiotherapy toxicity, or concomitant disease states (e.g., cardiac disease, renal dysfunction, chronic obstructive pulmonary disease, asthma, or diabetes). Depression is also common and sometimes persistent in patients with SCLC and NSCLC and should be treated. Identification, diagnosis, and treatment of the patient as a whole may improve the patient's overall quality of life and tolerance to cancer treatments.

9 The chemotherapy regimens used in the management of lung cancer are intensive and are associated with a wide variety of toxic effects. Nausea and vomiting may be severe. Cisplatin-containing regimens require the use of aggressive acute and delayed antiemetic regimens containing a serotonin antagonist, dexamethasone, and aprepitant.[91] Patients experiencing protracted nausea and vomiting may require IV hydration and nutritional support. Myelosuppression is often the dose-limiting toxicity associated with chemotherapy. Granulocytopenia places patients at a high risk for serious infections. Other toxic effects associated with these chemotherapy regimens include mucositis, anemia, nephrotoxicity, peripheral neuropathies, and ototoxicity.

About 30% to 65% of advanced-stage NSCLC patients will develop bone metastases, which may lead to significant bone pain, pathologic fractures, spinal cord compression, and hypercalcemia.[92] Zoledronic acid, an IV administered bisphosphonate, has been shown to reduce skeletal-related events in patients with bone metastases at a dose of 4 mg over 15 minutes infused every 3 weeks. Although the data do not show a significant reduction in skeletal-related events, time to first event is significantly increased (230 days vs. 163 days for placebo, $P = 0.023$), thereby making zoledronic acid a viable therapy for patients with bone metastases.

Patients receiving radiation therapy may experience complications including severe esophagitis, fatigue, radiation pneumonitis, and cardiac toxicity. These toxicities are usually more common and severe when radiation is combined with chemotherapy. The patient's baseline performance status and the degree of pulmonary dysfunction (e.g., chronic obstructive pulmonary disease from years of tobacco use) must be considered in decisions concerning radiation dosage and fractionation.

It is readily apparent that many lung cancer patients receive complex pharmacologic regimens that may include chemotherapeutic agents, antiemetics, antibiotics, analgesics, anticoagulants, bronchodilators, corticosteroids, anticonvulsants, and cardiovascular agents. Such regimens necessitate intensive therapeutic monitoring in order to avoid drug-related and radiotherapy-related toxic effects and to optimize therapeutic outcome for individual patients.

ABBREVIATIONS

AJCC	American Joint Committee on Cancer
ASCO	American Society of Clinical Oncology
CAV	cyclophosphamide, doxorubicin, and vincristine
CI	confidence interval
CT	computed tomography
ECOG	Eastern Cooperative Oncology Group
EGFR	epidermal growth factor receptor
EP	etoposide and cisplatin
ETS	environmental tobacco smoke
FLEX	First-Line ErbituX
LDCT	low-dose computed tomography
NCCN	National Comprehensive Cancer Network
NSAIDs	nonsteroidal antiinflammatory drugs
NSCLC	non–small cell lung cancer
PCI	prophylactic cranial irradiation
PET	positron emission tomography
SATURN	Sequential Tarceva in Unresectable NSCLC
SCLC	small cell lung cancer
SELECT	Selenium and Vitamin E Cancer Prevention Trial
TNM	tumor, node, and metastasis

REFERENCES

1. Siegel R, Naishadham D, Jemal A. Cancer statistics, 2013. CA Cancer J Clin 2013;62:11–30.
2. Couraud S, Cortot AB, Greillier L, et al. From randomized trials to the clinic: Is it time to implement individual lung-cancer screening in clinical practice? A multidisciplinary statement from French experts on behalf of the French intergroup (IFCT) and the Groupe d'Oncologie de langue Francaise (GOLF). Ann Oncol 2013;24:586–597.
3. Johnson DH, Blot WJ, Carbone DP, et al., eds. Cancer of the Lung: Non–Small Cell Lung Cancer and Small Cell Lung Cancer, 4th ed. Philadelphia: Churchill Livingstone Elsevier, 2008.
4. NCCN. NCCN Clinical Practice Guidelines in Oncology: Non-Small Cell Lung Cancer. In: National Comprehensive Cancer Network Inc; V1.2013.
5. NCCN. NCCN Clinical Practice Guidelines in Oncology: Small Cell Lung Cancer. V1.2013.
6. Azzoli CG, Temin S, Aliff T, et al. 2011 Focused Update of 2009 American Society of Clinical Oncology clinical practice guideline update on chemotherapy for Stage IV non-small-cell lung cancer. J Clin Oncol 2011;29: 3825–3831.
7. Dang P, Carbone DP. Cancer of the lung. In: DeVita VTJ, Lawrence TS, Rosenberg SA, eds. DeVita, Hellman, and Rosenberg's Cancer: Principles & Practice of Oncology, 8th ed. Philadelphia: Lippincott Williams & Wilkins, 2008.
8. Girard N. Crizotinib in ALK-positive lung cancer. Lancet Oncol 2012;13:962–963.
9. Alberts WM. Diagnosis and management of lung cancer executive summary: ACCP evidence-based clinical practice guidelines (2nd ed.). Chest 2007;132:1S–19S.
10. Centers for Disease Control and Prevention (CDC). Current cigarette smoking among adults—United States, 2011. MMWR Morb Mortal Wkly Rep 2012;61:889–894.
11. Travis WD. Pathology of lung cancer. Clin Chest Med 2011;32:669–692.
12. Detterbeck FC, Gibson CJ. Turning gray: The natural history of lung cancer over time. J Thorac Oncol 2008;3:781–792.
13. Johnson JL, Pillai S, Chellappan SP. Genetic and biochemical alterations in non-small cell lung cancer. Biochem Res Int 2012;2012:940405.
14. Bach PB, Mirkin JN, Oliver TK, et al. Benefits and harms of CT screening for lung cancer: A systematic review. JAMA 2012;307:2418–2429.
15. Keith RL. Lung cancer chemoprevention. Proc Am Thorac Soc 2012;9:52–56.
16. Kim ES, Lippman SM, Hong WK. Chemoprevention of lung cancer. In: Pass HI, Carbone DP, Johnson DH, eds. Lung Cancer: Principles and Practice, 3rd ed. Philadelphia: Lippincott, Williams & Wilkins, 2005.
17. Kushi LH, Doyle C, McCullough M, et al. American Cancer Society guidelines on nutrition and physical activity for cancer prevention: Reducing the risk of cancer with healthy food choices and physical activity. CA Cancer J Clin 2012;62:30–67.
18. Silvestri GA, Gould MK, Margolis ML, et al. Noninvasive staging of non-small cell lung cancer: ACCP evidenced-based clinical practice guidelines (2nd ed.). Chest 2007;132:178S–201S.
19. Kligerman S, Digumarthy S. Staging of non-small cell lung cancer using integrated PET/CT. AJR Am J Roentgenol 2009;193:1203–1211.
20. Goldstraw P, Crowley J, Chansky K, et al. The IASLC Lung Cancer Staging Project: Proposals for the revision of the TNM stage groupings in the forthcoming (seventh) edition of the TNM classification of malignant tumours. J Thorac Oncol 2007;2:706–714.
21. Pisters KM, Evans WK, Azzoli CG, et al. Cancer Care Ontario and American Society of Clinical Oncology adjuvant chemotherapy and adjuvant radiation therapy for stages I-IIIA resectable non–small cell lung cancer guideline. J Clin Oncol 2007;25:5506–5518.
22. Belani CP, Wang W, Johnson DH, et al. Phase III study of the Eastern Cooperative Oncology Group (ECOG 2597): Induction chemotherapy followed by either standard thoracic radiotherapy or hyperfractionated accelerated radiotherapy for patients with unresectable stage IIIA and B non-small-cell lung cancer. J Clin Oncol 2005;23:3760–3767.
23. Alam N, Darling G, Evans WK, Mackay JA, Shepherd FA. Adjuvant chemotherapy for completely resected non-small cell lung cancer: A systematic review. Crit Rev Oncol Hematol 2006;58:146–155.
24. Alam N, Shepherd FA, Winton T, et al. Compliance with post-operative adjuvant chemotherapy in non-small cell lung cancer. An analysis of National Cancer Institute of Canada and intergroup trial JBR.10 and a review of the literature. Lung Cancer 2005;47:385–394.
25. Arriagada R, Bergman B, Dunant A, Le Chevalier T, Pignon JP, Vansteenkiste J. Cisplatin-based adjuvant chemotherapy in patients with completely resected non-small-cell lung cancer. N Engl J Med 2004;350:351–360.
26. Arriagada R, Dunant A, Pignon JP, et al. Long-term results of the international adjuvant lung cancer trial evaluating adjuvant cisplatin-based chemotherapy in resected lung cancer. J Clin Oncol 2010;28:35–42.
27. Butts CA, Ding K, Seymour L, et al. Randomized phase III trial of vinorelbine plus cisplatin compared with observation

in completely resected stage IB and II non-small-cell lung cancer: Updated survival analysis of JBR-10. J Clin Oncol 2010;28:29–34.
28. Douillard JY, Rosell R, De Lena M, et al. Adjuvant vinorelbine plus cisplatin versus observation in patients with completely resected stage IB-IIIA non-small-cell lung cancer (Adjuvant Navelbine International Trialist Association [ANITA]): A randomised controlled trial. Lancet Oncol 2006;7:719–727.
29. Massard C, Tran Loc P, Haddad V, et al. Use of adjuvant chemotherapy in non-small cell lung cancer in routine practice. J Thorac Oncol 2009;4:1504–1510.
30. Scagliotti GV. The ALPI Trial: The Italian/European experience with adjuvant chemotherapy in resectable non-small lung cancer. Clin Cancer Res 2005;11: 5011s–5016s.
31. Winton T, Livingston R, Johnson D, et al. Vinorelbine plus cisplatin vs. observation in resected non-small-cell lung cancer. N Engl J Med 2005;352:2589–2597.
32. Burdett S, Stewart LA, Rydzewska L. Chemotherapy and surgery versus surgery alone in non-small cell lung cancer [review]. Cochrane Database Syst Rev 2009;1:1–24.
33. Gilligan D, Nicolson M, Smith I, et al. Preoperative chemotherapy in patients with resectable non-small cell lung cancer: Results of the MRC LU22/NVALT 2/EORTC 08012 multicentre randomised trial and update of systematic review. Lancet 2007;369:1929–1937.
34. van Meerbeeck JP, Kramer GWPM, Van Schil PEY, et al. Randomized controlled trial of resection versus radiotherapy after induction chemotherapy in stage IIIA-N2 non–small-cell lung cancer. J Natl Cancer Inst 2007;99: 442–450.
35. Tieu BH, Sanborn RE, Thomas CR Jr. Neoadjuvant therapy for resectable non-small cell lung cancer with mediastinal lymph node involvement. Thorac Surg Clin 2008;18: 403–415.
36. Non-Small Cell Lung Cancer Collaborative Group. Chemotherapy in non-small cell lung cancer: A meta-analysis using updated data on individual patients from 52 randomised clinical trials. BMJ 1995;311:899–909.
37. Spira A, Ettinger DS. Multidisciplinary management of lung cancer. N Engl J Med 2004;350:379–392.
38. Schiller JH, Harrington D, Belani CP, et al. Comparison of four chemotherapy regimens for advanced non-small-cell lung cancer. N Engl J Med 2002;346:92–98.
39. Bonomi P, Kim K, Fairclough D, et al. Comparison of survival and quality of life in advanced non-small-cell lung cancer patients treated with two dose levels of paclitaxel combined with cisplatin versus etoposide with cisplatin: Results of an Eastern Cooperative Oncology Group trial. J Clin Oncol 2000;18:623–631.
40. Kelly K, Crowley J, Bunn PA Jr, et al. Randomized phase III trial of paclitaxel plus carboplatin versus vinorelbine plus cisplatin in the treatment of patients with advanced non–small-cell lung cancer: A Southwest Oncology Group trial. J Clin Oncol 2001;19:3210–3218.
41. Kosmidis P, Mylonakis N, Nicolaides C, et al. Paclitaxel plus carboplatin versus gemcitabine plus paclitaxel in advanced non-small-cell lung cancer: A phase III randomized trial. J Clin Oncol 2002;20:3578–3585.
42. Georgoulias V, Ardavanis A, Tsiafaki X, et al. Vinorelbine plus cisplatin versus docetaxel plus gemcitabine in advanced non-small-cell lung cancer: A phase III randomized trial. J Clin Oncol 2005;23:2937–2945.
43. Gridelli C, Gallo C, Shepherd FA, et al. Gemcitabine plus vinorelbine compared with cisplatin plus vinorelbine or cisplatin plus gemcitabine for advanced non-small-cell lung cancer: A phase III trial of the Italian GEMVIN Investigators and the National Cancer Institute of Canada Clinical Trials Group. J Clin Oncol 2003;21:3025–3034.
44. Smit EF, van Meerbeeck JP, Lianes P, et al. Three-arm randomized study of two cisplatin-based regimens and paclitaxel plus gemcitabine in advanced non-small-cell lung cancer: A phase III trial of the European Organization for Research and Treatment of Cancer Lung Cancer Group—EORTC 08975. J Clin Oncol 2003;21:3909–3917.
45. Stathopoulos GP, Veslemes M, Georgatou N, et al. Front-line paclitaxel-vinorelbine versus paclitaxel-carboplatin in patients with advanced non-small-cell lung cancer: A randomized phase III trial. Ann Oncol 2004;15: 1048–1055.
46. Sandler A, Gray R, Perry MC, et al. Paclitaxel-carboplatin alone or with bevacizumab for non-small-cell lung cancer. N Engl J Med 2006;355:2542–2550.
47. Gatzemeier U, Pluzanska A, Szczesna A, et al. Phase III study of erlotinib in combination with cisplatin and gemcitabine in advanced non-small-cell lung cancer: The Tarceva Lung Cancer Investigation Trial. J Clin Oncol 2007;25:1545–1552.
48. Herbst RS, Prager D, Hermann R, et al. TRIBUTE: A phase III trial of erlotinib hydrochloride (OSI-774) combined with carboplatin and paclitaxel chemotherapy in advanced non-small-cell lung cancer. J Clin Oncol 2005;23: 5892–5899.
49. Pirker R, Pereira JR, Szczesna A, et al. Cetuximab plus chemotherapy in patients with advanced non-small-cell lung cancer (FLEX): An open-label randomised phase III trial. Lancet 2009;373:1525–1531.
50. Hirsch FR, Herbst RS. EGFR expression and the flexibility of FLEX. Lancet Oncol 2012;13:3–5.
51. Scagliotti G, Brodowicz T, Shepherd FA, et al. Treatment-by-histology interaction analyses in three phase III trials show superiority of pemetrexed in nonsquamous non-small cell lung cancer. J Thorac Oncol 2011;6:64–70.
52. Ardizzoni A, Boni L, Tiseo M, et al. Cisplatin- versus carboplatin-based chemotherapy in first-line treatment of advanced non-small-cell lung cancer: An individual patient data meta-analysis. J Natl Cancer Inst 2007;99:847–857.
53. Hotta K, Matsuo K, Ueoka H, Kiura K, Tabata M, Tanimoto M. Meta-analysis of randomized clinical trials comparing cisplatin to carboplatin in patients with advanced non-small-cell lung cancer. J Clin Oncol 2004;22:3852–3859.
54. Jiang J, Liang X, Zhou X, Huang R, Chu Z. A meta-analysis of randomized controlled trials comparing carboplatin-based to cisplatin-based chemotherapy in advanced non-small cell lung cancer. Lung Cancer 2007;57:348–358.
55. Rossi A, Di Maio M, Chiodini P, et al. Carboplatin- or cisplatin-based chemotherapy in first-line treatment of small-cell lung cancer: The COCIS meta-analysis of individual patient data. J Clin Oncol 2012;30:1692–1698.
56. D'Addario G, Pintilie M, Leighl NB, Feld R, Cerny T, Shepherd FA. Platinum-based versus non-platinum-based chemotherapy in advanced non-small-cell lung cancer: A meta-analysis of the published literature. J Clin Oncol 2005;23:2926–2936.
57. Rajeswaran A, Trojan A, Burnand B, Giannelli M. Efficacy and side effects of cisplatin- and carboplatin-based doublet chemotherapeutic regimens versus non-platinum-based doublet chemotherapeutic regimens as first line treatment of metastatic non-small cell lung carcinoma: A systematic review of randomized controlled trials. Lung Cancer 2008;59:1–11.

58. Azim HA Jr, Elattar I, Loberiza FR, Azim H, Mok T, Ganti AK. Third generation triplet cytotoxic chemotherapy in advanced non-small cell lung cancer: A systematic overview. Lung Cancer 2009;64:194–198.
59. Soon YY, Stockler MR, Askie LM, Boyer MJ. Duration of chemotherapy for advanced non-small-cell lung cancer: A systematic review and meta-analysis of randomized trials. J Clin Oncol 2009;27:3277–3283.
60. Smith IE, O'Brien ME, Talbot DC, et al. Duration of chemotherapy in advanced non-small-cell lung cancer: A randomized trial of three versus six courses of mitomycin, vinblastine, and cisplatin. J Clin Oncol 2001;19:1336–1343.
61. Socinski MA, Schell MJ, Peterman A, et al. Phase III trial comparing a defined duration of therapy versus continuous therapy followed by second-line therapy in advanced-stage IIIB/IV non-small-cell lung cancer. J Clin Oncol 2002;20:1335–1343.
62. Rosell R, Carcereny E, Gervais R, et al. Erlotinib versus standard chemotherapy as first-line treatment for European patients with advanced EGFR mutation-positive non-small-cell lung cancer (EURTAC): A multicentre, open-label, randomised phase 3 trial. Lancet Oncol 2012;13:239–246.
63. Kwak EL, Bang YJ, Camidge DR, et al. Anaplastic lymphoma kinase inhibition in non-small-cell lung cancer. N Engl J Med 2010;363:1693–1703.
64. Shaw AT, Kim DW, Nakagawa K, et al. Phase 3 randomized study of crizotinib versus pemetrexed or docetaxel chemotherapy in advanced, ALK-positive NSCLC (PROFILE 1007). Vienna, Austria: European Society for Medical Oncology, September 30, 2012. Abstract LBA1.
65. Johnson DH, Fehrenbacher L, Novotny WF, et al. Randomized phase II trial comparing bevacizumab plus carboplatin and paclitaxel with carboplatin and paclitaxel alone in previously untreated locally advanced or metastatic non-small-cell lung cancer. J Clin Oncol 2004;22: 2184–2191.
66. Reck M, von Pawel J, Zatloukal P, et al. Phase III trial of cisplatin plus gemcitabine with either placebo or bevacizumab as first-line therapy for nonsquamous non-small-cell lung cancer: AVAil. J Clin Oncol 2009;27: 1227–1234.
67. Ciuleanu T, Brodowicz T, Zielinski C, et al. Maintenance pemetrexed plus best supportive care versus placebo plus best supportive care for non-small-cell lung cancer: A randomised, double-blind, phase 3 study. Lancet 2009;374:1432–1440.
68. Paz-Ares L, de Marinis F, Dediu M, et al. Maintenance therapy with pemetrexed plus best supportive care versus placebo plus best supportive care after induction therapy with pemetrexed plus cisplatin for advanced non-squamous non-small-cell lung cancer (PARAMOUNT): A double-blind, phase 3, randomised controlled trial. Lancet Oncol 2012;13:247–255.
69. Barlesi F. AVAPERL Trial tests NSCLC maintenance regimens. Clin Oncol News 2011:12.
70. Patel J, Socinski MA, Garon E.B, et al. A randomized, open-label, phase 3, superiority study of pemetrexed (Pem) + carboplatin (Cb) + bevacizumab (B) followed by maintenance Pem + B versus paclitaxel (Pac) + Cb + B followed by maintenance B in patients (pts) with stage IIIB or IV non-squamous non-small cell lung cancer (NS-NSCLC) (abstract LBPL1). J Thorac Oncol 2012;9:s336.
71. Cappuzzo F, Ciuleanu T, Stelmakh L, et al. Erlotinib as maintenance treatment in advanced non-small-cell lung cancer: A multicentre, randomised, placebo-controlled phase 3 study. Lancet Oncol 2010;11:521–529.
72. Perol M, Chouaid C, Perol D, et al. Randomized, phase III study of gemcitabine or erlotinib maintenance therapy versus observation, with predefined second-line treatment, after cisplatin-gemcitabine induction chemotherapy in advanced non-small-cell lung cancer. J Clin Oncol 2012;30: 3516–3524.
73. Fidias PM, Dakhil SR, Lyss AP, et al. Phase III study of immediate compared with delayed docetaxel after front-line therapy with gemcitabine plus carboplatin in advanced non-small-cell lung cancer. J Clin Oncol 2009;27:591–598.
74. Shepherd FA, Dancey J, Ramlau R, et al. Prospective randomized trial of docetaxel versus best supportive care in patients with non-small-cell lung cancer previously treated with platinum-based chemotherapy. J Clin Oncol 2000;18:2095–2103.
75. Fossella FV, DeVore R, Kerr RN, et al. Randomized phase III trial of docetaxel versus vinorelbine or ifosfamide in patients with advanced non-small-cell lung cancer previously treated with platinum-containing chemotherapy regimens. The TAX 320 Non-Small Cell Lung Cancer Study Group. J Clin Oncol 2000;18:2354–2362.
76. Hanna N, Shepherd FA, Fossella FV, et al. Randomized phase III trial of pemetrexed versus docetaxel in patients with non-small-cell lung cancer previously treated with chemotherapy. J Clin Oncol 2004;22:1589–1597.
77. Shepherd FA, Rodrigues Pereira J, Ciuleanu T, et al. Erlotinib in previously treated non-small-cell lung cancer. N Engl J Med 2005;353:123–132.
78. Lilenbaum RC, Herndon JE 2nd, List MA, et al. Single-agent versus combination chemotherapy in advanced non-small-cell lung cancer: The cancer and leukemia group B (study 9730). J Clin Oncol 2005;23:190–196.
79. Hainsworth JD, Spigel DR, Farley C, et al. Weekly docetaxel versus docetaxel/gemcitabine in the treatment of elderly or poor performance status patients with advanced nonsmall cell lung cancer: A randomized phase 3 trial of the Minnie Pearl Cancer Research Network. Cancer 2007;110: 2027–2034.
80. Reynolds C, Obasaju C, Schell MJ, et al. Randomized phase III trial of gemcitabine-based chemotherapy with in situ RRM1 and ERCC1 protein levels for response prediction in non-small-cell lung cancer. J Clin Oncol 2009;27: 5808–5815.
81. Goffin J, Lacchetti C, Ellis PM, Ung YC, Evans WK. First-line systemic chemotherapy in the treatment of advanced non-small cell lung cancer: A systematic review. J Thorac Oncol 2010;5:260–274.
82. Kosmidis PA, Samantas E, Fountzilas G, Pavlidis N, Apostolopoulou F, Skarlos D. Cisplatin/etoposide versus carboplatin/etoposide chemotherapy and irradiation in small cell lung cancer: A randomized phase III study. Hellenic Cooperative Oncology Group for Lung Cancer Trials. Semin Oncol 1994;21:23–30.
83. Sundstrom S, Bremnes RM, Kaasa S, et al. Cisplatin and etoposide regimen is superior to cyclophosphamide, epirubicin, and vincristine regimen in small-cell lung cancer: Results from a randomized phase III trial with 5 years' follow-up. J Clin Oncol 2002;20: 4665–4672.
84. Auperin A, Arriagada R, Pignon JP, et al. Prophylactic cranial irradiation for patients with small-cell lung cancer in complete remission. Prophylactic Cranial Irradiation Overview Collaborative Group. N Engl J Med 1999;341:476–484.
85. Christodoulou C, Skarlos DV. Treatment of small cell lung cancer. Semin Respir Crit Care Med 2005;26:333–341.

86. Noda K, Nishiwaki Y, Kawahara M, et al. Irinotecan plus cisplatin compared with etoposide plus cisplatin for extensive small-cell lung cancer. N Engl J Med 2002;346: 85–91.
87. Hanna N, Bunn PA Jr, Langer C, et al. Randomized phase III trial comparing irinotecan/cisplatin with etoposide/cisplatin in patients with previously untreated extensive-stage disease small-cell lung cancer. J Clin Oncol 2006;24: 2038–2043.
88. Slotman BJ, Mauer ME, Bottomley A, et al. Prophylactic cranial irradiation in extensive disease small-cell lung cancer: Short-term health-related quality of life and patient reported symptoms: Results of an international phase III randomized controlled trial by the EORTC Radiation Oncology and Lung Cancer Groups. J Clin Oncol 2009;27:78–84.
89. von Pawel J, Schiller JH, Shepherd FA, et al. Topotecan versus cyclophosphamide, doxorubicin, and vincristine for the treatment of recurrent small-cell lung cancer. J Clin Oncol 1999;17:658–667.
90. Eckardt JR, von Pawel J, Pujol JL, et al. Phase III study of oral compared with intravenous topotecan as second-line therapy in small-cell lung cancer. J Clin Oncol 2007;25:2086–2092.
91. Basch E, Prestrud AA, Hesketh PJ, et al. Antiemetics: American Society of Clinical Oncology clinical practice guideline update. J Clin Oncol 2011;29:4189–4198.
92. Rosen LS, Gordon D, Tchekmedyian S, et al. Zoledronic acid versus placebo in the treatment of skeletal metastases in patients with lung cancer and other solid tumors: A phase III, double-blind, randomized trial—the Zoledronic Acid Lung Cancer and Other Solid Tumors Study Group. J Clin Oncol 2003;21:3150–3157.

107

Colorectal Cancer

Lisa E. Davis, Weijing Sun, and Patrick J. Medina

KEY CONCEPTS

1. Advancing age, inherited and acquired genetic susceptibilities, lifestyle choices, inflammatory bowel disease, type 2 diabetes mellitus, and environmental factors are associated with colorectal cancer risk.
2. Regular use of aspirin and other nonsteroidal antiinflammatory drugs, calcium intake, and higher blood vitamin D levels may reduce risk of colorectal cancer, but they are not currently recommended for routine cancer prevention.
3. Effective colorectal cancer screening programs incorporate regular examination of the entire colon starting at age 50 years for average-risk individuals. Colorectal adenomas can progress to cancer and should be removed.
4. The histologic stage of colorectal cancer upon diagnosis—determined by depth of bowel invasion, lymph node involvement, and presence of metastases—is the most important prognostic factor for disease recurrence and survival.
5. The treatment goal for stages I, II, and III colon cancer is cure; surgery should be offered to all eligible patients for this purpose. Six months of fluoropyrimidine-based adjuvant systemic therapy reduces the risk of cancer recurrence and overall mortality in patients with stage III and select populations with stage II colon cancer. An oxaliplatin-containing regimen further reduces risk as compared with fluoropyrimidine alone.
6. Combined modality neoadjuvant therapy consists of fluoropyrimidine-based chemosensitized radiation therapy and surgery for patients with stage II or III cancer of the rectum and is considered standard of care to decrease risk of local and distant disease recurrence.
7. Preoperative chemotherapy may reduce tumor size and convert unresectable disease to resectable disease in selected patients with metastatic colorectal cancer. This strategy offers the potential for prolonging overall survival and cure for metastatic disease.
8. Chemotherapy is palliative for metastatic disease. A fluoropyrimidine with oxaliplatin or irinotecan improves survival compared to fluoropyrimidine monotherapy and should be offered to patients who are candidates for aggressive treatment. The ability for patients to receive all active cytotoxic agents (e.g., fluoropyrimidine, oxaliplatin, irinotecan) during the course of their disease improves their overall survival.
9. Bevacizumab plus fluoropyrimidine-based chemotherapy as initial therapy for metastatic disease is considered standard of care and provides a survival benefit as compared with combination chemotherapy alone.
10. The addition of cetuximab or panitumumab to initial treatment for *KRAS* wild-type advanced or metastatic disease may improve tumor response rates and survival. Individuals who have disease progression after initial therapy not containing an epidermal growth factor receptor (EGFR) inhibitor may benefit from cetuximab or panitumumab, either alone as a single agent or combined with other drugs. However, patients with codon 12 or 13 *KRAS* gene mutations should not receive cetuximab or panitumumab as these tumor mutations predict lack of treatment response.

Colorectal cancer involves the colon, rectum, and anal canal. It is one of the three most common cancers occurring in adult men and women in the United States and accounts for about one in nine cancer diagnoses. In 2013, an estimated 142,820 new cases will be diagnosed, of which 102,480 will involve the colon and 40,340 the rectum.[1] An additional 7,060 new cases of cancer involve the anus, anal canal, or anorectum.[1]

For both adult men and women, colorectal cancer is the third leading cause of cancer-related deaths in the United States. An estimated 50,830 deaths will occur during 2013.[1]

Mortality and incidence rates associated with colorectal cancer in the United States have decreased steadily over the past two decades. Incidence rates vary worldwide, with the highest incidence rates in economically developed countries in North America, Europe, New Zealand, and Australia, whereas lowest rates are found in Central America, Africa, and South-Central Asia.[2] Colorectal cancer mortality rates have been decreasing in and are comparable between the United States and several Western countries; mortality rates continue to increase in less developed countries in eastern Europe and Central and South America.[2]

Multiple factors are associated with the development of colorectal cancer, including inherited susceptibility, environmental and lifestyle factors, and certain disease states. Overall, about 39% of affected individuals undergo a surgical procedure alone intended for cure. An additional 37% of individuals can potentially be cured with surgery followed by adjuvant radiation therapy (XRT), chemotherapy, or both. Curability is influenced primarily by the depth of tumor penetration, involvement of lymph nodes, and presence of metastatic disease. Five-year survival rates are about 91% and 88% for persons with early stages of colon and rectal cancer, respectively.[3] After the tumor has spread regionally to adjacent lymph nodes or tissues, 5-year survival rates drop to about 70% for both colon and rectal cancer; 5-year survival for individuals with metastatic disease is about 12%.

Treatment modalities for colorectal cancer include surgery, XRT, chemotherapy, and targeted molecular therapies (e.g., angiogenesis inhibitors, epidermal growth factor receptor inhibitors). Surgery is the important and definitive procedure associated with cure. XRT can improve curability following surgical resection in rectal cancer and may reduce symptoms and complications associated with advanced disease. Chemotherapy is used in the adjuvant setting to increase cure rates and in treatment for advanced stages of disease to prolong survival. Selected patients with advanced disease who receive aggressive preoperative chemotherapy and targeted therapies experience higher resection rates and can be potentially cured. Much progress has been made in the treatment of advanced disease, the ability to identify candidates for potentially curative surgical procedures, and the availability of active drug regimens that improve patients' survival.

EPIDEMIOLOGY

Colorectal cancer is the third most common malignancy worldwide, accounting for more than 1.2 million new cases annually.[2] The variation in colorectal cancer occurrence worldwide is at least 20-fold.[2] The highest incidence rates are found in Australia and New Zealand, Europe, and North America. The lowest incidence rates are seen in less-developed areas such as Africa, South Central Asia, and Central America. Most recently, incidence rates have rapidly increased in newer economically developed countries in eastern Europe and in Japan, Korea, and China.[2] The influence of environmental factors (e.g., increased intake of caloric-dense foods and physical inactivity) on colorectal cancer risk has become evident through studies of migrants, where the incidence of colorectal cancer increases rapidly within first-generation immigrants who migrate from low- to high-risk areas.[2] However, colorectal cancers are known to develop more frequently in certain families, and genetic predisposition to this disease is also well recognized.

The incidence of invasive colon cancer is greatest among males, who have an age-adjusted incidence rate of 37.4 per 100,000, as compared with females for whom the rate is 29.9 per 100,000.[3] Invasive cancer of the rectum occurs less frequently; the incidence rate is 16.5 and 10.3 per 100,000 for males and females, respectively. Differences in colorectal cancer incidence exist among ethnic groups in the United States, where incidence is highest among African Americans compared to white, American Indian/Alaska Native, Hispanic/Latino, and Asian American/Pacific Islander males and females.[1] Cultural and genetic factors, as well as disparities in access to healthcare services, may influence risk among population groups.[1]

The overall incidence of colon and rectal cancers in the United States continues to decline, with an annual percent decrease of 2.5% from 1975 to 2009.[3] Cancer incidence rates have declined in every major ethnic group since 1975, although less among American Indian/Alaska Natives. Most recent rapid declines in incidence rates are attributed to screening and polyp removal.[1] Figure 107-1 displays trends for incidence and mortality rates among white and African American males and females in the United States.

Cancer of the colon and rectum accounts for about 9% of all cancer deaths in the United States. The median age for death from cancer of the colon or rectum is 74 years.[3] It is estimated that 50,830 individuals will die of colorectal cancer in the United States in 2013, which represents a continued decline in overall combined mortality for both colon and rectal cancer by more than 30% observed during the last 20 years.[1] Overall mortality rates are highest among African American males and females, although a steep rate of decline began in the late 1990s.[3] Colorectal cancer death rates are decreasing among all ethnic groups; however, mortality rates are not statistically lower in American Indian/Alaska Natives.[3] Factors contributing to the overall decline in colorectal cancer mortality include decreasing incidence rates, screening programs with early polyp removal, and more effective and better tolerated treatments. Differences among different world geographic regions, and in population groups in the United States, may also reflect variations in underlying tumor biology, stage at diagnosis, access to screening programs, and availability of effective treatments.[1–3]

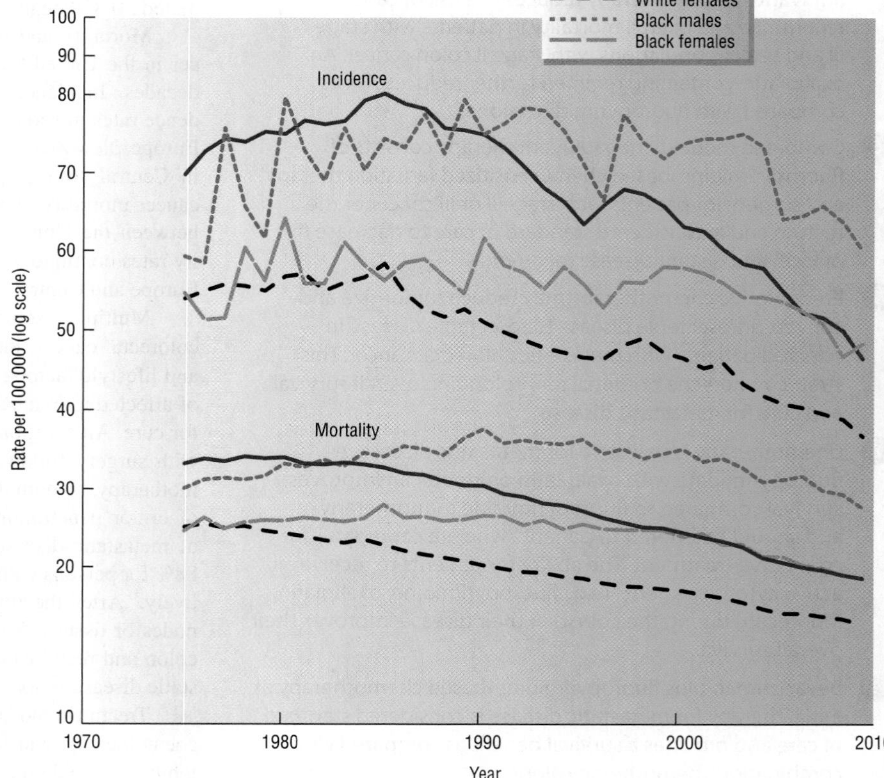

FIGURE 107-1 National Cancer Institute, Surveillance Epidemiology and End Results (SEER) incidence and mortality rates for invasive colon and rectum cancer, 1975–2009. SEER 9 areas and US Mortality Files (National Center for Health Statistics, CDC). Rates are age-adjusted to the 2000 U.S. standard population (19 age groups—Census P25-1103). *(From reference 3.)*

ETIOLOGY AND RISK FACTORS

Numerous studies suggest that the development of colorectal cancer is related to both uncontrollable and modifiable risk factors. Age, family history, clinical and genetic susceptibilities cannot be controlled by individuals. However, lifestyle choices, dietary and environmental factors that affect the bowel may influence an individual's risk of developing colorectal cancer.

Personal Medical History

Age

An individual's risk of developing cancer of the colon or rectum increases with advancing age, with the likelihood of cancer diagnosis increasing after 40 years of age and rising progressively after age 50.[3] The median age at diagnosis is 69 years.[3] Although fewer than 20% of patients are less than 50 years of age at the time of diagnosis, the incidence of colorectal cancer is increasing in this age group, in contrast to overall rates of decline among adults age 50 years and older. The reasons for this pattern are unclear, but may reflect increasing trends in obesity and detrimental dietary factors among younger people.[4]

Adenomatous Polyps or Colorectal Cancer

A prior history of high-risk adenomatous polyps, particularly multiple adenomas or size ≥10 mm, is associated with increased risk of colorectal cancer.[5] Individuals with a prior diagnosis of colon or rectal cancer have a greater risk of developing a new malignancy at another area in their colon or rectum as compared to individuals without a prior history of colorectal cancer.

Inflammatory Bowel Disease

1 Chronic ulcerative colitis, particularly when it involves the entire large intestine, predisposes individuals to colorectal cancer at a rate that is 5- to 10-fold greater than average.[6] The risk is even greater for young individuals and increases for all affected individuals with increasing extent of bowel involvement and disease duration. The cumulative risk of colorectal cancer is low early in life, but increases from 2% at 10 years after diagnosis to 8% and 18% at 20 and 30 years, respectively.[6] Chronic underlying inflammation, oxidative stress, and release of various cytokines, including nuclear factor-kappa B (NF-κB) and tumor necrosis factor-alpha (TNF-α), appear to promote tumorigenesis.[7] The progressive dysplastic changes that bowel mucosa undergo are similar to those observed in adenomatous polyps. Similarly, patients with Crohn's disease are also at increased risk, and the risk is believed to be about that of patients with ulcerative colitis.[6] As compared with sporadic colon cancer or cancer associated with ulcerative colitis, colon cancer in patients with Crohn's disease tends to arise in the proximal colon.[6] This is most likely related to the area of bowel affected by the chronic inflammatory process in individuals with Crohn's disease. Overall, persons diagnosed with either disease constitute about 1% to 2% of all new cases of colorectal cancer each year.

Type 2 Diabetes Mellitus

1 Type 2 diabetes mellitus, independent of body mass size and physical activity level, is associated with increased colorectal cancer risk, although glycosylated hemoglobin (HbA_{1c}) alone as an indicator of hyperglycemia and association with colorectal cancer is inconsistent.[8] Metabolic syndrome is associated with an elevated risk of colorectal cancer.[8] In a meta-analysis of 15 studies, diabetes was associated with a 30% increase in risk of colorectal cancer and increased risk of colorectal cancer mortality.[9] Features associated with type 2 diabetes, such as hyperinsulinemia and elevated levels of free insulin-like growth factor-1 (IGF-1), promote tumor cell proliferation.[8,10] Individuals diagnosed with colorectal cancer and type 2 diabetes have a higher risk of all-cause mortality compared to individuals without diabetes.[10] Risk of death from cardiovascular disease was higher among patients receiving insulin whereas colorectal cancer related mortality was lower with insulin use. Individuals with type 2 diabetes mellitus treated for colorectal cancer also have decreased disease-free survival and overall survival and experience a higher incidence of treatment-related diarrhea and risk of death.

Family History and Inherited Genetic Risk

Colorectal Cancer or Adenomatous Polyps

1 Three specific patterns of colon cancer occurrence are generally observed: sporadic, familial, and recognized hereditary syndromes. Although most cases of colon cancer are sporadic in nature, about 20% of patients who develop colorectal cancer will have a family history of colorectal cancer.[11,12] In these families, the frequency of colorectal cancer is too high to be considered sporadic, but the pattern is not consistent with an inherited syndrome. First-degree relatives of patients diagnosed with colorectal cancer have an increased risk of the disease, particularly if the relative was diagnosed at age 60 or younger.[12] Similarly, parents and siblings of relatives diagnosed with adenomatous polyps are at increased risk for developing colorectal cancer. The reasons for these associations are not established, but may be related to a combination of inherited genes and environmental factors.[12]

Hereditary Syndromes

1 Colorectal cancer is a consequence of several well-defined genetic syndromes.[11–15] The two most common forms of hereditary colon cancer are familial adenomatous polyposis (FAP) and hereditary nonpolyposis colorectal cancer (HNPCC). Both forms result from a specific germline mutation. FAP is a rare autosomal dominant trait caused by inactivating mutations of the adenomatous polyposis coli (*APC*) gene and accounts for 0.2% to 1% of all colorectal cancers. The disease is manifested by hundreds to thousands of tiny sessile adenomatous polyps that carpet the colon and rectum, typically arising during adolescence.[13] The polyps continue to proliferate throughout the colon, with eventual transformation to malignancy. The risk of developing colorectal cancer for individuals with untreated FAP is virtually 100%; most will develop colorectal cancer by the fourth and fifth decades of life.[12,13] Several variants of FAP exist and are associated with different extracolonic manifestations.[13]

HNPCC, also referred to as *Lynch syndrome*, is an autosomal dominant inherited syndrome and is the most common hereditary predisposition for colorectal cancer.[11] Germline mutations in one of the DNA mismatch-repair (MMR) genes, most commonly *MLH1*, *MSH2*, *MSH6*, or *PMS2*, are responsible for HNPCC, which accounts for 2% to 4% of overall colorectal cancer cases.[11] The estimated lifetime risk of developing colorectal cancer by age 70 years is about 66% and 43% for male and female carriers of germline MMR mutations, respectively.[14] Multiple generations within a family are affected, and colorectal cancer develops early in life, with a mean age at time of diagnosis of about 45 years of age.[13–15] About one-third of individuals with HNPCC develop another HNPCC-related extracolonic malignancy within the following 10 years.[15] In contrast to FAP, adenomatous polyps are not a primary manifestation of the HNPCC. Polyps that do form tend to be located primarily in the right-sided, or proximal colon. If HNPCC is suspected in a patient diagnosed with colorectal cancer, typically due to early age at diagnosis or family cancer history, the tumor is examined for evidence of deficient MMR to distinguish between sporadic or germline genetic mutations. Criteria for diagnosis of HNPCC have been established, and it is important to identify carriers of these MMR mutations so that they can be counseled and followed appropriately.[13–15]

Enzyme Polymorphisms

❶ Increasing evidence suggests that genetic polymorphisms in drug-metabolizing enzymes, such as *N*-acetyltransferases (NAT1 and NAT2), cytochrome P450 (CYP) isoenzymes, glutathione-*S*-transferase (GST) enzymes, methylenetetrahydrofolate reductase (MTHFR), and hemochromatosis gene mutations, may confer genetic susceptibility to colorectal cancer.[16] Individuals with certain variations in NAT1, NAT2, CYP1A2, CYP1A1, and CYP2E1 enzyme genotypes may be particularly susceptible to carcinogenic effects of a high dietary intake of meat, tobacco smoke, or other environmental factors.[16,17]

Lifestyle Factors

Nonsteroidal Antiinflammatory Drug and Aspirin Use

❷ Several lifestyle factors are known to affect colorectal cancer risk (Table 107-1). Observational studies have reported that regular (at least two doses per week) nonsteroidal antiinflammatory drug (NSAID) and aspirin use is associated with a reduced risk of colorectal cancer. In an average-risk individual, regular aspirin use is associated with a 13% to 28% reduction in the risk of colorectal adenoma, and the risk of colorectal cancer and mortality is reduced by 30% to 40%.[18,19] Regular daily aspirin use reduces colorectal adenoma recurrence, and colorectal cancer incidence and mortality in patients with prior adenomas or diagnosis of colorectal cancer.[8,18,19]

Benefit has also been seen with NSAID and cyclooxygenase-2 inhibitor (COX-2) use. NSAID use over a 10- to 15-year period is associated with protection against adenomas and colorectal cancer, with a 30% to 50% reduction in the risk of colorectal cancer.[19,20] The protective effects of these agents appear to be related to their inhibition of COX-2 and free radical formation. COX-2 overexpression is seen in precancerous and cancerous lesions in the colon and is associated with decreased colon cancer cell apoptosis and increased production of angiogenesis-promoting factors.[18,19] Up to 50% of colorectal adenomas and 85% of sporadic colon carcinomas have elevated levels of COX-2 and COX-2 overexpression in colorectal cancer is associated with a worse survival. COX-2 appears to play a role in polyp formation, and COX-2 inhibition suppresses polyp growth, restores apoptosis, and decreases expression of proangiogenic factors. Inhibition of COX-2 also downregulates the phosphatidylinositol 3-kinase (PI3K) signaling pathway, which plays an important role in carcinogenesis and cancer cell resistance to apoptosis.[21]

TABLE 107-1 Lifestyle Factors Associated with Colorectal Cancer Risk

Factor	Comments
Elevated Risk	
Sedentary lifestyle	Inverse relationship between physical activity and colon cancer risk; colon cancer risk 20–30% lower for physically active individuals compared to less active individuals
Overweight and obesity	Elevated BMI, waist circumference, and waist-to-hip ratio directly associated with increased cancer risk
Alcohol intake	Risk of colorectal cancer 23% higher with 2–4 alcohol drinks/day compared to <1 drink/day; risk association strongest for males
Cigarette smoking	Prolonged cigarette smoking increases risk of large adenomas and carcinoma; higher colorectal cancer mortality in current smokers; risk may be higher for rectal cancer than for colon cancer
Western diet	High caloric, saturated fat diet, red meat (especially fried and barbecued) and processed meat consumption increases cancer risk; influence of low dietary fiber intake not established
Reduced Risk	
Aspirin and nonaspirin NSAID use	Regular aspirin or NSAID use associated with 30–50% reduction in adenoma recurrence and colorectal cancer risk
Postmenopausal hormone use	Exogenous hormone intake decreases risk of adenomas, colon and rectal cancer by about 35%
Calcium and vitamin D intake	Vitamin D 400 international units and calcium intake of 1,000 mg/day (adults <50 years) or 1,200 mg/day (adults >50 years) may be sufficient to reduce colorectal cancer risk

BMI, body mass index; NSAID, nonsteroidal antiinflammatory drug.

Postmenopausal Hormone Replacement Therapy

Exogenous postmenopausal oral hormone replacement therapy is associated with a significant reduction in colorectal cancer risk.[22] Risk reduction is seen in postmenopausal women receiving both estrogen only and combined estrogen and progestin therapy, and persists for about 10 years after therapy is discontinued.

Several mechanisms for a protective effect of estrogens on the bowel have been identified.[8] Age-related declines in estrogen levels are associated with estrogen receptor hypermethylation, which is associated with reduced expression of the estrogen receptor gene and dysregulated colonic mucosal cell growth. Estrogen may also interact with bile acids, or alter levels of insulin and IGF-1, an important mitogen that influences cell-cycle progression in certain cells. However, because postmenopausal hormone replacement therapy increases breast cancer risk and harmful cardiovascular effects, its use is not recommended to prevent colorectal cancer.

Obesity and Physical Inactivity

❶ Physical inactivity and elevated body mass index (BMI), independent of level of physical activity, are associated with an elevated risk of colon adenoma, colon cancer, and rectal cancer.[8,12,23,24] Individuals with a higher level of activity throughout life have the lowest risk, which may be up to 50% lower than that of physically inactive individuals. Possible hypotheses are that physical activity stimulates bowel peristalsis, resulting in decreased bowel transit time; or that exercise-induced alterations in body glucose, insulin resistance, hyperinsulinemia, and possibly other hormones reduce tumor cell growth.[23]

In most studies, a 5-unit increase above a healthy BMI was associated with increased risk of colorectal cancer in men, but the relationship is weaker and less consistent for women, possibly because of interactions with age or hormone replacement therapy.[23,24] Differences in body composition and distribution of fat weight among men and women could contribute to this discrepancy.[8,22] Several mechanisms have been proposed to explain the association between body size and colorectal cancer risk, including insulin resistance, chronic inflammation, and alterations in growth factors or steroid hormones.[8]

Alcohol and Tobacco Use

❶ Alcohol consumption increases the risk of colorectal cancer, but stronger associations have been observed for men than for women, possibly because alcohol consumption is generally greater in men than in women.[8] Lifetime and baseline alcohol consumption increase risk of cancer of the colon and rectum, and an alcohol intake greater than 30 g/day (about two drinks/day) affects risk.[8,12] Proposed mechanisms include impaired folate metabolism, abnormal DNA methylation, suppressed tumor immune surveillance, and other procarcinogenic effects related to alcohol intake.[8]

Cigarette smoking is associated with an increased risk of colorectal cancer and mortality, with a stronger association for cancer of the rectum than for cancer of the colon.[8,12,25] A dose relationship with increasing number of pack-years and cigarettes smoked per day was also statistically significant but only among patients who had smoked for at least 30 years. As compared to never-smokers, the risks of colorectal cancer and mortality in smokers were 18% and 25% higher, respectively.[25] Early tobacco use may also influence risk of cancer recurrence and mortality among colon cancer survivors, possibly due to an increase in genetic alterations that influence tumor behavior.[26]

Dietary Intake and Nutrients

1 Epidemiologic studies of worldwide incidence of colorectal cancer suggest that economic development and dietary habits strongly influence its development. However, findings based on epidemiologic data are subject to potential biases and inconsistencies in how dietary factors are categorized and measured, and numerous studies have been able to clearly establish only a few specific dietary habits as independent risk factors for colorectal cancer development.

Fiber, Fruit, and Vegetables

1 Worldwide, high-fiber dietary patterns have been associated with a low incidence of colorectal cancer.[8,27,28] Dietary fiber is composed of both water-soluble and insoluble remnants of plant cells that are not processed by normal human digestive enzymes. Foods that are high in fiber include vegetables, fruits, grains, and cereals. Dietary fiber is postulated to reduce colonic mucosal cell exposure to carcinogens through the dilution or reduced absorption of carcinogens in the bowel, reduced fecal pH, reduced bowel transit time, alterations in bile acid metabolism, or increased production of short-chain fatty acids.[8] At present, the role of dietary fiber with regard to amount, source, and type and colorectal cancer risk requires further study.

Red Meat, Processed Meat, and Fat

1 Studies suggest that dietary fat intake may be associated with colorectal cancer risk.[8,27] This may have resulted from the use of dietary evaluations that focused on the quantity, origin, or type (saturated, monounsaturated, and polyunsaturated) of fat rather than on the source of dietary fat ingested. Dietary fat may promote cancer development as a result of its effect on fecal bile acid concentrations. Dietary fat ingestion stimulates the release of bile acids that are converted by colonic flora to secondary bile acids, which are associated with bowel mucosal irritation and cell proliferation responses and may promote tumor growth.[27]

The association between red, but not white, meat consumption and colorectal cancer is strongest, which may be related to the heterocyclic amines and polycyclic aromatic hydrocarbons formed during the cooking process, or the presence of specific fatty acids in red meat such as arachidonic acid.[8,27] Processed meat products containing certain preservatives may increase exogenous exposure to carcinogenic *N*-nitroso compounds.[27] Although red and processed meat and high saturated fat intake has been associated with increased risk of colorectal cancer, the exact nature and magnitude of these risks have not been determined.

Calcium and Vitamin D

2 Inverse associations between dietary calcium, vitamin D intake, and serum 25-hydroxyvitamin D_3 levels, and colorectal cancer risk have been reported in several observational studies.[8,27,29] Calcium may exert antiproliferative effects by binding to bile and fatty acids in the small intestine, thereby reducing colonic epithelial cell exposure to mutagens.[8] In addition, calcium induces differentiating, pro-apoptotic, and direct growth-restraining activities on both normal and tumor cells in the gastrointestinal tract.[8,27] Vitamin D has antiproliferative and differentiation and pro-apoptotic effects on colonic epithelial cells and on a variety of tumor cells.[8,29,30] Most of its actions are mediated through a high-affinity nuclear vitamin D receptor (VDR), and the expression of this receptor is altered during different phases of colon cancer development.[30] Other genes involved in key signaling pathways that influence colorectal cancer development, such as Wnt/β-catenin, are also regulated by the VDR transcription factor.[30] Thus, cellular responsiveness to vitamin D and associated cancer risk is unlikely limited to dietary intake alone. Vitamin D and calcium appear to interact synergistically to protect against adenoma recurrence and colorectal cancer.[8]

Folate and Other Micronutrients

Folate intake has been linked to colorectal cancer risk through epidemiologic and experimental studies in cell lines, animals, and humans.[8,31] However, the underlying basis for this is complex, particularly because alcohol use, smoking, genetic variants of the *MTHFR* gene, and other factors can interfere with folate metabolism.[8,31] Cellular folates act to accept and donate methyl groups in cellular processes that influence DNA synthesis and methylation of DNA, RNA, and proteins.[31] Variations in DNA methylation of gene promoter regions influence gene expression and DNA stability. Inappropriate hypermethylation leads to inactivation of tumor suppressor gene function and hypomethylation can result in oncogene activation.[31]

The relationship between the timing of folate exposure to the development of neoplastic foci may influence what appears to be a bimodal impact of folate on tumorigenesis.[8,31] Moderate folate supplementation, if initiated prior to the establishment of neoplastic foci, may be protective, whereas excessive or increased intake might enhance growth of established early neoplastic lesions.[8,31] Thus, an adequate dietary folate intake may be enough to lower the risk of colorectal cancer, and exceeding normal intake may not be beneficial.

Epidemiologic and animal model data suggest that deficiencies in other dietary micronutrients, including vitamin B_6, selenium, vitamin C, vitamin E, and carotenoids, may increase colorectal cancer risk, but there is no convincing evidence that the incidence of colorectal cancer is greater in patients with low serum levels than in patients with adequate levels.[8]

PATHOPHYSIOLOGY

Anatomy and Bowel Function

The large intestine consists of the cecum; the ascending, transverse, descending, and sigmoid colon; and the rectum (Fig. 107-2). In adults, it extends about 1.5 m and has a diameter ranging from 8 cm in the cecum to 2 cm in the sigmoid colon. The function of the large intestine is to receive 500 to 2,000 mL of ileal contents

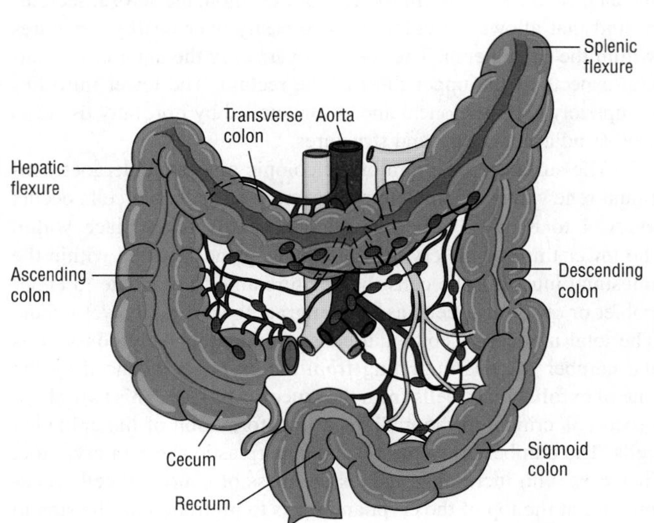

FIGURE 107-2 Colon and rectum anatomy.

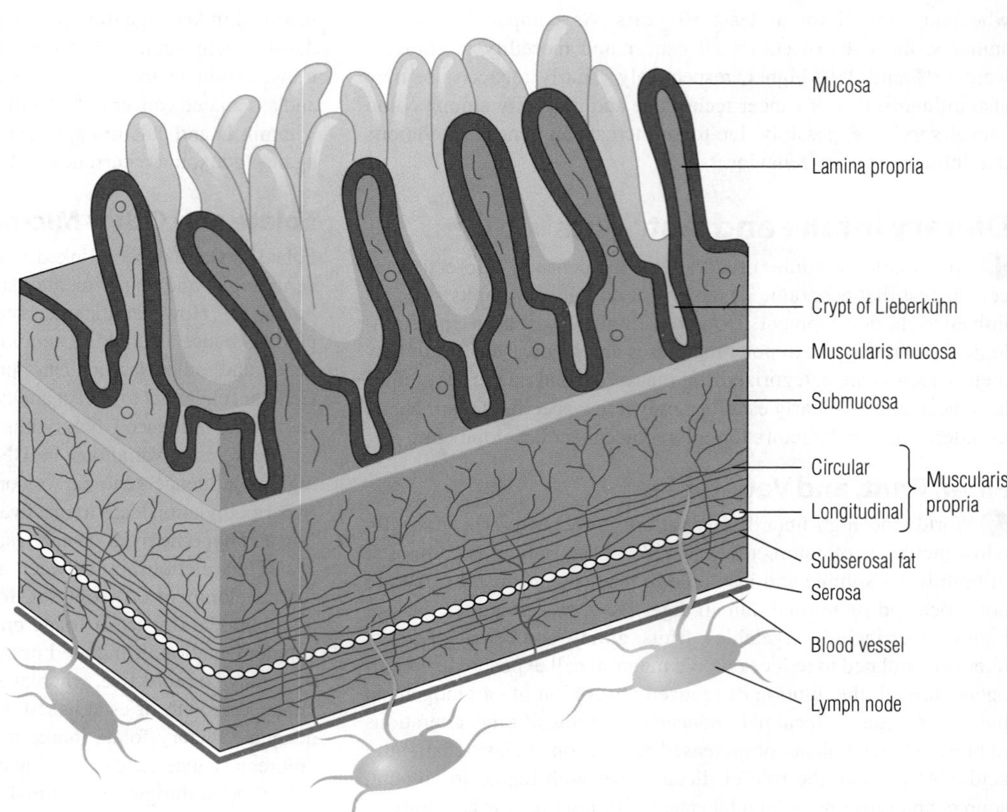

FIGURE 107-3 Cross-section of bowel wall.

per day. Absorption of fluid and solutes occurs in the right colon or the segments proximal to the middle of the transverse colon, with movement and storage of fecal material in the left colon and distal segments of the colon. Mucus secretion from goblet cells into the intestinal lumen lubricates the mucosal surface and facilitates movement of the dehydrated feces. It also serves to protect the luminal wall from bacteria and colonic irritants such as bile acids.

Four major tissue layers, from the lumen outward, form the large intestine: the mucosa, submucosa, muscularis propria, and serosa (Fig. 107-3). Embedded in the submucosa and muscularis propria is a rich lymphatic capillary system. Lymphatic channels do not extend into the mucosa. The muscularis propria consists of circular smooth muscle and outer longitudinal smooth muscle bands. Contraction of these muscle groups moves colonic material toward the anal canal. The outermost layer of the colon, the serosa, secretes a fluid that allows the colon to slide easily over nearby structures within the peritoneum. The serosa covers only the anterior and lateral aspects of the upper third of the rectum. The lower third lies completely extraperitoneal and is surrounded by fibrofatty tissue as well as adjacent organs and structures.

The surface epithelium of the colonic mucosa undergoes continual renewal, and complete replacement of epithelial cells occurs every 4 to 8 days. Cell replication normally takes place within the lower third of the crypts, the tubular glands located within the intestinal mucosa. The cells then mature and differentiate to either goblet or absorptive cells as they migrate toward the bowel lumen. The total number of epithelial cells remains relatively constant as the number of cells migrating from the crypts is balanced by the rate of exfoliation of cells from the mucosal surface. This two-phase process is critical to the malignant transformation of the epithelial cells. The number of dysplastic and hyperplastic aberrant crypt foci increases with increasing age; as the mass of abnormal cells accumulates at the top of the crypt and starts to protrude into the stream of fecal matter, their contact with fecal mutagens can lead to further cell mutations and eventual adenoma formation.

Colorectal Tumorigenesis

The development of a colorectal neoplasm is a multistep process involving several genetic and phenotypic alterations of normal bowel epithelium structure and function, leading to dysregulated cell growth, proliferation, and tumor development. Because most colorectal cancers develop sporadically, with no inherited or familial disposition, efforts have been directed toward identifying these alterations and learning whether detection of such changes may lead to improved cancer detection or treatment outcomes.

Features of colorectal tumorigenesis include genomic instability, activation of oncogene pathways, mutational inactivation or silencing of tumor-suppressor genes, and activation of growth factor pathways.[32,33] A genetic model has been proposed for colorectal tumorigenesis that describes a process of transformation from adenoma to carcinoma (Fig. 107-4). The adenoma to carcinoma sequence of tumor development reflects an accumulation of mutations within colonic epithelium that confers a selective growth advantage to the affected cells. Key elements of this process include hyperproliferation of epithelial cells to form a small benign neoplasm or adenoma in conjunction with acquisition of various genetic mutations.[32] These mutations occur early and frequently in sporadic cases of both adenomas and colorectal cancer. Somatic mutations must occur in multiple genes to produce the malignant transformation. Table 107-2 lists important genetic mutations that are associated with colorectal cancers.

Genomic Instability

Genomic instability plays an integral role in normal colonic or rectal mucosal transformation to carcinoma.[34] Three molecular pathways that lead to genomic instability are the microsatellite instability (MSI), CpG island methylator phenotype (CIMP), and chromosomal instability (CIN) pathways. The most common type is CIN, which leads to alterations in chromosomal structure and copy number.[32,34] Important consequences of CIN include imbalanced chromosome

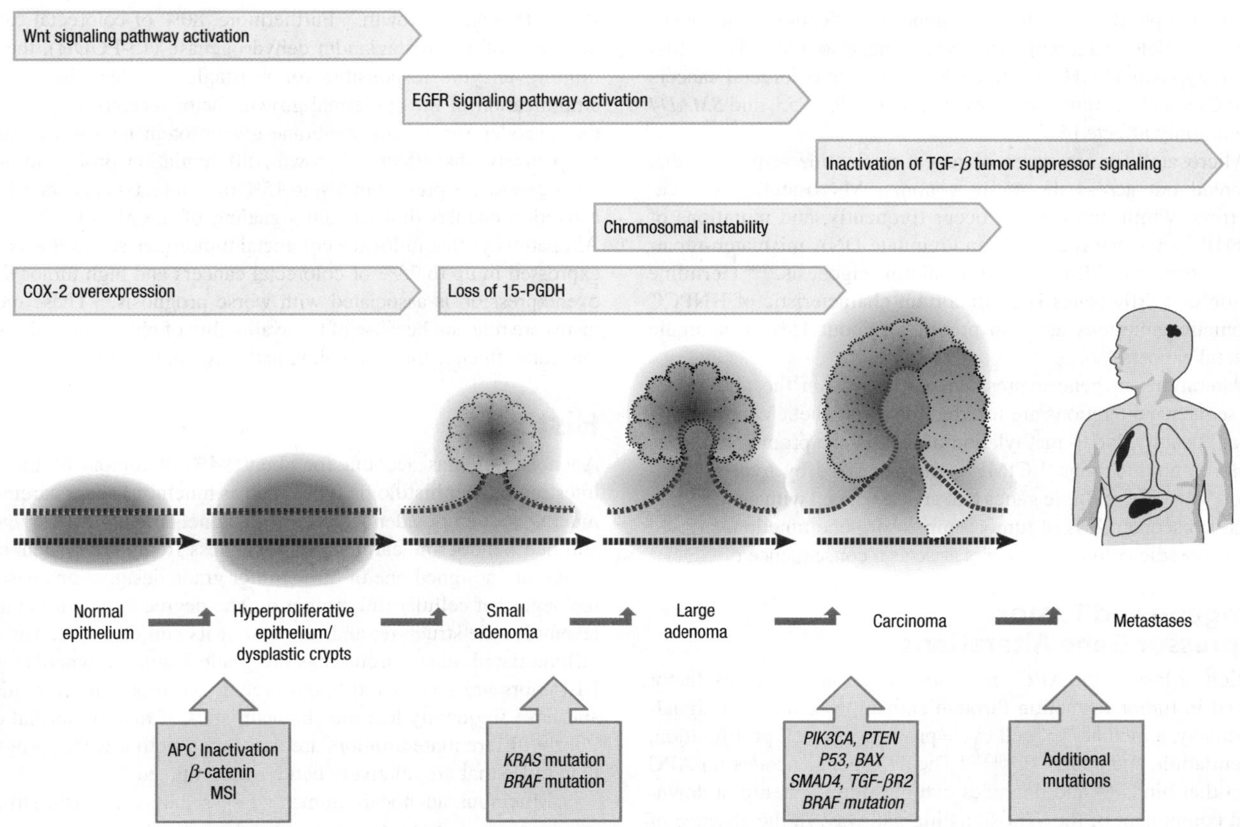

FIGURE 107-4 Genetic changes associated with the adenoma–carcinoma sequence in colorectal cancer. The accumulation of genetic changes in the pathogenesis of colorectal cancer includes microsatellite instability (MSI) initiated by aberrant DNA methylation or mismatch repair (MMR) gene mutation with subsequent disruption in transforming growth factor-β receptor type II (TGF-β2R) and BAX signaling; mutation in the adenomatous polyposis coli (APC) gene or abnormalities in β-catenin leading to inappropriate activation of the Wnt signaling pathway; mutational activation of cyclooxygenase-2 (COX-2) and impaired prostaglandin degradation from loss of 15-prostaglandin dehydrogenase (15-PGDH); *KRAS*, *PIK3CA*, or *BRAF* oncogene activation; increased epidermal growth factor receptor (EGFR) signaling; and deletions or mutations of tumor suppressor genes *SMAD4*, *PTEN*, *P53*. Chromosomal instability (CIN) is a common feature of sporadic disease, but causative factors are not defined. The sequence of molecular events may differ between somatic and inherited genetic alterations. *(Data from references 13, 32, 33, and 34.)*

TABLE 107-2 Genetic Mutations Associated with Colorectal Cancer

Type of Mutation	Disease	Genes	Comments
Germline	Familial adenomatous polyposis (FAP)	*APC*	Multiple adenomas and carcinomas in colon and rectum
	MYH-associated polyposis	*MYH*	Autosomal recessive syndrome; wide spectrum of degree of polyposis; frequent *KRAS* mutations
	Hereditary nonpolyposis colorectal cancer (HNPCC)	DNA MMR genes: *MSH2, MLH1, MSH6, PMS2*	Colorectal cancer in absence of extensive polyposis; predisposition for endometrial, ovarian, gastric, hepatobiliary, urothelial, pancreatic, brain, and skin cancers
Somatic	Sporadic colorectal cancer	Oncogenes:	
		KRAS	Mutations found in about 40% of cancers
		BRAF	*BRAF* V600E mutation found in 5–10% of cancers
		PIK3CA	Mutations found in 15–25% of cancers
		EGFR	Gene amplification in 5–15% of cancers
		Tumor suppressor genes:	
		P53	Loss or mutation in up to 55% of cancers
		SMAD4	Frequency of mutations 10–15% of cancers
		APC	Inactivated in 85% of sporadic cancers
		TGF-βR2	Inactivating mutations present in 10–25% of cancers; mutations in >90% of cancers with MSI
		PTEN	Frequency of inactivating mutations about 10% but loss of PTEN protein expression evident in 15–20% of cancers

APC, adenomatous polyposis coli; MMR, mismatch repair; EGFR, epidermal growth factor receptor; TGF-βR2, transforming growth factor-β receptor type II; MSI, microsatellite instability.

Data from references 13, 32, and 33.

number (aneuploidy), chromosomal gene amplifications, and loss of a wild-type allele of a tumor-suppressor gene, also referred to as loss of heterozygosity (LOH). Up to 85% of sporadic colorectal cancers exhibit CIN and the tumor suppressor genes *APC*, *P53*, and *SMAD4* are commonly affected.[32–34]

Microsatellites are series of repeat nucleotide sequences that are spread out across the entire genome. Microsatellite replication errors within tumor DNA occur frequently, and mutations of the MMR genes that recognize and regulate DNA mismatch-repair errors contribute to MSI and colorectal tumorigenesis.[32,34] Germline mutation of MMR genes is an important characteristic of HNPCC but somatic mutations are also present in about 15% of sporadic colorectal cancers.[34]

Alterations in gene expression or function in the absence of DNA sequence alterations are referred to as epigenetic changes, and these are usually due to methylation of DNA gene promotor regions or histone modifications.[34] CIMP is characterized by hypermethylation of a panel of multiple genes that are associated with gene silencing and subsequent loss of tumor suppressor gene function.[34] About 15% of sporadic colorectal cancers arise as a consequence of CIMP.

Oncogene and Tumor Suppressor Gene Alterations

Mutation or loss of the *APC* tumor suppressor gene is a key factor involved in tumor formation through activation of the Wnt signaling pathway, a mediator of cell cycle progression, cell proliferation, differentiation, and apoptosis.[10,32,34] The *APC* gene encodes for APC protein that binds to and degrades cytoplasmic β-catenin, a downstream component of the Wnt signaling pathway. In the absence of functional APC, β-catenin accumulates in the cytoplasm, then enters the nucleus and activates transcription of various genes, leading to constitutive activation of the Wnt signaling pathway. Inactivation of the *APC* gene is the single gene defect responsible for FAP, and is frequently an initiating event in sporadic colorectal cancer.[32]

Mutational inactivation of *P53* represents a frequent and second key step in colorectal tumorigenesis.[32] Normal *P53* gene expression is important for G_1 cell-cycle arrest to facilitate DNA repair during replication and to induce apoptosis. A third step in tumor progression is the mutational inactivation of the transforming growth factor-β (TGF-β) signaling pathway, which facilitates adenoma transition to high-grade dysplasia or carcinoma and also inactivates *SMAD4*.[32] In normal epithelium, TGF-β has an antiproliferative role and induces growth arrest and apoptosis. Alterations in *SMAD4* or TGF-β receptors lead to a loss of the normal growth inhibitory response to TGF-β.

Several oncogene activating mutations play an important role in promoting colorectal cancer.[32] Mutations in members of the Ras gene family—*KRAS*, *HRAS*, and *NRAS*—in addition to *BRAF*, activate the mitogen-activated protein kinase (MAPK) signaling pathway, which stimulates cell proliferation and other activities that promote carcinogenesis. Mutations of *PIK3CA*, which encodes the catalytic subunit of a PI3K survival pathway, increase production of phosphatidylinositol-3,4,5-triphosphate (PIP_3), which influences cell growth, proliferation, and survival.[34] Mutation or loss of *PTEN*, a tumor suppressor gene that antagonizes PI3K signaling, produces similar effects.[32,34] Multiple additional genetic alterations contribute to carcinoma formation and metastases by altering cellular growth, metabolism, migration and invasive capabilities, and angiogenesis.[34]

Growth Factor Signaling Pathways

Aberrant signaling of growth factor pathways plays an important role in colorectal tumorigenesis. Activation of prostaglandin signaling is an early step in the adenoma to carcinoma transformation process and is induced by upregulated expression of COX-2 and inflammation.[32] COX-2 mediates the synthesis of prostaglandin E_2, which stimulates cancer growth.[32] Furthermore, 80% of colorectal cancers have loss of 15-prostaglandin dehydrogenase (15-PGDH), the rate-limiting enzyme responsible for prostaglandin degradation. Gene amplification of the epidermal growth factor receptor (*EGFR*) gene that encodes for a transmembrane glycoprotein involved in signaling pathways that affect cell growth, differentiation, proliferation, and angiogenesis, is present in 5% to 15% of colorectal cancers.[33] EGFR activation enables downstream signaling of the MAPK, PI3K, and Akt pathways that influence colorectal tumorigenesis. EGFR is overexpressed in up to 75% of colorectal cancers and high tumor EGFR overexpression is associated with worse prognosis.[35] These mechanisms are relevant because of the availability of pharmacologic agents that can influence these signaling pathways and affect cell growth.

Histology

Adenocarcinomas account for about 94% of tumors of the large intestine.[3] Other histologic types such as mucinous adenocarcinoma, mucin-producing adenocarcinoma, signet-ring adenocarcinoma, and neuroendocrine carcinomas occur less frequently. Adenocarcinomas are assigned one of three tumor grade designations based on the degree of cellular differentiation, the degree to which the tumor resembles the structure, and function of its cell of origin. The most differentiated adenocarcinomas are grade I tumors, whereas grade III tumors are considered "high grade," the most undifferentiated, and have frequently lost the characteristics of mature normal cells. Poorly differentiated tumors are associated with a worse prognosis than those that are relatively better differentiated.[36]

Mucinous adenocarcinomas possess the same basic structure as adenocarcinomas but differ in that they secrete an abundant quantity of extracellular mucus. They account for only about 10% of colorectal carcinomas but tend to be frequent in patients with MMR mutations.[36] Signet-ring adenocarcinomas also have a characteristic appearance but are uncommon. Signet-ring histology occurs more frequently in individuals younger than 50 years of age, patients with ulcerative colitis, and tends to present at a more advanced stage of disease at diagnosis.[36] Both mucinous and signet-ring adenocarcinoma histologies confer a poor prognosis.[36]

PREVENTION AND SCREENING

Cancer prevention efforts can be considered as either primary or secondary. Primary prevention strategies aim to prevent the development of colorectal cancer in a population at risk. Secondary prevention approaches are undertaken to prevent malignancy in a population that has already manifested an initial disease process. Several promising primary and secondary prevention strategies are currently undergoing study (Table 107-3).[8,18,20,28,37–43]

Diet

❶ Although early studies suggest that a substantial increase in daily dietary fiber or decrease in dietary fat intake might significantly reduce colorectal cancer risk, results from prospective, controlled trials show no protective effects of fiber intake on colorectal adenoma or carcinoma risk. However, a recent meta-analysis suggests a 10% reduction in colorectal cancer risk with 10 g daily intake of total dietary and cereal fiber and up to a 20% risk reduction with three servings of whole grains daily.[27,28] There is insufficient evidence to support the use of fiber supplementation as a colorectal cancer prevention strategy at this time.

Chemoprevention

❷ The most widely studied agents for the chemoprevention of colorectal cancer are aspirin, nonaspirin NSAIDs, and COX-2

TABLE 107-3 Prevention Strategies for Colorectal Cancer

Prevention Strategy	Proposed Mechanism of Protective Effect
High-fiber diet supplementation	Decreases fecal bile acids; decreases bowel transit time; direct binding to fecal mutagens; dilution of fecal material
Aspirin, NSAIDs, and COX-2 selective inhibitors	Inhibit COX-2; downregulate PI3K signaling pathway; induce apoptosis
NO-NSAIDs	Nitrous-oxide release mimics effects of prostaglandins on gastrointestinal epithelium; suppress formation of aberrant colonic crypt foci
Calcium	Direct binding to bile and fatty acids; inhibits epithelial cell proliferation
Vitamin D	Antiproliferative effects; promotes cell differentiation; effects may be calcium-dependent
Probiotic bacteria	Alter intestinal microflora; inactivate carcinogens; improve host immune response; regulate cell proliferation by altering cell signaling pathways, apoptosis, and cell differentiation
HMG-CoA reductase inhibitors	Induce intestinal cell apoptosis and inhibit cell proliferation; suppress angiogenesis; synergistic COX-2 inhibition with NSAIDs
EGFR inhibitors	Downregulate COX-2; inhibit prostaglandin E_2 production
Difluoromethylornithine	Inhibits cellular proliferation through alterations in polyamine metabolism via inhibition of ornithine decarboxylase
Curcumin	Induces glutathione-*S*-transferase (GST) enzymes; inhibits COX-2 expression
Omega (ω)-3 polyunsaturated fatty acids (ω-3 PUFAs)	Inhibit COX-2 expression; COX-2 independent mechanisms
Metformin	Activates AMPK, thereby inhibiting the mTOR pathway and suppressing colonic epithelial proliferation
Vitamin B_6	Affects DNA synthesis and methylation; suppresses cell proliferation, angiogenesis, and may play a role in chronic inflammation
PPAR-γ agonists	Epigenetic modulation; induce cell-cycle arrest and/or colonic epithelial cell apoptosis
Resveratrol	Antiinflammatory and antioxidant effects; downregulates genes involved in cell cycle progression and proliferation
Green tea polyphenols	Enhance colonic epithelial cell apoptosis, inhibit cell proliferation and angiogenesis, possibly through inhibiting EGFR, IGF-1 receptor, and VEGF receptor kinase signaling pathways

AMPK, AMP-activated protein kinase; COX-2, cyclooxygenase-2; EGFR, epidermal growth factor receptor; HMG-CoA, β-hydroxy-β-methylglutaryl-coenzyme A; IGF-1, insulin-like growth factor 1; MAPK, mitogen-activated protein kinase; mTOR, mammalian target of rapamycin; NO-NSAIDs, nitrous oxide donating nonsteroidal antiinflammatory drugs; NSAIDs, nonsteroidal antiinflammatory drugs; PI3K; phosphatidylinositol 3-kinase; PPAR-γ, peroxisome proliferator-activated receptor-γ; TNF-α, tumor necrosis factor-alpha; VEGF, vascular endothelial growth factor.

Data from references 8, 20, 28, 31, and 37–43.

selective inhibitors, but current guidelines do not recommend their use as chemopreventive agents.[8,18,20,40] The effectiveness of these agents has been studied in high-risk individuals and within the general population.

In individuals with FAP, celecoxib, NSAIDs, and aspirin have been studied to delay development of adenomatous polyps and to reduce polyp recurrence following colectomy with a retained rectum, but they are not viewed as alternatives to surgery.[20] In randomized, controlled trials, celecoxib 400 mg orally twice daily as an adjunct to usual care significantly reduced the mean size and number of colorectal polyps after 6 to 9 months of treatment. However, FDA approval for celecoxib was withdrawn because of lack of data showing long-term benefit. Sulindac has been shown to induce adenoma regression, but does not appear to delay or prevent malignancy. The benefits of these agents are transient, because patients experience an increase in size and number of polyps within a few months after discontinuing treatment. Sulindac is not recommended as chemoprevention for individuals with FAP. These agents may be useful to reduce adenoma recurrence following surgery, but additional data with long-term use are needed.

Nonaspirin NSAIDs and COX-2 inhibitors were associated with reduced risk of sporadic and recurrent colorectal adenomas in cohort and case-control studies, and COX-2 inhibitors were also effective in controlled trials.[8] Celecoxib was associated with a 34% relative risk reduction in adenoma recurrence and 55% risk reduction in the incidence of advanced adenomas.[20] Optimal dosing, agents, and duration of treatment remain to be determined, and potential cardiovascular events in addition to risk of gastric ulceration and bleeding with these agents are of concern. Although NSAIDs may be appropriate for selected individuals at high risk for colorectal cancer but low risk for cardiovascular disorders, the United States Preventive Services Task Force has concluded that potential harms associated with their use outweigh benefits for prevention of colorectal cancer in the general population.[41]

Clinical **Controversy...**

Emerging data support the use of aspirin as colorectal cancer chemoprevention for patients with Lynch syndrome and regular long-term aspirin use modestly reduces colorectal cancer risk in individuals without Lynch syndrome. However, because of the small risk of serious bleeding associated with even low-doses, aspirin use is not recommended for cancer prevention in the general population. The role of aspirin chemoprevention in patients with Lynch syndrome and family history of colorectal cancer is undecided.

The use of aspirin as both a primary and a secondary chemopreventive agent remains controversial. Aspirin reduces of risk of sporadic and recurrent adenomas by about 17% and advanced adenomas by 28%.[20,42] Higher aspirin doses reduced the incidence of colorectal cancer over a 23-year follow-up period by 26% among the general population, but lower doses (75 to 300 mg) of daily aspirin for 5 years was also associated with a risk reduction in colorectal cancer incidence and in 20-year mortality from colorectal cancer by 34%.[20,40,42] Individuals with Lynch syndrome who received aspirin 600 mg daily for at least 2 years experienced a 59% reduction in colorectal cancer risk that became evident 5 years after the aspirin was first started and had been discontinued.[42] Although the optimal aspirin dose and treatment durations are unknown, increasing evidence supports a chemoprotective effect of aspirin in select high-risk individuals and in the general population. The extent of risk reduction appears to be inversely related to duration of therapy and the chemopreventive effects of aspirin may be delayed by several years. However, the balance of risks and benefits with long-term aspirin use is currently unclear, and aspirin is not recommended for colorectal cancer chemoprevention. *PIK3CA* mutations, which are present in up to 20% of colorectal cancers, may serve as a biomarker to identify patients diagnosed with colorectal cancer who may benefit from adjuvant aspirin therapy.[21]

Randomized controlled trials of calcium, vitamin D, and folate supplementation as chemoprevention have also been conducted, but findings do not support their use at this time.[8,20,43] Individuals at high risk of colorectal cancer may experience a moderate reduction in risk of recurrent colorectal adenomas with 5 years of calcium supplementation.[20] However, individuals with adequate vitamin D levels and no known increased risk of colorectal cancer do not appear to benefit from calcium or vitamin D supplementation. In two trials, folate supplementation was associated with a nonsignificant increase in adenoma recurrence. Based on these results, the use of folate supplementation to reduce colorectal cancer risk is not recommended at this time.[8] Several trials of difluoromethylornithine (DFMO), an irreversible inhibitor of the polyamine synthetic pathway, show promising activity as a chemopreventive agent, particular in combinations.[8] Additional intervention trials of various micronutrients, epigenetic modulators, and other chemopreventive agents have been completed or are ongoing.[8,18,20,28,29,31,37–39]

Surgical Resection

Surgical resection remains an option to prevent colon cancer in individuals at extremely high risk for its development. Despite the effects of NSAIDs and COX-2 selective inhibitors on adenoma development and recurrence in individuals with FAP, their effects are incomplete and surgical resection is necessary for cancer prevention for these high-risk individuals. Individuals with FAP who are found to have polyposis on lower endoscopy screening examinations should undergo total proctocolectomy and ileal pouch–anal anastomosis or subtotal colectomy with an ileorectal anastomosis, typically starting around age 20 years.[13] Because of the high incidence of metachronous cancers (45%) in patients with HNPCC, prophylactic subtotal colectomy with an ileorectal anastomosis is recommended for those individuals.[13] Colonoscopic polypectomy, removal of polyps detected during screening colonoscopy, is considered the standard of care for all individuals to prevent the progression of premalignant adenomatous polyps to adenocarcinomas.

Screening

3 Colorectal cancer screening decreases mortality by detecting cancers at an early, curable stage, and by detecting and removing adenomatous polyps. Multiple screening recommendations for early detection of colorectal cancer have been established; differences exist in specific screening guidelines published by various organizations.[5,44–49] Structural tests detect colorectal polyps and cancer whereas fecal-based tests detect early cancer. This section reviews available screening techniques for colon and rectal cancer.

Colonoscopy

3 Colonoscopy facilitates examination of the entire large bowel to the cecum in most patients, and allows for simultaneous removal of premalignant lesions. Although no randomized trials show that colonoscopy decreases colorectal cancer mortality, cohort and case control trials demonstrate a 56% to 77% decrease in the incidence in colorectal cancer with colonoscopy and polyp removal and about a 50% reduction in colorectal mortality.[46] Although it allows for greater visualization of the colon, colonoscopy involves sedation, complete bowel preparation, and is associated with greater risk and inconvenience to patients. However, it is the preferred screening method based on its superior ability to detect and remove lesions in the proximal as well as distal colon and colonoscopy is therefore considered the gold standard for colorectal screening.[45,46]

Flexible Sigmoidoscopy

3 Flexible sigmoidoscopy (FSIG) uses a 40 to 60 cm flexible sigmoidoscope to examine the lower half of the bowel to the splenic flexure for most patients, and is thus capable of detecting 50% to 60% of cancers.[44–46] Randomized trials show that FSIG decreases colorectal cancer incidence and mortality by 31% and 38%, respectively.[44–46] The combination of FSIG and a fecal-based test appears to improve sensitivity for lesions that will be missed by sigmoidoscopy alone, but the true benefit of this approach to general practice has not been established.[45] FSIG offers the advantage of not requiring sedation or extensive bowel preparation, but the entire colon cannot be examined with FSIG and suspicious lesions must be evaluated by colonoscopy.

Computed Tomography Colonography

3 Computed tomography colonography (CTC), also referred to as *virtual colonoscopy*, is an imaging procedure that creates two- or three-dimensional images of the colon by combining multiple helical computed tomography (CT) scans. Initial tests show high sensitivity and specificity for detecting adenomas at least 6 mm in size and sedation is not required.[46] However, the procedure requires complete bowel preparation, is associated with radiation exposure, and many individuals will still be referred for colonoscopy to remove detected lesions. Individuals who refuse to undergo invasive colonoscopy or FSIG may find this screening method more acceptable.

Double-Contrast Barium Enema

3 A double-contrast barium enema (DCBE) involves coating the interior bowel with barium and distending it with air to produce an image of the entire colon in most examinations, and the retained barium outlines small polyps and mucosal lesions. This approach is the least expensive method of examining the entire colon, but is considered inferior to colonoscopy for detecting polyps and colorectal cancer.[44,46] In addition, DCBE requires bowel preparation cleaning, is associated with radiation exposure, and a supplemental colonoscopy is required if suspicious lesions are identified. However, DCBE is considered an alternative for individuals who do not wish to undergo or are not suitable for colonoscopy.

Fecal Occult Blood Tests

3 Fecal occult blood tests (FOBTs) are used to detect occult blood in the stool that may be associated with bleeding adenomas or cancer. Results from randomized, controlled trials of annual FOBT screening show a reduction in colorectal cancer mortality by 33%.[44–46] Unlike structural tests, FOBTs are noninvasive and do not require bowel preparation. Two main methods are available to detect occult blood in the feces: guaiac-based FOBT (gFOBT) and fecal immunochemical tests (FITs), that is, the immunochemical fecal occult blood test (iFOBT). Several guaiac-based tests are available that detect peroxidase activity of heme when hemoglobin comes in contact with a guaiac-impregnated paper. When a solution containing hydrogen peroxide is poured over the paper, a blue color appears if the test is positive. The testing process is complex and requires specific patient counseling to avoid inaccurate results (Table 107-4).

Clinical guidelines have been developed for performing and interpreting results of gFOBT.[45] Several limitations associated with FOBT screening are of concern. Many early-stage tumors do not bleed, and therefore the false-negative rates are about 70% for cancer and 90% for polyps. In addition, the test results may not be valid

TABLE 107-4 Patient Counseling Points Prior to Guaiac-Based Stool Tests

To Avoid False Positives	To Avoid False Negatives
Dietary restrictions • Avoid red meat (beef, lamb, liver) and raw vegetables with peroxidase activity (turnips, broccoli, cauliflower, and radishes) for 3 days prior to testing[a] **Medical restrictions** • Avoid rectal enemas, rectal medications, and digital rectal examinations for 3 days prior to testing • Avoid aspirin and nonsteroidal antiinflammatory drugs for up to 7 days prior to testing • Avoid testing if blood from hemorrhoids is evident in stool • Delay testing until 3 days after menstrual bleeding has ended	• Avoid vitamin C in excess of 250 mg supplements and from citrus juices and fruit for 3 days prior to testing • Avoid testing dehydrated samples (rehydrating of samples is not recommended)
Procedure for Guaiac-Based Stool Testing	
Patient uses an applicator stick to apply stool to two test cards on three separate occasions, usually from different bowel movements on consecutive days (total of six test cards or samples). After the sample dries, the card is mailed or returned to the healthcare professional.	

[a]Test instructions for several products no longer contain dietary vegetable or fruit restrictions.

Data from reference 45.

because the test is often poorly performed both in the home and in physician office settings.[45,46] However, these concerns are addressed by testing three successive stool samples. False-positive results can prove to be very expensive and inconvenient for a patient because of the follow-up tests required to confirm a positive result. Annual screening, preferably using a high-sensitivity gFOBT (e.g., Hemoccult SENSA), is an acceptable option for individuals at average risk for colorectal cancer. It should be noted that FOBT conducted in conjunction with a digital rectal exam during an office visit is not considered adequate colorectal screening.

FITs (iFOBTs) were developed to reduce false-positive and false-negative test results associated with the gFOBT. FIT uses antibodies to detect the globin protein portion of human hemoglobin. Globin is degraded by enzymes in the upper gastrointestinal tract; therefore, FIT is more specific for lower gastrointestinal bleeding. Also, immunochemical tests do not produce false-negative results in the presence of vitamin C.[45] Moreover, testing involves a single stool sample collection annually. Comparative studies report that FIT is more accurate than gFOBT for detecting cancer and advanced adenomas, although colonoscopy identifies more adenomas.[50]

Stool DNA Screening Tests

Molecular screening strategies analyze stool samples for presence of potential markers of malignancy in cells that are shed from premalignant polyps or adenocarcinomas in the bowel.[44–46] Adenoma and carcinomas can contain certain DNA mutations and markers of MSI that can be detected using a multiple marker panel for stool DNA (sDNA) testing. However, no FDA-approved sDNA tests are currently commercially available.[46]

Screening Summary

3 Table 107-5 outlines current U.S. screening guidelines for early detection of colorectal cancer with the goal of cancer prevention. Men and women who are at average risk for colorectal cancer (their only risk factor is age ≥50 years) should begin regular screening starting at age 50 years with a colonoscopy every 10 years, annually using a sensitive gFOBT or FIT, or undergo FSIG every 5 years, alone or in conjunction with annual FOBT. Several screening methods are available, and because each method is associated with different benefits and potential harms, patient preferences and available resources should be considered for individual patients.[45] More rigorous (usually starting at an earlier age) screening recommendations are given for moderate- to high-risk individuals and colonoscopy is generally preferred for initial screening and surveillance following polyp removal in this population.[5,45,46,49] Most organizations recommend

TABLE 107-5 Guidelines for Colorectal Cancer Screening in the United States for Individuals at Average Risk, 50 Years of Age and Older

ACS	ACG	USPSTF	ACS-USMSTF-ACR	ACP	NCCN
gFOBT[a,e]	Colonoscopy[d]	gFOBT[a,e]	gFOBT[a,e]	gFOBT[a,e]	Colonoscopy[d]
Or	*Or*	*Or*	*Or*	*Or*	*Or*
FIT[a,e]	FIT[a]	gFOBT[a,e] + FSIG[c]	FIT[a]	FIT[a]	gFOBT[a,e]
Or	*Or*	*Or*	*Or*	*Or*	*Or*
sDNA[f]	FSIG[c–d]	Colonoscopy[d]	sDNA[e]	FSIG[c]	FIT[a]
Or	*Or*		*Or*	*Or*	*Or*
FSIG[c]	CTC[c]		FSIG[c]	Colonoscopy[d]	gFOBT[a,e] + FSIG[c]
Or	*Or*		*Or*	*Or*	*Or*
gFOBT[a,e] + FSIG[c]	gFOBT[a,e]		Colonoscopy[d]	sDNA[f]	FIT[a] + FSIG[c]
Or	*Or*		*Or*		
FIT[a,e] + FSIG[c]	sDNA[b]		DCBE[c]		
Or			*Or*		
DCBE[c]			CTC[c]		
Or					
Colonoscopy[d]					
Or					
CTC[c]					

ACG, American College of Gastroenterology; ACP, American College of Physicians; ACR, American College of Radiology; ACS, American Cancer Society; CTC, CT colonography; DCBE, double-contrast barium enema; FIT, fecal immunochemical testing; FSIG, flexible sigmoidoscopy; gFOBT, guaiac-based fecal occult blood testing; NCCN, National Comprehensive Cancer Network; USMSTF, U.S. Multi-Society Task Force on Colorectal Cancer; USPSTF, U.S. Preventive Services Task Force.

[a]Annually.
[b]Every 3 years.
[c]Every 5 years.
[d]Every 10 years.
[e]If >50% sensitivity for colorectal cancer.
[f]Interval uncertain.

Data from references 44–48, and 50.

discontinuing screening and surveillance in populations when risk may outweigh benefit.[5] The United States Preventive Services Task Force (USPSTF) recommends routine colorectal cancer screening for individuals age 50 to 75 years with different consideration given to adults 76 to 85 years and recommends against screening for adults older than 85 years.[5] The American College of Physicians recommends against screening adults older than age 75 years or with a life expectancy of less than 10 years.[44]

DIAGNOSIS

Signs and Symptoms

The signs and symptoms associated with colorectal cancer can be extremely varied and nonspecific. Patients with early-stage colorectal cancer are often asymptomatic, and lesions are usually found as a result of screening studies. Any change in bowel habits (e.g., constipation, diarrhea, or alteration in size or shape of stool), abdominal pain, or distension may all be warning signs of a malignant process. Obstructive symptoms and changes in bowel habits frequently develop with tumors located in the transverse and descending colon. Bleeding is the most common symptom of rectal cancer. Bleeding may be acute or chronic and can appear as bright red blood mixed with stool or melena. Iron-deficiency anemia, presenting as weakness and fatigue, frequently develops as a result of chronic occult blood loss.

About 20% of patients with colorectal cancer present with metastatic disease.[3] Metastatic spread occurs as a result of direct tumor invasion of adjacent tissues or by lymphatic or hematogenous spread. The venous drainage of the colon and rectum influences the pattern of metastases most commonly seen. The most common site of metastasis is the liver, often the only site of metastatic disease in 40% of patients, followed by the lungs and then bones, specifically the sacrum, coccyx, pelvis, and lumbar vertebrae. Liver metastases are present in 5% to 10% of patients at presentation.

Workup

When a patient is suspected of having colorectal carcinoma, a complete history and physical examination should be performed. The patient history should include a past medical history and family history, especially noting the presence of inflammatory bowel disease, colorectal cancer, polyps, and familial clustering of cancers to assess risk for an inherited colorectal cancer syndrome. A complete physical examination includes careful abdominal examination for the presence of masses or ascites, a rectal examination, and an assessment for possible hepatomegaly and lymphadenopathy. A breast and pelvic examination is recommended in all women.

An evaluation of the entire large bowel requires a total colonoscopy and allows for tissue collection for a histologic evaluation to provide a preliminary diagnosis following the procedure. Patients with invasive cancer of the colon or rectum require a complete staging workup with laboratory testing and CT scans of the abdomen, pelvis, and chest. Baseline laboratory tests should be obtained and include a complete blood cell count, platelet count, international normalized ratio (INR), prothrombin time, activated partial thromboplastin time, liver chemistries, renal function tests, and carcinoembryonic antigen (CEA) level. Abnormal liver chemistry test results may suggest liver involvement with tumor. However, patients with metastatic disease to the liver may have normal liver chemistries, and abnormal liver test results are not always indicative of metastatic disease. Iron studies (e.g., serum ferritin, serum iron, and total iron-binding capacity) may be useful to identify iron-deficiency in patients with anemia.

CEA belongs to a group of cell-surface glycoproteins termed *oncofetal proteins*, which are expressed during embryonic development and reexpressed on the cell surfaces of many carcinomas, particularly those originating from the gastrointestinal tract. CEA concentrations can be measured in the blood and can therefore potentially serve as a marker for colorectal cancer. Elevated CEA levels are more frequent in patients with metastatic disease but not all colorectal cancers produce CEA. It is important to recognize, however, that several concomitant disease states are associated with an elevated CEA: liver diseases, gastritis, peptic ulcer disease, diverticulitis, chronic obstructive pulmonary disease, chronic or acute inflammatory conditions, and diabetes.[51] Most commercially available assays list a value of less than 5 ng/mL as the upper limit of normal. Although CEA measurement is too insensitive and nonspecific to be used as a screening test for early-stage colorectal cancer, it is the surrogate marker of choice for monitoring colorectal cancer response to treatment, particularly if the pretreatment concentration is elevated.[51] The CEA test may have preoperative prognostic implications because it has been shown to correlate with the size and degree of differentiation of the carcinoma. Elevated preoperative CEA levels correlate with a poor survival and may predict likelihood of recurrence, regardless of tumor stage at diagnosis. However, it should not be used as an indication for adjuvant therapy. After a potentially curative resection, CEA levels should return to normal within 4 to 6 weeks. Persistently elevated CEA levels may indicate residual disease, while elevations after normalization may indicate relapsed disease.

CLINICAL PRESENTATION

General

- Patient symptoms are usually nonspecific and can vary drastically among patients.

Symptoms

- Change in bowel habits (generally an increase in frequency) or rectal bleeding.
- Constipation, depending on the location of the tumor.
- Nausea, vomiting, and abdominal discomfort.
- Fatigue may be present if anemia is severe.

Signs

- Blood in the stool is the most common sign.
- Hepatomegaly and jaundice in advanced disease.
- Leg edema as a consequence of lymph node involvement, thrombophlebitis, fistula formation, weight loss, and pain in the lower back or radiating down the legs may be indicative of widespread disease.

Laboratory Tests

- Positive guaiac stool test and anemia (iron deficiency) from blood loss.
- Elevated carcinoembryonic antigen (most patients).
- Elevated liver enzymes may be present with metastatic disease.

Radiographic imaging studies evaluate the extent of disease involvement. Contrast dye-enhanced CT scans of the chest, abdomen, and pelvis are performed to evaluate pulmonary, hepatic and retroperitoneal involvement and occult abdominal and pelvic disease, and to determine the depth of tumor penetration into the bowel wall and/or invasion to adjacent organs. In certain cases magnetic resonance imaging (MRI) of the abdomen and pelvis may be performed. If findings from CT or MRI scans are not sufficient to detect metastases, a glucose analog [^{18}F]-fluorodeoxyglucose-positron emission tomography (PET) scan may be performed to confirm metastatic disease. PET imaging can provide functional information to discriminate between benign and malignant disease by detecting tumor-related metabolic alterations in affected tissues. PET scans are commonly used for the detection of recurrent colorectal cancer in patients with rising CEA levels and inconclusive findings on standard imaging studies. A PET scan is often combined with or followed by a CT scan because anatomical localization of a lesion using PET alone can be difficult. For rectal cancer, assessment of the extent of tumor spread into the surrounding mesorectum and depth of invasion within the bowel wall may be performed using MRI or endorectal ultrasound (EUS), respectively.

Because of the increased likelihood of HNPCC in patients diagnosed with colorectal cancer younger than the age of 50 years, MMR protein testing on the cancer specimen is recommended.[49] The level of MMR protein expression can be determined by immunohistochemistry, which is decreased with MMR gene mutations. Gene sequencing can also be performed to detect MSI. If immunohistochemical analysis of the tumor reveals absence of MLHI protein expression, *BRAF* gene mutation testing is recommended to distinguish between somatic and germline *MLH1* gene mutation.[49] Individuals with abnormal MMR protein expression or MSI should be referred for genetic counseling as additional testing and cancer susceptibility risk assessment may be appropriate for themselves and family members.

STAGING

❹ The purpose of the staging examinations is to determine the extent of disease, which allows the oncologist to develop treatment options and estimate overall prognosis. The same TNM classification system is used for cancers of the colon and rectum since the categories reflect similar survival outcomes.[52,53] This classification takes three aspects of cancer growth: T (tumor penetration), N (lymph node involvement), and M (presence or absence of metastases) into account. The TNM classification also allows for various subdivisions within each of the three categories, which is then used for determining the disease stage. Table 107-6 summarizes the staging definitions used in the TNM system and corresponding 5-year survival rates.[52,54] Figure 107-5 shows the various stages of cancer based on cancer penetration through the bowel wall and extension to regional lymph nodes.

PROGNOSIS

❹ The stage of colorectal cancer upon diagnosis is the most important independent prognostic factor for survival and disease recurrence. Five-year relative survival is about 91% for individuals who present with a localized tumor stage at diagnosis as compared with about 12% for individuals with metastatic disease at diagnosis.[3]

Clinical factors present at the time of diagnosis that are associated with a poor prognosis and decreased survival include bowel obstruction or perforation, high preoperative CEA level, distant metastases, and location of the primary tumor in the rectum or rectosigmoid area.[55] Along with resection of the primary tumor, a minimum of 12 lymph nodes must be examined to accurately determine regional lymph node involvement and predict lymph node-negative disease.[55]

TABLE 107-6 Colon Cancer by TNM Classification and Associated 5-Year Relative Survival

Stage	T	N	M	Survival (%)
0	T_{is}	N_0	M_0	95.6
I	T_1	N_0	M_0	97.4
	T_2	N_0	M_0	96.8
IIA	T_3	N_0	M_0	87.5
IIB	T_{4a}	N_0	M_0	79.6
IIC	T_{4b}	N_0	M_0	58.4
IIIA	T_1–T_2	N_1/N_{1c}	M_0	71.1
	T_1	N_{2a}	M_0	68.5
IIIB	T_3–T_{4a}	N_1/N_{1c}	M_0	60.6–68.7
	T_2–T_3	N_{2a}	M_0	53.4–81.7
	T_1–T_2	N_{2b}	M_0	62.4
IIIC	T_{4a}	N_{2a}	M_0	40.9
	T_3–T_{4a}	N_{2b}	M_0	21.8–37.3
	T_{4b}	N_1–N_2	M_0	15.7
IVA	Any T	Any N	M_{1a}	
IVB	Any T	Any N	M_{1b}	11.5

Primary Tumor (T)

T_{is}, Carcinoma in situ: intraepithelial or invasion of lamina propia.[a]
T_1, Tumor invades submucosa.
T_2, Tumor invades muscularis propria.
T_3, Tumor invades through the muscularis propria into pericolorectal tissues.
T_{4a}, Tumor penetrates to the surface of the visceral peritoneum.[b]
T_{4b}, Tumor directly invades or is adherent to other organs or structures.[b,c]

Lymph Nodes (N)

N_0, no regional lymph node metastasis
N_1, metastasis in 1–3 lymph nodes
N_{1a}, metastasis in 1 lymph node
N_{1b}, metastasis in 2–3 lymph nodes
N_{1c}, tissue tumor deposits without lymph node metastasis
N_2, metastasis in >4 lymph nodes
N_{2a}, metastasis in 4–6 lymph nodes
N_{2b}, metastasis in >7 lymph nodes

Distant Metastasis (M)

M_0, no distant metastasis
M_{1a}, metastasis confined to one site or organ
M_{1b}, metastasis in peritoneum or > one site or organ

[a]T_{is} includes cancer cells confined within the glandular basement membrane (intraepithelial) or mucosal lamina propria (intramucosal) with no extension through the muscularis mucosae into the submucosa.

[b]Direct invasion in T_4 includes invasion of other organs or other segments of the colorectum as a result of direct extension through the serosa, as confirmed on microscopic examination (for example, invasion of the sigmoid colon by a carcinoma of the cecum) or, for cancers in a retroperitoneal or subperitoneal location, direct invasion of other organs or structures by virtue of extension beyond the muscularis propria (i.e., respectively, a tumor on the posterior wall of the descending colon invading the left kidney or lateral abdominal wall; or a mid or distal rectal cancer with invasion of prostate, seminal vesicles, cervix, or vagina).

[c]Tumor that is adherent to other organs or structures, grossly, is classified cT_{4b}. However, if no tumor is present in the adhesion, microscopically, the classification should be pT_{1-4a} depending on the anatomical depth of wall invasion. The V and L classifications should be used to identify the presence or absence of vascular or lymphatic invasion whereas the PN site-specific factor should be used for perineural invasion.

Data from references 52 and 54.

The pathologic assessment also includes determination of TNM stage, tumor type, and histologic grade, presence of venous and lymphatic invasion, and whether the resected margins are free of tumor.[56] Consideration of these factors plays an important role in determining optimal strategies for treatment and appropriate follow-up.

Additional morphologic tumor features that have negative prognostic value with regard to clinical outcome include infiltrative tumor border configuration, evidence of perineural invasion, extranodal tumor deposits, and presence of tumor budding, characterized by clusters of cells that possess properties of malignant stem cells and are associated with increased risk of local and distant spread.[56] A high density of tumor-infiltrating lymphocytes (TILs) in the tissue specimen is associated with a favorable outcome.[55,56]

Certain molecular markers, particularly MSI, 18q/*DCC* mutation or LOH, *BRAF* V600E mutation, and *KRAS* mutations, are also associated with colorectal cancer prognosis, although the pathologic stage of disease remains the primary prognostic assessment.[57]

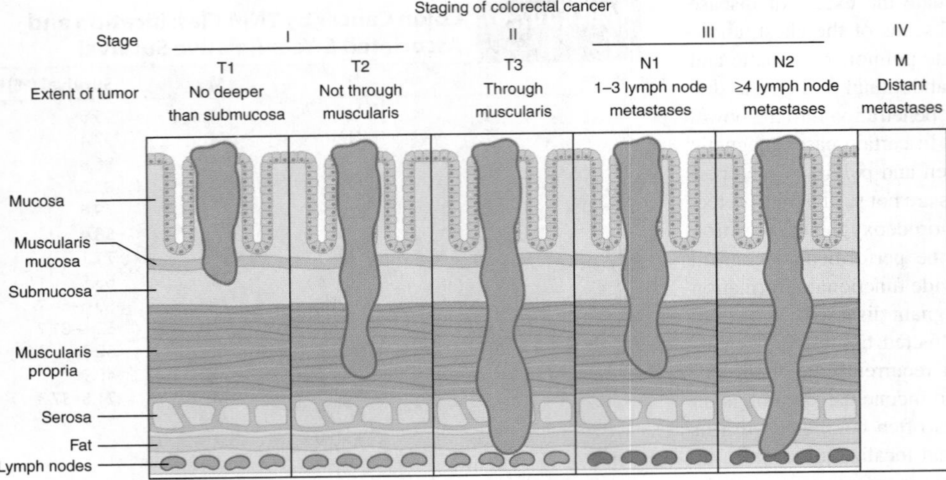

FIGURE 107-5 TNM staging for colorectal cancer. *(From Longo DL, Fauci AS, Kasper DL, Hauser SL, Jameson JL, Loscalzo J: Harrison's Principles of Internal Medicine, 18th ed. http://www.accessmedicine.com. Copyright © The McGraw-Hill Companies, Inc. All right reserved.)*

Colorectal cancers with allelic LOH on chromosome 18q or absent DCC protein are associated with a worse prognosis within stages II and III disease, but data are insufficient to warrant use of this test in practice at this time.[56,57] MSI can be determined through DNA sequencing or by immunohistochemistry staining for protein products of the MMR genes. Colorectal cancers that demonstrate high MSI (MSI-H) appear to be associated with a more favorable outcome and appear to predict the benefit of adjuvant fluoropyrimidines for early-stage disease.[55–57] Tumor DNA *BRAF* and *KRAS* mutation status appear to be linked to overall survival but are not used to determine prognosis.

Although multiple prognostic biomarkers for colorectal cancer have been identified, single molecular tests other than MSI are not used routinely in clinical practice. However, several multigene assays have been developed that provide prognostic information to assist in identifying individuals at high risk for cancer recurrence from early-stage disease.[57,58] The Onco*type* DX colon cancer assay is commercially available and has been validated in several trials as a prognostic test for stage II and III colon cancer.[57–59] Gene expression profiles classify risk of recurrence of low, intermediate, or high, and these scores are prognostic for recurrence, disease-free survival (DFS), and overall survival (OS). The ColoPrint gene expression assay characterizes risk of recurrence as low or high, and is undergoing further validation in clinical trials.[58] The ability for these and other gene signature assays in development to predict which patients may benefit from adjuvant chemotherapy has not been well established.

TREATMENT
Colorectal Cancer

Desired Outcomes

Treatment goals for cancer of the colon or rectum are based on the stage of disease at presentation. Stages I, II, and III disease are considered potentially curable and are managed with the goal of eradicating potential micrometastases after surgical resection. Based on the numbers and site(s) of metastases, about 20% to 30% of patients with metastatic colorectal cancer may be cured, if their metastases are considered resectable. Most patients with stage IV disease are not curable, and treatments for metastatic disease are considered palliative to reduce symptoms, avoid disease-related complications, and prolong survival. However, special attention should be given to those with oligo-lesions in the liver or lung since potential cure is still possible for some of these patients.

General Approach to Treatment

Performance status, concomitant disease states, lifestyle factors, patient preferences, and patient age (although advanced age is not an absolute contraindication for aggressive therapies) must be considered in the treatment planning process. Special or emergent conditions, such as bowel obstruction or perforation, severe pain, anemia, or other symptomatic problems, need to be addressed acutely, after which time a more long-term disease-specific plan can be developed. The treatment approaches for cancer of the colon or rectum reflect two primary treatment goals: curative therapy for localized disease and palliative therapy for metastatic cancer.

For patients for whom treatment intent is curative, surgical resection of the primary tumor is the most important component of therapy. Depending on the extent of disease and whether the tumor originated in the colon or rectum, further adjuvant chemotherapy or chemotherapy plus XRT (chemoradiation) may be appropriate. For selected patients with resectable metastases, surgical resection may be an option. However, for most patients with metastases, systemic chemotherapy is the mainstay of treatment; XRT may also be useful for disease palliation of localized symptoms. Patients with metastatic disease who are asymptomatic may benefit from initiation of therapy, and continuous treatment should be considered.

Operable Disease

Surgery

❺ Individuals with operable—stages I, II, and III—cancer of the colon or rectum should undergo complete surgical resection of the primary tumor mass with regional lymphadenectomy as a curative approach for their disease.[60] The surgical approach for colon cancer generally involves complete resection of the tumor with at least a 5 cm margin of tumor-free bowel and a regional lymphadenectomy.

The preferred surgical procedure for rectal cancer is a total excision of the mesorectum (TME), the surrounding tissue containing perirectal fat and draining lymph nodes.[60,61] If the distal margin clear of tumor is at least 1 cm, sphincter-preserving surgery may be possible for patients with cancers in the middle and lower portion of the rectum. Individuals who are not candidates for sphincter-sparing resections or have extensive local spread of tumor will require an abdominoperineal resection (APR). This involves removal of the distal sigmoid, rectosigmoid, rectum, and anus with the establishment of a permanent sigmoid colostomy.

Colectomies for colon cancer can be performed as open procedures or laparoscopically. Laparoscopic colectomy has become an accepted procedure for colon and rectal cancer.[60] This technique appears to produce similar results to conventional surgery, with the benefits of a smaller surgical incision, shorter hospital stay, shorter duration of ileus, and reduced pain. Complications associated with colorectal surgery include infection, anastomotic leakage, obstruction, adhesion formation, sexual dysfunction, and malabsorption syndromes, depending on the site and extent of resection. Complications affecting bowel function associated with surgery for rectal cancer increase as the level of anastomosis approaches the anus.

Adjuvant Therapy for Colon Cancer

Adjuvant therapy in colorectal cancer is administered to selected individuals after complete tumor resection in an attempt to eliminate residual micrometastatic disease, thereby decreasing tumor recurrence and improving survival rates. Because more than 90% of patients with stage I colon or rectal cancer are cured by surgical resection alone, adjuvant therapy is not indicated.[58,60,61]

Adjuvant chemotherapy is standard therapy for patients with stage III colon cancer. The presence of lymph node involvement with tumor places patients with stage III colon cancer at high risk for recurrence, and the risk of death within 5 years of surgical resection alone is as high as 70%, depending on the number of lymph nodes involved.[60] In this population of patients, adjuvant chemotherapy significantly decreases risk of cancer recurrence and death and is standard of care.

The role of adjuvant chemotherapy for all patients without lymph node involvement (stage II) colon cancer is controversial because early studies that showed improvements in survival included patients with both stage II and III colon cancer. However, the QUASAR trial, which included patients with mostly stage II disease, showed a significant improvement in OS with adjuvant fluorouracil and leucovorin as compared to observation alone.[60]

Patients with stage II disease who are at higher risk for relapse include those with inadequate lymph node sampling, perforation of the bowel at presentation, poorly differentiated tumors, perineural invasion, and T_4 lesions (stage IIB/IIC), and many practitioners offer this therapy to selected patients, with a detailed discussion with patients regarding the potential benefits versus treatment-related toxicities.[56,59] Individuals with MSI-H tumors have a better prognosis compared to those with MSI-L and may not benefit or even be harmed from adjuvant fluoropyrimidine chemotherapy.[59] In addition, subgroup analysis from the QUASAR trial indicated that individuals greater than 70 years of age did not appear to benefit from adjuvant chemotherapy.[60] Optimal dosing, administration schedule, and duration of therapy have yet to be determined, but most practitioners use the same treatment approach as that used for patients with stage III colon cancer.

Adjuvant Radiation Therapy Adjuvant XRT has a limited role in colon cancer because most recurrences are extrapelvic and occur in the abdomen. A subset of patients with recurrent disease or with T_4 tumors that have penetrated fixed structures may benefit from adjuvant fluorouracil-based chemoradiation, with consideration of intraoperative radiation.[58] Selected candidates may also be considered for preoperative fluorouracil-based chemoradiation to improve resectability. Adverse effects associated with XRT in colorectal cancer can be acute or chronic. Acute effects primarily include hematologic depression, dysuria, diarrhea, abdominal cramping, and proctitis. Chronic symptoms that sometimes persist for months following discontinuation of XRT include persistent diarrhea, proctitis or enteritis, small bowel obstruction, perineal tenderness, sexual dysfunction, and impaired wound healing.

Adjuvant Systemic Chemotherapy 5 Standard adjuvant chemotherapy regimens include a fluoropyrimidine (fluorouracil [with leucovorin] or capecitabine) as a single agent and in combination with oxaliplatin.[62–69] The addition of leucovorin increases the binding affinity of the active fluorouracil metabolite to thymidylate synthase (TS), thus enhancing its cytotoxic activity. Combinations of fluorouracil plus leucovorin have been studied extensively in the adjuvant setting, based on the observation that fluorouracil plus leucovorin substantially improves response rates as compared with fluorouracil alone for metastatic disease.[58,60] When leucovorin is unavailable, levoleucovorin, the active isomer of racemic leucovorin, can be substituted as an alternative. The recommended levoleucovorin dose is 50% of the leucovorin dose.[70]

Schedules of fluorouracil and leucovorin administration vary among the different regimens. Historically in the United States, the Roswell Park regimen and the Mayo Clinic regimen were once commonly used, while in Europe, treatments such as the de Gramont regimen favored a continuous IV schedule of fluorouracil (Table 107-7).

TABLE 107-7 Chemotherapy Regimens for the Adjuvant Treatment of Colorectal Cancer

Regimen	Agents	Comments
FOLFOX4[62]	Oxaliplatin 85 mg/m² IV day 1 Leucovorin 200 mg/m² per day IV over 2 hours days 1 and 2 Fluorouracil 400 mg/m² IV bolus, after leucovorin, then 600 mg/m² CIV over 22 hours days 1 and 2 Repeat every 14 days	Improved OS and DFS as compared with infusional fluorouracil-leucovorin–based regimens.
mFOLFOX6[63]	Oxaliplatin 85 mg/m² IV on day 1 Leucovorin 400 mg/m² IV on day 1 Fluorouracil 400 mg/m² IV bolus, after leucovorin on day 1, then 1200 mg/m²/day × 2 days CIV (total 2,400 mg/m² over 46–48 hours) Repeat every 14 days	Sensory neuropathy, neutropenia; easier administration as compared to FOLFOX4.
FLOX[64]	Oxaliplatin 85 mg/m² IV administered on weeks 1, 3, and 5 Fluorouracil 500 mg/m² IV bolus weekly × 6 Folinic acid 500 mg/m² IV weekly × 6 Each cycle lasts 8 weeks and is repeated for 3 cycles	Improved DFS as compared with bolus fluorouracil-leucovorin–based regimens. Increased toxicity compared to FOLFOX4.
Capecitabine[65]	Capecitabine 1,250 mg/m² PO twice daily on days 1 through 14 Each cycle lasts 14 days and is repeated every 21 days	Equivalent DFS as compared with the Mayo Clinic regimen with improved tolerability.
CapOx[66]	Oxaliplatin 130 mg/m² IV day 1 Capecitabine 850–1000 mg/m² twice daily orally for 14 days Each cycle lasts 14 days and is repeated every 21 days	Improved DFS in patients with stage III colon cancer compared to capecitabine alone.
Fluorouracil-Based Regimens		
Roswell Park regimen[67]	Fluorouracil 600 mg/m² IV day 1 Leucovorin 500 mg/m² IV day 1 over 2 hours Repeat weekly for 6 of 8 weeks	
Mayo Clinic regimen[68]	Fluorouracil 425 mg/m² per day IV, days 1–5 Leucovorin 20 mg/m² per day IV, days 1–5 Repeat every 4 to 5 weeks	
de Gramont regimen[69]	Fluorouracil 400 mg/m² per day IV bolus, followed by 600 mg/m² CIV over 22 hours, days 1 and 2 for 2 consecutive days Leucovorin 200 mg/m² per day IV over 2 hours, days 1 and 2 Repeat every 2 weeks	Improved safety as compared with the Mayo Clinic regimen.

CIV, continuous intravenous infusion; DFS, disease-free survival; OS, overall survival; PO, by mouth.

Clinical studies comparing the efficacy of bolus and continuous infusion schedules generally favor continuous infusion of fluorouracil, which is probably related to its short plasma half-life and S-phase specificity for optimal TS inhibition. Continuous IV infusions also permit increased fluorouracil dose intensity, which may account for the higher response rates observed with prolonged infusions of fluorouracil. In most common combination regimens, fluorouracil is administered by both IV bolus injection and continuous IV infusion. This method of administration is now the most common method of administration in the United States and has replaced the Roswell Park and Mayo Clinic regimens.

Clinically significant differences in toxicity occur based on the dose, route, and schedule of fluorouracil administration. Leukopenia is the primary dose-limiting toxicity of IV bolus fluorouracil, although diarrhea, stomatitis, and nausea and vomiting can also occur.[71] The incidence and severity of stomatitis can be significantly reduced with the use of oral cryotherapy. In this approach, the patient is instructed to chew and hold ice chips in the mouth during the period between 5 minutes prior to and 30 minutes following the bolus injection of fluorouracil. The protective effects of this procedure are probably related to the local vasoconstriction caused by the ice chips, which temporarily reduces blood flow to the oral mucosa, thereby reducing drug exposure to the oral mucosa.

Although continuous IV infusion fluorouracil is generally well tolerated, dose-limiting toxicities can be substantial. A distinct toxicity, palmar–plantar erythrodysesthesia ("hand–foot syndrome" or PPE), and stomatitis occur most frequently with this route of administration.[71] Hand–foot syndrome occurs in 24% to 40% of patients receiving extended continuous IV infusions and is characterized by painful swelling and erythroderma of the soles of the feet, palms of the hands, and distal fingers. The skin toxicity is fully reversible on interruption of therapy or dose reduction and is not life threatening, but it can be significant and acutely disabling. The incidence of stomatitis, diarrhea, and hematologic toxicity is not substantial at standard doses, but it increases with increasing fluorouracil doses. No significant difference is noted in the incidence of mucositis, diarrhea, nausea and vomiting, or alopecia between continuous and bolus IV fluorouracil administration.[71]

An additional determinant of fluorouracil toxicity, regardless of the method of administration, is related to its catabolism and pharmacogenomic factors. Dihydropyrimidine dehydrogenase (DPD) is the main enzyme responsible for the catabolism of fluorouracil to inactive metabolites. A rare pharmacogenetic disorder characterized by complete or near-complete deficiency of this enzyme has been identified in patients with cancer. Patients with this enzyme deficiency develop severe toxicity, including death, after fluorouracil administration. Molecular studies have identified a relationship between allelic variants in the *DPYD* gene (the gene that encodes DPD) and a deficiency in DPD activity.[57]

In summary, fluorouracil and leucovorin can be administered in a variety of treatment schedules, but none has proven superior with regard to overall patient survival. Table 107-7 lists examples of some of these regimens.

Fluorouracil Plus Oxaliplatin 5 Current National Comprehensive Cancer Network (NCCN) guidelines recommend oxaliplatin-containing regimens as the preferred treatment for patients with stage III colon cancer who can tolerate combination therapy, and most practitioners incorporate oxaliplatin into adjuvant treatment regimens.[58] These recommendations are based on results from the Multicenter International Study of Oxaliplatin/5-Fluorouracil/Leucovorin in the Adjuvant Treatment of Colon Cancer (MOSAIC) trial, where the addition of oxaliplatin resulted in a 20% risk reduction in disease recurrence and increased 5-year DFS (73% vs. 67%) as compared with fluorouracil plus leucovorin alone. With a median follow-up of 82 months, the addition of oxaliplatin resulted in a statistically significant absolute 6-year OS difference of 2.5%.[63] Oxaliplatin was associated with increased risk of paresthesia, neutropenia, and gastrointestinal toxicity (nausea, vomiting, diarrhea) that were manageable with supportive care. Further supporting the role of oxaliplatin in the adjuvant setting are the results of the National Surgical Adjuvant Breast and Bowel Project C-07 trial, which compared bolus fluorouracil and leucovorin, with or without oxaliplatin.[64] A significant risk reduction in disease recurrence by 20% was seen with oxaliplatin added to the fluorouracil backbone. As expected, neurotoxicity was increased with oxaliplatin. This method of administration, called the FLOX regimen (fluorouracil, leucovorin, oxaliplatin), is associated with increased diarrhea and neuropathies as compared with the aforementioned regimen used in the MOSAIC trial. Though listed as an option according to current NCCN guidelines, its use is limited by its toxicity.[58]

Further modifications of the FOLFOX4 (infusional fluorouracil and leucovorin, oxaliplatin) regimen may also improve tolerability. Capecitabine has been evaluated in adjuvant studies as a replacement for fluorouracil in an attempt to improve the safety and ease of administration of the chemotherapy regimen. The use of CapOx (capecitabine plus oxaliplatin) has been demonstrated to be superior to bolus fluorouracil alone in patients with stage III disease with regard to 3-year DFS (71% vs. 67%), but no difference in OS was observed. The toxicities differed for the two regimens, with increased risks of neuropathies and hand–foot syndrome with CapOx and increased risk of neutropenia/neutropenic fever with fluorouracil.[66]

Capecitabine 5 Capecitabine is FDA approved as a single agent in the adjuvant setting and has been shown to be noninferior to bolus fluorouracil and leucovorin in patients with stage III colon cancer.[65] Both regimens were given for 6 months. DFS between the groups was found to be equivalent. Secondary end points of relapse-free survival (hazard ratio [HR] 0.86; $P = 0.04$) and safety were improved with capecitabine. In particular, the incidence of diarrhea, stomatitis, and neutropenia was decreased with capecitabine, but the incidence of hand–foot syndrome was increased with capecitabine. This regimen is recommended when patients are considered unable to tolerate combination therapy.[58]

Investigational Approaches Despite its proven benefit in the metastatic setting, irinotecan has not shown a benefit in the adjuvant setting and should not be used outside of clinical trials. Three trials have evaluated the addition of irinotecan to bolus or continuous infusion fluorouracil and leucovorin, and all failed to demonstrate a DFS benefit. Cancer and Leukemia Group B (CALGB) 89803 compared the irinotecan, fluorouracil, and leucovorin (IFL) regimen to bolus fluorouracil and leucovorin; not only was there no DFS benefit, but the IFL regimen was associated with significant toxicity.[72] The Third Pan-European Trial in Adjuvant Colon Cancer (PETACC-3) and ACCORD studies, which used infusional regimens similar to fluorouracil, leucovorin, and irinotecan (FOLFIRI), also found no difference in DFS as compared with infusional fluorouracil and leucovorin.[69,73]

With the success of cetuximab and bevacizumab in the metastatic setting, adjuvant trials evaluating monoclonal antibodies in combination with the previously mentioned regimens were conducted. The final results of the NSABP-C08 trial that compared FOLFOX with or without bevacizumab did not meet its primary end point of DFS.[74] Also, results showed no benefit in 3-year DFS from the addition of cetuximab to the combination of infusional fluorouracil plus oxaliplatin (mFOLFOX6) as adjuvant therapy for patients with *KRAS* wild-type stage III colon cancer.[75] Therefore, there is no role for these agents in the adjuvant treatment setting at this time.

Selection of an Adjuvant Regimen Selecting a specific regimen from those listed in Table 107-7 requires an assessment of several patient-specific factors, including the performance status of the patient, comorbid conditions that may exist, and patient preferences for treatment based on lifestyle factors that are important to the patient. If a clinical trial is not an option, most patients with a good performance status will receive oxaliplatin in combination with fluorouracil and leucovorin. Single-agent capecitabine may be the preferred option for patients with preexisting neuropathies, such as diabetic patients, or those patients wishing not to receive IV chemotherapy for any other reason. Fluorouracil and leucovorin has limited use at this time but is an acceptable option for patients who cannot receive oxaliplatin and are unable to tolerate or take oral capecitabine. For example, patients who develop severe hand–foot syndrome may tolerate bolus fluorouracil/leucovorin because this toxicity is minimal with this administration method.

Patient age should also be considered when selecting an appropriate regimen. Subset analysis of the MOSAIC and NSABP-C07 trials have demonstrated no OS benefit from adding oxaliplatin to patients older than the age of 70 years and these patients may be appropriate for fluoropyrimidine-based therapy.[60,64]

Clinical **Controversy...**

Current guidelines discourage the use of age as a sole determining factor in choosing an adjuvant chemotherapy regimen. However, subset analysis of large clinical trials has shown that patients older than the age of 70 years may not benefit from adjuvant oxaliplatin and may need to be treated differently.

Adjuvant and Neoadjuvant Therapy for Rectal Cancer

6 Rectal cancer involves those tumors found below the peritoneal reflection in the most distal 15 cm of the large bowel, and as such is distinct from colon cancer in that it has a propensity for both local and distant recurrence. The higher incidence of local failure and overall poorer prognosis associated with rectal cancer is a result of anatomic limitations in excising adequate radial margins around the rectal tumor. Most patients with stage II or stage III rectal cancer should receive combined-modality therapy consisting of XRT and fluoropyrimidine-based chemotherapy perioperatively.[60]

Neoadjuvant Therapy 6 Neoadjuvant (preoperative) chemoradiation is considered standard of care for most patients with stage II or II rectal cancer because of significant reduction in local recurrence, fewer toxicities, and improved sphincter-preserving surgeries as compared to postoperative chemoradiation.[61] However, some patients are unable to tolerate a typical 5- to 6-week chemoradiation regimen and may be more appropriate candidates for a short course of preoperative radiation therapy alone. Chemotherapy combined with XRT typically involves continuous infusion fluorouracil, oral capecitabine, or bolus fluorouracil and leucovorin; the addition of oxaliplatin to either fluoropyrimidine was associated with increased toxicities without clear improvements in complete remission rates or survival benefit.[60] Although oxaliplatin and other agents continue to be evaluated in this setting, the addition of oxaliplatin or biologic agents (e.g., cetuximab, panitumumab, bevacizumab) is currently not recommended.[76]

Adjuvant Therapy 6 Current NCCN guidelines for rectal cancer indicate that preoperative fluoropyrimidine-based chemotherapy plus XRT is the preferred initial treatment for resectable T_3 N_0, any T, N_{1-2}, or T_4/locally unresectable lesions.[76] This should be followed by additional adjuvant chemotherapy after surgery to total 6 months of chemotherapy (combined total from preoperative and postoperative regimens). Postoperative treatment regimens include bolus fluorouracil and leucovorin, infusional fluorouracil, capecitabine, CapOx, or FOLFOX. Combined chemoradiation is preferred for patients that do not receive preoperative radiation therapy.[60,61,76]

Metastatic Disease: Initial Therapy

Multiple efficacious treatment options for metastatic colorectal cancer are available. Patients are generally considered as having resectable, potentially resectable, or unresectable metastatic disease. Surgery and XRT are used to manage isolated sites of tumor. Chemotherapy is for disseminated disease and the primary treatment modality for unresectable metastatic colorectal cancer. Patients with resectable or potentially resectable metastases are candidates for multimodality therapy.[77] Tumor *KRAS* genotyping for mutation status is recommended for patients at the time when metastatic disease is diagnosed to identify appropriate treatment options.[58] Testing can also be performed on archived tissue samples obtained when the cancer was initially diagnosed.

Resectable or Potentially Resectable Metastatic Colorectal Cancer

Surgery 7 Up to 25% of patients will present with hepatic metastases at the time of diagnosis, and 60% of patients with colorectal cancer will develop hepatic metastases sometime during the course of their disease.[78] The lung is the second most common site of cancer recurrence. Resection of colorectal cancer metastases (metastasectomy) can achieve 5-year OS rates between 20% and 50%, whereas 5-year OS in patients with unresectable metastatic disease is uncommon. Therefore, a primary goal is surgical resection of metastases with curative intent in those individuals for whom complete surgical resection is realistically possible. Patients with no significant general medical risk factors, fewer than four hepatic lesions, CEA levels less than 200 ng/mL, small tumor size, lack of extrahepatic tumor, and adequate surgical margins have the best opportunity for an improved long-term outcome.[78] The primary site of tumor should also be completely resected. Complete surgical resection of discrete metastases in extrahepatic sites, such as the lung, peritoneum, abdomen, and brain, has been less studied but appears to benefit patients with small numbers of metastases who are appropriate candidates for surgery. Adjuvant systemic chemotherapy is recommended to reduce the risk of recurrence following resection.[58]

Neoadjuvant (Conversional) and Adjuvant Chemotherapy

7 Patients that present with metastatic disease isolated to the liver or lung and who undergo resection of all metastatic and primary lesions have an increased probability of survival compared with those whose metastatic lesions remain unresected.[77] Therefore, strategies to increase the success rate of these resections (or convert unresectable lesions to resectable) is the primary goal in these patients. Neoadjuvant chemotherapy, also referred to as conversional chemotherapy, is the primary method to increase complete resection rates in both patients with resectable or potentially resectable liver or lung lesions. In some cases, individuals with metastatic disease initially deemed unresectable may achieve significant tumor regression following neoadjuvant chemotherapy to then be considered for surgery.[77]

The optimal sequencing of chemotherapy for patients with initially resectable metastatic disease is controversial, as treatment options include surgery followed by chemotherapy or perioperative (pre- and postoperative) chemotherapy with surgery.[58,78] Because of the high risk of recurrence following resection of metastases, postoperative chemotherapy is always recommended. Administration of both pre- and postoperative chemotherapy is common practice, but hepatotoxicity associated with preoperative chemotherapy should be considered. Steatohepatitis occurs in 4% to 8% of patients who receive irinotecan-containing regimens and vascular sinusoidal obstructive liver injury develops in 20% to 52% of patients receiving oxaliplatin.[78] Therefore, surgery is performed as soon as possible after the disease becomes resectable. Preoperative chemotherapy is limited to a 2-to-3-month time period and patients undergo close monitoring.

The choice of agents depends on patient-specific factors but may include regimens such as FOLFOX, FOLFIRI, FOLFOXIRI (infusional fluorouracil and leucovorin, oxaliplatin, irinotecan), CapOx, and FOLFOX alternating with FOLFIRI. Biologic agents have been added to the foregoing regimens.[79] If patients receive bevacizumab, surgery should not occur within 6 weeks of the last dose of therapy, and bevacizumab should not be restarted until 6 to 8 weeks after surgery. EGFR inhibitors should be considered only in patients that have tumors with wild-type *KRAS*. Postoperative chemotherapy should be administered to patients to complete a total of 6 months of chemotherapy (pre- and postoperative).[58]

Patients with unresectable lesions are eligible for the same chemotherapy regimens (Table 107-7). However, because the primary goal is surgical resection whenever possible, patients should be evaluated for possible resection after every 2 months of therapy. If resection occurs, adjuvant chemotherapy should be administered to complete a total of 6 months of chemotherapy.

Hepatic-Directed Therapies 7 Individuals with liver-only or liver-predominant metastatic disease may be considered for hepatic-directed therapy in addition to or as an alternative to surgical resection. Hepatic artery infusion (HAI) involves the placement of a permanent access catheter to the hepatic artery through which chemotherapy can be infused directly into the liver.[80] This approach offers the advantage of delivering high drug concentrations to tumors locally, thereby limiting systemic toxicities. Floxuridine and fluorouracil have undergone the most study for hepatic artery infusion, but other active agents such as irinotecan, oxaliplatin, and cetuximab have also been studied. Trials involving HAI have been conducted in patients with unresectable liver metastases to render the disease resectable and as adjuvant therapy following curative resection of isolated metastases. Overall objective tumor response rates range between 40% and 100%, but HAI is associated with potential biliary toxicity and the technical expertise required warrants use in selected patients by experienced practitioners.[58,80] XRT can be directed to sites of hepatic tumor using external beam radiation therapy (EBRT) or percutaneous arterial injection of micron-sized embolic particles loaded with a radioisotope (radioembolization). Tumor ablation procedures use radiofrequency ablation (RFA) or microwave energy to generate heat that destroys localized tumor cells. Cryoablation placement of a cryoprobe into the tumor, either percutaneously or intraoperatively, and then lowering the probe temperature to –20 to –40°C and rewarming it in cycles, resulting in formation of an ice ball that causes tumor destruction. These strategies may be useful for patients who have very small hepatic lesions and are unable to undergo liver resection surgery but they are less successful than surgical interventions.[80]

Unresectable Metastatic Colorectal Cancer

Unless the primary tumor is causing an obstruction, surgery in patients with established unresectable disease is rarely indicated. XRT may be useful to control localized symptoms in patients with metastatic colorectal cancer. Systemic chemotherapy palliates symptoms and improves survival in patients with unresectable disease. Common treatment regimens include combinations of cytotoxic and biologic agents.

Chemotherapy 8 Accepted initial chemotherapy regimens for metastatic colorectal cancer consist of oxaliplatin-containing regimens (FOLFOX, CapOx), irinotecan-containing regimens (FOLFIRI), oxaliplatin plus irinotecan plus fluorouracil plus leucovorin (FOLFOXIRI), infusional fluorouracil plus leucovorin alone, and capecitabine alone.[81–85] Current guidelines recommend the addition of bevacizumab to FOLFOX, CapOx, FOLFIRI, infusional fluorouracil plus leucovorin, and capecitabine alone, or an EGFR inhibitor added to FOLFOX or FOLFIRI, as appropriate.[58] Multiple treatment regimens are effective for metastatic disease.[62,67,81–113] The goals of therapy, history of prior chemotherapy, tumor *KRAS* mutation status, and risk of drug-related toxicities should be considered when an appropriate management strategy is defined for each individual. Treatment regimens are the same for metastatic cancer of the colon and rectum. Table 107-8 lists common chemotherapeutic regimens for metastatic disease.

TABLE 107-8 Chemotherapeutic Regimens for Metastatic Colorectal Cancer

Regimen	Agents	Major Dose-Limiting Toxicities	Comments
Oxaliplatin-Containing Regimens			
Oxaliplatin plus bimonthly infusional fluorouracil/leucovorin; FOLFOX4[62]	See Table 107-7	Sensory neuropathy, neutropenia	
Modified oxaliplatin plus bimonthly infusional fluorouracil/leucovorin; mFOLFOX6[81]	See Table 107-7	Sensory neuropathy, neutropenia; easier administration as compared to FOLFOX4	
FOLFOX plus bevacizumab[81]	Bevacizumab 5 mg/kg IV day 1 before mFOLFOX6 Repeat cycle every 2 weeks	Hypertension, thrombosis, proteinuria from bevacizumab added to toxicities of FOLFOX	
FOLFOX plus panitumumab[86]	Panitumumab 6 mg/kg IV day 1 before mFOLFOX6 Repeat cycle every 2 weeks	Rash, diarrhea, hypomagnesemia added to toxicities of FOLFOX	Only *KRAS* wild-type tumor.
Oxaliplatin plus capecitabine; CapOx[81]	Oxaliplatin 130 mg/m² IV day 1 Capecitabine 850 mg/m² orally twice a day, days 1–14 Repeat cycle every 3 weeks	Diarrhea, hand–foot syndrome, neuropathies	
CapOx plus bevacizumab[81]	Bevacizumab 7.5 mg/kg IV day 1 Capecitabine 850 mg/m² orally twice a day, days 1–14 Repeat cycle every 3 weeks	Hypertension, thrombosis, proteinuria from bevacizumab added to toxicities of CapOx	Reduced capecitabine dose better tolerated.
Irinotecan-Containing Regimens			
Irinotecan plus infusional fluorouracil/leucovorin; FOLFIRI[82]	Irinotecan 180 mg/m² IV day 1 Leucovorin 400 mg/m² IV day 1 Fluorouracil 400 mg/m² IV bolus, after leucovorin on day 1, then 1200 mg/m²/day × 2 days CIV (total 2,400 mg/m² over 46–48 hours) Repeat cycle every 14 days	Diarrhea, mucositis, neutropenia	
FOLFIRI plus bevacizumab[87]	Bevacizumab 5 mg/kg IV day prior to FOLFIRI Repeat cycle every 2 weeks	Hypertension, thrombosis, proteinuria from bevacizumab added to toxicities of FOLFIRI	

(*continued*)

TABLE 107-8 Chemotherapeutic Regimens for Metastatic Colorectal Cancer (*Continued*)

Regimen	Agents	Major Dose-Limiting Toxicities	Comments
FOLFIRI plus ziv-aflibercept[88]	Ziv-aflibercept 4 mg/kg IV prior to FOLFIRI Repeat cycle every 2 weeks	Hypertension, hemorrhage, thrombosis, proteinuria from ziv-aflibercept added to toxicities of FOLFIRI, with increased incidence of diarrhea, asthenia, and neutropenia	
FOLFIRI plus cetuximab[87,89]	Cetuximab (weekly or biweekly) IV before FOLFIRI Repeat cycle every 2 weeks	Toxicities from cetuximab added to toxicities of FOLFIRI	Only *KRAS* wild-type tumor.
FOLFIRI plus panitumumab[90]	Panitumumab 6 mg/kg IV day 1 before FOLFIRI Repeat cycle every 2 weeks	Toxicities from panitumumab added to toxicities of FOLFIRI	Only *KRAS* wild-type tumor.
FOLFOXIRI[83]	Irinotecan 165 mg/m² IV day 1 prior to oxaliplatin Oxaliplatin 85 mg/m² IV prior to leucovorin day 1 Leucovorin 400 mg/m² IV day 1 prior to fluorouracil Fluorouracil 1600 mg/m²/day × 2 days CIV (total 3,200 mg/m² over 48 hours) Repeat cycle every 2 weeks	Neutropenia, diarrhea, stomatitis, peripheral neurotoxicity, thrombocytopenia	More neutropenia and peripheral neurotoxicity compared to FOLFIRI.
IROX[91]	Oxaliplatin 85 mg/m² IV day 1 prior to irinotecan Irinotecan 200 mg/m² IV day 1 Repeat cycle every 3 weeks	Neutropenia, diarrhea, sensory disturbances	
Irinotecan Regimens			
Weekly irinotecan[92]	Irinotecan 125 mg/m² IV every week for 4 of 6 weeks	Neutropenia, diarrhea	
Biweekly irinotecan[89]	Irinotecan 180 mg/m² IV every 2 weeks	Neutropenia, diarrhea	
Every 3-week irinotecan[92]	Irinotecan 350 mg/m² IV every 3 weeks	Neutropenia, diarrhea (less-than-weekly irinotecan)	
Cetuximab plus irinotecan[89,92,93]	Cetuximab (weekly or biweekly) prior to irinotecan continued as previously dosed or as above	Asthenia, diarrhea, nausea, papulopustular and follicular rash	Only *KRAS* wild-type tumor. Cetuximab added to irinotecan following disease progression with irinotecan regimen.
Panitumumab plus irinotecan[94]	Panitumumab 6 mg/kg IV day 1 prior to irinotecan Irinotecan 180 mg/m² IV day 1 Repeat cycle every 2 weeks	Asthenia, diarrhea, nausea, papulopustular and follicular rash	Only *KRAS* wild-type tumor. Panitumumab added to irinotecan following disease progression with irinotecan regimen.
Fluoropyrimidine Regimens			
Simplified bolus plus infusional fluorouracil/leucovorin; (sLV5FU2)[84]	Fluorouracil 400 mg/m² IV bolus, after leucovorin on day 1, then 1200 mg/m²/day × 2 days CIV (total 2,400 mg/m² over 46–48 hours) Repeat cycle every 14 days	Neutropenia, mucositis	Easier to administer compared to de Gramont regimen.
Bolus fluorouracil plus leucovorin; Roswell Park regimen[67]	See Table 107-7	Neutropenia, diarrhea	
Bevacizumab plus fluorouracil/leucovorin[84,95]	Bevacizumab 5 mg/kg IV day 1 prior to fluorouracil and leucovorin, repeat every 2 weeks	Hypertension, bleeding, proteinuria, diarrhea, neutropenia	Infusional fluorouracil/leucovorin regimen preferred to bolus fluorouracil regimen.
Capecitabine[85]	Capecitabine 850-1250 mg/m² orally twice a day, days 1–14, repeated every 3 weeks	Hand-foot syndrome, diarrhea, hyperbilirubinemia	
Capecitabine plus bevacizumab[96]	Bevacizumab 7.5 mg/kg IV day 1 Capecitabine 850–1250 mg/m² orally twice a day, days 1–14 Repeat cycle every 3 weeks	Hypertension, thrombosis, proteinuria, hand–foot syndrome, diarrhea, asthenia	
EGFR-Inhibitors			
Cetuximab[97]	Cetuximab 400 mg/m² IV loading dose, then cetuximab 250 mg/m² IV weekly thereafter	Papulopustular and follicular rash, asthenia, constipation, diarrhea, allergic reactions, hypomagnesemia	Only *KRAS* wild-type tumor.
Biweekly cetuximab[93]	Cetuximab 500 mg/m² IV every 2 weeks		
Panitumumab[98]	6 mg/kg IV over 60 minutes every 2 weeks	Rash, hypomagnesemia, rare allergic reactions	Only *KRAS* wild-type tumor.
Regorafenib[99]	Regorafenib 160 mg orally once daily, days 1–21 Repeat cycle every 4 weeks	Hand-foot syndrome, fatigue, diarrhea, hypertension, rash	Can be given without regard to tumor *KRAS* genotype.

CIV, continuous intravenous; EGFR, epidermal growth factor receptor.

Currently, most metastatic colorectal cancers are incurable, and treatment goals are to control cancer growth, reduce patient symptoms, improve quality of life, and extend survival. The benefit of palliative chemotherapy for metastatic colorectal cancer as compared to observation or supportive care alone with regard to these treatment goals has been established. Results from multiple randomized trials and meta-analyses demonstrate that chemotherapy prolongs life and improves quality of life of patients with metastatic colorectal cancer.[60,114]

Most first-line chemotherapy regimens used for metastatic colorectal cancer incorporate a fluoropyrimidine. Irinotecan or oxaliplatin added to a fluoropyrimidine-based regimen significantly improves response rates, progression-free survival (PFS), and median survival.[60] Biologic agents further improve response rates and survival when combined with chemotherapy as compared to chemotherapy alone. Patients considered appropriate for initial intensive chemotherapy typically receive an oxaliplatin or irinotecan-containing regimen with infusional fluorouracil plus leucovorin and a biologic agent. Capecitabine can be substituted for fluorouracil and leucovorin. Patients that are not considered appropriate candidates for initial intensive therapy may be considered for fluoropyrimidine monotherapy, a fluoropyrimidine regimen combined with a biologic agent, or EGFR inhibitor monotherapy, as appropriate.[58] Patients may receive multiple different regimens, and the sequence of drugs used appears less important than exposure to all active agents during the course of cancer treatments.[60] Table 107-9 summarizes comparative outcome data from potentially useful chemotherapeutic treatments for metastatic colorectal cancer.

Fluorouracil-Based Regimens **8** Fluorouracil administered as a single agent by IV bolus induces response rates of only 10% to 20% and is therefore considered ineffective for metastatic colorectal cancer. Several continuous IV infusion fluorouracil regimens have been developed to increase the duration of drug exposure during the

TABLE 107-9 Comparative Outcomes from Selected Trials in Metastatic Colorectal Cancer

Trial	Number	Outcome Measures	Results
First-Line			
Goldberg[100]	795	Primary: TTP; secondary: OS, ORR, time to treatment discontinuation	Median TTP: IFL vs. FOLFOX 6.9 vs. 8.7 months ($P = 0.0014$). Median survival 15.0 months with IFL vs. 19.5 months with FOLFOX ($P = 0.001$). ORR with FOLFOX (45%) higher compared to IFL (31%; $P = 0.002$) and IROX (35%, $P = 0.03$). TTP and OS with IROX (6.5 and 17.4 months) no different from FOLFOX.
de Gramont[101]	420	Primary: PFS; secondary: ORR, OS, tolerability, QOL	Median PFS: 9.0 vs. 6.2 months ($P = 0.0003$); ORR: 50.7 vs. 22.3% ($P = 0.0001$), oxaliplatin plus LV5FU2 vs. LV5FU2 alone; no difference in OS (16.2 vs. 14.7 months) or QOL between oxaliplatin plus LV5FU2 vs. LV5FU2 alone.
Douillard[102]	387	Primary: ORR; secondary: TTP, response duration, TTF, OS, QOL	Significantly higher ORR with infusional IFL vs. infusional FU/LV alone (35 vs. 22%; $P < 0.005$) by ITT; TTP longer with IFL (6.7 vs. 4.4 months; $P < 0.001$) and OS longer with IFL vs. infusional FU/LV alone (17.4 vs. 14.1 months; $P = 0.031$).
Tournigand[82]	226	Test the best sequence of FOLFIRI vs. FOLFOX6; primary: second PFS; secondary: PFS, OS, ORR, safety	Median survival 21.5 months with FOLFIRI then FOLFOX6 vs. 20.6 months with FOLFOX6 then FOLFIRI; median PFS also no different (14.2 vs. 10.9 months), or ORR or median PFS with first treatment: FOLFOX6 54% and 8.0 months, vs. 56% and 8.5 months with FOLFIRI.
Masi[83]	244	Primary: ORR; secondary: PFS, OS, rate of surgical resection, QOL	FOLFOXIRI increased median PFS (9.8 months) vs. FOLFIRI (6.8 months; $P < 0.001$) and median OS (23.4 vs. 16.7 months; $P = 0.26$). Absolute 5-year survival benefit improved by 7% with FOLFOXIRI.
Hurwitz[103]	925	Primary: OS; secondary: PFS, ORR, response duration, QOL	Bevacizumab plus IFL increased median survival (20.3 months) vs. IFL alone (15.6 months; $P = 0.00003$), PFS (10.6 vs. 6.24 months; $P < 0.00001$), ORR (45% vs. 35%; $P = 0.0029$), and duration of response (10.4 vs. 7.1 months; $P = 0.0014$).
Twelves[85]	1,207	Primary: ORR; secondary: TTP, OS, response duration	Tumor response to capecitabine greater than with FU/LV (25.7 vs. 16.7%; $P < 0.0002$), but no difference in median TTP (4.6 vs. 4.7 months) or median survival (392 vs. 391 days).
Hochster[81]	360	Primary: toxicity; secondary ORR, TTP, OS	Grade 3/4 toxicity not increased with bevacizumab. TTP, ORR, and OS all greater when bevacizumab added to CapOx, FOLFOX, or bolus fluorouracil/leucovorin. Median survival with bevacizumab-containing regimens was 24.4 months vs. 18.4 months without bevacizumab (not a randomized trial).
Saltz[104]	1,401	Primary: PFS; secondary ORR, OS	PFS increased from 8 to 9.4 months with bevacizumab added to oxaliplatin-containing regimens (XELOX or FOLFOX). ORR and OS not different between groups.
Fuchs[105]	547	Primary: PFS; secondary ORR, OS, toxicity	PFS increased with FOLFIRI compared with IFL (7.6 vs. 5.9 months, $P = 0.004$); addition of bevacizumab improved OS (28 months for FOLFIRI + bevacizumab vs. 19.2 months for IFL + bevacizumab; $P = 0.037$). CapeIri equivalent to IFL and not included in final analysis and not recommended.
Bokemeyer[106]	337	Primary: ORR; secondary PFS, OS, toxicity	ORR and PFS increased in patients with wild-type *KRAS* treated with FOLFOX + cetuximab compared with FOLFOX alone; *KRAS* mutant patients had no benefit with cetuximab (ORR 33 vs. 49%, $P = 0.106$ in cetuximab + FOLFOX and FOLFOX treated patients, respectively).
Van Cutsem[107]	1,198	Primary: PFS	FOLFIRI + cetuximab increased PFS by 0.9 months and ORR by 8% compared with FOLFIRI alone. Similar to FOLFOX + cetuximab in that benefit limited to *KRAS* wild-type patients.
Maughan[108]	1,630	Primary: OS in *KRAS* wild-type tumors	Oxaliplatin-based chemotherapy + cetuximab had no effect on OS versus the control group of chemotherapy alone (17.9 months vs. 17.0 months, $P = 0.67$). Additionally, no difference was seen in PFS ($P = 0.60$).
Douillard[86]	1,183	Primary: PFS	656 patients had *KRAS* wild-type tumors. Panitumumab + FOLFOX improved PFS compared with FOLFOX (9.6 vs. 8.0 months, respectively; HR = 0.80; $P = 0.02$). A nonsignificant increase of 3.3 months OS was also observed for panitumumab + FOLFOX ($P = 0.072$).

(continued)

TABLE 107-9 Comparative Outcomes from Selected Trials in Metastatic Colorectal Cancer (*Continued*)

Trial	Number	Outcome Measures	Results
Second-Line			
Rougier[109]	267	Primary: OS; secondary: PFS, ORR, symptom-free survival, adverse effects, QOL	Irinotecan improved median PFS (4.2 vs. 2.9 months; $P = 0.030$) compared with infusion fluorouracil and 1-year survival (45% vs. 35%; $P = 0.035$) but not median OS (10.8 vs. 8.5 months). Median pain-free survival was similar ($P = 0.06$; 10.3 vs. 8.5 months) between irinotecan and fluorouracil, as was QOL.
Cunningham[110]	279	Primary: OS; secondary: performance status, body weight, tumor-related symptoms, QOL	Compared to best supportive care, OS was improved with irinotecan (13.8% 1-year survival vs. 36.2%; $P = 0.0001$); survival without deterioration in performance status, weight loss greater than 5%, and pain-free survival were also improved with irinotecan.
Cunningham[97]	329	Primary: PFS; secondary: ORR, OS, safety	Panitumumab plus BSC prolonged PFS compared to BSC alone, with a median PFS of 8 weeks with panitumumab (hazard ratio 0.54; 95% CI, 0.44–0.66).
Giantonio[111]	829	Primary: ORR; secondary: TTP, OS	Addition of cetuximab to continuing irinotecan associated with 22.9% ORR compared with 10.9% with cetuximab alone ($P = 0.0074$); median survival with cetuximab plus irinotecan similar to cetuximab alone (8.6 vs. 6.9 months; $P = 0.48$), but TTP was longer with cetuximab plus irinotecan (4.1 vs. 1.5 months; hazard ratio 0.54; 95% CI, 0.42–0.71).
Van Cutsem[98]	463	Primary: OS; secondary: PFS, ORR, toxicity	Addition of bevacizumab to FOLFOX4 in patients previously treated with irinotecan and a fluoropyrimidine improved median OS (12.2 vs. 10.8 months; $P = 0.001$), PFS (7.3 vs. 4.7 months; $P < 0.0001$), and ORR (22.7% vs. 8.6%, $P < 0.0001$) compared with FOLFOX4 alone.
Sobrero[93]	1,298	Primary: OS; secondary: PFS, RR, QOL	No difference in OS was seen between the cetuximab + irinotecan or irinotecan alone group (10.7 months vs. 10.0 months, respectively; HR = 0.975; $P = 0.71$). Cetuximab + irinotecan significantly improved PFS (median, 4.0 vs. 2.6 months; HR = 0.692; $P \leq 0.0001$) and QOL.
Peeters[112]	1,186	Primary: PFS and OS prospectively analyzed by *KRAS* status	In *KRAS* wild-type patients the addition of panitumumab to chemotherapy demonstrated a significant improvement in PFS (5.9 months for panitumumab + FOLFIRI vs. 3.9 months for FOLFIRI; HR = 0.73; $P = 0.004$). A nonsignificant increase of 2 months in OS was observed (HR = 0.85; $P = 0.12$).
Bennouna[113]	820	Primary: OS	Median OS was 11.2 months for bevacizumab plus chemotherapy and 9.8 months for chemotherapy alone (HR = 0.81; $P = 0.0062$). Second-line chemotherapy choice based on what was administered as first-line therapy (patients who received oxaliplatin-based chemotherapy in the first-line received irinotecan-based therapy in the second-line setting and vice versa).
Grothey[99]	753	Primary: OS	Median OS was 6.4 months for regorafenib and 5.0 months for placebo (HR 0.77; $P = 0.0052$). Median duration of treatment for regorafenib was 2.8 months.

BSC, best supportive care; Capelri, capecitabine plus irinotecan; CapOx: capecitabine plus oxaliplatin; CI: confidence interval; FOLFIRI, fluorouracil plus leucovorin plus irinotecan; FOLFOX, fluorouracil plus leucovorin plus oxaliplatin; FOLFOXIRI, fluorouracil plus leucovorin plus oxaliplatin plus irinotecan; FU/LV, fluorouracil plus leucovorin; LV5FU2, bolus plus infusional fluorouracil and leucovorin; HR, hazard ratio; IFL, irinotecan plus fluorouracil plus leucovorin; IROX, irinotecan plus oxaliplatin; ITT, intention to treat; ORR, overall response rate; OS, overall survival; PFS, progression-free survival; QOL, quality-of-life; TTF, time-to-treatment failure; TTP, time-to-tumor progression; XELOX, capecitabine plus oxaliplatin.

S-phase of the cell cycle and increase cytotoxicity. No clear survival advantages are observed for any particular regimen, but continuous infusion schedules of fluorouracil when combined with irinotecan or oxaliplatin are better tolerated and commonly used in clinical practice.

Leucovorin is frequently added to fluorouracil in an attempt to improve treatment outcomes. Response rates of 14% to 58% have been observed with a variety of fluorouracil doses in combination with leucovorin at doses ranging from 20 to 500 mg/m^2.[55] Leucovorin administration sequence and timing may be important factors in the efficacy of biochemical modulation of fluorouracil. Leucovorin administration prior to fluorouracil is the most effective approach to enable intracellular-reduced folates to accumulate prior to fluorouracil administration. Despite significantly higher response rates and improved PFS achieved with leucovorin-modulated fluorouracil regimens, their effect on OS is modest.

Bimonthly and weekly regimens of infusional fluorouracil plus leucovorin are the most common treatment schedules for metastatic disease. Increased response rates are noted in bimonthly regimens of fluorouracil administered first as an IV bolus infusion followed by a 22-hour continuous infusion in combination with high-dose leucovorin administered over 2 hours (de Gramont regimen).[69] A similar but simplified "high-dose infused regimen" includes IV bolus fluorouracil with leucovorin followed by 46-hour continuous infusion fluorouracil.[84] These regimens are considered superior to IV bolus regimens due to higher tumor response rates, lower toxicity, and improved PFS.[114]

In summary, a weekly or bimonthly schedule of leucovorin plus fluorouracil (either bolus or continuous infusion) may be more convenient for the patient in terms of fewer scheduled clinic appointments, less interference with work schedules, and ease of dose adjustments based on toxicity. However, the incorporation of newer agents into treatment regimens rather than continual adjustments of fluorouracil and leucovorin doses and administration schedules have led to the greatest advances in drug therapy for metastatic colorectal cancer and will be discussed in the following sections.

Fluorouracil and Leucovorin Plus Irinotecan (8) Irinotecan added to fluorouracil plus leucovorin as initial therapy for metastatic disease improves tumor response rates, time to progression, and OS. In a randomized trial of 387 previously untreated patients with advanced colorectal cancer, irinotecan plus fluorouracil and leucovorin was compared to fluorouracil plus leucovorin with regard to tumor response, survival, and quality of life (Table 107-9).[102] Patients randomized to fluorouracil plus leucovorin could receive weekly fluorouracil (2,600 mg/m^2) as a 24-hour IV infusion plus leucovorin (500 mg/m^2), or the de Gramont regimen of IV bolus and infusional fluorouracil. For the three-drug treatment, a weekly regimen of irinotecan (80 mg/m^2) with a 24-hour infusion of fluorouracil (2,300 mg/m^2) plus leucovorin 500 mg/m^2, or an every-2-week regimen consisting of irinotecan (180 mg/m^2) on day 1 with IV bolus fluorouracil (400 mg/m^2) followed by a 22-hour IV infusion (600 mg/m^2) plus leucovorin (200 mg/m^2 given on days 1 and 2) can be used. Tumor response, median time-to-disease progression, and OS were all greater in the irinotecan group. Diarrhea and neutropenia were the most common toxicities and were worse in the irinotecan-containing groups. Diarrhea was the most common reason for dose reduction or treatment discontinuation with the weekly regimens and led to hospital admission for 32% of patients receiving irinotecan as compared with 12% of patients who received only fluorouracil plus leucovorin. Neutropenia was the most common cause of dose reductions with the every-2-week regimens. Results from questionnaires indicated that quality of life consistently declined later in the irinotecan group.

A second randomized trial compared the addition of irinotecan to weekly IV bolus fluorouracil plus leucovorin (IFL regimen) to the Mayo Clinic regimen and to irinotecan alone as first-line therapy in 683 patients with metastatic colorectal cancer.[114] Although the combination of irinotecan, fluorouracil, and leucovorin resulted in significantly increased tumor response rates and improved PFS and OS as compared with fluorouracil plus leucovorin and irinotecan alone, respectively, the IFL regimen was associated with unacceptable toxicity. Modifications of the original IFL regimen have been made to give irinotecan on an every-2-weeks schedule with fluorouracil as a continuous infusion (FOLFIRI regimen). The median OS is improved by about 6 months with decreased toxicity by this method of administration, and irinotecan administered as IFL is not recommended.[58,105]

The most common adverse effects of irinotecan in these regimens are diarrhea, neutropenia, nausea and vomiting, dehydration, asthenia, abdominal pain, and alopecia; diarrhea and neutropenia are dose limiting.[102] Two distinct patterns of diarrhea have been described. Early-onset diarrhea occurs during or within 2 to 6 hours after irinotecan administration and is characterized by lacrimation, diaphoresis, abdominal cramping, flushing, and/or diarrhea. These cholinergic symptoms, thought to be caused by inhibition of acetylcholinesterase, respond to atropine 0.25 to 1 mg given IV or subcutaneously. About 10% of patients experience the acute symptoms during or shortly following the irinotecan. More commonly, late-onset diarrhea occurs 1 to 12 days after irinotecan administration and may last for 3 to 5 days. Late-onset diarrhea may require hospitalization or discontinuation of therapy, and fatalities have been reported. The incidence of late-onset diarrhea can be decreased with aggressive antidiarrheal intervention. Aggressive intervention with high-dose loperamide therapy should consist of 4 mg taken at the first sign of soft or watery stools, followed by 2 mg orally every 2 hours until symptom-free for 12 hours; this regimen can be modified to 4 mg taken orally every 4 hours during the night.

The severity of delayed diarrhea has been correlated with the systemic exposure (i.e., area under the concentration-versus-time curve) of irinotecan and SN-38 (irinotecan's active metabolite) and with genetic polymorphisms in the enzyme uridine diphosphate-glucuronosyltransferase (UGT1A1), which is responsible for the glucuronidation of SN-38 to inactive metabolites. Reduced or deficient levels of the UGT1A1 enzyme are observed in Gilbert syndrome, a familial hyperbilirubinemia disorder, and correlate with irinotecan-induced diarrhea and neutropenia.[115] An FDA-approved test for deficiency in this enzyme is available, and clinicians can consider obtaining these results for individual patients prior to initiating irinotecan-based therapy to see if a dose reduction is warranted.

Based on these studies, the addition of irinotecan to fluorouracil plus leucovorin (FOLFIRI) increases survival when compared to fluorouracil plus leucovorin in the first-line treatment of metastatic colorectal cancer. These data support the current consensus that the three-drug treatment regimen be considered a first-line option for metastatic colorectal cancer. Accordingly, irinotecan is FDA-approved as first-line therapy for metastatic colorectal cancer in combination with fluorouracil and leucovorin.

Fluorouracil and Leucovorin Plus Oxaliplatin 8 Oxaliplatin, in combination with infusional fluorouracil plus leucovorin, is FDA-approved for use in first-line and salvage regimens for metastatic colorectal cancer (Table 107-8). Oxaliplatin incorporation into fluorouracil-based regimens as first-line therapy for metastatic colorectal cancer is associated with higher response rates and improved PFS, with variable effects on OS.[101] Oxaliplatin is not effective as a single agent in colorectal cancer and is therefore only used in combination regimens.

Intergroup Trial N9741, a comparison of oxaliplatin plus fluorouracil and leucovorin (FOLFOX4) to weekly irinotecan plus IV bolus fluorouracil and leucovorin (IFL), and a combination of irinotecan plus oxaliplatin (IROX) in 795 patients with previously untreated metastatic colorectal cancer showed superior efficacy with FOLFOX4.[100] The IROX arm showed no advantage over either of the other two arms. Significant improvements in response rates, PFS, and median survival were seen with FOLFOX4 as compared with IFL (Table 107-9). However, because of the crossover study design and different methods of fluorouracil administration among treatment arms, it is not possible to evaluate the true contributions of oxaliplatin and irinotecan combined with fluorouracil plus leucovorin in this study.

In a phase III cooperative group study, a simplified combined bolus and infusional fluorouracil regimen with irinotecan (FOLFIRI) was compared with oxaliplatin combined with the same fluorouracil plus leucovorin schedule (FOLFOX6) in previously untreated patients with advanced colorectal cancer to determine whether the sequence of administration of both regimens differed with regard to efficacy and toxicities.[82] Patients were randomized to receive initial treatment with FOLFIRI or FOLFOX6, and at disease progression the patients then received the alternate regimen. Both sequences resulted in similar response rates, PFS, and median survival, but the grade 3 or 4 toxicity profiles were different. Neurotoxicity, neutropenia, and thrombocytopenia were more common with FOLFOX6, while febrile neutropenia, nausea/vomiting, mucositis, and fatigue were significantly more frequent with FOLFIRI. Therefore, based on this trial either FOLFOX or FOLFIRI are acceptable chemotherapy backbones for the first-line treatment of metastatic colorectal cancer.

Oxaliplatin has minimal renal toxicity, myelosuppression, and nausea and vomiting when compared with other platinum-based drugs. Oxaliplatin is associated with both acute and persistent neuropathies.[116] The acute neuropathies occur within 1 to 2 days of dosing and resolve within 2 weeks. The neuropathies usually occur peripherally, but may also occur in the jaw and tongue. A rare acute syndrome of pharyngolaryngeal dysesthesia (1% to 2% of patients) is characterized by subjective sensations of difficulty in swallowing and shortness of breath. Overall, acute neuropathies occur in about 90% of patients, and are precipitated or exacerbated by exposure to cold temperatures or cold objects. Thus, patients should be instructed to avoid cold drinks and use of ice, and to cover skin before exposure to cold or cold objects. Several prophylactic and treatment strategies have been studied with varying degrees of success. Carbamazepine, gabapentin, amifostine, and calcium and magnesium infusions have been used to both prevent and treat oxaliplatin-induced neuropathies.[116] Persistent neuropathy is typically a cumulative adverse effect, occurring after 8 to 10 cycles, and is seen mostly in patients who are responding to therapy.[100] The neuropathy is characterized by paresthesia, dysesthesia, and hypoesthesia, but may also include deficits in proprioception that can interfere with daily activities (e.g., writing, buttoning, swallowing, and difficulty walking as a result of impaired proprioception). Persistent neuropathy occurs in about one-half of patients receiving oxaliplatin but usually resolves with dosage reductions or cessation of oxaliplatin therapy.[114,116] Prophylaxis with calcium and magnesium infusions has not been proven effective. A "stop-and-go" approach where oxaliplatin is temporarily discontinued after 3 months of therapy (or sooner with significant neuropathic symptoms) with the other drugs continued, reduces neurotoxicity without compromising OS and has been advocated.[58,114,116] Oxaliplatin can be reinitiated at disease progression in those patients that experience near complete resolution of neurotoxicity. Anticonvulsant and antidepressant agents are potentially useful to treat symptoms.

Fluorouracil and Leucovorin plus Oxaliplatin plus Irinotecan 8 To further improve survival rates achieved with FOLFOX and FOLFIRI regimens, a four-drug regimen (FOLFOXIRI) was developed and has been compared with FOLFIRI.[83] FOLFOXIRI improved PFS and OS compared to FOLFIRI and a higher proportion of patients receiving FOLFOXIRI were able to undergo radical resection of metastases. As expected, FOLFOXIRI causes more neutropenia, neurotoxicity, diarrhea, and alopecia, but may be appropriate for medically fit individuals with diffuse aggressive disease to palliate symptoms and as potential conversion therapy.[58,83,114]

Capecitabine 8 Capecitabine is an oral, tumor-activated, and tumor-selective fluoropyrimidine carbamate. Capecitabine is converted to fluorouracil through a three-step activation process, the final step being activation by thymidine phosphorylase, which is present in greatest concentrations at the tumor site. These activation steps lead to about a threefold increase in tumor fluorouracil levels. Capecitabine was compared to fluorouracil plus leucovorin as first-line therapy for metastatic colorectal cancer in two randomized phase III trials. In a pooled analysis of 1,207 patients randomized to capecitabine (1,250 mg/m^2 orally twice daily for 14 days, repeated every 3 weeks) or the Mayo Clinic regimen, tumor response to capecitabine was superior to that of fluorouracil plus leucovorin (26% vs. 17%).[85] Time-to-tumor-progression and median survival, however, were no different. Hand–foot syndrome was more common with capecitabine, whereas grades 3 or 4 neutropenia and stomatitis were more common with fluorouracil plus leucovorin. The convenience of oral administration and different toxicity profile make capecitabine a useful substitution for infusional fluorouracil in regimens for metastatic disease.

Both irinotecan and oxaliplatin have been combined with capecitabine. In a study of more than 2,000 patients with metastatic colon cancer, FOLFOX was compared with the combination of capecitabine, fluorouracil, and leucovorin (CapOx) and found to have equivalent OS and PFS. Toxicity was as expected with increased grades 3 or 4 neutropenia (including neutropenic fever) and increased diarrhea and hand–foot syndrome seen with oxaliplatin and capecitabine-based regimens, respectively.[60,114] Based on these results, CapOx is an acceptable first-line option for the treatment of metastatic colorectal cancer.[58]

The combination of capecitabine with irinotecan resulted in no survival benefit compared with IFL and showed inferior results when compared with FOLFIRI in a randomized trial of 430 patients. Additionally, the combination of capecitabine with irinotecan had higher rates of nausea, vomiting, and dehydration and is not recommended for use outside of clinical trials.[105,114]

The current FDA-approved indication for capecitabine in metastatic colorectal cancer is when therapy with a fluoropyrimidine alone is desired. Replacement of fluorouracil-leucovorin with capecitabine in other regimens is not currently approved, although completed trials demonstrate that capecitabine is a suitable replacement for infusional fluorouracil in combination with oxaliplatin but not irinotecan.

Biologic Therapy 9 Current guidelines and clinical practice recommend the addition of biologic therapy to one of the chemotherapy backbones mentioned above.[58]

Bevacizumab 9 Bevacizumab is a recombinant, humanized monoclonal antibody that inhibits vascular endothelial growth factor (VEGF). Bevacizumab, in combination with IV fluorouracil-based chemotherapy, was FDA approved in 2004 for initial treatment of patients with metastatic colorectal cancer. Results from randomized trials show increased PFS and OS benefit as compared with chemotherapy alone.[114]

A phase III trial of bevacizumab in combination with IFL as first-line therapy in patients with metastatic colorectal cancer has also been completed. Patients were randomized to receive IFL and either placebo or bevacizumab 5 mg/kg every 2 weeks.[103] The addition of bevacizumab to IFL therapy resulted in an increase in response rate (35% vs. 45%) and median survival (15.6 vs. 20.3 months) and PFS (6.24 vs. 10.6 months) as compared with IFL alone. The frequency of typical adverse effects associated with IFL chemotherapy was not increased with the addition of bevacizumab. The risk of grade 3 hypertension was significantly increased in the bevacizumab group, but the risk of bleeding, thromboembolism, and proteinuria was similar in the bevacizumab and placebo groups. The hypertension is easily managed with oral antihypertensive agents. The risk of gastrointestinal perforation was increased by the addition of bevacizumab to IFL, and patients complaining of abdominal pain associated with vomiting or constipation should be considered for this rare but potentially fatal complication. Bevacizumab is also associated with a twofold increased risk of arterial thrombotic events, with patients who are older than age 65 or who have a prior history of arterial thrombotic events at greatest risk. Nevertheless, because these individuals derive the same survival benefits with bevacizumab as do other patients, they may be appropriate candidates to receive bevacizumab.

An infusional fluorouracil regimen should be used with the combination of bevacizumab and irinotecan. A randomized phase III trial demonstrated a median OS of 28 months compared with 19.2 months with FOLFIRI and IFL, respectively (HR 1.79; $P = 0.037$) when given in combination with bevacizumab.[105] A third arm of this trial replaced fluorouracil and leucovorin with capecitabine and was found to be inferior to FOLFIRI; during accrual the trial was amended to add bevacizumab to all treatment arms. The capecitabine arm remained inferior to FOLFIRI. Based on these results, capecitabine should not be administered with irinotecan, with or without bevacizumab.

Bevacizumab has also been combined with oxaliplatin in a variety of chemotherapy regimens for the initial treatment of metastatic colon cancer. In contrast to irinotecan-containing regimens, the method of fluorouracil administration (or substitution with capecitabine) does not appear to significantly affect outcomes. One trial, randomized one cohort of patients to one of three oxaliplatin-based regimens (TREE-1 [arm 1: oxaliplatin plus infusional fluorouracil {5-FU}; arm 2: oxaliplatin plus bolus 5-FU; arm 3: oxaliplatin plus oral capecitabine]) while the second cohort of patients (TREE-2) received the same chemotherapy regimens plus bevacizumab as their first-line treatment for metastatic colon cancer.[81] The addition of bevacizumab was associated with increased overall response rate and longer time-to-progression and median survival, although these differences were not significant as a consequence of the small sample size. Overall median survival was 18.2 months in the TREE-1 cohort and 23.7 months in the TREE-2 cohort with the addition of bevacizumab. In a separate phase III trial, the addition of bevacizumab to oxaliplatin-based chemotherapy (capecitabine and oxaliplatin [CapOx] or FOLFOX) significantly improved PFS but not OS.[104] Studies that compare the addition of bevacizumab to oxaliplatin- and irinotecan-containing combinations with bevacizumab are ongoing.

EGFR Inhibitors **10** EGFR inhibitors may also be used in combination with first-line chemotherapy. Results with cetuximab in the first-line metastatic setting combined with FOLFIRI suggest that the combination improves response rates and PFS to either chemotherapy regimen without adding substantial toxicity.[107]

The benefit of EGFR inhibitors is limited to patients with wild-type *KRAS* tumors and they should not be used in patients with tumor *KRAS* mutations.[114] Cetuximab combined with FOLFIRI demonstrated an increase in PFS of 1.2 months and improved median OS from 21 to 24.9 months (HR 0.84, P = NS) compared with FOLFIRI alone in the subset of patients with wild-type *KRAS*.[107] No benefit is seen in patients with mutant *KRAS*. Cetuximab is FDA-approved for administration in a weekly schedule, but bimonthly infusions have been used and may be more convenient.[89]

Conflicting results have been seen with the use of cetuximab in combination with FOLFOX. Initial reports demonstrated an increased response rate and a decreased PFS (HR 0.57; P = .0163) with the combination as compared with FOLFOX4 alone in patients with wild-type *KRAS*.[108] However, a large phase III trial failed to confirm the benefit of this regimen and demonstrated no difference in PFS or OS with the combination of FOLFOX and cetuximab and current NCCN guidelines do not recommend this combination.[58] This lack of benefit was seen in patients with both *KRAS* wild-type and mutant tumor types.

Panitumumab can be combined with either FOLFOX or FOLFIRI in patients with *KRAS* wild-type tumors. PFS was increased with the combination of FOLFOX plus panitumumab compared to FOLFOX alone in a randomized phase III trial (9.6 vs. 8 months; P = 0.02) in patients demonstrated to have *KRAS* wild-type tumors.[86] No benefit was seen, and a possible harmful effect was seen in patients with mutant *KRAS* tumors.

Panitumumab was also combined with FOLFIRI in a phase II trial and demonstrated activity without substantially increasing the toxicity of FOLFIRI.[90] In this trial, PFS was improved by 1.7 months with the combination of panitumumab and FOLFIRI in patients with KRAS wild-type tumors (8.9 vs. 7.2 months, respectively).

For reasons that are not well understood, the addition of panitumumab or cetuximab to bevacizumab plus irinotecan- or oxaliplatin-containing chemotherapy *reduces* PFS and is currently not recommended. The Panitumumab Advanced Colorectal Cancer Evaluation Study (PACCE) trial and the CAIRO2 demonstrated a decrease in PFS of 1.4 months when panitumumab and 1.3 months when cetuximab was added to bevacizumab-containing chemotherapy, respectively.[117,118] Both of these differences were clinically and statistically significant. The results from these trials demonstrate the potential pitfalls of treating patients with multiple biologic agents outside of the setting of a clinical trial and why this practice should be avoided.

Selection of an Initial Metastatic Regimen

Several factors should be considered when selecting first-line therapy for metastatic colorectal cancer when disease palliation is the primary treatment goal. Based on the comparable results of FOLFIRI versus mFOLFOX6, either of these regimens (FOLFOX or FOLFIRI) are considered the reference standard in metastatic colorectal cancer. Most patients will receive first- and second-line regimens and patient preference for either sequence of treatments based on their different toxicity profiles is important. Preexisting neuropathies may lead to FOLFIRI being chosen initially, whereas increased bilirubin or known UGT1A1 deficiency (known risk factors for delayed diarrhea) may lead to FOLFOX as the initial choice. Alopecia occurs much more frequently with irinotecan compared to oxaliplatin combinations. Because FOLFOX can cause persistent neuropathy, a rationale for starting with FOLFIRI is based on the observation that time to progression is longer with first-line treatment than in second line; therefore, the time to death during which some patients will have to live with neuropathy may be shorter.[114] Capecitabine is an appropriate substitute for IV fluorouracil in oxaliplatin combination regimens. Because of higher response rates and modest survival benefit with FOLFOXIRI, this four-drug combination may be useful for patients with initially aggressive and symptomatic disease. Although efficacy with IROX is inferior to FOLFOX or FOLFIRI, this regimen might be considered for patients that are not candidates for a fluoropyrimidine.

The 2013 NCCN guidelines recommend the addition of bevacizumab to any initial fluoropyrimidine-based regimen unless its use is contraindicated in an individual patient.[58] EGFR inhibitors are an alternative first-line option in patients with wild-type *KRAS* tumors only. Fluorouracil plus leucovorin alone or capecitabine monotherapy is also appropriate first-line treatment for those individuals who cannot tolerate three-drug combination regimens.

Metastatic Disease: Second-Line and Subsequent Therapy

Systemic chemotherapy represents the mainstay of therapy for patients whose disease progresses following initial treatment for metastatic disease. Table 107-10 lists treatment options for refractory metastatic disease. Treatment options are based on the type of and response to prior treatments, the site and extent of disease, and patient factors and treatment preferences.

Systemic Chemotherapy

On disease progression following standard initial therapy, appropriate treatment options depend primarily on the type of prior therapy received. Because most patients will have received a combination of a fluoropyrimidine with either irinotecan or oxaliplatin, second-line therapy with the alternate regimen should be considered. Patient

TABLE 107-10 Second-line and Salvage Chemotherapy Regimens for Metastatic Colorectal Cancer[a]

Disease Progression with Prior Regimen	Comments
Oxaliplatin-Based Regimen	
Options	
1. Single agent cetuximab or panitumumab	Only if *KRAS* wild-type; cetuximab improved OS compared to best supportive care
2. Panitumumab + FOLFIRI	Only if *KRAS* wild-type; increased PFS compared to FOLFIRI alone
3. Ziv-aflibercept + irinotecan	
Irinotecan-Based Regimen	
Options	
1. FOLFOX or CapOx ± bevacizumab	Bevacizumab FDA- approved to continue with second-line options
2. FOLFOX or CapOx ± cetuximab or panitumumab	Only if *KRAS* wild-type
3. Cetuximab ± irinotecan	Only if *KRAS* wild-type; response rates with combination greater than cetuximab monotherapy
4. Single-agent panitumumab	Only if *KRAS* wild-type
Therapy after second progression or third progression	
1. Regorafenib	

CapOx, capecitabine plus oxaliplatin; FOLFIRI, fluorouracil plus leucovorin plus irinotecan; FOLFOX, fluorouracil plus leucovorin plus oxaliplatin.

[a]Single-agent fluoropyrimidine-based therapy or clinical trials are also acceptable options depending on patient-specific factors.

survival can exceed 2 years with this approach and it is important for patients to receive all traditional chemotherapy options if possible. Targeted agents can either be added to the above regimens or used as single agents.

Irinotecan Irinotecan was initially FDA approved as a second-line treatment for recurrent or progressive disease following fluorouracil. Two phase III trials compared irinotecan to either best supportive care or continuous-infusion fluorouracil in patients who had progressed within 6 months of treatment with fluorouracil.[109,110] Both trials demonstrated an improvement in OS with irinotecan as compared to the control arms. However, this approach is rarely used since single agent fluorouracil is rarely given as first-line therapy.

The use of the FOLFIRI regimen after progression with first-line FOLFOX demonstrated an objective response rate of 4% with a median PFS of 2.5 months.[82] These results are consistent with observations that demonstrate improved outcomes in those patients who are able to receive all active cytotoxic agents during the course of their disease.[114]

Based on these results, irinotecan should be considered standard second-line therapy for patients with disease progression with first-line treatment with oxaliplatin-containing regimens. Continuous-infusion fluorouracil (FOLFIRI), with or without biologic therapy, is most commonly given.

Oxaliplatin Oxaliplatin plus fluorouracil and leucovorin should be considered for patients who received primary treatment with irinotecan plus fluorouracil. Despite the low activity of single-agent oxaliplatin against fluorouracil-refractory disease, when oxaliplatin has been administered in a bimonthly regimen with high-dose leucovorin and continuous fluorouracil infusion, a 21% response rate with a median survival in excess of 10 months has been reported.[114] The combination of oxaliplatin plus fluorouracil and leucovorin is also effective as salvage therapy after initial treatment with irinotecan plus fluorouracil and leucovorin, with a similar response rate.[114] Although irinotecan can be used effectively as a single agent in colorectal cancer, it should be noted that oxaliplatin does not have substantial activity alone, and should only be given in combination with a fluoropyrimidine.

Targeted Therapy

(10) EGFR inhibitors may be administered in combination with irinotecan but can be used as single agents in patients who cannot tolerate irinotecan-based chemotherapy. Angiogenesis inhibitors are also used in second-line and subsequent therapy. However, the monoclonal antibodies bevacizumab and ziv-aflibercept are not given as single agents.

EGFR Inhibitors (10) Cetuximab is active in chemotherapy-refractory disease as a single agent and in combination with continued irinotecan.[60] The combination of cetuximab plus irinotecan was compared with cetuximab monotherapy in 329 patients with colorectal cancer who had progressed on irinotecan.[97] Cetuximab was given 400 mg/m^2 IV as a loading dose, followed by weekly infusions of 250 mg/m^2 IV plus irinotecan or cetuximab alone until disease progression. The objective response rates, 23% and 11% with cetuximab plus irinotecan and cetuximab alone, respectively, were very encouraging, and resulted in the endorsement of cetuximab by the FDA via accelerated approval. Median survival was 8.6 months for the combination and 6.9 months with monotherapy (P = 0.48). Time-to-disease-progression was significantly longer with cetuximab plus irinotecan than with cetuximab alone (4.1 vs. 1.5 months; HR 0.54), even among patients who also had oxaliplatin-refractory disease. The incidence of grade 3 or 4 adverse effects was as anticipated based on previous trials; asthenia (14%) and a follicular rash (9%) occurred most commonly with cetuximab alone, and in addition to typical irinotecan-related side effects (e.g., nausea, vomiting, diarrhea, and neutropenia). Another phase III trial that compared single agent cetuximab to best supportive care in patients refractory to oxaliplatin or irinotecan-based regimens confirmed these results.[110] Cetuximab demonstrated a 23% improvement in OS compared with best supportive care (HR, 0.77; 95%; P = .0046).

The combination of cetuximab and irinotecan has also been evaluated in the second-line setting in patients' naïve to irinotecan after oxaliplatin-based failures. The trial referred to as the EPIC trial, randomized patients to cetuximab plus irinotecan (N = 648) or irinotecan alone (N = 650).[93] The trial failed to meet its primary end point of an improvement of OS (HR = 0.98; P = .71) but did demonstrate significant improvements in PFS and relative risk (RR) with cetuximab. An important caveat for most initial trials with cetuximab is that *KRAS* testing was not initially performed. Retrospective analyses of these studies show that antitumor effects are limited to patients with wild-type *KRAS*.[114]

Panitumumab is a fully human monoclonal antibody targeted to the EGFR that was FDA approved for use in patients with metastatic colorectal cancer that no longer responds to previous therapy. The approval was based on a comparison of panitumumab to best supportive care in patients who had experienced disease progression after standard chemotherapy, including a fluoropyrimidine, irinotecan, and oxaliplatin. Patients received best supportive care or panitumumab (6 mg/kg IV every 2 weeks) until tumor progression.[98] Those patients who received panitumumab showed a 46% decrease in the rate of tumor progression compared with those who only received best supportive care (HR 0.54, 95% confidence interval [CI] 0.44 to 0.66). Retrospective analysis of *KRAS* testing demonstrated that the benefit was limited to patients with wild-type *KRAS* in that no responses and a decreased PFS was reported in patients with *KRAS* mutations treated with panitumumab.[114] As expected, dermatologic toxicities were observed in patients receiving panitumumab, as well as fatigue, abdominal pain, nausea, and diarrhea. Only one hypersensitivity reaction was reported.

Panitumumab has also been studied in combination with FOLFIRI in the second-line setting. In one of the first trials to prospectively evaluate end points by *KRAS* status, a phase III trial randomized patients to FOLFIRI with or without panitumumab.[112] In the *KRAS* wild-type group, a 2-month improvement in PFS was demonstrated; OS was not statistically different, although there was a trend to improvement with the panitumumab. Both monotherapy with panitumumab or combination with chemotherapy regiments such as FOLFIRI are recommended by current NCCN guidelines as second-line options (Table 107-10).[58]

Current evidence does not support restricting the use of EGFR inhibitors to patients with immunohistochemical evidence of EGFR-positive staining but rather results stress the influence of *KRAS* mutations on the efficacy of EGFR inhibitors in treating colorectal cancer.[58] *KRAS* is located downstream from the EGFR receptor and is involved in the EGFR signaling cascade by activating the MAPK pathway that influences cellular proliferation. Activating mutations in exon 2 are able to activate *KRAS* independent of EGFR receptor activation.[57] Therefore, EGFR receptor inhibition strategies are not effective in controlling cancer proliferation and growth. Several studies have demonstrated that *KRAS* mutational status predicts response to EGFR inhibitors used in colorectal cancer and its status should be determined prior to starting therapy directed at the EGFR receptor. Therapy with an EGFR inhibitor is not recommended in patients with mutant *KRAS*.[58]

Tumors harboring *BRAF* mutations are also associated with a poor prognosis and a poor response to EGFR inhibitors in patients with wild-type *KRAS*.[57] Although *BRAF* mutation testing is not routinely recommended at this time, *BRAF* mutation status may be considered in patients with wild-type *KRAS*.[58] Individuals with *BRAF* mutations should not receive EGFR inhibitors.

Neither of the EGFR inhibitors should be used in the second-line setting if they were part of a patient's initial treatment regimen. Therefore, the initial first-line regimen determines whether cetuximab should be used as monotherapy or combined with irinotecan in the second-line setting (Table 107-10).

Angiogenesis Inhibitors Angiogenesis inhibitors are also used in the second-line setting. In patients who did not receive bevacizumab in their initial treatment, FOLFOX plus bevacizumab is recommended based on phase III data. Results from Eastern Cooperative Group 3200 demonstrated that bevacizumab, in combination with FOLFOX4, improved survival in patients with previously treated advanced colorectal cancer.[111] It should be noted that patients were excluded if they received prior oxaliplatin or bevacizumab and the dose of bevacizumab was 10 mg/kg instead of 5 mg/kg. Median survival was improved from 10.7 to 12.5 months ($P = 0.0018$). The FDA has also approved the use of bevacizumab after progression on first-line bevacizumab. In the Phase III registry trial, patients were randomized at progression to second-line treatment with chemotherapy plus bevacizumab or chemotherapy alone.[113] The chemotherapy regimen was switched in the second-line setting based on what they received in the first-line setting (e.g., if FOLFOX was given in the first-line setting, therapy was changed to FOLFIRI). The primary end point of OS was 1.4 months longer with bevacizumab and reached statistical significance.

Clinical **Controversy...**

Continuation of bevacizumab after disease progression has recently been FDA approved. Originally justified based on retrospective data that demonstrate improved survival, a confirmatory phase III trial demonstrated a small improvement in OS. Benefit of this strategy versus changing the antiangiogenic therapy to a new agent that targets the same pathway will need to be determined.

Ziv-aflibercept, a soluble recombinant fusion protein that was designed to block the angiogenic process, is also approved in the second-line setting. The agent was developed by fusing sections of the VEGFR-1 and VEGFR-2 immunoglobulin domains to the F_c portion of human immunoglobulin G1 (IgG1) and blocks VEGF-A, VEGF-B, and placental growth factor (PIGF) by "trapping" the ligands before they get to the native transmembrane receptors. In a phase III randomized trial, FOLFIRI plus ziv-aflibercept was compared to FOLFIRI after progression on an oxaliplatin-based regimen.[88] The trial met its primary end point with an improvement in OS (13.5 months for FOLFIRI/ziv-aflibercept vs. 12.1 months for FOLFIRI/placebo; HR, 0.82; $P = 0.003$). It is dosed at 4 mg/kg as an IV infusion over 1 hour every 2 weeks and is associated with similar adverse effects as bevacizumab.

Regorafenib, a small-molecule inhibitor of tumor angiogenesis (VEGFR-1, VEGFR-2, and VEGFR-3) and other downstream targets (C-KIT, RET, RAF1, and BRAF), is approved for the third- or fourth-line treatment of metastatic colorectal cancer. This oral agent is dosed 160 mg once daily for the first 21 days of each 28-day cycle. In a phase III trial of patients with metastatic colorectal cancer and progression during or within 3 months of last chemotherapy, regorafenib demonstrated a 1.4-month improvement in OS when compared to placebo.[99] Because this is an oral-only regimen, patients must be counseled on its use and potential toxicity. Regorafenib should be taken with a low-fat breakfast and may interact with CYP P4503A4 inducers and inhibitors. Toxicities include hypertension, hand–foot syndrome, and hepatotoxicity.

Hepatic-Directed Therapies

Patients with unresectable or nonablatable hepatic-predominant metastases or who are unable to undergo surgery may be candidates for chemoembolization, radioembolization, or HAI chemotherapy, as discussed previously.[80] Hepatic arterial chemoembolization delivers high concentrations of cytotoxic agents directly to the tumor and results in the embolization or devascularization of the liver, which blocks perfusion of the tumor and eliminates its blood supply. This procedure involves the instillation of a mixture that incorporates chemotherapeutic agents, radioactive contrast dye, and/or an embolic agent directly into the hepatic artery. Agents most commonly used include doxorubicin, mitomycin, and cisplatin, which are usually dissolved in about 10 to 15 mL of a radiographic contrast dye. Addition of an embolic agent to the mixture results in either a temporary or permanent occlusion of the hepatic artery. Local tumor response rates with these strategies are high and most patients will experience partial or complete relief of symptoms. Toxicities include postembolization syndrome characterized by nausea, fatigue, and transient elevations in hepatic enzymes and bilirubin, gastrointestinal ulcerations, and biliary toxicity. Although various hepatic-directed therapies offer potential disease palliation in select patients with unresectable, yet limited hepatic metastases, no conclusive survival advantage has been demonstrated.

New Strategies and Agents in Development

The number of active cytotoxic agents against cancers of the colon and rectum is limited. These traditional chemotherapy agents, which target rapidly dividing cells, kill both malignant and nonmalignant cells, and new cancer therapies are needed to improve therapeutic outcomes. In particular, targeted therapies aimed at the underlying cancer pathology are increasingly being developed and used in colorectal cancer treatment. A variety of agents targeted toward augmenting the host immune system response have undergone, or are currently undergoing, study for colorectal cancer, including monoclonal antibodies and tumor vaccines. Additional strategies include regulating tumor growth through the inhibition of various cell proliferation, survival, and death pathways, angiogenesis, and cancer stem cells. Agents that can alter microenvironmental factors that support angiogenesis and tumor metastases may also be of benefit.

PERSONALIZED PHARMACOTHERAPY

Drug therapy for patients diagnosed with colorectal cancers should be individualized based on several established tumor and patient pharmacogenetic factors that influence treatment response. In addition, various tumor characteristics, patient genetics, and molecular markers may predict prognosis and/or response to certain therapies and provide the rationale for pharmacogenomic strategies to select appropriate therapies for individual patients. Table 107-11 summarizes potential predictive markers for individualizing colorectal cancer treatment.

The most important development in biomarkers for colorectal cancer treatment has been validation of *KRAS* mutation status as a predictive marker for lack of tumor response to EGFR inhibitors.[60,119] Tumors should be tested for *KRAS* mutations at diagnosis of stage IV disease; patients with *KRAS* mutations on codons 12 and 13 on chromosome 12 are not candidates for EGFR inhibitors. However, not all *KRAS* mutations confer similar biology. In contrast to codon 2 mutations, *KRAS* G13D mutations may be associated with improved outcomes to cetuximab in first-line therapy, but additional studies are needed.[120] Because only about 60% of patients with *KRAS* wild-type tumors respond to treatment, additional factors

TABLE 107-11 Potential Predictive Markers for Personalized Pharmacotherapy for Colorectal Cancer

Biomarker	Relationship to response
Tumor Characteristics	
MSI (MSI-H)	Improved prognosis; may predict lack of benefit from adjuvant fluorouracil
KRAS mutations at codons 12 and 13 on chromosome 12	Predict lack of response to EGFR MoAb inhibitors
BRAF V600E mutation	May predict lack of response to EGFR MoAb inhibitors in *KRAS* wild-type tumors
Thymidylate synthase	Increased TS expression associated with reduced response to fluorouracil
PIK3CA mutation	May predict lack of response to EGFR inhibitors May predict patients likely to benefit from adjuvant aspirin or aspirin chemoprevention
EGFR copy number	Increased *EGFR* copy number may predict increased likelihood of response to EGFR inhibitors
PTEN mutation	May predict lack of response to EGFR inhibitors
ERCC1	Elevated mRNA expression or ERCC1 protein expression associated with resistance to platinum-based chemotherapy Decreased ERCC1 protein expression associated with improved survival with FOLFOX
TFAP2E-DKK4	*TFAP2E* hypermethylation associated with fluorouracil resistance
Patient Characteristics	
DPYD polymorphisms	Polymorphisms associated with DPD deficiency associated with risk of severe fluorouracil toxicities
Skin rash with EGFR inhibitor	Development of skin rash with EGFR inhibitors may predict response to treatment and improved treatment outcome
TS polymorphisms	Low TS expression associated with increased incidence of toxicity with fluorouracil
MTHFR polymorphisms	Polymorphisms linked to reduced intracellular folate pools associated with capecitabine toxicity
UTG1A1 polymorphisms	Homozygous 7-repeat allele (UGT1A1*28) associated with increased risk of severe diarrhea with irinotecan

DPYD, dihydropyrimidine dehydrogenase; EGFR, epidermal growth factor receptor; ERCC1, excision repair cross-complementing C1; FOLFOX, fluorouracil, leucovorin, and oxaliplatin; MoAb, monoclonal antibody; MSI, microsatellite instability; MTHFR, methylenetetrahydrofolate reductase; TS, thymidylate synthase; UGT1A1, uridine diphosphate-glucuronosyltransferase.

Data from references 21, 33, 57-60, 119.

have been explored for their ability to predict response to EGFR inhibitors, including *BRAF* V600E mutation, and mutation or loss of *PTEN* or *PIK3CA*.[33,60] Although the predictive value of *BRAF* mutation status has not been established, the presence of this mutation appears to be associated with lack of response to EGFR monoclonal antibody inhibitors.[119]

About 12% to 22% of stage II and III colorectal cancers show high-frequency microsatellite instability (MSI-H), which is associated with an improved prognosis.[60] Findings from pooled analyses of patients with MSI-H tumors who received adjuvant fluorouracil indicate a lack of response to treatment, perhaps due to an improved overall prognosis and/or additional factors. Nevertheless, some practitioners use MSI status to determine which patients with low-risk stage II colorectal cancer should not receive adjuvant fluorouracil. Current NCCN guidelines recommend MSI testing for stage II colon cancers because MSI-H status confers a good prognosis and those patients do not benefit from adjuvant fluorouracil.[58]

Of factors predictive for tumor sensitivity to fluorouracil, TS expression has been most studied. Tumors that overexpress TS, an enzyme that converts deoxyuridine monophosphate to deoxythymidine monophosphate, an essential step for DNA synthesis, are less sensitive to fluorouracil chemotherapy.[57] Patients whose cancers have higher levels of TS appear to have a significantly worse overall 5-year survival than patients whose cancers have a low level of TS.[55] However, no large cooperative group trial has identified a subgroup of patients who failed to benefit from fluorouracil plus leucovorin therapy based on tumor TS levels. Therefore, tumor testing for TS overexpression is not routinely used to select fluorouracil treatments.[57]

TFAP2E, a gene that encodes transcription factor AP-2 epsilon, is frequently hypermethylated in colorectal cancer.[121] *TFAP2E* hypermethylation and decreased expression is associated with nonresponse to fluorouracil chemotherapy, independent of MSI, mutations of key regulatory cancer genes, or genes known to affect fluorouracil metabolism. Additional studies are needed to confirm the role of *TFAP2E* mutation testing for optimal drug selection.

Tumors with *P53* mutations demonstrate a high degree of resistance to radiation, fluorouracil, and certain other chemotherapeutic agents and are associated with a less-favorable prognosis. However, because of difficulties with adequately sensitive and specific immunohistochemical analysis to identify *P53* mutations, widespread testing and application of this as a marker is unlikely.[57]

Patients that are homozygous for a *UGT1A1* 7-repeat allele (*UGT1A1*28*) are at increased risk for severe diarrhea with irinotecan. A FDA-approved test to determine UGT1A1 genotype is commercially available. Although some individuals advocate testing UGT1A1 genotype prior to starting irinotecan, widespread testing has not been adopted.[57] The package insert recommends an initial reduced dose in patients with *UGT1A1*28* genotype.

Although patients who are deficient in DPD experience severe and potentially life-threatening toxicities with conventional doses of fluorouracil, determination of DPD activity is relatively time consuming and the techniques are not amenable to routine clinical practice. However, genetic testing for *DPYD* polymorphisms can identify patients who would require lower fluorouracil doses to avoid severe toxicity. As an alternative, plasma ratio determinations of uracil and dihydrouracil, which are more easily obtainable, can identify individuals with DPD deficiency that are at risk of developing significant toxicities.[122]

Excision repair cross-complementing C1 (ERCC1) is a DNA excision repair protein that has been evaluated as a predictive test for response to platinum chemotherapy.[57] Certain *ERCC1* polymorphisms are associated with decreased ERCC1 protein expression, which may predict for response to and improved survival with FOLFOX chemotherapy.[57] Presently, there is a lack of consensus as to the preferred test for tumor ERCC1 expression, immunohistochemistry analysis or mRNA expression using reverse-transcription polymerase chain reaction (RT-PCR). However, testing approaches to aid in optimal drug selection may become available in the future.

Tests for other polymorphisms that may be useful to predict treatment toxicity have been established but are not routinely used. Germline polymorphisms that result in decreased TS expression are associated with an increased frequency of fluorouracil toxicities, including myelosuppression, diarrhea, and mucositis.[57] *MTHFR* polymorphisms that are linked to reductions in intracellular folate pools have been associated with increased capecitabine toxicity.[57]

Because of the wide inter- and intrapatient variability in fluorouracil pharmacokinetics and a narrow therapeutic range, pharmacokinetic optimization of fluorouracil represents a potential strategy to individualize dosing and optimize efficacy and minimize adverse effects.[123] Published data suggest that only 20% to 30% of patients treated with fluorouracil achieve therapeutic concentrations.[124] A prospective study that compared pharmacokinetically guided fluorouracil dosing with conventional dosing in patients with metastatic colorectal cancer demonstrated that pharmacokinetically guided dose adjustments reduced grade 3/4 toxicities, increased the objective tumor response rate, and provided a higher yet not significantly increased survival rate.[125] Valid assay methods that facilitate therapeutic drug monitoring are now available and are being used in some centers. Algorithms are available for specific treatment protocols that enable practitioners to determine doses based on patient physiological and pathophysiological characteristics.[123] Whether clinicians adopt this strategy and if it will indeed advance therapeutic outcomes have yet to be established.

EVALUATION OF THERAPEUTIC OUTCOMES

The goal of monitoring is to evaluate whether the patient is receiving any benefit from the management of the disease or to detect recurrence. Similarly, examinations help to determine whether preventive interventions or screening studies effectively reduce an individual's risk for developing colorectal cancer or presenting with an advanced stage of disease. During treatment for active disease, patients should undergo monitoring for measurable tumor response, progression, or new metastases; these tests may include chest CT scans or radiographs, abdominal or pelvic CT scans or radiographs, depending on the site of disease being evaluated for response, and CEA measurements every 3 months if the CEA is or was previously elevated. In addition, a complete blood cell count should be obtained prior to each course of chemotherapy administration to ensure that hematologic indices are adequate. Baseline liver function tests and an assessment of renal function should be evaluated prior to and periodically during therapy. These tests and other selected serum chemistries should also be evaluated with the development of any new symptoms or significant change in disease status. Patients should be evaluated during every treatment visit for the presence of anticipated side effects, which generally include loose stools or diarrhea, nausea or vomiting, mouth sores, fatigue, and fever, as well as other side effects such as neuropathy, skin rash, and hepatotoxicity that are typically associated with oxaliplatin, EGFR inhibitors, and regorafenib, respectively. Serum electrolytes, including magnesium, should be monitored for during treatment with EGFR inhibitors. Patients receiving bevacizumab, ziv aflibercept, or regorafenib should be evaluated for hypertension and proteinuria.

Symptoms of recurrence such as pain syndromes, changes in bowel habits, rectal or vaginal bleeding, pelvic masses, anorexia, and weight loss develop in less than 50% of patients. A greater percentage of recurrences are detected in asymptomatic patients because of increased serum CEA levels that lead to further examination. Although the value of CEA monitoring for asymptomatic disease recurrence is questioned by some because of the related expense and emotional stress associated with false-positive elevations, CEA monitoring plays an important role in postoperative follow-up studies for most individuals. A PET scan can be considered to identify localized sites of metastatic disease when a rising CEA level suggests metastatic disease but CT scans and other imaging studies are negative.

Patients who undergo curative surgical resection, with or without adjuvant therapy, require close follow-up based on the premise that early detection and treatment of recurrence could still render them cured. In addition, early treatment for asymptomatic metastatic colorectal cancer appears superior to delayed therapy. Specific practice guidelines for postoperative surveillance examinations following successful treatment for stage II or III disease were developed by NCCN and include: history, physical examination, and CEA test every 3 to 6 months for the first 2 years, then every 6 months for a total of 5 years; annual chest and abdominal and pelvic CT scans for up to 5 years following primary therapy; and colonoscopy at about 1 year after surgery. Repeat colonoscopies are recommended at 3 years, unless findings of polyps warrant closer follow-up. Less intensive surveillance is recommended for patients treated for stage I disease because of low risk of recurrence.[58]

Posttreatment surveillance should also include a survivorship care plan with immunizations for vaccine-preventable diseases, early detection of second primary cancers, and support systems that encourage smoking cessation, establish regular exercise and maintain a healthy BMI, and encourage healthy lifestyle and dietary choices.[58]

Recent advances in the treatment for cancer of the colon and rectum now offer the potential to improve patient survival, but for many patients, improved DFS and PFS represent equally important therapeutic outcomes. Although treatment approaches for metastatic colorectal cancer have been historically assessed by their ability to produce a measurable objective tumor response, which is generally believed necessary for any treatment to improve survival, the effects of therapies on survival are clinically more meaningful than their ability to induce a tumor response. However, with the availability of multiple active treatments for metastatic disease, and the likelihood that patients will receive more than one during the course of their treatment, improvements in OS with new therapies will be increasingly difficult to determine.

In the absence of the ability of a specific treatment to demonstrate improved survival, important outcome measures should include the effects of the treatment on patient symptoms, daily activities and performance status, and other quality-of-life indicators, as well as PFS and time-to-treatment failure. Because most metastatic colorectal cancers are incurable, a specific decision regarding an individual patient's care will ultimately be required. This decision should be based on a careful assessment of the balance between risks associated with treatment (or lack thereof) and benefits of treatment. Effort should also be made to ensure that the costs of screening, diagnostic tests, treatments, and procedures for colorectal cancer are consistent with their value in improving patient outcomes.

ABBREVIATIONS

APC	adenomatous polyposis coli (gene)
APR	abdominoperineal resection
BMI	body mass index
CALGB	Cancer and Leukemia Group B
CapOx	capecitabine plus oxaliplatin
CEA	carcinoembryonic antigen
CIN	chromosomal instability
CIMP	CpG island methylator phenotype
COX	cyclooxygenase
CT	computed tomography
CTC	computed tomography colonography
CYP	cytochrome P450 isoenzyme
DCBE	double-contrast barium enema
DFMO	difluoromethylornithine

DFS	disease-free survival
DPD	dihydropyrimidine dehydrogenase
EBRT	external beam radiation therapy
EGFR	epidermal growth factor receptor
ERCC1	excision repair cross-complementing C1
EUS	endorectal ultrasound
FAP	familial adenomatous polyposis
FDA	Food and Drug Administration
FIT	fecal immunochemical test
FLOX	fluorouracil, leucovorin, oxaliplatin
FOBT	fecal occult blood test
FOLFIRI	fluorouracil, leucovorin, and irinotecan
FOLFOX	fluorouracil, leucovorin, and oxaliplatin
FOLFOXIRI	infusional fluorouracil and leucovorin, oxaliplatin, irinotecan
FSIG	flexible sigmoidoscopy
5-FU	fluorouracil
LV5FU2	infusional fluorouracil and leucovorin
gFOBT	guaiac-based fecal occult blood test
GST	glutathione-*S*-transferase
HAI	hepatic artery infusion
HbA_{1c}	glycosylated hemoglobin
HNPCC	hereditary nonpolyposis colorectal cancer
HR	hazard ratio
IFL	irinotecan, fluorouracil, and leucovorin
iFOBT	immunochemical fecal occult blood test
IGF-1	insulin-like growth factor-1
IgG1	immunoglobulin G1
INR	international normalized ratio
IROX	irinotecan and oxaliplatin
LOH	loss of heterozygosity
MAPK	mitogen-activated protein kinase
MMR	mismatch-repair
MOSAIC	Multicenter International Study of Oxaliplatin/5-Fluorouracil/Leucovorin in the Adjuvant Treatment of Colon Cancer
MRI	magnetic resonance imaging
MTHFR	methylenetetrahydrofolate reductase
MSI	microsatellite instability
NAT	*N*-acetyltransferase
NCCN	National Comprehensive Cancer Network
NF-κB	nuclear factor kappa B
NSAID	nonsteroidal antiinflammatory drug
OS	overall survival
PACCE	Panitumumab Advanced Colorectal Cancer Evaluation Study
PET	positron emission tomography
PETACC-3	Third Pan-European Trial in Adjuvant Colon Cancer
PFS	progression-free survival
15-PGDH	15-prostaglandin dehydrogenase
PIGF	placental growth factor
PI3K	phosphatidylinositol 3-kinase
PIP_3	phosphatidylinositol-3,4,5-triphosphate
PPE	palmar–plantar erythrodysesthesia
RFA	radiofrequency ablation
RR	relative risk
RT-PCR	reverse-transcription polymerase chain reaction
sDNA	stool DNA
TGF-β	transforming growth factor-β
TIL	tumor-infiltrating lymphocyte
TME	total excision of the mesorectum
TNF-α	tumor necrosis factor-alpha
TS	thymidylate synthase
UGT1A1	uridine diphosphate-glucuronosyltransferase
USPSTF	United States Preventive Services Task Force
VDR	vitamin D receptor
VEGF	vascular endothelial growth factor
VEGFR	vascular endothelial growth factor receptor
XRT	radiation therapy

REFERENCES

1. Siegel R, Naishadham MA, Jemal A. Cancer statistics, 2013. CA Cancer J Clin 2013;63:11–30.
2. Jemal A, Bray F, Center MM, Ferlay J, Ward E, Forman D. Global cancer statistics. CA Cancer J Clin 2011;61:69–90.
3. Howlader N, Noone AM, Krapcho M, et al., eds. SEER Cancer Statistics Review, 1975–2009 (Vintage 2009 Populations). Bethesda, MD: National Cancer Institute. November 2011 SEER data submission; posted April 2012, *http://seer.cancer.gov/csr/1975_2009_pops09/*.
4. Siegel RL, Jemal A, Ward EM. Increase in incidence of colorectal cancer among young men and women in the United States. Cancer Epidemiol Biomarkers Prev 2009;18:1695–1698.
5. Lieberman DA, Rex DK, Winawer SJ, et al. Guidelines for colonoscopy surveillance after screening and polypectomy: A consensus update by the US Multi-Society Task Force on Colorectal Cancer. Gastroenterology 2012;143:844–857.
6. Collins P, Mpofu C, Watson A, Rhodes J. Strategies for detecting colon cancer and/or dysplasia in patients with inflammatory bowel disease. Cochrane Database Syst Rev 2006;2:CD000279.
7. Triantafillidis JK, Nasioulas G, Kosmidis PA. Colorectal cancer and inflammatory bowel disease: Epidemiology, risk factors, mechanisms of carcinogenesis and prevention strategies. Anticancer Res 2009;29:2727–2737.
8. Chan AT, Giovannucci EL. Primary prevention of colorectal cancer. Gastroenterology 2010;138:2020–2043.
9. Larsson SC, Orsini N, Wolk A. Diabetes mellitus and risk of colorectal cancer: A meta-analysis. J Natl Cancer Inst 2005;97:1679–1687.
10. Dehal AN, Newton CC, Jacobs EJ, et al. Impact of diabetes mellitus and insulin use on survival after colorectal cancer diagnosis: The Cancer Prevention Study-II Nutrition Cohort. J Clin Oncol 2011;30:53–59.
11. Patel SG, Ahnen DJ. Familial colon cancer syndromes: An update of a rapidly evolving field. Curr Gastroenterol Rep 2012;14:428–438.
12. Haggar FA, Boushey RP. Colorectal cancer epidemiology: Incidence, mortality, survival, and risk factors. Clin Colon Rectal Surg 2009;22:191–197.
13. Gala M, Chung DC. Hereditary colon cancer syndromes. Semin Oncol 2011;38:490–499.
14. Stoffel E, Mukherjee B, Raymond VM, et al. Calculation of risk of colorectal and endometrial cancer among patients with Lynch syndrome. Gastroenterology 2009;137:1621–1627.
15. Lynch HT, Lynch PM, Lanspa SJ, et al. Review of the Lynch syndrome: History, molecular genetics, screening, differential diagnosis, and medicolegal ramifications. Clin Genet 2009;76:1–18.
16. Reszka E, Wasowicz W, Gromadzinska J. Genetic polymorphism of xenobiotic metabolising enzymes, diet and cancer susceptibility. Br J Nutr 2006;96:609–619.
17. Goode EL, Potter JD, Bamlet WR, Rider DN, Bigler J. Inherited variation in carcinogen-metabolizing enzymes and risk of colorectal polyps. Carcinogenesis 2007;28:328–341.

18. Thun MJ, Jacobs EJ, Patrono C. The role of aspirin in cancer prevention. Nat Rev Clin Oncol 2012;9:259–267.
19. Rothwell PM. Aspirin in prevention of sporadic colorectal cancer: Current clinical evidence and overall balance of risks and benefits. Recent Results Cancer Res 2013;191:121–142.
20. Cooper K, Squires H, Carroll C, et al. Chemoprevention of colorectal cancer: Systematic review and economic evaluation. Health Technol Assess 2010;14:1–206.
21. Liao X, Lochhead P, Nishihara R, et al. Aspirin use, tumor *PIK3CA* mutation, and colorectal-cancer survival. N Engl J Med 2012;367:1596–1606.
22. Rennert G, Rennert HS, Pinchey M, et al. Use of hormone replacement therapy and the risk of colorectal cancer. J Clin Oncol 2009;27:4542–4547.
23. Ma Y, Yang Y, Wang F, et al. Obesity and risk of colorectal cancer risk: A systemic review of prospective studies. PLoS One 2013;8:e53916.
24. Campbell PT, Jacobs ET, Ulrich CM, et al. Case-control study of overweight, obesity, and colorectal cancer, overall and by tumor microsatellite instability status. J Natl Cancer Inst 2010;102:391–400.
25. Botteri E, Iodice S, Bagnardi V, et al. Smoking and colorectal cancer: A meta-analysis. JAMA 2008;300:2765–2778.
26. McCleary NJ, Niedzwiecki D, Hollis D, et al. Impact of smoking on patients with stage II colon cancer. Cancer 2010;116:956–966.
27. Vargas AJ, Thompson PA. Diet and nutrient factors in colorectal cancer risk. Nutr Clin Pract 2012;27:612–623.
28. Aune D, Chan DSM, Lau R, et al. Dietary fibre, whole grains, and risk of colorectal cancer: Systematic review and dose-response meta-analysis of prospective studies. BMJ 2011;343:d6617.
29. Ma Y, Zhang P, Wang F, et al. Association between vitamin D and risk of colorectal cancer: A systematic review of prospective studies. J Clin Oncol 2011;29:3775–3782.
30. Pend's-Franco N, Aguilera Ó, Pereira F, et al. Vitamin D and Wnt/β-catenin pathway in colon cancer: Role and regulation of *DICKKOPF* genes. Anticancer Res 2008;28: 2613–2624.
31. Hubner RA, Houlston RS. Folate and colorectal cancer prevention. Br J Cancer 2009;100:233–239.
32. Markowitz SD, Bertagnolli MM. Molecular basis of colorectal cancer. N Engl J Med 2009;361:2449–2460.
33. Fearon ER. Molecular genetics of colorectal cancer. Annu Rev Pathol 2011;6:479–507.
34. Al-Sohaily S, Biankin A, Leong R. et al. Molecular pathways in colorectal cancer. J Gastroenterol Hepatol 2012;27: 1423–1431.
35. Yarom N, Jonker DJ. The role of the epidermal growth factor receptor in the mechanism and treatment of colorectal cancer. Discov Med 2011;11:95–105.
36. Lanza G, Messerini L, Gafà R, Risio M; Gruppo Italiano Patologi Apparato Digerente (GIPAD); Società Italiana di Anatomia Patologica e Citopatologia Diagnostica/ International Academy of Pathology, Italian division (SIAPEC/IAP). Colorectal tumors: The histology report. Dig Liver Dis 2011(43 suppl 4):S344–S355.
37. Zhou P, Cheng SW, Yang R, et al. Combination chemoprevention: Future direction of colorectal cancer prevention. Eur J Cancer Prev 2012;21:231–240.
38. Uccello M, Malaguarnera G, Basile F, et al. Potential role of probiotics on colorectal cancer prevention. BMC Surg 2012;12(suppl 1):S35, DOI:10.1186/1471-2482-12-S1-S35. *http://www.biomedcentral.com/1471-2482/12/S1/S35.*
39. Hosono K, Endo H, Takahashi H, et al. Metformin suppresses azoxymethane-induced colorectal aberrant crypt foci by activating AMP-activated protein kinase. Mol Carcinog 2010;49:662–671.
40. Cuzick J, Otto F, Baron JA, et al. Aspirin and non-steroidal anti-inflammatory drugs for cancer prevention: an international consensus statement. Lancet Oncol 2009;10:501–507.
41. U.S. Preventive Services Task Force. Routine aspirin or nonsteroidal anti-inflammatory drugs for the primary prevention of colorectal cancer: U.S. Preventive Services Task Force Recommendation Statement. Ann Intern Med 2007;146:361–364.
42. Chan AT, Arber N, Burn J, et al. Aspirin in the chemoprevention of colorectal neoplasia: An overview. Cancer Prev Res (Phila) 2012;5:164–178.
43. Chung M, Lee J, Terasawa T, et al. Vitamin D with or without calcium supplementation for prevention of cancer and fractures: An updated meta-analysis for the U.S. Preventive Services Task Force. Ann Intern Med 2011;155:827–838.
44. Qaseem A, Denberg TD, Hopkins RH, et al. Screening for colorectal cancer: A guidance statement from the American College of Physicians. Ann Intern Med 2012; 156:378–386.
45. Levin B, Lieberman DA, McFarland B, et al. Screening and surveillance for the early detection of colorectal cancer and adenomatous polyps, 2008; a joint guideline from the American Cancer Society, the US Multi-Society on Colorectal Cancer, and the American College of Radiology. CA Cancer J Clin 2008;58:138–160.
46. Smith RA, Brooks D, Cokkinides V, et al. Cancer Screening in the United States, 2013: A review of current American Cancer Society guidelines, current issues in cancer screening, and new guidance on cervical cancer screening and lung cancer screening. CA Cancer J Clin 2013;63: 87–105.
47. Rex DK, Johnson DA, Anderson JC, et al. American College of Gastroenterology Guidelines for Colorectal Cancer Screening 2008. Am J Gastroenterol 2009;104:739–750.
48. U.S. Preventive Services Task Force. Screening for colorectal cancer: U.S. Preventive Services Task Force recommendation statement. Ann Intern Med 2008;149:627–637.
49. NCCN Guidelines—Colorectal Cancer Screening v.2.2012. 2013, *http://www.nccn.org/professionals/physician_gls/pdf/colorectal_screening.pdf.*
50. Quinter E, Castells A, Bujanda L, et al. Colonoscopy versus fecal immunochemical testing in colorectal-cancer screening. N Engl J Med 2012;366:697–706.
51. Locker GY, Hamilton S, Harris J, et al. ASCO 2006 update of recommendations for the use of tumor markers in gastrointestinal cancer. J Clin Oncol 2006;24:5313–5327.
52. Gunderson LL, Jessup JM, Sargent DJ, Greene FL, Stewart AK. Revised TN categorization for colon cancer based on national survival outcomes data. J Clin Oncol 2010;28: 264–271.
53. Gunderson LL, Jessup JM, Sargent DJ, Greene FL, Stewart AK. Revised tumor and node categorization for rectal cancer based on surveillance, epidemiology, and end results and rectal pooled analysis outcomes. J Clin Oncol 2010;28: 256–263.
54. Colon and rectum. In: Edge SB, Byrd DR, Compton CC, et al., eds.; American Joint Committee on Cancer. AJCC Cancer Staging Manual, 7th ed. New York: Springer, 2010:143–159.
55. Libutti KS, Saltz LB, Willett CG. Cancers of the gastrointestinal tract: Cancer of the colon. In: DeVita VT, Lawrence TS, Rosenberg SA, eds. Cancer: Principles and

Practice of Oncology, 9th ed. Philadelphia: Lippincott Williams & Wilkins, 2011:1084–1126.
56. Zlobec I, Lugli A. Prognostic and predictive factors in colorectal cancer. J Clin Pathol 2008;61:561–569.
57. Ross JS, Torres-Mora J, Wagle N, et al. Biomarker-based prediction of response to therapy for colorectal cancer. Am J Clin Pathol 2010;134:478–490.
58. NCCN Guidelines—Colon Cancer v.3.2013. 2013, *http://www.nccn.org/professionals/physician_gls/pdf/colon.pdf.*
59. Kelley RK, Venook AP. Prognostic and predictive markers in stage II colon cancer: Is there a role for gene expression profiling? Clin Colorectal Cancer 2011;10:73–80.
60. Cunningham D, Atkin W, Lenz HJ, et al. Colorectal cancer. Lancet 2010;375:1030–1047.
61. Phillips JG, Hong TS, Ryan DP. Multidisciplinary management of early-stage rectal cancer. J Natl Compr Canc Netw 2012;10:1577–1585.
62. Giantonio BJ, Catalano PJ, Meropol NJ, et al. Bevacizumab in combination with oxaliplatin, fluorouracil, and leucovorin (FOLFOX4) for previously treated metastatic colorectal cancer: Results from the Eastern Cooperative Oncology Group Study E3200. J Clin Oncol 2007;25:1539–1544.
63. Andre T, Boni C, Navarro M, et al. Improved overall survival with oxaliplatin, fluorouracil, and leucovorin as adjuvant treatment in stage II or III colon cancer in the MOSAIC trial. J Clin Oncol 2009;27:3109–3116.
64. Yothers G, O'Connell MJ, Allegra CJ, et al. Oxaliplatin as adjuvant therapy for colon cancer: Updated results of NSABP C-07 trial, including survival and subset analyses. J Clin Oncol 2011;29:3768–3774.
65. Twelves C, Scheithauer W, McKendrick J, et al. Capecitabine versus 5-fluorouracil/folinic acid as adjuvant therapy for stage III colon cancer: Final results from the X-ACT trial with analysis by age and preliminary evidence of a pharmacodynamic marker of efficacy. Ann Oncol 2012;23;1190–1197.
66. Haller DG, Tabernero J, Maroun J, et al. Capecitabine plus oxaliplatin compared with fluorouracil and folinic acid as adjuvant therapy for stage III colon cancer. J Clin Oncol 2011;29:1465–1471.
67. Wolmark N, Rockette H, Fisher B, et al. The benefit of leucovorin-modulated fluorouracil as postoperative adjuvant therapy for primary colon cancer: Results from National Surgical Adjuvant Breast and Bowel Project protocol C-03. J Clin Oncol 1993;11:1879–1887.
68. O'Connell MJ, Mailliard JA, Kahn MJ, et al. Controlled trial of fluorouracil and low-dose leucovorin given for 6 months as postoperative adjuvant therapy for colon cancer. J Clin Oncol 1997;15:246–250.
69. Van Cutsem E, Labianca R, Bodoky G, et al. Randomized phase III trial comparing biweekly infusional fluorouracil/leucovorin alone or with irinotecan in the adjuvant treatment of stage III colon cancer: PETACC-3. J Clin Oncol 2009;27:3117–3125.
70. Chuang VTG, Suno M. Levoleucovorin as replacement for leucovorin in cancer treatment. Ann Pharmacother 2012;46:1349–1357.
71. Meta-Analysis Group in Cancer. Toxicity of fluorouracil in patients with advanced colorectal cancer: Effect of administration schedule and prognostic factors. J Clin Oncol 1998;16:3537–3541.
72. Saltz LB, Niedzwiecki D, Hollis D, et al. Irinotecan fluorouracil plus leucovorin is not superior to fluorouracil plus leucovorin alone as adjuvant treatment for stage III colon cancer: Results of CALGB 89803. J Clin Oncol 2007;25:3456–3461.
73. Ychou M, Raoul J, Douillard J, et al. A phase III randomized trial of LV5FU2+CPT-11 vs. LV5FU2 alone in adjuvant high risk colon cancer (FNCLCC Accord02/FFCD9802). Ann Oncol 2009;20:674–680.
74. Allegra CJ, Yothers G, O'Connell MJ, et al. Phase III trial assessing bevacizumab in stages II and III carcinoma of the colon: results of NSABP protocol C-08. J Clin Oncol 2011;29:11–16.
75. Alberts SR, Sargent DJ, Nair S, et al. Effect of oxaliplatin, fluorouracil, and leucovorin with or without cetuximab on survival among patients with resected stage III colon cancer: A randomized trial. JAMA 2012;307:1383–1393.
76. NCCN Guidelines—Rectal Cancer v.4.2013. 2013, *http://www.nccn.org/professionals/physician_gls/pdf/rectal.pdf.*
77. Cai GX, Cai SJ. Multi-modality treatment of colorectal liver metastases. World J Gastroenterol 2012;18:16–24.
78. Chua TC, Morris DL. Therapeutic potential of surgery for metastatic colorectal cancer. Scand J Gastroenterol 2012;47:258–268.
79. Schwarz RE, Berlin JD, Lenz HJ. Systemic cytotoxic and biological therapies of colorectal liver metastases: expert consensus statement. HPB (Oxford) 2013;15:106–115.
80. Mahnken AH, Pereira PL, de Baère T. Interventional oncologic approaches to liver metastases. Radiology 2013;266:407–430.
81. Hochster HS, Hart LL, Ramanathan RK, et al. Safety and efficacy of oxaliplatin and fluoropyrimidine regimens with or without bevacizumab as first-line treatment of metastatic colorectal cancer: Results of the TREE study. J Clin Oncol 2008;26:3523–3529.
82. Tournigand C, Andre T, Achille E, et al. FOLFIRI followed by FOLFOX6 or the reverse sequence in advanced colorectal cancer: A randomized GERCOR study. J Clin Oncol 2004;22:229–237.
83. Masi G, Vasile E, Loupakis F, et al. Randomized trial of two induction chemotherapy regimens in metastatic colorectal cancer: An updated analysis. J Natl Cancer Inst 2011;103:21–30.
84. Ducreux M, Malka D, Mendiboure J, et al. Sequential versus combination chemotherapy for the treatment of advanced colorectal cancer (FFCD 2000-05): An open-label, randomised, phase 3 trial. Lancet Oncol 2011;12:1032–1044.
85. Twelves C. Capecitabine as first-line treatment in colorectal cancer. Eur J Cancer 2002;38:15–20.
86. Douillard JY, Siena S, Cassidy J, et al. Randomized, phase III trial of panitumumab with infusional fluorouracil, leucovorin, and oxaliplatin (FOLFOX4) versus FOLFOX4 alone as first-line treatment in patients with previously untreated metastatic colorectal cancer: The PRIME study. J Clin Oncol 2010;28:4697–4705.
87. Stintzing S, Fischer von Weikersthal L, Decker T, et al. FOLFIRI plus cetuximab versus FOLFIRI plus bevacizumab as first-line treatment for patients with metastatic colorectal cancer-subgroup analysis of patients with KRAS: Mutated tumours in the randomised German AIO study KRK-0306. Ann Oncol 2012;23:1693–1699.
88. Van Cutsem E, Tabernero J, Lakomy R, et al. Addition of aflibercept to fluorouracil, leucovorin, and irinotecan improves survival in a phase III randomized trial in patients with metastatic colorectal cancer previously treated with an oxaliplatin-based regimen. J Clin Oncol 2012;30:3499–3506.
89. Martín-Martorell P, Roselló S, Rodríguez-Braun E, et al. Biweekly cetuximab and irinotecan in advanced colorectal cancer patients progressing after at least one previous line of chemotherapy: Results of a phase II single institution trial. Br J Cancer 2008;99:455–458.

90. Kohne CH, Hofheinz R, Mineur L, et al. First-line panitumumab plus irinotecan/5-fluorouracil/leucovorin treatment in patients with metastatic colorectal cancer. J Cancer Res Clin Oncol 2012;138:65–72.
91. Haller DG, Rothenberg ML, Wong AO, et al. Oxaliplatin plus irinotecan compared with irinotecan alone as second-line treatment after single-agent fluoropyrimidine therapy for metastatic colorectal carcinoma. J Clin Oncol 2008;26: 4544–4550.
92. Fuchs CS, Moore MR, Harker G, et al. Phase III comparison of two irinotecan dosing regimens in second-line therapy of metastatic colorectal cancer. J Clin Oncol 2003;21: 807–814.
93. Sobrero AF, Maurel J, Fehrenbacher L, et al. EPIC: phase III trial of cetuximab plus irinotecan after fluoropyrimidine and oxaliplatin failure in patients with metastatic colorectal cancer. J Clin Oncol 2008;26:2311–2319.
94. André T, Blons H, Mabro M, Chibaudel B, et al. Panitumumab combined with irinotecan for patients with *KRAS* wild-type metastatic colorectal cancer refractory to standard chemotherapy: A GERCOR efficacy, tolerance, and translational molecular study. Ann Oncol 2013;24: 412–419.
95. Kabbinavar FF, Hambleton J, Mass RD, et al. Combined analysis of efficacy: The addition of bevacizumab to fluorouracil/leucovorin improves survival for patients with metastatic colorectal cancer. J Clin Oncol 2005;23: 3706–3712.
96. Feliu J, Safont MJ, Salud A, et al. Capecitabine and bevacizumab as first-line treatment in elderly patients with metastatic colorectal cancer. Br J Cancer 2010;102: 1468–1473.
97. Cunningham D, Humblet Y, Siena S, et al. Cetuximab monotherapy and cetuximab plus irinotecan in irinotecan-refractory metastatic colorectal cancer. N Engl J Med 2004;351:337–345.
98. Van Cutsem E, Peeters M, Siena S, et al. Open-label phase III trial of panitumumab plus best supportive care compared with best supportive care alone in patients with chemotherapy-refractory metastatic colorectal cancer. J Clin Oncol 2007;25:1658–1664.
99. Grothey A, Van Cutsem E, Sobrero A. Regorafenib monotherapy for previously treated metastatic colorectal cancer (CORRECT): an international, multicentre, randomised, placebo-controlled, phase 3 trial. Lancet 2013;381:303–312.
100. Goldberg RM, Sargent DJ, Morton RF, et al. A randomized controlled trial of fluorouracil plus leucovorin, irinotecan, and oxaliplatin combinations in patients with previously untreated metastatic colorectal cancer. J Clin Oncol 2004;22:23–30.
101. de Gramont A, Figer A, Seymour M, et al. Leucovorin and fluorouracil with or without oxaliplatin as first-line treatment in advanced colorectal cancer. J Clin Oncol 2000;18: 2938–2947.
102. Douillard J, Cunningham D, Roth A, et al. Irinotecan combined with fluorouracil compared with fluorouracil alone as first-line treatment for metastatic colorectal cancer: A multicentre randomised trial. Lancet 2000;355: 1041–1047.
103. Hurwitz H, Fehrenbacher L, Novotny W, et al. Bevacizumab plus irinotecan, fluorouracil, and leucovorin for metastatic colorectal cancer. N Engl J Med 2004;350:2335–2342.
104. Saltz L, Clark S, Diaz-Rubio E, et al. Bevacizumab in combination with oxaliplatin-based chemotherapy as first-line therapy in metastatic colorectal cancer: A randomized phase III study. J Clin Oncol 2008;26:2013–2039.
105. Fuchs CS, Marshall J, Barrueco J. Randomized, controlled trial of irinotecan plus infusional, bolus, or oral fluoropyrimidines in first-line treatment of metastatic colorectal cancer: Updated results from the BICC-C study. J Clin Oncol 2008;26:689–690.
106. Bokemeyer C, Bondarenko I, Makhson A, et al. Fluorouracil, leucovorin, and oxaliplatin with and without cetuximab in the first-line treatment of metastatic colorectal cancer. J Clin Oncol 2009;27:663–667.
107. Van Cutsem E, Kohne C-H, Hitre E, et al. Cetuximab and chemotherapy as initial treatment for metastatic colorectal cancer. N Engl J Med 2009;360:1408–1417.
108. Maughan TS, Adams RA, Smith CG, et al. Addition of cetuximab to oxaliplatin-based first-line combination chemotherapy for treatment of advanced colorectal cancer: results of the randomised phase 3 MRC COIN trial. Lancet 2011;377:2103–2114.
109. Rougier P, Van Cutsem E, Bajetta E, et al. Randomised trial of irinotecan versus fluorouracil by continuous infusion after fluorouracil failure in patients with metastatic colorectal cancer. Lancet 1998;352:1407–1412.
110. Cunningham D, Pyrhönen S, James R, et al. Randomised trial of irinotecan plus supportive care versus supportive care alone after fluorouracil failure for patients with metastatic colorectal cancer. Lancet 1998;352:1413–1418.
111. Giantonio BJ, Catalano PJ, Meropol NJ, et al. Bevacizumab in combination with oxaliplatin, fluorouracil, and leucovorin (FOLFOX4) for previously treated metastatic colorectal cancer: Results from the Eastern Cooperative Oncology Group Study E3200. J Clin Oncol 2007;25: 1539–1544.
112. Peeters M, Price TJ, Cervantes A, et al. Randomized phase III study of panitumumab with fluorouracil, leucovorin, and irinotecan (FOLFIRI) compared with FOLFIRI alone as second-line treatment in patients with metastatic colorectal cancer. J Clin Oncol 2010;28:4706–4713.
113. Bennouna J, Sastre J, Arnold D et al. Continuation of bevacizumab after first progression in metastatic colorectal cancer (ML18147): A randomised phase 3 trial. Lancet Oncol 2013;14:29–37.
114. Glimelius B, Cavalli-Björkman N. Metastatic colorectal cancer: current treatment and future options for improved survival. Scand J Gastroenterol 2012;47:296–314.
115. Benhaim L, Labonte MJ, Lenz HJ. Pharmacogenomics and metastatic colorectal cancer: Current knowledge and perspectives. Scand J Gastroenterol 2012;47: 325–339.
116. Weickhardt A, Wells K, Messersmith W. Oxaliplatin-induced neuropathy in colorectal cancer. J Oncol 2011;2011:201593, DOI:10.1155/2011/201593.
117. Hecht JR, Mitchell E, Chidiac T, et al. A randomized phase IIIB trial of chemotherapy, bevacizumab, and panitumumab compared with chemotherapy and bevacizumab alone for metastatic colorectal cancer. J Clin Oncol 2009;27: 672–680.
118. Tol J, Koopman M, Cats A, et al. Chemotherapy, bevacizumab, and cetuximab in metastatic colorectal cancer. N Engl J Med 2009;360:563–572.
119. Siena S, Sartore-Bianchi A, Nicolantonio FD, et al. Biomarkers predicting clinical outcome of epidermal growth factor receptor-targeted therapy in metastatic colorectal cancer. J Natl Cancer Inst 2009;101: 1308–1324.

120. Tejpar S, Celik I, Schlichting M, et al. Association of *KRAS* G13D tumor mutations with outcome in patients with metastatic colorectal cancer treated with first-line chemotherapy with or without cetuximab. J Clin Oncol 2012;30:3570–3577.
121. Ebert MPA, Tänzer M, Balluff B, et al. *TFAP2E-DKK4* and chemoresistance in colorectal cancer. N Engl J Med 2012;366:44–53.
122. Boisdron-Celle M, Remaud G, Traore S, et al. 5-Fluorouracil-related severe toxicity: A comparison of different methods for the pretherapeutic detection of dihydropyrimidine dehydrogenase deficiency. Cancer Lett 2007;249:271–282.
123. Boisdron-Celle M. Pharmacokinetic adaptation of 5-fluorouracil: Where are we and where are we going? Pharmacogenomics 2012;13:1437–1439.
124. Saif MW, Choma A, Salamone SJ, Chu E. Pharmacokinetically guided dose adjustment of 5-fluorouracil: A rational approach to improving therapeutic outcomes. J Natl Cancer Inst 2009;101: 1543–1552.
125. Gamelin E, Delva R, Jacob J, et al. Individual fluorouracil dose adjustment based on pharmacokinetic follow-up compared with conventional dosage: Results of a multicenter randomized trial of patients with metastatic colorectal cancer. J Clin Oncol 2008;26:2099–3105.

108

Prostate Cancer

LeAnn B. Norris and Jill M. Kolesar

KEY CONCEPTS

1. Prostate cancer is the most frequent cancer in men in the United States. African American ancestry, family history, and increased age are the primary risk factors for prostate cancer.
2. Prostate-specific antigen is a useful marker to detect prostate cancer at early stages, predict outcome for localized disease, define disease-free status, and monitor response to androgen-deprivation therapy or chemotherapy for advanced-stage disease.
3. The prognosis for prostate cancer patients depends on the histologic grade, the tumor size, and the disease stage. More than 85% of patients with stage A_1 disease but less than 1% of those with stage D_2 can be cured.
4. Androgen deprivation therapy with a luteinizing hormone-releasing hormone (LHRH) agonist plus an antiandrogen should be used prior to radiation therapy for patients with locally advanced prostate cancer to improve outcomes over radiation therapy alone.
5. Androgen deprivation therapy, with either orchiectomy, an LHRH agonist alone or an LHRH agonist plus an antiandrogen (combined hormonal blockade), can be used to provide palliation for patients with advanced (stage D_2) prostate cancer. The effects of androgen deprivation seem most pronounced in patients with minimal disease at diagnosis.
6. Antiandrogen withdrawal, for patients having progressive disease while receiving combined hormonal blockade with an LHRH agonist plus an antiandrogen, can provide additional symptomatic relief. Mutations in the androgen receptor have been documented that cause antiandrogen compounds to act like receptor agonists.
7. Chemotherapy, with docetaxel and prednisone improves survival in patients with castrate-refractory prostate cancer and is considered first-line therapy for these patients. Additional effective agents include cabazitaxel, enzalutamide, and abiraterone.

Prostate cancer is the most commonly diagnosed cancer in American men.[1] For most men, prostate cancer has an indolent course, and treatment options for early disease include expectant management, surgery, or radiation. With expectant management, patients are monitored for disease progression or development of symptoms. Localized prostate cancer can be cured by surgery or radiation therapy, advanced prostate cancer is not yet curable. Treatment for advanced prostate cancer can provide significant disease palliation for many patients for several years after diagnosis. The endocrine dependence of this tumor is well documented, and hormonal manipulation to decrease circulating androgens remains the basis for the treatment of advanced disease.

EPIDEMIOLOGY

1 Prostate cancer is the most frequent cancer among American men and represents the second leading cause of cancer-related deaths in all males.[1] In the United States alone, it is estimated that 238,590 new cases of prostatic carcinoma were diagnosed and more than 29,720 men died from this disease in 2013.[1] Although prostate cancer incidence increased during the late 1980s and early 1990s related to widespread prostate-specific antigen (PSA) screening, deaths from prostate cancer have been declining since 1995.[1]

ETIOLOGY

Table 108-1 summarizes the possible factors associated with prostate cancer.[2,3] The widely accepted risk factors for prostate cancer are age, race-ethnicity, and family history of prostate cancer.[2,3] The disease is rare in those younger than 40 years of age, but the incidence sharply increases with each subsequent decade, most likely because the individual has had a lifetime exposure to testosterone, a known growth signal for the prostate.[3]

Race and Ethnicity

The incidence of clinical prostate cancer varies across geographic regions. Scandinavian countries and the United States report the highest incidence of prostate cancer, whereas the disease is relatively rare in Japan and other Asian countries.[4] African American men have the highest rate of prostate cancer in the world, and in the United States, prostate cancer mortality in African Americans is more than twice that seen in white populations.[1] Hormonal, dietary, and genetic differences, and differences in access to healthcare may contribute to the altered susceptibility to prostate cancer in these populations.[2,3] Testosterone, commonly implicated in the pathogenesis of prostate cancer, is approximately 15% higher in African American men compared with white males. Activity of 5-α-reductase, the enzyme that converts testosterone to its more active form, dihydrotestosterone (DHT), in the prostate, is decreased in Japanese men compared with African Americans and whites.[2,3] In addition, genetic variations in the androgen receptor exist. Activation of the androgen receptor is inversely correlated with CAG repeat length. Shorter CAG repeat sequences have been found in African Americans. Therefore the combination of increased testosterone and increased androgen receptor activation may account for the increased risk of prostate cancer for African American men.[2,3] The Asian diet is generally considered to be low in fat and high in fiber with a high concentration of phytoestrogens, potentially explaining their decreased risk.[4,5]

TABLE 108-1 Risk Factors Associated with Prostate Cancer

Factor	Possible Relationship
Probable Risk Factors	
Age	More than 70% of cases are diagnosed in men older than 65 years old.
Race	African Americans have higher incidence and death rate.
Genetic	Familial prostate cancer inherited in an autosomal dominant manner. Mutations in *p53*, *Rb*, E-cahedrin, α-catenin, androgen receptor, *KAI1*, microsatellite instability, loss of heterozygocity at 1, 2q, 12p, 15q, 16p, and 16q, *BRCA1* and *BRCA2* mutation. Candidate prostate cancer gene locus identified on chromosome 1.
Possible Risk Factors	
Environmental	Clinical carcinoma incidence varies worldwide. Latent carcinoma similar between regions. Nationalized males adopt intermediate incidence rates between those of the United States and their native country.
Occupational	Increased risk associated with cadmium exposure.
Diet	Increased risk associated with high-meat and high-fat diets. Decreased intake of 1,25-dihydroxyvitamin D, lycopene, and β-carotene increases risk.
Hormonal	Does not occur in castrated men. Low incidence in cirrhotic patients. Up to 80% are hormonally dependent; African Americans have 15% increased testosterone. Japanese have decreased 5-α-reductase activities. Polymorphic expression of the androgen receptor.

Family History

Men with a brother or father with prostate cancer have twice the risk for prostate cancer as compared with the rest of the population.[5] Familial clustering of a prostate cancer syndrome has been reported, and genome-wide scans have identified potential prostate cancer susceptibility candidate genes. Male carriers of germline mutations of *BRCA1* and *BRCA2* are known to have an increased risk for developing prostate cancer.[6] Common exposure to environmental and other risk factors may also contribute to increased risk among patients with first-degree relatives with prostate cancer.[5,7]

Diet

Several epidemiologic studies support an association between high fat intake and risk of prostate cancer. A strong correlation between national per capita fat consumption and national prostate cancer mortality has been reported, and prospective case-control studies suggest that a high-fat diet doubles the risk of prostate cancer.[5] This relationship between high fat intake and prostate cancer may explain differences in insulin-like growth factor-1 (IGF-1). High-calorie and high-fat diets stimulate hepatic production of IGF-1, which is involved in the regulation of proliferation and apoptosis of cancer cells.[5] High levels of IGF-1 are associated with an increased risk for prostate cancer.[5]

Other dietary factors implicated in the development or prevention of prostate cancer include retinol, carotenoids, lycopene, and vitamin D consumption.[5,7] Retinol, or vitamin A, intake, especially in men older than 70 years, is correlated with an increased risk of prostate cancer, whereas intake of its precursor, β-carotene, has a protective or neutral effect. Lycopene, obtained primarily from tomatoes, decreases the risk of prostate cancer in small cohort studies. Men who developed prostate cancer in one cohort study had lower levels of 1,25$(OH)_2$-vitamin D than matched controls, although a prospective study did not support this. Clearly, dietary risk factors require further evaluation, and since fat and vitamins are modifiable risk factors, dietary intervention may be promising in prostate cancer prevention. Investigations of selenium and vitamin E supplementation are discussed further in the section titled chemoprevention.

Other Factors

Benign prostatic hyperplasia (BPH) is a common problem among elderly men, affecting more than 40% of men older than 70 years of age (see Chap. 67). BPH results in the urinary symptoms of hesitancy and frequency. Because prostate cancer affects a similar age group and often has similar presenting symptoms, the presence of BPH often complicates the diagnosis of prostate cancer, although it does not appear to increase the risk of developing prostate cancer.[2,7]

Smoking has not been associated with an increased risk of prostate cancer, but smokers with prostate cancer have an increased mortality resulting from the disease when compared with nonsmokers with prostate cancer (relative risk 1.5 to 2).[2,7] In addition, in a prospective cohort analysis, alcohol consumption was not associated with the development of prostate cancer.

CHEMOPREVENTION

Currently, the most promising agents for the prevention of prostate cancer are the 5-α-reductase inhibitors, finasteride, and dutasteride.[8–11] These drugs inhibit 5-α-reductase, an enzyme that converts testosterone to its more active form, DHT, which is involved in prostate epithelial proliferation. 5-α-reductase exists as two types, type I and type II, and both are implicated in the development of prostate cancer. Finasteride selectively inhibits the 5-α-reductase type II isoenzyme, whereas dutasteride inhibits both isoenzymes.[9] Both finasteride and dutasteride falsely lower the PSA by approximately 50% in patients, and this must be considered when one interprets PSA in patients on these medications.[12]

The efficacy of 5-α-reductase inhibitors in reducing the risk of prostate cancer was recently evaluated in a Cochrane review.[8] Eight randomized studies involving 41,638 men were included. Both the Reduction by Dutasteride of Prostate Cancer Events (REDUCE) study, which compared dutasteride to placebo and included more than 8000 subjects and the Prostate Cancer Prevention Trial (PCPT), which compared finasteride to placebo and enrolled more than 18,000 subjects in the analysis. The mean subject age in the analysis was 64 years; 92% of subjects were white and 15% had a family history of prostate cancer. The mean (range) baseline PSA level was 3.1 (1.2 to 9.8 ng/mL [1.2 to 9.8 mcg/L]). Compared with placebo, 5-α-reductase inhibitors reduced the risk of prostate cancers detected by 25% (relative risk 0.75, 95% confidence interval [CI] 0.67–0.83; 1.4% absolute risk reduction [3.5% vs. 4.9%]). Studies were not designed to evaluate prostate cancer mortality, and in the combined analysis, 5-α-reductase inhibitors did not improve mortality.

Subjects who discontinued therapy or were lost to follow-up were not different between the placebo and treatment arms, but adverse effects, including gynecomastia, decreased libido, and erectile dysfunction, were more common in patients treated with 5-α-reductase inhibitors than in placebo. In the REDUCE trial, the incidence of "cardiac failure," defined as congestive heart failure, cardiac failure, acute cardiac failure, ventricular failure, cardiopulmonary failure, or congestive cardiomyopathy, was greater in the dutasteride group (0.7%, $n = 30$) compared with the placebo group (0.4%, $n = 16$; $P = 0.03$), but deaths from cardiovascular events were not significantly different between groups.

The American Society of Clinical Oncology and the American Urological Association published a joint practice guideline for prostate cancer chemoprevention.[13] The guideline recommends that asymptomatic men with a PSA ≤3.0 ng/mL (3.0 mcg/L) who are regularly screened with PSA for early detection of prostate cancer may benefit from a discussion of both the benefits of dutasteride or finasteride for 7 years for the prevention of prostate cancer and the potential risks.[13]

The guideline does not recommend the use of finasteride or dutasteride for prostate cancer chemoprevention and noted that, while most panel members believed the higher risk of high-grade cancer in the finasteride group observed in the PCPT is most likely related to biases, cancer induction or promotion by finasteride cannot be excluded with certainty. In addition, while finasteride and dutasteride reduce the prevalence of prostate cancer, the impact of 5-α-reductase inhibitors on prostate cancer morbidity and mortality has not been demonstrated. Patients considering finasteride or dutasteride for prostate cancer chemoprevention or taking it for benign conditions such as BPH must weigh the risks and benefits of treatment. The primary benefit is that these agents reduce the incidence of prostate cancer by about 25%, and improve lower urinary tract symptoms of BPH, but the risks include the potential for more high-grade prostate cancers; the long-term benefit of these agents is not known; and reversible sexual adverse effects can occur.[13]

Selenium and vitamin E alone or in combination were evaluated in the *Sel*enium and Vitamin *E* *C*ancer Prevention *T*rial (SELECT), a clinical trial investigating their effects on the incidence of prostate cancer in healthy men. The data and safety monitoring committee found that after 5 years selenium or vitamin E taken alone or together did not prevent prostate cancer. Based on these data and safety concerns, the trial was halted. With longer follow-up of that trial, dietary supplementation with vitamin E significantly increased the risk of prostate cancer by 17% (P = 0.008).[14] Other agents, including vitamin D, lycopene, green tea, nonsteroidal antiinflammatory agents, isoflavones, and statins, are under investigation for prostate cancer and show promise; however, none are currently recommended for routine use outside of a clinical trial.[15]

SCREENING

Digital rectal examination (DRE) has been recommended since the early 1900s for the detection of prostate cancer. The primary advantage of DRE is its specificity, reported at greater than 85%, for prostate cancer. Other advantages of DRE include low cost, safety, and ease of performance. However, DRE is relatively insensitive and is subject to interobserver variability. DRE as a single screening method has poor compliance and showed little effect in preventing metastatic prostate cancer in one large observational study.[16]

2 PSA is a useful marker for detecting prostate cancer at early stages, predicting outcome for localized disease, defining disease-free status, and monitoring response to androgen-deprivation therapy or chemotherapy for advanced-stage disease. PSA is used widely for prostate cancer screening in the United States, with simplicity its major advantage and low specificity its primary limitation.[17] PSA may be elevated in men with acute urinary retention, acute prostatitis, and prostatic ischemia or infarction, as well as BPH, a nearly universal condition in men at risk for prostate cancer. PSA elevations between 4.1 and 10 ng/mL (4.1 and 10 mcg/L) cannot distinguish between BPH and prostate cancer, limiting the utility of PSA alone for the early detection of prostate cancer. Additionally, many men with clinically significant prostate cancer do not have a serum PSA outside the reference range.[18]

Early detection of potentially curable prostate cancers is the goal of prostate cancer screening. For cancer screening to be beneficial, it must reliably detect cancer at an early stage, when intervention would decrease mortality. Whether prostate cancer screening, with PSA, DRE or a combination fits these criteria has generated considerable controversy, and two recent studies have done little to resolve the controversy.[19–22] The European Randomized Study of Screening for Prostate Cancer (ERSPC) evaluated the effect of PSA screening on prostate cancer mortality. More than 182,000 men from seven different European countries were randomized between being offered screening with PSA to no screening. The frequency of screening and PSA threshold for a biopsy varied by country. Most centers used a PSA cutoff of 3 ng/mL (3 mcg/L), but Belgium allowed up to 10 ng/mL (10 mcg/L). Most centers screened every 4 years, although Sweden screened every 2 years. Eighty-two percent of men in the screening group had at least one PSA performed. With a median follow-up of 11 years, the cumulative incidence of prostate cancer was 9.6% in the screening group and 6.0% in the control group.[23] The rate ratio for death from prostate cancer in the screening group, compared with the control group, was 0.79 (95% CI, 0.68 to 0.91; adjusted P = 0.001), which corresponds to about one less death from prostate cancer per 1000 men (at a median follow-up of 11 years) in the screened group compared with the unscreened group. Of the 136,689 PSA tests performed, 16.6% of the tests were positive; biopsies were performed for 86% of men with elevated PSAs. Overall mortality was similar in the two study groups (rate ratio 0.99, 95% CI, 0.97 to 1.01).[23]

In the United States, the Prostate, Lung, Colon and Ovarian Screening (PLCO) study randomized 76,693 men to receive either annual screening (38,343 subjects) or usual care as the control (38,350 subjects). In the screening group, men were offered annual PSA testing for 6 years and DRE for 4 years. Compliance with screening was 85%. Men in the usual care group were able to receive screening, with the rate of PSA testing ranging from 40% to 52% and DRE from 41% to 46%. After 13 years of follow-up, the incidence of death per 10,000 person-years was not significantly different between the two groups with 3.7 (158 deaths total) in the screening group and 3.4 (145 deaths total) in the control group (relative risk, 1.09; 95% CI, 0.87 to 1.36).[24]

In the United States, clinicians believe that neither DRE nor PSA is sensitive or specific enough to be used alone as a screening test. Although the relative predictability of DRE and PSA is similar, the tumors identified by each method are different. The common approach to prostate cancer screening today involves offering a baseline PSA and DRE at age 40 years with annual evaluations beginning at age 50 to all men of normal risk with a 10-year or greater life expectancy. Men with an increased risk of prostate cancer, including men of African American ancestry and men with a family history of prostate cancer, may begin screening earlier, at age 40 to 45 years.

Despite this common practice, the benefits of prostate cancer screening remain controversial.[19,20,22] The ERSPC demonstrated that PSA testing every 4 years was better than no PSA testing, decreasing prostate cancer deaths in the screened group by about 1 per 1,000 men screened compared with the unscreened group, but the false-positive rate was 76%, resulting in more than 13,000 unnecessary biopsies. The PLCO screening study showed no reduction in prostate cancer death between the annual (PSA and DRE) screening group and the usual care group, which is not surprising given the small reduction in death expected and that about one-half of the patients in the usual screening groups had PSA and DRE screening performed. Both studies demonstrated that screening identifies more prostate cancers than not screening.[21,23,24] PSA measurements can identify small, subclinical prostate cancers, where no intervention may be required. Detecting prostate cancer in those not needing therapy not only increases the cost of care through unnecessary screening and workups, but also increases harm by subjecting some patients to unnecessary therapy. Based on this evidence, the United States Preventative Services Task Force (USPSTF) recommends against screening for prostate cancer (grade D recommendation), based on moderate or high certainty that screening has no net benefit or that the harms outweigh the benefits.[21,22] The American Cancer Society recommends that asymptomatic men who have at least a 10-year life expectancy have an opportunity to make to make an informed decision about prostate cancer screening, including discussion of the uncertainties, risks, and potential benefits associated with screening.[20]

Clinical **Controversy. . .**

Prostate cancer screening with prostate-specific antigen (PSA) tests is controversial. Recently completed trials of screening show no overall survival benefit in screened patients. However, usual clinical practice was allowed in the control arm, and control patients received PSA screening nearly as frequently as those in the screening arm. Overall, the trial compared screening annually to screening every 2 to 3 years, not to no screening.

Based on the available evidence, Gulati et al. recently evaluated the comparative effectiveness of alternative PSA screening strategies.[25] Examples of alternative screening strategies include the use of higher PSA thresholds for biopsy referral or longer screening intervals. Several of the screening scenarios were predicted to produce similar reductions in prostate cancer mortality and reduce harms.

PATHOPHYSIOLOGY

The prostate gland is a solid, rounded, heart-shaped organ positioned between the neck of the bladder and the urogenital diaphragm (Fig. 108-1). The normal prostate is composed of acinar secretory cells arranged in a radial shape and surrounded by a foundation of supporting tissue. The size, shape, or presence of acini is almost always altered in the gland that has been invaded by prostatic carcinoma. Adenocarcinoma, the major pathologic cell type, accounts for more than 95% of prostate cancer cases.[26,27] Much rarer tumor types include small cell neuroendocrine cancers, sarcomas, and transitional cell carcinomas.

Prostate cancer can be graded systematically according to the histologic appearance of the malignant cell and then grouped into well, moderately, or poorly differentiated grades.[27,28] Gland architecture is examined and then rated on a scale of 1 (well differentiated) to 5 (poorly differentiated). Two different specimens are examined, and the score for each specimen is added. Groupings for total Gleason score are 2 to 4 for well differentiated, 5 or 6 for moderately differentiated, and 7 to 10 for poorly differentiated tumors. Poorly differentiated tumors grow rapidly (poor prognosis), while well-differentiated tumors grow slowly (better prognosis).

Metastatic spread can occur by local extension, lymphatic drainage, or hematogenous dissemination.[28,29] Lymph node metastases are more common in patients with large, undifferentiated tumors that invade the seminal vesicles. The pelvic and abdominal lymph node groups are the most common sites of lymph node involvement (see Fig. 108-1). Skeletal metastases from hematogenous spread are the most common sites of distant spread. Typically, the bone lesions are osteoblastic or a combination of osteoblastic and osteolytic. The most common site of bone involvement is the lumbar spine. Other sites of bone involvement include the proximal femurs, pelvis, thoracic spine, ribs, sternum, skull, and humerus. The lung, liver, brain, and adrenal glands are the most common sites of visceral involvement, although these organs are not usually initially involved. About 25% to 35% of patients will have evidence of lymphangitic or nodular pulmonary infiltrates at autopsy. The prostate is rarely a site for metastatic involvement from other solid tumors.

Normal growth and differentiation of the prostate depend on the presence of androgens, specifically DHT.[29,30] The testes and the adrenal glands are the major sources of circulating androgens. Hormonal regulation of androgen synthesis is mediated through a series of biochemical interactions between the hypothalamus, pituitary, adrenal glands, and testes (Fig. 108-2). Luteinizing hormone-releasing hormone (LHRH) released from the hypothalamus stimulates the release of luteinizing hormone (LH) and follicle-stimulating hormone (FSH) from the anterior pituitary gland. LH complexes with receptors on the Leydig cell testicular membrane and stimulates the production of testosterone and small amounts of estrogen. FSH acts

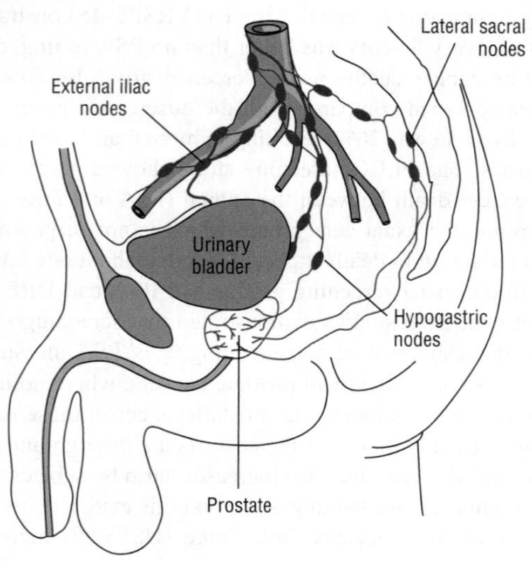

FIGURE 108-1 The prostate gland.

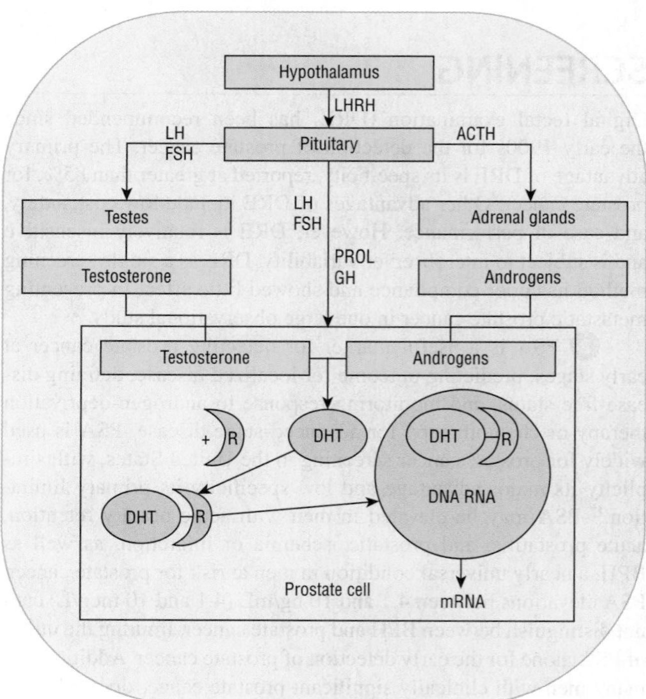

FIGURE 108-2 Hormonal regulation of the prostate gland. (ACTH, adrenocorticotropic hormone; DHT, dihydrotestosterone; FSH, follicle-stimulating hormone; GH, growth hormone; LH, luteinizing hormone; LHRH, luteinizing hormone-releasing hormone; PROL, prolactin; R, receptor).

TABLE 108-2 Hormonal Manipulations in Prostate Cancer

Androgen source ablation	Antiandrogens
Orchiectomy	Flutamide
Adrenalectomy	Bicalutamide
Hypophysectomy	Enzalutamide
LHRH or LH inhibition	Nilutamide
Estrogens	Cyproterone acetate[b]
LHRH agonists	Progesterones
Progesterones[a]	5-α-Reductase inhibition
Cyproterone acetate[b]	Finasteride[b]
Androgen synthesis inhibition	Dutasteride
Aminoglutethimide	
Ketoconazole	
Abiraterone Acetate	
Progesterones[a]	

LH, luteinizing hormone; LHRH, luteinizing hormone-releasing hormone.

[a]Minor mechanisms of action.

[b]Investigational compounds or use.

on the Sertoli cells within the testes to promote the maturation of LH receptors and to produce an androgen-binding protein. Circulating testosterone and estradiol influence the synthesis of LHRH, LH, and FSH by a negative feedback loop operating at the hypothalamic and pituitary level.[31] Prolactin, growth hormone, and estradiol appear to be important accessory regulators for prostatic tissue permeability, receptor binding, and testosterone synthesis.

Testosterone, the major androgenic hormone, accounts for 95% of the androgen concentration. The primary source of testosterone is the testes, but 3% to 5% of the testosterone concentration is derived from direct adrenal cortical secretion of testosterone or C19 steroids such as androstenedione.[28–30]

In early-stage prostate cancers, aberrant tumor cell proliferation is promoted by the presence of androgens. For these tumors, blockade of androgens induces tumor regression in most patients. Hormonal manipulations to ablate or reduce circulating androgens can occur through several mechanisms[29,30] (Table 108-2). The organs responsible for androgen production can be removed surgically (orchiectomy, hypophysectomy, or adrenalectomy). Hormonal pathways that modulate prostatic growth can be interrupted at several steps (see Fig. 108-2). Interference with LHRH or LH can reduce testosterone secretion by the testes (estrogens, LHRH agonists, progestogens, and cyproterone acetate). Estrogen administration reduces androgens by directly inhibiting LH release, by acting directly on the prostate cell, or by decreasing free androgens by increasing steroid-binding globulin levels.[28–30]

Isolation of the naturally occurring hypothalamic decapeptide hormone luteinizing hormone-releasing hormone or LHRH has provided another group of effective agents for advanced prostate cancer treatment. The physiologic response to LHRH depends on both the dose and the mode of administration. Intermittent pulsed LHRH administration, which mimics the endogenous release pattern, causes sustained release of both LH and FSH, whereas high-dose or continuous IV administration of LHRH inhibits gonadotropin release due to receptor downregulation.[23] Structural modification of the naturally occurring LHRH and innovative delivery have produced a series of LHRH agonists that cause a similar downregulation of pituitary receptors and a decrease in testosterone production.[31]

Androgen synthesis can also be inhibited in the testes or in the adrenal gland. Aminoglutethimide inhibits the desmolase-enzyme complex in the adrenal gland, thereby preventing the conversion of cholesterol to pregnenolone. Pregnenolone is the precursor substrate for all adrenal-derived steroids, including androgens, glucocorticoids, and mineralocorticoids. Ketoconazole, an imidazole antifungal agent, causes a dose-related reversible reduction in serum cortisol and testosterone concentration by inhibiting both adrenal and testicular steroidogenesis.[31] Megestrol is a synthetic derivative of progesterone that exhibits a secondary mechanism of action by inhibiting androgen synthesis. This inhibition appears to occur at the adrenal level, but circulating levels of testosterone are also reduced, suggesting that inhibition at the testicular level may also occur.[31]

Antiandrogens inhibit the formation of the DHT-receptor complex and therefore interfere with androgen activity at the cellular level.[31] The conversion of testosterone to DHT may be inhibited by 5-α-reductase inhibitors.[7]

In advanced stages of disease, prostate cancer cells may be able to survive and proliferate without the signals normally provided by circulating androgens.[31] When this occurs, the tumor is no longer sensitive to therapies that depend on androgen blockade. These tumors are often referred to as hormone refractory or androgen independent.

CLINICAL PRESENTATION

Prior to the implementation of routine screening, prostate cancers were frequently identified on the investigation of symptoms, including urinary hesitancy, retention, painful urination, hematuria, and erectile dysfunction. With the introduction of screening techniques, most prostate cancers are now identified prior to the development of symptoms.

The information obtained from the diagnostic tests is used to stage the patient (Table 108-3). There are two commonly recognized staging classification systems (Table 108-4). The formal international classification system (tumor, node, metastases [TNM]), adopted by the International Union Against Cancer in 1974, was last updated in 2002. The AUS classification is the most commonly used staging system in the United States. Patients are assigned to stages A through D and corresponding subcategories based on size of the tumor (T), local or regional extension, presence of involved lymph node groups (N), and presence of metastases (M). Based on men diagnosed with prostate cancer at Walter Reed Army Medical

CLINICAL PRESENTATION

Localized Disease

- Asymptomatic

Locally Invasive Disease

- Ureteral dysfunction, frequency, hesitancy, and dribbling
- Impotence

Advanced Disease

- Back pain
- Cord compression
- Lower extremity edema
- Pathologic fractures
- Anemia
- Weight loss

TABLE 108-3 Diagnostic and Staging Workup for Prostate Cancer

Initial tests	Digital rectal examination (DRE) Prostate-specific antigen (PSA) transrectal ultrasonography (TRUS) if either DRE is positive or PSA is elevated Biopsy
Staging tests	Gleason score on biopsy specimen Bone scan Complete blood count Liver function tests Serum phosphatases (acid/alkaline) Excretory urogram Chest x-ray
Additional staging tests (depends on tumor classification, PSA, and Gleason score)	Skeletal films Lymph node evaluation Pelvic computed tomography ^{111}In-labeled capromab pendetide scan Bipedal lymphangiogram Transrectal magnetic resonance imaging

TABLE 108-4 Staging and Classification Systems for Prostate Cancer

AUS[a] Stage (A–D)	AJCC-UICC[b] Classification (TNM)
A (occult, nonpalpable)	$T_xN_xM_x$ (cannot be assessed)
A_1: Focal	$T_0N_0M_0$ (nonpalpable)
A_2: Diffuse	T_0: Focal or diffuse
B (confined to prostate)	$T_1N_0M_0$, $T_2N_0M_0$
B_1: Single nodule in one lobe, less than 1.5 cm	T_1 (Clinically inapparent tumor not palpable or visible by imaging) T_{1a}: Tumor incidental histologic finding in 5% or less of tissue resected T_{1b}: Tumor incidental histologic finding in 5% or more of tissue resected T_{1c}: Tumor identified by needle biopsy (e.g., because of elevated PSA)
B_2: Diffuse involvement of whole gland, greater than 1.5 cm	T_2: (Tumor confined within the prostate[c]) T_{2a}: Tumor involves half of a lobe or less T_{2b}: Tumor involves more than half a lobe, but not both lobes T_{2c}: Tumor involves both lobes
C (localized to periprostatic area)	$T_3N_0M_0$, $T_4N_0M_0$
C_1: No seminal vesicle involvement, less than 70 g	T_3: (Tumor extends through the prostatic capsule[d]) T_{3a}: Unilateral extracapsular extension T_{3b}: Bilateral extracapsular extension T_{3c}: Tumor invades the seminal vesicle(s)
C_2: Seminal vesicle involvement, greater than 70 g	T_4: (Tumor is fixed or invades adjacent structures other than the seminal vesicles) T_{4a}: Tumor invades any of bladder neck, external sphincter, or rectum T_{4b}: Tumor invades levator muscles and/or is fixed to the pelvic wall
D (metastatic disease)	Any T, N_{1-4}, M_0, or N_{0-4}, M_1
D_1: Pelvic lymph nodes or ureteral obstruction	N_1: Metastasis in a single lymph node, 2 cm or less in greatest dimension
D_2: Bone, distant lymph node, organ, or soft tissue metastases	N_2: Metastasis in single lymph node more than 2 cm but not more than 5 cm in greatest dimension; or multiple lymph node metastases, none more than 5 cm in greatest dimension N_3: Metastasis in lymph node more than 5 cm in greatest dimension M_{1a}: Nonregional lymph node(s) M_{1b}: Bone(s) M_{1c}: Other site(s)

PSA, prostate-specific antigen.

[a]American Urologic System.
[b]American Joint Committee on Cancer–International Union Against Cancer.
[c]Note: Tumor found in one or both lobes by needle biopsy, but not palpable or visible by imaging, is classified as T_{1c}.
[d]Note: Invasion into the prostatic apex or into (but not beyond) the prostatic capsule is not classified as T_3 but as T_2.

Center from 1988 to 1998, including more than 2,042 prostate cancer diagnoses, localized prostate cancer (stage T_1 and T_2) was diagnosed more frequently (89% vs. 68%), and advanced disease (stages T_3, T_4, and D) was diagnosed less frequently (11% vs. 32%) in 1998 as compared to 1988.

3 The prognosis for patients with prostate cancer depends on the histologic grade, the tumor size, and the local extent of the primary tumor.[27] The most important prognostic criterion appears to be the histologic grade, because the degree of differentiation ultimately determines the stage of disease. Poorly differentiated tumors are highly associated with both regional lymph node involvement and distant metastases.[27]

From 1999 to 2005, 5-year overall survival rates were estimated at 100% for whites and 97% for African Americans.[1] For this same period, the survival rates for localized or regional disease (100%), and distant disease (30%) in white males were about the same as the survival rates for localized or regional disease (100%), and distant disease (29%) in African American males.[1] A 4.1% decline in age-adjusted mortality has been observed for the period 1994 to 2006. Ten-year cancer-specific survival is estimated as 95% for stage A_1, 80% for stages A_2 to B_2, 60% for stage C, 40% for stage D_1, and 10% for stage D_2. It is estimated that more than 85% of patients with stage A_1 can be cured, whereas less than 1% of patients with stage D_2 will be cured.

TREATMENT
Prostate Cancer

Desired Outcomes

The desired outcome in early-stage prostate cancer is to minimize morbidity and mortality caused by prostate cancer.[32,33] The most appropriate therapy of early-stage prostate cancer is a matter of debate. Early-stage disease may be treated with surgery, radiation, or expectant management. While surgery and radiation are curative, they are associated with significant morbidity and mortality. Because the overall goal is to minimize morbidity and mortality associated with the disease, watchful waiting is appropriate in selected individuals. Advanced prostate cancer (stage D) is not currently curable, and treatment should provide symptom relief and maintain quality of life. The mainstay of treatment for advanced prostate cancer is androgen deprivation therapy, with a goal of reducing testosterone to castrate levels, with either an orchiectomy or an LHRH agonist.

General Approach To Treatment

The initial treatment for prostate cancer depends primarily on the disease stage, the Gleason score, the presence of symptoms, and the life expectancy of the patient.[32] Prostate cancer is usually initially diagnosed by PSA and DRE and confirmed by a biopsy, where the Gleason score is assigned. Asymptomatic patients with a low risk of recurrence, those with a T_1 or T_{2a}, with a Gleason score of 2 through 6, and a PSA of less than 10 ng/mL (10 mcg/L) may be managed by observation, radiation, or radical prostatectomy (Table 108-5). As patients with asymptomatic early-stage disease generally have an

TABLE 108-5 Initial Management of Prostate Cancer Based on Expected Survival and Recurrence Risk

Recurrence Risk	Expected Survival (Years)	Initial Therapy
Very Low		
T_{1c}	Less than 20	Observation
T_{1c}	20 or more	Observation or Radical prostatectomy with or without pelvic lymph node dissection or Radiation therapy
Low		
T_1–T_{2a} and Gleason 2–6 and PSA less than 10 ng/mL (10 mcg/L) and less than 5% tumor in specimen	10 or more	Observation or Radical prostatectomy with or without pelvic lymph node dissection or radiation therapy
	Less than 10	Observation
Intermediate		
T_{2b}–T_{2c} or Gleason 7 or PSA 10–20 ng/mL (10–20 mcg/L)	10 or less	Observation or Radical prostatectomy with pelvic lymph node dissection or Radiation therapy with or without 4–6 months of neoadjuvant androgen deprivation therapy with or without brachytherapy
T_{2b}–T_{2c} or Gleason 7 or PSA 10–20 ng/mL (10–20 mcg/L)	10 or more	Radical prostatectomy with pelvic lymph node dissection or Radiation therapy with or without 4–6 months of neoadjuvant androgen deprivation therapy with or without brachytherapy
High		
T_{3a}, Gleason 8–10, PSA greater than 20 ng/mL (20 mcg/L)		Radiation therapy and ADT[a] (2-3 years) with or without brachytherapy or Radical prostatectomy and pelvic lymph node dissection
Very High		
T_{3b}–T_4		Radiation therapy and ADT (2-3 years) with or without brachytherapy or Radical prostatectomy and pelvic lymph node dissection or ADT
Very High		
Any T, N_1		ADT (2–3 years) or Radiation therapy and ADT (2–3 years)
Any T, Any N, M_1		ADT with Orchiectomy or LHRH agonist[b] + 7 days antiandrogen therapy or LHRH agonist + antiandrogen or LHRH agonist

ADT, androgen deprivation therapy; LHRH, luteinizing hormone-releasing hormone; PSA, prostate-specific antigen.

[a]Androgen deprivation therapy to achieve serum testosterone levels less than 50 ng/dL (1.7 nmol/L)

[b]LHRH agonist, medical castrations, or surgical are equivalent.

excellent 10-year survival, immediate morbidities of treatment must be balanced with the lower likelihood of dying from prostate cancer. In general, more aggressive treatment of early-stage prostate cancer is reserved for younger men, although patient preference is a major consideration in all treatment decisions. In a patient with a normal life expectancy of less than 10 years, observation or radiation therapy may be offered. In those with a normal life expectancy of equal to or greater than 10 years, either observation, radiation (external beam or brachytherapy), or radical prostatectomy with a pelvic lymph node dissection may be offered. Radiation and radical prostatectomy therapy are generally considered therapeutically equivalent for localized prostate cancer, although neither has been proven to be better than observation alone.[34]

Wilt and colleagues conducted a systematic review of 18 randomized trials and 473 observational studies to compare the effectiveness and potential complications from treatment options from prostate cancer. This study showed that the effectiveness of radiation, radical prostatectomy, and androgen deprivation therapy could not be compared because of the paucity of high-quality evidence available for analysis. Adverse effect profiles were similar, although severity varied among the treatments.[35] Complications from radical prostatectomy include blood loss, stricture formation, incontinence, lymphocele, fistula formation, anesthetic risk, and impotence. Nerve-sparing radical prostatectomy can be performed in many patients; 50% to 80% regain sexual potency within the first year. Although a recently published prospective study showed that even in patients with good preoperative sexual health, many do not return to baseline after surgery even with the assistance of erectile dysfunction treatments.[36] Acute complications from radiation therapy include cystitis, proctitis, hematuria, urinary retention, penoscrotal edema, and impotence (30% incidence).[27] Chronic complications include proctitis, diarrhea, cystitis, enteritis, impotence, urethral stricture, and incontinence.[27] In addition, androgen deprivation can also cause cognitive impairment, mood disturbances, and lack of initiative.[35] Because radiation and prostatectomy have significant and immediate mortality when compared with expectant management alone, many patients may elect to postpone therapy until symptoms develop.

Individuals with T_{2b} and T_{2c} disease or a Gleason score of 7 or a PSA ranging from 10 to 20 ng/mL (10 to 20 mcg/L) are considered at intermediate risk for prostate cancer recurrence.[32] Individuals with less than a 10-year expected survival may be offered observation or radical prostatectomy with pelvic lymph node dissection or radiation therapy with or without 4 to 6 months of neoadjuvant androgen deprivation therapy with or without brachytherapy, and those with a greater than or equal to 10-year life expectancy may be offered either radical prostatectomy with or without a pelvic lymph node dissection or radiation therapy with or without 4 to 6 months of neoadjuvant androgen deprivation therapy with or without brachytherapy (see Table 108-5).

The treatment of patients at high risk of recurrence (stage T_3, a Gleason score ranging from 8 to 10, or a PSA value greater than 20 ng/mL [20 mcg/L]) should be treated with androgen ablation for 2 to 3 years combined with radiation therapy with or without brachytherapy (see Table 108-5). Selected individuals with a low tumor volume may receive a radical prostatectomy with or without a pelvic lymph node dissection.

Patients with T_{3b} and T_4 disease have a very high risk of recurrence and are usually not candidates for radical prostatectomy because of extensive local spread of disease, although it may be possible for some individuals.[32] **4** Androgen deprivation therapy with a LHRH agonist plus an antiandrogen should be used prior to radiation therapy for patients with locally advanced prostate cancer to improve outcomes over radiation therapy alone. Recent evidence suggests that androgen ablation should be instituted at diagnosis rather than waiting for symptomatic disease or progression to occur. In a randomized clinical trial of 500 men with locally advanced prostate cancer who were randomized to either immediate initiation of androgen ablation (either orchiectomy or androgen ablation) or deferred hormonal therapy, patients who received immediate therapy had a median actuarial cause-specific survival duration of 7.5 years for immediate treatment as compared with 5.8 years for deferred treatment.[37]

5 Androgen deprivation therapy, with orchiectomy, an LHRH agonist alone, or an LHRH agonist plus an antiandrogen (combined androgen blockade), can be used to provide palliation for patients with advanced (stage D_2) prostate cancer.

Patients who develop metastatic disease often have tumor progression and develop castration resistant prostate cancer.[32] This may be described clinically by a rising PSA while on optimal androgen deprivation therapy, or the development of symptoms, typically related to bone metastases, including bone pain and fractures. Patients with metastatic disease may be continued on androgen deprivation therapy and denosumab (receptor activator of nuclear factor κ B [RANK] ligand inhibitor) or an IV bisphosphonate is added in patients with bone metastases. Importantly, further therapy is determined by the presence of symptomatic disease or whether the metastatic progression is manifested as only a rising PSA.

For clinically asymptomatic patients with a rising PSA, the recently approved sipuleucel-T is recommended as first-line treatment. Prior to the introduction of sipuleucel-T, standard therapy was a secondary hormonal manipulation, including the addition or withdrawal of antiandrogen therapy.

For those with symptomatic or disease involving internal organs, such as the liver, treatment with docetaxel is recommended as first-line therapy. For patients with symptomatic visceral disease who have a rising PSA following docetaxel chemotherapy, abiraterone acetate is recommended as first-line treatment. Other first-line treatment options following docetaxel chemotherapy include cabazitaxel, a microtubule inhibitor, in combination with prednisone, or the antiandrogen enzalutamide (Fig. 108-3).

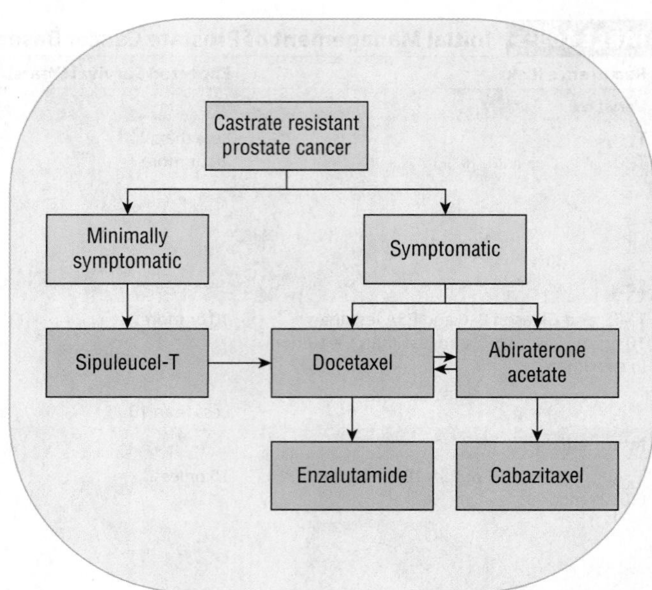

FIGURE 108-3 Treatment of castrate-resistant prostate cancer.

Nonpharmacologic Therapy

Observation

Observation is often referred to as expectant management, and active surveillance or watchful waiting. Observation involves monitoring the course of disease and initiating treatment if the cancer progresses. It is estimated that only about 10% of men who are eligible for observation choose this option.[34] A PSA and DRE are performed every 6 months, with a repeat biopsy at any sign of disease progression. The advantages of observation are avoiding the adverse effects associated with definitive therapies such as radiation and radical prostatectomy, and minimizing the risk of unnecessary therapies. The major disadvantage of observation is the risk that the cancer progresses and requires a more intensive therapy.

Orchiectomy

Bilateral orchiectomy, or removal of the testes, is a form of androgen deprivation therapy that rapidly reduces circulating androgens to castrate levels (less than 50 ng/dL [1.7 nmol/L]).[22] However, many patients are not surgical candidates because of advanced age, and other patients find this procedure psychologically unacceptable.[26] Orchiectomy is the preferred initial treatment in patients with impending spinal cord compression or ureteral obstruction.

Radiation

The two commonly used methods for radiation therapy are external beam radiotherapy and brachytherapy.[32] In external beam radiotherapy, doses of 70 to 75 Gy (7000 to 7500 rad) are delivered in 35 to 41 fractions in patients with low-grade prostate cancer and 75 to 80 Gy (7500 to 8000 rad) for those with intermediate- or high-grade prostate cancer. Brachytherapy involves the permanent implantation of radioactive beads of 145 Gy (14500 rad) ^{125}iodine or 124 Gy (12400 rad) of ^{103}palladium and is generally reserved for individuals with low-risk cancers. Radiation therapy may also be given after surgery in patients with localized disease. Acute complications from radiation therapy include cystitis, proctitis, hematuria, urinary retention, penoscrotal edema, and impotence (30% incidence).[16] Chronic complications include proctitis, diarrhea, cystitis, enteritis, impotence, urethral stricture, and incontinence.[26] Because radiation and prostatectomy have significant and immediate mortality when compared with observation alone, many patients may elect to postpone therapy until symptoms develop.

Radical Prostatectomy

Complications from radical prostatectomy include blood loss, stricture formation, incontinence, lymphocele, fistula formation, anesthetic risk, and impotence. Nerve-sparing radical prostatectomy can be performed in many patients; 50% to 80% regain sexual potency within the first year.

Pharmacologic Therapy

Drug Treatments of First Choice

Luteinizing Hormone-Releasing Hormone Agonists LHRH agonists are a reversible method of androgen ablation and are as effective as orchiectomy in treating prostate cancer.[38] Currently available LHRH agonists include leuprolide, leuprolide depot, leuprolide implant, triptorelin depot, triptorelin implant, and goserelin acetate implant. Leuprolide acetate is administered once daily, while leuprolide depot and goserelin acetate implant can be administered either once monthly, once every 12 weeks, or once every 16 weeks (leuprolide depot, every 4 months) (Table 108-7). The leuprolide depot formulation contains leuprolide acetate in coated pellets. The dose is administered intramuscularly, and the coating dissolves at different rates to allow sustained leuprolide levels throughout the dosing interval. Goserelin acetate implant contains goserelin acetate dispersed in a plastic matrix of D, L-lactic and glycolic acid copolymer and is administered subcutaneously. Hydrolysis of the copolymer material provides continuous release of goserelin over the dosing period. A leuprolide implant is a mini-osmotic pump that delivers 120 mcg of leuprolide daily for 12 months. After 12 months the implant is removed, and a different implant can be placed. Triptorelin LA is administered as an intramuscular injection of 11.25 mg every 84 days. Triptorelin depot is 3.75 mg once every 28 days.

Several randomized trials have demonstrated that leuprolide, goserelin, and triptorelin are effective agents when used alone in patients with advanced prostate cancer.[30] Response rates around 80% have been reported, with a lower incidence of adverse effects as compared with estrogens.[30] The currently available LHRH agonists or the dosage formulations have not been directly compared in clinical trials, but a meta-analysis showed no significant differences in efficacy or toxicity between leuprolide, goserelin, and orchiectomy.[39] Triptorelin is a more recent addition but is generally considered equally effective. Therefore the choice between the three agents is usually made based on cost and patient and physician preference for a dosing schedule.

The most common adverse effects reported with LHRH agonist therapy include a disease flareup during the first week of therapy, hot flashes, erectile impotence, decreased libido, and injection-site reactions.[30] The disease flareup is caused by an initial induction of LH and FSH by the LHRH agonist leading to an initial phase of increased testosterone production, and manifests clinically as either increased bone pain or increased urinary symptoms.[30] This flare reaction usually resolves after 2 weeks and has a similar onset and duration pattern for the depot LHRH products.[40,41] Tumor flare can be minimized by initiating an antiandrogen prior to the administration of the LHRH agonist and continuing for 2 to 4 weeks.[31]

LHRH agonist monotherapy can be used as initial therapy, with response rates similar to those for orchiectomy. The incidence of cardiovascular-related adverse effects is lower with LHRH therapy than with estrogen administration. Patients should be counseled to expect worsening symptoms during the first week of therapy. Appropriate pain and symptom management is required during this period, and a short course of concomitant antiandrogen therapy may need to be considered prior to initiating the LHRH agonist. Caution should be exercised if initiating LHRH agonist therapy in patients with widely metastatic disease involving the spinal cord or having the potential for ureteral obstruction because irreversible complications may occur.

Another potentially serious complication of androgen deprivation therapy (ADT) is a resultant decrease in bone mineral density leading to an increased risk for osteoporosis, osteopenia, and an increased risk for skeletal fractures. During initial therapy, bone mineral density of the hip and spine decreases by 2% to 3%.[42] Additionally, ADT has been associated with a 21% to 45% relative increase in fracture risk.[43–45] Therefore, most clinicians recommend that men starting long-term ADT should have a baseline bone mineral density and be initiated on a calcium and vitamin D supplement.[31,32]

In addition, an antiresorptive agent, either zoledronic acid or denosumab should be considered. A recent meta-analysis combined data from three identically designed double-blind randomized controlled trials that compared the efficacy and safety of denosumab at a dose of 120 mg with that of zoledronic acid at a dose of 4 mg administered IV.[46] Almost 6,000 patients with breast and prostate cancer and multiple myeloma were included in the meta-analysis. Denosumab reduced the risk of first skeletal-related event (SRE) by 17% (hazard ratio, 0.83 [95% CI: 0.76 to 0.90]; $P < 0.001$ for both noninferiority and superiority tests) as compared with zoledronic acid and the median time to first SRE was 27.66 (24.21 to not estimable) months for denosumab versus 19.45 (18.53 to 21.42) months for zoledronic acid. The benefits were consistent across tumor types evaluated and the incidence of adverse effects was not significantly different between the denosumab and zoledronic acid groups.

ADT has also been associated with a higher incidence of metabolic effects. In a landmark population-based trial, patients treated with an ADT and a gonadotropin-releasing hormone (GnRH) agonist had a greater risk of new-onset diabetes, coronary artery disease, and myocardial infarctions.[47] However, it is not clear whether ADT increases the risk of cardiovascular death. A recently published meta-analysis of eight trials with 4,141 patients treated with ADT evaluated prostate cancer specific mortality and all-cause mortality.[48] The trials included patients with nonmetastatic disease who were treated with immediate predominantly GnRH-agonist–based ADT versus no immediate ADT (control group). The incidence of cardiovascular deaths was 11.0% (95% CI, 8.3% to 14.5%) in the ADT group versus 11.2% (95% CI, 8.3% to 15.0%) in the control group. The risk of cardiovascular death for ADT versus control was not significantly different (relative risk 0.93; 95% CI, 0.79 to 1.10; $P = 0.41$) and these results suggest that ADT does not lead to increased cardiovascular mortality.[32] Patients receiving ADT should be screened for cardiovascular disease and diabetes and appropriate interventions to prevent and treat these complications should be initiated.[32]

Gonadotropin-Releasing Hormone Antagonists An alternative to LHRH agonists is the recently approved GnRH antagonist, degarelix. Degarelix works by binding reversibly to GnRH receptors in the pituitary gland, reducing the production of testosterone to castrate levels. The major advantage of degarelix over LHRH agonists is the rapidity at which it reduces testosterone levels. Castration levels are achieved in 7 days or less with degarelix, as compared with 28 days with leuprolide; tumor flare does not occur and antiandrogens are not required.

In a trial of 610 men with advanced prostate cancer, degarelix was shown to be equivalent to leuprolide in lowering testosterone levels for up to 1 year. Degarelix is available as a 40 mg/mL and a

20 mg/mL vial for subcutaneous injection, and the starting dose is 240 mg followed by 80 mg every 28 days. The starting dose should be divided into two 120 mg injections.[49] Degarelix has not been studied in combination with antiandrogens, and routine use of the combination cannot be recommended.

The most frequently reported adverse reactions were injection site reactions, including pain (28%), erythema (17%), swelling (6%), induration (4%), and nodule (3%). Most were transient and mild to moderate, leading to discontinuation in less than 1% of study subjects. Other adverse effects included elevations in liver function tests, which occurred in about 10% of study subjects. Osteoporosis may develop, and calcium and vitamin D supplementation should be considered.[49]

Antiandrogens Four antiandrogens, flutamide, bicalutamide, nilutamide, and enzalutamide, are currently available (Table 108-6). Cyproterone is another agent with antiandrogen activity, but it is not available in the United States. Antiandrogens have been used as monotherapy in previously untreated patients, but a recent meta-analysis determined that monotherapy with antiandrogens is less effective than LHRH agonist therapy.[41] Therefore, for advanced prostate cancer, flutamide, bicalutamide, and nilutamide are indicated only in combination with androgen-ablation therapy; flutamide and bicalutamide are indicated in combination with an LHRH agonist, and nilutamide is indicated in combination with orchiectomy.[50] Antiandrogens can reduce the symptoms from the flare phenomenon associated with LHRH agonist therapy.[31] Recently, the FDA approved the newest androgen receptor inhibitor, enzalutamide. Enzalutamide, also known as MDV3100, is currently approved as a single agent for patients with metastatic hormone-resistant prostate cancer who have previously received docetaxel.[51] As with the other antiandrogens, enzalutamide does not lower androgen levels but inhibits androgen-receptor signaling by competitively inhibiting the binding of androgens without stimulation of the androgen receptor. Enzalutamide may have an advantage over the currently available antiandrogen agents in that it inhibits nuclear translocation of the androgen receptor, DNA binding, and coactivator recruitment. It also has a greater affinity for the androgen receptor and has shown activity in patients resistant to other antiandrogens. There is also an ongoing trial in patients with advanced prostate cancer with enzalutamide prior to docetaxel.[52]

The most common antiandrogen-related adverse effects are listed in Table 108-7. In the only randomized comparison of bicalutamide plus an LHRH agonist versus flutamide plus an LHRH agonist, diarrhea was more common in flutamide-treated patients. The adverse effects of enzalutamide are similar to those of the other antiandrogens, but enzalutamide does have an increased risk of seizures.

Combined Androgen Blockade Although up to 80% of patients with advanced prostate cancer will respond to initial hormonal manipulation, almost all patients will progress within 2 to 4 years after initiating therapy.[26] Two mechanisms have been proposed to explain this tumor resistance. The tumor could be heterogeneously composed of cells that are hormone-dependent and hormone-independent, or the tumor could be stimulated by extratesticular androgens that are converted intracellularly to DHT. The rationale for combination hormonal therapy is to interfere with multiple hormonal pathways to completely eliminate androgen action. In clinical trials, combination hormonal therapy, sometimes also referred to as maximal androgen deprivation or total androgen blockade, or *combined androgen blockade (CAB)*, has been used. The combination of LHRH agonists or orchiectomy with antiandrogens is the most extensively studied combined androgen blockade approach.

A systematic review of six meta-analyses concluded that the best evidence for CAB came from the largest meta-analysis, conducted by the Prostate Cancer Trialists Collaborative Group including 8725 patients from 27 trials.[53] That analysis found no difference in overall survival between CAB and castration alone at 2 or 5 years, but a subgroup analysis showed that CAB with nonsteroidal antiandrogens, including flutamide, bicalutamide or nilutamide was associated with a statistically significant improvement in 5-year survival over castration alone (27.6% vs. 24.7%; $P = 0.005$). As expected, antiandrogens increased toxicity over placebo.

Although some clinicians consider CAB to be the initial hormonal therapy of choice for newly diagnosed patients, the clinician must weigh the costs of combined therapy against the modest survival benefit.[53] It is appropriate to use either LHRH agonist monotherapy or CAB as initial therapy for metastatic prostate cancer. CAB may be most beneficial for improving survival in patients with minimal disease and for preventing tumor flare, particularly in those with advanced metastatic disease. All other patients may be started on LHRH monotherapy, and an antiandrogen may be added after several months if androgen ablation is incomplete.

It is not clear when to start hormonal-deprivation therapy in patients with advanced prostate cancer.[30] The original recommendation to start therapy when symptoms appeared was based on the Veterans Administration Cooperative Urologic Research Group (VACURG) trials, in which no overall survival difference was demonstrated in patients who either started diethylstilbestrol (DES) initially or crossed over to active treatment when symptoms appeared; the excess mortality was attributed to estrogen administration.[54] Because LHRH agonists and antiandrogens are viable therapies with less cardiovascular toxicity, it is not clear whether delaying therapy is justified with these agents. Reanalysis of the original VACURG data[55] and recent combined androgen-deprivation trials[54] demonstrate a survival advantage for young, good-performance-status, minimal-disease patients treated initially with hormonal therapy, suggesting that early intervention before symptoms appear may be appropriate.[55]

Alternative Drug Treatments

Secondary or salvage therapies for patients who progress after their initial therapy depend on what was used for initial management.[32] For patients initially diagnosed with localized prostate cancer, radiotherapy can be used in the case of failed radical prostatectomy. Alternatively, androgen ablation can be used in patients who progress after either radiation therapy or radical prostatectomy.

Secondary Hormonal Manipulations In patients treated initially with one hormonal modality, secondary hormonal manipulations may be attempted. This may include adding an antiandrogen to a patient with incompletely supressed testosterone secretion with an LHRH agonist. In patients that have progression while receiving CAB, withdrawing antiandrogens, or using agents that inhibit androgen synthesis may be attempted. For patients who initially received an LHRH agonist alone, castration testosterone levels should be documented. Patients with inadequate testosterone suppression (greater than 20 ng/dL [0.7 nmol/L]) can be treated by adding an antiandrogen or performing an orchiectomy. If castration testosterone levels have been achieved, the patient is considered to have androgen-independent disease, and palliative androgen-independent salvage therapy can be used.

6 Antiandrogen withdrawal, for patients having progressive disease while receiving combined hormonal blockade with an LHRH agonist plus an antiandrogen, can provide additional symptomatic relief. Mutations in the androgen receptor have been documented that cause antiandrogens to act like receptor agonists.

If the patient initially received combined androgen blockade with an LHRH agonist and an antiandrogen, then androgen withdrawal is the first salvage manipulation.[32] Objective and subjective responses have been noted following the discontinuation of

TABLE 108-6 Hormonal Therapies for Prostate Cancer[65–72]

Drug (Brand Name)	Usual Dose	Toxicities	Hepatic/Renal Adjustments	Monitoring Parameters	Drug Interactions	Administration
Antiandrogens						
Flutamide (Eulexin)	750 mg/day	Gynecomastia Hot flashes Gastrointestinal disturbances (diarrhea) Loss of libido LFT abnormalities Breast tenderness Methemoglobinemia	Contraindicated in patients with hepatic impairment No dosage adjustment necessary in chronic renal impairment	Serum transaminases should be monitored prior to start of therapy and monthly for first 4 months, then periodically thereafter. Monitor for tumor reduction, testosterone/estrogen, and phosphatase serum levels.	Substrate of CYP1A2 and CYP3A4	Administered orally in three divided doses. Capsule may be opened into applesauce, pudding, or other soft foods.
Bicalutamide (Casodex)	50 mg/day (up to 150 mg/day—unlabeled use)	Gynecomastia Hot flashes Gastrointestinal disturbances (diarrhea) Decrease libido LFT abnormalities Breast tenderness	Discontinue if ALT >2 times upper limit of normal or patient develops jaundice	Serum transaminases should be monitored prior to start of therapy and monthly for first 4 months, then periodically thereafter. Periodic monitoring of CBC, EKG, echocardiograms, serum testosterone, luteinizing hormone, and PSA.	Inhibits CYP3A4 May increase concentration of vitamin K antagonists.	May be taken with or without food.
Nilutamide (Nilandron)	300 mg/day for first month then 150 mg/day	Gynecomastia Hot flashes Gastrointestinal Disturbances (constipation) LFT abnormalities Breast tenderness Visual disturbances (impaired dark adaptation) Alcohol intolerance Interstitial pneumonitis	Contraindicated in patients with hepatic impairment Discontinue if ALT >2 times upper limit of normal or patient develops jaundice	Serum transaminases should be monitored prior to start of therapy and monthly for first 4 months, then periodically thereafter. Chest x-ray at baseline and consideration of pulmonary function testing (at baseline)	Substrate of CYP2C19 and weak inhibitor of CYP2C19	May be taken with or without food.
Enzalutamide (Xtandi)	160 mg/day	Gastrointestinal disturbances (diarrhea) Musculoskeletal disorders (back pain, arthralgias, muscle pain, weakness) Asthenia Peripheral edema CNS (headache, dizziness) Seizures LFT abnormalities	No adjustment necessary for renal or hepatic impairment	Complete blood counts baseline and periodically. LFTs baseline and periodically.	Strong CYP3A4 and moderate CYP2C9 and CYP2C19 inducer. Avoid CYP3A4, CYP2C9 and CYP2C19 sensitive substrates. CYP2C8 substrate, avoid strong inducers and inhibitors of CYP2C8 If vitamin K antagonists necessary, conduct additional INR monitoring.	May be taken with or without food.
Androgen Synthesis Inhibitor						
Abiraterone acetate (Zytiga)	1000 mg/day + prednisone 5 mg BID	Gastrointestinal disturbances (diarrhea) Edema Hypokalemia Hypophosphatemia LFT abnormalities Hypertriglyceridemia	250 mg daily for Child Pugh Class B. Avoid use in Child Pugh Class C. Withhold treatment if LFTs >5 times the ULN or bilirubin >3 ULN	Serum transaminases should be monitored prior to start of therapy, every 2 weeks for 3 months, then monthly thereafter. Monitor for signs and symptoms of adrenocorticoid insufficiency; monthly for hypertension, hypokalemia, and fluid retention.	Substrate of CYP3A4. Use with caution with CYP3A4 inhibitors and inducers. Inhibits CYP1A2, CYP2C19, CYP2C8, CYP2C9, CYP2D6, CYP3A4, and P-glycoprotein. Use sensitive substrates with caution.	Administer on an empty stomach, at least 1 hour before and 2 hours after food.

(Continued)

TABLE 108-6 Hormonal Therapies for Prostate Cancer[65–72] ***(Continued)***

Drug (Brand Name)	Usual Dose	Toxicities	Hepatic/Renal Adjustments	Monitoring Parameters	Drug Interactions	Administration
Luteinizing-Hormone Agonists						
Leuprolide (Lupron)	7.5 mg IM every month 22.5 mg IM every 3 months 30 mg IM every 4 months 45 mg IM every 6 months	Hot flashes Decreased libido Gynecomastia Osteoporosis Fatigue Weight gain	No adjustment necessary for renal or hepatic impairment	Serum testosterone ~ 4 weeks after initiation, PSA, blood glucose, and $HgbA_{1c}$ prior to initiation and periodically thereafter.	May diminish the effects of antidiabetic agents.	Vary injection site.
Goserelin (Zoladex)	3.6 mg SQ implant every month 10.8 mg SQ implant every 3 months	Hot flashes Decreased libido Gynecomastia Osteoporosis Fatigue Weight gain	No adjustment necessary for renal or hepatic impairment	Monitor bone mineral density, serum calcium, and cholesterol/lipids.	May diminish the effects of antidiabetic agents.	Vary injection site.
Triptorelin (Trelstar)	3.75 mg IM every month 11.25 mg IM every 3 months 22.5 mg IM every 6 months	Hot flashes Decreased libido Gynecomastia Osteoporosis Fatigue Weight gain	No adjustment necessary for renal or hepatic impairment	Monitor serum testosterone levels and prostate specific antigen.	May diminish the effects of antidiabetic agents.	Vary injection site.
Gonadotropin-Releasing Hormone Antagonists						
Degarelix (Firmagon)	240 mg SQ loading dose 80 mg SQ every 28 days (following 28 days after loading dose)	Hot flashes Decreased libido Gynecomastia Osteoporosis Fatigue Weight gain	Use in caution with CL_{cr} <50 mL/min Do not use in patients with severe hepatic impairment	Prostate-specific antigen periodically, serum testosterone monthly until castration achieved then every other month, LFTs at baseline in addition to serum electrolytes and bone mineral density.	Use with caution with agents that may increase QTC interval.	Vary injection site.

ALT, alanine aminotransferase; BID, twice daily; CBC, complete blood count; CL_{cr}, creatinine clearance; CNS, central nervous system; CYP, cytochrome P450; EKG, electrocardiogram; $HgbA_{1c}$, hemoglobin A1c; IM, intramuscular injection; INR, international normalized ratio; LFT, liver function test; PSA, prostate-specific antigen; SQ, subcutaneous injection; ULN, upper limit of normal.

TABLE 108-7 Chemotherapy and Immunotherapy for Prostate Cancer[73–76]

Drug (Brand Name)	Usual Dose	Toxicities	Hepatic/Renal Adjustments	Monitoring Parameters	Drug Interactions	Administration
Antimicrotubule Agents						
Docetaxel (Taxotere)	75 mg/m² IV every 3 weeks	Fluid retention, alopecia, mucositis, myelosuppression, hypersensitivity	Aspartate transaminase/alanine transaminase >1.5 times the upper limit of normal and alkaline phosphatase >2.5 times the upper limit of normal do not administer.	CBC with differential, LFTs, bilirubin, alkaline phosphatase, renal function. Monitor for hypersensitivity reactions.	Avoid concomitant use of CYP3A4 inhibitors	Administer IV infusion over 1 hour. Premedication with corticosteroids for 3 days beginning the day before.
Cabazitaxel (Jevtana)	25 mg/m² IV every 3 weeks	Fluid retention, constipation, mucositis, myelosuppression, hypersensitivity	Discontinue if ALT >2 times upper limit of normal or patient develops jaundice.	CBC weekly during first cycle, then prior to each treatment. Monitor for hypersensitivity.	Avoid concomitant use of CYP3A4 inducers and inhibitors	Administer IV infusion over 1 hour.
Immunotherapy						
Sipuleucel-T (Provenge)	Each injection contains >50 million autologous CD54+ cells (obtained through leukapheresis) activated with PAP-GM-CSF. Dose is given ~ every 2 weeks for 3 total doses	Hypersensitivity, chills, fatigue, fever, headache, myalgias	No dosage adjustment necessary for renal or hepatic dysfunction.	No specific laboratory monitoring recommended.	Immunosuppressants may decrease the therapeutic effects of sipuleucel-T	Administer IV infusion over 1 hour. Observe patient for 30 minutes after the completion of the infusion. Premedicate with acetaminophen and an antihistamine 30 minutes prior to administration.

ALT, alanine aminotransferase; CBC, complete blood count; CYP, cytochrome P450; LFT, liver function test;. PAP-GM-CSF, prostatic acid phosphatase granulocyte-macrophage colony-stimulating factor.

flutamide,[56] bicalutamide,[57] or nilutamide[58] in patients receiving these agents as part of combined androgen ablation with an LHRH agonist. Mutations in the androgen receptor have been demonstrated that allow antiandrogens such as flutamide, bicalutamide, and nilutamide (or their metabolites) to become agonists and activate the androgen receptor.[59] Patient responses to androgen withdrawal manifest as significant PSA reductions and improved clinical symptoms. Androgen withdrawal responses lasting 3 to 14 months have been observed in up to 35% of patients, and predicting response seems to be most closely related to longer androgen exposure times. Incomplete cross-resistance has been noted in some patients who received bicalutamide after they had progressed while receiving flutamide.[60] The addition of an agent that blocks adrenal androgen synthesis, such as aminoglutethimide, at the time that androgens are withdrawn may produce a better response than androgen withdrawal alone.[59] Because of the potential for response immediately after antiandrogen withdrawal, a sufficient observation and assessment period (usually 4 to 6 weeks) is usually required before a patient can be enrolled on a clinical trial evaluating a new agent or therapy for advanced prostate cancer.

Androgen synthesis inhibitors, such as aminoglutethimide or ketoconazole, can provide symptomatic relief for a short time in approximately 50% of patients with progressive disease despite previous androgen-ablation therapy.[32] Adverse effects during aminoglutethimide therapy occur in about 50% of patients.[32] Central nervous system effects that include lethargy, ataxia, and dizziness are the major adverse reactions. A generalized morbilliform, pruritic rash has been reported in up to 30% of patients treated. The rash is usually self-limiting and resolves within 5 to 8 days with continued therapy. Adverse effects from ketoconazole include gastrointestinal intolerance, transient rises in liver and renal function tests, and hypoadrenalism. Ketoconazole is combined with replacement doses of hydrocortisone to prevent symptomatic hypoadrenalism.[32]

Abiraterone is the newest androgen synthesis inhibitor that targets cytochrome P450 (CYP)17A1, which results in a decrease in circulating levels of testosterone.[61] Abiraterone is indicated in patients with metastatic castration-resistant prostate cancer, either before or after docetaxel-based chemotherapy. The initial approval was based on the results of a phase III study of patients previously treated with a docetaxel-containing regimen. The combination of abiraterone and prednisone increased median overall survival by 3.9 months in comparison to placebo. Hypertension, hypokalemia, and edema may occur due to hypoadrenalism. Abiraterone is available as the prodrug, abiraterone acetate, and should be taken on an empty stomach as food increases bioavailability by up to 10-fold. Monitoring of liver function tests is recommended at baseline, every 2 weeks for the first 3 months, and then monthly thereafter. Since abiraterone is an inhibitor of CYP2D6, medication profiles should be reviewed for potential drug interactions prior to initiation of abiraterone therapy.

7 Chemotherapy Chemotherapy with docetaxel and prednisone improves survival in patients with castrate-refractory prostate cancer and is considered first-line therapy for these patients. Docetaxel 75 mg/m² every 3 weeks combined with prednisone 5 mg twice a day improves survival in hormone-refractory metastatic prostate cancer.[62] The most common adverse events with this regimen are nausea, alopecia, and bone marrow suppression. Other adverse effects of docetaxel include fluid retention and peripheral neuropathy. Docetaxel is metabolized in the liver; patients with hepatic impairment may not be eligible for treatment with docetaxel because of an increased risk for toxicity (Table 108-7).

Cabazitaxel is a taxane with demonstrated activity in docetaxel resistant cell lines and animal models of human cancer.[63] Cabazitaxel has lower affinity for P-glycoprotein multidrug resistance transporter than docetaxel, which may explain why cabazitaxel is active in the setting of docetaxel resistance. In patients previously treated with docetaxel and prednisone, treatment with cabazitaxel 25 mg/m^2 every 3 weeks with prednisone 10 mg daily significantly improved progression-free survival and overall survival as compared to mitoxantrone and prednisone. Neutropenia, febrile neutropenia, neuropathy, and diarrhea are the most significant toxicities. Hypersensitivity reactions may occur and premedication with an antihistamine, a corticosteroid and an H_2 antagonist is recommended. Cabazitaxel is extensively metabolized in the liver and should be avoided in patients with hepatic dysfunction (see Table 108-7).

Immunotherapy Sipuleucel-T is a novel autologous cellular immunotherapy that was FDA-approved in April 2010 for the treatment of asymptomatic or minimally symptomatic metastatic hormone-refractory prostate cancer.[64] Alternative treatment options for this patient population are secondary hormonal therapy, including antiandrogen therapy, withdrawal of antiandrogen therapy, ketoconazole, abiraterone acetate, steroids, estrogen, or enrollment on a clinical trial, although none of these options has been shown to improve overall survival. No clinical trials have compared sipuleucel-T to secondary hormonal therapies. Patients treated with sipuleucel-T undergo leukapheresis on day 1 to collect peripheral blood mononuclear cells, the cellular fraction that includes immune effector cells. These cells are incubated with a prostatic acid phosphatase (PAP)–granulocyte-macrophage colony-stimulating factor (GM-CSF) fusion protein; PAP is the specific tumor antigen, and GM-CSF is the immune cell activator. The cellular product is then infused IV into the patient on day 3 or 4, providing an autologous infusion of activated cells. Each course of sipuleucel-T consists of three infusions of activated cells, given every 2 weeks. In the pivotal trial, sipuleucel-T prolonged median survival by 4.1 months and reduced the risk of death by 22% (hazard ratio = 0.78, 95% CI, 0.61 to 0.98; $P = 0.03$).[64] Adverse effects related to sipuleucel-T were generally mild and nearly all patients were able to receive the entire course (i.e., 3 infusions). A course of sipuleucel-T costs about $93,000, and some insurers have questioned the value of the therapy.

Clinical **Controversy...**

The use of sipuleucel-T is controversial. The treatment is indicated for minimally symptomatic prostate cancer and has not been compared to standard second-line hormonal interventions.

PERSONALIZED PHARMACOTHERAPY

Prevention strategies for prostate cancer, specifically whether to undergo PSA screening for early detection or whether to start chemoprevention with finasteride or dutasteride in an effort to prevent prostate cancer, are highly personalized decisions and depend on an individual patient weighing the risks and benefits of either strategy. This is a major change from previous recommendations, which uniformly recommended screening regardless of age, health status or patient preference.

Prostate cancer therapy is personalized based on clinical factors, including stage of cancer, life expectancy of the patient, and a patient's fitness for surgical interventions (see Table 108-5). Agents used in the treatment of prostate cancer are often personalized with dose adjustments for organ dysfunction of other clinical characteristics (see Table 108-7). Although there are no current selection strategies, where individuals with a specific mutation receive a specific therapy, this remains an important area of research.

EVALUATION OF THERAPEUTIC OUTCOMES

Monitoring of prostate cancer depends on the stage of the cancer.[32] When definitive, curative therapy is attempted, objective parameters to assess tumor response include assessment of the primary tumor size, evaluation of involved lymph nodes, and the response of tumor markers such as PSA to treatment. Following definitive therapy, the PSA level is checked every 6 months for the first 5 years, then annually. Local recurrence in the absence of a rising PSA may occur, so the DRE is also performed. In the metastatic setting, chemotherapy and novel hormonal manipulations have been shown to prolong overall survival. In addition, clinical benefit responses can be documented by evaluating performance status changes, weight changes, quality of life, and analgesic requirements, in addition to the PSA or DRE at 3-month intervals.

ABBREVIATIONS

ADT	Androgen deprivation therapy
AUS	American Urologic System
BPH	benign prostatic hyperplasia
CAB	combined androgen blockade
CI	confidence interval
CYP	cytochrome P450
DES	diethylstilbestrol
DHT	dihydrotestosterone
DRE	digital rectal examination
ERSPC	European Randomized Study of Screening for Prostate Cancer
FDA	Food and Drug Administration
FSH	follicle-stimulating hormone
GM-CSF	granulocyte-macrophage colony-stimulating factor
GnRH	gonadotropin-releasing hormone
IGF-1	insulin-like growth factor
LH	luteinizing hormone
LHRH	luteinizing hormone–releasing hormone
PAP	prostatic acid phosphatase
PCPT	Prostate Cancer Prevention Trial
PLCO	Prostate, Lung, Colon and Ovarian Screening (study)
PSA	prostate-specific antigen
RANK	receptor activator of nuclear factor κ B
REDUCE	Reduction by Dutasteride of Prostate Cancer Events
SELECT	Selenium and Vitamin E Cancer Prevention Trial
SRE	skeletal-related event
TNM	tumor, node, metastases
USPSTF	United States Preventative Services Task Force
VACURG	Veterans Administration Cooperative Urologic Research Group

REFERENCES

1. Siegel R, Naishadham D, Jemal A. Cancer statistics, 2013. CA Cancer J Clin 2013;63:11–30.
2. Hsieh K, Albertsen PC. Populations at high risk for prostate cancer. Urol Clin North Am 2003;30:669–676.
3. Odedina FT, Ogunbiyi JO, Ukoli FA. Roots of prostate cancer in African-American men. J Natl Med Assoc 2006;98:539–543.
4. Denis L, Morton MS, Griffiths K. Diet and its preventive role in prostatic disease. Eur Urol 1999;35:377–387.
5. Crawford ED. Epidemiology of prostate cancer. Urology 2003;62:3–12.

6. Liede A, Karlan BY, Narod SA. Cancer risks for male carriers of germline mutations in BRCA1 or BRCA2: A review of the literature. J Clin Oncol 2004;22:735–742.
7. Gurel B, Iwata T, Koh CM, et al. Molecular alterations in prostate cancer as diagnostic, prognostic, and therapeutic targets. Adv Anat Pathol 2008;15:319–331.
8. Wilt TJ, Macdonald R, Hagerty K, et al. 5-α-Reductase inhibitors for prostate cancer chemoprevention: An updated Cochrane systematic review. BJU Int 2010;106: 1444–1451.
9. Thompson IM, Goodman PJ, Tangen CM, et al. The influence of finasteride on the development of prostate cancer. N Engl J Med 2003;349:215–224.
10. Andriole GL, Bostwick DG, Brawley OW, et al. REDUCE Study Group Effect of dutasteride on the risk of prostate cancer. N Engl J Med 2010;362:1192–1202.
11. Sandhu GS, Nepple KG, Tanagho YS, Andriole GL. Prostate cancer chemoprevention. Semin Oncol 2013;40(3):276–285.
12. Redman MW, Tangen CM, Goodman PJ, et al. Finasteride does not increase the risk of high-grade prostate cancer: A bias-adjusted modeling approach. Cancer Prev Res (Phila Pa) 2008;1:174–181.
13. Kramer BS, Hagerty KL, Justman S, et al. Use of 5-alpha-reductase inhibitors for prostate cancer chemoprevention: American Society of Clinical Oncology/American Urological Association 2008 Clinical Practice Guideline. J Urol 2009;181:1642–1657.
14. Klein EA, Thompson IM, Tangen CM, et al. Vitamin E and the risk of prostate cancer. The Selenium and Vitamin E Cancer Prevention Trial (SELECT). JAMA 2011;306: 1549–1556.
15. Thompson IM, Tangen CM, Goodman PJ, Lucia MS, Klein EA. Chemoprevention of prostate cancer. J Urol 2009;182:499–507.
16. Galic J, Karner I, Cenan L, et al. Role of screening in detection of clinically localized prostate cancer. Coll Antropol 2003;27(suppl 1):49–54.
17. Wilson SS, Crawford ED. Screening for prostate cancer: Current recommendations. Urol Clin North Am 2004;31:219–226.
18. Thompson IM, Pauler DK, Goodman PJ, et al. Prevalence of prostate cancer among men with a prostate-specific antigen level ≤4.0 ng per milliliter. N Engl J Med 2004;350:2239–2246.
19. Shteynshlyuger A, Andriole GL. Prostate cancer: to screen or not to screen? Urol Clin North Am 2010;37:1–9.
20. Wolf AMD, Wender RC, Etzioni RB, et al. American Cancer Society guideline for the early detection of prostate cancer. Update 2010. CA Cancer J Clin 2010;60:70–98.
21. Chou R, Croswell JM, Dana T, et al. Screening for prostate cancer: A review of the evidence for the U.S. Preventive Services Task Force. Ann Intern Med 2011;155:762–771.
22. Moyer VA on behalf of the USPSTF. Screening for prostate cancer: U.S. Preventive Services Task Force Recommendation Statement. Ann Intern Med 2012;157:120–134. *www.uspreventiveservicestaskforce.org/prostatecancerscreening/prostatefinalrs.pdf.*
23. Schröder FH, Hugosson J, Roobol MJ, et al. Prostate-cancer mortality at 11 years of follow-up. N Engl J Med 2012;366:981–990.
24. Andriole GL, Crawford ED, Grubb RL, et al. Prostate cancer screening in the randomized Prostate, Lung, Colorectal, and Ovarian Cancer Screening Trial: Mortality results after 13 years of follow-up. J Natl Cancer Inst 2012;104:125–132.
25. Gulati R, Gore JL, Etzioni R. Comparative effectiveness of alternative prostate-specific antigen-based prostate cancer screening strategies: model estimates of potential benefits and harms. Ann Intern Med 2013;158:145–153.
26. Khauli RB. Prostate cancer: Diagnostic and therapeutic strategies with emphasis on the role of PSA. J Med Liban 2005;53:95–102.
27. Iczkowski KA. Current prostate biopsy interpretation: Criteria for cancer, atypical small acinar proliferation, high-grade prostatic intraepithelial neoplasia, and use of immunostains. Arch Pathol Lab Med 2006;130:835–843.
28. De Marzo AM, Meeker AK, Zha S, et al. Human prostate cancer precursors and pathobiology. Urology 2003;62:55–62.
29. Culig Z. Role of the androgen receptor axis in prostate cancer. Urology 2003;62:21–26.
30. Marks LS. Luteinizing hormone-releasing hormone agonists in the treatment of men with prostate cancer: Timing, alternatives, and the 1-year implant. Urology 2003;62:36–42.
31. Sharifi N, Gulley JL, Dahut WL. Androgen deprivation therapy for prostate cancer. JAMA 2005;294:238–244.
32. National Comprehensive Cancer Network. National Comprehensive Cancer Network guidelines for the management of prostate cancer. 2012, *http://www.nccn.org/professionals/physician_gls/f_guidelines.asp* Prostate Cancer v.3.2012.
33. Scher HI. Prostate carcinoma: Defining therapeutic objectives and improving overall outcomes. Cancer 2003;97:758–771.
34. Ganz PA, Barry JM, Burke W, et al. National Institutes of Health State-of-the-Science Conference: role of active surveillance in the management of men with localized prostate cancer. Ann Intern Med 2012;156:591–595.
35. Wilt TJ, Macdonald R, Rutks I, et al. Systematic review: Comparative effectiveness and harms of treatments for clinically localized prostate cancer. Ann Intern Med 2008;148:435–448.
36. Dalkin BL, Christopher BA. Potent men undergoing radical prostatectomy: A prospective study measuring sexual health outcomes and the impact of erectile dysfunction treatments. Urol Oncol 2008;26:281–285.
37. Immediate versus deferred treatment for advanced prostatic cancer: Initial results of the Medical Research Council Trial. The Medical Research Council Prostate Cancer Working Party Investigators Group. Br J Urol 1997;79:235–246.
38. Novara G, Galfano A, Secco S, Ficarra V, Artibani W. Impact of surgical and medical castration on serum testosterone level in prostate cancer patients. Urol Int 2009;82:249–255.
39. Seidenfeld J, Samson DJ, Aronson N, et al. Relative effectiveness and cost-effectiveness of methods of androgen suppression in the treatment of advanced prostate cancer. Evid Rep Technol Assess (Summ) 1999 May;(4):i–x, 1–246.
40. Hedlund PO, Henriksson P. Parenteral estrogen versus total androgen ablation in the treatment of advanced prostate carcinoma: Effects on overall survival and cardiovascular mortality. The Scandinavian Prostatic Cancer Group (SPCG)-5 Trial Study. Urology 2000;55:328–333.
41. Seidenfeld J, Samson DJ, Hasselblad V, et al. Single-therapy androgen suppression in men with advanced prostate cancer: A systematic review and meta-analysis. Ann Intern Med 2000;132:566–577.
42. Smith MR, Finkelstein JS, McGovern FJ, et al. Changes in body composition during androgen deprivation therapy for prostate cancer. J Clin Endocrinol Metab 2002;87:599–603.
43. Shahinian VB, Kuo YF, Freeman JL, Goodwin JS. Risk of fracture after androgen deprivation for prostate cancer. N Engl J Med 2005;352:154–164.
44. Smith MR, Boyce SP, Moyneur E, et al. Risk of clinical fractures after gonadotropin-releasing hormone agonist therapy for prostate cancer. J Urol 2006;175:136–139.

45. Smith MR, Lee WC, Brandman W, et al. Gonadotropin-releasing hormone agonist and fracture risk: A claims-based cohort study of men with nonmetastatic prostate cancer. J Clin Oncol 2005;23:7897–7903.
46. Lipton A, Fizazi K, Stopeck AT, et al. Superiority of denosumab to zoledronic acid for prevention of skeletal-related events: A combined analysis of 3 pivotal, randomised, phase 3 trials. Eur J Cancer 2012;48:3082–3092.
47. Keating NL, O'Malley AJ, Smith MR. Diabetes and cardiovascular disease during androgen deprivation therapy for prostate cancer. J Clin Oncol 2006;24:4448–4456.
48. Nguyen PL, Je Y, Schutz FA, et al. Association of androgen deprivation therapy with cardiovascular death in patients with prostate cancer: A meta-analysis of randomized trials. JAMA 2011;306:2359–2366.
49. Klotz L, Boccon-Gibod L, Shore ND, et al. The efficacy and safety of degarelix: A 12-month, comparative, randomized, open-label, parallel group phase III study in patients with prostate cancer. BJU Int 2008 102:1531–1538.
50. Akaza H. Combined androgen blockade for prostate cancer: review of efficacy, safety and cost-effectiveness. Cancer Sci 2011;102:51–56.
51. Scher HI, Fizazi K, Saad F, et al. AFFIRM Investigators. Increased survival with enzalutamide in prostate cancer after chemotherapy. N Engl J Med 2012;367:1187–1197.
52. Vogelzang NJ. Enzalutamide—a major advance in the treatment of metastatic prostate cancer. N Engl J Med 2012;367:1256–1257.
53. Lukka H, Waldron T, Klotz L, Winquist E, Trachtenberg J; Genitourinary Cancer Disease Site Group; Cancer Care Ontario Program in Evidence-based Care. Maximal androgen blockade for the treatment of metastatic prostate cancer—a systematic review. Curr Oncol 2006;13:81–93.
54. Carcinoma of the prostate: Treatment comparisons. J Urol 1967;98:516–522.
55. Ryan CJ, Small EJ. Early versus delayed androgen deprivation for prostate cancer: New fuel for an old debate. J Clin Oncol 2005;23:8225–8231.
56. Scher HI, Kelly WK. Flutamide withdrawal syndrome: Its impact on clinical trials in hormone-refractory prostate cancer. J Clin Oncol 1993;11:1566–1572.
57. Small EJ, Srinivas S. The antiandrogen withdrawal syndrome: experience in a large cohort of unselected patients with advanced prostate cancer. Cancer 1995;76:1428–1434.
58. Huan SD, Gerridzen RG, Yau JC, et al. Antiandrogen withdrawal syndrome with nilutamide. Urology 1997;49:632–634.
59. Sartor O, Cooper M, Weinberger M, et al. Surprising activity of flutamide withdrawal, when combined with aminoglutethimide, in treatment of "hormone-refractory" prostate cancer. J Natl Cancer Inst 1994;86:222–227.
60. Scher HI, Liebertz C, Kelly WK, et al. Bicalutamide for advanced prostate cancer: The natural versus treated history of disease. J Clin Oncol 1997;15:2928–2938.
61. de Bona JS, Logothetis CJ, Molina A, et al. Abiraterone and increased survival in metastatic prostate cancer. N Engl J Med 2011;364:1995–2005.
62. Tannock IF, de Wit R, Berry WR, et al. Docetaxel plus prednisone or mitoxantrone plus prednisone for advanced prostate cancer. N Engl J Med 2004;351:1502–1512.
63. de Bono JS, Oudard S, Ozguroglu M, et al. Prednisone plus cabazitaxel or mitoxantrone for metastatic castration-resistant prostate cancer progressing after docetaxel treatment: A randomised open-label trial. Lancet 2010;376:1147–1154.
64. Kantoff PW, Higano CS, Shore ND, et al. Sipuleucel-T immunotherapy for castration-resistant prostate cancer. N Engl J Med 2010;363:411–442.
65. Flutamide [package insert]. Kenilworth, NJ: Schering Corporation, 2000.
66. Bicalutamide [package insert]. Wilmington, DE: AstraZeneca Pharmaceuticals LP, 2000.
67. Nilutamide [package insert]. Bridgewater, NJ: Sanofi-Aventis, 2006.
68. Enzalutamide [package insert]. Northbrook, IL: Astellas Pharma, 2012.
69. Abiraterone [package insert]. Horsham, PA: Janssen Biotech, 2012
70. Leuprolide [package insert]. Irvine, CA: SICOR Pharmaceuticals, 2005.
71. Goserelin [package insert]. Wilmington, DE: AstraZeneca Pharmaceuticals LP, 2012.
72. Triptorelin [package insert]. Kalamazoo, MI: Pharmacia & Upjohn Company, 2001.
73. Degarelix [package insert]. Parsippany, NJ: Ferring Pharmaceuticals, 2012.
74. Docetaxel [package insert]. Bridgewater, NJ: Sanofi-Aventis, 2011.
75. Cabazitaxel [package insert]. Bridgewater, NJ: Sanofi-Aventis, 2012.
76. Sipuleucel-T [package insert]. Seattle, WA: Dendreon Corporation, 2011.

109

Lymphomas

Alexandre Chan and Gary C. Yee

KEY CONCEPTS

1. Patients with Hodgkin lymphoma present with a painless, rubbery lymph node, which most commonly resides in the neck (cervical or supraclavicular nodes).
2. Patients with early stage Hodgkin lymphoma should be treated with combination chemotherapy with or without involved-field radiation.
3. Combination chemotherapy with doxorubicin (Adriamycin), bleomycin, vinblastine, and dacarbazine (ABVD) is the primary treatment for patients with advanced-stage Hodgkin lymphoma. Patients with advanced unfavorable disease may be treated with more aggressive regimens that have greater activity, but are associated with a higher risk of secondary malignancies.
4. Some patients with Hodgkin lymphoma will be refractory to initial therapy or will have a recurrence following a complete remission. Response to salvage therapy depends on the extent and site of recurrence, previous therapy, and duration of initial remission. High-dose chemotherapy and autologous hematopoietic stem cell transplantation should be considered in patients with refractory or relapsed disease.
5. The current classification system for non-Hodgkin lymphoma is the World Health Organization classification system, which is based on the principle that non-Hodgkin lymphomas can be classified into specific disease entities, defined by a combination of morphology, immunophenotype, genetic features, and clinical features.
6. As compared with Hodgkin lymphoma, the clinical presentation of non-Hodgkin lymphoma is more variable because of disease heterogeneity and more frequent extranodal involvement.
7. The Ann Arbor staging system correlates poorly with prognosis in non-Hodgkin lymphoma because the disease does not spread through contiguous lymph nodes and often involves extranodal sites.
8. Several prognostic models have been developed to estimate prognosis in patients with non-Hodgkin lymphoma. The International Prognostic Index (IPI) score is a well-established model for patients with aggressive non-Hodgkin lymphoma. The Follicular Lymphoma International Prognostic Index (FLIPI) is a similar model used for patients with follicular and other indolent lymphomas.
9. The clinical behavior and degree of aggressiveness can be used to categorize non-Hodgkin lymphoma into indolent and aggressive lymphomas. Patients with an indolent lymphoma usually have a relatively long survival, with or without aggressive chemotherapy. Although these lymphomas respond to a wide range of therapeutic approaches, few if any of these patients are cured of their disease. In contrast, aggressive lymphomas are rapidly growing tumors and patients have a short survival if appropriate therapy is not initiated. Most patients with aggressive lymphomas respond to intensive chemotherapy and many are cured of their disease.
10. Patients with localized follicular lymphoma can be cured with radiation therapy alone. Advanced follicular lymphoma is not curable, and there are many treatment options, including watchful waiting, extended-field radiation therapy, single-agent alkylating agents, anthracycline-containing combination chemotherapy, purine analogs, interferon-α, anti-CD20 monoclonal antibodies, and high-dose chemotherapy with hematopoietic stem cell transplantation.
11. Patients with localized aggressive lymphomas can be cured with several cycles of R-CHOP (rituximab, cyclophosphamide, doxorubicin, vincristine [Oncovin], prednisone) chemotherapy and involved-field irradiation. Patients with bulky stage II, stage III, or stage IV aggressive lymphomas can be cured of their disease with R-CHOP chemotherapy.
12. Conventional-dose salvage therapy can induce responses in patients with aggressive lymphomas who relapse, but long-term survival and cure is uncommon. Some patients with aggressive lymphoma who relapse and respond to salvage therapy can be cured with high-dose chemotherapy and autologous hematopoietic stem cell transplantation.

Lymphomas are a heterogeneous group of malignancies that arise from malignant transformation of immune cells that reside predominantly in lymphoid tissues. They most commonly present as a solid tumor, but can sometimes present as circulating tumor cells in peripheral blood. The differing histology of lymphoma cells has led to classification of Hodgkin lymphoma (Reed–Sternberg cells) or non-Hodgkin lymphoma (B- or T-cell lymphocyte markers). Non-Hodgkin lymphomas (NHLs) are further classified into distinct clinical entities, which are defined by a combination of morphology, immunophenotype, genetic features, and clinical features. Chemotherapy is the mainstay of treatment in patients with lymphoma, especially those with widespread disease. Overall cure rates are high for many subtypes of lymphomas, even when patients present with advanced disease.

HODGKIN LYMPHOMA

Hodgkin lymphoma is a form of lymphoma, named after Thomas Hodgkin, who first described seven cases of a mysterious disease of the lymph system more than 150 years ago. Hodgkin lymphoma is fatal in more than 90% of the patients who are untreated for 2 to 3 years, and the cause is still unknown. The prognosis with treatment is generally good, but is not well predicted by stage alone. The International Prognostic Index (IPI) score was created to better predict an individual's risk of recurrence, which in turn influences treatment decisions. Patients with Hodgkin lymphoma can be categorized into four prognostic groups: early favorable disease, early unfavorable disease, advanced favorable disease, and advanced unfavorable disease. These groups are defined by patient age, gender, tumor size and spread (tumor stage), presence or absence of systemic symptoms, and laboratory test results. When appropriate therapy is given, more than 75% of all newly diagnosed Hodgkin lymphoma patients can be cured. However, the success of treatment has not been without cost. The treatment programs are intense, technically demanding, and associated with considerable acute toxicity and long-term complications. The long-term effects, particularly secondary malignancies, account for a higher cumulative mortality than Hodgkin lymphoma 15 to 20 years after treatment. Long-term toxicities with standard chemotherapy regimens have been more fully documented in recent years and are shaping future therapies.[1–3]

Epidemiology and Etiology

Hodgkin lymphoma represents less than 1% of all known cancers in the United States. It is estimated that 9,290 new cases of Hodgkin lymphoma will be diagnosed in the United States in 2013, and there will be 1,180 deaths associated with Hodgkin lymphoma during this same period.[4] This disease occurs slightly more frequently in males than in females. Once thought to be a disease of the young, it is now recognized that Hodgkin lymphoma exhibits bimodal distribution in industrialized countries. The first peak occurs in the third decade of life, with a small peak occurring after age 50.[1,3] The 5-year overall survival for all stages of Hodgkin lymphoma is about 85%.[5] Death rates as a consequence of recurrent Hodgkin lymphoma are less than those from other causes 15 years after treatment.[6]

The etiology of Hodgkin lymphoma is currently unknown, but laboratory and epidemiologic evidence support infectious exposure as a potential cause.[7,8] Studies suggest an increased risk of Hodgkin lymphoma in patients who have been infected with the Epstein-Barr's virus (EBV); and many patients experience EBV activation even before the onset of Hodgkin lymphoma. EBV is found in about 40% of all classical Hodgkin lymphoma cases, and it is frequently observed in cases of mixed cellularity and lymphocyte-depleted Hodgkin lymphoma.[9] Reed–Sternberg cells (large, bilobate, multinuclear cells), the malignant cells in Hodgkin lymphoma, are linked to EBV. Immunosuppressed individuals are also at much higher risk to develop Hodgkin lymphoma. Such individuals include patients with congenital immunosuppression, solid-organ transplantation recipients, and human immunodeficiency virus (HIV)-infected patients. Although the risk of developing Hodgkin lymphoma is about sevenfold greater in patients with HIV, the level of CD4 may vary depending on the subtype of Hodgkin lymphoma.[7]

Genetic factors are also associated with an increased risk of Hodgkin lymphoma. The strongest evidence suggesting that genes are important in the etiology of Hodgkin lymphoma comes from identical twin studies, which show that the unaffected identical twin has almost a 100-fold increase in risk.[10]

Pathophysiology

Hodgkin lymphoma is a clonal malignant lymphoid disease of transformed lymphocytes. The malignant cell in Hodgkin lymphoma is known as the *Reed–Sternberg* cell named after Drs. Dorothy Reed and Carl Sternberg, who were credited with the first definitive microscopic description of Hodgkin lymphoma.[1,11] Procedures to isolate and analyze Reed–Sternberg cells remain a challenge to scientists, due to the relatively small percentage (1% to 2%) of Reed–Sternberg cells that are found in the Hodgkin lymphoma mass.[9] Fortunately, new laboratory techniques have led to significant progress in identifying the origin of the Reed–Sternberg cell. Single-cell polymerase chain reaction and DNA microarray analyses indicate that nearly all classic Hodgkin lymphoma cases and all nodular lymphocyte-predominant Hodgkin lymphomas have immunoglobulin gene rearrangements, which indicates a germinal center or postgerminal center B-cell origin.[9,12] Interestingly, nearly all Reed–Sternberg cells fail to express B-cell specific cell surface proteins.

B-cell transcriptional processes are disrupted during malignant transformation, which prevents B-cell surface marker expression and production of immunoglobulin messenger ribonucleic acid. The normal cellular consequence of failure to express immunoglobulin is apoptosis, but because of alterations in the normal apoptotic pathways, cell survival and proliferation are favored. Reed–Sternberg cells overexpress nuclear factor-κB, which is associated with cell proliferation and antiapoptotic signals. Infections with viral and bacterial pathogens upregulate nuclear factor-κB and consequently are hypothesized to be involved with the etiology of Hodgkin lymphoma.[1,9,12] This hypothesis is supported by the presence of EBV in many Hodgkin lymphoma tumors, but it is important to note that not all tumors are associated with EBV. Another signaling pathway, Janus kinase–signal transduction and transcription (JAK–STAT), has also been found to be active in Hodgkin lymphoma.[1,9] As molecular techniques continue to improve, our understanding of the pathophysiology of Hodgkin lymphoma will also improve.

The histopathologic classification of Hodgkin lymphoma has undergone numerous changes over the past three decades. The current classification system is the 2008 World Health Organization (WHO) classification (see Table 109-1).[13] This classification divides Hodgkin lymphoma into two major groups: classical Hodgkin lymphoma and nodular lymphocyte-predominant Hodgkin lymphoma, which constitute about 95% and 5% of cases, respectively. Classic Hodgkin lymphoma is further divided into four subtypes: nodular sclerosis, mixed cellularity, lymphocyte-depletion, and lymphocyte-rich. The subtypes in these classifications are based on characteristics of the Reed–Sternberg cell, the surrounding cells, and the connective tissue. Nodular sclerosis has features that make it distinct from the other three subtypes, which represent a continuum of background cellularity, with lymphocyte-predominance being the most cellular and lymphocyte-depletion being the least cellular. Nodular lymphocyte-predominant Hodgkin lymphoma is separated because of its distinct immunophenotype: $CD15^-$, $CD20^+$, $CD30^-$, and $CD45^+$ (the opposite of classical Hodgkin lymphoma). With the introduction of extensive staging, sophisticated radiotherapy, and effective combination chemotherapy, the prognostic value of these subtypes is becoming less clear. The true value of understanding these subtypes is likely tied to the pathogenesis of the disease and its potential prevention in the future.

Clinical Presentation

❶ Most patients with Hodgkin lymphoma present with a painless, rubbery, enlarged lymph node in the supradiaphragmatic area and commonly have mediastinal nodal involvement.[14] Hodgkin lymphoma is occasionally diagnosed in an asymptomatic patient who has a mediastinal mass found with chest radiography or another imaging procedure. Asymptomatic adenopathy of the inguinal and axillary regions may be present at diagnosis but is less common (Fig. 109-1).[1,14] Patients can also present with constitutional

TABLE 109-1 **WHO Classification of the Mature B-Cell, T-Cell, and NK-Cell Neoplasms (2008)**

B Cell	T Cell	Hodgkin Lymphoma
Precursor B-cell neoplasm	Precursor T-cell neoplasm	Nodular lymphocyte-predominant Hodgkin lymphoma
Precursor B lymphoblastic leukemia/lymphoma (precursor B-cell acute lymphoblastic leukemia)	**Precursor T lymphoblastic lymphoma/leukemia (precursor T-cell acute lymphoblastic leukemia)**	Classical Hodgkin lymphoma
Mature (peripheral) B-cell neoplasm	Mature (peripheral) T-cell neoplasm	Nodular sclerosis classical Hodgkin lymphoma
B-cell chronic lymphocytic leukemia/small lymphocytic lymphoma	T-cell prolymphocytic leukemia	Lymphocyte-rich classical Hodgkin lymphoma
	T-cell granular lymphocytic leukemia	Mixed cellularity classical Hodgkin lymphoma
B-cell prolymphocytic leukemia	Aggressive NK cell leukemia	Lymphocyte-depleted classical Hodgkin lymphoma
Lymphoplasmacytic lymphoma	Adult T-cell leukemia/lymphoma (HTLV-I+)	
Splenic marginal zone B-cell lymphoma (± villous lymphocytes)	Extranodal NK / T-cell lymphoma, nasal type	
	Enteropathy-associated T-cell lymphoma	
Hairy cell leukemia	Hepatosplenic $\gamma\delta$ T-cell lymphoma	
Plasma cell myeloma/plasmacytoma	Subcutaneous panniculitis-like T-cell lymphoma	
Extranodal marginal zone B-cell lymphoma of MALT type	**Mycosis fungoides/Sézary syndrome**	
	Anaplastic large cell lymphoma, primary cutaneous type	
Mantle cell lymphoma		
Follicular lymphoma	**Peripheral T-cell lymphoma, not otherwise specified (NOS)**	
Nodal marginal zone B-cell lymphoma (± monocytoid B cells)		
	Angioimmunoblastic T-cell lymphoma	
Diffuse large B-cell lymphoma (DLBCL)	**Anaplastic large cell lymphoma, primary systemic type**	
Burkitt's lymphoma		

HTLV, human T-cell lymphotropic virus; MALT, mucosa-associated lymphoid tissue; NK, natural killer; WHO, World Health Organization.

Note: Not all subtypes are listed. **Malignancies in bold occur in at least 1% of patients.**

From Longo DL. Malignancies of lymphoid cells. In: Longo DL, Fauci AS, Kasper DL, et al. eds. Harrison's Principles of Internal Medicine. 18th ed. New York, NY: McGraw-Hill, 2012.

symptoms (B symptoms) before the discovery of lymph node enlargement, and these symptoms include fever, drenching night sweats, and weight loss. At diagnosis, these symptoms may appear in about 25% of all patients and up to 50% of patients with advanced disease. Patients may also experience other nonspecific symptoms including pruritus, fatigue, and development of pain after alcohol consumption at sites where nodes are involved.[3] Extranodal manifestations, such as bowel and hepatic involvements, are much less common in Hodgkin lymphoma than NHL.[1]

Diagnosis, Staging, and Prognostic Factors

Diagnostic and staging procedures are based on recommendations made at the Ann Arbor and Cotswolds conferences and new scientific advances, as described in the National Comprehensive Cancer Network (NCCN) guidelines.[15] The diagnosis and pathologic classification of Hodgkin lymphoma can only be made by review of a biopsy (preferably an excisional biopsy) of the enlarged node by an expert hematopathologist.

In addition to a careful physical examination and routine laboratory tests, chest radiography and computed tomography (CT) scans of the chest, abdomen, and pelvis are routinely performed. Furthermore, positron emission tomography (PET) plays an important role in the initial staging of Hodgkin lymphoma, as it has shown high sensitivity and specificity in the staging of the disease.[16] The use of integrated PET-CT has further improved the staging of Hodgkin lymphoma given that it can provide more sensitive and specific imaging as compared with each imaging alone. The NCCN guideline recommends either an integrated PET-CT scan (preferred) or a PET scan with diagnostic CT for initial staging.[15] Bone marrow biopsy is also recommended in patients with advanced-stage disease.

Staging can be based on clinical or pathologic findings. The clinical stage is based on all noninvasive procedures (history, physical examination, laboratory tests, and radiologic findings), whereas

CLINICAL PRESENTATION Hodgkin Lymphoma

General

- Most patients with Hodgkin lymphoma may have lymph node in the supradiaphragmatic and mediastinal areas.

Symptoms

- About 25% of all patients present with fever, night sweats, and weight loss (i.e., B symptoms), and up to 50% of patients with advanced disease.
- Fatigue, malaise, and pruritus.

Signs

- Enlarged lymph node, which may present as painless and rubbery.

Laboratory Tests

- A complete blood count, tests of renal and liver function, and serum electrolytes should be obtained.
- Lactate dehydrogenase levels may be useful as prognostic factors and for monitoring response to therapy.

Other Diagnostic Tests

- Varies depending on sites of involvement.

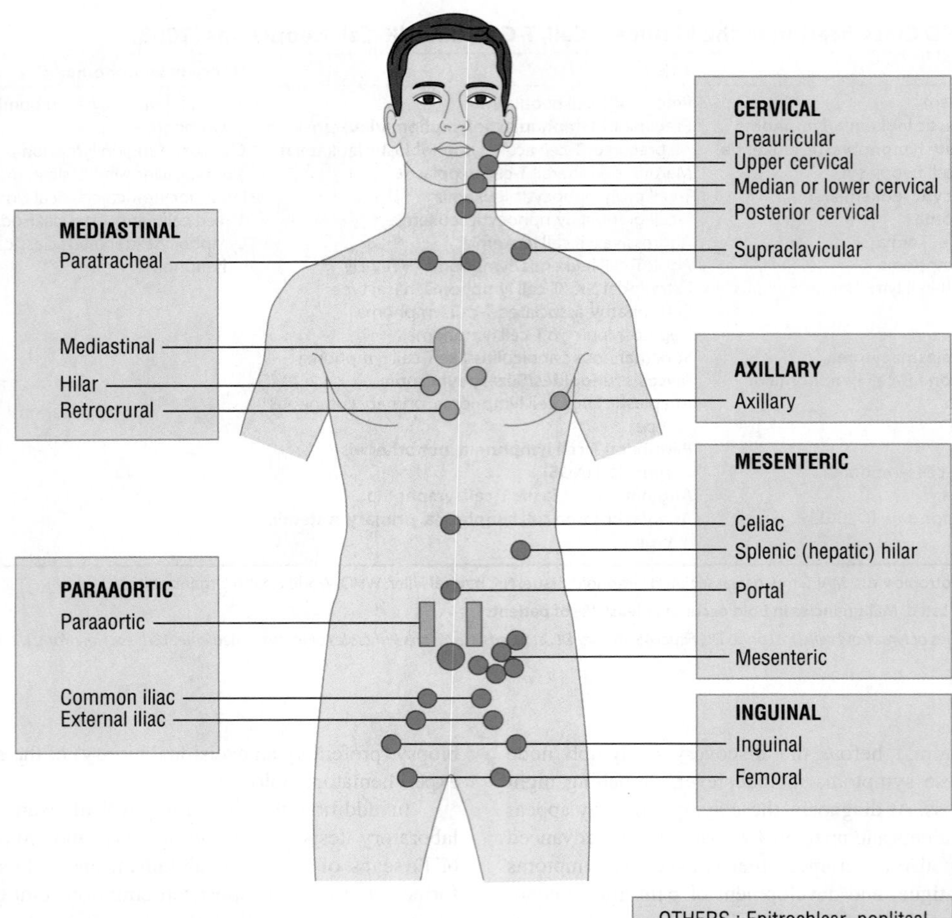

FIGURE 109-1 Areas of lymph nodes used in the staging of Hodgkin and non-Hodgkin lymphoma. Each rectangle corresponds to a nodal area.

the pathologic stage is based on the biopsy findings of strategic sites (muscle, bone, skin, spleen, and abdominal nodes) with an invasive procedure such as a laparoscopy or laparotomy. Patients with extranodal disease (muscle, skin, bone, or Waldeyer ring) contiguous to involved nodes are classified with the subscript "E" in the Cotswolds staging system.[15] As a result of improved imaging techniques, pathologic workup and staging that can be associated with toxicity is rarely performed.

The Ann Arbor staging classification, which was developed at the 1970 Ann Arbor conference, has proven to be a good workable scheme. At the Cotswolds meeting in 1989, the Ann Arbor classification was modified to account for new diagnostic techniques (e.g., CT and magnetic resonance imaging), and the understanding that prognosis is associated with the bulk of the disease and the number of involved nodal sites (see Table 109-2).[3] After careful staging, about one-half of patients have localized disease (stages I, II, and II_E) and the remainder have advanced disease (stage III or IV). About 10% to 15% present with metastatic disease (stage IV). It is important to note that Hodgkin lymphoma appears to follow a predictable pattern of nodal spread that is not seen with the NHLs.[14,15]

Patient prognosis is predominately driven by age and tumor stage. Patients older than ages 65 to 70 have a lower cure rate than younger patients. The difference in cure rates may be related to the frequent presence of comorbid diseases and decreased organ function in older patients, which impairs their ability to tolerate intensive chemotherapy.[17] Stage is the other dominant factor in predicting survival; patients with limited-stage disease (stages I to II) have a

TABLE 109-2 The Ann Arbor Staging Classification of Hodgkin Lymphoma

Stage I	Involvement of a single lymph node region or structure (I) or of a single extralymphatic organ or site (I_E)
Stage II	Involvement of two or more lymph node regions on the same side of the diaphragm (II) or localized involvement of an extralymphatic organ or site and of one or more lymph node regions on the same side of the diaphragm (II_E). The number of nodal regions involved should be indicated by a subscript (e.g., II_2)
Stage III	Involvement of lymph node regions on both sides of the diaphragm (III), which may also be accompanied by localized involvement of an extralymphatic organ or site (III_E) or by involvement of the spleen (IIIS) or both ($IIIS_E$). III_1: with or without splenic, hilar, celiac, or portal node involvement. III_2: with paraaortic, iliac, or mesenteric node involvement
Stage IV	Diffuse or disseminated involvement of one or more extralymphatic organs or tissues with or without associated lymph node enlargement A—No symptoms B—Fever, night sweats, weight loss (>10%) X—Bulky disease >One-third the width of the mediastinum >10 cm maximal dimension of nodal mass E—Involvement of extralymphatic tissue on one side of the diaphragm by limited direct extension from an adjacent, involved lymph node region S—Involvement of the spleen CS—Clinical stage PS—Pathologic stage

TABLE 109-3 The International Prognostic Factors Project Score for Advanced Hodgkin Lymphoma

Risk Factors		
Serum albumin (<4 g/dL [<40 g/L])		
Hemoglobin (<10.5 g/dL [<105 g/L; 6.52 mmol/L])		
Male gender		
Stage IV disease		
Age (≥45 years)		
White blood cell (WBC) count (≥15,000 cells/mm³ [≥15 × 10⁹/L])		
Lymphocytopenia (<600 cells/mm³ [<0.6 × 10⁹/L] or <8% of WBC count)		
Number of Factors	**Freedom from Progression**[a]	**Overall Survival**[a]
0	84 ± 4	89 ± 2
1	77 ± 3	90 ± 2
2	67 ± 2	81 ± 2
3	60 ± 3	78 ± 3
4	51 ± 4	61 ± 4
≥5	42 ± 5	56 ± 5

[a]Percentage of patients at 5 years.

Data from reference 18.

90% to 95% cure rate, while those with advanced disease (stages III to IV) have only a 60% to 80% cure rate.[3,15]

Seven adverse prognostic factors with similar impact on survival (each factor reduced survival by 7% to 8% per year) have been identified through an international collaborative effort. These factors can be combined to generate an International Prognostic Score (IPS) that can be used to predict progression-free and overall survival (see Table 109-3).[18]

TREATMENT
Hodgkin Lymphoma

Desired Outcomes

The current goal in the treatment of Hodgkin lymphoma is to maximize curability while minimizing short- and long-term treatment-related complications. According to the Surveillance, Epidemiology, and End Results (SEER) database, the 5-year age-adjusted relative survival is greater than 80%.[5] Therefore, the treatment goal of all stages of Hodgkin lymphoma should be cure.

General Approach to Treatment

Although multiple treatment modalities are used to treat Hodgkin lymphoma, surgery has a limited therapeutic role regardless of stage. It is, however, important for diagnosis (excisional biopsy), and on certain occasions, such as placement of a central line.

Combination chemotherapy is the primary treatment modality for most patients with Hodgkin lymphoma. In general, patients with early stage Hodgkin lymphoma are treated with combination chemotherapy and radiation, whereas patients with advanced-stage disease are treated with combination chemotherapy with or without radiation therapy. For patients with refractory or recurrent disease, salvage therapy consists of multiagent chemotherapy with or without high-dose chemotherapy and autologous hematopoietic stem cell transplantation (HSCT), which can be curative.[1,3,19]

Radiation is often an integral part of the treatment plan. Selected patients with early stage disease (usually nodular lymphocyte-predominant histology) can receive radiation as the only treatment modality, whereas most patients will receive chemotherapy and radiation. Although radiation is a local therapy, many patients with advanced disease will also receive radiation therapy to residual or bulky disease sites after chemotherapy. The major concern with radiation therapy is its long-term effects, such as cardiovascular disease and secondary malignancies, which commonly occur in the lung, breast, gastrointestinal tract, and connective tissue.[20] To avoid these toxicities, several studies have been completed and others are ongoing to determine the optimal extent (radiation field) and dose of radiation.[21,22] Radiation to a single field that contains Hodgkin lymphoma is called *involved-field radiation*; radiation to the involved field and a second uninvolved area is termed *extended-field radiation* or *subtotal nodal irradiation*; and radiation of all areas is called *total nodal irradiation*. When given with chemotherapy, involved-field radiation is usually used to avoid the increased toxicity associated with extended-field radiation.[21] The following sections review treatment of early stage favorable disease, early stage unfavorable disease, advanced-stage favorable disease, advanced-stage unfavorable disease, and salvage therapy.

Treatment of Early Stage Favorable Disease

Patients with early stage favorable disease have stage IA or IIA disease and no adverse risk factors (extranodal disease, bulky disease, three or more sites of nodal involvement, or an erythrocyte sedimentation rate of ≥50 mm/h [≥13.9 μm/s]). In the past, extended-field radiation was considered to be the treatment of choice for stages IA and IIA disease. Although most patients were cured of their disease, it is associated with long-term toxicities due to large radiation fields, such as heart disease, pulmonary dysfunction, and secondary malignancies.[3,20,23]

In an effort to avoid the long-term effects of extended-field radiation and improve treatment results, several studies have evaluated a combined modality approach that involves the use of short-duration chemotherapy and involved-field radiation. Based on favorable results of these studies, most patients with early stage favorable disease are no longer treated with radiation alone.

Clinical trials comparing radiation alone to radiation plus chemotherapy show lower relapse rates in patients treated with combined modality therapy (radiation and chemotherapy), but no change in overall survival because of the availability of effective salvage therapy.[22] Current trials focus on questions such as the optimal number of chemotherapy cycles, the volume of radiation that must be used to obtain optimal patient outcomes, and the role of PET scanning to individualize therapy. Emerging data also suggest that as few as two cycles of chemotherapy followed by involved-field radiation is sufficient in favorable, early stage disease patients. Different combination chemotherapy regimens have been used in these studies, and no one regimen is clearly superior to another.[21–23]

The current NCCN guidelines recommend that patients with early stage favorable disease be treated with two cycles of the Stanford V regimen (doxorubicin, vinblastine, mechlorethamine, etoposide, vincristine, bleomycin, and prednisone) or four cycles of the ABVD (doxorubicin [Adriamycin], bleomycin, vinblastine, and dacarbazine) regimen, followed by consolidative involved-field radiation.[24] With this approach, 5-year progression-free and overall survival rates of >90% can be achieved.

Investigators are now focusing on novel strategies to minimize the long-term toxicities of Hodgkin lymphoma treatment, particularly among those patients who have good treatment prognosis. One recently published study compared the efficacy of two versus four cycles of ABVD and involved-field radiation in early stage favorable disease Hodgkin lymphoma patients. It was shown that treatment with two cycles was as effective and less toxic than four cycles of chemotherapy followed radiation therapy at 5 years.[25] Such encouraging data would need to be confirmed with longer followup of the treatment.

Nodular lymphocyte-predominant Hodgkin lymphoma has been described as more indolent in nature, and better prognosis can be achieved when compared with classic Hodgkin lymphoma. The use of radiation alone for nodular lymphocyte-predominant Hodgkin lymphoma patients who choose to omit chemotherapy, or who cannot tolerate chemotherapy, does not appear to adversely affect survival.[15] The disadvantage of radiation therapy alone as compared with combination chemotherapy and radiation is the higher relapse rate. Patients who relapse after radiation alone (20% to 25%) can be successfully salvaged with chemotherapy. If the decision is made to use radiation alone, extended-field radiation appears to be superior to involved-field radiation.[26] It is shown that more extensive radiation reduces the risk of treatment failure at 10 years (31% vs. 43%), although it does not improve overall survival. However, the risk of long-term complications (such as secondary malignancies) is increased with the use of extended-field radiotherapy when compared with less extensive radiation fields.[20]

Treatment of Early Stage Unfavorable Disease

Patients with early stage disease who have certain features associated with a poor prognosis (B symptoms, extranodal disease, bulky disease, three or more sites of nodal involvement, or an erythrocyte sedimentation rate >50 mm/h [≥13.9 μm/s]) are defined as having unfavorable disease. Different groups or clinical trials have different definitions for unfavorable disease.[22] Current guidelines recommend combined modality therapy (combination chemotherapy and involved-field radiation) to reduce the relapse rate and avoid the toxicity associated with extended-field radiation.[15]

❷ Although randomized trials show that combined modality therapy reduces the relapse rate in patients with early stage unfavorable disease, questions concerning the appropriate radiation volume, most effective chemotherapy regimen, and number of chemotherapy cycles remain.[22] A number of studies have compared extended-field radiation to involved-field radiation. In one large trial conducted by the German Hodgkin Study Group (GHSG), patients with early stage unfavorable Hodgkin lymphoma treated with chemotherapy and involved-field radiation had similar freedom from treatment failure and overall survival as those treated with the same chemotherapy regimen and extended-field radiation.[27] Because toxicity was greater with extended-field radiation, the accepted standard is chemotherapy and involved-field radiation.

Different chemotherapy regimens and number of chemotherapy cycles were also compared in clinical trials. Mechlorethamine, vincristine, procarbazine, and prednisone (MOPP) was one of the first highly effective regimens introduced to treat Hodgkin lymphoma. MOPP or MOPP-like regimens were then given alternately or hybridized with a combination of ABVD. In advanced disease, ABVD was found to be less toxic than alternating MOPP/ABVD, and both were found to be superior to MOPP alone. Consequently, ABVD has now become the standard regimen used to treat patients with early stage unfavorable disease. It has established effectiveness in patients with advanced-stage disease and a favorable toxicity (both acute and chronic) profile.

Despite excellent results from treatment with ABVD and radiation, about 5% of patients do not respond to initial treatment and another 15% of patients will relapse following an initial response. Several studies have evaluated more aggressive regimens or more cycles of therapy. However, none of these regimens has proven to be more effective than ABVD, and each is associated with more toxicity. The current NCCN guideline lists the Stanford V regimen as an acceptable option, which also uses more drugs than the ABVD regimen.[15]

In summary, most patients with early stage disease will be treated with two to four cycles of ABVD chemotherapy and involved-field radiation. The number of cycles administered is based on the classification of favorable versus unfavorable disease. For patients who have unfavorable disease with bulky disease, ABVD followed by involved-field radiation. If patients attain complete remission after four cycles by restaging, they can be treated with involved-field radiation alone or two additional cycles of ABVD (total of six) followed by involved-field radiation. For patients who have unfavorable yet nonbulky disease, observation without involved-field radiation can be a treatment option after six cycles of ABVD.[15] Current trials are evaluating the use of PET scans as biomarkers to individualize therapy and minimize the amount of therapy necessary for cure.[16]

Treatment of Advanced-Stage Disease

Advanced-stage disease consists of stages III and IV disease. In some studies, stage IIB with a large mediastinal mass or extranodal disease is also considered advanced-stage disease (Table 109-2). By definition, patients with stages III and IV disease have tumors on both sides of the diaphragm, which almost always precludes the use of radiation alone as a therapeutic modality. Intensive combination chemotherapy is the mainstay of treatment, although some patients will benefit from radiation following chemotherapy. The prognosis of advanced-stage disease is excellent with 5-year overall survival rates ranging from less than 56% to 90%. Prognostic factors have been identified and standardized to provide a more accurate individual prognosis (Table 109-3).[18]

Patients with advanced-stage Hodgkin lymphoma can be classified into two groups based on the number of prognostic factors present from the IPI (Table 109-3). Advanced-stage patients with three or fewer poor prognostic factors are considered to have favorable disease and an about 60% likelihood of being failure-free at 5 years with traditional combination chemotherapy. Advanced-stage patients with four or more poor prognostic factors are considered to have unfavorable disease and a less than 50% likelihood of being failure-free at 5 years with traditional combination chemotherapy. Because of the high treatment failure rate, the therapeutic goal for this group of high-risk patients is to improve antitumor control.

Combination Chemotherapy

One of the initial combination chemotherapy regimens introduced in the early 1960s that was shown to cure advanced Hodgkin lymphoma was the MOPP regimen (Table 109-4). MOPP chemotherapy was a mainstay of treatment for patients with stages III and IV advanced Hodgkin lymphoma.

❸ The development of ABVD by Bonnadonna et al. at the Milan Cancer Institute about a decade later represents the next important step in the evolution of therapy for Hodgkin lymphoma (Table 109-4).[28] ABVD was initially shown to be effective in treating MOPP failures and was later compared directly to MOPP in advanced disease, where it produced an 82% complete response rate, as compared to a 67% complete response rate with MOPP. Improved failure-free survival was demonstrated with ABVD, but no significant differences in 5-year overall survival were noted.[29] Because ABVD was less toxic and provided similar or better outcomes than MOPP, it eventually replaced MOPP as the standard regimen for advanced-stage Hodgkin lymphoma.

In the early 1980s, the Goldie–Coldman hypothesis proposed that chemotherapy resistance was related to spontaneous mutation rates and the development of resistant clones. To test that hypothesis, researchers designed several clinical trials to evaluate the efficacy of alternating non–cross-resistant drug combinations in patients with Hodgkin lymphoma.[30] The initial approach adopted by investigators was to alternate or combine the MOPP and ABVD regimens. When MOPP and ABVD (or doxorubicin [Adriamycin], bleomycin, vinblastine [ABV]) are combined in a monthly cycle, it is referred to as a hybrid regimen. Besides a potential benefit in efficacy, another potential benefit of alternating or hybrid regimens is the decreased risk of long-term toxicities. In the alternating

TABLE 109-4 Combination Chemotherapy Regimens for Hodgkin Lymphoma

Drug	Dosage (mg/m²)	Route	Days
MOPP			
Mechlorethamine	6	IV	1, 8
Vincristine	1.4	IV	1, 8
Procarbazine	100	Oral	1–14
Prednisone	40	Oral	1–14
Repeat every 21 days			
ABVD			
Doxorubicin (Adriamycin®)	25	IV	1, 15
Bleomycin	10	IV	1, 15
Vinblastine	6	IV	1, 15
Dacarbazine	375	IV	1, 15
Repeat every 28 days			
MOPP/ABVD			
Alternating months of MOPP and ABVD			
MOPP/ABV hybrid			
Mechlorethamine	6	IV	1
Vincristine	1.4	IV	1
Procarbazine	100	Oral	1–7
Prednisone	40	Oral	1–14
Doxorubicin	35	IV	8
Bleomycin	10	IV	8
Vinblastine	6	IV	8
Repeat every 28 days			
Stanford V			
Doxorubicin	25	IV	Weeks 1, 3, 5, 7, 9, 11
Vinblastine	6	IV	Weeks 1, 3, 5, 7, 9, 11
Mechlorethamine	6	IV	Weeks 1, 5, 9
Etoposide	60	IV	Weeks 3, 7, 11
Vincristine	1.4[a]	IV	Weeks 2, 4, 6, 8, 10, 12
Bleomycin	5	IV	Weeks 2, 4, 6, 8
Prednisone	40	Oral	Every other day for 12 weeks; begin tapering at week 10
One course (12 weeks)			
BEACOPP (standard-dose)			
Bleomycin	10	IV	8
Etoposide	100	IV	1–3
Adriamycin (doxorubicin)	25	IV	1
Cyclophosphamide	650	IV	1
Oncovin® (vincristine)	1.4[a]	IV	8
Procarbazine	100	Oral	1–7
Prednisone	40	Oral	1–14
Repeat every 21 days			
BEACOPP (escalated-dose)			
Bleomycin	10	IV	8
Etoposide	200	IV	1–3
Adriamycin (doxorubicin)	35	IV	1
Cyclophosphamide	1250	IV	1
Oncovin® (vincristine)	1.4[a]	IV	8
Procarbazine	100	Oral	1–7
Prednisone	40	Oral	1–14
Granulocyte colony-stimulating factor		Subcutaneously	8+
Repeat every 21 days			

[a]Vincristine dose capped at 2 mg.

MOPP/ABVD regimen, the cumulative doses of procarbazine and mechlorethamine are reduced by 50%, and the cumulative doxorubicin dose is reduced by 50%. In the hybrid regimen, the cumulative doxorubicin dose is reduced by 33%, and the cumulative bleomycin dose is reduced by 50%.

Several clinical trials have been performed to evaluate the efficacy of alternating or hybrid MOPP/ABVD regimens. The results of these trials show that alternating and hybrid regimens are superior to MOPP but not to ABVD.[30] Another approach evaluated by researchers was the administration of sequential cycles of MOPP and ABVD (MOPP → ABVD). Results of an intergroup trial showed sequential MOPP and ABVD to be inferior to the MOPP/ABV hybrid regimen in terms of response and survival.[31] In another randomized comparison trial of the MOPP/ABV hybrid regimen and ABVD, the complete remission rate, failure-free survival, and overall survival were similar between the two regimens.[32] The latter trial was closed prematurely because of an increased number of treatment-related deaths and secondary malignancies in the patients who received the MOPP/ABV hybrid regimen.

More aggressive regimens such as Stanford V and bleomycin, etoposide, doxorubicin (Adriamycin), cyclophosphamide, vincristine (Oncovin), procarbazine, and prednisone (BEACOPP) have been evaluated as alternatives to MOPP or ABVD.[19] The Stanford V regimen generated considerable interest because of the results of phase II trials.[23,33] Stanford V, ABVD, and a MOPP/ABV hybrid-like regimen (mechlorethamine, vincristine, procarbazine, prednisone, epidoxorubicin, bleomycin, vinblastine, lomustine, doxorubicin, and vindesine [MOPPEBVCAD]) were compared in a randomized trial to determine the best regimen to support a reduced radiotherapy program.[34] Five-year failure-free and progression-free survival were significantly worse for the Stanford V regimen as compared to the other two regimens. However, no significant differences in projected

5-year progression-free and overall survival were observed between Stanford V and ABVD in a recently published randomized trial of patients with advanced Hodgkin lymphoma.[35] The investigators speculated that differences in the application of radiotherapy may explain the divergent results in the two randomized trials. More pulmonary toxicity occurred in the ABVD group, but other toxicities occurred more frequently in the Stanford V group.

The GHSG developed the BEACOPP regimens based on principles of dose density, dose intensity, and mathematical modeling. BEACOPP uses similar drugs as in the cyclophosphamide, vincristine, procarbazine, and prednisone (COPP)/ABVD regimen, but rearranges the drugs in a shorter 3-week cycle. Several different versions of BEACOPP have been developed: standard-dose BEACOPP, escalated-dose BEACOPP, and dose-dense BEACOPP (BEACOPP-14).[36] Granulocyte colony-stimulating factor support is required for the escalated-dose BEACOPP and BEACOPP-14 regimens.

Several randomized trials have compared BEACOPP to other regimens.[3,19] The GHSG conducted a randomized comparison of eight cycles of COPP/ABVD (alternating), BEACOPP, or an escalated-dose BEACOPP regimen in 1,201 patients with advanced Hodgkin lymphoma.[37] Most patients had advanced favorable disease, and all patients received radiation to sites of bulky or residual disease after chemotherapy. Escalated-dose BEACOPP appears to be the most active regimen in this study with 10-year freedom from treatment failure at 82% and overall survival at 86%, but this regimen also appeared to be more toxic.[38] Despite filgrastim support, 90% of patients in the escalated-dose BEACOPP group had grade IV leukopenia, as compared with 19% in patients in the COPP/ABVD arm and 37% in the standard-dose BEACOPP arm. The higher rate of acute toxicity did not translate into a higher risk of treatment-related fatalities (<2% for all three regimens). The risk of toxic deaths due to sepsis or acute cardiac events was higher in elderly patients receiving BEACOPP.[39] Furthermore, the higher rate of leukemia in patients receiving escalated-dose BEACOPP (2.5% at 5 years followup, and 3% at 10 years followup) as compared with those in the COPP/ABVD arm (0.4%) are of concern. In another study, 370 patients with advanced Hodgkin lymphoma were randomized to receive six cycles of ABVD, six cycles of CEC (cyclophosphamide, lomustine, vindesine, melphalan, prednisone, epirubicin, vincristine, procarbazine, vinblastine, bleomycin), or four cycles of escalated-dose BEACOPP with two cycles of standard-dose BEACOPP.[40] BEACOPP was superior to ABVD for 5-year failure-free survival (78% vs. 65%, $P = 0.036$) and progression-free survival (81% vs. 68%, $P = 0.038$), but 5-year overall survival was not significantly different between ABVD and BEACOPP. It appears that BEACOPP may be superior to ABVD in patients with high-risk advanced Hodgkin lymphoma (IPS ≥3). Higher rates of neutropenia and severe infections were observed with BEACOPP as compared with ABVD.

Finally, GHSG has conducted several trials to evaluate the optimal number and intensity of BEACOPP. In the HD12 study, eight cycles of escalated-dose BEACOPP were compared to four cycles of escalated-dose and four cycles of standard-dose BEACOPP (4 + 4 BEACOPP regimen) with or without radiation therapy. Freedom-from-treatment failure, progression-free survival, and overall survival were not different between the two treatment arms.[41] Although the 4 + 4 BEACOPP regimen resulted in less acute hematologic toxicities during cycles five to six, this difference did not translate into a lower risk of treatment-related mortality. In the recently published HD15 noninferiority trial, eight cycles of escalated-dose BEACOPP was compared with six cycles of escalated-dose BEACOPP and eight cycles of BEACOPP-14.[42] Freedom-from-treatment failure and overall survival were significantly better in the patients treated with six cycles of escalated-dose BEACOPP as compared with those treated with eight cycles of escalated-dose BEACOPP. No significant differences were observed between the eight cycles of escalated-dose BEACOPP versus BEACOPP-14. The risk of treatment-related mortality and secondary malignancies was also lower in patients treated with six cycles of escalated-dose BEACOPP. Of interest was the use of PET-guided radiotherapy in all of the treatment arms.

Clinical **Controversy. . .**

Some clinicians believe that escalated-dose BEACOPP is superior to ABVD in the treatment of patients with advanced-stage Hodgkin lymphoma. Escalated-dose BEACOPP has been shown to be superior to COPP/ABVD, which is similar to MOPP/ABVD. Other experts believe that ABVD is still the treatment of choice because escalated-dose BEACOPP has not been tested directly against it. They also express concern over the long-term toxicity with escalated-dose BEACOPP.

The results of these studies suggest that escalated-dose BEACOPP is superior to ABVD in the treatment of advanced Hodgkin lymphoma, but at the cost of more treatment-related toxicity. Some experts recommend that these more intensive regimens should only be considered in patients with high-risk disease because of the potentially higher risk of secondary malignancies. The NCCN guideline suggests that patients attaining a complete remission after four cycles of escalated-dose BEACOPP can be followed up with standard-dose BEACOPP and radiation therapy.[15]

Risk-Adapted Therapy

Patients with advanced-stage Hodgkin lymphoma can be classified into two groups based on the IPS (Table 109-3). Advanced-stage patients with three or fewer poor prognostic factors are considered to have favorable disease and an about 60% likelihood of being failure-free at 5 years with traditional combination chemotherapy.[18] Advanced-stage patients with four or more poor prognostic factors are considered to have unfavorable disease and a less than 50% likelihood of being failure-free at 5 years with traditional combination chemotherapy. Because of the high treatment failure rate, the therapeutic goal for high-risk patients is to improve antitumor control.

One recently published study has reported the feasibility of a risk-adapted treatment approach based on the IPS, with the goal of reducing cumulative doses of chemotherapy in patients with low-risk Hodgkin lymphoma.[43] Low-risk patients with early unfavorable disease and standard-risk patients with IPS of <3 were treated with two cycles of standard-dose BEACOPP, and high-risk patients with an IPS ≥3 were treated with two cycles of escalated-dose BEACOPP. After an interim gallium or PET/CT scan, patients with positive disease were given escalated-dose BEACOPP, while patients who had negative disease were given standard-dose BEACOPP. For all patients, the complete remission rate, 5-year event-free survival, and overall survival were 97%, 85%, and 90%, respectively. Although this was not a randomized study, the results support the use of a risk-adapted treatment modality in the treatment of advanced-stage Hodgkin lymphoma.

In summary, the NCCN guidelines suggest that ABVD or Stanford V should be considered for primary treatment for patients with advanced disease. Escalated-dose BEACOPP should be considered for patients with unfavorable disease because of increased efficacy. It is recommended that patients in advanced-stage disease with an IPS <4 should be treated with ABVD because of less acute toxicity, the absence of sterility, and a low risk of secondary acute myeloid leukemia/myelodysplastic syndrome.[15]

Radiation

The role of low-dose consolidative radiation when added to chemotherapy for the treatment of advanced-stage Hodgkin lymphoma is controversial.[19,23] The rationale for its use is based on the radiosensitivity of Hodgkin lymphoma, a 20% to 40% relapse rate, and the tendency of Hodgkin lymphoma to relapse at sites of initial involvement.[44] Many clinical trials have been conducted to evaluate the benefit of additional radiation in patients who have a complete response to combination chemotherapy. The results of these studies are inconsistent, and a meta-analysis of 14 randomized trials showed a modest improvement in disease control at 10 years, but no difference in overall survival.[45] In one study, patients with advanced disease were randomized to receive either involved-field radiation after MOPP/ABV hybrid chemotherapy or no further therapy. Eight-year event-free survival reported for patients achieving a complete response randomized to receive radiation, no radiation, and a group of partial responders who received radiation were 73%, 77% and 76%, respectively. These results suggest that radiation provides no benefit for patients who achieve a complete remission with chemotherapy. Furthermore, radiation was also associated with a higher risk of secondary cancers (12.9% vs. 5.6% in the radiation and no radiation arms, respectively). It does, however, show a significant role for consolidative radiation in patients who have a partial response after chemotherapy.[46]

Summary

In summary, the standard treatment of advanced-stage favorable Hodgkin lymphoma is six to eight cycles of ABVD chemotherapy. Escalated-dose BEACOPP should be considered for patients with unfavorable disease. This risk-adapted approach should result in 70% to >90% of patients achieving a complete remission and 60% to 80% of patients being cured of their disease. No further treatment is needed for patients attaining a complete remission. Patients achieving a partial remission should receive consolidative radiation to residual sites of disease.

Treatment of Refractory or Relapsed Disease

4 The goal of salvage therapy is cure regardless of the site(s) of recurrence or primary therapy. With the increasing use of chemotherapy with or without radiation, regardless of disease extent, the rate of primary refractory disease is decreasing. Patients who do not achieve a complete remission with the initial regimen are considered to have primary refractory disease. These patients have a poor prognosis when treated with salvage chemotherapy, and therefore should be offered autologous HSCT as a treatment option.[47,48]

Patients who relapse after an initial complete response can be treated with the same regimen, a different potentially non–cross-resistant regimen, radiation, or high-dose chemotherapy and autologous HSCT (often preceded by conventional-dose chemotherapy). There are no data available from randomized trials comparing the cytoreductive regimens that are used before transplantation. However, as most patients are now treated with ABVD, doxorubicin should be avoided in salvage chemotherapy regimens if the cumulative dose has reached >400 mg/m^2, particularly in those patients who have received mediastinal radiotherapy because they are at much higher risk of cardiotoxicity.

The response to salvage therapy depends on the extent and site of recurrence, previous therapy, and duration of initial remission. Patients who relapse after radiation therapy alone have a good chance of being cured with combination chemotherapy, although fewer patients are being treated with radiation alone. High response rates (60% to 87%) have been observed with salvage chemotherapy regimens.[49] Other patient groups who have a favorable prognosis following salvage therapy include patients who experience a local recurrence in a nonirradiated location and those who relapse more than 1 year after completion of their initial chemotherapy. Patients who experience late relapses can be cured with retreatment with the same chemotherapy regimen, treatment with a different, potentially non–cross-resistant regimen, or high-dose chemotherapy and autologous HSCT.

Patients who have an early relapse (<1 year after treatment) generally respond poorly to standard-dose salvage chemotherapy. High-dose chemotherapy and autologous HSCT is more effective, but also produces a higher risk of treatment-related mortality. Therefore, the choice of salvage treatment should consider the patient's tolerance for a particular set of chemotherapeutic agents and treatment approach (standard-dose chemotherapy vs. high-dose chemotherapy and autologous HSCT).[47]

High-dose therapy should be considered in patients who relapse within 12 months of initial remission and in those who are refractory to first-line chemotherapy.[47] Although no single preparative regimen has been shown to be superior to another, most regimens do not include total-body irradiation because of its potential pulmonary toxicity. Most patients are already at higher risk for pulmonary toxicity because of previous exposure to one or more of the following: bleomycin, thoracic radiation, and nitrosoureas. Long-term effects of high-dose chemotherapy and autologous HSCT were elucidated in a recent study. Among 218 Hodgkin lymphoma patients who were treated with high-dose chemotherapy and autologous HSCT, 70% survived over 2 years. A total of 15 patients were diagnosed with a second malignancy and the median time from autologous HSCT to secondary malignancy diagnosis was 9 years. The risk of secondary malignancy is possibly caused by high-dose etoposide in the rescue regimen, as well as those patients who were initially treated with MOPP chemotherapy.[50]

Brentuximab vedotin is an antibody-drug conjugate (ADC) comprising an anti-CD30 antibody conjugated by a protease cleavable linker to a potent antimicrotubule agent, monomethyl auristatin E (MMAE). After binding of the ADC to CD30 on the cell surface, the ADC-CD30 complex is internalized. This leads to the release of MMAE via proteolytic cleavage in the lysosomal compartment. Tubulin binding by MMAE disrupts the microtubule network, which can lead to apoptotic death of the cancer cells.[51] In a pivotal multicenter phase II study of 102 patients with relapsed or refractory Hodgkin lymphoma after HSCT, objective responses and complete remissions was observed in 75% and 34% patients, after a median followup of 9 months. Common toxicities associated with brentuximab vedotin include neuropathy, neutropenia, nausea, and fatigue.[52] Based on these results, the FDA recently approved brentuximab vedotin (Adcetris®) for the treatment of patients with Hodgkin lymphoma after failure of HSCT or in patients who have failed at least two prior chemotherapy regimens and are not candidates for HSCT.

Long-Term Complications

A variety of acute and chronic toxicities may occur as a result of treatment for Hodgkin lymphoma. Long-term complications of radiation therapy, chemotherapy, and combined modality therapy have become more evident as the curability and long-term survival of Hodgkin lymphoma patients has improved.[1–3,20] Gonadal dysfunction (including sterility and hypothyroidism), secondary malignancies, and cardiopulmonary diseases have become important considerations in the treatment of this malignancy. Almost all men and up to 50% of premenopausal women treated with six cycles of regimens containing alkylating agents become sterile. This appears to be a dose-related phenomenon. For men, even a single dose of nitrogen mustard or chlorambucil can cause sterility, so if fertility is a major concern, ABVD may be the best alternative.[50]

The risk of secondary malignancies is increased about threefold in long-term survivors of Hodgkin lymphoma. The risk of developing leukemia carries the highest increase in risk and is seen with radiotherapy, chemotherapy, and chemoradiotherapy. Solid tumors, including breast cancers, gastrointestinal cancers, and lung cancers are also likely to develop more than 10 years after the completion of treatment.[53–55] A recently published British cohort study suggested that unlike radiotherapy, which may increase the occurrence of cancer at almost all anatomic sites, chemotherapy is associated with an increased risk of leukemia, NHL, and lung cancer.[55] However, studies that evaluate the risk of secondary malignancies (and other complications) must be interpreted cautiously because many factors probably contribute to the development of secondary malignancies.[56] In addition, much of the long-term complication data are derived from patients who were treated with older regimens and extensive field radiotherapy, which are no longer commonly used in clinical practice. Furthermore, as minimal data are currently available on the appropriate followup duration and procedures to monitor for long-term effects, many of the recommendations in the NCCN guideline are based on clinical practice. Monitoring and followup should be personalized and patient-specific, after assessing a patient's risks for long-term complications.[15]

NON-HODGKIN LYMPHOMA

The NHLs are a heterogeneous group of lymphoproliferative disorders that affect individuals from early childhood to late adulthood. Advances in molecular biology techniques and our understanding of the human immune system have led to major progress in understanding the pathogenesis and treatment of the lymphomas. NHLs are classified into distinct clinical entities that are defined by a combination of morphology, immunophenotype, genetic features, and clinical features. These differences influence the natural history, and approach and response to treatment. The use of extensive combination chemotherapeutic regimens shows dramatic improvement in survival and cure in patients with a disease that was once considered incurable. The 5-year survival rate for patients with NHL has increased from 48% to 71% over the past 25 years, and the mortality rate actually *declined* from 1997 to 2004.[4,5] Further improvement in survival is anticipated with the continued expansion of our therapeutic armamentarium, including high-dose chemotherapy and biologic therapy.

Epidemiology and Etiology

NHL is the fifth most common cause of newly diagnosed cancer in the United States and accounts for about 4% of all cancers. An estimated 69,740 new cases will be diagnosed in 2013, and it is estimated that 19,020 people will die from NHL during this same period.[4] Although the average age of patients at the time of diagnosis is about 67 years, NHL can occur at any age. The incidence rate generally increases with age, and is higher in men than in women and in whites than in blacks.[5] The age-adjusted incidence rate of NHL increased by more than 80% in the United States since the early 1970s, from about 11 cases per 100,000 in 1975 to about 20 cases per 100,000 in 2003 and 2004.[5] The incidence of NHL increased by 3% to 4% from 1975 to 1991, but appears to have stabilized since reaching its peak in 1994. The increased incidence of NHL over the past three decades is second only to melanoma and has been referred to as an epidemic of NHL. Although the increase has been noted particularly among the elderly and patients with acquired immune deficiency syndrome (AIDS), much of it cannot be explained by known risk factors.

The etiology of NHL is unknown, although several genetic diseases, environmental agents, and infectious agents are associated with the development of NHL.[7,57] An increased incidence of NHL is seen in many congenital and acquired immunodeficiency states, supporting the role of immune dysregulation in the etiology of NHL.[57] Patients with congenital immunodeficiency disorders such as Wiskott-Aldrich's syndrome and ataxia telangiectasia, acquired immunodeficiency disorders such as AIDS, and those receiving chronic pharmacologic immunosuppression in the setting of solid-organ transplantation are predisposed to the development of NHL. Autoimmune diseases (Hashimoto's thyroiditis, Sjögren's syndrome) cause chronic inflammation in the mucosa-associated lymphoid tissue (MALT), which predisposes patients to subsequent lymphoid malignancies. Other autoimmune diseases, such as systemic lupus erythematosus and rheumatoid arthritis, are also associated with the development of NHL, but the use of immunosuppressive agents in these diseases makes the pathologic cause less clear.

Certain infections are associated with the development of lymphoma.[7] EBV was discovered in cell lines from tumors of patients with African (endemic) Burkitt lymphoma, and EBV DNA is associated with nearly all cases of endemic Burkitt lymphoma. However, EBV is associated with sporadic Burkitt lymphoma in 15% to 85% of cases. EBV is also associated with posttransplant lymphoproliferative disorders and some lymphomas in patients with AIDS or congenital immunodeficiencies. The human T-cell lymphotropic virus type 1 was the first human retrovirus associated with a malignancy. Infection with human T-cell lymphotropic virus type 1, especially in early childhood, is strongly associated with an aggressive form of T-cell lymphoma, known as adult T-cell leukemia/lymphoma. Human T-cell lymphotropic virus type 1 is endemic in parts of southern Japan, Africa, South America, and the Caribbean. In endemic areas, more than 50% of all NHL cases are adult T-cell leukemia/lymphoma. A third virus associated with NHL is human herpes virus 8 (also referred as Kaposi sarcoma–associated herpesvirus [KSHV]). This virus was originally isolated from Kaposi sarcoma lesions in AIDS patients. Gastric infection with *Helicobacter pylori*, a gram-negative bacteria that leads to chronic gastritis, is associated with gastric MALT lymphomas. Finally, hepatitis C virus has been associated with splenic and nodal marginal zone lymphomas.

A number of physical agents are also associated with the development of NHL.[57] Exposure to herbicides, particularly phenoxyl herbicides, is associated with the development of NHL. These observations may explain why certain occupations, such as farmers, forestry workers, and agricultural workers, are associated with a higher risk of NHL. Exposure to lawn-care pesticides is also increasing in the general population. A higher risk of NHL is also associated with exposure to other chemical solvents and dyes, exposure to radiation from nuclear explosions, and high intake of meats and dietary fats. Smoking or alcohol consumption is not strongly associated with an increased risk of NHL.

Molecular Abnormalities

Chromosomal translocations have become a hallmark of many lymphoid malignancies.[58,59] The presence of these specific translocations can be helpful in the diagnosis and classification of lymphoid malignancies. The mechanisms leading to the translocations are unknown, but they usually involve the antigen receptor loci. In contrast to most myeloid and some lymphoid leukemias, NHLs usually place a structurally intact cellular protooncogene under the regulatory influence of highly expressed immunoglobulin or T-cell receptor genes, leading to effects on cell growth, cellular differentiation, or apoptosis. The most common chromosomal translocations involve t(8;14), t(14;18), and t(11;14); each translocation involves the immunoglobulin heavy-chain gene locus on chromosome 14 at 14q32. The translocation t(8;14) that involves c-*MYC*, a well-characterized oncogene clearly associated with malignancy, is implicated in nearly all cases of Burkitt lymphoma. The translocation t(14;18) that involves *BCL*-2, one of several putative B-cell lymphoma–associated oncogenes, is found in about 90% of cases of follicular B-cell lymphomas. The translocation t(11;14) that involves *BCL*-1 is found in about 70% of patients with mantle cell lymphoma. Another putative B-cell lymphoma–associated oncogene, *BCL*-6, is found in about one-third of diffuse large B-cell lymphomas.

Although mutations in the *p53* tumor suppressor gene have been recognized in many human neoplasms, such mutations have not been consistently found in patients with lymphoma, which suggests that it may occur late in malignant evolution.

Because of their role in the pathogenesis of lymphoma, oncogenes are attractive molecular targets for the development of new and novel therapies.[60]

Pathology and Classification

NHLs are neoplasms derived from the monoclonal proliferation of malignant B or T lymphocytes and their precursors. About 85% to 90% of NHLs in the United States are of B-cell origin.[57] Proliferation of malignant cells results in the replacement of the normal cells and architecture of lymph nodes or bone marrow with a relatively uniform population of lymphoid cells. The classification of NHLs has evolved over the past five decades, as advances in immunology and genetics have allowed scientists to recognize a number of previously unrecognized subtypes of NHLs (Table 109-5).[61,62] The current classification schemes characterize the NHLs according to the cell of origin (B cell vs. T cell), clinical features, and morphologic features. Additional immunohistochemical markers, cytogenetic features, and genotypic characteristics may help to further classify NHL into subtypes.

Morphology

The macroscopic and microscopic appearance of the involved tissue remains one of the most important factors in the diagnosis and classification of NHLs.[61,62] In the 1950s, Rappaport et al. proposed a morphologic classification of malignant lymphomas based on two features: that the malignant cell would disrupt the nodal architecture in a *nodular* or *diffuse* manner, and that lymphomas of histiocytic origin existed. The Rappaport classification gained rapid acceptance in the United States because of its precision, simplicity, and prognostic significance. Application of the system divided NHLs into those with large (i.e., incorrectly called "histiocytes") or small cells, with or without a nodular (i.e., follicular) growth pattern.

Immunology

In the 1970s, it became apparent that NHLs were tumors of the immune system and were derived from B or T lymphocytes. With the availability of techniques using antibodies to antigens on the surface of lymphoid cells (i.e., immunophenotype) and cytochemical assays, expert pathologists independently developed new classification schemes for NHL in the 1970s and 1980s.[61,62] The Kiel classification was based primarily on the work of Lennert in Germany and became widely used in Europe. In North America, the Lukes and Collins classification scheme was used briefly, but was soon superseded by the Working Formulation. Like the Rappaport classification, divisions within the Working Formulation were based largely on cell size (large [histiocytic] vs. small [lymphocytic]), cell shape (round vs. not round), and growth pattern (follicular [nodular] vs. diffuse). Both the Kiel and Working Formulation classification schemes considered the histologic grade of the tumor, but only the Working Formulation considered actual survival curves of patients with the various subtypes of NHL. *Low-grade* indicated longer median survival (i.e., indolent) whereas *intermediate-grade* and *high-grade* indicated shorter median survival (i.e., aggressive). In the 1980s and early 1990s, the Working Formulation became the most widely used classification scheme in North America. It was based on the premise that NHL was a single disease with a range of histologic grades and clinical aggressiveness.

New Disease Entities

In the 1980s and early 1990s, rapid advances in immunology and genetics allowed scientists to recognize a number of previously unrecognized subtypes of NHLs. Cytogenetic and molecular genetic analyses identified the presence of many chromosomal translocations, oncogenes, and their gene products in patients with NHL (see Molecular Abnormalities later in this chapter). In addition, diseases that would have been lumped together as low-grade or intermediate/high grade in the Working Formulation showed marked differences in survival, which prompted scientists to reevaluate lymphoma classification schemes.

Information from these studies allowed scientists to further classify B-cell lymphomas as malignant expansions of cells from the germinal center, mantle zone, or marginal zone of normal lymph nodes.[61,63] Germinal centers are complex structures that form in the spleen and lymph nodes in response to antigenic challenge. In addition to B cells, germinal centers contain antigen-presenting cells and helper T cells that cooperate in mediating the B-cell changes that result in a more potent secondary immune response. Malignant transformation often occurs or is initiated in germinal center B cells. Follicular, Burkitt, and most large cell lymphomas are believed to be tumors of germinal center B cells. Three histologically distinct microenvironments have been described within the germinal center: a mantle zone surrounding interior, dark, and light zones. The mantle zone contains small resting B cells that have not been exposed to antigens (naïve). Tumors of cells from the mantle zone are usually clinically indolent and histologically low grade. Antigen-triggered activation of the densely packed B cells of the dark zone causes cells to proliferate and subjects genomic DNA to somatic hypermutation. Surviving clones from within the dark zone then enter the light zone where proliferation slows and affinity selection occurs. During affinity selection, only cells with surface immunoglobulin receptors with high affinity for the antigen survive. Antigen-specific B cells generated in the germinal center reaction leave the follicle and reappear in the outer mantle zone, to form a marginal zone. Marginal zones are particularly prominent in mesenteric lymph nodes, Peyer's patches, and the spleen. These postgerminal center B cells include memory B cells of the marginal zone and plasma cells. Marginal cell B-cell lymphomas tend to be indolent and may be either extranodal or nodal; extranodal marginal cell B-cell lymphomas are also referred to as MALT lymphomas.

T-cell lymphomas can be classified on the basis of antigen expression as either precursor (thymic) or mature (peripheral) in origin. These classifications clinically translate to precursor lymphoblastic lymphomas or to a heterogeneous group of peripheral

TABLE 109-5 Evolution in the Classification of Non-Hodgkin Lymphomas

Time	Classification System	Basis for Classification
1950s–1960s	Rappaport	Morphology
1970s–1980s	Luke–Collins	Morphology and immunophenotype
1970s–1980s	Kiel	Morphology and immunophenotype
1980s–1990s	International Working Formulation	Morphology and clinical behavior
1990s	REAL	Disease entities
2001	WHO	Disease entities

REAL, Revised European–American Classification of Lymphoid Neoplasms developed by the International Lymphoma Study Group; WHO, World Health Organization.

T-cell lymphomas. Tumors of natural killer or natural killer-like T cells are uncommon.

The International Lymphoma Study Group, an informal group of 19 hematopathologists from the United States, Europe, and Asia, adopted a new approach to lymphoma classification in 1993. Because it represented a revision of current or prior European and American lymphoma classifications, it was called the Revised European-American Classification of Lymphoid Neoplasms (REAL). The REAL classification system is based on the principle that a classification is a list of "real" disease entities, which are defined by a combination of morphology, immunophenotype, genetic features, and clinical features.[61,62] The relative importance of each of these criteria for both definition and diagnosis differs among different diseases. Morphology is always important, and some diseases are primarily defined by morphology alone (e.g., follicular lymphoma), although immunophenotype can be helpful in difficult cases. Some diseases have a specific immunophenotype (e.g., mantle cell lymphoma, small lymphocytic lymphoma) that is virtually diagnostic of that disease. A specific genetic abnormality is important in some lymphomas—t(11;14) in mantle cell lymphoma, t(8;14) in Burkitt lymphoma, and t(14;18) in follicular lymphoma—whereas other lymphomas lack specific genetic abnormalities (e.g., MALT lymphoma, diffuse large B-cell lymphoma). Finally, other lymphomas consider clinical features (e.g., extranodal vs. nodal presentation in marginal zone lymphoma and peripheral T-cell lymphoma).

Since 1995, members of the European and American Hematopathology societies have worked to develop a new WHO classification of hematologic malignancies. The final classification was published in 2001 and revised in 2008.[13,61,62] The WHO classification uses an updated version of the REAL classification and expands the principles of the REAL classification to the classification of myeloid and lymphoid malignancies.

5 The 2008 WHO classification categorizes lymphoid malignancies into two major categories: B-cell lymphomas and T-cell (and natural killer cell) lymphomas (Table 109-1).[13,61,62] B-cell lymphomas represent about 85% to 90% of all NHLs. Lymphomas within each category can be divided into malignancies of precursor or mature cells. Hodgkin lymphoma and multiple myeloma are now recognized as mature B-cell neoplasms. The WHO classification uses the term *grade* to refer to histologic parameters such as cell and nuclear size, density of chromatin, and proliferation fraction, and the term *aggressiveness* to denote clinical behavior of a tumor. This classification scheme includes both lymphomas and lymphoid leukemias because there is no distinction between the solid and circulating forms of these diseases. The WHO classification includes several previously unrecognized types of lymphomas, and new entities not specifically recognized in the Working Formulation account for about 20% to 25% of the cases.

The WHO classification has broad clinical implications. The WHO Clinical Advisory Committee has agreed that clinical groupings of lymphoid neoplasms into prognostic categories are neither necessary nor desirable because such arbitrary groupings are of no practical value and may be misleading.[64]

Clinical Presentation

6 Patients with NHL present with a wide variety of symptoms, depending on the site of involvement and whether tumor involvement is nodal or extranodal. Sites of involvement and dissemination of the malignant cells can sometimes be predicted based on the cell of origin and the tendency of tumors to frequently disseminate to areas where the normal counterparts of the lymphoma cells are located. For example, B-cell lymphomas involve areas of the lymphoid system normally populated by B-lymphocytes, such as lymph nodes, spleen, and bone marrow. T-cell lymphomas commonly disseminate to various extranodal sites, such as the skin and lungs.[59]

Most patients present with peripheral lymphadenopathy. The lymphadenopathy may be either localized or generalized, and the involved nodes are often painless, rubbery, and discrete, and usually located in the cervical and supraclavicular regions as in Hodgkin lymphoma (Fig. 109-1). Rapid and progressive lymphadenopathy is more characteristic of aggressive lymphomas. Waxing and waning of lymph nodes, including their complete disappearance and reappearance, is more characteristic of indolent lymphomas. Massive lymphadenopathy can sometimes lead to organ dysfunction. For example, patients with NHL may present with acute renal failure from retroperitoneal adenopathy causing ureteral obstruction or from metabolic abnormalities such as hyperuricemia with uric acid nephropathy.

About 40% of patients with NHL present with fever (temperature >38°C [100.4°F]), weight loss (unexplained weight loss of 10% of body weight over the past 6 months), or night sweats (drenching night sweats). If one or more of these symptoms is present, the patient is noted to have B symptoms, and a B is added to the stage of disease (discussed in the Diagnosis, Staging, and Prognostic Factors section under Hodgkin Lymphoma earlier in this chapter).

CLINICAL PRESENTATION Non-Hodgkin Lymphoma

General

- Patients with non-Hodgkin lymphoma present with a wide variety of symptoms, depending on the site of involvement and whether tumor involvement is nodal or extranodal.

Symptoms

- About 40% of patients present with fever, night sweats, and weight loss (i.e., B symptoms).
- Fatigue, malaise, and pruritus.

Signs

- More than two-thirds of patients present with peripheral lymphadenopathy.

Laboratory Tests

- A complete blood count, tests of renal and liver function, and serum electrolytes should be obtained.
- Serum β_2-microglobulin and lactate dehydrogenase levels may be useful as prognostic factors and for monitoring response to therapy.

Other Diagnostic Tests

- Varies depending on sites of involvement.

B symptoms are more commonly observed in patients with aggressive NHLs.

Patients with Hodgkin lymphoma rarely present with extranodal (i.e., extralymphatic) disease, but 10% to 35% of patients with NHL have primary extranodal disease at the time of diagnosis. The frequency of extranodal presentation varies dramatically among different subtypes. The most common extranodal sites are the gastrointestinal tract followed by the skin. The liver or spleen may be enlarged in patients with generalized adenopathy. Patients with mesenteric or gastrointestinal involvement may present with signs and symptoms of nausea, vomiting, obstruction, abdominal pain, a palpable abdominal mass, or gastrointestinal bleeding. Patients with bone marrow involvement may have symptoms related to anemia, neutropenia, or thrombocytopenia. Other sites of extranodal disease include the testes and bone. The incidence of solitary brain lymphoma is increasing, especially in patients with AIDS.

Diagnosis, Staging, and Prognostic Factors

As with Hodgkin lymphoma, the diagnosis of NHL must be established by pathologic review of tissue obtained by biopsy.[59,65] The preferred procedure is an excisional biopsy, where the entire involved lymph node is removed for review by an experienced hematopathologist. This procedure should be done carefully to prevent distortional artifact of the architecture, which could lead to an inaccurate diagnosis. Needle biopsy of the node can sometimes provide adequate tissue for pathologic diagnosis, if an excisional biopsy cannot be performed. When adenopathy is not present, diagnosis may be established by biopsy of cutaneous lesions, bone marrow biopsy and aspiration in patients with unexplained myelosuppression, liver biopsy in patients with hepatomegaly or elevated liver function tests, or biopsy of involved extranodal organs, such as bone, Waldeyer's ring, lung, and testis.

After the diagnosis is established, further workup is required to determine the extent of involvement.[59,65] Clinical staging always begins with a thorough history and physical examination. Patients should be questioned about the presence or absence and extent of fever, night sweats, and weight loss. A detailed history of lymphadenopathy should also be obtained, including when and where the lymph nodes were first noted, and their rate of growth. A complete physical examination is performed to assess the extent of disease involvement, with special attention given to all nodal areas (Fig. 109-1). All patients should have a complete blood count, serum chemistries including liver and renal profiles, a chest radiograph, and bone marrow aspiration and biopsy. The likelihood of bone marrow involvement varies among the different histologic types of lymphoma (Table 109-6). Lumbar puncture to evaluate the cerebrospinal fluid is recommended in patients who have histologic types of lymphoma that often spread to the CNS.

Imaging studies are usually important in the staging workup. CT scanning can identify both nodal and extranodal sites of disease, and has largely replaced lymphangiography for the evaluation of retroperitoneal lymphadenopathy. The abdominal and pelvic CT scan can identify mesenteric and retrocrural node involvement. CT scans can also detect tumor involvement of organs, including the kidneys, ovary, spleen, and liver. PET is currently not used routinely for staging of NHL.[65,66] Magnetic resonance imaging is of limited usefulness in the staging of NHL. Gallium scans are sometimes used as part of the staging workup. Other tests, such as liver–spleen scan, bone scan, upper gastrointestinal series, and IV pyelogram, are sometimes useful in patients with organ symptomatology or serum chemistry abnormalities.

Although staging laparotomy was widely used in the late 1960s and 1970s as part of the staging workup in patients with lymphoma, it is rarely used today because of technical improvements in imaging studies and the morbidity and potential mortality associated with the procedure.

The Ann Arbor staging classification developed for the clinical staging of Hodgkin lymphoma is also used to stage patients with NHL (Table 109-2). After completion of the staging workup, most patients will be found to have advanced disease (stages III and IV). The frequency of localized disease at the time of diagnosis varies depending on the histologic type of lymphoma (Table 109-6). Stage is a more important prognostic factor in Hodgkin lymphoma than in NHL.

7 The Ann Arbor system emphasizes the distribution of nodal disease sites because Hodgkin lymphoma usually spreads through contiguous lymph nodes and does not involve extranodal sites. But NHL is a disease with tremendous heterogeneity that does not spread through contiguous lymph nodes and that often involves extranodal sites. As a result of these clinical differences between Hodgkin lymphoma and NHL, Ann Arbor stage correlates poorly with prognosis.

8 This lack of accuracy with the Ann Arbor staging system in NHL has led to several international projects to develop prognostic models for the most common types of NHLs—diffuse large B-cell lymphomas and follicular lymphomas. The International Non-Hodgkin Lymphoma Prognostic Factors Project was based on more

TABLE 109-6 Clinical Characteristics of Patients with Common Types of Non-Hodgkin Lymphomas

Disease	Median Age (Years)	Frequency in Children	% Male	Stage I/II vs. III/IV (%)	B Symptoms (%)	BM Involvement (%)	GI Tract Involvement (%)	% Surviving 5 years
B-cell chronic lymphocytic leukemia/small lymphocytic lymphoma	65	Rare	53	9 vs. 91	33	72	3	51
Mantle cell lymphoma	63	Rare	74	20 vs. 80	28	64	9	27
Extranodal marginal zone B-cell lymphoma of MALT type	60	Rare	48	67 vs. 33	19	14	50	74
Follicular lymphoma	59	Rare	42	33 vs. 67	28	42	4	72
Diffuse large B-cell lymphoma	64	≈25% of childhood NHL	55	54 vs. 46	33	16	18	46
Burkitt lymphoma	31	≈30% of childhood NHL	89	62 vs. 38	22	33	11	45
Precursor T-cell lymphoblastic lymphoma	28	≈40% of childhood NHL	64	11 vs. 89	21	50	4	26
Anaplastic large T-/null cell lymphoma	34	Common	69	51 vs. 49	53	13	9	77
Peripheral T-cell non-Hodgkin lymphoma	61	≈5% of childhood NHL	55	20 vs. 80	50	36	15	25

BM, bone marrow; GI, gastrointestinal; MALT, mucosa-associated lymphoid tissue; NHL, non-Hodgkin lymphoma.

From Longo DL. Malignancies of Lymphoid Cells. In: Longo DL, Fauci AS, Kasper DL, et al. eds. Harrison's Principles of Internal Medicine. 18th ed. New York, NY: McGraw-Hill, 2012.

TABLE 109-7 Risk Factors and Survival According to the International Non-Hodgkin Lymphoma Prognostic Factors Project

All Patients	Patients ≤60 Years of Age
Age >60 years	Abnormal LDH level
Abnormal LDH level	Performance status ≥2
Performance status ≥2	Ann Arbor stage III or IV
Ann Arbor stage III or IV	
Extranodal involvement ≥2 sites	

LDH, lactic dehydrogenase.

Data from reference 67. Copyright © 1993 Massachusetts Medical Society.

TABLE 109-8 Risk Factors and Survival According to the Follicular Lymphoma International Prognostic Index

All Patients	
Age >60 years	
Ann Arbor stage III or IV	
Number of nodal sites ≥5	
Abnormal lactate dehydrogenase level	
Hemoglobin <12 g/dL [<120 g/L; 7.45 mmol/L]	
Risk Group (% of Patients)	**Number of Risk Factors**
Low (36)	0–1
Intermediate (37)	2
High (27)	≥3

than 2,000 patients with diffuse aggressive lymphomas treated with an anthracycline-containing combination chemotherapy regimen in the United States, Europe, and Canada.[67] The Project identified five risk factors that correlated with low complete response rate to chemotherapy and poor survival: age >60 years, reduced performance status ≥2, abnormal serum lactate dehydrogenase (LDH) levels, two or more extranodal sites of disease, and advanced tumor stage (Ann Arbor stages III or IV) (Table 109-7). In patients ≤60 years old, three risk factors correlated with low complete response rate to chemotherapy and poor survival: reduced performance status, abnormal serum LDH levels, and Ann Arbor stage. It is unclear whether the effect of serum LDH level is related to a tumor or a host event. LDH likely measures cellular catabolism (the enzyme is released from injured cells), or the product of tumor burden and proliferation. Because each of the factors has about the same impact (e.g., relative risk) on prognosis, the number of adverse risk factors is summed to provide the IPI. Patients could, therefore, have a score of 0 to 5. For patients ≤60 years old, a simplified IPI score can be developed based on Ann Arbor stage, serum LDH level, and performance status.

As prognosis improves as a result of more effective therapy, it is important to reevaluate prognostic factors. The IPI was based on patients treated from 1982 to 1987 with anthracycline-based combination chemotherapy; none of the patients received rituximab. In a reexamination of the IPI in a cohort of patients treated with rituximab-containing chemotherapy, Sehn et al. found that the IPI remained predictive, but it only identified two, rather than four, risk groups.[68] When the number of risk factors is redistributed, three risk groups are identified that correlate with prognosis. This revised IPI score may more accurately predict prognosis in patients treated with rituximab-containing combination chemotherapy, but needs to be validated in a larger group of patients.

Although the IPI is often used to predict prognosis in patients with other NHL subtypes, the IPI has several shortcomings when applied to patients with indolent lymphomas. Because only patients with diffuse aggressive lymphomas were used to develop the IPI system, some important prognostic factors may have been missed. Furthermore, the IPI system has limited discriminating power in follicular lymphoma because only about 10% of patients are categorized as high-risk in the IPI system. To address these concerns, an international cooperative study was designed to develop a prognostic model similar to the IPI in patients with follicular lymphoma. The results of that study, which was based on more than 4,000 patients with follicular lymphoma diagnosed between 1985 and 1992, were recently published.[69] Five factors were identified that correlated with poor survival: age >60 years, advanced tumor stage (Ann Arbor stage III or IV), low hemoglobin level (<12 g/dL [7.45 mmol/L]), five or more nodal sites of disease (Fig. 109-1), and an abnormal serum LDH level. Analogous to the IPI, the number of adverse risk factors is summed to provide the Follicular Lymphoma International Prognostic Index (FLIPI). Three prognostic groups were identified: low-risk (0 to 1 factors), intermediate-risk (2 factors), and high-risk (≥3 factors). FLIPI appeared to have higher discriminating power among groups as compared with the IPI system. Table 109-8 shows the correlation between the FLIPI score and overall survival. The survival data from FLIPI, however, may not reflect current treatment results because none of the patients in the cohort used to derive the FLIPI were treated with rituximab. In an updated prognostic model (FLIPI-2) derived from patients with newly diagnosed follicular lymphoma treated with rituximab-containing chemoimmunotherapy regimens, age >60 years, low hemoglobin level (<12 g/dL [7.45 mmol/L]), longest diameter of the largest lymph node >6 cm, abnormal β_2-microglobulin levels and bone marrow involvement were identified as adverse risk factors. FLIPI-2 was highly predictive of treatment outcomes and separated patients into three distinct risk groups: low-risk (0 factors), intermediate-risk (1 or 2 factors), and high-risk (≥3 factors). Three-year progression-free survival was 91%, 69%, and 51% and overall survival was 99%, 96%, and 84% in low-, intermediate-, and high-risk patients, respectively.[70]

Although IPI and FLIPI are clinically useful tools to estimate prognosis, the factors used to calculate these scores probably represent clinical surrogates for the biologic heterogeneity among NHLs and many researchers are interested in determining the prognostic importance of certain phenotypic and molecular characteristics of NHLs. For example, molecular markers of apoptosis, cell-cycle regulation, cell lineage, and cell proliferation are being evaluated as potentially clinically useful prognostic factors.[71]

Gene expression profiling with microarrays may also correlate with survival. Using gene expression profiling, investigators identified at least two molecularly distinct forms of diffuse large B-cell lymphomas based on gene expression patterns indicative of different stages of B-cell differentiation: germinal center B-cell–like (GCB) and activated B-cell–like (ABC).[72] The GCB subtype of diffuse large B-cell lymphoma probably arises from normal germinal center B-cells while the ABC subtype may arise from postgerminal center B-cells. Many oncogenic pathways are different for the GCB and ABC subtypes, and these differences may lead to the development of targeted therapies for each subtype.[63,71] Patients with the germinal center B-cell profile had significantly better overall survival independent of IPI score after treatment with cyclophosphamide, doxorubicin, vincristine (Oncovin®), prednisone (CHOP) or CHOP-like chemotherapy. In a recently published study of patients with diffuse large B-cell lymphoma treated with either CHOP or rituximab and CHOP (R-CHOP), Lenz et al. identified several gene expressions signatures that predicted survival in both CHOP and R-CHOP cohorts: GCB, stromal-1, and stromal-2.[73] The GCB and stromal-1 signatures were associated with a favorable prognosis while the stromal-2 signature was associated with an unfavorable prognosis. The stromal-1 signature reflects extracellular matrix deposition and histiocytic infiltration whereas the stromal-2 signature reflects tumor blood vessel density. The authors speculated that diffuse large B-cell lymphomas that express the stromal-2 signature may respond to antiangiogenic agents.

Another recently identified molecular subtype is double-hit diffuse large B-cell lymphoma, defined as the existence of both MYC gene arrangement and t(14;18) BCL2 translocation.[74] In one pathologic study that used immunohistochemical scoring, patients with high expression of both BCL2 and MYC protein had the worst prognosis. Double-hit NHL is associated with significantly lower complete response rate, shorter overall survival and shorter progression-free survival.[75] NCCN guidelines suggest that patients with double-hit lymphoma usually have a very poor prognosis, with a median overall survival that is 4 to 6 months even with highly aggressive chemotherapy. It is highly recommended that these patients be enrolled in clinical trials.[65]

Two molecularly distinct profiles of follicular lymphoma also have been identified; the first included genes encoding for T-cell markers and genes highly expressed in macrophages, and the second included genes that are preferentially expressed in macrophages, dendritic cells, or both.[76] Patients with the first molecular signature had a more favorable outcome than those with the second signature. These results suggest that molecular classification of tumors on the basis of gene expression may allow identification of clinically significant subtypes of cancer.

TREATMENT
Non-Hodgkin Lymphoma

Desired Outcomes

The primary goals in the treatment of NHL are to relieve symptoms, cure the patient of the disease whenever possible, and minimize the risk of serious toxicities. The treatment strategy depends on many factors, including the patient's age, concomitant disease, disease type, stage of disease, site of disease, and patient preference.

General Approach

9 Historically, both the clinical behavior and degree of aggressiveness are often used to describe NHLs. Indolent lymphomas, which make up about 25% to 40% of all NHLs, are characterized by their slow-growth behavior. Patients with an indolent lymphoma usually have a relatively long survival (measured in years), with or without aggressive chemotherapy. Although these lymphomas respond to a wide range of therapeutic approaches, there is no convincing evidence of a survival plateau, which indicates that patients are rarely cured of their disease. In contrast, aggressive lymphomas, which make up about 60% to 75% of all NHLs, are characterized by rapid growth rate and short survival (measured in weeks to months), if appropriate therapy is not initiated. Despite their more aggressive nature, many patients with aggressive lymphomas who respond to chemotherapy can experience prolonged disease-free survival and some are cured of their disease. Therefore, the terminology for the NHLs represents a paradox, where "indolent" is bad and "aggressive" is good in terms of the likelihood for cure.

Therapeutic approaches to NHL include radiation therapy, chemotherapy, and biologic agents. The role of radiation therapy in the treatment of NHL differs from its role in the treatment of Hodgkin lymphoma. Although the disease responds to radiation therapy, only a small percentage of patients with NHL present with truly localized disease that can be treated with local or regional radiation therapy. Radiation therapy is used more commonly in advanced disease, primarily as a palliative measure to control local bulky disease.

Effective chemotherapy for NHL ranges from single-agent therapy in indolent lymphomas to aggressive, complex chemotherapy regimens in aggressive lymphomas. The most active agents used in the treatment of NHL include the alkylating agents (e.g., cyclophosphamide, chlorambucil), bleomycin, doxorubicin, purine analogs, etoposide, methotrexate, vincristine, and corticosteroids (e.g., prednisone, dexamethasone). The most aggressive chemotherapy approaches are dose-dense chemotherapy or high-dose chemotherapy followed by autologous or allogeneic HSCT.

B-cell lymphomas have served as a model for immunotherapy with monoclonal antibodies for more than 20 years, beginning with the successful use of custom-made monoclonal antibodies targeted against the idiotype present on the patient's cancer cells.[77,78] These encouraging results lead to the development of monoclonal antibodies against a more generic target, a molecule on the surface of B cells that would be present on tumor cells. One potential target, the CD20 molecule, is present only on cells in the B-lymphocyte lineage. It is expressed on the surface of both normal and malignant B cells, but not on other normal tissues. Rituximab (Rituxan®) is a chimeric monoclonal antibody directed at the CD20 molecule. Its antitumor activity is mediated through complement-dependent cytotoxicity, antibody-dependent cytotoxicity, and induction of apoptosis.[78] With the availability of monoclonal antibodies and radioimmunoconjugates for the therapy of lymphoma, nearly all patients with NHL will receive one or more biologic agents during the course of their disease.

Objective response to therapy for NHL should be defined according to the International Workshop to Standardize Response Criteria for Non-Hodgkin Lymphoma, which was recently updated to incorporate the results of newer tests to monitor response such as PET, immunohistochemistry, and flow cytometry.[66] The revised guidelines describe criteria for response (e.g., complete response, partial response, and stable disease) and survival (e.g., overall, disease-free, event-free, progression-free).

Appropriate therapy for NHL depends on the patient's age, histologic type, stage of disease, site of disease, and presence of adverse prognostic factors (as measured by IPI or FLIPI score), and patient preferences. In general, treatment of lymphoma can be divided into limited disease and advanced disease. Limited disease includes those patients with localized disease (Ann Arbor stages I and II). Advanced disease is defined as all Ann Arbor stage III or IV patients, and also frequently includes Ann Arbor stage II patients with poor prognostic features (Tables 109-6 and 109-7).[67,69]

The following section discusses the clinical characteristics and therapy of the most common disease entities.

Indolent Lymphomas

Follicular Lymphomas

The combined group of follicular lymphomas makes up the second most common histologic type of NHL in the United States, comprising about 20% of all NHLs worldwide and up to 70% of indolent lymphomas reported in American and European clinical trials.[79] The WHO classification includes criteria for grading follicular lymphoma based on the number of centroblasts per high-power field: grade 1 to 2 (0 to 15 centroblasts/high-power field) and grade 3 (>15 centroblasts/high-power field).[13] The clinical behavior and treatment outcome of grades 1 and 2 follicular lymphoma are similar, and they are usually treated as indolent lymphomas. In contrast, grade 3 follicular lymphoma is synonymous with what is often referred to as follicular large cell lymphoma and is usually treated as an aggressive lymphoma.

Follicular lymphomas tend to occur in older adults, with a slight female predominance (Table 109-6). Most patients have advanced disease at diagnosis, but about 25% to 33% of patients have localized disease (clinical stage I or II) at diagnosis.[80] Extranodal disease, bulky disease, and B symptoms are uncommon features at diagnosis. Most patients with follicular lymphoma have the chromosomal translocation t(14;18) at the time of diagnosis.

The clinical course is generally indolent, with median survivals of 8 to 10 years. But the natural history of follicular lymphoma can be unpredictable. Spontaneous regression of objective disease has been noted in as many as 20% to 30% of patients.[81] There is also a high conversion rate of follicular lymphoma to a more aggressive histology over time that steadily increases after diagnosis and reaches about 30% at 10 years.[82] At autopsy, most patients with follicular lymphoma have some evidence of diffuse large B-cell lymphoma. Patients with transformed indolent lymphoma should be treated in the same way as patients with an aggressive lymphoma.

Most patients have dramatic responses to initial therapy, and their disease course is characterized by multiple relapses, with responses to salvage therapy becoming progressively shorter after every relapse, eventually leading to death from disease-related causes. This pattern of constant relapses over time without evidence of a survival plateau and the failure of randomized controlled trials to show a survival benefit with aggressive chemotherapy led to the conclusion that therapy does not prolong overall survival and patients are not cured of their disease. However, several recently published studies suggest that the use of biologic agents, particularly rituximab, has changed the natural history of the follicular lymphoma. In a study of patients enrolled in Southwest Oncology Group (SWOG) trials over a period of more than 20 years, patients treated with CHOP and a monoclonal antibody had a significantly longer 4-year overall survival than those treated with CHOP alone (91% vs. 69%).[83] Similar results were reported in patients treated over a 30-year period at the M.D. Anderson Cancer Center.[84] That study also showed an apparent plateau in the failure-free survival curve.

Certain subsets of patients with follicular lymphoma have a much better or worse prognosis. Some studies suggest that the natural history of follicular large cell lymphoma (i.e., grade 3 follicular lymphoma) is similar to that of other aggressive lymphomas and that treatment with intensive combination chemotherapy regimens may result in long-term disease-free survival, including a possible plateau in the survival curve.[79] The recent development of the FLIPI prognostic model should help clinicians to identify patients in different prognostic groups based on disease characteristics at the time of diagnosis.[69] Patients who are predicted to have a poor prognosis (i.e., high-risk) could then be offered aggressive or experimental therapy, whereas those who are predicted to have a good prognosis (i.e., low-risk) would be treated with standard therapy, avoiding unnecessary toxicity.

Treatment of Localized Disease (Stages I and II) Radiation therapy is the standard treatment for early stage follicular lymphoma. Involved-field, extended-field, and total nodal irradiation have been used. Carefully staged patients with either stage I or contiguous stage II disease treated with radiation therapy alone can achieve disease-free survival rates of 40% to 50% and overall survival rates of 60% to 70% at 10 years.[79] Late relapses are uncommon; only 10% of patients who reached 10 years without relapse subsequently experienced a recurrence.

Chemotherapy is not usually given in most patients with localized follicular lymphoma, but it may be helpful in some patients with high-risk stage II disease (e.g., multiple sites of involvement or bulky disease).[85]

⑩ About 40% to 60% of patients with clinical stage I or II follicular lymphoma are cured of their disease with radiation therapy alone.[65] Most centers use radiation at a dose of 30 to 40 Gy (3000 to 4000 rad) to either involved (i.e., local) or regional fields, which would consist of irradiation to the involved nodal region plus one additional uninvolved region on each side of the involved nodes. Extended-field irradiation is not usually used because of the absence of a survival benefit and possible increased risk of secondary malignancies. In addition, previous use of extended-field irradiation compromises the ability of that patient to receive subsequent chemotherapy. The current NCCN guidelines state that locoregional radiation therapy is preferred for most patients with early stage follicular lymphoma.[65] Immunotherapy (i.e., rituximab) with or without chemotherapy or radiation therapy is also listed as an option (category 2B).

Treatment of Advanced Disease (Stages III and IV) ⑩ The management of stages III and IV indolent lymphomas remains controversial because until recently, no therapeutic approaches had been shown to prolong overall survival despite the high complete remission rates to initial therapy. However, the results of recently published studies suggest that the initial use of biologic therapy such as rituximab is associated with longer overall survival.[83,84] More than 80% of patients with stage III or IV follicular lymphoma are alive at 5 years, and the median survival ranges between 7 and 10 years.

Therapeutic options for these patients are diverse and include watchful waiting, radiation therapy, single-agent chemotherapy, combination chemotherapy, biologic therapy, radioimmunotherapy, and combined-modality therapy.[86] Although complete remission can be achieved in 50% to 80% of patients with various treatments, the median time to relapse is usually only 18 to 36 months. About 20% of patients who have a complete response remain in remission for longer than 10 years. After relapse, patients are retreated, and high remission rates can be achieved. Unfortunately, response rates and duration of response both decrease with each retreatment.

Several different approaches can be used to treat follicular lymphoma. Carefully selected patients may receive no initial therapy followed by single-agent chemotherapy, rituximab, or radiation therapy when treatment is needed. Candidates for the conservative approach are usually older, asymptomatic, and have minimal tumor burden. Patients with symptoms, extensive extranodal involvement, bulky disease, cytopenia due to bone marrow involvement, or impaired end-organ function at the time of diagnosis are not candidates for conservative treatment. Alternatively, patients can be treated aggressively with combination chemotherapy, with or without rituximab, or radioimmunotherapy early in the disease course. Both conservative and aggressive approaches are listed as possible options in the current NCCN guidelines, but the guidelines recommend that initial therapy should include rituximab unless contraindicated.[65] Patients who respond to induction therapy may receive maintenance therapy with single-agent rituximab.

A recently published observational study of 2,728 patients with newly diagnosed follicular lymphoma treated in the United States from March 2004 to March 2007 showed that about two-thirds of patients were treated with rituximab, either alone (14%) or combined with chemotherapy (52%).[87] About 18% of patients were treated with observation.

At the time of relapse, many of the same treatment options are available, and the following factors must be considered: age, symptomatic status of the patient, tumor burden, rate of regrowth (based on previous assessment of active disease sites), presence or absence of characteristics suggesting transformation or biologic progression, prior therapy, degree and duration of response to prior therapy, availability of clinical trials, and patient preferences.[65]

Watch-and-Wait Because there are no convincing data that standard treatment approaches have improved survival, some clinicians have adopted a "watch-and-wait" approach for asymptomatic patients where therapy is delayed until the patient experiences systemic symptoms or disease progression such as rapidly progressive or bulky adenopathy, anemia, thrombocytopenia, or disease in threatening sites such as the orbit or spinal cord.[86,88] The median time until treatment is required is 3 to 5 years, and about 20% of patients do not require therapy for up to 10 years. The 10-year survival is 73%, which is not significantly different from patients who received therapy at the time of diagnosis. In a randomized study of asymptomatic patients with indolent lymphomas (mostly follicular), patients who underwent watchful waiting had similar cause-specific and overall survival as compared with those who received immediate chlorambucil.[88] With a median length of followup of 16 years, about 17% of patients who were randomized to the watchful waiting group died of other causes without receiving chemotherapy and an additional 9% are alive and have not yet had chemotherapy. As described above, patients with follicular lymphoma who are followed without therapy sometimes have spontaneous regressions that can be complete while the disease in other patients can convert to a more aggressive histology. If the watchful waiting approach is chosen, the patient should be evaluated at least every 2 months for the first year and quarterly thereafter, so that intervention can occur before serious problems occur.

Chemotherapy Oral alkylating agents, given either alone or combined with prednisone, have been the mainstay of treatment for follicular lymphoma. More intensive chemotherapy has not been shown to improve patient outcome. In a randomized trial of oral chlorambucil, oral cyclophosphamide, or cyclophosphamide, vincristine, and prednisone (CVP) in patients with indolent lymphoma, no significant difference in overall survival or freedom-from-relapse between the three groups was observed.[81] The dosage of single-agent chlorambucil or cyclophosphamide is usually adjusted to maintain a platelet count above 100,000 cells/mm^3 (100×10^9/L) and a white blood cell count above 3,000 cells/mm^3 (3×10^9/L). Although single-agent alkylating agents have a high initial complete remission rate, the time required to achieve a complete response is slow (median time is 9 to 12 months). Complete responses occur more rapidly with combination chemotherapy, particularly with doxorubicin-containing regimens. Many clinicians will therefore give CHOP or CHOP-like chemotherapy when a rapid response is necessary. The development of the CHOP regimen is described in more detail in the Aggressive Lymphomas section later in this chapter. Table 109-9 shows the CHOP regimen that is widely used in the treatment of NHL. In those who achieve a complete response, the duration of response is relatively short (about 2.5 years). There is no benefit of maintenance therapy with chemotherapy. After the "best" response is achieved, many experts will discontinue therapy and observe.

Both single-agent alkylating agents and CVP are well tolerated by most patients. The advantages of oral chlorambucil are no hair loss, little or no nausea, and minimal myelosuppression. Because of its mild side effect profile, oral chlorambucil is usually recommended for older patients who are minimally symptomatic or who have other comorbidities. There are some concerns with the risk of secondary acute leukemia in patients receiving continuous exposure to alkylating agents.

Anti-CD20 Monoclonal Antibodies The approval of rituximab is arguably the most important recent development in the treatment of NHL. Its initial approval in 1997 was based on an open-label multicenter study that enrolled 166 patients with relapsed or recurrent indolent lymphoma.[89] Rituximab, given IV at a dose of 375 mg/m^2 weekly for 4 weeks, resulted in an overall response of 48% (complete response: 6%, partial response: 42%). Median time to progression for responders was 13.2 months and median duration of response was 11.6 months. Other studies of single-agent rituximab in patients with relapsed or refractory indolent NHL have reported overall response rates of 40% to 60% and complete response rates of 5% to 10%.[90]

Based on the activity of rituximab in relapsed or refractory patients, it is currently being used as first-line therapy, either alone or in combination with chemotherapy.[77,90–92] When given as a single agent to patients with previously untreated indolent NHL, the overall response rate is 60% to 70% and the complete response rate is 20% to 30%. It is interesting to note that many of these patients remain in molecular remission (i.e., polymerase chain reaction–negative) at 12 months. Single-agent rituximab is listed as an acceptable option for first-line therapy of follicular lymphoma, particularly for patients who cannot tolerate more intensive chemotherapy regimens.[65]

The rationale for the use of rituximab in combination with conventional agents is based on clinical activity of both agents/regimens, non–cross-resistant mechanisms of action, nonoverlapping toxicities, and synergistic antitumor activity in vitro. Many clinical trials have evaluated the use of rituximab in combination with other chemotherapy agents. In a phase II trial of six courses of R-CHOP, the overall and complete response rate in 40 patients with previously untreated or relapsed indolent lymphoma was 95% and 55%, respectively.[93] More than 70% of patients were progression-free after 4 years of followup. In an updated analysis, median time-to-progression was reached at 82 months.[94] Based on these encouraging results, several randomized controlled trials have evaluated rituximab in combination with various chemotherapy regimens in first-line therapy for follicular or other indolent lymphomas.[77,91] In the R-CHOP versus CHOP trial, patients who were randomized to receive R-CHOP as initial therapy had significantly higher overall response rates (96% vs. 90%), reduced risk for treatment failure (relative risk 0.4), and longer time-to-treatment failure and overall survival.[95] In another randomized trial of R-CHOP versus CHOP in relapsed or resistant follicular lymphoma, patients treated with R-CHOP had higher overall and complete response rates (85% vs. 72% and 30% vs. 16%, respectively) and lower risk of treatment failure (hazard ratio [HR] 0.65), but no significant difference in overall survival was observed.[96] Similar results were reported when rituximab was added to other combination regimens.[77,78] In a meta-analysis of all randomized controlled trials, patients with indolent lymphoma treated with rituximab and chemotherapy had a significantly higher overall response rate and reduced risk of treatment failure (HR 0.62) and death (HR 0.65).[97] Rituximab is FDA-approved for first-line therapy for follicular lymphoma in combination with CVP chemotherapy. R-CHOP is listed as an acceptable option for first-line therapy of follicular lymphoma (category 1).[65]

Rituximab and CHOP chemotherapy can be combined in many different ways.[98] In the R-CHOP regimen developed by Czuczman et al., two doses of rituximab are given before the start of CHOP therapy; two more doses are given in the middle of the six cycles of CHOP; and two additional doses are given at the end of CHOP therapy.[93] However, in most NHL protocols and in clinical practice, rituximab is given on day 1 of CHOP chemotherapy.[98] In some protocols, rituximab is given on the day before chemotherapy (i.e., day 0) or rituximab is given on day 1 and the other drugs are given on day 3.

In patients who respond to rituximab, either alone or combined with chemotherapy, maintenance therapy with single-agent rituximab is often given to prolong the duration of remission. Rituximab is FDA approved as single-agent maintenance therapy in patients

TABLE 109-9 CHOP Regimen

Drug	Dose (mg/m^2)	Route	Treatment Days
Cyclophosphamide	750	IV	1
Doxorubicin	50	IV	1
Vincristine	1.4[a]	IV	1
Prednisone	100	Oral	1–5
One cycle is 21 days			

Another name for doxorubicin is hydroxydaunorubicin.

[a]Vincristine dose is typically capped at 2 mg/m^2.

achieving a complete or partial response following induction chemotherapy. The FDA approval was based on a randomized controlled trial in previously untreated patients with advanced-stage follicular lymphoma treated with maintenance rituximab after CVP chemotherapy.[99] Three-year progression-free survival was significantly longer in the maintenance rituximab group as compared with the observation group (68% vs. 33%). However, it is important to note that only about 3% of patients with newly diagnosed follicular lymphoma are treated with chemotherapy alone in the United States.[92] In another recently published randomized controlled trial, patients responding to first-line chemotherapy in combination with rituximab (such as R-CVP, R-CHOP or rituximab, fludarabine, cyclophosphamide, and mitoxantrone [R-FCM]) were randomized to receive rituximab maintenance (12 infusions of 375 mg/m^2 given IV, once every 8 weeks) or no maintenance.[100] After a median followup of 24 months, rituximab maintenance significantly improved progression-free survival compared to observation (75% vs. 58%). Interestingly, induction therapy with R-CHOP or R-FCM was associated with improved progression-free survival, which suggests that R-CVP was not beneficial in this study. Longer followup is needed to evaluate the effect of rituximab maintenance on overall survival.

The use of maintenance rituximab in newly diagnosed follicular lymphoma is controversial.[101,102] Although it improves progression-free survival, no overall survival benefit has been observed. And maintenance rituximab is expensive and may be associated with adverse effects, including an increased risk of grades 3 or 4 infections. The NCCN guideline lists maintenance therapy with rituximab (one dose every 8 weeks for up to 2 years) as an option following first-line therapy for patients initially presenting with high tumor burden.[65]

Clinical **Controversy. . .**

Maintenance rituximab is often used in patients with indolent lymphoma who respond to induction chemoimmunotherapy. While maintenance rituximab has been shown to prolong overall survival in patients with refractory or relapsed disease, no consistent survival benefit has been observed in newly diagnosed patients. Various dosing schedules have been used.

Rituximab maintenance following second-line therapy has also been evaluated in patients with relapsed or refractory disease. Two randomized trials have demonstrated a progression-free survival advantage with rituximab maintenance over observation for patients treated with induction chemotherapy.[103,104] In a recently published trial of patients with relapsed or resistant follicular lymphoma responding to CHOP or R-CHOP induction, maintenance rituximab significantly improved median progression-free survival as compared with observation alone (3.7 years vs. 1.3 years). The 5-year overall survival, however, was not significantly different between the study arms (74% vs. 64%).[104] It is also important to note that patients who develop progression of disease during or within 6 months of first-line maintenance rituximab will likely experience little, if any, benefit from maintenance therapy in the second-line setting. The NCCN guideline recommends optional maintenance therapy with rituximab (one dose every 12 weeks for 2 years) for patients who are in remission after second-line therapy.[65]

Most of the adverse effects of rituximab are infusion-related, particularly after the first infusion, and consist of fever, chills, respiratory symptoms, fatigue, headache, pruritus, and angioedema.[94] Premedication with oral acetaminophen 650 mg and diphenhydramine 50 mg is usually given 30 minutes before rituximab infusion. The package insert recommends a step-up infusion rate of rituximab to decrease the risk of infusion-related infusion. Duration of infusions, however, may take up to 5 hours. Studies have demonstrated that rapid infusion of rituximab (infused over 90 minutes) is feasible in patients who tolerate their first cycle of rituximab without increasing the risk of infusion-related reactions.[105–106] The FDA has approved rapid infusions of rituximab, but they are not recommended in patients with clinically significant cardiovascular disease and high circulating lymphocyte counts (greater than 5000 cells/mm^3 [5 x 10^9/L]). Reactivation of hepatitis B has been reported in patients receiving chemotherapy, either alone or combined with rituximab.[107] Hepatitis B testing is recommended in patients who are considering rituximab therapy.[65]

In addition to rituximab, other anti-CD20 antibodies are currently under research development.[78] Ofatumumab, a fully human antibody against CD20, is currently approved for treatment of refractory chronic lymphocytic leukemia. It binds to two sites on the CD20 molecule, which brings the antibody closer to the cell membrane and increases complement-dependent cytotoxicity.[108] Ofatumumab is being evaluated in randomized controlled trials against rituximab-based regimens for treatment of both indolent and aggressive lymphomas.

Bendamustine Bendamustine is an alkylating agent with structural similarities to both alkylating agents and purine analogs. The mechanism of action of bendamustine appears to be different from other alkylating agents and it does not show cross-resistance to other alkylating agents. When used as a single agent, bendamustine shows antitumor activity in relapsed or refractory indolent lymphomas. Overall and complete response rates of 70% to 80% and 30% to 35% have been reported, respectively, in phase II trials.[109]

The combination of bendamustine and rituximab (BR) has been shown to demonstrate better efficacy outcomes than R-CHOP in advanced follicular lymphoma. In a phase II trial, the overall and complete response rate to BR was 92% and 55%, respectively.[110] In a randomized controlled trial of first-line therapies for advanced indolent NHL, patients who received BR had a higher complete response rate (40% vs. 30%) and longer median progression-free survival (55 vs. 35 mo) as compared with those who received R-CHOP.[109] The BR regimen was tolerated better than R-CHOP. Based on these results, BR is listed as an acceptable option for first-line therapy of follicular lymphoma (category 2A).[65]

The combination of bendamustine, rituximab, and bortezomib (BVR) has also been evaluated in two recent studies in patients with relapsed or refractory follicular lymphoma. In both studies, overall response rate was high (>90%) with median progression-free survival ranging from 15 to 22 months.[111,112] Serious adverse events were reported in 34% of patients; the most common grade 3 or 4 adverse events were myelosuppression, gastrointestinal side effects, fatigue, and peripheral neuropathy. The NCCN guideline lists BVR as an option for second-line therapy for follicular lymphoma.[65]

Purine Analogs Several studies report encouraging results with two adenosine analogs, fludarabine phosphate in previously untreated and relapsed advanced follicular lymphoma.[87] The mechanism of action for both drugs is not well understood, but both agents accumulate in lymphocytes and are resistant to adenosine deaminase. In patients with relapsed or refractory indolent lymphoma, single-agent fludarabine has an overall response rate of almost 50% and a complete response rate of 10% to 15%. Response rates are higher in previously untreated patients, with overall and complete response rates of 70% and almost 40%, respectively. The median time to progression is less than 6 months for relapsed disease and more than 12 months for previously untreated patients. Although the response rates to 2-chlorodeoxyadenosine in previously untreated patients is similar to those with fludarabine, the duration of response appears to be shorter with 2-chlorodeoxyadenosine.

Combination regimens that include one of these purine analogs are also being investigated.[87] Fludarabine and mitoxantrone (FN) and fludarabine, mitoxantrone, and dexamethasone (FND), given with or without rituximab, are examples of fludarabine-containing regimens that show encouraging results in patients with indolent lymphoma.

Purine analogs usually do not cause nausea and vomiting or hair loss, but they are associated with cumulative and prolonged myelosuppression and profound immunosuppression, which increases the risk of opportunistic infections, such as fungal infections, *Pneumocystis jiroveci* pneumonia, and viral infections. Because the use of fludarabine-based regimens may impair stem cell mobilization and collection, some experts avoid fludarabine-based regimens for patients who are potential candidates for autologous HSCT.

Radioimmunotherapy Two anti-CD20 radioimmunoconjugates—^{131}I-tositumomab (Bexxar) and ^{90}Y-ibritumomab tiuxetan (Zevalin)—are currently available as treatment options for patients with indolent NHLs.[113] Both ^{131}I-tositumomab and ^{90}Y-ibritumomab tiuxetan are mouse antibodies linked to a radioisotope, either iodine-131 (^{131}I) or yttrium-90 (^{90}Y). Indolent lymphomas are known to be responsive to radiation therapy (i.e., radiosensitive), and the rationale of radioimmunotherapy is that the antibody will act as a guided missile to deliver its payload (i.e., radiation) to its target (i.e., lymphoma cells that express the CD20 antigen). The specificity of the monoclonal antibody allows delivery of the radiation selectively to the tumor (and adjacent normal tissues).

Radioimmunoconjugates have some advantages and disadvantages over unlabeled ("naked") monoclonal antibodies such as rituximab. Tumor cell kill following rituximab depends on binding of the antibody to the tumor cell and the host immune system. Therefore, tumor cells that do not express the target antigen are not accessible to the antibody, or those that are resistant to immune-mediated attacks may escape treatment. Radioimmunoconjugates, because of their ability to deliver radiation over a distance from a source, can not only kill tumor cells that are in contact with the antibody, but also adjacent tumor cells which may not have been in contact with the antibody or may not express the target antigen. This effect is sometimes referred to as the relevant bystander or crossfire effect. However, one disadvantage of radioimmunotherapy is that it can also damage adjacent normal tissues, such as bone marrow cells.

Both ^{131}I-tositumomab and ^{90}Y-ibritumomab tiuxetan have shown activity in relapsed and refractory patients with indolent or transformed lymphomas.[113] In patients who respond to radioimmunotherapy, the duration of remission can be more than several years. Although radioimmunotherapy is usually reserved for second-line therapy of follicular lymphoma, some clinicians consider radioimmunotherapy earlier in the disease course, including for patients with previously untreated disease. In a phase II study, patients with previously untreated follicular lymphoma were treated with six cycles of CHOP chemotherapy followed 4 to 8 weeks later by ^{131}I-tositumomab.[114] The overall response rate to the entire treatment regimen was 91%, including 69% complete remissions, and the 5-year progression-free survival is estimated to be 67%. Similar results were reported in a phase II trial of ^{131}I-tositumomab given without induction CHOP chemotherapy in previously untreated patients with advanced-stage follicular lymphoma.[115] Durable responses have also been reported with ^{131}I-tositumomab and CVP.[116]

Radioimmunotherapy is generally well-tolerated. The major acute toxicities with both radioimmunoconjugates are infusion-related reactions and myelosuppression. ^{131}I-tositumomab can also cause thyroid dysfunction. The primary concern with radioimmunotherapy is the development of treatment-related myelodysplastic syndrome or acute myelogenous leukemia.[117]

The decision to use radioimmunotherapy must be made carefully because of the complexity, risks, and costs of the treatment regimen. Because of safety concerns related to delivery of radiation to bone marrow, candidates for radioimmunotherapy usually have limited bone marrow involvement and adequate absolute neutrophil and platelet counts. Although medical oncologists usually select patients for therapy, the radioimmunotherapy regimen must be administered at a radiation oncology or nuclear medicine facility.

Hematopoietic Stem Cell Transplantation High-dose chemotherapy, followed by autologous or allogeneic HSCT, is another option for patients with relapsed follicular lymphoma.[118,119] In patients who are transplanted at the time of initial treatment failure, 5-year event-free survival is about 40% to 50%. Although the rate of recurrence is lower after allogeneic HSCT as compared with autologous HSCT, that benefit is offset by increased treatment-related mortality after allogeneic HSCT. The presence of a survival plateau after allogeneic HSCT suggests that some patients may be cured of their disease.

A panel of follicular lymphoma experts recently published their recommendations, which was based on an evidence-based review.[119] Their recommendations are: (1) autologous HSCT is recommended as salvage therapy based on pre-rituximab data, with a significant improvement in progression-free and overall survival; (2) autologous HSCT is not recommended as consolidation therapy after first-line chemotherapy for most patients because of no significant improvement in overall survival; (3) autologous HSCT is recommended for transformed follicular lymphoma patients; (4) reduced-intensity conditioning before allogeneic HSCT appears to be an acceptable alternative to myeloablative regimens; and (5) an human leukocyte antigen (HLA)-matched unrelated donor appears to be as effective as an HLA-matched related donor for reduced intensity conditioning allogeneic HSCT. There are insufficient data to make a recommendation on the use of autologous HSCT after rituximab-based salvage therapy.

Rituximab is being evaluated in the setting of autologous HSCT.[120] It is given pretransplant as an in vivo purging agent prior to stem cell collection. In other studies, rituximab is given as post-transplant consolidation.

Aggressive Lymphomas

Diffuse Large B-Cell Lymphoma

Diffuse large B-cell lymphomas (DLBCLs) are the most common lymphoma in the International NHL Classification Project, accounting for about 30% of all NHLs.[121] DLBCLs are characterized by the presence of large cells, which are similar in size to or larger than tissue macrophages and usually more than twice the size of normal lymphocytes. The median age at the time of diagnosis is in the seventh decade, but DLBCL can affect individuals of all ages, from children to the elderly. Patients often present with a rapidly enlarging symptomatic mass, with B symptoms in about 30% to 40% of cases.[121] About 30% to 40% of patients with DLBCL present with extranodal disease; common sites include the head and neck, gastrointestinal tract, skin, bone, testis, and CNS. DLBCL is the most common type of diffuse aggressive lymphomas, which are characterized by an aggressive clinical behavior that leads to death within weeks to months if the tumor is not treated. Diffuse aggressive lymphomas are also sensitive to many chemotherapeutic agents, and some patients treated with chemotherapy can be cured of their disease.

Several factors have been shown to correlate with response to chemotherapy and survival in patients with aggressive lymphoma.[71] Because the IPI was originally developed based on patients with aggressive lymphoma, IPI score correlates with prognosis (Table 109-7).[67] As described above, the revised IPI score may more accurately predict prognosis in patients receiving rituximab-containing combination chemotherapy.[68]

Therapy of DLBCL is based on the Ann Arbor stage, IPI (or revised IPI) score, and other prognostic factors.[121] About one-half of patients present with localized (stage I or II) disease. However, many patients present with large bulky masses (i.e., larger than 10 cm), and patients with bulky stage II disease are treated with the same approach used for patients with advanced disease (stage III or IV).

Treatment of Localized Disease (Stages I and II) Before 1980, radiation therapy was the primary treatment for patients with localized DLBCL. Five-year disease-free survival with radiation therapy alone was about 50% and 20% in patients with stage I and stage II disease, respectively.[121] Randomized trials in the 1980s showed that radiation therapy followed by chemotherapy resulted in significantly longer disease-free and overall survival as compared with radiation therapy alone. Other studies reported excellent results with a short course of chemotherapy (three cycles) followed by involved-field radiotherapy or six to eight cycles of CHOP chemotherapy, with or without consolidation radiotherapy. With either of these approaches, 5-year progression-free survival was >90% for patients with stage I disease and about 70% for patients with stage II disease.[121]

Because the more effective approach was not clear, the SWOG performed a randomized trial that compared three cycles of CHOP and involved-field radiotherapy or six cycles of CHOP in patients with stage I and nonbulky stage II aggressive lymphoma.[65] Patients treated with three cycles of CHOP plus radiotherapy had significantly better 5-year progression-free (77% vs. 64%) and overall (82% vs. 72%) survival than did patients treated with CHOP alone. The incidence of life-threatening toxicity was higher in patients who received CHOP alone. But with longer followup, more patients who received abbreviated chemotherapy experienced late relapses and the differences in progression-free or overall survival were no longer significant between the two arms. Further subgroup analysis of that trial identified several prognostic factors that led to the development of the stage-modified IPI score. Four adverse risk factors comprise the score: nonbulky stage II disease (bulky stage II disease is considered advanced disease), age >60 years, elevated LDH levels, or performance status ≥2.

The stage-modified IPI score is often used to identify patients with localized aggressive NHL who may have a poor prognosis. Based on the results of this trial, the current standard for therapy of most patients with localized nonbulky aggressive lymphoma without any adverse risk factors is three to four cycles of R-CHOP followed by locoregional radiation therapy (30 to 40 Gy [3000 to 4000 rad]).[121] Five-year median survival in this favorable group of patients exceeds 90%.

Five-year median survival is reduced to about 70% in patients with at least one adverse risk factor in the stage-modified IPI score. Patients in this high-risk subgroup may benefit from more aggressive chemotherapy (six cycles of R-CHOP) followed by locoregional radiation therapy.[65]

Treatment of Advanced Disease (Bulky Stage II, Stages III and IV) It has been known since the late 1970s that intensive combination chemotherapy can cure some patients with disseminated DLBCL.[121] Initial studies with cyclophosphamide, vincristine (Oncovin), and prednisone or prednisolone (COP; same as CVP) produced a plateau on the survival curve of just 10%, with a median survival of less than 1 year. Based on the activity of single-agent doxorubicin, McKelvey et al. developed the CHOP regimen (Table 109-9).[122] A few years later, a SWOG study showed that CHOP was more active than COP, and CHOP chemotherapy rapidly became the treatment of choice for patients with aggressive lymphomas.[123] Studies in larger numbers of patients showed that about 50% of patients had a complete remission to CHOP chemotherapy, and 50% to 75% of the patients who had a complete response (about one-third of all patients) experienced long-term disease-free survival and cure of their disease.

In an effort to improve these results, many investigators used several general approaches to develop second- and third-generation regimens in the 1980s.[121] Results of phase II trials suggested that these second- and third-generation regimens were more active than CHOP, with slightly higher complete response rates and improved disease-free survival rates. However, they were also more difficult to administer, more toxic, and more expensive. Based on these results, many oncologists adopted one of these second- or third-generation combination regimens as their standard regimen for patients with advanced aggressive lymphomas.

Many randomized studies have compared different combination regimens in patients with aggressive lymphoma. Although the results of these studies show that no one regimen is clearly superior to another, they demonstrate the superiority of anthracycline-containing regimens over those that do not contain an anthracycline. In the largest and most widely quoted study, the SWOG initiated a randomized trial in 1986 that compared CHOP to three of the most commonly used third-generation regimens in nearly 900 patients with bulky stage II, stage III, or stage IV aggressive NHL. At the time of the initial publication (median followup: 35 months), no differences in disease-free and overall survival were observed between the four groups.[124] Furthermore, no significant differences in disease-free or overall survival were observed in any subgroup of patients. But the risk of treatment-related mortality was higher in patients receiving one of the third-generation regimens. Extended followup of that trial shows that about 35% of patients who participated in that trial are probably cured of their disease, regardless of the initial combination chemotherapy regimen.[125] Interestingly, the overall survival is about 10% higher than the disease-free survival, which probably reflects the effectiveness of salvage high-dose chemotherapy with autologous HSCT (see the Treatment of Refractory or Relapsed Disease section later in this chapter).

Based on the lack of survival benefit with the newer combination chemotherapy regimens, the less complicated and less expensive CHOP regimen was considered as the treatment of choice for most patients with DLBCL and other aggressive NHLs for many years. Even with CHOP chemotherapy, however, less than 50% of patients with DLBCL were cured of their disease and most patients who relapse after an initial response do so in the first two years. New treatment approaches were clearly needed.

Several studies attempted to improve treatment results by increasing chemotherapy dose (i.e., dose-intensity), shortening the interval between chemotherapy cycles (i.e., dose-density), or both. Because of the increased risk of severe neutropenia, these approaches require growth factor support. Although results of these studies have not consistently shown improved survival, encouraging results from several recently published studies suggest that these approaches be evaluated in future randomized trials.[126,127]

Based on the encouraging results of R-CHOP in indolent lymphomas, several studies evaluated this combination in aggressive lymphomas.[91,125] The first randomized controlled trial that established the efficacy of R-CHOP in advanced-stage DLBCL showed that R-CHOP significantly increased complete response rates and overall survival in elderly (≥60 years old) patients as compared with CHOP alone (discussed in the Treatment of Elderly Patients with Advanced Disease section later in this chapter).[128,129] Although the results of that study established R-CHOP as standard therapy in older patients, the role of R-CHOP in the treatment of younger patients was not clear. That issue was recently addressed in the MabThera International Trial, which enrolled younger (18 to 60 years old) patients with good-prognosis DLBCL.[130] Patients randomized to receive rituximab plus CHOP-like chemotherapy had significantly higher complete response rates (86% vs. 68%) and longer

3-year event-free and overall survival (79% vs. 59% [HR 0.44] and 93% vs. 84% [HR 0.40], respectively). Furthermore, in a population-based study conducted in British Columbia, institution of a policy recommending R-CHOP for all patients with newly diagnosed advanced-stage DLBCL resulted in significant improvements in progression-free and overall survival.[131] Based on these trial results, rituximab received FDA approval for first-line treatment in combination with CHOP or CHOP-like chemotherapy and R-CHOP is recommended for all patients with advanced-stage DLBCL in the current NCCN guideline.[65]

Treatment outcomes for high-risk patients according to the IPI (or revised IPI) score are unsatisfactory. High-risk groups generally include all patients older than 60 years and those with an IPI score of ≥3 (or an age-adjusted IPI score of ≥2). Because progression-free survival is only about 50% in these high-risk patients treated with R-CHOP,[68,132] other more aggressive treatments, preferably as part of a clinical trial, should be considered in these patients. Examples of more aggressive approaches include dose-intense or dose-dense chemotherapy with growth factor support, usually combined with rituximab, or high-dose chemotherapy with autologous HSCT.[121,133]

One approach is to give high-dose chemotherapy with autologous HSCT as intensive consolidation in high-risk patients with DLBCL who achieve a remission with standard chemotherapy.[121] Several randomized controlled trials have been conducted in patients with aggressive NHLs, and no consistent survival advantage has been reported. A recently published meta-analysis of all randomized controlled trials of autologous HSCT as intensive consolidation in aggressive NHL concluded that there was no evidence that autologous HSCT improved outcomes in good-risk patients.[134] The evidence for high-risk patients was inconclusive.

Clinical **Controversy...**

Because of high relapse rate in patients who have a complete response to R-CHOP, some experts believe that high-dose chemotherapy with autologous HSCT should be considered as consolidation therapy in high-risk patients with aggressive NHLs who have a complete remission to R-CHOP chemotherapy. Other experts, however, believe that the evidence supporting high-dose chemotherapy with autologous HSCT in this setting is inconclusive and that autologous HSCT should be reserved for patients who relapse.

11 In summary, all patients with bulky stage II, stage III, or stage IV disease should be treated with R-CHOP or rituximab and CHOP-like chemotherapy until a complete response is achieved (usually four cycles).[65] Clinicians are encouraged to adopt the revised response criteria proposed by the International Working Group.[66] In patients who have a positive pretreatment PET scan, PET scanning can be useful in response assessment. A rapid response to chemotherapy (i.e., a complete response achieved in the first three treatment cycles) is associated with a more durable remission compared with patients requiring longer treatment cycles. Two or more cycles of chemotherapy should be given following attainment of a complete response (total of six to eight cycles). The use of long-term maintenance therapy following a complete response has not been shown to improve survival. Treatment outcomes for high-risk patients according to the IPI (or revised IPI) score are unsatisfactory and alternative treatment approaches, preferably as part of a clinical trial, should be considered in these patients.[65] High-dose chemotherapy with autologous HSCT should be considered in high-risk patients who respond to standard chemotherapy and are candidates for autologous HSCT.

Treatment of Elderly Patients with Advanced Disease More than one-half of patients with NHL are older than 60 years of age at diagnosis, and about one-third are older than age 70 years. The International Non-Hodgkin Lymphoma Prognostic Factors Project showed that patients older than 60 years of age had a significantly lower complete response rate and overall survival.[67] The reasons for the poorer outcome in elderly patients are not clear. Older patients do not tolerate intensive chemotherapy as well as younger patients, and some studies report that older patients have a higher risk of treatment-related mortality. As a result, many clinicians treat elderly patients with reduced dose or less-aggressive chemotherapy regimens. In general, these less-intensive regimens have used anthracyclines with less cardiotoxicity than doxorubicin, have substituted mitoxantrone for doxorubicin, or have used short-duration weekly therapy.[121]

Over the past few years, several nonrandomized and randomized trials have evaluated different treatment approaches in older patients with aggressive NHL.[121] The results of these studies suggest that carefully selected elderly patients with good performance status and without significant comorbidities can tolerate aggressive anthracycline-containing regimens as well as younger patients. These patients should be treated initially with full-dose R-CHOP or similar regimens; dosages can be reduced later if severe toxicity occurs. Hematopoietic growth factors may allow elderly patients to maintain dose intensity.

The combination therapy, R-CHOP, has replaced CHOP as standard treatment for elderly patients with aggressive lymphoma, based on the results of the Groupe d'Etude des Lymphomes de l'Adulte (GELA) study.[128,129] In that study of 399 elderly patients with DLBCL, patients who were randomized to receive R-CHOP had a significantly higher complete response rate (76% vs. 63%) and longer event-free and overall survival as compared with those who received CHOP. After 10 years of followup, progression-free survival was significantly longer among those who received R-CHOP than CHOP (36.5% vs. 20.1%).[129] A higher risk of death or development of secondary cancer was not observed with the additional of rituximab to CHOP after 10 years of followup. In another randomized controlled trial conducted primarily in the United States (Eastern Cooperative Oncology Group 4494), elderly (≥60 years old) patients who received rituximab, either as induction or maintenance with CHOP chemotherapy, had significantly longer failure-free survival as compared with those not given rituximab during their treatment course.[135] Maintenance therapy with single-agent rituximab did not provide any additional benefit in patients who received R-CHOP as induction therapy. It is important to note that rituximab is given differently in the two studies. In the GELA study, rituximab is given on day 1 (the same day that cyclophosphamide, doxorubicin, and vincristine are administered) with each cycle of CHOP chemotherapy.[128,129] In the Eastern Cooperative Oncology Group 4494 study,[135] R-CHOP was modeled after the regimen developed by Czuczman et al.: Two doses of rituximab are given before cycle 1, and one dose is given before cycles 3, 5, and 7 (if administered).[93] In most NHL protocols and in clinical practice, rituximab is given on day 1 of CHOP chemotherapy.[98]

Dose-dense chemotherapy, where the interval between cycles is shortened from 3 weeks to 2 weeks has been evaluated. Before the rituximab era, patients who were randomized to receive biweekly CHOP (CHOP-14) had significantly longer 5-year event-free and overall survival than patients who received standard CHOP every 21 days (CHOP-21).[136] All patients in the CHOP-14 group received prophylactic growth factors starting from day 4. Toxicity was similar between the two groups. In the next study, the same group of investigators evaluated the addition of rituximab (CHOP-14 vs. R-CHOP-14) and the number of treatment cycles (six vs. eight cycles).[137] Patients who received rituximab did better than those who did not, and eight cycles were not better than six cycles. The addition of rituximab to the CHOP-14 regimen resulted in significantly longer 3-year event-free and overall survival (67% vs. 47% and 78% vs. 68%, respectively). Emerging data in the rituximab era, however, suggested that R-CHOP-21 remains the standard treatment regimen when compared against R-CHOP-14 for treatment of DLBCL. The NCCN guideline does not recommend dose-dense R-CHOP (R-CHOP-14) as first-line therapy for DLBCL.[65]

Treatment of Refractory or Relapsed Disease Although many patients with aggressive NHL experience long-term survival and cure with intensive chemotherapy, about 10% to 20% of patients fail to achieve a complete remission and, of those patients who do achieve a complete remission, about 20% to 30% subsequently relapse. Therefore, about 30% to 40% of all patients with aggressive NHL will require salvage therapy at some point during their disease course. Response to salvage therapy depends on the initial responsiveness of the tumor to chemotherapy. Patients who achieve an initial complete remission and then relapse generally have a better response to salvage therapy than those who are primarily or partially resistant to chemotherapy.

Many conventional-dose salvage chemotherapy regimens have been used in patients with relapsed or refractory NHL. Many patients who respond to salvage therapy (i.e., chemosensitive relapse) will then receive high-dose chemotherapy with autologous HSCT. In an effort to avoid cross-resistance, most salvage regimens incorporate drugs not used in the initial therapy. Some of the more commonly used salvage regimens include dexamethasone, cytarabine, cisplatin (DHAP), etoposide, methylprednisolone, cytarabine, cisplatin (ESHAP), and mesna, ifosfamide, mitoxantrone, etoposide (MINE), and no one regimen appears to be clearly superior to any other regimen.[121] Rituximab is sometimes added to these salvage regimens. With these salvage regimens, about 30% to 50% of patients achieve a complete response, with a median duration of remission of 1 to 2 years. Only about 5% to 10% of patients will have long-term disease-free survival.

Ifosfamide, carboplatin, and etoposide (ICE) chemotherapy is a newer regimen that has been used in patients with refractory disease. Some clinicians believe that ICE is better tolerated than older cisplatin-based regimens, particularly in older patients. The combination of ICE and rituximab (RICE) is currently being evaluated as a salvage regimen, and early results are encouraging.[120] It is recommended, however, to exclude rituximab in second-line therapy if patient's disease is refractory or if the duration of remission is less than 6 months. One recent study (CORAL study) has compared two salvage regimens (R-ICE and R-DHAP) that are used for treatment of patients with relapsed or refractory DLBCL, followed by autologous HSCT.[138] No significant difference was detected between R-ICE and R-DHAP for 3-year event-free survival or overall survival. However, poor prognosis was observed among patients who have received prior rituximab treatment and if they have experienced early relapse (defined as less than 12 months after diagnosis). This suggests that new treatment strategies are needed in order to improve the response rates of salvage regimens.

⓬ To improve the cure rate, many studies have evaluated high-dose chemotherapy with autologous HSCT as intensive consolidation therapy in patients who respond to salvage therapy.[139] In the PARMA study, 215 patients with relapsed aggressive NHL who had a response to DHAP salvage therapy were randomized to receive either high-dose chemotherapy or continued DHAP therapy.[140] Patients who received high-dose chemotherapy had significantly longer 5-year disease-free survival (46% vs. 12%) and overall survival (53% vs. 32%) than those treated with conventional salvage therapy. Further analysis of that study showed that patients who relapsed within 12 months of their initial diagnosis were less likely to benefit from high-dose chemotherapy than patients who relapsed after 12 months. Based on a review of the available evidence, including the PARMA study, high-dose chemotherapy with autologous HSCT is considered to be the treatment of choice in younger patients with chemotherapy-sensitive relapse.[65] High-dose chemotherapy with autologous HSCT is not recommended in patients with untested or chemotherapy-refractory relapse.

Rituximab is being evaluated in the setting of autologous HSCT. It can be given pretransplant as an in vivo purging agent prior to stem cell collection and as posttransplant consolidation.[139]

Other Aggressive Lymphomas

Mantle cell lymphoma (MCL) is one of the new disease entities that was previously unrecognized by other classification systems.[141] This histologic type was found in 6% of cases in the International Lymphoma Classification Project.[80] The chromosomal translocation t(11;14) occurs in most cases of MCL. MCL usually occurs in older adults, particularly in men, and most patients have advanced disease at the time of diagnosis (Table 109-6). Extranodal involvement is found in about 90% of cases. The course of the disease is moderately aggressive; the median overall survival is about 3 years, with no evidence of a survival plateau.

Patients with disseminated MCL are usually treated with the same intensive combination chemotherapy regimens that are used in diffuse aggressive lymphomas. One widely used combination regimen is cyclophosphamide, vincristine, doxorubicin, dexamethasone alternating with methotrexate and cytarabine (hyperCVAD) with or without rituximab. Overall response rates to these regimens is about 90%, with about two-thirds of patients achieving a complete response.[141] Because MCL usually expresses CD20, rituximab, either alone or combined with CHOP and bendamustine, has been used with some success in patients with newly diagnosed and relapsed MCL.[97,142] In a meta-analysis of randomized controlled trials, the addition of rituximab to combination chemotherapy was associated with improved overall survival (HR 0.60).[97] Despite the high response rates, MCL is not considered curable with standard chemotherapy. Consequently, younger patients who have an initial response to chemotherapy often undergo autologous or allogeneic HSCT as consolidation therapy. The NCCN guideline recommends that patients with advanced-stage MCL be treated initially with rituximab and combination chemotherapy, followed by autologous HSCT as first-line consolidation therapy.[65] Unfortunately, most patients with MCL eventually relapse and are treated with salvage therapy or enrolled in trials of investigational agents, some of which are aimed at molecular targets. Bortezomib (Velcade®) is currently approved for treatment of patients with MCL that has relapsed after at least one prior therapy based on the results of a phase II study that showed a 33% response rate.[143] Ibrutinib, an oral Bruton tyrosine kinase (BTK) inhibitor is currently investigated for treatment of relapsed or refractory MCL. In a Phase 2 study, ibrutinib had demonstrated a high response rate of 68%, with majority of the patients receiving three prior therapies.[144]

Non-Hodgkin Lymphoma in Acquired Immune Deficiency Syndrome

The risk of NHL for patients with AIDS is increased more than 100-fold as compared with the general population.[145,146] AIDS-related lymphoma arises as a consequence of long-term stimulation and proliferation of B lymphocytes from HIV and the reactivation of prior EBV infection as a consequence of HIV-induced immunosuppression. AIDS-related lymphoma usually occurs late in the course of HIV infection and is the cause of death in about 15% of HIV-infected individuals. Although HIV infects T cells, more than 95% of AIDS-related lymphomas are B-cell neoplasms. Most cases of AIDS-related lymphomas are classified as Burkitt or DLBCL.

The clinical presentation is similar to that observed in other immunocompromised states. Most patients with AIDS-related lymphoma present with B symptoms and have advanced-stage

(III or IV) disease at the time of diagnosis.[145] Involvement of extranodal sites is common. The clinical course of AIDS-related lymphoma is usually aggressive and has improved with the availability of highly active antiretroviral therapy (HAART). Improved survival has been observed, primarily in patients with DLBCL. Patients with AIDS-related lymphoma treated with intensive therapy have a median survival that is similar to the survival of patients with HIV-negative NHLs.[146] In the post-HAART era, many of the prognostic factors have also changed and only lymphoma-related factors such as the IPI remain as independent predictors of prognosis.

The treatment of patients with AIDS-associated lymphomas is difficult because the immunocompromised state of these patients increases their risk of significant toxicity as a consequence of myelosuppressive therapy. Except for primary CNS lymphoma, AIDS-related lymphoma is never considered truly localized and systemic chemotherapy is indicated. For patients with adequate immune function and without a history of an opportunistic infection, chemotherapy regimens similar to that used for aggressive lymphomas may be used.[65] However, many patients with AIDS-related lymphoma were previously treated with less-intensive regimens because of the increased risk of treatment-related toxicity. In the post-HAART era, however, most clinicians believe that standard doses of chemotherapy can be safely administered to patients who achieve a virologic response to HAART.

The results of treatment with standard chemotherapy regimens have been disappointing, particularly in patients with Burkitt lymphoma. In patients with DLBCL, the complete response rate with combination chemotherapy is about 40% to 50%, with 5-year overall survival rates of about 20% to 30%. Newer approaches, such as the dose-adjusted etoposide, prednisone, vincristine, cyclophosphamide, and doxorubicin (EPOCH) regimen developed at the National Cancer Institute, appear promising. The role of rituximab in the treatment of AIDS-related DLBCL is not clear. In a randomized trial of CHOP versus R-CHOP, no significant differences in progression-free and overall survival were observed.[147] However, 14% of patients treated with R-CHOP died of treatment-related infection as compared with only 2% of those in the CHOP group. NCCN guidelines suggest omission of rituximab in patients at high risk for serious infectious complications.[65]

The optimal timing for HAART is not clear in patients with AIDS-related lymphoma.[145,146] If HAART is given concurrently with chemotherapy, patients should be monitored closely for possible pharmacokinetic interactions between HAART and chemotherapy. Some experts suggest that HAART should be withheld until the completion of chemotherapy to allow administration of full chemotherapy doses and to avoid the risk of pharmacokinetic interactions. Prophylactic antibiotics should be continued during chemotherapy and intrathecal chemotherapy should be administered to prevent CNS relapses.

PERSONALIZED PHARMACOTHERAPY

Molecular testing of the lymphoma cells at the time of diagnosis is an essential part of the diagnostic work-up. Molecular subtypes have been identified that predict for survival. For example, two molecular subtypes of DLBCL have been identified, and the ABC subtype appears to be less responsive to chemotherapy than the GCB subtype. Another molecular subtype associated with poor response is double-hit DLBCL, defined as the existence of both MYC gene arrangement and t(14;18) BCL2 translocation.

In addition to disease stage, several prognostic indices such as IPS, IPI and FLIPI are used clinically for predicting response to therapy and survival in individual patients. The results of these evaluations form the basis for risk-adapted therapy, where the intensity of the recommended therapy is tailored to the risk category of the patient. More intensive therapy is generally recommended for higher risk patients, particularly when long-term survival or cure is the treatment goal.

Age or comorbidities often limit the use of chemotherapy regimens. Patients with poor cardiac function may not be able to receive doxorubicin, an important component of combination regimens used to treat both Hodgkin lymphoma and NHL. Patients with preexisting diabetic neuropathy or who develop peripheral neuropathy during chemotherapy may not be able to receive all of their planned doses of vinca alkaloids, particularly vincristine. Most patients with NHL are elderly and these patients may not tolerate the toxicities of intensive chemotherapy regimens. Dosage adjustments or treatment delays may be required.

Interim PET scans are currently being investigated as a biomarker of early response in patients with advanced-stage Hodgkin lymphoma. If validated, PET scans may allow clinicians to decide which patients should receive treatment intensification and which patients should have their treatment discontinued.

EVALUATION OF THERAPEUTIC OUTCOMES

Hodgkin and NHLs tend to respond well to radiation, chemotherapy, and biologic therapy. The goal of therapy for patients with Hodgkin lymphoma and aggressive NHL is long-term survival and cure. The therapeutic goal in patients with indolent NHLs is less clear because of the indolent nature of the disease and the lack of convincing evidence showing that therapy prolongs survival. Therapeutic responses should be evaluated based on physical examination, radiologic evidence, PET/CT scanning, and other positive findings at baseline. Patients with Hodgkin lymphoma and aggressive NHLs are usually evaluated for response at the end of four cycles of therapy or at the end of treatment if fewer than four cycles of therapy are planned. If patients are treated with chemotherapy alone, two additional cycles of chemotherapy are given after the patient has achieved a complete remission. Recent studies have also shown that early interim PET scans may possess prognostic value in patients with advanced Hodgkin lymphoma. The rapidity of response to therapy in patients with indolent NHL depends on the choice of therapy. Responses occur slowly with therapy with oral alkylating agents, but occur much more rapidly with aggressive therapies such as combination chemotherapy with or without rituximab. If radiation alone is used, then a therapeutic evaluation should occur at the end of treatment.

ABBREVIATIONS

ABC	activated B-cell–like
ABV	doxorubicin (Adriamycin®), bleomycin, vinblastine
ABVD	doxorubicin (Adriamycin®), bleomycin, vinblastine, and dacarbazine
ADC	antibody-drug conjugate
AIDS	acquired immune deficiency syndrome
BEACOPP	bleomycin, etoposide, doxorubicin (Adriamycin®), cyclophosphamide, vincristine (Oncovin®), procarbazine, and prednisone
BR	bendamustine and rituximab
BVR	bendamustine, rituximab, and bortezomib
CEC	cyclophosphamide, lomustine, vindesine, melphalan, prednisone, epirubicin, vincristine, procarbazine, vinblastine, bleomycin

CHOP	cyclophosphamide, doxorubicin, vincristine (Oncovin®), prednisone
CNS	central nervous system
COP	cyclophosphamide, vincristine (Oncovin®), and prednisone or prednisolone
COPP	cyclophosphamide, vincristine, procarbazine, and prednisone
CT	computed tomography
CVP	cyclophosphamide, vincristine, and prednisone
DHAP	dexamethasone, cytarabine, cisplatin
DLBCL	diffuse large B-cell lymphoma
EBV	Epstein-Barr's virus
EPOCH	etoposide, prednisone, vincristine, cyclophosphamide, and doxorubicin
ESHAP	etoposide, methylprednisolone, cytarabine, cisplatin
FDA	Food and Drug Administration
FLIPI	Follicular Lymphoma International Prognostic Index
FN	fludarabine and mitoxantrone
FND	fludarabine, mitoxantrone, and dexamethasone
GCB	germinal center B-cell–like
GELA	Groupe d'Etude des Lymphomes de l'Adulte
GHSG	German Hodgkin Study Group
HAART	highly active antiretroviral therapy
HIV	human immunodeficiency virus
HLA	human leukocyte antigen
HR	hazard ratio
HSCT	hematopoietic stem cell transplantation
hyperCVAD	cyclophosphamide, vincristine, doxorubicin, dexamethasone alternating with methotrexate and cytarabine
ICE	ifosfamide, carboplatin, and etoposide
IPI	International Prognostic Index
IPS	International Prognostic Score
JAK–STAT	Janus kinase–signal transduction and transcription
KSHV	Kaposi sarcoma–associated herpesvirus
LDH	lactate dehydrogenase
MALT	mucosa-associated lymphoid tissue
MCL	mantle cell lymphoma
MINE	mesna, ifosfamide, mitoxantrone, etoposide
MMAE	monomethyl auristatin E
MOPP	mechlorethamine, vincristine, procarbazine, and prednisone
MOPPEBVCAD	mechlorethamine, vincristine, procarbazine, prednisone, epidoxorubicin, bleomycin, vinblastine, lomustine, doxorubicin, and vindesine
NCCN	National Comprehensive Cancer Network
NHL	non-Hodgkin lymphoma
PET	positron emission tomography
R-CHOP	rituximab, cyclophosphamide, doxorubicin, vincristine (Oncovin®), prednisone
R-FCM	rituximab, fludarabine, cyclophosphamide, and mitoxantrone
REAL	Revised European-American Classification of Lymphoid Neoplasms
RICE	rituximab, ifosfamide, carboplatin, and etoposide
SEER	Surveillance, Epidemiology, and End Results
SWOG	Southwest Oncology Group
WHO	World Health Organization

REFERENCES

1. Diehl V, Re D, Harris NL, Mauch PM. Hodgkin Lymphoma. In: DeVita VT, Jr., Hellman S, Rosenberg SA, eds. Cancer: Principles & Practice of Oncology. Philadelphia, PA: Lippincott Williams & Wilkins, 2008:2167–2220.
2. Townsend W, Linch D. Hodgkin's lymphoma in adults. Lancet 2012;380:836–847.
3. Horning SJ. Hodgkin's lymphoma. In: Abeloff MD, Armitage JO, Niederhuber JE, Kastan MB, McKenna WG, eds. Abeloff's Clinical Oncology. 4th ed. New York, NY: Churchill Livingstone, 2008:2353–2370.
4. Siegel R, Naishadham D, Jemal A. Cancer statistics, 2013. CA Cancer J Clin 2013;63:11–30.
5. Howlader N, Noone AM, Krapcho M, et al. SEER Cancer Statistics Review, 1975–2009. 2012, http://seer.cancer.gov/csr/1975_2009_pops09/.
6. Ng AK, Bernardo MP, Weller E, et al. Long-term survival and competing causes of death in patients with early-stage Hodgkin's disease treated at age 50 or younger. J Clin Oncol 2002;20:2101–2108.
7. Ambinder RF. Infectious etiology of lymphoma. In: Armitage JO, Mauch PM, Harris NL, Coiffier B, Dalla-Favera R, eds. Non-Hodgkin Lymphoma. 2nd ed. Philadelphia, PA: Lippincott Williams & Wilkins, 2010:83–101.
8. Hjalgrim H, Engels EA. Infectious aetiology of Hodgkin and non-Hodgkin lymphomas: A review of the epidemiological evidence. J Intern Med 2008;264:537–548.
9. Küppers R. New insights in the biology of Hodgkin lymphoma. Hematology Am Soc Hematol Educ Program 2012:328–334.
10. Mack TM, Cozen W, Shibata DK, et al. Concordance for Hodgkin's disease in identical twins suggesting genetic susceptibility to the young-adult form of the disease. N Engl J Med 1995;332:413–418.
11. Jaffe ES, Harris NL, Stein H, Isaacson PG. Classification of lymphoid neoplasms: The microscope as a tool for disease discovery. Blood 2008;112:4384–4399.
12. Papadaki T, Stamatopoulos K. Hodgkin disease immunopathogenesis: long-standing questions, recent answers, further directions. Trends Immunol 2003;24:508–511.
13. Swerdlow SH, Campo E, Harris NL, et al. WHO Classification of Tumours of Haematopoietic and Lymphoid Tissues. 4th ed. Lyon, France: IARC Press, 2008.
14. Mauch PM, Kalish LA, Kadin M, Coleman CN, Osteen R, Hellman S. Patterns of presentation of Hodgkin disease. Implications for etiology and pathogenesis. Cancer 1993;71:2062–2071.
15. Oncology NCPGi. Hodgkin Disease/Lymphoma, version 2.2012. 2012, *http://www.nccn.org*.
16. Connor JM. Positron emission tomography in the management of Hodgkin lymphoma. Hematology Am Soc Hematol Educ Program 2011:317–322.
17. Proctor SJ, Wilkinson J, Sieniawski M. Hodgkin lymphoma in the elderly: A clinical review of treatment and outcome, past, present and future. Crit Rev Oncol Hematol 2009;71:222–232.
18. Hasenclever D, Diehl V. A prognostic score for advanced Hodgkin's disease. International Prognostic Factors Project on Advanced Hodgkin's Disease. N Engl J Med 1998;339:1506–1514.
19. Advani R. Optimal therapy of advanced Hodgkin lymphoma. Hematology Am Soc Hematol Educ Program 2011:310–316.
20. Hodgson DC. Late effects in the era of modern therapy for Hodgkin lymphoma. Hematology Am Soc Hematol Educ Program 2011:323–329.

21. Meyer RM, Hoppe RT. Point/counterpoint: Early-stage Hodgkin lymphoma and the role of radiation therapy. Hematology Am Soc Hematol Educ Program 2012: 313–321.
22. Armitage JO. Early-stage Hodgkin lymphoma. N Engl J Med 2010;363:653–662.
23. Evens AM, Hutchings M, Diehl V. Treatment of Hodgkin lymphoma: The past, present, and future. Nat Clin Pract Oncol 2008;5:543–556.
24. Abuzetun JY, Loberiza F, Vose J, et al. The Stanford V regimen is effective in patients with good risk Hodgkin lymphoma but radiotherapy is a necessary component. Br J Haematol 2009;144:531–537.
25. Engert A, Plutschow A, Eich HT, et al. Reduced treatment intensity in patients with early-stage Hodgkin's lymphoma. N Engl J Med 2010;363:640–652.
26. Specht L, Gray RG, Clarke MJ, Peto R. Influence of more extensive radiotherapy and adjuvant chemotherapy on long-term outcome of early stage Hodgkin's disease: A meta-analysis of 23 randomized trials involving 3,888 patients. International Hodgkin's Disease Collaborative Group. J Clin Oncol 1998;16:830–843.
27. Engert A, Schiller P, Josting A, et al. Involved-field radiotherapy is equally effective and less toxic compared with extended-field radiotherapy after four cycles of chemotherapy in patients with early-stage unfavorable Hodgkin's lymphoma: Results of the HD8 trial of the German Hodgkin's Lymphoma Study Group. J Clin Oncol 2003;21:3601–3608.
28. Bonnadonna G, Zucali R, Monfardini S, De Lena M, Uslenghi C. Combination therapy of Hodgkin's disease with Adriamycin, bleomycin, vinblastine, and imidazole carboxamide versus MOPP. Cancer 1975;36:252–259.
29. Canellos GP, Anderson JR, Propert KJ, et al. Chemotherapy of advanced Hodgkin's disease with MOPP, ABVD, or MOPP alternating with ABVD. N Engl J Med 1992;327:1478–1484.
30. Goldie JH, Coldman AJ, Gudauskas GA. Rationale for the use of alternating non-cross-resistant chemotherapy. Cancer Treat Rep 1982;66:439–449.
31. Glick JH, Young ML, Harrington D, et al. MOPP/ABV hybrid chemotherapy for advanced Hodgkin's disease significantly improves failure-free and overall survival: The 8-year results of the intergroup trial. J Clin Oncol 1998;16:19–26.
32. Duggan DB, Petroni GR, Johnson JL, et al. Randomized comparison of ABVD and MOPP/ABV hybrid for the treatment of advanced Hodgkin's disease: Report of an intergroup trial. J Clin Oncol 2003;21:607–614.
33. Horning SJ, Hoppe RT, Breslin S, Bartlett NL, Brown BW, Rosenberg SA. Stanford V and radiotherapy for locally extensive and advanced Hodgkin's disease: Mature results of a prospective clinical trial. J Clin Oncol 2002;20:630–637.
34. Gobbi PG, Levis A, Chisesi T, et al. ABVD versus modified Stanford V versus MOPPEBVCAD with optional and limited radiotherapy in intermediate- and advanced-stage Hodgkin's lymphoma: Final results of a multicenter randomized trial by the Intergruppo Italiano Linfomi. J Clin Oncol 2005;23:9198–9207.
35. Hoskin PJ, Lowry L, Horwich A, et al. Randomized comparison of the Stanford V regimen and ABVD in the treatment of advanced Hodgkin's Lymphoma: United Kingdom National Cancer Research Institute Lymphoma Group Study ISRCTN 64141244. J Clin Oncol 2009;27:5390–5396.
36. Klimm B, Diehl V, Pfistner B, Engert A. Current treatment strategies of the German Hodgkin Study Group (GHSG). Eur J Haematol 2005 (suppl s66);75:125–134.
37. Diehl V, Franklin J, Pfreundschuh M, et al. Standard and increased-dose BEACOPP chemotherapy compared with COPP-ABVD for advanced Hodgkin's disease. N Engl J Med 2003;348:2386–2395.
38. Engert A, Diehl V, Franklin J, Lohri A, Dorken B. Escalated-dose BEACOPP in the treatment of patients with advanced-stage Hodgkin's Lymphoma: 10 Years of follow-up of the GHSG HD9 study. J Clin Oncol 2009;27:4548–4554.
39. Ballova V, Ruffer JU, Haverkamp H, et al. A prospectively randomized trial carried out by the German Hodgkin Study Group (GHSG) for elderly patients with advanced Hodgkin's disease comparing BEACOPP baseline and COPP-ABVD (study HD9 elderly). Ann Oncol 2005;16:124–131.
40. Federico M, Luminari S, Iannitto E, et al. ABVD compared with BEACOPP compared with CEC for the initial treatment of patients with advanced Hodgkin's lymphoma: Results from the HD2000 Gruppo Italiano per lo Studio dei Linfomi Trial. J Clin Oncol 2009;27:805–811.
41. Borchmann P, Haverkamp H, Diehl V, et al. Eight cycles of escalated-dose BEACOPP compared with four cycles of escalated-dose BEACOPP followed by four cycles of baseline-dose BEACOPP with or without radiotherapy in patients with advanced-stage Hodgkin's lymphoma: Final analysis of the HD12 trial of the German Hodgkin Study Group. J Clin Oncol 2011;29:4234–4242.
42. Engert A, Haverkamp H, Kobe C, et al. Reduced-intensity chemotherapy and PET-guided radiotherapy in patients with advanced stage Hodgkin's lymphoma (HD15 trial): A randomised, open-label, phase 3 non-inferiority trial. Lancet 2012;379:1791–1799.
43. Dann EJ, Bar-Shalom R, Tamir A, et al. Risk-adapted BEACOPP regimen can reduce the cumulative dose of chemotherapy for standard and high-risk Hodgkin lymphoma with no impairment of outcome. Blood 2007;109:905–909.
44. Prosnitz LR. Consolidation radiotherapy in the treatment of advanced Hodgkin's disease: Is it dead? Int J Radiat Oncol Biol Phys 2003;56:605–608.
45. Loeffler M, Brosteanu O, Hasenclever D, et al. Meta-analysis of chemotherapy versus combined modality treatment trials in Hodgkin's disease. International Database on Hodgkin's Disease Overview Study Group. J Clin Oncol 1998;16: 818–829.
46. Aleman BM, Raemaekers JM, Tomisic R, et al. Involved-field radiotherapy for patients in partial remission after chemotherapy for advanced Hodgkin's lymphoma. Int J Radiat Oncol Biol Phys 2007;67:19–30.
47. Brice P. Managing relapsed and refractory Hodgkin lymphoma. Br J Haematol 2008;141:3–13.
48. Majhail NS, Weisdorf DJ, Defor TE, et al. Long-term results of autologous stem cell transplantation for primary refractory or relapsed Hodgkin's lymphoma. Biol Blood Marrow Transplant 2006;12:1065–1072.
49. Seyfarth B, Josting A, Dreyling M, Schmitz N. Relapse in common lymphoma subtypes: salvage treatment options for follicular lymphoma, diffuse large B-cell lymphoma and Hodgkin disease. Br J Haematol 2006;133:3–18.
50. Kulkarni SS, Sastry PS, Saikia TK, et al. Gonadal function following ABVD therapy for Hodgkin's disease. Am J Clin Oncol 1997;20:354–357.
51. de Claro RA, McGinn KM, Kwitkowski VE, et al. U.S. Food and Drug Administration approval summary: Brentuximab vedotin for the treatment of relapsed Hodgkin lymphoma or relapsed systemic anaplastic large cell lymphoma. Clin Cancer Res 2012;18:5855–5859.
52. Younes A, Gopal AK, Smith SE, et al. Results of a pivotal phase II study of brentuximab vedotin for patients with

relapsed or refractory Hodgkin's lymphoma. J Clin Oncol 2012;30:2183–2189.
53. Dores GM, Metayer C, Curtis RE, et al. Second malignant neoplasms among long-term survivors of Hodgkin's disease: A population-based evaluation over 25 years. J Clin Oncol 2002;20:3484–3494.
54. Franklin J, Pluetschow A, Paus M, et al. Second malignancy risk associated with treatment of Hodgkin's lymphoma: Meta-analysis of the randomised trials. Ann Oncol 2006;17:1749–1760.
55. Swerdlow AJ, Higgins CD, Smith P, et al. Second cancer risk after chemotherapy for Hodgkin's lymphoma: A collaborative British cohort study. J Clin Oncol 2011;29:4096–4104.
56. Travis LB. Evaluation of the risk of therapy-associated complications in survivors of Hodgkin lymphoma. Hematology Am Soc Hematol Educ Program 2007: 192–196.
57. Wang SS, Hartge P. Epidemiology. In: Armitage JO, Mauch PM, Harris NL, Coiffier B, Dalla-Favera R, eds. Non-Hodgkin Lymphoma. 2nd ed. Philadelphia, PA: Lippincott Williams & Wilkins, 2010:64–82.
58. Dalla-Favera R, Pasqualucci L. Molecular genetics of lymphoma. In: Armitage JO, Mauch PM, Harris NL, Coiffier B, Dalla-Favera R, eds. Non-Hodgkin Lymphoma. 2nd ed. Philadelphia, PA: Lippincott Williams & Wilkins, 2010: 115–130.
59. Wilson WH, Armitage JO. Non-Hodgkin's lymphoma. In: Abeloff MD, Armitage JO, Niederhuber JE, Kastan MB, McKenna WG, eds. Abeloff's Clinical Oncology. 4th ed. New York, NY: Churchill Livingstone, 2008:2371–2404.
60. Reeder CB, Ansell SM. Novel therapeutic agents for B-cell lymphoma: developing rational combinations. Blood 2011;117:1453–1462.
61. Swerdlow S, Campo E, Harris NL, et al., eds. World Health Organization Classification of Tumours of Haematopoietic and Lymphoid tissues. Lyon: IARC Press, 2008.
62. Harris NL. History and classification of lymphoid malignancies. In: Armitage JO, Mauch PM, Harris NL, Coiffier B, Dalla-Favera R, eds. Non-Hodgkin Lymphoma. Philadelphia, PA: Lippincott Williams & Wilkins, 2010: xv–xxix.
63. Lenz G, Staudt LM. Aggressive lymphomas. N Engl J Med 2010;362:1417–1429.
64. Harris NL, Jaffe ES, Diebold J, et al. World Health Organization Classification of neoplastic diseases of the hematopoietic and lymphoid tissues: Report of the Clinical Advisory Committee meeting—Airlie House, Virginia, November 1997. J Clin Oncol 1999;17:3835–3849.
65. Oncology NCPGi. Non-Hodgkin's Lymphoma, version 1.2013. 2013, *http://www.nccn.org*.
66. Cheson BD, Pfistner B, Juweid ME, et al. Revised response criteria for malignant lymphoma. J Clin Oncol 2007;25: 579–586.
67. The International Non-Hodgkin's Lymphoma Prognostic Factors Project. A predictive model for aggressive non-Hodgkin's lymphoma. N Engl J Med 1993;329:987–994.
68. Sehn LH, Berry B, Chhanabhai M, et al. The revised International Prognostic Index (R-IPI) is a better predictor of outcome than the standard IPI for patients with diffuse large B-cell lymphoma treated with R-CHOP. Blood 2007;109:1857–1861.
69. Solal-Celigny P, Roy P, Colombat P, et al. Follicular lymphoma international prognostic index. Blood 2004;104:1258–1265.
70. Federico M, Bellei M, Marcheselli L, et al. Follicular lymphoma international prognostic index 2: a new prognostic index for follicular lymphoma developed by the international follicular lymphoma prognostic factor project. J Clin Oncol 2009;27:4555–4562.
71. Sehn LH. Paramount prognostic factors that guide therapeutic strategies in diffuse large B-cell lymphoma. Hematology Am Soc Hematol Educ Program 2012: 402–409.
72. Rosenwald A, Wright G, Chan WC, et al. The use of molecular profiling to predict survival after chemotherapy for diffuse large-B-cell lymphoma. N Engl J Med 2002;346:1937–1947.
73. Lenz G, Wright G, Dave SS, et al. Stromal gene signatures in large-B-cell lymphomas. N Engl J Med 2008;359: 2313–2323.
74. Aukema SM, Siebert R, Schuuring E, et al. Double-hit B-cell lymphomas. Blood 2011;117:2319–2331.
75. Green TM, Young KH, Visco C, et al. Immunohistochemical double-hit score is a strong predictor of outcome in patients with diffuse large b-cell lymphoma treated with rituximab plus cyclophosphamide, doxorubicin, vincristine, and prednisone. J Clin Oncol 2012;30:3460–3467.
76. Dave SS, Wright G, Tan B, et al. Prediction of survival in follicular lymphoma based on molecular features of tumor-infiltrating immune cells. N Engl J Med 2004;351: 2159–2169.
77. Cheson BD, Leonard JP. Monoclonal antibody therapy for B-cell non-Hodgkin's lymphoma. N Engl J Med 2008;359:613–626.
78. Maloney DG. Anti-CD20 antibody therapy for B-cell lymphomas. N Engl J Med 2012;366:2008–2016.
79. Freedman AS, Friedberg JW, Mauch PM, Dalla-Favera R, Harris NL. Follicular lymphoma. In: Armitage JO, Mauch PM, Harris NL, Coiffier B, Dalla-Favera R, eds. Non-Hodgkin's Lymphoma. 2nd ed. Philadelphia, PA: Lippincott Williams & Wilkins, 2010:266–283.
80. The Non-Hodgkin's Lymphoma Classification Project. A clinical evaluation of the International Lymphoma Study Group classification of non-Hodgkin's lymphoma. Blood 1997;89:3909–3918.
81. Horning SJ. Natural history of and therapy for the indolent non-Hodgkin's lymphomas. Semin Oncol 1993;20 (suppl 5): 75–88.
82. Bernstein SH, Burack WR. The incidence, natural history, biology, and treatment of transformed lymphoma. Hematology Am Soc Hematol Educ Program 2009:532–541.
83. Fisher RI, LeBlanc M, Press OW, et al. New treatment options have changed the survival of patients with follicular lymphomas. J Clin Oncol 2005;23:8477–8452.
84. Liu Q, Fayad L, Cabanillas F, et al. Improvement of overall and failure-free survival in stage IV follicular lymphoma: 25 Years of treatment experience at the University of Texas M.D. Anderson Cancer Center. J Clin Oncol 2006;24: 1582–1589.
85. Seymour JF, Pro B, Fuller LM, et al. Long-term follow-up of a prospective study of combined modality therapy for stage I–II indolent non-Hodgkin's lymphoma. J Clin Oncol 2003;21:2115–2122.
86. Gribben JG. How I treat indolent lymphoma. Blood 2007;109:4617–4626.
87. Freedman AS, Friedberg JW. Approach to the diagnosis of non-Hodgkin's lymphoma. In: Rose BD, ed. UpToDate. Waltham, MA, 2009.
88. Ardeshna KM, Smith P, Norton A, et al. Long-term effect of a watch and wait policy versus immediate systemic treatment for asymptomatic advanced-stage non-Hodgkin's lymphoma: A randomised controlled trial. Lancet 2003;362:516–522.

89. McLaughlin P, Grillo-Lopez AJ, Link BK, et al. Rituximab chimeric anti-CD20 monoclonal antibody therapy for relapsed indolent lymphoma: Half of patients respond to a four-dose treatment program. J Clin Oncol 1998;16:2825–2833.
90. Cohen Y, Solal-Celigny P, Polliack A. Rituximab therapy for follicular lymphoma: A comprehensive review of its efficacy as primary treatment, treatment for relapsed disease, re-treatment and maintenance. Haematologica 2003;88:811–823.
91. Cvetkovic RS, Perry CM. Rituximab: A review of its use in non-Hodgkin's lymphoma and chronic lymphocytic leukemia. Drugs 2006;66:791–820.
92. Friedberg JW, Taylor MD, Cerhan JR, et al. Follicular lymphoma in the United States: First report of the National LymphoCare Study. J Clin Oncol 2009;27:1202–1208.
93. Czuczman MS, Grillo-Lopez AJ, White CA, et al. Treatment of patients with low-grade B-cell lymphoma with the combination of chimeric anti-CD20 monoclonal antibody and CHOP chemotherapy. J Clin Oncol 1999;17:268–276.
94. Czuczman MS, Weaver R, Alkuzweny B, Berlfein J, Grillo-Lopez AJ. Prolonged clinical and molecular remission in patients with low-grade or follicular non-Hodgkin's lymphoma treated with rituximab plus CHOP chemotherapy: 9-Year follow-up. J Clin Oncol 2004;22:4711–4716.
95. Hiddemann W, Kneba M, Dreyling M, et al. Frontline therapy with rituximab added to the combination of cyclophosphamide, doxorubicin, vincristine, and prednisone (CHOP) significantly improves the outcome for patients with advanced-stage follicular lymphoma compared with therapy with CHOP alone: Results of a prospective randomized study of the German Low-Grade Lymphoma Study Group. Blood 2005;106:3725–3732.
96. van Oers MHJ, Klasa R, Marcus RE, et al. Rituximab maintenance improves clinical outcome of relapsed/resistant follicular lymphoma non-Hodgkin's lymphoma in patients both with and without rituximab during induction: Results of a prospective randomized phase 3 intergroup trial. Blood 2006;108:3295–3301.
97. Schulz H, Bohlius JF, Trelle S, et al. Immunochemotherapy with rituximab and overall survival in patients with indolent or mantle cell lymphoma: A systematic review and meta-analysis. J Natl Cancer Inst 2007;99:706–714.
98. Ghielmini M. Multimodality therapies and optimal schedule of antibodies: Rituximab in lymphoma as an example. Hematology Am Soc Hematol Educ Program 2005:321–328.
99. Hochster H, Weller E, Gascoyne RD, et al. Maintenance rituximab after cyclophosphamide, vincristine, and prednisone prolongs progression-free survival in advanced indolent lymphoma: Results of the randomized phase III ECOG1496 study J Clin Oncol 2009;27:1607–1614.
100. Salles G, Seymour JF, Offner F, et al. Rituximab maintenance for 2 years in patients with high tumour burden follicular lymphoma responding to rituximab plus chemotherapy (PRIMA): A phase 3, randomised controlled trial. Lancet 2011;377:42–51.
101. Cheson BD. Hematology: The case against rituximab maintenance. Nat Rev Clin Oncol 2009;6:622–624.
102. Seymour JF. Follicular lymphoma: Maintenance therapy is (often) indicated. Nat Rev Clin Oncol 2009;6:624–626.
103. Forstpointner R, Unterhalt M, Dreyling M, et al. Maintenance therapy with rituximab leads to a significant prolongation of response duration after salvage therapy with a combination of rituximab, fludarabine, cyclophosphamide, and mitoxantrone (R-FCM) in patients with recurring and refractory follicular and mantle cell lymphomas: Results of a prospective randomized study of the German Low Grade Lymphoma Study Group (GLSG). Blood 2006;108:4003–4008.
104. van Oers MH, Van Glabbeke M, Giurgea L, et al. Rituximab maintenance treatment of relapsed/resistant follicular non-Hodgkin's lymphoma: Long-term outcome of the EORTC 20981 phase III randomized intergroup study. J Clin Oncol 2010;28:2853–2858.
105. Al Zahrani A, Ibrahim N, Al Eid A. Rapid infusion rituximab changing practice for patient care. J Oncol Pharm Pract 2009;15:183–186.
106. Chiang J, Chan A, Shih V, Hee SW, Tao M, Lim ST. A prospective study to evaluate the feasibility and economic benefits of rapid infusion rituximab at an Asian cancer center. Int J Hematol 2010;91:826–830.
107. Yeo W, Chan TC, Leung NWY, et al. Hepatitis B virus reactivation in lymphoma patients with prior resolved hepatitis B undergoing anticancer therapy with or without rituximab. J Clin Oncol 2009;27:605–611.
108. Beers SA, Chan CH, French RR, et al. CD20 as a target for therapeutic type I and II monoclonal antibodies. Semin Hematol 2010;47:107–114.
109. Rummel MJ, Gregory SA. Bendamustine's emerging role in the management of lymphoid malignancies. Semin Hematol 2011;48:S24–S36.
110. Robinson KS, Williams ME, van der Jagt RH, et al. Phase II multicenter study of bendamustine plus rituximab in patients with relapsed indolent B-cell and mantle cell non-Hodgkin's lymphoma. J Clin Oncol 2008;26:4473–4479.
111. Fowler N, Kahl BS, Lee P, et al. Bortezomib, bendamustine, and rituximab in patients with relapsed or refractory follicular lymphoma: the phase II VERTICAL study. J Clin Oncol 2011;29:3389–3395.
112. Friedberg JW, Vose JM, Kelly JL, et al. The combination of bendamustine, bortezomib, and rituximab for patients with relapsed/refractory indolent and mantle cell non-Hodgkin lymphoma. Blood 2011;117:2807–2812.
113. Goldsmith SJ. Radioimmunotherapy of lymphoma: Bexxar and Zevalin. Semin Nucl Med 2010;40:122–135.
114. Press OW, Unger JM, Braziel RM, et al. Phase II trial of CHOP chemotherapy followed by tositumomab/iodine I-131 tositumomab for previously untreated follicular non-Hodgkin's lymphoma: Five-year follow-up of Southwest Oncology Group Protocol S9911. J Clin Oncol 2006;24:4143–4149.
115. Kaminski MS, Tuck M, Estes J, et al. ^{131}I-tositumomab therapy as initial treatment for follicular lymphoma. N Engl J Med 2005;352:441–449.
116. Link BK, Martin P, Kaminski MS, Goldsmith SJ, Coleman M, Leonard JP. Cyclophosphamide, vincristine, and prednisone followed by tositumomab and iodine-131-tositumomab in patients with untreated low-grade follicular lymphoma: Eight-year follow-up of a multicenter phase II study. J Clin Oncol 2010;28:3035–3041.
117. Armitage JO, Carbone PP, Connors JM, Levine AM, Bennett JM, Kroll S. Treatment-related myelodysplasia and acute leukemia in non-Hodgkin's lymphoma patients. J Clin Oncol 2003;21:897–906.
118. van Besien KW. Allogeneic stem cell transplantation in follicular lymphoma: recent progress and controversy. Hematology Am Soc Hematol Educ Program 2009:610–618.
119. Oliansky DM, Gordon LI, King J, et al. The role of cytotoxic therapy with hematopoietic stem cell transplantation in the treatment of follicular lymphoma: An evidence-based review. Biol Blood Marrow Transplant 2010;16:443–468.
120. Gisselbrecht C. Use of rituximab in diffuse large B-cell lymphoma in the salvage setting. Br J Haematol 2008;143:607–621.
121. Armitage JO, Mauch PM, Harris NL, Dalla-Favera R, Bierman PJ. Diffuse large B-cell lymphoma. In: Armitage JO,

Mauch PM, Harris NL, Coiffier B, Dalla-Favera R, eds. Non-Hodgkin Lymphoma. 2nd ed. Philadelphia, PA: Lippincott Williams & Wilkins, 2010:304–326.

122. McKelvey EM, Gottleib JA, Wilson HE, et al. Hydroxydaunomycin (Adriamycin) combination chemotherapy in malignant lymphoma. Cancer 1976;38:1484–1493.
123. Jones SE, Grozea PN, Metz EN, et al. Superiority of Adriamycin containing combination chemotherapy in the treatment of diffuse lymphoma: A Southwest Oncology Group study. Cancer 1979;43:417–425.
124. Fisher RI, Gaynor ER, Dahlberg S, et al. Comparison of a standard regimen (CHOP) with three intensive chemotherapy regimens for advanced non-Hodgkin's lymphoma. N Engl J Med 1993;328:1002–1006.
125. Fisher RI, Miller TP, O'Connor OA. Diffuse aggressive lymphoma. Hematology Am Soc Hematol Educ Program 2004:221–236.
126. Blayney DW, LeBlanc ML, Grogan T, et al. Dose-intense chemotherapy every 2 weeks with dose-intense cyclophosphamide, doxorubicin, vincristine, and prednisone may improve survival in intermediate- and high-grade lymphoma: A phase II study of the Southwest Oncology Group (SWOG 9349). J Clin Oncol 2003;21:2466–2473.
127. Coiffier B. Increasing chemotherapy intensity in aggressive lymphoma: A renewal? J Clin Oncol 2003;21:2457–2459.
128. Coiffier B, Lepage E, Briere J, et al. CHOP chemotherapy plus rituximab compared with CHOP alone in elderly patients with diffuse large-B-cell lymphoma. N Engl J Med 2002;346:235–242.
129. Coiffier B, Thieblemont C, Van Den Neste E, et al. Long-term outcome of patients in the LNH-98.5 trial, the first randomized study comparing rituximab-CHOP to standard CHOP chemotherapy in DLBCL patients: A study by the Groupe d'Etudes des Lymphomes de l'Adulte. Blood 2010;116:2040–2045.
130. Pfreundschuh M, Trumper L, Osterborg A, et al. CHOP-like chemotherapy plus rituximab versus CHOP-like chemotherapy alone in young patients with good-prognosis diffuse large B-cell lymphoma: A randomised controlled trial by the MabThera International Trial (MInT) Group. Lancet Oncol 2006;7:379–391.
131. Sehn LH, Donaldson J, Chhanabhai M, et al. Introduction of combined CHOP plus rituximab therapy dramatically improved outcome of diffuse large B-cell lymphoma in British Columbia. J Clin Oncol 2005;23:5027–5033.
132. Feugier P, Van Hoof A, Sebban C, et al. Long-term results of the R-CHOP study in the treatment of elderly patients with diffuse large B-cell lymphoma: A study by the Groupe d'Etude des Lymphomes de l'Adulte. J Clin Oncol 2005;23:4117–4126.
133. Held G, Schubert J, Reiser M, Pfreundschuh M. Dose-intensified treatment of advanced-stage diffuse large B-cell lymphomas. Semin Hematol 2006;43:221–229.
134. Greb A, Bohlius J, Trelle S, et al. High-dose chemotherapy with autologous stem cell support in first-line treatment of aggressive non-Hodgkin lymphoma—results of a comprehensive meta-analysis. Cancer Treat Rev 2007;33:338–346.
135. Habermann TM, Weller EA, Morrison VA, et al. Rituximab-CHOP versus CHOP alone or with maintenance rituximab in older patients with diffuse large B-cell lymphoma. J Clin Oncol 2006;24:3121–3127.
136. Pfreundschuh M, Trumper L, Kloess M, et al. Two-weekly or 3-weekly CHOP chemotherapy with or without etoposide for the treatment of elderly patients with aggressive lymphomas: Results of the NHL-B2 trial of the DSHNHL. Blood 2004;104:634–641.
137. Pfreundschuh M, Schubert J, Ziepert M, et al. Six versus eight cycles of bi-weekly CHOP-14 with or without rituximab in elderly patients with aggressive CD20$^+$ B-cell lymphomas: A randomised controlled trial (RICOVER-60). Lancet Oncol 2008;9:105–116.
138. Gisselbrecht C, Glass B, Mounier N, et al. Salvage regimens with autologous transplantation for relapsed large B-cell lymphoma in the rituximab era. J Clin Oncol 2010;28: 4184–4190.
139. Nademanee A, Forman SJ. Role of hematopoietic stem cell transplantation for advanced-stage diffuse large B-cell lymphoma. Semin Hematol 2006;43:240–250.
140. Philip T, Guglielmi C, Hagenbeek A, et al. Autologous bone marrow transplantation as compared with salvage chemotherapy in relapses of chemotherapy-sensitive non-Hodgkin's lymphoma. N Engl J Med 1995;333: 1540–1545.
141. Zain J, Bhagat G, O'Connor OA. Mantle cell lymphoma. In: Armitage JO, Mauch PM, Harris NL, Coiffier B, Dalla-Favera R, eds. Non-Hodgkin Lymphoma. 2nd ed. Philadelphia, PA: Lippincott Williams & Wilkins, 2010: 284–303.
142. Rummel MJ, Al-Batran SE, Kim SZ, et al. Bendamustine plus rituximab is effective and has a favorable toxicity profile in the treatment of mantle cell and low-grade non-Hodgkin's lymphoma. J Clin Oncol 2005;23: 3383–3389.
143. Fisher RI, Bernstein SH, Kahl BS, et al. Multicenter phase II study of bortezomib in patients with relapsed or refractory mantle cell lymphoma. J Clin Oncol 2006;24: 4867–4874.
144. Wang ML, Rule S, Martin P, et al. Targeting BTK with ibrutinib in relapsed or refractory mantle cell lymphoma. N Engl J Med 2013;369:507–516.
145. Levine AM, Said JW. Management of acquired immunodeficiency syndrome-related lymphoma. In: Armitage JO, Mauch PM, Harris NL, Coiffier B, Dalla-Favera R, eds. Non-Hodgkin Lymphoma. 2nd ed. Philadelphia, PA: Lippincott Williams & Wilkins, 2010: 507–526.
146. Mounier N, Spina M, Gisselbrecht C. Modern management of non-Hodgkin's lymphoma in HIV-infected patients. Br J Haematol 2007;136:685–698.
147. Kaplan LD, Lee JY, Ambinder RF, et al. Rituximab does not improve clinical outcome in a randomized phase III trial of CHOP with or without rituximab in patients with HIV associated non-Hodgkin's lymphoma: AIDS Malignancy Consortium trial 010. Blood 2005;106: 1538–1543.

110

Ovarian Cancer

Judith A. Smith and Judith K. Wolf

KEY CONCEPTS

1. Ovarian cancer is denoted "the silent killer" because of the nonspecific signs and symptoms that contribute to the delay in diagnosis. The few patients who present with disease still confined to the ovary will have a 5-year survival rate greater than 90%, but most patients present with advanced disease and have a 5-year survival rate of 10% to 30%.
2. Ovarian cancer is a sporadic disease with less than 10% of cases of ovarian cancer attributed to heredity. However, a history of two or more first-degree relatives with ovarian cancer increases a woman's risk of developing ovarian cancer by greater than 50%.
3. Considerable education efforts have been made to identify patients with the persistence, greater than 2 weeks, of nonspecific presenting symptoms of ovarian cancer including: abdominal pressure/pain, difficulty eating or feeling full quickly, urinary urgency/frequency, change in bowel habits, or unexplained vaginal bleeding.
4. CA-125 is a nonspecific antigen used as a tumor marker for diagnosis and monitoring epithelial ovarian carcinoma. If CA-125 is positive at the time of diagnosis, changes in CA-125 levels correlate with disease response and progression.
5. Although most patients will achieve a complete response to initial treatment, more than 50% of patients will have recurrence within the first 2 years. If recurrence is less than 6 months after completion of chemotherapy, tumor is defined to be platinum-resistant. The antitumor activity of second-line chemotherapy regimens is similar, and the choice of treatment for recurrent platinum-resistant ovarian cancer depends on residual toxicities, physician preference, and patient convenience. Participation in a clinical trial is also a reasonable option for these patients.
6. Ovarian cancer is staged surgically with the International Federation of Gynecology and Obstetrics (FIGO) staging algorithm. Tumor debulking and total abdominal hysterectomy–bilateral oophorectomy surgery are the primary surgical interventions for ovarian cancer. After the completion of the staging and primary surgical treatment, the current standard of care is six cycles of a taxane/platinum-containing chemotherapy regimen.
7. The interperitoneal (IP) route of chemotherapy administration has demonstrated a significant route of administration; however, it is dependent on appropriate patient selection.
8. A platinum-containing doublet chemotherapy regimen is the standard of care for the first recurrence of platinum-sensitive ovarian cancer.
9. Despite recent advances, enrollment still primary treatment recommendation for patients with recurrent platinum-resistant ovarian cancer.

Ovarian cancer is a gynecologic cancer that usually arises from disruption or mutations in the epithelium of the ovary.[1] It is associated with the highest mortality among the gynecologic cancers, primarily because most patients present with advanced disease. (1) Ovarian cancer is denoted "the silent killer" because of the nonspecific signs and symptoms that often lead to a delay in diagnosis. Ovarian cancers often metastasize via the lymphatic and blood systems to the liver and/or lungs. Common complications of advanced and progressive ovarian cancer include ascites and small bowel obstruction. The few patients who present with disease still confined to the ovary will have a 5-year survival rate greater than 90%, but most patients present with advanced disease and have a 5-year survival rate of 10% to 30%. Primary treatment includes tumor-debulking surgery followed by six cycles of a taxane-platinum chemotherapy regimen. Although 70% of patients achieve an initial complete response to chemotherapy, more than 50% of these patients will have recurrence within the first 2 years from diagnosis.[2]

ETIOLOGY AND EPIDEMIOLOGY

It is estimated that 22,240 new cases of ovarian cancer were diagnosed, and 14,030 women died of the disease in 2013.[3] Ovarian cancer is associated with the highest mortality rate among the gynecologic cancers and is the fifth leading cause of cancer-related deaths in women. Despite research efforts and recent advances, the mortality rate associated with ovarian cancer has not changed significantly over the past four decades. The high mortality rate is related to the insidious onset of nonspecific symptoms and the lack of adequate screening tools, which allows the disease to go undiagnosed until it has progressed beyond the pelvic cavity.

As with many other cancers, the risk of ovarian cancer increases with increasing age. A woman's risk increases from 15.7 to 54 per 100,000 as her age advances from 40 to 79 years, and the median age at diagnosis is 59.[3] Most cases of ovarian cancer are diagnosed during the peri- and postmenopausal phase of women's reproductive life span.[4]

(2) Heredity accounts for less than 10% of all ovarian cancer cases. Family history is an important risk factor in the development of ovarian cancer. If one family member has a diagnosis of ovarian cancer, the associated lifetime risk is 9%, but this risk increases to greater than 50% if there are two or more first-degree relatives (e.g., her mother and sister) with a diagnosis of ovarian cancer or multiple cases of ovarian and breast cancer within the same family.[1,2]

BRCA1 and *BRCA2* are the tumor suppressor genes thought to be involved in one or more pathways of DNA damage recognition and repair. The *BRCA1* gene is located on chromosome 17q12–21, and the *BRCA2* gene is located on chromosome 13q12–13. Both *BRCA1* and *BRCA2* mutations are associated with ovarian cancer. However, *BRCA1* is more prevalent, being associated with 90% of inherited and 10% of sporadic cases of ovarian cancer.[5] Patients with *BRCA1*-associated ovarian cancer are usually considerably younger than patients with *BRCA2* mutations, with a mean age of 54 years.[6] Patients usually present with advanced stage at diagnosis, and the *BRCA1*-linked ovarian cancers are more aggressive tumors that typically are serous histology, moderate to high grade. As *BRCA1* and *BRCA2* are thought to be involved in DNA damage or repair, their inactivation/mutations may be associated with an increased resistance of ovarian cancer cells to cytotoxic agents.

Hereditary breast and ovarian cancer syndrome is one of the two different forms of hereditary ovarian cancer and is associated with germline mutations in *BRCA1* and *BRCA2*.[5,7] The hereditary nonpolyposis colorectal cancer or Lynch syndrome is a familial syndrome with germline mutations causing defects in enzymes involved in DNA mismatch repair, which is associated with up to 12% of hereditary ovarian cancer cases.[5] This syndrome is associated with mutations in DNA mismatch repair genes such as *MSH2, MLH1, PMS1,* and *PMS2* and leads to microsatellite instability.

Hormone exposure, specifically estrogen, and reproductive history are also associated with the risk of developing ovarian cancer. Conditions that increase the total number of ovulations in women's reproductive history, such as nulliparity, early menarche, or late menopause, are associated with an increasing risk for epithelial ovarian cancers.[8,9] Conversely those conditions that limit ovulations are associated with a protective effect. Each time ovulation occurs, the ovarian epithelium is broken, followed by cellular repair. According to the *incessant ovulation hypothesis*, the risk of mutations and, ultimately, cancer increases each time the ovarian epithelium undergoes cell repair.

Finally, ovarian cancer is associated with certain dietary and environmental factors. A diet that is high in galactose, animal fat, and meat may increase the risk of ovarian cancer, whereas a vegetable-rich diet may decrease the risk of ovarian cancer.[7,10] Although controversial, exogenous factors such as asbestos and talcum powder use in the perineal area are also associated with an increased risk of ovarian cancer.[7,10]

PATHOLOGY AND CLASSIFICATION

Ovarian carcinomas can be separated into three major entities: epithelial carcinomas, germ cell tumors, and stromal carcinomas. Most ovarian tumors (85% to 90%) are derived from the epithelial surface of the ovary.[11] The classification of common epithelial tumors has been developed by the World Health Organization and the International Federation of Gynecology and Obstetrics (FIGO).[12] The nomenclature considers cell type, location of the tumor, and the degree of the malignancy, which ranges from benign tumors to tumors of low malignancy to invasive carcinomas. Epithelial tumors classified as low malignancy ("borderline malignancy") are characterized by epithelial papillae with atypical cell clusters, cellular stratification, nuclear atypia, and increased mitotic activity, and have a much better prognosis than those classified as invasive carcinomas. Malignant tumors are characterized by an infiltrative destructive growth pattern with malignant cells growing in a disorganized manner and dissection into stromal planes.

Invasive epithelial adenocarcinomas are characterized by histologic subtype and grade, which measures the degree of cellular differentiation. Although the histologic type of the tumor is not a significant prognostic factor, with the exception of clear cell, the histopathologic grade is an important prognostic factor. Undifferentiated tumors are associated with a poorer prognosis than those lesions that are considered to be well or moderately differentiated. A universal grading system for ovarian cancer was developed that combines mitotic score, nuclear atypia score, and architectural score based on the histologic pattern.[13]

The histologic subtypes of adenocarcinomas include papillary serous, mucinous, endometrioid, clear cell, mixed epithelial, transition-cell, and undifferentiated.[2,4,13] Papillary serous adenocarcinoma is the most common type of epithelial ovarian cancer and accounts for about 46% of cases. The peak age of diagnosis ranges from 45 to 65 years with 63 years as the median age of diagnosis.[14] Serous carcinomas typically display complex papillary and solid patterns and qualify as high-grade carcinomas. Endometrioid carcinomas are seen in women 40 to 50 years of age and comprise about 8% of ovarian carcinomas, of which about 6% are surface epithelial neoplasms.[14] Endometrioid tumors are usually diagnosed as stage I disease and have a better prognosis than tumors with serous histology. Mucinous carcinomas occur in women between 40 and 70 years of age and account for about 36% of all ovarian cancers. The overall prognosis for mucinous carcinoma is better than for serous carcinoma because most patients present with stage I disease. Clear cell carcinoma comprises about 3% of ovarian carcinomas in women, with a mean age of 57 years. Although clear cell carcinoma is the least common ovarian neoplasm, it is most commonly associated with paraneoplastic-related hypercalcemia.[14]

Germ cell tumors of the ovary, including malignant teratoma and dysgerminomas, are rare, comprising about 2% to 3% of all ovarian cancers in Western countries with an increased incidence in black and Asian women.[15,16] These tumors are highly curable and affect primarily young women. In contrast to epithelial tumors, about 60% to 70% of germ cell tumors are stage I at diagnosis, which is related to earlier detection and response to symptoms in this younger patient population.[16] Serum markers (human β-chorionic gonadotropin and α-fetoprotein) are helpful to confirm the diagnosis and monitor response to treatment.

Finally, ovarian sex cord-stromal tumors account for 7% of all ovarian cancers and tend to be diagnosed at stage I.[12] Sex cord-stromal tumors are associated with hormonal effects, such as precocious puberty, amenorrhea, and postmenopausal bleeding. Because these tumors are rare, the optimal treatment of ovarian sex cord-stromal tumors is not clear. The current recommended standard of care is surgery followed by treatment with a platinum-based chemotherapy regimen.

Ovarian cancer is usually confined to the abdominal cavity, but spread can occur to the lung, liver, and, less commonly, the bone or brain. Disease is spread by direct extension, peritoneal seeding, lymphatic dissemination, or bloodborne metastasis. Lymphatic seeding is the most common pathway and frequently causes ascites.

SCREENING AND PREVENTION

Screening

Ovarian cancer is an uncommon disease with no known preinvasive component, which has made it difficult to screen patients to detect early disease. In addition, the risk factors for developing ovarian cancer are not well understood, which also makes it difficult to identify a high-risk group of individuals. At the present time, there are no effective screening tools for early detection of ovarian cancer. (3) However, considerable education efforts have been made to help identify patients with the persistence (i.e., >2 weeks) of nonspecific presenting symptoms of ovarian cancer including: abdominal pressure/pain, difficulty eating or feeling full quickly, urinary urgency/frequency, change in bowel habits, or unexplained vaginal bleeding.

Pelvic examinations are noninvasive and well accepted and can detect large tumors with a sensitivity of 67% for detecting all tumors.[15] However, because pelvic examinations cannot detect minimal or microscopic disease, they do not usually detect ovarian cancer until it is in an advanced stage. As a result of these limitations, routine pelvic examinations are not an effective screening tool and do not decrease overall mortality.[15]

Transvaginal ultrasound (TVUS) creates an image of the ovary by releasing sound waves. It can be used to evaluate the size and shape and to detect the presence of cystic or solid masses or abdominal fluid. TVUS can also evaluate blood flow within an ovarian mass. Normal ovarian size cutoff parameters range from 1.25 cm^2 for women 55 to 59 years of age to 1.0 cm^2 for women older than age 65 to 69 years.[17,18] TVUS is sensitive in identifying ovarian lesions and abnormalities, but its use as a routine screening test is limited by a lack of specificity and an inability to detect peritoneal cancer or cancer in normal-size ovaries.[19,20]

Serum cancer antigen-125 (CA-125) is a nonspecific inflammatory antigen that can be elevated in numerous conditions associated with inflammation in the abdominal cavity. CA-125 has been extensively studied as a potential tumor marker for ovarian cancer based on the observation that CA-125 levels in a woman without ovarian cancer tend to stay the same or decrease over time, whereas levels associated with malignancy tend to gradually increase over time.[19] However, CA-125 is a nonspecific test that can be elevated in a number of benign conditions, including other gynecologic conditions, such as endometriosis, and many nongynecologic conditions, such as diverticulitis and peptic ulcer disease. Because of these limitations, CA-125 levels are not recommended as a routine screening test for detection of ovarian cancer. Numerous other serologic markers such as carcinoembryonic antigen and lipid-associated sialic acid have been evaluated but cannot be recommended for routine screening for ovarian cancer.

The United States Preventive Services Task Force found fair evidence to support screening with CA-125 or TVUS and concluded that earlier detection would likely have a small effect, at best, on mortality from ovarian cancer.[21] Unfortunately, because of the low prevalence of ovarian cancer and the invasive nature of diagnostic testing after a positive screening test, the United States Preventive Services Task Force also found fair evidence that screening could likely lead to important harms. The United States Preventive Services Task Force concluded that the potential harms outweigh the potential benefits and recommended against any form of routine screening with CA-125 or TVUS for ovarian cancer.

In high-risk women, as defined by family history, most clinicians use a multimodality approach for ovarian cancer screening that includes an annual TVUS in combination with a CA-125 blood test every 6 months. Changes in CA-125 are monitored over time, and changes such as a persistent elevation or consistent increases in CA-125 levels in conjunction with TVUS abnormalities are evaluated further.

Prevention

It is difficult to make recommendations for prevention for the general population because ovarian cancer is a sporadic disease with no established risk factors. Noninvasive measures, such as chemoprevention, have demonstrated some benefit in decreasing the risk of developing ovarian cancer. Ovulation itself is considered a potential insult to the ovarian epithelium, increasing its susceptibility to damage and, ultimately, to cancer. Interventions or reproductive conditions associated with decreasing the number of ovulations, including multiparity, may have a protective effect for the prevention of ovarian cancer. However, the more invasive prevention interventions, such as prophylactic surgery and genetic screening, should be reserved for those women identified to be at high risk based on their heredity for developing ovarian cancer.

Chemoprevention

Although a number of agents have been investigated as chemoprevention of ovarian cancer, including oral contraceptives, aspirin, nonsteroidal antiinflammatory agents, and retinoids, none of these agents is currently accepted as standard treatment for the prevention of ovarian cancer. Oral contraceptives inhibit ovulation, which reduces the opportunity for potential for damage to the ovarian epithelium. When taken for longer than 10 years, oral contraceptives decrease the relative risk to less than 0.4.[22,23] Because oral contraceptive use is associated with an increased risk of breast cancer, women with a family history of breast cancer are not candidates for this use of oral contraceptives as chemoprevention of ovarian cancer.[22,23]

Nonsteroidal antiinflammatory drugs, aspirin, and acetaminophen also have been suggested for use in the chemoprevention of different cancers, especially hereditary nonpolyposis colon cancer.[24] Although the results of observational studies show that the use of nonsteroidal antiinflammatory drugs, aspirin, and acetaminophen reduces the risk of ovarian cancer, these findings have not been confirmed in prospective clinical studies. The proposed mechanism of these agents is the antiinflammatory effect on normal ovulation and inhibition of ovulation.[24,25]

Prophylactic Surgery

Prophylactic surgical interventions for the prevention of ovarian cancer are reserved for patients with a significant family history and/or with known genetic mutations such as *BRCA1* and should be postponed until after childbearing is completed. The goal is to remove healthy, at-risk organs before any carcinogenic activity is initiated, ultimately reducing the risk of developing cancer. These surgeries include prophylactic oophorectomy or bilateral salpingo-oophorectomy and tubal ligation. These procedures will cause surgical menopause, which can be associated with severe hot flashes, vaginal dryness, sexual dysfunction, and increased risk for development of osteoporosis and heart disease in these women. Because of the potential impact on quality of life and increased health risks, prophylactic surgery is not recommended as a general prevention intervention for the general population.

Although prophylactic surgical interventions are associated with significant reduction in risk of developing ovarian cancer, patients who choose to have a prophylactic oophorectomy/bilateral salpingo-oophorectomy completed need to be informed that complete protection is not guaranteed.[15,23,26] Although a 67% risk reduction has been shown, a potential 2% to 5% risk of primary peritoneal cancer remains.[27,28] Primary peritoneal cancers have identical histology of ovarian tumors with diffuse involvement of peritoneal surfaces. Primary peritoneal cancers can often result from "seeding" during the prophylactic surgery. It is recommended for peritoneal washings to be completed during the prophylactic surgery to check for presence of peritoneal surfaces. If positive, then prophylactic surgery would change to staging and treatment surgery to determine extent of disease and remove any other possible lesions.

Tubal ligation is another procedure that can potentially reduce the risk for developing ovarian cancer. In a case-control study, Narod et al. reported that tubal ligation in *BRCA*-positive women was associated with a 63% reduction in risk of developing ovarian cancer.[29] However, it is not recommended as a sole procedure in prophylaxis. The mechanism for its protective effect is not clear, but it has been proposed that tubal ligation may limit exposure of the ovary to environmental carcinogens.

Genetic Screening

Genetic screening should be considered for those women with a significant family history of ovarian cancer. Patients should be

CLINICAL PRESENTATION

General

- Ovarian cancer is sometimes referred to as "the silent killer" because of the vague nonspecific signs and symptoms that contribute to the delay in diagnosis.

Symptoms

- The patient may complain of abdominal discomfort, nausea, dyspepsia, flatulence, bloating, fullness, early satiety, urinary frequency, change in bowel function (diarrhea or constipation), weight change, and digestive disturbances.

Signs

- Abdominal or pelvic mass may be palpable.
- Lymphadenopathy may be present.
- Vaginal bleeding may be irregular.
- Patient may have signs of ascites (abdominal distension, shifting, and dullness to percussion—may present like "pregnant abdomen").

Laboratory Tests

- CA-125 may be elevated (normal level is less than 35 units/mL [35 kU/L]).
- Abnormalities in liver function tests may suggest hepatic involvement.
- Abnormalities in renal function tests may suggest compression of the renal system by the tumor.

evaluated for the presence of genes such as *BRCA1*, *BRCA2*, or other genes such as those associated with hereditary nonpolyposis colorectal cancer or the hereditary breast ovarian cancer (hereditary breast and ovarian cancer syndrome) syndrome.[29–32] Prior to genetic screening, appropriate patient/family counseling and genetic counseling should be available to help women prepare and deal with the health and psychosocial implications of the genetic screening results.

CLINICAL PRESENTATION

Patients with early ovarian cancer are often asymptomatic and the ovarian mass is often detected incidentally during their annual pelvic examinations. Patients with ovarian cancer often present with nonspecific, vague symptoms such as abdominal bloating, pressure or pain, indigestion, or change in bowel movements.[2,4,33] These symptoms can easily be confused with symptoms of common benign gastrointestinal disorders. Patients will often not seek medical attention until these symptoms become unrelenting and bothersome, which allows the disease to progress undetected. Patients with advanced disease may report symptoms such as pain, abdominal distension, and ascites.[2,33]

Several groups have partnered together to educate women about early signs and symptoms of ovarian cancer. Goff et al. recently developed a symptom index, based on a comparison of symptoms experienced in patients with ovarian cancer and a matched control group.[34] Symptoms that were correlated with ovarian cancer were persistent or recurrent bloating, pelvic or abdominal pain, difficulty eating or feeling full quickly, and urinary symptoms (either urgency or frequency). The Gynecologic Cancer Foundation, Society of Gynecologic Oncologists, and American Cancer Society recommend that women who have any of those problems nearly every day for more than 2 weeks should see a gynecologist, especially if the symptoms are new and quite different from her usual state of health. Furthermore, healthcare professionals should keep ovarian cancer in the differential for women presenting with these persistent symptoms.

DIAGNOSIS

The diagnostic workup for suspected ovarian cancer includes a careful physical examination including a Papanicolaou (Pap) smear and a pelvic and rectovaginal examination.[7] The presence of a pelvic mass that is unilateral or bilateral, solid, irregular, fixed, or nodular is highly suggestive of ovarian cancer. Unfortunately, by the time a pelvic mass can be palpitated on physical exam, the disease is already advanced beyond the pelvic cavity. A detailed family history should be taken, especially noting the number and pattern of first-degree relatives with malignancies.

A complete blood count, chemistry profile (including liver and renal function tests), and CA-125, carcinoembryonic antigen, and CA19–9 levels should be performed. ❹ Although CA-125 is a nonspecific antigen, it is the best current tumor marker for epithelial ovarian carcinoma. A normal CA-125 value is less then 35 units/mL (35 kU/L). If CA-125 is elevated at the time of diagnosis, changes in CA-125 levels correlate with tumor burden. Rising CA-125 levels are often associated with disease progression, but CA-125 can be elevated in various other conditions such as different phases of the menstrual cycle, diverticulitis, endometriosis, as well as other nongynecologic cancers. When a patient presents with an abdominal mass, it is important to rule out other cancers in the abdominal cavity. Carcinoembryonic antigen and CA19–9 are markers for other gastrointestinal cancers and may be helpful in the differential diagnosis.

Other diagnostic tests should include a transvaginal or abdominal ultrasonography, chest radiography, computed tomography, magnetic resonance imaging, or positron emission tomography scan. An upper GI series, IV pyelogram, cystoscopy, proctoscopy, or barium enema is sometimes indicated to confirm diagnosis and extent of disease.

TREATMENT
Ovarian Cancer

Desired Outcomes

The goals of treatment of ovarian cancer are dependent upon the FIGO stage at diagnosis. While ideally "treatment for cure" is desired, it is important to set realistic expectations for the patient. ❺ Most patients will achieve a complete response to the initial multimodality treatment, but over 50% of these patients will present with recurrent disease within the first 2 years after completion of treatment. Although overall survival has not significantly changed for ovarian cancer patients, the progression-free survival has improved, which translates to less time on chemotherapy and overall improvement in quality of life for these patients.

In patients who present with metastatic disease or are not surgical candidates, the goal of treatment becomes focused on alleviating symptoms and prolonging survival as long as quality of life is acceptable. In the setting of recurrent platinum-resistant ovarian cancer, the treatment goal is also focused on alleviating symptoms and prolonging survival as long as quality of life is acceptable. (9) Phase I/investigational agent clinical trials should be considered because they may be the best treatment option for potential benefit due to the poor efficacy of the available chemotherapy agents for recurrent platinum-resistant ovarian cancer.

General Approach

(5) A multimodality approach that includes comprehensive surgery and chemotherapy is used for the initial treatment of ovarian cancer with curative intent. Although most patients will initially achieve a complete response, more than 50% will recur within the first 2 years.[2,35] A clinical complete response to treatment is defined as no evidence of disease by physical examination or diagnostic tests and a normal CA-125 level.

Chemotherapy regimens for ovarian cancer have evolved over the past several decades. Treatment regimens began with single-agent melphalan followed by single-agent cyclophosphamide. Shortly after cisplatin was introduced into clinical practice, it was added to cyclophosphamide, and this combination was the "standard of care" for more than a decade until the introduction of paclitaxel in the 1980s. Paclitaxel soon replaced cyclophosphamide, and paclitaxel plus cisplatin became the standard of care. Carboplatin was then substituted for cisplatin because of its improved toxicity profile, and paclitaxel plus carboplatin was adopted. During this same period, many researchers have conducted numerous clinical trials of intraperitoneal (IP) chemotherapy. In 2006, Armstrong and colleagues published the first IP therapy clinical trial to demonstrate a survival advantage over the standard IV regimen.[36] However, these advances in chemotherapy for the treatment of ovarian cancer have not yet translated into major changes in overall 5-year survival, which remains less than 20%.

Certain subgroups of patients have a better or worse response to chemotherapy. The histologic subtype of the tumor is a prognostic factor; clear cell histology is more likely to be poorly differentiated, faster growing, and have intrinsic drug resistance.[2,37] However, the extent of residual disease, size larger than 1 cm, and tumor grade are better predictors of response to chemotherapy and overall survival.[2]

In general, younger patients have a better performance status and tolerate chemotherapy better than elderly patients. For unknown reasons, white women tend to have a worse prognosis and response to therapy as compared with women of other ethnic backgrounds.[2,6,7]

In patients with recurrent ovarian cancer, the goals of treatment are to relieve symptoms such as pain or discomfort from ascites, slow disease progression, and prevent serious complications such as small bowel obstructions.

Surgery

Surgery is the primary treatment intervention for ovarian cancer.[37–41] Surgery may be curative for selected patients with limited stage IA disease.

Primary surgical treatment includes a total abdominal hysterectomy with bilateral salpingo-oophorectomy (TAH/BSO), omentectomy, and lymph node dissection (Fig. 110-1).[37–41] The primary objective of the surgery is to optimally debulk the tumor to less than 1 cm of residual disease.[42] Long-term followup studies confirm that

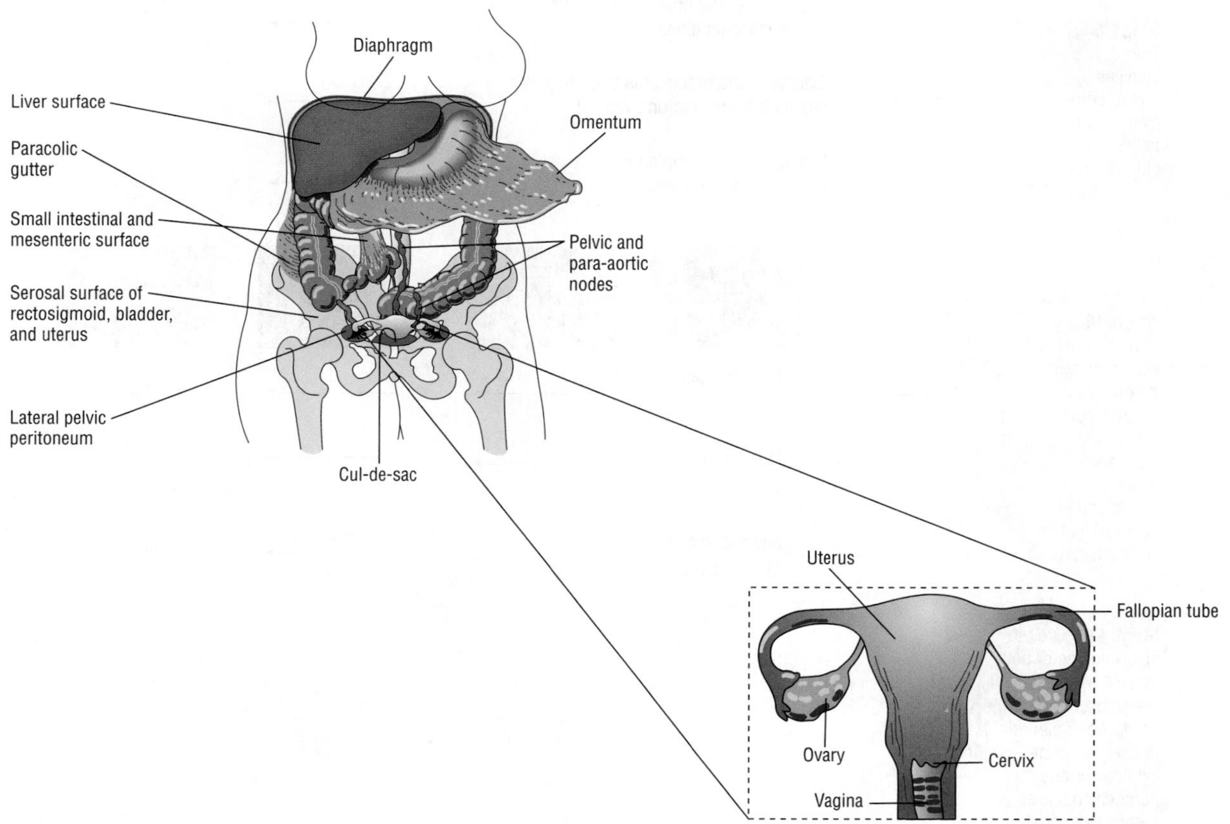

FIGURE 110-1 Staging laparotomy for ovarian cancer with diagram of female reproductive tract (uterus, fallopian tubes, ovaries, vagina). *Dashed line box* outlines what is removed during the total abdominal hysterectomy with bilateral salpingo-oophorectomy.

residual disease smaller than 1 cm correlates with higher complete response rates to chemotherapy and longer overall survival as compared to patients with bulky residual disease (>1 cm).[40,41]

A comprehensive exploratory laparotomy is vital for the accurate confirmation of diagnosis and staging of ovarian cancer.[37–39] 6 Unlike other cancers that are typically diagnosed by biopsy or laboratory results and clinically staged by results from imaging tests, gynecologic cancers, such as ovarian cancer, are surgically diagnosed and then staged according to the FIGO staging algorithm (Fig. 110-2). The FIGO staging system requires a fairly extensive surgery by an experienced gynecologic oncologist. The skill of the surgeon has a significant effect on prognosis, with definitive benefit of a trained gynecologic oncologist performing surgery as compared with a gynecologist or general surgeon.[43] The reasons for this approach include (a) pelvic tumors cannot be readily biopsied without risk of "tumor seeding," which can increase the risk of recurrence, and (b) surgical staging takes into account the presence of microscopic disease in samples obtained by pelvic washing and lymph node dissection and read by a pathologist during the surgical procedure. It is recommended that the initial surgical staging and tumor-debulking surgery be completed by a trained gynecologic oncology surgeon when ovarian cancer is suspected to prevent understaging and to optimize overall outcome.[44]

Secondary cytoreduction or interval debulking is when surgery is performed after completion of some or all chemotherapy to remove residual disease. Some protocols include additional cycles of chemotherapy after the surgical procedure. The importance of cytoreduction before, during, or after chemotherapy is still controversial,

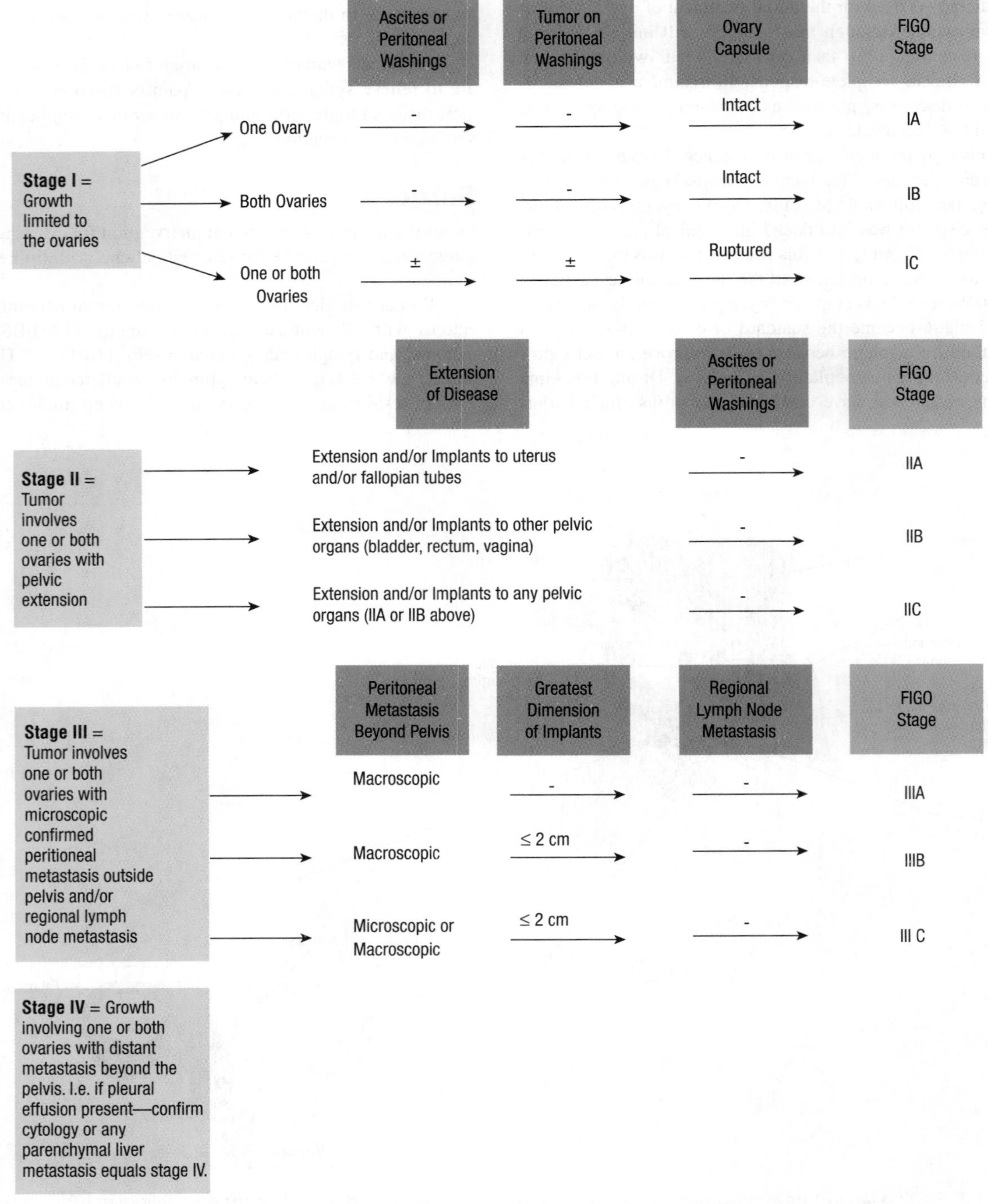

FIGURE 110-2 International Federation of Gynecology and Obstetrics (FIGO) staging algorithm.

but it has been recommended to facilitate response to chemotherapy and improve overall survival. Randomized trials of secondary surgical cytoreduction have reported conflicting results. In an older randomized trial, van der Burg et al. performed interval debulking surgery on 140 stage IIB to stage IV suboptimally debulked (<1 cm of residual disease) ovarian cancer patients after receiving three cycles of cisplatin plus cyclophosphamide.[45] Patients then received an additional three cycles of these same drugs after surgery. Patients randomized to the nonsurgical treatment arm received six cycles of chemotherapy. Interval debulking surgery significantly prolonged overall and progression-free survival and reduced the risk of death by 33%. However, in a recently published study of 550 women with stage III or IV disease treated with primary cytoreductive surgery and three cycles of paclitaxel and cisplatin, patients randomized to receive secondary cytoreductive surgery followed by three more cycles of chemotherapy had similar progression-free survival and overall survival as compared with those randomized to receive three more cycles of chemotherapy alone.[46]

The overall effect of interval debulking is influenced by several factors, including initial response to chemotherapy, the amount of residual disease before and after second-look surgery, and the presence of microscopic residual disease. The results of recent trials suggest that secondary surgical cytoreduction does not prolong survival in patients who are treated with maximal primary cytoreductive surgery followed by appropriate postoperative chemotherapy.

"Second-look surgery" is an elective surgical procedure performed in patients who achieve a clinical complete response after primary chemotherapy to determine if any visible or microscopic disease is present in the peritoneal cavity. The benefit of "second-look laparotomy" to evaluate residual disease after completing chemotherapy remains controversial because it has been difficult to establish any impact on overall survival. It has questionable benefit because approximately 50% of those with a negative second look still relapsed.[3] If visible or microscopic disease is detected during second look, then the clinician may decide to give additional chemotherapy. But if no visible or microscopic disease is detected during second look, the clinician may decide to observe and monitor the patient. Use of laparoscopic surgical techniques is controversial for initial surgery but is sometimes considered in debulking of recurrent or advanced disease when the intent is palliative rather than curative.[40] In patients with recurrent disease, the goal of debulking surgery is to relieve symptoms associated with complications such as small bowel obstructions and to help improve the patient's quality of life.

Radiation

Radiation has a limited role in the management of ovarian cancer. Use of radiation for treatment of early stage disease has had no benefit or impact on overall survival.[47] Radiation therapy is most beneficial for palliation of symptoms in patients with recurrent pelvic disease, often associated with small bowel obstructions. The two forms of radiation therapy used in ovarian cancer are external beam whole-abdominal irradiation and intraperitoneal isotopes such as phosphorus-32 (^{32}P). Alleviation of symptoms with external beam whole-abdominal irradiation is associated with a significant improvement in the patient's quality of life. The recommended dose ranges from 35 to 45 Gy (3500 to 4500 rad), depending on the treatment history and ability to tolerate radiation treatments.

First-Line Chemotherapy

The mainstay of ovarian cancer treatment is chemotherapy. It is used as a component of first-line treatment after completion of surgery and is the primary modality of treatment for recurrent ovarian cancer.

Systemic chemotherapy with a taxane and platinum regimen following optimal surgical debulking is the standard of care for treatment of epithelial ovarian cancer (Fig. 110-3). Table 110-1 summarizes the chemotherapeutic regimens used as the initial treatment of newly diagnosed epithelial ovarian cancer. More than 60 randomized, controlled clinical trials have evaluated combination chemotherapy regimens for the treatment of advanced ovarian cancer, and a meta-analysis of these trials confirmed the efficacy of platinum and taxane regimens over other regimens.[48,49]

Historically, single-agent alkylating agents such as melphalan, and later cyclophosphamide, were used for the treatment of advanced ovarian cancer until the introduction of cisplatin in the 1970s. Combination chemotherapy regimens containing cisplatin and cyclophosphamide achieved higher response rates and overall survival than regimens without cisplatin in patients with advanced ovarian cancer.[50] Based on the results of these trials, the combination of cisplatin plus cyclophosphamide remained the standard of care for the treatment of ovarian cancer until the early 1990s.

The next major advance in the therapy of advanced ovarian cancer occurred with the introduction of paclitaxel into chemotherapy regimens. McGuire et al. reported the results of a Gynecologic Oncology Group (GOG)-111 study that found the combination of paclitaxel 135 mg/m^2 over 24 hours and cisplatin 75 mg/m^2 achieved higher response rates and longer survival than did cyclophosphamide 750 mg/m^2 and cisplatin 75 mg/m^2 in patients with newly diagnosed, suboptimally debulked, stages III and IV ovarian cancer.[51] Survival improved significantly in the paclitaxel arm, with an increase in median progression-free survival (18 months vs. 13 months) and overall survival (38 months vs. 24 months). Neutropenia, alopecia, and peripheral neuropathy were more severe in the paclitaxel plus cisplatin group. Similar results were reported in a large European-Canadian Intergroup Phase III randomized trial study (OV10) that also confirmed superior response rates with the paclitaxel 135 mg/m^2 over 24 hours with cisplatin 75 mg/m^2 regimen as compared with cyclophosphamide 750 mg/m^2 with cisplatin 75 mg/m^2 regimen.[52] Based on the results of these studies, paclitaxel plus cisplatin was widely adopted and became the accepted standard of care.

The availability of carboplatin led to clinical trials to evaluate whether carboplatin could be substituted for cisplatin, which would spare patients from the significant neurotoxicity and nephrotoxicity associated with cisplatin. Several prospective randomized comparisons of carboplatin plus paclitaxel versus cisplatin plus paclitaxel in patients with advanced ovarian cancer have been conducted.[53–56] The results of these trials show that carboplatin plus paclitaxel is equally efficacious and better tolerated than cisplatin and paclitaxel. In the GOG-158 study, 840 previously untreated patients with optimally resected stage III disease (no residual tumor nodule >1 cm) were randomized to carboplatin (area under the curve [AUC] = 7.5) plus paclitaxel 175 mg/m^2 over 3 hours, or cisplatin 75 mg/m^2 plus paclitaxel 135 mg/m^2 over 24 hours administered every 21 days for six cycles.[53,55] The results of that trial showed no difference in progression-free survival between the two treatment arms with a median time-to-progression of 19.4 months in the paclitaxel plus cisplatin arm versus 20.7 months in the paclitaxel plus carboplatin arm. As expected, the incidence of leukopenia, fever, gastrointestinal toxicity, and metabolic toxicity was higher in patients in the cisplatin arm, whereas patients in the carboplatin arm experienced more thrombocytopenia and pain. Although the incidence of neurotoxicity was similar in the two treatment arms, it was more severe in the paclitaxel plus cisplatin arm. The results of this study showed that the substitution of carboplatin for cisplatin in the regimen does not compromise efficacy and improves tolerability. These findings were confirmed in two other large randomized, controlled studies.[55,56] Based on these results, paclitaxel plus carboplatin became the accepted standard of care.

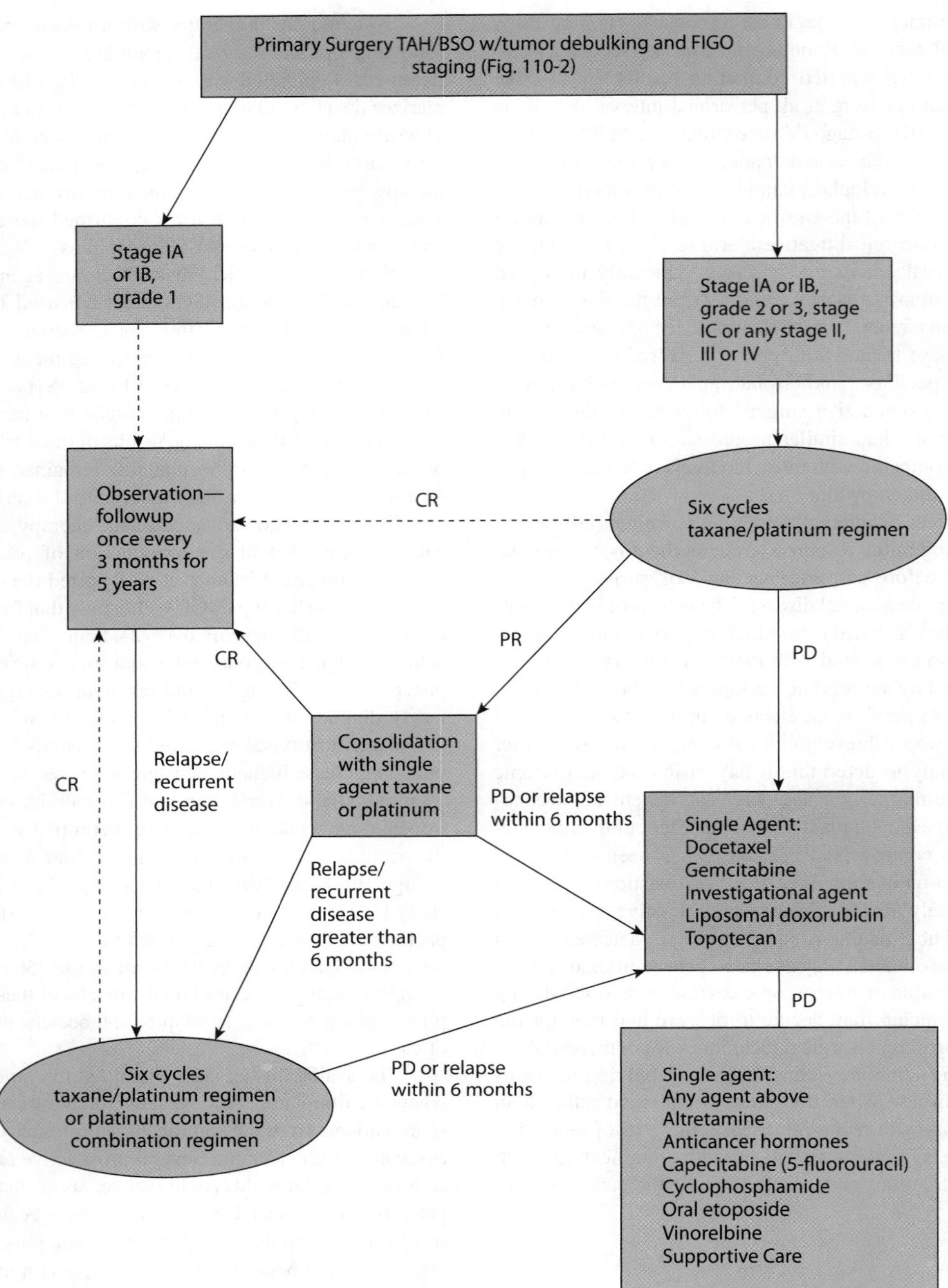

FIGURE 110-3 Management of newly diagnosed, refractory, and progressive epithelial ovarian cancer. All recommendations are category 2A unless otherwise indicated. (CR, complete response; PD, progression of disease; PR, partial response; TAH/BSO, total abdominal hysterectomy/bilateral salpingo-oophorectomy; USO, unilateral salpingo-oophorectomy.)

Other clinical trials have evaluated the use of docetaxel as a substitute for paclitaxel. In the Scottish Randomized Trial in Ovarian Cancer (SCOTROC), Vasey et al. compared carboplatin (AUC = 5) combined with either docetaxel (75 mg/m^2 over 1 hour) or paclitaxel (175 mg/m^2 over 3 hours) administered every 21 days for six cycles as first-line chemotherapy for stages IC to IV epithelial ovarian cancer.[57] The results of this study showed that the substitution of docetaxel for paclitaxel does not compromise efficacy and improves tolerability, particularly neurotoxicity. These findings were not confirmed in another randomized, controlled trial. However, based on the results of this study the combination of docetaxel plus carboplatin is considered a reasonable treatment option for patients with advanced ovarian cancer. Six cycles of paclitaxel plus carboplatin following tumor debulking surgery remain the current standard of care for treatment of advanced ovarian cancer.

Although the choice of taxane or platinum agent does not appear to have a major effect on antitumor activity, weekly paclitaxel administration ("dose density") may be superior to administration every 3 weeks.[58–60] In a phase III trial conducted in Japan, Katsumata et al. reported that patients randomized to six cycles of dose-dense weekly paclitaxel plus carboplatin every 3 weeks had longer progression-free survival as compared to the standard paclitaxel plus carboplatin every 3 weeks.[60] Overall survival at 3 years

TABLE 110-1 Initial Chemotherapeutic Regimens of Epithelial Ovarian Cancer

Drug(s)	Brand Name	Initial Dose(s)/Usual Range	Cycle Frequency
Paclitaxel + carboplatin	Taxol/Paraplatin	175 mg/m² IV (3-h infusion) day 1 Dosed to AUC 5–7.5 IV day 1	Every 21 days
Paclitaxel + cisplatin (IV)	Taxol/Platinol	135 mg/m² IV (24-h infusion) day 1 75 mg/m² IV day 1	Every 21 days
Paclitaxel + cisplatin (IP)	Taxol/Platinol	Day 1: Paclitaxel 135 mg/m² IV infused over 24 hours Day 2: Cisplatin 100 mg/m² IP infused over 1 hour Day 8: Paclitaxel 60 mg/m² IP infused over 1 hour.	Every 21 days
Cisplatin + cyclophosphamide	Platinol/Cytoxan	50–100 mg/m² IV day 1 500–1,000 mg/m² IV day 1	Every 21–28 days
Docetaxel + carboplatin	Taxotere/Paraplatin	75 mg/m² IV day 1	Every 21 days

AUC, area under the curve; IP, interperitoneal.

was also significantly longer in patients who received the dose-dense regimen (72% vs. 65%, $P = 0.03$). However, over 42% of the patients who received the dose-dense regimen dropped out of the study before completing six cycles because of treatment-related toxicities. A confirmatory GOG phase III trial is ongoing to confirm these results and address concerns regarding the feasibility of the dose-dense regimen in a larger group of patients as well as the elderly population.

IP chemotherapy was initially employed as palliative care in the management of ascites and uncontrolled intraabdominal tumors. In the late 1970s, IP chemotherapy administration as a primary treatment intervention was initiated based on the rationale that exposure of the tumor to high drug concentrations would increase tumor drug uptake by passive diffusion and ultimately cancer cell death.[61] The increase in AUC exposure in the peritoneal cavity was demonstrated, but the correlative increase in drug uptake in tumor tissue has yet to be validated in any preclinical or clinical study.

7 IP chemotherapy has demonstrated a benefit in the first-line treatment of patients with optimally debulked advanced-stage ovarian cancer.[49,62–64] In the most recent trial, Armstrong et al. reported the results of the GOG-172 study, which evaluated 415 patients randomized to receive either the combination regimen of paclitaxel 135 mg/m² over 24 hours and cisplatin 75 mg/m² or a new combination regimen that included paclitaxel 135 mg/m² IV infused over 24 hours followed by cisplatin 100 mg/m² IP infused over 1 hour on day 2, and then paclitaxel 60 mg/m² IP infused over 1 hour on day 8.[36] Both treatment regimens were given once every 21 days for a total of six cycles. Patients randomized to the IP chemotherapy arm had a 5.5-month increase in the median progression-free survival and a 15.9-month increase in overall survival.[36]

Since the publication of this study, there has been a resurgence of interest in the use of IP chemotherapy despite the limitation that only 42% of the patients on the IP treatment arm were able to complete the planned six cycles as a result of significantly more toxicity, including pain, fatigue, myelosuppression, gastrointestinal, metabolic, and neurotoxicity.[36,63,65,66] Because only 42% of patients were able to complete the planned six courses of IP chemotherapy, some experts have questioned whether the route of administration was an important contributing factor in the observed differences in overall survival.[36] The significant increase in systemic toxicity, primarily neurotoxicity, has led to the question of whether IP carboplatin could be substituted for IP cisplatin. Although these platinum agents have demonstrated equal efficacy when administered IV to ovarian cancer patients, based on the concept that drug passively diffuses into the tumor, the difference in molecular size of cisplatin versus carboplatin makes it difficult to extrapolate IP activity of cisplatin to carboplatin.

Clinical **Controversy...**

The use of interperitoneal (IP) chemotherapy as first-line treatment of advanced ovarian cancer has been recommended by the National Comprehensive Cancer Network (NCCN) guidelines. Most clinical trials have used platinum agents given IP until the Gynecologic Oncology Group (GOG)-172 trial that incorporated IP paclitaxel. Many clinicians are concerned about how to manage hypersensitivity reactions to either platinum or taxane agents when administered IP.

The National Comprehensive Cancer Network (NCCN) 2013 guidelines recommend that IP chemotherapy be considered and offered to appropriate patients as first-line treatment of optimally debulked, ≥1 cm residual disease, ovarian cancer.[67] The National Cancer Institute also released a position statement in January 2006 supporting the role of IP chemotherapy as first-line treatment for advanced ovarian cancer.[68] 7 Because of the significant toxicities associated with IP therapy, only carefully selected patients should receive IP therapy. Ideal candidates for IP therapy are younger patients with good performance status, minimal comorbidities, adequate renal and liver function, and optimally debulked disease without significant bowel resection.[62,66]

In patients who are poor surgical candidates because of comorbidities or bulky tumors, neoadjuvant chemotherapy can be given prior to any surgical interventions.[69] In patients with bulky disease, the goal of neoadjuvant chemotherapy is to reduce tumor burden to make surgery more feasible and optimal tumor debulking more likely. The typical regimen used in neoadjuvant chemotherapy is three cycles of a taxane combined with a platinum agent followed by surgery. After surgery, patients usually receive another three to six cycles, depending on their response to chemotherapy. In patients who are poor candidates for surgery because of comorbidities, the, primary intent of neoadjuvant chemotherapy is to relieve symptoms and slow disease progression. In this setting, palliative chemotherapy alone has not been curative for patients with advanced ovarian cancer.[69] If tolerated, these patients will receive the standard taxane plus platinum chemotherapy regimen once every 3 to 4 weeks. Another option for palliative neoadjuvant chemotherapy, especially in elderly patients, is single-agent carboplatin once every 4 weeks.

Neoadjuvant Chemotherapy

Neoadjuvant chemotherapy is first-line treatment for patients who are poor surgical candidates or patients with bulky or significant tumor burden.[35] The neoadjuvant chemotherapy regimen typically includes a combination of taxane with platinum agent is administered every 21 to 28 days as tolerated with intent to reduce tumor burden to point where it potentially could be surgically resected and ideally optimally debulking during surgery.[36] After surgery, patient will receive another three to six cycles depending on response to chemotherapy. The role of neoadjuvant chemotherapy for all patients presenting with advance ovarian cancer is being revisited in ongoing GOG clinical trials.

Consolidation Therapy

If patients do not achieve a clinical complete response after completion of six cycles of taxane-platinum regimen, then consolidation chemotherapy should be considered in an attempt to achieve a complete response (see Fig. 110-3). If the patient has a partial response to first-line chemotherapy, as measured by a greater than 50% decline in CA-125 (as compared with the presurgery level) or tumor regression, the cancer is still considered sensitive to the regimen. The typical regimens for consolidation chemotherapy are the taxane plus platinum regimen or single-agent therapy with either a taxane or platinum agent.[70] If the patient had a poor response to taxane and platinum, then alternative second-line agents can be considered.[67] Additional cycles of chemotherapy are given until complete response is achieved. Another alternative in the setting of no or minimal measurable disease after completion of primary chemotherapy is to just observe the patient and provide supportive care as indicated until disease progresses, then reinitiate chemotherapy at that time.[67]

Because the initial clinical complete response observed in first-line treatment has not been durable, optimization of first-line therapy is under investigation. Numerous options have been evaluated, including the use of additional cycles or maintenance chemotherapy and dose intensity.

Maintenance Chemotherapy

Maintenance chemotherapy is similar to consolidation chemotherapy except maintenance chemotherapy is given to those patients who have achieved a clinically complete response. The primary differences between consolidation and maintenance chemotherapy are the types of agents used and duration of therapy. Consolidation therapy usually consists of more aggressive combination regimens, whereas maintenance chemotherapy usually consists of single agents given less frequently (i.e., once monthly) to minimize adverse effects. The goal of maintenance chemotherapy is to eliminate any residual microscopic disease that may be present to extend progression-free and overall survival.

Maintenance chemotherapy has gained popularity after the publication of the results of the collaborative Southwest Oncology Group (SWOG) and GOG 178 study that compared single-agent paclitaxel 175 mg/m^2 over 3 hours once every 21 days for 3 additional cycles versus an additional 12 cycles.[71,72] Eligible patients had to have been in complete clinical remission after at least five to six cycles of a taxane-platinum regimen. This study was closed after the interim analysis by the SWOG Safety Monitoring Committee because patients receiving the additional 12 cycles had longer progression-free survival than those receiving 3 cycles of single-agent paclitaxel (28 vs. 21 months). After the results were reported, many patients randomized to the three-cycle arm chose to receive nine additional cycles of paclitaxel, which reduced the ability of the trial to show a difference in overall survival.[73] Because this study was closed early and did not demonstrate an overall survival benefit, another randomized, controlled trial through the GOG was initiated to confirm the improvement in progression-free survival and to attempt to determine the impact on overall survival. Until these confirmatory trials are completed, the role of maintenance chemotherapy is controversial in the management of advanced ovarian cancer patients. Maintenance chemotherapy is listed as an option in the 2013 NCCN guidelines (2B recommendation).[67]

High-Dose Chemotherapy with Hematopoietic Stem Cell Transplantation

High-dose chemotherapy with autologous or allogeneic hematopoietic stem cell transplantation (HSCT) is an option for selected patients with chemosensitive disease, few comorbidities, and good performance status. Although high response rates have been reported in patients with recurrent ovarian cancer treated with autologous HSCT, the duration of response is usually short and few patients have experienced long-term progression-free survival.[74,75] Allogeneic HSCT has also been evaluated in recurrent ovarian cancer to induce an immune response against the tumor ("graft-versus-tumor" effect).

Based on the activity of autologous HSCT in recurrent ovarian cancer, Goncalves et al. evaluated the modality for first-line treatment of patients with optimally debulked ovarian cancer. In this multicenter phase II study, 34 patients received two cycles of high-dose cyclophosphamide-epirubicin once every 21 days followed by two cycles of high-dose carboplatin (days 42 and 98).[76] Each dose of high-dose carboplatin was followed by hematopoietic stem cell infusion. The results of this study failed to show an improvement in the rate of pathologic complete response with upfront autologous HSCT as compared with standard taxane plus platinum chemotherapy. Additional studies are ongoing to determine the role of autologous or allogeneic HSCT in the treatment of advanced ovarian cancer.

Treatment of Recurrent Disease

5 Although most patients will achieve a complete response to initial treatment, most patients will eventually have recurrence of their disease within the first 2 years. When a patient relapses, the prognostic factors are similar to the factors after initial surgery except that the disease-free interval—defined as the length of time that has lapsed since the completion of chemotherapy—should be considered to determine if the tumor is likely to be drug resistant to agents used in first-line treatment, which included platinum and taxanes agents. If recurrence occurs less than 6 months after completion of chemotherapy, or if the patient progresses during platinum-based chemotherapy, the tumor is defined as platinum-resistant. Patients with platinum-sensitive disease generally have a better prognosis than platinum-resistant patients.

If the patient has a clinical complete response to first-line chemotherapy and the recurrence occurs more than 6 months after chemotherapy is completed, the tumor is considered platinum-sensitive. 8 In patients with platinum-sensitive ovarian cancer the standard of care is to treat the first recurrence with a doublet, platinum-containing chemotherapy regimen. Table 110-2 summarizes some of the chemotherapeutic regimens used in the treatment of recurrent or refractory ovarian cancer. Because the chemotherapy agents used for second-line treatment of recurrent or refractory platinum-resistant disease have similar response rates that average less than 30%, the selection of the agent is dependent on multiple factors including the toxicity profile of the agent, physician preference, patient performance status, residual toxicities, and patient convenience (see Fig. 110-3). In this setting, the intent of treatment is to prolong survival and alleviate symptoms, not necessarily to achieve another "complete response" to chemotherapy. 9 Because of poor response rates of the available agents, participation in a clinical trial of an investigational agent is often recommended for patients with recurrent platinum-resistant ovarian cancer.

Platinum-Sensitive Disease

9 Retreatment with a platinum-containing regimen should be considered in patients with platinum-sensitive disease. The International Collaborative Ovarian Neoplasm 4 and Arbeitsgemeinschaft Gynaekologische randomized 802 patients with recurrent

TABLE 110-2 Single-Agent Chemotherapeutic Regimens for Recurrent or Refractory Ovarian Cancer

Drug(s)	Brand Name(s)	Initial Dose(s)/Usual Range	Cycle Frequency
Docetaxel	Taxotere	75 mg/m² IV day 1	Every 21 days
Pegylated-liposomal doxorubicin	Doxil	40 mg/m² IV day 1	Every 28 days
Gemcitabine	Gemzar	800–1000 mg/m² IV days 1, 8, and 15	Every 28 days
Paclitaxel	Taxol	60–80 mg/m² IV (1-h infusion) day 1	Every week
Paclitaxel	Taxol	135–175 mg/m² IV day 1	Every 21 days
Carboplatin	Paraplatin	AUC 5 IV day 1	Every 21–28 days
Cisplatin	Platinol	75 mg/m² IV day 1	Every 21–28 days
Topotecan	Hycamtin	1.3–1.5 mg/m² IV once daily for 5 days	Every 21 days
Topotecan	Hycamtin	4 mg/m² IV once a week × 3 weeks, then 1 week off	Every 21 days
Etoposide	Vepesid	50 mg/m² orally once daily days 1–10 repeat every 21 days	Every 28 days
Capecitabine	Xeloda	1800–2000 mg/m² in divided dose twice a day for 2 weeks on, 1 week off	Every 21 days
Altretamine	Hexalen	260 mg/m² orally (total daily dose divided in four doses) for 14–21 days	Every 28 days
Tamoxifen	Nolvadex	20 mg orally twice a day	Continuous
Letrozole	Femara	2.5 mg orally once daily	Continuous

AUC, area under the curve.

platinum-sensitive ovarian cancer to either single-agent platinum, a non–taxane-platinum combination, or a taxane plus platinum combination.[75] Patients treated with the paclitaxel plus platinum regimen had significantly longer progression-free (29 vs. 24 months) and overall survival (hazard ratio = 0.82 [95% CI 0.69 to 0.97]) as compared with the other two treatment arms.[77,78] Although the taxane–platinum combination was clearly superior in this European study, it is difficult to extrapolate these results to patients treated in the United States because of differences in first-line treatment. At the time that International Collaborative Ovarian Neoplasm 4 (ICON4) was conducted, the standard of care in Europe for first-line treatment was single-agent carboplatin, so most patients enrolled in this study had no prior exposure to a taxane agent.[77] However, the standard of care in the United States has been a taxane-platinum combination since the early 1990s. Confirmatory data are needed to evaluate whether combination regimens would also be more beneficial in these patients for treatment of recurrent ovarian cancer.

Clinical **Controversy. . .**

In patients with recurrent ovarian cancer that is platinum-sensitive, some clinicians will recommend retreatment with a chemotherapy regimen including a platinum agent. Other clinicians suggest that the platinum-free interval for these patients should be extended and will recommend that recurrent disease first be treated with a non-platinum regimen (i.e., liposomal doxorubicin) and reserve the platinum agent until the next relapse.

TABLE 110-3 Combination Chemotherapy Regimens for Platinum-Sensitive Recurrent Ovarian Cancer

Drug(s)	Brand Name	Initial Dose(s)/Usual Range	Cycle Frequency
Gemcitabine + carboplatin	Gemzar/ Paraplatin	800 mg/m² IV day 1 & 8	Every 21 days
Gemcitabine + cisplatin	Gemzar/ Platinol	Dosed to AUC 5 IV day 1	Every 21 days
Liposomal doxorubicin + carboplatin	Doxil/ Paraplatin	Day 1 & day 8: gemcitabine 800 mg/m² & cisplatin 40 mg/m²	Every 28 days
Cyclophosphamide + bevacizumab	Cytoxan/ Avastin	30 mg/m² IV over 1–3 h & carboplatin AUC 5 50 mg PO once daily + bevacizumab 15 mg/kg q 3 weeks	Every 28 days

AUC, area under the curve; PO, by mouth.

The 2013 NCCN guidelines recommend the combination of platinum agent with gemcitabine, liposomal doxorubicin, or paclitaxel for treatment of platinum-sensitive recurrent ovarian cancer[67] (Table 110-3). In addition, the combination of gemcitabine plus cisplatin has demonstrated improvement in progression-free survival[78] (see Table 110-3). Carboplatin alone or any of the second-line agents is recommended for patients with platinum-sensitive disease who are unable to tolerate additional combination chemotherapy regimens because of residual toxicity or poor performance status.[67,79]

Platinum-Resistant Disease

Frequently patients present with recurrent drug-resistant disease after initial platinum-based therapy and cytoreductive surgery.[80,81] Patients who progress on a platinum agent or have no response are considered "platinum-refractory," whereas those patients who have recurrence within 6 months of completing a platinum-containing regimen are considered "platinum-resistant."[79] The 2013 NCCN guidelines list many possible treatment options for recurrent platinum-resistant or refractory ovarian carcinoma.[67] The optimal chemotherapeutic agent or regimen in the treatment of platinum-resistant disease is currently unclear. Ideally, the agent should be active in ovarian cancer and non–cross-resistant with taxanes or platinum agents. Regrettably, the response rate is low for all of the agents in platinum-refractory or resistant ovarian cancer.[82] Patients should typically be evaluated for response after treatment with at least three cycles of the chemotherapy agent or regimen. Because partial responses are rare, stable disease with relief of symptoms is considered a treatment success. If no response is observed, then an alternative chemotherapy regimen may be selected. Because all the potential agents have similar efficacy, the selection of agents and sequence used for treatment as the patient progresses will vary based on residual toxicity, dosing schedule, patient convenience, and physician preference.

Topotecan, an analog of the plant alkaloid 20(S)-camptothecin, is active in patients with metastatic ovarian cancer and is non–cross-resistant with platinum-based chemotherapy.[83] Preclinical studies suggest that protracted schedules of administration with low doses achieve the greatest antitumor response.[84] Topotecan has demonstrated activity in phase II trials as second-line and salvage therapy in patients who have relapsed after, or progressed during, platinum-based therapy.[83–85] A randomized phase III trial compared topotecan and paclitaxel in patients with advanced ovarian cancer who had failed one platinum-based regimen.[86] Patients were randomized to receive topotecan 1.5 mg/m² per day as a 30-minute infusion for 5 days repeated every 21 days or paclitaxel 175 mg/m² as a 3-hour infusion every 21 days. The overall response rate was 21% and 13% for the topotecan- and paclitaxel-treated groups, respectively. The median time-to-progression for topotecan-treated patients (32 weeks) was not significantly different from that for paclitaxel-treated patients (20 weeks). Median survival was 61 weeks in the topotecan-treated group and 43 weeks in the paclitaxel-treated group. Topotecan was well tolerated with minimal nonhematologic toxicities.[83,85,86]

Pegylated liposomal doxorubicin is one of the primary agents used for second-line therapy of recurrent ovarian cancer.[87–89] The drug tends to be better tolerated than topotecan, which is important for heavily pretreated patients with advanced disease. A large, randomized phase III study compared pegylated liposomal doxorubicin 50 mg/m^2 every 4 weeks to topotecan 1.5 mg/m^2 per day for 5 days repeated every 21 days in patients who failed first-line platinum therapy.[86] A total of 474 patients were randomized, 239 to pegylated liposomal doxorubicin and 235 to topotecan. The overall response rates for the pegylated liposomal doxorubicin and topotecan groups were 20% and 17%, respectively. Overall survival tended to favor pegylated liposomal doxorubicin, with a median of 108 weeks versus 71 weeks for topotecan. Differences in toxicity were observed between the arms, with more hematologic toxicity occurring in the topotecan arm and more palmar–plantar erythrodysesthesia (PPE) in the pegylated liposomal doxorubicin arm. However, the incidence of PPE has decreased in current clinical practice because the standard dose of pegylated liposomal doxorubicin used currently, 40 mg/m^2, is less than the dose that was used in the initial clinical trials and approved by the FDA.[90,91]

Gemcitabine, a novel pyrimidine antimetabolite, is also widely used in the treatment of recurrent platinum-resistant ovarian cancer. Although the overall response rate is only about 13% to 22% with single-agent gemcitabine in patients with platinum-refractory recurrent ovarian cancer, an additional 16% to 50% of patients have stable disease for a median of 7 months.[92,93] The main toxicities include myelosuppression, fatigue, myalgia, and skin rash. Because of its non–cross-resistant activity and in vivo synergy with platinum agents, gemcitabine is being evaluated in doublet regimens in patients with refractory disease and with carboplatin/taxane regimens in previously untreated patients.[93] The combination of gemcitabine with taxanes has demonstrated response rates from 36% to 90%, which if confirmed, are extremely encouraging.[93]

Other agents that have shown an overall response rate of 10% to 25% in patients with recurrent ovarian cancer include altretamine, etoposide, capecitabine, tamoxifen, letrozole, vinorelbine, and oxaliplatin.[94] Response rates tend to be higher in the platinum-sensitive subgroups. Most of these agents are available in oral formulations, which allows for outpatient administration in the palliative care setting.

Although there are no therapeutic guidelines for the selection of agents for the treatment of recurrent platinum-resistant ovarian cancer, the three most commonly used agents in clinical practice include pegylated liposomal doxorubicin, gemcitabine, and topotecan. These agents have demonstrated efficacy when used as a single agent and in combination with other agents. A phase II GOG study is ongoing to help define the optimal chemotherapy combination for treatment of recurrent or refractory platinum-resistant ovarian cancer. Selection of chemotherapy for treatment of recurrent disease is ultimately based on the patient's residual toxicities, scheduling and convenience, and physician preference.

Additional research continues to identify new agents and new targets for the treatment of ovarian cancer. Because platinum agents and taxanes have been identified as the most active classes of agents for treatment of ovarian cancer, drug development has focused on new platinum derivatives, taxanes and taxane analogs, and agents that exert cytotoxic activity by interacting with DNA directly. Specifically, new cytotoxic agents such as trabectedin, pemetrexed, and epothilones are currently being evaluated in clinical trials.

Biologic and Targeted Agents

Monoclonal antibodies such as bevacizumab and cetuximab and small-molecule tyrosine kinase inhibitors such as sunitinib, gefitinib, or sorafenib, are being evaluated to be incorporated into first-line and recurrent treatment regimens for ovarian cancer.[95–99] Although the biologic agents as single agents have not demonstrated significant activity, the results of several clinical trials show that the addition of agents such as bevacizumab into first-line and maintenance regimens improves progression-free survival. However, the impact on overall survival is controversial.

Bevacizumab

Bevacizumab is a recombinant humanized monoclonal antibody that targets vascular endothelial growth factor (VEGF), a key mediator of angiogenesis. In the setting of recurrent disease, single-agent bevacizumab produces a response rate similar to other therapies of 16% to 21%.[100,101] Response rates with combinations of bevacizumab range from 15% to 80%.[98,100–110] However, these phase II trials have also reported a higher risk of bowel perforation in patients treated with bevacizumab-containing regimens.[100,101,111] Bevacizumab should therefore not be given to patients who have had recent bowel surgery or a history of significant bowel resections. Recent efforts have focused on the integration of bevacizumab into first-line treatment regimens. Phase II studies confirmed the safety and feasibility of 6 cycles of paclitaxel, carboplatin plus bevacizumab, given every 3 weeks, followed by maintenance bevacizumab once every 3 weeks for 1 year.[107,108] Based on these encouraging results, the GOG initiated a confirmatory phase III study comparing six cycles of standard paclitaxel plus carboplatin to six cycles of the same regimen with bevacizumab to determine whether bevacizumab improves the efficacy of paclitaxel plus carboplatin. The duration of maintenance bevacizumab remains controversial. The results of these trials should determine the role of bevacizumab in the treatment of ovarian cancer.

Clinical **Controversy. . .**

Although bevacizumab has demonstrated some progression-free survival advantages when used in combination, its effect on overall survival is not clear. Therefore, it is not clear that the benefits justify the high cost of bevacizumab. As a result, health insurance companies do not consistently reimburse providers for bevacizumab when used for the treatment of ovarian cancer.

Targeted Agents

Tyrosine kinase inhibitors such as sorafenib, sunitinib, pazopanib, and cediranib inhibit angiogenesis by specifically targeting the VEGF receptor (VEGFR). When given as single agents, tyrosine kinase inhibitors have demonstrated some antitumor activity in ovarian cancer.[112,113] Ongoing trials have focused on combination regimens with cytotoxic agents for first-line treatment and also treatment of recurrent ovarian cancer. Another interesting targeted agent is VEGF Trap (aflibercept), a fusion protein that targets VEGF-A. Aflibercept has been beneficial in the treatment of malignant ascites and is currently being incorporated into first-line regimens. Epidermal growth factor receptor (EGFR) inhibitors such as erlotinib have not demonstrated activity either alone or combined with chemotherapy or bevacizumab for the treatment of ovarian cancer.[109] The newer classes of targeted therapies such as platelet-derived growth factor (PDGF) inhibitors and poly-ADP-ribose polymerase (PARP) inhibitors are being investigated in ongoing clinical trials.[114]

PERSONALIZED PHARMACOTHERAPY

Current research efforts are focused on identifying biomarkers which are predictive of response in ovarian cancer. The primary focus has been on response to first-line treatment agents, paclitaxel and platinum and the multidrug resistance (MDR) pathway, specifically ABC-transport protein P-glycoprotein (Pgp).[115]

Epigenetics is a potential source of drug resistance. Epigenetic changes are heritable changes outside of the "traditional" DNA coding sequence. Aberrant DNA methylation and histone acetylation are epigenetic events which can silence tumor suppression genes required for apoptosis or DNA repair and therefore lead to resistance. The acetylation of histones is required for active genes and deacetylation occurs in silenced genes. Histone acetyltransferases (HATs) add acetyl groups and histone deacetylases (HDACs) remove acetyl groups.[116]

Ovarian cancers upregulate a variety of factors involved in DNA repair, angiogenesis, proliferation, and migration; they also downregulate mismatch-repair (MMR), cell adhesion, and apoptotic genes.[116] Tumorigenesis can induce hypermethylation or hypomethylation, which leads to chromosomal instability.[117] Hypermethylation or deacetylation has been shown to silence specific genes such as *hMLH1*, which leads to tumor formation and progression in the ovaries. Deacetylation of p21, a cell cycle regulator, can occur in ovarian carcinomas. Epigenetics may downregulate Apaf-1 and p16 while potentially upregulating MDR1. Finally, resistance to a platinum and taxane regimen may be associated with *hMLH1* methylation.[116]

Genomic information is being gathered to help overcome resistance such as finding amplified or deleted sequences or determining whether single nucleotide polymorphisms (SNPs) are the cause of resistance. Proteomics can also be used to identify mechanisms of resistance by finding over- or underexpressed proteins. These methods could lead to personalized pharmacotherapy if any of these biomarkers are predictive of drug response or resistance.[118]

While most chemotherapy drugs used to treat ovarian cancer are dosed according to body surface area (BSA), carboplatin dosing is personalized based on each individual's renal function with the Calvert formula: carboplatin dose = AUC × (glomerular filtration rate [GFR] + 25).[119] When it was originally developed and validated, measured GFR was used in the Calvert equation. However, the estimated creatinine clearance (CL_{cr}) is now used in clinical practice in place of measured GFR. Despite more than 30 years of clinical use, it is still not clear which equation to use to estimate CL_{cr} and the best method to estimate CL_{cr} in certain patient subgroups. The use of personalized carboplatin dose has reduced potential toxicity such as thrombocytopenia, neuropathy, and nephrotoxicity.[119] Personalized dosing of carboplatin is one of the reasons why it is often the preferred platinum agent over cisplatin for primary treatment for ovarian cancer.[56]

EVALUATION OF THERAPEUTIC OUTCOMES

During chemotherapy patients may experience numerous side effects such as nausea and vomiting, myelosuppression, neuropathy, and changes in organ function. Patients receiving a taxane or platinum chemotherapy regimen should be monitored for signs of hypersensitivity or infusion-related reactions. Patients treated with paclitaxel often experience infusion-related reactions, which have been attributed to the polyethoxylated castor oil (Cremophor) diluent. Premedications including an H_1-blocker, H_2-blocker, and steroid should be administered prior to each chemotherapy administration to prevent hypersensitivity reactions. If a patient has a reaction, increasing the duration of the infusion from 3 to 6 hours may help with infusion-related reactions. For patients with a true taxane allergy, paclitaxel desensitization can be attempted with 24 hours of premedications (H_1-blocker, H_2-blocker, and steroids) followed by paclitaxel given as a titrated infusion (1:1000 → 1:100 → 1:10 → full dose) over 8 hours. With repeated exposure (i.e., seven cycles or more) to carboplatin, patients can develop a delayed hypersensitivity reaction. A similar protocol can be used for carboplatin desensitization.

Ovarian cancer patients receive multiple courses of chemotherapy that can have varying effects on kidney and liver function, often with a delayed onset. Appropriate laboratory tests should be ordered to assess organ function so that chemotherapy doses can be adjusted as indicated. Patients on platinum-containing regimens can often experience electrolyte wasting, so patients should be monitored for electrolyte replacement, IV or oral, as indicated. The use of myeloid growth factors should be considered to prevent treatment delays and/or dose reductions. Prevention of nausea and vomiting, both acute and delayed, is critical for patients receiving emetogenic chemotherapy regimens such as paclitaxel plus carboplatin.

During initial taxane plus platinum chemotherapy, a CA-125 level should be obtained with each cycle and monitored for at least a 50% reduction in CA-125 after completion of four cycles, which is related to an improved prognosis. Patients who achieve a complete response after completion of first-line treatment should have followup once every 3 months, including CA-125, physical examination, pelvic examination, and appropriate diagnostic scans (i.e., computed tomography, magnetic resonance imaging, or positron emission tomography), which should be evaluated for presence of disease. In addition to routine followup examinations, clinicians should monitor for resolution of any residual chemotherapy-related side effects, including neuropathies, nephrotoxicity, ototoxicity, myelosuppression, and nausea and vomiting.

In the progressive disease or recurrent setting, CA-125 levels can still be used to monitor for response and should be checked with each cycle, although no change in therapy is recommended until after completion of at least three cycles of the second-line chemotherapy. In addition to laboratory monitoring, appropriate diagnostic scans (i.e., computed tomography, magnetic resonance imaging, or positron emission tomography) should be done once every three cycles. Patients need to be monitored with each cycle of chemotherapy to evaluate for new or persistent toxicities such as neuropathies, fluid retention, PPE, myelosuppression, and nausea and vomiting. Another precaution to keep in mind for patients with significant ascites, the "dry weight" or an adjusted body weight should be used for dosing chemotherapy.

Eventually, most ovarian cancer patients will progress through all chemotherapy regimens and investigational treatment options, after which the best supportive care measures should be provided to maintain patient comfort and quality of life. A plan to treat common complications of progressive ovarian cancer, including thrombosis, ascites, uncontrollable pain, and small bowel obstruction should be developed. The primary goal at the end of life for patients with progressive ovarian cancer is to provide any measures necessary to maintain patient comfort and quality of life.

ABBREVIATIONS

AUC	area under the curve
BRCA1	breast cancer activator gene 1
BRCA2	breast cancer activator gene 2
BSA	body surface area
CA-125	cancer antigen 125
CA-19	cancer antigen 19
CI	confidence index
CL_{cr}	creatinine clearance
EGFR	epidermal growth factor receptor

FDA	Food and Drug Administration
FIGO	International Federation of Gynecology and Obstetrics
GFR	glomerular filtration rate
GI	gastrointestinal
GOG	Gynecologic Oncology Group
HAT	histone acetyltransferase
HDAC	histone deacetylase
HSCT	hematopoietic stem cell transplantation
ICON4	International Collaborative Ovarian Neoplasm 4
IP	intraperitoneal
MMR	mismatch-repair
MDR	multidrug resistance
NCCN	National Comprehensive Cancer Network
^{32}P	phosphorus-32
Pap	Papanicolaou
PARP	poly-ADP-ribose polymerase
PDGF	platelet-derived growth factor
Pgp	P-glycoprotein
PPE	palmar–plantar erythrodysesthesia
SCOTROC	Scottish Randomized Trial in Ovarian Cancer
SNP	single nucleotide polymorphism
SWOG	Southwest Oncology Group
TAH/BSO	total abdominal hysterectomy/ bilateral salpingo oophorectomy
TVUS	transvaginal ultrasound
VEGF	vascular endothelial growth factor
VEGFR	vascular endothelial growth factor receptor

REFERENCES

1. Bast RC, Brewer M, Zou, C, et al. Prevention and early detection of ovarian cancer: Mission impossible? Recent Results Cancer Res 2007;174:91–100.
2. Heintz APM, Odicino F, Maisonneuve P, et al. Carcinoma of the ovary. FIGO 6th annual report on the results of treatment in gynecological cancer. Int J Gynaecol Obstet 2006;95(suppl):S161–S192.
3. Siegel R, Naishadham D, Jemal A. Cancer statistics, 2013. CA Cancer J Clin 2013;63:11–30.
4. Colomob N, VanGorp T, Parma G, et al. Ovarian cancer. Crit Rev Oncol Hematol 2006;60:159–179.
5. Lux MP, Fashing PA, Beckmann MW. Hereditary breast and ovarian cancer: Review and future perspectives. J Mol Med 2006;84:16–28.
6. Pavelka JC, Li AJ, Karlan BY. Hereditary ovarian cancer-assessing risk and prevention strategies. Obstet Gynecol Clin North Am 2007;34:651–665.
7. Lancaster JM, Powell CB, Kauff ND, et al. Society of Gynecologic Oncologists Education Committee statement on risk assessment for inherited gynecologic cancer predispositions. Gynecol Oncol 2007;107:159–162.
8. RimMertens-Waler I, Baxter RC, Marsh DJ. Gonadotropin signaling in epithelial ovarian cancer. Cancer Letters 2012;324:152–159.
9. Aletti GC, Gallenberg MM, Cliby WA, et al. Current management strategies for ovarian cancer. Mayo Clin Proc 2007;82:751–770.
10. Permuth-Wey J, Sellers TA. Epidemiology of ovarian cancer. Methods Mol Biol 2009;472:413–437.
11. Bhoola S, Hoskins WJ. Diagnosis and management of epithelial ovarian cancer. Obstet Gynecol 2006;107: 1399–1410.
12. Cannistra SA, Gershenson, DM, Recht A. Ovarian cancer, fallopian tube carcinoma, and peritoneal carcinoma. In: Devita VT, Hellman S, Rosenberg SA, eds. Cancer: Principles and Practice of Oncology. 8th ed. Philadelphia: Lippincott Williams & Wilkins, 2008:1568–1592.
13. Silverberg SG, Histopathologic grading of ovarian carcinoma: A review and proposal. Int J Gynecol Pathol 2000;19:7–15.
14. Longuespee R, Boyon C, Desmons A, et al. Ovarian cancer molecular pathology. Cancer Metastat Rev 2012;31:713–732.
15. Krygiou M, Tsoumpou I, Martin-Hirsch P, et al. Ovarian cancer screening. Anticancer Res 2006;26:4793–4801.
16. Patterson DM, Rustin GJS. Controversies in the management of germ cell tumours of the ovary. Curr Opin Oncol 2006;18:500–506.
17. Sherman ME, Lacey JV, Buys SS, et al. Ovarian volume: Determinants and associations with cancer among postmenopausal women. Cancer Epidemiol Biomarkers Prev 2006;15:1550–1554.
18. Pavlik EJ, DePriest PD, Gallion HH, et al. Ovarian volume related to age. Gynecol Oncol 2000;77:410–412.
19. Edwards BK, Brown ML, Wingo PA, et al. Annual report to the nation on the status of cancer 1975–2002 featuring population-based trends in cancer treatment. J Natl Cancer Inst 2005;97:1407–1427.
20. Munkarah A, Chatterjee M, Tainsky MA. Update on ovarian cancer screening. Curr Opin Obstet Gynecol 2007;19:22–26.
21. Moyer VA. U.S. Preventive Services Task Force. Screening for ovarian cancer: Recommendation statement. Ann Intern Med 2012;157:900–904.
22. Chu CS, Rubin SC. Screening for ovarian cancer in the general population. Best Pract Res Clin Obstet Gynaecol 2006;20:307–320.
23. Dann JL, Zorn KK. Strategies for ovarian cancer prevention. Obstet Gynecol Clin North Am 2007;34:667–686.
24. Harris RE, Beebe-Donk J, Doss H, et al. Aspirin, ibuprofen, and other non-steroidal anti-inflammatory drugs in cancer prevention: A critical review of non-selective COX-2 blockade. Oncol Rep 2005;13:559–583.
25. Tavani A, Gallus S, La Vecchia C, et al. Aspirin and ovarian cancer: An Italian case-control study. Ann Oncol 2000;11:1171–1173.
26. Domchek SM, Rebbeck TR. Prophylactic oophorectomy in women at increased cancer risk. Curr Opin Obstet Gynecol 2007;19:27–30.
27. Meeuwissen PAM, Seynaeve C, Brekelmans CTM, et al. Outcome of surveillance and prophylactic salpingo-oophorectomy in asymptomatic women at high risk for ovarian cancer. Gynecol Oncol 2005;97:476–482.
28. Finch A, Beiner M, Lubinski J, et al. Salpingo-oophorectomy and the risk of ovarian, fallopian tube, and peritoneal cancers in women with a *BRCA1* or *BRCA2* mutation. JAMA 2006;296:185–192.
29. Narod SA, Sun P, Ghadirian P, et al. Tubal ligation and risk of ovarian cancer in carriers of *BRCA1* and *BRCA2* mutations: A case control study. Lancet 2001;357:1467–1470.
30. Lux MP, Fashing PA, Beckmann MW. Hereditary breast and ovarian cancer: Review and future perspectives. J Mol Med 2006;84:16–28.
31. Coukos G. Gene therapy for ovarian cancer. Oncology 2001;15:1197–1208.
32. Tait DL, Obermiller PS, Hatmaker AR, Relin-Frazier S, Holt JT. Ovarian cancer *BRCA1* gene therapy: Phase I and II trial differences in immune response and vector stability. Clin Cancer Res 1999;5:1708–1714.
33. Goff BA, Mandel LS, Melancon CH, Muntz HG. Frequency of symptoms of ovarian cancer in women presenting to primary care clinics. JAMA 2004;291:2705–2712.

34. Goff BA, Mandel LS, Drescher CW, et al. Development of an ovarian cancer symptom index. Cancer 2007;109:221–227.
35. Fung-Kee-Fung M, Oliver T, Elit L, Oza A, Kirte HW. Optimal chemotherapy treatment for women with recurrent ovarian cancer. Curr Oncol 2007;14:195–208.
36. Armstrong DK, Bundy B, Wenzel L, et al. Intraperitoneal cisplatin and paclitaxel in ovarian cancer. N Engl J Med 2006;354:34–43.
37. Cooper A, DePriest P. Surgical management of women with ovarian cancer. Semin Oncol 2007;34:226–233.
38. Schorge JO, McCann C, Del Carmen M. Surgical debulking of ovarian cancer: What difference does it make? Rev Obstet Gynecol 2010;3:111–117.
39. Stratton JF, Tidy JA, Paterson MEL. The surgical management of ovarian cancer. Cancer Treat Rev 2001;27:111–118.
40. Ibeanu OA, Bristow RW. Predicting the outcome of cytoreductive surgery for advanced ovarian cancer: a review. Int J Gynecol Cancer 2010;20(suppl 1):S1–S11.
41. Hoffman MS, Griffin D, Tebes S, et al. Sites of bowel resected to achieve optimal ovarian cancer cytoreduction: Implications regarding surgical management. Am J Obstet Gynecol 2005;193:582–588.
42. Bhoola S, Hoskins WJ. Diagnosis and management of epithelial ovarian cancer. Obstet Gynecol 2006;107:1399–1410.
43. Mayer AR, Chambers SK, Graves E, et al. Ovarian cancer staging: Does it require a gynecologic oncologist? Gynecol Oncol 1992;47:223–227.
44. Nguyen HN, Averette HE, Hoskins W, et al. National survey of ovarian carcinoma, V: The impact of physician's specialty on patients' survival. Cancer 1993;72:3663–3670.
45. Bristo RE, Eisenhauer EL, Santillan An, Chi DS. Delaying the primary surgical effort for advanced ovarian cancer: A systematic review of neoadjuvant chemotherapy and interval cytoreduction. Gynecol Oncol 2007;140:480–490.
46. Martinek IE, Kehoe S. When should surgical cytoreduction in advanced ovarian cancer take place? J Oncol 2010. DOI:10.1155/2010/852028.
47. Lorusso D, Mancini M, Di Rocco R, Fontanelli R, Raspagliesi F. The role of secondary surgery in recurrent ovarian cancer. Int J Surg Oncol 2012, in press.
48. Bohra U. Recent advances in management of epithelial ovarian cancer. Apollo Med 2012;9:212–218.
49. Kyrgiou M, Salanti G, Pavlidis N, Paraskevaidis E, Ioannidis JPA. Survival benefits with diverse chemotherapy regimens for ovarian cancer: Meta-analysis or multiple treatments. J Natl Cancer Inst 2006;98:1655–1663.
50. Ozols R. Systemic therapy for ovarian cancer: Current status and new treatments. Semin Oncol 2006;33(suppl 6):S3–S11.
51. McGuire WP, Hoskins WJ, Brady MF, et al. Cyclophosphamide and cisplatin compared with paclitaxel and cisplatin in patients with stage III and stage IV ovarian cancer. N Engl J Med 1996;334:1–6.
52. Piccart MJ, Bertelsen K, Stuart G, et al. Long-term follow-up confirms a survival advantage of the paclitaxel-cisplatin regimen over the cyclophosphamide-cisplatin combination in advanced ovarian cancer. Int J Gynecol Cancer 2003;13(suppl 2):144–148.
53. Bookman MA, Greer BE, Ozols RF. Optimal therapy of advanced ovarian cancer: Carboplatin and paclitaxel vs. cisplatin and paclitaxel (GOG 158) and an update on GOG0 182-ICON5. Int J Gynecol Cancer 2003;136:735–740.
54. Ozols RF, Bundy BN, Green BE, et al. Phase III trial of carboplatin and paclitaxel compared with cisplatin and paclitaxel in patients with optimally resected stage III ovarian cancer: A Gynecologic Oncology Group Study. J Clin Oncol 2003;21:3194–3200.
55. du Bois A, Luck HJ, Meier W, et al. A randomized clinical trial of cisplatin/paclitaxel versus carboplatin/paclitaxel as first-line treatment of ovarian cancer. J Natl Cancer Inst 2003;95:1320–1329.
56. Neijt JP, Engelholm SA, Tuxen MK, et al. Exploratory phase III study of paclitaxel and cisplatin versus paclitaxel and carboplatin in advanced ovarian cancer. J Clin Oncol 2000;18:3084–3092.
57. Vasey PA, Jayson GC, Gordon A, et al. Phase III randomized trial of docetaxel-carboplatin versus paclitaxel-carboplatin as first-line chemotherapy for ovarian carcinoma. J Natl Cancer Inst 2004;96:1682–1691.
58. Fennelly D, Aghajanian C, Shapiro F, et al. Phase I and pharmacologic study of paclitaxel administered weekly in patients with relapsed ovarian cancer. J Clin Oncol 1997;15:187–192.
59. Markman M, Blessing J, Rubin SC, et al. Phase II trial of weekly paclitaxel (80 mg/m^2) in platinum and paclitaxel-resistant ovarian and primary peritoneal cancers: A Gynecologic Group Study. Gynecol Oncol 2006;101:436–440.
60. Katsumata N, Yasuda M, Takahashi F, et al. Dose-dense paclitaxel once a week in combination with carboplatin every 3 weeks for advanced ovarian cancer: A phase 3, open-label, randomized controlled trial. Lancet 2009;374:1331–1338.
61. Fujiwara K, Armstrong D, Morgan M, Markman M. Principles and practice of intraperitoneal chemotherapy for ovarian cancer. Int J Gynecol Cancer 2007;17:1–20.
62. Jaaback K, Johnson N. Intraperitoneal chemotherapy for the initial management of primary epithelial ovarian cancer. Cochrane Database Syst Rev 2006;3:1–28.
63. Markman M, Bundy BN, Alberts DS, et al. Phase III trial of standard-dose intravenous cisplatin in small-volume stage III ovarian carcinoma: An intergroup study of the gynecologic oncology group, southwestern oncology group, and eastern cooperative oncology group. J Clin Oncol 2001;19:1001–1007.
64. Alberts DS, Liu PY, Hannigan EV, et al. Intraperitoneal cisplatin plus intravenous cyclophosphamide versus intravenous cisplatin plus intravenous cyclophosphamide for stage III ovarian cancer. N Engl J Med 1996;335:1950–1955.
65. Walker JL, Armstrong DK, Huang HQ, et al. Intraperitoneal catheter outcomes in a phase III trial of intravenous versus intraperitoneal chemotherapy in optimal stage III ovarian and primary peritoneal cancer: A Gynecologic Oncology Group Study. Gynecol Oncol 2006;100:27–32.
66. Markman M, Walker JL. Intraperitoneal chemotherapy of ovarian cancer: A review, with a focus on practical aspects of treatment. J Clin Oncol 2006;24:988–994.
67. National Comprehensive Cancer Network (NCCN) Practice Guidelines in Oncology—Ovarian Cancer, V1.2013. 2013, *http://www.nccn.org*.
68. NCI Clinical Announcement. Intraperitoneal Chemotherapy for Ovarian Cancer. January 5, 2006, *http://ctep.cancer.gov/highlights/clin_annc_010506.pdf*.
69. Salzberg M, Thurlimann B, Bonnefois H, et al. Current concepts of treatment strategies in advanced or recurrent ovarian cancer. Oncology 2005;68:293–298.
70. Gadducci A, Cosio S, Conte PF, Genazzani AR. Consolidation and maintenance treatments for patients with advanced epithelial ovarian cancer in complete response after first-line chemotherapy: A review of the literature. Crit Rev Oncol Hematol 2005;55:153–166.

71. Markman M, Liu PY, Wilczynski S, et al. Phase III randomized trial of 12 versus 3 months of maintenance paclitaxel in patients with advanced ovarian cancer who attained a clinically-defined complete response to platinum/paclitaxel-based chemotherapy: A Southwest Oncology Group and Gynecology Oncology Group trial. J Clin Oncol 2003;21:2460–2465.
72. Gadducci A, Cosio S, Conte PF, Genazzani AR. Consolidation and maintenance treatments for patients with advanced epithelial ovarian cancer in complete response after first-line chemotherapy: A review of the literature. Crit Rev Oncol Hematol 2005;55:153–166.
73. Markman M. Unresolved issues in the chemotherapeutic management of gynecologic malignancies. Semin Oncol 2006;33(suppl 6):S33–S38.
74. Mulder PO, Willemse PH, Aalders JG, et al. High-dose chemotherapy with autologous bone marrow transplantation in patients with refractory ovarian cancer. Eur J Cancer Clin Oncol 1989;25:645–649.
75. Stiff PJ, Veum-Stone J, Lazarus HM, et al. High-dose chemotherapy and autologous stem cell transplantation for ovarian cancer: An autologous blood and marrow transplant registry report. Ann Intern Med 2000;133:504–515.
76. Goncalves A, Delva R, Fabbro M, et al. Post-operative sequential high-dose chemotherapy with haematopoietic stem cell support as front-line treatment in advanced ovarian cancer: A multicenter study. Bone Marrow Transplant 2006;37:651–659.
77. ICON and AGO Collaborators. Paclitaxel plus platinum-based chemotherapy versus conventional platinum-based chemotherapy in women with relapsed ovarian cancer: The ICON4/AGO-OVAR-2.2 trial. Lancet 2003;361:2099–2106.
78. Bozas G, Bamias A, Koutsoukou, et al. Biweekly gemcitabine and cisplatin in platinum resistant/refractory, paclitaxel pre-treated, ovarian and peritoneal carcinoma. Gynecol Oncol 2007;104:580–585.
79. Gronlund B, Hogdall C, Hansen HH, Engelholm SA. Performance status rather than age is the key prognostic factor in second-line treatment of elderly patients with epithelial ovarian carcinoma. Cancer 2002;94:1961–1967.
80. Fung-Kee-Fung M, Oliver T, Elit L, et al. Optimal chemotherapy treatment for women with recurrent ovarian cancer. Curr Oncol 2007;14:195–208.
81. Inciura A, Simavicius A, Juozaityte E, et al. Comparison of adjuvant and neoadjuvant chemotherapy in the management of advanced ovarian cancer: A retrospective study of 574 patients. BMC Cancer 2006;6:153.
82. Herzog TJ, Pothuri B. Ovarian cancer: A focus on management of recurrent disease. Nat Clin Pract Oncol 2006;3:604–611.
83. Swisher EM, Mutch DG, Rader JS, et al. Topotecan in platinum- and paclitaxel-resistant ovarian cancer. Gynecol Oncol 1997;66:480–486.
84. Markman M. Topotecan: An important new drug in the management of ovarian cancer. Semin Oncol 1997;24:S5–S11.
85. ten Bokkel Huinink W, Gore M, Carmichael J, et al. Topotecan versus paclitaxel for the treatment of recurrent epithelial ovarian cancer. J Clin Oncol 1997;15:2183–2193.
86. Creemers GJ, Bolis G, Gore M, et al. Topotecan, an active drug in the second-line treatment of epithelial ovarian cancer: Results of a large European phase II study. J Clin Oncol 1996;14:3056–3061.
87. Muggia FM, Hainsworth JD, Jeffers S, et al. Phase II study of liposomal doxorubicin in refractory ovarian cancer: Antitumor activity and toxicity modification by liposomal encapsulation. J Clin Oncol 1997;15:987–993.
88. Gordon AN, Cranai CO, Rose PG, et al. Phase II study of liposomal doxorubicin in platinum- and paclitaxel refractory epithelial ovarian cancer. J Clin Oncol 2000;18:3093–3100.
89. Gordon AN, Fleagle JT, Guthrie D, et al. Recurrent epithelial ovarian carcinoma: A randomized phase III trial of pegylated liposomal doxorubicin versus topotecan. J Clin Oncol 2001;19:3312–3322.
90. Wilailk S, Linasmita V. A study of pegylated liposomal doxorubicin in platinum-refractory epithelial ovarian cancer. Oncology 2004;67:183–186.
91. Drake RD, Lin WM, King M, Farrar D, Miller DS, Coleman RL. Oral dexamethasone attenuates Doxil-induced palmer-plantar erythrodysesthesias in patients with recurrent gynecologic malignancies. Gynecol Oncol 2004;94:320–324.
92. Lund B, Hansen P, Theilade K, et al. Phase II study of gemcitabine (2′, 2′-difluorodeoxycytidine in previously treated ovarian cancer patients. J Natl Cancer Inst 1994;6:1530–1533.
93. Poveda A. Gemcitabine in patients with ovarian cancer. Cancer Treat Rev 2005;31(suppl 4):S29–S37.
94. Cannistra SA, Bast RC, Berek JS, et al. Progress in the management of gynecologic cancer: Consensus summary statement. J Clin Oncol 2003;21(suppl):129S–132S.
95. Ozols RF. Systemic therapy for ovarian cancer: Current status and new treatments. Semin Oncol 2006;33(suppl 6): S3–S11.
96. Kurzeder C, Sauer G, Deissler H. Molecular targets of ovarian carcinomas with acquired resistance to platinum/taxane chemotherapy. Curr Cancer Drug Targets 2006;6:207–227.
97. Cannistra SA, Bast RC, Berek JS, et al. Progress in the management of gynecologic cancer: Consensus summary statement. J Clin Oncol 2003;21(suppl):129s–132s.
98. Garcia AA, Hirte H, Fleming G, et al. Phase II Clinical Trial of Bevacizumab and Low-Dose Metronomic Oral Cyclophosphamide in Recurrent Ovarian Cancer: A Trial of the California, Chicago, and Princess Margaret Hospital Phase II Consortia. J Clin Oncol 2008;26:76–82.
99. Cohn DE, Valmadre S, Resnick KE, et al. Bevacizumab and weekly taxane chemotherapy demonstrates activity in refractory ovarian cancer. Gynecol Oncol 2006;102:134–139.
100. Cannistra SA, Matulonis UA, Penson RT, et al. Phase II study of bevacizumab in patients with platinum-resistant ovarian cancer or peritoneal serous cancer. J Clin Oncol 2007;25:5180–5186.
101. Burger RA, Sill MW, Monk BJ, Greer BE, Sorvosky JI. Phase II trial of bevacizumab in persistent or recurrent epithelial ovarian cancer or primary peritoneal cancer: A gynecologic oncology group study. J Clin Oncol 2007;25:5165–5171.
102. Monk BJ, Han E, Josephs-Cowan CA, Pugmire G, Burger RA. Salvage bevacizumab (rhuMAB VEGF)-based therapy after multiple prior cytotoxic regimens in advanced refractory epithelial ovarian cancer. Gynecol Oncol 2006;102:140–144.
103. Wright JD, Hagemann A, Rader JS, et al. Bevacizumab combination therapy in recurrent, platinum-refractory, epithelial ovarian carcinoma. Cancer 2006;107:83–89.
104. Chura JC, Van Iseghem K, Downs LS Jr, Carson IF, Judson PI. Bevacizumab plus cyclophosphamide in heavily pretreated patients with recurrent ovarian cancer. Gynecol Oncol 2007;107:326–330.
105. Simpkins F, Belinson JI, Rose PG, et al. Avoiding bevacizumab related gastrointestinal toxicity for recurrent ovarian cancer by careful patient screening. Gynecol Oncol 2007;107:118–123.

106. McGonigle KF, Muntz HG, Vuky J, et al. Combined weekly topotecan and biweekly bevacizumab in women with platinum-resistant ovarian, peritoneal, or fallopian tube cancer: Results of a phase 2 study. Cancer 2011;117:3731–3740.
107. Penson RT, Dizon DS, Cannistra SA, et al. Phase II study of carboplatin, paclitaxel, and bevacizumab with maintenance bevacizumab as first-line chemotherapy for advanced müllerian tumors. J Clin Oncol 2009;28:154–159.
108. Micha JP, Goldstein BH, Rettenmaier MA, et al. A phase II study of outpatient first-line paclitaxel, carboplatin, and bevacizumab for advanced-stage epithelial ovarian, peritoneal, and fallopian tube cancer. Int J Gynecol Cancer 2007;17:771–776.
109. Nimeiri HS, Oza AM, Morgan RJ, et al. Efficacy and safety of bevacizumab plus erlotinib for patients with recurrent ovarian, primary peritoneal, and fallopian tube cancer: A trial of the Chicago, PMH, and California Phase II consortia. Gynecol Oncol 2008;110:49–55.
110. Azad NS, Posadas EM, Kwitkowski, et al. Combination targeted therapy with sorafenib and bevacizumab results in enhanced toxicity and antitumor activity. J Clin Oncol 2008;26:3709–3714.
111. Richardson DL, Backes FJ, Seamon LG, et al. Combination gemcitabine, platinum, and bevacizumab for the treatment of recurrent ovarian cancer. Gynecol Oncol 2008;111: 461–466.
112. Matulonis UA, Berlin S, Ivy P, et al. Cediranib, an inhibitor of vascular endothelial growth factor receptor kinases, in an active drug in recurrent epithelial ovarian, fallopian tube and peritoneal cancer. J Clin Oncol 2009;27:5601–5606.
113. Biagi JJ, Oza AM, Chalchal HI, et al. A phase II study of sunitinib in patients with recurrent epithelial ovarian and primary peritoneal carcinoma: An NCIC Clinical Trials Group Study. Ann Oncol 2011;22:335–340.
114. Banerjee S, Kaye S. The role of targeted therapy in ovarian cancer. Eur J Cancer 2011;47(suppl 3):S116–S130.
115. Marsh S, Paul J, King CR, Gifford G, McLeod H, Brown R. Pharmacogenetic assessment of toxicity and outcome after platinum plus taxane chemotherapy in ovarian cancer: The Scottish Randomized Trial in Ovarian Cancer. J Clin Oncol 2007;25:4528–4535.
116. Glasspool RM, Teodoridis JM, Brown R. Epigenetics as a mechanism driving polygenic clinical drug resistance. Br J Cancer 2006;94:1087–1092.
117. Kanai Y. Alterations of DNA methylation and clinicopathological diversity of human cancers. Pathol Int 2008;58:544–558.
118. Schiavone MB, Bashir S, Herzog TJ. Biologic therapies and personalized medicine in gynecologic malignancies. Obstet Gynecol Clin North Am 2012;39:131–144.
119. Calvert AH, Newell DR, Gumbrell LA, et al. Carboplatin dosage: Prospective evaluation of a simple formula based on renal function. J Clin Oncol 1989;7:1748–1756.

111

Acute Leukemias

Betsy Bickert Poon and Amy Hatfield Seung

KEY CONCEPTS

1. Acute leukemias are the most common malignancies in children and the leading cause of cancer-related death in patients younger than age 35 years.
2. To establish a definitive diagnosis of acute leukemia, the following diagnostic components are required: bone marrow biopsy and aspirate (with >20% blasts), cytogenetics, and immunophenotyping.
3. Several risk factors correlate with prognosis for acute lymphoblastic leukemia (ALL). Poor prognostic factors include high white blood cell count at presentation, very young or very old age at diagnosis, delayed remission induction and presence of certain cytogenetic abnormalities (e.g., Philadelphia chromosome positive [Ph^+]).
4. For children with ALL, remission induction therapy includes vincristine, a corticosteroid, and asparaginase, with or without an anthracycline. For adults with ALL, vincristine, prednisone, and an anthracycline are given, and asparaginase is sometimes added.
5. All patients with ALL require prophylactic therapy to prevent CNS disease because of the high risk of central nervous system relapse. The choice for therapy includes a combination of the following: cranial irradiation, intrathecal chemotherapy, or high-dose systemic chemotherapy with drugs that cross the blood–brain barrier.
6. Long-term maintenance therapy for 2 to 3 years is essential to eradicate residual leukemia cells and prolong the duration of remission. Maintenance therapy consists of oral methotrexate and mercaptopurine, with or without monthly pulses of vincristine and a corticosteroid.
7. Disease-free survival is lower in adults with ALL and has been attributed to greater drug resistance, poor side effect tolerance with subsequent nonadherence, and possibly less-effective therapy. This population is also more likely to have Ph^+ ALL, which is associated with a worse outcome, but the use of tyrosine kinase inhibitors has improved treatment results.
8. There are several poor prognostic factors for adult acute myeloid leukemia (AML): older age, organ impairment, presence of extramedullary disease, and presence of certain cytogenetic and molecular abnormalities.
9. Therapy of AML usually includes induction therapy with an anthracycline and cytarabine. Postremission therapy is required in all patients and can include either consolidation chemotherapy with or without maintenance therapy, or hematopoietic stem cell transplantation.
10. It is estimated that up to 10^8 to 10^9 malignant cells remain following attainment of a complete remission. Postremission therapy with either chemotherapy or hematopoietic stem cell transplantation is essential in AML.
11. Treatment of acute promyelocytic leukemia consists of induction therapy, followed by consolidation and maintenance therapy. Induction includes tretinoin and an anthracycline; consolidation therapy consists of two to three cycles of anthracycline-based therapy; maintenance consists of pulse doses of tretinoin, mercaptopurine, and methotrexate for 2 years.
12. Hematopoietic growth factors can be safely and effectively used with myelosuppressive chemotherapy for acute leukemias. The benefits may include reduced incidence of serious infections, reduced hospital stays, and fewer treatment delays, but do not include prolonged disease-free survival or overall survival.

The leukemias are heterogeneous hematologic malignancies characterized by unregulated proliferation of the blood-forming cells in the bone marrow. These immature proliferating leukemia cells (blasts) physically "crowd out" or inhibit normal cellular maturation in bone marrow, resulting in anemia, neutropenia, and thrombocytopenia. Leukemic blasts may also infiltrate a variety of tissues such as lymph nodes, skin, liver, spleen, kidney, testes, and the central nervous system.

Historically, leukemia has been classified based on the cell of origin and cell line maturation, and as acute or chronic based on differences in clinical presentation, rapidity of progression of the untreated disease, and response to therapy. The four major leukemias are acute lymphoblastic (or lymphocytic) leukemia (ALL), acute myeloid leukemia (AML), chronic lymphocytic leukemia, and chronic myeloid leukemia. Undifferentiated immature cells that proliferate autonomously characterize acute leukemias. Chronic leukemias also proliferate autonomously, but the cells are more differentiated and mature. Untreated, acute leukemia is fatal within weeks to months.

EPIDEMIOLOGY

It is estimated that 20,660 new cases of acute leukemia—14,590 cases of AML and 6,070 cases of ALL—will be diagnosed in the United States in 2013, accounting for 1.2% of the total cancer incidence.[1] The incidence has been relatively stable for two decades. An estimated 11,800 deaths per year, representing about 2% of all cancer deaths, are caused by acute leukemias.[1] (1) Leukemia is the leading cause of cancer-related deaths in persons younger than age

20 years, but an uncommon cause of cancer-related death after age 40 years.[1] Among adults, acute and chronic leukemias occur at equal rates. More than 90% of the cases of acute and chronic leukemia occur in adults. AML accounts for most cases of acute leukemia in adults, and occurs with increasing frequency in elderly patients. There are about 3.6 cases of AML and 1.4 cases of ALL per 100,000 individuals.[2] The median age at diagnosis of patients with AML is about 67 years, whereas the peak age for ALL patients is 2 to 3 years.[1,2] The incidence of AML increases with age from 1.8 per 100,000 in individuals younger than age 65 years to 16 per 100,000 in those 65 years or older.[2,3] Acute leukemia is about 30% more common in males than in females. In the United States, acute leukemia is more common among whites than among African Americans, American Indians, and Hispanic ethnicities.[2]

Despite the low incidence, the acute leukemias are the most common malignancy in persons younger than 20 years of age, accounting for 26% of all childhood malignancies.[2] About 80% of children with leukemia have ALL and 15% AML.[2] Childhood ALL is about 30% more common in males than in females, peaks at 2 to 4 years of age, and is almost twice as likely to affect white children as African American children.[2] The incidence of childhood AML is highest in the Hispanic population and occurs throughout childhood without any peak age period. Acute leukemia during the first year of life (infant leukemia) slightly favors ALL over AML.[2,4]

Chemotherapy has dramatically improved the outlook of patients with acute leukemia. More than 85% of children and young adults with acute leukemia achieve an initial complete remission (CR) of their disease. Overall, 65% to 85% of adults achieve an initial CR.[3] For persons younger than 19 years of age, the 5-year survival rate is nearly 90% for ALL and 70% for AML.[2,5] The prognosis of adult acute leukemia is generally worse than that of childhood leukemia, with only 30% to 40% of patients becoming long-term survivors. When all ages are included, the 5-year relative survival rate in 2008 for ALL was 66% and 25% for AML.[2]

ETIOLOGY

The exact cause of the acute leukemias is unknown. A multifactorial process involving genetics, environmental and socioeconomic factors, toxins, immunologic status, and viral exposures is likely. Table 111-1 summarizes the major factors that have been linked to acute leukemias. Infectious and genetic factors have the strongest associations to date.[6] In pediatric ALL, a number of environmental factors are inconsistently linked to the disease: exposure to ionizing radiation, toxic chemicals, herbicides and pesticides; maternal use of contraceptives, diethylstilbestrol, or cigarettes; parental exposure to drugs (amphetamines, diet pills, and mind-altering medications), diagnostic radiographs, alcohol consumption, or chemicals before and during pregnancy; and chemical contamination of groundwater.[7,8] A growing body of evidence indicates that high birthweight is a risk for ALL.[6,9] Ionizing radiation and benzene exposure are the only environmental risk factors strongly associated with ALL or AML.[8] A few studies have reported a possible link between electromagnetic fields of high-voltage power lines and the development of leukemia, but larger studies could not confirm this association. In most patients who develop leukemia, a cause cannot be identified.

Childhood AML is associated with Hispanic ethnicity, prior exposure to alkylating agents or epipodophyllotoxins, and in utero exposure to ionizing radiation.[8] Maternal alcohol consumption, parental and child organophosphate pesticide exposure, and parental benzene exposure are also associated with childhood AML. AML has been associated with both low and high birth weight.[9] Adult AML has been associated with prior anthracycline exposure in addition to prior exposure to alkylating agents or epipodophyllotoxins.

TABLE 111-1 Risk Factors for Acute Leukemia

Drugs	**Chemical**
Alkylating agents	Benzene
Anthracyclines	**Pesticides**
Epipodophyllotoxins	**Pyrethroid-based shampoo**
Genetic conditions	**Radiation**
Amegakaryocytic thrombocytopenia	Ionizing radiation
Ataxia telangiectasia	**Virus**
Bloom syndrome	Epstein-Barr virus
Diamond-Blackfan anemia	Human T-lymphocyte virus (HTLV-1 and HTLV-2)
Down syndrome	
Dyskeratosis congenita	**Social habits**
Familial monosomy 7	Cigarette smoking
Fanconi anemia	Maternal marijuana use
Klinefelter syndrome	Maternal ethanol use
Kostmann syndrome	
Langerhans cell histiocytosis	
Li Fraumeni syndrome	
Neurofibromatosis type 1	
Noonan syndrome	
Shwachman syndrome	
Severe combined immunodeficiency syndrome	
Wiskott-Aldrich syndrome	

PATHOPHYSIOLOGY

A basic understanding of normal hematopoiesis is needed before one can understand the pathogenesis of leukemia. eChapter 20 has a detailed discussion of hematopoiesis. Normal hematopoiesis consists of multiple well-orchestrated steps of cellular development. A pool of pluripotent stem cells undergoes differentiation, proliferation, and maturation, to form the mature blood cells seen in the peripheral circulation. These pluripotent stem cells initially differentiate to form two distinct stem cell pools. The myeloid stem cell gives rise to six types of blood cells (erythrocytes, platelets, monocytes, basophils, neutrophils, and eosinophils). Lymphoid stem cells differentiate to form natural killer cells, B lymphocytes, and T lymphocytes. Leukemia may develop at any stage and within any cell line.

Two features are common to both AML and ALL: First, both arise from a single leukemic cell that expands and acquires additional mutations, culminating in a monoclonal population of leukemia cells. Second, there is a failure to maintain a relative balance between proliferation and differentiation, so that the cells do not differentiate past a particular stage of hematopoiesis. Cells (lymphoblasts or myeloblasts) then proliferate uncontrollably. Proliferation, differentiation, and apoptosis are under genetic control, and leukemia can occur when the balance between these processes is altered.

AML probably arises from a defect in the pluripotent stem cell or a more committed myeloid precursor, resulting in partial differentiation and proliferation of immature precursors of the myeloid blood-forming cells. In older patients, trilineage leukemia occurs suggesting that the cell of origin is probably a stem or very early progenitor cell. In younger patients, a more differentiated progenitor becomes malignant, allowing maturation of some granulocytic and erythroid populations. These two forms of AML exhibit different patterns of resistance to chemotherapy, with resistance more evident in the older adults with AML. ALL is a disease characterized by proliferation of immature lymphoblasts. In this type of acute leukemia, the defect is probably at the level of the lymphopoietic stem cell or a very early lymphoid precursor.

Leukemic cells have growth and/or survival advantages over normal cells, leading to a "crowding out" phenomenon in the bone marrow. This growth advantage is not caused by more rapid proliferation as compared with normal cells. Some studies suggest that it is caused by factors produced by leukemic cells that either inhibit normal cellular proliferation and differentiation, or reduce apoptosis as compared with normal blood cells.

The types of genetic alterations that lead to leukemia have only recently become evident. The genetic defects may include (a) activation of a normally suppressed gene (protooncogene) to create an oncogene that produces a protein product that signals increased proliferation; (b) loss of signals for the blood cell to differentiate; (c) loss of tumor suppressor genes that control normal proliferation; and (d) loss of signals for apoptosis. Most normal cells are programmed to die eventually through apoptosis, but the appropriate programmed signal is often interrupted in cancer cells, leading to continued survival, replication, and drug resistance. Signal transduction, RNA transcription, cell-cycle control factors, cell differentiation, and programmed cell death may all be affected.

LEUKEMIA CLASSIFICATION

In 2001, the World Health Organization (WHO), in collaboration with the Society for Hematopathology and the European Association of Haematopathology, proposed a new classification system for myeloid neoplasms. This new classification system incorporates not only morphologic findings, but also genetic, immunophenotypic, cytochemical, and clinical features. About 40% to 50% of adult patients with AML have no detectable chromosomal abnormality on standard cytogenetic analysis, but the percent increases with age.[10] The WHO classification attempts to formally incorporate the relationship between AML and myelodysplastic syndrome (MDS). In 2008, this classification was revised (Table 111-2) and is being used routinely for children and adults.[11] The WHO classification defines acute leukemias as more than 19% blasts in the marrow or blood.

Lymphoblast analysis is used to classify ALL. Immunophenotype is determined by flow cytometry that analyzes specific antigens, known as clusters of differentiation (often abbreviated "CD"), present on the surface of hematopoietic cells. Although no leukemia-specific antigens have been identified, the pattern of cell-surface antigen expression reliably distinguishes between lymphoid and myeloid leukemia. The immunophenotype defines the cell of origin. The major phenotypes are mature B-cell, precursor B-cell, and T-cell disease; however, the WHO classifies ALL as either B lymphoblastic or T lymphoblastic. About 80% of childhood ALL derives from precursor B cells and about 15% from T cells; the remainder is either mixed lineage or from mature B cells. T-cell ALL is more common in teenage males.

Leukemias may also be described by cytogenetic abnormalities. Chromosome alterations include numerical (hyperdiploidy and hypodiploidy), and structural abnormalities due to exchanges of genetic information within (inversion) or between (translocation) chromosomes. Unique translocations can identify specific subtypes of acute leukemia. Twenty-five percent of children with precursor B-cell ALL have the *ETV6-RUNX1* (formerly *TEL-AML1*) fusion gene generated by the t(12;21)(p13;q22) chromosomal translocation.[6,12] This translocation appears to endow the preleukemia cell with altered self-renewal and survival properties. The most common translocation in adult ALL, occurring in 25% of patients, is the t(9;22) or Philadelphia chromosome positive (Ph^+), which causes fusion of the BCR signaling protein to the ABL nonreceptor tyrosine kinase, resulting in constitutive tyrosine kinase activity. More than 50% of childhood T-cell ALL have activating mutations of the *NOTCH1* gene that encodes for a transmembrane receptor implicated in regulation of T cell development.[6,12] Acute promyelocytic leukemia (APL) is characterized by a specific translocation between chromosomes 15 and 17: t(15;17). Molecular tests may be used to identify products of specific translocations, such as promyelocytic leukemia (PML) retinoic acid receptor-α (RARα) in APL and *AML1-ETO* and *CBFβ/MYH 11* in other subtypes of AML.

A number of factors may affect the cytogenetics of AML in adults. First, in about 5% of patients, simultaneous blood and marrow samples demonstrate normal cytogenetics versus abnormal cytogenetics, respectively.[10] Second, central cytogenetic analysis is done in multicenter trials because of variability in specimen examination. A small number of patients may have a normal karyotype on standard review, but carry fusion genes, which are identical to those of translocations or inversions. These insertions of very small chromosome segments do not alter chromosome morphology but may affect outcome.

TABLE 111-2 World Health Organization Classification of Acute Myeloid Leukemia

Acute myeloid leukemia (AML) with recurrent genetic abnormalities
AML with t(8;21)(q22;q22), (AML1/ETO)
AML with abnormal bone marrow eosinophils and inv(16)(p13;q22) or t(16;16)(p13;q22), (CBFβ/MYH11)
Acute promyelocytic leukemia with t(15;17)(q22;q12), (PML/RARα) and variants
AML with 11q23 (MLL) abnormalities
Acute myeloid leukemia with multilineage dysplasia
Following MDS or MDS/MPD disorder
Without antecedent MDS or MDS/MPD, but with dysplasia in at least 50% of cells or two or more lineages
Acute myeloid leukemia and MDS, therapy-related
Alkylating agent/radiation-related type
Topoisomerase II inhibitor-related type (some may be lymphoid)
Others
Acute myeloid leukemia, not otherwise categorized, classify as
Acute myeloid leukemia, minimally differentiated
Acute myeloid leukemia without maturation
Acute myeloid leukemia with maturation
Acute myelomonocytic leukemia
Acute monoblastic/acute monocytic leukemia
Acute erythroid leukemia (erythroid/myeloid and pure erythroleukemia)
Acute megakaryocytic leukemia
Acute basophilic leukemia
Acute panmyelosis with myelofibrosis
Myeloid sarcoma

MDS, myelodysplastic syndrome; MLL, mixed lineage leukemia; MPD, myeloproliferative disease; PML, promyelocytic leukemia; RARα, retinoic acid receptor-α.

CLINICAL PRESENTATION AND DIAGNOSIS

Common signs and symptoms at presentation result from malignant cells that replace and suppress normal hematopoietic progenitor cells and infiltrate into extramedullary spaces. Many of the signs and symptoms result from low blood cells. Thrombocytopenia can result in bruising, petechiae, and bleeding; low red blood cells can result in fatigue and loss of energy; and low white blood cells can result in signs and symptoms of infection such as fever, chills, and rigors. Patients with ALL may rarely present with small blue-green collections of leukemia cells under the skin called *chloromas*.

❷ In addition to clinical presentation, laboratory and pathology evaluations are required for a definitive diagnosis of leukemia. An abnormal complete blood count is usually the diagnostic test that initiates a leukemia workup. The most important test is a bone marrow biopsy and aspirate, which is submitted to hematopathology for numerous evaluations. A lumbar puncture is performed to determine if there are blasts in the central nervous system (CNS). A chest radiograph is performed to screen for a mediastinal mass (most common in T-cell disease).

CLINICAL PRESENTATION

General

- Recent history of vague symptoms such as tiredness, lack of exercise tolerance, weight loss, and "feeling unwell," but in no obvious distress.

Signs and Symptoms

- Common: Patients with anemia present with pallor, malaise, palpitations, and fatigue. Patients with low platelet counts present with bruising, ecchymoses, and petechiae. Temperature is often elevated and may be caused by disease or infection. Patients may have bone pain from a hyperactive bone marrow.
- Other possible symptoms include epistaxis, dyspnea on exertion, seizures, or headache. Splenomegaly, hepatomegaly, and/or lymphadenopathy are common in patients presenting with acute lymphoblastic leukemia (ALL), but may also have painless testicular enlargement and rarely, small, blue-green collections of leukemia cells under the skin (chloromas). Patients with acute myeloid leukemia (AML) may present with gum hypertrophy and bleeding.

Laboratory Tests

- Complete blood count with differential. Anemia (43% <7 g/dL [4.34 mmol/L]) is normochromic and normocytic (without a compensatory increase in reticulocytes). Thrombocytopenia (severe, <20,000 cells/mm^3 [20×10^9/L]) is present in 28% of ALL and 50% of AML cases. Patients can present with leukopenia or leukocytosis; about 20% of patients will present with a white blood cell (WBC) count ≥50,000 cells/mm^3 (50×10^9/L) and 53% of ALL and 20% of AML cases with a WBC <10,000 cells/mm^3 (10×10^9/L). Even patients with elevated counts can be considered functionally neutropenic.
- Uric acid may be elevated because of rapid cellular turnover and is more common in patients presenting with elevated WBC count and with ALL.
- Electrolytes: potassium and phosphate may be elevated with a compensatory decrease in calcium, more common with ALL.
- Coagulation (more common with AML): elevated prothrombin time, partial thromboplastin time, D-dimers; hypofibrinogenemia.

Other Diagnostic Tests

- Bone marrow aspirate and biopsy: send for morphologic examination, cytochemical staining, immunophenotyping, and cytogenetic (chromosome) analysis. Molecular testing for FMS-like tyrosine kinase 3 (FLT3), nucleophosmin (NPM1), and CCAAT/enhancer binding-protein α (CEBPA) mutations is warranted for suspected AML.
- All children and adults with ALL should have a screening lumbar puncture performed to assess CNS involvement.

ACUTE LYMPHOBLASTIC LEUKEMIA

Risk Classification

Many clinical and biologic features at diagnosis are associated with response to treatment, as measured by the CR rate, duration of remission, and long-term survival. The patient's response to initial therapy is also strongly associated with response to treatment. Identification of these risk factors allows the clinician to better understand the disease and to tailor treatment according to risk of disease recurrence (i.e., risk-adapted therapy). For example, if a patient has many clinical and laboratory features that are associated with a good response to chemotherapy ("standard risk"), then the clinician may choose to give less-intensive therapy to reduce the risk of long-term adverse effects. Conversely, if a patient is unlikely to respond well to standard therapy (high-risk or very-high-risk disease), then the clinician may choose to give more intensive chemotherapy. The factors can be grouped as follows: patient characteristics at diagnosis, leukemic cell features at diagnosis, and patient response to initial therapy.

Patient Characteristics

3 The National Cancer Institute (NCI) developed an ALL risk stratification to create a standard for comparison in children.[13] Induction therapy is initially selected based on this classification, which divides children into standard- or high-risk categories based on age and initial white blood cell (WBC) count (Table 111-3a). Age remains an independent predictor of outcome with children aged 1 to 9 years having the best event-free survival (EFS). This is mostly explained by the more frequent occurrence of the *ETV6-RUNX1* translocation and hyperdiploidy (>51 chromosomes) in addition to increased drug sensitivity in this age group.[14] Presence of CNS disease at diagnosis is associated with a higher relapse rate. About 2% of males have testicular disease at diagnosis, but cooperative groups vary in whether this is an adverse prognostic factor. Patients with Down syndrome tend to have lower EFS, but this is mostly attributed to higher treatment-related morbidity and mortality.

Race is controversial, with older studies indicating worse outcomes for minorities. Male race and obesity have been associated with worse outcome in cooperative group studies, but not single-institution studies.[6] Hepatosplenomegaly and mediastinal mass are both associated with worse outcomes.

Leukemic Cell Characteristics

With current therapy, the cell of origin no longer has a prognostic significance as therapy is tailored to account for this historical

TABLE 111-3a National Cancer Institute (NCI) Risk Classification (Smith 1996)

Risk Group	Standard Risk	High Risk
Age (years)	1 to <10	<1 or ≥10
WBC count ($\times 10^3$ cells/mm^3 or 10^9/L)	<50	≥50
Karyotype	No t(9;22) or t(4;11)	t(9;22) or t(4;11)

WBC, white block cell.

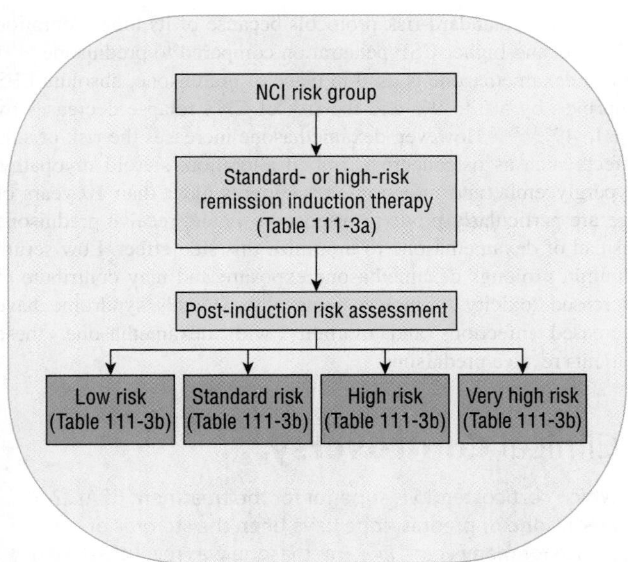

FIGURE 111-1 Pediatric precursor B-cell acute lymphoblastic leukemia risk classification. (NCI, National Cancer Institute.)

difference. Several chromosomal (cytogenetic) abnormalities are associated with prognosis. Children with ALL have an average of six DNA copy number alterations.[12] Favorable outcomes are associated with three copies of chromosomes 4 and 10, high hyperdiploidy (51-65 chromosomes), and the *ETV6-RUNX1* cryptic translocation, t(12;21).[12] *NOTCH1* and *FBXW7* mutations confer a favorable prognosis for patients with T-cell disease.[12] The Philadelphia chromosome is present in 3% to 5% of children and 25% of adults and is historically associated with a poor prognosis.[15] The mixed lineage leukemia (*MLL*) gene rearrangement (11q23), intrachromosomal amplification of chromosome 21 ($iAMLP_{21}$), and hypodiploidy (<44 chromosomes) are associated with a poorer prognosis.[16]

Initial Response to Therapy

The strongest prognostic factor for outcome for ALL is response to therapy. Both the rapidity of response and the level of residual disease at the end of induction therapy are associated with long-term outcome. Children with a reduction of bone marrow lymphoblasts within 14 days of initiating chemotherapy (rapid early responders) have a more favorable prognosis. Molecular measurement of subclinical minimal residual disease (MRD) by either flow cytometry or polymerase chain reaction has enabled detection of leukemic cells not visible on morphologic examination to assess treatment response and detect relapse in children and adults.[17] This technique allows detection of 1 leukemia cell in 10,000 normal cells, which is about 100-fold more sensitive than morphologic examination.[17] If MRD is detected at the end of induction therapy, the clinician may decide to give more intensive therapy to decrease the risk of relapse.

The Children's Oncology Group uses a risk- and response-based classification of childhood ALL (Fig. 111-1).[18] This classification system uses the NCI risk assignment to initially categorize patients into standard- or high-risk groups (Table 111-3a). Following induction therapy, risk is reclassified based on the rapidity and completeness of response to therapy, the presence or absence of cytogenetic abnormalities or CNS involvement (Table 111-3b). Patients are then reclassified as low risk, standard risk, high risk, or very-high risk (Fig. 111-1). Patients who are initially high risk do not have therapy reduced, but may have it intensified to very-high risk as discussed below.

Children are classified as low risk and will have therapy reduced if they have trisomy 4 and 10 or the *ETV6-RUNX1* cryptic translocation with less than 0.01% MRD on day 8 peripheral blood and day 29 bone marrow samples. Children with testicular disease, >5% blasts in the bone marrow by day 15, MRD ≥0.01% at day 29, or who received steroids prior to diagnosis have postinduction therapy intensified and are classified as high risk. Childhood precursor B-ALL with more than five WBCs and blasts present in the cerebrospinal fluid (CSF), Ph^+ disease, hypodiploidy, $iAMLP_{21}$, induction failure, or *MLL* gene rearrangement have therapy intensified and are considered very-high risk. Infant ALL, trisomy 21, or childhood T-cell ALL have unique risk classification schemas. Children with T-cell leukemia historically have an inferior response to standard-risk therapy and are automatically categorized as high risk to receive augmented therapy and T cell targeted therapy. T-cell and mature B-cell disease are favorable phenotypes in adults.[6] Age is inversely associated with prognosis in patients with Ph^+ ALL.[6]

TREATMENT
Acute Lymphoblastic Leukemia

Desired Outcomes

The short-term goal for ALL treatment is to rapidly achieve a complete clinical and hematologic remission. A CR is defined as the disappearance of all physical and bone marrow evidence (normal cellularity with <5% blasts) of leukemia, with restoration of normal hematopoiesis. After a CR is achieved, the goal is to maintain the patient in continuous CR. In general, a child is considered to be "cured" after being in continuous CR for 5 to 10 years.

Successful treatment of ALL was first developed in children. Current regimens induce clinical remission in 96% to 99% of children with ALL.[6] MRD is a strong predictor of relapse in ALL. Children with MRD in the bone marrow at the end of induction have a 5-year EFS of 59% versus 88% in children without.[19] Children with low-risk disease have a 5-year EFS of more than 95%.[21] The 5-year EFS for average-risk disease is 90 to 95%.[21] The 5-year EFS is nearly 90% for high-risk childhood B-precursor and T-cell ALL including rapid and slow responders. Children with very-high-risk disease have a 5-year EFS of less than 80%.[21] Response to treatment

TABLE 111-3b Pediatric Precursor B-Cell Acute Lymphoblastic Leukemia Risk Classification

	Low	Average		High			Very High			
NCI Risk[a]	SR	SR	SR	SR	SR	HR (age <13y)	SR	HR	HR (age >13y)	Any
Favorable Genetics	Yes	Yes	No	Yes	No	Any	No	Any	Any	Any
Unfavorable Characteristics	None	None	None	None	None	None	None	None	None	Yes
Day 8 PB MRD	<0.01%	≥0.01%	<1%	Any	≥1%	Any	Any	Any	Any	Any
Day 29 Marrow MRD	<0.01%	<0.01%	<0.01%	>0.01%	<0.01%	<0.01%	>0.01%	>0.01%	<0.01%	Any

HR, high-risk; MRD, minimal residual disease; NCI, National Cancer Institute; PB, peripheral blood; SR, standard-risk.

[a]See Table 111-3a for criteria used to categorize patients into risk categories.

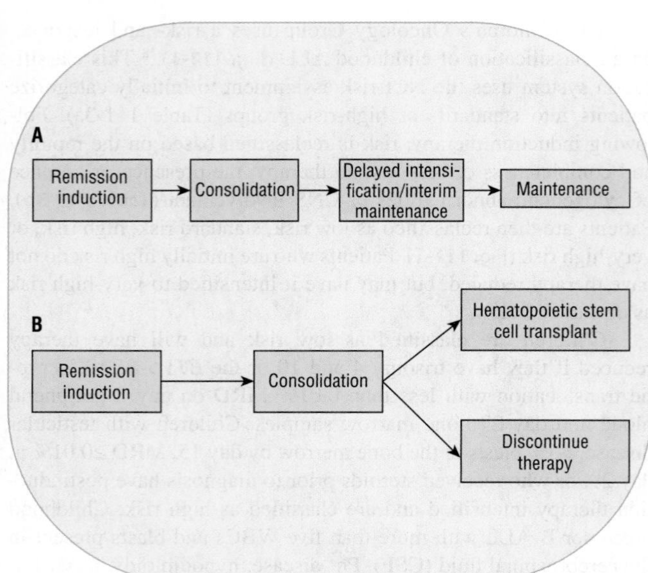

FIGURE 111-2 Treatment algorithm for (*A*) acute lymphoblastic leukemia and (*B*) acute myeloid leukemia.

is determined by intrinsic drug sensitivity and the patient's pharmacogenomics and pharmacodynamics, treatment received, and treatment adherence. Cure rates in children have risen from less than 5% with treatments used in the 1960s to about 90% by 2005.[22] The reason for this improvement lies largely in improved scheduling of existing drugs, as relatively few new drugs have come to the market since the 1960s.

Although treatment results with adult ALL are worse than those with childhood ALL, recent use of aggressive chemotherapy in adult ALL has increased the CR rate from 60% to 85%. Long-term EFS in this population, however, remains low (between 30% and 40%) because a higher proportion of adults present with poor-risk disease. CR rates and EFS vary according to a number of poor prognostic factors and certain types of ALL are associated with a very poor outcome.

Treatment Phases

Therapy for childhood ALL is divided into five phases: (a) induction, (b) consolidation therapy, (c) interim maintenance, (d) delayed intensification, and (e) maintenance therapy (Fig. 111-2). CNS prophylaxis is a mandatory component of ALL treatment regimens and is administered longitudinally during all phases of treatment. The total duration of treatment is 2 to 3 years.

Induction

The goal of induction is to rapidly induce a complete clinical and hematologic remission. ❹ The CR rate is 98% for standard-risk children treated with vincristine, a glucocorticoid (dexamethasone or prednisone), and asparaginase or pegaspargase.[22] Most treatment protocols add daunorubicin to induction (four-drug induction) for high-risk or very-high-risk ALL, while others add cyclophosphamide, methotrexate, or cytarabine. Most children achieve a CR in 4 weeks, which classifies them as rapid early responders. Those who have a M2 (5% to 25% blasts) or M3 (>25% blasts) marrow on day 15 of induction or have positive MRD at day 29 are classified as slow early responders and receive intensified therapy. Only 2% to 3% of children fail induction therapy, but the therapy results in a 10-year survival rate of 32%.[23]

Prednisone has historically been the primary glucocorticoid used in pediatric ALL regimens.[24] Dexamethasone is now being used in most standard-risk protocols because of its longer duration of action and higher CSF penetration compared to prednisone.[6,22,24] When dexamethasone is used in place of prednisone, absolute EFS improves by 5% to 9% and the risk of CNS relapse decreases by 2% to 4%.[14,24,25] However, dexamethasone increases the risk of side effects such as osteonecrosis, mood alteration, steroid myopathy, hyperglycemia, and infections.[24–26] Patients older than 10 years of age are particularly prone to osteonecrosis and receive prednisone instead of dexamethasone to minimize this side effect. Low serum albumin prolongs dexamethasone exposure and may contribute to increased toxicity.[14] Since patients with Down's syndrome have increased infections and mortality with dexamethasone, these patients receive prednisone.

Clinical **Controversy...**

Which corticosteroid is superior for the treatment of ALL? Prednisone or prednisolone have been the steroids of choice for many years. Dexamethasone was recently shown to have better CNS penetration than prednisone with a consequent decrease in CNS relapse rate. However, the incidence of debilitating side effects, such as osteonecrosis, is higher with dexamethasone. Many investigators have difficulty weighing the quality-of-life decrease from the side effects against the small increase in survival.

The incidence of transient hyperglycemia during pediatric ALL induction therapy has increased. In a recent study, 20% of children had transient hyperglycemia, defined as at least two random serum glucose levels greater than or equal to 200 mg/dL (11.1 mmol/L).[27] The incidence was higher (42%) in children older than 10 years of age. The risk was higher for patients with a body mass index (BMI) greater than or equal to the 95th percentile and those receiving asparaginase as compared to pegaspargase.

Asparaginase has historically been available in three forms. Asparaginase (no longer manufactured in the United States) and pegaspargase are isolated from *Escherichia coli* while *Erwinia* asparaginase is isolated from *Erwinia chrysanthemi*. A recombinant *E. coli* asparaginase and a pegylated form of recombinant *Erwinia* asparaginase are currently in clinical trials. Pegaspargase is pegylated *E. coli* asparaginase; pegylation prolongs its duration of activity and allows it to be given less frequently. Pegaspargase is used in most protocols and is preferred over asparaginase because of fewer intramuscular injections, decreased antibody formation, and superior response rates. Pegaspargase is also approved for IV administration. The use of prolonged intensive asparaginase treatment compared with shorter treatment increases absolute EFS by 4% to 17%.[28]

Asparaginase products are the chemotherapeutic agents most likely to cause hypersensitivity reactions. Depending on the product and coadministered steroid, 8% to 42% of patients develop antibodies to asparaginase. Reactions usually occur during postinduction phases of therapy when asparaginase has not been given for a prolonged period of time.[28] The reaction is delayed with pegaspargase and usually occurs 6 to 12 hours following a dose. The hypersensitivity reaction to pegaspargase may also be prolonged and frequently requires hospitalization for 5 to 7 days. *Erwinia* asparaginase is currently only used for patients who are allergic to other available forms. Patients may also have "silent hypersensitivity" in which they develop neutralizing antibodies that can rapidly inactivate the asparaginase, but the patient does not have a clinical hypersensitivity reaction. Therefore, many centers prefer switching from *E. coli* derived products to *Erwinia* asparaginase to avoid this scenario.

Central Nervous System Prophylaxis

CNS prophylaxis is incorporated throughout all phases of therapy. The rationale for CNS prophylaxis is based on two observations. First, many chemotherapeutic agents do not readily cross the blood–brain barrier. Second, results from early clinical trials of ALL showed that 50% to 85% of patients with ALL and no CNS involvement at diagnosis experienced a CNS relapse.[7] These observations indicate that the CNS is a potential sanctuary for leukemic cells and undetectable leukemic cells are present in the CNS in many patients at the time of diagnosis. Detectable CNS involvement at the time of diagnosis occurs in 3% of children with ALL.[14] Factors that are associated with an increased risk of CNS involvement at diagnosis in children include a high initial WBC count, T-cell phenotype, mature B-cell phenotype, age ≤1 year, African American race, thrombocytopenia, lymphadenopathy, and hepatomegaly or splenomegaly.[22]

The goal of CNS prophylaxis is to eradicate undetectable leukemic cells from the CNS while minimizing neurotoxicity and late effects. Leukemic meningitis is more easily prevented than treated. Once CNS relapse has occurred, patients are at increased risk of bone marrow relapse and death from refractory leukemia. Initial trials of childhood ALL in the 1960s established craniospinal irradiation as the standard for prevention of CNS relapse.[22] However, this approach is associated with long-term sequelae including neuropsychological deficits, precocious puberty, osteoporosis, decreased intellect, thyroid dysfunction, brain tumors, short stature, and obesity. Subsequent trials have demonstrated that irradiation may be replaced by frequent administration of intrathecal chemotherapy in children with ALL.[22] Some centers may treat children with CNS disease at diagnosis or very-high-risk disease with cranial radiation.

❺ The CNS prophylaxis regimen is selected based on efficacy, toxicity, and risk of CNS disease. Intrathecal chemotherapy, cranial irradiation, dexamethasone, and high-dose IV methotrexate or cytarabine can be used to treat or prevent CNS disease. Current treatment approaches have reduced isolated CNS relapses to less than 5% among children.[29] Risk factors for CNS relapse include male sex, hepatomegaly, T-cell phenotype, CNS2 disease (the presence of leukemic blasts in a CSF sample that contains <5 WBC/mm^3), age younger than 2 years or older than 6 years, and a bloody diagnostic lumbar puncture.[6,29] Intrathecal therapy consists of methotrexate and cytarabine, given either alone or in combination. When given together, hydrocortisone is commonly added (triple intrathecal therapy) to decrease the incidence of arachnoiditis. For standard-risk ALL, triple intrathecal therapy decreased relative CNS relapse rates by 30% in comparison to intrathecal methotrexate and no effect on EFS and worse overall survival (OS).[29] Triple intrathecal therapy is typically reserved for children with refractory CNS disease. The doses of intrathecal chemotherapy used for childhood ALL are age-based because of differences in the volume of CSF at various ages. For example, intrathecal methotrexate is dosed as 8 mg if <2 years, 10 mg for 2 to 2.99 years, 12 mg for 3 to 8.99 years, and 15 mg for ≥9 years. Liposomal cytarabine induces CNS remission in 57% of relapsed patients, but is associated with a high incidence of arachnoiditis and other CNS-related adverse effects.[30] Currently its use is limited to refractory or relapsed CNS disease in children.

Patients with T-cell leukemia have an increased incidence of CNS disease and usually receive systemic therapy that penetrates the CNS such as high-dose methotrexate.[26] A WBC count greater than 100,000 cells/mm^3 (100×10^9/L) is associated with an increased risk of CNS relapse.[6] Patients with T-cell disease have lower methotrexate polyglutamate accumulation and addition of high-dose methotrexate in these patients results in fewer CNS relapses and improves EFS.[14]

Consolidation Therapy

Consolidation therapy in ALL is started after a CR has been achieved, and refers to continued intensive chemotherapy in an attempt to eradicate clinically undetectable disease in order to secure (consolidate) the remission. Regimens usually incorporate either non–cross-resistant drugs that are different from the induction regimen, or more dose-intensive use of the same drugs.

Randomized trials show that consolidation therapy clearly improves patient outcome in children, but its benefit in adults is less clear.[22] The relative benefit of individual components of treatment regimens is difficult to demonstrate because of the overall complexity of therapy in ALL. Standard consolidation lasts 4 weeks and usually consists of vincristine, mercaptopurine, and intrathecal methotrexate. Children with testicular disease usually receive radiation during this phase of therapy if a complete clinical response in the testes is not achieved by the end of induction. In children, the intensity of consolidation therapy is based on the child's initial risk classification and response to induction therapy. Patients who respond slowly to induction therapy are at higher risk of relapse if they are not treated on more aggressive regimens. Children who are slow early responders or have high-risk disease benefit from intensified consolidation that includes the addition of vincristine and pegaspargase to standard therapy (cyclophosphamide, low-dose cytarabine, mercaptopurine).[20]

Children with Ph$^+$ ALL, infants with MLL, or children who only achieve a partial remission may undergo allogeneic hematopoietic stem cell transplantation (HSCT) in first remission if a suitable donor is available. Nelarabine is a prodrug of ara-G that preferentially accumulates in T lymphoblasts as ara-guanosine triphosphate (GTP). Children and young adults in first bone marrow relapse had a 55% complete or partial response in the phase II trial.[30] Nelarabine added to a high-risk backbone for initial therapy of childhood T-cell ALL in Children's Oncology Group (COG) AALL00P2 was well tolerated and had a 5-year EFS of 69% in slow early responders compared to 35% to 51% in historical controls.[31]

Reinduction (Delayed Intensification and Interim Maintenance)

One or two delayed intensification phases separated by low-intensity interim maintenance cycles can be added to maintain remission and to decrease cumulative toxicity. Delayed intensification usually consists of drugs used during induction and consolidation or agents that lack cross-resistance with those already received such as cyclophosphamide, methotrexate, and limited amounts of doxorubicin. The methotrexate dose is variable; standard-risk children generally receive 1 to 2 g/m^2 while those with T-cell disease generally receive 5 g/m^2. Interim maintenance usually consists of dexamethasone, vincristine, weekly methotrexate, mercaptopurine, and intrathecal methotrexate. Delayed intensification improves EFS for standard-risk children.[14,20] Delayed intensification with dose intensification improved EFS and decreased late relapses for high-risk childhood ALL, but there was no additional benefit for two delayed intensification cycles.[20] Children on the intensified arms of the study received significantly more antimicrobial drugs, blood products, and parenteral nutrition but had no increase in treatment-related mortality.[20] The antimetabolite-based regimens may have a reduced risk of late toxicities, but the more intensive regimens appear to result in better survival for some patients, especially those with higher risk disease.

Maintenance Therapy

❻ Maintenance therapy allows long-term drug exposure to slowly dividing cells, allows the immune system time to eradicate leukemia cells, and promotes apoptosis (programmed cell death). The goal of maintenance therapy is to further eradicate residual leukemic cells and prolong remission duration. Although maintenance therapy is clearly beneficial in childhood ALL, the benefit in adults has only recently been demonstrated.

Maintenance therapy usually consists of daily mercaptopurine and weekly methotrexate for 12-week courses, at doses that produce relatively little myelosuppression, with monthly "pulses" of vincristine and a steroid for 5 days per month. Based on the results of studies that show a trend toward an increase in late relapse (excluding isolated testicular relapse) among male children treated for 2 years versus 3 years, some centers treat female children for 2 years while males receive maintenance for a total of 3 years of therapy.

Interpatient variability in the pharmacokinetics of oral methotrexate and mercaptopurine may also be an important determinant of the effectiveness and toxicity of maintenance therapy. Patients who take oral methotrexate and mercaptopurine on an evening versus a morning schedule appear to have a superior outcome. Mercaptopurine cannot be given with milk or milk products because of the presence of xanthine oxidase. Children whose adherence rate taking mercaptopurine is less than 95% have a 2.5-fold higher risk of suffering a relapse.[32] Factors associated with nonadherence include single-parent household, adolescence, lower socioeconomic status, and Hispanic ethnicity.[32] To account for the interpatient variability, most clinicians will titrate the dose of either agent to maintain an absolute neutrophil count of 500 to 1,500 cells/mm^3 (0.5 to 1.5 × 10^9/L).[6] Some protocols overcome bioavailability and poor adherence issues by administering methotrexate IV or intramuscularly. The importance of these pharmacokinetic issues in adults is not well defined.

Philadelphia Chromosome Positive Acute Lymphoblastic Leukemia

Ph$^+$ ALL has a 45% 7-year EFS and has historically been treated as very-high-risk disease.[15] This includes a four-drug induction. The addition of continuous imatinib mesylate, a signal transduction inhibitor that inhibits *BCR-ABL* kinase, through all phases of treatment resulted in a 3-year EFS of 80% in comparison to 35% for historical controls.[33] The results for patients receiving chemotherapy with imatinib were equivalent to those receiving HSCT. Imatinib is currently incorporated into childhood treatment trials for Ph$^+$ ALL in Europe and the United States. Trials are ongoing with the more potent tyrosine kinase inhibitors, nilotinib and dasatinib. Imatinib has been incorporated into consolidation for children with Ph$^+$ disease.

Acute Lymphoblastic Leukemia in Infants

ALL and AML in infants younger than 1 year of age account for less than 5% of the reported acute leukemias in childhood, but they are associated with poor outcomes. OS in infant ALL is 30% to 50%.[34] About 70 to 80% of infants with acute leukemia have t(4;11) involving the *MLL* gene.[34] *MLL* gene rearrangements are associated with worse outcome, with only 18% to 34% 4- to 8-year EFS.[34] Infants with ALL are more likely to present with a high WBC count, hepatosplenomegaly, and CNS disease.[34] Age younger than 6 months at diagnosis and poor response to prednisone alone given prior to starting other agents are poor prognostic indicators.[34] Infants with *MLL* gene rearrangements are more likely to overexpress FLT3, a tyrosine kinase implicated in leukemogenesis. Current trials are testing the efficacy of FLT3 inhibitors in infants with *MLL* gene rearrangements. Patients with infant ALL may have greater drug resistance to asparaginase, vincristine, and corticosteroids, but increased sensitivity to cytarabine and cladribine.[34] Although intensive regimens such as high-dose methotrexate and high-dose cytarabine have improved survival rates they resulted in unacceptably high mortality rates. Lack of pharmacokinetic data for chemotherapy in infants has contributed to toxicity from inappropriate dosing of doxorubicin and vincristine. The use of allogeneic HSCT for infants with ALL remains controversial because of a lack of donors, concerns over the long-term toxicity of total body irradiation, and excessive mortality in some series. The Interfant-99 study showed a benefit for HSCT in a subset of infants with *MLL* gene rearrangement, age younger than 6 months of age, or WBC greater than 300,000 cells/mm^3 (300 × 10^9/L).[35]

Acute Lymphoblastic Leukemia in Adolescents and Young Adults

Although ALL is relatively uncommon in adolescents and young adults (AYA) (15 to 39 years AYA), the outcomes are generally worse than for childhood ALL. ALL in AYA has a higher frequency of T-cell immunophenotype and a lower frequency of the t(12;21)(p13;q22) cryptic translocation responsible for hyperdiploidy and the *ETV6-RUNX1* fusion gene; about 5% to 7% of ALL in AYA have Ph$^+$ disease (higher than children, but lower than older adults).[12,36] A retrospective comparison of 16- to 20-year-old patients treated on pediatric versus adult protocols in the United States resulted in identical CR rates, but the 7-year EFS favored the patients treated on pediatric regimens (64% vs. 34%).[36] Patients treated on the pediatric regimens also had a 10% lower CNS relapse rate. The adult regimens studied were more myelosuppressive, while the pediatric regimens intensified steroids and asparaginase and included earlier and more intensive CNS-directed therapy. The adult regimens also had a higher risk of late effects due to higher doses of daunorubicin and use of cyclophosphamide. A current adult intergroup study is using a pediatric regimen for AYA patients and will be able to evaluate some of the other potential reasons for the outcome disparity, such as adherence and psychosocial differences. AYA patients may receive treatment based on an adult or pediatric regimen depending on institutional preferences, but the trend is shifting toward pediatric regimens.[37]

Acute Lymphoblastic Leukemia in Adults

Treatment risk stratification for adult patients differs depending on age and Philadelphia chromosome status. The National Comprehensive Cancer Network (NCCN) guidelines recommend different strategies for adolescents and young adults (AYA) ages 15 to 39, adults 40 to 65, and adults older than 65 years with or without poor performance status.[37] While complete remission is achieved in 70% to 90% of adults with a four-drug induction regimen containing daunorubicin or doxorubicin, vincristine, an asparaginase formulation, and prednisone, long-term EFS is considerably lower and achieved in only 30% to 40% of patients.[38] **7** Poorer outcomes in adults have been attributed to differences in cytogenetic abnormalities, greater drug resistance, higher risk of treatment-related adverse effects with subsequent nonadherence, and possibly less effective therapy. The value of adding more agents to the basic four-drug induction regimen or higher doses of drugs in the remission induction regimen is not clear. Several different regimens are considered appropriate to use as first-line therapies in adults including the Cancer and Leukemia Group B (CALGB) 8811 (Larson regimen), Eastern Cooperative Oncology Group (ECOG) 2993, or Linker regimen.[39–41] Some studies suggest that high-dose methotrexate and cytarabine alternating with fractionated cyclophosphamide plus vincristine, doxorubicin, and dexamethasone (hyperCVAD) may improve response and survival in adults with ALL.[42] A considerable number of ALL cases occur in patients older than age 65 years, and treatment of this group of patients is an even greater challenge. The response to therapy and durability of response is less than in all other populations. Treatment-related mortality rates during remission induction therapy are also higher in this population.

While the overall incidence of Ph+ positive disease is 25% in adults, the incidence rises with increasing age to over 40% in adults older than the age of 50 years.[43] Traditionally, treatment outcomes for patients with Ph+ ALL has been extremely poor with reported OS rates of less than 20% and for those continuing to allogeneic HSCT a 2-year OS of 40% to 50%. As compared with historical control patients treated with standard chemotherapy alone, the addition of *BCR-ABL* tyrosine kinase therapy to chemotherapy was associated with an increased CR and OS.[44,45] No randomized trials have compared imatinib and conventional chemotherapy versus conventional chemotherapy alone. The CR rates seen with tyrosine kinase inhibitors appear to be more durable and allow more patients with Ph+ disease to proceed to allogeneic HSCT. This approach also appears to be tolerated in elderly patients.[46,47] For patients older than 65 years of age or for those with a poor performance status, induction regimens may include concurrent chemotherapy with a tyrosine kinase inhibitor, either alone or combined with corticosteroids. Based on these data, the combination of imatinib with concurrent chemotherapy is currently considered as the standard of care for first-line therapy.

Dasatinib has also been studied in combination with concurrent chemotherapy as first-line therapy with demonstrated efficacy.[48] Other newer *BCR-ABL* tyrosine kinase inhibitors, nilotinib, bosutinib, and ponatinib, have also been evaluated in patients with imatinib-resistant Ph+ leukemias. Responses can be achieved, but more data are needed to evaluate their specific role in the treatment of Ph+ ALL.[49–51] A primary concern with the tyrosine kinase inhibitors is the emergence of resistance, specifically T315I mutations. Ponatinib is the only *BCR-ABL* tyrosine kinase inhibitor available in the United States with known activity against T315I mutations.[52] The use of the *BCR-ABL* tyrosine kinase inhibitors other than imatinib for first-line therapy is not well established.

In adults with B-cell ALL, about 50% have leukemic cells that express CD20. CD20 expression has been associated with decreased CR rates and OS.[53] A phase II study has evaluated hyperCVAD and rituximab versus hyperCVAD alone and reported a higher CR rate (70% vs. 38%) and longer OS (75% vs. 47%) in patients treated with hyperCVAD and rituximab.[54] These results are encouraging and support the use of rituximab in patients who have cells that express CD20.

HSCT plays an important role in the treatment of adult patients with ALL. For patients with Ph+ ALL who have a CR after induction therapy, consolidation with allogeneic HSCT should be considered if a human leukocyte antigen (HLA)-matched sibling or matched unrelated donor is available. After HSCT, patients should continue with standard maintenance therapy that includes a tyrosine kinase inhibitor. For patients with Philadelphia chromosome negative (Ph−) disease who have MRD after induction therapy or have high-risk features for relapse, allogeneic HSCT should be considered if a matched donor is available.[55]

Relapsed Acute Lymphoblastic Leukemia

About 20% of children with ALL will relapse.[56] The most common site for relapse is the bone marrow (53%), although isolated relapses can occur in the CNS (19%) or testicles (5%), in addition to multiple sites of disease.[57] Because marrow relapse usually follows isolated CNS or testicular relapses, patients with isolated extramedullary relapses are treated with localized radiation (cranial or testicular) and aggressive systemic chemotherapy similar to that given to patients with a marrow relapse.[58]

Children who fail to achieve a CR by day 29 of initial remission induction therapy usually receive an additional 2 weeks of four-drug induction therapy. If the children do not achieve a CR with the additional therapy, they are usually treated for bone marrow relapse consisting of intensive induction therapy consisting of at least three cycles of chemotherapy. Examples of regimens include vincristine, pegaspargase, corticosteroid, and doxorubicin; etoposide, cyclophosphamide, and high-dose methotrexate; and high-dose cytarabine and asparaginase.

Patients who have completed treatment and have stayed in remission for longer periods are more likely to be reinduced into remission again. Patients with more favorable risk factors initially, and those who received less intensive initial treatments, are more likely to respond well to reinduction/salvage regimens. The second CR rate is 78% in children who were in continuous complete remission for less than 18 months, 78% if the duration of remission was 18 to 36 months, and 93% if the duration of remission was more than 36 months.[56] Three-year OS following bone marrow (28%), CNS (60%), and testicular (60%) relapse is not optimal.[58] Overall, 5-year disease-free survival rates are 27% for second complete remission (CR2) and 15% for third complete remission (CR3).[56] Clofarabine, a purine antimetabolite, is an option for patients on second or later relapses, but the duration of response is less than 6 months. Current trials are evaluating the place for clofarabine in combination with other agents.

Allogeneic HSCT has traditionally been the treatment of choice for early bone marrow relapse (continuous CR less than 36 months) while children who relapse more than 36 months after completion of initial therapy have traditionally received chemotherapy alone.[22] Some more recent analyses have shown HSCT to be an advantage to all relapsed children, while some have not shown a benefit.[56] Therefore, the question of who would benefit from HSCT continues to be investigated.

Most patients with relapsed or refractory disease are considered for an allogeneic HSCT with a matched sibling or unrelated donor if they achieve a CR2 following salvage chemotherapy. Most elderly patients are not candidates for standard allogeneic HSCT but are candidates for nonmyeloablative transplant (NMT). Patients who undergo a NMT receive a reduced intensity conditioning regimen. A NMT may produce similar outcomes with less treatment-related morbidity and mortality. The National Marrow Donor Program and the American Society for Blood and Marrow Transplantation have developed guidelines for transplant consultation based on current clinical practice and evidence-based medicine.[55,59]

For relapsed or refractory disease in Ph+ patients, leukemic cells should be tested for mutations to guide selection of the tyrosine kinase inhibitor. In addition, nelarabine may be an option for adults with relapsed or refractory T-cell disease.

Late Effects of Treatment

Certain late effects associated with cranial or craniospinal irradiation and corticosteroids were discussed earlier. The Childhood Cancer Survivor Study tracks the health status of adults treated for childhood cancer between 1970 and 1986 and has yielded invaluable information on how to monitor adult survivors.[60] Leukemia survivors are 3.7 times more likely to develop a severe or life-threatening chronic health condition as compared with healthy siblings, and 2.8 times more likely to report multiple chronic conditions.[60]

Older ALL regimens that incorporated intensive use of topoisomerase II inhibitors (etoposide and teniposide) are associated with unacceptably high risks of development of secondary leukemia.[22] High cumulative doses of anthracyclines used in high-risk or relapsed patients can cause cardiomyopathy. Cranial irradiation is also associated with learning deficits, especially in patients younger than 5 years of age at the time of treatment. Patients who received cranial radiation as children also have higher unemployment rates and lower marital rates among females two decades after diagnosis.[60] The Children's Oncology Group has developed long-term follow-up guidelines for survivors of childhood, adolescent, and young adult cancers (*www.survivorshipguidelines.org*).

ACUTE MYELOID LEUKEMIA

Risk Classification

Many clinical and laboratory features at diagnosis are associated with response to treatment, as measured by the CR rate, duration of remission, and long-term survival. Identification of these risk factors may allow the clinician to better understand the disease and to tailor treatment according to risk of disease recurrence. For example, if a patient has many clinical and laboratory features that are associated with a good response to chemotherapy ("good risk"), then the clinician may choose to give less intensive therapy to reduce the risk of long-term toxic effects. Conversely, if a patient is unlikely to respond well to therapy ("high risk"), then the clinician may choose to give more intensive chemotherapy that may include HSCT.

Several prognostic factors have been identified for adults with AML. ❽ The most important patient factor is age, with younger patients more likely to achieve a CR than patients older than age 60 years.[3,61] The lower CR rate in older patients results from an increased frequency of fatal infection and bleeding complications and resistance to conventional chemotherapy. The duration of remission is also shorter in older patients as compared to younger patients. Other patient-specific prognostic factors include concurrent infection and any major organ impairment.[3] Patients with extramedullary disease, CNS involvement, or underlying MDS have a worse prognosis. Other unfavorable prognostic factors in adult AML include: age older than 60 years, multidrug-resistance gene expression, WBC >100,000 cells/mm^3(100 × 10^9/L), and therapy-related AML.[62] Age must be evaluated as a continuous variable when looking at prognostic factors. The clinical difference between a patient 61 years old and one 71 years old, is much greater than a 59-year-old and a 61-year-old. Certain cytogenetic abnormalities are also known to worsen the response rate and survival of patients with AML (Table 111-4).[3,63] Chromosome 16 or translocations between chromosome 8 and 21 alter core-binding factor. Core-binding factor is associated with sensitivity to cytarabine.[64] In addition, patients who develop a "secondary" leukemia after treatment of another malignancy usually have a very poor response to antileukemic chemotherapy (i.e., therapy-related AML). Another factor that needs consideration for any cancer treatment is performance status. A bedridden patient with a new diagnosis of AML would not be a good candidate for treatment because of high treatment-related morbidity and mortality. Patients with poor performance status may be offered supportive care.

Cytogenetics may be the most important prognostic factor for a patient newly diagnosed with AML.[65] Molecular testing for FLT3-ITD, CEBPA, C-KIT, and *NPM1* is becoming more common in commercial laboratories and referral centers, and should be considered for all newly diagnosed AML patients.[66] Patients with core-binding factor with t(8;21)(q22;q22) or inv(16)(p13q22)/t(16;16)(p13;q22) treated with a cytarabine-based regimen have a relatively favorable prognosis. Adults and children with chromosomal deletions such as 3q[abn(3q)] or 5q[del(5q)], monosomies of chromosome 5 and/or 7(-5/-7) have a poor prognosis with standard chemotherapy for AML, and may benefit from experimental treatments. The limitations to karyotype as a risk stratification tool include failed cytogenetic analysis and presence of cryptic chromosomal rearrangements. About 40% of cases have a normal karyotype. Molecular mutations, such as FLT3, *NPM1* (nucleophosmin), C-KIT, and CEBPA (CCAAT/enhancer-binding protein α), can identify subsets of patients with differing outcome who have normal karyotypes. FLT3 is a receptor tyrosine kinase that is mutated in about one-third of patients with AML, including those with normal karyotype, and is associated with higher presenting WBC, decreased duration of CR, and a poorer prognosis. *NPM1* is present in about 30% of patients with AML, even in patients with normal karyotype, and commonly coexists with FLT3, and is associated with a higher CR and reduced relapse risk compared to patients without the mutation. C-KIT mutations have been observed in about 20% of patients with core-binding factor AML and are associated with decreased duration of CR and OS.[67] CEBPA is present in about 10% of patients with AML, and is associated with a favorable outcome. The area of cytogenetic and molecular abnormalities is complex and still evolving.

Prognostic factors associated with pediatric AML include response to the first course of remission induction therapy, cytogenetics, and molecular genetics. Poor prognostic factors include monosomy 7, age older than 10 years, black race, internal tandem duplications of FLT3, *MLL* gene rearrangements, and a diagnosis of AML secondary to prior chemotherapy or radiation therapy.[5] Conversely, inversion of chromosome 16, trisomy 21, CBF-AML, *PML-RARA*, *NPM1*, biallelic CEBPA, and *RUNX1-RUNX1T1* fusion transcript t(8;21) are associated with a favorable outcome.[5,10]

AML treatment in the future may be based on cytogenetic and molecular classification. Treatment algorithms based on these newer classifications have been proposed, but they are not currently incorporated into the initial remission induction therapy. These tests do provide prognostic information that may be incorporated into subsequent treatment decisions.[10]

TREATMENT
Acute Myeloid Leukemia

Desired Outcomes

The short-term goal of treatment for AML is to rapidly achieve a complete clinical and hematologic remission. In the absence of a CR, a rapid and fatal outcome is inevitable. CR is defined as the disappearance of all clinical and bone marrow evidence (normal cellularity >20% with <5% blasts) of leukemia, with restoration of normal hematopoiesis (neutrophils ≥1,000 cells/mm^3 [1 × 10^9/L] and platelets >100,000 cells/mm^3 [100 × 10^9/L]).[68] Partial remission is a significant response to treatment (a decrease of at least 50% of blasts), but evidence of residual disease in the bone marrow remains (5% to 25% blasts) and is considered a treatment failure requiring additional therapy. The definition of response for adult AML was

TABLE 111-4 Risk Category According to Cytogenetic and Molecular Abnormalities Present

	Risk Category		
Disease	***Good-Risk***	***Intermediate-Risk***	***High-Risk***
AML	t(8;21)(q22;q22); inv(16); t(15;17); t(9;11) trisomy 21 Mutated NPM1 without FLT3-ITD Mutated CEBPA	Normal karyotype; trisomy 8; 11q23; del(7q); del(9q); trisomy 22;t(9;11)	Complex karyoptype; –5; –7; del(5q); inv(3p) FLT3 ITD

AML, acute myeloid leukemia; CEBPA, CCAAT/enhancer binding-protein α; FLT3-ITD, Fms-like tyrosine kinase 3 internal tandem duplication; NPM1, nucleophosmin.

reevaluated in 2003, and changes in the definition of response were proposed to include not only CR (morphologic CR with restoration of normal hematopoiesis), but also CR with complete remission with incomplete hematological recovery (CRi), cytogenetic CR ([CRc] patient with normal cytogenetics in which cytogenetics were previously abnormal), and molecular CR ([CRm] molecular studies negative).[68] If there is a question of residual leukemia on bone marrow biopsy in adults, a bone marrow aspirate/biopsy should be repeated in one week.

After a CR is achieved, the goal is to maintain the patient in continuous CR. As discussed later, the occurrence of leukemic relapse in the bone marrow significantly reduces the likelihood of cure. Most patients who will die from acute leukemia die within the first 6 years; the survival curve (percentage alive versus time) beyond the sixth year after therapy does not continue to decline as rapidly ("survival plateau"), and at this time patients can be considered "cured."

With recent advances in chemotherapy and supportive care, 65% to 85% of all patients with AML achieve a CR, and 20% to 40% become long-term survivors.[3] Overall, the median duration of remission is 1 to 2 years. In patients 60 years of age or older, the CR rate is lower (39% to 64%), and the median duration of remission is shorter than one year.[69] In contrast to ALL, effective therapies used in AML cause severe and often prolonged myelosuppression. As a result, patients with AML, particularly patients older than 60 years of age, are at greater risk for treatment-related fatal infectious and bleeding complications.

The 5-year survival in children with AML has increased from 17% in 1976 to 50% in 2005.[26,70] Children with Down's syndrome and AML receive less intensive therapy and have a 83% EFS.[26,70] Treatment of childhood AML, unlike that of ALL, usually consists only of induction and intensive postremission therapy (Fig. 111-2). CNS prophylaxis and maintenance therapy are not routinely given to patients with AML.

Treatment Phases

Remission Induction

As with ALL, the goal of remission induction for AML is to rapidly induce a CR with associated restoration of normal hematopoiesis. Compared to ALL, however, fewer patients with AML achieve CR. Because the CR rate in AML is related to the intensity of the remission induction regimen, the drugs used in AML are given at doses that uniformly cause severe myelosuppression (except tretinoin). One reason for the lower CR rate in AML as compared to ALL is the inability to give optimal doses of chemotherapy because of marrow toxicity. With continued improvement of supportive care for patients undergoing chemotherapy, more intensive treatment regimens are being given in an effort to reduce the high rate of leukemic relapse and increase the proportion of long-term survivors. Most patients achieve a CR after 1 or 2 courses of chemotherapy. Patients who require additional chemotherapy to achieve a CR have been reported to have a poor prognosis, even if remission is ultimately achieved.

9 The most active single agents in AML are the anthracycline antibiotics (daunorubicin, doxorubicin, and idarubicin), mitoxantrone, and the antimetabolite cytarabine. The standard therapy for the treatment of adult AML has not changed in several decades. The most common regimen ("7+3") combines daunorubicin administered as a short infusion of 45 to 60 mg/m^2 per day on days 1 to 3, along with cytarabine administered as a continuous 24-hour infusion of 100 to 200 mg/m^2 per day on days 1 to 7.[3,71,72] The CR rate with the 7+3 regimen is 65% to 75% in patients 18 to 60 years old. Several trials have attempted to improve on conventional 7+3 therapy, but have shown no improvement by (a) increasing cytarabine to 10 days, (b) shortening cytarabine to 5 days, (c) substituting doxorubicin for daunorubicin, (d) adding thioguanine, or (e) increasing cytarabine dosage to 200 mg/m^2 per day (given by continuous infusion).[3] The most recent change to the standard 7+3 regimen is to increase the daunorubicin dose. Adults younger than 60 years old with AML who were randomized to receive higher daunorubicin dosages (90 mg/m^2 per day on days 1 to 3) in combination with 7 days of standard-dose cytarabine (100 mg/m^2 per day) had a significantly higher CR rate (71% vs. 57%) and longer overall median survival (23.7 vs. 15.7 months) as compared with those who received the standard 7+3 regimen of daunorubicin (45 mg/m^2 per day on days 1 to 3) and cytarabine.[73]

Idarubicin or mitoxantrone has been evaluated as alternatives to daunorubicin in combination with standard-dose continuous infusion cytarabine. Trials in younger patients reported improved CR rates with these newer anthracyclines (idarubicin) or anthracenediones (mitoxantrone), and one trial reported prolonged survival. Among older adults, the CR rate and OS do not appear to be different among the different anthracyclines or anthracenediones.[62,72] Therefore, the anthracycline of choice for the standard 7+3 regimen remains controversial, with many centers adopting idarubicin into the induction regimen in younger AML patients, and the choice in the elderly is based on individual clinician preference and institutional acquisition costs.

Clinical **Controversy...**

Is there a superior anthracycline to use as part of the induction regimen for acute myeloid leukemia (AML)? Some clinicians believe that idarubicin is superior in attaining a complete remission following one cycle of induction compared to alternative anthracyclines or anthracenediones. Randomized trials in the elderly show similar remission rates with all anthracyclines and anthracenediones. However, randomized trials in younger patients reported higher complete remission (CR) rates with idarubicin or mitoxantrone.

Other strategies that have been evaluated include adding another agent such as etoposide to the induction regimen.[3,71,72] A comparison of the standard 7+3 regimen with or without etoposide on days 1 to 7 ("7+3+7") in newly diagnosed AML patients ages 15 to 70 years showed no difference in CR rates or OS. A subset analysis of patients younger than 55 years of age showed a two-fold increase in the duration of remission and OS in the etoposide-containing arm. The 7+3+7 regimen was more toxic in patients older than 55 years of age. These results have been confirmed in other studies, but this regimen has not been adopted as standard therapy in the United States.

Based on experimental tumor models that showed a steep dose–response curve for cytarabine, higher cytarabine doses have also been evaluated as a means to increase the antileukemic activity of remission induction therapy. Several groups, including the Southwest Oncology Group and the Australian Leukemia Study Group, have evaluated the impact of adding high-dose cytarabine to induction therapy. This strategy does not improve the CR rate or OS, but does improve EFS. A retrospective study conducted by the European Group for Blood and Marrow Transplantation demonstrated that the cytarabine dose administered during induction and/or consolidation did not influence the outcome in patients who ultimately went on to receive allogeneic or autologous HSCT.[74] These data suggest that high doses of cytarabine during induction may not be needed in patients who receive HSCT as postremission therapy. In summary, the role of high-dose cytarabine during induction remains controversial. If used during induction, high-dose cytarabine is more appropriate in younger patients than in elderly patients because of poor tolerance by elderly patients. Additionally, it may be an option in patients unable to tolerate anthracyclines.

NCCN has published guidelines for the treatment of AML.[59,66] The classic 7+3 regimen may be inadequate in adults younger than 60 years of age because the duration of remission is less than that reported in some studies that employed high-dose cytarabine in induction. The NCCN guideline recommends that adults younger than 60 years of age without an antecedent hematologic disorder (i.e., no preexisting hematologic malignancy such as MDS) be treated with either the 7+3 regimen or more aggressive chemotherapy including high-dose cytarabine with an anthracycline or anthracenedione. In patients 60 years of age or older with good performance status, the conventional 7+3 regimen should be used or the patient should be enrolled in a clinical trial. The approach in patients with an antecedent hematologic disorder differs, and younger patients (<60 years) should be offered available clinical trials or proceed to allogeneic HSCT (provided a suitable donor is available).

Older patients (≥60 years) with an antecedent hematologic disorder or those with significant comorbidities unrelated to leukemia should be offered a low-intensity therapy with a hypomethylating agent such as azacitidine or decitabine, a clinical trial or best supportive care because of the dismal outcomes and toxicity risks associated with conventional chemotherapy. Azacitidine and decitabine are pyrimidine nucleoside analogs of cytidine that inhibit DNA methylation. While each agent has shown promising results versus conventional chemotherapy and best supportive care, the agents have not been compared to each other in trials. Azacitidine is usually given 75 mg/m^2/dose IV or subcutaneously for 7 days while decitabine is given 20 mg/m^2/dose IV for 5 days. Cycles are repeated about every 28 days. A minimum of 4 to 6 cycles of therapy must be given before evaluation of response. Azacitidine has resulted in OS rates of 50% as compared to 16% in those treated with usual care (chemotherapy, low-dose cytarabine, or best supportive care).[75,76] These agents are generally well-tolerated with the most significant adverse effect being myelosuppression. Best supportive care includes use of blood product transfusion support.

All adult patients who present with CNS symptoms, and all patients who present with asymptomatic monocytic disease, should have a diagnostic lumbar puncture, and if it is positive, should be treated for disease. Methotrexate 12 to 15 mg, with or without cytarabine, should be administered intrathecally twice a week until clearance of leukemic blasts from the CSF, and then weekly for 4 to 6 weeks. Continued secondary prophylaxis is recommended following treatment for CNS disease.

Intensive Postremission Therapy

Although most adults with AML achieve a CR, the duration of remission is short (6 to 9 months) if no further treatment is given. Relapse is presumably a consequence of the presence of residual, but clinically undetectable, leukemic cells after remission induction therapy. The goal of intensive postremission therapy is to eradicate these residual leukemic cells and to prevent the emergence of drug-resistant disease. (10) The need for postremission therapy is based on postmortem analysis and cell kinetic data suggesting that nearly 10^9 residual leukemic cells remain after effective remission induction therapy. Strategies evaluated as postremission therapy include (a) low-dose, prolonged maintenance therapy, (b) short-course intensive chemotherapy-alone regimens, and (c) high-dose chemotherapy with or without radiation therapy followed by allogeneic or autologous HSCT.

Chemotherapy In the treatment of AML, intensive postremission therapy is often referred to as *consolidation therapy*. Results of randomized controlled trials in adults clearly show that intensive postremission therapy following remission induction therapy prolongs survival versus no therapy, although the exact duration of postremission therapy is controversial.[3,71,72,77,78]

The intensity of postremission therapy is important. In a large CALGB trial, all patients who achieve a CR after standard 7+3 induction, were randomized to receive one of three cytarabine-based consolidation regimens: 100 mg/m^2 per day or 400 mg/m^2 per day as a continuous 24-hour infusion, or 3,000 mg/m^2 every 12 hours on days 1, 3, and 5.[79] For adults younger than age 60 years, the probability of remaining in CR after 4 years was significantly higher in patients who received high-dose cytarabine (25% vs. 29% vs. 44%, respectively).[79] Elderly patients had lower response rates in all arms and did not benefit from the administration of higher cytarabine doses, probably because they were unable to tolerate the high-dose regimen. Dose-limiting neurotoxicity in the high-dose arm was more common in elderly patients and those patients with impaired kidney function.[79]

It is not clear whether the same agents (cytarabine and an anthracycline) given for remission induction should be used for postremission therapy in higher doses, or whether different agents should be given. If leukemic relapse is caused by a resistant cell line, then the use of different agents that are non–cross-resistant with drugs used in induction might be beneficial.

High-dose cytarabine appears to be an important component of postremission therapy, particularly if it is not used in induction therapy. However, many questions remain, such as the optimal dose (g/m^2), number of doses per cycle, and number of cycles of high-dose cytarabine. Among patients with core-binding factor AML, defined as the presence of either t(8;21) or inv(16), it is clear that multiple cycles are beneficial, generally 3 to 4 cycles.[80] The NCCN guideline recommends four cycles of high-dose cytarabine for adults younger than 60 years of age and with good cytogenetics or, alternatively, one cycle of high-dose cytarabine followed by autologous HSCT.[66] Patients with intermediate-risk cytogenetics should receive 3 to 4 cycles of high-dose cytarabine, one to two cycles of high-dose cytarabine followed by autologous HSCT, or proceed directly to a matched allogeneic HSCT.[66] If a patient is 60 years of age or older, standard-dose cytarabine with or without anthracycline for one to two cycles, a reduced-dose high-dose cytarabine regimen (1 to 1.5 g/m^2 per day for 4 to 6 doses) for one to two cycles, continuation of low-intensity therapy such as azacitidine or decitabine, or enrollment in a clinical trial is recommended. Patients with high-risk cytogenetics, underlying MDS, or secondary AML should either be enrolled in a clinical trial or be referred for either a matched sibling or alternative donor allogeneic HSCT.[66]

Clinical **Controversy...**

Intensive postremission therapy is clearly necessary to prevent relapse and those regimens containing high-dose cytarabine appear to be a key part of postremission therapy. However, the optimal dose of high-dose cytarabine, the number of doses per cycle, and the number of cycles to give remain unknown.

Allogeneic Hematopoietic Stem Cell Transplantation Allogeneic HSCT represents the most aggressive postremission therapy in the management of AML. Much controversy surrounds this treatment approach, specifically the appropriateness, timing, treatment design, and donor selection.

The antileukemic activity of allogeneic HSCT is based on the administration of pretransplant high-dose chemotherapy (or chemoradiotherapy) and the development of a posttransplant immune-based antileukemic response. The immune-based response, referred to as a graft-versus-leukemia (GVL) effect, often accompanies the graft-versus-host disease (GVHD) reaction. The immune-based benefit of allogeneic HSCT has been demonstrated through the observation of consistently lower relapse rates with allogeneic HSCT as compared to autologous or syngeneic HSCT. This potential benefit of allogeneic HSCT can be offset by the risk of posttransplant complications such as GVHD, sinusoidal obstruction syndrome, graft failure, and infections.

Allogeneic HSCT was first evaluated as a treatment modality for AML in refractory patients, but because of initial success in small numbers of patients, it has also been evaluated as intensive postremission therapy in AML patients in first or subsequent remission. Nonrandomized trials of HLA-identical sibling allogeneic HSCT performed in AML patients in first complete remission (CR1) reported 5-year survival rates of 45% to 60% with relapse rates of 10% to 20%.[3,71,72,78] Transplant-related mortality following HLA-matched sibling allogeneic HSCT ranges from 15% to 25% in most series. As clinicians have gained more experience in this intensive form of therapy and been provided with more effective immunosuppressive and antibiotic regimens, transplant-related mortality rates have decreased and survival rates have increased. Bone marrow registry data indicate that long-term survival rates in AML patients who receive a matched sibling allogeneic HSCT while in first remission have increased from about 45% in the early 1980s to about 60% in the mid-1990s.

Allogeneic HSCT from an HLA-matched sibling donor for AML patients in CR1 results in long-term EFS in 43% to 55% of patients. Although the results vary, some of the studies show longer EFS and lower relapse rates with allogeneic HSCT in AML in CR1 as compared to chemotherapy-alone postremission regimens. Overall, single center prospective trials have not shown an OS advantage for allogeneic HSCT in all patients with AML CR1. Meta-analyses of clinical trials evaluating allogeneic HSCT versus other consolidation strategies in CR1 shows that allogeneic HSCT does provide an OS advantage for patients with intermediate- and high-risk AML.[78]

Myeloablative allogeneic HSCT is generally restricted to patients younger than 60 years of age, which limits the number of patients eligible for treatment of a disease that primarily affects older adults. NMT uses reduced intensity preparative regimens and is now being used in AML patients, particularly in older patients and those with comorbid illnesses that would limit their eligibility for conventional allogeneic HSCT. NMT is designed to provide enough immunosuppression in the preparative regimen to allow for engraftment of donor cells, and depends heavily on the development of a GVL effect as a means to treat and prevent relapse of AML. Initial results of NMTs in AML indicate that the procedure is well tolerated in a wide age range of patients, and that it is associated with low rates of regimen-related toxicity.[81] A larger trial evaluating 264 patients who had received a NMT from matched related and unrelated donors demonstrated a 5-year OS of 33% and disease-free survival of 32%.[82] Because only 30% of patients have an HLA-matched sibling donor, allogeneic HSCT is further restricted as a treatment alternative for AML patients.[83] Matched unrelated donor HSCT with a phenotypically HLA-matched donor identified from bone marrow registries is also a treatment option in young adults and pediatric AML patients. This approach is associated with long-term EFS rates of 30% to 40%, which are slightly lower than in AML patients undergoing HLA-matched sibling allogeneic HSCT because of a higher risk of treatment-related mortality with the procedure.[3,72]

The decision to transplant a patient depends a great deal on which prognostic risk group the patient belongs. Among patients with favorable-risk AML, allogeneic HSCT does not result in better outcomes as compared to high-dose cytarabine-based therapy. All patients with high-risk AML, including those with an antecedent hematologic disorder, treatment-related MDS, or induction failure, should undergo evaluation for HSCT. Similarly, patients in CR1 with high-risk cytogenetics and patients in CR2 and beyond should undergo evaluation for allogeneic HSCT.[59]

Autologous Hematopoietic Stem Cell Transplantation Compared to allogeneic HSCT, autologous HSCT has the advantage of a lower risk of posttransplant complications because of lack of immunosuppression and GVHD, and more broad applicability because of a lack of donor limitations and fewer age restrictions. Although the preparative regimen still provides antileukemic activity, autologous HSCT is associated with a higher risk of relapse because of a lack of a GVL effect and potential tumor contamination with autologous stem cells. EFS following autologous HSCT for adult AML in CR1 ranges from 40% to 60%, with treatment-related mortality of 5% to 15% and relapse rates of 30% to 50%.[84] Long-term response rates decrease proportionally as autologous HSCT is employed in second or subsequent CR. Controversies in autologous HSCT include the optimal timing of therapy, the amount of consolidation therapy needed prior to HSCT, the dose of stem cells needed, and the impact of posttransplant therapy.[84] In general, an autologous HSCT may be considered if an allogeneic HSCT is not possible.

Comparisons of Postremission Therapy Options Several randomized trials in AML patients in CR1 have compared outcomes following allogeneic HSCT, autologous HSCT, and/or intensive consolidation chemotherapy. In most trials, eligible patients based on age and donor availability received an allogeneic HSCT and the remaining patients were randomized between autologous HSCT and chemotherapy alone. The European Organization for Research and Treatment of Cancer-GIMEMA (Gruppo Italiano Malattie Ematologiche Maligne dell'Adulto) trial observed a EFS advantage and reduced relapse risk for allogeneic HSCT or autologous HSCT as compared to chemotherapy alone, but no differences in OS.[3,72] Survival rates were comparable because of a higher relapse rate in the chemotherapy group as compared to a higher treatment-related mortality rate in the allogeneic HSCT group. This is the only trial that has demonstrated superior 4-year EFS with HSCT versus chemotherapy. Interestingly, the response rates in the conventional chemotherapy arm in this trial were lower than those reported in other studies, which may account for the survival benefit in the transplant group. Several other trials have shown no difference in EFS or OS between autologous HSCT, allogeneic HSCT, and conventional chemotherapy. In aggregate, these trials show that either autologous HSCT or allogeneic HSCT can reduce the risk of relapse, although this has not translated into an OS benefit. One trial design issue that might explain this lack of survival benefit was the low percentage of patients who progressed to transplantation when randomized, thus diluting the effect of transplantation. The effect of stem cell source on EFS and OS is controversial. Several comparative trials of bone marrow versus peripheral blood have been completed in patients with hematologic malignancies, and a meta-analysis of nine randomized trials showed a lower relapse rate for those patients receiving peripheral blood stem cells.[85]

Most transplant centers base their decision to transplant on cytogenetic risk category.[3] Patients with high-risk cytogenetics do poorly with conventional chemotherapy or autologous HSCT (EFS <15%), making allogeneic HSCT the treatment of choice in this population. Patients with good-risk cytogenetics should not proceed to transplant in CR1, as neither autologous nor allogeneic HSCT is superior to conventional chemotherapy. The optimal treatment of choice in patients with intermediate-risk cytogenetics is not clear and is based on clinician preference. Many centers consider a relapse probability of 40% to 50% sufficiently high so as to justify the risk of transplant-related mortality. The decision to proceed with HSCT in this group may depend on the results of molecular testing. As discussed in Risk Classification above, several genetic molecular abnormalities have prognostic significance in adults with AML. Abnormalities that are associated with a poor outcome include FLT3 abnormalities; myeloid/lymphoid or MLL abnormalities; *BAALC*; and WT-1.

According to the NCCN guidelines, the decision to proceed to HSCT depends on unfavorable prognostic risk features including cytogenetics.[66] If the patient has a good-risk cytogenetic profile and is younger than age 60 years, then high-dose cytarabine for four cycles or one cycle of high-dose cytarabine-based therapy followed by autologous HSCT is preferred over allogeneic HSCT. If the patient has a high-risk cytogenetic profile and is younger than 60 years of age, then allogeneic HSCT transplantation should be considered early after remission induction. Patients with intermediate-risk cytogenetics should be entered into a clinical trial, but if a clinical trial is not available, either a matched sibling allogeneic HSCT or an autologous HSCT should be considered. Autologous HSCT can be used if a hematologic and cytogenetic remission is achieved. For patients 60 years and older, the NCCN guidelines do not favor HSCT and recommend either enrollment into a clinical trial, or consideration of conventional dose cytarabine with or without an anthracycline or intermediate-dose cytarabine. Clinicians increasingly consider autologous HSCT as a treatment option, and for selected patients older than 60 years of age, NMT is being used more frequently.[81,82,86] For the AML patient who relapses early after induction therapy, if a sibling or matched related donor is available, then allogeneic HSCT is the primary reinduction therapy because conventional chemotherapy offers little benefit. If the relapse occurs late, then HSCT can be used as postremission consolidation after conventional induction therapy.[66]

Acute Myeloid Leukemia in Children

The most effective induction regimens for children include 3 days of an anthracycline and 7 to 10 days of cytarabine yielding a CR of greater than 85% and a 5-year OS of 70%. The Children's Oncology Group is using risk-adapted therapy for childhood AML based on cytogenetics, molecular markers, and MRD results.[5] About 73% of children have t(8;21), no MRD at the end of induction, inversion 16, or other good risk factors leading to a low-risk classification and an 80% OS with chemotherapy alone.[87] Children with monosomy 7, 5q deletion, high FLT3-ITD to wild-type allelic ratio, or MRD at the end of induction are considered high risk with a 35% OS.[87] The use of intrathecal CNS prophylaxis varies by protocol because of the low CNS relapse rate.[70] Cranial radiation is only used for patients with refractory CNS disease.

Following induction therapy, patients should be evaluated for a response. Those not achieving a CR will require additional chemotherapy called *reinduction*. A bone marrow biopsy is usually performed 7 to 10 days after the completion of chemotherapy to document disease eradication. If there is persistent disease, a second course of therapy is administered. The second course may be identical to the initial induction regimen, or include high-dose cytarabine and asparaginase, or mitoxantrone and cytarabine. If the marrow is aplastic, a repeat marrow biopsy should be performed on hematologic recovery to document a CR.

Following induction, children go onto consolidation therapy. An evidence-based review of the role of HSCT in the treatment of pediatric AML concluded that HSCT was indicated in the following settings: (a) initial CR: matched sibling allogeneic HSCT is superior to autologous HSCT and chemotherapy, but are only available in 25% of children; (b) CR2: allogeneic HSCT is preferable to chemotherapy and autologous HSCT.[70,88] Children with high-risk disease and no suitable stem cell donor should receive consolidation chemotherapy including high-dose cytarabine. A recent international expert panel recommended no transplant for favorable risk children in CR1.[6] For other risk groups in first remission transplant risks must be weighed against potential benefit. Patients in CR2 generally receive an allogeneic HSCT. AML in children younger than 2 years of age is different from older children and are considered high risk. Poor prognostic factors include t(1;22), high WBC count, and CNS disease. Neonates with Down syndrome may develop transient myeloproliferative disease that usually spontaneously resolves without treatment within a few months. Infants with AML receive the same therapy as children of other ages, with the dosing per kilogram and not per body surface area.

Relapsed or Refractory Acute Myeloid Leukemia

The most common cause of treatment failure in AML patients receiving chemotherapy alone or undergoing HSCT is relapse. In addition, many patients, particularly elderly patients, have refractory disease as defined by the inability to achieve a CR after two courses of induction therapy. In most cases, the preferred method of treatment for relapsed or refractory disease is HSCT. Prolonged EFS is observed in 30% to 40% of patients receiving allogeneic or autologous HSCT in first relapse or CR2. Unfortunately, only a small percentage of relapsed or refractory adult patients will be eligible for HSCT, particularly allogeneic HSCT, because of age and donor restrictions. The role of NMT is also being evaluated in this setting.

The timing of HSCT to treat relapse is controversial. Some studies suggest that outcomes of HLA-matched, related allogeneic HSCT are similar regardless of whether the transplant is performed at the time of early first relapse or in CR2. The difficulty with this approach is identifying a patient in "early relapse," as often the patient will present in a florid relapse. While performing the allogeneic HSCT in first relapse eliminates the need for and toxicity of salvage chemotherapy, the feasibility of this approach is limited by the lead time required to activate a donor search. Allogeneic HSCT is superior to autologous HSCT in adults younger than age 55 years.

Patients who relapse following allogeneic HSCT have a poor outcome, with a median survival of about 3 to 4 months.[89] In this setting, treatment options depend on performance status, clinical condition, and the time since allogeneic HSCT. Patients relapsing less than 100 days following allogeneic HSCT are unlikely to respond to current therapies, and salvage attempts are often associated with a high treatment-related mortality. For selected patients relapsing more than 1 year after allogeneic HSCT, a second allogeneic HSCT may be an alternative, but the likelihood of prolonged survival is generally less than 10% with a second transplant. Other strategies being investigated for the treatment of relapse after allogeneic HSCT include immune manipulation to stimulate a GVL effect through donor lymphocyte infusions, and premature discontinuation of calcineurin inhibitors and other immunosuppressants.

Autologous HSCT is an option at the time of first relapse if cells have been previously collected and stored during first remission. If such cells were not collected, then it is necessary to achieve a CR2 in order to proceed to autologous HSCT. Prolonged EFS of 30% and 20% are reported when autologous HSCT is performed in CR2 and CR3, respectively. The advantages of autologous HSCT are the lack of donor limitations and fewer age-based restrictions; the disadvantage is the need to achieve a CR, which requires exposure to more cytotoxic chemotherapy. If patients relapse following autologous HSCT, allogeneic HSCT from a related or matched unrelated donor is preferred in selected younger patients. NMT or other investigational therapies can be considered for older patients who relapse after autologous HSCT.

If patients with relapsed or refractory disease are not candidates for HSCT, until recently the primary mode of treatment was salvage chemotherapy. The ability to achieve a CR2 with salvage chemotherapy is related to the duration of the first remission. About 50% to 60% of patients who relapse longer than 2 years after induction therapy will achieve a CR2, often with the same induction regimen.[3,72]

If the patient relapses 1 to 2 years after induction therapy, the CR2 rate decreases to 40%, and only 10% to 20% of patients who relapse within 6 to 12 months following induction are able to achieve a CR2 with alternate salvage chemotherapy regimens. Long-term survival at 3 years ranges from zero in patients who relapse early to 20% to 25% in those who experience a prolonged duration of initial remission. Based on these data, a risk-adapted approach should be taken when considering treatment options.

The most commonly used salvage regimens include high-dose cytarabine given at doses of 2,000 to 3,000 mg/m^2 every 12 hours for 8 to 12 doses. High-dose cytarabine schedules that use once-daily doses or alternate-day doses have also been used in an attempt to minimize toxicity.[72] Cytarabine has been administered alone or in combination with various agents, including etoposide, fludarabine, topotecan, clofarabine, and an anthracycline, as treatment of relapsed or refractory AML. Response rates to such salvage regimens range from 30% to 50%, but are often short-lived. Patients who received high-dose cytarabine during remission induction may be less likely to benefit from such a regimen for treatment of relapse, and thus require alternate salvage strategies. Patients with remission duration of longer than 1 year appear to benefit most from high-dose cytarabine regimens.[3,72] One additional option is clofarabine, a purine analog, which can be used either alone or combined with cytarabine. While studies have shown CR rates of about 50%, median OS is less than 12 months.[90]

Several classes of new agents are being investigated as alternate treatment approaches for relapsed or refractory AML, including the ubiquitin-proteasome pathway inhibitors (bortezomib), new novel nucleoside analogs (troxacitabine), histone deacetylase inhibitors (phenylbutyrate, vorinostat), and angiogenesis modulators (bevacizumab and thalidomide).[91] Arsenic trioxide, which is effective in the treatment of APL, is being investigated for the treatment of AML via its modulation of apoptotic and chromatin remodeling pathways.

In children with AML, about 5% have refractory disease and 30% experience a relapse.[6] About one-half the children relapse within 1 year of initial diagnosis and have a poor prognosis.[5] Therapy should include and anthracycline and antimetabolite followed by allogeneic HSCT if a CR2 is achieved.

Late Effects of Therapy

Because of the intense therapy received by children with AML, they are at risk for a variety of long-term sequelae. A recent study reported that more than 50% of survivors have growth abnormalities.[92] Other findings include neurocognitive deficits, transfusion-associated hepatitis, endocrine disorders, cataracts, and cardiomyopathy (median cumulative anthracycline dose 335 mg/m^2). The 20-year cumulative risk for a second malignancy is estimated to be 1.8%.

TREATMENT
Acute Promyelocytic Leukemia

APL is a subclass of AML that accounts for about 10% of all cases, and is the most curable of the AML subtypes. Most patients are diagnosed between the ages of 15 and 60 years. Five-year EFS rates of 70% to 80% are reported with APL.[93] APL is clinically unique from the other subclasses because of the common occurrence of severe coagulopathy (characterized by disseminated intravascular coagulation) at diagnosis and during induction therapy, which frequently resulted in intracerebral hemorrhage. In APL, differentiation and maturation arrest are caused by alterations in the retinoic acid receptor (RAR) because of the translocation of chromosomes 15 and 17. The discovery of t(15;17) provides a cytogenetic marker of the disease and is predictive of response to differentiation therapy with tretinoin (commonly referred to as all-*trans* retinoic acid or ATRA). This translocation leads to a fusion protein of the *PML* gene on chromosome 15 and the RARα on chromosome 17.

Prior to the availability of tretinoin in the late 1980s, treatment of APL consisted of the same combination chemotherapy regimens used in the treatment of other subclasses of AML. Such standard regimens produced CR rates of 50% to 60%, but were associated with a high treatment-related mortality rate caused by hemorrhagic complications. The introduction of molecularly targeted therapy with tretinoin allows for high CR rates with a significant reduction in life-threatening bleeding complications. Arsenic trioxide targets the PML moiety, resulting in apoptosis, and appears to be synergistic with tretinoin.

The WBC count at initial presentation is the most important prognostic factor in patients with APL. Risk stratification of patients at diagnosis based on WBC count has improved outcomes. Abnormal creatinine, increased peripheral blast count, and presence of coagulopathy are prognostic factors that predict for early death due to hemorrhage.[94]

Treatment Phases
Induction

Tretinoin, an oral vitamin A analog, is given orally in a dose of 45 mg/m^2 per day, as a single dose or divided into two doses, given after a meal. Tretinoin-based regimens achieve CR rates as high as 95% in APL patients within 1 to 3 months. Because tretinoin does not cross the blood–brain barrier, leukemic meningitis should be treated with conventional intrathecal chemotherapy.

Although it is not myelosuppressive, tretinoin therapy is associated with headache, skin and mucous membrane reactions, bone pain, nausea, and the retinoic acid syndrome. When tretinoin is started, rapid onset of differentiation of promyelocytes occurs, which can lead to leukocytosis and retinoic acid syndrome. The retinoic acid syndrome (fever, respiratory distress, interstitial pulmonary infiltrates, pleural effusions, and weight gain) is now referred to as the APL differentiation syndrome or APL hyperleukocytosis syndrome, because it is associated with other treatment modalities in the management of APL. The syndrome is fatal in 5% to 29% of cases. A combination of chemotherapy with tretinoin induction decreases the risk of APL differentiation syndrome, and rapid initiation of dexamethasone 10 mg (0.2 mg/kg per dose in children) twice daily on development of symptoms decreases associated mortality.[93]

A number of clinical trials have evaluated treatment regimens for APL since the discovery of tretinoin.[93] These trials show that tretinoin induction therapy, followed by consolidation chemotherapy, produces similar CR rates but decreased relapse and increased EFS and OS as compared to chemotherapy alone for remission induction and consolidation. However, a significant proportion of patients receiving tretinoin in that study relapsed by 4 years, and 25% of patients experienced the APL differentiation syndrome. In an effort to extend the duration of remission and decrease tretinoin-associated toxicity, other trials have evaluated the sequential and concurrent administration of tretinoin with chemotherapy during induction and consolidation therapy. Additionally, the stratification of therapies based on WBC at diagnosis has been used in trials. A combined analysis of the Programa para el Estudio de la Terapeutica en Hemopatıa Maligna (PETHEMA) 99 and the French APL 2000 trial showed that in patients with WBC <10,000/mm^3 (10×10^9/L), the regimen containing tretinoin with idarubicin for induction and tretinoin in consolidation produced similar CR rates with decrease relapse rates, whereas for patients with WBC >10,000/mm^3 (10×10^9/L), the induction regimen containing cytarabine resulted in higher CR rates and improved OS rates.[93] (11) Based on these data, the current NCCN guideline for induction therapy for newly diagnosed APL patients includes selection of one of three options based on WBC and ability to tolerate anthracyclines (tretinoin 45 mg/m^2 per day until a CR is achieved, in combination with an anthracycline (either daunorubicin 50 to 60 mg/m^2 per dose for 3 or 4 days, or idarubicin 12 mg/m^2 per dose every other day for four doses) or tretinoin plus arsenic trioxide for patients unable to tolerate anthracycline therapy.[66] Several of the induction regimens also contain cytarabine 200 mg/m^2 per dose for 7 days; similar CR rates are observed with daunorubicin or idarubicin. APL cells appear to be more sensitive to anthracyclines, possibly because of decreased P-glycoprotein expression. The NCCN guidelines also emphasize the use of one published regimen consistently throughout induction, consolidation, and maintenance phases.[66] Children should also be treated with tretinoin, an anthracycline, and cytarabine with results similar to those achieved in adults.

Another difference in the treatment of APL is the timing of bone marrow biopsy. Assessment of response to treatment of APL is done at the time of count recovery after induction therapy. A day 10 to 14 day bone marrow biopsy, which is usually done for monitoring the effect of induction chemotherapy for other types of AML, is not long enough because leukemic promyelocytes need more time for differentiation. Assessment of molecular remission should be made after consolidation.

Arsenic trioxide is a compound with demonstrated efficacy in relapsed APL. It has been evaluated as part of remission induction therapy in several studies. The concept of a "chemotherapy-free" regimen in this disease is attractive especially for patients unable to tolerate anthracyclines. A combination of tretinoin with arsenic trioxide for induction therapy resulted in CR of 95% of low-risk patients.[95]

Consolidation Therapy

Consolidation chemotherapy should be administered to patients with APL because of the high relapse rate. Consolidation therapy usually consists of an idarubicin or daunorubicin-based regimen in combination with tretinoin. Arsenic trioxide has also been evaluated in consolidation therapy.

Postconsolidation Therapy

Unlike other subtypes of AML, maintenance therapy is an important component of therapy for APL. Before the advent of tretinoin, nonrandomized trials suggested a benefit of continuous low-dose methotrexate and mercaptopurine in prevention of relapse of APL. Larger prospective randomized trials have demonstrated decreased relapse rates in patients who received maintenance therapy (either tretinoin or combination chemotherapy), and some trials have demonstrated increased EFS and OS.[93] In a study that compared maintenance with tretinoin, chemotherapy, or tretinoin plus chemotherapy versus observation, observation was associated with the highest relapse rate and tretinoin plus chemotherapy with the lowest relapse rate.[95] Current recommendations for maintenance therapy in adult APL patients include tretinoin 45 mg/m^2 per day for 15 days every 3 months, in addition to mercaptopurine 100 mg/m^2 orally daily and methotrexate 10 mg/m^2 per week, for 2 years in all patients. Although the use of maintenance therapy in patients with low-risk disease who have achieved a molecular remission at the end of consolidation is controversial.[93] The NCCN guidelines similarly recommend tretinoin maintenance therapy with or without mercaptopurine and methotrexate.[66]

Relapsed Acute Promyelocytic Leukemia

The incidence of relapsed APL is 10% to 15% overall with rates as high as 20% to 30% in high-risk disease. Most relapses occur in the first 3 years following induction therapy. Arsenic trioxide is the agent of choice for relapsed APL. Multiple studies have shown CR rates of about 85%. It is controversial as to whether adding tretinoin to arsenic therapy is better than just treating with arsenic monotherapy.[96]

Arsenic trioxide has induced clinical remissions in relapsed APL through its induction of apoptosis and differentiation.[96,97] The recommended dose is 0.15 mg/kg per day IV until bone marrow remission, not to exceed 60 doses, followed by consolidation beginning 3 to 6 weeks after completion of induction at the same dose for a total of 25 doses over a period up to 5 weeks. Arsenic trioxide therapy is associated with two specific toxicities. First, it can cause the APL differentiation syndrome, similar to that seen with tretinoin. Management is similar: corticosteroids at first signs of pulmonary distress or a rapidly rising WBC count. The second toxicity is a prolongation of the QT_c interval. Consequently, it is important to obtain a baseline 12-lead electrocardiogram prior to starting therapy with arsenic trioxide, and correct any electrolyte abnormalities, including potassium, calcium, and magnesium. Other medications known to prolong the QT_c interval should be avoided, if possible, during arsenic trioxide therapy. The QT_c interval should not exceed 500 milliseconds at baseline, and if it increases to more than 500 milliseconds during therapy, the patient should be reevaluated. Arsenic trioxide should not be restarted until the QT_c is less than 460 milliseconds. Following induction of a CR2 with arsenic trioxide in relapsed patients, postremission therapy with combination arsenic trioxide and chemotherapy can result in molecular remissions and improved EFS, as compared to chemotherapy or arsenic trioxide alone following remission.[96] Additional investigations are underway to evaluate the role of arsenic trioxide in multidrug postremission regimens.

It is recommended for patients to proceed to an autologous HSCT following hematologic and molecular remission after arsenic therapy. Outcomes with autologous HSCT depend on the disease status of the patient at the time of transplant. Autologous HSCT in CR2 (versus CR1) is associated with a lower OS, leukemia-free survival, and increased treatment-related mortality. Allogeneic HSCT is also an option for patients with a HLA-matched related donor in CR2 as consolidation after reinduction with arsenic trioxide.[98]

Patient Monitoring

In comparison to non-APL AML, molecular and cytogenetic testing at the end of remission induction therapy in APL has no prognostic value. Clinicians should not make decisions based on the presence or absence of any genetic abnormalities at this time. Because terminal differentiation of blasts in APL requires more than 40 days, results of a bone marrow biopsy obtained at the end of remission induction can be misleading because insufficient time has elapsed to determine response. Molecular and cytogenetic response assessment should occur after the completion of consolidation treatment.

Detection of residual PML/RARα transcripts in the bone marrow at the end of consolidation therapy is strongly associated with subsequent hematologic relapse. Achievement of PML/RARα-negative status is associated with a higher probability of cure. The use of this molecular technique allows the clinician to assess response to therapy and also detect relapse earlier, which might prevent the development of overt disease recurrence and is associated with improved outcome compared with delaying treatment until overt morphologic relapse.[93] Most experts recommend that APL patients should be routinely evaluated for continuous remission status. Suggested follow-up includes polymerase chain reaction for PML/RARα every 3 to 6 months for 2 years, and then every 6 months for 2 years.[66,93]

ROLE OF HEMATOPOIETIC GROWTH FACTORS IN ACUTE MYELOID LEUKEMIA

(12) Hematopoietic growth factors have been evaluated in AML patients to enhance chemotherapy cytotoxicity, shorten the duration of neutropenia, and reduce the incidence and severity of infection

following induction and consolidation chemotherapy. Most studies show limited benefit with the use of colony-stimulating factors as "priming" agents administered during remission induction therapy in an effort to recruit leukemia cells into the cycle to enhance susceptibility to cell-cycle–specific chemotherapy agents, leading to increased cell kill. Use of hematopoietic growth factors concurrently during chemotherapy administration is discouraged outside the setting of a clinical trial and is not recommended for this use in the American Society of Clinical Oncology guidelines.[99]

Both filgrastim and sargramostim are FDA approved to prevent neutropenic complications in adult AML patients receiving intensive chemotherapy. Myeloid blast cells have receptors for granulocyte colony-stimulating factor and granulocyte-macrophage colony-stimulating factor, and there was initial concern that the use of these factors would stimulate regrowth of the myeloid leukemia. Although subsequent studies have addressed these concerns, many clinicians do not initiate filgrastim until an initial remission is achieved.

A number of randomized trials, primarily in elderly patients, consistently demonstrate that filgrastim or sargramostim reduces the duration of neutropenia following AML induction chemotherapy.[99] While neutropenia can be reduced from 2 to 12 days depending on the trial, results vary in terms of improvements in infectious morbidity and mortality, resource use, and disease response rates. The American Society of Clinical Oncology Guidelines for the Use of White Blood Cell Growth Factors considers the use of hematopoietic growth factors after initial induction therapy reasonable, with the understanding that the effects on length of hospitalization and incidence of severe infection are modest.[99] Patients older than age 55 years appear to derive the greatest benefit, and use is appropriate in this population where more rapid marrow recovery might decrease the duration of hospitalization.[99] A recent review of 19 trials including a total of 5256 patients showed no difference in the incidence of bacteremias or invasive fungal infections with the use of hematopoietic growth factors.[100] It also concluded that the use of hematopoietic growth factors after consolidation did not affect CR duration, relapse rates or OS. Further pharmacoeconomic data are required in this setting, but the body of evidence supports their use following consolidation therapy in adults. Other controversial issues surrounding hematopoietic growth factor use in AML include which growth factor to use, what dose, which day to start after chemotherapy, how long to continue, and should the marrow be examined for leukemia prior to starting a colony-stimulating factor. All hematopoietic growth factors have been evaluated in patients with AML, including sargramostim, filgrastim, and pegfilgrastim. Although pegfilgrastim is not FDA approved for this indication, research supports using it in this setting.[101] The use of hematopoietic growth factors can also interfere with the interpretation of the day 14 bone marrow examination. Hematopoietic growth factors should be discontinued at least 7 days prior to a bone marrow aspirate and biopsy to avoid interfering with the interpretation of the results (i.e., may see immature myeloid forms that would suggest residual disease).

SUPPORTIVE CARE

The most common and significant toxic effect of antileukemic agents is marrow suppression. With the exception of corticosteroids, tretinoin, asparaginase/pegaspargase, and vincristine, antineoplastic agents used to treat acute leukemia cause myelosuppression. During AML remission and postremission therapy, daily monitoring of the complete blood count and the absolute neutrophil count is necessary to determine when red cell and platelet transfusions are needed and when neutropenia is achieved. Less frequent monitoring may be sufficient during ALL induction. Marrow hypoplasia from the myelosuppressive regimens usually reaches its lowest point (nadir) after 1 to 2 weeks of therapy and lasts for another 1 to 2 weeks. During this period of hypoplasia, infectious and bleeding complications are major causes of death in leukemic patients. As typical signs and symptoms of infection may be absent in the neutropenic host, frequent monitoring of vital signs (especially fever) and daily physical examination are important.[102] Infection control strategies often include routine hand washing; dietary restrictions; reverse isolation and laminar-air flow rooms; fungal, *Pneumocystis*, and bacterial prophylaxis; and the empiric use of broad-spectrum antibiotics when fever occurs (see Chap. 100).[102] In contrast to the practice at many institutions, the NCCN guidelines do not recommend prophylactic antimicrobials or gut decontamination during induction or consolidation, and leave the choice to the discretion of the treating facility based on local infection patterns and concerns.[103] Several groups have analyzed the evidence supporting the use of prophylactic antibacterials. In general, prophylactic antibacterials should be reserved for patients who are expected to have prolonged (more than 7 days) and profound (absolute neutrophil count <100 cells/mm^3 [100×10^6/L]) neutropenia. Based on these criteria, prophylaxis following induction chemotherapy is warranted and postconsolidation therapy is warranted on a case-by-case basis.

In children, prophylactic antibiotics have not proven useful and have resulted in increased resistance. Pediatric ALL patients on standard induction regimens, which generally are minimally myelosuppressive, often have recovered blood counts earlier and do not require very aggressive measures. However, they do require close monitoring of vital signs and blood counts until their counts recover. Pediatric AML patients are usually admitted for at least 1 month during induction and again for consolidation. Infectious complications, especially fungal, are a major cause of morbidity and mortality. The incidence of viridans streptococci has increased with the intensity of therapy and is most associated with high-dose cytarabine. These infections can lead to meningitis or delayed acute respiratory distress syndrome.

Pneumocystis jiroveci prophylaxis (usually trimethoprim-sulfamethoxazole) is begun in all adults and children with ALL by the end of induction and continues until 6 months after therapy is discontinued. Infants are at high risk for developing *Pneumocystis jiroveci* pneumonia early in therapy, so should start prophylaxis immediately.[34] These infants can receive trimethoprim-sulfamethoxazole despite the risk of kernicterus with careful monitoring.

Acute leukemia patients, particularly those patients with an initial elevated WBC count, are at risk for tumor lysis syndrome. Preventive measures include allopurinol or rasburicase, and adequate hydration (with or without sodium bicarbonate) prior to and during chemotherapy to prevent the development of urate nephropathy from rapid destruction of WBCs. Rasburicase, a recombinant urate-oxidase enzyme produced by genetic modification of *Saccharomyces cerevisiae*, catalyzes the enzymatic oxidation of uric acid into the inactive soluble metabolite, allantoin. In children, rasburicase more rapidly reduces uric acid levels in patients with aggressive malignancies compared to allopurinol, and reduces the need for dialysis.[104] Rasburicase has been evaluated in adults, and some studies in adults show that fixed dosing produces equivalent outcomes to a mg/kg dosing strategy.[105] Because of its cost, rasburicase is usually limited to patients with ALL who have a high WBC count or bulky extramedullary disease, aggressive lymphoma, or patients with AML with a high presenting WBC. Most institutions also include an elevated uric acid as part of the criteria for use. Rasburicase has a rapid onset of action and long duration of action, so many institutions also limit its use to a single dose and allow repeat doses as needed. Rasburicase is contraindicated in patients with glucose-6-phosphate dehydrogenase deficiency. Tumor lysis syndrome may lead not only to hyperuricemia, but also to hyperkalemia, hyperphosphatemia, hypocalcemia and subsequent renal insufficiency.[104]

Hematologic support consists primarily of platelet and packed red blood cell transfusions. Platelet transfusions are often given for peripheral counts below 10,000 cells/mm^3 (10×10^9/L) or clinical signs of bleeding. Transfusions of packed red cells may also be indicated for a hemoglobin less than 8 gm/dL (4.96 mmol/L), profound fatigue, shortness of breath, tachycardia, or chest pain. APL can release procoagulants that can cause disseminated intravascular coagulation, necessitating close monitoring and replacement of coagulation factors with cryoprecipitate. Because of the gastrointestinal toxic effects of chemotherapy, parenteral nutrition may be required. Patients are frequently receiving infusions of antibiotics, fluids, hyperalimentation, opioids, and blood products simultaneously. To provide the total support needed for these patients, a multiple-lumen central venous access device should be considered at the start of therapy.

PERSONALIZED PHARMACOTHERAPY

Treatment of acute leukemia is highly personalized. A risk-adapted approach is used in the treatment of ALL and AML. In ALL, patients are placed into risk categories based on age and disease characteristics. The initial risk category is sometimes changed based on the rapidity and completeness of response to remission induction therapy. The same risk-adapted approach is used in the treatment of AML, but age and cytogenetics are the most important factors in determining the risk category. Molecular mutations are becoming more important in both ALL and AML.

Genetic polymorphisms may affect drug metabolism, receptor expression, drug transportation, drug disposition, and pharmacologic response. These alterations may contribute to acute and chronic toxicity from ALL therapy and to treatment outcome.[6,106] The most studied polymorphism involves thiopurine metabolism. Cellular thiopurine *S*-methyltransferase (TPMT) inactivates thiopurines such as mercaptopurine and thioguanine. About 10% of the population has intermediate TPMT activity as a result of heterozygous polymorphisms in the gene encoding for TPMT, and 1 in 300 has extremely low activity as a result of homozygous presence of this TPMT polymorphism. Deficiency of TPMT activity can result in excessive myelosuppression from standard doses of thiopurines. Patients with low activity (homozygous mutant TPMT genotype) require 85% to 90% dose reductions. About 50% of the heterozygous patients will require dose reductions. TPMT deficiency is also associated with an increased risk of developing secondary AML and radiation-induced brain tumors. Prospective evaluation of TPMT status was complicated in the past, as many ALL patients receive transfusions prior to definitive diagnosis. TPMT status can now be determined directly by DNA-based testing, which may become a standard of care in the near future.

EVALUATION OF THERAPEUTIC OUTCOMES

Appropriate development of a pharmaceutical care plan for the acute leukemia patient begins with establishing the diagnosis and prognosis for the patient. Long-term therapeutic goals for the patient may include long-term EFS, although palliative care is a possibility in some patients. The desired short-term outcome is the establishment of remission. The return of hematologic values to normal and a repeat bone marrow biopsy that demonstrates no evidence of disease serve as documentation that remission has been achieved. Monitoring guidelines for induction or consolidation are similar (Table 111-5). After the appropriate postremission therapy has been completed, the patient may return monthly for 1 year, and then every 3 months, to check hematologic values. If no evidence of disease exists after 5 years from the diagnosis and the patient has been in continuous CR, the patient is considered cured.

Frequent monitoring of fevers, hematologic and chemistry laboratory values, microbiology reports, and the patient's physical condition are necessary to identify infection, risk of bleeding, and tumor lysis syndrome early. A coagulation screening panel will identify patients with ongoing disseminated intravascular coagulation, a particular risk with APL.

During therapy, the pharmacist can be an important provider of patient and caregiver education. Patients should receive information regarding acute and chronic toxicities of the chemotherapy being administered, as well as possible treatments for those toxicities. Pharmacists should follow patients during consolidation therapy for dosing adjustments and toxicities due to chemotherapy. For example, the pharmacist should make sure the patient is receiving corticosteroid and saline eye drops four times daily while the patient is receiving high-dose cytarabine to prevent the ocular toxicity of cytarabine. The pharmacist can also be an important resource for information regarding antibiotics, antiemetics, nutritional support, hematopoietic growth factors, and other supportive care issues.

Pharmacists should be involved in assessing drug doses and any dose modifications for organ dysfunction or prior toxicity.

TABLE 111-5 Acute Myeloid Leukemia Assessment and Monitoring

Baseline Workup	Monitoring During Therapy	Postremission Monitoring
History and physical examination CBC with differential, platelets Serum chemistries (creatinine, bilirubin, AST, ALT to assess organ function) Coagulation (PT, PTT, D-dimers, fibrinogen) Bone marrow biopsy and aspirate with cytogenetics Immunophenotyping and cytochemistry Human leukocyte antigen (HLA) typing Cardiac workup (MUGA or echocardiogram; ECG) Intravascular access Lumbar puncture (if symptomatic or monocytic disease) Chest radiography Height and weight Molecular testing for genetic aberrations (FLT3, NPM1)	Daily physical examination CBC with differential, platelets Serum chemistries (including uric acid, K^+, Ca^{+2}, PO_4, S_{cr} during tumor lysis syndrome risk period[a]) Coagulation (PT, PTT, D-dimers, fibrinogen [if APL]) Bone marrow biopsy and aspirate 7–10 days after end of chemotherapy. Repeat bone marrow biopsy and aspirate upon hematologic recovery to document complete response (with cytogenetics if initially abnormal) Temperature curve (initiate antibiotics when febrile) Lumbar puncture (with intrathecal chemotherapy) if initial lumbar puncture was positive for leukemia	Routine physical examination at clinic visit CBC with differential, platelets Bone marrow biopsy and aspirate at set intervals to evaluate ongoing remission and if peripheral blood counts are abnormal or if they fail to recover within 5 weeks of treatment PML/RARα monitoring [if APL]

ALT, alanine aminotransferase; APL, acute promyelocytic leukemia; AST, aspartate aminotransferase; CBC, complete blood cell count; ECG, electrocardiogram; FLT3, FMS-related tyrosine kinase 3; MUGA, multiple-gated acquisition (blood pool scan); NMP1, nucleophosmin; PML/RARα, promyelocytic-leukemia retinoic acid receptor-α; PT, prothrombin time; PTT, partial thromboplastin time; S_{cr}, serum creatinine.

[a]Risk for tumor lysis syndrome during induction therapy only.

Pharmacists are often in the best position to recognize the potential for medication errors and drug interactions and to help avoid them. Similarly, pharmacists are often able to identify the possibility that patient problems are secondary to drug treatments.

Numerous late sequelae from leukemia therapy have been recognized and should be included in the monitoring plan after therapy is completed. Chapter 117 discusses the long-term consequences of HSCT.

ABBREVIATIONS

ALL	acute lymphoblastic leukemia
AML	acute myeloid leukemia
APL	acute promyelocytic leukemia
ATRA	all-*trans* retinoic acid
AYA	adolescents and young adults
BMI	body mass index
CALGB	Cancer and Leukemia Group B
CEBPA	CCAAT/enhancer binding-protein α
CNS	central nervous system
COG	Children's Oncology Group
CR	complete remission
CR1	first complete remission
CR2	second complete remission
CR3	third complete remission
CRi	complete remission with incomplete hematological recovery
CRc	cytogenetic complete remission
CRm	molecular complete remission
CSF	cerebrospinal fluid
ECOG	Eastern Cooperative Oncology Group
EFS	event-free survival
FDA	Food and Drug Administration
GTP	guanosine triphosphate
GVHD	graft-versus-host disease
GVL	graft-versus-leukemia
HLA	human leukocyte antigen
HSCT	hematopoietic stem cell transplantation
hyperCVAD	high-dose methotrexate and cytarabine alternating with fractionated cyclophosphamide plus vincristine, doxorubicin, and dexamethasone
$iAMLP_{21}$	intrachromosomal amplification of chromosome 21
MDS	myelodysplastic syndrome
MLL	mixed lineage leukemia
MRD	minimal residual disease
NCCN	National Comprehensive Cancer Network
NCI	National Cancer Institute
NMT	nonmyeloablative transplant
NPM1	nucleophosmin
OS	overall survival
PETHEMA	Programa para el Estudio de la Terapeutica en Hemopatıa Maligna
Ph^+	Philadelphia chromosome positive
PML	Promyelocytic leukemia
RARα	retinoic acid receptor-α
TPMT	thiopurine *S*-methyltransferase
WBC	white blood cell
WHO	World Health Organization

REFERENCES

1. Siegel R, Naishadham D, Jemal A. Cancer statistics, 2013. CA Cancer J Clin 2013;63:11–30.
2. Howlader N, Noone A, Krapcho M, Neyman N, Aminou R. SEER Cancer Statistics Review, 1975–2009. Bethesda, MD: National Cancer Institute. September 29, 2012, *http://seer.cancer.gov/csr/1975_2009_pops09/*.
3. Estey E, Dohner H. Acute myeloid leukemia. Lancet 2006;368:1894–1907.
4. Linabery AM, Ross JA. Trends in childhood cancer incidence in the U.S. (1992–2004). Cancer 2008;112:416–432.
5. Creutzig U, van den Heuvel-Eibrink MM, Gibson B, Dworzak MN. Diagnosis and management of acute myeloid leukemia in children and adolescents: Recommendations from an international expert panel. Blood 2012;120:3187–3205.
6. Pui C-H, Robison LL, Look AT. Acute lymphoblastic leukemia. Lancet 2008;371:1030–1043.
7. Faderl S, Jeha S, Kantarjian H. The biology and therapy of adult acute lymphoblastic leukemia. Cancer 2003;98:1337–1354.
8. Belson M, Kingsley B, Holmes A. Risk factors for acute leukemia in children: A review. Environ Health Perspect 2007;115:138–145.
9. Caughey RW, Michels KB. Birth weight and childhood leukemia: A meta-analysis and review of the current evidence. Int J Cancer 2009;124:2658–2670.
10. Mrozek K, Marcucci G, Paschka P, Whitman S, Bloomfield C. Clinical relevance of mutations and gene-expression changes in adult acute myeloid leukemia with normal cytogenetics: Are we ready for a prognostically prioritized molecular classification. Blood 2007;109:431–448.
11. Vardiman JW, Thiele J, Arber DA, Brunning RD. The 2008 revision of the World Health Organization (WHO) classification of myeloid neoplasms and acute leukemia: Rationale and important changes. Blood 2009;114:937–951.
12. Pui C-H, Deqing P, Campana D, Bowman WP. Improved prognosis for older adolescents with acute lymphoblastic leukemia. J Clin Oncol 2011;29:386–391.
13. Smith M, Arthur D, Camitta B, et al. Uniform approach to risk classification and treatment assignment for children with acute lymphoblastic leukemia. J Clin Oncol 1996;14:18–24.
14. Seibel NL. Treatment of acute lymphoblastic leukemia in children and adolescents: Peaks and pitfalls. Hematology Am Soc Hematol Educ Program 2008;2008:374–80.
15. Arico M, Schrappe M, Hunger SP, et al. Clinical outcome of children with newly diagnosed Philadelphia chromosome positive acute lymphoblastic leukemia treated between 1995 and 2005. J Clin Oncol 2010;28:4755–4761.
16. Moorman AV, Ensor H, Richards S. Prognostic effect of chromosomal abnormalities in childhood B-cell precursor acute lymphoblastic leukaemia: Results from the UK Medical Research Council ALL97/99 randomised trial. Lancet Oncol 2010;11:429–438.
17. Campana D. Minimal residual disease in acute lymphoblastic leukemia. Semin Hematol 2009;46:100–106.
18. Schultz KR, Pullen DJ, Sather HN, et al. Risk- and response-based classification of childhood B-precursor acute lymphoblastic leukemia: A combined analysis of prognostic markers from the Pediatric Oncology Group (POG) and Children's Cancer Group (CCG). Blood 2007;109:926–935.
19. Borowitz MJ, Devidas M, Hunger SP, et al. Clinical significance of minimal residual disease in childhood acute lymphoblastic leukemia and its relationship to other prognostic factors: A Children's Cancer Group study. Blood 2008;111:5477–5485.
20. Seibel NL, Steinherz PG, Sather HN, Nachman JB, Cynthia D. Early postinduction intensification therapy improves survival for children and adolescents with high-risk acute lymphoblastic leukemia: A report from the Children's Oncology Group. Blood 2008;111:2548–2555.

21. Hunger SP, Loh ML, Whitlock JA, et al. Children's Oncology Group's 2013 blueprint for research: acute lymphoblastic leukemia. Pediat Blood Cancer 2013; 60:957–963.
22. Pui C-H, Evans WE. Treatment of acute lymphoblastic leukemia. N Engl J Med 2006;354:166–178.
23. Schrappe M, Hunger SP, Pui C-H, et al. Outcomes after induction failure in childhood acute lymphoblastic leukemia. N Engl J Med 2012;366:1371–1381.
24. Inaba H, Pui C-H. Glucocorticoid use in acute lymphoblastic leukemia. Lancet Oncol 2010;11:1096–1106.
25. Mitchell CD, Richards S, Kinsey S, et al. Benefit of dexamethasone compared with prednisolone for childhood lymphoblastic Leukaemia: Results of the UK Medical Research Council ALL97 randomised trial. Br J Haematol 2005;129:734–745.
26. Ravindranath Y. Recent advances in pediatric acute lymphoblastic and myeloid leukemia. Curr Opin Oncol 2003;15:23–35.
27. Lowas SR, Marks D, Malempati S. Prevalence of transient hyperglycemia during induction chemotherapy for pediatric acute lymphoblastic leukemia. Pediatr Blood Cancer 2009;52:814–818.
28. Pieters R, Hunger SP, Boos J, et al. L-asparaginase treatment in acute lymphoblastic leukemia. Cancer 2011;117:238–249.
29. Matloub Y, Lindemulder S, Gaynon PS, et al. Intrathecal triple therapy decreases central nervous system relapse but fails to improve event-free survival when compared with intrathecal methotrexate: Results of the Children's Cancer Group (CCG) 1952 study for standard-risk acute lymphoblastic leukemia, reported by the Children's Oncology Group. Blood 2006;108:1165–1173.
30. Bomgaars L, Geyer JR, Franklin JL, et al. Phase I trial of intrathecal liposomal cytarabine in children with neoplastic meningitis. J Clin Oncol 2004;22:3916–3921.
31. Dunsmore K, Devidas M, Linda S, et al. Pilot study of nelarabine in combination with intensive chemotherapy in high-risk T-cell acute lymphoblastic leukemia: A report from the Children's Oncology Group. J Clin Oncol 2012;30:2753–2759.
32. Bhatia S, Landier W, Shangguan M, et al. Nonadherence to oral mercaptopurine and risk of relapse in Hispanic and non-Hispanic white children with acute lymphoblastic leukemia: A report from the Children's Oncology Group. J Clin Oncol 2012;30:2094–2101.
33. Schultz KR, Bowman WP, Aledo A, et al. Improved early event-free survival with imatinib in Philadelphia chromosome-positive acute lymphoblastic leukemia: A Children's Oncology Group study. J Clin Oncol 2009;27:5175–5181.
34. Silverman LB. Acute lymphoblastic leukemia in infancy. Pediatr Blood Cancer 2007;49:1070–1073.
35. Mann G, Attarbaschi A, Schrappe M, et al. Improved outcome with hematopoietic stem cell transplantation in a poor prognostic subgroup of infants with mixed-lineage-leukemia (MLL)-rearranged acute lymphoblastic leukemia: Results from the Interfant-99 Study. Blood 2010;116:2644–2650.
36. Stock W, La M, Sanford B, Bloomfield CD, et al. What determines the outcomes for adolescents and young adults with acute lymphoblastic leukemia treated on cooperative group protocols? A comparison of Children's Cancer Group and Cancer and Leukemia Group B studies. Blood 2008;112:1646–1654.
37. National Comprehensive Cancer Network Clinical Practice Guidelines in Oncology. Acute Lymphoblastic Leukemia. Version 2.2012. December 24, 2012, *http://www.nccn.org/professionals/physician_gls/pdf/all.pdf.*
38. Bassan R, Hoelzer D. Modern therapy of acute lymphoblastic leukemia. J Clin Oncol 2011;29:532–543.
39. Larson RA, Dodge RK, Burns CP. A five-drug remission induction regimen with intensive consolidation for adults with acute lymphoblastic leukemia: Cancer and leukemia group B study 8811. Blood 1995;85:2025–2037.
40. Rowe JM, Buck G, Burnett AK. Induction therapy for adults with acute lymphoblastic leukemia: Results of more than 1500 patients from the international ALL trial: MRC UKALL XII/ECOG E2993. Blood 2005;106: 3760–3767.
41. Linker C, Damon L, Ries C, Navarro W. Intensified and shortened cyclical chemotherapy for adult acute lymphoblastic leukemia. J Clin Oncol 2002;20:2464–2471.
42. Kantarjian H, O'Brien S, Smith T. Results of treatment with hyper-CVAD, a dose-intensive regimen, in adult acute lymphocytic leukemia. J Clin Oncol 2000;18:547–561.
43. Burmeister T, Schwartz S, Bartrum CR. Patients' age and BCL-ABL frequency in adult-B precursor ALL: A retrospective analysis from the GMALL study group. Blood 2008;112:918–919.
44. de Labarthe A, Rousselot P, Huguet-Rigal F. Imatinib combined with induction or consolidation chemotherapy in patients with de novo Philadelphia chromosome-positive acute lymphoblastic leukemia: Results of the GRAAPH-2003 study. Blood 2007;109:1408–1413.
45. Bassan R, Rossi G, Pogliani EM. Chemotherapy-phased imatinib pulses improve long-term outcome of adult patients with Philadelphia chromosome-positive acute lymphoblastic leukemia: Northern Italy Leukemia Group protocol 09/00. J Clin Oncol 2010;28:3644–3652.
46. Ottmann O, Wassmann B, Pfeifer H. Imatinib compared with chemotherapy as frontline treatment of elderly patients with Philadelphia chromosome-positive acute lymphoblastic leukemia (Ph+ ALL). Cancer 2007;109:2068–2076.
47. Vignetti M, Fazi P, Cimino G. Imatinib plus steroids induces complete remissions and prolonged survival in elderly Philadelphia chromosome-positive patients with acute lymphoblastic leukemia without additional chemotherapy: Results of the Gruppo Italiano Malattie Ematologiche dell'Adulto (GIMEMA) LAL0201-B protocol. Blood 2007;109:3676–3678.
48. Ravandi F, O'Brien S, Thomas D. First report of phase 2 study of dasatinib with hyper-CVAD for the frontline treatment of patients with Philadelphia chromosome-positive (Ph+) acute lymphoblastic leukemia. Blood 2010;116:2070–2077.
49. Talpaz M, Shah N, Kantarjian H. Dasatinib in imatinib-resistant Philadelphia chromosome-positive leukemias. N Engl J Med 2006;354:2531–2541.
50. Kantarjian H, Giles F, L W. Nilotinib in imatinib-resistant CML and Philadelphia chromosome-positive ALL. N Engl J Med 2006;354:2542–2551.
51. Khoury HJ, Cortes J, Kantarjian HM. Bosutinib is active in chronic phase chronic myeloid leukemia after imatinib and dasatinib and/or nilotinib therapy failure. Blood 2012;119:3403–3412.
52. Cortes JE, Kantarjian HM, Shah NL. Ponatinib in refractory Philadelphia chromosome-positive leukemias. N Engl J Med 2012;367:2075–2088.
53. Thomas D, O'Brien S, Jorgenson J. Prognostic significance of CD20 expression in adults with de novo precursor B-lineage acute lymphoblastic leukemia. Blood 2009;113:6330–6337.

54. Thomas D, O'Brien S, Faderl S. Chemoimmunotherapy with a modified hyper-CVAD and rituximab regimen improves outcome in de novo Philadelphia chromosome-negative precursor B-cell lineage acute lymphoblastic leukemia. J Clin Oncol 2010;28:3880–3889.
55. Oliansky DM, Larson RA, Weisdorf DJ. The role of cytotoxic therapy with hematopoietic stem cell transplantation in the treatment of adult acute lymphoblastic leukemia: Update of the 2006 evidence-based review. Biol Blood Marrow Transplant 2012;18:16–17.
56. Ko RH, Ji L, Barnette P, Bostrom B, et al. Outcome of patients treated for relapsed or refractory acute lymphoblastic leukemia: A Therapeutic Advances in Childhood Leukemia Consortium study J Clin Oncol 2010;28:648–654.
57. Harned TM, Gaynon PS. Relapsed acute lymphoblastic leukemia: Current status and future opportunities. Curr Opin Oncol 2008;10:453–458.
58. Gaynon PS. Childhood acute lymphoblastic leukaemia and relapse. Br J Haematol 2005;131:579–587.
59. National Marrow Donor Program. 2013, *http://www/nmdp.org/*.
60. Mody R, Li S, Dover DC, et al. Twenty-five-year follow-up among survivors of childhood acute lymphoblastic leukemia: A report from the Childhood Cancer Survivor Study. Blood 2008;111:5515–5523.
61. Deschler B, M L. Acute myeloid leukemia: Epidemiology and etiology. Cancer 2006;107:2099–2107.
62. Kolitz JE. Acute leukemias in adults. Dis Mon 2008;54:226–241.
63. Byrd JC, Mrozek K, Dodge RK. Pretreatment cytogenetic abnormalities are predictive of induction success, cumulative incidence of relapse, and overall survival in adult patients with de novo acute myeloid leukemia: Results from Cancer and Leukemia Group B(CALGB 8461). Blood 2002;100:4325–4336.
64. Estey EH. Treatment of acute myeloid leukemia. Haematologica 2009;94:10–16.
65. Grimwade D, Hills R. Independent prognostic factors for AML outcome. Hematology Am Soc Hematol Educ Program 2009;2009:385–395.
66. National Comprehensive Cancer Network Clinical Practice Guidelines in Oncology. Acute Myeloid Leukemia. Version 2.2012. December 24, 2012, *http://www.nccn.org/professionals/physician_gls/pdf/aml.pdf*.
67. Paschka P, Marcucci G, Ruppert AS. Adverse prognostic significance of KIT mutations in adult acute myeloid leukemia with inv(16) and t(8;21): A Cancer and Leukemia Group B study. J Clin Oncol 2006;24:3904–3911.
68. Cheson B, Bennett J, Kopecky K. Revised recommendations of the International Working Group for diagnosis, standardization or response criteria, treatment outcomes, and reporting standards for therapeutic trials in acute myeloid leukemia. J Clin Oncol 2003;21:4642–4649.
69. Buchner T, Berdel W, Wormann B. Treatment of older patients with acute myeloid leukemia. Crit Rev Oncol Hematol 2005;56:247–259.
70. Rubnitz JE, Gibson B, Smith FO. Acute myeloid leukemia. Pediatr Clin North Am 2008;55:21–51.
71. Kolitz JE. Current therapeutic strategies for acute myeloid leukemia. Br J Haematol 2006;134:555–572.
72. Milligan DW, Grimwade D, Cullis J. Guidelines on the management of acute myeloid leukemia in adults. Br J Haematol 2006;135:450–474.
73. Fernandez HF, Sun Z, Yao X, et al. Anthracycline dose intensification in acute myeloid leukemia. N Engl J Med 2009;361:1249–1259.
74. Cahn JY, Labopin M, Sierra J. No impact of high-dose cytarabine on the outcome of patients transplanted for acute myeloblastic leukaemia in first remission. Acute Leukemia Working Party of the European group for Blood and Marrow Transplant (EBMT). Br J Haematol 2000;110:308–314.
75. Fenaux P, Mufti GJ, Hellstrom-Lindberg E. Azacitidine prolongs overall survival compared with conventional care regimens in elderly patients with low bone marrow blast count acute myeloid leukemia. J Clin Oncol 2010;28:562–569.
76. Al-Ali HK, Jaekel N, Junghanss C. Azacitidine in patients with acute myeloid leukemia medically unfit for or resistant to chemotherapy: a multicenter phase I/II study. Leuk Lymphoma 2012;53:110–117.
77. Burnett A, Wetzler M, Lowenberg B. Therapeutic advances in acute myeloid leukemia. J Clin Oncol 2011;29:487–494.
78. Dohner H, Estey E, Amadori S. Diagnosis and management of acute myeloid leukemia in adults: Recommendations from an international expert panel, on behalf of the European Leukemia Net. Blood 2010;115:453–474.
79. Mayer RJ, Davis RB, Schiffer CA. Intensive post-remission chemotherapy in adults with acute myeloid leukemia. Cancer and Leukemia Group B. N Engl J Med 1994;331:896–903.
80. Byrd JC, Ruppert AS, Mrozek K. Repetitive cycles of high-dose cytarabine benefit patients with acute myeloid leukemia and inv(16)(p13q22) or t(16;16)(p13;q22): Results from CALGB 8461. J Clin Oncol 2004;22:1087–1094.
81. Aoudjhane M, Labopin M, Gorin NC. Comparative outcome of reduced intensity and myeloablative conditioning regimen in HLA identical sibling allogeneic haematopoietic stem cell transplantation for patients older than 50 years of age with acute myeloblastic leukaemia: A retrospective survey from the Acute Leukemia Working Party (ALWP) of the European Group for Blood and Marrow Transplantation (EBMT). Leukemia 2005;18:2304–2312.
82. Gyurkocza B, Storb R, Stover BE. Nonmyeloablative allogeneic hematopoietic cell transplantation in patients with acute myeloid leukemia. J Clin Oncol 2010;28:859–867.
83. Estey E, de Lima M, Tibes R. Prospective feasibility analysis of reduced-intensity conditioning (RIC) regimens for hematopoietic stem cell transplantation (HSCT) in elderly patients with acute myeloid leukemia (AML) and high-risk myelodysplastic syndrome (MDS). Blood 2007;109:1395–1400.
84. Breems DA, Lowenberg B. Autologous stem cell transplantation in the treatment of adults with acute myeloid leukemia. Br J Haematol 2005;2005:825–833.
85. Group SCTC. Allogeneic peripheral blood stem-cell compared with bone marrow transplantation in the management of hematologic malignancies: an individual patient data meta-analysis of nine randomized trials. J Clin Oncol 2005;23:5074–5087.
86. Alyea EP, Kim HT, Ho V. Comparative outcome of nonmyeloablative and myeloablative allogeneic hematopoietic cell transplantation for patients older than 50 years of age. Blood 2005;105:1810–1814.
87. Pui C-H, Carroll WL, Meshinchi S, Arceci RJ. Biology, risk stratification, and therapy of pediatric acute leukemias: an update. J Clin Oncol 2011;29:551–565.
88. Oliansky DM, Rizzo JD, Aplan PD. The role of cytotoxic therapy with hematopoietic stem cell transplantation in the therapy of acute myeloid leukemia in children: An evidence-based review. Biol Blood Marrow Transplant 2007;13:1–25.

89. Michallet M, Thomas X, Vernant J-P. Long-term outcome after allogeneic hematopoietic stem cell transplantation for advanced stage acute myeloblastic leukemia: A retrospective study of 379 patients reported to the Societe Francaise de Greffe de Moelle (SFGM). Bone Marrow Transplant 2000;26:1157–1163.
90. Faderl S, Ravandi F, Huang X. A randomized study of clofarabine versus clofarabine plus low-dose cytarabine as front-line therapy for patients aged 60 years and older with acute myeloid leukemia and high-risk myelodysplastic syndrome. Blood 2008;112:1638–1645.
91. Brune M, Castaigne S, Catalano J. Improved leukemia-free survival after postconsolidation immunotherapy with histamine dihydrochloride and interleukin-2 in acute myeloid leukemia: Results of a randomized phase 3 trial. Blood 2006;108:88–96.
92. Leung W, Hudson MM, Strickland DK. Late effects of treatment in survivors of childhood acute myeloid leukemia. J Clin Oncol 2000;18:3273–3279.
93. Ades L, Sanz MA, Chevret S. Treatment of newly diagnosed acute promyelocytic leukemia (APL): A comparison of French-Belgian-Swiss and PETHEMA results Blood 2008;111:1078–1084.
94. DelaSerna J, Montesinos J, Vellenga E. Causes and prognostic factors of remission induction failure in patients with acute promyelocytic leukemia treated with all-trans retinoic acid and idarubicin. Blood 2008;111:3395–3402.
95. Estey E, Garcia-Manero G, Ferrajoli A. Use of all-trans retinoic acid plus arsenic trioxide as an alternative to chemotherapy in untreated acute promyelocytic leukemia. Blood 2006;107:3469–3473.
96. Soignet S, Frankel S, Douer D. United States multicenter study of arsenic trioxide in relapsed acute promyelocytic leukemia. J Clin Oncol 2001;19:3852–3860.
97. Soignet S, Maslak P, Wang Z. Complete remission after treatment of acute promyelocytic leukemia with arsenic trioxide. N Engl J Med 1998;339:1341–1348.
98. Nabhan C, Mehta J, Tallman MS. The role of bone marrow transplantation in acute promyelocytic leukemia. Bone Marrow Transplant 2001;28:219–226.
99. Smith TJ, Khatcheressian J, Lyman GH, et al. 2006 Update of recommendations for the use of white blood cell growth factors: An evidence-based clinical practice guideline. J Clin Oncol 2006;24:3187–3205.
100. Gurion R, Belnik-Plitman Y, Gafter-Gvili A. Colony-stimulating factors for prevention and treatment of infectious complications in patients with acute myelogenous leukemia. Cochrane Database Syst Rev 2012 Jun 13;6:CD008238.
101. Sierra J, Szer J, Kassis J, et al. A single dose of pegfilgrastim compared with daily filgrastim for supporting neutrophil recovery in patients treated for low-to-intermediate risk acute myeloid leukemia: results from a randomized, double-blind, phase 2 trial. BMC Cancer 2008;8:195.
102. Freifeld AG, Bow EJ, Sepkowitz KA. Clinical practice guideline for the use of antimicrobial agents in neutropenic patients with cancer: 2010 Update by the Infectious Diseases Society of America. Clin Infect Dis 2011;52:427–431.
103. NCCN. National Comprehensive Cancer Network Clinical Practice Guidelines in Oncology. Prevention and treatment of cancer-related infections. Version 1.2012. December 24, 2012, *http://www.nccn.org/professional/physician_gls/pdf/infections.pdf*.
104. Coiffier B, Altman A, Pui C-H, Younes A, Cairo MS. Guidelines for the management of pediatric and adult tumor lysis syndrome: An evidence-based review. J Clin Oncol 2008;26:2767–2778.
105. Trifilio S, Gordon L, Singhal S. Reduced-dose rasburicase (recombinant xanthine oxidase) in adult cancer patients with hyperuricemia. Bone Marrow Transplant 2006;37:997–1001.
106. Cheok MH, Pottier N, Kager L, Evans WE. Pharmacogenetics in acute lymphoblastic leukemia in children. Semin Hematol 2009;46:39–51.

112

Chronic Leukemias

Christopher A. Fausel and Patrick J. Kiel

KEY CONCEPTS

1. Chronic myelogenous leukemia (CML) is defined by the presence of the Philadelphia chromosome (Ph), a translocation between chromosomes 9 and 22. The resulting abnormal fusion protein, p210 *BCR-ABL*, phosphorylates tyrosine kinase residues and is constitutively active, resulting in uncontrolled hematopoietic cell proliferation.
2. The disease course of CML is characterized by a progressive increase in white blood cells over a period of years that ultimately transforms to an acute leukemia.
3. The four commercially available tyrosine kinase inhibitors, imatinib, dasatinib, nilotinib, and bosutinib, have demonstrated efficacy in treatment of newly diagnosed CML patients and in patients with either accelerated phase or blast crisis.
4. CML monitoring requires assessment of milestone throughout therapy such as hematologic, cytogenetic, and molecular responses, the ideal of which is a molecular response.
5. Allogeneic hematopoietic stem cell transplant (HSCT) is the only known curative treatment option for CML and is reserved for patients with a suitable donor and progression after treatment with tyrosine kinase-based therapy.
6. The management of CLL is highly individualized and includes observation in patients with early-stage disease and treatment with chemotherapy, biologic therapy, or both in patients with more advanced disease.
7. Alemtuzumab, ofatumumab, and rituximab monoclonal antibody therapy are all indicated for the treatment of CLL. Ofatumumab is reserved for patients that have progressed following fludarabine-based and alemtuzumab-based regimens.
8. Regimens such as fludarabine, cyclophosphamide, and rituximab are considered as first-line therapy for patients with CLL who are younger or have more aggressive disease, such as the presence of chromosome 17 deletion.
9. Allogeneic HSCT in patients with CLL appears to achieve long-term disease-free survival in some patients, but the older patient population diagnosed with the disease and donor availability preclude widespread use.

The chronic leukemias include chronic myeloid leukemia (CML), chronic lymphocytic leukemia (CLL), hairy cell leukemia, and prolymphocytic leukemia. The typical clinical presentation of the chronic leukemias is an indolent course in contrast to patients with acute leukemia who will die of their disease within weeks to months if not treated. This chapter focuses on the two most common types of chronic leukemia, CML and CLL.

CHRONIC MYELOGENOUS LEUKEMIA

Chronic myeloid leukemia is a myeloproliferative disease that results from malignant transformation of a subpopulation of pluripotent hematopoietic stem cells. Bone marrow hyperplasia and accumulation of differentiated myeloid cells in the peripheral blood are the initial presenting features of the disease. The terminal stage of CML is characterized by rapid accumulation of blast cells in the bone marrow and suppression of normal hematopoiesis that ultimately leads to death. CML was the first malignant disease identified with a consistent cytogenetic abnormality, namely the Philadelphia chromosome (Ph) that code for the *BCR-ABL* oncogene. This dominant cytogenetic abnormality has allowed CML to become the template for development of molecular targeted drug therapies.

Epidemiology and Etiology

It is estimated that 5,920 new cases of CML will be diagnosed in the United States in 2013, with 610 deaths.[1] The median age of diagnosis is 64 and are no currently known associations between the development of CML and hereditary, familial, geographic, ethnic, or economic status. An increased risk of CML has been noted with ionizing radiation exposure and in atomic bomb survivors from Hiroshima and Nagasaki.[2,3]

Pathophysiology

Chronic myeloid leukemia was first described in 1845, but extensive research into the genetic and molecular characteristics of the disease began with the discovery of the Ph in 1960 by Nowell and Hungerford.[4] Research in the 1980s identified the molecular changes that occur as a result of the Ph when an oncogenic protein was identified and implicated in the pathophysiology of CML.[4,5]

Ph is the first karyotypic abnormality specifically implicated in the pathogenesis of cancer, and its discovery has resulted in extensive research into the molecular biology of CML.[6] This chromosomal abnormality is characteristic of CML and is present in about 95% of patients with the disease.[7,8]

(1) Ph, identified as a shortened long arm of chromosome 22, is found in granulocyte and erythrocyte progenitors, macrophages, megakaryocytes, and lymphocytes. The Ph is the consequence of breaks in chromosomes 9 and 22 resulting in a transposition that relocates the 3′ end of *ABL* (Abelson proto-oncogene) from its normal site on chromosome 9 at band 34 to the 5′ end of *BCR* (breakpoint cluster region) on chromosome 22 at band 11 [symbolized as t(9;22)(q34;q11)].[8,9] This results in the formation of the hybrid *BCR-ABL* fusion gene (Fig. 112-1). Through this chromosomal translocation, the *ABL* protooncogene is able to escape the normal genetic controls

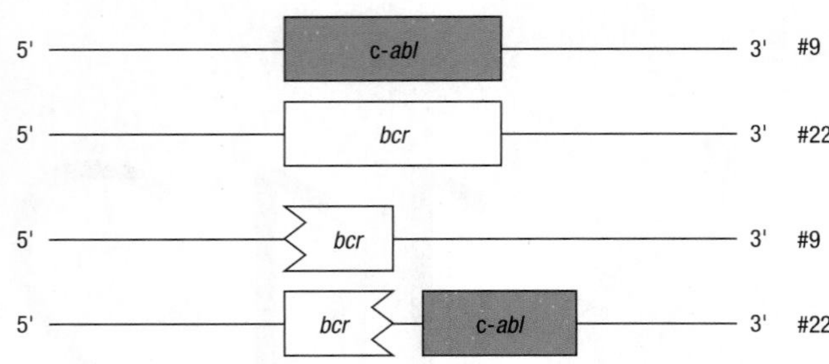

FIGURE 112-1 Diagram of the chromosomal translocation that results in the Philadelphia chromosome. *(Reprinted with permission from Fishleder AJ. Oncogenes and cancer: Clinical applications. Cleve Clin J Med 1990;57:721–726. Copyright © 1990 Cleveland Clinic. All rights reserved.)*

on its senescence and is activated into a functional oncogene, directing the transcription of an 8.5-kilobase messenger ribonucleic acid (mRNA) molecule. The mRNA is translated into a 210-kDa protein—p210 *BCR-ABL*—that is constitutively (constantly) activated compared to the 145-kDa protein translated by the normal *ABL* gene.[7,8] Although p210 *BCR-ABL* is the most common tyrosine kinase found in CML, variations in the breakpoints in the *ABL* gene encode different size proteins. For example, a smaller protein, p190 *BCR-ABL*, is involved in two-thirds of adults with Ph-positive acute lymphoblastic leukemia, but is rarely found in patients with CML.[8]

Because CML begins with the malignant transformation of a single cell, it is considered a clonal disease. The progeny from this transformed primitive hematopoietic stem cell results in a proliferative advantage over normal hematopoietic cells that displaces normal hematopoiesis. The Ph is found in both myeloid and lymphoid cells, which suggests that the transformed cell of CML is a pluripotent stem cell.[9] This alteration gives the transformed progenitor cell an inheritable growth advantage, leading to the proliferation of a neoplastic, monoclonal population of cells.[8] Disrupted maturation leads to additional divisions by CML progenitor cells before reaching a nonproliferative stage; the resulting number of circulating granulocytes may be many times higher than normal. In the advanced stages of CML, cytopenias may occur in association with fibrotic changes in the bone marrow.[8]

The *BCR-ABL* fusion gene encodes for a constitutively active tyrosine kinase that is involved in both the increased proliferation of the CML clone and the reduction in Fas-mediated apoptosis. Characterization of the adenosine triphosphate binding site on the *BCR-ABL* tyrosine kinase has provided a target for inhibition of tyrosine kinase activity. The first FDA-approved tyrosine kinase inhibitor (TKI), imatinib mesylate (Gleevec®), was indicated for patients in chronic phase who had failed interferon alpha (IFN-α) or for those with advanced disease. Imatinib received additional FDA approval in 2002 for first-line treatment in newly diagnosed CML. Second-generation TKIs with a higher binding affinity and selectivity for *ABL* kinase are approved as both frontline agents and salvage for patients with resistance or intolerance to imatinib.

Clinical Presentation

2 The three clinical phases of CML are: chronic phase (CP), accelerated phase (AP), and blast crisis (BC) (Table 112-1). Nearly 90% of patients present with CP at the time of diagnosis. Often the diagnosis of CML is found incidentally during routine examination or if a complete blood count is obtained for unrelated reasons because patients are often asymptomatic upon presentation. Signs and symptoms include fatigue, sweating, bone pain, weight loss, abdominal discomfort, and early satiety secondary to splenomegaly. Leukocytosis is the hallmark of CP, which can be as high as 1,000,000 cells/mm^3 (1,000 × 10^9/L) placing patients at risk for complications of leukostasis. Symptoms secondary to leukostasis include acute abdominal pain resulting from splenic infarctions, priapism, retinal hemorrhage, cerebrovascular accidents, confusion, hyperuricemia, and gouty arthritis.[8] Patients can survive several years in CP without treatment.

Initial laboratory workup includes complete blood count with differential, complete metabolic panel, and serum uric acid. A bone marrow aspiration and biopsy is required to confirm the diagnosis of CML. The differential diagnosis of CML includes infection, myeloproliferative disorders (i.e., polycythemia vera, essential thrombocythemia, myelofibrosis), and chronic myelomonocytic leukemia. Bone marrow is markedly hypercellular (75% to 90%)

CLINICAL PRESENTATION Chronic Myelogenous Leukemia[1]

General

- 90% of patients are diagnosed in chronic phase
- 50% are asymptomatic in chronic phase and often diagnosed following abnormal complete blood count

Signs and Symptoms

- Fatigue
- Left upper quadrant pain
- Abdominal pain or distension
- Weight loss
- Night sweats

Physical Examination

- Splenomegaly
- Hepatomegaly

Laboratory Tests

- Peripheral blood
  - Leukocytosis
  - Thrombocytosis
  - Basophilia
  - Low or undetectable leukocyte alkaline phosphatase
  - Elevated uric acid and lactate dehydrogenase
- Molecular testing
  - Presence of *BCR-ABL* by reverse-transcription polymerase chain reaction
- Bone marrow
  - Hypercellular
  - Fully mature myeloid cells
  - Increased megakaryocytes
  - <10% blasts in chronic phase
- Cytogenetics
  - Presence of the Philadelphia chromosome
  - Additional abnormalities

TABLE 112-1 Criteria for Different Phases of Chronic Myelogenous Leukemia

Chronic Phase	Accelerated Phase	Blast Crisis
• <10% blasts in peripheral blood or bone marrow	• 10–29% blasts in peripheral blood or bone marrow • Platelets <100,000 cells/mm³ or >1,000,000 cells/mm³ Additional findings • Cytogenetic evolution • Progressive splenomegaly	• >30% blasts in peripheral blood or bone marrow • Large clusters of blasts on bone marrow biopsy • Presence of extramedullary infiltrates Additional findings • Fever • Malaise • Splenomegaly

Data from Cortes JE, Talpaz M, O'Brien S, et al. Staging of chronic myeloid leukemia in the imatinib era. Cancer 2006;106:1306–1315.

with increased granulocyte/erythroid ratio increased (10 to 30:1), erythropoiesis increased megakaryocytes normal. Karyotyping (cytogenetic analysis) is required for a diagnosis. The bone marrow aspiration is analyzed with fluorescence in situ hybridization (FISH) to determine the presence of the Ph chromosome. Quantitative reverse-transcription polymerase chain reaction (RT-PCR) is also performed to assess the baseline *BCR-ABL* transcript levels.

AP is characterized by progressive myeloid maturation arrest and loss of efficacy of drug therapy directed to attenuate the increase in white blood cells. Clinical findings of AP include anemia, increasing peripheral blood and bone marrow blasts and basophils, clonal cytogenetic evolution, extramedullary disease sites (bone, breast, CNS, mucosal tissue, lymph nodes, and skin), exacerbation of splenomegaly, and either thrombocytosis or thrombocytopenia. Nonspecific findings such as bone pain, fever, night sweats, and weight loss may occur. The most commonly observed cytogenetic changes with disease progression are an additional Ph chromosome, trisomy 8, and isochromosome 17q. Survival typically will not exceed several months. The World Health Organization (WHO) classification defines AP CML as one or more of the following changes: 10% to 19% of blasts in the peripheral blood or bone marrow, persistent thrombocytopenia less than 100,000 cells/mm³ (100×10^9/L) (not related to drug therapy), thrombocytosis greater than 1,000,000 cells/mm³ ($1{,}000 \times 10^9$/L) despite drug therapy, peripheral basophilia >20%, increasing spleen size and white blood cell count despite drug therapy, bone marrow evidence of progression of the leukemic clone or new cytogenetic abnormalities.[10]

BC is the terminal stage of disease and clinically resembles acute leukemia where the leukemic clone overwhelmingly dominates the bone marrow at the expense of normal hematopoiesis. The WHO classification defines BC CML as the presence of one or more of the following: >20% blasts in the peripheral blood or bone marrow, extramedullary disease, or large clusters of blasts in the bone marrow.[10] Patients can present occasionally with BC without an apparent AP. One-third of patients present with BC of lymphoid lineage, while two-thirds present with BC of myeloid lineage or undifferentiated like phenotype. The increased proliferative rate in BC CML is the consequence of a number of factors in addition to *BCR-ABL*, such as the activation of the oncogene signaling pathways and loss of tumor suppressors such as p53. Duration of BC is typically days to weeks before death.

Prognosis

Several models have been proposed for estimating prognosis in patients with CML, but the one proposed by Sokal et al. has become the most widely used.[13] The Sokal algorithm uses spleen size, percentage of circulating blasts, platelet count, and age as prognostic factors for patients in CP. However, this scoring system was developed prior to the advent of TKI therapy and may have limited predictive value in the era of imatinib. The median overall survival for patients diagnosed with CP, AP, and BC CML was reported to be 47 months, 12 to 24 months, and 3 to 6 months respectively in the era prior to the introduction of TKIs.[11,12]

TREATMENT
Chronic Myelogenous Leukemia

Desired Outcomes

Without effective treatment, CML disease progression leads inexorably to a fatal outcome within 5 years. The overriding treatment goals for CML include the eradication of the leukemic clone from the bone marrow and maintenance of CP with minimal toxicity from treatment. The only proven therapy to eradicate the malignant clone from the bone marrow is an allogeneic hematopoietic stem cell transplantation (HSCT). Both immunotherapy with IFN-α and TKI-based therapies have demonstrated the ability to extend CP beyond the expected period of several years, but data to confirm the curative ability of these agents are lacking. The introduction of TKI therapy has dramatically changed the clinical course of CML where patients can now expect to maintain disease control for many years.[13] The current standard of practice is to initiate TKI therapy for newly diagnosed CML patients. Long-term follow-up from phase III trials have documented a response in excess of 85% of patients that receive imatinib as primary treatment.[14,15] Table 112-2 shows the effect of various treatment modalities on survival in CP CML.

Clinical response in CML is measured by hematologic, cytogenetic, and molecular indices, all of which have standardized criteria.[16] *Hematologic response* is defined as the normalization of peripheral blood counts and is the earliest type of response observed in CML patients. *Cytogenetic responses* are based on the percentage of cells positive for Ph in a bone marrow biopsy. *Complete cytogenetic response* is defined as the elimination of Ph from all cells in the marrow sample whereas *major cytogenetic response* is defined as fewer than 35% Ph-positive cells. Patients who have a major or complete cytogenetic response have an improved survival compared to those who fail to achieve a cytogenetic response.[17]

TABLE 112-2 Effect of Therapy on Survival in Patients with Early Chronic-Phase Chronic Myelogenous Leukemia

Therapy	5-Year Survival (%)	Median Survival (Months)
Busulfan[25]	30–40	40–50
Hydroxyurea[25]	40–50	50–60
IFN-α[1]	50–70	60–80
IFN-α + ara-C[1]	60–80	NR
Allogeneic transplantation		
Matched sibling[1,55]	60–80	NR
Matched unrelated[1,7]	40–70	NR
Imatinib[21]	89	NR
Dasatinib	NR	NR
Nilotinib	NR	NR
Bosutinib	NR	NR
Omacetaxine	NR	NR
Ponatinib	NR	NR

IFN, interferon; NR, not yet reached.

Because most patients on imatinib achieve a complete cytogenetic response, more sensitive tests to monitor disease status have become more prominently used. *Molecular responses* are determined by RT-PCR, which are several logs more sensitive than methods used to measure cytogenetic responses. A *complete molecular response* is the absence of *BCR-ABL* transcripts by RT-PCR. RT-PCR assays should be interpreted carefully because they have varying sensitivities and may show a complete molecular remission even when low levels of *BCR-ABL* transcripts are present.[17] A major molecular response is a ≥3-log reduction in *BCR-ABL* transcripts by RT-PCR assay. Quantitative RT-PCR should be performed on every patient prior to initiating therapy and throughout therapy to monitor residual disease. Because bone marrow and peripheral blood *BCR-ABL* mRNA levels are correlated, peripheral blood can often be used for this analysis.[16,17]

Conventional Chemotherapy

Conventional cytotoxic chemotherapy is used in CP CML to reduce and temporarily control high peripheral white blood cell (WBC) counts. Historically, the two agents used for leukoreduction are busulfan (Myleran) and hydroxyurea (Hydrea). Busulfan is no longer used because randomized trials have shown that hydroxyurea treatment provides a modest survival advantage, and busulfan has a risk of potentially life-threatening pulmonary fibrosis.[18]

Hydroxyurea rapidly lowers high circulating WBCs in CP CML by inhibiting ribonucleotide reductase, which inhibits DNA synthesis, eliminating cells in the S phase of the cell cycle, and synchronizing cells in the G_1 or pre-DNA synthesis phase. Hydroxyurea is initiated at 40 to 50 mg/kg/day in divided doses until the WBC count falls to about 10,000 cells/mm^3 (10×10^9/L). Hydroxyurea may be discontinued once adequate control of the WBC count is achieved and a TKI has been initiated. Hydroxyurea is not specifically active against Ph and will not change the natural progression of the disease to BC.

Interferon Alfa

The interferons are a family of glycoproteins involved in many of the functional aspects of the hematopoietic system. Prior to the introduction of imatinib, IFN-α was the preferred agent in the treatment of CML. The role of IFN-α has since been relegated to patients who fail TKIs and are not candidates for allogeneic HSCT.

❸ Use of IFN-α in the treatment of CP CML was based on reports that 20% to 50% of patients achieve a major cytogenetic response, which led to prolonged survival.[6] In the 10% to 15% of patients achieving a complete cytogenetic response, the median survival was more than 10 years. Patients enrolled on the IFN-α arm in the International Randomized Interferon vs. STI571 (IRIS) trial had a complete cytogenetic response of 14%, as compared with 76% of patients treated with imatinib.[14] The 2013 National Comprehensive Cancer Network (NCCN) guidelines recommend IFN-α only for posttransplant relapse.[15]

IFN-α use is also limited by its toxicity profile because it is associated with both short-term constitutional toxicities and potentially dose-limiting long-term toxicities. In the IRIS trial, 26% of patients discontinued IFN-α as a result of intolerable side effects.[14] The most predictable early toxicity is a flu-like syndrome characterized by fever, chills, myalgia, headache, and anorexia. These dose-dependent effects may be a result of IFN-α–induced leukocytosis and release of inflammatory cytokines. Cardiovascular toxicities (tachycardia, hypotension) are seen in approximately 15% of patients in the first few weeks. Long-term adverse effects include weight loss, alopecia, neurologic effects (paresthesia, cognitive impairment, depression), and immune-mediated complications (hemolysis, thrombocytopenia, nephrotic syndrome, systemic lupus erythematosus, hypothyroidism) occur in approximately 5% to 20% of patients.

Despite falling out of clinical favor, IFN-α still remains a disease-modifying agent and ongoing clinical trials are investigating the use of imatinib and IFN-α in combination for the treatment of CML. Imatinib has been combined with pegylated interferon-α_{2a} in newly diagnosed CP CML yielding improved major molecular response rate at 12 months compared with imatinib 400 mg daily alone (57% vs. 38%), but the 12-month complete cytogenetic response rate was similar (66% vs. 58%).[19]

Imatinib Mesylate (Gleevec®)

A transformative discovery in cancer therapeutics was the characterization of the adenosine triphosphate binding site on the *BCR-ABL* tyrosine kinase. This specific receptor established a novel drug discovery platform for molecular targeted therapy in CML. Numerous TKIs were in development in the 1990s and STI571 (STI stands for *signal transduction inhibitor*), subsequently named imatinib (Gleevec®), emerged as the drug with the best oral bioavailability and high binding affinity for the *BCR-ABL* tyrosine kinase.[20,21] In 2001, imatinib mesylate received FDA approval for patients in CP CML who had failed IFN-α treatment and in patients with AP or BC CML based on phase II studies. In 2002, it received FDA approval for first-line treatment in newly diagnosed CML on the basis of the 2-year follow-up in the IRIS phase III trial.[22]

Imatinib inhibits several other tyrosine kinases including *BCR-ABL*, C-Kit, and platelet-derived growth factor receptor (PDGFR). Imatinib competitively binds to the adenosine triphosphate (ATP)-binding site on *BCR-ABL*, which inhibits the phosphorylation of proteins involved with CML clone proliferation.[23] Table 112-3 summarizes the clinical results of imatinib in CML patients in CP, AP, and BC CML. Table 112-4 summarizes the dosing, food–drug interactions, and drug–drug interactions of TKIs. Early phase I and phase II studies of imatinib, designed to determine maximum tolerated dose and safety, showed higher than expected response rates in all stages of CML.[24]

TABLE 112-3 Cytogenetic and Molecular Response Associated with Tyrosine Kinase Inhibitor Therapy in Chronic Myelogenous Leukemia

Drug (Disease Status)	Daily Dose	CCyR	MMR	Median Follow-up
Imatinib (CP)	400 mg	82%	57%	70 months
	800 mg	90%	NR	30 months
Imatinib (AP)	600 mg	43%	NR	12 months
	400 mg	11%	NR	
Imatinib (BC)	400–800 mg	7.40%	NR	—
Dasatinib (CP)	100 mg	86%	64%	24 months
Dasatinib (AP)	140 mg	32%	NR	15 months
Nilotinib (CP)	600 mg	87%	73%	36 months
Nilotinib (AP)	800 mg	16%	NR	24 months
Bosutinib (CP–3rd line)	500 mg	24%	15%	28.5 months
Bosutinib	500 mg	70%	41%	12 months
Omacetaxine (CP–2nd line, T315I mutation)	2.5 mg	16%	NR	19.1 months
Ponatinib (CP-resistant/ intolerant disease)	45 mg	37%	NR	10 months
Ponatinib (CP-T315I mutation	45 mg	66%	NR	10 months

AP, accelerated phase; BC, blast crisis; CCyR, complete cytogenetic response; CML, chronic myelogenous leukemia; CP, chronic phase; MCyR, major cytogenetic response; MMR, major molecular response; NR, no response.

TABLE 112-4 Dosing of Tyrosine Kinase Inhibitors in Chronic Myelogenous Leukemia

Drug	Brand Name	Dose Range	Food–Drug Interactions	Drug–Drug Interactions
Imatinib	Gleevec	400 mg/day (CP) 600 mg/day (AP/BC) 400 mg/day (moderate hepatic impairment) 300 mg/day severe hepatic impairment	Take with food and a large glass of water	CYP3A4 inducers may decrease C_{max} and AUC CYP3A4 inhibitors may increase C_{max} and AUC Imatinib inhibits CYP3A4 and 2D6. Package labeling recommendations against using warfarin concurrently.
Dasatinib	Sprycel	100 mg/day (CP) 140 mg/day (AP/BC)	With or without meals; do not crush tablets	CYP3A4 inhibitors may increase dasatinib drug levels. CYP3A4 inducers may decrease dasatinib drug levels. H_2 antagonists/PPIs decrease dasatinib drug levels.
Nilotinib	Tasigna	300 mg BID (CP) 400 mg BID (AP/BC)	Take with water; avoid food 2 hours prior to a dose or 1 hour after	Avoid drugs concurrently known to prolong QT interval. CYP inducers may decrease nilotinib serum concentrations. CYP inhibitors may increase nilotinib serum concentrations. Nilotinib is an inhibitor of CYP3A4, CYP2C8, CYP2C9, and CYP2D6. Nilotinib is an inducer of CYP2B6, CYP2C8, and CYP2C9.
Bosutinib	Bosulif	500 mg/day; may increase to 600 mg/day in patients who do not clinically respond by weeks 8–12	Take with food; PPIs may decrease absorption	Concurrent use with CYP3A or Pgp inhibitors increase bosutinib plasma concentrations. Concurrent use with CYP3A inducers reduces bosutinib plasma concentrations.
Ponatinib	Iclusig	45 mg/day	With or without food	Concurrent use with CYP3A or Pgp inhibitors increase ponatinib plasma concentrations. Concurrent use with CYP3A inducers reduces ponatinib plasma concentrations.

AP, accelerated phase; AUC, area under the curve; BC, blast crisis; BID, twice daily; C_{max}, maximum concentration; CP, chronic phase; CYP, cytochrome P450; Pgp, P-glycoprotein; PPI, proton pump inhibitor.

Chronic Phase

The IRIS study compared imatinib 400 mg orally daily to IFN-α plus low-dose subcutaneous cytarabine in 1,106 patients with newly diagnosed CP CML.[22] After a median follow-up of 19 months, patients who received imatinib achieved a complete hematologic response of 96%, major cytogenetic response of 85%, and complete cytogenetic response of 69%. Six percent of patients had progressed to AP or BC and only 4% discontinued imatinib because of an adverse event. The study was designed to allow crossover to the opposite treatment arm for lack of response or intolerance. After 5 years of follow-up, only 3% of patients randomized initially to receive IFN-α remained on their initial regimen compared with 69% of patients in the imatinib arm. The 5-year follow-up data from the IRIS trial was published in December 2006 and 8-year follow-up data presented in December 2009.[14,25] Estimated 5-year and 8-year overall survival of the 553 patients who were originally randomized to receive imatinib is 89% and 85%, respectively. At 8 years, estimated event-free survival (EFS) was 81% and freedom-from-progression to AP or BC was 92% and annual rates of progression to AP or BC in years 4 through 8 were 0.9%, 0.5%, 0%, 0%, and 0.4%. Only 55% of patients remained on imatinib therapy at the 8-year time point.[25]

Cytogenetic and molecular responses secondary to imatinib are associated with EFS and risk of progression to AP or BC. Patients that do not achieve a hematologic response by 3 months, cytogenetic response by 6 months, or a major cytogenetic response by 12 months fare significantly worse compared to responders. In addition, patients with a complete cytogenetic response and at least a 3-log reduction in *BCR-ABL* levels via RT-PCR correlated with a 100% survival without disease progression at 18 months. The risk of disease progression according to the Sokal scoring system estimated the rates of disease progression to be 3%, 8%, and 17% in low-risk, intermediate-risk, and high-risk patients, respectively. However, the Sokal score was not associated with disease progression in patients who achieved a complete cytogenetic response.[14]

4 Although most patients attain a complete cytogenetic response on imatinib, very few patients achieve a complete molecular response. In a study of patients enrolled in the IRIS study, Hughes et al. reported that less than 5% of patients on imatinib have undetectable levels of *BCR-ABL* when analyzed by RT-PCR.[26] Recent data suggest that the level of residual disease is predictive of progression-free survival. A 3-log decline in *BCL-ABL* mRNA within 3 months after achieving a complete cytogenetic response is reported to be a predictor of longer progression-free survival.[27] Careful monitoring of *BCR-ABL* levels by RT-PCR is necessary to guide clinician decision making for therapy modification. The 2013 NCCN guidelines recommend imatinib 400 mg orally daily as one of several options for patients in CP CML (see Table 112-3).[15]

Higher imatinib doses have been evaluated in clinical trials. The European Leukemia Net conducted a randomized phase II trial in high-risk patients defined by the Sokal scoring system to imatinib 400 mg versus 800 mg daily and evaluated the proportion of patients achieving a complete cytogenetic response at 12 months.[28] Patients receiving the higher dose of imatinib achieved a 64% complete cytogenetic response compared to 58% of patients receiving standard dose with a median follow-up period of 12 months ($P = 0.435$). These study results do not justify the routine use of imatinib 800 mg daily as frontline therapy in high-risk patients with CP CML. A phase II trial evaluated imatinib 400 mg daily for 2 weeks, then titrated to 400 mg twice daily in patients with an intermediate-risk Sokal score appeared to have benefit with 88% and 91% of patients achieving a complete cytogenetic response at 12 and 24 months.[29] These data require validation with a phase III clinical trial before a widespread use of a higher dose can become standard of care in CP CML.

Accelerated Phase/Blast Crisis

Response rates for patients with AP or BC CML are reduced compared with those in CP CML. A phase II study evaluating imatinib 600 mg daily in patients with AP CML yielded complete hematologic and complete cytogenetic response rates of 71% and 19%, respectively.[30] Prior to protocol amendments, patients were able to receive imatinib 400 mg daily, but the rates of hematologic response, cytogenetic response, disease progression, and overall survival were inferior to imatinib 600 mg. The toxicity profile between imatinib 400 mg and 600 mg daily was similar.

Traditional therapy for BC CML has focused on administering cytotoxic chemotherapy in treatment programs similar to acute leukemia induction. Etoposide (VP-16) cytarabine (Ara-C), and carboplatin (VAC-regimen) has demonstrated efficacy in patients with BC CML with a median overall survival of 7 months.[31] Imatinib has demonstrated modest benefit in BC CML. An open-label, nonrandomized trial evaluated imatinib 400 mg daily with dose escalation to 600 mg daily and 400 mg twice daily (for patients not achieving a hematologic response after one month).[32] The primary objectives were to assess hematologic response, complete cytogenetic response, and the return to CP CML. Fifteen percent developed a complete hematologic response, 7.4% achieved a complete cytogenetic response, and 18% achieved a second CP. Imatinib 600 mg was associated with sustained hematologic response. The median overall survival was 6.9 months.

Imatinib Resistance

Despite having high cytogenetic response rates, some patients treated with imatinib will not respond to therapy or will relapse after an initial response.[33] The most prominent mechanism of imatinib resistance is the presence of point mutations in one or more areas on the ABL kinase. More than 100 different mutations have been discovered thus far. Many of these mutations can cause a conformational change in the ATP binding site, which greatly decreases the ability of imatinib to bind and inhibit kinase activity.[34] Imatinib binds to *BCR-ABL* by establishing a series of hydrogen bonds with side changes of amino acids within the kinase domain. Mutations which alter this surface can decrease the affinity of imatinib for *BCR-ABL*, potentially preventing binding entirely. The kinase domain of *BCR-ABL*, which encompasses amino acids 225 to 400, can be subdivided into ATP and imatinib binding site (P loop), the catalytic site where the phosphate from ATP is transferred to the substrate protein, and the activation domain that determines the state of the kinase (open or closed). The imatinib binding site is located in the region of amino acids 300 to 325. Resistance is caused by point mutations in one or more of several areas on the ABL kinase. The T315I mutation occurs directly within the imatinib binding site and completely disrupts imatinib binding.[35] This mutation has gained notoriety by conferring resistance not only to imatinib but also to second-generation *BCR-ABL* kinase inhibitors.

The other known clinically relevant mechanism of resistance is *BCR-ABL* gene amplification. The *BCR-ABL* gene is overexpressed to such an extent that the typical 400 mg daily dose of imatinib is insufficient to inhibit the activity of the kinase. Reports of clinically significant resistance have been published owing to *BCR-ABL* gene amplification, multiple copies of Ph, or both. The largest series published this far included 66 patients, in whom only 2 had confirmed *BCR-ABL* genomic amplification.[35] Other proposed mechanisms of resistance to imatinib include differential binding to α_1-acid glycoprotein in serum, overexpression of P-glycoprotein-induced drug efflux, and clonal evolution to acquisition of additional cytogenetic abnormalities.[36]

Imatinib Monitoring

Imatinib therapy should be frequently monitored to assess response or disease progression. Recommendations for monitoring include baseline molecular and cytogenetic assessment. Patients with CP CML who have an optimal response have a complete hematologic response within 3 months, partial cytogenetic response within 6 months, complete cytogenetic response within 12 months and major molecular response within 18 months of starting imatinib. *BCR-ABL* transcripts should be evaluated by RT-PCR every 3 months and bone marrow cytogenetics performed at 3 months if RT-PCR is unavailable or 12 months if neither complete cytogenetic response nor major molecular response is achieved. Bone marrow cytogenetics are repeated at 18 months if the patient is not in major molecular response or did not have a complete cytogenetic response at 12 months.[15–17] The loss of hematologic or cytogenetic responses or clonal evolution at any time should be considered a treatment failure warranting a change in therapy. *BCR-ABL* kinase domain mutation analysis is performed for patients who have an inadequate initial response at 3, 12, or 18 months, have any sign of loss of response, or demonstrate disease progression to AP or BC.[15]

Adverse Effects and Drug Interactions

Tables 112-4 and 112-5 summarize drug–drug interactions, adverse drug reactions, and monitoring of imatinib. Imatinib-induced myelosuppression is one of the most common adverse events. Moderate-to-severe myelosuppression occurs in about 5% to 10% of patients with CP CML and in 50% to 60% of patients in AP or BC.[14] The myelosuppression typically occurs within the first 4 weeks of therapy and is more common in patients with advanced disease (i.e., high blastic involvement of the bone marrow) and those with a low hemoglobin. Hematopoiesis in patients with CML depends on the amount of Ph-positive progenitors, although some degree of myelosuppression should be expected when the malignant clone is suppressed. However, imatinib also suppresses normal hematopoiesis, which suggests that myelosuppression associated with imatinib is probably related to effects on the Ph clone and normal hematopoietic cells.[3] Patients should have complete blood counts drawn every 1 to 2 weeks to assess for myelosuppression while receiving imatinib. Appropriate initial management of myelosuppression is to interrupt imatinib treatment, not dose reduce, as dose reductions below 300 mg daily do not fully inhibit *BCR-ABL* and may lead to the emergence of imatinib resistance.[15]

Nonhematologic toxicities associated with imatinib include gastrointestinal complications, fluid retention, myalgias and arthralgias, rash, and hepatotoxicity. Drug rash frequently occurs but is usually mild and can be managed with antihistamines or topical steroids. Severe rash, while uncommon, has been reported as an important cause for discontinuation of therapy. Algorithms for desensitization for patients that have experienced serious imatinib-associated rash have been published.[37] Hepatotoxicity can occur with imatinib, and the drug should be withheld if liver function tests exceed five times the upper limits of normal. After the liver function tests normalize, imatinib can be restarted at a reduced dose of not less than 300 mg per day. Imatinib is then dose escalated to the initial dose if liver function tests do not rise during 6 to 12 weeks of treatment. Death as a consequence of liver failure has been reported in a patient receiving large doses of acetaminophen concomitantly with imatinib. It is recommended that patients on imatinib limit their use of acetaminophen to 1,300 mg daily.[15] Other medications that are known to be hepatotoxic should be used with caution while patients are treated with imatinib.

Advanced-Generation Tyrosine Kinase Inhibitors

Dasatinib (Sprycel®) and nilotinib (Tasigna®) are approved second-generation TKIs used for the treatment of CML in patients who are resistant or intolerant to imatinib therapy; both drugs are also approved for first-line treatment of CP CML. Dasatinib is an oral *BCR-ABL* TKI that was FDA approved in 2006 for the treatment of imatinib-resistant CML. Dasatinib is an oral TKI of *BCR-ABL,* the SRC family, C-KIT, EPHA2, and PDGFR. Preclinical data show that dasatinib is 300 times more potent than imatinib and inhibits the growth of imatinib-resistant clones, with the exception of the T315I.[38] Dasatinib received accelerated approval based on hematologic and cytogenetic responses seen in imatinib-resistant or imatinib-intolerant patients.

Dasatinib has been evaluated in patients with imatinib-resistant or -intolerant CP, AP, and BC CML. In a phase II trial of 186 patients in CP CML receiving dasatinib 70 mg orally twice daily

TABLE 112-5 Monitoring of Tyrosine Kinase Inhibitors in Chronic Myelogenous Leukemia

Drug	Adverse Reactions	Monitoring Parameters	Comments
Imatinib	Common: • Myelosuppression • Fluid retention (pleural/pericardial effusion, ascites, periorbital and peripheral edema) • Nausea/vomiting • Rash • Fatigue • Hepatotoxicity • Hypothyroidism • Myalgias Rare but serious: • Congestive heart failure/left ventricular dysfunction • Hemorrhage • Bullous dermatologic reactions	• CBC for myelosuppression • CMP for hepatotoxicity • Consider baseline echocardiogram if preexisting cardiac dysfunction or risk factors for cardiac dysfunction, repeat if experiencing symptoms of cardiac dysfunction • Thyroid-stimulating hormone	Nausea and vomiting improved when drug is administered with food
Dasatinib	Common: • Myelosuppression • Myalgia • Fluid retention • Cardiotoxicity • Rash • Gastrointestinal toxicity • Hypophosphatemia • Hepatotoxicity Rare but serious: • Pleural effusion • QT prolongation • Congestive heart failure/left ventricular dysfunction • Pulmonary arterial hypertension • Hemorrhage	• CBC for myelosuppression • CMP for hypophosphatemia and hepatotoxicity • ECG if risk factors for QTc prolongation • Chest radiograph for signs and symptoms of pleural effusion • Evaluate for signs/symptoms of underlying cardiopulmonary disease for pulmonary arterial hypertension	Gastrointestinal hemorrhage reported to be fatal; severe pleural effusions requiring thoracentesis; fatal myocardial infarction are reported
Nilotinib	Common: • Myelosuppression • Rash • Gastrointestinal toxicity • Peripheral edema • Liver function abnormalities • Elevated serum lipase/amylase • Electrolyte abnormalities (hypophosphatemia, hypokalemia, hypocalcemia, and hyponatremia) Rare but serious: • Tumor lysis syndrome • Cardiotoxicity (QTc prolongation/sudden cardiac death/left ventricular dysfunction)	• CBC for myelosuppression • CMP for hypophosphatemia and hepatotoxicity • Serum amylase/lipase • ECG if risk factors for QTc prolongation at baseline, 7 days thereafter and then as clinically indicated	Sudden deaths reported with nilotinib; ventricular repolarization abnormalities may have been contributory
Bosutinib	Common: • Myelosuppression • Gastrointestinal toxicity • Fluid retention • Hepatotoxicity • Hypophosphatemia • Rash Rare but serious: • Embryofetal toxicity	• CBC for myelosuppression • CMP for hypophosphatemia and hepatotoxicity • Serum amylase/lipase • ECG if risk factors for QTc prolongation at baseline, 7 days thereafter and then as clinically indicated	Potential for additive risk of hepatotoxicity when given concurrently with letrozole
Ponatinib	Common: • Myelosuppression • Arthralgia • Headache • Fatigue • Fever • Pancreatitis • Elevated lipase • Hypertension • Gastrointestinal toxicity • Dermatologic toxicity • Electrolyte abnormalities • Fluid retention Rare but serious: • Arterial thrombosis • Hepatotoxicity • Cardiotoxicity (arrhythmia/congestive heart failure) • Embryofetal toxicity • Hemorrhage • Tumor lysis syndrome • Impaired wound healing/GI perforation	• CBC for myelosuppression • Serum lipase • CMP for hepatotoxicity, at baseline for tumor lysis syndrome • Blood pressure as clinically indicated	Deaths reported from hepatotoxicity, thrombosis including myocardial infarction and hemorrhage

CBC, complete blood count; CMP, comprehensive metabolic panel; ECG, electrocardiogram; GI, gastrointestinal.

a hematologic response and major cytogenetic response were noted in 90% and 52% of patients, respectively.[39] Kantarjian et al. evaluated imatinib 400 mg twice daily compared to dasatinib 70 mg twice daily in patients who developed resistance or were intolerant to imatinib 400 mg daily dosing. At 2 years follow-up, patients receiving dasatinib were more likely to achieve a complete hematologic response (93% vs. 82%; $P = 0.034$), major cytogenetic response (53% vs. 33%; $P = 0.023$), and an increased estimated progression-free survival at 2 years, which suggests that dasatinib is superior to imatinib dose escalation in disease progression.[40] A trial evaluating different dosing strategies of dasatinib showed that 100 mg once daily was as efficacious as dasatinib 70 mg twice daily, 50 mg twice daily or 140 mg once daily but with decreased adverse events such as pleural effusions.[41] The standard dose of dasatinib for patients with CP CML is now accepted to be 100 mg daily.

Dasatinib induces responses in patients who are resistant or intolerant to imatinib with advanced disease CML. Patients with AP CML were administered dasatinib 70 mg twice daily with 45% achieving a complete hematologic response, 39% achieved a complete cytogenetic response, 66% had progression-free survival, and 82% were alive at 2 years.[42] A phase III trial comparing dasatinib 70 mg twice daily to 140 mg once daily reported similar efficacy at 15 months follow-up, but an improved safety profile that established dasatinib 140 mg once daily as the preferred dosing in AP CML.[43] Dasatinib induced a hematologic response in 35% and a major cytogenetic response in 33% of patients with BC CML. Median overall survival for patients receiving dasatinib in BC CML is 11.8 months.[44]

Dasatinib has been evaluated as first-line therapy in a phase III trial of 519 patients with CP CML.[45] Patients were randomized to dasatinib 100 mg once daily or imatinib 400 mg once daily. The rate of complete cytogenetic response at 2 years was higher with dasatinib as compared with imatinib (86% vs. 82%, $P = 0.007$). The rate of major molecular response was also significantly higher in the dasatinib group (64% vs. 46%, $P < 0.0001$). At the time of analysis, 77% of dasatinib and 75% of imatinib patients remained on study with transformation to AP/BC occurring in 2.3% of dasatinib versus 5% of imatinib patients. Progression-free survival at 2 years was similar in the two groups. Adverse effects were similar between the two treatment groups, with the exception that 14% of dasatinib-treated patients developed grade 1 or 2 pleural effusions.

Nilotinib has 20 to 30 times the inhibitory activity of the *BCR-ABL* tyrosine kinase with activity against C-KIT and PDGFR (but not SRC kinases) due to a modification of the methylpiperazinyl structure of imatinib. Nilotinib has inhibitory activity against imatinib-resistant mutants with the exception of T315I. In a phase II trial of 280 patients with imatinib-resistant or -intolerant CP CML, 59% of patients treated with nilotinib 400 mg twice daily achieved a major cytogenetic response, with an estimated 4-year progression-free and overall survival of 57% and 78%, respectively.[46] In patients with AP CML treated with nilotinib 400 or 600 mg twice daily, 26% achieved a complete hematologic response and 29% achieve a major cytogenetic response.[47] For first-line treatment of CML, results of a randomized trial in 846 patients comparing nilotinib at two doses (300 or 400 mg twice daily) to imatinib 400 mg once daily have been published.[48] The primary end point of the trial was major molecular response. At 3 years, both nilotinib arms had a significantly higher major molecular response rate at 12 months (73% and 70% for nilotinib 300 and 400 mg twice daily, respectively) as compared to imatinib (53%, $P < 0.001$ for both comparisons). The nilotinib arms also had a significant improvement in the time-to-progression to the AP or BC, as compared to the imatinib arm. The number of patients discontinued from treatment was similar in all three treatment arms. Nilotinib provides an alternative to dasatinib in patients with imatinib-resistant or -intolerant CP or AP CML and is one of several options in frontline treatment of CP CML.[15] The phase III trial results for both dasatinib and nilotinib have made them viable alternatives to imatinib for first-line treatment for newly diagnosed CP CML.

Two other TKIs were approved for treatment of CML in 2012, bosutinib and ponatinib. Bosutinib has 15 to 100 times the inhibitory activity of the *BCR-ABL* tyrosine kinase as imatinib with activity against SRC kinases with minimal activity against C-KIT and PDGFR. In a phase I/II dose escalation study, bosutinib was evaluated in patients with CP CML with resistance or intolerance to imatinib.[49] Among the 288 patients previously treated with imatinib, 34% achieved a major cytogenetic response at 24 weeks. Among patients previously treated with imatinib followed by dasatinib or nilotinib, 27% achieved a major cytogenetic response at 24 weeks. Grade 3 or 4 nonhematologic adverse events included diarrhea (9%), rash (9%), and vomiting (3%). Based on this study, the bosutinib dose that was recommended for phase II trials was 500 mg daily. A major cytogenetic response was observed in 32% of patients and a complete cytogenetic response was observed in 24% of patients in the phase II trials.[50]

Bosutinib 500 mg daily was compared to imatinib 400 mg daily in a phase III randomized trial of 502 patients in newly diagnosed CP CML.[51] Although the primary end point of complete cytogenetic response rate at 12 months (70% with bosutinib vs. 68% with imatinib) was not significantly different observed, the rate of major molecular response was significantly higher in the bosutinib group (41% vs. 27%, $P < 0.001$). The incidence of adverse events was similar between the groups with the exception that bosutinib had a higher incidence of diarrhea (68% vs. 21%) and imatinib had a higher incidence of edema (38% vs. 11%).

Ponatinib is considered a third-generation TKI that contains a novel triple-bond linkage in its chemical structure that avoids the steric hindrance caused by the bulky isoleucine residue at position 315 in T315I *BCR-ABL* binding site cleft, providing clinical activity against this resistance phenotype. In a phase I trial, 65 patients had refractory CML in either CP, AP, BC or Ph positive ALL, the maximum tolerated dose of ponatinib was 45 mg with dose-limiting toxicities identified as pancreatitis and myelosuppression.[52] Of the 43 patients with CP CML, 63% achieved a complete cytogenetic response and 44% a major molecular response. The 22 patients with AP/BC CML or Ph positive acute lymphocytic leukemia (ALL), 14% achieved complete cytogenetic response and 9% major molecular response. In the 12 patients who harbored a T315I mutation, 92% attained a complete cytogenetic response and 67% a major molecular response. These data led to the design of a phase II study of 449 CML patients who were resistant or intolerant to dasatinib or nilotinib or had documented T315I mutation on study entry.[53] Patients were assigned to six cohorts: CP CML, AP CML or BC CML with each disease group further stratified by TKI resistance/intolerance or presence of T315I mutation. The patient population was heavily pretreated with 53% having received imatinib, dasatinib and nilotinib prior to enrollment. The primary end point was major cytogenetic response at 12 months. For patients with TKI resistant/intolerant disease, the primary end point was achieved in 50%, 58%, and 35% of patients with CP, AP, and BC CML, respectively. For patients with T315I mutations, major cytogenetic responses reported were 70% for CP CML, 50% for AP CML and 33% for BC CML. About one-third of patients experienced myelosuppression and/or cutaneous reaction and pancreatitis was reported in 5% of patients. The drug label contains a black box warning for arterial thrombosis including fatal myocardial infarction and stroke in 8% of patients in clinical trials.[54] Hepatotoxicity including reports of liver failure and death are also included in the black box warning, several of which occurred within 1 week of starting therapy. The manufacturer recommends specific dose modifications for myelosuppression, hepatotoxicity and elevated lipase.

Tables 112-4 and 112-5 summarize dosing, drug interactions, adverse drug reactions, and monitoring of advanced-generation TKIs. Edema and plural effusions can be managed by dasatinib drug holiday, diuretics, or short courses of steroids. Nilotinib can be associated with indirect bilirubin elevations in 10% to 15% of patients.[46,47] Nilotinib may prolong the QTc interval (block box warning) and patients should have an electrocardiogram at baseline, at 7 days following initiation of therapy, and periodically thereafter. Based on early clinical trial data, bosutinib appears to have similar adverse events of diarrhea, nausea and vomiting, rash, and abdominal discomfort.[49] Like imatinib, advanced-generation TKIs are metabolized by cytochrome P450 (CYP)3A4. Clinicians need to be aware of possible drug interactions with inducers and inhibitors of the CYP3A4 pathway such as phenytoin, azole antifungals, or macrolide antibiotics.

Omacetaxine

Omacetaxine was approved by the FDA in October 2012 for treatment of CP or AP CML with resistance or intolerance to two or more TKIs. Omacetaxine is a first-in-class cephalotaxine ester that inhibits protein synthesis independent of direct *BCR-ABL* binding. The putative mechanism is the reduction of *BCR-ABL* oncoproteins and Mcl-1, an anti-apoptotic Bcl-2 family member, via binding to A-site cleft in the peptidyl-transferase center of the large ribosomal subunits. Efficacy with omacetaxine has been demonstrated in two patients groups: CP or AP CML resistant to two or more TKIs and patients previously treated with imatinib harboring the T315I mutation. The former group was presented in a combined analysis of two phase II studies for CP and AP CML. Omacetaxine was administered at 1.25 mg/m^2 subcutaneously twice daily for 14 consecutive days every 28 days then for 7 days every 28 days as maintenance.[55] Of the 122 patients enrolled, 81 had CP CML of which 20% achieved a major cytogenetic response with a median duration of 18 months and a median overall survival of 34 months. In the AP CML group, no patients achieved a major cytogenetic response and 27% of patients had a major hematologic response with a median overall survival of 16 months.

A phase II trial of omacetaxine was conducted in 62 CP CML patients with a history of the T315I mutation.[56] Patients were treated with the induction regimen as above and transitioned to maintenance when the patient achieved a hematologic response. Hematologic response was attained in 77%, complete cytogenetic response in 16%, and major cytogenetic response in 23% of patients. The median number of cycles to gain a hematologic response was one, and for major cytogenetic response was 2.5 months. The median duration of complete hematologic response was 9.1 months, and major cytogenetic response was 6.6 months. Grade 3/4 toxicities reported in these trials was myelosuppression with occasional reports of myalgias and arthralgias and gastrointestinal toxicity.

Hematopoietic Stem Cell Transplantation

5 Allogeneic HSCT remains the only therapy proven to cure patients with CML, with many patients alive and disease-free decades after transplant. Patients undergoing allogeneic HSCT from a human leukocyte antigen (HLA)-matched sibling donor have 5-year survival rates ranging from 60% to 80% and long-term survival of approximately 50%.[54,55] In most long-term survivors, the *BCR-ABL* translocation is absent in all diagnostic tests including RT-PCR. Prognostic risk factors associated with survival outcomes include age, phase of disease, and disease duration. Increasing age is associated with poorer prognosis, with higher transplant-related mortality in patients older than age 50 years. Patients with CP who receive allogeneic HSCT have better outcomes than those in AP or BC. The time from diagnosis to transplantation also affects outcomes. Patients who undergo matched-sibling allogeneic HSCT within the first year of diagnosis have a better 5-year survival rate than those who undergo transplantation more than 1 year after their diagnosis (70% to 80% vs. 50% to 60%).[57,58] These data were reported prior to the use of imatinib as first-line therapy for CML.

The major limitation for broad application of HSCT is that fewer than 30% of patients who are transplant-eligible will have an HLA-matched sibling donor. The most practical approach is to use an HLA-matched unrelated donor, if available. Matched unrelated donor HSCT has an overall 5-year survival reported to be 40% to 70%, which approaches overall survival data results reported for matched-sibling donor HSCT.[9,57,58] The advent of TKI therapy has resulted in fewer transplants for CML. Data collected to date appear to show that imatinib use prior to transplantation does not negatively affect transplant-related mortality.[59]

Clinical **Controversy. . .**

The controversy of whether to use allogeneic hematopoietic stem cell transplantation (HSCT) or second-generation tyrosine kinase inhibitor (TKI) therapy as second-line treatment for patients that have progression or are intolerant to imatinib is ongoing. Dasatinib keeps 90% of chronic phase (CP) patients treated first-line with imatinib free from disease progression with a median follow-up of 15 months. For patients that have progressed to accelerated phase (AP), dasatinib and nilotinib can produce hematologic response in about one-half of patients and major cytogenetic responses in close to one-third of patients. At 1 year, about 75% of patients will still be alive. It is unknown what efficacy of second-generation TKIs will confer as a long-term treatment option. Allogeneic HSCT remains an option for patients with a suitable donor, younger age, and good performance status.

Treatment options in patients who relapse after transplantation are limited. Graft-versus-leukemia (GVL) effect, TKIs, omacetaxine, IFN-α, or a clinical trial are reasonable options. The infusion of donor lymphocytes function as a form of adoptive immunotherapy can induce a GVL effect. In relapsed CML, donor lymphocytes induce durable responses and these responses strongly correlate with the development of graft-versus-host disease (GVHD).[60] Tumor burden also predicts the likelihood of response to donor lymphocyte infusion in relapsed CML. The optimal method of administering donor lymphocytes remains unclear, but these data suggest it may be possible to partially separate the GVL effect from GVHD.

Imatinib has been used in patients who have residual disease after allogeneic HSCT. Most patients respond to imatinib with complete molecular response of 70%.[61] Use of imatinib or other TKI therapies require further study to determine the magnitude of benefit when applied in the post-HSCT setting.[62] The role of nonmyeloablative transplants in CML is evolving, but preliminary results suggest comparable outcomes to myeloablative transplants. The experience of German registry data suggests that 17% of all transplants for CML use a reduced-intensity conditioning regimen.[63]

Personalized Pharmacotherapy

Personalized treatment of CML is mostly directed following initiation of second-line therapy. Mutational analysis of binding sites that confer resistance to TKIs should be evaluated if initial response is inadequate, or the milestones of complete cytogenetic response or major molecular response are lost, or if any signs of disease progression in the form of AP or BC are noted.[64] The results of this analysis will guide selection of the appropriate TKI as second-line therapy.[65] In addition, with the advent of omacetaxine and ponatinib, two agents are now available that are active against the T315I mutation that confers resistance to the rest of the TKIs.

Preliminary data support the role of therapeutic drug monitoring of TKIs in CML. Trough imatinib levels of ≥1 mcmol/L have been associated in patients with a higher response than those with >1 mcmol/L.[66] Data on nilotinib and dasatinib are more limited. The clinical applicability of therapeutic drug monitoring is still to be determined because the drug assays are not yet commercially available

Evaluation of Therapeutic Outcomes

Current standard of care is for patients with newly diagnosed CP CML to receive imatinib or one of the second-generation TKI. The goal of disease monitoring in CML is to differentiate patients who have optimally responded to an initial course of TKI therapy from those at high risk for treatment failure. With imatinib, nilotinib, and dasatinib as appropriate options for frontline therapy for newly diagnosed CP CML, and bosutinib, ponatinib, and omacetaxine approved for salvage therapy, clinicians have a large number of treatment options to consider before allogeneic HSCT. Future research opportunities will focus on how to select second-, third-, and fourth-line therapies and whether combination therapy provides additional long-term benefit.

CHRONIC LYMPHOCYTIC LEUKEMIA

Epidemiology and Etiology

CLL is a lymphoproliferative disorder characterized by accumulation of functionally incompetent clonal B lymphocytes.[67] CLL is the most common form of leukemia in the United States, but is rare in other countries, such as Japan and China. It is estimated that 15,680 new cases of CLL will be diagnosed in the United States in 2013 with 4,580 deaths.[1] Occasional family clusters have been recognized, and first-degree relatives of patients with CLL are at three times the risk of developing a lymphoid malignancy as compared with the general population. CLL is a disease of the elderly, with a median age of 72 years, although 20% to 30% of CLL occurs in patients who are younger than 55 years of age. Male sex, white race, family history, and advanced age are known risk factors for the disease.

Pathophysiology

CLL cells are comprised of a neoplastic clone of CD5$^+$ cells, which express low levels of surface-membrane immunoglobulin M (IgM) and immunoglobulin D (IgD) compared to normal peripheral blood B cells. Normal CD5$^+$ B lymphocytes are present in the lymph nodes and in the blood. Neoplastic CD5$^+$ cells accumulate in the lymph nodes and spleen because of the loss of apoptosis by either the overexpression of an oncogene, such as *bcl-1* or *-2*, or loss of a tumor suppressor gene, such as *RB1*.[67] The bcl-2 protein is a major regulator of apoptosis or programmed cell death. Evidence is emerging that antigenic stimulation and cytokines drive the proliferation of the CLL cells.

A monoclonal population of B cells with a similar surface antigen phenotype as CLL cells has been recently identified in patients up to several years prior to diagnosis of the disease.[68] This phenomenon, termed monoclonal B-cell lymphocytosis (MBL) appears to be predictive as to whether a patient is at risk for developing CLL over time. In a cohort of 77,000 patients enrolled in a cancer screening trial, 45 patients were diagnosed with CLL throughout the duration of the study. Baseline blood samples collected on enrollment of the screening trial were analyzed for the patients who developed CLL. MBL was present in 44 of 45 of the patients by either flow cytometric or molecular analysis (i.e., RT-PCR assay) and confirmed in 41 of 45 of these patients by both methods. Samples predated the diagnosis of CLL in a time period ranging from 6 months to 6.4 years. This finding could lead to potentially earlier diagnosis and intervention for CLL.

Cytogenetic abnormalities correlate with disease progression in CLL. About 80% of patients with CLL have a karyotypic abnormality. The chromosomes that are most frequently involved include chromosomes 13, 12, 11, and 17.[69] Additional cytogenetic abnormalities may be acquired during therapy, particularly with deletions of chromosome 17, which have an adverse effect on survival.[70] Somatic point mutations have been identified in a cohort of 91 patients yielding nine mutated genes: *TP53*, *ATM*, *MYD88*, *NOTCH1*, *SF3B1*, *ZMYM3*, *MAPK1*, *FBXW7*, and *DDX3X*.[71] These mutations were associated with cell-cycle and DNA repair pathways, intracellular signaling, inflammatory pathways, and RNA splicing and processing. A correlation was identified with *SF3B1* and chromosome 11 deletions providing insight into how these mutations may impact clinical outcomes.

About 4% of patients with CLL will undergo transformation of their disease to an aggressive non-Hodgkin lymphoma (diffuse large B cell), which is termed *Richter's syndrome*. Richter's syndrome may be triggered by accumulation of additional cytogenetic

CLINICAL PRESENTATION Chronic Lymphocytic Leukemia

Constitutional Symptoms

- Fever, fatigue, weight loss

Physical Examination

- Lymphadenopathy (87%)
- Splenomegaly (54%)
- Hepatomegaly (14%)

Laboratory Tests

- Peripheral blood
  - Lymphocytosis
  - Coombs-positive autoimmune hemolytic anemia
  - Hyper- or hypogammaglobulinemia
  - Monoclonal gammopathy
  - Anemia
  - Thrombocytopenia
- Bone marrow
  - Hypercellular
  - Increased mature lymphocytes
  - Increased megakaryocytes
- Molecular markers
  - Cytogenetics (17p-)
  - ZAP-70 mutations

abnormalities in the malignant clone of lymphocytes or by viral infections, such as Epstein-Barr's virus.[72]

Staging and Prognosis

Survival times for patients with CLL are widely variable, with some patients succumbing to disease within 3 years and others living into a second decade from the time of diagnosis. The Rai and the Binet staging systems are commonly used in CLL with the Rai being favored in the United States and the Binet in Europe. The Rai staging system has been combined into a risk classification scheme: low risk (stage 0), intermediate risk (stages I and II), and high risk (stages III and IV) with median survivals of greater than 10 years, 7 years, and 2 to 4 years, respectively.[73]

The disease course for CLL varies within each stage such that one patient may have an indolent course with long survival time, while another patient may have more aggressive disease and a relatively short survival time. The Rai and Binet staging systems incompletely predict for individual patients who may experience more rapid disease progression. Patients with Richter's syndrome will have a rapidly advancing disease course that mimics diffuse large B-cell non-Hodgkin lymphoma. However, successful treatment of the diffuse large B-cell non-Hodgkin lymphoma with combination chemotherapy will not eradicate the underlying clone of CLL cells and patients will ultimately relapse.[72]

Biomarkers such as CD38 expression and ζ-associated protein 70 (ZAP-70) expression have been explored as prognostic factors for CLL. CD38 is a cell-surface antigen that is associated with early progression, significantly shorter overall survival, and a poor response to fludarabine.[74–76] ZAP-70 is an intracellular protein with tyrosine kinase activity. Once considered as simply a surrogate marker for the unmutated variable region of the immunoglobulin heavy chain gene (IGHV), elevated ZAP-70 expression appears to predict for rapid CLL disease progression and independently correlates with prognosis.[73,76,77]

Cytogenetic changes such as deletion of the short arm of chromosome 17 (17p-), which corresponds to p53 silencing, can be biomarkers of poor response to therapy. A prospective study showed that newly diagnosed patients with 17p- had a median time-to-progression following first-line therapy with either fludarabine or fludarabine and cyclophosphamide of 10 to 12 months.[70] Patients with chromosomal abnormalities of 13, 12, 11, and 17 have reported median survivals of 133 months, 114 months, 79 months, and 32 months, respectively.[69]

Clinical **Controversy...**

Certain molecular and cellular markers have been identified that may predict chronic lymphocytic leukemia (CLL) disease progression. ZAP-70 expression, CD38 expression, IGHV mutations, and 17p- are associated with a more aggressive clinical course of CLL. Controversy surrounds whether or not treatment should be based on these biologic markers alone. 17p- is the most consistent poor prognostic marker and results in a loss of the tumor suppressor gene, p53. Consensus guidelines now delineate treatment options for patients based on the presence of 17p-. If a patient has 17p- more aggressive regimens that contain immunotherapy and purine analogs (e.g., fludarabine, cyclophosphamide, and rituximab) are recommended as first-line treatments. For second-line therapy, regimens with multiagent chemotherapy combined with immunotherapy (e.g., oxaliplatin, fludarabine, cytarabine, and rituximab) are considered standard therapy.

TREATMENT
Chronic Lymphocytic Leukemia

Desired Outcomes

6 The primary goals of treatment for CLL are to achieve and maintain remission duration with minimize treatment-related toxicity. The management of patients with CLL is highly individualized with some patients receiving therapy on diagnosis, while other patients with early-stage disease are managed expectantly. Indications for starting treatment include disease-related symptoms (fatigue, night sweats, weight loss, fever), threatened end-organ function, bulky disease, doubling of lymphocyte doubling time in less than 6 months, progressive anemia, and platelet count less than 100,000/mm³ (100×10^9/L).[79–81] Consideration of initial treatment options is based on several factors including age of the patient, disease stage, and high-risk prognostic factors, such as deletion 17p or 11q.

Most stage 0 patients do not require treatment and can be managed with observation. In patients with stage I disease, treatment is controversial. A consistent survival benefit from early therapy has not been reported in asymptomatic patients.[79,81] Cytotoxic chemotherapy in early stage CLL is usually reserved for patients who have disease characteristics consistent with a more aggressive course, such as short lymphocyte doubling times and presence of biologic markers such as ZAP-70 or high-risk cytogenetics. In stages II through IV disease, treatment is required, with the goal of achieving a partial or complete remission. Table 112-6 shows the regimens used to treat newly diagnosed and previously treated CLL.[73,74,76,77]

Cytotoxic Chemotherapy

Orally administered alkylating agents such as chlorambucil and cyclophosphamide, given either alone or with corticosteroids,

TABLE 112-6 Treatment for Newly Diagnosed and Previously Treated Chronic Lymphocytic Leukemia

Treatment	Overall Response	Complete Response
Chlorambucil		
Untreated	37%	4%
Fludarabine alone		
Untreated	60–80%	20–30%
Previously treated	13–59%	3–37%
Fludarabine + cyclophosphamide		
Untreated	80–90%	25–40%
Previously treated	60–70%	10–15%
Rituximab alone		
Untreated	50–60%	10–20%
Previously treated	80–90%	20–40%
Fludarabine + rituximab		
Untreated	80–100%	30–50%
Previously treated	80–90%	20–40%
Fludarabine + cyclophosphamide + rituximab		
Untreated	95%	70%
Previously treated	73%	25%
Alemtuzumab alone		
Untreated	80–90%	20–30%
Previously treated	30–50%	0–20%
Alemtuzumab + fludarabine		
Previously treated	83%	17–30%
Bendamustine + rituximab	88%	23%
Previously treated	59%	9%

historically have been used as primary treatment for CLL. Results from a meta-analysis involving 2,048 patients from six randomized controlled studies evaluated low-dose alkylating agents in CLL.[82] That analysis showed that delayed treatment with alkylating agents in asymptomatic patients did not adversely affect 10-year survival. More importantly, if only deaths caused by CLL were considered, significantly longer survival was observed when treatment was deferred. Chlorambucil continues to be widely used in elderly, symptomatic patients as initial treatment for CLL, but its use is based on a small number of studies with no demonstrable survival advantage.[73] Commonly used dosing schedules for chlorambucil are intermittent pulse dosing of 15 to 40 mg/m^2 orally every 28 days or daily doses of 4 to 8 mg/m^2/day.[83] The dose of chlorambucil is often titrated to circumvent myelosuppression.

Cyclophosphamide produces a similar response rate as chlorambucil (overall response rate: 40% to 60%; complete response: 4%) and can be used in patients who cannot tolerate chlorambucil or in whom response is not optimal. Some patients who do not respond to chlorambucil will respond to single-agent cyclophosphamide. Cyclophosphamide is typically given orally at a daily dose of 1 to 3 mg/kg. Oral cyclophosphamide is less commonly used compared to chlorambucil because of the risk of hemorrhagic cystitis and bladder cancer with prolonged treatment.

Fludarabine-based therapy is a common initial treatment in CLL. It is particularly useful in younger patients and in those patients who can tolerate immunosuppressive chemotherapy. Fludarabine, along with the other purine analogs, 2-chlorodeoxyadenosine (cladribine) and 2-deoxycoformycin (pentostatin), are highly active in CLL, with fludarabine being the most widely studied agent in the class in the treatment of CLL.[83,84] Most patients receive fludarabine 25 to 30 mg/m^2 IV daily for 5 days when used as a single agent. Cladribine and pentostatin have similar activity, although head-to-head trials comparing these three nucleosides have not been conducted.[83,85,86]

Fludarabine was initially studied in CLL patients who were refractory to chlorambucil. Several trials reported overall response rates to fludarabine in previously treated patients ranging from 13% to 59% and complete response rates of 3% to 37%.[87] Fludarabine has higher overall response and complete remission rates than alkylating-based therapies in the frontline setting. In one of the randomized studies that compared fludarabine to chlorambucil in chemotherapy-naïve patients, fludarabine-treated patients had a higher complete remission rate as compared with chlorambucil (20% vs. 5%).[88] However, the higher complete remission rate did not translate into a significant difference in overall survival and patients treated with fludarabine had a higher rate of severe neutropenia and infection. The study allowed chlorambucil failures to cross over to fludarabine, which may have hampered the ability to show a survival advantage in the fludarabine arm. A recent review of younger patients enrolled in a large phase III trial showed that 33% of patients receiving fludarabine or fludarabine-based therapy had infectious complications.[89] An increase in *Pneumocystis* infections was not observed, but a 6% increase in herpes and varicella zoster infection was documented. Dose reductions occurred frequently as a result of the infectious episodes. Based on the increased risk of infectious complications, some practitioners recommend antiviral and antibacterial prophylaxis be given with treatment.[81]

Bendamustine is an alkylating agent that contains a purine-derivative benzimidazole ring in its chemical structure that yields a compound that is non–cross-resistant with other alkylating agents. Bendamustine induces cell death via single and double-stranded cross-links.[89] Efficacy of bendamustine was established as first-line agent in Binet stage B or C CLL in a phase III trial that randomized 319 patients to bendamustine or chlorambucil.[90] Complete response rates of 31% versus 2% and an overall response rate for 68% versus 31% were observed for bendamustine and chlorambucil respectively. The median progression-free survival was 21.6 versus 8.3 months favoring bendamustine. Adverse events reported for bendamustine includes hematologic toxicity in about 25% of patients, and gastrointestinal and cutaneous toxicity.

Biologic Therapy

Monoclonal antibodies, such as rituximab and alemtuzumab, are increasingly being used in the treatment of CLL. Rituximab is a chimeric monoclonal antibody that targets the CD20 antigen expressed on B lymphocytes. Rituximab was initially approved for patients with indolent non-Hodgkin lymphoma and later for aggressive non-Hodgkin lymphoma. Rituximab received FDA approval for the treatment of CD20-positive CLL in 2010. CLL cells have less prominent CD20 expression on their surface as compared to non-Hodgkin lymphoma, which may translate into lower clinical response. Efficacy with rituximab as a single agent in CLL is moderate with a 58% overall response rate reported with 9% complete responses.[91] Subsequent studies have used higher rituximab doses (up to 500 mg/m^2 per cycle) when given in combination with other agents.

7 Alemtuzumab is a monoclonal antibody that targets the CD52 antigen found on both B and T lymphocytes. This agent was initially FDA approved in 2001 for the treatment of patients with CLL who had been treated with alkylating agents and had failed fludarabine therapy and is now approved as a single agent for both frontline and salvage treatment of CLL. Alemtuzumab is titrated to a maintenance dose of 30 mg IV or subcutaneously given 3 times a week for 12 weeks. As a single agent, alemtuzumab has produced response rates from 33% to 53% in patients with refractory disease, but complete responses are infrequent.[92]

Results from a randomized phase III trial comparing alemtuzumab to chlorambucil in chemotherapy-naïve patients with symptomatic CLL showed higher complete response rates with alemtuzumab than with chlorambucil, 24% versus 2%, respectively.[93] These differences in response rate translated into a significant difference in progression-free survival (hazard ratio, 0.58; 95% confidence interval, 0.43 to 0.77, $P < 0.0001$).

Infusion-related reactions are one of the most frequently reported toxicities with alemtuzumab. The reactions experienced with IV administration include fever, rigors, and hypotension.[94] Alemtuzumab is associated with serious, potentially life-threatening toxicities, including pancytopenia, infusion reactions, and opportunistic infections. Because of alemtuzumab's profound immunosuppression, the 2013 NCCN guidelines recommend antibacterial and antiviral prophylaxis to prevent *Cytomegalovirus* reactivation and *Pneumocystis* infections.[80] Prophylaxis with trimethoprim-sulfamethoxazole and famciclovir or valacyclovir is recommended with the use of alemtuzumab.[91] Alemtuzumab is FDA-approved for IV administration, although the use of subcutaneous alemtuzumab has been evaluated to reduce the frequency of these reactions. In a study by Lundin et al., 41 patients received 30 mg of subcutaneous alemtuzumab three times a week for 12 weeks, which yielded a response rate of 87%.[95] Major adverse event were grades 1 and 2 skin reactions in 90% of patients; fever, rigors, and hypotension were infrequent. About 10% of patients had reactivation of *Cytomegalovirus* and required ganciclovir treatment. Similar to IV administration, antiviral and antibacterial prophylaxis is warranted when alemtuzumab is given via the subcutaneous route.[95]

Ofatumumab is a fully human monoclonal antibody to CD20 that was approved as single-agent therapy in 2009 for patients with CLL that is refractory to fludarabine and alemtuzumab. Ofatumumab is administered as an IV infusion with an initial dose of

300 mg then four weekly doses followed by four monthly doses of 2,000 mg. An overall response rate was reported of 58% in patients with fludarabine and alemtuzumab refractory disease and 47% in bulky fludarabine refractory disease.[96] Median time-to-progression was 5.7 and 5.9 months and median overall survival 13.7 and 15.4 months in the fludarabine, alemtuzumab refractory patients and bulky fludarabine refractory disease patients, respectively. Adverse events reported in greater than 10% of patients included infection and neutropenia. Infusion-related events were reported in approximately 60% of patients with the 40% during the first infusion and 25% with the second infusion. Serious toxicities such as fatal infections, progressive multifocal leukoencephalopathy, and hepatitis B reactivation have been reported.

Combination Therapy

The single-agent activity of fludarabine has led to incorporation of fludarabine in combination regimens in patients with CLL. The most widely studied combination is fludarabine with cyclophosphamide, which produces complete response rates between 25% and 40% in treatment-naïve patients as compared with 20% to 30% for single-agent fludarabine.[78,84] Although improved response rates and progression-free survival have been reported with fludarabine and cyclophosphamide combinations compared with fludarabine alone, no benefit in overall survival has yet been observed.

8 The combination of fludarabine and rituximab has promising activity. In vitro studies suggest that rituximab is synergistic with fludarabine and cyclophosphamide and has led investigators to evaluate this combination in clinical trials. Results from an uncontrolled trial of fludarabine, cyclophosphamide, and rituximab (FCR) reported a complete remission rate of 70% in previously untreated CLL patients.[97] FCR has documented a complete remission rate of 25% in previous treated patients. Results of two phase III trials comparing FCR with fludarabine and cyclophosphamide documented a progression-free survival benefit (30 vs. 20 months) in patients treated with FCR in patients with refractory disease and an overall survival benefit (87.2% vs. 82.5%) in patients with newly diagnosed disease.[98,99] The results of these phase III trials led to FDA approval of rituximab with fludarabine and cyclophosphamide in CLL.

Bendamustine and rituximab have been combined in two phase II studies in patients with CLL, in frontline and the relapsed setting. In the frontline setting, 117 patients were treated with bendamustine 90 mg/m^2 days 1 and 2 and rituximab 375 mg/m^2 IV on day 0 for cycle 1 and then 500 mg/m^2 IV on day 1 for subsequent cycles.[100] Overall, 88% of patients had a clinical response with 23% being complete responses. The median EFS was 34 months with 90% of patients reported being alive at the median follow-up time point of 27 months. Patients with 17p- responded less well, with a 37.5% overall response rate. Grade 3/4 myelosuppression was experienced in about 20% of patients. In the relapsed setting, a similar regimen as above was administered with the exception of a lower bendamustine dose of 70 mg/m^2 in 78 patients who had received a median of two prior treatments.[101] The overall response rate was 59%, with 9% of patients having a complete response. With a median follow-up of 24 months, the EFS was 14.7 months with a median overall survival of 34 months. About 25% of patients experienced grade 3/4 myelosuppression with three treatment-related deaths related to infection.

Hematopoietic Stem Cell Transplantation

9 There is limited experience with the use of HSCT in CLL. Patients treated with allogeneic HSCT achieve higher remission rates and appear to have a longer disease-free survival, but is associated with high treatment-related mortality, which approaches 40%. Contrary to the high mortality reported in most studies, a randomized phase II study of high-risk CLL patients comparing allogeneic and autologous HSCT reported 100-day mortality of 4% in both arms. After 6 years of follow-up, no difference in overall survival (58% autologous and 55% allogeneic) was observed.[102] This low early mortality must be interpreted carefully, given that only 25 carefully selected patients received allogeneic HSCT as compared with 137 who received autologous HSCT. T-cell depletion was performed on the allogeneic grafts, which may reduce 100-day mortality at the cost of increased relapse, infectious complications, or posttransplant lymphoproliferative disorders as a consequence of reduced GVL effect.[102]

Although allogeneic HSCT may offer the potential of cure in CLL, the advanced age of most patients, limited donor availability, and the high treatment-related mortality precludes the routine application in the management of this disease. Allogeneic HSCT is a more viable option for younger patients with aggressive disease. Older patients who are not candidates for full-intensity allogeneic HSCT may be candidates for nonmyeloablative allogeneic HSCT.

Gene Therapy

The use of gene therapy in CLL had been considered as a potential treatment strategy because of the presence of tumor specific antigens such as CD19. A preliminary report described the modification of autologous T cells expressing an anti-CD19 chimeric antigen receptor (CART19) in a single patient who had advanced CLL.[103] The patient's autologous T cells were collected via leukapheresis and treated with a self-inactivating lentiviral vector to express the CD19 specific chimeric antigen receptor concurrently with the costimulatory CD137 signaling domain. The patient received a preparative regimen of pentostatin 4 mg/m^2 and cyclophosphamide 600 mg/m^2 IV followed by reinfusion of 3×10^8 autologous T cells of which 5% were transduced over three separate daily infusions 96 hours following completion of chemotherapy.

The patient's clinical course was marked by low-grade fevers and chills 2 weeks following the first infusion. In the succeeding 5-day period, the patient experienced fevers, rigors, diaphoresis, anorexia, nausea, and diarrhea. The patient was diagnosed with tumor lysis syndrome on day 22 following the first infusion and was treated with rasburicase and supportively. By day 28, the patient had neither resolution of his adenopathy nor evidence of CLL from a bone marrow aspirate. At 3 and 6 months following infusion, the patient remained free of adenopathy and bone marrow studies continued to show no evidence of CLL by morphologic karyotypic or flow cytometric analysis. This clinical report represents the first sustained remission published in the medical literature with transduced autologous T cells in treatment of CLL.

Personalized Pharmacotherapy

Molecular biomarkers are important as predictors for disease time to progression, decision making for initiation of treatment, and prognosis. The most important are cytogenetic abnormalities such as deletion 17p and 11q, which are associated with more aggressive disease that is less responsive to treatment. Unmutated status of the immunoglobulin heavy chain variable gene locus and overexpression of ZAP-70 and CD38 expression are also predictive of poor prognosis.

The 2013 NCCN guidelines segregate treatment options based on the presence of deletion 17p- or 11q, age older or younger than 70 years, and first- and second-line regimens.[80] Preferred first-line therapy options for patients younger than 70 years without poor-risk cytogenetics or significant comorbidities are aggressive chemoimmunotherapy regimens such as fludarabine, cyclophosphamide, rituximab; and pentostatin, cyclophosphamide, and rituximab. Patients who are older than 70 years without poor-risk cytogenetics may be treated with chemotherapy (bendamustine, chlorambucil, and cyclophosphamide/prednisone), immunotherapy (rituximab), or milder chemoimmunotherapy (fludarabine and rituximab). Second-line therapeutic options for patients without poor-risk cytogenetics are again divided by the duration of response with first-line treatment, which is loosely defined as a long response greater than 36 months for fludarabine/cyclophosphamide and rituximab or greater than 18 months for chlorambucil. Regimens recommended for short responses consist of chemoimmunotherapy (fludarabine, cyclophosphamide, and rituximab; pentostatin, cyclophosphamide, and rituximab; and oxaliplatin, fludarabine, cytarabine, and rituximab) or traditional regimens used for aggressive non-Hodgkin lymphoma (cyclophosphamide, hydroxydaunorubicin, vincristine, prednisone [CHOP]) with rituximab. For patients who have poor-risk cytogenetics, first-line therapy options consist primarily of more aggressive chemoimmunotherapy treatment options (fludarabine, cyclophosphamide, and rituximab; fludarabine and rituximab; high-dose methylprednisolone and rituximab; bendamustine and rituximab; pentostatin, cyclophosphamide, and rituximab). Second-line regimens are similar to those outlined above for patients younger than as described above for short responses.

The next generation of prognostic data to incorporate into drug therapy decision making will likely come from the study of somatic gene mutations and whole genome sequencing from individual patients. A report identified specific somatic gene mutations that were associated with resistance to chemotherapy such as TP53 and others newly associated with CLL, such as SF3B1.[104] Tracking subclonal heterogeneity was performed in patients receiving therapy revealed that certain tumor subclones evolved over time in a heterogeneous fashion for each individual patient. These data may ultimately predict which patients will achieve a suboptimal response to therapy and guide the selection of salvage therapies.[105]

Evaluation of Therapeutic Outcomes

CLL is an incurable disease and the goal of therapy is to optimize remission duration while minimizing the burden of treatment-related adverse effects.

Supportive care for patients undergoing active treatment for CLL is crucial for ensuring a successful outcome. Patients may become hypogammaglobinemic as a consequence of disease progression or treatment will need routine monitoring of serum IgG. If the serum IgG falls below 500 mg/dL (5 g/L), then monthly replacement doses of 300 to 500 mg/kg of IV immune globulin is warranted. Antibiotic prophylaxis for patients receiving fludarabine-based regimens or chemoimmunotherapy should be considered for herpes virus and *Pneumocystis*. Patients who are treated with alemtuzumab will require monitoring for cytomegalovirus (CMV) antigen every 1 to 2 weeks while on therapy and for 2 months after or be given prophylaxis with valganciclovir.

ABBREVIATIONS

ALL	acute lymphocytic leukemia
AP	accelerated phase
ATP	adenosine triphosphate
BC	blast crisis
CHOP	cyclophosphamide, hydroxydaunorubicin, vincristine, prednisone
CLL	chronic lymphocytic leukemia
CML	chronic myelogenous leukemia
CMV	cytomegalovirus
CNS	central nervous system
CP	chronic phase
CYP	cytochrome P450
EFS	event-free survival
FCR	fludarabine, cyclophosphamide, rituximab
FDA	Food and Drug Administration
FISH	fluorescence in situ hybridization
GVHD	graft-versus-host disease
GVL	graft-versus-leukemia (effect)
HLA	human leukocyte antigen
HSCT	hematopoietic stem cell transplantation
Ig	immunoglobulin M
IGHV	immunoglobulin heavy chain gene
IFN-α	interferon alpha
IRIS	International Randomized study of Interferon vs STI571 trial
MBL	monoclonal B-cell lymphocytosis
mRNA	messenger ribonucleic acid
NCCN	National Comprehensive Cancer Network
Ph	Philadelphia chromosome
PDGFR	platelet-derived growth factor receptor
RT-PCR	reverse-transcription polymerase chain reaction
TKI	tyrosine kinase inhibitor
WBC	white blood cell
WHO	World Health Organization
ZAP-70	ζ-associated protein 70

REFERENCES

1. Siegel R, Naishadham MA, Jemal A, et al. Cancer statistics, 2013. CA Cancer J Clin 2013;63:11–30.
2. Corso A, Lazzarino M, Morra E, et al. Chronic myelogenous leukemia and exposure to ionizing radiation—a retrospective study of 443 patients. Ann Hematol 1995;70:79–82.
3. Ichimaru M, Ishimaru T, Belsky JL. Incidence of leukemia in atomic bomb survivors belonging to a fixed cohort in Hiroshima and Nagasaki, 1950-71. Radiation dose, years after exposure, age at exposure, and type of leukemia. J Radiat Res (Tokyo) 1978;19:262–282.
4. Druker BJ. Translation of the Philadelphia chromosome into therapy for CML. Blood 2008;112:4808–4817.
5. Borgaonkar DS. Philadelphia-chromosome translocation and chronic myeloid leukaemia. Lancet 1973;1:1250.
6. Stam K, Heisterkamp N, Grosveld G, et al. Evidence of a new chimeric bcr/c-abl mRNA in patients with chronic myelocytic leukemia and the Philadelphia chromosome. N Engl J Med 1985;313:1429–1433.
7. Goldman JM, Melo JV. Chronic myeloid leukemia—Advances in biology and new approaches to treatment. N Engl J Med 2003;349:1451–1464.
8. Quintas-Cardama A, Cortes JE. Chronic myelogenous leukemia: Diagnosis and treatment. Mayo Clin Proc 2006;81:973–988.
9. Fialkow PJ, Jacobson RJ, Papayannopoulou T. Chronic myelocytic leukemia: Clonal origin in a stem cell common to the granulocyte, erythrocyte, platelet, and monocyte/macrophage. Am J Med 1977;63:125–130.
10. Vardiman JW, Harris NL, Brunning RD. The World Health Organization (WHO) classification of myeloid neoplasms. Blood 2002;100:2292–2302.
11. Sokal JE, Cox EB, Baccarani M, et al. Prognostic discrimination in "good-risk" chronic granulocytic leukemia. Blood 1984;63:789–799.

12. Cortes JE, Kantargian HM. How I treat newly diagnosed chronic phase CML. Blood 2012;120:1390–1397.
13. Jabbour E, Kantarjian H. Chronic myeloid leukemia: 2012 Update on diagnosis, monitoring and management. Am J Hematol 2012;87:1038–1045.
14. Druker BJ, Guilhot F, O'Brien S, et al. Five-year follow-up of patients receiving imatinib for chronic myelogenous leukemia. N Engl J Med 2006;355:2408–2417.
15. National Comprehensive Cancer Network. The NCCN Chronic Myelogenous Leukemia Clinical Practice Guideline (Version 2.2013). 2013, *http://www.nccn.org.*
16. Baccarani M, Pane F, Saglio G. Monitoring treatment for CML. Haematologica 2008;93:161–169.
17. Radich JP. How I monitor residual diseases in chronic myeloid leukemia. Blood 2009;114:3376–3381.
18. Hehlmann R, Heimpel H, Hasford J, et al. Randomized comparison of busulfan and hydroxyurea in chronic myelogenous leukemia: Prolongation of survival by hydroxyurea. The German CML Study Group. Blood 1993;82:398–407.
19. Preudhamme C, Guillhot J, Nicolini FE, et al. Imatinib plus peginterferon alfa-2a in chronic myeloid leukemia. N Engl J Med 2010;363:2511–2521.
20. Deininger MWN, Druker BJ. Specific targeted therapy at chronic myelogenous leukemia with imatinib. Pharmacol Rev 2003;55:401–423.
21. Deininger M, Buchdunger E, Druker BJ. The development of imatinib as a therapeutic agent for chronic myeloid leukemia. Blood 2005;105:2640–2653.
22. O'Brien SG, Guilhot F, Larson RA, et al. Imatinib compared with interferon and low-dose cytarabine for newly diagnosed chronic-phase chronic myeloid leukemia. N Engl J Med 2003;348:994–1004
23. Kurzrock R, Kantarjian HM, Druker BJ, Talpaz M. Philadelphia chromosome-positive leukemias: From basic mechanisms to molecular therapeutics. Ann Intern Med 2003;138:819–830.
24. Druker BJ, Talpaz M, Resta DJ, et al. Efficacy and safety of a specific inhibitor of the *BCR-ABL* tyrosine kinase in chronic myeloid leukemia. N Engl J Med 2001;344:1031–1037.
25. Deininger M, O'Brien SG, Guilhot F, et al. International Randomized Study of Interferon vs. STI-571 (IRIS) 8 year follow-up: Sustained survival and low risk for progression or events in patients with newly diagnosed chronic myeloid leukemia in chronic phase treated with imatinib. Blood (ASH Annual Meeting Abstracts) 2009;116: Abstract 1126.
26. Hughes TP, Kaeda J, Branford S, et al. Frequency of major molecular responses to imatinib or interferon alfa plus cytarabine in newly diagnosed chronic myeloid leukemia. N Engl J Med 2003;349:1423–1432.
27. Press RD, Love Z, Tronnes AA, et al. *BCR-ABL* mRNA levels at and after the time of a complete cytogenetic response (CCR) predict the duration of CCR in imatinib mesylate-treated patients with CML. Blood 2006;107: 4250–4256.
28. Baccarani M, Rosti G, Castagnetti F, et al. Comparison of imatinib 400 mg and 800 mg daily in the front-line treatment of high-risk, Philadelphia-positive chronic myeloid leukemia: a European Leukemia Net study. Blood 2009;113:4497–4504.
29. Castagnetti F, Palandri F, Amabile M, et al. Results of high-dose imatinib mesylate in intermediate Sokal risk chronic myeloid leukemia in early chronic phase: a phase 2 trial of the GIMEMA CML Working Party. Blood 2009;113: 3428–3434.
30. Talpaz M, Silver RT, Druker BJ, et al. Imatinib induces durable hematologic and cytogenetic responses in patients with accelerated phase chronic myeloid leukemia: Results of a phase 2 study. Blood 2002;99: 1928–1937.
31. Amadori S, Picardi A, Fazi P, et al. A phase II study of VP-16, intermediate-dose Ara-C and carboplatin (VAC) in advanced acute myelogenous leukemia and blastic chronic myelogenous leukemia. Leukemia 1996;10:766–768.
32. Sawyers CL, Hochhaus A, Feldman E, et al. Imatinib induces hematologic and cytogenetic responses in patients with chronic myelogenous leukemia in myeloid blast crisis: results of a phase II study. Blood 2002;99:3530–3539.
33. Quintas-Cardama A, Cortes J. Molecular biology of bcr-abl1 positive chronic myeloid leukemia. Blood 2009;113: 1619–1630.
34. Milojkovic D, Apperly J. Mechanisms of resistance to imatinib and second-generation tyrosine kinase inhibitors in chronic myeloid leukemia. Clin Cancer Res 2009;15: 7519–7527.
35. Apperly JF. Part I: Mechanisms of resistance to imatinib in chronic myeloid leukemia. Lancet Oncol 2007;8: 1018–1029.
36. Krause DS, Van Etten RA. Tyrosine kinases as targets for cancer therapy. N Engl J Med 2005;353:172–187.
37. Nelson RP, Cornetta K, Ward KE, Ramanaju S, Fausel C, Cripe L. Desensitization to imatinib in patients with leukemia. Ann Allergy Asthma Immunol 2006;97:216–222.
38. Talpaz M. Shah NP, Kantarjian H, et al. Dasatinib in imatinib-resistant Philadelphia chromosome-positive leukemias. N Engl J Med 2006;354:2531–2541.
39. Hochhaus A, Kantarjian HM, Baccarani M, et al. Dasatinib induces notable hematologic and cytogenetic responses in chronic-phase chronic myeloid leukemia after failure of imatinib therapy. Blood 2007;109:2303–2309.
40. Kantarjian HM, Pasquini R, Levy V, et al. Dasatinib or high-dose imatinib for chronic-phase chronic myeloid leukemia resistant to imatinib at a dose of 400 to 600 milligrams daily. Cancer 2009;115:4136–4147.
41. Shah NP, Kantarjian HM, Kim DW, et al. Intermittent target inhibition with dasatinib 100 mg once daily preserves efficacy and improves tolerability in imatinib-resistant and –intolerant chronic-phase chronic myeloid leukemia. J Clin Oncol 2008;26:3204–3212.
42. Apperley JF, Cortes JE, Kim DW, et al. Dasatinib in the treatment of chronic myeloid leukemia in accelerated phase after imatinib failure: The START A trial. J Clin Oncol 2009;24:3472–3479.
43. Kantarjian HM, Cortes J, Kim DW, et al. Phase 3 study of dasatinib 140 mg once daily versus 70 mg twice daily in patients with chronic myeloid leukemia in accelerated phase resistant or intolerant to imatinib: 15-month median follow-up. Blood 2009;113:6322–6329.
44. Cortes J, Kim DW, Martinelli G, et al. Efficacy and safety of dasatinib in imatinib-resistant or –intolerant patients with chronic myeloid leukemia in blast phase. Leukemia 2008;22:2176–2183.
45. Kantarjian HM, Shah NP, Cortez JE, et al. Dasatinib or imatinib in newly diagnosed chronic-phase chronic myeloid leukemia: 2-Year follow-up from a randomized phase 3 trial. Blood 2012;119:1123–1129.
46. Giles FJ, le Coutre PD, Pinilla-Ibarz J, et al. Nilotinib in imatinib-resistant or imatinib-intolerant patients with chronic myeloid leukemia in chronic phase: 48-Month follow-up results of a phase II study. Leukemia 2013;27: 107–112.

47. Le Coutre P, Ottmann OG, Giles F, et al. Nilotinib (formerly AMN107), a highly selective BCR-ABL tyrosine kinase inhibitor, is active in patients with imatinib-resistant or -intolerant accelerated phase chronic myelogenous leukemia. Blood 2008;111:1834–1839.
48. Larson RA, Hochhaus A, Hughes TP, et al. Nilotinib vs imatinib in patients with newly diagnosed Philadelphia chromosome-positive chronic myeloid leukemia in chronic phase: ENESTnd 3-year follow-up. Leukemia 2012;26:2197–2203.
49. Cortes JE, Kantarjian HM, Brummendorf TH, et al. Safety and efficacy of bosutinib (SKI-606) in chronic phase Philadelphia chromosome positive chronic myeloid leukemia patients with resistance or intolerance to imatinib. Blood 2011;118:4567–4576.
50. Khoury HJ, Cortes JE, Kantarjian HG, et al. Bosutinib is active in chronic phase chronic myeloid leukemia after imatinib and dasatinib therapy failure. Blood 2012;119:3403–3412.
51. Cortes JE, Kim DW, Kantarjian HM, et al. Bosutinib versus imatinib in newly diagnosed chronic phase chronic myeloid leukemia: Results from the BELA trial. J Clin Oncol 2012;30:3486–3492.
52. Cortes JE, Kantarjian H, Shah NP, et al. Ponatinib in refractory Philadelphia chromosome-positive leukemias. N Engl J Med 2012;367:2075–2088.
53. Cortes JE, Kim DW, Ibarz JP et al. A pivotal phase II trial of ponatinib in patients with chronic myeloid leukemia and Philadelphia chromosome-positive acute lymphoblastic leukemia (Ph+ ALL) resistant or intolerant to dasatinib or nilotinib or with T315I BCR-ABL mutation: 12 month follow-up of the PACE trial. Blood (ASH Annual Meeting Abstracts) 2012:119:163.
54. Ponatinib (Iclusig) prescribing information. 2013, *http://iclusig.com/pi/*.
55. Cortes JE, Nicolini FE, Wetzler, et al. Subcutaneous omacetaxine in chronic or accelerated phase chronic myeloid leukemia resistant to two or more tyrosine kinase inhibitors including imatinib. Blood (ASH Annual Meeting Abstracts) 2011;118: Abstract 3761.
56. Cortes J, Lipton JH, Rea D, et al. Phase II study of subcutaneous omacetaxine mepesuccinate after tyrosine kinase inhibitor failure in patients with chronic phase chronic myeloid leukemia with the T315I mutation. Blood 2012;120:2573–2580.
57. Gratwohl A, Brand R, Apperly J, et al. Allogeneic hematopoietic stem cell transplantation for chronic myeloid leukemia in Europe 2006: Transplant activity, long-term data and current results. An analysis by the Chronic Leukemia Working Party of the European Group for the Blood and Marrow Transplantation (EBMT). Haematologica 2006;91:513–521.
58. van Rhee F, Szydlo RM, Hermans J, et al. Long-term results after allogenic bone marrow transplantation for chronic myelogenous leukemia in chronic phase: A report from the Chronic Leukemia Working Party of the European Group for Blood and Marrow Transplantation. Bone Marrow Transplant 1997;20:553–560.
59. Deininger M, Schleuning M, Greinix H, et al. The effect of prior exposure to imatinib on transplant-related mortality. Haematologica 2006;91:452–459.
60. Porter D, Levine JE. Graft-versus host disease and graft-versus leukemia after donor leukocyte infusion. Semin Hematol 2006;43:53–61.
61. Hess G, Bunjes D, Siegert W, et al. Sustained complete molecular remissions after treatment with imatinib mesylate in patients with failure after allogeneic stem cell transplantation for chronic myelogenous leukemia: Results of a prospective phase II open label multicenter study. J Clin Oncol 2005;23:7583–7593.
62. Klyuchnikov E, Kroger N, Brummendorf TH, et al. Current status and perspectives of tyrosine kinase inhibitor treatment in the post-transplant period in patients with chronic myeloid leukemia. Biol Blood Marrow Transplant 2010;16: 301–310.
63. Bacher U, Klyuchnikov E, Zabelina T, et al. The changing scene of allogeneic stem cell transplantation for chronic myeloid leukemia: a report from the German Registry covering the period from 1998-2004. Ann Hematol 2009;88:1237–1247.
64. Jabbour E, Kantarjian HM. Chronic Myeloid Leukemia: 2012 Update on diagnosis, monitoring, and management. Am J Hematol 2012;87:1038–1045.
65. Soverini S, Hochhaus A, Nicolini FE, et al. BCR-ABL kinase domain mutation analysis in chronic myeloid leukemia patients treated with tyrosine kinase inhibitors: recommendations from an expert panel on behalf of the European Leukemia. Blood 2011;118: 1208–1215.
66. Gao B, Yeap S, Clements A, et al. Evidence for therapeutic drug monitoring of targeted anticancer therapies. J Clin Oncol 2012;30:4017–4025.
67. Chiorazzi N, Rai KR, Ferarini M. Chronic lymphocytic leukemia. N Engl J Med 2005;352:804–815.
68. Landgren O, Albitar M, Ma W, et al. B-cell clones as early markers for chronic lymphocytic leukemia. N Engl J Med 2009;360:659–667.
69. Dohner H, Stilgenbauer S, Benner A, et al. Genetic aberrations and survival in chronic lymphocytic leukemia. N Engl J Med 2000;343:1910–1916.
70. Tam CS, Shanafelt TD, Wierda WG, et al. De novo deletion of 17p13.1 chronic lymphocytic leukemia shows significant clinical heterogeneity: The MD Anderson and Mayo Clinic experience. Blood 2009;114:957–964.
71. Wang, L, Lawrence MS, Wan Y, et al. SF3B1 and other novel cancer genes in chronic lymphocytic leukemia. N Engl J Med 2011;365:2497–2506.
72. Tsimberidou AS, O'Brien S, Khouri I, et al. Clinical outcomes and prognostic factors in patients with Richter's syndrome treated with chemotherapy or chemoimmunotherapy with or without stem cell transplantation. J Clin Oncol 2006;24: 2343–2351.
73. Eisele L, Haddad T, Sellmann L, Durhsen U, Durig J. Expression of CD38 on leukemic B-cells but not on non-leukemic T-cells are comparably stable over time and predict the course of disease in chronic lymphocytic leukemia. Leuk Res 2009;33:775–778.
74. Vroblova V, Smolej L, Vrbacky F, et al. Biological prognostic markers in chronic lymphocytic leukemia. Acta Medica (Hradec Kralove) 2009;52:3–8.
75. Deaglio S, Vaisitti T, Aydin S, Ferrero E, Malavasi F. In-tandem insight from basic science combined with clinical research: CD38 as both marker and key component of the pathogenetic network underlying chronic lymphocytic leukemia. Blood 2006;108:1135–1144.
76. Rassenti LZ, Huynh L, Toy TL, et al. ZAP-70 compared with immunoglobulin heavy-chain gene mutation status as a predictor of disease progression in chronic lymphocytic leukemia. N Engl J Med 2004;351:893–901.
77. Orchard J, Ibbotson R, Best G, Parker A, Oscier D. ZAP-70 in B cell malignancies. Leuk Lymphoma 2005;46: 1689–1698.

78. Zenz T, Mertens D, Kuppers R, Dohner H, Stilgenbauer S. From pathogenesis to treatment of chronic lymphocytic leukemia. Nat Rev Cancer 2010;10:37–50.
79. Shanafelt TD, Byrd JC, Call TG, Zent CS, Kay NE. Narrative review: Initial management of newly diagnosed, early-stage chronic lymphocytic leukemia. Ann Intern Med 2006;145:435–447.
80. National Comprehensive Cancer Network. The NCCN Non-Hodgkin's Lymphoma Clinical Practice Guideline (Version 1.2013). 2013, *http://www.nccn.org.*
81. CLL Trialists' Collaborative Group. Chemotherapeutic options in chronic lymphocytic leukemia: A meta-analysis of the randomized trials. J Natl Cancer Inst 1999;91: 861–868.
82. Lamanna N, Weiss MA. Purine analogue-based chemotherapy regimens for second-line therapy in patients with chronic lymphocytic leukemia. Semin Hematol 2006;43:S44–S49.
83. Gribben JG. How I treat CLL up front. Blood 2010;115: 187–197.
84. Robak T, Blonski JZ, Kasznicki M, et al. Cladribine with or without prednisone in the treatment of previously treated and untreated B-cell chronic lymphocytic leukaemia—Updated results of the multicentre study of 378 patients. Br J Haematol 2000;108:357–368.
85. Sorensen JM, Vena DA, Fallavollita A, et al. Treatment of refractory chronic lymphocytic leukemia with fludarabine phosphate via the group C protocol mechanism of the National Cancer Institute: Five-year follow-up report. J Clin Oncol 1997;15:458–465.
86. Rai KR, Peterson BL, Appelbaum FR, et al. Fludarabine compared with chlorambucil as primary therapy for chronic lymphocytic leukemia. N Engl J Med 2000;343: 1750–1757.
87. Eichhorst BF, Busch R, Schweighofer C, et al. Due to the low infection rates no routine anti-infective prophylaxis is required in younger patients with chronic lymphocytic leukemia during fludarabine-based first line therapy. Br J Haematol 2007;136:63–72.
88. Keating MJ, O'Brien S, Kontoyiannis D, et al. Results of first salvage therapy for patients refractory to a fludarabine regimen in chronic lymphocytic leukemia. Leuk Lymphoma 2002;43:1755–1762.
89. Cheson BD, Rummel MJ. Bendamustine: Rebirth of an old drug. J Clin Oncol 2009;27:1492–1501.
90. Knauf WU, Lissichkov T, Aldaoud A, et al. Phase III randomized study of bendamustine compared with chlorambucil in previously untreated patients with chronic lymphocytic leukemia. J Clin Oncol 2009;27:4378–4384.
91. Hainsworth JD, Litchey S, Barton JH. Single agent rituximab as first-line and maintenance for patients with chronic lymphocytic leukemia or small lymphocytic lymphoma. J Clin Oncol 2003;21:1746-1751.
92. Ravandi F, O'Brien S. Alemtuzumab in CLL and other lymphoid neoplasms. Cancer Invest 2006;24:718–725.
93. Hillmen P, Skotnicki AB, Robak T, et al. Alemtuzumab compared with chlorambucil as first-line therapy for chronic lymphocytic leukemia. J Clin Oncol 2007;35: 5616–5623.
94. Osterborg A, Karlsson C, Lundin J, Kimby E, Mellstedt H. Strategies in the management of alemtuzumab-related side effects. Semin Oncol 2006;33(suppl 5):S29–S35.
95. Lundin J, Kimby E, Bjorkholm M, et al. Phase II trial of subcutaneous anti-CD52 monoclonal antibody alemtuzumab (Campath-1H) as first-line treatment for patients with B-cell chronic lymphocytic leukemia (B-CLL). Blood 2002;100:768–773.
96. Weirda WG, Kipps TJ, Mayer J, et al. Ofatumumab as a single agent CD20 immunotherapy in fludarabine refractory chronic lymphocytic leukemia: A phase I/II study. J Clin Oncol 2010;28:1749-1755.
97. Keating MJ, O'Brien S, Albitar M, et al. Early results of a chemoimmunotherapy regimen of fludarabine, cyclophosphamide, and rituximab as initial therapy for chronic lymphocytic leukemia. J Clin Oncol 2005;23: 4079–4088.
98. Robak T, Dmoszynska A, Solal-Céligny P, et al. Rituximab plus fludarabine and cyclophosphamide prolongs progression-free survival compared with fludarabine and cyclophosphamide alone in previously treated chronic lymphocytic leukemia. J Clin Oncol 2010;28: 1756–1765.
99. Halleck M, Fischer K, Fingerle-Rowson G, et al. Addition of rituximab to fludarabine and cyclophosphamide in patients with chronic lymphocytic leukaemia: a randomized, open-labeled, phase 3 trial. Lancet 2010;376;1164–1174.
100. Fischer K, Cramer P, Busche R, et al. Bendamustine in combination with rituximab for previously untreated patients with chronic lymphocytic leukemia. A multicenter phase II trial of the German Chronic Lymphocytic Leukemia Study Group. J Clin Oncol 2012;30:3209–3216.
101. Fischer K, Cramer P, Busche R et al. Bendamustine combined with rituximab in patients with relapsed and/or refractory chronic lymphocytic leukemia. A multicenter phase II trial of the German Chronic Lymphocytic Leukemia Study Group. J Clin Oncol 2011;29:3559–3566.
102. Delgado J, Milligan DW, Dreger P. Allogeneic hematopoietic cell transplantation for chronic lymphocytic leukemia: ready for prime time? Blood 2009;114:2581–2588.
103. Porter DL, Levine BL, Kalos M, Bagg A, June CH. Chimeric antigen receptor-modified T cells in chronic lymphoid leukemia. N Engl J Med 2011;365:725–733.
104. Wang L, Lawrence MS, Wan Y, et al. SF3B1 and other novel cancer genes in chronic lymphocytic leukemia. N Engl J Med 2011;365:2497–2506.
105. Schuh A, Becq J, Humphray S, et al. Monitoring chronic lymphocytic leukemia progression by whole genome sequencing reveals heterogeneous clonal evolution patterns. Blood 2012;120:4191–4196.

113

Multiple Myeloma

Casey B. Williams and Timothy R. McGuire

KEY CONCEPTS

1. Multiple myeloma (MM) is a cancer that develops in plasma cells, leading to excessive production of a monoclonal immunoglobulin.
2. Most patients have skeletal involvement at the time of diagnosis with associated bone pain and fractures. Anemia, hypercalcemia, and renal failure may also be present. A bone marrow biopsy with 10% or more plasma cells and an M-protein spike on plasma or urine electrophoresis confirms the diagnosis.
3. Most patients require treatment after diagnosis, but treatment can be deferred in patients with smoldering (asymptomatic) MM. In patients with symptomatic disease, treatment produces benefits in various measures of survival and quality of life.
4. Thalidomide, lenalidomide, or bortezomib plus dexamethasone are commonly used induction regimens. They produce higher complete remission rates compared with the classic regimens of melphalan plus prednisone and VAD (vincristine, doxorubicin, and dexamethasone). The increased response rate is at the expense of significant grade III and IV toxicity, which can include myelosuppression, venous thromboembolism (VTE), and neuropathy depending on the regimen used. These novel agents can be added to chemotherapy (melphalan, liposomal doxorubicin, cyclophosphamide, or VAD-like chemotherapy) as part of induction and results in substantially higher response rates. Novel agents can also be combined to produce more active regimens.
5. Bortezomib-based regimens are commonly used to treat newly diagnosed patients with high-risk disease and patients with relapsed MM.
6. Lenalidomide is more potent and better tolerated than thalidomide and is the most commonly used immunomodulatory drug.
7. A host of new drugs are being studied and integrated into treatment of relapsed MM, including carfilzomib, pomalidomide, vorinostat, and bendamustine. Carfilzomib is a very active agent and is currently being studied as induction therapy in newly diagnosed patients.
8. Melphalan plus prednisone is not used in transplant candidates as part of induction but commonly used in transplant-ineligible patients combined with thalidomide, lenalidomide, or bortezomib.
9. Autologous hematopoietic stem cell transplantation (HSCT) is used after induction in patients with reasonably good performance status to maximize complete remissions and prolong survival. Combining autologous HSCT with allogeneic HSCT must be considered investigational and should be performed under clinical trial.
10. Maintenance therapies can be used in both transplant-eligible and -ineligible patients. Current regimens usually include lenalidomide or bortezomib with the intent of increasing response rates and progression-free survival.
11. Bisphosphonates are used to treat bone disease associated with MM, which results in decreased pain and skeletal-related events and improvement in quality of life.
12. Salvage therapy for patients with relapsed or refractory MM can include any of the prior listed therapies, depending on performance status of the patient, risk category of the patient, and prior treatments used for induction.

INTRODUCTION

Multiple myeloma (MM) is a genetically complex and an increasingly more common hematologic malignancy that develops in plasma cells or immunoglobulin-producing B lymphocytes.[1,2] The plasma cells produce excessive monoclonal immunoglobulins that can be measured in the plasma or urine. As a result of the various bone-mobilizing cytokines secreted from the MM clone and bone marrow stromal cells, patients often have skeletal involvement at diagnosis. MM is often sensitive to chemotherapy initially, but drug resistance develops relatively rapidly. Although therapy is not currently curative, MM has been a remarkable example of bench-to-bedside translation in new drug development. In particular, the proteasome inhibitor bortezomib and the immunomodulatory drugs (IMiDs) thalidomide and lenalidomide target MM cells in the bone marrow microenvironment and have improved outcomes.

EPIDEMIOLOGY AND ETIOLOGY

In the United States, it is estimated that 22,350 cases of MM will be diagnosed in 2013, with 10,710 deaths. It is a disease that affects older adults with a median age at diagnosis of 66 years. MM occurs more frequently in males and African Americans.[3] Additionally, individuals with a first-degree relative with MM have a 3.7-fold increased risk of developing this malignancy than those with unaffected relatives.[4,5]

Epidemiologic data from the United States have demonstrated associations with MM and individuals who work in agriculture.[6] Studies have shown an increased incidence of lymphohematopoietic cancers associated with lifetime exposure to alchalor, a commonly used pesticide. Other occupational groups associated with the development of MM include miners, carpenters and wood workers, sheet-metal workers, and furniture makers.[1,4] Radiation exposure has also been historically linked to the development of MM, but existing evidence is inconclusive.[7]

Although the pathogenesis of MM has not been fully elucidated and the role of antigen stimulation in the pathogenesis of the disease remains controversial, the understanding of the cellular events underlying the development of MM is becoming clearer. Decades of research and improved scientific techniques have enabled closer examination of the changes that occur during the development of normal and abnormal B cells.

PATHOPHYSIOLOGY

Multiple myeloma is a genetically heterogeneous disease that belongs to a group of related diseases called paraproteinemias that are characterized by abnormal clonal plasma cell infiltration in the bone marrow. A precursor condition called monoclonal gammopathy of undetermined significance (MGUS) is associated with monoclonal immunoglobulin in the blood (≤3 g/dL [≤30 g/L]) without clinical manifestations of the complications of MM.[8,9] The conversion rate of MGUS to MM is about 1% per year. The molecular changes associated with the conversion of MGUS to MM are not clear, but genome-wide studies have identified several candidate genes associated with disease progression.[2,9,10] Distinct from MGUS, which is a premalignant syndrome, smoldering MM is an asymptomatic disease with a low tumor burden and an indolent course.[1,4] In patients with smoldering MM, the risk of progression is about 10% per year for the first 5 years after diagnosis, about 3% per year for the next 5 years, and about 1% per year for the next 10 years.[11]

Although both MGUS and smoldering MM lack the clinical features of MM, they share many of the same genetic features. A characteristic feature of MM cells is the requirement for an intimate relationship with the bone marrow microenvironment, where plasma cells are nurtured in specialized niches that maintain and promote their long-term survival.[12] In early MM, the balance between apoptotic and antiapoptotic genes is disrupted with overexpression of antiapoptotic genes. As the disease progresses, a greater number of gene products that confer resistance, such as mutated *p53*, are overexpressed.[13] Molecules such as interleukin-6 (IL-6) and the transcriptional regulator nuclear factor kappa B (NF-κB) also stimulate clonal growth and promote resistance to therapy. Given their imprecise but important role in initiation and progression of MM, IL-6 and NF-κB are targets for both old and new therapies.[13,14]

❶ MM is characterized by the accumulation of malignant plasma cells in the bone marrow and the production of a monoclonal immunoglobulin (M protein). These proteins, secreted by the malignant clone, are frequently referred to as paraproteins.[1,4] Both MM and normal plasma cells are produced from differentiated B cells after antigen stimulation. Whereas normal plasma cells will die within days to weeks after differentiation, MM plasma cells are immortalized.[1,4] MM cells are seldom seen in large quantities in the peripheral blood because of their interaction with bone marrow stromal cells. This interaction between MM cells and bone marrow stroma is mediated by adhesion molecules within an abnormal bone marrow microenvironment and is required for growth and disease progression.[14] Figure 113-1 shows several of the factors involved in disease pathogenesis and progression and potential targets for thalidomide, lenalidomide, pomalidomide, bortezomib, and carfilzomib.

Over the next several years, our current understanding of the pathogenesis of MM and the tumor-specific mutations that drive tumor development and proliferation should improve dramatically. Whole-genome sequencing may lead to improvements in clinical practice. The sequencing of the MM genome in 38 patients was recently published and revealed that mechanisms previously suspected to have a role in the biology of MM like NF-κB may have

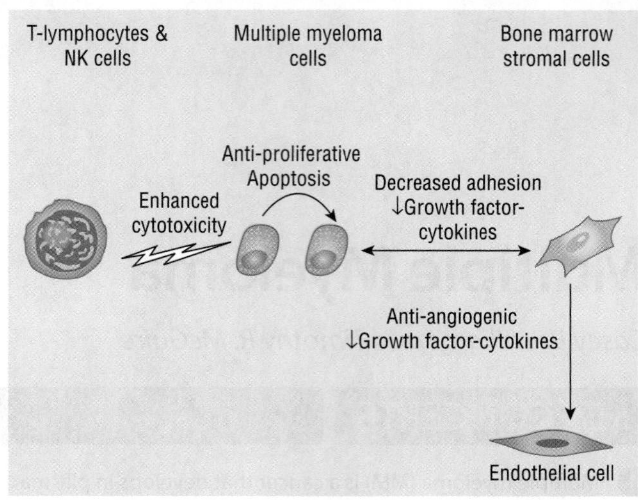

FIGURE 113-1 Sites of action for thalidomide, lenalidomide, pomalidomide, bortezomib, and carfilzomib.

much broader roles than previously suspected.[15] Additionally, the discovery of potential new mechanisms of transformation and progression such as mutations in the oncogenic kinase BRAF may lead to new therapeutic approaches in the future.[16,17]

CLINICAL PRESENTATION

❷ Most patients with MM present with complaints of bone pain and fatigue at diagnosis. About 10% to 20% of patients are asymptomatic at the time of diagnosis and have what is called smoldering MM.[4,11] Unfortunately, most patients show evidence of end-organ damage at the time of diagnosis. Initial laboratory evaluation often reveals hypercalcemia, renal insufficiency, anemia, and abnormalities in various disease markers, such as albumin and β_2-microglobulin. Skeletal evaluation shows gross abnormalities in most patients. Bone scans show abnormalities that often include lytic lesions, osteoporosis, and fractures. This group of findings (hypercalcemia, renal insufficiency, anemia, and bone lesions) is often referred by the acronym CRAB.[4,8] A bone marrow biopsy with 10% or more plasma cells and an M-protein spike on plasma or urine electrophoresis confirms the diagnosis.[8,18] Immunofixation is more sensitive and identifies the M-protein isotype being secreted. In a minority of patients, no M protein can be detected in the plasma but is found in the urine, requiring that urine be examined as part of a complete diagnostic workup. About 60% of patients have intact monoclonal immunoglobulin G (IgG), 20% have monoclonal IgA, and the remaining 20% secrete only monoclonal light chains. Antibodies are composed of two light chains where antigen binds and two heavy chains. Light-chain immunoglobulin alone can be secreted by the MM clone. Free monoclonal light chains in the urine are called Bence Jones proteins because they were first described by Dr. Henry Bence Jones and are primarily responsible for MM-associated renal failure.[1,4] In addition, serum IgG light chain can be measured with a free light chain assay (Freelite). This assay has several advantages compared with serum protein and urine electrophoresis, particularly increased sensitivity, and the free light chain ratio that may add valuable information on likelihood of disease progression.[19]

As discussed earlier, the skeleton is involved at the time of diagnosis in most patients with MM.[4,8] The effects of MM on the skeleton result from the abnormal production of cytokines, including IL-1, IL-6, tumor necrosis factor-α (TNF-α), and the receptor for activation of NF-κB ligand (RANK-L). Bone disease is the net effect of the activation of osteoclasts and inhibition of osteoblastogenesis.[20]

CLINICAL PRESENTATION Multiple Myeloma

General Criteria

- 80% of patients present with symptomatic disease

Signs and Symptoms

- Bone pain (fractures, lytic lesions)
- Fatigue (anemia)
- Infection (reduced polyclonal response)
- Neurologic symptoms (nerve compression)
- Polyuria (hypercalcemia)
- Nausea and vomiting (hypercalcemia)

Laboratory Parameters

- Elevated paraproteins
  - Plasma electrophoresis
  - Urine electrophoresis
  - Immunofixation
- Elevated serum creatinine
- Hypercalcemia
- Low hemoglobin
- Low albumin
- Elevated β_2-microglobulin
- Elevated C-reactive protein

Bone Marrow

- ≥10% plasma cells

Cytogenetics

- Chromosome 13 deletion
- Translocation (4;14)
- Del (17p)

In addition, patients are frequently anemic from infiltration of the bone marrow with the MM clone and poor erythropoietin response. Patients can have clinically important hypercalcemia, which results from calcium mobilization from the bone. Renal failure can occur as a result of high protein load from the monoclonal protein secretion as well as dehydration.

STAGING AND PROGNOSTIC FACTORS

Some patients with MM are asymptomatic and have no evidence of end-organ damage at the time of diagnosis. As discussed previously, these patients are categorized as having smoldering (asymptomatic) MM.[21] Most patients have evidence of end-organ damage (hypercalcemia [>10.5 g/dL (>2.63 mmol/L)], renal impairment [>2.0 mg/dL (>177 μmol/L)], anemia [<10 g/dL (<100 g/L; 6.21 mmol/L) or >2 g/dL (>20 g/L; 1.24 mmol/L) below normal]), or bone disease at the time of diagnosis and are categorized as having active (symptomatic) disease. Patients with asymptomatic disease have an indolent course with a median survival time of about 5 years.[11,21]

The International Staging System (ISS) uses serum β_2-microglobulin and albumin concentrations to stage patients.[22] These two routine laboratory tests are powerful prognostic discriminators. The ISS predicts survival in patients treated with either conventional treatment or autologous hematopoietic stem cell transplantation (HSCT). An older staging system, Durie-Salmon, uses hemoglobin, serum calcium, bone involvement, and M protein to categorize patients in one of three stages. Table 113-1 describes the ISS and median survival times for each of the three ISS stages.

TABLE 113-1 The International Staging System for Multiple Myeloma

Stage	Characteristics	Median Survival (mo)
I	Serum β_2-microglobulin <3.5 mcg/mL Serum albumin ≥3.5 g/dL	62
II	Not stage I or stage III	44
III	Serum β_2-microglobulin ≥5.5 mcg/mL	29

From Greipp PR, Miguel JS, Durie BG, et al. International staging system for multiple myeloma. J Clin Oncol 2005;23:3412–3420.

Several adverse prognostic factors have been proposed for MM, including chromosome 13 deletion and other cytogenetic abnormalities (e.g., 17p deletion, t(4,14)), elevated β_2-microglobulin, elevated C-reactive protein, high plasma cell labeling index, low albumin, and high bone marrow microvessel density.[1,4,8] These prognostic factors generally represent the underlying pathologic changes associated with MM, including genetic damage (chromosome 13 and 17 abnormalities), proinflammatory changes (C-reactive protein), tumor load (β_2-microglobulin), and dysregulated cellular growth (labeling index and marrow microvessel density).

TREATMENT

Desired Outcomes

❸ The current goal of therapy in MM is to prolong progression-free survival (PFS) and overall survival and improve quality of life. The initial goal of induction therapy in newly diagnosed patients with more active (symptomatic) and advanced disease (stages II and III) is to obtain at least a major response.[4,8,18] This is usually followed by consolidation and maintenance therapy, both of which can extend and often improve induction responses. With the integration of novel agents into therapy, PFS and overall survival have steadily improved, and responses have increased in frequency, depth, and duration. Unfortunately, there is no convincing evidence that patients are cured of their disease.

General Approach

In asymptomatic patients with smoldering MM, watchful waiting is the most common practice despite a systematic review that suggests early treatment with chemotherapy slows disease progression and may decrease vertebral compression.[11,21] The benefits of chemotherapy in this setting are generally offset by the absence of convincing evidence that early treatment improves overall survival and the risk of treatment-related adverse events. With the availability of new novel agents, progression of this form of MM may be delayed. The National Comprehensive Cancer Network (NCCN) guidelines currently recommend watchful waiting for smoldering MM.[23]

Initial management of symptomatic MM depends on the presence or absence of high-risk features of the disease (i.e., cytogenetics),

TABLE 113-2 Drug Therapy in Newly Diagnosed Multiple Myeloma

Induction Regimen	Level of Evidence
Regimens in Non–Autologous HSCT Candidates	**Category[a]**
Dexamethasone	2B
Vincristine plus doxorubicin plus dexamethasone	2B
Lenalidomide plus LD dexamethasone	1
Lipo doxorubicin + vincristine + dexamethasone (DVD)	2B
Thalidomide plus dexamethasone	2B
Bortezomib plus dexamethasone	2A
Melphalan + prednisone (MP)	2A
Melphalan + prednisone + thalidomide (MPT)	1
Melphalan + prednisone + bortezomib (MPB)	1
Melphalan + prednisone + lenalidomide (MPL)	1
Regimens in Autologous HSCT Candidates	
Dexamethasone	2B
Thalidomide + dexamethasone	2B
Liposomal doxorubicin + vincristine + dexamethasone (DVD)	2B
Lenalidomide + dexamethasone	1
Bortezomib + dexamethasone	1
Bortezomib + cyclophosphamide + dexamethasone	2A
Bortezomib + doxorubicin + dexamethasone	1
Bortezomib + thalidomide + dexamethasone	1
Bortezomib + lenalidomide + dexamethasone	2A

HSCT, hematopoietic stem cell transplantation.

[a]Category 1: Uniform National Comprehensive Cancer Network (NCCN) consensus based on high-level evidence. Category 2A: Uniform NCCN consensus based on lower evidence, including clinical experience. Category 2B: Nonuniform NCCN consensus but no major disagreement.

Data from NCCN Guidelines NCCN. Clinical Practice Guidelines in Oncology. Multiple Myeloma. Version 2014. 2014, http://www.NCCN.org.

TABLE 113-3 Definition of Clinical Response in Multiple Myeloma

Type of Response	Definition[a]
Partial response (PR)	• ≥50% decrease in serum M protein • Reduction in 24-hour urine light chain by ≥90%
Very good partial remission (vgPR)	• Serum and urine M protein detected on immunofixation but not electrophoresis
Complete remission (CR)	• Negative immunofixation on serum and urine • No soft tissue plasmacytomas
Stringent complete response (sCR)	• <5% plasma cells in the bone marrow • CR definition • Normal free light chain ratio • Absence of clonal cells in the bone marrow

[a]Maintained for a minimum of 6 weeks.

patient age, renal function, performance status, and whether autologous HSCT is planned. Although current treatments are not curative, the median survival time has increased significantly from about 7 months to 24 to 36 months in high-risk disease patients and 6 to 7 years or more in patients with standard-risk disease, primarily as a result of improved treatment of symptomatic MM and supportive care.[4,23]

All patients with symptomatic MM are treated with initial induction therapy. Although there is no standard initial or induction therapy, the regimens differ depending on whether the patient is a candidate for autologous HSCT (Table 113-2). The age restriction for autologous HSCT has changed because of low transplant-related mortality, but autologous HSCT is generally reserved for patients younger than 65 years of age.

For many years, the choice of induction therapy in autologous HSCT candidates included VAD (vincristine, doxorubicin, and dexamethasone) as the standard therapy. In the last 10 years, combination regimens such as dexamethasone combined with thalidomide, lenalidomide, or bortezomib and dexamethasone combined with bortezomib and lenalidomide or thalidomide have become common. The use of VAD chemotherapy before autologous HSCT is now obsolete given data that suggest superior outcomes in patients receiving newer drug combinations.[23,24]

The Mayo Clinic recommends a risk-adapted approach to initial therapy in which treatment is guided by cytogenetics and gene expression profiling.[25] In contrast to the single institution guidelines of Mayo Clinic, the NCCN recommendations are based on the opinions of experts from many nationally recognized cancer centers (Table 113-2).[23] The Mayo Clinic and NCCN guidelines both recommend the use of newer novel agents as initial therapy; these guidelines are discussed later in Recommendations for Initial Therapy section.

Induction therapy is usually continued until maximum response is achieved. Patients who are candidates for autologous HSCT then undergo hematopoietic stem cell collection. Most patients undergo autologous HSCT at that time, but some patients may decide to delay the procedure. Patients who are not candidates for autologous HSCT usually receive several cycles of consolidation therapy, although the optimal duration of therapy after maximum response is achieved is unknown. Single-agent maintenance therapy may be given in both transplant-eligible and -ineligible patients.

Clinical response to therapy is generally defined by a reduction in paraprotein in blood and urine.[4] Clinical complete remission (CR) is defined as elimination of plasma paraprotein as measured by electrophoresis and immunofixation and plasma cells (≤5%) in the bone marrow. A specialized type of complete remission, called stringent complete response (sCR), is defined by normal free light chain and negative immunofixation. Complete remissions are uncommon in MM, and lesser responses, including partial response (PR), near complete response (nCR), and very good partial response (VGPR), are more commonly attained. Although the nCR term is less commonly used in current trials, it was used in several important studies. These lesser responses can be important because they may correlate with improved survival. Table 113-3 describes the most common types of responses that are used clinically.[23]

Pharmacotherapy of Multiple Myeloma

The current treatment of MM relies heavily on integration of novel agents, including thalidomide, lenalidomide, bortezomib, carfilzomib, and pomalidomide. These novel agents have revolutionized the treatment of MM, greatly increasing responses and survival with acceptable but different toxicity profiles compared with conventional chemotherapy-based regimens previously used in MM. Tables 113-4 and 113-5 show dosing and monitoring parameters for the novel agents used in the treatment of MM. Dose reductions in elderly patients and in patients with adverse events are often required.[24]

Conventional Chemotherapy

As previously discussed, two of the common conventional chemotherapy regimens used historically to treat MM are melphalan plus prednisone (MP) and VAD.[4,26] Despite more active combinations, MP and VAD remain listed as options as initial therapy in patients with MM.[23] Because conventional-dose melphalan has an adverse effect on stem cell mobilization and subsequent autologous HSCT, the use of melphalan is limited to patients ineligible for autologous

TABLE 113-4 Dosing of Novel Agents in Multiple Myeloma

Drug (Brand Name)	Initial Dose	Usual Dose	Special Population
Thalidomide (Thalidomide®)	50–100 mg/day	200 mg/day	Start low in elderly adults; increase dose every 1–3 weeks
Lenalidomide (Revlimid®)	10–25 mg/day Days 1–21 (28-day cycle) Days 1–28 (35 day cycle)	25 mg/day	Adjust dose in renal impairment: 30–60 mL/min (10 mg every 24 h) <30 mL/min (15 mg every 48 h) <30 mL/min (dialysis) (5 mg every 24 h)
Bortezomib (Velcade®)	1.3 mg/m² Days 1, 4, 8, and 11 Every 21 days		Reduce initial dose in hepatic impairment (serum bilirubin >1.5x ULN) to 0.7 mg/m²
Carfilzomib (Kyprolis®)	20/m² given on days 1, 2, 8, 9, 15, and 16 of a 28-day cycle	27 mg/m²	
Pomalidomide (Pomalyst®)	4 mg/day for 21 days (28-day cycle)		

ULN, upper limit of the normal range.

HSCT. Melphalan has also been associated with the development of myelodysplastic syndromes.[27] The original use of VAD chemotherapy as initial treatment became more common because of these concerns with melphalan. However, the slightly higher response rates with VAD and similar combination chemotherapy did not translate into improved survival compared with MP, and VAD is now rarely used in MM.[23]

Because dexamethasone accounts for most of the antimyeloma activity of VAD (Table 113-6), dexamethasone was used alone as initial therapy. However, one study reported that MP produced similar response rates and survival compared with dexamethasone. The higher rate of infection and central nervous system toxicity in patients treated with dexamethasone led these investigators to conclude that high-dose dexamethasone be used with caution as initial therapy, particularly in older patients.[28] In current regimens, newer agents (thalidomide, bortezomib, lenalidomide, carfilzomib) are combined with dexamethasone or the MP backbone to maximize initial response rates.[4,8,23,26,29] Doxorubicin, which also is included in VAD chemotherapy, is recognized as highly active antimyeloma chemotherapy. Current regimens can combine doxorubicin in the liposomal form with various novel agents producing regimens with some of the highest responses seen in MM patients.

Thalidomide (Thalomid)

Thalidomide was first used clinically in Europe in the late 1950s as a sedative and antiemetic but its use was largely abandoned when teratogenicity was reported. Its immunomodulatory effects became evident with its use in Hansen disease (or leprosy), and it continues to be used for this rare indication. These clinical benefits are thought to be related to the anti-TNF activity of thalidomide. As a result of the role of inflammatory cytokines in the pathophysiology of MM, thalidomide was first studied in refractory MM in 1999. The observation that thalidomide had activity against myeloma rejuvenated it as an important therapeutic agent.[30]

Thalidomide and other IMiDs have multiple immune effects, including inhibition of inflammatory mediators, antiangiogenic activity, and T cell–modulating activity. Thalidomide destabilizes TNF-α messenger RNA, which leads to increased destruction of the transcripts and reduction in TNF-α production. One potential explanation for thalidomide's antimyeloma activity is inhibition of TNF-mediated NF-κB activation, which results in increased apoptosis of the MM clone. Thalidomide also has TNF-independent effects on NFκB; it protects the cytosolic inhibitor of NFκB (IκB) and prevents signal transduction to the nucleus, resulting in a decline in MM growth factors.[30,31]

Myeloma bone marrow has a high rate of neovascularization, which makes it susceptible to antiangiogenic therapy. Bone marrow microvessel density has been identified as an independent prognostic factor in MM.[32] One explanation for the angiogenesis that occurs in MM is the paracrine release of TNF-α by the myeloma clone and bone marrow stromal cells, which leads to the release of angiogenic factors, including vascular endothelial growth factor (VEGF), IL-8, basic fibroblast growth factor, and IL-1, through NF-κB induction. Thalidomide treatment can reduce bone marrow microvessel density, which may contribute to its antimyeloma activity.

The role of TNF-α inhibition is supported by the observation that TNF-α polymorphisms may predict for thalidomide response in patients with MM.[33] High producers of TNF-α had significantly

TABLE 113-5 Adverse Reactions and Monitoring Parameters for Novel Agents in Multiple Myeloma

Drug	Adverse Drug Reactions	Monitoring Parameters	Comments
Thalidomide	Neuropathy, sedations, constipation, VTE, rash, neutropenia, teratogenicity	Neurologic examination, active bowel sounds, CBC, STEPS Program	Evening dose to ↓ sedation Laxatives VTE prophylaxis
Lenalidomide	Myelosuppression, rash	CBC, renal function, REMS	Adjust dose in renal impairment VTE prophylaxis
Pomalidomide	Myelosuppression, rash, VTE, teratogenicity	CBC, REMS	
Bortezomib	Myelosuppression, neuropathy, infection gastrointestinal	CBC, neurologic examination	VZV prophylaxis
Carfilzomib	Myelosuppression, infection	CBC, fluid status, serum chemistries	Hydration to reduce risk of renal toxicity and TLS Dexamethasone premedication for infusion reactions VZV prophylaxis

CBC, complete blood count; REMS, Risk Evaluation and Mitigation Strategy; STEPS, System for Thalidomide Education and Prescribing Safety; TLS, tumor lysis syndrome; VTE, venous thromboembolism; VZV, varicella zoster.

TABLE 113-6 Initial Therapies for Multiple Myeloma

	Type of Response (%)		
Regimen	OR	CR	CR/nCR/VgPR
Melphalan + prednisone	40–50		5–10
Dexamethasone	40–50		
Thalidomide	34–40		
Thalidomide + dexamethasone	50–70	5–10	20–30
Melphalan, prednisone, and thalidomide	50–80	5–25	20–50
VAD chemotherapy	50–60		
Doxorubicin combinations + thalidomide	70–90		40–50
Single autoHSCT	80–90		40–50
Tandem autoHSCT	80–90		30–50
AutoHSCT followed by RI-alloHSCT	80–90		60
Bortezomib	40–50		12
Bortezomib + dexamethasone	80–90		20–30
Bortezomib + chemotherapy	80–98	10–30	43
Bortezomib + thalidomide + dexamethasone	85–95	20–35	50–60
Bortezomib + lenalidomide + dexamethasone	100		50–74
Lenalidomide + LD dexamethasone	70		40
Lenalidomide + high-dose dexamethasone	80		50
Clarithromycin + lenalidomide + dexamethasone	93	43	68
Lenalidomide + chemotherapy	80	15–25	
Carfilzomib + Lenalidomide + LD dexamethasone	98	42 (sCR)	81

alloHSCT, allogeneic hematopoietic stem cell transplantation; autoHSCT, autologous hematopoietic stem cell transplantation; CR, complete response; OR, overall response (at least partial response); RI, reduced intensity; LD, low dose; sCR, stringent complete response; VAD, vincristine, doxorubicin, and dexamethasone.

higher response rates and improved survival with thalidomide therapy compared with patients without the hypersecretory phenotype. These results may be explained by inhibition of TNF-α as a required growth factor in patients with the TNF-α hypersecretory phenotype. The authors commented that larger studies are required to confirm and explain these results. Figure 113-1 shows that thalidomide inhibits proliferation and angiogenesis, stimulates T lymphocytes, and modifies the cytokine-secreting ability of bone marrow stromal cells.

Single-agent thalidomide has been extensively evaluated in refractory MM in which it produces overall response rates (including minor responses) in about 30% of patients.[34] Although minor and partial responses are the most common types of responses, these end points are associated with improved survival.[35]

With the activity of thalidomide in refractory MM established, subsequent studies evaluated its activity in newly diagnosed patients and in combination with other therapies, including dexamethasone and chemotherapy. Partial response rates with single-agent thalidomide in untreated patients are about 30% to 40%.[36] When dexamethasone is added to thalidomide in untreated patients, response rates (≥PR) increase to about 70% to 80%.[37] The higher response rate with thalidomide plus dexamethasone has made this an attractive combination for initial therapy. However, the higher rate of thromboembolism with this combination (15%–20%) when used in newly diagnosed patients is a concern.[37,38]

❹ The addition of thalidomide to chemotherapy also increases response rates (Table 113-6). Three published randomized controlled trials in newly diagnosed MM showed that the addition of thalidomide to MP improved response.[39,40] In the first randomized trial, the overall CR rate with melphalan, prednisone, and thalidomide (MPT) was about 15% compared with 4% with MP. With a median follow-up time of about 3 years, patients in the MPT group had significantly improved PFS but not overall survival.[39] The second randomized trial was stopped early because MPT showed clear improvements over the other treatment arm. Results of this trial reported significantly improved median PFS (27.5 vs. 17.8 months) and overall survival (51.6 vs. 33.2 months) with MPT compared with MP.[40] A third trial compared MPT with MP in patients older than 75 years of age. Patients on MPT had superior PFS and overall survival at the cost of increased peripheral neuropathy and neutropenia.[41] Based on these impressive results, some have previously recommended that MPT be the new standard induction therapy in older patients ineligible for autologous HSCT. However, it is not possible to define a single standard regimen in this setting because of the number of highly active combination regimens and the lack of head-to-head comparative trials. The increased response rate of MPT is at the expense of higher rates of grades 3 and 4 toxicity, particularly venous thromboembolism (VTE), peripheral neuropathy, and infection.[40,41]

The combination of thalidomide, dexamethasone, and pegylated liposomal doxorubicin produces a high overall response rate of 98% and a complete remission rate of 34%. The major grades 3 and 4 toxicities were VTE (14%) and infection (22%). However, toxicity was acceptable, even in patients older than 65 years of age.[42] Although the activity of doxorubicin and thalidomide compares favorably with other combinations, one disadvantage of this regimen is that pegylated liposomal doxorubicin requires IV administration.

Thalidomide dose correlates with response and toxicity. In one large trial of single-agent thalidomide, a higher response rate was observed when more than 42 g of thalidomide was administered over a 3-month period, which is equivalent to a daily dose of about 450 mg.[35] As expected, the higher dose was associated with higher rates of thalidomide-related toxicity. When thalidomide is combined with chemotherapy, thalidomide doses of 100 mg/day are associated with high CR rates.[39,42,43] Neuropathy, one of the important dose-limiting toxicities, may correlate with cumulative thalidomide doses. Thalidomide-induced neuropathy is usually, but not always, reversible and is associated with demyelinating changes in peripheral neurons. About 10% to 20% of patients are unable to tolerate thalidomide, and neuropathy is often the toxicity associated with discontinuation of therapy.[35,41] Unfortunately, no effective methods have been identified to prevent or treat thalidomide-induced neuropathy.

Other common toxicities associated with thalidomide include constipation, sedation, and rash. Although these toxicities can be problematic, they rarely require discontinuation of thalidomide treatment. Stimulant laxatives can be used to prevent severe constipation. The severity of constipation and sedation declines over time in many patients.[44]

The rate of VTE with single-agent thalidomide is relatively low (<5%) and may not exceed the baseline incidence for MM patients. VTE prophylaxis is not recommended in patients receiving single-agent thalidomide.[44] When thalidomide is combined with dexamethasone, MP, or doxorubicin, the risk of thrombosis is elevated. The underlying mechanism for thrombosis in these patients is unknown, but rates in several studies of combination therapy were as high as 10% to 30%.[39–41,45] VTE prophylaxis is recommended and potential preventive strategies include therapeutic doses of warfarin, fixed-dose warfarin, low-molecular-weight heparin (LMWH), or aspirin depending on the patient's risk for VTE. Fixed-dose warfarin and 100 mg aspirin was recently compared with LMWH in MM patients on thalidomide combinations. Fixed-dose warfarin and 100 mg aspirin showed similar efficacy to LMWH in lowering a composite measure of VTE and cardiac events. However, when only grade 3 to 4 VTEs were evaluated, aspirin prophylaxis was similar to LMWH, but fixed-dose warfarin was inferior.[46] Warfarin is not a popular choice for VTE prophylaxis because fixed-dose warfarin remains controversial, and therapeutic warfarin is associated with bleeding complications. The evidence suggests low-dose aspirin is effective prophylaxis, but it should be reserved for patients in whom

LMWH is not feasible and in whom there is a low to moderate risk of developing VTE.[45–47]

Bortezomib (Velcade®)

5 Bortezomib is a proteasome inhibitor approved for use in newly diagnosed and relapsed or refractory MM. The proteasome is a protease complex responsible for degrading cytosolic proteins that are conjugated to ubiquitin. Ubiquitin is a 8.5-kD polypeptide that tags various proteins for destruction.[48] By reversibly binding to the chymotrypsin site in the catalytic core of the 26S proteasome, bortezomib inhibits the degradation of these targeted proteins.

In MM, NF-κB activity is increased, resulting in increased transcription of inflammatory cytokines such as IL-6 and TNF-α, which are involved in the pathogenesis and progression of MM. In the cytosol, NF-κB is bound to and inhibited by IκB. The proteasome degrades IκB. When the proteasome is inhibited with bortezomib, cytosolic concentrations of IκB remain high, and NF-κB is retained in the cytosol as an inactive complex. The resulting inhibition of the NF-κB signal leads to a reduction in cytokine production and growth inhibition of the MM clone. Other proteins involved in cell-cycle regulation and apoptotic signaling that may be affected by bortezomib include p53, JNK proteins, and caspase 3.[48]

In phase I studies in patients with refractory hematologic malignancies, bortezomib was administered twice weekly for 2 consecutive weeks followed by 1 week of rest. The responses observed in those studies included a CR in one of eight patients who completed the first course of therapy and minor responses in two patients. These responses were impressive for a phase I trial and confirmed the promising activity in preclinical studies.[49]

Patients with refractory MM were then enrolled in a phase II trial and received 1.3 mg/m^2 of bortezomib twice weekly for 2 weeks followed by 1 week of rest. Patients received up to 8 cycles. The overall response rate was 35% (includes minor responses) with seven (3.6%) patients achieving a CR.[50] Based on the phase I and II studies, bortezomib was approved in May 2003 under the Food and Drug Administration's (FDA's) accelerated approval process for relapsed or refractory MM in patients who had failed at least two prior therapies.

Subsequently, a large phase III study (Assessment of Proteasome Inhibition for Extending Remissions [APEX] trial) demonstrated that bortezomib had superior activity compared with high-dose dexamethasone in relapsed MM.[51] Bortezomib-treated patients had higher complete and partial response rates (38% vs. 18%), longer median time to progression (6.2 vs. 3.5 months), and improved 1-year overall survival (80% vs. 66%) compared with patients receiving dexamethasone. The differences in each of these end points were statistically significant. The results from this study led to expanded FDA approval in 2005 to include patients who had relapsed after one therapy.

Combination therapy with bortezomib has shown promising results in relapsed MM. It was reported that relapsed patients who had suboptimal response to bortezomib alone may respond after the addition of dexamethasone. Subsequent studies reported improved results with the combination of bortezomib and corticosteroids with the CR and nCR rate ranging between 5% and 15%.[52] The inclusion of bortezomib in three- to four-drug combinations, which may include doxorubicin, melphalan, thalidomide, and lenalidomide, produce CR and nCR rates of 10% to 50% in relapsed MM.[48,52]

A number of studies have investigated bortezomib in newly diagnosed patients (Table 113-6). Bortezomib alone produces about a 40% response rate with about 3% of patients obtaining a complete remission. When combined with dexamethasone, the overall response rate increases to about 90% (CR plus PR) with CR rates of 5% to 20%.[53,54] In a phase II study of bortezomib combined with MP (MPB) in newly diagnosed elderly MM patients, the overall response rates of 89% and CR rates of 32% are among the highest reported rates with induction therapies.[55] Subsequently, MPB was compared with MP in the large phase III VISTA (Velcade as Initial Standard Therapy in multiple myeloma) trial. The overall response and CR rates, time to progression, and overall survival were significantly better in the MPB group. Based on these results, bortezomib received FDA approval in 2008 as first-line therapy in newly diagnosed patients with MM. The improvement in response came at the expense of greater serious adverse effects, including neuropathy, gastrointestinal toxicity, and herpes zoster. However, treatment-related mortality was not different between MPB and MP groups.[56] An update of this study reported a continued survival benefit after 5 years of follow-up.[57]

Bortezomib can cause significant toxicity, the most common being mild to moderate fatigue and gastrointestinal toxicities. Neuropathy occurs frequently and is the most common cause of discontinuation of therapy. In the VISTA trial, the rate of neuropathy was 44% in the MPB group versus 5% in the MP group.[56] However, the MPB and MP groups had similar rates of therapy discontinuation at about 15%. Other important toxicities included thrombocytopenia, fever, neutropenia, and infection. An increased risk of shingles has been reported in bortezomib-treated patients, and the NCCN guidelines recommend that herpes zoster prophylaxis be considered.[23] VTE prophylaxis is not required with bortezomib when it is combined with MP based on the results of the VISTA trial, which reported low rates of VTE and nearly identical rates in the MPB versus MP group.[56]

Bortezomib plus dexamethasone has more recently been added to cyclophosphamide or lenalidomide, resulting in high response rates and improved PFS.[25] The use of bortezomib has become more convenient with the new subcutaneous regimens.[58] In a phase III trial in relapsed MM, therapeutic equivalence was found between IV and subcutaneous routes of administration.[58,59] In addition, subcutaneous administration offers the potential advantage of administration in patients without IV access and perhaps improved safety profile, particularly less peripheral neuropathy.

Lenalidomide (Revlimid®)

6 Lenalidomide is a thalidomide analog that shares a similar mechanism of action with thalidomide but is significantly more potent. Because of differences in the toxicity profile compared with thalidomide, the use of lenalidomide has increased. In phase I studies, patients with relapsed, refractory MM were found to have a maximum tolerated dose of lenalidomide of 25 mg/day, and this dose was the most commonly used dose in subsequent phase II and III studies.[60]

The addition of lenalidomide to high-dose dexamethasone has been shown to increase response rate and prolong survival in patients with relapsed MM. In 2006, lenalidomide received FDA approval in relapsed-refractory MM based on the results of two randomized controlled trials.[61,62] One trial was conducted in North America, and the other trial was conducted outside of North America. In both trials, patients were randomized to receive a combination of either lenalidomide (25 mg/day on days 1 to 21 of a 28-day cycle) and high-dose dexamethasone or an identical lenalidomide placebo and high-dose dexamethasone. In the North American trial, patients in the lenalidomide and dexamethasone group had overall and CR rates of 61% and 14% compared with 20% and 0.6% in the dexamethasone alone group ($P < 0.001$).[61] These improved response rates translated into longer median overall survival time in the lenalidomide and dexamethasone group (29.6 vs. 20.5 months). Similar results were reported in the trial conducted outside of the United States.[62]

Lenalidomide has been extensively studied as initial therapy in newly diagnosed MM (Table 113-6). Preliminary results of phase I and phase II studies of lenalidomide plus dexamethasone report an overall response rate of 90% and a CR rate of 18%.[63] These rates may be higher than those reported with thalidomide plus dexamethasone.

Lenalidomide causes less neurotoxicity and constipation but more myelosuppression than thalidomide.[64] When used as part of combination therapy, the risk of VTE with lenalidomide is similar to that observed with thalidomide, and VTE prophylaxis is recommended. Results from a phase III trial in newly diagnosed MM reported that patients randomized to lenalidomide plus high-dose dexamethasone had a 26% incidence of VTE compared with a 12% rate in those randomized to the lenalidomide plus low-dose dexamethasone arm.[65,66] That trial also reported a superior 2-year overall survival rate in the lenalidomide plus low-dose dexamethasone group (87% vs. 75%), and this regimen could become the new standard induction regimen for older patients ineligible for autologous HSCT. The improved survival in the low-dose dexamethasone arm is related to lower mortality from adverse events, particularly VTE. Excess deaths in the high-dose dexamethasone group usually occurred in the first 4 months and in elderly patients. The low risk of VTE in the lenalidomide plus low-dose dexamethasone arm may allow for VTE prophylaxis with low-dose aspirin alone.[65,66] These results have led to a category 1 NCCN recommendation in MM patients not eligible for transplant.[23]

Carfilzomib (Kyprolis®)

7 Carfilzomib is the first second-generation proteasome inhibitor to receive accelerated approval from the FDA in July 2012 as treatment for patients with MM who have received at least two prior therapies, including bortezomib and an immunomodulatory agent, and have demonstrated disease progression on or within 60 days of the completion of the last therapy.

The schedules for administration of carfilzomib are based on the results of preclinical and phase I and II studies and are different from those for bortezomib. Based on studies in preclinical murine models, which showed more potent, yet tolerable, proteasome inhibition with two consecutive daily doses, carfilzomib entered phase I clinical testing with two schedules: 5 consecutive days of 14-day cycle and 2 consecutive days weekly of a 28-day cycle.[67–69] The schedule that used 2 consecutive days of dosing showed better tolerability and allowed increases in carfilzomib doses. A subsequent multivariate analysis of three phase II trials showed a dose–response relationship in MM patients. The initial study used a 20 mg/m^2 fixed dose in every cycle and showed fourfold less response when compared with increasing to 27 mg/m^2 in the following cycle in patients who could tolerate the initial dose.[70] Collectively, subsequent clinical trials have generally adopted the administration schedule of day 1, 2, 8, 9, 15, 16, 22, and 23 of 28-day cycles with carfilzomib, starting at 20 mg/m^2 IV over 2 to 10 minutes on the first cycle/week and increased to 27 mg/m^2 or more afterward depending on tolerability. In addition, the results from phase Ib/II studies showed that prolonged infusion (30 min) is better tolerated and that the carfilzomib dose can be increased up to 56 mg/m^2.[71]

The most mature safety data for carfilzomib comes from the compiled results of three phase II studies. The most frequently reported adverse events included fatigue (55%), anemia (47%), nausea (45%), thrombocytopenia (36%), dyspnea (35%), diarrhea (33%), and pyrexia (30%). The most common grade 3 or greater adverse events were thrombocytopenia (23%), anemia (22%), lymphopenia (18%), pneumonia (11%), and neutropenia (10%). Grade 2 elevation of creatinine was reported in 25% of patients and was improved with the use of hydration and dexamethasone as premedication. Most of these events were manageable.[72]

The single-agent activity of carfilzomib is based on phase II studies of 266 relapsed and refractory MM patients who had received a median of five previous therapies.[73] Patients received carfilzomib 20 mg/m^2 IV over 2 to 10 minutes twice weekly on 2 consecutive days with dexamethasone premedication for 3 of 4 weeks in cycle 1 and then 27 mg/m^2 in subsequent cycles until disease progression, unacceptable toxicity, or completion of a maximum of 12 cycles. The primary end point of overall response rate (≥PR) was 22.9%, and the median duration of response was 7.8 months (95% confidence interval [CI] 5.6–9.2 months). In patients who were refractory or intolerant to both bortezomib and lenalidomide, 37% obtained clinical benefit. In patients refractory to both bortezomib and lenalidomide, the overall response rate (≥PR) was 15.4%. Moreover, unfavorable cytogenetic characteristics did not appear to adversely impact response rates. The median overall survival time was 15.6 months compared with the median of 9 months typically seen in this setting. An additional large multicenter trial in relapsed/refractory MM patients investigated variable dosing in bortezomib-naïve patients and those previously treated with bortezomib; the overall response rate reported as 52.2% in bortezomib-naïve patients in the 20/27 mg/m^2 dose cohort.[74] Importantly, these studies demonstrated that carfilzomib had a rapid time to response (0.5–1.0 months).[74,75]

The activity of carfilzomib combination regimens as first-line treatment is impressive. A phase I/II study of carfilzomib in combination with lenalidomide and dexamethasone enrolled 53 newly diagnosed patients treated with carfilzomib 20, 20/27, or 20/36 mg/m^2 in phase I and expansion to phase II at a 20/36 mg/m^2 dose.[76] The overall response rate (≥PR) was 94%. The responses were rapid and increased in depth with additional cycles of therapy, with 62% and 42% of patients achieving a CR and sCR, respectively. In 36 patients who completed induction, 78% reached at least nCR and 61% sCR. At a median follow-up time of 13 months, the estimated 24-month PFS was 92%. The three-drug regimen did not adversely affect stem cell collection, but was associated with peripheral neuropathy, which was predominately grade 1 or 2 and observed in 23% of patients.

Three randomized phase III trials are ongoing in relapsed myeloma. The **CA**rfilzomib, Lenalidomide, and Dexametha**S**one versus Lenalidomide and Dexamethasone for the treatment of **P**at**I**ents with **R**elapsed Multiple My**E**loma (ASPIRE) trial compares lenalidomide and dexamethasone with lenalidomide, dexamethasone, and carfilzomib; the Car**F**ilz**O**mib for Advan**C**ed Refractory M**U**ltiple Myeloma European **S**tudy (FOCUS) trial compares carfilzomib monotherapy to best supportive care; and the Randomiz**E**d, Ope**N**Label, Phase 3 Study of Carfilzomib Plus **DE**xameth**A**sone **V**s Bortezomib Plus Dexamethas**O**ne in Patients with **R**elapsed Multiple Myeloma (ENDEAVOR) trial compares carfilzomib and dexamethasone with bortezomib and dexamethasone.

Drugs in Development

7 Pomalidomide is the newest in the immunomodulatory class of antimyeloma drugs. It was recently granted accelerated approval by the FDA in relapsed MM. In a phase II trial, the combination of pomalidomide with dexamethasone produced good overall response rates (35%) in heavily pretreated relapsed and refractory MM. Toxicity profile was reasonable and consisted mainly of manageable myelosuppression. Pomalidomide is currently being evaluated in phase III trials.[77]

Recommendations for Initial Therapy

8 The Mayo Clinic Guidelines uses a risk-adapted approach that categorizes patients into risk groups based on cytogenetics and gene expression profiling. In high-risk patients, the combination of bortezomib, lenalidomide, and dexamethasone is recommended as induction therapy.[25] In intermediate-risk patients, the combination of bortezomib, cyclophosphamide, and dexamethasone is recommended as induction therapy. In both high- and intermediate-risk patients, induction therapy for 4 months is recommended in transplant-eligible patients and for 1 year in transplant-ineligible patients. In the largest group, standard-risk patients, lenalidomide and low-dose dexamethasone or bortezomib, cyclophosphamide, and dexamethasone are recommended for 4 cycles in transplant-eligible patients followed by transplant, but transplant can be delayed

depending on patient preference. Transplant-ineligible standard-risk patients should receive lenalidomide and low-dose dexamethasone, with dexamethasone dose reduction or discontinuation after 1 year Other options for induction therapy in these patients is MPT or a bortezomib-based regimen (in patients with renal insufficiency). Many patients receive maintenance therapy with bortezomib or lenalidomide after transplant (in transplant-eligible patients) or induction therapy (in transplant-ineligible patients).

Initial therapy in the NCCN guidelines is based on transplant eligibility. In patients ineligible for autologous HSCT, thalidomide, lenalidomide, or bortezomib is added to chemotherapy as initial therapy. MP forms the backbone to which these newer drugs are added if the patient is not a candidate for autologous HSCT. As previously discussed, MPT produces high response rates, and MPB produce equal or better results.[37] Based on the results of phase III trials demonstrating superiority of MPT over MP, many suggested that MPT was the preferred induction regimen in patients who were ineligible for autologous HSCT. However, the results of the VISTA trial, the continuous lenalidomide trial, in which MPL induction is followed by lenalidomide maintenance, and a phase II trial comparing MP with MPL in newly diagnosed patients supports the addition of MPB and MPL as two additional preferred induction regimens.[56,78,79] MPB, MPL, and MPT are listed as NCCN category 1 recommendations.[23] Bortezomib-containing regimens (i.e., MPB) may be particularly useful in MM patients with high-risk cytogenetics (t(4;14), 17p-). The preferred combination (MPT, MPB, or MPL) is currently unclear and will require randomized controlled trials that compare these combinations. Carfilzomib-based therapy will have an important role in heavily pretreated refractory MM and is being evaluated in ongoing phase III trials as induction therapy for newly diagnosed MM patients.

If autologous HSCT is planned after induction therapy, melphalan should be avoided, and thalidomide, bortezomib, or lenalidomide can be added to dexamethasone or VAD-like chemotherapy. The NCCN guidelines list several induction therapy options (Table 113-2). Because there is no standard induction regimen, clinicians can select from a wide range of possible induction regimens.[29] Many clinicians recommend lenalidomide or bortezomib and dexamethasone as two-drug induction regimens or bortezomib, dexamethasone, and either cyclophosphamide, doxorubicin, or lenalidomide as three-drug regimens for patients who are autologous HSCT candidates.

8 Patients with high-risk cytogenetics may benefit from bortezomib-containing induction regimens because of its activity in these high-risk patients.[14,25] Because patients with high-risk cytogenetics may have poorer outcomes after autologous HSCT, bortezomib-containing regimens should be considered in this group of patients.[14,25]

Clinical **Controversy. . .**

Novel agents, such as thalidomide, bortezomib, and lenalidomide, are now routinely used in combination with dexamethasone or chemotherapy as induction therapy. There is no standard induction therapy, and decisions are made based on physician preference and individual characteristics of the patient. Some experts recommend a risk-adapted approach that tailors the treatment-based cytogenetics and gene expression profiling.

Autologous Hematopoietic Stem Cell Transplantation

Although MM is a chemosensitive tumor with significant response rates after treatment with conventional chemotherapy, CR rates have historically been low, and response durations have been short. In an attempt to improve outcomes with chemotherapy, high-dose chemotherapy regimens with stem cell support have been used after initial induction therapy. The intent of the induction therapy before transplant is to reduce tumor burden. With the newer combinations being used as induction, higher rates of quality responses (CR, VGPR, nCR) can be obtained, and recent data suggest that obtaining quality responses during induction improves the outcomes associated with autologous HSCT.[80]

9 Several well-designed, randomized, controlled trials have evaluated the role of high-dose chemotherapy followed by autologous HSCT. In these trials, previously untreated patients were randomized to induction therapy alone versus the same induction therapy followed by high-dose chemotherapy and autologous HSCT. The results generally showed that autologous HSCT improved PFS with a more variable effect on overall survival.[81–83] No survival plateau was observed in the group treated with autologous HSCT, which suggests that few, if any, patients are cured of their disease. Despite this variable effect on overall survival, MM has become the leading indication for autologous HSCT in the United States.

A systematic review of autologous HSCT in newly diagnosed MM was published in 2007.[83] The review pooled results from nine studies comprising 2,411 patients randomized to either autologous HSCT or standard-dose chemotherapy. The combined hazard ratio for overall survival with autologous HSCT was 0.92 (95% CI, 0.74–1.13) and for PFS was 0.75 (95% CI, 0.59–0.96). These results indicate that high-dose therapy with autologous HSCT significantly improves PFS but does not significantly improve overall survival. This benefit in PFS was at the risk of greater transplant-related mortality. Patients who received autologous HSCT had a threefold higher risk of treatment-related death compared with conventional dose chemotherapy. The authors concluded that for every 26 patients who received a transplant, there would be one excess death from autologous HSCT compared with conventional chemotherapy. It should be noted that these trials used an induction of VAD or VAD-like chemotherapy, which is inferior to the modern induction therapies described previously.

Two of the randomized trials comparing autologous HSCT with standard therapy in newly diagnosed MM included in the systematic review were updated and illustrate the divergent results seen with autologous HSCT. Barlogie et al. reported that PFS and overall survival were equivalent between the high- and conventional-dose groups.[84] This is different than the conclusions of the systematic review, which reported a significant improvement in PFS. The contrary results of this study may be due to the use of total-body irradiation plus melphalan rather than the more commonly used high-dose melphalan alone. However, several other studies that used total-body irradiation in addition to melphalan have reported variable results, which suggest that the differences in the preparative regimen do not fully explain these negative results. In the second updated study, Fermand et al. reported a benefit in event-free survival (EFS) but no benefit in overall survival. These results were consistent with the systematic review. This study used standard high-dose melphalan and compared it with conventional therapy in previously untreated patients.[85]

Although the use of autologous HSCT as consolidation therapy has become standard of care in patients younger than age 65 years, it is associated with higher treatment-related mortality, and there is no convincing evidence that it improves overall survival. The widespread adoption of autologous HSCT as standard therapy is related to the significant improvement in PFS. But as conventional therapy continues to improve, response rates, PFS, and overall survival may equal or exceed results seen with autologous HSCT perhaps without the risk of transplant-related mortality.[86]

The role of autologous HSCT as consolidation therapy has been questioned because newer combinations produce results similar to transplantation with lower risk of mortality. However, many investigators continue to believe that the use of autologous HSCT as a scheduled sequential therapy after induction therapy is a logical approach to treating MM and offers the patient the greatest chance of prolonged PFS.

Induction regimens containing at least one of the novel agents may make a significant difference in outcomes after autologous HSCT.[87] Also, the use of these novel agents in induction may reduce the number of patients who require a second transplant because of the higher proportion of patients achieving major responses (CR, nCR, or VGPR) after the combination of novel induction regimen and the first transplant. A randomized phase III trial performed by the French group compared bortezomib in combination with dexamethasone with VAD as induction before autologous HSCT.[88] Patients were randomized to one of four arms, which included either bortezomib plus dexamethasone or VAD. All arms underwent autologous HSCT with melphalan preparation (200 mg/m^2). Postinduction CR and nCR rates were 15% in the bortezomib-containing arms compared to 6% in those receiving VAD. PFS was superior in the patients in whom autologous HSCT was preceded by bortezomib plus dexamethasone induction. Also, the proportion of patients requiring a second transplant was significantly lower in the bortezomib plus dexamethasone arm because of the higher rates of acquiring at least a VGPR in the bortezomib plus dexamethasone group. Two other studies that used bortezomib-based induction before autologous HSCT showed similar benefit.[87]

Most patients are treated with autologous HSCT as consolidation therapy after a short course of induction chemotherapy. However, a smaller number of patients receive autologous HSCT as salvage therapy after patients have failed conventional treatments. A study in the early 1990s compared autologous HSCT with chemotherapy in previously treated MM patients.[89] The results of that study showed that high-dose therapy was no better than VAD alone. However, other studies reported benefit from autologous HSCT in both primary treatment failures and relapsed MM.[90,91] The NCCN guidelines list autologous HSCT as one of the acceptable options in the salvage setting. Responses to autologous HSCT in the salvage setting can occur even in patients who have relapsed after prior successful autologous HSCT.[23]

The optimal timing of autologous HSCT (early vs. late) in MM was investigated in a randomized controlled trial. Patients were randomized to early (n = 91) or late transplantation (n = 94), and no significant difference in 5-year overall survival was observed between the groups.[92] EFS, however, was significantly longer in the early transplantation group (39 months vs. 13 months). In an analysis that factors in the time without symptoms, treatment, or treatment toxicity (TWisTT), patients receiving early transplantation had a longer time in a state associated with good quality of life (27.8 vs. 22.3 months). The results of this study support early autologous HSCT because of its effects on EFS and quality of life. The often long period of disease response after autologous HSCT without ongoing treatment must be considered as newer combinations are considered as upfront therapy to replace autologous HSCT. Although these new combinations may produce equivalent responses, they require prolonged treatment, which may lead to decline in quality of life and can make these therapies more expensive than autologous HSCT.

A specialized form of autologous HSCT, tandem transplantation, involves the use of two separate autologous HSCT procedures separated by a rest period of several months. In a meta-analysis, six randomized controlled trials (N = 1,803) were included, and the authors concluded that although overall response was superior with tandem transplant, overall survival was not superior compared with single transplant. Higher transplant-related mortality was observed in patients receiving tandem transplant.[93]

Transplant-related mortality is generally low for autologous HSCT but is higher in patients receiving tandem transplants (2.7% vs. 4.8%). About 10% to 15% of patients who did not achieve a CR with the first transplant attained it with the second transplant.[94] Because of this increased risk of mortality with tandem transplants, it would be helpful to identify patients who would benefit most from the second transplant. Two French studies reported that patients who did not achieve at least a VGPR after the first transplant benefited most from the second transplant.[95,96] One of these studies reported an estimated 7-year overall survival rate of 21% in the single-transplant arm and a 42% survival rate in the double-transplant arm.[95]

The primary conclusion from the current data on autologous HSCT as consolidation therapy in MM is that it should be used in younger patients with good performance status. Before transplant, all patients should receive induction therapy to reduce tumor burden. Because of higher transplant-related mortality, a second autologous HSCT should only be considered in patients who do not achieve a VGPR or better with the first autologous HSCT. However, a recent systematic review concluded that the evidence is sufficiently biased that no conclusion can be made regarding tandem versus single transplants. It is further limited by the fact that none of the trials used modern induction regimens. Definitive recommendations on tandem transplant will require well-designed trials that limit selection bias and use modern induction regimens.[97]

Because of the controversy surrounding the potential value of upfront autologous HSCT in an era of novel induction therapy, some experts recommend a risk-adapted approach to treatment. For example, the Mayo Clinic categorizes newly diagnosed patients as high risk, intermediate risk, or standard risk based on cytogenetics and gene expression profiling of the malignant clone. Transplant-eligible intermediate- and high-risk patients are offered autologous HSCT after bortezomib-based induction therapy, while standard-risk patients are given the option of autologous HSCT followed by maintenance therapy or induction followed by maintenance therapy.[25]

Maintenance Therapy

(10) Even with the advances in induction therapy and autologous HSCT, most patients eventually progress within 3 to 5 years, suggesting that effective maintenance therapy is needed to control or delay disease progression. The International Myeloma Working Group has published a consensus document on maintenance therapy in MM.[98]

Historically, variable efficacy and high toxicities have been reported with interferon-α (IFN-α) and dexamethasone maintenance, and neither drug can be recommended outside of a clinical trial.[23] IFN-α at one time was considered to be maintenance of choice after autologous HSCT based on data from a randomized trial showing superior PFS and overall survival after autologous HSCT.[99] A meta-analysis supports the benefit of IFN-α maintenance, but the benefit is limited by high toxicity and intolerance.[100] A randomized trial conducted by the Southwest Oncology Group evaluated the benefit of prednisone maintenance therapy in 125 patients.[101] Patients who received high-dose steroids had significantly longer PFS and overall survival but similar to IFN-α at the expense of high toxicity. Although IFN-α or corticosteroid maintenance has not been widely adopted because of toxicity, these therapies served as proof of principle and led to trials evaluating thalidomide, lenalidomide, and bortezomib.

Thalidomide has been studied as maintenance after autologous HSCT. Results of three separate phase III studies showed that thalidomide improves overall survival. In the largest study, 597 patients were randomized to receive no maintenance, pamidronate alone, or the combination of thalidomide plus pamidronate. Patients randomized to the thalidomide plus pamidronate group had significantly longer event-free and overall survival compared with those who received no thalidomide.[102] The median duration of thalidomide maintenance was 15 months, and the average dose was 200 mg/day. Nearly 40% of patients had to discontinue thalidomide as a consequence of toxicity. In a subgroup analysis, patients with deletion of chromosome 13 did not benefit, and other maintenance therapies need to be evaluated for this high-risk group. This effect of adverse cytogenetics predicting nonresponse to thalidomide maintenance was recently confirmed in a randomized study and accompanying meta-analysis.[103]

In another approach, investigators at the University of Arkansas used thalidomide in both induction and maintenance as part of the Total Therapy II trial.[104] Thalidomide increased CR and VGPR rates. In addition, EFS was improved in the thalidomide arm, including patients with adverse cytogenetics. The differences between the Arkansas group and other groups regarding response in patients with adverse cytogenetics may be related to different approaches to cytogenetic and molecular risk assessment. This group indicated that outcome with thalidomide was not related to cumulative dose, which may allow clinicians to limit the duration of thalidomide therapy and therefore reduce toxicity.[104]

Thalidomide maintenance has also been used after induction in elderly patients who were not candidates for autologous HSCT. The results in this setting are not clear and remain controversial. Despite evidence that thalidomide maintenance after autologous HSCT can improve outcomes, it is not widely used because of the adverse toxicity profile.[105]

Lenalidomide has largely replaced thalidomide as maintenance therapy because it is better tolerated than thalidomide. Two recently published randomized trials have investigated the use of lenalidomide maintenance after autologous HSCT. Both trials reported a significant improvement in PFS with lenalidomide maintenance compared with placebo.[106,107] Although lenalidomide was well tolerated, a significant increase in secondary malignancies was observed in the lenalidomide maintenance arm compared with placebo. In patients who are not candidates for autologous HSCT, lenalidomide maintenance has also been shown to improve PFS and was relatively well tolerated in this older group of patients.[79]

Bortezomib maintenance after autologous HSCT has been studied and compared with thalidomide maintenance, but interpretation of the data is complicated by the use of different induction therapies in the thalidomide (VAD) and bortezomib (PAD) maintenance arms.[108] The study did report a significant improvement in response rates in the bortezomib induction and maintenance arm compared with thalidomide induction and maintenance. Bortezomib was better tolerated than thalidomide, with 30% of the thalidomide group stopping therapy because of intolerance compared with 11% in the bortezomib group. The use of bortezomib maintenance in patients who are not candidates for autologous HSCT has not been extensively studied. Preliminary data indicate significantly improved response rates with bortezomib maintenance after the use of bortezomib-containing induction.

In summary, the NCCN guidelines do not strongly recommend the use of dexamethasone or IFN-α maintenance (category 2B). Thalidomide maintenance is given a category 1 recommendation in the NCCN guidelines, but it does not have a favorable adverse effect profile.[23] Lenalidomide maintenance is given a category 1 recommendation, both in patients who undergo autologous HSCT and those who are not transplant eligible. Bortezomib maintenance received a category 2A recommendation in both transplant-eligible and -ineligible patients. Both lenalidomide and bortezomib are relatively well tolerated. However, the clinical benefits of maintenance must be weighed against the risk of secondary malignancies for lenalidomide and infections for bortezomib.[23,109]

The Mayo Clinic guidelines recommend bortezomib-based maintenance in high- and intermediate-risk patients regardless of their eligibility for autologous HSCT.[25] Lenalidomide maintenance should be considered in standard-risk patients after autologous HSCT for a maximum of 2 years.

Allogeneic Hematopoietic Stem Cell Transplantation

Allogeneic HSCT uses a stem cell source other than the patient him- or herself and is therefore a transplant across immunologic barriers. The major posttransplant complications associated with transplanting across these barriers are graft failure and acute and chronic graft-versus-host disease (GVHD). Acute or chronic GVHD may be associated with a graft-versus-myeloma effect. The graft-versus-myeloma effect, which is mediated by antitumor effector cells from the GVHD reaction, reduces relapse risk and may offer the patient the best chance for long-term disease-free survival.[110] Unlike autologous HSCT, which is simply a method of increasing the dose intensity of chemotherapy, allogeneic HSCT is a form of immune therapy. This is best illustrated by nonmyeloablative allogeneic HSCT in which reduced-intensity preparation provides immunosuppression, so the graft is not rejected, but little or no antitumor activity yet long-term disease-free survival can be achieved as a result of graft-versus-tumor effect.[111]

Despite data reporting lower relapse rates in MM patients, myeloablative allogeneic HSCT is associated with high transplant-related mortality rates (20%–50%), leading to overall survival rates similar to those for autologous HSCT.[111] The reasons for the high transplant-related mortality rates in allogeneic HSCT are not entirely clear. One possible explanation is that MM patients come to transplantation heavily pretreated, at an older age, and with greater existing organ damage compared with patients with other cancers. However, a study was closed prematurely in MM patients younger than 55 years of age with minimal pretreatment because of an unacceptably high transplant-related mortality rate (~50%), suggesting that these explanations do not completely account for the high mortality rate.[94]

With the high transplant-related mortality rate associated with myeloablative allogeneic HSCT, the use of nonmyeloablative allogeneic HSCT is an attractive option to reduce early posttransplant mortality. Two conclusions can be made based on the available data regarding the use of nonmyeloablative allogeneic HSCT in MM patients. First, the transplant-related mortality rate associated with nonmyeloablative allogeneic HSCT is lower than that reported with myeloablative allogeneic HSCT. Second, the cytoreductive activity of the reduced-intensity preparation may be insufficient for the graft-versus-myeloma effect to have its full impact. Most immune therapies, including the graft-versus-myeloma reaction, are most effective when patients have minimal residual disease, and nonmyeloablative allogeneic HSCT may have insufficient antitumor activity to achieve important tumor reduction. The need for cytoreduction may be accomplished by autologous HSCT preceding the reduced-intensity allogeneic HSCT procedure. The trials investigating this novel approach have produced conflicting results. These studies compared tandem autologous HSCT with single autologous HSCT followed by reduced-intensity allogeneic HSCT. Three trials reported no differences in event-free or overall survival between tandem autologous HSCT and single autologous HSCT followed by reduced-intensity allogeneic HSCT.[112–114] Other trials reported significantly improved event-free and overall survival when autologous HSCT was combined with reduced-intensity allogeneic HSCT.[115,116] The conflicting results of these various trials may relate to the inclusion of particularly high-risk patients and the use of more aggressive immunosuppression in the negative trials. In most of the trials, the transplant-related mortality rate was higher in the combined autologous HSCT and reduced-intensity allogeneic HSCT arm compared with tandem autologous HSCT. Because of the variability of these results, the combined use of autologous and allogeneic HSCT should only be performed as part of an investigational protocol.

Supportive Care

Bisphosphonates

Along with anti-MM therapy, supportive care measures are aggressively used to stabilize skeletal abnormalities. Bisphosphonates have been used for more than a decade in the management of MM. The clinical benefits of bisphosphonates must be weighed against some of the serious adverse events such as osteonecrosis of the jaw (ONJ) and renal failure.

11 Bisphosphonates have a major role in the treatment of bone-related complications associated with MM. Bone resorption is a manifestation of the disease process and is mediated in part by inflammatory molecules, including IL-6, IL-1, and TNF-α.[1] Bone disease is not seen in MGUS but occurs in about 80% of MM patients at diagnosis. Although the classic cytokine mediators of bone loss are important, a newer view involves excessive production of RANK-L, which activates NF-κB through receptor activator of nuclear factor-κB (RANK).[117] As previously stated, NF-κB is a transcriptional regulator that increases the production of various inflammatory molecules. Normally, RANK-L–mediated activation is in equilibrium with osteoprotegerin, which inhibits NF-κB activation by serving as a decoy receptor for RANK-L.[117] In the bone marrow of MM patients, excess RANK-L is produced particularly from stromal cells, which, when coupled with a decline in osteoprotegerin from both stromal cells and osteoblasts, leads to osteoclast activation and bone destruction. Macrophage inflammatory protein α_1, macrophage colony-stimulating factor, and VEGF may also play important roles in MM bone disease by stimulating the production and activation of osteoclasts.[118] Macrophage inflammatory protein α_1 is also an important chemotactic factor released by MM cells; it attracts osteoclast precursors, enabling myeloma cells to influence the maturation and activation of osteoclasts, which suggests that antimyeloma drugs, particularly lenalidomide and bortezomib, can have a beneficial effect on MM bone disease.[119] Although MM bone disease may involve many cell types and many soluble and cell-bound molecules, it is useful to simplify its pathophysiology and consider it to be an imbalance between RANK-L and osteoprotegerin.

Activation of osteoclasts leads to a net loss of bone mass and to many of the common clinical features of MM, including fractures, hypercalcemia, and bone pain. The bone resorption is influenced by the MM cells in proximity to the osteolytic lesions and is associated with recruitment of osteoclasts.[120] The disruptive effect on skeletal integrity can lead to direct mortality but more commonly has a major impact on morbidity and quality of life.

Bisphosphonates are analogs of endogenous pyrophosphate but are more resistant to hydrolysis than pyrophosphate. Similar to endogenous pyrophosphate, the bisphosphonates bind to crystalline calcium in the bone and are then phagocytized by osteoclasts.[121] The best described effect of the bisphosphonates is the inhibition of osteoclast activity, which likely occurs by direct osteoclast cytotoxicity.[122] In addition to osteoclast inhibition, bisphosphonates may also promote apoptosis in MM cells. This effect may result from the inhibition of the mevalonic acid pathway, which produces several molecules required for growth of the MM clone.[123] In addition, other potential antimyeloma effects of bisphosphonates may include modifying the cytokine microenvironment, inhibiting the adhesion of MM cells to bone marrow matrix cells, and inhibiting angiogenesis.[124] Although it is possible that bisphosphonates have an antimyeloma effect, there is little direct clinical evidence to support this activity.

The use of bisphosphonates in MM is based on the results of several large, randomized, controlled trials. In the pamidronate study, the drug was compared with placebo in a group of MM patients undergoing their first or second course of chemotherapy.[125] Several clinical end points were found to be positively impacted by pamidronate therapy. The investigators reported that patients in the pamidronate group had a lower risk of skeletal-related events, lower pain scores, and improved quality of life. Importantly, a survival advantage was observed in the pamidronate-treated patients who had already received one or more courses of antimyeloma chemotherapy. This finding of improved survival in subgroup analysis is part of the circumstantial evidence to propose an antimyeloma effect for the bisphosphonates.

Guidelines for the use of zoledronic acid in MM are based partly on a randomized study in MM and breast cancer. In patients with bone metastases, zoledronic acid was compared with pamidronate with the intent of demonstrating clinical equipoise.[126] The study did show equivalence between pamidronate and zoledronic acid. The lack of a placebo arm because of ethical concerns complicates interpretation of this study. Despite this limitation, pamidronate and zoledronic acid appear to have equivalent clinical benefit in stabilizing the skeleton.

Other randomized, controlled trials have been conducted, and the results of these trials were pooled in a recent systematic review.[127] Twenty randomized trials were included, which accounted for 6,692 MM patients. The risk of vertebral fractures and pain was significantly lower in the bisphosphonate-treated patients, and there was no difference between zolendronic acid or pamidronate. Given that the aggregate data in the systematic review agreed with the large controlled studies described earlier, the effect on vertebral fractures and pain are well-supported benefits of bisphosphonate therapy. An overall survival benefit associated with bisphosphonate use in MM patients remains unclear, but this meta-analysis reported that zolendronic acid improved overall survival compared with placebo. In a recent randomized controlled trial comparing zolendronic and clodronate, there was a 16% reduction in mortality rate in the zolendronic arm which may suggest an antimyeloma effect associated with zolendronic acid.[128,129]

Osteonecrosis of the jaw is characterized by an area of exposed necrotic bone and often affects the mandible and the maxilla, but it can also affect the soft palate. Treatment of ONJ involves surgical debridement and antimicrobial therapy and is often suboptimal.[130] The development of ONJ may be related to dental disease and tooth extraction and appears to be more common with zoledronic acid than with pamidronate. The incidence of ONJ is unknown but may be as high as 10% in MM patients receiving zoledronic acid for extended periods of time. Because observational studies suggested the risk of ONJ during the first 2 years of pamidronate was low, the Mayo Clinic guidelines in 2006 recommended monthly infusions of pamidronate for 2 years after diagnosis of symptomatic MM.[131]

A subsequent longitudinal cohort study supported many of the conclusions of the Mayo Clinic recommendations. These investigators concluded that ibandronate and pamidronate were safer alternatives to zolendronic acid and that dental procedures and dentures were risk factors for the development of ONJ. They recommended a comprehensive dental examination with management of dental problems before initiating bisphosphonate therapy but made no recommendation on which agent is preferred.[132]

A strong recommendation on a preferred bisphosphonate based on ONJ incidence is likely not warranted. A recent meta-analysis found no difference between the bisphosphonate used and the risk of ONJ.[127]

Pamidronate and zoledronic acid are usually well tolerated. Flulike symptoms can occur after the administration of bisphosphonates. Acute renal impairment can occur with both agents and is related to both infusion time and dose. For zoledronic acid, the risk of acute renal impairment is higher with the 8-mg dose (vs. 4 mg) and when the duration of infusion is 5 minutes (vs. 15 minutes). Patients with moderate renal impairment (creatinine clearance: 30–60 mL/min [0.5–1.0 mL/s]) should have their dose of zoledronic acid adjusted downward by 25% (3 mg). This recommendation was included in the zoledronic acid package insert and is based on a greater renal toxicity in patients with preexisting renal impairment.[133] Randomized studies suggest that renal effects are similar between pamidronate and zoledronic acid, and patients on bisphosphonate therapy should have serum creatinine measured at baseline and then periodically thereafter.[134]

Clinical practice guidelines for the use of bisphosphonates in MM were published in 2007 by an expert panel under the auspices of the American Society of Clinical Oncology Health Services Research Committee.[129] The evidence-based guidelines remain relevant and recommend that symptomatic MM patients be placed on bisphosphonate therapy at the time of diagnosis to reduce pain and skeletal-related events and to improve quality of life. No firm recommendation was made on the duration of bisphosphonate therapy and whether pamidronate or zolendronic acid is preferred. However, the expert panel recommended a duration of bisphosphonate use of 2 years in patients with responsive or stable disease. Reinstituting bisphosphonate therapy at relapse or progression is at the discretion of the clinician.

Although the NCCN recommends upfront bisphosphonate therapy in symptomatic MM, many controversies remain, including whether an antimyeloma effect exists; how long patients should remain on this expensive therapy; and, most important, the risk of ONJ.

Clinical **Controversy...**

Although bisphosphonates are indicated in MM patients with bone disease, controversies surrounding the selection of the best agent and duration of therapy remain. Because of the risk of ONJ in MM patients, a cautious approach on bisphosphonate use is prudent. Some experts recommend that the duration of bisphosphonate therapy should be limited to 2 years. The preference of pamidronate over zoledronic acid is also controversial given that ONJ has also been reported with pamidronate, and the higher risk of ONJ with zoledronic acid is based on observational studies rather than head-to-head randomized comparisons.

Denosumab, a RANK-L antagonist, was recently compared with zolendronic acid in cancer patients with bone metastases, including a relatively small number of MM patients.[135] Denosumab was determined to be noninferior with rates of ONJ similar between the two groups. The authors concluded that denosumab was a reasonable therapy in cancer patients with bone disease and required no monitoring of renal function. However, this study was not sufficient evidence for the routine use of denosumab in MM patients given that MM patients were a relatively small subgroup in this study and outcomes were worse in the MM patients receiving denosumab. Although denosumab is FDA approved for use in patients with solid tumors, it is not approved for use in patients with MM.

Relapsed or Refractory Disease

12 A variety of factors must be considered when determining the most appropriate therapy for an individual who relapses, including the type and duration of previous therapies, presence or absence of adverse prognostic factors, toxicity of prior therapies (e.g., peripheral neuropathy), organ dysfunction (e.g., renal impairment), and how much time has elapsed from initial response to relapse.[26] The same drugs used to treat MM initially can also be used as salvage therapy in MM patients who have relapsed. Patients who relapse more than 6 months after initial induction therapy can have that induction therapy repeated.[25] Bortezomib is an effective salvage therapy. When bortezomib was compared with high-dose dexamethasone, response rates were 43% versus 18%, respectively.[51] The activity of bortezomib in patients with high-risk cytogenetics is particularly useful because high-risk patients are more likely to relapse and require salvage therapy. The addition of dexamethasone to patients who progress on single-agent bortezomib has been shown to improved response.[52]

The combination of bortezomib and pegylated liposomal doxorubicin is another active regimen in relapsed or refractory MM. In a phase III trial, patients randomized to the bortezomib and pegylated liposomal doxorubicin arm had significantly longer median time to progression (9.3 vs. 6.5 months; hazard ratio = 0.55; 95% CI, 0.43–0.71) and 15-month survival rate (76% vs. 65%) compared with patients randomized to receive bortezomib alone.[136] It is interesting to note that the overall (complete and partial) response rate was only slightly higher in the bortezomib and pegylated liposomal doxorubicin group (44% vs. 41%). Based on the results of this study, the combination of bortezomib and pegylated liposomal doxorubicin received FDA approval in 2007 for patients with previously treated MM and is listed as a category 1 recommendation in the NCCN guidelines.[23] As expected, patients who received the combination experienced more adverse effects. Prior use of IMiDs or high-dose chemotherapy does not appear to affect bortezomib activity in relapsed MM. A phase III trial reported that bortezomib with or without dexamethasone had activity in relapsed or refractory disease despite prior thalidomide therapy or autologous HSCT.[137]

Lenalidomide also has received a category 1 recommendation when combined with dexamethasone in relapsed or refractory patients.[61,62] The combination of lenalidomide plus dexamethasone increased response rate compared with dexamethasone alone but came at the cost of increased grade 3 and 4 hematologic toxicity. Based on the activity of bortezomib and lenalidomide in the setting of relapsed or refractory disease, a phase II trial of these two novel agents combined with dexamethasone showed good response rates and a relatively good toxicity profile (primarily grade 3 hematologic toxicity).[138]

As previously discussed, questions remain on the optimal timing for autologous HSCT. For patients who are eligible for autologous HSCT and did not receive transplant as part of initial therapy, it is appropriate to offer autologous HSCT at first relapse. It is important to emphasize that although higher quality of life was realized when autologous HSCT was used as consolidation therapy, there was no difference in overall survival based on timing of transplant.[92] The use of salvage autologous HSCT in patients who received a prior autologous HSCT seemed to be most beneficial in patients who had a response of greater than 24 months after initial autologous HSCT.[139] In patients with relapsed or refractory MM, autologous HSCT followed by nonmyeloablative allogeneic HSCT has potential benefit but at the expense of increased transplant-related mortality requiring treatment only be performed as part of a clinical protocol.

The treatment of relapsed-refractory patients can be with active agents in combination or single agents used sequentially. With the growing number of highly active agents, combination salvage therapy has become predominant. The NCCN has three category 1 recommendations: single-agent bortezomib, bortezomib plus liposomal doxorubicin, and lenalidomide plus dexamethasone. The combined use of bortezomib with lenalidomide has not yet been given a category 1 recommendation but remains a category 2A recommendation in the NCCN Guidelines.[23] Treatment decisions for individual patients with relapsed disease may potentially be improved by taking into account patient-specific information such as the type of previous therapies, adverse cytogenetics, and end-organ dysfunction. For example, in patients with relapsed MM, combined bortezomib and liposomal doxorubicin has shown improved time to progression compared with bortezomib alone, including in patients who had received prior anthracyclines, lenalidomide, and thalidomide.[136] In contrast, treatment with lenalidomide and dexamethasone resulted in a significantly shorter time to progression in patients who had previously been treated with thalidomide compared with thalidomide-naïve patients.[61,62]

Carfilzomib is indicated in patients who have received bortezomib and lenalidomide salvage and have progressive disease. The FDA approval in this group of relapsed or refractory patients was based on a phase II study in patients, 80% of whom were refractory to both bortezomib and lenalidomide, which showed an overall response rate of 25%.[23,73] Based on these impressive results, phase III trials comparing carfilzomib combinations with lenalidomide or bortezomib plus dexamethasone in a group of previously treated relapsed MM patients are ongoing. Single-agent carfilzomib is also being compared with supportive care in patients who had received at least three prior therapies.[23]

Bendamustine is a highly active chemotherapeutic agent in MM with overall response rates in variously treated relapsed patients of 30% to 55%. Toxicity has been largely hematologic and manageable.[23] Bendamustine has been combined with novel agents to further improve response. Bendamustine was added to lenalidomide and dexamethasone in a phase II trial that reported a more than 50% response rate with nearly half being VGPR.[140] The NCCN has given both single agent bendamustine and the bendamustine, lenalidomide, and dexamethasone combination a category 2A recommendation.[23]

Vorinostat is an inhibitor of histone deacetylase and modifies the expression of genes involved in tumor progression and has good activity in relapsed MM when combined with bortezomib. The results of phase II trials have been encouraging, and the NCCN has given vorinostat and bortezomib combinations a category 2A recommendation in relapsed MM.[23,141]

The NCCN guidelines offer many options for salvage therapy, including thalidomide, lenalidomide, or bortezomib with or without dexamethasone or chemotherapy (Table 113-7). Newer agents such as ponalidomide, carfilzomib, bendamustine, and vorinostat are being integrated into therapy. In addition, autologous HSCT has a role as salvage therapy.[23] Therapy should be selected based on disease and patient risk factors and previous treatment. Despite clear progress, most salvage therapies produce less than a 50% response rate, and new drugs and drug combinations are needed.

TABLE 113-7 Salvage Therapy in Multiple Myeloma

Regimen	Level of Evidence Category[a]
Bendamustine	2B
Bortezomib	1
Bortezomib + dexamethasone	2A
Bortezomib + lenalidomide + dexamethasone	2B
Bortezomib + liposomal doxorubicin	1
Pomalidomide + dexamethasone	2A
Carfilzomib	2A
Dexamethasone + cyclophosphamide + etoposide + cisplatin (DCEP)	2A
Dexamethasone + thalidomide + cisplatin + doxorubicin + cyclophosphamide + etoposide (DT-PACE)	2A
High-dose cyclophosphamide	2A
Lenalidomide + dexamethasone	1
Lenalidomide	2A
Repeat primary induction therapy (if relapse at >6 months)	2A
Thalidomide	2A
Thalidomide + dexamethasone	2A

[a]Category 1: Uniform National Comprehensive Cancer Network (NCCN) consensus based on high-level evidence. Category 2A: Uniform NCCN consensus based on lower evidence, including clinical experience. Category 2B: Nonuniform NCCN consensus but no major disagreement.

Data from NCCN Guidelines NCCN. Clinical Practice Guidelines in Oncology. Multiple Myeloma. v1.2014. 2014, http://www.NCCN.org.

PERSONALIZED PHARMACOTHERAPY

Therapy for MM is personalized based on staging (e.g., ISS), cytogenetics, gene expression profiling, performance status of the patient, age of the patient, and preexisting risk for drug toxicity. Personalized therapy has been driven by the explosion of new treatment options in MM and a better understanding of the MM biology and therapeutic targets. As described previously, the Mayo Clinic recommends a risk-adapted approach that tailors therapy based on risk category (e.g., high, intermediate, or standard).

The use of a risk-adapted approach is reasonable in newly diagnosed patients. MM is currently not curable, and the disease will evolve as the disease progresses, which will require evaluation of biomarkers at times of relapse and progression to tailor therapy in each stage of the disease.

In addition to molecular characteristics of the tumor, a number of patient-related factors guide personalized treatment. For example, older patients with poor performance status would not be candidates for autologous HSCT. Patients with preexisting severe peripheral neuropathy would be less likely to receive thalidomide or bortezomib because of neurotoxicity. Patients with risk factors for VTE would be more likely to receive bortezomib-containing combinations because the risk of VTE is lower compared with thalidomide or lenalidomide combinations. Patients with preexisting renal failure may be less likely to receive lenalidomide because it requires dose adjustment based on renal function. With personalized therapy, patients will have the opportunity to benefit from the use of novel agents.

EVALUATION OF THERAPEUTIC OUTCOMES

Because MM is currently not a curable disease, the goals of therapy are to prolong survival and to improve quality of life. Patients with asymptomatic MM are usually followed and not treated. Asymptomatic patients are assessed every 3 to 6 months for disease progression, which would then require therapy. Assessment involves measurement of M protein in blood and urine and laboratory tests that include complete blood count, serum creatinine, and calcium. Patients are treated as the disease produces symptoms. Disease response is defined by a decline in M protein. After completion of the initial course of therapy and response is obtained, patients should be monitored every 3 months. Bone surveys are performed yearly or as required because of changes in symptoms. Various other tests, including bone marrow biopsy, magnetic resonance imaging, and positron emission tomography, or computed tomography scan, are performed on an as-needed basis to evaluate disease status.

ABBREVIATIONS

CR	complete remission
EFS	event-free survival
IFN	interferon
IL	interleukin
IMiD	immunomodulatory drug
IκB	inhibitor of NF-κB
ISS	International Staging System
LMWH	low-molecular-weight heparin
MGUS	monoclonal gammopathy of undetermined significance
MM	multiple myeloma
MP	melphalan plus prednisone
MPB	melphalan, prednisone, and bortezomib

MPL	melphalan, prednisone, and lenalidomide
MPT	melphalan, prednisone, and thalidomide
NF-κB	nuclear factor kappa B
nCR	near complete response
ONJ	osteonecrosis of the jaw
PR	partial response
PFS	progression-free survival
RANK	receptor activator of nuclear factor-κB
RANK-L	receptor for activation of NF-κB ligand
sCR	stringent complete response
TNF-α	tumor necrosis factor-α
VAD	vincristine, doxorubicin, and dexamethasone
VEGF	vascular endothelial growth factor
VGPR	very good partial response
VTE	venous thromboembolism

REFERENCES

1. Mahindra A, Hideshima T, Anderson KC. Multiple Myeloma: biology of the disease. Blood Reviews 2010;S5–S11.
2. Morgan GJ, Walker BA, Davies FE. The genetic architecture of multiple myeloma. Nature Reviews 2012;12:335–348.
3. Siegel R, Naishadham D, Jemal A. Cancer statistics, 2013. CA Cancer J Clin 2013;63:11–30.
4. Munshi NC, Anderson KC. Plasma cell neoplasms. In: Devita VT, Hellman S, Rosenberg SA, eds. Cancer Principles and Practice of Oncology, 9th ed. Philadelphia, PA: Lippincott Williams & Wilkins, 2011:2305–2342.
5. Brown LM, Linet MS, Greenberg RS, et al. Multiple myeloma and family history of cancer among blacks and whites in the U.S. Cancer 1999;85:2385–2390.
6. Lee WJ, Hoppin JA, Blair A, et al. Cancer incidence among pesticide applicators exposed to alchalor in the Agricultural Health Study. Am J Epidemiol 2004;159:373–380.
7. Preston DL, Kusumi S, Tomonaga M, et al. Cancer incidence in atomic bomb survivors. Part III. Leukemia, lymphoma, and multiple myeloma, 1950–1987. Radiat Res 1994;137(2 Suppl):S68–S97.
8. Palumbo A, Anderson K. Multiple myeloma. N Engl J Med 2011;364:1046–1060.
9. Kyle RA, Therneau TM, Rajkumar SV, et al. Prevalence of monoclonal gammopathy of undetermined significance. N Engl J Med 2006;354:1362–1369.
10. Walker BA, Leone PE, Jenner MW, et al. Integration of global SNP-based mapping and expression arrays reveals key regions, mechanisms, and genes important to the pathogenesis of multiple myeloma. Blood 2006;108:1733–1743.
11. Kyle RA, Remstein ED, Thereau TM, et al. Clinical course and prognosis of smoldering (asymptomatic) multiple myeloma. N Engl J Med 2007;356:2582–2590.
12. Manier S, Sacco A, Leleu X, et al. Bone marrow microenvironment in multiple myeloma progression. J Biomed Biotech 2012;2012:157496.
13. Spets H, Stromberg T, Georgii-Hemming P, et al. Expression of the bcl-2 family of pro- and anti-apoptotic genes in multiple myeloma and normal plasma cells. Eur J Haematol 2002;69:76–89.
14. Mahindra A, Laubach J, Raje N, et al. Latest advances and current challenges in the treatment of multiple myeloma. Nat Rev Clin Oncol 2012;9:135–143.
15. Chapman MA, Lawrence, MS, Keats JJ, et al. Initial genome sequencing and analysis of multiple myeloma. Nature 2011;471:467–472.
16. Gertz MA, Ghobrial I, Luc-Harousseau J. Multiple myeloma: Biology, standard therapy, and transplant therapy. Biol Blood Marrow Transplant 2009;15:46–52.
17. Anderson KC. New insights into therapeutic targets in myeloma. Hematology Am Soc Hematol Educ Program 2011;2011:184–190.
18. Sirohi B, Powles R. Multiple myeloma. Lancet 2004;363: 875–887.
19. Dispenzieri A, Kyle R, Merlini G, et al. International myeloma working group guidelines for serum light chain analysis in multiple myeloma and related disorders. Leukemia 2009;23:215–224.
20. Roodman GD. Pathogenesis of myeloma bone disease. Leukemia 2009;23:435–441.
21. Agarwal A, Ghobrial IM. Monoclonal gammopathy of undetermined significance and smoldering multiple myeloma: A review of the current understanding of epidemiology, biology, risk stratification and management of myeloma precursor disease. Clin Cancer Res 2013;9(5):985–994.
22. Greipp PR, Miguel JS, Durie BG, et al. International staging system for multiple myeloma. J Clin Oncol 2005;23: 3412–3420.
23. National Comprehensive Cancer Network. The NCCN Multiple Myeloma Clinical Practice Guidelines in Oncology (Version 1.2013). 2013, http://www.NCCN.org.
24. Palumbo A, Attal M, Roussel M. Shifts in the therapeutic paradigm for patients newly diagnosed with multiple myeloma: Maintenance therapy and overall survival. Clin Cancer Res 2011;17:1253–1263.
25. Mikhael JR, Dingli D, Roy V, et al. Management of Newly Diagnosed Symptomatic Multiple Myeloma: Updated Mayo Stratification of Myeloma and Risk-Adapted Therapy (mSMART) Consensus Guidelines 2013. Mayo Clin Proc 2013;88:360–376.
26. Raab MS, Podar K, Breitkreutz I, Richardson PG, Anderson KC. Multiple myeloma. Lancet 2009;374:324–339.
27. Thomas A, Mailankody S, Korde N, et al. Second malignancies after multiple myeloma: From 1960s to 2010s. Blood 2012;119:2731–2737.
28. Facon T, Mary JY, Pegourie B, et al. Dexamethasone-based regimens versus melphalan prednisone for elderly multiple myeloma patients ineligible for high dose therapy. Blood 2006;107:1292–1298.
29. Rajkumar SV. Doublets, triplets, or quadruplets of novel agents in newly diagnosed myeloma? Hematology Am Soc Hematol Educ Program 2012;2012:354–361.
30. Gordan JN, Goggin PM. Thalidomide and its derivative emerging from the wilderness. Postgrad Med J 2003;79: 127–132.
31. Kotla V, Gold S, Nischal S, et al. Mechanism of action of lenalidomide in hematological malignancies. J Hematol Oncol 2009;2:36.
32. Rajkumar SV, Leong T, Roche PC, et al. Prognostic value of bone marrow angiogenesis in multiple myeloma. Clin Cancer Res 2000;6:3111–3116.
33. Neben K, Mytilineos J, Moehler TM, et al. Polymorphisms of the TNF-α gene promoter predict for outcome after thalidomide therapy in relapsed and refractory multiple myeloma. Blood 2002;100:2263–2265.
34. Reece DE, Leitch HA, Atkins H, et al. Treatment of relapsed and refractory myeloma. Leuk Lymphoma 2008;49:1470–1485.
35. Barlogie B, Desikan R, Eddlemon P, et al. Extended survival in advanced and refractory multiple myeloma after single-agent thalidomide: Identification of prognostic factors in a phase 2 study of 169 patients. Blood 2001;98:492–494.
36. Cavallo F, Boccadoro M, Palumbo A. Review of thalidomide in the treatment of newly diagnosed multiple myeloma. Ther Clin Risk Manag 2007;3:543–552.

37. Larocca A, Palumbo A. Evolving paradigms in treatment of newly diagnosed multiple myeloma. J NCCN 2011;9: 1186–1196.
38. Rajkumar SV, Blood E, Vesole D, et al. Phase III clinical trial of thalidomide plus dexamethasone compared with dexamethasone alone in newly diagnosed multiple myeloma: A clinical trial coordinated by Eastern Cooperative Oncology Group. J Clin Oncol 2006;24:431–436.
39. Palumbo A, Bringhen S, Liberati AM, et al. Oral melphalan with prednisone and thalidomide in elderly patients with multiple myeloma: Updated results of a randomized controlled trial. Blood 2008;112:3107–3114.
40. Facon T, Mary JY, Hulin C, et al. Melphalan and prednisone plus thalidomide versus melphalan and prednisone alone or reduced-intensity autologous stem cell transplantation in elderly patients with multiple myeloma (IFM 99–06): A randomised trial. Lancet 2007;370:1209–1218.
41. Hulin C, Facon T, Rodon P, et al. Efficacy of melphalan and prednisone plus thalidomide in patients older than 75 years with newly diagnosed multiple myeloma: IFM 01/01 Trial. J Clin Oncol 2009;27:3664–3670.
42. Offidani M, Corvatta L, Piersantelli M, et al. Thalidomide, dexamethasone, and pegylated liposomal doxorubicin for patients older than 65 years with newly diagnosed multiple myeloma. Blood 2006;108:2159–2164.
43. Dingli D, Rajkumar SV. How best to use new therapies in multiple myeloma. Blood Rev 2010;24:91–100.
44. Gleason C, Nooka A, Lonial S. Supportive therapies in multiple myeloma. J Natl Compr Canc Netw 2009;7:971–979.
45. Lyman GH, Khorana AA, Falanga A, et al. ASCO Guideline: Recommendations for venous thromboembolism prophylaxis and treatment in patients with cancer. J Clin Oncol 2007;25: 5490–5505.
46. Palumbo A, Cavo M, Bringhan S, et al. Aspirin, warfarin, or enoxaparin thromboprophylaxis in patients with multiple myeloma treated with thalidomide: A phase III open label randomized trial. J Clin Oncol 2011;29:986–993.
47. Larolla A, Cavallo F, Bringhen S, et al. Aspirin or enoxaparin thromboprophylaxis for patients with newly diagnosed multiple myeloma treated with lenalidomide. Blood 2012;119:933–939.
48. Shah JJ, Orlowski RZ. Proteasome inhibitors in the treatment of multiple myeloma. Leukemia 2009;23:1964–1979.
49. Orlowski RZ, Stinchcombe TE, Mitchell BS, et al. Phase 1 trial of the proteasome inhibitor PS341 in patients with refractory hematologic malignancies. J Clin Oncol 2002;20:4420–4427.
50. Richardson P, Barlogie B, Berenson J, et al. A phase II study of bortezomib in relapsed, refractory myeloma. N Engl J Med 2003;348:2609–2617.
51. Richardson PG, Sonneveld P, Schuster MW, et al. Bortezomib or high dose dexamethasone in relapsed multiple myeloma. N Engl J Med 2005;352:2487–2498.
52. Richardson PG, Mitsiades C, Ghobrial I, Anderson K. Beyond single agent bortezomib: Combination regimens in relapsed multiple myeloma. Curr Opin Oncol 2006;18:598–608.
53. Jagannath S, Durie BG, Wolf J, et al. Bortezomib therapy alone and in combination with dexamethasone for previously untreated symptomatic multiple myeloma. Br J Haematol 2005;129:776–783.
54. Harousseau JL, Attal M, Leleu X, et al. Bortezomib plus dexamethasone as induction treatment prior to autologous stem cell transplant in patients with newly diagnosed multiple myeloma: Results of an IFM Phase II study. Haematologica 2006;91:1498–1505.
55. Mateos MV, Hernandez JM, Hernandez MT, et al. Bortezomib plus melphalan and prednisone in elderly untreated patients with multiple myeloma: Results of a multivariate phase I/II study. Blood 2006;108:2165–2172.
56. San Miguel JF, Schlag R, Khuageva NK, et al. Bortezomib plus melphalan and prednisone for initial treatment of multiple myeloma. N Engl J Med 2008;359:906–917.
57. San Miguel JF, Schlag R, Khuageva NK, et al. Persistent overall survival benefit and no increased risk of secondary malignancies with bortezomib-melphalan-prednisone versus melphalan-prednisone in patients with previously untreated multiple myeloma. J Clin Oncol 2013;31:448–455.
58. Hoy SM. Subcutaneous bortezomib in multiple myeloma. Drugs 2013;73:45–54.
59. Arnulf B, Pylypenko H, Grosicki S, et al. Updated survival analysis of a randomized Phase III study of subcutaneous verus intravenous bortezomib in patients with relapsed multiple myeloma. Hematologica 2012;97:1925–1928.
60. Armoiry X, Auglagner G, Facon T. Lenalidomide in the treatment of multiple myeloma: A review. J Clin Pharm Ther 2008;33:219–226.
61. Weber DM, Chen C, Niesvizky R, et al. Lenalidomide plus dexamethasone for relapsed multiple myeloma in North America. N Engl J Med 2007;357:2133–2142.
62. Dimopoulous M, Spencer A, Attal M, et al. Lenalidomide plus dexamethasone for relapsed or refractory multiple myeloma. N Engl J Med 2007;357:2123–2132.
63. Lacy MQ, Gertz MA, Dispenzieri A, et al. Long-term results of response to therapy, time to progression, and survival with lenalidomide plus dexamethasone in newly diagnosed myeloma. Mayo Clin Proc 2007;82:1179–1184.
64. Rajkumar SV, Hayman SR, Lacy MQ, et al. Combination therapy with lenalidomide plus dexamethasone for newly diagnosed myeloma. Blood 2005;106:4050–4053.
65. Rajkumar SV, Jacobus S, Callander NS, et al. Lenalidomide plus high-dose dexamethasone versus lenalidomide plus low-dose dexamethasone as initial therapy for newly diagnosed multiple myeloma: an open-labeled randomized control trial. Lancet Oncol 2010;11:29–37.
66. Larocca A, Cavallo F, Bringhen S, et al. Aspirin or enoxaparin thromboprophylaxis for patients with newly diagnosed multiple myeloma treated with lenalidomide. Blood 2012;119:933–939.
67. Kuhn DJ, Chen Q, Voorhees PM, et al. Potent activity of carfilzomib, a novel, irreversible inhibitor of the ubiquitin-proteasome pathway, against preclinical models of multiple myeloma. Blood 2007;110:3281–3290.
68. Demo SD, Kirk CJ, Aujay MA, et al. Antitumor activity of PR-171, a novel irreversible inhibitor of the proteasome. Cancer Res 2007;67:6383–6391.
69. O'Connor OA, Stewart AK, Vallone M, et al. A phase 1 dose escalation study of the safety and pharmacokinetics of the novel proteasome inhibitor carfilzomib (PR-171) in patients with hematologic malignancies. Clin Cancer Res. 2009;15:7085–7091.
70. Moreau P, Richardson PG, Cavo M, et al. Proteosome inhibitors in multiple myeloma: 10 years later. Blood 2012;120:947–959.
71. Kortuem KM, Stewart AK. Carfilzomib. Blood 2013;121: 893–897.
72. Singhal S, Siegel DS, Martin T, et al. Integrated safety from phase 2 studies of monotherapy carfilzomib in patients with relapsed and refractory Multiple Myeloma (MM): an updated analysis. Blood 2011;118:1876 [abstract].
73. Siegel DS, Martin T, Wang M, et al. A phase 2 study of single agent carfilzomib (PX-171-003-A1) in patients with relapsed and refractory multiple myeloma. Blood. 2012;120:2817–2825.

74. Vij R, Wang M, Kaufman JL, et al. An open-label, single-arm, phase 2 (PX-171-004) study of single-agent carfilzomib in bortezomib-naive patients with relapsed and/or refractory multiple myeloma. Blood. 2012;119:5661–5670.
75. Wang L, Siegel DS, Jakubowiak AJ, et al. The speed of response to single-agent carfilzomib in patients with relapsed and/or refractory multiple myeloma: An exploratory analysis of results from 2 multicenter phase 2 clinical trials. Blood 2011;118:3969 [abstract]
76. Jakubowiak AJ, Dytfeld D, Griffith KA, et al. A phase 1/2 study of carfilzomib in combination with lenalidomide and low-dose dexamethasone as a frontline treatment for multiple myeloma. Blood 2012;120:1801–1809.
77. Leleu X, Attal M, Arnulf B, et al. Pomalidomide plus low-dose dexamethasone is active and well tolerated in bortezomib and lenalidomide refractory multiple myeloma: IFM 2009-02. Blood 2013;121(11):1968–1967.
78. Palumbo A, Falco P, Corradini P, et al. Melphalan, prednisone, lenalidomide treatment for newly diagnosed myeloma: A report from the GIMEMA Italian Multiple Myeloma Network. J Clin Oncol 2007;25:4459–4465.
79. Palumbo A, Hajek R, Delforge M, et al. Continuous lenalidomide treatment for newly diagnosed multiple myeloma. N Engl J Med 2012;366:1759–1769.
80. Rosinol L, Oriol A, Teruel AI, et al. Superiority of bortezomib, thalidomide, and dexamethasone (VTD) as induction pre-transplantation in multiple myeloma: A randomized Phase 3 PETHEMA/GEM study. Blood 2012;120:1589–1596.
81. Child JA, Morgan GJ, Davies FE, et al. High-dose chemotherapy with hematopoietic stem cell rescue for multiple myeloma. N Engl J Med 2003;348:1875–1883.
82. Attal M, Harousseau JL, Stoppa AM, et al. A prospective, randomized trial of autologous bone marrow transplantation and chemotherapy in multiple myeloma. N Engl J Med 1996;335:91–97.
83. Koreth J, Cutler CS, Djulbegovic B, et al. High-dose therapy with single autologous transplantation versus chemotherapy for newly diagnosed multiple myeloma: A systematic review and meta-analysis of randomized controlled trials. Biol Blood Marrow Transplant 2007;12:183–196.
84. Barlogie B, Kyle RA, Anderson KC, et al. Standard chemotherapy compared with high dose chemotherapy for multiple myeloma: Final results of phase III US Intergroup Trial S9321. J Clin Oncol 2006;24:929–936.
85. Fermand JP, Katsahian S, Divine M, et al. High dose therapy and autologous blood stem cell transplantation compared with conventional treatment in multiple myeloma patients aged 55 to 65 years: Long-term results of a randomized control trial from the Group Myeloma-Autograffe. J Clin Oncol 2005;23:9227–9233.
86. Moreau P, Rajkumar SV. Should all eligible patients with multiple myeloma receive autologous stem cell transplant as part of initial treatment. Leuk Res 2012;36: 677–681.
87. Giralt S. Stem cell transplantation for multiple myeloma: Current and future status. Hematology Am Soc Hematol Educ Program 2012;2012:191–196.
88. Harousseau JL, Avet-Loiseau H, Attal M, et al. Bortezomib plus dexamethasone is superior to VAD as induction treatment prior to ASCT in newly diagnosed multiple myeloma: Results of the IFM 2005-01 Phase III trial. J Clin Oncol 2010;28:4621–4629.
89. Alexanian R, Dimopoulos M, Smith T, et al. Limited value of myeloablative therapy for late multiple myeloma. Blood 1994;83:512–516.
90. Kumar S, Lacy MQ, Dispenzieri A, et al. High-dose therapy and autologous stem cell transplantation for multiple myeloma poorly responsive to initial therapy. Bone Marrow Transplant 2004;34:161–167.
91. Pant S, Copeland EA. Hematopoietic stem cell transplantation in multiple myeloma. Biol Blood Marrow Transplant 2007;13:877–885.
92. Fermand JP, Ravaud P, Chevaer S, et al. High dose therapy and autologous peripheral blood stem cell transplantation in multiple myeloma: Up-front or rescue treatment? Results of a multicenter sequential randomized clinical trial. Blood 1998;92:3131–3136.
93. Kumar A, Kharfan-Dabaja MA, Glasmacher A, Djulbegovic B. Tandem versus single autologous hematopoietic cell transplantation for treatment of multiple myeloma: A systematic review and meta-analysis. J Natl Cancer Instit 2009;101:100–106.
94. Vesole DH, Simic A, Lazarus HM. Controversy in multiple myeloma transplants: Tandem autotransplants and mini-allografts. Bone Marrow Transplant 2001;28:725–735
95. Attal M, Harousseau JL, Facon T, et al. Single versus double autologous stem cell transplantation for multiple myeloma. N Engl J Med 2003;349:2495–2502.
96. Harousseau JL, Avet-Loiseau H, Attal M, et al. Achievement of at least very good partial response is a simple and robust prognostic factor in patients with multiple myeloma treated with high-dose therapy: Long-term analysis of the IFM 99–02 and 99–04 trials. J Clin Oncol 2009;34:5720–5726.
97. Neumann-Winter F, Greb A, Borchmann P, et al. First-line tandem high-dose chemotherapy and autologous stem cell transplant versus single high-dose chemotherapy and autologous stem cell transplant in multiple myeloma, A systematic review of controlled studies. Cochrane Database Syst Rev 2012;10:CD004626.
98. Ludwig H, Durie BG, McCarthy P, et al. IMWG consensus on maintenance therapy in multiple myeloma. Blood 2012;119:3003–3015.
99. Mandelli F, Avvisati G, Amadori S, et al. Maintenance treatment with recombinant interferon-alpha 2b in patients with multiple myeloma responding to conventional induction chemotherapy. N Engl J Med 1990;322: 1430–1434.
100. Fritz E, Ludwig H. Interferon-alpha treatment in multiple myeloma: Meta-analysis of 30 randomized trials among 3948 patients. Ann Oncol 2000;11:1427–1436.
101. Berenson JR, Crowley JJ, Grogan TM, et al. Maintenance therapy with alternate-day prednisone improves survival in multiple myeloma patients. Blood 2002;99:3163–3168.
102. Attal M, Harousseau JL, Leyvraz S, et al. Maintenance therapy with thalidomide improves survival in patients with multiple myeloma. Blood 2006;108:3289–3294.
103. Morgan GJ, Gregory WM, Davies FE, et al. The role of maintenance thalidomide therapy in multiple myeloma: MRC Myeloma IX results and meta-analysis. Blood 2012;119:7–15.
104. Barlogie B, Pineda-Roman M, vanRhee F, et al. Thalidomide arm of total therapy II improve complete response duration and survival in myeloma patients with metaphase cytogenetic abnormalities. Blood 2008;112:3115–3121.
105. Ghobrial IM, Stewart AK. ASH evidence-based guidelines: What is the role of maintenance therapy in treatment of multiple myeloma? Hematology Am Soc Hematol Educ Program 2009;2009:587–589.
106. Attal M, Lauwers-Cances V, Marit G, et al. Lenalidomide maintenance after stem cell transplant for multiple myeloma. N Engl J Med 2012;366:1782–1791.

107. McCarthy PL, Owzar K, Hofmeister CC, et al. Lenalidomide after stem cell transplantation for multiple myeloma. 2012;366:1770–1781.
108. Sonneveld P, Schmidt-Wolf I, van der Holt B, et al. Bortezomib induction and maintenance treatment in patients with newly diagnosed multiple myeloma: Results of the randomized Phase III Hovon-65/GMMG-HD4 trial. J Clin Oncol 2012;30:2946–2955.
109. Palumbo A, Mina R. Part II: Role of maintenance therapy in transplant-ineligible patients. JNCCN 2013;11:43–49.
110. Laterveer L, Verdonck LF, Peeters T, et al. Graft-versus-myeloma may overcome the unfavorable effect of deletion of chromosome 13 in multiple myeloma. Blood 2003;101:1201–1202.
111. Bruno B, Giaccone L, Sorasio R, Boccadoro M. Role of allogeneic stem cell transplantation in multiple myeloma. Semin Hematol 2009;46:158–165.
112. Garban F, Attal M, Michallet M, et al. Prospective comparison of autologous stem cell transplantation followed by dose reduced allograft with tandem autologous stem cell transplant in high risk de novo multiple myeloma. Blood 2006;107:3474–3480.
113. Bruno B, Rotta M, Patriarcia F, et al. A comparison of allografting with autografting for newly diagnosed myeloma. N Engl J Med 2007;356:1110–1120.
114. Rosinol L, Perez-Simon JA, Sureda A, et al. A prospective study of tandem autologous transplant versus autologous transplant followed by reduced intensity conditioning allogeneic transplant in newly diagnosed multiple myeloma. Blood 2008;112:3591–3593.
115. Bjorkstrand B, Iacobelli S, Hegenbant U, et al. Tandem autologous reduced intensity allogeneic stem cell transplant versus autologous stem cell transplant in myeloma: long-term follow-up. J Clin Oncol 2011;29:3016–3022.
116. Krishnan A, Pasquini M, Logan B, et al. Autologous stem cell transplant followed by allogeneic or autologous stem cell transplant in patients with multiple myeloma: A phase 3 biologic assessment trial. Lancet Oncology 2011;12:1195–1203.
117. Sezer O, Heider U, Zavrski, et al. RANK ligand and osteoprotegerin in myeloma bone disease. Blood 2003;101:2094–2098.
118. Roodman GD. Pathogenesis of myeloma bone disease. Leukemia 2009;23:435–441.
119. Raje N, Roodman GD. Advances in the biology and treatment of bone disease in multiple myeloma. Clin Cancer Res 2011;17:1278–1286.
120. Andersen TL, Soe K, Sondergaard TE, et al. Myeloma cell-induced disruption of bone remodeling compartments leads to osteolytic lesions and generation of osteoclast-myeloma hybrid cells. Br J Hematol 2009;148:551–561.
121. Russell RG. Bisphosphonates: From bench to bedside. Ann N Y Acad Sci 2006;1068:367–401.
122. Papapoulos SE. Bisphosphonate actions: Physical chemistry revisited. Bone 2006;38:613–616.
123. Baulch-Brown C, Molloy TJ, Yeh SL, et al. Inhibitor of the mevalonate pathway as potential therapeutic agents in multiple myeloma. Leuk Res 2007;31:341–352.
124. Neville-Webbe HL, Holen I, Coleman RE. The anti-tumor activity of bisphosphonates. Cancer Treat Rev 2002;28:305–319.
125. Berenson JR, Lichtenstein A, Porter L, et al. Long-term pamidronate treatment of advanced multiple myeloma patients reduces skeletal events. Myeloma Aredia Study Group. J Clin Oncol 1998;16:593–602.
126. Rosen LS, Gordon D, Antonio BS, et al. Zoledronic acid versus pamidronate in the treatment of skeletal metastases in patients with breast cancer or osteolytic lesions of multiple myeloma: A phase III, double blind, comparative trial. Cancer J 2001;7:377–387.
127. Mhaskar R, Redzepovic J, Wheatley K, et al. Bisphosphonates in multiple myeloma: A network meta-analysis. Cochrane Database Syst Rev 2012;5:CD003188.
128. Morgan GJ, Davies FE, Gregory WM, et al. First-line treatment with zolendronic acid as compared with clodronic acid in multiple myeloma: A randomized control trial. Lancet 2010;376:1989–1999.
129. Kyle RA, Yee GC, Somerfield MR, et al. American Society of Clinical Oncology 2007 Clinical Practice Guideline update on the role of bisphosphonates in multiple myeloma. J Clin Oncol 2007;25:2462–2472.
130. Reid IR, Cornish J. Epidemiology and pathogenesis of osteonecrosis of the jaw. J Nat Rev Rheumatol 2012;8:90–96.
131. Lacy MQ, Dispenzieri A, Gertz MA, et al. Mayo clinic consensus statement for the use of bisphosphonates in multiple myeloma. Mayo Clin Proc 2006;81:1047–1053.
132. Vahtsevanos K, Kyrgidis A, Verrou F, et al. Longitudinal cohort study of risk factors in cancer patients of bisphosphonate-related osteonecrosis of the jaw. J Clin Oncol 2009;27:5356–5362.
133. Guarueri V, Donati S, Nicolini M, et al. Renal safety and efficacy of intravenous bisphosphonates in patients with skeletal metastases treated for up to ten years. Oncologist 2005;10:842–848.
134. Pozzi S, Raje N. The role of bisphosphonates in multiple myeloma: Mechanisms, side-effects, and future. Oncologist 2011;16:651–662.
135. Henry DH, Costa L. Goldwasser F, et al. Randomized double blind study of denosumab versus zolendronic acid in treatment of bone metastasis in patients with advanced cancer or multiple myeloma. J Clin Oncol 2011;29: 1125–1132.
136. Orlowski RZ, Nagler A, Sonnveld P, et al. Randomized phase III study of pegylated liposomal doxorubicin plus bortezomib compared with bortezomib alone in relapsed or refractory multiple myeloma: Combination therapy improves time to progression. J Clin Oncol 2007;25:3892–3901.
137. Mikhael JR, Belch AR, Prince HM, et al. High response rates to bortezomib with or without dexamethasone in patients with relapsed or refractory multiple myeloma: Results of a global phase IIIb expanded access programs. Br J Hematol 2009;144:169–175.
138. Richardson PG, Jagannath S, Jakubowiak AJ, et al. Phase II trial of lenalidomide, bortezomib, and dexamethasone in patients with relapsed and relapsed/refractory multiple myeloma: Updated efficacy and safety data after more than 2 years of follow-up. Blood 2010;116:3049 [abstract].
139. Lemieux E, Hulin C, Caillot D, et al. Autologous stem cell transplant: Effective salvage therapy in multiple myeloma. Biol Blood Marrow Transplant 2013;19(3):445–449.
140. Lentzch S, O'Sullivan A, Kennedy RC, et al. Combination of bendamustine, lenalidomide, and dexamethasone (BLD) in patients with relapsed or refractory multiple myeloma is feasible and highly effective: Results of Phase I/II open label, dose escalation study. Blood 2012;17: 4608–4613.
141. Siegel DS, Dimopoulos MA, Yoon SS, et al. Vorinostat in combination bortezomib in salvage multiple myeloma patients: Final study results of a global phase 2b trial. Blood 2011;118:480 [abstract].

114

Myelodysplastic Syndromes

Julianna A. Merten, Kristen B. McCullough, and Mrinal M. Patnaik

KEY CONCEPTS

1. Myelodysplastic syndromes (MDS) primarily affect elderly adults, with median age at diagnosis of 76 years.
2. MDS are associated with environmental, occupational, and therapeutic exposures to chemicals or radiation.
3. The clonal population of cells manifested as MDS results from enhanced self-renewal of a hematopoietic stem cell or acquisition of self-renewal in a progenitor cell, increased proliferative capacity in the abnormal clone, impaired cell differentiation, evasion of immune regulation, and antiapoptotic mechanisms in the disease-sustaining cell.
4. Most patients with MDS present with fatigue and lethargy or symptoms related to anemia-induced tissue hypoxia.
5. The prognosis of patients with MDS is variable. Overall survival time ranges from a few months to several years and can be estimated with the International Prognostic Scoring System (IPSS) or International Prognostic Scoring System—Revised (IPSS-R).
6. The primary goal of therapy is hematologic improvement for low-risk patients and alteration in the natural course of the disease for high-risk patients. Palliation of symptoms and improvement in quality of life are goals of therapy for all patients.
7. Current guidelines recommend erythropoietin (EPO) or darbepoetin for management of anemia in patients with MDS.
8. Hypomethylating agents are appropriate for patients with low-risk and intermediate-1-risk MDS with clinically significant neutropenia or thrombocytopenia, patients with anemia who are unlikely to respond to or have not responded to a trial of EPO, and patients who qualified for and failed immunosuppressive therapy.
9. Antithymocyte globulin is appropriate treatment for low or intermediate-1 IPSS risk, human leukocyte antigen DR15 positive expressing MDS in patients with symptomatic anemia that is unlikely to respond to erythropoietic agents.
10. Lenalidomide is the recommended initial treatment for low-risk 5q- syndrome accompanied by symptomatic anemia.
11. Allogeneic hematopoietic stem cell transplantation offers potentially curative therapy to patients with MDS who have a donor and are healthy enough for the procedure.

INTRODUCTION

Myelodysplastic syndromes (MDS) are clonal, heterogenous, stem cell disorders characterized by predominantly hypercellular bone marrows, anemia, thrombocytopenia, leukopenia, and an inherent predisposition toward evolution to acute myeloid leukemia (AML).[1–3] The diagnostic hallmark for MDS is the presence of bone marrow dysplasia in at least 10% of cells of a single myeloid lineage.[3] The clinical course of patients with MDS varies from a slowly progressing indolent disease to more aggressive disease characterized by excess bone marrow blasts and rapid progression to AML.[4]

Our understanding of MDS and the available treatment options have advanced in recent years. Based on new scientific and clinical information, the World Health Organization (WHO) revised its classification system in 2008 to refine diagnostic criteria and the subcategorization of MDS.[1] Genetic aberrations in hematopoietic transcription factors, methylation regulators, spliceosome components, and tumor suppressor genes have redefined the molecular landscape in MDS and have been incorporated into prognostic models predicting survival and leukemic transformation.[5–7] Between 2004 and 2006, three medications (azacitidine, decitabine, and lenalidomide) were approved by the FDA for the treatment of MDS. In 2009, the first randomized controlled clinical trial that showed a survival advantage for a therapeutic intervention in MDS was published, and several more randomized trials have been published or are ongoing.[8] The change in classification of MDS, improvement in risk stratification, and development of new treatment options represent important steps forward in MDS.

EPIDEMIOLOGY

1 MDS primarily affect elderly adults, with a median age at diagnosis of 76 years and a male predominance, with an estimated male-to-female ratio of about 1.75 to 1.[9,10] Overall, an estimated 3 to 12 cases of MDS are diagnosed per 100,000 persons per year. The incidence of MDS increases with age; in patients older than 65 to 70 years, an estimated 27 to 75 new cases occur per 100,000 persons per year.[11,12] The Surveillance, Epidemiology and End Results (SEER) Program estimates about 19,600 new cases of MDS are diagnosed in the United States each year.[10] Recent reports suggest that the incidence of MDS has been grossly underestimated, with an analysis of a Medicare claims database indicating it could be as high as 45,000 per year.[12] Many experts predict that the incidence of MDS will increase as the population of the United States ages and clinicians become more aware of MDS.[9]

ETIOLOGY

2 The exact cause of MDS is unknown and is probably multifactorial. MDS have been associated with environmental, occupational, and therapeutic exposures to chemicals or radiation.[13] Environmental exposure to agricultural chemicals has been associated with an increased risk of developing MDS.[13,14] MDS have also been linked in a dose-dependent relationship to ionizing radiation in atomic bomb survivors in Japan and have been reported in workers in the Chernobyl nuclear accident.[15] Occupational exposures to hair dyes, cereal dusts, exhaust gases, diesel fuel, and industrial solvents (including benzene and toluene) have been associated with development of MDS.[13,14] Individuals with a family history of a hematologic malignancy are at increased risk for developing MDS.[13,14] Modifiable risk factors for MDS include smoking and obesity.[16] Recent data suggest that chronic immune stimulation or therapy to manage infectious and autoimmune diseases increases the risk for development of MDS.[17]

About 10% to 15% of all cases of MDS are attributed to radiation, chemotherapy, or both and are termed *therapy-related MDS* (t-MDS).[18–20] More aggressive chemotherapy regimens and improved survival after cancer treatment are contributing to an increased incidence of t-MDS.[20,21] t-MDS have an increased likelihood of progression to AML and a poorer prognosis than de novo MDS.[19,20,22] Chromosomal abnormalities are found in about 90% of t-MDS compared with 50% to 60% of de novo MDS.[23–25]

The risk for developing t-MDS increases with age, higher doses of chemotherapy or radiation, longer duration of exposure, and exposure to both chemotherapy and radiation.[14,22,23] Several chemotherapeutic agents have been associated with t-MDS (Table 114-1). The contribution of a specific agent is difficult to assess because patients are usually exposed to multiple agents, often in combination with radiation.[22] The most frequently reported classes of chemotherapeutic agents associated with t-MDS are alkylating agents and topoisomerase II inhibitors.[18,19,23,24]

The role of alkylating agents in the development of t-MDS is well established in patients with cancer and those receiving high cumulative doses of alkylating agents for autoimmune disorders such as rheumatoid arthritis.[14,18,24] The latency period between exposure to alkylating agents and the development of t-MDS is about 4 to 7 years. Characteristic chromosomal abnormalities in t-MDS associated with alkylating agents include deletions on chromosome 5 and chromosome 7.[18]

Topoisomerase II inhibitors, including the epipodophyllotoxins (etoposide and teniposide), anthracyclines (daunorubicin, doxorubicin, epirubicin, idarubicin), and the anthracenedione mitoxantrone, are also associated with t-MDS. t-MDS associated with topoisomerase II inhibitors typically occurs a median of 2 to 3 years after exposure, and patients are more likely to present with AML at diagnosis.[14] Chromosomal abnormalities often found in patients with t-MDS associated with topoisomerase II inhibitors include balanced translocations involving the MLL gene 11q23 and 21q22.[18]

Radioimmunoconjugates, including ibritumomab tiuxetan and iodine-131 tositumomab, are monoclonal antibodies linked to radioactive isotopes. Radiation is delivered to the antibody-bound targeted cell and to neighboring cells through a "cross-fire" effect. t-MDS or AML is reported to occur in 5% to 10% of patients exposed to iodine-131 tositumomab and in 1% to 5% of patients exposed to ibritumomab tiuxetan.[26–30] About 8% of patients receiving myeloablative doses of ibritumomab tiuxetan as conditioning regimen before hematopoietic stem cell transplantation (HSCT) developed t-MDS or AML, similar to the rate in patients receiving myeloablative chemotherapy-based conditioning regimens.[31] Both agents are used to treat non-Hodgkin lymphoma, a patient population likely to receive other therapies associated with t-MDS, including alkylating agents, anthracyclines, and radiation. Therefore, it is difficult to determine the additional risk for t-MDS due solely to exposure to one of these agents.[26,28,30]

Granulocyte colony-stimulating factor (G-CSF) use during treatment of solid tumors and lymphoma in adults has been associated with an increased risk for t-MDS.[32] A systematic review of 25 randomized controlled trials comparing patients receiving filgrastim or lenograstim with placebo found an absolute risk increase of 0.41% for development of t-MDS or AML associated with use of a colony-stimulating factor.[32] The absolute risk of death was 3.4% lower in the group of patients randomized to a hematopoietic growth factor; the benefit was attributed to lower cancer-related mortality because of a greater chemotherapy dose intensity. This systematic review indicates the administration of hematopoietic growth factors to prevent complications associated with febrile neutropenia outweighs the increased t-MDS risk.[21] The risk of development of t-MDS may also be higher in patients with congenital neutropenia and aplastic anemia treated with long-term G-CSF.[18,33,34]

Patients undergoing autologous HSCT are at increased risk for development of t-MDS. Conditioning regimens given before HSCT usually include high doses of alkylating agents or etoposide, often in combination with total-body irradiation. As many as 8% to 20% of patients with non-Hodgkin lymphoma treated with autologous HSCT will be diagnosed with t-MDS within 10 years of transplantation.[35–37] Risk factors for development of t-MDS after autologous HSCT include antecedent conventional chemotherapy, prior radiation therapy, low stem cell dose, older age at time of transplant, and use of total-body irradiation in the conditioning regimen.[35,36,38]

TABLE 114-1 Therapies Associated with Therapy-Related Myelodysplastic Syndrome

Alkylating Agents	Topoisomerase II Inhibitors	Miscellaneous
Busulfan	Dactinomycin	Azathioprine
Carmustine	Daunorubicin	Carboplatin
Chlorambucil	Doxorubicin	Cladribine
Cyclophosphamide	Epirubicin	Cisplatin
Dacarbazine	Etoposide	Docetaxel
Ifosfamide	Idarubicin	Fludarabine
Lomustine	Mitoxantrone	Iodine-131 tositumomab
Mechlorethamine	Teniposide	Mercaptopurine
Melphalan		Methotrexate
Mitomycin		Paclitaxel
Procarbazine		Vinblastine
Temozolomide		Vincristine
Thiotepa		Yttrium-90 ibritumomab tiuxetan
		Radiation therapy

Data from Blaszkowsky and Erlichman[22] and Czader and Orazi.[18]

PATHOPHYSIOLOGY

3 Knowledge of normal hematopoiesis is needed to understand the pathophysiology of MDS (see eChap. 20 for a more detailed description of hematopoiesis). Progressive bone marrow failure is characteristic of patients with MDS and is the result of ineffective hematopoiesis. In addition to peripheral blood cytopenias, the terminally differentiated cells that are produced may have functional defects. Neutrophils may have reduced bactericidal and fungicidal activity despite a normal quantity of neutrophils.[39] Platelets may be normal in quantity but have impaired activation, secretion, and aggregation.[40] The diverse pathophysiology underlying MDS causes the heterogeneity in clinical presentation, pattern of disease progression,

and response to therapy and has not been fully elucidated.[41] A multistep model for the pathogenesis of MDS has been proposed, and it is likely that the disease can arise via multiple different pathways.[3,13,41] The clonal population of cells manifested as MDS results from enhanced self-renewal of a hematopoietic stem cell or acquisition of self-renewal in a progenitor cell, increased proliferative capacity in the abnormal clone, impaired cell differentiation, evasion of immune regulation, and antiapoptotic mechanisms in the disease-sustaining cell.[41] The abnormal clone proliferates or evades apoptosis because of genomic instability and abnormalities in cytokines and the bone marrow stroma.[3,41] These changes create a dysplastic, clonal population of cells in a milieu unable to support normal hematopoiesis.

Bone Marrow Microenvironment

The myelodysplastic clone is associated with cellular dysfunction, including excess secretion of cytokines, defective differentiation, genomic instability, and reduced response to regulatory cytokines.[3] In contrast to the peripheral blood cytopenias characteristic of MDS, bone marrow cells often have a paradoxically high rate of cellular division. Apoptosis, or programmed cell death, also is increased, leading to futile cycling of precursor cells and impaired production of mature peripheral blood cells.[13] Overproduction of proapoptotic and inflammatory cytokines and vascular endothelial growth factor may contribute to this process.[41] Bone marrow stromal cells from MDS patients show decreased ability to support normal hematopoietic cell function.[13]

Patients with MDS frequently have evidence of immune dysregulation, such as impaired immune surveillance and autoimmune reactions.[3] Cytopenias can be related to an autoimmune T-cell–mediated response. A subset of MDS patients characterized by younger age, refractory anemia of short duration, a hypocellular bone marrow, trisomy 8 as the sole cytogenetic abnormality, and expression of human leukocyte antigen (HLA) haplotype DR15 have a high likelihood of response to immunosuppressive therapy.[13,41] Immunosuppressive therapy with cyclosporine and antithymocyte globulin may induce durable responses in this subgroup of patients, confirming the role of immune dysregulation.[3] Whether B cells and T cells are a part of the MDS clonal population or a secondary reaction after the development of the malignant clone is unclear.[13]

Genomic Instability

In the multistep model for development of MDS, one or more transformations occur that confer a growth advantage to the dysplastic cell, leading to the emergence of a clonal population.[41] The inciting transformations in genetic material have not been identified. Chromosomal abnormalities, most often genomic losses and gains, are detected by cytogenetic analysis in about 50% of patients with de novo MDS and remain one of the strongest determinants of prognosis.[4,20,25,42–44] Multiple cytogenetic abnormalities that correlate with the clinical course of MDS were incorporated in the original International Prognostic Scoring System (IPSS) classification and prognostic assessment, including 5q or 20q deletions and chromosome 7 abnormalities.[4] The newly revised IPSS classification (International Prognostic Scoring System–Revised [IPSS-R]) includes several additional cytogenetic abnormalities, including trisomy 8 or 19, 12p or 11q deletions, and double abnormalities, that correlate with the clinical course of MDS.[7] Deletions on chromosome 5q occur in up to 12% of patients and are of particular interest because multiple genes involved in hematopoiesis are located there.[25] Additionally, MDS with 5q deletions as the sole genetic aberration are recognized as a distinct subtype of MDS with a favorable prognosis and a high likelihood of response to lenalidomide.[25,45]

High-resolution single nucleotide polymorphism array, a new type of karyotypic analysis that can detect molecular abnormalities that are too minute for traditional metaphase cytogenetics, has shown independent prognostic value for MDS.[6,46] One of the most frequently occurring molecular alterations, seen in 22% to 26% of MDS patients, is alteration of TET2 protein thought to be responsible for passive DNA methylation. Mutation in TET2 has been identified as a favorable prognostic factor, although results were not confirmed in larger confirmatory studies.[47–49] Transformations in additional tumor suppressor genes, transcription factors, and cell cycle regulators such as ASXL1, RUNX1, EZH2, DNMT3A, and several others are also thought to provide the dysplastic stem cell with a growth advantage and offer additional prognostic insight.[50]

Epigenetics

In addition to changes detected on chromosomal analysis, several transformations have been identified that may contribute to myelodysplasia that do not result from alteration of the nucleic acid sequence in DNA. The term *epigenetics* refers to mechanisms that regulate the expression of DNA without affecting its sequence. Epigenetic changes have been identified in numerous malignancies and are of particular importance in the context of MDS.[51]

DNA methylation is the best described and most common epigenetic marker. In the mammalian genome, only cytosine located 5′ to a guanosine (CpG) can be methylated (CpG pair). Clusters of CpG pairs, known as *CpG islands*, are near the promoter regions for many genes. These regions are unmethylated in normal cells, allowing for standard DNA expression to occur.[51] Increased methylation (hypermethylation) of *CpG* islands occurs via DNA methyltransferase and is associated with aberrant gene silencing, which may lead to further genetic instability and dysfunction of the cell cycle. Decreased methylation (hypomethylation) may lead to reexpression of previously silenced genes.[51] Hypermethylation and gene silencing have been identified in patients with MDS, and azacitidine and decitabine reverse this process.[51,52]

Histone acetylation, a second epigenetic marker, is also gaining significance in MDS.[53] Histones coil with DNA to form tightly wound complexes called chromatin. Posttranslational modifications of histones, by acetylation or deacetylation, can alter the structure of chromatin creating opportunities for gene suppression or expression, depending on the structural change of the chromatin.[53] Histone hypoacetylation has been documented in malignant cells and several histone deacetylase inhibitors have been studied in patients with MDS as monotherapy or in combination with hypomethylating agents in an attempt to promote histone acetylation and expression of previously suppressed tumor suppressor genes.[54,55]

CLASSIFICATION AND PROGNOSIS

Several classification systems and models for predicting risk in MDS have been developed. The French-American-British (FAB) and WHO are classification schemes for MDS. The FAB classification established subgroups of MDS based on morphology of bone marrow aspirates and peripheral blood blast percentage.[14] In the 2008 WHO classification system, MDS are categorized based on bone marrow and peripheral blood blast percentage, cytogenetics, and whether dysplasia or cytopenias affect a single cell lineage or multiple myeloid cell lines (Table 114-2).[56] The most significant changes in the WHO classification compared with the FAB classification include the following: patients with a single cell lineage affected are separated from those with multiple myeloid cell lines affected, patients with greater than 20% blasts in the marrow are now considered to have acute leukemia, patients with deletion on chromosome 5 are now in a distinct category, and chronic myelomonocytic leukemia is classified as a myelodysplastic/myeloproliferative disorder. Two studies showed the ability of the WHO classification to identify patient subgroups with differences in survival and responses to

CLINICAL PRESENTATION AND DIAGNOSIS Myelodysplastic Syndromes

General

- **4** Patients with MDS may develop isolated anemia (hemoglobin <11 g/dL), neutropenia (<1,500 cells/mm³), or thrombocytopenia (<100 × 10⁹/L) or multiple peripheral cytopenias.
- Patients may be asymptomatic, with cytopenia(s) discovered on complete blood count with differential.

Symptoms

- If symptomatic, the patient may report fatigue, lethargy, malaise, palpitations, dyspnea on exertion, or other symptoms associated with hypoxia secondary to anemia.
- Patients may have symptoms of infection, including cough or dysuria.
- Patients may present with complaints of easy bruising or bleeding.

Signs

- Pallor, tachycardia, or tachypnea related to anemia
- Fever, chills, rigors caused by infection and immune dysfunction
- Petechiae, bruising, epistaxis, gingival bleeding, excessive vaginal bleeding, bruising, or hematuria caused by thrombocytopenia

Laboratory Tests

- Complete blood count with differential
- Anemia often is macrocytic or normocytic with a low reticulocyte index
- Serum vitamin B_{12}, red blood cell (RBC) folate and copper levels
- Testing for the human immunodeficiency virus (HIV)
- Serum thyroid-stimulating hormone
- Serum EPO level
- Serum ferritin, iron, and total iron-binding capacity

Other Diagnostic Tests

- Bone marrow biopsy and aspirate: send for morphologic examination, cytochemical staining, immunophenotyping, and cytogenetics (chromosome analysis).
- Repeat bone marrow biopsy of patients with MDS often is required because dysplastic features may progress over time or the bone marrow may be unevenly distributed.

Criteria for Diagnosis

- Stable cytopenia for at least 6 months (2 months if accompanied by a specific karyotype associated with MDS or bilineage dysplasia)
- Exclusion of other causes of cytopenia or dysplasia
- One of the following:
  1. Dysplasia (>10% in one or more of three major bone marrow lineages)
  2. Blast cell count of 5% to 19%
  3. Specific MDS-associated karyotype (e.g., del(5q), del(20q), +8, or del(7q))

Data from Tefferi and Vardiman,[3] Faderl and Kantarjian,[14] Valent et al.,[161] and The NCCN Clinical Practice Guidelines in Oncology™.[61]

erythropoietin (EPO) and filgrastim. Patients with refractory anemia or refractory anemia with ringed sideroblasts (RARS) had prolonged overall and leukemia-free survival and improved response to therapy compared with those with refractory cytopenia with multilineage dysplasia or refractory anemia with excessive blasts.[57] This classification scheme may help predict the prognosis of MDS, but it has not been shown to predict response to a given therapy.

Models to predict overall survival and risk of transformation to AML continue to be developed and refined as new information about the genetic basis of MDS evolves. The IPSS is still used in clinical trials and continues to guide therapy as newer models are developed and validated.[3,5] **5** Based on an observational study of mostly untreated MDS patients, the IPSS was developed to identify factors that would predict progression of MDS.[4] Multivariate analyses identified four prognostic factors: cytogenetic abnormalities, percentage of bone marrow blasts, age, and number of cytopenias. Using these four factors, researchers were able to stratify patients into four risk groups that correlated with overall survival, which ranged from a few months to several years (Table 114-3).

The IPSS-R was developed after analysis of more than 7,000 patients whose disease had not been treated with disease-altering therapy (Table 114-4).[7] This model differs from the IPSS by identifying five risk categories by incorporating different categories for marrow blast percentage value and depth of cytopenias, expanding the cytogenetic risk groups from three to five groups and including a number of less common cytogenetic abnormalities. Patient age, performance status, and serum ferritin and lactate dehydrogenase levels were additional significant predictors for survival but not for AML transformation. Recent reports have demonstrated that recurrent somatic gene mutations predict prognosis independent of the IPSS score, and their incorporation into a risk classification scheme does enhance the model.[6,58] About half of patients with MDS have normal cytogenetics; therefore, after the full spectrum of somatic mutations in MDS has been defined, optimal prognostic scoring systems will need to include relevant molecular features. No single method of predicting risk of disease progression, overall survival, or response to therapy has been universally adopted.[5] The risk prognostic schemas are derived from patients with primary, untreated MDS and may not be applicable to patients who have t-MDS, those who received disease-modifying therapy, or those who have undergone karyotypic evolution in the course of their disease.

Clinical **Controversy...**

Several MDS risk scoring systems have been proposed in the past few years. The optimal method to predict overall survival, progression to AML, and likelihood of response to therapy continues to be debated.

TABLE 114-2 World Health Organization Classification of Myelodysplastic Syndromes

Classification	Blood	Bone Marrow
Refractory cytopenia with unilineage dysplasia (RCUD): refractory anemia [RA]; refractory neutropenia [RN]; refractory thrombocytopenia [RT]	Unicytopenia or bicytopenia No or rare blasts (<1%)	Unilineage dysplasia: ≥10% of the cells in one myeloid lineage <5% blasts <15% ringed sideroblasts
Refractory anemia with ringed sideroblasts (RARS)	Anemia No blasts	≥15% ringed sideroblasts Erythroid dysplasia only <5% blasts
Refractory cytopenia with multilineage dysplasia (RCMD)	Cytopenia(s) No or rare blasts (<1%) No Auer rods Monocytes <1,000 cells/mm³	Dysplasia in ≥10% of cells in ≥2 myeloid cell lines <5% blasts +15% ringed sideroblasts No Auer rods
Refractory anemia with excess blasts-1 (RAEB-1)	Cytopenia(s) <5% blasts No Auer rods Monocytes <1,000 cells/mm³	Unilineage or multilineage dysplasia 5–9% blasts No Auer rods
Refractory anemia with excess blasts-2 (RAEB-2)	Cytopenia(s) 5–19% blasts ±Auer rods Monocytes <1,000 cells/mm³	Unilineage or multilineage dysplasia ± Auer rods
Myelodysplastic syndrome, unclassified (MDS-U)	Cytopenias <1% blasts	Unequivocal dysplasia in <10% of cells in one or more myeloid lineage when accompanied by a cytogenetic abnormality considered as presumptive evidence for a diagnosis of MDS <5% blasts
Myelodysplastic syndrome associated with **isolated** deletion of 5q	Anemia Usually normal or increased platelet count No or rare blasts (<1%)	Normal to increased megakaryocytes with hypolobated nuclei <5% blasts No Auer rods Isolated del(5q) cytogenetic abnormality
Childhood myelodysplastic syndrome (provisional entity: refractory cytopenia of childhood [RCC])	Cytopenia(s) <2% blasts	<5% blasts Dysplasia in ≥10% of cells in ≥2 myeloid cell lines

Data from Vardiman et al.[1,56]

Currently, the FAB classification is used for coding and billing purposes, for drug indication languages approved by regulatory agencies, and for some clinical trial inclusion or evaluation criteria.[5] The WHO criteria are used by pathologists to describe MDS and in both clinical trial and off-study management of patients with MDS. The IPSS is the most widely used prognostic scoring system for MDS patients enrolling in clinical trials and is used to guide therapy in the United States.[3,5] The IPSS-R will likely be adopted by most centers until the role of molecular information in the prognosis of MDS is better defined.[59]

TREATMENT

Treatment of MDS has rapidly evolved during the last decade following discoveries in disease biology, introduction of new methods for predicting the natural history of the disease and response to a given therapy, and development of new treatment strategies (Fig. 114-1).

Desired Outcomes

6 The goals of treatment vary with disease-specific factors, including the type of MDS; cytogenetics; risk of progression to AML and death; rate of disease progression; and patient factors, including age, organ function, performance status, and presence of symptoms related to myelodysplasia.[60] The primary goal of therapy is hematologic improvement for low-risk patients and alteration in the natural course of the disease for high-risk patients.[61] Additional critical goals for all risk groups include symptom palliation and quality-of-life improvement. Lower-intensity treatment with a DNA hypomethylating agent or immunosuppressive therapy may improve overall survival, provide symptom palliation, and enhance quality of life without significant toxicity.[8,60,61] The only curative therapy for MDS is allogeneic HSCT, but most patients lack a suitable donor, are not healthy enough to undergo this intensive therapy, or may not be referred for HSCT because of advanced biologic age despite adequate health and organ function.[3,62]

TABLE 114-3 International Prognostic Scoring System for Myelodysplastic Syndromes

	Score Value				
Prognostic Variable	**0**	**0.5**	**1**	**1.5**	**2**
Bone marrow blasts (%)	5	5–10	—	11–20	21–30
Karyotype	Good	Intermediate	Poor		
Cytopenia	0 or 1	2 or 3			

Cytopenia: absolute neutrophil count <1,800 cells/mm³
Hemoglobin <10 g/dL
Platelet count <100,000 cells/mm³

Karyotype: Good: normal, isolated 5q deletion, isolated 20q deletion, -Y
Intermediate: any other abnormalities
Poor: trisomy 7, complex or >3

Score	Risk Group	Median Survival (years)
0	Low	5.7
0.5–1	Intermediate-1	3.5
1.5–2.0	Intermediate-2	1.2
≥2.5	High	0.4

Data from Greenberg et al.[4]

TABLE 114-4 International Prognostic Scoring System—Revised for Myelodysplastic Syndromes[a]

Prognostic Variable	0	0.5	1	1.5	2	3	4
Cytogenetics	Very good		Good		Intermediate	Poor	Very poor
Bone marrow blast (%)	≤2		>2 to <5		5–10	>10	
Hemoglobin (g/dL)	≥10		8 to <10	<8			
Platelets (cells/mm³)	≥100,000	50,000 to <100,000	<50,000				
Absolute neutrophil count (cells/mm³)	≥800	<800					

[a]Karyotype: very good: -Y, del(11q).
Good: normal, del(5q), del(12p), del(20q), double including del(5q).
Intermediate: del(7q), +8, +19, i(17q), any other single or double independent clones.
Poor: -7, inv(3)/t(3q)/del(3q), double, including -7/del(7q); complex: three abnormalities.
Very poor: Complex: >3 abnormalities.

Score	Risk Group	Median Survival (years)
<1.5	Very low	8.8
>1.5–3	Low	5.3
>3–4.5	Intermediate	3
>4.5–6	High	1.6
>6	Very high	0.8

Data from Greenberg et al.[7]

General Approach

Therapy for MDS is determined by symptoms, IPSS risk for progression to AML or death, patient age and comorbidities, likelihood of response to a given therapy and its effects on quality of life, and patients' treatment preferences.[2] Patients with extensive, life-limiting comorbidities or who are asymptomatic at diagnosis may warrant supportive care alone.[2] About 30% to 60% of patients with MDS receive supportive care alone.[25,63] Lower-risk patients are thought to have better prognoses, and thus less toxic therapies are used to manage MDS, including EPO, darbepoetin, lenalidomide, or DNA hypomethylating agents. Patients with intermediate-2 and high IPSS risk MDS have poorer prognoses and may be candidates for allogeneic HSCT; patients who are not HSCT candidates may benefit from a DNA hypomethylating agent.[8,61] As outcomes of therapeutic interventions for all risk categories are identified and genetic markers increase the ability of clinicians to stratify patients into even more specific risk categories, the line between therapies for high- and low-risk patients has been blurred.[20] Clinicians should recognize that the clinical course of MDS is not static. MDS may progress; comorbidities or symptoms may change over time along with the ability to create more personalized medicine, necessitating an adjustment in treatment strategy. Therapy for MDS is generally palliative, and enrollment in a suitable clinical trial is always a viable approach.[2,64]

Careful interpretation is necessary when comparing the results of clinical trials in MDS because patient characteristics and response criteria vary widely. Described previously, the clinical course and prognosis are affected by patient-specific characteristics.[4,65] Examples of different response criteria used include changes in hemoglobin, changes in RBC transfusion requirements, or effects on quality of life.[60] The use of RBC transfusion requirement as a primary end point is especially problematic because decisions concerning RBC transfusion needs are highly individualized and may not be consistent among clinicians. Additionally, the relationship between changes in hemoglobin or decreases in RBC transfusion requirements and improved quality of life is not clear. Some treatments for MDS can cause significant adverse effects, resulting in hospitalization or increased clinic visits, and may negatively impact quality of life regardless of their positive effects on hematologic parameters. The impact of treatment on quality of life is an important consideration when selecting therapy and should be assessed regularly with the use of validated instruments.

Supportive Care

All patients with MDS should receive supportive care, including clinical monitoring, psychosocial support, and quality-of-life assessment.[61] The National Comprehensive Cancer Network (NCCN) guidelines recommend that patients with symptomatic anemia should receive leukoreduced RBC transfusions, and those with bleeding caused by thrombocytopenia or platelet counts below 10,000 cells/mm³ (10×10^9/L) should receive platelet transfusions.[61] Hematopoietic growth factor support should be considered in patients with refractory, symptomatic cytopenias. Patients with evidence of infection should have an appropriate diagnostic evaluation based on history and physical examination followed by appropriate antimicrobial therapy. Routine antimicrobial or hematopoietic growth factor prophylaxis is not recommended in the absence of repeated infections. Iron chelation may be considered in low-risk and intermediate-1-risk patients and candidates for allogeneic HSCT who have received more than 20 to 30 RBC transfusions and are expected to continue to require transfusions.[61]

Infection

Patients with MDS may be neutropenic or have functional defects in neutrophils, predisposing them to infection.[39] In MDS, the most frequently isolated organisms are bacteria, and the most common sites of infection are the lungs, urinary tract, and bloodstream.[66] Patients with evidence of infection should have appropriate diagnostic evaluation based on history and physical examination and then appropriate antimicrobial therapy. Neutropenic patients with evidence of infection or fever of unknown origin should receive empiric broad-spectrum, IV antibiotics.[67]

Hematopoietic Growth Factors

Filgrastim (G-CSF) and sargramostim (granulocyte-macrophage colony-stimulating factor [GM-CSF]) are colony-stimulating factors that stimulate white blood cell production and may increase circulating neutrophils in 70% to 90% of patients, which may decrease risk of infection.[68] These agents have not been shown to be beneficial as chronic monotherapy because they do not reliably prevent infection and have no impact on survival.[68] G-CSF or GM-CSF should only be administered temporarily as monotherapy in the rare neutropenic MDS patient who develops recurrent severe infections.[2,3]

EPO is a protein produced by the kidney in response to hypoxia that stimulates proliferation and differentiation of erythroid cells. Anemic patients with MDS may have either a lower than expected endogenous serum EPO level relative to the degree of anemia present or an elevated EPO level. The mechanism of action of recombinant erythropoiesis-stimulating agents (ESAs) in MDS is not clear, but exogenous EPO may stimulate a normal clone of cells that is unresponsive to low endogenous levels of EPO, stimulate a dysplastic clone to differentiate that is less responsive to endogenous EPO, or induce apoptosis. An immunomodulatory effect of EPO, G-CSF, or GM-CSF has been proposed.

7 Current guidelines recommend use of ESAs for management of anemia in patients with MDS.[61,69] Unlike some solid tumors,[70] no detrimental effects on overall survival or progression

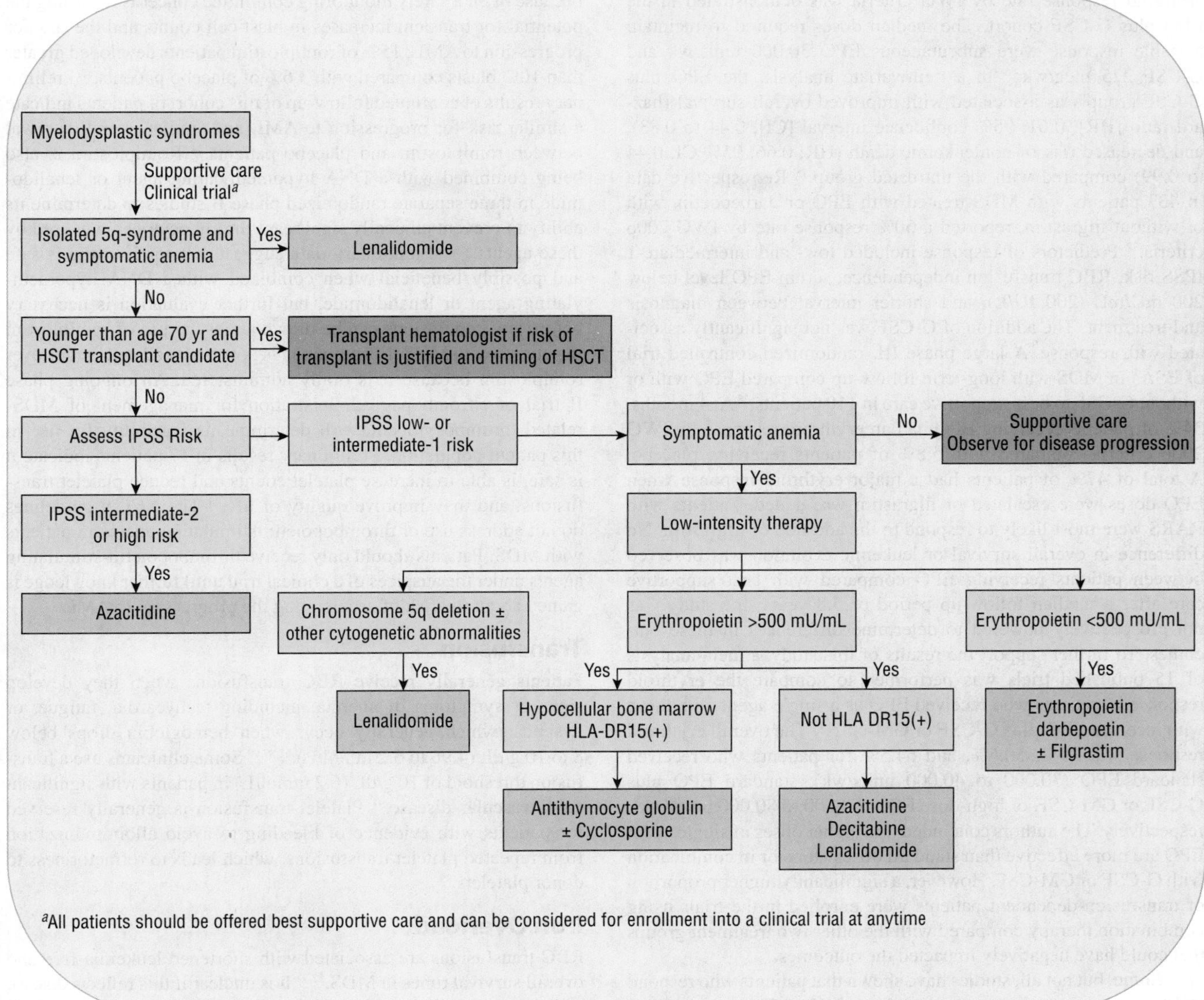

FIGURE 114-1 Myelodysplastic syndromes treatment algorithm. (HSCT, hematopoietic stem cell transplant; IPSS, International Prognostic Scoring System.)

to leukemia have been noted in patients with MDS. Treatment with ESAs alone may result in hematologic improvement and transfusion independence in low- and intermediate-1 IPSS risk patients. Two meta-analyses have evaluated the efficacy of ESAs in MDS. The first analysis, which included 2,106 patients from 59 studies reported between 1990 and 2005, found a hemoglobin response of about 30% based on the definition of hemoglobin response in the original publication.[71] A subsequent meta-analysis only included studies from 1990 to 2006 that reported results by International Working Group (IWG) criteria[60] to define erythroid response (an increase in hemoglobin of 2 g/dL [1.24 mmol/L] or transfusion independence). This report included 30 studies with 925 patients with MDS and found an overall erythroid response rate of 58% in patients receiving ESAs.[72] The latter report also suggests that EPO and darbepoetin can be used interchangeably for the management of MDS based on similar response rates achieved. The higher response rate compared with the previous meta-analysis likely reflects inclusion of a higher proportion of patients most likely to respond to ESAs. Patients with low- and intermediate-1 IPSS risk MDS who have a serum EPO level less than 500 mU/mL (500 IU/L) and a history of receiving fewer than 2 units of RBC transfusions per month have the best chance at responding to ESAs.[2,73] The doses required to achieve a response in MDS are higher than those used to treat renal causes of anemia, with EPO doses in the range from 40,000 to 60,000 units subcutaneously two to three times per week.[61] Darbepoetin doses ranging from 100 to 300 mcg subcutaneously weekly or every other week have also been used for MDS management.[2,72] Doses should be titrated up or down, as clinically indicated, to achieve a hemoglobin level of 10 to 12 g/dL (6.2 to 7.44 mmol/L).[74] Additionally, patients should receive at least 8 weeks of therapy before doses are adjusted or before patients are considered nonresponders because response to ESAs in MDS can be delayed.[2,61] The median response duration for ESAs in MDS is 1 to 2 years, and the ESA should be discontinued if there is no benefit or the response wanes.[2]

Several trials have evaluated if adding G-CSF to ESAs can enhance the hematologic response, and the conclusions have been inconsistent. Long-term follow-up of 121 patients from three uncontrolled phase II studies was retrospectively compared with that of 237 untreated patients who were matched for FAB classification, hemoglobin, and transfusion needs.[75] A 39% major erythroid response rate by IWG criteria was demonstrated in the EPO plus G-CSF cohort. The median doses required to maintain a stable response were subcutaneous EPO 30,000 units/wk and G-CSF 225 mcg/wk.[76] In a multivariate analysis, the EPO plus G-CSF group was associated with improved overall survival (hazard ratio [HR], 0.61; 95% confidence interval [CI], 0.44 to 0.83), and decreased risk of nonleukemic death (HR, 0.66; 95% CI, 0.44 to 0.99) compared with the untreated group.[75] Retrospective data in 433 patients with MDS treated with EPO or darbepoetin, with or without filgrastim, reported a 50% response rate by IWG 2006 criteria.[77] Predictors of response included low- and intermediate-1 IPSS risk, RBC transfusion independence, serum EPO level below 200 mU/mL (200 IU/L), and shorter interval between diagnosis and treatment. The addition of G-CSF was not significantly associated with response. A large phase III, randomized controlled trial of ESAs in MDS with long-term follow-up compared EPO with or without G-CSF to best supportive care in 110 patients.[78] At 4 months, 34% of patients receiving EPO had an erythroid response by IWG 2006 criteria compared with 5.8% of patients receiving placebo. A total of 47% of patients had a major erythroid response when EPO doses were escalated or filgrastim was added. Patients with RARS were most likely to respond to the addition of filgrastim. No difference in overall survival or leukemic evolution was observed between patients receiving EPO compared with best supportive care after a median follow-up period of 5.8 years; the study was not prospectively powered to determine differences in these outcomes. To further support the results of this study, a meta-analysis of 15 published trials was performed to compare the erythroid response in patients who received EPO as a single agent with those who received EPO plus G-CSF or GM-CSF.[79] The overall erythroid response was 49%, 50.6%, and 64.5% for patients who received standard EPO (30,000 to 40,000 units/wk), standard EPO plus G-CSF or GM-CSF, or high-dose EPO (60,000 to 80,000 units/wk), respectively. The authors concluded that higher doses of single agent EPO are more effective than standard doses alone or in combination with G-CSF or GM-CSF. However, a significantly higher proportion of transfusion-dependent patients were enrolled in the trials using combination therapy compared with the other two treatment groups that could have negatively impacted the outcomes.

Some, but not all, studies have shown that patients who respond to ESAs have improvements in quality of life.[78] The value of this costly intervention has not been proven, and long-term safety has not been evaluated in randomized controlled trials.[80] Although EPO, with or without G-CSF, does not improve overall survival, it does not shorten overall survival or time to development of leukemia and may decrease the need for RBC transfusions and improve quality of life. ESA therapy is well tolerated, and the NCCN recommends a trial in low- and intermediate-1 IPSS risk patients who have a serum EPO level less than 500 mU/mL (500 IU/L) and a limited transfusion history.[61]

Thrombopoietin is a hormone synthesized in the liver and secreted into the systemic circulation, where it binds to thrombopoietin receptors on stem cells, progenitor cells, and platelets, resulting in increased platelet production. Romiplostim and eltrombopag are novel drugs that stimulate the thrombopoietin receptor similarly to endogenous thrombopoietin, and are currently FDA approved for patients with chronic idiopathic thrombocytopenic purpura. Two small phase II open-label trials evaluating romiplostim in patients with low- and intermediate-1-risk MDS with platelets less than 50,000 cells/mm^3 (50×10^9/L) resulted in durable platelet responses in 30% to 46% of patients by IWG 2000 criteria.[81,82] Four of 45 patients developed a transient increase in the proportion of bone marrow blasts, and 2 patients developed AML in one of the studies[81]; in the other study 2 of 28 patients developed progression to AML.[82] A randomized, placebo-controlled trial evaluating romiplostim to manage thrombocytopenia in MDS was stopped early in 2011 because of data safety monitoring committee concerns regarding the potential for transient increases in blast cell counts and the risk for progression to AML; 15% of romiplostim patients developed greater than 10% blasts compared with 3.6% of placebo patients.[83] Preliminary results of continued follow-up of this cohort of patients indicate a similar risk for progression to AML and similar overall survival between romiplostim and placebo patients.[84] Romiplostim is also being combined with a DNA hypomethylating agent or lenalidomide in three separate randomized phase II studies to determine its ability to prevent clinically significant thrombocytopenia caused by these agents.[85–87] Preliminary data suggest that romiplostim is safe and possibly beneficial when combined with a DNA hypomethylating agent or lenalidomide, but further evaluation is necessary before any conclusions can be drawn about the use of romiplostim in patients with MDS. Eltrombopag is potentially advantageous over romiplostim because it is orally administered. An ongoing phase II trial of eltrombopag administration for management of MDS-related thrombocytopenia will determine its feasibility for use in this patient population. Preliminary results in 17 patients indicate it is safe, is able to increase platelet counts and reduce platelet transfusions, and may improve quality of life.[88] The NCCN guidelines do not address use of thrombopoietin-stimulating agents in patients with MDS. Patients should only receive thrombopoietin-stimulating agents under the auspices of a clinical trial until further knowledge is gained about the risk of accelerating the progression to AML.

Transfusion

Patients generally receive RBC transfusions when they develop signs or symptoms of anemia, including tachycardia, fatigue, or dyspnea, which generally occur when hemoglobin drops below 8 to 10 g/dL (4.96 to 6.2 mmol/L).[61,89,90] Some clinicians use a transfusion threshold of 10 g/dL (6.2 mmol/L) in patients with significant cardiovascular disease.[91] Platelet transfusion is generally reserved for patients with evidence of bleeding to avoid alloimmunization from repeated platelet transfusions, which leads to refractoriness to donor platelets.[89,91]

Iron Overload

RBC transfusions are associated with shortened leukemia-free and overall survival times in MDS.[57,92] It is unclear if this reflects disease severity or is a direct result of iron toxicity.[3,93] Recent data indicate MDS patients receiving RBC transfusions more frequently develop infections, cardiac, hepatic, and endocrine dysfunction compared with nontransfused MDS patients or the general population without MDS.[12,94] Prospective clinical trials in MDS demonstrate that iron chelation is able to decrease markers of iron overload.[95–99] Two studies suggest that patients receiving iron chelation experience hematologic improvement during iron chelation therapy in the absence of other therapy to treat MDS, and three studies suggest iron chelation may improve overall survival.[97,98,100–102] In a retrospective study of 18 low- or intermediate-1-risk patients, deferoxamine was associated with improved overall survival compared with matched control participants not receiving iron chelation therapy; the median overall survival time was not reached at 226 months in the deferoxamine group versus 40 months in the control group.[100] A prospective cohort of low- or intermediate-1-risk patients received iron chelation ($n = 53$) or no iron chelation ($n = 44$) and was shown to have a median overall survival time of 124 months versus 53 months in nonchelated patients.[101] A survival advantage persisted after adjustment for IPSS, age, World Health Organization Classification-based Scoring System (WPSS), level of transfusion requirement, and number of comorbidities. Neukirchen et al. conducted a retrospective, matched-pair analysis of registry data for 94 MDS patients undergoing long-term iron chelation therapy and 94 matched partners in the Düsseldorf MDS Registry; 83% of patients had low- or intermediate-1-risk MDS.[102] Patients received supportive care, including growth factors, but no other therapy for MDS other than iron chelation. Median survival time in the iron chelation group was 74 months versus 49 months in the supportive care alone group. It is unclear if the apparent survival benefit with iron chelation is truly a result of reducing iron overload or if confounding factors contributed to these results.[103] Preliminary results of a cohort of Medicare beneficiaries with MDS indicate longer duration of deferasirox use correlated with improved overall survival times, but deferasirox was not found to be associated with altered risk of heart failure or endocrine or renal disease.[104] It is hypothesized that iron chelation may lower infection risk, improve the outcome of allogeneic HSCT, and delay leukemic transformation in patients with MDS.[93] A prospective, randomized trial comparing deferasirox with placebo in low- and intermediate-1-risk MDS patients with transfusional iron overload with a primary outcome of event-free survival is ongoing (registered at *www.clinicaltrials.gov*; NCT00940602).

The potential toxicity, expense, and benefits of iron chelation should be carefully considered before initiating therapy.[103] Deferasirox and deferoxamine are FDA approved for use in patients with chronic iron overload caused by RBC transfusions. Deferiprone is FDA approved for patients with transfusional iron overload secondary to thalassemia when current chelation therapy is inadequate. The prescribing information for deferiprone has a black box warning regarding agranulocytosis, which may lead to serious infection and death. The prescribing information for deferasirox has a black box warning describing renal and hepatic impairment and GI hemorrhage; fatalities were reported. These reactions were more frequently observed in patients with advanced age, high-risk MDS, underlying renal or hepatic impairment, or thrombocytopenia (<50,000 cells/mm^3 [50×10^9/L]).

Clinical **Controversy. . .**

Initiation of iron chelation in patients with MDS is controversial because controlled trials of iron chelation have not been completed. It is unclear if iron chelation will impact the natural history of MDS despite the anticipated prevention or reversal of end-organ damage associated with iron overload.[159,160] Even though no prospective, randomized controlled trials have been completed, eight different clinical practice guidelines have been published regarding iron chelation in MDS.[159] These guidelines differ on whether or not to initiate chelation and at what threshold; which agent, dose, and duration to use; and how to monitor for the efficacy and toxicity of iron chelation.

Many clinicians recommend iron chelation be initiated after 20 to 30 RBC transfusions are administered or when serum ferritin levels exceed 1,000 to 2,500 ng/mL (1,000 to 2,500 mcg/L) in patients with low- or intermediate-1-risk MDS who have an anticipated survival of at least 1 year or in patients proceeding to allogeneic HSCT.[61,90,91,105–107] Patients receiving pharmacotherapy for iron chelation should be monitored for ocular toxicity, ototoxicity due to renal and hepatic dysfunction, and complete blood counts in addition to markers of iron overload.[106]

Pharmacologic Therapy

Pharmacotherapy of MDS is intended to change the natural history of MDS. Table 114-5 lists the responses reported in selected clinical trials of non-HSCT therapies. DNA hypomethylating agents may prolong overall survival, yet allogeneic HSCT remains the only curative option for patients. Because most patients with MDS are not candidates for HSCT, less toxic therapeutic modalities are being evaluated in an attempt to improve quality of life and disease-free survival.

Immunosuppressive Agents

Immunosuppressive agents that modulate T cells, including corticosteroids, antithymocyte globulin, and cyclosporine, have been evaluated in patients with MDS. Clinically significant adverse events and low response rates have limited the widespread use of corticosteroids as a therapeutic option for MDS, but antithymocyte globulin and cyclosporine continue to be studied alone and in combination for the treatment of patients with low-risk MDS.[108]

Antithymocyte globulin has been investigated primarily in patients with intermediate-1-risk and low-risk MDS. Treatment with antithymocyte globulin may not be beneficial for all patients because of the potential for infectious complications, serum sickness, and variations in response. Most studies have used equine antithymocyte globulin at a dose of 40 mg/kg/day IV for 4 consecutive days with corticosteroids to prevent serum sickness.[109,110] Responses generally occur within 8 months, and about one third of previously transfusion-dependent patients achieve durable transfusion independence.[109,110] Rabbit antithymocyte globulin has also been evaluated in daily doses ranging from 3.5 to 3.75 mg/kg administered IV for 5 days.[111,112] Response rates, although modest, appear to be similar and treatment with either horse or rabbit antithymocyte globulin is reasonable. Patient factors associated with response to immunosuppressive therapy include age younger than 60 years, hypocellular marrow, refractory anemia of short duration, trisomy 8 as the sole cytogenetic abnormality, and HLA DR15 positive expression.[41,113] A recent retrospective evaluation of patients enrolled on clinical trials

TABLE 114-5 Results from Pivotal Trials of Low-Intensity Treatment for Myelodysplastic Syndromes

Medication	Patients (*n*)	Median Age (years)	Percent of Patients by IPSS Risk Category: Low	Int-1	Int-2	High	Response Criteria	Complete Response (%)	RBC Transfusion Independence (%)	Overall Hematologic Improvement (%)
Azacitidine[125]	191	69	5[a]	53	23	17	Other	7	45	37
Decitabine[126]	170	70	—	31	43	26	IWG	9	NR	30
Antithymocyte globulin (equine) + cyclosporine[114]	88	62	18[b]	56	14	1	Other	NR	34	NR
Lenalidomide[158] (5q deletions)	148	71	37	44	5	—	IWG	NR	67	76
Lenalidomide[119]	214	72	43	36	4[c]	—	IWG	NR	26	43

Int, intermediate; IWG, International Working Group; NR, no response; RBC, red blood cell.

[a]Evaluated in 39 of 99 patients.
[b]International Prognostic Scoring System (IPSS) not evaluable because of missing cytogenetics in 11%.
[c]Intermediate-2- and high-risk patients.

at the National Institutes of Health demonstrated that the combination of equine antithymocyte globulin and cyclosporine was an independent factor associated with response to therapy compared with either agent administered alone.[113]

A survival benefit from therapy with antithymocyte globulin has not been demonstrated despite studying various regimens, including both formulations, with or without hematopoietic growth factor support, and cyclosporine or corticosteroids. A phase III randomized controlled trial compared equine antithymocyte globulin and cyclosporine versus best supportive care in all IPSS risk categories.[114] At 6 months, 29% of patients achieved a hematologic response in the immunotherapy cohort compared with 9% of those receiving best supportive care, but no difference was seen in overall, leukemia-free, or 2-year transformation-free survival. Notably, these patients were not evaluated for HLA DR15, and nearly 25% of patients in each group had undetermined risk, intermediate-2-risk, or high-risk IPSS.[114]

Alemtuzumab is a monoclonal antibody with immunosuppressive properties that is being evaluated in MDS. Preliminary data demonstrated hematologic improvement in 77% of intermediate-1 and 58% of intermediate-2 IPSS risk patients with HLA DR15 positivity.[115] Further evaluation will be needed to determine its role in therapy of MDS.

Immunomodulating Drugs

Thalidomide and lenalidomide are immunomodulating drugs, frequently referred to as *IMiDs*. Thalidomide was discovered to possess antiinflammatory, antiangiogenic, and antiapoptotic properties, prompting its investigation as a potential treatment of MDS. Initial response rates were encouraging, but few complete responses and high rates of discontinuation because of intolerable side effects have made thalidomide rarely used in MDS. Common side effects of thalidomide include fluid retention, peripheral neuropathy, thrombosis, sedation, and constipation.

Lenalidomide is structurally similar to thalidomide but offers a distinct side effect profile and potentially enhanced therapeutic effects. Lenalidomide is more potent in vitro than thalidomide with respect to T-cell modulation and inhibition of tumor necrosis factor-α, a proapoptotic and proinflammatory cytokine. Compared with thalidomide, lenalidomide causes less fluid retention, peripheral neuropathy, thrombosis, and constipation but more frequently induces neutropenia and thrombocytopenia. Pruritus, rash, diarrhea, and hypothyroidism have been reported with lenalidomide use but seldom require treatment discontinuation. Lenalidomide undergoes substantial renal elimination, and dose reduction in patients with renal insufficiency is recommended to decrease the likelihood of significant bone marrow suppression. Treatment-emergent thrombocytopenia and neutropenia during lenalidomide therapy are associated with response in low-risk MDS patients.[116] Careful consideration is necessary before reducing the dose or holding lenalidomide treatment in low-risk MDS patients who develop myelosuppression.

Lenalidomide gained recognition after an uncontrolled trial of 43 MDS patients reported a 56% overall response rate and 62% rate of transfusion independence. Patients with a clonal deletion of chromosome 5q demonstrated an 83% complete response rate.[117] A subsequent phase II trial of patients with a 5q deletion and transfusion-dependent anemia evaluated lenalidomide 10 mg orally once daily. Cytogenetic remission was seen in 45% of patients with 67% achieving transfusion independence.[45] The median time to response was 4 weeks. The results of this pivotal trial led to FDA approval of lenalidomide for treatment of low-risk MDS in patients with a 5q deletion.

Lenalidomide in Low- and Intermediate-1-Risk Myelodysplastic Syndromes A phase III randomized, placebo-controlled study of lenalidomide in low- and intermediate-1-risk MDS patients with a deletion 5q compared the efficacy and safety of lenalidomide 10 mg daily for 21 of 28 days or 5 mg daily with placebo in transfusion dependent patients with a primary end point of transfusion independence for at least 26 consecutive weeks.[118] Transfusion independence was significantly improved in both the lenalidomide 10- and 5-mg groups, 56% and 46%, respectively, versus placebo at 6%. The lenalidomide 10-mg group showed significantly better transfusion independence for patients with baseline EPO levels greater than 500 mU/mL (500 IU/L). Cytogenetic remission was achieved in 50% and 25% of the lenalidomide 10- and 5-mg patients, respectively. Overall survival was not significantly different between groups, although this may reflect the crossover of more than 80% of placebo patients beginning at week 16.

Lenalidomide has also been studied in a phase II trial of 214 patients with low- and intermediate-1-risk MDS without 5q deletions. Transfusion independence was achieved in 26% of patients who received lenalidomide after a median of 4.8 weeks, and 43% had hematologic improvement by IWG criteria.[119] Two trials have reported on the combination of lenalidomide and epoetin.[120,121] Evaluation of lenalidomide in 31 patients without deletion 5q and refractory to ESAs demonstrated transfusion independence in 37% of patients. Response was more robust in patients who remained on ESA therapy at 55% versus those on lenalidomide monotherapy at 36%. Median response duration was 24 months.[120] In the second trial, lower-risk MDS patients received lenalidomide 10 or 15 mg daily for 16 weeks; erythroid nonresponders were eligible to receive EPO 40,000 units/wk in addition to lenalidomide. Among 39 patients, 23 patients proceeded to combination therapy, with 6 (26%) achieving erythroid hematologic improvement. In 19 non-del(5q) patients, 4 (21%) showed erythroid hematologic improvement. A randomized, phase III study is currently underway to assess the effects of combination therapy in patients who have failed ESA monotherapy (*www.clinicaltrials.gov*; NCT00843882).

Lenalidomide in Intermediate-2- and High-Risk Myelodysplastic Syndromes Lenalidomide activity in low-risk MDS patients prompted its evaluation in patients with higher-risk MDS with 5q deletion. A phase II trial of lenalidomide in patients with higher-risk MDS with a 5q deletion and other cytogenetic abnormalities reported responses by IWG 2006 criteria in 13 of 47 patients (27%); significant myelosuppression was reported, and most patients (64%) required hospitalization.[122] Patients with thrombocytopenia or additional cytogenetic complexity progressed rapidly despite lenalidomide therapy.

Lenalidomide produces high rates of sustained transfusion independence in patients with low- and intermediate-1-risk MDS with 5q deletions. The response rate to lenalidomide is lower in patients with higher-risk MDS and those without a 5q deletion but may still be considered as a treatment option for patients who do not respond to initial therapy.[61]

DNA Hypomethylating Agents

Azacitidine and decitabine are nucleoside analogs structurally similar to cytosine and capable of being incorporated into DNA in place of cytosine. When these agents incorporate into DNA, substitution of carbon for nitrogen at the 5′ position prevents methylation by DNA methyltransferase. As a result, DNA methylation is decreased, and genes previously silenced by aberrant hypermethylation are activated. In vitro studies have confirmed that these agents can promote the reexpression of previously silenced genes.[51] The activity of both agents is concentration and time dependent, and trials are ongoing to evaluate the optimal dose, route, schedule, and duration of therapy.

The median time to response with DNA hypomethylating agents is 3 to 4 months.[2] Minimal evidence exists for appropriate duration of treatment. Long-term follow-up of high-risk MDS patients who responded to azacitidine therapy reported the median time to first response was two cycles, but responses improved in 48% of patients who continued therapy. Best response was achieved in 92% of responders by cycle 12.[123] Experts recommend continuing therapy until evidence of disease progression or unacceptable toxicity even in patients who only achieve stable disease.[2,124] The primary dose-limiting toxicity of both azacitidine and decitabine is myelosuppression, including leukopenia, granulocytopenia, and thrombocytopenia. Febrile neutropenia and other infectious complications have been reported with azacitidine and decitabine.[125,126] Nausea and vomiting may occur, and antiemetic prophylaxis is recommended. Azacitidine-induced erythema at the site of subcutaneous injection may occur; this can be minimized with the use of hot or cold compresses or topical corticosteroids. Rare hepatotoxicity is reported after either azacitidine or decitabine. Caution should be taken when using hypomethylating agents in patients with an estimated glomerular filtration rate of less than or equal to 29 mL/min because of a potential increased incidence of grade 3 or 4 myelosuppression, necessitating cycle delays and dose reductions.[127]

One important question about DNA hypomethylating agents is whether or not the degree of DNA methylation at baseline predicts response and survival after treatment with these agents. In a quantitative methylation analysis of patients who had received decitabine or supportive care only, Shen et al. showed that higher levels of methylation correlated with shorter median overall survival and progression-free survival (PFS) times.[128] The degree of methylation at baseline did not predict response to decitabine. However, changes in methylation levels over time were significantly correlated with the quality of the response; whereas the median decrease in methylation was 40.6% for those who achieved a complete or partial response and only 9.8% for those with hematologic improvement, methylation levels increased a median of 27.2% in patients with progressive disease.[128] Notably, methylation levels provided prognostic information regardless of the type of treatment provided and may help serve as a guide for clinicians when determining treatment approaches for individual patients.

DNA Hypomethylating Agents in Low- and Intermediate-1-Risk Patients Azacitidine was evaluated in a phase III, multicenter, randomized trial of patients diagnosed with any classification of MDS based on FAB criteria.[125] Patients in lower-risk categories of MDS, including refractory anemia and RARS, were required to meet additional criteria for significant bone marrow dysfunction. A total of 191 patients (median age, 68 years) were randomized to treatment with either supportive care alone or supportive care plus azacitidine 75 mg/m^2 subcutaneously once daily for 7 days, repeated every 28 days. Hematopoietic growth factor support was not permitted. Responses based on Cancer and Leukemia Group B criteria occurred in 60% of patients in the azacitidine group compared with 5% in the supportive care alone group. Almost half (45%) of the patients previously transfusion dependent who received azacitidine became transfusion independent. The rate of progression to AML was significantly lower with azacitidine (15%) compared with supportive care alone (38%), but azacitidine did not significantly improve overall survival. A quality-of-life analysis was also performed and identified a significant advantage for azacitidine therapy compared with supportive care alone, including improvements in physical functioning, fatigue, dyspnea, psychosocial distress, and affect.[129]

Decitabine was also evaluated in a multicenter, randomized phase III trial of patients diagnosed with MDS by FAB criteria.[126] Patients were required to have an IPSS risk of intermediate-1 or greater; two thirds of patients had intermediate-2- or high-risk MDS. A total of 170 patients were randomized to either supportive care alone or supportive care plus treatment with decitabine 15 mg/m^2 by IV infusion every 8 hours for 3 days repeated every 6 weeks. In contrast to the azacitidine trial, hematopoietic growth factor support was allowed. The overall response rate by IWG criteria was 17% in the decitabine group compared with 0% in the supportive care group. Thirteen percent of patients who received decitabine experienced hematologic improvement compared with 7% who received supportive care alone. Time to progression to AML or overall survival was not significantly different between groups. The patients with known clonal abnormalities at baseline who underwent follow-up cytogenetic evaluation were noted to have a complete cytogenetic response of 35% with decitabine compared with 10% with supportive care. Decitabine also improved quality-of-life measures, including global health status, fatigue, and dyspnea.

DNA Hypomethylating Agents in Intermediate-2- and High-Risk Patients An open-label, randomized, phase III study compared azacitidine with a conventional care regimen (CCR) in patients with higher-risk MDS.[8] Before randomization, treating physicians selected supportive care alone, low-dose cytarabine, or AML-type induction as the CCR for a given patient if randomized to the conventional care arm. Of the 340 patients receiving treatment, 175 received azacitidine, 102 received best supportive care, 44 received low-dose cytarabine, and 19 received AML-type induction. At 2 years, 51% of azacitidine patients were alive compared with 26% of patients who received a CCR, and median overall survival time was prolonged by 9 months. This is the only prospective, randomized controlled study to demonstrate therapy improves overall survival in MDS.

In attempt to better define which patients are most likely to respond to azacitidine, Itzykson et al. identified four factors that independently predicted overall survival in a cohort of 282 high- or intermediate-2-risk MDS patients who received azacitidine for a median six cycles in a compassionate use study.[130] Each factor was given a point-based score: performance status greater than or equal to 2 (1 point), intermediate- and poor-risk cytogenetics (1 and 2 points, respectively), presence of circulating blasts (1 point), and RBC transfusion dependency of at least 4 units within 8 weeks (1 point). Median overall survival was not reached in the low-risk (0 points), 15 months in intermediate-risk (1 to 3 points), and 6.1 months in high-risk (4 to 5 points) patients. This prognostic scoring system was independently validated in the azacitidine cohort of Fenaux and colleagues.[8]

Decitabine has also been compared with best supportive care in a phase III trial of 233 intermediate- or high-risk MDS patients older than 60 years who were ineligible for intensive chemotherapy.[131] Decitabine was more active than best supportive care, with a complete and partial response rate of 13% and 6%, respectively, versus 0% for best supportive care. Median PFS was significantly improved with decitabine compared with supportive care at 6.6 months versus 3 months, respectively. Progression to AML at 1 year was significantly reduced with decitabine to 22% versus 33% in the best supportive care arm. However, unlike the trial with azacitidine, no overall survival benefit was observed. Decitabine did demonstrate improvement in quality-of-life measures of fatigue and physical functioning.

Clinical **Controversy...**

Although both azacitidine and decitabine have demonstrated significant improvement in complete response, partial response, and hematologic improvement rates, only azacitidine has demonstrated overall survival benefit. The lack of survival improvement for decitabine remains under intense debate because it may reflect suboptimal administration because of the dosing interval (4 weeks vs. 6 weeks), schedule (3 days vs. 5 days), and number of cycles received.[124] Currently, the NCCN guidelines do not favor one agent over the alternative in low- or intermediate-1-risk patients but give a more favorable rating to azacitidine in high-risk MDS (intermediate-2 or higher).[61]

Despite moderate success with both hypomethylating agents, current data suggest that using decitabine after azacitidine failure is not effective. Bhatnagar and colleagues evaluated 22 MDS or AML patients with disease progression or lack of response to azacitidine who went on to receive decitabine.[132] After a median of two courses, all 22 patients demonstrated disease progression or lack of response to decitabine. Higher-risk MDS patients who fail hypomethylating therapy may require therapeutic intervention with an alternative mechanism of action or as part of a clinical trial.

The pivotal trials for azacitidine and decitabine led to the approval of these agents for the treatment of patients with MDS, but their FDA-approved administration schedules are inconvenient and impossible for many cancer centers whose outpatient clinics are not open for extended hours or are closed on weekends, necessitating hospitalization. A more convenient regimen for decitabine (20 mg/m^2 by IV infusion daily for 5 consecutive days every 4 weeks) demonstrated similar response rates and adverse events to the traditional regimen.[133] In early 2010, the FDA granted approval for this alternative dosing regimen. Preliminary results of an oral azacitidine formulation have been positive, particularly in extended dosing strategies of 14 or 21 days, which also correlated with higher achievement of demethylation.[104] Although a variety of dosing options have been studied, none of these approaches have been directly compared in prospective trials, and further evaluation is required to determine optimal azacitidine and decitabine treatment regimens.[133,134]

Intensive Chemotherapy

Patients with intermediate-2- or high-risk MDS may be candidates for intensive chemotherapy with AML-type induction combination chemotherapy regimens, including anthracyclines, cytarabine, fludarabine, and topotecan. AML-type induction therapy is described in detail in Chapter 111. Intensive chemotherapy offers complete remission rates of 40% to 60% but is associated with a median duration of response of only 10 to 12 months.[135] Treatment-related mortality in younger patients with current supportive care measures, including antibiotic and hematopoietic growth factor support, is less than 10%.[8,135] Patients younger than 55 years of age who have a normal karyotype and good performance status are most likely to benefit, but this approach cures fewer than 15% of patients.[135] Intensive chemotherapy can be used as a bridge to allogeneic HSCT to reduce tumor burden and control disease while a suitable donor is found and a referral is made to a transplant center.

Preliminary data suggest oral and IV clofarabine may have activity in patients with higher-risk MDS and those who experienced prior therapy failure with DNA hypomethylating agents.[136–139] The optimal dose, route, and schedule to balance activity and toxicity remain to be defined.

Hematopoietic Stem Cell Transplantation

Allogeneic HSCT offers potentially curative therapy to patients with MDS who have a suitable donor and are healthy enough for the procedure. Unfortunately, fewer than 5% of patients are referred for allogeneic HSCT.[140] Two large retrospective studies indicate that recipient age alone should not be considered a contraindication to allogeneic HSCT.[141,142] About 30% to 50% of patients with MDS treated with allogeneic HSCT have prolonged disease-free survival.[141,143–150] However, 20% to 50% of patients succumb to treatment-related mortality, and many of the remaining patients relapse. Outcomes vary based on patient comorbidities, time from diagnosis to transplant, FAB subtype of MDS, percentage of bone marrow blasts at the time of HSCT, IPSS risk category, type of conditioning regimen administered before HSCT, and dose and source of stem cells infused.[141,145] Complications of allogeneic HSCT are described in greater detail in Chapter 117. An HLA-matched allogeneic HSCT is recommended if an appropriate donor is available. An autologous HSCT can be considered in the context of a clinical trial if an allogeneic donor is not available, complete remission is achieved with chemotherapy, and adequate stem cells can be collected.[143]

Because of the high rate of treatment-related mortality in patients with MDS, allogeneic HSCT has not been recommended for lower-risk patients because these patients may have stable disease for several years, and early transplant may shorten overall survival. The International MDS Risk Assessment Workshop conducted a decision analysis based on clinical data from two international registries and a single center to identify the optimal time to recommend allogeneic HSCT for patients who have a donor and meet HSCT eligibility criteria.[151] The analysis showed that patients with low- and intermediate-1 IPSS risk scores should be closely observed and transplanted at the time of disease progression. Patients with intermediate-2 and high IPSS risk scores should be transplanted soon after diagnosis to confer the greatest benefit from allogeneic HSCT.[143] This model was developed in 2003 and included patients younger than 60 years of age who had undergone HSCT primarily in the 1990s. It did not incorporate treatment with novel agents for MDS, the use of reduced-intensity conditioning (RIC), or all of the known prognostic factors currently available and thus may not be applicable to contemporary patients being evaluated for HSCT.[152] The WPSS may enhance selection of patients likely to derive the most benefit from allogeneic HSCT based on recent retrospective data demonstrating patients with low-risk disease have low rates of treatment-related mortality and relapse and a 5-year overall survival rate of 80%.[153] Another retrospective series by de Witte et al. reported a 4-year overall survival rate of 52% in younger patients with lower risk refractory anemia after allogeneic HSCT,[154] remarkably similar to the median survival rate for untreated patients with refractory anemia.[4] The decision to proceed to allogeneic HSCT and optimal timing should be weighed carefully at diagnosis and subsequently at regular intervals for factors that might influence prognosis, such as degree of cytopenias, cytogenetic abnormalities, transfusion requirement, progression to a higher risk category, donor selection, comorbidities, and availability of effective nontransplant therapies.[62,154] A prospective study comparing allogeneic HSCT with azacitidine in patients aged 55 to 69 years is ongoing (available at *www.clinicaltrials.gov*; NCT01404741).

Retrospective comparisons of RIC and myeloablative conditioning regimens before allogeneic HSCT showed inconsistent results with some reporting a lower treatment-related mortality rate but a higher rate of disease relapse with RIC and others reporting no difference.[147,155] Comparison of the results from patients receiving RIC with myeloablative conditioning regimens is difficult because patients treated with RIC regimens tend to be older or have significant comorbid illnesses preventing them from receiving myeloablative conditioning regimens. A prospective, randomized controlled trial is underway to compare myeloablative and RIC in patients with MDS undergoing allogeneic HSCT (available at *www.clinicaltrials.gov*; NCT00682396); in the interim, comorbidities and risk of relapse are the main factors used to select the intensity of the conditioning regimen.[62]

Treatment Based on International Prognostic Scoring System Risk Group

All patients with MDS should receive appropriate supportive care and be encouraged to participate in clinical trials to determine the role of different approaches in the management of MDS.[61,64]

Low or Intermediate-1 International Prognostic Scoring System Risk

Patients with low- or intermediate-1-risk MDS may be managed with supportive care alone; those who are likely to respond to ESAs should be managed with this strategy because it is well tolerated.[61] Patients with endogenous EPO less than 500 mU/mL (500 IU/L) and a low transfusion requirement are most likely to respond to ESAs. Addition of low-dose G-CSF may benefit some patients who do not respond to EPO alone. Most patients eventually stop responding to ESAs and develop an increased need for transfusions; these patients may benefit from more intensive therapy.

8 The NCCN recommends DNA hypomethylating agents (azacitidine and decitabine) for treatment of low-risk and intermediate-1-risk MDS in patients with clinically significant neutropenia or thrombocytopenia and patients with anemia who are unlikely to respond to or have not responded to a trial of ESAs, and patients who qualified for and failed immunosuppressive therapy.[61] Small numbers of low-risk and intermediate-1-risk MDS patients were enrolled in the clinical trial that evaluated azacitidine, and further research is needed to determine its place in therapy for these patients. Responses often require 2 to 4 months of treatment, and the duration of response is generally less than 1 year. Clinical trials of azacitidine and decitabine enrolled different patient populations, used different response criteria, and administered therapy for different durations, making it difficult to determine if one agent is superior. A phase III open-label trial to compare decitabine with azacitidine in low- and intermediate-1-risk patients with MDS is underway in the United States (available at *www.clinicaltrials.gov*; NCT01720225). DNA hypomethylating agents are appropriate for low- and intermediate-1-risk MDS patients who are transfusion dependent or who are symptomatic despite management with best supportive care.[2,61,64]

9 The current NCCN treatment guideline for MDS recommends immunosuppressive therapy (antithymocyte globulin or cyclosporine) for select patients with low-risk MDS; young patients (60 years old or younger) with a hypocellular marrow, normal cytogenetics, expression of HLA DR15, or paroxysmal nocturnal hemoglobinuria are most likely to respond.[61] The potential benefit of transfusion independence must be considered carefully in the context of complications that can arise from immunosuppressive treatments.

10 Lenalidomide is currently recommended for patients with symptomatic anemia and low-risk MDS with a 5q deletion.[61,156] Patients with multiple cytogenetic abnormalities, in addition to a chromosome 5 deletion, may respond to lenalidomide but typically to a lower degree. Lenalidomide is also effective for some patients with low-risk and intermediate-1-risk MDS without a chromosome 5 deletion and is considered an alternative treatment approach by NCCN.[61,119]

Intermediate-2 or High International Prognostic Scoring System Risk

11 Patients with intermediate-2- or high-risk disease who are candidates for intensive therapy should receive an allogeneic HSCT, if possible, because it is the only curative option for MDS.[2,64] Patients may receive intensive chemotherapy with an AML-type induction regimen or a less intensive therapy with a DNA hypomethylating agent to reduce disease during the process of finding a donor and referral to a transplant center. They also may proceed directly to allogeneic HSCT without cytoreduction if they have fewer than 10% bone marrow blasts. The NCCN guidelines suggest that high-intensity chemotherapy without subsequent allogeneic HSCT be conducted as part of a clinical trial for intermediate-2- and high-risk MDS patients.[61] Azacitdine should be considered for intermediate-2- and high-risk MDS patients who are not eligible for allogeneic HSCT based on the observation that azacitidine prolongs survival in these patients.[2,8,61]

Although clinical trials are beginning to determine which therapies are effective in patients with different risk categories, none of the therapeutic options have been directly compared in a clinical trial. The optimal management of patients who progress or do not respond to initial therapy is not clear.

PERSONALIZED PHARMACOTHERAPY

Although many different genetic abnormalities and variances have been discovered in MDS, only two are used to personalize pharmacotherapy: deletion 5q syndrome and HLA DR15 positivity. Patients with an isolated deletion of chromosome 5q and no excess marrow blasts are a distinct WHO category of MDS termed *5q- syndrome*. This subtype of MDS is characterized by severe refractory anemia often requiring frequent RBC transfusions.[156] Patients with 5q- syndrome typically survive longer and have a lower risk for progression to AML than a similar IPSS risk patient. About 50% to 67% of 5q-syndrome patients become transfusion independent with lenalidomide therapy, and 45% to 50% achieve cytogenetic remission.[45,118] The NCCN guidelines recommend these patients receive lenalidomide as primary therapy before alternative treatments.[61] As discussed earlier (see Immunosuppressive Agents above), patients with HLA DR15 positivity have a superior response to immunosuppressive therapy as first-line management.[113] Patients with HLA DR15 are most likely to respond if they are younger than 60 years of age, have IPSS risk of intermediate-1 or lower, and have rapid initiation of immunosuppressive therapy on diagnosis.[113] More definitive studies are needed to determine if other recently discovered genetic abnormalities can be linked to treatment success.

EVALUATION OF THERAPEUTIC OUTCOMES

Standardized response criteria in clinical trials of MDS enable clinicians to evaluate study outcomes, compare results from different trials, and tailor therapy according to patient or disease characteristics.[60] The IWG for MDS guidelines for response criteria in MDS clinical trials categorize patient responses into categories that correlate with quality of life or morbidity.[60,157] Based on these criteria, the four treatment goals are altering the natural history of the disease, cytogenetic response, hematologic improvement, and quality of life. Changes in the WHO classification system and new therapies with novel mechanisms of action, time to response, and likelihood of treatment-related cytopenias have created a need for further refinement of these guidelines.[107] Patients with MDS should have regular follow-up with a history, physical examination, and complete blood counts. The frequency of follow-up varies with the natural history of each patient from weekly to every 6 months.

ABBREVIATIONS

AML	acute myeloid leukemia
CCR	conventional care regimen
CI	confidence interval
EPO	erythropoietin
ESAs	erythropoiesis-stimulating agents
FAB	French-American-British
G-CSF	granulocyte colony-stimulating factor
GM-CSF	granulocyte-macrophage colony-stimulating factor
HIV	human immunodeficiency virus
HLA	human leukocyte antigen

HR	hazard ratio
HSCT	hematopoietic stem cell transplantation
IMiD	immunomodulating drug
IPSS	International Prognostic Scoring System
IPSS-R	International Prognostic Scoring System—Revised
IWG	International Working Group
MDS	myelodysplastic syndromes
NCCN	National Comprehensive Cancer Network
PFS	progression-free survival
RARS	refractory anemia with ringed sideroblasts
RIC	reduced-intensity conditioning
RBC	red blood cell
SEER	Surveillance, Epidemiology and End Results
t-MDS	therapy-related MDS
WHO	World Health Organization
WPSS	World Health Organization Classification-based Scoring System

REFERENCES

1. Vardiman JW, Harris NL, Brunning RD. The World Health Organization (WHO) classification of the myeloid neoplasms. Blood 2002;100:2292–2302.
2. Stone RM. How I treat patients with myelodysplastic syndromes. Blood 2009;113:6296–6303.
3. Tefferi A, Vardiman JW. Myelodysplastic syndromes. N Engl J Med 2009;361:1872–1885.
4. Greenberg P, Cox C, LeBeau MM, et al. International scoring system for evaluating prognosis in myelodysplastic syndromes. Blood 1997;89:2079–2088.
5. Steensma DP. The changing classification of myelodysplastic syndromes: What's in a name? Hematology (Am Soc Hematol Educ Program) 2009;2009:645–655.
6. Bejar R, Stevenson KE, Caughey BA, et al. Validation of a prognostic model and the impact of mutations in patients with lower-risk myelodysplastic syndromes. J Clin Oncol 2012;27:3376–3382.
7. Greenberg PL, Tuechler H, Schanz J, et al. Revised International Prognostic Scoring System (IPSS-R) for myelodysplastic syndromes. Blood 2012;120:2454–2465.
8. Fenaux P, Mufti GJ, Hellstrom-Lindberg E, et al. Efficacy of azacitidine compared with that of conventional care regimens in the treatment of higher-risk myelodysplastic syndromes: A randomised, open-label, phase III study. Lancet Oncol 2009;10:223–232.
9. Ma X. Epidemiology of myelodysplastic syndromes. Am J Med 2012;125:S2–S5.
10. Howlader N, Noone AM, Krapcho M, et al. SEER Cancer Statistics Review, 1975–2010, National Cancer Institute. Bethesda, MD, http://seer.cancer.gov/csr/1975_2010/, based on November 2012 SEER data submission, posted to the SEER web site, April 2013.
11. Cogle CR, Craig BM, Rollison DE, et al. Incidence of the myelodysplastic syndromes using a novel claims-based algorithm: High number of uncaptured cases by cancer registries. Blood 2011;117:7121–7125.
12. Goldberg SL, Chen E, Corral M, et al. Incidence and clinical complications of myelodysplastic syndromes among United States Medicare beneficiaries. J Clin Oncol 2010;28: 2847–2852.
13. Jadersten M, Hellstrom-Lindberg E. Myelodysplastic syndromes: Biology and treatment. J Intern Med 2009;265:307–328.
14. Faderl S, Kantarjian HM. Myelodysplastic syndromes. In: Devita VT, Lawrence SL, Rosenberg SA, eds. Cancer: Principles and Practice of Oncology, 8th ed. Philadelphia, PA: Lippincott Williams & Wilkins, 2008:2292–2304.
15. Iwanaga M, Hsu WL, Soda M, et al. Risk of myelodysplastic syndromes in people exposed to ionizing radiation: A retrospective cohort study of Nagasaki atomic bomb survivors. J Clin Oncol 2011;29:428–434.
16. Ma X, Lim U, Park Y, et al. Obesity, lifestyle factors, and risk of myelodysplastic syndromes in a large US cohort. Am J Epidemiol 2009;169:1492–1499.
17. Kristinsson SY, Bjorkholm M, Hultcrantz M, et al. Chronic immune stimulation might act as a trigger for the development of acute myeloid leukemia or myelodysplastic syndromes. J Clin Oncol 2011;29:2897–2903.
18. Czader M, Orazi A. Therapy-related myeloid neoplasms. Am J Clin Pathol 2009;132:410–425.
19. Borthakur G, Estey AE. Therapy-related acute myelogenous leukemia and myelodysplastic syndrome. Curr Oncol Rep 2007;9:373–377.
20. Larson RA. Cytogenetics, not just previous therapy, determines the course of therapy-related myeloid neoplasms. J Clin Oncol 2012;30:2300–2302.
21. Sill H, Olipitz W, Zebisch A, et al. Therapy-related myeloid neoplasms: Pathobiology and clinical characteristics. Br J Pharmacol 2011;162:792–805.
22. Blaszkowsky LS, Erlichman EC, eds. Carcinogenesis of anticancer drugs. In: Chabner BA, Longo DL, eds. Cancer Chemotherapy and Biotherapy: Principles and Practice, 4th ed. Philadelphia: Lippincott Williams & Wilkins, 2006:70–90.
23. Armitage JO, Carbone PP, Connors JM, et al. Treatment-related myelodysplasia and acute leukemia in non-Hodgkin's lymphoma patients. J Clin Oncol 2003;21:897–906.
24. Smith SM, Le Beau MM, Huo D, et al. Clinical-cytogenetic associations in 306 patients with therapy-related myelodysplasia and myeloid leukemia: The University of Chicago series. Blood 2003;102:43–52.
25. Haase D, Germing U, Schanz J, et al. New insights into the prognostic impact of the karyotype in MDS and correlation with subtypes: Evidence from a core dataset of 2124 patients. Blood 2007;110:4385–4395.
26. Bennett JM, Kaminski MS, Leonard JP, et al. Assessment of treatment-related myelodysplastic syndromes and acute myeloid leukemia in patients with non-Hodgkin lymphoma treated with tositumomab and iodine I131 tositumomab. Blood 2005;105:4576–4582.
27. Czuczman MS, Emmanouilides C, Darif M, et al. Treatment-related myelodysplastic syndrome and acute myelogenous leukemia in patients treated with ibritumomab tiuxetan radioimmunotherapy. J Clin Oncol 2007;25:4285–4292.
28. Horning SJ, Younes A, Jain V, et al. Efficacy and safety of tositumomab and iodine-131 tositumomab (Bexxar) in B-cell lymphoma, progressive after rituximab. J Clin Oncol 2005;23:712–719.
29. Kaminski MS, Estes J, Zasadny KR, et al. Radioimmunotherapy with iodine (131)I tositumomab for relapsed or refractory B-cell non-Hodgkin lymphoma: Updated results and long-term follow-up of the University of Michigan experience. Blood 2000;96:1259–1266.
30. Witzig TE, White CA, Gordon LI, et al. Safety of yttrium-90 ibritumomab tiuxetan radioimmunotherapy for relapsed low-grade, follicular, or transformed non-Hodgkin's lymphoma. J Clin Oncol 2003;21:1263–1270.
31. Guidetti A, Carlo-Stella C, Ruella M, et al. Myeloablative doses of yttrium-90-ibritumomab tiuxetan and the risk of secondary myelodysplasia/acute myelogenous leukemia. Cancer 2011;117:5074–5084.

32. Lyman GH, Dale DC, Wolff DA, et al. Acute myeloid leukemia or myelodysplastic syndrome in randomized controlled clinical trials of cancer chemotherapy with granulocyte colony-stimulating factor: A systematic review. J Clin Oncol 2010;28:2914–2924.
33. Rosenberg PS, Alter BP, Bolyard AA, et al. The incidence of leukemia and mortality from sepsis in patients with severe congenital neutropenia receiving long-term G-CSF therapy. Blood 2006;107:4628–4635.
34. Socie G, Mary JY, Schrezenmeier H, et al. Granulocyte-stimulating factor and severe aplastic anemia: A survey by the European Group for Blood and Marrow Transplantation (EBMT). Blood 2007;109:2794–2796.
35. Brown JR, Yeckes H, Friedberg JW, et al. Increasing incidence of late second malignancies after conditioning with cyclophosphamide and total-body irradiation and autologous bone marrow transplantation for non-Hodgkin's lymphoma. J Clin Oncol 2005;23:2208–2214.
36. Metayer C, Curtis RE, Vose J, et al. Myelodysplastic syndrome and acute myeloid leukemia after autotransplantation for lymphoma: A multicenter case-control study. Blood 2003;101:2015–2023.
37. Milligan DW, Kochethu G, Dearden C, et al. High incidence of myelodysplasia and secondary leukaemia in the UK Medical Research Council Pilot of autografting in chronic lymphocytic leukaemia. Br J Haematol 2006;133:173–175.
38. Kalaycio M, Rybicki L, Pohlman B, et al. Risk factors before autologous stem-cell transplantation for lymphoma predict for secondary myelodysplasia and acute myelogenous leukemia. J Clin Oncol 2006;24:3604–3610.
39. Fianchi L, Leone G, Posteraro B, et al. Impaired bactericidal and fungicidal activities of neutrophils in patients with myelodysplastic syndrome. Leuk Res 2012;36:331–333.
40. Vladareanu AM, Vasilache V, Bumbea H, et al. Platelet dysfunction in acute leukemias and myelodysplastic syndromes. Rom J Intern Med 2011;49:93–96.
41. Bejar R, Levine R, Ebert BL. Unraveling the molecular pathophysiology of myelodysplastic syndromes. J Clin Oncol 2011;29:504–515.
42. Schanz J, Tuchler H, Sole F, et al. New comprehensive cytogenetic scoring system for primary myelodysplastic syndromes (MDS) and oligoblastic acute myeloid leukemia after MDS derived from an international database merge. J Clin Oncol 2012;30:820–829.
43. Schanz J, Steidl C, Fonatsch C, et al. Coalesced multicentric analysis of 2,351 patients with myelodysplastic syndromes indicates an underestimation of poor-risk cytogenetics of myelodysplastic syndromes in the international prognostic scoring system. J Clin Oncol 2011;29:1963–1970.
44. Belli CB, Bengio R, Aranguren PN, et al. Partial and total monosomal karyotypes in myelodysplastic syndromes: Comparative prognostic relevance among 421 patients. Am J Hematol 2011;86:540–545.
45. List A, Dewald G, Bennett J, et al. Lenalidomide in the myelodysplastic syndrome with chromosome 5q deletion. N Engl J Med 2006;355:1456–1465.
46. Tiu RV, Gondek LP, O'Keefe CL, et al. Prognostic impact of SNP array karyotyping in myelodysplastic syndromes and related myeloid malignancies. Blood 2011;117: 4552–4560.
47. Smith AE, Mohamedali AM, Kulasekararaj A, et al. Next-generation sequencing of the TET2 gene in 355 MDS and CMML patients reveals low-abundance mutant clones with early origins, but indicates no definite prognostic value. Blood 2010;116:3923–3932.
48. Ko M, Huang Y, Jankowska AM, et al. Impaired hydroxylation of 5-methylcytosine in myeloid cancers with mutant TET2. Nature 2010;468:839–843.
49. Kosmider O, Gelsi-Boyer V, Cheok M, et al. TET2 mutation is an independent favorable prognostic factor in myelodysplastic syndromes (MDSs). Blood 2009;114: 3285–3291.
50. Schlegelberger B, Gohring G, Thol F, et al. Update on cytogenetic and molecular changes in myelodysplastic syndromes. Leuk Lymphoma 2012;53:525–536.
51. Esteller M. Epigenetics in cancer. N Engl J Med 2008;358:1148–1159.
52. Lyko F, Brown R. DNA methyltransferase inhibitors and the development of epigenetic cancer therapies. J Natl Cancer Inst 2005;97:1498–1506.
53. Quintas-Cardama A, Santos FP, Garcia-Manero G. Histone deacetylase inhibitors for the treatment of myelodysplastic syndrome and acute myeloid leukemia. Leukemia 2011;25:226–235.
54. Cashen A, Juckett M, Jumonville A, et al. Phase II study of the histone deacetylase inhibitor belinostat (PXD101) for the treatment of myelodysplastic syndrome (MDS). Ann Hematol 2012;91:33–38.
55. Raza A, Galili N, Smith SE, et al. A phase 2 randomized multicenter study of 2 extended dosing schedules of oral ezatiostat in low to intermediate-1 risk myelodysplastic syndrome. Cancer 2012;118:2138–2147.
56. Vardiman JW, Thiele J, Arber DA, et al. The 2008 revision of the World Health Organization (WHO) classification of myeloid neoplasms and acute leukemia: Rationale and important changes. Blood 2009;114:937–951.
57. Malcovati L, Porta MG, Pascutto C, et al. Prognostic factors and life expectancy in myelodysplastic syndromes classified according to WHO criteria: A basis for clinical decision making. J Clin Oncol 2005;23:7594–7603.
58. Bejar R, Stevenson K, Abdel-Wahab O, et al. Clinical effect of point mutations in myelodysplastic syndromes. N Engl J Med 2011;364:2496–2506.
59. Garcia-Manero G. Myelodysplastic syndromes: 2012 update on diagnosis, risk-stratification, and management. Am J Hematol 2012;87:692–701.
60. Cheson BD, Greenberg PL, Bennett JM, et al. Clinical application and proposal for modification of the International Working Group (IWG) response criteria in myelodysplasia. Blood 2006;108:419–425.
61. The NCCN Clinical Practice Guidelines in Oncology™ Myelodysplastic Syndromes (Version 2.2013). National Comprehensive Care Network Inc. 2012, *http://www.NCCN.org*.
62. Kroger N. Allogeneic stem cell transplantation for elderly patients with myelodysplastic syndrome. Blood 2012;119:5632–5639.
63. Sekeres MA, Schoonen M, Kantarjian H, et al. Characteristics of US patients with myelodysplastic syndromes: Results of six cross-sectional physician surveys. J Natl Cancer Inst 2008;100:1542–1551.
64. Schiffer CA. Clinical issues in the management of patients with myelodysplasia. Hematology (Am Soc Hematol Educ Program) 2006;2006:205–210.
65. Malcovati L, Germing U, Kuendgen A, et al. Time-dependent prognostic scoring system for predicting survival and leukemic evolution in myelodysplastic syndromes. J Clin Oncol 2007;25:3503–3510.
66. Pomeroy C, Oken MM, Rydell RE, et al. Infection in the myelodysplastic syndromes. Am J Med 1991;90: 338–344.

67. Freifeld AG, Bow EJ, Sepkowitz KA, et al. Clinical practice guideline for the use of antimicrobial agents in neutropenic patients with cancer: 2010 update by the Infectious Diseases Society of America. Clin Infect Dis 2011;52:427–431.
68. Greenberg P, Taylor K, Larson RA. Phase III randomized multicenter trial of G-CSF vs observation for myelodysplastic syndromes (MDS). Blood 1993;82:196a.
69. Rizzo JD, Somerfield MR, Hagerty KL, et al. Use of epoetin and darbepoetin in patients with cancer: 2007 American Society of Clinical Oncology/American Society of Hematology clinical practice guideline update. J Clin Oncol 2008;26:132–149.
70. Bohlius J, Schmidlin K, Brillant C, et al. Recombinant human erythropoiesis-stimulating agents and mortality in patients with cancer: A meta-analysis of randomised trials. Lancet 2009;373:1532–1542.
71. Ross SD, Allen IE, Probst CA, et al. Efficacy and safety of erythropoiesis-stimulating proteins in myelodysplastic syndrome: A systematic review and meta-analysis. Oncologist 2007;12:1264–1273.
72. Moyo V, Lefebvre P, Duh MS, et al. Erythropoiesis-stimulating agents in the treatment of anemia in myelodysplastic syndromes: A meta-analysis. Ann Hematol 2008;87:527–536.
73. Hellstrom-Lindberg E, Gulbrandsen N, Lindberg G, et al. A validated decision model for treating the anaemia of myelodysplastic syndromes with erythropoietin + granulocyte colony-stimulating factor: Significant effects on quality of life. Br J Haematol 2003;120:1037–1046.
74. Sekeres MA. Treatment of MDS: Something old, something new, something borrowed. Hematology (Am Soc Hematol Educ Program) 2009;2009:656–663.
75. Jadersten M, Malcovati L, Dybedal I, et al. Erythropoietin and granulocyte-colony stimulating factor treatment associated with improved survival in myelodysplastic syndrome. J Clin Oncol 2008;26:3607–3613.
76. Jadersten M, Montgomery SM, Dybedal I, et al. Long-term outcome of treatment of anemia in MDS with erythropoietin and G-CSF. Blood 2005;106:803–811.
77. Park S, Grabar S, Kelaidi C, et al. Predictive factors of response and survival in myelodysplastic syndrome treated with erythropoietin and G-CSF: The GFM experience. Blood 2008;111:574–582.
78. Greenberg PL, Sun Z, Miller KB, et al. Treatment of myelodysplastic syndrome patients with erythropoietin with or without granulocyte colony-stimulating factor: Results of a prospective randomized phase 3 trial by the Eastern Cooperative Oncology Group (E1996). Blood 2009;114:2393–2400.
79. Mundle S, Lefebvre P, Vekeman F, et al. An assessment of erythroid response to epoetin alpha as a single agent versus in combination with granulocyte- or granulocyte-macrophage-colony-stimulating factor in myelodysplastic syndromes using a meta-analysis approach. Cancer 2009;115:706–715.
80. Steensma DP. Erythropoiesis-stimulating agents are effective in myelodysplastic syndromes, but are they safe? Am J Hematol 2009;84:3–5.
81. Kantarjian H, Fenaux P, Sekeres MA, et al. Safety and efficacy of romiplostim in patients with lower-risk myelodysplastic syndrome and thrombocytopenia. J Clin Oncol 2010;28:437–444.
82. Sekeres MA, Kantarjian H, Fenaux P, et al. Subcutaneous or intravenous administration of romiplostim in thrombocytopenic patients with lower risk myelodysplastic syndromes. Cancer 2011;117:992–1000.
83. Giagounidis A, Mufti GJ, Kantarjian HM, et al. Treatment with the thrombopoietin (TPO)-receptor agonist romiplostim in thrombocytopenic patients with low or intermediate-1 (Int-1) risk myelodysplastic syndrome (MDS): Results of a randomized, double-blind, placebo-controlled study [abstract]. Blood 2011;118:117a.
84. Kantarjian HM, Mufti GJ, Fenaux P, et al. Treatment with the thrombopoietin (TPO)-receptor agonist romiplostim in thrombocytopenic patients with low or intermediate-1 (Int-1) risk myelodysplastic syndrome (MDS): Follow-up AML and survival results of a randomized, double-blind, placebo-controlled study [abstract]. Blood 2012;120:421a.
85. Wang ES, Lyons RM, Larson RA, et al. A randomized, double-blind, placebo-controlled phase 2 study evaluating the efficacy and safety of romiplostim treatment of patients with low or intermediate risk myelodysplastic syndrome receiving lenalidomide. J Hematol Oncol 2012;5:71.
86. Greenberg PL, Garcia-Manero G, Moore MR, et al. A randomized controlled trial of romiplostim in patients with low or intermediate-risk myelodysplastic syndrome receiving decitabine. Leuk Lymphoma 2013;54:321–328.
87. Kantarjian HM, Giles FJ, Greenberg PL, et al. Phase 2 study of romiplostim in patients with low- or intermediate-risk myelodysplastic syndrome receiving azacitidine therapy. Blood 2010;116:3163–3170.
88. Oliva EN, Santini V, Zini G, et al. Efficacy and safety of eltrombopag for the treatment of thrombocytopenia of low and intermediate-1 IPSS risk myelodysplastic syndromes: Interim analysis of a prospective, randomized, single-blind, placebo-controlled trial (EQoL-MDS) [abstract]. Blood 2012;120:923a.
89. Jädersten M, Hellström-Lindberg E. Myelodysplastic syndromes: Biology and treatment, 2009;265:307–328.
90. Bennett JM. Consensus statement on iron overload in myelodysplastic syndromes. Am J Hematol 2008;83:858–861.
91. Balducci L. Transfusion independence in patients with myelodysplastic syndromes: Impact on outcomes and quality of life. Cancer 2006;106:2087–2094.
92. Sanz G, Nomdedeu B, Such E, et al. Independent impact of iron overload and transfusion dependency on survival and leukemic evolution in patients with myelodysplastic syndrome [abstract]. Blood 2008;112:640a.
93. Pullarkat V. Objectives of iron chelation therapy in myelodysplastic syndromes: More than meets the eye? Blood 2009;114:5251–5255.
94. Delea TE, Hagiwara M, Phatak PD. Retrospective study of the association between transfusion frequency and potential complications of iron overload in patients with myelodysplastic syndrome and other acquired hematopoietic disorders. Curr Med Res Opin 2009;25:139–147.
95. Gattermann N, Jarisch A, Schlag R, et al. Deferasirox treatment of iron-overloaded chelation-naive and prechelated patients with myelodysplastic syndromes in medical practice: Results from the observational studies eXtend and eXjange. Eur J Haematol 2012;88:260–268.
96. Greenberg PL, Koller CA, Cabantchik ZI, et al. Prospective assessment of effects on iron-overload parameters of deferasirox therapy in patients with myelodysplastic syndromes. Leuk Res 2010;34:1560–1565.
97. List AF, Baer MR, Steensma DP, et al. Deferasirox reduces serum ferritin and labile plasma iron in RBC transfusion-dependent patients with myelodysplastic syndrome. J Clin Oncol 2012;30:2134–2139.
98. Jensen PD, Heickendorff L, Pedersen B, et al. The effect of iron chelation on haemopoiesis in MDS patients with transfusional iron overload. Br J Haematol 1996;94:288–299.

99. Cermak J, Jonasova A, Vondrakova J, et al. Efficacy and safety of administration of oral iron chelator deferiprone in patients with early myelodysplastic syndrome. Hemoglobin 2011;35:217–227.
100. Leitch HA, Leger CS, Goodman TA, et al. Improved survival in patients with myelodysplastic syndrome receiving iron chelation therapy. Clin Leuk 2008;2:205–211.
101. Rose C, Brechignac S, Vassilief D, et al. Does iron chelation therapy improve survival in regularly transfused lower risk MDS patients? A multicenter study by the GFM (Groupe Francophone des Myelodysplasies). Leuk Res 2010;34: 864–870.
102. Neukirchen J, Fox F, Kundgen A, et al. Improved survival in MDS patients receiving iron chelation therapy: A matched pair analysis of 188 patients from the Dusseldorf MDS registry. Leuk Res 2012;36:1067–1070.
103. Leitch HA, Vickars LM. Supportive care and chelation therapy in MDS: Are we saving lives or just lowering iron? Hematology (Am Soc Hematol Educ Program) 2009;2009:664–672.
104. Zeidan AM, Hendrick F, Friedmann E, et al. Deferasirox is associated with reduced mortality risk in a Medicare population with myelodysplastic syndromes [abstract]. Blood 2012;120:426a.
105. Steensma DP. The role of iron chelation therapy for patients with myelodysplastic syndromes. J Natl Compr Canc Netw 2011;9:65–75.
106. Wells RA, Leber B, Buckstein R, et al. Iron overload in myelodysplastic syndromes: A Canadian consensus guideline. Leuk Res 2008;32:1338–1353.
107. Sekeres MA, Steensma DP. Defining prior therapy in myelodysplastic syndromes and criteria for relapsed and refractory disease: Implications for clinical trial design and enrollment. Blood 2009;114:2575–2580.
108. Calado RT. Immunologic aspects of hypoplastic myelodysplastic syndrome. Semin Oncol 2011;38:667–672.
109. Sauntharajah Y, Nakamura R, Nam JM, et al. HLA-DR15 (DR2) is overrepresented in myelodysplastic syndrome and aplastic anemia and predicts a response to immunosuppression in myelodysplastic syndrome. Blood 2002;100:1570–1574.
110. Sauntharajah Y, Nakamura R, Wesley R, et al. A simple method to predict response to immunosuppressive therapy in patients with myelodysplastic syndrome. Blood 2003;102:3025–3027.
111. Garg R, Faderl S, Garcia-Manero G, et al. Phase II study of rabbit anti-thymocyte globulin, cyclosporine and granulocyte colony-stimulating factor in patients with aplastic anemia and myelodysplastic syndrome. Leukemia 2009;23:1297–1302.
112. Stadler M, Germing U, Kliche KO, et al. A prospective, randomised, phase II study of horse antithymocyte globulin vs rabbit antithymocyte globulin as immune-modulating therapy in patients with low-risk myelodysplastic syndromes. Leukemia 2004;18:460–465.
113. Sloand EM, Wu CO, Greenberg P, et al. Factors affecting response and survival in patients with myelodysplasia treated with immunosuppressive therapy. J Clin Oncol 2008;26:2505–2511.
114. Passweg JR, Giagounidis AA, Simcock M, et al. Immunosuppressive therapy for patients with myelodysplastic syndrome: A prospective randomized multicenter phase III trial comparing antithymocyte globulin plus cyclosporine with best supportive care—SAKK 33/99. J Clin Oncol 2011;29:303–309.
115. Sloand EM, Olnes MJ, Shenoy A, et al. Alemtuzumab treatment of intermediate-1 myelodysplasia patients is associated with sustained improvement in blood counts and cytogenetic remissions. J Clin Oncol 2010;28:5166–5173.
116. Sekeres MA, Maciejewski JP, Giagounidis AA, et al. Relationship of treatment-related cytopenias and response to lenalidomide in patients with lower-risk myelodysplastic syndromes. J Clin Oncol 2008;26:5943–5949.
117. List A, Kurtin S, Roe DJ, et al. Efficacy of lenalidomide in myelodysplastic syndromes. N Engl J Med 2005;352: 549–557.
118. Germing U, Lauseker M, Hildebrandt B, et al. Survival, prognostic factors and rates of leukemic transformation in 381 untreated patients with MDS and del(5q): A multicenter study. Leukemia 2012;26:1286–1292.
119. Raza A, Reeves JA, Feldman EJ, et al. Phase 2 study of lenalidomide in transfusion-dependent, low-risk, and intermediate-1 risk myelodysplastic syndromes with karyotypes other than deletion 5q. Blood 2008;111:86–93.
120. Sibon D, Cannas G, Baracco F, et al. Lenalidomide in lower-risk myelodysplastic syndromes with karyotypes other than deletion 5q and refractory to erythropoiesis-stimulating agents. Br J Haematol 2012;156:619–625.
121. Komrokji RS, Lancet JE, Swern AS, et al. Combined treatment with lenalidomide and epoetin alfa in lower-risk patients with myelodysplastic syndrome. Blood 2012;120: 3419–3424.
122. Ades L, Boehrer S, Prebet T, et al. Efficacy and safety of lenalidomide in intermediate-2 or high-risk myelodysplastic syndromes with 5q deletion: Results of a phase 2 study. Blood 2009;113:3947–3952.
123. Silverman LR, Fenaux P, Mufti GJ, et al. Continued azacitidine therapy beyond time of first response improves quality of response in patients with higher-risk myelodysplastic syndromes. Cancer 2011;117:2697–2702.
124. Garcia-Manero G. Treatment of higher-risk myelodysplastic syndrome. Semin Oncol 2011;38:673–681.
125. Silverman LR, Demakos EP, Peterson BL, et al. Randomized controlled trial of azacitidine in patients with the myelodysplastic syndrome: A study of the cancer and leukemia group B. J Clin Oncol 2002;20:2429–2440.
126. Kantarjian H, Issa JP, Rosenfeld CS, et al. Decitabine improves patient outcomes in myelodysplastic syndromes: Results of a phase III randomized study. Cancer 2006;106:1794–1803.
127. Batty GN, Kantarjian H, Issa JP, et al. Feasibility of therapy with hypomethylating agents in patients with renal insufficiency. Clin Lymphoma Myeloma Leuk 2010;10: 205–210.
128. Shen L, Kantarjian H, Guo Y, et al. DNA methylation predicts survival and response to therapy in patients with myelodysplastic syndromes. J Clin Oncol 2009;28:605–613.
129. Kornblith AB, Herndon JE 2nd, Silverman LR, et al. Impact of azacytidine on the quality of life of patients with myelodysplastic syndrome treated in a randomized phase III trial: A Cancer and Leukemia Group B study. J Clin Oncol 2002;20:2441–2452.
130. Itzykson R, Thepot S, Quesnel B, et al. Prognostic factors for response and overall survival in 282 patients with higher-risk myelodysplastic syndromes treated with azacitidine. Blood 2011;117:403–411.
131. Lubbert M, Suciu S, Baila L, et al. Low-dose decitabine versus best supportive care in elderly patients with intermediate- or high-risk myelodysplastic syndrome (MDS) ineligible for intensive chemotherapy: Final results of the randomized phase III study of the European Organisation for Research and Treatment of Cancer Leukemia Group and the German MDS Study Group. J Clin Oncol 2011;29:1987–1996.

132. Bhatnagar B, Zandberg DP, Vannorsdall EJ, et al. Lack of response of myelodysplastic syndrome (MDS) and acute myeloid leukemia (AML) to decitabine after failure of azacitidine [abstract]. Blood 2012;120:3858.
133. Steensma DP, Baer MR, Slack JL, et al. Multicenter study of decitabine administered daily for 5 days every 4 weeks to adults with myelodysplastic syndromes: The alternative dosing for outpatient treatment (ADOPT) trial. J Clin Oncol 2009;27:3842–3848.
134. Lyons RM, Cosgriff TM, Modi SS, et al. Hematologic response to three alternative dosing schedules of azacitidine in patients with myelodysplastic syndromes. J Clin Oncol 2009;27:1850–1856.
135. Beran M, Shen Y, Kantarjian H, et al. High-dose chemotherapy in high-risk myelodysplastic syndrome: Covariate-adjusted comparison of five regimens. Cancer 2001;92:1999–2015.
136. Faderl S, Garcia-Manero G, Ravandi F, et al. A randomized study of low dose oral clofarabine 10 mg versus 20 mg (flat dose) daily × 5 for patients with higher-risk myelodysplastic syndrome (MDS) [abstract]. Blood 2012;120:3851a.
137. Faderl S, Garcia-Manero G, Estrov Z, et al. Oral clofarabine in the treatment of patients with higher-risk myelodysplastic syndrome. J Clin Oncol 2010;28: 2755–2760.
138. Faderl S, Garcia-Manero G, Jabbour E, et al. A randomized study of 2 dose levels of intravenous clofarabine in the treatment of patients with higher-risk myelodysplastic syndrome. Cancer 2012;118:722–728.
139. Lim SH, McMahan J, Zhang J, et al. A phase II study of low dose intravenous clofarabine for elderly patients with myelodysplastic syndrome who have failed 5-azacytidine. Leuk Lymphoma 2010;51:2258–2261.
140. Sekeres MA, Schoonen WM, Kantarjian H, et al. Characteristics of US patients with myelodysplastic syndromes: Results of six cross-sectional physician surveys. J Natl Cancer Inst 2008;100:1542–1551.
141. Lim Z, Brand R, Martino R, et al. Allogeneic hematopoietic stem-cell transplantation for patients 50 years or older with myelodysplastic syndromes or secondary acute myeloid leukemia. J Clin Oncol 2010;28:405–411.
142. McClune BL, Weisdorf DJ, Pedersen TL, et al. Effect of age on outcome of reduced-intensity hematopoietic cell transplantation for older patients with acute myeloid leukemia in first complete remission or with myelodysplastic syndrome. J Clin Oncol 2010;28:1878–1887.
143. Oliansky DM, Antin JH, Bennett JM, et al. The role of cytotoxic therapy with hematopoietic stem cell transplantation in the therapy of myelodysplastic syndromes: An evidence-based review. Biol Blood Marrow Transplant 2009;15:137–172.
144. Tauro S, Craddock C, Peggs K, et al. Allogeneic stem-cell transplantation using a reduced-intensity conditioning regimen has the capacity to produce durable remissions and long-term disease-free survival in patients with high-risk acute myeloid leukemia and myelodysplasia. J Clin Oncol 2005;23:9387–9393.
145. Kindwall-Keller T, Isola LM. The evolution of hematopoietic SCT in myelodysplastic syndrome. Bone Marrow Transplant 2009;43:597–609.
146. Castro-Malaspina H, Harris RE, Gajewski J, et al. Unrelated donor marrow transplantation for myelodysplastic syndromes: Outcome analysis in 510 transplants facilitated by the National Marrow Donor Program. Blood 2002;99:1943–1951.
147. Martino R, Iacobelli S, Brand R, et al. Retrospective comparison of reduced-intensity conditioning and conventional high-dose conditioning for allogeneic hematopoietic stem cell transplantation using HLA-identical sibling donors in myelodysplastic syndromes. Blood 2006;108:836–846.
148. Sierra J, Perez WS, Rozman C, et al. Bone marrow transplantation from HLA-identical siblings as treatment for myelodysplasia. Blood 2002;100:1997–2004.
149. Sutton L, Chastang C, Ribaud P, et al. Factors influencing outcome in de novo myelodysplastic syndromes treated by allogeneic bone marrow transplantation: A long-term study of 71 patients Societe Francaise de Greffe de Moelle. Blood 1996;88:358–365.
150. Barrett AJ, Savani BN. Allogeneic stem cell transplantation for myelodysplastic syndrome. Semin Hematol 2008;45: 49–59.
151. Cutler CS, Lee SJ, Greenberg P, et al. A decision analysis of allogeneic bone marrow transplantation for the myelodysplastic syndromes: Delayed transplantation for low-risk myelodysplasia is associated with improved outcome. Blood 2004;104:579–585.
152. Giralt SA, Horowitz M, Weisdorf D, et al. Review of stem-cell transplantation for myelodysplastic syndromes in older patients in the context of the Decision Memo for Allogeneic Hematopoietic Stem Cell Transplantation for Myelodysplastic Syndrome emanating from the Centers for Medicare and Medicaid Services. J Clin Oncol 2011;29: 566–572.
153. Alessandrino EP, Della Porta MG, Bacigalupo A, et al. WHO classification and WPSS predict posttransplantation outcome in patients with myelodysplastic syndrome: A study from the Gruppo Italiano Trapianto di Midollo Osseo (GITMO). Blood 2008;112:895–902.
154. de Witte T, Brand R, van Biezen A, et al. Allogeneic stem cell transplantation for patients with refractory anaemia with matched related and unrelated donors: Delay of the transplant is associated with inferior survival. Br J Haematol 2009;146:627–636.
155. Luger SM, Ringden O, Zhang MJ, et al. Similar outcomes using myeloablative vs reduced-intensity allogeneic transplant preparative regimens for AML or MDS. Bone Marrow Transplant 2012;47:203–211.
156. Nimer SD. Clinical management of myelodysplastic syndromes with interstitial deletion of chromosome 5q. J Clin Oncol 2006;24:2576–2582.
157. Cheson BD, Bennett JM, Kantarjian H, et al. Report of an international working group to standardize response criteria for myelodysplastic syndromes. Blood 2000;96:3671–3674.
158. Fenaux P, Giagounidis A, Selleslag D, et al. A randomized phase 3 study of lenalidomide versus placebo in RBC transfusion-dependent patients with low-/intermediate-1-risk myelodysplastic syndromes with del5q. Blood 2011;118:3765–3776.
159. Steensma DP. Myelodysplasia paranoia: Iron as the new radon. Leuk Res 2009;33:1158–1163.
160. Steensma DP. The relevance of iron overload and the appropriateness of iron chelation therapy for patients with myelodysplastic syndromes: A dialogue and debate. Curr Hematol Malig Rep 2011;6:136–144.
161. Valent P, Horny HP, Bennett JM, et al. Definitions and standards in the diagnosis and treatment of the myelodysplastic syndromes: Consensus statements and report from a working conference. Leuk Res 2007;31:727–736.

115

Renal Cell Carcinoma

Christine M. Walko and Ashley E. Simmons

KEY CONCEPTS

1. Renal cell carcinoma (RCC) predominantly occurs later in life, with 70% of all cases diagnosed between the ages of 55 and 84 years.
2. The most established risk factors for RCC are smoking, obesity, and hypertension.
3. Inactivation of the von Hippel-Lindau (VHL) tumor suppressor gene is the hallmark of the most common type of RCC, the clear cell subtype.
4. More than 50% of RCC cases are diagnosed by incidental findings on routine imaging for unrelated reasons.
5. The Memorial Sloan-Kettering Cancer Center Prognostic Factors Model for Survival classifies patients into low-, intermediate-, and high-risk groups based on five clinical factors and can predict survival in untreated patients and those treated with immunotherapy and targeted agents.
6. Surgical removal of the primary tumor, either by total or partial nephrectomy, is the preferred initial treatment for all stages of RCC.
7. Immunotherapy used to be considered first-line therapy for metastatic RCC but has largely been replaced by targeted agents because of their improved efficacy and tolerability.
8. Sunitinib and pazopanib are oral small molecule inhibitors of vascular endothelial growth factor (VEGF) and platelet-derived growth factor and are each treatment options as first-line therapy for metastatic RCC.
9. The VEGFR–tyrosine kinase inhibitor axitinib and the mammalian target of rapamycin (mTOR) inhibitor everolimus are both second-line therapy options for metastatic RCC patients who progress on a targeted therapy or cytokine-based therapy first-line regimen.
10. Temsirolimus is an IV administered mTOR inhibitor indicated for first-line therapy in patients with high-risk metastatic RCC.

INTRODUCTION

Renal cell carcinoma (RCC) is a less common malignancy that, until recently, had few treatment options that were poorly tolerated and resulted in few positive outcomes for patients. However, treatment for the disease has been revolutionized by an increased understanding of the pathophysiology of RCC. Clear cell is the predominant subtype of RCC and is the result of inactivation of the von Hippel-Lindau (VHL) tumor suppressor gene on chromosome 3p25, which leads to increased production of growth factors such as vascular endothelial growth factor (VEGF), transforming growth factor (TGF), platelet-derived growth factor (PDGF), and others responsible for angiogenesis and cell growth.[1] Before 2005, the primary therapy option for patients with advanced RCC after nephrectomy was immunotherapy with few responses and high toxicity. However, seven new drugs have been approved as first- or second-line therapy for RCC: sorafenib, sunitinib, temsirolimus, bevacizumab (in combination with interferon-α [IFN-α]), everolimus, pazopanib, and axitinib.[2–7] Each drug is an example of targeted therapy against growth factors important in the pathophysiology of RCC and has yielded much needed progress in a disease with few therapeutic options. RCC serves as an example of rational development of targeted agents based on knowledge of tumor biology for the treatment of other malignancies.

EPIDEMIOLOGY

About 65,000 new cases of kidney and renal pelvis cancer are diagnosed each year in the United States, with two-thirds of these cases occurring in men. More than 13,000 people in the United States will die of kidney cancer each year.[8] RCC is the fifth most commonly occurring cancer in men, and the number of new cases diagnosed each year is similar to non-Hodgkin lymphoma and melanoma. In women, kidney cancer is the sixth most common cancer, occurring at a rate similar to the rates for ovarian and pancreatic cancers. The incidence of RCC has increased over the past three decades. The rate has increased more rapidly in blacks than whites and in women than men. In the United States, between 2002 and 2006, the age-adjusted incidence rate in black men was 21.3, white men 19.2, black women 10.3, and white women 9.9 per 100,000 person years.[9] This increase may be related to improved imaging techniques and greater use of these imaging modalities, although the higher prevalence of some risk factors may also explain the increased incidence.

Kidney cancer is most commonly diagnosed between the ages of 40 and 70 years, with a peak in the sixth and seventh decades of life. Nearly 70% of all cases of kidney cancer are diagnosed in people between the ages of 55 and 84 years, with less than 3% of all cases diagnosed in patients younger than 34 years.[9] (1)

One of the primary factors influencing overall survival (OS) is the extent of disease spread. When the tumor is confined to the kidney at the time of diagnosis, surgical resection can result in a 5-year OS rate of about 85%. That figure falls to 64% when localized spread has occurred beyond the kidney and to less than 23% when metastatic disease is present.[10] The 5-year relative survival rate of kidney cancer in general improved from 40% in the early 1960s to nearly 70% in 2005.[9] Survival is expected to improve with the growing availability of numerous targeted agents.

ETIOLOGY

The incidence rates of RCC vary more than 10-fold worldwide, with the highest incidence rates in Western and European countries and the lowest in Asia and Africa, which suggests that lifestyle and possibly the environment are important factors. The most established risk factors associated with RCC are smoking, obesity, and hypertension.

❷ Smoking remains the most consistently established risk factor and is estimated to be responsible for 20% to 30% and 10% to 20% of RCC cases diagnosed in men and women, respectively.[11,12] Smoking is associated with a relative risk of 1.54 for men and 1.22 for women with a strong dose-dependent relationship. Heavy smoking, defined as 21 or more cigarettes per day, was associated with an increased relative risk of 2.03 and 1.58 for men and women, respectively.[13] Smoking cessation has been demonstrated to reduce the risk of RCC with a 15% to 30% decrease after 10 to 15 years after cessation and a 50% decrease for those who quit for 30 years or more.[13,14]

Obesity is also linked to RCC development in observational studies and appears to be equally associated in men and women. Compared with a body mass index (BMI) of 20.75 kg/m^2 or less, men with a BMI between 22.86 and 27.75 kg/m^2 had a relative risk of 1.3 to 1.7, and those with a BMI of 27.76 kg/m^2 or greater had a relative risk of 1.9.[15] A separate analysis reported a relative risk of 2.5 for those with a BMI of 30 kg/m^2 or greater.[16] It is estimated that 30% to 40% of RCC cases may be attributed to obesity, which suggests that increasing rates of obesity in the United States may be partially responsible for the increased incidence seen over the past 3 decades.[12] Numerous mechanisms explaining the link between obesity and the development of RCC have been proposed. Obesity has been linked to increased lipid peroxidation, which can result in carcinogenesis of the proximal renal tubules. Byproducts of the lipid peroxidation pathway have also been shown to result in DNA adducts in the kidney, which can result in oncogene and tumor suppressor gene mutations and eventually malignancy.[17] Adipose tissue, when stimulated, can release numerous substances to regulate energy balance and lipid metabolism. Insulin resistance and compensatory elevated insulin levels result in increased levels of insulin-like growth factor-1 (IGF-1), which regulates cell proliferation and can inhibit cellular apoptosis.[16] Finally, the kidneys of obese men and women are more susceptible to carcinogenesis because of higher glomerular filtration rates, renal perfusion, and atrophic scarring of the kidneys.[12]

The risk of RCC is associated with increased duration and severity of elevated blood pressure. Patients with a diastolic blood pressure (DBP) greater than 90 mm Hg had a relative risk of 2.1 compared with DBP less than 70 mm Hg. A systolic blood pressure (SBP) greater than 150 mm Hg was associated with a relative risk of 1.6 compared with SBP less than 120 mm Hg.[15] The exact mechanism explaining the causality of hypertension to RCC is unknown, but it is believed to be related to hypertension-induced renal injury and lipid peroxidation.[12,17] Medications commonly used to treat hypertension do not appear to be associated with RCC.

The analgesic phenacetin has a historical link to RCC. The drug was introduced in 1887 and used until the 1970s, when increased concerns for carcinogenesis resulted in replacement with safer analgesics, such as the major metabolite of phenacetin, acetaminophen. Despite its association with the known carcinogen, acetaminophen has not been associated with an increased risk of RCC.[12]

A well-defined genetic link has also been described. Although most RCC cases are not associated with hereditary factors and are considered "sporadic," 2% to 3% of cases are secondary to inherited syndromes.[18,19] Kidney tumors arising from a genetic etiology are most commonly the result of an autosomal dominant transmission of the diseased gene from a carrier to the offspring. Initially, one carrier parent has one healthy chromosome and one chromosome with the diseased gene. When this carrier has offspring with a healthy individual with two healthy chromosomes, the offspring each have a 50% chance of also being a carrier. These carriers with one healthy chromosome and one chromosome with the diseased gene are then more sensitive to developing RCC after being exposed to additional somatic mutations that can affect the remaining healthy chromosome.

SUBTYPES AND PATHOPHYSIOLOGY

About 85% of kidney cancers affect the parenchyma of the kidney and are classified as RCC. The renal pelvis is less commonly affected, making up 12% of the cases of kidney cancer diagnosed each year, with other rare malignancies affecting other parts of the kidney and making up the remaining 3%. The subtypes of RCC include clear cell, papillary (also known as chromophilic), chromophobic, and oncocytic. Each subtype has a unique genetic pathophysiology that results in a different clinical course and response to therapy.[18]

Clear Cell Renal Cell Carcinoma: The Role of the von Hippel-Lindau Gene

Clear cell is the predominant subtype responsible for most cases of RCC. These tumors typically affect the proximal tubule of the kidney and are more likely to metastasize than other subtypes. The initial finding of an association between clear cell histology and losses in the short arm of chromosome 3 eventually led to the gene responsible for this subtype being mapped to the location 3p24-25 and termed the VHL gene in 1993.[20–22] Inactivation of this tumor suppressor gene is now recognized as the hallmark of clear cell RCC. The Knudson and Strong two-hit model explains the development of clear cell RCC after inactivation of both copies of the tumor suppressor gene VHL.[22] In patients with sporadic disease, the two copies of VHL present in a healthy kidney can be inactivated via loss of chromosome 3p, gene silencing via hypermethylation, missense mutations, and premature truncation or nonsense mutations. Additional mutations can result in a single, unilateral tumor. In patients with hereditary disease, one copy of VHL has already been deleted via a germline mutation. Fewer events are then needed to delete the remaining gene copy, which explains why patients with hereditary disease are more likely to present with multicentric, bilateral tumors.[18,19]

The VHL gene produces the VHL protein (pVHL), which is expressed ubiquitously throughout the body and is part of the complex that selects substances for ubiquitination and subsequent destruction by the proteasome.[23] Because of this role, VHL regulates cellular response to oxygen. In a normal oxygen environment, the target for proteasome destruction is hypoxia-inducible factor (HIF)-1α. Hydroxylated HIF-1α binds to pVHL and is destroyed by the proteasome (Fig. 115-1). When the cellular environment is hypoxic, HIF-1α is not hydroxylated and does not bind to pVHL. The unbound HIF-1α can then initiate transcription of hypoxia-inducible genes in the cell nucleus, which enables the cell to adapt and survive a hypoxic insult[23,24] (Fig. 115-2). ❸ In the case of clear cell RCC, when VHL is mutated or silenced, pVHL is unable to bind and target HIF-1α for degradation regardless of the oxygen presence in the environment. HIF-1α therefore becomes abundant and activates transcription of hypoxia-inducible genes, including VEGF, PDGF, TGF, glucose transporters, erythropoietin, and other factors that promote angiogenesis and tumor development[23,24]

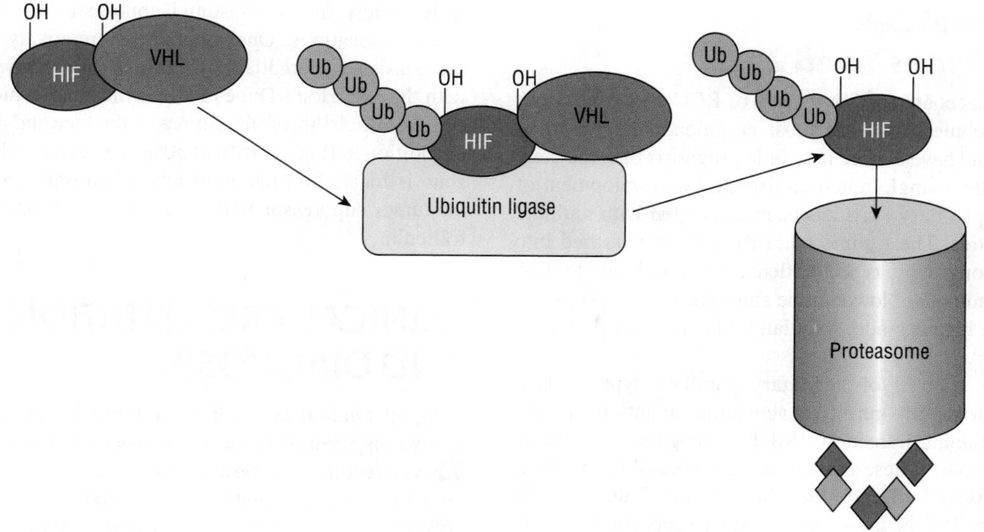

FIGURE 115-1 The role of von Hippel-Lindau (VHL) protein and hypoxia-inducible factor (HIF): normal oxygen, normal VHL. In a normal oxygen environment, HIF is hydroxylated. This enables binding of the VHL protein and subsequent attachment of a polyubiquitin chain, a process called ubiquitination. This allows the ubiquitin-tagged HIF to be recognized for destruction by the proteasome. The proteasome acts as a garbage disposal for compounds labeled by the ubiquitination process.

(Fig. 115-3). Numerous therapies for RCC target these hypoxia-inducible genes that are activated by HIF and are discussed later in the chapter.

In addition to VHL, other growth factors and cell adhesion pathways control HIF-1α activity.[23] TGF is a ligand for the epidermal growth factor receptor (EGFR) and, upon binding, activates the phosphatidylinositol 3-kinase (PI3K)/AKT/mammalian target of rapamycin (mTOR) pathway, in addition to other protein kinase pathways. Activation of the mTOR pathway increases production of HIF-1α, which can drive the oncogenic process described earlier.[23,25,26] The mTOR is another pathway targeted for the therapy of RCC.

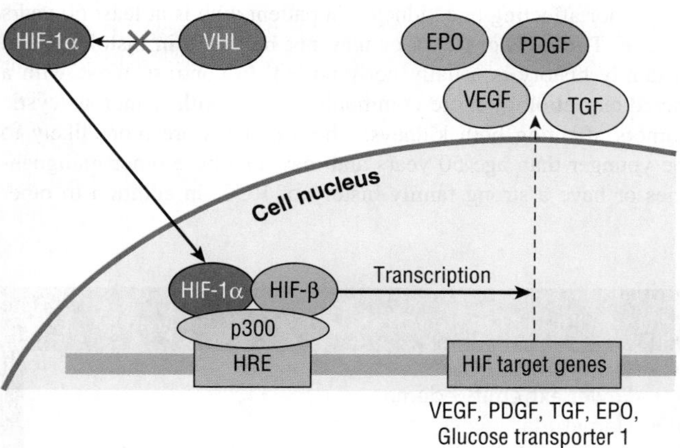

FIGURE 115-2 The role of von Hippel-Lindau (VHL) and hypoxia-inducible factor (HIF)-1α: low oxygen, normal VHL. In a low oxygen environment, the cell wants to increase production of substances to promote a switch to anaerobic metabolism, including enzymes involved in glycolysis and glycerol metabolism. In this situation, HIF-1α is not hydroxylated and cannot bind to VHL. HIF-1α is then able to translocate into the nucleus of the cell. In the nucleus, HIF-1α combines with the HIF-β subunit and the p300 transcriptional cofactor on the hypoxia response element (HRE) that promotes the transcription of HIF-1α target genes. More than 100 genes can be activated by this complex and include vascular endothelial growth factor (VEGF), platelet-derived growth factor (PDGF), transforming growth factor (TGF), erythropoietin (EPO), and glucose transporter 1.

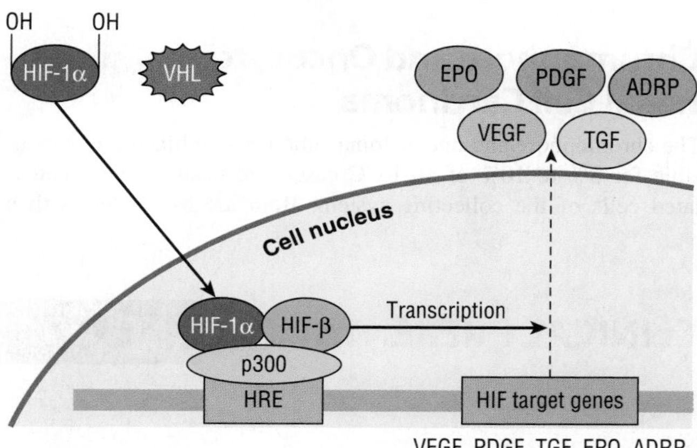

FIGURE 115-3 The role of von Hippel-Lindau (VHL) and hypoxia-inducible factor (HIF)-1α: normal oxygen, mutated VHL. When VHL is mutated, it is not able to bind to the hydroxylated HIF-1α regardless of the presence of oxygen in the environment. Because HIF-1α is not bound to VHL, it is not destroyed by the proteasome and is thus free to translocate into the nucleus, combine with the HIF-β subunit and the p300 transcriptional cofactor on the HRE, and initiate gene transcription. Because a hypoxia situation is not present, production of these genes involved in angiogenesis, cellular survival, and glucose metabolism can result in an oncogenic process. (ADRP, adipose differentiation-related protein [responsible for neutral lipid accumulation in the cell cytoplasm, resulting in the clear cell appearance]; EPO, erythropoietin; PDGF, platelet-derived growth factor; TGF, transforming growth factor; VEGF, vascular endothelial growth factor.)

Papillary Renal Cell Carcinoma Types 1 and 2

Papillary subtypes account for 5% to 10% of RCC cases and occur in the proximal tubule. They are most commonly diagnosed as localized disease and have a more favorable prognosis than the clear cell subtype. Unlike a single mutation driving the development of clear cell disease, papillary RCC has been associated with multiple genetic abnormalities. These tumors are further subclassified into types 1 and 2. Chromophilic type 1 patients are more likely to have multiple, bilateral tumors of lower grade and have a better prognosis compared with the higher grade, singular, unilateral poor prognosis type 2 tumors.[17,19,23]

The majority (>80%) of hereditary papillary type 1 RCC cases are associated with germline activating mutations in the mesenchymal–epithelial transition (MET) oncogene, located at chromosome 7q31-34.[27] These mutations are responsible for about 13% of sporadic type 1 disease, but chromosome 7 duplications have been found in 75% of these cases, further supporting the role of MET.[23] Activation of the c-MET receptor results in increased cell proliferation and motility and decreased cellular apoptosis.[26] Stabilization of HIF can also play a role in the oncogenic potential of the c-MET receptor.[28]

The papillary type 2 subtype occurs in patients with hereditary leiomyomatosis, which initially presents as multiple skin and uterine leiomyomas when patients are in their 20s and 30s and eventually results in formation of RCC. The associated gene for this subtype is the fumarase hydratase (FH) gene, located at chromosome 1q42.3-45. FH is a tumor suppressor gene that encodes the enzyme FH responsible for catalyzing fumarate to malate in the Krebs cycle. The gene is predominantly inactivated by loss-of-function mutations, which ultimately results in stabilization of HIF and subsequent oncogenesis.[29,30]

Chromophore and Oncocytoma Renal Cell Carcinoma

The chromophore and oncocytoma subtypes combined are responsible for 5% to 10% of all RCC cases and occur in the intercalated cells of the collecting system. Both are associated with a wide variety of chromosomal abnormalities, including deletions and translocations. Oncocytomas are relatively benign and rarely metastasize.[31] Hereditary forms of these subtypes are associated with the Birt-Hogg-Dube (BHD) syndrome, which is characterized by hair follicle fibrofolliculomas of the face and neck and lung cysts in addition to RCC in 15% to 30% of affected individuals. The BHD gene is located on the short arm of chromosome 17 and encodes the tumor suppressor BHD gene that is responsible for the protein folliculin.[17]

CLINICAL PRESENTATION AND DIAGNOSIS

Imaging modalities, such as computed tomography (CT) scans, are widely used in the medical work-up of numerous conditions. (4) As a result, most cases of RCC are now diagnosed incidentally after radiographic imaging for unrelated reasons compared with 10% in 1970.[32] Fewer than 10% of patients currently present with the classic triad of flank pain, hematuria, and a palpable abdominal mass. Incidentally diagnosed tumors, or those diagnosed in the absence of signs and symptoms commonly associated with RCC, are usually smaller in size, of a lower stage, and more localized than those seen in patients who present with symptoms such as the classic triad. In addition to the classic triad, common presenting complaints are nonspecific signs and symptoms, including fatigue, weight loss, anemia, hypertension, fever, and lower extremity edema. Bone pain, adenopathy, and pulmonary symptoms are indicators of metastatic disease spread to the mediastinum or lung parenchyma.[32]

As noted earlier, RCC can be either sporadic or hereditary. Several differences exist between the two etiologies in terms of patterns of development. Sporadic RCC most often presents as a single tumor affecting one kidney in a patient who is at least 60 years of age. These lesions may or may not be cystic in histology, and a family history is usually not reported. In contrast, those with a hereditary etiology more commonly present with numerous cystic tumors affecting both kidneys. These patients are more likely to be younger than age 50 years and may also have other malignancies or have a strong family history of RCC, in addition to other

CLINICAL PRESENTATION

Symptoms

- Flank pain
- Fatigue
- Absence of symptoms is often seen with early disease
- Lower extremity edema
- Hematuria
- Palpable abdominal mass

Symptoms of Disease Progression

- Bone pain
- Pulmonary symptoms, including shortness of breath and cough
- Types of symptoms differ depending on location of disease spread

Signs

- Weight loss
- Anemia
- Hypertension
- Fever

Sign of Advanced Disease

- Adenopathy

Diagnostic Tests

- Complete blood count
- Serum calcium
- Serum creatinine
- Liver function tests
- Lactate dehydrogenase
- Coagulation profile
- Urinalysis
- Contrast and non-contrast CT or MRI of the chest, abdomen pelvis
- Fine-needle biopsy only in select cases

malignancies, including retinal angiomas, hemangioblastomas, and pheochromocytomas.[19,32]

Laboratory evaluation should include a complete blood count, serum calcium, serum creatinine, liver function tests, lactate dehydrogenase (LDH), coagulation profile, and urinalysis. Imaging studies, including contrast and noncontrast CT or magnetic resonance imaging (MRI) of the chest, abdomen, and pelvis, are also performed to further characterize the renal tumor, assess involvement of the inferior vena cava, and determine the patient's disease stage. Fine-needle biopsy is used only in rare selected cases.

STAGING AND PROGNOSIS

The factors associated with prognosis are positive margins after surgery, evidence of metastatic spread, presence of sarcomatoid architecture, tumor subtype, tumor grade, and tumor stage, with the latter being the most powerful prognostic indicator.[33] The Union Internationale Contre le Cancer/International Union Against Cancer (UICC) and the American Joint Committee for Cancer Staging and End Results Reporting (AJCC) introduced the tumor–nodes–metastasis (TNM) staging system for RCC in 1978. The 7th edition was published most recently in 2010.[34,35] The AJCC staging classification considers tumor size, number of lymph nodes involved, and the presence or absence of distant metastases. Subdivisions in the tumor (T) classification further describe the structures of the kidney that have been invaded by the tumor, including the adrenal gland, Gerota's fascia (the layer of connective tissue surrounding the kidneys), and perinephric fat that lies between the fascia and renal capsule.[35] Table 115-1 summarizes the AJCC TNM staging definitions, and Table 115-2 shows the TNM stage and corresponding 5-year OS rates.

5 In patients with metastatic disease, the Memorial Sloan-Kettering Cancer Center (MSKCC) Prognostic Factors Model was developed from a retrospective analysis of 670 patients with advanced RCC from 24 different trials at MSKCC between 1975 and 1996. The model identified five factors associated with poor prognosis: Karnofsky performance status (KPS), LDH, hemoglobin, corrected serum calcium, and nephrectomy status (later interchanged with duration of time from diagnosis to initial treatment). Patients with none of the poor prognostic risk factors are considered low risk, one or two factors are intermediate risk, and three or more factors are high risk (Table 115-3). In this analysis, 25% of patients were classified as low risk and had a median OS of 20 months, 53% were intermediate risk with a median OS of 10 months, and 22% were high risk with a median OS of 4 months. Three-year OS for the low-, intermediate-, and high-risk groups was 31%, 7%, and 0%, respectively.[36] This model has been validated externally and can be used to predict survival outcomes for patients treated with IFN-based therapy.[37] Another retrospective study in 353 patients with untreated RCC confirmed the MSKCC model but identified two additional independent prognostic factors: prior radiation and number of metastatic sites (none or one compared with two or more). Low risk was defined as the presence of no or one risk factor, intermediate risk as two risk factors, and high risk as the presence of three or more risk factors. Based on these

TABLE 115-1 American Joint Committee for Cancer Staging and End Results Reporting Sixth Edition Staging

Primary Tumor (T)	
T_x	Primary tumor cannot be assessed
T_0	No evidence of primary tumor
T_1	Tumor ≤7 cm in greatest dimension, limited to the kidney
T_{1a}	Tumor ≤4 cm in greatest dimension, limited to the kidney
T_{1b}	Tumor >4 cm but not >7 cm in greatest dimension, limited to the kidney
T_2	Tumor >7 cm in greatest dimension, limited to the kidney
T_3	Tumor extends into major veins or invades adrenal gland or perinephric tissues but not beyond Gerota's fascia
T_{3a}	Tumor directly invades the adrenal gland or perirenal and/or renal sinus fat but not beyond Gerota's fascia
T_{3b}	Tumor grossly extends into the renal vein or its segmental (muscle-containing) branches or vena cava below the diaphragm
T_{3c}	Tumor grossly extends into vena cava above the diaphragm or invades the wall of the vena cava
T_4	Tumor invades beyond Gerota's fascia
Regional Lymph Nodes (N)	
N_x	Regional lymph nodes cannot be assessed
N_0	No regional lymph node metastases
N_1	Metastases in a single regional lymph node
N_2	Metastases in more than one regional lymph node
Distant Metastasis (M)	
M_x	Distant metastasis cannot be assessed
M_0	No distant metastasis
M_1	Presence of distant metastasis

Used with the permission of the American Joint Committee on Cancer (AJCC), Chicago, Illinois. The original source for this material is the AJCC Cancer Staging Manual, 7th ed. (2010) published by Springer Science and Business Media LLC, www.springer.com.

TABLE 115-2 American Joint Committee for Cancer Staging and End Results Reporting Stage Grouping

Stage	T	N	M	5-Year Overall Survival (%)
I	T_1	N_0	M_0	96
II	T_2	N_0	M_0	82
III	T_1	N_1	M_0	64
	T_2	N_1	M_0	
	T_3	N_0	M_0	
	T_3	N_1	M_0	
	T_{3a}	N_0	M_0	
	T_{3a}	N_1	M_0	
	T_{3b}	N_0	M_0	
	T_{3b}	N_1	M_0	
	T_{3c}	N_0	M_0	
	T_{3c}	N_1	M_0	
IV	T_4	N_0	M_0	23
	T_4	N_1	M_0	
	Any T	N_2	M_0	
	Any T	Any T	M_1	

M, metastasis; N, node; T, tumor.

From Linehan WM, Rini BI, Yang JC. Cancer of the kidney. In: DeVita VT Jr HS, Rosenberg SA, eds. Cancer Principles and Practice of Oncology, 8th ed. Philadelphia, PA: Lippincott Williams & Wilkins, 2008:1331–1357.

Used with the permission of the American Joint Committee on Cancer (AJCC), Chicago, Illinois. The original source for this material is the AJCC Cancer Staging Manual, 7th ed. (2010) published by Springer Science and Business Media LLC, www.springer.com.

TABLE 115-3 Memorial Sloan-Kettering Cancer Center Poor Prognostic Factors

- Karnofsky performance status (KPS) <80%
- Low serum hemoglobin (<13 g/dL [<130 g/L; 8.07 mmol/L] for men and <11.5 g/dL [<115 g/L; 7.14 mmol/L] for women)
- Elevated corrected calcium (>10 mg/dL [2.50 mmol/L])
- Elevated serum LDH (≥300 U/L [≥5.00 μkat/L] or 1.5 × ULN)
- Absence of prior nephrectomy (has been shown to be a function of duration of time between diagnosis and start of therapy, with >1 year delay being considered a poor prognostic factor)

Expanded criteria in untreated patients include

- Two or more sites of metastatic disease
- Prior radiotherapy

LDH, lactate dehydrogenase; ULN, upper limit of normal.

criteria, 37% of the patients were classified as low risk (median OS, 26 months), 35% as intermediate risk (median OS, 14.4 months), and 28% as high risk (median OS, 7.3 months).[38] In an updated analysis of metastatic RCC patients treated with targeted agents, the MSKCC model confirmed the importance of hemoglobin, corrected serum calcium, KPS, and time from diagnosis to treatment as prognostic factors for OS. Elevated neutrophil and platelet counts were also independent survival prognostic factors. Of the 586 evaluable patients treated with targeted agents (sunitinib, sorafenib, or bevacizumab), 23% were low risk with an OS that was not reached after a median follow up of 24.5 months, 51% were intermediate risk with a median OS of 27 months, and 26% were high risk with a median OS of 8.8 months. Corresponding 2-year OS rates for the low-, intermediate-, and high-risk groups were 75%, 53%, and 7%, respectively.[39]

Clinical **Controversy...**

Traditionally, the Response Evaluation Criteria in Solid Tumors (RECIST) model has been used to evaluate treatment response rates in solid tumors. Whether this remains the optimal method of assessing response rates in patients receiving targeted therapies is unknown because the drugs may result in tumor death and internal tumor necrosis without much change in the tumor size itself.

The MSKCC criteria, with minor additions as discussed earlier, are currently used in practice to determine optimal therapy for patients and are incorporated into the National Comprehensive Cancer Network (NCCN) guidelines. For example, temsirolimus is currently recommended for patients with high-risk disease. Additionally, the criteria are used to determine eligibility or stratification for clinical trials in an effort to further individualize and optimize patient therapy.

Current efforts have focused on the identification of predictive biologic biomarkers for therapy. In contrast to the prognostic factors discussed earlier that correlate with survival regardless of intervention, predictive biomarkers correlate with response to a specific therapy. Predictive biomarkers can help clinicians to optimize therapy choices for patients. No clinically validated biomarkers for RCC are available, but numerous factors are under investigation, including the HIF target carbonic anhydrase IX; angiogenic proteins linked to HIF-associated signaling; and biologic participants in the mTOR signaling pathway, such as phosphorylated-AKT, phosphorylated-S6 kinase, phosphatase and tensin homologue (PTEN), and cytoplasmic p27.[40–43]

Clinical **Controversy...**

The VEGFR inhibitors are recommended as first-line therapy for treatment of advanced or metastatic RCC. A known adverse effect of VEGF and VEGFR inhibition is hypertension and is commonly reported with both bevacizumab and the tyrosine kinase inhibitors of this pathway. Preliminary data have suggested that development of treatment-associated hypertension may be associated with improved response rates of VEGF-directed therapy. However, prospective correlations are needed to determine the degree of hypertension and magnitude of PFS benefit before this can be translated into clinical practice.

TREATMENT

Surgical excision of the renal tumor remains the primary method of local disease control and is performed in patients with stage I, II, or III disease.[44] In patients with advanced disease, treatment options for patients after nephrectomy had historically been limited to immunotherapy approaches with IFN-α, interleukin-2 (IL-2), or both. However, novel VEGFR-targeted tyrosine kinase inhibitors (TKIs), including sunitinib, sorafenib, pazopanib, and axitinib, in addition to the mTOR inhibitors temsirolimus and everolimus have provided numerous therapy options and remain the cornerstone of therapy for advanced and metastatic disease.

Desired Outcomes

The goal of therapy for RCC depends on the stage of disease at diagnosis and other patient-specific factors, including age, performance status, and comorbidities. In patients with localized disease confined to the kidney (stages I, II, and III), the initial treatment recommendation is surgical removal with curative intent. In patients with initially localized disease who undergo nephrectomy, 20% to 30% will relapse, with most relapses occurring in the first 2 years after surgery. When patients have developed metastatic disease, the goal of therapy is to control disease burden and prolong survival while maximizing quality of life.[44] Even within patients with metastatic disease, survival outcomes depend on patient specific factors, including the MSKCC-adapted model for targeted agents and the specific therapy chosen.[39] The selection of each line of therapy and even agents within the same line of therapy should be weighed against the risks and benefits for each individual patient.

Regardless of the first-line and subsequent therapies, optimizing quality of life is always a goal of treatment. Symptoms differ based on disease stage, sites of distant disease, and treatment. Patients with bone involvement may experience pain in the areas of metastatic disease that can be addressed with the use of bone modifying agents, such as bisphosphonates or denosumab, or palliative radiation therapy, along with optimizing daily pain medication regimens. Adherence with oral targeted therapies should be emphasized with patients, both in terms of taking the medication regularly as prescribed but also following administration recommendations such as taking medication with or without food and avoiding interacting medications. Treatment-related toxicities should also be aggressively addressed to optimize the benefits of therapy. Hypertension, skin related effects, and diarrhea are common toxicities of the VEGFR-TKIs, and hypercholesterolemia and hyperglycemia are common with the mTOR inhibitors. These effects should be anticipated with preventative treatment when appropriate or close monitoring and therapeutic intervention when needed to improve tolerability to these agents and optimize patient quality of life. The subjective nature of many of these treatment-related and disease-related effects can make consistent assessment challenging, but trials incorporating quality of life outcomes using validated patient-reported assessments will improve our ability to optimize survival as well as quality of outcomes for patients with RCC.

Surgery

6 Surgery represents the initial therapy for most patients with RCC regardless of stage. Surgical options include total nephrectomy and nephron-sparing surgery and depend on numerous patient-specific factors, including the size and location of the renal tumor, whether multiple tumors are present, and whether the patient has a single kidney or has a concurrent disease with a risk of multiple kidney tumors, such as a known genetic predisposition. Radical nephrectomy involves excision of the total kidney, Gerota's fascia, and

ipsilateral adrenal gland after ligation of the renal vein and artery. Nephrectomy is preferred for patients with large tumors (4–7 cm), depending on the location of the tumor. Centrally located tumors are more amenable to total resection than partial nephrectomy.[44,45] Regardless of the functional capacity of the remaining kidney, total nephrectomy has been associated with a higher risk of developing chronic kidney disease, which explains why nephron-sparing techniques have become more common.[46]

Nephron-sparing surgery usually refers to partial nephrectomy, but it can also be used to describe probe-based thermal ablation procedures such as radiofrequency ablation (RFA) and cryoablation. The long-term efficacy of these two techniques has not yet been established, with some reports suggesting higher local recurrence rates than actual surgical excision.[47] Because RFA and cryoablation can result in localized fibrotic reactions, surgical salvage after relapse can be compromised, and these procedures are typically reserved for patients who are not surgical candidates but still desire aggressive localized therapy. The most common nephron-sparing procedure is partial nephrectomy, which has been shown, in appropriately selected patients, to have equivalent outcomes as those seen in patients receiving total nephrectomy.[48] Partial nephrectomy candidates are those with smaller lesions (usually less than 4 cm) that are located in the cortical region of the kidney. Patients with bilateral tumors and those with already compromised renal function are also partial nephrectomy candidates.

In addition to surgical removal of the tumor, some surgeons recommend extended lymphadenectomy. The procedure is controversial if there is no known lymph node involvement, but supporters suggest the procedure can be prognostic because positive nodal findings on lymphadenectomy can indicate systemic involvement, which often results in distant metastatic disease even after lymph nodes removal.[44,49] Although nearly one-third of patients relapse after surgery, adjuvant therapy does improve relapse-free survival in patients who initially present with localized disease. Radiation therapy is not recommended. As a result, observation is the recommended strategy, with imaging of the chest and abdomen every 4 to 6 months after surgery and then as clinically indicated.[44,50]

Surgery is still used for patients with distant (stage IV) disease and may consist of surgical resection of the renal tumor, metastectomy (or removal of metastatic sites), or both. Ideal candidates are those who have minimal regional lymphadenopathy and a solitary site of metastatic disease. Metastatic sites amenable to resection include the lung, bone, brain, and soft tissue.[44,49] The benefits of surgical resection in patients with metastatic disease treated with IFN-α have been demonstrated in two randomized trials. Patients with metastatic RCC in both studies were randomized to nephrectomy followed by IFN-α or IFN-α alone. In a combined analysis, the median OS was 13.6 months for the nephrectomy followed by IFN-α group as compared with 7.8 months for the IFN-α alone group (hazard ratio = 0.69; 95% confidence interval = 0.55–0.87; $P = 0.002$).[51–53] Patients with metastatic disease only involving the lung, good prognostic features, and a performance status of 0 or 1 appear to benefit the most from nephrectomy followed by IFN-α. The mechanism for the apparent improved OS is unknown, but nephrectomy may reduce total tumor burden and increase the time for tumor burden to develop or may eliminate the primary source of immunosuppressive cytokines and tumor-producing growth factors. The benefit of newer targeted therapies is also being evaluated in this setting.[50] Finally, palliative nephrectomy may be an option for patients with symptoms related to their primary tumor when removal can provide symptom relief.

Chemotherapy

Traditional cytotoxic therapy has demonstrated minimal efficacy in the treatment of RCC. Numerous agents have been investigated, the most active being gemcitabine, vinblastine, and 5-fluorouracil. However, response rates of more than 4% to 6% were rarely observed with single agents.[19] Intrinsic resistance to chemotherapy may be partially explained by increased expression of the multidrug resistance gene (*mdr1*), which encodes for a P-glycoprotein (Pgp) transmembrane pump involved in drug efflux. Variable expression of the *mdr1* gene has been found throughout many normal human tissues and in a number of different tumor types. Normal kidney tissue and various carcinomas of the kidney express high levels the *mdr1* gene.[54,55] A number of different chemotherapeutic agents have shown high levels of resistance in RCC tumors expressing the Pgp drug transporter. Overexpression of other drug transporter proteins, including the multidrug-resistance–associated proteins, may also play a role in the development of resistance, along with other mechanisms, such as alterations in glutathione metabolism and proteins involved with regulation of apoptosis, ultimately leading to failure of cells to undergo programmed cell death.[56]

Immunotherapy

Patients with RCC occasionally experience spontaneous regression of their disease, which has led researchers to hypothesize that RCC evokes a host immune response and to study immunotherapy for RCC.[57] 7 IFN-α and IL-2 have been investigated in numerous trials and combinations and were the standard of care for patients with metastatic RCC until the recent emergence of targeted therapy. Their low response rates and high toxicity have resulted in their current roles being limited, with ongoing trials to determine their potential in combination regimens.

Interleukin-2 (aldesleukin) is a glycoprotein primarily produced by helper T lymphocytes that stimulates the growth and cytotoxicity of T lymphocytes. IL-2 has been associated with response rates of 6% to 30%. Although the complete response rate is only about 4% to 6%, some of these complete responses are durable.[50,58] The FDA-approved dose of IL-2 is 600,000 international units/kg IV over 15 minutes given every 8 hours for a maximum of 14 doses. After this initial treatment, the schedule is repeated 9 days later for an additional 14 doses as tolerated. Because of the significant toxicity of IL-2, treatment delays and discontinuations are frequent. The most common reported toxicities are hypotension (71%), diarrhea (67%), chills (52%), vomiting (50%), dyspnea (43%), and peripheral edema (28%) in addition to increases in bilirubin (40%), serum creatinine (33%), and electrolyte abnormalities.[59] Many of these effects are related to capillary leak syndrome. Inpatient administration and intensive monitoring and supportive care are required, and many institutions administer IL-2 in an intensive care setting. Many patients are not candidates for IL-2 therapy because of their age (>60 years), comorbidities, organ function, and poor performance status.

Interferons are naturally occurring glycoproteins produced by macrophages and lymphocytes in response to foreign antigens as part of the host immunity. They exert their antitumor effects by activating cytotoxic T and natural killer cells, enhancing expression of cell surface antigens (i.e., major histocompatibility class I), and modulating gene expression.[60,61] A number of different IFNs have been studied for the treatment of metastatic RCC, including IFN-α, -β, and -γ. The response rates are similar among the different IFNs, but IFN-α is most commonly used to treat RCC.

Although IFN has been used to treat RCC for 2 decades, it is not approved by the FDA for the treatment of advanced or metastatic RCC. Overall response rates to IFN generally range from 5% to 20%.[58,60,62] Two randomized trials demonstrated a survival benefit with IFN. IFN-α plus vinblastine was compared with vinblastine alone in 160 patients with advanced RCC. Both groups received vinblastine at 0.1 mg/kg IV every 3 weeks, and the

TABLE 115-4 Comparison and Dosing of Targeted Agents in Patients with Metastatic Renal Cell Carcinoma

		Drug Dosing Table			
Targeted Agent	**Brand Name**	**Initial Dose**	**Maintenance Dose**	**Special Population Dose**	**Drug Interactions**
Tyrosine Kinase Inhibitors/Vascular Endothelial Growth Factor Inhibitors					
Sunitinib[5,66a]	Sutent	50 mg orally daily × 4 weeks; then off 2 weeks	None	Hemodialysis: no adjustment to starting dose; subsequent doses may be increased up to twofold	CYP 3A4 inducers may decrease sunitinib exposure CYP 3A4 inhibitors may increase sunitinib exposure
Sorafenib[69b]	Nexavar	400 mg orally twice daily	None	No data	UGT1A1 and UGT1A9 substrates may have increased exposure when coadministered with sorafenib because of inhibition of glucuronidation Docetaxel and doxorubicin exposure may increase when coadministered with sorafenib CYP 3A4 inducers may decrease sorafenib exposure
Pazopanib[9c]	Votrient	400 mg orally daily	800 mg orally daily	Moderate hepatic impairment, 200 mg orally once a day Do not use in severe hepatic impairment	CYP 3A4 inducers may decrease pazopanib exposure CYP 3A4 inhibitors may increase pazopanib exposure
Axitinib[d]	Inlyta	5 mg orally twice daily	Increase every 2 weeks to 7 mg orally twice daily and then 10 mg orally twice daily	Hepatic impairment (Child-Pugh class B), reduce dose by half	CYP3A4/5 inhibitors may increase exposure; reduce dose of axitinib by half if a strong CYP3A4/5 inhibitor is administered CYP3A4/5 inducers may decrease exposure
Monoclonal Antibody Vascular Endothelial Growth Factor Inhibitor					
Bevacizumab[7,71e]	Avastin	10 mg/kg IV every 2 weeks	None	No data	No known drug interactions
mTOR Kinase Inhibitors					
Everolimus[8f]	Afinitor	10 mg orally daily	None	Hepatic impairment (Child-Pugh class B), reduce dose to 5 mg orally daily	CYP3A4 and Pgp inhibitors may increase exposure CYP3A4 inducers may decrease exposure
Temsirolimus[6g]	Torisel	25 mg IV once weekly	None	If mild hepatic impairment, reduce dose to 15 mg IV once weekly Do not use if bilirubin is greater than 1.5 times the ULN	CYP3A4 inhibitors may increase exposure CYP3A4 inducers may decrease exposure

ULN, upper limit of normal.

[a]Sunitinib (Sutent) prescribing information: Pfizer, Inc. New York, NY. Revised February 2010.
[b]Sorafenib (Nexavar) prescribing information: Bayer Healthcare Pharmaceuticals, Inc. Wayne, NJ. Revised February 2009.
[c]Pazopanib (Votrient) prescribing information: GlaxoSmithKline, Inc. Research Triangle Park, NC. Revised October 2009.
[d]Axitinib (Inlyta) prescribing information: Pfizer, Inc. New York, NY. Issued January 2012.
[e]Bevacizumab (Avastin) prescribing information: Genentech, Inc. San Francisco, CA. Revised July 2009.
[f]Everolimus (Afinitor) prescribing information: Novartis Pharmaceuticals Corp. East Hanover, NJ. Revised March 2009.
[g]Temsirolimus (Torisel) prescribing information: Wyeth Pharmaceuticals Inc. Philadelphia, PA. Revised September 2008.

combination group also received IFN at a dose of 3 million units subcutaneously or intramuscularly 3 times a week for the first week and then 18 million units subcutaneously 3 times a week thereafter. The median OS was significantly improved in the combination group compared with the vinblastine alone group at 67.6 weeks and 37.8 weeks ($P = 0.005$), respectively.[63] In another study, IFN-α was compared with medroxyprogesterone acetate 300 mg/day in 350 patients with metastatic RCC. IFN-α was dosed at 5 million units for two doses and then increased to 10 million units 3 times a week for a total of 12 weeks. The median OS was 8.5 months compared with 6 months for IFN-α and medroxyprogesterone, which translated into a 28% reduction in the risk of death in the IFN-α group ($P = 0.017$).[64] Based on these studies, IFN remains the comparator for novel treatments in metastatic RCC. It is better tolerated than IL-2 and can be self-administered at home. However, more than 90% of patients experience chills, fever, asthenia, fatigue, headache, diarrhea, and liver function abnormalities, and some patients develop depression and other neuropsychiatric symptoms.

Targeted Therapy

8 Since 2005, seven new drugs have been approved either as first- or second-line therapy: sunitinib, sorafenib, pazopanib, axitinib, bevacizumab (in combination with IFN), temsirolimus, and everolimus (Table 115-4 and Fig. 115-4).

Sunitinib

Sunitinib is an orally administered antiangiogenic agent that inhibits multiple tyrosine kinases, including VEGFR and platelet-derived growth factor receptor (PDGFR).[65] Sunitinib is approved for the first-line treatment of metastatic RCC (NCCN guidelines, category I).[44] That approval was based on a randomized, phase III clinical trial, which compared sunitinib with IFN-α_{2a} as first-line therapy in 750 patients with clear cell metastatic RCC.[66] Sunitinib was administered in a 6-week cycle at 50 mg orally given daily for 4 weeks followed by 2 weeks without treatment. IFN was administered subcutaneously 3 times weekly on nonconsecutive days, with a gradual dose increase from 3 million units to 9 million units over a 3-week

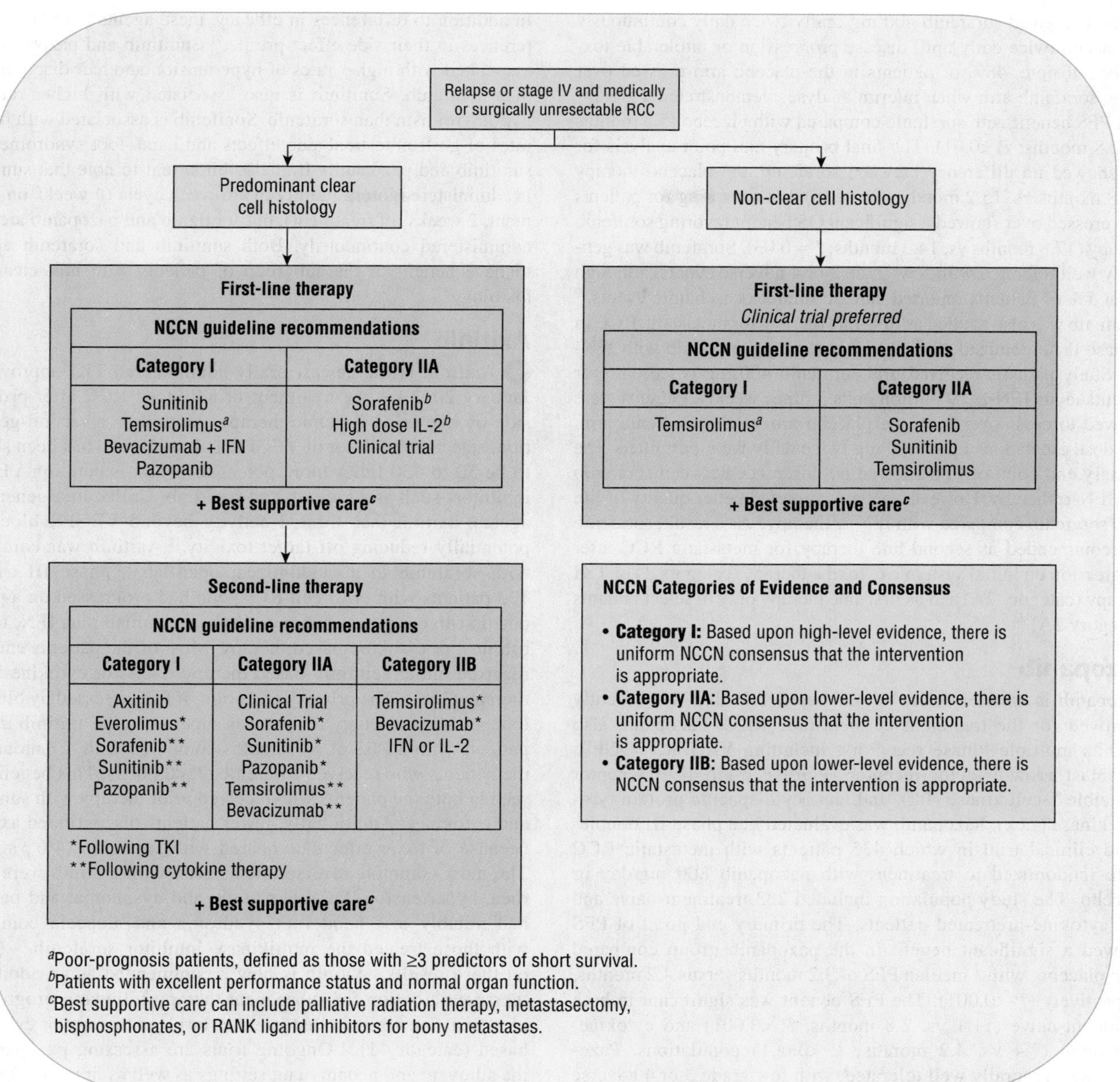

Relapse or stage IV and medically or surgically unresectable RCC
Predominant clear cell histology
Non-clear cell histology
First-line therapy
NCCN guideline recommendations
Category I
Sunitinib
Temsirolimus[a]
Bevacizumab + IFN
Pazopanib
Category IIA
Sorafenib[b]
High dose IL-2[b]
Clinical trial
+ Best supportive care[c]
First-line therapy
Clinical trial preferred
NCCN guideline recommendations
Category I
Temsirolimus[a]
Category IIA
Sorafenib
Sunitinib
Temsirolimus
+ Best supportive care[c]
Second-line therapy
NCCN guideline recommendations
Category I
Axitinib
Everolimus*
Sorafenib**
Sunitinib**
Pazopanib**
Category IIA
Clinical Trial
Sorafenib*
Sunitinib*
Pazopanib*
Temsirolimus**
Bevacizumab**
Category IIB
Temsirolimus*
Bevacizumab*
IFN or IL-2
*Following TKI
**Following cytokine therapy
+ Best supportive care[c]
NCCN Categories of Evidence and Consensus
• Category I: Based upon high-level evidence, there is uniform NCCN consensus that the intervention is appropriate.
• Category IIA: Based upon lower-level evidence, there is uniform NCCN consensus that the intervention is appropriate.
• Category IIB: Based upon lower-level evidence, there is NCCN consensus that the intervention is appropriate.
[a]Poor-prognosis patients, defined as those with ≥3 predictors of short survival.
[b]Patients with excellent performance status and normal organ function.
[c]Best supportive care can include palliative radiation therapy, metastasectomy, bisphosphonates, or RANK ligand inhibitors for bony metastases.

FIGURE 115-4 First and second line therapy recommendations for relapsed or Stage IV and medically or surgically unresectable RCC. (IFN, interferon; IL, interleukin; NCCN, National Comprehensive Cancer Network; RANK, receptor activator of nuclear factor-κB.)

period. Sunitinib was found to be superior to IFN, with median progression-free survival (PFS) of 11 months and 5 months (P <0.001), respectively. The improved PFS with sunitinib was observed regardless of baseline characteristics and prognostic factors. Both treatments were generally well tolerated with a low incidence of grade 3 or 4 adverse events. The sunitinib group had higher rates of diarrhea, vomiting, hypertension, hand–foot syndrome, hair discoloration, and myelosuppression than IFN-treated patients. Health-related quality of life was significantly better in the sunitinib group (P <0.001) compared with the IFN group. Sunitinib-treated patients also had prolonged OS as compared with IFN-treated patients (26 vs. 22 months; P = 0.05) even though 25 patients in the IFN group crossed over to the sunitinib group.[5] Sunitinib has been evaluated in three clinical trials as either first- or second-line therapy after progression on cytokine therapy, with response rates of 30% to 45%, which was considerably higher than the response rates observed for cytokines.[50,66–68] In addition to the high response rate, sunitinib was relatively well tolerated, with most adverse events managed by supportive care or dose modification and fewer than 10% requiring treatment discontinuation. As a result, the NCCN guidelines recommend sunitinib for first-line therapy in patients with metastatic RCC who have never received systemic therapy (category 1) and for second-line therapy in patients who have progressed on cytokine (category 1) or TKI (category 2A) therapy.[44] 8

Sorafenib

Sorafenib is another orally administered antiangiogenic agent that inhibits multiple tyrosine kinases, including VEGFR, PDGFR, Raf-1, fms-like tyrosine kinase receptor-3 (Flt-3), and c-kit. Sorafenib is approved for second-line treatment of metastatic RCC after progression on cytokine therapy. The approval was based on a phase III double-blind clinical trial in which 903 patients with metastatic RCC who had progressed after first-line systemic therapy were randomized to treatment with sorafenib or placebo. Study patients received sorafenib 400 mg orally twice daily continuously or placebo twice daily until disease progression or intolerable toxicities. Of note, 48% of patients in the placebo arm crossed over to the sorafenib arm when interim analyses demonstrated a significant PFS benefit with sorafenib compared with placebo (5.5 months vs. 2.8 months; P <0.01). The final primary end point analysis for OS showed no difference between sorafenib and placebo therapy (17.8 months vs. 15.2 months; $P = 0.15$), but censoring for patients who crossed over showed a significant OS benefit favoring sorafenib therapy (17.8 months vs. 14.3 months; $P = 0.03$). Sorafenib was generally well tolerated with few grade 3 or 4 adverse events, although about 5% of patients reported cardiac infarct or ischemic events.[69] Sorafenib was also studied as first-line therapy for metastatic RCC in a phase II randomized clinical trial comparing sorafenib with IFN-α_{2a}. Study patients received oral sorafenib 400 mg twice daily or subcutaneous IFN-α_{2a} 9 million units 3 times weekly. Patients were allowed to cross over from the placebo arm to the sorafenib arm, and dose escalations up to 600 mg twice daily were permitted. The primary end point of PFS showed no difference between sorafenib and IFN-α therapy. However, patients reported better quality of life with sorafenib compared with IFN-α therapy.[4] As a result, sorafenib is recommended as second-line therapy for metastatic RCC after progression on initial systemic cytokine therapy (category 1) or TKI therapy (category 2A) and as first-line therapy only in select patients (category 2A).[44]

Pazopanib

Pazopanib is another orally administered TKI that was recently approved for the treatment of metastatic RCC. Pazopanib also inhibits multiple kinase receptors, including VEGFR, PDGFR, fibroblast growth factor receptor (FGFR), c-kit, IL-2 receptor inducible T-cell kinase (Itk), and leukocyte-specific protein tyrosine kinase (Lck). Pazopanib was evaluated in a phase III double-blind clinical trial in which 435 patients with metastatic RCC were randomized to treatment with pazopanib 800 mg/day or placebo. The study population included 233 treatment-naive and 202 cytokine-pretreated patients. The primary end point of PFS showed a significant benefit in the pazopanib group compared with placebo, with a median PFS of 9.2 months versus 4.2 months, respectively (P <0.001). The PFS benefit was significant in both treatment-naive (11.1 vs. 2.8 months; P <0.001) and cytokine-pretreated (7.4 vs. 4.2 months; P <0.001) populations. Pazopanib was generally well tolerated, with few grade 3 or 4 adverse events.[9] It is an option for the first-line treatment of metastatic RCC (category 1) and as second-line therapy after progression on cytokines (category 1) or TKI (category 3).[44] A randomized, double-blind, placebo-controlled cross-over trial in patients with metastatic RCC assessing patient preference between pazopanib and sunitinib demonstrated that 70% of patients preferred pazopanib compared with 22% who preferred sunitinib and 8% who had no preference. The most common reasons patients gave for pazopanib preference were improved quality of life and less fatigue.[70] A phase III clinical trial comparing the efficacy of these two agents as first-line treatment of metastatic RCC was anticipated to complete data collection in 2012 with final results available in 2014. Pazopanib is also being studied for neoadjuvant therapy and in a single-arm phase II clinical trial as second-line therapy in patients who have progressed on sunitinib or bevacizumab therapy.

Although sunitinib, sorafenib, and pazopanib are all orally administered antiangiogenic multikinase inhibitors, clinical studies have clearly demonstrated that these agents have different efficacy and toxicity profiles (Tables 115-4 and 115-5). Whereas sunitinib and pazopanib have been reported to improve PFS in both first- and second-line treatment settings, sorafenib has demonstrated improved PFS only in the second-line treatment setting. In addition to differences in efficacy, these agents have subtle differences in their side effect profile.[71] Sunitinib and pazopanib are associated with higher rates of hypertension and hair discoloration than sorafenib. Sunitinib is also associated with higher rates of hypothyroidism than sorafenib. Sorafenib is associated with higher rates of gastrointestinal side effects and hand–foot syndrome than sunitinib and pazopanib. It is also important to note that sunitinib is administered intermittently in a 6-week cycle (4 weeks on treatment, 2 weeks off treatment), but sorafenib and pazopanib are both administered continuously. Both sunitinib and sorafenib appear to have benefit in the subgroup of patients with non–clear cell histology.

Axitinib

9 Axitinib is the newest orally administered TKI approved in January 2012 for the treatment of advanced RCC after progression on one prior systemic therapy. Axitinib is a second-generation, selective inhibitor of VEGFR 1, 2, and 3 and has been shown to be 50 to 450 times more potent than first-generation VEGFR inhibitors such as sorafenib and sunitinib. Unlike first-generation agents, axitinib has limited activity beyond VEGFR blockade, potentially reducing off-target toxicity.[72] Axitinib was compared with sorafenib in a randomized, open-label, phase III trial in 723 patients with clear cell RCC who had progressed on a previous first-line regimen of sunitinib, bevacizumab plus IFN, temsirolimus, or cytokine-based therapy. Most of the patients enrolled received either sunitinib-based therapy (54%) or cytokine-based therapy (35%). The primary end point of PFS assessed by blinded, independent radiology review was superior in the axitinib treated patients with a PFS of 6.7 months compared with 4.7 months in the patients who received sorafenib (P <0.0001). This benefit was seen in both the patients who received prior therapy with sunitinib and cytokines. Additionally, fewer patients discontinued axitinib because of toxic effects compared with sorafenib (4% vs. 8%). The most common adverse effects seen with axitinib were diarrhea, hypertension, fatigue, nausea, and dysphonia, and patients had notably less hand–foot syndrome and alopecia compared with those treated the multikinase inhibitor sorafenib.[73] Based on these results, axitinib is now recommended as an additional therapeutic option for subsequent therapy following progression on a first-line regimen that is either targeted therapy or cytokine-based (category 1).[44] Ongoing trials are assessing pazopanib in the adjuvant and neoadjvuant settings as well as first-line for poor risk patients with metastatic disease.

Bevacizumab

Bevacizumab is a humanized monoclonal antibody that binds circulating VEGF and thus inhibits the effects of VEGF.[65] Bevacizumab was studied in a phase III double-blind clinical trial in which 649 treatment-naive patients with metastatic disease were randomized to receive bevacizumab plus IFN-α_{2a} or placebo plus IFN-α_{2a}. Bevacizumab was administered IV at 10 mg/kg every 2 weeks until disease progression or intolerable toxicity; no dose reductions were allowed. IFN was administered subcutaneously at 9 million units three times weekly with dose reduction to 6 million or 3 million units for treatment-related toxicity.[7] The primary end point of OS was not statistically different between the two treatment groups, 23.3 months versus 21.3 months for bevacizumab plus IFN and placebo plus IFN, respectively ($P = 0.13$).[71] However, the secondary end points showed a significant benefit with the addition of bevacizumab to IFN therapy, with a PFS of 10.2 months as compared with 5.4 months with IFN plus placebo therapy ($P = 0.0001$). In addition, objective response rates were higher with the addition of bevacizumab to IFN, 31% compared with 13% in the placebo plus IFN group. The most common adverse effects were related to IFN therapy, and the addition

TABLE 115-5 Drug Monitoring Recommendations for Renal Cell Carcinoma Therapy

	Drug Monitoring Table		
Targeted Agent	**Adverse Drug Reactions**	**Monitoring Parameters**	**Comments**
Tyrosine Kinase Inhibitors/ Vascular Endothelial Growth Factor Inhibitors			
Sunitinib[5,66a]	Leukopenia, thrombocytopenia, diarrhea, nausea, vomiting, anorexia, constipation, mucositis, hypertension, hand–foot syndrome, hair discoloration, hypothyroidism, decreased LVEF	Adrenal insufficiency, CBC with platelets, electrolytes, liver function, thyroid function, urinalysis, blood pressure, ECG, for hemorrhagic events, for signs and symptoms of CHF or TLS	Discontinue sunitinib if clinical manifestations of CHF occur. Delay or reduce dose if no clinical manifestations of CHF but EF <50% and >20% below baseline.
Sorafenib[69b]	Diarrhea, nausea, vomiting, anorexia, fatigue, hand–foot syndrome, desquamating rash, hypertension, fatigue, cardiac ischemia, hemorrhagic events	Electrolytes, blood pressure, liver function tests, ECG for QT interval prolongation in patients with CHF, bradyarrhythmias, or electrolyte abnormalities	Consider discontinuing therapy if clinical manifestations of cardiac ischemia or hemorrhagic event occur.
Pazopanib[9c]	ALT elevation, leukopenia, thrombocytopenia, diarrhea, nausea, vomiting, hypertension, hair discoloration, QT prolongation, hemorrhage, thromboembolism, hypothyroidism	Hepatic function, electrolytes, thyroid function, urinalysis, ECG, blood pressure	Temporarily discontinue therapy in patients undergoing surgery.
Axitinib[d]	Diarrhea, hypertension, fatigue, decreased appetite, nausea, dysphonia, hand-foot syndrome, weight loss, vomiting, asthenia, constipation, hypothyroidism, stomatitis, arthralgia, proteinuria, rash, dry skin, headache, dyspepsia, cough Laboratory abnormalities: anemia, lymphopenia, thrombocytopenia, hyperkalemia, hyperglycemia, hypocalcemia, decreased bicarbonate, increased lipase, amylase, serum creatinine, ALP, AST, and ALT	Blood pressure, for thromboembolism, hemorrhage, GI perforation or fistula, thyroid function, wound healing, RPLS, proteinuria, hepatic impairment, pregnancy	None
Monoclonal Antibody/Vascular Endothelial Growth Factor Inhibitor			
Bevacizumab[7,71e]	Epistaxis, hemorrhage, delayed wound healing, hypertension, thromboembolic events, proteinuria, GI perforation, dry skin, rhinitis, taste alteration	Blood pressure, urine protein	Do not administer within 4 weeks of surgery
mTOR Kinase Inhibitors			
Everolimus[8f]	Abdominal pain, asthenia, cough, dehydration, diarrhea, dyspnea, fatigue, infections, pneumonitis, and stomatitis Laboratory abnormalities: anemia, hypercholesterolemia, hypertriglyceridemia, hyperglycemia, lymphopenia, and increased serum creatinine	Blood glucose, serum cholesterol, serum creatinine, triglycerides, liver function tests, chemistry, and hematologic parameters	Avoid live vaccinations and close contact with those who received live vaccines.
Temsirolimus[6g]	Anorexia, asthenia, edema, hypersensitivity reactions, infections, interstitial lung disease, mucositis, nausea, rash, wound healing complications Laboratory abnormalities: anemia, hyperglycemia, hyperlipidemia, hypertriglyceridemia, hypophosphatemia, leukopenia, lymphopenia, thrombocytopenia, and elevated ALP, aspartate transaminase, and serum creatinine	Blood glucose, serum cholesterol, serum creatinine, triglycerides, liver function tests, chemistry, and hematologic parameters	Avoid live vaccinations and close contact with those who received live vaccines.

ALP, alkaline phosphatase; ALT, alanine aminotransferase; AST, aspartate aminotransferase; CBC, complete blood count; CHF, congestive heart failure; ECG, electrocardiogram; GI, gastrointestinal; LVEF, left ventricular ejection fraction; RPLS, reversible posterior leukoencephalopathy syndrome; TLS, tumor lysis syndrome.

[a]Sunitinib (Sutent) prescribing information: Pfizer, Inc. New York, NY. Revised February 2010.
[b]Sorafenib (Nexavar) prescribing information: Bayer Healthcare Pharmaceuticals, Inc. Wayne, NJ. Revised February 2009.
[c]Pazopanib (Votrient) prescribing information: GlaxoSmithKline, Inc. Research Triangle Park, NC. Revised October 2009.
[d]Axitinib (Inlyta) prescribing information: Pfizer, Inc. New York, NY. Issued January 2012.
[e]Bevacizumab (Avastin) prescribing information: Genentech, Inc. San Francisco, CA. Revised July 2009.
[f]Everolimus (Afinitor) prescribing information: Novartis Pharmaceuticals Corp. East Hanover, NJ. Revised March 2009.
[g]Temsirolimus (Torisel) prescribing information: Wyeth Pharmaceuticals Inc. Philadelphia, PA. Revised September 2008.

of bevacizumab did not significantly increase the toxicity of IFN. However, treatment discontinuations because of adverse events occurred more often in the bevacizumab group, with proteinuria, hypertension, and gastrointestinal perforation as the most common causes.[7,74] Bevacizumab plus IFN-α_{2a} was studied in another clinical trial (Cancer and Leukemia Group B 90206), which compared it with IFN-α_{2a} monotherapy as first-line treatment.[75] The results of this study were similar, with improvements in PFS and objective response rates but no difference in OS. The combination of bevacizumab plus IFN-α_{2a} is an option for the first-line treatment of metastatic RCC (category 1), and bevacizumab monotherapy is an option as second-line therapy (category 2B).[44]

Temsirolimus

10 Temsirolimus is an IV administered agent that inhibits mTOR. As discussed previously, mTOR is a downstream component of the PI3K/AKT pathway that ultimately results in HIF regulation.[23,27] Temsirolimus was compared with IFN-α_{2a} or the combination of the two agents in a phase III multicenter trial of 626 treatment-naive patients with higher risk metastatic RCC. About 75% of patients were considered high risk (three or four of five factors), and 25% were considered intermediate risk (one or two of five factors), based on the MSKCC risk classification. The IFN-α_{2a} group received 3 million units subcutaneously 3 times weekly for

the first week, 9 million units the second week, and 18 million units thereafter. The temsirolimus group received 25 mg IV once weekly, and the combination group received IFN-α_{2a} at 3 million units subcutaneously 3 times weekly for the first week and 6 million units subcutaneously 3 times weekly and temsirolimus 15 mg IV once weekly. The study was discontinued early after the second interim analysis based on temsirolimus benefit.[6] Single-agent temsirolimus was found to be superior for the primary end point, with an OS of 10.9 months compared with 7.3 months for IFN alone and 8.4 months for the combination. The median PFS for the temsirolimus, IFN, and combination groups was 5.5, 3.1, and 4.7 months, respectively. Serious adverse effects were more common in the IFN groups than in the temsirolimus group, resulting in fewer dose reductions and dose delays compared with the IFN and combination groups. Patients receiving temsirolimus were more likely to experience hyperlipidemia, hyperglycemia, and hypercholesterolemia, which were expected based on the role of mTOR in the regulation of glucose and lipid metabolism. The results of this study support the use of temsirolimus for first-line treatment of patients with poor prognostic features, making it the first therapy specifically approved for this patient population. Historical data on patients with three or more poor-risk features, such as those in this study, have resulted in a median OS of 4 to 8 months compared with 7.3 months in this study.[38,76–78] Based on these results, temsirolimus is recommended by NCCN for first-line treatment in patients with metastatic RCC with poor prognosis (category 1) and as an option for select patients of other risk groups (category 2B).[44]

Everolimus

9 Everolimus is another mTOR inhibitor, but it is available in an oral formulation. A phase II trial of everolimus in patients with predominantly clear cell histology metastatic RCC with no more than one prior therapy resulted in a modest number of partial responses or stable disease.[79] Based on these data, everolimus was compared with placebo in 410 patients who experienced disease progression within 6 months of stopping sunitinib or sorafenib. This international, multicenter, double-blind, phase III trial randomized patients to everolimus or placebo. Those randomized to the everolimus group received everolimus 10 mg orally once daily continuously while in the fasting state or with a light, fat-free meal. The trial was halted after the second interim analysis based on benefit seen in the everolimus group.[8] Everolimus was found to be superior to placebo for the primary endpoint, with a median PFS of 4 months as compared with 1.9 months (P <0.0001). Patients in the everolimus group had a 26% probability of being progression free at 6 months compared with 2% in the placebo group. At the time of analysis, median OS had not been reached in the everolimus group and was 8.8 months in the placebo group. Partial responses were rare and were seen in only three patients in the everolimus group and none in the placebo group. Health-related quality of life was assessed using the European Organization for the Research and Treatment of Cancer (EORTC) QLQ-30 and Functional Assessment of Cancer Therapy Kidney Symptom Index—Disease-Related Symptoms (FKSI-DRS) questionnaires.[80,81] Although the time to definitive deterioration of patient-reported outcomes was not different between the two groups, quality of life was sustained during treatment with everolimus relative to placebo as assessed by the EORTC QLQ-C30 and FKSI-DRS questionnaires. All adverse events occurred more frequently in the everolimus group than in the placebo group, but severe adverse effects were uncommon.[8] Elevations in glucose and lipids were seen because of everolimus' ability to inhibit mTOR.[82] Based on these results, the NCCN guidelines recommend everolimus for patients with metastatic RCC who have failed treatment with sunitinib, sorafenib, or both (category 1).[44]

Clinical **Controversy. . .**

The majority of patients with advanced or metastatic RCC will receive first-line therapy with a VEGFR–tyrosine kinase inhibitor; however, disease progression will inevitably occur, and therapy with a different VEGFR-targeted agent or mTOR inhibitor will be initiated. This raises the question of optimal therapy sequencing because few head-to-head studies have been done addressing this problem. The AXIS trial demonstrated superior PFS with the selective VEGFR tyrosine kinase inhibitor axitinib compared with sorafenib in the second-line setting, and RECORD-1 reported superiority of the oral mTOR inhibitor everolimus compared with placebo in the same patient population.[6,73] Both axitinib and everolimus are classified as category 1 level recommendations by NCCN in patients progressing on a first-line tyrosine kinase inhibitor regimen.[44] Ongoing trials are needed to determine the optimal sequencing of these distinct agents beyond the first-line setting.

Temsirolimus and everolimus are both mTOR inhibitors, but they have several important differences. First, everolimus is administered orally once daily, but temsirolimus is administered as an IV infusion once weekly. Second, although most patients in the temsirolimus trial had clear cell histology (80%), the trial also included patients with other histologies (20%). Everolimus was studied only in patients with RCC exhibiting clear cell histology. Third, whereas temsirolimus was studied in the first-line setting in patients with poor prognosis based on clinical features, everolimus was studied in the second-line setting in patients who had progressed after sorafenib or sunitinib.

PERSONALIZED PHARMACOTHERAPY

Given the numerous treatment options for advanced and metastatic RCC, the utilization of patient-related factors to guide treatment selection would be beneficial, but no validated predictors of treatment response have been determined. The use of therapeutic drug monitoring (TDM) for the TKIs and mTOR inhibitors is an attractive option given the numerous factors that can cause variation in drug exposures. For example, differences in first-pass liver metabolism, variation in activation and deactivation pathways, and drug interactions can result in differences in the pharmacokinetics of these agents. Barriers of implementation in current practice are numerous and include a well-defined and validated therapeutic target concentration and availability of reliable analytic assays that can be implemented into clinical practice.[83] However, there is some evidence with sunitinib and everolimus that this may be a future possibility.[82]

A meta-analysis of sunitinib in patients with RCC or gastrointestinal stromal tumors was performed to explore the relationship between exposures of sunitinib and its active metabolite, SU12662, and clinical outcomes. Steady-state area under the curve (AUC) of sunitinib and SU12662 were associated with time to progression, OS, and toxicity. Higher AUC was associated with longer time to progression and OS; increased response rate; and increased incidence of fatigue, hypertension, and neutropenia.[84] This type of analysis may help to select agents that may be included in prospective dose-targeting trials.

Everolimus is a derivative of sirolimus, an immunosuppressant agent used in the prevention of solid organ transplant rejection. TDM is commonly used in clinical practice to optimize dosing of sirolimus, which suggests that the same may be possible and beneficial with everolimus. In a phase I pharmacodynamic trial in solid tumor patients, plasma trough concentrations of everolimus were correlated with inhibition of mTOR as evidenced by decreased concentrations of downstream mTOR pathway proteins.[85] The linear pharmacokinetics of everolimus also makes pharmacokinetic-directed therapy an attractive and feasible future option.[85]

In summary, current clinical applications of personalized therapy for RCC are limited, but properties of the agents currently used for management of the disease make them attractive options for future pharmacodynamic studies.

EVALUATION OF THERAPEUTIC OUTCOMES

The outcome of treatment in patients with RCC depends on the extent of disease at the time of diagnosis. Whereas localized RCC has a 5-year OS of about 85%, metastatic RCC has a 5-year OS of less than 23%.[10] The standard of care in patients with localized RCC (stage I–III) is surgical removal with a goal of long-term survival and cure. However, 20% to 30% of patients will relapse within 3 years, and 50% to 60% of these patients will have distant recurrence to the lungs. The NCCN Kidney Cancer Panel recommends that patients undergo a medical history; physical examination; comprehensive metabolic panel (including blood urea nitrogen, serum creatinine, calcium levels, and liver function tests); and abdominal, pelvic, and chest imaging every 6 months for the first 2 years after surgery and annually thereafter.[44] For patients with stage IV and unresectable RCC, the goal of treatment is to control disease burden and prolong survival while maximizing quality of life. Current treatment options depend on RCC histology, comorbidities, patient performance status, and prognosis and include enrollment in a clinical trial; immunotherapy (IFN-α, IL-2); or targeted therapy with VEGFR-TKIs (sunitinib, sorafenib, pazopanib, axitinib), mTOR inhibitors (everolimus, temsirolimus), or a monoclonal antibody VEGF inhibitor (bevacizumab). If a patient has disease progression on the initial treatment regimen, subsequent treatment from a different medication class should be considered. At each patient visit, adherence to medication regimens must be strongly emphasized, and treatment-related toxicities should be closely monitored and prevented, if possible. Because optimizing quality of life is usually the therapeutic end point in metastatic RCC, best supportive care should be given to all patients, which may include palliative radiation, metastasectomy, and bisphosphonates or receptor activator of nuclear factor-κB ligand inhibitors for the treatment of bony metastases.[44]

ABBREVIATIONS

AUC	area under the curve
BHD	Birt-Hogg-Dube syndrome
BMI	body mass index
CI	confidence interval
CT	computed tomography
DBP	diastolic blood pressure
EGFR	epidermal growth factor receptor
Flt3	fms-like tyrosine kinase receptor-3
HR	hazard ratio
HIF	hypoxia-inducible factor
IFN	interferon
IFN-α	interferon alfa
IGF-1	Insulin-like growth factor-1
IL-2	Interleukin-2
KPS	Karnofsky performance status
LDH	lactate dehydrogenase
Mdr1	multidrug resistance gene
MET	mesenchymal–epithelial transition
MRI	magnetic resonance imaging
MSKCC	Memorial Sloan-Kettering Cancer Center
mTOR	mammalian target of rapamycin
NCCN	National Comprehensive Cancer Network
OS	overall survival
PDGF	platelet-derived growth factor
PDGFR	platelet-derived growth factor receptor
PFS	progression-free survival
Pgp	P-glycoprotein
PI3K	phosphatidylinositol 3-kinase
PTEN	phosphatase and tensin homologue
RCC	renal cell carcinoma
RFA	radiofrequency ablation
SBP	systolic blood pressure
TCE	trichloroethylene
TDM	therapeutic drug monitoring
TGF	transforming growth factor
TKI	tyrosine kinase inhibitor
ULN	upper limit of normal
VEGF	vascular endothelial growth factor
VEGFR	vascular endothelial growth factor receptor
VHL	von Hippel-Lindau

REFERENCES

1. Iliopoulos O. Molecular biology of renal cell cancer and the identification of therapeutic targets. J Clin Oncol 2006;24:5593–5600.
2. Escudier B, Eisen T, Stadler WM, et al. Sorafenib for treatment of renal cell carcinoma: Final efficacy and safety results of the phase III treatment approaches in renal cancer global evaluation trial. J Clin Oncol 2009;27:3312–3318.
3. Motzer RJ, Hutson TE, Tomczak P, et al. Overall survival and updated results for sunitinib compared with interferon alfa in patients with metastatic renal cell carcinoma. J Clin Oncol 2009;27:3584–3590.
4. Hudes G, Carducci M, Tomczak P, et al. Temsirolimus, interferon alfa, or both for advanced renal cell carcinoma. N Engl J Med 2007;356:2271–2281.
5. Escudier B, Pluzanska A, Koralewski P, et al. Bevacizumab plus interferon alpha-2a for treatment of metastatic renal cell carcinoma: A randomized, double-blind, phase III trial. Lancet 2007;370:2103–2111.
6. Motzer RJ, Escudier B, Oudard S, et al. Efficacy of everolimus in advanced renal cell carcinoma: A double-blind, randomised, placebo-controlled phase III trial. Lancet 2008;372:449–456.
7. Sternberg CN, Davis ID, Mardiak J, et al. Pazopanib in locally advanced or metastatic renal cell carcinoma: Results of a randomized phase III trial. J Clin Oncol 2010;28:1061–1068.
8. Siegel R, Naishadham D, Jermal A. Cancer statistics, 2013. CA Cancer J Clin 2013;63:11–30.
9. Horner MJ, Ries LAG, Krapcho M, et al., eds. SEER Cancer Statistics Review, 1975–2006. National Cancer Institute. 2006, *http://seer.cancer.gov/csr/1975_2006/*.
10. Linehan WM, Rini BI, Yang JC. Cancer of the kidney. In: DeVita VT Jr, Lawrence TS, Rosenberg SA, eds. Cancer Principles and Practice of Oncology, 8th ed. Philadelphia, PA: Lippincott Williams & Wilkins, 2008:1331–1357.
11. McLaughlin JK, Lipworth L, Tarone RE. Epidemiologic aspects of renal cell carcinoma. Semin Oncol 2006;33:527–533.
12. Lipworth L, Tarone RE, McLaughlin JK. The epidemiology of renal cell carcinoma. J Urol 2006;176:2353–2358.

13. Hunt JD, van der Hel OL, McMillian GP, et al. Renal cell carcinoma in relation to cigarette smoking: Meta-analysis of 24 studies. Int J Cancer 2005;114:101–108.
14. Parker AS, Cerhan JR, Janney CA, et al. Smoking cessation and renal cell carcinoma. Ann Epidemiol 2003;13:245–251.
15. Chow WH, Gridley G, Fraumeni JF Jr, et al. Obesity, hypertension, and the risk of kidney cancer in men. N Engl J Med 2000;343:1305–1311.
16. Calle EE, Kaaks R. Overweight, obesity and cancer: Epidemiological evidence and proposed mechanisms. Nat Rev Cancer 2004;4:5795–5797.
17. Gago-Dominguez M, Castelao JE, Yuan JM, et al. Lipid peroxidation: A novel and unifying concept of the etiology of renal cell carcinoma (United States). Cancer Causes Control 2002;13:287–293.
18. Linehan WM, Walther MM, Zbar B. The genetic basis of cancer of the kidney. J Urol 2003;170:2163–2172.
19. Cohen HT, McGovern FJ. Medical progress: Renal cell carcinoma. N Engl J Med 2005;353:2477–2490.
20. Latif F, Tory K, Gnarra J, et al. Identification of the von Hippel-Lindau disease maps to the region of chromosome 3 associated with renal cell carcinoma. Nature 1988;332: 268–269.
21. Seizinger BR, Rouleau GA, Ozelius LJ, et al. Von Hippel-Lindau disease maps to the region of chromosome 3 associated with renal cell carcinoma. Nature 1988;332;268–269.
22. Knudson AG Jr, Strong LC. Mutation and cancer: Neuroblastoma and pheochromocytoma. Am J Hum Gen 1972;24:514–532.
23. Clifford SC, Astuti D, Hooper L, et al. The pVHL-associated SCF ubiquitin ligase complex: Molecular genetic analysis of elongin B and C, Rbx1 and HIF-1alpha in renal cell carcinoma. Oncogene 2001;20:5067–5074.
24. Giaccia AJ, Simon MC, Johnson R, et al. The biology of hypoxia: The role of oxygen sensing in development, normal function, and disease. Genes Dev 2004;18:2183–2194.
25. Ananth S, Knebelmann B, Gruning W, et al. Transforming growth factor beta1 is a target for the von Hippel-Lindau tumor suppressor and a critical growth factor for clear cell renal carcinoma. Cancer Res 1999;59:2210–2216.
26. Boccaccio C, Comoglio PM. Invasive growth: A MET-driven genetic programme for cancer and stem cells. Nat Rev Cancer 2006;6:637–645.
27. Duh FM, Scherer SW, Tsui LC, et al. Gene structure of the human MET proto-oncogene. Oncogene 1997;15:1583–1586.
28. Pennacchietti S, Michieli P, Galluzzo M, et al. Hypoxia promotes invasive growth by transcriptional activation of the met protooncogene. Cancer Cell 2003;3:347–361.
29. Alam NA, Olpin S, Leigh IM. Fumarate hydratase mutations and predisposition to cutaneous leiomyomas, uterine leiomyomas and renal cancer. Br J Dermaol 2005;153:11–17.
30. Isaacs JS, Jung YJ, Mole DR, et al. HIF overexpression correlates with biallelic loss of fumarate hydratase in renal cell cancer: Novel role of fumarate in regulation of HIF stability. Cancer Cell 2005;8:143–153.
31. Cheville JC, Lohse CM, Zincke H, et al. Comparisons of outcome and prognostic features among histologic subtypes of renal cell carcinoma. Am J Surg Pathol 2003;27: 612–624.
32. DeCastro GJ, McKiernan JM. Epidemiology, clinical staging, and presentation of renal cell carcinoma. Urol Clin North Am 2008;35:581–592.
33. Henson De, Fielding LP, Grignon DJ, et al. College of American Pathologists Conference XXVI on clinical relevance of prognostic markers in solid tumors. Arch Pathol Lab Med 1995;119:1109–1112.
34. Delahunt B. Advanced and controversies in grading and staging of renal cell carcinoma. Mod Pathol 2009;22:S24–S36.
35. Edge SB, Byrd DR, Compton CC, et al., eds. AJCC Cancer Staging Manual, 7th ed. New York, NY: Springer, 2010: 479–489.
36. Motzer RJ, Mazumdar M, Bacik J, et al. Survival and prognostic stratification of 670 patients with advanced renal cell carcinoma. J Clin Oncol 1999;17: 2530–2540.
37. Motzer RJ, Bacik J, Murphy BA, et al. Interferon-alfa as a comparative treatment for clinical trials of new therapies against advanced renal cell carcinoma. J Clin Oncol 2002;20:289–296.
38. Mekhail TM, Abou-Jawde RM, BouMerhi G, et al. Validation and extension of the Memorial Sloan-Kettering Prognostic Factors Model for survival in patients with previously untreated metastatic renal cell carcinoma. J Clin Oncol 2005;23:832–841.
39. Heng DYC, Xie W, Regan MM, et al. Prognostic factors for overall survival in patients with metastatic renal cell carcinoma treated with vascular endothelial growth factor-targeted agents: Results from a large, multicenter study. J Clin Oncol 2009;27:5794–5799.
40. Bui MH, Seligson D, Han KR, et al. Carbonic anhydrase IX is an independent predictor of survival in advanced renal cell carcinoma: Implications for prognosis and therapy. Clin Cancer Res 2003;9:802–811.
41. Atkins M, Regan M, McDermott D, et al. Carbonic anhydrase IX expression predicts outcome of interleukin 2 therapy for renal cell cancer. Clin Cancer Res 2005;11: 3714–3721.
42. Deprimo SE, Bello CL, Smeraglia J, et al. Circulating protein biomarkers of pharmacodynamic activity of sunitinib in patients with metastatic renal cell carcinoma: Modulation of VEGF and VEGF-related proteins. J Transl Med 2007;5: 32–43.
43. Pantuck AJ, Seligson DB, Klatte T, et al. Prognostic relevance of the mTOR pathway in renal cell carcinoma: Implications for molecular patient selection for targeted therapy. Cancer 2007;109:2257–2267.
44. The NCCN Clinical Practice Guidelines in Oncology™ Kidney Cancer (Version 1.2013). 2013, *http://www.NCCN.org*.
45. Uzzo R, Novick AC. Nephron-sparing surgery for renal tumors: Indications, techniques and outcomes. J Urol 2001; 166:6–18.
46. Huang WC, Levey AS, Serio AM, et al. Chronic kidney disease after nephrectomy in patients with renal cortical tumours: A retrospective cohort study. Lancet Oncol 2006;7:735–740.
47. Kunkle DA, Egleston BL, Uzzo RG. Excise, ablate or observe: The small renal mass dilemma. A meta-analysis and review. J Urol 2008;179:1227–1233.
48. Lerner SE, Hawkins CA, Blute ML, et al. Disease outcome in patients with low stage renal cell carcinoma treated with nephron-sparing or radical surgery. J Urol 1996;155: 1868–1873.
49. Lam JS, Breda A, Belldegrun AS, Figlin RA. Evolving principles of surgical management and prognostic factors for outcome in renal cell carcinoma. J Clin Oncol 2006;24: 5565–5575.
50. Rini BI, Campbell SC, Escudier B. Renal cell carcinoma. Lancet 2009;373:1119–1132.
51. Flanigan RC, Salmon SE, Blumenstein BA, et al. Nephrectomy followed by interferon alfa-2b compared with interferon alfa-2b alone for metastatic renal cell cancer. N Engl J Med 2001;345:1655–1659.

52. Mickisch GH, Garin A, von Poppel H, et al. Radical nephrectomy plus interferon alfa-based immunotherapy compared with interferon alfa alone in metastatic renal cell carcinoma: A randomised trial. Lancet 2001;358:966–970.
53. Flanigan RC, Mickisch G, Sylvester R, et al. Cytoreductive nephrectomy in patients with metastatic renal cell cancer: A combined analysis. J Urol 2004;171:1071–1076.
54. Fojo AT, Shen DW, Mickley LA, et al. Intrinsic drug resistance in human kidney cancer is associated with expression of a human multidrug-resistance gene. J Clin Oncol 1987;5:1922–1927.
55. Kakehi Y, Kanamaru H, Yoshida O, et al. Measurement of multidrug-resistance messenger RNA in urogenital cancers: Elevated expression in renal cell carcinoma is associated with intrinsic drug resistance. J Urol 1988;139:862–865.
56. Mickisch GH, Roehrich K, Koessig J, et al. Mechanisms and modulation of multidrug resistance in primary human renal cell carcinoma. J Urol 1990;144:755–759.
57. Oliver RT, Nethersell AB, Bottomley JM. Unexplained spontaneous regression and alpha-interferon as treatment for metastatic renal carcinoma. Br J Urol 1989;63:128–131.
58. Motzer RJ, Bukowski RM. Targeted therapy for metastatic renal cell carcinoma. J Clin Oncol 2006;24: 5601–5608.
59. Proleukin (aldesleukin) prescribing information. East Hanover, NJ: Novartis Pharmaceuticals, 2008.
60. Motzer RJ, Bander NH, Nanus DM. Renal cell carcinoma. N Engl J Med 1996;335:865–875.
61. Jonasch E, Haluska FG. Interferon in oncological practice: A review of interferon biology, clinical applications and toxicities. Oncologist 2001;6:35–55.
62. Parton M, Gore M, Eisen T. Role of cytokine therapy in 2006 and beyond for metastatic renal cell cancer. J Clin Oncol 2006;24:5584–5592.
63. Pyrhonen S, Salminen E, Ruutu M, et al. Prospective randomized trial of interferon-alfa 2a plus vinblastine versus vinblastine alone in patients with advanced renal cell carcinoma. J Clin Oncol 1999;17:2859–2867.
64. Inteferon-alpha and survival in metastatic renal cell carcinoma: Early results of a randomised controlled trial. Medical Research Council Renal Cell Collaborators. Lancet 1999;353:14–17.
65. Rini BI. Vascular endothelial growth factor-targeted therapy in metastatic renal cell carcinoma. Cancer 2009;115: 2306–2312.
66. Motzer RJ, Hutson TE, Tomczak P, et al. Sunitinib versus interferon alfa in metastatic renal cell carcinoma. N Engl J Med 2007;356:1115–1124.
67. Motzer RJ, Michaelson MD, Redman BG, et al. Activity of SU11248, a multitargeted inhibitor of vascular endothelial growth factor receptor and platelet-derived growth factor receptor, in patients with metastatic renal cell carcinoma. J Clin Oncol 2006;24:15–24.
68. Motzer RJ, Rini BI, Bukowski RM, et al. Sunitinib in patients with metastatic renal cell carcinoma. JAMA 2006;295:2516–2524.
69. Escudier B, Eisen T, Stadler WM, et al. Sorafenib in advanced clear-cell renal-cell carcinoma. N Engl J Med 2007;356:125–134.
70. Escudier BJ, Porta C, Bono P, et al. Patient preference between pazopanib and sunitinib: Results of a randomized, double-blind, placebo-controlled, cross-over study in patients with metastatic renal cell carcinoma—PISCES study. J Clin Oncol 2012;30(Suppl):abstr CRA4502.
71. Rini BI. Metastatic renal cell carcinoma: Many treatment options, one patient. J Clin Oncol 2009;27:3225–3234.
72. Sonpavde G, Hutson TE, Rini BI. Axitinib for renal cell carcinoma. Expert Opin Investig Drugs 2008;17: 741–748.
73. Rini BI, Escudier B, Tomczak P, et al. Comparative effectiveness of axitinib versus sorafenib in advanced renal cell carcinoma (AXIS): A randomized phase 3 trial. Lancet 2011;378:1931–1939.
74. Escudier BJ, Bellmunt J, Negrier S, et al. Phase III trial of bevacizumab plus interferon alfa-2a in patients with metastatic renal cell carcinoma (AVOREN): final analysis of overall survival. J Clin Oncol 2010;28:2144–2150.
75. Rini BI, Halabi S, Rosenberg J, et al. Phase III trial of bevacizumab plus interferon alfa versus interferon alfa monotherapy in patients with metastatic renal cell carcinoma: Final results of CALGB 90206. J Clin Oncol 2010;28:2137–2143.
76. Motzer RJ, Bacik J, Murphy BA, et al. Interferon-alfa as a comparative treatment for clinical trials of new therapies against advanced renal cell carcinoma. J Clin Oncol 2002;20:289–296.
77. Negrier S, Escudier B, Gomez F, et al. Prognostic factors of survival and rapid progression in 782 patients with metastatic renal carcinomas treated by cytokines: A report from the Groupe Français d'Immunotherapie. Ann Oncol 2002;13:1460–1468.
78. Bukowski RM, Negrier S, Elson P. Prognostic factors in patients with advanced renal cell carcinoma: Development of an international kidney cancer working group. Clin Cancer Res 2004;10:6310S–6314S.
79. Amato RJ, Jac J, Giessinger S, et al. A phase II study with a daily regimen of the oral mTOR inhibitor RAD001 (everolimus) in patients with metastatic clear cell renal cell cancer. Cancer 2009;115:2438–2446.
80. Aaronson NK, Ahmedzai S, Bergman B, et al. The European Organization for Research and Treatment of Cancer QLQ-C30: A quality-of-life instrument for use in international clinical trials in oncology. J Natl Cancer Inst 1993;85:365–376.
81. Cella D, Yount S, Brucker PS, et al. Development and validation of a scale to measure disease-related symptoms of kidney cancer. Value Health 2007;104:285–293.
82. Busaidy NL, Farooki A, Dowlati A, et al. Management of metabolic effects associated with anticancer agents targeting the PI3K-Akt-mTOR pathway. J Clin Oncol 2012;30: 2919–2928.
83. Gao B, Yeap S, Clements A, et al. Evidence for therapeutic drug monitoring of targeted anticancer therapies. J Clin Oncol 2012;30:4017–4025.
84. Houk BE, Bello CL, Poland B, et al. Relationship between exposure to sunitinib and efficacy and tolerability endpoints in patients with cancer: results of a pharmacokinetic/ pharmacodynamics meta-analysis. Cancer Chemother Pharmacol 2010;66:357–371.
85. Tabernero J, Rojo F, Calvo E, et al. Dose- and schedule-dependent inhibition of the mammalian target of rapamycin pathway with everolimus: A phase I tumor pharmacodynamics study in patients with advanced solid tumors. J Clin Oncol 2008;26:1603–1610.

116

Melanoma

Cindy L. O'Bryant and Jamie C. Poust

KEY CONCEPTS

1. Cutaneous melanoma is an increasingly common malignancy, but it is a cancer that can be cured if detected early. Public education about screening and early detection is one strategy for controlling the increase in incidence and the mortality associated with cutaneous melanoma.
2. Surgical resection can cure patients with early-stage melanoma.
3. The toxicities associated with interferon-α_{2b} (IFN-α_{2b}) therapy are significant and require patient education, close patient monitoring, and appropriate dose modification based on toxicity.
4. Patients with locally advanced disease should be evaluated for adjuvant therapy; recommended options include IFN-α_{2b} or participation in a clinical trial.
5. Metastatic melanoma remains a clinical challenge. At this time, there is not a single standard treatment approach for individuals with metastatic disease. Dacarbazine and temozolomide are considered the most active chemotherapies and can be used as single agents. Combination chemotherapy has not been shown to be superior to single-agent therapy with dacarbazine.
6. As the biology of melanoma has been further delineated, a growing number of potential targets for drug therapy have been identified. BRAF mutations appear in up to 70% of melanoma patients. Vemurafenib is a BRAF inhibitor that has been shown to improve overall survival in patients with this mutation.
7. Ipilimumab is an option for some individuals with metastatic melanoma. The immune-related toxicities associated with the use of this drug are significant and warrant close patient selection. Individuals require close monitoring and management by an experienced healthcare team. Clinical trials using this drug showed a significant improvement in overall survival.
8. Treatment of melanoma is determined by many factors. As the number of treatment options for patients with metastatic melanoma grows, it will be important to consider disease- and patient-related aspects when determining appropriate therapy.

INTRODUCTION

Melanoma is the seventh most common cancer in the United States. The incidence of melanoma has steadily increased from the 1970s, and today it is increasing at a faster rate than most other cancer types.[1] Although nonmelanoma skin cancers (NMSCs) are the most common malignancies of the skin, cutaneous melanoma accounts for up to 75% of all skin cancer–related deaths. With the rise in the number of melanoma skin cancer and the associated mortality, it is essential to consider issues of care beyond that of disease treatment. Skin cancer prevention and screening have a major impact on public health and on the success of treatment for those individuals diagnosed with both NMSC and melanoma. Skin cancers tend to occur more frequently in older individuals. Therefore, as the population continues to age, effective strategies to prevent, detect, and treat individuals with these cancers are needed.

The incidence of melanoma varies worldwide with the highest rates found in Australia, New Zealand, North America, and Northern Europe. In the United States, about one in every 50 Americans will be diagnosed with melanoma in their lifetime. The lifetime risk is greater in men (2.9%) than women (1.8%) and varies with ethnicity.[1,2] The median age at diagnosis is 61 years old.[3] In 2013, it was estimated that 76,690 new cases of melanoma would be diagnosed in the United States. Unfortunately, this estimate may not be accurate because many superficial and in situ melanomas are managed in facilities that do not routinely report their cases to cancer registries.[4] Childhood and adolescent melanoma is rare with 2% of cases being diagnosed in individuals younger than 20 years old. The incidence in this age group is increasing by 2.9% per year. Young adults between the ages of 15 and 19 years account for about 75% of childhood melanomas. Different than the adult population, the incidence of melanoma appears to be the same between genders except in the 10- to 19-year-old age group in which the incidence is higher in girls than boys.[5]

The estimated number of individuals expected to die of melanoma in 2013 in the United States is 9,480.[4] Survival rates have gradually increased over the past 4 decades. At present, the 5- and 10-year relative survival rates are 91% and 89%, respectively, but survival rates decline with more advanced disease. The overall mortality rate has remained stable.[1] Men older than 65 years old have the highest mortality rates from melanoma. Death rates have declined in younger patients. The stabilization of mortality rates appears to be related to efforts at both primary and secondary prevention of melanoma in addition to advances in the treatment and management of melanoma patients.

ETIOLOGY AND EPIDEMIOLOGY

The etiology of melanoma, similar to most other malignancies, is not fully understood. A number of patient-specific factors and environmental factors have been identified (Table 116-1), and it is likely that these factors alone or in combination increase the occurrence of cutaneous melanomas.

Individual physical characteristics can determine responses to ultraviolet (UV) radiation. Caucasians with fair-colored hair (red or blond), light-colored eyes (blue or green), high degrees of freckling,

TABLE 116-1 Risk Factors for Melanoma

Patient-Specific Risk Factors
Adulthood (age older than 15 years)
History of cutaneous melanoma
Dysplastic nevi
High density of common nevi and atypical nevi
Cutaneous melanoma in first-degree relative
Immunodeficiency or immunosuppression
High degree of freckling
Sunburns easily or tans rarely
Blonde or red hair
Blue, green, or gray eyes
Socioeconomic status (higher > lower)
Race (Caucasians > Hispanics > African Americans)
External Risk Factors
Intense intermittent sun exposures
History of sunburn
More than four painful sunburns before age 15 years
Recreational sun exposure

and those who have a tendency to burn and rarely tan with exposure to sunlight appear especially at risk.[5] Clinical and epidemiologic research shows a higher rate of melanoma in those who have extensive or repeated intense sun exposure.[5] Intermittent intense sun exposure, blistering sunburns, and the time of life of exposure to the sun now are believed to be critical factors for development of cutaneous melanoma. Individuals with a history of these are at this highest risk. The risk is lower in individuals who had chronic sun exposure without a history of burning and those with occupational exposure. The risk with sunlight and UV radiation seems to be greatest during childhood and adolescence and is more hazardous than exposure during adult life.

One of the most important risk factors for melanoma is the number of melanocytic nevi (pigmented lesions or moles) on the body. The formation of these nevi has been shown to be directly related to cumulative sun exposure. The relative risk of developing melanoma increases with the greater number of typical nevi an individual has. A second risk factor is the presence of atypical melanocytic nevi. Atypical nevi may progress from a normal nevus or be dysplastic from the onset. Up to 20% of melanomas develop from atypical nevi, and individuals with these have an increased risk of developing melanoma compared with the general population. Small congenital melanocytic nevi may be present at birth or within the first few months after birth. About 1% to 3% of newborns are born with pigmented lesions, and the lifetime risk of developing melanoma is related to the size of the nevus.[6]

Immunocompromised patients are at an increased risk for development of cutaneous melanoma.[5,6] Immunodeficiency includes individuals with ataxia telangiectasia, chronic lymphocytic leukemia, Hodgkin lymphoma, and immunosuppression after organ transplant. Acquired immunodeficiency syndrome has been shown to increase the risk of developing cutaneous melanoma and the disease often is more aggressive.[7] A personal history of nonmelanoma or melanoma skin cancers is a risk factor for subsequent melanoma and may be associated with a poor prognosis. Xeroderma pigmentosum is a rare skin disorder but does carry an increased risk for melanoma.

A rare but important risk for melanoma is maternal–fetal transfer of melanoma. Although melanoma is not the most common cancer in pregnancy, it is the cancer most likely to metastasize to the placenta and the fetus.[6] Maternal–fetal transmission of melanoma is commonly lethal. However, neonates delivered with concomitant placental involvement but without clinical evidence of disease still are considered to be at increased risk for development of disease.

A number of genes have been implicated in melanoma development and progression, and molecular profiling studies have identified several distinct molecular subclasses of melanoma.[8] Familial atypical multiple mole syndrome (FAMMS) or dysplastic nevus syndrome is a hereditary disease characterized by a predisposition to develop dysplastic nevi and cutaneous melanoma. About 8% to 10% of cases of melanoma are associated with a family history or hereditary dysplastic nevus syndrome. Patients with FAMMS suggest a risk for melanoma of 400- to 1,000-fold higher than that seen in the general population. The mode of inheritance is somewhat controversial and is believed to be polygenic.

Genetic studies of this heritable trait in families led to the identification of *CDKN2A* as the familial melanoma gene, located at chromosome 9p21. *CDKN2A* encodes two distinct proteins: inhibitor of cyclin-dependent kinase 4 (INK4A [inhibitor of cyclin-dependent kinase 4] or $p16^{INK4a}$) and ARF (alternative reading frame; p14ARF). INK4A regulates cell cycle progression at the G_1/S checkpoint by inhibiting the G_1 cyclin-dependent kinases that phosphorylate and inactivate the retinoblastoma protein. ARF inhibits p53 degradation; therefore, loss of ARF inactivates p53. The frequencies of *CDKN2A* mutations vary in melanoma but are found more commonly in individuals with familial inheritance patterns and are associated with multiple cases of melanoma in a family, young age at diagnosis, multiple primary melanomas among family members, and pancreatic cancer.[9]

One of the major signaling pathways found to be associated with the development of melanoma is the mitogen-activated protein kinase pathway (MAPK), which mediates receptor tyrosine kinases, resulting in activation of RAS and downstream BRAF. Activating *BRAF* mutations are the most common somatic genetic event in human melanoma, occurring in 25% to 70% of melanoma patients and primarily noted by a single point mutation *BRAF* (V600E). *BRAF* does not appear to be an inherited disposition gene, but the high prevalence of *BRAF* mutations in cutaneous melanoma appears to be an epidemiologic link between UV radiation and melanoma. *BRAF* mutations are common in melanomas arising from skin with intermittent sun exposure and not as common in melanomas in chronically sun-exposed areas. This may be an early event in the damage to the melanocytes because these mutations are also found in benign and dysplastic nevi.[5]

Upstream of BRAF, mutations in *NRAS* and c-*Kit* have also been found as molecular drivers in the development of melanoma. Mutations in *NRAS* are found in 15% to 20% of patients. These tumors are associated with more advanced disease at diagnosis, high growth rates, and shorter survival times than those with *BRAF* mutations.[10] c-*Kit* is a transmembrane receptor tyrosine kinase that when activated signals the MAPK and phosphatidyl-inosital-3-OH kinase (PI3K) pathways, resulting in transcription and cell proliferation. Mutations in c-*Kit* are commonly found in acral and mucosal melanomas.[10]

Other genetic alterations involved with the development of melanoma include *MITF* (microphthalmia-associated transcription factor), a gene that is important to the survival of melanocytes and has been shown to play a key role in melanoma signaling. The melanocortin 1 receptor gene (*MC1R*), which is associated with the red hair and fair skin phenotype, is involved in melanin synthesis and is more prevalent in individuals with melanoma. *NEDD9* modulates metastatic activity and has been found to be unregulated in melanoma. These melanoma-specific pathways give better understanding of the biology of the disease and may lead to better more directed treatment. A variety of other molecular pathways and receptor tyrosine kinases are also being studied to identify their role in the development of melanoma.[5]

Sunlight is one of the most important environmental factors in the pathogenesis of melanoma. The incidence of melanoma has been associated with latitude and the intensity of solar exposure among susceptible populations. Radiation in the ultraviolet B (UVB) range (280–320 nm) is historically considered to be the critical factor linking sunlight and melanoma, although prolonged exposure to ultraviolet A (UVA) radiation (320–400 nm) also may be important. Use of older UVB-blocking sunscreens may not be as protective as once thought because they allow more sustained sun exposure without any clinical symptoms of burn (e.g., erythema or pain), ultimately resulting in intense irradiation of the skin by UVA light.

PATHOGENESIS

Melanomas most often arise within epidermal melanocytes of the skin, although they can also arise from noncutaneous melanocytes. Human melanocytes are dendritic pigmented cells that arise from the neural crest tissue during early fetal development and migrate over a predictable route to a variety of sites within the body including the skin, uveal tract, meninges, and ectodermal mucosa. In adults, most melanocytes are located at the epidermal–dermal junction of the skin and the choroid of the eye, but they can also be found in other tissues such as the meninges and the alimentary and respiratory tracts. Primary melanoma can arise in any area of the body with melanocytes. The skin is the most frequent site of melanoma; cutaneous melanoma constitutes 90% of all melanomas. Primary melanoma can arise in the eye (ocular melanoma) and less frequently the mucosa and metastatic disease with unknown primary site.[5]

Normal melanocytes arise from melanoblasts. They undergo a series of differentiation events before reaching a final end-cell differentiation state and can be arrested in their differentiation process at any given state of maturation without loss of their proliferation capacity. Melanocytes adhere to the basement membrane of the epidermis and, despite a resting state, maintain a lifelong proliferation potential. The existence of melanoma stem cells has been suggested from work with melanoma cell lines.[8]

Melanocytes synthesize melanin to protect various tissues, such as the skin, from UV radiation–induced damage and reach the keratinocytes in the upper layers of the epidermis via dendrites. Tyrosinase is an essential enzyme within melanosomes that synthesizes melanin. They are resistant to severe UV radiation, unlike keratinocytes, and their survival leads to the proliferation of mutated genes.[5]

Skin melanocytes transform from preexisting nevocellular nevi in the development of melanoma. A series of distinct steps are involved in the development and progression of melanoma from melanocytes. The pathologic components of the progression in human melanoma involve a series of morphologic stages: melanocytic atypia, atypical melanocytic hyperplasia, radial growth phase in which limited growth and radial expansion of the nevi may occur without metastatic competence, primary melanoma in the vertical growth phase with or without in-transit metastases, regional lymph node metastatic melanoma, and distant metastatic melanoma.[5] Primary melanoma is characterized by radial growth and limited vertical thickness (<0.75 mm). Primary melanoma demonstrates little tendency to metastasize. Melanoma has a potential for metastasis formation with the onset of a vertical growth phase. Therefore, the thickness of a primary melanoma is an important prognostic factor and is used in the staging classification of cutaneous melanoma. Of note, melanomas can skip steps in this development pathway.

Normal melanocytes require growth factors for proliferation, but melanoma cells can proliferate without growth factors. Melanoma cells secrete a variety of growth autocrine and paracrine factors that may facilitate proliferation. Additionally, with disease progression, melanoma cells increase production of certain growth factors and cytokines. The PI3K–AKT pathway often is overactive in melanoma. Integrins and growth factors promote growth and survival of melanoma through these pathways.

Basic fibroblast growth factors (bFGFs) are thought to be important mediators of growth stimulation and cell survival, act as motility factors for melanoma cells, and upregulate serine proteinases and metalloproteinases. Melanoma cells are strong producers of chemoattractive proteins such as interleukin-8. Vascular endothelial growth factor (VEGF) can be triggered in the vertical growth phase.[11] Most of these changes occur between the radial growth phase and vertical growth phase of primary melanoma, and metastatic cells often show the highest cytokine production.

Understanding the biology of melanoma has provided potential targets for drug therapy.[12] For example, the role of bFGF in the pathogenesis of melanoma has led to investigation of antisense oligonucleotides to block bFGF. Other pathways, such as MAPK pathway, have been targeted by RAF and MEK inhibitors and the PI3K/AKT pathway by mTOR (mammalian target of rapamycin) inhibitors. As pathways are identified and as agents that inhibit these pathways enter clinical trials and practice, there is growing excitement about the opportunities to impact treatment of melanoma in new and effective ways.

Immune factors appear to be involved in the progression of melanoma more often than in most other solid tumors.[5] Spontaneous cancer regressions are rare but are a well-documented phenomenon seen in melanoma. Focal regression in primary melanoma has been reported. Tumor regression appears to be associated with host immunity.

A number of different tumor antigens have been identified in the cellular membrane and cytoplasm of melanoma cells and are referred to as melanoma-associated antigens. Ganglioside antigens have been of particular interest in the development of immunotherapy for melanoma. A large number of monoclonal antibodies to melanoma-associated antigens have been developed and are being evaluated in clinical trials for diagnosis of and therapy for melanoma.

The humoral and cellular responses of individuals with melanoma that express melanoma-associated antigens have been described and provide the rationale for immunotherapy in the management of metastatic melanoma.[5] Melanoma-directed antibodies have been isolated in the sera of patients with melanoma. The presence of antimelanoma antibodies in the sera of patients correlates with the clinical status of the patients, and the antibodies gradually disappear from the serum as the disease progresses. This phenomenon may be explained by the possible formation of anti-idiotype antibodies directed against the antimelanoma antibodies, an increase in the circulation of soluble tumor antigens that saturate all antibody combining sites, increased levels of immunosuppression, or absorption of antibodies on the tumor mass.

Interest has focused on the role of cell-mediated immune response in melanoma. Specific cell-mediated responses may play a role in tumor regression, but the role of specific cells, such as cytotoxic T lymphocytes (CTLs), is not fully understood. Tumor-infiltrating lymphocytes (TILs) have been shown in vivo and in vitro to possess antitumor reactivity. TILs contain a large number of mature tumor-specific lymphocytes and have been a target for manipulation in immunotherapeutic approaches for melanoma.[5] Two identified targets are cytotoxic T lymphocyte antigen 4 (CTLA-4) and toll-like receptor 9 (TLR9). CTLA-4 is a glycoprotein expressed on the surface of activated T cells that appears to have an inhibitory effect on T cells. Blocking the effect of CTLA-4 is an effective strategy for increasing the T-cell antitumor response.

HISTOLOGIC SUBTYPES

Cutaneous melanomas are categorized by growth patterns. Four major histologic subtypes or growth patterns of primary cutaneous melanoma have been identified: superficial spreading melanoma, nodular melanoma, lentigo maligna melanoma, and acral lentiginous melanoma. Clinical outcomes of the four major melanoma subtypes are similar if the comparison controls for depth of penetration or tumor thickness. Any of the four subtypes can present as an amelanotic variant. Amelanotic melanomas appear to be devoid of clinically apparent pigmentation. Two less common types of melanoma include desmoplastic melanoma and lentiginous melanoma. Desmoplastic melanoma is more commonly seen in older individuals, and its clinical presentation is similar to that seen in NMSCs. If a biopsy of the lesion is not obtained, the disease may be mismanaged. Lentiginous melanoma is histologically different than the four major subtypes. Uveal melanoma is considered a separate disease from cutaneous melanoma.

Superficial spreading melanoma is the most common morphologic type of cutaneous melanoma, accounting for about 70% of all melanomas.[5] The lesions usually arise from a preexisting nevus, known as a *precursor lesion*, and evolve slowly over 1 to 5 years. At some point, superficial spreading melanoma may progress to a more rapid growth phase. Early in lesion development, the superficial spreading melanoma is flat, but the surface becomes irregular and asymmetrical as the lesion progresses. The lesion enlarges when it enters into a rapid growth phase, and the edges appear notched or lacy. The lesions can be blue, black, or pink. Areas within the lesion may be hypopigmented. These patches of color variation, specifically the hypopigmented areas, are thought to be associated with tumor regression within the lesion or pigment inconsistency. The clinical differential diagnosis of superficial spreading melanoma includes both benign and malignant skin disease. This subtype is sometimes confused with seborrheic keratoses or pigmented basal cell carcinoma. Superficial spreading melanomas may occur at any anatomic site on the body, but they are more commonly seen on the back in men and on the legs in women. This subtype of melanoma is more common in women. The mean age of diagnosis of superficial spreading melanoma is 51 years, which is earlier than that seen for other subtypes. Superficial spreading melanoma usually occurs after puberty.

Lentigo maligna melanoma represents 10% to 20% of melanomas and is commonly found on the head and neck. It is unique from other histologic subtypes; because of its prolonged radial growth phase, it does not have the same propensity to metastasize.[5] Lentigo maligna melanoma arises on chronically sun-exposed sites in older individuals and presents as a freckle-like lesion. Lentigo maligna melanomas are generally large (>3 cm), flat, and tan-colored lesions with shades of brown and black. The lesions gradually grow and develop darker, with asymmetric flecks in areas. Lentigo maligna melanoma is uncommon before age 50 years and may have been present for more than 5 years. Only about 5% to 8% of lentigo maligna melanomas evolve into invasive melanoma, which is characterized by nodular development within the flat precursor lesion. Lentigo maligna melanoma can be difficult to distinguish from solar lentigo, which typically is a smaller and evenly pigmented flat-appearing lesion.

Nodular melanoma is the second most common growth pattern of melanoma, occurring in 15% to 30% of patients. Nodular melanoma is a pure vertical growth phase disease. In nodular melanoma, a small, expansive nodule in the papillary dermis invades the reticular dermis and subcutis. The radial growth phase is absent at all times. Nodular melanomas are more aggressive and develop more rapidly than superficial spreading melanoma. Nodular melanomas are dark blue–black and often uniform in color with a shiny surface, although a small percentage of nodular melanomas are amelanotic and have a fleshy appearance. Nodular melanomas are raised and often symmetric. They can occur at any age, typically around 50 years of age, and are most common on the trunk, head, and neck. Nodular melanomas are more common in men. Of note, nodular melanomas can resemble traumatized nevi.

Acral lentiginous melanoma makes up about 5% of melanomas and is most likely not related to UV exposure. It presents as three distinct clinical subtypes: melanoma on the palms of the hands or soles of the feet, subungual melanoma, and mucosal melanoma.[6] Most acral lentiginous melanomas are located on the soles of the feet and look like a large tan or brown stain. The lesions often have irregular convoluted borders. The initial macular component of palmar/plantar melanomas can be masked by the thickened stratum corneum at these sites. Many of these lesions look verrucous in appearance making them difficult to distinguish from warts by the untrained eye. Suspicious lesions on the palms or soles of the feet should be evaluated. Acral lentiginous melanoma includes subungual melanoma, which arises in the nail matrix or nail bed. The most common presentation is a brown or black line in the great toe or the thumbnail. Mucosal melanoma is rare but can occur on any mucosal surface. Mucosal melanoma occurs most commonly in the oropharyngeal mucosa followed by the anal and rectal mucosa, genital mucosa, and urinary mucosa. Unfortunately, mucosal melanoma often does not become clinically apparent until the mass is large or the lesion bleeds. Acral lentiginous melanoma occurs in fewer than 10% of Caucasians with melanoma but is the most common type of melanoma reported in individuals with a dark complexion (e.g., African Americans, Asians, and Hispanics). Similar to lentigo maligna melanomas, this subtype is characterized by a protracted radial growth phase.

Uveal melanoma is the most common primary intraocular malignancy seen in adults but is an uncommon tumor.[13] Unlike cutaneous melanoma, the frequency and mortality rates of uveal melanoma have remained steady. This melanoma arises from the pigmented epithelium of the choroid. Iris melanoma is a subset of uveal melanoma and tends to have a more benign course. The risk of metastasis varies with the histologic type and size of the tumor as well as the location in the eye. Metastases occur most frequently in the liver but have been documented in a variety of tissues.

The ability to predict the metastatic potential of melanomas would be a valuable prognostic tool. An attempt to predict the likelihood for metastasis is based on radial and vertical growth phases. Radial growth phase describes the early stage of melanoma when the tumor is thin and primarily intraepidermal in location. By definition, malignant melanoma in situ is a form of radial growth phase melanoma. Vertical growth phase is the stage of melanoma with clear metastatic potential.

CLINICAL PRESENTATION

Benign nevi often occur in sun-exposed areas and typically are 4 to 6 mm in diameter (about the size of a pencil eraser), raised or flat, uniform in color and round in shape. Dysplastic nevi are believed to be a link between benign nevi and melanoma. Dysplastic nevi tend to be larger than common nevi (>5 mm), appear as flat macules with asymmetry, have a fuzzy or ill-defined shape, and vary in color. Compared with melanoma lesions, dysplastic nevi appear less evolved.

The initial clinical presentation of melanoma often is a cutaneous lesion and depends on the histologic subtype and the stage of development of the lesion. The lesion can be located anywhere on the body but is most commonly discovered on the lower extremities in women and on the back and trunk in men. The cardinal clinical feature of a cutaneous melanoma is a pigmented skin lesion that changes over a period of time. Any changes in the skin surrounding a nevus, including redness or swelling, are important clinical signs. Uncommonly, the sensation of the lesion may become itchy or tender and painful. Friability of the lesion, resulting in bleeding or oozing, is a danger sign. Perhaps the most important warning sign

CLINICAL PRESENTATION

General

- Any lesion that changes in appearance over time.

Local Signs and Symptoms

- The clinical features used to describe questionable lesions are highlighted with the mnemonic "ABCDE."
  - (A) Asymmetry: Melanoma lesions are often asymmetric.
  - (B) Border: Melanoma lesions have irregular boarders.
  - (C) Color: Color is often variegated in a melanoma ranging from tan, blue-black, red, purple, or white.
  - (D) Diameter: Melanoma lesions are frequently greater than 6 mm.
  - (E) Enlargement or evolution: A sudden enlargement or change in lesion is concerning for melanoma.
- Other signs of melanoma include a lesion that swells, bleeds, or oozes.

Systemic Disease Signs and Symptoms

- Palpable lymph nodes.
- Depending on the site of metastases, shortness of breath, abdominal pain, bone pain, headache, and mental status changes.

Laboratory Tests

- In addition to a comprehensive metabolic panel, LDH should be evaluated.

Other Diagnostic Tests

- Biopsy and pathology review for staging with molecular testing for BRAF and c-Kit.
- When applicable, SLNB.
- Systemic staging should include chest, abdomen, and pelvic CT scan or CT/PET bone scan, and brain MRI.

CT, computed tomography; LDH, lactate dehydrogenase; MRI, magnetic resonance imaging; PET, positron emission tomography; SLNB, sentinel lymph node biopsy.

of danger is the evolution in any characteristic of a lesion. A biopsy of the lesion is critical to establish diagnosis of melanoma. Subsequent pathologic interpretation of the biopsy will help provide information on prognosis and treatment options. An excisional biopsy with a 1- to 2-mm margin of normal-appearing skin is recommended for a suspicious lesion and should include a portion of underlying subcutaneous fat for microstaging. For larger lesions with which an excisional biopsy is impractical, an incisional or punch biopsy can be performed and should include a core of full-thickness skin and subcutaneous tissue. When excisional biopsies are not appropriate, as with the face or palmar surface of the hands, a full-thickness incisional or punch biopsy is preferred. A shave biopsy is never appropriate because it can underestimate the thickness of the lesion and may not fully remove the lesion. Additionally scarring may mask the remaining tumor.

Evaluation of any individual with a suspected melanoma includes a complete history and total-body skin examination. The focus of the patient history is identifying potential risk factors. Risk-related questions include an assessment of family history of melanoma, personal history of skin cancer or nevus excisions, sun exposure, and phenotype. Total dermatologic examination is necessary to determine melanoma risk factors (e.g., mole pattern, mole type, or freckling) and for staging. Melanoma commonly spreads to the lymph nodes; therefore, individuals suspicious for advanced disease should have their lymph nodes examined for lymphadenopathy. Lactate dehydrogenase (LDH) should be measured because elevated serum levels have been shown to be an independent predictor of decreased survival.[14] In addition, any other signs or symptoms suggestive of metastatic disease should be completely evaluated.

The diagnosis of melanoma is complicated by the number of pigmented moles (melanocytic nevi) and nonmelanocytic lesions that resemble melanoma. An average of 10 to 40 ordinary nevi can be found on the skin of white adults. Nonmelanocytic pigmented lesions, such as seborrheic keratoses, pigmented basal cell carcinoma, and vascular lesions, also can appear similar to a melanoma lesion. In childhood melanoma, commonly the lesions are thicker at the time of diagnosis. This may be in part due to the low level of suspicion by pediatricians, the fact that many melanomas associated with congenital nevi develop in the dermis rather than the epidermis, and histologic uncertainty.[6]

1 Improved survival rates for melanoma have been attributed to the identification and treatment of disease at an early stage when the disease is limited and has not yet metastasized. It follows that one strategy to improve survival rates would be to increase efforts to identify early-stage melanoma. The cost effectiveness of massive screening for all adults by a physician has never been demonstrated. However, routine examination of the skin by physicians is recommended for individuals, adults, and children who are at high risk. The entire cutaneous surface, including the scalp, should be examined.

It has been estimated that about 50% of the initial melanoma lesions found are discovered by self-examination. Therefore, one of the most direct strategies to improve early detection would be a method to increase effective skin self-examination (SSE) by the individual, the individual's partner, or a caregiver. Identification of early melanoma allows the opportunity to treat the lesions when they are thin and curable. Persons who perform SSE present for care at an earlier stage in the disease process and have 50% less advanced melanoma and lower mortality rate from the disease.[5] Healthcare individuals who routinely work with the public, such as community pharmacists, have an opportunity to increase public awareness concerning the benefits and appropriate methods for SSE. Educational pamphlets describing SSE (Table 116-2) for the public are widely available through the American Cancer Society, American Academy of Dermatology, and Skin Cancer Foundation. If a newly discovered pigmented lesion is identified or if a preexisting pigmented

TABLE 116-2 Self-Examination of Suspicious Moles

1. Examine your body front and back in the mirror and then the right and left sides with the arms raised.
2. Bend the elbows and look carefully at the forearms and upper arms and palms.
3. Look at the backs of the legs and feet. Look specifically in the spaces between toes and at the soles of the feet.
4. Examine the back of the neck and scalp with the help of a hand-held mirror; part the hair (or use a blow dryer) to lift the hair and give yourself a closer look.
5. Check the back and buttocks with a handheld mirror.

Derived from publications of the American Academy of Dermatology.

lesion changes, the individual should be evaluated by a physician immediately.

Skin self-examination is of special interest in elderly adults. As the population of older adults (≥65 years of age) increases, it is expected that the mortality rate from melanoma also will increase. Barriers to successful SSE in elderly adults, such as failing eyesight, lack of partners, and poor memory, impact older adults in detecting new or changing lesions. These barriers, coupled with the higher incidence of melanoma in men, present challenges and opportunities for healthcare professionals to target education on this growing segment of our population.

STAGING AND PROGNOSTIC FACTORS

The size of a primary melanoma lesion is associated with the likelihood of metastases. As such, Breslow tumor thickness of the primary melanoma lesion is commonly used as prognostic factor to determine predicated outcomes.[15] Tumor thickness is quantified to the nearest tenth of a millimeter with an ocular micrometer, measuring from the top of the granular layer of the overlying epidermis to the deepest contiguous invasive melanoma cell. The correlation between tumor thickness and probability of tumor metastases is strong but does not include aspects such as tumor satellites, defined rather arbitrarily as skin involvement within 2 cm of the primary lesion, and vascular invasion. It was once thought that the presence of satellite nodule(s) had the same impact on prognosis as a high-risk primary lesion (tumor thickness >4 mm). It is now known that patients with satellitosis have a worse prognosis than patients with thick primary lesions, and prognosis is more similar to that of patients with nodal metastases. Mitotic rate has now emerged as another important prognostic factor for developing metastatic disease. Mitotic rate is defined as the number of mitosis per square millimeters. Increasing mitotic rate represents a more aggressive lesion and is associated with a poorer survival rate despite tumor size. Ten-year survival rates drop by 8% for a nonulcerated T_1 melanoma with a mitotic rate of less than 1/mm^2 compared with a lesion with a mitotic rate of greater than 1/mm^2.[16] The American Joint Committee on Cancer (AJCC) developed a staging system for melanoma that divides patients with localized melanoma into four stages according to microstaging criteria of Breslow.[17] In addition to consideration of the primary lesion, the AJCC staging system includes aspects of the tumor satellite, extent of lymph node involvement, and presence of metastatic disease.[17] Analysis of several large databases worldwide identified areas in which the AJCC staging system, which was published in 1997, did not reflect the natural history of melanoma. Issues such as the appropriate cutoff values for primary tumor thickness, ulceration of the melanoma, and satellite lesions of the primary tumor should be considered when making decisions about therapy.[17] The cutoff values initially proposed by Breslow for primary tumor thickness were initially used in the AJCC staging system, but it appears that cutoff depths of 1, 2, and 4 mm of thickness may better predict overall survival. Melanoma ulceration and increased mitotic rate within a primary melanoma are both associated with decreased survival and thus are the most considerable prognostic factors in patients with localized disease.[14] The revised AJCC staging system for cutaneous melanoma was published in 2002 and updated in 2009.[14,17] It is important to carefully examine older clinical trials to determine which staging system was used to determine patient inclusion and exclusion criteria, as results may differ based on these patient criteria. Revisions of the new melanoma staging system include (a) principal prognostic factors for localized disease includes melanoma thickness, ulceration, and mitotic rate; (b) mitotic rate replaces invasion as primary criterion for T_{1b} tumors ; (c) number of metastatic nodes, tumor burden, and ulceration define the nodes (N) category for patients with regional metastasis; (d) presence of microscopic nodal metastasis classifies a patient as stage III; and (e) two dominant components are site of distant metastases and presence of elevated serum LDH for metastatic disease.[14] Clinical staging includes microstaging of the primary melanoma and clinical and radiologic evaluation. It is used after complete excision of the primary melanoma with clinical assessment for regional and distant metastasis. Pathologic staging includes microstaging of the primary melanoma and pathologic information about the regional nodes after partial or complete lymphadenectomy. At this time, it appears that patients with very limited disease (in situ or stage 0) do not require pathologic evaluation of lymph nodes (Tables 116-3 and 116-4). As with other solid tumors, the presence of regional

TABLE 116-3 Melanoma Tumor, Node, Metastasis Classification

T Classification	Thickness	Ulcerative Status
T_X	Primary tumor cannot be addressed (e.g., shave biopsy)	
T_0	No evidence of primary tumor	
T_{is}	Melanoma in situ	
T_1	≤1 mm	A: No ulceration and mitosis <1/mm^2 B: With ulceration or mitosis ≥1/mm^2
T_2	1.01–2 mm	A: No ulceration B: With ulceration
T_3	2.01–4 mm	A: No ulceration B: With ulceration
T_4	>4 mm	A: No ulceration B: With ulceration
N Classification	**No. of Metastatic Nodes**	**Nodal Metastatic Mass[a]**
N_X	Regional lymph nodes cannot be assessed	
N_0	No regional lymph nodes	
N_1	1 node	A: Micrometastasis B: Macrometastasis
N_2	2–3 nodes	A: Micrometastasis B: Macrometastasis C: In-transit metastases or satellite(s) without metastatic nodes
N_3	≥4 metastatic lymph nodes or matted nodes or in-transit metastases or satellite(s) with metastatic node(s)	
M Classification	**Site**	**Serum Lactate Dehydrogenase**
M_X	Distant metastases cannot be assessed	
M_0	No detectable distant metastasis	
M_{1a}	Distant skin, subcutaneous tissue, or nodal metastatic disease	Normal
M_{1b}	Lung metastases	Normal
M_{1c}	All other visceral metastases	Normal
	Any distant metastasis	Elevated

M, metastasis; N, node; T, tumor.

[a]Micrometastases are diagnosed after sentinel or elective lymphadenectomy. Macrometastases are defined as clinically detectable lymph node metastases confirmed by therapeutic lymphadenectomy or when any lymph node metastasis exhibits extracapsular extension.

Data from Balch CM, Gershenwald JE, Soong SJ, et al. Final version of 2009 AJCC melanoma staging and classification. J Clin Oncol 2009;27:6199–6206.

TABLE 116-4 American Joint Committee on Cancer Tumor (T), Node (N), Metastasis (M) Stage Grouping for Cutaneous Melanoma

Pathologic Stage	T	N	M	Clinical Stage	T	N	M
0	T_{is}	N_0	M_0	0	T_{is}	N_0	M_0
IA	T_{1a}	N_0	M_0	IA	T_{1a}	N_0	M_0
IB	T_{1b}	N_0	M_0	IB	T_{1b}	N_0	M_0
	T_{2a}	N_0	M_0		T_{2a}	N_0	M_0
IIA	T_{2b}	N_0	M_0	IIA	T_{2b}	N_0	M_0
	T_{3a}	N_0	M_0		T_{3a}	N_0	M_0
IIB	T_{3b}	N_0	M_0	IIB	T_{3b}	N_0	M_0
	T_{4a}	N_0	M_0		T_{4a}	N_0	M_0
IIC	T_{4b}	N_0	M_0	IIC	T_{4b}	N_0	M_0
IIIA	T_{1-4a}	N_{1a}	M_0	III	Any	$>N_1$	M_0
	T_{1-4a}	N_{2a}	M_0				
IIIB	T_{1-4a}	N_{1b}	M_0				
	T_{1-4a}	N_{2b}	M_0				
	T_{1-4a}	N_{2c}	M_0				
	T_{1-4b}	N_{1a}	M_0				
	T_{1-4bb}	N_{2a}	M_0				
IIIC	T_{1-4b}	N_{1b}	M_0				
	T_{1-4b}	N_{2b}–N_{2c}	M_0				
	Any T	N_3	M_0				
IV	Any T	Any N	M_1	IV	Any T	Any N	M_1

lymph node involvement is a powerful predictor of tumor burden and patient outcome. In the past, the primary method for determining nodal status was surgical resection and analysis of the lymph nodes via a regional lymph node dissection. The extent of lymph node dissection was determined by the anatomy of the area of the lesion. In recent years, preoperative lymphoscintigraphy and intraoperative sentinel node mapping have become more widely used methods for identifying the first or sentinel lymph node in the direct pathway of lymph drainage from the primary cutaneous melanoma. Sentinel lymph node biopsy (SLNB) is a minimally invasive procedure that determines if a patient is a candidate for a complete lymph node dissection. The rationale for lymphatic mapping and subsequent SLNB is based on the observation that regions of the skin have patterns of lymphatic drainage to specific lymph nodes in the regional lymphatic basin. The sentinel lymph node is believed to be the first node in the lymphatic basin into which the primary melanoma drains. Unlike other solid tumors, melanoma appears to progress in an orderly nodal distribution. Evaluation of sentinel nodes has been used for detection of micrometastases in breast cancer and in melanoma. SLNB allows for more thorough examination of a single sentinel node than is possible when examining multiple lymph nodes with a lymph node dissection and may be most useful for melanomas located in ambiguous drainage sites such as the head and neck areas. SLNB is associated with low false-negative rates and low complication rates.[18] Detection of clinically undetectable disease in a lymph node basin that is not directly adjacent to the primary lesion may allow for upstaging of patients who initially are believed to have node-negative disease. The American Society of Clinical Oncology and Society of Surgical Oncology joint clinical practice guidelines now recommend SLNB for patient with any intermediate-thickness melanoma.[19]

The stage of melanoma at the time of diagnosis is one of the primary indicators of the natural history of the disease and contributes to prognosis. Tumor thickness, level of tumor invasion, and ulceration all contribute to the stage of a patient and the overall outcome. Other factors such as tumor growth pattern or histological subtype, mitotic rate, density of TILs infiltrating the tumor tissue, elevated LDH level, satellite lesions, angiolymphatic invasion, gender, and age also have been reported to influence survival (Table 116-5). The location of the primary tumor on the skin is also important because individuals with tumors of the extremities have an increased survival compared with those with axial, neck, head, and trunk tumors. In addition, a number of additional prognostic factors have been identified in patients with advanced disease. The number of metastatic sites, disease involvement of the gastrointestinal tract, liver, pleura, or lung, Eastern Cooperative Oncology Group (ECOG) performance status of 1 or greater, male sex, and prior immunotherapy have been associated with poor prognosis.[20]

TREATMENT

Desired Outcomes

Treatment of cutaneous melanoma depends on the stage of disease. Local disease is managed and often cured with surgical ablation. Regional disease is treated with surgical resection of the primary lesion and, depending on the risk of recurrence, possibly adjuvant therapy in an effort to eradicate any residual disease and cure the patient. The use of adjuvant therapy after surgical resection and the role of interferon-α (IFN-α) as adjuvant therapy remain

TABLE 116-5 Prognostic Factors for Cutaneous Melanoma

Tumor-Related Factors
Tumor thickness
Level of tumor invasion
Ulceration
Histologic subtype
Anatomic site of primary tumor
Mitotic rate
Lymphangitic invasion
Occurrence of microsatellites
Presence of tumor-infiltrating lymphocytes
Patient-Related Factors
Age
Gender

controversial. When disease becomes metastatic, the treatment goals are to slow tumor progression, prolong life, and improve quality of life. The approvals of ipilumumab and vemurafenib have dramatically changed the management of metastatic melanoma. Both agents are more efficacious than standard chemotherapy treatment options, dacarbazine and temozolomide. Numerous clinical trials have evaluated single-agent and combination chemotherapy, immunotherapy, targeted therapy, and biochemotherapy regimens. Patients with advanced disease should have their tumors tested to document mutational status in an effort to direct appropriate therapy.

Surgery

❷ Patients who present with a suspicious pigmented lesion should undergo a full-thickness excisional biopsy, if possible. Sites for which excisional biopsy is inappropriate include the face, palm of the hand, sole of the foot, distal digit, and subungual lesions. A full-thickness incisional or punch biopsy is preferred in these cases to provide microstaging and ultimately to determine therapy.

Localized cutaneous melanoma can often be cured with surgical excision. The cure rates for melanomas smaller than 1 mm are as high as 98%.[5] The extent of the excision margin is important in preventing local recurrence and ultimate survival. For melanoma in situ, excision of the visible lesion or biopsy site with a 0.5 to 1 cm border of clinically normal skin and a layer of subcutaneous tissue with confirmation of histologically negative peripheral margins is recommended. The recommended clinical margin for invasive melanoma depends on the tumor thickness. Excision with a 1 cm margin of clinically normal skin and underlying subcutaneous tissue is recommended for invasive melanomas 1 mm or smaller thick.[20,21] The appropriate margin of excision for melanomas between 1 and 2 mm in thickness is controversial. A study suggests the risk of locoregional recurrence is higher when melanomas that are at least 2 mm thick are excised with a 1-cm margin rather than a 2 cm margin.[22] Current National Comprehensive Cancer Network (NCCN) guidelines recommend a 1 to 2 cm margin for melanoma with tumor thickness of 1.01 to 2 mm.[20] Lesions that are 2 to 4 mm thick should be excised with a 2 cm margin. Primary tumors more than 4 mm thick require at least a 2 cm margin, but whether a larger margin is beneficial is not clear. Surgical management of lentigo maligna melanoma is problematic because subclinical extension of atypical junctional melanocytic hyperplasia may extend beyond the visible margins. Complete excision of these lesions is important.

When isolated regional lymph nodes are detected via physical examination in the absence of distant disease, therapeutic lymphadenectomy is recommended. The extent of therapeutic lymph node dissection often is modified according to the anatomic area of the lymphadenopathy. Prophylactic lymphadenectomy in all patients is not recommended. Although a subgroup of patients with early-stage melanoma will have microscopic metastatic disease in nonpalpable lymph nodes, prophylactic regional lymph node dissection does not prolong survival or decrease time to relapse in randomized clinical trials.[5,23] Selective regional lymphadenectomy performed after scintigraphic and dye lymphographic identification of the affected sentinel draining lymph node(s) is the standard of care for melanomas more than 1 mm thick. If the sentinel node is found to have micrometastatic melanoma, regional dissection of the involved nodal basin is performed. If the lesion is 0.75 to 1 mm in thickness with ulceration or is Clark level IV or V, lymphatic mapping with SLNB may be considered based on patient characteristics such as ulceration of the tumor.[24] Of note, the likelihood of detecting metastatic disease in the sentinel lymph node depends on tumor thickness. The likelihood of detecting metastatic disease is about 1% in tumors that are smaller than 0.8 mm but increases to more than 30% in tumors 4 mm thick.[24] The Multicenter Selective Lymphadenectomy Trial II is currently enrolling patients to assess whether or not a complete lymph node dissection after a positive SLNB improves overall survival. SLNB results are important for accurate staging, for therapeutic lymphadenectomy, and to aid in the decision to offer adjuvant treatment.[18,23]

One of the most important aspects of surgical management of cutaneous melanoma is the role of patient follow-up.[20] Postsurgical follow-up of patients who have had a melanoma excised is essential to monitor for undetected metastatic disease and the development of a second primary cutaneous melanoma or nonmelanoma primary malignancy. Scheduled screening in addition to routine surgical follow-up is required for any patient with a melanoma; the recommended frequency and duration depend on the stage of melanoma. The optimal duration of follow-up remains controversial. Most patients who develop recurrent disease do so in the first 5 years after treatment, but late recurrences more than 10 years after surgery have been observed. The increased lifetime risk of developing a second primary melanoma supports lifetime dermatologic surveillance for all patients.

Curative surgery usually is limited to patients with early-stage disease. A patient with stage III melanoma commonly has lymph node involvement, but in-transit metastases also may occur. In-transit metastasis is the clinical manifestation of tumor that develops in lymphatics between the primary melanoma and the regional lymph node basin.[5] In-transit metastases are more than 2 cm from the original lesion. In-transit metastases are more common in individuals with thick, ulcerated lesion. Surgery is used for management of in-transit lesions, and the goal is complete resection. Unfortunately, subsequent recurrence in the same extremity often occurs after initial resection of in-transit metastases.

The role of surgery beyond that of cure is less clear, although surgery may offer palliation for patients with isolated metastases.[23] Resection of isolated lesions in the brain and lungs may be appropriate in certain cases and should be evaluated based on individual patient criteria. Surgery can be an option when the lesion is accessible and when the lesion may cause problems if not removed. Surgery can extend survival time in select patients with metastatic disease. Patients whose metastases can be completely resected may experience improved quality of life, improved overall survival, and occasionally long-term disease control.[23]

Brain metastasis is a frequent complication of advanced melanoma. About 20% to 50% of patients with stage IV disease develop clinically apparent central nervous system (CNS) involvement. Surgical resection, with or without radiation, has been used in select individuals. More recently, high control rates of brain metastases have been achieved with focal radiation therapy such as linear accelerator–based stereotactic radiosurgery or gamma-knife technologies.[25] Melanoma in the gastrointestinal tract can lead to bowel obstruction, and appropriate resection or bypass may provide significant relief of symptoms. Despite the lack of controlled clinical trials, the impact on palliative surgery should be evaluated in the context of a patient's comfort and quality of life. Surgery may be an appropriate option if the perceived outcome is to provide patient comfort. On the other hand, surgery may constitute a significant physical challenge or financial burden to a patient with a limited life expectancy. The clinical scenarios involving surgical resection should be fully evaluated in terms of overall quality of life.

The risk of relapse and death after resection of a local or regional cutaneous melanoma is the primary determinant for use of adjuvant therapy after primary resection. Adjuvant trials have focused on patients at intermediate or high risk for recurrence.

Immunotherapy

Melanoma is considered one of the most immunogenic solid tumors, and it appears to interact with and respond to the immune system of the host in which it arises. Spontaneous regressions of melanoma suggest the importance of the immune system in disease modulation. Lymphoid infiltration into the primary melanoma also suggests that immunomodulation may impact the biology of melanoma. Early work showed that nonspecific immunomodulators, such as levamisole and bacillus Calmette-Guérin (BCG), for treatment of melanoma were associated with some regression of the tumor, although many of these responses were limited and short-lived. Because melanoma is generally resistant to traditional treatment modalities such as radiation and chemotherapy, immunotherapy offers an avenue of treatment. Although the complete response rate seen in patients with melanoma treated with biotherapy is relatively low, the durability of responses in individuals who respond can be significant. Remaining unanswered questions include what is the best approach to biotherapy in a patient with melanoma and can biotherapy be combined with other available and emerging antineoplastic therapy.

Interferon

One of the oldest, and most controversial, immunotherapy approaches for the treatment of melanoma is the use of IFNs. The IFN*s* are a group of proteins with diverse immunomodulatory and antiangiogenic properties. A number of studies have evaluated various doses and schedules of recombinant IFN for treatment of metastatic melanoma. Response rates in metastatic melanoma range from 10% to 30%, and overall response rates are about 15% for IFN-α. Unfortunately, the optimal dose, treatment schedule, and treatment combinations and regimens have not been established for management of metastatic melanoma.[5]

In clinical trials of IFN therapy for patients with metastatic melanoma, response rates were highest in patients with minimal disease. Responses were seen at all sites of disease but were most frequent in subcutaneous, lymph node, and pulmonary metastases. The success of IFN in patients with minimal disease encouraged investigators to evaluate the role of adjuvant IFN after curative surgical resection in patients who were at high risk for recurrent disease (bulky disease or regional lymph node involvement). Early trials of short-term or low-dose regimens of IFN-α did not demonstrate a survival benefit in the adjuvant setting. In an attempt to optimize response in the adjuvant setting, maximum tolerated doses of IFN-α were administered for 1 month followed by prolonged therapy of IFN-α at more tolerable doses for 48 weeks. The rationale for the intensive induction phase was to provide peak IFN levels sufficient to inhibit tumor growth and avoid the development of anti-IFN antibodies. A large, multicenter cooperative group trial (E1684) of adjuvant IFN-α_{2b} versus observation was designed for 287 patients with high-risk (stages IIB and III disease based on the 1997 AJCC staging criteria) melanoma after curative surgical resection. IFN-α_{2b} was given IV as an induction therapy at maximum tolerated doses of 20 million IU/m^2 per dose 5 days per week for 4 weeks in an outpatient setting; treatment was continued for 48 weeks with subcutaneous IFN-α_{2b} 10 million IU/m^2 per dose 3 times per week at home. This therapy now is often referred to as *high-dose interferon* (HDI). With a median followup period of 6.9 years, patients treated with HDI had significantly longer relapse-free and overall survival compared with patients who were observed after surgical resection (1.72 vs. 0.98 years and 3.8 vs. 2.8 years, respectively).[26] Both the 5-year relapse-free and overall survival rates were higher with HDI. With longer follow-up (median, 12.6 years), however, the difference in overall survival was no longer significant.[27] Further analysis showed that the greatest reduction in melanoma recurrence occurred during the first few months of treatment. Subgroup analysis of this study indicated that patients with large primary tumors and node-negative disease ($T_4N_0M_0$) did not receive the same benefit from therapy, but the small number of patients in this group made it difficult to draw definite conclusions about the role of IFN for adjuvant therapy in this setting.

Pegylated IFN-α_{2b} has also been evaluated in the adjuvant setting. The European Organization for Research and Treatment of Cancer (EORTC) 18991 trial evaluated 1,256 patients with resected stage III melanoma. Patients were randomized to observation or pegylated IFN. Pegylated IFN was given less frequently (once weekly) compared with nonpegylated IFN. Updated results demonstrated an improvement in relapse-free survival but no difference in overall survival or distant metastasis-free survival.[28] Based on these data, the Food and Drug Administration (FDA) approved pegylated IFN-α_{2b} (Sylatron) as an option for adjuvant treatment.

High-dose interferon treatment is associated with multiple toxicities, including flulike syndrome. Other toxicities include depression, nausea, weight loss, fatigue, myelosuppression, elevations in liver function tests, and renal insufficiency. Toxicities of IFN therapy in the adjuvant HDI trials were common and severe, and most patients required dose reductions or delays at some point during treatment. Dose modifications were required for dose-limiting constitutional symptoms, myelosuppression, and hepatic toxicities. Approximately three-quarters of patients were able to complete the year of therapy in an outpatient setting.

One of the strategies for reducing the toxicities associated with IFN was to modify the dose and duration. A subsequent ECOG trial (E1690) of low-dose IFN (LDI; 3 million IU per dose given subcutaneously three times weekly) for 24 months compared with the HDI regimen described earlier versus observation did not demonstrate an overall survival advantage of HDI versus observation.[29] At a median followup period of 52 months, the 5-year estimated relapse-free survival rates for HDI, LDI, and observation were 44%, 40%, and 35%, respectively. Relapse-free survival was significantly longer in the HDI group, prolonging the median time to relapse by 10 months compared with observation and LDI. With longer follow-up, however, the difference in relapse-free survival was no longer significant.[29] A significant overall survival benefit was not seen for HDI or LDI compared with observation, although the investigators speculated that this analysis of survival was affected by the number of patients in the observation arm who received IFN therapy after disease progression.[29]

The use of IFN in the adjuvant setting remains controversial. Although the HDI regimen is used in the United States, the LDI strategy remains standard in many European countries. In a pooled analysis of 713 patients who participated in two randomized controlled trials (E1684 and E1690), HDI was associated with a significant reduction in relapse-free survival compared with observation ($P < 0.006$).[27] No benefit in overall survival was observed in the pooled analysis. The results of nine randomized clinical trials of adjuvant HDI or LDI versus observation in melanoma were included in a systematic review. The systematic review observed a trend toward reduced risk of recurrence of melanoma and of death among the IFN-treated patients in nearly all studies.[30] Because of differences in dose, frequency, and duration of IFN-α treatment in the various trials, the review was not able to compare LDI versus HDI. Furthermore, the wide variability in number of patients enrolled, end points, patient selection, quality, type of therapy, duration of treatment, and follow-up precluded statistical analysis of the pooled results. Although the differences in overall survival were not always statistically significant, HDI remains the only adjuvant treatment shown to prolong survival in prospective randomized trials. IFN-α_{2b} is approved by the United States FDA for treatment of patients with primary melanomas larger than 4 mm (stages IIB and IIC) and in patients with melanoma involving regional lymph nodes who are disease-free after lymph node dissection (stage III).

Although IFN is widely used in the adjuvant setting, there are concerns over the considerable treatment toxicities and the lack of consistent overall survival advantage of a toxic and expensive regimen. In addition, whether the results from the HDI trials should be extrapolated to patients with local recurrences, satellite lesions, or in-transit metastases is not clear. Remaining questions include the following: (a) Are the toxicities associated with HDI treatment worth the potential benefits for patients? (b) What are the mechanism(s) and best approaches to managing IFN toxicity? (c) Is the regimen or schedule of IFN used in the initial positive trial necessary to achieve the benefits seen in this study? Aggressive toxicity evaluation and individualized management are essential to help preserve quality of life in individuals receiving IFN therapy.

❸ A mechanism for optimizing the care of patients receiving IFN is to effectively prevent and manage treatment-related toxicities. A common syndrome seen with IFN-α therapy is a diverse group of side effects referred to as *constitutional symptoms*, which can include acute symptoms such as fever, chills, myalgia, and fatigue, and can encompass some of the more chronic toxicities such as fatigue, anorexia, and depression.[31] Acetaminophen can be used to prevent or minimize acute dose-related symptoms such as fever, myalgia, and chills. Opiates, such as meperidine, are often required when patients experience severe chills or rigors, most commonly during the initial month of the HDI induction phase. Nonsteroidal antiinflammatory drugs (NSAIDs) have been used to manage IFN-related myalgia but may have overlapping side effects with IFN, such as a decrease in renal blood flow. Some NSAIDs, such as acetaminophen, may mask fevers that occur in patients who experience neutropenia while undergoing therapy. Additionally, NSAIDs may increase the risk of bleeding in the setting of thrombocytopenia caused by IFN. Fatigue is one of the most frequently observed dose-limiting toxicities seen with IFN therapy, occurring in 70% to 100% of patients.[31] The mechanisms of IFN-induced fatigue are not fully understood and may be multifactorial in individual patients. IFN-induced fatigue appears to be dose related and may worsen with continued therapy. Pharmacologic (e.g., methylphenidate) and nonpharmacologic (e.g., exercise, psychosocial techniques, distraction, energy management, and dietary modifications) interventions for treatment of cancer-related fatigue and now IFN-related fatigue are being evaluated.[31] Depression is common and should be fully evaluated. Contributing factors such as IFN-induced hypothyroidism or concomitant IFN symptoms (e.g., nausea and fatigue) should be evaluated concurrently with depression symptoms to optimize treatment decisions.[32] Antidepressants, such as selective serotonin reuptake inhibitors, have been studied in IFN-induced depression with notable benefit.[31] Anorexia was reported in about 70% of patients receiving adjuvant IFN therapy for melanoma and is thought to be mediated through direct effects on hypothalamic neurons, modification of normal hypothalamic neurotransmitters or neuropeptides, or effects from stimulation of other cytokines.[31] Taste alterations may contribute to anorexia. Investigational strategies for ameliorating IFN-induced anorexia include nutritional intervention, use of appetite stimulants such as megestrol acetate, and patient education. Glucocorticoids should not be used for appetite stimulation or as part of an antiemetic therapy because they may adversely impact the immunomodulatory effects of IFN. Other toxicities such as hematologic or hepatic toxicities require monitoring and appropriate dose modification.

Because of the associated toxicity and adverse effects seen with IFN-α therapy, many experts have questioned the usefulness of intensive adjuvant therapy for melanoma despite the possible benefits in relapse-free and overall survival. A subsequent report from the cooperative group study demonstrated a quality-of-life benefit with IFN therapy based on the quality-of-life–adjusted survival analysis.[33] This analysis calculates the quality-of-life–adjusted years gained as a result of IFN-α treatment or the clinical benefit of time without toxicities and without disease. Another approach that has been investigated is the use of a pegylated product. Unfortunately, pegylated IFN has been evaluated in an attempt to improve the benefit-toxicity ratio without much success.[34]

❹ The role of IFN as adjuvant therapy is not clear at this time. If adjuvant IFN is given, it is not clear what product (e.g., pegylated IFN), dose, and duration of therapy should be used. The issues of patient side effects and cost must be carefully weighed against the potential disease-free survival benefit. Because HDI is the only therapy to demonstrate benefit in large comparative trials, it should be considered for patients with high-risk disease. The 2013 NCCN guidelines for melanoma list IFN-α as one of several options for select patients with high-risk disease.[20] Other options include observation and probably, most importantly, clinical trials. Individuals should be prescreened for potential problems associated with therapy; relative contraindications to HDI therapy include autoimmune diseases, immunosuppression, decompensated liver disease, severe neuropsychiatric diseases, and life-threatening infection.[31] Efforts continue to better define the optimal treatment regimen for HDI versus other strategies in well-designed clinical trials.

Clinical **Controversy...**

The role of IFN-α as adjuvant therapy for high-risk patients after surgical resection of melanoma is controversial. Assessment of patient risk factors, availability of clinical trials, and cost of therapy should be evaluated before initiation of therapy.

The role of IFN in advanced disease is even less clear, especially for patients whose disease has recurred after treatment with adjuvant IFN therapy. IFN-α has been used as a single agent in patients with metastatic disease who have not received adjuvant therapy and in combination with chemotherapy or other biotherapy for metastatic melanoma. The challenges of combination therapy are that many of the toxicities seen with IFN can be exacerbated by concomitant chemotherapy (e.g., nausea, vomiting, and neutropenia).

Interleukin-2

Interleukin-2 (IL-2) is a glycoprotein produced by activated lymphocytes.[35] IL-2 was first identified as a T-cell growth factor, but now IL-2 clearly is a growth factor for a variety of cells, including lymphocytes, T cells, and natural killer (NK) cells. IL-2 also may be immunosuppressive. The role of each of these effects of IL-2 on disease control in melanoma is not clear.

The precise mechanism of cytotoxicity of IL-2 is unknown. High IL-2 concentrations have not been shown to have a direct antitumor effect on cancer cells in vitro. In vitro and in vivo, IL-2 stimulates the production and release of many secondary monocyte-derived and T-cell–derived cytokines, including IL-4, IL-5, IL-6, IL-8, tumor necrosis factor (TNF)-α, granulocyte-macrophage colony-stimulating factor, and IFN-γ, which may have direct or indirect antitumor activity. In addition, IL-2 stimulates the cytotoxic activities of NK cells, monocytes, lymphokine-activated killer (LAK) cells, and CTLs. IL-2 also appears to activate endothelial cells, which results in increased expression of adhesion molecules.[35]

Based on preclinical studies that demonstrated a dose–response relationship between recombinant IL-2 (aldesleukin) and tumor response, initial clinical trials of aldesleukin in patients with melanoma used relatively high doses of the drug as a single agent or in combination with LAK cells. The response rates seen in these trials ranged from 15% to 25%, and 2% to 5% of patients achieved complete responses, some of which were durable (median response, 70 months).[35] Responses were seen at a number of metastatic sites such as the lung, liver, bone, lymph nodes, and subcutaneous tissue. Based on reevaluation of early clinical trials, aldesleukin received FDA approval for treatment of metastatic melanoma. Overall, objective response rates were about 16%, but 4% to 6% of responses were durable and were observed in patients with large tumor burdens.[36] The high doses of aldesleukin used in the initial clinical trials and recommended in the drug label are associated with serious toxicities and may limit the practicality of therapy for individual patients and broad application in certain healthcare systems. The high-dose aldesleukin regimen used for treatment of metastatic melanoma is 600,000 IU/kg per dose every 8 hours for 14 doses maximum in a 5-day period given for two cycles, with a 10- to 14-day rest period between cycles. At these doses, cytokine-induced capillary leak syndrome is a common problem and often is accompanied by significant hypotension, visceral edema, dyspnea, tachycardia, and arrhythmias. Increased permeability of capillary walls allows for a fluid shift from the intravascular space into tissue. As the patient becomes intravascularly dehydrated, hypotension may occur, resulting in reflex tachycardia and arrhythmias. In addition, the decrease in blood volume may result in decreased renal blood flow and urine output, manifesting as increases in blood urea nitrogen, serum creatinine, edema, and weight gain and a decrease in urine output (input greater than output). Visceral edema can result in pulmonary congestion, pleural effusions, and edema. The management of patients receiving high-dose aldesleukin requires extensive supportive care medications, careful monitoring, and a staff trained in aspects of critical care such as hypotension management. Although patients initially receiving high-dose aldesleukin are treated in an intensive care unit, most patients can be managed on a designated oncology unit if the staff is familiar with the toxicities and management strategies of the toxicities. Constitutional symptoms are a frequent complication of aldesleukin therapy and become more intense as therapy progresses. Additional side effects seen with aldesleukin include pruritus, eosinophilia, bone marrow suppression (including thrombocytopenia), increased liver function test results, neurologic disturbances, diarrhea, and nausea.

In an attempt to reduce treatment-related toxicities, a number of studies have evaluated continuous-infusion aldesleukin and lower doses of aldesleukin given either alone or combined with chemotherapy and IFN therapy. Although initial reports were encouraging, survival has not been significantly affected. At this time, direct comparisons of various dosing schedules and regimens are needed to determine the optimum approach to aldesleukin therapy in metastatic melanoma. Coadministration of LAK cells with aldesleukin does not appear to significantly improve clinical response.

One of the greatest treatment challenges in treatment of metastatic melanoma is determining the role of aldesleukin therapy for each patient. Pretreatment factors such as performance status, site of metastases, and LDH may predict who will respond and are currently being assessed in clinical trials. Based on reports of long-term responses (>10 years) experienced by some patients, the risk certainly is worth the benefit for those individuals. Unfortunately, at this time, it is difficult to determine which individuals will respond to aldesleukin therapy because no biologic or immunologic parameters have been found to correlate with response. The decision to treat an individual with high-dose aldesleukin should be based on an analysis of an individual patient's risk versus potential benefit. Patients with inadequate pulmonary function, cardiac function, renal insufficiency, active infection, or poor performance status are poor candidates for this therapy. Aldesleukin can be safely administered with a properly trained healthcare team and is one of only two approved therapies for treatment of metastatic melanoma.

Clinical **Controversy. . .**

Although aldesleukin has been associated with long-term durable responses in a small subset of patients with metastatic melanoma, the toxicity profile, intensity of therapy, and cost have limited its acceptance in the United States. Patients should be evaluated for treatment before initiation of therapy.

Chemotherapy

5 A number of antineoplastic agents have demonstrated in vitro activity against melanoma, but only a few drugs have consistently shown a response rate greater than 10% in individuals with metastatic melanoma. Most clinical trials of new agents in melanoma measure antitumor activity in terms of response rates, which usually include complete and partial response rates. It is important to understand that these response rates do not always correlate with survival and do not evaluate benefit to the patient. Complete responses can be durable in a small number of patients.

Dacarbazine, a cytotoxic drug thought to exert its antitumor effect through alkylation, currently is the most effective single agent for treatment of melanoma. Dacarbazine remains the only FDA-approved chemotherapeutic agent for treatment of metastatic melanoma in the United States.[37] Prospective controlled clinical trials have observed response rates of 10% to 25%, with an average duration of response of 5 to 7 months. Randomized trials in large numbers of patients have confirmed that response rates are closer to 7%.[38] Complete responses are uncommon, with fewer than 5% of patients treated with single-agent dacarbazine sustaining long-term complete responses. There does not appear to be a survival benefit for dacarbazine relative to other treatments or supportive care. Patients with skin, subcutaneous tissue, and lymph node involvement respond most frequently, but patients with metastatic disease to the liver, bone, and CNS often are unresponsive. The optimum dose schedule of dacarbazine has never been determined; therefore, single-dose regimens are often preferred for patient convenience. Doses of 250 mg/m^2/day for 5 days or 800 to 1,000 mg/m^2 every 3 weeks are seen in practice. Common adverse effects of dacarbazine therapy include myelosuppression, severe nausea and vomiting, and a flulike syndrome after high doses. Nausea and vomiting can be prevented and managed with available antiemetics and is not a major complication. At this time, dacarbazine has no defined role in the adjuvant setting.

Temozolomide is one of a series of imidazole tetrazine derivatives that was developed as a potential alternative to dacarbazine.[37] Temozolomide is an oral prodrug of the active metabolite of dacarbazine. Dacarbazine requires hepatic transformation to its active intermediate, but at physiologic pH, temozolomide chemically degrades to the cytotoxic monomethyltriazenoimidazole carboxamide (MTIC). Temozolomide is administered orally and appears to be less emetogenic than dacarbazine, although nausea can be a challenging chronic toxicity. Temozolomide appears to cross into the CNS and so initially was thought to have benefit for patients with CNS metastases. In a phase III trial of chemotherapy-naïve individuals with metastatic melanoma, temozolomide showed efficacy at least equivalent to that of dacarbazine in terms of objective response rates, time to progression, and overall and disease-free survival.[39] Temozolomide appeared to be associated with improvement in some aspects of quality of life, although overall disease control was similar to dacarbazine.[40]

A potential advantage of temozolomide is the convenience of oral dosing, which allows a potentially more effective dosing schedule. Low-dose intermittent dosing schedules with a rest period are being evaluated. This schedule allows for a threefold increase in drug exposure and may overcome some drug resistance mechanisms. The active metabolite of dacarbazine and temozolomide, MTIC, methylates guanine residues in DNA at the O^6 position. Resistance to agents that produce O^6 methylation is partly due to increased levels of O^6-alylguanine-DNA alkyltransferase. Temozolomide administration results in the depletion of the DNA repair protein O^6-methylguanine-DNA methyltransferase (MGMT), which is a major mechanism of tumor resistance.[40] Clinical evaluations of prolonged administration of temozolomide are ongoing, often in combination with other agents such as IFN.

The *nitrosoureas* are active against melanoma. Nitrosoureas, such as carmustine and lomustine, have antitumor activity similar to that of dacarbazine, with reported response rates between 10% and 20%. Sites of responses are similar to those seen with dacarbazine. It was initially hoped that use of the lipophilic nitrosoureas would provide added benefit against a malignancy that can metastasize to the brain. Unfortunately, despite the ability of these agents to cross the blood–brain barrier, the commercially available nitrosoureas have not been shown to have increased activity against melanoma in the CNS. Fotemustine, a nitrosourea available in Australia and some European countries, appears to cross the blood–brain barrier more rapidly than do other nitrosoureas. Response rates of 30% have been reported in previously untreated patients, with response rates of 25% of patients who had cerebral metastases. Fotemustine is considered standard therapy in some countries.[41] The most common toxicities of the nitrosoureas are nausea and vomiting and delayed myelosuppression, particularly thrombocytopenia. Leukopenia and thrombocytopenia may be seen as long as 3 to 5 weeks after drug administration and may limit the inclusion of these agents to multidrug regimens.

Cisplatin and related compounds have been evaluated in the management of metastatic melanoma. The effectiveness of platinum compounds as single agents is limited, with reported response rates of 10% to 15% with a short median duration. The activity of cisplatin in melanoma may be dose dependent, and higher response rates have been seen with higher doses of cisplatin in single-institution studies.[42] The toxicities of cisplatin can be problematic, especially in higher doses, and include acute and delayed nausea and vomiting, renal toxicity, and neurotoxicity. Carboplatin, another platinum analog, has been evaluated in small trials for treatment of melanoma. Results demonstrated similar response rates to cisplatin with differing toxicities.[39] Carboplatin has been studied in combination with paclitaxel for treatment of melanoma in the second-line setting and this combination as has shown activity.[43,44]

Taxanes have demonstrated encouraging results in initial trials of metastatic melanoma. Response rates of 15% to 17% have been seen in initial phase II trials with paclitaxel and docetaxel. In a small phase II trial, the albumin-bound nanoparticle formulation of paclitaxel (Abraxane®), showed encouraging results.[45] A phase III trial comparing Abraxane with dacarbazine in chemotherapy-naïve melanoma patients reported an increase in progression-free survival (PFS) and a trend in overall survival in patients receiving Abraxane. As would be expected, neuropathy and neutropenia were more common in the Abraxane arm.[46] At this time, these agents are not routinely used as single-agent therapy for melanoma but are being incorporated into multidrug strategies against metastatic melanoma.

In an attempt to improve the limited responses seen with single-agent chemotherapy, a variety of combination chemotherapy regimens (Table 116-6) have been evaluated in both small and large clinical trials. Response rates as high as 30% to 50% were reported in single-institution phase II trials of patients with metastatic melanoma. The combination of dacarbazine with other chemotherapy, most commonly cisplatin, increased the response rates reported with dacarbazine alone, but the survival benefit has been minimal. Responses often were limited to metastases in soft tissue, lymph nodes, and the lung, the sites most likely to

TABLE 116-6 Combination Chemotherapy Regimens for Metastatic Melanoma

CVD: Repeated every 3 weeks
Cisplatin 20 mg/m² IV daily × 4 (days 2, 3, 4, and 5)
Vinblastine 1.6 mg/m² IV daily × 5 (days 1, 2, 3, 4, and 5)
Dacarbazine 800 mg/m² IV daily × 1 (day 1)
CP: Repeated every 3 weeks
Carboplatin AUC 6 IV daily × 1 (day 1)
Paclitaxel 225 mg/m² IV daily × 1 (day 1)

AUC, area under the curve.

respond to single-agent dacarbazine therapy. The concern with combination chemotherapy is increased toxicity, and any reports of increased response rates should be weighed against the effect of toxicities on overall quality of life. The initial reports with the cisplatin, vinblastine, and dacarbazine (CVD) regimen were exciting, with reported response rates greater than 50%, a 4% complete response rate, a median response duration of 9 months, and acceptable toxicities.[47] Comparisons of this regimen to dacarbazine alone have been conflicting. Subsequent reports showed no difference in response rates or survival.

The Dartmouth regimen is a combination that includes carmustine, dacarbazine, cisplatin, and tamoxifen. Initial reports from uncontrolled phase II trials of this combination have demonstrated high response rates of 20% to 50%, but few patients achieve long-term survival. The benefit of tamoxifen to this regimen is controversial, but a controlled clinical trial from the National Cancer Institute of Canada demonstrated no benefit in response or survival from tamoxifen in this combination.[48] Careful analysis of the initial studies demonstrates that the criteria used to measure response were not the same as those used in large multicenter studies. Phase III trials showed no benefit of the Dartmouth regimen compared with single-agent dacarbazine.[49,50] Response rates were 15%, and median survival was about 7 months in both studies. Of concern, toxicities were higher with the combination study and included bone marrow suppression, nausea, vomiting, and fatigue.

Biochemotherapy

Low overall response rates and toxicity have limited the routine use of chemotherapy alone or immunotherapy alone in the management of metastatic disease. Over the past decade, the strategy of a combination of chemotherapy (dacarbazine, platinum agents, or vinca alkaloids) and cytokines, aldesleukin, or IFN, often termed *biochemotherapy*, has been a major focus of investigation in the management of metastatic melanoma and more recently in the adjuvant setting. The primary rationale is to combine two therapies with some biologic activity to increase overall activity and perhaps response rates. In addition, some preclinical trials suggest potential synergistic interactions between cytokines and some chemotherapy agents. As with other treatment strategies in melanoma, the results from initial trials suggested a higher response rate with biochemotherapy than the rates seen with either chemotherapy or biotherapy alone. Although several studies have suggested an increase in response rate with the addition of IFN-α to chemotherapy, results of most studies have shown that the addition of IFN-α does not increase the antitumor effect of dacarbazine but does increase toxicity and cost. Similarly, the combination of aldesleukin to chemotherapy has not been consistently shown to increase response or survival. The most encouraging results have been seen with combination chemotherapy and combination biotherapy, but the results of phase III studies have not demonstrated a clear advantage of biochemotherapy compared with chemotherapy alone.[51] A recently published meta-analysis of 18 randomized trials of chemotherapy versus biochemotherapy showed that biochemotherapy was associated with a significantly higher response rate in treatment of metastatic melanoma. However, these differences in response rates did not translate into a significant difference in overall survival. Toxicities can be severe and are consistent with the individual agents in the regimen.[52]

One of the problems with most studies of biochemotherapy is the relatively short duration of response. Recurrence rates among patients who respond to therapy are as high as 50% within 18 to 24 months. Strategies such as subcutaneous low-dose aldesleukin are being investigated in an effort to prolong overall survival and time to progression in patients who do respond to treatment. Initial response rates, durable complete remission, and activity in patients in whom HDI therapy was not successful have stimulated interest in evaluating biochemotherapy in the adjuvant setting for high-risk patients with node-positive disease compared with HDI.

Biochemotherapy has also been evaluated in the adjuvant setting. Phase II data in a neoadjuvant approach provided promising results in terms of response rates, relapse-free survival, and overall survival.[51] Results from a phase III study that compared biochemotherapy with IFN as adjuvant therapy in high-risk stage III disease were recently published. This trial demonstrated that biochemotherapy significantly improved relapse-free survival, but no difference in overall survival was observed.[53]

Vaccines

The rationale for vaccination as a therapeutic modality is based on the observation that antigens expressed on the surface of tumor cells differ from normal cells and the hope that vaccines might induce effective tumor-specific immune responses with fewer toxicities than conventional chemotherapy or other immunotherapies. Greater knowledge about tumor antigens and the mechanism of antigen presentation and immune response to antigens has led to the development of several vaccination strategies for treatment of early and advanced melanoma.

A variety of melanoma vaccines based on whole tumor cells, peptides, proteins, and tumor lysates have been evaluated for treatment of patients with metastatic disease and for intermediate- and high-risk patients after surgical resection of disease.[54,55] Although tumor responses with some of these approaches have been observed in phase I and II trials, none of the vaccine responses have been confirmed in phase III trials.[55] These early trials have focused on the safety, feasibility, and immunogenicity of the vaccine. Vaccines are a promising but still experimental approach in the treatment of melanoma.

Vaccination is a form of active specific immunotherapy directed against a particular cellular target or specific membrane antigen. The ideal tumor vaccine would generate an active, systemic, long-lived immune response in the cancer-bearing host against tumors; protect against primary development or subsequent relapse of cancer; or induce regression of established cancer. Obstacles in the development of a vaccine include identifying appropriate antigens to target and generating immune responses against tumor antigens to which the immune system has been already exposed.

Whole-cell tumor vaccines can be derived from cell lines that are already established (allogeneic vaccines) or from the patient's own tumor cells (autologous). Whole-cell vaccines are challenging to produce for several reasons: a new vaccine must be prepared for each patient, patients must have sufficient tumor available to provide adequate material, and considerable delay may exist between time of tumor removal and vaccine administration. In addition, there are technical challenges to producing the vaccine in a laboratory.[54] Currently, no autologous tumor cell vaccine has been successfully studied in a phase III randomized clinical trial. An example of a whole-cell tumor vaccine that is being studied is Canvaxin. Canvaxin™ (CancerVax, Carlsbad, CA) is an allogeneic whole-cell vaccine that uses BCG as an immune adjuvant. Small trials have shown improvements in survival compared with historical control participants, and some objective clinical responses have been seen in patients with metastatic melanoma. The results from two large phase III trials that compared Canvaxin with observation in stage III and IV melanoma demonstrated a survival disadvantage for patients who received the vaccine.[56]

Antigen vaccines use individual antigens to stimulate immune responses compared with whole-cell vaccines, which contain many thousands of antigens.[55] These antigens usually are proteins or pieces of proteins called *peptides*. Antigen vaccines may be specific for a certain type of cancer, but they are not made for a specific patient. Vaccines against GM2 ganglioside, a glycolipid expressed on most melanomas, are examples of vaccines targeted against an antigen. Two randomized controlled trials with anti-GM2 vaccines have failed to show any benefit with the vaccine.[55]

Peptide antigen vaccines match the patient's haplotype with the spectrum of immunity that he or she expresses. T cells recognize antigens as peptide epitopes on the surface of major histocompatibility complex (MHC) molecules. Antigenic peptides can be mixed with an immunologic adjuvant and administered with the goal of loading empty MHC molecules in vivo. To date, the most commonly used peptides have shown activity only in patients who express human leukocyte antigen (HLA)-A2. However, many patients would not be eligible for this vaccine because not all patients express this HLA antigen. Additional peptide antigens that are compatible in other haplotypes have been identified, and eventually this disadvantage may be overcome. Peptide vaccination can generate quantifiable and functional tumor-reactive T cells, but clinical responses are rare and do not consistently correlate with CTL response.

Because protein antigen vaccines have a slightly broader spectrum of antigen diversity, all patients with melanoma potentially could be eligible for vaccination with this particular type of vaccine. Whereas proteins intrinsically produced by the cell are presented only to $CD8^+$ T cells, proteins taken up by antigen-presenting cells (APCs) are presented only to $CD4^+$ T cells. Under certain conditions, APCs can present protein-derived antigens to both $CD4^+$ and $CD8^+$ in a process known as *cross-presentation*.[55]

Tumor lysates can be generated from tumor cells by mechanical disruption or enzymatic digestion. Tumor cells that shed antigens in culture can be purified and used as an antigen source for vaccines. Production of a vaccine from these sources raises concern because standardization of production and verification of purity and biological activity are more difficult.

Vaccines in combination with other biologic therapies are being evaluated. In a randomized trial of 604 patients with resected stage III cutaneous melanoma, LDI combined with an allogeneic melanoma lysate vaccine (2 years) was compared with HDI alone (1 year).[57] The median overall survival was not significantly different between the two treatment arms. Five-year relapse-free and overall survival were similar in the two treatment arms. The incidence of serious treatment-related adverse events was similar in the two arms, but more severe neuropsychiatric toxicity was observed in patients receiving HDI. Although the results of this trial suggest that the vaccine has some activity in melanoma, the study was not powered sufficiently to show either equivalency or small differences in efficacy. HLA typing was optional based on whether the centers were able to perform the typing. With ongoing research, additional trials performed with this vaccine, specifically in patients with certain HLA types, may prove promising.

Occasional clinical responses have been observed in clinical trials of melanoma vaccines, which demonstrate the potential of this form of treatment. Many clinical trials with vaccine therapy in melanoma patients are ongoing. The results of completed clinical trials have not yet shown definitive evidence of improved survival. Further research is needed to improve vaccine responses and to determine how to apply treatment to melanoma patients.

Targeted Therapy

6 The role of protein kinases in the regulation and proliferation signals in cancer cells is becoming a key focus for anticancer agents. The role of protein kinase inhibitors has emerged as standard therapy for malignancies such as renal cell carcinoma, chronic myelogenous leukemia, and gastrointestinal stromal tumors. As the biology of melanoma continues to unfold, there is increasing excitement about the development of targeted therapies against targets important for the development and progression of melanoma.[58] There now is greater interest in identifying potential targets in melanoma and determining the applicability in specific patients or patient subsets.

The MAPK pathway and Akt pathway are involved in tumor cell growth and differentiation and are activated in melanoma. BRAF is downstream in the MAPK pathway. Mutations of BRAF have been described in melanoma cell lines, and it appears that about 70% of melanomas exhibit BRAF alteration.[59] In a phase I/II trial, vemurafenib, an orally available inhibitor of mutated BRAF, showed activity in patients with melanoma that had BRAF with the V600E mutation. In the V600E mutation, a valine is substituted for glutamic acid at codon 600. Among the 16 patients with melanoma that had BRAF with the V600E mutation and who received 240 mg or more of vemurafenib twice daily, 10 had a partial response, and one had a complete response.[60] In a phase III trial comparing vemurafenib with dacarbazine in patients with unresectable, previously untreated stage IIIC or IV melanoma with a *BRAF* V600E mutation, vemurafenib significantly improved response rate and overall survival.[61] Patients treated with vemurafenib 960 mg orally twice a day demonstrated an overall survival rate at 6 months of 84% as compared with 64% in the dacarbazine arm. The estimated median PFS times were 5.3 months with vemurafenib and 1.6 months with dacarbazine. The vemurafenib arm showed a significant higher objective response rate of 48% compared with 5% in the dacarbazine arm. The median time to response was also shorter with vemurafenib than dacarbazine (1.45 months vs. 2.7 months). Vemurafenib was associated with cutaneous squamous cell carcinoma or keratoacanthoma in 18% of the patients. Unfortunately, patients developed resistance to vemurafenib, typically after 5 to 6 months of therapy. Resistance is potentially caused by mutations in *MEK,* dependency on MEK/ERK antiapoptotic signaling, PI3/AKT pathway involvement, *NRAS* mutation, or MAPK pathway reactivation.[61,62] The use of intermittent, rather than continuous, dosing has been shown to delay resistance to vemurafenib in animal models, and studies of combination therapy to minimize resistance are ongoing.[61–63] Dabrafenib, another oral selective *BRAF* inhibitor, demonstrated similar responses in profession-free survival and response rates in a phase II study in patients with previously untreated *BRAF* V6000E mutated melanoma. The incidence of cutaneous squamous cell carcinoma was much lower at 6%.[64]

Other drugs targeted toward mutated *BRAF* have not reported encouraging results. Sorafenib is a multikinase inhibitor that inhibits both wild-type and mutant *BRAF* in addition to other tyrosine kinases involved in angiogenesis and tumor progression. Preclinical studies demonstrated activity against human melanoma tumor xenografts in preclinical trials, but minimal activity was observed in phase I and II clinical trials in refractory metastatic melanoma. However, sorafenib may be active when given in combination with chemotherapy. In phase I to II studies, 27% of patients responded to sorafenib when given in combination with carboplatin and paclitaxel, and 73% of patients maintained a response at a 6-month follow-up.[59] However, results from two phase III trials with this same combination failed to show an improvement in PFS and overall survival.[43,44] But the trials did report a higher than expected response rate for the chemotherapy only (carboplatin and paclitaxel) arm, thus making this combination a viable treatment option for this patient population.

Another agent of interest is imatinib mesylate, an oral agent that inhibits c-*Kit* and platelet-derived growth factor receptor. c-*Kit* is expressed primarily on acral and mucosal melanomas. Imatinib suppressed melanoma cell growth in preclinical studies. In phase II trials, imatinib was shown to be inactive in metastatic melanoma despite downregulation of phosphorylated c-*Kit*, but this patient population was not selected for c-*Kit* mutations.[59] A phase II trial in patients with c-*Kit* mutations reported partial response in 23% of patients, 30% with stable disease, and a PFS of 3.5 months.[10]

Other targeted therapies such as MEK inhibitors have been studied in the treatment of metastatic melanoma and have shown modest activity. Trametinib is an inhibitor of MEK1/2. Compared with chemotherapy (dacarbazine or paclitaxel) in *BRAF*-mutated patients in a phase II trial, patients treated with trametinib had improved progression-free survival, overall survival, and response rates. MEK162 is also a MEK1/2 inhibitor but preclinically showed activity against *NRAS*-mutated melanomas. In patients with *NRAS* mutations, more than half of the patients had a response (partial response or stable disease) when given MEK-162.[10] Both of these agents are currently being studied in combination with other BRAF and PI3K inhibitors.

Other Approaches

Dendritic cells are potent APCs that initiate antigen-specific immune responses. Dendritic cells express high levels of MHC class I and class II molecules, which are essential in antigen presentation. Activation of T cells and recruitment of non–antigen-specific effectors, such as NK cells and macrophages, result in a broad immune response. One strategy that uses dendritic cells for inducing antitumor immune responses is peptide-pulsed dendritic cells. Antimelanoma CTLs can be generated from healthy donors and patients with melanoma with dendritic cells pulsed with melanoma-derived peptides. A number of clinical trials have evaluated dendritic cell–based immunotherapy, and its clinical benefit is yet to be substantiated. The immunosuppressive role of regulatory T cells may be affecting the success of these agents. Trials with dendritic cells given with high dose IL-2, chemotherapy, and anti-inflammatory agents demonstrated disease stabilization in patients with metastatic melanoma.[65]

7 *Monoclonal antibodies* have been used for diagnosis and treatment of melanoma. Monoclonal antibodies can be used to target biologic pathways that are associated with tumor progression and as a delivery system for antineoplastic drugs. Monoclonal antibodies have been conjugated to cytotoxic agents, radioisotopes, and toxins. More recently, monoclonal antibodies have been developed to target processes that are involved in the host immune response to melanoma. CTLA-4 is a transmembrane protein expressed on T lymphocytes that is a homodimer that functions as an inhibitory receptor for the costimulatory molecule B7. Crosslinking of CTLA-4 by B7 inhibits T-cell activation, transcription, translation, and transduction. CTLA-4 blockage overcomes this inhibition and results in activation and proliferation of T cells.[66] CTLA-4 blockade may represent a novel approach to enhance the immune response against melanoma antigens. Ipilimumab and tremelimumab are two fully human monoclonal antibodies against CTLA-4. Preliminary results of clinical trials showed promising activity in malignant melanoma. Results from phase I and II trials with ipilimumab and tremelimumab demonstrate up to 20% response rates in advanced disease.[67] In a phase III trial of 676 HLA-A*0201-positive patients with refractory

metastatic melanoma, ipilumumab (3 mg/kg) plus a glycoprotein 100 (gp100) peptide vaccine was compared with ipilumumab (3 mg/kg) alone or gp100 alone.[68] The median overall survival time was significantly longer in patients treated with ipilumumab either alone or combined with gp100 as compared with patients treated with gp100 alone (10.0 or 10.1 months vs. 6.4 months). No difference in overall survival was observed between the two ipilimumab groups. Another phase III trial compared a higher dose of ipilimumab (10 mg/kg) plus dacarbazine with dacarbazine alone in patients previously untreated for metastatic melanoma.[69] Ipilimumab plus dacarbazine demonstrated significantly longer overall survival (11.2 vs. 9.1 months) and higher survival rates at 1 year (47.3% vs. 36.3%), 2 years (28.5% vs. 17.9%), and 3 years (20.8% vs. 12.2%) than dacarbazine alone. The potential role of ipilimumab in the adjuvant setting was evaluated in a phase II trial that reported encouraging results; a phase III trial is ongoing to further assess its role in this setting.[70] Unfortunately, a phase III study of tremelimumab reported no difference in overall survival compared with dacarbazine or temozolamide.[71] CTLA-4 antibodies produce several immune-mediated adverse events that are distinct from the typical adverse events associated with conventional cancer treatments. Many of these adverse effects are autoimmune in nature and can occur in up to 40% of patients.[66] Antibodies against CTLA-4 may cause autoimmune-mediated adverse events by promoting the activation of self-reactive T cells. The most common serious adverse events included dermatitis, enterocolitis, and diarrhea. Less common adverse effects include autoimmune thyroiditis, adrenal disease, or hepatitis.[67–68] Close monitoring for immune-related adverse events and participation in a risk evaluation and mitigation strategy (REMS) program while on therapy is necessary.[20] Ipilimumab therapy should be held for moderate immune-related events. High-dose systemic corticosteroids are initiated for patients who do not improve from withholding therapy or for grade 3 immune-related events. Ipilimumab can be restarted when adverse events improve to grade 0 or 1 and systemic corticosteroid doses have been minimized. Infliximab can be used for patients who do not respond to steroids.[68] In cases of severe or life-threatening immune-related adverse events, permanent discontinuation of therapy is recommended. In the clinical studies reported to date, patients who experienced grade 3 or 4 autoimmune toxicities were also the most likely to exhibit tumor regression and increased time to relapse.[66] The timing of adverse effects is variable and may occur several months after the cessation of treatment.

Clinical **Controversy...**

The optimal dose of ipilumumab for the treatment of metastatic melanoma is currently unknown. The FDA-approved dosing is 3 mg/kg IV every 3 weeks for a total of four doses. Clinical studies that dosed ipilumumab at 10 mg/kg have shown slightly higher response rates but also greater toxicity. An ongoing clinical trial comparing the outcomes of the 3 mg/kg and 10 mg/kg dosing will help to answer this question.

Antibodies directed against programmed death 1 (PD-1), which is upregulated on activated T cells, block the binding of program death-ligand 1 and 2 to the receptor on tumor cells, thus allowing T cells to remain stimulated and the immune response to continue.[10] Early-stage clinical trials with these agents show potential, and they are associated with less frequent immune-related adverse events compared to ipilumumab.[10]

Gene therapy of human melanoma is in its infancy but suggests several exciting approaches to management of metastatic melanoma. Several strategies for gene therapy are under investigation for the treatment of melanoma. One approach to gene therapy for melanoma is adoptive therapy. In this process, T lymphocytes are removed from the patient and are genetically altered to target specific antigens on the cancer cell. They are then expanded to large numbers and given back to the patient along with IL-2 after receiving an immunosuppressive preparative chemotherapy regimen.[10] In a very small clinical trial in which T cells were engineered with a receptor against the cancer-testis antigen NY-ESO-1, found in about 25% of melanoma patients, response rates of 45% were seen in patients with treatment refractory metastatic melanoma.[72] The challenges to this type of therapy are determining a patient population that can tolerate the intensity of treatment and who do not need immediate treatment because cell processing takes several week to complete.[10]

Antiangiogenic agents are also being evaluated for the management of metastatic melanoma. Thalidomide, given either as a single agent or in combination with chemotherapy or cytokines, was the initial agent studied. Thalidomide analogs are now being studied in an attempt to avoid toxicities associated with the parent compound. The thalidomide analogs are grouped into two classes: selective cytokine inhibitory drugs and immunomodulatory derivatives. Both classes appear to have antiangiogenic and antiinflammatory properties, but the selective cytokine inhibitory drugs are phosphodiesterase inhibitors. Immunomodulatory derivatives also have effects on T-cell stimulation and inhibition of TNF-α. Other antiangiogenic agents such as integrins and VEGF inhibitors are also being investigated. As seen in other cancer using these therapies, disease stabilization rather than tumor response is most likely to be the best outcome.[5]

Radiation

The role of radiation for the adjuvant treatment of melanoma is being investigated based on retrospective data that suggest that patients treated with therapeutic lymphadenectomy for lymph node field relapse benefit from postoperative adjuvant radiation to the nodal basins. Overall, these data demonstrate improvement in locoregional control with reasonable toxicity but with no impact on overall survival. A recently completed phase III trial reported that adjuvant radiotherapy reduced the risk of lymph node field relapse in patients who had undergone therapeutic lymphadenectomy for metastatic melanoma in regional lymph nodes.[73] No difference in relapse-free survival was observed. For patients with metastatic melanoma, radiation is limited to the palliative setting to symptomatic areas of disease progression.

Limb Perfusion and Limb Infusion

Isolated limb perfusion is a surgical procedure of regional intravascular delivery of chemotherapy or biotherapy (or both) into an extremity with cutaneous melanoma.[74] When in-transit metastases occur in extremities, local therapy with isolated limb perfusion or isolated limb infusion has been used.[5] Isolated limb perfusion is a method for escalating the dose of chemotherapeutic drugs to a specific region of the body while limiting the systemic toxicities of the agent. Most perfusions can be performed with drug exposures of less than 2%. The most significant side effect of isolated limb perfusion is regional toxicity; all of the skin, subcutaneous tissue, and tissue of the extremity receives the same dose and is subjected to the same perfusion conditions as the tumor located within the extremity. After regional perfusions, objective response rates greater than 50% in treated limbs have been reported, with overall response rates possibly as high as 80%. The role of hyperthermia (39°C to 40°C [102°F to 104°F]) with regional isolated perfusion is not clearly defined. Although most clinical trials have used melphalan, whether the combination of melphalan with other agents may improve results is not known.[75] Agents that have been combined with melphalan include actinomycin D, nitrogen mustard, thiotepa, and cisplatin. Work with biologic response modifiers, such as TNF-α, has been encouraging.[76] A simplified form of isolated limb perfusion, called isolated limb infusion, is a low-flow isolated limb perfusion performed under hypoxic conditions via small-caliber arterial and venous catheters. It has been proposed that the hypoxia that develops during isolated limb infusion may be beneficial with certain cytotoxic agents such as melphalan.

PREVENTION AND DETECTION

The results of early treatment emphasize the role of early detection and prevention. There are three different strategies for chemoprevention for melanoma. Primary chemoprevention is used to prevent occurrences of melanoma in healthy individuals. Secondary chemoprevention is used to prevent premalignant melanoma precursors from becoming melanoma. Tertiary chemoprevention is used to prevent melanoma recurrence in individuals who were treated for melanoma and have no evidence of disease. The mainstay of melanoma prevention remains strategies to protect individuals from harmful effects of the sun[77] (Table 116-7).

Ultraviolet light exposure plays a major role in melanoma development. Childhood sunburns and intermittent sun exposure correlate positively with melanoma risk. Studies have shown that a decrease in recreational sun exposure is associated with a reduction of a second primary melanoma in individuals diagnosed with primary melanoma.[78] Education and reeducation about the importance of sun protection have the potential to help decrease the rising incidence of this disease. Strategies, such as sun avoidance, especially during peak hours of sun intensity (10 AM to 4 PM), and staying in the shade when outdoors, are important education concepts for individuals who are in the sun for prolonged periods or who are at high risk for burning. Skiers and winter sports enthusiasts should be cautioned about exposure to UV radiation because the reflection off snow and high altitude contribute to increased UV exposure. There is also the use of protective clothing to minimize damage to the skin for individuals who spend time in the sun. Clothing designed to protect an individual from sun exposure but allows for physical activities such as water sports and hiking is widely available. The clothes are designed for skin protection, but it is important to realize that not all clothing provides sufficient protection from UV radiation. Clothes with tight weaves provide the greatest protection. In addition to protective clothing, wide-brimmed hats to protect ears, the neck, and the nose as wells as sunglasses with both UVA and UVB protection are important. Additionally, the use of tanning beds over the past 3 decades has led to an increased exposure of individuals to UVA light. Observational studies show that individuals who spent time in tanning devices before the age of 35 years have a 75% increase in risk of melanoma.[79] As a result, the World Health Organization International Agency for Research on Cancer declared in 2009 that UV light emitted from tanning beds was a human carcinogen.[80] A recent report from the Centers for Disease Control and Prevention found that 5.6% of people in the United States reported indoor tanning in the last 12 months. The highest rates, 12.3%, were seen in young women 18 to 25 years old. Evidence suggests that behavioral counseling in the primary care setting can decrease UV exposure, including tanning beds, in younger patients. To aid in the prevention skin cancers, laws such as bans or requiring parental consent have been put in place to restrict minors' access to indoor tanning in 33 states.[81]

TABLE 116-7 Options for Sun Protection Sunscreens

	Sunscreens	
Behavioral	**Physical Blockers (Reflectants)**	**Chemical Absorbers**
Protective clothing and accessories Seek shade (avoid peak sun hours) Avoid tanning equipment	Zinc oxide Talc Titanium dioxide Red petrolatum	Ultraviolet B absorbers Salicylates Cinnamates Camphor derivatives Aminobenzoates Ultraviolet A absorbers Benzopehnone-6 Dibenzoylmethanes

It is important to counsel patients about the appropriate use of sunscreens to optimize benefits from these products. Sunscreens should be applied 15 to 30 minutes before going into the sun and should be reapplied every 2 hours, after swimming, and after perspiring heavily. About 1 oz of sunscreen (a "palmful") should be used to cover the arms, legs, neck, and face of the average adult. Sun protection must be used regularly and not limited to times of recreation or anticipated "prolonged" exposure. Times of season changes, when the potential for sun exposure can be perceived as erratic, are possible times for the "first-of-the-season sunburn."

Historically, patients have been counseled that the risk of skin cancer can be limited by the use of sunscreens with a sun protection factor (SPF) of 15 or greater. SPF is a measure of protection from UVB radiation only. Although some studies have found a decreased risk of melanoma in sunscreens users, others have demonstrated no association and even increased melanoma risk with sunscreen use. Methodologic difficulties may explain the discrepancy in study results. Factors that include variables in sun exposure, sunscreen use, and sun sensitivity are very difficult to control in these trials. In addition, all sunscreens are not the same. It is important that people understand that no sunscreen provides complete protection and that the SPF scale is not linear; the higher the SPF, the smaller the difference in sun protection. For example, whereas SPF 15 sunscreens filter out about 93% of UVB rays, SPF 30 sunscreens filter out about 97%, SPF 50 sunscreens about 98%, and SPF 100 about 99%.

Sunscreens traditionally have been designed to prevent erythema by blocking UVB, leaving users relatively unprotected from wavelengths such as UVA. As a result, the use of sunscreens, especially those with higher SPFs, may lead to the ability of individuals to increase their time in the sun without clinical indication of sunburn. Newer forms of sunscreens combine protection for UVA and UVB. Unfortunately, no currently approved system rates products for UVA protective capabilities, but the FDA has proposed new sunscreen rules that will establish an UVA testing and labeling system. It is unclear when this system will be put into place. The impact of the use of high-potency sunscreens on the incidence of melanoma is not clear at this time because the lag time for melanoma is about 2 decades, and high-potency sunscreens have only been popular for about 10 years.

Thickness and stage of the disease are inversely related to melanoma survival. Early detection can play a large part in the secondary prevention of melanoma. Many healthcare organizations and skin cancer groups recommend monthly SSE to serve as a mechanism for recognizing moles or marks on the skin that may be melanoma. Patients with a strong family history should additionally have a clinical examination and, in some cases, screening photography to document the size, shape, and location of moles. Both patients and clinicians need to be properly educated in the clinical features of the disease to ensure more appropriate diagnosis. Currently, there are no consistent recommendations for the screening and early detection of melanoma.

PERSONALIZED PHARMACOTHERAPY

8 Treatment of cutaneous melanoma is determined by many factors including disease-related and patient-related issues. Most available reviews and guidelines provide treatment recommendations based on stage of disease.[20] Most patients present with localized disease.[20] Treatment of localized disease is surgical excision, with the extent of excision based on the tumor size. Wide excision is recommended for in situ melanoma and wide excision with SLNB for stage IA, IB, and II disease. The long-term survival of individuals with early-stage disease and thin tumors (<1 mm) is good, but survival is negatively impacted as tumor thickness increases.

The role of adjuvant therapy in the management of individuals at high risk for recurrence remains controversial. One controversy is determination of which patients are appropriate candidates for treatment after resection of the primary tumor. Although adjuvant therapy has been considered historically in patients with locally advanced disease (stages II and III), it is increasingly being considered after surgical resection of an isolated distant metastases.

Another controversy with adjuvant therapy is the choice of therapy. HDI has the most evidence supporting its use and is FDA approved for this indication. The challenges with this therapy have been discussed, and the therapy has limited worldwide acceptance. With the encouraging data of ipilimumab in the metastatic setting, clinical trials are now underway as an adjuvant treatment option. New therapies and combinations must be evaluated to help answer the questions that remain about adjuvant therapy in melanoma. The most appropriate option is a clinical trial, if available. Clinical trials of chemotherapy, immunotherapy, vaccines, and emerging therapies are ongoing.

Another treatment challenge is the management of patients with advanced disease. The 2013 NCCN guidelines list a variety of preferred systemic therapies for advanced or metastatic melanoma, including ipilimumab, vemurafenib, high-dose aldesleukin, and clinical trial. Dacarbazine, temozolomide, combination chemotherapy, or biochemotherapy are also included as treatment options.[20] The choice of drug therapy should be based on BRAF mutational status, the aggressiveness of the disease, and disease-related symptoms. Patients with a more indolent clinical picture may respond better to immunotherapy. Patients with a documented BRAF mutation are candidates for vemurafenib. Vemurafenib may be particularly beneficial in patients with BRAF mutations who are symptomatic from their disease because of the rapid response rates that are seen. In patients who harbor the *c-KIT* mutation, imatinib can be offered as first-line therapy.[20] Combination chemotherapy or biochemotherapy provides a treatment option for most patients. Furthermore, these modalities may be particularly beneficial in patients with rapid disease progression. Patients who have predominantly visceral disease and have appropriate organ function may be eligible for high-dose aldesleukin therapy. Best supportive care is also an option in some individuals. Data suggest that surgical treatment of metastatic melanoma should be considered in select individuals based on the extent and location of disease and performance status.

In patients who develop brain metastases, treatment of CNS disease is independent of systemic therapy. Depending on the size and location of metastases, surgical resection can be offered as the first-line treatment modality in patients with a favorable prognosis. Stereotactic radiosurgery is an acceptable alternative for patients who are unable to undergo resection. Whole-brain radiotherapy is generally reserved for patients with a large volume of metastases because of the concern of cognitive decline.[82] In many cases, after brain metastases have been treated, patients can continue with their systemic treatment. As previously mentioned, temozolamide may also be a treatment option for patients with brain metastases. An important consideration for treatment of melanoma is the presentation of the disease. As discussed, treatment of melanoma isolated to the limb may be most appropriately treated with regional therapy. Treatment options for metastatic uveal melanoma include strategies for managing hepatic metastasis, such as chemoembolization to the liver and intrahepatic chemotherapy.[13]

EVALUATION OF THERAPEUTIC OUTCOMES

The outcome of patients treated with melanoma depends on the stage of disease at presentation. The prognosis of patients with thin tumors (<1 mm in thickness) and localized disease is good with long-term survival in more than 90% of patients. The risk of regional nodal involvement increases with increasing tumor thickness, so survival rates decrease in patients with nodal involvement. Long-term survival in patients with distant metastases is even lower. Therefore, early diagnosis and appropriate treatment of early disease are essential. Patients with suspicious pigmented lesions should be evaluated and the lesion excised whenever possible. Treatment is determined by patient factors and stage of disease.

Clinical practice guidelines published by the NCCN and ESMO provide some guidance for follow-up of patients with melanoma.[20,83] Intensive surveillance has the benefit of early detection of recurrent disease, which may lead to better options of surgical resection. Emphasis on evaluation of locoregional areas is important. For patients with in situ melanoma, periodic skin examinations for life are recommended, although frequency is determined based on patient risk factors. Local recurrence is associated with aggressive tumor biology and frequently is a manifestation of an aggressive primary tumor. If a local recurrence occurs after inadequate primary disease, the patient should undergo a workup based on the lesion thickness of the original melanoma. Patients with nodal recurrence should be evaluated for lymph node metastases. Patients with systemic recurrence should be evaluated and treated in a fashion similar to patients presenting with systemic disease.

ABBREVIATIONS

AJCC	American Joint Committee on Cancer
ARF	alternative reading frame
bFGF	basic fibroblast growth factor
CTL	cytotoxic T lymphocyte
CTLA-4	cytotoxic T lymphocyte antigen 4
ECOG	Eastern Cooperative Oncology Group
EORTC	The European Organization for Research and Treatment of Cancer
ESMO	European Society of Clinical Oncology
FDA	Food and Drug Administration
HDI	high-dose interferon
HLA	human leukocyte antigen
IFN	interferon
IL-2	interleukin-2
INK4A	inhibitor of cyclin-dependent kinase 4
LAK	lymphokine-activated killer
LDH	lactate dehydrogenase
LDI	low-dose interferon
MAPK	mitogen-activated protein kinase pathway
MHC	major histocompatibility complex
MTIC	monomethyltriazenoimidazole carboxamide
mTOR	mammalian target of rapamycin
NCCN	National Comprehensive Cancer Network
NK	natural killer
NMSC	nonmelanoma skin cancer
NSAID	nonsteroidal antiinflammatory drug

PET	positron emission tomography
PI3K	phosphatidyl-inosital-3-OH kinase
SLNB	sentinel lymph node biopsy
SPF	sun protection factor
SSE	skin self-examination
TNF	tumor necrosis factor
TIL	tumor-infiltrating lymphocyte
TLR9	toll-like receptor 9
UV	ultraviolet
UVA	ultraviolet A
UVB	ultraviolet B
VEGF	vascular endothelial growth factor

REFERENCES

1. Rigel DS. Trends in dermatology: melanoma incidence. Arch Dermatol 2010;146:318.
2. American Cancer Society. Cancer Facts & Figures 2013. Atlanta. American Cancer Society; 2013.
3. U.S. National Center for Health Statistics (NCHS) and the Surveillance, Epidemiology, and End Results (SEER) database, 1975–2010. *http://seer.cancer.gov/canques/.*
4. Siegel R, Naishadham, Jemal A. Cancer statistics, 2013. CA Cancer J Clin 2013;63:11–30.
5. Slinluff CL, Flaherty K, Rosenberg SA, Read PW. Cutaneous melanoma. In: DeVita VT, Hellman S, Rosenberg SA, eds. Cancer: Principles and Practice of Oncology, 9th ed. Philadelphia, PA: Lippincott Williams & Wilkins, 2011:1643–1692.
6. Jen M, Murphy M, Grant-Kels J. Childhood melanoma. Clin Dermatol 2009;27:529–536.
7. Wilkins K, Turner R, Dolev JC, et al. Cutaneous malignancy and human immunodeficiency virus disease. J Am Acad Dermatol 2006;54:189–206.
8. Chin L, Garraway LA, Fisher DE. Malignant melanoma: Genetics and therapeutics in the genomic era. Genes Dev 2006;20:2149–2182.
9. Goldstein AM, Cahn M, Harland M, et al. Features associated with germline CDKN2A mutations: A GenoMEL study of melanoma-prone families from three continents. J Med Genet 2007;44:99–106.
10. Amaria RN, Gonzalez R. Updated approach to the patient with metastatic melanoma. Emerg Cancer Ther 2012;3:583–602.
11. Mahabeleshwar GH, Byzova TV. Angiogenesis in melanoma. Semin Oncol 2007;34:555–565.
12. Gray-Schopfer V, Wellbrock C, Marais R. Melanoma biology and new targeted therapy. Nature 2007;445:851–857.
13. Albert DM, Kulkarni AD. Intraocular melanoma. In: DeVita VT, Hellman S, Rosenberg SA, eds. Cancer: Principles and Practice of Oncology, 9th ed. Philadelphia, PA: Lippincott Williams & Wilkins, 2011:2090–2099.
14. Balch CM, Gershenwald JE, Soong SJ, et al. Final version of 2009 AJCC melanoma staging and classification. J Clin Oncol 2009;27:6199–6206.
15. Breslow A. Thickness, cross-sectional areas and depth of invasion in the prognosis of cutaneous melanoma. Ann Surg 1970;172:1902–1908.
16. Davar D, Tarhini AA, Kirkwood JM. Adjuvant therapy for melanoma. J Cancer 2012;18:192–202.
17. Greene FL, Page DL, Flemming ID, et al., eds. AJCC Cancer Staging Manual, 6th ed. Philadelphia, PA: Lippincott-Raven, 2002:209.
18. Morton DL, Thompson JF, Cochran AJ, et al. Sentinel-node biopsy or nodal observation in melanoma. N Engl J Med 2006;355:1307–1317.
19. Wong SL, Balch CM, Hurley P, et al. Sentinel lymph node biopsy for melanoma: American Society of Clinical Oncology and Society of Surgical Oncology Joint Clinical Practice Guideline. J Clin Oncol 2012;30:2912–2918.
20. National Comprehensive Cancer Network. NCCN Melanoma Clinical Practice Guidelines in Oncology, version 2. 2013, *http://www.nccn.org*.
21. Balch CM, Urist MM, Karakousis CP, et al. Efficiency of 2-cm surgical margins for intermediate-thickness melanomas (1–4 mm): Results of a multi-institutional randomized surgical trial. Ann Surg 1993;218:262–269.
22. Meirion Thomas K, Newton-Bishop J, A'Hern R, et al. Excision margins in high-risk malignant melanoma. N Engl J Med 2004;350:757–766.
23. Wargo JA, Tanabe K. Surgical management of melanoma. Hematol Oncol Clin North Ame 2009;23:565–581.
24. Tsao H, Atkins MB, Sober AJ. Management of cutaneous melanoma. N Engl J Med 2004;351:998–1012.
25. Kondziolka D, Martin JJ, Flickinger JC, et al. Long-term survivors after gamma knife radiosurgery for brain metastases. Cancer 2005;104:2784–2791.
26. Kirkwood JM, Straderman MH, Ernstoff MS, et al. Interferon alfa-2b adjuvant therapy of high-risk resected cutaneous melanoma: The Eastern Cooperative Oncology Group Trial EST 1684. J Clin Oncol 1996;14:7–17.
27. Kirkwood JM, Manola J, Ibrahim J, et al. A pooled analysis of Eastern Cooperative Oncology Group and Intergroup trials of adjuvant high-dose interferon for melanoma. Clin Cancer Res 2004;10:1670–1677.
28. Eggermont AM, Suciu S, Testori A, et al. Long-term results of the randomized phase III trial EORTC 18991 of adjuvant pegylated interferon alfa-2b versus observation in resected stage III melanoma. J Clin Oncol 2012;30:3810–3818.
29. Kirkwood JM, Ibrahim JG, Sondak VK, et al. High- and low-dose interferon alfa-2b in high risk melanoma: First analysis of intergroup trial E1690/S9111/C9190. J Clin Oncol 2000;18:2444–2458.
30. Lens MB, Dawes M. Interferon alfa therapy for malignant melanoma: A systematic review of randomized controlled trials. J Clin Oncol 2002;20:1818–1825.
31. Hauschild A, Gogas H, Tarhini A, et al. Practical guidelines for the management of interferon-alpha-2b side effects in patients receiving adjuvant treatment for melanoma. Cancer 2008;112:982–994.
32. Myint AM, Schwarz MJ, Steinbusch HW, et al. Neuropsychiatric disorders related to interferon and interleukins treatment. Metab Brain Dis 2009;24:55–68.
33. Cole BF, Gelber RD, Kirkwood JM, et al. A quality-of-life-adjusted survival analysis of interferon alfa-2b adjuvant treatment for high-risk resected cutaneous melanoma: An Eastern Cooperative Oncology Group Study (E1684). J Clin Oncol 1996;14:2666–2673.
34. Bottomley A, Coens C, Suciu S, et al. Adjuvant therapy with pegylated interferon alfa-2b versus observation in resected stage III melanoma: a phase III randomized controlled trial of health-related quality of life and symptoms by the European Organisation for Research and Treatment of Cancer Melanoma Group. J Clin Oncol 2009;27:2916–2923.
35. Petrella T, Quirt I, Verma S, et al. Single-agent interleukin-2 in the treatment of metastatic melanoma: A systematic review. Cancer Treat Rev 2007;33:484–496.
36. Schadendorf D, Algarra SM, Bastholt L, et al. Immunotherapy for distant metastatic disease. Ann Oncol 2009;20(Suppl 6):41–50.

37. Gogas HJ, Kirkwood JM, Sondak VK. Chemotherapy for metastatic melanoma. Time for a change? Cancer 2007;109:455–464.
38. Agarwala SS. Metastatic melanoma: an AJCC review. Community Oncol 2008;5:441–445.
39. Yang AS, Chapman PB. The history and future of chemotherapy for melanoma. Hematol Oncol Clin North Am 2009;23:583–597.
40. Quirt I, Verma S, Petrella T, et al. Temozolomide for the treatment of metastatic melanoma: A systematic review. Oncologist 2007;12:1114–1123.
41. Jacquillat C, Khayat D, Banzet P, et al. Final report of the French multicenter phase II study of the nitrosourea fotemustine in 153 evaluable patients with disseminated malignant melanoma including patients with cerebral metastases. Cancer 1990;66:1873–1878.
42. Glover D, Ibrahim J, Kirkwood J, et al. Phase II randomized trial of cisplatin and WR-2721 versus cisplatin alone for metastatic melanoma: An Eastern Cooperative Oncology Group study (E1686). Melanoma Res 2003;13:619–626.
43. Hauschild A, Agarwala SS, Trefzer U, et al. Results of a phase III randomized, placebo controlled study of sorafenib in combination with carboplatin and paclitaxel as second line therapy in patients with unresectable stage II or stage IV melanoma. J Clin Oncol 2009;27:2823–2830.
44. Flaherty KT, Lee SJ, Fengmin Z, et al. Phase III trial of carboplatin and paclitaxel with or without sorafenib in metastatic melanoma. J Clin Oncol 2013;31:373–379.
45. Hersch E, O'Day SJ, Ribas A, et al. A phase 2 clinical trial of nab-paclitaxel in previously treated and chemotherapy naïve patients with metastatic melanoma. Cancer Res 2010;116:155–163.
46. Hersh E, DelVecchio M, Brown M, et al. Phase 3, randomized, open-label, multicenter trial of nab-paclitaxel vs dacarbazine in previously untreated patients with metastatic malignant melanoma. Society for Melanoma Research 2012 Congress. Pigment Cell Melanoma Res 2012;25:836–903.
47. Legha SS, Ring S, Papadopoulos N, et al. A prospective evaluation of a triple-drug regimen containing cisplatin, vinblastine and DTIC (CVD) for metastatic melanoma. Cancer 1989;64:2024–2029.
48. Rusthoven JJ, Quirt IC, Iscoe NA, et al. Randomized, double-blind, placebo-controlled trial comparing the response rates of carmustine, dacarbazine, and cisplatin with and without tamoxifen in patients with metastatic melanoma. National Cancer Institute of Canada clinical trials group. J Clin Oncol 1996;14:2083–2090.
49. Chapman PB, Einhorm L, Meyeres ML, et al. Phase III multicenter randomized trial of the Dartmouth regimen versus dacarbazine in patients with metastatic melanoma. J Clin Oncol 1999;17:2745–2751.
50. Middleton MR, Lorigan P, Owen J, et al. A randomized phase III study comparing dacarbazine, BCNU, cisplatin and tamoxifen with dacarbazine and interferon in advanced melanoma. Br J Cancer 2000;82:1158–1162.
51. Hamm C, Verna S, Petrella T, et al. Biochemotherapy for the treatment of metastatic melanoma: a systemic review. Cancer Treat Rev 2007;34:145–156.
52. Ives NJ, Stowe RL, Lorigan P, Whearley K. Chemotherapy compared with biochemotherapy for the treatment of metastatic melanoma. A meta-analysis of 18 trials involving 2,621 patients. J Clin Oncol 2007;25:5426–5434.
53. Flaherty LE, Moon J, Atkins MB, et al. Phase III trial of high-dose interferon alpha-2b versus cisplatin, vinblastine, DTIC plus IL-2 and interferon in patients with high risk melanoma (SWOG S0008): An intergroup study of CALGB, COG, ECOG and SWOG [abstract]. J Clin Oncol 2012;30:541s (suppl; abstr 8504).
54. Terando AM, Faries MB, Morton DL. Vaccine therapy for melanoma: Current status and future directions. Vaccine 2007;25(Suppl 2):B4–B16.
55. Chapman PB. Melanoma vaccines. Semin Oncol 2007;34: 516–523.
56. Kirkwood JM, Tarhini AA, Panelli MC, et al. Next generation of immunotherapy for melanoma. J Clin Oncol 2008;26:3445–3455.
57. Mitchell MS, Abrams J, Thompson JA, et al. Randomized trial of allogeneic melanoma lysate vaccine with low-dose interferon alfa-2b compared with high-dose interferon alfa-2b for resected stage III cutaneous melanoma. J Clin Oncol 2007;25:2078–2085.
58. Becker JC, Kirkwood JM, Agarwala SS, et al. Molecularly targeted therapy for melanoma. Cancer 2006;107:2317–2327.
59. Jilaveanu LB, Aziz S, Kluger HM. Chemotherapy and biologic therapies for melanoma: do they work? Clin Dermatol 2009;27:614–625.
60. Flaherty KT, Puzanov I, Kim KB, et al. Inhibition of mutated, activated BRAF in metastatic melanoma. N Engl J Med 2010;363:809–819.
61. Chapman PB, Hauschild A, Robert C, et al. Improved survival with vemurafenib in melanoma with BRAF V600E mutation. N Engl J Med 2011;364:2507–2516.
62. Luke JJ, Hodi FS. Vemurafenib and BRAF inhibition: A new class of treatment for metastatic melanoma. Clin Cancer Res 2012;18:9–14.
63. Thakur MD, Slangsang F, Lansman AS, et al. Modeling vemurafenib resistance in melanoma reveals strategy to forestall drug resistance. Nature 2013;494(7436):251–255.
64. Hauschild A, Grob JJ, Demidov LV, et al. Dabrafenib in BRAF-mutated metastatic melanoma: A multicentre, open-label, phase 3 randomized controlled trial. Lancet 2012;380:358–365.
65. Ellenbaek E, Engell-Noerregaard L, Iversen TZ, et al. Metastatic melanoma patients treated with dendritic cell vaccine, interleykien-2, and metronomic dosing of cyclophosphamide: results from a phase II trial. Cancer Immunol Immunother 2012;61:1791–1804.
66. Sarnaik AA, Weber JS. Recent advances using anti-CTLA-4 for the treatment of melanoma. Cancer J 2009;15:169–173.
67. O'Day SJ, Hamid O, Urba WJ. Targeting cytotoxic T-lymphocyte antigen-4 (CTLA-4): A novel strategy for the treatment of melanoma and other malignancies. Cancer 2007;110:2614–2627.
68. Hodi FS, O'Day SJ, McDermott DF, et al. Improved survival with ipilimumab in patients with metastatic melanoma. N Engl J Med 2010;363:711–723.
69. Robert C, Thomas L, Bondarenko I, et al. Ipilimumab plus dacarbazine for previously untreated metastatic melanoma. N Engl J Med 2011;364:2517–2526.
70. Sarnaik AA, Yu B, Yu D, et al. Extended dose ipilimumab with a peptide vaccine: immune correlates associated with clinical benefit in patients with resected high risk stage IIIc/IV melanoma. Clin Cancer Res 2011;17:896–906.
71. Ribas AA, Kefford R, Marshall MA, et al. Phase III randomized clinical trial comparing tremelimumab with standard-of-care chemotherapy in patients with advanced melanoma. J Clin Oncol 2013;31(5):616–622.
72. Robbins PF, Morgan RA, Feldman SA, et al. Tumor regression in patients with metastatic synovial cell sarcoma and melanoma using genetically engineered lymphocytes reactive with NY-ESO-1. J Clin Oncol 2011;29:917–924.

73. Burmeister BH, Henderson MA, Ainslie J, et al. Adjuvant radiotherapy versus observation alone for patients at risk of lymph-node field relapse after therapeutic lymphadenectomy for melanoma: A randomised trial. Lancet Oncol 2012;13:589–597.
74. Coleman A, Augustine CK, Beasely G, et al. Optimizing regional infusion treatment strategies for melanoma extremities. Expert Rev Anticancer Ther 2009;9:1599–1609.
75. Sanki A, Kam PCA, Thompson JF. Long-term results of hyperthermic isolated limb perfusion for melanoma. Ann Surg 2007;245:591–596.
76. Lejeune FJ, Eggermont AMM. Hyperthermic isolated limb perfusion with tumor necrosis factor is a useful therapy for advanced melanoma of the limbs. J Clin Oncol 2007;25:1449–1450.
77. Francis SO, Mahlberg MJ, Johnson KR, et al. Melanoma chemoprevention. J Am Acad Dermatol 2006;55:849–861.
78. Kricker A, Armstrong BK, Goumas C, et al. Ambient UV, personal sun exposure and risks of multiple primary melanomas. Cancer Causes Control 2007;18:295–304.
79. The International Agency for Research on Cancer Working Group on artificial ultraviolet (UV) light and skin cancer. The association of use of sunbeds with cutaneous malignant melanoma and other skin cancers: A systematic review. Int J Cancer 2007;120:1116–1122.
80. El Ghissassi F, Baan R, Straif K, et al. A review of human carcinogens-part D: Radiation. Lancet Oncol 2009;10: 751–752.
81. Centers for Disease Control and Prevention. Use of indoor tanning devices by adults—United States 2010. Morbid Mortal Wkly Rep 2012;61(18):323–326.
82. Gibney GT, Forsyth PA, Sondak VK. Melanoma of the brain: biology and therapeutic options. Melanoma Res 2012;22:144–183.
83. Dummer R, Hauschild A, Guggenheim M, et al. Cutaneous malignant melanoma: ESMO clinical practice guidelines for diagnosis, treatment and follow-up. Ann Oncol 2012;23:vii86–vii91.

117

Hematopoietic Stem Cell Transplantation

Susanne Liewer and Janelle Perkins

KEY CONCEPTS

1. Hematopoietic stem cell transplantation (HSCT) is a process that involves IV infusion of hematopoietic stem cells from a donor into a recipient, after the administration of chemotherapy with or without radiation. The rationale is to increase tumor cell kill by increasing the dose of chemotherapy. Immune-mediated effects also contribute to the tumor cell kill observed after allogeneic HSCT.
2. Hematopoietic stem cells used for transplantation can come from the recipient (autologous) or from a related or unrelated donor (allogeneic). If the related donor is a twin, the transplant is referred to as a syngeneic transplant.
3. Human leukocyte antigen (HLA) mismatching of allogeneic donor–recipient pairs at either class I or class II loci increases the risk of graft failure, graft-versus-host disease (GVHD), and worse survival. The ideal donor is one that is matched at HLA-A, -B, -C, and DRB1.
4. Hematopoietic stem cells are found in the bone marrow, peripheral blood, and umbilical cord blood. Because of the rarity and similarity to other cells, hematopoietic stem cells are difficult to isolate and measure. These stem cells express the CD34 antigen, and measurement of the number of $CD34^+$ cells is a clinically useful measure of the number of hematopoietic stem cells.
5. Because of clinical and economic advantages, peripheral blood has replaced bone marrow as the source of hematopoietic stem cells in the autologous and adult allogeneic HSCT setting.
6. The purpose of the preparative (or conditioning) regimen in traditional myeloablative transplants is twofold: (a) maximal tumor cell kill and (b) immunosuppression of the recipient to reduce the risk of graft rejection (allogeneic HSCT only).
7. Reduced-intensity conditioning regimens (including those that are nonmyeloablative) have been developed in order to reduce early posttranslant morbidity and mortality while maximizing the GVT effect of the allogeneic graft. The advantage to this approach is that patients who would otherwise not be eligible for allogeneic HSCT can now be offered a potentially curative therapy.
8. The transplant-related mortality rate associated with allogeneic HSCT ranges from 10% to 80% depending mostly on age and donor and disease status. Major causes of death include infection, organ toxicity, and GVHD. The most common cause of death after autologous HSCT is disease relapse; the transplant-related mortality rate is usually less than 5%, depending on the conditioning regimen, age, and disease status.
9. Patients undergoing allogeneic HSCT are given prophylactic immunosuppressive therapy, which inhibits T-cell activation, proliferation, or both. The most commonly used GVHD prophylaxis regimens are cyclosporine or tacrolimus and methotrexate.
10. Initial treatment of both acute and chronic GVHD consists of prednisone, either alone or combined with cyclosporine or tacrolimus. Treatment of patients with steroid-refractory GVHD is unsatisfactory.

INTRODUCTION

1 Hematopoietic stem cell transplantation (HSCT) is a process that involves IV infusion of hematopoietic stem cells from a compatible donor into a recipient, usually after administration of high-dose chemotherapy with or without radiation (called conditioning or preparative regimens). The original rationale for HSCT for treatment of malignant disease is based on studies showing that most anticancer drugs have a steep dose–response relationship and that myelosuppression limits the chemotherapy dosage that can be safely administered. Although standard-dose chemotherapy can prolong survival in many cancer patients, most patients are not cured of their disease with this strategy alone. Infusion of hematopoietic stem cells allows administration of very high doses of chemotherapy (as much as 10-fold higher) by reestablishing hematopoiesis. If tumor cells that are resistant to standard doses are sensitive to higher doses of chemotherapy, then tumor cell kill will be greatly increased, and the likelihood of cure would be higher with HSCT compared with standard dose chemotherapy. However, the chemotherapy dose cannot be escalated indefinitely because of the risk for death caused by nonhematologic toxicity (Fig. 117-1). The success of reduced-intensity conditioning (RIC) regimens shows that immune-mediated effects of the donor cells also contribute to the antitumor effect of allogeneic HSCT.

HSCT is an important modality for treatment of a variety of malignant and nonmalignant diseases. More than 16,000 transplants were performed in the United States in 2009, primarily for malignant diseases.[1] The most common malignancies treated with HSCT are multiple myeloma, lymphoma, and leukemia. The number of transplants has grown steadily over the past decade because of an increase in the number of patients receiving umbilical cord blood (UCB) transplants and patients older than 60 years undergoing transplantation.

Although HSCT is most commonly used for treatment of malignant diseases, many nonmalignant hematologic disorders, including aplastic anemia, thalassemia, and sickle cell anemia; immunodeficiency disorders; and other genetic disorders are also potentially curable with allogeneic HSCT. Transplantation is also

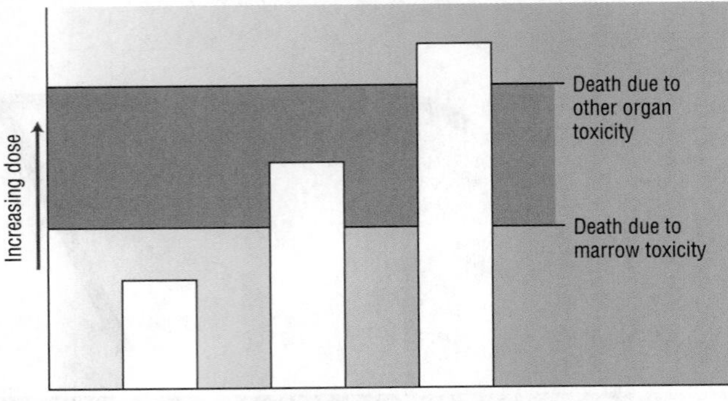

FIGURE 117-1 Patients represented by the middle column are the best candidates for hematopoietic stem cell transplantation because the technique allows for administration of chemotherapy or radiation in doses that otherwise would be intolerable because of severe myelosuppression.

being investigated as a treatment modality for patients with life-threatening autoimmune diseases, such as rheumatoid arthritis, systemic and multiple sclerosis, and systemic lupus erythematosus.

This chapter summarizes the procedures involved in HSCT and the common complications associated with HSCT. More detailed information on HSCT can be found in published reviews and books.[2–5] Information on HSCT also can be found on several websites, including *http://www.cibmtr.org* (Center for International Blood and Marrow Transplant Research [CIBMTR]) and *http://www.marrow.org* (National Marrow Donor Program).

DONORS AND HISTOCOMPATIBILITY TESTING

❷ Different types of donors are used in HSCT. The choice of donor depends on the diagnosis and disease status of the recipient as well as his or her age and comorbidities. The role and indications for HSCT are discussed in detail within individual disease chapters of this text. In *autologous* transplants, patients receive their own hematopoietic stem cells, which were collected and stored before administration of the transplant conditioning regimen. In *syngeneic* transplants, an identical twin serves as the donor. In *allogeneic* transplants, the donor is genetically not identical to the recipient but shares some common cell surface antigens called human leukocyte antigens (HLAs). These antigens are encoded by the major histocompatibility complex (MHC), a cluster of genes located on the sixth chromosome.[6] The MHC contains three distinct regions designated as class I, class II, and class III. Class I and class II genes encode for HLA; products of class III genes have other important roles in the immune system. Class I and class II HLA antigens differ in their tissue distribution, structure, and function. Their primary function is to aid the immune system in recognizing cells or tissues as "self" or "nonself." The genes (and the corresponding antigens they encode for) important in HSCT are HLA-A, HLA-B, and HLA-C (class I) and HLA-DRB1 (class II). Because of the polymorphism of the HLA system, there are many different HLA antigens within each different class of HLA. To reduce the chance of graft rejection and graft-versus-host disease (GVHD), a donor is chosen based on how many of these HLA antigens are the same as those of the recipient.

To identify a suitable allogeneic donor, both the recipient and potential donors are HLA typed (specific HLA antigens are identified); the potential donor who is most closely matched (has the most similar HLA antigens to the recipient) is generally chosen to be the transplant donor. HLA typing is accomplished by DNA-based techniques that use polymerase chain reaction (PCR) amplification of specific HLA genes from genomic DNA. DNA typing methods are categorized by the level of discrimination they provide in defining the sequence of an HLA gene. Low-resolution methods provide limited sequence information about a particular HLA gene and are typically used to identify sibling donors. However, low-resolution techniques cannot distinguish the extremely polymorphic nature of many of the HLA antigens. HLA antigens are characterized by thousands of genetic variations (alleles), and each allele may correspond to a unique HLA molecule. Different alleles can be distinguished only by high-resolution typing techniques; high-resolution methods are used to identify suitable unrelated donors.

❸ The degree of HLA mismatching correlates with the risk of graft rejection, GVHD, and survival.[6] In an analysis of 1,874 patients who received HLA-matched unrelated bone marrow donor transplants under the auspices of the National Marrow Donor Program (NMDP), low-resolution mismatches at HLA-A, HLA-B, HLA-C, and HLA-DRB1 were similarly associated with increased risk of GVHD and mortality.[7] The observation concerning the prognostic value of HLA-C was particularly important because until that time, the locus was omitted from most matching algorithms. Based on these results, HLA-C typing is now included in standard typing protocols. High-resolution mismatches, particularly at HLA-A and HLA-DRB1, also were associated with increased mortality. These findings were confirmed in an analysis of more than 3,800 unrelated bone marrow donor–recipient pairs in which high-resolution matching for HLA-A, -B, -C, and DRB1 was associated with the overall survival.[8]

In the search for an allogeneic donor, the patient's siblings are typed first. The odds that any one full sibling will match a patient are one in four. About 30% of Americans have an HLA-identical sibling. In an effort to offer allogeneic HSCT to patients who lack an HLA-identical sibling donor, alternative donors are being used. Rarely, a parent is HLA identical with his or her child. Although some patients who receive transplants from mismatched related donors experience long-term survival, their risks of graft failure and acute GVHD are higher than for recipients of matched-sibling transplants. It is estimated that only another 10% of patients will have a closely HLA-matched related donor.

The most common type of alternative donor is an individual unrelated to the recipient who is fully or closely HLA matched. To facilitate identification of these donors, the NMDP (*http://www.marrow.org*) was started in 1986 with initial funding from a U.S. Navy contract. To date, the NMDP has registered more than 10 million donors in the United States and has facilitated more than 50,000 unrelated donor transplants. Donors outside the United States can also be accessed by the NMDP through agreements with international cooperative registries. About one-third of the allogeneic HSCTs performed worldwide are from unrelated donors.[1] The NMDP currently requires that the recipient be typed by high-resolution methodology at HLA-A, -B, -C, and -DRB1. Although it is the transplant center's responsibility to select the donor, the NMDP recommends that selected donor and recipient be matched at HLA-A, -B, -C, and -DRB1 by high-resolution typing when possible for bone marrow or peripheral blood HSCT; matching criteria are less stringent for UCB transplant.[9] If more than one suitable HLA-matched unrelated donor is identified, other factors can be used to select the donor, such as younger age, being male or a nulliparous female, and negative cytomegalovirus (CMV) serostatus.

The likelihood of a recipient finding an HLA-matched donor ranges from one in 100 to one in 1,000,000, depending on the prevalence of the recipient's HLA type, race, and ethnic background. With the current size of the NMDP registry, the matching likelihood is higher than 80% for whites. Because most minorities are not as well represented in the program, the likelihood of finding a donor for patients from some racial or ethnic groups is lower. Agreements between NMDP and international registries may improve the likelihood of finding donors for these patients. Another limitation is the time needed to search for a potential donor. Some donor searches take up to 3 to 4 months, and patients with acute leukemia can relapse while waiting for completion of the search. Cost is also a concern, with the cost for donor search and procurement ranging from $25,000 to $50,000. With improved HLA typing techniques and better supportive care, most reported outcomes with matched unrelated donors are no longer significantly different than those reported with related sibling donors.[10,11]

HEMATOPOIETIC STEM CELLS

Hematopoietic stem cells serve as "mother" cells for all blood cells, including erythrocytes, leukocytes, and platelets (see eChap. 20). Stem cells have varying degrees of "stemness." True pluripotent stem cells are capable of replicating indefinitely and can give rise to stem and progenitor cells of all tissues. Multipotent stem cells, such as hematopoietic stem cells, have the capacity for self-renewal and can differentiate into more than one cell type in a particular tissue lineage. Because of their capacity for self-renewal, hematopoietic stem cells are capable of repopulating the recipient's marrow, which has been "emptied" by administration of high-dose chemotherapy, either alone or combined with radiation.

4 Hematopoietic stem cells are rare cells, comprising less than 0.01% of all bone marrow cells. Isolation and quantitative measurement of hematopoietic stem cells are extremely difficult because of their rarity and their similar appearance to other cells. For these reasons, surrogate markers are used to measure the number of stem cells. CD34 is an antigen expressed on hematopoietic stem cells and other early progenitor cells. Determination of the number of cells expressing the CD34 antigen (CD34$^+$ cells), as determined by flow cytometry, has become the standard method of measuring hematopoietic stem cell content.

Hematopoietic stem cells are found in the bone marrow, peripheral blood, and UCB. Hematopoietic stem cells from the bone marrow are obtained by multiple aspirations from the anterior and posterior iliac crests while the donor is under general anesthesia. The procedure takes about 1 hour and yields 200 to 1,500 mL, depending on the size of the donor. The marrow is transferred into tissue culture medium containing preservative-free heparin. The pooled marrow is passed through a series of stainless steel screens to break up aggregated particles, resulting in an essentially single-cell suspension. In allogeneic HSCT, the marrow stem cells are given to the recipient 12 to 24 hours after harvest. In autologous HSCT, the marrow is frozen and stored until needed. After IV infusion, the marrow stem cells enter the systemic circulation and find their way to the bone marrow cavity, where they reseed and grow in the bone marrow microenvironment. Although the donor experiences local soreness for a few days, the procedure usually is well tolerated, with no delayed complications resulting from the marrow aspiration. The major risk of serving as a marrow donor is the risk of undergoing general anesthesia.

Hematopoietic stem cells in peripheral blood (peripheral blood stem cells [PBSCs]) are found in the mononuclear fraction of white blood cells (lymphocytes and monocytes) and are collected by a procedure called leukapheresis (or apheresis). This is an outpatient procedure that involves withdrawal of blood from a vein (through a specialized IV catheter), selective removal of mononuclear cells by an apheresis machine, and reinfusion of the unneeded blood components back to the patient. During this process, about 9 to 14 L of blood is processed over several hours during each daily apheresis session. Most of the blood cells are returned to the donor, and each apheresis yields about 200 mL of cells.

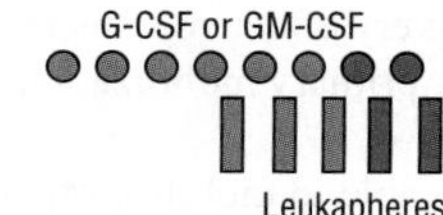

FIGURE 117-2 Schema for collection of peripheral blood progenitor cells after hematopoietic growth factor administration (top) or after chemotherapy and hematopoietic growth factor administration (bottom). Symbols with darker shading represent procedures performed only if adequate numbers of CD34$^+$ cells have not been collected. (G-CSF, granulocyte colony-stimulating factor; GM-CSF, granulocyte-macrophage colony-stimulating factor.)

The number of hematopoietic stem cells that circulate in peripheral blood normally is too low for apheresis to be technically feasible. Without mobilization techniques, at least six aphereses usually are required to collect a sufficient number of PBSCs. Several methods have been used clinically to "mobilize" hematopoietic stem cells from the bone marrow into peripheral blood for use in autologous transplantation.[12] Figure 117-2 shows representative schemas for mobilization and collection of PBSCs. One type of mobilization method is administration of chemotherapy, which can briefly increase the number of PBSCs as much as 100-fold. The more commonly used method is administration of a recombinant hematopoietic growth factor such as granulocyte colony-stimulating factor (G-CSF; filgrastim) or granulocyte-macrophage colony-stimulating factor (GM-CSF; sargramostim). Each agent has its own potential advantages and disadvantages.[12] Both agents are approved by the Food and Drug Administration (FDA) for this indication, but filgrastim is the most commonly used growth factor. Dosages are 10 mcg/kg/day (5–32 mcg/kg/day) for filgrastim and 250 mcg/m^2/day for sargramostim. The combination of chemotherapy followed by a hematopoietic growth factor increases the number of PBSCs to a greater extent than either method alone. This approach is more expensive and is associated with more adverse effects than a growth factor alone, but the number of aphereses is reduced, and the additional chemotherapy may further reduce the tumor burden before transplant, which may reduce the likelihood of tumor cell contamination in the apheresis collection. Pegfilgrastim (pegylated filgrastim) has also been evaluated in the mobilization setting, either alone or after chemotherapy. Pegylation prolongs the half-life of filgrastim from 3 to 4 hours to 33 hours, allowing for single-dose administration. Both the 6- and 12-mg doses appear to be safe and at least as effective as filgrastim.[13,14] Based on these studies, pegfilgrastim may be used in place of filgrastim for stem cell mobilization for patient convenience.

Plerixafor is a novel inhibitor of the CXCR4 chemokine receptor that is FDA approved as a mobilizing agent in combination with filgrastim. Its approval was based on two multicenter, randomized, double-blinded trials that compared filgrastim plus plerixafor or placebo as primary mobilization in patients with multiple myeloma or non-Hodgkin lymphoma.[15,16] In both studies, patients received filgrastim 10 mcg/kg/day for 4 days; on the evening of the fourth day, they received either 240 mcg/kg of plerixafor or placebo. In both studies, a significantly larger proportion of the filgrastim plus plerixafor–treated patients were able to collect the target number of CD34$^+$ cells in no more than two aphereses procedures compared with the filgrastim plus placebo group. These initial trials demonstrated that plerixafor is very effective in increasing the number of CD34+ cells available for primary mobilization of hematopoietic stem cells.

Because most patients are able to mobilize efficiently with filgrastim alone and plerixafor is expensive, transplant centers generally use some type of risk-adapted approach to identify which patients are appropriate candidates for plerixafor. One approach is to give plerixafor to patients with certain characteristics that have been associated with a high risk of poor mobilization.[17,18] These characteristics include previous exposure to extensive chemotherapy, lenalidomide, or radiation, older age, hypocellular bone marrow, or low platelet counts. Another approach is to monitor CD34+ cell counts in the peripheral blood on day 4 or 5 of filgrastim administration because low numbers of CD34+ cells after filgrastim have been associated with mobilization failure. Patients who do not have a minimal number of CD34+ cells receive plerixafor.[19–21] In general, these individualized approaches limit plerixafor administration to patients at high risk for poor mobilization.

In about 20% to 30% of autologous transplant candidates, an optimal number of CD34+ cells will not be obtained after the first attempt with standard mobilization regimens.[22] Several strategies for overcoming the obstacle of poor mobilization have been evaluated, including remobilization with the same or higher doses of the same hematopoietic growth factor, a combination of hematopoietic growth factors (i.e., filgrastim and sargramostim), or a combination of chemotherapy and a hematopoietic growth factor. Bone marrow harvest is an option but often is of limited value. Plerixafor has been evaluated in patients who have failed primary mobilization. In a study of 115 patients who had failed at least one previous mobilization attempt, plerixafor and filgrastim were given with the objective of collecting at least 2×10^6 CD34+ cells/kg.[23] Depending on diagnosis, about 60% to 75% of patients successfully mobilized with this regimen, which compares favorably with other secondary mobilization strategies. Although plerixafor with filgrastim may be effective for remobilization, it has been associated with a higher cost compared with other strategies, especially if multiple doses of plerixafor are required.[24] The decision on which secondary mobilization regimen to be used should be based on patient-specific factors and clinician judgment.

Several studies show that the number of CD34+ cells infused correlates significantly with the rate of neutrophil and platelet recovery after high-dose chemotherapy.[12] Rapid neutrophil recovery usually is observed in patients who receive at least 2×10^6 CD34+ cells/kg (body weight of recipient). More rapid platelet recovery is observed when at least 5×10^6 CD34+ cells/kg is transplanted compared with lower cell doses. As a result, most transplant centers use 2×10^6 CD34+ cells/kg as a minimum number to collect for autologous transplant, with an optimal target of 5×10^6 CD34+ cells/kg. For patients with multiple myeloma undergoing tandem transplants, cells for both transplants are collected before the first transplant. A minimum of 4×10^6 CD34+ cells/kg is required, and generally the entire cell dose collected is divided into two equal aliquots, one for each transplant.

5 Use of peripheral blood instead of bone marrow as a source of hematopoietic stem cells offers several clinical and economic advantages. The most clinically important advantage is that patients who receive mobilized PBSCs experience more rapid hematopoietic engraftment. Although engraftment of all lineages is more rapid when PBSCs are used, the most significant effect is observed with platelet recovery. Patients who receive mobilized PBSCs experience platelet recovery as much as 2 to 3 weeks earlier and require fewer platelet transfusions than those who receive bone marrow stem cells. As a result, patients usually are discharged earlier from the hospital, so the overall cost of autologous HSCT is reduced with the use of PBSCs. Another advantage is that the donor does not experience the discomfort associated with marrow aspirations and is not exposed to the risk associated with general anesthesia. PBSCs may be less likely to be contaminated with malignant cells compared with marrow stem cells. Finally, because PBSCs are collected from the mononuclear cell fraction, a fraction that also contains immunocompetent cells (e.g., natural killer [NK] cells and T lymphocytes), some investigators believe that infusion of PBSCs represents a form of "adoptive immunotherapy." In this model, NK cells and lymphocytes targeted against tumor cells help to kill residual tumor cells. As a result of these clinical and economic advantages, peripheral blood has replaced bone marrow as the source of stem cells in the autologous setting.

Peripheral blood has also become the predominant source of hematopoietic stem cells in adult allogeneic HSCT.[1,25] About 75% of allogeneic HSCTs performed in adults currently come from PBSCs harvested from normal donors. Concerns were raised initially over the safety and ethics of administering filgrastim to normal individuals volunteering as donors. Filgrastim is generally well tolerated. Short-term effects are similar to those seen in cancer patients receiving filgrastim (e.g., bone pain, headache, fever, arthralgias, malaise). Although there are concerns about increased risk of acute myelogenous leukemia (AML) in healthy subjects given filgrastim, no higher risk has been observed thus far.[26] Because of the long latent period of drug-related AML and the very low incidence of AML in the general population, longer follow-up of thousands of healthy donors will be required to definitively conclude that an association between filgrastim and AML does not exist.

Randomized controlled trials and large registry studies show that patients who received allogeneic PBSC transplants from HLA-identical siblings experienced more rapid hematopoietic recovery and required fewer transfusions compared with patients receiving bone marrow.[27] The difference in the rate of engraftment may be related to the threefold higher numbers of CD34+ cells infused in recipients of PBSC transplants. Although most of these studies did not report an increased risk of acute GVHD or transplant-related mortality in patients receiving allogeneic PBSC transplants, a higher risk of chronic GVHD has been observed. In a meta-analysis of nine randomized trials evaluating HLA-matched sibling donor transplants in adult patients, the risk of chronic GVHD was nearly twofold higher for patients who received allogeneic PBSC transplants compared with those who received bone marrow transplantation (BMT). However, the risk of relapse was higher in the patients receiving BMT, and no significant difference in overall survival was observed in the meta-analysis, although in some individual studies, disease-free and overall survival were improved with PBSC. When patients were analyzed based on disease status at the time of transplant, patients with hematologic malignancies at high risk of relapse had a better overall survival when transplanted with PBSC as compared with those who received BMT, which may be related in part to the lower risk of relapse in patients who received PBSC transplants.[27] The Blood and Marrow Transplant Clinical Trials Network recently reported the results of a trial that randomized 551 patients to allogeneic PBSC or bone marrow from matched unrelated donors.[28] At 2 years after transplant, there were no differences in overall survival, relapse, or mortality not related to relapse. Neutrophil and platelet engraftment were more rapid, and the risk of graft failure was reduced in the PBSC transplants compared with patients receiving BMT. The risk of acute GVHD was similar, but a higher incidence of chronic GVHD was reported in patients who received PBSC transplants. Two-year survival is an early outcome, and further follow-up will need to be done to determine if these results are maintained over time. Selection of the optimal source of hematopoietic stem cells for an individual patient should be based on the risk of relapse, chronic GVHD, graft failure, and donor preference. It is also important to note that most patients treated in the randomized trials of bone marrow versus peripheral blood transplants received myeloablative conditioning (MAC) regimens (discussed later), and it is unknown whether these results can be extrapolated to RIC regimens.

Several small studies have reported the engraftment and outcomes of patients receiving allogeneic bone marrow from donors who received filgrastim for 3 to 4 days before harvest. The use of the filgrastim was hypothesized to increase the yield of bone marrow from healthy donors. A meta-analysis of studies comparing filgrastim stimulated bone marrow to PBSCs showed similar rates of engraftment, acute GVHD, relapse, and overall survival but a greater risk of chronic GVHD with PBSCs. These initial studies suggest that filgrastim-stimulated bone marrow may result in early engraftment similar to PBSCs without the higher risk of GVHD.[29] A large prospective randomized trial is comparing filgrastim–mobilized PBSCs with filgrastim-stimulated bone marrow.

In addition to bone marrow and peripheral blood, hematopoietic stem cells are found in UCB. UCB is an attractive source for several reasons.[30] Because the stem cells are collected from placental blood, there is no risk to the mother or the baby and a very low risk of transmissible infectious diseases, such as cytomegalovirus and Epstein-Barr virus. The cells are available immediately because the donor does not have to be located and the stem cells harvested. UCB initially was obtained from siblings, but now recipients of transplants from unrelated donors account for almost all patients who receive UCB transplants. More than 600,000 UCB grafts are available in more than 100 UCB banks, and more than 20,000 unrelated UCB transplants have been performed worldwide.[30]

Recipients of UCB transplants usually receive a $CD34^+$ cell dose more than 1 log lower than that given to recipients of BMT, and this difference in $CD34^+$ cell dose may explain the delayed engraftment in recipients of UCB transplants. The number of infused total nucleated and $CD34^+$ cells correlates with outcomes after UCB transplantation. Although no randomized comparisons have been performed, many retrospective studies have compared outcomes of UBC transplantation with more traditional stem cell sources such as bone marrow or PBSCs. Analysis of data from the CIBMTR and the New York Blood Center showed similar survival in children with acute leukemia who underwent either unrelated HLA-mismatched UCB transplantation or unrelated HLA-matched BMT. Children who received HLA-matched UCB transplants had better outcomes than those who received HLA-matched BMTs. However, higher transplant-related mortality was observed in children transplanted with a low UCB cell dose and a mismatched UCB graft.[31] Similar studies of adults with hematologic malignancies have been conducted. The CIBMTR compared outcomes for adults with acute leukemia who were transplanted with unrelated BM or PBSC versus UCB. Both overall survival and leukemia-free survival were similar in all transplant groups. The risk of both acute and chronic GVHD was lower in UCB recipients compared with PBSC, and the risk of chronic GVHD was lower in UCB compared with bone marrow. However, transplant-related mortality was higher after UCB as compared with other stem cell sources. These data support the use of UBCs as a source of stem cells when matched PBSCs or bone marrow are not immediately available.[32]

A major limitation of UCB transplants is the small volume of blood collected, usually 60 to 150 mL with resultant low numbers of $CD34^+$ cells. Although the relatively low numbers of hematopoietic cells may be adequate for hematopoietic engraftment in children and small adults, it may not be adequate for larger recipients. Efforts to expand the number of hematopoietic stem cells include "pooling" 2 or more units of UCB for one recipient (referred to as double cord transplant). The Seattle and Minnesota groups recently published their experience in more than 500 patients older than 10 years of age who received a matched related donor, matched unrelated donor, mismatched unrelated donor, or double cord transplant. Leukemia-free survival was similar in all groups, but the double cord transplant recipients had a higher risk of transplant-related mortality. Although the role of double cord transplantation has not yet been fully defined, the results of this study suggest that pooled UBCs may provide an option for patients in which no other appropriate donors are available.[33]

APPROACHES TO ERADICATE MALIGNANT CELLS

Conditioning Regimens

6 The purpose of the pretransplant conditioning regimen (also called the preparative regimen) depends on the type of transplant and the indication for its use. In the autologous setting, pretransplant conditioning is used to eradicate malignant cells. This is also the case in allogeneic transplantation for malignant diseases, but the conditioning regimen also serves a dual purpose to suppress the recipient's immune system to allow for donor cell engraftment. Two types of conditioning regimens are used, myeloablative and reduced intensity. Myeloablative conditioning (MAC) regimens contain very high doses of chemotherapy with or without radiation that would lead to life-threatening or fatal myelosuppression if hematopoietic stem cells were not infused. Patients undergoing autologous transplantation receive MAC regimens. Reduced-intensity conditioning (RIC) regimens consist of lower doses or different types of chemotherapy or lower doses of radiation than used in MAC regimens. RIC regimens were developed after the observation was made that some of the antitumor effect of the allogeneic transplant was mediated by a reaction between the donor's immune system and the recipient's cancer cells. This meant that very high doses of chemotherapy, radiation, or both may not be needed. Because RIC regimens use lower doses of chemotherapy or radiation or less toxic drugs, older patients and those with comorbidities are now able to undergo allogeneic transplant. Both types of regimens are discussed in detail below.

Myeloablative Regimens

MAC regimens usually include at least one anticancer drug with a relatively steep dose-response curve and myelosuppression as their dose-limiting toxicity, such as alkylating agents. Cyclophosphamide, melphalan, busulfan, and carmustine are examples of chemotherapy agents commonly used in MAC regimens. Other agents are usually added that have additive or synergistic effects with these alkylating agents in specific types of cancers; other alkylating agents have also been used. Table 117-1 lists chemotherapeutic agents that are frequently used in MAC regimens as well as the doses used and their dose-limiting toxicity in the transplant setting.

Total-body irradiation (TBI) is also used in some pretransplant conditioning regimens. In patients with malignant disease, the rationale of TBI is to eradicate malignant cells located in areas inaccessible to the systemic circulation and thus to the chemotherapeutic agents. TBI also has significant immunosuppressive activity. TBI doses for MAC regimens range from 10 to 15 Gy (1,000–1500 rads), which is more than twice the lethal dose of radiation for a normal person. TBI in these doses is typically fractionated (split over several days, once or twice a day) rather than given as a single-dose. Fractionated TBI has an improved therapeutic ratio compared with single-dose administration, that is, destruction of more leukemic cells and marrow stem cells while sparing other normal tissues. The acute toxicities of TBI consist of fever, nausea, vomiting, diarrhea, mucositis, and tender swelling of the parotid gland. Long-term complications of TBI-containing regimens include cataract formation, growth retardation, carcinogenesis, permanent reproductive sterility, and secondary malignancies.

Two of the most commonly used MAC regimens for allogeneic transplant are cyclophosphamide and TBI (CyTBI) or busulfan and

TABLE 117-1 Dose-Limiting Nonhematologic Toxicities for Selected Chemotherapeutic Agents Included in Myeloablative Conditioning Regimens in Hematopoietic Stem Cell Transplantation

Drug	Conventional Dose[a] (mg/m^2)	HSCT Dose (mg/m^2)	Dose-Limiting Toxicity
Busulfan (oral)	2	450	Hepatic
Carboplatin	400	2,000	Hepatic, renal
Carmustine	200	1,200	Pulmonary, hepatic
Cisplatin	100	200	Renal, peripheral neuropathy
Cyclophosphamide	1,000	7,500	Cardiomyopathy
Etoposide	300–600	2,400	Mucositis
Ifosfamide	5,000	18,000	Renal
Melphalan	40	225	Mucositis
Thiotepa	20–50	1125	Mucositis, central nervous system

HSCT, hematopoietic stem cell transplantation.

[a]Doses are approximate and are for drugs used as single agents. When combinations are used, doses may need to be decreased.

Eder JP, Elias A, Shea TC, et al. A phase I–II study of cyclophosphamide, thiotepa, and carboplatin with autologous bone marrow transplantation in solid tumor patients. J Clin Oncol 1990;8:1242. Reprinted with permission.

cyclophosphamide (BuCy). When given with TBI, cyclophosphamide is usually given first as two doses of 60 mg/kg/day followed by TBI. In the original BuCy regimen, busulfan was given orally at a dosage of 1 mg/kg orally every 6 hours for 16 doses on days –9 to –6 (4 mg/kg/day for 4 days; day 0 being the day of transplant) followed by four doses of cyclophosphamide given IV once daily at a dosage of 50 mg/kg on days –5 to –2. In one widely used modification of the regimen (BuCy2), the total cyclophosphamide dosage is reduced from 200 (50 × 4) to 120 (60 × 2) mg/kg. Plasma busulfan concentrations are monitored at some centers because studies suggest that systemic exposure correlates with outcome, and use of a targeted busulfan and cyclophosphamide preparative regimen may improve patient outcome.[34] The IV form of busulfan (Busulfex®) reduces some of the interpatient variability in systemic exposure and may also reduce the risk of hepatotoxicity. The dose of IV busulfan approved for pretransplant conditioning regimens is 0.8 mg/kg every 6 hours for 4 days, although once-daily dosing regimens have also been developed.

Several prospective randomized studies have compared CyTBI with BuCy in patients with acute or chronic myeloid leukemia (CML) undergoing allogeneic matched related donor HSCT.[35,36] Early results of these studies showed that BuCy had similar or greater antileukemic activity than CyTBI in patients with CML and that CyTBI was associated with slightly better disease-free survival in patients with AML. However, with longer follow-up, similar survival rates were observed. In a large retrospective analysis of the CIBMTR in patients with myeloid malignancies receiving unrelated donor transplants, overall and disease-free survival were not significantly different between the two regimens.[37] Long-term toxicities between the two regimens appear to be comparable. Since the publication of these studies, several improvements in clinical practice have been made (e.g., better supportive care, more specific HLA typing methodologies, use of PBSCs) that may have some effect on the comparison of these two commonly used regimens. For example, use of the IV form and pharmacokinetic monitoring of busulfan may optimize its use, giving an advantage to the use of BuCy. In addition, other MAC regimens have been developed that may be safer or more effective. Without definitive data showing the superiority of one regimen over another, the choice of regimens before allogeneic transplant generally is based on the experience of the transplant center, patient characteristics, diagnosis, and disease status.

Conditioning regimens used in autologous HSCT are exclusively myeloablative and generally include at least one alkylating agent with other agents added that may have specific activity against the tumor type being treated. TBI usually is not included in the conditioning regimen in patients who have received prior radiotherapy. MAC regimens used in patients with lymphoma generally include different combinations of cyclophosphamide, carmustine, etoposide, and cytarabine. Rituximab is commonly added to the high-dose chemotherapy regimen in patients with CD20-positive lymphomas. Many transplant treatment regimens also use rituximab at the time of stem cell collection to reduce the number of CD20-positive lymphoma cells in the stem cell product being collected. The availability of anti-CD20–radiolabeled monoclonal antibodies, iodine-131 tositumomab and yttrium-90 ibritumomab, offers the potential to deliver targeted radiation to CD20-positive tumor cells and less to normal organs. Based on the results of several promising phase II studies with these two agents, the Blood and Marrow Transplant Clinical Trials Network conducted a prospective comparative trial randomizing patients with diffuse large B cell lymphoma to receive high-dose chemotherapy with rituximab or iodine-131 tositumomab followed by autologous HSCT.[38] Progression-free survival (PFS) and overall survival were not significantly different between the two groups, and thus these agents are not used routinely as part of conditioning for patients with lymphoma undergoing autologous HSCT. Single-agent melphalan (200 mg/m^2) is the standard conditioning regimen for patients undergoing autologous HSCT for myeloma. Studies are ongoing evaluating the addition of newer agents (e.g., bortezomib).

Reduced-Intensity Conditioning Regimens

7 Donor T cells contribute to the tumor cell kill and prevention of relapse observed after allogeneic HSCT, an effect referred to as the graft-versus-malignancy (GVM) effect. Evidence for the GVM effect is based on retrospective studies showing that patients who developed GVHD had a lower risk of leukemic relapse than those who did not develop GVHD. However, the overall survival rate was not different because of the increased nonrelapse mortality associated with GVHD. Other anecdotal evidence supporting a T cell–mediated GVM effect was the increased risk of relapse found with T cell–depleted transplants compared with unmodified transplants and the efficacy of donor lymphocyte infusions (DLIs) in producing responses in patients who have relapsed after allogeneic HSCT.

RIC regimens containing lower doses of chemotherapy or radiation or less toxic agents were developed to take advantage of the GVM effect but with a lower incidence of regimen-related toxicity than that of MAC regimens. Animal data demonstrated that MAC was not required for engraftment of donor cells (the other important role of conditioning in allogeneic HSCT), thus paving the way for the evaluation of RIC in humans.[39,40] The major advantage of RIC is that potentially curative transplants can be offered to patients who typically would not be considered for allogeneic HSCT because of their unacceptably high risk of transplant-related complications because of increased age or moderately compromised organ function. Use of RIC regimens has steadily increased in patients aged 50 and older.[1] In addition, because of the lower rate of toxicity, allogeneic HSCT with RIC can be offered to patients who have relapsed after traditional myeloablative autologous or allogeneic transplants. About 30% of allogeneic transplants are now being performed with RIC regimens.[1]

Because RIC regimens may not be completely myeloablative, host hematopoiesis can persist and lead to mixed chimerism (blood cells from both donor and recipient are present) (Fig. 117-3).[39]

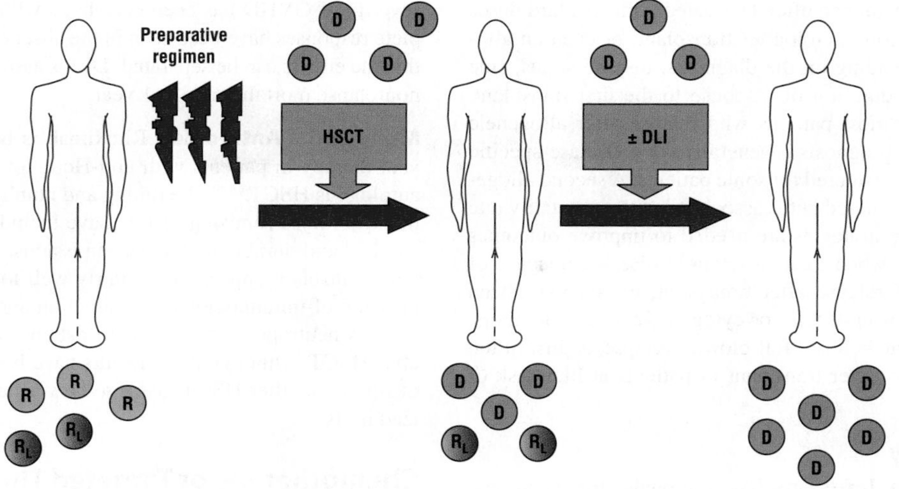

FIGURE 117-3 Schema for nonmyeloablative transplantation for hematologic malignancy. Recipients (R) receive a reduced-intensity conditioning regimen and an allogeneic hematopoietic stem cell transplant (HSCT). Initially, mixed chimerism is present with the coexistence of donor (D) cells and recipient-derived normal and leukemia/lymphoma (R_L) cells. Donor-derived T cells mediate a graft-versus-host hematopoietic effect that eradicates residual recipient-derived normal and malignant hematopoietic cells. Donor lymphocyte infusions (DLIs) can be administered to enhance graft-versus-malignancy effects.

Several studies have reported significant correlations between donor T-cell chimerism levels and the risk of graft rejection, GVHD, and relapse. For example, a low percentage of donor T and NK cells present on day 14 has been associated with graft rejection, but high T-cell donor chimerism on day 28 has been associated with acute GVHD. Achievement of full donor chimerism was associated with better PFS. These data suggest that monitoring donor chimerism after transplant may allow early interventions to prevent graft rejection or relapse.

A number of RIC regimens that vary in their cytotoxic, myelosuppressive, and immunosuppressive activity have been developed.[39,40] Most regimens include fludarabine (125–240 mg/m^2) because of its potent immunosuppressive activity, combined with either low-dose TBI (at doses up to 8 Gy [800 rad]) or an alkylating agent, such as cyclophosphamide (2–3.6 g/m^2 or 120–200 mg/kg), busulfan (up to 10 mg/kg), or melphalan (up to 180 mg/m^2). Antithymocyte globulin or alemtuzumab is sometimes given for additional immunosuppression, and other purine analogs (e.g., pentostatin or clofarabine) are sometimes used instead of fludarabine. Rituximab has also been included in patients with CD20-positive lymphoid malignancies.[41] Many of these regimens are myeloablative but are defined as RIC because of the reduced doses of chemotherapy.[42]

Some RIC regimens are considered nonmyeloablative because they result in little to no myelosuppression and do not require hematopoietic cell support for recovery of hematopoiesis. Nonmyeloablative regimens are associated with very little regimen-related toxicity but, similar to other RIC regimens, are immunosuppressive enough to result in full engraftment of important donor immune effector cells.[42] Two of the most common nonmyeloablative regimens are fludarabine (25 mg/m^2/day for 3–5 days) combined with cyclophosphamide (60 mg/kg/day × 2 days) or with TBI (≤2 Gy [<200 rad]). Although these regimens are clearly nonmyeloablative, the distinction may be more difficult with other regimens as definitions remain somewhat arbitrary.

Progression-free and overall survival varies depending on the specific RIC regimen, disease type and status at the time of transplant, donor type, and patient age and comorbidities. Patients with indolent lymphoid malignancies generally have the lowest relapse rate after RIC transplants; those with advanced myeloid and lymphoid malignancies have higher relapse rates.[43] Patients transplanted while in remission have lower relapse rates than those who were not in remission at the time of transplant. Studies evaluating "disease-targeted" therapy (radiolabeled monoclonal antibody, imatinib, or rituximab) combined with RIC transplants to improve outcomes in specific malignancies are ongoing.[39] Several large retrospective registry-based studies have reported the results of RIC regimens.[39,40,44] In general, regimen-related toxicity and nonrelapse mortality have been reported to be lower than that of historical or concurrent control participants receiving MAC regimens in nonrandomized comparisons. This is remarkable considering the older age and higher incidence of comorbidities in patients receiving RIC transplants. Of concern, however, has been an increased rate of relapse seen in some comparisons, resulting in similar overall survival being reported regardless of regimen intensity. Prospective randomized trials are needed to more fully define the role of RIC regimens in specific patient populations and to determine their relative safety and efficacy compared with standard MAC regimens. Until the results of those trials are available, most centers will continue to use RIC regimens because of better tolerability, especially in older patients and those with significant comorbidities.

Clinical **Controversy...**

Although RIC regimens reduce transplant-related mortality, whether this approach results in improved survival compared with MAC regimens is not clear. Direct comparison of the results of RIC versus MAC transplants is difficult because patients undergoing RIC transplants tend to be older and have more comorbidities. Randomized controlled trials addressing these questions are ongoing, and the results of these studies should better define the role of RIC transplants.

Posttransplant Therapy

Relapse of primary disease remains the most common cause of death for both allogeneic and autologous transplant patients. Several posttransplant therapies have been evaluated, including immunotherapy, conventional chemotherapy, and targeted therapy. Relapse after autologous transplant can often be treated with standard doses of chemotherapy, a second autologous transplant, or even an allogeneic transplant, depending on the diagnosis, disease status, side effects, response, and duration of response to the first transplant. Treatment options for most patients who relapse after allogeneic HSCT are limited, and prognosis is generally poor. Disease-specific chemotherapy can be considered for some patients. A second allogeneic HSCT may be considered but is associated with a mortality rate of up to 45%.[45] Newer strategies are needed to improve outcomes while limiting toxicity when treating relapsed disease. Because of the poor prognosis of relapse after transplant, efforts have been focused on treatment of molecular or cytogenetic disease markers, which generally appear before "full-blown" relapse or institution of maintenance therapy after transplant in patients at high risk of relapse.

Immunotherapy

Donor Lymphocyte Infusions The rationale for posttransplant immunotherapy after allogeneic HSCT is based on the GVM effect. To take advantage of the GVM effect in patients who relapse after allogeneic HSCT, immunosuppressive therapy being used for GVHD is withdrawn as quickly as possible without inducing a serious GVHD flare. In rare cases, this is enough to reinduce a remission, but in the majority of cases, further therapy is required. Perhaps the most commonly used form of posttransplant immunotherapy is DLIs.[46,47] Lymphocytes are collected from the same donor who provided hematopoietic stem cells for the original transplant. Response to DLI is disease specific. More than 80% of patients with CML who are in cytogenetic or molecular relapse respond to DLI. The response rate of patients in more advanced phases is about 15% to 30%. Although the time to response is delayed (median, 3–4 months), patients often have a durable molecular remission to DLI. Response rates to DLI of patients with other myeloid malignancies, such as AML and myelodysplasia, are generally lower (25%–30%) than the rates of patients with CML.[46,47] This may be related to the rapid proliferation of acute leukemia within the often prolonged time to response after DLI or to the lack of suitable target antigens on non-CML cells for recognition by donor cytotoxic T cells. Patients with relapsed AML after HSCT are more likely to achieve a complete response to DLI if they had a longer remission period after transplant and had some GVHD after the DLI; low tumor burden, remission at the time of DLI, and good-risk cytogenetics have also been shown to be favorable characteristics. Administration of induction chemotherapy before DLI administration may improve the antitumor activity of DLI in patients with AML, but this method has not been tested in a randomized study. DLI has been shown to have limited benefit in patients with relapsed acute lymphocytic leukemia (ALL) after transplant.

Donor lymphocyte infusion appears to be effective in patients with multiple myeloma who relapse after allogeneic HSCT, with reported response rates of 40% to 50%. Because it is relatively uncommon for a patient with multiple myeloma to be a candidate for allogeneic HSCT and patients have the option of treatment with lenalidomide or bortezomib after HSCT, the role of DLI in this population remains unclear. Chemotherapy followed by DLI may induce a GVM effect in patients with relapsed lymphoma. The highest response rates were reported in patients with indolent lymphoma while more aggressive malignancies had lower response rates.

The most serious complications of DLI are pancytopenia and GVHD, and DLI is not usually given to patients with GVHD. The cytopenias generally are transient and can be treated with hematopoietic growth factors. Some patients may have a more prolonged course of aplasia with associated risk of infection, bleeding, and anemia, and these patients may benefit from another infusion of donor hematopoietic stem cells. Acute GVHD (grade II or greater) occurs in 40% to 60% of patients receiving DLI. Although the severity of GVHD has been correlated with the GVM effect, complete responses have been seen in the absence of GVHD, suggesting that the effects can be separated. DLI is associated with 10% to 15% nonrelapse mortality rate at 1 year.

Monoclonal Antibodies Rituximab is being evaluated as adjuvant therapy in patients with non-Hodgkin lymphoma treated with autologous HSCT.[48,49] The timing and number of doses of rituximab therapy vary. Promising results have included increased event-free survival and durable molecular remissions. Rituximab after autologous transplant appears to be fairly well tolerated. Prolonged suppression of immunoglobulin production and hematologic toxicities such as neutropenia can occur in patients who received rituximab after HSCT. Although these results have been encouraging, the use of rituximab after HSCT needs to be verified within large randomized trials.

Chemotherapy or Targeted Therapy

Tyrosine kinase inhibitors (TKIs), such as imatinib, have been shown to be effective in the prevention and treatment of relapse after allogeneic HSCT in patients with CML and Philadelphia chromosome–positive (Ph+) ALL.[50] In patients with CML who experience hematologic relapse (presence of leukemic blasts in blood or bone marrow) after allogeneic HSCT, imatinib has been reported to induce complete hematologic responses (disappearance of leukemic blasts) and complete cytogenetic responses (disappearance of cytogenetic markers of disease) in a majority of these patients. Outcomes in patients with Ph+ ALL have also been encouraging. Second-generation TKIs, dasatinib and nilotinib, have also been used in both patient populations with relapsed disease. These agents appear to be effective with acceptable toxicity profiles.[50] TKIs are also given soon after transplant to prevent relapse (maintenance therapy) or to treat early relapse described as minimal residual disease (preemptive therapy; i.e., appearance of molecular or cytogenetic markers of disease before appearance of leukemic blast in the bone marrow or peripheral blood).[50,51] Patients with Ph+ ALL and CML without evidence of disease after transplant who are treated with imatinib to prevent relapse appear to have sustained cytogenetic remissions (without evidence of cytogenetic markers of disease). In a preemptive study of patients with Ph+ ALL, 50% of patients who had minimal residual disease detected after stem cell transplant had a complete response to TKI therapy.[51] TKIs are generally well tolerated after transplant. Commonly reported side effects include neutropenia, thrombocytopenia, liver function abnormalities, edema, and muscle pain. Larger comparative studies will be required to clearly define the benefit of TKIs after transplant, as well as the optimal dosing, timing, and duration of therapy.

Based on its activity in AML and MDS, 5-azacitidine is being evaluated in the posttransplant setting to prevent or treat relapse in patients with these diagnoses. Investigators at the MD Anderson Cancer Center performed a dose and schedule finding study with 5-azacitidine in patients who were in a complete remission after HSCT. The dose-limiting toxicity was thrombocytopenia, and the optimal dose was 32 mg/m^2 given subcutaneously for 5 days for 4 cycles. This study demonstrated that low-dose azacitidine may be administered in this population safely, and it may prolong event-free survival and overall survival, justifying further studies to optimize outcomes.[52]

Posttransplant therapy is also being evaluated in patients with multiple myeloma. Previous studies showed a potential benefit of thalidomide to prevent relapse after transplant, but its use is limited by neurotoxicity and other bothersome adverse effects. When given after autologous transplant in patients with nonprogressing disease, lenalidomide has been shown to prolong PFS compared with patients receiving placebo.[53,54] However, a small but significant increased incidence of second primary cancers was reported in the lenalidomide-treated patients. Further study is needed to better define the risk of second malignancies. Patients should be aware of this potential safety issue when discussing treatment with lenalidomide after autologous HSCT. Bortezomib maintenance therapy after autologous HSCT has also been associated with prolonged PFS.[55]

TRANSPLANT-RELATED COMPLICATIONS

8 Although many patients with cancer who are treated with high-dose chemotherapy and autologous or allogeneic HSCT experience long-term survival and cure of their disease, this modality is associated with many serious and potentially life-threatening complications. In the early 1970s, the posttransplant mortality rate was extremely high, and most allogeneic HSCT patients did not survive beyond 100 days because of infection, GVHD, organ toxicities, and leukemic relapse. Today, largely because of the availability of improved broad-spectrum antiinfective agents, immunosuppressive drugs, and hematopoietic growth factors, the transplant-related mortality rate after allogeneic HSCT with HLA-matched sibling donors has been reduced to less than 30%. The mortality rate is even lower with the use of RIC regimens. Causes of death are still related to transplant-related organ toxicity, GVHD, or immunosuppression. Until recently, allogeneic HSCT usually was restricted to patients younger than 50 years with an HLA-identical sibling donor and younger than 40 years with an HLA-matched unrelated donor. With advances in the prevention and treatment of transplant-related complications and the availability of RIC regimens, allogeneic HSCT now is being offered to patients up to the age of 70 years. The risk of transplant-related mortality after high-dose chemotherapy with autologous HSCT generally is less than 5%, depending on patient population and conditioning regimen. The mortality rate is lower with autologous transplants because of the lack of GVHD and associated complications of immunosuppression. Transplant-related mortality in autologous HSCT usually is caused by regimen-related toxicity or infection.

Table 117-1 lists the dose-limiting nonhematologic toxicities for several drugs that are commonly included in MAC regimens. These toxicities may be uncommon or rare with administration of conventional doses of specific drugs. When these agents are given in high doses, the toxicities seen with conventional doses (e.g., mucositis, enteritis, nausea, vomiting, hematuria) can be more frequent or severe. Several unusual and severe manifestations of regimen-related toxicities are discussed in this section.

Sinusoidal Obstruction Syndrome

Sinusoidal obstruction syndrome (SOS), formerly known as hepatic venoocclusive disease, occurs as a result of chemotherapy-induced damage to the sinusoidal endothelial cells of the liver, which leads to release of proinflammatory cytokines and further damage to the endothelium. Gaps develop between the endothelial cells allowing cellular debris to accumulate, causing the sinusoids to narrow and eventually become occluded. In addition, injury to the endothelial cells produces fibrin deposition and clot formation, further narrowing the sinusoids.[56] These histologic changes can lead to obstruction of sinusoidal flow, reduced hepatic venous outflow, portal hypertension, and hepatic failure. Clinical signs of SOS include fluid retention (resulting in sudden weight gain and ascites), hepatomegaly (sometimes painful), and hyperbilirubinemia or jaundice. SOS usually occurs within the first 4 weeks after transplant, and the incidence of SOS ranges from 5% to 20% in most published series. Severe SOS is fatal in 50% to 75% of cases. Factors that have been reported to increase the risk of SOS include use of TBI-containing conditioning regimens (dose dependent), use of sirolimus for the prevention of GVHD, increased systemic exposure to busulfan, individual variability in cyclophosphamide metabolism, chronic viral hepatitis, and elevated liver function test results before transplant. Pretransplant exposure to gemtuzumab ozogamicin (Mylotarg®) has been implicated in the development of SOS in patients undergoing allogeneic HSCT, especially when given within a few months of transplant.

The pharmacokinetics of busulfan or cyclophosphamide may correlate with the risk of SOS.[57] Because busulfan concentrations have been correlated with the risk of SOS, many HSCT centers adjust busulfan doses based on plasma concentrations. Exposure to the O-carboxymethyl-phosphoramide mustard metabolite of cyclophosphamide has been reported to correlate with the risk of SOS and nonrelapse mortality. In addition, when busulfan and cyclophosphamide are given in combination, the order in which they are given may contribute to the risk of SOS. Presumably because of the effect of busulfan on cyclophosphamide pharmacokinetics (increased exposure to active or toxic metabolites), liver toxicity appears to be worse when busulfan is given first, as traditionally given in the BuCy regimen. This effect appears to be ameliorated by reversing the order or delaying cyclophosphamide administration to 24 to 48 hours after busulfan.[58]

Some studies suggest that prostaglandin E_1, unfractionated low-molecular-weight heparin, or ursodiol may be partially effective in preventing SOS.[57] In a systematic review of three randomized trials comparing prophylactic ursodiol versus no treatment, Tay et al.[59] found a reduced risk of SOS (relative risk [RR], 0.34; 95% confidence interval [CI], 0.17–0.66) with prophylactic ursodiol. These studies were conducted in patients undergoing myeloablative transplants. The transplant-related mortality rate was reduced (RR, 0.58; 95% CI, 0.35–0.95). Other outcomes, such as relapse and overall survival, were not affected. Defibrotide, a polydisperse oligonucleotide with fibrinolytic properties, is another agent that has been used successfully in the prophylaxis of SOS, mostly in pediatric transplant patients.[56]

Treatment is generally supportive, including fluid and electrolyte management. Mild to moderate disease generally resolves without specific therapy. Recombinant tissue plasminogen activator has been given to patients with severe SOS because of the possible role of the coagulation cascade in the pathogenesis of SOS. Responses have been reported, but patients also experienced a higher risk of bleeding.[57] Some evidence supports the use of defibrotide in the treatment of patients with severe SOS, demonstrating improved response rates and lower mortality compared with historical control participants.[56]

Pulmonary Complications

Pulmonary complications after HSCT can be categorized as infectious and noninfectious (infectious complications are discussed in Chap. 100). Noninfectious complications can be caused by direct damage to the pulmonary tissue by chemotherapy or radiation used in the conditioning regimen, immune effects of the graft, or other causes not clearly understood. Early complications include diffuse alveolar hemorrhage, engraftment syndrome, and idiopathic interstitial pneumonitis. Diffuse alveolar hemorrhage is characterized by dyspnea, hypoxia, dry cough, and fever; chest radiography usually shows diffuse infiltrates in an alveolar pattern. Diffuse alveolar hemorrhage is diagnosed by examination of bronchoalveolar lavage fluid via bronchoscopy, which reveals progressively bloodier fluid with each instilled aliquot and negative findings on microbiologic analysis. Although the condition can be life-threatening or fatal, prompt treatment with high doses of corticosteroids is sometimes beneficial. A few patients have been treated successfully with recombinant human activated factor VIIa, desmopressin, or aminocaproic acid.[60]

Engraftment syndrome is characterized by fever, erythrodermatous skin rash, and noncardiogenic pulmonary edema can occur during neutrophil recovery after HSCT.[61] The incidence of engraftment syndrome is not known because of the lack of uniform diagnostic criteria, although some series report that about 10% of patients who receive autologous HSCT develop the syndrome. Engraftment syndrome can progress to life-threatening respiratory failure with or without multiple organ failure. Corticosteroids are effective in some patients.

Idiopathic interstitial pneumonitis (also called idiopathic pneumonia syndrome) is defined as widespread alveolar injury in the absence of active lower respiratory tract infection after HSCT.[62] Patients with idiopathic interstitial pneumonitis are clinically indistinguishable from patients with interstitial pneumonitis related to infection. Idiopathic interstitial pneumonitis is postulated to have a multifactorial etiology, including toxic effects of MAC, immunologic cell-mediated injury, inflammatory cytokine-induced lung damage, and occult pulmonary infections. The risk is similar in recipients of autologous or allogeneic HSCT but appears to be higher in patients who are conditioned with a TBI-containing regimen or who have acute GVHD. A mortality rate as high as 70% has been reported, and treatment consists of supportive care only. Etanercept has been beneficial in some patients with idiopathic interstitial pneumonitis.[63]

Late pulmonary complications cover a wide spectrum of disorders and include both obstructive and restrictive lung diseases.[64] The most well-described of these disorders is bronchiolitis obliterans with or without organizing pneumonia. Although bronchiolitis obliterans is thought to be a result of chronic GVHD affecting the lungs, its pathogenesis has not been completely elucidated. Therapy consists of corticosteroids, which are approximately 50% effective. Patients with mild to moderate airflow impairment appear to have the best response. The survival rate at 5 years from diagnosis of bronchiolitis obliterans is less than 20%.

Graft Failure

Initial engraftment after high-dose chemotherapy conditioning regimens usually occurs in the first 2 to 4 weeks after transplant. Engraftment is evidenced by rising peripheral blood counts and the presence of hematopoietic precursor cells in the marrow. In allogeneic HSCT, the presence of donor cells (i.e., chimerism) is confirmed by PCR-based analysis of polymorphic DNA sequences of cells from the bone marrow and peripheral T cells. Full chimerism is defined as greater than 95% of cells of donor origin. In most patients, engraftment is sustained with complete recovery of hematopoiesis.

However, graft failure (loss of bone marrow function with resultant lose in peripheral blood counts) can occur. It can be the result of heavy pretreatment with chemotherapy or radiation therapy (or both); infusion of insufficient numbers of hematopoietic stem cells; viral infection; recurrence of primary hematologic malignancy; drug reaction (e.g., to ganciclovir); development of a secondary myelodysplasia; or in the allogeneic setting, an immunologic reaction between the donor and recipient caused by inadequate immunosuppression of the recipient (i.e., graft rejection). Two syndromes have been observed. Whereas early graft failure occurs when the rate of hematopoietic recovery is delayed or does not occur at all (primary graft failure or delayed engraftment), late graft failure is characterized by a decline in peripheral blood counts after initial engraftment (secondary graft failure). With widespread use of PBSCs and posttransplant growth factors, primary graft failure is rare after autologous and HLA-matched allogeneic HSCT but is not uncommon after UCB transplant. Graft failure that occurs after allogeneic HSCT, characterized by regrowth of immunocompetent recipient cells and a simultaneous loss of donor cells, is referred to as *graft rejection*. Graft rejection occurs rarely after HLA-matched allogeneic HSCT. An increased risk of graft rejection has been observed in recipients of hematopoietic stem cells from HLA-mismatched donors, recipients of T cell–depleted marrow, and patients with severe aplastic anemia. The long-term prognosis of patients with graft failure is poor. Despite supportive care and treatment with hematopoietic growth factors, death may result from infection or bleeding. In some patients with an allogeneic donor, a second infusion of stem cells can be attempted.

Hematopoietic growth factors usually are given after transplant to patients who receive autologous HSCT, although some clinicians believe that posttransplant filgrastim or sargramostim is unnecessary because of the already rapid engraftment seen after mobilized PBSC transplants.[65,66] Sargramostim is dosed at 250 mcg/m^2/day, and filgrastim is usually dosed at 5 or 10 mcg/kg/day. Growth factors can be initiated the day of, the day after, or as late as 7 days after the infusion of stem cells and are continued until neutrophil recovery to greater than an arbitrary number of neutrophils (500–1,000 cells/mm^3 [$0.5–1.0 \times 10^9$]). Pegfilgrastim appears to be equally efficacious to filgrastim in this setting.

Hematopoietic growth factors accelerate the rate of hematopoietic recovery in patients undergoing allogeneic HSCT. In a meta-analysis of 34 randomized controlled trials, no increased risk of acute GVHD or treatment-related mortality was observed when filgrastim or sargramostim was used after allogeneic HSCT.[67] In another retrospective analysis of 2,719 patients from the CIBMTR, no association between filgrastim use and acute or chronic GVHD, transplant-related mortality, or survival was observed in recipients of HLA-identical sibling bone marrow, recipients of HLA-identical sibling peripheral blood, and recipients of HLA-matched unrelated donor bone marrow.[68] Filgrastim is most commonly used in patients receiving UCB transplants who are at increased of delayed engraftment and graft failure.

Results of studies with platelet growth factors, such as thrombopoietin and interleukin-11 (IL-11), given posttransplant have been disappointing. Platelet transfusions remain the standard of care in patients with thrombocytopenia below a given threshold (e.g., 10,000 cells/mm^3 [10×10^9]) and in patients with significant bleeding.

Anemia may be problematic in the posttransplant setting, especially in patients receiving allogeneic HSCT. The etiology is unclear and most likely is multifactorial. Although erythropoietin administration may be useful in reducing the need for red blood cell transfusions, its use in cancer patients is associated with an increased risk of adverse events and is limited by FDA warnings and restrictions.

Graft-versus-Host Disease

GVHD is caused by immunocompetent allogeneic donor T cells reacting against recipient/host antigens presented by antigen-presenting cells (APCs). In that setting, donor T cells recognize unmatched major or minor histocompatibility antigens of the host as genetically foreign, become activated, proliferate, and attack recipient tissue, thereby producing the clinical syndrome of GVHD.

Two different clinical GVHD syndromes (acute and chronic) are recognized, depending on the time of onset and clinical presentation.[69,70] Acute GVHD usually presents before day 100 after transplant (classic acute GVHD), but it can be persistent, recurrent, or late onset with clinical manifestations occurring after day 100. Acute GVHD observed after day 100 usually is the result of immunosuppression withdrawal for relapsed or persistent malignancy or administration of DLI or occurs in the setting of RIC. Chronic GVHD usually occurs after day 100, either with or without concurrent acute GVHD. Chronic GVHD without characteristics of acute GVHD (classic chronic GVHD) occurs after resolution of acute GVHD or de novo (no prior acute GVHD). An "overlap syndrome" may occur in which features of both acute and chronic GVHD are

TABLE 117-2 Consensus Grading of Acute Graft-versus-Host Disease

	Organ/Extent of Involvement		
	Skin	**Liver**	**Intestinal Tract**
Stage			
1	Rash on <25% of skin[a]	Bilirubin 2–3 mg/dL (34.2–51.3 μmol/L)[b]	Diarrhea >500 mL/day[c] or persistent nausea[d]
2	Rash on 25%–50% of skin	Bilirubin 3–6 mg/dL (51.3–102.6 μmol/L)	Diarrhea >1,000 mL/day
3	Rash on >50% of skin	Bilirubin 6–15 mg/dL (102.6–256.5 μmol/L)	Diarrhea >1,500 mL/day
4	Generalized erythroderma with bulla formation	Bilirubin >15 mg/dL (>256.5 μmol/L)	Severe abdominal pain with or without ileus
Grade			
0	None	None	None
I	Stage 1–2	None	None
II	Stage 3	or Stage 1	or Stage 1
III	—	Stage 2–3	or Stage 2–4
IV[e]	Stage 4	or Stage 4	—

[a]Use the "rule of nines" to determine body surface area involvement.
[b]Range given as total bilirubin. Downgrade one stage if an additional cause of elevated bilirubin has been documented.
[c]Volume of diarrhea applies to adults. For pediatric patients, the volume of diarrhea should be based on body surface area.
[d]Persistent nausea with histologic evidence of graft-versus-host disease in the stomach or duodenum.
[e]Grade IV may include lesser organ involvement but with extreme decrease in performance status.

Reprinted from Semin Hematol, Vol. 43, Deeg HJ, Artin JH. The clinical spectrum of acute graft-verus-host disease, pages 24–31. Copyright © Elsevier 2006 with permission from Elsevier.

present simultaneously, usually when chronic GVHD develops before resolution of acute GVHD (also called progressive onset). Whereas acute GVHD usually is limited to the gastrointestinal tract, skin, and liver, signs and symptoms of chronic GVHD resemble an autoimmune disorder and can affect many organ systems.

A "hyperacute" form of GVHD may occur in patients with multiple HLA mismatches and in patients who receive T cell–replete transplants without adequate GVHD prophylaxis, especially after MAC regimens.[71] Descriptions of hyperacute GVHD vary but usually include fever, generalized erythroderma, desquamation, and edema. More severe forms with accompanying organ failure have been seen in haploidentical donors. Hyperacute GVHD typically occurs about 1 week after transplant before engraftment of neutrophils. The response rate to first-line therapy appears to be lower in patients with hyperacute GVHD compared with patients who develop GVHD later after transplant, but no difference in survival has been observed.

Acute Graft-versus-Host Disease

The pathophysiology of acute GVHD has been described as a three-step process.[72] In step 1, the conditioning regimen causes damage to the intestinal mucosa, leading to release of lipopolysaccharides into the systemic circulation. This stimulates secretion of inflammatory cytokines such as IL-1 and tumor necrosis factor-α (TNF-α). These cytokines upregulate MHC gene products and host APCs such as dendritic cells, which play a critical role in this immune response. In step 2, donor T cells are activated, and secretion of other cytokines (IL-2 and interferon-γ) by activated T cells results in recruitment of macrophages and alteration of target cells in the gastrointestinal tract and skin so that they are more susceptible to damage. In step 3, multiple cytotoxic effector cells (T cells and macrophages) are generated and contribute to target tissue injury by secreting more inflammatory cytokines that cause target cell apoptosis. The term "cytokine storm" is sometimes used to describe the critical role of inflammatory cytokines in this process.

Based on this three-step model, three general approaches have been used to prevent GVHD in humans. The first is to reduce host tissue damage with the use of RIC regimens. The second and most widely used approach is to modulate donor T cells by reducing T-cell numbers (T-cell depletion), activation (most immunosuppressive agents), or proliferation (antiproliferative agents). The third approach is to block inflammatory stimulation and effectors (e.g., TNF-α inhibition, IL-1 receptor blockade).

The principal target organs in acute GVHD are the skin, liver, and gastrointestinal tract.[72] Acute GVHD is classified into four grades, depending on the number of organs involved and the degree of involvement of each organ (Table 117-2). Grade I disease involves only the skin. Grades II through IV involve the skin and the liver, gastrointestinal tract, or both. Acute skin GVHD usually is manifested as a generalized maculopapular rash that initially involves the face, ears, palms, soles, and upper trunk. The skin rash can spread to the rest of the body and, if untreated or refractory to treatment, will progress to bullae formation and desquamation similar to a burn injury. Gastrointestinal GVHD presents as a secretory diarrhea but may progress to abdominal pain or cramping and ileus; hemorrhage may also occur. GVHD of the upper intestinal tract appears as persistent nausea, vomiting, anorexia, and dyspepsia. The diagnosis of gastrointestinal GVHD should be made by biopsy of the intestinal tract (stomach, duodenum, or rectum). Hepatic GVHD usually is asymptomatic, consisting of hyperbilirubinemia and elevated alkaline phosphatase levels; increases in serum transaminases occur less consistently. The diagnosis can be made by biopsy, if possible.

The overall incidence of moderate to severe (grades II–IV) acute GVHD ranges from 10% to more than 80%.[72] Mortality directly attributable to acute GVHD or its treatment occurs in 10% to 20% of patients. The incidence of GVHD is related to the degree of histocompatibility, number of T cells in the graft, donor and recipient age and gender, intensity of the conditioning regimen, source of hematopoietic cells (bone marrow vs. peripheral blood), and prophylactic regimen. The most severe acute GVHD is observed in allogeneic HSCT with non–HLA-identical donors. In these settings, the incidence of grades II to IV acute GVHD can exceed 50% despite aggressive GVHD prophylaxis. Severe acute GVHD is a major cause of mortality with the risk of death increasing as the grade of GVHD increases. This risk is further increased if initial therapy is not effective.

Multiorgan acute GVHD and the drugs given to prevent or treat the disease are associated with delayed immunologic recovery and increased susceptibility to infections. Infection is often the primary cause of death in patients with GVHD. Patients with GVHD treated with an immunosuppressive regimen should receive prophylactic antiviral, antibacterial, and antifungal therapy and be monitored routinely for the occurrence of these infections.

Prevention of Acute Graft-versus-Host Disease 9 Because treatment of established acute GVHD often is unsatisfactory, aggressive preventive measures usually are taken. The most common strategy used to prevent acute GVHD is to block the activation of T cells by administration of immunosuppressive agents.[72] Several immunosuppressive agents have been used, including methotrexate, cyclosporine, tacrolimus, sirolimus, mycophenolate mofetil, antithymocyte globulin, corticosteroids, and monoclonal antibodies directed at T cells. Table 117-3 shows the doses, toxicities, and monitoring of immunosuppressive agents used to prevent or treat GVHD. Most GVHD prophylaxis regimens combine immunosuppressive agents that affect different stages of T-cell activation. The most commonly used GVHD prophylaxis regimens are cyclosporine or tacrolimus and methotrexate. Another strategy is removing or depleting most T cells from donor bone marrow ex vivo before transplant by physical separation or by treatment with monoclonal antibodies directed at T cells.

Despite standard prophylaxis with cyclosporine or tacrolimus and methotrexate, grade II to IV acute GVHD occurs in 30% to 50% in matched related donor transplants and 40% to 70% in matched unrelated donor transplants. IV cyclosporine or tacrolimus usually is started a few days before or on the day of transplant. Cyclosporine is given at an initial dosage of 3 to 5 mg/kg/day and tacrolimus at 0.02 to 0.03 mg/kg/day. Dosages are adjusted based on trough concentrations. Patients are converted to oral formulations when they can be tolerated. Cyclosporine and tacrolimus typically are given at full doses until days 50 to 100, gradually tapered in the absence of GVHD, and discontinued by day 180. Methotrexate is given IV on days 1, 3, 6, and 11 after transplant. The methotrexate dose is 10 mg/m^2 except for the first dose given on day 1 (15 mg/m^2). Alternatively, some centers use 5 mg/m^2 (same schedule). The day 11 dose is sometimes omitted because of severe mucositis or hepatotoxicity or development of conditions that may prolong methotrexate systemic exposure (e.g., renal failure or third spacing). For patients

TABLE 117-3 Immunosuppression for the Prevention and Treatment of GVHD

Agent	Dose	Drug Monitoring
Prevention		
Tacrolimus[73,74]	0.02–0.03 mg/kg/day IV beginning 1–3 days before transplant; change to PO when able to tolerate	Check serum levels ~72 hours after start and then 2–3 times/wk until stable (trough serum levels, 5–15 mcg/L); serum creatinine for renal toxicity, CBC for hematologic toxicity, blood pressure for hypertension, and BMP for electrolyte abnormalities
Cyclosporine[73,74]	3–5 mg/kg/day IV beginning 1–3 days before transplant; change to PO when able to tolerate	Check blood levels ~72 hours after start and then 2–3 times/wk until stable (trough blood levels, 150–450 mcg/L); serum creatinine for renal toxicity, CBC for hematologic toxicity, blood pressure for hypertension, and BMP for electrolyte abnormalities
Sirolimus[75]	Loading dose 12 mg PO on day +1 followed by 4 mg PO daily starting on day +2	Check serum levels ~24 hours after start and then 2–3 times/wk until stable (trough serum levels, 3–12 mcg/L); serum creatinine for renal toxicity and CBC for hematologic toxicity
Methotrexate[72,73]	15 mg/m^2 IV on day +1 followed by 10 mg/m^2 IV on days +3, 6, and 11 *or* 5 mg/m^2 IV on days +1, 3, 6, and 11	Monitor for toxicity: mucositis, LFTs for hepatic dysfunction, serum creatinine for renal impairment, fluid retention, and CBC for hematologic toxicity; methotrexate levels are not routinely monitored unless the patient develops renal dysfunction or third spacing; doses may be omitted if severe mucositis or hepatotoxicity develops
Mycophenoloate[77]	15 mg/kg/dose IV twice daily beginning on day 0; change to PO when able to tolerate	Monitor for toxicity: CBC for neutropenia and severe GI symptoms
Pentostatin[81]	1.5 mg/m^2 IV weekly × 4 doses beginning day +8	Monitor for toxicity: BMP for renal impairment and CBC for thrombotic thrombocytopenic purpura
Cyclophosphamide[79]	50 mg/kg/day IV on days +3 and +4	Monitor for toxicity: BMP for renal impairment, LFTs for hepatic toxicity (including SOS), urinalysis for hemorrhagic cystitis, vital signs and possible cardiac workup for pericarditis (only for symptomatic patients)
Rabbit anti-thymocyte globulin (ATG)[72]	2.5–5 mg/kg/day IV beginning 3 days before transplant	Monitor for toxicity: frequent vital signs during infusion for fever, rash, cardiovascular and GI dysfunction, anaphylaxis and serum sickness
Alemtuzumab[72]	10–20 mg/day IV daily beginning 4–5 days before transplant	Monitor for toxicity: fever, chills, infection, anaphylaxis
Treatment		
Methylprednisolone[a] *or* Prednisone[a,87]	1–2 mg/kg/day	Monitor for toxicity: glucose for hyperglycemia, blood pressure for hypertension, labile mood, bone osteopenia, avascular bone necrosis, impaired wound healing, adrenal insufficiency
Mycophenolate[87]	1.5–2 g PO daily in divided doses	As above
Sirolimus[87]	1–2 mg/day; then adjust based on levels	As above
Denileukin diftitox[87]	9 mcg/kg on days 1, 3, 5, 15, 17, and 19	Monitor for toxicity: LFTs for hepatic toxicity
Infliximab[87]	10 mg/kg/wk for at least 4 doses	Monitor for toxicity: anaphylaxis (rare)
Etanercept[87]	0.4 mg/kg/dose (maximum dose, 25 mg) SC twice weekly for 8 weeks	Monitor for toxicity; generally well tolerated
Rabbit ATG[87]	0.5 mg/kg for first dose followed by 1–1.5 mg/kg for subsequent doses	As above
Pentostatin[87]	1.5 mg/m^2 IV on days 1–3 and 15–17	As above

BMP, basic metabolic panel; CBC, complete blood count; GI, gastrointestinal; LFT, liver function test; PO, orally; SC, subcutaneous; SOS, sinusoidal obstruction syndrome.

[a]Considered 1st line therapy.

who experience significant toxicity from methotrexate, monitoring of methotrexate levels with leucovorin rescue may be warranted.

Two large multicenter randomized trials, one in HLA identical sibling donors and the other matched unrelated donors, compared cyclosporine and methotrexate with tacrolimus and methotrexate.[73,74] Both studies found the tacrolimus combination to be significantly superior to the cyclosporine combination in preventing grades II to IV acute GVHD. Survival did not differ between the two acute GVHD prophylaxis strategies, but the risk of renal impairment and need for hemodialysis were higher in patients receiving tacrolimus. The authors suggested that lowering the target blood levels to less than 20 ng/mL (20 mcg/L [24.8 nmol/L]) may reduce the renal toxicity of tacrolimus, and most centers currently use target trough tacrolimus levels of 5 to 15 ng/mL (5–15 mcg/L [6.2–18.6 nmol/L]). Based on the results of these two studies, many transplant centers use tacrolimus and methotrexate as first-line acute GVHD prophylaxis.

Because of the gastrointestinal and hematologic toxicities of methotrexate, other prophylactic regimens have been evaluated. Sirolimus has been successfully used for the prevention of rejection in solid organ transplant patients and has theoretical advantages for patients when used as prophylaxis of GVHD. This agent has been reported to have antiviral properties against CMV and Epstein-Barr virus and antitumor activity against some hematologic malignancies.[75] Several studies have shown encouraging results with sirolimus when combined with a calcineurin inhibitor (tacrolimus or cyclosporine) in the prevention of GVHD, but the combination of tacrolimus and sirolimus is thought to be less toxic and more efficacious than cyclosporine and sirolimus. A typical dosing strategy for sirolimus includes a loading dose of 12 mg for 1 day followed the next day by 4 mg/day with further doses based on serum levels. In the initial studies evaluating tacrolimus and sirolimus, with the majority of patients receiving matched related donor transplants, the incidence of grade II to IV acute GVHD was 20% to 40% and grade III to IV was 5% to 15%.[75] A phase III randomized trial was conducted through the Blood and Marrow Clinical Trials Network to compare tacrolimus and sirolimus versus tacrolimus and methotrexate as GVHD prophylaxis. Neutrophil and platelet engraftment were more rapid in the tacrolimus and sirolimus group. The incidence of grade II to IV and grade III to IV acute GVHD at 100 days were lower in the tacrolimus and sirolimus group (26 vs. 34%, $P = 0.17$; 8 vs. 15%, $P = 0.05$), but the primary end point of 114-day acute GVHD-free survival was not statistically different. Neither treatment-related mortality nor relapse at 2 years from transplantation was different between groups. Chronic GVHD was more common in the tacrolimus and sirolimus arm (54 vs. 43%, $P = 0.044$). Oral mucositis scores were lower in the tacrolimus and sirolimus arm, but the risk of SOS and thrombotic microangiopathy was higher in the tacrolimus and sirolimus arm. At 2 years from transplantation, disease-free and overall survival rates were not different between study arms. Tacrolimus and sirolimus can be used as an alternative to tacrolimus and methotrexate, but careful monitoring to minimize the risk of toxicities is required for both agents.[76]

Other methotrexate-sparing strategies have been evaluated for GVHD prophylaxis. Mycophenolate mofetil with tacrolimus was compared with tacrolimus and methotrexate in recipients of matched related and unrelated donors. The results of two small randomized trials have shown less toxicity with mycophenolate mofetil but little to no improvement in the rate of acute GVHD or overall survival.[77,78] Single-agent cyclophosphamide (50 mg/kg on days 3 and 4 after transplant) also has been tested in patients receiving MAC. With single-agent cyclophosphamide posttransplant prophylaxis, 43% developed grade II to IV GVHD, and 10% had grade III to IV. The incidence of chronic GVHD was 10% at 26 months.[79]

Another novel GVHD prophylaxis regimen includes bortezomib given on days 1, 4, and 7 after transplant in addition to standard tacrolimus and methotrexate in RIC mismatched unrelated donor transplants. The incidence of grade II to IV GVHD was comparable to patients who received HLA-matched transplants.[80] The MD Anderson Cancer Center reported its results with the addition of pentostatin 1.5 mg/m^2 weekly for 4 weeks combined with a calcineurin inhibitor and methotrexate. The addition of pentostatin to the standard GVHD prophylaxis regimen increased the proportion of patients alive without GVHD at day 100 compared with control participants.[81] Although the addition of these novel agents is intriguing, it is difficult to compare outcomes because of different populations and study design. The CIBMTR is conducting a phase II trial evaluating the addition of agents like cyclophosphamide or bortezomib to standard prophylaxis regimens.

A reduction in the number of donor T cells in the stem cell donation decreases the risk of GVHD, but the role of ex vivo T-cell depletion is controversial.[72] Earlier reports of this technique were associated with an increased risk of graft failure, delayed immune reconstitution, leukemic relapse, CMV reactivation, and Epstein-Barr virus–related lymphoproliferative disorders. Most of these studies occurred when bone marrow was the preferred stem cell source. The role of T-cell depletion is not well studied in patients who receive PBSC as a graft source. A recent study reported outcomes of a comparative analysis of among patients who received ex vivo T-cell depletion or the standard calcineurin inhibitor and methotrexate prophylaxis. Patients who received the T cell–depleted stem cells had lower rates of chronic GVHD. No differences in rates of graft rejection, leukemia relapse, treatment-related mortality, or overall survival rates were reported.[82] Another approach is infusion of the T cells originally depleted from the graft later in the posttransplant period to prevent leukemic relapse. Because of the higher risk of GVHD in allogeneic HSCT with HLA-mismatched donors, T-cell depletion is sometimes included as part of the GVHD prophylaxis regimen in that setting.

Treatment of Acute Graft-versus-Host Disease (10) Patients with mild skin-only acute GVHD (grade I) can be treated with topical corticosteroid preparations and counseled on the appropriate use of sunscreen. If a patient develops grades II to IV GVHD, prophylactic agents are continued, and high-dose corticosteroids in the form of IV methylprednisolone are given.[72] The usual dosage is 1 to 2 mg/kg/day given in two divided doses; higher dosages have not been shown to be more efficacious. About 25% to 40% of patients with established acute GVHD respond to high-dose corticosteroids. If the patient responds, the corticosteroid dose is tapered gradually over several weeks to months, depending on response. In patients who experience a flare in GVHD during the taper phase, therapy consists of increasing the corticosteroid dose and then tapering more slowly. Oral beclomethasone dipropionate, a topically active corticosteroid, has been shown to reduce the frequency of gastrointestinal GVHD relapses when continued after prednisone taper.[83] Administration of beclomethasone has been associated with a better survival at 200 days and 1 year after transplant. Budesonide, another nonabsorbable corticosteroid, has also been evaluated in uncontrolled studies and may also help to reduce the need for sustained use of high-dose systemic corticosteroid administration.[84]

GVHD-associated mortality is strongly correlated to response to initial treatment and ranges from about 25% in patients who had a complete response to about 80% in patients who had no response or progressive disease. Several randomized trials have evaluated other agents combined with methylprednisolone in an effort to improve response to initial therapy for acute GVHD.[72] The combination of methylprednisolone and the anti–TNF-α monoclonal antibody infliximab has not been shown to increase response rate compared to methylprednisolone alone.[85] The Blood and Marrow Transplant Clinical Trials Network randomized 180 patients to methylprednisolone 2 mg/kg/day combined with etanercept, mycophenolate mofetil, denileukin diftitox, or pentostatin.[86] After 28 days of treatment, complete response rates were 60% for mycophenolate mofetil, 53% for denileukin diftitox, 38% for pentostatin, and 26% for etanercept. Efficacy and toxicity data suggested that the use of mycophenolate mofetil plus corticosteroids was the most promising regimen to compare with corticosteroids alone in a definitive phase III trial. This trial was halted early when a futility rule was met at a planned interim analysis. GVHD-free survival 56 days after randomization was not different between the groups. Based on the current published data, the use of glucocorticoid treatment with an additional agent for initial therapy of acute GVHD should only be done within the confines of a clinical trial.[87]

The mortality rate of patients with steroid-refractory GVHD is high. Criteria and indications for initiating secondary therapy for steroid-refractory acute GVHD have not been well defined in the literature. Although different centers may have varying criteria, in general, if the manifestations of acute GVHD in any organ worsen over 3 days of corticosteroid treatment or symptoms do not improve by 5 days, the patient likely will not respond to corticosteroids, and secondary therapy should be considered.[87] From the available data, there is no standard treatment of patients with steroid-refractory acute GVHD because very few prospective comparative studies have been conducted to assess the efficacy of individual agents. Second-line therapy has consisted of continuation of corticosteroids with the addition of one or more of the following: antithymocyte globulin, mycophenolate mofetil, sirolimus, infliximab, etanercept, denileukin diftitox, alemtuzumab, or pentostatin.[87,88] One approach that has shown benefit as corticosteroid-sparing therapy is extracorporeal photopheresis. During this procedure, the patient's blood is exposed extracorporeally to 8-methoxypsoralen followed by ultraviolet A radiation and then returned to the patient. This process is thought to result in suppression of T-cell reactivity and induction of regulatory T cells. Clinical results have been positive, especially in patients with skin GVHD.[89] The choice of a second-line regimen for acute GVHD should be based on the risk of potential toxicities, interactions with other agents, convenience, and cost.

Clinical **Controversy. . .**

Optimal treatment of steroid-refractory GVHD is unclear. Comparative trials are needed to determine a standard approach to this difficult condition.

Chronic Graft-versus-Host Disease

Chronic GVHD is the major determinant of late transplant-related morbidity and mortality.[69,90] The pathophysiology of chronic GVHD is poorly understood but is generally thought to be a result of a persistence of pathogenic donor T cells that are responsible for tissue damage through direct cytolytic attack, lack of immune tolerance, stimulation of inflammatory cytokines, or B-cell activation and antibody production.[90] Chronic GVHD is often considered an autoimmune disease because of its similarity to other autoimmune disorders.

The incidence of chronic GVHD in patients who survive more than 150 days ranges from 20% to 70%.[91] The risk of chronic GVHD increases with increasing donor and recipient age and is higher in patients who receive transplants from HLA-nonidentical donors and in patients who receive PBSC transplants (especially with higher $CD34^+$ cell doses). The incidence of chronic GVHD is rising because of increasing use of alternative donors, use of PBSCs as the graft source, use of DLI for treatment of recurrence, and older recipient age. Previous acute GVHD increases the risk of chronic GVHD, but about 20% to 30% of patients who develop chronic GVHD after HLA-matched allogeneic HSCT have no history of acute GVHD. Unlike acute GVHD, prophylactic immunosuppression does not appear to reduce the incidence or severity of chronic GVHD.

Chronic GVHD resembles autoimmune diseases and can affect any organ or tissue of the body. The most common sites involved are the skin, mouth, liver, and eye, but other sites include the gastrointestinal tract, joints, muscles, and lungs. The National Institutes of Health (NIH) Consensus Development Project developed standardized criteria for the diagnosis of chronic GVHD and proposed a clinical scoring system for the evaluation of patients with chronic GVHD based on the extent of organ damage and degree of functional impairment.[70] The Working Group recommends that the diagnosis of chronic GVHD be made with the presence of at least one diagnostic clinical sign of chronic GVHD (e.g., poikiloderma or esophageal web) or a distinctive manifestation (e.g., keratoconjunctivitis sicca) confirmed by biopsy or other test (e.g., Schirmer test).

The clinical scoring system categorizes chronic GVHD into mild, moderate, and severe.[70] Mild chronic GVHD involves only one or two organs or sites (except the lung) with no clinically significant functional impairment. Moderate chronic GVHD involves at least one organ or site with clinically significant but no major disability, three or more organs or sites with no clinically significant functional impairment, or mild lung involvement. Severe chronic GVHD indicates major disability caused by chronic GVHD or at least moderate lung involvement.

Patients with mild skin-only chronic GVHD can be treated with a variety of topical preparations, such as clobetasol, tacrolimus, and pimecrolimus.[90] Initial treatment of patients with more severe or systemic involvement of chronic GVHD consists of prednisone 1 mg/kg/day followed by taper with or without a calcineurin inhibitor. Although calcineurin inhibitors do not conclusively improve outcomes, it is often considered to reduce toxicities of prolonged steroid therapy, especially in patients who may be at high risk for prednisone-related complications.[90] Prospective randomized trials evaluating the addition of mycophenolate mofetil to prednisone for initial therapy have shown limited to no benefit compared to prednisone alone.[92] Treatment is continued until signs and symptoms of the disease have resolved and then are tapered gradually over an extended period of time. Patients with chronic GVHD may require prolonged immunosuppressive treatment for an average of 2 to 3 years from the initial diagnosis.

In addition to treatment specifically for chronic GVHD, ancillary therapies should be recommended to lessen the symptoms of chronic GVHD.[93] Patients should be educated on the use of sunscreens (and avoidance of sun exposure) to reduce skin injury and exacerbation of GVHD skin lesions. Nonsclerotic skin lesions without erosions or ulcerations may respond well to emollients in addition to topical corticosteroids. Patients should be advised to maintain good oral hygiene with routine dental care. Saliva substitutes can be given for dry mouth symptoms, and topical corticosteroid gels can be used for localized and symptomatic oral lesions. Artificial tears or, if necessary for more severe symptoms, cyclosporine or corticosteroid eye drops are useful for patients with chronic GVHD manifesting as dry eyes or conjunctivitis. Physical therapy is recommended to reduce functional loss as a result of steroid myopathy, joint contractures, and deconditioning.

Patients who do not respond to initial therapy have a very poor prognosis. Uncontrolled trials have investigated several therapies with varying degrees of success. When choosing initial salvage therapy, clinicians should consider agents with documented activity and an adequate safety profile as well as agents that are steroid sparing.[94] Agents with reported activity in refractory chronic GVHD include thalidomide, extracorporeal photophoresis, tacrolimus, sirolimus, pentostatin, mycophenolate mofetil, hydroxychloroquine, rituximab, imatinib and others.[94–96] The Blood and Marrow Clinical Trials Network has initiated a randomized phase II/III trial comparing the following three treatment strategies: sirolimus and prednisone; sirolimus, prednisone, and extracorporeal photophoresis; and sirolimus, prednisone, and a calcineurin inhibitor. Eligible subjects must have chronic GVHD, as diagnosed by NIH consensus criteria, and must be either untreated and high risk or not responding to standard therapy. The outcomes of this trial may help guide clinicians in the treatment of chronic GVHD.

Monitoring for long-term drug toxicities and infectious complications is critical during long-term immunosuppression. Infection is the primary cause of death in patients with chronic GVHD, and antimicrobial prophylaxis is an important component of the care of patients being treated for chronic GVHD.[93,94] Patients should receive oral trimethoprim–sulfamethoxazole, penicillin, an antifungal azole agent, and acyclovir to prevent infections commonly seen in immunocompromised patients. Routine monitoring for CMV reactivation should be performed. Some HSCT centers also administer IV immunoglobulin to patients with low serum immunoglobulin G levels. Patients who remain on long-term steroids should be monitored for steroid-induced osteoporosis and diabetes mellitus. Other potential long-term complications of chronic GVHD therapies include hyperlipidemia, cataracts, myelosuppression, elevated blood pressure, and renal dysfunction.

Infection

Patients undergoing high-dose chemotherapy with autologous or allogeneic HSCT are severely immunocompromised and therefore are at high risk for bacterial, fungal, and viral infections. Management of these infections is discussed in detail in Chapters 99 and 100.

Late Complications

With the success of HSCT, the number of long-term survivors has grown. Many survivors experience delayed complications of transplantation and treatments used to prevent or treat those complications, including restrictive and obstructive pulmonary disease, bone and joint disease (including osteoporosis and avascular necrosis), cataract formation, endocrine dysfunction (including sterility and thyroid dysfunction), impaired growth and development, infections, cardiovascular disease, chronic renal and hepatic dysfunction, and secondary malignancies. These effects are more frequent after allogeneic compared with autologous and among allogeneic transplant patients, those with chronic GVHD tend to have a higher prevalence of multiple health conditions than those without chronic GVHD.[97,98] Physical recovery tends to occur earlier than psychological or work recovery. Full recovery usually takes several years, and about two thirds of patients are without major limitations by 5 years. The Bone Marrow Transplant Survivor Study compared late mortality (2 years after HSCT) in allogeneic and autologous patients with that of the general population.[99,100] Both types of transplants were associated with a several-fold increase in risk of premature death; relative mortality decreased with time but remained significantly elevated even 10 years after transplant. The leading cause of death was relapse of primary disease in both allogeneic and autologous patients, but allogeneic HSCT patients also continued to die from complications of chronic GVHD, but autologous HSCT patients frequently succumbed to secondary malignancies. Long-term monitoring of HSCT patients is required, both by transplant clinicians and primary care providers who are knowledgeable in the care of these patients, to prevent and treat late complications when such therapies are available.

ABBREVIATIONS

ALL	acute lymphocytic leukemia
AML	acute myelogenous leukemia
APC	antigen-presenting cell
BMT	bone marrow transplantation
CIBMTR	Center for International Blood and Marrow Transplant Research
CML	chronic myeloid leukemia
CMV	cytomegalovirus
DLI	donor lymphocyte infusion
G-CSF	granulocyte colony-stimulating factor; filgrastim
GM-CSF	granulocyte-macrophage colony-stimulating factor; sargramostim
GVHD	graft-versus-host disease
GVM	graft-versus-malignancy (effect)
HLA	human leukocyte antigen
HSCT	hematopoietic stem cell transplantation
IL	interleukin
MAC	myeloablative conditioning
MHC	major histocompatibility complex
NK	natural killer (cells)
NMDP	National Marrow Donor Program
PCR	polymerase chain reaction
Ph+	Philadelphia chromosome positive
PBSC	peripheral blood stem cell
RIC	reduced-intensity conditioning
SOS	sinusoidal obstruction syndrome
TBI	total-body irradiation
TNF-α	tumor necrosis factor-α
TKI	tyrosine kinase inhibitor
UCB	umbilical cord blood

REFERENCES

1. Pasquini MC, Wang Z. Current use and outcome of hematopoietic stem cell transplantation: CIBMTR Summary Slides. 2011, *http://www.cibmtr.org.*
2. Wingard JA, Gastineau DA, Leather HL, Szczepiorkowski ZM, Snyder EL, eds. Hematopoietic Stem Cell Transplantation: A Handbook for Clinicians. Bethesda, MD: AABB, 2009.
3. Appelbaum F, Forman S, Negrin R, Blume K, eds. Thomas' Hematopoietic Cell Transplantation. Oxford, UK: Wiley-Blackwell, 2009.
4. Gyurkocza B, Rezvani A, Storb RF. Allogeneic hematopoietic cell transplantation: the state of the art. Expert Rev Hematol 2010;3:285–299.
5. Copelan EA. Hematopoietic stem-cell transplantation. N Engl J Med 2006;354:1813–1826.
6. Nowak J. Role of HLA in hematopoietic SCT. Bone Marrow Transplant 2008;42(Suppl):S71–S76.
7. Flomenberg N, Baxter-Lowe LA, Confer D, et al. Impact of HLA class I and class II high resolution matching on outcomes of unrelated donor bone marrow transplantation: HLA-C mismatching is associated with a strong adverse effect on transplant outcome. Blood 2004;104:1923–1930.
8. Lee SJ, Kline J. Haagenson M, et al. High resolution donor-recipient HLA matching contributes to the success of unrelated donor marrow transplantation. Blood 2007;110: 4576–4583.
9. Spellman SR, Eapen M, Logan BR, et al. A perspective on the selection of unrelated donors and cord blood units for transplantation. Blood 2012;120:259–265.
10. Ringden O, Pavletic SZ, Anasetti C, et al. The graft-versus-leukemia effect using matched unrelated donors is not

superior to HLA-identical siblings for hematopoietic stem cell transplantation. Blood 2009;113:3110–3118.
11. Moore J, Nivison-Smith I, Goh K, et al. Equivalent survival for sibling and unrelated donor allogeneic stem cell transplantation for acute myelogenous leukemia. Biol Blood Marrow Transplant 2007;13:601–607.
12. Bensinger W, DiPersio JF, McCarty JM. Improving stem cell mobilization strategies: Future directions. Bone Marrow Transplant 2009;43:181–195.
13. Kobbe G, Bruns I, Fenk R, Czibere A, Haas R. Pegfilgrastim for PBSC mobilization and autologous haematopoietic SCT. Bone Marrow Transplant 2009;43:669–677.
14. Herbert KE, Gambell P, Link EK, et al. Pegfilgrastim compared with filgrastim for cytokine-alone mobilization of autologous haematopoietic stem and progenitor cells. Bone Marrow Transplant 2013;48(3):351–356.
15. DiPersio JF, Stadtmauer EA, Nademanee A, et al. Plerixafor and G-CSF versus placebo and G-CSF to mobilize hematopoietic stem cells for autologous stem cell transplantation in patients with multiple myeloma. Blood 2009;113:5720–5726.
16. DiPersio, Micallef IV, Stiff PJ, et al. Phase III prospective randomized double-blind placebo-controlled trial of plerixafor plus granulocyte colony stimulating factor compared with placebo plus granulocyte colony stimulating factor for autologous stem cell mobilization and transplantation for patients with non-Hodgkin's lymphoma. J Clin Oncol 2009;27:4767–4773.
17. Stiff P, Micallef I, McCarthy P, et al. Treatment with plerixafor in non-Hodgkin's lymphoma and multiple myeloma patients to increase the number of peripheral blood stem cells when given a mobilizing regimen of G-CSF: Implications for the heavily pretreated patient. Biol Blood Marrow Transplant 2009;15:249–256.
18. Tricot G, Cottler-Fox MH, Calandra G. Safety and efficacy assessment of plerixafor in patient with multiple myeloma proven or predicted to be poor mobilizers, including assessment of tumor cell mobilization. Bone Marrow Transplant 2010;45:63–68.
19. Micallef IN, Sinha S, Gastineau DA, et al. Cost-effectiveness analysis of a risk-adapted algorithm of plerixafor use for autologous peripheral blood stem cell mobilization. Biol Blood Marrow Transplant 2013;19(1):87–93.
20. Abhyankar S, DeJarnette S, Aljitawi O, et al. A risk-based approach to optimize autologous hematopoietic stem cell (HSC) collection with the use of plerixafor. Blood Marrow Transplant 2012;47:483–487.
21. Costa LJ, Alexander ET, Hogan KR, et al. Development and validation of a decision-making algorithm to guide the use of plerixafor for autologous hematopoietic stem cell mobilization. Bone Marrow Transplant 2011;46:64–69.
22. Wuchter P, Ran D, Bruckner T, et al. Poor mobilization of hematopoietic stem cells—definitions, incidence, risk factors and impact on outcomes of autologous transplantation. Biol Blood Marrow Transplant 2010;16:490–499.
23. Calandra G, McCarty J, McGuirk J, et al. AMD3100 plus G-CSF can successfully mobilize CD34+ cells from non-Hodgkin's lymphoma, Hodgkin's disease and multiple myeloma patients previously failing mobilization with chemotherapy and/or cytokine treatment: compassionate use data. Bone Marrow Transplant 2008;41:331–338.
24. Perkins JB, Shapiro JF, Bookout RN, et al. Retrospective comparison of filgrastim plus plerixafor to other regimens for remobilization after primary mobilization failure: clinical and economic outcomes. Am J Hematol 2012;87:673–677.
25. Korbling M, Freireich EJ. Twenty-five years of peripheral blood stem cell transplantation. Blood 2011;117:6411–6416.
26. Avalos BR, Lazaryan A, Copelan EA. Can G-CSF cause leukemia in hematopoietic stem cell donors? Biol Blood Marrow Transplant 2011;17:1739–1746.
27. Stem Cell Trialists' Collaborative Group. Allogeneic peripheral blood stem-cell compared with bone marrow transplantation in the management of hematologic malignancies: An individual patient data meta-analysis of nine randomized trials. J Clin Oncol 2005;23:5074–5087.
28. Anasetti C, Logan Br, Lee SJ, et al. Peripheral blood stem cells versus bone marrow from unrelated donors. N Engl J Med 2012;367:1487–1496.
29. Chang YJ, Huang XJ. Use of G-CSF-stimulated marrow in allogeneic hematopoietic stem cell transplantation settings: a comprehensive review. Clin Transplant 2011;25:13–23.
30. Gluckman E, Ruggeri A, Volt F, Cunha R, Boudjedir K, and Rocha V. Milestones in umbilical cord blood transplantation. Br J Haematol 2011;154:441–447.
31. Eapen M, Rubinstein P, Zhang MJ, et al. Outcomes of transplantation of unrelated donor umbilical cord blood and bone marrow in children with acute leukaemia: A comparison study. Lancet 2007;369:1947–1954.
32. Eapen M, Rocha V, Sanz G, et al. Effect of graft source on unrelated donor haemopoietic stem-cell transplantation in adults with acute leukaemia: A retrospective analysis. Lancet Oncol 2010;11:653–660.
33. Ballen KK, Koreth J, Chen YB, Dey BR, Spitzer TR. Selection of optimal alternative graft source: Mismatched unrelated donor, umbilical cord blood, or haploidentical transplant. Blood 2012;119:1972–1980.
34. Ciurea SO, Andersson BS. Busulfan in hematopoietic stem cell transplantation. Biol Blood Marrow Transplant 2009;15:523–536.
35. Socie G, Clift RA, Blaise D, et al. Busulfan plus cyclophosphamide compared with total-body irradiation plus cyclophosphamide before marrow transplantation for myeloid leukemia: Long-term follow-up of 4 randomized studies. Blood 2001;98:3569–3574.
36. Gupta V, Lazarus HM, Keating A. Myeloablative conditioning regimens for AML allografts: 30 years later. Bone Marrow Transplant 2003;32:969–978.
37. Uberti JP, Agovi M-A, Tarima S, et al. Comparative analysis of BU and CY versus CY and TBI in full intensity unrelated marrow donor transplantation for AML, CML, and myelodysplasia. Bone Marrow Transplant 2011;46:34–43.
38. Vose JM, Carter SL, Burns LJ, et al. Randomized phase III trial of 131iodine-tositumomab (Bexxar)/carmustine, etoposide, cytarabine, melphalan (BEAM) vs rituximab/BEAM and autologous stem cell transplantation for relapsed diffuse large B-cell lymphoma (DLBCL): No difference in progression-free (PFS) or overall survival (OS). 53rd ASH Annual Meeting and Exposition, December 10–13, 2011, San Diego, CA. Abstract 661. 2011, *http://ash.confex.com/ash/2011/webprogram/Paper39888.html*.
39. Sandmaier BM, Mackinnon S, Childs RW. Reduced intensity conditioning for allogeneic hematopoietic cell transplantation: Current perspectives. Biol Blood Marrow Transplant 2007;13:87–97.
40. Pollack SM, O'Connor TP, Hashash J, Tabbara IA. Nonmyeloablative and reduce-intensity conditioning for allogeneic hematopoietic stem cell transplantation: A clinical review. Am J Clin Oncol 2009;32:618–628.
41. Kharfan-Dabaja MA, Barzarbachi A. Emerging role of CD20 blockade in allogeneic hematopoietic cell transplantation. Biol Blood Marrow Transplant 2010;16:1347–1354.

42. Bacigalupo A, Ballen K, Rizzo D, et al. Defining the intensity of conditioning regimens: Working definitions. Biol Blood Marrow Transplant 2009;15:1628–1633.
43. Kahl C, Storer BE, Sandmaier BM, et al. Relapse risk in patients with malignant disease given allogeneic hematopoietic cell transplantation after nonmyeloablative conditioning. Blood 2007;110:2744–2748.
44. Horwitz ME. Reduced intensity versus myeloablative allogeneic stem cell transplantation for the treatment of acute myeloid leukemia, myelodysplastic syndrome and acute lymphoid leukemia. Curr Opin Oncol 2011;23: 197–202.
45. van den Brink MR, Porter DL, Giralt S, et al. Relapse after allogeneic hematopoietic cell therapy. Biol Blood Marrow Transplant 2010;16(1 Suppl):S138–S145.
46. Tomblyn M, Lazarus HM. Donor lymphocyte infusions: The long and winding road: should it be traveled? Bone Marrow Transplantation 2008;42:569–579.
47. Kolg HJ. Graft-versus leukemia effects of transplantation and donor lymphocytes. Blood 2008;112:4371–4383.
48. Tsirigotis P, Dray L, Resnick IB, et al. Post-autologous stem cell transplantation administration of rituximab improves the outcome of patients with aggressive B cell non-Hodgkin's lymphoma. Ann Hematol 2010;89:263–272.
49. Haioun C, Mounier N, Emile JF, et al Rituximab versus observation after high-dose consolidative first-line chemotherapy with autologous stem-cell transplantation in patients with poor-risk diffuse large B-cell lymphoma Ann Oncol 2009;20:1985–1992.
50. Klyuchnikov E, Kroger N, Brummendorf TH, et al. Current status and perspectives of tyrosine kinase inhibitor treatment in the posttransplant period in patients with chronic myelogenous leukemia. Biol Blood Marrow Transplant 2010;16:301–310.
51. Lee HJ, Thompson JE, Wang ES, Wetzler M. Philadelphia chromosome-positive acute lymphoblastic leukemia. Cancer 2011;117:1583–1594.
52. de Lima M, Giralt S, Thall PF, et al. Maintenance therapy with low-dose azacitidine after allogeneic hematopoietic stem cell transplantation for recurrent acute myelogenous leukemia or myelodysplastic syndrome. Cancer 2010;116:5420–5433.
53. Attal M, Lauwers-Cances V, Marit G, et al. Lenalidomide maintenance after stem-cell transplantation for multiple myeloma. N Engl J Med 2012;366:1782–1791.
54. McCarthy PL, Owzar K, Hofmeister CC, et al. Lenalidomide after Stem-cell transplantation for multiple myeloma. N Engl J Med 2012;366:1770–1781.
55. Sonneveld P, Schmidt-Wolf IG, van der Holt B, et al. Bortezomib induction and maintenance treatment in patients with newly diagnosed multiple myeloma: Results of the randomized phase III HOVON-65/ GMMG-HD4 trial. J Clin Oncol 2012;30:2946–2955.
56. Richardson PG, Ho VT, Cutler C, Glotzbecker B, Antin JH, Soiffer R. Hepatic veno-occlusive disease after hematopoietic stem cell transplantation: Novel insights to pathogenesis, current status of treatment, and future directions. Biol Blood Marrow Transplant. 2013 Jan; 19(1 suppl):S88–S90.
57. Ho VT, Revta C, Richardson PG. Hepatic veno-occlusive disease after hematopoietic stem cell transplantation: Update on defibrotide and other current investigational therapies. Bone Marrow Transplant 2008;41:229–237.
58. McCune JS, Batchelder A, Deeg HJ, et al. Cyclophosphamide following targeted oral busulfan as conditioning for hematopoietic cell transplantation: pharmacokinetics, liver toxicity, and mortality. Biol Blood Marrow Transplant 2007;13:853–862.
59. Tay J, Timmouth A, Fergusson D, Huebsch L, Allan DS. Systematic review of controlled clinical trials on the use of ursodeoxycholic acid for the prevention of hepatic venoocclusive disease in hematopoietic stem cell transplant. Biol Blood Marrow Transplant 2007;13:206–217.
60. Gupta S, Jain A, Warneke CL, et al. Outcome of alveolar hemorrhage in hematopoietic stem cell transplant. Bone Marrow Transplant 2007;40:71–78.
61. Gorak E, Geller N, Srinivasan R, et al. Engraftment syndrome after nonmyeloablative allogeneic hematopoietic stem cell transplantation: Incidence and effects on survival. Biol Blood Marrow Transplant 2005;11:542–550.
62. Panoskaltsis-Mortari A, Griese M, Madtes DK, et al. An official American Thoracic Society research statement: Noninfectious lung injury after hematopoietic stem cell transplantation: Idiopathic pneumonia syndrome. Am J Respir Crit Care Med 2011;183:1262–1279.
63. Yanik GA, Ho VT, Levine JE, et al. The impact of soluble tumor necrosis factor receptor etanercept on the treatment of idiopathic pneumonia syndrome after allogeneic hematopoietic stem cell transplantation. Blood 2008;112:3073–3081.
64. Bacigalupo A, Chien J, Barisione G, Pavletic S. Late pulmonary complications after allogeneic hematopoietic stem cell transplantation: Diagnosis, monitoring, prevention and treatment. Semin Hematol 2012;49:15–24.
65. Trivedi M, Martinez S, Corringham S, Medle K, Ball ED. Optimal use of G-CSF administration after hematopoietic SCT. Bone Marrow Transplant 2009;43:895–908.
66. Smith TJ, Khatcheressian J, Lyman GH, et al. 2006 update of recommendations for the use of white blood cell growth factors: An evidence-based clinical practice guidelines. J Clin Oncol 2006;24:3187–3205.
67. Dekker A, Bulley S, Beyene J, et al. Meta-analysis of randomized controlled trials of prophylactic granulocyte colony-stimulating factor and granulocyte-macrophage colony-stimulating factor after autologous and allogeneic stem cell transplantation. J Clin Oncol 2006;24:5207–5215.
68. Khoury HJ, Loberiza FR, Ringden O, et al. Impact of posttransplantation G-CSF on outcomes of allogeneic hematopoietic stem cell transplantation. Blood 2006;107: 1712–1716.
69. Reddy P, Arora M, Guimond M, Mackall CL. GVHD: A continuing barrier to the safety of allogeneic transplantation. Biol Blood Marrow Transplant 2009;15:162–168.
70. Filipovich AH, Weisdorf DJ, Pavletic S, et al. National Institutes of Health consensus development project on criteria for clinical trials in chronic graft-versus-host disease: I. Diagnosis and staging working group report. Biol Blood Marrow Transplant 2005;11:945–955.
71. Saliba RM, deLima M, Giralt S, et al. Hyper-acute GVHD. Risk factors, outcomes, and clinical applications. Blood 2007;109:2751–2758.
72. Ferrara JLM, Levine JE, Reddy P, Holler E. Graft-versus-host disease. Lancet 2009;373:1550–1561.
73. Ratanatharathorn V, Nash RA, Przepiorka D, et al. Phase III study comparing methotrexate and tacrolimus (Prograf, FK506) with methotrexate and cyclosporine for graft-versus-host disease prophylaxis after HLA-identical sibling bone marrow transplantation. Blood 1998;92: 2303–2314.
74. Nash RA, Antin JH, Karanes C, et al. Phase 3 study comparing methotrexate and tacrolimus with methotrexate and cyclosporine for prophylaxis of acute graft-versus-host

disease after marrow transplantation from unrelated donors. Blood 2000;96:2062–2068.

75. Abouelnasr A, Cohen S, Kiss T, Roy J, Lachance S. Defining the role of sirolimus in the management of graft-versus-host disease: From prophylaxis to treatment. Biol Blood Marrow Transplant 2013;19(1):12–21.
76. Tacrolimus/Sirolimus vs. Tacrolimus/Methotrexate for Graft-vs.-Host Disease Prophylaxis After HLA-Matched, Related Donor Hematopoietic Stem Cell Transplantation: Results of Blood and Marrow Transplant Clinical Trials Network Trial 0402. *https://ash.confex.com/ash/2012/webprogram/Paper47941.html*.
77. Perkins J, Field T, Kim J, et al. A randomized phase II trial comparing tacrolimus and mycophenolate mofetil to tacrolimus and methotrexate for acute graft-versus-host disease prophylaxis. Biol Blood Marrow Transplant 2010:16:937–947.
78. Bolwell B, Sobecks R, Pohlman B, et al. A prospective randomized trial comparing cyclosporine and short course methotrexate with cyclosporine and mycophenolate mofetil for GVHD prophylaxis in myeloablative allogeneic bone marrow transplantation. Bone Marrow Transplant 2004;34:621–625.
79. Luznik L, Bolanos-Meade J, Zahurak M, et al. High-dose cyclophosphamide as single agent, short-course prophylaxis of graft-versus-host disease. Blood 2010;115:3324–3230.
80. Koreth J, Stevenson KE, Kim HT, et al. Bortezomib-based graft-versus-host disease prophylaxis in HLA-mismatched unrelated donor transplantation. J Clin Oncol 2012;30: 3202–3208.
81. Parmar S, Andersson BS, Couriel D, et al. Prophylaxis of graft-versus-host disease in unrelated donor transplantation with pentostatin, tacrolimus, and mini-methotrexate: A phase I/II controlled, adaptively randomized study. J Clin Oncol 2011;29:294–302.
82. Pasquini MC, Devine S, Mendizabal A, et al. Comparative outcomes of donor graft CD34+ selection and immune suppressive therapy as graft-versus-host disease prophylaxis for patients with acute myeloid leukemia in complete remission undergoing HLA-matched sibling allogeneic hematopoietic cell transplantation. J Clin Oncol 2012;30(26):3194–3201.
83. Hockenbery DM, Cruickshank S, Rodell TC, et al. A randomized, placebo-controlled trial of oral beclomethasone dipropionate as a prednisone-sparing therapy for gastrointestinal graft-versus-host disease. Blood 2007;109:4557–4563.
84. Ibrahim RB, Abidi MH, Cronin SM, et al. Nonabsorbable corticosteroid use in the treatment of gastrointestinal graft-versus-host disease. Biol Blood Marrow Transplant 2009;15:395–405.
85. Couriel DR, Saliba R, de Lima M, et al. A phase III study of infliximab and corticosteroids for the initial treatment of acute graft-versus-host disease. Biol Blood Marrow Transplant 2009;15:1555–1562.
86. Alousi AM, Weisdorf DJ, Logan BR, et al. Etanercept, mycophenolate, denileukin, or pentostatin plus corticosteroids for acute graft-versus-host disease: A randomized phase 2 trial from the Blood and Marrow Transplant Clinical Trials Network. Blood 2009;114: 511–517.
87. Martin PJ, Rizzo JD, Wingard JR, et al. First- and second-line systemic treatment of acute graft-versus-host disease: Recommendations of the American Society of Blood and Marrow Transplantation. Biol Blood Marrow Transplant 2012;18(8):1150–1163.
88. Pidala J, Anasetti C. Glucocorticoid-refractory acute graft-versus-host disease. Biol Blood Marrow Transplant 2010;16:1504–1518.
89. Knobler R, Barr ML. Couriel DR, et al. Extracorporeal photopheresis: Past, present, and future. J Am Acad Dermatol 2009;61:652–665.
90. Wolff D, Gerbitz A, Ayuk F, et al. Consensus conference on clinical practice in chronic graft-versus-host disease (GVHD): First-line and topical treatment of chronic GVHD. Biol Blood Marrow Transplant 2010;16:1611–1628.
91. Lee SJ. Have we made progress in the management of chronic graft-vs-host disease? Best Pract Res Clin Hematol 2010;23:529–535.
92. Martin PJ, Storer BE, Rowley SD, et al. Evaluation of mycophenolate mofetil for initial treatment of chronic graft-versus-host disease. Blood 2009;113:5074–5082.
93. Couriel D, Carpenter PA, Cutler C, et al. Ancillary Therapy and supportive care of chronic graft-versus-host disease: National Institutes of Health consensus development project on criteria for clinical trials in chronic graft-versus host disease: V. Ancillary therapy and supportive care working group report. Biol Blood Marrow Transplant 2006;12: 375–396.
94. Dignan FL, Scarisbrick JJ, Cornish J, et al. Organ-specific management and supportive care in chronic graft-versus-host disease. Br J Haematol 2012;158(1):62–78.
95. Wolff D, Schleuning M, von Harsdorf S, et al. Consensus conference on clinical practice in chronic GVHD: Second-line treatment of chronic graft-versus-host disease. Biol Blood Marrow Transplant 2011;17:1–17.
96. Magro L, Mohty M, Catteau, et al. Imatinib mesylate as salvage therapy for refractory sclerotic chronic graft-versus-host disease. Blood 2009;114:719–722.
97. Savani B, ed. Late effects after allogeneic stem cell transplantation. Semin Hematol 2012;49:1–110.
98. Sun C-L, Francisco L, Kawashima T. et al. Prevalence and predictors of chronic health conditions after hematopoietic cell transplantation: A report from the Bone Marrow Transplant Survivor Study. Blood 2010;116:3129–3139.
99. Bhatia S, Robison LL, Francisco L, et al. Late mortality in survivors of autologous hematopoietic cell transplantation: Report from the Bone Marrow Transplant Survivor Study. Blood 2005;105:4215–4222.
100. Bhatia S, Francisco L, Carter A, et al. Late mortality after allogeneic hematopoietic cell transplantation and functional status of long-term survivors: Report from the Bone Marrow Transplant Survivor Study. Blood 2007;110:3784–3792.

Assessment of Nutrition Status and Nutrition Requirements

118

Katherine Hammond Chessman and Vanessa J. Kumpf

KEY CONCEPTS

1. Malnutrition is a consequence of nutrient imbalance, overnutrition or undernutrition, and has a high prevalence in the United States.
2. Nutrition screening is distinct from assessment and should be designed to quickly and reliably identify those who are at risk of nutrition-related poor outcomes.
3. A comprehensive nutrition assessment is the first step in formulating a nutrition care plan for a patient who is found to be nutritionally at risk.
4. A nutrition-focused medical, surgical, and dietary history and a nutrition-focused physical examination are key components of a comprehensive nutrition assessment.
5. Appropriate evaluation of anthropometric measurements (e.g., weight, height) is essential in nutrition assessment and should be based on published standards.
6. Laboratory assessment of visceral proteins is essential for a comprehensive nutrition assessment and must be interpreted in the context of physical findings, medical and surgical history, and the patient's clinical status.
7. The presence of micronutrient or macronutrient deficiencies or risk factors for these deficiencies can be identified by a comprehensive nutrition assessment.
8. Patient-specific goals should be established using evidence-based criteria considering the patient's clinical condition and the need for maintenance or repletion in adults or continued growth and development in children.
9. Indirect calorimetry is the most accurate method to determine energy requirements, but because of cost and availability, validated predictive equations are most often used to determine energy requirements.
10. Drug–nutrient interactions can affect nutrition status and the response to and adverse effects seen with drug therapy and must be considered when developing or assessing a patient's nutrition care plan.

INTRODUCTION

Nutrition is a vital component of quality patient care. No single clinical or laboratory parameter is an absolute indicator of nutrition status, so data from a number of areas must be analyzed. This chapter reviews the tools most commonly used for accurate, relevant, and cost-effective nutrition screening and assessment. The various methods used to determine patient-specific macro- and micronutrient requirements and potential drug–nutrient interactions are also discussed.

CLASSIFICATION OF NUTRITION DISEASE

❶ Malnutrition is a consequence of nutrient imbalance. In general, deficiency states can be categorized as those involving protein and calories or single nutrients such as individual vitamins or trace elements. Starvation-associated malnutrition, marasmus, results from prolonged inadequate intake, absorption, or utilization of protein and energy. It occurs in patients with an inadequate food supply, anorexia nervosa, major depression, and malabsorption syndromes. Somatic protein (skeletal muscle) and adipose tissue (subcutaneous fat) wasting occurs, but visceral protein (e.g., albumin [ALB] and transferrin [TFN]) production is usually preserved. Weight loss may exceed 10% of usual body weight (UBW; typical weight). With severe marasmus, cell-mediated immunity and muscle function are impaired. Patients with marasmus commonly have a prototypical starved, wasted appearance.[1,2] Kwashiorkor is a specific form of starvation-associated malnutrition that develops when there is inadequate protein intake and usually develops in areas where there is famine, limited food supply, or low educational levels. Although rarely reported in the United States, children who are abused or neglected and elderly individuals can develop this condition. Often patients with kwashiorkor do not appear malnourished because of relative adipose tissue sparing, especially with mild undernutrition, but visceral (and to some degree somatic) protein stores are depleted, resulting in severe hypoalbuminemia and edema in more advanced cases. In patients with marasmus or kwashiorkor, enhancing nutritional intake or bypassing impaired absorption with specialized nutrition support can reverse the malnutrition.[1,2]

Malnutrition can also result from chronic mild-to-moderate inflammation when there is heightened cellular substrate demand or use, such as in patients with chronic inflammatory diseases, organ failure, or cancer. In patients with severe acute disease or injury (e.g., major infections, burns, trauma, traumatic brain injury), malnutrition can develop because of increased metabolic demands. Individuals with mild-to-moderate marasmus or kwashiorkor can develop marked malnutrition when severe injury or inflammation occurs. In patients with inflammation or injury-associated malnutrition, simply providing nutrients in usual or even increased amounts may not be sufficient to reverse the nutrient imbalance caused by hypermetabolism. Regardless of the cause, undernutrition can result in changes in subcellular, cellular, or organ function that increase the individual's risks of morbidity and mortality.

Obesity (overnutrition) is a major healthcare concern worldwide. In 2009 to 2010, approximately 69% of American adults were overweight (defined as a body mass index [BMI] ≥25 kg/m^2), and about 36% (78 million) were obese (BMI ≥30 kg/m^2).[3] In 2010, obesity prevalence ranged from 21% in Colorado to 34% in Mississippi.[4] Additionally, 17% (12.5 million) of all U.S. children and adolescents (age 2–19 years) were obese (BMI ≥95th percentile for age on the gender-appropriate BMI-for-age Centers for Disease Control and Prevention's [CDC's] 2000 growth chart).[5,6] Many more children (~32%) were overweight (BMI ≥85th percentile for age).[5] Although the Healthy People 2010 goals of 15% obesity in adults and 5% obesity in children[7] were not met, there was no change in obesity prevalence among U.S. adults or children in 2009 to 2010 compared with 2003 to 2008[3] or 2007 to 2008,[5] respectively. This leveling trend is encouraging after a steady increase in prevalence since 1999. Nutrition assessment allows identification of overweight and obese individuals and those at risk of becoming obese. The consequences of obesity are numerous and include type 2 diabetes mellitus, cardiovascular disease, and stroke.

Poor nutritional status is associated with higher morbidity and mortality in many settings. An effective nutrition screening program will identify patients at nutrition-related risk. Clinicians trained to perform a comprehensive nutrition assessment will accurately characterize the at-risk patient's baseline nutrition status, allowing an appropriate estimate of an individual's nutrition needs and development of a patient-specific nutrition care plan. Diligent monitoring of ongoing nutrition status will ensure that nutrition-related goals are being met and patient outcomes are improved.

NUTRITION SCREENING

2 Nutrition screening is distinct from nutrition assessment.[8,9] It is neither practical nor warranted to conduct a comprehensive nutrition assessment on every individual; thus, nutrition screening protocols are useful to provide a reliable, systematic method to identify persons for whom a detailed nutrition assessment is needed. A nutrition screen can be used to detect those who are overweight, obese, malnourished, or at risk for malnutrition; predict the probability of their outcome as a result of nutritional factors; and identify those who would benefit from nutritional treatment. Ideally, potential nutrition-related issues can be identified and addressed before complications develop.

The ideal nutrition screen is quick, simple, and noninvasive and can be done by lay and healthcare providers in many settings, including homes, long-term care facilities, ambulatory care clinics, and hospitals. The Joint Commission includes nutrition screening and assessment in its performance standards for accredited healthcare institutions.[10] Each entity must have a written process by which a nutrition screen is done and criteria that determine when a more in-depth assessment will be performed. In hospitals, a nutrition screen must be completed within 24 hours of admission. A comprehensive nutrition assessment, if needed, should be completed within 48 to 72 hours. For outpatients, nutrition screening should occur ideally at the first visit with a new provider and thereafter as warranted by the patient's condition. Nutrition screening is a cost-effective way to decrease complications and length of hospital stay.

Appropriate screening is based on risk factor identification. Risk factors for undernutrition include recent weight loss, presence of chronic disease states, disease severity, complicating conditions, treatments, and socioeconomic factors that may result in a decreased nutrient intake or altered nutrient metabolism, utilization, or malabsorption. Risk factors for obesity include BMI, family history of obesity, certain medical diagnoses, poor dietary habits, lack of exercise, and some drug therapies. Various rating and classification systems have been proposed to screen for nutrition risk and guide subsequent interventions.[8,11–14] Checklists are used to quantify a person's food and alcohol consumption habits; ability to buy, prepare, and eat food; weight history; diagnoses; and medical and surgical procedures. Nutrition screens for children most often evaluate growth parameters against the CDC or World Health Organization (WHO) growth charts[6,15] and medical conditions known to increase nutrition risk. Screening programs should also identify patients receiving specialized nutrition support (enteral or parenteral nutrition). In any setting, patients determined to be "at nutrition risk" should receive a timely comprehensive nutrition assessment by a trained nutrition professional to verify nutrition-related risk and to formulate a nutrition care plan.

ASSESSMENT OF NUTRITION STATUS

3 A comprehensive nutrition assessment is the first step in formulating a patient-specific nutrition care plan. Nutrition assessment has four major goals: (a) identification of the presence of factors associated with an increased risk of developing malnutrition, including disorders resulting from macro- or micronutrient deficiencies (undernutrition), obesity (overnutrition), or impaired nutrient metabolism or utilization; (b) determination of the risk of malnutrition-associated complications; (c) estimation of nutrition needs; and (d) establishment of baseline nutrition status with parameters against which to measure nutrition therapy outcomes. Nutrition assessment should include a nutrition-focused medical, surgical, and dietary history; a nutrition-focused physical examination, including anthropometrics; and laboratory measurements. A comprehensive nutrition assessment provides a basis for determining the patient's nutrition requirements and the optimal type and timing of nutrition intervention.

Nutrition-Focused History and Physical Examination

4 The nutrition-focused medical, surgical, and dietary history provides information regarding factors that predispose to malnutrition (e.g., prematurity, chronic diseases, gastrointestinal [GI] dysfunction, alcohol abuse, acute or chronic inflammation, cancer, surgery, trauma), and overnutrition (e.g., poor dietary habits, limited exercise, chronic diseases, family history). The clinician should direct the interview to elicit any history of weight gain or loss, anorexia, vomiting, diarrhea, and decreased or unusual food intake (Table 118-1).

The nutrition-focused physical examination takes a systems approach to assess lean body mass (LBM) and findings of deficiencies or excesses of vitamins, trace elements, or essential fatty acids. The degree of muscle wasting, edema, or loss of subcutaneous fat, if present, should be documented. The presence of findings suggestive of malnutrition (e.g., dermatitis, glossitis, cheilosis, jaundice) should be noted. Additionally, nonspecific indicators of ongoing inflammation or stress (e.g., fever, tachycardia) should be noted because these are important findings (Table 118-2).

The Subjective Global Assessment, a simple, reproducible, cost-effective, bedside approach to nutrition assessment, has been

TABLE 118-1 Pertinent Data from a Nutrition-Focused Medical, Surgical, and Dietary History

Nutrition intake and dietary habits
Anorexia
Unusual or absent taste
Dietary intake, including vegetarianism
Special diets, including enteral or parenteral nutrition
Supplemental vitamin, mineral, or herbal intake
Food allergies or intolerance
Underlying pathology with nutritional effects
Chronic infections or inflammatory states
Neoplastic diseases
Endocrine disorders
Chronic illness, including pulmonary disease, liver cirrhosis, and kidney failure
Hypermetabolic states, such as trauma, burns, and sepsis
Digestive or absorptive disease, nausea, vomiting, diarrhea, and constipation
Hyperlipidemia
End-organ effects
Weight changes
Skin or hair changes
Exercise intolerance or fatigue
Gastrointestinal tract symptoms such as diarrhea, vomiting, and constipation
Gastrointestinal surgery
Bariatric surgery
Small bowel or colon resection
Gastrectomy
Miscellaneous
Catabolic medications or therapies, including corticosteroids, immunosuppressive agents, radiation, or chemotherapy
Other medications, including diuretics, laxatives, antipsychotics, or anabolic steroids
Genetic background, including body habitus of parents, siblings, and family
Alcohol or drug abuse

Data from references 8–14 and 16–18.

TABLE 118-2 Physical Examination Findings Suggestive of Malnutrition

General appearance
Edema (especially ankle and sacral)
Cachexia or obesity
Ascites
Signs and symptoms of dehydration, including poor skin turgor, sunken eyes, orthostasis, or dry mucous membranes
Muscle wasting or loss of subcutaneous fat
Fever
Tachycardia
Skin and mucous membranes
Thin, shiny, dry, or scaly skin
Decubitus ulcers
Ecchymoses or perifollicular petechiae
Poor healing of surgical or traumatic wounds
Pallor or redness of gums or fissures at mouth edge
Glossitis, stomatitis, or cheilosis
Musculoskeletal
Retarded growth or short stature
Bone pain or tenderness or epiphyseal swelling
Muscle mass less than expected for habitus, exercise level
Neurologic
Ataxia, positive Romberg test result,[a] or decreased vibratory or position sense
Nystagmus
Seizures or paralysis
Encephalopathy
Failure to meet age-appropriate developmental milestones
Hepatic
Jaundice
Hepatomegaly

[a]The Romberg test is a neurologic test used to detect problems with balance.

Data from references 8 to 14 and 16 to 18.

used in a variety of patient populations.[2,12,16,17] Five aspects of the medical and dietary history comprise the Subjective Global Assessment: weight changes in the previous 6 months, dietary changes, GI symptoms, functional capacity, and the presence of disease states known to affect nutrition status. Weight loss of less than 5% of UBW is considered a "small" loss, 5% to 10% loss is "potentially significant," and more than a 10% loss is "definitely significant." Dietary intake is characterized as normal or abnormal, and the duration and degree of abnormal intake are noted. The presence of daily GI symptoms (e.g., anorexia, nausea, vomiting, diarrhea) for longer than 2 weeks is significant. Functional capacity assesses the patient's energy level and whether the patient is active or bedridden. Finally, disease states are assessed as to their impact on metabolic demands (i.e., no, low, moderate, or high stress). Four physical examination findings are rated as normal, mild, moderate, or severe: loss of subcutaneous fat (triceps and chest), muscle wasting (quadriceps and deltoids), edema (ankle and sacral), and ascites. The patient's nutrition status is then rated as adequately nourished, moderately malnourished or suspected of being malnourished, or severely malnourished. Critics of the Subjective Global Assessment find it time-consuming and complex.[2] Another tool, the Mini Nutritional Assessment, has been used extensively in geriatric patients and found to be useful for elderly living in the community, subacute care facilities, and nursing homes.[2,18]

Anthropometric Measurements

5 Anthropometric measurements, which are physical measurements of the size, weight, and proportions of the human body, are also used to assess nutrition status. Common measurements are weight, stature (standing height or recumbent length depending on age), head circumference (for children younger than 3 years of age), and waist circumference. Measurements of limb size, such as skinfold thickness, midarm muscle circumference, and wrist circumference, may be useful in selected individuals. Bioelectrical impedance analysis (BIA) is also an anthropometric assessment tool. An individual's body measurements can be compared with normative population standards or repeated at various intervals to monitor response to a nutrition care plan. In adults, nutrition-related changes in anthropometric measurements occur slowly; several weeks or more are usually required before detectable changes are noted. In infants and young children, changes may occur more quickly. Acute changes in weight and skinfold thickness usually reflect changes in hydration, which must be considered when interpreting these parameters, particularly in hospitalized patients.

Weight, Stature, and Head Circumference

Body weight is a nonspecific measure of body cell mass, representing skeletal mass, body fat, and the energy-using component (i.e., LBM). Change in weight over time, particularly in the absence of edema, ascites, or voluntary losses, is an important indicator of altered LBM. Actual body weight (ABW) interpretation should include consideration of ideal weight for height, referred to as ideal body weight (IBW), UBW, fluid status, and age (Table 118-3). The UBW describes an individual's typical weight. Dehydration will result in decreased ABW but not a loss in LBM. After the patient is rehydrated, rechecking the weight is important to establish a baseline to use for nutrition evaluation. Edema and ascites increase total body water (TBW), thereby increasing ABW. Thus, the ABW of patients with severe edema and ascites should not be used for nutrition assessment; practitioners often use a "dry weight" to account for this increase in TBW. Both acute and chronic changes in fluid status can affect the ABW; these changes often can be detected by monitoring the patient's daily fluid intake and output. Accurate weight measurement can be difficult in critically ill patients because of their clinical condition and stress-related water retention.

TABLE 118-3 Evaluation of Body Weight

Parameter	Interpretation
ABW compared with IBW	
ABW <69% IBW	Severe malnutrition
ABW 70%–79% IBW	Moderate malnutrition
ABW 80%–89% IBW	Mild malnutrition
ABW 90%–120% IBW	Normal
ABW >120% IBW	Overweight
ABW ≥150% IBW	Obese
ABW ≥200% IBW	Morbidly obese
ABW compared with UBW	
ABW 85%–95% UBW	Mild malnutrition
ABW 75%–84% UBW	Moderate malnutrition
ABW <75% UBW	Severe malnutrition
BMI (kg/m²)	
Adults	
<16	Severe malnutrition
16–16.9	Moderate malnutrition
17–18.9	Mild malnutrition
19–24.9	Healthy
25–29.9	Overweight
30–40	Moderate obesity
>40	Severe or morbid obesity
Children	
BMI for age <5th percentile	Underweight
BMI for age 5th–84th percentile	Healthy
BMI for age 85th–94th percentile	Overweight
BMI for age ≥95th percentile	Obese

ABW, actual body weight; BMI, body mass index; IBW, ideal body weight; UBW, usual body weight.

Data from references 6, 7, and 12.

The IBW provides one population reference standard against which the ABW can be compared to detect both over- and undernutrition states. Numerous IBW-for-height reference tables have been generated. In clinical practice, mathematical equations based on gender and height (e.g., Hamwi method) are used commonly. IBW is calculated as 48 kg + (2.7 × [inches over 5 feet]) or 48 kg + (1.06 × [cm over 152 cm]) for adult men and for adult women as 45 kg + (2.3 × [inches over 5 feet]) or 45 kg + (0.906 × [cm over 152 cm]). For both equations, a range of ± 4.5 kg for large or small frame size is used for interpretation purposes. For obese adults, use of an adjusted ABW has been recommended for nutrition-related calculations, where adjusted ABW = ([ABW – IBW] × 0.25) + IBW. However, the use of this adjusted ABW is not evidence-based because most of the metabolic rate equations were developed with a mix of obese and nonobese individuals, and ABW was used to formulate the equations.[19] The IBW of a child can be calculated as ([height in cm]^2 × 1.65)/1,000. Alternatively, IBW for height can be determined by identifying the body weight corresponding to the same growth channel as the child's measured stature on the appropriate CDC or WHO growth chart. Comparison with the 50th percentile weight-for-age has been suggested but can be misleading if the child's height is not also at the 50th percentile.

Change in weight over time can be calculated as the percentage of UBW, where percent UBW = (ABW/UBW) × 100 (Table 118-3). Use of UBW as a reference point provides a more accurate reflection of clinically significant weight changes over time. However, determining UBW depends on patient or family recall, which may be inaccurate. The use of UBW avoids the problems associated with normative tables and documents comparative changes in body weight. Weight changes should be interpreted relative to time. Unintentional weight loss, especially rapid weight loss (i.e., 5% of UBW in 1 month or 10% of UBW in 6 months), increases the risk of poor clinical outcomes.[12]

Stature is determined by both genetics and nutrition. In infants, recumbent length is measured; in older children and adults, a standing height is preferred. If a standing height cannot be measured, the measurement of demispan can be used to estimate height. Demispan is determined in a seated patient by measuring the distance from the sternal notch to the web between the middle and ring fingers along a horizontally outstretched arm with the wrist in neutral rotation and zero extension or flexion. Demispan may more accurately assess stature in elderly adults, especially those with kyphosis or vertebral collapse. After the demispan is measured, height is estimated using the following equations: women: height (cm) = 1.35 × demispan (cm) + 60.1; men: height (cm) = 1.4 × demispan (cm) + 57.8.[20] Knee height may also be used to estimate stature and is especially helpful in patients with limb contractures, such as patients with cerebral palsy.[20–23] Knee height is measured from just under the heel to the anterior surface of the thigh just proximal to the patella. Using the average of two measurements rounded to the nearest 0.1 cm, height can be estimated using the following equations: women: height (cm) = 84.88 (0.24 × age [years]) + (1.83 × knee height [cm]); men: height (cm) = 64.19 (0.04 × age [years]) + (2.02 × knee height [cm]).[23]

The best indicator of adequate nutrition in a child is appropriate growth. At each medical encounter, weight, stature, head circumference (until 3 years), and BMI (after 2 years) should be plotted on the WHO (younger than 2 years) or CDC gender- and age-specific growth curves. Specialized charts are available for assessment of short- and long-term growth of premature infants,[24,25] children with Down's syndrome,[26] and children with other specific conditions. For premature infants with corrected postnatal age of 40 weeks or more, the WHO growth charts can be used; however, weight-for-age and length-for-age should be plotted according to corrected postnatal age until 2 years and 3.5 years of age, respectively.

Recommended intervals between measurements in young children are weight, 7 days; length, 4 weeks; height, 8 weeks; and head circumference, 7 days in infants and 4 weeks in children until 3 years of age. Growth velocity can be used to assess growth at intervals too close to plot accurately on a growth chart (Table 118-4). In newborns, average weight gain is 10 to 20 g/kg/day (24–35 g/day in term infants and 10–25 g/day in preterm infants). The rate of weight gain declines considerably after 3 months of age. Head growth (measured by head circumference), usually 0.5 cm/week (0.2 inches/week) during the first year of life, can be compromised during periods of critical illness or malnutrition. Rapid head growth, especially at a rate faster than expected, suggests hydrocephalus and should be further evaluated.

Failure to thrive (growth failure) is defined as weight-for-age or weight-for-height (or length) below the 5th percentile or a falloff

TABLE 118-4 Expected Growth Velocities in Term Infants and Children

Age	Weight (g/day)	Height (cm/mo)[a]
0–3 mo	24–35	2.8–3.4
4–6 mo	15–21	1.7–2.4
7–12 mo	10–13	1.3–1.6
1–3 yr	5–9	0.6–1
4–6 yr	5–6	0.5–0.6
7–10 yr	7–11	0.4–0.5

Example of growth assessment

Age: 2 mo; weight: 3.2 kg; weight at 1 mo of age, 3.1 kg; time since last weight was obtained: 30 days

Growth velocity = ([3.2 kg–3.1 kg] × 1,000 g/kg)/30 days = 3.3 g/day

Interpretation: suboptimal growth; comprehensive nutrition assessment needed

[a]Growth velocity of 1 cm/mo is equivalent to 0.4 inches/mo.

Data from references 6 and 15.

of two or more major percentiles (major percentiles are defined as 97th, 95th, 90th, 75th, 50th, 25th, 10th, 5th, and 3rd). Weight-for-height evaluation is age independent and helps differentiate a stunted child (chronic malnutrition) from a wasted child (acute malnutrition). Short stature, which can be associated with chronic disease, is a manifestation of chronic undernutrition. Short stature in the absence of poor weight gain suggests another etiology, such as growth hormone deficiency or constitutional growth delay.

Body Mass Index

Body mass index can be calculated as either body weight in kilograms divided by the patient's height in meters squared (kg/m^2) or body weight in pounds multiplied by 703 divided by the patient's height in inches squared (lb/in^2). A BMI of 25 kg/m^2 or higher is considered a risk factor for premature death and disability. Health risks increase as the BMI increases. Although BMI correlates strongly with total body fat, individual variation, especially in very muscular persons, may lead to erroneous classification of nutrition status. BMI should be interpreted based on characteristics such as gender, frame size, and age. For example, at the same BMI, a woman tends to have more body fat than a man, and an older adult would have more body fat than a younger one.

In general, a BMI between 18.5 and 24.9 kg/m^2 is indicative of a healthy weight, between 25 kg/m^2 and 29.9 kg/m^2 signifies being overweight, and 30 kg/m^2 or higher indicates obesity (Table 118-3).[12,27] These BMI classifications may not be appropriate for older subjects, especially those older than 60 years, where a BMI between 27 kg/m^2 and 30 kg/m^2 has not been associated with the same increased nutrition-related risks seen in younger individuals.[28] BMI has also been used to assess undernutrition (<18.5 kg/m^2 indicates undernutrition), but this relationship is not as well established.[12] Children 2 years of age and older are considered overweight if their BMI is at or above the 85th percentile on the age- and gender-specific CDC BMI chart and obese if the BMI is at or above the 95th percentile.[6] Use of these charts at each medical encounter helps to heighten awareness of children whose BMI and family history put them at risk for adult obesity and its associated complications.

Clinical **Controversy...**

Clinicians often debate whether nutrition needs for overweight and obese patients should be calculated using IBW, ABW, or adjusted ABW.

Skinfold Thickness and Mid-Arm Muscle Circumference

More than 50% of the body's fat is subcutaneous; thus, changes in subcutaneous fat reflect changes in total body fat. Whereas skinfold thickness measurement provides an estimate of subcutaneous fat, mid-arm muscle circumference, which is calculated using the skinfold thickness and mid-arm circumference, estimates skeletal muscle mass. Although simple and noninvasive, these anthropometric measurements are not used commonly in clinical practice but can be used for both population analysis and long-term monitoring of individuals. Triceps skinfold thickness is used most commonly, but reference standards also exist for subscapular and iliac sites. Careful technique in the use of pressure-regulated calipers is essential for reproducibility and reliability in measuring triceps skinfold thickness. Results should be interpreted cautiously because standards do not account for variation in bone size, muscle mass, hydration, or skin compressibility, and they do not consider obesity, ethnicity, illness, and increased age. Furthermore, these parameters change slowly in adults, often requiring weeks before significant alterations from baseline can be detected.

Waist Circumference

Waist circumference is a simple measurement used to assess abdominal (visceral) fat. Excess abdominal fat, rather than excess peripheral (subcutaneous) fat, is an independent predictor of obesity-related complications, especially diabetes mellitus and cardiovascular disease.[29,30] Waist circumference is determined by measuring the distance around the smallest area below the rib cage and the top of the iliac crest. Men are at increased risk (beyond the BMI-related risk) if the waist circumference is greater than 40 inches (102 cm); women are at increased risk if the waist circumference is greater than 35 inches (89 cm); and children are at risk if the waist circumference is at the 75th percentile or greater (16–17-year-old girls) or 90th percentile (all others) according to age- and gender-specific standards.[31]

Waist-to-Hip and Waist-to-Height Ratios

Extra weight around the waist confers a greater health risk than extra weight around the hips and thighs. The waist-to-hip ratio is determined by dividing the waist circumference by the hip circumference (maximal posterior extension of the buttocks). In adults, a waist-to-hip ratio of greater than 0.9 in men and 0.85 in women is considered an independent risk factor for adverse health consequences.[29] Waist-to-height ratio (both measured in centimeters) has been used to evaluate children at risk for the metabolic syndrome because, unlike waist circumference, it is independent of age and gender. A child with a waist-to-height ratio of more than 0.5 is at risk for developing the metabolic syndrome.[32]

Bioelectrical Impedance

Bioelectrical impedance is a simple, noninvasive, portable, and relatively inexpensive technique used to measure body composition.[33,34] The technology is based on the fact that lean tissue has a higher electrical conductivity (less resistance) than fat, which is a poor current conductor because of its lower water and electrolyte content. When a small electric current is applied to two appendages (wrist and ankle or both feet), impedance (resistance) to flow is measured. Assessment of LBM, TBW, and water distribution can be determined with BIA. Increased TBW decreases impedance; thus, it is important to evaluate hydration along with BIA. Other potential limitations of BIA include variability with electrolyte imbalance and interference by large fat masses, environment, ethnicity, menstrual cycle phase, and underlying medical conditions. Although BIA equations have high validity when used in the population in which they were developed (mostly young healthy adults), BIA calculations are subject to considerable errors if applied to other populations. Although BIA measures body fat accurately in controlled trials, accuracy in clinical practice is inconsistent. The lack of reference standards that reflect variations in individual body size and clinical condition also limits BIA use in clinical practice. BIA is not superior to BMI as a predictor of overall adiposity in the general population and is currently used primarily as a research tool.

OTHER NUTRITION ASSESSMENT TOOLS

Diminished skeletal muscle function can be a useful indicator of malnutrition because muscle function is an end-organ response. Muscle function also recovers more rapidly in response to initiation of nutrition support than anthropometric measurements. Hand-grip strength (forearm muscle dynamometry), respiratory muscle strength, and muscle response to electrical stimulation have been used. Measuring hand-grip strength is a relatively simple, noninvasive, and inexpensive procedure that correlates with patient outcome.[35–37] Normative standards supplied by the manufacturer of the measuring device can be used to establish the presence of a deficiency state. Ulnar nerve stimulation causes measurable muscle contraction and is used in most intensive care units to monitor neuromuscular blockade. In malnourished patients, increased fatigue and a slowed muscle relaxation rate are noted; these indices return to normal with refeeding.

A number of methods have been used to determine body composition in the research setting, including bioimpedance spectroscopy, dual energy x-ray absorptiometry (DXA), quantitative CT, air displacement plethysmography, three-dimensional photonic scanning, MRI, quantitative MRI, and positron emission tomography.[38,39] These methods are generally complex and require expensive technology. DXA, best known for its use in measuring bone density in patients with osteoporosis, is one of the most promising methods for routine clinical practice. It can be used to quantify the mineral, fat, and LBM compartments of the body and is available in most hospitals and many outpatient facilities. Equipment for a central DXA scan requires a fair amount of space, and the cost depends on the complexity of the scanner. Portable (or peripheral) DXA devices that use ultrasound and infrared interactance can be used to measure bone density in peripheral bones, such as the wrist, fingers, or heel, and have also been used to assess subcutaneous fat. These portable DXA scanners are much less expensive and can be used in community screenings in malls, health fairs, and pharmacies. Further research is needed to determine if DXA will be useful clinically in nutrition assessment. MRI and CT can measure subcutaneous, intraabdominal, and regional fat distribution and thus have the potential to be useful clinical tools.

Laboratory Assessment

6 Biochemically, LBM can be assessed by measuring the serum visceral proteins, albumin (ALB), transferrin (TFN), and prealbumin (also known as transthyretin). C-reactive protein (CRP) is useful as a marker of inflammation. Creatinine-height index has historically been calculated to assess LBM but is seldom done today because of the lack of evidence to support its usefulness.

Visceral Proteins

Measurement of serum proteins synthesized by the liver can be used to assess the visceral protein compartment. It is assumed that in undernutrition states, a low serum protein concentration reflects diminished hepatic protein synthetic mass and indirectly reflects the functional protein mass of other organs (heart, lung, kidney, intestines). Visceral proteins with the greatest relevance for nutrition assessment are serum ALB, TFN, and prealbumin. Many factors other than nutrition affect the serum concentration of these proteins, including age, abnormal kidney (nephrotic syndrome), GI tract (protein-losing enteropathy) or skin (burns) losses, hydration (dehydration results in hemoconcentration, overhydration in hemodilution), liver function (the synthetic site), and metabolic stress and inflammation (e.g., sepsis, trauma, surgery, infection). Assessing visceral proteins is of greatest value in the presence of uncomplicated semi-starvation and recovery. Thus, visceral protein concentrations must be interpreted relative to the individual's overall clinical condition (Table 118-5). During severe acute stress (trauma, burns, sepsis), these proteins are relatively poor markers of nutrition status because of increased vascular permeability with dramatic fluid shifts and reprioritizing of liver protein synthesis increasing the production of acute-phase reactants such as CRP, ferritin, fibrinogen, and haptoglobin.[40] CRP can be used in these cases to assess the degree of inflammation present: if CRP is elevated and ALB and prealbumin are decreased, then inflammation is a likely contributing factor. Assessing trends is most useful in these cases.

Albumin is the most abundant plasma protein and is involved in maintenance of colloid oncotic pressure and binding and transport of numerous hormones, anions, drugs, and fatty acids. It is widely used as a marker of chronic malnutrition. It is, however, a relatively insensitive index of early protein malnutrition because there is a large amount normally in the body (4–5 g/kg of body weight), it is extensively distributed in the extravascular compartment (60%), and it has a long half-life (18–20 days). However, chronic protein deficiency in the setting of adequate nonprotein calorie intake leads to marked hypoalbuminemia because of a net ALB loss from the intravascular and extravascular compartments. Serum ALB concentrations also are affected by moderate-to-severe calorie deficiency and liver, kidney, and GI disease. ALB is an acute-phase reactant, and serum concentrations decrease with inflammation, infection, trauma, stress, and burns. Decreased serum ALB concentrations are associated with poorer clinical outcomes in most of the above-mentioned settings. Additionally, serum ALB concentrations less than 2.5 g/dL (25 g/L) can be expected to exacerbate ascites and peripheral, pulmonary, and GI mucosal edema as a result of decreased colloid oncotic pressure. Hypoalbuminemia will also affect the interpretation of serum calcium concentrations as well as serum concentrations of highly protein bound drugs (e.g., phenytoin, valproic acid).

Transferrin is a glycoprotein that binds and transports ferric iron to the liver and reticuloendothelial system for storage. Because it has a shorter half-life (8–9 days) and there is less of it in the body (<100 mg/kg of body weight), TFN will decrease in response to protein and energy depletion before the serum ALB concentration decreases. Serum TFN concentrations are commonly measured directly. In rare situations when a direct measure is not available, TFN concentration can be estimated indirectly from measurement of total iron-binding capacity (in mcg/dL), where TFN (in mg/dL) = (total iron-binding capacity × 0.8) – 43. TFN is also an acute-phase

TABLE 118-5 Visceral Proteins Used for Assessment of Lean Body Mass

Serum Protein	Half-Life (Days)	Function	Factors Resulting in Increased Values	Factors Resulting in Decreased Values
Albumin	18–20	Maintains plasma oncotic pressure; transports small molecules	Dehydration, anabolic steroids, insulin, infection	Overhydration; edema; kidney dysfunction; nephrotic syndrome; poor dietary intake; impaired digestion; burns; congestive heart failure; cirrhosis; thyroid, adrenal, or pituitary hormones; trauma; sepsis
Transferrin	8–9	Binds Fe in plasma; transports Fe to bone	Fe deficiency, pregnancy, hypoxia, chronic blood loss, estrogens	Chronic infection, cirrhosis, burns, enteropathies, nephrotic syndrome, cortisone, testosterone
Prealbumin	2–3	Binds T_3 and, to a lesser extent, T_4; retinol-binding protein carrier	Kidney dysfunction	Cirrhosis, hepatitis, stress, surgery, inflammation, hyperthyroidism, cystic fibrosis, burns, kidney dysfunction, zinc deficiency

T_3, triiodothyronine; T_4, thyroxine.

reactant, and its concentration is increased in the presence of critical illness. Iron stores also affect serum TFN concentrations: in iron deficiency, hepatic TFN synthesis is increased, resulting in increased serum TFN concentrations irrespective of the patient's nutrition status.

Prealbumin (transthyretin) is the transport protein for thyroxine and a carrier for retinol-binding protein. Prealbumin stores are low (10 mg/kg of body weight), and it has a very short half-life (2–3 days). The serum prealbumin concentration may be reduced after only a few days of a significant reduction in calorie and protein intake or in patients with severe metabolic stress (e.g., trauma, burns). It is most useful in monitoring the short-term, acute effects of nutrition support or deficits, as it responds very quickly in both situations. As with ALB and TFN, prealbumin synthesis is decreased in liver disease. Increased prealbumin concentrations may be seen in patients with kidney disease because of impaired excretion.

Immune Function Tests

Nutrition status affects immune function either directly, via actions on the lymphoid system, or indirectly by altering cellular metabolism or organs that are involved with immune system regulation. Immune function tests most often used in nutrition assessment are the total lymphocyte count and delayed cutaneous hypersensitivity (DCH) reactions. Both tests are simple, readily available, and inexpensive.

Total lymphocyte count reflects the number of circulating T and B lymphocytes. Tissues that generate T cells are very sensitive to malnutrition, undergoing involution resulting in decreased T-cell production and eventually lymphocytopenia. A total lymphocyte count less than 1,500 cells/mm^3 ($<1.5 \times 10^9$ cells/L) has been associated with nutrition depletion.[2] DCH is commonly assessed using recall antigens to which the patient was likely previously sensitized, such as mumps and *Candida albicans*. Anergy is associated with severe malnutrition, and response is restored with nutrition repletion. Other immune function tests used in nutrition-related research include lymphocyte surface antigens (CD4, CD8, and the CD4:CD8 ratio), T-lymphocyte responsiveness, and various serum interleukin concentrations.

Total lymphocyte count is reduced in the presence of infection (e.g., human immunodeficiency virus [HIV], other viruses, tuberculosis), immunosuppressive drugs (e.g., corticosteroids, cyclosporine, tacrolimus, sirolimus, chemotherapy, antilymphocyte globulin), leukemia, and lymphoma. A number of factors affect DCH, including fever, viral illness, recent live virus vaccination, critical illness, irradiation, immunosuppressive drugs, diabetes mellitus, HIV, cancer, and surgery. Thus, a lack of specificity limits the usefulness of these tests as nutrition status markers. Nutrients such as arginine, omega-3 fatty acids, and nucleic acids given in pharmacologic doses may improve immune function. Monitoring efficacy of a nutrition care plan that includes these potentially immune-modulating nutrients may include immune function assessment with these or other immune function indicators.[41,42]

SPECIFIC NUTRIENT DEFICIENCIES AND TOXICITIES

7 A comprehensive nutrition assessment should include an evaluation for possible trace element, vitamin, and essential fatty acid deficiencies. Because of their key role in metabolic processes (as coenzymes and cofactors), a deficiency of any of these nutrients may result in altered metabolism and cell dysfunction. An accurate history to identify symptoms and risk factors for a specific nutrient deficiency is critical. A nutrition-focused physical examination for signs of deficiencies and biochemical assessment to confirm a suspected deficiency should be done in all at-risk patients. Ideally, biochemical assessment would be based on the nutrient's function (e.g., metalloenzyme activity) rather than simply measuring the serum concentration. Unfortunately, few practical methods to assess micronutrient function are available; thus, the nutrient's serum concentration is most often measured.

Trace Elements

Clinical syndromes are associated with a deficiency of the essential trace elements zinc, copper, manganese, selenium, chromium, iodine, fluoride, molybdenum, and iron in children and adults.[43–46] A deficiency state has not been recognized for tin, nickel, vanadium, cobalt, gallium, aluminum, arsenic, boron, bromine, cadmium, germanium, or silicon. Each trace element is involved in a variety of biologic functions and is necessary for normal metabolism, serving as a coenzyme or playing a role in hormonal metabolism or erythropoiesis. Toxicities can occur with excess intake of some trace elements. With the current public interest in complementary medicine, clinicians must ask patients about their use of dietary supplements and assess for signs and symptoms of toxicities as well as deficiencies (Table 118-6).

Zinc, the second most prevalent trace element, is a component of many enzymes and proteins and is involved in the regulation of gene expression, wound healing, and liver regeneration.[47] Excess zinc intake is usually eliminated by the kidneys and GI tract; thus, zinc toxicity is uncommon except in overdose settings. Zinc deficiency is characterized by several signs and symptoms, including a moist eczematous dermatitis that is most apparent in the nasolabial folds and around orifices (Table 118-6). Recovery is rapid with oral zinc supplementation; severe dermatitis can remit in as little as 4 to 5 days.[41] Zinc deficiency can be documented by the presence of low plasma zinc concentrations.[48] However, plasma zinc concentrations decrease during acute stress states (trauma, surgery, burns, sepsis) and generally remain depressed until the stress resolves. Also, because zinc is a normal contaminant of most blood collection tubes, special zinc-free collection tubes must be used for plasma assays. Hair zinc analysis and urinary zinc excretion can also be used as biomarkers of zinc status.[48]

Copper is a component of ceruloplasmin and key metalloenzymes involved in iron metabolism (ceruloplasmin), electron transport and energy metabolism (cytochrome oxidase), connective tissue and collagen cross-linking (lysyl oxidase, elastase, and monamine oxidase), and free radical scavenging (superoxide dismutase). Copper intake in excess of metabolic requirements is excreted through the bile. Signs and symptoms of copper deficiency include hypochromic anemia, neutropenia, neurologic dysfunction, skeletal demineralization, and hypercholesterolemia (Table 118-6). In severe cases, such as in Menkes' syndrome, copper deficiency is further manifested as hypothermia, hair and skin depigmentation, progressive mental deterioration, and growth retardation. Factors predisposing to copper deficiency include malabsorption states, protein-losing enteropathy, nephrotic syndrome, and copper-free parenteral nutrition.[49] The chronic ingestion of too much copper or inadequate elimination can result in cirrhosis as seen in Wilson's disease, an autosomal-recessive genetic disorder. Copper deficiency is best assessed using serum copper concentrations, which appear to reflect changes in copper status in both copper-depleted and copper-replete individuals.[50] Serum copper concentrations may not accurately reflect total body copper status because serum concentrations may be altered by a variety of conditions (Table 118-6).

Trivalent chromium is an important cofactor, along with insulin, in the maintenance of normal blood glucose concentrations. Recent data indicate that a low-molecular-weight chromium binding substance, sometimes referred to as the glucose tolerance factor, may enhance the response of the insulin receptor to insulin.[51] Chromium

TABLE 118-6 Assessment of Trace Element Status

Trace Element	Signs of Deficiency	Signs of Toxicity	Factors Associated with Altered Plasma Concentrations
Chromium	Impaired glucose/protein utilization, peripheral neuropathy, low RQ, weight loss, increased LDL-C, increased free fatty acid concentrations	Industrial exposure: skin or nasal septum lesions, allergic dermatitis, increased incidence of lung cancer	Decreased: long-term inadequate intake Increased: kidney failure
Copper	Menkes' syndrome: progressive mental deterioration, vomiting, diarrhea, protein-losing enteropathy, hypopigmentation, bone and hair changes Deficiency: neutropenia, hypochromic anemia, pallor, dermatitis, neurological dysfunction	Wilson's disease: cirrhosis, Kayser-Fleischer rings,[a] kidney dysfunction, neurologic or psychiatric symptoms (tremors, slow speech, inappropriate behavior, personality changes) Mild chronic toxicity: fatigue, anemia, thrombocytopenia Acute toxicity: nausea, vomiting, diarrhea	Decreased: high zinc, iron, or vitamin C intake, corticosteroid use Increased: infection, rheumatoid arthritis, pregnancy, oral contraceptives, decreased biliary excretion
Iodine	Hypothyroid goiter, neuromuscular impairment, deaf-mutism, increased embryonic and postnatal mortality, cognitive impairment, impaired fertility, congenital hypothyroidism (severe cases)	Thyrotoxicosis: nodular goiter, weight loss, tachycardia, muscle weakness, warm skin	Decreased: long-term inadequate intake
Iron	Microcytic, hypochromic anemia (weakness, pallor, fatigue), glossitis, headache, dysphasia, nail changes, gastric atrophy, paresthesia, decreased cognitive function	Cirrhosis, cardiomyopathy, pancreatic damage, skin pigmentation changes	Increased: blood transfusion Decreased: blood loss
Manganese	Nausea; vomiting; dermatitis; hair color changes; hypocholesterolemia; growth retardation; defective carbohydrate, lipid, and protein metabolism	Parkinsonian-like symptoms, hyperirritability, hallucinations, libido disturbances, ataxia, mental confusion, lack of attention, memory loss	Increased: decreased biliary excretion, high iron or vitamin C intake
Molybdenum	Tachycardia, tachypnea, altered mental status, visual changes, headache, nausea, vomiting	Gout-like syndrome, increased urinary copper	Decreased: low birth weight, excessive GI losses
Selenium	Muscle weakness or pain, cardiomyopathy, skin and hair pigmentation changes	Nausea, vomiting, hair or nail loss, tooth decay, skin lesions, irritability, fatigue, peripheral neuropathy	Decreased: malignancy, liver failure, pregnancy Increased: reticuloendothelial neoplasia
Zinc	Dermatitis (scaly, hyperpigmented skin lesions), altered taste and smell, alopecia, diarrhea, apathy, depression, growth retardation, impaired wound healing, anorexia, confusion, immunosuppression, delayed sexual maturation, hypogonadism (decreased sperm count and function)	Acute: diarrhea, vomiting, nausea, dizziness, garlic-smelling breath; death with large IV doses Chronic: immunosuppression, decreased HDL-C, copper deficiency	Decreased: infection, burns, stress, hypoalbuminemia, corticosteroids, pregnancy, inflammation Increased: tissue injury, hemolysis, contaminated collection tube

GI, gastrointestinal; HDL-C, high-density-lipoprotein cholesterol; LDL-C, low-density-lipoprotein cholesterol; RQ, respiratory quotient.

[a]Kayser-Fleischer rings are dark rings that appear to encircle the iris of the eye.

Data from references 12 and 38 to 41.

deficiency is characterized by glucose intolerance, impaired protein utilization, and increased insulin requirements. Patients with chromium deficiency also may have increased free fatty acid concentrations and a low respiratory quotient (RQ) (Table 118-6). Chromium deficiency has only been identified in patients receiving long-term parenteral nutrition with inadequate chromium intake. Plasma chromium concentrations do not accurately reflect total body chromium status, presumably because the biologically active form of chromium is the low-molecular-weight chromium binding substance. Toxicity from trivalent chromium is not a common clinical concern, and chromium toxicity has been reported only with contaminated drinking water or industrial exposure. Chromium supplementation as an adjunct for weight loss has not been proven effective.

Manganese is important in the function of many enzymes, including arginase (amino acid metabolism via the urea cycle), pyruvate carboxylase and phosphoenolpyruvate carboxykinase (carbohydrate and cholesterol metabolism), superoxide dismutase (mitochondrial antioxidant), glycosyltransferases (bone formation via proteoglycans), and prolidase (wound healing).[43,46,52] Excess manganese is eliminated via the bile. Manganese deficiency has only been reported in association with the ingestion of chemically defined manganese-deficient oral diets. Table 118-6 lists common symptoms associated with manganese deficiency. Manganese toxicity is more concerning and has been described in industrial exposures via inhaled manganese and in patients receiving long-term parenteral nutrition supplemented with manganese (standard trace element preparation) in the setting of chronic cholestasis.[43,46,52–55] Manganese can accumulate in brain tissue, and the newborn brain may be more susceptible to the effects of manganese toxicity.[46,53] Whole-blood manganese concentrations can be obtained to assess manganese status. MRI with intensity and T1 values in the globus pallidus may be useful for assessing manganese toxicity.[54,55] Clinical toxicity is evidenced primarily by extrapyramidal symptoms mimicking Parkinson's disease, such as tremors, ataxia, and facial muscle spasms. These symptoms may be preceded by psychiatric symptoms, including irritability, aggressiveness, and hallucinations. In most reported cases, manganese removal from the parenteral nutrition solution resulted in resolution of neurologic symptoms in 6 months with partial or total normalization of the MRI after 1 to 2 years.

Selenium is incorporated into at least 25 enzymes known as selenoproteins, about half of which have a defined metabolic function. Important selenoproteins include selenoprotein P (antioxidant activity), glutathione peroxidases (antioxidant activity), iodothyronine deiodinase (thyroid hormone regulation), thioredoxin reductase (vitamin C), selenoprotein V (spermatogenesis), and selenoprotein S (inflammation and immune response).[43–45,56] Selenoprotein P is the major (60%) circulating form of selenium in plasma. A key metabolic function of selenium has been attributed to its role in the enzymatic cofactor selenocysteine, the 21st amino acid.[56] Prematurity, critical illness, chronic GI losses, and long-term selenium-free parenteral nutrition are associated with low serum selenium concentrations and decreased glutathione peroxidase activity.[43–45,56] The clinical significance of reduced serum selenium concentrations is unclear, but low selenium concentrations may make individuals more susceptible to physiologic stressors. Although higher selenium intakes are suggested for critically ill patients, the optimal intake is unknown. Current recommendations range from 20 to 1000 mcg/day.[56] Low plasma selenium concentrations in critically ill patients correlate with low triiodothyronine (T_3) concentrations.[56] Serum selenium concentrations reflect acute distribution between tissues rather than selenium stores. Selenium deficiency is associated with muscle pain, wasting, and weakness (Table 118-6), but severe biochemical deficiency is not always accompanied by these symptoms. Fatal cardiomyopathy has been reported in several cases. Plasma, serum, erythrocyte, and whole-blood selenium, plasma selenoprotein P, and plasma, platelet, and whole-blood glutathione peroxidase activity respond to changes in selenium intake, but the response is heterogeneous.[57] Decreased plasma selenium concentrations may indicate selenium deficiency, but reductions have been observed in patients with malignancies, liver failure, pregnancy, alcoholism, and HIV; in patients receiving statins or corticosteroids; and in smokers. Selenium toxicity or selenosis generally occurs only in those with long-term exposure to foods grown in selenium-rich soil (e.g., U.S. Great Plains area) and may occur when intake exceeds 400 mcg/day for prolonged periods; although, the lowest observed adverse event intake is 850 mcg/day. Selenium toxicity results in hair and nail brittleness and loss, GI disturbance, skin rash, garlic breath odor, fatigue, irritability, and nervous system abnormalities.

Molybdenum is a cofactor for enzymes involved in catabolism of sulfur amino acids, purines, and pyrimidines (i.e., xanthine, aldehyde, and sulfite oxidases).[43–45] Molybdenum deficiency is rare, but an inborn error of metabolism resulting in molybdenum deficiency has been identified. One case of molybdenum deficiency has been reported in a patient receiving long-term parenteral nutrition who presented with symptoms that included tachycardia, tachypnea, headache, night blindness, nausea, vomiting, central scotomas, lethargy, disorientation, and ultimately coma (Table 118-6). Symptoms were reversed when molybdenum was added to the parenteral nutrition solution.[58] Factors predisposing to molybdenum deficiency appear to be low birth weight,[59] excessive GI losses, and long-term inadequate intake, such as with molybdenum-free parenteral nutrition. Biochemical abnormalities expected in molybdenum deficiency include very low serum and urine uric acid concentrations (low xanthine oxidase activity) and low urine inorganic sulfate concentrations with high urine inorganic sulfite concentrations (low sulfate oxidase activity).[43–45] Molybdenum toxicity has not been described.

Deficiency of iodine, a component of thyroid hormones, may result in goiter formation (see Chap. 58). However, not everyone with an iodine-deficient diet will develop a goiter. Measurement of thyroxine (T_4) and T_3 can be used to assess iodine status (Table 118-6). IV iodine supplementation is not necessary except during long-term parenteral nutrition with minimal enteral intake. Iodine needs may be met by cutaneous absorption of iodine from germicides (e.g., povidone–iodine) used in catheter care or consumption of iodized salt.[43–45] Use of povidone–iodine as a topical antiseptic has decreased with the increased use of chlorhexidine for catheter care; thus, the need for iodine supplementation must be individualized. Iodine excess is rarely a clinical concern when thyroid and kidney function are normal.

Iron is the most abundant trace element and is an important component of hemoglobin, myoglobin, and cytochrome enzymes; it is important in oxygen transport and cellular energy production. Patients with iron-deficiency anemia generally present with fatigue, weakness, and pallor, but they may have other symptoms (see Chap. 80).[43–45] Inadequate iron intake, malabsorption, and blood loss are the principal causes of iron-deficiency anemia. Iron toxicity (overload) with possible organ damage can occur when chronic iron intake exceeds requirements, such as in patients receiving chronic blood transfusions. Iron deficiency or overload is confirmed by assessment of body iron stores, as reflected indirectly by measurement of hemoglobin, serum iron, total iron-binding capacity, and serum ferritin or directly by bone marrow staining or liver biopsy. Direct methods are the most accurate but are invasive and rarely necessary. Because indirect parameters may be altered by acute or chronic illness independent of iron stores, concomitant illness must be considered in their interpretation.

Vitamins

Vitamins act as both catalysts (cofactors) and substrates in essential metabolic reactions. A comprehensive nutrition-focused history and physical examination is the most valuable means of assessing patients for vitamin deficiency or toxicity (Table 118-7). A thorough review of vitamins and their complex effects on nutrition and metabolism is beyond the scope of this chapter.[43–45,60,61] Multiple vitamin deficiencies may be associated with generalized malnutrition; however, single vitamin deficiencies occur. Thiamine deficiency results in lactic acidosis and encephalopathy. Pernicious anemia caused by vitamin B_{12} (cyanocobalamin) deficiency can occur after ileal resection and has been reported with increasing frequency as a consequence of decreased gastric acidity, especially in elderly adults.[62]

The increasing prevalence of vitamin D deficiency is a growing U.S. healthcare concern, especially in children and elderly adults.[63–65] Laboratory assessment can confirm the clinical suspicion of a deficiency or toxicity state. The most common assessment is measurement of 25-OH-vitamin D, the storage form of vitamin D, in plasma or serum. Because 1,25-$(OH)_2$-vitamin D is not stored and usually found in low concentrations in the blood because it is produced only when needed, it is not a useful marker of vitamin D deficiency (Table 118-7). The first indication of a deficiency is usually a decrease in circulating serum concentrations of 25-OH-vitamin D. Subsequently, there is a decrease in urinary excretion of vitamin D, which is followed by diminished tissue concentrations.

Vitamin toxicity can occur, especially with fat-soluble vitamins (A, D, E, and K), which are stored in the body. Excessive dietary vitamin A intake (hypervitaminosis A) is linked to an increased risk of hip fractures in both men and women.[66,67] With the exception of cyanocobalamin, which is stored in the liver, water-soluble vitamins are not stored in the body; consequently, the risk of toxicity is minimal unless ingested in very high doses. Recent evidence, however, suggests that even water-soluble vitamins may be associated with adverse events when taken chronically in high doses. Although folic acid administration is definitively associated with a reduction in neural tube defects, its effect on some cardiac outcomes (as a result of its effect on homocysteine concentrations) is not established.[68] The administration of folic acid, vitamin B_6 (pyridoxine), and vitamin B_{12} after coronary artery stenting has been associated with an increased risk of stent restenosis.[69] With Americans' current use of nutrition supplements, clinicians should be alert for signs of hypervitaminosis (Table 118-7) and inappropriate vitamin use and discuss rational supplement use with all patients.

Essential Fatty Acids

The human body can synthesize all fatty acids except the essential fatty acids, linoleic acid (an omega-6 fatty acid) and α-linolenic acid (an omega-3 fatty acid). A deficiency state or essential fatty acid deficiency (EFAD) can be prevented if approximately 5% of total calories are ingested as these fatty acids.[70,71] EFAD is rare in adults and children but can occur with prolonged use of lipid-free parenteral nutrition, severe fat malabsorption, very low-fat enteral feeding formulations or diets, high medium chain triglyceride-containing diets,

TABLE 118-7 Assessment of Vitamin Status

Vitamin	Signs of Deficiency	Laboratory Assay	Comments
Water-Soluble Vitamins			
Thiamine (B_1)	Early: anorexia, fatigue, depression, impaired memory or concentration Late: paresthesia, nystagmus, GI beriberi (nausea, vomiting, abdominal pain, lactic acidosis), beriberi (congestive heart failure, edema), Wernicke's encephalopathy, Korsakoff's psychosis, peripheral neuropathy	Whole blood or erythrocyte transketolase activation test Blood thiamine pyrophosphate Erythrocyte glutathione reductase activity coefficient	Increased need with hemo- and peritoneal dialysis, alcoholism, malabsorption, hypermetabolism
Riboflavin (B_2)	Mucositis, dermatitis, cheilosis, glossitis, photophobia, corneal vascularization, lacrimation, decreased vision, impaired wound healing and growth, normocytic anemia	Urinary riboflavin	
Pantothenic acid	Fatigue, malaise, headache, insomnia, vomiting, abdominal cramps	Serum pantothenic acid	
Niacin	Pellagra: dermatitis, dementia, glossitis, diarrhea, memory loss, headaches	Urinary niacin and N_1-methylnicotinamide Erythrocyte NAD and NADP concentrations to determine "niacin number"	Flushing, nausea, and vomiting seen with hyperlipidemia treatment; increased need with hemo- and peritoneal dialysis
Pyridoxine (B_6)	Pellagra, dermatitis, glossitis, cheilosis, distal limb numbness or paresthesia, convulsions, microcytic anemia	Plasma pyridoxal 5-phosphate Urinary 4-pyridoxic acid	Sensory neuropathy and seizures with very high doses (>2 g/day)
Folic acid	Macrocytic anemia, diarrhea, glossitis, cheilosis, angular stomatitis, fatigue, difficulty concentrating, irritability, headache, palpitations, shortness of breath, heart failure, tachycardia, postural hypotension, lactic acidosis, neural tube defects, impaired cellular immunity, paranoid behavior	Serum or plasma folate (acute) Red blood cell folate (chronic) Serum homocysteine	Decreased with increased cellular/tissue turnover (pregnancy, malignancy, hemolytic anemia); masks diagnosis of vitamin B_{12} deficiency; decreases risks of neural tube defects
Cyanocobalamin (B_{12})	Pernicious anemia, glossitis, spinal cord degeneration, peripheral neuropathy	Serum cobalamin Plasma homocysteine Urinary or plasma methylmalonic acid	Decreased absorption in the elderly, distal ileal resection, loss of gastric intrinsic factor due to gastrectomy or long-term gastric acid suppression
Biotin	Dermatitis, depression, lassitude, somnolence	Urinary biotin	
Ascorbic acid (C)	Enlargement or keratosis of hair follicles, impaired wound healing, anemia, lethargy, depression, bleeding, ecchymosis, scurvy	Plasma ascorbic acid Leukocyte ascorbate	GI disturbances, hyperoxaluria and kidney stones, excess iron absorption with excess intake; smokers need 35 mg/day more than nonsmokers; rebound scurvy with abrupt discontinuation after long-term high doses
Fat-Soluble Vitamins			
Vitamin A (includes retinol, retinal, retinoic acid, and retinyl esters)	Dermatitis, night blindness, xerophthalmia, Bitot spots,[a] pruritus, follicular hyperkeratosis, excessive deposition of periosteal bone, hair changes, poor growth and wound healing, impaired resistance to infection Irreversible: punctate keratopathy, keratomalacia, corneal perforation	Serum retinol Serum retinol-binding protein Serum retinyl esters (toxicity)	Teratogenic, liver toxicity with excessive intake; alcohol intake, liver disease, hyperlipidemia, and severe protein malnutrition increase susceptibility to adverse effects of high intake; β-carotene supplements recommended only for those at risk of deficiency (fat malabsorption); can reverse corticosteroid-induced poor wound healing
D	Rickets, osteomalacia, osteoporosis, muscle weakness, poor growth, hypocalcemia, immune dysfunction, cardiomyopathy	Serum 25-hydroxy-vitamin D	Elevated intake causes hypercalcemia, nephrocalcinosis, azotemia, poor growth; decreased in uremia, elderly (especially in winter), fat malabsorption
α-Tocopherol (E)	Hemolysis	Serum α-tocopherol Ratios of serum α-tocopherol to total lipids	Excess intake: hemorrhagic toxicity; increased risk of bleeding with anticoagulants; impaired leukocyte function
K	Bleeding (ecchymosis, petechiae, hematomas)	Prothrombin time INR	Anticoagulant therapy can be affected by supplements or diet

GI, gastrointestinal; INR, international normalized ratio; NAD, nicotinamide adenine dinucleotide; NADP, nicotinamide adenine dinucleotide phosphate.

[a]Bitot spots are spots located superficially in the conjunctiva, which are oval, triangular, or irregular in shape.

Data from references 12, 38 to 40, and 55 to 58.

and severe malnutrition, especially in stressed patients.[71] Although the time course to develop EFAD is variable, overt EFAD has been shown to occur after 4 weeks of lipid-free parenteral nutrition, and biochemical evidence can occur within 1 week.[71] Because newborns, especially those born prematurely, have limited fat stores, they may develop EFAD more rapidly than adults. Biochemical evidence of EFAD has been noted within 72 hours after birth in preterm infants receiving fat-free IV solutions.[72] Symptoms reported with EFAD include dermatitis (dry, cracked, scaly skin), alopecia, impaired wound healing, growth failure, thrombocytopenia, and anemia.

Linoleic acid is converted to arachidonic acid (a tetraene fatty acid). When linoleic acid is unavailable, oleic acid is substituted, resulting in production of eicosatrienoic acid (a triene fatty acid) as the metabolic end product. Thus, EFAD can be detected by decreased tetraene production and increased triene production. The usual ratio of trienes to tetraenes is less than 0.4; when the ratio is greater than 0.4, the diagnosis of EFAD is established. Analysis of plasma fatty acids is expensive and not widely available; therefore, EFAD diagnosis is generally made based on risk assessment and clinical findings.

Carnitine

Carnitine is a quaternary amine required for transport of long-chain fatty acids into the mitochondria for β-oxidation and energy production. Carnitine also binds acyl residues aiding in their elimination (detoxification), thereby decreasing the number conjugated with coenzyme A and increasing the ratio of free to acetylated coenzyme A. Carnitine is available from a wide variety of dietary sources (especially meats) and can be synthesized by the liver and kidneys from lysine and methionine. Hepatic synthesis is decreased in premature infants, and low plasma carnitine concentrations and overt carnitine deficiency have been documented in premature infants receiving carnitine-free parenteral nutrition or diets, as well as in those with inborn errors of metabolism.[73] Other predisposing factors for carnitine deficiency include chronic kidney[74] or liver disease, chronic valproic acid and zidovudine use,[75] and a vegetarian diet. The clinical presentation of carnitine deficiency includes generalized skeletal muscle weakness, fatty liver, and fasting hypoglycemia.[73]

In clinical practice, carnitine status is most often assessed by measurement of plasma total and free carnitine concentrations and acylcarnitine, although tissue concentrations, especially muscle, are higher than plasma concentrations.[73] Plasma and urine carnitine concentrations are most helpful in primary carnitine deficiency (an inborn error of metabolism); acylcarnitine concentrations are more helpful in secondary causes of carnitine deficiency. When only total and free concentrations are available, the free is subtracted from the total to give the acylcarnitine concentration.

NUTRIENT REQUIREMENTS

8 Nutrient requirements vary with age, gender, size, disease state, and clinical condition. Nutrition status, physical activity, and the need for continued maintenance of adequate nutrition or repletion in those with ongoing metabolic stress dictate the nutrient requirements for an individual. For obese patients, usual nutrition requirements may be altered because of the need for weight loss. In children, there is the added consideration of sustaining or reestablishing normal growth and development. Organ function (e.g., intestine, kidney, liver, pancreas) may affect nutrient utilization. Nutrient requirements can be estimated using guidelines interpreted in the context of patient-specific factors.

Recommended Dietary Allowances

The recommended daily allowances (RDAs) were initially established in 1941, but in 1997, the Food and Nutrition Board introduced a new family of nutrition reference values, the dietary reference intakes (DRIs).[76] The four DRI categories are estimated average requirements (EARs), RDAs, adequate intakes (AIs), and tolerable upper intake levels (ULs). EARs, defined as the nutrient intake that meets the needs of 50% of persons in a given population, can be used for planning nutrient intakes for groups. The RDA, the nutrient intake that meets the needs of almost all persons in a designated group, is approximately 2 standard deviations above the EAR for nutrients for which the requirement is well defined and 1.2 times the EAR for other nutrients. To evaluate an individual's daily intake, the RDA is the most appropriate comparator. AIs, defined as the average intake for the designated group that appears to sustain a particular nutrition state, growth, or other functional indicator of health, is reserved for nutrients for which no EAR or RDA has been determined. Finally, the UL is the maximum nutrient intake unlikely to pose adverse effects in almost all persons in a designated group.[76]

Dietary reference intakes have been established for six nutrient groups: calcium, phosphorus, magnesium, vitamin D, and fluoride; folate and other B vitamins; antioxidants (e.g., selenium and vitamins C and E); trace elements; macronutrients (e.g., protein, fat, carbohydrates, and fiber); and electrolytes and water.[76] Because of the increased prevalence of vitamin D deficiency, calcium and vitamin D recommendations were revised in 2010.[77] The U.S. Department of Agriculture's website includes an Interactive DRI for Healthcare Professionals, which calculates a generally healthy individual's DRI-based nutrition needs.[78]

According to the DRIs, adults should consume 45% to 65% of their total calories as carbohydrates (RDA, 130 g), 20% to 35% as fat, and 10% to 35% as protein.[70] The recommendations for children are similar: carbohydrate, 45% to 65%; fat, 30% to 40%; and protein, 10% to 30%. Infants, especially premature infants, require a higher proportion of calories from fat (~40%–50% of total calories) to ensure normal neurological development.

Energy

9 Energy requirements of individuals can be estimated using published, validated equations or can be measured directly. The most appropriate method is determined by a variety of factors, including severity of illness and resource availability.

Estimating Energy Expenditure

Daily energy expenditure consists of the basal energy expenditure (BEE), diet-induced thermogenesis (10%), and energy used for physical activity. In sick or injured patients, the BEE is increased because of stress-related hypermetabolism, but the physical activity and the energy needed for metabolism are usually reduced. For example, continuous infusion enteral feeding, often used in critically ill patients, results in minimal diet-induced thermogenesis (5%) when overfeeding is not present.[19] Failure to account for these changes can result in overfeeding.

More than 200 methods for determining an individual's daily energy requirement have been published. These methods use population estimates of calories per kilogram of body weight (kcal/kg), equations that estimate energy expenditure (kcal/day or kJ/day; 1 kcal is equivalent to 4.186 kJ), or indirect calorimetry. The simplest method to determine energy requirements is to use population estimates of calories required per kilogram of body weight. This method assumes standard values for health or the energy requirements associated with various disease states or clinical conditions, as well as the additional requirements for repletion of a malnourished individual. Most do not take into consideration age- or gender-related differences in energy needs. No stress or activity modifiers are used with these equations because the effect of the clinical condition (hypermetabolism) is already captured in the calculation. Daily adult requirements by this method can be estimated as shown below.[2,19,79–81]

1. Healthy, normal nutrition status, minimal illness severity: 20 to 25 kcal ABW/kg/day (84–105 kJ ABW/kg/day)
2. Illness, metabolic stress (BMI <30 kg/m^2): 25 to 30 kcal ABW/kg/day (105–126 kJ ABW/kg/day)
3. Illness, metabolic stress (BMI ≥30 kg/m^2): 11 to 14 kcal ABW/kg/day (46–59 kJ ABW/kg/day) or 22 to 25 kcal IBW/kg/day (92–105 kJ ABW/kg/day)
4. Major burn injury (≥50% total body surface area) or repletion: 30 kcal ABW/kg/day or greater (≥126 kJ ABW/kg/day)

TABLE 118-8 Dietary Reference Intakes for Energy and Protein in Healthy Children

Age (Reference age/weight)	Estimated Energy Requirement (kcal/day)[a] Boys	Girls	Protein RDA (g/kg/day)[b]
0–6 mo (3 mo/6 kg)	570	520	1.52[c]
7–12 months (9 mo/9 kg)	743	676	1.5
1–2 yr (24 mo/12 kg)	1,046	992	
1–3 yr (24 mo/12 kg)			1.1
3–8 yr (6 yr/20 kg)	1,742	1,642	
4–8 yr (6 yr/20 kg)			0.95
9–13 yr (11 yr/M: 36 kg; W: 37 kg)	2,279	2,071	0.95
14–18 yr (16 yr/M: 61 kg; W: 54 kg)	3,152	2,368	0.85

M, men; RDA, recommended dietary allowance; W, women.
[a]One kcal is equal to approximately 4.19 kJ.
[b]Protein requirements in children with moderate to severe stress increase by 50% or more.
[c]Adequate intake.
Data from reference 65.

When equation 3 is used for patients with a BMI of 30 kg/m^2 or more, the calories provided allow for permissive underfeeding (provision of approximately 80% of estimated or measured energy needs), which decreases infection rates and hospital length of stay.[79] Table 118-8 shows suggested calorie intakes (kcal/kg) for maintenance and normal growth of healthy infants and children.[70,71] These maintenance energy requirements are approximately 150% of the basal metabolic rate, with the additional calories provided to support usual activity and growth. For all ages, energy requirements increase with fever, sepsis, major surgery, trauma, burns, and long-term growth failure and in the presence of chronic conditions such as bronchopulmonary dysplasia, congenital heart disease, and cystic fibrosis. Energy needs may decrease with obesity and neurologic disability (e.g., cerebral palsy).[22]

Numerous equations are available to estimate energy expenditure in adults and children (Tables 118-9 and 118-10, respectively).[2,19,70,71,79,81,82] The Harris-Benedict equations, derived in 1919 in a study of 239 individuals, are still used for assessing energy requirements in adults. They have the advantage of incorporating the patient's age, height, weight, gender, and clinical condition into the estimation. These equations were derived from oxygen consumption measurements made on normally nourished healthy individuals who were in a fasting and resting state. Although these equations are commonly referred to as the "BEE equations," they actually estimate resting energy expenditure (REE), the amount of energy expended at rest by a fasting, awake individual in a temperature-controlled environment performing only basal functions such as breathing, circulation, and metabolic processes.

Because these equations approximate REE, their results must be modified by a factor that adjusts for the individual's clinical condition. For example, whereas an individual who is confined to bed may require a calorie intake that is only 20% to 30% above the REE, a person who has sustained a severe burn injury may require 150% to 200% of the calculated REE. Some clinicians multiply the calculated REE by both a stress factor and an activity factor. Because validation studies in healthy subjects have shown that these equations overestimate REE by 6% to 15%, the calculated REE should be multiplied by either a stress factor or an activity factor to avoid further overestimation of the individual's energy needs.[2] It should also be noted that ABW (up to a BMI of 57 kg/m^2 in men and 40 kg/m^2 in women), not IBW or adjusted body weight, was used to generate the original data with these equations and should be used for these calculations.[81] Overestimation of energy needs with the Harris-Benedict equations is well documented.[19,81] The Mifflin-St Jeor equations are more accurate in healthy adults than the Harris-Benedict equations (Table 118-9): the accuracy rate is

TABLE 118-9 Estimates of Energy Expenditure in Adults[a]

Healthy Adults

Harris-Benedict[b] Equations (kcal/day)
Men: BEE = 66 + (13.75W [kg] + 5H [cm]) – (6.8A)
Women: BEE = 655 + (9.6W [kg] + 1.8H [cm]) – (4.7A)

DRI Equations (kcal/day)[c]
Men: EER = 662 – 9.53A + (PA × 15.91W) + 539.6H (m)
Women: EER = 354 – 6.91A + (PA × 9.36W) + 726H (m)
PA = 1 if sedentary; 1.12 if low active; 1.27 if active; and 1.45 if very active

Mifflin-St Jeor Equations
Men: 10W + 6.25H (cm) – 5A + 5
Women: 10W + 6.25H (cm) – 5A – 16

Critically Ill Adults

Penn State Equations
Age ≥60 years with BMI ≥30 kg/m^2: Mifflin(0.71) + Tmax(85) + Ve(64) – 3085
All others: Mifflin(0.96) + Tmax(167) + Ve(31) – 6212

A, age in years; BEE, basal energy expenditure; BMI, body mass index; DRI, dietary reference intakes; EER, estimated energy requirement; H, height in centimeters or meters, as indicated; PA, physical activity factor; Tmax, maximum body temperature in the previous 24 hours in degrees centigrade; Ve, minute ventilation in L/min; W, actual body weight in kilograms.
[a]No real consensus exists as to which formula is best in all situations. Many clinicians use more than one equation and calculate a range of acceptable intakes.
[b]The common practice of using an adjusted body weight for obesity in these calculations is not supported by the original data that used actual body weight in all cases up to a BMI of 56 kg/m^2 in men and 40 kg/m^2 in women.[19,81]
[c]One kcal is equal to approximately 4.19 kJ.
Data from references 2, 19, 65, 79, and 81.

TABLE 118-10 Equations to Estimate Energy Expenditure in Children[a,b]

FAO/WHO/UNU 2001 (kcal/day)[b]

0–12 Months

Breastfed
TEE (kcal/day) = –152 + 92.8W
TEE (MJ[c]/day) = –0.635 + 0.388W

Formula fed
TEE (kcal/day) = –29 + 82.6W
TEE (MJ[c]/day) = –0.122 + 0.346W

Boys 1–17 Years
TEE (kcal/day) = 310.2 + 63.3W – 0.263W^2
TEE (MJ[c]/day) = 1,298 + 0.265W – 0.0011W^2

Girls 1–17 Years
TEE (kcal/day) = 263.4 + 65.3W – 0.454W^2
TEE (MJ[c]/day) = 1,102 + 0.273W – 0.0019W^2

DRI Equations (kcal/day)

Birth through 2 years of age
EER = (89W – 100) + GF
GF = 175 kcal if 0–3 months; 56 kcal if 4–6 months; 22 kcal if 7–12 months; 20 kcal if 13–35 months

3–18 years of age
Boys: EER = 88.5 – (61.9A) + PA (26.7W + 903H) + GF
Girls: EER = 135.3 – (30.8A) + PA (10W + 934H) + GF
GF = 20 kcal if 3–8 years; 25 kcal if 9–18 years
PA = 1 if sedentary; 1.13–1.16 if low activity; 1.26–1.31 if normal activity; and 1.42–1.56 if very active

A, age in years; DRI, dietary reference intakes; EER, estimated energy requirement; FAO/WHO/UNU, Food and Agriculture Organization/World Health Organization/ United Nations University; GF, growth factor, H, height in meters; PA, physical activity factor; TEE, total energy expenditure; W, actual body weight in kilograms.
[a]No real consensus exists as to which formula is best in all situations. Many clinicians use more than one equation and calculate a range of acceptable intakes.
[b]Additional daily calories are needed for growth; about 2 kcal/g of weight gain desired.
[c]One kcal is equivalent to approximately 4.19 kJ; 1 MJ = 1000 kJ.
Data from references 65 and 82.

TABLE 118-11 Stress Factors for Use in Adults and Children

Condition	Factor
No Stress	
Confined to bed	1.2
Out of bed: normal activity	1.3
Catch-up growth	1.5
Mild Stress[a]	
Postoperative recovery: uncomplicated surgery	1–1.15
Trauma: mild (e.g., long-bone fracture)	1.2
Moderate Stress[a]	
Sepsis (moderate)	1.2–1.4
Trauma: CNS (sedated)	1.3
Trauma: moderate to severe	Children: 1.5 Adults: 1.3–1.4
Severe Stress[a]	
Sepsis (severe)	Children: 1.6 Adults: 1.3
Trauma: CNS (severe)	Children: up to 2.0 Adults: up to 1.3
Burns (proportionate to burned area)[b]	Up to 2.0

CNS, central nervous system.

[a]Assumes decreased activity during periods of stress.

[b]Formulas specifically for estimating energy needs in burned children and adults have been published and are likely to be more accurate. See reference 80.

Data from reference 2.

80% in patients who are not obese (BMI ≤30 kg/m^2) and 70% in obese patients (BMI >30 kg/m^2).[19]

There is no individual method proven to accurately determine the energy needs of all critically ill patients. The Penn State equations are more accurate in critically ill adults receiving mechanical ventilation[19] (Table 118-9). There is no consensus as to the best equation for critically ill adults who are not mechanically ventilated. Likewise, there is insufficient evidence to support the use of one equation over another in estimating the energy expenditure of critically ill children.[83,84] The metabolic response to stress in children appears to be similar to that seen in critically ill adults; thus, "stress factors" used in adults, shown in Table 118-11, are often used in children after the energy expenditure has been estimated using one of the predictive equations shown in Table 118-10.

Clinical **Controversy...**

Numerous equations and "stress" factors have been published for estimating energy requirements. None is superior in all situations. Practitioners vary as to which equation they choose to use for any given patient.

Measuring Energy Expenditure

The most accurate method to determine energy expenditure is to measure it using indirect calorimetry (metabolic gas monitoring); however, because of lack of access to necessary equipment, it is used in only a small fraction of patients receiving nutrition support. The indirect calorimetry methodology is based on pulmonary gas exchange: when a substrate (carbohydrate, fat, protein) is oxidized, heat is produced, oxygen is consumed, and carbon dioxide is expired in specific amounts depending on the substrate being oxidized. Indirect calorimetry is a noninvasive procedure in which oxygen consumption (VO_2, mL/min) and carbon dioxide production (VCO_2, mL/min) are measured, and the measured resting energy expenditure (MREE; kcal/day) is calculated using the abbreviated Weir equation as $MREE = ([3.94\ VO_2 + 1.11\ VCO_2] + [2.17\ uN_2]) \times 1.44$.[85,86] The urinary nitrogen component (uN_2) is often omitted when calculating energy expenditure because it accounts for less than 4% of the energy expenditure in critically ill patients, and its omission results in only a 1% to 2% calculation error.[19,86] Excluding the nitrogen component obviates the need for a 24-hour urine collection, which can be problematic in many patients.

The MREE represents the total energy expended during the time period over which the measurements were taken. It is often extrapolated to a 24-hour period to approximate daily energy requirements. MREE reflects alterations in energy requirements as a result of disease or clinical condition, but it does not include energy required for repletion of a malnourished individual or growth in a child. The energy intake required for these functions is accounted for by multiplying MREE by a metabolic or activity factor: mechanically ventilated, critically ill, 1; critically ill, no mechanical ventilation, 1 to 1.1; adult acute, not critically ill, 1.1 to 1.4, depending on activity; adult needing repletion or a child, 1.3 to 2; adult outpatient, 1.1 to 2, depending on activity; and adult depletion (weight loss), less than 1.[87]

Indirect calorimetry can be used to determine the patient's RQ, which reflects substrate oxidation, characterizes substrate utilization, and is calculated as VCO_2/VO_2. RQ values for nutrient substrates are fat, 0.7; carbohydrate, 1; protein, 0.8; and mixed substrate (fat, carbohydrate, and protein), 0.85. RQ values of greater than 1 represent either lipogenesis or hyperventilation; less than 0.7 may indicate a ketogenic diet, fat gluconeogenesis, or ethanol oxidation. Values outside the physiologic range of 0.67 to 1.3 suggest an invalid test. Clinically, the RQ is used to determine if a patient is being overfed, which is likely if the RQ value is greater than 1.

Indirect calorimetry is a respiratory measurement that does not reflect metabolism in all clinical situations.[81,85–87] Calibration errors are common, and indirect calorimetry overestimates REE for patients with hyperventilation, metabolic acidosis, overfeeding, and if there are air leaks anywhere in the system. Underestimation of REE is likely with hypoventilation, metabolic alkalosis, underfeeding, and gluconeogenesis. Mechanically ventilated patients are technically easier to study because the indirect calorimeter circuit can be integrated into the ventilator circuit. However, the patient must be at complete rest for 1 hour, must not receive bolus feedings either by feeding tube or orally for 4 hours, should have no changes in substrate delivery for 12 hours, and must be on a fraction of inspired O_2 of less than 0.6 with a positive end-expiratory pressure less than 5 cm H_2O to ensure a steady-state reading. Unfortunately, many of the patients in whom indirect calorimetry would be most useful will not meet these requirements. Indirect calorimetry should be considered in any patient in whom uncertainty in estimating energy requirements needs to be minimized, such as severely malnourished patients (BMI <18.5 kg/m^2) or obese patients (BMI >30 kg/m^2), patients with unexplained high partial arterial pressure of carbon dioxide ($PaCO_2$) concentrations or minute ventilation, patients with spinal cord injuries, and patients who experience weight loss despite apparently receiving adequate protein and energy intakes.[19,79,85] In the outpatient setting, the availability of portable, less expensive devices has allowed an increase in indirect calorimetry use in weight management.[88]

Protein

Daily protein requirements are based on age, gender, nutrition status, disease state, and clinical condition. Table 118-8 lists the RDAs for protein for children; for individuals older than 18 years of age, the RDA is 0.8 g/kg/day, which is significantly less than most Americans typically consume.[70] In adults older than 60 years of age, protein needs are increased to 1 to 1.5 g/kg/day to help reduce loss of LBM that occurs with aging, and 1.5 to 2 g/kg/day or more may be needed in states of metabolic stress (infection, trauma, surgery) to prevent loss of LBM.[70,79,89] Protein requirements are also higher in pregnant and lactating women (1.1 g/kg/day or 6–10 g protein per day above the usual RDA).[70,90]

Protein metabolism depends on both kidney and liver function. Critical illness results in a hypercatabolic state in which there is increased protein synthesis and degradation. The goal of protein administration is to minimize catabolism by maximizing protein synthesis. Consequently, protein requirements are increased to 1.2 to 2 g/kg/day in critically ill patients. For obese critically ill patients, protein needs are 2 g/kg IBW or more if the BMI is between 30 and 40 kg/m^2 and 2.5 g/kg IBW or more if the BMI is greater than 40 kg/m^2.[79] Adults with significant total body surface area burns have protein requirements as high as 2.5 to 3 g/kg ABW/day. In children with significant burns, between 20% and 25% of their total calorie needs should be provided as protein.[80] Soft tissue defects and large stool or ileostomy losses also increase protein requirements. Liver failure typically results in the need for protein restriction (0.5 g/kg/day) unless a hypercatabolic state is also present, which will increase requirements to 1.5 g/kg/day. Protein needs in patients with kidney failure are variable and affected by the various renal replacement therapies available. The application of these protein intake guidelines requires both clinical judgment and frequent monitoring of kidney and liver function, serum chemistries, clinical condition, and nutrition outcomes.

Nitrogen is found only in protein and at a relatively constant ratio of 1 g nitrogen per 6.25 g of protein. This ratio may vary somewhat for enteral and parenteral feeding formulations, depending on the biologic value of the protein source. The adequacy of protein intake can be assessed clinically by a nitrogen balance study—measuring urinary nitrogen excretion and comparing it with nitrogen intake. Nitrogen balance indirectly reflects protein use or protein catabolic rate, which increases with hypercatabolism. As the stress level increases, a concomitant increase in protein catabolism results in an increase in urinary nitrogen excretion. Usually the amount of urine urea nitrogen (UUN) is measured in a 24-hour urine collection. In healthy individuals, UUN accounts for 80% to 90% of the total urine nitrogen (TUN) excreted. Nitrogen output (g/day) can be approximated as 24-hour UUN + 4, where 4 is a factor representing usual skin, fecal, and respiratory nitrogen losses. Alternatively, if available, TUN can be measured and may be more accurate, especially in critically ill patients. If TUN is used, then the best estimate of nitrogen output is TUN × 1.05.[91] In patients with kidney failure, in which case neither UUN nor TUN accurately represents net protein degradation, nitrogen balance can be approximated with equations based on urea nitrogen appearance.[92]

Fat

The daily AI for men and women for α-linolenic acid is 1.6 and 1.1 g, respectively; for linoleic acid, it is 14 to 17 g/day for men and 11 to 12 g/day for women.[70] Overall, for adults, fat should represent no more than 10% to 35% of total calories, with the recommendation that saturated fatty acids, *trans* fatty acids, and dietary cholesterol intake be kept as low as possible while a nutritionally adequate diet is consumed. Fat should constitute 30% to 40% of energy in children 1 to 3 years of age and 25% to 35% of energy in children 4 to 18 years of age.[70] Fat intake in children younger than 3 years of age is critical for proper central nervous system growth and development; generally, fat-restricted diets (e.g., skim milk) should not be imposed until after the age of 2 to 3 years except under medical supervision. A lower limit of 15% of total energy intake has been suggested as the minimum fat intake in children when fat restriction is warranted.[93]

Fiber

Lower blood pressure and serum cholesterol concentrations as well as maintenance of normal bowel habits have been attributed to dietary fiber intake. Fiber intake may also have a role in the prevention of colon cancer and may promote weight control through its effect on satiety. Men and women 50 years of age and younger should ingest 38 g/day and 25 to 26 g/day, respectively, of total fiber. For men and women older than 50 years of age, the recommended intakes are 30 g/day and 21 g/day, respectively.[70,94] The AI for fiber has not been set for children younger than 1 year of age. For older children, the recommended fiber intake is 19 g/day for children 1 to 3 years of age, 24 g/day for children 4 to 8 years of age, and 26 to 31 g/day for children 9 to 13 years of age.[70] Another method to determine fiber need in children is the "age + 5" rule. The recommended daily intake of fiber is calculated by adding 5 g to the child's age in years.[95] Using this rule, a 6-year-old child would need 11 g/day of dietary fiber.

TABLE 118-12 Factors That Alter Fluid Requirements

Increased Requirements	Decreased Requirements
Fever	Fluid overload
Radiant warmers	Cardiac failure
Diuretics	Decreased urinary output
Vomiting	Heat shields
Nasogastric suction	Relatively high humidity
Ostomy or fistula drainage	Humidified air via endotracheal tube
Diarrhea	Kidney failure
Glycosuria	Hypoalbuminemia with starvation
Phototherapy	Syndrome of inappropriate secretion of antidiuretic hormone (SIADH)
Diabetes insipidus	
Increased ambient temperatures	
Hyperventilation	
Prematurity	
Excessive sweating	
Increased metabolism (e.g., hyperthyroidism)	

Fluid

The daily fluid requirement for an adult depends on many factors but is generally estimated to be 30 to 35 mL/kg, 1 mL for each kcal ingested, or 1,500 mL/m^2. Fluid requirements per kilogram of body weight are higher for children and even higher for preterm infants because of their higher percentage of TBW and basal energy needs. Additionally, premature neonates have increased fluid requirements because of greater insensible losses and the kidneys' inefficiency in concentrating urine. The Holliday-Segar method is a commonly used, quick, and simple method for estimating minimum daily fluid needs of children and adults. Children weighing less than 10 kg should receive at least 100 mL/kg per day. An additional 50 mL/kg/day should be provided for each kilogram of body weight between 11 kg and 20 kg and 20 mL/kg/day for each kilogram above 20 kg. Thus, whereas minimum daily fluid needs for a child weighing 8 kg would be 800 mL/day; 1,350 mL/day would be needed for a 17-kg child, and 2000 mL/day is needed for a 50-kg individual.

Table 118-12 lists factors that alter fluid needs for both adults and children. All sources of fluid intake should be assessed (e.g., fluid vehicles for IV medications and IV or feeding tube flushes) when determining fluid requirements. Urine output and specific gravity as well as serum electrolytes and weight changes can be used to assess fluid status. A urine output of at least 1 mL/kg/hr (in children) and approximately 40 to 50 mL/hr (in adults) is considered adequate to ensure tissue perfusion. Urine output should be higher if large fluid volumes or high renal solute loads (e.g., parenteral nutrition or concentrated enteral feeding formulations) are being administered. Urine specific gravity depends on the kidney's concentrating and diluting capabilities. Concomitant diuretic therapy, as a result of increased solute excretion, limits the usefulness of urine specific gravity as an index of fluid status.

Micronutrients

Requirements for micronutrients (i.e., electrolytes, minerals, trace elements, and vitamins) vary with age, gender, and the route by which the nutrient is ingested (Table 118-13; see Chaps. 34 to 36).[43–46,60,61,77,96] Oral and parenteral requirements vary as a result

TABLE 118-13 Recommended Daily Electrolytes, Trace Elements, and Vitamins Intakes[a]

	Adult (≥19 yr of age)		Pediatric	
Nutrient	**Enteral**	**Parenteral**	**Enteral**	**Parenteral**
Electrolytes and Minerals				
Acetate[b]	—	—	—	—
Calcium	1,000–1,200 mg	0–15 mEq (0–7.5 mmol)	0–12 mo: 210–270 mg 1–3 yr: 700 mg 4–8 yr: 1000 mg 9–18 yr: 1,300 mg	Premature: 2–4 mEq/kg (1–2 mmol/kg) Other: 1–2.5 mEq/kg (0.5–1.25 mmol/kg)
Chloride[b]		—	—	2–6 mEq/kg (2–6 mmol/kg)
Magnesium	M: 400–420 mg W: 310–320 mg	10–20 mEq (5–10 mmol)	0–6 mo: 30 mg 7–12 mo: 75 mg 1–3 yr: 80 mg 4–8 yr: 130 mg 9–18 yr: 240–410 mg	0.25–1 mEq/kg (0.12–0.5 mmol/kg)
Phosphorus	700 mg	20–45 mmol	0–6 mo: 100 mg 7–12 mo: 275 mg 1–8 yr: 460–500 mg 9–18 yr: 1,250 mg	Premature: 1–2 mmol/kg Others: 0.5–1 mmol/kg
Potassium[c,d]	4,700 mg	60–100 mEq (60–100 mmol) (1–2 mEq/kg [1–2 mmol/kg])	0–6 mo: 400 mg 7–12 mo: 700 mg 1–8 yr: 3,000–3,800 mg 9–18 yr: 4,500–4,700 mg	2–5 mEq/kg (2–5 mmol/kg)
Sodium[c,d]	1,200–1,500 mg	60–100 mEq (60–100 mmol) (1–2 mEq/kg [1–2 mmol/kg])	0–6 mo: 120 mg 7–12 mo: 370 mg 1–8 yr: 1,000–1,200 mg 9–18 yr: 1,500 mg	2–6 mEq/kg (2–6 mmol/kg)
Trace Elements				
Chromium[e] (mcg)	20–35	10–15	0–6 mo: 0.2 7–12 mo: 5.5 1–8 yr: 11–15 9–18 yr: 21–35	0.14–0.2 mcg/kg (maximum, 5 mcg)
Copper[f] (mcg)	900	0.3–1.5	0–12 mo: 200–220 1–8 yr: 340–440 9–18 yr: 700–890	20 mcg/kg (maximum, 300 mcg)
Fluoride	3–4 mg	—	0–6 mo: 0.01 mg 7–12 mo: 0.5 mg 1–8 yr: 0.7–1 mg 9–18 yr: 2–3 mg	—
Iodine[g] (mcg)	150	70–140 (not well defined)	0–12 mo: 110–130 1–8 yr: 90 9–18 years: 120–150	1 mcg/kg
Iron (mg)	M: 8 W (≤50 yr): 18 W (>50 yr): 8	Varies	0–6 mo: 0.27 7 mo–8 yr: 7–11 M (9–18 yr): 8–11 F (9–13 yr): 8 F (14–18 yr): 15	Varies
Manganese[f] (mg)	1.8–2.3	0.15–1	0–6 mo: 0.003 7–12 mo: 0.6 1–8 yr: 1.2–1.5 9–18 yr: 1.6–2.2	1 mcg/kg (maximum, 50 mcg)
Molybdenum (mcg)	45	100–200	0–12 mo: 2–3 1–8 yr: 17–22 9–18 yr: 34–43	0.25 mcg/kg (maximum, 5 mcg)
Selenium (mcg)	55	20–60[h]	0–12 mo: 15–20 1–8 yr: 20–30 9–18 yr: 40–55	1.5–3 mcg/kg (maximum, 30 mcg)
Zinc[i] (mg)	8–11	2.5–5[h]	0–12 mo: 2–3 1–8 yr: 3–5 9–18 yr: 8–11	Premature: 300–400 mcg/kg Other: 50–250 mcg/kg
Vitamins				
Ascorbic acid (mg) (Vitamin C)	75–90	100	0–12 mo: 40–50 1–8 yr: 15–25 9–18 yr: 45–75	80
Biotin (mcg)	30	60	0–12 mo: 5–6 1–8 yr: 8–12 9–18 yr: 20–25	20

(continued)

TABLE 118-13 Recommended Daily Electrolytes, Trace Elements, and Vitamins Intakes[a] (Continued)

	Adult (≥19 yr of age)		Pediatric	
Nutrient	**Enteral**	**Parenteral**	**Enteral**	**Parenteral**
Cobalamin (mcg) (vitamin B_{12})	2.4	5	0–12 mo: 0.4–0.5 1–8 yr: 0.9–1.2 9–18 yr: 1.8–2.4	1
Folic acid (mcg)	400	400	0–12 mo: 65–80 1–8 yr: 150–200 9–18 yr: 300–400	140
Niacin (mg NE)	14–16	40	0–12 mo: 2–4 1–8 yr: 6–8 9–18 yr: 12–16	17
Pantothenic acid (mg)	5	15	0–12 mo: 1.7–1.8 1–8 yr: 2–3 9–18 yr: 4–5	5
Pyridoxine (mg) (vitamin B_6)	1.3–1.7	4	0–12 mo: 0.1–0.3 1–8 yr: 0.5–0.6 9–18 yr: 1–1.3	1
Riboflavin (mg)	1.1–1.3	3.6	0–12 mo: 0.3–0.4 1–8 yr: 0.5–0.6 9–18 yr: 0.9–1.3	1.4
Thiamine (mg)	1.1–1.2	3	0–12 mo: 0.2–0.3 1–8 yr: 0.5–0.6 9–18 yr: 0.9–1.2	1.2
Vitamin A (mcg RE) (retinol)	700–900	600–1,000 (3,300–5,500 international units)	0–12 mo: 400–500 1–8 yr: 300–400 9–18 yr: 600–900	700 (2,300 international units)
Vitamin D (mcg)	≤70 yr: 15 (600 international units) >70 yr: 20 (800 international units)	5 (200 international units)	All ages: 15 (600 international units)	5–10 (200–400 international units)
Vitamin E (mg TE) (α-tocopherol)	15 (15 international units)	10 (10 international units)	0–12 mo: 4–5 (4–5 international units) 1–8 yr: 6–7 9–18 yr: 11–15	7 (7 international units)
Vitamin K (mcg)	90–120	0.7–2.5 mg	0–12 mo: 2–2.5 1–8 yr: 30–55 9–18 yr: 60–75	200

M, men; NE, niacin equivalents; RE, retinol equivalents; TE, tocopherol equivalent; W, women.

[a]Data represent either the recommended dietary allowance (RDA) or the adequate intake (AI) for each nutrient where established.
[b]Not established; as needed to maintain acid–base balance.
[c]Newborns and low-birth-weight or very-low-birth-weight infants or with concomitant disease (e.g., necrotizing enterocolitis) may have higher requirements. Intake in nonhealthy children must be individualized.
[d]No RDA or AI has been established.
[e]An additional 20 mcg/day is recommended in patients with significant intestinal losses.
[f]May accumulate in cholestasis.
[g]Long-term parenteral nutrition only if no topical preparations containing iodide or iodized table salt are used.
[h]Higher doses may be required in patients with short bowel syndrome receiving long-term parenteral nutrition.
[i]Additional intake needed with small bowel losses, which can be 12 mg zinc/L or 17 mg zinc/kg of stool or ileostomy output; an additional 2 mg/day needed for acute catabolic stress.

Data from references 38 to 41, 55, 56, 77, and 92.

of bioavailability considerations. Micronutrients poorly absorbed via the GI tract usually are required in greater amounts enterally than parenterally. However, many water-soluble micronutrients are excreted more rapidly via the kidneys when administered IV. In these situations, the IV dose is greater than the oral dose. Other factors that affect micronutrient requirements include GI losses through diarrhea, vomiting, or high-output fistula; wound healing; and hypermetabolism or hypercatabolism. Cutaneous micronutrient losses (e.g., zinc, copper, selenium) also may be significant after major burn injury. Sodium, potassium, magnesium, and phosphorus excretion are particularly dependent on kidney function, and in the setting of kidney failure, intake will likely need to be restricted. Calcium needs, on the other hand, may be increased in these patients. (See Chaps. 28 and 29.) Patients who are severely malnourished will have increased electrolyte requirements during early refeeding owing to preexisting deficiencies or rapid intracellular uptake with anabolism. Failure to provide adequate electrolyte replacement, especially phosphorus, and vitamin supplementation before delivery of full calories during refeeding has resulted in death from the refeeding syndrome.[97,98]

DRUG–NUTRIENT INTERACTIONS

10 Drug-induced nutrient deficiency, poor therapeutic response, enhanced drug toxicity, and failure to achieve desired nutrition outcomes can occur if either nutrition support or drug therapy is stopped as a consequence of adverse effects. Patient outcomes may be enhanced when an effective screening method to identify significant drug–nutrient interactions is coupled with a patient counseling program. An important part of the screening process is to recognize risk factors that influence drug–nutrient interactions. The potential for drug–nutrient interactions is greatest in pediatric and elderly individuals, those with poor nutrition status (obesity and marasmus), and those receiving multiple drug therapies or tube feedings.[99–103]

Mineral and electrolyte serum concentrations may change because of drug therapy. For example, with loop diuretics, urine sodium, potassium, calcium, and magnesium wasting may occur, causing a reduction in their respective serum concentrations (see Chaps. 34 to 36). Alternatively, calcium excretion is reduced with thiazide diuretics. Serum electrolyte concentrations also may increase as a direct result of the drug's mechanism (e.g., potassium-sparing diuretics) or because of the drug's salt form. Corticosteroids and cyclosporine are known to cause hyperglycemia; other drugs are prescribed to pharmacologically lower blood glucose concentrations (e.g., insulin and oral hypoglycemics) (see Chap. 57).

Vitamin status also may be affected by drugs (Table 118-14). For example, sulfasalazine therapy causes a decrease in folic acid, isoniazid therapy causes pyridoxine deficiency, and furosemide therapy may result in decreased thiamine concentrations. Drug therapy outcomes also may be affected by vitamin intake. Whereas the ingestion of high folic acid doses may decrease methotrexate's therapeutic effect, changes in an individual's usual vitamin K or vitamin E intake may cause variability in warfarin's anticoagulant effects.

Drug-delivery vehicles also may contain nutrients. Most IV therapies (maintenance IV fluids, drugs, and electrolyte replacements) are delivered using either dextrose (e.g., dextrose 5% or 10% in water) or sodium (e.g., 0.9% normal saline) in the admixture. Lipid emulsion (10%) is used as the vehicle for the anesthetic agent propofol and the IV calcium channel blocker clevidipine and contributes fat calories (1.1 kcal/mL or 4.6 kJ/mL) when continuous infusions are used. In these instances, nutrition support regimens must be adjusted to accommodate these calories and other nutrients delivered through these therapies to avoid overfeeding and other complications.

TABLE 118-14 Drug and Vitamin Interactions

Drug	Effect
Antacids	Thiamine deficiency
Antibiotics	Vitamin K deficiency
Aspirin	Folic acid deficiency; increased vitamin C excretion
Cathartics	Increased requirements for vitamins D, C, and B_6
Cholestyramine	Vitamins A, D, E, and K and β-carotene malabsorption
Colestipol	Vitamins A, D, E, and K and β-carotene malabsorption
Corticosteroids	Decreased vitamins A, D, and C
Diuretics (loop)	Thiamine deficiency
Efavirenz	Vitamin D deficiency caused by increased metabolism of 25(OH)-vitamin D and 1,25$(OH)_2$-vitamin D
Histamine$_2$ antagonists	Vitamin B_{12} malabsorption (reduced acid results in impaired release of B_{12} from food)
Isoniazid	Vitamin B_6 and niacin deficiency
Isotretinoin	Vitamin A increases toxicity
Mercaptopurine	Niacin deficiency
Methotrexate	Folic acid inhibits effect
Orlistat	Vitamins A, D, E, and K malabsorption caused by fat malabsorption
Pentamidine	Folic acid deficiency
Phenobarbital	Increased vitamin D metabolism
Phenytoin	Increased vitamin D metabolism folic acid concentrations decrease
Primidone	Folic acid deficiency
Protease inhibitors	Vitamin D deficiency (impaired renal hydroxylation)
Proton pump inhibitors	Vitamin B_{12} malabsorption (reduced acid results in impaired release of B_{12} from food)
Sulfasalazine	Folic acid malabsorption
Trimethoprim	Folic acid depletion
Warfarin	Vitamin K inhibits effect; vitamins A, C, and E may affect prothrombin time
Zidovudine	Folic acid and B_{12} deficiencies increase myelosuppression

Data from references 99 to 103.

PRACTICAL GUIDELINES FOR NUTRITION ASSESSMENT

The value of any marker used for nutrition assessment is only as good as its ability to accurately identify the patient with malnutrition and to correlate with nutrition-related complications. The response of the various nutrition status markers to nutrition therapy and the correlation between improvement in these markers and decreased morbidity and mortality support their validity. However, when applied to an individual, most of these markers lack specificity and sensitivity, which makes the development of a clinically useful, cost-effective approach to an individual patient nutrition assessment challenging.

The importance of the nutrition-focused history and physical examination in both nutrition screening and nutrition assessment cannot be overemphasized. The minimum amount of objective data that can further substantiate the clinical impression and provide a baseline for subsequent monitoring is markers that show the best correlation with outcome: weight and serum ALB concentration. The cost effectiveness of the addition of other biochemical parameters is unknown. The assessment of other anthropometric measures is most useful in the setting of anticipated long-term nutrition support in which these measurements will serve as a longitudinal marker of response to the nutrition care plan.

Initially, nutrition requirements are determined on the basis of assumptions made about the patient's clinical condition and the nutrition needs associated with repletion or growth, if needed. After a nutrition intervention has been initiated, periodic reassessment of nutrition status is critical to determine the accuracy of the initial estimate of nutrition requirements. Nutrition requirements are dynamic in the setting of acute or critical illness—as the patient's clinical status changes, so will protein and energy requirements, further emphasizing the need for continued reassessment.

Better markers of nutrition status and methods for determining patient-specific nutrition requirements are needed to allow further refinement of estimates of an individual's nutrition needs. Functional tests and simple, noninvasive tests for body composition analysis hold promise for the future. However, until better methods of assessment become available clinically and are demonstrated to be cost effective, the currently available battery of tests will continue to be the mainstay of nutrition assessment.

ABBREVIATIONS

ABW	actual body weight
AI	adequate intake
ALB	albumin
BEE	basal energy expenditure
BIA	bioelectrical impedance analysis
BMI	body mass index
CDC	Centers for Disease Control and Prevention
CRP	C-reactive protein
DCH	delayed cutaneous hypersensitivity
DRI	dietary reference intake
DXA	dual-energy x-ray absorptiometry

EAR	estimated average requirement
EFAD	essential fatty acid deficiency
GI	gastrointestinal
HIV	human immunodeficiency virus
IBW	ideal body weight
LBM	lean body mass
MREE	measured resting energy expenditure
MRI	magnetic resonance imaging
RDA	recommended dietary allowance
REE	resting energy expenditure
RQ	respiratory quotient
TBW	total body water
TFN	transferrin
TUN	total urine nitrogen
UBW	usual body weight
UL	tolerable upper intake level
UUN	urine urea nitrogen
VCO_2	carbon dioxide production
VO_2	oxygen consumption
WHO	World Health Organization

REFERENCES

1. Jensen GL, Hsiao PY, Wheeler D. Adult nutrition assessment tutorial. J Parenter Enteral Nutr 2012;36:267–274.
2. DeLegge MH, Drake LM. Nutritional assessment. Gastroenterol Clin North Am 2007;36:1–22.
3. Flegal KM, Carroll MD, Kit BK, Ogden CL. Prevalence of obesity and trends in the distribution of body mass index among US adults, 1999–2010. JAMA 2012;307:491–497.
4. Centers for Disease Control and Prevention. Overweight and Obesity: Adult Obesity Facts. 2013, *http://www.cdc.gov/obesity/data/adult.html*.
5. Ogden CL, Carroll MD, Kit BK, Flegal KM. Prevalence of obesity and trends in body mass index among US children and adolescents, 1999–2010. JAMA 2012;307:483–490.
6. Centers for Disease Control and Prevention. Growth Charts. 2010, *http://www.cdc.gov/growthcharts/*.
7. Food and Drug Administration and National Institutes of Health. Final review. Healthy People 2010: Nutrition and Overweight. 2013, *http://www.cdc.gov/nchs/healthy_people/hp2010/hp2010_final_review.htm*.
8. Charney P. Nutrition screening vs nutrition assessment: How do they differ? Nutr Clin Pract 2008;23:366–372.
9. Soeters PB, Reijven PLM, van Bokhorst-de van der Schueren MAE, et al. A rational approach to nutritional assessment. Clin Nutr 2008;27:706–716.
10. Joint Commission on Accreditation of Healthcare Organizations. Comprehensive Accreditation Manual for Hospitals: 2012 (Edition). Oakbrook Terrace, IL: Joint Commission Resources. 2012, *http://www.jointcommission.org*.
11. Kondrup J, Allison SP, Elia M, et al. ESPEN guidelines for nutrition screening 2002. Clin Nutr 2003;22:415–421.
12. Jensen GL, Hsiao PY, Wheeler D. Nutrition screening and assessment. In: Mueller C, ed. The A.S.P.E.N. Adult Nutrition Support Core Curriculum, 2nd ed. Silver Spring, MD: American Society for Parenteral and Enteral Nutrition, 2012:155–169.
13. Skipper A, Ferguson M, Thompson K, et al. Nutrition screening tools: An analysis of the evidence. J Parenteral Enteral Nutr 2012;36:292–298.
14. Anthony PS. Nutrition screening tools for hospitalized patients. Nutr Clin Pract 2008;23:373–382.
15. Centers for Disease Control and Prevention. Use of World Health Organization and CDC growth charts for children aged 0-59 months in the United States. Morbid Mortal Week Report 2010;59(RR-9):1–16.
16. Makhija S, Baker J. The subjective global assessment: A review of its use in clinical practice. Nutr Clin Pract 2008;23:405–409.
17. Keith J. Bedside nutrition assessment past, present, and future: A review of the subjective global assessment. Nutr Clin Pract 2008;23:410–416.
18. Bauer JM, Kaiser MJ, Anthony P, et al. The Mini Nutritional Assessment®: Its history, today's practice, and future perspectives. Nutr Clin Pract 2008;23:388–396.
19. Frankenfield DC, Ashcraft CM. Estimating energy needs in nutrition support patients. J Parenter Enteral Nutr 2011;35: 563–570.
20. Hickson M, Frost G. A comparison of three methods for estimating height in the acutely ill elderly population. J Hum Nutr Diet 2003;16:13–20.
21. Bell KL, Davies PS. Prediction of height from knee height in children with cerebral palsy and non-disabled children. Ann Hum Biol 2006;33:493–499.
22. Marchand V, Motil KJ, and the NASPGHAN Committee on Nutrition. Nutrition support for neurologically impaired children: A clinical report of the North American Society for Pediatric Gastroenterology, Hepatology, and Nutrition. J Pediatr Gastroenterol Nutr 2006;43:123–135.
23. Chumlea WC, Guo SS, Steinbaugh ML. Prediction of stature from knee height for black and white adults and children with application to mobility-impaired or handicapped persons. J Am Diet Assoc 1994;94:1385–1388.
24. Fenton TR. A new growth chart for preterm babies: Babson and Benda's chart updated with recent data and a new format. BMC Pediatrics 2003;3:13.
25. Rao SC, Tompkins J, World Health Organization. Growth curves for preterm infants. Early Human Dev 2007;83: 643–651.
26. Cronk C, Crocker AC, Pueschel SM, et al. Growth charts for children with Down syndrome: 1 month to 18 years of age. Pediatrics 1988;81:102–110.
27. Centers for Disease Control and Prevention. Body Mass Index. 2011, *http://www.cdc.gov/healthyweight/assessing/bmi*.
28. Cook Z, Kirk S, Lawrenson S, Sandford S. Use of BMI in the assessment of undernutrition in older subjects: Reflecting on practice. Proc Nutr Soc 2005;64:313–317.
29. Ness-Abramof R, Apovian CM. Waist circumference measurement in clinical practice. Nutr Clin Pract 2008;23:397–404.
30. Klein S, Allison DB, Heymsfield SB, et al. Waist circumference and cardiometabolic risk: A consensus statement from Shaping American's Health: Association for Weight Management and Obesity Prevention; NAASO, The Obesity Society; the American Society for Nutrition; and the American Diabetes Association. Diabetes Care 2007;30:1647–1652.
31. Fernández JR, Redden DT, Pietrobelli A, Allison DB. Waist circumference percentiles in nationally representative samples of African-American, European-American, and Mexican-American children and adolescents. J Pediatr 2004;145:439–444.
32. Maffeis C, Banzato C, Talamini G, on behalf of the Obesity Study Group of the Italian Society of Pediatric Endocrinology and Diabetology. Waist-to-height ratio, a useful index to identify high metabolic risk in overweight children. J Pediatr 2008;152:207–213.

33. Buchholz AC, Bartok C, Schoeller DA. The validity of bioelectrical impedance models in clinical populations. Nutr Clin Pract 2004;19:433–446.
34. Willett K, Jiang R, Lenart E, et al. Comparison of bioelectrical impedance and BMI in predicting obesity-related medical conditions. Obesity (Silver Spring) 2006;14:480–490.
35. Schlüssel MM, dos Anjos LA, de Vasconcellos MTL, et al. Reference values of handgrip dynamometry of healthy adults: A population-based study. Clin Nutr 2008;27:601–607.
36. Budziareck MB, Duerte RRP, Barbosa-Silva MCG. Reference values and determinants for handgrip strength in healthy subjects. Clin Nutr 2008;27:357–362.
37. Kerr A, Syddall HE, Cooper C, et al. Does admission grip strength predict length of stay in hospitalized older patients? Age Ageing 2006;35:82–84.
38. Lee SY, Gallagher D. Assessment methods in human body composition. Curr Opin Clin Nutr Metab Care 2008;11: 566–572.
39. Baracos V, Caserotti P, Earthman CP, et al. Advances in the science and application of body composition measurement. J Parenter Enteral Nutr 2012;36:96–107.
40. Crook MA. Hypoalbuminemia: The importance of correct interpretation. Nutrition 2009;25:1004–1005.
41. Grimble RF. Immunonutrition. Curr Opin Gastroenterol 2006;21:216–222.
42. Kudsk KA. Immunonutrition in surgery and critical care. Annu Rev Nutr 2006;26:463–479.
43. Food and Nutrition Board, Institute of Medicine, National Academy of Sciences. Dietary Reference Intakes: Elements. 2009, *http://www.iom.edu/Home/Global/News%20 Announcements/~/media/48FAAA2FD9E74D95BBDA2236E 7387B49.ashx*.
44. Clark SF. Vitamins and trace elements. In: Mueller C, ed. The A.S.P.E.N. Adult Nutrition Support Core Curriculum. Silver Spring, MD: American Society for Parenteral and Enteral Nutrition, 2012:121–154.
45. Sriram K, Lonchyna VA. Micronutrient supplementation in adult nutrition therapy: Practical considerations. J Parenter Enteral Nutr 2009;33:548–562.
46. Kleinman RE, ed. Trace elements. In: Pediatric Nutrition Handbook, 6th ed. Elk Grove Village, IL: American Academy of Pediatrics, 2009:423–451.
47. Mohommad MA, Zhou Z, Cave M, et al. Zinc and liver disease. Nutr Clin Prac 2012;27:8–20.
48. Lowe NM, Fekete K, Decsi T. Methods of assessment of zinc status in humans: A systematic review. Am J Clin Nutr 2009;89(Suppl):2040S–2051S.
49. Hurwitz M, Garcia MG, Poole RL, Kerner JA. Copper deficiency during parenteral nutrition: A report of four pediatric cases. Nutr Clin Pract 2004;19:305–308.
50. Harvey LJ, Ashton K, Hooper L, et al. Methods of assessment of copper status in humans: A systematic review. Am J Clin Nutr 2009;89(Suppl):2009S–2024S.
51. Vincent JB. Quest for the molecular mechanism of chromium action and its relationship to diabetes. Nutr Rev 2000;58:67–72.
52. Dickerson RN. Manganese intoxication and parenteral nutrition. Nutrition 2001;17:689–693.
53. Erikson KM, Thompson K, Aschner J, Aschner M. Manganese neurotoxicity: A focus on the neonate. Pharmacol Ther 2007;113:369–377.
54. Iinuma Y, Kubota M, Uchiyama M, et al. Whole-blood manganese levels and brain manganese accumulation in children receiving long-term home parenteral nutrition. Pediatr Surg Int 2003;19:268–272.
55. Takagi Y, Okada A, Sando K, et al. Evaluation of indexes of in vivo manganese status and the optimal intravenous dose for adult patients undergoing home parenteral nutrition. Am J Clin Nutr 2002;75:112–118.
56. Hardy G, Hardy I, Manzanares W. Selenium supplementation in the critically ill. Nutr Clin Prac 2012;27:21–33.
57. Ashton K, Hooper L, Harvey LJ, et al. Methods of assessment of selenium status in humans: A systematic review. Am J Clin Nutr 2009;89(Suppl):2025S–2039S.
58. Sardesai VM. Molybdenum: An essential trace element. Nutr Clin Pract 1993;8:277–281.
59. Friel JK, MacDonald AC, Mercer CN, et al. Molybdenum requirements in low-birth-weight infants receiving parenteral and enteral nutrition. J Parenter Enteral Nutr 1999;23:155–159.
60. Food and Nutrition Board, Institute of Medicine, National Academy of Sciences. Dietary Reference Intakes: Vitamins. 2009, *http://www.iom.edu/Home/Global/News%20 Announcements/~/media/48FAAA2FD9E74D95BBDA2236E 7387B49.ashx*.
61. Kleinman RE, ed. Vitamins. In: Pediatric Nutrition Handbook, 6th ed. Elk Grove Village, IL: American Academy of Pediatrics, 2009:453–495.
62. Allen LH. How common is vitamin B-12 deficiency? Am J Clin Nutr 2009;89(Suppl):693S–696S.
63. Wagner CL, Greer FR. American Academy of Pediatrics Section on Breastfeeding and Committee on Nutrition. Prevention of rickets and vitamin D deficiency in infants, children, and adolescents. Pediatrics 2008;122:1142–1152.
64. Reis JR, von Mühlen D, Miller ER, et al. Vitamin D status and cardiometabolic risk factors in the United States adolescent population. Pediatrics 2009;124:e371–e379.
65. Holick MF. Vitamin D deficiency. N Engl J Med 2007;357:266–281.
66. Peskanich D, Singh V, Willett WC, Colditz GA. Vitamin A intake and hip fractures among postmenopausal women. JAMA 2002;287:47–54.
67. Michaëlsson K, Lithell H, Vessby B, Melhus H. Serum retinol levels and the risk of fracture. N Engl J Med 2003;348:287–294.
68. The Heart Outcomes Prevention Evaluation (HOPE) 2 Investigators. Homocysteine lowering with folic acid and B vitamins in vascular disease. N Engl J Med 2006;354: 1567–1577.
69. Lange H, Suryapranata H, De Luca G, et al. Folate therapy and in-stent restenosis after coronary stenting. N Engl J Med 2004;350:2673–2681.
70. Food and Nutrition Board, Institute of Medicine, National Academy of Sciences. Dietary Reference Intakes for Energy, Carbohydrate, Fiber, Fat, Fatty Acids, Cholesterol, Protein, and Amino Acids. 2005, *http://www.nap.edu/ books/0309085373/html/R2.html*.
71. Hise M, Brown JC. Lipids. In: Mueller C, ed. The A.S.P.E.N. Adult Nutrition Support Core Curriculum. Silver Spring, MD: American Society for Parenteral and Enteral Nutrition, 2012:63–82.
72. Foote KD, MacKinnon MJ, Innis SM. Effect of early introduction of formula versus fat-free parenteral nutrition on essential fatty acid status of preterm infants. Am J Clin Nutr 1991;54:93–97.
73. Crill CM, Helms RA. The use of carnitine in pediatric nutrition. Nutr Clin Prac 2007;22:204–213.
74. Schreiber B. Levocarnitine and dialysis: A review. Nutr Clin Prac 2005;20:218–243.
75. Scruggs ER, Dirks Naylor AJ. Mechanisms of zidovudine-induced mitochondrial toxicity and myopathy. Pharmacology 2008;82:83–88.

76. Food and Nutrition Board, Institute of Medicine, National Academy of Sciences. Dietary Reference Intakes (DRIs): The Development of DRIS 1994-2004: Lessons Learned and New Challenges. 2008, *http://books.nap.edu/openbook.php?record_id=12086&page=R1*.
77. Food and Nutrition Board. Committee to Review Dietary Reference Intakes for Vitamin D and Calcium. Dietary Reference Intakes for Calcium and Vitamin D. Report brief. November 2010, *http://www.iom.edu/vitamind*.
78. United States Department of Agriculture, National Agriculture Library. Interactive DRI for Healthcare Professionals. 2013, *http://fnic.nal.usda.gov/interactiveDRI/*.
79. McClave SA, Martindale RG, Vanek VW, et al. Guidelines for the provision and assessment of nutrition support therapy in the adult critically ill patient: Society of Critical Care Medicine (SCCM) and American Society for Parenteral and Enteral Nutrition (A.S.P.E.N.). J Parenter Enter Nutr 2009;33:277–316.
80. Chan MM, Chan GM. Nutrition therapy for burns in children and adults. Nutrition 2009;25:261–269.
81. Wooley JA, Frankenfield D. Energy. In: Mueller C, ed. The A.S.P.E.N. Adult Nutrition Support Core Curriculum. Silver Spring, MD: American Society for Parenteral and Enteral Nutrition, 2012:22–35.
82. FAO/WHO/UNU Expert Consultation. Food and Nutrition Technical Report Series. Human Energy Requirements. October 2001;1–103, *ftp://ftp.fao.org/docrep/fao/007/y5686e/y5686e00.pdf*.
83. Meyer R, Kulinskaya E, Briassoulis G, et al. The challenge of developing a new predictive formula to estimate energy requirements in ventilated critically ill children. Nutr Clin Pract 2012;27:669–676.
84. Mehta NM, Compher C, A.S.P.E.N. Board of Directors. A.S.P.E.N. clinical guidelines: Nutrition support of the critically ill child. J Parenter Enteral Nutr 2009;33:260–276.
85. Haugen HA, Chan L-N, Li F. Indirect calorimetry: A practical guide for clinicians. Nutr Clin Pract 2007;22:377–388.
86. Moreira de Rocha EE, Alves VGF, da Fonseca RBV. Indirect calorimetry: Methodology, instruments and clinical application. Curr Opin Clin Nutr Metab Care 2006;9: 247–256.
87. Holdy KE. Monitoring energy metabolism with indirect calorimetry: Instruments, interpretation, and clinical application. Nutr Clin Pract 2004;19:447–454.
88. Rubenbauer JR, Johannsen DL, Baier SM, et al. The use of a handheld calorimetry unit to estimate energy expenditure during different physiological conditions. J Parenter Enteral Nutr 2006;30:246–250.
89. Wolfe RR, Miller SL, Miller KB. Optimal protein intake in the elderly. Clin Nutr 2008;27:675–684.
90. Duggleby SL, Jackson AA. Protein, amino acid and nitrogen metabolism during pregnancy: How might the mother meet the needs of her fetus? Curr Opin Clin Nutr Metab Care 2002;5:503–509.
91. Velasco N, Long CL, Otto DA, et al. Comparison of three methods for the estimation of total nitrogen losses in hospitalized patients. J Parenter Enteral Nutr 1990;14: 517–522.
92. Wolk R, Foulks C. Renal disease. In: Mueller C, ed. The A.S.P.E.N. Adult Nutrition Support Core Curriculum. Silver Spring, MD: American Society for Parenteral and Enteral Nutrition, 2012:491–510.
93. Kleinman RE, ed. Fats and fatty acids. In: Pediatric Nutrition Handbook, 6th ed. Elk Grove Village, IL: American Academy of Pediatrics, 2009:357–386.
94. American Dietetic Association. Position of the American Dietetic Association: Health implications of dietary fiber. J Am Diet Assoc 2002;102:993–1000.
95. Dwyer JT. Dietary fiber for children: How much? Pediatrics 1995;96:1019–1022.
96. Greene HL, Hambidge KM, Schanler R, Tsang RC. Guidelines for the use of vitamins, trace elements, calcium, magnesium, and phosphorus in infants and children receiving total parenteral nutrition: Report of the Subcommittee on Pediatric Parenteral Nutrient Requirements from the Committee on Clinical Practice Issues of the American Society for Clinical Nutrition. Am J Clin Nutr 1988;48:1324–1342.
97. Kraft MD, Btaiche IF, Sacks GS. Review of the refeeding syndrome. Nutr Clin Pract 2005;20:625–633.
98. Skipper A. Refeeding syndrome or refeeding hypophosphatemia: A systematic review of cases. Nutr Clin Prac 2012;27:34–40.
99. Jefferson JW. Drug and diet interactions: Avoiding therapeutic paralysis. J Clin Psychiatry 1998;59:31–39.
100. Saito M, Hirata-Koizumi M, Matsumoto M, et al. Undesirable effects of citrus juice on the pharmacokinetics of drugs: focus on recent studies. Drug Saf 2005;28: 677–694.
101. Santos CA, Boullata JI. An approach to evaluating drug-nutrient interactions. Pharmacotherapy 2005;25:1789–1800.
102. McCabe BJ. Prevention of food–drug interactions with special emphasis on older adults. Curr Opin Clin Nutr Metab Care 2004;7:21–26.
103. Hester EK. HIV medications: An update and review of metabolic complications. Nutr Clin Prac 2012;27:51–64.

119

Parenteral Nutrition

Todd W. Mattox and Catherine M. Crill

KEY CONCEPTS

1. Four steps to developing a successful nutrition plan include definition of nutrition goals, determination of nutrition requirements, determination of appropriate route of delivery of nutrients, and subsequent monitoring of the nutrition regimen to evaluate suitability of the regimen as a patient's clinical condition changes and to minimize or treat complications.
2. The appropriate route of nutrition support depends on the functional condition of the patient's gastrointestinal (GI) tract, risk of aspiration, expected duration of nutrition therapy, and clinical condition.
3. Identifying the patient who is most likely to benefit from parenteral nutrition (PN) therapy includes consideration of the patient's age, nutrition status, expected duration of GI dysfunction, and potential risks of initiating therapy.
4. PN formulations include IV sources of protein, dextrose, fat, water, electrolytes, vitamins, trace elements, and other additives.
5. PN solutions may be appropriately formulated for administration by peripheral or central venous access.
6. PN solutions may be infused continuously or intermittently.
7. Biochemical and clinical measurements considered necessary for effective monitoring of patients receiving PN include serum chemistries, vital signs, weight, total daily fluid intake and losses, and nutritional intake.
8. Non–catheter-related complications of PN therapy are minimized with application of age-appropriate nutrient dosing guidelines, frequent monitoring, and rational adjustments to the PN regimen when metabolic abnormalities occur.
9. Individualized PN therapy is based on goals determined from a patient-specific nutrition assessment, type of available IV access, and macronutrient and micronutrient requirements. Nutrient requirements are affected by age, degree of metabolic demand, organ function, other drug therapy, exogenous losses, acid–base status, and enteral intake in patients with recovering GI function.

INTRODUCTION

Maintenance of adequate nutrition status during illness has been recognized for more than 50 years as an integral part of the medical treatment plan for patients who are unable to use normal physiologic means of nourishment. Successful techniques for providing IV nutrition support were introduced to clinical practice in adults and subsequently, infants in the late 1960s.[1] Use of central venous access was investigated to reduce risk of metabolic complications associated with fluid overload and electrolyte imbalances. The use of larger vessels permitted infusion of concentrated formulas, which decreased the fluid volume required and avoided the phlebitis that commonly occurred when hypertonic infusions were given peripherally.

Further clinical experience and research fostered development of protocols that promoted better patient care and resulted in a decline in complications associated with parenteral nutrition (PN) therapy.[2] The scope of practice for nutrition support clinicians has broadened as a result of increasing knowledge regarding the metabolic consequences associated with acute injury and chronic disease states. The pharmacist's role in providing safe and effective nutrition-support care requires knowledge of the principles of patient selection, initial therapy design, preparation and dispensing of the nutritional formulations, outcome monitoring, and strategies for providing therapy during PN product shortages.[3] Other responsibilities of the nutrition support pharmacist may include development of policy and procedures as well as quality improvement activities for patient care and operational processes associated with providing parenteral and enteral nutrition.[4–6] However, the role of other healthcare professionals may be similar because of the evolving interprofessional approach to nutritional support.[7–9] This chapter reviews indications for PN, components of PN formulations, routes of IV administration, practical aspects of regimen design, solution admixture, outcome monitoring, and management of complications for both adult and pediatric (neonates, infants, and children) patients.

DESIRED OUTCOMES

1 The primary objective of nutrition support therapy is to promote positive clinical outcomes of an illness and improve a patient's quality of life. Four fundamental steps are key to providing optimal care for patients who require nutrition support. They are definition of nutrition goals, determination of nutrient requirements for achievement of the nutrition goals, delivery of the required nutrients, and subsequent assessment of the nutrition regimen.[5,6]

A patient's nutrition goals can be established after a thorough nutritional assessment (see Chap. 118). Nutrient requirements and an appropriate route for delivery of the required nutrients can then be determined. Nutrition support goals include correction of the patient's caloric and nitrogen imbalances and any fluid or electrolyte abnormalities or known vitamin or trace element abnormalities. An additional goal is to lessen the metabolic response to injury by minimizing oxidant stress and favorably modulating immune response. These interventions should not cause or worsen other metabolic complications.

2 The gastrointestinal (GI) tract is the optimal route for providing nutrients unless obstruction or other GI complications are present (see Chap. 120).[10,11] Other considerations that may impact determination of an appropriate route for delivery of nutrition support include expected duration of nutrition therapy and risk of aspiration. Patients who have nonfunctional GI tracts or are otherwise not candidates for enteral nutrition may benefit from PN.

INDICATIONS FOR PARENTERAL NUTRITION SUPPORT

The association between malnutrition and development of complications and mortality is well documented for adult and pediatric patients.[11,12] Although improvement in nutrition status as defined by various clinical nutrition markers has been reported for patients who received PN, the impact on clinical outcome is difficult to demonstrate in many adult populations. Several investigations have reported a positive effect of PN on complications and mortality, but others have failed to demonstrate any difference.[10,13] Early studies have been criticized for defects in study design, such as small sample sizes, inappropriate randomization, and inconsistent baseline nutrition status among the study group, which hindered demonstration of the effectiveness of PN therapy. The impact of PN on clinical outcome has been more successfully demonstrated for critically ill infants and children, particularly those with acquired or congenital GI tract anomalies.[14] Consensus guidelines for PN use for adults (Table 119-1) and pediatric (Table 119-2) patients are based on clinical experience and investigations in specific patient populations.[10,11,13–18] Unfortunately, conflicting data have resulted in a lack of consistency in published guidelines from different sources, which complicates identification of the patient who is most likely to benefit from PN. However, these published reports may serve as resources for development of institution-specific standards.

3 The decision to initiate PN is based on the assessment that the patient cannot meet his or her nutritional requirements through the GI tract. This assessment must include an evaluation of the patient's nutrition status, clinical status, age, and potential risks of initiating therapy (e.g., infection and other metabolic abnormalities). The appropriate length of time to wait before starting PN therapy depends on patient age and clinical status.[10,11,13–18] Adult PN therapy is not an emergent intervention and should not be initiated until the patient is hemodynamically stable.[10] In general, previously well-nourished, clinically stable adults who are not candidates for enteral nutrition should be considered candidates for PN after 7 to 14 days of suboptimal nutritional intake.[10,13] Guidelines for use in infants and children are primarily influenced by age. The most appropriate time to initiate therapy for infants and children varies with age and nutritional status. Early PN within the first 24 hours of life has been recommended for extremely low-birth-weight infants whose protein loss can be twofold higher than in term infants and frequently results in a negative nitrogen balance that cannot be corrected by glucose as a sole nutrient.[19] Early aggressive PN in neonates can enhance protein accretion and somatic growth.[19,20] Although there has been some concern regarding protein tolerance with early initiation of PN, most clinicians now support the practice. Withholding PN for 2 to 3 days after birth, coupled with a slow advancement of substrate, only appears to contribute to the acute semistarvation and growth failure seen for many neonates.[19,20] PN should be initiated within 5 to 7 days for other pediatric patients who are unable to meet their nutrient requirements with enteral nutrition.[14] Earlier intervention should be considered for term infants (within 2–3 days), critically ill children (within 3–5 days), and children

TABLE 119-1 Indications for Adult Parenteral Nutrition

1. Inability to absorb nutrients via the GI tract because of one or more of the following:
   a. Massive small bowel resection: usually patients with less than 100 cm of small bowel distal to the ligament of Treitz without a colon or less than 50 cm of small bowel with an intact colon
   b. Intractable vomiting when adequate EN is not expected for 7–14 days.
   c. Severe diarrhea
   d. Bowel obstruction
   e. GI fistulae: PN is indicated in patients with prolonged inadequate nutritional intake longer than 5–7 days who are not candidates for EN
2. Cancer: antineoplastic therapy, radiation therapy, or HSCT
   a. PN may be used in moderately to severely malnourished patients receiving active anticancer treatment who are not candidates for EN.
   b. PN is not routinely indicated for well-nourished or mildly malnourished patients undergoing surgery, chemotherapy, or radiation therapy.
   c. PN is unlikely to benefit patients with advanced cancer whose malignancy is unresponsive to treatment. However, use may be appropriate for carefully selected patients who have failed trials of less invasive medical therapies and have good performance status, an estimated life expectancy of longer than 40–60 days, and strong social and financial support.
   d. PN is appropriate in patients undergoing HSCT who are malnourished and who are anticipated to be unable to ingest or absorb adequate nutrients for 7–14 days. PN should be discontinued as soon as toxicities have resolved after stem cell engraftment.
3. Pancreatitis: PN may be used in patients with severe pancreatitis with prolonged inadequate nutritional intake longer than 5–7 days who are not candidates for EN. PN should be used when EN exacerbates abdominal pain, ascites, or fistula output.
4. Critical care
   a. PN should be used in malnourished patients in whom EN is contraindicated or is unlikely to provide adequate nutritional requirements as soon as possible after ICU admission and adequate resuscitation.
   b. PN should be reserved and initiated only after the first 7 days of hospitalization for previously well-nourished patients.
   c. Organ failure (liver, renal, or respiratory): PN should be used in patients with moderate to severe catabolism when EN is contraindicated.
   d. Burns: PN should be used in those patients in whom EN is contraindicated or is unlikely to provide adequate nutritional requirements within 4–5 days.
5. Perioperative PN
   a. Preoperative: for 5–7 days for patients with moderate to severe malnutrition who are undergoing major GI surgery if the operation can be safely postponed
   b. Postoperative: PN should be used in patients in whom EN is contraindicated or is unlikely to provide adequate nutritional requirements within 7–14 days after surgery.
6. Hyperemesis gravidarum: when EN is not tolerated
7. Eating disorders: PN should be considered for patients with anorexia nervosa and severe malnutrition who are unable or unwilling to ingest adequate nutrition.

EN, enteral nutrition; GI, gastrointestinal; HSCT, hematopoietic stem cell transplantation; ICU, intensive care unit; PN, parenteral nutrition; SBS, short-bowel syndrome.

From references 10, 13, 17, and 18.

TABLE 119-2 Indications for Pediatric Parenteral Nutrition

1. When enteral nutrition is unlikely to provide adequate nutritional requirements
   a. Premature infant within 24–48 hours
   b. Other pediatric patients within 5–7 days
2. When the GI tract is not functional or cannot be assessed
   a. Massive small bowel resection resulting in short-bowel syndrome
   b. Neonatal necrotizing enterocolitis
   c. Congenital anomalies of the GI tract
   d. Severe inflammatory bowel disease
   e. Intractable diarrhea or vomiting
   f. Graft-versus-host disease
   g. After chemotherapy
3. Infants and children requiring extracorporeal membrane oxygenation
4. Organ failure (liver, renal, pulmonary, pancreas) or congenital heart disease when enteral nutrition is contraindicated and the child is catabolic

GI, gastrointestinal.

From references 11, and 14 to 16.

with preexisting malnutrition. Guidelines for older children are similar to those for adults.

Clinical **Controversy...**

Some guidelines advocate for early PN use to correct the resulting protein-energy deficit that has been associated with worse clinical outcome in some studies, but others recommend withholding PN support in previously healthy patients until at least 7 days after admission to the intensive care unit.

COMPONENTS OF PARENTERAL NUTRITION

4 Parenteral nutrition formulations include IV sources of protein, dextrose, fat, water, electrolytes, vitamins, trace elements, and other additives. PN solutions should provide the optimal combination of macro- and micronutrients to provide a patient's specific nutritional requirements. Macronutrients include water, protein, dextrose, and IV fat emulsion (IVFE) (Table 119-3). Micronutrients include vitamins, trace elements, and electrolytes. Both macronutrients and micronutrients are necessary for maintenance of normal metabolism. In general, macronutrients are used for energy (dextrose and fat) and as structural substrates (protein and fat). Micronutrients are required to support a variety of metabolic activities necessary for cellular homeostasis such as enzymatic reactions, fluid balance, and regulation of electrophysiologic processes.

Parenteral nutrition component availability has been adversely affected by intermittent product shortages. Over the past several years, shortages of all PN components except concentrated dextrose have been reported.[3] The unavailability of these products has resulted in delays in PN therapy, restricted or precluded nutrient dosing, and had negative effects on all steps of the PN process that have compromised patient safety. Strategies for providing safe therapy during PN product shortages can be challenging for PN patients and practitioners. Conservation recommendations and alternative therapy measures are available.[3]

Amino Acids

Protein in PN solutions is provided in the form of crystalline amino acids (CAAs), which are used primarily for protein synthesis. When

TABLE 119-3 Macronutrient Components of Parenteral Nutrition Solutions

Nutritional Substrate	IV Source	Description
Fluid	Sterile water for injection USP	
Nitrogen	Crystalline amino acids	
	Standard solutions	Contain a balanced profile of essential, semi-essential, and nonessential L-amino acids
	Disease-specific solutions	
	Hepatic encephalopathy	Amino acid profile includes higher BCAA concentrations and lower AAA and methionine concentrations
	Renal failure	Amino acid profile includes higher EAA and histidine concentrations
	Metabolic stress or trauma	Amino acid profile provides standard essential, semi-essential, and nonessential amino acids with higher BCAA concentrations
	Pediatrics	Amino acid profile includes standard essential, semi-essential, and nonessential amino acids with lower methionine, phenylalanine, and glycine concentrations; these solutions also contain taurine, glutamate, and aspartate
Energy		
Carbohydrate	Dextrose	
	Glycerol	Used in ProcalAmine (B. Braun Medical, Inc.)
Fat	IV fat emulsion	Fatty acid source
	LCT emulsions	Soybean
	Alternative fat emulsions (investigational)	MCT-LCT Olive oil Fish oil Mixed fat emulsions: SMOF (soybean oil, MCT, olive, and fish oils) MSF (MCT, soybean, and fish oils)

AAA, aromatic amino acids (includes phenylalanine and tyrosine); BCAA, branched-chain amino acids (leucine, isoleucine, and valine); EAA, essential amino acids (leucine, isoleucine, valine, phenylalanine, tryptophan, methionine, threonine, and lysine); LCT, long-chain triglycerides; MCT, medium-chain triglycerides; PN, parenteral nutrition.

oxidized for energy, 1 g of protein yields 4 cal (or ~17 J). However, including the caloric contribution from protein when calculating calories provided by the PN regimen is controversial.[21]

Commercially available CAA solutions may be categorized as standard amino acid solutions or modified amino acid solutions. Standard CAA solutions are designed for patients with "normal" organ function and nutritional requirements (see Table 119-3). Although standard CAA solutions differ in the proportion of specific amino acids, they contain a balanced profile of essential, semi-essential, and nonessential L-amino acids. Despite these differences, similar effects on markers of protein use have been reported.[22] The protein concentration, total nitrogen, and electrolyte content are also different among products. Because the nitrogen concentration of dietary protein is approximately 16%, 6.25 (100 g protein/16 g nitrogen) is commonly accepted as the conversion figure for calculating the nitrogen amount provided by CAA protein. Differences in nitrogen content per gram of amino acids among CAA products may affect calculation of nitrogen amounts infused when determining nitrogen balance.[22,23] The clinical significance of these differences in determining nitrogen balance for routine clinical use is unknown.[23]

Electrolyte composition of standard CAA solutions varies from small, obligatory amounts to the provision of maintenance requirements of most electrolytes for an adult. Electrolytes provided by CAA solutions must be considered when determining a patient's individual requirements. CAAs are available in several different concentrations, which facilitates compounding of patient-specific PN regimens. Use of highly concentrated products (15%–20%) is attractive for critically ill patients who typically require fluid restriction but have large protein needs. Modified amino acid solutions are designed for patients who have altered protein requirements, such as those with hepatic encephalopathy, renal failure, and metabolic stress or trauma, as well as for neonates and pediatric patients (see Table 119-3). These solutions tend to be more expensive than standard CAA solutions. The rationale for and clinical efficacy of modified amino acids in disease-specific PN regimens is controversial.[10,17,24–27]

Several commercially available CAA solutions are designed to provide conditionally essential amino acids, which are considered nonessential during health because they are produced from other amino acids. However, under certain physiologic conditions, such as prematurity or sepsis, these amino acids cannot be synthesized in sufficient quantities.[22] CAA solutions specifically designed for neonates and pediatric patients contain increased amounts of taurine, aspartic acid, and glutamic acid. Other conditionally essential amino acids, such as cysteine, carnitine, and glutamine, are not available in commercial CAA solutions in pharmacologic amounts because they are relatively unstable or poorly soluble.[22]

Clinical **Controversy...**

Exclusive use of standardized, commercially prepared premixed IV products has been advocated for use to improve medication safety. However, American Society for Parenteral and Enteral Nutrition (A.S.P.E.N.) has reported that patient safety data do not support the general use of standardized PN formulations across healthcare organizations.

Consequently, PN solutions may need to be modified to provide the desired amount of supplemental conditionally essential amino acids. For example, cysteine is a conditionally essential amino acid for preterm and term infants because of their enzymatic immaturity of the trans-sulfuration pathway. Cysteine may be added to PN solutions at the time of compounding as a supplement to CAA solutions and to enhance calcium and phosphate solubility by decreasing solution pH.[24] Carnitine is a quaternary amine required for long-chain fatty acid transport into the mitochondria for β-oxidation and energy production. Newborns are at risk for carnitine deficiency because of their immature biosynthetic capacity. Decreased plasma carnitine concentrations have been reported for infants and children receiving PN without carnitine.[28] Supplemental carnitine may be added to the PN solution at the time of compounding. Although the benefit of carnitine supplementation in PN has not been clearly identified, positive effects on nutritional markers, including improved fatty acid oxidation, weight gain, and nitrogen balance, have been documented. In general, carnitine supplementation is reserved for neonates expected to receive PN support for 7 days or longer.[28]

Glutamine is the most abundant free amino acid in the body and is an important intermediate for many metabolic processes. Glutamine is reported to have an important role in maintaining intestinal integrity, immune function, and protein synthesis during conditions of metabolic stress.[29] Investigations in humans and animals have reported positive effects on nutritional markers such as nitrogen balance, but others have reported significant improvement in other outcome markers, such as decreased length of hospitalization, incidence of infections, and GI toxicities associated with chemotherapy or radiation.[29] However, the best adult candidate for response to glutamine therapy has not been clearly identified.[29] The clinical usefulness of glutamine in neonates and infants is less clear.[29–31] Plasma glutamine concentrations increase with supplementation, but no beneficial effect on sepsis, enteral feeding tolerance, necrotizing enterocolitis, growth, or mortality has been reported.[29–31] The clinical use of glutamine is further complicated because there is no parenteral glutamine formulation commercially available in the United States. Currently available CAA solutions do not contain glutamine because of poor solubility and instability. Use of parenteral glutamine requires special manufacturing techniques not readily available in many institutional pharmacies.[29] However, parenteral glutamine is available from several licensed pharmacies that extemporaneously compound L-glutamine crystalline powder under sterile conditions either as a separate parenteral solution or as a part of a CAA solution.

Dextrose

The primary energy source in PN solutions is carbohydrate, usually in the form of dextrose monohydrate, which is available in concentrations ranging from 5% to 70%. When oxidized, each gram of hydrated dextrose provides 3.4 kcal (14.2 kJ). The appropriate IV dextrose dose depends on the patient's age, estimated caloric requirements, and clinical condition. For example, minimum dextrose requirements for neonates are estimated to be approximately 6 to 10 mg/kg/min.[16,20] However, IV dextrose infusion rates should not exceed 14 to 18 mg/kg/min for infants or 4 to 7 mg/kg per minute for adults.[16,32] The recommended dextrose dose for routine clinical care rarely exceeds 5 mg/kg per minute for older critically ill children (1–11 years old) and adults.[16,32] Maintaining an age-appropriate dextrose infusion rate is necessary to minimize risk of adverse effects. If the dextrose infusion rate exceeds the glucose oxidation rate, metabolically expensive pathways, such as glycogen repletion and lipid synthesis, are favored, resulting in increased energy expenditure, increased oxygen consumption, and increased carbon dioxide production. Excessive dextrose infusion rates also may contribute to the development of hyperglycemia and an increase in the concentration biochemical markers for liver function associated with fatty infiltration of the liver.[32,33]

Carbohydrate sources that are not insulin dependent have been investigated as an alternative to dextrose to improve glycemic control for patients with impaired insulin secretion or activity who require PN. Glycerol, a sugar alcohol that provides 4.3 kcal/g (18 kJ/g), is the only dextrose alternative commercially available. It is available as an isotonic, 3% solution in combination with 3% amino acids and supplemental electrolytes (ProcalAmine, B. Braun Medical, Irvine, CA). Although the solution may be peripherally infused, a major disadvantage of this formula is the dilute amino acid and carbohydrate concentrations. Most adult patients require up to 3 to 4 L/day of ProcalAmine solution together with IVFE as a caloric source to provide minimum energy requirements.[34] IV glycerol use for catabolic adults is safe and effective, but similar data are not available for infants and children.[35]

IV Fat Emulsion

IVFE is used as a concentrated source of calories and essential fatty acids. Although commercially available IVFE products have traditionally contained soybean oil or a combination of soybean oil and safflower oil, IVFE products containing safflower oil are no longer manufactured. Soybean oil–based IVFE products are available in various concentrations (10%, 20%, and 30%) and contain egg phospholipids as an emulsifying agent and glycerol to make the emulsion isotonic. Although the caloric contribution of fat is 9 kcal/g (38 kJ/g), the caloric content of IVFE is 1.1 kcal/mL (4.6 kJ/mL) for 10% emulsion, 2 kcal/mL (8.4 kJ/mL) for 20% emulsion, and 3 kcal/mL (12.6 kJ/mL) for 30% emulsion because of the caloric contribution of the egg phospholipid and glycerol.[16] The fatty acid composition of soybean oil–based IVFEs is approximately 44% to 62% linoleic acid and 4% to 11% linolenic acid.[36] Linolenic acid, an omega-3 fatty acid, and linoleic acid, an omega-6 fatty acid, are both polyunsaturated long-chain triglycerides (LCTs).[36] IVFE products differ in phospholipid and triglyceride concentrations. Higher concentrated IVFEs (20% and 30%) have a lower phospholipid-to-triglyceride ratio compared with 10% IVFE.[16,37] Because higher amounts of circulating phospholipids are associated with impaired triglyceride clearance in neonates and infants, 20% IVFE is the preferred product for this population.[16,37]

Soybean oil–based IVFE is effective for treatment or prevention of essential fatty acid deficiency (EFAD). EFAD is the result of a biochemical deficiency of linoleic acid and arachidonic acid, which are considered essential for humans.[38] Linoleic and linolenic acids are important for a variety of functions such as cellular integrity, platelet function, postnatal brain development, and wound healing.[38] Normally, linoleic acid is converted to the tetraenearachidonic acid. When linoleic acid is not present in sufficient amounts, oleic acid is converted to the triene 5,8,11-eicosatrienoic acid, a fatty acid of lesser physiologic integrity, and EFAD occurs. EFAD may be prevented by providing 2% to 4% of total calories as linoleic acid and 0.25% to 0.5% of total calories as linolenic acid.[39] This may be achieved for most adult patients by giving approximately 100 g IVFE weekly.[32,39] Neonates and infants require a minimum of 0.5 to 1 g/kg daily.[16,37]

Plasma IVFE clearance is directly related to gestational age of infants and appears to be influenced by the infusion rate and the patient's clinical status.[37,40] The risk of developing hypertriglyceridemia decreases with longer infusion times.[37,39,40] Rapid IVFE infusions are reported to contribute to decreased oxygenation for neonates.[40,41] Adverse pulmonary effects are thought to be caused by polyunsaturated fatty acid (PUFA)–driven prostaglandin production, which results in altered vascular tone. Although the association between IVFE and pulmonary dysfunction is not clear, a black box warning appears in the Food and Drug Administration (FDA) labeling for soybean oil–based IVFE that acknowledges deaths in preterm infants associated with pulmonary fat accumulation thought to be related to IVFE infusions.[40,42] In addition, data for animals and humans also suggest that rapid infusion of long-chain fatty acid formulations may have a negative impact on immunocompetence by saturating the reticuloendothelial system.[32,43]

As a caloric source, IVFE use may facilitate provision of adequate calories and minimize complications of nutrition therapy such as hyperglycemia, hepatotoxicity, or increased carbon dioxide production.[32] Although the frequency of acute adverse effects is reported to be less than 1% with current formulations, patients receiving their first IVFE dose should be monitored for dyspnea, chest tightness, palpitations, and chills. Headache, nausea, and fever also have been reported and might be associated with a rapid infusion rate. In general, IVFE use is contraindicated for patients with an impaired ability to clear fat emulsion, such as patients with pathologic hyperlipidemia, lipoid nephrosis, and hypertriglyceridemia associated with pancreatitis.[42] Finally patients with a reported egg allergy should be evaluated carefully for the nature and severity of the reaction before deciding to initiate a fat-based PN regimen.

Commercially available 10% and 20% IVFE products may be administered by either the central or the peripheral route. They may be added directly to the PN solution as a total nutrient admixture (TNA), also referred to as a three-in-one system (lipids, protein, glucose, and additives), or they may be piggybacked with the CAA-dextrose solution, commonly referred to as a two-in-one solution.[39,42] The more concentrated 30% IVFE is only approved for use in the preparation of TNA and is not intended for direct IV administration.

Soybean oil–based IVFEs have negative effects on immune function as the result of omega-6 PUFA influence on proinflammatory eicosanoid production. These negative effects on immune function have stimulated a search for alternative IVFE sources that provide adequate essential fatty acids but lower amounts of omega-6 FA.[36,43] Medium-chain triglycerides (MCTs) may offer several advantages, especially for critically ill patients. MCTs are hydrolyzed and cleared more rapidly than LCTs, and they do not accumulate in the liver. In addition, MCTs do not require carnitine for entrance into mitochondria for oxidation. However, MCTs are not a source of essential fatty acids. Subsequent studies of IV MCT-LCT mixtures in a number of patients demonstrate safety and efficacy comparable with standard LCT emulsions.[36,43] Several MCT-LCT products are available in Europe, although no IV MCT formulations are currently available commercially in the United States. Other IVFE that are available outside the United States include a fish oil-based emulsion, an olive oil– and soybean oil–based emulsion and mixed fat source emulsions, including a soybean, MCT, olive oil, and fish oil combination and a soybean, MCT, and fish oil combination.[36,43] Fish oil–based IVFE contain predominantly omega-3 PUFAs, which are metabolized to cytokine mediators that may be less inflammatory and immunosuppressive than those derived from omega-6 PUFAs. Olive oil–based IVFEs provide essential fatty acids, are a rich source of vitamin E, and may have a neutral effect on immune function. The clinical effect of IVFE administration on immune function, as well as on patient morbidity and mortality, is not clear.[36,43] However, investigations of enteral solutions with a higher concentration of omega-3 PUFAs have reported decreased infections and improvement of in vitro immunologic indices in critically ill patients.[38,44] Recent evidence suggests that soybean-based IVFE, which contains phytosterols and predominantly omega-6 PUFAs, may play a greater role in the development of PN-associated liver disease (PNALD). Investigations of fish oil–based IVFE have reported improvement in or reversal of PNALD.[36,45]

Clinical **Controversy...**

The association between soybean oil–based IVFE and PNALD has stimulated modifications to standard clinical practice, including soybean oil–based IVFE restriction and the replacement of soybean oil–based IVFE with fish oil–based IVFE. When reducing or eliminating soybean oil–based IVFE from the parenteral diet, debate exists with respect to whether the decreased amount of long-chain fats provided is sufficient to prevent essential fatty acid deficiency.

Although IVFE products remain the most common source of parenteral fat, a number of drugs have been introduced that contain lipid either as a vehicle for delivery or as a portion of the drug molecular formulation. Propofol, an IV anesthetic, is delivered in a soybean-oil-in-water emulsion that has essentially the same composition and caloric concentration as 10% IVFE. This agent is used commonly for continuous sedation of ventilated patients and should be considered a potentially significant source of calories that may require adjustment of a patient's nutrition regimen.[46] The antifungal amphotericin B is available in several lipid-containing combinations such as liposomal and lipid complex formulations. The caloric contribution from these products when used in standard doses generally is small and is not relevant clinically.

Vitamins

Maintenance guidelines for daily parenteral vitamin supplements were initially established in 1975 by the Nutrition Advisory Group of the American Medical Association (NAG-AMA) for adults, children, and infants.[47] The NAG-AMA identified 13 essential vitamins that include four fat-soluble vitamins and nine water-soluble vitamins based on requirements for healthy people. Revised recommendations to these original guidelines were made in 1985 and again in 1988 based on clinical experience and research for specific adult and pediatric patient groups who required PN.[47]

For example, the NAG-AMA guidelines for infants and children were later revised to primarily reflect changes for preterm infants requiring PN.[47] In addition, the U.S. FDA mandated reformulation of adult parenteral multiple-vitamin product guidelines to include 150 mcg of vitamin K in addition to higher doses of vitamins B_1, B_6, and C compared with the original AMA-NAG recommendations.[47]

Vitamin K was not included in previous parenteral multiple-vitamin formulations to minimize the risk of a drug–nutrient interaction for patients receiving anticoagulants, which antagonize vitamin K–dependent coagulation factors. The NAG-AMA recommendation for vitamin K for adults is 2 to 4 mg weekly. Other practitioners recommend larger doses of 0.5 to 1 mg/day or 5 to 10 mg weekly.[39] An investigation of patients receiving long-term IVFE-containing PN with vitamin K–free parenteral multivitamins at home suggests that supplemental vitamin K may not be necessary to maintain normal prothrombin times and plasma vitamin K concentrations.[48] Soybean oil used in IVFEs is a natural source of phylloquinone (vitamin K_1). However, the vitamin K concentration is dependent on the soybean oil concentration in the IVFE.[48–50] Mean concentrations of 30.9 and 67.5 mcg/100 mL were reported for 10% and 20% Intralipid (Baxter Healthcare Corporation, Deerfield, IL), a soybean oil–based IVFE. The bioavailability of vitamin K1 from IVFEs is unknown. Although hospitalized patients who received no additional vitamin K supplementation during short-term PN that included a low vitamin K–containing IVFE experienced minimal effects on international normalized ratio, supplemental vitamin K may be given intramuscularly or subcutaneously or added to the PN solution if needed.[49] Current recommendations suggest supplemental vitamin K is unnecessary when a vitamin K–containing multiple-vitamin product is used.[39]

Adult parenteral multiple-vitamin products formulated to comply with the FDA-mandated changes to the NAG-AMA guidelines are available commercially. In addition, a parenteral multiple-vitamin formulation containing no vitamin K is commercially available for adult patients receiving home PN and warfarin anticoagulation (MVI-12, multivitamin infusion without vitamin K; Hospira, Inc. Lake Forest, IL). Two parenteral multiple-vitamin products are commercially available for use for pediatric patients. MVI-Pediatric (Hospira Inc.) and Infuvite Pediatric (Baxter Healthcare Corporation) are formulated to meet the revised NAG-AMA guidelines for infants weighing less than 1 kg (<2.2 lb) to children up to 11 years old. However, there are no commercially available IV multivitamin products designed to specifically meet the unique requirements of premature infants, including higher vitamin A and lower doses of vitamins B_1, B_2, B_6, and B_{12} compared with recommendations for term infants and older children.

Vitamin requirements may be altered in malnutrition and other specific disease states or with certain drug therapies. Individual and combination products are available to provide additional or tailored supplementation, which may be necessary to prevent development of vitamin toxicities or deficiencies caused by altered metabolism or drug therapy.

The 2012 A.S.P.E.N. recommendations question whether the vitamin D content of parenteral multivitamins is adequate to meet current RDAs and advocate for a parenteral vitamin D product for PN-dependent patients who are unresponsive to additional enteral vitamin D supplementation.[47] In addition, the recommendations support the continued production of adult multivitamin products with and without vitamin K and for the supplementation of carnitine (2–5 mg/kg/day) in neonatal PN and choline in all patients receiving PN.[47]

Trace Elements

Many trace elements are an important part of metalloenzymes and function as cofactors in a variety of regulatory metabolic pathways.[51,52] Although 17 trace elements have demonstrated biologic importance, clear deficiency syndromes in humans have been described only for cobalt (as vitamin B_{12}), copper, iodine, iron, and zinc.[52–54] In 1979, the NAG-AMA recommended chromium, copper, manganese, and zinc supplementation for patients receiving PN.[47,52] Recommendations followed in 1984 to also supplement with selenium.[47,52] Although a clear deficiency syndrome for manganese has not been reported in humans, the NAG-AMA considered manganese essential based on case reports of patients receiving PN with metabolic complications that corrected after manganese supplementation. Reports of syndromes associated with selenium and molybdenum deficiency suggest that they also may be essential.[52,53] Although iodine deficiency has not been reported for patients receiving short-term PN, it has been observed for patients receiving long-term PN and may be related to the use of chlorhexidine for central-line care instead of povidone–iodine.[55]

IV trace elements are available as single-trace element solutions and as multiple-trace element combinations. Most products for adults provide the daily requirements for the trace elements considered essential by the NAG-AMA (i.e., chromium, copper, manganese, selenium, and zinc). Currently available combination products for neonates and pediatric patients contain only chromium, copper, manganese, and zinc. Combination products containing iodide and molybdenum are no longer commercially available in the United States. Single-entity IV products are available that allow for individualization of trace mineral supplementation of chromium, copper, iodine, manganese, selenium, and zinc; however, recent shortages have threatened the supply of these single-entity products.

Requirements for trace elements also change depending on the clinical condition of the patient. For example, higher doses of supplemental zinc likely are necessary for patients with high-output ostomies or diarrhea because the GI tract is the predominant excretion route for zinc. Whereas manganese and copper are excreted through the biliary tract, chromium, molybdenum, and selenium are excreted renally. Hence, these trace elements should be restricted or withheld from PN solutions for patients with cholestatic liver disease and renal failure, respectively.

A.S.P.E.N. recommended formulation changes to the available multiple-trace element preparations for PN patients.[47] The recommendations support overall decreased contamination of trace elements in large- and small-volume PN products.[47] The recommendations advocate for decreased copper and manganese, no (or decreased) chromium, and inclusion and increased dose of selenium in all adult multiple-trace products.[47] The recommendations also support products with no chromium, decreased manganese, and the inclusion of selenium in all pediatric multiple-trace products.[47]

Electrolytes

Electrolytes such as sodium, potassium, calcium, magnesium, phosphorus, chloride, and acetate are necessary PN components for the maintenance of numerous cellular functions. Electrolytes may be given to maintain normal serum concentrations or to correct deficits. Patients who have "normal" organ function and relatively normal serum concentrations of any electrolyte should receive normal maintenance electrolyte doses when PN is initiated and daily thereafter. Specific electrolyte requirements vary according to the patient's age, disease state, organ function, previous and current drug therapy, nutrition status, and extrarenal losses. Electrolytes are available commercially as single- and multiple-nutrient solutions. Multiple-electrolyte solutions are useful for stable patients with normal organ function who are receiving PN. Concentrated multiple-electrolyte solutions designed for addition to PN solutions generally contain only sodium, potassium, calcium, and magnesium. Phosphorus must be added as a separate additive. Further information regarding metabolism and requirements of vitamins, trace elements, and electrolytes is given elsewhere.[39,56]

TABLE 119-4 Osmolarities of Selected Parenteral Nutrients

Nutrient	Osmolarity
Amino acid	100 mOsm/%
Dextrose	50 mOsm/%
Lipid emulsion (20%)	1.3–1.5 mOsm/g
Sodium (acetate, chloride)	2 mOsm/mEq
Sodium phosphate	3 mOsm/mEq sodium
Potassium (acetate, chloride)	2 mOsm/mEq
Potassium phosphate	1.7–2.7 mOsm/mEq potassium
Magnesium sulfate	1 mOsm/mEq
Calcium gluconate	1.4 mOsm/mEq

DESIGNING A PARENTERAL NUTRITION REGIMEN

5 Several factors, including the patient's venous access, fluid status, and macronutrient and micronutrient requirements, are important considerations when designing the PN regimen. A patient's venous access and fluid status determines how concentrated the PN solution may be compounded and hence have an impact on the nutrient amount that may be provided. PN solutions may be administered by central or peripheral venous access. The patient's clinical condition determines which route is most appropriate.

Parenteral nutrition solutions may be provided as a two-in-one formulation that contains dextrose, CAA, and other necessary micronutrients or as a three-in-one formulation or TNA that contains dextrose, CAA, and IVFE, as well as other necessary micronutrients. Use of TNA solutions offers several potential advantages, including reduced inventory (infusion pumps, tubing, and other related supplies), decreased time for compounding and administration, a potential decrease in manipulations of the infusion line (which should correspond with a decreased risk of catheter contamination), and ease of delivery and storage for patients receiving home PN.[57] Potential disadvantages include increased risk of infections and stability and compatibility concerns. For example, the stability of TNA solutions is less predictable than that of two-in-one solutions, which makes their use less desirable in specific patient populations such as neonates and infants.[39]

Routes of Parenteral Nutrition Administration

Peripheral Route

Peripheral parenteral nutrition (PPN) is an option for mild to moderately stressed patients for whom central access is unavailable or undesirable and function of their GI tract is expected to return within 10 to 14 days.[58] Potential PPN candidates should not be fluid restricted or require large nutrient amounts. Lower concentrations of amino acid (3%–5% final concentration), dextrose (5%–10% final concentration), and micronutrients compared with central parenteral nutrition (CPN) are necessary for peripheral administration. Because PPN solutions are relatively dilute, larger volumes are usually necessary to provide nutrient requirements. Additionally, many patients who receive PPN likely will require the use of IVFE to increase caloric support to levels more consistent with CPN regimens. The primary advantages of PPN include a lower risk of infectious, metabolic, and technical complications.[58] However, several other factors may complicate PPN use in many patient populations. Patients who have received multiple courses of chemotherapy, malnourished patients, premature infants, elderly patients, and others with an illness of long duration who have already been subjected to multiple venous accesses for fluid and medication administration are likely to have limited peripheral venous access. PPN use is also limited by relatively poor peripheral vein tolerance to hypertonic solutions. Thrombophlebitis is a commonly reported complication for patients receiving PPN. Although the risk of developing phlebitis is greater with solution osmolarities greater than 600 to 900 mOsm/L (>600–900 mmol/L), peripherally administered TNA with much higher osmolarities has been associated with low infusion-site complications in some centers.[58] Efforts to minimize development of phlebitis or infiltration sequelae for patients receiving PPN include addition of IVFE to the regimen as a possible venous lumen protectant, subtherapeutic heparin doses (0.5–1 unit/mL) to prevent thrombus formation, or small doses of hydrocortisone (5 mg/L) to minimize access site inflammation.[58] However, heparin is not compatible for use in TNA formulations. Midline catheter use may offer some advantage and has been associated with a reduced risk of thrombophlebitis.[59] Although these catheters are not central venous access devices, they are longer and infuse into larger venous vessels that may dilute the PN solution to a more tolerable osmolarity. The osmolarity of a PN solution may be estimated by using the guidelines for osmolarities of selected PN components in Table 119-4.

Central Route

Central parenteral nutrition is the preferred choice for PN delivery and is used predominantly for patients who require PN for periods of more than 7 to 14 days during hospitalization or indefinitely at home.[39,60] These patients may have large nutrient requirements; poor peripheral venous access; or fluctuating fluid requirements, such as metabolically stressed patients with extensive surgery, trauma, sepsis, multiple-organ failure, or malignancy. CPN solutions are highly concentrated hypertonic solutions that must be administered through a large central vein. Unlike peripheral veins, central veins have a higher blood flow, which quickly dilutes the hypertonic solutions. Disadvantages of CPN include risks associated with catheter insertion, routine catheter use, and care of the access site. Relative to peripheral venous access, central venous catheter (CVC) access is associated with a greater potential for infection. In addition, the risk of more serious catheter-induced trauma and related sequelae and other serious technical or mechanical problems is greater than that with peripheral access.

The choice of central venous access site depends on a number of factors, including the patient's age and anatomy. CVCs vary in composition, lumen size, number of injection ports, and other special features that affect ease or convenience of care and maintenance. CVCs for short-term use for adults are commonly inserted percutaneously into the subclavian vein and advanced so that the tip is at the superior vena cava.[59] If this approach is not possible, the internal jugular vein can be used. Frequently, short-term central venous access is obtained for critically ill neonates via a catheter placed in the umbilical vein. Other sites for central venous access in infants and older children are similar to those in adults. When therapy is expected to last longer than 4 weeks, the catheter usually is tunneled subcutaneously before entering the central vessel, secured initially with retaining sutures, and anchored in place with a felt cuff that promotes subcutaneous fibrotic tissue growth around the catheter. The injection port may remain external or may be concealed entirely beneath the skin. Implanted CVCs have a larger port or reservoir that is surgically placed beneath the skin surface and anchored in the chest wall muscle. Peripherally inserted central catheters (PICCs) are venous access devices that are inserted into a peripheral vein (basilic, cephalic, or brachial) and advanced so that the tip is at the superior vena cava.[59] PICCs are increasingly used for both short- and long-term central venous access in acute or home care settings because of ease and economy of bedside placement.[39,60]

Constructing a Parenteral Nutrition Regimen

After the route of delivery is chosen, components of the PN regimen are determined based on the patient's nutritional assessment. Some healthcare systems may require the entire PN formula to be written in individual components and additives without the use of a standard order form. More commonly, the ordering process has been simplified by the use of order forms designed specifically for PN. These standardized order forms promote education of practitioners by providing brief guidelines for initiating PN and foster cost-efficient nutrition support by minimizing errors in ordering, compounding, and administration.[39] Standardized order forms also may include options for ordering certain related procedures, laboratory tests, protocols for patient management, or consultations with other medical services related to the patient's nutrition support. Standardized forms and protocols should be reviewed and updated periodically to reflect changes in the practices and patient population of a practice setting and advances in technology that may affect provision of nutrition support.

Adult Parenteral Nutrition Solutions

In general, there are two methods for ordering adult PN. The "standard formula approach" offers a variety of base formulations with a fixed nonprotein-calorie-to-nitrogen ratio. This method usually includes different formulas designed for mild to moderately stressed patients, renal failure patients, fluid-restricted patients, and liver failure patients. Because the nonprotein-calorie-to-nitrogen ratio is fixed, the daily amount of nutrient delivered depends solely on the volume infused. Standard institutional PN formulations may be compounded; however, standardized commercial PN products or "premixed" solutions are available from manufacturers.[61] Use of a standard institutional formula may promote clinician prescribing of a complete, balanced formulation. Their use may also promote consistent provision of stable, compatible admixtures. However, efficiencies associated with use of the standard formula approach may be hindered if there is a frequent need to modify the PN formulation. Finally, standard PN formulations may be difficult to use in potentially complicated patients, such as neonatal or pediatric patients, and those with severe malnutrition, organ failure, glucose intolerance, large GI losses, or critical illness.[61]

The "individualized formula approach" permits compounding of patient-specific solutions. Compounding of the PN solution is limited only by the concentrations of stock solutions and stability of the additives. The nutrient amount delivered depends on the daily volume of the PN solution infused and the nutrient amounts in the PN solution. The total daily amount of PN solution may be prepared in multiple bags or more cost effectively in a single container.[39]

Traditionally, adult PN solutions have been ordered by expressing the final concentrations of each component in the solution. For example, CAA and dextrose are ordered commonly in final percentage, electrolytes in milliequivalents per liter, and other additives in amount (milliliters or units) per day. This inconsistency may promote confusion and misinterpretation of PN solution contents that may result in harm, especially when patients are transferred between health system environments. To ensure that PN labels in all health system environments clearly and accurately reflect the PN solution contents, guidelines for standardized adult PN labeling have been recommended.[39] In addition to including a variety of other information on the label such as dosing weight and administration route, the guidelines recommend expressing PN ingredients in amounts per total volume, which minimizes the need for pharmaceutical calculations to determine the nutrient value of the admixture. Computer software for calculating PN solutions is widely available, and several programs have adapted the recommended labeling guidelines. Pharmaceutical calculations of a two-in-one PN regimen are briefly reviewed (Fig. 119-1).

Several guidelines or clinical rules of thumb are available to help simplify calculation of a PN regimen after a patient's nutritional requirements have been decided. For example, adult patients receiving only PN therapy may need larger volumes of fluid to provide maintenance requirements and replace extrarenal losses. However, patients requiring other IV drug therapy may receive adequate fluid from an additional IV maintenance solution (e.g., 0.45% NaCl in 5% dextrose) or piggybacked medications (or both). Depending on individual institutional practices, maximally concentrating the PN solution and using an inexpensive maintenance fluid to manage hydration may provide a cost-effective regimen that requires fewer adjustments. Another guideline that may be helpful in designing a PN regimen is to allow a volume of approximately 100 to 150 mL/L of base solution (approximately 200–300 mL/day) for electrolytes and other additives. PN regimens for patients who require very small amounts of additives, such as patients with renal failure, may be further concentrated.

Pediatric Parenteral Nutrition Solutions

Pediatric PN solutions are typically ordered using an individualized approach because clinical practice guidelines often recommend nutrient intakes based on the patient's weight. To simplify pediatric PN ordering, many institutions use a pediatric-specific PN order form that expresses daily nutrient amount based on weight. For example, protein and fat are ordered as grams per kilogram per day, dextrose as milligrams per kilogram per minute, and electrolytes as milliequivalents per kilogram per day. However, some institutions may order macronutrients by expressing the final concentration of each component in the solution. Current safe practice guidelines suggest that the pediatric PN label identify components as an "amount per day" with a secondary expression of components as "amount per kilogram per day."[39] Auxiliary labels may be needed when the format between PN ordering and PN labeling is different. Calculations for determining a pediatric PN solution are reviewed to illustrate fundamental concepts for ordering pediatric PN solutions (Fig. 119-2). Additional features of the pediatric PN label include the dosing weight, administration date and time, expiration date, infusion rate, and duration of infusion. Because infants and children generally receive daily maintenance fluid from the PN regimen, supplemental IV solutions are rarely needed. Pediatric PN may be provided as a two-in-one or TNA formulation. However,

Calculation of an Adult Parenteral Nutrition (PN) Regimen

Patient case: A patient's daily nutritional requirements have been estimated to be 100 g protein and 2,000 total kcal. The patient has central venous access and reports no history of hyperlipidemia or egg allergy. The patient is not fluid restricted. The PN solution will be compounded as an individualized regimen using a single-bag, 24-h infusion of a two-in-one solution with IV fat emulsion (IVFE) piggybacked into the PN infusion line. Determine the total PN volume and administration rate by calculating the macronutrient stock solution volumes required to provide the desired daily nutrients. The stock solutions used to compound this regimen are 10% crystalline amino acids (CAA), 70% dextrose, and 20% IVFE.

1. Determine the daily IVFE calories and volume.

- 2,000 kcal/day × 30%–40% of total calories as fat = 600–800 kcal/day
  Choose IVFE 20% 250 mL/day × 2 kcal/mL = 500 kcal/day

2. Determine the 70% dextrose stock solution volume.

- Determine dextrose calories:
  Dextrose calories = Total – IVFE – Protein
  2,000 kcal – 500 kcal IVFE – (4 kcal/g × 100 g CAA) = 1,100 kcal
  - Calculate required dextrose (grams):
    1,100 kcal ÷ 3.4 kcal/g dextrose = 324 g dextrose
  - Determine 70% dextrose volume:
    70 g/100 mL = 324 g/X mL 70% dextrose; X = 463 mL 70% dextrose

3. Calculate the 10% CAA stock solution volume.

   10 g/100 mL = 100 g/X mL 10% CAA; X = 1,000 mL 10% CAA

4. Determine the two-in-one PN volume and administration rate.

- Calculate CAA/dextrose volume:
  463 mL 70% dextrose + 1,000 mL 10% CAA = 1,463 mL CAA–dextrose
- Add 100–200 mL for additives:
  Total two-in-one volume = approximately 1,600–1,700 mL/day
- Calculate the administration rate:
  1,600–1,700 mL/day ÷ 24 h = 67–71 mL/h; round to 65–70 mL/h

5. Choose final two-in-one PN regimen and determine provided nutrient amounts.

- Final two-in-one regimen
  100 g CAA/324 gm dextrose in 1,680 mL/day to infuse at 70 mL/h
  + 20% IVFE 250 mL to infuse at 20 mL/h
- Calculate macronutrient calories

20% IVFE calories:	250 mL × 2 kcal/mL =	500 kcal
Dextrose calories:	324 g × 3.4 kcal/g =	1,102 kcal
Protein calories:	100 g × 4 kcal/g =	400 kcal
Total kcal:		2,002 kcal
Nonprotein kcal:		1,602 kcal

FIGURE 119-1 Calculation of an adult parenteral nutrition (PN) regimen. To convert to energy units of kilojoules (kJ) multiply values with kilocalories as the numerator (kcal, kcal/mL, kcal/kg, kcal/g) by 4.18 to give the corresponding value in kilojoules (kJ, kJ/mL, kJ/kg, kJ/g).

the TNA system is not recommended for compounding neonatal and infant PN because of IVFE instability with the often needed higher calcium and phosphorus concentrations.[39] The IVFE labeling guidelines for pediatric PN are similar to adult IVFE labeling recommendations.

Administration Techniques

Parenteral nutrition solutions should be administered with an infusion pump. The IV administration line for CAA-dextrose solutions should include a 0.22-μm inline filter to remove particulate matter, air, and any microorganisms that may be present in the solution. IVFEs administered separately from the CAA-dextrose solution must be infused into the PN line by utilizing a y-site port beyond the inline filter because the average size of IVFE particles is approximately 0.5 μm.[39] The FDA recommends use of a 1.2-μm filter with TNA solutions, which may be effective in preventing catheter occlusion caused by precipitates or lipid aggregates.[39] This filter size is also reported to remove *Candida albicans*.

Calculation of a Pediatric Parenteral Nutrition (PN) Regimen

Patient case: A 30-week gestational age infant (weight 2 kg) with an estimated nutrition goal of 3 g/kg/day protein, 3 g/kg/day IV fat emulsion (IVFE), and 100 nonprotein kcal/kg/day. The infant has central venous access and no history of hyperlipidemia or egg allergy. The PN regimen will be compounded as an individualized regimen using a single-bag, 24-h infusion of a two-in-one solution with 20% IVFE piggybacked into the PN infusion line. Determine the macronutrient calculations to deliver this infant's nutrition goals; 10% crystalline amino acids (CAA) and 70% dextrose stock solutions will be used to compound the solution.

1. Determine the goal daily IVFE amount, volume, and administration rate.
   - 3 g/kg/day IVFE × 2 kg = 6 g/kg
   - Calculate 20% IVFE volume:
20 g/100 mL = 6 g/X mL X = 30 mL/day of 20% IVFE
   - Calculate the IVFE administration rate:
30 mL 20% IVFE ÷ 24 hs = 1.25 mL/h
2. Determine the goal two-in-one PN volume and administration rate.
   - PN volume based on maintenance fluid requirements:
120 mL/kg/day × 2 kg = 240 mL/day
   - PN infusion rate is 240 mL/day ÷ 24 hs/day = 10 mL/h
3. Determine the daily protein amount and the corresponding 10% CAA volume.
   - Calculate the goal protein amount:
3 g/kg/day × 2 kg = 6 g/day
   - Calculate the 10% CAA stock solution volume:
10 g/100 mL = 6 g/X mL 10% CAA X = 60 mL10% CAA
4. Determine the daily dextrose amount, corresponding 70% dextrose volume, and final dextrose concentration in the two-in-one PN solution.
   - Goal is to provide approximately 14 mg/kg/min dextrose:
14 g × 2 kg × 1440 min/day ÷ 1000 mg/g = 40.3 g dextrose
   - Calculate the 70% dextrose volume:
70 g/100 mL = 40.3 g/X mL 70% dextrose X = 57.6 mL 70% dextrose
   - Calculate the final dextrose concentration of the PN solution:
40.3 g dextrose/240 mL = X g/100 mL X = 16.8% dextrose
5. Determine available volume for additives.
   - 240 mL – 60 mL (10% CAA) – 57.6 mL (70% dextrose) = ~122 mL
Sterile water for injection may be necessary to QS to total volume of 240 mL.
6. Determine the final PN regimen and provided nutrient amounts.
   - Final PN regimen:
3 g/kg/day CAA and 16.8% dextrose to infuse at 10 mL/h
3 g/kg/day (or 30 mL) 20% IVFE to infuse at 1.25 mL/h
   - Macronutrient calories

20% IVFE:	30 mL × 2 kcal/mL =	60 kcal
Dextrose:	40.3 g × 3.4 kcal/g =	137 kcal
Protein:	6 g × 4 kcal/g =	24 kcal
Total kcal (kcal/kg):		221 kcal (111 kcal/kg)
Nonprotein kcal (kcal/kg):		197 kcal/kg (99 kcal/kg)

FIGURE 119-2 Calculation of a pediatric parenteral nutrition (PN) regimen. To convert to energy units of kilojoules, multiply values with kcal as the numerator (kcal, kcal/mL, kcal/kg, kcal/g) by 4.18 to give the corresponding value in kilojoules (kJ, kJ/mL, kJ/kg, kJ/g).

INITIATING AND ADVANCING THE PARENTERAL NUTRITION INFUSION

Adult Parenteral Nutrition

The patient's nutrition status, current clinical status, history of glucose tolerance, and dextrose concentration in the formula will dictate the infusion rate at which the adult PN solution should be initiated. Stable patients with normal organ function and stable baseline serum glucose concentrations have demonstrated minimal effect on serum glucose concentrations when abruptly initiating or discontinuing PN therapy.[62,63] However, another approach is to begin the PN infusion and increase the rate gradually over 12 to 24 hours to the desired rate. The infusion rate is likewise reduced in a stepwise fashion, such as decreasing the rate by 50% for 1 hour before discontinuation, when the PN therapy ends.[62] This approach should prevent development of hyperglycemia and rebound hypoglycemia, respectively. Alternatively, the PN regimen may be initiated at the goal infusion rate but with a hypocaloric dextrose dose. The dextrose dose can be increased daily to the goal based on patient response. Tapered initiation and cessation should be considered for patients receiving intermittent subcutaneous regular insulin; patients with severe renal or hepatic disease; and patients with other disease states that may increase the risk for development of hyperglycemia or hypoglycemia, such as severe diabetes or pancreatic malignancy.

Although the IVFE dose should not exceed 2.5 g/kg per day or 60% of total daily calories, lower doses of 1 g/kg per day not to exceed 30% of calories have been recommended to minimize negative effects associated with long-chain fatty acids.[39] Manufacturer's information recommends IVFE infusion over 4 to 8 hours for adults. However, infusion over 12 to 24 hours appears to be the best clinical strategy to promote IVFE clearance and minimize risk of negative effects on pulmonary and immune function.[39,40]

The manufacturer's guidelines recommend initiating IVFE for adults with a test dose of 0.5 to 1 mL/min for the first 15 to 30 minutes because of the potential for an immediate hypersensitivity reaction. For most patients, this is probably not necessary because of the relatively low incidence and benign nature of acute adverse reactions. In addition, infusion over 12 to 24 hours eliminates the need for a test dose because the infusion rate is within the range of the test dose rates recommended by the manufacturer. Appropriate electrolytes should be provided to patients with normal organ function based on standard nutrient ranges.[39] Adjustments may be necessary depending on the patient's clinical condition. Adults and children older than 11 years of age should receive daily amounts of trace elements and an adult vitamin formulation.

Pediatric Parenteral Nutrition

Pediatric PN solutions are typically initiated with a volume calculated to provide the patient's daily maintenance fluid requirements on the first day of therapy. Individual substrates are then advanced daily as tolerated with the goal PN regimen generally being achieved by day 3 of therapy. PN should be initiated with the goal protein dose. The initial dextrose dose for older infants and children is based on previous glucose tolerance. Although practices may vary, one approach is to start with 10% dextrose and advance the concentration in 5% increments daily as tolerated to goals of 8 to 12 mg/kg/min in infants, 8 to 10 mg/kg/min in children, or 5 to 6 mg/kg/min in adolescents.[16] Initial dextrose doses for premature infants should approximate fetal nutrient delivery rates of 5 to 6 mg/kg per minute. Frequently, this mathematically translates into a final concentration range of 5% to 10% dextrose. The dextrose concentration for the neonatal PN should be advanced daily by 1% to 2.5% or by 2 to 4 mg/kg/min increments to a goal of 8 to 12 mg/kg/min (maximum, 14–18 mg/kg/min).[16] IVFE is usually initiated at 0.5 g/kg/day for neonates and 0.5 to 1 g/kg/day for older children and increased daily by 0.5 to 1 g/kg/day. Incremental increases of IVFE dose allow daily serum triglyceride evaluation and early detection of those with impaired fat clearance. The IVFE dose should not exceed 60% of total daily calories for neonates and 30% of total calories for children, and the maximum IVFE dose should not exceed 3 g/kg/day (~30 kcal/kg/day [126 kJ/kg/day]) for infants and children.[37] The best clinical strategy for minimizing the risk of adverse effects associated with rapid IVFE administration and promoting IVFE clearance is to infuse IVFE over 20 to 24 hours or at a rate of 0.15 g/kg/h.[37,40] This slow infusion also eliminates the need for a test dose because the infusion rate is less than the test-dose rate recommended by the manufacturer.

IV electrolytes, vitamins, and trace elements should be initiated on the first day of therapy and continued as a daily component of the PN solution.[39] Children younger than age 11 years should receive a vitamin product formulated for pediatric patients. Two multivitamin dosing schemas have been suggested for infants and children.[39] One method recommends 2 mL/kg/day for infants weighing less than 2.5 kg (<5.5 lb) and 5 mL/day for infants and children weighing 2.5 kg (5.5 lb) or greater. The other suggests 30% of a vial (1.5 mL/day) for infants weighing less than 1 kg (<2.2 lb), 65% of a vial (3.25 mL/day) for infants weighing 1 to 3 kg (2.2–6.6 lb), and 100% of the vial (5 mL/day) for children weighing more than 3 kg (6.6 lb) (up to 11 years of age). Adult IV vitamin formulations should not be used for infants because of potential neurotoxicity from accumulation of polysorbate and propylene glycol preservatives. Weight-based dosage recommendations for pediatric multiple trace element formulations are 0.3 mL/kg for children weighing less than 3 kg (<6.6 lb) and 0.2 mL/kg for children weighing 3 kg (6.6 lb) or greater (maximum, 5 mL/day). Children weighing more than 25 kg (55 lb) should receive an adult trace element formulation. Weight-based doses of the multiple trace element formulations do not provide the recommended daily intake for all trace elements, so additional supplementation or individual dosing with single-entity products may be necessary. Individualized dosing allows for dose adjustment based on serum trace element assessment, individual patient characteristics (e.g., cholestasis, stool losses, wounds), and the need to minimize administration of trace elements that accumulate in patients receiving chronic PN such as chromium and manganese. Pediatric patients receiving PN commonly transition from PN support to enteral nutrition by gradually, over a period of days to weeks, decreasing the PN infusion rate while increasing the enteral intake. The PN infusion rate should be reduced for 1 to 2 hours before stopping the infusion for neonates and infants because of their immature counter-regulatory mechanisms that contribute to an increased risk for developing rebound hypoglycemia.[14] Blood glucose concentrations should be checked within 15 to 60 minutes after the PN infusion ends.

Continuous versus Cyclic Infusions

❻ Use of continuous infusions is attractive for patients with unstable fluid balance or glucose control. The intermittent or cyclic infusion of PN over a period of time less than 24 hours, usually for 12 to 18 hours each day, is useful for hospitalized patients with limited venous access in whom administration of multiple other medications requires interruption of the PN infusion.[62] Cyclic PN also may prevent or treat hepatotoxicities associated with continuous PN therapy. In addition, this delivery mode allows patients receiving PN at home the ability to resume a relatively normal lifestyle.[62] Various protocols have been reported that suggest incremental increases to the maximum infusion rate for a desired period of time followed by a gradual taper to discontinue the solution.[14,62] However, metabolically stable adults and older children (older than age 2 years) receiving fat-based PN regimens are likely candidates for abrupt initiation and discontinuation of their intermittent PN regimen.[14,62–64] Cyclic PN is not optimal for all patients and should be used with caution for those with severe glucose intolerance, diabetes, or unstable fluid balance.

EVALUATION OF THERAPEUTIC OUTCOMES

7 Thorough and consistent monitoring of patients who are receiving PN is necessary to ensure that the desired nutritional outcomes are achieved and to prevent the occurrence of adverse effects or complications. Routine evaluation should include the assessment of the patient's clinical condition with a focus on nutritional and metabolic effects of the PN regimen. Serial documentation of a patient's response to a particular regimen is a helpful guide for determining appropriate adjustments in fluid, electrolyte, and nutrient therapies.

Several biochemical and clinical measurements are necessary for effective monitoring of patients receiving PN. Serum concentrations of electrolytes, hematologic indices, and biochemical markers for renal function, liver function, and nutrition status should be measured before PN initiation and periodically thereafter depending on the patient's age, nutrition status, and clinical condition. The frequency of blood laboratory measurements for neonates and infants tends to be more conservative because of their smaller circulating blood volumes and, in some cases, lack of central vascular access. Other important clinical measurements include vital signs, weight, total fluid intake and losses, and nutritional intakes. Weekly measurements of height, length, and head circumference are helpful for monitoring nutritional changes in neonates. Monitoring parameters considered important for patients receiving PN; the suggested frequency of measurement for each are outlined in Figure 119-3. Appropriate assessment and evaluation of patient

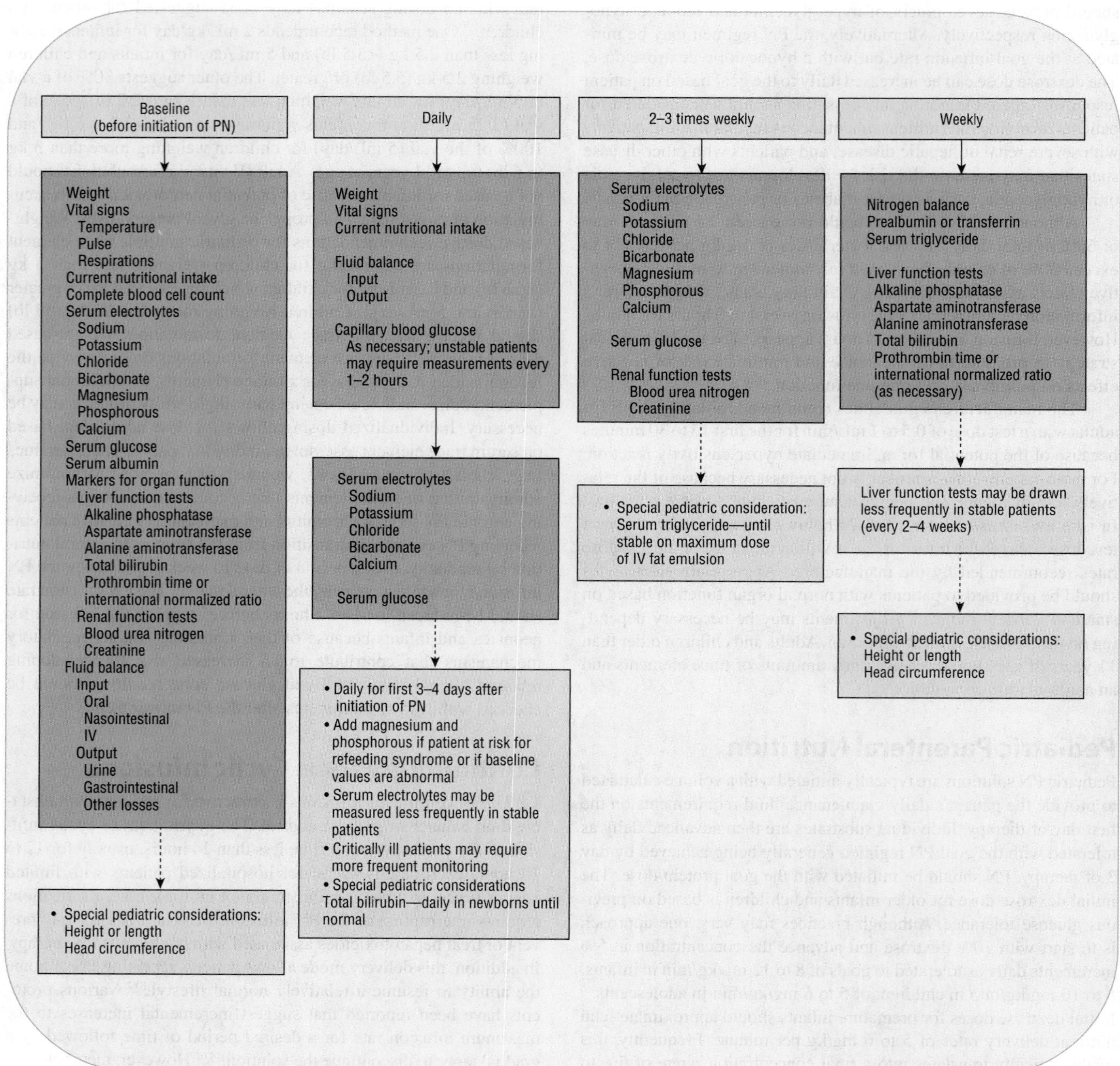

FIGURE 119-3 Monitoring strategy for patients receiving parenteral nutrition (PN).

data can identify potential complications that may be avoided or treated early. Monitoring protocols should be developed and tailored for the patient population, medical practices, and resources of individual practice settings.

COMPOUNDING, STORAGE, AND INFECTION CONTROL

The United States Pharmacopeia (USP) Chapter 797 details the procedures and requirements for compounding sterile preparations, including PN formulations.[65] These standards apply to all healthcare settings in which sterile preparations are compounded and are used by boards of pharmacy, the FDA, and accreditation organizations such as The Joint Commission. Compounded sterile preparations are defined by risk level (immediate use, low, low with 12-hour beyond-use date, medium, and high) based on the probability of microbial, chemical, or physical contamination. PN solutions are classified as a medium-risk compounded sterile preparation. In general, PN solutions should be prepared using aseptic technique in a device or room that meets International Organization for Standardization (ISO) class 5 standards that is located in an ISO class 7 buffer area with an ISO class 8 ante area.[65] Personnel must be trained adequately for personnel cleansing and garbing procedures and aseptic manipulations. Supervision by a pharmacist experienced in compounding IV solutions and knowledgeable about the stability, compatibility, and storage of PN solutions is necessary. Quality assurance procedures should be developed to maintain safe and accurate admixture preparation. A standardized process for PN ordering, labeling, determining nutrient requirements, screening of the PN order, PN administration, and monitoring has been recommended to minimize risk of potentially life-threatening compounding errors.[39,61,66] The potential risk of infectious complications associated with PN solution contamination can be decreased greatly when pharmacy-based admixture programs follow specific guidelines developed to ensure proper compounding of PN solutions.[65]

In general, the type of solution being prepared dictates the methods of compounding, storage, and infusion. Currently, the two most commonly used types of PN solutions are two-in-one solutions with or without IVFE piggybacked into the PN line and TNAs. Methods for compounding PN solutions vary based on a healthcare system's patient population and medical practices and the number of PN solutions that need to be prepared. PN base solutions may be prepared by using gravity-driven transfer of CAA stock solutions to partially filled bags of concentrated dextrose stock solutions.[39,67] Other practice settings may use standardized commercial PN products with CAA and dextrose separated within a single bag that must be mixed before use.[39,61] Advances in compounding technology have facilitated the use of automated compounders for preparing PN solutions. Automated compounders are computer-based systems that perform the calculations necessary to determine volumes of nutrient stock solutions for PN formulations. In addition, most automated compounder systems include software that communicates the determined calculations directly to a transfer pump device that delivers fluid from the source container to the final container by either a volumetric or gravimetric fluid pumping system.[67] Advantages associated with automated compounders include reduced personnel time and compounding materials and improved compounding accuracy. Disadvantages include the potential for equipment failure and power outages.

Assurance of solution sterility during compounding, storage, and administration is necessary to reduce the risk of infection and related complications. Because of their acidic pH and hypertonicity, two-in-one PN formulations are poor media for microbial growth.[39,68] However, several characteristics of IVFE, such as isoosmotic tonicity, near neutral to alkaline pH, and glycerol content favor microbial growth, particularly at room temperature.[39] When IVFEs are added to dextrose-CAA solutions to make TNAs, the growth potential is decreased, presumably because of the protective effects of the hypertonic dextrose-CAA solution and decreased pH.[69]

CAA-dextrose solutions generally are stable for 30 days if refrigerated at 4°C (39°F) and protected from light.[24] However, because of the risk for microbial contamination, manufacturers recommend storage of PN solutions for as little time as possible after preparation. The USP 797 standards recommend storage times of not more than 30 hours at controlled room temperature (20°–25°C [68°–77°F]) and not more than 9 days at cold temperatures (2°–8°C [36°–46°F]) for all medium-risk compounded sterile preparations, including PN solutions.[65]

Because IVFEs support growth of gram-positive and gram-negative bacteria as well as fungi, the appropriate hang time for IVFE has been largely debated. Some recommend that infusion time for IVFE administered as a separate infusion should not exceed 12 hours and infusion time for IVFE administered as a component of TNA should not exceed 24 hrs.[39] The Centers for Disease Control and Prevention (CDC) guidelines do not address infusion times for IVFE.[59] Instead, the guidelines recommend IV tubing replacement every 24 hours for both IVFE infused separately or when given as part of a TNA. IV tubing used continuously for infusion of IV solutions other than blood, blood products, or IVFE should be changed no more frequently than at 96-hour intervals but at least every 7 days.[59] Compliance with recommendations for safe IVFE administration to pediatric patients is challenging. First, the maximum recommended rate of IVFE infusion for infants typically requires an infusion time longer than 12 hours, the recommended infusion time to minimize the risk of IVFE contamination. For example, an infant receiving the maximum recommended IVFE dose (3 g/kg/day) at the maximum recommended rate of 0.15 g/kg/h would require at least a 20-hour infusion.[37] Some institutions attempt to comply with a 12-hour hang time by dividing the daily dose into two unit volumes and infusing them over 12 hours each. Second, commercially available IVFE products are not manufactured in unit volumes consistent with the daily volumes usually prescribed to infants, which may be as low as 2 mL/day. Infants receiving unit volumes larger than those prescribed are at risk for adverse events associated with IVFE infusion–related errors.[41] Finally, use of TNA formulations, which would allow IVFE infusion over 24 hours with decreased contamination risk, are not an option because they are not recommended for neonates and infants.[39] Because of these reasons, some institutions aseptically transfer IVFE into plastic syringes for syringe pump infusion to improve safety and to comply with IVFE administration rate recommendations.[41,69] Use of repackaged IVFE preparations, however, has been associated with increased risk of contamination during compounding or infusion because of IV line manipulation.[69] There are no consistent recommendations for an acceptable infusion time of repackaged IVFE preparations for non-TNA use. In fact, the CDC recommendations do not address use of repackaged IVFE preparations.[59] Given the well-documented risk of microbial contamination with IVFE manipulation, however, a 12-hour maximum infusion time for repackaged IVFE seems prudent.

Clinical **Controversy...**

Repackaging IVFE before administration to neonates and infants has been heavily debated. Although some clinicians maintain that the benefits of cost effectiveness and increased patient safety with administering smaller IVFE units outweigh the risks of microbial contamination, others clinicians continue to advocate for the delivery of IVFE direct from the manufacturer's container to decrease infection risk.

Stability and Compatibility

Comprehensive current information regarding compatibility and stability of PN solutions can be found in several reference sources such as Handbook on Injectable Drugs[68] and King Guide to Parenteral Admixtures.[70] In many cases, the answer to a compatibility question may not be readily available, and a review of the primary literature may be necessary. When information is not available, clinical judgment and experience must be used carefully to resolve the situation.

The stability of a PN formulation is determined by the rate or degree of component degradation and any resulting changes in chemical integrity or pharmacologic activity that may render the formulation unsuitable for safe administration. In general, the sterile combination of PN components accelerates the rate of physicochemical destabilization of all of the components in the formulation; certain amino acids, vitamins, and IVFE are the most susceptible nutrients.[39] When compounded and stored appropriately, the degree of degradation is usually not clinically relevant for most patients receiving short-term PN because many patients have sufficient stores of those susceptible nutrients to support any short-term periods of suboptimal intake, thereby minimizing the risk of clinical symptoms of deficiency. However, nutrient degradation that is more extensive may be problematic for patients with marginal nutrient stores who receive long-term PN. TNAs present additional stability challenges because of the presence of IVFE in the solution. IVFE stability in TNAs is affected by amino acid and dextrose concentration, solution pH, order of mixing, electrolyte amounts, and final TNA volume as well as container material, storage conditions, and addition of nonnutrient drugs. Stability studies on the effect of specific electrolyte concentrations on TNA stability are limited. In general, IVFE stability is affected by the PN cation content. Divalent and trivalent cation additives such as calcium and magnesium have a greater destabilizing potential compared with monovalent cation additives such as sodium and potassium. However, when given in sufficiently high concentrations, monovalent cation additives may also produce instability. Cations act to reduce the surface potential of the emulsion droplet, thereby enhancing tendency to aggregate and ultimately, in some cases, destabilize the solution to coalescence or a "cracked" admixture.[24,39,71] When a cracked IVFE occurs, the oil phase separates from the water phase, resulting in the appearance of free oil fat globules. Early stages may appear as subtle changes in the uniformly white appearance of the TNA, which may progress to yellow oil streaks throughout the bag or development of an amber oil layer at the top of the admixture bag. TNA formulations with any visible free oil should be considered unsafe for parenteral administration because infusion of circulating fat globules may be of sufficient size to accumulate in the pulmonary vasculature and potentially compromise respiratory function. In general, the likelihood of preparing an unstable TNA formulation can be minimized by maintaining the final concentrations of CAA greater than 4%, dextrose greater than 10%, and IVFE greater than 2%.[71] Specific guidelines for compounding TNA formulations are reviewed elsewhere.[24]

Because of differences in pH among various CAA products and in phospholipid content among IVFE products, the manufacturer of each product should be consulted for compatibility and stability information before routine mixing of components. One approach to compounding TNA formulations manually is to first combine CAA, dextrose, and sterile water (if necessary). Electrolytes, vitamins, and trace elements are added, and then the solution is visually inspected for precipitate or other particulates. Finally, IVFE is added, and the solution is visually inspected to ensure a uniform emulsion exists.[24,42] However, mixing components in this specific order and time sequence may not be possible with the use of automated compounders. Although CAA, dextrose, and IVFE may be simultaneously transferred to an admixture container, the compounder's manufacturer should be consulted for the optimal mixing sequence to ensure safe compounding of TNA solutions.

The precipitation of calcium and phosphorus is a common interaction that is potentially life-threatening.[24,39,72] Factors that enhance the risk of precipitate formation include high concentrations of calcium and phosphorus salts, use of the chloride salt of calcium, decreased amino acid and dextrose concentrations, increased solution temperature, increased solution pH, use of an improper sequence when mixing calcium and phosphorus salts, and the presence of other additives (including IVFEs).[24,39,72] In general, steps to minimize risk of calcium and phosphate precipitation in PN formulations include the use of calcium gluconate instead of calcium chloride because it is less reactive, adding phosphate salts early in the mixing sequence, adding calcium last or nearly last, and agitating the mixture throughout the admixture process to achieve homogeneity. PN formulations with a lower final pH should be used when clinically appropriate. Higher final concentrations of dextrose and CAA and lower final concentrations of IVFE favor a lower admixture pH. CAA product-specific solubility curves that are available from the manufacturer or primary literature should be used for determining solubility. Use of a calculation to derive a sum or product of calcium and phosphate concentrations should not be used as the sole criterion for determining solubility because products of calcium and phosphate concentrations vary inconsistently as calcium concentration decreases and phosphate concentration increases.[72]

Electrolyte stability in TNA solutions is difficult to assess because of poor visualization of a precipitate if one occurs. PN solutions for neonates and infants tend to have larger calcium and phosphorus amounts, as well as other divalent cations, that limit the use of TNA formulations. Because of the relatively limited amount of published stability information, the use of a two-in-one formulation with separate administration of IVFEs is recommended for neonates and infants.[39] In general, alternative methods of delivering electrolytes or other medications should be pursued in any clinical situation in which compatibility information involving a TNA solution is lacking. Because the addition of bicarbonate to acidic PN solutions may result in the formation of carbon dioxide gas and insoluble calcium and magnesium carbonates, sodium bicarbonate use in PN solutions is not recommended.[39] Use of a bicarbonate precursor salt such as acetate usually is preferred.

Vitamins may be affected adversely by changes in solution pH, presence of other additives, storage time, solution temperature, and exposure to light.[24] Because of variable stabilities of individual vitamins, IV vitamin solutions should be added to the PN solution as near to the time of administration as is clinically feasible and should not be in the PN solution longer than 24 hours.

Increased peroxide concentrations have been reported in IVFE and dextrose–amino acid solutions after addition of IV multivitamins or exposure to air or light.[73] Multiple in vitro experiments have reported negative effects of peroxides and associated metabolites on organ and immune function. Peroxides are associated with neonatal hypoxic–ischemic encephalopathy, intraventricular hemorrhage, periventricular leukomalacia, chronic lung disease, retinopathy of prematurity, and necrotizing enterocolitis.[73] Neonates and infants are at increased risk for harmful effects of peroxides because they receive a higher daily peroxide load from PN solutions and they have lower endogenous antioxidant levels. Protecting PN and IVFE solutions from light is therefore recommended to minimize peroxide formation.[73]

Many patients receiving PN also receive other IV medications. The compatibility of these medications and other IV solutions is an important concern. Although some medications may be added directly to the PN solution and administered at the same rate as the PN infusion, most are administered as a separate admixture piggybacked in the PN line. Several criteria should be considered before medications are added directly to the PN solution because of the potential for ineffective drug therapy or other complications associated with physiochemical incompatibility and stability of the PN solution.[39] First, the drug should be stable for at least 24 hours and should have pharmacokinetic properties appropriate for continuous infusion. Second, there should be documented chemical and physical compatibility of the medication with PN mixture components and other medications that may be piggybacked concomitantly into the PN line. Advantages of using PN admixtures as drug vehicles include consolidation of dosage units, improved pharmacodynamics for certain drugs, conservation of fluid in volume-restricted patients, fewer venous catheter violations, and decreased compounding and administration times. However, a major disadvantage to the use of PN solutions as drug-delivery vehicles is the lack of compatibility and stability data for the PN solutions that are used commonly in clinical practice. Medications frequently added to PN solutions include regular insulin and histamine-2 receptor antagonists.[39,68,70]

COMPLICATIONS OF PARENTERAL NUTRITION

Mechanical and Technical Complications

Mechanical and technical complications include malfunctions in the system used for IV delivery of the solution, such as infusion pump failure, problems with administration sets or tubing, and problems with the catheter. Although problems associated with infusion pumps and administration sets can be decreased by appropriate equipment selection and routine care and monitoring, catheter-related complications are potentially life-threatening. Pneumothorax, catheter misdirection or migration into the wrong vein or improperly positioned within the cardiac chambers, arterial puncture, bleeding, and hematoma formation may occur during surgical placement of the catheter. Many of these complications, in addition to venous thrombosis and air embolism, can occur after insertion. Catheters occasionally occlude or break during use. If these problems cannot be rectified easily, the catheter may need to be surgically replaced.

Infectious Complications

Infectious complications can be a major hazard for patients receiving CPN because of the increased risk associated with the presence of an indwelling CVC. The source of a CVC infection may be skin organisms at the catheter insertion site, contamination of the catheter hub, or hematogenous seeding of the catheter from a distant site. In addition, patients receiving PN therapy are often predisposed to infection because of compromised immunity or concomitant infection. Frequent use of broad-spectrum antibiotic therapy and malnutrition are also predisposing factors for development of infection. The risk of catheter infection is increased for those who require multiple manipulations of the line used for PN administration. The risks for infection are also increased for those who experience failure of in-line bacterial filter, poor catheter placement technique, and poor CVC and insertion site care.[59]

Infection rarely develops secondary to solution contamination.[59,74] Strict adherence to protocols for preparation of PN solutions should minimize this occurrence.[39,65] Catheter-related bloodstream infections (CRBSIs), defined as the presence of clinical manifestations of infection (e.g., fever, chills, hypotension) associated with bacteremia or fungemia resulting from no apparent source other than the catheter, are common sources of systemic infection.[74] Before this diagnosis can be made, there should be evidence of more than one positive blood culture result obtained from the peripheral vein with growth of the same organism from a blood culture obtained from the catheter or catheter segment. When a CRBSI is suspected or confirmed, appropriate antimicrobial therapy is initiated. Retention or removal of the central catheter depends on the patient's severity of illness, the suspected or identified pathogen, and the type of catheter involved. The catheter may be removed and replaced in the same site, the catheter may be removed and replaced at a different anatomic location, or it may not be replaced.[74] Filling the catheter with antimicrobials such as vancomycin or antiseptics such as 70% alcohol and allowing the solution to dwell for a period of time while the catheter is not in use is referred to as a catheter lock.[59] Antimicrobial catheter locks have been used to prevent and treat CRBSI in patients with long-term catheters such as those receiving home PN.[59,75] Specific guidelines for treatment of CRSBI have been recently reviewed.[74]

Clinical **Controversy. . .**

Ethanol catheter lock therapy has offered promise for the prevention and treatment of CRBSI. The best method for ethanol removal from the CVC after ethanol catheter lock is not known. If the ethanol is withdrawn from the CVC, blood is introduced into the CVC, which may increase the risk of biofilm formation. Alternatively, clearing the catheter by flushing the ethanol into the patient is concerning because the safe amount of ethanol to routinely infuse into patients, particularly neonates and infants, is not known.

Metabolic and Nutritional Complications

8 Metabolic and nutritional complications associated with PN therapy are numerous; frequently multifactorial in origin; and if left untreated, potentially fatal. Metabolic abnormalities related to substrate intolerance, fluid and electrolyte disorders, and acid–base disorders are summarized in multiple review articles.[32,33,38,39,56,62]

Parenteral Nutrition–Associated Liver Disease

Parenteral nutrition–associated liver disease as evidenced by elevations in total bilirubin, aspartate aminotransferase, alanine aminotransferase, and alkaline phosphatase is well documented.[33,76] No single etiology has been identified, although several risk factors have been reported. Risk factors for children include degree of prematurity, sepsis, hypoxia, lack of enteral nutrition, small bowel bacterial overgrowth, GI conditions requiring surgical intervention, duration of PN therapy, and long-term administration of excessive calories.[33,76,77] PNALD in infants is characterized clinically by a serum direct bilirubin concentration greater than 2 mg/dL (>34.2 μmol/L).[33] Taurine deficiency has been proposed as an etiology of cholestasis for preterm infants and neonates.[33,76] Taurine is a conditionally essential amino acid that is not present in standard CAA solutions but is important for neonatal and infant bile metabolism. However, the effectiveness of PN regimens with CAA solutions containing supplemental taurine is unclear. Recent studies have focused on the potential relationship between IVFE and the development of PNALD.[45] Soybean oil–based IVFEs contain large concentrations of plant sterols or phytosterols, which are inefficiently metabolized to bile acids by the liver. Experimental data suggest parenteral phytosterols may impair bile flow. Improvement or reversal of PNALD has been reported for patients who received a fish oil–based IVFE that is not currently commercially available in the United States.[45] Other PNALD treatments that have been investigated include providing reduced doses of soybean oil–based IVFE and use of enteral fish oil in patients with limited oral intake.[78]

Risk factors for PNALD in adults include preexisting liver diseases, sepsis, preexisting malnutrition, extensive bowel resection, prolonged duration of PN therapy, lack of enteral intake, nutrient deficiencies such as choline deficiency, and long-term administration of excessive calories.[33,76] PNALD in adults typically presents as steatosis and steatohepatitis on biopsy. Clinically, PNALD is characterized by mild elevations in serum liver enzymes, usually less than three times the upper limit of normal, with peak enzyme levels usually occurring between 1 and 4 weeks after initiating PN. In many cases, the liver abnormalities improve or resolve with manipulation of substrate intake or discontinuation of PN therapy. However, in severe cases, liver dysfunction may progress to overt failure and death despite use of traditional therapies such as using cyclic PN, ursodiol, and oral antibiotics for bacterial overgrowth; maximizing enteral feeding; and avoiding sepsis and parenteral overfeeding.[33,76] Intestinal transplant with or without liver transplantation has become a treatment option for PN-dependent patients who have progressive PNALD.

Hypertriglyceridemia

Hypertriglyceridemia, defined as serum triglyceride concentrations greater than 400 mg/dL (>4.52 mmol/L) for adults and 150 mg/dL (1.70 mmol/L) to 200 mg/dL (2.26 mmol/L) for preterm infants, neonates, and older pediatric patients, may occur for patients receiving IVFE-based PN. Risk factors include preexisting liver or pancreatic dysfunction, sepsis, multiple-organ failure, degree of prematurity, IVFE infusion rate, and dose.[39,40]

IVFE–associated hypertriglyceridemia is generally thought to be caused by defective lipid clearance or an excessive rate of IVFE administration.[37,39] Premature infants and neonates have relatively slower lipid clearance than do adults because of immature metabolic pathways, including decreased lipoprotein lipase activity.[37,40] Reducing the IVFE infusion rate or dose or withholding IVFE therapy should be considered when patients present with hypertriglyceridemia or lipemic serum.[37,39] Use of low-dose heparin (1 unit/mL of two-in-one PN formulation) to stimulate lipoprotein lipase activity has been suggested as a potential therapeutic intervention to treat IVFE-associated hypertriglyceridemia in neonates.[14,37] However, others have suggested that the risk associated with heparin delivery via PN outweighs the clinical benefits because of the potential for compounding errors associated with heparin and insulin confusion.[79] The role of carnitine for treatment of IVFE-associated hypertriglyceridemia is not clear.[14,37]

Hyperglycemia

Hyperglycemia is one of the most common complications associated with PN administration and is associated with a history of diabetes, metabolic stress, adverse effects of medications such as glucocorticoids, and excessive carbohydrate administration. In the pediatric population, additional risks for hyperglycemia include prematurity and surgery. The optimal blood glucose concentration for acutely ill hospitalized patients receiving PN is not known. However, a target range of 140 to 180 mg/dL (7.8–10 mmol/L) has been suggested for adults, and less than 150 mg/dL (8.3 mmol/L) has been suggested for neonates.[80,81] Clinical management of PN patients with hyperglycemia has not been well studied and is largely empiric. Blood glucose concentrations can be controlled with regular insulin, which may be given subcutaneously or added to the PN formulation. One approach for adult PN patients requiring insulin or oral hypoglycemic agents before starting PN therapy is to initiate PN with approximately 100 to 200 g of dextrose and add 0.05 to 0.1 units of regular insulin per gram of dextrose in the PN solution for those patients with mild hyperglycemia (130–150 mg/dL [7.2–8.3 mmol/L]). The insulin dose may be increased to 0.15 to 0.2 units per gram of dextrose for patients with moderate hyperglycemia (151–200 mg/dL [8.4–11.1 mmol/L]).[39,82] Blood glucose concentrations should be monitored every 4 to 6 hours. Blood glucose measurements above the goal range should be treated with regular insulin administered subcutaneously according to an appropriate sliding scale. The insulin dose is modified daily by adding 60% to 100% of the sliding-scale insulin given over the previous 24 hours to the PN formulation daily until blood glucose concentrations are stable and within the target range. When blood glucose measurements are stable, the dextrose dose may be advanced. The frequency of monitoring blood glucose concentrations may be decreased after blood glucose concentrations are stable within the target range at the goal dextrose dose. Use of a separate IV insulin infusion is most commonly used for pediatric patients, but it may also provide better and safer glycemic control for patients with very large insulin requirements or unstable marked fluctuations in their blood glucose concentrations.

Refeeding Syndrome

Severe and rapid declines in serum phosphate, potassium, and magnesium concentrations; fluid retention; and other micronutrient deficiencies are common features of the refeeding syndrome.[83,84] Individuals at risk for refeeding syndrome include those who are severely malnourished with significant weight loss and who receive aggressive nutritional supplementation. Other examples of patients receiving PN therapy who may be at risk for developing refeeding syndrome abnormalities include those who are unfed for 7 to 10 days with evidence of stress or nutritional depletion; those with chronic diseases causing undernutrition such as cancer, cardiac cachexia, chronic obstructive pulmonary disease, or cirrhosis; and individuals who were previously morbidly obese and have experienced massive weight loss.[84] The mechanism of the electrolyte abnormalities appears to be related to acute provision of macronutrient substrates that promote anabolism in an environment of depleted total body stores of phosphorus, potassium, and magnesium. Recommendations for initiating PN in adults at risk for refeeding syndrome include providing 25% to 50% of the calculated nonprotein caloric requirements initially. The dextrose dose should be initiated at approximately 100 to 200 g/day. Calories should be advanced over 3 to 4 days to the desired goal. Because the metabolic abnormalities described with refeeding syndrome appear to be related primarily to acute provision of large amounts of dextrose, the goal protein dose may be provided with the initial PN infusion. Pediatric PN regimens are usually advanced over several days as a general practice for all pediatric patients. Additional recommendations for minimizing the risk of refeeding syndrome for pediatric patients include provision of additional phosphorus and potassium above standard nutrient requirements at the time PN is initiated.[85]

Complications Associated with Long-Term Parenteral Nutrition

Other nutritional complications of PN therapy may develop over a prolonged course of therapy (weeks to months) as a result of inappropriate intake of a particular nutrient. Certain conditions, such as metabolic stress in a previously malnourished patient, may elicit symptoms of deficiency much earlier if a nutrient is not appropriately provided. For example, lactic acidosis and other life-threatening complications associated with severe thiamine deficiency have been reported for patients who received PN solutions without multivitamin supplementation.[86] Maintenance doses of vitamins, trace elements, and essential fatty acids should be provided to all patients with normal age-related organ function receiving PN.

Essential Fatty Acid Deficiency

Patients receiving PN regimens without IVFEs for extended periods (weeks to months) are at risk for development of EFAD. Clinical signs of EFAD include hair loss, desquamative dermatitis, thrombocytopenia, and malabsorption and diarrhea resulting from changes in intestinal mucosa.[38,39] EFAD also may be diagnosed by evaluating plasma fatty acid profiles. Although this assessment is not routinely available, it can be provided by several larger regional labs. A triene-to-tetraene ratio more than 0.4 is biochemical evidence for EFAD. Although the time in which EFAD may develop depends on the patient's nutrition status, disease state, and age, these manifestations may occur 2 to 4 weeks after initiation of fat-free PN in adults and within 48 hours in newborn infants.[38,40]

Metabolic Bone Disease

Metabolic bone disease has been reported for adults and children receiving long-term home PN.[33] This disorder in adults is characterized by osteomalacia with or without osteoporosis that may present without associated clinical, radiologic, or biochemical abnormalities. The diagnosis may not be made for premature infants until after the development of bone fractures or overt rickets. The etiology is poorly understood and likely multifactorial. Treatment options include pharmacologic intervention, calcium and vitamin D supplementation, and exercise. Because excessive vitamin D has also been implicated in the development of metabolic bone disease, others have recommended removal of vitamin D from the PN for patients with a normal 25-hydroxyvitamin D concentration and low serum parathyroid hormone and 1,25-hydroxyvitamin D concentrations.[14,33]

Trace Elements and Vitamin Complications

Clinical symptoms of trace element deficiencies, although rare, have been reported for patients receiving PN. More commonly, decreased serum trace element concentrations have been reported in a variety of patient populations. However, the clinical significance of decreased concentrations of many trace elements is not known because serum concentrations often do not correlate with total body stores.[47] Occasionally, patients may develop clinical toxicities from elevated vitamin or trace element intakes or decreased metabolism. These abnormalities are frequently associated with an underlying disease state such as severe renal or hepatic failure and may necessitate reduction in vitamin and trace element intake.

Many trace elements are present in PN components as contaminants.[47] Some investigations of patients with normal organ function who were receiving PN supplemented with commercially available parenteral multiple trace element solutions have reported concern with elevated serum concentrations of trace elements such as chromium and manganese.[47,87] Aluminum is a common contaminant of many sterile IV solutions, including those used for compounding PN. Calcium and phosphorus solutions are among those components with higher levels of aluminum contamination.[88,89] Aluminum accumulation may occur during long-term PN therapy, especially for patients with renal insufficiency, and is associated with abnormal neurologic and hematologic function and metabolic bone disease in adults and premature infants.[33,88,89] Preterm infants are at higher risk of aluminum toxicities because they receive larger doses (micrograms per kilogram) from PN solutions than adults.[88] Preterm infants are also more likely to retain aluminum because of immature renal function. Although the maximum safe level of IV aluminum intake is unknown, the FDA has reported that parenteral doses of 4 to 5 mcg/kg/day were associated with central nervous system and bone toxicity for patients with impaired renal function, including premature neonates.[90] Even smaller amounts may result in tissue accumulation but no documented toxicity.

Recent data suggest that the aluminum content of sterile solutions used for compounding PN has declined as a result of awareness of toxicity and improvements in industrial PN component preparation.[88] However, in 2004, the FDA implemented a restriction of aluminum content in large-volume PN stock solutions (CAA, dextrose, sterile water for injection, IVFE) to a maximum of 25 mcg/L and a requirement for manufacturers to indicate the maximum aluminum concentration at expiration for both large- and small-volume parenteral products used for PN.[90] Recent investigations of aluminum content in PN component products have reported differences in actual aluminum amounts in stock solutions and expected amounts based on the manufacturer's label, but measured levels in PN solutions exceed FDA guidelines.[89,91] In addition, the aluminum content of PN stock solutions appears to vary considerably during the shelf life of the products and tends to increase with time because of leaching from glass containers. The amount of aluminum contamination delivered to patients receiving long-term parenteral therapy, such as chronic PN patients or dialysis patients, is substantially reduced if newer stock is used for their therapy.[89]

HOME PARENTERAL NUTRITION

Advances in technology for the delivery of IV solutions have allowed medically stable patients who require extended PN therapy to be maintained indefinitely on IV nutrition. An increasing concern for cost containment of healthcare services has fostered use of sophisticated infusion devices to provide PN at home. Numerous programs are now available outside the traditional healthcare setting to support patients with various long-term or permanent medical conditions. Standards have been developed to promote safe and effective care.[92] Home PN services may be coordinated and administered through a hospital or by a commercial home care company.

Many factors are considered in selecting candidates for home PN therapy. Significant benefit must be expected from the therapy. Examples of patients who have been maintained successfully with home PN include those with severe GI dysfunction secondary to Crohn's disease, ischemic bowel disease, severe GI motility disorders, extensive intestinal obstruction, and congenital bowel dysfunction.[93] The patient and the patient's caregiver must be willing to complete training and assume numerous responsibilities for managing the new daily routine in the home. Other logistics such as funding, procurement of solutions and supplies, and clinical management and followup must be evaluated, resolved, and individualized for each patient in order to achieve the desired outcomes.[92]

Patients commonly receive PN solutions from the home care provider. IV vitamins or other additives may be added daily by the patient or caregiver, depending on the arrangement with the home care provider. The solution generally is administered through the night by infusion pump over 10 to 12 hours.[62] A cycled regimen allows the patient time away from the pump during daylight hours and provides many patients with the freedom to have a reasonably normal daily routine. Clinical management and follow up are performed periodically according to the needs of the patient and the protocol of the home care provider or the managing healthcare team. A coordinated effort among several healthcare professionals, including physicians, pharmacists, nurses, social workers, and the patient and the patient's caregiver, as well as the suppliers, is paramount to providing safe and effective management. Home PN affords some patients the potential for an ambulatory lifestyle while maintaining an IV feeding regimen that was previously only available in the hospital setting. For others, home PN may contribute to a better quality of life in the comfort of their homes.[93]

PERSONALIZED PHARMACOTHERAPY

9 Considerations for individualizing a patient's PN regimen include goals determined from a patient-specific nutrition assessment, type of available vascular access, and macronutrient and micronutrient requirements. In general, both macronutrient and

micronutrient doses are age and weight based but are also affected by degree of metabolic demand, organ function, other drug therapy, exogenous losses, and acid–base status. Nutrient amounts provided by the PN may also require adjustment based on enteral intake either orally or by feeding tube in patients with recovering GI tract function.

Patient-specific caloric goals include (a) adequate energy intake to promote normal growth and development in neonates, infants, and children; (b) energy equilibrium and preservation of fat calorie stores in well-nourished adults; and (c) positive energy balance in malnourished patients with depleted endogenous fat stores. Overweight patients with a body mass index above 30 kg/m^2 may require less caloric support than nonobese patients with the same clinical condition.[10] Critically ill adults may also benefit from a hypocaloric regimen.[10] Specific nitrogen goals are positive nitrogen balance or nitrogen equilibrium and improvement in the serum concentration of visceral protein markers such as transferrin or prealbumin in patients without systemic inflammation. Routine monitoring is necessary to ensure that the nutrition regimen is suitable for a given patient as the patient's clinical condition changes and to minimize or treat complications. The PN component doses usually require individualized adjustments as the patient's clinical condition affects further changes in metabolic stress, organ function, fluid and electrolyte balance, and acid–base status.

Appropriate patient selection, assessment, and monitoring are key to successful PN therapy and the prevention of unnecessary complications. Because pharmacists are actively involved in the provision of PN at many levels, including direct patient care, education, and research, nutrition support is recognized as a pharmacy practice specialty.[94] In addition, as the interprofessional approach to specialized nutrition support has evolved, standards of practice have been defined for pharmacists as well as for other healthcare professionals who provide nutrition support care.[4,7–9] Standardized order forms and monitoring protocols are useful tools to ensure safe administration and monitoring of PN therapy. The future of PN therapy and the role of nutrition-support clinicians will be affected primarily by new insights from clinical research and economic challenges in the healthcare environment.

ABBREVIATIONS

AAP	American Academy of Pediatrics
A.S.P.E.N.	American Society for Parenteral and Enteral Nutrition
CAA	crystalline amino acid
CDC	Centers for Disease Control and Prevention
CPN	central parenteral nutrition
CRBSI	catheter related bloodstream infection
CVC	central venous catheter
EFAD	essential fatty acid deficiency
FDA	Food and Drug Administration
GI	gastrointestinal
IVFE	IV fat emulsion
LCT	long-chain triglyceride
MCT	medium-chain triglyceride
NAG-AMA	Nutrition Advisory Group of the American Medical Association
PICC	peripherally inserted central catheter
PN	parenteral nutrition
PNALD	parenteral nutrition–associated liver disease
PPN	peripheral parenteral nutrition
PUFA	polyunsaturated fatty acid
TNA	total nutrient admixture

REFERENCES

1. Dudrick SJ. History of Parenteral Nutrition. J Am Coll Nutr 2009;28:243–251.
2. Schneider PJ. Nutrition support teams: An evidence-based practice. Nutr Clin Pract 2006;21:62–67.
3. Mirtallo JM, Holcombe B, Kochevar M. Parenteral nutrition product shortages: The A.S.P.E.N. strategy. JPEN J Parenter Enter Nutr 2012;27:385–391.
4. Rollins C, Durfee SM, Holcombe BJ, et al. Standards of practice for nutrition support pharmacists. Nutr Clin Pract 2008;23:189–194.
5. Ukleja A, Freeman KL, Gilbert K, et al; Task Force on Standards for Nutrition Support: Adult Hospitalized Patients, and the American Society for Parenteral and Enteral Nutrition Board of Directors. Standards for nutrition support: Adult hospitalized patients. Nutr Clin Pract 2010;25:403–414.
6. American Society for Parenteral and Enteral Nutrition Board of Directors and Task Force on Standards for Specialized Nutrition Support for Hospitalized Pediatric Patients. Standards for specialized nutrition support: Hospitalized pediatric patients. Nutr Clin Pract 2005;20:103–116.
7. Task Force of A.S.P.E.N; American Dietetic Association Dietitians in Nutrition Support Dietetic Practice Group, Russell M, Stieber M, et al. American Society for Parenteral and Enteral Nutrition (A.S.P.E.N.) and American Dietetic Association (ADA): Standards of practice and standards of professional performance for registered dietitians (generalist, specialty, and advanced) in nutrition support. Nutr Clin Pract 2007;22:558–586.
8. American Society for Parenteral and Enteral Nutrition (A.S.P.E.N.) Board of Directors and Nurses Standards Revision Task Force, DiMaria-Ghalili RA, Bankhead R, Fisher AA, Kovacevich D, Resler R, Guenter PA. Standards of practice for nutrition support nurses. Nutr Clin Pract 2007;22:458–465.
9. Mascarenhas MR, August DA, DeLegge MH, et al; Task Force on Standards for Nutrition Support Physicians; American Society for Parenteral and Enteral Nutrition Board of Directors; American Society for Parenteral and Enteral Nutrition. Standards of practice for nutrition support physicians. Nutr Clin Pract 2012;27:295–299.
10. McClave SA, Martindale RG, Vanek VW, et al. Guidelines for the provision and assessment of nutrition support therapy in the adult critically ill patient: Society of Critical Care Medicine (SCCM) and American Society for Parenteral and Enteral Nutrition (A.S.P.E.N.). JPEN J Parenter Enteral Nutr 2009;33:277–316.
11. Mehta NM, Compher C, and A.S.P.E.N. Board of Directors. A.S.P.E.N. Clinical guidelines: Nutrition support of the critically ill child. JPEN J Parenter Enteral Nutr 2009;33;260–276.
12. White JV, Guenter P, Jensen G, Malone A, Schofield M; Academy of Nutrition and Dietetics Malnutrition Workgroup, A.S.P.E.N. Malnutrition Task Force, A.S.P.E.N. Board of Directors. Consensus statement: Academy of Nutrition and the American Society for Parenteral and Enteral Nutrition: Characteristics recommended for the identification and documentation of adult malnutrition (undernutrition). JPEN J Parenter Enteral Nutr 2012;36: 275–283.
13. August DA, Huhmann MB; American Society for Parenteral and Enteral Nutrition (A.S.P.E.N.) Board of Directors. A.S.P.E.N. clinical guidelines: Nutrition support therapy during adult anticancer treatment and in hematopoietic cell

transplantation. JPEN J Parenter Enteral Nutr 2009;33:472–500.
14. A.S.P.E.N. Board of Directors and the Clinical Guidelines Taskforce. Administration of specialized nutrition support—Issues unique to pediatrics. JPEN J Parenter Enteral Nutr 2002;26(Suppl A):97SA–110SA.
15. A.S.P.E.N. Board of Directors and the Clinical Guidelines Taskforce. Specific guidelines for disease—Pediatrics. JPEN J Parenter Enteral Nutr 2002;26(Suppl A):111SA–138SA.
16. Carney LN, Nepa A, Cohen SS, Dean A, Yanni C, Markowitz. Parenteral and enteral nutrition support: Determining the best way to feed. In: The A.S.P.E.N. Pediatric Nutrition Support Core Curriculum. Corkins MR, ed. Silver Spring, MD: American Society for Parenteral and Enteral Nutrition (A.S.P.E.N.), 2010:433–447.
17. Brown RO, Compher C; American Society for Parenteral and Enteral Nutrition Board of Directors. A.S.P.E.N. clinical guidelines: Nutrition support in adult acute and chronic renal failure. JPEN J Parenter Enteral Nutr 2010;34:366–377.
18. A.S.P.E.N. Board of Directors and the Clinical Guidelines Taskforce. Specific guidelines for disease—Adults. JPEN J Parenter Enteral Nutr 2002;26(Suppl A):61SA–96SA.
19. Denne SC, Poindexter BB. Evidence supporting early nutritional support with parenteral amino acid infusion. Semin Perinatol 2007;31:56–60.
20. Hay WW Jr. Strategies for feeding the preterm infant. Neonatology 2008;94:245–254.
21. Van Way CW. Editorial: Total calories vs nonprotein calories. Nutr Clin Pract 2001;16:271–272.
22. Furst P, Stehle P. Are intravenous amino acid solutions unbalanced? New Horizons 1994;2:215–223.
23. Dickerson RN. Using nitrogen balance in clinical practice. Hosp Pharm 2005;40:1081–1085.
24. Trissel LA. Amino acid injection In: Trissel LA, ed. Handbook on Injectable Drugs, 15th ed. Bethesda, MD: American Society of Health-System Pharmacists, 2009: 49–95.
25. Kocoshis SA, Wieman RA. Hepatic disease. In: The A.S.P.E.N. Pediatric Nutrition Support Core Curriculum. Corkins MR, ed. Silver Spring, MD: American Society for Parenteral and Enteral Nutrition (A.S.P.E.N.) 2010: 302–311.
26. Nelms CL, Juarez M, Warady BA. Renal disease. In: The A.S.P.E.N. Pediatric Nutrition Support Core Curriculum. Corkins MR, ed. Silver Spring, MD: American Society for Parenteral and Enteral Nutrition (A.S.P.E.N.), 2010:256–282.
27. Squires RH. Intestinal Failure. In: The A.S.P.E.N. Pediatric nutrition support core curriculum. Corkins MR, ed. Silver Spring, MD: American Society for Parenteral and Enteral Nutrition (A.S.P.E.N.), 2010:311–322.
28. Crill CM, Helms RA. The use of carnitine in pediatric nutrition. Nutr Clin Pract 2007;22:204–213.
29. Vanek VW, Matarese LE, Robinson M, Sacks GS, Young LS, Kochevar M; Novel Nutrient Task Force, Parenteral Glutamine Workgroup; American Society for Parenteral and Enteral Nutrition (A.S.P.E.N.) Board of Directors. A.S.P.E.N. position paper: Parenteral nutrition glutamine supplementation. Nutr Clin Pract 2011;26:479–494.
30. Moe-Byrne T, Wagner JV, McGuire W. Glutamine supplementation to prevent morbidity and mortality in preterm infants. Cochrane Database Syst Rev 2012;(3):CD001457.
31. Wagner JV, Moe-Byrne T, Grover Z, McGuire W. Glutamine supplementation for young infants with severe gastrointestinal disease. Cochrane Database Syst Rev 2012;(7):CD005947.
32. Btaiche IF, Khalidi N. Metabolic complications of parenteral nutrition in adults, part 1. Am J Health Syst Pharm 2004;61:1938–1949.
33. Btaiche IF, Khalidi N. Metabolic complications of parenteral nutrition in adults, part 2. Am J Health Syst Pharm 2004;61:2050–2057.
34. Waxman K, Day AT, Stellin GP, et al. Safety and efficacy of glycerol and amino acids in combination with lipid emulsion for peripheral parenteral nutrition support. JPEN J Parenter Enteral Nutr 1992;16:374–378.
35. ProcalAmine. Product information. Irvine, CA: B. Braun Medical, 2012.
36. Vanek VW, Seidner DL, Allen P, et al; Novel Nutrient Task Force, Intravenous Fat Emulsions Workgroup; American Society for Parenteral and Enteral Nutrition (A.S.P.E.N.) Board of Directors. A.S.P.E.N. position paper: Clinical role for alternative intravenous fat emulsions. Nutr Clin Pract 2012;27:150–192.
37. Parenteral Nutrition. In: Kleinman RE, ed. American Academy of Pediatrics Committee on Nutrition. Pediatric Nutrition Handbook, 6th edition. Elk Grove, IL: American Academy of Pediatrics, 2009:519–540.
38. Bistrian BR. Clinical aspects of essential fatty acid metabolism: Johnathon Rhoads Lecture. JPEN J Parenter Enteral Nutr 2003;27:168–175.
39. Task Force for the Revision of Safe Practices for Parenteral Nutrition. Safe practices for parenteral nutrition. JPEN J Parenter Enteral Nutr 2004;28:539–570.
40. Kerner JA Jr, Poole RL. The use of IV fat in neonates. Nutr Clin Pract 2006;21:374–380.
41. Hicks RW, Becker SC, Chuo J. A summary of NICU fat emulsion medication errors and nursing services. Data from MEDMARX. Adv Neonatal Care 2007;7:299–310.
42. Intralipid. Product information. Uppsala, Sweden: FresniusKabi, 2007.
43. Waitzberg DL, Torrinhas RS. Fish oil based lipid emulsions and immune response: What clinicians need to know. Nutr Clin Pract 2009;24:487–499.
44. Marik PE, Zaloga GP. Immunonutrition in critically ill patients: A systematic review and analysis of the literature. Intensive Care Med 2008;11:1980–1990.
45. de Meijer VE, Gura KM, Le HD, Meisel JA, Puder M. Fish oil-based lipid emulsions prevent and reverse parenteral nutrition-associated liver disease: The Boston experience. JPEN J Parenter Enteral Nutr 2009;33:541–547.
46. Diprivan. Product information. Schaumburg, IL: APP Pharmaceuticals, LLC, 2009.
47. Vanek VW, Borum P, Buchman A, et al; Novel Nutrient Task Force, Parenteral Multi-Vitamin and Multi–Trace Element Working Group; American Society for Parenteral and Enteral Nutrition (A.S.P.E.N.) Board of Directors. A.S.P.E.N. Position paper: Recommendations for changes in commercially available parenteral multivitamin and multi-trace element products. Nutr Clin Pract 2012;27:440–491.
48. Chambrier C, Lellerq M, Saudin F, et al. Is vitamin K_1 supplementation necessary in long-term parenteral nutrition? JPEN J Parenter Enteral Nutr 1998;22:87–90.
49. Helphingstine CJ, Bistrian BR. New food and drug administration requirements for inclusion of vitamin K in adult parenteral multivitamins. JPEN J Parenter Enteral Nutr 2003;27:220–224.
50. Lennon C, Davidson KW, Sandowski JA, Mason JB. The vitamin K content of intravenous lipid emulsion. JPEN J Parenter Enteral Nutr 1993;17:142–144.
51. Demling RH, DeBiasse MA. Micronutrients in critical illness. Crit Care Clin 1995;11:651–673.

52. Green HL, Hambidge KM, Schanler R, Tsang RC. Guidelines for the use of vitamins, trace elements, calcium, magnesium, and phosphorus in infants and children receiving total parenteral nutrition: Report of the Subcommittee on Pediatric Parenteral Nutrient Requirements from the Committee on Clinical Practice Issues of the American Society for Clinical Nutrition. Am J Clin Nutr 1988;48:1324–1342.
53. Misra S, Kirby DF. Micronutrient and trace element monitoring in adult nutrition support. Nutr Clin Pract 2000;15:120–126.
54. Aggett PJ. Trace elements of the micropremie. ClinPerinatol 2000;27:119–129.
55. Zimmermann MB, Crill CM. Iodine in enteral and parenteral nutrition. Best Pract Res Clin Endocrinol Metab 2010;24:143–158.
56. Kraft MD, Btaiche IF, Sacks GS, Kudsk KA. Treatment of electrolyte disorders in adult patients in the intensive care unit. Am J Health Syst Pharm 2005;62:1663–1682.
57. Parenteral Nutrition Formulations. In: Canada T, Crill C, Guenter P, eds. A.S.P.E.N. Parenteral Nutrition Handbook. Silver Spring, MD: The American Society for Parenteral and Enteral Nutrition, 2009.
58. Anderson ADG, Palmer D, MacFie J. Peripheral parenteral nutrition. Br J Surg 2003;90:1048–1054.
59. O'Grady NP, Alexander M, Burns LA, et al; Healthcare Infection Control Practices Advisory Committee. Guidelines for the prevention of intravascular catheter-related infections. Am J Infect Control 2011;39(Suppl):S1–S34.
60. A.S.P.E.N. Board of Directors and The Clinical Guidelines Taskforce. Access for administration of nutrition support. JPEN J Parenter Enteral Nutr 2002;26(Suppl A): 33SA–41SA.
61. A.S.P.E.N. Board of Directors and Task Force on Parenteral Nutrition Standardization, Kochevar M, Guenter P, Holcombe B, Malone A, Mirtallo J. A.S.P.E.N. Statement on Parenteral Nutrition Standardization. JPEN J Parenter Enteral Nutr 2007;31:441–448.
62. Speerhas R, Wang J, Seidner D, Steiger E. Maintaining normal blood glucose concentrations with total parenteral nutrition: Is it necessary to taper total parenteral nutrition? Nutr Clin Pract 2003;18:414–416.
63. Krzyda EA, Andris DA, Whipple JK, et al. Glucose response to abrupt initiation and discontinuation of total parenteral nutrition. JPEN J Parenter Enteral Nutr 1993;17:64–67.
64. Stout ST, Cober MP. Metabolic effects of cyclic parenteral nutrition infusion in adults and children. Nutr Clin Pract 2010;25:277–281.
65. USP <797> Guidebook to Pharmaceutical Compounding—Sterile Preparations. Rockville, MD: United States Pharmacopeia Convention, 2008.
66. Cohen MR. Safe practices for compounding of parenteral nutrition. JPEN J Parenter Enteral Nutr 2012;36(Suppl): 14S–19S.
67. American Society for Health-System Pharmacists. ASHP guidelines on the safe use of automated compounding devices for the preparation of parenteral nutrition admixtures. Am J Health Syst Pharm 2000;57:1343–1348.
68. Trissel LA, ed. Handbook on Injectable Drugs, 17th ed. Bethesda, MD: American Society of Health-System Pharmacists, 2012.
69. Crill CM, Hak EB, Robinson LA, Helms RA. Evaluation of microbial contamination associated with different preparation methods for neonatal intravenous fat emulsion infusion. Am J Health-Syst Pharm 2010;67:914–918.
70. King JC, Catania PN, ed. King Guide to Parenteral Admixtures, Napa, CA: King Guide Publications, 2012.
71. Driscoll DF. Lipid injectable emulsions: 2006. Nutr Clin Pract 2006;21:381–386.
72. Newton DW, Driscoll DF. Calcium and phosphate compatibility: Revisited again. Am J Health-Syst Pharm 2008;65:73–80.
73. Hoff DS, Michaelson AS. Effects of light exposure on total parenteral nutrition and its implications in the neonatal population. J Pediatr Pharmacol Ther 2009;14:132–143.
74. Mermel LA, Allon M, Bouza E, et al. Clinical practice guidelines for the diagnosis and management of intravascular catheter-related infection: 2009 Update by the Infectious Diseases Society of America. Clin Infect Dis 2009;49:1–45.
75. Maiefski M, Rupp ME, Hermsen ED. Ethanol lock technique: Review of the literature. Infect Control Hosp Epidemiol 2009;30:1096–1108.
76. Buchman AL, Iyore K, Fryer J. Parenteral nutrition-associated liver disease and the role for isolated intestine and intestine/liver transplantation. Hepatology 2006;43: 9–19.
77. Rangel SJ, Calkins CM, Cowles RA, et al; 2011 American Pediatric Surgical Association Outcomes and Clinical Trials Committee. Parenteral nutrition-associated cholestasis: An American Pediatric Surgical Association Outcomes and Clinical Trials Committee systematic review. J Pediatr Surg 2012;47:225–240.
78. Tillman EM, Helms RA. Omega-3 long chain polyunsaturated Fatty acids for treatment of parenteral nutrition-associated liver disease: A review of the literature. J Pediatr Pharmacol Ther 2011;16:31–38.
79. ISMP Medication Safety Alert!® Acute Care. Action needed to prevent dangerous heparin-insulin confusion. May 3, 2007, *http://www.ismp.org/Newsletters/acutecare/articles/20070503.asp.*
80. McMahon MM, Nystrom E, Braunschweig C, Miles J, Compher C; American Society for Parenteral and Enteral Nutrition (A.S.P.E.N.) Board of Directors. A.S.P.E.N. Clinical guidelines: nutrition support of adult patients with hyperglycemia. JPEN J Parenter Enteral Nutr 2012;37(1):23–36.
81. Arsenault D, Brenn M, Kim S, Gura K, Compher C, Simpser E; American Society for Parenteral and Enteral Nutrition Board of Directors, Puder M. A.S.P.E.N. Clinical Guidelines: Hyperglycemia and hypoglycemia in the neonate receiving parenteral nutrition. JPEN J Parenter Enteral Nutr 2012;36:81–95.
82. Marie E., McDonnell ME, Apovian CM. Diabetes mellitus. In: Gottschlich MM, ed. The A.S.P.E.N. Nutrition Support Core Curriculum. A Case-Based Approach—The Adult Patient. Silver Spring, MD: American Society for Parenteral and Enteral Nutrition (A.S.P.E.N.), 2007;676–694.
83. Mehanna HM, Moledina J, Travis J. Refeeding syndrome: What it is, and how to prevent and treat it. BMJ 2008;336;1495–1498.
84. Kraft MD, Btaiche IF, Sacks F. Review of the refeeding syndrome. Nutr Clin Pract 2005;20:625–633.
85. Schmidt GL. Fluid and electrolytes. In: The A.S.P.E.N. Pediatric Nutrition Support Core Curriculum. Corkins MR, ed. Silver Spring, MD: American Society for Parenteral and Enteral Nutrition (A.S.P.E.N.), 2010:87–102.
86. Centers for Disease Control and Prevention. Lactic acidosis traced to thiamine deficiency related to nationwide shortage of multivitamins for total parenteral nutrition—United States, 1997. MMWR Morb Mortal Wkly Rep 1997;46: 523–528.

87. Krishnan Sriram K, Lonchyna VA. Micronutrient supplementation in adult nutrition therapy: Practical considerations. JPEN J Parenter Enteral Nutr 2009;33:548.
88. Gura KM, Puder M. Recent developments in aluminum contamination of products used in parenteral nutrition. Curr Opin Clin Nutr Metab Care 2006;9:239–246.
89. Speerhas RA, Seidner DL. Measured versus estimated aluminum content of parenteral nutrient solutions. Am J Health Syst Pharm 2007;64:740–746.
90. Food and Drug Administration. Aluminum in large and small volume parenterals used in total parenteral nutrition. Fed Regist 2000;65:4103–4111.
91. Poole RL, Schiff L, Hintz SR, Wong A, Mackenzie N, Kerner JA Jr. Aluminum content of parenteral nutrition in neonates: Measured versus calculated levels. J Pediatr Gastroenterol Nutr 2010;50:208–211.
92. American Society for Parenteral and Enteral Nutrition Board of Directors and the Standards for Specialized Nutrition Support Task Force. Standards for specialized nutrition support: Home care patients. Nutr Clin Pract 2005;20:579–590.
93. Howard L. Home parenteral nutrition: Survival, cost, and quality of life. Gastroenterology 2006;130(Suppl):S52–S59.
94. Mirtallo JM. Advancement of nutrition support in clinical pharmacy. Ann Pharmacother 2007;41:869–872.

120

Enteral Nutrition

Vanessa J. Kumpf and Katherine Hammond Chessman

KEY CONCEPTS

1. The GI tract defends the host from toxins and antigens by both immunologic and nonimmunologic mechanisms, collectively referred to as the gut barrier function. Whenever possible, enteral nutrition (EN) is preferred over parenteral nutrition (PN) because it is as effective, may reduce metabolic and infectious complications, and is less expensive.
2. Candidates for EN are those with a sufficiently functioning GI tract to allow adequate nutrient absorption who cannot or will not eat and in whom enteral access can be safely obtained.
3. The most common route for both short- and long-term EN access is directly into the stomach. The method of delivery may be either continuously via an infusion pump, intermittently via a pump or gravity drip, or by gravity or syringe bolus administration.
4. Patients unable to tolerate feeding directly into the stomach because of impaired gastric motility and for those at high risk of aspiration, feeding tube tip placement into the duodenum or jejunum may be indicated. When feeding into the small bowel, the continuous method of delivery via an infusion pump is required to enhance tolerance.
5. Selection of the enteral feeding formulation depends on nutritional requirements, the patient's primary disease state and related complications, and nutrient digestibility and absorption. A standard polymeric formulation will meet the needs of the majority of adults and children.
6. Measurement of gastric residual volumes can be used to monitor GI tolerance in patients receiving gastric feeding. Although not always reliable, excessive residual volumes may be associated with nausea, abdominal distension, and increased aspiration risk.
7. Management of diarrhea in patients receiving EN should focus on identification and correction of the most likely cause(s). Tube feeding-related causes include too rapid delivery or advancement, intolerance to the formula composition, and occasionally formula contamination.
8. Prior to administering medications through a feeding tube, the feeding tube tip location should be verified (stomach or small bowel) and the most suitable dosage form selected. Medications that should not be crushed and administered through a tube include enteric-coated or sustained-release capsules or tablets and sublingual or buccal tablets.
9. The coadministration of medications with EN can result in alterations in bioavailability and/or changes in the desired pharmacologic effects. Medications known to interact with EN include phenytoin, warfarin, selected antibiotics, antacids, and proton-pump inhibitors.

INTRODUCTION

Enteral nutrition (EN) is defined as the delivery of nutrients by tube or by mouth into the GI tract. This chapter focuses on nutrient delivery through a feeding tube rather than the oral ingestion of food. The terms enteral nutrition and tube feeding are thus used interchangeably in this context. The goal of EN is to provide calories, macronutrients, and micronutrients to those patients who are unable to achieve these requirements from an oral diet. Improvements in enteral access techniques and feeding formulations over the past 20 to 30 years and the recognition of methods to prevent and manage complications have resulted in an increased use of EN across all healthcare settings.

In this chapter, principles and practices related to the successful use of EN support are described. Digestive and absorptive physiology is reviewed, and the beneficial effects of EN are presented. The indications for EN and descriptions of various enteral access and administration methods are also summarized. Characteristics of commercially available enteral feeding formulations are presented, as well as administration and monitoring guidelines. Strategies to prevent and manage complications are discussed, and clinical therapeutic controversies are highlighted. In addition, issues of drug compatibility, drug–nutrient interactions, and drug administration via feeding tubes are discussed. Finally, the effectiveness and pharmacoeconomics of EN in enhancing nutrition and disease outcome goals are reviewed.

GASTROINTESTINAL TRACT PHYSIOLOGY

The GI tract plays a key role in the processing of ingested foods many of which are modifiable by the presence of acute and chronic illnesses.

Digestion and Absorption

Digestion and absorption are GI processes that generate the body's usable fuels.[1,2] Digestion consists of the stepwise conversion of a complex chemical and physical nutrient into a molecular form that is absorbable by the intestinal mucosa. Absorption from the GI tract is a multistep process that includes the transfer of a nutrient across the intestinal cell membrane. The nutrient ultimately reaches the systemic circulation through the portal venous or splanchnic lymphatic systems, provided that the GI or biliary tract does not excrete it. Ingested nutrients are primarily large polymers that cannot be absorbed by the intestinal cell membrane unless they are transformed into an absorbable molecular form. In addition, a coordinated interplay of GI motility and neurohormonal secretion is required to facilitate adequate digestion and absorption.

TABLE 120-1 Gastrointestinal Enzymes and Hormones

Enzyme/Hormone	Site of Secretion	Main Actions
Amylase	Salivary glands, pancreas	Converts carbohydrates, starch, and glycogen to simple disaccharides
Cholecystokinin	Duodenum, jejunum	Stimulates pancreatic enzyme secretion and gallbladder contraction
Chymotrypsinogen	Pancreas	Breaks down proteins into peptides
Enteroglucagon	Duodenum, small intestine	Inhibits pancreatic enzyme secretion and bowel motility
Gastric inhibitory peptide	Small intestine	Decreases gastric motility and stimulates insulin secretion
Gastrin	Stomach, duodenum	Stimulates gastric acid secretion and mucosal growth
Glucagon	Pancreas	Stimulates hepatic glycogenolysis and inhibits motility
Lipase	Pancreas	Hydrolyzes dietary fat to release fatty acids
Pancreatic polypeptide	Pancreas	Inhibits gallbladder contraction and pancreatic and biliary secretion
Pepsinogen	Stomach	Converts large proteins into polypeptides
Secretin	Small intestine	Stimulates hepatic and pancreatic water and bicarbonate release
Trypsinogen	Pancreas	Breaks down proteins into peptides
Vasoactive inhibitory peptide	Small intestine, pancreas	Vasodilator; stimulates water and bicarbonate secretion, insulin and glucagon release, and small bowel secretions

Nutrient digestion involves the complex coordination of multiple mechanical, enzymatic, and physiochemical processes.[1,2] Mechanical dissolution of food occurs by chewing, then mixing and grinding the stomach contents. Food stimulates the secretion of numerous hormones and enzymes from the salivary glands, stomach, liver and biliary system, pancreas, and intestines (see Table 120-1). As food passes along the gut lumen, these hormones modulate GI motility and the secretions from subsequent organs of the digestive system. Nutrient digestion and absorption occurs within the gut lumen and is a specific function of the intestinal cell membrane, which is comprised of fingerlike projections called villi. Each individual villus is made up of epithelial cells called enterocytes. The enterocyte surface contains special luminal projections called microvilli, which provide an increased surface area that is referred to as the brush-border membrane.

The digestion and absorption of carbohydrate, fat, and protein within the small intestine are illustrated in Figure 120-1. Carbohydrates are presented to the small intestine in either a digestible or a nondigestible form. Polysaccharides (starches) and oligosaccharides (sucrose and lactose) undergo enzymatic digestion within the small intestine to produce simple sugars. The simple sugars are absorbed via active and passive transport mechanisms and are eventually released into the portal vein. Polysaccharides, such as cellulose complexes and other fiber components, pass undigested to the colon, where they are digested by bacteria and enzymes to form short-chain fatty acids. Absorption of short-chain fatty acids by the colon stimulates sodium and water reabsorption, serves as an energy source, and provides nourishment to the colonic mucosa cells.

Fat is presented to the small intestine as long-chain triglycerides. Its digestion requires pancreatic enzyme release and formation of mixed bile salt micelles, the end product, which is then absorbed across the intestinal enterocyte. Within the enterocyte, triglycerides are reesterified and packaged into chylomicrons for release into

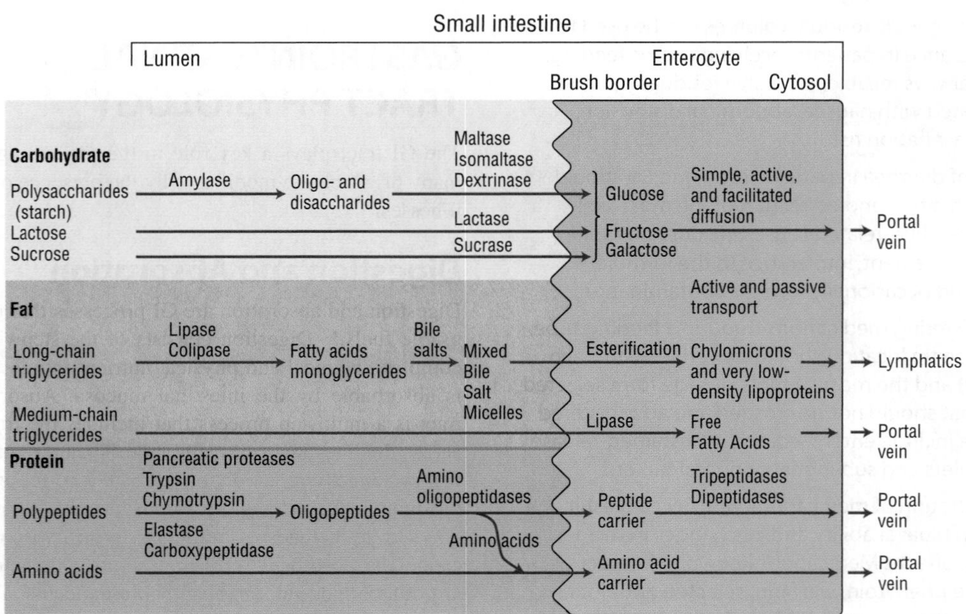

FIGURE 120-1 Schematic of carbohydrate, fat, and protein digestion.

the lymphatic system. Medium-chain triglycerides (MCTs) can be absorbed intact by the mucosal membrane and are acted on by intracellular lipase within the enterocyte to release free fatty acids that pass directly into the portal vein.[3]

Protein is presented to the small intestine primarily as large polypeptides and to a small extent as free amino acids because of the denaturation of protein within the stomach. Luminal polypeptide digestion generates oligopeptides, which are further hydrolyzed to dipeptides and tripeptides. Absorption of peptides occurs via a peptide transport system; free amino acids are carried via specific amino acid transport systems. The carriers for the peptides are very efficient, whereas absorption of free amino acids appears to be more limited and less efficient.[2]

Understanding the mechanisms of digestive and absorptive physiology can greatly enhance the rational use of EN during conditions of normal or altered GI anatomy and/or function. Various circumstances may alter the efficacy of nutrient digestion and absorption. For example, the functional immaturity of the neonatal gut may lead to clinical problems associated with inadequate digestion and absorption of EN. These factors, as they relate to successful EN practice, are discussed in detail throughout this chapter.

Gut Host Defense Mechanisms

❶ Besides digesting and absorbing nutrients to maintain nutritional health, the GI tract is actively involved in defending the host from toxins and antigens by means of both immunologic and nonimmunologic mechanisms.[4] These gut host defense mechanisms are collectively referred to as the gut barrier function. The gut barrier acts to prevent the spread of intraluminal bacteria and endotoxins to systemic organs and tissues. Hydrochloric acid secreted by the stomach kills most of the bacteria ingested with food. Under normal circumstances, a mucus layer coats the intestinal epithelium and thereby alters the adherence of bacteria to the cells of the GI tract but provides a favorable environment for anaerobic bacteria. Anaerobic bacteria, which normally colonize the mucus layer, aid in preventing tissue colonization by potential pathogens. Small bowel peristalsis further prevents bacterial stasis and overgrowth. The gut barrier function is also maintained by the intestinal immune system, known as the gut-associated lymphoid tissue (GALT). GALT regulates the local immune response to antigens within the GI tract. Specific immunoglobulins are secreted to kill the remaining organisms and neutralize any toxins they produce. The liver Kupffer cells help to maintain gut barrier function by clearing the portal blood of gut-derived bacteria and endotoxins. The integrity of gut barrier function may be affected negatively by numerous pathogenic insults, such as physiologic stress and ischemia, and a variety of drugs, including chemotherapeutic agents. The administration of certain probiotics can modify intestinal flora and may have beneficial effects in various disease states and patient populations by positively affecting the maintenance of gut barrier function and intestinal immune function.[5,6]

INDICATIONS FOR ENTERAL NUTRITION

❷ The decision to initiate EN is based on a variety of factors. Suitable candidates are those who cannot or will not eat a sufficient amount to meet nutritional requirements, those who exhibit a sufficient functioning GI tract to allow the absorption of nutrients, and those in whom a method of enteral access can be safely obtained.[7–9] EN may be indicated in a variety of conditions or disease states (Table 120-2). For example, patients who have neurologic disorders, such as a cerebrovascular accident, and have difficulty swallowing often require EN. Patients unable to eat because of conditions such

TABLE 120-2 Potential Indications for Enteral Nutrition

Neoplastic disease	**GI disease**
Chemotherapy	Inflammatory bowel disease
Radiation therapy	Short bowel syndrome
Upper GI tumors	Esophageal motility disorder
Cancer cachexia	Pancreatitis
Organ dysfunction	Fistulas
Liver disease/failure	Gastroesophageal reflux disease (severe)
Kidney insufficiency/failure	Esophageal or intestinal atresia
Cardiac cachexia	**Neurologic impairment**
ARDS/ALI	Comatose state
Bronchopulmonary dysplasia	Cerebrovascular accident
Congenital heart disease	Demyelinating disease
Organ transplantation	Severe depression
	Cerebral palsy
Hypermetabolic states	**Other indications**
Closed head injury	AIDS
Burns	Anorexia nervosa
Trauma	Complications during pregnancy
Postoperative major surgery	Failure-to-thrive
Sepsis	Geriatric patients with multiple chronic diseases
	Extreme prematurity
	Inborn errors of metabolism
	Cystic fibrosis

AIDS, acquired immune deficiency syndrome; ALI, acute lung injury; ARDS, acute respiratory distress syndrome.

as facial or jaw injuries, lesions of the oral cavity or esophagus, esophageal stricture, or head and neck cancer may also be candidates for EN delivered distal to the affected site. Extreme prematurity necessitates tube feeding because the suck–swallow mechanism has not yet developed sufficiently to allow safe oral intake.

Critically ill patients who are endotracheally intubated for mechanical ventilation represent a large percentage of patients requiring EN. Traditionally, EN in the critically ill population was regarded as supportive care designed to provide nutrients during the period of time the patient was unable to maintain oral dietary intake. Recently, the use of EN has been initiated to modulate the stress response to critical illness and improve patient outcomes. Nutrition guidelines support the initiation of EN in critically ill adults[10–12] and children[13] who are unable to maintain volitional intake. Some of these patients may have reduced gastric emptying caused by sepsis, GI surgery, anesthetic agents, opioid analgesics, and underlying pathology, such as diabetic gastroparesis and burns. However, successful EN can often be achieved by bypassing the stomach and placing the tip of the feeding tube beyond the pylorus into the duodenum, or preferably into the jejunum. Small bowel feeding may also be appropriate for patients with gastric outlet obstruction, those with pancreatitis, those with moderate to severe gastroesophageal reflux, or those with high risk of aspiration.

The only absolute contraindications for EN are distal mechanical intestinal obstruction[12] and necrotizing enterocolitis.[14] However, conditions such as severe diarrhea, protracted vomiting, enteric fistulas, severe GI hemorrhage, and intestinal dysmotility may result in significant challenges to the successful use of EN.

BENEFITS OF ENTERAL NUTRITION

The importance of maintaining nutrient delivery through the GI tract in patients without a contraindication to its use is well supported. The beneficial effects of EN, specifically in the critically ill patient, are further enhanced if EN is initiated within 24 to 48 hours of admission to an intensive care unit (ICU).[10]

Enteral Versus Parenteral Nutrition

Clinical studies comparing EN and parenteral nutrition (PN) in the critically ill patient demonstrate a decrease in infectious complications and thus improved outcomes with the use of EN.[15–19] Infectious complications are less common with EN in part because EN supports the functional integrity of the gut by stimulating bile flow and the release of endogenous trophic agents, such as cholecystokinin, gastrin, and bile salts. Provision of enteral nutrients appears to help maintain the villous height of the intestinal mucosa and support the mass of secretory immunoglobulin A (IgA)-producing immunocytes that comprise the GALT. In the setting of critical illness or injury, adverse changes in gut permeability and gut barrier function that result in increased risk for systemic infection and multiorgan dysfunction syndrome have been noted. By supporting gut integrity, the enteral route of feeding is more likely than the parenteral route to lower the risk of infection and minimize organ failure.[10]

Critical reviews of available prospective randomized, controlled trials comparing EN with PN in the critically ill adult patient with an intact GI tract suggest a significant reduction in infectious complications associated with EN.[10,11] Decreased infectious complications have been documented in patients with abdominal trauma, burns, severe head injury, major surgery, and acute pancreatitis. The reduced infectious complications are primarily the result of a lower incidence of pneumonia and catheter-related bloodstream infections in most of these patient populations and a decrease in abdominal abscess in trauma patients. EN is thus preferred over PN for the feeding of critically ill adult patients requiring specialized nutrition support.[10,11] There are no randomized, controlled trials that compare the use of EN and PN in children.[13]

EN is more physiologic than PN in terms of nutrient utilization and therefore is generally associated with fewer metabolic complications, such as glucose intolerance and elevated insulin requirements.[20] Enteral formulations contain both complex and simple carbohydrates, which results in slower carbohydrate absorption compared with the simple carbohydrate, dextrose, used in PN. In addition, enteral formulations that contain fiber and/or a high fat content will further slow carbohydrate absorption and decrease any elevation in blood sugar by delaying gastric emptying. This may account for better blood glucose control when carbohydrate is given via the enteral route. An additional physiologic benefit of enteral feeding is that it stimulates bile flow through the biliary tract and thus reduces the risk of developing cholestasis, gallbladder sludge, and gallstones, conditions that have been associated with long-term PN and bowel rest.[21] Also, EN avoids the potential infectious and technical complications associated with the placement and use of a central venous access device required for PN. Finally, EN is less costly than PN when all factors are considered.

Early Versus Delayed Initiation

The timing of initiation of EN in the critically ill patient is of clinical significance. Initiating EN in the first 24 to 72 hours following admission appears to attenuate the stress response and may reduce disease severity and infectious complications when compared with the initiation of feedings after 72 hours.[10,11] Early EN has also been associated with a decrease in the release of inflammatory cytokines and fewer alterations in gut permeability.[22] Clinical studies demonstrating a decrease in infectious complications with the use of EN compared with PN in the critically ill patient initiated feeding within 24 to 48 hours of hospital admission.[10,11,15,22,23] The benefits of decreased infectious complications are not apparent when the initiation of EN is delayed. A review of available studies comparing early versus delayed EN in critically ill patients showed a trend toward a reduction in infectious complications with early EN.[10,11] In addition, a trend toward reduction in mortality associated with early EN has been noted.[10,11,24]

In critically ill patients who are hemodynamically unstable, early EN may result in gut ischemia because of poor gut blood flow and increased oxygen demand. Consequently, it is recommended that initiation of EN be delayed until the patient is fluid resuscitated and has an adequate perfusion pressure. Once this goal is achieved, often within 6 hours of hospitalization, the initiation of EN at a low administration rate is considered appropriate, along with clinical monitoring to ensure GI tolerance.[25,26] Therefore, early EN (within 24 to 48 hours after hospital admission) is recommended in critically ill adult patients.[10,11] Although no randomized, controlled trials have assessed early EN in critically ill children, initiation of EN within 48 to 72 hours of admission is common.[13] Early initiation of EN is not warranted for the mild to moderately stressed adult patient who is otherwise well nourished. It is reasonable to delay the initiation of EN in these patients until oral intake is inadequate for 7 to 14 days.[7] In the mild to moderately stressed adult patient with inadequate oral intake who is malnourished, it is unclear when to initiate EN, but most clinicians would wait no longer than 7 days.

ENTERAL ACCESS

Advances in enteral access techniques have contributed to the expanded use of EN for conditions in which PN had previously been used. In particular, improved methods of achieving jejunal access for feeding have allowed for the use of EN during the early postoperative and postinjury period when gastric motility is typically impaired. As outlined in Table 120-3, various factors influence the selection of enteral access site and device, including anticipated duration of use (short- or long-term) and whether to feed into the stomach or small bowel. Figure 120-2 illustrates the predominant enteral access options.

Short-Term Access

3 Short-term enteral access is easier to initiate, less invasive, and less costly than the establishment of long-term access.[27] The most frequently used routes for short-term enteral access are established by inserting a tube through the nose and passing the tip into the stomach (nasogastric [NG]), duodenum (nasoduodenal), or jejunum (nasojejunal). In general, these tubes are used in the hospitalized patient when the anticipated tube feeding duration is less than 4 to 6 weeks. The orogastric route is generally reserved for patients in whom the nasopharyngeal area is inaccessible or in young infants who are obligate nasal breathers. Because these routes do not require surgical intervention, they are the least invasive. The feeding tube is frequently held in place only by a piece of tape on the nose or face; therefore, it can be inadvertently pulled out relatively easily.

NG tubes vary in diameter size and stiffness. Large-bore (≥14F) rigid NG tubes are used primarily to decompress the stomach but can also be used for feeding. There is a low incidence of clogging with these tubes, and they provide a reliable way to measure gastric residual volumes (GRVs). The major disadvantage associated with the use of these tubes is patient discomfort. Small-bore nasal tubes designed solely for feeding are available in varying lengths (16 to 60 inches [41 to 152 cm]) and diameter sizes (4F to 12F) to accommodate both pediatric (including neonates) and adult patients. The tip of the tube can be placed into the stomach, duodenum, or jejunum. These tubes consist of a lightweight, pliable silicone or polyurethane material that is more comfortable for the patient. A disadvantage of the small-bore tubes is that they may become easily occluded, often as a result of improper medication administration or tube-flushing technique.

4 In general, the stomach is the least expensive and the least labor-intensive access site to use for enteral feeding; however,

TABLE 120-3 Options and Considerations in the Selection of Enteral Access

Access	EN Duration/Patient Characteristics	Tube Placement Options	Advantages	Disadvantages
Nasogastric or orogastric	Short term Intact gag reflex Normal gastric emptying	Manually at bedside	Ease of placement Allows for all methods of administration Inexpensive Multiple commercially available tubes and sizes	Potential tube displacement Potential increased aspiration risk
Nasoduodenal or nasojejunal	Short term Impaired gastric motility or emptying High risk of GER or aspiration	Manually at bedside Fluoroscopically Endoscopically	Potential reduced aspiration risk Allows for early postinjury or postoperative feeding Multiple commercially available tubes and sizes	Manual transpyloric passage requires greater skill Potential tube displacement or clogging Bolus or intermittent feeding not tolerated
Gastrostomy	Long term Normal gastric emptying	Surgically Endoscopically Radiologically Laparoscopically	Allows for all methods of administration Low-profile buttons available Large-bore tubes less likely to clog Multiple commercially available tubes and sizes	Attendant risks associated with each type of procedure Potential increased aspiration risk Risk of stoma site complications
Jejunostomy	Long term Impaired gastric motility or gastric emptying High risk of GER or aspiration	Surgically Endoscopically Radiologically Laparoscopically	Allows for early postinjury or postoperative feeding Potential reduced aspiration risk Multiple commercially available tubes and sizes Low-profile buttons available	Attendant risks associated with each type of procedure Bolus or intermittent feeding not tolerated Risk of stoma site complications

EN, enteral nutrition; GER, gastroesophageal reflux.

feeding into the stomach is not always tolerated. Patients with impaired gastric motility may be predisposed to aspiration and pneumonia when feedings are delivered into the stomach. Many critically ill, injured, and postoperative patients exhibit delayed gastric emptying, limiting their ability to tolerate gastric feeding. In addition, patients with diabetic gastroparesis or patients with severe gastroesophageal reflux disease or intractable vomiting are at a higher risk for aspiration of gastric contents, resulting in pneumonia. In these patients, placing the tip of the tube into the duodenum or jejunum (also referred to as transpyloric placement) has been suggested as a method to decrease risk for aspiration.[12] Nasoduodenal feeding has been associated with a lower rate of vomiting and ventilator-associated pneumonia when compared to NG feeding.[28] However, the evidence to support the difference in aspiration and aspiration pneumonia risk associated with gastric and small bowel feeding is inconclusive. In general, small bowel feeding may be beneficial in patients who do not tolerate gastric feeding and offers an alternative to PN.[10–13] Nasoenteric feeding tubes can be inserted at the patient's bedside by trained medical personnel. However, greater skill is required to advance the tip of the feeding tube beyond the pylorus. Several techniques have been described in the literature to help facilitate bedside placement. Variable success rates have been reported with these techniques and are largely dependent on clinician experience. Electromagnetic tube placement devices that can be used at the bedside to guide tip position into the small bowel have been shown to be safe and cost-effective for small bowel feeding tube placement.[29,30] Alternatively, a variety of endoscopic and fluoroscopic techniques have been described to insert transpyloric

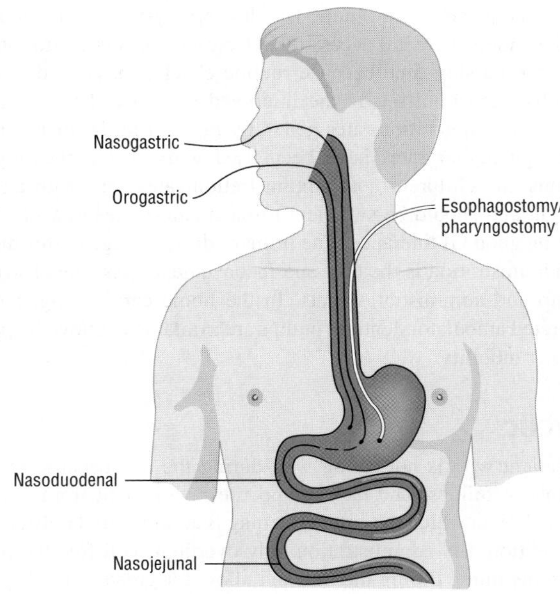

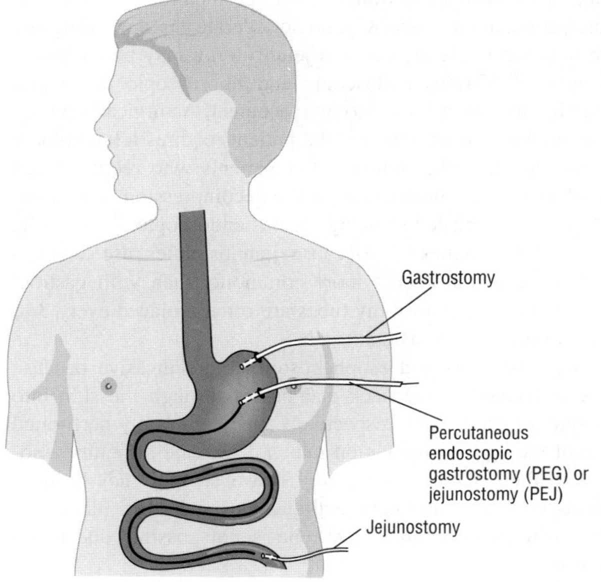

FIGURE 120-2 Access sites for tube feeding.

tubes.[12,27] Radiographic confirmation of appropriate tip placement should be obtained prior to use for all feeding tubes inserted by bedside techniques.[7,8]

Long-Term Access

Feeding tubes used for short-term enteral access are usually not optimal for long-term use because of patient discomfort, complications, and mechanical failures that develop over time. Long-term access should generally be considered when EN is anticipated for longer than 4 to 6 weeks. Many techniques can be used to establish long-term enteral access, including laparotomy, laparoscopy, endoscopic and image guidance (e.g., fluoroscopy, ultrasound).[12] The ability to perform the various techniques will be somewhat dependent on the expertise and facilities available within each institution. Long-term enteral access options include gastrostomy and jejunostomy tubes.

A gastrostomy is the most common type of long-term enteral access. It eliminates the nasal irritation and discomfort associated with nasoenteric feeding tubes and inadvertent removal is uncommon. In addition, because feeding gastrostomies use large-bore tubes, clogging is less of a problem. The most common technique for placement is the percutaneous endoscopic gastrostomy (PEG). It is minimally invasive and can be performed safely and cost-effectively in an endoscopy suite or at the bedside using conscious sedation and local anesthesia. Young children, however, will usually require general anesthesia for the procedure. Gastrostomy tubes are available in various sizes (12F to 28F; 1 to 4.5 cm shaft lengths), material (e.g., silicone, polyurethane), and have different retention mechanisms. Since smaller-diameter tubes are prone to more frequent occlusion and dysfunction, the larger diameter size is usually preferred. For patient convenience and comfort, a low-profile skin-level gastrostomy device may be placed in 2 to 3 months, once the gastrostomy tract has matured, if this type of device was not placed initially. This "gastric button" consists of a short, silicone, self-retaining conduit with either a mushroom tip or a balloon at the internal end and a one-way valve and small flange at the skin surface. Because this averts the external tube presence, it tends to be preferred in children or ambulatory adults who are receiving intermittent feedings. The exit site of all gastrostomies requires general stoma care to prevent inflammation and infection. Routine replacement of the gastrostomy tube at defined intervals (usually 3 to 6 months) is a standard of practice of many clinicians to prevent failure of the retention mechanism that can occur over time.[12]

In patients with a functional bowel but impaired gastric motility, pancreatitis, or who otherwise do not tolerate gastric feeding and require long-term enteral access, a jejunostomy may be an appropriate option.[27] Various endoscopic and fluoroscopic techniques are available for direct jejunostomy placement. A surgically placed jejunostomy may be an option if the patient requires a laparotomy or laparoscopy for other reasons. For patients who require small bowel feeding with simultaneous gastric decompression, a gastrojejunal tube may be placed utilizing various endoscopic, fluroscopic, and surgical techniques.[12,27] Because jejunostomies use smaller-bore tubes, occlusion occurs more commonly than with gastrostomy tubes. Gastrojejunostomy tubes are often replaced every 3 to 6 months to prevent occlusion.

Pharyngostomies and esophagostomies are invasive because the tube is located in the neck and passes through the skin into the pharynx or esophagus, respectively. They are rarely performed because of the high complication rate and extreme difficulty associated with their maintenance care.[31] However, they may be used in patients with head and neck malignancies and when placement of a gastrostomy or jejunostomy tube is not possible due to GI obstruction.

There are ethical implications regarding determination of appropriate candidates for long-term feeding tube placement.[12,31,32] Because a gastrostomy is relatively easy to place and many patients, families, and nonspecialist clinicians overestimate the benefits of EN, it is prone to inappropriate use. In certain patient populations, such as those with end-stage cancer or advanced dementia, the placement of a gastrostomy is controversial. Artificial nutrition and hydration (ANH) has not been shown to promote the healing of pressure ulcers, increase patient comfort or functional status, or prolong survival when compared to hand feeding in patients with advanced dementia.[32] From a clinical standpoint, ANH does not increase a patient's comfort or improve nutrition parameters of most terminally ill people and can result in medical complications.[33] Placement of a feeding tube resulted in a higher 1-year mortality rate in a group of 5,266 nursing home residents with dysphagia.[34] Evaluation by a multidisciplinary team is warranted for patients near end of life to establish whether the benefit outweighs the risk of feeding tube placement.[8,32]

ADMINISTRATION METHODS

EN may be administered by continuous, cyclic (continuous rate over a portion of the day), intermittent (infused over 20 to 60 minutes), or bolus (generally given in 5 to 10 minutes) methods and may be accomplished by syringe, gravity, or pump-controlled techniques. The method of delivery depends on the location of the tip of the feeding tube, the patient's clinical condition and intestinal function, the environment in which the patient resides, and the patient's tolerance to the tube feeding.

Continuous

Pump-assisted continuous administration of EN is generally the method of choice for feeding patients who are critically ill, have poor glycemic control, are being fed via jejunostomy tube, or have demonstrated intolerance to intermittent or bolus feeding.[9,35] When EN is delivered into the small intestine, the continuous method is preferred because it is associated with enhanced tolerance. The rapid delivery of feeding into the small intestine, especially hyperosmotic formulations, may contribute to abdominal distension, cramping, hyperperistalsis, and diarrhea. Therefore, conversion to intermittent or bolus administration is not recommended for those with jejunostomy tubes.

The delivery system for continuous administration generally includes a feeding reservoir or bag attached to an extension set that is connected to a pump. The delivery system is then attached to the patient's enteral access tube. Continuous administration may increase nursing time because routine checks are needed, but this disadvantage is offset by the improved tolerance. For adults, target EN administration rates generally range from 50 to 125 mL/h, although higher rates have been used without complications. In infants and children, goal administration rates vary with age and weight and should be sufficient to meet caloric needs while maintaining good GI tolerance. The primary disadvantage to this method of administration is the cost and inconvenience associated with the pump and administration sets. In the home care setting, battery-operated ambulatory enteral pumps are available to allow the patient greater mobility.

Cyclic

A patient who is not eating well during the day because of complaints of fullness and lack of appetite may benefit from a trial of cyclic EN, in which the enteral feeding is administered only at night. In addition, EN administration only overnight will free the patient from the pump during the day and allow for greater mobility. This increased mobility may be particularly useful for the home patient or patient requiring rehabilitation. Because a pump controls the rate of administration, this method may be used in patients with either gastric or small bowel access.

Bolus

The bolus administration of EN is commonly used for patients in long-term care settings who have a gastrostomy. This administration technique involves the delivery of the enteral feeding formulation over 5 to 10 minutes. Essentially, the only equipment needed is a syringe to instill the feeding volume into the tube. Depending on the patient's nutritional requirements, an instillation volume of 240 to 500 mL is generally used and repeated four to six times daily. From a convenience standpoint, it is generally preferable to adjust the bolus volume in increments of the feeding formulation container size (usually 240 to 250 mL). Bolus volumes given to infants and children vary with age and weight (usually 30 to 240 mL) and should be sufficient to meet the calorie needs of most patients. In neonates, the bolus regimen is usually begun with an every 3-hour schedule; as the child grows, feedings may be given less frequently.[36] In patients with duodenal or jejunal access, bolus delivery may result in cramping, nausea, vomiting, aspiration, and diarrhea. Bolus administration also should be avoided in patients with delayed gastric emptying and in patients who are at high risk of aspiration.

Intermittent

If a patient is experiencing intolerance to bolus administration over 5 to 10 minutes, it may be helpful to administer the prescribed volume over a longer time period, generally 20 to 60 minutes. For this method, the desired volume of feeding formulation is emptied into a reservoir bag or container and administered by an enteral pump or via gravity drip using a roller clamp. The bolus method of administration is more consistent physiologically with normal eating patterns than the continuous method. One study in infants demonstrated that normal gallbladder emptying did not occur with continuous feedings but was present in those infants receiving bolus feedings.[37] Thus, those patients who need long-term EN and PN, especially children, may benefit when this approach is used because it may minimize the development of cholestatic liver disease.

INITIATION AND ADVANCEMENT PROTOCOL

Guidelines for the initiation and advancement of enteral feeding formulations vary greatly and are primarily tailored to patient tolerance. The typical recommendation for continuous EN administration for adults is to start at 20 to 50 mL/h and advance by 10 to 25 mL/h every 4 to 8 hours until the desired goal is achieved. For intermittent administration, the typical recommendation is to start with 120 mL every 4 hours and advance by 30 to 60 mL every 8 to 12 hours.[8,35] In children, the recommendation for continuous administration is initiation at a rate of 1 to 2 mL/kg per hour (no more than 25 to 30 mL/h) or 2 to 4 mL/kg per bolus (no more than 30 to 90 mL) with advancement by similar amounts every 4 to 24 hours. In premature infants, feedings may be initiated at lower rates usually 10 to 20 mL/kg per day and advanced by similar rates daily. Schedules for progression of tube feeding from initial to target rates are important and may influence tolerance. If the protocol is too conservative, it may take an excessively long period of time to reach nutrient goals. The practice of diluting enteral feeding formulations is not routinely recommended unless necessary to increase fluid intake.[8,35] The development of an EN protocol within an institution that outlines initiation and advancement criteria may be a useful strategy to optimize achievement of nutrient goals.[10,11] Such a protocol should allow nursing to advance the rate (e.g., 25 mL/h every 4 hours until the goal rate is achieved) based on GI tolerance. Clinical signs of intolerance include abdominal distension, abdominal cramping, high GRVs, aspiration, and diarrhea.

ENTERAL FEEDING FORMULATION SELECTION

Historically, enteral formulas were created to provide essential nutrients. Over the years, enhancements have been made to meet specific patient needs and improve tolerance. For example, nutrient composition has been enhanced by changing the content of the amino acids (e.g., glutamine and arginine), changing the omega-3 polyunsaturated fatty acid content, and adding RNA to enhance immune function and improve therapeutic outcomes. These specific nutrients have been called nutraceuticals or pharmaconutrients because of the intent to use them to modify disease processes and improve clinical outcomes. Currently, enteral feeding formulations are categorized by the FDA as medical foods.[8] They are considered components of supportive care and are simply regulated to ensure sanitary manufacture. Unfortunately, they are not subject to rules governing health claims, and promotion of medical foods for therapeutic intent is currently not regulated by the FDA.[38]

The macronutrient content of enteral formulas (namely, protein, carbohydrate, and fat) varies in nutrient complexity (Table 120-4). Nutrient complexity refers to the amount of hydrolysis and digestion a substrate requires prior to intestinal absorption. Polymeric or intact substrates are of similar molecular form as the foods we eat. Enteral formulas that contain partially hydrolyzed or elemental substrates are characterized as elemental or defined-formula diets. The caloric contribution of each of the macronutrients is as follows: carbohydrates, 4 kcal/g (17 kJ/g); protein, 4 kcal/g (17 kJ/g); and fat, 9 kcal/g (38 kJ/g).

Protein Composition

The essential amino acid content of the protein source determines the quality of the protein, and most commercially available enteral feeding formulations contain proteins of high quality. The form of the protein source in enteral formulas will determine the amount of digestion that is required for absorption within the small bowel. Polymeric or intact protein sources require digestion to smaller peptides and free amino acids before absorption from the GI tract. Therefore,

TABLE 120-4 Enteral Formula Nutrient Complexity

Nutrient	Polymeric or Intact	Partially Hydrolyzed or Elemental
Carbohydrate	Starches Fruit, vegetable, cereal solids Glucose polymers Corn syrup solids Polysaccharides	Oligosaccharides Maltodextrins Disaccharides Maltose, sucrose, lactose Monosaccharides Glucose Galactose
Fat	Long-chain triglycerides Polyunsaturated fatty acids Corn oil Safflower oil Soybean oil Canola oil Marine oils	Medium-chain triglycerides Coconut oil Palm kernel oil Free fatty acids Linoleic
Protein	Whole Egg, milk, wheat, whey Isolates Caseinate salts Lactalbumin	Oligopeptides Dipeptides Tripeptides L-amino acids

enteral formulation protein sources such as meat, milk, eggs, and caseinates require digestion by hydrochloric acid, specific protein enzymes, and pancreatic proteases. Enteral formulations may also contain protein sources that are partially hydrolyzed to peptides or L-amino acids. As the molecular form of protein is reduced in size, the osmotic load of the enteral formulation is increased. Many commercially available enteral feeding formulations contain combinations of intact and partially hydrolyzed protein sources.

Conditionally Essential Amino Acids

Glutamine and arginine are generally considered nonessential amino acids. However, during periods of high physiologic stress, the need for these nutrients may be increased beyond the body's synthetic ability; consequently, these amino acids are characterized as conditionally essential. Because they are usually present in low amounts in most enteral feeding formulations, those formulations targeted for the critically ill may be supplemented with glutamine and/or arginine.

Glutamine serves as a key fuel for rapidly dividing cells, including enterocytes, endothelial cells, lymphocytes, and fibroblasts. The primary site of glutamine production is skeletal muscle. During critical illness, the catabolism of skeletal muscle provides an increased glutamine supply, but this may not be enough to meet the high rate of glutamine use by cells of the immune system and other cells involved in recovery and repair. Glutamine depletion may develop, particularly during prolonged periods of metabolic stress. Favorable outcomes have been documented in critically ill patients when enteral formulations have been supplemented with glutamine.[10,39,40]

Arginine has been added to some immune-modulating enteral formulations in concentrations that range from 4.5 to 14 g/L. However, arginine supplementation remains controversial, especially in patients with sepsis.[40,41] Many of the physiologic effects of arginine are mediated by its conversion to nitric oxide, which, in turn, modulates immune function, inflammation, vasodilation, and response to sepsis. Some of these effects may be potentially harmful in the patient with sepsis, especially when higher arginine intakes are used.[10,11]

Carbohydrate Composition

The carbohydrate component of enteral feeding formulations usually provides the major source of calories. Polymeric or intact enteral formulations contain starches and numerous types of glucose polymers, which require digestion to monosaccharide moieties prior to intestinal absorption (see Fig. 120-1). As the hydrolysis of carbohydrate increases within an enteral formulation, the osmolality of the formulation increases. Simple sugars, such as glucose and galactose, contribute significantly to the osmolality of enteral formulations. Consequently, polymeric entities, rather than elemental sugars, are preferred in enteral formulas. Glucose polymers provide a useful carbohydrate source that is tolerated by most individuals (see Table 120-4). The polymers are large chains that provide minimal osmotic load, yet are absorbed easily in the intestine. The one shortcoming of glucose polymers and oligosaccharides is that they are not as sweet as simple glucose and thus may decrease the palatability of orally consumed products. Finally, almost all commercially available enteral feeding formulations used in adults and older children are lactose-free because disaccharidase production within the gut lumen is reduced during illness and periods of prolonged bowel rest. Additionally, there is a high incidence of lactose intolerance in those of certain ethnic decent: rates range from 5% in white northern Europeans, North Americans, and Australians to over 50% in people from South America, Africa, and Asia.[42] By adulthood, 15% of Caucasian, 40% of Asians, 50% to 80% of Hispanics, and 85% of African Americans have lactase deficiency. Infant formulas are available with or without lactose.[36]

Fat and Fatty Acid Composition

Fat is an important constituent in the diet because it provides a concentrated calorie source and serves as a carrier for fat-soluble vitamins. Sufficient linoleic acid is required to prevent essential fatty acid deficiency and should approximate at least 1% to 3% of total daily calories. The most common sources of fat in enteral feeding formulations are vegetable oils (soy or corn) rich in polyunsaturated fatty acids. The concentration of fat varies between less than 2% and 45% of total calories. High fat content of the diet is associated with delayed gastric emptying. Enteral feeding formulations can also contain fat in the form of MCTs derived from palm kernel or coconut oils. Because MCTs do not contain linoleic acid, enteral formulations that contain MCTs will also have a source of long-chain triglycerides to provide essential fatty acids. Potential advantages of MCTs compared to long-chain triglycerides are that they are more water soluble, undergo rapid hydrolysis, require no pancreatic lipase or bile salts for absorption, and do not require carnitine for transport into the mitochondria, where they are converted to energy. They also do not require chylomicron formation for small bowel enterocyte absorption and are not transported via the lymphatic system.

The source of long-chain fat within some enteral formulations has been modified from omega-6 to omega-3 fatty acids in an effort to modulate the inflammatory response in patients with acute respiratory distress syndrome (ARDS), acute lung injury (ALI), and sepsis.[43] The omega-6 fatty acids serve as precursors to certain cytokines that are potent inflammatory mediators and also decrease cell-mediated immune response. The omega-6 fatty acids are high in linoleic acid and are derived from vegetable oil, whereas the omega-3 fatty acids, derived from coldwater fish oils, are high in linolenic acid. It has been proposed that if the dietary proportion of omega-3 fatty acids is increased and omega-6 fatty acids is decreased, less inflammation and immunosuppression may occur during metabolic stress due to an alteration in the type and quantity of cytokines produced.

Docosahexaenoic acid (DHA) and arachidonic acid (ARA) are two fatty acids abundant in human milk, but until recently, they were not contained in commercial infant formulas. Although the role of ARA supplementation is unclear, DHA is important in brain and eye development. In some studies, DHA and ARA supplementation provided benefits to a child's visual function and/or cognitive and behavioral development.[44] The FDA has classified plant-based fatty acid blends of DHA and ARA as generally recognized as safe (GRAS), and most infant formulas, as well as some products for pregnant and lactating women, are supplemented with these fatty acids.

Fiber Content

Fiber, in both soluble and insoluble forms, is added to several adult and pediatric enteral feeding formulations in amounts ranging from 5.9 to 24 g/L. Infant formulas generally do not contain fiber; however, at least one formula intended for use in infants with diarrhea contains soy fiber. Fiber supplementation is common in clinical practice, primarily because fiber-free enteral formulations are implicated as a contributing factor to both diarrhea and constipation. Soluble fiber undergoes bacterial degradation within the colon to produce short-chain fatty acids. Potential benefits of soluble fiber are its trophic effects on the colonic mucosa and promotion of sodium and water absorption within the colon. Insoluble fiber is undigested and may help decrease GI transit time by increasing fecal weight. Fiber supplementation may help regulate bowel function in both normal individuals and those with altered colonic motility. In addition, the resulting short-chain fatty acids are an excellent energy source. Although beneficial effects of fiber supplementation have not been clearly proven in clinical studies, there is experimental evidence that fiber may play an integral role in normal nutrition, and risk is generally minimal.[45] Fiber supplementation may be beneficial when long-term EN is required or in patients who experience diarrhea or constipation while receiving a fiber-free enteral formulation. Soluble fiber may also be beneficial in the critically ill patient who is hemodynamically stable and develops diarrhea while receiving EN.[10,46] Insoluble fiber should be avoided in all critically ill patients due to case reports of bowel obstruction.[10]

Osmolality and Renal Solute Load

Osmolality and renal solute load can affect tolerance to enteral feeding formulations. The osmolality of a given enteral formulation is a function of the size and quantity of ionic and molecular particles, primarily related to the protein, carbohydrate, electrolyte, and mineral content within a given volume. The unit of measure of osmolality is milliosmoles per kilogram (mOsm/kg) or millimoles per kilogram (mmol/kg). Iso-osmolar is considered to be ~300 mOsm/kg (300 mmol/kg). Enteral formulations with greater amounts of partially hydrolyzed or elemental substrates have a higher osmolality than formulations containing polymeric or intact substrate forms. Therefore, formulations that contain sucrose or glucose, dipeptides and tripeptides, and amino acids are generally hyperosmolar. Increased caloric density also increases the osmolality of an enteral formulation. In general, the osmolality of commercially available enteral feeding formulations ranges from 300 to 900 mOsm/kg (300 to 900 mmol/kg). The American Academy of Pediatrics recommends that enteral formulations for use in infants have an osmolality of 450 mOsm/kg (450 mmol/kg) or less.

Symptoms of gastric retention, diarrhea, abdominal distension, nausea, and vomiting have been attributed to enteral formulations having high osmolality based on the assumption that a higher osmolality will draw water into the gut lumen. However, clinical evidence to support the relationship between osmolality and GI tolerance is lacking. The practice of diluting hyperosmolar formulations has not been shown to enhance tolerance and should be discouraged unless dilution is done to increase fluid intake.[8] Factors such as concurrent antibiotic therapy, method of enteral feeding administration, and the formulation's composition are likely to play a greater role in GI tolerance than the osmolality.

The renal solute load is determined by the protein, sodium, potassium, and chloride content of the enteral formulation. Formulations that contain a greater solute load increase the obligatory water loss via the kidney. It is estimated that 40 to 60 mL of water is the minimal amount necessary to excrete 1 g of nitrogen. Those receiving high-protein enteral formulations unable to ingest more water, such as a geriatric patient and a patient with altered mental status, may be at risk for significant dehydration.

CLASSIFICATION OF ENTERAL FEEDING FORMULATIONS

5 Although most patients' needs can probably be met using three or four different formulations, certain disease states or clinical conditions may warrant the use of a specialty feeding formulation. Development of an evidence-based, effective formulary system should focus on clinically significant characteristics of available formulations and avoid duplicate feeding formulations. Categorizing enteral feeding formulations according to therapeutic class is necessary in developing a formulary system for adults (Table 120-5) and children (Table 120-6).

TABLE 120-5 Adult Enteral Feeding Formulation Classification System

Category	Features	Indications
Standard polymeric	Isotonic 1–1.2 kcal/mL (4.2–5 kJ/mL) NPC:N 125:1 to 150:1 May contain fiber	Designed to meet the needs of the majority of patients Patients with functional GI tract Not suitable for oral use
High protein	NPC:N <125:1 May contain fiber	Patients with protein requirements >1.5 g/kg/day, such as trauma patients and those with burns, pressure sores, or wounds Patients receiving propofol
High caloric density	1.5–2 kcal/mL (6.3–8.4 kJ/mL) Lower electrolyte content per calorie Hypertonic	Patients requiring fluid and/or electrolyte restriction, such as kidney insufficiency
Elemental	High proportion of free amino acids Low in fat	Patients who require low fat Use has generally been replaced by peptide-based formulations
Peptide-based	Contains dipeptides and tripeptides Contains MCTs	Indications/benefits not clearly established Trial may be warranted in patients who do not tolerate intact protein due to malabsorption
Disease-specific		
Kidney	Caloric dense Protein content varies Low electrolyte content	Alternative to high caloric density formulations, but generally more expensive
Liver	Increased branched-chain and decreased aromatic amino acids	Patients with hepatic encephalopathy
Lung	High fat, low carbohydrate Antiinflammatory lipid profile and antioxidants	Patients with ARDS and severe ALI
Diabetes mellitus	High fat, low carbohydrate	Alternative to standard, fiber-containing formulation in patients with uncontrolled hyperglycemia
Immune-modulating	Supplemented with glutamine, arginine, nucleotides, and/or omega-3 fatty acids	Patients undergoing major elective GI surgery, trauma, burns, head and neck cancer, and critically ill patients on mechanical ventilation Use with caution in patients with sepsis Select nutrients may be beneficial or harmful in subgroups of critically ill patients
Oral supplement	Sweetened for taste Hypertonic	Patients who require supplementation to an oral diet

ALI, acute lung injury; ARDS, acute respiratory distress syndrome; MCT, medium-chain triglyceride; NPC:N, nonprotein calorie-to-nitrogen ratio.

TABLE 120-6 Pediatric Enteral Feeding Formulation Classification System

Formula Type	Features	Indications
Infants		
Cow's milk-based	Standard energy density for feeding: 20–24 kcal/oz (2.8–3.3 kJ/mL); also available in concentrate (40 kcal/oz [5.6 kJ/mL]) and powder forms Standard formulation contains lactose, but also available as lactose-free	Normal, healthy infant
Soy protein-based	Standard energy density for feeding: 20 kcal/oz (2.8 kJ/mL); also available in concentrate (40 kcal/oz [5.6 kJ/mL]) and powder forms Lactose free May contain added soy fiber	Lactase deficiency or lactose intolerance, galactosemia, diarrhea (fiber added)
Prematurity	Standard energy density for feeding: 24 kcal/oz (3.3 kJ/mL); also available in 20 (2.8 kJ/mL) and 30 kcal/oz (4.2 kJ/mL) forms	Preterm infants weighing <2–3 kg (4.4–6.6 lb)
Transition	Standard energy density for feeding: 22 kcal/oz (3.1 kJ/mL) Provide higher calcium and phosphorus content compared with term infant formulas	Preterm infants weighing <3 kg (6.6 lb) and ready for discharge
Semi-elemental/elemental	Standard energy density for feeding: 20 kcal/oz (2.8 kJ/mL) Hydrolyzed protein and free amino acids May contain ARA and DHA Lactose free Typically contain MCTs ranging from 5% to 86% of fat content	Malabsorption, cow's milk protein allergy, chylothorax, cystic fibrosis, biliary atresia, short bowel syndrome, food allergies
Special diets	Low electrolyte/mineral content	Kidney disease
Children Ages 1–10 Years		
Standard	Standard energy density for feeding: 30 or 45 kcal/oz (1 or 1.5 kcal/mL [4.2 or 6.3 kJ/mL]) Intact protein; 30–38 g/L May contain added fiber	Functioning GI tract requiring tube feedings
Semi-elemental/elemental	Standard energy density for feeding: 20–30 kcal/oz (2.8–4.2 kJ/mL) Hydrolyzed protein and free amino acids Lactose-free MCTs range from 33% to 87% of fat content	Malabsorption, cow's milk protein allergy, chylothorax, cystic fibrosis, biliary atresia, short bowel syndrome, food allergies

ARA, arachidonic acid; DHA, docosahexaenoic acid; MCT, medium-chain triglyceride.

Standard Polymeric

A large number of commercially available enteral feeding formulations fall within the category of a standard polymeric formulation. These formulations are approximately isotonic (300 mOsm/L [300 mmol/L]), provide 1 to 1.2 kcal/mL (4.2 to 5 kJ/mL), and are composed of intact nutrients in a nutritionally balanced mix of carbohydrate, fat, and protein. They are provided with or without dietary fiber. The nonprotein calorie-to-nitrogen ratio of these products is ~125:1 to 150:1. This ratio is a useful parameter for assessing protein density in relation to calories provided. Certain feeding formulations in this category may be promoted as high nitrogen but fall within standard protein amounts. To maintain their isotonicity, many products within this category are not sweetened, making them unpalatable and generally suited only for tube feeding and not oral supplementation; however, flavored products are available. The nutrient requirements of the majority of adult patients and children older than 1 year receiving EN can generally be met using feeding formulations in this category. Many infant formulas will also fall into this category because they provide 20 to 30 kcal/oz (2.8 to 4.2 kJ/mL).[36]

High Protein

Enteral feeding formulations with a nonprotein calorie-to-nitrogen ratio less than 125:1 can be categorized as high protein. The lower the ratio, the higher the protein density in relation to calories provided. In patients with high protein requirements, it is generally unacceptable to use a feeding formulation with standard protein amounts because the volume necessary to meet protein requirements will result in excessive calorie intake. Patients who may be candidates for a high-protein feeding formulation are critically ill patients and those with pressure sores, surgical wounds, and high output enterocutaneous fistula. In general, adult patients with estimated protein requirements exceeding 1.5 g/kg per day may benefit from a high-protein formulation. High-protein formulations may also be beneficial in mechanically ventilated patients who are receiving propofol for sedation. The vehicle for propofol is a soybean fat emulsion that contains 1.1 kcal/mL (4.6 kJ/mL). At therapeutic dosages, the use of propofol can significantly contribute to caloric intake, and a high protein formulation may be beneficial in allowing for the provision of protein requirements while minimizing the risk of overfeeding.

High Caloric Density

High caloric density formulations are concentrated to provide less fluid and electrolyte intake in comparison to a standard polymeric formulation. They provide ~2 kcal/mL (8.4 kJ/mL) and will achieve similar calorie and protein intake as a standard polymeric formulation, using half the volume. High caloric density formulations are often necessary for patients who require fluid and/or electrolyte restriction, such as those with kidney insufficiency or congestive heart failure. Although specialty enteral formulations targeted for acute and chronic kidney failure are also available, many patients with kidney failure can be managed using a product in this category.

Elemental/Peptide Based

Formulations in this category contain protein and/or fat components that are hydrolyzed into smaller, predigested forms. Traditionally, enteral formulations in this category were referred to as elemental and contained a high proportion of protein in the form of free amino acids and a low amount of fat. Although still commercially available, many of the formulations in this category have been reformulated to provide a portion of the protein in the form of dipeptides and tripeptides and fewer free amino acids because dipeptides and tripeptides are more readily absorbed than an equivalent mixture of free amino acids.[47] These peptide-based formulations, may be beneficial in patients with impaired digestion or absorption. Peptide-based formulations are generally higher in fat than the older, elemental formulations and use MCTs in varying proportions as the fat source.

Evidence to support the use of elemental or peptide-based formulations is limited, and their routine use is generally not recommended. Patients who do not tolerate standard, intact nutrient formulations as a result of malabsorption or short bowel syndrome might be candidates for a trial of a peptide-based formulation. In addition, elemental or peptide-based products that have higher percentages of MCTs and small amounts of long-chain triglycerides may be beneficial for patients with severe pancreatic insufficiency, such as chronic pancreatitis and cystic fibrosis; severe abnormalities of the intestinal mucosa, such as untreated celiac disease; biliary tract disease, such as biliary atresia or severe cholestasis; or chylothorax.

Disease Specific

Newer enteral feeding formulations have been designed to meet unique nutrient requirements and manage metabolic abnormalities associated with specific disease states. Conditions for which specialized enteral feeding formulations exist include kidney and liver failure, lung disease, including ARDS, diabetes mellitus, wound healing, and metabolic stress. Specialized enteral formulations designed to modulate the inflammatory response in patients with severe metabolic stress have been referred to as immune-modulating formulations or immunonutrition. These specialized formulations are supplemented with nutrients such as glutamine, arginine, branched-chain amino acids, nucleotides, and omega-3 polyunsaturated fatty acids, as a result of their potential role in regulating immune function; guidelines for their use in critically ill patients have been published.[10,11,48] Positive results have been reported in patients undergoing major elective GI surgery and major cancer surgery of the head and neck, patients with severe trauma or burns, and critically ill patients on mechanical ventilation. Multiple meta-analyses have shown that the use of immune-modulating enteral formulations in these select patient populations is associated with significant reductions in infectious complications, hospital length of stay, and duration of mechanical ventilation.[49,50] However, use of immune-modulating formulations has been associated with increased mortality in patients with preexisting severe sepsis and should therefore not be used or used with caution in these patients and in those who become septic while receiving these products.[10] Because of the lack of evidence to support their use, immune-modulating formulations are not currently recommended for use in children.[13]

Clinical **Controversy...**

Although there appears to be a role for immune-modulating enteral formulations in critically ill patients, the optimal pharmaconutrient composition and type of critically ill patient most likely to benefit are unclear. Available literature has been criticized for the heterogeneity of studies, including a wide range of patient populations and a variety of enteral formulations. The specific effects and optimal dose of individual nutrient components contained in immune-modulating enteral formulations also remain unclear. Caution is suggested in patients with severe sepsis due to arginine content, but available evidence is conflicting.

In patients with ARDS, improved outcomes from using a low carbohydrate formulation supplemented with specific fatty acids (eicosapentaenoic acid and γ-linolenic acid) and antioxidants have been documented.[43,51] When compared with a high fat formulation, the specialized diet was associated with fewer days of ventilatory support, fewer ICU days, and fewer new organ failures. Consequently, it is recommended that this specialized formulation be used for patients with ARDS and severe ALI.[10,11,48]

There are no disease-specific enteral products currently marketed for use in infants or children younger than 10 years of age. The use of modular supplements may be necessary in children with special nutrition needs (see Modular Products below).

Oral Supplements

In general, oral supplements are not intended for tube feeding but to enhance an oral diet. They are sweetened to improve taste and therefore are hypertonic (~450 to 700 mOsm/kg [~450 to 700 mmol/kg]). Osmolality is generally not a problem in the patient with a functioning GI tract. However, in the tube-fed patient, a sweetened product is unnecessary and may contribute to GI intolerance, particularly diarrhea. Powder supplements that are mixed with milk should be avoided in lactose-intolerant patients. In addition to liquid supplements, puddings, gelatins, bars, and milkshake-like supplements are available.

Modular Products

A module is a powder or liquid form of a nutrient (e.g., protein, carbohydrate, and fat) that is used to supplement nutrition intake when the diet or commercially available enteral formulation does not fully meet a patient's needs.[36,52] Alternatively, formulations available in powder or concentrate can be mixed with less water than needed for the standard dilution to deliver more nutrients in less volume. Infant formulas generally are concentrated beyond their standard concentration in this way. The mixing process required for modular components increases the potential for bacterial contamination and incorrect preparation. Contamination is a particular concern with the use of blenders and reconstitution of powders.[8,53] Human milk fortifiers are available for supplementation of human milk so that it meets the needs of a premature infant. Human milk fortifiers add calories, protein, and minerals and have been shown to improve nutritional outcomes in human milk-fed premature infants.[36,54–57]

Rehydration

Oral rehydration formulations are useful in maintaining hydration or treating dehydration in adult and pediatric patients with high GI output. Such formulations are available commercially in powder or liquid form or can be extemporaneously compounded. They can be administered orally or given via a feeding tube. The glucose content of oral rehydration solutions is important because it stimulates active transport systems, which, in turn, stimulate passive sodium and water uptake simultaneously with the glucose. Therefore, oral or enteral administration of rehydration solutions may decrease fecal water loss and generate a positive electrolyte balance.[58,59]

FORMULARY AND DELIVERY SYSTEM CONSIDERATIONS

For an institution's formulary considerations, generally no more than one product is necessary per category of enteral feeding formulation, and it may be possible to omit certain categories based on the specific patient population within a given institution. Additional selection criteria include container size and type, liquid or powder form, shelf life, ease of use, and cost.

Most enteral products are available as ready-to-use, prepackaged liquids, and a few are available in the powdered state and require reconstitution prior to use. Advantages of ready-to-use liquid formulations are convenience and lower susceptibility to microbiologic contamination. One disadvantage is that more storage space is required. The ease or convenience of a ready-to-use liquid is especially important for self-care patients, the disabled, and those who have difficulty reading or following printed instructions. Ready-to-use liquid enteral formulations are generally available in rigid plastic containers, cans, or closed, ready-to-hang bags. Bolus administration of EN is usually achieved using formulas available in cans. However, when formula from a can is used for continuous or cyclic administration, it must first be poured into a bag or bottle to allow for administration via a pump. This "open system" has a higher risk of microbial contamination than closed, ready-to-hang containers. The use of a powder formula is also considered an open delivery system.

Contaminated enteral feeding formulations are a potential source of infectious complications.[8,58] The GI tract may serve as a portal of entry for bacteria into the systemic circulation, especially in patients who are receiving multiple antibiotics, have undergone a surgical procedure, are immunosuppressed, or have GI tract stasis from a variety of causes. The contamination of enteral feeding formulations is associated with a lack of attention to proper handling techniques, inability to disinfect preparation equipment, and nonsterile or contaminated tube-feeding additives. Unlike liquid formulations, powdered products are not guaranteed by the manufacturer to be sterile because of the inability to properly sterilize the powder without destruction of some of its components. Contamination of milk powder and consequently powdered infant formulas with *Enterobacter sakazakii* (*Cronobacter* species) has been reported.[53] Contamination of one infant formula with *E. sakazakii* at the manufacturing site was implicated in the death of an infant in a neonatal ICU, prompting FDA warnings regarding the use of powdered formulations in premature neonates and other immunocompromised infants. Because powder formulations require reconstitution, often in a blender that is difficult to sterilize, they are also more susceptible to contamination at the time of preparation. To minimize contamination risk, stringent handling procedures should be followed during all stages of enteral feeding preparation and delivery. The closed-system containers supply a ready-to-hang, prefilled, sterile supply of formula in volumes of 1 to 1.5 L. Most but not all enteral formulations intended for use in adults and some pediatric formulations are available in the closed-administration system. The closed-administration system also offers the advantage of not requiring refrigeration and allowing hang times beyond 24 to 36 hours, whereas the conventional open-delivery system necessitates hang times of generally 4 to 8 hours.

COMPLICATIONS AND MONITORING

The majority of complications associated with EN are metabolic, GI, and mechanical. The early detection and management of potential complications is necessary to allow for the successful use of EN. In addition, measures to avoid complications should be incorporated into the management of all patients receiving EN (Table 120-7).

Metabolic Complications

Metabolic complications associated with EN are similar to those associated with PN, but the incidence tends to be lower. EN is associated with a lower incidence of hyperglycemia than PN.[20,60] Complications related to hydration and electrolyte imbalance and altered glucose control are observed more frequently in critically ill patients, especially those with underlying organ dysfunction. The micronutrient and water contents within enteral feeding formulations are in fixed amounts intended to meet recommended dietary allowances for the average person. Consequently, the frequency of clinical and laboratory assessment to monitor hydration, electrolyte, organ function, and glucose control adequately for a patient who is critically ill is greater than for a stable patient or patients residing in rehabilitation units or at home. Patients receiving long-term EN at home may require laboratory monitoring only every 2 to 3 months, depending on their clinical status. Besides macronutrient content, it is important to evaluate the actual content of water

TABLE 120-7 Suggested Monitoring for Patients on Enteral Nutrition

Parameter	During Initiation of EN Therapy	During Stable EN Therapy
Vital signs	Every 4–6 hours	As needed with suspected change (i.e., fever)
Clinical assessment		
Weight	Daily	Weekly
Length/height (children)	Weekly–monthly	Monthly
Head circumference (<3 years of age)	Weekly–monthly	Monthly
Total intake/output	Daily	As needed with suspected change in intake/output
Tube-feeding intake	Daily	Daily
Enterostomy tube site assessment	Daily	Daily
GI tolerance		
Stool frequency/volume	Daily	Daily
Abdomen assessment	Daily	Daily
Nausea or vomiting	Daily	Daily
Gastric residual volumes	Every 4–8 hours (varies)	As needed when delayed gastric emptying suspected
Tube placement	Prior to starting, then ongoing	Ongoing
Laboratory		
Electrolytes, blood urea nitrogen/serum creatinine, glucose	Daily	Every 1–3 months
Calcium, magnesium, phosphorus	3–7 times/week	Every 1–3 months
Liver function tests	Weekly	Every 1–3 months
Trace elements, vitamins	If deficiency/toxicity suspected	If deficiency/toxicity suspected

EN, enteral nutrition.

and micronutrients provided by the enteral formulation, especially in critically ill patients at high risk of metabolic complications. Supplemental fluid, electrolytes, and minerals may be required in some patients. Conversely, for patients who have fluid retention or increased serum electrolytes, the enteral formulation may need to be changed to one that is more concentrated or provides less of a particular nutrient.

Gastrointestinal Complications

6 The GI complications associated with tube feeding include nausea, vomiting, abdominal distension, cramping, aspiration, diarrhea, and constipation. GRV refers to the volume of contents in the stomach and is measured by using a syringe and aspirating from a large-bore NG or gastrostomy tube. For patients receiving tube feeding into the stomach, GRV is widely used to assess tolerance. Although not well documented, patients with high GRVs may be at higher risk of vomiting and/or aspiration. The frequency of measuring GRV generally varies between 4 and 8 hours, and most institutions follow a protocol that directs the frequency of monitoring and at what volume and for how long to hold feedings.[61] In critically ill patients receiving gastric feeding, GRVs should be measured every 4 hours.[10]

If high GRVs occur, the response is often to hold the next scheduled bolus or stop or decrease the rate if feeding is continuous. However, frequent interruptions in EN delivery can adversely affect the attainment of nutrition outcome goals. Because GRV is an unreliable measure of EN tolerance, symptoms such as abdominal distension, fullness, bloating, and discomfort are generally more reliable indicators of EN intolerance and should be assessed frequently. A trend toward increased GRV is generally more important than one isolated high measurement. Generally, in the absence of other signs of intolerance, EN should not be held when the GRV is less than 500 mL.[10] If symptoms are present, and GRVs are elevated, a decrease in the tube-feeding rate or discontinuation may be warranted. Measures to reduce aspiration risk should be implemented when GRVs are consistently elevated, including elevating the head of the patient's bed to a 30° to 45° angle and consideration of postpyloric continuous feeding. In addition, it may be beneficial to initiate a prokinetic agent such as metoclopramide or erythromycin to increase the gastric emptying rate.[10,62,63] Other interventions include minimizing the use of narcotics, sedatives, or other agents that may delay gastric emptying and correcting underlying fluid imbalance and electrolyte disturbances that can impair GI motility.[64] Unless GRVs are excessive (greater than 500 mL in adults), they should generally be reinstilled (refed) through the tube to minimize nutrient, fluid, and electrolyte losses.[8,65]

Aspiration pneumonia is considered the most serious complication associated with tube feeding and is potentially life-threatening. Although aspiration is a fairly common event for critically ill patients receiving tube feeding, progression to aspiration pneumonia is difficult to predict. Risk factors for aspiration include a previous aspiration episode, decreased consciousness, neuromuscular disease, structural airway or GI tract abnormalities, endotracheal intubation, vomiting, persistently high GRVs, and prolonged supine positioning.[65] Identification of these risk factors, along with close monitoring of GRV, is recommended for all critically ill patients receiving tube feeding. Historically, blue food coloring had been added to enteral formulations in an attempt to detect aspiration. However, because of its low sensitivity for detection and association with several serious adverse events, including death, the addition of blue food dye to enteral formulations is no longer advised.[10,66] There are currently no reliable methods available to detect aspiration in enterally fed patients.[10,67]

Clinical **Controversy...**

Some clinicians use low-dose "trickle" or trophic EN (10 to 20 mL/h) early in the course of critical illness to maintain gut integrity and function while decreasing risk of GI complications. However, the necessary volume of EN required to maintain intestinal integrity remains unknown. There is some evidence that providing initial trophic EN in mechanically ventilated patients with acute respiratory failure results in similar clinical outcomes to those of full energy EN with fewer episodes of GI intolerance.

Diarrhea develops in 20% to 70% of patients receiving EN. Because of the lack of a standard definition and the number of contributing factors, the true incidence is unknown.[20,35] When monitoring for diarrhea, stool frequency, consistency, and volume should be evaluated, and previous bowel habits should be considered. Diarrhea has been defined as more than three liquid stools daily or a stool volume of more than 250 to 500 mL/day (10 to 25 mL/kg per day in children) for at least two consecutive days.[20] Therefore, the occurrence of one or two loose stools does not constitute diarrhea or require intervention.

7 Diarrhea in patients receiving tube feeding may be caused by a number of factors, and management should be directed at identifying and correcting the most likely cause(s). Tube feeding-related factors that may contribute to diarrhea include too rapid delivery or advancement of formula, intolerance to the formula composition, administration of large volumes of feeding into the small bowel, and formula contamination. Thus, measures to prevent or manage diarrhea related directly to the tube feeding should address these potential causes.[20,58,64] If diarrhea occurs when using a fiber-free formulation, consider switching to a fiber-containing formulation. If using a high-fat formulation, it may be beneficial to switch to a formulation lower in fat or having a proportion of the fat supplied as MCTs. Finally, it is important to assess the risk of bacterial contamination of the formula and take steps to minimize any potential risk factors. Once infectious etiologies have been excluded, severe diarrhea may require pharmacologic treatment with loperamide, diphenoxylate/atropine, or opioids.

Drug therapy, particularly the use of broad-spectrum antibiotics, is a common cause of diarrhea that is unrelated to tube feeding. Sorbitol, used as a sweetening agent in many liquid formulations to enhance palatability, is an osmotic laxative that can cause diarrhea. In addition, many drugs available in a liquid form are hyperosmolar, which may contribute to diarrhea, especially when these medications are not diluted properly before administration. Because many patients receiving tube feeding also receive medications in a liquid form, all medications should be evaluated for their potential contribution. Infectious causes, such as antibiotic-induced bacterial overgrowth by *Clostridium difficile* or other intestinal flora, need to be considered when diarrhea develops. Malabsorption, secondary to the underlying disease state or condition, may also cause diarrhea.

Mechanical Complications

Mechanical complications of EN are those associated with the feeding tube, including tube occlusion or malposition, and nasopulmonary intubation. Feeding tube occlusion usually results from the improper administration of medications and/or flushing technique. Kinking of the tube also may cause occlusion. The tube should be flushed with at least 30 mL of water before and after administering any medication. The recommended volume used in children is generally less than 30 mL and depends on the size of the tube. The frequency of flushing should be at least every 8 hours during continuous feeding and before and after each intermittent feeding. If tube occlusion occurs, an attempt to irrigate the tube with warm water should be made. Other fluids such as colas and cranberry juice have been used to irrigate occluded tubes but have not been shown to be any better than warm water. Some success in reestablishing patency has been shown with the use of pancreatic enzymes mixed in sodium bicarbonate.[68] Declogging devices that are specifically designed to unclog feeding tubes are available. They have been designed to either mechanically break through or remove the occlusion or provide an applicator and syringe prefilled with pancreatic enzymes and various powders targeted to restore patency.

Inadvertent nasoenteric tube removal or displacement has been reported in ~40% of patients receiving EN.[69] An agitated or confused patient may pull at the feeding tube and cause its removal or malposition. Measures to decrease agitation and confusion should be attempted. Various manipulations done to the patient may also cause malposition. Securing the tube with tape may be helpful, as well as marking the tube with permanent ink at the exit site to assess for position change. A recently developed nasal bridle that uses a magnetic retrieval system has proven to be a simple and effective method for securing nasoenteric feeding tubes and preventing accidental removal.[69]

When a feeding tube is inserted nasally or orally, there is a risk that the tube may inadvertently enter the tracheobronchial tree. The risk may be higher in patients who have an impaired cough or gag reflex and when a stylet is used for tube insertion. Proper positioning of the tube should always be confirmed by radiography prior to feeding initiation and routinely reassessed to avoid inadvertent administration of enteral formula into the lung.

Other Complications

Infectious complications of feeding tube placement include sinusitis (with nasoenteric placement), exit site-related infections (e.g., cellulitis, subcutaneous abscess, and necrotizing fasciitis), and intraabdominal infections (e.g., peritonitis and abscess). Leaking and bleeding around the exit site can also occur.[12,31] Formation of excessive granulation tissue around the exit site is often the cause of leaking and bleeding and can be managed by applying silver nitrate.

A unique complication of tube feedings in children, especially in the first year of life, is the development of feeding disorders as a consequence of oral hypersensitivity, poor oral/motor skills, and food aversion. In these children, transitioning from tube to oral nutrition is often difficult and protracted. The involvement of an occupational or speech therapist, behavioral psychologist, or other trained individual, as well as perseverance by the family, often is necessary to improve oral intake. Avoidance of a strict nothing by mouth (NPO) status, if possible, and oral stimulation programs for those children who must remain NPO are recommended to avoid this complication.[70]

DRUG DELIVERY VIA FEEDING TUBE

Using enteral feeding tubes to deliver drugs is a common practice and offers an alternative for patients unable to take drugs by the oral route. However, in addition to tube occlusion, effects on drug bioavailability and other potential interactions need to be considered when using this route. Medications have been given as a concomitant bolus administration via the feeding tube or admixed with the enteral feeding formulation.

Concomitant Drug Administration

8 Concomitant administration of medications with enteral feedings requires awareness of certain limitations. Medications delivered directly into the stomach allow for the normal process of drug dissolution. Medications delivered into the small bowel may result in alterations of drug dissolution because the stomach is bypassed. In addition, therapeutic effect designed to occur within the stomach, such as with antacids and sucralfate, may be influenced by the feeding tube route. Because many drugs are best absorbed in the fasting state, they should be administered on an empty stomach whenever possible. Patients on bolus gastric feeding may receive medications appropriately spaced between the feedings, but patients on continuous feeding will require interruption for drug administration.

Selecting the proper medication dosage form for coadministration with the tube feeding is another important consideration. Medications in sublingual form, sustained-release capsules or tablets, and enteric-coated tablets should not be crushed and therefore should not be administered via enteral feeding tubes.[8,68] Solid dosage forms that are appropriate to crush should be prepared as a very fine powder and mixed with 15 to 30 mL of water or other appropriate solvent before administering through the tube. In addition, many capsules may be opened and the contents administered in the same manner. Pellets contained inside microencapsulated dosage forms should generally not be crushed. It may be acceptable to administer intact pellets through feeding tubes, provided that the pellets are small enough and drug absorption is not compromised.[69,71,72] To avoid the need to crush a solid dosage form and mix with water, liquid dosage forms are used commonly for administration through feeding tubes. However, the risk of GI intolerance should be considered because of the hyperosmolality of many liquid formulations and possible sorbitol content.[68,71] Although the use of a liquid dosage preparation may be more convenient than a solid dosage form, it may not be the best choice if GI intolerance is an issue.

As previously mentioned, adherence to the proper flushing technique is necessary to prevent occlusion when administering medication through a feeding tube. At least 15 mL of water should be given before and after each medication administration to clear the drug through the tube and help get the drug into the stomach.[8] If more than one medication is scheduled for a given time, each should be administered separately, and the tube should be flushed with 5 to 15 mL of water between them.[8,68] Flush volume will be less for children but generally should be at least 5 mL to ensure adequate flushing of the tube.[8]

Clinical **Controversy. . .**

The source of water used to flush the feeding tube and maintain patient hydration via the feeding tube is controversial. Tap water is adequate for the otherwise healthy, immunocompetent patient. However, the acute or chronically ill patient receiving EN may be at higher risk from exposure to nonsterile tap water and may benefit from the use of purified water. Nosocomial infections from contaminated tap water sources have been reported in critically ill patients. The use of purified water for tube-feeding flushes in at-risk patients has been recommended by some clinicians.

Admixture of Drugs with Enteral Feeding

Mixing liquid medications with certain enteral feeding formulations is associated with several types of physical incompatibilities, including granulation, gel formation, separation, and precipitation.[68,71] Not only can these physical incompatibilities inhibit drug absorption, but gel formation potentially may clog small-bore feeding tubes. Physical incompatibility with medications is more common in formulations that contain intact protein than in those with hydrolyzed protein. Also, medication and enteral formula incompatibilities are

TABLE 120-8 Medications with Special Considerations for Enteral Feeding Tube Administration

Drug	Interaction	Comments
Phenytoin	Reduced bioavailability in the presence of tube feedings Possible phenytoin binding to calcium caseinates or protein hydrolysates in enteral feeding	To minimize interaction, holding tube feedings 1–2 hours before and after phenytoin has been suggested; this has no proven benefit Adjust tube-feeding rate to account for time held for phenytoin administration Monitor phenytoin serum concentration and clinical response closely Consider switching to IV phenytoin if unable to reach therapeutic serum concentration
Fluoroquinolones Tetracyclines	Potential for reduced bioavailability because of complexation of drug with divalent and trivalent cations found in enteral feeding	Consider holding tube feeding 1 hour before and after administration Avoid jejunal administration of ciprofloxacin Monitor clinical response
Warfarin	Decreased absorption of warfarin because of enteral feeding; therapeutic effect antagonized by vitamin K in enteral formulations	Adjust warfarin dose based on INR Anticipate need to increase warfarin dose when enteral feedings are started and decrease dose when enteral feedings are stopped Consider holding tube feeding 1 hour before and after administration
Omeprazole Lansoprazole	Administration via feeding tube complicated by acid-labile medication within delayed-release, base-labile granules	Granules become sticky when moistened with water and may occlude small-bore tubes Granules should be mixed with acidic liquid when given via a gastric feeding tube An oral liquid suspension can be extemporaneously prepared for administration via a feeding tube

INR, International Normalized Ratio.

more common with the use of acidic pharmaceutical syrups. The most prudent recommendation is to avoid the routine admixture whenever possible, especially for nonaqueous preparations and syrups. In the clinical setting, exceptions do exist, such as adding electrolyte injections of potassium or sodium to enteral formulas to assist in maintaining or repleting electrolytes.

Drug–Nutrient Interactions

9 The most significant drug–nutrient interactions that can occur during continuous enteral feeding are those in which the bioavailability of the drug is reduced, and the desired pharmacologic effect is not achieved (Table 120-8). Unfortunately, limited clinical studies are available to document the extent of this problem with enteral feeding. Most of the observations are anecdotal case reports involving few patients. One of the most well-documented interactions is between phenytoin and enteral feeding. Phenytoin serum concentrations may decrease by 50% to 75% when phenytoin is given concomitantly with EN, possibly as a result of the binding of phenytoin to calcium caseinates or protein hydrolysates in the enteral formulation. Patients typically require higher than normal phenytoin doses while receiving EN.[68,71] The patient's clinical response and phenytoin serum concentrations should be monitored closely if phenytoin is given enterally during continuous enteral feeding and after its discontinuation.

Decreased bioavailability of certain antibiotics, particularly quinolones, has been documented when coadministered with enteral feeding due to complexation with multivalent cations such as calcium, magnesium, and iron contained in the feeding.[68,71] Although the practice of holding tube feeding for 30 minutes before and 30 minutes after quinolone administration has been recommended, it has not been shown to improve drug absorption. Another option is to increase the quinolone dose when given concurrently with EN. There is evidence to suggest that ciprofloxacin absorption is significantly decreased when given via a jejunostomy tube, so this practice should be avoided, if possible.[68]

Warfarin resistance has been documented during enteral feeding, possibly as a consequence of decreased absorption or the antagonist effects of vitamin K. Before 1980, it was thought that the content of vitamin K (up to 1,330 mcg/1,000 kcal [or 317 mcg/1,000 kJ] of enteral feeding formula) was contributing to the pharmacologic interaction with warfarin. Subsequently, the vitamin K content within formulas intended for use in adults was reduced to less than 200 mcg/1,000 kcal (or 48 mcg/1,000 kJ). However, warfarin resistance continues to be reported, and a warfarin dosage increase may be required in patients receiving EN.[68,73] The International Normalized Ratio should be closely monitored in patients receiving both warfarin and enteral feedings. Conversely, when EN is discontinued, a reduction in warfarin dose may be required.

Desired Outcomes

Desired outcome goals of EN are to promote an adequate nutritional state in adults and to promote growth and development of infants and children. Assessing the outcome of EN includes monitoring objective measures of body composition, protein and energy balance, and subjective outcome for physiologic muscle function and wound healing. In addition to optimizing nutrition, the goal of EN is to reduce disease-related morbidity and mortality. Measures of disease-related morbidity include length of hospital stay, infectious complications, and the patient's sense of well-being. Such clinical outcome goals are extremely difficult to document with the use of EN, in part because other factors, such as age, underlying comorbidities, extent of injury, immunocompetence, and end-organ complications, also affect disease outcome. The successful use of EN can minimize the need for PN in patients unable to meet nutrient requirements with an oral diet. Ultimately, no disease process can improve with prolonged starvation and malnutrition.

PERSONALIZED PHARMACOTHERAPY

A nutrition care plan that incorporates nutrition assessment and therapy goals should be developed for all EN patients. The EN goals are individualized to each patient and based on meeting estimated fluid, calorie, protein, and micronutrient requirements. The desired end point should be included in the care plan. The end point may be resolution of a disease or condition that impairs ability to eat, such as a critically ill trauma patient who is expected to transition back to an oral diet. EN may be considered a lifelong therapy for those with a permanent impairment that restricts or limits eating, such as gastroparesis. Selection of appropriate enteral access device should be individualized based on anticipated duration of therapy, expected tolerance to gastric or jejunal feeding, and patient lifestyle preferences. For example, a low-profile gastrostomy tube may be a good option for active adult or pediatric patients who do not want the presence of an external tube. The method of EN administration should be individualized based on route of enteral access and patient tolerance. A patient with a gastrostomy tube who does not tolerate bolus feedings may do better when switched to slower, intermittent feedings. A patient with a jejunostomy tube may prefer nocturnal feeding to continuous, around-the-clock feeding. A target weight should be established for each patient and energy content from the EN regimen adjusted as needed to safely achieve target weight (i.e., no more than 1 to 2 pound [~0.45 to 0.9 kg] per week weight gain or loss). EN may be used to supplement an oral diet when oral intake is inadequate and should be modified as needed based on changes in tolerance to the diet. A monitoring plan should be developed for each patient to identify potential complications and assess response to therapy.

CLINICAL BOTTOM LINE

Identifying appropriate candidates for EN and designing a personalized EN regimen and monitoring plan is a complex process that is often under-appreciated. A.S.P.E.N. has identified safety issues related to the administration and management of EN and created practice recommendations based on evidence-based research and expert opinion.[9] Evidence-based practice guidelines for the provision and assessment of nutrition support therapy, including EN, are also available for the adult critically ill patient.[10] All healthcare professionals should be knowledgeable in EN therapy because it is provided to a diverse patient population across various healthcare settings. A multidisciplinary approach, either as a formal nutrition support service or as a team of caregivers within the practice setting, is recommended to optimize patient outcomes.

ABBREVIATIONS

ALI	acute lung injury
ANH	artificial nutrition and hydration
ARA	arachidonic acid
ARDS	acute respiratory distress syndrome
DHA	docosahexaenoic acid
EN	enteral nutrition
GALT	gut-associated lymphoid tissue
GRV	gastric residual volume
ICU	intensive care unit
IgA	immunoglobulin A
MCT	medium-chain triglyceride
NG	nasogastric
NPO	nothing by mouth
PEG	percutaneous endoscopic gastrostomy
PN	parenteral nutrition

REFERENCES

1. Colaizzo-Anas T. Nutrient intake, digestion, absorption, and excretion. In: Mueller CM, ed. The A.S.P.E.N. Adult Nutrition Support Core Curriculum. Silver Spring, MD: American Society for Parenteral and Enteral Nutrition, 2012:3–21.
2. Farrell JJ. Digestion and absorption of nutrients and vitamins. In: Feldman M, Friedman LS, Brandt LJ, eds. Sleisenger & Fordtran's Gastrointestinal and Liver Disease: Pathophysiology/Diagnosis/Management, 9th ed. Philadelphia, PA: Saunders Elsevier, 2010: 1695–1733.
3. Hise ME, Brown JC. Lipids. In: Mueller CM, ed. The A.S.P.E.N. Adult Nutrition Support Core Curriculum. Silver Spring, MD: American Society for Parenteral and Enteral Nutrition, 2012:63–82.
4. Dotan I, Mayer L. Mucosal immunity. In: Feldman M, Friedman LS, Brandt LJ, eds. Sleisenger & Fordtran's Gastrointestinal and Liver Disease: Pathophysiology/Diagnosis/Management, 9th ed. Philadelphia, PA: Saunders Elsevier, 2010:21–30.
5. Minocha A. Probiotics for preventive health. Nutr Clin Prac 2009;24:227–241.
6. Wallace B. Clinical use of probiotics in the pediatric population. Nutr Clin Prac 2009;24:50–59.
7. A.S.P.E.N. Board of Directors and the Clinical Guidelines Task Force. Guidelines for the use of parenteral and enteral nutrition in adult and pediatric patients. JPEN J Parenter Enteral Nutr 2002;26(1 Suppl):1SA–138SA.
8. Bankhead R, Boullata J, Brantley S, et al. A.S.P.E.N. enteral nutrition practice recommendations. JPEN J Parenter Enteral Nutr 2009;33:122–167.
9. Brantley SL, Mills ME. Overview of enteral nutrition. In: Mueller CM, ed. The A.S.P.E.N. Adult Nutrition Support Core Curriculum. Silver Spring, MD: American Society for Parenteral and Enteral Nutrition, 2012:170–184.
10. McClave SA, Martindale RG, Vanek VW, et al. Guidelines for the provision and assessment of nutrition support therapy in the adult critically ill patient: Society of Critical Care Medicine (SCCM) and American Society for Parenteral and Enteral Nutrition (A.S.P.E.N.). JPEN J Parenter Enteral Nutr 2009;33:277–316.
11. Heyland DK, Dhaliwal R, Drover JW, et al. Canadian clinical practice guidelines for nutrition support in mechanically ventilated, critically ill adult patients. JPEN J Parenter Enteral Nutr 2003;27:355–373.
12. Itkin M, DeLegge MH, Fang JC, et al. Multidisciplinary practical guidelines for gastrointestinal access for enteral nutrition and decompression from the Society of Interventional Radiology and American Gastroenterological Association (AGA) Institute, with endorsement by Canadian Interventional Radiological Association (CIRA) and Cardiovascular and Interventional Radiological Society of Europe (CIRSE). Gastroenterology 2011;141:742–765.
13. Mehta NM, Compher C, A.S.P.E.N. Board of Directors. A.S.P.E.N. clinical guidelines: Nutrition support of the critically ill child. JPEN J Parenter Enteral Nutr 2009;33:260–276.
14. Thompson AM, Bizzarro MJ. Necrotizing enterocolitis in newborns: Pathogenesis, prevention and management. Drugs 2008;68:1227–1238.
15. Dhaliwal R, Heyland DK. Nutrition and infection in the intensive care unit: What does the evidence show? Curr Opin Crit Care 2005;11:461–467.
16. Braunschweig CL, Levy P, Sheean PM, Wang X. Enteral compared with parenteral nutrition: A meta-analysis. Am J Clin Nutr 2001;74:534–542.
17. Simpson F, Doig GS. Parenteral vs. enteral nutrition in the critically ill patient: A meta-analysis of trials using the intention to treat principle. Intensive Care Med 2005;31:12–23.

18. Gramlich L, Kichian K, Pinilla J, et al. Does enteral nutrition compared to parenteral nutrition result in better outcomes in critically ill adult patients? A systematic review of the literature. Nutrition 2004;20:843–848.
19. Peter JV, Moran JL, Phillips-Hughes J. A meta-analysis of treatment outcomes of early enteral versus early parenteral nutrition in hospitalized patients. Crit Care Med 2005;33:213–220.
20. Malone A, Seres D, Lord L. Complications of enteral nutrition. In: Mueller CM, ed. The A.S.P.E.N. Adult Nutrition Support Core Curriculum. Silver Spring, MD: American Society for Parenteral and Enteral Nutrition, 2012:218–233.
21. Kumpf VJ. Parenteral nutrition-associated liver disease in adult and pediatric patients. Nutr Clin Pract 2006;21: 279–290.
22. McClave SA, Heyland DK. The physiologic response and associated clinical benefits from provision of early enteral nutrition. Nutr Clin Pract 2009;24:305–315.
23. Artinian V, Krayem H, DiGiovine B. Effects of early enteral feeding on the outcome of critically ill mechanically ventilated medical patients. Chest 2006;129:960–967.
24. Doig GS, Heighes PT, Simpson F, et al. Early enteral nutrition, provided within 24 h of injury or intensive care unit admission, significantly reduces mortality in critically ill patients: A meta-analysis of randomized controlled trials. Intensive Care Med 2009;35:2018–2027.
25. McClave SA, Wei-Kuo Chang. Feeding the hypotensive patient: Does enteral feeding precipitate or protect against ischemic bowel? Nutr Clin Pract 2003;18:279–284.
26. Zaloga GP, Roberts PR, Marik P. Feeding the hemodynamically unstable patient: A critical evaluation of the evidence. Nutr Clin Pract 2003;18:285–293.
27. Fang JC, Bankhead R, Kinikini M. Enteral access devices. In: Mueller CM, ed. The ASPEN Adult Nutrition Support Core curriculum. Silver Spring, MD: American Society for Parenteral and Enteral Nutrition, 2012:206–217.
28. Hsu CW, Sun SF, Lin SL, et al. Duodenal versus gastric feeding in medical intensive care patients: A prospective, randomized, clinical study. Crit Care Med 2009;37: 1866–1872.
29. Koopmann MC, Kudsk KA, Szotkowski MJ, Rees SM. A team-based protocol and electromagnetic technology eliminate feeding tube placement complications. Ann Surg 2011;253:297–302.
30. Rivera RJ, Campana J, Seidner D, Hamilton C. Small bowel feeding tube placement using an electromagnetic tube placement device: Accuracy of tip placement [abstract]. JPEN J Parenter Enteral Nutr 2009;33:225.
31. Vanek VW. Ins and outs of enteral access: 2. Long-term access—Esophagostomy and gastrostomy. Nutr Clin Pract 2003;18:50–74.
32. Barrocas A, Geppert C, Durfee SM, et al. A.S.P.E.N. ethics position paper. Nutr Clin Pract 2010;25: 672–679.
33. Dorner B, Posthauer ME, Friedrich EK, Robinson GE. Enteral nutrition in older adults in nursing facilities. Nutr Clin Pract 2011;26:261–272.
34. Finucane TE, Christmas C, Travis K. Tube feeding with advanced dementia. A review of the evidence. JAMA 1999;282:1365–1370.
35. Parrish CR. Enteral feeding: The art and the science. Nutr Clin Pract 2003;18:76–85.
36. Chessman KH. Infant nutrition and special nutritional needs of children. In: Berardi RR, Kroon LA, McDermott JH, et al., eds. Handbook of Nonprescription Drugs, 15th ed. Washington, DC: American Pharmacists Association, 2006:521–552.
37. Jawaheer G, Shaw NJ, Pierro A. Continuous enteral feeding impairs gallbladder emptying in infants. J Pediatr 2001;138:822–825.
38. Cresci G, Lefton J, Esper DH. Enteral formulations. In: Mueller CM, ed. The A.S.P.E.N. Adult Nutrition Support Core Curriculum. Silver Spring, MD: American Society for Parenteral and Enteral Nutrition, 2012:185–205.
39. Wishmeyer PE. Glutamine: Role in critical illness and ongoing clinical trials. Curr Opin Gastroenterol 2008;24:190–197.
40. Chen Y, Peterson SJ. Enteral nutrition formulas: Which formula is right for your adult patient? Nutr Clin Pract 2009;24:344–355.
41. Marik PE, Zaloga GP. Immunonutrition in critically ill patients: A systematic review and analysis of the literature. Intensive Care Med 2008;34:1980–1990.
42. Lomer MCE, Parkes GC, Sanderson JD. Review article: Lactose intolerance in clinical practice—Myths and realities. Aliment Pharmacol Ther 2009;27:93–103.
43. Singer P, Theilla M, Fisher H, et al. Benefit of an enteral diet enriched with eicosapentaenoic acid and gamma-linolenic acid in ventilated patients with acute lung injury. Crit Care Med 2006;34:1033–1038.
44. Koletzko B, Lien E, Agostoni C, et al. The roles of long-chain polyunsaturated fatty acids in pregnancy, lactation and infancy: Review of current knowledge and consensus recommendations. J Perinat Med 2008; 36:5–14.
45. Roy CC, Kien L, Bouthillier L, Levy E. Short-chain fatty acids: Ready for prime time? Nutr Clin Pract 2006;21: 351–366.
46. Rushdi TA, Pichard C, Khater YH. Control of diarrhea by fiber-enriched diet in ICU patients on enteral nutrition: A prospective randomized controlled trial. Clin Nutr 2004;23:1344–1352.
47. Young LS, Kearns LR, Schoefel SL, Clark NC. Protein. In: Mueller CM, ed. The A.S.P.E.N. Adult Nutrition Support Core Curriculum. Silver Spring, MD: American Society for Parenteral and Enteral Nutrition, 2012: 83–97.
48. Kreymann KG, Berger MM, Deutz NEP, et al. ESPEN guidelines on enteral nutrition: Intensive care. Clin Nutr 2006;25:210–223.
49. Waitzberg DL, Saito H, Plank LD, et al. Postsurgical infections are reduced with specialized nutrition support. World J Surg 2006;30:1592–1604.
50. Montejo JC, Zarazaga A, Lopez-Martinez J, et al. Immunonutrition in the intensive care unit: A systematic review and consensus statement. Clin Nutr 2003;22: 221–233.
51. Doley J, Mallampalli A, Sandberg R. Nutrition management for the patient requiring prolonged mechanical ventilation. Nutr Clin Pract 2011;26:232–241.
52. Davis A, Baker S. The use of modular nutrients in pediatrics. JPEN J Parenter Enteral Nutr 1996;20:228–236.
53. Chenu JW, Cox JM. Cronobacter (*Enterobacter sakazakii*): Current status and future prospects. Lett Appl Microbiol 2009;49:153–159.
54. Groh-Wargo S, Sapsford A. Enteral nutrition support of the preterm infant in the neonatal intensive care unit. Nutr Clin Prac 2009;24:363–376.
55. Berseth CL, Van Aerde JE, Gross S, et al. Growth, efficacy, and safety of feeding an iron-fortified human milk fortifier. Pediatrics 2004;114:e699–e706.

56. Porcelli P, Schanler R, Greer F, et al. Growth in human milk-fed very low birth weight infants receiving a new human milk fortifier. Ann Nutr Metab 2000;44:2–10.
57. Reis BB, Hall RT, Schanler RJ. Enhanced growth of preterm infants fed a new powdered human milk fortifier: A randomized controlled trial. Pediatrics 2000;106:581–588.
58. Corkins MR, Scolapio J. Diarrhea. In: Merritt R, ed. The A.S.P.E.N. Nutrition Support Practice Manual, 2nd ed. Silver Spring, MD: A.S.P.E.N., 2005:203–210.
59. Kelly DG, Nadeau J. Oral rehydration solution: A "low-tech" oft neglected therapy. Pract Gastroenterol 2004;10:51–62.
60. Zaloga GP. Parenteral nutrition in adult inpatients with functioning gastrointestinal tracts: Assessment of outcomes. Lancet 2006;367:1101–1111.
61. Williams TA, Leslie GD. A review of the nursing care of enteral feeding tubes in critically ill adults: Part 1. Intensive Crit Care Nurs 2004;20:330–343.
62. Fraser RJL, Bryant L. Current and future therapeutic prokinetic therapy to improve enteral feed tolerance in the ICU patient. Nutr Clin Pract 2010;25:26–31.
63. Nguyen NQ, Chapman MJ, Fraser RJ, Bryant LK, Holloway RH. Erythromycin in more effective than metoclopramide in the treatment of feed intolerance in critical illness. Crit Care Med 2007;35:483–489.
64. Btaiche IF, Chan LN, Pleva M, Kraft MD. Critical illness, gastrointestinal complications, and medication therapy during enteral feeding in critically ill adult patients. Nutr Clin Pract 2010;25:32–49.
65. McClave SA, Lukan JK, Stefater JA, et al. Poor validity of residual volumes as a marker for risk of aspiration in critically ill patients. Crit Care Med 2005;33:324–330.
66. Maloney JP, Ryan TA, Brasel KJ, et al. Food dye use in enteral feedings: A review and a call for a moratorium. Nutr Clin Pract 2002;17:168–181.
67. Maloney JP, Ryan TA. Detection of aspiration in enterally fed patients: A requiem for bedside monitors of aspiration. JPEN J Parenter Enteral Nutr 2002;26(6 Suppl):S34–S42.
68. Williams NT. Medication administration through enteral feeding tubes. Am J Health Syst Pharm 2008;65:2347–2357.
69. Gunn SR, Early BJ, Zenati MS, Ochoa JB. Use of a nasal bridle prevents accidental nasoenteral feeding tube removal. JPEN J Parenter Enteral Nutr 2009;33:50–54.
70. Rommel N, DeMeyer AM, Feenstra L, Veereman-Wauters G. The complexity of feeding problems in 700 infants and young children presenting to a tertiary care institution. J Pediatr Gastroenterol Nutr 2003;37:75–84.
71. Wohlt PD, Zheng L, Gunderson S, et al. Recommendations for the use of medications with continuous enteral nutrition. Am J Health Syst Pharm 2009;66:1458–1467.
72. Magnuson BL, Clifford TM, Hoskins LA, Bernard AC. Enteral nutrition and drug administration, interactions, and complications. Nutr Clin Pract 2005;20:618–624.
73. Dickerson RN, Garmon WM, Kuhl DA, Minard G, Brown RO. Vitamin K-independent warfarin resistance after concurrent administration of warfarin and continuous enteral nutrition. Pharmacotherapy 2008;28:308–313.

121

Obesity

Amy Heck Sheehan, Judy T. Chen, Jack A. Yanovski, and Karim Anton Calis

KEY CONCEPTS

1. Two clinical measures of excess body fat, regardless of sex, are the body mass index (BMI) and the waist circumference (WC). BMI and WC provide a better assessment of total body fat than weight alone and are independent predictors of obesity-related disease risk.
2. Excessive central adiposity increases risk for development of type 2 diabetes, hypertension, and dyslipidemia.
3. Weight loss of as little as 5% of total body weight can significantly improve blood pressure, lipid levels, and glucose tolerance in overweight and obese patients. Sustained, large weight losses (e.g., after bariatric surgery) are associated with long-term improvements in many of the complications associated with obesity and a lower risk of both myocardial infarction and death.
4. Bariatric surgery may be considered in patients with extreme obesity with a BMI ≥ 40 kg/m^2 or ≥ BMI ≥ 35 kg/m^2 with significant comorbidities.
5. Pharmacotherapy may be considered in patients with a BMI ≥ 30 kg/m^2 and/or a WC ≥ 40 inches (≥ 102 cm) for men or 35 inches (89 cm) for women, or BMI of 27 to 30 kg/m^2 with concurrent risk factors if 6 months of diet, exercise, and behavioral modification fail to achieve weight loss.
6. Long-term pharmacotherapy with centrally acting appetite suppressants should be discontinued if weight loss of at least 5% is not achieved after 12 weeks of maximum-dose therapy.
7. There is a high probability of weight regain when obesity pharmacotherapy is discontinued.
8. The Food and Drug Administration does not regulate labeling of herbal and food supplement diet agents, and content is not guaranteed.

INTRODUCTION

It is now estimated that more than 140 million or two of every three adults are overweight or obese in the United States.[1] Additionally, the number of children and adolescents who are overweight has been increasing at an alarming rate in the last 40 years,[2] with one of every three adolescents currently considered overweight or obese.[3] Based on the national trend, this epidemic is projected to affect about 80% of the U.S. adults by 2020, and the prevalence of overweight among children is expected to double by 2030.[4] The presence of obesity and overweight is associated with a significantly increased risk for the development of many diseases (Table 121-1),[5–17] poorer outcomes of comorbid disease states, and increased healthcare costs. Prospective cohort studies show that overall mortality parallels increases in adiposity.[18,19] The evidence is strongest for middle-aged adults. In older individuals, excess body weight and adiposity increase the risk of death, but the degree of impact diminishes with age.[18,19] As of 2008, it was estimated that obesity accounts for 9.1% of total medical expenditures in the United States, and the cost of treating obesity-related illnesses in adults approached national health spending of $147 billion annually.[20] National initiatives to reverse the obesity epidemic have been established through prevention strategies, consensus guidelines, and best practices.[21–25] This chapter reviews the epidemiology, pathophysiology, and therapeutic approaches for the management of obesity. Although nonpharmacologic treatment modalities are discussed, the pharmacotherapy of obesity is highlighted, and the role of pharmacotherapy relative to the other therapeutic options is critically reviewed.

EPIDEMIOLOGY

Obesity in the United States has increased in prevalence since the 1960s. The National Health and Nutrition Examination Survey (NHANES) II data (1976–1980) estimated the prevalence of obesity among adults in the United States at 15%.[2] During NHANES 1999 to 2000, the prevalence increased twofold to 30.9%,[2] and by 2010 obesity affected 35.9% of the adult population,[1] making the prevention of obesity a public health priority.[23] This is further emphasized by the continued pursuit of safe and effective long-term therapies for obesity. Existing evidence consistently suggests that children who are overweight are at least twice as likely to remain overweight as adults compared with normal-weight children.[26] Furthermore, overweight or obese children and adolescents have a higher risk of premature mortality and morbidity as adults.[27] Therefore, childhood and early adulthood are critical intervention periods for prevention of obesity in the future. The prevalence of obesity varies by sex among racial and ethnic minorities within the United States.[2] The highest prevalence is observed among non-Hispanic black women (58.5% obese and 17.8% with extreme obesity) compared with values of 38.8% and 7.4% for non-Hispanic black men, respectively.[1] This gender disparity is also associated with the level of parental education. Young black women from the lowest educated families are at greater risk of obesity compared with young black men.[28] The prevalence of obesity also increases with age, reaching a maximum by the eighth decade.[2] After the age of 80 years, the prevalence falls progressively for both genders. Socioeconomic status clearly affects the prevalence of obesity among non-Hispanic white adults; a strong inverse association is observed among non-Hispanic white women from lower socioeconomic classes.[2] Educational achievement, which is linked to socioeconomic status, is also correlated with the fraction of people who are overweight; the prevalence of overweight is greatest in those with less than a high school education.

TABLE 121-1 Conditions More Prevalent Among Patients with Obesity

Cancer	Genitourinary
Breast cancer (postmenopausal)	Chronic kidney disease
Colorectal cancer	Increased serum urate
Gallbladder cancer	End-stage renal disease
Endometrial cancer	Obesity-related glomerulopathy
Esophageal carcinoma	Urinary stress incontinence
Hepatic cancer	**Metabolic**
Kidney cancer	Diabetes mellitus
Ovarian cancer	Hyperlipidemia
Pancreatic cancer	Hyperinsulinemia
Prostate cancer	Hypertriglyceridemia
Rectal cancer	Low high-density lipoprotein
Cardiovascular	Impaired glucose tolerance
Atrial fibrillation	Metabolic syndrome
Cerebral vascular accidents	**Musculoskeletal**
Congestive heart failure	Degenerative joint disease
Coronary artery disease	Diffuse idiopathic skeletal hyperostosis
Cor pulmonale	Disc disease
Hypertension	Gait disturbance
Left ventricular hypertrophy	Gout and hyperuricemia
Myocardial infarction	Fibromyalgia
Peripheral vascular disease	Immobility
Peripheral venous insufficiency	Low back pain/back strain
Pulmonary embolism	Osteoarthritis (knee, hips, ankles, feet)
Thrombophlebitis	Plantar fasciitis
Varicose veins	**Neurologic**
Venous thromboembolism	Carpal tunnel syndrome
Dermatologic	Idiopathic intracranial hypertension
Acanthosis nigricans	Meralgia paresthetica
Cellulitis	Pseudotumor cerebri
Intertrigo, carbuncles	Stroke
Lymphedema	**Oral Health**
Skin tags	Dental caries
Status pigmentation of legs	Loss of teeth
Striae distensae (stretch marks)	Periodontitis
Psoriasis (women)	Xerostomia
Endocrine and Reproductive	**Psychological**
Amenorrhea and other menstrual disorders	Affective disorders
Congenital anomalies	Body image disturbance
Fetal abnormalities	Depression
Hirsutism	Eating disorders
Hypogonadism (male)	Low self-esteem
Infertility	Social stigmatization
Polycystic ovarian syndrome	**Respiratory**
Hyperandrogenism	Asthma
Pregnancy complications	Chronic obstructive pulmonary disease
Sexual dysfunction	Dyspnea
Gastrointestinal	Hypoventilation syndrome
Cholelithiasis	Obstructive sleep apnea
Gastroesophageal reflux disease	Pickwickian syndrome
Hepatic cirrhosis	Pneumonia
Hernias	Pulmonary hypertension
Nonalcoholic fatty liver disease	

Data from references 5 to 17.

ETIOLOGY

Obesity occurs when there is increased energy storage resulting from an imbalance between energy intake and energy expenditure over time. The specific etiology for this imbalance in the vast majority of individuals is multifactorial, with genetic and environmental factors contributing to various degrees. In a small minority of individuals, excess weight may be attributed to an underlying medical condition or an unintended effect of a medication.

Genetic Influences

Observational studies in humans and experimental studies in animal models have demonstrated the strong role of genetics in determining both obesity and distribution of body fat. In some individuals, genetic factors are the primary determinants of obesity, whereas in others, obesity may be caused primarily by environmental factors. The genetic contribution to the actual variance in body mass index (BMI) and body fat distribution is estimated to be up to 80%.[29] The increase in the prevalence of obesity that has taken place in the United States over the past 40 years is without doubt the result of alterations in our environment that readily allow obesity-promoting genotypes to cause excessive adiposity.

The role of genetic influences in the development of obesity is an area of extensive research. A number of single-gene mutations producing extreme obesity have been identified, but such mutations are rare and account for an extremely small number of the total cases of obesity.[30] Some common alleles—for instance, the rs9939609 obesity-risk allele in the *FTO* (fat mass and obesity associated) gene that is found in almost 70% of people—increases BMI by about 2 kg/m^2.[31] The total number and identity of contributing genes are still being determined, as is the means by which the many potential so-called "obesity" genes interact with each other and with the environment to produce the obese phenotype.

Environmental Factors

Many of the societal changes associated with economic development over the past 40 years have been implicated as potential causes for the increase in the prevalence of obesity. These include an abundant and easily accessible food supply and the material comforts of modern life in Western civilizations, which have contributed to a reduction in physical activity.[32] Advances in technology and automation have resulted in more sedentary lifestyles during both work and leisure time for most individuals. At the same time, there has been a significant increase in the availability and portion size of high-fat foods, which are aggressively marketed and are often more convenient and less expensive than healthier alternatives. This modern environment has been described by some as "obesogenic" because it is likely to result in a state of positive energy balance in many individuals (Fig. 121-1).[33] Obesity has also been reported more frequently among individuals within close social networks (e.g., siblings, spouses, and friends), with a person's risk of becoming obese increasing significantly if a friend in his or her social network is obese.[34] Finally, it should be noted that cultural factors, socioeconomic status, and religious beliefs may influence eating habits and body weights.

Medical Conditions

Occasionally, patients present with obesity secondary to an identifiable medical condition. Conditions associated with weight gain include iatrogenic and idiopathic Cushing's syndrome, growth hormone deficiency, insulinoma, leptin deficiency, and various psychiatric disorders, such as depression, binge-eating disorder, and schizophrenia. Hypothyroidism is often included in this list, but it mostly causes fluid retention (myxedema) and is generally not a cause of significant obesity. Genetic syndromes that have obesity as a major component are extremely rare and include Prader-Willi's, WAGR (Wilms' tumor, aniridia, genitourinary abnormalities or gonadoblastoma, and mental retardation), Simpson-Golabi-Behmel's, Cohen's, Bardet-Biedl's, Carpenter's, Börjeson's, and Wilson-Turner's syndromes. The clinician evaluating a patient for obesity needs to be aware of these potential conditions. The physical examination of obese patients always should include an assessment for secondary causes of obesity, including genetic syndromes.

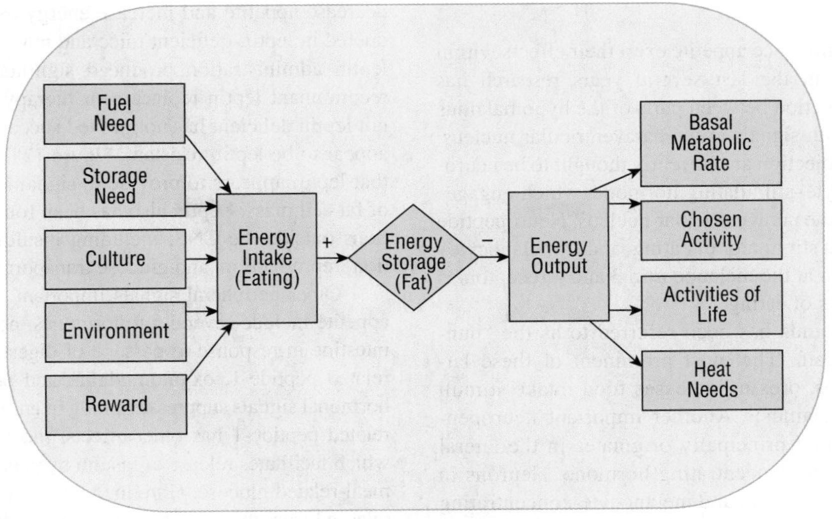

FIGURE 121-1 Net energy stores are determined by various inputs and outputs. Simply stated, obesity occurs when there is an imbalance between energy intake and expenditure.

Medications

An increasing number of medications are associated with unintended weight gain.[35] These include several anticonvulsants (e.g., carbamazepine, gabapentin, pregabalin, and valproic acid), antidepressants (e.g., mirtazapine and tricyclic antidepressants), atypical antipsychotics (e.g., clozapine, olanzapine, quetiapine, and risperidone), conventional antipsychotics (e.g., haloperidol), and hormones (e.g., corticosteroids, insulin, and medroxyprogesterone). Although the pharmacologic mechanism responsible for weight gain is usually drug-specific, in most cases the precise mechanism is unknown.

PATHOPHYSIOLOGY

The pathophysiology of obesity involves numerous factors that regulate appetite, energy storage, and energy expenditure. Disturbance of these homeostatic functions results in an imbalance between energy intake and energy expenditure.

Appetite

Human appetite is a complex process that is the net result of many inputs within a neural network involving principally the hypothalamus, limbic system, brainstem, hippocampus, and elements of the cortex.[36] Within this neural network, many neurotransmitters and neuropeptides have been identified that can stimulate or inhibit the brain's appetite network and thereby affect total caloric intake.

Biogenic Amines

The first receptor systems found to alter food intake in animals and humans were the biogenic amines. These neurotransmitters are the foundation from which the most robust pharmacologic interventions for obesity have been developed. Serotonin, also known as 5-hydroxytryptamine (5-HT), and cells known to respond to 5-HT are found throughout the central nervous system (CNS) and the periphery. Currently, two major noradrenergic receptor subtypes are recognized (α and β), each with multiple subtypes. Histamine and dopamine also demonstrate multiple receptor subtypes, but their role in the regulation of human eating behaviors and food intake is less well documented. Direct stimulation of 5-HT_{1A} and noradrenergic α_2-receptors increases food intake; the opposite occurs with 5-HT_{2C} and noradrenergic α_1- or β_2-receptor activation. Table 121-2 summarizes the major effects of direct receptor stimulation, inhibition, and changes in synaptic cleft amine concentrations on food intake.

TABLE 121-2 Effects of Various Neurotransmitters, Receptors, and Peptides on Food Intake[36,37]

Anatomic Region	Increased Eating	Decreased Eating
Arcuate nucleus of hypothalamus	Ghrelin	Leptin Insulin GLP-1 PYY
Paraventricular nucleus of hypothalamus	NPY AgRP Opioids (especially μ) Galanin	MSH, melanocortin CRH CCK
Lateral hypothalamus	Orexin MCH	
Hypothalamus	Norepinephrine α_2 Serotonin 5-HT_{1A}	Norepinephrine α_1 and β_2 Serotonin 5-HT_{1B} and 5-HT_{2C} Histamine H_1 and H_3
Nucleus accumbens	Dopamine	
Amygdala	Opioids (especially μ)	
Brainstem (hindbrain)	NPY AgRP Opioids (especially μ)	Leptin MSH, melanocortin CCK
Vagus nerve	Ghrelin	Leptin CCK GLP-1 PYY
Various or undetermined	Cannabinoid CB_1	Dopamine D_1 and D_2

AgRP, agouti-related protein; CCK, cholecystokinin; CRH, corticotropin-releasing hormone; GLP-1, glucagon-like peptide-1; MCH, melanocyte concentration hormone; MSH, melanocyte-stimulating hormone; NPY, neuropeptide Y; PYY, peptide YY.

Neuropeptides

Many neuropeptides that influence appetite exert their effects within the hypothalamus. Thus, in the last several years research has focused on the neural projection between parts of the hypothalamus and the arcuate nucleus with signals to the paraventricular nucleus. The key peptides in this projection are currently thought to be neuropeptide Y and α-melanocyte–stimulating hormone, which engages melanocortin receptors in the paraventricular nucleus. Neuropeptide Y is the most potent known stimulator of eating, and α-melanocyte–stimulating hormone action at the melanocortin 3 and 4 receptors is one of the crucial inhibitors of eating.[36,37]

The lateral hypothalamus has been referred to as the "hunger" center within the brain. The most prominent of these lateral hypothalamic peptides, orexin, increases food intake stimuli within the lateral hypothalamus.[36] Another important neuropeptide stimulator of eating that principally originates in the lateral hypothalamus is melanocyte-concentrating hormone. Neurons in the lateral hypothalamus use orexin and melanocyte-concentrating hormone to communicate with other neurons throughout the brain and thereby affect a number of functions beyond appetite.[36,37] Table 121-2 summarizes the major effects of various neuropeptides on food intake. Although hunger and satiety functions are thought to be primarily regulated by the hypothalamus, humans eat in response to a broad set of stimuli, including reward, pleasure, learning, and memory.

Peripheral Appetite–Related Signals to the Brain

Peripheral appetite signals also dramatically affect food intake. Leptin, a hormone that is secreted by adipose cells, acts on the arcuate nucleus of the hypothalamus and elsewhere in the brain to decrease appetite and increase energy expenditure.[38,39] Studies conducted in leptin-deficient mice and humans revealed that exogenous leptin administration produced significant weight loss. However, recombinant leptin replacement therapy in obese humans who are not leptin deficient has not proved successful because obese humans appear to be leptin resistant. Figure 121-2 shows the peripheral link that leptin appears to provide in signaling the CNS about the status of fat cell mass. Leptin also has been found to regulate various functions outside the CNS, including insulin and glucocorticoid secretion, reproduction, and glucose transport within the small intestine.[38]

Other peripheral signals important to the brain's processing of appetite include several gut hormones, notably those released by the intestine in response to passage of digesting food such as glucagon-related peptide-1, oxyntomodulin, and peptide YY.[40] Each of these hormonal signals suppresses eating in animals and humans. Glucagon-related peptide-1 has other effects, most importantly as an incretin, which facilitates release of insulin by pancreatic β cells in response to meal-related glucose. Ghrelin, another important gut hormone that is released from the distal stomach and duodenum, stimulates appetite.

An understanding of the relationships among the brain, its many neurotransmitters and neuropeptides, environmental stimulation of brain activities, and other hormones is still evolving. Dysfunction in any of these factors can upset the homeostatic functions regulating energy balance. Exogenous manipulation of neural signals and associated peripheral hormones may provide future pharmacotherapeutic targets for obesity management.

Energy Balance

The net balance of energy ingested relative to energy expended by an individual over time determines the degree of obesity (see Fig. 121-1). An individual's metabolic rate is the single largest

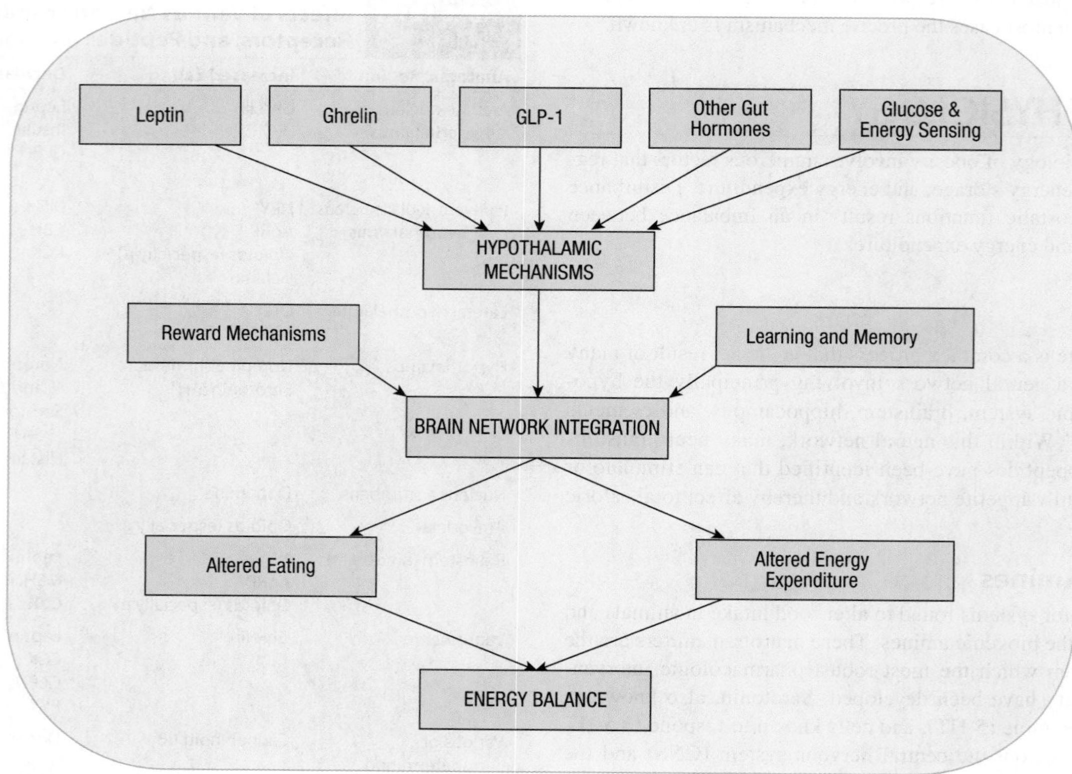

FIGURE 121-2 Intrinsic hypothalamic hunger and satiety mechanisms are modified by input from fat tissue via leptin, and from the gut via ghrelin, glucagon-like peptide-1 (GLP-1), and other hormones. Additional input is derived by direct sensing of prevailing glucose and other energy signals. The hypothalamus generates signals that are integrated within brain networks, which also receive additional signals. The brain network effects change in energy balance by modifying food intake and energy expenditure.

determinant of energy expenditure. Resting energy expenditure (REE) is defined as the energy expended by a person at rest under conditions of thermal neutrality. Basal metabolic rate (BMR) is defined as the REE measured soon after awakening in the morning at least 12 hours after the last meal. Metabolic rate increases after eating based on the size and composition of the meal. It reaches a maximum approximately 1 hour after the meal is consumed and returns to basal levels 4 hours after the meal. This increase in metabolic rate is known as the *thermogenic effect of food.* The REE measures the energy costs of the wakeful state and may include the residual thermogenic effect of a previous meal; it is thus usually higher than the metabolic rate measured during quiet sleep. Physical activity is the other major factor that affects total energy expenditure and is the most variable component.

Peripheral Storage and Thermogenesis

There are two major types of adipose tissue, white and brown. The primary function of white adipose tissue is lipid manufacture, storage, and release. Brown adipose tissue, once believed to be found only in infants, is now recognized to exist in most adults.[41] It is more commonly identified in lean than obese individuals, but its importance for human obesity remains unclear. Whereas lipid storage occurs in response to insulin, lipid release is seen during periods of calorie restriction. Brown adipose tissue is notable for its ability to dissipate energy via uncoupled mitochondrial respiration.[42] Both white and brown adipose tissues are highly innervated by the sympathetic nervous system, and adrenergic stimulation via β-adrenergic receptors (β_1, β_2, and β_3) is known to activate lipolysis in fat cells as well as increase energy expenditure in adipose tissue and skeletal muscle. Genetic polymorphisms have been identified in both the β_2- and β_3-receptor systems that are associated with obesity or excess weight gain.[43] Thus, genetic susceptibility for excess weight status may in part be related to adrenergic dysfunction.

CLINICAL PRESENTATION

Although obesity is readily apparent, most obese patients seek healthcare only when obesity-associated comorbidities become problematic. A consistent and reproducible description of weight status is essential in the diagnosis and management of obesity. Evidence-based guidelines issued by many groups, notably the World Health Organization and the National Institutes of Health (NIH), have established a stratification of weight excess based on associated medical risks.[44] The first increment of excess weight is termed *overweight*, with the term *obesity* reserved for the higher levels of weight excess. These levels of excess weight are defined on the basis of BMI, a measure of total body weight relative to height. Adults with a BMI of 18.5 to 24.9 are considered to have "normal" weight; the terms *overweight*, *obese*, and *extreme obese* are reserved for those with a BMI of 25 to 29.9, 30 to 39.9, and 40 and over, respectively. Children and adolescents ages 2 to 18 years with a BMI at the 95th percentile or above are considered obese, and those with a BMI between the 85th and 94th percentiles are considered overweight.[45] Using metric units, BMI (kg/m^2) is defined as weight in kilograms divided by height in meters squared (kg/m^2). Using pounds and inches, BMI (kg/m^2) is estimated as (Weight [lb]/Height [inches^2]) × 703. Because BMI may overestimate the degree of excess body fat in some clinical situations (e.g., edematous states, extreme muscularity, muscle wasting, and short stature), the assessment of body composition in such cases often requires clinical judgment.

❶ Body mass index is an acceptable measure of obesity and is the practical method of defining obesity in the clinic and epidemiologic studies; however, it does not always correspond to excess fat. There are well-established differences in the relationship between BMI and obesity-related risks among disparate racial and ethnic groups. For examples, BMI overestimates adiposity among non-Hispanic blacks and underestimates risk among Asians.[46–49] Ideally, obesity refers to a state of excess body fat as determined by measures of adiposity. Research techniques that can accurately measure fat mass separately from the body's fat-free mass include determination of body density using underwater body weight or air displacement plethysmography, dual-energy x-ray absorptiometry, computed tomography (CT), and magnetic resonance imaging (MRI).[50] These measurement techniques are currently too expensive and time-consuming to be used routinely in the clinical setting. Furthermore, all fat is not equal in its metabolic function or danger to health. Whereas brown adipose tissue promotes energy expenditure and has a weak association with metabolic markers of insulin production, release, and resistance, visceral white adipose tissue accumulation promotes energy storage and demonstrates a strong relationship with insulin resistance.[42] Central obesity reflects high levels of intraabdominal or visceral fat, and this pattern of obesity is associated with an increased propensity for the development of hypertension, dyslipidemia, type 2 diabetes, and cardiovascular disease (sometimes referred to as the "metabolic syndrome"). Thus, in addition to the absolute excess fat mass, the distribution of this fat regionally in the body has important clinical effects. Intraabdominal fat is best estimated by imaging techniques such as CT and MRI but can be approximated through measurement of the waist circumference (WC). Clinically, WC is the narrowest circumference measured in the area between the last rib and the top of the iliac crest.[51] The current definition for high-risk WC is greater than 40 inches (102 cm) in men and greater than 35 inches (89 cm) in women.[51] Notably, epidemiologic studies demonstrate that WC adds little in terms of risk prediction after a patient's BMI reaches 35 kg/m^2. Thus, routine determination of WC should be implemented in those with BMIs between 25 and 34.9 kg/m^2.

❷ Although BMI and WC are related, each measure independently predicts disease risk. Both measurements should be assessed and monitored during therapy for obesity.[52] The risks for development of type 2 diabetes, hypertension, or cardiovascular disease at various stages of obesity based on BMI or WC are outlined in Table 121-3. Note that increased WC confers increased risk even in normal-weight individuals.

TABLE 121-3 Classification of Overweight and Obesity by Body Mass Index, Waist Circumference, and Associated Disease Risk

	BMI (kg/m^2)	Obesity Class	Disease Risk^a (Relative to Normal Weight and Waist Circumference): Men ≤40 in (≤102 cm) / Women ≤35 in (≤89 cm)	Men >40 in (>102 cm) / Women >35 in (>89 cm)
Underweight	<18.5		—	—
Normal weight^b	18.5–24.9		—	High
Overweight	25.0–29.9		Increased	High
Obesity	30.0–34.9	I	High	Very high
	35.0–39.9	II	Very high	Very high
Extreme obesity	≥40	III	Extremely high	Extremely high

BMI, body mass index.

^{a}Disease risk for type 2 diabetes, hypertension, and cardiovascular disease.

^{b}Increased waist circumference can also be a marker for increased risk even in persons of normal weight.

Adapted from Preventing and Managing the Global Epidemic of Obesity. Report of the World Health Organization Consultation on Obesity. Geneva: World Health Organization, 1997. Reprinted with permission from National Institutes of Health, National Heart, Lung and Blood Institute. 1997, http://www.nhlbi.nih.gov/guidelines/obesity/ob_home.htm.

Comorbidities

Although overall mortality rate is not increased among those classified as overweight, those who are obese have serious health risks and increased mortality rates,[52] particularly adults with BMIs greater than 35 kg/m^2.[53] Substantial reductions in life expectancy have been predicted in adults with BMIs greater than 35 kg/m^2.[53] Further reduction in life span has been observed in obese individuals who are current or former smokers.[53] Several disease states and conditions are more prevalent in obese patients (see Table 121-1).[5–17] Increased body fat, increased total body weight, and a central distribution of body fat all are associated with an increased incidence of mortality, primarily as a result of cardiovascular disease. Hypertension, hyperlipidemia, insulin resistance, and glucose intolerance are all known cardiac risk factors that tend to cluster in obese individuals. Therefore, obese individuals are exposed to multiple risk factors. Some of the earliest studies from Framingham have confirmed the relationship between obesity and increased risk of stroke and coronary heart disease in both men and women.[54] Blood pressure frequently is elevated in obese individuals and may in part explain the increased incidence of stroke and cardiovascular disease observed with obesity. Hypertension in lean individuals is associated with concentric cardiac hypertrophy as a consequence of an increased afterload, which increases the risk of cardiac ischemia. In contrast, eccentric dilation is observed in obesity, leading to an increased volume load. This dilated cardiomyopathy is associated with a reduction in ventricular ejection fraction and a high-output cardiac state. The combination of obesity and hypertension is associated with thickening of the ventricular wall, ischemia, and increased heart volume. This leads more rapidly to heart failure, an association that has been recognized for more than 2 decades.[55,56] Alterations in pulmonary function are common in patients with obesity. Sleep apnea, which is more common in men, is a significant and costly condition that is associated with increased morbidity and mortality in obese individuals.[55,56] The exact mechanism by which obesity leads to sleep apnea is unknown, but weight loss often results in significant and sometimes dramatic improvements in the condition.

Impaired glucose tolerance and Type 2 diabetes are associated with insulin resistance and obesity. As insulin response becomes impaired, the pancreatic β cells respond by increasing insulin production and release, resulting in a state of relative hyperinsulinemia. Although hyperinsulinemia is known to be associated with an increased risk of cardiovascular disease, it is not known whether the increased insulin levels contribute directly to cardiac disease or if they are a marker for the underlying defect of insulin resistance and glucose intolerance. Insulin resistance, in turn, also frequently leads to impaired lipid metabolism (increased cholesterol, increased triglycerides, and low circulating high-density lipoprotein) and hypertension. As with cardiovascular disease, central obesity is an important factor in determining the risk of developing type 2 diabetes.

Osteoarthritis in weight-bearing joints, such as the knees, may be related directly to the mechanical effects of excess body weight and the resulting forces exerted on these joint surfaces. The increase of osteoarthritis in non–weight-bearing joints, however, suggests that obesity may lead to altered cartilage, collagen, and even bone metabolism.[8] Increasing evidence has suggested proinflammatory adipocytokines, such as tumor necrosis factor-α and leptin, may play an important role in the metabolic influence of overweight on osteoarthritis.[57] Osteoarthritis and its symptoms, such as pain, are significant barriers to physical activity and key impediments to sustained weight loss.

Obesity affects the human reproductive system in a number of ways. Obesity is associated with earlier menarche in girls and hyperandrogenism, hirsutism, and anovulatory menstrual cycles in women. In some women, this disorder manifests as overt polycystic ovary syndrome, a condition in which insulin resistance is common.[58] Weight loss therapy with an insulin sensitizer such as metformin has been shown to restore normal ovulation in some women.[58] These observations suggest that insulin resistance plays a part in the causation of polycystic ovary syndrome associated with obesity.

TREATMENT

Available treatment options for the chronic management of obesity include reduced caloric intake, increased physical activity, behavioral modification, pharmacotherapy, and bariatric surgery.

Desired Outcomes

Weight management is commonly considered successful when a predefined amount of weight has been lost such that a final goal is achieved. However, desired outcomes are fully dependent on the clinical situation. The ultimate goals of treatment must be defined clearly. These goals may be absolute weight loss if obesity is present without other comorbid conditions. If improvement in blood glucose, blood cholesterol, and hypertension are primary goals, then these must be defined appropriately and may include setting target levels for low-density lipoprotein cholesterol, glycosylated hemoglobin, or blood pressure. Per current national guidelines, the recommended weight loss goal for adults is 10% of initial weight gradually over 6 months of therapy to achieve a reasonable rate of weight loss of about 1 to 2 lb (0.5–0.9 kg) per week.[6] Success may also include end points of decreasing the rate of weight gain or maintaining a weight-neutral status. All too often patients expect to lose weight overnight, only to be disappointed. Thus, it is important to set a time course for the plan. A significant number of web-based resources for supporting both patient and practitioner weight management activities are available.[22,23,51]

General Approach to Treatment

The success of weight loss intervention has been measured most often as weight loss over a defined study period. Successful obesity treatment plans have incorporated an integrated dietary intervention, exercise, behavior modification (with or without pharmacologic therapy), and/or surgical intervention. Specific weight goals should be established that are consistent with medical needs and the patient's personal desire. For most obese patients, a weight loss goal of 5% to 10% of initial weight is reasonable. Patients should not be allowed to attain an abnormally low body weight (i.e., less than their estimated ideal body weight).

Patients seeking help for obesity do so for many reasons, including improvement in their quality of life, a reduction in associated morbidity, and increased life expectancy. Unfortunately, numerous individuals seek therapy for obesity primarily for cosmetic purposes and often have unrealistic goals and expectations. Aggressive marketing of weight loss programs, therapies, and diets—parallel to the fashion industry's standards of desirable body profiles—has led many individuals to set impossible goals and expectations. In some cases, these individuals will go to extreme measures to achieve weight loss. Consequently, clinicians must be careful to fully discuss the risks of therapies and to clearly define the achievable benefits and magnitude of weight loss. Obese patients should be redirected away from trying to achieve an "ideal weight" to the more reasonable goals of modest (e.g., loss of 5%–10% of body weight) but sustained, medically relevant weight loss. In practice, the goal has to be set based on many factors, including initial body weight, patient motivation and desire, presence of comorbid conditions, and age. For example, in patients with diabetes, even modest weight loss can improve glucose control and may reduce mortality rates,[59–62] yet in individuals with osteoarthritis, significantly more weight reduction may be required to improve symptoms. Indeed, dietary modification and exercise have been shown to ameliorate hyperglycemia, hyperlipidemia, and hypertension with weight loss of less than 5% of initial body weight. The Look AHEAD (Action for Health in Diabetes) study found that patients with diabetes who maintained weight loss with lifestyle modifications for a period of 11 years did not experience a reduced incidence of cardiovascular events, but they did have a reduced need for diabetes medications and other positive health benefits.[63] These data emphasize the importance of defining end points and measures of success in any weight loss plan.

3 Weight loss interventions must be founded on lifestyle changes, such as a modification in eating practices; complemented by drug therapy, if indicated; and in some cases, surgery (Fig. 121-3). Before recommending any therapy, the clinician must evaluate the patient for the presence of secondary causes of obesity. If a secondary cause is suspected, then a more complete diagnostic workup and the initiation of appropriate therapy may be warranted. The next step in patient evaluation is to determine the presence and severity of other medical conditions that are either directly associated with obesity (e.g., diabetes) or that have an impact on therapeutic decision making (e.g., history of liver disease or cardiac arrhythmia). Appropriate laboratory tests to exclude or quantify the degree of specific conditions such as diabetes, liver dysfunction, and nephropathy should be performed as indicated by the history and physical examination. Based on the outcome of this medical evaluation, the patient should be counseled on treatment options, benefits, and risks. No matter what the treatment options are, they all require significant effort on the part of the patient to change lifestyle and comply with the management plan. If the patient is not yet ready to meet these expectations, then early counseling will reduce the chance of frustration for the patient; clinician; and in some cases, other family members. Providing basic education can lead to a significant change in motivation and desire to lose weight and improved compliance. Ultimately, lifelong therapeutic goals should consist of maintenance of reduced body weight and prevention of weight gain.

Nonpharmacologic Therapy

Nonpharmacologic therapy, including reduced caloric intake, increased physical activity, and behavioral modification, is the mainstay of obesity management. This combination is recommended as first-line therapy in current evidence-based clinical guidelines for the treatment of overweight and obesity in adults set forth by the NIH.[6]

Reduced Caloric Intake

Current adult guidelines recommend reduced caloric intake through adherence to a low-calorie diet (LCD).[6] The LCD should provide a daily caloric deficit of 500 to 1,000 kcal (2,093–4,486 kJ),

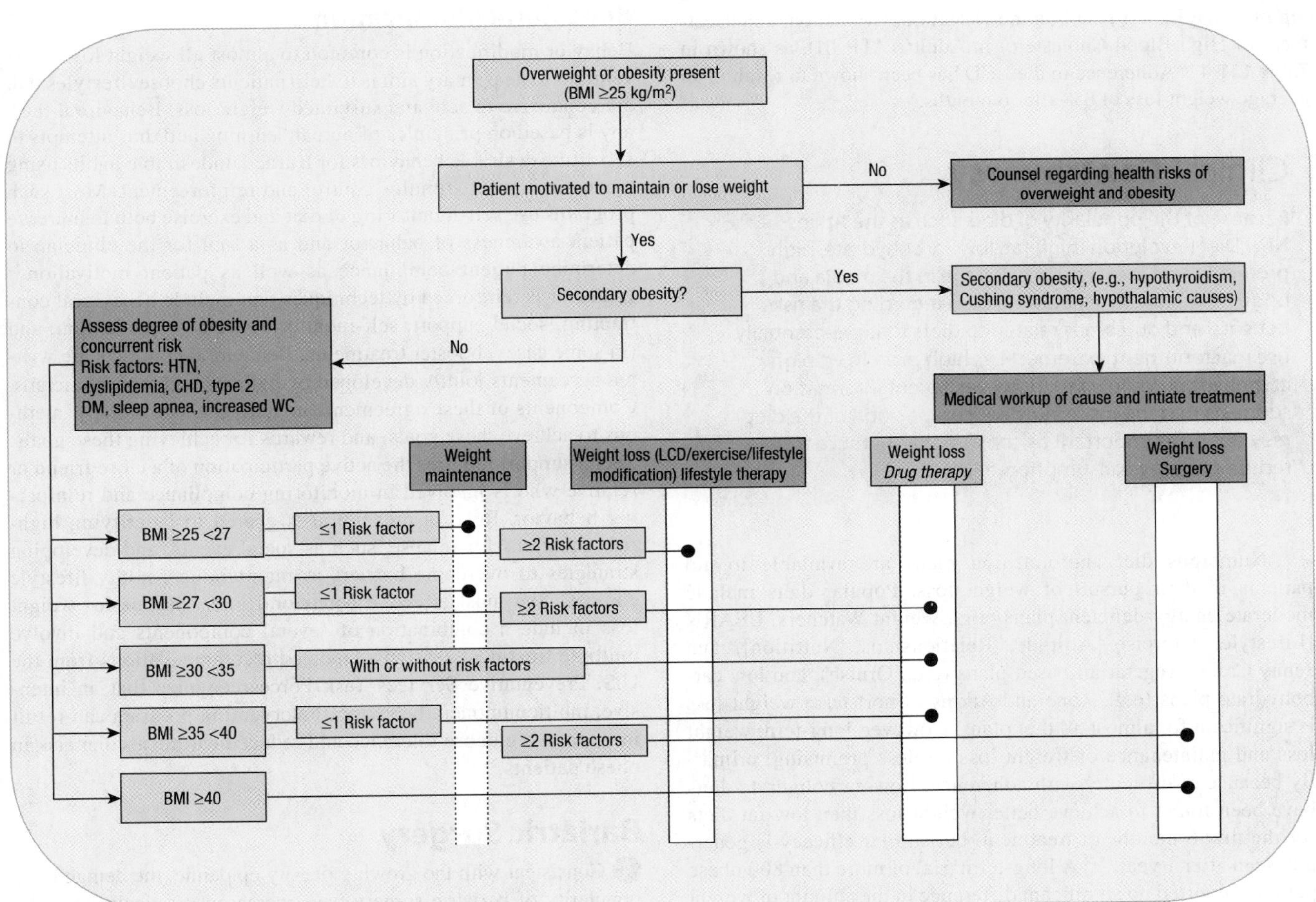

FIGURE 121-3 Treatment algorithm. Candidates for pharmacotherapy are selected on the basis of body mass index and waist circumference criteria along with consideration of concurrent risk factors. Medication therapy is always used as an adjunct to a comprehensive weight-loss program that includes diet, exercise, and behavioral modification. CHD, coronary heart disease; DM, diabetes mellitus; HTN, hypertension; LCD, low-calorie diet; WC, waist circumference (≥40 inches [≥102 cm] for men and ≥35 inches [≥89 cm] for women).

TABLE 121-4 Recommended Composition of the Step I Low-Calorie Diet

Nutrient	Recommended Intake
Total fat	25%–35% or less of total calories
Saturated fat	<7% of total calories
Monounsaturated fat	≤20% of total calories
Polyunsaturated fat	≤10% of total calories
Cholesterol	<200 mg/day
Protein	~15% of total calories
Carbohydrate	50%–60% or more of total calories
Fiber	20–30 g
Calories	*Overall daily intake reduced by 500–1,000 kcal (2,093–4,186 kJ)*
Total caloric intake	*1,000–1,200 kcal/day (4,186–5,023 kJ/day) for most women; 1,200–1,600 kcal/day (5,023–6,697 kJ/day) for most men*

Adapted from Third report of the National Cholesterol Education Program (NCEP) Expert Panel on Detection, Evaluation, and Treatment of High Blood Cholesterol in Adults (Adult Treatment Panel III) final report. Circulation 2002;106(25):3143–3421.

which generally correlates to a total intake of 800 to 1,200 kcal/day (3,349–5,024 kJ/day). Severely obese individuals will require more energy, at least at the start of dietary restriction. The composition of the LCD is outlined in the Step I Diet recommended by the third report of the Expert Panel on the Detection, Evaluation, and Treatment of High Blood Cholesterol in Adults (ATP III), as shown in Table 121-4.[64] Adherence to the LCD has been shown to result in an average weight loss of 8% after 6 months.[6]

Clinical **Controversy. . .**

Because of the popularity of diets such as the Atkins New Diet Revolution (high fat, low carbohydrate, high protein), there is extensive coverage in the media and ongoing debate in academic circles regarding the risks, benefits, and outcomes related to diets that preferentially use macronutrient extremes (i.e., high protein vs. high carbohydrate vs. low fat). However, recent information suggests that the macronutrient composition of the diet may not be as important as consistent adherence to reduced energy consumption.

Numerous diet and nutrition plans are available to aid patients in their pursuit of weight loss. Popular diets include moderate energy-deficient plans (e.g., Weight Watchers, LEARN [Lifestyle, Exercise, Attitude, Relationships, Nutrition], and Jenny Craig), vegetarian-based plans (e.g., Ornish), and low carbohydrate plans (e.g., Zone and Atkins). Short-term weight loss is significant for almost all diet plans. However, long-term weight loss and maintenance of weight loss are less promising, primarily because of difficulty with adherence. Low-carbohydrate diets have been found to achieve better weight loss than low-fat diets for the first 6 months of treatment, but similar efficacy is generally seen after 1 year.[65,66] A long-term trial of more than 800 obese patients reported no significant difference in the amount of weight loss achieved with adherence to various types of reduced-calorie diets.[67] Therefore, the macronutrient composition of the diet may not be as important as consistent adherence to reduced energy consumption.

Very-low-calorie diets, providing less than 800 kcal/day (3,349 kJ/day), are generally not recommended.[6] Although very-low-calorie diets can often result in early weight loss, long-term results have been disappointing because it is difficult for individuals to maintain compliance.[68] Additionally, very-low-calorie diets require intensive medical monitoring and should only be used in certain situations under the supervision of an experienced clinician. Regardless of the diet program, it is clear that energy consumption must be less than energy expenditure to achieve weight loss (see Fig. 121-1). The challenge is to develop a diet plan that leads to consistent adherence by the patient and sustained weight loss and maintenance.

Increased Physical Activity

Increased physical activity is an important component in achieving the state of greater energy expenditure than energy intake that is necessary to lose weight and maintain weight loss. When increased physical activity is attempted as monotherapy, only modest weight loss has been reported.[69] However, when it is combined with reduced calorie intake and behavior modification, it can augment weight loss and improve obesity-related comorbidities and cardiovascular risk factors.[6,69] Current adult recommendations suggest at least 150 minutes of moderate physical activity per week.[70] However, 1 hour of moderate physical activity per day may be required to augment weight loss. Patients should be advised to start slowly and gradually increase intensity. All obese patients should receive a medical examination before embarking on a physical activity program.

Behavioral Modification

Behavior modification is common to almost all weight loss interventions. The primary aim is to help patients choose lifestyles that are conducive to safe and sustained weight loss. Behavioral therapy is based on principles of human learning and thus attempts to substitute desirable behaviors for learned undesirable habits using a combination of stimulus control and reinforcement. Most such programs use self-monitoring of diet and exercise both to increase patient awareness of behavior and as a tool for the clinician to determine patient compliance as well as patient motivation.[24] Behavior is reinforced by techniques that include behavioral contracting, social support, self-monitoring, relapse prevention, and (in some cases) booster treatments. Behavioral contracts are written agreements jointly developed by patients and their clinicians. Components of these agreements include goals of therapy, methods to achieve these goals, and rewards for achieving these goals. Social support requires the active participation of a close friend or relative who is involved in monitoring compliance and reinforcing behavior. Relapse prevention is geared to identifying high-risk situations for relapse, such as social events, and developing strategies to overcome barriers to maintaining healthy lifestyle choices. The most effective behavioral interventions for weight loss include a combination of several components and involve multiple treatment sessions. Updated recommendations from the U.S. Preventative Services Task Force recognize that an intensive, multicomponent behavioral intervention program can result in improved glucose tolerance and reduced cardiovascular risk in obese patients.[24]

Bariatric Surgery

❹ Consistent with the growing obesity epidemic, the demand and popularity of bariatric surgery have increased drastically over the past 2 decades. Between 1990 and 2000, the annual prevalence of bariatric procedures grew nearly sixfold, from 2.4 to 14.1 per 100,000 adults.[71] Each year, there are approximately 344,000 bariatric procedures performed worldwide.[72] From 2004 to 2007, an increase of 148% in laparoscopic bariatric surgical procedures has been observed, and this number continues to rise.[73]

Clinical **Controversy. . .**

Current practice guidelines state that bariatric surgery may be considered in patients with a BMI of 40 kg/m^2 or above or BMI of 35 kg/m^2 with significant comorbidities. Although the popularity of bariatric surgery has increased drastically over the past couple decades, the long-term outcomes on the duration of comorbidity remission remain uncertain with the procedure. Researchers are also beginning to study the effects of bariatric procedures among patients with BMIs below 35 kg/m^2 for remediation of comorbid conditions such as diabetes, but the long-term benefits and cost effectiveness of this approach remain unclear.

The American Association of Clinical Endocrinologists, the Obesity Society, and the American Society for Metabolic and Bariatric Surgery issued clinical practice guidelines for the perioperative management of bariatric surgical patients.[74] Surgery remains the most effective intervention for the treatment of obesity. However, because of its related morbidity and mortality, this intervention is reserved for patients with extreme obesity (BMI greater than or equal to 40 kg/m^2) or BMI greater than 35 kg/m^2 with significant comorbidities.[6,74,75] Surgical weight loss options should only be considered in patients who have met the eligibility criteria and have failed other recommended methods for weight loss. It is critical for bariatric surgical candidates to fully understand the associated surgical risks and be able to adhere to the extensive postoperative care, follow-ups, and necessary lifelong dietary and lifestyle adjustments to ensure the long-term success of the procedure. Careful patient selection and choice of procedure are critical to achieving a successful outcome. The input of an experienced surgeon working with a multidisciplinary team is invaluable in the care of these patients.

All bariatric surgical procedures achieve weight loss and maintenance through two principle mechanisms: (a) restriction or reduction of food intake by reducing stomach volume or (b) malabsorption by reducing the absorptive surface of the alimentary tract. Currently, the four major types of procedures are adjustable gastric banding, vertical banded gastroplasty, biliopancreatic diversion with duodenal switch, and conventional Roux-en-Y gastric bypass. Gastroplasty and adjustable gastric banding are designed to reduce the volume of the stomach and thus restrict the rate of nutrient intake. The biliopancreatic diversion with duodenal switch is primarily malabsorptive in nature, and the length of the diversion determines the extent of nutrient malabsorption. The conventional roux-en-Y gastric bypass is the most common procedure currently performed in the United States. It combines a restrictive approach with a degree of malabsorption induced by excluding 90% to 95% of the stomach, the entire duodenum, and a portion of the proximal jejunum from the effective alimentary tract. Conventional roux-en-Y gastric bypass yields greater and longer lasting weight loss than the other purely restrictive methods.[5] Ultimately, reductions in excess body weight of about 48% to 85% can be achieved within the first 1 or 2 years, and weight loss maintenance of 25% to 68% of presurgery weight has been reported after 7 to 10 years with this procedure.[5,72,74]

Improvements in the peri- and postoperative care of gastric surgery patients have reduced morbidity and mortality associated with bariatric surgeries. The operative 30-day mortality rate is about 0.3% with conventional bypass or laparoscopic gastric banding[76] and 1.1% with malabsorptive procedures.[74] Some of the most common early complications of conventional gastric bypass are deep venous thrombosis, pulmonary emboli, anastomotic leaks, bleeding, and wound infections. Approximately one third of patients who do not receive vitamin supplementation will develop significant vitamin B_{12} and iron deficiency, with a large proportion demonstrating microcytic anemia.[74] Empiric supplementation with one or two tablets of daily multivitamin, 1,200 to 2,000 mg/day of calcium citrate with 400 to 800 IU/day of vitamin D, 400 mcg/day of folic acid, 40 to 65 mg/day of elemental iron, and at least 350 mcg/day of oral vitamin B_{12} (or 500 mcg intranasally once weekly) is essential to prevent nutritional deficiencies in bariatric recipients.[74] Dumping syndrome, characterized by abdominal pain and cramping, nausea, diarrhea, and bloating, tachycardia, and syncope, can occur in more than 70% of patients after roux-en-Y gastric bypass procedures[74] and may complicate the provision of drug therapy in some cases. Dietary changes such as eating small, frequent meals; avoiding refined sugars; and increasing intake of fiber, complex carbohydrates, and protein can help alleviate the symptoms associated with dumping syndrome.[77] Weight losses resulting from bariatric surgery are often accompanied by dramatic improvements, and sometimes complete resolution, of many obesity-related complications.[78,79] With improved glycemic control and reduced insulin resistance, remission rates for type 2 diabetes mellitus have been as high as 95% after biliopancreatic diversion and 80% after gastric bypass.[79,80] Such dramatic improvements of diabetes after bariatric surgery have been attributed to mechanisms that are additive to, and independent of, the weight loss effect.[81] Other clinical benefits are improvements in hypertension (which may be transitory), hypertriglyceridemia, high-density lipoprotein cholesterol, cardiomyopathy, cardiac function, degenerative joint diseases, mobility, nonalcoholic fatty liver disease, respiratory functions, obstructive sleep apnea, obesity–hypoventilation syndrome, polycystic ovary syndrome, infertility, pregnancy complications, and positive psychosocial changes, as well as enhanced quality of life.[78] Reduced risk of cancer-related mortality[82] and cardiovascular deaths and events[83] have also been documented after bariatric surgery. Furthermore, data from the prospective controlled Swedish Obese Subjects study have demonstrated a significant 29% reduction in overall mortality for patients who underwent bariatric surgery compared with those who received conventional treatments (ranging from lifestyle or behavioral modifications to no intervention) after an average follow-up duration of 10.9 years.[84]

After experiencing weight loss, many gastric surgery patients are able to discontinue pharmacotherapy for glucose lowering, dyslipidemia, and hypertension. Frequently, however, antihypertensive medications must be restarted after surgery even though the patient has not experienced marked weight regain. It is imperative for clinicians to recognize that bariatric interventions not only alter nutrient absorption but also may impede drug absorption.[85,86] Achlorhydria and reduced surface area for intestinal and gastric absorption after bariatric surgery can lead to altered dissolution of certain pH-dependent medications, such as ketoconazole, enalapril, simvastatin, tacrolimus, sirolimus, and mycophenolic acid.[85,87] Furthermore, medications with narrow therapeutic windows, such as cyclosporine, thyroxine, phenytoin, and rifampin, have consistently demonstrated reduced drug absorption after bariatric surgery.[86] Close therapeutic monitoring of any orally administered medication after surgery is highly recommended because dosage form selection, dose conversion, or therapeutic interchange may be necessary to avoid or minimize absorption problems and ensure bariatric surgery success.

Pharmacologic Therapy

5 The debate regarding the appropriateness of obesity pharmacotherapy remains heated, fueled by the recognized national need to treat a growing epidemic and the medical and litigious fallout from the adverse effects of dexfenfluramine (Redux) and sibutramine (Meridia). Strategies for the pharmacologic management of

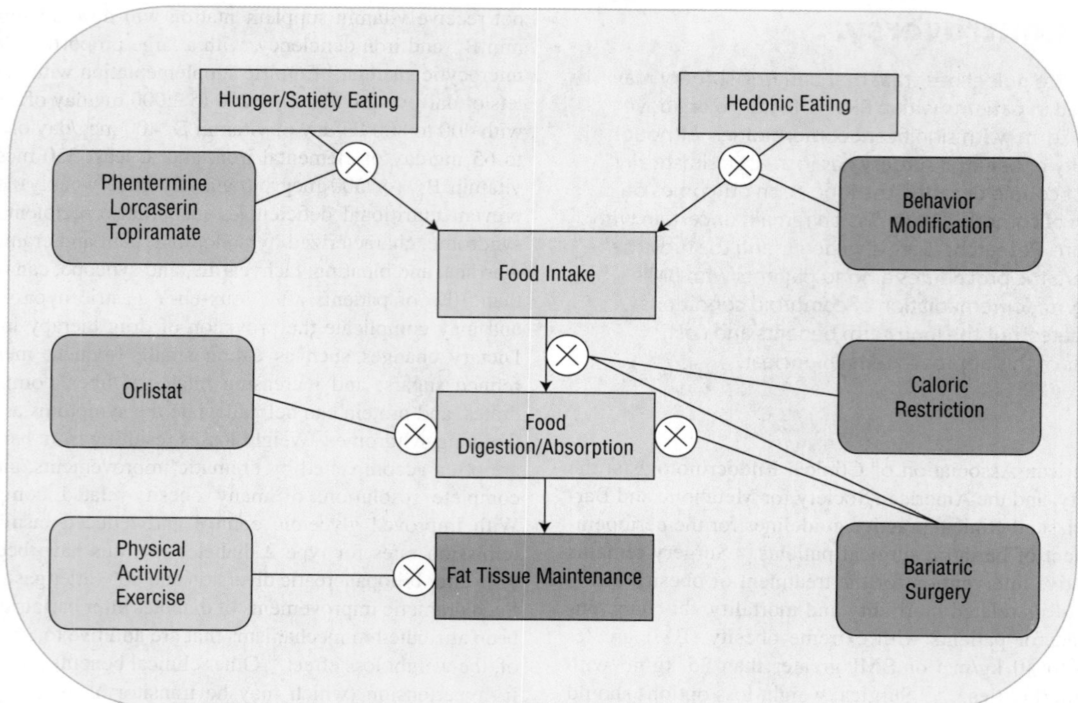

FIGURE 121-4 Sites of action for obesity treatments are represented by a circled X. Most appetite suppressants act on hunger and satiety mechanisms. Traditional diets and bariatric surgery act by limiting food intake. Whereas orlistat interferes with fat absorption in the gut, gastric bypass surgery interferes with absorption more generally.

obesity have historically focused on modulating central or peripheral sites that regulate energy balance. Figure 121-4 depicts the sites of action of these therapies within the energy intake, storage, and expenditure cycle. Short-term use of anorexic agents is difficult to justify because of the predictable weight regain that occurs with discontinuation of therapy. Long-term pharmacotherapy may have a place in the treatment of obesity for patients who have no obvious contraindications to approved drug therapy.[51,88] According to the NIH guidelines for the treatment of overweight and obese patients, pharmacotherapy may be considered in adults with BMIs of 30 kg/m^2 or greater or a WC of 40 inches (102 cm) or greater for men or 35 inches (89 cm) for women or BMI of 27 to 30 kg/m^2 with at least two concurrent risk factors if 6 months of diet, exercise, and behavioral modification failed to achieve weight loss.[6] A pharmacotherapy treatment algorithm based on these treatment guidelines is shown in Figure 121-3. Table 121-5 lists the status of the most common classes of agents currently available.

A multidisciplinary team approach to the management of obesity is necessary to ensure long-term success. It is common for patients to use a combination of nonprescription, prescription, and other complementary and alternative therapies to attain the desired weight loss goal. Therefore, clinicians should maintain a high degree of sensitivity toward the potential polypharmacy practices of patients with obesity. Finally, it is prudent to consider specific patient factors and characteristics along with the efficacy and safety profiles of individual therapies when determining if use of a pharmacologic intervention is warranted.

Agents Approved for Long-Term Use

There are currently three products approved in the United States for the chronic management of obesity. These include the lipase inhibitor orlistat (Xenical, Alli), the serotonin 2C receptor agonist lorcaserin (Belviq), and the combination product phentermine–topiramate extended release (Qsymia).

Clinical **Controversy. . .**

Obesity is considered a chronic disease. Agents currently approved by the FDA for the long-term management of obesity have limited data regarding morbidity and mortality outcomes, and the optimal treatment duration is unknown. Because discontinuation of drug treatment tends to result in weight regain, continuation of an effective and well-tolerated drug regimen is common practice.

Lipase Inhibitor: Orlistat Excessive intake of dietary fat is one of the contributing factors in the development of obesity. Gastrointestinal (GI) (gastric, pancreatic, and carboxyl ester) lipases are essential in the absorption of the long-chain triglycerides. Additionally, lipase is known to play a role in facilitating gastric emptying and secretion of other pancreaticobiliary substances. Orlistat (Xenical) is a synthetic derivative of lipstatin, a natural lipase inhibitor produced by *Streptomyces toxytricini*. The drug is minimally absorbed and induces weight loss by persistent lowering of dietary fat absorption through selective inhibition of the GI lipase. Furthermore, lower luminal free fatty acid concentrations result in malabsorption of cholesterol. Up to 30% reduction in fat absorption occurred with daily doses of 120 mg three times daily with meals.[89] A nonprescription formulation of orlistat (Alli) is approved in the United States at a reduced daily dose of 60 mg three times daily.[90] The drug must be taken within 1 hour of consuming foods that contain fat in order to exert its effect. If a meal is skipped or contains no fat, the dose of orlistat can be omitted.

6 Clinical studies using orlistat as an adjunct to diet therapy demonstrate dose-dependent reductions in fat absorption. Overall, results from clinical trials demonstrate that orlistat modestly increases the amount of weight lost and decreases the amount of weight regained during medically supervised weight loss

TABLE 121-5 Pharmacotherapeutic Agents for Weight Loss

Drug	Brand Name	Initial Dose	Usual Range	Special Population Dose	Comment
Gastrointestinal Lipase Inhibitor					
Orlistat	Xenical	120 mg three times daily with each main meal containing fat	120 mg three times daily with each main meal containing fat		Approved for long-term use Take during or up to 1 hour after the meal. Omit dose if meal is occasionally missed or contains no fat
Orlistat	Alli[a]	60 mg three times daily with each main meal containing fat	60 mg three times daily with each main meal containing fat		Same as Xenical
Serotonin 2C Receptor Agonist					
Lorcaserin	Belviq	10 mg twice daily	10 mg twice daily	Use with caution in moderate renal impairment and severe hepatic impairment; not recommended in patients with end state renal disease	Approved for long-term use Controlled substance: C–IV
Phentermine–Topiramate Combination					
Phentermine and topiramate extended release	Qsymia	3.75 mg of phentermine and 23 mg of topiramate once daily for 14 days; then increase to 7.5 mg of phentermine and 46 mg of topiramate once daily	7.5 mg of phentermine and 46 mg of topiramate once daily to a maximum dose of phentermine 15 mg and topiramate 92 mg	Maximum dose for patients with moderate or severe renal impairment or patients with moderate hepatic impairment is 7.5 mg of phentermine and 46 mg of topiramate	Approved for long-term use Take dose in the morning to avoid insomnia Controlled substance: C–IV
Noradrenergic Agents					
Phendimetrazine	Bontril PDM; Bontril Slow-Release	Conventional tablet: start at 17.5 mg two or three times daily, given 1 hour before meals Extended-release capsule: 105 mg once daily 30–60 minutes before morning meal	70–105 mg/day	Use caution in patients with renal impairment	Approved for short-term monotherapy Controlled substance: C–III Prescriptions should be written for the smallest quantity to minimize possibility of overdose
Phentermine	Adipex-P, Suprenza	Orally disintegrating tablet: 15 or 30 mg once every morning Phentermine hydrochloride: 15–37.5 mg/day given in one or two divided doses; administer before breakfast or 1–2 hours after breakfast	Orally disintegrating tablet: 15 or 30 mg once every morning Phentermine hydrochloride: 15–37.5 mg/day given in one or two divided doses; administer before breakfast or 1–2 hours after breakfast	Use with caution in patients with renal impairment	Approved for short-term monotherapy Controlled substance: C–IV Prescriptions should be written for the smallest quantity to minimize possibility of overdose Individualize to achieve adequate response with lowest effective dose
Diethylpropion	Tenuate, Tenuate Dospan	Immediate release: 25 mg three times daily administered 1 hour before meals Controlled release: 75 mg once daily administered at midmorning	75 mg/day	Use with caution in patients with renal impairment	Approved for short-term monotherapy Dose should not be administered in the evening or at bedtime Controlled substance: C–IV

[a]Available without a prescription.

programs.[89,91] The longest trial that evaluated the safety and efficacy of orlistat is XENDOS (XENical in the prevention of Diabetes in Obese Subjects), a 4-year, double-blind, randomized, placebo-controlled prospective study.[92] Although weight regain was observed with continual therapy beyond the first year of orlistat therapy, results from this study show moderate weight loss sustained after 4 years of treatment compared with placebo, 12.8 lb (5.8 kg) and 6.6 lb (3.0 kg), respectively. Weight loss using orlistat also decreased the rate of development of type 2 diabetes by 37.3% in patients with impaired glucose tolerance. Improved glycemic control can be attained in patients with type 2 diabetes by inducing or increasing weight loss with orlistat in addition to diet management.[89,91] In some cases, dosages or the number of antidiabetic medications may be reduced or discontinued.[89] Significant improvements in lipid profile (reduction in total and low-density lipoprotein [LDL] cholesterol), glucose control, and other markers of metabolism are seen when using orlistat in addition to the diet.[89,91] Orlistat is approved for the chronic treatment of obesity in adults and adolescents ages 12 to 16 years. The recommended dose is 120 mg three times daily taken within 1 hour of consuming a fat-containing meal.

At least one GI complaint (soft stools, abdominal pain or colic, flatulence, fecal urgency, or incontinence) has been reported in up to 80% of individuals using prescription-strength orlistat. These complaints are most common in the first 1 to 2 months of therapy, are mild to moderate in severity, and tend to improve with continued orlistat use. Limiting dietary fat before initiation of orlistat therapy may be beneficial in decreasing initial GI complaints. Severe diarrhea secondary to orlistat use can affect the absorption of orally administered drugs, such as oral contraceptives, fat-soluble vitamins (A, D, E, and K) and β-carotene.[89,91] Therefore, supplementation with a multivitamin should be considered during therapy. In the presence of severe diarrhea, women receiving oral contraceptives should be advised of the need to use alternative backup methods because absorption of oral contraceptive may be reduced.[89] Although orlistat does not appear to alter the pharmacokinetic profiles of other agents, including digoxin, glyburide, metformin, phenytoin, fluoxetine, amitriptyline, phentermine, losartan, nifedipine, captopril, atenolol, furosemide, alcohol, or atorvastatin, reduced fat absorption can potentially affect the absorption of lipophilic drugs, such as lamotrigine, valproic acid, gabapentin, and amiodarone.[93] Decreased vitamin K absorption has also been noted and can alter the patient's warfarin dosage needs.[93] Clinicians should also be aware that orlistat may directly interfere with the absorption of other narrow therapeutic range drugs, such as cyclosporine and levothyroxine.[93] In patients requiring concomitant therapies with orlistat, close monitoring is warranted to ensure an adequate therapeutic response. Separation of the administration times of the medications may minimize these potential drug interactions.

In 2009 to 2010, the FDA performed a complete safety review for the possible risk of a rare liver damage with the use of orlistat. Between 1999 and August 2009, there were one U.S. case with Alli and 12 foreign cases with Xenical, including two patients who died from liver failure and three who required liver transplantation, in patients using orlistat.[94] Although causality has not been definitively linked to orlistat, patients are advised to monitor for any signs and symptoms of liver injury, such as development of itching, yellow eyes or skin, dark urine, loss of appetite, or light-colored stools, to their healthcare providers.

Serotonin Receptor Agonist: Lorcaserin Lorcaserin (Belviq) is a selective serotonin (5-HT_{2C}) receptor agonist, recently approved by the FDA for chronic weight management in patients who are obese (BMI ≥30 kg/m^2) or overweight (BMI >27 kg/m^2) with at least one weight-related comorbidity.[95] At the recommended dose of 10 mg twice daily, lorcaserin selectively activates central 5-HT_{2C} receptors on hypothalamic anorexigenic pro-opiomelanocortin neurons. Activation of central 5-HT_{2C} receptors results in appetite suppression, leading to reduced energy intake and enhanced satiety.

Clinical trials evaluating the efficacy of loracaserin, used in combination with a low-calorie diet and exercise counseling, have reported a modest but significantly greater weight loss compared with placebo.[96,97] The Behavioral Modification and Lorcaserin for Overweight and Obesity Management (BLOOM) trial was a 2-year, randomized, placebo-controlled, double-blind, prospective trial that enrolled more than 3,000 obese and overweight patients.[96] Mean weight loss at 1 year was 5.8 kg (12.8 lb) in the lorcaserin group compared with 2.2 kg (4.8 lb) in the placebo group. Patients in the lorcaserin-treated group also experienced significant improvements in fasting glucose, insulin, total cholesterol, LDL cholesterol, and triglyceride concentrations at the end of the first year. Although weight regain was observed during the second year of the trial, 68% of the patients who had previously achieved 5% weight loss during the first year were able to maintain this level of weight loss by the end of the second year. The efficacy of lorcaserin has also been shown in patients with type 2 diabetes, with an average weight loss of 4.5% and significant improvements in hemoglobin A_{1c} (HbA_{1c}) and fasting glucose after 1 year of treatment.[98] Based on data from clinical trials, the approved label states that lorcaserin therapy should be discontinued if 5% weight loss not is not achieved by week 12 because it is unlikely that a benefit will be seen.[95]

The most common adverse effects associated with the use of lorcaserin in clinical trials were headache, dizziness, constipation, fatigue, and dry mouth.[96] Previous serotonergic agents (e.g., dexfenfluramine) used for weight loss have been associated with cardiac valvulopathy.[99] The mechanism for this toxicity is thought to be related to stimulation of $5HT_{2B}$ receptors on cardiac cells. At therapeutic doses, lorcaserin is selective for central $5HT_{2C}$ receptors. During clinical trials, the incidence of cardiac valvulopathy was not significantly different between patients who received lorcaserin (2.4%) and those who received placebo (2%).[95] However, patients should be counseled to contact their healthcare providers if they experience signs or symptoms cardiac valve disease such as dyspnea or edema. Lorcaserin should not be used in combination with other serotonergic and dopaminergic drugs because of the increased risk of serotonin syndrome or neuroleptic malignant syndrome–like reactions. Lorcaserin should be used cautiously in patients with congestive heart failure because these patients may be at an increased risk for cardiac valvulopathy. Additional rare adverse effects that clinicians should be aware of include psychiatric disorders, priapism, and elevated serum prolactin concentrations. Lorcaserin is classified as a controlled substance in class IV due to potential for abuse.

Phentermine–Topiramate Extended Release A combination product containing phentermine and topiramate extended release (Qsymia) is approved by the FDA for chronic weight management in patients who are obese (BMI ≥30 kg/m^2) or overweight (BMI >27 kg/m^2) with at least one weight-related comorbidity.[100] Phentermine is structurally similar to amphetamine, but it has less severe CNS stimulation and a lower abuse potential. Its mechanism of action centers on its ability to enhance norepinephrine (NE) and dopamine neurotransmission, resulting in appetite suppressing effects. Topiramate is an antiepileptic drug. Although the exact mechanism for its efficacy in weight management is not known, it may decrease appetite and increase satiety through multiple pathways, including effects on γ-aminobutyrate, voltage-gated ion channels, excitatory glutamate receptors, or carbonic anhydrase.[100] The doses of phentermine (3.75–15 mg) and topiramate (23–92 mg) in this combination are significantly lower than the therapeutic doses of each separate product when used as monotherapy for obesity (37.5 mg) and epilepsy (400 mg), respectively. The recommended dosing strategy for phentermine–topiramate extended release involves gradual titration, staring with 3.75 mg of phentermine and 23 mg of topiramate once daily for 14 days and then increasing the dose to 7.5 mg of phentermine and 46 mg of topiramate once daily.[100] After 12 weeks of therapy, the dose may be increased again to 11.25 mg of phentermine and 69 mg of topiramate for 14 days and then to a maximum dose of 15 mg of phentermine and 92 mg of topiramate daily. Likewise, when discontinuing therapy, the dose should be gradually decreased by taking a dose every other day for at least 1 week to prevent the possible precipitation of seizures.

Clinical trials evaluating the efficacy of phentermine–topiramate, when used as an adjunct to a reduced-calorie diet and lifestyle changes, have reported dose-dependent weight loss and significant reductions in blood pressure, total cholesterol, LDL cholesterol, triglycerides, fasting glucose, and HbA_{1c}.[101,102] The CONQUER trial was a randomized, placebo-controlled, double-blind, prospective trial of 2,487 overweight or obese patients with two or more obesity-related comorbidities.[101] After a 4-week dose titration phase, subjects were randomized to receive (a) placebo, (b) 7.5 mg of phentermine with 46 mg of topiramate, or (c) 15 mg of phentermine with 92 mg of topiramate daily. Weight loss at 1 year was significantly greater than placebo in both of the treatment groups, with a mean weight loss of 8.1 kg (17.8 lb) in the 7.5-mg phentermine and 46-mg topiramate group and a mean weight loss of 10.2 kg (22.4 lb) in the 15-mg phentermine and 92-mg topiramate group. The efficacy of phentermine–topiramate has also been documented in patients with class II and class III obesity (mean BMI, 42 kg/m^2), with a reported mean weight loss of 10.9% after 1 year of treatment.[102]

The most common adverse effects associated with the use of phentermine–topiramate in clinical trials were constipation, dry mouth, paraesthesia, dysgeusia, and insomnia.[101,102] Because topiramate is a known teratogen, this drug is contraindicated in pregnancy because fetal exposure in the first trimester increases the risk of cleft lip or cleft palate. To manage the potential risk of teratogenicity, the drug is only available through a limited distribution process under a risk evaluation and mitigation strategy (REMS).[100] All women of childbearing age must have a documented negative pregnancy test result before beginning treatment and then monthly to continue therapy. Topiramate has been associated with acute myopia associated with secondary angle-closure glaucoma, and phentermine can cause mydriasis from adrenergic stimulation. Therefore, this product is also contraindicated in patients with glaucoma. The potential for hypertensive crisis with coadministration of phentermine and monoamine oxidase inhibitors (MAOIs) exists; therefore, patients should have stopped an MAOI for at least 14 days before use of any adrenergic agent. Phentermine–topiramate is also contraindicated in patients with untreated hyperthyroidism.

Monitoring parameters and drug interactions that clinicians should be aware of include known issues related to both components of the formulation. Of note, increases in heart rate greater than 10 beats/min were observed in approximately 50% of patients receiving phentermine–topiramate during clinical trials.[100] In patients receiving the highest dose, 19% experienced increases in heart rate that were greater than 20 beats/min. Therefore, heart rate should be monitored in all patients, particularly those with preexisting cardiovascular disease. Decreases in serum bicarbonate were also noted in clinical trials, which were generally mild with peak decreases observed after 4 weeks of therapy. Decreases in serum potassium and increases in serum creatinine were also reported. Therefore, monitoring of serum electrolytes and creatinine is recommended at baseline and during therapy. Clinicians should be aware that concomitant use of non–potassium-sparing diuretics may potentiate the risk for hypokalemia. Although pregnancy risk is not expected, use of phentermine–topiramate concomitantly with oral contraceptives may result in breakthrough bleeding because of increased exposure to progestin and decreases exposure to estrogen. Phentermine–topiramate is classified as a controlled substance in schedule IV because of the abuse potential of phentermine. Similarly to lorcaserin, therapy should be discontinued if 5% weight loss is not achieved after 12 weeks.[100]

7 Combination Therapy Theoretically, combination therapy including any of the currently available agents would be expected to produce synergistic effects because each agent works through different mechanisms of action to induce weight loss. However, no studies are currently available evaluating the efficacy and safety of combination therapy. The concomitant use of these drugs may lead to increased adverse effects without improved therapeutic outcomes. Therefore, combination therapy is not recommended over the use of either product individually at this time.

Agents Approved for Short-Term Use

Several noradrenergic agents are currently approved by the FDA for short-term weight loss. Because short-term therapy is not consistent with current national guidelines for the chronic management of obesity, these agents have limited clinical utility in practice.

Phentermine Phentermine is available in both immediate-release and sustained-release formulations. However, the value of sustained-release formulations is questionable based on the reported phentermine plasma half-life of 12 to 24 hours.[103] Phentermine is an effective adjunct to diet, exercise, and behavior modification for producing weight loss in excess of that seen with placebo.[104] Intermittent phentermine therapy appears to elicit comparable weight loss as that seen with continuous use. However, most individuals experience weight regains during therapy and generally always after discontinuing use.[103] A single dose of 30 mg once daily in the morning provides effective appetite suppression throughout the day. Divided doses of 8 mg immediately before meals, however, are common. Doses greater than 30 mg daily do not improve effectiveness.[104] Evening or nighttime dosing should be avoided because of insomnia. Significant increases in blood pressure, palpitations, and arrhythmias can occur with phentermine administration. Use is not advisable in hypertensive patients and those with underlying cardiac abnormalities.

The potential for hypertensive crisis with coadministration of phentermine and MAOIs is noted in the product labeling of each agent; therefore, patients should be off an MAOI for at least 14 days before use of any adrenergic agent to avoid excessive adrenergic stimulation syndromes.[105] Phentermine use is contraindicated in patients with hyperthyroidism or agitated states and in those who are abusers of substances such as cocaine, phencyclidine, and methamphetamine, again because of the potential for excessive adrenergic stimulation syndromes and abuse potential. Mydriasis from adrenergic stimulation can worsen glaucoma, and patients diagnosed with glaucoma should not receive phentermine. Patients with diabetes may experience altered insulin or oral hypoglycemic dosage requirements soon after beginning therapy and before any substantial weight loss. Phentermine remains the most widely prescribed weight management medication by obesity specialists despite product labeling that indicates short-term (a few weeks), monotherapy use only.[106] This usage pattern deviates from the current national recommendations that promote only long-term drug intervention when obesity pharmacotherapy is appropriate.[51]

Diethylpropion Diethylpropion stimulates NE release from presynaptic storage granules. Increased adrenergic neurotransmitter concentrations activate hypothalamic centers, which result in decreased appetite and food intake. This drug undergoes extensive first-pass hepatic metabolism. Active metabolites are eliminated renally and account for about 70% of the administered dose. The elimination half-life of these metabolites is about 8 hours.[104] Less than 10% of the parent compound is recovered in urine. No specific dosing recommendations exist for use in patients with renal or hepatic insufficiency. Diethylpropion can be taken in divided daily doses, generally 25 mg three times daily before meals. An extended-release formulation is also used by some clinicians, usually as 75 mg taken once daily in the morning or midmorning. Both dosing regimens are effective in achieving short-term weight loss in excess of placebo.[107] Complaints of insomnia increase if late afternoon dosing is used. Diethylpropion causes less stimulation of the CNS than mazindol and generally causes less insomnia than phentermine. Patients with severe hypertension or significant cardiovascular disease should not receive diethylpropion. Patients with diabetes may experience decreased insulin or oral hypoglycemic dosage requirements soon after beginning therapy and before any substantial weight loss. More frequent blood glucose self-monitoring and medical follow-up are warranted when treating diabetic patients with diethylpropion.

Amphetamines Appetite suppressant effects of the amphetamines were well recognized in the 1930s. Amphetamines activate central noradrenergic receptor systems as well as dopaminergic pathways at higher doses by stimulating neurotransmitter release. Increases in blood pressure and mild bronchodilation are attributed to peripheral α- and β-receptor activation. Amphetamines are no longer widely used for the treatment of obesity because of their powerful stimulant effects and addictive potential.

Other Agents Used for Weight Management

Off-Label Use of Serotonergic Agents Serotonin is an important neurotransmitter involved in many human physiologic systems such as sleep–wake cycles, sensitivity to pain, blood pressure, mood, and eating behaviors. Increasing central serotonin levels disrupts the body's natural development of satiety by decreasing the amount of food consumed and prolongs the time between food intake.[108] Some serotonergic agents increase central serotonin concentrations via stimulating release of presynaptic stores or inhibition of reuptake into storage granules. Additionally, either the parent compound or metabolites of these agents may stimulate postsynaptic 5-HT receptors directly. Peripheral serotonin effects that have an impact on appetite, such as slowing gastric motility, have been described. A major distinction between serotonergic and noradrenergic anorexiants is that serotonergic agents lack the central stimulant effects and thus the abuse potential seen with the noradrenergic compounds.[107] Conversely, decreased wakefulness, altered sleep patterns, and changes in affect can be seen. Some of the serotonergic agents were first studied as antidepressants (see Chap. 51), and when weight loss was noted in some patients, they began to be used as weight management agents. These drugs are not approved by the FDA as weight management agents and are currently not recommended for the treatment of obesity. Nonetheless, some practitioners have prescribed these agents for the treatment of obesity "off label" either alone or in combination with phentermine.

Fluoxetine is a serotonergic agent that has been prescribed as an appetite-suppressing agent. Higher doses of fluoxetine (60 mg) were generally used for weight loss as opposed to the lower doses (20 mg) frequently used for the treatment of depression. A meta-analysis of five fluoxetine trials in patients with diabetes resulted in weight loss of 4.3 kg (9.4 lb) compared with placebo over periods of up to 1 year.[109] Evidence also demonstrates sustained benefits in fasting blood glucose, HbA_{1c}, and triglycerides in patients with poor glycemic control. However, weight regain was noted to occur with discontinuation of medication.

The safety and efficacy of phentermine–serotonin reuptake inhibitor combinations is limited. A case report of adverse experiences (e.g., impaired mentation, tremor, hyperreflexia, and GI symptoms) with unintentional concurrent use of phentermine and fluoxetine reinforces the need for caution by prescribers of this unapproved combination therapy.[110] Although cases of pulmonary hypertension have been reported in patients exposed to fluoxetine,[111] serious adverse effects such as cardiac valve abnormalities in excess of baseline prevalence have not been reported in relation to selective serotonin reuptake inhibitor use for obesity therapy.[112]

Noradrenergic–Serotonergic Agents Until 2010, sibutramine was available as Meridia in the United States for long-term use for weight loss. This agent induced weight loss by decreasing appetite and maintaining or increasing thermogenesis via increasing the synaptic concentration of serotonin, NE, and dopamine through reuptake inhibition. The STORM (Sibutramine Trial of Obesity Reduction and Maintenance) was the longest randomized, double-blind study to evaluate the effectiveness of sibutramine, lasting up to 2 years.[113] The group receiving sibutramine achieved more weight loss than the placebo group (22.4 lb [10.2 kg] vs. 10.3 lb [4.7 kg], respectively) and had more subjects who retained at least 80% of the weight loss. Common adverse effects associated with sibutramine were increase in blood pressure and heart rate, dry mouth, anorexia, insomnia, constipation, dizziness, and nausea.[91] The SCOUT (Sibutramine Cardiovascular OUTcomes) study—the first prospective trial that evaluated the potential benefits of sibutramine on cardiovascular outcomes in obese or overweight individuals with preexisting cardiovascular disease, type 2 diabetes mellitus, or both, failed to provide any reassurance regarding sibutramine's safety.[114] Although individuals taking sibutramine had modest weight loss, improvement in cardiovascular outcomes was not seen. Conversely, subjects with preexisting cardiovascular disease actually had an increased risk of nonfatal myocardial infarction and nonfatal stroke. Because of concerns that the effectiveness of sibutramine on weight loss is counterbalanced by increased rather than decreased cardiovascular risk, the drug was voluntarily withdrawn from the U.S. market.

Complementary and Alternative Therapies

8 Many complementary and alternative therapy products are currently promoted for weight loss. A nationwide survey of U.S. consumers reported that about 34% of adults reported that they had used "dietary supplements" specifically for the purposes of weight loss.[115] It is important for clinicians to be aware that the regulation of dietary supplements is less rigorous than that of prescription and over-the-counter drug products. As such, a manufacturer of a dietary supplement does not have to prove the safety or effectiveness of the product before it is marketed. Of concern, some herbal and food supplement diet agents contain pharmacologically active substances that should be used with caution or avoided in obese patients with conditions such as diabetes, hypertension, and significant cardiovascular disease. In addition, many marketed products have been reported to lack consistency in labeling versus actual product content. More recently, a number of dietary supplements have been found to contain undeclared prescription drugs.[116] Clinicians may access the FDA Dietary Supplement Alerts and Safety Information website to keep informed of these issues.[117] Table 121-6 lists some of the common herbal and natural products used for weight loss and the constituents found in many of these products.

Bitter Orange

Bitter orange (*Citrus aurantium*) contains m-synephrine, a sympathomimetic amine with structural similarities to ephedrine.[118] After the FDA banned the sale of ephedra-containing dietary supplements in 2004, several manufacturers replaced the ephedra constituents within their products with bitter orange. Bitter orange–containing products are commonly promoted as "ephedra free." Although bitter orange has been shown to effectively promote weight loss, it may also increase heart rate and blood pressure, potentially causing the same adverse cardiovascular effects that were observed with ephedra.[118]

Chromium

Chromium is considered an essential nutrient and experimentally in animals is an insulin cofactor active in carbohydrate, protein, and lipid metabolism. In humans, insulin resistance has been reported in a few cases of apparent severe chromium deficiency during long-term total parenteral nutrition (see Chap. 119). Currently, there is no reliable means of assessing total body chromium status, making diagnosis of deficiency difficult. The tryptophan metabolite, picolinic acid, forms a complex with trivalent chromium, which improves bioavailability. Food sources with highly available chromium include brewer's yeast, calves' liver, American cheese, and wheat germ. Clinical trials assessing chromium picolinate as a supplement to aerobic exercise in the treatment of obesity have failed to demonstrate any effectiveness.[119,120]

Chitosan

Chitosan is a cationic polysaccharide, specifically a partially *N*-deacetylated form of chitin. This nonhydrolyzable fiber exhibits properties similar to those of cellulose. In vitro and preclinical data indicate that chitosan may be effective in blocking absorption of fat from the gut. It has been suggested that orally administered chitosan may be an effective weight reduction agent by blocking calories ingested as fat. Chitosan is a major constituent in several heavily advertised weight management food supplements and nonprescription preparations. Although a small number of short-term investigations have reported that oral chitosan is more effective than placebo

TABLE 121-6 Drug Monitoring

Drug	Brand Name	Adverse Reactions	Monitoring Parameters	Comments
Gastrointestinal Lipase Inhibitor				
Orlistat	Xenical, Alli[a]	Soft stools, diarrhea, abdominal pain or colic, flatulence, fecal urgency, incontinence, liver damage (rare)	BMI; calorie and fat intake; serum glucose in patients with diabetes; thyroid function in patients with thyroid disease; liver function tests in patients exhibiting symptoms of hepatic dysfunction	Supplement with a multivitamin during therapy to prevent vitamin deficiency
Serotonin 2C Receptor Agonist				
Lorcaserin	Belviq	Headache, dizziness, fatigue, nausea, dry mouth, constipation, hypoglycemia in patients with diabetes, psychiatric disorders, priapism, elevated serum prolactin level	BMI; calorie and fat intake; serum glucose in patients with diabetes; complete blood count, depression or suicidal thoughts; signs or symptoms of serotonin syndrome; signs or symptoms of valvular heart disease	Discontinue if 5% weight loss not achieved by week 12
Phentermine–Topiramate Combination				
Phentermine and topiramate extended release	Qsymia	Constipation, dry mouth, paraesthesia, dysgeusia, insomnia, hypoglycemia in patients with diabetes	BMI; calorie and fat intake; serum glucose in patients with diabetes; pregnancy; depression or suicidal thoughts; mood or sleep disorders; heart rate; serum electrolytes and creatine at baseline and during treatment	Discontinue or escalate dose if 3% weight loss not achieved by week 12 on phentermine 7.5 mg and topiramate 46 mg Discontinue if 5% weight loss not achieved by week 12 on phentermine 15 mg and topiramate 92 mg Gradually discontinue phentermine 15 mg and topiramate 92 mg to prevent possible seizure
Noradrenergic Agents				
Phendimetrazine Phentermine Diethylpropion	Bontril PDM; Bontril Slow-Release Adipex-P, Suprenza Tenuate, Tenuate Dospan	Increased blood pressure, ischemic events, palpitations, tachycardia, valvular disease, urticaria, agitation, dizziness, headache, insomnia, overstimulation, psychosis, restlessness, dry mouth, constipation, thirst, diarrhea	Baseline cardiac evaluation (for preexisting valvular heart disease, pulmonary hypertension); echocardiogram during therapy; weight, waist circumference; blood pressure	Discontinue if satisfactory weight loss has not occurred within the first 4 weeks of treatment or if tolerance develops Abrupt discontinuation after prolonged high doses may be associated with extreme fatigue and depression

BMI, body mass index.

[a]Available without a prescription.

for weight loss, the degree of weight loss has not been clinically significant.[121]

Ephedra Alkaloids

Based on the known effects of ephedrine, dietary supplements claiming weight management effects have used plant sources of ephedra alkaloids. Various parts of the Ephedraceae, ma huang, *Sida cordifolia,* and *Pinellia ternata* plants are known to produce ephedra alkaloids, including L-ephedrine, D-pseudoephedrine, L-norephedrine, D-norpseudoephedrine, L-*N*-methylephedrine, and D-*N*-methylpseudoephedrine.[122] Common names routinely included in dietary supplement labeling for these alkaloid sources include joint fir, popotillo, country mallow, sea grape, and yellow horse. From 1994 through July 1997, the FDA received more than 800 reports of serious adverse events; including seizures, stroke, and death, coincident with ephedrine alkaloid–containing dietary supplement use. An in-depth review of 140 reports of adverse events related to ephedrine alkaloid–containing dietary supplements demonstrated that approximately half the reports involved cardiovascular symptoms.[123] In 2004, the FDA determined that all sources of ephedra alkaloids must be excluded from dietary supplements because they present an unreasonably high health risk.[124]

Guarana Extract and Various Tea Extracts

Guarana and tea are sources of caffeine that have inherent adrenergic properties and increase the effects of stimulant substances, such as ephedrine and ephedra alkaloids. Guarana and various tea extracts are commonly found in energy drinks and combination weight loss products that contain other substances with stimulant properties.[125]

Hoodia

Hoodia is a desert cactus of the Apocynaceae plant family. Natives indigenous to the Kalahari Desert are purported to consume the stems and roots of this plant for their appetite suppressant effects.[126] Other names appearing on product labels are Kalahari cactus, Hoodia cactus or extract, *Hoodia gordonii* cactus, and Kalahari diet. Hoodia extract, sometimes referred to as P57, is rumored to elicit weight loss; however, only one short-term, randomized, placebo-controlled trial evaluating the efficacy and safety of a purified extract is available. In this 15-day study, overweight women did not experience a change in energy intake, and the purified Hoodia extract was associated with nausea, vomiting, and changes in skin sensation.[127]

Pyruvate

Pyruvate is a commonly listed ingredient in many herbal weight management preparations. Multiple salt forms are used, including sodium, magnesium, potassium, and calcium. Other names are α-ketopropionic acid, 2-oxypropanoic acid, and acetylformic acid. Pyruvate is a three-carbon intermediate formed during normal glucose metabolism or during glycolysis. It is advertised in the lay press for its ability to "increase metabolism" and thus promote weight loss.

Objective data documenting these effects are lacking.[128,129] Although most pyruvate nutritional weight management supplements contain less than 2 g per dose, large exposures (>20 g) are known to cause noticeable GI side effects, including bloating and diarrhea.

Agents Under Investigation

Several investigational pharmacologic agents are currently being evaluated for weight management. Tesofensine is a monoamine reuptake inhibitor that enhances activity of serotonin, NE, and dopamine, resulting in significant reduction in appetite.[99] A randomized, double-blind, placebo-controlled, phase 2 trial of tesofensine in 203 obese patients reported dose-dependent weight loss ranging from 4.5% to 10.6% after 6 months of treatment.[130]

Another agent under development for obesity treatment is cetilistat, a lipase inhibitor. A randomized, double-blind, placebo-controlled trial involving 612 obese subjects with type 2 diabetes reported an average weight loss of 3.9 kg (8.5 lb) and 4.3 kg (9.5 lb) over 12 weeks in patients who received 80 mg and 120 mg, respectively, of cetilistat three times daily in combination with a hypocaloric diet.[131] This trial also included an orlistat treatment arm. Orlistat-treated patients lost a similar amount of weight at 12 weeks but also reported significantly more GI adverse effects than patients who received cetilistat, suggesting that cetilistat may be better tolerated than orlistat.

After the unsuccessful use of rimonabant, a potent central and peripheral inhibitor of the cannabinoid receptor CB_1 that was withdrawn from the European Union in 2008 because of serious psychiatric concerns, a selective peripheral CB_1 receptor antagonist is in development.[132] Although rimonabant effectively promoted weight loss, it was associated with an increased risk of serious neurologic side effects, including seizures, depression, anxiety, aggressiveness, and suicidal thoughts. These adverse effects are related to central antagonism of CB_1 receptors. Development of central CB_1 antagonists has been suspended, with focused research now on peripheral CB_1 antagonists, to retain the weight loss efficacy reported with rimonabant, while reducing the adverse effects. Other products currently being studied for weight management include several drug combinations: bupropion and naltrexone, bupropion and zonisamide, and pramlintide and metreleptin.[133]

PERSONALIZED PHARMACOTHERAPY

Genetic influences are estimated to contribute to as much as 80% of the actual variance in body weight and fat distribution.[29] As such, identifying specific genes involved in the development of obesity is an area of extensive research. Several gene variants have been identified over the past 15 years that are associated with the development of obesity.[134] However, the use of personalized pharmacotherapy to treat obesity has only been documented in patients with congenital leptin deficiency.[135] This is an extremely rare condition in which administration of recombinant human leptin results in significant improvement in body weight and other associated abnormalities of leptin deficiency. Recommendations regarding how currently available medications can be individualized to maximize patient benefit are not yet available.

EVALUATION OF THERAPEUTIC OUTCOMES

The evaluation and management of a patient with obesity requires careful clinical; biochemical; and, if necessary, psychological evaluation. This evaluation should include an assessment of the patient's current medical condition and medication regimen. A multidisciplinary team including, but not limited to, a physician, nutritionist, psychologist, and pharmacist should be involved in the care of obese individuals.

Monitoring the Pharmaceutical Care Plan

Assessment of patient progress should be documented once or twice monthly for 1 to 2 months and then monthly thereafter.[6] Each encounter should document weight, WC, BMI, blood pressure, medical history, and patient assessment of obesity medication tolerability.[6] Chronic use of obesity medications should be consistent with the approved product labeling, and medication therapy should be discontinued after 3 to 4 months if the patient has failed to demonstrate weight loss or maintenance of prior weight. To achieve optimal weight loss, patients should be instructed about the importance of adherence to prescribed medication and lifestyle changes. Numerous tools for the patient and practitioner are readily available from the Department of Health and Human Services, including the National Heart Lung and Blood Institute Obesity Education Initiative.[136] The Short Form 36 (SF-36) also has been used as a quality-of-life evaluation tool for obese patients undergoing programmatic weight loss. Quarterly assessments of well-being and quality of life using validated assessment tools can be helpful in objectively quantifying the effectiveness of therapy.

Patients with diabetes receiving weight loss medication require more intense medical monitoring and self-monitoring of blood glucose. Insulin therapy may need to be adjusted with the start of obesity medication therapy. Some patients with diabetes may require daily telephone contact with a healthcare provider to assist in adjusting their hypoglycemic therapy. Weekly patient visits to a healthcare setting may be necessary for 1 to 2 months until the effects of diet, exercise, and weight loss medication become more predictable. As frequent as quarterly assessment of HbA_{1c} may be appropriate in patients with type 2 diabetes who lose weight to aid in adjustment of hypoglycemic therapy. Lipid profiles can normalize or improve with weight loss. Lipid status should be assessed semiannually or annually in patients with hyperlipidemia to determine the need for continued hyperlipidemia therapies. Weight loss also can result in normalization of blood pressure in hypertensive obese patients. Assessment of appropriateness of antihypertensive therapy should occur with each followup visit.

CONCLUSION

Obesity is a chronic disease with a prevalence that has increased dramatically over the past 30 years. Increased body weight is a consequence of increased energy storage resulting from an imbalance between energy intake and energy expenditure over time, which is influenced by many factors, including genetics and the environment. Nonpharmacologic therapy, including reduced caloric intake, increased physical activity, and behavioral modification, is currently the mainstay of obesity management. Drug therapy may be considered as an adjunct for patients who fail to achieve adequate weight loss after 6 months of diet, exercise, and behavioral modification. Currently, three products—orlistat, lorcaserin, and phentermine–topiramate extended release—are approved by the FDA for the long-term treatment of overweight and obesity. Bariatric procedures have evidence for long-term efficacy for weight reduction, but they also introduce surgical comorbidities and, for the most efficacious procedures, may cause significant nutritional deficiencies. Treatment of obesity should be individualized, considering factors such as patient desires, age, degree and duration of obesity, and the presence or absence of medical conditions both directly related to obesity and those that may have an impact on the therapeutic decisions. Regardless of the chosen treatment plan, the management of obesity is a lifelong process requiring patient support and careful monitoring for safety and efficacy.

ACKNOWLEDGMENT

This research was supported in part by the Intramural Research Program of the National Institute of Child Health and Human Development, National Institutes of Health.

ABBREVIATIONS

AHEAD	Action for Health in Diabetes
ATP III	Third Report of the Expert Panel on the Detection, Evaluation, and Treatment of High Blood Cholesterol in Adults
BLOOM	Behavioral Modification and Lorcaserin for Overweight and Obesity Management
BMI	Body mass index
BMR	basal metabolic rate
CNS	central nervous system
CT	computed tomography
FDA	Food and Drug Administration
5-HT	5-hydroxytryptamine (serotonin)
GI	gastrointestinal
HbA_{1c}	hemoglobin A_{1c}
HDL	high-density lipoprotein
LCD	low-calorie diet
LDL	low-density lipoprotein
MAOI	monoamine oxidase inhibitor
MRI	magnetic resonance imaging
NE	norepinephrine
NHANES	National Health and Nutrition Examination Survey
NIH	National Institutes of Health
REE	resting energy expenditure
REMS	risk evaluation and mitigation strategy
SCOUT	Sibutramine Cardiovascular OUTcomes
SF-36	Short Form 36
STORM	Sibutramine Trial of Obesity Reduction and Maintenance
WAGR	Wilms' tumor, aniridia, genitourinary abnormalities or gonadoblastoma, and mental retardation
XENDOS	XENical in the prevention of Diabetes in Obese Subjects
WC	waist circumference

REFERENCES

1. Flegal KM, Carroll MD, Kit BK, Ogden CL. Prevalence of obesity and trends in the distribution of body mass index among US Adults, 1999–2010. JAMA 2012;307(5):491–497.
2. Ogden CL, Yanovski SZ, Carroll MD, Flegal KM. The epidemiology of obesity. Gastroenterology 2007;132(6):2087–2102.
3. Ogden CL, Carroll MD, Kit BK, Flegal KM. Prevalence of obesity and trends in body mass index among US children and adolescents 1999–2010. JAMA 2012;307:483–490.
4. Wang Y, Beydoun MA, Liang L, Caballero B, Kumanyika SK. Will all Americans become overweight or obese? Estimating the progression and cost of the US obesity epidemic. Obesity 2008;16(10):2323–2330.
5. Picot J, Jones J, Colquitt JL, et al. The clinical effectiveness and cost-effectiveness of bariatric (weight loss) surgery for obesity: A systematic review and economic evaluation. Health Technol Assess 2009;13(41):1–190, 215–357, iii–iv.
6. U.S. Department of Health and Human Services. National Heart Lung and Blood Institute. Obesity Initiative Expert Panel on the Identification, Evaluation, and Treatment of Overweight and Obesity in Adults. Washington, DC: U.S. Public Health Service, 1998.
7. Anand RG, Peters RW, Donahue TP. Obesity and dysrhythmias. J Cardiometab Syndr 2008;3(3):149–154.
8. Anandacoomarasamy A, Caterson I, Sambrook P, Fransen M, March L. The impact of obesity on the musculoskeletal system. Int J Obes 2008;32(2):211–222.
9. Esposito K, Giugliano F, Ciotola M, De Sio M, D'Armiento M, Giugliano D. Obesity and sexual dysfunction, male and female. Int J Impot Res 2008;20(4):358–365.
10. Guh DP, Zhang W, Bansback N, Amarsi Z, Birmingham CL, Anis AH. The incidence of co-morbidities related to obesity and overweight: A systematic review and meta-analysis. BMC Public Health 2009;9:88.
11. Kushner RF, Roth JL. Assessment of the obese patient. Endocrinol Metab Clin North Am 2003;32(4):915–933.
12. Mathus-Vliegen EM, Nikkel D, Brand HS. Oral aspects of obesity. Int Dent J 2007;57(4):249–256.
13. Murugan AT, Sharma G. Obesity and respiratory diseases. Chron Respir Dis 2008;5(4):233–242.
14. Nguyen S, Hsu CY. Excess weight as a risk factor for kidney failure. Curr Opin Nephrol Hypertens 2007;16(2):71–76.
15. Pan SY, DesMeules M. Energy intake, physical activity, energy balance, and cancer: Epidemiologic evidence. Methods Mol Biol 2009;472:191–215.
16. Setty AR, Curhan G, Choi HK. Obesity, waist circumference, weight change, and the risk of psoriasis in women: Nurses' Health Study II. Arch Intern Med 2007;167(15):1670–1675.
17. Stothard KJ, Tennant PW, Bell R, Rankin J. Maternal overweight and obesity and the risk of congenital anomalies: A systematic review and meta-analysis. JAMA 2009;301(6):636–650.
18. Janssen I, Bacon E. Effect of current and midlife obesity status on mortality risk in the elderly. Obesity 2008;16(11):2504–2509.
19. Reis JP, Macera CA, Araneta MR, Lindsay SP, Marshall SJ, Wingard DL. Comparison of overall obesity and body fat distribution in predicting risk of mortality. Obesity 2009;17(6):1232–1239.
20. Trogdon JG Finkelstein EA, Feagan CW, Cohen JW. State- and payer-specific estimates of annual medical expenditures attributable to obesity. Obesity 2012;20(1):214–220.
21. U.S. Preventative Services Task Force. Screening and interventions for overweight in children and adolescents: Recommendations and rationale. Pediatrics 2005;116(1):205–209.
22. U.S. Department of Health and Human Services. Healthy People 2020 Summary of Objectives: Nutrition and Weight. *http://healthypeople.gov/2020/topicsobjectives2020/pdfs/NutritionandWeight.pdf.*
23. U.S. Department of Health and Human Services, NIH-NHLBI. Obesity Education Initiative. 2003, *http://www.nhlbi.nih.gov/about/oei/oei_pd.htm.*
24. Moyer VA. Screening for and management of obesity in adults: US Preventative Services Task Force Recommendation Statement. Ann Intern Med 2012;157 (5):373–378.
25. Institute of Medicine Committee on Prevention of Obesity in Children and Youth. Preventing Childhood Obesity: Health in the Balance. Washington, DC: National Academies Press, 2005.
26. Singh AS, Mulder C, Twisk JW, van Mechelen W, Chinapaw MJ. Tracking of childhood overweight into adulthood: A systematic review of the literature. Obes Rev 2008;9(5): 474–488.

27. Reilly JJ, Kelly J. Long-term impact of overweight and obesity in childhood and adolescence on morbidity and premature mortality in adulthood: Systematic review. Int J Obes 2011;35(7):891–898.
28. Robinson WR, Gordon-Larsen P, Kaufman JS, Suchindran CM, Stevens J. The female-male disparity in obesity prevalence among black American young adults: Contributions of sociodemographic characteristics of the childhood family. Am J Clin Nutr 2009;89(4):1204–1212.
29. Lee YS. The role of genes in the current obesity epidemic. Ann Acad Med Singapore 2009;38(1):45–43.
30. Rankinen T, Zuberi A, Chagnon YC, et al. The human obesity gene map: The 2005 update. Obesity 2006;14(4):529–644.
31. Frayling TM, Timpson NJ, Weedon MN, et al. A common variant in the FTO gene is associated with body mass index and predisposes to childhood and adult obesity. Science 2007;316(5826):889–894.
32. French SA, Story M, Jeffery RW. Environmental influences on eating and physical activity. Annu Rev Public Health 2001;22:309–335.
33. Hill JO, Peters JC. Environmental contributions to the obesity epidemic. Science 1998;280(5368):1371–1374.
34. Christakis NA, Fowler JH. The spread of obesity in a large social network over 32 years. N Engl J Med 2007;357(4):370–379.
35. Sheehan AH. Weight gain. In: Tisdale JE, Miller DA, eds. Drug-Induced Diseases: Prevention, Detection and Management, 2nd ed. Bethesda, MD: American Society of Health-System Pharmacists; 2010.
36. Dhillo WS. Appetite regulation: An overview. Thyroid 2007;17(5):433–445.
37. Valassi E, Scacchi M, Cavagnini F. Neuroendocrine control of food intake. Nutr Metab Cardiovasc Dis 2008;18(2): 158–168.
38. Farooqi IS, O'Rahilly S. Leptin: A pivotal regulator of human energy homeostasis. Am J Clin Nutr 2009;89(3):980S–984S.
39. Friedman JM. Leptin at 14 years of age: An ongoing story. Am J Clin Nutr 2009;89(3):973S–979S.
40. Small CJ, Bloom SR. Gut hormones and the control of appetite. Trends Endocrinol Metab 2004;15(6):259–263.
41. Cypess AM, Lehman S, Williams G, et al. Identification and importance of brown adipose tissue in adult humans. N Engl J Med 2009;360(15):1509–1517.
42. Gil A, Olza J, Gil-Campos M, Gomez-Llorente C, Aguilera CM. Is adipose tissue metabolically different at different sites? Int J Pediatr Obes 2011;6(Suppl 1):13–20.
43. Arner P, Hoffstedt J. Adrenoceptor genes in human obesity. J Intern Med 1999;245(6):667–672.
44. Clinical guidelines on the identification, evaluation, and treatment of overweight and obesity in adults: The Evidence Report. National Institutes of Health. Obes Res 1998; 6(Suppl 2):51S–209S.
45. Barlow SE and Expert Committee. Expert committee recommendations regarding the prevention, assessment, and treatment of child and adolescent overweight and obesity: Summary report. Pediatrics 2007;120(Suppl 4): S164–S192.
46. Carroll JF, Chiapa AL, Rodriquez M, et al. Visceral fat, waist circumference, and BMI: Impact of race/ethnicity. Obesity 2008;16(3):600–607.
47. Cheng CY, Reich D, Coresh J, et al. Admixture mapping of obesity-related traits in African Americans: The Atherosclerosis Risk in Communities (ARIC) Study. Obesity 2010;18(3):563–572.
48. Cossrow N, Falkner B. Race/ethnic issues in obesity and obesity-related comorbidities. J Clin Endocrinol Metab 2004;89(6):2590–2594.
49. Rahman M, Temple JR, Breitkopf CR, Berenson AB. Racial differences in body fat distribution among reproductive-aged women. Metabolism 2009;58(9):1329–1337.
50. Lee SY, Gallagher D. Assessment methods in human body composition. Curr Opin Clin Nutr Metab Care 2008;11(5): 566–572.
51. U.S. Department of Health and Human Services. National Heart Lung and Blood Institute: Clinical guidelines on the identification, evaluation, and treatment of overweight and obesity in adults–Practical guide. 2003, *http://www.nhlbi.nih.gov/guidelines/obesity/ob_home.htm.*
52. Pischon T, Boeing H, Hoffmann K, et al. General and abdominal adiposity and risk of death in Europe. N Engl J Med 2008;359(20):2105–2120.
53. Finkelstein EA, Brown DS, Wrage LA, Allaire BT, Hoerger TJ. Individual and aggregate years-of-life-lost associated with overweight and obesity. Obesity 2010;18(2):333–339.
54. Hubert HB, Feinleib M, McNamara PM, Castelli WP. Obesity as an independent risk factor for cardiovascular disease: A 26-year follow-up of participants in the Framingham Heart Study. Circulation 1983;67(5): 968–977.
55. Poirier P, Giles TD, Bray GA, et al. Obesity and cardiovascular disease: Pathophysiology, evaluation, and effect of weight loss–An update of the 1997 American Heart Association Scientific Statement on Obesity and Heart Disease from the Obesity Committee of the Council on Nutrition, Physical Activity, and Metabolism. Circulation 2006;113(6):898–918.
56. Poirier P, Giles TD, Bray GA, et al. Obesity and cardiovascular disease: Pathophysiology, evaluation, and effect of weight loss. Arterioscler Thromb Vasc Biol 2006;26(5):968–976.
57. Rai MF, Sandell LJ. Inflammatory mediators: Tracing links between obesity and osteoarthritis. Crit Rev Eukaryot Gene Expr 2011;21(2):131–142.
58. Vrbikova J, Hainer V. Obesity and polycystic ovary syndrome. Obesity Facts 2009;2:26–35.
59. Gregg EW, Gerzoff RB, Thompson TJ, Williamson DF. Trying to lose weight, losing weight, and 9-year mortality in overweight U.S. adults with diabetes. Diabetes Care 2004; 27(3):657–662.
60. Klein S, Sheard NF, Pi-Sunyer X, et al. Weight management through lifestyle modification for the prevention and management of type 2 diabetes: Rationale and strategies. A statement of the American Diabetes Association, the North American Association for the Study of Obesity, and the American Society for Clinical Nutrition. Diabetes Care 2004;27(8):2067–2073.
61. Wing RR, Lang W, Wadden TA, et al. Benefits of modest weight loss in improving cardiovascular risk factors in overweight and obese individuals with type 2 diabetes. Diabetes Care 2011;34(7):1481–1486.
62. Johnson WD, Brashear MM, Gupta AK, Rood JC, Ryan DH. Incremental weight loss improves cardiometabolic risk in extremely obese adults. Am J Med 2011;24(10): 931–938.
63. NIH News. National Institute of Diabetes and Digestive and Kidney Diseases. Weight loss does not lower heart disease risk of type 2 diabetes. *http://www.nih.gov/news/health/oct2012/niddk-19.htm.*
64. Third report of the National Cholesterol Education Program (NCEP) Expert Panel on Detection, Evaluation, and Treatment of High Blood Cholesterol in Adults

(Adult Treatment Panel III) final report. Circulation 2002;106(25):3143–3421.
65. Gardner CD, Kiazand A, Alhassan S, et al. Comparison of the Atkins, Zone, Ornish, and LEARN diets for change in weight and related risk factors among overweight premenopausal women: The A TO Z Weight Loss Study–A randomized trial. JAMA 2007;297(9):969–977.
66. Nordmann AJ, Nordmann A, Briel M, et al. Effects of low-carbohydrate vs low-fat diets on weight loss and cardiovascular risk factors: A meta-analysis of randomized controlled trials. Arch Intern Med 2006;166(3):285–293.
67. Sacks FM, Bray GA, Carey VJ, et al. Comparison of weight-loss diets with different compositions of fat, protein, and carbohydrates. N Engl J Med 2009;360(9): 859–873.
68. Franz MJ, VanWormer JJ, Crain AL, et al. Weight-loss outcomes: A systematic review and meta-analysis of weight-loss clinical trials with a minimum 1-year follow-up. J Am Diet Assoc 2007;107(10):1755–1767.
69. Shaw K, Gennat H, O'Rourke P, Del Mar C. Exercise for overweight or obesity. Cochrane Database Syst Rev 2006;(4):CD003817.
70. Donnelly JE, Blair SN, Jakicic JM, et al. American College of Sports Medicine Position Stand. Appropriate physical activity intervention strategies for weight loss and prevention of weight regain for adults. Med Sci Sports Exerc 2009;41(2):459–471.
71. Trus TL, Pope GD, Finlayson SR. National trends in utilization and outcomes of bariatric surgery. Surg Endosc 2005;19(5):616–620.
72. Dumon KR, Murayama KM. Bariatric surgery outcomes. Surg Clin North Am 2011;91(6):1313–1338.
73. Hinojosa MW, Varela JE, Parikh D, et al. National trends in use and outcome of laparoscopic adjustable gastric banding. Surg Obes Relat Dis 2009;5(2):150–155.
74. Mechanick JI, Kushner RF, Sugerman HJ, et al. American Association of Clinical Endocrinologists, the Obesity Society, and the American Society for Metabolic and Bariatric Surgery medical guidelines for clinical practice for the perioperative nutritional, metabolic, and nonsurgical support of the bariatric surgery patient. Obesity 2009;17(Suppl 1):S1–S70.
75. Rubino F, Kaplan LM, Schauer PR, Cummings DE; Diabetes Surgery Summit Delegates. The Diabetes Surgery Summit consensus conference: Recommendations for the evaluation and use of gastrointestinal surgery to treat type 2 diabetes mellitus. Ann Surg 2010;251(3):399–405.
76. Flum DR, Belle SH, King WC, et al. Perioperative safety in the longitudinal assessment of bariatric surgery. N Engl J Med 2009;361(5):445–454.
77. Heber D, Greenway FL, Kaplan LM, Livingston E, Salvador J, Still C; Endocrine Society. Endocrine and nutritional management of the post-bariatric surgery patient: An Endocrine Society Clinical Practice Guideline. J Clin Endocrinol Metab 2010;95(11):4823–4843.
78. Schauer PR, Kashyap SR, Wolski K, et al. Bariatric surgery versus intensive medical therapy in obese patients with diabetes. N Engl J Med 2012;366(17): 1567–1576.
79. Buchwald H, Estok R, Fahrbach K, et al. Weight and type 2 diabetes after bariatric surgery: Systematic review and meta-analysis. Am J Med 2009;122(3):248–256.
80. Mingrone G, Panunzi S, De Gaetano A, et al. Bariatric surgery versus conventional medical therapy for type 2 diabetes. N Engl J Med 2012;366(17): 1577–1585.
81. Dirksen C, Jørgensen NB, Bojsen-Møller KN, et al. Mechanisms of improved glycaemic control after Roux-en-Y gastric bypass. Diabetologia 2012;55(7):1890–901.
82. Sjöström L, Gummesson A, Sjöström CD, et al. Effects of bariatric surgery on cancer incidence in obese patients in Sweden (Swedish Obese Subjects Study): A prospective, controlled intervention trial. Lancet Oncol 2009;10(7): 653–662.
83. Sjöström L, Peltonen M, Jacobson P, et al. Bariatric surgery and long-term cardiovascular events. JAMA 2012;307(1): 56–65.
84. Sjostrom L, Narbro K, Sjostrom CD, et al. Effects of bariatric surgery on mortality in Swedish obese subjects. N Engl J Med 2007;357(8):741–752.
85. Miller AD, Smith KM. Medication and nutrient administration considerations after bariatric surgery. Am J Health Syst Pharm 2006;63(19):1852–1857.
86. Padwal R, Brocks D, Sharma AM. A systematic review of drug absorption following bariatric surgery and its theoretical implications. Obes Rev 2010;11(1):41–50.
87. Rogers CC, Alloway RR, Alexander JW, Cardi M, Trofe J, Vinks AA. Pharmacokinetics of mycophenolic acid, tacrolimus and sirolimus after gastric bypass surgery in end-stage renal disease and transplant patients: A pilot study. Clin Transplant 2008;22(3):281–291.
88. Yanovski SZ. Pharmacotherapy for obesity: Promise and uncertainty. N Engl J Med 2005;353(20):2187–2189.
89. McClendon KS, Riche DM, Uwaifo GI. Orlistat: Current status in clinical therapeutics. Expert Opin Drug Saf 2009;8(6):727–744.
90. Anderson JW. Orlistat for the management of overweight individuals and obesity: A review of potential for the 60-mg, over-the-counter dosage. Expert Opin Pharmacother 2007;8(11):1733–1742.
91. Rucker D, Padwal R, Li SK, Curioni C, Lau DC. Long term pharmacotherapy for obesity and overweight: Updated meta-analysis. BMJ 2007;335(7631):1194–1199.
92. Torgerson JS, Hauptman J, Boldrin MN, Sjostrom L. XENical in the prevention of diabetes in obese subjects (XENDOS) study: A randomized study of orlistat as an adjunct to lifestyle changes for the prevention of type 2 diabetes in obese patients. Diabetes Care 2004;27(1): 155–161.
93. Filippatos TD, Derdemezis CS, Gazi IF, Nakou ES, Mikhailidis DP, Elisaf MS. Orlistat-associated adverse effects and drug interactions: A critical review. Drug Saf 2008;31(1):53–65.
94. FDA Drug Safety Communication: Completed safety review of Xenical/Alli (orlistat) and severe liver injury. 2010, *http://www.fda.gov/Drugs/DrugSafety/PostmarketDrugSafetyInformationforPatientsandProviders/ucm213038.htm?utm_campaign=Google2&utm_source=fdaSearch&utm_medium=website&utm_term=Early communication about an ongoing safety review of orlistat&utm_content=2*.
95. Belviq® [package insert]. Zofingen, Switzerland: Arena Pharmaceuticals, 2012.
96. Smith SR, Weissman NJ, Anderson CM, et al. Multicenter, placebo-controlled trial of lorcaserin for weight management. N Engl J Med 2010;363:245–256.
97. Fidler MC, Sanchez M, Raether B, Weissman NJ, et al. A one-year randomized trial of lorcaserin for weight loss in obese and overweight adults: The BLOSSOM trial. J Clin Endocrinol Metab 2011;96(10):3067–3077.
98. O'Neil PM, Smith SR, Weissman NJ, et al. Randomized placebo-controlled clinical trial of lorcaserin for weight loss

in type 2 diabetes mellitus: The BLOOM-DM study. Obesity 2012;20(7):1426–1436.

99. Halford JC, Boyland EJ, Lawton CL, et al. Serotonergic anti-obesity agents: Past experience and future prospects. Drugs 2011;71(17):2247–2255.
100. Qsymia™ [package insert]. Mountain View, CA: Vivus Inc, 2012.
101. Gadde KM, Allison DB, Ryan DH, Peterson CA, et al. Effects of low-dose, controlled-release, phentermine plus topiramate combination on weight and associated comorbidities in overweight and obese adults (CONQUER): A randomized, placebo-controlled, phase 3 trial. Lancet 2011;377:1341–1352.
102. Allison DB, Gadde KM, Garvey WT, et al. Controlled-release phentermine/topiramate in severely obese adults: A randomized controlled trial (EQUIP). Obesity 2012;20(2)330–342.
103. Bray GA, Greenway FL. Current and potential drugs for treatment of obesity. Endocr Rev 1999;20(6):805–875.
104. Silverstone T. Appetite suppressants: A review. Drugs 1992;43(6):820–836.
105. Adipex-P (phentermine hydrochloride) product information. Sellersville, PA: Teva Pharmaceuticals, 2005.
106. Hendricks EJ, Rothman RB, Greenway FL. How physician obesity specialists use drugs to treat obesity. Obesity 2009;17(9):1730–1735.
107. Li Z, Maglione M, Tu W, et al. Meta-analysis: pharmacologic treatment of obesity. *Ann Intern Med.* 2005;142(7):532–546.
108. Halford JC, Harrold JA, Boyland EJ, Lawton CL, Blundell JE. Serotonergic drugs: Effects on appetite expression and use for the treatment of obesity. Drugs 2007;67(1):27–55.
109. Ye Z, Chen L, Yang Z, et al. Metabolic effects of fluoxetine in adults with type 2 diabetes mellitus: A meta-analysis of randomized placebo-controlled trials. PLoS One 2011; 6(7):e21551.
110. Bostwick JM, Brown TM. A toxic reaction from combining fluoxetine and phentermine. J Clin Psychopharmacol 1996;16(2):189–190.
111. Anchors M. Fluoxetine is a safer alternative to fenfluramine in the medical treatment of obesity. Arch Intern Med 1997;157(11):1270.
112. Whigham LD, Dhurandhar NV, Rahko PS, Atkinson RL. Comparison of combinations of drugs for treatment of obesity: Body weight and echocardiographic status. Int J Obes 2007;31(5):850–857.
113. James WP, Astrup A, Finer N, et al. Effect of sibutramine on weight maintenance after weight loss: A randomised trial. STORM Study Group. Sibutramine Trial of Obesity Reduction and Maintenance. Lancet 2000;356(9248):2119–2125.
114. James WPT, Caterson ID, Coutinho W, et al. Effect of sibutramine on cardiovascular outcomes in overweight and obese subjects. N Engl J Med 2010;363(10):905–917.
115. Pillitteri JL, Shiffman S, Rohay JM, et al. Use of dietary supplements for weight loss in the United States: results of a national survey. Obesity 2008;16(4):790–796.
116. Cohen PA. American roulette: Contaminated dietary supplements. N Engl J Med 2009;361(16):1523–1525.
117. United States Food and Drug Administration. Dietary Supplement Alerts and Safety Information. *http://www.fda.gov/Food/DietarySupplements/Alerts/default.htm2*.
118. Haaz S, Fontaine KR, Cutter G, Limdi N, Perumean-Chaney S, Allison DB. Citrus aurantium and synephrine alkaloids in the treatment of overweight and obesity: An update. Obes Rev 2006;7(1):79–88.
119. Lukaski HC, Siders WA, Penland JG. Chromium picolinate supplementation in women: Effects on body weight, composition, and iron status. Nutrition 2007;23(3):187–195.
120. Yazaki Y, Faridi Z, Ma Y, et al. A pilot study of chromium picolinate for weight loss. J Altern Complement Med 2010; 16(3):291–299.
121. Jull AB, Ni Mhurchu C, Bennet DA, Dunshea-Mooij CA, Rodgers A. Chitosan for overweight or obesity. Cochrane Database Syst Rev 2008;(3):CD003892.
122. Betz JM, Gay ML, Mossoba MM, Adams S, Portz BS. Chiral gas chromatographic determination of ephedrine-type alkaloids in dietary supplements containing Ma Huang. J AOAC Int 1997;80(2):303–315.
123. Haller CA, Benowitz NL. Adverse cardiovascular and central nervous system events associated with dietary supplements containing ephedra alkaloids. N Engl J Med 2000;343(25): 1833–1838.
124. Department of Health and Human Services, Food and Drug Administration. Final rule declaring dietary supplements containing ephedrine alkaloids adulterated because they present an unreasonable risk. Fed Regist 2004;69(28):6787–6854.
125. Clauson KA, Shields KM, McQueen CE, Persad N. Safety issues associated with commercially available energy drinks. J Am Pharm Assoc 2008;48(3):e55–e63.
126. Van Heerden FR. Hoodia gordonii: A natural appetite suppressant. J Ethnopharmacol 2008;119(3):434–437.
127. Blom WA, Abrahamse SL, Bradford R, et al. Effects of 15-d repeated consumption of Hoodia gordonii purified extract on safety, ad libitum energy intake, and body weight in healthy, overweight women: A randomized controlled trial. Am J Clin Nutr 2011;94(5):1171–1181.
128. Koh-Banerjee PK, Ferreira MP, Greenwood M, et al. Effects of calcium pyruvate supplementation during training on body composition, exercise capacity, and metabolic responses to exercise. Nutrition 2005;21(3):312–319.
129. Pittler MH, Ernst E. Dietary supplements for body-weight reduction: A systematic review. Am J Clin Nutr 2004;79(4): 529–536.
130. Astrup A, Madsbad S, Breum L, et al. Effect of tesofensine on bodyweight loss, body composition, and quality of life in obese patients: A randomized, double-blind, placebo-controlled trial. Lancet 2008;372(9653):1906–1913.
131. Kopelman P, Groot G, Rissanen A, et al. Weight loss, HbA_{1C} reduction, and tolerability of cetilistat in a randomized, placebo-controlled phase 2 trial in obese diabetics: Comparison with orlistat (Xenical). Obesity 2010;18(1):108–115.
132. Kirilly E, Gonda X, Bagdy, G. CB1 receptor antagonists: New discoveries leading to new perspectives. Acta Physiol 2012;205(1):41–60
133. Klonoff DC, Greenway F. Drugs in the pipeline for the obesity market. J Diabetes Sci Technol 2008;2(5):913–918.
134. Choquet H, Meyre D. Genetics of obesity: What have we learned? Curr Genomics. 2011;12(3):169–179.
135. Farooqi IS, Matarese G, Lord GM, et al. Beneficial effects of leptin on obesity, T cell hyporesponsiveness, and neuroendocrine/metabolic dysfunction of human congenital leptin deficiency. J Clin Invest 2002;110(8):1093–103.
136. National Heart Lung and Blood Institute. Obesity Education Initiative. 1991, *http://www.nhlbi.nih.gov/about/oei*.

Glossary

2,3-Bisphosphoglycerate: An intermediate in the Rapoport-Luebering shunt, formed between 1,3-bisphosphoglycerate and 3-phosphoglycerate; an important regulator of the affinity of hemoglobin for oxygen.

5-α-Reductase: Enzyme responsible for conversion of testosterone to its active metabolite dihydrotesterone. Two types of this enzyme exist. Type 2 is predominant in prostate cells.

α-Amino-3-hydroxy-5-methyl-4 isoxazolepropionate (AMPA)/kainate receptors: Two of three types of ionotropic post-synaptic glutamate receptors. These receptors are similar and are often considered together. Upon binding glutamate, these receptors permit the influx of Na^+ ions and result in brain excitation. These are one of the two primary receptors for excitatory neurotransmission in the brain.

α-Amino-3-hydroxy-5-methylisoxazole-4-propionate: See *AMPA*.

α-Hydroxy acids: Exfoliating products such as lactic, glycolic, malic, mandelic, and tartaric acid used in cosmetics.

β-Hydroxy acid: Salicylic acid.

γ-Aminobutyric acid (GABA): The major inhibitory neurotransmitter in the central nervous system.

γ-Aminobutyric acid ($GABA_A$) receptors: Postsynaptic ionotropic receptors that bind to GABA and result in Cl^- influx and neuronal hyperpolarization. GABA is the main inhibitory neurotrasmitter in the brain and $GABA_A$ receptors mediate fast CNS inhibitory neurotransmission.

Abscess: A purulent collection of fluid separated from surrounding tissue by a wall comprised of inflammatory cells and adjacent organs. It usually contains necrotic debris, bacteria, and inflammatory cells.

Abstinence: Refraining from the indulgence in something, as sexual intercourse or substances, by one's own choice. The absence of genital contact that could permit a pregnancy (i.e., penile penetration into the vagina).

Acanthosis: Increased thickness of the prickle cell layer of the skin.

Acculturation: The process by which individuals from one cultural group adopt or change behaviors, attitudes, and/or beliefs through contact with a different culture.

Acetabular: Relating to the acetabulum, the hollow, cuplike portion of the pelvis into which the head of the thigh bone (femur) fits.

Achalasia: Problem that occurs when a ring of muscle fibers, such as a sphincter of the esophagus, fail to relax.

Acne: Inflammatory eruption of the sebaceous gland.

Acnegenicity: Product effect that causes irritation of follicles resulting in papules and pustules.

Acquired resistance: See *Secondary resistance*.

Acromegaly: A pathologic condition characterized by excessive production of growth hormone.

Activities of daily living: Dressing, bathing, getting around inside the home, feeding, toileting, and grooming. See also *Instrumental activities of daily living*.

Acute bacterial pharyngitis: Acute bacterial infection of the oropharynx or nasopharynx.

Acute bacterial sinusitis: Acute bacterial infection of the paranasal sinuses lasting less than 30 days.

Acute coronary syndrome (ACS): Ischemic chest discomfort at rest most often accompanied by ST-segment elevation, ST-segment depression, or T-wave inversion on the 12-lead electrocardiogram; further, it is caused by plaque rupture and partial or complete occlusion of the coronary artery by thrombus. Acute coronary syndromes include myocardial infarction and unstable angina. Former terms used to describe types of ACS include Q-wave myocardial infarction, non–Q-wave myocardial infarction, and unstable angina.

Acute kidney injury (AKI): Abrupt decrease in kidney function resulting in an increase in serum creatinine and/or decrease in urine output. AKI is usually classified as prerenal, instrinsic, or postrenal type.

Acute otitis media: Acute inflammation of the middle ear.

Acute pain: Can be a useful physiologic process warning individuals of disease states and potentially harmful situations. Severe, unremitting, undertreated, acute pain, when it outlives its biologic usefulness, can produce many deleterious effects (e.g., psychological problems). It usually subsides when the healing process decreases the pain-producing stimuli.

Acute pancreatitis: Acute inflammation of the pancreas that can be mild with minimal or no organ dysfunction or severe with organ failure and local complications.

Acute stress disorder: A disorder characterized by anxiety, dissociative, and other symptoms that occurs within 1 month after exposure to an extreme traumatic stressor.

Adaptive functioning: Individual effectiveness coping with everyday stressors compared to a peer with similar background, and socioeconomic and psychosocial opportunities.

Adaptive inflammation: Inflammatory pain that promotes the shifting from prevention of tissue damage to promotion of healing.

Addiction: A primary, chronic, neurobiologic disease, with genetic, psychosocial, and environmental factors influencing its development and manifestations. It is characterized by behaviors that include one or more of the following five Cs: *c*hronicity, impaired *c*ontrol over drug use, *c*ompulsive use, *c*ontinued use despite harm, and *c*raving.

Adjuvant analgesics: Agents that are useful in the treatment of pain but are usually not classified as analgesics.

Adjuvant therapy: Any therapy administered after primary surgical resection of the tumor or cancer, with the intent to eradicate micrometastes and cure the disease.

Administrative burden: The demands placed on those who administer an instrument.

Adolescents: Pediatric patients who are 12 to 16 years of age.

Adoptive immunotherapy: Administration of immune cells for the treatment of cancer.

Adrenergic: Neuronal or neurologic activity caused by neurotransmitters such as epinephrine, norepinephrine, and dopamine.

Adrenocorticotropic hormone (ACTH): A polypeptide hormone secreted by the anterior pituitary that controls secretion of cortisol from the adrenal glands.

Adverse drug events: Injuries resulting from administration of a drug or other circumstances surrounding use of the drug but not necessarily caused by the drug itself. See also *Adverse drug reaction*.

Adverse drug reaction: Any noxious, unintended, and undesired effect of a drug that occurs at doses used in humans for prophylaxis, diagnosis, or therapy.

Aerophagia: Excessive swallowing of air.

Affect: Pattern of behaviors that a clinician can observe that expresses a person's current state of emotion.

Afterload: The pressure or the "load" the heart must generate to eject blood into the systemic circulation. Although approximated by the systemic vascular resistance, it is a complex measure that includes blood viscosity, aortic impedance, and ventricular wall thickness. Along with preload, it is an important determinant of cardiac output.

Aganglionosis: The state of being without ganglia.

Agnosia: Cardinal symptom of Alzheimer's disease; inability to recognize or identify a familiar object in the absence of impaired sensory function.

Agoraphobia: Anxiety about, or avoidance of, places or situations from which escape might be difficult (or embarrassing) or in which help might not be available in the event of having a panic attack or panic-like symptoms.

Akathisia: The sensation of inner restlessness resulting in the need to make movements such as pacing or moving the legs. Akathisia has subjective and objective components.

Albumin: The major protein in plasma, with a molecular weight of 65 kDa.

Albuminuria: A condition where a large amount of albumin (>300 mg/day) is present in the urine, often indicating glomerular damage in the kidney.

Alcohol ablation: Alcohol ablation of the septum is a nonsurgical procedure to improve outflow tract obstruction. It is a percutaneous catheter-based method to decrease septal thickness by therapeutic myocardial infarction.

Alcoholism: A chronic, progressive, and potentially fatal biogenic and psychosocial disease characterized by tolerance and physical dependence and manifested by a total loss of control, as well as diverse personality changes and social consequences.

Algorithm (treatment algorithm): Identifies and specifies sequences for treatment alternatives, with specific options and tactics for care. Based on scientific data and on expert consensus in areas where there are little scientific data, algorithms are divided into stages so that the simplest, most efficacious, and best-tolerated treatments available are tried first. If results are not optimal, treatment advances to the next stage. Unless a patient's illness fails to improve sufficiently with early-stage treatments, he or she is spared treatments that are more complex, that might be less well tolerated, or that have more potential for drug interactions or serious side effects. Algorithms recommend key decision points in treatment decision making.

Allergic interstitial nephritis: Inflammation of the interstitial region of the kidney often associated with acute onset of renal insufficiency.

Allergic salute: Constant upward rubbing of the nose as a result of allergies.

Allergic shiners: Dark circles under the eyes as a result of nasal congestion leading to venous pooling.

Allodynia: Painful response to normally non-noxious stimuli.

Allogeneic transplantation: Transfer of cells between genetically nonidentical individuals.

Allograft: An organ or tissue transplant from one human being to another.

Allokinesis: A phenomenon whereby pruritic skin affects the surrounding normally nonpruritic skin area, whether inflamed or noninflamed. The nonpruritic skin becomes very sensitive, reacts to light stimuli, and begins itching.

Alloimmunization: Rapid consumption of transfused platelets through an immune-mediated reaction.

Alternate forms: All modes of administration other than the mode for which the instrument was originally developed.

Amenorrhea: Lack of menstruation or the abnormal ending of the female menstrual cycle.

American Urological Association (AUA) Symptom Index: A validated questionnaire of seven questions that can be used by patients to assess the bothersomeness of their voiding symptoms. The total score range is 0 to 35. Higher scores are consistent with severely bothersome symptoms.

Amnesia: A pathologic impairment of memory.

AMPA/kainate receptors: Two of three types of ionotropic postsynaptic glutamate receptors. These receptors are similar and are often considered together. On binding glutamate, these receptors permit the influx of sodium ions (Na^+) and results in brain excitation. These are one of the two primary receptors for excitatory neurotransmission in the brain.

Amygdala: A small almond-shaped temporal lobe structure that plays a role in emotions and fear control.

Anaphylactoid: Anaphylaxis-like reactions that do not involve immunoglobulin E (IgE)-mediated mechanisms.

Anaphylaxis: Acute, life-threatening allergic reaction involving multiple organ systems.

Anastomosis: The surgical connection of two tubular structures, such as blood vessels, in a transplanted organ.

Andropause: Refers to a number of symptoms associated with decreased testosterone production by the testes in aging men. The symptoms include decreased libido, increased body fat, depressed mood, and osteoporosis. The symptoms of andropause generally worsen as the patient ages. Andropause in men parallels menopause in women.

Anemia of chronic disease: Mild-to-moderate anemia not associated with blood loss or hemolysis. Usually with normal cell size. Can be seen with chronic inflammation (e.g., rheumatoid arthritis, chronic infection) or malignancy.

Anemia of chronic kidney disease: A decrease in red blood cell production caused by a deficiency in the hormone erythropoietin normally produced by progenitor cells of the kidney. As kidney function declines, less erythropoietin is available to stimulate red blood cell production (erythropoiesis) in the bone marrow. Contributing factors include iron deficiency and a shortened, red blood cell life span.

Aneuploid: Deviation by a whole number in the total number of chromosomes in a cell compared to normal (46 in humans).

Angioedema: An allergic reaction characterized by edema of a tissue such as the lips, eyes, mouth, joints, or other structures because of leak of fluid from blood vessels.

Anhedonia: A lack of pleasure or interest in usual activities.

Anisocytosis: Considerable variation in the size of cells that are normally uniform, especially with reference to red blood cells.

Ankylosis: Bony fusion resulting from chronic joint inflammation.

Anomia: Cardinal symptom of Alzheimer's disease; inability to name objects or to recognize names.

Anorexia nervosa: A psychiatric disorder in which patients present with a fear of being obese. These patients often express a dislike or lack of interest in food; it is most common in young females and can disrupt normal menstrual cycles. It is associated with poor medication treatment response and can result in fatal medical complications.

Anosognosia: Lack of self-awareness or ignorance, real or feigned, of the presence of disease.

Antenatal: Time between conception and birth; same as prenatal.

Anterograde amnesia: Inability to remember events or actions that occur after taking a sedative hypnotic medication.

Antibiogram: A summary of antimicrobial susceptibilities.

Anticipatory anxiety: The fear of having an anxiety attack, which is often a trigger by itself; "fear of fear."

Anticoagulant: Any substance that inhibits, suppresses, or delays the formation of blood clots. These substances occur naturally and regulate the clotting cascade. Several anticoagulants have been identified in a variety of animal tissues and have been commercially developed for medicinal use.

Antigenic drift: The creation of antigenic variants by point mutations in the surface antigens, hemagglutinin and/or neuraminidase, of a particular subtype of influenza.

Antigenic shift: Occurs when an influenza virus acquires a new hemagglutinin and/or neuraminidase.

Antimicrobial cycling: A predetermined change in an antimicrobial recommendation for empiric therapy of a specific infection at a predetermined time.

Antimycotic: Inhibiting fungal growth.

Antithrombotic: A pharmacologic agent that prevents thrombus/clot formation. This category includes both antiplatelet agents and anticoagulants.

Anuria: Production of less than 50 mL of urine/day.

Anxiety: A state of apprehension, uncertainty, and fear resulting from the anticipation of a realistic or fantasized threatening event or situation that often impairs physical and psychological functioning.

Aortic stenosis: Aortic stenosis is the obstruction of blood flow across the aortic valve. This disorder has several etiologies: congenital unicuspid or bicuspid valve, rheumatic fever, and degenerative calcific changes of the valve.

Aphasia: Cardinal symptom of Alzheimer's disease; inability to generate or comprehend spoken language.

Aphthous ulcer: A small superficial area of ulceration within the gastrointestinal mucosa, typically found in the oral cavity.

Apical pulse: Point at the apex (bottom portion) of the heart impacts the chest wall.

Apoptosis: Programmed cell death.

Appendageal: Referring to hair, sweat glands, and nails.

Apraxia: Cardinal symptom of Alzheimer's disease; inability to carry out a motor task in the absence of impaired motor function.

Aromatase: Enzyme responsible for conversion of estrogens (estradiol and estrone) to androgens (androstenedione and testosterone).

Arteriovenous (AV) fistula: In hemodialysis, a vascular access surgically created by connection of an artery directly to a vein, usually in the forearm.

Arteriovenous (AV) graft: In hemodialysis, a vascular access surgically created using a synthetic tube to connect an artery to a vein.

Arteriovenous malformations: A tangle of blood vessels, both arterial and venous, that can rupture and cause hemorrhage in the brain.

Arthrodesis: The surgical immobilization of a joint (i.e., joint fusion).

Arthropathy: Disease of the joints.

Ascites: Accumulation of serous fluid in the peritoneal cavity.

Asherman's syndrome: A cause for menstrual flow obstruction; often resulting from infection or surgery affecting the endometrium.

Asperger's disorder: A type of pervasive developmental disorder characterized by severe and sustained impairment in social interaction, restricted and repetitive patterns of behavioral/interested activities—similar to autism but without clinically significant delays in language and cognitive development or age-appropriate self-help skills.

Aspiration pneumonitis: The inflammation of lung tissue caused by the aspiration of fluids and gastric contents that often leads to dyspnea, pulmonary edema, secondary infections, and adult respiratory distress syndrome. Hydrocarbon pneumonitis is caused by the pulmonary aspiration of hydrocarbons such as kerosene and gasoline.

Assertive community treatment: A treatment program for the care of individuals with schizophrenia in which teams provide comprehensive wraparound services for the patient, including going to the home to provide support for daily living skills, housing, and supported employment. Team members are available 24 hours daily if needed to meet the patient's comprehensive care needs.

Asystole: The presence of a flat line on the electrocardiogram monitor.

Ataxia: Loss of the ability to coordinate muscular movement.

Atelectasis: Pulmonary parenchymal collapse caused by alveolar or bronchial obstruction.

Atopic dermatitis: Skin inflammation that causes itching, scales, and erythema.

Atopic pleat (Dennie–Morgan fold): An extra fold of skin that develops under the eye, characteristic of atopic dermatitis.

Atopy: An allergic syndrome characterized by asthma, hay fever, and urticaria or eczema.

Atrial fibrillation: Rapid beating of the atria that results in variable ventricular rates.

Atropinism: Symptoms of poisoning by atropine or belladonna.

Aura: Sensory or somatosensory alteration without loss of consciousness.

Augmentation: Addition of a medication not usually used as monotherapy for a disorder to a core medication for a disorder in an attempt to enhance the patient's clinical response.

Auscultation: Listening to the heart or other organs with a stethoscope.

Autism/Autistic disorder: A type of pervasive developmental disorder with a neurobiologic etiology, characterized by impaired reciprocal social interaction, impaired communication skills, and a limited range of activities and interests; frequently associated with mental retardation; sometimes referred to as early infantile autism, childhood autism, or Kanner autism.

Autologous transplantation: Readministration of the same person's cells that were previously collected.

Autosomal: Pertaining to a chromosome.

Axonal transaction: Destroying or severing the axon so that electrical impulses are impeded along the nerve sheath or across the nerve synapse. Axonal damage is not reversible and leads to long-term disability and the formation of black holes.

Azotemia: Term referring to elevated levels of urea in the serum or blood.

Azotorrhea: An excessive loss of protein in the feces.

Bacteremia: Presence of viable bacteria (fungi) in the bloodstream.

Bacterial prostatitis: An inflammation of the prostate gland and surrounding tissue as a result of infection.

Bacteriuria: The presence of bacteria in the urine.

Barrett esophagus: Inflammatory changes in the esophagus resulting in replacement of epithelial lining by columnar-type cells that can lead to stricture or adenocarcinoma.

Basal ganglia and striatum: Parts of the brain regulating movements.

Behavioral phenotype: The actions or reactions of a person to internal or external environmental influences.

Benign prostatic hyperplasia: Nonmalignant enlargement of the prostate gland in elderly men.

Bilateral salpingo-oophorectomy: Surgical excision (removal) of both ovaries.

Biliverdin: A green bile pigment formed from the oxidation of heme.

Binge eating: Excessive intake of calorie-laden food over a short period of time.

Bioavailability: The fraction of drug absorbed into the systemic circulation after extravascular administration.

Biochemical markers: Intracellular macromolecules released into the peripheral circulation from necrotic myocytes as a result of myocardial cell death (infarction). These laboratory tests are used in the diagnosis of myocardial infarction. Examples include troponin I, troponin T, creatinine kinase myocardial band (MB), and myoglobin.

Biofilm: A population or community of microorganisms adhering to a surface by a secreted coating. This coating also reduces microorganism vulnerability to antibiotics.

Biopsy: A procedure in which a tiny piece of a body part, such as the kidney or bladder, is removed for examination under a microscope.

Bioterrorism agents: Organisms or toxins that can cause disease and death in humans, animals, or plants for the purpose of eliciting terror.

Bipolar I disorder: Characterized by one or more manic episodes. The manic episode may have been preceded by and may be followed by hypomanic or major depressive episodes.

Bipolar II disorder: Characterized by at least one hypomanic episode and at least one major depressive episode.

Bleeding diathesis: A condition in which there is an unusual susceptibility or predisposition to bleeding.

Blood urea nitrogen (BUN): A waste product in the blood that comes from the breakdown of food protein. The kidneys filter blood to remove urea and thus maintain homeostasis. As kidney function decreases, the BUN level increases.

Blood–brain barrier: The relative lack of permeability of large molecules (and those molecules lacking lipid solubility) into the central nervous system because of the nonfenestrated capillary beds of the cerebral vasculature.

Borborygmi: Rumbling or gurgling noises produced by movement of gas, fluid, or both in the alimentary canal and audible at a distance.

Brachytherapy: A procedure in which radioactive material sealed in needles, seeds, wires, or catheters is placed directly into or near a tumor. Also called internal radiation, implant radiation, or interstitial radiation therapy.

Bradykinesia: Delay or slowness in initiating and performing purposeful, voluntary movement as seen in Parkinsonism.

Breakthrough bleeding: The unpredictable and irregular bleeding associated with hormone therapy.

Bronchiectasis: Dilation of a bronchus or bronchi, usually related to excessive secretions.

Bronchioles: A subdivision of bronchi; smaller in diameter and without cartilage.

Bronchiolitis: Inflammation of the bronchioles.

Bronchoalveolar lavage: Instilling and then removing a lavage fluid to reveal the secretory and/or cellular contents from deep in the lung.

Bronchorrhea: Excessive bronchial secretions that can impair pulmonary ventilation.

Bruit: An abnormal and often harsh sound heard over a blood vessel, usually an artery, on examination with a stethoscope caused by turbulent blood flow.

B-type natriuretic peptide: B-type natriuretic peptide is a 32-amino-acid polypeptide secreted by the ventricles in response to excessive myocyte stretching. Elevated levels are typically seen in patients with left ventricular dysfunction and can correlate with both the heart failure severity and the prognosis.

Bulimia nervosa: A psychiatric disorder manifested by episodes of consuming a large caloric load over a short period of time (binge eating), with subsequent self-induced vomiting, use of cathartics or diuretics, fasting, or excessive exercise to prevent weight gain.

BUN (blood urea nitrogen): A waste product in the blood that comes from the breakdown of food protein. The kidneys filter blood to remove urea. As kidney function decreases, the BUN level increases.

Bursitis: Inflammation of the bursa, a fluid-filled soft tissue structure that usually results in pain and swelling.

Caffeinism: A clinical syndrome produced by acute or chronic overuse of caffeine characterized by anxiety, psychomotor alterations, sleep disturbances, mood changes, and psychophysiologic complaints.

Calcimimetic: A class of agents that stimulate calcium-sensing receptors on the parathyroid gland and *mimic* the effects of extracellular calcium. They suppress parathyroid hormone (PTH) release and increase the sensitivity of the receptor to extracellular calcium.

Calcium-sensing receptor: The calcium receptor on the chief cells of the parathyroid gland, activation of which leads to suppression of PTH release.

Candidiasis: Fungal infection involving *Candida* species.

Carbuncles: Broad, swollen, erythematous, deep, and painful, follicular masses commonly associated with fever, chills, and malaise.

Carcinoid: A carcinoid is a slow-growing tumor usually located in the gastrointestinal system and sometimes in the lungs or other sites. Carcinoids can spread to the liver and can secrete serotonin or prostaglandins.

Cardiac arrest: The sudden cessation of cardiac mechanical activity as confirmed by the absence of signs of circulation.

Cardiac index: Cardiac output standardized for body surface area. Mathematically, cardiac index = cardiac output/body surface area.

Cardiac output: The volume of blood pumped by the heart per unit of time. Cardiac output is the product of heart rate and stroke volume.

Cardioembolic stroke: An ischemic stroke thought to be caused by an embolism arising from the heart. Cardioembolic stroke can be assumed in patients with significant cardiovascular disease including atrial fibrillation, dilated cardiomyopathy, prosthetic valves, recent myocardial infarction (MI), and patent foramen ovale.

Cardiopulmonary bypass: The use of extracorporeal devices to pump blood and oxygenate the blood while the heart or lungs are not functional. Extracorporeal membrane oxygenation (ECMO) is a form of long-term cardiopulmonary bypass that is typically used for days to weeks.

Cardiopulmonary resuscitation: The attempt to restore spontaneous circulation by performing chest compressions with or without ventilations.

Carotid Doppler: A technique that provides information about the presence and severity of atherosclerosis of the carotid artery using noninvasive sound wave technology.

Carotid endarterectomy: Removal of the atherosclerotic plaque from the inside of a stenotic carotid artery by a surgical technique. The vessel is surgically opened and sewn and/or patched after removal of the plaque.

Carpal tunnel syndrome: A medical condition in which the median nerve is compressed at the wrist, leading to parethesias, numbness, and muscle weakness in the hand.

Case-control study: An observational study of persons with the disease of interest (cases) and a suitable control group of persons without the disease to establish the extent of association between exposure(s) of interest and disease.

Castration: Removal of the ovaries or testicles.

Cataplexy: A sudden loss of muscle control with retention of clear consciousness that follows a strong emotional stimulus (e.g., elation, surprise, or anger) and is a characteristic symptom of narcolepsy.

Catheter lock therapy: A method for preventing or treating catheter-related bloodstream infections by instilling a highly concentrated antimicrobial solution into a catheter lumen and allowing the solution to dwell for a specified time period for the purpose of sterilizing the lumen.

Cellulitis: An acute, infectious process that initially affects the epidermis and dermis and can subsequently spread within the superficial fascia.

Central parenteral nutrition: Parenteral nutrition delivered into a large-diameter vein, usually the superior vena cava adjacent to the right atrium.

Central venous catheter: A venous access device inserted percutaneously, or tunneled beneath the skin and terminating in a central vein such as the subclavian, internal jugular, or femoral veins.

Centrilobular: Affecting the central portion of the lobe.

Cerebral autoregulation: The process by which cerebral blood flow is maintained in a tight range over a wide range of peripheral blood pressures. It is accomplished by reactive dilation and constriction of cerebral arteries.

Cerebral blood flow (CBF): The volume of blood perfusing a given brain mass as a function of time.

Cerebral blood volume (CBV): The total volume of blood within the cerebral vasculature at a given point in time.

Cerebral microdialysis: A sampling method that allows continuous acquisition of a small volume of cerebral extracellular fluid specimens using a microdialysis probe inserted into the brain.

Cerebral oxygen consumption ($CMRo_2$): The cerebral metabolic rate for oxygen consumption calculated as the mean hemispheric CBF and the arteriovenous oxygen content difference ($AVDo_2$).

Cerebral oxygen delivery (CDo_2): The product of CBF and arterial oxygen content.

Cerebral perfusion pressure: A critical monitoring parameter in traumatic brain injury patients defined as the difference between the mean arterial pressure and the intracranial pressure.

Cerebrospinal fluid: The clear, colorless fluid that bathes and cushions the brain and spinal cord.

Cervical cap: A thimble-shaped latex rubber device that is held on the cervix by suction, thus acting as a barrier to reduce the risk of pregnancy.

Cervical effacement: During the first stage of labor, as the cervix is opening, it is also thinning. The thinning of the cervix is termed *effacement*.

Cervical ripening: Prior to inducing labor, the cervix must be favorable, approximately 2 cm dilated and 80% thinned out. If this is not the case, an agent must be used to induce histochemical changes to make the cervix more favorable.

Cervical stenosis: A cause for menstrual flow obstruction; often caused by surgical interventions for cervical dysplasia.

Cervicitis: Inflammation of the cervix.

Chancre: A sore or ulcer, the dermal lesion of primary syphilis.

Chancroid: A venereal dermal lesion caused by agents other than syphilis.

Cheilitis: Inflammation of the lips; can be related to retinoid use.

Children: Pediatric patients who are 1 to 11 years of age.

Cholelithiasis: A solid formation in the gallbladder or bile duct composed of cholesterol and bile salts. Also known as gallstone.

Cholestatic hepatitis: Rare form of hepatitis marked by stopped or suppressed flow of bile; characterized by pruritus, dark urine, light-colored stools, elevated alkaline phosphatase, and conjugated bilirubin.

Cholinesterase inhibitors: Class of medication that inhibits enzymatic activity of acetylcholinesterase, butyrylcholinesterase, or both to prevent the degradation of acetylcholine.

Chronic condition: An illness or impairment that cannot be cured.

Chronic kidney disease (CKD): Slow and progressive loss of kidney function that takes several years, often resulting in permanent kidney failure requiring dialysis or transplantation.

Chronic pain/persistent pain: Pain persisting for months to years.

Chronic pancreatitis: Chronic inflammation of the pancreas caused by the many sequelae of long-standing pancreatic injury leading to irreversible pancreatic damage.

Chvostek's sign: A facial twitch produced by tapping on the cheek over the branches of the facial nerve.

Circumstantial speech: Speech pattern whereby the expressed ideas are characterized by unnecessary detail. The speaker ultimately makes their point, but in a very roundabout manner.

Clearance: The volume of blood per unit time (e.g., L/h, mL/min) completely cleared of a drug.

Clinical inertia: A clinical situation in which no therapeutic move was made to treat a medical condition in a patient that is not considered adequately treated, or at their treatment goal.

Clinical outcomes: Medical events that occur as a result of the condition or its treatment.

Clinical pharmacokinetics: The discipline that describes the absorption, distribution, metabolism, and elimination of drugs in patients.

Clinical proteinuria: Total protein in the urine in amounts greater than 300 mg/day.

Clinical resistance: Refers to failure of an antifungal agent in the treatment of a fungal infection that arises from factors other than microbial resistance, such as failure of the antifungal agent to reach the site of infection, or inability of a patient's immune system to eradicate a fungus whose growth is retarded by an antifungal agent; applicable to many other drugs.

Clinically isolated syndrome: The first attack of multiple sclerosis characterized by a neurologic syndrome such as optic neuritis and generally seen with silent or asymptomatic white matter lesions (seen on magnetic resonance imaging) suggestive of demyelination. Individuals that experience a clinically isolated syndrome are at high risk of developing definite multiple sclerosis.

Clotting cascade: A series of enzymatic reactions by clotting factors leading to the formation of a blood clot. The clotting cascade is initiated by several thrombogenic substances. Each reaction in the cascade is triggered by the preceding one, and the effect is amplified by positive feedback loops.

Clotting factor: Plasma proteins found in the blood that are essential to the formation of blood clots. Clotting factors circulate in inactive forms but are activated by their predecessor in the clotting cascade or a thrombogenic substance. Each clotting factor is designated by a Roman numeral (e.g., factor VII) and by the letter "a" when activated (e.g., factor VIIa).

Cluster headache: A primary headache disorder characterized by attacks of severe unilateral headache that occurs in series of weeks or months (cluster periods) separated by remission periods usually lasting months or years.

Cluster period: The time during which cluster-headache attacks occur regularly and at least once every other day.

Codon: A sequence of three consecutive nucleotides that specify an amino acid or amino acid chain termination.

Coelomic metaplasia: Transformation of normal cells into endometrial cells.

Cognitive behavioral therapy: A form of psychotherapy designed to replace distorted or inappropriate ways of thinking with healthy, more realistic thoughts to alter maladaptive moods and behavior. It is instructional in approach and is based on the theory that thoughts (not external influences such as people, situations, and events) cause feelings and behaviors. Patients learn to identify the thinking that causes the negative feelings and behaviors and then learn how to replace that thinking with thoughts that lead to more desirable feelings and behaviors.

Cogwheeling: A ratchet-like movement in the joints, characteristic of Parkinson disease.

Cohort study: Assembly of a group of persons without a disease(s) of interest at the onset of the study, determination of the exposure status of each person, and observation of the cohort over time to determine the development of disease in exposed and nonexposed persons.

Colectomy: Surgical removal of the colon.

Colonization resistance: Preservation of anaerobic flora by selective gut decontamination to prevent colonization by potentially pathogenic gram-negative organisms.

Colony-stimulating factors: Proteins that regulate the proliferation, maturation, and differentiation of stem cells to red blood cells, white blood cells, or platelets; may be classified into myeloid growth factors, erythropoietic agents, and thrombopoietic agents.

Coma: A state of unconsciousness whereby a patient is not opening his or her eyes, not obeying commands, and not uttering understandable words.

Comedo, comedones (pl.): Plug of sebum and keratinous material in a hair follicle; blackhead.

Comedogenicity: Product effect that causes follicular plugging resulting in comedones.

Comedolytic: Prevents shed keratinocytes from aggregating in follicle and clogging pores.

Communities: Organized groups of people with a shared identity or relationship that may be based on history, culture, context, or geography.

Comorbidity: A concomitant but unrelated pathologic or disease process.

Complementary and alternative medicine (CAM): Any practice for the prevention and treatment of disease that is not usual conventional medicine.

Complex partial seizure: A seizure beginning in one hemisphere of the brain. It is manifested by automatisms, periods of memory loss, or aberrations of behavior.

Compulsion: Repetitive ritualistic behavior such as ordering or hand washing or a mental act such as repeating words silently with the intent of preventing or reducing distress or some dreaded event or situation.

Conceptual model: The rationale for and description of the concepts that a measurement instrument is intended to assess and the interrelationships of those concepts.

Condom: A sheath, usually made of thin rubber, used to cover the penis during sexual intercourse to prevent conception or infection.

Confounding: A situation in which the effects of two processes are not separated. The distortion of the apparent effect of an exposure on risk brought about by the association of other factors that can influence the outcome.

Constrictive pericarditis: Constrictive pericarditis is a disorder caused by inflammation of the pericardium with subsequent thickening, scarring, and contracture of the pericardium. The pericardium cannot stretch during contraction, thereby preventing chamber filling.

Construct validity: The strength of the relationship between measures purporting to measure or reflect the same underlying theoretical construct.

Content validity: Refers to how adequately the questions/items capture the relevant aspects of the domain or concept being measured.

Continuation therapy: The second phase in drug therapy during which the goal is to eliminate any remaining symptoms and prevent a relapse.

Continuous-combined estrogen-progestogen therapy: Daily administration of both estrogen and a progestogen.

Continuous long-cycle estrogen-progestogen therapy: Estrogen is given daily and a progestogen is given six times a year (every other month for 12 to 14 days).

Contralateral: Of or pertaining to the opposite side of the body.

Convection: The movement of solutes, or metabolic waste products, by bulk flow in association with fluid removal. Convective clearance is not dependent on concentration gradients, and the magnitude of its contribution to total clearance is directly related to the ultrafiltration (fluid removal) rate.

Convulsion: Specific seizure type where the seizure is manifested by involuntary muscle contractions.

Cor pulmonale: Right-sided heart failure caused by lung disease.

Corneocytes: Flattened, dead, keratin-filled epidermal cells.

Coronary artery bypass graft (CABG) surgery: Thoracic surgery where parts of a saphenous vein from a leg or internal mammary artery from the axilla (armpit) are placed as conduits to restore blood flow between the aorta and one or more coronary arteries to "bypass" the coronary artery stenosis (occlusion).

Corpus cavernosum: Two chambers on the dorsal side of the penis. Chambers composed of sinusoidal tissue, which can fill with arterial blood to produce an erection.

Corpus luteum: The small yellow endocrine structure that develops within a ruptured ovarian follicle and secretes progesterone and estrogen.

Corpus spongiosum: One chamber on the ventral side of the penis. Chamber is composed of sinusoidal tissue, which can fill with arterial blood to produce an erection. The urethra passes through the corpus spongiosum.

Cortical necrosis: Acute renal failure secondary to ischemic necrosis of the renal cortex usually caused by significantly diminished renal arterial perfusion.

Corticotropin-releasing hormone (CRH): A trophic hormone released by the hypothalamus that stimulates release of adrenocorticotropic hormone (ACTH).

Cost-effectiveness ratio: The outcome of cost-effective analysis. The numerator of the ratio summarizes the costs and financial savings associated with the therapy, including the costs of the therapy itself, side effects, medical costs, and savings from avoided illness and disability. The denominator of the cost-effectiveness ratio reflects the health effect of the intervention. The year of life saved is probably the most commonly used measure of the health effect.

Cranial nerve palsy: Paralysis of one or more of the 12 cranial (brain) nerves.

Craniectomy (for stroke): Removal of part of the skull overlying an area of injury to relieve the pressure of cerebral edema.

C-reactive protein: An endogenous marker released by the body in response to inflammation.

Creatine kinase, creatine kinase myocardial band: Creatine kinase (CK) enzymes are found in many isoforms, with varying concentrations depending on the type of tissue. Creatine kinase is a general term used to describe the nonspecific total release of all types of CK, including that found in skeletal muscle (MM), brain (BB), and heart (MB). Creatine kinase–MB is released into the blood from necrotic myocytes in response to infarction and is a useful laboratory test for diagnosing myocardial infarction. If the total CK is elevated, then the relative index (RI), or fraction of the total that is composed of CK-MB, is calculated as follows:

$$RI = \frac{\text{CK-MB}}{\text{CK total}} \times 100$$

A RI greater than 2 is typically diagnostic of infarction.

Creatinine (serum): A protein metabolic by-product obtained from the diet or generated from muscles of the body. Creatinine is removed from blood by the kidneys; as kidney disease progresses, the level of creatinine in the blood increases.

Creatinine clearance: A test that measures how efficiently the kidneys filter creatinine and other waste products from the blood. Low creatinine clearance (<60 mL/min) usually indicates the presence of kidney damage.

Crepitus: A crinkly, crackling, or grating feeling or sound in the joints, skin, or lungs.

Cronbach α-coefficient: Commonly used statistical measure to quantify internal consistency reliability for multi-item scales or tests.

Crossmatch: A test to determine if a recipient has antibodies against donor antigens. A positive crossmatch indicates that the recipient has antibodies against the donor, and the two are incompatible. A negative crossmatch means the recipient does not have antibodies against the donor, and the two are considered compatible.

Crust: Dried exudate, secretion, or hemorrhage; scab.

Crypt abscess: Neutrophilic infiltration of the intestinal glands (Crypts of Lieberkuhn); a characteristic finding for patients with UC.

Cultural competency: The attitudes, knowledge, skills, and values that an individual and/or an organization acquires, develops, and uses to work effectively in a cross-cultural environment.

Culture: The acquired and shared attitudes, beliefs, knowledge, and values that individuals and/or groups use to influence their actions and behavior.

Culture negative endocarditis: Describes a patient in whom a clinical diagnosis of infective endocarditis is likely, but blood cultures do not yield a pathogen.

Cutaneous: Pertaining to the skin.

Cutis: Skin.

Cyanopsia: A condition when a patient sees a blue halo around objects, or objects appear to be blue-colored.

Cyanosis: Bluish tint to the skin or mucous membranes because of lack of oxygen.

Cyclic estrogen-progestogen therapy: Estrogen is taken continuously, with a progestogen added cyclically the last 10 to 14 days during each 28-day cycle.

Cyst: Sac or closed cavity containing fluid, semifluid, or solid material.

Cystitis: Inflammation of the bladder, usually caused by infection.

Cytokines: Protein molecules that are released by one cell (e.g., T-lymphocytes) that can have an influence on other cells. These proteins are important in numerous cell functions, such as regulating the immune response and cell-to-cell communication.

Dactylitis: Erythema and swollen hands, feet, fingers, and toes. Also known as *hand-and-foot syndrome*.

Deep vein thrombosis: A disorder of thrombus formation causing obstruction of a deep vein in the leg, pelvis, or abdomen.

Defibrillation: The therapeutic use of electric current in attempt to completely depolarize the myocardium and provide an opportunity for the natural pacemaker centers of the heart to resume normal activity.

Delayed cerebral ischemia: A worsening in neurologic function in a subarachnoid hemorrhage patient, occurring several days after the initial bleed, not due to another cause.

Delusion: Fixed, false beliefs that are not based in reality or consistent with the patient's religion or culture. Delusions can be classified as paranoid, somatic, or grandiose in nature. Delusions are often unshakable in spite of evidence to the contrary.

Dementia: A chronic progressive neurodegenerative syndrome characterized by a decline in memory and at least one other cognitive function.

Demyelination: Destruction of myelin in the spinal cord and brain leading to the formation of plaques that impair communication between neurons. Demyelination is classically found in the central nervous system of patients with multiple sclerosis and may be reversible.

Depersonalization: A change in an individual's self-awareness, such that one feels detached from his or her own experiences, with the self, body, and mind seeming alien or distant. Persistent or recurrent experiences as if one is an outside observer of one's mental processes or body (e.g., feeling like one is in a dream).

Derealization: A feeling of estrangement or detachment from one's environment.

Dermatitis: Inflammation of the skin.

Dermatophyte: Fungal infection of the skin.

Dermis: The inner layer of skin between the epidermis and hypodermis.

Desensitization: Administration of increasing doses of drug to achieve patient tolerance and avoidance of hypersensitivity reactions.

Detoxification programs: A medically supervised treatment program for alcohol or drug addiction designed to purge the body of intoxicating or addictive substances. Such a program is used as a first step in overcoming physiologic or psychologic addiction.

Detumescence: Process by which an erect penis becomes flaccid.

Diagnostic overshadowing: Underestimating the significance of the emotional disturbances because of the presence of significant cognitive deficits.

Dialysate: The cleansing solution used in dialysis to remove excess fluids and waste products from the blood.

Dialysis: The process of removing toxic substances and fluid across a semipermeable membrane to maintain fluid, electrolyte, and acid–base balance.

Diaphragm: (1) A flexible ring covered with rubber or other plastic material, fitted over the cervix of the uterus to prevent pregnancy. (2) Muscular membrane separating the abdominal and thoracic cavities, used for respiration.

Diaphoresis: Perspiration.

Diastolic blood pressure: The arterial BP that occurs after cardiac contraction when the cardiac chambers are filling.

Diastolic heart failure: A condition caused by increased resistance to the filling of one or both ventricles; this leads to symptoms of congestion from the inappropriate upward shift of the diastolic pressure-volume relation.

Diffuse idiopathic skeletal hyperostosis (DISH): A form of degenerative arthritis caused by calcification or a bony hardening of ligaments alongside the vertebrae of the spine. Also known as Forestier disease.

Diffuse idiopathic skeletal hyperostosis (DISH): Abnormal bone formation with calcifications and ossifications along the anterolateral aspect of vertebral bodies. A variant of Forestier disease.

Diffusion-weighted imaging: A type of magnetic resonance imaging (MRI) that can sensitively detect changes in water movement in tissue. It is particularly sensitive to the early changes seen during brain ischemia.

Digital clubbing: Rounded and swollen tip of finger usually associated with long-term pulmonary disease.

Dihydrotestosterone: The active androgen metabolite, which is formed inside various cells. In the case of benign prostatic hyperplasia (BPH), dihydrotestosterone is formed inside prostate cells by the action of 5-α-reductase, which converts testosterone to dihydrotestosterone. Dihydrotestosterone stimulates the glandular portion of the prostate to undergo hyperplasia.

Disinhibition: A physiologic effect that occurs during psychoactive substance use characterized by a loss of normal, executive functioning and normal behavior. An increase in behaviors with the propensity to harm the individual is common.

Dissociative amnesia: Inability to remember some important aspect of an event.

Diverticulitis: Inflammation of a diverticulum, especially of the small pockets in the wall of the colon that fill with stagnant fecal material and become inflamed; rarely, they can cause obstruction, perforation, or bleeding.

Dopamine: A monoamine neurotransmitter formed in the brain by the decarboxylation of dopa and essential to the normal functioning of the central nervous system.

Doppler imaging: With Doppler imaging, a probe generates sound waves typically at 2.5 MHz. When encountering an object, sound waves are scattered or reflected back toward the probe from the object's interface with adjacent structures; this is repeated in many times per second to build up a moving real-time image of the heart.

Drug abuse: A maladaptive pattern of substance use indicated by repeated adverse consequences related to the repeated use of the substance. Examples include failure to fulfill important obligations at work, school, or home; repeated use in situations in which it is physically dangerous, such as driving under the influence; legal problems; and social or interpersonal problems such as arguments and fights.

Drug addiction: A chronic disorder characterized by the compulsive use of a substance resulting in physical, psychologic, or social harm to the user and continued use despite that harm.

Dual diagnosis: A developmentally disabled person comorbid with a psychiatric disorder.

Dumping syndrome: A condition characterized by weakness, dizziness, flushing/warmth, nausea, and palpitation immediately or shortly after eating and produced by abnormally rapid emptying of the stomach, particularly in individuals who have had part of the stomach removed.

Dysentery: Diarrhea characterized by blood, mucus, and leukocytes in the stool with tenesmus and fever.

Dyskinesia: Choreiform abnormal involuntary movements involving usually the face, neck, trunk, and extremities.

Dysmenorrhea: Crampy pelvic pain occurring with or just prior to menses. *Primary* dysmenorrhea implies pain in the setting of normal pelvic anatomy, whereas *secondary* dysmenorrhea is secondary to underlying pelvic pathology.

Dyspareunia: Painful sexual intercourse.

Dyspepsia: Literally means "bad digestion" but refers to persistent or recurrent pain or discomfort centered in the upper abdomen. Symptoms may include epigastric pain, bloating, abdominal distention, postprandial fullness, early satiety, and nausea.

Dysphagia: Difficulty swallowing.

Dysphoria or dysphoric: A feeling of discomfort or an unpleasant mood, such as sadness, anxiety, or irritability.

Dyspnea: Dyspnea is referred to as shortness of breath or difficulty or distress in breathing.

Dystonia: Sustained muscular spasm or abnormal postures.

Early empirical therapy: The administration of systemic antifungal agents at the onset of fever and neutropenia.

Economic outcomes: The direct, indirect, and intangible costs compared with the consequences of a medical intervention.

Edema: Accumulation of fluid in tissues.

Effective renal plasma flow (ERPF): The flow of plasma through the kidneys; often measured by *p*-aminohippurate (PAH) clearance and expressed in volume per unit of time (mL/min). The ERPF is less than the true renal plasma flow (RPF) because plasma flow through renal connective and adipose tissue is not measured and the extraction of PAH, although high (>0.9), is not complete.

Ejaculatory dysfunction: This is a type of sexual dysfunction that can present as premature ejaculation (before orgasm has occurred), anejaculation (failure of emission), or retrograde ejaculation (when ejaculate moves backward into the bladder as opposed to forward and out of the body during orgasm). In some cases, ejaculatory dysfunction can decrease sexual enjoyment in the patient.

Ejection fraction: The ejection fraction is the percentage of blood ejected from the left ventricle with each heart beat.

Elation: An exaggerated feeling of well-being, euphoria, or elation.

Electroconvulsive therapy: A treatment for severe mental illness in which a precisely calculated electric stimulus is administered in a controlled medical setting to produce a generalized seizure.

Electroencephalograph (EEG): Used to evaluate brain electrical activity.

Electroencephalography: A test that measures electrical brain wave activity through the use of multiple scalp electrodes.

Electromyography: Test of muscle function because of either primary muscle disease or secondary to nerve injury.

Embolism: The sudden blockage of a vessel caused by a blood clot or foreign material that has been brought to the site by the flow of blood.

Embolization: The process by which a blood clot or foreign material dislodges from its site of origin, flows in the blood, and blocks a distant vessel.

Emergency contraception: Any method of contraception that acts after intercourse to prevent pregnancy.

Emesis: See *Vomiting*.

Empirical therapy: With systemic antifungal agents is administered to granulocytopenic patients with persistent or recurrent fever despite the administration of appropriate antimicrobial therapy.

Enanthem: Eruption on a mucous membrane (as the inside of the mouth) occurring as a symptom of a disease.

Encephalitis: Inflammation of the brain tissue.

Encephalopathy: An altered brain state that may occur with altered brain structure. Many etiologies are associated with encephalopathy (toxins, cancer, metabolic disorders, CNS infections, increased cranial pressure, radiation, alcohol, psychotropic drugs, trauma, inadequate nutrition, decreased brain oxygen, and CNS injury). Consciousness is impaired with patients having a decreased/altered mental state and diffuse slowing of the EEG.

End-stage kidney disease: Glomerular filtration rate (GFR) <15 mL/min/1.73 m^2 (<0.14 mL/s/m^2) or need for renal replacement therapy.

Endobronchitis: Inflammation of the epithelial lining of the bronchi.

Endocarditis: An infection of the endocardial surface of the heart, which can include one or more heart valves, the mural endocardium, or a septal defect.

Endocrine therapy: A group of drugs used to treat cancer that target the production or action of endogenous hormones.

Endometriosis: Presence of endometrial tissue outside the uterus.

Endoscopy: A diagnostic tool used to examine the inside of the body using a lighted, flexible instrument called an endoscope.

Enkephalins: Pentapeptide endorphins, found in many parts of the brain, that bind to specific receptor sites, some of which can be pain-related opiate receptors.

Enteric fever: Intestinal inflammation and ulceration with high fever and abdominal complaints caused by infection.

Enterocolitis: Inflammation of the small intestine and colon.

Enterotoxin: A cholera-like disease that produces secretory diarrhea.

Enuresis: Urinary incontinence, especially at night.

Enzymuria: Presence of enzymes in the urine.

Epidermis: The outer layer of skin.

Epigenetic: A change in the genome that is heritable and potentially reversible that does not alter the nucleotide sequence of DNA.

Epilepsy: Two or more unprovoked seizures; symptoms of disturbed electrical activity in the brain.

Epilepsy syndrome: The combination of seizure type with other components of the patient history such as age of onset, intellectual development, findings on neurologic examination, and results of neuroimaging.

Episodic: Recurring and remitting in a regular or irregular pattern.

Epistaxis: Nose bleed.

Epithelial cells: Cells that make up epithelium.

Epithelial tissue of the prostate: Also known as glandular tissue. This portion of the prostate is responsible for producing prostatic secretions, and this comprises only approximately 25% of the total volume of the enlarged prostate gland in patients with benign prostatic hyperplasia. Epithelial tissue is androgen dependent.

Epithelium: Layer of avascular cells covering body surfaces.

Erectile dysfunction: Also known as *impotence*. This is a failure of the penis to become rigid enough to allow for vaginal penetration of the sexual partner.

Erysipelas: Infection of the more superficial layers of the skin and cutaneous lymphatics.

Erythema: Redness.

Erythema multiforme: Symmetrical patches of raised, red skin.

Erythema nodosum: Raised, red, tender nodules on the skin that vary in size from 1 cm.

Erythroderma: Generalized redness of the skin.

Erythropoiesis: The production of erythrocytes (red blood cells) within the bone marrow.

Erythropoietic agents: Agents developed with recombinant DNA technology that have the same biologic activity as endogenous erythropoietin to stimulate red blood cell production. Available agents in the United States include epoetin alfa and darbepoetin alfa.

Erythropoietin: A hormone made by the kidneys that is required for red blood cell formation in the bone marrow. Lack of this hormone leads to anemia.

Eschar: Black, painless skin ulcer characteristic of cutaneous anthrax.

Esophageal: Involving the esophagus.

Esophageal stricture: A narrowing of the esophageal lumen because of acid reflux into the lower esophagus.

Esophagitis: Inflammation of the esophagus.

Essential hypertension: Persistently elevated BP that results from unknown pathophysiological etiology.

Essential or primary hypertension: Persistently elevated blood pressure that results from unknown pathophysiological etiology.

Estrogen therapy: Unopposed estrogen regimens administered to postmenopausal women following hysterectomy.

Euphoria: A mood state characterized by an exaggerated, superficial sense of well-being, characterized extreme happiness, sometimes more than is reasonable in a particular situation.

Euthymia or euthymic: A mood in a *normal* range without depression or mood elevation.

Evidence-based medicine (EBM): Evidence-based medicine emphasizes the consideration of results from clinical research as the basis for clinical decision making. Under this practice approach, unless individual patient-specific factors dictate otherwise, treatment should generally be guided by those approaches that have the best research evidence for efficacy, tolerability, and patient acceptance.

Evoked potentials: EEG-based technique involving measurement of brain-wave activity in response to stimuli, usually visual or auditory.

Exanthema: An eruption on the skin occurring as a symptom of a disease.

External beam radiotherapy: Treatment by radiation emitted from a source located at a distance from the body; also called beam therapy and external beam therapy.

Extrapyramidal: Regarding involuntary motor movement.

Extrapyramidal system: Neurotransmitter tracts in the midbrain with dopamine as the primary ascending neurotransmitter, with cell bodies in the substantial nigra and axons terminating in the basal ganglia (e.g., caudate nucleus, putamen). The extrapyramidal system is largely involved in the control of fine motor movements, and with some degree of emotional expression as well.

Fasciculations: The localized contractions of muscle groups, often visible through the skin, because of excessive neuronal discharge.

Fear: A direct, focused response to a specific event or object of which an individual is consciously aware.

Felty syndrome: Rheumatoid arthritis associated with splenomegaly and neutropenia.

Fibrin: An insoluble protein that is one of the principle ingredients of a blood clot. Fibrin strands bind to one another to form a fibrin mesh. The fibrin mesh often traps platelets and other blood cells.

Fibromyalgia: A syndrome characterized by chronic widespread pain, multiple tender points, abnormal pain, sleep disturbances, fatigue, and psychological distress.

Fibrosis: Formation of fibrous tissue as a reparative or reactive process.

First-degree relative (FDR): A close blood relative, including the individual's parents, full siblings, and children.

First-generation (typical or traditional) antipsychotic: An antipsychotic medication with a mechanism of action thought to be primarily caused by the blockade of dopamine-2 (D_2) receptors. D_2-blockade is associated with hyperprolactinemia and extrapyramidal side effects.

Fistula: A communicating tube-like passage from one organ to another or from an organ to an external surface; often seen in severe cases of Crohn's disease.

Flight of ideas: An accelerated flow of speech with thoughts that change rapidly from one topic to another.

Focal seizures: Partial seizures.

Follicle-stimulating hormone (FSH): A polypeptide hormone secreted by the anterior pituitary gland that promotes ovarian follicle development and stimulates estradiol and progesterone.

Fragile X syndrome: A genetic disorder commonly associated with mental retardation in which the tip of the long arms of the X chromosome separates from the rest of the genetic material; most males and 30% of females with fragile X syndrome have mental retardation; males develop enlarged testicles, enlarged ears, and a prominent jaw.

Freezing: Intermittent immobility lasting a few seconds, particularly in walking, seen in Parkinsonism.

Fulminant hepatitis: Acute hepatic failure; rare complication of viral hepatitis, it can also result from hepatotoxins, or drug sensitivity and causes massive necrosis of the liver; marked by a high fatality rate.

Functional analysis: Evaluation performed by a psychologist qualified in applied behavioral analysis to determine if a behavior is caused by some environmental factor.

Functional pain: Pain due to abnormal operation of the nervous system.

Functional psychiatric disorder: A mental disorder that is primarily defined by a constellation of symptoms and behaviors and for which the pathophysiologic etiology is still largely unknown.

Fungemia: The presence of fungi in the blood.

Gastroesophageal reflux disease (GERD): Symptomatic clinical condition or histologic alteration that results from episodes of gastroesophageal reflux.

Gene: Series of codons that specify a particular protein.

Generalized anxiety disorder (GAD): Excessive anxiety and worry about a number of events or activities occurring more days than not for a period of at least 6 months.

Generalized convulsive status epilepticus (GCSE): Most common and dangerous type of status epilepticus. It consists of bilateral (both brain hemispheres) electrical seizure activity that manifests as tonic and/or clonic motor activity. The convulsions and/or brain discharges can be symmetrical or asymmetrical (i.e., parts of body and brain mirroring or not mirroring each other in activity). Consciousness is not maintained during the seizures episodes. The duration is sufficient enough in length to meet the definition of status epilepticus.

Generalized seizures: Seizures occurring in both hemispheres of the brain. They can be primary or secondarily generalized.

Generic/general measures: Instruments designed to be applicable across a wide variety of conditions/diseases, medical interventions, and populations.

Germ-line mutations: Inherited variations in germ cells that are transmitted to offspring compared with variations in somatic cells, which are not passed on to offspring.

Genotype: The genetic constitution of an individual.

Genu valgum: A deformity marked by lateral angulation of the leg in relation to the thigh.

Genu varum: A deformity marked by medial angulation of the leg in relation to the thigh; an outward bowing of the legs.

Gestation: Time from fertilization of egg until birth.

Gigantism: Excess secretion of growth hormone prior to epiphyseal closure in children.

Glasgow coma scale: The most widely used system to grade the arousal and functional capacity of the cerebral cortex consisting of eye opening, motor responses, and verbal responses.

Glaucoma: Any of a group of ocular disorders that lead to an optic neuropathy characterized by changes in the optic nerve head (optic disk) that is associated with loss of visual sensitivity and field. Open angle and closed angle are the two major types of glaucoma.

Glomerular filtration rate (GFR): The primary index of overall kidney function; the volume of plasma that is filtered by the glomerulus per unit of time; often reported in mL/min or mL/min/1.73 m^2.

Glomerulonephritis: Glomerular lesions characterized by inflammation of the capillary loops in the glomerulus caused by immunologic, vascular, and other idiopathic diseases (may be diffuse or membranoproliferative).

Glomerulosclerosis: Fibrosis of the glomeruli.

Glomerulus: A coiled capillary bed in the kidney that is responsible for filtering water and small molecular weight substances from the blood.

Gonadotropin: A sex hormone that promotes gonadal growth and functioning in both males and females.

Gonadotropin-releasing hormone (GnRH): A trophic hormone released by the hypothalamus that stimulates release of follicle-stimulating hormone (FSH) and luteinizing hormone (LH).

Gout: A disease spectrum that includes hyperuricemia, recurrent attacks of acute arthritis associated with monosodium urate crystals in leukocytes found in synovial fluid, deposits of monosodium urate crystals in tissues (tophi), interstitial renal disease, and uric acid nephrolithiasis.

gp120: The glycoprotein structure on the surface of human immunodeficiency virus (HIV) that binds to CD4 on human cells.

Grandiosity: An inflated self-appraisal of one's status, power, or identity.

Granuloma inguinale: Granuloma lesions affecting the genital area.

Growth hormone (GH): A polypeptide hormone secreted by the anterior pituitary gland that stimulates insulinlike growth factor-1 (IGF-1) production and promotes growth of all body cells.

Growth hormone-releasing hormone (GHRH): A trophic hormone released by the hypothalamus that stimulates release of growth hormone.

Guillain-Barré's syndrome: A disorder characterized by progressive symmetrical paralysis and loss of reflexes, usually beginning in the legs. The paralysis typically involves more than one limb, is progressive, and usually proceeds from the end of an extremity toward the torso. Areflexia or hyporeflexia can occur in the limbs. It typically occurs after recovery from a viral infection.

Gumma: A granulomatous lesion found in organs or tissues as a result of syphilis.

Gynecomastia: Gynecomastia is the abnormal development of large breasts in men.

Half-life: The time required for serum concentrations to decrease by one-half after absorption and distribution are complete.

Hallucination: A sensory perception (e.g., auditory, gustatory, olfactory, somatic, tactile, visual) that occurs without external stimulation of the relevant sensory organ.

Haplotype: Set of polymorphisms that are inherited together.

Haptocorrin: A group of carrier proteins that bind with vitamin B_{12} in the blood and aid in its transport.

Haptoglobin: A group of α_2-globulins in human serum, so called because of their ability to combine with hemoglobin, preventing loss in the urine; levels are decreased in hemolytic disorders and increased in inflammatory conditions or with tissue damage.

Hay fever: See *Rhinitis.*

Health literacy: The degree to which individuals have the capacity to obtain, process, and understand basic health information and services needed to make appropriate health decisions (as defined by the Institute of Medicine).

Health outcomes: The consequences or ends results of a disease and/or its treatment.

Health profiles: Generic instruments that provide an array of scores representing individual dimensions or domains of health-related quality of life (HRQOL) or health status.

Health-related quality of life (HRQOL): A person's perception of how health impacts his or her physical, social, and psychologic functioning and well-being.

Health state preference: The perceived relative desirability of a health state measured on a scale where 1.0 equals full health, and 0.0 equals dead.

Heart failure: A clinical syndrome that can result from any disorder that impairs the ability of the heart to fill with or eject blood. Although heart failure may be caused by numerous cardiac disorders, the primary clinical signs and symptoms of dyspnea, fatigue, and volume overload are similar regardless of the initial cause.

Heinz bodies: Intracellular inclusions usually attached to the red cell membrane composed of denatured hemoglobin.

Hemagglutinin: The major antigenic determinant of the influenza virus; a surface antigen that allows the influenza virus to enter host cells by attaching to sialic acid receptors.

Hematemesis: Vomiting up blood that can be bright red or similar to coffee grounds in appearance.

Hematochezia: The presence of visible bright red blood in the stool.

Hematopoiesis: The formation and maturation of blood cells and their derivatives.

Hematopoietic growth factors: See *Colony-stimulating factors.*

Hematopoietic stem cell: An immature cell capable of self-renewal and subsequent differentiation into mature blood cells.

Hematuria: Presence of red blood cells in the urine.

Hemetemesis: Vomiting up blood that may be bright red or appear like coffee grounds. The digestive action of acid and enzymes may cause blood in the stomach to darken and appear like coffee grounds in the vomitus.

Hemochromatosis: Hemochromatosis is a disorder that interferes with iron metabolism, which results in excess iron deposition throughout the body.

Hemodialysis: A dialysis procedure during which blood is pumped outside the body through a dialyzer that acts like an artificial kidney; the dialyzer removes extra fluids and wastes from the blood and returns the clean blood to the body.

Hemolytic uremic syndrome: A condition characterized by the breakup of red blood cells (hemolysis) and kidney failure. Platelets clump together within the kidney's small blood vessels resulting in ischemia leading to kidney failure.

Hemosiderin: A golden yellow or yellow-brown insoluble protein produced by phagocytic digestion of hematin; found in most tissues, especially in the liver, spleen, and bone marrow, in the form of granules much larger than ferritin molecules (of which they are believed to be aggregates) but with a higher content, as much as 37%, of iron.

Heparin-induced thrombocytopenia: A clinical syndrome of IgG antibody production against the heparin–platelet factor 4 complex occurring in approximately 1% to 5% of patients exposed to either heparin or low-molecular-weight heparin. Heparin-induced thrombocytopenia results in excess production of thrombin, platelet aggregation, and thrombocytopenia (due to platelet clumping), often leading to venous and arterial thrombosis, amputation of extremities, and death.

Hepatosplenic candidiasis: Clinical presentation often manifested only as fever while a patient remains neutropenic (<1,000 white blood cells/mm^3). When the white blood cell (WBC) count increases to >1000 cells/mm^3, imaging studies can detect the presence of abscess or microabscesses in the liver and spleen, often found with acute suppurative and granulomatous reactions. Infection can persist for months and ultimately cause the patient's death despite aggressive systemic therapy with antifungal agents.

Heterozygous: Presence of different (alleles) genes at one location.

Hippocampal sclerosis: A condition in which there is histopathological changes in the hippocampus that have been associated with patients with a history of prolonged status epilepticus. There is an association with hippocampal sclerosis and temporal lobe epilepsy.

Hippocampus: A sea horse–shaped structure located within the brain that is an important part of the limbic system. The hippocampus is involved in some aspects of memory, in the control of the autonomic functions, and in emotional expression.

Hirsutism: Heavy, abnormal growth of hair on the face or body; excess body hair appearing on the lower abdomen, around the nipples, around the chin and upper lip, between the breasts, and on the lower back.

HLA (human leukocyte antigen): See *Human leukocyte antigen*.

Hollenhorst plaque: Cholesterol emboli that usually dislodges from the carotid arteries, or calcific fragments from a stenosed aortic valve that can be visualized on a retinal exam.

Homocysteine: A homolog of cysteine, produced by the demethylation of methionine, and an intermediate in the biosynthesis of 1-cysteine from 1-methionine through 1-cystathionine. Elevated levels of homocysteine have been associated with certain forms of heart disease.

Homozygous: Presence of identical genes (alleles) at one location.

Hormone therapy: Either estrogen-only therapy or combined estrogen and progestogen therapy.

Hot flashes/flushes: A sensation of warmth, frequently accompanied by skin flushing and perspiration.

Human leukocyte antigen (HLA): The *self antigens* are the histocompatibility antigens found on human leukocytes and tissues that enable the body to differentiate *self* from *foreign* cells. The HLA antigens are used in histocompatibility testing to determine the suitability of an organ for transplant.

Humanistic outcomes: Patient-reported outcomes such as patient satisfaction and health-related quality of life.

Hydrocephalus: An uncharacteristic increase in the amount of cerebrospinal fluid within the skull, causing dangerous expansion of the cerebral ventricles.

Hyperalgesia: Exaggerated painful response to normally noxious stimuli.

Hyperarousal: A state of elevated or increased alertness, awareness, or wakefulness.

Hypercapnia: Elevation of carbon dioxide gas in the blood.

Hypercoagulable state: A disorder or state of excessive or frequent thrombus formation; also known as *thrombophilia*.

Hypereosinophilic syndrome: Hypereosinophilic syndrome is a group of leukoproliferative disorders characterized by an overproduction of eosinophils resulting in organ damage.

Hyperkalemia: Serum potassium concentration above 5.5 mEq/L.

Hyperlinear palms: Increased number of skin creases on the palms.

Hypermagnesemia: Serum magnesium concentration above 1.8 mEq/L or 2.3 mg/dL.

Hyperpigmentation: Excess pigment in skin causing an area of darker color than surrounding skin.

Hyperprolactinemia: A state of persistent serum prolactin elevation characterized by prolactin concentrations greater than 20 mcg/L observed on multiple occasions.

Hyperresponsiveness: In the airways, the characteristic of an exaggerated response to stimuli.

Hypertensive crises: Clinical situations where BP values are very elevated, typically greater than 180/120 mm Hg. They are categorized as either a hypertensive emergency or hypertensive urgency depending on the clinical presentation.

Hypertensive emergency: A clinical situation in which a patient has extremely high BP values, typically greater than 180/120 mm Hg that is also accompanied by the presence of acute and/or progressing target-organ damage. Immediate but gradual reduction in BP using intravenous antihypertensive agents is needed to prevent acute morbidity and/or mortality.

Hypertensive urgency: A clinical situation in which a patient has extremely high BP values, typically >180/120 mm Hg, that is not accompanied by acuter or progressing target-organ injury. These situations require oral antihypertensive therapy to reduce BP to Stage 1 values over a period of several hours to several days.

Hypertrichosis: Abnormal hair growth on the body in areas where hair does not usually grow.

Hypertrophic cardiomyopathy: Hypertrophic cardiomyopathy is a genetic disorder characterized by disproportionate hypertrophy of the left ventricle, and occasionally of the right ventricle.

Hypervigilance: An enhanced state of sensory sensitivity accompanied by an exaggerated intensity of behaviors whose purpose is to detect threats.

Hypnagogic hallucinations: Dreamlike experiences on the threshold of sleep that intrude into wakefulness.

Hypnopompic hallucinations: Dreamlike experiences on the threshold of awakening that intrude into wakefulness.

Hypochlorhydria: Presence of an abnormally small amount of hydrochloric acid in the stomach.

Hypogonadism: Little or no hormone production by the testes (in men) or ovaries (in women).

Hypokalemia: Serum potassium concentration below 3.5 mEq/L.

Hypomagnesemia: Serum magnesium concentration below 1.4 mEq/L or 1.7 mg/dL.

Hypomania: An abnormally and persistently elevated, expansive, or irritable mood resembling mania, but of lesser intensity and which does not cause marked impairment in functioning.

Hypomimia: Decreased facial expression often associated with decreased blink rate.

Hypophonia: Decreased volume of speech.

Hypothalamus: A small region at the base of the brain that controls the release of hormones from the anterior and posterior regions of the pituitary gland and regulates limbic functions, fluid balance, body temperature, cardiovascular function, respiratory function, and diurnal rhythms.

Hysterectomy: Excision of the uterus.

Hysteresis: A situation in which concentration-effect curves do not always follow the same pattern when serum concentrations increase as they do when serum concentrations decrease. Can result from tolerance to a drug (clockwise hysteresis) or accumulation of active metabolites (counterclockwise hysteresis).

Iatrogenesis or iatrogenic disease: A disease produced as a consequence of medical or surgical treatment.

Ichthyosis: Dry, rectangular scales on the skin.

Ictal: The period during a seizure.

Icteric: Relating to or marked by jaundice.

Idiopathic: Unknown etiology of status epilepticus, often considered a genetic etiology for the prolonged seizure; definition specific to seizures, but really applies to any disease.

Ileitis: Inflammation of the ileus.

Illusions: Visual perceptions that are misinterpreted but have a real sensory stimulus.

Immunocompromised host: A patient with defects in host defenses that predispose him or her to infection (risk factors can include neutropenia, immune system defects from disease or immunosuppressive drug therapy, compromise of natural host defenses, environmental contamination, and changes in normal flora of the host).

Immunoglobulin: Structurally related glycoproteins that function as antibodies and are divided into classes on the basis of structure/biologic activity.

Impaction: An immovable packing; a lodgment of something in a strait or passage of the body; as, impaction of the fetal head in the strait of the pelvis; impaction of food or feces in the intestines of man or beast.

Impedance-pH monitoring: New technique used to detect reflux by measuring changes in intraluminal resistance determined by the presence of liquid or gas inside the esophagus. When combined with pH monitoring, it can differentiate between acid and nonacid reflux.

Impending status epilepticus: Any seizure that does not stop automatically within 5 minutes has been termed impending status epilepticus. This is a fairly new term that was created to recognize the importance of early treatment of status epilepticus. Pharmacologic and nonpharmacologic treatment of status epilepticus should be initiated for those seizures that do not spontaneously terminate within 5 minutes.

Impetigo: A superficial skin infection that is seen most commonly in children.

Implantable cardioverter-defibrillator (ICD): The ICD is a surgically implanted electronic device that monitors, detects, and treats potentially life-threatening ventricular tachycardia with rate-responsive ventricular pacing.

Inanition: Severe weakness and wasting as occurs from lack of food, defect in assimilation, or neoplastic disease.

Incubation period: The time between exposure of a biologic (i.e., pathogen), chemical, or radiologic substance and when symptoms first start to appear (also known as latency).

Induction: Administration of a highly intense level of immunosuppression in the perioperative period or use of antibody therapy to provide enough immunosuppression to delay administration of nephrotoxic calcineurin inhibitors.

Infant mortality: Deaths occurring in those younger than the age of 1 year per 1,000 live births.

Infants: Pediatric patients who are 1 month to 1 year of age.

Infarction: The formation of an infarct, an area of tissue death due to a local lack of oxygen.

Infection: Inflammatory response to invasion of host tissue by microorganisms.

Information bias: A flaw in measuring exposure or outcome data that results in systematic differences in the quality of information gathered for study and comparison groups. See also *Selection bias.*

Instrumental activities of daily living: Housekeeping chores, shopping, going outside, medication management. See also *Activities of daily living.*

Insulin-like growth factor-1: An anabolic peptide that acts as a direct stimulator of cell proliferation and growth in all body cells.

Integumentary system: Skin, subcutaneous tissue, and skin appendages.

Intravenous fat emulsion: An intravenous oil-in-water emulsion of oil(s), egg phosphatides, and glycerin.

Interleukin: A type of cytokine, usually influencing a white blood cell.

Intermittent-combined estrogen-progestogen therapy: A regimen that combines a daily estrogen with a progestogen administered intermittently in cycles of 3 days on and 3 days off (which is then repeated without interruption).

International normalized ratio (INR): A measure of coagulation calculated from the patient's prothrombin time (PT) measurement compared to the laboratory's mean normal control measurement and takes into account the sensitivity of the thromboplastin used to perform the test.

Interpersonal psychotherapy: A psychologic intervention that focuses on interpersonal relationships and psychosocial functioning.

Interpretability: The degree to which one can assign qualitative meaning to an instrument's quantitative scores.

Intertriginous areas: Body fold areas (e.g., between buttocks, beneath breasts, between toes, under arms).

Intertrigo: An inflammatory condition of skinfolds induced or aggravated by heat, moisture, maceration, friction, and lack of air circulation.

Intoxication: The development of a substance-specific syndrome after recent ingestion and presence in the body of a substance; associated with maladaptive behavior during the waking state caused by the effect of the substance on the central nervous system.

Intracavernosal injection: Injection into the corpus spongiosum.

Intracranial hypertension: Excessive pressure (>20 mm Hg) within the nondistensible intracranial cavity (i.e., skull) that can develop following traumatic brain injury.

Intracranial pressure: The pressure of the cerebral spinal fluid that is essentially the same as the pressure within the brain tissue (i.e., intraparenchymal pressure).

Intraperitoneal: Within the peritoneal cavity.

Intrauterine device: A device inserted in the uterus to prevent pregnancy, either through spermicidal action (copper device) or thickening cervical mucus to inhibit sperm penetration and migration (progesterone device).

Intrinsic resistance: See *Primary resistance.*

Intussusception: Invagination of one portion of the intestine into an adjacent part of the intestines.

Inulin: A fructose polysaccharide that is filtered by the glomerulus; its clearance is often used as an index of GFR.

Iothalamate: A nonradiolabeled or radiolabeled iodinated contrast agent that is filtered by the glomerulus; its clearance is often used as an index of GFR.

Ipsilateral: Of or pertaining to the same side of the body.

Irritable: Easily annoyed and provoked to anger.

Irritative voiding symptoms: Urinary urgency and frequency. This results from detrusor muscle decompensation that results from long-standing bladder outlet obstruction.

Isolated systolic hypertension: Patients with DBP values that are less than or equal to 90 mm Hg and SBP values that are greater than or equal to 140 mm Hg.

Janeway lesion: These lesions appear as flat, painless, red to bluish-red spots on the palms and soles of patients with acute bacterial endocarditis.

Jarisch-Herxheimer reaction: An increase in symptoms of spirochetal disease caused by the initiation of treatment.

J-curve phenomenon (in hypertension): A theoretical situation where lowering BP provides a reduced risk of cardiovascular events, but when BP is lowered too much, can paradoxically increase the risk of cardiovascular events.

Jugular venous oxygen saturation ($Sjvo_2$): Oxygen hemoglobin saturation of blood in the jugular bulb, which is a key element in estimating $CMRo_2$.

Just culture of patient safety: An approach to analysis and prevention of medication errors that relies on encouragement of internal risk transparency, coaching and consoling of employees, avoiding negative retribution for errors, and gathering then using information to prevent error recurrence.

K complexes: Electronegative waves followed by electropositive waves seen on the EEG during sleep.

Karyotyping: Chromosomal analysis.

Keratinization: Keratin formation.

Keratinized: Skin that has developed thicker areas of keratin in the stratum corneum.

Keratinocyte: Cell of the epidermis that produces keratin.

Keratoconjunctivitis sicca: Dry, itchy eyes that result from atrophy of the lacrimal ducts, which can be seen in inflammatory arthritis.

Keratolytic: Agent that solubilizes intracellular cement of keratin cells in the stratum corneum.

Keratosis pilaris: Small, rough bumps, generally on the face, upper arms, and thighs.

Ketogenic diet: A special antiseizure diet that is high in fat and low in carbohydrates and protein.

Kleptomania: An impulse control disorder characterized by frequent and repeated theft.

Köbner phenomenon: De novo lesion psoriasis appearing at the site of cutaneous trauma.

Kt/V: A measurement of how much urea is being removed from the blood during dialysis. The measurement takes into account the efficiency of the dialyzer (clearance, K), the treatment time (t), and the volume of distribution of urea (V).

Kussmaul sign: Kussmaul sign is a rise in jugular venous pressure on inspiration. Kussmaul sign is seen in conditions in which there is right ventricular filling.

Kwashiorkor: Starvation-associated malnutrition associated with inadequate protein intake.

Lactation: Production and secretion of breast milk.

Lanugo: Fine body hair normally found on a fetus. The hair develops in patients with anorexia nervosa when they are very underweight and malnourished.

Laparoscopic: Abdominal exploration or surgery employing a type of endoscope called laparoscope.

Laparotomy: Surgical opening of the abdominal cavity.

Laryngospasm: The spasmodic closure of the larynx because of a variety of causes such as allergic reactions, response to irritants, and pharmacologic actions.

Lavage: Washing out.

Laxative: A medication or agent used to produce a bowel movement.

Left ventricular ejection fraction: Also known simply as the ejection fraction, it is the fraction or percentage of the end-diastolic blood volume ejected by the left ventricle during systole. It is a measurement of cardiac systolic function with a normal ejection being >60% (>0.60). It can be determined noninvasively by an echocardiogram; it is really institution dependent and highly variable. It now states that >60% is normal, but in our institution, >50% is considered normal.

Left ventricular end diastolic volume: Left ventricular end diastolic volume refers to the volume of blood found in the left ventricular at the end of heart relaxation or diastole.

Left ventricular hypertrophy: Enlargement of the left ventricle, which is seen in heart failure and can give rise to arrhythmias.

Lentigines, PUVA: Brown to black macules resulting from long-term use of psoralens plus ultraviolet A light.

Leptospirosis: A bacterial disease that affects humans and animals caused by the genus Leptospira.

Lewy bodies: Pink-staining spheres found inside neuronal cells of the substantia nigra and other brain regions, considered to be a histopathologic marker for Parkinson's disease.

Lichenification: Thick, leathery skin, usually the result of constant scratching and rubbing.

Linear pharmacokinetics: The situation when changes in long-term daily doses of drugs result in proportional changes in steady state serum drug concentrations. Most drugs follow this pattern.

Linguistic competency: The ability of individuals and organizations to communicate effectively with people from diverse language backgrounds.

Linkage disequilibrium: Two or more polymorphisms that are inherited together more frequently than would be expected based on chance.

Lipid peroxidation: A pathophysiologic process involving the iron-catalyzed attack of lipid membranes by reactive oxygen species.

Liposomes: Spherical amphiphilic vesicles capable of sustained release of water-soluble substances.

Locus ceruleus: A small area in the brainstem containing norepinephrine neurons that is considered to be a key brain center for anxiety and fear.

Low-glycemic-load diet: A low-glycemic-load diet emphasizes consuming carbohydrates with a low glycemic index. To eat a low-glycemic-load diet, avoid foods such as white bread, refined cereal, cookies, and sugary drinks. Emphasize fruits, vegetables, legumes, and minimally processed grains.

Low glycemic index: The term low glycemic index refers to the quality of carbohydrates and how fast they are absorbed. Foods with a low glycemic index are absorbed more slowly, thus keeping insulin levels more stable.

Lumbar puncture: The procedure used to withdraw cerebrospinal fluid through a needle inserted in the lumbar region of the spinal column.

Luteinizing hormone (LH): A polypeptide hormone secreted by the anterior pituitary gland that stimulates ovulation and maintains the corpus luteum.

Luteolysis: Death of the corpus luteum.

Lymphangitis: An inflammation involving the subcutaneous lymphatic channels.

Lymphocytosis: Increased blood concentration of lymphocytes ($>4 \times 10^9$ cells/mm^3) commonly observed in mononucleosis, pertussis, measles, chickenpox, or lymphoid malignancies.

Lymphedema: A lymphatic obstruction of localized fluid retention and tissue swelling caused by compromised lymphatic system.

Lymphogranuloma venereum: Inflammation of the lymph nodes caused by *Chlamydia trachomatis* resulting in destruction and scarring of tissue.

Macule: Flat, nonpalpable, variable-colored lesion.

Maculopapular: Skin eruption containing both macules and papules.

Magnetic resonance angiography (MRA): A noninvasive method to evaluate the patency of blood vessels using magnetic resonance imaging.

Magnetic resonance imaging (MRI): An imaging technique based on the magnetic properties of the hydrogen atom. It provides an accurate, computer-processed image that can be more sensitive than computed tomography.

Major depression: A psychiatric disorder in which the patient can present with symptoms of depressed mood, a lack of interest in usual activities or inability to experience pleasure, changes in sleep and eating habits, guilt, reduced energy, thoughts of self-harm, and a sense of helplessness or hopelessness.

Major histocompatibility complex (MHC): A set of genes responsible for most of the proteins on the surface of cells in the body that are responsible for recognition of *self*.

Mania: An abnormally and persistently elevated, expansive, or irritable mood with increased activity or energy which causes marked impairment in functioning.

Marasmus: Starvation-associated malnutrition.

Masked hypertension: Patients that have elevated BP measurements based on home measurements but have normal BP measurements when measured in a clinical setting. These patients have chronic hypertension but either may not be diagnosed or may have a diagnosis of hypertension that is undertreated.

Mass effect: Distortion or displacement of the brain anatomy because of an implied or apparent mass (such as stroke or tumor).

Mastalgia or mastodynia: Pain in the breast.

Mean arterial pressure: The mean arterial pressure is the product of the cardiac output and systemic vascular resistance. Since the cardiac output is pulsatile, rather than continuous, and since 2/3 of the normal cardiac cycle is spent in diastole, the mean arterial pressure is not the arithmetic mean of the systolic and diastolic blood pressures. Mean arterial pressure = diastolic blood pressure + 1/3 (systolic blood pressure − diastolic blood pressure).

Measurement model: An instrument's scale and subscale structure and the procedures followed to create scale and subscale scores.

Meconium ileus: Intestinal obstruction caused by meconium.

Medication error: Any preventable event that may cause or lead to inappropriate medication use or patient harm while the medication is in the control of the healthcare professional, patient, or consumer (per the National Coordinating Council for Medication Error Reporting and Prevention).

Megakaryocytes: Precursors of platelets.

Melanin: Dark pigment that is part of determining skin color.

Melena: Dark-colored stools resulting from upper gastrointestinal bleed.

Membrane stripping: When the cervix is dilated, a practitioner can use a hand to separate the amniotic membranes from the uterus. This technique has been shown to reduce the need for labor induction.

Menarche: The time of the first menstrual period or flow.

Meningitis: Inflammation, usually infectious, of the meninges, a covering of the brain.

Menopause: The permanent cessation of menses following the loss of ovarian follicular activity.

Menorrhagia: Menstrual blood loss of greater than 80 mL per cycle; a more practical definition is heavy menstrual flow associated with problems of containment of flow, unpredictably heavy flow days, or other associated symptoms.

Menses: Periodic bloody discharge from the uterus.

Mental status examination: An objective patient evaluation conducted through a direct patient interview and used to make a diagnosis, assess the course of illness, or determine treatment response.

Meralgia parethetica: A disorder characterized by tingling, numbness, and burning pain in the outer side of the thigh. The disorder is caused by compression of the lateral femoral cutaneous nerve, a sensory nerve to the skin, as it exits the pelvis.

Mesolimbic pathway: A dopaminergic pathway in the brain that connects the ventral tegmental area in the midbrain to the nucleus accumbens in the striatum and is involved in motivation and reward.

Metabolic syndrome: A constellation of metabolic and cardiovascular changes consisting of at least three of the following: obesity, low high-density lipoprotein (HDL), elevated triglycerides, hypertension, and elevated fasting blood glucose.

Metastasis: Movement or spread of disease from one organ or part to new location not directly connected.

Methemoglobin: A form of hemoglobin that occurs when its iron is oxidized to the +3 state, which decreases oxygen binding.

Methionine: The 1-isomer is a nutritionally essential amino acid and the most important natural source of *active methyl* groups in the body, hence usually involved in methylations in vivo.

Michaelis–Menten kinetics: the situation where changes in steady state serum drug concentrations of drugs are disproportional to changes in long-term daily doses due to alterations in drug metabolism.

Microalbuminuria: A condition in which a small amount of albumin (30–300 mg/day) is present in the urine; often indicates an early stage of chronic kidney disease (CKD).

Microcephalic: Abnormally small head.

Microcomedo: Microscopic lesion formed from the combination of sloughed, clumping keratinocytes reacting with sebum and fatty acids from the sebaceous gland.

Micrographia: Handwriting that is small, trails off in size, or very slow.

Micrometastases: Spread of microscopic cancer cells to secondary sites distant from the primary site.

Midsystolic: Middle of systole.

Migraine aura: Early symptom of an attack of migraine with aura, which is the manifestation of focal cerebral dysfunction. The aura typically precedes the headache.

Mild cognitive impairment: A syndrome characterized by cognitive impairment that is not of sufficient severity to warrant a diagnosis of dementia.

Milia: Small, white cysts containing keratin.

Mixed states: Rapidly alternating mood states (mania and major depressive episodes) that last at least 1 week, and cause marked impairment in functioning.

Molds: Fungal organisms that grow as multicellular branching, thread-like filaments (hyphae) that are either *septate* (divided by transverse walls) or *coenocytic* (multinucleate without cross walls). On agar media, molds grow outward from the point of inoculation by extension of the tips of filaments, and then branch repeatedly, interweaving to form fuzzy, matted growths called *mycelium.* Germ tubes are the beginning of *hyphae*, which arise as perpendicular extensions from the yeast cell, with no constriction at their point of origin.

Molybdenum (Mo): A bioelement found in a number of proteins.

Monoamine neurotransmitters: Neurotransmitters that contain one amino group and are derived from amino acids such as tyrosine and tryptophan. Include, among others, the catecholamines (dopamine and norepinephrine) and an indoleamine (serotonin).

Mood: A more pervasive and sustained emotional state that colors a person's perception of the world.

Morbilliform: Maculopapular lesions that become confluent on the face and body.

Mucolytic: The ability to break down mucus.

Mucositis: Inflammation of the mucosa.

Multiattribute health status classification systems: Preference-based HRQOL instruments for which health-state preferences have been derived from population studies. The instruments assess respondents' health status, and then population preferences are applied to produce the index score.

Multiparity: Condition of having given birth to multiple children.

Multiple-organ dysfunction syndrome (MODS): Presence of altered organ function requiring intervention to maintain homeostasis.

Multiple sclerosis (MS): A demyelinating disease, caused by inflammation, leading to neurologic deficits and often, disability.

Mutism: A state in which a person either has the inability or refuses to speak or vocalize sounds.

Mycotic: A fungal infection.

Myectomy: A surgical removal of the overgrown septal muscle to decrease the outflow tract obstruction.

Myocarditis: Inflammation of the cardiac muscle.

Myoclonic seizures: Brief shock-like muscular contractions of the face, trunk, and extremities. They usually begin in adolescence and are referred to as *juvenile myoclonic epilepsy* (JME).

Myoclonus: A sudden twitching of muscles or parts of muscles, without any rhythm or pattern.

Myositis: Inflammation of the muscle, characterized by pain, tenderness, and sometimes spasm in the affected area.

Narrowband UVB (NB-UVB): 311 nm ultraviolet B light.

National Kidney Foundation (NKF): A major voluntary health organization that seeks to prevent kidney and urinary tract diseases, improve the health and well-being of individuals and families affected by these diseases, and increase the availability of all organs for transplantation.

Nausea: An unpleasant sensation associated with an awareness of the urge to vomit.

Necrosis: Local death of cells or tissue.

Necrotizing fasciitis: A rare, but very severe infection of the subcutaneous tissue that can be caused by aerobic and/or anaerobic bacteria and results in progressive destruction of the superficial fascia and subcutaneous fat.

Negative symptoms: Those symptoms of schizophrenia that are largely associated with a deficit in psychosocial functioning, emotional expression, and interpersonal interactions. Examples include blunted affect, alogia, decreased interest and involvement in social and occupational activities, and decreased grooming and hygiene.

Neoadjuvant therapy: Any therapy administered before surgical resection of the tumor or cancer, providing benefits related to tumor shrinkage and eradication of micrometastases.

Neonatal: Within the first 4 weeks (28 days) of life.

Neonates: Newborns who are 1 day to 1 month of age.

Nephritis: Inflammation of the kidney.

Nephrolithiasis: Presence of one or more stones in the renal pelvis, collecting system, or ureters.

Nephron: The working unit of the kidney that is comprised of a glomerulus and tubule. Each kidney is made up of approximately 1 million nephrons, which collectively remove drugs, toxins, and fluid from the blood.

Nephropathy: Refers to a pathologic alteration of the kidney.

Nephrotic range proteinuria: Proteinuria >3 g/day associated with glomerular disease and nephrotic syndrome.

Nephrotoxicity: Toxic insult to the kidney.

Nerve conduction studies: Measurement of the speed of electrical conduction through a nerve.

Neuraminidase: The second major antigenic determinant of the influenza virus; a surface antigen that allows the release of new viral particles from host cells by catalyzing the cleavage of linkages to sialic acid.

Neuritic plaques: Hallmark pathologic marker of Alzheimer's disease comprised of β-amyloid protein and masses of broken neurites.

Neurofibrillary tangles: Hallmark pathologic marker of Alzheimer's disease derived from abnormal phosphorylation of τ-protein filaments.

Neuropathic pain: Pain due to nervous system damage.

Neuropsychological: Pertaining to a specialty of psychology concerned with the study of the relationships between the brain and behavior, including the use of psychological tests and assessment techniques to diagnose specific cognitive and behavioral deficits and to prescribe rehabilitation strategies for their remediation.

Neutropenia: An abnormally reduced number of neutrophils circulating in peripheral blood; although exact definitions of neutropenia often vary, an absolute neutrophil count of <1000 cells/mm^3 indicates a reduction sufficient to predispose patients to infection.

New York Heart Association classification: The New York Heart Association classification provides a simple way of classifying the extent of heart failure. It places patients in one of four categories based on how much they are limited during physical activity.

***N*-methyl-D-aspartate antagonists:** Class of medications that decreases the activity of synaptic glutamate, thus decreasing the likelihood of cell death.

***N*-methyl-D-aspartate (NMDA) receptors:** One of three types of ionotropic postsynaptic glutamate receptors. Upon binding glutamate, these receptors permit the influx of Ca^{+2} ions and results in brain excitation. These are one of the two primary receptors for excitatory neurotransmission in the brain.

Nociceptive pain: Pain due to physiologic processes that involve transduction, transmission, perception, and modulation.

Nocturia: Frequent nighttime urination (>2 micturitions per night).

Nodule: Elevated, palpable, solid, round or oval lesion more than 0.5 cm in diameter.

Non–ST-segment elevation: A type of myocardial infarction that is limited to the subendocardial myocardium and is smaller and less extensive than an ST-segment MI, and usually there is no pathologic Q wave on the ECG.

Nonalcoholic fatty liver disease (NAFLD): Refers to a wide spectrum of liver disease ranging from simple fatty liver (steatosis), to nonalcoholic steatohepatitis (NASH), to cirrhosis (irreversible, advanced scarring of the liver). All of the stages of NAFLD have in common the accumulation of fatty infiltration in the liver cells.

Nonarteritic, anterior, ischemic optic neuropathy: A disorder caused by an acute decrease of blood flow to the optic nerve, which results in sudden vision loss. If persistent, it can lead to permanent vision loss.

Nonconvulsive status epilepticus (NCSE): Believed to be less common and have a better prognosis than GCSE. The most common two types are absence status epilepticus and complex partial status epilepticus. Both are associated with an impairment in consciousness. For the more common of the two, absence status, the patient appears in a twilight state to lethargy, there is no return to consciousness as occurs in complex partial status epilepticus. For complex partial status epilepticus partial return to consciousness can occur. It may or may not be associated with motor activity or automatisms. The duration is sufficient enough in length to meet the definition of status epilepticus.

Nonoliguria: Production of >500 mL urine/day.

Nonpolyposis: Absence of polyps.

Nonulcer dyspepsia: Ulcer-like dyspepsia that has been investigated, but endoscopic findings yield no evidence of mucosal injury (ulcer).

Norepinephrine (NE): A hormone secreted by the adrenal medulla and also released at synapses.

Nosocomial infection: An infection acquired in a healthcare facility.

NSAID: Nonsteroidal antiinflammatory drug.

***N*-terminal proBNP:** The biologically inactive fragment of B-type natriuretic peptide (BNP). Compared to BNP, *N*-terminal proBNP circulates at higher plasma concentrations and has a longer half-life.

Nulliparity: Condition of not having given birth to a child.

Obesity–hypoventilation syndrome: Also known as Pickwickian syndrome.

Oblique lie: The fetus is at an angle to the cervix. The head is not the presenting part, and often the patient will need to be delivered by cesarean section.

Obsession: Recurrent and persistent thoughts, images, or impulses experienced as intrusive and distressing.

Obsessive–compulsive disorder (OCD): An anxiety disorder characterized by obsessions and/or compulsions that are time-consuming and interfere significantly with normal routine, social or occupational functioning, or relationships.

Obstructive voiding symptoms: Decreased force of the urinary stream, hesitancy, incomplete bladder emptying, urinary dribbling. This results from bladder outlet obstruction as could be caused by benign prostatic hyperplasia.

Odynophagia: Painful swallowing.

Oligoanovulation: The condition of having few to no ovulatory menstrual cycles.

Oligomenorrhea: Reduced frequency of menses with a time interval between periods greater than 40 days but less than 6 months.

Oliguria: Production of <500 mL urine/day.

Omentumectomy: Excision of the double fold of peritoneum attached to the stomach and connecting it with abdominal viscera (omentum).

Onychomycosis: Fungal infection of the nail apparatus.

Open prostatectomy: In this surgical procedure, an enlarged prostate is removed in its entirety. Access to the prostate can be achieved by cutting through the bladder and reaching down to the prostate, or by cutting through the perineum (between the legs).

Ophthalmia neonatorum: Inflammation of the conjunctiva resulting from acquisition of gonococcal infection at birth.

Opioid addiction: A behavioral pattern manifesting as loss of control over opioid use, compulsive use, and continued use despite harm.

Opioid dependence: State that occurs subsequent to extended exposure to an opioid and manifests as withdrawal symptoms after abrupt dose reduction, discontinuation or after the administration of an opioid antagonist.

Opioid tolerance: Decreased effectiveness of opioid over time due to opioid exposure.

Opportunistic infection (OI): Infection with microorganism that occurs because of altered physiologic state of the patient.

Orchiectomy: The surgical removal of the testicles.

Organic erectile dysfunction: Term used to refer to erectile dysfunction that is caused by vascular, neurologic, and/or hormonal causes.

Orthopnea: Difficulty breathing after lying down.

Orthostatic hypotension: A significant drop in BP, defined as a SBP decrease of greater than 20 mm Hg or a DBP decrease of greater than 10 mm Hg, that occurs when changing from a supine to a standing position.

Osler nodes: Osler nodes are red, raised tender nodules usually 5 mm in diameter on the pulps of toes or fingers. Seen in patients with endocarditis, they are thought to be caused by the deposition of immune complexes.

Osteogenesis imperfecta: Genetic disorder characterized by low trabecular and cortical bone density.

Osteomalacia: Abnormal bone mineralization, referred to as rickets in children.

Osteomyelitis: Infection involving the bone.

Osteopenia: Low bone density, dual-energy x-ray absorptiometry (DXA) T-score of –1 to –2.5.

Osteophyte: A bony outgrowth or protuberance.

Osteoporosis: Very low bone density, DXA T-score less than –2.5, with or without a low trauma fracture. National Osteoporosis Foundation definition: "A chronic, progressive disease characterized by low bone mass, microarchitectural deterioration and decreased bone strength, bone fragility and a consequent increase in fracture risk."

Osteotomy: The surgical cutting of a bone.

Otitis media: Inflammation of the middle ear.

Ovarian ablation: Removal or irradiation of the ovaries, rendering them nonfunctional.

Ovarian suppression: Medical castration in women through the use of medications.

Ovulation: Periodic ripening and rupture of mature follicle and the discharge of ovum from the cortex of the ovary.

Oxytocin: A polypeptide hormone secreted by the posterior pituitary gland that stimulates uterine contraction.

Paget's disease: Disorder of bone remodeling in discrete sections of bone; also a disorder of the breast (primarily nipple complex) associated with breast cancer and/or bone changes.

PAH: *p*-Aminohippurate, a small molecule that is completely secreted from the tubules into urine, so that blood leaving the kidney is virtually free of PAH; a marker that is often used to measure renal plasma flow (RPF).

Pain: An unpleasant sensory and emotional experience associated with actual or potential tissue damage or described in terms of such damage.

Palpation: Touching the skin to feel the outline of an organ.

Pan- or holosystolic: Throughout the end time of systole.

Pancolitis: Inflammation that involves the majority of the colon for patients with inflammatory bowel disease.

Pancreatitis: An acute or chronic inflammation of the pancreas with variable involvement of local tissues and remote organs.

Panel reactive antibody (PRA): The percentage of cells from a panel of donors with which a potential recipient's bloodstream reacts. The more antibodies in the recipient's bloodstream, the higher the PRA. The higher the PRA, the higher the risk for a positive crossmatch.

Panhypopituitarism: A condition of complete or partial loss of anterior and posterior pituitary function resulting in a complex disorder characterized by multiple pituitary-hormone deficiencies.

Panic attack: A discrete period in which there is the sudden onset of intense apprehension, fearfulness, or terror, often associated with feelings of impending doom.

Panic disorder: The presence of recurrent, unexpected panic attacks followed by at least 1 month of persistent concern about having another panic attack, worry about the possible implications or consequences of the panic attacks, or a significant behavioral change related to the attacks.

Panlobular: Affecting the entire lobe.

Papillary: Upper layer of the dermis.

Papilledema: Swelling around the optic nerve, usually caused by pressure on the nerve by a tumor or stroke.

Papule: Solid, elevated, lesion more than 0.5 cm in diameter.

Papules: Small raised bumps that may open when scratched and become crusty and infected.

Papulosquamous: Raised plaque or papule with scaling.

***p*-Aminohippurate (PAH):** A small molecule that is completely secreted from the tubules into urine, so that blood leaving the kidney is virtually free of PAH; a marker that is often used to measure renal plasma flow (RPF).

Paranoia: Ideation involving suspiciousness or the belief that one is being harassed, persecuted, or unfairly treated.

Parenchyma: Specific cells or tissue of an organ.

Parenteral nutrition: The intravenous administration of nutrients.

Paresthesia: An abnormal sensation, such as burning, pricking, tickling, or tingling.

Peripherally inserted central catheter (PICC): A venous access device usually inserted into the basilic, cephalic, or brachial veins that terminates at the superior vena cava.

Peripheral parenteral nutrition: Parenteral nutrition delivered into a peripheral vein, usually of the hand or forearm.

Parkinsonism: A constellation of symptoms with atypical features such that a diagnosis of idiopathic Parkinson disease cannot be made.

Parous: Having borne one or more children.

Paroxysmal nocturnal dyspnea: Onset of difficulty breathing after lying down for several hours.

Partial agonist: A drug with high binding affinity to a receptor that elicits a weaker response than the endogenous neurotransmitter. At least theoretically, this causes an agonist effect in states of decreased endogenous neurotransmitter tone and an antagonist effect in the endogenous state of heightened neurotransmitter activity.

Partial seizure: A seizure that begins in one hemisphere of the brain. It can be simple, complex, or secondarily generalized.

Patch: Large macule (more than 2 cm in diameter).

Patient-reported outcomes: The consequences of the disease and/or its treatment as perceived and reported by the patient.

Pelvic inflammatory disease (PID): Infection of the lining of the uterus, the fallopian tubes, or the ovaries.

Penumbra (ischemic): The area of brain tissue around the core of the infarct that has decreased function but remains viable. It is proposed that reperfusion of this tissue will allow survival of the affected neurons and other brain cells.

Peptic ulcer: Cellular distribution of the gastrointestinal mucosa, submucosa, and muscular layer. Chronic peptic ulcers usually occur as a "single hole" and are found most often in the stomach and duodenum.

Percussion: Tapping on a structure to elicit a sound.

Percussion and postural drainage: Tapping on the thorax to physically loosen pulmonary secretions and posturing the body to facilitate expectoration.

Percutaneous coronary intervention (PCI): A minimally invasive procedure whereby access to the coronary arteries is obtained through the femoral artery up the aorta to the coronary os. Contrast media is used to visualize the coronary artery stenosis using a coronary angiogram. A guidewire is used to cross the stenosis and a small balloon is inflated and/or stent is deployed to break up atherosclerotic plaque and restore coronary artery blood flow. The stent is left in place to prevent acute closure and restenosis of the coronary artery. Newer stents are coated with antiproliferative drugs, such as paclitaxel and sirolimus, which further reduce the risk of restenosis of the coronary artery.

Pericarditis: Inflammation of the pericardium, which is the fibroserous sac enclosing the heart.

Perimenopause: The period immediately prior to the menopause and the first year after menopause. Reflects the transition to menopause (with irregular menstrual cycles) and includes the 3 to 5 years before and 1 year after the cessation of menstrual flow.

Perinatal: Time shortly before and after birth.

Periodontitis: A serious gum infection caused by inflammation and infection of the ligaments that support the teeth.

Perioral dermatitis: Rash around the mouth. In patients with anorexia nervosa or bulimia nervosa, the rash is secondary to repeated vomiting that creates skin irritation from exposure to the gastric contents.

Peripheral arterial disease (PAD): Atherosclerotic occlusive disease of the extremities, usually diagnosed by symptoms (claudication) or assessment of the blood flow to an extremity.

Peripheral blood progenitor cells: Immature blood cells, which are capable of producing white blood cells, platelets, and red blood cells.

Peritoneal dialysis (PD): A dialysis procedure performed in the peritoneal cavity in which the peritoneum acts as the semipermeable membrane.

Peritonitis: The acute, inflammatory response of the peritoneal lining to microorganisms, chemicals, irradiation, or foreign body injury.

Periungual pyogenic granulomas: Benign vascular lesion around the fingernails or toenails; can relate to acitretin use.

Perseveration: Persistent repetition of the same verbal or motor response despite differing stimuli.

Pervasive developmental disorder: A group of disorders described in the DSM-IV-TR characterized by severe and pervasive impairments in the development of socialization and communication skills, as well as behavioral repertoire, with a typical diagnosis younger than age 3 years; includes autistic disorder, Rett syndrome, pervasive development disorder not otherwise specified, childhood disintegrative disorder, and Asperger disorder. The term pervasive developmental disorder is not used in the DSM-5.

Petechiae: Pinpoint, flat, round, red spots under the skin caused by intradermal hemorrhage.

Peyronie's disease: Disease of the penis associated with fibrous tissue scarring along the inside of the penile shaft resulting in significant and abnormal curvature of the erect penis. Associated with penile pain; deformity makes sexual intercourse difficult or impossible.

P-glycoprotein: An adenosine triphosphatase (ATPase)-dependent membrane transporter efflux pump coded for by the multidrug-resistance gene 1 (MDR1 or ABCB1 or PGY1) found in the human blood-brain barrier and intestine as well as other tissues; lipophilic molecules are good substrates for the ABCB1 efflux transport system at the blood–brain barrier.

Pharmacodynamics: The study of the relationship between the concentration of a drug and the response obtained in a patient.

Pharmacoepidemiology: The study of the use of and the effects of drugs in large numbers of people with the purpose of supporting safe and effective drug therapies. This type of observational research is useful when more rigorous, experimental designs are not feasible.

Pharmacogenetics: Genetic basis for interindividual differences in drug response.

Pharmacovigilance: The science and activities relating to the detection, assessment, understanding, and prevention of adverse effects or any other drug-related problems.

Pharyngitis: An acute infection of the oropharynx or nasopharynx.

Phase I reactions: Metabolic changes by the body that generally make the drug molecule more polar and water soluble so that it is prone to elimination by the kidney, such as oxidation, hydrolysis, and reduction.

Phase II reactions: Metabolic changes by the body that generally make the drug molecule more prone to elimination by the kidney, such as conjugation to form glucuronides, acetates, or sulfates.

Phenotype: Outward expression of the genotype.

Phenotypes: How a gene is expressed (e.g., eye color, height, drug metabolism capacity). The expression of genetic alleles (genotype) as an observable physical or biochemical trait.

Phobia: A persistent, abnormal, and irrational fear of a specific thing or situation that compels one to avoid it, despite the awareness and reassurance that it is not dangerous.

Phonophobia: Hypersensitivity to sound, usually causing avoidance.

Photic stimulation: Stimulation of the visual cortex through visual stimulation with bright and alternating light.

Photoallergy: Photosensitivity disorder of skin (light and photoallergic agent).

Photophobia: Hypersensitivity to light, usually causing avoidance.

Phototoxicity: Photosensitivity disorder of skin (light and phototoxic agent).

Physical dependence: A state of adaptation that is manifested by a drug class–specific withdrawal syndrome that can be produced by abrupt cessation, rapid dose reduction, decreasing blood level of the drug, and/or administration of an antagonist.

Pickwickian syndrome: Excess load of excess body fat on the chest tissues resulting in a constellation of syndromes that include excessive daytime sleepiness, shortness of breath due to elevated blood carbon dioxide pressure, disturbed sleep at night, and flushed face.

Pilonidal: Hair-containing cyst.

Pilosebaceous: Sebaceous gland and adjacent hair follicle.

Placenta accreta: Attachment of placental villi to the muscle of the uterine wall causing abnormally firm placental adherence. Complications include intractable postpartum hemorrhage.

Placenta previa: Placental implantation at or near the opening of the cervix. Severe maternal hemorrhage can occur because the placenta precedes the infant during birth.

Plantar fasciitis: A condition that causes heel and arch pain as a result of irritation and inflammation of the plantar fascia, the connective tissues that form the arch of the foot.

Plaque: Raised, flat lesion (more than 2 cm in diameter).

Pneumonitis: Inflammation of lung tissue.

Podagra: Intense pain in the foot, often in the great toe as a symptom of gout.

Poikilocytosis: The presence of irregularly shaped red blood cells in the peripheral blood.

Poikilothermia: Inability to maintain normal body temperature.

Polyarteritis nodosa: A systemic necrotizing vasculitis of small and medium-sized arteries.

Polycystic ovarian syndrome: An endocrine disorder with a constellation of symptoms with excessive androgen activity, including irregular or no menstrual periods, acne, excessive hair growth, and infertility.

Polycythemia: An increase in the number of red cells present in the blood.

Polymorphism: Genetic variations occurring at a frequency of at least one percent in the human population.

Porphyria: A group of disorders involving heme biosynthesis, characterized by excessive excretion of porphyrins or their precursors; can be inherited or can be acquired, as from the effects of certain chemical agents.

Porphyrins: Pigments widely distributed throughout nature (e.g., heme, bile pigments, cytochromes) consisting of four pyrroles joined in a ring (porphin) structure.

Positive symptoms: Those symptoms of schizophrenia, largely based on perceptual and thought disturbances, that are typically associated with psychosis. Examples are suspiciousness, paranoia, delusions, hallucinations, and disorganized thought processes.

Positron emission tomography (PET): Specialized nuclear scanning technique that allows the measurement of regional blood flow and glucose metabolism. With radiolabeled ligands, it also allows for the measurement of the binding of drugs to receptors.

Posterior fossa: The cavity in the back part of the skull that contains the cerebellum, brainstem, and cranial nerves 5–12.

Postexposure prophylaxis: Dispensing or administering a medication (including a vaccine) to start immediately after exposure to a disease or organism, to prevent the disease from developing or spreading.

Postictal: The recovery period after a seizure, when a patient can be lethargic or confused. Duration can be variable.

Posttraumatic seizures: Seizure event(s) that can occur following a traumatic brain injury within the first 7 days postinjury (early) or beyond 7 days postinjury (late).

Posttraumatic stress disorder: An anxiety disorder in which exposure to an exceptional mental or physical stressor is followed by persistent reexperiencing of the event, avoidance of reminders of the event, and arousal symptoms.

Postvoid residual urine volume: Urine left in the bladder after the patient has been asked to completely empty urine out of the bladder. Normally, the postvoid residual urine volume should be zero. A high postvoid residual urine volume is associated with recurrent urinary tract infection.

PRA (panel reactive antibody): The percentage of cells from a panel of donors with which a potential recipient's bloodstream reacts. The more antibodies in the recipient's bloodstream, the higher the PRA. The higher the PRA, the higher the risk for a positive crossmatch.

Preexposure vaccination: Administration of a protective vaccine to the public, military troops, or high-risk individuals prior to the potential exposure to an infectious disease.

Preference-based measures: Measures that provide an overall HRQOL index score based on a scale anchored by 1.0 (full health) and 0.0 (dead).

Prefrontal cortex: Part of the brain that integrates thought, emotion, and motivation.

Preload: Along with afterload, it is an important determinant of cardiac output. It is the degree of stretch of the myocardial fibers (sarcomeres) at the end of diastole. As the sarcomeres are stretched, the force of contraction increases. Preload is approximated by the left ventricular end diastolic volume or pressure.

Premature infants: Those born before 37 weeks of gestational age.

Premature ovarian failure: Amenorrhea, sex-steroid deficiency, and infertility in women younger than 40 years of age.

Premenstrual dysphoric disorder (PMDD): Severe psychiatric mood disorder with marked affective symptoms causing significant interference in work or relationships temporally associated with the final week before the onset of menses and not caused by an underlying psychiatric disturbance. The diagnostic criteria require prospective documentation of symptoms, a specific constellation of symptoms, and functional impairment.

Premenstrual molimina: Includes premenstrual symptoms such as breast tenderness, pelvic heaviness or bloating, and food cravings that are not distressing and do not interfere with daily functioning.

Premenstrual syndrome (PMS): A constellation of symptoms including mild mood disturbance and physical symptoms that occur prior to the menses and resolve with initiation of menses.

Premonitory migraine symptoms: Symptoms preceding and forewarning of a migraine attack by 2 to 48 hours, occurring before the aura in migraine with aura and before the onset of pain in migraine without aura.

Presbycusis: Progressive bilateral loss of hearing that occurs in the aged.

Pressured speech: More and faster speech that is difficult or impossible to interrupt.

Preterm: Before 37 weeks of gestation.

Priapism: Painful prolonged erection.

Primary amenorrhea: Absence of menses by age 16 years in the presence of normal secondary sexual development or absence of menses by age 14 years in the absence of normal secondary sexual development.

Primary hypertension: Same as essential hypertension; persistently elevated BP that results from unknown pathophysiological etiology.

Primary hypogonadism: Failure of the testes to produce an adequate supply of testosterone to meet physiologic needs.

Primary lesion: Basic skin lesion that appears at the beginning of skin disorder.

Primary resistance: Refers to resistance recorded prior to drug exposure in vitro or in vivo, as determined by in-vitro susceptibility testing using standardized methodology.

Proctitis: Inflammation confined to the rectum for patients with inflammatory bowel disease.

Prodrome: Early symptom indicating that disease or further symptoms are imminent.

Progestins: Formulations of synthetic progesterone.

Progestogen: A term referring to progesterone and the synthetic progestational compounds (sometimes referred to as *progestins*).

Progressive multifocal leukoencephalopathy (PML): Rapidly progressive neuromuscular disease caused by opportunistic infection of brain cells by the JC virus.

Prolactin: A polypeptide hormone secreted by the anterior pituitary gland that stimulates lactation.

Proprioception: A sense or perception, usually at a subconscious level, of the movements and position of the body and especially its limbs, independent of vision; this sense is gained primarily from input from sensory nerve terminals in muscles and tendons and the fibrous capsule of joints combined with input from the vestibular apparatus.

Prostate-specific antigen (PSA): A clinical laboratory test; PSA is a tumor marker that is used to screen for, monitor response to treatment of, and determine degree of spread of prostate cancer. Normally, PSA blood levels should be low as PSA is passed out of the body in the ejaculate.

Prostatectomy: Removal of all or part of the prostate gland. There are two main types: (1) transurethral resection of the prostate (TURP)—removes part of the tissue surrounding the urethra that can be blocking the flow of urine; and (2) radical prostatectomy, which removes all of the prostate and the seminal vesicles.

Protease: An enzyme in HIV that cleaves large precursor polypeptides into functional proteins that are necessary to produce a complete virus.

Proteinuria: A condition in which the urine contains large amounts of protein (>150 mg/day); often a sign of glomerular or tubular damage in the kidney.

Proteolytic: The ability to break down protein.

Prothrombin: A clotting factor that is converted to thrombin; also known as factor II.

Prothrombin time (PT): A measure of coagulation representing the amount of time required to form a blood clot after the addition of thromboplastin to the blood sample; also known as Quick's test.

Pruritus: Itching.

Pseudoaddiction: A behavior pattern reflective of seeking relief of pain and resembling that of addictive behavior.

Pseudoallergic: Adverse reactions that appear like allergic reactions but do not have an immunologic mechanism.

Pseudocyst: Collection of pancreatic juice and tissue debris enclosed by a wall of fibrous or granulation tissue.

Pseudohypertension: A falsely elevated BP measurement that is usually because of rigid, calcified brachial arteries; this can be seen in patients who are elderly, have longstanding diabetes, or have chronic kidney disease.

Pseudomembranous colitis: Inflammation of the colon caused by the toxin of *Clostridium difficile* and resulting in bloody diarrhea.

Pseudopolyps: An area of hypertrophied gastrointestinal mucosa that resembles a polyp and contains nonmalignant cells.

Pseudotumor cerebri: Increased intracranial pressure caused by decreased venous drainage from the brain as a result of increased intraabdominal pressure. Symptoms usually include severe headache, bilateral pulsatile auditory tinnitus, and visual field cuts. Also known as idiopathic intracranial hypertension.

Pseudoxanthoma elasticum: Pseudoxanthoma elasticum is a chronic degenerative disease of connection tissues of the skin, eyes, and cardiovascular system resulting from fragmentation and calcification of elastic fibers.

Psoriasis: A chronic, noncontagious autoimmune disease that affects the skin in the form of thick, red, scaly patches.

Psychoeducation: Education geared toward patients becoming more informed about their mental illness and treatment. Additional goals include self-monitoring, efforts to improve treatment adherence, interactions between patient and clinicians, and empowerment.

Psychogenic erectile dysfunction: Erectile dysfunction because of failure of central nervous system to perceive or process sexually stimulating information.

Psychometrics: The measurement of psychologic constructs, such as quality of life.

Psychomotor: Movement or muscular activity related to mental processes.

Psychomotor retardation: A slowing or limitation of motor functioning or muscular movements.

Psychosocial functioning: A person's level of functioning on a daily basis that encompasses all the domains of life experience (e.g., interpersonal relationships, work, school, recreation).

Psychosocial rehabilitation programs: Care programs oriented toward improving patient's daily adaptive functioning. Includes such interventions as basic living skills, social skills training, basic education, work programs, and supported housing.

Psychosocial stressor: Any significant life event or change that can be associated with the onset, occurrence, or exacerbation of a mental disorder.

Psychotherapy: A general term used to describe a form of treatment based on talking with a therapist. Psychotherapy aims to relieve distress by discussing and expressing feelings, to help the patient to change attitudes, behavior, and habits and to develop better ways of coping.

Pulmonary artery occlusion pressure: It is usually determined by a balloon-tipped Swan-Ganz catheter that is advanced into a distal branch of the pulmonary artery. Inflation of the balloon at the catheter tip occludes the pulmonary artery and allows measurement of the left atrial pressure which reflects the left ventricular diastolic pressure. Therefore, it is a measure of the left ventricular preload.

Pulmonary aspiration: The inhalation of fluids and gastric contents into the lungs that can cause aspiration pneumonitis.

Pulmonary capillary wedge pressure: It is usually determined by a balloon-tipped Swan-Ganz catheter that is advanced into a distal branch of the pulmonary artery (PA). Inflation of the balloon at the catheter tip occludes the PA and allows measurement of the left atrial pressure which reflects the left ventricular diastolic pressure. Therefore, it is a measure of the left ventricular preload.

Pulmonary embolism: A disorder of thrombus formation causing obstruction of a pulmonary artery or one of its branches and results in pulmonary infarction.

Pulsating: Throbbing or beating with a rhythm.

Pulseless electrical activity: The absence of a detectable pulse and the presence of some type of electrical activity other than VF or PVT.

Purgatives: An agent used for purging the bowels.

Purpura: Discoloration of skin because of a hemorrhagic spot more than 0.5 cm in diameter.

Pustule: Small, raised lesion containing pus or exudates.

Pyelonephritis: An infection involving the kidneys and representing upper tract infection.

Pyoderma: Purulent skin disease.

Pyoderma gangrenosum: Skin ulceration with necrotic edges.

Pyuria: Presence of pus or white blood cells in the urine.

Quality-adjusted life-years (QALY): A health outcome summary measure in which quantity of life is adjusted for its quality. A year in full health is equivalent to 1.0 QALY. A year in a health state considered worse than full health, such as 0.5, would equal 0.5 QALY, which is equivalent to living half a year in full health.

Radionuclide ventriculography: Radionuclide ventriculography, also known as contrast ventriculography, provides imaging of a ventricle of the heart after the injection of a radioactive contrast medium. The technique is less invasive than cardiac catheterization and is used to assess ventricular function.

Rales: The clicking, rattling, or crackling noises heard on auscultation of the lungs during inhalation.

Rating scales: Tools used to objectively describe, assess, and measure subjective findings common in psychiatric illnesses. Rating scales are also used to diagnose specific psychiatric conditions.

Rational polytherapy: The concurrent use of two or more drugs for patients not responding to monotherapy. The combination of drugs is based on a consideration of mechanism of action, clinical pharmacokinetics, adverse reactions, and drug interactions.

Rebound insomnia: Sleep that is worsened compared with patient's baseline sleep for a few days after discontinuation of a sedative hypnotic medication.

Rebound vasodilation or congestion: See *Rhinitis medicamentosa*.

Refractory status epilepticus: Status epilepticus is considered refractory when adequate doses of a benzodiazepine, hydantoin, or barbiturate have failed to terminate the seizures, that is, a patient must have failed two first line therapies to be considered refractory.

Rejection: The response of the immune system, usually involving T- or B-lymphocytes, to the recognition of foreign antigens in transplanted tissue, which destroys the cells in the transplanted organ and ultimately leads to organ failure, if not treated successfully.

Relapse in multiple sclerosis: New or old multiple sclerosis symptoms lasting 24 hours or longer often associated with demyelination or inflammation in the brain or spinal cord. Relapses are also referred to as an attack, exacerbation, or flare-up of multiple sclerosis.

Relapsing-remitting multiple sclerosis: The most common form of multiple sclerosis at the time of diagnosis. It is characterized by attacks usually with full or partial recovery and no disease progression between attacks.

Relative risk reduction: The amount of risk reduced when compared to a control. When one sees a 5% event rate in the control group and a 4% event rate in the treatment group, the relative risk reduction is 20%. The absolute risk reduction is 1%.

Reliability: The extent to which measures give consistent or accurate results.

Remote symptomatic: When the cause of the status epilepticus is from a previous neurological injury or anatomical malformation, e.g., a patient with a prior stroke, head trauma or brain tumor.

Renal osteodystrophy (ROD): The condition resulting from sustained metabolic changes that occur with chronic kidney disease including secondary hyperparathyroidism, hyperphosphatemia, hypocalcemia, and vitamin D deficiency. The skeletal complications associated with ROD include osteitis fibrosa cystica (high bone turnover disease), osteomalacia (low bone turnover disease), adynamic bone disease, and mixed bone disorders.

Renal replacement therapy: Any form of dialysis or hemofiltration used to support patients without adequate kidney function. Goals of renal replacement therapy are to remove excess fluid; remove waste products and toxins; and control electrolyte concentrations.

Renal: General term referring to the kidneys.

Renin-angiotensin-aldosterone system: A complex endogenous humoral mediated system that is involved with most of the regulatory components involved with arterial BP.

Renovascular: Pertaining to blood vessels located within the kidney, such as the afferent and efferent arterioles, and renal arteries.

Resistant hypertension: Patients with hypertension who have not achieved their goal BP value despite treatment with three or more antihypertensive drugs.

Respiratory disturbance index: A summary measure that quantifies the number of apneas, hypopneas, and respiratory effort-related arousals per hour of sleep.

Respondent burden: The time, energy, and other demands placed on those to whom the instrument is administered.

Responsiveness: The ability or power of a measure to detect clinically important change when it occurs.

Resting tremor: Tremor that occurs or exacerbates when the affected body part is at rest; it decreases or disappears with active motions.

Restrictive cardiomyopathy: Restrictive cardiomyopathy is characterized by nondilated ventricles with impaired ventricular filling. Hypertrophy is typically absent, although the infiltrative and storage diseases can cause a left ventricular wall thickness elevation.

Retching: Contractions of the diaphragm, thoracic, and abdominal muscles without expulsion of gastric contents.

Retinitis: Inflammation of the retina, often caused by infection with cytomegalovirus.

Retinoid dermatitis: Erythematous scaly patches with superficial skin fissuring.

Retrograde pyelography: A procedure where radiocontrast dye is injected into the ureter to produce detailed radiographs of the ureter and kidneys.

Rett's syndrome: A type of pervasive developmental disorder (DSM-IV) typically associated with severe to profound mental retardation, seen in females only, with the development of significant multiple progressively worsening deficits following a period of normal development (microcephaly, loss of purposeful hand motor skills, and acquisition of stereotyped hand movements, diminished social interests, and appearance of poorly coordinated gait or trunk movements). This disorder falls within Austism Spectrum Disorder in the DSM-5.

Reverse transcriptase: The enzyme in HIV that synthesizes a complementary strand of DNA.

Reversible posterior leukoencephalopathy syndrome (RPLS): Rare, life-threatening condition affecting the brain. Symptoms include headaches, seizures, confusion, and vision problems. Prognosis good with early identification and treatment.

Reye's syndrome: Acute encephalopathy characterized by fever, vomiting, fatty infiltration of the liver, disorientation, and coma, occurring mainly in children and usually following a viral infection, such as chicken pox or influenza.

Rhabdomyolysis: The breakdown of muscle tissue and release of myoglobin and intracellular electrolytes into the circulation because of a variety of causes such as crush injuries, drug-induced immobilization, and status epilepticus. It often leads to acute renal failure.

Rheumatoid arthritis: A systemic, symmetric autoimmune disease with swelling, pain, and inflammation of joints as a key finding.

Rhinitis: Inflammation of the nasal mucous membrane. Can be seasonal (*hay fever*) or perennial (increasingly called *intermittent* or *persistent*).

Rhinitis medicamentosa: Nasal congestion associated with tolerance to and resulting overuse of topical decongestants. Also known as *rebound vasodilation* or *rebound congestion*.

Rickets: See *Osteomalacia*.

Rigidity: Increased resistance detectable with the passive movement of a limb.

Roth spots: A hemorrhage in the retina with a white center. Roth spots are often associated with bacterial endocarditis.

Russell sign: Callus on dorsum of the hand secondary to self-induced vomiting.

S_4 gallop: An S_4 gallop is a presystolic atrial sound that immediately precedes the first heart sound (S_1). This finding on auscultation of the heart can be indicative of myocardial disease.

Salicylism: Poisoning by salicylic acid or any of its compounds.

Salpingo-oophorectomy: Surgical removal of the ovaries and fallopian tubes.

Sarcoidosis: Sarcoidosis is a multisystem granulomatous disorder of unknown etiology characterized histologically by noncaseating epithelioid granulomas involving various organs or tissues, with symptoms dependent on the site and degree of involvement.

Scale: Flake of stratum corneum.

Scar: Fibrous tissue formed during healing of injury to skin.

Schizophrenia: A chronic disorder of thought and affect encompassing different constellations of symptoms (i.e., positive symptoms, negative symptoms, cognitive dysfunction), with the individual having a significant disturbance in interpersonal relationships and ability to function in society on a daily basis.

Scleritis: Inflammation of the white portion of the eyeball, which can be superficial (episcleritis) or involve deeper layers of the eye.

Scleroderma: Scleroderma is a diffuse connective tissue disease characterized by changes in the skin, blood vessels, skeletal muscles, and internal organs.

Sebaceous gland: Gland that secretes sebum.

Sebosuppressive: Decreasing amount of sebum produced by the sebaceous gland.

Sebum: Oil produced by the sebaceous gland.

Second-degree relative (SDR): A blood relative, including the individual's grandparents, grandchildren, aunts, uncles, nephews, nieces, and half-siblings.

Second-generation antipsychotic (atypical antipsychotic): An antipsychotic medication that has pharmacodynamic and clinical properties different than the first generation (typical or traditional) antipsychotics that act primarily by having high levels of binding to dopamine-2 (D_2) receptors. Although definitions of atypicality vary, all second-generation antipsychotics share the property of causing a much lower incidence of extrapyramidal side effects.

Secondary amenorrhea: Cessation of menses in a woman previously menstruating for 6 months or more.

Secondary brain injury: A complex sequence of pathophysiologic events precipitated by the initial or primary brain injury that disrupts the normal central nervous system balance between oxygen supply and demand resulting in a worsened patient outcome.

Secondary hypertension: Persistently elevated BP that results from a known pathophysiological etiology or drug-induced cause.

Secondary hypogonadism: Failure of hypothalamus or pituitary gland to produce adequate amount of luteinizing hormone-releasing hormone (LHRH) or luteinizing hormone (LH). Thus, testicular production of testosterone is reduced.

Secondary prophylaxis (or suppressive therapy): Refers to administration of systemic antifungal agents (generally prior to and throughout the period of granulocytopenia) to prevent relapse of a documented invasive fungal infection that was treated during a previous episode of granulocytopenia.

Secondary resistance: Develops on exposure to an antifungal agent and can be either reversible, because of transient adaptation, or acquired as a result of one or more genetic alterations.

Secondary-progressive multiple sclerosis: Often follows relapsing-remitting multiple sclerosis whereby attacks become continuously progressive over time. It is sometimes accompanied by acute relapses.

Seizure: Paroxysmal disorder of central nervous system, characterized by abnormal neuronal discharges with or without loss of consciousness. They vary in cause, presentation, consequences, duration, and management.

Selection bias: Systematic differences in characteristics between those selected for study and those who are not. See also *Information bias.*

Sepsis: The systemic inflammatory response syndrome (SIRS) secondary to infection. See also *Systemic inflammatory response syndrome.*

Septic arthritis: Infection involving a joint.

Septic shock: Sepsis with persistent hypotension despite fluid resuscitation, along with the presence of perfusion abnormalities. Patients who are on inotropic or vasopressor agents might not be hypotensive at the time perfusion abnormalities are measured.

Serotonin (5-hydroxytryptamine [5-HT]): An inhibitory neurotransmitter present in the raphe nucleus of the brainstem, platelets, carcinoid tumors, and other tissues. It is a vasoconstrictor and neurochemical involved in mood and sleep.

Serum urea nitrogen (SUN): See *Blood urea nitrogen.*

Severe sepsis: Sepsis associated with organ dysfunction, hypoperfusion, or hypotension. Hypoperfusion and perfusion abnormalities can include, but are not limited to, lactic acidosis, oliguria, or acute alteration in mental status.

Short stature: A broad term describing a condition commonly defined by a physical height that is more than two standard deviations below the population mean and lower than the third percentile for height in a specific age group.

Sickle cell disease: A group of inherited red blood cell (RBC) disorder in which sickle cell hemoglobin (HbS) is present. Hemolytic anemia and painful vasoocclusion are the main features.

Simple partial seizure: A seizure beginning in one hemisphere of the brain. It is manifested by alterations in motor functions, sensory or somatosensory symptoms without loss of consciousness. It can progress to a complex partial seizure or to a secondarily generalized seizure with loss of consciousness.

Single-nephron GFR (SNGFR): The rate of filtration through a single glomerulus of a nephron; often reported in nL/min.

Sinus ostia: The pathways that drain the sinuses.

Sinusitis: An inflammation and/or infection of the paranasal sinus mucosa.

Sjögren's syndrome: An inflammatory process affecting the mucous membranes. Can cause dry mouth with difficulty swallowing. Can occur secondary to autoimmune diseases such as rheumatoid arthritis or systemic lupus erythematosus.

Sleep latency: The amount of time it takes to fall asleep.

Sleep spindles: Brief burst of electrical activity seen on the EEG, 12 to 14 Hz.

Slipped capital femoral epiphysis (SCFE): Increased width of the femoral plate observed during GH treatment resulting in hip or knee pain.

Social anxiety disorder (SAD): A disorder characterized by clinically significant anxiety provoked by exposure to certain types of social or performance situations, often leading to avoidance behavior.

Social determinants of health: Include the socioeconomic, culture, and environmental conditions as well as social and family networks that influence individual health.

Social phobia: See *Social anxiety disorder*.

Somatic pain: Pain arising from skin, bone, joint, muscle, or connective tissue.

Specific measures: Instruments intended to provide greater detail concerning particular outcomes, in terms of functioning and well-being, uniquely associated with a condition and/or its treatment.

Specific phobia: A phobia characterized by clinically significant anxiety provoked by exposure to a specific feared object or situation, often leading to avoidance behavior.

Spermicide: A substance (nonoxynol-9 in the United States) placed in the vagina to inhibit the activity of sperm, thus reducing the risk of pregnancy; available as vaginal creams, films, foams, gels, suppositories, sponges, and tablets.

Spiculated: With spikes or points on the surface.

Spirochete: The class of microorganism that is the agent of syphilis (*Treponema pallidum*).

ST-segment elevation: A type of myocardial infarction that typically results in an injury that transects the thickness of the myocardial wall. Following an ST-elevation MI, pathologic Q waves are frequently seen on the ECG, indicating transmural myocardial infarction.

Standard gamble: An approach to health-state preference elicitation in which the respondent is offered a choice between two alternatives: choice A—living in health state i (a health state between full health and death) with certainty, or choice B—taking a gamble on a new treatment for which the outcome is uncertain.

Status epilepticus: Defined as any recurrent or continuous seizure activity lasting longer than 30 minutes in which the patient does not regain baseline mental status. The two most common types are generalized convulsive status epilepticus and nonconvulsive status epilepticus.

Steatorrhea: Excessive fat in stool.

Stereotypy: Persistent repetition of senseless acts or words.

Stevens–Johnson syndrome: A serious dermatologic reaction characterized by blistering of the mucous membranes (mouth, eyes, vagina) with patchy rashes that can cover most of the body. Patients can also experience fever, headache, and cough.

Stress-related mucosal damage: Superficial gastritis-like lesions associated with critical illness in hospitalized patients.

Striae: Linear, atrophic, pink, purple, or white lesions of skin secondary to changes in connective tissue.

Stricture: An area of narrowing or constriction in the gastrointestinal tract due to buildup of fibrotic tissue; often a result of longstanding inflammation.

Stroke: A sudden onset, focal neurologic deficit, of presumed vascular origin, lasting longer than 24 hours.

Stroke volume: The volume of blood ejected from the heart during systole.

Stromal tissue of the prostate: This portion of the prostate is composed of smooth muscle tissue, which is embedded with α-adrenergic receptors. When stimulated, the muscle contracts around the urethra. This comprises approximately 75% of the total volume of the enlarged prostate gland in patients with benign prostatic hyperplasia.

Subarachnoid hemorrhage: Accumulation of blood in the space (subarachnoid space) surrounding the brain that usually contains the cerebrospinal fluid. It is usually caused by rupture of an intracranial aneurysm or trauma. It is a type of hemorrhagic stroke and can cause focal neurologic deficits.

Substance abuse: A maladaptive pattern of substance use indicated by repeated adverse consequences related to the repeated use of the substance. Examples include failure to fulfill important obligations at work, school, or home; repeated use in situations in which it is physically dangerous, such as driving under the influence; legal problems; and social or interpersonal problems such as arguments and fights.

Substance dependence: A state of adaptation that is manifested by a drug class-specific withdrawal syndrome that can be produced by abrupt cessation, rapid dose reduction, decreasing blood level of the drug, and/or administration of an antagonist. The continued use of the substance despite adverse substance-related problems.

Substantia nigra: Area of the brain (basal ganglia) where cells produce dopamine; characterized by neuromelanin deposits.

Subtle status epilepticus: For patients with prolonged refractory status epilepticus. The electrographical seizures persist; however, the motor manifestations of the seizures may not be apparent. In such cases the patient is considered in subtle status epilepticus.

Sudden death: Also known as sudden cardiac death; an unexpected death because of cardiac causes occurring in a short time period (generally within 1 hour of symptom onset) in a person with known or unknown cardiac disease in whom no previously diagnosed fatal condition is apparent. Most cases are related to cardiac arrhythmias, particularly ventricular fibrillation.

SUN (serum urea nitrogen): See *Blood urea nitrogen*.

Suppressive therapy: See *Secondary prophylaxis*.

Surge capacity: A term that refers to a healthcare system's ability to handle a large influx of patients in the event of an epidemic or disaster.

SV2A: A presynaptic vesicle protein found in the hippocampus as well as other areas of the brain believed to be important in the mechanism of action of levetiracetam.

Swan–Ganz catheter: A catheter (tube) inserted into the heart to measure pressure and cardiac output.

Symptomatic intracerebral hemorrhage: Collection of blood in the brain, usually after an ischemic stroke, that is associated with neurologic worsening.

Symptomatic status epilepticus: Status epilepticus occurring during the time of an acute neurological injury. This etiology is associated with a poorer prognosis.

Systemic vascular resistance: The resistance to blood flow that is primarily determined by the vascular tone of the arteriolar blood vessels.

Syncope: Fainting.

Synechiae: A *creeping* angle closure that sometimes occurs in patients between attacks of closed-angle glaucoma.

Synergism: The combination of two drugs (such as antibiotics) that produces an effect greater than the sum of the two drugs if used alone.

Synesthesias: The overflow of one sensory modality to another. For example, colors are heard, sounds are seen.

Synovitis: Inflammation of the synovial lining of the joint.

Synovium: Synovial membrane, the inner of the two layers of the articular capsule of a synovial joint, composed of loose connective tissue and having a free smooth surface that lines the joint cavity. It secretes the synovial fluid.

Systemic inflammatory response syndrome (SIRS): Systemic inflammatory response to a variety of clinical insults, which can be of infectious or noninfectious etiology.

Systemic vascular resistance (SVR): The resistance to blood flow that is primarily determined by the vascular tone of the arteriolar blood vessels.

Systolic blood pressure: The arterial BP that occurs during cardiac contraction.

Systolic heart failure: Systolic heart failure is a condition characterized by a decrease in myocardial contractility, which results in a reduction in the cardiac output and left ventricular ejection fraction.

Tachy-brady syndrome: Tachy-brady syndrome, also known as sick sinus syndrome, is a condition in which the sinoatrial node is unable to perform as the pacemaker of the heart.

Tangential speech: Speech pattern whereby the connections between expressed ideas are unrelated or have little relationship to each other.

Taper: To gradually decrease the dosage of a drug over a period of time.

Tardive: A modifier used to describe movement disorders secondary to chronic antipsychotic treatment (duration of treatment must be greater than 3 months). The disorder must persist for greater than 4 weeks and exhibit masking and unmasking characteristics. Tardive dyskinesia, tardive chorea, tardive dystonia, and tardive akathisia are examples of tardive movement disorders.

Telangiectases: Spidery red skin lesions caused by dilated blood vessels.

Tendonitis: Inflammation of tendons.

Tenesmus: Difficulty with bowel evacuation despite the urgency to defecate.

Teratogenicity: Ability of an agent to cause a defect or malformation in a fetus.

TEWL (transepidermal water loss): The rate of water loss by evaporation from the skin.

Thalassemia: Any of a group of inherited disorders of hemoglobin metabolism in which there is impaired synthesis of one or more of the polypeptide chains of globin.

Third-spacing: The shift of fluid and protein into the peritoneal cavity and bowel wall lumen that occurs as a result of peritonitis.

Thought blocking: Interruption of a train of thought whereby the person stops speaking suddenly and without warning, even in the middle of a sentence. Person may report that the thoughts were taken out of his or her head.

Thought broadcasting: Belief that one's thoughts are audible to others.

Thrombin: The enzyme formed from prothrombin that converts fibrinogen to fibrin. It is the principle driving force in the clotting cascade.

Thrombogenesis: The process of forming a blood clot.

Thrombolysis: The process of enzymatically dissolving or breaking apart a blood clot.

Thrombolytic: An enzyme that dissolves or breaks apart blood clots.

Thromboplastin: A substance that triggers the coagulation cascade. Tissue factor is a naturally occurring thromboplastin and used in the prothrombin time (PT) test.

Thrombopoiesis: The process of platelet production from immature cells.

Thrombosis: The process of forming a thrombus.

Thrombotic thrombocytopenic purpura: A life-threatening disease involving embolism and thrombosis of the small blood vessels in the brain and kidney.

Thrombus: An aggregation of fibrin and platelets within a blood vessel. A thrombus often causes vessel obstruction, inflammation, and injury.

Thrush: Fungal infection of the oral mucosa.

Thyroid-stimulating hormone (TSH): A polypeptide hormone secreted by the anterior pituitary gland that stimulates iodine uptake and thyroid hormone synthesis.

Thyrotropin-releasing hormone (TRH): A trophic hormone released by the hypothalamus that stimulates release of thyroid-stimulating hormone (TSH).

Time trade-off: An approach to health-state preference elicitation in which the respondent is asked to trade off years of life in less than full health for a shorter number of years in full health.

Tinea barbae: Fungal infection of the hair follicles of the beard or mustache.

Tinea capitis: Fungal infection of the scalp, hair follicles, or adjacent skin.

Tinea corporis: Fungal infection of the glabrous skin of the trunk and extremities.

Tinea cruris: Fungal infection of the proximal thighs and buttocks.

Tinea manuum: Fungal infection of the palmar surface of the hands.

Tinea pedis: Fungal infection of the feet.

Tinnitus: A noise in the ears, as ringing, buzzing, roaring, clicking, etc.

Tocolytic: Agent that stops labor contractions.

Tolerance: (1) A state of adaptation in which exposure to a drug induces changes that result in a diminution of one or more of the drug's effects over time. (2) The ability of the immune system to accept a transplanted allograft as part of *self*.

Tonic-clonic seizures: Sharp tonic contraction of muscles followed by a period of rigidity and clonic movement.

Tophi: Urate deposits.

Total nutrient admixture: A parenteral nutrition formulation containing intravenous fat emulsion as well as the other components of parenteral nutrition (dextrose, amino acids, vitamins, minerals, water, and other additives) in a single container.

Toxic epidermal necrolysis: A syndrome similar to Stevens-Johnson syndrome characterized by blistering of skin and mucous membranes in response to administration of a drug. Large areas of skin may peel off.

Toxic megacolon: A segmental or total colonic distension of >6 cm with acute colitis and signs of systemic toxicity.

Toxic shock syndrome: Sudden onset of fever, muscle ache, vomiting and diarrhea, accompanied by a peeling rash and followed by low body temperature and shock; caused by staphylococcal endotoxin, especially from infection of the vagina associated with tampon use.

Toxoplasmosis: Clinical infection with *Toxoplasma gondii.*

Transmural: Across the wall of an organ or structure; in the case of CD, inflammation may extend through all four layers of the intestinal wall.

Transurethral incision of the prostate: In this surgical procedure, the bladder neck opening is widened by making incisions at various locations around the bladder neck with a resectoscope, which is inserted into the penis. Excess prostate tissue is not removed.

Transurethral prostatectomy: In this surgical procedure, an enlarged prostate core is removed from the inside out. That is, a resectoscope is inserted into the penis. A cutting blade at the end shaves out excess prostate tissue.

Transverse lie: The fetus is perpendicular to the mother. Usually the shoulder is the presenting part. Fetuses in this position must be delivered by cesarean section.

Transverse myelitis: Inflammation of the full width of the spinal cord that disrupts communication to the muscles, resulting in pain, weakness, and muscle paralysis.

Traveler's diarrhea: Diarrhea caused by contaminated food or water and usually attributed to enterotoxigenic *Escherichia coli* (ETEC), *Shigella*, *Campylobacter*, *Salmonella* species, or viruses.

Triple-negative breast cancer (TNBC): Breast cancer cells lacking estrogen, progesterone, and HER2 receptor protein overexpression.

Troponins T or I: Proteins found predominately in cardiac and not skeletal muscle that regulates calcium-mediated interaction of actin and myosin. Troponin I and T are released into the blood from the myocytes at the time of myocardial cell necrosis secondary to infarction. These biochemical markers become elevated and are used in the diagnosis of myocardial infarction. Troponin I and T are more sensitive and specific for infarction than creatine kinase, which is found in both skeletal and myocardial cells. The exact value of troponin I or T, which is diagnostic of infarction, differs based on assay.

Trousseau's sign: A hand spasm produced by placing a blood pressure cuff over the forearm and inflating the pressure above the systolic pressure for 3 minutes.

Tubule: Section of the nephron that is responsible for secretion and reabsorption of water, electrolytes, and drugs.

Tumor: Elevated, solid lesion.

Tumor necrosis factor-α (TNF-α): A proinflammatory cytokine.

Type I reaction: An immediate, immunoglobulin E (IgE)-mediated allergic reaction.

Ulcer: Loss of epidermis and dermis caused by sloughing of necrotic tissue.

Ultradian sleep–wake rhythm: Is a cycle of sleep and wake that repeats in less than 24 hours. Babies have an ultradian sleep–wake rhythm with multiple sleep and wake periods in a 24-hour period.

Ultrafiltration: The process of removing water from the blood during dialysis.

Ultraviolet A light: 315–400 nm ultraviolet A light.

Ultraviolet A light 1: 340–400 nm ultraviolet A light.

Ultraviolet B light, broadband: 280–315 nm ultraviolet B light.

Ultraviolet B light, narrow band: 311 nm ultraviolet B light.

Umbilication: Slight, navel-like depression, or dimpling, of the center of a rounded body.

Unilateral: On either the right or left side, not crossing the midline. When used for defining sensory or motor disturbances of migraine aura, it includes complete or partial hemi-distribution; not just applicable to migraines, but to just about any disease related to anatomical structure(s).

Upper respiratory tract infection: Otitis media, sinusitis, pharyngitis, laryngitis (croup), rhinitis, or epiglottitis.

Urea: A waste product found in the blood and caused by the normal breakdown of protein in the body.

Uremia: An array of symptoms associated with accumulation of metabolic by-products and endogenous toxins in the blood due to impaired kidney function. Symptoms include nausea, vomiting, loss of appetite, weakness, and mental confusion.

Urethritis: Inflammation of the urethra.

Urinalysis: The diagnostic analysis of urine and its components; can be microscopic or macroscopic in nature.

Urinary incontinence: Involuntary leakage of urine; can result from urethral underactivity (stress urinary incontinence), urethral overactivity (overflow incontinence), or mixed pathophysiologic mechanisms.

Urine: Fluid waste resulting from filtration of blood by the kidneys; transferred to the bladder by ureters and expelled from the body through the urethra by the act of voiding or urinating.

Urticaria: Hives (red, raised bumps) that may occur after exposure to an allergen.

USP Chapter 797: A chapter of the United States Pharmacopeia (USP) that details the procedures and requirements for compounding sterile preparations and sets standards that are applicable to all practice settings in which sterile preparations are compounded.

Vacuum erection device: Medical device used to manually induce an erection.

Vagal nerve stimulator (VNS): A medical device that is surgically implanted in patients with refractory epilepsy.

Validity: An estimation of the extent to which an instrument is measuring what it is purported to be measuring.

Valsalva maneuver: The Valsalva maneuver is the expiratory effort against a closed glottis, which increases thoracic cavity pressure, which impedes venous return to the heart. This maneuver results in blood pressure and heart rate changes and is used to diagnose treat various cardiac conditions.

Vasculitis: Inflammation of blood vessels.

Vasopressin: A posterior pituitary hormone that controls fluid balance by acting on the renal collecting ducts to prevent water loss.

Vector: Carrier (person, animal, or insect) of disease.

Vegetation: Bacterial growth on heart valves.

Ventricular remodeling: Alterations in myocardial cells and the extracellular matrix that result in changes in the size, shape, structure, and function of the heart. The remodeling process leads to reductions in myocardial systolic and/or diastolic function that, in turn, leads to further myocardial injury, perpetuating the remodeling process and the decline in ventricular dysfunction and progression of heart failure.

Vesicle: Clear blister (<0.5 cm in diameter) filled with fluid.

Visceral pain: Pain arising from internal organs such as the large intestine or pancreas.

Visual analog scale: A response scale that is a line with the end points well defined (e.g., 0 = worst imaginable health state, and 100 = best imaginable health state).

Visuospatial: Denoting the ability to comprehend visual representations and spatial relationships in learning and performing a task.

Volume of distribution: A proportionality constant that relates the amount of drug in the body to its serum concentration.

Vomiting: Contraction of the abdominal muscles, descent of the diaphragm, and opening of the gastric cardia resulting in expulsion of stomach contents from the mouth.

Vulgaris: Ordinary, common.

Wearing-off phenomena: Also known as end-of-dose wearing-off or motor fluctuations. The waning of the effects of a dose of levodopa prior to the scheduled time for the next dose, resulting in return of parkinsonian features, such as, tremor, slowness, and rigidity.

Wernicke's encephalopathy: A serious neurologic disorder caused by thiamine deficiency.

White coat hypertension: Patients have normal BP measurements based on home measurements but have elevated BP measurements when measured in a clinical setting.

Withdrawal: The development of a substance-specific syndrome after cessation of or reduction in intake of a substance that was used regularly by the individual to induce a state of intoxication. Withdrawal causes significant distress to the individual and is associated with impairment in social, occupational, or other areas of functioning. Withdrawal is usually associated with substance dependence. Withdrawal generally is also associated with a craving to readminister the drug to relieve the symptoms.

Withdrawal bleeding: The predictable bleeding that results from cessation of a progestogen.

Withdrawal syndrome: The onset of a predictable constellation of signs and symptoms involving the central nervous system after the abrupt discontinuation of, or rapid decrease in, dosage of a drug.

Xerosis: Dry skin.

Xerostomia: Dry mouth caused by decreased salivary production.

Yeasts: Oval or spherically shaped unicellular forms that generally produce pasty or mucoid colonies on agar media, similar to those observed with bacterial cultures. Yeasts have rigid cell walls that reproduce by budding, a process in which daughter cells arise from pinching off a portion of the parent cell.

Zeitgeber: Environmental cue.

Zollinger–Ellison syndrome: Gastric acid hypersecretory disease caused by a gastrin-secreting tumor and leading to multiple, severe duodenal ulcers.

Index

Page numbers followed by *f*, *t*, or *b* indicate figures, tables, or clinical presentation boxes, respectively.

B

C

D

F

G

H

M

N

O

P

INDEX

S

INDEX

T

U

INDEX

V

W

X

Y

Z